An Index to Literature in the Health Sciences

MEDICAL AND HEALTH CARE

BOOKS AND SERIALS IN PRINT

2002

Volume 2
Books—Title Index
Publisher Symbol Index
Wholesaler & Distributor Symbol Index
Serials—Subject Index
Serials—Online Service Index
Serials—Title Index

Bowker™

New Providence, New Jersey

Published by
R.R. Bowker LLC,
630 Central Avenue, New Providence, NJ 07974

Michael Cairns, President

Telephone: 908-464-6800, Toll-free: 1-888-BOWKER2 (1-888-269-5372); Fax: 908-665-3502
E-mail address: info@bowker.com
URL: http://www.bowker.com

Readers may send any corrections and/or updates to the information in this work to R.R. Bowker through the corrections option on the Bowker Web site at http://www.bowker.com or may send e-mail directly to the address: corrections@bowker.com

Publishers may update their own listings in the Books In Print and Ulrich's databases using the BowkerLink Publisher Access System at www.bowkerlink.com

No payment is either solicited or accepted for the inclusion of entries in this publication.
R.R. Bowker has used its best efforts in collecting and preparing material for inclusion in this publication, but does not warrant that the information herein is complete or accurate, and does not assume, and hereby disclaims any liability to any person for the loss or damage caused by errors or omissions in **Medical and Health Care Books & Serials In Print 2002** whether such errors or omissions result from negligence, accident or any other cause.

International Standard Book Numbers
Set: 0-8352-4483-0
Volume 1: 0-8352-4484-9
Volume 2: 0-8352-4485-7

International Standard Serial Number
0000-085X

Library of Congress Control Number
77-94389

Printed and bound in the United States of America

ISBN 0-8352-4483-0

9 780835 244831

CONTENTS

PREFACE

The 2002 edition of *Medical and Health Care Books and Serials In Print* constitutes the thirty-first annual cumulation of titles in the highly specialized health sciences and allied health fields. The indexes to books list titles which are in-print and have been or will be published or distributed in the United States. The coverage of the serials indexes is international and contains selected titles of periodicals issued more frequently than once a year and usually published at regular intervals, plus irregular serials and annuals. This definition has been adopted in order not to overlook any important sources of information because of periodicity.

CLASSIFICATION

Medical and Health Care Books and Serials In Print covers a wide range of books and serials related to the major health sciences disciplines, e.g., medicine, dentistry, human health, nursing, nutrition, veterinary medicine, psychiatry, psychology, behavioral sciences and other associated health sciences. Entries for the biomedical sciences are equally comprehensive. An effort has been made to include titles of historic and biographical interest. Some scientific and technical publications, peripherally related to these subjects and therefore of possible interest to the user, have also been included. Most titles have been selected for the professional or college student audience; however, in the areas of career development and vocational guidance, some titles of interest to high school students have been included. Beyond its immediate usefulness to the health sciences community, this reference work should thus be of value to the staff and users of public and school libraries, and to book publishers and suppliers.

The reader will find certain advantages in *Medical and Health Care Books and Serials In Print.* Rather than the mere identification of material, each entry has been listed under several indexes and is accompanied by essential data.

COMPILATION

Medical and Health Care Books and Serials In Print 2002 is excerpted from the Books In Print database of R.R. Bowker's Database Publishing Group. Citations for books in the health sciences field have been retrieved from the same database used in compiling Bowker's *Books In Print, Books In Print Supplement, Subject Guide To Books In Print, Forthcoming Books,* and other bibliographies in the In-Print line. The database has been updated to conform with the latest information received from publishers for the production of *Books In Print* 2001-2002 and its Subject Index. Entries from the serials indexes have been selected from the database used to produce *Ulrich's Periodicals Directory.*

DATA ACQUISITION AND EDI

Bowker receives bibliographic information from publishers in many different formats: catalogs, Advance Book Information forms, checklists, and phoned or faxed information. Publishers may also update their listings using the BowkerLink Publisher Access System at www.bowkerlink.com.

Larger publishing houses are urged to use Electronic Data Interchange (EDI). EDI is a process by which participating publishers can submit their bibliographic information to Books In Print from their own databases. Bowker's EDI system accepts publisher data 24 hours a day, 7 days a week. Methods of data transmission include the Internet (FTP), modem transfer, diskette, and magnetic tape. The benefits to these methods are: no paper intervention, reduced costs, increased timeliness, and less chance of human error that can occur when re-keying information.

Bowker's EDI system is an outstanding tool for updating titles presently included in the Books In Print database (backlist especially), most notably price and status information. However, to communicate new title information to Books In Print via EDI, the quality of the publishers textual data must be up to or extremely close to reference book standards. This is very true as it pertains to title and contributor information.

Publishers wishing more information concerning Bowker's EDI system are encouraged to contact the EDI group at 908-790-2117.

CONTENT

Author and title indexes to books include more than 92,100 entries for titles available from some 6,097 publishers. The subject index follows the headings assigned by the Library of Congress. Headings and cross-references were selected from the latest CDMARC Subjects and CDMARC Names disks produced by the Library of Congress. In this edition, the 92,100 entries appear 155,000 times under 5,120 populated subject headings.

SERIALS INFORMATION

The periodicals were chosen for their subject-matter. The simple arrangements of the subject and titles indexes allows the user a direct approach to those titles to be considered for possible selection and acquisition. The subject index to serials contains entries with complete information listed under the primary subject of the serials, with cross-references to the entry appearing under secondary subjects and in the title index. Actually 19,975 entries appear under 532 subject headings.

ISBN AGENCY

Each title included in *Medical and Health Care Books and Serials In Print* and other Books In Print products has been assigned an International Standard Book Number (ISBN) by the publisher. All ISBNs listed in these volumes have been validated by using the check digit control, ensuring accuracy. ISBNs allow order transmission and bibliographic information updating using the Book Industry System Advisory Committee's (BISAC) standard format for data transmission. Publishers not currently participating in the ISBN system may request the assignment of an ISBN Publisher Prefix from the ISBN Agency by calling 877-310-7333, fax 908-665-2895, or through the ISBN/SAN web site at www.isbn.org/. Please note: The ISBN prefix 0-615 is for decentralized use by the U.S. ISBN Agency and has been assigned to many publishers. It is not for use by one publisher.

SAN AGENCY

Another listing feature in *Medical and Health Care Books and Serials In Print* and other Books in Print products is the Standard Address Number (SAN) assigned to each address of each organization in/or served by the book industry. SANs are assigned by the SAN Agency, R.R. Bowker, to booksellers, publishers, distributors, wholesalers, libraries, schools/school systems, book manufacturers and service organizations providing a business function for each of these organizations.

The SAN functions in its application to activities such as purchasing, billing, shipping, receiving, paying, crediting, and refunding, and can be used for any other communication or transaction between participating organizations. For more information related to the SAN, please contact Diana Luongo, SAN Senior Editor, R.R. Bowker, by calling 908-771-7755, fax 908-665-2895, or visit the ISBN/SAN web site at www.isbn.org/.

Every effort has been made to ensure that this index will serve as an effective and useful reference tool, providing information to a large number of clientele interested in health sciences literature.

It is hoped that the present edition of *Medical and Health Care Books and Serials In Print* proves to be a valuable tool for those who are interested in publications in all areas of health and biomedical sciences, and that it will help to fill the need for easy access to the rapidly growing body of specialized data in these fields.

How To Use MEDICAL AND HEALTH CARE BOOKS & SERIALS IN PRINT 2002

BOOK INDEXES

GENERAL EDITORIAL POLICIES

In order to ensure that the essential information in these listings is uniform, complete, and easy to find, the following editorial policies have been maintained:

Every effort is made by most contributing publishers to prepare their material with consideration for its accuracy throughout the life of this edition of *Medical and Health Care Books and Serials In Print*. Most publishers anticipate price changes when they revise their material, list forthcoming books even if publication dates and prices are not set, and for the most part, try not to list books that may shortly become unavailable before the new edition is published. All prices are subject to change without notice.

Most prices are retail prices. Lack of uniformity in the individual catalogs prohibits indicating trade discounts. However, all publishers do not uniformly supply this information, and Bowker can only make its best efforts to transmit this information when it is provided.

An asterisk (*) at the beginning of the title indicates titles added since the last publiscation of *Medical and Health Care Books & Serials In Print*.

ALPHABETICAL ARRANGEMENT OF ENTRIES

Each entry is filed alphabetically by word, with the following exceptions:

Initial articles in English, French, German, Italian and Spanish are deleted from both author and title entries.

Proper names beginning with Mc and Mac are filed in strict alphabetical order. For example, entries for contributor's names such as MacAdam, MacAvory, MacCarthy, MacDonald, and MacLean are located prior to the pages with entries for names such as McAdams, McCarthy, McCoy, and McDermott.

In the Books-Author Index, compound names are listed under the first part of the name and cross-references appear under the last part of the name.

Entries beginning with initial letters (whether authors' given names or titles) are filed first: Smith, H.C. comes before Smith, Harold A.; J.B. Priestley: The Man and His Ideas comes before Jade.

Numerals, including year dates are filed alphabetically:

SEVEN YEARS
SEVENTEEN
SEVENTEEN FAMOUS INVENTIONS
SEVENTEEN-FIFTEEN TO THE PRESENT
17 PAST YEARS
SEVENTEEN READER
SEVENTEETH CENTURY

INFORMATION INCLUDED IN ENTRIES

Entries include the following bibliographic information, when available: author, co-author, editor, co-editor, translator, title, number of volumes, edition, Library of Congress control number, series information, whether or not illustrated, number of pages, year of publication, price with type of binding if other than cloth over boards, publisher's order number, International Standard Book Number, and Publisher's name.

(Information on the International Standard Book Numbering System in the United States and other English-speaking countries is available from R.R. Bowker. See page viii.)

If more than two authors are responsible for a certain publication, only the name of the first is given followed by *et al.*

BOOKS—SUBJECT INDEX

Entries are arranged alphabetically by author within subject. If no author is given, the entry is filed alphabetically by title within the author arrangement.

Headings and cross-references were updated to conform to the most recent edition of Library of Congress Subject Headings and its supplements.

Whenever official LC classification was unavailable, headings were assigned provisional subjects. Among these fall most of the titles now in preparation or to be published sometime in 2002. As LC headings for such books become available, the provisional headings will be verified or changed in future editions of *Medical and Health Care Books and Serials In Print.*

ALPHABETICAL ARRANGEMENT OF SUBJECT HEADINGS

Subject headings are arranged alphabetically:

ABDOMEN
ABORTION
ACIDOSIS
ACRIDINE

Many of the main headings are broken down still further:

CANCER
CANCER–BIBLIOGRAPHY
CANCER–CHEMOTHERAPY
CANCER–DIAGNOSIS

There are also many cross-references:

ABBREVIATIONS, MEDICAL
see MEDICINE–ABBREVIATIONS

ABDOMEN
see also GROIN; INTESTINES; KIDNEYS; LIVER STOMACH

Headings, patterned after those used in the card catalog in the Library of Congress, are explicit rather than general. Thus, books on pediatric gynecology are under PEDIATRIC GYNECOLOGY, not under GYNECOLOGY.

In looking for books on psychiatry, search past the main entry to various subheadings:

PSYCHIATRY
PSYCHIATRY–BIBLIOGRAPHY
PSYCHIATRY–COLLECTED WORKS
PSYCHIATRY–DICTIONARIES
PSYCHIATRY–HISTORY
PSYCHIATRY–RESEARCH
PSYCHIATRY, CHILD
PSYCHIATRY, FORENSIC
PSYCHIATRY, MILITARY
PSYCHIATRY, SOCIAL

Note the sequence of the above cited headings and subheadings. The editors of this book took as a guideline the Filing Rules for the Dictionary Catalogs of the Library of Congress as prepared by the Processing Department of the Library of Congress.

Other typical examples of the sequence used are:

AIR–POLLUTION
AIR, IONIZED
AIR MYELOGRPAHY

CHILDREN
CHILDREN–ASYLUMS
CHILDREN–DISEASES
CHILDREN–DISEASES–DIAGNOSIS
CHILDREN, APHASIC
CHILDREN, DEAF
CHILDREN, DEAF–EDUCATION
CHILDREN AND DEATH

Although a constant effort is made to maintain consistency and to avoid splitting entries on a given subject among several headings, a certain amount is inevitable. The Library of Congress updates its subject headings constantly but cannot make such updating retroactive to cards and catalogs previously issued. For example, LC recently added the subject heading KIRLIAN PHOTOGRAPHY. If previously published titles which appear under the heading PHOTOGRAPHY did not indicate by their titles that they should have been moved to KIRLIAN PHOTOGRAPHY, they may have been left under PHOTOGRAPHY.

SAMPLE ENTRY
BOOKS-TITLE INDEX

(1) Adult-Child Research & Experience: (2) Personal & Professional Legacies of a Dysfunctional, Co-Dependent Family. (3) Sheldon I. London. (4) Developments in Clinical Psychology Ser. (5) 3rd ed. (6) (C.) (7) 1998. (8) (illus.). (9) 200p. (10) pap. (11) 39.95 o.p. (12) *(0-9657352-9-X)* (13) 4th (14) rev. ed. (15) 1999. (16) 200p. (17) pap. (18) 41.95 o.s.i. (19) *(0-9657352-9-X)* (20) 5th (21) rev. ed. (22) 2000. (23) 240p. (24) (C). (25) pap. (26) 45.00 (27) *(0-9657352-5-7)* (28) Elsie & Darcy (29) GBR (30) *Dist.* Harbison

Note: Sample entry shows three separate backlist editions linked, or joined, by their common title, subtitle, contributor and publisher. Pertinent information for each edition appears prior to its ISBN, followed by a semi-colon. Items containing distributor information should be ordered from the distributor, not the publisher.

KEY

1. Title
2. Subtitle
3. Contributor
4. Series
5. Edition Number
6. Audience Code
7. Publication year
8. Illustrated
9. Number of pages
10. Binding type
11. Price & title status
12. International Standard Book Number
13. Additional edition number
14. Additional edition information
15. Corresponding backlist publication year
16. Corresponding number of pages
17. Corresponding binding type
18. Corresponding price
19. Corresponding ISBN
20. Additional edition number
21. Additional edition information
22. Corresponding backlist publication year
23. Corresponding number of pages
24. Corresponding audience code
25. Corresponding binding type
26. Corresponding price
27. Corresponding ISBN
28. Publisher's symbol
29. Foreign publisher ISO code
30. U.S.A. distributor's symbol

PUBLISHER SYMBOL INDEX

A key to the publisher symbols (e.g. "Kluwer Ac") used in the book bibliographic entries of *Medical and Health Care Books and Serials In Print* can be found in the Book Publisher Symbol Index at the end of Volume 2. Entries in this index contain each publisher's symbol, followed by its abbreviated name, ISBN prefix(es), business affiliation when available (e.g., "Div. of International Publishing"), ordering address(es), SAN (Standard Address Number), telephone number(s), fax and toll-free numbers. Editorial address(es) (and associated contact numbers) follows.

Abbreviations used to identify publishers' imprints are followed by the full name of the imprint. E-mail and Web site addresses are then supplied. A listing of distributors associated with the publisher concludes each entry; each distributor symbol is in bold type, followed by its abbreviated name. Full information on these distributors and wholesalers can be found in the Wholesaler & Distributor Symbol Index (also in volume two). Note that publishers who also serve as distributor may be listed both here and in the Publisher Symbol Index.

A dagger preceding an entry and the note "CIP" at the end of the entry both indicate that the publisher participates in the Cataloging in Publication Program of the Library of Congress.

Foreign publishers with US distributors are also listed, followed by their three-character ISO (International Standards Organization) country code ("GBR", "CAN", etc.), ISBN prefix(es), and a cross-reference to their US distributor, as shown below:

Millvres Bks (GBR) *(1-873741) Dist by* **LPC InBook**

Publishers with like or similar names are referenced by a "Do not confuse with..." notation at the end of the entry. In addition, cross references are provided from imprints and former company names to the new name.

SAMPLE ENTRY
PUBLISHER SYMBOL INDEX

❶ † ❷ **Mosby Inc.** ❸ *Mosby, Inc.;* ❹ *0-323; 0-7234; 0-8016; 0-8151; 0-88416; 0-941158; 1-55664; 1-56815),* ❺ Div. of Harcourt, Inc., A Harcourt Health Sciences Co., ❻ Orders Addr.: 6227 Sea Harbor Dr., Orlando, FL 32887 ❼ (SAN 200-2280) ❽ Toll Free Fax: 800-235-0256 ❾ Toll Free: 800-543-1918 ❿ Edit Addr.: 11830 Westline Industrial Dr., Saint Louis, MO 63146 ⓫ Toll Free: 800-325-4177 ⓬ Web site: http://www.mosby.com/ ⓭ Dist(s): **PennWell Corp** *(PennWell Corp.);* ⓮ *CIP.*

KEY
❶ CIP Identifier
❷ Publisher Symbol
❸ Publisher Name
❹ ISBN Prefixes
❺ Division of
❻ Orders Address
❼ SAN
❽ Orders Fax
❾ Orders toll-free
❿ Editorial Address
⓫ Toll-Free
⓬ Web site
⓭ Distributors
⓮ Cataloguing in Publication

SAMPLE ENTRY
WHOLESALER & DISTRIBUTOR
SYMBOL INDEX

❶ **New Leaf Dist.,** ❷ *(New Leaf Distributing Co., Inc.;* ❸ *0-9627209),* ❹ Div. of Al-Wali Corp., ❺ 401 Thornton Rd., Lithia Springs, GA 30122-1557 ❻ (SAN 169-1449) ❼ Tel: 770-948-7845; ❽ Fax: 770-944-2313; ❾ Toll Free Fax: 800-326-1066; ❿ Toll Free: 800-326-2665 ⓫ Email: NewLeaf@NewLeaf-dist.com ⓬ Web site: http://www.NewLeaf-dist.com

KEY
❶ Distributor Symbol
❷ Distributor Name
❸ ISBN Prefix
❹ Division of
❺ Editorial Address
❻ SAN
❼ Telephone
❽ Fax
❾ Toll Free Fax
❿ Toll Free
⓫ E-mail
⓬ Website

SERIAL INDEXES

SERIALS—SUBJECT INDEX

Entries with bibliographic and buying information for selected, current serials which are published periodically or irregularly are arranged alphabetically by title within subject category. The complete entry is listed under one subject heading. If a serial covers more than one subject, cross-references direct the user from related subjects to the subject under which the complete entry is listed. Subheadings on "Abstracting, Bibliographies & Statistics" are also included in 21 subject categories.

SERIALS—TITLE INDEX

Title Index entries include the following: title, ISSN, and country code, name of issuing body if main entry title contains only the initials of the issuing body. Cross-references of variant titles, parallel language titles, and former titles are included. The page number where the complete entry appears is printed in **boldface** type; page numbers in Roman type indicate pages of related subject listings.

FULL ENTRY CONTENT DESCRIPTION

Basic Information

The following elements are mandatory for listing and appear in all entries: main entry title, frequency of publication, publisher address, country code, and Dewey Decimal Classification number.

Certain electronic journals may not have a physical mailing address; the URL and/or E-mail address provide a means of contacting the publication.

Dewey Decimal Classification Number

The Dewey Decimal number is printed at the top left of each entry. More than one Dewey number may have been assigned if a serial covers several subjects.

LC Classification Number

The Library of Congress classification number, if known, appears directly below the Dewey Decimal number. Shelf numbers are not included.

Country Code

The ISO Country Code is printed at the top center of each entry following the Dewey Decimal number. A complete list of country codes used will be found on p. xxi of volume two.

ISSN

The ISSN for the main entry title is printed to the right of the country code. Not all publications have been assigned an ISSN, and lack of a number does not render a publication ineligible for listing.

CODEN

The CODEN designation, if known, is printed directly below the country code and ISSN. The CODEN is an alphanumeric code, applied uniquely to a specific publication. Devised by the American Society for Testing and Materials, it is used primarily for scientific and technical titles. New CODEN are assigned by Chemical Abstracts Service.

Title Information

The main title is printed in **boldface** and upper case as the first item in the entry. Titles are catalogued according to rules described below in the "Cataloging Rules for Main Entry Title" section. For multi-language publications, the parallel language title is also printed in upper case, immediately following the main entry title, and is separated from it by a slash.

A triangle symbol (▼) printed before the title indicates that the title began publishing within the past three years. This symbol also appears before titles announced for publication in the coming year. An asterisk (✱) printed after the title indicates that the address in the entry was not verified by the publisher for this edition.

The subtitle is printed in lower case after the title. Variant titles are given within the entry and are labeled as such. The Key Title, which is assigned at the time of ISSN assignment by the responsible center of the International Serials Data System, is given only if it is different from the main entry title. Former titles are given at the end of the bibliographic data. See the paragraph below.

Language

The language or languages is given, even if a serial is written in the main language of the country of publication. The order of languages is generally alphabetical and does not represent prominence. If a serial includes abstracts, summaries or sections in additional language(s), that information will be provided as well.

Year First Published

The year first published is given if provided by the publisher. If a title has been suspended and later resumed publication, these dates may be provided as well. If volume numbering was restarted, the notation "N.S." denoting new series precedes the date. If information is lacking, a volume number and specific year may be provided to indicate the approximate age of the publication.

SAMPLE ENTRY

1 362 2 USA 3 ISSN 1234-5678 4 RA1 5 CODEN: MDLCBD
6 **MEDICAL CARE FOR BURNS;** 7 short articles on caring for burns and burn victims. 8 Key title: Burn Care 9 (In 3 sections.) 10 Text in French, English. 11 1987. 12 24/yr. (in 2 vols.)
13 USD 136 in US and Canada; USD 148 elsewhere (effective 2001) 14 bk.rev. abstr, illus. cum. index: 1987-1997. 15 back issues avail.; reprint service avail. From HZI, LMI 16 8 cols./p., 20 p./no. 17 *Refereed.* 18 **Document type:** *Academic/scholarly.* 19 **Description:** Analyzes, critiques, and synthesizes relevant literature and research in the field of health care.
20 **Supersedes in part** (in 1989): Medical Care 21 (0000-8888); Which was formerly: Aide Medicale
22 **Media:** Online – full text (from Hooper, Inc.) 23 **Related titles:** CD-ROM ed.: Burns Medical Care on Disc. 1992. q. USD 32. (from Healthcare Institute (File no.42), Platter Corp.); Microform ed. (from SMI); French ed.: ISSN 5678-2345. Supplement: Annual Burns Medical Review. ISSN 4567-2345. 24 **Indexed:** Med.Sci.& Tech.Abstr. 25 (1995-), Med.Packag.Ind. 26 – BLDSC (3645.7365333), CISTI, GNLM. 27 **CCC** 28 **Published by:** (Health Care Research Institute) 29 Medi-Care Publishing Inc., 30 1480 US Rte.46, Parsippany, NJ-07084. 31 TEL 973-273-4415, 32 FAX 973-283-4416, 33 Telex 9735 PARV TH,
34 Burnscare@medi.com 35 http://www. medi.com/burnscare. 36 Eds. Shawn Kent, Brian Mathews. 37 Pub. Judy Smith. 38 R & P Eve Brown, TEL 908-773-7745. 39 Adv. contact. Lara Sankar. 40 adv.: B&W page USD 2300, color page USD 3500; trim 8 x 10. 41 Circ. 5,000 (paid); 3,200 (controlled). 42 Wire service: SP. 43 **Subscr. in the Americas to:** Medical Science Research Centre, Regional Sales Office, PO Box 435, New York, NY 10159-0945. TEL 212-555-7645, FAX 212-576-4785; 44 **Dist. by:** Bio-Medical Distributors, 3423 St. Denis, Montreal, Quebec C0N 4R1, Canada. TEL 234-123-4523, FAX 243-465-7654. 45 **Co-sponsors:** Burns Medical Association; Burn Science Society. **Affiliate:** United States Burns Research Society.

KEY

1 Dewey Decimal Classification
2 ISO Country Code
3 ISSN
4 LC Classification
5 CODEN
6 Main Entry Title
7 Subtitle
8 Key Title
9 Bibliographic Note
10 Language
11 First Published
12 Frequency
13 Price
14 Special Features
15 Back Issues & Reprint
16 Page format
17 Refereed
18 Document Type
19 Brief Description
20 Title Changes
21 Former ISSN
22 Media
23 Related Editions
24 Abstracting & Indexing
25 Years of Coverage
26 Document Suppliers
27 Copyright Clearance Center
28 Corporate Author
29 Publishing Company
30 Address
31 Telephone
32 Fax
33 Telex
34 E-mail
35 URL
36 Editor
37 Publisher
38 Rights & Permission Contact
39 Advertising Contact
40 Advertising Rates
41 Circulation
42 Wire Service
43 Subscription
44 Distributor
45 Co-sponsors and other bodies

Frequency

The frequency of publication is given in abbreviated form, such as "a." for annual, "irreg." for irregular, "m." for monthly, "3/yr." for three times per year. All abbreviations used are listed in the "General Abbreviations and Special Symbols" on p. xix of volume two.

Price

Unless otherwise indicated, the price given is the annual price for an individual subscription in the currency of the country of origin. The price in U.S. dollars may also be given if it is provided by the publisher. No attempt is made to convert foreign currency to U.S. dollars. Separate postage information is not given, since postal rates vary widely. A complete list of ISO currency codes used will be found on p. xxv of volume two.

Special Features

A listing of special features may include such items as book or other types of reviews, advertising (usually meaning commercial, not classified advertising), charts, illustrations, bibliography section, article abstracts, and an annual index to the periodical's contents.

Reprint Services

If a serial is known to be available from a reprint service, a code referring to the service appears in the entry. More than one code may be listed. For a list of reprint services and a translation of the codes, please refer to p. xxxv of volume two.

Pages Per Issue; Columns Per Page

When known, the number of pages per issue (p./no.:) and/or columns per page (cols./p.:) is/are noted.

Refereed Serial

The manuscript peer review and evaluation system is utilized to protect, maintain and raise the quality of scholarly material published in serials. If a serial is known to be refereed or juried, the notation "*Refereed*" appears in italics towards the end of the bibliographic data. This information is generally provided by the serial publisher.

Document Type

Notations are included to indicate type of publication, e.g. trade, newsletter, or abstract/index. The words "**Document type:**" appcar in boldface, followed by the document type description, in entries where this information is known. More than one document type may be listed for a single publication, if applicable.

Brief Description

A brief description of the contents and editorial focus of the publication may be provided, preceded by the word "**Description:**" at the end of the bibliographic data. These descriptions were submitted by the publisher or were written by editorial staff after examination of sample copies or publisher catalogs.

Former Titles

Title changes are common phenomena in serials publishing. Entries may contain former title information, providing a history of changes which may be useful for bibliographic record-keeping. Previous titles for the serial are given, along with their ISSN, if known. ISSN are assigned to specific titles and therefore change with the title. The former titles are preceded by a description of the type of title change. Simple title changes are noted by the words "Formerly" or "Former titles." Other types may include mergers, incorporations or supersessions. Dates provided are generally the date that the change became effective. For mergers and incorporations, date ranges indicate the years of publication for that previous title.

Media

The primary medium is specified for other than the traditional print on paper, with the exception of the notation "Duplicated." Common media listed include Online, CD-ROM, Diskette, Microfilm, and Microfiche. Online - full text denotes that the entire text of all the articles of a serial is available online, while Online - full content denotes that the entire content including graphics is available. If a serial is primarily available in Braille or Large Type, that notation will be found here.

Related Titles

This section provides information on all available formats, editions, and related publications. Often the title and ISSN are provided. The diamond symbol (♦) indicates that there is a complete listing elsewhere in the CLASSIFIED LIST OF SERIALS. Please refer to the TITLE INDEX for the page number of that listing. When no complete record is available, data such as start year, frequency, or price may be provided.

Information on alternate media editions, such as online, CD-ROM or microform editions, is provided here. Online providers and CD-ROM producer names are given if known. Complete address and contact information for these companies is provided in the ONLINE SERVICE LISTING on page 4571. For publications available in microform, a three-letter code for the vendor or micropublisher is provided. A list of names, addresses, and contact information begins on p. xxxi of volume two.

Abstracting and Indexing

The notation "**Indexed:**" precedes a list of abbreviations for all abstracting and indexing services known to cover the serial on a regular basis. Years of coverage immediately follow each abstracting and indexing service code, if known. The complete names of the abstracting and indexing services are listed with their abbreviations on p. xxxix of volume two. This section also includes status information and related titles. Consult the TITLE INDEX for page references to entries in the CLASSIFIED LIST OF SERIALS for active services.

Document Suppliers

These notations are preceded by an em-dash (–). The presence of a notation indicates the availability of articles from that serial through the specified service, by permission from the copyright holder. Such permissions are subject to change without notice. Articles may be available in paper and/or electronic format, depending on the service. The full names and complete address and contact information for these companies are listed beginning on p. xxix of volume two.

The British Library Document Supply Centre shelfmark number, a unique identifier of each serial, appears in parentheses after that organization's code, ex. "BLDSC (0000.000000)." The format of the shelfmark is four digits, a decimal point, then six digits.

The *Medical and Health Care Books and Serials In Print* Database and the individual databases of document suppliers were matched on the presence of ISSNs. When a match was successful, the appropriate document supplier code was noted. Not all serials titles in general or in these individual databases, have ISSNs. Therefore, the absence of one or any document supplier codes in an ***Medical and Health Care Books & Serials In Print*** listing does not necessarily mean the title is not available from one or any of these suppliers.

Copyright Clearance Center, Inc.

Copyright Clearance Center, Inc. (CCC), the largest licenser of text reproduction rights in the world, was formed in 1978 to facilitate compliance with U.S. Copyright law. CCC provides licensing systems for reproduction and distribution of copyrighted materials in print and electronic formats. CCC manages rights for over 1.75 million works and represents over 9,600 publishers and hundreds of thousands of authors and other creators, directly or through their representatives. CCC-licensed customers in the U.S. Number over 10,000 corporations and subsidiaries, and thousands of government agencies, law firms, document suppliers, libraries, academic institutions, copy shops, and bookstores.

The boldfaced **CCC** notation appears in the entries of titles for which the CCC has been authorized by the publisher to grant photocopy permissions on any of their works. Contact them at 222 Rosewood Dr., Danvers, MA 01923, USA; tel: 978-750-8400; fax: 978-750-4470; URL: http://www.copyright.com.

Publishing Company Information

This section begins with the bold phrase "Published by," or "Address" if the company name is the same as the titles.

Many serials are editorially controlled by a sponsoring organization or corporate author and published by a commercial publisher. In these instances, the commercial publishing company's name and address are given, and the name of the corporate author is given in parentheses immediately preceding. In other instances, either a sponsoring organization or a commercial publishing company has sole responsibility, and only one name is given. We avoid listing printers as publishing companies, preferring the name and address of someone with editorial responsibility. For the same reason, we avoid listing distributors as publishing companies.

Telephone, Fax, Telex Numbers, E-mail, and Web Site Addresses

Telephone, fax, telex numbers, and e-mail as well as web site addresses (URLs) are given when provided by the publisher. U.S. and Canadian numbers are given in standard North American format. Toll-free numbers within U.S. and Canada are also included, when available. Numbers in other countries are provided in the same format as supplied by the publisher, resulting in some inconsistencies (e.g. sometimes with a country and/or city code, sometimes without). Users are advised to consult an international operator before placing calls.

Editor

Only one or two names are given when known, preceded by the notation "Ed." or "Eds." Advanced degrees and titles are omitted, except for medical, military, and religious titles; absence of a title does not mean that the editor has none.

Publisher

Only one or two names are given when known, preceded by the notation "Pub." or "Pubs." Advanced degrees and titles are omitted, except for medical, military, and religious titles; absence of a title does not mean that the publisher has none.

If the publisher is also the editor, and no publishing company name is available, the person's name is given in place of company name with the notation "Ed. & Pub."

Rights and Permissions Contact

A name is given when supplied, preceded by the notation "R&P contact." The telephone number information follows, when known and different from the main number.

Advertising Rates and Contact

When provided by the publisher, the name of the advertising contact, as well as full-page advertising rates and size are indicated. Most dimensions are listed in millimeters, except for U.S. publications, the dimensions of which are usually in inches.

Circulation

All circulation figures used are approximate. Circulation is given only if provided by the publisher. The notation "controlled" indicates that the publication is available only to qualified persons, usually members of a particular trade or profession. The notation "paid" indicates that subscribers pay to receive the publication, while the notation "free" indicates that the title is freely distributed.

Wire Services

If a newspaper is known to use one or more news or photo wire services, abbreviations or names of the services used are listed in the entry. Such information is preceded by the words "Wire Service(s):." Abbreviations for wire services used are listed on p. xxxvii of volume two.

Subscription or Distribution Information

A second address is given only if the address for ordering subscriptions is different from the publishing company's address. Distributors are listed only if we have been informed that a particular organization is the exclusive distributor. Additional subscription and/or distribution offices of international publishers are listed, if known. Telephone and fax numbers and e-mail and URL addresses for subscription and/or distribution offices appear if provided by the publisher.

Other related organizations and companies such as co-sponsors, affiliates, or co-publishers may be noted here.

Newspaper Ownership

The name of the owner(s) of a newspaper is listed, usually accompanied by the owner(s) address, and telephone and fax numbers. The owner address may differ from the newspaper location address. Owner information is preceded by the notation "Owner(s):."

CATALOGING RULES FOR MAIN ENTRY TITLE

The majority of titles in the Ulrich's database were cataloged according to *Anglo-American Cataloging Rules* prior to 1978, the date of the new edition of *Anglo-American Cataloging Rules*. The new *AACR II* reflects a trend toward the Key Title concept of cataloging as used by the International Serials Data System (ISDS) and published in its *International Standard Bibliographic Description for Serials* (1974).

Because recataloging a database the size of Bowker's was not feasible, our cataloging rules were modified but not radically changed. Cross-references are provided in the TITLE INDEX from variant forms of title, such as Key Title, to aid users searching by other methods.

Whenever possible, main entry title cataloging is done from a sample of the title page of the most recent issue, according to the following rules:

Articles at the beginning of titles are omitted, or are bypassed in filing.

Serials with distinctive titles are usually entered under title. For Example:

> *Annual Bulletin of Historical Literature*
> *Business Week*
> *Milton Studies*

If a title consists only of a generic term followed by the name of the issuing body, or if the name of the issuing body clarifies the content of the publication, entry is under the name of the issuing body. For example:

> *Newsletter of the American Medical Library Association*

would be entered as

> *American Medical Library Association. Newsletter*

> *Medical Prospects,* issued by the Medical Development Corporation of the Philippines

would be entered as

> *Medical Development Corporation of the Philippines.*
> *Medical Prospects*

A title which consists of a subject modified generic term followed by the name of the issuing body is considered nondistinctive and is entered under the name of the isssuing body. For example:

> *Annual Meeting Scientific Proceedings of the American Animal Hospital Association*

would be entered as

> *American Animal Hospital Association. Annual Meeting Scientific Proceedings*

Government publications with nondistinctive titles are entered under the name of the government jurisdiction of the issuing body, although distinctive titles of government organizations may be entered directly under title. For example:

> *Great Britain. Pharmacological Research Council.*
> *Annual Report*

but

> *Medical Abstract of Iceland*

Titles which begin with the initials of the issuing body are entered under the initials. Cross-references from the full name are provided in the TITLE INDEX.

If a geographic name is part of the name of the issuing body, entry will be under the common form of the name of the body. For example:

> *University of the West Indies. Vice-Chancellor's Report*

not

> *West Indies. University. Vice-Chancellor's Report*

Note, however, that government publications retain similar cataloging as government jurisdiction:

Canada. Statistics Canada. Field Research Reporting Series

Multilingual titles are entered under the first title given on the title page, or the first title reported by the publisher if the title page is not available. Titles in other languages are entered directly after the main entry title. Cross-references are provided in the TITLE INDEX for each language title.

FILING RULES

Due to the restrictions imposed by computer filing of titles, the following special filing rules should be noted. The majority of punctuation marks are treated as spaces. A combination of punctuation and spaces is treated as one space.

Acronyms and initials are treated as such and are listed at the beginning of each letter of the alphabet.

D H Lawrence Review
D.L.A.N.Y. Newsletter
D N R
Dade County Teacher

Hyphenated words are treated as separate words:

Pre-Text

precedes

Preaching

Initial articles may be provided for a title, but do not affect their alphabetization. Articles and prepositions within titles are alphabetized as words:

Journal of the West

precedes

Journal of Theological Studies

Diacritical marks have been omitted. The German and Scandinavian umlaut has been replaced by the letter "e" following the vowels a, e, o, and u. In Danish, Norwegian and Swedish, the letter D is sequenced as "aa" and the letter r as "oe."

Key to Abbreviations

General

a.	annual
abr.	abridged
abstr.	abstracts
adpt.	adapted
adv.	advertising
aft.	afterword
Amer.	American
anno.	annotated by
annot.	annotation(s)
ans.	answer(s)
app.	appendix
Apple II	Apple II disk
approx.	approximately
ARA	Arabic
assn.	association
audio	analog audio cassette
auth.	author
avail.	available
Ave.	Avenue
bd.	bound
bdg.	binding
bds.	boards
bi-m.	bimonthly (every two months)
bibl(s).	bibliography (ies)
bi-w.	biweekly (every two weeks)
bk(s).	book(s)
bk.rev.	book reviews
bklet(s).	booklet(s)
BLDSC	British Library Document Supply Center
Blvd.	Boulevard
boxed	boxed set, slipcase, or caseboard
Bro.	Brother
C	college audience level
CAT	Catalan
CCC	Copyright Clearance Center
CHI	Chinese
c/o	care of
circ.	circulation
coll.	college
cols./p.	columns per page
co.	company
comm.	Commission, committee
comment.	commentaries
comp.	compiled
cond.	condensed
contr.	controlled
corp.	corporation
CRO	Croatian
cum.index	cumulative index
Cy.	county
CZE	Czech
d.	daily
DAN	Danish
dance rev.	dance reviews
dept.	department
des.	designed
diag(s).	diagram(s)
digital audio	digital audio cassette
Dir.	Director
disk	software disk or diskette
dist.	distributed
Div.	Division
doz.	dozen
Dr.	Drive
DUT	Dutch
ea.	each
ed.	edited, edition, editor
eds.	editions, editors
Ed.Bd.	Editorial Board
educ.	education
elem.	elementary
ency.	encyclopedia
ENG	English
enl.	enlarged
epil.	epilogue
exp.	expurgated
expr.	experiments
fac.	facsimile
fasc.	fascicle
fict.	fiction
fig(s).	figure(s)
film rev.	film reviews
FIN	Finnish
5.25 hd	1.2M, 5.25″ disk, DOS
5.25 ld	360K, 5.25″ disk, DOS
flmstrp.	filmstrip
footn.	footnotes
for.	foreign
fortn.	fortnightly (every two weeks)
FRE	French
frwd.	foreward
gen.	general
GER	German
GRE	Greek
gr.	grade, grades
hdbk.	handbook
HEB	Hebrew
HUN	Hungarian
i.t.a.	initial teaching alphabet
Illus.	Illustrated, Illustration(s), Illustrator(s)
in prep.	in preparation
incl.	includes, including
info.	information
inst.	institute
intro.	introduction
irreg.	irregular
ISBN	International Standard Book Number
ISSN	International Standard Serial Number

KEY TO ABBREVIATIONS

ITA	Italian
J	juvenile audience level
JPN	Japanese
Jr.	Junior
jt. auth.	joint author
jt. ed.	joint editor
k	kindergarten audience level
KOR	Korean
lab.	laboratory
LC	Library of Congress
lang(s).	language(s)
LAT	Latin
lea.	leather
lib.	library
lib. bdg.	library binding
lit.	literature, literary
lp	record, album, long playing
ltd. ed.	limited edition
m.	monthly
mac hd	144M, Mac
mac ld	800K, Mac
mass mkt.	mass market paperbound
math.	mathematics
mic. film	film microfilm
mic form	microform
mkt.	market prices
mod.	modern
mor	Morocco
MS(S)	Manuscript(s)
music rev.	music reviews
natl.	national
NOR	Norwegian
no(s).	number(s)
N.S.	New Series
o.p.	out of print
orig.	original text, not a reprint (paperback)
o.s.i.	out of stock indefinitely
p.	pages
pap.	paper
pat.	patents
per.	perfect binding
PER	Persian (Modern)
photos.	photographer, photographs
play rev.	play reviews (theater reviews)
PLB	publisher's library binding
P.O.	Post Office
POL	Polish
pop. ed.	popular edition
POR	Portuguese
pp./issue	pages per issue
prep.	preparation
probs.	problems
Prof.	Professor
prog. bk.	programmed book
ps	preschool audience level
pseud.	pseudonym
pt(s).	part(s)
pub.	published, publisher, publishing
pubn.	publication
R&P	Rights & Permissions
q.	quarterly
record rev.	record reviews
ref(s).	reference(s)
repr.	reprint
reprod(s).	reproduction(s)
ret.	retold by
rev.	revised
rpm.	revolution per minute (photo records)
RUS	Russian
s-a.	semiannually (twice annually)
SAN	Standard Address Number
S&L	Signed and Limited
scp	single copy (Direct to Consumer Price)
SER	Serbian
s-m.	semimonthly (twice monthly)
s.p.	school price
s-w.	semiweekly (twice weekly)
SWE	Swedish
sec.	section
sel.	selected
ser.	series
s & l	signed & limited
Soc.	Society
sols.	solutions
SPA	Spanish
Sr. (after given name)	Senior
Sr. (before given name)	Sister
St.	Saint, Street
stat.	statistics
subs.	subsidiary
subscr.	subscription
suppl.	supplement
tech.	technical
tele. rev.	television reviews
text ed.	text edition
3.5 hd	1.44M, 3.5″ disk, DOS
3.5 ld	720K, 3.5″ disk, DOS
3/m.	3 times a month
3/yr.	3 times a year
tr.	translator, translated, translation
tr.lit.	trade literature (manufacturers' catalogs, etc.)
tr.mk.	trade marks
trans.	transparencies
univ.	university
URL	Uniform Resource Locator
vdisk	videodisc
VHS	video, VHS format
video rev.	video reviews
vol(s).	volume(s)
w.	weekly
wkbk.	workbook
x (after price)	short discount (20 or less)
YA	young adult audience level
yrbk.	yearbook
✶	not updated/unverified
●	online and / or CD-ROM availability
▼	new serial
(†)	ceased
♦	complete listing available
➤	refereed

Country of Publication Codes

This list of countries and their codes is the International Standards Organization (ISO) set of 3-letter country abbreviations. This is the complete list of ISO codes, though not all countries may be represented in **Medical and Health Care Books and Serials In Print**. The codes are mnemonic in most cases. The country names listed here may have been shortened to a more common usage form. Country names no longer in use remain on the list to represent any titles that may have ceased while that country name was still in use.

Code Sequence

ABW	Aruba
AFG	Afghanistan
AGO	Angola
AIA	Anguilla
ALB	Albania
AND	Andorra
ANT	Netherlands Antilles
ARE	United Arab Emirates
ARG	Argentina
ARM	Armenia
ASM	American Samoa
ATA	Antarctica
ATF	French Southern Territories
ATG	Antigua & Barbuda
AUS	Australia
AUT	Austria
AZE	Azerbaijan
BDI	Burundi
BEL	Belgium
BEN	Benin
BFA	Burkina Faso
BGD	Bangladesh
BGR	Bulgaria
BHR	Bahrain
BHS	Bahamas
BIH	Bosnia & Herzegovina
BLR	Belarus
BLZ	Belize
BMU	Bermuda
BOL	Bolivia
BRA	Brazil
BRB	Barbados
BRD	West Germany
BRN	Brunei Darussalam
BTN	Bhutan
BVT	Bouvet Island
BWA	Botswana
CAF	Central African Republic
CAN	Canada
CCK	Cocos (Keeling) Islands
CHE	Switzerland
CHL	Chile
CHN	China
CIV	Cote' D'Ivoire
CMR	Cameroon
COD	Congo, Democratic Republic of
COG	Congo
COK	Cook Islands
COL	Colombia
COM	Comoros
CPV	Cape Verde
CRI	Costa Rica
CSK	Czechoslovakia
CUB	Cuba
CXR	Christmas Island
CYN	Cayman Islands
CYP	Cyprus
CZE	Czech Republic
DDR	East Germany
DEU	Germany
DJI	Djibouti
DMA	Dominica
DNK	Denmark
DOM	Dominican Republic
DZA	Algeria
ECU	Ecuador
EGY	Egypt
ERI	Eritrea
ESH	Western Sahara
ESP	Spain
EST	Estonia
ETH	Ethiopia
FIN	Finland
FJI	Fiji
FLK	Falkland Islands
FRA	France
FRO	Faeroe Islands
FSM	Fed. States of Micronesia
GAB	Gabon
GBR	United Kingdom
GEO	Georgia
GHA	Ghana
GIB	Gibraltar
GIN	Guinea
GLP	Guadeloupe
GMB	Gambia
GNB	Guinea-Bissau
GNQ	Equatorial Guinea
GRC	Greece
GRD	Grenada
GRL	Greenland
GTM	Guatemala
GUF	French Guiana
GUM	Guam
GUY	Guyana
HKG	Hong Kong
HMD	Heard Island & Mcdonald Islands
HND	Honduras
HRV	Croatia
HTI	Haiti
HUN	Hungary
IDN	Indonesia
IND	India
IOT	British Indian Ocean Territory
IRL	Ireland
IRN	Iran
IRQ	Iraq
ISL	Iceland
ISR	Israel
ITA	Italy
JAM	Jamaica
JOR	Jordan
JPN	Japan
KAZ	Kazakstan
KEN	Kenya
KGZ	Kyrgyzstan
KHM	Cambodia
KIR	Kiribati
KNA	Saint Kitts & Nevis
KOR	Korea, Republic of
KWT	Kuwait
LAO	Laos
LBN	Lebanon
LBR	Liberia
LBY	Libya
LCA	St. Lucia
LIE	Liechtenstein
LKA	Sri Lanka
LSO	Lesotho
LTU	Lithuania
LUX	Luxembourg
LVA	Latvia
MAC	Macau
MAR	Morocco
MCO	Monaco
MDA	Moldova
MDG	Madagascar
MDV	Maldive Islands
MEX	Mexico
MHL	Marshall Islands
MKD	Macedonia
MLI	Mali
MLT	Malta
MMR	Myanmar
MNG	Mongolia
MNP	Northern Mariana Islands
MOZ	Mozambique
MRT	Mauritania
MSR	Monteserrat
MTQ	Martinique
MUS	Mauritius
MWI	Malawi
MYS	Malaysia
MYT	Mayotte
NAM	Namibia
NCL	New Caledonia
NER	Niger
NFK	Norfolk Island
NGA	Nigeria
NIC	Nicaragua
NIU	Niue
NLD	Netherlands
NOR	Norway
NPL	Nepal
NRU	Nauru
NZL	New Zealand
OMN	Oman
PAK	Pakistan
PAN	Panama
PCN	Pitcairn
PER	Peru
PHL	Philippines
PLW	Palau
PNG	Papua New Guinea
POL	Poland
PRI	Puerto Rico
PRK	Korea, Democratic People's Rep. of
PRT	Portugal
PRY	Paraguay
PSE	Occupied Palestinian Territory
PYF	French Polynesia
QAT	Qatar
REU	Reunion
ROM	Romania
RUS	Russia
RWA	Rwanda
SAU	Saudi Arabia
SDN	Sudan
SEN	Senegal

SGP	Singapore
SGS	South Georgia & Sandwich Islands
SHN	Saint Helena
SJM	Svalbard & Jan Mayen
SLB	Solomon Islands
SLE	Sierra Leone
SLV	El Salvador
SMR	San Marino
SOM	Somalia
SPM	Saint Pierre & Miquelon
STP	Sao Tome e Principe
SUN	U.S.S.R.
SUR	Suriname
SVK	Slovakia
SVN	Slovenia
SWE	Sweden
SWZ	Swaziland
SYC	Seychelles
SYR	Syrian Arab Republic
TCA	Turks & Caicos Islands
TCD	Chad
TGO	Togo
THA	Thailand
TJK	Tajikistan
TKL	Tokelau
TKM	Turkmenistan
TNP	East Timor
TON	Tonga
TTO	Trinidad & Tobago
TUN	Tunisia
TUR	Turkey
TUV	Tuvalu
TWN	Taiwan
TZA	Tanzania
UGA	Uganda
UKR	Ukraine
UMI	US Minor Islands
URY	Uruguay
USA	United States
UZB	Uzbekistan
VAT	Vatican City
VCT	St. Vincent & Grenadines
VEN	Venezuela
VGB	Virgin Islands, British
VIR	Virgin Islands, U.S.
VNM	Viet Nam
VUT	Vanuatu
WLF	Wallis & Futuna
WSM	Somoa
YEM	Yemen
YUG	Yugoslavia
ZAF	South Africa
ZAR	Zaire
ZMB	Zambia
ZWE	Zimbabwe

Country Sequence

AFGHANISTAN	AFG
ALBANIA	ALB
ALGERIA	DZA
AMERICAN SAMOA	ASM
ANDORRA	AND
ANGOLA	AGO
ANGUILLA	AIA
ANTARCTICA	ATA
ANTIGUA & BARBUDA	ATG
ARGENTINA	ARG
ARMENIA	ARM
ARUBA	ABW
AUSTRALIA	AUS
AUSTRIA	AUT
AZERBAIJAN	AZE
BAHAMAS	BHS
BAHRAIN	BHR
BANGLADESH	BGD
BARBADOS	BRB
BELARUS	BLR
BELGIUM	BEL
BELIZE	BLZ
BENIN	BEN
BERMUDA	BMU
BHUTAN	BTN
BOLIVIA	BOL
BOSNIA & HERCEGOVINA	BIH
BOTSWANA	BWA
BOUVET ISLAND	BVT
BRAZIL	BRA
BRITISH INDIAN OCIAN TERRITORY	IOT
BRUNEI DARUSSALAM	BRN
BULGARIA	BGR
BURKINA FASO	BFA
BURUNDI	BDI
CAMBODIA	KHM
CAMEROON	CMR
CANADA	CAN
CAPE VERDE	CPV
CAYMAN ISLANDS	CYM
CENTRAL AFRICAN REPUBLIC	CAF
CHAD	TCD
CHILE	CHL
CHINA	CHN
CHRISTMAS ISLAND	CXR
COCOS (KEELING) ISLANDS	CCK
COLOMBIA	COL
COMOROS	COM
CONGO	COG
CONGO, DEMOCRATIC REPUBLIC OF	COD
COOK ISLANDS	COK
COSTA RICA	CRI
COTE' D'IVOIRE	CIV
CROATIA	HRV
CUBA	CUB
CYPRUS	CYP
CZECH REPUBLIC	CZE
CZECHOSLOVAKIA	CSK
DENMARK	DNK
DJIBOUTI	DJI
DOMINICA	DMA
DOMINICAN REPUBLIC	DOM
EAST GERMANY	DDR
EAST TIMOR	TMP
ECUADOR	ECU
EGYPT	EGY
EL SALVADOR	SLV
EQUATORIAL GUINEA	GNQ
ERITREA	ERI
ESTONIA	EST
ETHIOPIA	ETH
FAEROE ISLANDS	FRO
FALKLAND ISLANDS	FLK
FED. STATES OF MICRONESIA	FSM
FIJI	FJI
FINLAND	FIN
FRANCE	FRA
FRENCH GUIANA	GUF
FRENCH POLYNESIA	PYF
FRENCH SOUTHERN TERRITORIES	ATF
GABON	GAB
GAMBIA	GMB
GEORGIA	GEO
GERMANY	DEU
GHANA	GHA
GIBRALTAR	GIB
GREECE	GRC
GREENLAND	GRL
GRENADA	GRD
GUADELOUPE	GLP
GUAM	GUM
GUATEMALA	GTM
GUINEA	GIN
GUINEA-BISSAU	GNB
GUYANA	GUY
HAITI	HTI
HEARD ISLAND & MCDONALD ISLANDS	HMD
HONDURAS	HND
HONG KONG	HKG
HUNGARY	HUN
ICELAND	ISL
INDIA	IND
INDONESIA	IDN
IRAN	IRN
IRAQ	IRQ
IRELAND	IRL
ISRAEL	ISR
ITALY	ITA
JAMAICA	JAM
JAPAN	JPN
JORDAN	JOR
KAZAKHSTAN	KAZ
KENYA	KEN
KIRIBATI	KIR
KOREA, DEMOCRATIC PEOPLE'S REP. OF	PRK
KOREA, REPUBLIC OF	KOR
KUWAIT	KWT
KYRGYZSTAN	KGZ
LAOS	LAO
LATVIA	LVA
LEBANON	LBN
LESOTHO	LSO
LIBERIA	LBR
LIBYA	LBY
LIECHTENSTEIN	LIE
LITHUANIA	LTU
LUXEMBOURG	LUX
MACAO	MAC
MACEDONIA	MKD
MADAGASCAR	MDG
MALAWI	MWI
MALAYSIA	MYS
MALDIVE ISLANDS	MDV
MALI	MLI
MALTA	MLT
MARSHALL ISLANDS	MHL
MARTINIQUE	MTQ
MAURITANIA	MRT
MAURITIUS	MUS
MAYOTTE	MYT
MEXICO	MEX
MOLDOVA	MDA
MONACO	MCO
MONGOLIA	MNG
MONTSERRAT	MSR
MOROCCO	MAR
MOZAMBIQUE	MOZ
MYANMAR	MMR
NAMIBIA	NAM
NAURU	NRU
NEPAL	NPL
NETHERLANDS	NLD
NETHERLANDS ANTILLES	ANT
NEW CALEDONIA	NCL
NEW ZEALAND	NZL
NICARAGUA	NIC
NIGER	NER
NIGERIA	NGA
NIUE	NIU
NORFOLK ISLAND	NFK
NORTHERN MARIANA ISLANDS	MNP
NORWAY	NOR
OCCUPIED PALESTINIAN TERRITORY	PSE
OMAN	OMN
PAKISTAN	PAK
PALAU	PLW
PANAMA	PAN
PAPUA NEW GUINEA	PNG
PARAGUAY	PRY
PERU	PER
PHILIPPINES	PHL
PITCAIRN	PCN
POLAND	POL
PORTUGAL	PRT
PUERTO RICO	PRI
QATAR	QAT
REUNION	REU
ROMANIA	ROM
RUSSIA	RUS
RWANDA	RWA
SAINT HELENA	SHN
SAINT KITTS-NEVIS	KNAI
SAINT PIERRE & MIQUELON	SPM
SAMOA	WSM
SAN MARINO	SMR
SAO TOME E PRINCIPE	STP
SAUDI ARABIA	SAU
SENEGAL	SEN
SEYCHELLES	SYC
SIERRA LEONE	SLE
SINGAPORE	SGP
SLOVAKIA	SVK
SLOVENIA	SVN

SOLOMON ISLANDS	SLB	TANZANIA	TZA	US MINOR ISLANDS	UMI
SOMALIA	SOM	THAILAND	THA	UZBEKISTAN	UZB
SOUTH AFRICA	ZAF	TOGO	TGO	VANUATU	VUT
SOUTH GEORGIA & SANDWICH ISLAND	SGS	TOKELAU	TKL	VATICAN CITY	VAT
SPAIN	ESP	TONGA	TON	VENEZUELA	VEN
SRI LANKA	LKA	TRINIDAD & TOBAGO	TTO	VIET NAM	VNM
ST. LUCIA	LCA	TUNISIA	TUN	VIRGIN ISLANDS, BRITISH	VGB
ST. VINCENT & GRENADINES	VCT	TURKEY	TUR	VIRGIN ISLANDS, U.S.	VIR
SUDAN	SDN	TURKMENISTAN	TKM	WALLIS & FUTUNA	WLF
SURINAM	SUR	TURKS & CAICOS ISLANDS	TCA	WEST GERMANY	BRD
SVALBARD & JAN MAYEN	SJM	TUVALU	TUV	WESTERN SAHARA	ESH
SWAZILAND	SWZ	U.S.S.R.	SUN	YEMEN	YEM
SWEDEN	SWE	UGANDA	UGA	YUGOSLAVIA	YUG
SWITZERLAND	CHE	UKRAINE	UKR	ZAIRE	ZAR
SYRIAN ARAB REPUBLIC	SYR	UNITED ARAB EMIRATES	ARE	ZAMBIA	ZMB
TAIWAN	TWN	UNITED KINGDOM	GBR	ZIMBABWE	ZWE
TAJIKISTAN	TJK	UNITED STATES	USA		
		URUGUAY	URY		

Currency Codes

This list of world currencies and their codes is the International Standards Organization (ISO) set of 3-letter currency abbreviations. This is the complete list of ISO codes, though not all currencies may be present in **Medical and Health Care Books and Serials In Print**. The codes are mnemonic in most cases, with the first 2 letters representing the country name and the third representing the currency name.

CODE	CURRENCY
ADP	Andorran Peseta
AED	United Arab Emirates Dirham
AFA	Afghanistan Afghani
ALL	Albanian Lek
AMD	Armenian Dram
ANG	Netherlands Antillian Guilder
AON	Angolan New Kwanza
ARS	Argentinean Peso
ATS	Austrian Schilling
AUD	Austrialian Dollars
AWG	Aruban Florin
AZM	Azerbaijan Manat
BAD	Bosnian Dinar
BBD	Barbados Dollar
BDT	Bangladeshi Taka
BEF	Belgian Franc
BGL	Bulgarian Lev
BHD	Bahraini Dinar
BIF	Burundi Franc
BMD	Bermudan Dollar
BND	Brunei Dollar
BOB	Bolivian Boliviano
BPS	British Pounds Sterling
BRL	Brazilian Real
BSD	Bahamian Dollar
BTN	Bhutan Ngultrum
BWP	Botswanan Pula
BYB	Belarus Ruble
BZD	Belize Dollar
CHF	Swiss Franc
CLP	Chilean Peso
CND	Canadian Dollars
CNY	Yuan (Chinese) Renminbi
COP	Colombian Peso
CRC	Costa Rican Colon
CUP	Cuban Peso
CVE	Cape Verde Escudo
CYP	Cyprus Pound
CZK	Czech Koruna
DEM	Deutsche Mark
DJF	Djibouti Franc
DKK	Danish Krone
DOP	Dominican Peso
DZD	Algerian Dinar
ECS	Ecuador Sucre
EEK	Estonian Kroon
EGP	Egyptian Pound
ERB	Eritrean Birr
ESP	Spanish Peseta
ETB	Ethiopian Birr
FIM	Finnish Markka
FJD	Fiji Dollar
FKP	Falkland Islands Pound

CODE	CURRENCY
FRF	French Franc
GBP	British Pound
GEL	Georgian Lari
GHC	Ghanaian Cedi
GIP	Gibraltar Pound
GMD	Gambian Dalasi
GNF	Guinea Franc
GNS	Guinea Syli
GRD	Greek Drachma
GTQ	Guatemalan Quetzal
GWP	Guinea-Bissau Peso
GYD	Guyanan Dollar
HKD	Hong Kong Dollar
HNL	Honduran Lempira
HRK	Croatian Kuna
HTG	Haitian Gourde
HUF	Hungarian Forint
IDR	Indonesian Rupiah
IEP	Irish Punt
ILS	Israeli Shekel
INR	Indian Rupee
IQD	Iraqi Dinar
IRR	Iranian Rial
ISK	Iceland Krona
ITL	Italian Lira
JMD	Jamaican Dollar
JOD	Jordanian Dinar
JPY	Japanese Yen
KES	Kenyan Schilling
KGS	Kyrgyzstan Som
KHR	Cambodian New Riel
KMF	Comoros Franc
KPW	North Korean Won
KRW	South Korean Won
KWD	Kuwaiti Dinar
KYD	Cayman Islands Dollar
KZT	Kazakhstani Tenge
LAK	Lao Kip
LBP	Lebanese Pound
LKR	Sri Lanka Rupee
LRD	Liberian Dollar
LSL	Lesotho Loti
LTL	Lithuanian Litas
LUF	Luxembourg Franc
LVL	Latvian Lat
LYD	Libyan Dinar
MAD	Moroccan Dirham
MDL	Moldova Leu
MGF	Malagasy Franc
MKD	Macedonian Denar
MLF	Mali Franc
MMK	Myanmar Kyat
MNT	Mongolian Tugrik

CURRENCY CODES

MOP	Macao Pataca
MRK	German Marks
MRO	Mauritanian Ouguiya
MTL	Maltese Lira
MUR	Mauritius Rupee
MVR	Maldive Rufiyaa
MWK	Malawi Kwacha
MXP	Mexican New Peso
MYR	Malaysian Ringgit
MZM	Mozambique Metical
NAD	Namibian Dollar
NGN	Nigerian Naira
NIC	Nicaraguan Gold Cordoba
NLG	Dutch Guilder
NOK	Norwegian Kroner
NPR	Nepalese Rupee
NZD	New Zealand Dollar
OMR	Omani Rial
PAB	Panamanian Balboa
PEN	Peruvian New Sol
PGK	Papua New Guinea Kina
PHP	Philippine Peso
PKR	Pakistan Rupee
PLZ	Polish Zloty
PTE	Portuguese Escudo
PYG	Paraguay Guarani
QAR	Qatari Rial
ROL	Romanian Leu
RUR	Russian Ruble
RWF	Rwanda Franc
SAR	Saudi Arabian Riyal
SBD	Solomon Islands Dollar
SCR	Seychelles Rupee
SDP	Sudanese Pound
SEK	Swedish Krona
SGD	Singapore Dollar
SHP	St. Helena Pound
SIT	Slovenian Tolar
SKK	Slovakian Koruna
SLL	Sierra Leone Leone
SOS	Somali Schilling
SRG	Suriname Guilder
STD	Sao Tome and Principe Dobra
SVC	El Salvador Colon
SYP	Syrian Pound
SZL	Swaziland Lilangeni
THB	Thai Bhat
TJR	Tajikistan Rubl
TMM	Turkemenistan Manat
TND	Tunisian Dinar
TOP	Tongan Pa'anga
TPE	East Timor Escudo
TRL	Turkish Lira
TTD	Trinidad and Tobago Dollar
TWD	Taiwan Dollar
TZS	Tanzanian Schilling
UAK	Ukraine Hryvnia
UGX	Uganda Shilling
USD	US Dollars
UYP	Peso Uruguayo
UZS	Uzbek Som
VEB	Venezuelan Bolivar
VND	Vietnamese Dong
VUV	Vanuatu Vatu
WST	Somoan Tala
XAF	CFA Franc
XDR	Special Drawing Rights
XEC	Eastern Caribbean Dollar
XEU	Euro
XOF	CFA Franc
XPF	French Polynesian Franc
YER	Yemeni Rial
YUN	Yugoslavian New Dinar
ZAR	South African Rand
ZMK	Zambian Kwacha
ZWD	Zimbabwe Dollar

Language Codes

ACE	Acholi
AFR	Afrikaans
AFA	Afro-Asiatic
AKK	Akkadian
ALB	Albanian
ALE	Aleut
ALG	Algonquin
AMH	Amharic
ANG	Anglo-Saxon
APA	Apache
ARA	Arabic
ARC	Aramaic
ARP	Arapaho
ARN	Araucanian
ARW	Arawak
ARM	Armenian
ASM	Assamese
AVA	Avar
AVE	Avesta
AYM	Aymara
AZE	Azerbaijani
BAT	Baltic
BAL	Baluchi
BAM	Bambara
BAK	Bashkir
BAQ	Basque
BEJ	Beja
BEL	Belorussian
BEM	Bemba
BEN	Bengali
BER	Berber Group
BIH	Bihari
BLA	Blackfoot
BRE	Breton
BUL	Bulgarian
BUR	Burmese
CAD	Caddo
CAM	Cambodian
CAR	Carib
CAT	Catalan
CAU	Caucasian
CEL	Celtic Group
CAI	Central American Indian
CHE	Chechen
CHR	Cherokee
CHY	Cheyenne
CHB	Chibcha
CHI	Chinese
CHN	Chinook
CHO	Choctaw
CHU	Church Slavic
CHV	Chuvash
COP	Coptic
COR	Cornish
CRE	Cree
CRP	Creoles and Pidgins
CRO	Croatian
CUS	Cushitic
CZE	Czech
DAK	Dakota
DAN	Danish
DEL	Delaware
DIN	Dinka
DOI	Dogri
DRA	Dravidian
DUA	Duala
DUT	Dutch
EFI	Efik
EGY	Egyptian
ELX	Elamite
ENG	English
ENM	English, Middle
ESK	Eskimo
ESP	Esperanto
EST	Estonian
ETH	Ethiopic
EWE	Ewe
FAN	Fang
FAR	Faroese
FIJ	Fijian
FIN	Finnish
FIU	Finno-Ugrian
FLE	Flemish
FON	Fon
FRE	French
FEM	French, Middle
FRO	French, Old
FRI	Frisian
GAA	Ga
GAE	Gaelic
GAL	Galla
GAG	Gallegan
GEO	Georgian
GER	German
GEH	German, Middle High
GOH	German, Old High
GEM	Germanic
GON	Gondi
GOT	Gothic
GRE	Greek
GEC	Greek, Classical
GUA	Guarani
GUJ	Gujarati
HAU	Hausa
HAW	Hawaiian
HEB	Hebrew
HER	Herero
HIL	Hiligaynon
HIN	Hindi
HUN	Hungarian
HUP	Hupa
IBA	Iban
ICE	Icelandic
IBO	Igbo
ILO	Ilocano
INC	Indic
INE	Indo-European
IND	Indonesian
INT	Interlingua
IKU	Inuktitut
IRA	Iranian
IRI	Irish
IRO	Iroquois
ITA	Italian
JPN	Japanese
JAV	Javanese
KAC	Kachin
KAM	Kamba
KAN	Kannada
KAU	Kanuri
KAA	Karakalpak
KAR	Karen
KAS	Kashmiri
KAZ	Kazakh
KHA	Khasi
KIK	Kikuyu
KIN	Kinyarwanda
KIR	Kirghiz
KON	Kongo
KOK	Konkani
KOR	Korean
KPE	Kpelle
KRO	Kru
KUR	Kurdish
KRU	Kurukh
KUA	Kwanyama
LAD	Ladino
LAH	Lahnda
LAM	Lamba
LAO	Laotian
LAP	Lapp
LAT	Latin
LAV	Latvian
LIN	Lingala
LIT	Lithuanian
LOL	Lolo
LUB	Luba
LUG	Luganda
LUI	Luiseno
MAC	Macedonian
MAI	Maithili
MLA	Malagasy
MAY	Malay
MAL	Malayalam
MAP	Malayo-Polynesian
MLT	Maltese
MAN	Mandingo
MNO	Manobo
MAO	Maori
MAR	Marathi
MAS	Masai
MYN	Mayan
MEN	Mende
MIC	Micmac
MIS	Miscellaneous
MOL	Moldavian
MON	Mongol
MOS	Mossi
MUL	Multiple languages
MUS	Muskogee
NAV	Navaho
NDE	Ndebele, Northern
NBL	Ndebele, Southern
NEP	Nepali
NEW	Newari
NIC	Niger-Congo
NAI	North American Indian
NOR	Norwegian
NUB	Nubian
NYM	Nyamwezi
NYA	Nyanja
NYO	Nyoro Group
OJI	Ojibwa
ORI	Oriya
OSA	Osage
OES	Ossetic
OTO	Otomi
PAH	Pahari
PAL	Pahlavi
PLI	Pali
PAN	Panjabi
PAA	Papuan-Australian
PER	Persian, Modern
PEO	Persian, Old
POL	Polish
POR	Portuguese
PRO	Provencal
PUS	Pushto
QUE	Quechua
RAJ	Rajasthani

ROA	Romance
RUM	Romanian
ROH	Romansh
ROM	Romany
RUN	Rundi
RUS	Russian
SAM	Samaritan
SAO	Sampan
SAD	Sandawe
SAG	Sango
SAN	Sanskrit
SRD	Sardinian
SCO	Scots
SEL	Selkup
SEM	Semitic
SER	Serbian
SBC	Serbo-Croatian
SRR	Serer
SHN	Shan
SHO	Shona
SID	Sidamo
SND	Sindhi
SNH	Singhalese
SIT	Sino-Tibetan
SIO	Siouan languages
SLA	Slavic
SLO	Slovak
SLV	Slovenian
SOG	Sogdian
SOM	Somali
SON	Songhai
NSO	Sotho, Northern
SOT	Sotho, Southern
SAI	South American Indian
SPA	Spanish
SSA	Sub-Saharan African
SUK	Sukuma
SUX	Sumerian
SUN	Sundanese
SUS	Susu
SWA	Swahili
SWE	Swedish
SYR	Syriac
TAG	Tagalog
TAJ	Tajik
TAM	Tamil
TAR	Tatar
TEL	Telugu
TEM	Temne
TER	Tereno
THA	Thai
TIB	Tibetan
TIG	Tigre
TIR	Tigrinya
TOG	Tonga, Nyasa
TON	Tonga, Tonga Islands
TSI	Tsimshian
TSO	Tsonga
TSW	Tswana
TUR	Turkish
TUK	Turkmen
TUT	Turko-Tataric
TWI	Twi
UGA	Ugaritic
UIG	Uigur
UKR	Ukrainian
UMB	Umbundu
UND	Undetermined
URD	Urdu
UZB	Uzbek
VIE	Vietnamese
VOT	Votic
WAL	Walamo
WAS	Washo
WEL	Welsh
WEN	Wendic
WOL	Wolof
XHO	Xhosa
YAO	Yao
YID	Yiddish
YOR	Yoruba
ZAP	Zapotec
ZEN	Zenaga
ZUL	Zulu
ZUN	Zuni

Document Suppliers

ADONIS **ADONIS BV**
Molenwerf 1, Amsterdam 1014 AG, Netherlands
TEL 31-20-485-3870, FAX 31-20-485-3871
E-mail info@adonis.nl
URL http://www.adonis.nl
PO Box 765, Framingham, MA 01701
TEL 508-877-6400, 800-944-6415, FAX 508-877-6464
E-mail infousa@adonis.nl

AskIEEE **AskIEEE**
10850 Wilshire Blvd., 8th Fl. Los Angeles, CA 90024
TEL 800-422-4633
E-mail service@infotrieve.com, info@infotrieve.com
URL http://ieee.org/services/askieee

BLDSC **British Library Document Supply Centre**
Boston Spa, Wetherby LS23 7BQ, United Kingdom
TEL 44-1937-546060
FAX 44-1937-5463336
TELEX 557381
E-mail dsc-customer-service@bl.uk

CASDDS **Chemical Abstracts Service Document Detective Service**
2540 Olentangy River Rd, PO Box 3012, Columbus, OH 43210-0012
TEL 614-447-3670, 800-678-4337
FAX 614-447-3648
E-mail dds@cas.org
URL http://www.cas.org/support/dds.html

CINDOC **CINDOC Suministro de Documentos Service**
Joaquin Costa, 22, Madrid 28002, Spain
TEL 91-563-5482
FAX 91-564-2644
E-mail bib-icytfot@cindoc.csic.es
URL http://www.cindoc.csic.es/

CIS **Congressional Information Service, Incorporated**
(Subsidiary of: LexisNexis)
4520 East-West Hwy., Suite 800, Bethesda, MD 20814
TEL 301-654-1550, 800-638-8380
FAX 301-657-3203
E-mail academicinfo@lexisnexis.com
URL http://www.lexis-nexis.com/academic/

CISTI **CISTI**
(Canada Institute for Scientific and Technical Information)
(Subsidiary of: National Research Council of Canada)
1200 Montreal Rd., Bldg, M-55, Ottawa, ON K1A 0S2, Canada
TEL 613-993-9251, 800-668-1222, FAX 613-993-7619
E-mail cisti.producthelp@nrc.ca
URL http://www.nrc.ca/cisti

CatchWord **CatchWord Ltd.**
23-28 Hythe Bridge St., Ground Fl., Oxford OX1 2ET, United Kingdom
TEL 44-1865-799000, FAX 44-1865-799111
E-mail sales@catchword.com
URL http://www.catchword.com.

EMDOCS **EMDOCS: The EMBASE Document Delivery Service**
Suspended

East View **East View Publications, Incorporated**
3020 Harbor Ln., N., Minneapolis, MN 55447
TEL 763-550-0961, 800-477-1005, FAX 763-559-2931, 800-800-3839
E-mail eastview@eastview.com
URL http://www.eastview.com

Ei **Engineering Information, Incorporated**
see Linda Hall Library Document Services

DOCUMENT SUPPLIERS

GNLM — **German National Library of Medicine**
Joseph-Stelzman-Str. 9, D-50924, Koeln, Germany
TEL 49-221-4785600, FAX 49-221-4785697
E-mail zbmed.zbmed@uni-koeln.de
URL http://www.zbmed.de

Haworth — **Haworth Press, Incorporated, The**
10 Alice St., Binghamton, NY 13904-1580
TEL 607-722-5857, 800-429-6784, FAX 607-771-0012, 607-722-1424, 800-895-0582, TELEX 49 325 99 HAWORTH
FAX 800-895-0582
E-mail orders@haworthpressinc.com
URL http://www.haworthpressinc.com

IDS — **Institute for Scientific Information**
3501 Market St., Philadelphia, PA 19104
TEL 215-386-0100, 800-336-4474 ext. 4900
FAX 215-222-0840, 212-386-4343
E-mail ids@isinet
URL http://www.isinet.com/isi/products/ids/ids

ingenta — **ingenta**
44 Brattle St., 4th Fl., Cambridge, MA 02138
TEL 617-395-4000, 800-296-2221, FAX 617-395-4099, 617-395-4099
E-mail help@ingenta.com
URL http://www.ingenta.com

Infotrieve — **Infotrieve**
10850 Wilshire Blvd 8th Fl, Los Angeles, CA 90024
TEL 800-422-4633, FAX 310-208-5971
E-mail info@infotrieve.com
URL http://www3.infotrieve.com

KNAW — **NIWI (Netherlands Institute of Scientific Information Services)**
Customer Service, 95180, Amsterdam 1090 HD, Netherlands
TEL 31-20-462-8628, FAX 31-20-663-9257
E-mail info@niwi.knaw.nl
URL http://www.niwi.knaw.nl/us/docdel/docdel.htm

Linda Hall — **Linda Hall Library Document Services**
5109 Cherry St, Kansas City, MO 64110-2498
TEL 816-363-4600, 800-662-1545, FAX 816-926-8785
E-mail requests@lindahall.org
URL http://www.lindahall.org/docserv/

PADDS — **Petroleum Abstracts**
600 S. College Ave., Tulsa, OK 74104
TEL 918-631-2296, 800-247-8678, FAX 918-599-9361
University of Tulsa, McFarlin Library, 2933 E. Sixth St., Tulsa, OK 74104-3123
TEL 918-631-2231, 800-247-8678, FAX 918-631-3823
E-mail question@TUred.pa.utulsa.edu
URL http://www.pa.utulsa.edu

Micropublishers and Distributors

ADL **Advanced Library Systems, Inc.**
30 Massachusetts Ave, N. Andover, MA 01845
TEL 978-682-7561
FAX 978-682-3457
E-mail advlibsy@shore.net

AGU **American Geophysical Union**
2000 Florida Ave., NW, Washington, DC 20009
TEL 202-462-6900, 800-966-2481, FAX 202-328-0566
E-mail service@agu.org
URL http://www.agu.org

AIP **American Institute of Physics**
1 Physics Ellipse, College Park, MD 20740-3843
TEL 301-209-3100, FAX 301-209-0843
E-mail aipinfo@aip.org
URL http://www.aip.org/

AJP **American Jewish Periodical Center**
3101 Clifton Ave., Cincinnati, OH 45220
TEL 513-221-1875, FAX 513-221-0519

ALP **Alpha Com**
Sportallee 6, Hamburg 22335, Germany
TEL 49-40-51302-123, FAX 49-40-51302-111
URL http://www.alpha-com.de

AMP **Adam Matthew Publications Ltd.**
Pelham House, London Rd, Marlborough, Wiltshire SN8 2AA, United Kingdom
TEL 44-1672-511921, FAX 44-1672-511663
E-mail adam-matthew@msn.com
URL http://www.ampltd.co.uk

BHP **Brookhaven Press**
(Subsidiary of: N M T Corporation)
2004 Kramer St., LaCrosse, WI 54603
TEL 608-781-0850, 800-236-0850, FAX 608-781-3883
E-mail brookhaven@nmt.com
URL http://www.brookhavenpress.com

BIO **BIOSIS**
(BioSciences Information Service of Biological Abstracts)
Two Commerce Square, 2001 Market Street, Suite 700, Philadelphia, PA 19103-7095
TEL 800-523-4806
FAX 215-578-2016
E-mail info@mail.biosis.org
URL http://www.biosis.org

BLI **Balch Institute for Ethnic Studies, The**
18 S. Seventh St., Philadelphia, PA 19106
TEL 215-925-8090, FAX 215-925-8195
E-mail info@balchinstitute.org, balchlib@balchinstitute.org
URL http://www.balchinstitute.org

BNB **British Library National Bibliographic Service**
Boston Spa, Weyherby, W. Yorkshire LS23 7BQ, United Kingdom
TEL 44-1937-546585, FAX 44-1937-546586
E-mail nbs-info@bl.uk
URL http://www.bl.uk/

BNQ **Bibliotheque Nationale du Quebec (B N Q)**
2275 Rue Holt, Montreal, PQ H2G 3H1, Canada
TEL 514-873-1100 ext.158, 800-363-9028, FAX 514-873-7510
E-mail web@biblinat.gouv.qc.ca
URL http://www.biblinat.gouv.qc.ca/

CDS **Current Digest of the Soviet Press**
3857 N. High St., Columbus, OH 43214
TEL 614-292-4234, FAX 614-267-6310
E-mail fowler.40@osu.edu
URL http://www.cohums.ohio-state.edu/

CHL **Chadwyck-Healey Limited**
see Proquest Information & Learning

CIS **Congressional Information Service, Incorporated**
(Subsidiary of: LexisNexis)
4520 East-West Hwy., Suite 800, Bethesda, MD 20814
TEL 301-654-1550, 800-638-8380
FAX 301-657-3203
E-mail academicinfo@ @lexisnexis.com
URL http://www.lexisnexis.com/academic

CMC **M.R. Technology**
3655 Wheeler Ave, Alexandria, VA 22304
TEL 703-461-4400, FAX 703-461-0042

CML **Commonwealth Microfilm Products**
543 Richmond St., W. Ste 119, 201, Toronto, ON M5V 1Y6, Canada
TEL 416-703-3755, FAX 416-703-3753
URL http://www.westcanadian.com

EEE **Institute of Electrical & Electronics Engineers, Incorporated**
445 Hoes Ln., Piscataway, NJ 08855
TEL 732-562-3967, 800-678-4333, FAX 732-981-9334, TELEX 236411
E-mail ieeepress@ieee.org
URL: http://www.ieee.org/organizations/pubs/press

EVP **East View Publications, Incorporated**
3020 Harbor Ln., N., Minneapolis, MN 55447
TEL 612-550-0961, 800-477-1005, FAX 612-559-2931, 800-800-3839
E-mail micro@eastview.com
URL http://www.eastview.com

FCM **Fairchild Books**
7 W. 34th St., New York, NY 10001
TEL 212-286-2948, 800-932-4724, FAX 212-286-3122, , TELEX 232666 FAPB
URL http://www.fairchildbooks.com

GCS **Preston Publications, Incorporated (Division of Preston Industries, Inc.)**
6600 W. Touhy Ave., Niles, IL 60714-4588
TEL 847-647-2900, FAX 847-647-1155
URL http://www.prestonpub.com

IAM **SIAM Publications**
3600 University City Science Center, Philadelphia, PA 19104-2688
TEL 215-382-9800, FAX 215-386-7999
E-mail service@siam.org
URL http://www.siam.org

IDC **IDC Microform Publishers bv**
PO Box 11205, Leiden 2301 EE, Netherlands
TEL 31-71-5142700, FAX: 31-71-5142700
E-mail info@idc.nl
URL http://www.idc.nl

IFA **International Federation of Film Archives (FIAF)**
1 rue Defacqz, Bruxelles 1000, Belgium
TEL 32-2-534-6130
FAX 32-2-534-4774
E-mail pip@fiafnet.org
URL http://www.cinema.ucla.edu/fiaf/

ILO **ILO Publications**
PO Box 753, Waldorf, MD 20604-0753
TEL 301-638-3152, FAX 301-843-0159
E-mail icopubs@tasco1.com
URL http://www.ilo.org

IMI **Irish Microforms Limited**
Unit 18, Southern Cross, Business Park, Bray, Wicklow, Ireland
TEL 353-1-2867055, FAX 353-1-2867095
E-mail griffiths@imagenow.ie

IPC **Institute of Paper Science & Technology**
500 Tenth St., NW, Rm. 258, Atlanta, GA 30318-5794
TEL 404-894-5726, FAX 404-894-9596
E-mail sharon.kirkes@ipst.edu
URL http://www.ipst.edu/

ISI **Institute for Scientific Information**
3501 Market St., Philadelphia, PA 19104
TEL 215-386-0100, 800-523-1850, FAX 215-386-6362, TELEX 84-5305
E-mail sales@isinet.com, webmaster@isinet.com
URL http://www.isinet.com

LCP **The Library of Congress Photoduplication Service**
101 Independence Ave SE, Washington, DC 20540-5230
TEL 202-707-5640
FAX 202-707-1771
E-mail photoduplication@loc.gov
URL http://www.loc.gov/preserve-pds

LIB **Library Microfilms**
(Subsidiary of: BMI Imaging Systems)
1115 E. Arques Ave., Sunnyvale, CA 94086
TEL 408-736-7444, 800-359-3456, FAX 408-736-4397
E-mail info@bmiimaging.com
URL http://www.bmiimaging.com

MIM **Elsevier Science, Limited**
84 Theobold's Rd. London WC!X 8RR, United Kingdom
TEL 44-207-611-4400
FAX 44-207611-4001
URL http://www.elsevier.com

MIS **Moody's Investors Service**
Sales Department, 99 Church St., New York, NY 10007
TEL 212-553-0300, FAX 212-553-4700
URL http://www.moodys.com

MML **Micromedia, Limited**
(Subsidiary of: IHS Canada)
20 Victoria St., Toronto, ON M5C 2N8, Canada
TEL 416-362-5211, 800-387-2689, FAX 416-362-6161
E-mail info@micromedia.on.ca
URL http://www.micromedia.on.ca

MMP **McLaren Micropublishing Limited**
PO Box 972, Sta. F, Toronto, ON M4Y 2N9, Canada
TEL 416-960-4801, FAX 416-964-3745
E-mail mmicro@interlog.com
URL http://www.mclarenmicropublishing.com

MUE **University Music Editions**
(Subsidiary of: High Density Systems, Incorporated)
Box 192, Fort George Sta., New York, NY 10040
TEL 212-569-5340, 800-448-2805, FAX 212-569-1269
E-mail ume@valueweb.net
URL http://www.universitymusicedition.com

NBI **Newsbank, Incorporated**
5020 Tamiami Trail North, Suite 1190, Naples, FL 34013
TEL 941-263-6004
FAX 41-263-6108
E-Mail sales@newsbank.com
URL http://www.newsbank.com

NRP **Norman Ross Publishing, Incorporated**
330 W. 58th St., Suite 214, New York, NY 10019
TEL 212-765-8200, 800-648-8850, FAX 212-765-2393
E-mail info@nross.com
URL http://www.nross.com

NTI **National Technical Information Service, U. S. Department of Commerce**
5285 Port Royal Rd., Springfield, VA 22161
TEL 703-605-6000, 800-553-6847, FAX 703-605-6900, TELEX 89-9405
E-mail orders@ntis.gov, info@ntis.gov
URL http://www.ntis.gov

NYL **American Lawyer Media, Incorporated**
345 Park Ave, S., New York, NY 10010
TEL 212-779-9200, FAX 212-481-8161, 212-481-8110
E-mail catalog@amlaw.com
URL http://www.americanlawyermedia.com

OEC **Organization for Economic Cooperation & Development**
2001 L St., NW, Suite 650, Washington, DC 20036-4922
TEL 202-785-6323, 800-456-6323, FAX 202-785-0350
E-mail washington.contact@oecd.org
URL http://www.oecdwash.org

OMN **OmniSys Corporation**
see Norman Ross Publishing, Incorporated

PMC **Princeton Microfilm Corporation**
43 Hightstown Rd., Princeton Junction, NJ 08550
TEL 609-452-2066, 800-257-9502, FAX 609-275-6201
E-mail info@princetonmicro.com
URL http://www.princetonmicro.com

PQC **ProQuest Information & Learning**
300 N. Zeeb Rd., Ann Arbor, MI 48106-1346
TEL 734-761-4700, 800-521-0600, FAX 734-997-4040
E-mail info@proquest.com
URL http://www.umi.com

PSL **The Pretoria State Library**
PO Box 397, Pretoria 0001, South Africa
TEL 27-12-3218931, FAX 27-12-3255984
E-mail statelib@statelib.pwv.gov.za

RPI **Primary Source Microfilm**
(Subsidiary of: Gale Group)
12 Lunar Dr., Woodbridge, CT 06525
TEL 203-397-2600, 800-444-0799
FAX 203-397-3893
E-Mail sales@galegroup.com
URL http://www.galegroup.com/psm

SAL **South African Library**
P.O. Box 496, Queen Victoria St., Cape Town, 8000, South Africa
TEL 27-21-246320
FAX 27-21-244848

SAS **Society for Applied Spectroscopy**
201-B Broadway St., Frederick, MD 21701-6501
TEL 301-694-8122, FAX 301-694-6860
E-mail orders@press.com, sasoffice@aol.com.
URL http://www.s-a-s.org, http://www.s-a-s.org

SOC **Societe Canadienne du Microfilm Inc. /Canadian Microfilming Company Limited**
464 rue Saint-Jean, Suite 110, Montreal, PQ H2Y 2S1, Canada
TEL 514-288-5404, FAX 514-843-4690
E-mail info@socami.qc.ca
URL http://www.socami.qc.ca

SWZ **Swets & Zeitlinger Publishers**
P.O. Box 825, 2160 SZ Lisse, Heereweg, Netherlands
TEL 31-252-435-111
FAX 31-252-415-888
E-mail orders@swets.nl, pub@swets.nl
URL http://www.swets.nl, http://www.szp.swets.nl

TMI **Tennessee Microfilms Incorporated**
PO Box 23075, Nashville, TN 37202
TEL 615-895-0535, 615-242-3632

VCI **VCH Publishers, Incorporated**
605 3rd Ave, New York, NY 10158
TEL 212-629-6200

VFN **Voltaire Foundation Limited**
99 Banbury Rd., Oxford 0X2 6JX, United Kingdom
TEL 44-1865-284600, FAX 44-1865-284610
E-mail vfweb.mail@wwwserver.volt.ox.oc.uk
URL http://www.voltaire.ox.ac.uk

WDS **RoweCom UK, Limited**
Cannon House., Park Farm Rd., Folkestone, Kent CT19 5EE, United Kingdom
TEL 44-1303-850101, FAX 44-1303-850440, TELEX 96392
E-mail info@rowecom.co.uk
URL http://www.rowecom.co.uk

WMP **World Microfilm Publications Limited**
3 Pinewood Rd., Hordle, Lymington, Hampshire SO41 0GN, United Kingdom
FAX 44-870-7411-313
E-mail sales@microworld.co.uk
URL http://www.microworld.co.uk

WSH **William S. Hein & Company, Incorporated**
1285 Main St., Buffalo, NY 14209-1987
TEL 716-882-2600, 800-828-7571, FAX 716-883-8100
E-mail mail@wshein.com
URL http://www.wshein.com

WWS **Lippincott Williams & Wilkins (Baltimore)**
(Subsidiary of: Wolters Kluwer N.V.)
351 W Camden St, Baltimore, MD 21201-2436
TEL 410-528-4000
P.O. Box 1600, Hagerstown, MD 21741
TEL 223-2300, 800-638-3030
FAX 301-223-2320
E-mail customerservice@lww.com
URL http:/www.lww.com

Reprint Services

CIS **Congressional Information Service, Incorporated**
(Subsidiary of: LexisNexis)
4520 East-West Hwy., Suite 800, Bethesda, MD 20814
TEL 301-654-1550, 800-638-8380
FAX 301-657-3203
E-mail academicinfo@lexis-nexis.com
URL http://www.lexisnexis.com/academic

CMC **M.R. Technology**
3655 Wheeler Ave, Alexandria, VA 22304
TEL 703-461-4400, FAX 703-461-0042

HAW **Haworth Press, Incorporated, The**
10 Alice St., Binghamton, NY 13904-1580
TEL 607-722-5857, 800-429-6784, FAX 607-771-0012, 800-895-0582
TELEX 49 325 99 HAWORTH
FAX 800-895-0582
E-mail orders@haworthpressinc.com
URL http://www.haworthpressinc.com

IRC **International Reprint Corporation**
287 East H St, Benicia, CA 94510
TEL 707-746-8740, FAX 707-746-1643
E-mail irc@intlreprints.com
URL http://www.intlreprints.com

ISI **Institute for Scientific Information**
3501 Market St., Philadelphia, PA 19104
TEL 215-386-0100, 800-336-4474 ext 4900
FAX 215-222-0840, 212-386-4343
E-mail ids.isinet.com
URL http://www.isinet.com/isi/products/ids/ids

NRP **Norman Ross Publishing, Incorporated**
330 W. 58th St., Suite 214, New York, NY 10019
TEL 212-765-8200, 800-648-8850, FAX 212-765-2393
E-mail info@nross.com
URL http://www.nross.com

NTI **National Technical Information Service, U. S. Department of Commerce**
5285 Port Royal Rd., Springfield, VA 22161
TEL 703-605-6000, 800-553-6847, FAX 703-605-6900, TELEX 89-9405
E-mail info@ntis.gov
URL http://www.ntis.gov

PQC **ProQuest Information & Learning**
300 N. Zeeb Rd., Ann Arbor, MI 48106-1346
TEL 734-761-4700, 800-521-0600, FAX 734-997-4270
E-mail info@il.proquest.com
URL http://www.il.proquest.com

PSC **Periodicals Service Company**
11 Main St., Germantown, NY 12526
TEL 518-537-4700, FAX 518-537-5899
E-mail psc@backsets.com
URL http://www.backsets.com

RPI **Primary Source Microfilm**
(Subsidiary of: Gale Group)
12 Lunar Dr., Woodbridge, CT 06525
TEL 203-397-2600, 800-444-0799
FAX 203-397-3893, 203-389-0484
E-mail sales@galegroup.com
URL http://www.galegroup.com/psm

SCH **Schmidt Periodicals GmbH**
Ortsteil Dettendorf, Bad Feilnbach D 83075, Germany
TEL 49-8064221, FAX 49-8064557
E-mail schmidt@backsets.com
URL http://www.backsets.com

SWZ **Swets & Zeitlinger Publishers**
P.O. Box 825, 2160 SZ Lisse, Heereweg, Netherlands
TEL 31-252-435-111
FAX 31-252-415-888
E-mail orders@swets.nl, pub@swets.nl
URL http://www.swets.nl, http://www.szp.swets.nl

WDS **RoweCom UK, Limited**
Cannon House., Park Farm Rd., Folkestone, Kent CT19 5EE, United Kingdom
TEL 44-1303-850101, FAX 44-1303-850440,
E-mail info@rowecom.co.uk
URL http://www.rowecom.co.uk

WSH **William S. Hein & Company, Incorporated**
1285 Main St., Buffalo, NY 14209-1987
TEL 716-882-2600, 800-828-7571, FAX 716-883-8100
E-mail mail@wshein.com
URL http://www.wshein.com

Wire Services

AAP **Australian Associated Press**
9 Lang St, Sydney, NSW 2000, Australia
TEL 02-9322-8000, 1800-676-868
E-mail helpdesk@aap.com.au
URL http://aap.com.au

AFP **Agence France-Presse**
Service Communication, 11-13, place de la Bourse, Paris 75002, France
TEL 33-1-40414865, FAX 33-1-40414632
E-mail communication@afp.com
URL http://www.afp.com

ANP **Algemeen Nederlands Persbureau /Netherlands Press Agency**
Handelskade 49, Rijswijk, 1, Den Haag 2501 AA, Netherlands
TEL 70-414-1414
E-mail marketing@anp.nl
URL http://www.anp.nl

AP **Associated Press**
50 Rockefeller Plaza, New York, NY 10020
TEL 212-621-1500
E-mail info@ap.org
URL http://www.ap.org

APP **Associated Press of Pakistan**
Mashkoor Mahal, I.I. Chundrigar Rd, Karachi, Pakistan
TEL 2635695, FAX 2628118

BNS **Baltic News Service**
Parnu mnt 105, Tallinn 15043, Estonia
TEL 372-6-108-800, FAX 372-610-8811
E-mail bns@bns.ee
URL http://bnsnews.bns.ee

CanP **Canadian Press, The**
36 King St., E., Toronto, ON M5C 2L9, Canada
TEL 416-364-0321, 800-434-7578, FAX 416-364-0207

EFE **Agencia EFE**
C/Espronceda, 32, Madrid 28003, Spain
TEL 346-74-00, FAX 346-71-13
E-mail mailto:efe@efe.es
URL http://www.efe.es

KR **Knight Ridder**
50 W. San Fernando St.,, Suite 1200, 1500, San Jose, CA 95113
TEL 408-938-7700, FAX 408-938-7938

LAT-WAT **Los Angeles Times-Washington Post News Service**
1150 15th St., N.W., Washington, DC 20071
TEL 202-334-6173, FAX 202-334-5096
E-mail latwp@newsservice.com
URL http://www.newsservice.com

NYT **New York Times News Service**
229 W. 43rd St., Rm. 943, New York, NY 10036
TEL 212-556-1927, FAX 212-556-3535

PPI **Pakistan Press International**
Press Centre, Shahrah-e-Kamal Attaturk, Karachi, Pakistan
TEL 210680, FAX 2631125
Press Centre, Shahrah-e-Kamal Ataturk, Karachi, Pakistan
Press Centre, Dr. Ziauddin Ahmed Rd., Karachi, Pakistan
TEL 92-21-2627850, FAX 92-21-2631125, TELEX 23868 PPI PK
E-mail owais.ali@ihm.net

RN **Reuters Group, PLC**
85 Fleet St., London EC4P 4AJ, United Kingdom
TEL 44-170-250-1122, FAX 44-170-542-8006, TELEX 44-71-250-1122
URL http://www.reuters.com

SHNA **Scripps-Howard Newspaper Alliance - Scripps-Howard News Service**
1090 Vermont Ave., N.W., Suite 1000, Washington, DC 20005
TEL 202-408-1484
E-mail copelandp@shns.com
URL http://www.shns.com

UPI **United Press International**
1510 H St. N.W., Washington, DC 20005
TEL 202-898-8046, FAX 202-898-8138
E-mail jugo@upi.com
URL http://www.upi.com

Abstracting and Indexing Services

This list contains the full names of all abstracting and indexing services whose abbreviations are used in entries in the CLASSIFIED LIST OF SERIALS. For all currently published abstracting and indexing services, please consult the TITLE INDEX for page references to full entries in the CLASSIFIED LIST OF SERIALS. (Bibliographic information on titles for which cessations were noted more than three years ago are not listed in this book. To view information on such titles, one must refer to Ulrich's™ on Disc, Ulrich's Online, or ulrichsweb.com™

A

ABSEARCH - ASHA ABSEARCH A S H A (American Speech - Language - Hearing Association)

A.D.& D. †Alcohol, Drugs and Driving (Formerly: Alcohol, Drugs and Driving: Abstracts and Reviews)

AIDS & Cancer Res. AIDS & Cancer Research
consists of:
Immunology Abstracts
Oncogenes and Growth Factors Abstracts
Virology and AIDS Abstracts

AIDS Abstr. AIDS Abstracts (Formerly (until 1993): AIDS Information)

AIM †Abridged Index Medicus
consists of:
†Cumulated Abridged Index Medicus

AMED A M E D

API Hlth.& Environ. Technical Literature Abstracts: Health & Environment (Former titles: Literature Abstracts: Health and Environment; (until 1991): A P I Abstracts - Health and Environment)

ASCA Research Alert (Philadelphia) (Former titles (until 1989): Automatic Subject Citation Alert; A S C A Topics)

Abstr.Bulg.Sci. Med.Lit. Abstracts of Bulgarian Scientific Medical Literature

Abstr.Crim.& Pen. †Criminology, Penology & Police Science Abstracts (Formed by the merger of: Police Science Abstracts; Which was formerly: Abstracts on Police Science; Criminology and Penology Abstracts; Abstracts on Criminology and Penology; Excerpta Criminologica)

Abstr.Health Care Manage.Stud. †Abstracts of Health Care Management Studies (Formerly: Abstracts of Hospital Management Studies)

Abstr.Hyg. Abstracts on Hygiene and Communicable Diseases (Former titles: Abstracts on Hygiene; Bulletin of Hygiene)

Abstr.Inter.Med. †Abstracts in Medicine and Key Word Index (Formerly: Abstracts in Internal Medicine)

Abstr.Soc. Geront. Abstracts in Social Gerontology (Formerly (until 1990): Current Literature on Aging)

Addic.Abstr. Addiction Abstracts

Adol.Ment.Hlth. Abstr. †Adolescent Mental Health Abstracts

AgBiotech AgBiotech News and Information

AgeLine AgeLine

Agroforest.Abstr. Agroforestry Abstracts

Anim.Behav. Abstr. Animal Behavior Abstracts (Formerly: Behavioural Biology Abstracts, Section A: Animal Behaviour)

Anim.Breed. Abstr. Animal Breeding Abstracts

Artemisa Artemisa

B

BBCI Biochemistry and Biophysics Citation Index

B.R.I. Biological Abstracts - R R M (Reports, Reviews, Meetings) (Formerly (until 1980): BioResearch Index)

BSL Biol. †Abstracts of Bulgarian Scientific Literature. Biology (Formerly: Abstracts of Bulgarian Scientific Literature. Biology and Biochemistry)

Behav.Abstr. †Behavioural Abstracts

Behav.Med.Abstr. Annals of Behavioral Medicine (Incorporates (in 1991): Behavioral Medicine Abstracts; Formerly: Behavioral Medicine Update)

ABSTRACTING AND INDEXING

Bibl.Dev.Med.& Child Neur. †Bibliography of Developmental Medicine and Child Neurology. Books and Articles Received

Bibl.Repro. Human Reproduction Update (Formed by the 1995 merger of: Oxford Review of Reproductive Biology; Bibliography of Reproduction)

Bibliogr.Bras. Odontol. Bibliografia Brasileira de Odontologia

Bio-Contr.News & Info. Biocontrol News and Information

Biodet.Abstr. †Biodeterioration Abstracts

Biol.& Agr.Ind. Biological & Agricultural Index (Formerly: Agricultural Index)

Biol.Abstr. Biological Abstracts (Formed by the 1926 merger of: Abstracts of Bacteriology; Botanical Abstracts)

Biol.Dig. Biology Digest (Incorporates: Environmental Quality Abstracts)

Biostat. Biostatistica

Brit.Nur.Ind. British Nursing Index (Former titles (until 1997): Nursing and Midwifery Index; (until Dec. 1995): Nursing Bibliography)

C

C.C.I.Ob.Gyn. Combined Cumulative Index to Obstetrics and Gynecology

C.C.I.P. Combined Cumulative Index to Pediatrics

CHNI †Consumer Health and Nutrition Index

CINAHL Cumulative Index to Nursing & Allied Health Literature (Incorporates: Nursing and Allied Health Index; Which was formerly (1956-1976): Nursing Literature Index; (until 1977): Cumulative Index to Nursing Literature; Incorporates: C I N A H L'S List of Subject Headings; Which was formerly (until 1977): Cumulative Index to Nursing Literature, Nursing Subject Headings)

C.I.S. Abstr. Safety and Health at Work (Former titles: C I S Abstracts; Occupational Safety and Health Abstracts)

CSNB Chemical Safety NewsBase
consists of:
Chemical Hazards in Industry
Hazards in the Office
Laboratory Hazards Bulletin

Cal.Tiss.Abstr. Calcium and Calcified Tissue Abstracts (Formerly (until 1994): Calcified Tissue Abstracts)

Chicago Psychoanal. Lit.Ind. †Chicago Psychoanalytic Literature Index

Child Devel. Abstr. †Child Development Abstracts and Bibliography

Clin-Alert Clin-Alert

Community Ment. Health Rev. Journal of Prevention and Intervention in the Community (Former titles (until 1996): Prevention in Human Services; (until 1981): Community Mental Health Review)

Curr.Adv. Biochem. Current Advances in Protein Biochemistry (Formerly (until 1992): Current Advances in Biochemistry)

Curr.Adv.Cancer Res. Current Advances in Cancer Research

Curr.Adv.Cell & Devel.Biol. Current Advances in Cell & Developmental Biology

Curr.Adv.Gen.& Molec.Biol. Current Advances in Genetics and Molecular Biology

Curr.Adv. Immunol. Current Advances in Immunology & Infectious Diseases (Formerly (until 1992): Current Advances in Immunology)

Curr.Adv. Microbiol. Current Advances in Applied Microbiology & Biotechnology (Formerly (until 1992): Current Advances in Microbiology)

Curr.Adv. Pharmacol.& Toxicol. Current Advances in Toxicology (Formerly (until 1992): Current Advances in Pharmacology and Toxicology)

Curr.Biotech. Abstr. Current Biotechnology (Incorporates (in 2000): Biotechnology: Apparatus, Plant, and Equipment; Formerly (until 1990): Current Biotechnology Abstracts)

Curr.Lit.Fam. Plan. †Current Literature in Family Planning

Curr.Tit.Dent. †Current Titles in Dentistry

D

DNP Digest of Neurology & Psychiatry

DSH Abstr. †D S H Abstracts (Deafness, Speech and Hearing)

Dent.Abstr. Dental Abstracts

Dent.Ind. †Index to Dental Literature

Derwent Biotech. Abstr. Biotechnology Abstracts

Diab.Cont. †Diabetes Contents

Diar.Dis.Res. Journal of Health Population and Nutrition (Supersedes (in 2000): Journal of Diarrhoeal Diseases Research)

Dok.Arbeitsmed. †Arbeitsmedizin (Former titles: Beruf und Gesundheit - Occupational Health; (until 1985): Dokumentation Arbeitsmedizin - Documentation Occupational Health)

E

E & P Hlth. E & P Health, Safety and Environment (Exploration and Production)

Entomol.Abstr. Entomology Abstracts

Environ.Abstr. Environment Abstracts (Incorporates (1985-1991): Acid Rain Abstracts; Formerly: Environment Information Access)

Ergon.Abstr. Ergonomics Abstracts

Except.Child Educ.Abstr.	Exceptional Child Education Resources (Formerly (until May 1977): Exceptional Child Education Abstracts)
Excerp.Med.	Excerpta Medica. Abstract Journals *consists of:* Excerpta Medica. Section 10: Obstetrics and Gynecology Excerpta Medica. Section 11: Otorhinolaryngology Excerpta Medica. Section 12: Ophthalmology †Excerpta Medica. Section 130: Clinical Pharmacology Excerpta Medica. Section 13: Dermatology and Venereology Excerpta Medica. Section 14: Radiology Excerpta Medica. Section 15: Chest Diseases, Thoracic Surgery and Tuberculosis Excerpta Medica. Section 16: Cancer Excerpta Medica. Section 17: Public Health, Social Medicine and Epidemiology Excerpta Medica. Section 18: Cardiovascular Diseases and Cardiovascular Surgery Excerpta Medica. Section 19: Rehabilitation and Physical Medicine Excerpta Medica. Section 1: Anatomy, Anthropology, Embryology & Histology Excerpta Medica. Section 20: Gerontology and Geriatrics Excerpta Medica. Section 21: Developmental Biology and Teratology Excerpta Medica. Section 22: Human Genetics Excerpta Medica. Section 23: Nuclear Medicine Excerpta Medica. Section 24: Anesthesiology Excerpta Medica. Section 25: Hematology Excerpta Medica. Section 26: Immunology, Serology and Transplantation Excerpta Medica. Section 27: Biophysics, Bio-Engineering and Medical Instrumentation Excerpta Medica. Section 28: Urology and Nephrology Excerpta Medica. Section 29: Clinical and Experimental Biochemistry Excerpta Medica. Section 2: Physiology Excerpta Medica. Section 30: Clinical and Experimental Pharmacology Excerpta Medica. Section 31: Arthritis and Rheumatism Excerpta Medica. Section 32: Psychiatry Excerpta Medica. Section 33: Orthopedic Surgery †Excerpta Medica. Section 34: Plastic Surgery Excerpta Medica. Section 35: Occupational Health and Industrial Medicine Excerpta Medica. Section 36: Health Policy, Economics and Management †Excerpta Medica. Section 37: Drug Literature Index Excerpta Medica. Section 38: Adverse Reactions Titles Excerpta Medica. Section 3: Endocrinology Excerpta Medica. Section 40: Drug Dependence, Alcohol Abuse and Alcoholism Excerpta Medica. Section 46: Environmental Health and Pollution Control Excerpta Medica. Section 48: Gastroenterology Excerpta Medica. Section 49: Forensic Science Abstracts Excerpta Medica. Section 4: Microbiology: Bacteriology, Mycology, Parasitology and Virology Excerpta Medica. Section 50: Epilepsy Abstracts †Excerpta Medica. Section 51: Mycobacterial Diseases: Leprosy, Tuberculosis and Related Subjects Excerpta Medica. Section 52: Toxicology †Excerpta Medica. Section 54: AIDS Excerpta Medica. Section 5: General Pathology and Pathological Anatomy Excerpta Medica. Section 6: Internal Medicine Excerpta Medica. Section 7: Pediatrics and Pediatric Surgery Excerpta Medica. Section 8: Neurology and Neurosurgery Excerpta Medica. Section 9: Surgery
ExtraMED	ExtraMED

F

FAMLI	†F A M L I (Family Medicine Literature Index)
Fam.Ind.	Family Index
Focus on: Mol. Med.	Focus On: Molecular Medicine
Focus on: Psychophar.	Focus On: Psychopharmacology
Focus on: Sports Sci.& Med.	Focus On: Sports Science and Medicine

Focus on: Vet. Sci.& Med.	Focus On: Veterinary Science and Medicine

G

Genet.Abstr.	Genetics Abstracts
Ger.J.Psych.	European Psychologist (Formerly (until 1995): German Journal of Psychology)

H

Hlth.Dev.Alerts	Health Devices System (Formerly: Health Devices Alerts)
Hlth.Ind.	†Health Index
Hosp.Abstr.	Health Service Abstracts (Incorporates (in May 1985): Hospital Abstracts; Current Literature on Health Services; Current Literature on General Medical Practice)
Hosp.Lit.Ind.	†Hospital and Health Administration Index (Former titles (until 1995): Hospital Literature Index; Hospital Periodical Literature Index)
Hum.Gen.Abstr.	†Human Genome Abstracts

I

I.P.A.	International Pharmaceutical Abstracts
Immun.Abstr.	Immunology Abstracts
Ind.Hyg.Dig.	Industrial Hygiene Digest
Ind.Imag.Lit.	R S N A Index to Imaging Literature (Radiological Society of North America, Inc.)
Ind.Med.	Index Medicus
Ind.Med.Esp.	Indice Medico Espanol
Ind.Vet.	Index Veterinarius
Indian Psychol. Abstr.	Indian Psychological Abstracts and Reviews (Formerly (until 1994): Indian Psychological Abstracts)
Inpharma	Inpharma Weekly (Formerly: Inpharma)
Int.Abstr.Biol.Sci.	Current Awareness in Biological Sciences (Formerly (until 1983): International Abstracts of Biological Sciences)
Int.Nurs.Ind.	†International Nursing Index
InterActions Bibl.	†Humans & Other Species (Former titles (until 1997): InterActions Bibliography; (until vol.3, 1992): Interactions of Man and Animals)

J

Jrnl.Watch	Journal Watch
Jrnl.Watch Card.	Journal Watch Cardiology
Jrnl.Watch Derm.	Journal Watch Dermatology
Jrnl.Watch Emer. Med.	Journal Watch Emergency Medicine
Jrnl.Watch Gastr.	Journal Watch Gastroenterology
Jrnl.Watch Inf. Dis.	Journal Watch Infectious Diseases
Jrnl.Watch Neuro.	Journal Watch Neurology
Jrnl.Watch Psych.	Journal Watch Psychiatry
Jrnl.Watch Wom. Hlth.	Journal Watch Women's Health

K

Kidney	Kidney (New York, 1992)

L

Lab.Haz.Bull.	Laboratory Hazards Bulletin

M

MEDOC	†Medoc: Index to U S Government Publications in the Medical and Health Sciences
Med.& Pharm. Biotech.Abstr.	Medical & Pharmaceutical Biotechnology Abstracts (Supersedes in part (in 1993): Biotechnology Research Abstracts)
Med.& Surg. Dermat.	Medical & Surgical Dermatology
Med.Care Rev.	Medical Care Research and Review (Former titles (until Mar. 1995): Medical Care Review; Public Health Economics and Medical Care Abstracts)
Mult.Ed.Abstr.	Multicultural Education Abstracts
Mycol.Abstr.	Abstracts of Mycology

N

NBA	Notiziario Bibliografico di Audiologia O R L e Foniatria (Formerly: Notiziario Bibliografico di Audiologia)
NRN	Nutrition Research Newsletter (Incorporates (1981-1998): Food Safety Notebook)
Neuropsych. Abstr.	Neuropsychology Abstracts (Formerly: PsychSCAN: Neuropsychology)
Neurosci.Abstr.	C S A Neurosciences Abstracts (Cambridge Scientific Abstracts) (Incorporates: Endocrinology Abstracts)
Neurosci.Cit.Ind.	Neuroscience Citation Index
Nuc.Acids Abstr.	Nucleic Acids Abstracts (Former titles (until 1994): Cambridge Scientific Biochemistry Abstracts: Part 2. Nucleic Acids; Biochemistry Abstracts: Part 2. Nucleic Acids; Nucleic Acids Abstracts)
Nurs.Abstr.	†Nursing Abstracts

O

Oncog.G.F.Abstr.	Oncogenes and Growth Factors Abstracts
Oncol.Abstr.	†Oncology Abstracts
Ophthal.Lit.	Ophthalmic Literature

P

P.N.I.	†P N I (Pharmaceutical News Index)
Pharm.&Out. News	Pharmacoeconomics and Outcomes News (Formerly: PharmacoResources)
Phys.Ed.Ind.	Physical Education Index
Plant Breed. Abstr.	Plant Breeding Abstracts
Protozool.Abstr.	Protozoological Abstracts
PsycInfo	PsycINFO
Psychoanal. Abstr.	Psychoanalytic Abstracts (Former titles: PsycSCAN: Psychoanalysis; Psychoanalysis Abstracts)
Psychol.Abstr.	Psychological Abstracts
Psychol.R.G.	†Psychological Reader's Guide
Psychopharmacol.Abstr.	†Psychopharmacology Abstracts
Psycscan A.P.	PsycSCAN: Applied Psychology
Psycscan B.A.& T.	PsycSCAN: Behavior Analysis and Therapy
Psycscan C.P.	PsycSCAN: Clinical Psychology
Psycscan D.P.	PsycSCAN: Developmental Psychology
Psycscan L.D.& M.R.	PsycSCAN: Learning Disorders and Mental Retardation (Former titles: PsycSCAN: Learning and Communication Disorders and Mental Retardation; PsycSCAN: Learning Disabilities - Mental Retardation)

R

Reac.	Reactions Weekly (Formerly (until 1990): Reactions)
Rehabil.Lit.	†Rehabilitation Literature
Repindex	Repindex
Rev.Arom.& Med. Plants	Review of Aromatic and Medicinal Plants
Rev.Med.& Vet. Mycol.	Review of Medical and Veterinary Mycology
Rev.Plant Path.	Review of Plant Pathology (Formerly: Review of Applied Mycology)
Risk Abstr.	Risk Abstracts

S

Saf.Sci.Abstr.	Health and Safety Science Abstracts (Former titles: Safety Science Abstracts Journal; Safety Science Abstracts)
Sage Fam.Stud. Abstr.	Sage Family Studies Abstracts
Small Anim. Abstr.	†Small Animals (Formerly (until 1991): Small Animal Abstracts)
Sp.Ed.Needs Abstr.	Special Educational Needs Abstracts

T

THA	†Tobacco & Health Abstracts (Formerly: Tobacco and Health)
Telegen	†Telegen Abstracts (Formerly: Telegen Reporter)
Tob.Abstr.	Tobacco Abstracts
Tox.Abstr.	Toxicology Abstracts
Trop.Dis.Bull.	Tropical Diseases Bulletin

V

Vet.Bull.	Veterinary Bulletin
Viol.& Abuse Abstr.	Violence & Abuse Abstracts
Virol.Abstr.	Virology and AIDS Abstracts (Formerly: Virology Abstracts)

Y

Yrbk.Assoc. Educ.& Rehab. Blind	†Association for Education and Rehabilitation of the Blind and Visually Impaired. Yearbook (Incorporates (1976-1982): Blindness, Visual Impairment, Deaf-Blindness; Which was formerly (until 1983): Blindness)

Z

Zoo.Rec.	Zoological Record
e-psyche	E-psyche

TITLE INDEX

A

***A & l Review for Physician Assistants.** Anthony Miller & Albert Simon. 4th ed. 2002. 386p. 39.95 incl. audio compact disk (0-07-137544-9) McGraw-Hill Prof.

A B C of Clinical Haematology. Ed. by Drew Provan & Andrew Henson. 1997. 80p. pap. text (0-7279-1206-2) BMJ Pub GBR. *Dist:* AIDC.

A-Bomb Radiation Effects Digest. Ed. by Itsuzo Shigematsu et al. Tr. by Brian Harrison. 1995. 44p. pap. text 33.00 (3-7186-5463-6) Gordon & Breach.

A. D. A. M.'s Student Atlas: Animated Dissection of Anatomy for Medicine. Todd R. Olson. 1996. LC 95 11593. (Illus.). 544p. pap. text 39.95 (0-683-00042-X) Lppncott W & W.

A. D. D. & A. D. H. D. Diet: Attention Deficit Disorder & Hyperactivity. Rachel Bell & Howard Peiper. Ed. by Nina Anderson. 1997. LC 97-66518. 96p. pap. 9.95 (1-884820-29-8) SAFE GOODS.

A. D. D. Book: New Understanding, New Approaches to Parenting. William Sears & Lynda Thompson. 1998. LC 97-29504. (Illus.). 320p. pap. 17.95 (0-316-77873-7, Back Bay) Little.

A. D. D. from A to Z: A Comprehensive Guide to Attention Deficit Disorder. University of Georgia Staff. Ed. by William N. Bender & Phillip J. McLaughlin. 1994. 76p. pap. text, tchr. ed. 195.00 incl. VHS (1-57035-016-7, 60KIT) Sopris.

A. D. D., the Natural Approach: Help for Attention Deficit Disorder & Hyperactivity. Nina Anderson & Howard Peiper. 1996. 40p. pap. 4.95 (1-884820-19-0) SAFE GOODS.

A. Edward Maumenee, M. D. The Wilmer Ophthalmological Institute at the Johns Hopkins University & the Stanford Medical School. A. Edward Maumenee. 1994. (Ophthalmology Oral History Ser.). (Illus.). xxx, 267p. pap. 45.00 (1-56055-068-6) FAAO.

A Is for Allergies. Frank Kwong & Bruce Cook. 2001. 256p. pap. 12.95 (0-89087-973-7) Celestial Arts.

A to Z Drug Facts, 2000. Facts and Comparisons Staff. 2nd ed. 2000. LC 00-702913. (Illus.). 1,300p. pap. text 36.95 (1-57439-068-6) Lppncott W & W.

***A to Z Drug Reference.** Ed. by Facts and Comparisons Staff. 3rd ed. 2001. 1300p. per. 39.95 (1-57439-106-2) Facts & Comparisons.

A to Z of Pathology. M. J. Wilkinson. 1997. pap. text (0-443-03536-9) Church.

A-Z Counseling Theory & Practice. William Stewart. 2nd ed. 1997. 496p. 57.50 (1-56593-938-7, 1858) Singular Publishing.

A-Z Guide to Healing Herbal Remedies. Shelagh R. Masline. 1995. 320p. mass mkt. 5.99 (0-440-22061-0) Dell.

A-Z of Childhood Health Problems. Patricia Gilbert. 2nd ed. 1999. (Illus.). 224p. pap. (0-7487-3716-2) Nelson Thornes GBR. *Dist:* Intl Spec Bk.

A-Z of Counselling Theory & Practice. William Stewart. 1992. LC 92-23363. 57.50 (1-56593-055-X, 0363) Thomson Learn.

A-Z of Dog Diseases & Health Problems. Dick Lane. 1997. 288p. pap. 24.95 (0-87605-042-9, Howell) Hungry Minds.

A-Z of Horse Diseases & Health Problems: Signs-Diagnoses-Causes-Treatment. Tim Hawcroft. 1990. (Illus.). 312p. pap. 24.95 (0-87605-884-5, Howell) Hungry Minds.

A-Z of Medical Statistics: A Companion for Critical Appraisal. Filomena Pereira-Maxwell. 1998. LC 99-173194. (Arnold Publication). (Illus.). 128p. (Orig.). pap. 26.50 (0-340-71940-0) OUP.

A-Z of Medical Writing. Ed. by Tim Albert. 2000. 145p. pap. (0-7279-1487-1) BMJ Pub GBR. *Dist:* AIDC.

A-Z of Natural Therapies. Judy Jacka. 1995. 333p. pap. (0-85091-293-8) Lothian Pub AUS. *Dist:* Seven Hills Bk.

***A-Z of Orthopaedic Radiology.** Martin Watson et al. 2000. (Illus.). 240p. text (0-7020-2492-9) W B Saunders GBR. *Dist:* Saunders.

A-Z of Practical Advice for Women after Breast Cancer Surgery. Maria Hussain & E. Mayer-Spitzweck. 5th ed. 1993. (Illus.). 121p. (Orig.). pap. text (3-88603-473-9) W Zuckschwerdt DEU. *Dist:* Scholium Intl.

A-Z of Women's Health. Derek Llewellyn-Jones. 2nd ed. 1990. (Oxford Paperback Reference Ser.). (Illus.). 272p. pap. 16.95 (0-19-286112-3) OUP.

A-Z Reference Book of Childhood Conditions. Patricia Gilbert. 1995. 208p. (Orig.). (C). pap. text 49.95 (1-56593-332-X, 0662) Singular Publishing.

A-Z Reference Book of Syndromes & Inherited Disorders. Patricia Gilbert. 2nd ed. 1996. LC 95-70015. (Illus.). 394p. pap. 55.00 (1-56593-611-6, 1268) Thomson Learn.

A-Z Reference of Syndromes & Inherited Disorders. Patricia Gilbert. 2nd ed. 1995. 378p. pap. (0-7487-3474-0) Nelson Thornes GBR. *Dist:* Intl Spec Bk.

A.A. Comes of Age see A.A. Llega a Su Mayor Edad

A.A. Llega a Su Mayor Edad. 1975.Tr. of A.A. Comes of Age. (SPA.). 338p. pap. 3.15 (0-916856-10-0) AAWS.

AABB Blood Bank Operations Manual: Complete Manual with 'Standards Blood Banks & Transfusion Services' American Association of Blood Banks Staff. 1998. 18th rev. ed. ring bd. (3-8055-6752-9); 19th rev. ed. ring bd. (3-8055-6943-2) S Karger.

AABB Blood Bank Operations Manual: Without 'Standards Blood Banks & Transfusion Services' American Association of Blood Banks Staff. rev. ed. 1998. ring bd. (3-8055-6819-3) S Karger.

AACN Handbook of Critical Care Nursing. Marianne Chulay. 1997. 752p. (C). pap. 44.95 incl. audio (0-8385-0346-2, A-0346-5) McGraw-Hill Prof.

AACN Pocket Handbook of Critical Care Nursing. Marianne Chulay et al. 1997. LC 97-71823. 240p. (C). spiral bd. 25.95 (0-8385-0322-5, A-0322-6) McGraw-Hill Prof.

AACN Procedure Manual for Critical Care. American Association for Critical Care Nurses Staff. Ed. by Rochelle L. Boggs & Maribeth Wooldridge-King. 3rd ed. 1993. (Illus.). 984p. pap. text 65.00 (0-7216-3073-1) Saunders.

AACN Procedure Manual for Critical Care. AACN Staff. 4th ed. 2000. (Illus.). 890p. pap. text 60.00 (0-7216-8268-5) Saunders.

AACN Tissue & Organ Transplantation: Implications for Professional Nursing Practitioners. Ed. by Susan L. Smith. 1990. (Illus.). 384p. (C). (gr. 13). text 49.95 (0-8016-5526-9, 05526) Mosby Inc.

Aacn's Clinical Reference for Critical Care Nursing. Contrib. by Marguerite Rodgers Kinney & American Association of Critical-Care Nurses Staff. 4th ed. 1998. LC 98-10709. (Illus.). 1344p. (C). (gr. 13). text 85.00 (0-8151-1323-4, 29596) Mosby Inc.

AACP Roster of Faculty & Professional Staff in Colleges of Pharmacy: Annual. 100.00 (0-937526-00-2) AACP Alexandria.

AAHA Directory of Members, 1995. American Association of Homes for the Aging Staff. rev. ed. 1986. LC 78-641009. 214p. (Orig.). pap. text 50.00 (0-943774-31-4) Am Assn Homes.

AAHE Scholar Presentations, 1981-1995. Des. by Kerry Redican & Linda Moore. 1997. (Illus.). 180p. pap. 21.95 (0-88314-606-1) AAHPERD.

AAMI: Hemodialyzers. AAMI Staff. 2nd ed. 1996. (Illus.). 18p. pap. 70.00 (1-57020-059-9, RD16-209) Assn Adv Med Instrn.

AAMI Electrical Safety Manual. 1996. (Illus.). (Orig.). pap. 95.00 (1-57020-050-5, ESMI-209) Assn Adv Med Instrn.

AAMI Medical Equipment Management Manual. 1996. (Illus.). (Orig.). pap. 75.00 (1-57020-051-3, MEM1-209) Assn Adv Med Instrn.

AAMT Book of Style for Medical Transcription. Claudia Tessier. 1995. LC 95-141685. 519p. (Orig.). (C). pap. text 79.00 (0-935229-22-1) Am Assoc Med.

A&L Pract. TST Preventive. Richard Hart. 2nd ed. 1998. pap. text 19.95 (0-8385-0356-X, Medical Exam) Appleton & Lange.

A&l Review General Patholgy. Lewis & Barton. 4th ed. 1999. pap. text 34.95 (0-8385-0396-9) Appleton & Lange.

AAOA Homestudy Course in Otolaryngic Allergy. Jacquelynne Corey. 2nd ed. 1995. 416p. pap. text, stu. ed. 135.00 (1-887064-01-X) J M Ryan.

AAOHN - Core Curriculum for Occupational Health Nursing. American Association of Occupational Health Nurses. Ed. by Thomas Eoyang. 1997. LC 97-7112. 288p. pap. text 51.50 (0-7216-6904-2) Saunders.

AAOS Instructional Course Lectures, Vol. 37. Ed. by Frank H. Bassett, III. 1988. LC 43-17054. (Illus.). 299p. 45.00 (0-89203-022-4) Amer Acad Ortho Surg.

AAOS Instructional Course Lectures, Vol. 38. Ed. by Joseph S. Barr, Jr. 1989. LC 43-17054. (Illus.). 502p. 45.00 (0-89203-028-3) Amer Acad Ortho Surg.

AAOS Instructional Course Lectures, Vol. 39. Ed. by Walter B. Greene et al. 1990. LC 43-17054. (Illus.). 600p. 45.00 (0-89203-032-1) Amer Acad Ortho Surg.

AAOS Instructional Course Lectures, Vol. 41. Ed. by Robert E. Eilert. 1992. (Illus.). 538p. 85.00 (0-89203-057-7) Amer Acad Ortho Surg.

AAOS Instructional Course Lectures, Vol. 43. Ed. by Michael F. Schafer. 1994. (Illus.). 644p. 85.00 (0-89203-102-6) Amer Acad Ortho Surg.

AAOS Instructional Course Lectures, Vol. 44. Ed. by Douglas Jackson. 1995. (Illus.). 400p. 90.00 (0-89203-115-8) Amer Acad Ortho Surg.

AAOS Instructional Course Lectures Vol. 40: 15 Year Cumulative Index. Ed. by Hugh S. Tullos. 1991. LC 43-17054. (Illus.). 368p. 45.00 (0-89203-043-7) Amer Acad Ortho Surg.

Aaron T. Beck. Marjorie Weishaar. 1993. (Key Figures in Counselling & Psychotherapy Ser.). (Illus.). 160p. (C). 57.95 (0-8039-8564-9, 9151); pap. 21.50 (0-8039-8565-7, 9152) Sage.

ABA Criminal Justice Mental Health Standards. 1989. 530p. pap. 15.00 (0-89707-450-5, 509-0041-001) Amer Bar Assn.

Abandoned to Their Fate: Social Policy & Practice Toward Severely Retarded People in America, 1820-1920. Philip M. Ferguson. 1994. LC 93-21887. (Health, Society, & Policy Ser.). 232p. 44.95 (1-56639-154-7) Temple U Pr.

Abandonment of the Patient: The Impact of Profit-Driven Health Care on the Public. Ed. by Ellen D. Baer et al. 1996. LC 96-271. 132p. text 31.95 (0-8261-9470-2) Springer Pub.

Abating Treatment with Critically Ill Patients: Ethical & Legal Limits to the Medical Prolongation of Life. Robert F. Weir. 1989. (Illus.). 472p. text 39.50 (0-19-504528-9) OUP.

Abbott Labs: What's Not in the Annual Report. Market Intelligence Staff. 1992. 321p. (Orig.). 995.00 (1-56753-378-7) Frost & Sullivan.

ABC de las Hierbas (The ABC Herbal) Una Guia Simplificada Para el Cuidado de los Ninos por Medio de la Salud Natural. Steven H. Horne. Tr. by Rosina E. Moreira de Roberts. 1996. (SPA.). 96p. pap. 9.95 (1-885653-06-9) W W Whitman.

ABC Herbal: A Simplified Guide to Natural Health Care for Children. Steven H. Horne. 1995. 80p. (Orig.). reprint ed. pap. 7.95 (1 885653-04-2) W W Whitman.

ABC of Acid-Base Chemistry: The Elements of Physiological Blood-Gas Chemistry for Medical Students & Physicians. Horace W. Davenport. 6th rev. ed. 1974. LC 79-88230. 132p. pap. text 21.00 (0-226-13703-1) U Ch Pr.

***ABC of AIDS.** M. W. Adler. 5th ed. 2001. (ABC Ser.). (Illus.). 118p. pap. (0-7279-1503-7) BMJ Pub GBR. *Dist:* AIDC.

ABC of AIDS, Vol. 4. Ed. by Michael W. Adler. 4th rev. ed. 1997. (Illus.). 102p. pap. (0-7279-1137-6) BMJ Pub GBR. *Dist:* AIDC.

ABC of Alcohol. Alex Paton. 3rd ed. 1994. 48p. pap. text (0-7279-0812-X) BMJ Pub GBR. *Dist:* AIDC.

ABC of Antenatal Care. Geoffrey Chamberlain. 1992. (Illus.). 84p. pap. text (0-7279-0313-6); 2nd ed. 1994. 92p. pap. text (0-7279-0884-7) BMJ Pub GBR. *Dist:* AIDC.

***ABC of Antenatal Care.** Chamberlain & Morgan. 4th ed. 2002. (ABC Ser.). 96p. pap. (0-7279-1692-0) BMJ Pub.

ABC of Arterial & Venous Diseases. Donelly & London. 2001. (ABC Ser.). (Illus.). 72p. pap. text (0-7279-1561-4) BMJ Pub GBR. *Dist:* AIDC.

ABC of Asthma. John Rees & John Price. 3rd ed. 1997. (Illus.). 49p. (C). pap. (0-7279-0882-0) BMJ Pub GBR. *Dist:* AIDC.

ABC of Asthma Allergies & Lupus: Eradicate Asthma - Now! F. Batmanghelidj. 2000. (Illus.). 237p. pap. 17.00 (0-9629942-6-X) Global Hlth.

ABC of Atrial Fibrillation. Ed. by G. Y. Lip. 1996. 48p. pap. text (0-7279-1070-1) BMJ Pub GBR. *Dist:* AIDC.

ABC of Breast Diseases. Ed. by J. Michael Dixon. (Illus.). 1995. 80p. pap. text (0-7279-0915-0); 2nd ed. 2001. 120p. pap. text (0-7279-1461-8) BMJ Pub GBR. *Dist:* AIDC.

ABC of Child Abuse. Ed. by Roy Meadow. 3rd ed. 1997. 100p. pap. text (0-7279-1106-6) BMJ Pub GBR. *Dist:* AIDC.

ABC of Clinical Genetics. Helen M. Kingston. (Illus.). 1989. 62p. pap. (0-7279-0263-6); 2nd ed. 1994. 84p. pap. (0-7279-0846-4) BMJ Pub GBR. *Dist:* AIDC.

***ABC of Colorectal Cancer.** Kerr & Hobbs. 2001. (ABC Ser.). 48p. pap. (0-7279-1526-6) BMJ Pub GBR. *Dist:* AIDC.

ABC of Colorectal Diseases. Ed. by D. J. Jones & M. H. Irving. 1993. (Illus.). 112p. pap. (0-7279-0755-7) BMJ Pub GBR. *Dist:* AIDC.

ABC of Complementary Medicine. Ed. by Catherine Zollman & Andrew Vickers. 2000. 50p. (0-7279-1237-2) BMJ Pub GBR. *Dist:* AIDC.

ABC of Dermatology. Ed. by P. K. Buxton. 2nd ed. 1993. 104p. (C). pap. text (0-7279-0777-8); 3rd ed. 1998. (Illus.). 114p. pap. text (0-7279-1150-3) BMJ Pub GBR. *Dist:* AIDC.

ABC of Diabetes. Peter J. Watkins. 3rd ed. 1993. (Illus.). 56p. pap. text (*0-7279-0763-8*) BMJ Pub GBR. *Dist:* AIDC.

ABC of Diabetes. Ed. by Peter J. Watkins. 4th ed. 1998. (Illus.). 80p. pap. text (*0-7279-1189-9*) BMJ Pub GBR. *Dist:* AIDC.

ABC of Emergency Radiology. Ed. by David Nicholson & Peter Driscoll. 1995. (Illus.). 120p. (Orig.). pap. text (*0-7279-0832-4*) BMJ Pub GBR. *Dist:* AIDC.

***ABC of Emergency Radiology.** Nicholson & Driscoll. 2nd ed. 2002. (ABC Ser.). 130p. pap. (*0-7279-1528-2*) BMJ Pub GBR. *Dist:* AIDC.

ABC of Eyes. A. R. Elkington & P. T. Khaw. 2nd ed. 1994. (Illus.). 68p. pap. (*0-7279-0766-2*) BMJ Pub GBR. *Dist:* AIDC.

ABC of Healthy Travel. Eric Walker. Ed. by Glyn Williams & Fiona Raeside. 4th ed. 1993. (Illus.). 56p. pap. text (*0-7279-0762-X*) BMJ Pub GBR. *Dist:* AIDC.

ABC of Heart Failure. Ed. by C. R. Gibbs et al. 2000. (Illus.). 46p. pap. text (*0-7279-1457-X*) BMJ Pub GBR. *Dist:* AIDC.

ABC of Hypertension. E. T. O'Brien et al. 3rd ed. 1997. (Illus.). 79p. pap. (*0-7279-0769-7*) BMJ Pub GBR. *Dist:* AIDC.

***ABC of Liver, Pancreas & Gall Bladder.** Ed. by I. J. Beckingman. 2001. (ABC Ser.). (Illus.). 54p. pap. text (*0-7279-1531-2*) BMJ Pub GBR. *Dist:* AIDC.

ABC of Major Trauma. Ed. by David Skinner et al. 2nd ed. 1996. (Illus.). 140p. pap. text (*0-7279-0917-7*) BMJ Pub GBR. *Dist:* AIDC.

ABC of Medical Computing. Ed. by Nicholas Lee & Andrew Millman. 1996. 85p. pap. text (*0-7279-1046-9*) BMJ Pub GBR. *Dist:* AIDC.

ABC of Monitoring Drug Therapy. J. K. Aronson et al. 1993. 48p. pap. text (*0-7279-0791-3*) BMJ Pub GBR. *Dist:* AIDC.

ABC of Natural Beauty Recipes. Dian Dincin Buchman. Ed. by Cheryl Hirsch. 1996. (Good Health Guides). 48p. pap. 3.95 (*0-87983-680-6*, 36806K, Keats Pubng) McGraw-Hill Trade.

ABC of Nutrition. Ed. by A. Stewart Truswell. 2nd ed. 1992. (Illus.). 116p. pap. text (*0-7279-0315-2*) BMJ Pub GBR. *Dist:* AIDC.

ABC of One to Seven. H. B. Valman. 3rd ed. 1993. 152p. pap. text (*0-7279-0768-9*) BMJ Pub GBR. *Dist:* AIDC.

ABC of Oral Health. Ed. by Crispian Scully. 2001. (ABC Ser.). (Illus.). 64p. pap. text (*0-7279-1551-7*) BMJ Pub GBR. *Dist:* AIDC.

ABC of Otolaryngology. Harold Ludman. 3rd ed. 1993. (Illus.). 68p. pap. text (*0-7279-0765-4*) BMJ Pub GBR. *Dist:* AIDC.

ABC of Otolaryngology. Harold Ludman. 4th ed. 1997. (Illus.). 57p. pap. text (*0-7279-1205-4*) BMJ Pub GBR. *Dist:* AIDC.

ABC of Palliative Care. Ed. by Marie Fallon & Bill O'Neill. 1998. 68p. pap. text (*0-7279-0793-X*) BMJ Pub GBR. *Dist:* AIDC.

ABC of Poisoning. John Henry & Glyn Volans. 1985. (Illus.). 76p. pap. (*0-7279-0142-7*) BMJ Pub GBR. *Dist:* AIDC.

ABC of Resuscitation. Ed. by M. C. Colquhoun & A. J. Handley. 3rd ed. 1995. (Illus.). 95p. pap. text (*0-7279-0839-1*) BMJ Pub GBR. *Dist:* AIDC.

ABC of Rheumatology. Ed. by Michael L. Snaith. 1996. 95p. (Orig.). (C). pap. text (*0-7279-0997-5*) BMJ Pub GBR. *Dist:* AIDC.

ABC of Sexually Transmitted Diseases. Ed. by Michael W. Adler. 3rd ed. 1995. (Illus.). 75p. pap. (*0-7279-0889-8*) BMJ Pub GBR. *Dist:* AIDC.

ABC of Sleep Disorders. Colin M. Shapiro. 1993. 104p. pap. text (*0-7279-0794-8*) BMJ Pub GBR. *Dist:* AIDC.

ABC of Spinal Cord Injury. Ed. by David Grundy & Andrew Swain. 3rd ed. 1996. (Illus.). 80p. pap. text (*0-7279-1049-3*) BMJ Pub GBR. *Dist:* AIDC.

***ABC of Spinal Cord Injury.** Grundy & Swain. 4th ed. 2002. (ABC Ser.). 96p. pap. 27.95 (*0-7279-1518-5*) BMJ Pub GBR. *Dist:* AIDC.

ABC of Sports Medicine. Ed. by G. McLatchie et al. 1995. (Illus.). 144p. (Orig.). pap. text (*0-7279-0844-8*) BMJ Pub GBR. *Dist:* AIDC.

ABC of Transfusion. Marcela Contreras. 2nd ed. 1992. (Illus.). 76p. pap. text (*0-7279-0754-9*) BMJ Pub GBR. *Dist:* AIDC.

ABC of Vascular Diseases. Ed. by John H. Wolfe et al. 1992. (Illus.). 79p. pap. text (*0-7279-0259-8*) BMJ Pub GBR. *Dist:* AIDC.

ABC's for Inner Strength & Well-Being. Robin E. Inwald. 1999. 64p. (Orig.). pap. 5.95 (*1-885738-13-7*) Hilson Res.

ABCs of Behavior Change: Skills for Working with Behavior Problems in Nursing Homes. Margaret Cohn et al. 1994. LC 94-61218. 246p. spiral bd. 29.95 (*0-910251-69-X*, ABC72) Venture Pub PA.

ABC's of Coronary Heart Disease. James J. Maciejko. 2001. LC 00-12249. (Illus.). 160p. pap. 24.95 (*1-886947-99-6*) Sleepng Bear.

ABCs of Dementia. Kathryn A. Bayles & Cheryl K. Tomoeda. 1993. (Orig.). pap. text 35.00 (*0-9639381-1-8*) Canyonlnds Pubng.

ABCs of HMOs: How to Get the Best from Managed Care. John J. Connolly. 1997. LC 95-70353. 228p. pap. 11.95 (*1-883769-74-4*) Castle Connolly Med.

ABCs of Hormones. Jack Challem. 1999. (Good Health Guides). 48p. pap. 3.95 (*0-87983-902-3*, 39023K, Keats Pubng) McGraw-Hill Trade.

ABC's of Nutrition & Supplements for Prostate Cancer. Mark A. Moyad. 2000. LC 99-18425. (Illus.). 286p. pap. 24.95 (*1-886947-69-4*) Sleepng Bear.

ABCs of Prenatal Diagnosis: A Guide to Pregnancy Testing & Issues. Keith Wexler & Laurie Wexler. Ed. by Paul Wexler. 1995. 124p. pap. 7.00 (*0-9644243-0-4*) Genassist.

ABCs of Prostate Cancer. Mark A. Moyad & Joseph E. Oesterling. 1996. (Illus.). 196p. pap. text 19.95 (*1-886569-06-1*) J W Edwards.

ABCs of Sports Medicine. Ed. by James H. McMaster. 1982. LC 80-20636. 400p. lib. bdg. 38.00 (*0-88275-890-X*) Krieger.

ABCs of Stress: A Submarine Psychologist's Perspective. Benjamin B. Weybrew. 1992. LC 92-11956. 240p. 64.00 (*0-275-94233-3*, C4233, Praeger Pubs) Greenwood.

ABCs to Better Hearing. John G. Clark. 1992. (Illus.). 87p. pap. text 9.95 (*0-9632001-0-0*) Hearcare.

ABDO Frame Rule. Association of British Opticians Staff. 1989. (C). (*0-89771-749-X*) Assn Brit Dispen Opticians GBR. *Dist:* St Mut.

Abdomen, Vol. 3. 1972. (*0-443-00810-8*) Church.

Abdominal Access in Open & Laparoscopic Surgery. Ed. by Edmund K. Tsoi & Claude H. Organ. 1996. LC 95-49690. 194p. 152.00 (*0-471-13352-3*) Wiley.

Abdominal & Pelvic MRI. Ed. by Andreas Heuck et al. 1998. LC 97-29286. (Medical Radiology Ser.). (Illus.). 338p. 225.00 (*3-540-61450-8*) Spr-Verlag.

Abdominal & Pelvic MRI. Ed. by Andreas Heuck & M. Reiser. 2000. (Medical Radiology Ser.). (Illus.). 330p. pap. 75.00 (*3-540-67216-8*) Spr-Verlag.

Abdominal Aortic Aneurysm: Genetics, Pathophysiology & Molecular Biology. M. David Tilson & Charles D. Boyd. 1996. LC 96-36001. (Annals of the New York Academy of Sciences Ser.). pap. 80.00 (*1-57331-051-4*); 80.00 (*1-57331-050-6*) NY Acad Sci.

Abdominal C. T. A Source for Resident & Clinician. Richard A. Sorgen & Robert D. Russo, Jr. 1982. 192p. 39.50 (*0-87527-289-4*) Green.

Abdominal Plain Film. Stephen R. Baker. 1990. (Illus.). 431p. (C). pap. text 149.00 (*0-8385-7896-9*, A7896-2) Appleton & Lange.

Abdominal Plain Film. Stephen R. Baker. 2nd ed. 1998. LC 98-6879. 431p. text 169.00 (*0-8385-0275-X*) McGraw-Hill Prof.

Abdominal Radiology: Syllabus. M. S. Joshi. 1998. LC 98-33963. (Bracco Education in Diagnostic Imaging Ser.). (*88-470-0033-5*) Spr-Verlag.

Abdominal Radiology I, Tomo I. Miguel Stoopen Rometti. 1998. LC 98-27737. (Illus.). 384p. pap. text 80.00 (*0-7817-1665-9*) Lppncott W & W.

Abdominal Radiology Ii, Tomo III. Kenji Kimura Fujikami. 1999. LC 98-27737. (Illus.). 376p. pap. text 80.00 (*0-7817-1664-0*) Lppncott W & W.

Abdominal Sonography. Mordecai Koenigsberg & Janet Hoffman-Tretin. 1991. (Illus.). 144p. (C). (gr. 13). text 75.00 (*1-56375-006-6*, GM0195) Mosby Inc.

Abdominal Sonography. Eric E. Sauerbrei et al. 1992. 304p. text 129.00 (*0-88167-917-8*) Lppncott W & W.

Abdominal Sonography Review. Cindy Owen. Ed. by Edward G. Grant. 1999. (Illus.). 214p. pap. 55.00 (*0-941022-46-3*, 11023) Davies Pubng.

Abdominal Surgery of Infancy & Childhood, Set. Ed. by William L. Donnellan et al. 1996. 1424p. text 375.00 (*3-7186-5409-1*, Harwood Acad Pubs) Gordon & Breach.

Abdominal Trauma: Surgical & Radiologic Diagnosis. H. M. Delaney & R. Jason. 1981. (Illus.). 224p. 142.00 (*0-387-90502-2*) Spr-Verlag.

Abdominal Ultrasound. Ed. by Kathryn A. Gill. Date not set. LC 00-56232. 474p. text (*0-7216-8131-X*) Saunders.

Abdominal Ultrasound. Mike Stocksley. 2001. (Medical Media Ser.). (Illus.). 286p. pap. text (*1-900151-66-9*) Greenwich Med GBR. *Dist:* JAMCO Dist.

***Abdominal Ultrasound: How, Why & When.** Jane A. Bates. 1999. (Illus.). 261p. text (*0-443-06007-X*) Church GBR. *Dist:* Saunders.

Abdominal Ultrasound Study Guide & Exam Review. Sandra L. Hagen-Ansert. 1995. LC 95-40123. (Illus.). 464p. (C). (gr. 13). pap. text, stu. ed. 45.95 (*0-8151-4176-9*, 26271) Mosby Inc.

Abdominal Wall Hernias. Madden. 1989. 368p. text 145.00 (*0-7216-1288-1*) Saunders.

Abdominal Wall Hernias: Principles & Management. Robert Bendavid. 2000. LC 00-20620. (Illus.). xxxiv, 792p. (C). 198.00 (*0-387-95004-4*) Spr-Verlag.

Abdominal Wall Lifting & Advanced Techniques in Laparoscopic Surgery. Daijo Hashimoto et al. Ed. by Subhash S. Erram & Zhong Ren Xu. 1995. LC 95-14347. 350p. text 78.00 (*981-02-2208-4*); pap. text 28.00 (*981-02-2247-5*) World Scientific Pub.

Abdominal Wound Infections. Richard J. Casey et al. 1994. (Illus.). 164p. text 19.95 (*1-880906-01-5*) IDI Pub.

Abdominal X-Rays Made Easy. James D. Begg. 1999. LC 99-27853. 192p. pap. (*0-443-06205-6*) Saunders.

Abdominal X-rays Made Easy. James D. Begg. 1999. LC 99-27853. 192p. (*0-443-06206-4*) Church.

Abernathy's Surgical Secrets: Questions You Will Be Asked on Rounds, in the OR, on Oral Ezams. Ed. by Alden H. Harken & Ernest E. Moore. 4th rev. ed. 2000. LC 99-50332. (Secrets Ser.). 300p. (C). pap. 39.95 (*1-56053-363-3*) Hanley & Belfus.

Abilities, Motivation, & Methodology: The Minnesota Symposium on Learning & Individual Differences. Ed. by R. Kanfer et al. 1989. 536p. (C). pap. 55.00 (*0-8058-0496-X*); text 99.95 (*0-8058-0495-1*) L Erlbaum Assocs.

Abilities of Man, Their Nature & Measurement. Charles E. Spearman. LC 73-121291. reprint ed. 49.50 (*0-404-06174-5*) AMS Pr.

Ability to Mourn: Disillusionment & the Social Origins of Psychoanalysis. Peter Homans. 1989. LC 88-4656. 404p. 41.95 (*0-226-35111-4*) U Ch Pr.

Able Lives: Women's Experience of Paralysis. Ed. by Jenny Morris. pap. (*0-7043-4155-7*) Womens Press GBR. *Dist:* Trafalgar.

ABM Business Certification Training Manual. Wyatt Woodsmall. 1998. (Advanced Neuro Linguistic Programming Applications Ser.). 170p. spiral bd. 50.00 (*1-892876-01-9*) Next Step Pr.

ABMS Handbook on Board Certification & the Americans with Disabilities Act. Ed. by Philip G. Bashook & J. Lee Dockery. 1992. LC 92-73098. 68p. pap. 20.00 (*0-934277-16-8*) Am Bd Med Spec.

Abnormal Behavior David Sue. 1993. (C). pap., tchr. ed., suppl. ed. 7.96 (*0-395-69079-X*); pap., stu. ed. 20.36 (*0-395-69104-4*); pap., tchr. ed. 5.96 (*0-395-69078-1*); 4th ed. LC 93-78705. text 70.36 (*0-395-67659-2*) HM.

Abnormal Behavior: Perspectives in Conflict. Richard R. Price. 2nd ed. 1978. LC 77-20504. (C). pap. text 32.00 (*0-03-089964-8*) Harcourt Coll Pubs.

Abnormal Behavior & the Criminal Justice System. Robert G. Meyer. 1992. LC 91-3702. 312p. 45.00 (*0-669-24450-3*) Lxngtn Bks.

Abnormal Child Psychology. Wolfe. 1998. (Psychology Ser.). 550p. spiral bd. 84.95 (*0-534-34290-6*) Brooks-Cole.

***Abnormal Child Psychology.** David A. Wolfe & Eric J. Mash. 2nd ed. 2001. 612p. 81.95 (*0-534-55417-2*) Duxbury.

Abnormal Cortical Development & Epilepsy. Ed. by Roberto Spreafico et al. 1999. 336p. (*0-86196-579-5*) J Libbey Med GBR. *Dist:* Buttrwrth-Heinemann.

Abnormal Fetal Growth. M. Divon. 1991. (Illus.). 408p. (C). (gr. 13). text 83.95 (*0-412-04541-9*) Chapman & Hall.

Abnormal Illness Behaviour. Issy Pilowsky. 1997. LC 96-38645. 278p. 83.95 (*0-471-96573-1*) Wiley.

Abnormal Morphology of Bovine Spermatozoa. A. D. Barth & R. J. Oko. 1989. LC 89-1770. (Illus.). 294p. (C). text 74.95 (*0-8138-0112-5*) Iowa U Pr.

***Abnormal Pap Smears: What Every Woman Needs to Know.** Lynda Rushing & Nancy Joste. 2001. LC 2001-31619. (Illus.). 274p. pap. 21.00 (*1-57392-929-8*) Prometheus Bks.

Abnormal Psychology. 1998. (C). (*0-205-28692-5*, Macmillan Coll) P-H.

Abnormal Psychology. David H. Barlow. 1994. (Psychology Ser.). pap., stu. ed. 17.00 (*0-534-20360-4*) Brooks-Cole.

Abnormal Psychology. Richard Halgin & Susan K. Whitbourne. 1993. LC 92-70918. (Illus.). 640p. (C). text 61.00 (*0-03-093761-2*) Harcourt Coll Pubs.

Abnormal Psychology Kendall. (C). Date not set. pap. 11.96 (*0-395-87694-X*); 1994. pap., tchr. ed. 11.96 (*0-395-62185-2*); 1994. pap., tchr. ed., suppl. ed. 11.96 (*0-395-62186-0*); 1994. pap. text, stu. ed. 20.36 (*0-395-62184-4*); 1994. LC 94-76520. text 69.56 (*0-395-62183-6*) HM.

Abnormal Psychology. Michael T. Nietzel et al. 1997. (C). text, tchr. ed. (*0-205-26281-3*, T6281-4); pap. text, stu. ed. 19.00 (*0-205-27327-0*, T7327-4); LC 96-52617. 764p. 102.00 (*0-205-14721-6*) Allyn.

Abnormal Psychology. Susan Nolen-Hoeksema & Robert Davis. 1997. 256p. (C). pap., stu. ed. 25.94 (*0-697-25271-X*, WCB McGr Hill) McGrw-H Hghr Educ.

Abnormal Psychology. Thomas F. Oltmanns & Robert E. Emery. 1994. LC 94-35274. 704p. text 88.00 (*0-13-007295-8*) P-H.

Abnormal Psychology. Susanna M. Perry. 1997. LC 98-23395. (Test Yourself Ser.). (Illus.). 192p. pap. 14.95 (*0-8442-2384-0*, 23840) NTC Contemp Pub Co.

Abnormal Psychology. Jack Rudman. 1994. (ACT Proficiency Examination Program Ser.: PEP-53). pap. 23.95 (*0-8373-5903-1*) Nat Learn.

Abnormal Psychology. Sexton. 2000. pap. text 11.97 net. (*0-395-97198-5*) HM.

Abnormal Psychology. Ronald J. Comer. 2nd ed. 1994. LC 94-30148. (Illus.). 816p. (C). (gr. 11-12). text 69.95 (*0-7167-2494-4*) McGraw.

Abnormal Psychology. Susan Nolen-Hoeksema. 2nd ed. 2000. 50.25 net. (*0-697-36193-4*) McGraw.

Abnormal Psychology. Susan Nolen-Hoeksema & Hoeksema. 2nd ed. 2000. pap. text 13.80 (*0-697-36197-7*) McGraw.

Abnormal Psychology. Ronald J. Comer. 3rd ed. 1997. pap. text, stu. ed. 23.95 (*0-7167-3205-X*); LC 97-25100. 896p. text 77.95 (*0-7167-3089-8*) W H Freeman.

Abnormal Psychology. Halgin. 3rd ed. 1999. 360p. pap., stu. ed. 23.44 (*0-07-232387-6*) McGrw-H Hghr Educ.

Abnormal Psychology. David S. Holmes. 3rd ed. 1997. 446p. (C). pap. text, stu. ed. 28.00 (*0-673-98472-9*) Addison-Wesley.

Abnormal Psychology. 4th ed. 2000. tchr. ed. (*0-205-32754-0*) Allyn.

Abnormal Psychology. Ronald J. Comer. 4th ed. 2000. pap. text, stu. ed. 22.95 (*0-7167-3853-8*) Worth.

***Abnormal Psychology.** Lauren B. Alloy. 8th ed. 84.06 (*0-07-240255-5*) McGrw-H Hghr Educ.

Abnormal Psychology. Lauren B. Alloy. 8th ed. 1998. 320p. (C). pap., stu. ed. 20.31 (*0-07-303469-X*) McGrw-H Hghr Educ.

Abnormal Psychology. Robert S. Carson & James Neal Butcher. 9th ed. 1991. LC 91-20863. (C). pap. text 10.00 (*0-673-46617-5*, Harper Ref) HarperCollins Pubs.

Abnormal Psychology. Barbara R. Sarason. 9th ed. 1998. (C). pap. text, stu. ed. 21.33 (*0-13-080444-4*) P-H.

Abnormal Psychology, Vol. 1. Clark. 3rd ed. 1997. pap. 24.00 (*0-7167-3131-2*) St Martin.

Abnormal Psychology, Vol. 1. Ronald J. Comer. 3rd ed. 1997. tchr. ed. 24.00 (*0-7167-3202-5*) W H Freeman.

Abnormal Psychology: A Discovery Approach. Steven Schwartz. 2000. LC 99-46116. (Illus.). (C). 72.95 (*1-55934-266-8*) Mayfield Pub.

Abnormal Psychology: An Integrated Approach. David H. Barlow & V. Mark Durand. 1994. LC 94-35287. 806p. pap. 61.00 (*0-534-20358-2*) Brooks-Cole.

Abnormal Psychology: An Integrative Approach with InfoTrac. David H. Barlow. 2nd ed. 1998. (Psychology Ser.). 53.25 incl. cd-rom (*0-534-36330-X*) Brooks-Cole.

Abnormal Psychology: An Introduction. V. Mark Durand & David H. Barlow. 1996. (Psychology Ser.). (C). 550p. mass mkt. 53.25 (*0-534-20364-7*); mass mkt., stu. ed. 14.75 (*0-534-34295-7*) Brooks-Cole.

Abnormal Psychology: An Introduction (Casebound with CD-ROM) V. Mark Durand. 2nd ed. 1999. LC 99-42478. (Psychology). (Illus.). 608p. (C). text 91.95 (*0-534-35427-0*) Brooks-Cole.

Abnormal Psychology: Case History. Harold S. Zamansky. 1991. 88p. pap. text 23.00 (*0-536-57881-8*) Pearson Custom.

Abnormal Psychology: Casebook. 8th ed. 1998. 288p. (C). 31.25 (*0-07-303473-8*) McGrw-H Hghr Educ.

Abnormal Psychology: Current Perspectives. Richard R. Bootzin et al. rev. ed. 1994. (C). text 57.74 net. incl. audio (*0-07-911953-0*); 6th ed. 1993. LC 92-49206. (*0-07-006536-5*) McGraw.

Abnormal Psychology: Current Perspectives. Lauren B. Alloy et al. 7th ed. 1996. (C). text 65.25 net. (*0-07-844963-4*); 7th rev. ed. 1996. LC 95-16246. text (*0-07-006615-9*); 8th ed. 1998. LC 98-4014. 74.25 (*0-07-292838-7*) McGraw.

***Abnormal Psychology: Essential Cases & Readings.** Ed. by Thomas Bradbury & Cindy Yee-Bradbury. 2001. LC 2001-30727. pap. (*0-393-97730-7*) Norton.

Abnormal Psychology: Integrating Perspectives. G. Terence Wilson et al. 1995. LC 95-40374. 778p. stu. ed. 109.00 (*0-205-17578-3*) Allyn.

Abnormal Psychology: Its Experience & Behavior. Peter McKellar. 1989. 352p. 49.95 (*0-415-02812-4*, A3869); pap. 14.95 (*0-415-03132-X*, A3873) Routledge.

Abnormal Psychology: Presentation Manager. 1998. (C). pap., tchr. ed. 15.63 incl. cd-rom (*0-07-039655-8*) McGrw-H Hghr Educ.

Abnormal Psychology: The Human Experience of Psychological Disorders with DSM-IV. Richard P. Halgin & Susan K. Whitbourne. 1994. (C). 540p. text 51.00 net. (*0-697-27385-7*); 311p. text, stu. ed. 22.50 (*0-697-27388-1*) Brown & Benchmark.

Abnormal Psychology: The Problem of Maladaptive Behavior. Jeffrey S. Nevid. 9th ed. 1999. (C). 76.00 (*0-13-084953-7*) P-H.

Abnormal Psychology: The Problem of Maladaptive Behavior. Irwin G. Sarason & Barbara R. Sarason. 9th ed. 1998. LC 98-2836. 665p. (ps). 90.00 (*0-13-080186-0*) P-H.

Abnormal Psychology & Modern Life. Robert C. Carson & James Neal Butcher. 8th ed. 1997. (C). pap. text 21.00 (*0-673-18933-3*) Addson-Wesley Educ.

Abnormal Psychology & Modern Life 1998. Robert C. Carson. 10th ed. 1997. (C). pap. text, stu. ed. 30.00 (*0-321-02459-1*) Addison-Wesley.

Abnormal Psychology & Study Guide, 2 bks. Michael T. Nietzel. 1998. text 67.95 net. (*0-205-28947-9*) Allyn.

Abnormal Psychology Case Studies. Archipelag. 1998. (C). 77.50 (*0-15-503092-2*) Harcourt Coll Pubs.

Abnormal Psychology Casebook. Lauren B. Alloy. 7th ed. 1995. 63.00 net. (*0-07-911861-5*) McGraw.

Abnormal Psychology in a Changing World. 4th ed. 1999. (*0-13-030009-8*) P-H.

Abnormal Psychology with Study Cards. Halgin-Whitbourn. 2nd ed. 1996. 16.25 net. (*0-697-38084-X*) McGrw-H Hghr Educ.

Abnormal Psychology. Gerald C. Davison & John M. Neale. 7th ed. 1998. 1088p. text, stu. ed. 131.90 (*0-471-29821-2*) Wiley.

Abnormal States of Brain & Mind. Allan J. Hobson. 1988. (Readings from the Encyclopedia of Neuroscience Ser.). 135p. 41.00 (*0-8176-3397-9*) Birkhauser.

Abnormalities of IgG Glycosylation & Immunological Disorders. Ed. by D. A. Isenberg & T. W. Rademacher. 1996. LC 95-45453. 280p. 285.00 (*0-471-96260-0*) Wiley.

Abnormalities of Personality: Within & Beyond the Realm of Treatment. Michael H. Stone. 1993. LC 93-7704. 350p. 50.00 (*0-393-70127-1*) Norton.

Abortion. Lawrence Lader. 1966. LC 66-18592. 5.95 (*0-672-50601-7*, Bobbs) Macmillan.

Abortion: A Positive Decision. Patricia W. Lunneborg. 1992. LC 91-27946. 232p. 31.50 (*0-89789-243-7*, H243, Bergin & Garvey) Greenwood.

Abortion: An Annotated Indexed Bibliography. Ed. by Maureen Muldoon. 1980. LC 79-91622. (Studies in Women & Religion: Vol. 3). 167p. lib. bdg. 79.95 (*0-88946-972-5*) E Mellen.

Abortion: Medical Progress & Social Implication - Symposium No. 115, No. 115. CIBA Foundation Staff. 1985. (CIBA Foundation Symposia Ser.). 320p. 128.00 (*0-471-91084-8*) Wiley.

Abortion: Understanding Differences. Ed. by Sidney Callahan & Daniel Callahan. 1984. LC 84-9965. (Hastings Center Series in Ethics). (Illus.). 360p. (C). text 65.00 (*0-306-41640-9*, Kluwer Plenum) Kluwer Academic.

Abortion - the American Holocaust. Kent Kelly. 1981. LC 81-65240. (Illus.). 149p. (Orig.). pap. 2.95 (*0-9604138-1-2*) Calvary Pr.

Abortion & Divorce in Western Law. Mary Ann Glendon. 1989. 224p. pap. 21.50 (*0-674-00161-3*) HUP.

Abortion & Family Planning Bibliography for 1987. Compiled by Bonnie L. Clements. 1990. LC 72-78877. Orig. Title: Abortion Bibliography. xxii, 199p. 30.00 (*0-87875-404-0*) Whitston Pub.

Abortion & Family Planning Bibliography for 1988. Compiled by Bonnie L. Clements. 1991. LC 72-78877. Orig. Title: Abortion Bibliography. xxii, 190p. 35.00 (*0-87875-407-5*) Whitston Pub.

Abortion & Family Planning Bibliography for 1989-1990. Compiled by Bonnie L. Clements. 1992. 500p. 55.00 (*0-87875-420-2*) Whitston Pub.

Abortion & RU-486 - Mifepristone - Index of New Information & Research Bible. Karl J. Cominsky. 1995. LC 95-17205. pap. 47.50 (*0-7883-0685-5*) ABBE Pubs Assn.

Abortion & RU-486 (Mifepristone) Index of New Information & Research Bible. Karl J. Cominsky. 1995. LC 95-17205. 57.50 (*0-7883-0684-7*) ABBE Pubs Assn.

Abortion & RU-486 (Mifepristone) Index of New Information & Research Bible. Karl J. Cominsky. 1994. 150p. 57.50 (*0-7883-0216-7*); pap. 47.50 (*0-7883-0217-5*) ABBE Pubs Assn.

Abortion Bibliography see Abortion & Family Planning Bibliography for 1988

Abortion Bibliography for 1970. Compiled by Mary K. Floyd. 1972. LC 72-78877. xiv, 125p. 7.50 (*0-87875-024-X*) Whitston Pub.

Abortion Bibliography for 1971. Compiled by Mary K. Floyd. 1973. LC 72-78877. xxii, 250p. 11.00 (*0-87875-030-4*) Whitston Pub.

Abortion Bibliography for 1972. Compiled by Mary K. Floyd. 1973. LC 72-78877. xx, 226p. 11.00 (*0-87875-044-4*) Whitston Pub.

Abortion Bibliography for 1976. Compiled by Mary K. Floyd. 1978. LC 72-78877. 390p. 17.00 (*0-87875-126-2*) Whitston Pub.

Abortion Bibliography for 1979. Whitston Publishing Company Inc. Staff. 1982. LC 72-78877. xxxiv, 502p. (C). 38.50 (*0-87875-225-0*) Whitston Pub.

Abortion Bibliography for 1980. Whitston Publishing Company Inc. Staff. 1982. xxx, 445p. 38.50 (*0-87875-260-9*) Whitston Pub.

Abortion Bibliography for 1984. Compiled by Polly T. Goode. 1986. LC 72-78877. xxviii, 386p. 40.00 (*0-87875-329-X*) Whitston Pub.

Abortion Bibliography for 1981. Compiled by Polly T. Goode. 1983. LC 72-78877. xxx, 405p. 38.50 (*0-87875-278-1*) Whitston Pub.

Abortion Bibliography for 1983. Compiled by Polly T. Goode. 1986. LC 72-78877. xxx, 360p. 40.00 (*0-87875-294-3*) Whitston Pub.

Abortion Bibliography for 1986. Compiled by Polly T. Goode. 1989. LC 72-78877. 285p. 35.00 (*0-87875-369-9*) Whitston Pub.

Abortion Bibliography for 1973. Compiled by Mary K. Floyd. 1974. LC 72-78877. xviii, 237p. 11.00 (*0-87875-056-8*) Whitston Pub.

Abortion Bibliography for 1974. Compiled by Mary K. Floyd. 1974. LC 72-78877. 360p. 15.00 (*0-87875-079-7*) Whitston Pub.

Abortion Controversy. Ed. by Charles P. Cozic & Jonathan S. Petrikin. 1995. (Current Controversies Ser.). 288p. pap. text 16.20 (*1-56510-228-2*, 2282); lib. bdg. 26.20 (*1-56510-229-0*, 2290) Gale (Greenhaven Pr).

Abortion Decisions of the Supreme Court, 1973 Through 1989: A Comprehensive Review with Historical Commentary. Dan Drucker. 1990. LC 89-43620. 220p. lib. bdg. 42.50 (*0-89950-459-0*) McFarland & Co.

Abortion Dispute & the American System. Gilbert Y. Steiner. 1983. LC 82-45978. 103p. pap. text 10.95 (*0-8157-8125-3*) Brookings.

Abortion Facts & Feelings: A Handbook for Women & the People Who Care about Them. Nada L. Stotland. 1998. LC 97-35435. 224p. 24.95 (*0-88048-740-2*, 8740) Am Psychiatric.

Abortion in Nineteenth Century America. 1976. LC 73-20643. (Sex, Marriage & Society Ser.). 234p. reprint ed. 30.42 (*0-405-05791-1*) Ayer.

Abortion Is a Blessing. Anne N. Gaylor. 1976. LC 75-24775. 140p. 7.95 (*0-88437-006-2*) Psych Dimensions.

Abortion Laws: A Survey of Current World Legislation. 1970. (International Digest of Health Legislation Offprints: Vol. 21, No. 3). 78p. reprint ed. pap. text 12.00 (*92-4-169213-8*, 1957001) World Health.

Abortion Laws in Commonwealth Countries. R. Cook & B. Dickens. 1979. (International Digest of Health Legislation Offprints: Vol. 30, No. 3). 108p. 14.00 (*92-4-169303-7*) World Health.

Abortion Policy: An Evaluation of the Consequences for Maternal & Infant Health. Jerome S. Legge, Jr. 1985. LC 84-16356. 182p. (C). text 64.50 (*0-87395-958-2*); pap. text 21.95 (*0-87395-959-0*) State U NY Pr.

Abortion Practice. Warren M. Hern. 1990. LC 83-18744. (Illus.). 368p. reprint ed. 35.00 (*0-9625728-0-2*) Alpenglo Graphics.

Abortion Practice in Britain & the United States. Colin Francome. 1986. 224p. pap. text 16.95 (*0-04-179004-9*) Routledge.

Abortion Privacy Doctrine, A Compendium & Critique of Federal Abortion Cases, 1980. Lynn D. Wardle. 1980. LC 80-80930. 337p. lib. bdg. 40.00 (*0-89941-059-6*, 301860) W S Hein.

Abortion Regimes. Kerry A. Petersen. 1993. (Medico-Legal Issues Ser.). 201p. (*1-85521-159-9*) Dartmth Pub GBR. *Dist:* Ashgate Pub Co.

Abortion Resource Handbook. K. Kaufmann. 1997. LC 97-10262. 144p. per. 11.00 (*0-684-83076-0*, Fireside) S&S Trade Pap.

Abortion to Zoophilia: A Sourcebook of Sexual Facts. Anne Mandetta & Patricia Gustaveson. 1975. LC 75-31909. (Illus.). pap. text 3.00 (*0-89055-114-6*) Carolina Pop Ctr.

About AIDS. 1993. LC 93-34109. (For Your Information Ser.). 9.50 (*1-56420-019-1*) New Readers.

About Alcoholism: A Common Sense Perspective. Donald A. Staccia. Ed. by Kathryn R. Anderson. 1986. (Illus.). 176p. (Orig.). pap. 6.95 (*0-9616402-1-9*) Acosep Corp.

About Behaviorism. B. F. Skinner. 1976. 304p. mass mkt. 12.00 (*0-394-71618-3*) Vin Bks.

About Cancer. Cynthia Moritz. 1993. LC 93-37166. (For Your Information Ser.). 9.50 (*1-56420-031-0*) New Readers.

About Dyslexia: Unravelling the Myth. Priscilla L. Vail. Ed. by Linda Skladal. 1990. 48p. pap. 7.95 (*0-935493-34-4*) Modern Learn Pr.

About Ependymoma. 1991. (*0-944093-10-8*) Am Brain Tumor.

About Epilepsy. Donald F. Scott. rev. ed. 1973. LC 73-5255. 189p. 30.00 (*0-8236-0016-5*); pap. 24.95 (*0-8236-8000-2*, 20016) Intl Univs Pr.

About Glaucoma. E. Jaeger. Tr. & Intro. by Donald Blanchard. 1989. 80p. (C). text 20.00 (*0-9624399-0-8*) Blanchards Brook.

About Glioblastoma Multiforme & Anaplastic Astrocytoma. 1993. (*0-944093-25-6*) Am Brain Tumor.

About Glioblastoma Multiforme & Malignant Astrocytoma. rev. ed. 1990. (*0-944093-09-4*) Am Brain Tumor.

About Herbs: Nature's Medicine. Benedict Lust. 1983. pap. 2.95 (*0-87904-045-9*) Lust.

About Looking. John Berger. 1992. LC 91-50099. (Vintage International Ser.). (Illus.). 224p. pap. 13.00 (*0-679-73655-7*) Vin Bks.

About Medulloblastoma - PNET (Medulloblastoma) 1994. (*0-944093-33-7*) Am Brain Tumor.

About Medulloblastoma, Medulloblastoma (PNET) rev. ed. 1991. (*0-944093-17-5*) Am Brain Tumor.

About Medulloblastoma-PNET. rev. ed. 1990. (*0-944093-11-6*) Am Brain Tumor.

About Meningioma. rev. ed. 1992. (*0-944093-24-8*); 1988. (*0-944093-01-9*) Am Brain Tumor.

About Oligodendroglioma & Mixed Glioma. 1992. (*0-944093-23-X*) Am Brain Tumor.

About Pituitary Tumors. 1993. (*0-944093-22-1*) Am Brain Tumor.

About Prostate Trouble. Benedict Lust. 1983. pap. 2.95 (*0-87904-042-4*) Lust.

About Raw Juices. John B. Lust. 1982. pap. 2.95 (*0-87904-047-5*) Lust.

About Your Heart Medication. U. S. Pharmacopeia Staff. 1999. pap. 10.95 (*0-452-27434-6*, Plume) Dutton Plume.

About Your Medicines. U. S. Pharmacopeia Staff. 7th ed. 1993. 1088p. pap. 7.95 (*0-913595-74-8*, 940334) US Pharmacopeia.

***Above & Beyond: 365 Meditations for Transcending Chronic Pain & Illness.** J. S. Dorian. 2001. 500p. pap. 10.00 (*0-7881-9817-3*) DIANE Pub.

Abrams' Angiography, Vols. I, II & III. Ed. by Stanley Baum. 4th ed. 1996. 3,000p. text 550.00 (*0-316-08226-0*) Lppncott W & W.

Abrams' Angiography, Vols. 1-3. Stanley A. Baum. 4th ed. 1996. 3,000p. 650.00 (*0-7817-2902-5*) Lppncott W & W.

Abrams' Angiography: Vascular & Interventional Radiology. Herbert L. Abrams & Stanley Baum. 4th ed. 1996. LC 96-24525. (*0-316-08467-0*, Little Brwn Med Div) Lppncott W & W.

Abridgement of Mental Philosophy. Thomas Upham. 1979. LC 79-10925. (History of Psychology Ser.). reprint ed. lib. bdg. 75.00 (*0-8201-1331-X*) Schol Facsimiles.

Absent Fathers, Lost Sons: The Search for Masculine Identity. Guy Corneau. Tr. by Larry Shouldice from FRE. 1991. LC 90-53373. (C. G. Jung Foundation Bks.). 208p. (Orig.). pap. 17.95 (*0-87773-603-0*) Shambhala Pubns.

Absent Mothers & Orphaned Fathers: Narcissism & Abjection in Lessing's Aesthetic & Dramatic Production. Susan E. Gustafson. 1995. LC 94-38323. (Kritik: German Literary Theory & Cultural Studies). 316p. text 39.95 (*0-8143-2503-3*) Wayne St U Pr.

Absite Combat Manual: Clinical Surgery. Hratch L. Karamanoukian. Ed. by Jacob Bergsland & Raffy Leon Karamanoukian. 2nd ed. 2000. 386p. ring bd. 89.00 (*0-9663292-6-0*) Magalhaes Sci Pr.

Absorbent Mind. Maria Montessori. 1995. LC 95-18404. 302p. pap. 17.00 (*0-8050-4156-7*, Owl) H Holt & Co.

Absorption & Utilization of Amino Acids Ed. by Mendel Friedman. 1989. Vol. I. 272p. lib. bdg. 225.00 (*0-8493-6006-4*, QP561); Vol. II. 304p. lib. bdg. 225.00 (*0-8493-6007-2*, QP566); Vol. III. 304p. lib. bdg. 225.00 (*0-8493-6008-0*, QP561) CRC Pr.

Abstinence: Members of Overeaters Anonymous Share Their Experience, Strength, & Hope. Overeaters Anonymous, Inc. Staff. 1994. LC 94-67576. pap. 8.35 (*0-9609898-7-0*) Overeaters Anym.

Abstinence in Action: Food Planning for Compulsive Eaters. Barbara McFarland & Ann M. Erb. 1989. LC 88-81269. 140p. pap. 16.95 (*0-89486-538-2*, 5045A) Hazelden.

Abstraction & Aging: A Social Psychological Analysis. J. S. Lee. 1990. (Recent Research in Psychology Ser.). (Illus.). 113p. 88.95 (*0-387-97433-4*) Spr-Verlag.

Abstracts Vol. 23, Pts. 1 & 2: Society for Neuroscience 27th Annual Meeting New Orleans, La. October 25-29, 1997. Society for Neuroscience Staff. 1997. LC 75-7761. 1440p. pap. 18.00 (*0-916110-53-2*) Society for Neuroscience.

Abstracts from Extramural Grant Program Meeting: Abstracts. Ed. by Debra Adenau. 1996. (Journal: Vol. 14, Suppl. 1, 1996). (Illus.). viii, 112p. pap., suppl. ed. 36.50 (*3-8055-6284-5*) S Karger.

Abstracts from the 1993 ASHA Conference on Cochlear Implants: The State-of-the-Art. Ed. by Maureen Thompson. 1994. 35p. pap. text 27.00 (*0-910329-77-X*, 0111849) Am Speech Lang Hearing.

Abstracts from the Asia/Pacific Clinical Symposium (CarboMedics) Ed. by Silent Partners, Inc. Staff. 1992. 38p. (Orig.). pap. (*1-878353-25-X*) Silent Partners.

Abstracts from the Fifth International CarboMedics Clinical Symposium. 1996. 36p. (Orig.). pap. (*1-878353-40-3*) Silent Partners.

Abstracts of the Collected Works of C. G. Jung. Ed. by Carrie L. Rothgeb. 1993. LC 78-603478. 150p. pap. text (*1-85575-035-X*) Karnac Bks GBR. *Dist:* Other Pr LLC.

Abstracts of the International Association of Logopedics & Phoniatrics 18th Congress, Washington, D.C. August, 1980. International Association of Logopedics and Phoniatr. Ed. by E. Loebell. 1980. (Journal: Vol. 32, No. 3). 110p. 28.75 (*3-8055-1249-X*) S Karger.

Abstracts of the International Conference on Gastrointestinal Cancer, Tel Aviv, Israel, November 1977. International Conference on Gastrointestinal Cancer Staff. Ed. by P. Rozen. 1978. (Journal: Vol. 16, No. 3). pap. 18.50 (*3-8055-2843-4*) S Karger.

Abstracts of the International Conference on Renal Transport of Organic Substances Held in Innsbruck, July, 1980. Ed. by S. Silbernagel. 1980. (Journal: Vol. 2, No. 3). (Illus.). 66p. pap. 24.50 (*3-8055-1641-X*) S Karger.

Abstracts of the Proceedings of the 5th Conference of the Japan Life Support Technology Society. H. Funakubo. 1991. 123p. pap. text 444.00 (*2-88124-810-1*) Gordon & Breach.

Abstracts of the Standard Edition of the Complete Psychological Works of Sigmund Freud. Ed. by Carrie L. Rothgeb. 1973. LC 73-2144. 770p. (C). 85.00 (*0-8236-0030-0*) Intl Univs Pr.

Abstracts of the Standard Edition of the Complete Works of Sigmund Freud. Ed. by Carrie L. Rothgeb. 1987. LC 94-70895. 315p. 35.00 (*0-87668-135-6*) Aronson.

Abstracts - XVII International Congress of Allergology & Clinical Immunology: Syndey, October 15-20, 2000. Ed. by International Association of Allergology and Clinica. 2000. ix, 261p. 49.00 (*0-88937-231-4*) Hogrefe & Huber Pubs.

Abuse & Victimization Across the Life Span. Ed. by Martha B. Straus. 1990. LC 87-46306. (Johns Hopkins Series in Contemporary Medicine & Public Health Ser.). (Illus.). 280p. reprint ed. pap. text 17.95 (*0-8018-3637-9*) Johns Hopkins.

Abuse During Pregnancy: A Protocol for Prevention & Intervention. Judith McFarlane & Barbara J. Parker. Ed. by Karla Damus & Margaret C. Freda. 1994. LC 94-34250. (*0-86525-059-6*) March of Dimes.

Abuse, Neglect, & Exploitation of Older Persons: Strategies for Assessment & Intervention. Ed. by Lorin A. Baumhover & S. Colleen Beall. 1996. LC 95-42646. (Illus.). 288p. (Orig.). pap. 29.00 (*1-878812-29-7*) Hlth Prof Pr.

***Abuse of Men: Trauma Begets Trauma.** Ed. by Barbara Jo Brothers. 2001. LC 2001-24317. 140p. pap. text 17.95 (*0-7890-1379-7*); text 34.95 (*0-7890-1378-9*) Haworth Pr.

Abused Boys: The Neglected Victims of Sexual Abuse. Mic Hunter. 1991. pap. 12.00 (*0-449-90629-9*) Fawcett.

Abused Child: Psychodynamic Understanding & Treatment. Toni V. Heineman. 1998. LC 98-15497. 243p. text 31.00 (*1-57230-375-1*) Guilford Pubns.

Abused Women & Survivor Therapy: A Practical Guide for the Psychotherapist. Lenore E. A. Walker. 1994. LC 93-50591. 529p. text 34.95 (*1-55798-229-5*) Am Psychol.

Abusing Cancer Science: The Truth about NMR & Cancer. Donald P. Hollis. 1987. LC 87-60046. 200p. (Orig.). pap. (*0-942033-15-9*) Strawberry Fields Pr.

Abusing Family. Ed. by Blair Justice & Rita Justice. rev. ed. LC 89-26659. (Illus.). 312p. (C). 25.95 (*0-306-43441-5*) Da Capo.

Abusive Elder: Service Considerations. Ed. by Vera R. Jackson. 1996. LC 96-30431. (Activities, Adaptation & Aging Ser.: Vol. 21, No. 1). 102p. (C). 29.95 (*1-56024-845-9*) Haworth Pr.

Abusive Head Trauma Quick Reference for Healthcare Professionals, Social Services & Law Enforcement. Rauth-Farley & Frasier. 2002. (Illus.). 300p. 39.95 (*1-878060-57-0*) GW Medical.

ACA: Pain Management, Vol. 6. Miller. 1998. text 195.00 (*0-443-07513-1*) Saunders.

ACA: Pediatric Anesthesia, Vol. 7. Miller. 1998. LC 98-21386. text 135.00 (*0-443-07964-1*) Harcourt.

ACA: Subspecialty Care, Vol. 5. Miller. 1998. LC 97-47123. (C). text 135.00 (*0-443-07905-6*) Saunders.

Academic Health Centers in the Managed Care Environment. Ed. by David Korn et al. 1995. 250p. pap. 20.00 (*1-879694-10-7*) AAH Ctrs.

Academic Paths: Career Decisions & Experiences of Psychologists. Ed. by Peter A. Keller. 1994. 184p. pap. 19.95 (*0-8058-1371-3*); text 36.00 (*0-8058-1370-5*) L Erlbaum Assocs.

Academic Recovery after Head Injury. Dinah Russell & Anita Sharratt. 1992. (Illus.). 110p. (C). text 26.95 (*0-398-05788-5*) C C Thomas.

Academic Skills Problems: Direct Assessment & Intervention. Edward S. Shapiro. 2nd ed. 1996. LC 96-28. (Guilford School Practitioner Ser.). 315p. text 35.00 (*1-57230-093-0*, 0093) Guilford Pubns.

Academy Guide to on-Site Medical Staff Training: You Can Do It, We Can Help. 1995. (*1-56055-033-3*) Am Acad Ophthal.

Academy of Sciences & Technology in Berlin see Akademie der Wissenschaften zu Berlin: Jahrbuch Yearbook, 1990-1992

Acarbose for the Treatment of Diabetes Mellitus. Ed. by W. Creutzfeldt. 1989. (Illus.). 208p. 58.00 (*0-387-19145-3*) Spr-Verlag.

Acarology Six, Set. D. A. Griffiths & C. E. Bowman. 1984. LC 79-17386. (Acarology Ser.). 645p. 155.00 (*0-470-27410-7*) P-H.

Accelerating CNS Drug Development. Neal R. Cutler. 1998. LC 97-50438. 194p. 95.00 (*0-471-98128-1*) Wiley.

Accent on Living Reprint Series, No. 1. Ed. by Raymond C. Cheever. 1975. 26p. pap. text 1.95 (*0-915708-01-9*) Cheever Pub.

Acceptability of Cell Substrates for Production of Biologicals. 1987. (Technical Reports: No. 747). (ENG & RUS.). 29p. pap. text 5.00 (*92-4-120747-7*, 1100747) World Health.

Acceptance & Change in Couple Therapy. Stephen Jacobson. 1999. LC 98-19060. 304p. text 25.00 (*0-393-70290-1*) Norton.

Acceptance & Commitment Therapy: An Experiential Approach to Behavior Change. Steven C. Hayes et al. 1999. LC 99-32741. 304p. 36.00 (*1-57230-481-2*, C0481) Guilford Pubns.

Acceptance Testing of Radiological Imaging Equipment: Proceedings of the Symposium Held on October 1-2, 1981. Ed. by Pei-Jan P. Lin et al. 1982. (American Association of Physicists in Medicine Symposium Ser.: No. 1). 310p. 40.00 (*0-88318-400-1*) Am Inst Physics.

Accepting Criticism. 1986. (Pocket Power Ser.). 16p. (Orig.). pap. 1.25 (*0-89486-367-3*, 5366B) Hazelden.

Access Health Brief. Krenz. 2nd ed. 1993. pap. text, stu. ed. 19.00 (*0-13-007808-5*) P-H.

Access Surgery. G. Kootstra & P. J. Jorning. 1982. 350p. text 179.50 (*0-85200-453-2*) Kluwer Academic.

Access to Cadaveric Kidney Transplantation. Joel D. Kallich et al. 1993. LC 93-8688. pap. text 9.00 (*0-8330-1408-0*, MR-202-HCFA) Rand Corp.

Access to Experimental Drugs in Terminal Illness: Ethical Issues. Udo Schuklenk. 1998. LC 98-4689. 288p. (C). 49.95 (*0-7890-0563-8*, Pharmctl Prods) Haworth Pr.

Access to Health. Rebecca J. Donatelle & Lorraine G. Davis. 6th ed. 1999. LC 99-35425. 670p. pap. text 67.00 incl. cd-rom (*0-205-30502-4*) P-H.

***Access to Health.** Donatelle. 7th ed. 2001. suppl. ed. 16.00 (*0-205-35054-2*) Allyn.

Access to Health Care. Center for Health Economics Research Staff. 1993. (Key Indicators for Policy Ser.). (Illus.). 96p. (Orig.). pap. (*0-942054-09-1*) R W Johnson Found.

A
B

Access to Health Care, Pt. 1. Barbara Bloom & National Center for Health Statistics Staff. 1997. LC 97-21807. (Vital & Health Statistics Ser.). (*0-8406-0528-5*) Natl Ctr Health Stats.

Access to Health Care, Pt. 2. Robin A. Cohen & National Center for Health Statistics Staff. 1997. LC 97-21778. (Vital & Health Statistics Ser.). (*0-8406-0529-3*) Natl Ctr Health Stats.

Access to Health Care: States Respond to Growing Crisis. 1993. (Illus.). 94p. (Orig.). (C). pap. text 30.00 (*1-56806-327-X*) DIANE Pub.

Access to Health Care Services in Rural Areas: Delivery & Financing Issues. Ed. by Sheldon Weisgrau. 1999. (Illus.). 146p. (C). reprint ed. pap. text 25.00 (*0-7881-7684-6*) DIANE Pub.

Access to Health Services for Vulnerable Populations. Ed. by Linda F. Wolf. 1996. (Illus.). 288p. (C). reprint ed. pap. text 40.00 (*0-7881-3384-5*) DIANE Pub.

Access to Primary Health Care for Children with HIV: A Guide for Pediatricians, Family Physicians & Nurse Practitioners. Robert H. Parrott & Mary Rathlev. 1993. pap. 9.95 (*0-9634295-1-5*) Childs Hosp.

Access to Primary Health Care in Texas. Sophia Wright. 1995. (Working Papers Ser.: Vol. 81). 39p. pap. 5.50 (*0-89940-560-6*) LBJ Sch Pub Aff.

Accessing Community Resources: Discharge Planning. Ed. by William H. Burke. 2nd ed. 1996. (Professional Series on Traumatic Brain Injury: Vol. 13). 80p. pap. 9.50 (*1-882855-48-5*) HDI Pubs.

Accessories for the Light Microscope, Vol. 16. Robert B. McLaughlin. 1975. LC 74-79374. (Illus.). 30.00 (*0-904962-00-8*) Microscope Pubns.

Accessory Cells in HIV & Other Retroviral Infections. Ed. by P. Racz et al. 1991. (Illus.). viii, 212p. 172.25 (*3-8055-5323-4*) S Karger.

Accident & Emergency: Diagnosis & Management. Anthony F. Brown. 3rd ed. 1996. LC 96-3796. 432p. pap. text (*0-7506-2233-4*) E A GBR. *Dist:* OUP.

Accident & Emergency Care. Ed. by Brian Dolan & Lynda Holt. 1999. 564p. pap. text 25.00 (*0-7020-2239-X*) Saunders.

Accident & Emergency Data & Drug Guide. Francis Morris et al. 1995. 119p. pap. text 30.00 (*0-7506-2035-8*) Buttrwrth-Heinemann.

Accident & Emergency Departments: Health Care Needs Assessment: The Epidemiologically Based Needs Assessment Review, Second Series. Andrew Stevens et al. 1997. LC 97-13346. (*1-85775-290-2*) Radcliffe Med Pr GBR. *Dist:* Balogh.

Accident & Emergency Management: Problems & Solutions. Ed. by Louis Theodore et al. 1991. 187p. (Orig.). (C). pap., stu. ed. 49.50 (*1-56081-094-7*, Wiley-VCH) Wiley.

Accident & Emergency Medicine. Roger Evans. 1997. (Medico-Legal Practitioner Ser.). 163p. (*1-85941-216-5*) Cavendish Pubng GBR. *Dist:* Gaunt.

Accident & Emergency Medicine. David G. Ferguson & David I. Fodden. 1993. LC 92-49913. (Colour Guide Ser.). pap. text 24.00 (*0-443-04512-7*) Saunders.

Accident & Emergency Medicine. G. S. Laing. 1988. 164p. 32.95 (*0-387-19508-4*) Spr-Verlag.

Accident & Emergency Medicine: Survival. Ashis Banerjee. 1996. pap. text 31.50 (*0-7020-2210-1*) Saunders.

Accident & Emergency Nursing. Mike Walsh & Andrew Kent. 4th ed. 2001. LC 2001-278394. (Illus.). 203p. pap. text 40.00 (*0-7506-4317-X*) Buttrwrth-Heinemann.

Accident & Emergency Nursing: A New Approach. Mike Walsh. 3rd ed. 1996. LC 95-44139. 360p. pap. text 47.00 (*0-7506-2443-4*) Buttrwrth-Heinemann.

Accident & Emergency Nursing: A Nursing Model. Lynn Sbaih. 1992. LC 92-22808. pap. 34.95 (*0-412-41180-6*) Chapman & Hall.

Accident & Emergency Nursing: A Nursing Model. Lynn Sbaih. 1992. 192p. 38.25 (*1-56593-031-2*, 0279) Thomson Learn.

Accident & Emergency Radiology: A Survival Guide. Nigel Raby et al. 1995. (Illus.). 262p. pap. text (*0-7020-1905-4*) W B Saunders GBR. *Dist:* Saunders.

Accident Prevention Bulletin, No. 17.01. Myers, S. D., Inc. Staff. 1977. (Illus.). 97p. 15.00 (*0-939320-04-5*) Myers Inc.

Accidental Falls: Their Causes & Their Injuries. Alvin S. Hyde. 1996. LC 97-120331. (Illus.). 251p. 127.00 (*0-9637057-1-7*) Hyde Assocs.

Accidental Injury: Biomechanics & Prevention. Alan M. Nahum & John W. Melvin. 2nd ed. 2000. LC 00-24950. (Illus.). 624p. 165.00 (*0-387-98820-3*) Spr-Verlag.

Accidental Logics: The Dynamics of Change in the Health Care Arena in the United States, Britain, & Canada. Carolyn H. Tuohy. 1999. LC 98-28698. 328p. text 45.00 (*0-19-512821-4*) OUP.

***Accident/Incident Prevention Techniques.** Charles D. Reese. 2001. (Illus.). 544p. (C). text 95.00 (*0-415-25019-6*) Routledge.

Accidents & Emergencies in Children. Rosemary Morton & Barbara Phillips. 2nd ed. 1996. LC 96-1308. (Handbooks in Emergency Medicine Ser.: No. 15). (Illus.). 282p. text 84.50 (*0-19-262720-1*); pap. text 47.50 (*0-19-262719-8*) OUP.

Accidents in Childhood & Adolescence: The Role of Research. Ed. by M. Manciaux & C. J. Romer. 1991. (ENG & FRE.). xiii, 217p. pap. text 35.00 (*92-4-156119-X*, 1150313) World Health.

Accidents in the Year 2000. Ed. by R. M. Labre. 1989. (C). pap. text 90.50 (*0-7923-0475-6*) Kluwer Academic.

Accommodating Disability. Marsha Saxton. 1987. pap. 2.00 (*0-913937-23-1*) Rational Isl.

Accommodation & Refraction of the Eye. F. C. Donders. 1979. LC 78-27045. (Classics in Ophthalmology Ser.). 656p. reprint ed. lib. bdg. 49.50 (*0-88275-839-X*) Krieger.

Accommodation for Day Care Day Surgery Unit, Vol. 1. 1993. (Health Building Note Ser.: No. 52). 65p. pap. (*0-11-321423-5*, HM14235) Statnry Office GBR. *Dist:* Bernan Associates.

Accommodation Nearwork & Myopia. Editha Ong & Kenneth J. Ciuffreda. 1997. LC 96-51078. (Illus.). (C). lib. bdg. 21.00 (*0-943599-88-1*) OEPF.

Accompany Nursing Research: Principles & Methods. Denise F. Polit & Bernadette P. Hungler. 6th ed. 1998. pap. text, stu. ed. 19.95 (*0-7817-1563-6*) Lppncott W & W.

Account of the Foxglove & Its Medical Uses 1785-1985. J. K. Aronson. 1986. (Illus.). 420p. text 45.00 (*0-19-261501-7*) OUP.

Accountability in Nursing Practice. Ed. by R. Watson. 1995. LC 95-71225. 288p. pap. 41.50 (*1-56593-172-6*, 0493) Singular Publishing.

Accountable Systems of Behavioral Health Care: A Provider's Guide. Howard A. Savin & Susan Soldivera Kiesling. 2000. LC 00-8479. 304p. pap. 49.95 (*0-7879-5005-X*) Jossey-Bass.

Accounting for Aggression: Perspectives on Aggression & Violence. Gerda Siann. 1985. 260p. pap. text 19.95 (*0-04-301188-8*) Routledge.

Accounting for Transsexualism & Transhomosexuality. Bryan Tully. 1992. 300p. text (*1-871177-08-1*) Whiting & Birch GBR. *Dist:* Paul & Co Pubs.

Accounts Receivable, Financial Arrangements & Collections, Vol. 1: A Complete How-to Manual for the Doctor & Staff. Robert D. Westerman. 1993. 436p. 295.00 (*0-9629983-1-1*) R Westerman.

ACCP Pulmonary Board Review, 2000. 2000. 650p. pap. 55.00 (*0-916609-20-0*) Am Chest Phys.

ACCP-Seek, Vol. X. 2000. (Illus.). 213p. pap. 250.00 (*0-916609-21-9*) Am Chest Phys.

ACCP Seek Vol. VI: Critical Care Medicine. R. S. Irwin et al. Ed. by American College of Chest Physicians Staff. 1996. (Illus.). 204p. pap. text 350.00 (*0-916609-10-3*) Am Chest Phys.

ACCP SEEK Critical Care Medicine: Assessment in Critical Care & Pulmonology: Self-Education & Evaluation of Knowledge, Set. John G. Weg et al. Ed. by American College of Chest Physicians Staff. 1994. (ACCP SEEK Annual Self-Assessment Ser.). (Illus.). 110p. pap. 150.00 (*0-916609-03-0*) Am Chest Phys.

ACCP Seek Pulmonary Medicine: Assessment in Critical Care & Pulmonology: Self-Education & Evaluation of Knowledge, Vol. V. R. S. Irwin et al. Ed. by American College of Chest Physicians Staff. 1995. (Illus.). 204p. (Orig.). pap. 350.00 (*0-916609-07-3*) Am Chest Phys.

ACCP SEEK Pulmonary Medicine, 1994-95 John G. Weg et al. rev. ed. 1993. (Illus.). (*0-916609-02-2*) Am Chest Phys.

Accreditation: Protecting the Professional or the Consumer? Ellie Scrivens. 1995. LC 94-44778. (State of Health Ser.). 200p. (*0-335-19492-3*); pap. (*0-335-19491-5*) OpUniv Pr.

Accreditation Handbook. 2000. 162p. ring bd. 35.00 (*1-887759-18-2*, E-1) Am Phys Therapy Assn.

ACCSAP - Adult Clinical Cardiology Self Assessment Program. American College of Cardiology Staff. Ed. by Richard P. Lewis. 1993. LC 93-70707. (Illus.). 300p. text 395.00 (*1-882764-01-3*) Am Coll Cardiology.

ACCSAP, 1997-98: Adult Clinical Cardiology Self-Assessment Program. Date not set. LC 97-74437. pap. 390.00 (*1-882764-18-8*) Am Coll Cardiology.

Accu.Net: Dosage Calculations System CD (3) Delmar Publishing Staff & Kip Summerlin. 1998. 1255.95 incl. cd-rom (*0-7668-0722-3*) Delmar.

Accupril (Quinapril) Review of Preclinical & Clinical Data. 1991. LC 91-75285. (Illus.). 189p. text 28.95 (*0-924428-04-X*) Phys Sci Pub.

Accurate Coding for Critical Care Services & Pulmonary Medicine. Patricia Booth. Ed. by Walter J. O'Donohue, Jr. et al. 1996. 75p. (*0-916609-08-1*) Am Chest Phys.

Ace: Behavoral Science. Steven Cody. 1996. (Illus.). 192p. pap. text 30.00 incl. mac hd (*0-8151-1487-7*, 28955) Mosby Inc.

Ace: Histology. E. Robert Burns & M. Donald Cve. 1996. (Illus.). 272p. text 30.00 incl. disk (*0-8151-1335-8*, 28954) Mosby Inc.

Ace Clinical Sciences. Alfred Jay. Bollett. 1996. (Illus.). 522p. text 37.00 (*0-8151-1054-5*, 28976) Mosby Inc.

ACE-Inhibition: State of the Art. Ed. by Hans R. Brunner. 1989. (Journal: Vol. 76, Suppl. 2, 1989). (Illus.). iv, 68p. pap. 22.75 (*3-8055-5062-6*) S Karger.

ACE Inhibitors at the Kidney. Ed. by K. Arakawa et al. 1990. (Journal: Vol. 54, Supl. 1, 1990). (Illus.). iv, 100p. pap. 43.50 (*3-8055-5180-0*) S Karger.

ACE Inhibitors in Heart Failure: Advancing Clinical Practice. Ed. by M. K. Davies & T. Giles. 1996. (Journal: Vol. 87, Suppl. 1, 1996). (Illus.). iv, 44p. pap., suppl. ed. 21.75 (*3-8055-6272-1*) S Karger.

Ace Micro Immunology. Kenneth S. Rosenthal. 1996. (Illus.). 344p. pap. text 30.00 incl. disk (*0-8151-8670-3*, 28951) Mosby Inc.

Ace Pathology. Mosby Staff. 1997. (Illus.). 624p. pap. text 29.95 incl. disk (*0-8151-9428-5*, 28948) Mosby Inc.

Ace Step 3 (Mac) Mosby Staff. 1996. (Illus.). 416p. (C). (gr. 13). pap. text 38.00 incl. mac hd (*0-8151-2756-1*, 28975) Mosby Inc.

Ace the Boards: Anatomy (Mac) 1996. (Illus.). 480p. pap. text 29.95 incl. mac hd (*0-8151-8671-1*, 28952) Mosby Inc.

Ace the Boards: Mosby's USMLE Step 1 Review for Behavioral Science. Steven Cody. 1996. (Illus.). 192p. (C). (gr. 13). pap. text 30.00 (*0-8151-1844-9*, 27043) Mosby Inc.

Ace the Boards Pharmacology (Mac) Mosby Staff. 1996. 450p. (C). (gr. 13). 30.00 incl. mac hd (*0-8151-3152-6*, 28953) Mosby Inc.

Acetabular Dysplasia-Skeletal Dysplasias in Childhood. Ed. by U. H. Weil. 1978. (Progress in Orthopedic Surgery Ser.: Vol.2). (Illus.). 199p. 41.95 (*0-387-08400-2*) Spr-Verlag.

Acetaldehyde. 1995. (Environmental Health Criteria Ser.: No. 167). (FRE & SPA.). 129p. (C). pap. text 29.00 (*92-4-157167-5*, 1160167) World Health.

Acetaminophen: Index of New Information with Authors & Subjects. American Health Research Institute Staff. rev. ed. 1996. 57.50 (*0-7883-0840-8*); 1996. pap. 47.50 (*0-7883-0841-6*); 1994. 57.50 (*0-7883-0158-6*); 1994. pap. 47.50 (*0-7883-0159-4*) ABBE Pubs Assn.

Acetonitrile. Ed. by World Health Organization Staff. 1993. (Environmental Health Criteria Ser.: No. 154). (ENG, FRE & SPA.). 110p. pap. text 26.00 (*92-4-157154-3*, 1160154) World Health.

Acetylene—Index of New Information & Medical Research Bible. Kathryn P. Schumburg. 1994. 150p. 57.50 (*0-7883-0084-9*); pap. 47.50 (*0-7883-0085-7*) ABBE Pubs Assn.

Achieve Maximum Health: Colon Flora the Missing Link in Immunity, Health & Longevity. David Webster. 1995. (Illus.). 240p. (Orig.). pap. 22.95 (*0-9647537-1-5*) Hygeia Pubng.

Achievement & Addiction: A Guide to the Treatment of Professionals. Edgar P. Nace. 1995. LC 95-2834. 272p. text 34.95 (*0-87630-753-5*) Brunner-Routledge.

Achievement & Motivation: A Social-Developmental Perspective. Ed. by Ann K. Boggiano & Thane S. Pittman. 1993. (Illus.). 303p. (C). text 59.95 (*0-521-32220-0*) Cambridge U Pr.

Achievement & Task Motivation. Ed. by J. H. Van den Bercken et al. 1986. vi, 276p. (Orig.). pap. (*90-265-0739-9*) Swets.

Achievement Motive. David C. McClelland. LC 75-34465. (Illus.). 42.50 (*0-8290-1167-6*) Irvington.

Achievement-Related Motives in Children. Ed. by Charles P. Smith. 1969. LC 75-81045. 264p. 29.95 (*0-87154-811-9*) Russell Sage.

Achievements in Gynecology. Ed. by S. Mancuso. 1989. (Contributions to Gynecology & Obstetrics Ser.: Vol. 17). (Illus.). vi, 130p. 85.25 (*3-8055-4825-7*) S Karger.

Achievements in Gynecology 1989-90. Ed. by S. Mancuso. 1991. (Contributions to Gynecology & Obstetrics Ser.: Vol. 18). (Illus.). x, 186p. (C). 156.75 (*3-8055-5122-3*) S Karger.

Achieving Equitable Access: Studies of Health Care Issues Affecting Hispanics & African Americans. Ed. by Marsha Lillie-Blanton et al. 1996. (Illus.). 186p. (C). pap. text 28.00 (*0-7618-0378-5*) U Pr of Amer.

Achieving Equitable Access: Studies of Health Care Issues Affecting Hispanics & African Americans. Ed. by Marsha Lillie-Blanton et al. 2001. (Illus.). 186p. (C). lib. bdg. 58.50 (*0-7618-0377-7*) U Pr of Amer.

Achieving Evidence-Based Practice: A Handbook for Practitioners. Contrib. by Susan Hamer & Gill Collinson. 1999. LC 99-31334. xiv, 221p. (*0-7020-2349-3*) Bailliere Tindall.

Achieving Health for All by the Year 2000: Midway Reports of Country Experiences. Ed. by E. Tarimo & A. Creese. 1990. (ENG, FRE & SPA.). v, 262p. pap. text 46.00 (*92-4-156132-7*, 1150341) World Health.

Achieving Patient Compliance: Psychology of the Medical Practitioner's Role. M. Robin DiMatteo & D. Dante DiNicola. 1982. (General Psychology Ser.). (Illus.). 300p. text 65.00 (*0-08-027552-4*); pap. text 25.00 (*0-08-027551-6*) Elsevier (Pergamon Pr).

Achieving Profitability with a Medical Office System. James Allen. 1993. (Illus.). 150p. ring bd. 59.95 (*0-07-600633-6*, ME101) Practice Mgmt Info.

Achieving Sterility in Medical & Pharmaceutical Products. Nigel A. Halls. 1994. LC 94-6372. (Drugs & the Pharmaceutical Sciences Ser.: Vol. 64). (Illus.). 296p. text 135.00 (*0-8247-9014-6*) Dekker.

Achieving Unlimited Health: The Elusive Fountain of Youth. James P. Cima. 1997. 150p. (Orig.). pap. 19.95 (*0-9659476-0-2*) JPC Pubng.

Acid: LSD Today. Jennifer James. 1999. pap. 0.50 (*0-89230-181-3*) Do It Now.

Acid-Base. Horacio J. Adrogue & Donald E. Wesson. 1994. LC 94-18243. (Basics of Medicine Ser.). 224p. pap. 10.95 (*0-86542-428-4*) Blackwell Sci.

Acid-Base. Horacio J. Adrogue & Donald E. Wesson. 1991. LC 91-75540. (& W Basics in Medicine Ser.). 204p. (C). text 29.95 (*0-9630670-0-1*) Libra & Gemini.

Acid-Base. Jordan J. Cohen & Jerome P. Kassirer. 1982. 79.95 (*0-316-15011-8*, Little Brwn Med Div) Lppncott W & W.

Acid-Base & Electrolyte Disorders. Horacio Adrogue. 1991. (Contemporary Management in Critical Care Ser.: Vol. 1, No. 2). (Illus.). 240p. text (*0-443-08829-2*) Church.

Acid-Base Balance. Alan Y. Cohen. 1990. (Illus.). 127p. pap. text 16.95 (*0-910271-01-1*) Critical Care Pr.

Acid Base Balance: A Manuel for Clinicians. Jorge A. Quintero. 2nd ed. 1981. LC 77-81798. (Illus.). 138p. 12.50 (*0-87527-148-0*) Green.

Acid-Base Reaction Cements: Their Biomedical & Industrial Applications. Alan D. Wilson & John W. Nicholson. 1993. (Chemistry of Solid State Materials Ser.: No. 2). (Illus.). 418p. (C). text 100.00 (*0-521-37222-4*) Cambridge U Pr.

Acid Deposition. Ed. by S. Beilke & A. J. Elshout. 1983. text 106.00 (*90-277-1588-2*) Kluwer Academic.

Acid-Peptic Disorders of the Upper Gastrointestinal Tract: Diagnosis & Management. Harris R. Clearfield. 1995. pap. 27.95 (*1-884065-04-X*) Assocs in Med.

Acid-Related Diseases: Improving the Treatment Options - Journal: Digestion, Vol. 51, Suppl. 1, 1992. Ed. by J. Dent & N. D. Yeomans. 1992. (Illus.). vi, 126p. pap. 41.00 (*3-8055-5685-3*) S Karger.

Acidophilus & Your Health. Frank Murray. 1997. LC 98-202883. 48p. pap. 3.95 (*0-87983-807-8*, 38078K, Keats Pubng) McGraw-Hill Trade.

Acidosis—Index of New Information & Medical Research Bible. Timmy R. Laforre. 1994. 150p. 57.50 (*0-7883-0086-5*); pap. 47.50 (*0-7883-0087-3*) ABBE Pubs Assn.

Acinetobacter: Microbiology, Epidemiology, Infections, Management. Ed. by E. Bergogne-Berezin et al. 1995. LC 95-30812. 288p. 189.95 (*0-8493-9223-3*, 4833) CRC Pr.

Ackerman's Histopathologic Diagnosis of Adnexal Neoplasms. Luis Requena et al. 1998. (Illus.). 1,184p. text 199.00 (*0-397-58793-7*) Lppncott W & W.

Ackerman's Surgical Pathology. Juan Rosai. 1999. 439.00 incl. cd-rom (*0-323-00534-9*); 8th ed. 1995. (Illus.). 2896p. (C). (gr. 13). text 315.00 (*0-8016-7004-7*, 07004) Mosby Inc.

ACL Deficient Knee. Ed. by Edward M. Wojtys. 1994. 140p. pap. 38.00 (*0-89203-118-2*) Amer Acad Ortho Surg.

ACL Teaching Kit: An Instructor's Resource. Ken Grauer. 1989. (C). (gr. 13). 175.00 (*0-8016-0174-6*) Mosby Inc.

ACLS: Quick Review Study Cards. Barbara Aehlert. 1994. pap. 18.00 (*0-8151-0343-3*) Mosby Inc.

ACLS: Quick Review Study Guide. Barbara Aehlert. 1993. (Illus.). 320p. (C). (gr. 13). pap. text 13.95 (*0-8151-0007-8*) Mosby Inc.

ACLS for EMTBs. Mike Smith. Ed. by American Academy of Orthopaedic Surgeons Staff. 2002. (Illus.). 128p. (C). pap. text 25.00 (*0-7637-1505-0*, 1505-0) Jones & Bartlett.

ACLS Pearls of Wisdom: Over 500 Questions. Plantz. 1999. (Pearls of Wisdom Ser.). pap. 12.00 (*1-58409-004-9*) Boston Medical.

***ACLS Quick Review Study Guide: And Study Cards Package.** Barbara Aehlert. 1994. 29.00 (*0-8151-0050-7*) Mosby Inc.

***ACLS Quick Reviews Study Guide.** Barbara Aehlert. 2nd ed. 2001. (*0-323-00892-5*) Mosby Inc.

ACLS Rapid Reference. Ken Grauer. 1997. (Illus.). 176p. (gr. 13). spiral bd. 12.00 (*0-8151-3831-8*, 30971) Mosby Inc.

ACLS Rapid Review & Case-Based Scenarios. Ken Grauer & Daniel Cavallaro. 4th ed. 1996. (Illus.). 400p. (gr. 13). pap. text 21.00 (*0-8151-3623-4*, 28155) Mosby Inc.

ACLS Scenarios: Core Concepts for Case-Based Learning. Richard O. Cummins. 2nd ed. 1995. (Illus.). 320p. (C). (gr. 13). pap. text 25.00 (*0-8151-1517-2*, 25095) Mosby Inc.

ACLS Scenarios Review Study Case: Rapid Study Card Review. Ken Grauer & Dan Cavallaro. 3rd ed. 1996. 350p. pap. text 28.00 (*0-8151-3576-9*) Mosby Inc.

ACLS Skills Review. Mosby Staff. rev. ed. 1992. tchr. ed. (*0-8016-7826-9*) Mosby Inc.

***Acne.** John Cunliffe & Thiboutot. 2003. (Fast Facts Ser.). (Illus.). 80p. pap. (*1-899541-73-X*) Health Pr GBR. *Dist:* JAMCO Dist.

Acne & Related Disorders: International Meeting, Ardiff, Held March, 1988. Marks & Gerd Plewig. 1989. 98.00 (*0-948269-94-4*) CRC Pr.

ACOEM Occupational Medicine Practice Guidelines: Evaluation & Management of Common Health Problems & Functional Recovery in Workers. Ed. by Jeffrey S. Harris. 1998. LC 00-690007. 354p. ring bd. 199.00 (*1-883595-14-2*, 23039, OEM Pr) OEM Health.

ACOG Guide to Planning for Pregnancy, Birth, & Beyond see Planning for Pregnancy, Birth, & Beyond

Acoustic Neuroma: Trends & Controversies. Ed. by R. Filipo & M. Barbara. 1999. (Illus.). vii, 177p. (*90-6299-176-9*) Kugler.

Acoustic Immittance Measures in Clinical Audiology: A Primer. Terry L. Wiley & Cynthia Fowler. 1997. LC 97-2454. (Illus.). 264p. (Orig.). pap. text 39.95 (*1-56593-693-0*, 1358) Thomson Learn.

Acoustic Mirror: The Female Voice in Psychoanalysis & Cinema. Kaja Silverman. 1988. LC 87-45834. (Theories of Representation & Difference Ser.). 268p. pap. 14.95 (*0-253-20474-7*, MB-474) Ind U Pr.

Acoustic Neuroma. Leonard I. Malis. 1998. 152p. 184.50 (*0-444-82976-8*) Elsevier.

Acoustic Neuroma & Skull Base Surgery: Proceedings of the 2nd International Conference on Acoustic Neuroma Surgery & 2nd European Skull Base Society Congress, Paris, France, April 22-26, 1995. Jean-Marc Sterkers et al. 1996. LC 96-25536. (*90-6299-128-9*) Kugler NLD. *Dist:* Lib Res.

Acoustic Theory of Speech Production. Gunnar Fant. rev. ed. 1970. (D A C S R Ser.: No. 2). text (*90-279-1600-4*) Mouton.

Acoustical Signal Processing in the Central Auditory System: Proceedings of an International Symposium Held in Prague, Czech Republic, September 4-7, 1996. Ed. by Josef L. Syka. 1997. LC 97-25247. (Illus.). 630p. 179.00 (*0-306-45608-7*, Kluwer Plenum) Kluwer Academic.

Acoustics of Crime: The New Science of Forensic Phonetics. H. Hollien. 1990. (Applied Psycholinguistics & Communication Disorders Ser.). (Illus.). 380p. (C). 65.00 (*0-306-43467-9*, Plenum Trade) Perseus Pubng.

ACPA Workbook Manual see From Patient to Person - First Steps: A Workbook for People with Chronic Pain

ACP/ALA/Med Basic Statistics. Eurostat Staff. 1997. 280p. pap. (*92-827-6197-5*, CA92-95-683-ENC) Comm Europ Commun BEL. *Dist:* Bernan Associates.

Acquired Aphasia in Children. Ed. by Isabel P. Martins et al. 1991. 328p. text 171.00 (*0-7923-1315-1*) Kluwer Academic.

Acquired Brain Injury in Childhood & Adolescence: A Team & Family Guide to Educational Program Development & Implementation. Ed. by Alan L. Goldberg. 1996. (Illus.). 262p. 60.95 (*0-398-06589-6*); pap. 41.95 (*0-398-06590-X*) C C Thomas.

Acquired Colour Vision Deficiencies: Proceedings of the International Research Group on Colour Vision Deficiencies Symposium, 1st, Ghent, Belgium, 1971. International Research Group on Colour Vision Deficiencies. Ed. by Guy Verriest. 1972. (Modern Problems in Ophthalmology Ser.: Vol. 11). (Illus.). 64.50 (*3-8055-1303-8*) S Karger.

Acquired Hearing Loss: Psychological & Psychosocial Implications. Alan J. Thomas. 1985. text 120.00 (*0-12-687920-6*) Acad Pr.

Acquired Immune Deficiency Syndrome: Reprint from Pathobiology, Vol. 60, No. 4, 1992. Ed. by David B. Weiner. 1992. (Illus.). 80p. 36.75 (*3-8055-5680-2*) S Karger.

Acquired Immune Deficiency Syndrome (AIDS) A Source Guide. 1991. lib. bdg. 250.00 (*0-8490-4888-5*) Gordon Pr.

Acquired Immune Deficiency Syndrome (AIDS) & Chemical Dependency. 1990. lib. bdg. 250.00 (*0-87700-894-9*) Revisionist Pr.

Acquired Immune Deficiency Syndrome & Chemical Dependency. Peter Petrakis. 1997. (Illus.). 78p. reprint ed. pap. text 25.00 (*0-7881-4693-9*) DIANE Pub.

Acquired Immunodeficiency Syndrome. Ed. by Eva Klein. 1986. (Progress in Allergy Ser.: Vol. 37). (Illus.). x, 398p. 239.25 (*3-8055-4156-2*) S Karger.

Acquired Immunodeficiency Syndrome: Current Issues & Scientific Studies. Ed. by Pascal J. Imperato. 1989. (Illus.). 166p. (C). text 65.00 (*0-306-43188-2*, Kluwer Plenum) Kluwer Academic.

Acquired Immunodeficiency Syndrome: Legal & Regulatory Policy. William J. Curran & Lawrence O. Gostin. 1988. (Special Studies on AIDS). 400p. text 45.00 (*1-55572-008-0*) Univ Pub Group.

Acquired Resistance of Micro-Organisms to Chemotherapeutic Drugs. Ed. by H. Schoenfeld et al. 1975. (Antibiotics & Chemotherapy Ser.: Vol. 20). (Illus.). 121.00 (*3-8055-2198-7*) S Karger.

Acquired Speech & Language Disorders: A Neuroanatomical & Functional Neurological Approach. Bruce E. Murdoch. 1990. 300p. pap. (*0-412-33440-2*, A4422) Chapman & Hall.

Acquiring Critical Thinking Skills. Marilyn Meltzer & Susan M. Palau. 1996. pap. text 26.95 (*0-7216-6151-3*) Saunders.

Acquiring Interpersonal Skills: A Handbook of Experimental Learning for Health Professionals. Philip Burnard. 2nd ed. 1996. pap. 38.25 (*1-56593-767-8*, 1492) Singular Publishing.

Acquiring Optimal Health. Gary P. Todd. 1994. LC 94-215154. 128p. pap. 8.95 (*1-878901-92-3*) Hampton Roads Pub Co.

Acquisition & Use of Physiologic Waveform Databases for Testing of Medical Devices: AAMI TIR 24:1999. 2000. (Illus.). 53p. pap. 100.00 (*1-57020-132-3*) Assn Adv Med Instrn.

Acquisition of American Sign Language. Ed. by Slobin Newport & Meier. 1986. (Crosslinguistic Study of Language Acquisition Ser.: Vol. 1). 80p. pap. 14.95 (*0-89859-849-4*) L Erlbaum Assocs.

Acquisition of Two Languages from Birth: A Case Study. Annick De Houwer. 1990. (Cambridge Studies in Linguistics: Supplementary Volumes). (Illus.). 407p. (C). text 100.00 (*0-521-36652-6*) Cambridge U Pr.

Acquisition of Verb Placement: Functional Categories & V2 Phenomena in Language Acquisition. Ed. by Jurgen M. Meisel. 1992. LC 92-23956. (Studies in Theoretical Psycholinguistics: Vol. 16). 464p. (C). text 212.00 (*0-7923-1906-0*) Kluwer Academic.

Acquisitions in Health Sciences Libraries. Ed. by David H. Morse & Alison Bunting. 1996. LC 96-46948. (Current Practice in Health Sciences Librarianship Ser.: Vol. 5). 256p. 42.00 (*0-8108-3052-3*) Scarecrow.

Acquisitions of Physician Practices. 1997. 99.00 incl. audio PA Bar Inst.

Acre of Light: Living with Cancer. Mark Nepo. 1994. pap. 9.95 (*0-87886-138-6*) Ithaca House.

Acres of Skin: Human Experiments at Holmesburg Prison. Allen M. Hornblum. 1999. LC 98-43691. 320p. pap. 16.00 (*0-415-92336-0*) Routledge.

Acres of Skin: The Human Guinea Pigs of Holmesburg Prison. Allen M. Hornblum. 1998. LC 97-41755. 320p. reprint ed. 31.95 (*0-415-91990-8*) Routledge.

Acrolein. 1992. (Environmental Health Criteria Ser.: No. 127). (ENG, FRE & SPA.). 119p. pap. text 24.00 (*92-4-157127-6*, 1160127) World Health.

Acromegaly. Ed. by G. Michael Besser. 1990. (Journal: Vol. 33, Suppl. 1, 1990). (Illus.). vi, 36p. pap. 19.25 (*3-8055-5207-6*) S Karger.

Across This Doctor's Horizons: My Own Mission Field. James F. Crenshaw. 1995. (Illus.). 176p. (Orig.). pap. text 9.95 (*0-87651-937-0*) Southern U Pr.

Acrylamide. 1985. (Environmental Health Criteria Ser.: No. 49). 121p. pap. text 20.00 (*92-4-154189-X*, 1160049) World Health.

ACSM Clinical Study Kit. American College of Sports Medicine Staff. 2000. pap. text 82.95 (*0-7817-2816-9*) Lppncott W & W.

ACSM Clinical Track Certification Study Guide, 1997. American College of Sports Medicine Educational Ma. 1997. 48p. pap., stu. ed. 13.95 (*0-683-30354-6*) Lppncott W & W.

ACSM Clinical Track Certification Study Guide, 1998. American College of Sports Medicine Educational Ma. 1998. LC 98-145935. iii, 48 p. pap. 13.95 (*0-683-30600-6*) Lppncott W & W.

ACSM Clinical Track Certification Study Guide, 2000. Ed. by American College of Sports Medicine Staff. 2000. 42p. pap. text 14.95 (*0-7817-2526-7*) Lppncott W & W.

ACSM Health & Fitness Track Certification Study Guide, 1998. American College of Sports Medicine Health, Fitnes. 1998. 59p. pap. 13.95 (*0-683-30601-4*) Lppncott W & W.

ACSM Health/Fitness Study Kit. Ed. by American College of Sports Medicine Staff. 2000. pap. text 82.95 (*0-7817-2815-0*) Lppncott W & W.

ACSM Health/Fitness Track Certification Study Guide, 2000. Ed. by American College of Sports Medicine Staff. 2000. 69p. pap. text 14.95 (*0-7817-2527-5*) Lppncott W & W.

ACSM's Essentials of Sports Medicine. Ed. by Robert E. Sallis & Ferdy Massimino. 1997. LC 96-6180. (Illus.). 646p. (C). pap. text 73.00 (*0-8151-0157-0*, 25353) Mosby Inc.

ACSM's Exercise Management for Persons with Chronic Diseases & Disabilities. American College of Sports Medicine Staff. Ed. by J. Larry Durstine. 1997. LC 96-48817. 269p. 45.00 (*0-87322-798-0*, BACS0798) Human Kinetics.

ACSM's Guidelines for Clinical Exercise Physiology: Exercise Testing & Prescription for Special Populations. American College of Sports Medicine Staff. 2001. pap. text (*0-7817-2348-5*) Lppncott W & W.

ACSM's Guidelines for Exercise Testing & Prescription. American College of Sports Medicine Staff. 6th ed. 2000. (Illus.). 368p. spiral bd. 29.95 (*0-683-30355-4*) Lppncott W & W.

ACSM's Handbook for the Team Physician. Ed. by W. Ben Kibler. 6th ed. 1996. LC 95-25993. 512p. 29.95 (*0-683-00028-4*) Lppncott W & W.

ACSM's Resource Manual for Guidelines for Exercise Testing & Prescription. American College of Sports Medicine Staff et al. 3rd ed. 1998. LC 97-50181. (Illus.). 715p. pap. text 49.95 (*0-683-00026-8*) Lppncott W & W.

ACSM's Sports Medicine Review. Ed. by Robert E. Sallis et al. 1997. LC 96-6218. (Illus.). 309p. (C). pap. text 49.95 (*0-8151-0392-1*, 25197) Mosby Inc.

Act Smart. American Red Cross Staff. 1995. (gr. 13). 6.00 (*0-8151-0918-0*) Mosby Inc.

Act Step 1 Exam Review WIN: Basic Sciences. Ed. by Emma D. Underdown. 1996. LC 96-6191. (Ace the Boards Ser.). (Illus.). 256p. (C). (gr. 13). pap. text 32.00 incl. 3.5 hd (*0-8151-6904-3*, 27050) Mosby Inc.

Acta Medicinae Legalis 1994: Proceedings of the XVIIth Congress of the International Academy of Legal Medicine. P. Mangin & B. Ludes. 1996. 560p. pap. 159.00 (*3-540-58847-7*) Spr-Verlag.

ACTH & LPH in Health & Disease. Ed. by Lesley H. Rees & T. Van Wimersma Greidanus. 1981. (Frontiers of Hormone Research Ser.: Vol. 8). (Illus.). x, 210p. 115.00 (*3-8055-1977-X*) S Karger.

Acting for Real: Drama Therapy Process, Technique, & Performance. Renee Emunah. 1994. LC 93-44042. 336p. text 54.95 (*0-87630-747-0*); pap. text 27.95 (*0-87630-730-6*) Brunner-Routledge.

Acting-In: Practical Applications of Psychodramatic Methods. Adam Blatner. 3rd rev. ed. 1996. LC 95-49848. (Illus.). 224p. pap. 32.95 (*0-8261-1402-4*) Springer Pub.

Acting Out: The Workbook: A Guide to the Development & Presentation of Issue-Oriented, Audience-Interactive, Improvisational Theatre. Mario Cossa et al. 1996. LC 96-15842. 115p. pap. text 14.95 (*1-56032-534-8*) Accel Devel.

Acting Out: Theoretical & Clinical Aspects. Ed. by Lawrence E. Abt. 1996. LC 96-126930. (Master Work Ser.). 352p. pap. 50.00 (*1-56821-778-1*) Aronson.

Acting Out: Theoretical & Clinical Aspects. Ed. by Lawrence E. Abt & Stuart L. Weissman. 2nd ed. 1976. LC 76-53942. 336p. reprint ed. 50.00 (*0-87668-287-5*) Aronson.

Actinomycosis of the Thorax. George E. Farrell. 1981. (Illus.). 104p. 22.50 (*0-87527-205-3*) Green.

Action Control. Ed. by Julius Kuhl & J. Beckmann. 1985. (Social Psychology Ser.). 320p. 86.95 (*0-387-13445-X*) Spr-Verlag.

Action for Children Affected by AIDS: Programme Profiles & Lessons Learned. 128p. pap. 14.95 (*92-806-3149-7*) UN.

Action for Mental Health. Joint Commission on Mental Illness and Health. Ed. by Gerald N. Grob. 1980. LC 78-22569. (Historical Issues in Mental Health Ser.). reprint ed. lib. bdg. 30.95 (*0-405-11922-4*) Ayer.

Action Guide for Emergency Service Personnel. Rescue Training Association Staff. 1985. 656p. pap. text 39.00 (*0-89303-301-4*) P-H.

Action in Affirmation: Towards an Unambiguous Profession of Nursing. Jerome P. Lysaught. 1981. (Illus.). 224p. text 27.95 (*0-07-039271-4*) McGraw.

Action in Social Context: Perspectives on Early Development. Ed. by J. J. Lockman & N. L. Hazen. 1989. (Perspectives in Developmental Psychology Ser.). (Illus.). 326p. (C). 65.00 (*0-306-43139-4*, Plenum Trade) Perseus Pubng.

Action Methods in Group Psychotherapy: Practical Aspects. Daniel J. Tomasulo. 1997. LC 98-30865. 234p. 49.95 (*1-56032-658-1*); 175p. pap. text 24.95 (*1-56032-659-X*) Hemisp Pub.

Action Modality Couples Therapy: Using Psychodramatic Techniques in Helping Troubled Relationships. Joyce A. Hayden-Seman. 1997. LC 96-53646. 50.00 (*0-7657-0064-6*) Aronson.

Action on AIDS: National Policies in Comparative Perspective, 28. Ed. by Barbara A. Misztal & David Moss. 1990. LC 89-26034. (Contributions in Medical Studies Ser.: No. 28). 280p. 59.95 (*0-313-26369-8*, MZA/, Greenwood Pr) Greenwood.

Action Plan for Women's Health. 1995. (Illus.). 165p. (Orig.). (C). reprint ed. pap. text 35.00 (*0-7881-1789-0*) DIANE Pub.

Action Research in Health Care. Alison Morton-Cooper. 2000. LC 99-87086. pap. 41.95 (*0-632-04091-2*) Blackwell Sci.

Action Speaks Louder. Remocker. 6th ed. 1998. LC 98-40030. (C). pap. text (*0-443-05865-2*) Church.

Action Speaks Louder: A Handbook of Structured Group Techniques. A. Jane Remocker & Elizabeth T. Storch. 5th ed. 1992. (Illus.). 190p. (Orig.). pap. text (*0-443-04364-7*) Church.

Action Therapy & Adlerian Theory: Selected Papers. Walter E. O'Connell. 1975. LC 75-16932. 253p. (Orig.). pap. text 8.00 (*0-918560-06-3*) Adler Sch Prof Psy.

Actions for Health: Grade 1. Mary S. Garzino. 1992. LC 92-461. (Contemporary Health Ser.). (Illus.). 49.95 (*1-56071-095-0*) ETR Assocs.

Actions for Health: Grade 3. 1992. LC 92-8719. (Contemporary Health Ser.). 49.95 (*1-56071-097-7*) ETR Assocs.

Actions, Styles, & Symbols in Kinetic Family Drawings (KFD) An Interpretative Manual. R. C. Burns & S. H. Kaufman. 1987. LC 70-186854. 320p. pap. text 23.95 (*0-87630-228-2*) Brunner-Routledge.

***Actions to Protect California Citizens from Exposure to Cryptosporidium & Other Waterborne Pathogens.** Ed. by Rufus Howell. 2001. 58p. (C). pap. 25.00 (*0-7567-1223-8*) DIANE Pub.

Activated Charcoal in Medical Applications. David O. Cooney. 2nd ed. 1995. LC 94-40860. (Illus.). 584p. text 225.00 (*0-8247-9300-5*) Dekker.

Activated Prothrombin Complex Concentrates: Managing Hemophilia With Factor VIII Inhibitor. Ed. by G. Mariani. 1982. LC 81-23358. 239p. 75.00 (*0-275-91373-2*, C1373, Praeger Pubs) Greenwood.

Activation to Acquisition: Functional Aspects of the Basal Forebrain Cholinergic System. R. T. Richardson. 1991. (Illus.). 392p. 119.00 (*0-8176-3467-3*) Birkhauser.

Activator Methods Chiropractic Techniques. Ed. by Arlan Fuhr. 1996. (Illus.). 480p. (C). (gr. 13). text 82.95 (*0-8151-3684-6*, 29990) Mosby Inc.

Activators & Inhibitors of Complement. Ed. by R. B. Sim. 1992. LC 92-14814. (C). text 205.50 (*0-7923-1819-6*) Kluwer Academic.

Active Analytic Group Therapy. Evans. 1998. LC 98-151087. (International Library of Group Analysis: Vol. 6). 236p. pap. 26.95 (*1-85302-616-6*) Taylor & Francis.

***Active & Passive Movement Testing.** Cheryl M. Petersen & Russell A. Foley. 2002. LC 2001-31560. pap. 45.00 (*0-07-137033-1*) McGraw-Hill Prof.

Active Birth: The New Approach to Giving Birth Naturally. Janet Balaskas. Ed. by Linda Ziedrich. rev. ed. 1992. LC 91-32334. (Illus.). 272p. 19.95 (*1-55832-037-7*); pap. 14.95 (*1-55832-038-5*) Harvard Common Pr.

Active Communities: Healthy Families. Gay M. Gross. 1987. 100p. (Orig.). pap. 20.00 (*0-932622-11-9*) Ctr Public Rep.

Active Hearing. Ed. by A. Flock et al. 1995. LC 94-41161. (Wenner-Gren International Ser.: Vol. 65). (Illus.). 394p. 173.50 (*0-08-042514-3*, Pergamon Pr) Elsevier.

Active Psychotherapy. Harold Greenwald. 2nd ed. 1984. LC 84-45026. (Active Psychotherapy Ser.). 384p. reprint ed. 50.00 (*0-87668-663-3*) Aronson.

Active Techniques & Group Psychotherapy. Theodore Saretsky. 1978. LC 77-88834. 270p. 50.00 (*0-87668-272-7*) Aronson.

Active Treatment of Depression. Richard O'Connor. 2001. LC 00-64724. (Illus.). 250p. 35.00 (*0-393-70322-3*) Norton.

Actively Seeking Nutrition. Richard Duquet. 1978. 27p. pap. 2.00 (*0-934332-20-7*) LEpervier Pr.

***Actividades de Emergencia.** Ed. by Seth Lindstromberg. 2001. pap. text (*84-8323-119-0*) Cambridge U Pr.

Actividades Diarias Despues de Tu Reemplazo Total de Rodilla. Janet V. Platt et al. Tr. by Dyhalma Irizarry. 1993. (Illus.). (C). pap. text (*1-56900-005-0*) Am Occup Therapy.

Activism & Marginalization in the AIDS Crisis. Ed. by Michael A. Hallett. 1997. LC 97-700. (Research on Homosexuality Ser.: Vol. 32, Nos. 3-4). 228p. (C). 49.95 (*0-7890-0004-0*); pap. text 19.95 (*1-56023-090-8*, Harrington Park) Haworth Pr.

Activist Cancer Patient: How to Take Charge of Your Treatment. Beverly Zakarian. 1996. LC 96-4984. 240p. pap. 15.95 (*0-471-12026-X*) Wiley.

Activites de Formation a la Vitamine a pour la Sante et le Developpement Communautaires. Helen Keller International Staff. 1993. LC 93-395669. (FRE., Illus.). 72p. (Orig.). 10.00 (*0-915173-27-1*) Helen Keller Intl.

Activities: Reality & Symbol. Gail Fidler & Beth Velde. 1999. LC 98-45928. (Illus.). xii, 177p. 35.00 (*1-55642-383-7*, 33837) SLACK Inc.

Activities for Adolescents in Therapy: A Handbook of Facilitating Guidelines & Planning Ideas for Group Therapy with Troubled Adolescents. Susan T. Dennison. 2nd ed. 1998. LC 97-25317. 264p. pap. 41.95 (*0-398-06807-0*) C C Thomas.

Activities for Daily Living. 1995. 17.00 (*0-8342-0721-4*); VHS 94.00 (*0-8342-0722-2*) Aspen Pub.

Activities for the Aged & Infirm: A Handbook for the Untrained Worker. Toni Merrill. 1979. (Illus.). 392p. 64.95 (*0-398-01294-6*) C C Thomas.

Activities Handbook for the Teaching of Psychology. Ed. by Vivian P. Makosky et al. LC 81-1648. (Activities Handbook for the Teaching of Psychology Ser.: Vol. 2). Vol. 2. 1988. 345p. pap. 24.95 (*1-55798-030-6*, 4280050); Vol. 3. 1981. (Illus.). 372p. (C). 24.95 (*1-55798-081-0*) Am Psychol.

Activities Program for Senior Citizens. H. Fish & E. Fish. 2000. 12.95 (*0-13-003590-4*, Parker Publishing Co) P-H.

Activities with Developmentally Disabled Elderly & Older Adults. Ed. by M. Jean Keller. 1991. LC 90-5310. (Activities, Adaptation & Aging Ser.). (Illus.). 154p. text 44.95 (*1-56024-092-X*) Haworth Pr.

Activity Analysis: A Primer. Haru Hirama. 1992. 106p. (C). pap. text 22.95 (*0-935273-05-0*) Chess Pub.

Activity Analysis & Application: Building Blocks of Treatment. Nancy K. Lamport et al. 3rd ed. 1996. (Illus.). 264p. pap. text 29.00 (*1-55642-321-7*, 33217) SLACK Inc.

Activity & Volunteer Service Policies & Procedures. Pamela Sander. 3rd ed. 1993. (Illus.). 187p. pap. 39.50 (*1-877735-10-8*, 2112PP) Prof Prnting & Pub.

Activity Anorexia: Theory, Research, & Treatment. Ed. by W. Frank Epling & W. David Pierce. 1996. LC 97-17916. (Illus.). 240p. text 49.95 (*0-8058-1929-0*) L Erlbaum Assocs.

Activity-Based Costing & Activity-Based Management for Health Care. Judith J. Baker. 1998. LC 97-38539. 416p. 96.00 (*0-8342-1115-7*) Aspen Pub.

Activity Care Plans for LTC: If You Didn't Write It down, It Wasn't Done! Pamela Sander. 4th rev. ed. 1999. 212p. (C). 28.50 (*1-877735-05-1*, 2106pp) Prof Prnting & Pub.

Activity Experiments & Programming Within Long-Term Care. Ted Tedrick & Elaine R. Green. 1995. LC 95-60643. 252p. (C). text 32.95 (*0-910251-74-6*, AEX77) Venture Pub PA.

Activity Measurement in Psychology & Medicine. Warren W. Tryon. 1991. (Applied Clinical Psychology Ser.). (Illus.). 268p. (C). 55.00 (*0-306-43786-4*, Plenum Trade) Perseus Pubng.

***Activity of Tumor-Antigens in Polyomavirus Replication.** Hongyun Li. 2001. (Comprehensive Summaries of Uppsala Disertations from the Faculty of Medicine: No. 985). (Illus.). 49p. (Orig.). pap. (*91-554-4904-2*) Uppsala Universitet SWE. *Dist:* Coronet Bks.

Activity of Young Children During Sleep: An Objective Study, Vol. 18. Chester R. Garvey. 1970. LC 76-44474. (Illus.). 102p. reprint ed. lib. bdg. 48.00 (*0-8371-8073-2*, CWGY, Greenwood Pr) Greenwood.

Actrion & Mechanism of Action of 1,25: Dihydroxyvitamin D3 on the Proliferation & Differentiation of Malignant Cells. Lieve Verlinden. 2000. (Acta Biomedica Lovaniensia Ser.: No. 211). (Illus.). 158p. pap. (*90-5867-012-0*) Leuven Univ BEL. *Dist:* Coronet Bks.

Acts of Meaning. Jerome S. Bruner. 1992. (Jerusalem Lectures). 208p. pap. text 14.00 (*0-674-00361-6*) HUP.

Acts of Meaning: Four Lectures on Mind & Culture. Jerome S. Bruner. 1990. LC 90-40485. (Jerusalem-Harvard Lectures). 160p. text 25.00 (*0-674-00360-8*) HUP.

Acts of Will: The Life & Work of Otto Rank. E. James Lieberman. 2nd ed. 1993. LC 93-28227. (Illus.). 536p. reprint ed. pap. 21.95 (*0-87023-871-X*) U of Mass Pr.

Actual Problems in Pediatric Surgery: Proceedings of the 7th Congress of the Hungarian Pediatric Surgeons, Budapest, Hungary, August 25-28, 1982. Tibor Verebely. 1983. 331p. (*963-05-3392-8*) Akade Kiado HUN. *Dist:* St Mut.

Actual Trends in Thyroid Physiopathology. Ed. by T. Lemarchand-Beraud & L. Vanhaelst. 1987. (Journal: Vol. 26, No. 1-4, 1987). ii, 230p. 168.75 (*3-8055-4582-7*) S Karger.

Actualites de Chimie Therapeutique 1995. 1996. 140p. pap. 42.50 (*2-906077-74-7*) Elsevier.

Actualizations: You Don't Have to Rehearse to Be Yourself. Stewart Emery. Ed. by Neal Rogin. 1980. 237p. (C). reprint ed. 18.95 (*0-8290-0222-7*); pap. 6.95 (*0-8290-0965-5*) Irvington.

Actualizing Therapy: Foundations for a Scientific Ethic. Everett L. Shostrom. Ed. by Lila Knapp & Robert R. Knapp. 1976. LC 75-17255. 18.00 (*0-912736-14-3*) EDITS Pubs.

Actuarial Issues in the Fee-for-Service Prepaid Medical Group. Harry L. Sutton, Jr. & Allen J. Sorbo. 2nd ed. 1993. (Going Prepaid Ser.). (Orig.). (C). pap. 32.00 (*0-933948-33-6*, 3296) MGMA Ctr.

Acuenergy. Patti Lloyd. 1982. 208p. 12.95 (*0-89557-060-2*) Woodland UT.

Acumoxa Therapy Vol. 1: Reference & Study Guide. Paul Zmiewski. Ed. by Richard Feit. 1993. 208p. pap. text 28.00 (*0-912111-22-4*) Paradigm Publns.

Acumoxa Therapy, Vol. 2: Treatment of Disease. Paul Zmiewski & Richard Feit. 2nd ed. 1993. 160p. (Orig.). (C). pap. text 26.00 (*0-912111-27-5*) Paradigm Publns.

Acupinch Cramp Relief...in Seconds. Milton F. Allen. 1981. (Illus.). 64p. pap. 1.95 (*0-9607456-0-2*) Acupinch.

Acupoint Exercises for the Six Senses: Professional Edition. Ralph Alan Dale. 1996. (Illus.). 53p. spiral bd. 15.00 (*1-877589-10-1*) Dialectic Pubng.

Acupoint Pocket Reference. Bob Flaws. 1997. (Illus.). 135p. pap. 9.95 (*0-936185-93-7*) Blue Poppy Pr.

Acupressure: Clinical Applications in Musculoskeletal Conditions. John R. Cross. 2000. LC 99-58724. (Illus.). 192p. pap. text 47.50 (*0-7506-4054-5*) Buttrwrth-Heinemann.

Acupressure: Index of New Information for Health, Disease & Therapy with Authors, Subjects & References. Alice M. Frames. 1998. 150p. 57.50 (*0-7883-1370-3*); pap. 47.50 (*0-7883-1371-1*) ABBE Pubs Assn.

Acupressure & Reflextherapy: Clinical Application. John R. Cross. 2001. 224p. pap. 39.99 (*0-7506-4962-3*) Buttrwrth-Heinemann.

Acupressure for Athletes. David J. Nickel. 2nd rev. ed. 1987. LC 86-12097. (Illus.). 176p. pap. 10.95 (*0-8050-0128-X*, Owl) H Holt & Co.

Acupressure for Common Ailments: A Gaia Original. Chris Jarmey & John Tindall. 1991. (Illus.). 96p. (Orig.). pap. 12.95 (*0-671-73135-1*, Fireside) S&S Trade Pap.

Acupressure for Everybody: Gentle, Effective Techniques for Healing & Relaxing. Cathryn Bauer. 1991. 160p. (Orig.). pap. 14.00 (*0-8050-1579-5*, Owl) H Holt & Co.

Acupressure for the Boater: Alternative Emergency Medical Procedures. Michael Friedman. Ed. by Liz Jacobsen. 1983. (Illus.). 43p. (Orig.). pap. 14.95 (*0-912561-01-7*) Counsel & Stress.

Acupressure for the Boater & Backpacker. Michael Friedman. 1989. (Illus.). 43p. (Orig.). pap. 16.95 (*0-912561-09-2*) Counsel & Stress.

Acupressure Warmup: A System of Athletic Preparation & Injury Prevention. Marc Coseo. Ed. by Robert L. Felt. 1993. (Illus.). 144p. (Orig.). pap. text 18.00 (*0-912111-34-8*) Paradigm Publns.

Acupressure Way of Health: Jin Shin Do. Iona M. Teeguarden. 1978. (Illus.). 160p. (Orig.). pap. 17.00 (*0-87040-421-0*) Japan Pubns USA.

Acupressure's Potent Points: A Guide to Self-Care for Common Ailments. Michael R. Gach. 1990. LC 90-464. (Illus.). 272p. pap. 17.95 (*0-553-34970-8*) Bantam.

Acupuncture & Moxibustion Formulas & Treatments. Cheng Dan-an. Ed. & Tr. by Wu Ming from CHI. 1996. LC 95-83248. (Great Masters Ser.). 225p. (Orig.). pap. 22.95 (*0-936185-68-6*) Blue Poppy Pr.

Acupuncture. Gabriel Stux. 1995. 4p. 19.00 (*3-540-59455-8*); 1987. (Illus.). 342p. 120.00 (*0-387-17331-5*) Spr-Verlag.

Acupuncture. Felix Mann. rev. ed. 1973. (Illus.). 256p. pap. 10.00 (*0-394-71727-9*) Vin Bks.

Acupuncture: A Comprehensive Text. Shanghai College of Traditional Chinese Medicine Staff. Ed. & Tr. by John O'Connor & Dan Bensky from CHI. 1981. LC 81-65416. (Illus.). 741p. 65.00 (*0-939616-00-9*) Eastland.

Acupuncture: A Scientific Appraisal. Adrian White & E. Ernst. 1999. LC 99-27351. 168p. pap. text 40.00 (*0-7506-4163-0*) Buttrwrth-Heinemann.

Acupuncture: A Viable Medical Alternative. Marie Cargill. 1994. LC 94-12069. 200p. pap. 18.95 (*0-275-94881-1*, Praeger Pubs) Greenwood.

Acupuncture: An Introductory Guide to the Technique & Its Benefits. Michael Nightingale. 1997. (Illus.). 122p. pap. 13.95 (*0-09-181518-5*) Trafalgar.

Acupuncture: Cure of Many Diseases. Felix Mann. 2nd ed. 1992. LC 92-20085. (Illus.). 140p. pap. text 37.50 (*0-7506-0700-9*) Buttrwrth-Heinemann.

Acupuncture: Everything You Ever Wanted to Know. Gary F. Fleischman. 1997. LC 95-9171. 160p. pap. text 13.95 (*1-886449-09-0*) Barrytown Ltd.

Acupuncture: How It Works, How It Cures. Peter Firebrace et al. 1994. LC 93-46610. 160p. pap. 19.95 (*0-87983-639-3*, 36393K, Keats Pubng) McGraw-Hill Trade.

Acupuncture: Textbook & Atlas. Gabriel Stux & Bruce Pomeranz. 1987. 342p. 96.00 (*3-540-17331-5*) Spr-Verlag.

Acupuncture: Treatment of Musculo-Skeletal Conditions. Christopher M. Norris. 2001. 208p. pap. 44.99 (*0-7506-5173-3*) Buttrwrth-Heinemann.

Acupuncture - The Five Element-Phases: The Theory, Command Points, Clinical Applications & Comprehensive Index. Ralph Alan Dale. 2001. (Illus.). 400p. 95.00 (*1-877589-14-4*) Dialectic Pubng.

Acupuncture - The One Thousand New Points: A Comprehensive Manual & Prescription Index. Ralph Alan Dale. 2001. (Illus.). 500p. 125.00 (*1-877589-07-1*) Dialectic Pubng.

Acupuncture - The Special Function Points. Ralph Alan Dale. 1996. (Illus.). 205p. pap. 39.00 (*1-877589-12-8*) Dialectic Pubng.

Acupuncture & Moxibustion: A Guide to Clinical Practice. B. Auteroche et al. 1992. (Illus.). 164p. text (*0-443-04556-9*) Church.

Acupuncture & Oriental Medicine Laws: 1999 Edition. Barbara B. Mitchell. 1999. v, 181p. 27.00 (*0-9670262-0-2*) Natl Acup Fndt.

Acupuncture & Related Techniques in Physical Therapy. Val Hopwood et al. 1997. LC 96-44086. text (*0-443-05593-9*) Church.

Acupuncture, Art & Science: Index of Modern Authors & Subjects with Guide for Rapid Research. Stanley X. Garrett. 1994. LC 94-35175. 57.50 (*0-7883-0358-9*); pap. text 47.50 (*0-7883-0359-7*) ABBE Pubs Assn.

Acupuncture Case Histories from China. Ed. by Jirui Chen & Nissi Wang. 1988. (Illus.). 300p. text 35.00 (*0-939616-07-6*) Eastland.

Acupuncture Cases from China: A Digest of Difficult & Complicated Case Histories. Ed. by Oran Kivity & Richard James. 1996. LC 93-43057. text (*0-443-04788-X*) Church.

Acupuncture Certification Examination Review Book of Questions & Answers. Ralph Alan Dale. 1985. 87p. stu. ed., spiral bd. 25.00 (*1-877589-03-9*) Dialectic Pubng.

Acupuncture Comprehensive Prescription Index. Ralph Alan Dale. rev. ed. 1997. (Illus.). 550p. pap. 95.00 (*1-877589-15-2*) Dialectic Pubng.

Acupuncture Directory. 1974. (Orig.). pap. 2.50 (*0-914322-00-1*) Chans Corp.

Acupuncture, Electropuncture Anaesthesia. Pedro Chan. 1972. pap. 4.95 (*0-87505-149-9*) Borden.

Acupuncture Energetics: A Clinical Approach for Physicians. Joseph M. Helms. 1995. (Illus.). 800p. 175.00 (*1-57250-706-3*) Med Acupuncture.

Acupuncture Energetics: A Workbook for Diagnosis & Treatment. Mark D. Seem. 1987. (Illus.). 144p. (C). pap., wbk. ed. 14.95 (*0-89281-435-7*, Heal Arts VT) Inner Tradit.

Acupuncture, Expertise & Cross-Cultural Medicine. Roberta E. Bivins. 2000. LC 00-33326. (Science, Technology, & Medicine in Modern History Ser.). (Illus.). (*0-312-23761-8*) St Martin.

Acupuncture for Everyone: What It Is, Why It Works & How It Can Help You. Ruth Kidson. 2001. LC 00-56729. (Illus.). 224p. pap. 12.95 (*0-89281-899-9*, Heal Arts VT) Inner Tradit.

Acupuncture for Pets. Shawn Messonnier. 1998. (Pet Care Naturally Ser.). 64p. pap. 4.95 (*0-87983-924-4*, Keats Pubng) McGraw-Hill Trade.

Acupuncture Imaging: A Guide for Practitioners & Their Patients. Mark D. Seem. 1991. (Illus.). 96p. 19.95 (*0-89281-375-X*, Heal Arts VT) Inner Tradit.

Acupuncture in Holistic Practice Vol. 5: Selected Journal Articles, 1976-2000. Ralph Alan Dale. 2001. (Illus.). 600p. 125.00 (*1-877589-08-X*) Dialectic Pubng.

Acupuncture in Obstetrics & Gynecology. Valentin Tureanu & Luminita Tureanu. 1999. LC 2001-265426. xii, 390p. pap. 42.50 (*0-87527-525-7*) Green.

Acupuncture in Practice. Luc De Schepper. 1994. (Illus.). 350p. (Orig.). (C). pap. 39.95 (*0-942501-03-9*) Full of Life.

Acupuncture in Practice: Case Histories from the West. Hugh MacPherson & Ted J. Kaptchuk. 1996. LC 96-26153. text (*0-443-05049-X*) Church.

Acupuncture in Pregnancy & Childbirth. Zita West. 2000. (Illus.). 280p. pap. text 42.00 (*0-443-06138-6*) Saunders.

Acupuncture in the Treatment of Children. Julian Scott & Teresa Barlow. 3rd ed. 1999. LC 98-74564. (Illus.). xii, 628p. (C). 65.00 (*0-939616-30-0*) Eastland.

Acupuncture Is & Is Not. Pedro Chan. 1974. (Illus.). pap. 0.95 (*0-914322-01-X*) Chans Corp.

Acupuncture Manual Vol. 1: Points, Conduits, Functions & Indications. Ralph Alan Dale. 2001. (Illus.). 600p. 125.00 (*1-877589-13-6*) Dialectic Pubng.

Acupuncture Medicine: Its Historical & Clinical Background. Yoshiaki Omura. 1996. (Illus.). 288p. pap. 42.50 (*1-882345-09-6*) Cognizant Comm.

Acupuncture, Meridian Theory & Acupuncture Points. Li Ding. Tr. by You Benlin & Wang Zhaorong from CHI. 1992. (Illus.). 414p. (C). reprint ed. text 60.00 (*0-8351-2143-7*) China Bks.

Acupuncture on Midwifery. Yelland. 2001. LC 97-105713. 88p. text 29.99 (*1-898507-40-6*) Buttrwrth-Heinemann.

Acupuncture Patterns & Practice. Xuemai Li & Jingyi Zhao. 1993. LC 92-85309. (Illus.). 205p. text 35.00 (*0-939616-16-5*) Eastland.

Acupuncture Point Combinations: The Key to Clinical Success. Jeremy Ross. 1995. LC 94-43497. text (*0-443-05006-6*) Church.

Acupuncture Points: Images & Functions. Arnie Lade. 1989. LC 88-82703. 363p. (C). text 29.50 (*0-939616-08-4*) Eastland.

***Acupuncture Response: Balance Energy & Restore Health: A Western Doctor Tells You How.** Glenn S. Rothfield & Suzanne LeVert. 2001. LC 2001-37146. (Illus.). 256p. pap. 14.95 (*0-8092-9759-0*, Contemporary) McGraw-Hill Trade.

Acupuncture, the Ancient Chinese Art of Healing. Felix Mann. 1990. (Illus.). 24.00 (*0-8446-4583-4*) Peter Smith.

Acupuncture Treatment for Paralysis. Ed. by Yaoqi Kong et al. Tr. by Huan Ye & Guiying Lu. 1996. (Illus.). 210p. pap. 24.50 (*1-880132-24-9*) Sci Pr NY.

Acupuncture Treatment of Pain: Safe & Effective Methods for Using Acupuncture in Pain Relief. Leon Chaitow. 1990. 192p. pap. text 19.95 (*0-89281-383-0*, Heal Arts VT) Inner Tradit.

Acupuncture, Trigger Points & Muscloskeletal Pain: A Scientific Approach to Acupuncture for Use by Doctors & Physiotherapists in the Diagnosis & Management of Myofascial Trigger Point Pain. P. E. Baldry. 2nd ed. 1995. LC 92-17401. text (*0-443-04580-1*) Church.

Acupuncture with Your Fingers: An 18-Point Healing System. Ralph Alan Dale. (Illus.). 55p. 6th rev. ed. 1988. 12.00 (*1-877589-00-4*); 7th rev. ed. 2000. LC 99-161906. pap. 6.75 (*1-877589-01-2*) Dialectic Pubng.

Acupuncturist's Handbook - A Practical Encyclopedia, Vol. 1. Kuen-Shii Tsay. 1995. (Illus.). 500p. (C). 45.00 (*0-9647445-0-3*) CPM Whole Hlth.

Acupuntura Con Sus Dedos: Sistema Curativo de Dieciocho Puntos. Ralph Alan Dale. Tr. by Ronald Lorenzana. rev. ed. 1987. (SPA., Illus.). 55p. (Orig.). pap. 6.75 (*1-877589-02-0*) Dialectic Pubng.

***Acupunture in Practice: Beyond Points & Meridians.** Anthony Campbell. 2001. 192p. pap. 24.99 (*0-7506-5242-X*) Buttrwrth-Heinemann.

Acute Abdomen: Diagnostic Imaging in the Clinical Context. G. P. Krestin. 1995. (Illus.). 285p. pap. text 65.00 (*0-86577-606-7*) Thieme Med Pubs.

Acute Alcoholic Intoxication: A Critical Review. Henry W. Newman. 1941. x, 207p. 29.50 (*0-8047-0995-5*) Stanford U Pr.

Acute & Chronic Liver Diseases: Molecular Biology & Clinics: Proceedings of the 87th Falk Symposium (X International Congress of Liver Diseases 1995), Held in Basel, Switzerland, October 19-21, 1995. Ed. by R. Schmid et al. 1996. LC 96-17378. (Basel Liver Week Ser.: Pt. II). text 176.50 (*0-7923-8701-5*) Kluwer Academic.

Acute & Chronic Wound: Nursing Management. Ruth Bryant & Dorothy Doughty. 2nd ed. 1998. 558p. (C). 48.00 (*1-55664-410-8*) Mosby Inc.

Acute & Recurrent Unconsciousness. Caronna. Date not set. text 15.99 (*0-7506-9542-0*) Buttrwrth-Heinemann.

Acute & Secretory Otitis Media. Ed. by J. Sade. 1986. LC 86-20940. (Illus.). 574p. lib. bdg. (*90-6299-023-1*) Kugler NLD. *Dist:* Lib Res.

Acute Aneurysm Surgery. T. Asano et al. 1987. (Illus.). 300p. 175.00 (*0-387-81987-8*) Spr-Verlag.

Acute Appendicitis: Standard Treatment or Laparoscopic Surgery? International Meeting, Bern, May 1997. Ed. by L. Kraehenbuehl et al. 1998. LC 98-9426. (Progress in Surgery Ser.: Vol. 25, 1998). (Illus.). viii, 192p. 170.50 (*3-8055-6641-7*) S Karger.

Acute Asthma. Jesse B. Hall et al. 2000. LC 99-88571. (Illus.). 378p. text 65.00 (*0-07-026026-5*) McGraw-Hill Prof.

Acute Cardiac Care: Community & Hospital Management of Myocardial Infarction. Kevin Jennings. 1994. (Illus.). 222p. pap. text 39.50 (*0-19-263006-7*) OUP.

Acute Care: Based on the Proceedings of the Sixth International Symposium on Critical Care Medicine, Rio De Janeiro, 1977. Ed. by B. M. Tavares. 1979. (Anaesthesiologie und Intensivmedizin Ser.: Vol. 116). (Illus.). 345p. 61.00 (*0-387-09210-2*) Spr-Verlag.

Acute Care Gynecology. Thomas G. Stovall. 1998. (Illus.). 248p. pap. 49.00 (*0-387-94970-4*) Spr-Verlag.

Acute Care Handbook for Physical Therapists. Jaime Paz et al. 1997. LC 97-8765. (Illus.). 698p. pap. text 65.00 (*0-7506-9822-5*) Buttrwrth-Heinemann.

Acute Care Handbook for Physical Therapists. Michele P. West & Paz. 2001. 768p. pap. 59.99 (*0-7506-7300-1*) Buttrwrth-Heinemann.

Acute Care Hospital Challenge: Product Line Management, Matrix Management or Functional Management...Its Implications for the Future of Addication Treatment. Ronald J. Hunsicker. 1992. LC 92-80717. 70p. (C). pap. text (*0-9632545-0-2*) The Terraces.

***Acute Care in the Community: Intensive Home Treatment as an Alternative to Psychiatric Admission.** Neil Brimblecombe. 2001. 250p. (C). pap. (*1-86156-189-X*) Whurr Pub GBR. *Dist:* Taylor & Francis.

Acute Care 1995 (CHKS) 1996. (*1-57372-049-6*); 1995. (*1-899666-01-X*) Solucient.

Acute Care Nurse in Transition. American Nurses Association Staff & Research in Marketing, Incorporated Staff. 1996. LC 96-20009. 72p. pap. 19.95 (*1-55810-127-6*, EC-152) Am Nurses Pub.

Acute Care Nurse Practitioner. Ed. by Barbara Daly. 1997. LC 96-46566. 192p. 34.95 (*0-8261-9480-X*) Springer Pub.

Acute Care Nurse Practitioner: Clinical Reference & Certification Review. American Association of Critical-Care Nurses Staff. Ed. by Thomas Eoyang. 1998. LC 98-4059. (Illus.). xvii, 1033p. (C). text 65.00 (*0-7216-7311-2*) Saunders.

***Acute Care Nurse Practitioner Certification Examination: Review Questions & Strategies.** Barbara Todd. 2001. LC 2001-47102. 304p. per. 69.95 (*0-8036-0957-4*) Davis Co.

Acute Care Nurse Practitioner Certification Study Question Book. Ed. by Sally K. Miller. 1998. LC 99-10079. 300p. pap. text 35.00 (*1-878028-25-1*) Hlth Lead Assoc.

Acute Care Nursing in the Home: A Holistic Approach. Catheric Malloy & Edward A. Hartshorn. 1988. (Illus.). 606p. text 36.50 (*0-397-54661-0*) Lppncott W & W.

Acute Care of the Abdomen. Mitchell J. Spirt. 1998. LC 97-13638. 505p. pap. 65.00 (*0-683-18149-1*) Lppncott W & W.

Acute Care Psychiatry: Diagnosis & Treatment. Lloyd I. Sederer & Anthony J. Rothschild. 1997. LC 96-39069. (Diagnosis & Treatment). 577p. 99.00 (*0-683-30006-7*) Lppncott W & W.

Acute Catabolic State. A. Revhaug. 1996. LC 95-10442. (Illus.). 299p. 134.00 (*3-540-58445-5*) Spr-Verlag.

Acute Catabolic State. Ed. by A. Revhaug. 1995. LC 95-10442. (Update in Intensive Care & Emergency Medicine Ser.: Vol. 21). (*0-387-58445-5*) Spr-Verlag.

Acute Cervical Spinal Column & Cord Injury. David A. Herz & Janice E. Looman. Ed. by Oliver D. Grin & Dorothy L. Bouwman. 1990. (Patient Education Ser.). (Illus.). 22p. (Orig.). pap. text 4.00 (*0-929689-38-0*) Ludann Co.

Acute Childhood Leukemia. Ed. by Carl Pochedly. 1975. (Modern Problems in Pediatrics Ser.: Vol. 16). (Illus.). viii, 214p. 81.75 (*3-8055-2065-4*) S Karger.

Acute Cocaine Intoxication: Current Methods of Treatment. 1994. lib. bdg. 259.95 (*0-8490-9040-7*) Gordon Pr.

Acute Continuous Renal Replacement Therapy. Ed. by Emil P. Paganini. 1986. (Developments in Nephrology Ser.). (C). text 120.50 (*0-89838-793-0*) Kluwer Academic.

Acute Coronary Care, 1986. Ed. by Robert M. Califf & Galen S. Wagner. 1985. text 132.50 (*0-89838-762-0*) Kluwer Academic.

Acute Coronary Care, 1987. Ed. by Robert M. Califf & Galen S. Wagner. 1986. text 177.00 (*0-89838-842-2*) Kluwer Academic.

Acute Coronary Care in the Thrombolytic Era. Ed. by Robert M. Califf et al. 2nd ed. 1994. (Illus.). 984p. (C). (gr. 13). text 108.00 (*0-8016-6753-4*, 06753) Mosby Inc.

***Acute Coronary Ischemia & Myocardial Infarction.** Davies et al. 2003. (Fast Facts Ser.). (Illus.). pap. (*1-903734-00-2*) Health Pr GBR. *Dist:* JAMCO Dist.

Acute Coronary Syndromes. Eric J. Topol. 1998. LC 97-45853. (Illus.). 640p. text 99.75 (*0-8247-0140-2*) Dekker.

Acute Coronary Syndromes Monograph Series 2000: Unstable Angina - Non-Q-Wave Myocardial Infarction. International Cardiology Staff. 2000. (Illus.). 81p. pap. (*0-9665523-1-8*) Exeter Grp.

Acute Diseases, Pts. I-II: Their Uniform Treatment by Natural Methods: Mental, Emotional & Psychic Disorders. Henry Lindlarh. 1996. 54p. spiral bd. 9.00 (*0-7873-0562-6*) Hlth Research.

Acute Disorders of the Abdomen: Diagnosis & Treatment. V. Sreenivas. 1980. (Illus.). 200p. 60.00 (*0-387-90483-2*) Spr-Verlag.

Acute Drug Therapy. Barsan. 1999. text 59.00 (*0-7216-6517-9*) Saunders.

Acute Effects on Health of Smog Episodes. 1992. (WHO Regional Publications, European Ser.: No. 43). (ENG, FRE, GER & RUS.). 74p. pap. text 14.00 (*92-890-1306-0*, 1310043) World Health.

Acute Emergencies & Critical Care of the Geriatric Patient. Thomas T. Yoshikawa & Dean C. Norman. 2000. LC 00-22915. (Illus.). xiv, 519p. text 135.00 (*0-8247-0345-6*) Dekker.

Acute General Medicine: Self Assessment Workbook. Michael Clark & Parveen Kumar. 2000. 188p. pap. text 19.99 (*1-873207-07-7*) Buttrwrth-Heinemann.

Acute General Medicine, Brief learning materials: The Essentials. Michael Clark & Parveen Kumar. 2000. (Illus.). 512p. pap. text 44.99 (*1-873207-02-6*) Buttrwrth-Heinemann.

Acute Grief: Loss of an Adult Child, 8. Otto S. Margolis. 1988. LC 87-18315. 201p. 55.00 (*0-275-91304-X*, C1304, Praeger Pubs) Greenwood.

Acute Hand. Benisse Lester. 1998. LC 97-11816. 600p. text 85.00 (*0-8385-0258-X*, A-0258-2, Apple Lange Med) McGraw.

Acute Head Injury. Ruth Garner. Ed. by Jo Campling. 2nd ed. 1990. (Therapy in Practice Ser.: No. 13). 152p. pap. 33.95 (*0-412-32420-2*, A4419) Chapman & Hall.

Acute Heart Failure. Ed. by J. L. Vincent & Claude Perret. 1988. (Update in Intensive Care & Emergency Medicine Ser.: Vol. 6). (Illus.). 423p. 113.00 (*0-387-19169-0*) Spr-Verlag.

Acute Heart Failure in Intensive Care: A New Approach. Ed. by P. Foex & I. A. Davidson. 1990. (Journal: Vol. 77, Suppl. 3, 1990). (Illus.). iv, 68p. pap. 22.75 (*3-8055-5255-6*) S Karger.

Acute Hemorrhagic Conjunctivitis: Etiology, Epidemiology & Clinical Manifestations. Ed. by K. Ishii et al. 1989. (Illus.). xiv, 438p. 278.50 (*3-8055-4997-0*) S Karger.

Acute Leukemia: Approach to Diagnosis. Harold R. Schumacher. 1990. LC 89-24618. (Illus.). 312p. 78.00 (*0-89640-170-7*) Igaku-Shoin.

Acute Leukemia: Difficult, Controversial, Automated Diagnosis. Harold R. Schumacher. 1997. LC 97-34124. 170p. 51.95 (*0-683-30505-0*) Lppncott W & W.

Acute Leukemias: Biologic, Diagnostic & Therapeutic Determinants. Sanford A. Stass. 1987. (Hematology Ser.: Vol. 6). (Illus.). 496p. text 210.00 (*0-8247-7766-2*) Dekker.

Acute Leukemias - Pharmacokinetics: Pharmacokinetics & Management of Relapsed & Refractory Disease. Ed. by W. Hiddemann et al. 1992. (Illus.). 670p. 198.00 (*0-387-53949-2*) Spr-Verlag.

Acute Leukemias VIII: Prognostic Factors & Treatment Strategies. Ed. by T. Buechner et al. 2001. LC 00-46996. (Haematology & Blood Transfusion Ser.). (Illus.). 1200p. 225.00 (*3-540-41123-2*) Spr-Verlag.

Acute Leukemias 4: Prognostic Factors & Treatment Strategies. T. Buchner et al. 1996. LC 93-27989. (Haematology & Blood Transfusion Ser.: No. 36). (Illus.). 839p. 225.00 (*0-387-56951-0*) Spr-Verlag.

Acute Leukemias VII: Experimental Approaches & Novel Therapies. Ed. by W. Hiddemann et al. 1997. LC 97-31478. (Haematology & Blood Transfusion Ser.: Suppl. 39). (Illus.). 1198p. 289.00 (*3-540-63504-1*) Spr-Verlag.

Acute Leukemias V: Experimental Approaches & Management of Refractory Disease. Ed. by W. Hiddemann et al. 1995. (Haematology & Blood Transfusion Ser.: Vol. 37). (*3-540-57852-8*) Spr-Verlag.

Acute Leukemias VI: Prognostic Factors & Treatment Strategies - Haematology & Blood Transfusion (Hamatologie und Bluttransfusion), Suppl. 38. Ed. by T. Buchner et al. 1996. LC 97-120581. (Illus.). 784p. 236.00 (*3-540-60763-3*) Spr-Verlag.

Acute Liver Failure. Ed. by William M. Lee & Roger Williams. 1996. (Illus.). 296p. (C). text 120.00 (*0-521-55381-4*) Cambridge U Pr.

Acute Low Back Problems in Adults. 1995. lib. bdg. 260.00 (*0-8490-6846-0*) Gordon Pr.

Acute Lung Injury. Ed. by John J. Marini & Timothy W. Evans. 1997. LC 97-26537. (Update in Intensive Care & Emergency Medicine Ser.: Vol. 30). (Illus.). 463p. 112.00 (*3-540-62582-8*) Spr-Verlag.

Acute Management of Autonomic Disreflexia: Adults with Spinal Cord Injury Presenting to Health-Care Facilities. Consortium for Spinal Cord Medicine Staff. 1997. (Clinical Practice Guidelines Ser.). 18p. pap. (*0-929819-07-1*) Paralyzed Vets.

Acute Medical Emergencies. Ursula Guly & Drew Richardson. 1996. LC 95-45956. (Oxford Handbooks in Emergency Medicine Ser.: Vol. 14). (Illus.). 240p. text 79.50 (*0-19-262559-4*); 232p. pap. text 45.00 (*0-19-262558-6*) OUP.

***Acute Medical Emergencies: A Nursing Guide.** Richard Harrison. 2001. (Illus.). 320p. (*0-443-06422-9*) Church GBR. *Dist:* Saunders.

Acute Medical Emergencies: The Practical Approach. Ed. by Advanced Life Support Group Staff. 2001. (Illus.). 464p. pap. text (*0-7279-1464-2*) BMJ Pub GBR. *Dist:* AIDC.

Acute Medical Illness in Old Age. Ed. by Alan J. Sinclair & Ken W. Woodhouse. 1995. LC 94-74703. (Illus.). 304p. (C). (gr. 13). 131.95 (*0-412-56920-5*, Chap & Hall NY) Chapman & Hall.

Acute Medicine: A Practical Guide to the Management of Medical Emergencies. David Springings et al. 2nd ed. 1995. LC 94-3731. (Illus.). 448p. pap. 34.95 (*0-632-03652-4*) Blackwell Sci.

Acute Medicine: A Practical Guide to the Management of Medical Emergencies. David Sprigings & John Chambers. 3rd ed. 2001. LC 00-45449. (Illus.). ix, 518p. pap. 36.95 (*0-632-05455-7*) Blackwell Sci.

Acute Medicine Algorithms. Mervyn Singer & Andrew R. Webb. 1995. (Illus.). 182p. text 57.50 (*0-19-262460-1*); pap. text 37.50 (*0-19-262459-8*) OUP.

Acute Myocardial Infarction. Ed. by David McCall. 1992. (Contemporary Management in Internal Medicine Ser.: Vol. 2, No. 2). (Illus.). 213p. text (*0-443-08838-1*) Church.

Acute Myocardial Infarction. Bernard Gersh & Shahbudin H. Rahimtoola. 2nd ed. 1996. LC 96-16761. (Current Topics in Cardiology Ser.). (Illus.). 884p. (*0-412-07341-2*) E A GBR. *Dist:* OUP.

Acute Myocardial Infarction: Emerging Concepts of Pathogenesis & Treatment. Ed. by Robert H. Cox. 1989. LC 88-27576. 218p. 77.00 (*0-275-92438-6*, C2438, Praeger Pubs) Greenwood.

Acute Myocardial Infarction: Setting Priorities for Effectiveness Research. Institute of Medicine Staff. 1991. 72p. (C). pap. text 15.00 (*0-309-04380-8*) Natl Acad Pr.

***Acute Myocardial Infarction & Other Acute Ischemic Syndromes.** Robert M. Califf. 2nd ed. 2001. LC 00-69425. (Atlas of Heart Diseases Ser.). (Illus.). (*1-57340-159-5*) Current Med.

Acute Myocardial Infarction (Heart Attack) Robert C. Davidson & Denise Busman. Ed. by Oliver D. Grin & Dorothy L. Bouwman. 1992. (Patient Education Ser.). (Illus.). 30p. (Orig.). pap. text 4.00 (*0-929689-47-X*) Ludann Co.

Acute Neuroscience Nursing: Concepts & Care. Jane Lundgren. 1986. (Illus.). 400p. (C). text 59.95 (*0-86720-355-2*, 355-2) Jones & Bartlett.

Acute Non-Traumatic Intracranial Bleedings. B. P. Jensen et al. 1983. (Advances in Neurosurgery Ser.: Vol. 11). (Illus.). 405p. 94.00 (*0-387-12538-8*) Spr-Verlag.

Acute Obstetrics. Evan Wallace & Andrew Calder. 1997. (Illus.). 250p. (Orig.). pap. text 44.95 (*0-86542-941-3*) Blackwell Sci.

Acute Obstetrics: A Practical Guide. Martha C. Heppard & Thomas J. Garite. 2nd ed. 1996. LC 95-26682. (Illus.). 464p. (C). (gr. 13). pap. text 34.95 (*0-8151-4083-5*, 24640) Mosby Inc.

***Acute Paediatric Pain Management: A Practical Guide.** Ed. by Neil S. Morton. 1998. (Illus.). 296p. pap. (*0-7020-2219-5*) W B Saunders GBR. *Dist:* Saunders.

Acute Pain. Raymond S. Sinatra. 1992. 672p. 74.00 (*0-8016-7495-6*) Mosby Inc.

Acute Pain: Mechanisms & Management. Ed. by Raymond S. Sinatra et al. 1992. LC 92-8611. (Illus.). 656p. (C). (gr. 13). text 95.00 (*0-8016-4677-4*, 04677) Mosby Inc.

Acute Pain: Pathophysiology & Treatment. Jay B. Forrest. 1998. (Illus.). 256p. pap. 29.00 (*1-896918-03-4*) Manticore Pubs.

Acute Pain Management: Operative or Medical Procedure & Trauma. 1995. lib. bdg. 252.95 (*0-8490-6802-9*) Gordon Pr.

Acute Pain Management: Operative or Medical Procedures & Trauma. 1994. lib. bdg. 260.00 (*0-8490-9032-6*) Gordon Pr.

Acute Pain Management: Operative or Medical Procedures & Trauma Clinical Practice Guideline. Daniel B. Carr & Ada K. Jacox. 1997. (Illus.). 145p. (C). reprint ed. pap. text 30.00 (*0-7881-4611-4*) DIANE Pub.

Acute Pain Management in Infants, Children & Adolescents: Operative & Medical Procedures. 1994. lib. bdg. 250.00 (*0-8490-8541-1*) Gordon Pr.

Acute Pancreatitis. Markus Bucheler. 1998. 400p. 54.95 (*3-89412-376-1*) Blackwell Sci.

Acute Pancreatitis: Novel Concepts in Biology & Therapy. Ed. by M. W. Buchler. 1999. 497p. 78.95 (*0-632-05339-9*) Blackwell Sci.

Acute Pediatrics. Steven W. Ryan & Elizabeth Molyneux. 1996. (Illus.). 240p. pap. 49.95 (*0-86542-624-4*) Blackwell Sci.

Acute Perinatal Asphyxia in Term Infants: Report of the Workshop. Ed. by Linda L. Wright et al. 1997. (Illus.). 206p. (Orig.). (C). pap. text 40.00 (*0-7881-4544-4*) DIANE Pub.

Acute Peripheral Vascular Surgery. M. Staudacher. enl. rev. ed. 1985. LC 85-17328.Tr. of Akute Periphere GefaBchirurgie. (Illus.). 170p. 74.00 (*0-387-81874-X*) Spr-Verlag.

Acute Phase of Ischemic Heart Disease & Myocardial Infarction. A. J. Adgey. 1982. text 162.50 (*90-247-2675-1*) Kluwer Academic.

Acute Phase Proteins in the Acute Phase Response. Ed. by M. B. Pepys. 1989. (Argenteuil Symposia Ser.). (Illus.). 210p. 118.00 (*0-387-19582-3*, 3483) Spr-Verlag.

Acute Psychiatric Care: An Occupational Therapy Guide to Exercises in Daily Living Skills. Patricia L. Simmons & Linda Mullins. 1991. LC 80-54633. 166p. reprint ed. pap. 26.00 (*1-55642-210-5*, 30186) SLACK Inc.

***Acute Psychosis, Schizophrenia & Comorbid Disorders Vol. 1: Recent Topics from Advances in Psychiatric Treatment.** Ed. by Alan Lee. 1998. 152p. pap. (*1-901242-16-1*) Royal Coll Psych GBR. *Dist:* Balogh.

Acute Pulmonary Embolism: A Challenge for Hemostasiology. A. Geibel et al. 2000. 260p. (C). (*3-7985-1167-5*) D Steinkopff DEU. *Dist:* Spr-Verlag.

Acute Pulmonary Insufficiency: The Role of Haemostatic, Fibrinolytic & Related Mechanisms. Ed. by Tom Saldeen. 1985. (Illus.). viii, 147p. pap. 75.40 (*3-11-010567-5*) De Gruyter.

Acute Renal Disorders & Renal Emergencies. Ed. by Jose Strauss. 1984. (Developments in Nephrology Ser.). text 132.50 (*0-89838-663-2*) Kluwer Academic.

Acute Renal Failure. Ed. by Vittorio E. Andreucci. 1984. text 266.00 (*0-89838-627-6*) Kluwer Academic.

Acute Renal Failure. Barry M. Brenner & J. Michael Lazarus. 1983. (Illus.). 837p. text 179.00 (*0-7216-1964-9*) Saunders.

Acute Renal Failure. Ed. by U. Gessler & David Seybold. 1982. (Illus.). viii, 268p. pap. 35.75 (*3-8055-3579-1*) S Karger.

Acute Renal Failure: New Concepts & Therapeutic Strategies. Ed. by Michael S. Goligorsky. 1995. LC 95-9523. (Contemporary Issues in Nephrology Ser.: Vol. 31). text (*0-443-07580-8*) Church.

Acute Renal Failure in the Critically Ill. Ed. by R. Bellomo & C. Ronco. 1995. LC 94-42307. (Update in Intensive Care & Emergency Medicine Ser.: Vol. 20). (Illus.). 438p. 135.00 (*3-540-58401-3*) Spr-Verlag.

Acute Renal Insufficiency Made Ridiculously Simple. Carlos Rotellar. 1999. (Illus.). 56p. pap. text 12.95 (*0-940780-09-7*) MedMaster.

Acute Respiratory Care of the Neonate. Debbie F. Askin. 2nd rev. ed. 1997. LC 97-17399. (Illus.). 200p. pap. text 24.95 (*1-887571-01-9*) NICU Ink.

Acute Respiratory Distress Syndrome: A Comprehensive Clinical Approach. Ed. by James A. Russell & Keith R. Walley. 1999. LC 98-46408. (Illus.). 368p. (C). pap. text 49.95 (*0-521-65410-6*) Cambridge U Pr.

Acute Respiratory Distress Syndrome: Cellular & Molecular Mechanisms & Clinical Management. Ed. by Sadis Matalon & Jacob I. Sznajder. 1998. LC 98-17227. (NATO Advanced Science Institutes Ser.: No. 297). (Illus.). 448p. (C). text 129.50 (*0-306-45830-6*, Kluwer Plenum) Kluwer Academic.

Acute Respiratory Failure. Ed. by Roger C. Bone et al. 1987. (Illus.). 473p. (*0-443-08366-5*) Church.

Acute Respiratory Failure in Chronic Obstructive Pulmonary Disease. Ed. by Jean-Philippe Derenne et al. 1996. LC 96-2512. (Lung Biology in Health & Disease Ser.: No. 92). (Illus.). 952p. text 275.00 (*0-8247-9487-7*) Dekker.

Acute Rheumatic & Immunological Disease: Management of the Critically Ill Patient. Ed. by Brain F. Mandell. 1994. (Infectious Disease & Therapy Ser.). (Illus.). 640p. text 250.00 (*0-8247-9125-8*) Dekker.

Acute Stroke Therapy: Optimal Care of the Stroke Patient: Plenary Session to the 3rd World Stroke Congress & the 5th European Stroke Conference, Munich, September, 1996. Ed. by Nils G. Wahlgren & Takenori Yamaguchi. 1997. (Cerebrovascular Diseases Ser.: Vol. 7, Suppl. 3, 1997). (Illus.). iv, 30p. pap. 21.75 (*3-8055-6478-3*) S Karger.

Acute Stroke Treatment. Julien Bogousslavsky. 1997. 328p. (*1-85317-413-0*) Martin Dunitz GBR. *Dist:* Mosby Inc.

Acute Toxicities of Organic Chemicals to Fathead Minnows (Pimephales promelas) Ed. by N. J. Chinoy. 1984. (Advances in Agricultural Biotechnology Ser.). text 160.50 (*90-247-2908-4*) Kluwer Academic.

Acute Toxicities of Organic Chemicals to Fathead Minnows (Pimephales promelas), Vol. 1. Ed. by L. T. Brooke et al. 1984. LC 85-116909. (Toxicity of Organic Chemicals Ser.). (Illus.). 414p. (Orig.). pap. 75.00 (*0-9614968-0-0*) Lke Superior Res.

Acute Toxicity Testing. Ed. by Alan M. Goldberg. 1984. (Alternative Methods in Toxicology Ser.: Vol. 2). 292p. text 185.00 (*0-913113-03-4*) M Liebert.

Acute Toxicology Testing: Perspectives & Horizons. Shayne C. Gad & Christopher P. Chengelis. 1988. (Illus.). 530p. lib. bdg. 89.95 (*0-936923-06-7*) Telford Pr.

Acute Virus Infections of Poultry. Ed. by J. B. McFerran & M. S. McNulty. 1986. (Current Topics in Veterinary Medicine & Animal Science Ser.). text 175.00 (*0-89838-809-0*) Kluwer Academic.

Acutely Traumatized Small Animal Patient. Timothy H. Brasmer. 1984. (Major Problems in Veterinary Medicine Ser.: Vol. 2). (Illus.). 192p. text 69.00 (*0-7216-1917-7*) Saunders.

Acyclische Kohlenwasserstoffe, Hydroxy-Verbindungen und Oxo-Verbindungen. Beilstein Institut fur Literatur der Organischen Chemie. 1975. (Beilstein's Handbuch der Organischen Chemie Ser.: Vol. 1, Pt. 6). 569p. 695.00 (*0-387-07221-7*) Spr-Verlag.

Acyclische Verbindungen. Beilstein Institut fur Literatur der Organischen Chemie. Ed. by H. G. Boit. 1975. LC 72-95756. (Beilstein's Handbuch der Organischen Chemie Ser.: Vol. 2, Pt. 1). 692p. 795.00 (*0-387-07311-6*) Spr-Verlag.

Acyclovir Therapy for Herpes Virus Infections. Ed. by David A. Baker. 1989. (Infectious Disease & Therapy Ser.: Vol. 4). (Illus.). 344p. text 165.00 (*0-8247-8091-4*) Dekker.

***ADA Complete Guide to Carb Counting.** Hope S. Warshaw & Karmen Kulkarni. 2001. LC 2001-22562. (Illus.). 256p. pap. 16.95 (*1-58040-046-9*) Am Diabetes.

ADA Guide to Dental Therapeutics. Sebastian G. Ciancio. 1998. LC 98-194771. (Illus.). 600p. pap. text 59.00 (*1-891748-00-9*) ADA Publng.

Adalat: A Comprehensive Review. Ed. by P. R. Lichtlen & A. Reale. 1991. (Illus.). 248p. 62.95 (*0-387-54033-4*) Spr-Verlag.

***A.D.A.M. Interactive Anatomy: Student Lab Guide.** Mark Lafferty & Samuel Panella. 2nd ed. 2001. LC 2001-17329. (Illus.). 250p. 26.60 (*0-8053-5049-7*) Benjamin-Cummings.

Adam Principle: Genes, Genitals, Hormones & Gender - Selected Readings in Sexology. John Money. 1993. LC 93-1384. (New Concepts in Human Sexuality Ser.). 364p. (C). 51.00 (*0-87975-804-X*) Prometheus Bks.

***Adams & Victor's Manual of Neurology.** Maurice Victor & Allan H. Ropper. 7th ed. 2001. 570p. pap. 39.95 (*0-07-137351-9*) McGraw-Hill Prof.

Adams & Victor's Principles of Neurology. Maurice Victor & Allan H. Ropper. 7th ed. 2000. LC 00-52688. (Illus.). 1692p. text 89.95 (*0-07-067497-3*) McGraw-Hill Prof.

***Adams & Victor's Principles of Neurology.** Maurice Victor et al. 7th ed. 2001. LC 00-52688. (Illus.). xi, 1692p. (*0-07-116333-6*) McGraw-Hill Med Pub.

Adams' Heart Disease in Infants, Children, & Adolescents see Moss & Adams' Heart Disease in Infants, Children & Adolescents: Including the Fetus & Young Adult

Adams' Lameness in Horses. Ed. by Ted S. Stashak. 4th ed. 1987. LC 85-5787. (Illus.). 906p. text 105.00 (*0-8121-0980-5*) Lppncott W & W.

Adams' Lameness in Horses. O. R. Adams. 5th ed. 1998. LC 98-7679. 1,008p. text 110.00 (*0-683-07981-6*) Lppncott W & W.

Adaptability in Somatic Cell Specialization, set. M. A. DiBerardino & L. D. Etkin. 1989. LC 85-3406. (Developmental Biology Ser.). (Illus.). 256p. (C). text 85.00 (*0-306-43177-7*, Kluwer Plenum) Kluwer Academic.

Adaptability of Human Gait: Implications for the Control of Locomotion. Ed. by Aftab E. Patla. 1991. (Advances in Psychology Ser.: No. 78). 456p. 181.00 (*0-444-88364-9*, North Holland) Elsevier.

***Adaptable Brain Vol. II: Decade of the Brain.** Ed. by Sherry Levy-Reiner. 2001. 84p. (C). reprint ed. pap. 25.00 (*0-7567-0995-4*) DIANE Pub.

Adaptation & Human Behavior: An Anthropological Perspective. Ed. by Lee Cronk et al. 2000. LC 99-26821. (Evolutionary Foundations of Human Behavior Ser.). xv, 512p. lib. bdg. 69.95 (*0-202-02043-6*) Aldine de Gruyter.

Adaptation & Intelligence: Organic Selection & Phenocopy. Jean Piaget. Tr. by Steward Eames. LC 79-25592. vi, 124p. (C). 1997. pap. text 8.95 (*0-226-66778-2*); 1980. 11.00 (*0-226-66777-4*) U Ch Pr.

Adaptation & Natural Selection: A Critique of Some Current Evolutionary Thought. George C. Williams. 1974. 320p. pap. 19.95 (*0-691-02357-3*) Princeton U Pr.

Adaptation Nursing: Assessment & Intervention. Beverly J. Rambo. 1984. (Illus.). tchr. ed. (*0-7216-2031-0*); 432p. pap. text 52.00 (*0-7216-1048-X*) Saunders.

Adaptation to Changing Health: Response Shift in Quality-of-Life Research. Ed. by Carolyn E. Schwartz & Mirjam A. G. Sprangers. 2000. LC 00-25296. 264p. 39.95 (*1-55798-710-6*, 431-8950) Am Psychol.

Adaptation to Chronic Childhood Illness. Robert J. Thompson, Jr. & Kathryn E. Gustafson. 1995. LC 95-42008. 382p. pap. 29.95 (*1-55798-619-3*) Am Psychol.

Adaptation to Loss Through Short-Term Group Psychotherapy. William E. Piper et al. 1992. LC 92-1424. 219p. 40.00 (*0-89862-796-6*) Guilford Pubns.

Adaptation to Malaria: The Interaction of Biology & Culture. Ed. by Lawrence S. Greene & Maria E. Danubio. 1998. 336p. text (*90-5700-504-2*) GBSP NLD. *Dist:* Gordon & Breach.

Adaptational Psychodynamics. Ed. by Sandor Rado et al. 1995. LC 70-82528. (Master Work Ser.). 306p. reprint ed. pap. 45.00 (*1-56821-505-3*) Aronson.

Adaptations to Salinity & Dehydration. Ed. by R. Kirsch & B. Lahlou. 1987. (Comparative Physiology of Environmental Adaptations Ser.: Pt. I). (Illus.). viii, 204p. 155.00 (*3-8055-4470-7*) S Karger.

Adapted Aquatics Programming: A Professional Guide. Monica Lepore et al. 1998. LC 98-22953. (Illus.). 328p. text 42.00 (*0-88011-695-1*, BLEP0695) Human Kinetics.

Adapted Physical Activity: Health & Fitness. International Symposium on Adapted Physical Activity Staff. Ed. by K. Yabe et al. 1995. LC 94-31606. 133.00 (*0-387-70143-5*) Spr-Verlag.

Adapted Physical Education for Students with Autism. Kimberly Davis. 1990. (Illus.). 142p. (C). text 38.95 (*0-398-05688-9*) C C Thomas.

Adapted Physical Education in the Mainstream. Bryant J. Cratty. 2nd ed. 1989. LC 86-82896. (Illus.). 574p. text 48.00 (*0-89108-130-5*, 8826) Love Pub Co.

Adapting Activities for Therapeutic Recreation Service: Concepts & Applications. Jesse T. Dixon. 1981. (Illus.). 100p. (Orig.). pap. 14.50 (*0-916304-48-5*) SDSU Press.

Adapting to Life Threatening Illness. Andrew E. Slaby & Arvin S. Glicksman. 1985. LC 85-6421. 246p. 72.50 (*0-275-91324-4*, C1324, Praeger Pubs) Greenwood.

Adaptive Design of the Human Psyche: Psychoanalysis, Evolutionary Biology & the Therapeutic Process. Malcolm O. Slavin & Daniel Kriegman. 1992. LC 92-49856. 336p. 48.00 (*0-89862-795-8*) Guilford Pubns.

A B

***Adaptive Dynamics of Infectious Diseases.** U. Dieckmann et al. 2001. (Studies in Adaptive Dynamics). 500p. text 69.95 (*0-521-78165-5*) Cambridge U Pr.

Adaptive Language Disorders of Young Adults with Learning Disabilities. Carol Weller et al. 1992. LC 92-16006. (Illus.). 238p. (Orig.). (C). pap. text 39.95 (*1-879105-82-9*, 0345) Thomson Learn.

Adaptive Play for Special Needs Children: Strategies to Enhance Communication & Learning. Caroline R. Musselwhite. 1986. LC 90-52761. (Illus.). 249p. (C). pap. text 29.00 (*0-89079-303-4*, 1751) PRO-ED.

Adaptive Protection of the Heart: Protecting Against Stress & Ischemic Damage. Felix Z. Meerson. 1990. (Illus.). 312p. 139.00 (*0-8493-5150-2*, QP114) CRC Pr.

Adaptive User Support: Ergonomic Design of Manually & Automatically Adaptable Software. Ed. by Reinhard Oppermann. 1994. LC 94-21630. (Computers, Cognition, & Work Ser.). 272p. text 49.95 (*0-8058-1655-0*) L Erlbaum Assocs.

Adaptors & Innovators: Styles of Creativity & Problem-Solving. Ed. by Michael J. Kirton. 1989. 304p. 65.00 (*0-415-02424-2*) Routledge.

ADD: The Facts, the Fables, Hope for Your Family. Theresa Lamson. 1996. LC 96-60585. 208p. pap. 11.99 (*1-56384-121-5*, Vital Issue Pr) Huntington Hse.

***ADD & ADHD.** Judith Peacock. 2000. LC 00-12936. (Perspectives on Mental Health Ser.). (J). (gr. 5-12). lib. bdg. 23.93 (*0-7368-1029-3*, LifeMatters Bks) Capstone Pr.

ADD Brain: Diagnosis, Treatment & Science of Attention Deficit Disorder (ADD/ADHD) Monroe A. Gross. 1997. LC 97-182572. (Illus.). 207p. lib. bdg. 39.00 (*1-56072-436-6*) Nova Sci Pubs.

ADD Brain: Diagnosis, Treatment & Science of Attention Deficit Disorder (ADD/ADHD) in Adults, Teenagers & Children. Monroe A. Gross. 1997. 210p. (Orig.). pap. 18.95 (*1-56072-430-7*, Nova Kroshka Bks) Nova Sci Pubs.

ADD Children: A Handbook for Parents. John N. Blair. 1999. (Illus.). xii, 154p. pap. 12.95 (*0-9674306-0-7*) JB Enterp.

ADD Hyperactivity Handbook for Schools: Effective Strategies for Identifying & Teaching ADD Students in Elementary & Secondary Schools. Harvey C. Parker. 1992. (Illus.). 330p. pap. 29.00 (*0-9621629-2-2*) Spec Pr FL.

ADD in the Workplace: Choices, Changes, & Challenges. Kathleen G. Nadeau. 1997. LC 97-1312. (Illus.). 248p. pap. 23.95 (*0-87630-847-7*) Brunner-Routledge.

A.D.D. Quest for Identity: Inside the Mind of Attention Deficit Disorder. George H. Green. 4th ed. 1999. 195p. pap. 13.95 (*1-890669-01-6*, ADQ) Biofeedback Ctr.

ADD Success Stories: A Guide to Fulfillment for Families with Attention Deficit Disorder. Thom Hartmann. 1995. 228p. 24.95 (*1-887424-04-0*); 276p. pap. 11.95 (*1-887424-03-2*) Underwood Bks.

ADD/ADHD Behavior-Change Resource Kit: Ready-to-Use Strategies & Activities for Helping Children with Attention Deficit Disorder. Grad L. Flick. 1997. LC 97-42870. (Ready-To-Use Ser.). 392p. pap., tchr. ed. 29.95 (*0-87628-144-7*) Ctr Appl Res.

ADD/ADHD Checklist: An Easy Reference for Parents & Teachers. Sandra F. Rief. 1997. LC 97-37991. 272p. (C). pap. 11.95 (*0-13-762395-X*) P-H.

Added Dimension. Kate Kelly & Peggy Ramundo. 1997. LC 97-13536. 192p. 20.00 (*0-684-83224-0*) S&S Trade.

Added Value of Geographical Information Systems in Public & Environmental Health. Ed. by Marion J. De Lepper. 1995. (Geojournal Library). 370p. (C). lib. bdg. 169.00 (*0-7923-1887-0*) Kluwer Academic.

Addict Aftercare: Recovery Training & Self-Help. 1986. lib. bdg. 250.00 (*0-8490-3502-3*) Gordon Pr.

Addicted. Joan Morrone. 1986. LC 85-82145. 125p. (Orig.). pap. 6.00 (*0-9616771-0-4*) J & R Pub.

Addicted? A Guide to Understanding Addiction. Tom O'Connell. 1990. LC 90-91803. 204p. (Orig.). pap. text 19.00 (*0-9620318-0-1*) Sanctuary Unltd.

Addicted, in Their Own Words: Kids Talking about Drugs. Joel Engel. 1990. mass mkt. 3.95 (*0-8125-9446-0*, Tor Books) T Doherty Assocs.

Addicted to Love: Facts about Sexual Addictions. Jennifer James. rev. ed. 1999. pap. 0.50 (*0-89230-223-2*) Do It Now.

Addicted to Suicide: A Woman Struggling to Live. Mary Savage. 1979. LC 79-4695. 144p. pap. text 14.95 (*0-87073-907-7*) Schenkman Bks Inc.

Addiction. Deepak Chopra. 1997. pap. (*0-609-80077-9*) Harmony Bks.

Addiction: Entries & Exits. Ed. by Jon Elster. 1999. LC 99-31479. (Illus.). xx, 310p. 39.95 (*0-87154-235-8*) Russell Sage.

Addiction: The High-Low Trap. Irving Cohen. 1995. pap. 13.95 (*0-929173-10-4*) Health Press.

Addiction & Antisocial Behavior Process Prevention Education Counseling System. Arthur J. Stovall. 1997. (Illus.). 106p. tchr. ed., ring bd. 20.00 (*0-9660855-0-7*) Prevention Educ.

Addiction & Co-Dependency: HP 605. Eberhart. 1989. 49p. (C). stu. ed. (*0-933195-60-5*) CA College Health Sci.

Addiction & Pregnancy: Empowering Recovery Through Peer Counseling. Ed. by Barry R. Sherman & Laura M. Sanders. 1998. LC 98-21641. 216p. 72.50 (*0-275-95976-7*, Praeger Pubs) Greenwood.

Addiction & Recovery of Gay & Lesbian Persons. Ed. by Robert J. Kus. 1995. 97p. 34.95 (*1-56024-668-5*); LC 95-1683. 118p. pap. 9.95 (*1-56023-055-X*, Harrington Park) Haworth Pr.

Addiction & Sigmund Freud: Freud's Psychology Applied to Addiction. Dan Rivers. 1995. LC 94-79564. 350p. (Orig.). pap. 29.95 (*0-9644355-2-7*) Mercie Pub.

Addiction & the Vulnerable Self: Modified Dynamic Group Therapy for Substance Abusers. Edward J. Khantzian et al. 1990. LC 90-3821. (Substance Abuse Ser.). 176p. 30.00 (*0-89862-172-0*) Guilford Pubns.

Addiction Concept: Working Hypothesis or Self-Fulfilling Prophecy? Glenn D. Walters. 1998. LC 98-23863. 273p. (C). pap. text 67.00 (*0-205-28642-9*) Allyn.

Addiction Counselor. Jack Rudman. 1994. (Career Examination Ser.: C-2150). pap. 29.95 (*0-8373-2150-6*) Nat Learn.

Addiction-Free Pain Management. Stephen Grinstead & Terence T. Gorski. 1997. 72p. pap. 9.00 (*0-8309-0786-6*) Herald Pub Hse.

Addiction-Free Pain Management: Professional Guide: An Exiciting New Approach to Managing Pain Disorders for Those Who Suffer from Addictive Disorders. Stephen F. Grinstead & Terence T. Gorski. 1999. LC 00-502224. 204p. (*0-8309-0840-4*) Herald Pub Hse.

Addiction in America Series Ed. by Gerald N. Grob et al. 1981. 1419.00 (*0-405-13555-6*) Ayer.

Addiction in Human Development: Developmental Perspectives on Addiction & Recovery. Jacqueline Wallen. 1993. LC 91-32981. (Illus.). 176p. lib. bdg. 49.95 (*1-56024-246-9*); 170p. pap. 14.95 (*1-56024-247-7*) Haworth Pr.

Addiction Intervention: Strategies to Motivate Treatment-Seeking Behavior. Ed. by Robert K. White & Deborah G. Wright. 1998. LC 97-37000. (Haworth Addictions Treatment Ser.). (Illus.). 154p. 29.95 (*0-7890-0433-X*); pap. 19.95 (*0-7890-0434-8*) Haworth Pr.

Addiction Nursing. Hussein Rassool. 1997. (Illus.). 240p. (Orig.). pap. 39.95 (*1-56593-824-0*, 1618) Singular Publishing.

Addiction Potential of Abused Drugs & Drug Classes. Carlton K. Erickson et al. 1994. LC 90-4639. (Advances in Alcohol & Substance Abuse Ser.: Vol. 9, Nos. 1 & 2). 201p. text 39.95 (*0-86656-975-8*) Haworth Pr.

Addiction Psychiatry: Current Diagnosis & Treatment. Norman S. Miller. 1995. LC 94-32386. 300p. 92.50 (*0-471-56201-7*) Wiley.

Addiction Reform in the Progressive Age: Scientific & Social Responses to Drug Dependence in the United States 1870 to 1930. Arnold Jaffe. Ed. by Gerald N. Grob. 1981. LC 80-1269. (Addiction in America Ser.). (Illus.). lib. bdg. 37.95 (*0-405-13556-4*) Ayer.

Addiction Specialist. Jack Rudman. 1994. (Career Examination Ser.: C-1075). pap. 29.95 (*0-8373-1075-X*) Nat Learn.

Addiction, Stress & Amino Acid Deficiencies. 1996. lib. bdg. 250.95 (*0-8490-5886-4*) Gordon Pr.

Addiction Treatment: Avoiding Pitfalls—A Case Approach. Group for the Advancement of Psychiatry Staff. 1998. LC 97-48628. (Group for the Advancement of Psychiatry Ser.: Vol. 142). 272p. text 38.00 (*0-87318-210-3*, 7210) Am Psychiatric.

Addiction Treatment: Theory & Practice. Sandra Rasmusser. 2000. LC 00-8183. xii, 435p. 69.95 (*0-7619-0842-0*, 81291) Sage.

Addiction Workbook: A Step-By-Step Guide to Quitting Alcohol & Drugs. Patrick Fanning & John O'Neill. 1996. LC 97-162432. (Workbooks Ser.). 160p. pap. 17.95 (*1-57224-043-1*) New Harbinger.

Addictionary: A Primer of Recovery Terms & Concepts from Abstinence to Withdrawal. Jan R. Wilson & Judith A. Wilson. 1992. 410p. pap. 14.95 (*1-56838-116-6*) Hazelden.

Addictions: A Nutritional Approach to Recovery. John Finnegan. 1989. 144p. (Orig.). pap. 10.00 (*0-927425-05-X*) Elysian Arts.

Addictions: Concepts & Strategies for Treatment. Ed. by Judith A. Lewis. 1990. LC 94-9159. 414p. 68.00 (*0-8342-0563-7*) PRO-ED.

Addictions: Multidisciplinary Perspectives & Treatments. Ed. by Harvey B. Milkman & Howard J. Shaffer. 1984. LC 84-47871. 204p. 39.95 (*0-669-08739-4*) Lxngtn Bks.

Addictions: Personal Influences & Scientific Movement. Griffith Edwards. 1991. 384p. (C). text 49.95 (*0-88738-343-2*) Transaction Pubs.

Addictions & Substance Abuse: Strategies for Advanced Practice Nursing. Carolyn E. D'Avanzo & Madeline Naegle. 2000. LC 00-29857. 400p. (C). pap. 50.00 (*0-8385-8676-7*) P-H.

Addictions & Trauma Recovery. Dusty Miller. 2001. LC 2001-30353. (Professional Book Ser.). (Illus.). 240p. pap. 25.00 (*0-393-70368-1*) Norton.

Addictions Curriculum for Nurses & Other Helping Professionals, Vol. 1: The Undergraduate Level. Ed. by Elizabeth M. Burns et al. 1993. LC 93-18559. (Teaching of Nursing Ser.: Vol. 14). 288p. 46.95 (*0-8261-8190-2*) Springer Pub.

Addictions Curriculum for Nurses & Other Helping Professionals, Vol. 2: The Graduate Level - Advanced Knowledge & Practice. Ed. by Elizabeth M. Burns et al. 1993. LC 93-18559. (Teaching of Nursing Ser.: Vol. 15). 392p. pap. 49.95 (*0-8261-8191-0*) Springer Pub.

Addictions in the Gay & Lesbian Community. Ed. by Jeffrey R. Guss & Jack Drescher. 2000. LC 00-46152. 191p. text 70.00 (*0-7890-1037-2*); pap. text 24.95 (*0-7890-1038-0*) Haworth Pr (Hawrth Medical).

Addictions Treatment for Older Adults: Evaluation of an Innovative Client-Centered Approach. Kathryn Graham et al. 1995. LC 93-29334. (Illus.). 244p. text 49.95 (*1-56024-856-4*); 245p. pap. 19.95 (*1-56024-857-2*) Haworth Pr.

Addictive Behaviors. Ed. by Howard J. Shaffer. 1984. LC 83-18619. (Advances in Alcohol & Substance Abuse Ser.: Vol. 3, Nos. 1 & 2). 172p. text 44.95 (*0-86656-243-5*) Haworth Pr.

Addictive Behaviors: Prevention & Early Intervention. T. Loberg. 1989. 304p. (*90-265-0934-0*) Swets.

Addictive Behaviors: Readings on Etiology, Prevention, & Treatment. Ed. by G. Alan Marlatt & Gary R. VandenBos. 1997. LC 97-37315. 930p. pap. 39.95 (*1-55798-468-9*) Am Psychol.

Addictive Behaviors in Women. Ed. by Ronald R. Watson. 1994. LC 93-48458. (Drug & Alcohol Abuse Reviews Ser.: Vol. 5). (Illus.). 536p. text 99.50 (*0-89603-257-4*) Humana.

Addictive Behaviour: Cue Exposure Theory & Practice. Ed. by D. Colin Drummond et al. 1995. LC 94-23956. (Clinical Psychology & Personality Ser.). 268p. 175.00 (*0-471-94454-8*) Wiley.

Addictive Disease: A Basic Primer on America's #1 Health Problems. D. R. Blanks. Ed. by Thomas Chapman. 1999. 180p. pap. (*0-7392-0249-9*, PO3303) Morris Pubng.

Addictive Disorders. E. Fleming. 1994. (SPA.). (gr. 13). text 44.00 (*84-8086-066-9*) Mosby Inc.

Addictive Disorders in Arctic Climates: Theory, Research & Practice at the Novosibirsk Institute. Bernard Segal & Caesar Korolenko. 1991. LC 90-4611. (Drugs & Society Ser.: Vol. 4, Nos. 3-4). 125p. text 3.95 (*1-56024-036-9*) Haworth Pr.

Addictive Disorders Update: Alcoholism, Drug Abuse, Gambling. Stanley F. Yolles. Ed. by Pasquale A. Carone et al. 1982. LC 81-6880. (Problems of Industrial Psychiatric Medicine Ser.: Vol. 7). 192p. 35.95 (*0-89885-034-7*, Kluwer Acad Hman Sci) Kluwer Academic.

Addictive Organization: Why We Overwork, Cover up, Pick up the Pieces, Please the Boss, & Perpetuate Sick Organizations. Anne W. Schaef & Diane Fassel. 1990. LC 87-45720. 240p. pap. 15.00 (*0-06-254874-3*) Harper SF.

Addictive Personality: Understanding Compulsion in Our Lives. Craig Nakken. 1988. LC 88-45140. 128p. (Orig.). pap. 12.00 (*0-06-255488-3*) Harper SF.

Addictive Thinking: Understanding Self-Deception. 1990. LC 89-84785. pap. 12.00 (*0-06-255397-6*) Harper SF.

Addictive Thinking: Understanding Self-Deception. Abraham J. Twerski. 1997. LC 97-1857. 140p. pap. 11.95 (*1-56838-138-7*) Hazelden.

Adding Value to Long-Term Care: An Administrator's Guide to Improving Staff Performance, Patient Care. Dianne Lazer. 2000. LC 00-35740. (Illus.). 384p. pap. 75.00 (*0-7879-5170-6*) Jossey-Bass.

Addison Wesley Manual of Nursing Practice. Delores F. Saxton et al. 1983. text 27.96 (*0-201-07145-2*, Health Sci) Addison-Wesley.

Addison-Wesley Photo-Atlas of Nursing Procedures. Pamela L. Swearingen. 3rd ed. 1995. LC 95-40797. (Illus.). 628p. (C). pap. text 67.00 (*0-8053-8789-7*) Benjamin-Cummings.

Addison-Wesley's Nursing Examination. Sally L. Lagerquist. 2nd ed. 1982. pap. 26.50 (*0-201-14190-6*, Health Sci) Addison-Wesley.

Additional Protocol to the Agreement on the Temporary Importation, Free of Duty, of Medical, Surgical & Laboratory Equipment for Use on Free Loan in Hospitals & Other Medical Institutions for Purposes of Diagnosis or Treatment. Council of Europe Staff. 1983. (Conventions & Agreements Ser.: No. 110). (ENG & FRE.). (*92-871-0195-7*) Council of Europe FRA. *Dist:* Manhattan Pub Co.

Additional Protocol to the European Agreement on the Exchange of Tissue-Typing Reagents. Council of Europe Staff. 1976. (Conventions & Agreements Ser.: No. 89). (ENG & FRE.). (*92-871-0135-3*) Council of Europe FRA. *Dist:* Manhattan Pub Co.

Additional Protocol to the European Agreement on the Exchanges of Blood-Grouping Regeants. Council of Europe Staff. 1983. (Conventions & Agreements Ser.: No. 111). (ENG & FRE.). (*92-871-0196-5*) Council of Europe FRA. *Dist:* Manhattan Pub Co.

Additives to Blood Collection Devices: Heparin: Tentative Standard (1988), Vol. 8. National Committee for Clinical Laboratory Standards. rev. ed. 1988. 75.00 (*1-56238-053-2*, H24-T) NCCLS.

Additives to Blood Collective Devices: EDTA; Tentative Guideline (1992) Contrib. by Erwin Coyne. 1992. 75.00 (*1-56238-162-8*, H35-T) NCCLS.

Addressing Staffing Needs for Patient Care: Solutions for Hospital Leaders. Joint Commisson on Accreditation of Healthcare Organizations. 1998. LC 97-76553. (Illus.). 195p. 40.00 (*0-86688-521-8*, PC-100) Joint Comm Hlthcare.

Adenomatous Polyps of the Colon. R. Lev. 1989. (Illus.). 136p. 96.00 (*0-387-96985-3*, 2730) Spr-Verlag.

Adenosine & Adenine Nucleotides: From Molecular Biology to Integrative Physiology. International Symposium on Adrenosine and Adenine Staff. Ed. by Luiz Belardinelli et al. 1995. LC 94-40345. 576p. (C). text 333.00 (*0-7923-3190-7*) Kluwer Academic.

Adenosine & Adenine Nucleotides as Regulators of Cellular Function. John W. Phillis. 1991. (Illus.). 456p. 250.00 (*0-8493-6928-2*, QP625) CRC Pr.

Adenosine & Adenosine Receptors. Ed. by Michael Williams. 1990. LC 90-4000. (Receptors Ser.). (Illus.). 528p. 145.00 (*0-89603-163-2*) Humana.

Adenosine, Cardioprotection, & Its Clinical Application. Robert M. Mentzer. 1997. LC 97-14689. (Developments in Cardiovascular Medicine Ser.). 256p. text 55.00 (*0-7923-9954-4*) Kluwer Academic.

Adenosine in the Nervous System. Ed. by Trevor W. Stone. 1991. (Neuroscience Perspectives Ser.). (Illus.). 296p. text 78.00 (*0-12-672640-X*) Acad Pr.

Adenovirus Methods & Protocols. William S. M. Wold. 1998. LC 98-29395. (Methods in Molecular Medicine Ser.: Vol. 21). (Illus.). 368p. 99.50 (*0-89603-551-4*) Humana.

***Adenovirus Vector Systems Permitting Regulated Protein Expression & Their Use for "in vivo" Splicing Studies.** Magnus Molin. 2001. (Comprehensive Summaries of Uppsala Dissertations from the Faculty of Medicine Ser.: No. 994). (Illus.). 64p. pap. (*91-554-4926-3*) Uppsala Universitet SWE. *Dist:* Coronet Bks.

Adenoviruses. Ed. by Harold S. Ginsberg. 1984. LC 84-8264. (Viruses Ser.). (Illus.). 622p. (C). text 135.00 (*0-306-41592-5*, Kluwer Plenum) Kluwer Academic.

Adequacy of Access to Investigative Drugs for Seriously Ill Patients: Hearing Before the Subcommittee on Oversight & Investigations of the Committee on Commerce, House of Representatives, One Hundred Fifth Congress, First Session, September 23, 1997. U. S. Government Staff. 1997. LC 98-133492. iii, 78 p. (*0-16-055759-3*) USGPO.

Adequacy of the Comprehensive Clinical Evaluation Program: A Focused Assessment. Institute of Medicine Staff. 1997. 140p. pap. text 28.00 (*0-309-05949-6*) Natl Acad Pr.

Adequacy of the Comprehensive Clinical Evaluation Program: Nerve Agents. Institute of Medicine Staff. 1997. 64p. pap. text 15.00 (*0-309-05743-4*) Natl Acad Pr.

ADHD: How to Deal with Very Difficult Children. Alan Train. 1997. 208p. pap. (*0-285-63311-2*) Souvenir Pr Ltd GBR. *Dist:* IPG Chicago.

ADHD: The Great Misdiagnosis. Julian Stuart Haber. 2000. LC 00-42590. xiv, 210p. pap. 14.95 (*0-87833-181-6*) Taylor Pub.

ADHD - A Path to Success: A Revolutionary Theory & New Innovation in Drug-Free Therapy. Lawrence Weathers. 1998. LC 97-92384. (Illus.). 313p. pap. 16.95 (*0-9659513-1-6*) Ponderosa Press.

ADHD - Hyperactivity: A Consumer's Guide for Parents & Teachers. Michael Gordon. 1990. 178p. (Orig.). pap. 14.95 (*0-9627701-0-8*) GSI Pubns.

ADHD & the Nature of Self-Control. Russell A. Barkley. 1997. LC 97-25931. 410p. 46.00 (*1-57230-250-X*, 0250) Guilford Pubns.

***ADHD-Autism Connection: A Step Toward More Accurate Diagnoses & Effective Treatments.** Diane Kennedy. 2002. LC 2001-55754. pap. 14.95 (*1-57856-498-0*) Waterbrook Pr.

ADHD Day - With & Without Modifications & Accommodations: A How to for a Day of Positive Results. Jan Hunt & Bonnie L. Carpenter. 2000. 60p. pap. 19.95 (*1-892869-05-5*) Cambridge Cottage.

ADHD in Adolescents: Diagnosis & Treatment. Arthur L. Robin. 1998. LC 98-36026. 461p. text 46.95 (*1-57230-391-3*, 0391) Guilford Pubns.

ADHD in Adulthood: A Guide to Current Theory, Diagnosis & Treatment. Margaret Weis et al. 1999. LC 98-42934. (Illus.). 376p. 58.00 (*0-8018-6141-1*) Johns Hopkins.

ADHD in the Young Child: Driven to Redirection - A Guide for Parents & Teachers of Young Children with ADHD. Cathy Reimers & Bruce A. Brungers. 1999. LC 99-388861. (Illus.). 202p. pap. 18.95 (*1-886941-32-7*) Spec Pr FL.

ADHD Rating Scale IV: Checklists, Norms & Clinical Interpretation. George J. Du Paul et al. 1998. LC 98-35857. 80p. pap. text 38.00 (*1-57230-423-5*, 0423) Guilford Pubns.

Adherence to Pediatric Medical Regimens. M. A. Rapoff. 1999. LC 98-43927. (Clinical Child Psychology Library). (Illus.). 184p. (C). pap. text 24.95 (*0-306-46083-1*, Kluwer Plenum) Kluwer Academic.

Adherence to Pediatric Medical Regimens. M. A. Rapoff. 1999. LC 98-43927. (Clinical Child Psychology Library). (Illus.). 184p. (C). 75.00 (*0-306-46082-3*, Plenum Trade) Perseus Pubng.

Adherence to Treatment in Medical Conditions. Ed. by Lynn Myers & Kenny Midence. 1998. 517p. text 71.00 (*90-5702-264-8*); LC 00-500761. pap. text 28.00 (*90-5702-265-6*) Gordon & Breach (Harwood Acad Pubs).

Adhering to Medical Regimens: Pilot Experiments in Patient Education & Social Support. Robert D. Caplan et al. 1976. LC 76-620035. 284p. pap. 14.00 (*0-87944-207-7*) Inst Soc Res.

Adhesion in Leukocyte Homing & Differentiation. Ed. by D. Dunon et al. 1993. (Current Topics in Microbiology & Immunology Ser.: Vol. 184). (Illus.). 260p. (*3-540-56756-9*) Spr-Verlag.

Adhesion in Leukocyte Homing & Differentiation. D. Dunon et al. 1993. (Current Topics in Microbiology & Immunology Ser.: Vol. 184). (Illus.). 260p. 154.00 (*0-387-56756-9*) Spr-Verlag.

Adhesion Molecules in Allergic Disease. Ed. by Bruce S. Bochner. 1997. LC 97-7152. (Illus.). 440p. text 199.00 (*0-8247-9836-8*) Dekker.

Adhesion Molecules in Health & Disease. Ed. by Leendert C. Paul & Thomas B. Issekutz. 1997. LC 97-12034. (Illus.). 776p. text 225.00 (*0-8247-9824-4*) Dekker.

Adhesion Molecules in Hematology. Ed. by Elio Cacciola et al. 1996. (Acta Haematologica Ser.: Vol. 97, Nos. 1-2, 1997). (Illus.). 126p. pap. 101.00 (*3-8055-6393-0*) S Karger.

Adhesion Molecules in Renal Disease. Ed. by M. S. Goligorsky. 1999. (Experimental Nephrology Ser.: Vol. 7, No. 2 (1999)). (Illus.). 126p. pap. 39.25 (*3-8055-6886-X*) S Karger.

Adhesion of Porphyromonas Gingivalis & Periodontitis. William Papaioannou. 1998. (Acta Biomedica Lovaniensia Ser.). (Illus.). 128p. pap. (*90-6186-896-3*) Leuven Univ BEL. *Dist:* Coronet Bks.

Adhesive Metal-Free Restorations: Current Concepts for the Esthetic Treatment of Posterior Teeth. Didier Dietschi & Roberto Spreafico. 1997. LC 96-46353. 220p. text 98.00 (*0-86715-328-8*) Quint Pub Co.

Adipose Child. Ed. by Zvi Laron. 1976. (Pediatric & Adolescent Endocrinology Ser.: Vol.1). 250p. 77.50 (*3-8055-2343-2*) S Karger.

Adipose Tissue. Ed. by L. Robert. 1976. (Frontiers of Matrix Biology Ser.: Vol. 2). (Illus.). 200p. 79.25 (*3-8055-2223-1*) S Karger.

Adipose Tissue & Reproduction. Ed. by Rose E. Frisch. 1990. (Progress in Reproductive Biology & Medicine Ser.: Vol. 14). (Illus.). x, 142p. 121.00 (*3-8055-5066-9*) S Karger.

Adipose Tissue in Childhood. F. P. Bonnet. 1981. 192p. 108.00 (*0-8493-5771-3*, QP88, CRC Reprint) Franklin.

Adipose Tissues—For Clinical & Scientific Research: Index of New Information. John C. Bartone. 1998. 160p. 57.50 (*0-7883-1716-4*); pap. 47.50 (*0-7883-1717-2*) ABBE Pubs Assn.

Adjudication of Utilitarianism & Rights in the Sphere of Health Care. Harry L. Moore. 2000. LC 99-51663. (International Healthcare Ethics Ser.: Vol. 4). (Illus.). viii, 137p. text 46.95 (*0-8204-4933-4*) P Lang Pubng.

Adjunctive Medical Therapy of Acromegalic Patients. J. W. Nortier. 1984. (Clinical Research Ser.: No. 2). x, 91p. (Orig.). (C). pap. text (*3-11-013365-2*) Mouton.

Adjunctive Therapy: 1985 Edition. Frank T. Langilotti. 1985. (Illus.). 152p. 30.00 (*0-938470-03-5*) NY Chiro Coll.

Adjustment & Competence: Concepts & Applications. Tony Grasha & Daniel Kirschenbaum. 1986. LC 85-22702. (Illus.). 511p. (C). text 56.00 (*0-314-93183-X*); pap. text, tchr. ed. (*0-314-96629-3*) West Pub.

Adjustment & Growth. Rathus. 6th ed. 1994. LC 94-77536. (C). text 72.50 (*0-15-501670-9*) Harcourt Coll Pubs.

Adjustment & Growth: Challenges of Life. Spencer A. Rathus. 6th ed. 1994. (C). pap. text, tchr. ed., suppl. ed. 44.50 (*0-15-502440-X*); pap. text, stu. ed. 28.00 (*0-15-502439-6*) Harcourt Coll Pubs.

Adjustment & Growth: Challenges of Life. Spencer A. Rathus & William Kornblum. 6th ed. 1994. (C). pap. text, tchr. ed. 35.00 (*0-15-502438-8*) Harcourt Coll Pubs.

Adjustment & Growth in a Changing World. Vincent Napoli et al. Ed. by Marshall. 4th ed. 1992. 514p. (C). mass mkt. 38.25 (*0-314-93372-7*) West Pub.

Adjustment of Adolescents: Cross-Cultural Similarities & Differences. Ruth Scott & William A. Scott. 1998. LC 97-48935. (International Series in Social Psychology). 176p. (C). 78.95 (*0-415-18532-7*); pap. 26.95 (*0-415-18533-5*) Routledge.

Adjustment to Adult Hearing Loss. Ed. by Harold Orlans. 1991. (Illus.). 217p. (C). reprint ed. pap. 32.95 (*1-879105-47-0*, A056) Thomson Learn.

Adjuvant Nutrition in Cancer Treatment. Ed. by Patrick Quillin. 1993. (Illus.). 400p. (C). (*0-9638263-0-1*) Cancer Treatment.

Adjuvant Therapy for Colon & Rectum Cancer. 1991. lib. bdg. 250.00 (*0-8490-4222-4*) Gordon Pr.

Adjuvant Therapy of Breast Cancer. Ed. by I. Craig Henderson & William L. McGuire. 1992. (Cancer Treatment & Research Ser.). 480p. (C). text 265.00 (*0-7923-1656-8*) Kluwer Academic.

Adjuvant Therapy of Breast Cancer V. Ed. by H. J. Senn et al. 1996. (Recent Results in Cancer Research Ser.: Vol. 140). (Illus.). 342p. 158.00 (*3-540-58454-4*) Spr-Verlag.

Adjuvant Therapy of Breast Cancer IV. Ed. by H. J. Senn et al. 1993. LC 92-49032. (Recent Results in Cancer Research Ser.: Vol. 127). (Illus.). 300p. 145.00 (*0-387-55304-5*) Spr-Verlag.

Adjuvant Therapy of Cancer. Charles G. Salmon. 6th ed. 1990. (Illus.). 672p. text 85.00 (*0-7216-3630-6*) Saunders.

Adjuvant Therapy of Primary Breast Cancer. Ed. by Hansjorg Senn et al. 1989. (Recent Results in Cancer Research Ser.: Vol. 115). (Illus.). 296p. 137.00 (*0-387-18810-X*, 2887) Spr-Verlag.

Adjuvant Therapy of Primary Breast Cancer, Vol. 152. Hansjorg Senn. 1998. LC 98-36644. (Recent Results in Cancer Research Ser.). (Illus.). 522p. 129.00 (*3-540-64085-1*) Spr-Verlag.

Adjuvant Treatment in Urological Cancer. Ed. by Antoine S. Abi-Aad. 1997. LC 97-9163. (Illus.). 384p. ring bd. (*1-85070-917-3*, Parthenon Pbng) CRC Pr.

Adlerian Counseling: A Practical Approach for a New Decade. Thomas J. Sweeney. 3rd ed. 1989. LC 88-82676. 508p. (C). 32.95 (*0-915202-84-0*) Accel Devel.

Adlerian Counseling: A Practitioner's Approach. Thomas J. Sweeney. 4th ed. 1998. LC 98-20911. (Accelerated Development Ser.). 490p. 39.95 (*1-56032-510-0*) Hemisp Pub.

Adlerian Family Counseling: A Manual for Counselor, Educator & Psychotherapist. Ed. by Oscar C. Christensen. rev. ed. 1998. LC 93-70537. 270p. pap. 12.95 (*0-932796-56-7*) Ed Media Corp.

Adler's Physiology of the Eye. William M. Hart, Jr. 1995. (SPA.). (C). (gr. 13). text 156.00 (*84-8086-070-7*) Mosby Inc.

Adler's Physiology of the Eye: Clinical Application. Ed. by William M. Hart, Jr. 9th ed. 1992. LC 92-12791. (Illus.). 904p. (C). (gr. 13). text 110.00 (*0-8016-2107-0*, 02107) Mosby Inc.

Administering Medications. Phyllis Theiss Bayt. 1982. (Health Occupations Ser.). (Illus.). 384p. (*0-672-61538-X*, 61538); pap. 17.55 (*0-672-61522-3*, 61522) Macmillan.

Administering Medications: A Competency-Based Program for Health Occupations. Phyllis Theiss Bayt. 3rd ed. 1993. LC 93-16412. tchr. ed. (*0-02-800887-1*); text (*0-02-800886-3*) Glencoe.

Administering Nursing Service. Marie DiVincenti. 2nd ed. 1977. 350p. 20.50 (*0-316-18651-1*, Little Brwn Med Div) Lppncott W & W.

Administration of a Public Health Agency: A Case Study of the New York City Department of Health. Pascal J. Imperato. 1983. 226p. 35.95 (*0-89885-122-X*, Kluwer Acad Hman Sci) Kluwer Academic.

Administration of Environmental Health Programmes: A Systems View. M. Schaefer. 1974. (Public Health Papers: No. 59). pap. text 12.00 (*92-4-130059-0*, 1110059) World Health.

Administration of Imaging Pharmaceuticals. Marianne R. Tortorici. Ed. by Lisa Biello. 1996. LC 96-6051. (Illus.). 192p. pap. text 26.00 (*0-7216-4813-4*) Saunders.

Administrative Dental Assistant. Gaylor. 1999. (C). pap. text, wbk. ed. (*0-7216-7385-6*) Saunders.

Administrative Laboratory Management. 1996. ring bd. 250.00 (*1-56238-293-4*, SC16-L) NCCLS.

Administrative Manual, Vol. 1. Ed. by AABB Administrative Section Coordinating Committee. 3rd ed. 1985. LC 85-11061. (Illus.). 253p. pap. text 20.00 (*0-915355-08-6*) Am Assn Blood.

Administrative Manual, Vol. 2. Ed. by Ronald G. Wilkins. 1987. (Illus.). 220p. pap. text 20.00 (*0-915355-53-1*) Am Assn Blood.

Administrative Manual, Vol. III. Allan Ross, Jr. 1990. 134p. 25.00 (*0-915355-79-5*) Am Assn Blood.

Administrative Manual, Vol. IV. Ed. by Edmund N. Smith. 1993. (Illus.). 210p. (C). pap. text 30.00 (*1-56395-026-X*) Am Assn Blood.

Administrative Medical Assessing. Fordney. 1989. (Medical Assisting Ser.). tchr. ed. 15.00 (*0-8273-4243-8*) Delmar.

Administrative Medical Assistant. Mary E. Kinn. 3rd ed. 1993. (Illus.). pap., tchr. ed. (*0-7216-3404-4*); LC 93-259. 432p. pap. text 29.95 (*0-7216-3627-6*); pap. text, stu. ed. 15.95 (*0-7216-3628-4*) Saunders.

Administrative Medical Assistant. Mary E. Kinn. Ed. by Adrianne Williams. 4th ed. 1999. LC 99-17457. (Illus.). 365p. (C). pap. text 31.95 (*0-7216-7293-0*) Saunders.

Administrative Medical Assisting. Marilyn Takahashi Fordney & Joan J. Follis. 3rd ed. 1993. LC 92-49233. 429p. pap. 62.95 (*0-8273-5902-0*); 437p. (C). mass mkt., wbk. ed. 25.95 (*0-8273-4944-0*); LC 92-49233. 429p. (C). mass mkt. 48.95 (*0-8273-4942-4*) Delmar.

Administrative Medical Assisting. Marilyn Takahashi Fordney. 4th ed. 1997. LC 97-33446. 448p. pap. text 57.95 (*0-8273-7894-7*); 512p. (C). pap. text, wbk. ed. 19.00 (*0-8273-7895-5*) Delmar.

Administrative Procedures for Medical Assisting: A Patient-Centered Approach. Barbara Prickett-Ramutkowski. 1999. LC 98-26411. (Illus.). (YA). (gr. 6-12). stu. ed. 29.31 (*0-02-804863-6*) Glencoe.

Administrative Psychiatry. William A. Bryan. 1958. LC 58-14143. reprint ed. 46.00 (*0-8154-0034-9*) Cooper Sq.

Administrative Review. Ed. by Edmund N. Smith. 1990. 157p. (C). pap. 25.00 (*1-56395-028-6*) Am Assn Blood.

Administrator's Handbook for Community Health & Home Care Services. Anne S. Smith. 1988. 514p. 175.00 (*0-88737-400-X*, 21-2220) Natl League Nurse.

Admisiones Hospitalarias. Cosialls. 1995. (C). text 25.50 (*84-8174-080-2*) Mosby Inc.

Adobe Whitewater Club of New Mexico's Handbook of River Safety & Rescue. Charles Hammersley. 1985. (AWC Ser.). (Illus.). 29p. (Orig.). pap. 3.95 (*0-910467-03-X*) Heritage Assocs.

Adolescence. Robert Coles. 1996. (*0-201-19898-3*) Addison-Wesley.

Adolescence. Rhoda Woods Cummings. 1994. (C). pap. text, tchr. ed. 33.75 (*0-15-502971-1*); pap. text, stu. ed. 30.50 (*0-15-500393-3*) Harcourt Coll Pubs.

Adolescence. Laurence D. Steinberg. 3rd ed. 1993. LC 92-15734. (C). text 53.00 net. (*0-07-061218-8*) McGraw.

Adolescence. Laurence D. Steinberg. 5th ed. 1998. LC 97-52369. 544p. text 78.44 (*0-07-001323-3*) McGrw-H Hghr Educ.

Adolescence. John W. Santrock. 8th ed. 2000. 46.74 net. (*0-07-231671-3*); stu. ed. 15.00 net. (*0-07-231672-1*); LC 99-89722. (Illus.). xxix, 497p. 46.74 net. (*0-07-232349-3*) McGraw.

Adolescence. John W. Santrock. 6th ed. 1995. text (*0-697-34588-2*, WCB McGr Hill); 8th ed. 2000. 340p. pap., stu. ed. 25.00 (*0-07-232350-7*) McGrw-H Hghr Educ.

Adolescence: A Contemporary View. Nielsen. 3rd ed. 1995. (C). pap. text, suppl. ed. 44.50 (*0-15-503548-7*) Harcourt Coll Pubs.

Adolescence: A Developmental Transition. Douglas C. Kimmel & Irving B. Weiner. 2nd ed. 1994. LC 94-28382. 620p. 74.95 (*0-471-58264-6*) Wiley.

Adolescence: An Ethological Perspective. Ritch C. Savin-Williams. 1986. (Illus.). 249p. 84.00 (*0-387-96369-3*) Spr-Verlag.

Adolescence: Biological & Psychosocial Perspectives, 35. Benjamin B. Wolman. 1998. LC 97-14466. (Contributions in Psychology Ser.: Vol. 35). 152p. 62.50 (*0-313-30311-8*, Greenwood Pr) Greenwood.

Adolescence: From Crisis to Coping: A Thirteen Nation Study. Ed. by Janice G. Cline. 1998. LC 95-25382. (Social Psychology Ser.). (Illus.). 336p. pap. 27.95 (*0-7506-2604-6*) Routledge.

Adolescence: Its Social Psychology. Charlotte M. Fleming. 1969. reprint ed. pap. 24.95 (*0-8236-8004-5*, 020060) Intl Univs Pr.

Adolescence: Opportunities & Challenges. Ed. by Dante Cicchetti & Sheree L. Toth. 1996. LC 96-28192. (Rochester Symposium on Developmental Psychopathology Ser.: Vol. 7). 440p. 95.00 (*1-878822-67-5*) Univ Rochester Pr.

Adolescence: Theories, Research, Applications. Larry C. Jensen. 1985. (Illus.). 573p. (C). mass mkt. 45.75 (*0-314-85251-4*); pap. text, tchr. ed. (*0-314-87100-4*) West Pub.

Adolescence & Character Disturbance. James B. McCarthy. LC 94-16770. 218p. (C). reprint ed. 1995. lib. bdg. 61.50 (*0-8191-9582-0*); 1994. pap. text 30.50 (*0-8191-9583-9*) U Pr of Amer.

Adolescence & Developmental Breakdown: A Psychoanalytic View. Moses Laufer. 1995. 240p. pap. text (*1-85575-108-9*) Karnac Bks GBR. *Dist:* Other Pr LLC.

Adolescence & Myalgic Encephalomyelitis/Chronic Fatigue Syndrome: Journeys with the Dragon. Naida Edgar Brotherston. 2000. LC 00-38836. 280p. pap. 24.95 (*0-7890-1208-1*) Haworth Pr.

Adolescence & Myalgic Encephalomyelitis/Chronic Fatigue Syndrome: Journeys with the Dragon. Ed. by Naida Edgar Brotherston. 2000. LC 00-38836. (Illus.). xv, 185p. 49.95 (*0-7890-0874-2*) Haworth Pr.

Adolescence & Self-Esteem. Patricia Wellingham-Jones. 1984. (Illus.). 54p. (Orig.). pap. 10.00 (*0-939221-01-2*) PWJ Pubg.

Adolescence & Youth. Conger. 4th ed. 1991. (C). pap., stu. ed. 21.00 (*0-06-044579-3*) Addson-Wesley Educ.

Adolescence-Its Psychology & Its Relation to Physiology, Anthropology, Sociology, Sex, Crime, Religion & Education G. Stanley Hall. LC 79-89183. (American Education: Its Men, Institutions, & Ideas. Series 1). reprint ed. 1970. 71.95 (*0-405-01421-X*); Vol. 1. 1975. 42.95 (*0-405-01422-8*); Vol. 2. 1975. 38.95 (*0-405-01423-6*) Ayer.

Adolescent. Rice & Lemme. 9th ed. 1999. 143.40 (*0-205-31695-6*) Allyn.

Adolescent: Development, Relationships, & Culture. F. Philip Rice. 9th ed. 1998. LC 98-5164. 517p. 80.00 (*0-205-27617-2*) Allyn.

Adolescent Alone: Decision Making in Health Care in the United States. Ed. by Jeffrey Blustein et al. 1999. LC 98-48330. (Illus.). 288p. pap. text 19.95 (*0-521-65891-8*); text 54.95 (*0-521-65240-5*) Cambridge U Pr.

Adolescent & Adult Psychoeducational Profile: A Comprehensive Evaluation of the Autistic & Developmentally Disabled. Eric Schopler et al. pap. (*0-8290-1792-5*) Irvington.

Adolescent & His Environment. Ed. by H. Thomae & T. Endo. 1974. (Contributions to Human Development Ser.: Vol. 1). (Illus.). 109p. 38.50 (*3-8055-1651-7*) S Karger.

Adolescent & Mood Disturbance. Harvey Golombek & Barry D. Garfinkel. 1983. LC 82-13044. xvi, 285p. 45.00 (*0-8236-0085-8*) Intl Univs Pr.

Adolescent Anger Control: Cognitive-Behavioral Techniques. Eva L. Feindler & Randolph B. Ecton. 1987. (Psychology Practitioner Guidebooks). text 30.00 (*0-08-032374-X*); pap. text 15.95 (*0-08-032373-1*) Elsevier (Pergamon Pr).

Adolescent Art Therapy. Debra G. Linesch. 1988. LC 87-21866. 256p. text 37.95 (*0-87630-486-2*) Brunner-Routledge.

Adolescent As Decision-Maker: Applications to Development & Education. Ed. by Judith Worell & Fred Danner. 1989. (Educational Psychology Ser.). 320p. text 89.95 (*0-12-764052-5*) Acad Pr.

*__Adolescent Assessment/Referral System Manual.__ Elizabeeth R. Rahdert. 2001. 170p. reprint ed. 35.00 (*0-7567-0609-2*) DIANE Pub.

*__Adolescent Behavior: Readings & Interpretations.__ Elizabeth Aries. 2000. 22.50 (*0-07-244813-X*) McGrw-H Hghr Educ.

Adolescent Behavior & Society: A Book of Readings. Rolf E. Muuss. 4th ed. 1990. (C). text 27.25 net. (*0-07-044164-2*) McGraw.

Adolescent Breakdown & Beyond. Moses Laufer. 1997. 168p. pap. (*1-85575-149-6*) Karnac Bks GBR. *Dist:* Other Pr LLC.

Adolescent Coping: Theoretical & Research Perspectives. Erica Frydenberg. 1997. LC 96-14317. (Adolescence & Society Ser.). 256p. (C). pap. 27.95 (*0-415-11212-5*); (Illus.). 80.00 (*0-415-11211-7*) Routledge.

Adolescent Development. John S. Dacey & Maureen E. Kenny. (C). 1994. 560p. text, stu. ed. 21.87 (*0-697-20997-0*); 2nd ed. 1996. LC 95-83236. 592p. text 38.50 net. (*0-697-21012-X*) Brown & Benchmark.

Adolescent Development & the Biology of Puberty: Summary of a Workshop on New Research. National Research Council Staff & Institute of Medicine Staff. Ed. by Michele D. Kipke. 1999. 44p. pap. 12.00 (*0-309-06582-8*) Natl Acad Pr.

Adolescent Development, Psychopathology, & Treatment. H. Spencer Bloch. 1995. 417p. 55.00 (*0-8236-0065-3*) Intl Univs Pr.

Adolescent Endocrinology. R. Stanhope-Palmer. 1998. pap. text 49.95 (*1-901978-01-X*) Blackwell Sci.

Adolescent Fertility in Kenya. Benjamin Gyepi-Garbrah. 1985. (Adolescent Fertility in Sub-Sahara Africa Ser.: Vol. 4). 62p. (Orig.). (*0-933853-03-3*) Pathfinder Fund.

Adolescent Fertility in Liberia. Benjamin Gyepi-Garbrah. 1985. (Adolescent Fertility in Sub-Sahara Africa Ser.: Vol. 2). 55p. (Orig.). (*0-933853-01-7*) Pathfinder Fund.

Adolescent Fertility in Nigeria. Benjamin Gyepi-Garbrah. 1985. (Adolescent Fertility in Sub-Sahara Africa Ser.: Vol. 3). 69p. (Orig.). (*0-933853-02-5*) Pathfinder Fund.

Adolescent Fertility in Sub-Sahara Africa: An Overview. Benjamin Gyepi-Garbrah. 1985. (Adolescent Fertility in Sub-Sahara Africa Ser.: Vol. 1). 51p. (Orig.). (*0-933853-00-9*) Pathfinder Fund.

*__Adolescent Forensic Psychiatry.__ Susan Bailey & Odon. text 155.00 (*0-7506-4090-1*) Buttrwrth-Heinemann.

Adolescent Group Psychotherapy, No. 4. Ed. by Fern J. Azima & Lewis H. Richmond. LC 89-1972. xiv, 246p. 37.50 (*0-8236-0082-3*, BN 00082) Intl Univs Pr.

Adolescent Group Therapy: A Social Competency Model. George R. Holmes et al. 1991. LC 91-2693. 208p. 52.95 (*0-275-94024-1*, C4024, Praeger Pubs) Greenwood.

Adolescent Gynecology: A Guide for Clinicians. Ed. by Alfred M. Bongiovanni. 1983. LC 82-22396. 276p. 55.00 (*0-306-41203-9*, Kluwer Plenum) Kluwer Academic.

Adolescent Gynecology & Endocrinology. George Creatsas. 1999. (Annals of the New York Academy of Sciences Ser.). 488p. pap. text 24.95 (*0-8018-6215-9*) Johns Hopkins.

Adolescent Health: Abstracts of Active Projects FY 1994. National Center for Education in Maternal and Child. 1994. 350p. pap. text (*1-57285-004-3*) Nat Ctr Educ.

Adolescent Health: Reassessing the Passage to Adulthood. Judith Senderowitz. 1995. LC 94-48163. (Discussion Paper Ser.: No. 272). 64p. pap. 22.00 (*0-8213-3157-4*, 13157) World Bank.

Adolescent Health: The Role of Individual Differences. Patrick Haven. 1996. LC 95-35603. (Adolescence & Society Ser.). 224p. (C). 84.95 (*0-415-11578-7*); pap. 27.95 (*0-415-11579-5*) Routledge.

Adolescent Health Care: A Practical Guide. Lawrence S. Neinstein. (Illus.). rev. ed. 1990. 1112p. pap. 59.00 (*0-683-06373-1*); 2nd rev. ed. 1990. 1112p. 82.00 (*0-683-06374-X*); 3rd ed. 1996. LC 95-47009. 1,138p. pap. 79.00 (*0-683-06375-8*) Lppncott W & W.

Adolescent Health Care: Program Designs & Services. Ed. by John S. Wodarski et al. 1997. LC 96-38928. (Journal of Prevention & Intervention in the Community Ser.: Vol. 14, Nos. 1/2). 140p. (C). 29.95 (*0-7890-0020-2*) Haworth Pr.

Adolescent Health Issues: State Actions 1992-1994. Melissa Hough-Savage. 1995. 76p. 10.00 (*1-55516-610-5*, 6132) Natl Conf State Legis.

Adolescent Health Issues: State Actions 1995. Compiled by Melissa Hough-Savage & Joanne Ourada. 1996. 62p. pap. 20.00 (*1-55516-654-7*, 6656) Natl Conf State Legis.

Adolescent Health Problems: Behavioral Perspectives. Ed. by Jan L. Wallander & Lawrence J. Siegel. 1995. LC 95-10042. (Advances in Pediatric Psychology Ser.). 314p. 40.00 (*0-89862-113-5*) Guilford Pubns.

Adolescent in Family Therapy: Breaking the Cycle of Conflict & Control. Joseph A. Micucci. 1998. LC 98-37859. (Guilford Family Therapy Ser.). 336p. text 40.00 (*1-57230-389-1*) Guilford Pubns.

Adolescent in Group & Family Therapy. Ed. by Max Sugar. 2nd ed. 1997. LC 86-16157. xx, 320p. (C). pap. text 17.00 (*0-226-77964-5*) U Ch Pr.

A B

Adolescent in the Family: A Study of Personality Development in the Home Environment. White House Conference on Child Health and Protectio. 1979. LC 79-169401. (Family in America Ser.). 478p. reprint ed. 28.95 (*0-405-03878-X*) Ayer.

Adolescent in Turmoil. Ed. by Allan Z. Schwartzberg. 1998. LC 97-43958. 208p. 72.50 (*0-275-96048-X*, Praeger Pubs) Greenwood.

Adolescent Medicine. Ronald Shenker. 1994. LC 93-45850. (Monographs in Clinical Pediatrics: Vol. 7). (Illus.). 306p. text 80.00 (*3-7186-5509-8*) Gordon & Breach.

Adolescent Medicine. Adele D. Hofmann & Donald Greydanus. 3rd ed. 1997. LC 96-40179. 913p. (C). pap. text 99.00 (*0-8385-0067-6*, A0067-7, Apple Lange Med) McGraw.

Adolescent Medicine: A Practical Guide. Victor C. Strasburger & Robert T. Brown. 2nd ed. 1997. text 125.00 (*0-7817-1474-5*) Lppncott W & W.

Adolescent Medicine: A Practical Guide. Victor C. Strasburger et al. 2nd ed. 1997. LC 97-20889. 528p. pap. text 75.00 (*0-316-81875-5*, Little Brwn Med Div) Lppncott W & W.

Adolescent Medicine Residency Training Resources. American Academy of Pediatrics Staff. 1995. 238p. ring bd. 34.95 (*0-910761-74-4*) Am Acad Pediat.

Adolescent Molester. William Breer. 2nd ed. 1996. LC 95-47296. (Illus.). 234p. pap. 38.95 (*0-398-06572-1*); 55.95 (*0-398-06571-3*) C C Thomas.

Adolescent Nutrition: Assessment & Management. Ed. by Vaughn I. Rickert. 1995. LC 95-7376. (Series in Clinical Nutrition). 677p. (C). 92.00 (*0-412-05661-5*) Aspen Pub.

Adolescent Nutritional Disorders: Prevention & Treatment. Marc S. Jacobson. 1997. LC 97-13183. (Annals of the New York Academy of Sciences Ser.). pap. 110.00 (*1-57331-021-2*) NY Acad Sci.

Adolescent Nutritional Disorders: Prevention & Treatment. Ed. by Marc S. Jacobson et al. 1997. LC 97-13183. (Annals of the New York Academy of Sciences Ser.: Vol. 817). 110.00 (*1-57331-020-4*) NY Acad Sci.

Adolescent-Parental Separation. Michael Bloom. 1980. LC 79-13928. text 24.95 (*0-89876-035-6*) Gardner Pr.

Adolescent Passage: Developmental Issues. Peter Blos. 1979. LC 78-61245. 538p. (Orig.). 80.00 (*0-8236-0095-5*) Intl Univs Pr.

Adolescent Peer Pressure: Theory, Corelates, & Program Implications for Drug Abuse Prevention. 1986. lib. bdg. 300.00 (*0-8490-3503-1*) Gordon Pr.

Adolescent Period: A Graphic Atlas. Frank K. Shuttleworth. 1949. (SRCD Ser.: Vol. 14, No. 1). 25.00 (*0-527-01547-4*) Periodicals Srv.

Adolescent Period: A Pictorial Atlas. Frank K. Shuttlworth. 1949. (SRCD Ser.: Vol. 14, No. 2). 25p. pap. 10.00 (*0-527-01548-2*) Periodicals Srv.

Adolescent Portraits: Identity, Relationships, & Challenges. Andrew Garrod et al. 3rd ed. 1998. LC 98-6091. 294p. pap. text 36.00 (*0-205-27779-9*) Allyn.

Adolescent Pregnancy: The Challenge: A Framework for Prevention & Parenting. 1993. (Illus.). 150p. (Orig.). (C). pap. text 30.00 (*0-7881-0083-1*) DIANE Pub.

Adolescent Pregnancy in an Urban Environment: Issues, Programs, & Evaluation. Janet B. Hardy & Laurie S. Zabin. 1991. (Illus.). 492p. (C). pap. text 51.50 (*0-87766-520-6*) Urban Inst.

Adolescent Problem Behaviors: Issues & Research. Ed. by Robert D. Ketterlinus & Michael E. Lamb. 1994. 240p. pap. 27.50 (*0-8058-1157-5*); text 49.95 (*0-8058-1156-7*) L Erlbaum Assocs.

Adolescent Psyche: Jungian & Winnicottian Perspectives. Richard Frankel. 1998. LC 97-29591. (Illus.). 264p. (C). 89.95 (*0-415-16798-1*); pap. 26.95 (*0-415-16799-X*) Routledge.

Adolescent Psychiatry, Vol. 7. Ed. by Sherman C. Feinstein & Peter L. Giovacchini. 1979. LC 70-147017. (Adolescent Psychiatry Ser.: Vol. 7). 582p. lib. bdg. 33.00 (*0-226-24052-5*) U Ch Pr.

Adolescent Psychiatry, Vol. 8. Sherman C. Feinstein & Peter L. Giovacchini. 1981. LC 70-147017. (Adolescent Psychiatry Ser.: Vol. 8). 544p. lib. bdg. 33.00 (*0-226-24053-3*) U Ch Pr.

Adolescent Psychiatry, Vol. 9. Ed. by Sherman C. Feinstein & Peter L. Giovacchini. 1982. LC 70-147017. 670p. lib. bdg. 40.00 (*0-226-24054-1*) U Ch Pr.

Adolescent Psychiatry. Ed. by Sherman C. Feinstein et al. LC 70-147017. (Adolescent Psychiatry Ser.: Vol. 10). Vol. 10. 1983. 580p. lib. bdg. 40.00 (*0-226-24056-8*); Vol. 12. 1985. 594p. (C). lib. bdg. 39.00 (*0-226-24058-4*) U Ch Pr.

Adolescent Psychiatry, Vol. 14. Ed. by Sherman C. Feinstein. 1987. 648p. (C). lib. bdg. 45.00 (*0-226-24060-6*) U Ch Pr.

Adolescent Psychiatry, Vol. 15. Ed. by Sherman C. Feinstein & Aaron H. Esman. 1988. 624p. lib. bdg. 48.00 (*0-226-24061-4*) U Ch Pr.

Adolescent Psychiatry, Vol. 17. Ed. by Sherman C. Feinstein. 1990. (Adolescent Psychiatry Ser.: Vol. 17). 584p. lib. bdg. 48.00 (*0-226-24063-0*) U Ch Pr.

Adolescent Psychiatry, Vol. 19. Ed. by Sherman C. Feinstein & Richard C. Marohn. 1993. 532p. lib. bdg. 44.95 (*0-226-24065-7*) U Ch Pr.

Adolescent Psychiatry: The Annuals of the American Society for Adolescent Psychiatry, Vol. 11. Ed. by Max Sugar. 1984. LC 70-147017. (Adolescent Psychiatry Ser.: Vol. 11). 256p. (C). lib. bdg. 30.00 (*0-226-77962-9*) U Ch Pr.

Adolescent Psychiatry Vol. 6: Developmental & Clinical Studies. Ed. by Sherman C. Feinstein & Peter L. Giovacchini. 1979. (Adolescent Psychiatry Ser.). 532p. lib. bdg. 33.00 (*0-226-24051-7*) U Ch Pr.

Adolescent Psychiatry Vol. 13: Developmental & Clinical Studies. Ed. by Sherman C. Feinstein et al. 1986. LC 70-147017. xii, 608p. (C). lib. bdg. 42.00 (*0-226-24059-2*) U Ch Pr.

Adolescent Psychiatry Vol. 16: Developmental & Clinical Studies. Ed. by Sherman C. Feinstein. 1989. LC 70-147017. 588p. lib. bdg. 48.00 (*0-226-24062-2*) U Ch Pr.

Adolescent Psychiatry Vol. 18: Developmental & Clinical Studies. Ed. by Sherman C. Feinstein. 1991. 592p. lib. bdg. 49.50 (*0-226-24064-9*) U Ch Pr.

Adolescent Psychiatry Vol. 20: Developmental & Clinical Studies: The Annals of the American Society for Adolescent Psychiatry. Ed. by Richard C. Marohn. 1995. 456p. 49.95 (*0-88163-194-9*) Analytic Pr.

Adolescent Psychiatry Vol. 21: Developmental & Clinical Studies. Ed. by Lois T. Flaherty & Harvey Horowitz. 1997. 520p. 49.95 (*0-88163-195-7*) Analytic Pr.

Adolescent Psychiatry Vol. 22: Developmental & Clinical Studies: The Annals of the American Society for Adolescent Psychiatry. Ed. by Aaron H. Esman. 1998. 49.95 (*0-88163-196-5*) Analytic Pr.

Adolescent Psychiatry Vol. 23: The Annuals of the American Society for Adolescent Psychiatry. Ed. by Aaron H. Esman. 1998. (Adolescent Psychiatry Ser.: Vol. 23). 312p. 49.95 (*0-88163-197-3*) Analytic Pr.

Adolescent Psychiatry Vol. 24: Developmental & Clinical Studies:The Annuals of the American Society for Adolescent Psychiatry. Ed. by Aaron H. Esman. 1999. 396p. 55.00 (*0-88163-198-1*) Analytic Pr.

Adolescent Psychiatry in Clinical Practice. Ed. by Simon G. Gowers. 2000. (Illus.). 448p. text (*0-7506-4118-5*) E A GBR. *Dist:* OUP.

Adolescent Psychology. Michael L. Jaffe. 1997. LC 97-24350. 688p. pap. 44.95 (*0-471-57190-3*) Wiley.

***Adolescent Psychology: A Collection of Readings.** Ed. by Deborah L. Browning. 2001. 320p. pap. 31.90 (*0-8236-5769-8*, 20061, Psychosocial) Intl Univs Pr.

Adolescent Psychology: A Developmental View. Norman A. Sprinthall. 3rd ed. 1994. LC 94-25518. 600p. (C). text 74.06 (*0-07-060544-0*) McGrw-H Hghr Educ.

Adolescent Psychology: A Developmental View. Norman A. Sprinthall. 2nd ed. 1990. 47.50 (*0-394-37516-5*) Random.

Adolescent Psychology 1997-1998. annuals Anita M. Meehan & Eileen Astor-Stetson. 1996. (Annual Editions Ser.). (Illus.). 256p. (C). text 12.25 net. (*0-697-35417-2*, Dshkn McG-Hill) McGrw-H Hghr Educ.

Adolescent Psychology, 2001-2002. annuals Eileen Astor-Stetson & Anita M. Meehan. 3rd ed. 2000. (Annual Editions Ser.). 240p. pap. 18.44 (*0-07-242572-5*) McGrw-H Hghr Educ.

Adolescent Psychotherapy. Ed. by Marcia Slomowitz. 1991. LC 90-871. (Clinical Practice Ser.: No. 16). 206p. text 12.95 (*0-88048-181-1*, 8181) Am Psychiatric.

Adolescent Relations with Mothers, Fathers, & Friends. James Youniss & Jacqueline Smollar. 1987. LC 84-28067. viii, 210p. reprint ed. pap. text 12.00 (*0-226-96488-4*) U Ch Pr.

Adolescent Reproductive Behavior. 1988. 178p. 22.00 (*92-1-151173-9*, E. 88. XIII.8) UN.

Adolescent Reproductive Health. Peggy Smith & David Mumford. 1985. LC 83-20492. text 31.95 (*0-89876-096-8*) Gardner Pr.

Adolescent Reproductive Health: An Approach to Planning Health Services Research. H. Friedman. 1983. (WHO Offset Publications: No. 77). 53p. 8.00 (*92-4-170077-7*) World Health.

Adolescent Rheumatology. David A. Isenberg & John J. Miller, III. 1999. 362p. 115.00 (*1-85317-553-6*, M Dunitz) Scovill Paterson.

Adolescent Risk Taking. Nancy J. Bell & Robert W. Bell. 1993. LC 92-35561. (Illus.). 192p. pap. 36.95 (*0-8039-5065-9*, 3284) Sage.

Adolescent Rorschach Responses: Developmental Trends from 10 to 16 Years. Louise B. Ames et al. 2nd rev. ed. 1995. LC 94-49579. (Master Work Ser.). (Illus.). 340p. pap. 60.00 (*1-56821-466-9*) Aronson.

Adolescent Self. David B. Wexler. 1991. 192p. 22.95 (*0-393-70114-X*) Norton.

Adolescent Sex & Love Addicts. Eric Griffin-Shelley. 1994. LC 94-1149. 184p. 59.95 (*0-275-94681-9*, Praeger Pubs) Greenwood.

Adolescent Sexual Behavior & Childbearing. Laurie S. Zabin & Sarah C. Hayward. 1993. (Developmental Clinical Psychology & Psychiatry Ser.: Vol. 26). (Illus.). 140p. (C). pap. 34.95 (*0-8039-4259-1*, 7570) Sage.

Adolescent Sexuality. Thomas P. Gullotta et al. 1992. (Advances in Adolescent Development Ser.: Vol. 5). (Illus.). 248p. (C). pap. 37.95 (*0-8039-4773-9*, 4376); 86.95 (*0-8039-4772-0*, 4375) Sage.

Adolescent Sexuality & Teenage Pregnancy: A Selected, Annotated Bibliography with Summary Forewords. Ed. by Karen R. Stewart. 1976. pap. 2.00 (*0-89055-117-0*) Carolina Pop Ctr.

Adolescent Siblings in Stepfamilies: Family Functioning & Adolescent Adjustment. Ed. by E. Mavis Hetherington et al. 2000. (Monographs of the Society for Research in Children Development). 200p. pap. 32.95 (*0-631-22155-7*) Blackwell Pubs.

Adolescent Spine. Ed. by N. A. Keim. 2nd ed. 1981. (Illus.). 254p. 88.00 (*0-387-90612-6*) Spr-Verlag.

Adolescent Stress. Ed. by Mary E. Colten & Susan Gore. 1991. (Social Institutions & Social Change Ser.). 342p. pap. text 26.95 (*0-202-30421-3*); lib. bdg. 51.95 (*0-202-30420-5*) Aldine de Gruyter.

Adolescent Struggle for Selfhood & Identity. John J. Mitchell. 1992. 218p. (C). pap. text 18.95 (*1-55059-050-2*) Temeron Bks.

Adolescent Subcultures & Delinquency. Herman Schwendinger & Julia S. Schwendinger. 1985. LC 84-26329. 544p. 95.00 (*0-275-90161-0*, C0161); pap. 24.95 (*0-275-91656-1*, B1656) Greenwood (Praeger Pubs).

Adolescent Substance Abuse: A Comprehensive Guide to Theory & Practice. Y. Kaminer. 1994. (Critical Issues in Psychiatry Ser.). (Illus.). 280p. (C). text 42.50 (*0-306-44692-8*, Kluwer Plenum) Kluwer Academic.

Adolescent Substance Abuse: A Guide to Prevention & Treatment. Ed. by Mark Singer & Richard E. Isralowitz. 1983. LC 83-13015. (Child & Youth Services Ser.: Vol. 6, Nos. 1 & 2). 123p. text 39.95 (*0-86656-185-4*) Haworth Pr.

Adolescent Substance Abuse: An Empirical-Based Health Paradigm. John S. Wodarski & Marvin D. Feit. 1995. LC 94-29995. (Illus.). 220p. lib. bdg. 39.95 (*1-56024-879-3*) Haworth Pr.

Adolescent Substance Abuse: Assessment, Prevention & Treatment. Oscar G. Bukstein. 1995. LC 94-40264. (Personality Processes Ser.). 260p. 99.95 (*0-471-55080-9*) Wiley.

Adolescent Substance Abuse: Etiology, Treatment & Prevention. Gary W. Lawson & Ann W. Lawson. 1998. LC 92-11363. 576p. pap. 55.00 (*0-8342-0254-9*) PRO-ED.

Adolescent Substance Abuse Intervention Workbook: Taking a First Step. Steven L. Jaffe. 2000. 38p. pap., wbk. ed. 54.95 (*1-58562-006-8*, 62006) Am Psychiatric.

Adolescent Suicide. Group for the Advancement of Psychiatry Staff & Committee on Adolescence Staff. 1996. LC 95-47286. (Group for the Advancement of Psychiatry Ser.: No. 140). 212p. text 28.00 (*0-87318-208-1*, 7208) Am Psychiatric.

Adolescent Suicide. Andre Haim. 1975. LC 73-9250. 310p. 47.50 (*0-8236-0090-4*) Intl Univs Pr.

Adolescent Suicide: Assessment & Intervention. Alan L. Berman & David A. Jobes. 1991. 277p. 24.95 (*1-55798-107-8*); pap. text 19.95 (*1-55798-114-0*) Am Psychol.

Adolescent Suicide: Identification & Intervention. 1987. 40p. (Orig.). (gr. 10-12). pap. text 3.95 (*0-9613416-5-3*, 104P) Comm Intervention.

Adolescent Suicide: Recognition, Treatment & Prevention. Ed. by Gordon Northrup & Barry Garfinkel. 1994. LC 89-19773. (Residential Treatment for Children & Youth Ser.: Vol. 7, No. 1). (Illus.). 116p. text 39.95 (*0-86656-949-9*) Haworth Pr.

Adolescent Suicide: With a New Preface. Jerry Jacobs. 1980. 26.50 (*0-8290-0113-1*); pap. text 12.95 (*0-8290-0114-X*) Irvington.

Adolescents: Theoretical & Helping Perspectives. Inger P. Davis. 1985. LC 84-20175. lib. bdg. 91.00 (*0-89838-165-7*) Kluwer Academic.

Adolescents, Alcohol & Drugs: A Practical Guide for Those Who Work with Young People. Judith H. Jaynes & Cheryl A. Rugg. 1987. 210p. (C). text 41.95 (*0-398-05393-6*) C C Thomas.

Adolescents & ADD: Gaining the Advantage. Patricia O. Quinn. 1995. LC 95-25301. 128p. (YA). (gr. 8-12). pap. 12.95 (*0-945354-70-3*) Am Psychol.

Adolescents & AIDS: Stopping the Time Bomb. 1990. (State Legislative Reports: Vol. 15, No. 12). 11p. 15.00 (*1-55516-268-1*, 7302-1512) Natl Conf State Legis.

Adolescents & Sexuality Transmitted Diseases. Ed. by Penelope J. Hitchcock et al. 2000. (Illus.). 400p. 50.00 (*0-19-512067-1*) OUP.

Adolescents & the HIV-AIDS Epidemic: Stemming the Tide. Susan S. Messina. 1993. 41p. 15.00 (*1-55516-646-6*, 6646) Natl Conf State Legis.

Adolescents & the Media: Medical & Psychological Impact. Victor C. Strasburger. 1995. LC 94-45245. (Developmental Clinical Psychology & Psychiatry Ser.: Vol. 33). 144p. pap. 34.95 (*0-8039-5500-6*, 3870) Sage.

Adolescents & Their Families: Paths of Ego Development. Stuart T. Hauser et al. 1991. LC 90-25215. 285p. 35.00 (*0-02-914260-1*) Free Pr.

Adolescents in Psychiatric Hospitals: A Psychodynamic Approach to Evaluation & Treatment. Richard W. Brunstetter. 1998. LC 98-10206. 208p. text 47.95 (*0-398-06860-7*); pap. text 34.95 (*0-398-06861-5*) C C Thomas.

Adolescents, Literature & Work with Youth. Ed. by Pamela J. Weiner & Ruth M. Stein. 1985. LC 84-29001. (Child & Youth Services Ser.: Vol. 7, Nos. 1 & 2). 137p. text 4.95 (*0-86656-120-X*) Haworth Pr.

Adolescents Psychological Development: Rationality, Morality, & Identity. David Moshman. 1999. LC 98-54349. (Illus.). 152p. pap. 16.50 (*0-8058-2858-3*) L Erlbaum Assocs.

Adolescents, Sex & Contraception. Ed. by D. Byrne & W. A. Fisher. 1983. 336p. 59.95 (*0-89859-217-8*) L Erlbaum Assocs.

Adolescents with Down Syndrome. Siegfried M. Pueschel & Maria Sustrova. 1997. LC 96-52748. 416p. 35.95 (*1-55766-281-9*) P H Brookes.

Adolescents with Emotional & Behavioral Disabilities: Transition to Adulthood. Mieko K. Smith. 1998. LC 98-25028. (Studies in Health & Human Services). 108p. text 59.95 (*0-7734-8286-5*) E Mellen.

Adoleszentenpsychosen. M. H. Friedrich. 1983. (Bibliotheca Psychiatrica Ser.: No. 163). (Illus.). xii, 144p. pap. 60.00 (*3-8055-3640-2*) S Karger.

Adopting New Medical Technology Vol. IV, Vol. 4. Institute of Medicine Staff. Ed. by Annetine C. Gelijns & Holly V. Dawkins. 1994. LC 94-7852. (Medical Innovation at the Crossroads Ser.: Vol. 4). 240p. (Orig.). (C). pap. text 27.00 (*0-309-05035-9*) Natl Acad Pr.

Adopting Older Children. Alfred Kadushin. 1970. LC 71-125918. 245p. text 46.00 (*0-231-03322-2*) Col U Pr.

***Adoption of an Opinion on Ethical Aspects of Human Stem Cell Research & Use.** Ed. by Anne McLaren & Goran Hermeren. rev. ed. 2002. 259p. (C). pap. text 45.00 (*0-7567-1942-9*) DIANE Pub.

Adoptive Cellular Immunotherapy of Cancer. Ed. by Henry C. Stevenson. 1989. (Immunology Ser.: Vol. 48). (Illus.). 264p. text 155.00 (*0-8247-8111-2*) Dekker.

ADP-Ribosylation, DNA Repair & Cancer: Proceedings of the 13th International Symposium of the Princess Takamatsu Cancer Research Fund, Japan, 1982. Ed. by M. Miwa et al. 1983. 354p. lib. bdg. (*90-6764-003-4*) VSP NLD. *Dist:* Coronet Bks.

Adrenal & Endocrine Tumors in Children: Adrenal Cortical Carcinoma & Multiple Endocrine Neoplasia. Ed. by G. Bennett Humphrey et al. 1983. text 213.00 (*0-89838-590-3*) Kluwer Academic.

Adrenal Diseases in Childhood. Ed. by Maria I. New & Leonore S. Levine. 1984. (Pediatric & Adolescent Endocrinology Ser.: Vol. 13). (Illus.). viii, 236p. 143.50 (*3-8055-3777-8*) S Karger.

Adrenal Disorders. Ed. by Andrew N. Margioris & George P. Chrousos. 2001. LC 2001-24380. (Contemporary Endocrinology Ser.). (Illus.). 416p. 145.00 (*0-89603-411-9*) Humana.

Adrenal Gland. C. R. Kannan. 1988. LC 88-19690. (Clinical Surveys in Endocrinology Ser.: Vol. 2). (Illus.). 516p. (C). text 139.50 (*0-306-42886-5*, Kluwer Plenum) Kluwer Academic.

Adrenal Glands, Vascular System & Hypertension. Gavin P. Vinson & D. C. Anderson. 1996. 338p. 99.95 (*1-898099-07-3*) Blackwell Sci.

Adrenal Steroid Antagonism: Proceedings Satellite Workshop of the VII International Congress of Endocrinology, July 7, 1984. International Congress of Endocrinology Staff. Ed. by M. K. Agarwal. 1984. LC 84-19947. (Illus.). viii, 399p. 134.65 (*3-11-010090-8*) De Gruyter.

Adrenergic Activators & Inhibitors. Ed. by L. Szekeres. 1980. (Handbook of Experimental Pharmacology Ser.: Vol. 54, Pt. 1). (Illus.). 1160p. 424.00 (*0-387-09797-X*) Spr-Verlag.

Adrenoceptors: Structure, Function & Pharmacology. Ed. by Robert R. Ruffolo, Jr. 1995. 280p. text 105.00 (*3-7186-5644-2*, Harwood Acad Pubs) Gordon & Breach.

Adrenoceptors: Structure, Mechanisms, Function. Ed. by E. Szabadi & Chris M. Bradshaw. 1991. (Advances in Pharmacological Sciences Ser.). 408p. 127.50 (*0-8176-2518-6*) Birkhauser.

Adrenocortical Hormones: Their Origin, Chemistry, Physiology, & Pharmacology Ed. by H. W. Deane & Betty L. Rubin. (Handbook of Experimental Pharmacology Ser.: Vol. 14). (ENG, FRE & GER., Illus.). Pt. 2. 1964. 214p. 72.95 (*0-387-03146-4*); Pt. 3. 1968. 452p. 144.00 (*0-387-04147-8*) Spr-Verlag.

Adrenocortical Hormones Pt. 1: Their Origin, Chemistry, Physiology, & Pharmacology Ed. by H. W. Deane & Betty L. Rubin. 1962. (Handbook of Experimental Pharmacology Ser.: Vol. 14). (ENG, FRE & GER., Illus.). 738p. 232.00 (*0-387-02830-7*) Spr-Verlag.

Adriamycin & Derivatives in Gastrointestinal Cancer. Ed. by W. Weber-Stadelmann. 1983. (Beitraege Zur Onkologie, Contributions to Oncology Ser.: Vol. 15). (Illus.). vi, 90p. pap. 57.50 (*3-8055-3689-5*) S Karger.

Adriamycin-Symposium. Ed. by D. Fuellenbach et al. 1981. (Beitraege Zur Onkologie, Contributions to Oncology Ser.: Vol. 9). (Illus.). x, 462p. pap. 68.75 (*3-8055-2966-X*) S Karger.

Adsorption Processes on Semiconductor & Dielectric Surfaces I. V. F. Kiselev & Oleg V. Krylov. 1985. (Chemical Physics Ser.: Vol. 32). (Illus.). 295p. 91.95 (*0-387-12416-0*) Spr-Verlag.

Adult Abnormal Psychology. Edgar Miller & Peter J. Cooper. 1988. (Illus.). 400p. text (*0-443-03513-X*) Church.

Adult ADD: A Reader Friendly Guide to Identifying, Understanding, & Treating Adult Attention Deficit Disorder. Thomas Whiteman et al. 1995. LC 95-12685. (Illus.). 269p. pap. 14.00 (*0-89109-906-9*) Pinon Press.

Adult Age Differences in Memory. Alison M. Mackenzie. 1991. (C). (*1-85041-037-2*) Univ Nottingham GBR. *Dist:* St Mut.

Adult Analysis & Childhood Sexual Abuse. Ed. by Howard B. Levine. 1998. 248p. reprint ed. pap. 29.95 (*0-88163-306-2*) Analytic Pr.

Adult & Pediatric Dermatology: A Color Guide to Diagnosis & Treatment. Lowell A. Goldsmith et al. 1996. LC 96-26032. (Illus.). 627p. pap. 62.95 (*0-8036-0146-8*) Davis Co.

***Adult & Pediatric Urology.** Jay Y. Gillenwater et al. 2001. (Illus.). 3000p. (*0-323-01132-2*) Mosby Inc.

Adult & Pediatric Urology. Jay Y. Gillenwater et al. 3rd ed. 1995. (Illus.). 3136p. (C). (gr. 13). text 340.00 (*0-8151-4008-8*, 24424) Mosby Inc.

Adult Aphasia Rehabilitation. Gloriajean L. Wallace. 1996. 393p. text 59.99 (*0-7506-9535-8*) Buttrwrth-Heinemann.

Adult Art Psychotherapy: Issues & Applications. Ed. by Helen B. Landgarten & Darcy Lubbers. 1991. LC 90-15103. (Illus.). 224p. text 32.95 (*0-87630-593-1*) Brunner-Routledge.

Adult Attachment. Judith Feeney & Patricia Noller. 1996. LC 96-4527. (Series on Close Relationships: Vol. 14). 192p. 64.95 (*0-8039-7223-7*, 1089); pap. 36.95 (*0-8039-7224-5*, 1090) Sage.

***Adult Attachment & Couple Psychotherapy: A Secure Base in Practice & Research.** Christopher Clulow. 2000. LC 00-44648. (Illus.). 240p. (C). (gr. 13). pap. 29.95 (*0-415-22416-0*) Routledge.

***Adult Attachment & Couple Psychotherapy: The 'Secure Base' in Practice & Research.** Christopher Clulow. 2000. LC 00-44648. (Illus.). 240p. (C). (gr. 13). lib. bdg. 69.95 (*0-415-22415-2*) Routledge.

Adult Attention Deficit Disorder: Brain Mechanisms & Life Outcomes. Ed. by Jeanette Wasserstein et al. 2000. LC 2001-30123. (Annals of the New York Academy of Sciences Ser.: Vol. 931). 350p. 90.00 (*1-57331-255-X*) NY Acad Sci.

***Adult Attention Deficit Disorder: Brain Mechanisms & Life Outcomes.** Jeanette Wasserstein & F. F. LeFever. 2001. (Annals of the New York Academy of Sciences Ser.). 350p. pap. text 30.00 (*0-8018-6836-X*) NY Acad Sci.

Adult Audiology, Vol. 2. Dafydd Stephens. 6th ed. 1996. (Scott Brown's Otolaryngology Ser.: Vol. 2). 640p. (*0-7506-0596-0*) E A GBR. *Dist:* OUP.

Adult Behavior Therapy Casebook. C. G. Last & M. Hersen. 1994. LC 93-6252. 324p. (C). pap. 41.00 (*0-306-44459-3*, Kluwer Plenum) Kluwer Academic.

Adult Behavior Therapy Casebook. Ed. by Cynthia G. Last & Michel Herson. 1993. LC 93-6252. (Illus.). 324p. (C). 65.00 (*0-306-44451-8*, Kluwer Plenum) Kluwer Academic.

Adult Bullying: Perpetrators & Victims. Peter Randall. 1997. LC 96-1856. 192p. (C). 78.95 (*0-415-12672-X*); pap. 24.95 (*0-415-12673-8*) Routledge.

Adult-Child Interaction & the Promise of Language Acquisition. Jean A. Rondal. 1985. 236p. 67.00 (*0-275-90157-2*, C0157, Praeger Pubs) Greenwood.

Adult-Child Relations. Rudolf Dreikurs. 1972. reprint ed. pap. 6.00 (*0-918560-13-6*) Adler Sch Prof Psy.

Adult-Child Research & Experience: Personal & Professional Legacies of a Dysfunctional, Co-Dependent Family. Robert E. Haskell & University of New England Staff. Ed. by Glenn R. Caddy. 1993. LC 92-21896. (Developments in Clinical Psychology Ser.). 276p. (C). 77.00 (*0-89391-755-9*); pap. 39.50 (*1-56750-077-3*) Greenwood (Ablex).

Adult Children of Dysfunctional Families: Prevention, Intervention, & Treatment for Community Mental Health Promotion. Barbara C. Wallace. 1996. LC 95-45415. 328p. 72.50 (*0-275-94475-1*, Praeger Pubs) Greenwood.

Adult Cognition: An Experimental Psychology of Human Aging. Timothy A. Salthouse. 1982. (Cognitive Development Ser.). (Illus.). 253p. 92.00 (*0-387-90728-9*) Spr-Verlag.

Adult Critical Care. SCCM Staff. 1999. 170p. pap. text 175.00 (*0-7872-5755-9*, 41575501) Kendall-Hunt.

Adult Day Care: A Practical Guide. Carole L. O'Brien. 1982. LC 81-16212. (Nursing-Health Science Ser.). (Illus.). 400p. (C). text 42.95 (*0-8185-0506-0*, 506-0) Jones & Bartlett.

Adult Day Care: A Practical Guidebook & Manual. Intro. by Lenore A. Tate. 1989. LC 88-2773. (Activities, Adaptation & Aging Ser.: Vol. 11, No. 2). (Illus.). 144p. text 39.95 (*0-86656-711-9*) Haworth Pr.

Adult Developing & Aging. Cavanaugh. 2nd ed. 1993. (Psychology Ser.). pap., stu. ed. 19.95 (*0-534-17253-9*) Brooks-Cole.

Adult Development. Rybash et al. 3rd ed. 1995. tchr. ed. 14.68 (*0-697-10504-0*) McGraw.

Adult Development: A New Dimension in Psychodynamic Theory & Practice. Calvin A. Colarusso & Robert A. Nemiroff. 1981. LC 80-20250. (Critical Issues in Psychiatry Ser.). (Illus.). 320p. (C). 49.50 (*0-306-40619-5*, Plenum Trade) Perseus Pubng.

Adult Development: Models & Methods in the Study of Adolescent & Adult Thought, Vol. 2. Ed. by Michael L. Commons et al. 1990. LC 88-27425. 304p. 72.50 (*0-275-92755-5*, C2755, Praeger Pubs) Greenwood.

Adult Development & Aging. John C. Cavanaugh. 1989. 587p. (C). mass mkt. 45.50 (*0-534-11640-X*) Brooks-Cole.

Adult Development & Aging. Diane E. Papalia et al. 1995. LC 95-39802. 609p. (C). text 72.50 (*0-07-048756-1*) McGrw-H Hghr Educ.

Adult Development & Aging. John C. Cavanaugh. 2nd ed. 1993. LC 92-2316. (C). text 47.50 (*0-534-17250-4*) Brooks-Cole.

Adult Development & Aging. Marion Perlmutter & Elizabeth Hall. 2nd ed. 1992. 608p. (C). 77.95 (*0-471-51846-8*) Wiley.

Adult Development & Aging. Rybash. 5th ed. 2000. pap. text 37.75 (*0-697-36202-7*) McGraw.

Adult Development & Aging: Myths & Emerging Realities. Schulz et al. 3rd ed. 1998. LC 98-30673. 421p. (C). 82.67 (*0-13-080766-4*) P-H.

Adult Development of Career Army Officers. Jeffrey A. McNally. 1991. LC 91-8028. 296p. 72.95 (*0-275-93698-8*, C3698, Praeger Pubs) Greenwood.

Adult Development, Therapy, & Culture: A Postmodern Synthesis. Gerald D. Young. 1997. LC 96-38958. (Series in Adult Development & Aging). (Illus.). 396p. (C). 55.00 (*0-306-45353-3*, Plenum Trade) Perseus Pubng.

Adult Dyslexic: Interventions & Outcomes. David McLoughlin et al. 1997. 150p. 39.95 (*1-56593-914-X*, 1810) Singular Publishing.

Adult Emergency Nursing Procedures. Jean A. Proehl. 1993. (Nursing-Health Science Ser.). (Illus.). 619p. (C). text 62.95 (*0-86720-328-5*, 328-5) Jones & Bartlett.

Adult Health Case Studies: Nurse Practitional Certification Review. Kathleen M. Shurpin et al. 1999. LC 99-19658. (Nurse Practitioner Certification Review Ser.). 176p. pap. 40.00 (*0-8385-0392-6*) P-H.

Adult Health Nursing. Ed. by Bullock. 1990. (C). text (*0-321-01538-X*) Addson-Wesley Educ.

Adult Health Nursing. Ignatavici. 1997. text (*0-7216-4266-7*) Saunders.

Adult Health Nursing. Patricia Gauntlett Beare & Judith L. Myers. 3rd ed. 1998. (Illus.). 1920p. (*84-8174-372-0*) Mosby-Doyma Libros ESP. *Dist:* Mosby Inc.

Adult Health Nursing. Barbara L. Christensen & Elaine O. Kockrow. 3rd ed. 1998. (C). stu. ed. (*0-323-00315-X*); tchr. ed. (*0-323-00156-4*) Mosby Inc.

Adult Health Nursing. Barbara L. Christensen et al. 3rd ed. 1998. (Illus.). 768p. stu. ed. (*0-323-00153-X*); (C). pap. text 39.00 (*0-323-00157-2*) Mosby Inc.

Adult Health Nursing: A Study Guide. Carol R. Kneisl. 1986. (C). pap. text, stu. ed. 20.25 (*0-201-12651-6*) Addison-Wesley.

Adult Health Nursing: Includes Testbank. Patricia G. Beare & Judith L. Myers. 3rd ed. 1998. tchr. ed. (*0-8151-1008-1*) Mosby Inc.

Adult Health Nursing: Nursing Drug Guide Package. Patricia G. Beare & Judith L. Myers. 3rd ed. 1998. (Illus.). 1920p. (*0-323-00497-0*) Mosby Inc.

Adult Hemiplegia: Evaluation & Treatment. Berta Bobath. 3rd ed. 1990. 208p. pap. text 42.50 (*0-7506-0168-X*) Buttrwrth-Heinemann.

Adult Hip Ed. by John Callaghan et al. 1997. LC 97-28141. (Illus.). 1,712p. text 359.00 (*0-397-51704-1*) Lppncott W & W.

Adult Hip. John J. Callaghan et al. 1997. LC 97-28141. 1,712p. text 499.00 (*0-7817-1429-X*) Lppncott W & W.

Adult Leukemia: A Comprehensive Guide for Patients & Families. Barb Lackritz. 2001. LC 00-46478. (Patient-Centered Guides Ser.). (Illus.). 500p. pap. 29.95 (*0-596-50001-7*, Patient-Centered) OReilly & Assocs.

Adult Leukemias. Clara D. Bloomfield. 1982. text 226.00 (*90-247-2478-3*) Kluwer Academic.

***Adult Limb Fractures.** Siddiqui & Rushton. 2001. (Illus.). 102p. pap. (*1-84110-078-1*) Greenwich Med GBR. *Dist:* JAMCO Dist.

Adult Motor Speech Disorders Research Guide. Roth. 2001. pap. 40.00 net. (*0-7693-0113-4*) Singular Publishing.

Adult Neurogenic Language Disorders: Assessment & Treatment - A Comprehensive Ethnobiological Approach. Joan C. Payne. 1997. LC 97-6441. 405p. pap. text 65.95 (*1-56593-729-5*, 1418) Thomson Learn.

Adult Neurology. Jody Corey-Bloom. 4th ed. 1997. LC 97-27321. (Neurology Psychiatry Access Ser.). (Illus.). 456p. (C). (gr. 13). text 64.95 (*0-8151-1854-6*, 28571) Mosby Inc.

Adult Nurse Practitioner. Jack Rudman. 1994. (Certified Nurse Examination Ser.: CN-1). 47.95 (*0-8373-6151-6*); pap. 27.95 (*0-8373-6101-X*) Nat Learn.

Adult Nurse Practitioner Certification. JoAnn Zerwekh & Jo C. Claborn. Ed. by Robin Carter. 1999. LC 98-34769. 235p. (C). pap. text 40.00 (*0-7216-7744-4*) Saunders.

Adult Nurse Practitioner Certification Prep Exams. Amelie Hollier et al. 1998. 300p. (C). pap. text (*1-892418-04-5*) APEA.

Adult Nurse Practitioner Certification Review Guide. Ed. by Virginia L. Millonig & Sally Miller. 3rd ed. 1998. LC 98-30168. 700p. (C). pap. text 52.00 (*1-878028-16-2*) Hlth Lead Assoc.

Adult Nurse Practitioner Certification Study Question Book. Sally K. Miller. 1999. LC 99-22641. 300p. pap. text 35.00 (*1-878028-20-0*) Hlth Lead Assoc.

Adult Nurse Practitioner Review Course, Set. Anne Nichols & Michael Gibbs. 2000. (Illus.). 199.95 (*0-9679170-1-8*) NPeducationcom.

Adult Nurses Practitioner Certification Review. John's Hopkins University Staff. 1998. LC 2001-32641. (Illus.). 800p. 47.95 (*1-55664-429-9*) Mosby Inc.

Adult Nursing. Jack Rudman. (Regents College Proficiency Examination Ser.: Vol. 35). 43.95 (*0-8373-5485-4*); (ACT Proficiency Examination Program Ser.: Vol. 39). 43.95 (*0-8373-5589-3*); 1994. (ACT Proficiency Examination Program Ser.: PEP-39). pap. 23.95 (*0-8373-5539-7*); 1994. (Regents College Proficiency Examination Ser.: Vol. CPEP-35). pap. 23.95 (*0-8373-5435-8*) Nat Learn.

Adult Nursing: Acute & Community Care. Lenette O. Burrell et al. 2nd ed. 1996. LC 96-12365. (Illus.). 2064p. (C). 100.00 (*0-8385-0174-5*, A0174-1) P-H.

***Adult Nursing: Care Plans Value Pack.** Burrell & Jaffe. 2nd ed. (Illus.). 1997. suppl. ed. 124.67 (*0-8385-0192-3*); 1996. stu. ed., suppl. ed. 151.87 (*0-8385-0191-5*) Appleton & Lange (Medical Exam).

Adult Nursing in Hospital & Community Settings. Mary Jo Gerlach. 2nd ed. 1996. (C). pap. text, stu. ed. 21.95 (*0-8385-0180-X*) P-H.

Adult Obesity Therapy. Michael D. Lebow. 1989. (Psychology Practitioner Guidebooks). 160p. text 28.00 (*0-08-035556-0*); pap. text 14.95 (*0-08-035555-2*) Elsevier (Pergamon Pr).

Adult Orthopaedics Ed. by Richard L. Cruess & William R. Rennie. 1992. (Illus.). 1566p. text (*0-443-08107-7*) Church.

Adult Pain Management & Sedation Handbook. Myron Yaster et al. 2000. (Illus.). 600p. (YA). (gr. 13). pap. text 36.95 (*0-8151-9675-X*, 29471) Mosby Inc.

Adult Personality Development: Applications, Vol. 2. Lawrence S. Wrightsman. 1994. 272p. (C). pap. 34.95 (*0-8039-4402-0*, 3324) Sage.

Adult Personality Development, Vol. 1: Theories & Concepts, Vol. 1. Lawrence S. Wrightsman. 1994. 250p. (C). 67.95 (*0-8039-4399-7*, 3321); pap. 34.95 (*0-8039-4400-4*, 3322) Sage.

Adult Personality Development, Vol. 2: Applications, Vol. 2. Lawrence S. Wrightsman. 1994. 272p. (C). 67.95 (*0-8039-4401-2*, 3323) Sage.

Adult Personality-Inventory Manual. Samuel E. Krug. 1984. pap. text 25.00 (*0-918296-18-8*) Inst Personality & Ability.

Adult Play: A Reversal Theory Approach. Ed. by J. H. Kerr & Michael J. Apter. 1991. 194p. (*90-265-1014-4*) Swets.

Adult Primary Care. Pamela Meredith & Nancy Mathes Horan. 1999. LC 99-26387. (Illus.). 750p. text 65.00 (*0-7216-6037-1*) Saunders.

Adult Psychiatry. Ed. by Samuel B. Guze. 1996. LC 96-15338. (Neurology Psychiatry Access Ser.). (Illus.). 544p. (C). (gr. 13). text 66.95 (*0-8151-3993-4*, 26880) Mosby Inc.

Adult Psychological Problems: An Introduction. Ed. by Michael J. Power & Lorna A. Champion. 1992. LC 92-226724. 224p. 85.00 (*0-7507-0037-8*); pap. 29.95 (*0-7507-0038-6*) Taylor & Francis (Falmer Pr).

Adult Psychopathology: A Social Work Perspective. Ed. by Francis J. Turner. 1984. LC 83-48127. 704p. (C). 39.95 (*0-02-933000-9*) Free Pr.

Adult Psychopathology & Diagnosis. Ed. by Samuel M. Turner & Michel Hersen. 3rd ed. 1997. LC 96-42980. 640p. 103.00 (*0-471-11716-1*) Wiley.

Adult Psychotherapy Progress Notes Planner. Arthur E. Jongsma. 2000. (Practice Planners Ser.). 304p. pap. 100.00 incl. disk (*0-471-38105-5*) Wiley.

Adult Rehabilitation: A Team Approach for Therapists. Martha K. Logigian. 1982. 31.50 (*0-316-53083-2*, Little Brwn Med Div) Lppncott W & W.

Adult Relationships: Critical Issues & Analyses. William G. Emener. 1998. LC 98-27524. lib. bdg. 59.00 (*1-56072-590-7*) Nova Sci Pubs.

Adult Respiratory Distress Syndrome. Ed. by Warren M. Zapol & Francois LeMaire. 2nd ed. 1990. (Lung Biology in Health & Disease Ser.: Vol. 50). (Illus.). 616p. text 215.00 (*0-8247-8359-X*) Dekker.

Adult Respiratory Distress Syndrome: An Aspect of Multiple Organ Failure Results of a Prospective Clinical Study. Ed. by J. A. Sturm. 1991. (Illus.). 320p. 118.00 (*0-387-52180-1*) Spr-Verlag.

Adult Rheumatic Diseases. Ed. by Jeanne Melvin & Victoria Gall. 2000. (Rheumatologic Rehabilitation Ser.: Vol. 2). (Illus.). pap. (*1-56900-139-1*) Am Occup Therapy.

Adult Scoliosis. Ed. by P. Bartolozzi et al. 1990. (Progress in Spinal Pathology Ser.). (Illus.). 170p. 54.95 (*0-387-82201-1*) Spr-Verlag.

***Adult Severe Mental Illness.** Alain Gregoire. 2000. (Greenwich Medical Media Ser.). (Illus.). 410p. text (*1-900151-52-9*) Greenwich Med GBR. *Dist:* JAMCO Dist.

Adult Spine: Principles & Practice, Set. Ed. by John W. Frymoyer et al. 2nd ed. 1996. LC 95-23863. (Illus.). 2,590p. text 399.00 (*0-7817-0329-8*, 2927) Lppncott W & W.

Adult Survivors of Child Sexual Abuse. Christine A. Courtois. 1993. LC 93-18434. (Workshop Models for Family Life Education Ser.). 144p. pap. 18.95 (*0-87304-247-6*) Manticore Pubs.

Adult Survivors of Sexual Abuse: Treatment Innovations. Mic Hunter. 1995. LC 94-49383. 152p. 61.95 (*0-8039-7192-3*, 1063); pap. 31.95 (*0-8039-7193-1*, 1064) Sage.

Adult T-Cell Leukaemia. Ed. by Kiyoshi Takatsuki. 1995. (Illus.). 288p. 98.00 (*0-19-262284-6*) OUP.

Adult T-Cell Leukemia in Japan. Ed. by M. Corn & Stuart Roath. 1990. (Hematology Reviews & Communications Ser.: Vol. 3, No. 4). 102p. pap. text 225.00 (*3-7186-4933-0*) Gordon & Breach.

Adult Years: Continuity & Change. Ed. by Martha Storandt & Gary R. VandenBos. 1989. (APA Master Lectures: Vol. 8). 167p. pap. 24.95 (*1-55798-061-6*) Am Psychol.

Adulthood & Aging. Gisela Labouvie-Vief. 1996. text (*0-7167-2931-8*) W H Freeman.

Adulthood & Aging: An Interdisciplinary Developmental View. Douglas C. Kimmel. 3rd ed. 1989. LC 89-38339. 656p. 77.95 (*0-471-63580-4*) Wiley.

Adults with Autism: A Guide to Theory & Practice. Ed. by Hugh Morgan. 1996. (Illus.). 312p. (C). text 110.00 (*0-521-45070-5*); pap. text 41.95 (*0-521-45683-5*) Cambridge U Pr.

***Adults with Autism & Mental Retardation.** Bengt Akerstrom. 2001. (Studia Psychologica Upsaliensia: No. 20). (Illus.). 156p. pap. (*91-554-4977-8*) Uppsala Universitet SWE. *Dist:* Coronet Bks.

Adults with Developmental Disabilities: Current Approaches to Occupational Therapy. Ed. by Mildred Ross & Susan Bachner. 1998. 360p. pap. text 37.00 (*1-56900-084-0*, 1140) Am Occup Therapy.

Adults with Learning Difficulties: Curriculum, Choice & Empowerment: A Handbook of Good Practice. Jeannie Sutcliffe. 1990. 144p. pap. (*0-335-09609-3*) OpUniv Pr.

Adults with Learning Disabilities: A Practical Approach for Health Professionals. Jean O'Hara & Anthea Sperlinger. 1997. LC 97-17410. 256p. 100.00 (*0-471-97665-2*) Wiley.

Adults with Self Concepts about Health, Disorders & Disease: Index of New Information. Roger Z. Bronston. 1998. 57.50 (*0-7883-1808-X*); pap. 47.50 (*0-7883-1809-8*) ABBE Pubs Assn.

Advance Cardiac Life. Mistovich & Benner. 1997. 1p. (C). pap., tchr. ed. 295.00 (*0-8359-5145-6*) P-H.

Advance Directives. Joint Commission on Accreditation of Healthcare Organizations. 1999. (Topics in Clinical Care Improvement Ser.). (Illus.). 76p. pap. 19.95 (*0-86688-607-9*, CC-900) Joint Comm Hlthcare.

Advance Directives: Making End of Life Decisions. Linda O'Brien. 1996. 64p. (C). (gr. 13). text 99.00 incl. VHS (*0-8151-3709-5*, 30522) Mosby Inc.

Advance Directives - Making End of Life Decisions - Resource Guide & Photo Package. Linda A. O'Brien. 1996. 64p. (*0-8151-3628-5*) Mosby Inc.

Advance Directives & End of Life Discussions - A Manual for Instructors. Robert McCann et al. 1997. 11p. 80.00 (*1-892273-00-4*) U Rchstr Med & Dntstry.

Advance Directives & Surrogate Decision Making in Health Care: United States, Germany, & Japan. Hans-Martin Sass et al. 1998. LC 98-2598. 328p. 52.00 (*0-8018-5831-3*) Johns Hopkins.

Advance Directives & the Pursuit of Death with Dignity. Norman L. Cantor. 1993. LC 92-46072. (Medical Ethics Ser.). 228p. 29.95 (*0-253-31304-X*) Ind U Pr.

Advance Directives in Medicine. Ed. by Chris Hackler et al. 1989. LC 89-3562. 202p. 62.50 (*0-275-93233-8*, C3233, Praeger Pubs) Greenwood.

Advance in Stereotactic & Functional Neurosurgery: Proceedings of the Sixth Meeting of the European Society for Stereotatic & Functional Neurisurgery, Rome 1983. Ed. by J. M. Gybels et al. 1984. (Acta Neurochirurgica Ser.: No. 33). (Illus.). 583p. 219.00 (*0-387-81773-5*) Spr-Verlag.

Advance Medical Life Support: A Practical Approach to Adult Medical Emergencies. Alice L. Dalton et al. 1998. LC 98-21745. 480p. pap. 57.00 (*0-8359-5179-0*) P-H.

Advance of American Nursing. Philip A. Kalisch & Beatrice J. Kalisch. 2nd ed. 1986. (Illus.). 851p. (C). text 34.50 (*0-673-39392-5*) Lppncott W & W.

Advance of American Nursing. Philip A. Kalisch. 3rd ed. 1995. 560p. text 52.95 (*0-397-55089-8*) Lppncott W & W.

Advance Practice of Psychiatric Nursing. Ann Wolbert Burgess. 1997. LC 97-11817. 560p. 65.00 (*0-8385-0181-8*, A-0181-6) P-H.

Advanced Abnormal Child Psychology. Ed. by Michel Hersen & Robert T. Ammerman. 1995. 464p. text 99.95 (*0-8058-1203-2*) L Erlbaum Assocs.

Advanced Abnormal Psychology. Ed. by Michel Hersen & Vincent B. Van Hasselt. 2nd ed. 2000. LC 00-46624. (Illus.). xviii, 627p. 65.00 (*0-306-46381-4*, Kluwer Plenum) Kluwer Academic.

Advanced Abnormal Psychology. Ed. by Michel Hersen & Vincent B. Van Hasselt. 1994. 558p. 45.00 (*0-306-44547-6*, Plenum Trade) Perseus Pubng.

Advanced Aerohemodynamics. 1984. 17.95 (*0-930835-04-2*) Med Res Assocs.

Advanced & Critical Care Oncology Nursing: Managing Primary Complications. Cynthia C. Chernecky & Barbara J. Berger. Ed. by Barbara N. Cullen. 1997. LC 97-7109. 624p. pap. 39.95 (*0-7216-6860-7*) Saunders.

Advanced & Specialist Nursing Practice. George Casteldine & Paula McGee. 1998. LC 98-25008. pap. 49.95 (*0-632-04248-6*) Blackwell Sci.

Advanced Applications of Law & Ethics: A Workbook for Master-Level Clinicians. 4th rev. ed. 1998. 200p. pap. text, wbk. ed. 47.00 (*0-9654534-1-3*) F C Grosso.

Advanced Arrhythmias. Louise A. Smith. 1987. (Orig.). pap. (*0-932491-80-4*) Res Appl Inc.

A
B

Advanced Arthritis Study Guide. Competence Assurance Systems Staff. 1986. pap. text 235.00 (*0-89147-068-9*) CAS.

Advanced Arthroscopy. Ed. by J. C. Y. Chow. 2000. LC 99-31870. (Illus.). 768p. 250.00 (*0-387-98808-4*) Spr-Verlag.

Advanced Assessment & Clinical Diagnosis. Joyce Dains et al. 1998. LC 98-14984. (Illus.). 464p. (C). (gr. 13). pap. text 49.95 (*0-8151-3627-7*, 30504) Mosby Inc.

Advanced Atlas of Histology. W. H. Freeman & Brian Bracegirdle. 1976. (Heinemann Educational Bks.). (C). text 25.00 (*0-435-60317-5*, 60317) Heinemann.

Advanced Breast Cancer: A Guide to Living with Metastatic Disease. Musa Mayer. Ed. by Linda Lamb. 2nd ed. 1998. LC 98-38919. (Patient-Centered Guides Ser.). (Illus.). 540p. pap. 27.95 (*1-56592-522-X*) OReilly & Assocs.

Advanced Cancer: Living Each Day. rev. ed. 1995. (Illus.). 32p. pap. text 15.00 (*0-7881-2469-2*) DIANE Pub.

Advanced Cardiac Care in the Streets. Taylor. 1997. pap. text (*0-316-83353-3*) Lppncott W & W.

Advanced Cardiac Care in the Streets. Raymond V. Taylor. 1997. LC 97-36819. 320p. pap. text 27.95 (*0-7817-1462-1*) Lppncott W & W.

Advanced Cardiac Life Support. Householde. 1997. pap. text (*0-7216-4726-X*) Harcourt.

Advanced Cardiac Life Support. Advanced Life Support Group. 2nd ed. 1997. (Illus.). 272p. pap. text (*0-412-71090-0*) E A GBR. *Dist:* OUP.

Advanced Cardiac Life Support: Certification Preparation & Review. Bruce R. Shade et al. 1985. (Illus.). 640p. pap. text 26.95 (*0-89303-272-7*) P-H.

Advanced Cardiac Life Support: The Practical Approach. Advanced Life Support Group. 1993. LC 92-49023. 224p. (gr. 13). pap. 44.95 (*0-412-48390-4*) Chapman & Hall.

Advanced Cardiac Life Support Algorithms & Drugs: A Handbook for Adult & Pediatric Providers, 1993. Subcommittee on Advanced Cardiac Life Support Staf. 1993. (Illus.). 54p. (Orig.). pap. text (*0-87493-625-X*) Am Heart.

Advanced Cardiac Life Support Manual for Course Preparation & Review. Joseph J. Mistovich et al. 1997. LC 97-8217. 448p. (C). pap. text 42.00 (*0-8359-5050-6*) P-H.

Advanced Cardiac Life Support, 1997. 1997. (Emergency Cardiovascular Care Programs Ser.). (Illus.). 376p. pap., tchr. ed. 25.00 (*0-87493-623-3*); 375p. pap. 25.00 (*0-87493-617-9*) Am Heart.

Advanced Cardiac Treatment System (ACTS) David P. Doernbach. 1996. (Illus.). 20p. (Orig.). pap., spiral bd. 65.00 (*0-9638043-4-0*) Vital Signs.

Advanced Case Management: Outcomes & Beyond. Suzanne K. Powell. 1999. LC 99-40665. 352p. pap. text 42.95 (*0-7817-2234-9*) Lppncott W & W.

Advanced Clinical Skills & Physical Diagnosis. Dale D. Berg. 1998. LC 98-27856. (Illus.). 471p. pap. 39.95 (*0-86542-544-2*) Blackwell Sci.

Advanced Concepts & Applications, Vol. II. Ed. by Robert W. Broyles & Colin Lay. 1980. LC 79-23280. 557p. 88.00 Aspen Pub.

Advanced Concepts for Geriatric Nursing Assistants. Carolyn A. MacDonald. 1994. LC 94-61648. (Illus.). 224p. (gr. 11-12). pap. 28.95 (*0-910251-71-1*, ACG73) Venture Pub PA.

Advanced Concepts in Alcoholism: Proceedings of the Symposium on Alcoholism from the International Congress on Applied Psychology, Edinburgh, July 1982. H. G. Tittmar. 1984. LC 83-22155. (Advances in Biosciences Ser.: Vol. 47). 189p. 37.00 (*0-08-030777-9*, Pergamon Pr) Elsevier.

Advanced Concepts in Arrhythmias, No. 3. Henry J. L. Marriott & Mary B. Conover. 3rd ed. 1998. LC 97-15127. (Advanced Concepts in Arrhythmias Ser.: Vol. 3). (Illus.). 416p. (C). (gr. 13). text 42.95 (*0-8151-2090-7*, 28310) Mosby Inc.

Advanced Controlled Delivery Technology, No. C-010X. 1994. 245p. 2650.00 (*1-56965-008-X*) BCC.

Advanced Core Curriculum for Oncology Nursing. Ed. by Rose M. Carroll-Johnson. 1998. LC 2001-20398. (Illus.). 430p. pap. 39.95 (*0-7216-7394-5*) Saunders.

Advanced Dermatologic Diagnosis. Walter P. Shelley & E. Dorinda Shelley. 1992. (Illus.). 1315p. text 255.00 (*0-7216-3433-8*) Saunders.

Advanced Dermatology Study Guide. Competence Assurance Systems Staff. 1980. pap. text 235.00 (*0-89147-062-X*) CAS.

Advanced Design in Nursing Research. Pamela J. Brink & Marilynn J. Wood. 2nd ed. 1998. LC 97-33824. 69.95 (*0-8039-5800-5*, 8495) Sage.

***Advanced Diabetes Management Review & Resource Manual.** Contrib. by American Association of Diabetes Educators Staff & Aleksandar Institute for Research, Education and Consultation and ANCC Staff. 2001. 250p. (C). pap. text 54.00 (*1-55810-158-6*) Am Nurses Pub.

Advanced Diving: Technology & Techniques. National Association of Underwater Instructors Staff. 1994. (Illus.). 304p. (gr. 13). pap. text 35.95 (*0-8151-6286-3*, 25366) Mosby Inc.

Advanced Electrocardiography. Stanley Anderson et al. 1992. (Biophysical Measurement Ser.). (Illus.). 120p. (Orig.). (C). 28.00 (*0-9627449-4-8*) SpaceLabs.

Advanced Emergency Medicine. J. Douglas White. 1997. (Illus.). 750p. text 85.00 (*0-07-069724-8*) McGraw.

Advanced Endoscopic Sinus Surgery. Nikhil J. Bhatt. 2001. 192.95 (*0-7693-0155-X*) Singular Publishing.

Advanced Evoked Potentials. Ed. by Hans Luders. 1989. (Topics in Neurosurgery Ser.). (C). text 155.00 (*0-89838-963-1*) Kluwer Academic.

Advanced First Aid. Susan Landers. 1993. (C). stu. ed. 14.00 (*1-881592-00-6*) Hayden-McNeil.

Advanced First Aid Afloat. Peter F. Eastman. 4th ed. 1996. pap. text 14.95 (*0-07-018839-4*) McGraw.

Advanced Glycation End Products in Nephrology: Meeting on Advanced Glycosylation End Products in Nephrology: Much More Than Diabetic Nephropathy, Padua, January 2000. Ed. by A. D'Angelo et al. 2000. LC 00-43440. (Contributions to Nephrology Ser.: Vol. 131). viii, 148p. 198.25 (*3-8055-7135-6*) S Karger.

Advanced Gynecological Laparoscopy: A Practical Guide. P. G. Cusumano & Jan A. Deprest. 1995. LC 95-25586. (Illus.). 244p. 97.95 (*1-85070-655-7*, Parthenon Pbng) CRC Pr.

Advanced Health & Social Care. Liam Clarke et al. 2nd ed. 1995. 448p. (Orig.). pap. (*0-7487-2225-4*) Nelson Thornes GBR. *Dist:* Trans-Atl Phila.

Advanced Health Assessment of Women: Clinical Skills & Procedures. Helen N. Carcio. 1999. LC 98-44544. 496p. spiral bd. 42.50 (*0-7817-1826-0*) Lppncott W & W.

Advanced Health Physics Library, Set. 1983. (Illus.). 1300p. 595.00 (*0-87683-692-9*) GP Courseware.

Advanced Human Nutrition. Denis M. Medeiros & Robert E. Wildman. 1999. LC 00-501620. (Modern Nutrition Ser.). (Illus.). 608p. 79.95 (*0-8493-8566-0*) CRC Pr.

Advanced Imaging in Coronary Artery Disease: PET, SPECT, MRI, IVUS, EBCT. E. Van der Wall. 1998. LC 98-17190. (Developments in Cardiovascular Medicine Ser.). 348p. 130.00 (*0-7923-5083-9*) Kluwer Academic.

Advanced Immunoassays in Rheumatology. Marius Teodorescu. 1994. 400p. lib. bdg. 180.95 (*0-8493-5974-0*, RC934) CRC Pr.

Advanced Immunology. David Male et al. 3rd ed. 1996. 54.00 (*0-7234-2059-9*) Mosby Inc.

Advanced Interpretation of Clinical Laboratory Data. Ed. by Camille Heusghem et al. 1982. (Clinical & Biochemical Analysis Ser.: Vol. 13). (Illus.). 448p. text 189.00 (*0-8247-1744-9*) Dekker.

Advanced Intraoperative Technologies in Neurosurgery. Ed. by V. A. Fasano. 1986. (Illus.). 330p. 89.00 (*0-387-81880-4*) Spr-Verlag.

Advanced IPA Management: Direct Contracting. William J. DeMarco. 1999. LC 99-19184. (*0-07-134320-2*) McGraw.

Advanced IPA Management: Opportunities under the New Medicare. Contrib. by Jenifer Marx. 1998. LC 98-53664. (HFMA Healthcare Financial Management Ser.). (Illus.). viii, 119p. (*0-07-134321-0*) McGraw.

***Advanced Laboratory Methods in Haematology.** R. M. Rowan. Ed. by O. W. van Assendelft & F. E. Preston. 2001. (Arnold Publication). 256p. text (*0-340-80617-6*) E A GBR. *Dist:* OUP.

Advanced Laparoscopic Technique. M. Katkhouda. 1997. (Illus.). 250p. (C). text 125.00 (*0-7020-2039-7*) Harcourt.

Advanced Life Support for the Boards. Matt Flynn. 2nd ed. 1999. LC 99-20849. 160p. pap. text 19.95 (*0-7817-1976-3*) Lppncott W & W.

Advanced Life Support Skills. Jackson E. Allison et al. 1993. LC 93-19346. (Illus.). 304p. (YA). (gr. 13). pap. text 22.95 (*0-8016-7426-3*, 00200) Mosby Inc.

Advanced Medical Radiation Dosimetry. K. N. Govinda Rajan. 1992. 522p. pap. 23.95 (*0-87692-706-1*) Med Physics Pub.

Advanced Medical Terminology. Stiles. 1999. pap. text (*0-7216-4733-2*) Saunders.

***Advanced Medical Transcription SUM Program.** Health Professions Institute Staff. 2001. pap. 296.00 (*0-13-071833-5*) P-H.

Advanced Medicine. Ed. by Bellingham. 1975. 32.00 (*0-8464-4455-0*) Beekman Pubs.

Advanced Medicine. Ed. by Harper & Muir. 1972. 32.00 (*0-8464-4454-2*) Beekman Pubs.

Advanced Medicine: Topics in Therapeutics. A. M. Breckenridge. (Pitman Medical Conference Reports). (Illus.). No. 1. 1975. 200p. pap. 32.00 (*0-8464-0114-2*); No. 3. 1976. pap. 32.00 (*0-8464-0115-0*); No. 4. 1977. 32.00 (*0-8464-0116-9*) Beekman Pubs.

Advanced Medicine, Eleven: Proceedings of the 11th Annual Symposium on Advanced Medicine 1975. Ed. by A. F. Lant. 1975. (Illus.). 450p. (Orig.). 42.00 (*0-8464-0112-6*) Beekman Pubs.

Advanced Medicine Twelve: Proceedings of the 12th Annual Symposium of Advanced Medicine, 1976. Ed. by D. K. Peters. 1976. (Illus.). 32.00 (*0-8464-0117-7*) Beekman Pubs.

Advanced Methods of Pharmacokinetic & Pharmacodynamic Systems Analysis. Ed. by David Z. D'Argenio. 1991. (Illus.). 220p. (C). text 85.00 (*0-306-44028-8*, Kluwer Plenum) Kluwer Academic.

Advanced Methods of Pharmacokinetic & Pharmacodynamic Systems Analysis Vol. 2: Proceedings of a Meeting Held in Los Angeles, California, May 21-22, 1993, Vol. 2. Ed. by David Z. D'Argenio. 1995. (Illus.). 228p. (C). text 85.00 (*0-306-45018-6*, Kluwer Plenum) Kluwer Academic.

Advanced Methods of Physiological System Modeling, Vol. 2. Ed. by Vasilis Z. Marmarelis. 1989. (Illus.). 310p. (C). text 85.00 (*0-306-43259-5*, Kluwer Plenum) Kluwer Academic.

Advanced Methods of Physiological System Modeling, Vol. I. Intro. by Vasilis Z. Marmarelis. 1987. (Illus.). 344p. (C). reprint ed. text 35.00 (*0-941639-01-0*) USC Biomedical.

Advanced Models of Cognition for Medical Training & Practice. Ed. by D. A. Evans & V. I. Patel. 1992. (NATO ASI Ser.: Vol. 97). (Illus.). 372p. 133.00 (*0-387-55884-5*) Spr-Verlag.

Advanced Molecular Genetics. K. N. Timmis. Ed. by A. Puhler. 1986. (Illus.). 347p. 142.00 (*0-387-12740-2*) Spr-Verlag.

***Advanced Neurobiology of Physical Activity.** Phillip F. Gardiner. 2001. LC 00-54203. (Illus.). xvii, 237p. (*0-7360-0126-3*) Human Kinetics.

Advanced Neurosurgical Navigation. Eben Alexander & Robert J. Maciunas. 1998. LC 98-21792. (Illus.). 624p. 199.00 (*0-86577-767-5*) Thieme Med Pubs.

Advanced Nursing & Health Care Research. McLaughlin. 1990. (Illus.). 393p. text 69.00 (*0-7216-3098-7*) Saunders.

Advanced Nursing Practice. Suzanne Rita et al. Ed. by Linda Larson & Darcy Egging. unabr. ed. 1997. 113p. (Orig.). pap. 33.00 (*0-935890-09-2*) Emerg Nurses IL.

Advanced Nursing Practice: An Intergrated Approach. Ann B. Hamric & Judith A. Spross. Ed. by Thomas Eoyang. 1996. (Illus.). 654p. text 42.00 (*0-7216-5894-6*) Saunders.

***Advanced Nursing Skills: Principles & Practice.** Molly Courtenay. 2000. (Illus.). 136p. pap. (*1-84110-036-6*) Greenwich Med.

Advanced Nutrition: Macronutrients. Carolyn D. Berdanier. 1994. LC 94-11519. (Modern Nutrition Ser.). (Illus.). 304p. 104.95 (*0-8493-8500-8*, 8500) CRC Pr.

Advanced Nutrition: Micronutrients. Carolyn D. Berdanier. 1997. (Modern Nutrition Ser.). 256p. (C). 94.95 (*0-8493-2664-8*) CRC Pr.

Advanced Nutrition & Human Metabolism. Jim Groff & Sareen Gropper. 2nd ed. 1995. LC 94-24711. 550p. (C). 58.00 (*0-314-04467-1*) West Pub.

Advanced Nutrition & Human Metabolism. James L. Groff & Sareen S. Gropper. 3rd ed. 1999. LC 99-27331. (Health Sciences Ser.). 575p. spiral bd. 98.95 (*0-534-55521-7*) Wadsworth Pub.

Advanced Nutritional Therapies: Evaluates Hundreds of Foods, Supplements, & Nutrients, & Shows How to Use Them to Achieve Maximal Health & Long Life. Kenneth Cooper. 1998. 368p. pap. 12.99 (*0-7852-7073-6*) Thomas Nelson Pubs.

Advanced Obstetrics & Gynecology Study Guide. Competence Assurance Systems Staff. 1980. pap. text 235.00 (*0-89147-111-1*) CAS.

Advanced Oncologic Surgery. Ed. by Mark S. Roh. 1993. LC 92-49490. (gr. 13). (*1-56375-021-X*) Gower-Mosby.

Advanced Operative Dentistry. Luiz N. Baratieri et al. Tr. by Sylvio Monteiro, Jr. & Fernando J. Volkmer from SPA. 1993. (POR., Illus.). 510p. text 126.00 (*85-7288-002-X*, B9997) Quint Pub Co.

Advanced Ophthalmic Investigative Techniques. C. B. James & Larry Benjamin. 2002. 160p. pap. 60.00 (*0-7506-4953-4*) Buttrwrth-Heinemann.

Advanced Osseointegration Surgery: Maxillfacial Applications. Philip Worthington & P. I. Branemark. 1992. LC 91-40446. (Illus.). text 148.00 (*0-86715-242-7*) Quint Pub Co.

Advanced Paediatric Life Support: The Practical Approach. 2nd ed. 1993. 320p. pap. text (*0-7279-1069-8*) BMJ Pub GBR. *Dist:* AIDC.

***Advanced Paediatric Life Support: The Practical Approach.** Advanced Life Support Group Staff. 3rd ed. 2001. 288p. pap. (*0-7279-1554-1*) BMJ Pub GBR. *Dist:* AIDC.

***Advanced Pediatric ER Nursing.** Emergency Nurses Association Staff. 2001. (Illus.). (C). pap. text 59.95 (*0-7637-1910-2*, 1910-2) Jones & Bartlett.

Advanced Personality. Ed. by David F. Barone et al. 1998. LC 98-21499. (Plenum Series in Social-Clinical Psychology). (Illus.). 406p. (C). 49.50 (*0-306-45745-8*, Plenum Trade) Perseus Pubng.

Advanced Pharmaceutical Solids. Jens T. Carstensen. 2000. LC 00-60192. (Drugs & the Pharmaceutical Sciences Ser.: Vol. 110). (Illus.). viii, 518p. text 195.00 (*0-8247-0431-2*) Dekker.

Advanced Practice in Cancer Nursing. Ed. by N. Jodrell et al. 1998. (Illus.). 280p. pap. (*0-443-06040-1*) Church.

***Advanced Practice in Nurses: Education, Roles & Trends.** Ada Romaine-Davis. 2nd ed. 2002. (Illus.). (C). pap. text 44.95 (*0-7637-1805-X*, 1805-X) Jones & Bartlett.

Advanced Practice Nurses: Education, Roles, Trends. Ada Romaine-Davis. 1997. (Nursing Ser.). (Illus.). 232p. (C). pap. text 44.95 (*0-7637-0370-2*, 0370-2) Jones & Bartlett.

Advanced Practice Nurses: Education, Roles, Trends. Ada Romaine-Davis. 1997. LC 97-1397. (*0-07-637037-2*) McGraw.

Advanced Practice Nurse's Legal Handbook. Rebecca F. Cady. 2002. 320p. pap. text 29.95 (*0-7817-2337-X*) Lppncott W & W.

Advanced Practice Nursing. Ed. by Mariah Snyder & Michaelene Mirr. 1995. (Illus.). 312p. 37.95 (*0-8261-8850-8*) Springer Pub.

Advanced Practice Nursing: A Guide to Professional Development. Ed. by Mariah Snyder & Michaelene Mirr. 2nd ed. 1999. LC 99-27973. (Illus.). 344p. text 37.95 (*0-8261-1281-1*) Springer Pub.

Advanced Practice Nursing: Emphasizing Common Roles. Christine M. Sheehy & Marianne C. McCarthy. 1998. LC 97-34612. (Illus.). 329p. pap. 34.95 (*0-8036-0234-0*) Davis Co.

Advanced Practice Nursing: Roles & Clinical Applications. Joanne V. Hickey et al. 2nd ed. 1999. LC 99-17499. 512p. text 41.95 (*0-7817-1754-X*) Lppncott W & W.

Advanced Practice Nursing in Psychiatric & Mental Health Care. American Psychiatric Nursing Association Staff. Ed. by Carole A. Shea et al. 1999. LC 99-29231. 704p. (C). text (*0-323-00352-4*) Mosby Inc.

Advanced Practice Nursing in the Community. Carl O. Helvie. 1997. LC 97-4752. 716p. 96.95 (*0-7619-0034-9*, 1657); pap. 46.95 (*0-7619 0035-7*, 1658) Sage.

Advanced Practice Nursing with Older Adults. Ed. by Neville E. Strumpf & Valerie T. Cotter. 2001. LC 00-54888. 576p. pap. 49.95 (*0-07-134157-9*) McGraw-Hill Prof.

Advanced Practitioner Exam Review for Respiratory Care: Guidelines for Success. William V. Wojciechowski. 1995. LC 94-10939. (Respiratory Care Ser.). 486p. (C). pap. text 64.95 (*0-8273-7270-1*) Delmar.

Advanced Practitioner Respiratory Care Review: Written Registry & Clinical Simulation Exam. Gary Persing. 1994. LC 93-20774. pap. text 43.00 (*0-7216-4963-7*) Saunders.

Advanced Precautions for Today's O. R. The Operating Room Professional's Handbook for the Prevention of Sharps Injuries & Bloodborne Exposures. Contrib. by Mark S. Davis. 1999. LC 98-60981. (*0-9664873-5-4*) Sweinbinder.

Advanced Professional Skin Care. Peter T. Pugliese. Ed. by Susan Pugliese et al. 1991. (Illus.). 428p. (C). text 119.95 (*0-9630211-0-9*) P T Pugliese.

Advanced Psychodiagnostic Interpretation of the Bender Gestalt Test: Adults & Children. Norman Reichenberg & Alan J. Raphael. 1992. LC 91-37456. 176p. 47.95 (*0-275-94163-9*, C4163, Praeger Pubs) Greenwood.

Advanced Psychosomatic Research in Obstetrics & Gynecology. Ed. by D. Richter et al. 1991. (Illus.). 262p. 107.00 (*0-387-52500-9*) Spr-Verlag.

Advanced Radiographic & Angiographic Procedures with an Introduction to Specialized Imaging. Marianne R. Tortorici & Patrick J. Apfel. 1995. LC 95-13456. (Illus.). 361p. (C). text 51.95 (*0-8036-8571-8*) Davis Co.

Advanced Reference Guide to the Transactional Analysis Literature. Theodore B. Novey. 1987. 80p. pap. 12.00 (*0-9617020-1-X*) TA Assocs.

Advanced Respiratory Education Course. Competence Assurance Systems Staff. 1985. (Illus.). pap. text 75.00 (*0-89147-106-5*) CAS.

Advanced Respiratory Therapy Exam Guide. Sills. 2nd ed. 2000. 456p. pap. text 45.00 (*0-323-00784-8*) Mosby Inc.

Advanced Skills & Compentency. Francine Wolgin. 1997. LC 97-34821. (Advanced Skills & Competency Assessments for Caregivers Ser.). 256p. (C). pap. text 35.20 (*0-8359-5167-7*) P-H.

Advanced Skills for Health Care Providers. Contrib. by Barbara Acello. 1999. LC 99-50248. 316p. pap. text 30.95 (*0-7668-1437-8*) Delmar.

Advanced Social Psychology. Abraham Tesser. 1994. LC 94-30982. 416p. (C). text 69.38 (*0-07-063392-4*) McGrw-H Hghr Educ.

Advanced Sport Diver: Instructor's Guide. Clinchy. 2nd ed. 1993. 32p. pap. text 7.95 (*0-8016-9033-1*) Mosby Inc.

Advanced Sport Diver: Workbook. Clinchy. 2nd ed. 1993. 35p. pap. text 6.95 (*0-8016-9032-3*) Mosby Inc.

***Advanced Strategies for Evaluation & Medical Management of Lower Respiratory Tract Infections: Daiichi-Sponsored Symposium Held in Conjunction with the 7th Western Pacific Congress of Chemotherapy & Infectious Diseases, Hong Kong, December 2000: Proceedings.** Ed. by Wah Kit Lam. 2001. (Illus.). 56p. pap. 25.25 (*3-8055-7323-5*) S Karger.

Advanced Surgical Recall. Lorne H. Blackbourne & Kirk J. Fleischer. 1997. LC 96-35097. (Illus.). 1,403p. pap. text 34.95 (*0-683-00834-X*) Lppncott W & W.

Advanced Techniques for Radiotherapy. Ed. by Marco Castiglioni & Argeo A. Benco. 1992. LC 92-49636. (Eurocourses Ser.: Vol. 2). 144p. (C). text 95.00 (*0-7923-1588-X*) Kluwer Academic.

Advanced Techniques in Central Nervous System Metastases. Ed. by Robert J. Maciunas. 1998. 323p. 95.00 (*1-879284-47-2*) Am Assn Neuro.

Advanced Techniques in Chromosome Research. Ed. by Kenneth W. Adolph. 1991. (Illus.). 472p. text 215.00 (*0-8247-8430-8*) Dekker.

Advanced Technologies in Research, Diagnosis & Treatment of AIDS & in Oncology. Ed. by G. Giraldo et al. 1994. LC 94-28616. (Antibiotics & Chemotherapy Ser.: Vol. 46). (Illus.). viii, 70p. 165.25 (*3-8055-5970-4*) S Karger.

Advanced Technology in Critical Care Nursing. John M. Clochesy. 1988. 203p. 73.00 (*0-8342-0023-6*, 20023) Aspen Pub.

Advanced Test Anxiety Research, Vol. 6. A. R. Schwarzer et al. 1989. viii, 312p. pap. (*90-265-0964-2*) Swets.

Advanced Therapeutic Endoscopy. Ed. by Jamie S. Barkin & Cesar A. O'Phelan. 2nd ed. 1994. 434p. text 175.00 (*0-7817-0155-4*) Lppncott W & W.

Advanced Therapist, Vol. 34, No. 1. Sarah Cobb et al. 1992. (Vision Therapist Ser.: Vol. 1). (Illus.). 156p. (Orig.). pap. text 18.00 (*0-943599-51-2*) OEPF.

Advanced Therapy in Cardiac Surgery. Kenneth L. Franco & Edward D. Verrier. 1999. 543p. incl. cd-rom (*1-55009-052-6*) DEKR.

Advanced Therapy in Thoracic Surgery. Kenneth L. Franco & Joe B. Putnam, Jr. 1998. (Illus.). 527p. incl. cd-rom (*1-55009-044-5*) DEKR.

Advanced Therapy of Breast Disease. S. Eva Singletary & Geoffrey L. Robb. 1999. 400p. incl. cd-rom (*1-55009-106-9*) DEKR.

Advanced Therapy of Inflammatory Bowel Disease. Theodore M. Bayless & Stephen B. Hanauer. 2000. 400p. (*1-55009-122-0*) DEKR.

Advanced Therapy of Prostatic Disease. Martin I. Resnick & Ian M. Thompson. 1999. 672p. incl. cd-rom (*1-55009-102-6*) DEKR.

Advanced Traditional Chinese Medicine Series Date not set. (*90-5199-319-6*) IOS Pr NLD. *Dist:* IOS Press.

Advanced Training Skills for Reproductive Health Professionals see Competences Avancees en Formation pour les Professionnels en Sante de la Reproduction

Advanced Training Skills for Reproductive Health Professionals. Rick Sullivan et al. 2000. (Illus.). 224p. (Orig.). pap. 15.00 (*0-929817-29-X*) JHPIEGO.

Advanced Trauma Life Support Course. American College of Surgeons Staff. 1994. (Illus.). (Orig.). (SPA.). stu. ed. (*1-880696-05-3*); stu. ed. (*1-880696-06-1*) Am Coll Surgeons.

Advanced Trauma Skills. Smith. 2000. pap. text 35.50 (*0-7216-6808-9*) Saunders.

Advanced Tutorials for the Biomedical Sciences: Animations, Simulations, & Calculations Using Mathematica. Ed. by Charles Pidgeon. 1996. LC 96-1059. (Illus.). 304p. pap. 79.95 incl. 3.5 ld, mac hd (*1-56081-950-2*, Wiley-VCH) Wiley.

Advancement in Iron Nutrition Research. A. Hemant Ranjan. 1994. pap. (*0-7855-2750-8*) Scientific Pubs IND. *Dist:* St Mut.

Advancement of Veterinary Science Vol. 1: Veterinary Medicine Beyond 2000, Vol. 1. A. R. Michell. 1993. (Advancement of Veterinary Science Ser.). (Illus.). 288p. text 100.00 (*0-85198-759-1*) OUP.

Advancement of Veterinary Science Vol. 2: Veterinary Education - The Future, Vol. 2. A. R. Michell. 1993. (Advancement of Veterinary Science Ser.). (Illus.). 240p. text 100.00 (*0-85198-760-5*) OUP.

Advancement of Veterinary Science Vol. 3: History of the Healing Professions, Vol. 3. Ed. by A. R. Michell. 1993. (Advancement of Veterinary Science Ser.). (Illus.). 160p. text 80.00 (*0-85198-761-3*) OUP.

Advancement of Veterinary Science, Vol. 4: Veterinary Science - Growth Points & Comparative Medicine, Vol. 4. Ed. by A. R. Michell. 1993. (Illus.). 240p. text 100.00 (*0-85198-762-1*) OUP.

Advances & Progress in Oral Health Through Oral Care Education: Scientific Proof of the Effectiveness of a Global Oral Health Education Initiative. Ed. by Stephen M. Siegel. 1998. (Illus.). 48p. pap. text (*0-9662849-0-9*) Prof Audience.

Advances & Technical Standards in Neurosurgery, Vol. 1. Ed. by H. Krayenbuhl et al. 1978. LC 74-10499. (Illus.). 210p. 96.00 (*0-387-81218-0*) Spr-Verlag.

Advances & Technical Standards in Neurosurgery. Ed. by H. Krayenbuhl. LC 74-10499. (Illus.). Vol. 2. 1975. 217p. 112.00 (*0-387-81293-8*); Vol. 3. 1976. 154p. 96.00 (*0-387-81381-0*) Spr-Verlag.

Advances & Technical Standards in Neurosurgery, Vol. 4. N. A. Lassan. 1977. LC 74-10499. 96.00 (*0-387-81423-X*) Spr-Verlag.

Advances & Technical Standards in Neurosurgery, Vol. 5. Ed. by H. Krayenbuehl et al. 1978. LC 74-10499. (Illus.). 224p. 132.00 (*0-387-81441-8*) Spr-Verlag.

Advances & Technical Standards in Neurosurgery, Vol. 6. H. Krayenbuehl et al. 1979. LC 74-10499. (Illus.). 112.00 (*0-387-81518-X*) Spr-Verlag.

Advances & Technical Standards in Neurosurgery, Vol. 6. Ed. by L. Symon et al. 1979. 191p. 107.00 (*3-211-81518-X*) Spr-Verlag.

Advances & Technical Standards in Neurosurgery, Vol. 7. Ed. by H. Krayenbuehl et al. 1980. (Illus.). 247p. 132.00 (*0-387-81592-9*) Spr-Verlag.

Advances & Technical Standards in Neurosurgery, Vol. 7. Ed. by L. Symon et al. 1980. 247p. 126.00 (*3-211-81592-9*) Spr-Verlag.

Advances & Technical Standards in Neurosurgery, Vol. 8. Ed. by H. Krayenbuehl et al. 1981. (Illus.). 328p. 145.00 (*0-387-81665-8*) Spr-Verlag.

Advances & Technical Standards in Neurosurgery. Ed. by L. Symon et al. Vol. 8. 1981. 328p. 138.00 (*3-211-81665-8*); Vol. 9. 1983. 177p. 99.95 (*3-211-81718-2*) Spr-Verlag.

Advances & Technical Standards in Neurosurgery, Vol. 10. Ed. by H. Krayenbuhl et al. 1984. (Illus.). 231p. 132.00 (*0-387-81750-6*) Spr-Verlag.

Advances & Technical Standards in Neurosurgery. Ed. by L. Symon et al. Vol. 10. 1984. 231p. 126.00 (*3-211-81750-6*); Vol. 11. 1985. 248p. 126.00 (*3-211-81806-5*); Vol. 11. 1985. (Illus.). 248p. 132.00 (*0-387-81806-5*); Vol. 12. 1986. 186p. 109.00 (*3-211-81877-4*) Spr-Verlag.

Advances & Technical Standards in Neurosurgery, Vol. 12. Ed. by L. Symon. 1986. (Illus.). 186p. 114.00 (*0-387-81877-4*) Spr-Verlag.

Advances & Technical Standards in Neurosurgery, Vol. 13. Ed. by L. Symon et al. 1986. 179p. 112.00 (*3-211-81885-5*) Spr-Verlag.

Advances & Technical Standards in Neurosurgery, Vol. 13. Ed. by L. Symon. 1986. (Illus.). 200p. 112.00 (*0-387-81885-5*) Spr-Verlag.

Advances & Technical Standards in Neurosurgery. Ed. by L. Symon et al. Vol. 14. 1987. (Illus.). 230p. 150.00 (*0-387-81930-4*); Vol. 14. 1986. 230p. 140.00 (*3-211-81930-4*); Vol. 15. 1988. (Illus.). 180p. 139.00 (*0-387-82013-2*); Vol. 15. 1987. 180p. 132.00 (*3-211-82013-2*); Vol. 16. 1989. (Illus.). 215p. 145.00 (*0-387-82060-4*); Vol. 16. 1988. 215p. 138.00 (*3-211-82060-4*); Vol. 17. 1990. 255p. 157.00 (*3-211-82117-1*); Vol. 17. 1990. (Illus.). 255p. 165.00 (*0-387-82117-1*, 3829); Vol. 18. 1991. 209p. 136.00 (*3-211-82243-7*); Vol. 18. 1991. (Illus.). 209p. 143.00 (*0-387-82243-7*); Vol. 19. 1992. 224p. 149.00 (*3-211-82287-9*); Vol. 19. 1992. (Illus.). 224p. 160.00 (*0-387-82287-9*); Vol. 20. 1993. 250p. 192.00 (*3-211-82383-2*); Vol. 20. 1993. (Illus.). 308p. 199.00 (*0-387-82383-2*); Vol. 21. 1995. 286p. 166.00 (*3-211-82482-0*); Vol. 22. 1995. (Illus.). 400p. 210.00 (*3-211-82634-3*) Spr-Verlag.

Advances & Technical Standards in Neurosurgery. Ed. by F. Cohadon et al. (Illus.). Vol. 23. 1997. 330p. 179.00 (*3-211-82827-3*); Vol. 24. 1999. 304p. 159.00 (*3-211-83064-2*); Vol. 26. 2000. 362p. 139.00 (*3-211-83424-9*) Spr-Verlag.

Advances & Technical Standards in Neurosurgery, Vol.9. Ed. by H. Krayenbuehl et al. 1983. (Illus.). 177p. 105.00 (*0-387-81718-2*) Spr-Verlag.

Advances in ABC Relaxation Research. Jonathan C. Smith. 2001. LC 00-52657. (*0-8261-1397-4*) Springer Pub.

Advances in Abdominal Surgery. Ed. by Everardo Zanella. 1999. 249p. 130.00 (*0-7923-5988-7*) Kluwer Academic.

Advances in Acoustic Microscopy, Vol. 2. Ed. by Andrew Briggs & Walter Arnold. 1996. (Illus.). 287p. (C). text 90.00 (*0-306-45344-4*, Kluwer Plenum) Kluwer Academic.

Advances in Adolescent Mental Health, Vol. 4: Contraception, Pregnancy & Parenting. Ed. by Arlene R. Stiffman & Ronald A. Feldman. 1990. 300p. 88.00 (*1-85302-088-5*) Taylor & Francis.

Advances in Adult T-Cell Leukemia & HTLV-I Research. Ed. by Kiyoshi Takatsuki et al. 1992. (Gann Monographs on Cancer Research: No. 39). 83.95 (*0-8493-7746-3*, RC643) CRC Pr.

Advances in African American Psychology. Ed. by Reginald L. Jones. 1997. LC 98-20669. (Illus.). xvii, 380p. (C). lib. bdg. 35.00 (*0-943539-09-9*) Cobb & Henry Pubs.

Advances in Anesthesia, 15. Carol L. Lake. 1997. (Illus.). 464p. (C). (gr. 13). text 81.00 (*0-8151-5278-7*, 23021) Mosby Inc.

Advances in Anesthesia, 16. Lake. 1998. (Illus.). 352p. text 81.00 (*0-8151-9802-7*, 25039) Mosby Inc.

Advances in Anesthesia. Carol L. Lake. 18. 18th ed. 2000. (Illus.). 350p. text 81.00 (*0-8151-1216-5*, 31772); 19. 19th ed. 2000. 81.00 (*0-8151-1217-3*, 31773); 20. 2002. 81.00 (*0-8151-1218-1*, 31774) Mosby Inc.

Advances in Anesthesia, Vol. 17. 1999. (Illus.). 350p. text 84.00 (*0-8151-9803-5*, 25040) Mosby Inc.

***Advances in Anesthesia**, Vol. 21. Ed. by Carol L. Lake. 2003. (Illus.). 250p. (*0-323-01534-4*) Mosby Inc.

Advances in Animal Alternatives for Safety & Efficacy Testing. Harry Salem & Sidney A. Katz. 1997. LC 97-5402. 456p. 135.00 (*1-56032-623-9*) Hemisp Pub.

Advances in Animal Welfare Science 1984. Michael A. Fox. Ed. by Linda D. Mickley. 1985. 228p. lib. bdg. (*0-89838-699-3*) M Nijhoff NLD. *Dist:* Kluwer Academic.

Advances in Anti-Rheumatic Therapy. Ed. by Kim D. Rainsford. 1995. 252p. 149.95 (*0-8493-4937-0*, 4937) CRC Pr.

Advances in Anticalcific & Antidegenerative Treatment of Heart Valve Bioprostheses. International Association for Cardiac Biological Implantation Staff. Ed. by Shlomo Gabbay & David J. Wheatley. 1998. (Illus.). xx, 236p. (*1-878353-42-X*) Silent Partners.

Advances in Anticoagulant, Antithrombotic, & Thrombolytic Therapeutics. Ed. by George Zavoico. 1996. (Biomedical Library). 708p. pap. 895.00 (*1-57936-000-9*) Drug & Market Dev.

Advances in Antiviral Drug Design. Ed. by Erik De Clercq. Vol. 1. 1993. 329p. 109.50 (*1-55938-155-8*); Vol. 2. 1996. 244p. 90.00 (*1-55938-693-2*) Jai Pr.

Advances in Applied Developmental Psychology, Vol. 1. Ed. by Irving E. Sigel & Educational Testing Service Staff. 1985. (Advances in Applied Developmental Psychology Ser.). 227p. 77.00 (*0-89391-090-2*, Ablex) Greenwood.

Advances in Applied Psycholinguistics. Ed. by Sheldon Rosenberg. 1987. (Cambridge Monographs & Texts in Applied Psycholinguistics). (Illus.). Vols. 1. 318p. pap. text 29.95 (*0-521-31732-0*); Vols. 1 & 2. 656p. text 120.00 (*0-521-30027-4*) Cambridge U Pr.

Advances in Applied Social Psychology, Vol. 1. Ed. by Robert F. Kidd & Michael J. Saks. 1980. LC 80-17650. (Illus.). 272p. text 55.00 (*0-89859-027-2*) L Erlbaum Assocs.

Advances in Applied Social Psychology Vol. 3, Vol. 3. Ed. by Michael J. Saks & Leonard M. Saxe. 1986. 264p. text 49.95 (*0-89859-669-6*) L Erlbaum Assocs.

Advances in Art Therapy. Harriet Wadeson et al. 1989. LC 88-17350. (Personality Processes Ser.). 461p. 150.00 (*0-471-62894-8*) Wiley.

Advances in Assisted Reproductive Technologies. Ed. by Zion Ben-Rafael et al. 1990. (Illus.). 1094p. (C). text 270.00 (*0-306-43665-5*, Kluwer Plenum) Kluwer Academic.

Advances in Behavior Research & Therapy, Vol. 1, Pt. 1. Ed. by Hans J. Eysenck & Stanley J. Rachman. 1977. pap. 23.00 (*0-08-022257-9*, Pergamon Pr) Elsevier.

Advances in Behavior Research & Therapy, Vol. 2. Ed. by Stanley J. Rachman. 1980. (Illus.). 186p. 100.00 (*0-08-027110-3*, Pergamon Pr) Elsevier.

Advances in Behavior Research & Therapy. Ed. by Stanley J. Rachman & T. Wilson. (Illus.). Vol. 3. 1982. 206p. 125.00 (*0-08-029671-8*); Vol. 4. 1984. 282p. 125.00 (*0-08-031502-X*); Vol. 5. 1985. 258p. 145.00 (*0-08-032327-8*) Elsevier (Pergamon Pr).

Advances in Behavioral Medicine for Children & Adolescents. Philip Firestone et al. 1983. 184p. (C). text 39.95 (*0-89859-326-3*) L Erlbaum Assocs.

Advances in Behavioral Pharmacology, Vol. 6. Ed. by Travis Thompson et al. 1987. 336p. text 69.95 (*0-89859-599-1*) L Erlbaum Assocs.

Advances in Behavioral Pharmacology, Vol. 7. Ed. by J. E. Barrett et al. 1989. 216p. (C). text 59.95 (*0-8058-0351-3*) L Erlbaum Assocs.

Advances in Behavioral Pharmacology, Vol. V: Developmental Behavior Pharmacology. Ed. by Norman A. Krasnegor et al. 1986. 328p. (C). text 59.95 (*0-89859-676-9*) L Erlbaum Assocs.

Advances in Behaviour Research & Therapy, Vols. 3 & 4. Rachman. 1983. pap. 33.00 (*0-08-030465-6*, Pergamon Pr) Elsevier.

Advances in Biochemical Engineering, Vol. 3. Ed. by Tarum K. Ghose et al. 1974. LC 73-152360. (Illus.). 290p. 59.95 (*0-387-06546-6*) Spr-Verlag.

Advances in Bioclimatology, Vol. 4. G. Stanhill. 1996. (Illus.). 288p. 197.00 (*3-540-60819-2*) Spr-Verlag.

Advances in Bioengineering, 1997 n: Proceedings, ASME International Mechanical Engineering Congress & Exposition, Dallas, TX, 1997. Ed. by Bruce Simon. 1997. (BED Ser.: Vol. 36). 384p. pap. 60.00 (*0-7918-1823-3*, R856) ASME Pr.

Advances in Bioethics: New Essays on Abortion & Bioethics, Vol. 2. Ed. by Rem B. Edwards. 1997. LC 98-122024. 346p. 128.50 (*0-7623-0194-5*) Jai Pr.

Advances in Bioethics: Values, Ethics & Alcoholism, Vol. 3. Ed. by Wayne Shelton & Rem B. Edwards. 1997. LC 98-195128. 314p. 128.50 (*0-7623-0219-4*) Jai Pr.

Advances in Bioethics Vol. 4: Critical Reflections of Medical Ethics. Rem B. Edwards & E. Edward Bittar. 1998. LC 99-221486. 300p. 128.50 (*0-7623-0298-4*) Jai Pr.

Advances in Biological Psychiatry. Ed. by Jaak Panksepp. Vol. 1. 1991. 312p. 128.50 (*0-7623-0026-4*); Vol. 2, 1996. 1996. (Illus.). 250p. 90.00 (*0-7623-0170-8*) Jai Pr.

Advances in Biomedical Alcohol Research: Proceedings of the 6th ISBRA Congress, Bristol, U. K., 21-26 June 1992. Ed. by P. V. Taberner & A. A. Badawy. 1993. 528p. 118.75 (*0-08-041981-X*, Pergamon Pr) Elsevier.

Advances in Biomedical Engineering: Results of the 4th EC Medical & Health Research Programme (1987-1991) Ed. by J. E. W. Beneken & V. Thevin. 1993. LC 92-75336. (Studies in Health Technology & Informatics: Vol. 7). 364p. 130.00 (*90-5199-119-3*) IOS Press.

Advances in Bladder Research. Ed. by Laurence S. Baskin & Simon W. Hayward. 1999. LC 99-31871. (Advances in Experimental Medicine & Biology Ser.). (*0-306-46112-9*, Kluwer Plenum) Kluwer Academic.

Advances in Blood Substitutes: Industrial Opportunities & Medical Challenges. Ed. by Robert M. Winslow et al. 1997. LC 97-22453. (Advances in Blood Substitutes Ser.: Vol. 3). 230p. 99.00 (*0-8176-3980-2*) Birkhauser.

Advances in Blood Substitutes: Industrial Opportunities & Medical Challenges. Robert M. Winslow et al. 1997. LC 97-22453. (*3-7643-3980-2*) Birkhauser.

Advances in Body Composition Assessment. Timothy G. Lohman. 1992. LC 92-1476. (Current Issues in Exercise Science Ser.: Vol. 3). (Illus.). 160p. pap. text 19.00 (*0-87322-327-6*, BLOH0327) Human Kinetics.

***Advances in Brain Imaging.** Ed. by John M. Morihisa. 2001. (Review of Psychiatry Ser.: Vol. 20). 224p. pap. 29.95 (*1-58562-028-9*, 62028) Am Psychiatric.

Advances in Brain Resuscitation. Ed. by J. D. Miller et al. 1991. (Illus.). 344p. 141.00 (*0-387-70067-6*) Spr-Verlag.

Advances in Brain Vasopressin. Ivan J. Urban et al. 1998. LC 98-42188. (Progress in Brain Research Ser.). 664p. 207.00 (*0-444-50080-4*) Elsevier.

Advances in Breast Cancer Detection. Ed. by S. Brunner et al. 1990. (Recent Results in Cancer Research Ser.: Vol. 119). (Illus.). 195p. 106.00 (*0-387-52089-9*) Spr-Verlag.

Advances in Brucellosis Research. Ed. by L. Garry Adams. 1990. LC 90-11118. (Illus.). 542p. 39.95 (*0-89096-447-5*) Tex A&M Univ Pr.

Advances in Cancer Research, Vol. 6. Ed. by George F. Vande Woude & George Klein. 1995. (Illus.). 355p. text 83.00 (*0-12-006666-1*) Acad Pr.

Advances in Cancer Research. Ed. by George F. Vandewoude & George Klein. (Illus.). Vol. 62. 1993. 280p. text 94.00 (*0-12-006662-9*); Vol. 63. 1994. 357p. text 94.00 (*0-12-006663-7*) Acad Pr.

Advances in Cancer Research. Ed. by George F. Vande Woude & George Klein. (Illus.). Vol. 64. 1994. 305p. text 83.00 (*0-12-006664-5*); Vol. 65. 1994. 235p. text 83.00 (*0-12-006665-3*); Vol. 69. 1996. 256p. text 69.00 (*0-12-006669-6*); Vol. 70. 1996. 229p. text 79.00 (*0-12-006670-X*) Acad Pr.

Advances in Cancer Research, Vol. 71. George Klein. Ed. by George F. Vande Woude. 1997. (Advances in Cancer Research Ser.: Vol. 71). (Illus.). 385p. text 89.00 (*0-12-006671-8*) Morgan Kaufmann.

Advances in Cancer Research, Vol. 72. Ed. by George F. Vande Woude & George Klein. 1997. (Illus.). 242p. text 89.95 (*0-12-006672-6*) Morgan Kaufmann.

Advances in Cancer Research, Vol. 74. Ed. by George F. Vandewoude & George Klein. 1998. (Illus.). 223p. 89.95 (*0-12-006674-2*) Morgan Kaufmann.

Advances in Cancer Research, Vol. 75. Ed. by George F. Vande Woude & George Klein. 1998. (Illus.). 282p. (C). text 89.95 (*0-12-006675-0*) Acad Pr.

Advances in Cancer Research, Vol. 76. George F. Vandewoude & George Klein. 1999. (Advances in Cancer Research Ser.: Vol. 76). (Illus.). 264p. (C). text 89.95 (*0-12-006676-9*) Acad Pr.

Advances in Cancer Research, Vol. 79. Ed. by George F. Vande Woude & George Klein. 2000. (Advances in Cancer Research Ser.: Vol. 79). (Illus.). 320p. 89.95 (*0-12-006679-3*) Acad Pr.

***Advances in Cancer Research**, Vol. 81. Ed. by George Vande Woude & George Klein. 2001. 264p. 129.95 (*0-12-006681-5*) Acad Pr.

Advances in Cancer Research Vol. 73: Cumulative Index, Vols. 50-72, Vol. 73. Ed. by George F. Vande Woude & George Klein. 1997. (Illus.). 237p. text 89.95 (*0-12-006673-4*) Morgan Kaufmann.

Advances in Cancer Screening. Ed. by Anthony B. Miller. 1996. LC 97-17047. (Cancer Treatment & Research Ser.: Vol. 86). (Illus.). 208p. (C). text 212.00 (*0-7923-4019-1*) Kluwer Academic.

Advances in Carbohydrate Chemistry & Biochemistry. Ed. by Derek Horton. (Illus.). (C). Vol. 51. 1995. 348p. text 95.00 (*0-12-007251-3*); Vol. 53. 1998. 466p. 99.95 (*0-12-007253-X*) Acad Pr.

Advances in Carbohydrate Chemistry & Biochemistry, Vol. 52. Ed. by Derek Horton. 1997. (Illus.). 491p. (C). text 99.95 (*0-12-007252-1*) Morgan Kaufmann.

Advances in Cardiac & Pulmonary Rehabilitation. Ed. by Mary C. Singleton & Eleanor F. Branch. 1990. LC 89-24754. (Physical Therapy in Health Care Ser.: Vol. 3, Nos. 1-2). (Illus.). 78p. text 3.95 (*0-86656-986-3*) Haworth Pr.

Advances in Cardiac Surgery. Robert Karp. (Illus.). 12th ed. 2000. 210p. text 89.95 (*0-8151-2726-X*, 31330); 13th ed. 2001. 210p. text 89.95 (*0-8151-2719-7*, 31331); 14th ed. 2002. 210p. text 89.95 (*0-8151-2720-0*, 31332); 10. 10th ed. 1998. 312p. text 89.95 (*0-8151-9804-3*, 25041) Mosby Inc.

Advances in Cardiac Surgery, 11. 1999. (Illus.). 224p. text 89.95 (*0-8151-2728-6*, 31329) Mosby Inc.

Advances in Cardiomyopathies: Proceedings of the II Florence Meeting on Advances on Cardiomyopathies, April 24-26, 1997. F. Ting Camerini et al. 1998. LC 98-10658. xv, 317p. (C). (*88-470-0009-2*) Spr-Verlag ITA. *Dist:* Spr-Verlag.

Advances in Cardiopulmonary Rehabilitation. Ed. by Jean-Louis Jobin et al. 2000. LC 99-59589. (Illus.). 336p. text 44.00 (*0-7360-0312-6*) Human Kinetics.

Advances in Cardiopulmonary Resuscitation. Ed. by Peter Safar & J. O. Elam. 1980. (Illus.). 302p. 106.00 (*0-387-90234-1*) Spr-Verlag.

Advances in Cardiovascular Engineering. Ed. by N. H. Hwang et al. 1993. (NATO Advanced Science Institutes Ser.: Vol. 235). (Illus.). 452p. (C). text 135.00 (*0-306-44313-9*, Kluwer Plenum) Kluwer Academic.

Advances in Cell Aging & Gerontology, Vol. 1. Ed. by Paola S. Timiras & E. Edward Bittar. 1996. 258p. 90.00 (*1-55938-631-2*) Jai Pr.

Advances in Chemotherapy of AIDS. Robert B. Diasio & Jean-Pierre Sommadossi. 1990. (Illus.). 160p. 44.00 (*0-08-040315-8*) McGraw.

Advances in Child Development & Behavior. Ed. by Hayne W. Reese. (Illus.). (C). Vol. 24. 1993. 317p. text 94.95 (*0-12-009724-9*); Vol. 25. 1994. 385p. text 84.95 (*0-12-009725-7*) Acad Pr.

***Advances in Child Development & Behavior**, Vol. 28. Ed. by Hayne W. Reese & Robert Kail. 2001. 250p. 79.95 (*0-12-009728-1*) Acad Pr.

Advances in Child Health Psychology. Ed. by James H. Johnson & Suzanne B. Johnson. 1990. 480p. (C). 49.95 (*0-8130-1007-1*); pap. 29.95 (*0-8130-1019-5*) U Press Fla.

Advances in Child Neuropsychology, Vol. 1. Ed. by M. G. Tramontana & S. R. Hooper. 1991. (Illus.). 239p. 93.00 (*0-387-97611-6*) Spr-Verlag.

Advances in Child Neuropsychology. M. G. Tramontana & S. R. Hooper. 1994. (Illus.). Vol. 2. 247p. 90.00 (*0-387-94130-4*); Vol. 3. 185p. 104.00 (*0-387-94302-1*) Spr-Verlag.

Advances in Chinese Medicinal Materials Research: Proceedings of the International Symposium, Hong Kong, June 12-14, 1985. Ed. by A. Koo et al. 1985. 742p. text 139.00 (*9971-966-71-9*) World Scientific Pub.

Advances in Chiropractic. Dana J. Lawrence. (C). (gr. 13). 4. 4th ed. 1997. (Illus.). 688p. text 83.00 (*0-8151-5309-0*, 23097); Vol. 5. 5th ed. 1998. text 79.95 (*0-8151-5310-4*) Mosby Inc.

Advances in Chromatography. J. Calvin Giddings et al. (Illus.). Vol. 23. 1984. 272p. text 195.00 (*0-8247-7075-7*); Vol. 27. 1987. 384p. text 195.00 (*0-8247-7770-0*) Dekker.

Advances in Chromatography, Vol. 31. Ed. by J. Calvin Giddings. 1991. (Illus.). 416p. text 225.00 (*0-8247-8568-1*) Dekker.

Advances in Chronic Lymphocytic Leukemia. Ed. by Aaron Polliack. 1992. 150p. text 114.00 (*3-7186-5213-7*, Harwood Acad Pubs) Gordon & Breach.

Advances in Cirrhosis, Hyperammonemia & Hepatic Encephalopathy: Proceedings of an International Symposium Held in Valencia, Spain, December 2-4, 1996. Ed. by Vicente Felipo & Santiago Grisolia. 1997. LC 97-4391. (Advances in Experimental Medicine & Biology Ser.: Vol. 420). (Illus.). 290p. 114.00 (*0-306-45598-6*, Kluwer Plenum) Kluwer Academic.

Advances in Cladistics Vol. 2: Proceedings of the Second Meeting of the Willi Hennig Society. Ed. by Norman I. Platnick & Vicki A. Funk. 1983. 288p. text 71.50 (*0-231-05646-X*) Col U Pr.

Advances in Clinical Andrology. Ed. by Christopher L. Barratt & I.D. Cooke. 1988. (C). text 95.50 (*0-7462-0034-X*) Kluwer Academic.

Advances in Clinical Chemistry, Vol. 31. Ed. by Herbert E. Spiegel. 1994. (Illus.). 283p. text 94.00 (*0-12-010331-1*) Acad Pr.

Advances in Clinical Chemistry Vol. 34: Cumulative Subject & Author Indexes & Tables of Contents for Volumes 1-33, Vol.34. Ed. by Herbert E. Spiegel. 1999. (Advances in Chemical Engineering Ser.: Vol. 34). (Illus.). 432p. 120.00 (*0-12-010334-6*) Acad Pr.

Advances in Clinical Child Psychology. Ed. by Thomas H. Ollendick & Ronald J. Prinz. 1998. (Clinical Child Psychology Ser.: Vol. 20). (Illus.). 330p. (C). 85.00 (*0-306-45667-2*, Plenum Trade) Perseus Pubng.

Advances in Clinical Child Psychology. Ed. by Benjamin B. Lahey & Alan E. Kazdin. Vol. 4. 1981. LC 77-643411. 380p. 65.00 (*0-306-40705-1*); Vol. 10. 1987. LC 77-643411. 378p. 65.00 (*0-306-42536-X*); Vol. 11. 1988. LC 77-643411. (Illus.). 414p. (C). 102.00 (*0-306-42892-X*); Vol. 12. 1989. (Illus.). 270p. (C). 102.00 (*0-306-43271-4*); Vol. 13. 1990. LC 77-643411. (Illus.). 426p. (C). 85.00 (*0-306-43479-2*); Vol. 14. 1991. (Illus.). 325p. (C). 85.00 (*0-306-43957-3*) Perseus Pubng (Plenum Trade).

Advances in Clinical Child Psychology. Ed. by Thomas H. Ollendick & Ronald J. Prinz. Vol. 17. 1994. LC 77-643411. (Illus.). 422p. (C). 85.00 (*0-306-44799-1*); Vol. 19. 1997. 388p. 85.00 (*0-306-45447-5*) Kluwer Academic (Kluwer Plenum).

Advances in Clinical Child Psychology. Ed. by Thomas H. Ollendick & Ronald J. Prinz. (Illus.). (C). Vol. 15. 1993. 360p. 85.00 (*0-306-44273-6*); Vol. 16. 1993. 332p. 85.00 (*0-306-44552-2*); Vol. 18. 1996. 388p. 85.00 (*0-306-45143-3*) Perseus Pubng (Plenum Trade).

Advances in Clinical Neuropsychology, Vol. 1. Ed. by Gerald Goldstein. 1984. LC 84-645578. 198p. 75.00 (*0-306-41502-X*, Plenum Trade) Perseus Pubng.

Advances in Clinical Neuropsychology, Vol. 2. Ed. by Ralph E. Tarter & Gerald Goldstein. 1984. LC 84-645578. 248p. 75.00 (*0-306-41722-7*, Plenum Trade) Perseus Pubng.

Advances in Clinical Phonetics. Ed. by Martin J. Ball & Martin Duckworth. 1996. LC 96-28906. (Studies in Speech Pathology & Clinical Linguistics: Vol. 6). xiv, 258p. lib. bdg. 76.00 (*1-55619-393-9*) J Benjamins Pubng Co.

Advances in CNS Drug-Receptor Interactions, Vol. 1. Ed. by Joseph G. Cannon. 1991. 178p. 109.50 (*1-55938-163-9*) Jai Pr.

Advances in Cognitive Science: Theory & Applications, Vol. 2. Guy Tiberghien. 1989. 206p. 59.95 (*0-470-21436-8*) P-H.

Advances in Comparative & Environmental Physiology, Vol. 5. 1989. (Illus.). 238p. 97.00 (*0-387-50825-2*, 2701) Spr-Verlag.

Advances in Comparative & Environmental Physiology Vol. 11: Mechanics of Animal Locomotion. Ed. by R. E. Weber et al. 1992. (Illus.). 304p. 167.00 (*0-387-54119-5*) Spr-Verlag.

Advances in Controlled Clinical Inhalation Studies. Ed. by D. V. Mohr et al. 1993. (ILSI Monographs). (Illus.). 430p. 211.00 (*0-387-54958-7*) Spr-Verlag.

Advances in Controlled Delivery of Drugs. Ed. by Melvyn A. Kohudic. 1994. LC 94-60629. 154p. 84.95 (*1-56676-194-8*) CRC Pr.

Advances in Corneal Research No. 4: Selected Transactions of the World Congress on the Cornea: Proceedings of the World Congress on the Cornea IV Held in Orlando, Florida, April 17-19, 1996. World Congress on the Cornea Staff. Ed. by Jonathan H. Lass. 1998. LC 97-42705. (Illus.). 648p. (C). text 191.00 (*0-306-45763-6*, Kluwer Plenum) Kluwer Academic.

Advances in Corticosteroids: A Seminar in Print. Ed. by Stephen M. Krane. (Illus.). 80p. (Orig.). pap. (*0-941741-04-4*) Adis Pr Intl.

Advances in Critical Care Testing: The IFCC-AVL Award 1996. Ed. by Matthew J. McQueen et al. 1997. LC 97-12403. (Illus.). 180p. pap. 69.00 (*3-540-62590-9*) Spr-Verlag.

Advances in Cryosurgery: Proceedings of the Seventh International Congress of Cryosurgery, Beijing, 11-14 October, 1989. Ed. by Chinese Association of Refrigeration Staff et al. 1990. LC 89-20117. (International Academic Publishers Ser.: No. 13). 626p. (*0-08-037503-0*) IAP GBR. *Dist:* Elsevier.

Advances in CT IV: 4th International Scientific User Conference, SOMATOM PLUS, CT, Rotterdam, March 1998. Ed. by Gabriel P. Krestin & Gary M. Glazer. 1998. LC 98-18291. (Illus.). 350p. 129.00 (*3-540-64348-6*) Spr-Verlag.

Advances in Dementia Research. Ed. by Kurt A. Jellinger et al. 2000. LC 00-34451. (Journals of Neural Transmission: Suppl. 59). (Illus.). 200p. 99.00 (*3-211-83513-X*); viii, 336p. pap. 108.00 (*3-211-83512-1*) Spr-Verlag.

Advances in Dermatology, Vol. 13. William James. 13th ed. 1997. (Illus.). 568p. (C). (gr. 13). text 83.00 (*0-8151-9808-6*, 25045) Mosby Inc.

Advances in Dermatology,Vol. 16. William James. 16th ed. 2000. (Illus.). 350p. text 83.00 (*0-8151-0989-X*, 31771) Mosby Inc.

Advances in Dermatology, Vol. 14. Date not set. 79.95 (*0-8151-9810-8*) Mosby Inc.

Advances in Dermatology, Vol. 17. Ed. by William James. 2001. (Illus.). 580p. (*0-323-01535-2*) Mosby Inc.

***Advances in Dermatology.** Ed. by William James. Vol. 18. 2002. 250p. (*0-323-01536-0*); Vol. 19. 2003. (Illus.). 580p. (*0-323-01537-9*) Mosby Inc.

Advances in Dermatology, Vol.14. Williams James. 1998. (Illus.). 512p. (C). (gr. 13). text 83.00 (*0-8151-0731-5*, 31769) Mosby Inc.

Advances in Dermatology, Vol.15. 1999. 79.95 (*0-8151-6516-1*, 26101); (Illus.). 350p. text 83.00 (*0-8151-0913-X*, 31770) Mosby Inc.

Advances in Descriptive Psychology, Vol. 1. Ed. by Keith E. Davis. 1981. 389p. 40.00 (*0-89232-179-2*) Descriptive Psych Pr.

Advances in Descriptive Psychology. Ed. by Keith E. Davis & Thomas O. Mitchell. Vol. 2. 1982. 289p. 40.00 (*0-89232-225-X*); Vol. 3. 1983. 311p. 40.00 (*0-89232-293-4*); Vol. 4. 1985. 310p. 40.00 (*0-89232-358-2*) Descriptive Psych Pr.

Advances in Descriptive Psychology, Vol. 5. Ed. by Anthony O. Putman & Keith E. Davis. 1990. 320p. 70.00 (*0-9625661-0-1*) Descriptive Psych Pr.

Advances in Descriptive Psychology, Vol. 7. Ed. by H. Joel Jeffrey & Raymond M. Bergner. 1998. 351p. 70.00 (*1-891700-01-4*) Descriptive Psych Pr.

Advances in Descriptive Psychology Vol. 6: Clinical Topics: Adolescent-Family Problems, Bulimia, Chronic Mental Illness, & Mania. Ed. by Mary K. Roberts & Raymond M. Bergner. 1991. 316p. (C). 70.00 (*0-9625661-1-X*) Descriptive Psych Pr.

Advances in Developmental & Behavioral Pediatrics, Vol. 9. Ed. by Mark L. Wolraich & Donald K. Routh. 1990. 300p. 88.00 (*1-85302-071-0*) Taylor & Francis.

Advances in Developmental & Behavioral Pediatrics, Vol. 10. Ed. by Mark L. Wolraich. 1992. 270p. 99.00 (*1-85302-150-4*) Taylor & Francis.

Advances in Developmental Disorders, Vol. 2. Ed. by Rowland P. Barrett & Johnny L. Matson. 1993. 320p. 85.00 (*1-85302-093-1*) Taylor & Francis.

Advances in Developmental Psychology. Ed. by Michael E. Lamb & Ann L. Brown. (Advances in Developmental Psychology Ser.). Vol. 1. 1981. 256p. text 49.95 (*0-89859-103-1*); Vol. 2. 1982. 224p. (C). text 49.95 (*0-89859-244-5*) L Erlbaum Assocs.

Advances in Developmental Psychology. Ed. by Michael E. Lamb et al. Vol. 3. 1984. 312p. (C). text 59.95 (*0-89859-366-2*); Vol. 4. 1986. 376p. 79.95 (*0-89859-675-0*) L Erlbaum Assocs.

Advances in Diagnostic Visual Optics. Ed. by C. M. Breinin & I. M. Siegel. 1983. (Series in Optical Sciences: Vol. 41). (Illus.). 247p. 64.95 (*0-387-13079-9*) Spr-Verlag.

***Advances in Discovery & Development of Drugs for Cognitive Aging & Alzheimers Disease.** Ed. by Howard Fillit & Alan O'Connell. 2001. LC 2001-49760. (*0-8261-1542-X*) Springer Pub.

Advances in Disease. Ed. by Kerry F. Harris. 1988. (Vector Research Ser.: Vol. 5). (Illus.). 300p. 219.00 (*0-387-96738-9*) Spr-Verlag.

Advances in Disease Vector Research, Vol. 6. Ed. by Kerry F. Harris. 1989. (Illus.). 363p. 248.00 (*0-387-97080-0*, 3108) Spr-Verlag.

Advances in Disease Vector Research. Ed. by K. F. Harris. (Illus.). Vol. 7. 1990. 211p. 190.00 (*0-387-97335-4*); Vol. 8. 1991. 209p. 190.00 (*0-387-97478-4*); Vol. 9. 1992. 367p. 321.00 (*0-387-97791-0*); Vol. 10. 1993. 412p. 290.00 (*0-387-94073-1*) Spr-Verlag.

Advances in DNA Damage & Repair: Oxygen Radical Effects, Cellular Protection & Biological Consequences. Ed. by M. Dizdaroglu & A. E. Karakaya. 1999. LC 98-47311. (NATO ASI Ser.: 302). (Illus.). 524p. (C). text 185.00 (*0-306-46042-4*) Plenum.

Advances in Drug Delivery Systems 6: Proceedings of the Sixth International Symposium on Recent Advances in Drug Delivery Systems, Salt Lake City, UT, U. S. A., 21-24 February 1993. Ed. by J. M. Anderson et al. 1994. 350p. text 227.25 (*0-444-82027-2*) Elsevier.

Advances in Drug Metabolism in Man. G. M. Pacific & G. N. Fracchia. 1995. 1044p. (*92-827-3982-1*) Comm Europ Commun BEL. *Dist:* Bernan Associates.

Advances in Drug Research. Bernard Testa. 1986. text 104.00 (*0-12-013315-6*) Acad Pr.

Advances in Drug Research, Vol. 13. Ed. by N. J. Harper & A. B. Simmonds. 1984. (Serial Publication Ser.). text 104.00 (*0-12-013313-X*) Acad Pr.

Advances in Drug Research. Ed. by Bernard Testa. (Serial Publication Ser.). Vol. 18. 1989. 549p. text 104.00 (*0-12-013318-0*); Vol. 19. 1990. 581p. text 104.00 (*0-12-013319-9*); Vol. 23. 1992. (Illus.). 233p. text 104.00 (*0-12-013323-7*); Vol. 24. 1993. (Illus.). 288p. text 104.00 (*0-12-013324-5*) Acad Pr.

Advances in Drug Research, Vol. 25. Ed. by Bernard Testa & Urs A. Meyer. 1994. (Illus.). 309p. text 104.00 (*0-12-013325-3*) Acad Pr.

Advances in Drug Research, Vol. 26. Ed. by Bernard Testa. 1995. (Illus.). 279p. text 79.00 (*0-12-013326-1*) Acad Pr.

Advances in Drug Research, Vol. 28. Ed. by Bernard Testa & Urs A. Meyer. 1996. (Illus.). 384p. text 97.50 (*0-12-013328-8*) Acad Pr.

Advances in Drug Research. Ed. by Bernard Testa & Urs A. Meyer. 1997. (Illus.). Vol. 29. 336p. text 99.95 (*0-12-013329-6*); Vol. 30. 352p. text 89.95 (*0-12-013330-X*) Morgan Kaufmann.

Advances in Drug Therapy of Gastroesophageal Reflux Disease. Ed. by C. Scarpignato. 1991. (Frontiers of Gastrointestinal Research Ser.: Vol. 20). (Illus.). xii, 372p. 259.25 (*3-8055-5360-9*) S Karger.

Advances in Echo Imaging Using Contrast Enhancement. Ed. by Navin C. Nanda. 1993. LC 92-46545. 408p. (C). text 178.50 (*0-7923-2137-5*) Kluwer Academic.

Advances in Educational & Psychological Testing: Theory & Applications. Ed. by Ronald K. Hambleton. 1991. 480p. (C). lib. bdg. 153.00 (*0-7923-9070-9*) Kluwer Academic.

Advances in End-Stage Renal Diseases, 2000: International Conference on Dialysis II, Tarpon Springs (Florida), January 2000. Ed. by N. W. Levin & C. Ronco. 2000. (Blood Purification Ser.: Vol. 18, No. 4). (Illus.). iv, 120p. 97.50 (*3-8055-7080-5*) S Karger.

***Advances in End-Stage Renal Diseases, 2001: International Conference on Dialysis III, Miami Beach, Fla., January 2001.** C. Ronco. Ed. by N. W. Levin. 2001. (Blood Purification Ser.). vi, 132p. 97.50 (*3-8055-7186-0*) S Karger.

Advances in Endocrinology & Metabolism, Vol. 7. Ernest L. Mazzaferri. 1996. 300p. 64.95 (*0-8151-6153-0*) Mosby Inc.

Advances in Environment, Behavior & Design, Vol. 2. Ed. by Ervin H. Zube & G. T. Moore. 1989. LC 88-649861. (Illus.). 366p. (C). 79.50 (*0-306-42953-5*, Plenum Trade) Perseus Pubng.

Advances in Environmental Psychology Vol. 2: Applications of Personal Control. Ed. by Andrew Baum & Jerome E. Singer. 1980. 208p. 49.95 (*0-89859-018-3*) L Erlbaum Assocs.

Advances in Environmental Psychology Vol. 5: Methods & Environmental Psychology. Ed. by Andrew Baum & Jerome E. Singer. 1985. 232p. (C). text 49.95 (*0-89859-680-7*) L Erlbaum Assocs.

Advances in Enzyme Regulation: Eld at Titisee, FRG, May 2-4 1985, Vol. 24. George Weber. 1985. LC 63-19609. 500p. 167.00 (*0-08-031986-6*, Pergamon Pr) Elsevier.

Advances in Enzyme Regulation: Proceedings of the 17th Symposium on Regulation of Enzyme Activity & Synthesis in Normal & Neoplastic Tissues, Indiana University School of Medicine, Indianapolis, 2-3 October 1978, Vol. 17. Ed. by George Weber. 1979. (Illus.). 155.00 (*0-08-024424-6*, Pergamon Pr) Elsevier.

Advances in Enzyme Regulation: Proceedings of the 20th Symposium on Regulation of Activity & Synthesis in Normal & Neoplastic Tissues Held at Indiana University School of Medicine, Indianapolis, October 5-6, 1981, Vol. 20. Ed. by George Weber. 1982. LC 63-19609. (Illus.). 420p. 145.00 (*0-08-028898-7*, Pergamon Pr) Elsevier.

Advances in Enzyme Regulation: Proceedings of the 21st Symposium on Regulation of Activity & Synthesis in Normal & Neoplastic Tissues, Held at Indiana University School of Medicine, Indianapolis, October 4-5, 1982. George Weber. 1983. LC 63-19609. (Advances in Enzyme Regulation Ser.: Vol. 21). (Illus.). 448p. 90.00 (*0-08-030430-3*, Pergamon Pr) Elsevier.

Advances in Enzyme Regulation: Proceedings of the 34th Symposium on Regulation of Enzyme Activity & Synthesis in Normal & Neoplastic Tissues Held at Indiana University School of Medicine, Indianapolis, IN, 4-5 October, 1993, Vol. 34. Ed. by George Weber. 1994. (Illus.). 498p. 543.00 (*0-08-042482-1*) Elsevier.

Advances in Enzyme Regulation: Proceedings of the 36th International Symposium on Regulation of Enzyme Activity & Synthesis in Normal & Neoplastic Tissues Held at Indiana University School of Medicine, Indianapolis, Indiana, Oct. 2 & 3, 1995, Vol. 36. Ed. by G. Weber. 1996. 466p. 643.00 (*0-08-042894-0*, Pergamon Pr) Elsevier.

Advances in Enzyme Regulation: Proceedings of the Symposium Regulation of Enzyme Activity & Synthesis in Normal & Neoplastic Tissues, 22nd, Held at Indiana University School of Medicine, Indianapolis, U. S. A., 3-4 October 1983. Ed. by George Weber. 1984. LC 63-19609. (Advances in Enzyme Regulation Ser.: Vol. 22). (Illus.). 578p. 90.00 (*0-08-031498-8*, Pergamon Pr) Elsevier.

Advances in Enzyme Regulation: Proceedings of the Thirtieth Symposium on Regulation of Enzyme Activity & Synthesis in Normal & Neoplastic Tissues Held at Indiana University School of Medicine, Indianapolis, Indiana, 2-3 October 1989. Ed. by George Weber. 1990. (Advances in Enzyme Regulation Ser.: No. 30). (Illus.). 472p. 344.00 (*0-08-040172-4*, Pergamon Pr) Elsevier.

Advances in Ergometry. Ed. by N. Bachl et al. 1991. (Illus.). 544p. 65.00 (*0-387-53684-1*) Spr-Verlag.

Advances in Exercise Adherence. Ed. by Rod K. Dishman. 1994. LC 93-47608. (Illus.). 416p. text 35.00 (*0-87322-664-X*, BDIS0664) Human Kinetics.

Advances in Exercise Physiology: Proceedings of the International Symposium of Physiology, New Delhi-Patiala, Oct., 1974. International Symposium of Physiology Staff. Ed. by E. Jokl et al. 1976. (Medicine & Sport Science Ser.: Vol. 9). 160p. 82.75 (*3-8055-2291-6*) S Karger.

Advances in Experimental Social Psychology. Ed. by Mark P. Zanna. (Serial Publication Ser.). Vol. 23. 1990. 350p. text 89.95 (*0-12-015223-1*); Vol. 28. 1996. (Illus.). 468p. text 65.00 (*0-12-015228-2*) Acad Pr.

Advances in Experimental Social Psychology, Vol. 30. Ed. by Mark P. Zanna. 1998. (Illus.). 402p. text 75.00 (*0-12-015230-4*) Morgan Kaufmann.

Advances in Family Psychiatry. Ed. by John G. Howells. 1980. LC 78-13895. Vol. 1. 559p. 82.50 (*0-8236-0097-1*); Vol. 2. 565p. 82.50 (*0-8236-0101-3*) Intl Univs Pr.

Advances in Fertility & Sterility. D. Healey. 2001. LC 2001-55370. (Illus.). 300p. lib. bdg. 119.95 (*1-84214-036-1*, Parthenon Pbng) CRC Pr.

Advances in Field Theory. Susan A. Wheelan. 1991. 344p. (C). 56.95 (*0-8039-3979-5*, 3145) Sage.

Advances in Food & Nutrition Research, Vol. 37. Ed. by John E. Kinsella. 1993. (Illus.). 437p. (C). text 104.00 (*0-12-016437-X*) Acad Pr.

Advances in Food & Nutrition Research Vol. 40: Mathematical Modeling in Experimental Nutrition: Vitamins, Proteins, Methods, Vol. 40. Ed. by Steve Taylor et al. 1996. (Illus.). 362p. (C). text 85.00 (*0-12-016440-X*) Acad Pr.

Advances in Forensic Psychology & Psychiatry, Vol. 1. Ed. by Robert W. Rieber. 1984. (Advances in Forensic Psychology & Psychiatry Ser.). 186p. 77.00 (*0-89391-191-7*, Ablex) Greenwood.

Advances in Genetic Information: A Guide for State Policy Makers: Employment Issues, Insurance, Criminal Justice, Health Care, Genetic Testing, Civil Liberties. Ed. by Steven R. Brown & Karen Marshall. 1995. LC 94-225447. 123p. pap. 10.00 (*0-87292-983-3*) Coun State Govts.

Advances in Genetics, Vol. 38. Ed. by Jeffrey C. Hall et al. 1998. (Illus.). 225p. (C). text 89.95 (*0-12-017638-6*) Acad Pr.

Advances in Genetics, Vol. 39. Jeffrey C. Hall. 1999. 608p. (C). 89.95 (*0-12-017639-4*) Acad Pr.

Advances in Gerontological Nursing Vol. 1: Issues for the 21st Century. Ed. by Elizabeth A. Swanson & Toni Tripp-Reimer. 1996. (Advances in Gerontological Nursing Ser.). (Illus.). 296p. 46.95 (*0-8261-9110-X*) Springer Pub.

Advances in Glucuronide Conjugation. Ed. by Matern Siegfried et al. 1985. text 242.50 (*0-85200-901-1*) Kluwer Academic.

Advances in Group Processes, Vol. 4. Ed. by Edward J. Lawler et al. 1987. 315p. 73.25 (*0-89232-733-2*) Jai Pr.

Advances in Group Psychotherapy: Integrating Research & Practice. Ed. by Robert R. Dies & K. Roy MacKenzie. 1985. LC 83-206. (American Group Psychotherapy Association Monographs). xvii, 226p. 32.50 (*0-8236-0107-2*, 00107) Intl Univs Pr.

Advances in Gynaecological Pathology. Ed. by D. Lowe & H. Fox. 1992. (Illus.). 384p. text (*0-443-04377-9*) Church.

Advances in Gynaecological Surgery. Ed. by Ellisa Downes & P. J. O'Donovan. 2002. (Medical Media Ser.). (Illus.). 208p. text (*1-900151-49-9*) Greenwich Med GBR. *Dist:* JAMCO Dist.

Advances in Gynecological Endocrinology. A. R. Genazzani & F. Petraglia. 2001. (Illus.). 400p. lib. bdg. 86.95 (*1-84214-071-X*, Parthenon Pbng) CRC Pr.

Advances in Hadron Therapy: Proceedings of the 2nd International Symposium on Hadrontherapy, PSI & CERN, Switzerland, 9-13 September, 1996, Vol. 1144. U. Amaldi et al. 1997. LC 97-41613. (International Congress Ser.). 572p. 215.50 (*0-444-82782-X*) Elsevier.

Advances in Head & Neck Oncology. K. Thomas Robbins. 1998. LC 97-36322. (Illus.). 300p. pap. 99.95 (*1-56593-840-2*, 1640) Thomson Learn.

Advances in Headache Research. F. Clifford Rose. 1987. (Current Problems in Neurology Ser.: Vol. 4). 288p. (*0-86196-097-1*) J Libbey Med GBR. *Dist:* Bks Intl VA.

Advances in Health Care Research: 1982 Proceedings. Ed. by Scott M. Smith & M. Venkatesan. 1988. pap. text 15.00 (*0-945769-00-8*) AAAHCR.

Advances in Health Care Research: 1983 Proceedings. Ed. by Scott M. Smith & M. Venkatesan. 1988. pap. text 15.00 (*0-945769-01-6*) AAAHCR.

Advances in Health Care Research: 1984 Proceedings. Ed. by Scott M. Smith & M. Venkatesan. 1988. pap. text 15.00 (*0-945769-02-4*) AAAHCR.

Advances in Health Care Research: 1985 Proceedings. Ed. by Scott M. Smith & M. Venkatesan. 1988. pap. text 15.00 (*0-945769-03-2*) AAAHCR.

Advances in Health Care Research: 1986 Proceedings. Ed. by M. Venkatesan & Wade Lancaster. 1988. 90p. pap. text 15.00 (*0-945769-04-0*) AAAHCR.

Advances in Health Care Research: 1987 Proceedings. Ed. by M. Venkatesan & Wade Lancaster. 1988. 63p. pap. text 15.00 (*0-945769-05-9*) AAAHCR.

Advances in Health Care Research: 1988 Proceedings. Ed. by George T. Baker et al. 1988. 92p. pap. text 15.00 (*0-945769-06-7*) AAAHCR.

Advances in Health Care Research: Conference Proceedings 1991. 1991. (*0-945769-08-3*) AAAHCR.

Advances in Health Economics & Health Services Research. Ed. by Richard M. Scheffler et al. Vol. 2. 1981. 280p. 73.25 (*0-89232-100-8*); Vol. 3. 1982. 326p. 73.25 (*0-89232-222-5*); Vol. 4. 1983. 367p. 73.25 (*0-89232-260-8*); Vol. 5. 1984. 337p. 73.25 (*0-89232-487-2*); Vol. 13. 1993. 241p. 73.25 (*1-55938-466-2*); Vol. 15. 1995. 224p. 72.00 (*1-55938-873-0*) Jai Pr.

Advances in Health Economics & Health Services Research, Vol. 16. Ed. by Richard M. Scheffler & Louis F. Rossiter. Date not set. 73.25 (*0-7623-0028-0*) Jai Pr.

Advances in Health Economics & Health Services Research: An Annual Compilation of Research, Vol. 1. Ed. by Richard M. Scheffler et al. 1979. 401p. 73.25 (*0-89232-042-7*) Jai Pr.

Advances in Health Education: Current Research 1988-1993, Vols. 1-4. Ed. by James H. Humphrey. 1988. LC 86-47857. (*0-404-63550-4*) AMS Pr.

Advances in Health Education & Promotion, Vol. 3. Ed. by William B. Ward & Frances M. Lewis. 1991. 300p. 88.00 (*1-85302-074-5*) Taylor & Francis.

Advances in Health Telematics Education: A Nightingale Perspective. Ed. by J. Mantas. 1998. (Studies in Health Technology & Informatics: Vol. 51). 257p. (YA). (gr. 12 up). 70.00 (*90-5199-389-7*) IOS Press.

Advances in Hearing Research: Proceedings of the 10th International Symposium on Hearing. G. A. Manley et al. 1995. 580p. text 147.00 (*981-02-2260-2*) World Scientific Pub.

Advances in Hematological Methods: The Blood Count. O. W. van Assendelft & J. M. England. 1982. 272p. 152.00 (*0-8493-6596-1*, RB45, CRC Reprint) Franklin.

Advances in Hematopoietic Stem Cell Transplantation & Molecular Therapy, Vol. 144. R. Haas & R. Kronenwett. 1997. LC 97-11989. (Recent Results in Cancer Research Ser.). (Illus.). 150p. 119.00 (*3-540-62626-3*) Spr-Verlag.

Advances in Hemodynamics & Hemorheology. Ed. by T. V. How. Vol. 1. 1996. 444p. 90.00 (*1-55938-634-7*); Vol. 2. Date not set. 128.50 (*0-7623-0384-0*) Jai Pr.

Advances in Hepatic Encephalopathy & Metabolic Nitrogen Exchange. Livio Capocaccia. 1994. 672p. lib. bdg. 229.00 (*0-8493-8964-X*) CRC Pr.

Advances in Hepatic Enecephalopathy & Urea Cycle Diseases. Ed. by G. Kleinberger et al. 1985. (Illus.). xii, 770p. pap. 138.50 (*3-8055-3995-9*) S Karger.

Advances in Hepatobiliary & Pancreatic Diseases: Special Clinical Topics: Proceedings of the Falk Symposium No. 83, Held in Bolzano, Italy, April 7-8, 1995. Ed. by G. Dobrilla et al. 1995. LC 95-24716. 288p. (C). text 118.00 (*0-7923-8892-5*) Kluwer Academic.

Advances in Histamine Research. 1995. 345p. 121.00 (*4-431-70137-0*) Spr-Verlag.

Advances in Histamine Research: Proceedings of a Satellite Symposium to the 8th International Congress of Pharmacology, July 26-27, 1981, Okayama, Japan. Ed. by B. Uvnas & Kenji Tasaka. 1982. (Illus.). 260p. 69.50 (*0-08-028006-4*, H130, Pergamon Pr) Elsevier.

Advances in Human Ecology, Vol. 3. Ed. by Lee Freese. 1994. 247p. 78.50 (*1-55938-760-2*) Jai Pr.

Advances in Human Genetics. Harry Harris & Kurt Hirschhorn. (Illus.). (C). Vol. 19. 1989. 358p. text 95.00 (*0-306-43298-6*); Vol. 20. 1991. 308p. text 95.00 (*0-306-43998-0*) Kluwer Academic (Kluwer Plenum).

Advances in Human Genetics, Vol. 22. Ed. by Harry Harris & Kurt Hirschhorn. 1995. (Illus.). 288p. (C). text 95.00 (*0-306-44845-9*, Kluwer Plenum) Kluwer Academic.

Advances in Human Genetics, Vol. 23. Kurt Hirschhorn & R. J. Desnick. 1999. (*0-306-45170-0*, Kluwer Plenum) Kluwer Academic.

Advances in Human Nutrition, Vol. 2. Ed. by Edward J. Calabrese & George H. Scherr. 1985. LC 81-82478. 300p. 35.00 (*0-930376-35-8*) Chem-Orbital.

Advances in Human Nutrition, Vol. 3. Ed. by Jon J. Kabara & George H. Scherr. 1986. LC 81-83797. 286p. 23.00 (*0-930376-39-0*) Chem-Orbital.

Advances in Human Reproduction: Proceedings of the 8th World Congress on Human Reproduction Jointly with the 4th World Conference on Fallopian Tube in Health & Disease, Bali, Indonesia, April 1993. Ed. by F. A. Moeloek et al. 1994. LC 94-21471. (International Congress, Symposium, & Seminar Ser.: vol. 7). 554p. lib. bdg. 96.95 (*1-85070-521-6*, Parthenon Pbng) CRC Pr.

Advances in Humor & Psychotherapy. Ed. by William F. Fry, Jr. & Waleed A. Salameh. 1993. LC 93-17202. 332p. 39.95 (*0-943158-78-8*, AHPBP, Prof Resc Pr) Pro Resource.

Advances in Hybridization Techniques for Gene & Genome Mapping & Sequencing. Jorg Hoheisel. 1997. (Molecular Biology Intelligence Unit Ser.). 200p. 89.95 (*0-412-13171-4*) Chapman & Hall.

Advances in Hypertension. Ed. by M. A. Weber. 1996. (American Journal of Nephrology: Vol. 16, No. 3). (Illus.). 86p. pap. 32.25 (*3-8055-6289-6*) S Karger.

Advances in Imaging & Electron Physics, Vol. 103. Ed. by Peter W. Hawkes et al. 1998. (Illus.). 398p. 130.00 (*0-12-014745-9*) Acad Pr.

Advances in Imaging Techniques in Ischemic Heart Disease, Vol. 171. Ed. by Johan H. Reiber et al. 1995. LC 95-23084. (Developments in Cardiovascular Medicine Ser.). 168p. (C). text 73.50 (*0-7923-3620-8*) Kluwer Academic.

Advances in Immunity & Cancer Therapy, Vol. 1. 1985. (Illus.). 220p. 127.00 (*0-387-96083-X*) Spr-Verlag.

Advances in Immunity & Cancer Therapy, Vol. 2. P. K. Ray. 1986. (Illus.). 301p. 91.00 (*0-387-96258-1*) Spr-Verlag.

Advances in Immunohistochemistry. Ronald A. De Lellis. 1984. (C). (gr. 13). 87.00 (*0-89352-215-5*) Mosby Inc.

Advances in Immunology. Dixon. 1999. (Advances in Immunology Ser.: Vol. 74). (Illus.). 344p. (C). text 99.95 (*0-12-022474-7*) Acad Pr.

Advances in Immunology. Ed. by Frank J. Dixon. 2000. (Advances in Immunology Ser.: Vol. 76). 119.95 (*0-12-022476-3*); 325p. 119.95 (*0-12-022475-5*) Acad Pr.

Advances in Immunology. Frank J. Dixon. 400p. 1999. 89.95 (*0-12-022472-0*); 1998. (Advances in Immunology Ser.: Vol. 71). (Illus.). (C). text 89.95 (*0-12-022471-2*) Acad Pr.

Advances in Immunology. Ed. by Frank J. Dixon. (Illus.). Vol. 50. 1991. 343p. (C). text 104.00 (*0-12-022450-X*); Vol. 51. 1992. 397p. text 104.00 (*0-12-022451-8*); Vol. 53. 1993. 342p. text 104.00 (*0-12-022453-4*); Vol. 54. 1993. 443p. text 104.00 (*0-12-022454-2*); Vol. 55. 1993. 456p. text 104.00 (*0-12-022455-0*); Vol. 57. 1994. 391p. text 94.00 (*0-12-022457-7*); Vol. 60. 1995. 388p. text 85.00 (*0-12-022460-7*); Vol. 61. 1996. 416p. text 85.00 (*0-12-022461-5*); Vol. 62. 1996. 316p. text 79.00 (*0-12-022462-3*, Vol. 62); Vol. 69. 1998. 462p. 89.95 (*0-12-022469-0*) Acad Pr.

*__Advances in Immunology__, Vol. 78. Ed. by Frank J. Dixon. 2001. 400p. 119.95 (*0-12-022478-X*) Acad Pr.

Advances in Immunology, Vol. 70. Frank J. Dixon. 1998. (Illus.). 574p. (C). text 89.95 (*0-12-022470-4*) Harcourt.

Advances in Immunology. Ed. by Frank J. Dixon. (Illus.). Vol. 64. 1997. (Advances in Immunology Ser.: Vol. 64). 365p. text 89.00 (*0-12-022464-X*); Vol. 65. 1997. 408p. text 89.00 (*0-12-022465-8*); Vol. 66. 1997. 322p. text 89.95 (*0-12-022466-6*); Vol. 68. 1998. 432p. text 89.95 (*0-12-022468-2*) Morgan Kaufmann.

Advances in Infancy Research. Ed. by Lewis P. Lipsitt & Carolyn Rovee-Collier. (Advances in Infancy Research Ser.). Vol. 1. 1981. 290p. 85.00 (*0-89391-045-7*); Vol. 2. 1983. 344p. 85.00 (*0-89391-113-5*) Greenwood (Ablex).

Advances in Infancy Research, Vol. 3. Ed. by Lewis P. Lipsett & Carolyn Rovee-Collier. 1984. 296p. 85.00 (*0-89391-208-5*, Ablex) Greenwood.

Advances in Infancy Research. Ed. by Carolyn Rovee-Collier & Lewis P. Lipsitt. Vol. 5. 1988. 240p. 85.00 (*0-89391-378-2*); Vol. 6. 1990. 336p. (C). 85.00 (*0-89391-512-2*) Greenwood (Ablex).

Advances in Infancy Research, Vol. 8. Lois Bloom et al. 1993. 376p. 85.00 (*0-89391-827-X*, Ablex) Greenwood.

Advances in Infancy Research, Vol. 9. Ed. by Carolyn Rovee-Collier & Lewis P Lipsitt. 1995. (Illus.). 424p. 85.00 (*1-56750-126-5*, Ablex) Greenwood.

Advances in Infancy Research, Vol. 11. Ed. by Lewis P. Lipsitt & Carolyn Rovee-Collier. 1997. 281p. 78.50 (*1-56750-287-3*, Ablex) Greenwood.

Advances in Inflammatory Bowel Diseases. Ed. by P. Rutgeerts et al. 1999. (Falk Symposium Ser.: Vol. 106). 316p. 190.00 (*0-7923-8750-3*) Kluwer Academic.

Advances in Instructional Psychology, Vol. 3. Robert Glaser. 1986. 240p. (C). text 59.95 (*0-89859-706-4*) L Erlbaum Assocs.

Advances in Internal Medcine, 1999. (Illus.). 500p. text 78.00 (*0-8151-2817-7*, 29317) Mosby Inc.

Advances in Internal Medicine. 1992. 152.00 (*0-387-54235-3*); 1988. 128.00 (*0-387-19124-0*) Spr-Verlag.

Advances in Internal Medicine Robert W. Schrier. (Illus.). 1998. 456p. (C). text 79.00 (*0-8151-2816-9*, 29316); 46th ed. 2000. 500p. text 75.95 (*0-8151-2818-5*, 29318) Mosby Inc.

Advances in Internal Medicine, 43. Peter F. Abboud et al. 1997. (Illus.). 608p. (C). (gr. 13). text 79.00 (*0-8151-8317-8*, 21992) Mosby Inc.

Advances in Internal Medicine, Vol. 43. Robert W. Schrier. 43rd ed. 1998. (C). (gr. 13). pap. text 139.95 (*0-8151-9815-9*) Mosby Inc.

Advances in Internal Medicine, Vol. 47. Ed. by Robert W. Schrier. 2001. (Illus.). 500p. (*0-323-01538-7*) Mosby Inc.

*__Advances in Internal Medicine.__ Ed. by Robert W. Schrier. (Illus.). 500p. Vol. 48. 2002. (*0-323-01539-5*); Vol. 49. 2003. (*0-323-01540-9*) Mosby Inc.

Advances in Internal Medicine & Pediatrics, Vol. 44. 1980. (Illus.). 175p. 71.95 (*0-387-09869-0*) Spr-Verlag.

Advances in Internal Medicine & Pediatrics, Vol. 50. Ed. by P. Frick et al. 1982. (Illus.). 189p. 93.00 (*0-387-11445-9*) Spr-Verlag.

Advances in Interventional Neuroradiology & Intravascular Neurosurgery: Proceedings of the International Congress on Interventional Neuroradiology & Intravascular Neurosurgery, Kyoto, Japan, 19-22 November 1995. Ed. by Waro Taki et al. 1996. LC 96-22330. (International Congress Ser.). 524p. 185.00 (*0-444-82319-0*) Elsevier.

Advances in Lactoferrin Research. Ed. by G. Spik et al. 1998. LC 98-28776. (Advances in Experimental Medicine & Biology Ser.: Vol. 443). (Illus.). 364p. (C). text 95.00 (*0-306-45926-4*, Kluwer Plenum) Kluwer Academic.

Advances in Laparoscopic Surgery. Dirk Fahlenkamp. 1996. (Illus.). 900p. text 125.00 (*0-86542-901-4*) Blackwell Sci.

Advances in Laryngology in Europe: Proceedings of the First Scientific Conference of the European Laryngological Society, Marburg, Germany, 26-29 September, 1996. European Laryngological Society Staff et al. 1997. LC 97-8886. (International Congress Ser.: No. 1128). 506p. 185.00 (*0-444-82543-6*) Elsevier.

Advances in Learning & Behavioral Disabilities: Method Issues in Human Psychopharmacology. Ed. by Thomas E. Scruggs et al. Vol. 1. 1982. 472p. 78.50 (*0-89232-209-8*); Vol. 2. 1983. 312p. 78.50 (*0-89232-285-3*); Vol. 3. 1985. 272p. 78.50 (*0-89232-333-7*); Vol. 4. 1985. 347p. 78.50 (*0-89232-532-1*) Jai Pr.

Advances in Learning & Behavioral Disabilities: Methodological Issues in Human Psychopharmacology, Supp. No. 1. Ed. by Thomas E. Scruggs et al. 1986. 368p. suppl. ed. 78.50 (*0-89232-643-3*) Jai Pr.

Advances in Long-Term Care. Ed. by Paul R. Katz et al. 1992. 288p. Vol. I. text 44.95 (*0-8261-6830-2*); Vol. II. 47.95 (*0-8261-6831-0*) Springer Pub.

Advances in Luminesince Spectroscopy - STP 863. Ed. by L. J. Cline Love & Delyle Eastwood. 1985. LC 84-71320. (Illus.). 129p. pap. text 26.00 (*0-8031-0412-X*, STP863) ASTM.

Advances in Lymphoma Research. Ed. by Fernando Cabanillas & M. Alma Rodriguez. 1997. LC 96-4655. (Cancer Treatment & Research Ser.: Vol. 85). 184p. (C). text 214.50 (*0-7923-3929-0*) Kluwer Academic.

Advances in Macromolecular Carbohydrate Research, Vol. 1. Ed. by Robert J. Sturgeon. 1997. 211p. 85.00 (*1-55938-323-2*) Jai Pr.

Advances in Magnesium Research. Smetana. 1997. 600p. (*0-86196-555-8*) J Libbey Med GBR. *Dist:* Buttrwrth-Heinemann.

Advances in Magnetic Resonance Imaging, Vol. 1. Ed. by Ephraim Feig. 1989. 272p. (C). 78.50 (*0-89391-445-2*, Ablex) Greenwood.

Advances in Malaria Chemotherapy: Report of a WHO Scientific Group, 1984. WHO Staff. 1984. (Technical Report Ser.: No. 711). 218p. 20.00 (*92-4-120711-6*) World Health.

Advances in Materials Science & Implant Orthopedic Surgery: Proceedings of the NATO Advanced Study Institutes on Materials Science & Implant Orthopaedic Surgery II, Chinia, Crete, Greece, June 19-July 2, 1994. Ed. by Ram Kossowsky & Nir Kossovsky. 1995. LC 95-11082. (NATO Advanced Science Institutes Ser.: No. 294). 332p. text 174.00 (*0-7923-3558-9*) Kluwer Academic.

Advances in Maxillofacial Imaging: Selected Proceedings of the 11th Congress of the International Association of Dentomaxillofacial Radiology & the 3rd International Congress & Exposition on Computed Maxillofacial Imaging, Louisville, Kentucky, June 21-27, 1977. International Association of Dentomaxillofacial Ra & Allan G. Farman. 1997. LC 97-11875. (International Congress Ser.: 1143). 502p. 185.00 (*0-444-82542-8*) Elsevier.

Advances in Medical Biology, Vol. 1. Ed. by E. Edward Bittar. Date not set. 128.50 (*0-7623-0386-7*) Jai Pr.

Advances in Medical Biology: Results of the 4th EC Medical & Health Research Program. Ed. by C. Baya. 1994. LC 93-80284. (Biomedical & Health Research Ser.: Vol. 3). 276p. 117.00 (*90-5199-146-0*) IOS Press.

Advances in Medical Education. 1997. LC 97-41297. 832p. lib. bdg. 301.00 (*0-7923-4149-X*) Kluwer Academic.

Advances in Medical Informatics: Results of the AIM Exploratory Action. Ed. by Jaap N. Van Goor & Jens P. Christensen. 1992. LC 91-75447. (Studies in Health Technology & Informatics: Vol. 2). 444p. (YA). (gr. 12 up). 110.00 (*90-5199-058-8*) IOS Press.

Advances in Medical Information. P. L. Kerkhof & S. Vinkelstein. 1992. 108p. pap. text 335.00 (*2-88124-862-4*) Gordon & Breach.

Advances in Medical Oncology, Research & Education: Proceedings of the 12th International Cancer Congress, Buenes Aires, 1978, Set. A. Canonoico & O. Estevez. 1979. LC 79-40032. (*0-08-023777-0*) Pergamon Repr GBR. *Dist:* Franklin.

Advances in Medical Social Science, Vol. 2. Julio L. Ruffini. 1984. xii, 402p. text 196.00 (*0-677-06490-X*) Gordon & Breach.

Advances in Medical Sociology, Vol. 1. Ed. by Gary L. Albrecht. 1990. 329p. 78.50 (*1-55938-092-6*) Jai Pr.

Advances in Medical Sociology, Vol. 2. Ed. by Gary L. Albrecht & Judith A. Levy. 1991. 322p. 78.50 (*1-55938-252-X*) Jai Pr.

Advances in Medicinal Chemistry. Ed. by Bruce E. Maryanoff & Cynthia A. Maryanoff. Vol. 1. 1992. 288p. 90.00 (*1-55938-170-1*); Vol. 2. 1993. 272p. 90.00 (*1-55938-581-2*); Vol. 3. 1995. 188p. 90.00 (*1-55938-798-X*) Jai Pr.

Advances in Medicinal Chemistry, Vol. 4. Bruce E. Maryanoff & Allen Reitz. 1999. 336p. 90.00 (*0-7623-0064-7*) Jai Pr.

Advances in Medicine. Richard E. Edlich. 2000. 145.00 (*1-886236-27-5*) ABI Prof Pubns.

Advances in Mental Health Research. Ed. by Janet B. Williams & Kathleen Ell. 1998. LC 98-11120. 1124p. pap. text 27.95 (*0-87101-291-X*) Natl Assn Soc Wkrs.

Advances in Mental Retardation & Developmental Disabilities, Vol. 4. Ed. by Robert A. Gable & Steven F. Warren. 1991. 300p. 79.00 (*1-85302-075-3*) Taylor & Francis.

Advances in Mental Retardation & Developmental Disabilities: Strategies for Teaching Students with Mild Mental Retardation, Vol. 5. Ed. by Robert A. Gable. 1993. 300p. 85.00 (*1-85302-141-5*) Taylor & Francis.

Advances in Metabolic Mapping Techniques for Brain Imaging of Behavioral & Learning Functions: Proceedings of the NATO Advanced Research Workshop, Austin, Texas, U. S. A. 7-9 November 1991. Ed. by F. Gonzalez-Lima. 1992. (NATO Advanced Science Institutes Ser.). 552p. (C). text 316.50 (*0-7923-1947-8*) Kluwer Academic.

Advances in Metals in Medicine, Vol. 1. Ed. by M. J. Abrams & Barry A. Murrer. 1993. 196p. 128.50 (*1-55938-352-6*) Jai Pr.

Advances in Metals in Medicine, Vol. 2. Ed. by Michael J. Abrams et al. 1999. 78.50 (*0-7623-0090-6*) Jai Pr.

Advances in Methods of Fertility Regulation: Proceedings of the WHO Scientific Group, Geneva, 1972. WHO Staff. (Technical Reports: No. 575). 1975. pap. text 6.00 (*92-4-120575-X*, 1100575); 1973. (ENG & RUS.). pap. text 4.00 (*92-4-120527-X*, 1100527) World Health.

Advances in Microbial Physiology, Vol. 22. Ed. by A. H. Rose & J. Gareth Morris. 1981. (Serial Publication Ser.). text 104.00 (*0-12-027722-0*) Acad Pr.

Advances in Microbial Physiology. Ed. by A. H. Rose. (Illus.). Vol. 33. 1992. 424p. text 104.00 (*0-12-027733-6*); Vol. 35. 1993. 352p. text 104.00 (*0-12-027735-2*) Acad Pr.

*__Advances in Microbial Physiology__, Vol. 44. Ed. by Robert K. Poole. 2001. 288p. 129.95 (*0-12-027744-1*) Acad Pr.

Advances in Microcirculation. Ed. by H. Harders. Vol. 3. 1970. 57.50 (*3-8055-0453-5*); Vol. 4. 1972. (Illus.). 75.75 (*3-8055-1353-4*); Vol. 5. 1973. (Illus.). 106p. 47.00 (*3-8055-1337-2*); Vol. 6. 1975. (Illus.). 250p. 85.25 (*3-8055-1608-8*) S Karger.

Advances in Microcirculation, Vol. 7. Ed. by H. Harders et al. 1977. (Illus.). 74.00 (*3-8055-2247-9*) S Karger.

Advances in Migraine Management. Ed. by J. G. Edmeads & K. M. Welch. 1994. (Journal: Vol. 34, Supplement 2, 1994). (Illus.). iv, 44p. pap. 21.00 (*3-8055-6067-2*) S Karger.

Advances in Modern Human Nutrition, Vol. 1. Ed. by Richard B. Tobin & Myron A. Mehlman. 1980. 365p. 37.00 (*0-930376-07-2*) Chem-Orbital.

Advances in Molecular & Cell Biology Vol. 13: Cell Cycle. Ed. by Michael Whitaker et al. 1995. 240p. 97.50 (*1-55938-949-4*, Plenum Trade) Perseus Pubng.

Advances in Molecular & Cell Biology Vol. 25: Oxyradicals in Medical Biology. Ed. by Joe M. McCord. 1998. 200p. 90.00 (*0-7623-0379-4*) Jai Pr.

Advances in Molecular & Cellular Immunology. Ed. by Bhagirath Singh. Vol. 1, Pts. A & B. 1993. 440p. 257.00 (*1-55938-353-4*); Vol. 2. Date not set. 128.50 (*0-7623-0088-4*) Jai Pr.

Advances in Molecular Biology & Targeted Treatment for AIDS. Ed. by A. Kumar. 1991. (GWUMC Department of Biochemistry & Molecular Biology Annual Spring Symposium Ser.). (Illus.). 366p. (C). text 138.00 (*0-306-43901-8*, Kluwer Plenum) Kluwer Academic.

Advances in Motivation & Achievement: Motivation & Adulthood, Vol. 4. Ed. by Martin L. Maehr et al. 1985. 408p. 78.50 (*0-89232-544-5*) Jai Pr.

Advances in Motivation & Achievement: Motivation Enhancing Environments, Vol. 6. Ed. by Martin L. Maehr et al. 1989. 312p. 78.50 (*0-89232-889-4*) Jai Pr.

AB

Advances in Motivation & Achievement: The Effects of School Desegregation on Motivation & Achievement, Vol. 1. Ed. by Martin L. Maehr et al. 1984. 344p. 78.50 (*0-89232-290-X*) Jai Pr.

Advances in Motivation & Achievement: Women in Science, Vol. 2. Ed. by Martin L. Maehr et al. 1984. 400p. 78.50 (*0-89232-288-8*) Jai Pr.

Advances in Motor Development Research, Vol. 4. Ed. by Jane E. Clark & James H. Humphrey. 1992. 37.50 (*0-404-63454-0*) AMS Pr.

Advances in MRI. L. Heuser & Matthijs Oedkerk. 1996. 176p. 95.00 (*0-632-04177-3*) Blackwell Sci.

Advances in Mucosal Immunology. Ed. by T. C. MacDonald et al. 1990. (C). text 418.00 (*0-7462-0113-3*) Kluwer Academic.

Advances in Mucosal Immunology Pts. A & B: Proceedings of the Seventh International Congress of Mucosal Immunology, Held in Prague, Czechoslovakia, August 16-21, 1992, Pts. A & B. J. Mestecky et al. 1995. (Advances in Experimental Medicine & Biology Ser.: Vol. 371). (Illus.). 1724p. (C). text 265.00 (*0-306-45012-7*, Kluwer Plenum) Kluwer Academic.

Advances in Mutagenesis Research, Vol. 2. Ed. by G. Obe. 1991. (Illus.). 326p. 159.00 (*0-387-52428-2*) Spr-Verlag.

Advances in Mutagenesis Research. Ed. by G. Obe et al. (Illus.). Vol. 3. 1991. 197p. 149.00 (*0-387-53359-1*); Vol. 5. 1994. 193p. 220.00 (*0-387-56641-4*) Spr-Verlag.

Advances in Nd: YAG Laser Surgery. Ed. by S. N. Joffe & Yanao Oguro. 1987. (Illus.). 368p. 265.00 (*0-387-96506-8*) Spr-Verlag.

Advances in Nephrology, Vol. 29. Jean-Pierre Grunfeld et al. 1999. (Illus.). 350p. (C). text (*0-323-00744-9*) Mosby Inc.

Advances in Nephrology, Vol. 30. Grunfeld. 2000. text 92.00 (*0-323-00745-7*) Mosby Inc.

Advances in Nephrology, Vol.28. 1998. (Illus.). 520p. text 84.00 (*0-8151-3933-0*, 25758) Mosby Inc.

Advances in Nephrology: Proceedings of the International Congress, 6th, Florence, June, 1975. Ed. by Sergio Giovannetti & V. Bonomini. 1976. (Illus.). 784p. 155.75 (*3-8055-2287-8*) S Karger.

Advances in Nephrology & Dialysis. Ed. by G. Colasanti. 1990. (Contributions to Nephrology Ser.: Vol. 77). (Illus.). vi, 202p. 155.75 (*3-8055-5064-2*) S Karger.

Advances in Nephrology & Dialysis. Ed. by G. D'Amico & G. Colasanti. 1985. (Contributions to Nephrology Ser.: Vol. 45). (Illus.). x, 214p. 113.25 (*3-8055-3963-0*) S Karger.

Advances in Neural Information Processing Systems 9, Vol. 9. Ed. by Michael I. Jordan et al. 1997. (Advances in Neural Information Processing Systems 9 Ser.: Vol. 9). (Illus.). 1120p. 80.00 (*0-262-10065-7*) MIT Pr.

Advances in Neural Science, Vol. 1. Ed. by Sudarshan Malhotra & G. D. Das. 1993. 238p. 90.00 (*1-55938-356-9*) Jai Pr.

Advances in Neural Science. Ed. by Sudarshan Malhotra. Vol. 2. 1995. 254p. 90.00 (*1-55938-625-8*); Vol. 3. Date not set. 128.50 (*0-7623-0087-6*) Jai Pr.

Advances in Neuro-Oncology II. Ed. by Paul L. Kornblith & Michael D. Walker. 1997. LC 97-543. (Illus.). 584p. 125.00 (*0-87993-603-7*) Futura Pub.

Advances in Neurobehavioral Toxicology: Applications in Environmental & Occupational Health. Ed. by Barry L. Johnson et al. 1990. (Illus.). 536p. lib. bdg. 129.00 (*0-87371-374-5*, L374) Lewis Pubs.

Advances in Neuroblastoma Research: Proceedings of the Sixth Symposium on Advances in Neuroblastoma Research, Held in Philadelphia, Pennsylvania, May 13-15, 1993. Ed. by Audrey E. Evans et al. 1994. (Progress in Clinical & Biological Research Ser.: No. 385). 470p. 357.00 (*0-471-01454-0*, Wiley-Interscience) Wiley.

Advances in Neurodegenerative Disorders Vol. 1: Parkinson's Disease. Ed. by Joe Marwah & Herman Teitelbaum. 1999. LC 98-68496. (Illus.). 400p. (C). text 60.00 (*0-9668997-0-9*) Prominnt Pr.

Advances in Neurodegenerative Disorders Vol. 2: Alzheimer's & Aging, Vol. 2. Ed. by Joe Marwah & Herman Teitelbaum. 1999. LC 98-68496. (Illus.). 400p. (C). text 60.00 (*0-9668997-1-7*) Prominnt Pr.

Advances in Neuroendocrine Physiology. Ed. by K. B. Ruf & George Tolis. 1982. (Frontiers of Hormone Research Ser.: Vol. 10). (Illus.). vi, 142p. 85.25 (*3-8055-2949-X*) S Karger.

Advances in Neuroscience & Schizophrenia. Ed. by A. Hussain Tuma et al. 1992. (Journals of Neural Transmission: Suppl. 36). (Illus.). 160p. 86.95 (*0-387-82347-6*) Spr-Verlag.

Advances in Neurosurgery: Intracerebral Hemorrhages Hydrocephalus Malresorptivus Peripheral Nerves, Vol. 21. Ed. by R. Lorenz et al. 1993. (Illus.). 360p. 79.00 (*0-387-56304-0*) Spr-Verlag.

Advances in Neutron Capture Therapy. A. H. Soloway et al. 1993. (Illus.). 860p. (C). text 179.50 (*0-306-44567-0*, Kluwer Plenum) Kluwer Academic.

Advances in Neutron Capture Therapy: Proceedings of the 17th International Symposium on Neutron Capture Therapy for Cancer, Zurich, Switzerland, 4-7 September, 1996, Vol. 1132. Borje Larsson et al. 1997. LC 97-42036. 1356p. 312.50 (*0-444-82781-1*) Elsevier.

Advances in Nitrate Therapy. Adam Schneeweiss & M. Weiss. 2nd enl. rev. ed. 1990. 232p. 72.95 (*0-387-52798-2*) Spr-Verlag.

Advances in Non-Verbal Communication: Sociocultural, Clinical, Esthetic & Literary Perspectives. Ed. by Fernando Poyatos. 1992. LC 92-599. xxiv, 412p. 130.00 (*1-55619-121-9*) J Benjamins Pubng Co.

Advances in Noninvasive Cardiology. Ed. by J. Meyer et al. 1983. (Developments in Cardiovascular Medicine Ser.). text 141.50 (*0-89838-576-8*) Kluwer Academic.

Advances in Nutrition & Cancer. V. Zappia et al. 1993. LC 93-49575. (Advances in Experimental Medicine & Biology Ser.: Vol. 348). (Illus.). 170p. (C). text 79.50 (*0-306-44670-7*, Kluwer Plenum) Kluwer Academic.

Advances in Nutrition & Cancer: Proceedings of the 2nd International Conference on Nutrition & Cancer, Held October 20-23, 1998, in Naples, Italy. Vincenzo Zappia. 2nd ed. 2000. LC 99-49491. (Advances in Experimental Medicine & Biology Ser.). 312p. 95.00 (*0-306-46306-7*, Kluwer Plenum) Kluwer Academic.

Advances in Nutritional Research, Vol. 8. H. H. Draper. 1990. LC 78-640645. (Illus.). 162p. (C). text 78.00 (*0-306-43512-8*, Kluwer Plenum) Kluwer Academic.

Advances in Ocular Immunology & Immunopathology of the Eye: Proceedings of the Sixth International Symposium on the Immunology & Immunopathology of the Eye, Bethesda, U. S. A. Ed. by Robert B. Nussenblatt et al. 1995. LC 94-35302. (International Congress Ser.). 496p. 240.25 (*0-444-81742-5*) Elsevier.

Advances in Ocular Toxicology: Proceedings of the Fifth Congress of the International Society of Ocular Toxicology Held in Asheville, North Carolina, October 13-17, 1996. Ed. by Keith Green et al. 1997. LC 97-16694. 292p. 105.00 (*0-306-45614-1*, Kluwer Plenum) Kluwer Academic.

Advances in Old Age Psychiatry: Chromosomes to Community Care. Ed. by Clive Holmes & Robert Howard. 1997. LC 96-52925. 256p. (*1-871816-34-3*) Wrightson Biomed GBR. *Dist:* Taylor & Francis.

Advances in Oncology. M. Ghione et al. 1988. xiv, 278p. text 198.00 (*3-7186-0464-7*) Gordon & Breach.

Advances in Ophthalmic Genetic & Heritable Eye Diseases. Frederick A. Jakobiec. 1993. 39.00 (*0-316-45596-2*, Little Brwn Med Div) Lppncott W & W.

Advances in Ophthalmic Plastic & Reconstructive Surgery. Ed. by Stephen L. Bosniak & Byron C. Smith. 1989. Vol. 6, Pt. 1. 419p. 75.00 (*0-08-036842-5*); Vol. 7, Pt. 2. 351p. 75.00 (*0-08-036843-3*) Elsevier (Pergamon Pr).

Advances in Ophthalmic Plastic & Reconstructive Surgery, Vol. 5: History & Tradition. S. L. Bosniak. 1986. 464p. 78.00 (*0-08-033170-X*, Pergamon Pr) Elsevier.

Advances in Ophthalmology, Vol. 26. Ed. by Michael J. Roper-Hall et al. 1972. 116.75 (*3-8055-1354-2*) S Karger.

Advances in Ophthalmology. Ed. by E. B. Streiff et al. Vol. 29. 1975. 200p. 94.00 (*3-8055-1709-2*); Vol. 32. 1976. (Illus.). 212p. 111.50 (*3-8055-2222-3*); Vol. 34. 1977. 112.25 (*3-8055-2406-4*) S Karger.

Advances in Ophthalmology. Ed. by Michael J. Roper-Hall et al. (Illus.). Vol. 35. 1978. (GER.). 115.00 (*3-8055-2657-1*); Vol. 39. 1979. 163.50 (*3-8055-3030-7*) S Karger.

Advances in Ophthalmology, Vol. 40. Ed. by Michael J. Roper-hall et al. 1979. (Illus.). 136.75 (*3-8055-3031-5*) S Karger.

Advances in Ophthalmology. Ed. by E. B. Streiff. (Illus.). Vol. 41. 1980. xvii, 216p. 139.25 (*3-8055-0375-X*); Vol. 42. 1981. 164p. 85.25 (*3-8055-1025-X*) S Karger.

*__Advances in Optics & Laser Research.__ Ed. by William T. Arkin. 2002. lib. bdg. 89.00 (*1-59033-154-0*) Nova Sci Pubs.

Advances in Organ Biology Vol. 4, Pts. A & B: Heart Metabolism in Failure, Vol. 4. Ruth Altschuld & Robert Haworth. 1998. 257.00 (*0-7623-0389-1*) Jai Pr.

Advances in Organ Biology Vol. 7: Coronary Angiogenesis. Ed. by Karel Rakusan. 1999. 294p. 90.00 (*0-7623-0392-1*) Jai Pr.

Advances in Osteoarthritis. Ed. by R. A. White & C. Hamanishi. 1999. LC 98-46286. (Illus.). 308p. 129.00 (*4-431-70245-8*) Spr-Verlag.

Advances in Oto-Rhino-Laryngology, 58. Ed. by Tran Ba Huy & M. Toupet. 2001. LC 00-49737. (Advances in OtoRhinoLaryngology Ser.: Vol. 58). (Illus.). viii,132p. 148.00 (*3-8055-7130-5*) S Karger.

Advances in Otolaryngology. Eugene N. Myers. 2002. text 85.95 (*0-323-00939-5*) Harcourt.

Advances in Otolaryngology. Eugene N. Myers. 2000. text 85.95 (*0-323-00937-9*) Harcrt Hlth Sci Grp.

Advances in Otolaryngology. Eugene N. Myers. 2001. text 85.95 (*0-323-00938-7*); 12. 1998. (Illus.). 344p. text 89.00 (*0-8151-9821-3*, 25056); 13. 1999. (Illus.). 248p. text 89.00 (*0-8151-9822-1*, 25057) Mosby Inc.

Advances in Pain Therapy II. J. Chrubasik et al. 1993. (Illus.). 230p. pap. (*3-540-56917-0*) Spr-Verlag.

Advances in Pain Therapy One. Ed. by J. Chrubasik et al. 1992. (Illus.). 96p. 49.95 (*0-387-55536-6*) Spr-Verlag.

Advances in Parapsychological Research, Vol. 3. Ed. by Stanley Krippner. 1982. LC 77-9518. 352p. 59.50 (*0-306-40944-5*, Plenum Trade) Perseus Pubng.

Advances in Parapsychological Research Vol. 1: Psychokinesis. Ed. by Stanley Krippner. 1977. LC 77-9518. 246p. 59.50 (*0-306-32501-2*, Plenum Trade) Perseus Pubng.

Advances in Parasitology. John R. Baker. 1999. (Advances in Parasitology Ser.: Vol. 42). 448p. (C). 109.95 (*0-12-031742-7*) Acad Pr.

Advances in Parasitology, Vol. 31. Ed. by John R. Baker & Ralph L. Muller. 1992. (Illus.). 444p. text 104.00 (*0-12-031731-1*) Acad Pr.

Advances in Parasitology, Vol. 33. Ed. by John R. Baker & J. R. Muller. 1994. (Illus.). 299p. text 104.00 (*0-12-031733-8*) Acad Pr.

Advances in Parasitology. Ed. by John R. Baker et al. (Illus.). Vol. 34. 1994. 299p. text 104.00 (*0-12-031734-6*); Vol. 35. 1995. 387p. text 90.00 (*0-12-031735-4*); Vol. 36. 1995. (Advances in Parasitology Ser.: Vol. 36). 440p. text 95.00 (*0-12-031736-2*); Vol. 41. 1998. 352p. (C). text 99.95 (*0-12-031741-9*) Acad Pr.

Advances in Parasitology, Vol. 39. Ed. by John R. Baker et al. 1997. (Illus.). 368p. text 99.95 (*0-12-031739-7*) Morgan Kaufmann.

*__Advances in Parasitology,__ Vol. 49. David Rollinson. Ed. by John R. Baker & Ralph Muller. 2001. 397p. 139.95 (*0-12-031749-4*) Acad Pr.

Advances in Pathology (Anatomic & Clinical) Laboratory Medicine: Proceedings of the Triennial World Congress of the World Association of Societies of Pathology, 11th, Jerusalem, Israel, Sept. 20-25, 1981, Set. World Association of Societies of Pathology Staff & E. Levy. 1982. LC 82-11202. (Illus.). 542p. (*0-08-029777-3*) Pergamon Repr GBR. *Dist:* Franklin.

Advances in Pediatric Heart Rate Variability Analysis. I. Valimaki & K. J. Antila. 1985. 114p. (Orig.). pap. 34.50 (*951-642-757-X*) Coronet Bks.

Advances in Pediatric Infectious Disease, Vol. 15. Stephen C. Aronoff. 1999. 400p. text 79.95 (*0-8151-0958-X*) Mosby Inc.

Advances in Pediatric Infectious Diseases, Vol.14. Stepen C. Aronoff. 1998. (Illus.). 320p. (C). (gr. 13). text 83.00 (*0-8151-0961-X*, 29140) Mosby Inc.

Advances in Pediatric Pulmonology. Ed. by Eitan Kerem et al. 1997. LC 97-11160. (Pediatric & Adolescent Medicine Ser.: Vol. 7, 1997). (Illus.). viii, 172p. 172.25 (*3-8055-6382-5*) S Karger.

Advances in Pediatrics, Vol. 28. Lewis A. Barness. 1981. 54.50 (*0-8151-0500-2*) Mosby Inc.

Advances in Pediatrics, Vol. 48. Ed. by Lewis A. Barness. 2001. (Illus.). 500p. (*0-323-01526-3*) Mosby Inc.

*__Advances in Pediatrics,__ Vol. 49. Ed. by Lewis A. Barness. 2002. (Illus.). 500p. (*0-323-01527-1*) Mosby Inc.

*__Advances in Pediatrics,__ Vol. 50. Lewis A. Barness. 2003. (Illus.). 500p. (*0-323-01528-X*) Mosby Inc.

Advances in Pediatrics. Lewis A. Barness. (Illus.). Vol.45. 1998. 432p. text 74.95 (*0-8151-8401-8*, 25062); Vol.46. 1999. 514p. text 78.00 (*0-8151-8402-6*, 25063) Mosby Inc.

Advances in Peptic Ulcer Pathogenesis. W. D. Rees. 1988. 250p. text 155.00 (*0-7462-0062-5*) Kluwer Academic.

Advances in Perinantal Medicine, Vol. 1. Ermelando V. Cosmi et al. 1988. x, 314p. text 129.00 (*3-7186-0463-9*) Gordon & Breach.

Advances in Perinatal Medicine. Ed. by Aubrey Milunsky et al. LC 80-20701. Vol. 1. 1981. 456p. 85.00 (*0-306-40482-6*); Vol. 2. 1982. 400p. (C). 85.00 (*0-306-40763-9*); Vol. 3. 1983. 272p. 85.00 (*0-306-41208-X*); Vol. 4. 1985. 350p. 95.00 (*0-306-41840-1*) Kluwer Academic (Kluwer Plenum).

Advances in Perinatal Medicine: Proceedings of the XV European Congress of Perinatal Medicine. Ed. by Forrester Cockburn. 1997. LC 97-23209. (Illus.). 420p. lib. bdg. 121.95 (*1-85070-944-0*, Parthenon Pbng) CRC Pr.

Advances in Perinatal Thyroidology. Ed. by Barry B. Bercu & D. I. Shulman. 1991. (Advances in Experimental Medicine & Biology Ser.: Vol. 299). (Illus.). 280p. (C). text 107.00 (*0-306-44006-7*, Kluwer Plenum) Kluwer Academic.

Advances in Periodontics. Ed. by Thomas Wilson et al. 1992. LC 91-32558. (Illus.). 384p. text 126.00 (*0-86715-250-8*) Quint Pub Co.

Advances in Personal Construct Psychology. Ed. by Greg J. Neimeyer & Robert A. Neimeyer. Vol. 1. 1990. 287p. 78.50 (*1-55938-081-0*); Vol. 2. 1992. 272p. 78.50 (*1-55938-194-9*); Vol. 3. 1995. 336p. 78.50 (*1-55938-593-6*) Jai Pr.

Advances in Personal Relationships. Ed. by Warren H. Jones & Daniel Perlman. 300p. Vol. 2. 1990. 79.00 (*1-85302-077-X*); Vol. 3. 1991. 79.00 (*1-85302-078-8*) Taylor & Francis.

Advances in Personality Assessment, Vol. 1. Ed. by Charles D. Spielberger & James Neal Butcher. 1982. 256p. text 49.95 (*0-89859-151-1*) L Erlbaum Assocs.

Advances in Personality Assessment, Vol. 2. Ed. by James Neal Butcher & Charles D. Spielberger. 1983. 208p. (C). text 49.95 (*0-89859-216-X*) L Erlbaum Assocs.

Advances in Personality Assessment, Vol. 3. Charles D. Spielberger & James Neal Butcher. 1983. 216p. (C). text 49.95 (*0-89859-313-1*) L Erlbaum Assocs.

Advances in Personality Assessment, Vol. 4. Ed. by James Neal Butcher & Charles D. Spielberger. 1985. 288p. (C). text 69.95 (*0-89859-341-7*) L Erlbaum Assocs.

Advances in Personality Assessment, Vol. 5. Ed. by Charles D. Spielberger & James Neal Butcher. 1985. 224p. (C). text 49.95 (*0-89859-559-2*) L Erlbaum Assocs.

Advances in Personality Assessment, Vol. 6. Ed. by James Neal Butcher & Charles D. Spielberger. 1987. 176p. text 39.95 (*0-89859-660-2*) L Erlbaum Assocs.

Advances in Personality Assessment, Vol. 7. Ed. by Charles D. Spielberger & James Neal Butcher. 1988. 248p. 49.95 (*0-8058-0217-7*) L Erlbaum Assocs.

Advances in Personality Assessment, Vol. 8. Ed. by James Neal Butcher & Charles D. Spielberger. 1990. 296p. (C). text 69.95 (*0-8058-0503-6*) L Erlbaum Assocs.

Advances in Personality Assessment, Vol. 9. Ed. by Charles D. Spielberger & James Neal Butcher. 1992. 232p. text 49.95 (*0-8058-1226-1*) L Erlbaum Assocs.

Advances in Pharmaceutical Science, Vol. 7. Ed. by Trevor Jones et al. 1995. (Advances in Pharmaceutical Science Ser.: Vol. 7). (Illus.). 288p. text 111.00 (*0-12-032307-9*) Acad Pr.

Advances in Pharmacology Ed. by Kuan-Teh Jeang. 2000. LC 2001-274050. (Advances in Pharmacology Ser.: Vol. 49). (Illus.). 500p. 109.95 (*0-12-032950-6*) Acad Pr.

Advances in Pharmacology. J. Thomas August. Vol. 3. 1996. 426p. text 89.00 (*0-12-032938-7*); Vol. 4. 1998. (C). text 99.95 (*0-12-032945-X*) Acad Pr.

Advances in Pharmacology. Ed. by J. Thomas August et al. (Illus.). Vol. 28. 1994. 361p. text 104.00 (*0-12-032928-X*); Vol. 30. 1994. 399p. text 104.00 (*0-12-032931-X*); Vol. 32. 1995. 583p. text 104.00 (*0-12-032933-6*); Vol. 35. 1996. 409p. text 95.00 (*0-12-032936-0*) Acad Pr.

Advances in Pharmacology. Ed. by J. Thomas August et al. 1997. (Illus.). Vol. 4. 614p. (C). text 99.95 (*0-12-032942-5*); Vol. 39. 505p. text 99.00 (*0-12-032940-9*) Morgan Kaufmann.

Advances in Pharmacology: Conjugation-Dependent Carcinogenicity & Toxicity of Foreign Compounds, Vol. 27. Ed. by J. Thomas August et al. 1994. (Illus.). 519p. text 104.00 (*0-12-032927-1*) Acad Pr.

Advances in Pharmacology: Cumulative Subject Index, Vol. 4. Ed. by J. Thomas August et al. 1998. (Advances in Pharmacology Ser.: Vol. 45). (Illus.). 198p. (C). 99.95 (*0-12-032946-8*) Acad Pr.

Advances in Pharmacology: Cyclic GMP: Synthesis, Metabolism, & Function, Vol. 26. Ed. by J. Thomas August et al. 1994. (Illus.). 335p. text 104.00 (*0-12-032926-3*) Acad Pr.

Advances in Pharmacology: Intracellular Signal Transduction, Vol. 36. Ed. by M. W. Anders et al. 1996. (Illus.). 310p. text 69.00 (*0-12-032937-9*); (Advances in Pharmacology Ser.: Vol. 36). pap. text 39.00 (*0-12-513805-9*) Acad Pr.

Advances in Pharmacology Vol. 31: Anesthesia & Cardiovascular Disease. Ed. by Zeljko J. Bosnjak et al. 1994. (Illus.). 666p. text 104.00 (*0-12-032932-8*); pap. text 63.00 (*0-12-118860-4*) Acad Pr.

Advances in Pharmacology Vol. 34: Nitric Oxide: Biochemistry, Molecular Biology, & Therapeutic Implications, Vol. 34. Ed. by Louis Ignarro et al. 1995. (Illus.). 530p. text 94.00 (*0-12-032935-2*) Acad Pr.

Advances in Pharmacology Vol. 38: Antioxidants in Disease Mechanisms & Therapeutic Strategies, Vol. 38. Ed. by Helmut Sies. 1996. (Illus.). 707p. text 99.00 (*0-12-032939-5*) Acad Pr.

Advances in Pharmacology Vol. 40: Gene Therapy. Ed. by J. Thomas August et al. 1997. (Advances in Pharmacology Ser.). (Illus.). 508p. text 95.00 (*0-12-032941-7*) Morgan Kaufmann.

Advances in Pharmacology Vol. 42: Catecholamines: Bridging Basic Science with Clinical Medicine. Ed. by David S. Goldstein et al. 1997. LC 00-500755. (Illus.). 1084p. text 99.95 (*0-12-032943-3*) Morgan Kaufmann.

Advances in Pharmacology Vol. 43: Drug - Drug Interactions: Scientific & Regulatory Perspectives. Ed. by Albert P. Li. 1997. (Illus.). 304p. text 89.95 (*0-12-032944-1*) Morgan Kaufmann.

Advances in Pharmacology & Therapeutics: Proceedings of the Eight International Congress of Pharmacology, Tokyo, Japan, 19-24 July 1981, Ser. 2, Vol. 3. Ed. by H. Hagihara Yoshida & Setsuro Ebashi. 1982. (Illus.). 346p. (*0-08-028023-4*) Pergamon Repr GBR. *Dist:* Franklin.

Advances in Pharmacology & Therapeutics 2, Set. H. Hagihara Yoshida & Yoshida Hagihara. 1982. (*0-08-027975-9*) Pergamon Repr GBR. *Dist:* Franklin.

Advances in Phenylketonuria Research. Ed. by V. Romano. 1993. (Journal: Vol. 6, Nos. 1-3, 1993). (Illus.). 192p. pap. 85.25 (*3-8055-5759-0*) S Karger.

Advances in Photoreception: Proceedings of a Symposium on Frontiers of Visual Science. National Research Council Staff. 1990. 160p. pap. text 16.00 (*0-309-04240-2*) Natl Acad Pr.

Advances in Physical & Biological Radiation Detectors. International Atomic Energy Agency Staff. 1971. (Proceedings Ser.). (Illus.). 742p. pap. (*92-0-020171-7*, ISP269) IAEA AUT. *Dist:* Bernan Associates.

Advances in Physiological Sciences: Prostaglandins—Immunopharmacology, Vol. 4. Ed. by B. B. Vargaftig. 1979. LC 78-41029. 230p. pap. (*0-08-023208-6*) Pergamon Repr GBR. *Dist:* Franklin.

Advances in Physiological Sciences, Vol. 10: Chemotherapy. Ed. by M. Adolphe. ltd. ed. 1979. LC 78-41032. (Illus.). 220p. 40.00 (*0-08-023214-0*) Franklin.

Advances in Pituitary Adenoma Research: Proceedings of the 4th European Workshop on Pituitary Adenomas, University of Zurich-Irchel, Zurich, Switzerland, September 13-16, 1987. Ed. by A. M. Landolt et al. 1988. (Advances in the Biosciences Ser.: Vol. 69). 498p. 92.50 (0-08-035596-X, Pergamon Pr) Elsevier.

Advances in Plastic & Reconstructive Surgery, 15. Mutaz B. Habal. 15th ed. 1998. (Illus.). 272p. (C). (gr. 13). text 98.00 (0-8151-8404-2, 25065) Mosby Inc.

Advances in Plastic & Reconstructive Surgery, Vol. 16. 1999. 94.95 (0-8151-8405-0) Mosby Inc.

Advances in Population Vol. 2: Psychosocial Perspectives. Ed. by Lawrence J. Severy. 1994. 288p. 99.00 (1-85302-217-9) Taylor & Francis.

Advances in Pregnancy-Related Protein Research: Functional & Clinical Applications. Gabor N. Than et al. 1993. 352p. 208.00 (0-8493-4962-1, QP552) CRC Pr.

Advances in Progressive Supranuclear Palsy. Ed. by E. Tolosa et al. (Journals of Neural Transmission: Vol. 42). (Illus.). 1995. LC 94-8136. 88.00 (0-387-82523-1); 1994. 302p. 116.00 (0-387-82541-X) Spr-Verlag.

Advances in Projective Drawing Interpretation. Ed. by Emanuel F. Hammer. 1997. LC 96-47845. (Illus.). 476p. text 99.95 (0-398-06742-2); pap. text 72.95 (0-398-06743-0) C C Thomas.

***Advances in Protein Chemistry: Prion Proteins**, Vol. 57. Ed. by Bryan Caughey. 2001. (Biomedical Sciences Ser.). 405p. 119.95 (0-12-034257-X) Acad Pr.

Advances in Psychological Assessment, Vol. 7. Paul McReynolds et al. 1990. LC 78-647160. (Illus.). 330p. (C). 65.00 (0-306-43399-0, Plenum Trade) Perseus Pubng.

Advances in Psychological Assessment, Vol. 8. J. C. Rosen & Paul McReynolds. 1992. (Illus.). 282p. (C). 65.00 (0-306-44251-5, Plenum Trade) Perseus Pubng.

Advances in Psychology & Education, Vol. 1. Ed. by Charles A. Maher. Date not set. 78.50 (0-89232-842-8) Jai Pr.

Advances in Psychology & Law: International Contributions. Ed. by Santiago Redondo et al. 1997. LC 97-22521. 542p. 132.00 (3-11-015615-6) De Gruyter.

***Advances in Psychology Research.** Ed. by Serge P. Shohov. 2002. Vol. 9. lib. bdg. 59.00 (1-59033-139-7); Vol. 10. lib. bdg. 69.00 (1-59033-162-1) Nova Sci Pubs.

Advances in Psychoneuroimmunology. Ed. by Istvan Berczi & Judith Szelenyi. 1995. LC 94-47537. (Hans Selve Symposia on Neuroendocrinology & Stress Ser.: Vol. 3). 390p. text 110.00 (0-306-44883-1, Kluwer Plenum) Kluwer Academic.

Advances in Psychopharmacology: Predicting & Improving Treatment Response. Ed. by Mark S. Gold et al. 1984. 344p. 189.00 (0-8493-5680-6, RC483) CRC Pr.

Advances in Psychophysiology, Vol. 4. Ed. by J. Richard Jennings. 1991. 300p. 99.00 (1-85302-079-6) Taylor & Francis.

Advances in Psychophysiology, Vol. 5. Ed. by J. Richard Jennings et al. 1993. 300p. 99.00 (1-85302-191-1) Taylor & Francis.

Advances in Psychosomatic Obstetrics & Gynecology, Berlin 1980: Proceedings. Ed. by H. J. Prill & M. Stauber. 1982. (Illus.). 525p. 59.00 (0-387-11710-5) Spr-Verlag.

Advances in Qualitative Psychology: Themes & Variations. F. J. Van Zuuren et al. 1987. xii, 210p. pap. (90-265-0849-2) Swets.

Advances in Quantitative Coronary Arteriography. Ed. by Johan H. Reiber & Patrick W. Serruys. 1993. LC 92-20819. (Developments in Cardiovascular Medicine Ser.: Vol. 137). text 414.50 (0-7923-1863-3) Kluwer Academic.

Advances in Radiation Biology Vol. 18: Relative Radiation Sensitivities of Human Organ Systems, Vol. 18. Ed. by John T. Lett et al. 1994. (Illus.). 232p. 110.00 (0-12-034518-8) Acad Pr.

Advances in Radiation Oncology Physics: Dosimetry, Treatment Planning, & Brachytherapy. Ed. by James A. Purdy. 1993. LC 92-81653. (American Association of Physicists in Medicine Symposium Ser.: No. 19). 1099p. 75.00 (1-56396-054-0) Am Inst Physics.

Advances in Radiation Protection. Ed. by Martin Oberhofer. 1991. (C). text 185.50 (0-7923-1232-5) Kluwer Academic.

Advances in Radiation Research: Physics & Chemistry Ed. by J. F. Duplan & A. Chapiro. 1973. LC 72-92724. 668p. 238.00 (0-677-15780-0) Gordon & Breach.

Advances in Radiation Therapy. Ed. by Bharat B. Mittal et al. 1997. LC 97-24461. (Cancer Treatment & Research Ser.: No. 93). 320p. 290.00 (0-7923-9981-1) Kluwer Academic.

Advances in Radiation Therapy Treatment Planning: Proceedings of the AAPM Summer School Held at Southeastern Louisiana University, Hammond, Louisiana, July 26-30, 1982. Ed. by Ann E. Wright & Arthur L. Boyer. 1983. (American Association of Physicists in Medicine Symposium Ser.: No. 9). 635p. 60.00 (0-88318-423-0) Am Inst Physics.

Advances in Regional Cancer Therapy. Ed. by J. Kreidler et al. 1988. (Illus.). x, 228p. 58.50 (3-8055-4842-7) S Karger.

Advances in Renal Medicine. Ed. by A. E. Raine. 1993. LC 92-49499. (Oxford Medical Publications). 504p. 69.50 (0-19-262102-5) OUP.

Advances in Research on Cholera & Related Diarrheas. Ed. by S. Kuwahara. 1983. (New Perspectives in Clinical Microbiology Ser.). text 176.50 (0-89838-592-X) Kluwer Academic.

Advances in Research on Cholera & Related Diarrheas, Vol. 2. Ed. by S. Kuwahara & N. F. Pierce. 1985. (New Perspectives in Clinical Microbiology Ser.). text 203.00 (0-89838-680-2) Kluwer Academic.

Advances in Research on Neurod. 1997. (Illus.). 300p. 169.00 (3-211-82935-0); 280p. text 79.00 (3-211-82934-2) Spr-Verlag.

Advances in Research on Neurodegeneration. Ed. by Werner Poewe & Gerhard Ransmayr. 1999. (Journals of Neural Transmission: Vol. 6). (Illus.). 150p. 109.00 (3-211-83262-9) Spr-Verlag.

***Advances in Research on Neurodegeneration.** Ed. by Werner Poewe & Gerhard Ransmayr. 1999. (Journals of Neural Transmission: Suppl. 55). (Illus.). 150p. pap. 85.00 (3-211-83261-0) Spr-Verlag.

Advances in Research on Neurodegeneration, Vol. 8. Ed. by P. Riederer et al. 2001. (Journals of Neural Transmission). 400p. 124.00 (3-211-83538-5) Spr-Verlag.

Advances in Research on Neurodegeneration Vol. II: Etiopathogenesis. Ed. by Y. Mizuno et al. 1994. (Illus.). xiii, 221p. 104.50 (0-8176-3762-1) Birkhauser.

Advances in Research on Neurodegeneration 5. P Riederer. 1997. LC 96-51004. (Journals of Neural Transmission). (Illus.). 215p. 124.00 (3-211-82898-2) Spr-Verlag.

Advances in Research on Neurodegeneration 5. P. Riederer. 1997. LC 96-51004. (Journals of Neural Transmission). (Illus.). 250p. 164.00 (3-211-82933-4) Spr-Verlag.

Advances in Research on Neurodegeneration, I: Definitions, Clinical Features, & Morphology. Ed. by P. Riederer et al. 1993. (Advances in Research on Neurodegeneration Ser.). (Illus.). 280p. 109.50 (0-8176-3631-5) Birkhauser.

Advances in Reversal Theory. Ed. by John H. Kerr et al. 1993. LC 93-12666. 374p. pap. (90-265-1202-3) Swets.

Advances in School Psychology, Vol. 1. Thomas R. Kratochwill. 1981. 368p. text 79.95 (0-89859-076-0) L Erlbaum Assocs.

Advances in School Psychology. Ed. by Thomas R. Kratochwill. Vol. 4. 1985. 336p. text 69.95 (0-89859-454-5); Vol. 5. 1986. 264p. text 59.95 (0-89859-708-0); Vol. 7. 1990. 192p. 59.95 (0-8058 0350-5); Vol.3. 1983. 384p. text 79.95 (0-89859-280-1) L Erlbaum Assocs.

Advances in Sexually Transmitted Diseases: Diagnosis & Treatment. Ed. by R. Morisset & Edward Kurstak. 1986. 237p. lib. bdg. (90-6764-059-X) VSP NLD. Dist: Coronet Bks.

Advances in Some Aspects of Osteoporosis. Ed. by J. L. Ambrus et al. 1985. pap. 35.00 (0-915340-13-5) PJD Pubns.

Advances in Space Biology & Medicine, Vol. 1. Sjoerd L. Bonting. 1991. 348p. 90.00 (1-55938-296-1) Jai Pr.

Advances in Space Biology & Medicine. Ed. by Sjoerd L. Bonting. Vol. 2. 1992. 314p. 90.00 (1-55938-409-3); Vol. 6. 1997. 332p. 90.00 (0-7623-0147-3) Jai Pr.

Advances in Space Biology & Medicine, Vol. 7. Ed. by Sjoerd L. Bonting & Augusto Cogoli. 1999. 251p. 90.00 (0-7623-0393-X) Jai Pr.

Advances in Space Biology & Medicine Vol. 3: European Isolation & Confinement Study. Ed. by Sjoerd L. Bonting. 1993. 286p. 90.00 (1-55938-410-7) Jai Pr.

Advances in Space Biology & Medicine Vol. 5: European Isolation & Confinement Study: EXEMSI. Ed. by Sjoerd L. Bonting. 1996. 418p. 90.00 (1-55938-970-2) Jai Pr.

Advances in Spatial Reasoning. Ed. by Su-shing Chen. 1991. 312p. (C). Vol. I. 73.25 (0-89391-572-6); Vol. 2. 73.25 (0-89391-573-4) Greenwood (Ablex).

Advances in Sports Cardiology. A. Pelliccia et al. 1997. 161p. pap. 69.00 (3-540-75036-3) Spr-Verlag.

Advances in Stereotactic & Functional Neurosurgery, Vol. 8. Ed. by G. Broggi et al. 1989. (Illus.). 130p. 112.00 (0-387-82120-1) Spr-Verlag.

Advances in Stereotactic & Functional Neurosurgery, Vol. 10. Ed. by C. Ostertag et al. 1993. LC 93-41431. (Illus.). 200p. 158.00 (0-387-82478-2) Spr-Verlag.

Advances in Stereotactic & Functional Neurosurgery 11, No. 64. Ed. by B. Meyerson & C. Ostertag. 1996. (Acta Neurochirurgica Ser.: Vol. 64). 152p. 150.00 (3-211-82720-X) Spr-Verlag.

Advances in Stereotactic & Functional Neurosurgery 12. Ed. by C. B. Ostertag et al. 1997. LC 97-20848. (Acta Neurochirurgica Ser.: Suppl. 68). (Illus.). 144p. 85.00 (3-211-82978-4) Spr-Verlag.

Advances in Stereotactic & Functional Neurosurgery, No. 9: Proceedings of the 9th Meeting of the European Society for Stereotactic & Functional Neurosurgery, Malaga 1990, Acta Naurochirurgica - Supplementum, No. 52. Ed. by E. R. Hirchcock et al. 1991. (Illus.). 160p. 128.00 (0-387-82283-6) Spr-Verlag.

Advances in Steroid Analysis. S. Gorog. 1991. 492p. (C). (0-89771-834-8) Collets GBR. Dist: St Mut.

Advances in Steroid Analysis '87: Proceedings of the Symposium on the Analysis of Steroids, Sopron, Hungary, October 20-22, 1987. S. Gorog. Ed. by E. Heftmann. 1988. (Illus.). 583p. (C). (963-05-5229-9) Akade Kiado HUN. Dist: Intl Spec Bk, St Mut.

Advances in Strategic Management, Vol. 3. Ed. by Paul Shrivastava et al. 1985. 322p. 78.50 (0-89232-506-2) Jai Pr.

Advances in Stroke Prevention: New Outlooks. Ed. by J. M. Orgogozo & Charles P. Warlow. 1995. (Journal: Vol. 6, Suppl. 1, 1996). (Illus.). iv, 40p. pap., suppl. ed. 21.75 (3-8055-6278-0) S Karger.

Advances in Stroke Prevention: Sanofi-Winthrop Symposium, Second European Stroke Conference, Lausanne, June 1992. Ed. by J. M. Orgogozo & M. Dyken. 1993. (Journal: Vol. 3, Suppl. 1, 1993). (Illus.). iv, 44p. pap. 21.00 (3-8055-5787-6) S Karger.

Advances in Stroke Rehabilitation. Ed. by Wayne A. Gordon et al. 1993. LC 94-40389. 307p. text 49.50 (1-56372-035-3) Buttrwrth-Heinemann.

Advances in Substance Abuse, Vol. 4. Ed. by Nancy K. Mello. 1991. 300p. 88.00 (1-85302-080-X) Taylor & Francis.

Advances in Surgery. Ed. by John Cameron. 2001. (Illus.). 500p. (0-323-01529-8) Mosby Inc.

Advances in Surgery, 32. Cameron. 32nd ed. 1998. (Illus.). 432p. text 73.00 (0-8151-8407-7, 25068) Mosby Inc.

***Advances in Surgery.** Ed. by John Cameron. (Illus.). 500p. Vol. 36. 2002. (0-323-01530-1); Vol. 37. 2003. (0-323-01531-X) Mosby Inc.

Advances in Surgery, Vol.33. 1999. (Illus.). 342p. text 75.95 (0-8151-8408-5, 25069) Mosby Inc.

Advances in Swine in Biomedical Research. M. E. Tumbleson. 1997. LC 96-38650. (Illus.). (C). Vol. 1. 462p. 155.00 (0-306-45495-5); Vol. 2. 520p. 167.00 (0-306-45496-3) Kluwer Academic (Kluwer Plenum).

Advances in Test Anxiety Research, Vol. 1. Ed. by R. Schwarzer et al. 1982. xii, 164p. pap. (90-265-0414-4) Swets.

Advances in Test Anxiety Research. Ed. by H. M. Van der Ploeg et al. Vol. 2. 1983. x, 222p. pap. (90-265-0454-3); Vol. 3. 1984. xii, 286p. pap. (90-265-0556-6); Vol. 4. 1985. xiv, 262p. pap. (90-265-0596-5) Swets.

Advances in Test Anxiety Research, Vol. 5. Ed. by R. Schwarzer et al. 1986. xii, 278p. pap. (90-265-0673-2) Swets.

Advances in Thanatology, Vol. 5. 19.95 (0-405-12641-7); 19.95 (0-405-14221-8, 745) Ayer.

Advances in Thanatology, Vol. 4. 1978. 15.00 (0-8422-7305-0) Irvington.

Advances in the Behavioral Assessment of Children & Families, Vol. 5. Ed. by Ronald J. Prinz. 1991. 320p. 85.00 (1-85302-069-9) Taylor & Francis.

Advances in the Biomechanics of the Hand & Wrist. F. Schuind et al. 1994. LC 93-43655. (NATO Advanced Science Institutes Ser.: Vol. 256). (Illus.). 534p. (C). text 167.00 (0-306-44580-8, Kluwer Plenum) Kluwer Academic.

Advances in the Control of Theileriosis: Current Topics in Veterinary Medicine & Animal Science, No. 14. Ed. by A. D. Irvin et al. 1981. xiv, 428p. text 176.50 (90-247-2575-5) Kluwer Academic.

Advances in the Diagnosis & Treatment of Alzheimer's Disease. Ed. by Vinod Kumar & Carl Eisdorfer. 1998. LC 97-41352. (Series in Psychiatry). (Illus.). 400p. 55.95 (0-8261-1167-X) Springer Pub.

Advances in the Neurobiology of Anxiety Disorders. Ed. by H. G. Westenberg et al. 1997. LC 96-4645. (Clinical & Neurobiological Advances in Psychiatry Ser.: Vol. 2). 456p. 245.00 (0-471-96124-8) Wiley.

Advances in the Neurobiology of Schizophrenia. Ed. by J. A. Den Boer et al. 1995. LC 94-22397. 482p. 255.00 (0-471-95287-7) Wiley.

Advances in the Prevention of Occupational Respiratory Diseases: Proceedings of the 9th International Conference on Occupational Respiratory Diseases, Kyoto, 13-16 October, 1997. Keizo Chiyotani & Yutaka Hosoda. 1998. LC 98-27177. (International Congress Ser.). 1264p. 245.50 (0-444-82791-9) Elsevier.

Advances in the Psychology of Human Intelligence. Ed. by Robert J. Sternberg. Vol. 2. 1984. 408p. (C). text 79.95 (0-89859-287-9); Vol. 3. 1986. 400p. (C). text 79.95 (0-89859-655-6); Vol. 4. 1987. 272p. 59.95 (0-8058-0070-0); Vol. 5. 1989. 248p. 49.95 (0-8058-0454-4) L Erlbaum Assocs.

Advances in the Radiotherapeutic Management of Carcinoma of the Prostate. Anthony V. D'Amico & Gerald E. Hanks. 1998. LC 97-42594. 200p. pap. 0.00 (0-412-12211-1, Chap & Hall NY) Chapman & Hall.

Advances in the Study of Behavior. Peter J. Slater. 1999. 392p. (C). 99.95 (0-12-004528-1) Acad Pr.

Advances in the Study of Behavior. Ed. by Peter J. Slater et al. (Illus.). (C). Vol. 21. 1992. 303p. text 94.95 (0-12-004521-4); Vol. 22. 1993. 330p. text 89.95 (0-12-004522-2); Vol. 23. 1994. 284p. text 79.95 (0-12-004523-0); Vol. 24. 1995. 372p. text 74.95 (0-12-004524-9); Vol. 26. 1997. (Advances in the Study of Behavior Ser.: Vol. 26). 484p. text 95.00 (0-12-004526-5) Acad Pr.

Advances in the Study of Behavior Vol. 27: Stress & Behavior, Vol. 27. Ed. by Anders P. Moller et al. 1998. (Illus.). 552p. (C). text 99.95 (0-12-004527-3) Morgan Kaufmann.

Advances in the Study of Entrepreneurship, Innovation, & Economic Growth Vol. 4: Health Care Issues & American Economic Growth. Ed. by Gary D. Libecap. 1990. 235p. 78.50 (1-55938-191-4) Jai Pr.

Advances in the Study of Mammalian Behavior. Ed. by J. F. Eisenberg & D. G. Kleiman. 1983. (American Society of Mammalogists Special Publications: No.7). 753p. 45.00 (0-943612-06-3) Am Soc Mammalogists.

***Advances in the Treatment of Atrial Tachyarrhythmias: Pacing, Cardioversion & Defibrillation.** Ed. by Carsten W. Israel & S. Serge Barold. 2001. (Illus.). 480p. text (0-87993-497-2) Futura Pub.

Advances in the Treatment of Radiation Injuries: Proceedings of the 2nd Consensus Development Conference on the Treatment of Radiation Injuries, Held in Bethesda, Maryland, U. S. A. on 14-17 April 1993, No. 94. Ed. by T. J. MacVittie et al. 1996. LC 95-48288. (Advances in the Biosciences Ser.: Vol. 94). 350p. 141.50 (0-08-042497-X, Pergamon Pr) Elsevier.

Advances in the Treatment of Superficial Bladder Cancer: Optimizing BCG Immunotherapy. Ed. by D. L. Lamm. 1995. (Journal: Vol. 27, Suppl. 1, 1995). (Illus.). iv, 34p. pap. 21.75 (3-8055-6137-7) S Karger.

Advances in Tissue Banking, Vol. 1. G. O. Phillips et al. 1997. LC 97-37807. 340p. 82.00 (981-02-3190-3) World Scientific Pub.

Advances in Transplant Procedure, Vol. 8. Arun S. Mujumdar. 1993. (0-8493-9320-5) CRC Pr.

Advances in Transplantation. Emanual Hackel et al. 1993. (Illus.). 147p. (C). text 9.00 (1-56395-023-5) Am Assn Blood.

Advances in Trauma, Vol. 11. Kimball I. Maull. 1996. 270p. 69.95 (0-8151-6203-0) Mosby Inc.

Advances in Tuberculosis Research, Vol. 18. Ed. by H. Birkhaeuser et al. 1972. 85.25 (3-8055-1301-1) S Karger.

Advances in Tuberculosis Research, Vol. 19. Ed. by G. Urbanczik. 1976. (Illus.). 184p. 110.50 (3-8055-2215-0) S Karger.

Advances in Tuberculosis Research, Vol. 20. Ed. by H. Birkhaeuser & W. Fox. 1980. (Illus.). 61.00 (3-8055-2954-6) S Karger.

Advances in Ultrasound Techniques & Instrumentation. Ed. by Peter N. Wells. 2nd ed. 1993. LC 92-48481. (Clinics in Diagnostic Ultrasound Ser.: Vol. 28). (Illus.). 208p. text (0-443-08853-5) Church.

Advances in Understanding Genetic Changes in Cancer: Impact on Diagnosis & Treatment Decisions in the 1990's (Research Briefings) Institute of Medicine Staff. 1992. 96p. (C). pap. text 19.00 (0-309-04688-2) Natl Acad Pr.

Advances in Vaccination Against Virus Diseases. Ed. by R. Purtschert. 1979. (Monographs in Pediatrics: Vol. 11). (Illus.). pap. 27.25 (3-8055-3046-3) S Karger.

Advances in Vascular Pathology 1997: Selected Papers from the European Congress of Angiology, 11th Meeting of the European Chapter, EUROCHAP '97, Rome 23-26, October 1997. Andrew N. Nicolaides & Salvatore Novo. 1997. LC 97-41394. (International Congress Ser.: Vol. 115). 194p. 137.50 (0-444-82833-8) Elsevier.

***Advances in Vascular Surgery.** Ed. by James S. T. Yao & William H. Pearce. 2001. LC 2001-5545. (0-944496-69-5) Precept Pr.

Advances in Vascular Surgery. Anthony D. Whittemore. 10th ed. 2002. (Illus.). 320p. text 81.00 (0-8151-2730-8, 31327) Mosby Inc.

Advances in Vascular Surgery, 5. Ed. by Anthony D. Whittemore. 1997. (Illus.). 288p. (C). (gr. 13). text 81.00 (0-8151-9409-9, 21989) Mosby Inc.

Advances in Vascular Surgery. Anthony D. Whittemore. (Illus.). 8. 8th ed. 2000. 320p. text 81.00 (0-8151-2732-4, 31325); Vol.6. 1998. 312p. text 81.00 (0-8151-8415-8, 25076); Vol.7. 1999. 243p. text 83.00 (0-8151-8416-6, 25077) Mosby Inc.

Advances In Vascular Surgery, V9. Anthony D. Whittmore. 2001. (Illus.). 320p. text 81.00 (0-8151-2731-6, 31326) Mosby Inc.

Advances in Veterinary Dermatology. Claudia Von Tscharner & Heinemann Staff. Date not set. (0-08-042522-4, Pergamon Pr) Elsevier.

Advances in Veterinary Dermatology, Vol. 1. Ed. by Claudia Von Tscharner & R. E. Halliwell. 1990. (Illus.). 520p. (0-7020-1494-X) W B Saunders GBR. Dist: Saunders.

Advances in Veterinary Dermatology, Vol. 2. P. J. Ihrke. 1993. 100.00 (0-08-041997-6, Pergamon Pr) Elsevier.

Advances in Veterinary Medicine Vol. 41: Veterinary Vaccines & Diagnostics. Ed. by W. Jean Dodds & Ronald D. Schultz. 1999. LC 98-233668. (Illus.). xxxviii, 815p. (C). 149.95 (0-12-039242-9) Acad Pr.

Advances in Veterinary Science & Comparative Medicine Vol. 38A: Comparative Vertebrate Exercise Physiology: Unifying Physiological Principles. Ed. by R. R. Marshak et al. 1994. LC 94-209987. (Advances in Veterinary Science & Comparative Medicine Ser.: Vol. 38). (Illus.). 291p. text 104.00 (0-12-039238-0) Acad Pr.

Advances in Veterinary Science & Comparative Medicine Vol. 39: Veterinary Medical Specialization: Bridging Science & Medicine, Vol. 39. Ed. by W. Jean Dodds. 1995. (Illus.). 303p. (C). text 84.00 (0-12-039240-2) Acad Pr.

Advances in Veterinary Science & Comparative Medicine Vol. 40: From Molecular Genetics to Gene Transfer & Therapy. Ed. by W. Jean Dodds & James E. Womack. 1997. LC 97-201498. (Illus.). 227p. text 90.00 (0-12-039241-0) Morgan Kaufmann.

Advances in Veterinary Science & Comparative Medicine, Vol. 37: Animal Models in Liver Research. Ed. by Charles E. Cornelius et al. 1993. (Illus.). 512p. (C). text 104.00 (*0-12-039237-2*) Acad Pr.

Advances in Viral Hepatitis: Report of the WHO Expert Committee on Viral Hepatitis, 1977. 1977. (Technical Report Ser.: No. 602). 62p. pap. text 8.00 (*92-4-120602-0*, 1100602) World Health.

Advances in Virus Research. Ed. by Karl Maramorosch et al. (Illus.). 1998. (Advances in Virus Research Ser.: Vol. 51). 358p. (C). 89.95 (*0-12-039851-6*); Vol. 44. 1994. 473p. text 104.00 (*0-12-039844-3*); Vol. 45. 1995. 347p. text 79.00 (*0-12-039845-1*); Vol. 46. 1996. (Advances in Virus Research Ser.: Vol. 46). 512p. text 99.00 (*0-12-039846-X*); Vol. 47. 1996. 435p. text 99.00 (*0-12-039847-8*) Acad Pr.

Advances in Virus Research. Ed. by Karl Maramorosch et al. (Illus.). Vol. 48. 1997. 408p. text 89.95 (*0-12-039848-6*); Vol. 50. 1998. 455p. text 89.95 (*0-12-039850-8*) Morgan Kaufmann.

Advances in Virus Research, Vol. 52. Karl Maramorosch et al. 1999. (Advances in Virus Research Ser.: Vol. 52). (Illus.). 475p. 99.95 (*0-12-039852-4*) Acad Pr.

*__Advances in Virus Research: Neurovirology__, Vol. 56. Ed. by Michael Buchmeier & Ian Campbell. 2001. (Biomedical Sciences Ser.). 645p. 119.95 (*0-12-039856-7*) Acad Pr.

Advances in Virus Research Vol. 49: Cumulative Index, Volumes 25-47, Vol. 49. Ed. by Karl Maramorosch et al. 1997. (Illus.). 211p. text 89.95 (*0-12-039849-4*) Morgan Kaufmann.

Advances in World Diabetes Research. F. Belfiore & Silvia Iannello. 1984. (Frontiers in Diabetes Ser.: Vol. 5). x, 258p. 143.50 (*3-8055-3810-3*) S Karger.

Advances in X-Ray Analysis. Ed. by Charles S. Barrett et al. LC 58-35928. Vol. 29. 1986. 618p. 110.00 (*0-306-42287-5*); Vol. 30. 1987. (Illus.). 620p. 110.00 (*0-306-42690-0*) Perseus Pubng (Plenum Trade).

Advances in X-Ray Analysis, Vol. 32. Charles S. Barrett et al. 1989. (Illus.). 708p. 125.00 (*0-306-43236-6*, Plenum Trade) Perseus Pubng.

Advances in X-Ray Analysis. Ed. by Charles S. Barrett et al. (Illus.). (C). Vol. 34. 1991. 764p. text 162.00 (*0-306-44003-2*); Vol. 35. 1992. 1334p. text 234.00 (*0-306-44249-3*) Kluwer Academic (Kluwer Plenum).

Advances in X-Ray Analysis Vol. 38: Proceedings of the 43rd Annual Conference Held in Steamboat Springs, Colorado, August 1-5, 1994, Vol. 38. P. Predecki et al. 1995. LC 58-35928. (Illus.). 814p. (C). text 159.50 (*0-306-45045-3*, Kluwer Plenum) Kluwer Academic.

Advances in X-Ray Contrast: Collected Papers. Ed. by P. Dawson & W. Clauss. 1998. 114p. 50.00 (*0-7923-8741-4*) Kluwer Academic.

Advances of Diabetes Mellitus in East Asia: Proceedings of the 5th China-Japan Symposium on Diabetes Mellitus, Xian, China, 5-8 September 1996. Ed. by G. Mimura et al. 1997. LC 97-18023. (International Congress Ser.: No. 1141). 300p. 148.00 (*0-444-82664-5*, Excerpta Medica) Elsevier.

Advancing a Solution: Ending American Healthcare Crisis. Richard L. Scott. 1997. (Illus.). 160p. (Orig.). pap. (*0-9656835-0-8*) Columbia HCA Hlthcare.

*__Advancing Clinical Governance.__ Myriam Lugon & Jonathan Secker-Walker. 2001. 220p. pap. (*1-85315-471-7*) Royal Soc of Medicine Pr Ltd GBR. *Dist:* Balogh.

Advancing from the Ventral Striatum to the Extended Amygdala: Implications for Neuropsychiatry & Drug Abuse. Ed. by Jacqueline F. McGinty. 1999. LC 99-34750. (Annals of the New York Academy of Sciences Ser.: Vol. 877). (Illus.). xv, 835p. text 140.00 (*1-57331-178-2*) NY Acad Sci.

Advancing Health in Developing Countries: The Role of Social Research. Ed. by Lincoln C. Chen et al. 1992. LC 91-26133. 248p. 60.00 (*0-86569-034-0*, T034, Auburn Hse) Greenwood.

Advancing King's Conceptual Framework & Theory for Nursing. Maureen A. Frey & Christina L. Sieloff. 1995. 272p. 63.95 (*0-8039-5131-0*, 3173); pap. 32.95 (*0-8039-5132-9*, 3174) Sage.

Advancing Nursing Education Worldwide. Ed. by Doris M. Modly et al. 1995. LC 94-35282. (Illus.). 200p. 35.95 (*0-8261-8650-5*) Springer Pub.

Advancing Prescription Medicine Compliance: New Paradigms, New Practices. Ed. by Jack E. Fincham. LC 95-52198. (Journal of Pharmacoepidemiology: Vol. 3, No. 2). 148p. (C). 1997. pap. 19.95 (*0-7890-0220-5*); 1996. 39.95 (*1-56024-813-0*) Haworth Pr (Pharmctl Prods).

Advancing Professional Nursing Practice: Innovations at Boston's Beth Israel Hospital. Ed. by Joyce Clifford & Kathy Horvath. 1990. LC 90-9463. 384p. 48.95 (*0-8261-7180-X*) Springer Pub.

Advancing Quality: Total Quality Management in the NHS. Richard Joss & Maurice Kogan. 1995. LC 95-15493. (Health Services Management Ser.). 192p. (*0-335-19396-X*); pap. (*0-335-19395-1*) OpUniv Pr.

*__Advancing the Practice of Patient & Family-Centered Geriatric Care.__ 126p. ring bd. 30.00 (*0-9677733-5-0*) Inst Fmly Ctr.

Advancing Your Career: Concepts of Professional Nursing. Rose K. Nunnery. 1997. LC 96-29493. (Illus.). 424p. pap. 36.95 (*0-8036-0235-9*) Davis Co.

Advancing Your Career: Concepts of Professional Nursing. Rose Kearney. 2nd ed. 2001. LC 2001-28153. (Illus.). xxi, 528p. (C). pap. text 39.95 (*0-8036-0807-1*) Davis Co.

Advantages & Problems with Non-Opioids in Pain Management: Vancouver, Canada, August 19th, 1996. Michael J. Parnham. 1997. LC 97-511. (Illus.). 20p. pap. (*0-8176-5678-2*); pap. (*3-7643-5678-2*) Birkhauser.

Advantraz: The Natural Alternative for Weight Loss. Carl Germano. 1997. LC 98-208317. 128p. mass mkt. 5.99 (*1-57566-322-8*) Kensgtn Pub Corp.

Adventure of Self-Discovery: Dimensions of Consciousness & New Perspectives in Psychotherapy & Inner Exploration. Stanislav Grof. 1988. LC 87-17967. (Series in Transpersonal & Humanistic Psychology). 321p. (C). pap. text 20.95 (*0-88706-541-4*) State U NY Pr.

Adventure Therapy: Therapeutic Applications of Adventure Programming. Michael A. Gass. 1993. 528p. 29.95 (*0-8403-8272-3*) Assn Exper Ed.

Adventures in Consciousness: An Introduction to Aspect Psychology. Jane Roberts. 1978. 7.95 (*0-13-013953-X*) P-H.

Adventures in Fast Forward: Life, Love, & Work for the ADD Adult. Kathleen G. Nadeau. 1996. 224p. pap. 18.95 (*0-87630-800-0*) Brunner-Routledge.

Adventures in Food & Nutrition! Carol Byrd-Bredbenner. annot. ed. 1997. (Illus.). 654p. tchr. ed. 55.00 (*1-56637-325-5*) Goodheart.

Adventures in Food & Nutrition! Student Activity Guide. Carol Byrd-Bredbenner. 1997. (Illus.). 144p. stu. ed. 11.60 (*1-56637-326-3*) Goodheart.

Adventures in Food & Nutrition! Teacher's Resource Binder. Carol Byrd-Bredbenner. 1997. (Illus.). 300p. tchr. ed., ring bd. 112.00 (*1-56637-328-X*) Goodheart.

Adventures in Food & Nutrition! Teacher's Resource Guide. Carol Byrd-Bredbenner. 1997. (Illus.). 276p. tchr. ed. 49.00 (*1-56637-327-1*) Goodheart.

Adventures in Healing. Parnell Bradbury. 1969. 22.50 (*0-89979-000-3*) British Am Bks.

Adventures in Scuba Diving: A Text for the Beginning Diver. National Association of Underwater Instructors Staff. 1994. (Illus.). 240p. (C). (gr. 13). pap. text 25.95 (*0-8151-6277-4*, 25356) Mosby Inc.

Adventures in Successful Thinking. Richard A. Gunnell. 2nd ed. 1982. reprint ed. pap. text 5.95 (*0-939530-01-5*) Burtis Ent.

Adventures of a Nineteenth-Century Medic: The Life & Times of Dr. William Hunt, 1810-1882. Alice L. Howell. 1998. LC 98-65356. (Illus.). 64p. pap. 9.95 (*1-57736-080-X*, Hillsboro Pr) Providence Hse.

Adventurous Male: Chapters in the History of the White Male Mind. Martin Green. 1993. LC 92-26085. 256p. (C). text 42.50 (*0-271-00875-X*) Pa St U Pr.

Adventurous Years: Leaders in Action. Nell J. Watts. 1997. (Monographs). (Illus.). 187p. pap. text 30.00 (*0-9656391-2-6*) Sigma Theta Tau.

Adverse Cutaneous Reactions to Medication. Sanford M. Goldstein & Bruce U. Wintroub. 1996. LC 96-4660. (Illus.). 160p. pap. 14.95 (*0-683-18042-8*) Lppncott W & W.

Adverse Diagnostic Methods in Pathology. O'Leary. 2000. 800p. Price not set. (*0-7216-4976-9*) Saunders.

Adverse Drug Reaction Terms: Definition of Terms & Minimum Requirements for Their Use Respiratory & Skin Disorders. 1996. pap. text 9.00 (*92-9036-064-X*) World Health.

*__Adverse Drug Reactions.__ Lee. 2001. 312p. pap. (*0-85369-460-5*) Pharmaceutical Pr GBR. *Dist:* Rittenhouse.

Adverse Drug Reactions: Diagnosis & Reporting of Adverse Drug Reactions. Ed. by Christian Benichou. 1994. LC 94-6102. 320p. pap. 148.95 (*0-471-94211-1*) Wiley.

Adverse Drug Reactions & the Skin. S. M. Breathnach & H. Hintner. 1992. (Illus.). 408p. 165.00 (*0-632-03349-5*) Blackwell Sci.

Adverse Effects: Women & the Pharmaceutical Industry. Ed. by Kathleen McDonnell. 1986. 220p. reprint ed. pap. (*0-88961-108-4*) Womens Pr CAN. *Dist:* U of Toronto Pr.

Adverse Effects of Herbal Drugs. Ed. by P. A. De Smet et al. Vol. 1. 1992. 264p. pap. 72.00 (*0-387-53100-9*); Vol. 2. 1993. (Illus.). 348p. 78.95 (*0-387-55800-4*); Vol. 3. 1996. (Illus.). 208p. pap. 79.95 (*3-540-60181-3*) Spr-Verlag.

Adverse Effects of Pertussis & Rubella Vaccines. Ed. by Christopher P. Howson et al. 1991. 382p. text 39.95 (*0-309-04499-5*) Natl Acad Pr.

*__Adverse Event Reporting for Dietary Supplements: An Inadequate Safety Valve.__ Michael F. Mangano. 2001. 100p. pap. 25.00 (*0-7567-1236-X*) DIANE Pub.

Adverse Events Associated with Childhood Vaccines: Evidence Bearing on Causality. Institute of Medicine Staff. Ed. by Kathleen R. Stratton et al. 1993. LC 93-32099. 480p. (C). text 49.95 (*0-309-04895-8*) Natl Acad Pr.

Adverse Health Consequences of Cocaine Abuse. Ed. by A. Arif. 1987. (ENG & RUS.). 47p. pap. text 9.00 (*92-4-156107-6*, 1150272) World Health.

Adverse Neurological Effects of Cancer Therapy. 1995. lib. bdg. 251.95 (*0-8490-7585-8*); 1994. lib. bdg. 250.75 (*0-8490-8517-9*) Gordon Pr.

Adverse Reactions to Drug Formulations Agents: A Handbook of Excipients. Murray Weiner & I. Leonard Bernstein. 1989. (Clinical Pharmacology Ser.: Vol. 14). (Illus.). 480p. text 225.00 (*0-8247-7944-4*) Dekker.

Adverse Reactions to Drugs. O. L. Wade & Linda Beeley. 2nd ed. 1976. LC 76-676968. ix, 230p. (*0-433-34551-9*) Buttrwrth-Heinemann.

Adverse Reactions to Food. Therese Beaudette. 1991. LC 91-31708. pap. 7.65 (*0-88091-093-3*, 0154) Am Dietetic Assn.

Adverse Reactions to Non-Steroidal Anti-Inflammatory Drugs: Clinical Pharmacoepidemiology. Ed. by M. Kurowski. 1992. LC 92-17629. (Advances in Pharmacological Sciences Ser.). 103p. (C). (*0-8176-2628-X*) Birkhauser CHE. *Dist:* Spr-Verlag.

Adverse Reproductive Outcomes in Families of Atomic Veterans: The Feasibility of Epidemiologic Studies. Institute of Medicine Staff. Ed. by Committee to Study the Feasibility of, and Need for,. 1995. LC 95-70761. 108p. (Orig.). (C). pap. text 27.00 (*0-309-05340-4*, RA1231) Natl Acad Pr.

Adversity, Stress & Psychopathology. Ed. by Bruce P. Dohrenwend. 1998. LC 97-41525. (Illus.). 584p. text 89.50 (*0-19-512192-9*) OUP.

Advertising Handbook for Health Care Services. Ed. by William J. Winston. 1986. LC 85-27013. (Health Marketing Quarterly Ser.: Supplement No. 1). 287p. text 8.95 (*0-86656-390-3*) Haworth Pr.

Advice for a Young Investigator. Santiago Ramon Y Cajal. 1999. LC 98-26036. (Illus.). 120p. 24.95 (*0-262-18191-6*, Bradford Bks) MIT Pr.

Advice from a Pregnant Obstetrician: An Insider's Guide. Shari E. Brasner. 1998. LC 97-36475. 241p. pap. 12.95 (*0-7868-8339-1*) Hyperion.

Advice from the Diamond Headache Clinic. Seymour Diamond & Judi Diamond-Falk. 1982. LC 82-8973. ix, 194p. 30.00 (*0-8236-0119-6*) Intl Univs Pr.

Advice to Clever Children. Celia Green. 1989. (C). 65.00 (*0-900076-07-0*) St Mut.

Advice to Doctors & Other Big People from Kids. Gerald G. Jampolsky. Ed. by Center for Attitudinal Healing Staff. 1995. (Illus.). 112p. (Orig.). (YA). (gr. 2-8). pap. 7.95 (*0-89087-618-5*) Celestial Arts.

Advice to Parents of a Cleft Palate Child. Donna K. Wicka & Mervyn L. Falk. 2nd fac. ed. 1982. (Illus.). 80p. 24.95 (*0-398-04704-9*) C C Thomas.

Advising Premedical Students: Symposium, Friday, October 11, 1991. 1992. LC 92-48380. (C). 19.95 (*0-924143-02-9*) NY Acad Med.

Advising the Public about Radiation Emergencies: A Document for Public Comment. Intro. by Charles B. Meinhold. 1994. LC 94-37114. (NCRP Commentaries Ser.: No. 10). (Illus.). 29p. (Orig.). pap. text 20.00 (*0-929600-38-X*) NCRP Pubns.

Advisory Committee on Human Radiation Experiments: Executive Summary & Guide to Final Report. 1996. 36p. reprint ed. pap. text 15.00 (*0-7881-3053-6*) DIANE Pub.

Advisory Committee on Human Radiation Experiments: Interim Report. 1998. (Illus.). 140p. (C). reprint ed. pap. text 30.00 (*0-7881-3278-4*) DIANE Pub.

Advisory Panel on Alzheimer's Disease: Third Report. 1994. (Illus.). 75p. (Orig.). (C). pap. text 35.00 (*0-7881-0527-2*) DIANE Pub.

Advocacy in Health Care. Kevin Teasdale. 1999. LC 98-56109. pap. 38.95 (*0-632-04977-4*) Blackwell Sci.

Advocacy in Health Care: The Power of a Silent Constituency. Ed. by Joan H. Marks. 1986. LC 86-283. (Contemporary Issues in Biomedicine, Ethics & Society Ser.). 160p. 59.50 (*0-89603-092-X*) Humana.

Advocate's Guide to Home Care for the Elderly. Peter Komlos-Hrobsky. 1988. 132p. 15.00 (*0-941077-18-7*, 43,200) NCLS Inc.

Advocate's Guide to Medicaid Case Management Programs. 1988. 15.00 (*0-941077-20-9*, 44,300) NCLS Inc.

Advocate's Guide to the Medicaid Program. Roger Schwartz. 1985. 66p. (Orig.). pap. 8.00 (*0-941077-00-4*, 40,200) NCLS Inc.

Advocate's Guide to the Medically Needy Program. Jane Perkins & Lucien Wulsin. 1985. (Illus.). 120p. pap. 10.00 (*0-941077-01-2*, 40,250) NCLS Inc.

Advocating for Self: Women's Decisions Concerning Contraception. Peggy Matteson. 1995. LC 95-14297. (Haworth Innovations in Feminist Studies). (Illus.). 146p. (C). lib. bdg. 49.95 (*1-56024-948-X*) Haworth Jrnl Co-Edits.

Aehlert's EMT-Basic Instructor's Kit. Barbara Aehlert et al. 1998. LC 98-6576. 1,323p. 40.95 (*0-683-30581-6*) Lppncott W & W.

Aehlert's EMT-Basic Study Guide. Barbara Aehlert. 1997. LC 97-38043. (Illus.). 760p. 28.95 (*0-683-30217-5*) Lppncott W & W.

AEPS Curriculum for Birth to Three Years. Ed. by Juliann J. Cripe et al. 1992. LC 92-6690. (AEPS; Assessment, Evaluation, & Programming System Ser.: Vol. 2). 496p. (C). spiral bd. 59.95 (*1-55766-096-4*) P H Brookes.

Aequanimitas: With Other Addresses to Medical Students, Nurses & Practitioners of Medicine. William Osler. 3rd ed. 1932. 421p. text 60.00 (*0-07-047915-1*) McGraw-Hill Prof.

Aero Nursing News. Ed. by Darlene M. Sredl. 1985. pap. 2.50 (*0-930835-02-6*) Med Res Assocs.

Aeromedical Transportation: A Clinical Guide. Terence Martin & Howard Rodenberg. 1996. 288p. text (*0-291-39842-1*) Avebury Technical GBR. *Dist:* Ashgate Pub Co.

Aerosol Inhalation - Recent Research Frontiers: Proceedings of the International Workshop on Aerosol Inhalation, Lung Transport, Deposition & the Relation to the Environment: Recent Research Frontiers. Ed. by J. C. Marijnissen & L. Gradon. 1996. LC 96-17686. 320p. (C). text 140.00 (*0-7923-4058-2*) Kluwer Academic.

Aerosol Therapy. Lonny J. Ashworth. 1998. (CPG Mentor - Patient Cases in Respiratory Care Ser.: Unit 3). (*0-8151-2285-3*) Mosby Inc.

Aerosols in Medicine: Principles, Diagnosis, & Therapy. Ed. by F. Moren et al. 2nd ed. 1993. LC 93-36576. 450p. 227.25 (*0-444-81332-2*) Elsevier.

Aerosols in Science, Medicine & Technology: Proceedings of the Tenth Annual Conference of the Association for Aerosol Research (Gesellschaft fur Aerosolforschung), Bologna, Italy, 14-17 September 1982. Ed. by H. Fissan. 1983. 225p. pap. 32.00 (*0-08-030260-2*, Pergamon Pr) Elsevier.

Aerospace Medicine: Index of Modern Authors & Subjects with Guide for Rapid Research. Vasnil S. Sokov. 1994. LC 94-35176. 159p. 57.50 (*0-7883-0392-9*); pap. 47.50 (*0-7883-0393-7*) ABBE Pubs Assn.

Aerospace Software Engineering. Christine Anderson & Merlin Dorfman. 1991. (Progress in Astronautics & Aeronautics Ser.: Vol. 136). (Illus.). 630p. 79.95 (*1-56347-005-5*, V-136) AIAA.

Aesculapian. Dan Cloud. 2000. LC 97-36389. 368p. pap. 19.95 (*1-929490-08-9*) Beil.

Aesculapius in Latin America. Aristides A. Moll. 1969. LC 76-101589. (Illus.). reprint ed. 25.00 (*0-87266-022-2*) Argosy.

Aesthetic & Reconstructive Breast Surgery. John Bostwick, III. 1983. LC 82-8306. (Illus.). 748p. (C). (gr. 13). text 180.00 (*0-8016-0731-0*, 00731) Mosby Inc.

Aesthetic & Reconstructive Eyelid Surgery. Jelks. 1996. text (*0-7216-4369-8*) Saunders.

Aesthetic & Reconstructive Otoplasty. J. Davis. 1987. (Illus.). 581p. 357.00 (*0-387-96308-1*) Spr-Verlag.

Aesthetic Blepharoplasty. Ed. by Francis G. Wolfort & William R. Kanter. 1995. LC 94-21952. (Illus.). 256p. text 225.00 (*0-316-95091-2*, Little Brwn Med Div) Lppncott W & W.

Aesthetic Body Contour Surgery. Lockwood. 1999. text (*0-7216-5608-0*) Saunders.

Aesthetic Contouring of the Craniofacial Skeleton. Ousterhou. 1991. 350.00 (*0-316-67410-9*, Little Brwn Med Div) Lppncott W & W.

Aesthetic Dentistry: Color Atlas of Dental Medicine. J. Schmidseder. 2000. (Dental Medicine Ser.). (Illus.). 250p. 199.00 (*0-86577-923-6*) Thieme Med Pubs.

Aesthetic Facial Plastic Surgery: A Multidisciplinary Approach. Thomas Romo, III & Arthur L. Millman. 2000. (Illus.). 320p. 179.00 (*0-86577-807-8*) Thieme Med Pubs.

Aesthetic Facial Restoration. Elliott H. Rose. 1998. LC 97-29602. 384p. text 225.00 (*0-316-75646-6*, Little Brwn Med Div) Lppncott W & W.

Aesthetic Facial Surgery. Peter McKinney & Bruce L. Cunningham. 1992. (Illus.). 234p. text (*0-443-08703-2*) Church.

Aesthetic Facial Surgery. John Q. Owsley. 1993. LC 93-2826. (Illus.). 416p. text 185.00 (*0-7216-3364-1*) Saunders.

Aesthetic Laser Surgery: A Text & Video Atlas. Brooke R. Seckel. 1995. 162p. pap. text 240.00 incl. VHS (*0-316-78006-5*); (Illus.). pap. text 240.00 (*0-316-78007-3*) Lppncott W & W.

Aesthetic Laser Surgery, Resurfacing - Blepharoplasty Set. Roberts & Weinstein. 1996. 160p. text incl. VHS (*0-8151-8651-7*) Mosby Inc.

Aesthetic Perspectives in Jaw Surgery. Harvey M. Rosen. 1998. LC 97-26331. (Illus.). 302p. 192.00 (*0-387-98304-X*) Spr-Verlag.

Aesthetic Plastic Surgery M. Gonzalez-Ulloa et al. 1988. 1765p. text (*1-57235-007-5*) Piccin Nuova.

Aesthetic Plastic Surgery, Set. Thomas D. Rees & Gregory S. LaTrenta. 2nd ed. 1994. (Illus.). 1384p. text 450.00 (*0-7216-3712-4*) Saunders.

Aesthetic Plastic Surgery. M. Gonzalez-Ulloa et al. 1988. Vol. I. 322p. text (*1-57235-002-4*); Vol. IV. 353p. text (*1-57235-005-9*); Vol. V. 308p. text (*1-57235-006-7*) Piccin Nuova.

Aesthetic Plastic Surgery. M. Gonzalez-Ulloa et al. 1988. Vol. II. 334p. text (*1-57235-003-2*); Vol. III. 448p. text (*1-57235-004-0*) Piccin Nuova ITA. *Dist:* Scholium Intl.

Aesthetic Plastic Surgery: Principles & Techniques. Paule Regnault & Rollin K. Daniel. 1984. 800p. 230.00 (*0-316-73851-4*, Little Brwn Med Div) Lppncott W & W.

Aesthetic Plastic Surgery of Head & Body. I. Pitanguy. 1981. (Illus.). 412p. 719.00 (*0-387-08706-0*) Spr-Verlag.

Aesthetic Restoration of Nasal Defects. Burget & Menick. (Illus.). 1993. 615p. (C). (gr. 13). text 195.00 (*0-8016-7443-3*, 00909); 1992. 304p. text 160.00 (*0-8016-0909-7*) Mosby Inc.

Aesthetic Rhinoplasty. Nicolle. 1995. text 105.00 (*0-7020-1776-0*) Saunders.

Aesthetic Rhinoplasty G. Zaoli. 1994. 590p. text (*1-57235-065-2*) Piccin Nuova.

Aesthetic Rhinoplasty. Jack H. Sheen & Anitra P. Sheen. 2nd ed. 1997. LC 97-30275. 1544p. 250.00 (*1-57626-087-9*) Quality Med Pub.

Aesthetic Surgery Eyelids. 1989. (Illus.). 155p. 284.00 (*0-387-96912-8*) Spr-Verlag.

Aesthetic Surgery of the Craniofacial Skeleton. John J. Coleman, III et al. 1996. LC 96-13192. (Illus.). 187p. 137.00 (*0-387-94757-4*) Spr-Verlag.

Aesthetic Surgery of the Upper One-Third of the Face. Brian K. Howard & Joseph L. Leach. 1998. LC 98-27598. (Self-Instructional Package Ser.). (Illus.). 79p. pap. text 25.00 (*1-56772-067-6*, 5506335) AAO-HNS.

Aesthetics for the Therapist. Ann Hagman. 1991. 224p. pap. (*0-7487-0566-X*) Nelson Thornes GBR. *Dist:* Trans-Atl Phila.

Aesthetics of Change. Bradford P. Keeney. 1983. LC 82-15720. (Family Therapy Ser.). 217p. 30.00 (*0-89862-043-0*, 2043) Guilford Pubns.

Aesthetics of Movement. Paul Souriau. Ed. & Tr. by Manon Souriau. 1983. LC 83-10366. Orig. Title: L' Esthetique du Mouvement. (Illus.). 184p. lib. bdg. 25.00 (*0-87023-412-9*) U of Mass Pr.

Aetiological Studies of Isolated Common Congenital Abnormalities in Hungary. E. Czeizel & G. Tusnady. 1984. 358p. (C). (*963-05-3223-9*) Akade Kiado HUN. *Dist:* St Mut.

Aetiology - Idiopathic Scoliosis. Ed. by Gordon C. Robin. 1990. 83.00 (*0-8493-6722-0*, R) CRC Pr.

Affect: Psychoanalytic Perspectives. Ed. by Theodore Shapiro & Robert N. Emde. 1992. LC 92-49359. 514p. (C). 75.00 (*0-8236-0116-1*) Intl Univs Pr.

Affect & Accuracy in Recall: Studies of "Flashbulb" Memories. Ed. by Eugene Winograd & Ulric Neisser. 1992. (Emory Symposia in Cognition Ser.: No. 4). (Illus.). 327p. (C). text 64.95 (*0-521-40188-7*) Cambridge U Pr.

Affect & Attachment in the Family: A Family-Based Treatment of Major Psychiatric Disorder. Jeri A. Doane & Diana Diamond. 1998. (Illus.). 224p. (C). text 30.00 (*0-7881-5278-5*) DIANE Pub.

Affect & Creativity: The Role of Affect & Play in the Creative Process. Sandra Russ. 1993. (Spielberger: Personality Assessment Ser.). 160p. text 36.00 (*0-8058-0986-4*) L Erlbaum Assocs.

Affect & Emotion Journal: Psychopathology, Vol. 21, No. 2-3, 1988. Ed. by P. Berner & E. Gabriel. 1989. (Illus.). 92p. pap. 64.50 (*3-8055-5005-7*) S Karger.

Affect & Social Behavior. Bert S. Moore & Alice M. Isen. 1990. (Studies in Emotion & Social Interaction). (Illus.). 287p. (C). text 80.00 (*0-521-32768-7*) Cambridge U Pr.

Affect, Cognition & Social Behavior: New Evidence & Integrative Attempts. Ed. by Klaus Fiedler & J. P. Forgas. 1988. LC 87-26602. 392p. (C). text 59.00 (*0-88937-016-8*) Hogrefe & Huber Pubs.

Affect, Cognition, & Stereotyping: Interactive Processes in Group Perception. Ed. by Diane Mackie & David Hamilton. 1993. LC 92-28250. (Illus.). 389p. text 69.95 (*0-12-464410-4*) Acad Pr.

Affect, Conditioning & Cognition: Essays on the Determinants of Behavior. Robert Brush & Bruce J. Overmier. 1985. LC 85-15862. 400p. (C). text 79.95 (*0-89859-586-X*) L Erlbaum Assocs.

Affect, Creative Experience & Psychological Adjustment. Sandra W. Russ. 1998. LC 98-22837. (Series in Clinical & Community Psychology). 59.95 (*0-87630-917-1*); 225p. pap. 31.95 (*0-87630-918-X*) Brunner-Routledge.

Affect, Imagery, & Consciousness: The Negative Affects, Vol. 2. Silvan S. Tomkins. 1963. LC 62-16410. (Illus.). 580p. 69.95 (*0-8261-0542-4*) Springer Pub.

Affect, Imagery, & Consciousness: The Positive Affects, Vol. 1. Silvan S. Tomkins. 1962. LC 62-16410. (Illus.). 533p. 69.95 (*0-8261-0541-6*) Springer Pub.

Affect, Imagery, Consciousness: The Negative Affects: Anger & Fear, Vol. 3. Silvan S. Tomkins. 1991. 592p. 74.00 (*0-8261-0543-2*) Springer Pub.

Affect in Psychoanalysis: A Clinical Synthesis. Charles Spezzano. 1993. LC 92-48881. (Relational Perspectives Bks.: Vol. 2). 272p. 45.00 (*0-88163-128-0*) Analytic Pr.

Affect Regulation & the Origin of Self: The Neurobiology of Emotional Development. Allan N. Schore. 1994. 693p. text 135.00 (*0-8058-1396-9*) L Erlbaum Assocs.

***Affective & Non-Psychotic Disorders Vol. 2: Recent Topics from Advances in Psychiatric Treatment.** Ed. by Alan Lee. 1999. 159p. pap. (*1-901242-17-X*) Royal Coll Psych GBR. *Dist:* Balogh.

Affective & Schizoaffective Disorders: Similarities & Differences. Ed. by Andreas Marneros & Ming T. Tsuang. 1990. (Illus.). 292p. 108.00 (*0-387-52071-6*) Spr-Verlag.

Affective Disorders: Psychoanalytic Contributions to Their Study. Ed. by Phyllis Greenacre. 1961. LC 53-11058. 211p. 32.50 (*0-8236-0100-5*) Intl Univs Pr.

Affective Disorders & the Family: Assessment & Treatment. Ed. by John F. Clarkin et al. 1988. LC 87-28175. (Family Therapy Ser.). 263p. 37.95 (*0-89862-101-1*) Guilford Pubns.

Affective Disorders Reassessed, 1983. Ed. by Frank Ayd et al. 1983. 250p. (Orig.). text 35.00 (*0-931858-05-4*) Ayd Medical Comm.

Affective Neuroscience: The Foundations of Human & Animal Emotions. Jaak Panksepp. 1998. LC 98-15955. (Series in Affective Science). (Illus.). 480p. text 75.00 (*0-19-509673-8*) OUP.

Affects as Process: An Inquiry into the Centrality of Affect in Psychological Life. Joseph M. Jones. 1995. LC 94-46492. (Psychoanalytic Inquiry Book Ser.: Vol. 14). 296p. text 45.00 (*0-88163-125-6*) Analytic Pr.

Affinity Techniques Enzyme Purification, Pt. B. Ed. by William B. Jacoby & Meir Wilchek. 1974. (Methods in Enzymology Ser.: Vol. 34). text 199.00 (*0-12-181897-7*) Acad Pr.

Affirmative Dynamic Psychotherapy with Gay Men. Ed. by Carlton Cornett. 1993. LC 93-12886. 264p. 50.00 (*1-56821-001-9*) Aronson.

Affirming the Darkness: An Extended Conversation about Living with Prostate Cancer. Chuck Wheeler & Martha Wheeler. Ed. by Gretchen Hirsch. 1996. (Illus.). 218p. (Orig.). pap. 17.95 (*1-889833-00-2*) Memoirs Unltd.

Affordable Step Toward Universal Coverage: A Report by the Minnesota Health Care Commission. 1995. (Illus.). 51p. (Orig.). (C). pap. text 25.00 (*0-7881-2366-1*) DIANE Pub.

Afghanistan to France Afghanistan to France: A Global Review, Vol. I. LC 92-233111. (Abortion Policies Ser.: No. 129). 158p. 25.00 (*92-1-151246-8*, E.92.XIII.8) UN.

AFIP Advanced Laboratory Methods in Histology & Pathology. Mikel et al. 1994. (Illus.). 254p. pap. text 45.00 (*1-881041-13-1*) Am Registry Path.

AFIP Atlas of Tumor Pathology: Tumors of the Adrenal Gland & Extra Adrenal Paraganglia. Lack. 1997. (Illus.). 468p. pap. text 70.00 (*1-881041-28-X*) Am Registry Path.

AFIP Atlas of Tumor Pathology: Tumors of the Pancreas. Solcia et al. 1997. (Illus.). 264p. pap. text 50.00 (*1-881041-29-8*) Am Registry Path.

AFIP Laboratory Methods in Histotechnology see AFIP Methodos Histotecnologicos

AFIP Laboratory Methods in Histotechnology. Armed Forces Institute of Pathology Staff. 1992. 35.00 (*1-881041-00-X*) Am Registry Path.

AFIP Methodos Histotecnologicos. Prophet et al. Tr. by Mullick Heffes. 1995. Orig. Title: AFIP Laboratory Methods in Histotechnology. (SPA., Illus.). 280p. pap. text 35.00 (*1-881041-21-2*) Am Registry Path.

Aflatoxins & Human Health. Ed. by Ivana Dvorackova. 1989. 274p. lib. bdg. 166.00 (*0-8493-4628-2*, RA1242) CRC Pr.

Afraid to Ask: A Book for Families to Share about Cancer. Judylaine Fine. 1986. LC 85-28386. (Illus.). 172p. pap. 6.95 (*0-688-06196-6*, Wm Morrow) Morrow Avon.

African American Daughters & Elderly Mothers: Examining Experiences of Grief, Loss & Bereavement. Sharon H. Smith. rev. ed. 1998. LC 98-28996. (Studies on the Elderly in America). (Illus.). 191p. 53.00 (*0-8153-3177-0*) Garland.

African American Mental Health. Ed. by Reginald L. Jones. 1997. LC 97-20436. (C). lib. bdg. 45.00 (*0-943539-12-9*) Cobb & Henry Pubs.

African-American Perspectives on Biomedical Ethics. Ed. by Harley E. Flack & Edmund D. Pellegrino. 1992. LC 92-17638. 224p. (Orig.). pap. text 26.95 (*0-87840-532-1*) Georgetown U Pr.

African-American Pharmacists. 2000. (My Ancestors—My Heroes Ser.: Vol. 29). (J). (gr. 3-4). (*1-893091-28-7*) F R Parker.

African American Psychology: Theory, Research & Practice. A. Kathleen Burlew et al. 1992. LC 92-20394. (Illus.). 400p. (C). pap. 42.95 (*0-8039-4766-6*, 4224) Sage.

African American Task Force Report on the Year 2000: Health Promotion Objectives & Recommendations for California. 1993. 77p. (Orig.). (C). pap. text 40.00 (*0-7881-0090-4*) DIANE Pub.

African American Voices: African American Health Educators Speak Out. Ed. by Ruth W. Johnson. 1995. LC 95-151953. 212p. pap. 38.95 (*0-88737-625-8*) Natl League Nurse.

African American Voices: African American Health Educators Speak Out. Ruth W. Johnson & NLN Staff. 1999. (Illus.). 224p. (C). pap. text 34.95 (*0-7637-1084-9*, 1084-9, N L N Bart) Jones & Bartlett.

African American Women's Health & Social Issues. Otha Richard Sulllivan. Ed. by Catherine F. Collins. 1996. LC 96-10376. 248p. (J). (gr. 3-7). 67.00 (*0-86569-250-5*, Auburn Hse) Greenwood.

African Fever: A Study of British Science, Technology, & Politics in West Africa, 1787-1864. Dennis G. Carlson. 1984. LC 81-5621. 15.95 (*0-88202-196-6*) Watson Pub Intl.

African Health & Healing Systems: Proceedings of a Symposium. Ed. by P. Stanley Yoder. 1982. 252p. 30.00 (*0-918456-34-7*, Crossroads) African Studies Assn.

African Herbal Healing: An A-Z Guide for Everyday Use. A. Williams. 2001. (Illus.). 208p. pap. 12.00 (*0-8065-2103-1*, Citadel Pr) Kensgtn Pub Corp.

African Holistic Health. Llaila O. Afrika. Ed. by T. Nokwari Adesegun. rev. ed. 1989. (Illus.). 300p. pap. 14.95 (*1-877610-00-3*) Sea Island.

***African Power Dieting: Is America on the Wrong Path? You Decide!** African Missionary Surgeon Staff. 2001. LC 00-112299. (Illus.). 448p. pap. 18.98 (*1-931386-14-5*, 1062) A A D U P A Y Publng.

African Psychology in Historical Perspective & Related Commentary. Ed. by Daudi A. Ya Azibo. 1996. LC 95-50998. 288p. 69.95 (*0-86543-292-9*) Africa World.

African Sleeping Sickness: Political Ecology, Colonialism, & Control in Uganda. Jonathan Musere. 1990. LC 90-44199. (Studies in African Health & Medicine: Vol. 5). 224p. lib. bdg. 89.95 (*0-88946-280-1*) E Mellen.

African Swine Fever Virus. W. R. Hess. 1971. (Virology Monographs: Vol. 9). 26.00 (*0-387-81006-4*) Spr-Verlag.

African Trypanosomiases: A Report of the FAO-WHO Expert Committee, Geneva, 1968. FAO-WHO Expert Committee. 1979. (Technical Reports: No. 635). 96p. pap. text 7.00 (*92-4-120635-7*, 1100635) World Health.

African Trypanosomiasis: A Report of the FAO-WHO Expert Committee, Geneva, 1968. FAO-WHO Expert Committee. 1969. (Technical Reports: No. 434). 79p. pap. 5.00 (*92-4-120434-6*, 1541) World Health.

Africanized Honeybees in California, Vol. 2. Kenneth Umbach. 1999. 9p. pap. (*1-58703-105-1*, CRB Note 6) CA Res Bureau.

Africa's Changing Markets for Health & Veterinary Services. David K. Leonard. 2000. LC 99-88269. xxxix, 320p. pap. 25.00 (*0-312-23267-5*) St Martin.

Africa's Changing Markets for Health & Veterinary Services: The New Institutional Issues. David K. Leonard. 2000. LC 99-88269. xxxix, 320p. 79.95 (*0-312-23266-7*) St Martin.

After a Diagnosis of Cancer: Taking Charge. Michael Kelly & Renee Shaker. 2nd ed. 1998. 160p. pap. 15.95 (*1-893865-01-0*) Life Care.

After a Funeral. Diana Athill. 1986. 176p. 15.45 (*0-89919-454-0*) HM.

After a Stroke: A Support Book for Patients, Caregivers, Families & Friends. Geoffrey A. Donnan & Carol Burton. 2nd ed. 1992. LC 92-241764. (Family Health Ser.). (Illus.). 144p. reprint ed. pap. 11.95 (*1-55643-130-9*) North Atlantic.

After Anesthesia. Kay E. Fraulini. 1992. (Illus.). 448p. (C). text 54.95 (*0-8385-0078-1*, A0078-4) McGraw-Hill Educ Grp.

After Any Diagnosis: How to Take Action Against Your Illness Using the Best & Most Current Medical Information Available. Carol Svec. 2001. LC 00-67303. (Illus.). xii, 308p. pap. 15.00 (*0-609-80669-6*, Three Riv Pr) Harmony Bks.

After Cancer: A Guide to Your New Life. Wendy S. Harpham. 1995. LC 95-18918. 240p. pap. 13.50 (*0-06-097678-0*, Perennial) HarperTrade.

After Fifteen Years: Artificial Liver & Artificial Pancreas. K. N. Matsumura & William L. Hamilton. 2nd ed. 1978. LC 78-56092. (Illus.). 19.95 (*0-9606924-0-1*) Alin Found Pr.

After Oedipus: Shakespeare in Psychoanalysis. Julia R. Lupton & Kenneth Reinhard. 1993. LC 92-54975. (Illus.). 288p. 47.50 (*0-8014-2407-0*); pap. 18.95 (*0-8014-9687-X*) Cornell U Pr.

After Plastic Surgery: Adaptation & Adjustment. Francis C. MacGregor. 1979. 160p. (C). 45.00 (*0-03-052131-9*) Phoenix Soc.

After Residency: The Young Physician's Guide to the Universe. Joan Anderson. 1998. pap. 19.95 (*1-890114-01-4*) Physicians Pr.

After Restructuring: Empowerment Strategies at Work in America's Hospitals. Thomas G. Rundall et al. 1998. LC 98-17784. (Business & Management Ser.). 296p. 49.00 (*0-7879-4029-1*) Jossey-Bass.

After Shock: The Emotional Impact of Providing Emergency Care. EMP International Inc., Staff. 2000. 24.95 (*0-940430-90-8*, 1031) EMP Intl.

After Stroke. David M. Hinds. 2000. pap. (*0-7225-3885-5*) Thorsons GBR. *Dist:* Natl Bk Netwk.

After Stroke: Enhancing Quality of Life. Ed. by Wallace Sife. 1998. LC 98-16152. 281p. 49.95 (*0-7890-0321-X*); pap. 24.95 (*0-7890-0341-4*) Haworth Pr.

After Suicide. John H. Hewett. Ed. by Wayne E. Oates. 1980. LC 79-24373. (Christian Care Bks.: Vol. 4). 118p. pap. 13.00 (*0-664-24296-0*) Westminster John Knox.

After the Beyond: Human Transformation & the Near-Death Experience. Charles P. Flynn. 1985. LC 85-16720. 14.95 (*0-13-018359-8*) P-H.

After the Crash: Assessment & Treatment of Motor Vehicle Accident Survivors. Edward B. Blanchard & Edward J. Hickling. 1997. LC 97-5336. (Illus.). 353p. 39.95 (*1-55798-424-7*) Am Psychol.

After the Death of a Child: Living with Loss Through the Years. Ann K. Finkbeiner. 1998. LC 97-47017. 288p. reprint ed. pap. 16.95 (*0-8018-5914-X*) Johns Hopkins.

After the Fight: Using Your Disagreements to Build a Stronger Relationship. Daniel B. Wile. 1993. LC 93-4846. 326p. 42.00 (*0-89862-754-0*) Guilford Pubns.

After the Stork: Owner's Manual for the 1998 Model Year Baby. Elizabeth Morelli et al. Ed. by Bink Stiles. 1997. (Illus.). 240p. pap. 19.95 (*0-9658297-1-5*) Bink Productions.

After the Stroke: Coping with America's Third Leading Cause of Death. Evelyn Shirk. 1991. LC 91-3902. (Golden Age Bks.). 114p. 33.00 (*0-87975-693-4*); pap. 20.00 (*0-87975-694-2*) Prometheus Bks.

After You've Tried Everything Else: A "More Excellent Way" to Freedom from Addictions. Chuck Makela. 1987. 32p. (Orig.). pap. 1.00 (*0-9618532-0-4*) Just Pub Hse.

Aftermath: Survive & Overcome Trauma. Mariann Hybels-Steer. 1995. 256p. pap. 11.00 (*0-671-88389-5*, Fireside) S&S Trade Pap.

Aftermath of Stroke: The Experience of Patients & Their Families. Robert Anderson. 1992. 272p. (C). text 74.95 (*0-521-40196-8*) Cambridge U Pr.

Against All Odds Vol. 1: The Story of My Battle with Sickle Cell Anemia. 1997. pap. 10.00 (*0-9660549-0-3*) Janice Prodn.

Against Instinct: From Biology to Philosophical Psychology. Dennis M. Senchuk. 1991. 200p. 54.95 (*0-87722-815-9*) Temple U Pr.

Against Relativism: Cultural Diversity & the Search for Ethical Universals in Medicine. Ruth Macklin. 1999. LC 98-44063. 304p. text 32.95 (*0-19-511632-1*) OUP.

Against the Odds: Blacks in the Profession of Medicine in the United States. Wilbur Watson. 1998. LC 98-34953. (Illus.). xi, 198p. text 34.95 (*1-56000-376-6*) Transaction Pubs.

Against Therapy. Jeffrey M. Masson. LC 93-26695. reprint ed. 1994. lib. bdg. 29.95 (*1-56751-023-X*); 1993. 340p. pap. 15.95 (*1-56751-022-1*) Common Courage.

Agar Gel Electrophoresis in Neurology. A. Lowenthal. 1964. pap. 22.00 (*0-444-40377-9*) Elsevier.

Age-Associated Neurological Diseases. Ed. by L. Deecke & P. Dal-Bianco. 1991. (Journals of Neural Transmission: Suppl. 33). (Illus.). 180p. pap. 59.00 (*3-211-82261-5*) Spr-Verlag.

Age-Associated Neurological Diseases L. Deecke & P. Dal-Bianco. 1991. LC 91-5013. (Journals of Neural Transmission). viii, 165 p. (*0-387-82261-5*) Spr-Verlag.

Age Between Adolescence & Therapy. Derek Miller. 1995. LC 83-3893. 460p. pap. text 50.00 (*1-56821-732-3*) Aronson.

Age Between Adolescence & Therapy. Derek Miller. rev. ed. 1986. LC 83-3893. (Age Between Adolescence & Therapy C Ser.: Vol. 1). 456p. 50.00 (*0-87668-639-0*) Aronson.

Age-Dependent Doses to Members of the Public from Intake of Radionuclides, Pt. 1: A Report of a Task Group of Committee 2 of the International Commission on Radiological Protection. ICRP Staff. 1990. (International Commission on Radiological Protection Ser.: No. 56). (Illus.). 134p. pap. 40.00 (*0-08-040763-3*, Pergamon Pr) Elsevier.

Age, Health & Employment. James E. Birren et al. 1986. 192p. (C). text 49.00 (*0-13-018524-8*) P-H.

Age Markers in the Human Skeleton. Ed. by M. Yasar Iscan. 1989. (Illus.). 378p. pap. 58.95 (*0-398-06174-2*); (C). text 87.95 (*0-398-05614-5*) C C Thomas.

Age of Agony: The Art of Healing 1700-1800. Guy Williams. 1996. (Illus.). 230p. reprint ed. pap. 14.00 (*0-89733-203-2*) Academy Chi Pubs.

Age of Information: An Interdisciplinary Survey of Cybernetics. T. C. Helvey. 1971. LC 78-125870. 224p. 39.95 (*0-87778-008-0*) Educ Tech Pubns.

Age of Miracles: Medicine & Surgery in the Nineteenth Century. Guy Williams. 1987. (Illus.). 256p. pap. 14.00 (*0-89733-285-7*) Academy Chi Pubs.

Age of the Earth. G. Brent Dalrymple. 1994. xviii, 474p. pap. 30.95 (*0-8047-2331-1*) Stanford U Pr.

Age Proof Muscles & Joints. Lang. 1997. (C). text 25.95 (*0-13-593021-9*) P-H.

Age-Related Dopamine-Dependent Disorders. Ed. by M. Segawa & Y. Nomura. 1995. (Monographs in Neural Sciences: Vol. 14). (Illus.). x, 256p. 208.75 (*3-8055-5960-7*) S Karger.

Age-Related Factors in Radionuclide Metabolism & Dosimetry. Ed. by Georg B. Gerber et al. 1987. (Developments in Nuclear Medicine Ser.). (C). text 256.00 (*0-89838-953-4*) Kluwer Academic.

Age-Related Macular Degeneration. Jeffrey W. Berger et al. 1998. LC 98-39679. 175.00 (*0-323-00200-5*) Mosby Inc.

Age-Related Macular Degeneration: Current Treatment Concepts. Ed. by W. E. Alberti et al. 2000. LC 00-55661. (Medical Radiology Ser.). (Illus.). 150p. 75.00 (*3-540-66643-5*) Spr-Verlag.

Age, Work & Automation. Ed. by P. M. Paillat & M. E. Bunch. 1970. (Interdisciplinary Topics in Gerontology Ser.: Vol. 6). 26.25 (*3-8055-0507-8*) S Karger.

Aged in the Community: Managing Senility & Deviance. Dwight Frankfather. 1977. LC 77-8327. (Praeger Special Studies). 221p. 62.00 (*0-275-90264-1*, C0264, Praeger Pubs) Greenwood.

Ageing & Dementia. Burns. 1993. 320p. 55.00 (*0-340-56838-0*) Trafalgar.

***Ageing & Executive Control.** Ed. by Ulrich Mayr et al. 2001. 288p. (*1-84169-908-X*) Psychol Pr GBR. *Dist:* Taylor & Francis.

Ageing, Autonomy & Resources. Ed. by A. Harry Lesser. 1999. LC 99-72599. (Avebury Series in Philosophy). 256p. text (*1-84014-971-X*) Ashgate Pub GBR. *Dist:* Ashgate Pub Co.

Ageing of Asian Populations. LC 94-209500. 144p. 25.00 (*92-1-151267-0*, E.94.XIII.10) UN.

Ageless: Living Younger Longer. Ben H. Douglas. 1990. LC 89-70325. 204p. 14.95 (*0-937552-33-X*) Quail Ridge.

Ageless Bodies, Timeless Minds see Cuerpos Sin Edad, Mentes Sin Tiempo

A
B

Ageless Body, Timeless Mind: The Quantum Alternative to Growing Old. Deepak Chopra. 1994. LC 94-19236. 352p. pap. 14.00 (*0-517-88212-4*, Three Riv Pr) Crown Pub Group.

Ageless Exercise: A Gentle Approach for the Inactive or Physically Limited. Joan Laird. 1994. LC 93-60903. (Illus.). 64p. spiral bd. 10.95 (*0-9638390-0-4*) Angelwood Pr.

Ageless Remedies from Mother's Kitchen. Hanna Kroeger. 1981. 92p. pap. 6.00 (*1-883713-04-8*) Hanna Kroeger.

Agency for Health Care Policy & Research Role in Health Care Quality Improvement: Congressional Hearing. Ed. by Bill First. 1999. 75p. (C). reprint ed. pap. text 20.00 (*0-7881-8411-3*) DIANE Pub.

***Agency for Toxic Substances & Disease Registry: FY 2000 Profile & Annual Report.** Frwd. by Jeffrey P. Koplan. 2001. 82p. (C). pap. text 20.00 (*0-7567-1626-8*) DIANE Pub.

Agenda for Continuing Education: A Challenge to Health Care Institutions. Daniel S. Schechter. 1974. LC 74-83051. (Illus.). 96p. 12.00 (*0-87914-027-5*, 549605) Hosp Res & Educ.

Agenda for Solving America's Health Care Crisis: Task Force Report. 1990. 41p. pap. 10.00 (*0-943802-54-7*, 151) Natl Ctr Pol.

Agent of Trachoma: Recent Studies of the Biology, Biochemistry & Immunology of a Prokaryotic Obligate Parasite of Eukaryocytes. Y Becker. 1974. (Monographs in Virology: Vol. 7). (Illus.). 99p. 55.75 (*3-8055-1657-6*) S Karger.

Agent Orange on Trial: Mass Toxic Disasters in the Courts. Peter H. Schuck. 1988. LC 87-19613. 375p. reprint ed. pap. 22.50 (*0-674-01026-4*) HUP.

Agents in My Brain: How I Survived Manic Depression. Bill Hannon. 1997. LC 97-2782. 258p. pap. 18.95 (*0-8126-9346-9*) Open Court.

Agents of Apocalypse: Epidemic Disease in the Colonial Philippines. Ken De Bevoise. 1995. LC 94-19328. 274p. 47.50 (*0-691-03486-9*) Princeton U Pr.

Agents Stimulating Gonadal Function in the Human: Proceedings of the WHO Scientific Group, Geneva, 1972. WHO Staff. 1973. (Technical Reports: No. 514). pap. text 4.00 (*92-4-120514-8*, 1100514) World Health.

Agents Transmissible from Simians to Man. M. Brack. 1987. (Illus.). 454p. 135.00 (*0-387-17559-8*) Spr-Verlag.

Ages & Stages, New & Revised: Developmental Descriptions & Activities, Birth Through Eight Years. Karen Miller. 2nd ed. 2001. 227p. (C). pap. 16.95 (*0-910287-16-3*, RJ131.M54) TelShare Pub Co.

***Ages & Stages Questionnaires: Social-Emotional (ASQ:SE): A Parent-Completed, Child-Monitoring System for Social-Emotional Behaviors.** Jane Squires et al. 2001. 125.00 (*1-55766-534-6*) P H Brookes.

Agglutination Analyses: Antibody Characteristics, Methodology, Limitations, & Clinical Validation; Approved Guideline (1993) Contrib. by Robert M. Nakamura. 1993. 75.00 (*1-56238-195-4*, D13-A) NCCLS.

Aggression. 1996. 20.00 (*3-540-60550-9*) Spr-Verlag.

Aggression: Biological, Developmental, & Social Perspectives. Ed. by Seymour Feshbach & Jolanta Zagrodzka. 1997. LC 96-38783. (Series in Social/Clinical Psychology). 254p. 49.50 (*0-306-45497-1*, Plenum Trade) Perseus Pubng.

Aggression: Its Causes, Consequences, & Control. Leonard Berkowitz. 1993. LC 92-31862. 496p. text 59.95 (*1-56639-033-8*) Temple U Pr.

Aggression: Its Causes, Consequences & Control. Leonard Berkowitz. 1992. LC 92-33589. (Series in Social Psychology). 512p. (C). pap. 45.31 (*0-07-004874-6*) McGrw-H Hghr Educ.

Aggression & Anti-Social Behavior in Childhood & Adolescence No. 1: Book Supplement to the Journal of Child Psychology & Psychiatry. Ed. by Lional A. Hersov et al. 1978. LC 77-30484. suppl. ed. (*0-08-021810-5*) Pergamon Repr GBR. *Dist:* Franklin.

Aggression & Behavior Change: Biological & Social Processes. Ed. by Seymour Feshbach & Adam Fraczek. 1979. LC 79-17934. (Praeger Special Studies). (Illus.). 299p. 68.50 (*0-275-90352-4*, C0352, Praeger Pubs) Greenwood.

Aggression & Repression in the Individual & Society. Hans E. Lauer. Tr. by K. Castelliz & Saunders Davies from GER. 1981.Tr. of Aggression und Repression im individuellen und Sozialen Berich. 111p. pap. (*0-85440-359-0*) R Steiner Pr GBR. *Dist:* Anthroposophic.

Aggression & Violence: Social Interactionist Perspectives. Ed. by Richard B. Felson & James T. Tedeschi. 1993. LC 92-36152. (Illus.). 265p. text 24.95 (*1-55798-190-6*) Am Psychol.

Aggression, Family Violence & Chemical Dependency. Ed. by Ronald T. Potter-Efron & Patricia S. Potter-Efron. 1990. LC 89-24737. (Journal of Chemical Dependency Treatment Ser.: Vol. 3, No. 1). (Illus.). 226p. text 49.95 (*0-86656-964-2*); pap. text 17.95 (*0-86656-977-4*) Haworth Pr.

Aggression in Children & Youth. Ed. by Robert M. Kaplan et al. 1983. lib. bdg. 228.00 (*90-247-2903-3*) Kluwer Academic.

Aggression in Our Children: Coping with It Constructively. Henri Parens. 1993. LC 87-19547. 224p. pap. 27.50 (*1-56821-076-0*) Aronson.

Aggression in Personality Disorders & Perversions. Otto F. Kernberg. 1993. LC 92-18118. 384p. (C). 50.00 (*0-300-05003-8*) Yale U Pr.

Aggression und Repression im individuellen und Sozialen Berich see Aggression & Repression in the Individual & Society

Aggressive & Defiant Behavior: The Latest Assessment & Treatment Strategies for the Conduct Disorders. J. Mark Eddy. 2nd ed. 2001. (Condensed Reviews for Professionals Ser.). 120p. (C). pap. 14.95 (*1-887537-15-5*) Compact Clinicals.

Aggressive Behavior: Assessment & Modification. Arnold P. Goldstein & Harold Keller. 1987. (Psychology Practitioner Guidebooks). 200p. text 32.50 (*0-08-034320-1*); pap. text 16.95 (*0-08-034319-8*) Elsevier (Pergamon Pr).

Aggressive Behavior: Current Perspectives. Ed. by L. R. Huesmann. 1994. (Social-Clinical Psychology Ser.). (Illus.). 326p. (C). 49.50 (*0-306-44553-0*, Plenum Trade) Perseus Pubng.

Aggressive Behavior: Genetic & Neural Approaches. Ed. by Edward C. Simmel et al. 1983. 224p. text 49.95 (*0-89859-253-4*) L Erlbaum Assocs.

Agile at Eighty. Robert L. Whiteside. 1989. LC 89-90278. (Illus.). 128p. (Orig.). pap. 7.95 (*0-9623385-0-8*) R L Whiteside.

Agility in Health Care: Strategies for Mastering Turbulent Markets. Ed. by Steven Goldman & Carol Graham. 1998. LC 98-40111. (Health Care Management Ser.). (Illus.). 228p. 49.00 (*0-7879-4211-1*) Jossey-Bass.

Aging: A Source Guide. 1991. lib. bdg. 250.00 (*0-8490-4850-8*) Gordon Pr.

Aging: An Introduction to Gerontology. Lewis R. Aiken. 1994. 450p. 86.95 (*0-8039-5445-X*, 4659) Sage.

Aging: Genetic & Environmental Influences. C. S. Bergeman. 1997. LC 97-4592. (Individual Differences & Development Ser.). 160p. 76.95 (*0-8039-7377-2*, 1359); pap. 31.95 (*0-8039-7378-0*, 1360) Sage.

Aging: Issues & Policies for the 1980's. Ed. by Ted Tedrick. 1985. LC 84-26328. 243p. 64.00 (*0-275-90173-4*, C0173, Praeger Pubs) Greenwood.

Aging: Its History & Literature. Joseph T. Freeman. 1979. LC 79-11839. 161p. 29.95 (*0-87705-251-4*, Kluwer Acad Hman Sci) Kluwer Academic.

Aging: The Facts. Nicholas Coni et al. 2nd ed. 1992. (Facts Ser.). (Illus.). 214p. text 19.95 (*0-19-262150-5*) OUP.

Aging: The Health Care Challenge. Carole B. Lewis. 3rd ed. 1995. LC 95-460. (Illus.). 494p. (C). pap. text 43.95 (*0-8036-0042-9*) Davis Co.

Aging & Age Related Ocular Diseases. E. Lutjen-Drecoll. 2000. (Opthalmologica Ser.: Vol. 214, No. 1). (Illus.). 104p. pap. 34.00 (*3-8055-7038-4*) S Karger.

Aging & Biography: Explorations in Adult Development. Ed. by James E. Birren et al. 1995. LC 95-2876. (Illus.). 368p. 52.95 (*0-8261-8980-6*) Springer Pub.

Aging & Blood Stasis: A New TCM Approach to Geriatrics. Yan De-Xin. Ed. & Tr. by Bob Flaws from CHI. Tr. by Tang Guo-Shun from CHI. 1995. LC 95-77296. 255p. (Orig.). pap. 25.95 (*0-936185-63-5*) Blue Poppy Pr.

Aging & Cancer. F. F. Holmes. 1983. (Recent Results in Cancer Research Ser.: Vol. 87). (Illus.). 75p. 46.00 (*0-387-12656-2*) Spr-Verlag.

Aging & Cell Structure, Vol. 1. Ed. by John E. Johnson, Jr. 1981. LC 81-17886. 402p. (C). 89.50 (*0-306-40695-0*, Plenum Trade) Perseus Pubng.

Aging & Cellular Defense Mechanisms. Ed. by Claudio Franceschi et al. 1992. LC 92-49531. 150.00 (*0-89766-729-8*); pap. 150.00 (*0-89766-730-1*) NY Acad Sci.

Aging & Cognitive Processes. Ed. by Fergus Craik & Sandra E. Trehub. 1982. LC 82-18129. (Advances in the Study of Communication & Affect Ser.: Vol. 8). 396p. 80.00 (*0-306-40946-1*, Plenum Trade) Perseus Pubng.

Aging & Communication. Ed. by Barbara B. Shadden & Mary A. Toner. 1997. LC 96-38710. (For Clinicians by Clinicians Ser.). pap. 34.00 (*0-89079-711-0*, 8283) PRO-ED.

Aging & Dementia. Ed. by K. Jellinger et al. 1998. (Illus.). 380p. 159.00 (*3-211-83115-0*) Spr-Verlag.

***Aging & Development.** Peter Coleman et al. 2001. (Arnold Publication). 256p. pap. text 24.95 (*0-340-75894-5*) OUP.

Aging & Developmental Disability: Current Research, Programming & Practice Implications. Ed. by Joy Hammel & Susan M. Nochajski. 2000. LC 00-49890. (Illus.). 100p. pap. text 22.95 (*0-7890-1040-2*) Haworth Pr.

Aging & Ethics. Ed. by Nancy S. Jecker. 1991. LC 91-10792. (Contemporary Issues in Biomedicine, Ethics & Society Ser.). 408p. pap. 39.50 (*0-89603-255-8*) Humana.

Aging & Family Therapy: Practitioner Perspectives on Golden Pond. George A. Hughston et al. 1989. LC 88-39357. (Journal of Psychotherapy & the Family Ser.: Vol. 5, Nos. 1-2). (Illus.). 244p. text 49.95 (*0-86656-778-X*) Haworth Pr.

Aging & Health: Linking Research & Public Policy. Steven J. Lewis. 1989. (Illus.). 492p. lib. bdg. 119.00 (*0-87371-160-2*, L160) Lewis Pubs.

Aging & Health Care: Social Science & Policy Perspectives. Marcia G. Ory. 1993. 284p. pap. 95.00 (*1-56593-576-4*, 0684) Singular Publishing.

Aging & Health Care: Social Science & Policy Perspectives. Ed. by Marcia G. Ory & Kathleen Bond. 1989. (Contemporary Issues in Health, Medicine, & Social Policy Ser.). 320p. 49.95 (*0-415-01716-5*); pap. 19.95 (*0-415-01717-3*) Routledge.

Aging & Human Longevity. Marie-Francoise Schulz-Aellen. 1996. LC 96-17985. 290p. 89.95 (*0-8176-3875-X*); 283p. pap. 49.95 (*0-8176-3964-0*) Birkhauser.

Aging & Later Life. Julia Johnson & Robert Slater. 2nd ed. 1993. 336p. (C). pap. 27.95 (*0-8039-8966-0*, 9538) Sage.

Aging & Leisure. Robert W. Kleemeier. Ed. by Robert J. Kastenbaum. 1979. LC 78-22205. (Aging & Old Age Ser.). reprint ed. lib. bdg. 39.95 (*0-405-11820-1*) Ayer.

Aging & Life-Prolonging Processes. V. V. Frolkis. 1983. (Illus.). 380p. 71.95 (*0-387-81685-2*) Spr-Verlag.

Aging & Lifelong Disabilities: Partnership for the Twenty First Century: Wingspread Report. Edward F. Ansello & Thomas Rose. 1989. (C). pap. 10.00 (*0-924840-00-5*) E Lewis Found.

Aging & Menopause Among Indian South African Women. Brian M. Du Toit. 1990. LC 89-26107. (SUNY Series in Medical Anthropology). (Illus.). 343p. (C). pap. text 24.95 (*0-7914-0390-4*) State U NY Pr.

Aging & Mental Disorders: Psychological Approaches to Assessment & Treatment. Steven H. Zarit. 1983. LC 79-6768. 454p. (C). pap. 21.00 (*0-02-935980-5*) Free Pr.

Aging & Mental Health. Michael A. Smyer & Sara H. Quails. 1998. LC 98-20919. (Understanding Aging Ser.). (Illus.). xxiv, 335p. pap. 38.95 (*1-55786-557-4*) Blackwell Pubs.

Aging & Mental Health: A Comprehensive Guide to Working with the Elderly. Joseph M. Casciani & Stanley M. Rest. 1988. LC 87-73536. 520p. (C). pap. text 94.95 (*0-9619913-0-5*) Alliance Pr.

Aging & Mental Health: Positive Psychosocial & Biomedical Approaches. Robert N. Butler et al. 5th ed. 1998. LC 97-30861. 530p. pap. 66.00 (*0-205-19336-6*) P-H.

Aging & Mental Retardation: Extending the Continuum. M. Seltzer & M. Krauss. 1987. LC 87-27406. (Monographs of the American Association on Mental Retardation: No. 9). 200p. (Orig.). (C). pap. 18.00 (*0-940898-18-7*) Am Assn Mental.

Aging & Musculoskeletal Disorders. Ed. by Horace M. Perry, III et al. 1993. LC 93-1426. 392p. 48.95 (*0-8261-7930-4*) Springer Pub.

Aging & Neuropsychological Assessment. Asenath La Rue. 1991. (Critical Issues in Neuropsychology Ser.). (Illus.). 361p. (C). text 54.00 (*0-306-44062-8*, Kluwer Plenum) Kluwer Academic.

Aging & Old Age. Richard A. Posner. 1997. (Illus.). 384p. pap. 16.95 (*0-226-67568-8*) U Ch Pr.

Aging & Old Age Series, Set. Ed. by Robert J. Kastenbaum. 1979. (Illus.). reprint ed. lib. bdg. 835.00 (*0-405-11800-7*) Ayer.

Aging & Osteoporosis in Native Americans from Pecos Pueblo, New Mexico: Behavioral & Biomechanical Effects. Christopher Ruff. 1991. LC 91-2397. (Evolution of North American Indians Ser.: Vol. 20). 435p. text 10.00 (*0-8240-2515-6*) Garland.

Aging & Our Families: Handbook for Family Caregivers. D. P. Couper. 1989. (Illus.). 120p. pap. 18.95 (*0-89885-441-5*, Kluwer Acad Hman Sci) Kluwer Academic.

Aging & Our Families: Leader's Guide to Caregiver Programs. D. P. Couper. 1989. (Illus.). 140p. pap. 20.95 (*0-89885-440-7*, Kluwer Acad Hman Sci) Kluwer Academic.

Aging & Personality: A Study of Eighty-Seven Older Men. Suzanne Reichard et al. Ed. by Leon Stein. 1980. LC 79-8680. (Growing Old Ser.). (Illus.). reprint ed. lib. bdg. 25.95 (*0-405-12797-9*) Ayer.

Aging & Posttraumatic Stress Disorder. Ed. by Paul E. Ruskin & John A. Talbot. 1996. 288p. text 39.50 (*0-88048-513-2*, 8513) Am Psychiatric.

Aging & Prevention: New Approaches for Preventing Health & Mental Health Problems in Older Adults. Ed. by Sharon Simson et al. 1983. LC 83-17172. (Prevention in Human Services Ser.: Vol. 3, No. 1). 150p. text 4.95 (*0-86656-188-9*) Haworth Pr.

Aging & Public Policy. Ed. by Neal Cutler. 1984. (Orig.). pap. 15.00 (*0-918592-76-3*) Pol Studies.

Aging & Quality of Life. Ed. by Ronald P. Abeles et al. 1994. LC 94-6081. (Life Styles & Issues in Aging Ser.). 392p. 49.95 (*0-8261-8430-8*) Springer Pub.

Aging & Skilled Performance: Advances in Theory & Applications. Ed. by Wendy A. Rogers et al. 1996. LC 96-17205. 272p. text 59.95 (*0-8058-1909-6*); 288p. pap. text 29.95 (*0-8058-1910-X*) L Erlbaum Assocs.

Aging & Society Vol. 1: An Inventory of Research Findings. Matilda W. Riley & Anne Foner. 1968. LC 68-54406. 636p. 55.00 (*0-87154-718-X*) Russell Sage.

Aging & Society, Vol. 2: Aging & the Professions. John W. Riley, Jr. & Marilyn E. Johnson. Ed. by Matilda W. Riley et al. 1969. LC 68-54406. 410p. 55.00 (*0-87154-719-8*) Russell Sage.

Aging & Society, Vol. 3: A Sociology of Age Stratification. Matilda W. Riley et al. 1972. LC 68-54406. 652p. 55.00 (*0-87154-720-1*) Russell Sage.

Aging & the Auditory System: Anatomy, Physiology & Psychophysics. James F. Willott. 1991. (Illus.). 295p. (C). pap. text 65.00 (*1-879105-11-X*, 0075) Thomson Learn.

Aging & the Care of Older People in Europe. Richard Hugman. 1994. LC 94-7205. 199p. text (*0-312-12193-8*) Macmillan GBR. *Dist:* Trans-Atl Phila, St Martin.

Aging & the Human Condition, Vol. II. Ed. by Gari Lesnoff-Caravaglia. 1982. LC 81-6630. (Frontiers in Aging Ser.). 160p. 32.95 (*0-89885-029-0*, Kluwer Acad Hman Sci) Kluwer Academic.

Aging & the Immune Function. Takashi Makinodan et al. 1974. 227p. text 31.50 (*0-8422-7228-3*) Irvington.

Aging & Working Capacity: Report of a WHO Study Group. Ed. by World Health Organization Staff. 1993. (Technical Reports: No. 835). (ENG, FRE & SPA.). vi, 49p. pap. text 10.00 (*92-4-120835-X*, 1100835) World Health.

Aging Artfully: Health Benefits of Art & Dance. 1994. lib. bdg. 250.00 (*0-8490-8543-8*) Gordon Pr.

Aging Body. S. Krauss Whitbourne. 1985. (Illus.). 305p. 119.00 (*0-387-96157-7*) Spr-Verlag.

Aging Cardiovascular System: Physiology & Pathaology. Vladimir V. Frolkis et al. 1996. (Illus.). 256p. 55.95 (*0-8261-9050-2*) Springer Pub.

Aging Dimension: Perspectives in Behavioral Medicine. Ed. by Matilda W. Riley et al. 1987. 208p. text 39.95 (*0-89859-927-X*) L Erlbaum Assocs.

Aging Eye. Harvard Medical School Staff. 2001. LC 2001-40894. (Illus.). 256p. pap. 13.00 (*0-7432-1503-6*, Fireside) S&S Trade Pap.

Aging Eye: A Guide for Nurses. Marla J. Kapperud. 1983. LC 83-62321. (Illus.). 55p. (Orig.). pap. 6.95 (*0-9612370-5-8*) Sight & Hearing.

Aging Eye & Low Vision: Independent Study Guide for Physicians. Ed. by Cynthia Stuen. 1992. (Illus.). 100p. pap. text (*0-9603444-8-9*) Lighthouse NYC.

Aging Face. M. Gonzalez-Ulloa. 1987. 514p. text (*1-57235-008-3*) Piccin Nuova.

Aging-Face Surgery with Emphasis on Face-Lift. Terence M. Davidson. 2nd ed. 1998. LC 98-21889. (Self-Instructional Package Ser.). (Illus.). 179p. (Orig.). reprint ed. pap. text 25.00 (*1-56772-066-8*, 5506510) AAO-HNS.

Aging Gametes-Their Biology & Pathology: Proceedings of the International Symposium on Aging Gametes, Seattle, June, 1973. International Symposium on Aging Gametes Staff. Ed. by R. J. Blandeau. 1975. (Illus.). xii, 415p. 104.50 (*3-8055-1842-0*) S Karger.

Aging, Health, & Competence: The Next Generation of Longitudinal Research. Ed. by Johannes J. Schroots. 1992. LC 92-49891. 432p. 245.25 (*0-444-89340-7*) Elsevier.

Aging, Health, & Healing. Ed. by Manfred Bergener et al. 1995. LC 94-23930. (Illus.). 648p. 79.00 (*0-8261-8620-3*) Springer Pub.

Aging, Health Behaviors, & Health Outcomes. Ed. by K. Warner Schaie et al. 1991. 208p. text 39.95 (*0-8058-0780-2*) L Erlbaum Assocs.

Aging, Immunity, & Infection. Ed. by Douglas C. Powers et al. 1994. LC 93-42177. 328p. 47.95 (*0-8261-8180-5*) Springer Pub.

Aging in America. Sandra Zins. 1987. (LPN/LVN Nursing Ser.). 368p. (gr. 12). pap., stu. ed. 15.95 (*0-8273-2827-3*) Delmar.

Aging in America: An Introduction to Gerontology. Sandra Zins. 1987. 368p. (C). (gr. 12). pap. 29.95 (*0-8273-2825-7*) Delmar.

Aging in Chinese Society: A Holistic Approach to the Experience of Aging in Taiwan & Singapore. Homer L. Jernigan & Margaret B. Jernigan. 1992. LC 92-13222. (Journal of Religious Gerontology: Vol. 8, No. 3). 130p. text 39.95 (*1-56024-273-6*) Haworth Pr.

Aging in Cold Blooded Animals, Vol. 2. A. Comfort et al. 1974. 236p. text 24.50 (*0-8422-7209-7*) Irvington.

Aging in East & Southeast Asia. Ed. by David R. Phillips. 1992. (Research Studies in Gerontology). 272p. (*0-340-54367-1*, A9633) E A GBR. *Dist:* Routldge.

Aging in Europe. Ed. by Johannes J. F. Schroots et al. 1997. LC 97-77021. (Biomedical & Health Research Ser.: Vol. 17). 184p. 92.00 (*90-5199-382-X*) IOS Press.

Aging in Good Health: A Complete Essential Medical Guide for Men & Women Over Fifty & Their Families. Mark Beers & Steven Urice. Ed. by Claire Zion. 1992. 368p. (Orig.). pap. 10.00 (*0-671-72822-9*) PB.

Aging in Good Health: Multidiscinplinary Perspectives. Sue Levkoff & Yeon Kyung Chee. 2000. LC 00-30091. (Illus.). xiii, 371p. (*0-8261-1366-4*) Springer Pub.

Aging in Liver & Gastrointestinal Tract. Ed. by L. Bianchi et al. 1988. (Falk Symposium Ser.). (C). text 209.50 (*0-7462-0066-8*) Kluwer Academic.

Aging in Place: Supporting the Frail Elderly in Residential Environments. American Association Homes for the Aging Staff. 1990. 352p. (C). 36.66 (*0-673-24945-X*) Addson-Wesley Educ.

Aging in the Designed Environment. Margaret A. Christenson. 1990. LC 90-4421. (Physical & Occupational Therapy in Geriatrics Ser.: Vol. 8, Nos. 3 & 4). 133p. text 39.95 (*1-56024-031-8*) Haworth Pr.

Aging in the Western Pacific: A Four-Country Study. G. R. Andrews et al. 1986. (Western Pacific Reports & Studies: No. 1). 165p. pap. text 25.00 (*92-9061-161-8*, 1530001) World Health.

Aging Lung: Normal Function. J. R. Edge et al. 1974. LC 73-1458. 22.00 (*0-8422-7165-1*) Irvington.

Aging Medicine: A Guide to Geriatric Problems. Kae Ferber. Ed. by Kae Ferber & Tom Cook. 1999. 40p. pap. 12.95 (0-9700076-0-4, 608-833-8855) TC Enter.

Aging Mind: Opportunities in Cognitive Research. Ed. by Paul C. Stern & Laura L. Carstensen. 2000. LC 00-8630. (Illus.). xii, 271p. pap. 35.00 (0-309-06940-8) Natl Acad Pr.

Aging Mouth. Ed. by D. B. Ferguson. 1987. (Frontiers of Oral Physiology Ser.: Vol. 6). (Illus.). viii, 176p. 103.50 (3-8055-4513-4) S Karger.

Aging, Neuropsychology & the New Dementias: Definitions, Explanations & Practical Approaches. Una P. Holden. 1995. 176p. pap. 42.99 (1-56593-423-7, 1090) Singular Publishing.

Aging of Cells, Humans & Societies. Ian K. Ross. 1994. LC 93-73882. 240p. (C). pap. 60.94 (0-697-20327-1) McGrw-H Hghr Educ.

Aging of Connective Tissues-Skin: Proceedings of the International Colloquium of Dermo-Chemistry on Aging of Skin, Paris. International Colloquium of Dermo-Chemistry on Aging Staff. Ed. by L. Robert & Barbara Robert. 1973. (Frontiers of Matrix Biology Ser.: Vol. 1). (Illus.). 250p. 85.25 (3-8055-1633-9) S Karger.

Aging of Reproductive Organs. Ed. by Y. Taketani & S. Kawagoe. 1993. (Journal: Vol. 39, Suppl. 1, 1993). (Illus.). vi, 38p. pap. 19.25 (3-8055-5797-3) S Karger.

Aging of the Autonomic Nervous System. Ed. by Francesco Amenta. 1993. 368p. lib. bdg. 225.00 (0-8493-6981-9, QP368) CRC Pr.

Aging of the Central Nervous System. Vladislav V. Bezrukov & V. V. Frokis. 1979. (Interdisciplinary Topics in Gerontology Ser.: Vol. 16). (Illus.). pap. 57.50 (3-8055-2995-3) S Karger.

Aging Parents. Sybervision Staff. 1996. text 102.00 (0-8151-8357-7, 30434) Mosby Inc.

Aging Pigment: Current Research, Vol. 1. B. S. Nanda et al. 1974. 191p. text 28.50 (0-8422-7197-X) Irvington.

Aging Pigment: Current Research, Vol. 2. William B. Weglicki et al. 1974. 268p. text 31.50 (0-8422-7198-8) Irvington.

Aging Population: Opposing Viewpoints. Ed. by Charles P. Cozic. 1996. LC 95-49646. (Opposing Viewpoints Ser.). 216p. lib. bdg. 26.20 (1-56510-395-5, Greenhaven Pr) Gale.

Aging Population in the Twenty-First Century: Statistics for Health Policy. National Research Council Staff. 1988. 340p. pap. text 27.95 (0-309-03881-2) Natl Acad Pr.

Aging Process: Implications for ACE Inhibition: Proceedings of a Symposium Held in Montreux, March 1987. Ed. by Hans R. Brunner. 1988. (Journal: Vol. 33, Suppl. 1). (Illus.). x, 56p. pap. 18.50 (3-8055-4729-3) S Karger.

Aging Sensory Systems & Perception. John F. Corso. 1981. LC 80-39579. 302p. 68.50 (0-275-90599-3, C0599, Praeger Pubs) Greenwood.

Aging Skin: Properties & Functional Changes. Jean-Luc Leveque & Pierre G. Agache. 1992. (Basic & Clinical Dermatology Ser.: Vol. 4). (Illus.). 320p. text 189.00 (0-8247-8791-9) Dekker.

Aging, Some Social & Biological Aspects: Proceedings of the American Association for the Advancement of Science, Symposia presented at the Chicago Meeting. American Association for the Advancement of Science Staff. Ed. by Nathan W. Shock. 1977. LC 73-167305. (Essay Index Reprint Ser.). reprint ed. 38.95 (0-8369-2735-4) Ayer.

Aging, Stress & Amino Acid Therapy. 1996. lib. bdg. 250.95 (0-8490-5897-X) Gordon Pr.

Aging, the Individual, & Society. Georgia M. Barrow & Guy Shuttlesworth. Ed. by LaMarre. 5th ed. 1993. 380p. (C). pap. text 47.25 (0-314-93332-8) West Pub.

Aging Two Thousand: Our Health Care Destiny, Vol. 2. Ed. by C. M. Gaitz et al. 1985. (Illus.). 395p. 88.00 (0-387-96070-8) Spr-Verlag.

Aging Well: A Selected, Annotated Bibliography, 31. Tanya F. Johnson & Jennifer C. Solomon. 1995. LC 95-20888. (Bibliographies & Indexes in Gerontology Ser.: No. 31). 168p. lib. bdg. 57.95 (0-313-28771-6, Greenwood Pr) Greenwood.

Aging Well: The Complete Guide to Physical & Emotional Health. Jeanne Wei & Sue Levkoff. 2000. LC 99-50257. (Illus.). 373p. 29.95 (0-471-32678-X) Wiley.

***Aging Well: The Complete Guide to Physical & Emotional Health.** Jeanne Wei & Sue Levkoff. 2001. 384p. pap. 17.95 (0-471-08206-6) Wiley.

Aging with a Disability. Roberta B. Trieschmann. 2nd ed. 1987. LC 86-72100. (Illus.). 158p. 29.95 (0-939957-01-9) Demos Medical.

Aging with Spinal Cord Injury. Gale G. Whiteneck et al. Ed. by Scott Manley. 1992. 374p. 99.95 (0-939957-48-5) Demos Medical.

Agnosia & Apraxia: Selected Papers of Liepman, Lange, & Potzl. Ed. by Jason W. Brown. 1988. (Institute for Research in Behavioral Neuroscience Ser.). 336p. 69.95 (0-8058-0286-X) L Erlbaum Assocs.

Agoraphobia: A Clinical & Personal Account. J. C. Clarke. 1985. (Illus.). 202p. text 39.00 (0-08-029866-4); pap. text 21.00 (0-08-029846-X) Elsevier.

Agoraphobia: Fear of Fear. Adele Paolino. 1985. 256p. pap. text 8.95 (0-9611448-1-5) Adele Roberts.

Agoraphobia: How I Overcame This Crippling Disease. Adele Paolino. 1983. 80p. pap. 5.95 (0-9611448-0-7) Adele Roberts.

Agrammatic Aphasia: A Cross-Language Narrative Sourcebook Ed. by Lise Menn & Loraine K. Obler. LC 89-18418. 1989. 759.00 (1-55619-024-7); 1. 1990. 2100p. (1-55619-025-5); 2. 1990. 2100p. (1-55619-026-3); 3. 1990. 2100p. (1-55619-027-1) J Benjamins Pubng Co.

Agrammatism. Ed. by Harry A. Whitaker. 1997. LC 97-1040. 386p. 65.00 (1-56593-744-9, 1446) Thomson Learn.

Agreement on the Temporary Importation, Free of Duty, of Medical, Surgical & Laboratory Equipment for Use on Free Loan in Hospitals & Other Medical Institutions for Purposes of Diagnosis or Treatment. Council of Europe Staff. 1976. (Conventions & Agreements Ser.: No. 33). (ENG & FRE.). (92-871-0086-1) Council of Europe FRA. *Dist:* Manhattan Pub Co.

Agricultural Uses of Antibiotics. Ed. by William A. Moats. 1986. LC 86-20614. (ACS Symposium Ser.: No. 320). (Illus.). ix, 200p. 43.95 (0-8412-0996-0) Am Chemical.

Agriculture & Health Sciences: Index of Modern Information. Lyton L. Springer. 1997. 175p. 57.50 (0-7883-1634-6); pap. 47.50 (0-7883-1635-4) ABBE Pubs Assn.

Agriculture, Food & Nutrition in Four South Pacific Archipelagos: New Caledonia, Vanuatu, French Polynesia, Wallis & Futuna. J. P. Doumenge et al. 1988. pap. 12.00 (979-8059-05-0) Intl Spec Bk.

Agrobacterium Protocols. Ed. by Kevan M. A. Gartland & Michael R. Davey. 1995. LC 95-15031. (Methods in Molecular Biology Ser.: Vol. 44). (Illus.). 432p. 109.50 (0-89603-302-3) Humana.

AHA Annual Survey of Hospitals Product Line. Date not set. (0-87258-718-5) AHPI.

AHA Clinical Cardiac Consult. Joseph S. Alpert & Gerard P. Aurigemma. 2001. LC 00-65518. (Illus.). xiii, 311p. text 59.95 (0-7817-2420-1) Lppncott W & W.

AHA Guide. Healthcare Infosource Staff. 1998. pap. 330.75 (0-87258-733-9) Am Hospital.

AHA Guide to Health Care Field, 1996. American Hospital Association Staff. 1996. pap. text 250.00 (0-87258-706-1) Am Hospital.

***AHA Guide to the Health Care Field.** 2000. (AHA Guide to the Health Care Ser.). pap. 383.75 (0-87258-757-6) AHPI.

AHA Guide to the Health Care Field. American Hospital Association Staff. 1997. (Orig.). pap. 275.00 (0-87258-717-7) AHPI.

AHA Hospital Stat: Emerging Trends in Hospitals: 1995-1996 Edition. American Hospital Association Staff. 1996. (Illus.). 178p. (Orig.). pap. 95.00 (0-87258-682-0) Am Hospital.

AHFS Drug Information, 1997. Ed. by Gerald K. McEvoy. 39th rev. ed. 1997. 2900p. pap. text 132.00 (1-879907-69-0) Am Soc Hlth-Syst.

AHFS Drug Information, 1998. Ed. by Gerald K. McEvoy. 40th rev. ed. 1998. 3000p. pap. text 139.00 (1-879907-76-3) Am Soc Hlth-Syst.

AHFS Drug Information, 1999. Ed. by Gerald K. McEvoy. 40th rev. ed. 1999. 3300p. pap. text 155.00 (1-879907-91-7) Am Soc Hlth-Syst.

AHFS Drug Information 2001. Ed. by Gerald K. McEvoy. 43rd rev. ed. 2001. LC 59-7620. 3800p. pap. text (1-58528-018-6) Am Soc Hlth-Syst.

AHNA Standards of Holistic Nursing Practice: Guidelines for Caring & Healing. Barbara Montgomery Dossey et al. 2000. LC 00-25297. 330p. pap. 49.00 (0-8342-1045-2, 10452) Aspen Pub.

AHPAT - Allied Health Professions Admissions Test: Comprehensive Manual for Self Study. David M. Tarlow. 2nd rev. ed. 1999. (Illus.). 150p. (C). pap. text 19.95 (1-57732-067-0) Datar Pub.

AHPAT - Allied Health Professions Admissions Test No. 1: Practice Exam Annotated Answers. Contrib. by David M. Tarlow. 2nd rev. ed. 1999. 20p. (C). pap. text 6.95 (1-57732-069-7) Datar Pub.

AHPAT - Allied Health Professions Admissions Test No. 1: Practice Examination. David M. Tarlow. 2nd rev. ed. 1999. 40p. (C). pap. text 18.95 (1-57732-068-9) Datar Pub.

AHPAT - Allied Health Professions Admissions Test No. 2: Practice Exam Annotated Answers. Contrib. by David M. Tarlow. 2nd rev. ed. 1999. 20p. (C). pap. text 6.95 (1-57732-071-9) Datar Pub.

AHPAT - Allied Health Professions Admissions Test No. 3: Practice Exam Annotated Answers. Contrib. by David M. Tarlow. 2nd rev. ed. 1999. 20p. (C). pap. text 6.95 (1-57732-073-5) Datar Pub.

AHPAT - Allied Health Professions Admissions Test No. 3: Practice Examination. David M. Tarlow. 2nd rev. ed. 1999. 40p. (C). pap. text 18.95 (1-57732-072-7) Datar Pub.

AHPAT - Allied Health Professions Admissions Test No. 4: Practice Exam Annotated Answers. Contrib. by David M. Tarlow. 2nd rev. ed. 1999. 20p. (C). pap. text 6.95 (1-57732-075-1) Datar Pub.

AHPAT - Allied Health Professions Admissions Test No. 4: Practice Examination. David M. Tarlow. 2nd rev. ed. 1999. (C). pap. text 18.95 (1-57732-074-3) Datar Pub.

AHPAT - Allied Health Professions Admissions Test No. 5: Practice Exam Annotated Answer. Contrib. by David M. Tarlow. 2nd rev. ed. 1999. 20p. (C). pap. text 6.95 (1-57732-077-8) Datar Pub.

AHPAT - Allied Health Professions Admissions Test No. 5: Practice Examination. David M. Tarlow. 2nd rev. ed. 1999. (C). pap. text 18.95 (1-57732-076-X) Datar Pub.

AHPAT - Allied Health Professions Admissions Test - Core Content. David M. Tarlow. 2nd rev. ed. 1999. (Illus.). 400p. pap. 49.95 (1-57774-010-6) Educ Tsting Cnslts.

AHPAT (Allied Health Professions Admissions Test) Comprehensive Review. David M. Tarlow. 7th ed. 1996. (Illus.). (Orig.). pap., stu. ed. 19.95 (1-57732-055-7) Datar Pub.

AHPAT Exam No. 1 Annotated Answers (Allied Health Professions Admissions Test) David M. Tarlow. 7th ed. 1996. (Orig.). pap. 5.95 (1-57732-061-1) Datar Pub.

AHPAT Exam No. 3 (Allied Health Professions Admissions Test) David M. Tarlow. 7th ed. 1996. (Illus.). (Orig.). pap. 19.95 (1-57732-058-1) Datar Pub.

AHPAT Exam No. 3 Annotated Answers (Allied Health Professions Admissions Test) David M. Tarlow. 7th ed. 1996. pap. 5.95 (1-57732-063-8) Datar Pub.

AHPAT Exam No. 4 (Allied Health Professions Admissions Test) David M. Tarlow. 7th ed. 1996. (Illus.). (Orig.). pap. 19.95 (1-57732-059-X) Datar Pub.

AHPAT Exam No. 4 Annotated Answers (Allied Health Professions Admissions Test) David M. Tarlow. 7th ed. 1996. pap. 5.95 (1-57732-064-6) Datar Pub.

AHPAT Exam No. 5 (Allied Health Professions Admissions Test) David M. Tarlow. 7th ed. 1996. (Illus.). (Orig.). pap. 19.95 (1-57732-060-3) Datar Pub.

AHPAT Exam No. 5 Annotated Answers (Allied Health Professions Admissions Test) David M. Tarlow. 7th ed. 1996. pap. 5.95 (1-57732-065-4) Datar Pub.

AHPAT Exam No. 1 (Allied Health Professions Admissions Test) David M. Tarlow. 7th ed. 1996. (Illus.). (Orig.). pap. (1-57732-056-5) Datar Pub.

AHPAT Exam No. 2 (Allied Health Professions Admissions Test) David M. Tarlow. 7th ed. 1996. (Illus.). (Orig.). pap. (1-57732-057-3) Datar Pub.

AHPAT Exam No. 2 Annotated Answers (Allied Health Professions Admissions Test) David M. Tarlow. 7th ed. 1996. pap. (1-57732-062-X) Datar Pub.

Aid to Pediatric Surgery. Ed. by Robert A. MacMahon. 2nd ed. 1991. (Illus.). 272p. (Orig.). pap. text (0-443-04185-7) Church.

Aid to Radiology for the MRCP. K. K. Ray et al. 2000. LC 98-51790. (At a Glance Ser.). (Illus.). xi, 348p. pap. 49.95 (0-632-04912-X) Blackwell Sci.

***Aid to the Clinical MRCS/AFRCS.** Wong. 2001. (Illus.). 195p. pap. (0-7020-2574-7) W B Saunders GBR. *Dist:* Saunders.

Aid to the MRCP Short Cases. R. E. J. Ryder et al. 2nd ed. 1999. LC 98-42252. (Illus.). 400p. pap. 52.95 (0-632-03067-4) Blackwell Sci.

Aid to the MRCP VIVA. Afzal Mir et al. 1992. (Illus.). 332p. (Orig.). pap. text (0-443-04659-X) Church.

***Aid to the MRCP Viva.** Afzal Mir et al. 2001. 359p. pap. (0-443-06467-9) Church GBR. *Dist:* Saunders.

***Aid to the MRCPCH Viva.** Alan Cade et al. 2nd ed. 2001. LC 2001-32588. (Illus.). 245p. pap. (0-443-06494-6) Church GBR. *Dist:* Saunders.

Aid to the Pediatric MRCP. Alan Cade et al. 1995. pap. text 24.00 (0-443-05246-8) Saunders.

***Aide Tested Techniques to Improve Long-Term Resident Care.** Anthony Antoville, Jr. 2001. LC 2001-30170. (Studies in Health & Human Services: Vol. 42). (Illus.). 96p. 49.95 (0-7734-7443-9) E Mellen.

Aiding & Aging: The Coming Crisis in Support for the Elderly by Kin & State, 17. Ed. by John H. Mogey. 1990. LC 89-25670. (Contributions to the Study of Aging Ser.: No. 17). 304p. 72.50 (0-313-27315-4, MOD/, Greenwood Pr) Greenwood.

Aiding Older Adults with Memory Complaints. Forrest Scogin & Mark Prohaska. 1993. LC 93-13672. (Practitioner's Resource Ser.). 66p. pap. 15.95 (0-943158-92-3, AOABP, Prof Resc Pr) Pro Resource.

AIDS. Ed. by Gerald L. Mandell & Donna Mildvan. 2nd ed. 1997. LC 96-38725. (Atlas of Infectious Diseases Ser.: Vol. 1). (Illus.). 336p. text (0-443-07946-3) Church GBR. *Dist:* Saunders.

AIDS: A Basic Guide for Clinicians. Peter Ebbesen et al. 1985. (Illus.). 313p. text 97.00 (0-7216-1584-8) Saunders.

AIDS: A Catholic Educational Approach to HIV. Ed. by Carleen Reck. rev. ed. 1992. (Illus.). 176p. pap. 5.00 (1-55833-112-3); pap., tchr. ed. 16.00 (1-55833-111-5) Natl Cath Educ.

AIDS: A Cause for Concern. Patrick J. McLaughlin. (Orig.). pap. text (0-938279-01-7) W P Smedley.

AIDS: A Christian Response. Howard E. Mueller. 1996. LC 96-173150. (Master's Touch Bible Study Ser.). 58p. pap. 4.50 (0-570-09552-2, 20-2593) Concordia.

AIDS: A Communications Perspective. Ed. by Timothy Edgar et al. 1992. (Communication Ser.). 248p. text 49.95 (0-8058-0998-8) L Erlbaum Assocs.

AIDS: A Complete Guide to Psychosocial Intervention. Ed. by Helen Land. 1992. LC 92-18565. 318p. pap. 25.95 (0-87304-258-1) Manticore Pubs.

AIDS: A Multimedia Sourcebook. John J. Miletich. 1993. LC 92-39121. 232p. pap. 21.95 (0-89789-362-X, Greenwood Pr) Greenwood.

AIDS: A Multimedia Sourcebook, 10. Compiled by John J. Miletich. 1993. LC 93-10830. (Bibliographies & Indexes in Medical Studies: No. 10). 288p. lib. bdg. 68.50 (0-313-28669-8) Greenwood.

AIDS: A Nutritional Approach. Louise Tenney. 1987. (Today's Health Ser.: No. 6). 30p. pap. 3.95 (0-913923-62-1) Woodland UT.

AIDS: A Pocket Book of Diagnosis & Management. Ed. by Adrian Mindel & Robert Miller. 2nd ed. 1996. (Illus.). 384p. pap. text (0-340-58609-5) E A GBR. *Dist:* OUP.

AIDS: A Problem for Sociological Research. Michael Pollak. Ed. by Genevieve Paicheler & Janine Pierret. 1993. (Special Issue of Current Sociology Ser.). (Illus.). 144p. (C). 69.95 (0-8039-8841-9, 9225) Sage.

AIDS: A Problem for Sociological Research. Michael Pollak. Ed. by Genevieve Paicheler et al. 1992. (Special Issue of Current Sociology Ser.). (Illus.). 144p. (C). pap. 22.95 (0-8039-8840-0, 9226) Sage.

AIDS: A Second Opinion. Gary Null. 2001. LC 00-51013. 400p. 34.95 (1-58322-062-3) Seven Stories.

AIDS: A Special Issue of the "New England Journal of Public Policy" Ed. by Padraig O'Malley. 1988. 526p. pap. 21.95 (0-87023-657-1) U of Mass Pr.

AIDS: A Study. Loretta H. Kurban. 1991. pap. 8.00 (0-938863-23-1) HCI Pr.

AIDS: Abstracts of the Psychological & Behavioral Literature, 1983-1991. Ed. by John R. Anderson et al. 3rd ed. 1991. LC 91-22115. (Bibliographies in Psychology Ser.: No. 1). 301p. pap. 19.95 (1-55798-148-5) Am Psychol.

AIDS: An African Perspective. A. Olufemi Williams. 1991. 384p. 189.00 (0-8493-6437-X, RA644) CRC Pr.

AIDS: Blunt Talk on How to Avoid It. Randolph Norman. 1985. 32p. pap. 5.95 (0-86668-057-8) ARCsoft.

AIDS: CDC's Investigation of HIV Transmissions by a Dentist. 1993. (Illus.). 50p. (Orig.). (C). pap. text 40.00 (1-56806-908-1) DIANE Pub.

AIDS: Crisis in Professional Ethics. Ed. by Elliot D. Cohen & Michael Davis. 1994. 320p. (C). pap. 22.95 (1-56639-165-2); text 69.95 (1-56639-164-4) Temple U Pr.

AIDS: Cultural Analysis, Cultural Activism. Ed. by Douglas Crimp. 1988. (October Bks.). 275p. pap. text 18.95 (0-262-53079-1) MIT Pr.

AIDS: Diagnostic, Monitoring & Therapeutic Markets: Technology Assessment & Financial Impact. Market Intelligence Staff. 1993. LC 97-197205. 211p. 2495.00 (1-56753-519-4) Frost & Sullivan.

AIDS: Effective Health Communicaton for the 90's. Ed. by Scott C. Ratzan. 1992. LC 92-17933. 44.95 (1-56032-273-X) Hemisp Pub.

AIDS: Ending an Epidemic. Jim Parker. rev. ed. 2000. pap. 0.50 (0-89230-166-X) Do It Now.

AIDS: Etiology, Diagnosis, Treatment & Prevention. Ed. by Vincent T. DeVita, Jr. et al. 4th ed. 1996. LC 96-17611. 770p. text 120.00 (0-397-51538-3) Lppncott W & W.

AIDS: Facts & Issues for Health Professionals. Walton. (Allied Health Ser.). 1991. pap., tchr. ed. 8.00 (0-8273-4554-2); 1990. pap. 24.95 (0-8273-4553-4) Delmar.

AIDS: Foundations for the Future. Ed. by Peter Aggleton et al. 1994. LC 94-14183. (Social Aspects of AIDS Ser.). 240p. pap. 34.95 (0-7484-0228-4) Taylor & Francis.

AIDS: Images of the Epidemic. WHO Staff. 1994. LC 95-169804. (ARA, CHI, ENG, FRE & RUS., Illus.). x, 142p. pap. text 32.00 (92-4-156163-7, 1150406) World Health.

AIDS: Impact on Public Policy: An International Forum - Policy, Politics & AIDS. Ed. by Robert F. Hummel et al. 1987. LC 86-30516. (Illus.). 180p. (C). text 90.00 (0-306-42540-8, Kluwer Plenum) Kluwer Academic.

AIDS: Impact on Schools. Roberta Weiner. 1986. LC 86-81456. 274p. (Orig.). 45.50 (0-937925-02-0, AIDS) Capitol VA.

AIDS: Individual, Cultural & Policy Dimensions. Ed. by Peter Aggleton et al. 1990. 262p. pap. 39.95 (1-85000-764-0, Falmer Pr) Taylor & Francis.

AIDS: Insights & Strategies. 12.00 (0-8074-0742-9) UAHC.

AIDS: Intervening with Hidden Grievers. Barbara O. Dane & Samuel O. Miller. 1992. LC 92-10959. 240p. 57.50 (0-86569-028-6, T028, Auburn Hse) Greenwood.

AIDS: Meeting the Community Challenge. Ed. by Vicky Cosstick. 1989. 190p. pap. (0-86217-288-8) Veritas Pubns IRL. *Dist:* St Mut.

AIDS: Myths, Facts & Ethics. Elizabeth Prior-Jonson. 1989. 165p. pap. text 17.00 (0-08-034434-8, Pergamon Pr) Elsevier.

AIDS: No Nonsense Answers to a Company. Sizerwhitney. 1996. VHS 56.95 (0-314-09824-0) Wadsworth Pub.

AIDS: One Thousand Full-Text Statistical Abstracts from the "A Matter of Fact" Database, 1984-1992. Ed. by C. Edward Wall et al. 1993. (Statistical Perspectives Ser.). 112p. pap. 15.00 (0-87650-329-6) Pierian.

AIDS: Origins, Prevention & Cure 1987. (AIDS Ser.). lib. bdg. 800.00 (0-8490-3958-4) Gordon Pr.

AIDS: Papers from Science, 1982-1985. Ed. by Ruth Kulstad. 1986. LC 85-28776. 654p. 51.00 (0-87168-313-X, 85-23S) AAAS.

A
B

AIDS: Pathogenesis & Treatment. Levy. 1988. (Immunology Ser.: Vol. 44). (Illus.). 720p. text 165.00 (*0-8247-7684-4*) Dekker.

AIDS: Prevention & Treatment. Peterson & David Seligson. 1991. pap. 29.95 (*1-56032-093-1*) Hemisp Pub.

AIDS: Prevention Through Education, a World View. Ed. by Jaime Sepulveda et al. 1993. LC 92-49655. 384p. (C). 29.95 (*0-19-506882-3*) OUP.

AIDS: Principles, Practices & Politics. Ed. by Inge B. Corless & Mary Pittman-Lindeman. abr. ed. 1987. (Death Education, Aging & Health Care Ser.). 400p. 63.95 (*0-89116-795-1*, 66-57001); pap. 29.95 (*0-89116-772-2*, 66-56813) Hemisp Pub.

AIDS: Profile of an Epidemic. 1989. (PAHO Scientific Publication Ser.: No. 514). 382p. text 60.00 (*92-75-11514-1*) World Health.

AIDS: Public Health & Legal Dimensions. D. C. Jayasuriya. 1988. (C). lib. bdg. 81.00 (*90-247-3686-2*) Kluwer Academic.

AIDS: Rage & Reality: Why Silence Is Deadly. Gene Antonio. 1992. 336p. (Orig.). pap. 19.95 (*0-9634774-3-9*) Anchor Bks.

AIDS: Readings on a Global Crisis. Elizabeth R. Bethel. 1994. (Illus.). 448p. pap. 38.00 (*0-02-309192-4*, Macmillan Coll) P-H.

AIDS: Responses, Interventions & Care. Ed. by Peter Aggleton et al. 1991. (Social Aspects of AIDS Ser.). 256p. 69.95 (*1-85000-871-X*); pap. 39.95 (*1-85000-872-8*) Taylor & Francis (Falmer Pr).

AIDS: Rights, Risk & Reason. Peter Aggleton et al. Ed. by Peter M. Davies & Graham Hart. 1992. LC 92-112687. (Social Aspects of AIDS Ser.). 224p. pap. 34.95 (*0-7507-0040-8*, Falmer Pr) Taylor & Francis.

AIDS: Safety, Sexuality & Risk. Ed. by Peter Aggleton et al. 1995. (Social Aspects of AIDS Ser.). 240p. (*0-7484-0291-8*); pap. (*0-7484-0292-6*) Tay Francis Ltd GBR. *Dist:* Taylor & Francis.

AIDS: Science & Society. Hung Fan et al. 1995. LC 95-9108. (Health Science Ser.). (Illus.). 264p. (C). pap. text 33.75 (*0-86720-913-5*, 913-5) Jones & Bartlett.

AIDS: Science & Society. Hung Fan et al. 2nd ed. 1997. LC 97-38992. (Health Science Ser.). (Illus.). 288p. pap. text 30.95 (*0-7637-0415-6*, 0415-6) Jones & Bartlett.

AIDS: Science & Society. Ed. by Hung Fan et al. 3rd ed. 2000. LC 99-59504. (AIDS Ser.). (Illus.). 320p. (C). pap. text 32.95 (*0-7637-1117-9*, 1117-9) Jones & Bartlett.

AIDS: Scientific & Social Issues. Peter Aggleton et al. 1989. (Illus.). 132p. pap. text (*0-443-04182-2*) Church.

AIDS: Setting a Feminist Agenda. Ed. by Lesley Doyal et al. 1994. LC 94-4132. (Gender & Society Ser.). (*0-7484-0162-8*) Tay Francis Ltd GBR. *Dist:* Taylor & Francis.

AIDS: Setting a Feminist Agenda. Ed. by Lesley Doyal et al. 1994. LC 94-4132. (Gender & Society Ser.). pap. 29.95 (*0-7484-0163-6*) Taylor & Francis.

AIDS: Silent Killer. Don Boys. 1991. pap. 10.00 (*1-879805-00-6*) Freedom FL.

AIDS: The American Roads of Denial. Richard Carper. Ed. by Joella Ewing. 1990. (Illus.). 200p. (Orig.). pap. 11.50 (*0-930693-05-1*) Cross-Cultrl NY.

AIDS: The Biological Basis. I. Edward Alcamo. 304p. (C). 1992. text 38.50 net. (*0-697-12061-9*); 2nd ed. 1996. LC 96-83692. text 69.38 (*0-697-15882-9*) McGrw-H Hghr Educ (WCB McGr Hill).

AIDS: The Burdens of History. Ed. by Elizabeth Fee & Daniel M. Fox. 340p. 1992. pap. text 17.95 (*0-520-06396-1*); 1988. text 55.00 (*0-520-06395-3*) U CA Pr.

AIDS: The Challenge: Understanding, Education, & Care. Neil Small. 1993. LC 93-24408. 192p. (*1-85628-455-7*) Avebry GBR. *Dist:* Ashgate Pub Co.

AIDS: The Epidemic of Kaposi's Sarcoma & Opportunistic Infections. Ed. by Alvin E. Friedman-Kien & Linda J. Laubenstein. 1984. LC 83-25578. (Illus.). 371p. (C). text 68.00 (*0-89352-217-1*) Mosby Inc.

AIDS: The Facts. John J. Langone. 1988. 192p. pap. 8.95 (*0-316-51412-8*, Little Brwn Med Div) Lppncott W & W.

AIDS: The Good News is HIV Doesn't Cause It. Peter Duesberg & John Yiamonylannis. 1995. (Illus.). 200p. (Orig.). pap. 15.00 (*0-913571-05-9*) Health Act Pr.

AIDS: The Making of a Chronic Disease. Ed. by Elizabeth Fee & Daniel M. Fox. 1992. LC 91-731. (Illus.). 417p. text 55.00 (*0-520-07569-2*); pap. text 17.95 (*0-520-07778-4*) U CA Pr.

AIDS: The Mystery & the Solution. Alan Cantwell. 1987. (AIDS Ser.). lib. bdg. 250.00 (*0-8490-3924-X*) Gordon Pr.

AIDS: The Mystery & the Solution. Alan Cantwell, Jr. Ed. by Jim Highland. rev. ed. 1984. LC 86-1210. (Illus.). 210p. pap. 9.95 (*0-917211-16-2*) Aries Rising.

AIDS: The Pathology of the Nervous System. Ed. by Francesco Scaravilli. 1993. LC 92-2222. (*3-540-19739-7*); (Illus.). 271p. 319.00 (*0-387-19739-7*) Spr-Verlag.

AIDS: The Politics of Survival. Ed. by Nancy Krieger & Glen Margo. 1994. LC 94-372. (Policy, Politics, Health & Medicine Ser.). 296p. pap. text 28.50 (*0-89503-123-X*) Baywood Pub.

AIDS: The Second Decade. Ed. by Peter Aggleton et al. 1993. LC 93-16013. (Social Aspects of AIDS Ser.). 85.00 (*0-7507-0131-5*, Falmer Pr) Taylor & Francis.

AIDS: The Second Decade. Ed. by Heather G. Miller et al. 1990. 512p. pap. 39.95 (*0-309-04287-9*) Natl Acad Pr.

AIDS: The Ultimate Challenge. Elisabeth Kubler-Ross. 1997. 352p. pap. 12.00 (*0-684-83940-7*, Touchstone) S&S Trade Pap.

AIDS: Toward Long-Term Treatment Options: Hearing Before the Subcommittee on Human Resources of the Committee on Government Reform & Oversight, House of Representatives, 105th Congress, 2nd Session, February 20, 1998. USGPO Staff. 1998. LC 98-211357. iii, 144p. pap. (*0-16-057195-2*) USGPO.

AIDS: Virus or Drug Induced? Ed. by Peter H. Duesberg. 1996. (Contemporary Issues in Genetics & Evolution Ser.). 365p. (C). pap. text 55.50 (*0-7923-3961-4*); LC 95-17475. lib. bdg. 227.50 (*0-7923-3552-X*) Kluwer Academic.

AIDS: What Every Student Needs to Know. Spencer A. Rathus & Susan Boughn. 2nd ed. 1994. LC 93-80577. 106p. (C). pap. text 25.00 (*0-15-501700-4*) Harcourt.

AIDS: What the Government Isn't Telling You. Lorraine Day. 1991. LC 91-75346. (Illus.). 301p. pap., per. 22.95 (*0-9630940-0-9*) Rockford Pr.

AIDS: Women, Drugs & Social Care. Ed. by Nicholas Dorn et al. 1992. LC 90-20419. (Social Aspects of AIDS Ser.: Vol. 1). 224p. pap. 29.95 (*1-85000-874-4*, Falmer Pr) Taylor & Francis.

AIDS - Accepted in My Imperfection, Delivered from My Sin & Shame. Johnie Grainger. Ed. by Valerie M. Bailey. 1996. 125p. (Orig.). pap. 6.95 (*0-945641-07-9*) Castle Hills.

AIDS - From Fear to Hope: Channeled Teachings Offering Insight & Inspiration. Ed. by Spirit Speaks Staff. 1987. LC 87-61682. 275p. (Orig.). pap. 9.95 (*0-934619-02-6*) New Age FL Pub.

AIDS - The End of Civilization: The Greatest Biological Disaster in the History of Mankind. William C. Douglass. 1992. 256p. reprint ed. pap. text 9.95 (*1-881316-00-9*) A&B Bks.

AIDS - Today, Tomorrow: An Introduction to the HIV Epidemic in America. Robert S. Walker. 2nd rev. ed. 1994. LC 94-17975. 240p. (C). pap. 14.95 (*0-391-03859-1*) Brill Academic Pubs.

AIDS - Zmowa Milczenia. Gene Antonio. Tr. by Jacek Szacki from ENG. 1992. (POL.). 190p. (Orig.). pap. text 8.50 (*0-9632313-1-6*) Global Comm Netwk.

AIDS, 1981-1983: An Annotated Bibliography. Rhoda Garoogian. 1984. LC 84-1736. (CompuBibs Ser.: No. 2). 92p. pap. 15.00 (*0-914791-05-2*) Vantage Info.

AIDS, a Moral Issue: The Ethical, Legal, & Social Aspects. Ed. by Brenda Almond. 2nd ed. 1997. LC 96-10822. 224p. pap. 17.95 (*0-312-16153-0*) St Martin.

AIDS-Acquired Immune Deficiency Syndrome. 1985. 31.95 (*0-387-81902-9*) Spr-Verlag.

AIDS, Africa, & Racism. Richard Chirimuta & Rosalind Chirimuta. 1989. 192p. pap. 16.00 (*1-85343-077-3*) Col U Pr.

AIDS Agenda: Emerging Issues in Civil Rights. Nan D. Hunter. 1992. LC 91-66863. 610p. text 27.95 (*1-56584-001-1*) New Press NY.

AIDS Allergy & Rheumatology. Ed. by Nancy E. Lane. 1997. LC 97-138074. (Allergy & Immunology Ser.: Vol. 3). (Illus.). 112p. 89.50 (*0-89603-502-6*) Humana.

AIDS & Accusation: Haiti & the Geography of Blame. Paul Farmer. (Comparative Studies of Health Systems & Medical Care). 338p. 1997. (C). pap. text 17.95 (*0-520-08343-1*); 1994. LC 91-48206. text 50.00 (*0-520-07701-6*) U CA Pr.

AIDS & Adolescents. Linda Thayer. 90p. pap. 2.00 (*0-8198-0744-3*) Pauline Bks.

AIDS & African Americans. Pamela Blackwell-Johnson. 2000. LC 00-91405. 217p. pap. 24.95 (*0-9679718-0-2*, 0011) N C D Pubg.

AIDS & AIDS-Risk Patient Care. Hans Jager. 1988. 224p. 51.95 (*0-470-21101-6*) P-H.

AIDS & Alcohol-Drug Abuse: Psychosocial Research. Ed. by Dennis G. Fisher. 1991. LC 90-5311. (Drugs & Society Ser.). (Illus.). 109p. text 39.95 (*1-56024-041-5*); pap. text 9.95 (*0-918393-85-X*) Haworth Pr.

AIDS & Associated Cancers in Africa. Ed. by G. Giraldo et al. 1988. (Illus.). x, 346p. 259.25 (*3-8055-4701-3*) S Karger.

AIDS & Biological Warfare. 1991. (Nikola Tesla Ser.). lib. bdg. 250.00 (*0-8490-4328-X*) Gordon Pr.

AIDS & Chemical Dependency. 1991. lib. bdg. 250.00 (*0-8490-4367-0*) Gordon Pr.

AIDS & Chinese Medicine. Qingkai Zhang. 1993. pap. 19.95 (*0-941942-31-7*) Orient Heal Arts.

AIDS & Community-Based Drug Intervention Programs: Evaluation & Outreach. Ed. by Dennis G. Fisher. 1993. LC 93-23471. (Drugs & Society Ser.). (Illus.). 233p. pap. text 19.95 (*1-56023-050-9*, Harrington Park); lib. bdg. 39.95 (*1-56024-510-7*) Haworth Pr.

AIDS & Complinary & Alternatives. Standish. 2000. 360p. (C). text (*0-443-05831-8*) Church.

AIDS & Development in Africa: A Social Science Perspective. Ed. by Kempe R. Hope. 1999. LC 98-41560. 232p. lib. bdg. 39.95 (*0-7890-0638-3*, RA664.A25A3435) Haworth Pr.

AIDS & Ethics. Ed. by James M. Humber & Robert F. Almeder. 1989. LC 84-640015. (Biomedical Ethics Reviews Ser.: No. 1988). 180p. 49.50 (*0-89603-153-5*) Humana.

AIDS & Ethics. Frederic G. Reamer. 1993. LC 91-21477. 317p. pap. 21.00 (*0-231-07359-3*) Col U Pr.

AIDS & Ethics. Ed. by Frederic G. Reamer. 1991. 384p. text 50.00 (*0-231-07358-5*) Col U Pr.

AIDS & Families. Eleanor Macklin. 1994. LC 89-32929. pap. 19.95 (*0-918393-60-4*, Harrington Park) Haworth Pr.

AIDS & Health Care: Is Reform HIV-Positive? Neal A. Dickerson. 1995. LC 95-25564. (Politics of AIDS Ser.: Vol. 7). xii,65p. pap. 5.00 (*0-930383-45-1*) Monument Pr.

AIDS & Health Insurance. 1991. lib. bdg. 159.95 (*0-8490-4980-6*) Gordon Pr.

***AIDS & HIV: The Nursing Response.** Jean Faugier. 1995. pap. 34.95 (*0-412-56090-9*) Chapman & Hall.

AIDS & HIV: The Nursing Response. Jean Faugier & I. Hicken. 1995. 256p. pap. 34.95 (*1-56593-585-3*, 1192) Singular Publishing.

AIDS & HIV Essentials. Cynthia G. Carmichael. 1999. LC 00-500439. (Illus.). 83p. pap. text 22.00 (*1-879772-13-2*) Health Studies.

***AIDS & HIV Essentials.** Cynthia G. Carmichael. 2nd rev. ed. 2001. (Illus.). 86p. pap. text 22.00 (*1-879772-16-7*) Health Studies.

AIDS & HIV in Perspective: A Guide to Understanding the Virus & Its Consequences. Barry D. Schoub. (Illus.). (C). 1994. LC 93-21269. 288p. text 74.95 (*0-521-45231-7*); 1994. LC 93-21269. 288p. pap. text 27.95 (*0-521-45874-9*); 2nd ed. 1999. LC 98-11707. 296p. text 85.00 (*0-521-62150-X*); 2nd ed. 1999. LC 98-11707. 296p. pap. text 29.95 (*0-521-62766-4*) Cambridge U Pr.

AIDS & HIV Infection - The Wider Perspective. Ed. by A. J. Pinching et al. 1988. (Illus.). 234p. text (*0-443-03978-X*) Church.

***AIDS & HIV Long Term Survivors - Analysis & Results: Information & Guide-Book for Consumers, Reference & Research.** Silvester V. Polanta. 2002. 180p. 57.50 (*0-7883-2444-6*); pap. text 47.50 (*0-7883-2445-4*) ABBE Pubs Assn.

AIDS & HIV Programs & Services for Libraries. W. Bernard Lukenbill. 1994. xvi, 262p. lib. bdg. 32.00 (*1-56308-175-X*) Libs Unl.

AIDS & HIV-Related Diseases: An Educational Guide for Professionals & the Public. Josh Powell. 1996. (Illus.). 243p. (C). 24.95 (*0-306-45085-2*) Plenum.

AIDS & Ignorance: Selected Essays. 1992. lib. bdg. 250.00 (*0-8490-8797-X*) Gordon Pr.

AIDS & Intravenous Drug Use. 1990. lib. bdg. 250.00 (*0-8490-4040-X*) Gordon Pr.

AIDS & Intravenous Drug Use: Community Intervention & Prevention. C. G. Leukefeld et al. 1990. 300p. 42.95 (*1-56032-141-5*) Hemisp Pub.

AIDS & Intravenous Drug Use: Future Directions for Community-Based Prevention Research. 1991. lib. bdg. 300.00 (*0-8490-4348-4*) Gordon Pr.

AIDS & Intravenous Drug Use: The Influence of Morality, Politics, Social Science, & Race in the Making of a Tragedy. M. Daniel Fernando. 1993. LC 92-46557. 184p. 47.95 (*0-275-94245-7*, C4245, Praeger Pubs) Greenwood.

AIDS & Its Early, Late & Final Symptoms for Death: Index of New Information. Wallace W. Dakins. 1997. 160p. 57.50 (*0-7883-1658-3*); pap. 47.50 (*0-7883-1659-1*) ABBE Pubs Assn.

AIDS & Its Psychological Influences on the Public & Patients: Index of New Information. Alber G. Horner. 1998. 160p. 57.50 (*0-7883-1872-1*); pap. 47.50 (*0-7883-1873-X*) ABBE Pubs Assn.

AIDS & Malignancies: Current Concepts & Prospectives. Basil C. Golematis & Vincent T. Devita. 1996. LC 96-2979. 348p. 170.95 (*0-471-96714-9*) Wiley.

AIDS & Men: Taking Risks or Taking Responsibility? Martin Foreman. 1999. LC 00-302856. xii, 238p. (*1-85649-744-5*) Zed Books GBR. *Dist:* St Martin.

AIDS & Mental Health Practice: Clinical & Policy Issues. Michael Shernoff. 2000. LC 98-39347. 382p. pap. 24.95 (*0-7890-0624-3*, Harrington Park) Haworth Pr.

AIDS & Mental Health Practice: Clinical & Policy Issues. Ed. by Michael Shernoff. 1998. LC 98-39347. (Illus.). 392p. lib. bdg. 34.95 (*0-7890-0464-X*) Haworth Pr.

AIDS & Neurology. Michael J. Harrison. 1995. LC 94-14559. text (*0-443-04896-7*) Church.

AIDS & Other Manifestations of HIV Infection. Ed. by Gary P. Wormser. 3rd ed. 1997. LC 97-13738. (Illus.). 864p. text 180.00 (*0-397-58760-0*) Lppncott W & W.

AIDS & Other Sexually Transmitted Disease. Richmond. 1993. text 65.00 (*0-7295-0351-8*) Saunders.

***AIDS & Other STDs.** 2001. (YA). (gr. 6-12). pap. text 9.50 (*0-8359-0766-X*) Globe Fearon.

AIDS & People with Severe Mental Illness: A Handbook for Mental Health Professionals. Ed. by Francine Cournos & Nicholas Bakalar. 1996. LC 96-10948. 384p. 50.00 (*0-300-06757-7*) Yale U Pr.

AIDS & Persons with Developmental Disabilities: The Legal Perspective. 1990. 113p. pap. 10.00 (*0-89707-540-4*, 549-0207) Amer Bar Assn.

AIDS & Reproduction. Ed. by F. Melica. 1992. (Illus.). xii, 196p. 147.00 (*3-8055-5481-8*) S Karger.

AIDS & Respiratory Medicine. A. Zumla et al. 1996. (Illus.). 448p. (*0-412-60140-0*) E A GBR. *Dist:* OUP.

AIDS & Substance Abuse. Ed. by Larry Siegel. 1988. (Advances in Alcohol & Substance Abuse Ser.: Vol. 7, No. 2). (Illus.). 206p. LC 88-2733. text 49.95 (*0-86656-819-0*); LC 88-948. text 14.95 (*0-918393-59-0*, Harrington Park) Haworth Pr.

AIDS & Syphilis: The Hidden Link. Harris L. Coulter. 1987. LC 87-21961. (Orig.). 132p. 20.00 (*1-55643-025-6*); 80p. pap. 8.95 (*1-55643-021-3*) North Atlantic.

AIDS & the Body Politic: Biomedicine & Sexual Difference. Catherine Waldby. 1996. (Writing Corporealities Ser.). 192p. (C). LC 98-138830. pap. 22.95 (*0-415-14130-3*); (Illus.). 80.00 (*0-415-14129-X*) Routledge.

AIDS & the Construction of Meaning: Research=Care. Jean F. McGuire. 1998. (Health Care Policy in the United States Ser.). 250p. 60.00 (*0-8153-3130-4*) Garland.

AIDS & the Courts. Ed. by Clark C. Abt & Kathleen M. Hardy. 1990. (Illus.). 400p. 40.00 (*0-89011-615-6*); pap. 30.00 (*0-89011-616-4*); text 40.00 (*0-89011-640-7*) Abt Bks.

AIDS & the Demography of Africa. LC 94-198306. (Population Studies: No. 137). 72p. pap. 17.50 (*92-1-151268-9*, E.94.XIII.11) UN.

AIDS & the Doctors of Death: An Inquiry into the Origin of the AIDS Epidemic. Alan Cantwell, Jr. Ed. by Suzanne Henig & Jon Rappaport. 1988. LC 87-37355. 239p. reprint ed. pap. 14.95 (*0-917211-25-1*) Aries Rising.

AIDS & the Education of Our Children: A Guide for Parents & Teachers. 1993. (Illus.). 28p. (Orig.). (C). pap. text 15.00 (*1-56806-895-6*) DIANE Pub.

AIDS & the Health Care System. Lawrence O. Gostin. 1990. LC 89-25039. 336p. (C). 47.00 (*0-300-04719-3*); pap. 18.00 (*0-300-04720-7*) Yale U Pr.

AIDS & the Heterosexual. J. L. Denser. 1991. LC 91-92002. 128p. (Orig.). pap. 7.95 (*0-9629513-0-7*) J L Denser.

AIDS & the Heterosexual Population. Ed. by Lorraine Sherr. 1994. LC 93-29061. 300p. text 59.00 (*3-7186-5459-8*); pap. text 19.00 (*3-7186-5460-1*) Gordon & Breach.

AIDS & the Hospice Community. Ed. by Madalon O. Amenta. 1991. LC 91-20825. (Hospice Journal). (Illus.). 190p. pap. text 17.95 (*1-56023-011-8*); lib. bdg. 54.95 (*1-56024-184-5*) Haworth Pr (Harrington Park).

AIDS & the Impact of Cognitive Impairment: A Treatment Guide for Mental Health Providers. Penelope Zeifert et al. 1995. LC 95-35959. (UCSF AHP Monograph Ser.: No. 1). pap. (*1-879168-01-4*) AIDS Hlth Project.

AIDS & the Law. David W. Webber. 3rd ed. 1997. LC 97-11007. (Civil Rights Library). 1394p. 150.00 (*0-471-13542-9*) Wiley.

AIDS & the Law: A Basic Guide for the Non-Lawyer. Allan H. Terl. 1992. LC 91-38449. 175p. 59.95 (*1-56032-218-7*); pap. 29.95 (*1-56032-219-5*) Taylor & Francis.

AIDS & the Law: An Outline Guide. 1991. lib. bdg. 355.95 (*0-8490-5097-9*) Gordon Pr.

AIDS & the Law, 1999. David W. Webber. 3rd ed. 1999. pap. text, suppl. ed. 79.00 (*0-7355-0543-8*) Aspen Pub.

AIDS & the Lung. David M. Mitchell. Ed. by Ashley A. Woodcock et al. 1990. (Illus.). 110p. pap. text (*0-7279-0289-X*) BMJ Pub GBR. *Dist:* AIDC.

AIDS & the Lung. Stephen J. Semple & Robert Miller. 1997. LC 96-44118. (Illus.). 384p. 131.95 (*0-632-03623-0*) Blackwell Sci.

AIDS & the Positive Alternatives. Margaret White. 1988. pap. 7.95 (*0-310-55871-9*, 19095P) Zondervan.

AIDS & the Privacy Act in Canada - Le Sida et la Loi Sur la Protection des Renseignments Personnels. 1993. (ENG & FRE.). 160p. (Orig.). (C). pap. text 50.00 (*1-56806-523-X*) DIANE Pub.

AIDS & the Public Debate: Historical & Contemporary Perspectives. Ed. by Caroline Hannaway et al. 1995. LC 94-7847. 216p. 70.00 (*90-5199-190-8*) IOS Press.

AIDS & the Public Work Force: Local Government Preparedness in Managing the Epidemic. James D. Slack. 1991. LC 91-2769. 200p. (C). pap. text 17.95 (*0-8173-0548-3*) U of Ala Pr.

AIDS & the Social Sciences: Common Threads. Ed. by Richard Ulack & William F. Skinner. 1991. LC 91-13348. (Illus.). 192p. text 24.95 (*0-8131-1760-7*) U Pr of KY.

AIDS & Women's Reproductive Health. L. C. Chen et al. 1992. (Reproductive Biology Ser.). (Illus.). 216p. (C). text 79.50 (*0-306-44200-0*, Kluwer Plenum) Kluwer Academic.

AIDS & Your Church: Materials to Help Your Ministry Meet the Challenge. Jerry Thacker. Ed. by Cindy G. Spear. 1997. 142p. ring bd. 69.95 (*1-57052-075-5*, 445) Chrch Grwth VA.

AIDS Anthology: Essays, Poems, & Articles for & about Persons with HIV/AIDS. Ed. by Carol A. Mutzebaugh. 1996. (Illus.). 130p. pap. (*1-891814-04-4*) Found Care Mgmt.

AIDS Benefits Handbook: Everything You Need to Know to Get Social Security, Welfare, Medicaid, Medicare, Food Stamps, Housing, Drugs, & Other Benefits. Thomas P. McCormack. 1990. 240p. (C). 37.50 (*0-300-04736-3*); pap. 14.00 (*0-300-04721-5*) Yale U Pr.

AIDS Bibliography for 1987. Whitston Publishing Company Inc. Staff. 1990. 461p. 55.00 (*0-87875-373-7*) Whitston Pub.

AIDS Bibliography for 1988. Whitston Publishing Company Inc. Staff. 1992. 630p. 75.00 (*0-87875-411-3*) Whitston Pub.

AIDS Biological Warfare. T. E. Bearden. 1988. (Illus.). 484p. pap. 19.50 (*0-914119-04-4*) Tesla Bk Co.

AIDS Blindness & Low Vision: A Guide for Service Providers. Ed. by Mary A. Lang et al. 1996. 36p. reprint ed. pap. text 15.00 (*0-7881-3128-1*) DIANE Pub.

AIDS Book: Creating a Positive Approach. Louise L. Hay. (Orig.). (SPA.). 285p. pap. 10.00 (*84-86344-90-5*, 138); 1988. LC 88-81685. 288p. pap. 10.00 (*0-937611-32-8*, 108) Hay House.

AIDS Booklet. Frank D. Cox. 4th ed. 1995. 80p. (C). pap. 10.31 (*0-697-26261-8*, WCB McGr Hill) McGrw-H Hghr Educ.

AIDS Bureaucracy. Sandra Panem & Samuel O. Thier. 1988. LC 87-22972. 208p. pap. text 11.95 (*0-674-01271-2*) HUP.

AIDS Bureaucracy: Why Society Failed to Meet the AIDS Crisis & How We Might Impove Our Response. Sandra Panem & Samuel O. Thier. 1988. LC 87-22972. (Illus.). 208p. 39.50 (*0-674-01270-4*) HUP.

AIDS, Cancer & the Medical Establishment. R. K. Brown. 1986. (Illus.). 240p. 16.95 (*0-8315-0196-0*) Speller.

AIDS Capitation. Ed. by David Alex Cherin & George J. Huba. 1998. LC 98-33964. (Home Health Care Services Quarterly Ser.: Vol. 17, No. 1). 115p. pap. 54.95 (*0-7890-0654-5*, Hawrth Medical) Haworth Pr.

AIDS Care at Home: A Guide for Patients, Caregivers, & Loved Ones & People with AIDS. Judith Grief et al. 1994. LC 94-174599. (Illus.). 384p. pap. 17.95 (*0-471-58468-1*) Wiley.

AIDS Caregiver's Handbook. Ed. by Ted Eidson. rev. ed. 1993. LC 92-49770. (Illus.). 384p. pap. 14.95 (*0-312-08129-4*) St Martin.

AIDS Challenge: Breaking Through the Boundaries. Mary E. O'Brien. 1995. LC 94-43170. 176p. 58.00 (*0-86569-247-5*, Auburn Hse) Greenwood.

AIDS Challenge: Prevention Education for Young People. Ed. by Marcia Quackenbush et al. 526p. 1995. pap. 24.95 (*0-941816-53-2*); 1988. 29.95 (*0-941816-54-0*) ETR Assocs.

AIDS Clinical Chemistry. Reynolds. 1986. pap. text 22.00 (*0-443-03145-2*) Saunders.

AIDS Clinical Pharmacology. Rogers. 1989. pap. text 31.00 (*0-443-03971-2*) Saunders.

AIDS Clinical Review, 1997-1998. Ed. by Paul A. Volberding & Mark A. Jacobson. 1997. (Aids Clinical Review Ser.: Vol. 7). (Illus.). 416p. text 150.00 (*0-8247-0112-7*) Dekker.

AIDS Clinical Trials. Ed. by Dianne M. Finkelstein & David A. Schoenfeld. 1995. LC 95-7528. 458p. 94.95 (*0-471-58823-7*) Wiley.

AIDS, Communication, & Empowerment: Gay Male Identity & the Politics of Public Health Messages. Ed. by Roger Myrick. 1996. LC 95-45914. 141p. (C). 34.95 (*1-56023-884-4*, Haworth Pastrl) Haworth Pr.

AIDS Counselling: Institutional Interaction & Clinical Practice. Anssi Perakyla. 1996. (Studies in Interactional Sociolinguistics: No. 11). 380p. (C). text 74.95 (*0-521-45463-8*) Cambridge U Pr.

AIDS Counselor. Jack Rudman. 1994. (Career Examination Ser.: C-3619). pap. 29.95 (*0-8373-3619-8*) Nat Learn.

AIDS Cover-Up? The Real & Alarming Facts about AIDS. Gene Antonio. 2nd ed. 1986. LC 86-81935. 267p. (Orig.). pap. 9.95 (*0-89870-129-5*) Ignatius Pr.

AIDS Crisis: A Documentary History. Douglas A. Feldman & Julia W. Miller. 1998. LC 97-26891. (Primary Documents in American History & Contemporary Issues Ser.). 312p. 49.95 (*0-313-28715-5*, GR8715, Greenwood Pr) Greenwood.

AIDS Crisis: Impact On the Gay Subculture, Pt. 1. Kevin Michaels. 1986. 130p. ring bd. 11.95 (*0-939020-77-7*) MLP Ent.

AIDS Crisis: Voices from & to African-American Communities. Larry M. Gant & Patricia A. Stewart. 1998. LC 98-21658. 176p. pap. 19.95 (*0-275-96094-3*, Praeger Pubs) Greenwood.

AIDS Crisis & the Contraceptive Mentality. Eugene F. Diamond & Orville N. Griese. 1988. 69p. pap. 3.95 (*0-935372-22-9*) NCBC.

AIDS Crisis in America: A Reference Handbook. Mary E. Hombs. 1992. LC 92-48841. (Contemporary World Issues Ser.). 268p. lib. bdg. 39.50 (*0-87436-648-8*) ABC-CLIO.

AIDS Crisis in America: A Reference Handbook. Eric K. Lerner & Mary E. Hombs. 2nd ed. 1998. LC 98-25764. (Contemporary World Issues. Ser.). 344p. lib. bdg. 45.00 (*1-57607-070-0*) ABC-CLIO.

AIDS Demo Graphics. Douglas Crimp & Adam Rolston. 1990. LC 89-81756. (Illus.). 144p. pap. 13.95 (*0-941920-16-X*) Bay Pr.

AIDS, Dentistry, & the Illusion of Infection Control: Questioning the HIV Hypothesis. John Hardie. 1995. LC 95-44398. 356p. text 99.95 (*0-7734-4234-0*) E Mellen.

AIDS Diagnosis & Control - Current Situation: Report on a WHO Meeting. 1987. pap. text 5.00 (*92-890-1051-7*) World Health.

AIDS Dictionary. Sarah B. Watstein & Karen Chandler. 1998. 400p. LC 97-8114. 45.00 (*0-8160-3149-5*); pap. 24.95 (*0-8160-3754-X*) Facts on File.

AIDS Directory. Ed. by William H. Feldman. 2nd ed. 1995. 800p. (Orig.). pap. 250.00 (*1-882594-00-2*) LRP Publications.

AIDS Disaster: The Failure of Organizations in New York & the Nation. Charles Perrow & Mauro F. Guillen. 1990. 208p. (C). pap. 15.00 (*0-300-04880-7*) Yale U Pr.

AIDS Dissidents: An Annotated Bibliography. Ian Young. 1993. LC 93-23958. 272p. 40.00 (*0-8108-2675-5*) Scarecrow.

AIDS Doctors: Voices from the Epidemic - An Oral History. Ronald Bayer & Gerald M. Oppenheimer. 2000. LC 00-20913. 320p. 25.00 (*0-19-512681-5*) OUP.

AIDS Drug Assistance Program (ADAP) A Resource Guide for Women Living with HIV/AIDS. Patricia Nalls & Cathleen M. Maine. 1996. 36p. pap. 5.00 (*1-877966-38-X*) Ctr Women Policy.

AIDS Drugs & Prevention: Perspectives on Individual & Community Action. Ed. by Tim Rhodes & Richard Hartnoll. 1996. (Illus.). 256p. (C). pap. 29.95 (*0-415-10204-9*) Routledge.

AIDS, Drugs & Sexual Risk: Lives in the Balance. Neil McKeganey & Marina U. Barnard. 1992. 160p. pap. (*0-335-09970-X*) OpUniv Pr.

AIDS, Drugs of Abuse & the Neuroimmune Axis. Ed. by Herman Friedman et al. 1996. LC 96-25725. (Advances in Experimental Medicine & Biology Ser.: Vol. 402). (Illus.). 246p. 95.00 (*0-306-45375-4*, Kluwer Plenum) Kluwer Academic.

AIDS Education. Mark Hochhauser. 1991. pap. text, tchr. ed. 14.06 (*0-697-14164-0*) McGraw.

AIDS Education. Mark Hochhauser & James H. Roth. 1991. 240p. (YA). (gr. 10-12). pap. 32.19 (*0-697-11166-0*) McGrw-H Hghr Educ.

AIDS Education: Interventions in Multi-Cultural Societies. I. I. Schenker et al. 1997. LC 96-40882. (Illus.). 276p. 102.00 (*0-306-45489-0*, Kluwer Plenum) Kluwer Academic.

AIDS Education: Reaching Diverse Populations. Ed. by Melinda K. Moore & Martin L. Forst. 1996. LC 95-49715. (Illus.). 248p. 62.50 (*0-275-94904-4*, Praeger Pubs) Greenwood.

AIDS 88 Summary: A Practical Synopsis of the IV International Conference. Bruce Wallace & J. Lasker. 1988. (Illus.). 156p. (Orig.). pap. 75.00 (*0-924236-00-0*) Phila Scis Group.

AIDS 89 Summary: A Practical Synopsis of the V International Conference. Bruce Wallace & J. Lasker. 1989. (Illus.). 350p. (Orig.). pap. 85.00 (*0-924236-02-7*) Phila Scis Group.

AIDS Epidemic: How You Can Protect Yourself & Your Family, Why You Must. James I. Slaff & John K. Brubaker. 1985. mass mkt. 3.95 (*0-446-30143-4*) Warner Bks.

AIDS Epidemic & Its Demographic Consequences. 1991. 140p. 37.50 (*92-1-151224-7*, 91.XIII.5) UN.

AIDS Epidemiology: A Quantitative Approach. Ron Brookmeyer & Mitchell H. Gail. 1994. LC 92-48337. (Monographs in Epidemiology & Biostatistics: Vol. 22). (Illus.). 376p. (C). text 54.50 (*0-19-507641-9*) OUP.

AIDS Epidemiology: Methodological Issues. Ed. by Nicholas P. Jewell et al. 1994. LC 92-17877. xvi, 402p. 125.00 (*0-8176-3632-3*) Birkhauser.

AIDS, Fear & Society: Challenging the Dreaded Disease. Kenneth J. Doka. 1997. LC 96-44899. (Death Education, Aging & Health Care Ser.). 69.95 (*1-56032-248-9*) Hemisp Pub.

AIDS File. George Jacobs & Joseph Kerrins. Ed. by Julie Doohan. 1987. LC 87-70217. (Illus.). 128p. (Orig.). (YA). (gr. 8 up). pap. 7.95 (*0-9618059-0-0*) Cromlech Bks.

AIDS, Health, & Mental Health: A Primary Sourcebook. Judith Landau-Stanton & Colleen D. Clements. 1993. LC 92-30578. 360p. text 41.95 (*0-87630-688-1*) Brunner-Routledge.

AIDS Health Crisis: Psychological & Social Interventions. J. A. Kelly et al. 1988. LC 88-17881. (Applied Clinical Psychology Ser.). (Illus.). 222p. (C). text 42.50 (*0-306-42896-2*, Kluwer Plenum) Kluwer Academic.

AIDS Health Services at the Crossroads: Lessons for Community Care. Pref. by June E. Osborn. 1991. LC 91-67786. 136p. (Orig.). pap. (*0-942054-04-0*) R W Johnson Found.

AIDS, Herpes & Everything You Should Know about V. D. in Australia. David Bradford. 2nd ed. 1985. 300p. pap. 14.95 (*0-522-84311-5*) Intl Spec Bk.

AIDS-HIV: A Prescription for Cure. T. R. Shantha. 1991. (Illus.). 29.95 (*1-879144-00-X*) Internatl Pub Hse.

AIDS-HIV Vol. 1: A Prescription for Survival: Hyperthermia, Autoimmune Therapy & Drugs. T. R. Shantha. 1991. (Illus.). 317p. 29.95 (*1-879144-01-8*) Internatl Pub Hse.

AIDS Home Care Handbook. 1994. (Illus.). 178p. (Orig.). (C). pap. text 40.00 (*0-7881-1011-X*) DIANE Pub.

AIDS Hysteria. Arthur F. Ide. (Illus.). (Orig.). 1986. LC 85-29651. 117p. pap. 5.00 (*0-930383-08-7*); 2nd ed. 1988. LC 88-9166. 154p. (C). pap. 7.00 (*0-930383-12-5*) Monument Pr.

AIDS in Africa: A Manual for Physicians. P. Piot et al. 1992. (ENG & FRE., Illus.). viii, 125p. pap. text 16.00 (*92-4-154435-X*, 1150381) World Health.

AIDS in Africa: Its Present & Future Impact. Tony Barnett & Piers Blaikie. 1992. LC 91-77918. 200p. pap. 20.95 (*0-89862-880-6*) Guilford Pubns.

AIDS in Africa: The Social Impact & Policy Issues. Ed. by Norman Miller. 1989. LC 88-12750. (Studies in African Health & Medicine: Vol. 1). 350p. lib. bdg. 99.95 (*0-88946-187-2*) E Mellen.

AIDS in Africa: The Social Work Response. Rodreck Mupedziswa. 1998. LC 99-890976. (Illus.). (*0-7974-1937-3*) S African Res & Doc.

AIDS in Africa & the Caribbean. Ed. by George Bond et al. 1997. LC 97-9642. 256p. (C). pap. text 28.00 (*0-8133-2879-9*) Westview.

AIDS in America. C. H. Russell. 1991. 147p. 97.00 (*0-387-97462-8*) Spr-Verlag.

AIDS in America: Our Chances, Our Choices. Robert E. Lee. 1987. LC 87-51105. vi, 208p. 49.50 (*0-87875-355-9*); pap. 25.00 (*0-87875-357-5*) Whitston Pub.

AIDS in an Aging Society: What We Need to Know. Ed. by Matilda W. Riley et al. 1989. 240p. 32.95 (*0-8261-7060-9*) Springer Pub.

AIDS in Global Perspective. Hraf. 1996. 14.95 (*0-8161-1614-8*, Macmillan Ref) Gale.

AIDS in India: Myth & Reality. Gracious Thomas. 1994. (C). (*81-7033-218-4*) Rawat Pubns IND. *Dist:* S Asia.

AIDS in Jewish Thought & Law. Gad Freudenthal. 1998. LC 97-36232. 29.50 (*0-88125-610-2*) Ktav.

AIDS in Post Communist Russia & Its Successor States. Christopher Williams. 1995. 240p. (C). (*1-85628-570-7*) Avebry GBR. *Dist:* Ashgate Pub Co.

***AIDS in South Africa: The New Apartheid.** Zia Jaffrey. 2001. 160p. 20.00 (*1-85984-632-7*) Verso.

AIDS in South Africa & on the African Continent. Lorenzo S. Togni. 1997. LC 98-135350. (Illus.). (*0-7986-4214-9*) Kagiso Pub.

AIDS in the Dental Office? The Story of Kimberly Bergalis & Dr. David Acer. Robert R. Runnells. Ed. by Katherine Newman. 1993. (Illus.). 325p. 29.95 (*0-936751-11-8*) Infection Control.

AIDS in the Healthcare Workplace. Douglas. 1990. (Education Ser.). 24.95 (*0-8273-3597-0*); tchr. ed. 8.00 (*0-8273-3598-9*) Delmar.

AIDS in the Industrialized Democracies: Passions, Politics, & Policies. Ed. by David L. Kirp & Ronald Bayer. 1992. LC 91-40630. 406p. (C). text 45.00 (*0-8135-1821-0*); pap. text 18.95 (*0-8135-1822-9*) Rutgers U Pr.

AIDS in the Nervous System. Richard Lechtenberg & Joan H. Sher. 1988. (Illus.). 136p. text (*0-443-08616-8*) Church.

AIDS in the Netherlands up to the Year 2000. Scenario Committee on AIDS Staff. 1992. (Future Health Scenarios Ser.). pap. text 141.50 (*0-7923-1895-1*) Kluwer Academic.

AIDS in the U. K. The Making of a Policy, 1981-1994. Virginia Berridge. 1996. LC 95-38985. (Illus.). 404p. (C). pap. text 24.95 (*0-19-820473-6*) OUP.

AIDS in the Workplace: Here Are the Answers You Must Have. 1988. (C). pap. text 9.95 (*0-13-202714-3*, Macmillan Coll) P-H.

AIDS in the Workplace: Legal Questions & Practical Answers. William F. Banta. enl. rev. ed. 1993. LC 86-46309. 422p. 45.00 (*0-669-28056-9*) Lxngtn Bks.

AIDS in the World II: Global Dimensions, Social Roots & Responses. Ed. by Jonathan Mann & Daniel J. Tarantola. 2nd ed. 1996. LC 96-20008. (Illus.). 648p. pap. text 34.50 (*0-19-509097-7*) OUP.

AIDS in the World, 1992. Ed. by Jonathan Mann et al. 1992. LC 92-1545. (Illus.). 800p. text 62.00 (*0-674-01265-8*); 352p. pap. text 26.95 (*0-674-01266-6*) HUP.

AIDS Inc. Scandal of the Century. Jon Rappoport. 1988. LC 88-80560. (Illus.). 275p. pap. 13.95 (*0-941523-03-9*) Human Energy Pr.

AIDS Is for Death. Jack Van Impe. 1988. 266p. pap. 9.00 (*0-934803-67-6*) J Van Impe.

AIDS Issues in the Workplace: A Response Model for Human Resource Management. Dale A. Masi. 1990. LC 90-8912. 232p. 62.95 (*0-89930-516-4*, MAQ/, Quorum Bks) Greenwood.

AIDS Knowledge Base: A Textbook on HIV Disease from the University of California, San Francisco School of Medicine, & San Francisco General Hospital. University of California, San Francisco Staff et al. Ed. by P. T. Cohen et al. 3rd ed. 1999. LC 98-38890. (Illus.). xxiii, 966p. text 169.00 (*0-316-14903-9*, Little Brwn Med Div) Lppncott W & W.

AIDS Law. Margaret C. Jasper. 1996. LC 96-214382. (Legal Almanac Ser.). 103p. text 25.50 (*0-379-11227-2*) Oceana.

***AIDS Law.** Margaret C. Jasper. 2nd ed. 2000. LC 00-136420. (Legal Almanac Ser.). (Illus.). x, 261p. 25.50 (*0-379-11350-3*) Oceana.

AIDS Law & Litigation Reporter, Set. 2000. ring bd. 4000.00 (*1-55572-003-X*) Univ Pub Group.

AIDS Law in a Nutshell. Robert M. Jarvis et al. (Nutshell Ser.). 1992. 349p. reprint ed. pap. 17.50 (*0-314-80908-2*); 2nd ed. 1996. LC 96-31130. 301p. (C). pap. 22.50 (*0-314-06782-5*) West Pub.

AIDS Law Today: A New Guide for the Public. Ed. by Yale AIDS Law Project Staff et al. 2nd ed. 1993. LC 92-35572. 464p. (C). pap. 20.00 (*0-300-05512-9*) Yale U Pr.

AIDS Legal & Ethical Considerations: A Special Issue of Social Casework. 1988. 112p. 8.95 (*0-87304-229-8*) Manticore Pubs.

AIDS Litigation Digest 1995. Ed. by Zahna L. Ellis & Jennifer F. Vaughan. 1995. 117p. pap. text 34.50 (*0-9616858-9-1*) Strafford Pubns.

AIDS, Macrobiotics, & Natural Immunity. Michio Kushi & Martha C. Cottrell. 1989. LC 86-81560. (Illus.). 359p. pap. 34.00 (*0-87040-680-9*) Japan Pubns USA.

AIDS Memoir: Journal of an HIV-Positive Mother. Catherine Wyatt-Morley. 1997. LC 96-37848. (Illus.). 216p. (Orig.). pap. 14.95 (*1-56549-067-3*) Kumarian Pr.

AIDS Mirage. Hiram Caton. 1995. (Frontlines Ser.). 64p. pap. (*0-86840-342-3*) New South Wales Univ Pr AUS. *Dist:* Intl Spec Bk.

AIDS Movie: Representing a Pandemic in Film & Television. Kylo-Patrick Hart. 2000. LC 00-38879. xiii, 120p. 39.95 (*0-7890-1107-7*); pap. 17.95 (*0-7890-1108-5*) Haworth Pr.

AIDS 99: A Year in Review. Shinji Harada et al. 1999. 279p. pap. text 99.00 (*0-7817-2424-4*) Lppncott W & W.

AIDS 91 Summary: A Practical Synopsis of the VII International Conference. J. Arbeit et al. 1992. (Illus.). 350p. pap. 85.00 (*0-924236-07-8*) Phila Scis Group.

AIDS Ninety Summary: A Practical Synopsis of the VI International Conference. J. Arbeit et al. 1991. (Illus.). 350p. (Orig.). pap. 85.00 (*0-924236-05-1*) Phila Scis Group.

AIDS Notebooks. Stephen Schecter. 1990. LC 89-21824. (SUNY Series in the Philosophy of the Social Sciences). 166p. (C). pap. text 20.95 (*0-7914-0334-3*) State U NY Pr.

AIDS Pandemic: A Global Emergency. Ed. by R. Bolton. 1989. xii, 118p. pap. text 43.00 (*2-88124-374-6*) Gordon & Breach.

AIDS Pandemic: Social Perspectives, 38. Yole G. Sills. 1993. LC 93-25064. (Contributions in Medical Studies Ser.: No. 38). 264p. 67.00 (*0-313-28606-X*, ZAP/, Greenwood Pr) Greenwood.

AIDS Pastoral Care: An Introductory Guide. Sean Connolly. 1994. LC 94-70579. 96p. (Orig.). pap. 7.95 (*0-9636183-1-8*) Arc Res.

AIDS Pathogenesis. Ed. by Hanneke Schuitemaker & F. Miedema. 2000. LC 00-21827. (Immunology & Medicine Ser.). 294p. 133.00 (*0-7923-6196-2*) Kluwer Academic.

AIDS, Philosophy & Beyond: Philosophical Dilemmas of a Modern Pandemic. Joseph W. Smith. 1991. (Avebury Series in Philosophy). 347p. (*1-85628-138-8*) Avebry GBR. *Dist:* Ashgate Pub Co.

AIDS Phobia Disease Pattern & Possibilities of Treatment. Hans Jager. 1988. 104p. 29.95 (*0-470-21225-X*) P-H.

AIDS Plague. 1987. (AIDS Ser.). lib. bdg. 250.00 (*0-8490-3923-1*) Gordon Pr.

AIDS Practice Manual. Ed. by Paul Albert et al. 3rd ed. 1990. pap. (*0-9602188-7-4*) Natl Lawyers Guild.

AIDS Prevention & Control: Invited Presentations & Papers from the World Summit of Ministers of Health. WHO Staff. 1988. 191p. 30.00 (*92-4-156115-7*) World Health.

AIDS Prevention & Control: Invited Presentations & Papers from the World Summit of Ministers of Health on Programmes for AIDS Prevention - Jointly Organized by the WHO & the UK Government, London, 26-28 January, 1988. World Health Organization Staff. 1988. 192p. 65.00 (*0-08-036142-0*, Pergamon Pr) Elsevier.

AIDS Prevention & Services: Community Based Research. Ed. by Johannes P. Van Vugt. 1993. LC 93-207. 296p. 72.95 (*0-89789-264-X*, Bergin & Garvey); pap. 21.95 (*0-89789-265-8*) Greenwood.

AIDS Prevention in the Community: Lessons from the First Decade. Ed. by Nicholas Freudenberg & Marc A. Zimmerman. 1995. LC 96-148008. 238p. pap. 48.00 (*0-87553-219-5*, 053) Am Pub Health.

AIDS Prevention Through Educations: A World View. Ed. by Jaime Sepulveda et al. 1993. LC 92-49655. 384p. pap. text 29.95 (*0-19-508207-9*) OUP.

AIDS Prevention Through Health Promotion: Facing Sensitive Issues. 1991. (CHI, ENG, FRE & SPA.). viii, 78p. pap. text 14.40 (*92-4-156144-0*, 1150367) World Health.

AIDS Public Policy Dimensions. Ed. by John Griggs. 1987. 304p. 30.00 (*0-934459-35-5*) United Hosp Fund.

AIDS Reader, Vol. I. Loren K. Clarke & Malcolm Potts. 1988. 350p. pap. 17.95 (*0-8283-1918-9*) Branden Bks.

AIDS Reader: Privacy, Poverty, Community. Ed. by Nancy F. McKenzie. 1990. pap. 9.95 (*0-452-01048-9*, Mer) NAL.

AIDS Reference Guide: A Sourcebook for Planners & Decision Makers, set. Ed. by Frances Fernald. 2001. 2400p. ring bd. 448.00 (*0-929156-01-3*) Atlantic Info Services Inc.

AIDS-Related Neoplasis. Ed. by L. Schmid & H. J. Senn. 1988. (Recent Results in Cancer Research Ser.: Vol. 112). (Illus.). 97p. 76.00 (*0-387-19227-1*) Spr-Verlag.

AIDS-Related Psychotherapy. Mark G. Winiarski. 1991. 256p. (C). 68.00 (*0-205-14511-6*, H4511, Longwood Div) Allyn.

AB

AIDS-Related Psychotherapy. Mark G. Winiarski. 1991. (General Psychology Ser.). 220p. (*0-08-037913-3*) PPI GBR. *Dist:* Elsevier.

AIDS Research at E. C. Level: Results of the 4th E. C. Biomedical & Health Research Program. Ed. by Andre E. Baert et al. 1995. LC 94-7542. (Biomedical & Health Research Ser.: Vol. 6). 371p. 99.00 (*90-5199-159-2*) IOS Press.

AIDS Research Program of the National Institutes of Health. Institute of Medicine Staff. 1991. 156p. pap. text 24.00 (*0-309-04436-7*) Natl Acad Pr.

AIDS Scam: Science & Hoax, How Special Interests Benefit. 1994. lib. bdg. 250.00 (*0-8490-5623-3*) Gordon Pr.

AIDS, Sexual Behavior, & Intravenous Drug Use. Ed. by Charles F. Turner et al. 1989. 608p. 39.95 (*0-309-03976-2*) Natl Acad Pr.

AIDS, Social Change & Theater: Performance As Protest. Cindy J. Kistenberg. 1995. LC 95-34639. (Studies in American Popular History & Culture). 209p. text 44.00 (*0-8153-2159-7*) Garland.

AIDS Sourcebook: Basic Consumer Health Information about AIDS & HIV Infection. Ed. by Karen Bellenir. 2nd ed. 1999. LC 98-53294. (Health Reference Ser.: Vol. 48). (Illus.). xiii, 751p. lib. bdg. 78.00 (*0-7808-0225-X*) Omnigraphics Inc.

AIDS Sourcebook: Basic Information about AIDS & HIV Infection. Ed. by Peter D. Dresser & Karen Bellenir. 1995. LC 95-5997. (Health Reference Ser.: Vol. 4). 831p. lib. bdg. 78.00 (*0-7808-0031-1*) Omnigraphics Inc.

AIDS, Stories of Living Longer. Ed. by C. Ray. 1991. 32p. (Orig.). pap. 3.25 (*0-9616792-9-8*) Taterhill.

AIDS Summary: In-Depth Review & Update. Bruce Wallace & J. Lasker. 1989. (Illus.). 156p. (Orig.). pap. 55.00 (*0-924236-01-9*) Phila Scis Group.

AIDS Testing: A Comprehensive Guide to Technical, Medical, Social, Legal, & Management Issues. Ed. by G. Schochetman & J. R. George. 2nd ed. 1994. LC 94-7986. (Illus.). 411p. 74.95 (*0-387-94291-2*) Spr-Verlag.

AIDS Testing with Its Uses & Abuses: Index of New Information with Authors & Subjects. American Health Research Institute Staff. 1994. LC 94-31244. 57.50 (*0-7883-0438-0*) ABBE Pubs Assn.

AIDS the Expanding Epidemic - What the Public Needs to Know: A Multicultural Overview. Valiere Alcena. 1994. 204p. (Orig.). 24.99 (*0-9633365-1-7*) Alcena Med Comms.

AIDS the Last Great Plague. 1992. lib. bdg. 250.00 (*0-8490-8707-4*) Gordon Pr.

AIDS-The True Story: A Comprehensive Guide. Balamurali Ambati & Jayakrishna Ambati. 1989. 176p. (Orig.). (C). pap. 14.95 (*0-924385-00-6*) B J Pubns MD.

AIDS, the Unnecessary Epidemic: America under Seige. Stanley Monteith. 1995. 392p. reprint ed. pap. 14.95 (*0-925591-17-3*) Covenant Hse Bks.

AIDS Therapeutics in HIV Disease. A. Palfreeman. 2nd ed. 1998. LC 97-43724. 124p. pap. 45.00 (*0-471-97063-8*) Wiley.

AIDS Therapies: 1992 Edition. Daniel J. DeNoon & Charles W. Henderson. 1992. 350p. reprint ed. stu. ed. 899.00 (*0-9631698-0-7*) C W Henderson.

AIDS Therapy. Raphael Dolin et al. Ed. by Marc Staruss. 1999. LC 98-34773. 715p. (C). text (*0-443-07592-1*) Church.

Aids to Anaesthesia No. 1: Basic Sciences. T. E. Healy et al. 3rd ed. 1991. (Illus.). 272p. (Orig.). pap. (*0-443-04231-4*) Church.

Aids to Anaesthesia Vol. 2: Clinical Practice. M. J. Harrison et al. 22nd ed. 1999. (Illus.). 224p. (Orig.). (C). pap. (*0-443-04233-0*) Saunders.

Aids to Anatomy. Simon Paterson-Brown & Rupert Eckersley. 1988. (Illus.). 288p. pap. text (*0-443-03624-1*) Church.

Aids to Clinical Examination. Peter C. Hayes & Ronald S. McWalter. 2nd ed. 1992. (Illus.). 144p. (Orig.). pap. text (*0-443-04572-0*) Church.

Aids to Clinical Haematology. J. A. Child. 2nd ed. 1992. (Illus.). 194p. (Orig.). pap. text (*0-443-04192-X*) Church.

Aids to Clinical Pharmacology & Therapeutics. John Rees et al. 3rd ed. 1993. LC 92-49325. (Illus.). 350p. pap. text (*0-443-04698-0*) Church.

***Aids to Examination of the Peripheral Nervous System.** Contrib. by Mosby Staff. 2nd ed. 2000. pap. 23.25 (*0-7020-2512-7*) Mosby Inc.

Aids to General Practice. Michael Mead. 2nd ed. 1991. (Illus.). 170p. pap. text (*0-443-04589-5*); 3rd ed. 1995. LC 94-43949. pap. text (*0-443-05277-8*) Church.

Aids to Microbiology & Infectious Diseases. R. A. Benn. 1986. 208p. (Orig.). pap. text (*0-443-03127-4*) Church.

Aids to Obstetrics & Gynaecology. Gordon M. Stirrat. 2nd ed. 1987. (Illus.). 296p. pap. text (*0-443-03447-8*, Irwn Prfssnl) McGraw-Hill Educ Grp.

Aids to Obstetrics & Gynecology: For MRCOG. Gordon M. Stirrat. 4th ed. 1997. LC 96-39913. (Aids to... Ser.). (*0-443-05535-1*) Church.

Aids to Obstetrics & Gynecology: For MRCOG Part 2. Gordon M. Stirrat. 3rd ed. 1991. 306p. (Orig.). pap. text (*0-443-04382-5*) Church.

Aids to Operative Surgery. Graeme J. Poston. 1987. LC 86-8320. (Illus.). 224p. (Orig.). (C). pap. (*0-443-03566-0*) Church.

Aids to Ophthalmology. P. T. Khaw et al. 1989. (Illus.). 296p. pap. text (*0-443-04012-5*) Church.

Aids to Pathology. Michael F. Dixon & Philip Quirke. 4th ed. 1993. LC 93-18262. text (*0-443-04442-2*) Church.

Aids to Pediatrics Undergrads. Habel. 2nd ed. 1995. pap. text 18.95 (*0-443-05206-9*) Saunders.

Aids to Pharmacology. Steven Sacks & Roy Spector. 3rd rev. ed. 1993. LC 92-21013. pap. text (*0-443-04695-6*) Church.

Aids to Physiology. T. Scratcherd & J. I. Gillespie. 3rd ed. 1997. LC 97-8020. (AIDS Ser.). pap. text (*0-443-05451-7*) Church.

Aids to Physiotherapy. Ed. by Jennifer M. Lee. 2nd ed. 1988. (Illus.). 216p. pap. text (*0-443-03438-9*) Church.

Aids to Postgraduate Medicine. J. L. Burton. 5th ed. 1988. (Illus.). 272p. pap. text (*0-443-03548-2*); 6th ed. 1994. pap. text (*0-443-04913-0*) Church.

Aids to Postgraduate Surgery. Roger M. Watkins & J. Meirion Thomas. 3rd ed. 1989. 276p. pap. text (*0-443-03807-4*) Church.

Aids to Psychiatry. H. G. Morgan. 3rd ed. 1989. (Illus.). 224p. pap. text (*0-443-03928-3*) Church.

Aids to Radiological Differential Diagnosis. Chapman. 3rd ed. 1995. pap. text 32.00 (*0-7020-1895-3*) Saunders.

Aids to Undergrad Medicine. Burton. 7th ed. 1997. (C). pap. text 25.00 (*0-443-05692-7*) Saunders.

Aids to Undergraduate Obstetrics & Gynaecology. Christopher Sinclair & J. Beverley Webb. 2nd ed. 1993. LC 92-49138. (Illus.). 224p. pap. text (*0-443-04785-5*) Church.

Aids to Undergraduate Surgery. Peter M. Mowschenson. 4th ed. 1994. LC 93-34955. pap. text (*0-443-04966-1*) Church.

AIDS Trivia: Update for 90's Updated. Ed. by Thomas J. Rundquist. 3rd ed. 1995. disk 39.95 (*1-884239-02-1*); (Illus.). 42p. pap. text, tchr. ed. 14.95 (*1-884239-01-3*) Nova Media.

AIDS TV: Identity, Community, & Alternative Video. Alexandra Juhasz. 1995. LC 95-20385. (Console-ing Passions Ser.). (Illus.). 352p. text 54.95 (*0-8223-1683-8*) Duke.

AIDS under Pressure: Hyperbaric Medicine in the Management of HIV Disease. Michelle Reillo. 1997. LC 97-12032. 39.50 (*0-88937-153-9*) Hogrefe & Huber Pubs.

AIDS Update 1999. Gerald J. Stine. 1998. 458p. pap. text 34.67 (*0-13-080352-9*) P-H.

***AIDS Update 2002.** Gerald J. Stine. 2001. 528p. pap. 36.67 (*0-13-066429-4*) P-H.

AIDS War: Propaganda, Profiteering & Genocide from the Medical-Industrial Complex. John Lauritsen. 1993. LC 93-71717. (Illus.). 480p. (Orig.). pap. 20.00 (*0-943742-08-0*, Asklepios) Pagan Pr.

AIDS, Women, & the Next Generation: Towards a Morally Acceptable Public Policy for HIV Testing of Pregnant Women & Newborns. Ed. by Ruth R. Faden et al. 1991. (Illus.). 400p. text 42.50 (*0-19-506572-7*) OUP.

AIDS World Newsletter. Peter A. Mozeleski. Ed. by Paul M. Mozeleski. Ed. & Tr. by Rosie Dominguez. 1991. (YA). (gr. 6-12). Vol. 1, No. 1. pap. 2.50 (*1-880058-56-1*); Vol. 1, No. 1. (SPA.). pap. 2.50 (*1-880058-57-X*); Vol. 1, No. 2. pap. 2.50 (*1-880058-58-8*); Vol. 1, No. 2. (SPA.). pap. 2.50 (*1-880058-59-6*) Rubbers Bros Comics.

Aidsassault: A Role Playing Conceptual Game Pitting HIV-1 Against the Human Immune System. Darrell D. Barnes. 2nd rev. ed. 1998. (Illus.). 71p. pap. text 29.95 (*0-9654168-1-X*, 23846 Frey); 3rd ed. 2000. 78p. spiral bd. 29.95 (*0-9654168-2-8*) Barnes Publns.

AIDS/HIV & Confidentiality. 1991. 132p. pap. 25.00 (*0-89707-651-6*, 344-0018) Amer Bar Assn.

AIDS/HIV Reference Guide for Medical Professionals. John L. Fahey & Diana S. Flemmig. 4th ed. 1997. LC 95-52143. (Illus.). 360p. pap. 36.95 (*0-683-02960-6*) Lppncott W & W.

Ailing Spine: A Holistic Approach to Rehabilitation. Hans Tilscher & Manfred Eder. 1991. (Manuelle Medizin Ser.). (Illus.). 176p. 71.95 (*0-387-53008-8*) Spr-Verlag.

Aim of the Game. Armand Lauffer. 1974. LC 73-84873. 132p. 9.95 (*0-88437-052-6*) Psych Dimensions.

AIME '89. Ed. by J. Hunter et al. 1989. (Lecture Notes in Medical Informatics: Vol. 38). 330p. 64.95 (*0-387-51543-7*, 3394) Spr-Verlag.

Aiming for Quality Results: An Improvement Primer for Healthcare Organizations. Patrice L. Spath. 1994. (Illus.). 43.50 (*1-929955-00-6*) Brown Spath.

AIMS: Developmental Indicators of Emotional Health. Susan Partridge. 1991. (*0-939561-10-7*) Univ South ME.

Aims & Motives in Clinical Medicine: A Practical Approach to Medical Ethics. B. P. Bliss & A. G. Johnson. 1975. 150p. pap. 25.00 (*0-8464-0123-1*) Beekman Pubs.

AIN Symposium Proceedings, Nutrition '87. Ed. by Orville A. Levander. 1987. (Illus.). 157p. (Orig.). pap. 15.00 (*0-943029-01-5*) Am Soc Nutr Sci.

Air Analysis for Health & Dangers at Home, Work or Play in the U. S. A. Index of New Information with Authors & Subjects. Arlene A. Slattner. 1993. 180p. 47.50 (*1-55914-892-6*); pap. 44.50 (*1-55914-893-4*) ABBE Pubs Assn.

Air Pollutants. Ed. by Sagar V. Krupa & Allan H. Legge. 1986. LC 85-6461. (Advances in Environmental Science & Technology Ser.). 662p. 235.00 (*0-471-08312-7*) Wiley.

Air Pollutants & the Repiratory Tract. D. L. Swift. 1999. LC 98-49286. (Lung Biology in Health & Disease Ser.: Vol. 128). (Illus.). 404p. text 175.00 (*0-8247-9521-0*) Dekker.

Air Pollution. Vol. 5. Arthur C. Stern. 3rd ed. 1977. (Environmental Science Ser.). text 199.00 (*0-12-666605-9*) Acad Pr.

Air Pollution: A Survey of Existing Legislation. WHO Staff. 1963. (International Digest of Health Legislation Offprints: Vol. 14, No. 2). 45p. 3.00 (*92-4-169142-5*) World Health.

***Air Pollution: Air Quality & Respiratory Problems in & Near the Great Smoky Mountains.** John B. Stephenson. 2001. 51p. (C). pap. text 20.00 (*0-7567-1548-2*) DIANE Pub.

Air Pollution: Environmental Issues & Health Effects. Ed. by Shyamal K. Majumdar et al. 1991. LC 91-61996. (Illus.). x, 496p. (C). text 45.00 (*0-945809-05-0*) Penn Science.

Air Pollution: Its Effect on the Urban Man & His Adaptive Strategies. Kaiman Lee. 1974. LC 74-182905. 52p. 12.00 (*0-915250-13-6*) Environ Design.

Air Pollution - Health Management: Proceedings of the Joint IIASA-WHO-EURO Workshop, Laxenburg, Austria, 27-30 July, 1982. Michael J. Suess. Ed. by W. Klug et al. 1984. 176p. pap. 46.00 (*0-08-031429-5*, Pergamon Pr) Elsevier.

Air Pollution & Community Health: A Critical Review & Data Sourcebook. Frederick W. Lipfert. 1994. (Industrial Health & Safety Ser.). 576p. 150.00 (*0-471-28560-9*, VNR) Wiley.

Air Pollution & Lung Diseases in Adults. Philip A. Witorsch. 1994. 336p. lib. bdg. 210.00 (*0-8493-0181-5*) CRC Pr.

Air Pollution & the Lung: Proceedings of the "Oholo" Biological Conference, 20th Annual. Ed. by E. Ahronson et al. 1975. 328p. 3.5 hd 82.50 (*0-7065-1553-6*) Coronet Bks.

Air Pollution & the Politics of Control. Elliot Goldstein et al. 1973. 182p. (C). text 26.50 (*0-8422-7136-8*) Irvington.

Air Pollution of Humans with Bacteria, Fungus & Molds in Homes, Offices & Hospitals: Index of New Information with Authors & Subjects. George R. Bonadio. rev. ed. 1995. 157p. 57.50 (*0-7883-0404-6*); LC 95-19207. pap. 47.50 (*0-7883-0405-4*) ABBE Pubs Assn.

Air Polution & Health. R. E. Hester. 1998. (Issues of Environmental Science Technology Ser.). 250p. pap. text (*0-85404-245-8*) Royal Soc Chem GBR. *Dist:* Spr-Verlag.

Air Quality Guidelines for Europe. 1987. (WHO Regional Publications European Ser.: No. 23). 439p. text 60.00 (*92-890-1114-9*) World Health.

Air Quality Permitting. Mohan Balagopalan. Date not set. 55.00 (*1-56670-152-X*) Lewis Pubs.

Air Sampling Instrument Selection Guide: Indoor Air Quality. Ed. by Chuck McCammon. 1998. LC 00-501206. 56p. pap. text 25.00 (*1-882417-27-5*, 9852) Am Conf Govt Indus Hygienist.

Air Toxics & Risk Assessment. Edward J. Calabrese et al. 1991. LC 90-13404. (Toxicology & Environmental Health Ser.). (Illus.). 688p. lib. bdg. 110.00 (*0-87371-165-3*, L165) Lewis Pubs.

Airborne Care of the Ill & Injured. E. L. McNeil. 1982. (Illus.). 208p. 51.00 (*0-387-90754-8*) Spr-Verlag.

***Airborne Infections: Protesting Your Patients & Yourself.** Dennis James Cleri. 2001. 160p. pap. text 29.00 (*1-879772-17-5*) Health Studies.

Airborne Patient Care Management: A Multidisciplinary Approach. Darlene M. Sredl. LC 84-60070. (Illus.). 331p. (Orig.). pap. text 27.95 (*0-930835-00-X*) Med Res Assocs.

Aircraft Structural Maintenance & Repair. Lloyd Dingle. 2002. 547p. pap. 59.95 (*0-7506-5017-6*, Newnes) Buttrwrth-Heinemann.

Aircrafts & Air Transportation in Commerce & Medicine: Index of New Information for Research & Progress. John L. Klingenhagen. 1996. LC 96-12487. 57.50 (*0-7883-1038-0*); pap. 47.50 (*0-7883-1039-9*) ABBE Pubs Assn.

Airline Medical Manual. Ed. by P. Chapman. 1990. (Illus.). 192p. (Orig.). (C). (gr. 13). pap. 47.95 (*0-412-31290-5*) Chapman & Hall.

Airway Care. Mosby Staff. 1995. (Respiratory Care Workbook Ser.: No. 8). (C). wbk. ed. (*0-8151-6311-8*, 26029) Mosby Inc.

Airway Epithelium: Physiology, Pathophysiology & Pharmacology. Ed. by Stephen G. Farmer & Douglas W. Hay. 1991. (Lung Biology in Health & Disease Ser.: Vol. 55). (Illus.). 680p. text 275.00 (*0-8247-8510-X*) Dekker.

Airway Management. Bainton. 1994. 39.00 (*0-316-07673-2*) Little.

Airway Management: Principles & Practice. Ed. by Jonathan L. Benumof. 1995. (Illus.). 952p. (C). (gr. 13). text 150.00 (*0-8151-0625-4*, 24614) Mosby Inc.

Airway Mucus: Basic Mechanisms & Clinical Perspectives. Ed. by D. F. Rogers et al. 1997. LC 97-8040. (Respiratory Pharmacology & Pharmacotherapy Ser.). (Illus.). 370p. 175.00 (*3-7643-5691-X*) Spr-Verlag.

Airway Mucus: Basic Mechanisms & Clinical Perspectives. D. F. Rogers & M. I. Lethem. 1997. LC 97-8040. (Respiratory Pharmacology & Pharmacotherapy Ser.). (*0-8176-5691-X*) Birkhauser.

Airway Obstruction & Inflammation: Present Status & Perspectives. Ed. by D. Olivieri & S. Bianco. 1990. (Progress in Respiratory Research Ser.: Vol. 24). (Illus.). viii, 288p. 242.75 (*3-8055-5006-5*) S Karger.

Airway Pressure Release Ventilation: A Systematic Experimental Approach. Peter Neumann. 2000. (Comprehensive Summaries of Uppsala Dissertations from the Faculty of Medicine Ser.: No. 929). (Illus.). 57p. pap. (*91-554-4723-6*) Uppsala Universitet SWE. *Dist:* Coronet Bks.

Airway Remodeling. Peter Howarth. 2000. LC 00-47596. (Lung Biology in Health & Disease Ser.: Vol. 155). (Illus.). xviii, 293p. text 175.00 (*0-8247-0448-7*) Dekker.

Airway Secretions. Ed. by Tamotsu Takishima & Sanae Shimura. 1994. (Lung Biology in Health & Disease Ser.: Vol. 72). (Illus.). 744p. text 255.00 (*0-8247-8843-5*) Dekker.

Airway Smooth Muscle: Mod of Receptors & Response. Ed. by Devendra K. Agrawal. 1990. 312p. lib. bdg. 202.00 (*0-8493-5904-X*, QP121) CRC Pr.

Airway Smooth Muscle in Health & Disease. R. F. Coburn. 1989. (Illus.). 834p. (C). text 89.50 (*0-306-43120-3*, Kluwer Plenum) Kluwer Academic.

Airway Wall Remodelling in Asthma. Ed. by Alastair G. Stewart. 1996. LC 96-13125. (Pharmacology & Toxicology Ser.). 600p. 169.95 (*0-8493-7813-3*) CRC Pr.

Airways: Neural Control in Health & Disease. Michael A. Kaliner & Peter J. Barnes. 1987. (Lung Biology in Health & Disease Ser.: Vol. 33). (Illus.). 688p. text 255.00 (*0-8247-7779-4*) Dekker.

Airways & Vascular Remodelling in Asthma & Cardiovascular Disease: Implications for Therapeutic Intervention. Ed. by Clive Page & Judith Black. 1994. (Illus.). 189p. text 87.00 (*0-12-543540-1*) Acad Pr.

Airways Hyperresponsiveness. C. P. Page & P. J. Gardiner. 1993. (Illus.). 352p. 145.00 (*0-632-03061-5*) Blackwell Sci.

Airways Smooth Muscle: Biochemical Control of Contraction & Relaxation. Ed. by David Raeburn & Mark A. Giembycz. 1994. LC 94-20775. (Respiratory Pharmacology & Pharmacotherapy Ser.). viii, 351p. 207.00 (*0-8176-5043-1*) Birkhauser.

Airways Smooth Muscle: Development, & Regulation of Contractility. Ed. by D. Raeburn & Mark A. Giembycz. 1994. LC 94-8800. (Research Reports in Physics). 350p. 219.50 (*0-8176-5011-3*) Spr-Verlag.

Airways Smooth Muscle: Modelling the Asthmatic Response in Vivo. Mark A. Giembycz. Ed. by D. Raeburn. 1996. 276p. 208.00 (*3-7643-5300-7*) Birkhauser.

Airways Smooth Muscle: Modelling the Asthmatic Response in Vivo. Mark A. Giembycz. Ed. by David Raeburn. 1996. (*0-8176-5300-7*) Birkhauser.

Airways Smooth Muscle: Neurotransmitters, Amines, Lipid Mediators, & Signal Transduction. Ed. by David Raeburn & Mark A. Giembycz. LC 95-19812. (Respiratory Pharmacology & Pharmacotherapy Ser.). 1996. 351p. 209.00 (*3-7643-5141-1*); 1995. 230.00 (*0-8176-5141-1*) Birkhauser.

Airways Smooth Muscle: Peptide Receptors, Ion Channels & Signal Transduction. 1995. (Respiratory Pharmacology & Pharmacotherapy Ser.). 288p. 169.00 (*3-7643-5140-3*) Birkhauser.

Airways Smooth Muscle: Peptide Receptors, Ion Channels & Signal Transduction. David Raeburn & Mark A. Giembycz. 1995. LC 94-48621. (Respiratory Pharmacology & Pharmacotherapy Ser.). (Illus.). 288p. 169.00 (*0-8176-5140-3*) Birkhauser.

Airways Smooth Muscle: Structure, Innervation & Neurotransmission. David Raeburn & Mark A. Giembycz. 1994. LC 94-11899. (Respiratory Pharmacology & Pharmacotherapy Ser.). 336p. 194.00 (*0-8176-5010-5*) Birkhauser.

AIT/Preceptor Program for Health Care Administration. Robert Hacker. 1991. 65.00 (*0-929442-26-1*, 2211PP) Prof Prnting & Pub.

AIUM Quality Assurance Manual for Gray-Scale Ultrasound Scanners: Stage 2. 1995. (Illus.). 61p. pap. 45.00 (*1-930047-22-3*, QA) Am Inst Ultrasound.

AIUM 2000 Proceedings. 2000. (Illus.). pap. (*1-930047-57-6*, OP00) Am Inst Ultrasound.

Akademie der Wissenschaften zu Berlin: Jahrbuch Yearbook, 1990-1992. 1993.Tr. of Academy of Sciences & Technology in Berlin. (GER., Illus.). xii, 814p. (C). lib. bdg. 198.50 (*3-11-013891-3*) De Gruyter.

Akathisia & Restless Legs. Perminder Sachdev. 1995. (Illus.). 441p. (C). text 100.00 (*0-521-44426-8*) Cambridge U Pr.

AKPAT - Allied Health Professions Admissions Test No. 2: Practice Examination. David M. Tarlow. 2nd rev. ed. 1999. 40p. (C). pap. text 18.95 (*1-57732-070-0*) Datar Pub.

Aktuelle Aspekte der Hormonalen Kontrazeption. Ed. by P. J. Keller. 1991. (GER., Illus.). 104p. pap. 39.25 (*3-8055-5264-5*) S Karger.

Aktuelle Aspekte der Perioperativen Ernahrung und Des Ernahrungsaufbaus. Ed. by K. H. Jauch. 2000. (Chirurgische Gastroenterologie Ser.). (GER.). 58p. pap. 36.50 (*3-8055-7067-8*) S Karger.

Aktuelle Entwicklung und Standard der kuenstlichen Ernaehrung. Ed. by R. Doelp & D. Loehlein. 1986. (Beitraege zur Infusionstherapie und Klinische Ernaehrung Ser.: Vol. 16). (GER., Illus.). viii, 156p. 50.50 (*3-8055-4353-0*) S Karger.

Aktuelle Klinische Zytologie. Ed. by U. E. Bonk. 1990. (Beitraege Zur Onkologie, Contributions to Oncology Ser.: Vol. 38). (GER., Illus.). x, 350p. 68.75 (*3-8055-5230-0*) S Karger.

Aktuelle Probleme der Haematologie und Onkologie. Ed. by W. Wilmanns & Reiner W. Hartenstein. 1982. (Beitraege Zur Onkologie, Contributions to Oncology Ser.: Vol. 13). (GER., Illus.). xii, 388p. pap. 68.75 (*3-8055-3506-6*) S Karger.

Aktuelle Probleme der Paediatrischen Hepatologie. Ed. by R. Landolt. 1977. (Paediatrische Fortbildungskurse fuer die Praxis Ser.: Band 44). (GER., Illus.). 17.50 (*3-8055-2662-8*) S Karger.

Aktueller Stand der Diagnostik und Therapie von Hodentumoren. Ed. by N. J. Jaeger & J. H. Hartlapp. 1990. (Beitraege Zur Onkologie, Contributions to Oncology Ser.: Vol. 40). (GER., Illus.). viii, 264p. 68.75 (*3-8055-5232-7*) S Karger.

***Akupunktur Fur Schwangerschaft, Geburt und Wochenbett: Entsprechend A. L. F. (Akupunktur Leitlinie Fur Frauenarzte) der Deutschen Gesellschaft Fur Gynakologie und Geburtshilfe.** Claus Schulte-Uebbing. 2000. (GER., Illus.). xiv, 264p. 39.00 (*3-11-016397-7*) De Gruyter.

Akute Pankreatitis. Ed. by E. Klar et al. 1999. (Chirurgische Gastroenterologie Ser.: Band 15, No. 4). (GER.). 104p. pap. 44.50 (*3-8055-6832-0*) S Karger.

Akute Periphere GefaBchirurgie see Acute Peripheral Vascular Surgery

Al-Aqrabadhin al-Saghir: Dispensatorium Parvum. Sabur ibn Sahl. 1994. LC 93-47287. (Islamic Philosophy, Theology & Science Ser.: Vol. 16). (ARA & ENG.). x, 260p. 134.00 (*90-04-10004-0*) Brill Academic Pubs.

Al-Insan Kallan wa-'Adlan. Jawdat Sa'id. 1993. (Taghyir al-Nafs wa-al-Mujtama Ser.). 64p. pap. 1.95 (*1-57547-042-X*) Dar Al-Fikr.

Al-Junun: Mental Illness in the Islamic World. Ed. by Ihsan Al-Issa et al. 2000. LC 99-41683. (Illus.). xv, 382p. 48.00 (*0-8236-3337-3*, 03337) Intl Univs Pr.

Alabama Health Care in Perspective 1999. Ed. by Kathleen O'Leary Morgan & Scott E. Morgan. 1999. 21p. spiral bd. 19.00 (*0-7401-0050-5*) Morgan Quitno Corp.

Alabama Health Care in Perspective 2000. Ed. by Kathleen O'Leary Morgan & Scott E. Morgan. 2000. 21p. spiral bd. 19.00 (*0-7401-0200-1*) Morgan Quitno Corp.

Alabama Health Care Perspective, 1998. Ed. by Kathleen O'Leary Morgan & Scott E. Morgan. 1998. 20p. pap. 19.00 (*1-56692-800-1*) Morgan Quitno Corp.

Alarming History of Famous & Difficult Patients: An Alarming History Maladies Malingerers. Richard Gordon. 1997. LC 96-44844. 224p. 20.95 (*0-312-15048-2*) St Martin.

Alarming History of Medicine. Richard Gordon. 1997. 256p. pap. 12.95 (*0-312-16763-6*) St Martin.

Alaryngeal Speech Rehabilitation: For Clinicians by Clinicians. Ed. by Shirley J. Salmon & Kay H. Mount. 1991. LC 90-9164. 286p. pap. text 31.00 (*0-89079-415-4*, 1817) PRO-ED.

Alaska Health Care in Perspective 2000. Ed. by Kathleen O'Leary Morgan & Scott E. Morgan. 2000. 21p. spiral bd. 19.00 (*0-7401-0201-X*) Morgan Quitno Corp.

Alaska Health Care Perspective, 1998. Ed. by Kathleen O'Leary Morgan & Scott E. Morgan. 1998. 20p. pap. 19.00 (*1-56692-801-X*) Morgan Quitno Corp.

Alaska's Search for a Killer: A Seafaring Medical Adventure 1946-1948. Susan Meredith. 1998. (Illus.). xv, 273p. pap. (*0-9659849-1-5*) Alaska Pub Hlth.

Alaska's Wilderness Medicines: Healthful Plants of the Far North. Eleanor Gl Viereck. 1994. LC 87-1427. (Illus.). 116p. pap. 10.95 (*0-88240-322-2*, Alaska NW Bks) Gr Arts Ctr Pub.

Alateen: A Day at a Time. Al-Anon Family Group Headquarters, Inc. Staff. 1983. LC 83-70348. 379p. 7.00 (*0-910034-53-2*) Al-Anon.

Alateen's Fourth Step Inventory. Al-Anon Family Group Headquarters, Inc. Staff. 1989. 48p. pap. 3.50 (*0-910034-60-5*) Al-Anon.

Albanian Escape: The True Story of U. S. Army Nurses Behind Enemy Lines. Agnes Jensen Mangerich et al. 1999. LC 98-48348. (Illus.). xiii, 220p. 25.00 (*0-8131-2109-4*) U Pr of KY.

Albany Medical Center Inaugural Theses, 1839-1891. Ed. by Mary E. Morrison. 1989. (Guide to the Microfiche Collection). 218p. 20.00 (*0-8357-0870-5*) Univ Microfilms.

Alba's Medical Technology Board Examination Review Vol. 1: Complete Clinical Laboratory Text. Ed. by James I. Mangels et al. 12th rev. ed. 1996. LC 72-172446. (Illus.). 747p. text 42.00 (*0-910224-18-8*) Berkeley Sci.

Alba's Medical Technology Board Examination Review Vol. 2: Questions & Answers. Ed. by James I. Mangels et al. 8th rev. ed. 1996. (Illus.). 550p. text 38.00 (*0-910224-19-6*) Berkeley Sci.

Albert Bandura: The Man & His Ideas - a Dialogue. Richard I. Evans. 1989. LC 89-32273. (Dialogues in Contemporary Psychology Ser.). 130p. 55.00 (*0-275-93352-0*, C3352, Praeger Pubs) Greenwood.

Albert Ellis. Joseph Yankura & Windy Dryden. 1994. (Key Figures in Counselling Ser.). 160p. pap. 21.50 (*0-8039-8529-0*, 9224) Sage.

Albert Ellis: Passionate Skeptic. Daniel N. Wiener. 1988. LC 87-22494. 220p. 62.00 (*0-275-92751-2*, C2751, Praeger Pubs) Greenwood.

Albert Schweitzer. Helen R. Neinast. 1989. pap. 2.95 (*0-687-60015-4*) Abingdon.

Albert Schweitzer: A Biography. George Marshall & David Poling. rev. ed. 1991. (Illus.). 346p. pap. text 4.00 (*1-881815-26-9*) Albert Schweitzer.

Albert Schweitzer Jubilee Book. Ed. by Abraham A. Roback. 1971. LC 79-97392. (Illus.). 508p. reprint ed. lib. bdg. 65.00 (*0-8371-2670-3*, ASJB, Greenwood Pr) Greenwood.

Alberta Infant Motor Scale (AIMS) Martha C. Piper & Johanna Darrah. 1994. (Illus.). 25.00 (*0-7216-4721-9*) Saunders.

Albumin & Systematic Circulation. Ed. by P. Lundsgaard-Hansen & B. Blauhut. 1986. (Current Studies in Hematology & Blood Transfusion: No. 53). (Illus.). xiv, 234p. 154.00 (*3-8055-4367-0*) S Karger.

Alchemist's Handbook. Frater Albertus. 1987. LC 74-21127. (Illus.). 128p. (Orig.). reprint ed. pap. 12.50 (*0-87728-655-8*) Red Wheel ME.

Alchemy of Health: Herbal Medicines & Herbal Aromatherapy. Amira A. Sravesh. 1998. LC 98-90646. 220p. pap. 20.00 (*0-9666688-0-4*) Amira Alchemy.

Alco-Calculator: An Educational Instrument. 1983. 4.95 (*0-911290-04-4*); 0.95 (*0-911290-16-8*) Rutgers Ctr Alcohol.

Alcohol, Vol. 2. N. S. Miller & M. S. Gold. 1991. LC 91-2391. (Drugs of Abuse: Vol. 2). (Illus.). 290p. (C). text 51.00 (*0-306-43641-8*, Kluwer Plenum) Kluwer Academic.

Alcohol: How Drinking Affects Health & Nutrition. Christina Dye. rev. ed. 2000. pap. 0.50 (*0-89230-191-0*) Do It Now.

Alcohol: Minimizing the Harm. Ed. by Martin A. Plant et al. 1997. 220p. (C). pap. (*1-85343-349-7*) Free Assoc Bks GBR. *Dist:* NYU Pr.

***Alcohol: Mode of Actions & Clinical Perspectives.** Ed. by A. Sun et al. 2001. (Journal of Biomedical Science: Vol. 8, No. 1). (Illus.). 150p. 39.25 (*3-8055-7192-5*) S Karger.

Alcohol: The Beloved Enemy. Jack Van Impe. 1980. 190p. pap. 7.00 (*0-934803-07-2*) J Van Impe.

Alcohol Abuse in Indians of North & South America: Cultural Difference in the Conflict with Western Civilization - Journal: Confinia Psychiatrica, Vol. 21, No. 4. 1979. (Illus.). pap. 10.50 (*3-8055-3043-9*) S Karger.

Alcohol Abuse Treatment. Ed. by Ronald R. Watson. 1992. LC 92-1569. (Drug & Alcohol Abuse Reviews Ser.: No. 3). (Illus.). 336p. 89.50 (*0-89603-242-6*) Humana.

Alcohol Addiction & Chronic Alcoholism. E. M. Jellinek. Ed. by Gerald N. Grob. 1981. LC 80-1272. (Addiction in America Ser.). reprint ed. lib. bdg. 37.95 (*0-405-13593-9*) Ayer.

Alcohol & Aggression: Proceedings of the Symposium on Alcohol & Aggression Held at the Center of Alcohol Studies, Rutgers University, October 1992. Ed. by Larissa A. Pohorecky et al. 1993. (Journal of Studies on Alcohol: Suppl. No. 11). 200p. pap. 26.95 (*0-911290-52-4*, AJS-106) Rutgers Ctr Alcohol.

Alcohol & Aging. Ed. by Thomas P. Beresford & Edith S. Gomberg. 1995. LC 94-32853. (Illus.). 360p. text 65.00 (*0-19-508090-4*) OUP.

Alcohol & Alcohol Problems. Edwards. 1994. text 95.00 (*0-443-05151-8*) Saunders.

Alcohol & Alcoholism: Effects on Brain & Development. Ed. by John H. Hannigan et al. 1999. LC 98-17719. (Illus.). xv, 282p. 69.95 (*0-8058-2686-6*) L Erlbaum Assocs.

Alcohol & Brain Development. James R. West. 1986. (Illus.). 456p. text 60.00 (*0-19-503706-5*) OUP.

Alcohol & Cancer. Ronald R. Watson. 1992. 288p. 125.00 (*0-8493-7938-5*, RC268) CRC Pr.

Alcohol & Cardiovascular Disease. Ed. by J. Veenstra & D. G. Van der Heij. 1992. 120p. (*90-220-1060-0*, PDC0600) Bernan Associates.

Alcohol & Cardiovascular Disease, Vol. 216. Timothy Peters. 1998. LC 98-27198. (Novartis Foundation Symposium Ser.). 280p. 125.00 (*0-471-97769-1*) Wiley.

Alcohol & Conflict. U. G. Ahlfors. 1969. 4.00 (*951-9192-06-9*) Rutgers Ctr Alcohol.

Alcohol & Disease. Ed. by Niels Tygstrup & Rolf Olsson. 1985. (Illus.). 290p. text 87.50 (*91-22-00786-5*) Coronet Bks.

Alcohol & Drug Abuse as Encountered in Office Practice. Frank L. Iber & Edward Hines, Jr. 1990. (Illus.). 336p. 110.00 (*0-8493-0166-1*, RC564) CRC Pr.

Alcohol & Drug Abuse Funding: An Analysis of Foundation Grants, 1983-1987. Foundation Center Staff. Ed. by Loren Renz. 1989. pap. text 45.00 (*0-87954-286-1*) Foundation Ctr.

Alcohol & Drug Abuse Handbook. Roland E. Herrington. 1987. (Allied Health Professions Monograph). 516p. 55.00 (*0-87527-274-6*) Green.

Alcohol & Drug Abuse in the Affluent. Ed. by Barry Stimmel. 1984. LC 84-19164. (Advances in Alcohol & Substance Abuse Ser.: Vol. 4, No. 2). 106p. text 3.95 (*0-86656-332-6*) Haworth Pr.

Alcohol & Drug Abuse in the Workplace: The Complete Resource Guide. 2nd ed. 1989. ring bd. 95.00 (*1-55871-143-0*, BSP 132) BNA PLUS.

Alcohol & Drug Wildcard: Substance Use & Psychiatric Problems in People with HIV. Joan E. Zweben & Patt Denning. 1998. LC 98-39293. (UCSF AIDS Health Project Monograph Ser.). 9.95 (*1-879168-02-2*) AIDS Hlth Project.

Alcohol & Drugs Are Women's Issues Vol. 1: A Review of the Issues. Ed. by Paula Roth. 1991. LC 90-49988. (Copublished with Women's Action Alliance Ser.). (Illus.). 202p. 37.50 (*0-8108-2360-8*) Scarecrow.

Alcohol & Health. 1991. lib. bdg. 250.00 (*0-8490-4373-5*) Gordon Pr.

Alcohol & Health: Seventh Special Report to the U. S. Congress. Louis W. Sullivan. 1997. (Illus.). 289p. (C). reprint ed. pap. text 50.00 (*0-7881-4183-X*) DIANE Pub.

Alcohol & Highway Safety: Proceedings of the North American Conference on Alcohol & Highway Safety. Ed. by T. B. Turner et al. 1985. (Journal of Studies on Alcohol: Suppl. No. 10). pap. 20.00 (*0-911290-17-6*) Rutgers Ctr Alcohol.

Alcohol & Hormones. Ed. by Ronald R. Watson. 1995. LC 94-38231. (Drug & Alcohol Abuse Reviews Ser.: Vol. 6). 352p. text 119.50 (*0-89603-290-6*) Humana.

Alcohol & Illness: Health & Society. Ed. by John Duffy. 1992. LC 92-224214. 224p. text (*0-7486-0353-0*) Edinburgh U Pr GBR. *Dist:* Col U Pr.

Alcohol & Longevity. Raymond Pearl. Ed. by Gerald N. Grob. 1981. LC 80-1245. (Addiction in America Ser.). (Illus.). reprint ed. lib. bdg. 32.95 (*0-405-13615-3*) Ayer.

Alcohol & Man: The Effects of Alcohol on Man in Health & Disease. Ed. by Haven Emerson & Gerald N. Grob. 1981. LC 80-1227. (Addiction in America Ser.). reprint ed. lib. bdg. 43.95 (*0-405-13585-8*) Ayer.

Alcohol & Neurobiology: Brain Development & Hormone Regulation. Ed. by Ronald R. Watson. 1992. 416p. 125.00 (*0-8493-7935-0*, QP801) CRC Pr.

Alcohol & Neurobiology: Receptors, Membranes/ Channels. Ronald R. Watson. 1992. 336p. 120.00 (*0-8493-7936-9*) CRC Pr.

Alcohol & Other Drugs. (Orig.). (YA). (gr. 6-12). pap. text 9.50 (*0-8359-0763-5*) Globe Fearon.

Alcohol & Other Drugs: Self Responsibility. Ruth C. Engs. 1987. (C). reprint ed. pap. text 22.95 (*0-89917-473-6*) Tichenor Pub.

Alcohol & Pregnancy: A Retrieval Index & Bibliography of the Fetal Alcohol Syndrome. Leslie P. Gartner. 1984. LC 84-11311. 80p. pap. text 35.00 (*0-910841-03-9*) Jen Hse Pub Co.

Alcohol & Reproduction: A Bibliography. Compiled by Ernest L. Abel. 1982. LC 82-6202. 219p. lib. bdg. 62.50 (*0-313-23474-4*, AAR/, Greenwood Pr) Greenwood.

Alcohol & Sexuality: Effects on the Physiological & Psychological Components. 1991. (Illus.). 72p. pap. text 40.00 (*1-57979-134-4*) DIANE Pub.

Alcohol & Sexuality: The Effects of Alcohol on Both the Physiological & the Psychological Components of Sexuality & Reproduction. 1992. (Illus.). 168p. (C). pap. text 30.00 (*1-56806-002-5*) DIANE Pub.

Alcohol & Sport. Robert D. Stainback. 1997. LC 96-48332. 232p. text 32.00 (*0-87322-531-7*, BSTA0531) Human Kinetics.

Alcohol & Substance Abuse in Adolescence. Ed. by Judith S. Brook et al. 1985. LC 84-29004. (Advances in Alcohol & Substance Abuse Ser.: Vol. 4, Nos. 3 & 4). 206p. text 49.95 (*0-86656-333-4*) Haworth Pr.

Alcohol & Substance Abuse in Women & Children. Barry Stimmel. 1986. LC 86-251. (Advances in Alcohol & Substance Abuse Ser.: Vol. 5, No. 3). 148p. 49.95 (*0-86656-575-2*) Haworth Pr.

Alcohol & the Addictive Brain: New Hope for Alcoholics from Biogenetic Research. Kenneth Blum & James E. Payne. 1991. LC 90-14144. 336p. 29.95 (*0-02-903701-8*) Free Pr.

Alcohol & the Brain. 1993. (Illus.). 87p. (Orig.). (C). pap. text 30.00 (*0-7881-0032-7*) DIANE Pub.

Alcohol & the Brain: Chronic Effects. Ed. by Ralph E. Tarter & David H. Van Thiel. 1985. LC 85-12068. (Illus.). 366p. (C). text 90.00 (*0-306-41998-X*, Kluwer Plenum) Kluwer Academic.

Alcohol & the Cardiovascular System. 1993. (Illus.). 86p. (Orig.). (C). pap. text 30.00 (*1-56806-418-7*) DIANE Pub.

Alcohol & the Community: A Systems Approach to Prevention. Harold D. Holder. 1998. LC 97-20455. (International Research Monographs in the Addictions). (Illus.). 197p. (C). text 74.95 (*0-521-59187-2*) Cambridge U Pr.

Alcohol & the Constitution of Man. Edward L. Youmans. Ed. by Gerald N. Grob. 1981. LC 80-1255. (Addiction in America Ser.). reprint ed. lib. bdg. 19.95 (*0-405-13625-0*) Ayer.

Alcohol & the Elderly: A Comprehensive Bibliography. Grace M. Barnes et al. 1980. LC 80-1786. 138p. lib. bdg. 59.00 (*0-313-22132-4*, BAE/, Greenwood Pr) Greenwood.

Alcohol & the Family: A Comprehensive Bibliography, 9. Compiled by Grace M. Barnes & Diane K. Augustino. 1987. LC 86-27112. (Bibliographies & Indexes in Sociology Ser.: No. 9). 474p. lib. bdg. 85.00 (*0-313-24782-X*, BFA/, Greenwood Pr) Greenwood.

Alcohol & the Family: Research & Clinical Perspectives. Ed. by R. Lorraine Collins et al. 1990. LC 89-37204. (Substance Abuse Ser.). 386p. 45.00 (*0-89862-169-0*) Guilford Pubns.

Alcohol & the Fetus: A Clinical Perspective. Henry L. Rosett & Lyn Weiner. 1984. LC 84-919. (Illus.). 220p. text 37.50 (*0-19-503458-9*) OUP.

Alcohol & the Gastrointestinal Tract. Ed. by Victor R. Preedy & Ronald R. Watson. 1995. LC 95-24883. 368p. 199.95 (*0-8493-2480-7*, 2480) CRC Pr.

Alcohol & the Mass Media. J. Partanen & M. Montonen. 1988. (Euro Reports & Studies Ser.: No. 108). 73p. pap. text 8.00 (*92-890-1274-9*) World Health.

Alcohol & the Media. 1996. LC 97-103195. (WHO Regional Publications, European Ser.: No. 62). 165p. pap. 35.10 (*92-890-1326-5*, 1310062) World Health.

Alcohol & Primary Health Care. 1996. LC 97-103282. (WHO Regional Publications, European Ser.: No. 64). 90p. pap. 20.00 (*92-890-1328-1*, 1310064) World Health.

Alcohol & the Workplace. 1996. LC 97-103184. (WHO Regional Publications, European Ser.: No. 67). 100p. pap. 20.70 (*92-890-1331-1*, 1310067) World Health.

Alcohol & Tobacco: From Basic Science to Clinical Practice. Ed. by Joanne B. Fertig & John P. Allen. 2000. (Illus.). 323p. (C). pap. text 35.00 (*0-7881-7004-X*) DIANE Pub.

Alcohol, Cell Membranes & Signal Transduction in Brain. C. Alling et al. 1993. (Illus.). 334p. (C). text 105.00 (*0-306-44583-2*, Kluwer Plenum) Kluwer Academic.

Alcohol, Cocaine & Accidents. Ed. by Ronald R. Watson. 1995. LC 94-45440. (Drug & Alcohol Abuse Reviews Ser.: Vol. 7). 224p. 99.50 (*0-89603-294-9*) Humana.

Alcohol Disabilities, & Rehabilitation. Susan A. Storti. 1997. LC 97-12959. (Illus.). 240p. pap. 34.95 (*1-56593-690-6*, 1340) Thomson Learn.

Alcohol Disabilities Primer: A Guide to Physical & Psychological Disabilities Caused by Alcohol Use. Bozena-Eva Robertson. 1993. LC 93-22609. 208p. lib. bdg. 69.95 (*0-8493-8966-6*, RC565, CRC Reprint) Franklin.

***Alcohol Drinking for Pleasure, Sickness, Disease, Reproductive Abnormalities & Cancer Liability: Index of New Information & Guide-Book for Reference & Research.** Ed. by Research and Development Division Staff & John C. Bartone. 2001. (Illus.). 180p. 47.50 (*0-7883-2338-5*); pap. 44.50 (*0-7883-2339-3*) ABBE Pubs Assn.

Alcohol, Drugs & Driving: Proceedings of the Satellite Symposium, Helsinki, July, 1975. Satellite Symposium on Alcohol, Drugs and Driving Staff. Ed. by Markku Mattila. 1976. (Modern Problems of Pharmacopsychiatry Ser.: Vol. 11). (Illus.). 150p. 42.75 (*3-8055-2349-1*) S Karger.

Alcohol, Drugs of Abuse, & Immune Functions. Ed. by Ronald R. Watson. 1995. (Physiology of Drug Abuse Ser.). 288p. 179.95 (*0-8493-8312-9*) CRC Pr.

Alcohol, Drugs of Abuse & Immunomodulation. Ronald R. Watson. 1993. (Advances in Biosciences Ser.: Vol. 86). 718p. 197.75 (*0-08-042038-9*, Pergamon Pr) Elsevier.

Alcohol Education & Offenders. Steve Baldwin. 1990. 144p. 29.95 (*0-7134-6244-2*) Trafalgar.

Alcohol Education & Young Offenders: Medium & Short Term Effectiveness of Education Programs. S. Baldwin. 1991. (Recent Research in Psychology Ser.). (Illus.). 152p. 79.95 (*0-387-97507-1*) Spr-Verlag.

Alcohol (Ethanol)—Its Adverse, Harmful & Delayed Health Damage Including Cancer: Index of New Information with References. ABBE Research Department Staff. 1999. 150p. 57.50 (*0-7883-2216-8*) ABBE Pubs Assn.

***Alcohol Home Detoxification & Assessment.** David B. Cooper. 1994. 144p. pap. (*1-85775-060-8*) Radcliffe Med Pr GBR. *Dist:* Balogh.

***Alcohol, Illicit Drugs & the Global Burden of Disease No. 3: Special Issue European Addiction Research 2001,**, 7. Ed. by J. Rehm & G. Gmel. 2001. (Illus.). 68p. pap. 25.25 (*3-8055-7290-5*) S Karger.

Alcohol in America: Taking Action to Prevent Abuse. Steve Olson et al. 1985. LC 85-13667. (Illus.). 125p. pap. 14.95 (*0-309-03449-3*) Natl Acad Pr.

Alcohol in Human Violence. Kai Pernanen. 1991. LC 91-16338. (Substance Abuse Ser.). 279p. 40.00 (*0-89862-171-2*) Guilford Pubns.

Alcohol, Infectious Diseases, & Immunity. 1993. (Illus.). 92p. (Orig.). (C). pap. text 30.00 (*1-56806-442-X*) DIANE Pub.

Alcohol Interactions with Drugs & Chemicals. Edward J. Calabrese. 1991. 96p. lib. bdg. 79.95 (*0-87371-403-2*, L403) Lewis Pubs.

Alcohol Interventions: Historical & Sociocultural Approaches. Ed. by David L. Strug et al. 1986. LC 85-16405. (Supplement to Alcoholism Treatment Quart Ser.: Vol. 1). 218p. text 49.95 (*0-86656-359-8*); pap. text 19.95 (*0-86656-426-8*) Haworth Pr.

Alcohol Intoxication: Psychiatric, Psychological, Forensic Issues. Eric W. Fine. 1996. 156p. (Orig.). pap. text 30.00 (*0-935645-07-1*) AJFP.

Alcohol - Less Is Better. 1996. (WHO Regional Publications, European Ser.: No. 70). 39p. pap. 17.10 (*92-890-1334-6*, 1310070) World Health.

Alcohol, Medications, & Older Adults: A Guide for Families & Other Caregivers. Charles Vandeputte. 1991. 44p. pap. 4.95 (*1-56246-010-2*, 3262, HazeldenJohnson Inst) Hazelden.

Alcohol Metabolism & Alcoholism: The Role of Enzymes. Ed. by J. P. Von Wartburg. 1987. (Enzyme Ser.: Vol. 37, No. 1-2, 1987). (Illus.). 108p. pap. 68.00 (*3-8055-4551-7*) S Karger.

Alcohol on Immunity & Cancer. Raz Yirmiya. 1992. 320p. lib. bdg. 189.00 (*0-8493-5761-6*, RC268) CRC Pr.

Alcohol Patterns & Problems. Marc A. Schuckit. 1985. (Psychosocial Epidemiology Ser.: Vol. 5). 240p. (C). pap. text 15.00 (*0-8135-1061-9*) Rutgers U Pr.

Alcohol Poisoning Mortality in Four Nordic Countries. Kari Poikolainen. 1977. (Finnish Foundation for Alcohol Studies: Vol. 28). 8.00 (*951-9191-47-X*) Rutgers Ctr Alcohol.

Alcohol Policies. Ed. by M. Grant. 1985. (WHO Regional Publications, European Ser.: No. 18). (ENG & RUS.). 153p. pap. text 19.00 (*92-890-1109-2*, 1310018) World Health.

Alcohol, Pregnancy & the Developing Child. Ed. by Hans-Ludwig Spohr & Hans-Christoph Steinhausen. 1996. (Illus.). 325p. (C). text 85.00 (*0-521-56426-3*) Cambridge U Pr.

Alcohol Problem Intervention in the Workplace: Employee Assistance Programs & Strategic Alternatives. Ed. by Paul M. Roman. 1990. LC 89-27239. 432p. 90.00 (*0-89930-459-1*, RAD/, Quorum Bks) Greenwood.

Alcohol Problems among Adolescents: Current Directions in Prevention Research. Ed. by Gayle M. Boyd et al. 1995. 264p. text 39.95 (*0-8058-1915-0*) L Erlbaum Assocs.

Alcohol Problems & Alcohol Control in Europe. Phil Davies & Dermot Walsh. 1983. 320p. 31.95 (*0-89876-090-9*) Gardner Pr.

Alcohol Problems & Alcoholism: A Comprehensive Survey. James E. Royce. 2nd rev. ed. 1989. 480p. 35.00 (*0-02-927541-5*) Free Pr.

Alcohol Problems & Treatment: Follow-Up Studies of Problem-Drinkers with Special Reference to Drinking Behaviour. Fanny Duckert. 1993. 154p. (Orig.). pap. 47.50 (*82-7171-166-0*) Coronet Bks.

Alcohol Problems of Minority Youth in America: A Sociological Study in Causes, Treatment & Prevention. Ed. by Roosevelt Wright & Thomas D. Watts. 1990. LC 89-12508. (Interdisciplinary Studies in Alcohol & Drug Use & Abuse: Vol. 2). 232p. lib. bdg. 89.95 (*0-88946-297-6*) E Mellen.

Alcohol-Related Medicosocial Problems & Their Prevention. D. Walsh. 1982. (Public Health in Europe Ser.: No. 17). 87p. pap. text 8.00 (*92-890-1153-X*) World Health.

Alcohol-Related Problems in High Risk Groups. M. Plant. 1989. (Euro Reports & Studies Ser.: No. 109). 122p. pap. text 11.00 (*92-890-1275-7*) World Health.

Alcohol, Science & Society. Yale University Center of Alcohol Studies Staff. 1972. LC 72-4688. 473p. reprint ed. lib. bdg. 35.00 (*0-8371-6435-4*, ALSS, Greenwood Pr) Greenwood.

Alcohol, Tobacco & Other Drugs May Harm the Unborn. Paddy S. Cook et al. Ed. by Tineke B. Haase. 1993. 80p. (Orig.). (C). pap. text 20.00 (*1-56806-548-5*) DIANE Pub.

Alcohol Tolerance & Social Drinking: Learning the Consequences. Muriel Vogel-Sprott. 1992. LC 91-35422. (Substance Abuse Ser.). 221p. 35.00 (*0-89862-191-7*) Guilford Pubns.

***Alcohol Use.** Ed. by David B. Cooper. 2000. 312p. pap. (*1-85775-121-3*) Radcliffe Med Pr GBR. *Dist:* Balogh.

Alcohol Use - Abuse among Latinos: Issues & Examples of Culturally Competent Services. Ed. by Melvin Delgado. 1998. LC 97-46407. (Alcohol Treatment Quarterly Monograph: Vol. 16, Nos. 1-2). 208p. pap. 24.95 (*0-7890-0500-X*) Haworth Pr.

Alcohol Withdrawal Treatment Manual. Paolo B. DePetrillo & Mark K. McDonough. 1999. LC 00-301258. (Alcohol & Drug Abuse Treatment Ser.: No. 1). xii, 244p. 75.00 (*0-9661673-0-9*) Focused Treat.

Alcohol/Drug Dependant Women: New Insights into Their Problems, Treatment, & Recovery. Sheila B. Blume. 1988. pap. 4.95 (*0-935908-45-5*, 3273, HazeldenJohnson Inst) Hazelden.

Alcoholic Beverages - Health Effects & Risks: Index of New Information. Alice J. Jacobs. 1998. 160p. pap. 47.50 (*0-7883-1865-9*) ABBE Pubs Assn.

Alcoholic Beverages-Health Effects & Risks: Index of New Information. Alice J. Jacobs. 1998. 160p. 57.50 (*0-7883-1864-0*) ABBE Pubs Assn.

Alcoholic Inebriety from a Medical Standpoint. Joseph Parrish. Ed. by Gerald N. Grob. 1981. LC 80-1243. (Addiction in America Ser.). reprint ed. lib. bdg. 19.95 (*0-405-13613-7*) Ayer.

Alcoholic Man: What You Can Learn from the Heroic Journeys of Recovering Alcoholics. Sylvia Cary & Jokichi Takamine. 1991. 216p. pap. 9.95 (*0-929923-39-1*) Lowell Hse.

Alcoholic Patient: Emergency Medical Intervention. David Fassler. 1991. LC 87-21108. 196p. (C). text 29.95 (*0-89876-130-1*) Gardner Pr.

Alcoholic Psychoses in Finland. K. A. Achte et al. 1969. (Finnish Foundation for Alcohol Studies: Vol. 19). 4.00 (*951-9192-08-5*) Rutgers Ctr Alcohol.

Alcoholic Society: Addiction & Recovery of the Self. Norman K. Denzin. 1993. LC 92-35675. 355p. (C). pap. text 29.95 (*1-56000-669-2*) Transaction Pubs.

Alcoholics Anonymous. Ed. by Alcoholics Anonymous World Services, Inc., Staff. 1991. (TUR.). 9.90 (*0-916856-36-4*) AAWS.

Alcoholics Anonymous. Alcoholics Anonymous World Services, Inc., Staff. 1990. (CHI.). (*0-916856-35-6*) AAWS.

Alcoholics Anonymous. Ed. by Alcoholics Anonymous World Services, Inc., Staff. 1990. (ARA.). pap. 4.00 (*0-916856-34-8*) AAWS.

Alcoholics Anonymous. Alcoholics Anonymous World Services, Inc., Staff. 1989. (RUS.). 181p. pap. 2.75 (*0-916856-25-9*); 1939. LC 76-4029. 400p. 3.60 (*0-916856-00-3*) AAWS.

Alcoholics Anonymous Comes of Age: A Brief History of Alcoholic Anonymous. Alcoholics Anonymous World Services, Inc., Staff. 1957. LC 57-10949. 333p. 3.70 (*0-916856-02-X*) AAWS.

Alcoholism. Ed. by H. N. Barnes et al. 1989. (Frontiers of Primary Care Ser.). (Illus.). 231p. 68.95 (*0-387-96545-9*) Spr-Verlag.

Alcoholism. Kathleen Ross. 1993. 32p. pap. 1.00 (*0-87784-090-3*) InterVarsity.

Alcoholism: A Matter of Choice: A Twenty First Century View of Addiction. Jim Hewitt. 1999. LC 97-27008. 250p. 29.95 (*0-87047-107-4*) Schenkman Bks Inc.

Alcoholism: A Merry-Go-Round Named Denial. Joseph L. Kellermann. 1975. 20p. (Orig.). pap. 2.00 (*0-89486-022-4*, 1140) Hazelden.

Alcoholism: A Molecular Perspective. Ed. by T. Norman Palmer. 1991. (NATO Advanced Science Institutes Ser.: Vol. 206). (Illus.). 376p. (C). text 138.00 (*0-306-43926-3*, Kluwer Plenum) Kluwer Academic.

Alcoholism: A Perspective. Ed. by Tyner & F. S. Messiha. 1980. LC 80-80209. 512p. 49.95 (*0-915340-02-X*) PJD Pubns.

Alcoholism: A Source Book for the Priest. rev. ed. 2000. 408p. 29.95 (*0-912141-89-1*) Roman Cath Bks.

Alcoholism: A Source Guide. 1991. lib. bdg. 250.00 (*0-8490-4908-3*) Gordon Pr.

Alcoholism: A Treatment Manual. Wayne Poley et al. 1979. LC 78-13455. text 25.00 (*0-89876-063-1*) Gardner Pr.

Alcoholism: Biomedical & Genetic Aspects. H. Werner Goedde & Dharam P. Agarwal. 1989. (Illus.). 376p. 67.00 (*0-08-035763-6*, Pergamon Pr) Elsevier.

Alcoholism: Causes, Effects, & Treatment. Joseph F. Perez. 1992. LC 92-53191. 312p. pap. text 23.95 (*1-55959-039-4*) Accel Devel.

Alcoholism: The Curse, the Causes & the "Cures" William A. Sanderson. 1985. LC 85-70769. (Illus.). 180p. (Orig.). pap. 12.95 (*0-9614833-0-X*) Azure Zephyr.

Alcoholism: Treatment, Vol. 2. Cedric M. Smith. 1980. (Alcohol Research Review Ser.). 107p. reprint ed. 30.95 (*0-87705-968-3*, Kluwer Acad Hman Sci) Kluwer Academic.

Alcoholism - a Terminal Disease. Richard Kay. 1989. (C). text (*0-902662-92-9*) R K Pubns GBR. *Dist:* St Mut.

Alcoholism - The Genetic Inheritance. Kathleen W. Fitzgerald. rev. ed. (Illus.). 234p. reprint ed. pap. 14.95 (*1-882195-01-9*) Whales Tale Pr.

Alcoholism, a Multidisciplinary Approach: Proceedings of the Symposium on Alcoholism, Amsterdam, May 1978. Alcoholism Symposium Staff. Ed. by Julien Mendlewicz & Herman M. Van Praag. 1979. (Advances in Biological Psychiatry Ser.: Vol. 3). (Illus.). pap. 48.00 (*3-8055-2977-5*) S Karger.

Alcoholism & Aging: Advances in Research. Ed. by W. Gibson Wood & Merrill F. Elias. 1982. 240p. 92.00 (*0-8493-5832-9*, HV5138) CRC Pr.

Alcoholism & Depression. Sheila B. Blume. 1984. 32p. pap. 3.50 (*0-935908-25-0*, 3256, HazeldenJohnson Inst) Hazelden.

Alcoholism & Drug Abuse in the Workplace: Managing Care & Costs Through Employee Assistance Programs. Walter F. Scanlon. 2nd ed. 1991. LC 90-49202. 208p. 55.00 (*0-275-93675-9*, C3675); pap. 17.95 (*0-275-93676-7*, B3676) Greenwood (Praeger Pubs).

Alcoholism & Drug Addiction. Raistrick. 1986. text 53.00 (*0-443-03092-8*) Saunders.

Alcoholism & Homosexuality. Ed. by Thomas O. Ziebold & John E. Mongeon. 1982. LC 82-9217. (Journal of Homosexuality Ser.: Vol. 7, No. 4). 107p. text 39.95 (*0-917724-93-3*) Haworth Pr.

Alcoholism & Human Sexuality. Gary G. Forrest. 1994. LC 94-37991. (Master Work Ser.). 412p. pap. text 50.00 (*1-56821-404-9*) Aronson.

Alcoholism & Other Drug Problems. James E. Royce & David Scratchley. 1996. LC 95-44546. (Illus.). 400p. 35.00 (*0-684-82314-4*) Free Pr.

Alcoholism & Pathological Gambling: Similarities & Differences. Arthur G. Herscovitch. 1999. LC 00-551466. 166p. pap. 21.95 (*1-55691-146-7*, 467) Learning Pubns.

Alcoholism & Problem Drinking: Treating Addiction or Modifying Bad Habits? J. C. Clarke. 1988. 152p. text 24.51 (*0-08-034432-1*); pap. text 28.00 (*0-08-034433-X*) Elsevier (Pergamon Pr).

Alcoholism & Related Problems: Issues for the American People. Ed. by Louis J. West. 1984. LC 84-13451. 224p. pap. 6.95 (*0-13-021478-7*) Am Assembly.

Alcoholism & Sexual Dysfunction: Issues in Clinical Management. Ed. by David J. Powell. 1984. LC 89-1998. (Alcoholism Treatment Quarterly Ser.: Vol. 1, No. 3). 145p. text 49.95 (*0-86656-365-2*) Haworth Pr.

Alcoholism & Substance Abuse in Special Populations. Gary W. Lawson & Ann W. Lawson. 1992. LC 88-7600. 390p. (C). 79.00 (*0-8342-0007-4*) PRO-ED.

Alcoholism & the Family. Saturo Saitoh et al. 1992. LC 90-2644. 324p. text 28.95 (*0-87630-626-1*) Brunner-Routledge.

***Alcoholism & the Family: A Guide to Treatment & Prevention.** Gary Lawson. 1988. tchr. ed. (*0-8342-1279-X*) PRO-ED.

Alcoholism & the Family: A Guide to Treatment & Prevention. Gary Lawson & Ann W. Lawson. 2nd ed. 1998. LC 97-51270. 400p. pap. 48.00 (*0-8342-1058-4*) PRO-ED.

Alcoholism As a Medical Problem. Ed. by H. D. Kruse & Gerald N. Grob. 1981. LC 80-1266. (Addiction in America Ser.). reprint ed. lib. bdg. 16.95 (*0-405-13600-5*) Ayer.

Alcoholism Chemical Dependency & the College Student. Intro. by Timothy M. Rivinus. LC 88-9443. (Journal of College Student Psychotherapy Ser.: Vol. 2, Nos. 3-4). (Illus.). 257p. (Orig.). 1995. pap. text 14.95 (*0-86656-812-3*); 1988. text 49.95 (*0-86656-734-8*) Haworth Pr.

Alcoholism Counselor. Jack Rudman. 1994. (Career Examination Ser.: C-2145). pap. 29.95 (*0-8373-2145-X*) Nat Learn.

Alcoholism Facts Explored. Gary Stone. 1984. (Illus.). 164p. spiral bd. 15.95 (*0-930427-00-9*) G Stone Servs.

Alcoholism for Beginners. David Berger. 1994. (Illus.). 176p. pap. 9.95 (*0-86316-163-4*) Writers & Readers.

Alcoholism in the United States: Racial & Ethnic Considerations. Committee on Cultural Psychiatry & Group for the Advancement of Psychiatry Staff. 1996. LC 95-49241. (Group for the Advancement of Psychiatry Ser.: No. 141). 142p. text 26.00 (*0-87318-209-X*, 7209) Am Psychiatric.

Alcoholism, Narcissism & Psychopathology. Gary G. Forrest. 1994. LC 94-34542. 324p. pap. text 50.00 (*1-56821-377-8*) Aronson.

Alcoholism Problems: Selected Issues. Sidney Cohen. 1983. LC 83-179. 193p. text 6.95 (*0-86656-209-5*); pap. text 3.95 (*0-86656-179-X*) Haworth Pr.

Alcoholism Programs in Industry: The Patient's View. Margaret M. Heyman. 1978. LC 77-620066. (Monographs: No. 12). 7.50 (*0-911290-45-1*) Rutgers Ctr Alcohol.

Alcoholism Rehabilitation: Methods & Experiences of Private Rehabilitation Centers. Ed. by Vincent Groupe. 1978. LC 78-620026. (NIAAA-RUCAS Alcoholism Treatment Ser.: No. 3). pap. 6.00 (*0-911290-49-4*) Rutgers Ctr Alcohol.

Alcoholism Rehabilitation Consultant. Jack Rudman. 1994. (Career Examination Ser.: C-2772). pap. 29.95 (*0-8373-2772-5*) Nat Learn.

Alcoholism Sourcebook: Basic Consumer Health Information about the Physical & Mental Consequences of Alcohol Abuse... Ed. by Karen Bellenir. 2000. LC 00-34024. (Health Reference Ser.). (Illus.). xiii, 613p. lib. bdg. 78.00 (*0-7808-0325-6*) Omnigraphics Inc.

Alcoholism Syndrome in Finland. P. Kiviranta. 1969. (Finnish Foundation for Alcohol Studies: Vol. 17). 5.50 (*951-9192-07-7*) Rutgers Ctr Alcohol.

Alcoholism Treatment: Context, Process, & Outcome. Rudolf H. Moos et al. 1990. (Illus.). 304p. text 49.95 (*0-19-504362-6*) OUP.

Alcoholism Treatment for Impaired Drivers: An Evaluation. Paul C. Whitehead et al. 1990. LC 90-6104. (Interdisciplinary Studies in Alcohol & Drug Use & Abuse: Vol. 3). 150p. lib. bdg. 69.95 (*0-88946-284-4*) E Mellen.

Alcoholism Treatment Matching Research: Methodological & Clinical Approaches. Dennis M. Donovan & Margaret E. Mattson. 1994. (Journal of Studies on Alcohol: Suppl. No. 12). pap. 26.95 (*0-911290-53-2*, AJS-107) Rutgers Ctr Alcohol.

Aldicarb. 1991. (Environmental Health Criteria Ser.: No. 121). (ENG, FRE & SPA.). 130p. pap. text 26.00 (*92-4-157121-7*, 1160121) World Health.

Aleen Cust Veterinary Surgeon: Britain's First Woman Vet. Connie M. Ford. 1990. (Illus.). 109p. pap. (*0-948737-11-5*) Biopress GBR. *Dist:* Balogh.

Alexander A. Potebnja's Psycholinguistic Theory of Literature: A Metacritical Inquiry. John Fizer. 1990. LC 87-80688. (Harvard Ukrainian Research Institute Monograph Ser.). (Illus.). 164p. (C). text 19.95 (*0-916458-16-4*) Harvard Ukrainian.

Alexander Technique. Jeremy Chance. 2001. (Illus.). pap. (*0-00-711035-9*) Thorsons GBR. *Dist:* Natl Bk Netwk.

Alexander Technique: A Complete Course in How to Hold & Use Your Body for Maximum Energy. John Gray. 5th ed. 1991. LC 91-19993. (Illus.). 176p. (Orig.). pap. 13.95 (*0-312-06494-2*) St Martin.

Alexander Technique: An Introductory Guide to the Technique & Its Benefits. Chris Stevens. 1997. (Illus.). 128p. pap. (*0-09-180979-7*) Random GBR. *Dist:* Trafalgar.

Alexander's Care of the Patient in Surgery. Edythe Louise Alexander et al. 11th ed. 1999. LC 98-37345. 1248p. 68.00 (*0-323-00134-3*) Mosby Inc.

Alexander's Care of the Patient in Surgery: Includes Testbank. Margaret H. Meeker & Jane C. Rothrock. 11th ed. 1998. (Illus.). tchr. ed. (*0-323-00135-1*) Mosby Inc.

Alexis Carrel: The Perfectibility of Man. David Le Voy. unabr. ed. 1996. (Illus.). 402p. 79.50 (*1-57529-022-7*) Kabel Pubs.

Alexis Carrel: Visionary Surgeon. W. Sterling Edwards & Peter D. Edwards. 1974. (Illus.). 160p. 19.95 (*0-398-03130-4*) C C Thomas.

Alex's Journey: The Story of a Child with a Brain Tumor. 1994. (*0-944093-29-9*) Am Brain Tumor.

Alfred Adler: As We Remember Him. Ed. by Genevieve Painter et al. 2nd ed. 1998. (Illus.). 122p. reprint ed. pap. (*0-926164-00-7*) N Am Soc Adlerian.

Alfred Adler, the Forgotten Prophet: A Vision for the 21st Century. Loren Grey. 1998. LC 97-40885. 168p. 58.00 (*0-275-96072-2*, Praeger Pubs) Greenwood.

Alfred Adler's Basic Concepts & Implications. Robert W. Lundin. 1989. LC 88-71464. 166p. (Orig.). pap. text 18.95 (*0-915202-83-2*) Accel Devel.

Algebra of Conscience. Vladimir A. Lefebvre. 1982. 224p. text 126.50 (*90-277-1301-4*) Kluwer Academic.

Algebraic Mind: Integrating Connectionism & Cognitive Science. Gary F. Marcus. 2000. LC 00-38029. (Learning, Development & Conceptual Change Ser.). (Illus.). xiii, 224p. (C). pap. 27.95 (*0-262-13379-2*, Bradford Bks) MIT Pr.

Algebras in Genetics. A. Woerz-Busekros. 1980. (Lecture Notes in Biomathematics: Vol. 36). 237p. 27.00 (*0-387-09978-6*) Spr-Verlag.

Algodystrophy. P. Doury et al. 1981. (Illus.). 165p. 166.00 (*0-387-10624-3*) Spr-Verlag.

Algorithm for the Identification of Hemoglobin Variants: Proposed Guidelines (1997) 1997. 25.00 (*1-56238-327-2*, H33-P) NCCLS.

Algorithmic Approach to Treatment. R. Douglas Collins. 1997. LC 96-49629. 600p. (*0-89640-336-X*); 568p. pap. text (*0-89640-291-6*) Igaku-Shoin.

Algorithmic Approach to Treatment. R. Douglas Collins. 1997. LC 96-49629. 640p. pap. 45.00 (*0-683-30303-1*) Lppncott W & W.

Algorithmic Diagnosis of Symptoms & Signs: Cost Effective Approach. R. Douglas Collins. 1995. LC 95-1040. 616p. pap. 45.00 (*0-89640-283-5*) Igaku-Shoin.

Algorithmic Selection & Interpretation of Diagnostic Tests. R. Douglas Collins. 1997. LC 97-31730. 744p. 45.00 (*0-683-30426-7*) Lppncott W & W.

Algorithms for Rational Prescribing in the Critically Ill. Neal Evans & G. R. Park. 1997. LC 97-11638. (*0-632-04916-2*, Blackwell Hlthcare) Blackwell Sci.

Algorithms in Chemical Pathology. Martin Crook. 1997. LC 97-26208. (Illus.). 128p. pap. text (*0-7506-2780-8*) E A GBR. *Dist:* OUP.

Alienations in Perversions. R. Khan & M. Masud. 1977. LC 76-46811. 246p. (C). 37.50 (*0-8236-0135-8*) Intl Univs Pr.

Aliens & Alienists: Ethnic Minorities & Psychiatry. Ronald Littlewood & Maurice Lipsedge. 2nd ed. 1989. 256p. 40.00 (*0-04-445317-5*); pap. 15.95 (*0-04-445316-7*) Routledge.

Alignment: A Provider's Guide to Managing the Practice of Health Care. Paul A. Sommers. 1999. LC 98-39594. (Haworth Marketing Resources Ser.). (Illus.). xii, 331p. 49.95 (*0-7890-0635-9*) Haworth Pr.

Alimentary Tract. Ed. by Basil C. Morson. 3rd ed. 1987. (Symmers Systemic Pathology Ser.: Vol. 3). (Illus.). 472p. text (*0-443-03095-2*) Church.

Alimentation Clinique des Petits Animaux, No. III. Lon D. Lewis et al. Tr. by Philippe Moreau from ENG. 3rd ed. 1989. (Illus.). 470p. (C). 18.00 (*0-945837-00-3*) M Morris Assocs.

Alimentos Que Eliminan la Artritis. Lauri M. Aesoph. 2000. (SPA.). 365p. pap. 14.00 (*0-7352-0193-5*) PH Pr.

Aliphatic, Alicyclic, & Saturated Heterocyclic Chemistry: 1970-1971 Literature, Pt. 1. Ed. by W. Parker. 1973. LC 72-83454. 29.00 (*0-85186-502-X*) Am Chemical.

Aliphatic Derivatives. Vassil St. Georgiev. 1982. (Survey of Drug Research in Immunologic Disease Ser.: Vol. 1). (Illus.). x, 542p. 426.25 (*3-8055-3503-1*) S Karger.

Alive & Well: A Path of Healing in a Time of HIV. Peter A. Hendrickson. 1990. (Illus.). 150p. 24.95 (*0-8290-2450-6*); pap. 19.95 (*0-8290-2475-1*); pap. 12.95 (*0-8290-2460-3*) Irvington.

Alive & Well? A Research & Policy Review of Health Programs for Poor Young Children. Lorraine V. Klerman. 1991. LC 90-20002. (Illus.). 132p. (Orig.). pap. 11.95 (*0-926582-02-X*) NCCP.

Alive & Well in the Fast Lane. Carolyn Coats & Pamela Smith. 1987. (Illus.). 156p. pap. 10.00 (*1-878722-03-4*) C Coats Bestsellers.

***Alive at 25: How I'm Beating Cystic Fibrosis.** Andy Lipman. 2002. 256p. 24.95 (*1-56352-681-6*) Longstreet.

Alkaloids: Biochemistry, Ecology & Medicinal Applications. M. F. Roberts & M. Wink. 1998. LC 98-17602. (Illus.). 452p. (C). text 115.00 (*0-306-45465-3*, Kluwer Plenum) Kluwer Academic.

Alkaloids Vol. 48: Chemistry & Pharmacology. Ed. by Geoffrey A. Cordell. 1996. (Illus.). 374p. text 99.95 (*0-12-469548-5*) Acad Pr.

Alkaloids Vol. 49: Chemistry & Pharmacology, Vol. 49. Ed. by Geoffrey A. Cordell. 1997. (Illus.). 405p. text 120.00 (*0-12-469549-3*) Morgan Kaufmann.

Alkalosis—Index of New Information & Medical Bible of Research. Timmy R. Laforre. 1994. 150p. pap. 47.50 (*0-7883-0089-X*) ABBE Pubs Assn.

Alkohol, Tabak und Drogen im Leben des jungen Mannes. Ed. by G. Ritzel. 1976. (Sozialmedizinische und Paedagogische Jugendkunde Ser.: Band 14). (Illus.). 42.75 (*3-8055-2381-5*) S Karger.

Alkoholkonsum und Alkoholismus als didaktisches Problem. F. Kicherer. 1980. (Psychologische Praxis Ser.: Band 54). (Illus.). vi, 146p. pap. 25.25 (*3-8055-0957-X*) S Karger.

Alkylphosphocholines: New Drugs in Cancer Therapy. Ed. by H. Eibl et al. 1992. (Progress in Experimental Tumor Research Ser.: Vol. 34). (Illus.). x, 174p. 161.00 (*3-8055-5464-8*) S Karger.

All About A. D. D. Understanding Attention Deficit Disorder. Mark Selikowitz. 1995. (Illus.). 208p. pap. text 24.95 (*0-19-553684-3*) OUP.

All about A. D. H. D. Linda Pfiffner. 1996. pap. 16.95 (*0-590-25108-2*) Scholastic Inc.

All about AIDS. Jay S. Roth. 1989. xviii, 300p. (C). pap. text 49.00 (*3-7186-0488-4*) Gordon & Breach.

All about Arthritis. Derrick Brewerton. (Illus.). (C). 1995. 328p. pap. 15.95 (*0-674-01616-5*); 1992. LC 92-11557. 320p. text 29.95 (*0-674-01615-7*) HUP.

All about Asthma: Stop Suffering & Start Living. Irwin J. Polk. 1997. LC 96-49124. (Illus.). 252p. (C). 27.95 (*0-306-45569-2*, Plen Insight) Perseus Pubng.

All about Asthma & Its Treatment Without Drugs. David Potterton. 1996. (All about Ser.). 96p. pap. text (*0-572-02153-4*) W Foulsham GBR. *Dist:* Trans-Atl Phila.

All about Birth Control. Planned Parenthood Federation Staff. 1998. LC 98-13643. (Illus.). 352p. pap. 12.00 (*0-517-88506-9*) Random Hse Value.

***All about Breast Cancer.** Fred Stephens. 2001. (Illus.). 160p. (Orig.). pap. text 19.95 (*0-19-551396-7*) OUP.

All about Cancer. Jay S. Roth. 1985. LC 85-50. (Illus.). 341p. (Orig.). text 24.95 (*0-397-53068-4*) Lppncott W & W.

All about Child Care. Marilyn Segal. rev. ed. 1991. (Illus.). 155p. pap. text 16.95 (*1-879744-00-7*) Nova U Fam Ctr.

All about Childbirth: A Manual for Prepared Childbirth. Alice T. MacMahon. 4th ed. 1994. LC 94-27717. (Illus.). 208p. pap. 6.95 (*0-931128-04-8*) Family Pubns.

All about Hip Replacement: A Patient's Guide. Richard Trahair. 1998. LC 99-160758. (Illus.). 192p. pap. text 21.95 (*0-19-554112-X*) OUP.

***All about Joints: A User's Guide.** Irwin M. Siegel. 2001. 224p. pap. 19.95 (*1-888799-56-0*) Demos Medical.

All about Me... A Personal Emergency Medical Guide. 1998. 26p. wbk. ed. 9.95 (*0-9672076-0-6*) K S H Pubns.

All about Muscle: An Owner's Manual. Irwin M. Siegel. 2000. LC 00-35860. 224p. pap. 19.95 (*1-888799-42-0*) Demos Medical.

All about Prostate Cancer. Fred Stephens. 2001. (Illus.). 152p. pap. 19.95 (*0-19-551404-1*) OUP.

All about Raising Children. Helen Andelin. 1981. 410p. 18.00 (*0-911094-07-5*) Pacific Santa Barbara.

All about Sex Therapy. Peter R. Kilmann & Katherine H. Mills. 1983. LC 82-2257. (Illus.). 228p. (C). 18.95 (*0-306-41317-5*, Plenum Trade) Perseus Pubng.

All-American Medical Hall of Fame: Recognition by U. S. States & Medical Specialties of American Physicans from the Past. Hollister S. Smith. Ed. by Hollister S. Smith. unabr. ed. 1996. LC 95-924188. (Illus.). 153p. (Orig.). pap. 24.95 (*0-9650659-3-6*, 1000) An All American.

All Creatures Great & Small. James Herriot. 1998. LC 72-79632. 448p. reprint ed. mass mkt. 7.99 (*0-312-96578-8*, Tor Books) T Doherty Assocs.

All God's Mistakes: Genetic Counseling in a Pediatric Hospital. Charles L. Bosk. 1992. LC 91-36938. 222p. 27.50 (*0-226-06681-9*) U Ch Pr.

All I Want Is a Good Night's Sleep. Sonia Ancoli-Israel. 1996. LC 96-201. (Illus.). 144p. (C). (gr. 13). pap. text 9.95 (*0-8151-4843-7*, 26864) Mosby Inc.

All-in-One Guide to ADD & Hyperactivity. Elvis Ali et al. 2001. LC 00-48476. (All-in-One Guide Ser.: Vol. 3). (Illus.). 401p. pap. 14.95 (*1-886508-29-1*, Ages Pubns) Adi Gaia Esalen.

All-in-One Guide to Herbs, Vitamins & Minerals: The Quick & Easy Reference for Everything You Need to Know. Victoria Hogan. 1998. LC 96-910520. (Illus.). 60p. pap. 5.95 (*0-920470-99-8*) Alive Bks.

All Kinds of Love: Experiencing Hospice. Carolyn Jaffe & Carol H. Ehrlich. 1997. LC 96-48015. (Death, Value & Meaning Ser.). 364p. pap. text 29.95 (*0-89503-147-7*) Baywood Pub.

All of a Piece: A Life with Multiple Sclerosis. Barbara D. Webster. 1989. LC 88-29343. 152p. pap. text 26.95 (*0-8018-6162-4*) Johns Hopkins.

All Patients Sick & Crazy: The Madcap Memoirs of a Family Doctor. Philip H. Smith. 1993. 256p. (Orig.). pap. 4.99 (*1-56171-235-3*) SPI.

All Sickness Is Homesickness. Diane M. Connelly. 1987. (Illus.). 167p. (Orig.). pap. 12.00 (*0-912379-02-2*) Ctr Traditional Acupuncture.

All Stings Considered: First Aid & Medical Treatment of Hawai'i's Marine Injuries. Craig Thomas & Susan Scott. 1997. LC 96-44254. (Illus.). 248p. pap. 29.95 (*0-8248-1900-4*, Latitude Twenty) UH Pr.

All the Mothers Are One: Hindu India & the Cultural Reshaping of Psychoanalysis. Stanley S. Kurtz. 1994. LC 92-8190. 306p. pap. 21.00 (*0-231-07869-2*) Col U Pr.

All Things Bright & Beautiful. James Herriot. 1998. (All Things Bright & Beautiful Ser.: Vol. 1). 438p. mass mkt. 7.99 (*0-312-96619-9*, Tor Books) T Doherty Assocs.

All Things to All People: The Catholic Church Confronts the AIDS Crisis. Mark R. Kowalewski. 1994. LC 93-37730. 167p. (C). text 57.50 (*0-7914-1777-8*); pap. text 18.95 (*0-7914-1778-6*) State U NY Pr.

All Things Work for Good: A Book of Encouragement for People with Cancer, Their Family & Friends. Gavin Sinclair. 1997. (Illus.). 176p. (Orig.). pap. 9.95 (*0-9655381-0-9*) Positive Pr AZ.

All You Ever Wanted to Know about Herbs for Pets. Gregory L. Tilford & Mary Wulff-Tilford. 1999. LC 99-42466. (Illus.). 384p. 49.95 (*1-889540-46-3*) Bowtie Press.

All You Need to Know about DNA, Genes & Genetic Engineering: A Concise, Comprehensive Outline. Gordon R. Carter & Stephen M. Boyle. 1998. LC 98-3519. (Illus.). 146p. pap. text 23.95 (*0-398-06870-4*) C C Thomas.

All You Really Need to Know to Interpret Arterial Blood Gases. Lawrence Martin. 1992. (Illus.). 224p. pap. 25.00 (*0-8121-1572-4*) Lppncott W & W.

Allegheny General: Portrait of an Urban Medical Center. Ed. by Mary J. Bent et al. 1991. 40.00 (*0-9628790-0-2*) Allegheny Health.

Allen's Compounded Formulations: The U. S. Pharmacist Collection, 1995 to 1998. Loyd V. Allen, Jr. 1999. LC 99-47778. ix, 141p. pap. text 49.00 (*0-917330-99-4*) Am Pharm Assn.

Allen's Fertility & Obstetrics in the Dog. C. W. England et al. 2nd ed. 1998. LC 97-31975. (Library of Veterinary Practice). (Illus.). 208p. 44.95 (*0-632-04806-9*) Blackwell Sci.

Allen's Fertility & Obstetrics in the Horse. Rev. by Gary C. England. 2nd rev. ed. 1996. LC 96-24286. (Library of Veterinary Practice). (Illus.). 192p. (C). pap. text (*0-632-04084-X*) Blckwell Science GBR. *Dist:* Iowa U Pr.

Allergen-Free Living: How to Create a Healthy, Allergen-Free Home & Lifestyle. Anita Reid & Peter Howarth. 2000. LC 00-690793. (Illus.). 144p. (*1-84000-233-6*) Mitchell Beazley GBR. *Dist:* Antique Collect.

Allergen Immunotherapy. Richard F. Lockey & Samuel C. Bukantz. 2nd ed. 1998. LC 98-39465. (Illus.). 632p. text 225.00 (*0-8247-0188-7*) Dekker.

Allergic & Non-Allergic Rhinitis: Clinical Aspects. Ed. by Niels Mygind & Robert M. Naclerio. 1993. (Illus.). 200p. text 57.95 (*0-7216-5146-1*) Saunders.

Allergic & Respiratory Disease in Sports Medicine. J. M. Weiler. 1997. LC 97-5181. (Clinical Allergy & Immunology Ser.: Vol. 11). (Illus.). 472p. text 185.00 (*0-8247-9890-2*) Dekker.

Allergic & Vasmotor Rhinitis: Clinical Aspects. Ed. by Niels Mygind & Bent Weeke. 1988. 194p. 57.50 (*87-16-09878-1*) Coronet Bks.

Allergic Bronchopulmonary Aspergillosis. Ed. by Paul A. Greenberger et al. 1994. LC 94-67244. (Illus.). 96p. (C). 57.50 (*0-936587-05-9*) OceanSide Pubns.

***Allergic Contact Dermatitis: Chemical & Metabolic Mechanisms.** Camilla K. Smith & Sharon Hodgkiss. 2001. LC 00-64911. (Illus.). 336p. (C). (gr. 13). text 115.00 (*0-415-25047-1*) Routledge.

Allergic Contact Dermatitis: The Molecular Basis. Ed. by J. P. Lepoittevin & A. T. Karlberg. 1997. LC 97-28047. (Illus.). 186p. 65.00 (*3-540-61833-3*) Spr-Verlag.

Allergic Contact Dermatitis to Ingredients Used in Topically Applied Pharmaceutical Products & Cosmetics. A. Dooms-Goossens. 1993. 212p. (Orig.). pap. (*90-6186-147-0*) Leuven Univ BEL. *Dist:* Coronet Bks.

Allergic Diseases: Diagnosis & Management. Leslie C. Grammer & Paul A. Greenberger. 5th ed. 1997. LC 96-49540. 656p. text 129.00 (*0-397-51609-6*) Lppncott W & W.

Allergic Diseases: Diagnosis & Treatment. Ed. by Phil Lieberman & John A. Anderson. 1997. LC 96-38857. (Current Clinical Practice Ser.). (Illus.). 416p. 99.50 (*0-89603-367-8*) Humana.

Allergic Diseases: Diagnosis & Treatment. Ed. by Phil Lieberman & John A. Anderson. 2nd ed. 2000. LC 00-20615. (Current Clinical Practice Ser.). 496p. 99.50 (*0-89603-685-5*) Humana.

Allergic Diseases: Symposium in Immunology IV. Ed. by M. M. Eibl et al. 1995. LC 94-35638. (Illus.). 196p. 108.00 (*3-540-58769-1*) Spr-Verlag.

Allergic Diseases of the Eye. Mark B. Abelson. 2000. LC 99-23446. (Illus.). xiii, 270p. text (*0-7216-8679-6*) Saunders.

Allergic Disorders. William F. Jackson et al. 1997. 39.95 (*0-7234-2480-2*) Mosby Inc.

Allergic Mechanisms & Ummonotherapeutic Strategies. A. M. Roberts & M. R. Walker. 1997. LC 96-35332. 212p. 170.00 (*0-471-96999-0*) Wiley.

Allergic Reactions to Anaesthetics: Clinical & Basic Aspects. Ed. by E. S. K. Assem. 1992. (Monographs in Allergy: Vol. 30). (Illus.). xii, 236p. 256.75 (*3-8055-5489-3*) S Karger.

Allergic Reactions to Drugs. Ed. by Alain L. De Weck & H. Rundgaard. 1983. (Handbook of Experimental Pharmacology Ser.: Vol. 63). (Illus.). 752p. 393.00 (*0-387-12399-7*) Spr-Verlag.

Allergic Skin Diseases of Dogs & Cats. Lloyd Reedy. 2nd ed. 1997. 267p. text (*0-7020-1974-7*) Bailliere Tindall.

Allergic Travelers Passport to Worry-Free Vacations. Dolores J. Sloan. 1992. LC 92-13088. 12.00 (*0-943685-10-9*) Essential Science.

Allergies. Deepak Chopra. 1997. pap. (*0-609-80078-7*) Harmony Bks.

Allergies. Bridget McConville & Rajendra Sharma. 1999. LC 98-52354. (Your Child Ser.). 128p. pap. 9.95 (*1-86204-499-6*) Element MA.

Allergies. Lisa Newman. 1999. LC 99-37387. (Crossing Press Pocket Ser.). 96p. mass mkt. 6.95 (*1-58091-002-5*) Crossing Pr.

Allergies: A Guide for Patients. David Tinkleman. Ed. by Archie Wilson. 1996. (Allergy Ser.). (Illus.). 32p. (Orig.). pap. 2.95 (*1-885274-35-1*) Health InfoNet Inc.

Allergies: A Nutritional Approach. Louise Tenney. 1997. (Woodland Health Ser.: No. 4). 32p. pap. 3.95 (*0-913923-31-1*) Woodland UT.

Allergies: Questions You Have...Answers You Need. Jennifer Hay. 1997. LC 96-29512. 192p. pap. 12.95 (*1-882606-71-X*) Peoples Med Soc.

Allergies: The Complete Guide To Diagnosis, Treatment & Daily Management. Margaret Miner et al. 1999. LC 98-50350. 352p. pap. 13.95 (*0-452-27966-6*) Dutton Plume.

Allergies: What You Need to Know. Mark Giuliucci. 1999. LC 99-26955. (Johns Hopkins Health Ser.). 181p. (YA). (gr. 9-12). pap. 9.95 (*0-7370-1609-4*, Time Life) Henninger Prod.

Allergies A-Z. Myron A. Lipkowitz & Tova Navarra. 1997. (Illus.). 368p. pap. 19.95 (*0-8160-3654-3*) Facts on File.

Allergies A-Z: Practical Advice on Living with Allergies. Myron A. Lipkowitz & Tova Navarra. 2nd ed. 2001. LC 00-49490. (Library of Health & Living). (Illus.). 384p. pap. 19.95 (*0-8160-4405-8*, Checkmark) Facts on File.

Allergies & Asthma: A Natural Approach. Ed. by Christine Murphy. 2000. 96p. pap. 10.00 (*1-930051-08-5*) Booklight Inc.

Allergies & Candida: With the Physicist's Rapid Solution. Steven Rochlitz. 3rd ltd. ed. 1991. LC 91-3199. (Towards a Science of Healing Ser.: Vol. I). (Illus.). 272p. (Orig.). text 50.00 (*0-945262-20-5*) HEBS.

***Allergies & Candida: With the Physicist's Rapid Solution.** Illus. by Ken Vatter. 4th rev. ed. 2000. LC 2001-24120. (Towards a Science of Healing Ser.: Vol. 1). 272p. (C). pap. 19.95 (*0-945262-48-5*) HEBS.

Allergies & Chinese Herbal Medicine. Pi-Kwang Tsung & Hong-Yen Hsu. 1987. (Educational Series on Chinese Medicine: No. 3). 40p. (Orig.). (C). pap. text 5.95 (*0-941942-26-0*) Orient Heal Arts.

Allergies & Holistic Healing. Skye Weintraub. 1997. 414p. pap. text 12.95 (*1-885670-61-3*) Woodland UT.

Allergies & Your Family. Doris J. Rapp. 1990. 352p. reprint ed. pap. 12.95 (*0-9616318-2-1*) Practical Allergy.

Allergies in Childhood: A Guide for Parents. Frank A. Oski & David G. Tinkelman. 1999. (Pediatrics Ser.). (Illus.). 32p. pap. 2.95 (*1-885274-07-6*) Health InfoNet Inc.

Allergies Sourcebook: Basic Consumer Health Information about the Causes of Allergies. Ed. by Allan R. Cook. 1997. LC 96-30992. (Health Reference Ser.: Vol. 19). xi, 611p. lib. bdg. 78.00 (*0-7808-0036-2*) Omnigraphics Inc.

Allergy. Ed. by Stephen T. Holgate & Martin K. Church. 1992. LC 92-1576. (gr. 13). (*0-397-44725-6*) Gower-Mosby.

Allergy. Allen P. Kaplan. Ed. by Ray Kersey. 2nd ed. 1997. LC 96-29737. 880p. text 125.00 (*0-7216-4974-2*) Saunders.

***Allergy: An Illustrated Colour Text.** S. H. Arshad. 2001. (Illus.). 115p. pap. (*0-443-06271-4*) Church GBR. *Dist:* Saunders.

Allergy: Detection & Therapy. Robert P. Sundel. 1995. (Illus.). 78p. (Orig.). pap. text 22.00 (*1-879772-08-6*) Health Studies.

Allergy: Immunological & Clinical Aspects. M. H. Lessof et al. 2nd ed. 1987. 670p. 142.50 (*0-471-90927-0*) Wiley.

Allergy: The Facts. Robert J. Davies & Susan Ollier. 1989. (Illus.). 208p. 19.95 (*0-19-261439-8*) OUP.

Allergy: Theory & Practice. Philip E. Korenblat & H. James Wedner. 2nd ed. 1992. (Illus.). 596p. text 121.00 (*0-7216-7244-2*) Saunders.

Allergy Set: Principles & Practice Elliott Middleton, Jr. 5th ed. 1998. LC 98-173984. (Illus.). 2016p. (YA). (gr. 13). text 275.00 (*0-8151-0072-8*, 27204) Mosby Inc.

Allergy - a Disease of Modern Society: 21st Collegium Internationale Allergologicum, Salzburg, September 1996. Ed. by Dietrich Kraft & Johannes Ring. 1997. (Journal: Vol. 113, No. 1-3 (1997)). (Illus.). 396p. pap. 161.75 (*3-8055-6502-X*) S Karger.

***Allergy & Allergic Disease.** Ed. by A. Barry Kay. 2001. (BMB Ser.). 1107p. pap. (*1-85315-459-8*) Royal Soc of Medicine Pr Ltd GBR. *Dist:* Balogh.

Allergy & Allergic Diseases. A. Barry Kay. 1997. LC 96-13727. (Illus.). 1200p. 295.00 (*0-86542-867-0*) Blackwell Sci.

Allergy & Allergic Diseases: The New Mechanisms & Therapeutics. Judah A. Denburg. 1998. LC 98-17728. (Illus.). 608p. 155.00 (*0-89603-404-6*) Humana.

Allergy & Asthma: A Source Guide. 1991. lib. bdg. 250.00 (*0-8490-4820-6*) Gordon Pr.

Allergy & Immunity to Helminths: Common Mechanisms or Divergent Pathways? Ed. by Redwan Moqbel. 1992. LC 92-26365. 110.00 (*0-7484-0022-2*) Taylor & Francis.

Allergy & Immunology: A Practical Guide for Health Care Professionals. Judith G. Brooks. 1997. LC 96-39477. 150p. text 44.95 (*0-398-06735-X*); pap. text 31.95 (*0-398-06736-8*) C C Thomas.

Allergy & Inflammation. Ed. by A. Barry Kay. 1987. text 167.00 (*0-12-402745-8*) Acad Pr.

Allergy & Inflammation Nineteen Eighty-Eight: From Gene Cloning to Clinical Practice - Journal: International Archives of Allergy & Applied Immunology, Vol. 88, Nos. 1 & 2. Alec H. Sehon. 1989. (Illus.). 260p. pap. 104.50 (*3-8055-4988-1*) S Karger.

Allergy, Asthma, & Immunology from Infancy to Adulthood: Management in Infants, Children, & Adults. David S. Pearlman et al. 3rd ed. 1995. (Illus.). 784p. text 125.00 (*0-7216-5587-4*) Saunders.

Allergy Cures Your Allergist Never Mentioned. Sterling R. Booth, Jr. 1989. LC 80-20698. 22.95 (*0-87949-191-4*) Ashley Bks.

Allergy Free Living: The Birds & Bees Guide To. Scott E. Seargeant. 1998. (Illus.). 190p. pap. (*0-9657867-0-6*) Seargeant Pub.

***Allergy Free Naturally: 1,000 Nondrug Solutions for More Than 50 Allergy-Related Problems.** Rick Ansorge & Eric Metcalf. Ed. by Prevention Health Books Staff. 2001. LC 2001-2695. (Illus.). 544p. pap. 19.95 (*1-57954-392-8*) Rodale Pr Inc.

***Allergy Free Naturally: 1,000 Nondrug Solutions for More Than 50 Allergy-Related Problems.** Rick Ansorge & Eric Metcalf. 2001. LC 2001-2695. (*1-57954-327-8*) Rodale Pr Inc.

Allergy in ENT Practice: A Basic Guide. Hueston C. King et al. 1998. LC 98-9595. 452p. 59.00 (*0-86577-798-5*); 59.00 (*3-13-112761-9*) Thieme Med Pubs.

***Allergy in the 21st Century - New Answers to Old Questions: 23rd Symposium of the Collegium Internationale Allergologicum, Hakone, Japan, May 2000.** Ed. by T. Ishikawa et al. 2001. (International Archives of Allergy & Immunology Ser.: Vol. 124, No. 1-3). (Illus.). 422p. pap. 161.75 (*3-8055-7223-9*) S Karger.

Allergy Made Simple. R. Wahl. 1996. LC 95-81930. (GER., Illus.). 120p. pap. text 19.50 (*0-88937-157-1*) Hogrefe & Huber Pubs.

Allergy Methods & Protocols. Susan Gordon & Menir G. Jones. 2001. (Methods in Molecular Medicine Ser.). 500p. 99.50 (*0-89603-896-3*) Humana.

Allergy Plants. Mary Jelks. 1990. LC 86-50367. 64p. pap. 9.95 (*0-911977-04-X*) Wrld Tampa.

Allergy Prevention & Relief: A Doctor's Complete Guide to Treatment & Self-Care. Jacqueline Krohn et al. 3rd rev. ed. 2000. LC 00-53531. (Illus.). xi, 500p. pap. 24.95 (*0-88179-194-6*) Hartley & Marks.

Allergy Primary Care. Ed. by Stephen T. Holgate et al. 2nd ed. 1999. (Illus.). 350p. 69.95 (*0-7234-3066-7*) Mosby Inc.

Allergy Products Directory. 1992. lib. bdg. 75.00 (*0-8490-5321-8*) Gordon Pr.

Allergy Self-Help Cookbook. Marjorie Jones. 2001. LC 00-12347. (Illus.). xv, 416p. pap. 16.95 (*1-57954-276-X*) Rodale Pr Inc.

Allergy Solution for Dogs: Natural & Conventional Therapies to Ease Discomfort. Shawn Massonnier. 4th ed. 2000. LC 00-29132. (Natural Vet Ser.). 224p. pap. 14.00 (*0-7615-2672-2*) Prima Pub.

***Allergy Solutions.** Suzannah Olivier. 2001. pap. (*0-7432-1863-9*) Simon & Schuster GBR. *Dist:* Distican.

Allergy Sourcebook: Everything You Need to Know. Merla Zellerbach. 264p. 1996. pap. 16.00 (*1-56565-432-3*); 1995. LC 94-43948. 25.00 (*1-56565-208-8*) Lowell Hse.

Allergy Sourcebook: Everything You Need to Know. Merla Zellerbach & Vincent A. Marinkovich. 2nd rev. ed. 1998. 288p. pap. 16.00 (*1-56565-864-7*, 08647W) Lowell Hse.

Allgemeine Krankheitsbezeichnungen im Corpus Hippocraticum: Bedeutung und Gebrauch von Nousos und Nosema. Gerd Preiser. 1976. (Ars Medica, Abt. 2, Griechisch Lateinische Medizin Ser.). (C). text 101.55 (*3-11-001830-6*) De Gruyter.

Alliance for Change: A Plan for Community Action on Adolescent Drug Abuse. James F. Crowley. 1984. LC 84-71356. (Illus.). 226p. (Orig.). pap. 8.95 (*0-9613416-0-2*, 102B) Comm Intervention.

Alliances: Strategies for Building Integrated Delivery Systems. Douglas E. Goldstein. 1994. 316p. ring bd. 241.00 (*0-8342-0602-1*, 20602) Aspen Pub.

Allied Health: California. LearningExpress Staff. 1997. LC 97-3651. (Learning Express Allied Health Ser.). 288p. pap. 35.00 (*1-57685-064-1*) LrningExprss.

Allied Health: Florida. 1997. LC 97-296. (Learning Express Allied Health Ser.). 288p. pap. 32.50 (*1-57685-067-6*) LrningExprss.

Allied Health: New Jersey. LearningExpress Staff. 1997. LC 97-876. (Learning Express Allied Health Ser.). 288p. pap. 35.00 (*1-57685-068-4*) LrningExprss.

Allied Health: New York. Learning Express Staff. 1997. LC 97-875. (Learning Express Allied Health Ser.). 288p. pap. 35.00 (*1-57685-065-X*) LrningExprss.

Allied Health: Texas. Learning Express Staff. 1997. LC 97-874. (Learning Express Allied Health Ser.). 288p. pap. 32.50 (*1-57685-066-8*) LrningExprss.

Allied Health Aptitude Tests (AHAT) Jack Rudman. 1994. (Admission Test Ser.: ATS-78). pap. 27.95 (*0-8373-5078-6*) Nat Learn.

Allied Health Entrance Examination (AHEE) Jack Rudman. 1994. (Admission Test Ser.: ATS-79). pap. 27.95 (*0-8373-5079-4*) Nat Learn.

Allied Health Entrance Exams. LearningExpress Staff. 1998. LC 97-43306. (Allied Health Entrance Exams Ser.). 368p. pap. 20.00 (*1-57685-100-1*) LrningExprss.

Allied Health Guide to Risk Management: Risk-Management for the Allied Health Practitioner. Ricardo A. Scott. 1994. 110p. 25.95 (*1-883427-11-8*) Crnerstone GA.

Allied Health Professional Admission Test (AHPAT) - Core Content. David M. Tarlow. 1996. (Medical Examinations Ser.). 578p. (Orig.). (C). pap. 49.95 (*1-57774-005-X*) Educ Tsting Cnslts.

Allied Health Professions. Arco Editorial Staff. 1993. LC 92-48351. 176p. per. 18.00 (*0-671-84708-2*, Arc) Hungry Minds.

Allied Health Professions Admission Test (AHPAT) Jack Rudman. (Admission Test Ser.: Vol. 99). 47.95 (*0-8373-5199-5*) Nat Learn.

Allied Health Professions Admissions Test (AHPAT) Practice Examination Number 1. David M. Tarlow. 1992. (Practice Examination Ser.). 40p. pap. 16.95 (*0-931572-30-4*) Datar Pub.

Allied Health Professions Admissions Test (AHPAT) Practice Examination Number 2. David M. Tarlow. 1992. (Practice Examination Ser.). pap. 16.95 (*0-931572-31-2*) Datar Pub.

Allied Health Professions Admissions Test (AHPAT) Student Guide. David M. Tarlow. 1993. (Student Guide Ser.). 140p. pap. 15.95 (*0-931572-29-0*) Datar Pub.

Allied Heath & Rehabilatation. 1996. (*5-550-69278-3*) Nairi.

Allies & Adversaries: The Impact of Managed Care on Mental Health Services. Ed. by Robert K. Schreter et al. 1994. LC 94-368. 231p. text 38.00 (*0-88048-677-5*, 8677) Am Psychiatric.

Allies in Healing: When the Person You Love Was Sexually Abused As a Child, a Support Book for Partners. Laura Davis. 1991. LC 90-56423. 368p. pap. 16.00 (*0-06-096883-4*, Perennial) HarperTrade.

Alloantigen Systems of Human Leucocytes & Platelets. L. Fulop-Aszodi. 1979. 336p. (C). (*963-05-1721-3*) Akade Kiado HUN. *Dist:* St Mut.

Allocating Health Care Resources. Ed. by James M. Humber & Robert F. Almeder. 1995. LC 84-640015. (Biomedical Ethics Reviews Ser.). 230p. 49.50 (*0-89603-260-4*) Humana.

*__Allocating Scarce Medical Resources: Roman Catholic Perspectives.__ Ed. by H. Tristram Engelhardt & Mark J. Cherry. 2002. LC 2001-40800. 352p. pap. 39.95 (*0-87840-882-7*) Georgetown U Pr.

Allocation of Health Care Resources: An Ethical Evaluation of the "QALY" Approach. John McKie et al. 1998. LC 97-42927. (Medico-Legal Ser.). 151p. text (*1-85521-953-0*) Ashgate Pub GBR. *Dist:* Ashgate Pub Co.

Allografts in Orthopaedic Practice. Andrei A. Czitrom & Allan E. Gross. 1992. (Illus.). 240p. 75.00 (*0-683-02300-4*) Lppncott W & W.

*__Alloimmune Disorders of Pregnancy: Anaemia, Thrombocytopenia, & Neutropenia in the Fetus & Neonate.__ Ed. by Andrew Hadley & Peter Soothill. 2001. LC 2001-25639. 300p. text 80.00 (*0-521-78120-5*) Cambridge U Pr.

Alloimmunity: 1993 & Beyond. Ed. by Sandra T. Nance. 1993. 212p. text 9.00 (*1-56395-025-1*) Am Assn Blood.

Alloy Compounds, Aldehydes, Epoxides & Peroxides. 1985. (IARC Scientific Publications Ser.: No. 36). 369p. pap. text 77.00 (*92-832-1536-2*, 1710036) World Health.

Allyn & Bacon Molecular Model Set for Organic Chemistry. 2nd ed. 1997. pap. text 45.00 (*0-205-08136-3*, 688136) P-H.

Allyn & Bacon Quick Guide to the Internet for Psychology: 1999 Edition. 3rd ed. 1998. (C). (*0-205-28745-X*, Macmillan Coll) P-H.

Almanac of Back Pain Treatments. Julie Zimmerman. 1991. LC 90-85650. (Illus.). 190p. (Orig.). pap. 9.95 (*1-879418-03-7*) Biddle Pub.

Almanach des Dyspepsies. A. L. Blum et al. 1992. LC 92-28887. 57.95 (*0-387-55674-5*) Spr-Verlag.

Almost a Revolution: Mental Health Law & the Limits of Change. Paul S. Appelbaum. 1994. LC 93-37337. 248p. text 45.00 (*0-19-506880-7*) OUP.

Almost Coping. Terri Auchter. 1983. LC 83-61876. (Illus.). 160p. pap. 2.95 (*0-931762-20-0*) Phunn Pubs.

Aloe Vera, Jojoba & Yucca. John Heinerman. 1982. (Good Health Guides). 32p. pap. 3.95 (*0-87983-269-X*, 3269XK, Keats Pubng) McGraw-Hill Trade.

Alone in the Crowd: One Man's Struggle with Obsessive Compulsive Disorder. Joe H. Vaughan. 1993. 136p. (Orig.). pap. text 9.95 (*0-9636863-6-4*, 566369) J Vaughan Assocs.

Alopecia & Vitiligo in Autoimmune Polyendocrine Syndrome Type 1. Hakan Hedstrand. 2000. (Comprehensive Summaries of Uppsala Dissertations from the Faculty of Medicine Ser.: No. 935). (Illus.). 44p. pap. (*91-554-4733-3*) Uppsala Universitet SWE. *Dist:* Coronet Bks.

Alpha- & Beta-Hexachlorocyclohexanes. 1992. (Environmental Health Criteria Ser.: No. 123). (ENG, FRE & SPA.). 170p. pap. text 29.00 (*92-4-157123-3*, 1160123) World Health.

Alpha-Adrenoceptors: Molecular Biology, Biochemistry & Pharmacology. Ed. by R. R. Ruffolo. 1991. (Progress in Basic & Clinical Pharmacology Ser.: Vol. 8). (Illus.). xiv, 226p. 205.25 (*3-8055-5390-0*) S Karger.

Alpha Adrenoceptors: Signal Transduction, Ionic Channels & Effector Organs. Ed. by M. Fujiwara et al. 1993. (Current Clinical Practice Ser.: vol. 63). x, 284p. 156.25 (*0-444-89727-5*, Excerpta Medica) Elsevier.

Alpha & Gamma Motor Systems: Proceedings of a Symposium Held in London, England, July 11-14, 1994. Ed. by Anthony Taylor et al. 1995. LC 95-25924. (Illus.). 656p. 167.00 (*0-306-45186-7*, QP369, Kluwer Plenum) Kluwer Academic.

Alpha Book on Cancer & Living: For Patients, Family & Friends. Brent G. Ryder. 1993. pap. 18.95 (*0-9632360-9-1*) Alpha Inst.

Alpha Book on Cancer & Living: For Patients, Family, & Friends. Alpha Institute Staff & Brent G. Ryder. rev. ed. 1993. LC 93-71332. (Illus.). 448p. reprint ed. pap. 16.95 (*0-9632360-1-6*) Alpha Inst.

Alpha Book on Cancer & Living: For Patients, Family, & Friends. Brent G. Ryder. rev. ed. 1993. LC 93-71332. (Illus.). 448p. reprint ed. 24.95 (*0-9632360-0-8*) Alpha Inst.

Alpha Children: Right Brained & Gifted. Jack L. Fadely & Virginia Hosler. 1985. (Illus.). 141p. pap. text 7.00 (*0-934293-04-X*) Huber-Copeland Pub.

Alpha-Cypermethrin. 1992. (Environmental Health Criteria Ser.: No. 142). (ENG, FRE & SPA.). 112p. pap. text 26.00 (*92-4-157142-X*, 1160142) World Health.

Alpha-Emitting Particles in Lungs. 1975. LC 75-17147. (Report Ser.: No. 46). 28p. pap. text 20.00 (*0-913392-28-6*) NCRP Pubns.

Alpha-Glucosidease Inhibition: Potential Use in Diabetes: Proceedings of the First Preclinical Workshop on Acarbose. Ed. by C. A. Maggio & A. Scriabine. 1994. (Drugs in Development Ser.). (Illus.). 285p. (Orig.). pap. text 75.00 (*0-9637603-0-0*) Neva Pr.

Alpha1: Pre-Congress Satellite Symposium, Paris, July 1998, in Connection with the XIIIth International Congress of Pharmacology, Munich, July 1998. Ed. by S. Z. Langer. 3rd ed. 1999. (European Urology Ser.). (Illus.). iv, 100p. pap. 34.00 (*3-8055-6904-1*) S Karger.

Alpha 1-Antitrypsin Deficiency. Ed. by Ronald G. Crystal. 1995. LC 95-41834. (Lung Biology in Health & Disease Ser.: Vol. 88). (Illus.). 472p. text 199.00 (*0-8247-8848-6*) Dekker.

Alpha-1 Adrenergic Receptors. Ed. by Robert R. Ruffolo, Jr. 1988. LC 87-17006. (Receptors Ser.). 568p. 155.00 (*0-89603-110-1*) Humana.

Alpha-2 Adrenergic Receptors. Ed. by Lee E. Limbird. 1988. LC 88-6833. (Receptors Ser.). (Illus.). 377p. 145.00 (*0-89603-135-7*) Humana.

Alphabet & the Brain. Ed. by D. De Kerdhove. 1988. (Illus.). 455p. 135.00 (*0-387-18122-9*) Spr-Verlag.

Alphard: Form & Content. Ed. by Mary Shaw. 1981. 321p. 49.00 (*0-387-90663-0*) Spr-Verlag.

Alpha2-Agents in Animals Sedation, Analgesia & Anaesthesia. Charles E. Short. 1993. LC 92-64484. 85p. (Orig.). pap. text 25.00 (*0-9603534-2-9*) Vet Practice.

Alphita, a Medico-Botanical Glossary. Ed. by J. L. Mowat. 1988. (Anecdota Oxoniensia Ser.: No. 2). reprint ed. 67.40 (*0-404-63952-6*) AMS Pr.

Alpine Skiing. Ed. by Robert E. Leach. 2nd ed. 1994. LC 93-26993. (Handbook of Sports Medicine & Science Ser.). (Illus.). 144p. pap. 34.95 (*0-632-03033-X*, BLEA3033) Blackwell Sci.

ALS 1996 & Beyond: New Hopes & Challenges - Manual for Patients, Families & Friends. Carmel Armon. 2nd rev. ed. 1996. (Illus.). 18p. pap. (*0-9655186-0-4*) Loma Lnda U Neur.

Altenative Health & Medicine Encyclopedia. James Marti. 2nd ed. 1997. LC 97-34696. (Illus.). 480p. 15.95 (*1-57859-020-5*, GML14099-111198) Visible Ink Pr.

Alter und Altern: Ein Interdisziplinaerer Studientext zur Gerontologie. Ed. by Paul B. Baltes et al. 1994. (Sonderausgabe des 1992 Ershienenen 5. Forschungsberichtes der Akademie der Wissenschaft zu Berlin Ser.). (GER.). 822p. (C). pap. text 36.95 (*3-11-014408-5*) De Gruyter.

Alterations in the Neuronal Cytoskeleton in Alzheimer's Disease. Ed. by G. Perry. 1987. LC 87-29256. (Advances in Behavioral Biology Ser.: Vol. 34). 240p. 69.50 (*0-306-42766-4*, Plenum Trade) Perseus Pubng.

Alterations of Excitation-Contraction Coupling in the Failing Human Heart. Ed. by G. Hasenfuss & H. Just. 1998. (Illus.). 108p. (C). (*3-7985-1047-4*) D Steinkopff DEU. *Dist:* Spr-Verlag.

Alterations of Personality. 5. Alfred Binet. Tr. by Helen G. Baldwin from FRE. 1977. LC 77-72191. (Contributions to the History of Psychology Ser.). 346p. reprint ed. lib. bdg. 79.50 (*0-313-26944-0*, U6944, Greenwood Pr) Greenwood.

Altered Body Image: The Nurse's Role. Mave Salter. 2nd ed. 1998. 270p. pap. (*1-873853-40-8*) Saunders.

Altered Conditions: Disease, Medicine, & Storytelling. Julia Epstein. 320p. (C). 1995. 80.00 (*0-415-90717-9*, A9837); 1994. (gr. 13). pap. 26.99 (*0-415-90718-7*, A9841) Routledge.

Altered Fates: Gene Therapy & the Retooling of Human Life. Jeff Lyon. 1996. LC 00-4533. 636p. pap. 15.95 (*0-393-31528-2*) Norton.

Altered Fates: The Genetic Re-Engineering of Human Life. Jeff Lyon & Peter Gorner. 1995. LC 95-179610. 800p. 27.50 (*0-393-03596-4*) Norton.

Altered Proteins & Aging. Ed. by Richard C. Adelman & George S. Roth. 1983. 192p. 104.00 (*0-8493-5812-4*, QP86) CRC Pr.

Altered Sensation & Pain. Ed. by M. R. Dimitrijevic et al. 1990. (Recent Achievements in Restorative Neurology Ser.: Vol. 3). (Illus.). xiv, 214p. 172.25 (*3-8055-5036-7*) S Karger.

Altered States: Alcohol & Other Drugs in America. Patricia M. Tice. 1992. LC 92-36241. (*0-940365-05-7*) Strong Mus.

Altered States of Consciousness & Mental Health. Colleen A. Ward. 1989. (Cross-Cultural Research & Methodology Ser.: Vol. 12). 320p. 86.95 (*0-8039-3277-4*, 5174) Sage.

Altered States of Consciousness & PSI: An Historical Survey & Research Prospectus. Edward F. Kelly & Ralph G. Locke. 1981. LC 81-82545. (Parapsychological Monographs: No. 18). 91p. (Orig.). (C). pap. text 8.00 (*0-912328-34-7*) Parapsych Foun.

Altering the Image of AIDS. Maria De Bruyn. 1994. LC 95-122826. 96p. pap. (*90-5383-259-9*) VU Univ Pr NLD. *Dist:* Paul & Co Pubs.

Alternate Cite Acute Care Equipment & Supply Markets: Quest for Cost Reductions Foster Ambulatory Center Group. Market Intelligence Staff. 1993. 260p. 1695.00 (*1-56753-495-3*) Frost & Sullivan.

Alternate Conceptions of Work & Society: Implications for Professional Nursing. Ed. by Carol A. Lindeman. 1988. 225p. (Orig.). pap. 20.00 (*0-922148-00-7*) AACN.

Alternate Healing Methods: An Overview. Angela Plum. 1993. LC 93-85295. (Illus.). 128p. (Orig.). pap. 8.50 (*1-56664-051-2*) WorldComm.

Alternate Methods in the Treatment of Benign Prostatic Hyperlasia. Ed. by Nicholas A. Romas & E. Darracott Vaughan. 1993. LC 92-48354. (*3-540-56389-X*); 205p. 109.00 (*0-387-56389-X*) Spr-Verlag.

Alternate-Site Anesthesia: Clinical Practice Outside the Operating Room. Garfield B. Russell. 1997. LC 97-11403. (Illus.). 472p. text 79.99 (*0-7506-9817-9*) Buttrwrth-Heinemann.

Alternate Site Care Standards, Policies & Procedures: Cleveland Clinic Health Care Ventures, Inc. Charlene Szunyog. 1994. 366p. pap. 51.00 (*0-8342-0765-6*) PRO-ED.

Alternative Advisor: Natural Therapies & Alternative Treatments. Time-Life Books Editors. 1999. LC 96-49614. (Illus.). 400p. pap. 24.95 (*0-7835-4907-5*) Time-Life.

Alternative Advisor: The Complete Guide to Therapies New & Old. Time-Life Books Editors. 1999. 400p. (gr. 11). pap. 14.95 (*0-7370-0045-7*) Time-Life Educ.

Alternative & Complementary Diabetes Care: How to Combine Natural & Traditional Therapies. Diana W. Guthrie. 2000. LC 99-50258. 256p. pap. 14.95 (*0-471-34784-1*) Wiley.

Alternative & Complementary Therapies in Veterinary Medicine. Allen M. Schoen. Ed. by Susan G. Wynn. 1997. LC 97-10210. (Illus.). 840p. (C). (gr. 13). text 84.95 (*0-8151-7994-4*, 26585) Mosby Inc.

*__Alternative & Complementary Treatment in Neurologic Illness.__ Michael I. Weintraub. 2001. LC 00-65686. (Illus.). xvi, 325p. (*0-443-06558-6*) Church.

Alternative & Holistic Health Care for AIDS & Its Prevention: A Sourcebook of Descriptions, Bibliography, & Practitioners in the Washington, D.C.-Baltimore, Maryland Area. Paul N. Van Ness. 1988. 76p. (Orig.). pap. 5.00 (*0-9619604-0-X*) Whitman Walker.

Alternative Approach to Allergies: The New Field of Clinical Ecology Unravels the Environmental Causes of Mental & Physical Ills. Theron G. Randolph & Ralph W. Moss. rev. ed. 1990. LC 88-45902. 352p. reprint ed. pap. 14.00 (*0-06-091693-1*, Perennial) HarperTrade.

Alternative Approaches to Human Blood Resources in Clinical Practice: Proceedings of the 22nd International Symposium on Blood Transfusion, Groningen 1997. Ed. by C. Smith Sibinga et al. 1998. LC 98-44091. (Developments in Hematology & Immunology Ser.). 257p. (*0-7923-8305-2*) Kluwer Academic.

Alternative Bearing Surfaces in Total Joint Replacement. Ed. by Joshua J. Jacobs & Thomas L. Craig. 1998. LC 98-47496. (STP Ser.: No. 1346). (Illus.). 280p. 59.00 (*0-8031-2490-2*, STP1346) ASTM.

Alternative Birth: The Complete Guide. Carl Jones. 1965. 240p. (*0-87477-615-5*, Tarcher Putnam) Putnam Pub Group.

Alternative Bypass Conduits & Methods for Surgical Coronary Revascularization. Ed. by Ronald K. Grooters & Hiroshi Nishida. 1994. (Illus.). 336p. 65.00 (*0-87993-577-4*) Futura Pub.

Alternative Care Programs in Hospice. National Hospice Organization, Alternative Care Ta. 1991. 29p. 10.50 (*0-931207-11-8*) Natl Hospice.

*__Alternative Choices for the Management of Migraine Pain.__ Ed. by Seymour Diamond. 28p. pap. 25.00 (*0-8236-0056-4*, BN 00056) Intl Univs Pr.

Alternative Dictionary of Symptoms & Cures: A Comprehensive Guide to Diseases & Their Orthodox & Alternative Remedies. Caroline M. Shreeve. 1999. (Illus.). 504p. reprint ed. text 25.00 (*0-7881-6551-8*) DIANE Pub.

Alternative Healing Gift Set. Scott Cunningham et al. 1996. (Illus.). (Orig.). pap. 12.89 (*1-56718-894-X*) Llewellyn Pubns.

Alternative Healing Secrets. Random House Value Publishing Staff. 1999. LC 97-52140. 176p. 8.99 (*0-517-16047-1*) Random Hse Value.

Alternative Health & Medicine Encyclopedia 1: The Authoritative Guide to Holistic & Nontraditional Health Practices. James E. Marti. 2nd ed. 1997. LC 97-31144. 400p. 65.00 (*0-7876-0073-3*, GML14099-108800) Gale.

Alternative Health Care: Medicine, Miracle or Mirage? Michael S. Goldstein. 1999. LC 98-27769. viii, 278p. 59.50 (*1-56639-677-8*) Temple U Pr.

Alternative Health Care: Medicine, Miracle, or Mirage? Michael S. Goldstein. 1999. LC 98-27769. viii, 278p. pap. 19.95 (*1-56639-678-6*) Temple U Pr.

Alternative Health Care for Women: A Women's Guide to Self-Help Treatments & Natural Therapies. Patsy Wescott et al. 1987. LC 87-19432. 192p. pap. 12.95 (*0-89281-245-1*, Heal Arts VT) Inner Tradit.

Alternative Health Maintenance & Healing Systems for Families. Ed. by Doris Y. Wilkinson & Marvin B. Sussman. 1988. LC 87-31198. (Marriage & the Family Ser.: Vol. 11, Nos. 3-4). (Illus.). 171p. text 5.95 (*0-86656-701-1*) Haworth Pr.

Alternative Healthcare: A Comprehensive Guide. Jack Raso. 1994. LC 93-48260. (Consumer Health Library). 275p. (C). 34.00 (*0-87975-891-0*) Prometheus Bks.

Alternative Medical Secrets. Gitlow. 1999. (*1-56053-312-9*) Mosby Inc.

Alternative Medicine. Consumer Guide Editors. 1997. LC 97-200293. pap. 6.99 (*0-451-19272-9*, Sig) NAL.

Alternative Medicine, Vol. 1. Howard Facklam. 1996. (*0-8050-5274-7*) H Holt & Co.

Alternative Medicine: Expanding Medical Horizons. 1995. (Illus.). 365p. (Orig.). (C). pap. text 50.00 (*0-7881-1820-X*) DIANE Pub.

Alternative Medicine: Expanding Medical Horizons. 1997. (Orig.). lib. bdg. 259.99 (*0-8490-6220-9*) Gordon Pr.

Alternative Medicine: Expanding Medical Horizons in Alternative Medical Systems & Practices. 1996. lib. bdg. 349.95 (*0-8490-6895-9*) Gordon Pr.

Alternative Medicine: The Definitive Guide. Burton Goldberg. 1998. pap. 29.95 (*1-887299-33-5*); (SPA.). 1,120p. pap. 29.95 (*1-887299-34-3*) AlternMed Bks.

Alternative Medicine 2 Vols. Expanding Medical Horizons, Set. 1996. lib. bdg. 600.95 (*0-8490-5867-8*) Gordon Pr.

Alternative Medicine & Ethics. Ed. by James M. Humber & Robert F. Almeder. 1998. (Biomedical Ethics Reviews Ser.: Vol. 15). 232p. 49.50 (*0-89603-440-2*) Humana.

Alternative Medicine & Multiple Sclerosis. Allen C. Bowling. 2001. 266p. pap. 24.95 (*1-888799-52-8*) Demos Medical.

Alternative Medicine Definitive Guide to Cancer. W. John Diamond et al. 1997. LC 96-6580. (Illus.). 1,120p. 49.95 (*1-887299-01-7*) AlternMed Bks.

Alternative Medicine for Dummies. James Dillard & Terra Ziporyn. 1998. LC 98-88391. (For Dummies Ser.). (Illus.). 432p. pap. 19.99 (*0-7645-5109-4*) Hungry Minds.

Alternative Medicine Guide to Chronic Fatigue, Fibromyalgia & Environmental Illness. Burton Goldberg & Alternative Medicine Digest Editors. 1998. LC 97-48756. (Alternative Medicine Guide Ser.). (Illus.). 366p. pap. 18.95 (*1-887299-11-4*) AlternMed Bks.

Alternative Medicine Handbook: The Complete Reference Guide to Alternative & Complementary Therapies. Barrie Cassileth. 1998. LC 97-16268. (Illus.). 352p. 25.00 (*0-393-04566-8*) Norton.

Alternative Medicine Handbook: The Complete Reference Guide to Alternative & Complementary Therapies. Barrie R. Cassileth. 1999. LC 97-16268. (Illus.). 352p. pap. 19.95 (*0-393-31816-8*, Norton Paperbks) Norton.

Alternative Medicine in Britain. Ed. by Mike Saks. 1992. 282p. text 75.00 (*0-19-827278-2*) OUP.

Alternative Medicine Home Remedies. Jay Gordon. 1998. 72p. pap. 29.95 incl. VHS (*0-9636334-7-3*) AlternMed Bks.

Alternative Medicine Online: A Guide to Natural Remedies on the Internet. Ralph W. Moss. 1997. LC 97-22650. 208p. pap. 12.95 (*1-881025-10-1*) Equinox Pr.

Alternative Medicine or Magical Healing: The Trick Is to Know the Difference. George A. Ulett. 1996. pap. 24.95 *(0-87527-519-2)* Green.

Alternative Medicine Ratings Guide: An Expert Rates the Best Treatments & for over 80 Conditions. Steven Bratman. 1998. LC 97-38074. (Illus.). 408p. pap. 19.95 *(0-7615-1278-0*, Prima Health) Prima Pub.

Alternative Medicine Resource Guide. Francine Feuerman & Marsha J. Handel. 1997. LC 96-49534. 335p. 49.50 *(0-8108-3284-4)* Scarecrow.

Alternative Medicine Sourcebook: A Realistic Evaluation of Alternative Healing Methods. Steven Bratman. 1998. LC 96-49550. (Illus.). 272p. reprint ed. 27.00 *(1-56565-626-1)* Lowell Hse.

Alternative Medicine Sourcebook: A Realistic Evaluation of Alternative Healing Methods. Steven Bratman. 2nd ed. 1999. LC 99-41600. 272p. pap. 17.95 *(0-7373-0247-X*, 0247XW) NTC Contemp Pub Co.

Alternative Medicine Sourcebook: Basic Consumer Health Information about Alternatives to Conventional Medicine. Ed. by Allan R. Cook. 1999. LC 99-37612. (Health Reference Ser.). xiii, 736p. 78.00 *(0-7808-0200-4)* Omnigraphics Inc.

Alternative Medicine That Works. Adriane Fugh-Berman. 1997. 256p. pap. 14.95 *(0-683-30407-0)* Lppncott W & W.

Alternative Path: The Making & Remaking of Hahnemann Medical College & Hospital. Naomi Rogers. 1998. LC 97-43595. (Illus.). 360p. (C). text 50.00 *(0-8135-2535-7)*; pap. text 20.00 *(0-8135-2536-5)* Rutgers U Pr.

Alternative Perspectives in Assessing Children's Language & Literacy. Ed. by David Bloome et al. 1994. 240p. (C). 77.00 *(0-89391-864-4)*; pap. 39.50 *(0-89391-914-4)* Greenwood (Ablex).

Alternative Pharmacy. Ellen Hodgson Brown & Lynne P. Walker. 1998. LC 98-21512. 400p. pap. text 22.00 *(0-7352-0021-1)* PH Pr.

Alternative Pharmacy: Break the Drug Cycle with Safe, Natural Alternative Treatments for Over 200 Common Health Conditions. Ellen Hodgson Brown & Lynn P. Walker. 1998. LC 98-21512. 432p. (C). text 27.95 *(0-13-907254-3)* P-H.

Alternative Remedies. Karen Sullivan. 1994. (Collins Gem Ser.). 256p. pap. *(0-00-470536-X)* Collins.

Alternative Remedies for Common Ailments. Ed. by Time-Life Books Editors. 1999. LC 98-2853. (Time-Life Medical Guides). (Illus.). 144p. (gr. 11). pap. 6.95 *(0-7370-1105-X*, Time Life) Henninger Prod.

Alternative Social Agencies: Administrative Strategies. Intro. by Felice D. Perlmutter. 1989. LC 88-4414. (Administration in Social Work Ser.: Vol. 12, No. 2). (Illus.). 128p. text 39.95 *(0-86656-783-6)* Haworth Pr.

Alternative Systems in Oral Care Delivery. 1987. (Technical Reports: No. 750). (ENG, FRE, RUS & SPA.). 58p. pap. 9.00 *(92-4-120750-7*, 1100750) World Health.

Alternative Therapies: Exploring Options in Health Care. Ed. by Rena J. Gordon et al. 1998. LC 97-41351. (Illus.). 275p. 44.95 *(0-8261-1164-5)* Springer Pub.

Alternative Therapies for Cancer & Arthritis. E. Weisenburger & Irv Boichuk. 1996. 160p. pap. *(0-88982-154-2)* Oolichan Bks CAN. *Dist:* General Distrib Services.

Alternative Therapies for Pregnancy & Birth: Your Guide to Normal, Natural Pregnancy & Birth. Pat Thomas. 2000. (Illus.). 336p. pap. 16.95 *(1-86204-727-8)* Element MA.

Alternative Therapy: Lifestyle & Medical Paradigms. Ed. by Soren Gosvig et al. 4th ed. 1997. 222p. pap. *(87-7838-207-6)* Odense Univ DNK. *Dist:* Intl Spec Bk.

Alternatives to Animal Testing II: Proceedings of the Second International Conference Organized by the European Cosmetic Industry, Brussels, Belgium, 1999. Ed. by D. G. Clark et al. 1999. (Illus.). 304p. *(1-872691-12-9*, CPL Pr) CPL Sci Pub.

Alternative Treatments for Common Conditions. Howard Hassman. 1999. LC 00-699007. (Illus.). ix, 191p. pap. 16.95 *(1-57626-114-X)* Quality Med Pub.

Alternative Treatments for HIV Infection. Magnolia Goh & Tang Zhaoliang. 1994. 247p. (Orig.). pap. 24.95 *(1-880132-12-5)* Sci Pr NY.

Alternative vs. Orthodox Treatment of Leukemia. Lana C. Cantrell. 1999. LC 98-93567. 214p. pap. *(0-9620749-1-8)* L C Cantrell.

Alternatives: New Developments in the War on Breast Cancer. Rose Kushner. 1985. 448p. mass mkt. 4.95 *(0-446-32882-0)* Warner Bks.

Alternatives & Animal Use in the Life Sciences. Vol. 11. Alan M. Goldberg. 1994. 800p. 185.00 *(0-913113-66-2)* M Liebert.

Alternatives for Women with Endometriosis: A Guide by Women for Women. Ed. by Ruth Carol. 1994. LC 94-10122. 176p. (Orig.). pap. 12.95 *(1-879427-12-5)* Third Side Pr.

Alternatives in Cancer Therapy: The Complete Guide to Current Alternative Treatments. Ross Pelton & Lee C. Overholser. 1994. LC 93-30140. 304p. pap. 13.00 *(0-671-79623-2*, Fireside) S&S Trade Pap.

Alternatives in Health Care Delivery: Emerging Roles for Physician Assistants. Reginald Carter & Henry B. Perry. 1984. (Allied Health Professions Monograph). 412p. 42.50 *(0-87527-327-0)* Green.

Alternatives in Jewish Bioethics. Noam J. Zohar. 1997. LC 96-17494. (SUNY Series in Jewish Philosophy). 165p. (C). text 49.50 *(0-7914-3273-4)*; pap. text 18.95 *(0-7914-3274-2)* State U NY Pr.

Alternatives in Rehabilitating the Handicapped: A Policy Analysis. Ed. by Jeffrey Rubin & Valerie LaPorte. 1982. LC 81-4144. 244p. 35.95 *(0-89885-010-X*, Kluwer Acad Hman Sci) Kluwer Academic.

Alternatives to Alcoholism's Grand Conspiracy. Don Boone. Ed. by Ralph Roberts. 1992. (Illus.). 64p. pap. 6.95 *(1-56664-001-6)* WorldComm.

Alternatives to Animal Testing: New Ways in the Biomedical Sciences, Trends, & Progress. Ed. by Christoph A. Reinhardt. 1994. LC 93-44359. pap. 90.00 *(1-56081-831-X*, Wiley-VCH) Wiley.

Alternatives to Cognition: A New Look at Explaining Human Social Behavior. Christina Lee. 1997. LC 97-12615. *(0-8058-2654-8)* L Erlbaum Assocs.

Alternatives to Psychiatric Hospitalization: With Annotated Readers Guide. Harry Gottesfeld. 1977. 24.95 *(0-89876-057-7)* Gardner Pr.

Alternatives to the Hospital for Acute Psychiatric Treatment. Ed. by Richard Warner. 1995. LC 95-34. (Clinical Practice Ser.: No. 32). 272p. text 16.95 *(0-88048-484-5*, 8484) Am Psychiatric.

Altitude-Rated Places: A Medical Atlas, Vol. 1. Blake Mooney. Ed. by Juliette Landry. 2nd rev. ed. 1994. (Illus.). 225p. (Orig.). pap. 16.95 *(0-9638226-0-8)* Med-Travel Bks.

Alton Ochsner, Surgeon of the South. John Wilds & Ira Harkey. 1990. LC 89-13524. (Southern Biography Ser.). (Illus.). 264p. 24.95 *(0-8071-1564-9)* La State U Pr.

Altschul's Psychiatric & Mental Health Nursing. Margaret McGovern & Sarah Witcher. 7th ed. 1995. (Nurses' Aids Ser.). (Illus.). 383p. pap. text *(0-7020-1412-5)* W B Saunders GBR. *Dist:* Saunders.

Alum Official Proceedings, 1997. 1997. (Alum Official Proceedings Ser.: No. 1). (Illus.). pap. *(1-930047-32-0*, OP97) Am Inst Ultrasound.

Alum Official Proceedings, 1998. 1998. (Alum Official Proceedings Ser.: No. 2). (Illus.). pap. *(1-930047-33-9*, OP98) Am Inst Ultrasound.

Alum Official Proceedings, 1999. 1999. (Alum Official Proceedings Ser.: No. 3). (Illus.). pap. *(1-930047-34-7*, OP99) Am Inst Ultrasound.

Aluminium Toxicity in Infants' Health & Disease. P. F. Zatta & A. C. Alfrey. 1997. LC 98-206409. 300p. 54.00 *(981-02-2914-3)* World Scientific Pub.

Aluminum—Index of New Information & Medical Research Bible. Anita E. Funstun. 1994. 150p. 57.50 *(0-7883-0082-2)*; pap. 47.50 *(0-7883-0083-0)* ABBE Pubs Assn.

Aluminum & Renal Failure. Ed. by Marc E. De Broe. 1990. (C). lib. bdg. 226.00 *(0-7923-0347-4)* Kluwer Academic.

Aluminum, Drinking Water, & Alzheimer's Disease. Steven H. Reiber & Walter A. Kukull. 1996. LC 97-107408. (Illus.). 93p. pap. 125.00 *(0-89867-858-7*, 90683) Am Water Wks Assn.

Aluminum in Drinking Water & Alzheimer's Disease: A Resource Guide. 1993. (Illus.). 134p. pap. 63.00 *(0-89867-674-6*, 90623) Am Water Wks Assn.

Alveolar Interstitium of the Lung: Pathological & Physiological Aspects: Proceedings of the International Symposium on Pulmonary Interstitium, Paris, May, 1974. International Symposium on Pulmonary Interstitium. Ed. by F. Basset & Robert Geovges. 1975. (Progress in Respiratory Research Ser.: Vol. 8). viii, 245p. 133.25 *(3-8055-2193-6)* S Karger.

Always Aware. James S. Cusack. Ed. & Pref. by J. Colby. Pref. by Jeanne B. Ewing. 1995. LC 95-75583. (Self-Help Ser.). 200p. pap. text 9.95 *(1-883283-07-8*, 1-800-68-BRICK) Brick Tower.

Alyce's Fat Chance: How to Take off 100 Pounds & Keep It Off! Alyce P. Cornyn-Selby. 1989. 72p. (Orig.). pap. text 8.95 *(0-941383-13-X)* Beynch Pr.

Alzheimer Disease: From Molecular Biology to Therapy. Ezio Giacobini. Ed. by Robert E. Becker. 1996. LC 96-30911. (Advances in Alzheimer's Disease Therapy Ser.). 620p. 98.50 *(0-8176-3879-2)*; *(3-7643-3879-2)* Birkhauser.

Alzheimer Disease: The Changing View. Robert Katzman. 2000. LC 00-101589. (Illus.). xiii, 387p. 69.95 *(0-12-401955-2)* Acad Pr.

Alzheimer's. 1993. 27.95 *(0-387-56932-4)* Spr-Verlag.

Alzheimer's: A Handbook for the Caretaker. Eileen H. Driscoll. 1996. LC 94-4805. pap. 12.95 *(0-8283-1962-6)* Branden Bks.

Alzheimer's: Answers to Hard Questions for Families. James L. Nelson & Hilde Lindemann Nelson. 1997. 224p. pap. 12.95 *(0-385-48534-4*, Main St Bks) Doubleday.

Alzheimer's: Does "the System" Care? Ted Valenti. 1989. LC 89-90878. 208p. pap. 14.95 *(0-914984-17-9)* Starburst.

Alzheimer's: Finding the Words. Harriet Hodgson. 1995. 240p. pap. 14.95 *(0-471-34657-8)* Wiley.

Alzheimer's: Finding the Words: A Communication Guide for Those Who Care. Harriet Hodgson. 1995. LC 95-12869. 240p. pap. 10.95 *(1-56561-071-7)* Wiley.

Alzheimers: The Answers You Need. Helen Davies & Mike Jensen. 1997. LC 97-60630. 140p. (Orig.). per. 10.95 *(0-943873-46-0)* Elder Bks.

Alzheimer's: The Last Childhood. Carrie Knowles. Ed. by Bonnie Tilson. 1997. LC 97-65321. 192p. (Orig.). pap. 9.95 *(1-884570-67-4)* Research Triangle.

Alzheimer's & Dementia. Jennifer Hay. 1996. (Questions You Have...Answers You Need Ser.). 192p. pap. 12.95 *(1-882606-57-4)* Peoples Med Soc.

Alzheimer's & Parkinson's Disease: Strategies for Research & Development. Ed. by Abraham Fisher et al. 1986. LC 85-32056. (Advances in Behavioral Biology Ser.: Vol. 29). 726p. 125.00 *(0-306-42232-8*, Plenum Trade) Perseus Pubng.

Alzheimer's & Parkinson's Diseases: Recent Advances in Research & Clinical Management. Ed. by H. J. Altman & B. N. Altman. (Illus.). 628p. (C). 198.00 *(0-306-43482-2*, Kluwer Plenum) Kluwer Academic.

Alzheimer's & Parkinson's Diseases: Recent Advances in Research & Clinical Management. Ed. by H. J. Altman & B. N. Altman. 1990. LC 90-7241. (Illus.). 604p. 145.00 *(0-306-83482-0*, Plenum Trade) Perseus Pubng.

Alzheimer's & Parkinson's Diseases - Recent Developments: Proceedings of the Third International Conference on Alzheimer's & Parkinson's Diseases: Basic & Therapeutic Strategies Held in Chicago, Illinois, November 1-6, 1993. International Conference on Alzheimer's and Parkinson's Diseases Staff. Ed. by Israel Hanin et al. 1995. LC 95-14255. (Advances in Behavioral Biology Ser.: Vol. 44). (Illus.). 744p. (C). text 165.00 *(0-306-45004-6*, Kluwer Plenum) Kluwer Academic.

Alzheimer's Caregiver: Dealing with the Realities of Dementia. Harriet Hodgson. 1997. 240p. (Orig.). LC 98-231229. pap. 12.95 *(1-56561-125-X)*; pap. 12.95 *(0-471-34656-X)* Wiley.

Alzheimer's Challenged & Conquered? Louis Blank. 1996. 185p. *(0-572-02196-8)* W Foulsham GBR. *Dist:* Trans-Atl Phila.

Alzheimer's Chronicle: Letters to My Aunt. Penny A. Petersen. 1997. (Illus.). 224p. (Orig.). pap. 14.00 *(0-9655969-0-7)* Desert State.

Alzheimers Complete Guide MA. Howard Greutzner. rev. ed. 1997. 272p. pap. 5.99 *(0-471-19825-0)* Wiley.

Alzheimer's Dementia: Dilemmas in Clinical Research. Ed. by Vijaya L. Melnick & Nancy N. Dubler. 1985. LC 85-11740. (Contemporary Issues in Biomedicine, Ethics & Society Ser.). 312p. 89.50 *(0-89603-067-9)* Humana.

Alzheimer's Disease. Elwood Cohen. 1999. LC 99-13014. xvii, 253p. pap. 16.95 *(0-87983-964-3*, 39643K, Keats Pubng) McGraw-Hill Trade.

Alzheimer's Disease. Richards T. Woods. 1991. 232p. pap. 17.95 *(0-285-65038-6)* Paul & Co Pubs.

Alzheimer's Disease. Paul Aisen et al. 2nd ed. 1999. (Questions & Answers Ser.). (Illus.). 154p. pap. 26.95 *(1-873413-52-1)* Merit Pub Intl.

*__Alzheimer's Disease: A Compendium of Current Theories.__ Zaven S. Khachaturian & Eva Friedlander. 2001. (Annals of the New York Academy of Sciences Ser.). 195p. pap. text 19.95 *(0-8018-6834-3)* NY Acad Sci.

*__Alzheimer's Disease: A Guide for Families.__ Lenore S. Powell & Katie Courtice. 2001. 416p. pap. text 18.00 *(0-7382-0598-2)* Perseus Bks Grp.

Alzheimer's Disease: A Guide for Families. Lenore S. Powell. 2nd rev. ed. 2000. LC 92-35473. 362p. pap. 18.00 *(0-201-63201-2)* Perseus Bks Grp.

Alzheimer's Disease: A Guide to Diagnosis, Treatment & Management. James E. Soukup. 1996. LC 95-49687. 208p. 62.50 *(0-275-95460-9*, Praeger Pubs) Greenwood.

Alzheimer's Disease: A Guide to Federal Programs. 1995. 113p. (Orig.). (C). pap. text 35.00 *(0-7881-1564-2)* DIANE Pub.

Alzheimer's Disease: A Handbook for Caregivers. Ed. by R. C. Hamdy et al. 3rd ed. 1997. LC 97-14558. (Illus.). 480p. (C). (gr. 13). text 41.95 *(0-8151-2606-9*, 31076) Mosby Inc.

Alzheimer's Disease: A Medical Companion. Alistair Burns et al. 1995. LC 94-37632. 232p. pap. 39.95 *(0-632-03731-8)* Blackwell Sci.

*__Alzheimer's Disease: A Primer for Caregivers.__ Fructuoso Irigoyen. Tr. by Diana Schoefied-Melendez from SPA. rev. ed. 2001.Tr. of Enfermedad de Alzheimer. (Illus.). 64p. pap. 6.48 *(0-9709558-0-4)* Don Quixote Ed.

Alzheimer's Disease: A Source Guide. 1991. lib. bdg. 250.00 *(0-8490-4898-2)* Gordon Pr.

Alzheimer's Disease: Abstracts of the Psychological & Behavioral Literature. Ed. by Paul T. Costa, Jr. et al. 1989. (Bibliographies in Psychology Ser.: No. 4). 149p. pap. 25.00 *(1-55798-049-7)* Am Psychol.

Alzheimer's Disease: Activities That Work. Catherine Abrignani & Bill Messenger. 1991. (Illus.). 123p. (C). 19.50 *(1-877735-34-5*, 2182PP) Prof Prnting & Pub.

Alzheimer's Disease: Activity-Focused Care. Carly R. Hellen. 1992. (Illus.). 155p. spiral bd. 37.50 *(1-56372-018-3)* Buttrwrth-Heinemann.

*__Alzheimer's Disease: Advances in Etiology, Pathogenesis & Therapeutics.__ Khalid Iqbal et al. 2001. LC 00-67218. (Illus.). 888p. 295.00 *(0-471-52176-0)* Wiley.

Alzheimer's Disease: Aetiological Mechanisms & Therapeutic Possibilities. Ed. by J. D. Turner et al. 1996. LC 96-17823. (Ernst Schering Research Foundation Ser.: Vol. 17). *(0-387-60909-1)* Spr-Verlag.

Alzheimer's Disease: Aetiological Mechanisms & Therapeutic Possibilities. J. D. Turner et al. 1996. LC 96-17823. (Ernst Schering Research Foundation Ser.). (Illus.). 200p. 59.95 *(3-540-60909-1)* Spr-Verlag.

Alzheimer's Disease: Amyloid Precursor Proteins, Signal Transduction, & Neuronal Transplantation. Ed. by Roger M. Nitsch et al. 1993. LC 93-26927. (Annals Ser.: Vol. 695). 339p. 100.00 *(0-89766-853-7)*; pap. 100.00 *(0-89766-854-5)* NY Acad Sci.

Alzheimer's Disease: An Annotated Bibliography. Betty Weiner. 1986. (CompuBibs Ser.: No. 15). pap. 15.00 *(0-914791-14-1)* Vantage Info.

Alzheimer's Disease: Basic Mechanics Diagnosis & Therapeutic Strategies. Ed. by Khalid Iqbal et al. 1991. LC 90-13135. 676p. 687.95 *(0-471-92927-1)* Wiley.

Alzheimer's Disease: Biology, Diagnosis, & Therapeutics. Khalid Iqbal et al. 1997. LC 96-45760. 862p. 369.95 *(0-471-96964-8)* Wiley.

Alzheimer's Disease: Caregiver Practices, Programs & Community-Based Strategies. E. Pfeiffer et al. 1989. LC 89-60347. 103p. pap. 15.00 *(0-9622070-0-4)* USF SGC.

Alzheimer's Disease: Cause(s), Diagnosis, Treatment, & Care. Ed. by Zaven S. Khachaturian & Teresa S. Radebaugh. 1996. LC 96-16043. 368p. 129.95 *(0-8493-8997-6)* CRC Pr.

Alzheimer's Disease: Clinical & Treatment Perspectives. Ed. by Neal R. Cutler et al. 1995. LC 94-22396. 198p. 225.95 *(0-471-95039-4)* Wiley.

Alzheimer's Disease: Courage for Those Who Care. Martha O. Adams. 1999. LC 98-48409. xvi, 149p. pap. 16.95 *(0-8298-1304-7)* Pilgrim OH.

Alzheimer's Disease: Current Research in Early Diagnosis. Ed. by Robert E. Becker & Ezio Giacobini. 1990. 300p. 85.00 *(0-8448-1659-0*, Crane Russak) Taylor & Francis.

Alzheimer's Disease: Diagnosis, Cause & Treatment. Margaret Strock. rev. ed. 1996. (Illus.). 34p. (Orig.). pap. text 15.00 *(0-7881-2783-7)* DIANE Pub.

Alzheimer's Disease: Estimates of Prevalence in the United States. Ed. by Donald M. Keller. 1999. (Illus.). 45p. (C). pap. text 15.00 *(0-7881-7691-9)* DIANE Pub.

Alzheimer's Disease: Everything You Need to Know. Paul Caldwell & William Molloy. 1998. (Illus.). 216p. pap. 14.95 *(1-55209-241-0)* Firefly Bks Limited.

Alzheimer's Disease: Frequently Asked Questions: Making Sense of the Journey. Frena Gray-Davidson. rev. ed. 1999. 272p. pap. 15.95 *(0-7373-0079-5)* McGraw-Hill Prof.

Alzheimer's Disease: Legal & Financial Facts You Should Know. 1994. (Illus.). 20p. pap. 2.00 *(1-930181-02-7)* A H A F.

Alzheimer's Disease: Lessons from Cell Biology. Ed. by Kenneth S. Kosik et al. 1995. LC 94-41048. (Research & Perspectives in Alzheimer's Disease Ser.). 280p. 114.00 *(0-387-58744-6)* Spr-Verlag.

Alzheimer's Disease: Methods & Protocols. Ed. by Nigel M. Hooper. 2000. LC 00-61334. (Methods in Molecular Medicine Ser.: Vol. 32). (Illus.). xv, 287p. 125.00 *(0-89603-737-1)* Humana.

Alzheimer's Disease: New Treatment Strategies. Ed. by Khachaturian & John P. Blass. 1992. (Dementia Reviews Ser.: Vol. 1). (Illus.). 248p. text 145.00 *(0-8247-8620-3)* Dekker.

Alzheimer's Disease: Optimizing Drug Development Strategies. Neal R. Cutler et al. 1994. LC 94-10062. 178p. 195.00 *(0-471-95145-5)* Wiley.

Alzheimer's Disease: Optimizing the Development of the Next Generation of Therapeutic Compounds. Michael F. Murphy et al. 1999. LC 00-500877. (Greenwich Medical Media Ser.). (Illus.). 208p. text 98.50 *(1-84110-006-4)* OUP.

*__Alzheimer's Disease: Policy & Practice.__ Ed. by Morton Warner et al. 2001. 144p. pap. *(1-85775-416-6)* Radcliffe Med Pr GBR. *Dist:* Balogh.

Alzheimer's Disease: Problems, Prospects, & Perspectives. Ed. by H. J. Altman. 1987. LC 87-15374. (Illus.). 412p. 95.00 *(0-306-42662-5*, Plenum Trade) Perseus Pubng.

Alzheimer's Disease: Progress Report (1995) 1996. 28p. reprint ed. pap. text 20.00 *(0-7881-3133-8)* DIANE Pub.

Alzheimer's Disease: The ABCs of Diagnosis. 1994. (Illus.). 20p. pap. 2.00 *(1-930181-04-3)* A H A F.

Alzheimer's Disease: The Clinical Syndrome. Barry Reisberg. 1994. 19.18 *(0-02-926050-7)* S&S Trade.

*__Alzheimer's Disease: The Family Journey.__ Wayne A. Caron et al. 2001. 240p. pap. 22.00 *(0-9629614-2-6)* North Ridge Pr.

Alzheimer's Disease: The Physician's Guide to Practical Management. Ed. by Ralph W. Richter & John P. Blass. 2001. (Current Clinical Practice Ser.). 300p. 89.50 *(0-89603-891-2)* Humana.

Alzheimer's Disease: The Reference Text. Barry Reisberg. 1994. 67.50 *(0-02-926235-6)* S&S Trade.

Alzheimer's Disease: Therapeutic Strategies. Ed. by Ezio Giacobini et al. 1994. LC 94-34494. (Advances in Alzheimer's Disease Therapy Ser.). 509p. 95.50 *(0-8176-3757-5)* Birkhauser.

Alzheimer's Disease: Towards an Understanding of the Aetiology & Pathogenesis. Ed. by D. C. Davies. 1989. (Current Problems in Neurology Ser.: Vol. 11). 140p. *(0-86196-166-8)* J Libbey Med GBR. *Dist:* Bks Intl VA.

Alzheimer's Disease: Unraveling the Mystery. Caroline McNeil. 1997. (Illus.). 48p. reprint ed. pap. text 30.00 *(0-7881-3793-X)* DIANE Pub.

A B

Alzheimer's Disease Vol. I of II: Index of Modern Authors & Scientific Reviews for Inclusions in Current Research. Michael R. Scarborough. rev. ed. 1994. LC 90-56307. 213p. 57.50 (*0-7883-0414-3*); pap. 47.50 (*0-7883-0415-1*) ABBE Pubs Assn.

Alzheimer's Disease - From Basic Research to Clinical Applications. Ed. by H. J. Gertz & T. Arendt. 1998. (Illus.). 300p. 99.00 (*3-211-83113-4*) Spr-Verlag.

Alzheimer's Disease - Questions & Answers. Kenneth Davis et al. 1997. (Questions & Answers Ser.). (Illus.). 136p. (Orig.). pap. text 14.95 (*1-873413-36-X*) Merit Pub Intl.

Alzheimer's Disease - Radiation & Nutrition: Alzheimer's Aluminum Causation Thoughts. Marina Zokala et al. Ed. by Elena Plummer. 2nd rev. ed. 1998. (Illus.). 600p. 35.00 (*0-9665962-1-8*); pap. 25.00 (*0-9665962-0-X*) Life Ext Terres.

Alzheimer's Disease, Activity Focused Care. Carly R. Hellen. 2nd ed. 1998. LC 98-20819. 436p. pap. text 44.99 (*0-7506-9908-6*) Buttrwrth-Heinemann.

Alzheimer's Disease & Marriage. Lore K. Wright. 1993. LC 92-48987. (Clinical Nursing Research Ser.). 64.95 (*0-8039-4521-3*, 3357); pap. 27.95 (*0-8039-4522-1*, 3358) Sage.

Alzheimer's Disease & Related Disorders. Ed. by Marino Nicolini et al. 1993. (Advances in the Biosciences Ser.: Vol. 87). 526p. 190.25 (*0-08-042330-2*, Pergamon Pr) Elsevier.

Alzheimer's Disease & Related Disorders: 6th International Conference on Alzheimer's Disease. Khalid Iqbal. 1999. LC 98-44809. 878p. (C). 350.00 (*0-471-98683-6*) Wiley.

Alzheimer's Disease & Tacrine (Tetra-Hydro-9-Aminoacridine) Index of New Information with Authors, Subjects & References. Klaus J. Glauber. 1996. 150p. 57.50 (*0-7883-1268-5*); pap. 47.50 (*0-7883-1269-3*) ABBE Pubs Assn.

Alzheimer's Disease & the Dementias: An Alternative Perspective: Based on the Readings of Edgar Cayce. David McMillin. 1997. LC 96-54001. (Edgar Cayce Health Ser.). 96p. pap. 12.95 (*0-87604-380-5*, 494) ARE Pr.

Alzheimer's Disease Epidemiology, Neuropathology, Neurochemistry, & Clinics: Proceedings, International Congress on Alzheimer's Disease, Wurzburg, June 1989. Ed. by Konrad Maurer et al. 1990. (Key Topics in Brain Research Ser.). (Illus.). 581p. 127.95 (*0-387-82197-X*) Spr-Verlag.

Alzheimer's Disease from Care to Caring. Elinor Ringland. rev. ed. 1988. LC 85-81657. (Illus.). 112p. pap. 12.00 (*0-9613775-3-4*) Healthcare Pr.

Alzheimer's Disease Handbook. Cornelius Kelly. 2000. (Illus.). 100p. pap. 19.95 (*1-873413-37-8*) Merit Pub Intl.

Alzheimer's Disease Sourcebook: Basic Information about Alzheimer's Disease, Related Disorders & Other Dementias. Ed. by Karen Bellenir. 2nd ed. 1999. LC 98-51624. (Health Reference Ser.: Vol. 46). (Illus.). 600p. lib. bdg. 78.00 (*0-7808-0223-3*) Omnigraphics Inc.

Alzheimer's Disease Treatment & Family Stress: Directions for Research. Enid Light & Barry Liebowitz. 1990. 500p. 60.95 (*1-56032-137-7*) Hemisp Pub.

Alzheimer's Science & God. Hanna Kroeger. 1990. 15p. reprint ed. pap. text 1.25 (*1-883713-10-2*) Hanna Kroeger.

Alzheimer's, Stroke & Twenty-Nine Other Neurological Disorders: A Sourcebook Containing Basic Information on Types, Symptoms, Causes, Diagnostic Methods, & Treatments. Frank E. Bair. 1993. (Health Reference Ser.: Vol. 2). 600p. lib. bdg. 78.00 (*1-55888-748-2*) Omnigraphics Inc.

Alzheimer's...Another Opportunity To Love. Grayce B. Confer. 1992. LC 92-191581. 64p. pap. 6.99 (*0-8341-1403-8*) Beacon Hill.

Am I Crazy, or Is It My Shrink? Larry E. Beutler et al. 1998. LC 97-43546. 224p. 24.00 (*0-19-510780-2*) OUP.

***Am I Crazy, or Is It My Shrink? How to Get the Help You Need.** Larry E. Beutler et al. 2001. 214p. reprint ed. 24.00 (*0-7567-5119-5*) DIANE Pub.

Am I Fat? Abby Aronowitz. 2000. 92p. pap. 8.95 (*0-9703713-0-6*) A Aronowitz.

Am I My Brother's Keeper? The Ethical Frontiers of Biomedicine. Arthur L. Caplan. Ed. by David H. Smith & Robert M. Veatch. 1998. LC 97-19268. (Medical Ethics Ser.). 232p. 29.95 (*0-253-33358-X*) Ind U Pr.

AMA Drug Evaluations Annual 1994. Ed. by American Medical Association Staff. 1994. 2400p. 98.95 (*0-89970-602-9*, 932347) US Pharmacopeia.

AMA Essential Guide to Depression. Angela Perry. 1998. LC 98-19507. (American Medical Association Ser.). (Illus.). 256p. per. 14.00 (*0-671-01016-6*) PB.

AMA Guide to Your Family's Symptoms. 1993. 30.00 (*0-679-41370-7*) Random.

AMA Handbook of First Aid & Emergency Care. American Medical Association Staff. Ed. by James A. Hill & Stanley M. Zydlo, Jr. rev. ed. 2000. LC 99-14152. (Illus.). 352p. pap. 16.95 (*0-375-75486-5*) Random Hse Chldrns.

AMA Handbook of Project Management. Paul C. Dinsmore. 1993. LC 93-6947. 452p. 85.00 (*0-8144-0106-6*) AMACOM.

AMA Marketing Encyclopedia: Issues & Trends Shaping the Future. Jeffrey Heilbrunn. Ed. by Anne Knudsen. 1995. LC 94-17747. (Illus.). 360p. 47.95 (*0-8442-3593-8*, NTC Business Bks) NTC Contemp Pub Co.

AMA Medicolegal Forms with Legal Analysis. 1990. 32.00 (*0-89970-402-6*, OP630290) AMA.

Amador Study on Aging, Nutrition, & Stress. Effraim Alvi. 1984. LC 84-51500. (Illus.). 116p. pap. 39.95 (*0-918493-02-1*) Sierra Pub Co.

Amalgam Illness: Diagnosis & Treatment: What You Can Do to Get Better, How Your Doctor Can Help You. Andrew Hall Cutler. 1999. (Illus.). vi, 226p. pap. 35.00 (*0-9676168-0-8*, Andrew Hall Cutler) Minerva Labs.

Amaurosis Fugax. Ed. by E. F. Bernstein. 1988. (Illus.). 310p. 109.00 (*0-387-96601-3*) Spr-Verlag.

Amazing Brain. Robert E. Ornstein & Richard F. Thompson. 1991. (Illus.). 224p. pap. 15.95 (*0-395-58572-4*) HM.

Amazing Honey, Garlic & Vinegar Home Remedies: A Doctor's Guide to Using These Natural Remedies. Patrick Quillin. 1996. LC 98-127845. (Illus.). 250p. pap. 14.95 (*1-886898-03-0*) Leader OH.

Amazing Medicines the Drug Companies Don't Want You to Discover. Hans J. Kugler. 1999. LC 00-697971. (Illus.). viii, 390p. mass mkt. 6.99 (*0-425-16943-X*) Berkley Pub.

Amazon Healer: The Life & Times of an Urban Shaman. Marlene D. De Rios. 1992. 192p. (Orig.). (C). pap. (*1-85327-076-8*) Prism Pr GBR. *Dist:* Assoc Pubs Grp.

Amazonian Ethnobotanical Dictionary. James A. Duke & Rodolfo V. Martinez. 1994. LC 94-390. 224p. per. 57.95 (*0-8493-3664-3*) CRC Pr.

Ambiguity in Psycholinguistics. Joseph F. Kess & Ronald A. Hoppe. 1981. (Pragmatics & Beyond Ser.: Vol. II: 4). vi, 124p. pap. 32.00 (*90-272-2514-1*) J Benjamins Pubng Co.

Amblyopia: A Multidisciplinary Approach. Alistair Fielder & Merrick Moseley. 2001. 160p. 44.99 (*0-7506-4691-8*) Buttrwrth-Heinemann.

Ambroise Pare: Surgeon of the Renaissance. Wallace Hamby. 1967. LC 67-19384. (Illus.). 250p. 15.00 (*0-87527-039-5*) Green.

Ambulance: The Story of Emergency Transportation of Sick & Wounded Through the Centuries. Katherine T. Barkley. 1990. LC 90-62107. 25.00 (*0-9626357-2-3*) Load N Go Pr.

Ambulance Attendant. Jack Rudman. 1994. (Career Examination Ser.: C-1088). pap. 34.95 (*0-8373-1088-1*) Nat Learn.

Ambulance Calls: Review Problems in Emergency Care. Nancy L. Caroline. 2nd ed. 1987. pap. text 22.00 (*0-316-12871-6*, Little Brwn Med Div) Lppncott W & W.

Ambulance Corpsman. Jack Rudman. 1994. (Career Examination Ser.: C-2650). pap. 34.95 (*0-8373-2650-8*) Nat Learn.

Ambulance Driver. Jack Rudman. 1994. (Career Examination Ser.: C-1089). pap. 27.95 (*0-8373-1089-X*) Nat Learn.

Ambulances. Leslie Geary. 1991. (Illus.). 80p. (*0-86025-879-3*) I Henry Pubns GBR. *Dist:* Empire Pub Srvs.

Ambulante Rehabilitation nach Herzinfarkt. Karl-Ernst Schenk. 1979. pap. 21.00 (*3-8055-2965-1*) S Karger.

Ambulatory & Inpatient Procedures in the United States, 1994. Robert Pokras et al. 1998. (Illus.). 116p. (C). pap. text 30.00 (*0-7881-7424-X*) DIANE Pub.

Ambulatory & Inpatient Procedures in the United States, 1994. Robert Pokras et al. 1998. LC 97-42743. (Vital & Health Statistics Ser.: Series 13, No. 132). (*0-8406-0535-8*) Natl Ctr Health Stats.

Ambulatory Anesthesia & Surgery. Paul F. White. 1996. text 131.00 (*0-7020-1799-X*) Saunders.

Ambulatory Anesthesia Handbook. Rebecca S. Twersky. 1996. (Volume in the Year Book Handbooks Ser.). (Illus.). 464p. pap. 30.60 (*84-8174-124-8*) Mosby Inc.

Ambulatory Anesthesia Handbook. Ed. by Rebecca S. Twersky. 1994. LC 94-32505. (Illus.). 464p. (C). (gr. 13). pap. text 40.95 (*0-8151-8847-1*, 23620) Mosby Inc.

Ambulatory Anorectal Surgery. Ed. by H. Randolph Bailey & Michael J. Snyder. 1999. LC 98-52782. (Illus.). 240p. 110.00 (*0-387-98603-0*) Spr-Verlag.

Ambulatory Assessment: Computer-Assisted Psychological & Psychophysiological Methods in Monitoring & Field Studies. Ed. by Jochen Fahrenberg & Michael Myrtek. 1996. LC 96-3243. (Illus.). 432p. text 49.50 (*0-88937-167-9*) Hogrefe & Huber Pubs.

Ambulatory Blood Pressure Recording. Ed. by Bernard Waeber et al. 1992. LC 94-23214. 208p. 58.00 (*0-7817-0242-9*) Lppncott W & W.

Ambulatory Care: Organization & Management. Austin Ross et al. 1989. LC 83-16709. (Health Services Ser.: No. 1-456). 453p. text 41.95 (*0-8273-4349-3*) Delmar.

Ambulatory Care & Outpatient Services: Forms, Checklist & Guidelines. Aspen Reference Group Staff. rev. ed. 1997. ring bd. 220.00 (*0-8342-0804-0*, S285) Aspen Pub.

Ambulatory Care & Outpatient Services Manual: Includes Facility Design, Operations, Case Costing, Contracting, Integrated Delivery Systems, Reimbursement. Harvey E. Billig. 1997. LC 96-40918. 340p. (C). text 250.00 (*1-55738-641-2*, Irwn Prfssnl) McGraw-Hill Educ Grp.

Ambulatory Care Clinical Skills Program: Anticoagulation Management Module. Mary T. Pasko & Denise Komorowski-Swiatek. 2000. 250p. pap. text (*1-58528-015-1*) Am Soc Hlth-Syst.

Ambulatory Care Clinical Skills Program: Asthma Management Module. 1999. 250p. ring bd. (*1-879907-94-1*) Am Soc Hlth-Syst.

Ambulatory Care Clinical Skills Program: Core Module. Wendy P. Munroe et al. 1998. 464p. text 219.00 (*1-879907-88-7*) Am Soc Hlth-Syst.

Ambulatory Care Clinical Skills Program: Dyslipidemia Management Module. Geneva Clark Briggs. 2000. 250p. pap. text (*1-58528-010-0*) Am Soc Hlth-Syst.

Ambulatory Care Clinical Skills Program: Practice Management Module. 1999. 250p. pap. 50.00 (*1-879907-92-5*) Am Soc Hlth-Syst.

Ambulatory Care Clinical Skills Program: Type 2 Diabetes Mellitus Management Module. 1999. 250p. pap. (*1-879907-93-3*) Am Soc Hlth-Syst.

Ambulatory Care Clinics. Ed. by Peter Allen. 1989. 200p. pap. 1495.00 (*0-941285-42-1*) FIND-SVP.

Ambulatory Care Documentation. AHIMA, Ambulatory Care Section Staff. 1997. (Illus.). 252p. pap. text 48.00 (*1-58426-009-2*, AB101597) Am Hlth Info.

Ambulatory Care in Integrated Delivery Systems. Alan M. Zuckerman. 1998. LC 98-17780. 137p. pap. 40.00 (*1-55648-226-4*) AHPI.

Ambulatory Care in New York City 1984, Set. Compiled by Division of Research, Analysis, and Planning Staff. 1985. 60.00 (*0-934459-16-9*) United Hosp Fund.

Ambulatory Care Management. Austin Ross. 2nd ed. 1991. 432p. text 44.00 (*0-8273-4613-1*) Delmar.

Ambulatory Care Management. Austin Ross et al. 3rd ed. 1997. LC 96-47935. (Health Services Administration Ser.). 448p. (C). 82.95 (*0-8273-7664-2*) Delmar.

Ambulatory Care Management & Practice. Ed. by Albert E. Barnett & Gloria G. Mayer. 1992. 526p. 114.00 (*0-8342-0313-8*, 20313) Aspen Pub.

Ambulatory Care Procedures for the Nurse Practitioner. Margaret R. Colyar & Cynthia Ehrhardt. 1998. LC 98-42191. (Illus.). 472p. (C). pap. text 39.95 (*0-8036-0364-9*) Davis Co.

Ambulatory Care Services & the Prospective Payment System. Norbert Goldfield & William P. Kelly. 1995. LC 99-26845. 292p. pap. 76.00 (*0-8342-1640-X*) Aspen Pub.

Ambulatory Care Visits to Physician Offices, Hospital Outpatient Departments & Emergency Departments: United States, 1995. National Center for Health Statistics Staff & Susan M. Schappert. 1997. LC 97-10617. (Vital & Health Statistics Ser.: Series 13, No. 129). iv, 37p. (*0-8406-0525-0*) Natl Ctr Health Stats.

Ambulatory Esophageal PH Monitoring: Practical Approach & Clinical Applications. Joel E. Richter. 2nd ed. 1997. LC 97-2003. (*4-260-14343-3*); (*0-89640-343-2*) Igaku-Shoin.

Ambulatory Family Practice Protocols. Matthew M. Cohen & Anni Lanigan. 1994. 264p. pap. 55.00 (*0-924381-18-3*); ring bd. 85.00 (*0-924381-20-5*); 3.5 hd (*0-924381-19-1*) Sunbelt Med Pubs.

Ambulatory Gynecologic Surgery. Purvis L. Martin. 1979. LC 78-55286. (Illus.). 394p. 50.00 (*0-88416-209-5*) Mosby Inc.

Ambulatory Health Care: Case Studies for the Health Services Executive. Ed. by Austin Ross & Mary Richardson. 1996. LC 96-12939. 352p. (Orig.). pap. 46.00 (*1-56793-044-1*) Health Admin Pr.

Ambulatory Health Care Units by Children: Principal Diagnosis & Place of Visit. Virginia M. Freid et al. 1998. LC 98-15148. (DHHS Publication Statistics). 2.50 (*0-8406-0546-3*) Natl Ctr Health Stats.

Ambulatory Medicine. Mengel & Schwiebert. 3rd ed. 2000. (Lange Medical Bks.). (Illus.). 770p. pap. 49.95 (*0-8385-0387-X*) McGraw-Hill Prof.

Ambulatory Monitoring: Cardiovascular System & Applied Applications. Ed. by Carlo Marchesi. 1984. (Developments in Cardiovascular Medicine Ser.). text 219.50 (*0-89838-642-X*) Kluwer Academic.

Ambulatory Obstetrics. Washington Hill. 1998. LC 2001-50214. text 59.95 (*0-397-51855-2*) Lppncott W & W.

Ambulatory Obstetrics. Winifred Star et al. 3rd rev. ed. 1999. 1248p. pap. text 85.00 (*0-943671-18-3*) UCSF Schl Nursing.

Ambulatory Obstetrics: Protocols for Nurse Practitioners - Nurse-Midwives. Winifred Star et al. 2nd enl. ed. 1990. 432p. (C). 62.00 (*0-943671-07-8*) UCSF Schl Nursing.

Ambulatory Patient Care. Linda B. Chitwood. 1994. 250p. (Orig.). (C). pap. 49.95 (*1-878025-63-5*) Western Schls.

Ambulatory Patient Group Operations Manual. Duane C. Abbey. 1996. 360p. (C). text 195.00 (*0-7863-0842-7*, Irwn Prfssnl) McGraw-Hill Educ Grp.

Ambulatory Pediatric Care. Robert A. Dershewitz. 3rd ed. 1998. LC 98-35195. 1,136p. text 89.95 (*0-7817-1014-6*) Lppncott W & W.

Ambulatory Pediatrics. Ed. by James A. Stockman, III & Jacob A. Lohr. 1999. LC 99-50226. xxxvi, 472p. (C). text 67.25 (*0-7216-5845-8*) Saunders.

Ambulatory Pediatrics. Morris Green. 4th ed. 1990. text 92.00 (*0-7216-4240-3*) Saunders.

Ambulatory Pediatrics. Morris Green et al. Ed. by Judy Fletcher. 5th ed. 1999. LC 98-50611. (Illus.). xxii, 581p. (C). text 79.00 (*0-7216-7401-1*) Saunders.

Ambulatory Peritoneal Dialysis. M. M. Avram & C. Giordano. 1990. (Illus.). 356p. (C). text 95.00 (*0-306-43351-6*, Kluwer Plenum) Kluwer Academic.

Ambulatory Phlebectomy: A Practical Guide for Treating Varicose Veins. Stefano Ricci et al. 1995. (Illus.). 256p. (C). (gr. 13). text 138.00 (*0-8151-7045-9*, 24829) Mosby Inc.

Ambulatory Prenatal Nursing Care: Practice Standards for Positive Pregnancy Outcomes. Marjorie R. Berg et al. 1986. LC 85-27649. 224p. pap. 29.95 (*0-8261-5330-5*) Springer Pub.

Ambulatory Surgery. Joseph Schirmer. 1998. LC 97-41327. text 95.00 (*0-7216-5889-X*) Saunders.

Ambulatory Surgery Patient Education Manual. Aspen Reference Group Staff. Ed. by Sara N. Di Lima & Simon B. Weavers. 1997. LC 97-10866. ring bd. 99.00 (*0-8342-0877-6*, S314) Aspen Pub.

Ambulatory Surgical Nursing. Nancy Burden. 1993. (Illus.). 754p. text 73.50 (*0-7216-2897-4*) Saunders.

Ambulatory Surgical Nursing. Nancy Burden et al. 2nd ed. 1999. LC 99-31873. (Illus.). xix, 898p. text 60.00 (*0-7216-6847-X*) Saunders.

Ambulatory Surgical Nursing: Clinical. Nancy Burden. 2002. pap. text (*0-7216-5696-X*) Saunders.

Ambulatory Surgical Nursing Core Curriculum. American Society of PeriAnesthesia Nurses Staff. Ed. by Maura Connor. 1998. LC 98-34732. (Illus.). 635p. (C). pap. text 47.00 (*0-7216-6522-5*) Saunders.

Ambulatory Treatment of Venous Disease: An Illustrative Guide. Ed. by Mitchel P. Goldman & John J. Bergan. 1995. (Illus.). 192p. (C). (gr. 13). text 144.00 (*0-8151-3758-3*, 25193) Mosby Inc.

Ambulatory Women's Health Care Nursing. Jack Rudman. (Certified Nurse Examination Ser.: CN-24). 47.95 (*0-8373-6174-5*); pap. 27.95 (*0-8373-6124-9*) Nat Learn.

AmbuQual Data Guide: A System for Collecting, Organizing & Scoring Data. Judi Cagiano. 1993. (AmbuQual Ser.). pap. 78.00 (*1-884742-00-9*) Clarian Hlth.

AmbuQual II: An Ambulatory Quality Assessment & Quality Management System. Dale S. Benson & Jane A. Miller. 2nd ed. 1993. (AmbuQual Ser.). 345p. pap. 148.00 (*0-9603164-8-5*) Clarian Hlth.

AMDP System in Pharmacopsychiatry. Ed. by D. P. Bobon et al. 1983. (Modern Problems of Pharmacopsychiatry Ser.: Vol. 20). (Illus.). vi, 234p. 115.00 (*3-8055-3637-2*) S Karger.

Amebiasis Infection & Disease by Entamoeba Histolytica. Ed. by Roberto R. Kretschmer. 1990. LC 89-70837. 288p. 148.00 (*0-8493-5342-4*, RC121, CRC Reprint) Franklin.

Amelioration of the Human Environment: IGU Congress, Moscow, 1976, Proceedings, Pt. 1. Ed. by Yuri Medvedkov. 1977. pap. 23.00 (*0-08-021322-7*, Pergamon Pr) Elsevier.

America Exhausted Vol. 1: Breakthrough Treatments of Fatigue & Chronic Fatigue Syndrome. Edward J. Conley. 1997. LC 96-60868. 256p. (Orig.). pap. 14.95 (*0-9652544-0-2*) Vitality Pr.

America Living with AIDS: Transforming Anger, Fear, & Indifference into Action: Report of the National Commission on AIDS. 1992. 165p. (Orig.). (C). pap. text 30.00 (*1-56806-106-4*) DIANE Pub.

American Academy of Family Physicians: Family Health & Medical Guide. AAFP Staff. 1996. LC 95-46003. (Illus.). 608p. 39.99 (*0-8499-0839-6*) W Pubng Grp.

American Academy of Orthopaedic Surgeons Instructional Course Lectures, Vol. 42. Ed. by James D. Heckman. 1993. (Illus.). 570p. 85.00 (*0-89203-071-2*) Amer Acad Ortho Surg.

American Academy of Pediatrics Guide. American Academy of Pediatrics Staff. 1997. 125.00 (*0-676-53162-8*) Villard Books.

American Academy of Pediatrics Guide to Your Child's Allergies & Asthma: Breathing Easy & Bringing Up Healthy, Active Children. Michael Welsh. 2000. LC 99-57263. (Illus.). xii, 191p. pap. 12.95 (*0-679-76982-X*) Villard Books.

American Armamentarium Chirurgicum. George Tiemann. 1989. (Illus.). 846p. reprint ed. 165.00 (*0-930405-23-4*) Norman SF.

American Association of Oriental Medicine's Complete Guide to Chinese Herbal Medicine. David Molony. 1998. LC 98-150436. (Illus.). 288p. pap. 13.00 (*0-425-15705-9*) Berkley Pub.

American Association of Physicists in Medicine 1996 Membership Directory. rev. ed. 1995. 156p. (*1-888340-00-2*) AAPM.

American Association of Physicists in Medicine 1997 Membership Directory. rev. ed. 1996. 170p. (*1-888340-07-X*) AAPM.

American Bibliographic Notes: Three Massachusetts Broadsides; Earliest Medical Broadsides. William S. Reese & Morris H. Saffron. 1983. 25p. pap. 4.00 (*0-944026-79-6*) Am Antiquarian.

American Cancer Society: A Thorough & Compassionate Resource for Patients & Their Families. Carolyn Runowitz et al. 1999. LC 98-39231. (American Cancer Society Ser.). (Illus.). 336p. pap. 14.95 (*0-679-77814-4*) Random.

American Cancer Society - Colorectal Cancer: Cancer: A Thorough & Compassionate Resource for Patients & Their Families. Bernard Levin. 1999. LC 98-35323. (American Cancer Society Ser.). (Illus.). 336p. pap. 14.95 (*0-679-77813-6*) Random.

American Cancer Society Consumers Guide to Cancer Drugs. Gail M. Wilkes et al. 1999. (Illus.). 480p. (C). pap. text 21.95 (*0-7637-1170-5*, 1170-5) Jones & Bartlett.

American Cancer Society Cookbook. Anne Lindsay. 1990. 9.98 (*0-671-07484-9*) S&S Trade.

American Cancer Society Patient Education Guides to Oncology Drugs. Ed. by Gail M. Wilkes et al. 1999. LC 99-47122. (Illus.). 480p. (C). pap. text 93.95 (*0-7637-1173-X*, 1173-x) Jones & Bartlett.

American Cancer Society Prostate Cancer: Resource for Patients & Their Families. American Cancer Society Staff and Volunteers et al. rev. ed. 1999. LC 99-230190. (American Cancer Society Ser.). (Illus.). 336p. pap. 14.95 (*0-375-75319-2*) Villard Books.

American Cancer Society Textbook of Clinical Oncology. Ed. by Gerald P. Murphy et al. 2nd ed. 1995. LC 95-132. 766p. (*0-944235-10-7*) Am Cancer NY.

American Cancer Society's Informed Decisions: The Complete Book of Cancer Diagnosis, Treatment, & Recovery. Gerald P. Murphy. 1999. 40.00 (*0-525-93999-7*) NAL.

American Chamber of Horrors: The Truth about Food & Drugs. Ruth D. Lamb. 1976. LC 75-39255. (Getting & Spending: The Consumer's Dilemma Ser.). (Illus.). reprint ed. 35.95 (*0-405-08028-X*) Ayer.

American Civil War Medical Series 1991. reprint ed. 595.00 (*0-930405-45-5*) Norman SF.

American Civil War Surgery Series 1993. reprint ed. 495.00 (*0-930405-46-3*) Norman SF.

American College of Cardiology Guide to CPT 2000. Ed. by Douglas L. Wood. 2000. (Illus.). 176p. pap. 60.00 (*1-58397-006-1*, CPT00) Am Coll Cardiology.

American College of Cardiology Guide to CPT-4, 1994. 1993. 161p. (Orig.). (C). pap. text (*1-882764-07-2*) Am Coll Cardiology.

American College of Legal Medicine Foundation Medicolegal Primer, 1991 Edition. 1991. 400p. (*0-9629575-0-X*) Amer Coll Legal.

American College of Physicians Ethics Manual. American College of Physicians Staff & Lloyd W. Kitchens. 4th ed. 1998. LC 98-15901. 10.00 (*0-943126-67-3*) Amer Coll Phys.

American College of Physicians Home Care Guide for HIV & AIDS: For Family & Friends Giving Care at Home. Peter Houts. 1997. LC 96-37121. (Home Care Guides Ser.). 260p. (Orig.). (C). pap. text 24.95 (*0-943126-54-1*) Amer Coll Phys.

American College of Physicians Home Medical Guide: Asthma. Jon Ayres. 2000. LC 98-44067. (ACP Home Medical Guides Ser.). (Illus.). 96p. pap. 6.95 (*0-7894-4162-4*, D K Ink) DK Pub Inc.

American College of Radiology: The First 75 Years. Otha W. Linton. 1997. LC 97-24700. (*1-55903-140-9*) Am Coll Radiology.

American College of Sports Medicine 40th Anniversary Lectures. American College of Sports Medicine Staff. anniv. ltd. ed. 1994. LC 94-71614. (Illus.). 120p. (Orig.). pap. 10.00 (*1-885377-00-2*) Am Coll Sports Med.

American Cool: Constructing a Twentieth-Century Emotional Style. Peter N. Stearns. 1994. LC 93-42152. (History of Emotions Ser.). 368p. (C). text 47.50 (*0-8147-7979-4*) NYU Pr.

American Daughter Gone to War: On the Front Lines with an Army Nurse in Vietnam. Winnie Smith. Ed. by Julie Rubenstein. 1994. LC 93-27366. 352p. reprint ed. per. 12.00 (*0-671-87048-3*) PB.

American Dentist: A Pictorial History with a Presentation of Early Dental Photography in America. Richard A. Glenner. 1990. LC 90-60363. (Illus.). 202p. 24.95 (*0-929521-05-6*) Pictorial Hist.

American Diabetes Association & American Dietetic Association Family Cookbook, Vol. II. American Diabetes Association. 1984. 448p. 23.00 (*0-13-024910-6*, CCBF2) Am Diabetes.

American Diabetes Association & American Dietetic Association Family Cookbook: The American Tradition, Vol. IV. American Diabetes Association & American Dietetic Association Staff. 4th ed. 1991. (Illus.). 403p. 23.00 (*0-13-024092-3*, CCBF4) Am Diabetes.

American Diabetes Association Complete Guide to Diabetes. American Diabetes Association. 1996. LC 96-19104. 446p. 29.95 (*0-945448-64-3*, 4808-01); 2nd ed. 1999. LC 99-49617. (Illus.). 454p. pap. 23.95 (*1-58040-038-8*, 00388Q) Am Diabetes.

American Diabetes Association Complete Guide to Diabetes. Ed. by American Diabetes Association. 2nd ed. 2000. (Illus.). 544p. mass mkt. 6.99 (*0-553-58300-X*) Bantam.

American Diabetes Association Guide to Diabetes Coding. American Diabetes Association. 1999. LC 98-52396. (*1-58040-034-5*) Am Diabetes.

American Diabetes Association Holiday Cookbook. Betty Wedman. 1986. (Illus.). 206p. pap. 19.95 (*0-13-024894-0*) Am Diabetes.

American Diabetes Association Special Celebrations & Parties Cookbook. Betty Wedman. 1989. 243p. pap. 19.95 (*0-13-004219-6*) Am Diabetes.

American Diabetes Association's Guide to Medical Nutrition Therapy for Diabetes. Marion J. Franz et al. 1999. LC 98-47839. (Clinical Education Ser.). (Illus.). vii, 399p. (*1-58040-006-X*) Am Diabetes.

American Diabetes Association/The American Dietetic Association Family Cookbook, Vol. III. American Diabetes Association & American Dietetic Association Staff. 1987. 434p. 23.00 (*0-88091-035-6*, 0842) Am Diabetes.

American Dietetic Association Family Cookbook. American Diatetic Association Staff. 1989. 9.98 (*0-13-024980-7*) P-H.

American Dietetic Association's Complete Food & Nutrition Guide. American Dietetic Association Staff et al. 1998. 656p. pap. 24.95 (*0-471-34659-4*) Wiley.

American Dietetic Association's Complete Food & Nutrition Guide: The Most Comprehensive & Up-to-Date Resource on Healthy Food Choices from the World's Foremost Experts. Roberta L. Duyff. 1996. (Illus.). 644p. 39.95 (*1-56561-098-9*) Wiley.

American Doctors of Destiny. Frank J. Jirka. 1977. LC 76-121482. (Essay Index Reprint Ser.). 31.95 (*0-8369-1759-6*) Ayer.

American Drinking Practices: A National Study of Drinking Behavior & Attitudes. Don Cahalan et al. 1969. LC 70-626701. (Monographs: No. 6). pap. 10.95 (*0-911290-37-0*) Rutgers Ctr Alcohol.

American Experience with Alcohol: Contrasting Cultural Perspectives. L. A. Bennett & G. M. Ames. 1985. LC 85-9302. (Illus.). 514p. (C). 102.00 (*0-306-41945-9*, Plenum Trade) Perseus Pubng.

American Folk Healing: An A-Z Guide to Traditional American Remedies. Reader's Digest Editorial Staff. 1998. LC 97-23574. (*0-7621-0009-5*) RD Assn.

American Folk Medicine. Clarence Meyer. 1985. LC 85-155364. 320p. reprint ed. pap. 9.95 (*0-916638-10-3*) Meyerbooks.

American General Hospital: Communities & Social Contexts. Ed. by Diana E. Long & Janet Golden. 1989. LC 89-7264. (Illus.). 216p. pap. 18.95 (*0-8014-9604-7*) Cornell U Pr.

American Health Care: Government, Market Processes & the Public Interest. Ed. by Roger D. Feldman. 2000. LC 00-20662. (Illus.). xi, 444p. pap. text 24.95 (*0-7658-0676-2*) Transaction Pubs.

American Health Care: Realities, Rights, & Reforms. Charles J. Dougherty. 1988. 240p. text 35.00 (*0-19-505271-4*); pap. text 19.95 (*0-19-505272-2*) OUP.

American Health Care Blues: Blue Cross, HMOs & Pragmatic Reform. Irwin Miller. 1996. LC 96-17334. 125p. 32.95 (*1-56000-265-4*) Transaction Pubs.

American Health Care Delivery Systems. Joseph A. Snoe. 1998. LC 98-12665. (American Casebook Ser.). 800p. 65.00 (*0-314-22835-7*) West Pub.

American Health Care in Transition: A Guide to the Literature, 14. Barbara A. Haley & Brian Deevey. 1997. LC 97-5305. (Bibliographies & Indexes in Medical Studies: Vol. 14). 352p. lib. bdg. 82.95 (*0-313-27323-5*, Greenwood Pr) Greenwood.

***American Health Dilemma: Race, Medicine, & Health Care in the United States 1900-2000**, Vol. 2. W. Michael Byrd & Linda A. Clayton. 2001. (Illus.). 624p. 35.00 (*0-415-92737-4*) Routledge.

American Health Law. Law and Business Inc. Staff & George J. Annas. 1990. 54.00 (*0-316-04309-5*) Aspen Law.

American Health Policy: Critical Issues for Reform. Robert Helms. 1993. LC 92-22281. 200p. 39.75 (*0-8447-3818-2*) Am Enterprise.

***American Healthcare Resource Directory: The First Place to Look for Medical Help & Information.** Stephen K. Greer. 2001. LC 2001-19597. 412p. 29.95 (*0-9652442-2-9*) Preston Publng.

American Heart Association 365 Ways to Get Out the Fat. American Heart Association Staff. 1997. LC 97-28430. (Illus.). 128p. mass mkt. 4.99 (*0-8129-6385-7*, Crown) Crown Pub Group.

American Heart Association Clip Strip Program. American Heart Association Staff. 1995. pap. 29.94 (*0-8129-2669-2*, Crown) Crown Pub Group.

American Heart Association Low-Fat, Low Cholesterol Cookbook: Heart-Healthy, Easy-to-Make Recipes that Taste Great. American Heart Association Staff. 2nd rev. ed. 1997. LC 97-17099. (American Heart Association Cookbook Ser.). (Illus.). 384p. 25.95 (*0-8129-2684-6*, Crown) Crown Pub Group.

American Heart Association Meals in Minutes: Over 200 All-New Quick & Easy Low-Fat Recipes. American Heart Association Staff. 2000. LC 99-52989. (Illus.). 368p. 26.95 (*0-8129-3332-X*, Crown) Crown Pub Group.

American Herbal Medicine: The Country Doctor's Legacy. Thomas Squier. 1998. LC 97-27236. (Illus.). 228p. pap. 14.95 (*0-8050-3724-1*, Owl) H Holt & Co.

American Herbal Products Association's Botanical Safety Handbook: Guidelines for the Safe Use & Labeling for Herbs in Commerce. American Herbal Products Association Staff & Michael McGuffin. 1997. LC 97-17162. 256p. 44.95 (*0-8493-1675-8*) CRC Pr.

American Heritage Stedman's Medical Dictionary. American Heritage Publishing Staff. 1995. LC 95-10806. (Illus.). 960p. 27.00 (*0-395-69955-X*) HM.

American Holistic Health Association Complete Guide to Alternative Medicine. William Collinge. 1997. LC 95-10201. (American Holistic Health Association Complete Guide Ser.). 384p. pap. (*0-446-67258-0*) Warner.

American Holistic Medical Association Guide to Holistic Health: Healing Therapies for Optimal Wellness. Larry Trivieri, Jr. 2001. 448p. 29.95 (*0-471-32743-3*) Wiley.

American Indian Healing Arts: Herbs, Rituals & Remedies for Every Season of Life. E. Barrie Kavasch & Karen Baar. 1999. LC 98-43985. (Illus.). 336p. pap. 17.95 (*0-553-37881-3*) Bantam.

American Indian Health: Innovations in Health Care, Promotion & Policy. Ed. by Everett R. Rhoades. 2000. LC 99-50740. (Illus.). 484p. 65.00 (*0-8018-6328-7*) Johns Hopkins.

American Indian Medicine. Virgil J. Vogel. 1990. LC 69-10626. (Civilization of the American Indian Ser.: Vol. 95). (Illus.). pap. 24.95 (*0-8061-2293-5*) U of Okla Pr.

American Indian Task Force Report on the Year 2000: Health Promotion Objectives & Recommendations for California. 1993. 41p. (Orig.). (C). pap. text 30.00 (*0-7881-0091-2*) DIANE Pub.

American Jury on Trial: Psychological Perspectives. Saul M. Kassin & Lawrence S. Wrightsman. 1988. 232p. pap. 29.95 (*0-89116-856-7*) Hemisp Pub.

American Lung Association 7 Steps to a Smoke-Free Life. Edwin B. Fisher, Jr. & Toni L. Goldfarb. 1998. LC 97-38826. (Illus.). 240p. pap. 14.95 (*0-471-24700-6*) Wiley.

American Lung Association's Family Guide to Asthma & Allergies. American Lung Association Staff. 1998. LC 96-53497. (Illus.). 256p. pap. 13.95 (*0-316-03815-6*, Back Bay) Little.

American Lung Association's Family Guide to Asthma & Allergies. Norman Edelman & American Lung Association Staff. 1997. LC 96-53497. (Illus.). 256p. (gr. 8). 19.95 (*0-316-21271-7*) Little.

American Materia Medica Therapeutics & Pharmacognosy. Ed. by Kathryn Rosson. 1919. 564p. reprint ed. text 98.00 (*1-888483-05-9*) Eclectic Med.

American Medical Association & Organized Medicine: A Commentary & Annotated Bibliography. James A. Johnson & Walter J. Jones. 1993. LC 93-7145. (Organizations & Interest Groups Ser.: Vol. 8). 288p. 42.00 (*0-8240-3535-6*, SS722); text 15.00 (*0-8153-0049-2*, SS713) Garland.

***American Medical Association Complete Guide to Men's Health.** American Medical Association Staff. 2001. LC 2001-17905. (Illus.). 512p. 34.95 (*0-471-41411-5*) Wiley.

American Medical Association Encyclopedia of Medicine. American Medical Association Staff. 1989. (Illus.). 1184p. 45.00 (*0-394-56528-2*) Random.

American Medical Association Essential Guide to Asthma. Angela Perry. 1998. LC 98-15733. (American Medical Association Ser.). (Illus.). 320p. pap. 14.00 (*0-671-01013-1*, Pocket Books) PB.

American Medical Association Essential Guide to Asthma. AMA Staff. 2000. reprint ed. mass mkt. 6.99 (*0-7434-0357-6*, Pocket Books) PB.

American Medical Association Essential Guide to Depression. AMA Staff. 2000. reprint ed. mass mkt. 6.99 (*0-7434-0359-2*, Pocket Books) PB.

American Medical Association Essential Guide to Hypertension. AMA Staff. 2000. reprint ed. mass mkt. 6.99 (*0-7434-0360-6*, Pocket Books) PB.

American Medical Association Essential Guide to Menopause. Angela Perry. 1998. LC 98-15034. (American Medical Association Ser.). (Illus.). 256p. pap. 14.00 (*0-671-01014-X*, Pocket Books) PB.

American Medical Association Essential Guide to Menopause. AMA Staff. 2000. reprint ed. mass mkt. 6.99 (*0-7434-0358-4*, Pocket Books) PB.

American Medical Association Family Medical Guide. American Medical Association Staff. 1982. 29.45 (*0-394-53013-6*) Random.

American Medical Association Family Medical Guide. American Medical Association Staff. rev. ed. 1987. LC 86-17659. (Illus.). 832p. 35.00 (*0-394-55582-1*) Random.

American Medical Association Family Medical Guide. Charles B. Clayman. 3rd ed. 1994. (*0-679-44906-X*) McKay.

American Medical Association Family Medical Guide. Ed. by Charles B. Clayman. 3rd rev. ed. 1994. LC 94-2116. (AMA Family Medical Guide Ser.). (Illus.). 880p. 39.95 (*0-679-41290-5*) Random.

***American Medical Association Guide to Home Caregiving.** American Medical Association Staff. 2001. LC 2001-24710. (Illus.). 256p. pap. 14.95 (*0-471-41409-3*) Wiley.

***American Medical Association Guide to Talking to Your Doctor.** American Medical Association Staff. 2001. LC 2001-24711. (Illus.). 256p. pap. 14.95 (*0-471-41410-7*) Wiley.

American Medical Association Guide to Your Family's Symptoms. American Medical Association Staff. 1992. pap. 15.00 (*0-8129-2037-6*, Crown) Crown Pub Group.

American Medical Association Health Care Almanac. American Medical Association Staff. 2nd ed. 1997. LC 00-500759. 27.95 (*0-89970-900-1*) AMA.

American Medical Association Pocket Guide to Emergency First Aid. American Medical Association Staff. 1993. LC 92-56798. 96p. pap. 4.99 (*0-679-74672-2*) Random.

American Medical Education: The Formative Years, 1765-1910. Martin Kaufman. 1976. LC 75-35346. 210p. 60.00 (*0-8371-8590-4*, KME/, Greenwood Pr) Greenwood.

American Medical Education in the 20th Century. Kenneth M. Ludmerer. 1997. 352p. 22.95 (*0-465-00167-X*) Basic.

American Medical Imprints, 1820-1910: A Checklist of Publications Illustrating the History & Progress of Medical Science, Medical Education & the Healing Arts in the United States: A Preliminary Contribution, Set. Francesco Cordasco. 1985. 1654p. 275.00 (*0-940198-01-0*) St Aedans Pr & Bk.

American Medical Research Past & Present. Richard H. Shryock. Ed. by I. Bernard Cohen. 1980. LC 79-7989. (Three Centuries of Science in America Ser.). reprint ed. lib. bdg. 34.95 (*0-405-12571-2*) Ayer.

American Medicinal Plants: An Illustrated & Descriptive Guide to Plants Indigenous to & Naturalized in the United States Which Are Used in Medicine. Charles F. Millspaugh. 1974. LC 73-91487. (Illus.). 450p. reprint ed. pap. 18.95 (*0-486-23034-1*) Dover.

American Medicine: The Power Shift. Eli Ginzberg. 1985. LC 85-8173. 224p. text 59.00 (*0-8476-7439-8*) Rowman.

American Medicine: The Quest for Competence. Mary-Jo DelVecchio Good. 1998. 278p. pap. text 17.95 (*0-520-21653-9*) U CA Pr.

American Medicine & Statistical Thinking, 1800-1860. James H. Cassedy. 1984. LC 83-12831. (Illus.). 312p. 44.00 (*0-674-02560-1*) HUP.

American Medicine & the Public Interest: A History of Medical Specialization. Rosemary Stevens. rev. ed. 1998. LC 97-24102. 600p. pap. text 22.50 (*0-520-21009-3*) U CA Pr.

American Medicine in Transition, 1840-1910. John S. Haller, Jr. 1981. LC 80-14546. (Illus.). 461p. text 39.95 (*0-252-00806-5*) U of Ill Pr.

American Medicine, the Quest for Competence. Mary-Jo DelVecchio Good. 1995. LC 94-36162. 278p. text 45.00 (*0-520-08896-4*) U CA Pr.

American Midwife Debate: A Sourcebook on Its Modern Origins, 18. Judy B. Litoff. 1986. LC 85-17694. (Contributions in Medical Studies Ser.: No. 18). (Illus.). 251p. 68.00 (*0-313-24191-0*, LMD/, Greenwood Pr) Greenwood.

American Nervousness, Its Causes & Consequences: A Supplement to Nervous Exhaustion. George M. Beard. 1972. LC 72-180552. (Medicine & Society in America Ser.). 382p. reprint ed. 24.95 (*0-405-03932-8*) Ayer.

American Nurses Association Model Practice Act. American Nurses Association Staff. 1996. 64p. pap. 16.95 (*1-55810-128-4*, NP-110) Am Nurses Pub.

American Nursing: A Biographical Dictionary Ed. by Vern L. Bullough et al. 2000. LC 87-29076. (Illus.). 360p. text 69.95 (*0-8261-1296-X*) Springer Pub.

American Nursing: From Hospitals to Health Systems. Joan E. Lynaugh. 1997. LC 96-45993. 100p. pap. 28.95 (*1-57718-046-1*) Blackwell Pubs.

American Nursing Review: Questions & Answers for NCLEX-PN. Phyllis F. Healy & William Balkie. 1996. LC 95-42551. 192p. pap. 26.95 (*0-87434-800-5*) Springhouse Corp.

American Nursing Review: Questions & Answers for NCLEX-RN. Phyllis F. Healy. 1994. LC 93-50592. 224p. pap. 25.95 (*0-87434-688-6*) Springhouse Corp.

American Nursing Review: Questions & Answers for NCLEX-RN. Phyllis F. Healy & Kathleen M. Maher. 2nd ed. 1999. LC 98-49377. 224p. pap. 27.95 (*0-87434-983-4*) Springhouse Corp.

American Nursing Review for Critical Care Nursing Certification. Joseph T. Catalano. 2nd ed. 1998. LC 97-46905. 320p. pap. 37.95 (*0-87434-928-1*) Springhouse Corp.

American Nursing Review for Medical-Surgical Nursing Certification. Phyllis F. Healy. 2nd ed. 1998. LC 97-46904. 368p. pap. 37.95 (*0-87434-919-2*) Springhouse Corp.

American Nursing Review for NCLEX-PN. Leona A. Mourad. 3rd ed. 1997. LC 97-25002. 560p. pap. 29.95 (*0-87434-924-9*) Springhouse Corp.

American Nursing Review for NCLEX-RN. Phyllis E. Healy et al. 4th ed. 1997. LC 97-17857. 704p. pap. 34.95 (*0-87434-905-2*) Springhouse Corp.

American Nursing Review for Psychiatric & Mental Health Nursing Certification. Nancy S. Randolph. 2nd ed. 1998. LC 97-46587. 256p. pap. 37.95 (*0-87434-907-9*) Springhouse Corp.

American Patented Brace, 1829-1924: An Illustrated Directory of Patents. Ronald W. Pearson. 1994. (Illus.). 192p. (Orig.). pap. 22.95 (*1-879335-48-4*) Astragal Pr.

American Pediatric Urology. Frank Hinman. 1991. (Illus.). 287p. 75.00 (*0-930405-44-7*) Norman SF.

American Pediatrics: The Social Dynamics of Professionalism, 1880-1980. Sydney A. Halpern. 1988. 256p. (C). text 45.00 (*0-520-05195-5*) U CA Pr.

American Perceptions of Drug Addiction: Five Studies, 1872 to 1912. Ed. by Gerald N. Grob. 1981. LC 80-1209. (Addiction in America Ser.). lib. bdg. 35.95 (*0-405-13558-0*) Ayer.

American Pharmaceutical Association Drug Treatment Protocols. Ed. by Daniel H. Albrant. (Illus.). 1999. LC 99-72581. 457p. (C). text 100.00 (*0-917330-98-6*); 2nd ed. 2001. LC 2001-280059. 480p. 99.00 (*1-58212-006-4*) Am Pharm Assn.

American Pharmaceutical Association's Guide to Prescription Drugs. Donald Sullivan. 1998. LC 00-500194. 576p. pap. 7.99 (*0-451-18843-8*, Sig) NAL.

American Pharmaceutical Association's Parent's Guide to Childhood Medications. Ed. by Andrea Peirce & American Pharmaceutical Association Staff. 1997. 624p. (Orig.). pap. 16.95 (*0-8362-2138-9*) Andrews McMeel.

American Physician in Turkey: A Narrative of Adventures in Peace & in War. Clarence D. Ussher & Grace H. Knapp. 1990. LC 96-140437. xiii, 338 p. (*0-941567-16-8*) J C & A L Fawcett.

American Physicians in the Nineteenth Century: From Sects to Science. William G. Rothstein. 1992. 256p. reprint ed. pap. text 19.95 (*0-8018-4427-4*) Johns Hopkins.

American Pie, Myth Representation. Coleman et al. 1992. (Illus.). 16p. pap. 3.00 (*0-939784-22-X*) CEPA Gall.

American Popular Psychology: An Interdisciplinary Research Guide. Stephen B. Fried. 1994. LC 94-13412. 272p. text 15.00 (*0-8153-0402-1*, SS785) Garland.

American Psychiatric Association Capitation Handbook: Actuarially Determined Capitation Rates for Mental Health Benefits. American Psychiatric Association Staff et al. 1995. 112p. pap. text 37.00 (*0-89042-277-X*, 2277) Am Psychiatric.

American Psychiatric Association Practice Guideline for Major Depressive Disorder in Adults. American Psychiatric Association Staff. 1993. 51p. pap. text 24.50 (*0-89042-301-6*, 2301) Am Psychiatric.

American Psychiatric Association Practice Guideline for the Treatment of Patients with Alzheimer's Disease. American Psychiatric Association Staff. 1997. (American Psychiatric Association Practice Guidelines Ser.). 96p. pap. text 24.50 (*0-89042-310-5*, 2310) Am Psychiatric.

American Psychiatric Association Practice Guideline for the Treatment of Patients with Bipolar Disorder. Ed. by American Psychiatric Association Staff. 1995. LC 95-181188. (American Psychiatric Association Practice Guidelines Ser.). 88p. pap. text 24.50 (*0-89042-302-4*, 2302) Am Psychiatric.

***American Psychiatric Association Practice Guideline for the Treatment of Patients with Boderline Personality Disorder.** American Psychiatric Association Staff. 2001. (*0-89042-319-9*, 2309) Am Psychiatric.

American Psychiatric Association Practice Guideline for the Treatment of Patients with Eating Disorders. American Psychiatric Association Staff. 2nd ed. 2000. LC 00-702923. (American Psychiatric Association Practice Guidelines Ser.). vii, 76p. pap. 24.50 (*0-89042-314-8*, 2314) Am Psychiatric.

American Psychiatric Association Practice Guideline for the Treatment of Patients with Major Depressive Disorder. American Psychiatric Association Staff. 2nd ed. 2000. LC 00-698004. (American Psychiatric Association Practice Guidelines Ser.). 98p. pap. 24.50 (*0-89042-316-4*, 2316) Am Psychiatric.

American Psychiatric Association Practice Guideline for the Treatment of Patients with Panic Disorder. American Psychiatric Association Staff. 1998. LC 98-163059. (American Psychiatric Association Practice Guidelines Ser.). 80p. pap. text 24.50 (*0-89042-311-3*, 2311) Am Psychiatric.

American Psychiatric Association Practice Guideline for the Treatment of Patients with Schizophrenia. American Psychiatric Association Staff. 1997. LC 97-152812. (American Psychiatric Association Practice Guidelines Ser.). 145p. pap. text 24.50 (*0-89042-309-1*, 2309) Am Psychiatric.

American Psychiatric Association Practice Guideline for the Treatment of Patients with Substance Use Disorders: Alcohol, Cocaine, Opioids. American Psychiatric Association Staff. 1995. 126p. pap. text 24.50 (*0-89042-303-2*, 2303) Am Psychiatric.

American Psychiatric Association Practice Guidelines: Includes Psychiatric Evaluation of Adults, Eating Disorders, Bipolar Disorder, Etc. Ed. by APA, Office of Research Staff. 1996. LC 96-213131. 361p. pap. text 46.50 (*0-89042-306-7*, 2306) Am Psychiatric.

American Psychiatric Association Practice Guidelines: Includes Psychiatric Evaluation of Adults, Eating Disorders, Bipolar Disorder, Etc. Ed. by APA Staff. 1996. LC 96-213131. 361p. text 56.95 (*0-89042-305-9*, 2305) Am Psychiatric.

American Psychiatric Association Practice Guidelines for the Treatment of Psychiatric Disorders: Compendium 2000. American Psychiatric Association Staff. 2000. LC 00-24850. (American Psychiatric Association Practice Guidelines Ser.). xvi, 768p. 64.95 (*0-89042-312-1*, 2312); pap. 49.95 (*0-89042-315-6*, 2315) Am Psychiatric.

American Psychiatric Glossary. Ed. by Jane E. Edgerton & Robert J. Campbell, III. 7th ed. 1994. LC 94-5700. 224p. text 29.50 (*0-88048-526-4*, 8526); 274p. pap. text 20.50 (*0-88048-508-6*, 8508) Am Psychiatric.

American Psychiatric Press Review of Clinical Psychiatry & the Law. Ed. by Robert I. Simon. Vol. 1. 1990. 383p. text 19.95 (*0-88048-375-X*, 8375); Vol. 2. 1991. 472p. text 19.95 (*0-88048-376-8*, 8376) Am Psychiatric.

American Psychiatric Press Review of Psychiatry, Vol. 7. Ed. by Allen J. Frances & Robert E. Hales. 1988. 697p. 15.00 (*0-88048-245-1*, 8245) Am Psychiatric.

American Psychiatric Press Review of Psychiatry. Ed. by Allan Tasman et al. Vol. 8. 1989. 641p. text 15.00 (*0-88048-247-8*, 8247); Vol. 9. 1990. 699p. text 15.00 (*0-88048-248-6*, 8248) Am Psychiatric.

American Psychiatric Press Review of Psychiatry, Vol. 10. Ed. by Allan Tasman & Stephen M. Goldfinger. 1991. 675p. 15.00 (*0-88048-436-5*, 8436) Am Psychiatric.

American Psychiatric Press Review of Psychiatry, Vol. 11. Ed. by Allan Tasman & Michelle B. Riba. 1992. 630p. text 15.00 (*0-88048-437-3*, 8437) Am Psychiatric.

American Psychiatric Press Review of Psychiatry, Vol. 12. Ed. by John M. Oldham et al. 1993. 872p. text 15.00 (*0-88048-439-X*, 8439) Am Psychiatric.

American Psychiatric Press Review of Psychiatry, Vol. 13. Ed. by John M. Oldham & Michelle B. Riba. 1994. 804p. 15.00 (*0-88048-440-3*, 8440) Am Psychiatric.

American Psychiatric Press Review of Psychiatry. Ed. by Leah J. Dickstein et al. Vol. 15. 1996. 657p. 59.95 (*0-88048-442-X*, 8442); Vol. 16. 1997. 928p. text 59.95 (*0-88048-443-8*, 8443) Am Psychiatric.

American Psychiatric Press Textbook of Consultation-Liaison Psychiatry. Ed. by James R. Rundell & Michael G. Wise. 1996. LC 95-37954. 1184p. text 145.00 (*0-88048-336-9*, 8336) Am Psychiatric.

American Psychiatric Press Textbook of Geriatric Psychiatry. Ed. by Ewald W. Busse & Dan G. Blazer. 2nd ed. 1996. LC 95-33558. 560p. text 92.95 (*0-88048-713-5*, 8713) Am Psychiatric.

American Psychiatric Press Textbook of Neuropsychiatry. Ed. by Stuart C. Yudofsky & Robert E. Hales. 3rd ed. 1997. LC 97-2445. 1149p. text 175.00 (*0-88048-787-9*, 8787) Am Psychiatric.

American Psychiatric Press Textbook of Psychopharmacology. Alan F. Schatzberg & Charles B. Nemeroff. 2nd ed. 1998. LC 98-10616. (Illus.). 1095p. 155.00 (*0-88048-817-4*) Am Psychiatric.

American Psychiatric Press Textbook of Substance Abuse Treatment. Ed. by Marc Galanter & Herbert D. Kleber. 2nd ed. 1999. LC 98-32242. 608p. text 99.00 (*0-88048-820-4*, 8820) Am Psychiatric.

American Psychiatrists Abroad: An Original Anthology. Isaac Ray & Pliny Earle. 1976. LC 75-16679. (Classics in Psychiatry Ser.). 32.95 (*0-405-07411-5*) Ayer.

American Psychiatry after World War II (1944-1994) Ed. by Roy W. Menninger & John C. Nemiah. 2000. LC 00-24629. 656p. 49.00 (*0-88048-866-2*, 8866) Am Psychiatric.

American Psychological Association: A Historical Perspective. Ed. by Rand B. Evans et al. 1992. (Illus.). 415p. text 29.95 (*1-55798-136-1*) Am Psychol.

American Psychologist Special Issue Vol. 47, No. 2: The History of American Psychology. Ed. by Ludy T. Benjamin, Jr. 1992. 263p. pap. 20.00 (*1-55798-170-1*) Am Psychol.

American Psychology since World War II: A Profile of the Discipline. Albert R. Gilgen. 1982. LC 81-23740. (Illus.). 272p. 68.00 (*0-313-23027-7*, GAM/, Greenwood Pr) Greenwood.

American Red Cross Adult CPR. American Red Cross Staff. 1992. LC 92-583. 96p. (C). (gr. 13). pap. text 9.70 (*0-8016-7062-4*) Mosby Inc.

American Red Cross Babysitter's Handbook. American Red Cross Staff. 1998. LC 98-11145. (J). 9.75 (*0-8151-3685-4*) Mosby Inc.

American Red Cross Child Story Activity Book. American Red Cross Staff. 1992. 20p. (J). (ps-3). pap. text 43.00 (*0-8016-6509-4*) Mosby Inc.

American Red Cross Community CPR. American Red Cross Staff. 1992. 124p. (C). (gr. 13). pap. text 12.50 (*0-8016-7066-7*) Mosby Inc.

American Red Cross Community First Aid & Safety. American Red Cross Staff. (gr. 13). 1994. 256p. (C). pap. text 13.50 (*0-8016-7538-3*); 1992. 240p. pap. text 13.50 (*0-8016-7064-0*) Mosby Inc.

American Red Cross CPR for the Professional Rescue. Rescue American Red Cross Staff. 1993. 160p. (gr. 13). pap. text 11.90 (*0-8016-7067-5*) Mosby Inc.

American Red Cross First Aid & Safety Handbook. American Red Cross Staff & Kathleen A. Handal. 1992. 320p. pap. 17.95 (*0-316-73646-5*, Back Bay) Little.

American Red Cross Oxygen Administration. American Red Cross Staff. 1993. 24p. (gr. 13). pap. text 50.00 (*0-8016-7276-7*) Mosby Inc.

American Red Cross Preventing Disease Transmissions. American Red Cross Staff. 1993. 24p. (C). (gr. 13). pap. text 31.25 (*0-8016-7272-4*) Mosby Inc.

American Red Cross Standard First Aid. American Red Cross Staff. 1992. LC 92-581. 231p. (gr. 13). pap. text 13.50 (*0-8016-7065-9*) Mosby Inc.

American Red Cross until Help Arrives Booklet. American Red Cross Staff. 16p. (gr. 13). 1993. (SPA.). pap. text 18.75 (*0-8016-7756-4*); 1992. LC 92-39673. pap. text 18.75 (*0-8016-7063-2*) Mosby Inc.

American Saga: The Story of Helen Thomas & Simon Flexner. James T. Flexner. 2nd ed. 1993. LC 93-12573. (Illus.). xviii, 494p. 35.00 (*0-8232-1520-2*); pap. 20.00 (*0-8232-1521-0*) Fordham.

American Self-Dosage Medicines: An Historical Perspective. James H. Young. Ed. by Robert P. Hudson. 1974. (Logan Clendening Lectures: No. 1). pap. 5.00 (*0-87291-068-7*) Coronado Pr.

American Sign Language. Martin L. Sternberg. 1981. (ENG, FRE, GER, ITA & JPN., Illus.). 1184p. 95.00 (*0-8288-0192-4*, M9827) Fr & Eur.

American Society for Stereotactic & Functional Neurosurgery. 1981. (Journal: Vol. 43, Nos. 3-5, 1980). (Illus.). 184p. pap. 91.50 (*3-8055-3458-2*) S Karger.

American Society for Stereotactic & Functional Neurosurgery: Meeting, Snowbird, Utah, July 1999, Proceedings, Pt. I. Ed. by M. P. Heilbrun et al. 2000. (Stereotactic & Functional Neurosurgery Ser.: Vol. 72, No. 2-4). (Illus.). vi, 180p. pap. 45.25 (*3-8055-7071-6*) S Karger.

American Society for Stereotactic & Functional Neurosurgery Pt. I: Proceedings of the Meeting of the American Society, Marina del Rey, Calif., March 1995. Ed. by D. W. Roberts et al. 1996. (Journal: Vol. 65, Nos. 1-4, 1995). (Illus.). x, 212p. pap. 144.50 (*3-8055-6364-7*) S Karger.

American Society for Stereotactic & Functional Neurosurgery Pt. II: Proceedings of the Meeting of the American Society, Marina del Rey, Calif., March 1995. Ed. by D. W. Roberts et al. 1996. (Journal: Vol. 66, Nos. 1-3, 1996). (Illus.). viii, 160p. pap. 108.00 (*3-8055-6365-5*) S Karger.

American Society for Stereotactic & Functional Neurosurgery, Montreal, Quebec, June 1987: Journal: Applied Neurophysiology, Vol. 50, Nos. 1-6, 1987. Ed. by A. Olivier et al. 1988. xii, 512p. pap. 205.25 (*3-8055-4756-0*) S Karger.

American Society of Ophthalmic Plastic & Reconstructive Surgery (ASOPRS) History of Ophthalmic Plastic Surgery, 2500 BC-1995 AD: The First Twenty-Five Years 1969-1994. Ed. by David M. Reifler. 1994. LC 94-7908. (Illus.). 493p. 75.00 (*0-930405-64-1*) Norman SF.

American Statistical Association 1994 Proceedings of the Biopharmaceutical Section. 1995. (Illus.). (Orig.). pap. 50.00 (*1-883276-05-5*) Amer Statist.

American Surgery: An Illustrated History. Ira M. Rutkow & Williams and Wilkins Review Staff. 1999. LC 97-17654. (Illus.). 656p. text 99.00 (*0-316-76352-7*) Lppncott W & W.

American Surgical Instruments: An Illustrated History of Their Manufacture & a Directory of Instrument Makers to 1900. James M. Edmonson. 1997. LC 97-9009. (Illus.). 352p. 165.00 (*0-930405-70-6*, NP31378) Norman SF.

***American Urological Association Centennial History: 1902-2002.** American Urological Association Staff. 2002. LC 2001-7497. (Illus.). xi, 864p. 100.00 (*0-9649702-9-5*, CHAUAC) Am Urological.

American Urological Association Erectile Dysfunction Clinical Guidelines Panel Report on the Treatment of Organic Erectile Dysfunction. L. Levine et al. 1996. 80p. pap. 67.00 (*0-9649702-1-X*) Am Urological.

American Urological Association Pediatric Vesicoureteral Reflux Clinical Guidelines Panel: Report on the Management of Pediatric Vesicoureteral Reflux in Children. R. Weiss et al. 1997. (Illus.). 94p. pap. text 49.00 (*0-9649702-2-8*) Am Urological.

American Urological Association Prostate Cancer Guidelines Panel Report on the Management of Clinically Localized Prostate Cancer. Richard G. Middleton et al. 1995. 88p. pap. text 67.00 (*0-9649702-0-1*) Am Urological.

American Urological Association Report on the Management of Non-Muscle-Invasive Bladder Cancer (Stages Ta, T1 & Tis) J. A. Smith et al. 1999. 60p. pap. text 35.00 (*0-9649702-5-2*) Am Urological.

American Urological Association Ureteral Stones Clinical Guidelines Panel: Report on the Management of Ureteral Calculi. J. W. Segura et al. 1997. 80p. pap. text 69.00 (*0-9649702-4-4*) Am Urological.

American Vegetarian Resource Directory: Some Signposts on the Journey Towards a Healthier, More Ethically & Environmentally Balanced Lifestyle. Georgia Wheatley. 1998. 94p. (Orig.). reprint ed. pap. text 7.00 (*0-7881-5222-X*) DIANE Pub.

Americans! Their Attitudes, Beliefs, Behaviors, Disease, Emotions, Fears, Gifts, Health, Life, Violence, Sex & Work: Index of New Information. Science and Life Consultants Staff. 1997. 160p. pap. 47.50 (*0-7883-1719-9*) ABBE Pubs Assn.

Americans View Their Mental Health. Gerald Gurin et al. Ed. by Gerald N. Grob. 1980. LC 78-22564. (Historical Issues in Mental Health Ser.). (Illus.). reprint ed. lib. bdg. 37.95 (*0-405-11918-6*) Ayer.

Americans View Their Mental Health, 1976. Joseph Veroff et al. 1982. LC 82-80684. (*0-89138-939-3*) ICPSR.

Americans with Disabilities Act: A Guide to Provisions Affecting Persons with Seizure Disorders. Epilepsy Foundation of America Staff. 1992. 46p. pap. 9.95 (*0-916570-01-0*) Epilepsy Foundation of America.

America's Best Hoax: How Doctors Get Fat on Fitness. John LeMarr. 1993. LC 93-77223. (Illus.). 160p. (Orig.). pap. 12.95 (*0-9632923-7-4*) HealthMasters.

America's Best Hospitals. U. S. News and World Report Staff. 1995. LC 95-39977. 508p. pap. 19.95 (*0-471-12614-4*) Wiley.

America's Botanico-Medical Movements: Vox Populi. Alex Berman. Ed. by Michael Flannery. 2000. LC 00-33660. 359p. 69.95 (*0-7890-0899-8*, Pharmctl Prods) Haworth Pr.

America's Botanico-Medical Movements: Vox Populi. Ed. by Alex Berman & Michael Flannery. 2000. LC 00-33660. 359p. pap. 24.95 (*0-7890-1235-9*, Pharmctl Prods) Haworth Pr.

America's Care of the Mentally Ill: A Photographic History. William E. Baxter & David W. Hathcox, III. 1994. LC 93-48732. (Illus.). 176p. text 31.95 (*0-88048-539-6*, 8539) Am Psychiatric.

America's Children: Health Insurance & Access to Care. Institute of Medicine Staff & National Research Council Staff. Ed. by Margaret Edmunds & Molly J. Coye. 1998. LC 98-25491. 180p. pap. text 44.95 (*0-309-06560-7*) Natl Acad Pr.

America's Children: Triumph or Tragedy. Charles N. Oberg et al. 1994. LC 96-147980. 94p. pap. 22.50 (*0-87553-218-7*, 071) Am Pub Health.

America's Foods Health Messages & Claims: Scientific, Regulatory, & Legal Issues. 1993. LC 93-9594. (Series in Contemporary Food Science). 304p. 98.00 (*0-8493-8001-4*, TX551) CRC Pr.

America's Forgotten Pandemic: The Influenza of 1918. Alfred W. Crosby. 1990. (Illus.). 351p. (C). pap. text 19.95 (*0-521-38695-0*) Cambridge U Pr.

America's Future Work Force: A Health & Education Policy Issues Handbook. Carl W. Stenberg & William G. Colman. 1994. LC 93-25070. 640p. lib. bdg. 120.00 (*0-313-27980-2*, SXB/, Greenwood Pr) Greenwood.

America's Managed Care Revolution. Gollaher. 1995. (Health Services Administration Ser.). text 41.95 (*0-8273-6267-6*) Delmar.

America's Most Successful Cardiovascular Health Program: Vitamin Program. Matthias Rath. 1995. pap. text 12.95 (*0-9638768-2-1*) Health Now.

America's Newcomers: Health Care Issues for New Americans. Jonathan C. Dunlap. 1993. 18p. 10.00 (*1-55516-928-7*, 9359) Natl Conf State Legis.

America's Religions: An Educator's Guide to Beliefs & Practices. Benjamin J. Hubbard et al. 1997. LC 97-13949. xxiv, 162p. pap., tchr. ed. 25.00 (*1-56308-469-4*) Teacher Ideas Pr.

***America's Top Doctors.** 2nd ed. 2001. pap. 29.95 (*1-883769-26-4*) Castle Connolly Med.

America's Vital Interest in Global Health: Protecting Our People, Enhancing Our Economy, & Advancing Our International Interests. Institute of Medicine Staff. 1997. LC 97-206903. 72p. (C). pap. text 15.00 (*0-309-05834-1*) Natl Acad Pr.

America's Welfare State: From Roosevelt to Reagan. Edward D. Berkowitz. 1991. LC 90-46424. (American Moment Ser.). 240p. pap. text 16.95 (*0-8018-4128-3*) Johns Hopkins.

Amerikos Lietuviu Gydytoju Vardynas: Lithuanian-American Medical Directory (1884-1984) Milda Budrys. 1991. LC 90-64053. 139p. 15.00 (*0-929700-06-6*) Lith Res & Studies.

Ameslan - An Introduction to American Sign Language. Louie J. Fant, Jr. LC 72-90793. 11.95 (*0-917002-37-7*) Joyce Media.

Ameu en el Tratamiento del Aborto Incompleto: Experiencia Clinica y Programatica. Traci L. Baird et al. 1996. Orig. Title: MVA in the Treatment of Incomplete Abortion. (SPA.). 24p. (Orig.). pap. 4.00 (*1-882220-10-2*, INCMON-S95) IPAS.

Amiloride & Its Analogs: Unique Cation Transport Inhibitors. Ed. by Edward J. Cragoe, Jr. et al. 1992. LC 92-24492. 115.00 (*1-56081-056-4*, Wiley-VCH) Wiley.

Amine Oxidases: Function & Dysfunction: Proceedings of the Fifth International Amine Oxidase Workshop, Galway, Ireland, August 22-25, 1992. Keith F. Tipton. 1995. (Journals of Neural Transmission: Vol. 41). (Illus.). 129.00 (*0-387-82521-5*) Spr-Verlag.

Amino Acid & Peptides, Vol. 24. J. S. Davies. 1993. 286p. 200.00 (*0-85186-224-1*, R6224) CRC Pr.

Amino-Acid Biosynthesis & Genetic Regulation. Klaus Herrmann & Ronald Somerville. 1983. (Biotechnology Ser.: No. 3). (Illus.). 330p. (C). text (*0-201-10520-9*) Addison-Wesley.

Amino Acid Products & Technology. Business Communications Co., Inc. Staff. 1991. 120p. pap. 1750.00 (*0-89336-448-7*, C-056R) BCC.

Amino Acids & Peptides. Ed. by J. S. Davies. 1985. 800p. ring bd. (*0-412-26950-3*, NO. 6569, Chap & Hall CRC) CRC Pr.

Amino Acids & Proteins for the Athlete: The Anabolic Edge. Mauro G. Di Pasquale. 1997. LC 97-4307. (Nutrition in Exercise & Sport Ser.). 272p. 74.95 (*0-8493-8193-2*) CRC Pr.

Amino Acids for Stress, Pain & Anxiety. 1996. lib. bdg. 251.95 (*0-8490-5901-1*) Gordon Pr.

Amino Acids in Critical Care & Cancer. Ed. by Rifat Latifi. 1994. 118p. 94.00 (*1-57059-027-3*, LN9027) CRC Pr.

Amino Acids in Therapy: A Guide to the Therapeutic Application of Protein Constituents. Leon Chaitow. 1985. 112p. pap. 14.95 (*0-89281-287-7*, Heal Arts VT) Inner Tradit.

Amino Revolution: The Breakthrough Program That Will Change the Way You Feel. Robert Erdmann & Meirion Jones. 1989. 272p. 11.00 (*0-671-67359-9*, Fireside) S&S Trade Pap.

Aminoacidopathies, Immunoglobinopathies Neuro-Genetics & Neuro-Ophthalmology: Proceedings of the International Congress on Neuro-Genetics & Neuro-Ophthalmology, 3rd,

Brussels, 1970. International Congress on Neuro-Genetics and Neuro-O. Ed. by J. Francois. 1972. (Monographs in Human Genetics: Vol. 6). (Illus.). 56.75 (3-8055-1280-5) S Karger.

Aminoglycoside Antibiotics: Guide to Therapy. W. Barnes & G. Hodges. 1983. LC 83-2558. 248p. 142.00 (0-8493-5426-9, CRC Reprint) Franklin.

Aminopyridines & Similarly Acting Drugs: Effects on Nerves, Muscles & Synapses. Ed. by P. Lechat et al. 1982. LC 82-533. (Advances in the Biosciences Ser.: Vol. 35). (Illus.). 352p. (0-08-028000-5) Pergamon Repr.

Amiodarone Profile: Report XIII of the Senate Commission for Clinical-Toxicological Analysis. Ed. by David W. Holt et al. 1990. (DFG Ser.). 45p. pap. 49.95 (3-527-27378-6, Wiley-VCH) Wiley.

Amipaque Vascular. Ed. by J. Valk & F. L. Peeters. 1979. (Journal: Vol. 48, No. 4, 1979). (Illus.). pap. 20.00 (3-8055-0196-X) S Karger.

Amish Folk Medicine: Home Remedies Using Foods, Herbs & Vitamins. Patrick Quillin. 1995. (Illus.). 248p. pap. 14.95 (1-886898-01-4) Leader OH.

Amish Folk Remedies for Plain & Fancy Ailments. Ed. by William R. McGrath. 1988. 104p. pap. 9.95 (0-9617405-8-2) S Schupp.

Amitrole. 1994. (Environmental Health Criteria Ser.: No. 158). (ENG, FRE & SPA.). 123p. pap. text 28.00 (92-4-157158-6, 1160158) World Health.

AMIU No Atendimento ao Abortamento Incompleto: Experiencia Clinica e Programatica. Traci L. Baird et al. 1996. (POR.). 21p. (Orig.). pap. (1-882220-09-9) IPAS.

Amlodipine. W. G. Nayler. 1997. LC 93-23381. (Illus.). 277p. 137.00 (0-387-56698-8) Spr-Verlag.

Amma Therapy: A Complete Textbook of Oriental Bodywork & Medical Principles. Tina Sohn & Robert Sohn. 1997. LC 96-21032. (Illus.). 448p. 45.00 (0-89281-488-8, Heal Arts VT) Inner Tradit.

Ammonia. 1986. (Environmental Health Criteria Ser.: No. 54). (ENG & FRE.). 210p. pap. text 29.00 (92-4-154194-6, 1160054) World Health.

Amniotic Fluid Compartment: The Fetal Habitat. Walter Schmidt. Ed. by F. Beck et al. 1992. LC 92-2225. (Advances in Anatomy, Embryology & Cell Biology Ser.: Vol. 127). (Illus.). 100p. 104.00 (0-387-55162-X); vi, 100p. pap. 89.00 (3-540-55162-X) Spr-Verlag.

Amobarbital Effects & Lateralized Brain Function: The Wada Test. D. W. Loring et al. Ed. by D. W. King. 1991. (Illus.). 138p. 99.00 (0-387-97738-4) Spr-Verlag.

Amoebiasis: Proceedings of the WHO Expert Committee, Teheran, 1968. WHO Staff. 1969. (Technical Reports: No. 421). (ENG & RUS.). 52p. pap. text 5.00 (92-4-120421-4, 1100421) World Health.

AMOK Journal: Senssurround Edition, a Compendium of Physio-Psychological Investigations. Ed. by Stuart Swezey. 1993. (Illus.). 360p. (Orig.). (C). pap. 17.95 (1-878923-03-X) Amok Bks.

Among Friends: Hospice Care for the Person with AIDS. Robert W. Buckingham. 1992. LC 91-45568. 191p. (C). 32.00 (0-87975-720-5); pap. 20.00 (0-87975-759-0) Prometheus Bks.

Among the Heavens: The Human Side of Spaceflight. Patricia Allen. 1989. (Illus.). 200p. (Orig.). (0-9622456-0-7, 001); pap. (0-9622456-1-5) HFSI Inc.

Amoral Thoughts about Morality: The Intersection of Science, Psychology & Ethics. Howard H. Kendler. 2000. LC 99-53074. xi, 198p. 42.95 (0-398-07028-8); pap. 29.95 (0-398-07029-6) C C Thomas.

Amorolfine, A Breakthrough in Topical Antimyocotic Therapy. Ed. by R. J. Hay. 1992. (Journal: Vol. 184, Suppl. 1, 1992). (Illus.). vi, 30p. pap. 15.75 (3-8055-5573-3) S Karger.

Amphetamine & Its Analogs: Psychopharmacology, Toxicology, & Abuse. Ed. by Arthur K. Cho & David S. Segal. 1994. LC 93-38062. (Illus.). 503p. text 99.00 (0-12-173375-0) Acad Pr.

Amphetamine Misuse: International Perspectives on Current Trends. Hilary Klee. 1997. 336.p. text (90-5702-079-3) GBSP NLD. *Dist:* Gordon & Breach.

Amphetamine Misuse: International Perspectives on Current Trends. Ed. by Hilary Klee. 1997. 336.p. pap. text 22.00 (90-5702-081-5, Harwood Acad Pubs) Gordon & Breach.

Amphetamines & Other Stimulants. Lawrence Clayton. 1998. LC 94-573. (Drug Abuse Prevention Library). 64p. (YA). (gr. 7 up). reprint ed. pap. 6.95 (1-56838-210-3) Hazelden.

Amphetamines & PH-Shift Agents for Brain Imaging: Basic Research & Clinical Results. Ed. by Hans J. Biersack & C. Winkler. 1986. (Illus.). 208p. 119.25 (3-11-010772-4) De Gruyter.

Amphetamines & Related Stimulants, Vol. 1. John Caldwell, pseud. 1981. 216p. 121.00 (0-8493-5347-5, RM666, CRC Reprint) Franklin.

Amphibian in Transplantation Immunity. Ed. by E. P. Volpe. 1980. (Monographs in Developmental Biology: Vol. 14). (Illus.). x, 150p. pap. 108.00 (3-8055-1087-X) S Karger.

Amphibians. J. F. Frazer & O. H. Frazer. 1972. (Wykeham Science Ser.: No. 25). 128p. (C). 18.00 (0-8448-1152-1, Crane Russak) Taylor & Francis.

Amphizoic Amoebae: Human Pathology. E. G. Rondanelli. 1988. (Infectious Diseases Color Atlas Monographs: No. 1). 276p. text (1-57235-028-8) Piccin Nuova.

Amphotericin B Colloidal Dispersion: An Advance in Antifungal Therapy. Ed. by R. Herbrecht. 3rd ed. 1999. (Chemotherapy Ser.: Vol. 45, Suppl. 1 (1999)). (Illus.). iv, 78p. pap. 34.00 (3-8055-6845-2) S Karger.

Amplification for Children with Auditory Deficits. Ed. by Fred H. Bess et al. 1996. LC 95-78697. (Illus.). 500p. 55.00 (0-9631439-3-X) Vanderbilt Wilkerson.

Amplitude-Phase Patterns in Dynamic Scintigraphic Imaging. A. Bossuyt & F. Deconinck. 1984. (Developments in Nuclear Medicine Ser.). text 141.50 (0-89838-641-1) Kluwer Academic.

Amputation: Surgical Practice & Patient Management. G. M. Murdoch & A. Bennett Wilson. 1996. LC 95-6470. (Illus.). 391p. text (0-7506-0843-9) E A GBR. *Dist:* OUP.

Amputations & Prosthetics: A Case Study Approach. Bella J. May. 1996. LC 96-15601. (Illus.). 246p. (C). pap. text 34.95 (0-8036-0043-7) Davis Co.

Amputees & Devotees. Grant Riddle. 1989. 29.95 (0-8290-1824-7) Irvington.

AMRA-AHIMA Medical Record Administrator National Registration Examination (RRA) Jack Rudman. (Admission Test Ser.: Vol. 84). 49.95 (0-8373-5184-7) Nat Learn.

AMRA-AHIMA Medical Record Technician National Registration Examination (ART) Jack Rudman. (Admission Test Ser.: Vol. 85). 49.95 (0-8373-5185-5) Nat Learn.

AMRA/AHIMA Medical Record Administrator National Registration Examination (RRA) Jack Rudman. 1994. (Admission Test Ser.: ATS-84). pap. 29.95 (0-8373-5084-0) Nat Learn.

AMRA/AHIMA Medical Record Technician National Registration Examination (ART) Jack Rudman. 1994. (Admission Test Ser.: ATS-85). pap. 29.95 (0-8373-5085-9) Nat Learn.

Amsterdam Growth Study: A Longitudinal Analysis of Health, Fitness, & Lifestyle. Ed. by Han C. Kemper. 1995. LC 94-33964. (Sport Science Monographs: Vol. 6). (Illus.). 288p. pap. text 20.00 (0-87322-507-4, BKEM0507) Human Kinetics.

Amy Spangler Lactania Una Guia para los Padres. Illus. by Abby Drue. 6th ed. 1995. LC 96-92059. (SPA.). 108p. (Orig.). pap. 5.75 (0-9627450-8-1) A Spangler.

Amy Spangler's Breastfeeding: A Parent's Guide. Amy Spangler. 6th rev. ed. 1990. LC 90-63214. (Illus.). 108p. 5.75 (0-9627450-9-X) A Spangler.

Amy Spangler's Breastfeeding: A Parent's Guide. Amy Spangler et al. 7th rev. ed. 1999. LC 99-93780. (Illus.). 168p. pap. 8.50 (0-9627450-7-3) A Spangler.

Amyloid & Amyloidosis. Ed. by T. Isobe et al. 1988. LC 88-22425. (Illus.). 906p. 165.00 (0-306-42997-7, Plenum Trade) Perseus Pubng.

Amyloid & Amyloidosis, 1993. Ed. by R. Kisilevsky & M. D. Benson. 1994. (Illus.). 726p. lib. bdg. 93.95 (1-85070-579-8, Parthenon Pbng) CRC Pr.

Amyloid Protein Precursor in Development, Aging, & Alzheimer's Disease. C. L. Masters. 1994. LC 94-4461. (Research & Perspectives in Alzheimer's Disease Ser.). (Illus.). 257p. 132.00 (0-387-57788-2) Spr-Verlag.

Amyloidogenesis & the Cholinergic System in Alzheimer's Disease: From in Vitro Analysis to Transgenic Mice Models. Francisca C. Bronfman. 2000. LC 00-691820. (Acta Biomedica Lovaniensia Ser.: No. 221). (Illus.). 124p. pap. (90-5867-048-1) Leuven Univ BEL. *Dist:* Coronet Bks.

Amyloidosis. Ed. by George G. Glenner et al. 1986. LC 86-4889. 876p. 155.00 (0-306-42261-1, Plenum Trade) Perseus Pubng.

Amyloidosis. Jan Marrink. 1986. text 221.50 (0-89838-844-9) Kluwer Academic.

Amyloids, Part II. Ed. by S. Battaglia. 1986. (Journal: Vol. 3, Nos. 1-2). (Illus.). 116p. pap. 55.75 (3-8055-4458-8) S Karger.

Amyloids, Prions & Other Protein Aggregates. Sidney P. Colowick. 1999. (Methods in Enzymology Ser.: Vol. 309). (Illus.). 589p. 99.95 (0-12-182210-9) Acad Pr.

Amyloids, Pt. 1. Ed. by S. Battaglia. 1986. (Journal: Vol. 2, No. 6, 1984). (Illus.). vi, 86p. pap. 41.75 (3-8055-4351-4) S Karger.

Amyotrophic Lateral Sclerosis. Hiroshi Mitsumoto et al. 1998. LC 97-194. (Contemporary Neurology Ser.: No. 49). (Illus.). 512p. 140.00 (0-8036-0269-3) OUP.

Amyotrophic Lateral Sclerosis: A Comprehensive Guide to Management. Hiroshi Mitsumoto & Forbes H. Norris. 1994. 360p. pap. 39.95 (0-939957-58-2) Demos Medical.

Amyotrophic Lateral Sclerosis: A Guide for Patients & Families. Hiroshi Mitsumoto & Theodore L. Munsat. 2nd ed. 2000. (Illus.). 400p. pap. 34.95 (1-888799-28-5) Demos Medical.

Amyotrophic Lateral Sclerosis: A Synthesis of Research & Clinical Practice. Andrew Eisen & Charles Krieger. 1998. (Illus.). 323p. (C). text 74.95 (0-521-58103-6) Cambridge U Pr.

Amyotrophic Lateral Sclerosis: Diagnosis & Management for the Clinician. Ed. by Jerry M. Belsh & Philip L. Schiffman. 1996. (Illus.). 408p. 90.00 (0-87993-628-2) Futura Pub.

Amyotrophic Lateral Sclerosis: Progress & Perspectives in Basic Research & Clinical Application: Proceedings of the 11th Tokyo Metropolitan Institute for Neuroscience (TMIN) International Symposium, Tokyo, October 25-27, 1995. Ed. by Imaharu Nakano & Asao Hirano. 1996. LC 96-7789. (International Congress Ser.: No. 1104). 420p. 162.50 (0-444-82286-0) Elsevier.

Amyotrophic Lateral Sclerosis: Therapeutic, Psychological & Research Aspects. Ed. by V. Cosi et al. 1987. LC 87-1748. (Advances in Experimental Medicine & Biology Ser.: Vol. 209). 372p. 89.50 (0-306-42546-7, Plenum Trade) Perseus Pubng.

Anabaptists. Hans-Jurgen Goertz. Tr. by Trevor Johnson from GER. 1996. LC 96-12032. (Christianity & Society in the Modern World Ser.). (Illus.). 240p. (C). 85.00 (0-415-08238-2) Routledge.

Anabolic Muscle Mass: The Secrets of Anabolic Reinforcement Without Steroids. Dennis B. Weis. 1995. (Illus.). 240p. pap. (1-55210-000-6) MuscleMag Intl CAN. *Dist:* BookWorld.

Anabolic Steroid Abuse. 1992. lib. bdg. 99.95 (0-8490-8741-4) Gordon Pr.

Anabolic Steroids & Sports: A Selective Bibliography with Annotations. Compiled by Ellen R. Paterson. 1991. LC 90-83684. x, 67p. 25.00 (0-87875-389-3) Whitston Pub.

Anabolic Steroids & Sports & Drug Testing, 1991-1997: An Annotated Bibliography. Compiled by Ellen R. Paterson. 1998. LC 97-62104. xii, 90p. 29.50 (0-87875-499-7) Whitston Pub.

Anabolic Steroids & the Athlete. William N. Taylor. 1982. LC 82-17269. 128p. pap. 25.00 (0-89950-055-2) McFarland & Co.

Anabolic Treatments for Osteoporosis. James F. Whitfield & Paul Morley. 1997. LC 97-15242. (Pharmacology & Toxicology Ser.). 288p. lib. bdg. 99.95 (0-8493-8556-3) CRC Pr.

Anabolics 2002. William Llewellyn. 2nd ed. 2002. 220p. pap. 49.95 (0-9679304-1-3) W Llewellyn.

ANAC's Core Curriculum for HIV-AIDs Nursing. Kathleen M. Casey et al. 1995. (Illus.). 500p. (Orig.). pap. 40.00 (0-9637042-2-2) Nursecom Inc.

Anaerobic Digestion - Results of Research & Demonstration Projects: Proceedings of a Workshop Organized by the CEC, Directorate-General Science, Research & Development & Directorate-General Energy, Held in Villeneuve-d'Ascq, France, 4-6 March, 1986. Ed. by M. P. Ferranti et al. 1987. 277p. pap. (1-85166-027-5) Elsevier GBR. *Dist:* Elsevier.

Anaerobic Fungi: Biology, Ecology & Function. Ed. by Douglas O. Mountfort & Colin G. Orpin. 1994. LC 94-19072. (Mycology Ser.: Vol. 12). (Illus.). 304p. text 150.00 (0-8247-8948-2) Dekker.

Anaerobic Threshold: Physiological & Clinical Significance. Ed. by Luigi Tavazzi & Pietro Di Prampero. 1987. (Advances in Cardiology Ser.: Vol. 35). (Illus.). x, 158p. 124.50 (3-8055-4395-6) S Karger.

Anaesthesia. Walter S. Nimmo. 1989. 205.00 (0-632-02257-4) CRC Pr.

Anaesthesia. T. M. Craft & P. M. Upton. 2nd ed. 1995. (Key Topics Ser.). 360p. pap. (1-85996-075-8) Bios Sci GBR. *Dist:* Coronet Bks.

Anaesthesia Walter S. Nimmo & D. Rowbotham. 2nd ed. 1994. (Illus.). 2072p. 345.95 (0-632-03244-8) Blackwell Sci.

*__Anaesthesia: A Concise Handbook.__ Graham Arthurs. 2001. (Illus.). 160p. pap. (1-84110-080-3) Greenwich Med GBR. *Dist:* JAMCO Dist.

Anaesthesia: Essays on Its History. Ed. by J. Rupreht et al. 1985. (Illus.). 409p. 94.00 (0-387-13255-4) Spr-Verlag.

*__Anaesthesia: Fundamental Principles & Practice.__ Hutton et al. 2001. (Illus.). 800p. pap. (1-899066-57-8) Isis Med GBR. *Dist:* Bks Intl VA.

Anaesthesia, Analgesia & Intensive Care. Adams. 1991. 320p. pap. 19.95 (0-340-54927-0) Trafalgar.

Anaesthesia & Analgesia in Emergency Medicine. Karen Illingworth & Karen Simpson. 2nd ed. 1998. LC 97-41376. (Oxford Handbooks in Emergency Medicine Ser.). (Illus.). 406p. pap. text 59.95 (0-19-262908-5) OUP.

Anaesthesia & Emergency Situations: A Complete Management Guide. Garry D. Phillips & Gajinder Oberoi. 2000. (Illus.). 256p. 64.95 (0-07-470767-1) McGraw-Hill Educ Grp.

Anaesthesia & Intensive Care A-Z: An Encyclopaedia of Principles & Practice. S. M. Yentis et al. 2nd ed. 2000. LC 99-51561. (Illus.). 577p. pap. text 82.00 (0-7506-3249-6) Buttrwrth-Heinemann.

Anaesthesia & Intensive Care for the Neurosurgical Patient. Ed. by Frank J. Walters et al. 2nd ed. 1993. LC 93-19830. (Illus.). 480p. 165.00 (0-632-03715-6) Blackwell Sci.

Anaesthesia & Pediatric Diseases. Ed. by Jordan Katz & David J. Steward. 2nd ed. 1993. LC 92-48754. (Illus.). 752p. text 140.00 (0-7216-6681-7) Saunders.

Anaesthesia & Resuscitation: A Houseman's Guide. R. D. Jones & R. B. Holland. 1997. LC 97-5630. 320p. pap. text 40.00 (0-7506-2960-6) Buttrwrth-Heinemann.

Anaesthesia at the District Hospital. M. B. Dobson. 1988. (ENG, FRE & SPA., Illus.). 143p. pap. text 20.00 (92-4-154228-4, 1150289) World Health.

*__Anaesthesia Databook: A Perioperative & Peripartum Manual.__ Mason. 3rd ed. 2001. 624p. pap. (1-84110-067-6) Greenwich Med GBR. *Dist:* JAMCO Dist.

Anaesthesia for Burns, Maxillofacial & Plastic Surgery. 256p. (0-340-55302-2) E A GBR. *Dist:* Routldge.

Anaesthesia for Children. T. C. Brown & G. C. Fisk. 2nd ed. 1992. (Illus.). 560p. 199.00 (0-632-03023-2) Blackwell Sci.

*__Anaesthesia for the High Risk Patient.__ Ian McConachie. 2002. (Illus.). 256p. pap. (1-84110-072-2) Greenwich Med GBR. *Dist:* JAMCO Dist.

Anaesthesia for Thoracic Surgery. J. W. Gothard. 2nd ed. 1993. (Illus.). 264p. 110.00 (0-632-03275-8) Blackwell Sci.

Anaesthesia of the Cat. L.W. Hall. 1994. (C). text 84.00 (0-7020-1665-9) Harcourt.

Anaesthesia, Pain, Intensive Care, & Emergency Medicine . . . APICE: Proceedings of the 12th Postgraduate Course in Critical Care Medicine, Trieste, Italy, November 19-21, 1997. A. Gullo. 1998. LC 98-15946. 1000p. 129.00 (88-470-0007-6) Spr-Verlag.

Anaesthesia Review 8. Ed. by Leon Kaufman. 1991. (Illus.). 320p. (Orig.). pap. text (0-443-04384-1) Church.

Anaesthesia Review 11. Leon Kaufman. 1994. (Orig.). pap. text 61.00 (0-443-05015-5) Saunders.

Anaesthesia Review 4. Ed. by Leon Kaufman. 1987. (Illus.). 256p. (Orig.). (C). pap. text (0-443-03450-8) Church.

Anaesthesia Review 14. Leon Kaufman & R. N. Ginsburg. 1998. (Illus.). 216p. pap. (0-443-06018-5) Church.

Anaesthesia Review 9. Ed. by Leon Kaufman. 1992. (Illus.). 284p. text (0-443-04564-X) Church.

Anaesthesia Review 7. Ed. by Leon Kaufman. 1990. (Illus.). 240p. pap. text (0-443-04216-0) Church.

*__Anaesthesia Review 16.__ Leon Kaufman & Robert Ginsburg. 2001. (Illus.). 205p. pap. (0-443-06456-3) Church GBR. *Dist:* Saunders.

Anaesthesia Review 10. Ed. by Leon Kaufman. 1993. (Illus.). 276p. (Orig.). pap. text (0-443-04853-3) Church.

Anaesthesia Review 12. Leon Kaufman. 1996. (Orig.). pap. text 58.00 (0-443-05242-5) Saunders.

Anaesthetic Algorithms. Rodney F. Armstrong et al. 1996. LC 96-3406. (Illus.). 92p. pap. text 39.50 (0-19-262595-0) OUP.

Anaesthetic & Sedative Techniques for Aquatic Animals. Lindsay Ross et al. 2nd ed. 1999. (Illus.). 160p. pap. text (0-8138-2130-4) Blckwell Science GBR. *Dist:* Iowa U Pr.

Anal Fistula: Surgical Evaluation & Management. Ed. by R. Phillips & P. Lunniss. 1995. (Illus.). 204p. (0-412-54430-X) E A GBR. *Dist:* OUP.

*__Analgesia & Anaesthesia in Pregnancy.__ S. Yentis et al. 2000. (Illus.). 500p. (0-7020-2322-1) W B Saunders GBR. *Dist:* Saunders.

Analgesic & NSAID-Induced Kidney Disease. Ed. by J. H. Stewart. 1993. LC 92-22709. (Oxford Clinical Nephrology Ser.). (Illus.). 304p. text 69.50 (0-19-261956-X) OUP.

Analgesic Drugs. 1986. (Medical Ser.). lib. bdg. 79.95 (0-8490-3803-0) Gordon Pr.

Analogical Mind: Perspectives from Cognitive Science. Ed. by Dedre Gentner et al. 2001. LC 00-57889. (Illus.). xii, 541p. (C). 85.00 (0-262-07206-8); pap. 39.95 (0-262-57139-0) MIT Pr (Bradford Bks).

Analyses of Hazardous Substances in Biological Materials, Vol. 1, Vol. 1. Ed. by J. Angerer & K. H. Schaller. 2nd ed. 1992. 222p. 135.00 (3-527-27024-8, Wiley-VCH) Wiley.

Analysing Health Policy: Sociological Approaches. Judith Green & Nicki Thorogood. 1998. LC 97-44039. pap. (0-582-29801-6) Addison-Wesley.

Analysis & Assessment of Cardiovascular Function. Ed. by Gary M. Drzewiecki & John K. Li. 1997. LC 97-22078. (Illus.). 387p. 84.95 (0-387-98282-5) Spr-Verlag.

Analysis & Characterization of Steroids. Henryk Lamparczyk. 1992. 176p. lib. bdg. 179.00 (0-8493-3008-4, QP752) CRC Pr.

Analysis & Evaluation of Conceptual Models of Nursing. Jacqueline Fawcett. 3rd ed. 1994. LC 94-10087. (Illus.). 576p. (C). text 35.95 (0-8036-3411-0) Davis Co.

Analysis & Evaluation of Health Care Systems: An Integrated Approach to Managerial Decision Making. Thomas T. Wan. 1995. LC 95-5138. 256p. (C). 49.95 (1-878812-23-8) Hlth Prof Pr.

Analysis & Evaluation of Nursing Theories. Jacqueline Fawcett. 1993. LC 93-9610. (Illus.). 281p. (C). text 33.95 (0-8036-3413-7) Davis Co.

Analysis & Modeling of Neural Systems. Ed. by Frank H. Eeckman. 1991. 432p. (C). text 142.50 (0-7923-9217-5) Kluwer Academic.

Analysis & Simulation of the Cardiac System Ischemia. Ed. by Samuel Sideman & Rafael Beyar. 1989. 464p. lib. bdg. 153.00 (0-8493-5355-6, RC685) CRC Pr.

Analysis & Valuation of Health Care Enterprises. Arthur E. Gimmy & Charles R. Baumbach. 1996. LC 96-31795. 39.00 (0-922154-32-5) Appraisal Inst.

Analysis for Drugs & Metabolites. Eric Reid & Ian D. Wilson. 1990. 400p. (0-85186-956-4) Royal Soc Chem GBR. *Dist:* Spr-Verlag.

Analysis for Drugs of Abuse. T. Ryan. Date not set. (Illus.). text (0-8247-9853-8) Dekker.

Analysis, Networks, Peptides. 1984. (Advances in Polymer Science Ser.: Vol. 65). (Illus.). 230p. 79.95 (0-387-13656-8) Spr-Verlag.

Analysis of Addictive & Misused Drugs. John A. Adamovics. 1994. LC 94-22885. (Illus.). 800p. text 225.00 (0-8247-9238-6) Dekker.

Analysis of Amyloid Precursor Protein in Cells & Brain of Transgenic Mice as the Biochemical Correlat for their Phenotype. Ilse Dewachter. 1999. (Illus.). 164p. (*90-5867-006-6*) Leuven Univ BEL. *Dist:* Coronet Bks.

Analysis of Antibiotic & Drug Residues in Food Products of Animal Origin. V. K. Agarwal. 1992. (Illus.). 272p. (C). text 89.00 (*0-306-44199-3*, Kluwer Plenum) Kluwer Academic.

Analysis of Biological Material for Trace Elements Using X-Ray Spectroscopy. Vlado Valkovic. 1980. 256p. 129.00 (*0-8493-5723-3*, QP534, CRC Reprint) Franklin.

Analysis of Completion Sentences & Arithmetical Problems As Items for Intelligence Tests. Henry D. Rinsland. LC 73-177192. (Columbia University. Teachers College. Contributions to Education Ser.: No. 666). reprint ed. 37.50 (*0-404-55666-3*) AMS Pr.

Analysis of Cortical Connectivity. Malcolm P. Young et al. 1995. LC 95-37885. (Neuroscience Intelligence Unit Ser.). 157p. 89.95 (*1-57059-307-8*) Landes Bioscience.

Analysis of Delinquency & Aggression. Ed. by Albert Bandura & Emilio Ribes-Inesta. 1976. 256p. text 59.95 (*0-89859-360-3*) L Erlbaum Assocs.

Analysis of Doubly Censored Survival Data: An Application to Data Collected from the Amsterdam Cohort Studies on HIV Infection & AIDS. Lai Sing Lam. 1997. (WBBM Reports: No. 36). (Illus.). 75p. pap. (*90-407-1561-0*) Delft U Pr NLD. *Dist:* Coronet Bks.

Analysis of Drugs in Biological Fluids. Joseph Chamberlain. 1985. 320p. 161.00 (*0-8493-5144-8*, RB52); 2nd ed. 1995. LC 95-19022. 368p. 139.95 (*0-8493-2492-0*, 2492) CRC Pr.

Analysis of Drugs of Abuse. Ed. by T. A. Gough. 1991. LC 90-13149. (Separation Science Ser.). 648p. 620.00 (*0-471-92267-6*) Wiley.

Analysis of Emergency Medical Services in Austin, Texas David J. Eaton. Incl. Analysis of Emergency Medical Services in Austin, Texas Vol .1: Results. 164p. pap. 8.50 (*0-89940-641-6*); Analysis of Emergency Medical Services in Austin, Texas Vol. 2: Analytical Methods. 96p. pap. 7.95 (*0-89940-642-4*); (Policy Research Project Report Ser.: Vol. 41). 1980. Set pap. 16.45 (*0-89940-643-2*) LBJ Sch Pub Aff.

Analysis of Emergency Medical Services in Austin, Texas Vol .1: Results David J. Eaton. 1980. (Policy Research Project Report Ser.: Vol. 41A). 164p. pap. 8.50 (*0-89940-641-6*) LBJ Sch Pub Aff.

Analysis of Emergency Medical Services in Austin, Texas Vol. 2: Analytical Methods David J. Eaton. 1980. (Policy Research Project Report Ser.: Vol. 41B). 96p. pap. 7.95 (*0-89940-642-4*) LBJ Sch Pub Aff.

Analysis of Forages & Fibrous Foods. Peter J. Van Soest & James B. Robertson. 1999. 52.95 (*0-8493-8761-2*) CRC Pr.

Analysis of Free Radicals in Biological Systems. Ed. by Alain E. Favier et al. 1995. LC 95-21845. 312p. 139.00 (*3-7643-5137-3*) Spr-Verlag.

Analysis of Free Radicals in Biological Systems. Alan E. Favier. 1995. LC 95-21845. x, 312p. 139.00 (*0-8176-5137-3*) Birkhauser.

Analysis of Health Indicators for California's Minority Populations. James A. McCullough et al. 1998. (Illus.). 92p. (C). reprint ed. pap. text 20.00 (*0-7881-4319-0*) DIANE Pub.

Analysis of Human Behavior: A Psychological Laboratory Manual. Sonja Grover. 1985. 130p. pap. text 8.95 (*0-8290-0725-3*) Irvington.

Analysis of Human Genetic Linkage. Jurg Ott. 3rd ed. 1999. LC 98-37347. (Illus.). 405p. 59.95 (*0-8018-6140-3*) Johns Hopkins.

Analysis of Human Mandibular Movement. J. M. Goodson & E. L. Johansen. 1975. (Monographs in Oral Science: Vol. 5). 51.50 (*3-8055-1416-6*) S Karger.

Analysis of Human Motion: A Textbook in Kinesiology. M. Gladys Scott. 2nd ed. 1963. LC 63-13839. (Illus.). 22.95 (*0-89197-023-1*); pap. text 9.50 (*0-89197-024-X*) Irvington.

Analysis of Infectious Disease Data. N. G. Becker. 1989. (Monographs on Statistics & Applied Probability). 240p. (gr. 13). 62.95 (*0-412-30990-4*, A2802, Chap & Hall CRC) CRC Pr.

Analysis of Medical Data Using Mixed Models. Helen Brown & Robin Prescott. 2000. LC 99-14216. 428p. 110.00 (*0-471-96554-5*) Wiley.

Analysis of Medical Savings Accounts: Do Two Wrongs Make a Right? Pauly. 1994. 50p. (Orig.). pap. 9.95 (*0-8447-7027-2*) Am Enterprise.

Analysis of Mortality & Other Actuarial Statistics. B. Benjamin & J. H. Pollard. 1980. 212p. (*0-434-90137-7*) Trafalgar.

Analysis of Multifactorial Diseases. Tim Bishop & Pak Sham. 2000. (Human Molecular Genetics Ser.). 320p. 125.00 (*0-12-101610-2*) Acad Pr.

Analysis of Multivariate Survival Data. P. Hougaard. 2000. LC 00-40047. (Statistics for Biology & Health Ser.). 560p. 84.95 (*0-387-98873-4*) Spr-Verlag.

Analysis of Neural Networks. U. Heiden. 1980. (Lecture Notes in Biomathematics: Vol. 35). (Illus.). 159p. 41.95 (*0-387-09966-2*) Spr-Verlag.

Analysis of Neuronal Microcircuits & Synaptic Interactions, No. 8: Handbook of Chemical Neuroanatomy. Ed. by Anders T. Bjorklund et al. 1990. 548p. 280.00 (*0-444-81231-8*) Elsevier.

Analysis of Pesticides in Water: Significance, Principles, Techniques, & Chemistry of Pesticides, Vol. I. B. K. Afghan. Ed. by S. Y. Chau. 1982. 216p. 144.00 (*0-8493-5210-X*, TP248) CRC Pr.

Analysis of Psychiatric Drugs. Ed. by Alan A. Boulton et al. 1988. LC 88-13342. (Neuromethods Ser.: Vol. 10). (Illus.). 564p. 159.50 (*0-89603-121-7*) Humana.

Analysis of Psychological Theory: Meta-Psychological Perspectives. Ed. by Henderikus J. Stam. 1987. 300p. 79.95 (*0-89116-597-5*) Hemisp Pub.

Analysis of Quality of Care for Patients Who Are Black or Poor in Rural & Urban Settings. Katherine L. Kahn et al. 1994. LC 93-29147. pap. text 13.00 (*0-8330-1433-1*, MR-292-HCFA) Rand Corp.

Analysis of Radiographic Quality: Lab Manual & Workbook. Daniel P. Donohue. 3rd ed. 2000. 544p. pap. 65.00 (*0-8342-0678-1*) PRO-ED.

Analysis of Self: A Systematic Approach to the Psychoanalytic Treatment of Narcissistic Personality Disorders. Heinz Kohut. 1971. LC 70-143392. (Psychoanalytic Study of the Child Monographs: No. 4). 368p. 57.50 (*0-8236-0145-5*) Intl Univs Pr.

Analysis of Species-Specific Molar Adaptations in Strepsirhine Primates. D. Seligsohn. 1977. (Contributions to Primatology Ser.: Vol. 11). (Illus.). 44.50 (*3-8055-2634-2*) S Karger.

Analysis of the Administration's Health Proposal. Ed. by Paul Van De Water. 1994. (Illus.). 81p. (Orig.). (C). pap. text 50.00 (*0-7881-0539-6*) DIANE Pub.

Analysis of the California Syllabus on Radiation Protection: Radiology Student Workbook. Robert J. Parelli. 1996. (Illus.). 179p. (Orig.). (C). pap., wbk. ed. 35.00 (*1-880359-09-X*) Par Rad.

Analysis of the Cost Savings of the Medicare Hospice Benefit. 1995. 22p. pap. 11.85 (*0-931207-41-X*) Natl Hospice.

Analysis of the Managed Competition Act. Ed. by Paul Van De Water. 1994. (Illus.). 53p. (Orig.). (C). pap. text 35.00 (*0-7881-0832-8*) DIANE Pub.

Analysis of the Transference in the Here & Now. Gregory P. Bauer. 1993. LC 92-49521. 248p. 50.00 (*0-87668-143-7*) Aronson.

Analysis of Three Hundred & Thirty-Three Necro-Kidney-Allografts. G. K. Uhlschmid. 1979. (European Surgical Research Ser.: Vol. 11, Suppl. 1). (Illus.). pap. 21.75 (*3-8055-3004-8*) S Karger.

Analysis of Transference: Theory & Technique, Vol. 1. Merton M. Gill. 1981. LC 81-23654. (Psychological Issues Monographs: No. 53). 200p. 35.00 (*0-8236-0139-0*) Intl Univs Pr.

***Analysis of WNT/B-Catenin Signaling in Desmoid Tmors.** Sabine Tejpar. 2001. (Acta Biomedica Lovaniensia Ser.: No. 237). (Illus.). 116p. pap. (*90-5867-141-0*) Leuven Univ BEL. *Dist:* Coronet Bks.

Analysis Repair & Individuation. K. Lambert. 1981. 250p. (*1-85575-083-X*) Karnac Bks GBR. *Dist:* Other Pr LLC.

Analysis, Understanding, & Presentation of Cases Involving Traumatic Brain Injury. Ed. by Charles N. Simkins. 1994. LC 93-44705. 200.00 (*0-927093-01-4*) Brain Injury Assoc.

Analyst & the Mystic: Psychoanalytic Reflections on Religion & Mysticism. Sudhir Kakar. 1992. LC 90-29159. 96p. 18.95 (*0-226-42283-6*) U Ch Pr.

Analyst & the Working Alliance: The Reemergence of Convention in Psychoanalysis. Heinrich Deserno. Tr. by Andrew Jenkins from ENG. 1998. LC 98-10469. xii, 167p. 30.00 (*0-8236-0134-X*, 00134) Intl Univs Pr.

Analyst in the Inner City: Race, Class & Culture Through a Psychoanalytic Lens. Neil Altman. 1995. LC 95-23629. (Relational Perspectives Bks.: Vol. 3). 208p. 36.00 (*0-88163-173-6*) Analytic Pr.

Analyst-Patient Interaction: Collected Papers on Technique. Michael S. Fordham. Ed. by Sonu Shamdasani. 1995. LC 95-8618. 224p. (C). 78.95 (*0-415-12184-1*) Routledge.

Analysts at Work: Practice, Principles & Techniques. Ed. by Joseph Reppen. 1995. LC 94-36490. 268p. pap. text 50.00 (*1-56821-423-5*) Aronson.

Analytic Life: Personal & Professional Aspects of Being a Jungian Analyst. New England Society Of Jungian Analysts Staff. 1988. 78p. pap. 11.95 (*0-938434-28-4*) Sigo Pr.

Analytic Process. Ed. by Joseph B. Wheelwright. 1971. LC 74-142160. (Illus.). 12.00 (*0-913430-10-2*) C G Jung Foun.

Analytical & Quantitative Cardiology: Proceedings of the Tenth Goldberg Workshop Held in Haifa, Israel, December 2-5, 1996. Ed. by Samuel Sideman et al. 1997. LC 97-36238. (Advances in Experimental Medicine & Biology Ser.: Vol. 430). 388p. (C). text 110.00 (*0-306-45762-8*, Kluwer Plenum) Kluwer Academic.

Analytical Aspects of Drug Testing. Ed. by Dale G. Deutsch. 1989. LC 88-17291. (Chemical Analysis Monographs). 304p. 225.00 (*0-471-85309-7*) Wiley.

Analytical Control of Radiopharmaceuticals. 1970. (Panel Proceedings Ser.). (Illus.). 228p. (Orig.). pap. (*92-0-141070-0*, ISP253) IAEA AUT. *Dist:* Bernan Associates.

Analytical Hypnotherapy: Principles & Practice. Edgar Barnett. 1989. 510p. reprint ed. 32.50 (*0-930298-30-6*) Westwood Pub Co.

Analytical Instrumentation Handbook. Galen W. Ewing. 2nd ed. 1997. LC 96-51434. (Illus.). 1470p. text 275.00 (*0-8247-9455-9*) Dekker.

Analytical Instrumentation Markets: Product Sophistication Meets Tough Environmental Regulations & Biotech Research Demands. Market Intelligence Staff. 1992. 255p. (Orig.). 2295.00 (*1-56753-059-1*) Frost & Sullivan.

Analytical Lung Pathology. Klaus Kayser. 1992. LC 92-2154. (Illus.). 404p. 163.00 (*0-387-54263-9*) Spr-Verlag.

Analytical Methods for Materials Investigation. George A. Kirkendale. 1971. (Illus.). x, 264p. text 348.00 (*0-677-14500-4*) Gordon & Breach.

Analytical Methods in Clinical Chemistry. Ed. by Larry J. Kricka. 1984. (Illus.). 96p. pap. 28.00 (*0-08-031453-8*, Pergamon Pr) Elsevier.

Analytical Methods/T. Q. M. in Health Care. Pivnicny. 1998. (Health Services Administration Ser.). pap. 34.95 (*0-8273-7381-3*) Delmar.

Analytical Profiles of Drug Substances, Vol. 10. Ed. by Klaus Florey et al. 1981. text 157.00 (*0-12-260810-0*) Acad Pr.

***Analytical Profiles of Drug Substances & Excipients.** Ed. by Harry G. Brittain. 2001. (Analytical Profiles of Drug Substances & Excipients Ser.: Vol. 27). 382p. 125.00 (*0-12-260827-5*) Acad Pr.

Analytical Profiles of Drug Substances & Excipients, Vol. 23. Ed. by Harry G. Brittain. (Illus.). 1994. 611p. text 105.00 (*0-12-260823-2*); 1993. 691p. text 116.00 (*0-12-260822-4*) Acad Pr.

Analytical Profiles of Drug Substances & Excipients Vol. 26. Ed. by Harry G. Brittain. 1999. 650p. 99.00 (*0-12-260826-7*) Acad Pr.

Analytical Psychology: A Modern Science. Ed. by M. Fordham et al. 1973. 220p. (*1-85575-077-5*) Karnac Bks GBR. *Dist:* Other Pr LLC.

Analytical Psychology: Notes of the Seminar Given in 1925. Carl Gustav Jung. Ed. by William McGuire. 1991. (Bollingen Ser.: No. XCIX: 3). (Illus.). 199p. pap. 19.95 (*0-691-01918-5*) Princeton U Pr.

Analytical Techniques in Immunochemistry. Ed. by Terry M. Phillips. 1991. (Illus.). 364p. text 195.00 (*0-8247-8477-4*) Dekker.

Analytical Techniques in Occupational Health Chemistry. Ed. by Donald D. Dollberg & Allen W. Verstuyft. 1980. LC 79-28460. (ACS Symposium Ser.: No. 120). 318p. 43.95 (*0-8412-0539-6*) Am Chemical.

Analytical Toxicology for Clinical, Forensic & Pharmaceutical Chemists: For Clinical, Forensic, & Pharmaceutical Chemists. Ed. by Hans Brandenberger & Robert A. Maes. 1997. LC 97-2360. (Clinical Biochemistry Ser.: Vol. 5). (Illus.). 784p. (C). lib. bdg. 369.00 (*3-11-010731-7*) De Gruyter.

Analytical Transport Economics: An International Perspective. J. B. Polak & Arnold Heertje. 2000. LC 00-33171. (Transport Economics, Management & Policy Ser.). (Illus.). xx, 418p. 120.00 (*1-85898-786-5*) E Elgar.

Analytical Use of Fluorescent Probes in Oncology: Proceedings of a NATO ARW Held in Miami, Florida, October 14-18, 1995. Ed. by Elli Kohen & Joseph G. Hirschberg. 1997. (NATO Advanced Science Institutes Ser.: Vol. 286). (Illus.). 458p. 150.00 (*0-306-45369-X*, Kluwer Plenum) Kluwer Academic.

Analytika: Analytical Testing & Training Lists. Geoff Plant. 1994. 400p. ring bd. 110.00 (*1-56593-677-9*, 1332); ring bd. 135.00 incl. disk (*1-56593-678-7*, 1334) Singular Publishing.

Analyzing & Recording a Drug Information Request: Module 1. Kimberly A. Galt. 1994. (Clinical Skills Program Drug Information Ser.). (Illus.). (C). 50.00 (*1-879907-44-5*) Am Soc Hlth-Syst.

Analyzing Behavioral Problems. 1977. 2.00 (*0-939418-34-7*) Ferguson-Florissant.

Analyzing Cleft Palate Speech. Grunwell. 1993. pap. 62.25 (*1-56593-251-X*, 0466) Singular Publishing.

***Analyzing Criminal Behavior.** Michael R. King & Gregory M. Cooper. 2001. (Illus.). 216p. pap. text 24.95 (*0-615-11937-9*) IQ Design.

Analyzing Discourse in Communicatively Impaired Adults. Leora R. Cherney et al. 1995. LC 98-18602. (Rehabilitation Institute of Chicago Publication Ser.). 251p. 60.00 (*0-8342-0632-3*) PRO-ED.

Analyzing Food for Nutrition Labeling & Hazardous Contaminants. Ed. by Ike J. Jeon & William G. Ikins. 1994. LC 94-41547. (Food Science & Technology Ser.: Vol. 65). (Illus.). 520p. text 195.00 (*0-8247-9349-8*) Dekker.

Analyzing Neurological Status. Kathy A. Hausman et al. 1985. (Illus.). 125p. pap. text 14.95 (*0-932491-24-3*) Res Appl Inc.

Analyzing Psychotheraphy: A Social Role Interpretation. Melvyn L. Fein. 1992. LC 91-28650. 240p. 67.00 (*0-275-93966-9*, C3966, Praeger Pubs) Greenwood.

Analyzing Quantitative Behavioral Observation Data. H. K. Suen & D. Ary. 1989. 376p. 75.00 (*0-89859-945-8*) L Erlbaum Assocs.

Analyzing Within-Subjects Experiments. John W. Cotton. 1997. LC 97-8624. (*0-8058-2804-4*) L Erlbaum Assocs.

Anamnese en Lichamelijk Onderzoek bij Gezelschapsdieren see Medical History & Physical Examination in Companion Animals

Anamu. Woodland Publishing Staff. 1999. (Woodland Health Ser.). (SPA.). 14p. pap. text 3.95 (*1-58054-038-4*) Woodland UT.

Anaphylactic Reactions in Anesthesia & Intensive Care. Jerrold H. Levy. 2nd ed. 1992. LC 91-47872. 266p. text 74.99 (*0-7506-9064-X*) Buttrwrth-Heinemann.

Anaphylactoid Edema. Hans Selye. 1968. LC 67-26017. (Illus.). 344p. 26.50 (*0-87527-071-9*) Green.

Anarchist AIDS Medical Formulary: A Guide to Guerrilla Immunology. Charles R. Caulfield & Billi Goldberg. 1994. LC 93-43598. (Illus.). 155p. (Orig.). (C). pap. 12.95 (*1-55643-175-9*) North Atlantic.

Anarchist Critique of the Politics of AIDS. 1991. lib. bdg. 69.00 (*0-8490-4609-2*) Gordon Pr.

***Anatomia de Gray (Gray's Anatomy)**, Set Peter L. Williams. 38th ed. 1995. (SPA., Illus.). (*84-8174-384-4*) Mosby-Doyma Libros ESP. *Dist:* Saunders.

Anatomia de las Estruc Orofaci. Brand. 6th ed. 1999. (C). text 46.93 (*84-8174-381-X*) Mosby Inc.

Anatomia Oral. B. K. Berkovitz. 2nd ed. 1996. (C). text 88.40 (*84-8174-139-6*) Mosby Inc.

Anatomic Basis of Tumor Surgery. William C. Wood & John E. Skandalakis. 1999. LC 98-51163. (Illus.). xi, 912p. text 195.00 (*1-57626-003-8*) Quality Med Pub.

Anatomic Exposures in Vascular Surgery. Gary G. Wind & R. James Valentine. 1991. (Illus.). 512p. text 199.00 (*0-683-09140-9*) Lppncott W & W.

Anatomic Foundations in Plastic Surgery. Shaw. 1998. text (*0-7216-4070-2*) Saunders.

Anatomic Localization for Needle EMG. Steve R. Geiringer. 2nd rev. ed. 1999. LC 99-14491. (Illus.). 175p. pap. 31.95 (*1-56053-314-5*) Hanley & Belfus.

Anatomic Variations of the Upper Extremity. Chris P. Tountas & Ronald A. Bergman. 1992. (Illus.). 286p. text (*0-443-08771-7*) Church.

Anatomical Acupuncture. Hou Chi Dung. 1997. (Illus.). 550p. text 96.00 (*0-9663588-0-5*) Antarctic Pr.

Anatomical & Physiological Bases of Speech. David Dickson & Wilma Maue-Dickson. 1982. LC 90-21191. (Illus.). 338p. (C). text 54.99 (*0-7506-9760-1*, 1645) Buttrwrth-Heinemann.

Anatomical Atlas. Maud Jepson. 1993. 24p. reprint ed. spiral bd. 8.00 (*0-7873-0475-1*) Hlth Research.

Anatomical Atlas of the Temporomandibular Joint. Y. Ide & K. Nakazawa. 1991. (Illus.). 116p. text 148.00 (*4-87417-362-4*) Quint Pub Co.

Anatomical Basis of Dentistry. Bernard Liebgott. (Illus.). 1986. 511p. (C). 61.95 (*0-941158-88-8*); 2nd ed. 2000. LC 00-66437. x, 546p. 61.95 (*0-323-01013-X*) Mosby Inc.

Anatomical Dissections for Use in Neurosurgery. Wolfgang Seeger. Vol. 1. 1987. 313p. 165.00 (*3-211-81998-3*); Vol. 1. 1987. (Illus.). 313p. 181.00 (*0-387-81998-3*); Vol. 2. 1989. (Illus.). 314p. 194.00 (*0-387-82069-8*); Vol. 2. 1988. 314p. 165.00 (*3-211-82069-8*) Spr-Verlag.

Anatomical Exercises: De Motu Cordis & de Circulatione Sanguinis in English Translation. William Harvey. Ed. by Geoffrey L. Keynes. unabr. ed. 1995. LC 95-17389. 224p. reprint ed. pap. text 8.95 (*0-486-68827-5*) Dover.

Anatomical Guide for the Electromyographer: The Limbs & Trunk. Aldo O. Perotto. 3rd ed. 1994. (Illus.). 328p. (C). text 53.95 (*0-398-05900-4*) C C Thomas.

Anatomical Neuroendocrinology: Proceedings of the International Conference, Chapel Hill, 1974. International Conference on Neuroendocrinology, of. Ed. by L. D. Grant & Walter E. Stumpf. 1976. 300p. 112.25 (*3-8055-2154-5*) S Karger.

Anatomical Texts of the Earlier Middle Ages. George W. Corner. LC 75-23700. (Carnegie Institution of Washington. Publications: No. 364). reprint ed. 47.50 (*0-404-13250-2*) AMS Pr.

Anatomie-Chirurgie Encyclopedie Ou Dictionnaire Raissonne des Sciences. Denis Diderot. 2nd ed. 1977. (FRE.). 75.00 (*0-7859-0857-9*, M-7053) Fr & Eur.

Anatomie of the Bodie of Man, Pt. 1. Thomas Vicary. Ed. by F. J. Furnivall & Percey Furnivall. 1972. (EETS, ES Ser.: No. 53). reprint ed. 54.00 (*0-527-00259-3*) Periodicals Srv.

Anatomist at Large. George W. Corner. 1977. LC 76-86743. (Essay Index Reprint Ser.). 22.95 (*0-8369-1176-8*) Ayer.

Anatomy. Nikos M. Linardakis. 1999. LC 99-24495. (Digging Up the Bones Ser.). (Illus.). 117p. pap. 19.95 (*0-07-038415-0*) McGraw-Hill Prof.

Anatomy. Mosby Staff. 1997. pap. text 2.00 (*0-8151-8601-0*) Mosby Inc.

Anatomy. John Tesoriero. 1994. (Blond's Medical Guides Ser.). (Illus.). 282p. (Orig.). (C). pap. text 19.99 (*0-945819-20-X*) Sulzburger & Graham Pub.

Anatomy. George W. Corner. LC 75-23652. (Clio Medica Ser.: 3). (Illus.). reprint ed. 29.50 (*0-404-58903-0*) AMS Pr.

Anatomy: A Regional Atlas of the Human Body. Carmine D. Clemente. 1987. 49.50 (*0-8121-1723-9*); 3rd ed. 1987. LC 85-11157. (Illus.). 444p. (C). 52.00 (*0-683-01723-3*); 4th ed. 1997. LC 96-47623. (Illus.). 580p. pap. text 59.95 (*0-683-01733-0*) Lppncott W & W.

Anatomy: A Revision Companion. S. H. Jacob. 1995. LC 95-6578. pap. text (*0-443-04973-4*) Church.

Anatomy: Embryology, Gross Anatomy, Neuroanatomy, Microanatomy. Ed. & Contrib. by Raymond E. Papka. 1995. LC 94-45449. (Oklahoma Notes). 231p. 24.95 (*0-387-94395-1*) Spr-Verlag.

Anatomy: MedCharts. Thomas P. Gest. 1995. 17.95 (*1-882531-01-9*) ILOC.

Anatomy: Palpation & Surface Markings. Derek Field. 1995. (Illus.). 214p. pap. text 42.50 (*0-7506-0062-4*) Buttrwrth-Heinemann.

Anatomy Step 1: Review for USMLE. Kurt E. Johnson. 2nd ed. 1998. LC 98-65379. 275p. pap. text 25.00 (*1-888308-03-6*) J & S Pub VA.

Anatomy Step 1: Review for USMLE. Kurt E. Johnson et al. 2nd ed. 1998. (Illus.). 275p. pap. 25.00 (*0-8036-0711-3*) Davis Co.

Anatomy & Function. W. Rall. 1990. 75.00 (*0-8176-3502-5*) Birkhauser.

Anatomy & Imaging of the Cranial Nerves see Cranial Nerves: Anatomy, Imaging, Vascularisation

Anatomy & Physics. Anne B. Donnersberger & Anne E. Lesak. 7th ed. 1999. (Illus.). 128p. (C). pap. text, tchr. ed., lab manual ed. 19.95 (*0-7637-1053-9*, 1053-9) Jones & Bartlett.

Anatomy & Physiology. Contrib. by M. Fogiel. 2000. LC 00-130285. (Super Reviews; All You Need to Know Ser.). (Illus.). viii, 296p. pap. 9.95 (*0-87891-179-0*) Res & Educ.

Anatomy & Physiology. Cecelia G. Grindel et al. 1997. LC 97-65156. (Springhouse Notes Ser.). 352p. pap. 26.95 (*0-87434-901-X*) Springhouse Corp.

Anatomy & Physiology. Stanley E. Gunstream. 1992. text, tchr. ed., wbk. ed. 32.50 (*0-697-10053-7*) McGraw.

Anatomy & Physiology B. J. Melloni et al. 1971. 100.00 (*0-07-076420-4*) McGraw.

Anatomy & Physiology B. John Melloni et al. 1971. text 100.00 (*0-07-076421-2*); text 100.00 (*0-07-076422-0*); text 100.00 (*0-07-076423-9*); text 100.00 (*0-07-076424-7*) McGraw.

Anatomy & Physiology. Jack Rudman. 1994. (ACT Proficiency Examination Program Ser.: PEP-4). pap. 23.95 (*0-8373-5504-4*); (Regents College Proficiency Examination Ser.: Vol. CPEP-37). pap. 23.95 (*0-8373-5437-4*) Nat Learn.

Anatomy & Physiology. SPC Staff. 1997. LC 97-27723. (Healthcare Professional Guides: Vol. 2). (Illus.). 240p. spiral bd. 26.95 (*0-87434-912-5*) Springhouse Corp.

Anatomy & Physiology. Eva L. Weinreb. 1982. 896p. (C). text (*0-201-08852-5*) Addison-Wesley.

Anatomy & Physiology. Rodney Seeley. 2nd ed. 1992. suppl. ed. 28.12 (*0-8016-6847-6*) Mosby Inc.

Anatomy & Physiology. Rodney Seeley & Philip D. Tate. 3rd ed. 1995. LC 95-113469. 624p. (C). text, stu. ed. 25.62 (*0-8151-8823-4*, WCB McGr Hill) McGrw-H Hghr Educ.

Anatomy & Physiology. Gary A. Thibodeau & Kevin T. Patton. 3rd ed. 1996. (Illus.). tchr. ed., spiral bd., lab manual ed. 42.95 (*0-8151-8826-9*); text, stu. ed. 100.00 (*0-8151-8808-0*) Mosby Inc.

Anatomy & Physiology. Kevin T. Patton. 4th ed. 1998. (Illus.). 456p. stu. ed. (*0-323-00193-9*); 528p. lab manual ed. (*0-323-00195-5*) Mosby Inc.

Anatomy & Physiology. Gary A. Thibodeau & Kevin T. Patton. 4th ed. 1998. tchr. ed. (*0-323-00194-7*) Mosby Inc.

Anatomy & Physiology. Harold J. Benson et al. 5th ed. 1992. text, tchr. ed. 18.75 (*0-697-08692-5*); 6th ed. 1994. text, tchr. ed., lab manual ed. 10.93 (*0-697-16015-7*) McGraw.

Anatomy & Physiology, No. 2. Gary A. Thibodeau & Kevin T. Patton. 2nd ed. 1993. (Illus.). (C). (gr. 13). 464p. spiral bd., lab manual ed. 35.95 (*0-8016-7268-6*, 07268); 360p. pap. text, stu. ed. 19.95 (*0-8016-7269-4*, 07269) Mosby Inc.

Anatomy & Physiology. Rodney Seeley. Set A. 2nd ed. 1992. 289.06 (*0-8016-5013-5*); Set B. 2nd ed. 1992. 145.00 (*0-8016-6642-2*); Set B. 3rd ed. 1995. (*0-8151-7893-X*) Mosby Inc.

Anatomy & Physiology: A Dynamic Approach. Anthony N. Chee. 4th ed. 1991. (Illus.). 344p. pap. text 33.95 (*0-89641-198-2*) American Pr.

Anatomy & Physiology: A Laboratory Manual. James E. Crouch & Micheline H. Carr. 1989. LC 76-56507. (Illus.). 369p. (C). reprint ed. stu. ed. 25.00 (*0-87484-356-1*) Circle Pr CA.

Anatomy & Physiology: A Self Instructional Course Cambridge Communication, Ltd. Staff. 2nd ed. 1997. LC 84-4977. (Illus.). text (*0-443-03170-3*); text (*0-443-03206-8*); text (*0-443-03207-6*); text (*0-443-03208-4*); text (*0-443-03209-2*) Church.

Anatomy & Physiology: An Easy Learner. Ethel Sloane. 1994. LC 93-44843. (Illus.). 400p. (C). pap. text 37.95 (*0-86720-832-5*, 832-5) Jones & Bartlett.

Anatomy & Physiology: Complete Version, Lab Manual. Harold J. Benson et al. 6th ed. 1994. 664p. (C). text 44.00 net. (*0-697-16016-5*, WCB McGr Hill) McGrw-H Hghr Educ.

Anatomy & Physiology: Essentials Version. Stanley E. Gunstream. 2nd ed. 1995. text, tchr. ed., lab manual ed. 9.68 (*0-697-11312-4*) McGraw.

Anatomy & Physiology: Plus Quick Reference. Gary Thibodeau & Kevin T. Patton. 3rd ed. 1996. (Illus.). tchr. ed., lab manual ed. (*0-8151-8816-1*); tchr. ed. (*0-8151-8778-5*); wbk. ed. (*0-8151-8829-3*) Mosby Inc.

Anatomy & Physiology 3. Rodney Seeley. 3rd ed. 1995. stu. ed., lab manual ed. 113.95 (*0-8151-7774-7*); lab manual ed. (*0-8151-7772-0*) Mosby Inc.

Anatomy & Physiology & Lab Manual & Student Survival Guide (PKG) Gary Thibodeau & Kevin T. Patton. 4th ed. 1999. 105.00 (*0-323-00191-2*) Mosby Inc.

Anatomy & Physiology & Quick Reference: Student Survival Guide. Gary A. Thibodeau & Kevin T. Patton. 4th ed. 1998. LC 99-180801. (Illus.). 1280p. stu. ed. 90.00 (*0-323-00192-0*) Mosby Inc.

Anatomy & Physiology & Student Survival Guide. Gary A. Thibodeau & Kevin T. Patton. 4th ed. 1999. (Illus.). 1200p. 95.82 (*84-8174-449-2*) Mosby Inc.

Anatomy & Physiology Applied to Nursing. Janet T. Riddle. 6th ed. 1985. LC 84-21413. (Churchill Livingstone Nursing Text Ser.). (Illus.). 196p. pap. text (*0-443-03030-8*) Church.

Anatomy & Physiology Applied to Obstetrics. Sylvia Verralls. 3rd ed. 1995. LC 92-20055. 240p. pap. text (*0-443-04211-X*) Church.

Anatomy & Physiology Essentials Study Guide. Rodney R. Seeley. 1990. 336p. (C). text 23.12 (*0-8016-4419-4*) Mosby Inc.

Anatomy & Physiology for Emergency Care. Bryan Bledsoe. 1998. (C). 36.00 (*0-8359-4992-3*) P-H.

Anatomy & Physiology for Lawyers. Mike A. Rothenberg. 1998. pap. text, suppl. ed. 65.00 (*1-56706-834-0*) Aspen Pub.

Anatomy & Physiology for Medical Assistants. Dahma Jarrell. 2000. (Medical Assisting Ser.). (C). pap. 28.00 net. (*0-7668-1068-2*) Delmar.

Anatomy & Physiology for Midwives. Linda Wylie. 2000. 241p. pap. text 38.95 (*0-443-05998-5*) Saunders.

Anatomy & Physiology for Physiotherapists. D. B. Moffat & R. F. Mottram. 2nd ed. 1987. (Illus.). 680p. pap. 47.95 (*0-632-01464-4*) Blackwell Sci.

Anatomy & Physiology for Speech, Language, & Hearing. John A. Seikel et al. exp. ed. 1997. LC 97-30733. (Textbook Ser.). 720p. pap. 72.50 (*1-56593-949-2*, 1878) Thomson Learn.

***Anatomy & Physiology for the Emergency Care.** Brian E. Bledsoe & X. Martini. 2001. 350p. 49.33 (*0-13-042298-3*) P-H.

Anatomy & Physiology in Focus: Laboratory Workbook. Stephen G. Davenport. 1993. 473p. (C). pap. (*0-9637670-0-3*) Link Pub.

Anatomy & Physiology in Respiratory Care. Beachey. 1997. LC 97-1309. (Illus.). 409p. (gr. 13). pap. text, wbk. ed. 40.00 (*0-8151-1198-3*, 27684) Mosby Inc.

Anatomy & Physiology Intermediate. Harold J. Benson et al. 4th ed. 1995. text, tchr. ed., lab manual ed. 7.81 (*0-697-21931-3*, WCB McGr Hill) McGrw-H Hghr Educ.

Anatomy & Physiology Lab Manual Dutchess Cc. 1999. 276p. (C). 49.00 (*0-201-67719-9*) Addison-Wesley.

Anatomy & Physiology Laboratory Textbook, Complete Version. Harold J. Benson et al. 5th ed. 640p. (C). 1992. text 38.50 net. (*0-697-08689-5*); 1991. text 44.00 net. (*0-697-08691-7*) McGrw-H Hghr Educ (WCB McGr Hill).

Anatomy & Physiology Laboratory Textbook, Short Version. Harold J. Benson et al. 6th ed. 1994. 512p. (C). text 38.50 net. (*0-697-16014-9*, WCB McGr Hill) McGrw-H Hghr Educ.

***Anatomy & Physiology Learning System.** Edith Applegate. 2nd ed. 2000. (Illus.). pap., tchr. ed. (*0-7216-8021-6*) Saunders.

***Anatomy & Physiology Learning System: ExaMaster.** Edith Applegate. 2000. 500.00 (*0-7216-9024-6*) Saunders.

***Anatomy & Physiology Learning System: ExaMaster.** Edith J. Applegate. 1995. (Illus.). 507p. pap. (*0-7216-6045-2*) Saunders.

Anatomy & Physiology Learning System: Textbook. Edith J. Applegate. 1995. (Illus.). pap., tchr. ed. (*0-7216-6636-1*); 1994. LC 93-44258. (*0-7216-6835-6*); 1994. LC 93-44258. (Illus.). 507p. pap. text 32.50 (*0-7216-6635-3*, A0242); 1994. (Illus.). 214p. pap. text, wbk. ed. 17.95 (*0-7216-6638-8*); Textbook/Workbook Package. 1994. (Illus.). 507p. text, wbk. ed. 45.00 (*0-7216-5903-9*) Saunders.

Anatomy & Physiology Made Incredibly Easy. Springhouse Publishing Company Staff. 2001. LC 00-41973. (Made Incredibly Easy Ser.). (Illus.). vi, 326p. 32.95 (*1-58255-043-3*) Springhouse Corp.

Anatomy & Physiology Notebook. Eugene P. Rutheny. 1993. 272p. (C). text 16.00 net. (*0-697-20349-2*, WCB McGr Hill) McGrw-H Hghr Educ.

Anatomy & Physiology of Farm Animals. Banks. 1994. 32.50 (*0-8016-6395-4*) Mosby Inc.

Anatomy & Physiology of Farm Animals. R. D. Frandson & T. L. Spurgeon. 5th ed. 1992. LC 91-25246. (Illus.). 572p. text 62.00 (*0-8121-1435-3*) Lppncott W & W.

Anatomy & Physiology of Speech: Laboratory Textbook. Harold M. Kaplan. 1981. LC 80-82927. (Illus.). 180p. text 42.95 (*0-932126-04-9*); pap. text 37.95 (*0-932126-05-7*) Graceway.

Anatomy & Physiology of the Peripheral Hearing Mechanism. J. Donald Harris. 1974. LC 73-12474. (Studies in Communicative Disorders). (C). pap. text (*0-672-61304-2*, Bobbs) Macmillan.

Anatomy & Physiology of the Speech Mechanism. Boyd Sheets. 1973. LC 72-81499. (Studies in Communicative Disorders). (C). pap. text (*0-672-61275-5*, Bobbs) Macmillan.

Anatomy & Physiology Quiz Art. Gary A. Thibodeau & Kevin T. Patton. 1993. 13.95 (*0-8016-7531-6*) Mosby Inc.

Anatomy & Physiology Text Plus. Gary A. Thibodeau & Kevin T. Patton. 2nd ed. 1993. (C). (gr. 13). 73.95 (*0-8016-7709-2*, 07709) Mosby Inc.

Anatomy & Physiology the Easy Way. I. Edward Alcamo. 1996. LC 95-45605. (Barron's Easy Way Ser.). 496p. pap. 13.95 (*0-8120-9134-5*) Barron.

Anatomy & Positioning. Bontrager. 2nd ed. 1995. Nos. 1-18. stu. ed. (*0-8016-6283-4*); Nos. 19-25. stu. ed. (*0-8016-6282-6*) Mosby Inc.

Anatomy & Psychology. Seeley. 2nd ed. 1992. lab manual ed. 28.75 (*0-697-40350-5*); 1991. 28.75 (*0-697-40336-X*) McGrw-H Hghr Educ (WCB McGr Hill).

Anatomy & Surgery of the Cavernous Sinus. V. V. Dolenc. 1989. (Illus.). 344p. 264.00 (*0-387-82155-4*, 3503) Spr-Verlag.

Anatomy As a Basis for Clinical Medicine. E. C. Hall-Craggs. 2nd enl. rev. ed. 1990. (Illus.). 616p. text 49.00 (*0-683-03831-1*) Lppncott W & W.

***Anatomy at a Glance.** Omar Faiz & David Moffat. 2001. LC 2001-52646. (At a Glance Ser.). (Illus.). 158p. pap. 24.95 (*0-632-05934-6*) Blackwell Sci.

***Anatomy Atlas.** American Map Publishing Staff. (SPA.). pap. 2.95 (*0-8416-9554-7*) Am Map.

Anatomy Charts for Reflexology. Sandra B. Rogers. Ed. by Christine Issel. 1994. (Illus.). 21p. stu. ed. (*0-9638862-0-7*) B J Scott.

Anatomy Charts for Reflexology: Student Edition. Sandra B. Rogers. Ed. by Christine Issel. 1994. (Illus.). 55p. stu. ed. (*0-9638862-1-5*) B J Scott.

Anatomy Charts for Reflexology: Teacher's Edition. Sandra B. Rogers. Ed. by Christine Issel. 1994. (Illus.). 56p. tchr. ed. (*0-9638862-2-3*) B J Scott.

Anatomy Coloring Book. I. Edward Alcamo. 1997. (Princeton Review Ser.). (Illus.). 291p. pap. 18.00 (*0-679-77849-7*) Random.

***Anatomy Coloring Book.** Wynn Kapit & Lawrence M. Elson. 2nd ed. 2001. LC 2001-17095. 400p. 19.99 (*0-8053-5086-1*) Addison-Wesley.

Anatomy for Anaesthetists. Harold Ellis & Stanley A. Feldman. 7th ed. 1996. LC 96-18956. (Illus.). 168.95 (*0-86542-721-6*) Blackwell Sci.

Anatomy for Attorneys. Thomas H. Quinn et al. 2000. LC 99-10719. 295.00 (*1-57626-030-5*) Quality Med Pub.

Anatomy for Dental Students. D. R. Johnson & W. J. Moore. 3rd ed. 1996. (Illus.). 296p. pap. text 69.50 (*0-19-262673-6*) OUP.

Anatomy for Surgeons Vol. 1: The Head & Neck, Volume I. W. Henry Hollinshead. 3rd ltd. ed. 1982. (Illus.). 551p. text 129.00 (*0-06-141264-3*, 14-12642, Lippncott) Lppncott W & W.

***Anatomy, Histology & Cell Biology: Self-Assessment & Review.** Robert M. Klein & James C. MacKenzie. 4th ed. 2001. (Pretest Self-Assessment & Review Ser.). (Illus.). 368p. pap. 24.95 (*0-07-137087-0*) McGraw-Hill Prof.

Anatomy in Diagnostic Imaging. James Fleckenstein. 1993. pap. text 53.00 (*0-7216-4000-1*) Saunders.

Anatomy in Diagnostic Imaging (Bases Anatomicas del Diagnostico por Imagen), Vol. 2. Peter Fleckenstein & Jorgen Tranum-Jensen. 2000. (ENG & SPA., Illus.). 340p. (*84-8086-162-2*) Mosby-Doyma Libros ESP. *Dist:* Mosby Inc.

Anatomy in Outline. George Furman. 2000. LC 00-33674. (Illus.). v, 361p. (C). 26.95 (*0-86542-592-2*) Blackwell Sci.

Anatomy in Surgery. P. Thorek. 3rd ed. 1985. (Illus.). 938p. 355.00 (*0-387-90978-8*) Spr-Verlag.

Anatomy Lesson: Art & Medicine. 1992. (Illus.). 157p. pap. (*0-903162-66-0*) Art Bks Intl GBR. *Dist:* Partners Pubs Grp.

Anatomy of a Food Addiction: The Brain Chemistry of Overeating. Anne Katherine. 3rd ed. 1996. LC 90-20433. (Illus.). 244p. reprint ed. 13.95 (*0-936077-13-1*, AFA) Gurze Bks.

Anatomy of a Job Search: A Nurse's Guide to Finding & Landing the Job You Want. Jeanna Bozell. 1999. LC 98-48422. 160p. pap. 24.95 (*0-87434-950-8*) Springhouse Corp.

Anatomy of a Merger: BJC Health System. Ed. by Wayne M. Lerner. 1997. LC 96-37336. pap. 44.00 (*1-56793-052-2*) Health Admin Pr.

Anatomy of a Splitting Borderline: Description & Analysis of a Case History. Rene J. Muller. 1994. LC 94-16995. 240p. 77.00 (*0-275-94975-3*, Praeger Pubs) Greenwood.

Anatomy of an Illness: As Perceived by the Patient. Norman Cousins. 20th anniv. ed. 1995. 176p. text 18.95 (*0-393-03887-4*) Norton.

Anatomy of an Illness as Perceived by the Patient. Norman Cousins. 1991. 176p. pap. 13.95 (*0-553-34365-3*) Bantam.

Anatomy of Anatomy: In Images & Words. Meryl Levin. 2000. LC 00-191693. (Illus.). 133p. pap. 20.00 (*0-9702744-0-8*) Third Rail Pr NY.

***Anatomy of Diagnostic Imaging.** Peter Fleckenstein. 2nd ed. 2001. (Illus.). 400p. 84.00 (*87-16-12336-0*) Blackwell Sci.

Anatomy of Disgust. William I. Miller. 1997. LC 96-35420. 320p. 24.95 (*0-674-03154-7*) HUP.

Anatomy of Epileptogenesis. Ed. by Brian S. Meldrum et al. 1988. (Current Problems in Epilepsy Ser.: Vol. 6). 187p. (*0-86196-155-2*) J Libbey Med GBR. *Dist:* Bks Intl VA.

Anatomy of General Surgical Operations. G. G. Jamieson. 1992. (Illus.). 236p. text (*0-443-04458-9*) Church.

Anatomy of Loneliness. Ed. by Joseph Hartog et al. 1980. LC 79-53591. 617p. 82.50 (*0-8236-0146-3*) Intl Univs Pr.

Anatomy of Madness Ed. by Roy Porter et al. 1988. 352p. text 65.00 (*0-415-00859-X*) Routledge.

Anatomy of Madness Ed. by Roy Porter et al. 1985. 528p. (*0-422-60350-3*, 9688) Tavistock GBR. *Dist:* Routldge.

Anatomy of Madness Vol. 2: Institutions & Society. Ed. by Roy Porter et al. 1985. 264p. (*0-422-79440-6*, 9618) Tavistock GBR. *Dist:* Routldge.

Anatomy of Manual Dexterity: The New Connectivity of the Primate Sensorimotor Thalamus & Cerebral Cortex. J. Darian-Smith et al. 1996. LC 96-17837. (Advances in Anatomy, Embryology & Cell Biology Ser.: Vol. 133). (Illus.). 142p. pap. 99.50 (*3-540-61111-8*) Spr-Verlag.

Anatomy of Melancholy, Vol. IV. Robert Burton. Ed. by J. B. Bamborough & Martin Dodsworth. 1998. (Oxford English Texts). 384p. text 110.00 (*0-19-812332-9*) OUP.

Anatomy of Mirages: A Psychiatrist Reflects on Life & the Mind. John Ellard. 1994. LC 95-168380. 290p. pap. (*0-86840-014-9*) New South Wales Univ Pr AUS. *Dist:* Intl Spec Bk.

Anatomy of Movement: Exercises. Blandine Calais-Germain & Andree Lamotte. Ed. by Stephen Anderson. Tr. by Nicole Commarmond from FRE. 1996. LC 94-61964. (Illus.). 282p. (C). pap. text 29.95 (*0-939616-22-X*) Eastland.

Anatomy of Orofacial Structures. Richard W. Brand & Donald E. Isselhard. 6th ed. (Illus.). 1998. stu. ed. (*0-8151-1219-X*); 1997. LC 99-204440. 576p. (C). (gr. 13). pap. text 42.00 (*0-8151-1000-6*, 29800) Mosby Inc.

Anatomy of Psychiatric Administration: The Organization in Health & Disease. M. Greenblatt. 1992. (Topics in Social Psychiatry Ser.). (Illus.). 400p. (C). 54.00 (*0-306-44143-8*, Plenum Trade) Perseus Pubng.

Anatomy of Psychotherapy. Lawrence Friedman. 1988. 616p. text 65.00 (*0-88163-053-5*) Analytic Pr.

Anatomy of Psychotherapy: Viewer's Guide to the APA Psychotherapy Videotape Series. Gary R. VandenBos et al. 1995. LC 95-212922. 194p. pap. 11.95 (*1-55798-335-6*, 431-0340) Am Psychol.

Anatomy of Suicide: Silence of the Heart. Louis Everstine. 1998. LC 97-25594. (Illus.). 170p. text 44.95 (*0-398-06802-X*); pap. text 29.95 (*0-398-06803-8*) C C Thomas.

Anatomy of the Dog. Budras & Fricke. 1994. text 115.00 (*0-7234-1920-5*) Mosby Inc.

Anatomy of the Domestic Birds. R. Nickel et al. 1977. 71.00 (*0-387-91134-0*) Spr-Verlag.

***Anatomy of the Domestic Mammals (Viscera Domesticanimals)** Nickel. 2nd ed. 1985. (C). 97.00 (*0-387-91139-1*) Spr-Verlag.

Anatomy of the Guinea Pig. Gale Cooper & Alan L. Schiller. 1975. LC 74-81866. (Commonwealth Fund Publications). (Illus.). 392p. 70.00 (*0-674-03159-8*) HUP.

Anatomy of the Horse. Budras & N. P. Rock. 1994. text 115.00 (*0-7234-1921-3*) Mosby Inc.

Anatomy of the Horse. Ed. by William E. Jones. 1973. (Horse Health & Care Ser.). (Illus.). pap. 9.95 (*0-912830-07-7*) Printed Horse.

Anatomy of the Horse. George Stubbs. Ed. by J. C. McCunn & C. W. Ottaway. 1976. LC 76-17945. (Illus.). 121p. pap. 14.95 (*0-486-23402-9*) Dover.

Anatomy of the Horse. George Stubbs. 1999. (Illus.). 140p. reprint ed. pap. text 28.00 (*0-7881-6580-1*) DIANE Pub.

Anatomy of the Human Orbit & Accessory Organs of Vision. Ernest S. Whitnall. 1979. LC 78-27070. 480p. 37.50 (*0-88275-840-3*) Krieger.

Anatomy of the Human Skeleton: A Question & Answer Tutorial Text. Eric E. Denman. 1991. (Illus.). 240p. (Orig.). pap. text (*0-443-04498-8*) Church.

Anatomy of the Next Century: New Technologies, Materials & Their Applications in Medicine. George Cristino. 1997. 200p. pap. text 640.00 (*1-886974-15-2*) Inst Knowledge.

Anatomy of the Paranasal Sinuses: A Correlative Approach. J. B. Anon et al. 1996. (Illus.). 214p. 149.00 (*0-86577-517-6*) Thieme Med Pubs.

Anatomy of the Spirit: The Seven Stages of Power & Healing. Caroline Myss. 1997. LC 96-220328. (Illus.). 352p. pap. 14.00 (*0-609-80014-0*) Random Hse Value.

Anatomy of the Temporal Bone with Surgical Implications. A. Julianna Gulya & Harold F. Schuknecht. 2nd ed. 1994. (Illus.). 350p. 98.95 (*1-85070-586-0*, Parthenon Pbng) CRC Pr.

Anatomy of Vertebrates Fishes & Reptiles. R. Owen. 1984. 650p. pap. (*0-7855-0340-4*) Intl Bks & Periodicals IND. *Dist:* St Mut.

Anatomy of Workers Compensation Medical Costs & Utilization: A Reference Book. Stacey M. Eccleston et al. 2000. 300p. pap. 95.00 (*0-935149-94-5*, WC-00-8) Workers Comp Res Inst.

Anatomy Physiology. Eva L. Weinreb. 1982. 896p. (C). pap. text, tchr. ed. 12.75 net. (*0-201-08854-1*) Addison-Wesley.

Anatomy, Physiology & Hygiene. Janet K. Raeburn & H. A. Raeburn. 4th ed. 1975. pap. text 7.95 (*0-7195-3213-2*) Transatl Arts.

Anatomy, Physiology & Microbiology. Jack Rudman. 1994. (College Level Examination Ser.: CLEP-38). pap. 27.95 (*0-8373-5338-6*) Nat Learn.

Anatomy, Radiology & Kinesiology of Hand-Unit. Hosein A. Motamed. 2nd ed. 2001. LC 81-90206. (Illus.). 344p. reprint ed. 250.00 (*0-910161-06-2*) Motamed Med Pub.

Anatomy Review. Larsen. 2000. pap. text (*0-7216-4648-4*) Saunders.

Anatomy 10B. Waggener. 3rd ed. 1998. 176p. (C). pap. text, lab manual ed. 31.20 (*0-536-01224-5*) Pearson Custom.

Anatomy to Color & Study. Ray Poritsky. 1989. (Illus.). 544p. (Orig.). stu. ed. 26.95 (*0-932883-18-4*) Hanley & Belfus.

***Anatomy Trains: The Role of the Fascia in Health & Dysfunction.** Thomas W. Myers. 2001. (Illus.). 221p. pap. (*0-443-06351-6*) Church GBR. *Dist:* Saunders.

Anatomy/Physiology Learning System Examaster. Edith J. Applegate. 2nd ed. Date not set. (*0-7216-8784-9*) Saunders.

Anca-Associated Vasculitides: Immunological & Clinical Aspects. W. L. Gross. 1993. (Advances in Experimental Medicine & Biology Ser.: Vol. 336). (Illus.). 572p. (C). text 155.00 (*0-306-44573-5*, Kluwer Plenum) Kluwer Academic.

Ancestor Syndrome: Transgenerational Psychotherapy & the Hidden Links in the Family Tree. Anne Utzenberger. 1998. LC 98-20148. (Illus.). 202p. (C). 68.95 (*0-415-19186-6*); pap. 22.95 (*0-415-19187-4*) Routledge.

Anchors Health Network Resource Book. American Health Network Staff. 1995. 100p. (Orig.). pap. 10.50 (*0-9634399-9-5*) Funmakers.

Ancienne Medicine. Hippocrates. Ed. by W. R. Connor. 1979. LC 78-18573. (Greek Texts & Commentaries Ser.). (Illus.). reprint ed. lib. bdg. 22.95 (*0-405-11417-6*) Ayer.

Ancient & Healing Art of Chinese Herbalism. Anna Selby. 1998. LC 98-84045. (Illus.). 96p. pap. 14.95 (*1-56975-139-0*) Ulysses Pr.

Ancient Cymric Medicine. Henry Wellcome. 1988. reprint ed. pap. 8.95 (*1-55818-109-1*, Sure Fire) Holmes Pub.

Ancient Egyptian Medicine. John F. Nunn. 1996. LC 95-39770. (Illus.). 240p. 39.95 (*0-8061-2831-3*) U of Okla Pr.

Ancient Egyptian Medicine: The Papyrus Ebers. Cyril Bryan. 1991. 208p. pap. 25.00 (*0-89005-004-X*) Ares.

Ancient Eugenics. Allen G. Roper. 1982. 98p. reprint ed. 16.00 (*0-941694-05-4*) Inst Study Man.

Ancient Medicine. Ludwig Edelstein. Ed. by Owsei Temkin. Ed. & Tr. by C. Lilian Temkin from GER. 1987. LC 67-12425. (Softshell Bks.). 480p. reprint ed. pap. text 24.95 (*0-8018-3491-0*) Johns Hopkins.

Ancient Medicine, Airs, Waters, Places, Epidemics 1 & 2. Oath, Precepts, Nutriment, Vol. 1. Tr. by W. H. Jones. 1923. (Ancient Medicine, Airs, Waters, Places, Epidemics 1 & 2. Oat Ser.: No. 147). 432p. 19.95 (*0-674-99162-1*) HUP.

Ancient Ophthamological Agents. Harald Nielsen. 1974. (Acta Historica Scientarium Ser.: No. 31). 117p. (Orig.). pap. (*87-7492-108-8*) Odense Univ.

Ancillary (Bedside) Blood Glucose Testing in Acute & Chronic Care Facilities. 1994. (Tentative Guideline Ser.: Vol. 9). 75.00 (*1-56238-126-1*, C30-A) NCCLS.

And a Time to Die. Mark Pelgrin. Ed. by Sheila Moon & Elizabeth Howes. 1976. LC 75-26836. 159p. reprint ed. pap. 5.25 (*0-8356-0305-9*, Quest) Theos Pub Hse.

And Now What Do We Do? A Guide for the Selection of the Right Care Facility for You or Your Loved One. Robin Schroeder & Loranelle Schroeder. 1997. 100p. pap. 19.95 (*0-9659200-0-3*) EMMPS.

And the Band Played On: Politics, People & the AIDS Epidemic. Randy Shilts. 1993. 672p. pap. 15.00 (*0-14-023221-4*, Penguin Bks) Viking Penguin.

And They Shall Walk. Elizabeth Kenny & Martha Ostenso. Ed. by Janet Rosenberg & William R. Phillips. 1980. LC 79-6907. (Physically Handicapped in Society Ser.). (Illus.). reprint ed. lib. bdg. 30.95 (*0-405-13117-8*) Ayer.

And Where Were You, Dr. Spock? Mary P. Riedley. 1990. pap. 9.95 (*0-925928-08-9*) Tiny Thought.

And Yet We Are Human & Kierkegaard: The Cripple Finn Carling & Theodor Haecker. Ed. by William R. Phillips & Janet Rosenberg. Tr. by C. V. Bruyn from NOR. 1980. LC 79-6897. (Physically Handicapped in Society Ser.). (Illus.). reprint ed. lib. bdg. 25.95 (*0-405-13108-9*) Ayer.

***And You Shall Live By Them: Contemporary Jewish Medical Ethics.** Louis Flancbaum. 2001. 424p. pap. 34.95 (*0-9648508-4-2*) Mirkov Pubns.

Anderson's Pathology. Ivan Damjanov & James Linder. 10th ed. 1995. (Illus.). 3014p. (C). (gr. 13). text 295.00 (*0-8016-7236-8*, 07236) Mosby Inc.

Andover Project: Staffed Housing for Adults with Severe or Profound Mental Handicaps. David Felce. 1989. (C). 39.00 (*0-906054-70-2*) St Mut.

Andrenergic Mechanisms in Myocardial Ischemia. G. Heusch & J. Ross. 1991. 250p. 70.00 (*0-387-91370-X*) Spr-Verlag.

Andreoli's Comprehensive Cardiac Care. Marguerite Kinney. 8th ed. 1995. LC 95-9243. (Illus.). 528p. (C). (gr. 13). pap. text 45.95 (*0-8016-7887-0*, 07887) Mosby Inc.

Andrew Boorde: Healing Through Mirth. Robert Van de Weyer. 1997. (Teachers of Healing & Wholeness Ser.). pap. (*0-85305-414-2*, 6303) Arthur James GBR. *Dist:* Morehouse Pub.

Andrew Taylor Still: 1828-1917. Carol Trowbridge. 1991. (Illus.). 233p. 30.00 (*0-943549-06-X*) Truman St Univ.

Andrews' Deskbook: Aids. Ed. by Mary Rhoads. 1998. 50p. pap. 85.00 (*1-890155-06-3*) Andrews Pubns.

Andrew's Diseases of the Skin. Timothy G. Berger et al. 9th ed. 2000. LC 99-58324. (Illus.). x, 1135p. text (*0-7216-5832-6*) Saunders.

Andrews' Diseases of the Skin: Clinical Dermatology. Harry L. Arnold, Jr. et al. 8th ed. 1990. (Illus.). 1058p. text 153.00 (*0-7216-2424-3*) Saunders.

Androgen Deficiency in the Aging Male: Causes, Diagnosis & Treatment. M. Carruthers. 2001. 300p. 79.95 (*1-84214-032-9*, Parthenon Pbng) CRC Pr.

Androgen Disorders in Women: The Most Neglected Hormone Problem. Theresa Cheung. 1999. LC 99-26580. (Illus.). 208p. 23.95 (*0-89793-260-9*); pap. 13.95 (*0-89793-259-5*) Hunter Hse.

Androgenetic Alopecia: Modern Concepts of Pathogenesis & Treatment. M. Inaba & Y. Inaba. 1996. (Illus.). 338p. 279.00 (*4-431-70158-3*) Spr-Verlag.

Androgens: Pathophysiological & Behavioural Aspects. Ed. by T. Lemarchand-Beraud & P. Fossati. 1983. (Journal: Vol. 18, No. 1-3). (Illus.). 152p. pap. 71.50 (*3-8055-3728-X*) S Karger.

Androgens 11 & Antiandrogens. R. K. Wagner et al. 1974. (Handbook of Experimental Pharmacology Ser.: Vol. 35, Pt. 2). (Illus.). x, 625p. 318.00 (*0-387-06883-X*) Spr-Verlag.

Androgens & Prostate Cancer. Labrie. 1992. 14.95 (*0-8493-5824-8*) CRC Pr.

Androgens & the Aging Male: The Proceedings of a Workshop Organized by the International Health Foundation, Geneva, Switzerland, December 1995. Ed. by B. J. Oddens & A. Vermeulen. 1996. LC 96-29358. (Illus.). 260p. lib. bdg. 75.95 (*1-85070-763-4*, Parthenon Pbng) CRC Pr.

Androgens in Childhood: Biological, Physiological, Clinical & Therapeutic Aspects. Ed. by M. G. Forest. 1989. (Pediatric & Adolescent Endocrinology Ser.: Vol. 19). (Illus.). viii, 282p. 195.00 (*3-8055-4850-8*) S Karger.

Andrology: Basic & Clinical Aspects of Male Reproduction & Infertility. Ed. by J. Bain et al. 1978. (Progress in Reproductive Biology & Medicine Ser.: Vol. 3). (Illus.). 85.25 (*3-8055-2807-8*) S Karger.

Andrology: Male Reproductive Health & Dysfunction. E. Nieschlag et al. 1997. LC 96-45653. (*0-387-61616-0*) Spr-Verlag.

Andrology: Male Reproductive Health & Dysfunction. Ed. by Eberhard Nieschlag & Hermann Behrens. 2nd ed. 2000. LC 00-59578. (Illus.). 500p. 99.00 (*3-540-67224-9*) Spr-Verlag.

Ane Breve Description of the Pest. John Skene. 1971. LC 72-38109. (English Experience Ser.: No. 415). reprint ed. 20.00 (*90-221-0415-X*) Walter J Johnson.

Anesthesia. Ed. by Ronald D. Miller & Roy F. Cucchiara. 1999. LC 99-19722. (*0-443-07996-X*) Church.

Anesthesia. Ronald D. Miller. Ed. by Allan Ross. 5th ed. 1999. LC 99-19722. (Illus.). 2525p. text (*0-443-07988-9*) Saunders.

Anesthesia: A Comprehensive Review. Brian A. Hall et al. 2nd ed. 1997. LC 96-45302. (Illus.). 432p. (C). (gr. 13). pap. text 54.95 (*0-8151-4192-0*, 25696) Mosby Inc.

Anesthesia: Biologic Foundations. Julien Biebuyck. 1997. LC 97-23913. 1,528p. text 259.00 (*0-397-58742-2*) Lppncott W & W.

Anesthesia & Analgesia for Companion & Laboratory Animals: A Bibliography—January 1988-January 1994. Ed. by Tim Allen. 1994. 81p. (Orig.). (C). pap. text 40.00 (*0-7881-1074-8*) DIANE Pub.

Anesthesia & Analgesia for Companion & Laboratory Animals: Bibliography January 1989-January 1995. Tim Allen. 1995. 98p. (Orig.). (C). pap. text 25.00 (*0-7881-1969-9*) DIANE Pub.

Anesthesia & Analgesia in Laboratory Animals. Ed. by Dennis F. Kohn et al. 1997. LC 96-47584. (American College of Laboratory Animal Medicine Ser.). (Illus.). 426p. text 99.00 (*0-12-417570-8*) Morgan Kaufmann.

Anesthesia & Co-Existing Disease. Robert K. Stoelting et al. 2nd ed. 1988. (Illus.). 936p. text (*0-443-08555-2*) Church.

Anesthesia & Co-Existing Disease. Robert K. Stoelting & Stephen F. Dierdorf. 3rd ed. 1993. (Illus.). 648p. text (*0-443-08813-6*) Church.

Anesthesia & Critical Care Manual. Sorin Brull & Anthony Cunningham. 3rd ed. 2003. pap. text 39.00 (*0-683-30607-3*) Lppncott W & W.

Anesthesia & Gas Monitoring Equipment Markets: Rapid Transition to Multi Parameter Integration & Open Systems. Market Intelligence Staff. 1992. 224p. 1895.00 (*1-56753-389-2*) Frost & Sullivan.

Anesthesia & Intensive Care for Organ Transplantation. Ed. by J. R. Klinck & M. J. Lindhop. 1997. (Illus.). 412p. (*0-412-56820-9*) E A GBR. *Dist:* OUP.

Anesthesia & Intensive Care for the Patients with Liver Disease. Gilbert R. Park et al. 1994. LC 94-11812. 340p. text 110.00 (*0-7506-9554-4*) Buttrwrth-Heinemann.

Anesthesia & Neurosurgery. James E. Cottrell. Ed. by David S. Smith. 3rd ed. 1994. (Illus.). 704p. (C). (gr. 13). text 134.00 (*0-8016-6573-6*, 06573) Mosby Inc.

Anesthesia & Neurosurgery, Vol. 4. Contrib. by Mosby Staff. 4th ed. 1999. (Illus.). 864p. text 139.00 (*0-8151-0321-2*, 30636) Mosby Inc.

Anesthesia & Organ Transplantation. Ed. by Simon Gelman. 1987. (Illus.). 254p. text 85.00 (*0-03-011504-3*) Saunders.

Anesthesia & Pain Management for the Pediatrician. Lynne R. Ferrari. 1999. LC 98-37282. 224p. 60.00 (*0-8018-6076-8*); (Illus.). pap. text 24.95 (*0-8018-6077-6*) Johns Hopkins.

Anesthesia & Perioperative Complications. Jonathan L. Benumof & Lawrence J. Saidman. 1991. (Illus.). 704p. (C). (gr. 13). text 120.00 (*0-8016-0586-5*, 00586) Mosby Inc.

Anesthesia & Perioperative Complications. Ed. by Jonathan L. Benumof & Lawrence J. Saidman. 2nd ed. 1999. LC 99-22920. (Illus.). 640p. text 129.00 (*0-8151-2619-0*, 31640) Mosby Inc.

Anesthesia & the Brain: Clinical, Functional, Metabolic, & Vascular Correlates. John D. Michenfelder. 1988. (Illus.). 215p. text (*0-443-08628-1*) Church.

Anesthesia & the Cardiovascular System. Ed. by Theodore H. Stanley & W. Clayton Petty. 1984. (Developments in Critical Care, Medicine, & Anesthesiology Ser.). text 129.50 (*0-89838-626-8*) Kluwer Academic.

Anesthesia & the Central Nervous System: Papers Presented at the 38th Annual Postgraduate Course in Anesthesiology, February 19-23, 1993. Ed. by Richard J. Sperry et al. 1993. LC 92-49081. (Developments in Critical Care, Medicine, & Anesthesiology Ser.: No. 28). 412p. text 174.50 (*0-7923-2083-2*) Kluwer Academic.

Anesthesia & the Lung: DCCA. Ed. by Theodore H. Stanley. 1988. (C). text 173.50 (*0-7923-0075-0*) Kluwer Academic.

Anesthesia & the Lung, 1992. Ed. by Theodore H. Stanley & Richard J. Sperry. 1992. (DCCA Ser.). 340p. (C). text 185.00 (*0-7923-1563-4*) Kluwer Academic.

Anesthesia & Transplantation. Adrian W. Gelb & Michael D. Sharpe. 1999. LC 98-32026. 526p. pap. text 130.00 (*0-7506-9664-8*) Buttrwrth-Heinemann.

Anesthesia & Uncommon Diseases. Jonathan L. Benumof. Ed. by Lesley Day. 4th ed. 1997. LC 97-28926. (Illus.). 672p. text 95.00 (*0-7216-8673-7*) Saunders.

Anesthesia Drug Manual. Paul F. White. Ed. by Thomas Eoyang. 1996. (Illus.). 395p. pap. text 38.00 (*0-7216-6221-8*) Saunders.

Anesthesia Drug Markets: Patent Expirations Have Players Scrambling to Develop Short Duration Drugs. Market Intelligence Staff. 1992. 233p. 1995.00 (*1-56753-419-8*) Frost & Sullivan.

Anesthesia Drugs Handbook. Contrib. by Sota Omoigui. 3rd ed. 1999. LC 99-24987. 628p. pap. 39.95 (*0-632-04421-7*) Blackwell Sci.

Anesthesia Equipment: Principles & Applications. Jan Ehrenwerth & James B. Eisenkraft. 1992. LC 92-48755. (Illus.). 736p. (C). (gr. 13). text 110.00 (*0-8016-1556-9*, 01556) Mosby Inc.

Anesthesia Equipment: Principles & Applications, No. 2. Jan Ehrenwerth & James Eisenkraft. 2nd ed. 2000. (Illus.). 784p. (C). (gr. 13). text 95.00 (*0-8151-2538-0*, 30303) Mosby Inc.

Anesthesia for Ambulatory Surgery. White. 1994. 39.00 (*0-316-93623-5*, Little Brwn Med Div) Lppncott W & W.

Anesthesia for Aortic Surgery. Joseph I. Simpson. 1997. LC 96-50468. 394p. text 110.00 (*0-7506-9578-1*) Buttrwrth-Heinemann.

Anesthesia for Cardiac Surgery. Dinardo. 2nd ed. 1997. LC 97-8137. 417p. (C). text 125.00 (*0-8385-0253-9*, A-0253-3) McGraw-Hill Prof.

Anesthesia for Extracranial Surgery of the Head & Neck. Ed. by Allan C. Brown. Date not set. (Illus.). 352p. text 59.00 (*0-07-008312-6*) McGraw-Hill Med Pub.

Anesthesia for Obstetrics. Sol M. Shnider & Gershon Levinson. 3rd ed. 1993. (Illus.). 768p. text 125.00 (*0-683-07751-1*) Lppncott W & W.

Anesthesia for Ophthalmic & Otolaryngologic Surgery. Ed. by Kathryn E. McGoldrick. 1991. (Illus.). 336p. text 69.00 (*0-7216-2837-0*) Saunders.

Anesthesia for Ophthalmic Surgery. R. K. Mirakhur. 2000. (Illus.). 240p. (C). pap. 78.95 (*0-412-61760-9*, Chap & Hall NY) Chapman & Hall.

Anesthesia for Renal Transplantation. Ed. by Gwendolyn B. Graybar & Lois L. Bready. 1986. 288p. (C). text 138.00 (*0-89838-837-6*) Kluwer Academic.

Anesthesia for the New Millennium: Modern Anesthetic Clinical Pharmacology. Theodore H. Stanley & Talmage D. Egan. 1999. LC 99-13443. (Developments in Critical Care, Medicine, & Anesthesiology Ser.). (*0-7923-5632-2*) Kluwer Academic.

Anesthesia for Thoracic Surgery. Jonathan L. Benumof. 2nd ed. 1994. LC 93-42770. (Illus.). text 115.00 (*0-7216-4467-8*) Saunders.

Anesthesia for Vascular Surgery. Michael F. Roizen. 1989. (Illus.). 518p. text (*0-443-08567-6*) Church.

Anesthesia Guide. Richard P. Dutton. 1994. LC 94-27187. 416p. pap. text 39.95 (*0-316-19958-3*, Little Brwn Med Div) Lppncott W & W.

Anesthesia Handbook. D. Rogers. 1993. 27.95 (*0-8016-7997-4*) Mosby Inc.

Anesthesia History Association Newsletters: 1982-1995. Ed. by Doric K. Cope et al. 1996. (Illus.). 664p. lib. bdg. (*0-88135-172-5*) Watson Pub Intl.

Anesthesia in Clinical Practice. J. S. Gravenstein. 1996. (C). text 145.00 (*0-443-04552-6*) Harcourt.

Anesthesia in Emergency Medicine. Glenn Vanstrum. 1989. 67.95 (*0-316-89730-2*, Little Brwn Med Div) Lppncott W & W.

Anesthesia Keywords, 1992. Gregory A. Smith. pap. text (*0-9635538-1-X*) MEDTEXT Med.

Anesthesia Review. Michelle Bowman-Howard. 1999. LC 99-24538. (Illus.). 400p. pap. text 49.95 (*0-683-30671-5*) Lppncott W & W.

Anesthesia Review: A Study to Anesthesia & Basics of Anesthesia. Lorraine Sdrales & Ronald D. Miller. 5th ed. 2001. LC 00-65746. x, 572p. (*0-443-07978-1*) Church.

Anesthesia Secrets. Ed. by James C. Duke. 2nd ed. 2000. LC 99-48700. (Secrets Ser.). 450p. pap. 39.95 (*1-56053-354-4*) Hanley & Belfus.

Anesthesie Locoregionale de la Naissance a L'age Adulte **see Local & Regional Anesthesia from Birth to Adulthood**

Anesthesiologische und Intensivmedizinische Aspekte in der Kinderheilkunde. Ed. by U. Nordmeyer et al. 1987. (Beitraege zur Intensiv und Notfallmedizin Ser.: Vol. 6). (Illus.). xi, 208p. 61.75 (*3-8055-4589-4*) S Karger.

Anesthesiologist. Jack Rudman. 1994. (Career Examination Ser.: C-1090). pap. 49.95 (*0-8373-1090-3*) Nat Learn.

Anesthesiologist's Manual of Surgical Procedures. Richard A. Jaffe & Stanley I. Samuels. 2nd ed. 1999. LC 98-34027. 1,200p. text 125.00 (*0-7817-1471-0*) Lppncott W & W.

Anesthesiology: A Comprehensive Study Guide. Ed. by Jeffrey Katz. 1997. LC 96-15289. 700p. pap. 59.00 (*0-07-033986-4*) McGraw-Hill Educ Grp.

Anesthesiology: Pretest Self Assessment & Review. Saundra Curry. 2nd ed. 1997. LC 97-25675. (Illus.). 264p. pap. 45.00 (*0-07-015102-4*) McGraw-Hill Prof.

Anesthesiology: Problem-Oriented Patient Management. Fun-Sun F. Yao & Joseph F. Artusio, Jr. 2nd ed. 1988. LC 65-9657. (Illus.). text 65.00 (*0-397-50800-X*, Lippnctt) Lppncott W & W.

Anesthesiology: Problem-Oriented Patient Management. Fun-Sun F. Yao. 4th ed. 1998. LC 97-45061. (Illus.). 1,088p. text 110.00 (*0-397-58759-7*) Lppncott W & W.

Anesthesiology: Today & Tomorrow. Ed. by Theodore H. Stanley & W. Clayton Petty. 1984. (Developments in Critical Care, Medicine, & Anesthesiology Ser.). text 73.50 (*0-89838-705-1*) Kluwer Academic.

Anesthesiology, 1986. Ed. by Theodore H. Stanley & W. Clayton Petty. 1986. (Developments in Critical Care, Medicine, & Anesthesiology Ser.). text 140.00 (*0-89838-779-5*) Kluwer Academic.

Anesthesiology & Pain Control in the Geriatric Patient. Ed. by R. Brian Smith et al. 1995. LC 94-27066. (Illus.). 608p. text 69.00 (*0-07-058642-X*) McGraw-Hill Educ Grp.

Anesthesiology & Pain Management. Ed. by Theodore H. Stanley. 1991. (Developments in Critical Care, Medicine, & Anesthesiology Ser.). 396p. text 221.50 (*0-7923-1073-X*) Kluwer Academic.

Anesthesiology & Pain Management. Ed. by Theodore H. Stanley & M. A. Ashburn. 1994. LC 93-44398. (Developments in Critical Care, Medicine, & Anesthesiology Ser.: No. 29). text 166.50 (*0-7923-2662-8*) Kluwer Academic.

Anesthesiology & the Cardiovascular Patient. Ed. by Theodore H. Stanley & P. L. Bailey. 1996. (Developments in Critical Care, Medicine, & Anesthesiology Ser.: Vol. 31). 293p. text 118.00 (*0-7923-3895-2*) Kluwer Academic.

Anesthesiology & the Heart. Ed. by Theodore H. Stanley & Richard J. Sperry. 1990. (DCCA Ser.). (C). text 204.50 (*0-7923-0634-1*) Kluwer Academic.

Anesthesiology Boards: A Survival Guide. Michelle Starr. 1999. LC 99-33417. (C). text 55.00 (*0-443-07619-7*) Saunders.

Anesthesiology Pearls of Wisdom. DeMello. 1999. (Pearls of Wisdom Ser.). pap. 88.00 (*1-890369-08-X*) Boston Medical.

Anesthesiology Review. Ronald J. Faust. 2nd ed. 1994. pap. (*0-443-08983-3*); pap. text (*0-443-08986-8*) Church.

***Anesthesiology Review.** Ed. by Ronald J. Faust & Roy F. Cucchiara. 3rd ed. 2001. LC 2001-17365. (Illus.). xx, 595p. (*0-443-06601-9*) Church.

Anesthetic & Obstetric Management of High-Risk Pregnancy. Datta. 2nd ed. 1996. (Illus.). 656p. (C). (gr. 13). text 99.00 (*0-8151-2280-2*, 27531) Mosby Inc.

Anesthetic Complications. Kenneth Sugioka. 1992. LC 91-65079. (Illus.). x, 227p. 45.00 (*0-87875-415-6*); pap. 20.00 (*0-87875-414-8*) Whitston Pub.

Anesthetic Considerations in Plastic & Aesthetic Surgery. Gevirtz. 1993. 75.00 (*0-8385-0142-7*) Appleton & Lange.

Anesthetic Management of Acute Head Injury. Ed. by Arthur M. Lam. 1994. LC 93-49496. (Illus.). 304p. text 59.00 (*0-07-036127-4*) McGraw-Hill Med Pub.

Anesthetic Management of Carotid Endarterectomy. Leonard C. Jenkins & David H. Wong. 1988. 196p. (*0-683-13048-X*) E A GBR. *Dist:* Williams & Wilkins.

Anesthetic Management of Difficult & Routine Pediatric Patients. Frederic A. Berry. 2nd ed. 1990. (Illus.). 457p. text (*0-443-08678-8*) Church.

Anesthetic Pharmacology & Physiology. William McCaughey. 1997. LC 97-9202. text (*0-443-05203-4*) Church.

Aneuploidy: Etiology & Mechanisms. Ed. by Vicki L. Dellarco et al. 1985. LC 85-25696. (Basic Life Sciences Ser.: Vol. 36). 576p. 110.00 (*0-306-42118-6*, Plenum Trade) Perseus Pubng.

Aneurysm Surgery. Irwin Fairs et al. 1995. (Practice of Surgery Ser.). text (*0-443-04641-7*) Church.

Aneurysms: New Findings & Treatment. James S. Yao & William H. Pearce. 1994. (Illus.). 532p. (C). pap. text 169.00 (*0-8385-0172-9*, A0172-5, Apple Lange Med) McGraw.

Angel Dust: New Facts about PCP. Christina Dye. rev. ed. 2000. pap. 0.50 (*0-89230-165-1*) Do It Now.

Angel of Ashland: Practicing Compassion & Tempting Fate, a Biography of Robert Spencer, M. D. Vincent J. Genovese. 2000. LC 00-55263. (Illus.). 150p. 23.00 (*1-57392-831-3*) Prometheus Bks.

Angel of Bethesda. Cotton Mather. Ed. by Gordon W. Jones. 1972. LC 72-185323. 384p. 30.00 (*0-8271-7220-6*) Oak Knoll.

Angelhead: My Brother's Descent into Madness. Greg Bottoms. 2000. LC 00-21353. 206p. 20.00 (*0-609-60626-3*) Crown Pub Group.

***Angelhead: My Brother's Descent into Madness.** Greg Bottoms. 2001. 208p. pap. 12.00 (*0-609-80714-5*, Three Riv Pr) Harmony Bks.

Angelical Conjunction: The Preacher-Physicians of Colonial New England. Patricia A. Watson. 1991. LC 90-22214. 200p. (C). text 29.95 (*0-87049-696-4*) U of Tenn Pr.

Angels & Citizens: British Women As Military Nurses, 1854-1914. Anne R. Summers. 1988. (Illus.). 320p. text 35.00 (*0-7102-1479-0*, Routledge Thoemms) Routledge.

Angels & Ministers of Grace: An Ethno-Psychiatrist's Contribution to Biblical Criticism. M. J. Field. 1971. LC 77-876245. xv, 135 p. (*0-582-12662-2*) Longman.

Angels Dark & Light. Gary Kinnaman. 1994. LC 94-25610. 220p. pap. 10.99 (*0-89283-846-9*, Vine Bks) Servant.

Angels in Africa: A Memoir of Colonial Nursing. Bridget M. Robertson. 1993. 200p. text (*1-85043-527-8*) I B T GBR. *Dist:* St Martin.

Anger. Leo Madow. 1974. LC 75-162773. 132p. pap. 6.95 (*0-684-13688-0*, Macmillan Ref) Gale.

Anger: Deal with It, Heal with It, Stop It from Killing You. Bill DeFoore. 1991. 180p. (Orig.). pap. 8.95 (*1-55874-162-3*) Health Comm.

Anger: The Misunderstood Emotion. Carol Tavris. rev. ed. 1989. 384p. pap. 14.00 (*0-671-67523-0*, Touchstone) S&S Trade Pap.

Anger, Alcoholism & Addiction: Treating Anger in a Chemical Dependency Setting. Ronald T. Potter-Efron & Patricia S. Potter-Efron. 1992. LC 91-39083. 304p. 332.95 (*0-393-70126-3*) Norton.

Anger & Addiction: Breaking the Relapse Cycle - A Teaching Guide for Professionals. Jo Clancy. 1996. LC 96-7939. 200p. 29.50 (*1-887841-02-4*, BN 60155, Psychosocial) Intl Univs Pr.

Anger & Aggression. Ed. by Robert S. Wyer, Jr. & Thomas K. Srull. 1993. (Advances in Social Cognition Ser.). 216p. pap. 21.50 (*0-8058-1327-6*); text 45.00 (*0-8058-1326-8*) L Erlbaum Assocs.

Anger & Aggression: An Essay on Emotion. James R. Averill. 1982. (Social Psychology Ser.). (Illus.). 402p. 66.00 (*0-387-90719-X*) Spr-Verlag.

***Anger & Rage - Analysis & Conclusions of Life in Modern Times: Index of New Information for Consumers, Reference & Research.** Tr. by American Health Research Institute Staff. 2002. 180p. 57.50 (*0-7883-2342-3*) ABBE Pubs Assn.

Anger Disorders: Definition, Diagnosis & Treatment. Ed. by Howard Kassinove. 1995. 160p. 73.95 (*1-56032-352-3*); pap. 31.95 (*1-56032-353-1*) Taylor & Francis.

Anger, Hostility, & the Heart. Ed. by Aron W. Siegman & Timothy W. Smith. 1994. 296p. 69.95 (*0-8058-1194-X*) L Erlbaum Assocs.

Anger in Young Children, Vol. 9. Florence L. Goodenough. 1975. LC 77-141547. (University of Minnesota Institute of Child Welfare Monographs: No. 9). (Illus.). 278p. reprint ed. lib. bdg. 58.00 (*0-8371-5894-X*, CWGA, Greenwood Pr) Greenwood.

Anger Is a Choice. Tim F. LaHaye & Bob Phillips. 1982. 160p. (Orig.). pap. 9.99 (*0-310-27071-5*, 18335P) Zondervan.

Anger Kills: Seventeen Strategies for Controlling the Hostility That Can Harm Your Health. Redford Williams & Virginia Williams. 1994. LC 94-2624. (Illus.). 256p. reprint ed. pap. 13.00 (*0-06-097623-3*, Perennial) HarperTrade.

Anger, Madness, & the Daimonic: The Psychological Genesis of Violence, Evil, & Creativity. Stephen A. Diamond. 1999. LC 96-27865. (SUNY Series in the Philosophy of Psychology). 402p. (C). pap. text 20.95 (*0-7914-3076-6*) State U NY Pr.

Anger Management for Youth: Stemming Aggression & Violence. Leona L. Eggert. 1994. 156p. pap. 24.95 (*1-879639-29-7*) Natl Educ Serv.

Anger Therapy. Lisa Engelhardt et al. 1995. LC 95-79169. (Elf-Help Bks.). 88p. pap. 4.95 (*0-87029-292-7*) Abbey.

Angina. Bruce B. Brintnall & Ruth A. Brintnall. Ed. by Oliver D. Grin & Dorothy L. Bouwman. 1992. (Patient Education Ser.). (Illus.). 22p. (Orig.). pap. text 4.00 (*0-929689-19-4*) Ludann Co.

Angina Pectoris: Learn about Coronary Heart Disease & How to Prevent It. Julia A. Purcell et al. rev. ed. 1994. LC 84-26382. (Illus.). 32p. pap. text 5.50 (*0-939838-17-6*) Pritchett & Hull.

Angina Pectoris: Management Strategies & Guide to Interventions. Thomas Graboys & Charles Blatt. 2nd rev. ed. 1997. (Illus.). 240p. per. 21.95 (*1-884735-11-8*) Prof Comms.

Angina Pectoris: Management Strategies & Guide to Interventions see Angine de Poitrine: Demarch et Guide Therapeutiques

Angina Pectoris with Normal Coronary Arteries: Syndrome X. Ed. by Juan C. Kaski. 1994. LC 93-43083. (Developments in Cardiovascular Medicine Ser.: Vol. 152). 304p. (C). text 187.50 (*0-7923-2651-2*) Kluwer Academic.

Angine de Poitrine: Demarch et Guide Therapeutiques. Thomas B. Graboys & Charles M. Blatt. 2nd rev. ed. 1997.Tr. of Angina Pectoris: Management Strategies & Guide to Interventions. (FRE.). 263p. per. 19.95 (*1-884735-20-7*) Prof Comms.

Angiogenesis. Ed. by F. Hammersen. 1984. (Mikrozirkulation in Forschung und Klinik Ser.: Vol. 4). (Illus.). vi, 90p. pap. 52.25 (*3-8055-3883-9*) S Karger.

Angiogenesis: From the Molecular to Integrative Pharmacology. Michael E. Maragoudakis. 2000. LC 00-22405. (Advances in Experimental Medicine & Biology Ser.: Vol. 476). (Illus.). x, 382p. 95.00 (*0-306-46375-X*, Kluwer Plenum) Kluwer Academic.

Angiogenesis: Key Principles: Science - Technology - Medicine. Ed. by R. Steiner et al. 1992. (Experientia Supplementum Ser.: Vol. 61). 528p. 219.00 (*0-8176-2674-3*) Birkhauser.

Angiogenesis: Models, Modulators & Clinical Applications. Ed. by Michael E. Maragoudakis. 1998. LC 98-17558. (NATO Advanced Science Institutes Ser.: No. 298). (Illus.). 584p. (C). text 159.50 (*0-306-45833-0*, Kluwer Plenum) Kluwer Academic.

Angiogenesis: Molecular Biology & Clinical Aspects. Ed. by M. E. Maragoudakis et al. 1994. (NATO Advanced Science Institutes Ser.: Vol. 263). (Illus.). 382p. (C). text 115.00 (*0-306-44713-4*, Kluwer Plenum) Kluwer Academic.

Angiogenesis & Cardiovascular Disease. J. Anthony Ware. 1999. LC 98-22176. (Illus.). 376p. text 67.50 (*0-19-511235-0*) OUP.

Angiogenesis in Health & Disease. M. E. Maragoudakis et al. 1992. (NATO ASI Series A, Life Sciences: Vol. 227). (Illus.). 416p. (C). text 125.00 (*0-306-44196-9*) Plenum.

Angiogenesis in Health & Disease: Basic Mechanisms & Clinical Applications. Contrib. by Gabor M. Rubanyi et al. 1999. LC 99-47750. (Illus.). 576p. text 195.00 (*0-8247-8102-3*) Dekker.

Angiogenesis Inhibitors & Stimulators: Potential Therapeutic Implications. Shaker A. Mousa. 1999. (Medical Intelligence Unit Ser.). 194p. 89.00 (*1-57059-613-1*) Landes Bioscience.

Angiogenesis Protocols. J. Clifford Murray. 2001. (Methods in Molecular Medicine Ser.: Vol. 46). (Illus.). 276p. 99.50 (*0-89603-698-7*) Humana.

Angiographic Practice in a General Hospital. Kaz Kikkawa. 1979. LC 78-50158. (Illus.). 320p. 32.50 (*0-87527-146-4*) Green.

Angiography: Principles & Procedures. Joseph E. Whitley & Nancy O. Whitley. Ed. by Lewis Etter. 1971. LC 76-111804. (Modern Concepts of Radiology Ser.). (Illus.). 132p. 22.50 (*0-87527-089-1*) Green.

Angiology in Practice. Ed. by Abdul-Majeed Salmasi. 1996. LC 96-30909. (Developments in Cardiovascular Medicine Ser.). 544p. (C). text 313.00 (*0-7923-4143-0*) Kluwer Academic.

Angiotensin & the Heart. Ed. by H. Grobecker et al. 1993. (Illus.). viii, 224p. 47.00 (*0-387-91432-3*) Spr-Verlag.

Angiotensin II Receptors: Medicinal Chemistry, Vol. II. Ed. by Robert R. Ruffolo, Jr. 1994. 240p. 149.00 (*0-8493-8545-8*) CRC Pr.

Angiotensin-Konversionsenzyme-Hemmer Bei Hypertonie, Teil 2 (Angiotensin Converting Inhibitors in Treatment of Hypertension, Pt. 2) Schwerpunkt auf Cilazapril (Emphasis on Cilazapril) Ed. by J. Rosenthal & K. O. Stumpe. 1993. (Journal: Vol. 82, Suppl. 2, 1993). (Illus.). iv, 84p. pap. 35.00 (*3-8055-5772-8*) S Karger.

Angiotensin II Receptor Blockade: Physiological & Clinical Implications. Naranjan S. Dhalla. 1998. LC 98-15948. (Progress in Experimental Cardiology Ser.). (*0-7923-8147-5*) Kluwer Academic.

Anglais Medical: Medical English. Mireille Mandelbrojt-Sweeney. 1992. (ENG & FRE.). 168p. 49.95 (*0-8288-6918-9*, 2225827028) Fr & Eur.

Anglais Medical: Spoken & Written Medical English. C. Coude et al. 1983. (ENG & FRE.). 272p. pap. 79.95 (*0-8288-0561-X*, M14533) Fr & Eur.

Angle-Closure Glaucoma. Stanley Hyams. 1990. LC 90-4179. (Illus.). 186p. lib. bdg. (*90-6299-059-2*) Kugler NLD. *Dist:* Lib Res.

Anglo-Norman Medicine Vol. 1: Roger Frugard's Chirurgia & the Practica Brevis of Platearius. Ed. by Tony Hunt. 1994. 336p. (C). 99.00 (*0-85991-401-1*) Boydell & Brewer.

Anglo-Norman Medicine Vol. II: Shorter Treatises. Ed. by Tony Hunt. 1997. 296p. 90.00 (*0-85991-523-9*) Boydell & Brewer.

Anglo-Saxon Leechcraft. Henry S. Wellcome. abr. ed. 1992. (Illus.). 100p. (C). reprint ed. pap. 6.95 (*1-877934-04-6*) Rose & Nefr Pr.

Anglo-Saxon Medicine. M. L. Cameron. 1993. LC 92-29974. (Studies in Anglo-Saxon England: No. 7). 223p. (C). text 59.95 (*0-521-40521-1*) Cambridge U Pr.

Angry Gut: Coping with Colitis & Crohn's Disease. W. G. Thompson. 1993. LC 92-48259. (Illus.). 364p. (C). 26.95 (*0-306-44470-4*) Da Capo.

Angry Heart: Overcoming Borderline & Addictive Disorders. Joseph Santoro & Ronald J. Cohen. 1997. LC 97-66074. 272p. pap. 14.95 (*1-57224-080-6*) New Harbinger.

Angry Self: A Comprehensive Approach to Anger Management. Miriam M. Gottlieb. 1999. LC 98-27880. (Illus.). 143p. pap. 22.95 (*1-891944-07-X*) Zeig Tucker Theisen.

Angstlichkeit, Selbstregulation und Problemlosen Im Vorschulalter. Katja Mackowiak. 1998. (Psychologie Ser.: Bd. 609). (Illus.). 313p. 51.95 (*3-631-32802-8*) P Lang Pubng.

Anima: An Anatomy of a Personified Notion. James Hillman. 1985. LC 85-18320. (Illus.). 344p. pap. 14.50 (*0-88214-316-6*) Spring Pubns.

Animal Anatomy: An Illustrated Reference to Drawing Animals. Gottfried Bammes. 1994. 144p. 14.98 (*0-7858-0055-7*) Bk Sales Inc.

Animal Anatomy & Physiology. Jesse F. Bone. 2nd ed. 1981. (C). text 38.00 (*0-8359-0216-1*) P-H.

Animal Anatomy on File: An Internal & External Guide. Diagram Group Staff. (Illus.). 1990. 288p. ring bd. 165.00 (*0-8160-2244-5*); 1999. LC 98-55740. 316p. ring bd. 165.00 (*0-8160-3875-9*, Checkmark) Facts on File.

Animal Applications of Research in Mammalian Development. Ed. by Roger A. Pedersen et al. 1991. (Current Communications in Cell & Molecular Biology Ser.: No. 4). (Illus.). 334p. (C). pap. text 44.00 (*0-87969-333-9*) Cold Spring Harbor.

Animal Behavior. David J. McFarland. 1985. 576p. text 43.25 (*0-8053-6790-X*) Benjamin-Cummings.

Animal Behavior. John P. Scott. 2nd rev. ed. 1995. LC 76-188823. 328p. pap. text 9.95 (*0-226-74337-3*, P480) U Ch Pr.

Animal Biology & Care. Sue Dallas. 2000. LC 99-38885. (Illus.). 256p. pap. text (*0-632-05054-3*) Blckwell Science GBR. *Dist:* Iowa U Pr.

Animal Biotechnology: Comprehensive Biotechnology. Ed. by L. A. Babiuk et al. 1989. (Comprehensive Biotechnology Supplement Ser.: No. 1). (Illus.). 250p. 116.00 (*0-08-034730-4*, Pergamon Pr) Elsevier.

Animal Body Fluids & Their Regulation. Antony P. Lockwood. 1963. LC 64-9913. (Illus.). 184p. 25.50 (*0-674-03700-6*) HUP.

Animal Breeding & Infertility. Ed. by Michael J. Meredith. 1996. (Illus.). 508p. 125.00 (*0-632-04038-6*) Blackwell Sci.

Animal Brucellosis. Ed. by Klaus Nielsen & J. Robert Duncan. 1990. 464p. lib. bdg. 259.00 (*0-8493-5878-7*, SF809) CRC Pr.

Animal Cell Technology from Vaccines to Genetic Medicine. Ed. by Manuel J. Carrondo. 1996. LC 96-48832. 816p. text 441.50 (*0-7923-4321-2*) Kluwer Academic.

Animal Cells As Bioreactors. Terence Cartwright. 1994. LC 93-33980. (Studies in Biotechnology: No. 11). (Illus.). 192p. (C). text 59.95 (*0-521-41258-7*) Cambridge U Pr.

Animal Clinic for Cats. Jim Humphries. 1998. LC 97-29143. 256p. 8.99 (*0-517-18905-4*) Random Hse Value.

Animal Clinic for Dogs. Jim Humphries. 1998. LC 97-29101. 304p. 8.99 (*0-517-18906-2*) Random Hse Value.

Animal Clinical Biochemistry: The Future. Ed. by D. J. Blackmore et al. 1988. 398p. (C). text 95.00 (*0-521-35518-4*) Cambridge U Pr.

Animal Clinical Chemistry. Ed. by G. O. Evans. 1996. 224p. 99.95 (*0-7484-0350-7*); 192p. pap. 44.95 (*0-7484-0351-5*) Taylor & Francis.

Animal Cognition. Ed. by Herbert L. Roitblat et al. 1984. (Comparative Cognition & Neuroscience Ser.). 696p. pap. text 99.95 (*0-89859-334-4*) L Erlbaum Assocs.

Animal Cognition: A Tribute to Donald A. Riley. Ed. by Thomas R. Zentall. 1993. (Comparative Cognition & Neuroscience Ser.). 376p. text 79.95 (*0-8058-1183-4*) L Erlbaum Assocs.

Animal Cognition: A Tribute to Donald A. Riley. Inc. Ed. by Thomas R. Zentall & William S. Maki. 1993. (Comparative Cognition & Neuroscience Ser.). 376p. pap. 39.95 (*0-8058-1184-2*) L Erlbaum Assocs.

Animal Connection: Link Between Cancer & Other Diseases from Animals & Foods of Animal Origin. Agatha M. Thrash & Calvin L. Thrash, Jr. 1983. 126p. (Orig.). pap. 4.95 (*0-942658-04-3*) NLB.

Animal Diversity: A Textbook of Invertebrate Zoology. Eylers. 1991. 38.95 (*0-8016-2558-0*) Mosby Inc.

Animal Doctor's Answer Book see New Animal Doctor's Answer Book

Animal Doctor's Answer Book. Michael W. Fox. 1991. LC 84-6973. (Illus.). 320p. (Orig.). 14.95 (*0-937858-37-4*) Newmarket.

Animal Drugs & Human Health. Ed. by Lester M. Crawford & Donald A. Franco. 1994. LC 93-61759. 234p. 84.95 (*1-56676-102-6*) CRC Pr.

Animal Ecology: Special Reference to Insects. Royal N. Chapman. Ed. by Frank N. Egerton, 3rd. 1978. LC 77-74208. (History of Ecology Ser.). reprint ed. lib. bdg. 40.95 (*0-405-10379-4*) Ayer.

Animal ER: Extraordinary Stories of Hope & Healing from One of the World's Leading Veterinary Hospitals. Tufts University School of Veterinary Medicine Staff & Vicki Croke. l.t. ed. 2000. LC 00-26287. (G. K. Hall Nonfiction Ser.). (Illus.). 258p. 27.95 (*0-7838-9020-6*, Macmillan Ref) Gale.

Animal ER: Extraordinary Stories of Hope & Healing from One of the World's Leading Veterinary Hospitals. Tufts University School of Veterinary Medicine Staff & Vicki Croke. 2000. LC 99-32017. 208p. reprint ed. pap. 12.00 (*0-452-28101-6*, Plume) Dutton Plume.

Animal Euthanasia: Bibliography, January 1990-November 1997. Ed. by Michael A. Kreger. 1999. 46p. (C). pap. text 15.00 (*0-7881-7570-X*) DIANE Pub.

Animal Experimentation: A Guide to the Issues. Vaughan Monamy. 2000. LC 00-27642. 122p. (C). text, stu. ed. 42.95 (*0-521-66093-9*); pap. text 15.95 (*0-521-66786-0*) Cambridge U Pr.

Animal Experimentation: A Harvest of Shame. Moneim A. Fadali. 288p. pap. 14.95 (*1-885113-55-2*) Hidden Springs.

Animal Experimentation: Cruelty or Science? Nancy Day. 1994. LC 93-46996. (Issues in Focus Ser.). (Illus.). 128p. (YA). (gr. 6-12). lib. bdg. 20.95 (*0-89490-578-3*) Enslow Pubs.

Animal Experimentation & Human Health. Al Frazza. 1994. 52p. pap. 2.95 (*1-886605-00-9*) People for Reason.

Animal Experimentation & the Future of Medical Research. Ed. by J. Botting. 1993. (Portland Press Proceedings Ser.: Vol. 3). (Illus.). 107p. (Orig.). (C). (*1-85578-038-0*) Portland Pr Ltd GBR. *Dist:* Ashgate Pub Co.

Animal Genetics & Evolution: Selected Papers. Ed. by J. M. Van Brink & N. N. Vorontsov. 1980. (Illus.). 393p. text 278.00 (*90-6193-602-0*) Kluwer Academic.

Animal Health. David Sainsbury. 2nd rev. ed. 1998. LC 97-34605. (Illus.). 256p. (C). pap. text (*0-632-03888-8*) Blckwell Science GBR. *Dist:* Iowa U Pr.

Animal Health. Nancy S. Jackson et al. 3rd ed. 2000. LC 99-75340. (Illus.). x, 396p. 62.50 (*0-8134-3169-7*) Interstate.

Animal Health, 1995. HMSO Staff. 1996. 113p. pap. (*0-11-243012-0*, HM430082) Statnry Office GBR. *Dist:* Bernan Associates.

Animal Health, 1996. TSO Staff. 1997. 113p. pap. (*0-11-243030-9*, HM30309) Statnry Office GBR. *Dist:* Bernan Associates.

Animal Health Aide. Jack Rudman. 1994. (Career Examination Ser.: C-75). pap. 29.95 (*0-8373-0075-4*) Nat Learn.

Animal Health Care Products. June Santon & Anna Crull. 1997. LC 98-143141. (Report Ser.: No. C-108R). 123p. 3150.00 (*1-56965-385-2*) BCC.

Animal Health Care Training - Nepal's Animal Health Improvement Training Programme. John Young et al. 1994. 64p. pap. (*1-85339-245-6*) Intermed Tech GBR. *Dist:* Stylus Pub VA.

Animal Health Technician Licensing Examination. Jack Rudman. 1994. (Career Examination Ser.: C-3039). pap. 39.95 (*0-8373-3039-4*) Nat Learn.

Animal Health Technology. Ed. by E. J. Catcott. 2nd ed. 1991. LC 77-85491. (Illus.). 480p. text 44.95 (*0-939674-10-6*) Am Vet Pubns.

Animal Health Yearbook, 1990. 1991. (Animal Production & Health Papers: No. 30). 298p. (*92-5-003063-0*, F0630) FAO ITA. *Dist:* Bernan Associates.

Animal Health Yearbook, 1992. 1993. 328p. pap. (*92-5-003345-1*, F33451) FAO ITA. *Dist:* Bernan Associates.

Animal Health Yearbook, 1993. 1994. (Animal Production & Health Ser.: No. 33). 249p. (*92-5-003527-6*, F35276) FAO ITA. *Dist:* Bernan Associates.

Animal Health Yearbook, 1994. F. A. O. Staff. 1995. 248p. pap. text (*92-5-003693-0*, F36930) FAO ITA. *Dist:* Bernan Associates.

Animal Hospital. Stephen Sawicki. (Illus.). 1997. 252p. pap. 14.95 (*1-55652-281-9*); 1996. LC 96-5732. 240p. 22.00 (*1-55652-274-6*) Chicago Review.

Animal Husbandry: Animal Diseases, How Animals Reproduce. rev. ed. 1976. (Economic & Social Development Papers: No. 9). (Illus.). 33p. pap. (*92-5-100148-0*, F67) FAO ITA. *Dist:* Bernan Associates.

Animal Husbandry: Directory of Authors of New Medical & Scientific Reviews with Subject Index. Science and Life Consultants Association Staff. rev. ed. 1996. LC 96-3121. 135p. pap. 47.50 (*0-7883-1031-3*) ABBE Pubs Assn.

Animal Learning: An Introduction. Stephen Walker. 1987. (Introduction to Modern Psychology Ser.). (Illus.). 288p. (C). lib. bdg. 57.50 (*0-7102-0482-5*, Routledge Thoemms) Routledge.

Animal Learning: Survey & Analysis. Ed. by M. E. Bitterman et al. 1979. LC 78-9894. (NATO ASI Series A, Life Sciences: Vol. 19). 522p. 115.00 (*0-306-40061-8*, Plenum Trade) Perseus Pubng.

Animal Life As Affected by the Natural Conditions of Existence. Karl Semper. Ed. by Frank N. Egerton, 3rd. 1978. LC 77-74251. (History of Ecology Ser.). (Illus.). reprint ed. lib. bdg. 41.95 (*0-405-10420-0*) Ayer.

Animal Life Cycle Feeding & Nutrition. Tilden W. Perry. 1984. (Animal Feeding & Nutrition Ser.). text 79.00 (*0-12-552060-3*) Acad Pr.

Animal Locomotion: The Muybridge Work at the University of Pennsylvania. University of Pennsylvania Staff. 1978. LC 72-9239. (Literature of Photography Ser.). reprint ed. 18.95 (*0-405-04944-7*) Ayer.

Animal Magnetism: Mesmerism & Its Phenomena. William Gregory. 5th ed. 1975. LC 75-7384. (Perspectives in Psychical Research Ser.). reprint ed. 23.95 (*0-405-07032-2*) Ayer.

Animal Magnetism—Unmasked. Max Kappeler. Tr. by Kathleen Lee from GER. 1975. LC 76-362585.Tr. of Tierischer Magnetismus—Entlarvt. 169p. pap. 14.00 (*0-85241-097-2*) Kappeler Inst Pub.

Animal Management in Disasters: Handbook for Emergency Responders & Animal Owner. Sebastian E. Heath. 1998. LC 99-197350. (Illus.). 352p. (C). 41.95 (*1-55664-419-1*) Mosby Inc.

Animal Migration & Navigation. Philip Street. 1976. LC 75-30276. (Illus.). 9.95 (*0-684-14516-2*, Macmillan Ref) Gale.

Animal Mind, Human Voices: Provings of Eight New Animal Remedies. Nancy Herrick. unabr. ed. 1998. (Illus.). 420p. pap. text 39.95 (*0-9635368-1-8*) Hahnemann Clinic.

Animal Minds. Donald R. Griffin. 1994. LC 92-6538. x, 320p. (C). pap. 14.95 (*0-226-30864-2*) U Ch Pr.

Animal Modelling in Surgical Research. Ed. by Bengt Jeppsson. 1997. 464p. text 230.00 (*90-5702-213-3*, Harwood Acad Pubs) Gordon & Breach.

Animal Models for Cystic Fibrosis: The Reserpine-Treated Rat. Ed. by J. R. Martinez & B. J. Barbero. 1985. (Illus.). 20.00 (*0-911302-54-9*) San Francisco Pr.

Animal Models for Intestinal Disease. Ed. by Carl J. Pfeiffer. 1985. 320p. 179.00 (*0-8493-6215-6*, RC860, CRC Reprint) Franklin.

Animal Models for Psychiatry. J. D. Keehn. 1986. (Illus.). 237p. (C). 45.00 (*0-7102-0562-7*, 05627, Routledge Thoemms) Routledge.

Animal Models in Biomedical Research: Swine-A Bibliography. Ed. by Cynthia P. Smith. 1994. 118p. (Orig.). (C). pap. text 45.00 (*0-7881-1075-6*) DIANE Pub.

Animal Models in Cardiovascular Research. David R. Gross. 1985. text 329.00 (*0-89838-711-6*); 2nd rev. ed. 1994. LC 93-50932. (Developments in Cardiovascular Medicine Ser.: Vol. 153). 560p. (C). text 228.00 (*0-7923-2712-8*) Kluwer Academic.

Animal Models in Chronic Renal Failure. Ed. by N. Gretz & M. Strauch. 1988. (Contributions to Nephrology Ser.: Vol. 60). (Illus.). viii, 268p. 208.00 (*3-8055-4619-X*) S Karger.

Animal Models in Medical Mycology. Ed. by Makoto Miyaji. 1987. 176p. 105.00 (*0-8493-5844-2*, RC117, CRC Reprint) Franklin.

Animal Models in Orthopedic Research. Yuehuei H. An & Richard J. Friedman. 1998. LC 98-39579. (Illus.). 624p. 139.95 (*0-8493-2115-8*) CRC Pr.

Animal Models in Psychiatry I. Ed. by Alan A. Boulton et al. 1991. LC 91-7076. (Neuromethods Ser.: Vol. 18). (Illus.). 430p. 145.00 (*0-89603-198-5*) Humana.

Animal Models in Psychiatry II. Ed. by Alan A. Boulton et al. 1991. LC 91-7076. (Neuromethods Ser.: Vol. 19). (Illus.). 406p. 145.00 (*0-89603-177-2*) Humana.

Animal Models in Psychopharmacology. Ed. by B. Olivier et al. 1991. (Advances in Pharmacological Sciences Ser.). 476p. 146.00 (*0-8176-2503-8*) Birkhauser.

Animal Models in the Evaluation of Chemotherapeutic Agents Against HIV: Journal: Intervirology, Vol. 30, Suppl. 1. Ed. by H. D. Schlumberger & E. Schrinner. 1989. (Illus.). iv, 72p. pap. 23.50 (*3-8055-4982-2*) S Karger.

Animal Models in the Neurosciences. Michael G. Nosko. 2000. 99.95 (*0-8493-7683-1*) CRC Pr.

Animal Models in Toxicology. Ed. by A. Gad & Christopher P. Chengelis. 1992. (Drug & Chemical Toxicology Ser.: Vol. 8). (Illus.). 928p. text 295.00 (*0-8247-8456-1*) Dekker.

Animal Models of Depression. George Koob et al. 1989. 304p. 104.00 (*0-8176-3407-X*) Birkhauser.

Animal Models of Diabetes: A Primer. Anders F. Sima & Eleazar Shafrir. 2000. (Frontiers in Animal Diabetes Research Ser.: Vol. 2). 368p. 85.00 (*90-5823-096-1*, Harwood Acad Pubs) Gordon & Breach.

Animal Models of Disease: Bibliography. January 1988-January 1994. Ed. by Cynthia P. Smith & Jean A. Larson. 1996. 74p. (Orig.). (C). pap. text 30.00 (*0-7881-2730-6*) DIANE Pub.

Animal Models of HIV & Other Retroviral Infections. Ed. by P. Racz et al. 1993. (Illus.). viii, 200p. 172.25 (*3-8055-5677-2*) S Karger.

Animal Models of Human Emotion & Cognition. Ed. by Marc Haug & Richard E. Whalen. 1999. LC 99-30612. 341p. text 39.95 (*1-55798-583-9*, 431-8880) Am Psychol.

Animal Models of Human Pathology: A Bibliography of a Quarter Century of Behavioral Research, 1967-1992. Ed. by J. Bruce Overmier & Patricia D. Burke. 1992. 322p. pap. 19.95 (*1-55798-184-1*) Am Psychol.

Animal Models of Human Psychology: Critique of Science, Ethics & Policy. Kenneth J. Shapiro. 1998. LC 97-26436. (Illus.). 344p. 39.50 (*0-88937-189-X*) Hogrefe & Huber Pubs.

Animal Models of Neurological Disease I: Neurodegenerative Diseases. Ed. by Alan A. Boulton et al. 1992. LC 91-35401. (Neuromethods Ser.: Vol. 21). (Illus.). 388p. 145.00 (*0-89603-208-6*) Humana.

Animal Models of Neurological Disease II: Metabolic Encephalopathies & the Epilepsies. Ed. by Alan A. Boulton et al. 1992. LC 91-35401. (Neuromethods Ser.: Vol. 22). (Illus.). 380p. 145.00 (*0-89603-211-6*) Humana.

Animal Nutrition. J. W. Lassiter & Hardy M. Edwards. 1982. (C). tchr. ed. (*0-8359-0223-4*); text 46.20 (*0-8359-0222-6*) P-H.

Animal Nutrition: You May Be Poisoning Your Pet Unknowingly, a Little Each Day. John D. Rowe. 1997. (Illus.). 200p. pap. 12.95 (*0-9655196-0-0*) Setter Pubns.

Animal Nutrition & Feeding. James R. Gillespie. LC 86-8982. 576p. (C). 1987. text 53.95 (*0-8273-2354-9*); 1986. tchr. ed. 12.00 (*0-8273-2355-7*) Delmar.

Animal Nutrition in Tropics. S. K. Ranjhan. 1980. 446p. 19.95 (*0-7069-1005-2*) Asia Bk Corp.

Animal Origin Drugs Used in Unani Medicine. S. B. Vohra. 1979. 137p. 19.95 (*0-7069-0768-X*) Asia Bk Corp.

Animal Pain. Short. 1992. text 108.00 (*0-7216-5937-3*) Saunders.

Animal Pain: Perception & Alleviation. Ed. by Ralph L. Kitchell & Howard H. Erickson. 1988. (Animal Welfare Ser.). (Illus.). 231p. text 39.95 (*0-19-520695-9*) OUP.

Animal Physiologic Surgery. Ed. by C. Max Lang. 2nd ed. 1981. (Illus.). 180p. 35.50 (*0-387-90620-7*) Spr-Verlag.

Animal Physiology. Eckert. 4th ed. 1997. tchr. ed. 57.00 (*0-7167-3293-9*) W H Freeman.

Animal Physiology: Adaptations in Function. F. Reed Hainsworth. 1981. (Life Sciences Ser.). (Illus.). 600p. text (*0-201-03401-8*) Addison-Wesley.

Animal Production & Environmental Health. Ed. by D. Strauch. 1987. (World Animal Science Ser.: Vol. B6). 324p. 242.50 (*0-444-42731-7*) Elsevier.

Animal Psysiological Surgery. Ed. by C. M. Lang. 1976. LC 76-15020. (Illus.). 180p. 17.00 (*0-387-90187-6*) Spr-Verlag.

Animal Quarantine in Asia & the Pacific. Animal Production Organization Staff. 1994. 309p. pap. (*92-833-2145-6*, APO321456) Asian Prod Organ JPN. *Dist:* Bernan Associates.

Animal Reproductive Physiology. 1997. 112p. tchr. ed. (*0-02-305184-1*) P-H.

Animal Research & Ethical Conflict. M. T. Phillips & J. A. Sechzer. 1989. (Illus.). 251p. 135.00 (*0-387-96935-7*, 2512) Spr-Verlag.

Animal Rhythms. Orland A. Soave. 1999. LC 99-10334. 224p. 74.95 (*1-57292-140-4*); 102p. pap. 57.95 (*1-57292-139-0*) Austin & Winfield.

Animal Science. James R. Gillespie. 1998. (Agriculture Ser.). 152p. pap. text, tchr. ed. 12.00 (*0-8273-7780-0*); LC 97-13862. 1152p. (C). 99.95 (*0-8273-7779-7*); (C). pap. text, lab manual ed. 21.50 (*0-8273-8116-6*) Delmar.

Animal Science. Horne. 1998. (Agriculture Ser.). (C). pap., lab manual ed. 18.25 net. (*0-8273-8117-4*) Delmar.

Animal Science Anatomy & Physiology. Gillespie & Colverson. 1998. 160p. pap. text, lab manual ed. 28.95 (*0-7668-0190-X*) Delmar.

Animal Social Behavior: Index of New Information with Authors, Subjects & Bibliography. Richard F. Pinecrest. rev. ed. 1995. 173p. 57.50 (*0-7883-0716-9*); pap. 47.50 (*0-7883-0717-7*) ABBE Pubs Assn.

Animal Specialist. 1992. lib. bdg. 300.00 (*0-8490-8870-4*) Gordon Pr.

Animal Species & Evolution. Ernst W. Mayr. 1963. LC 63-9552. (Illus.). 811p. text 56.00 (*0-674-03750-2*, Belknap) HUP.

Animal Stress. Ed. by Gary P. Moberg. 1988. (American Physiological Society Book). (Illus.). 332p. text 42.50 (*0-19-520696-7*) OUP.

Animal Structure & Function. Cecie Starr & Ralph Taggart. 6th ed. 1993. (Biology Ser.). pap. 12.75 (*0-534-30478-8*) Wadsworth Pub.

Animal Testing Alternatives in Health Sciences: Index of New Information with Authors, Subjects & Bibliography. Ruth C. Mahoney. rev. ed. 1994. 147p. 57.50 (*0-7883-0368-6*); pap. 47.50 (*0-7883-0369-4*) ABBE Pubs Assn.

Animal Testing & Consumer Products. Heidi J. Welsh. 1990. 167p. pap. 25.00 (*0-931035-39-2*) IRRC Inc DC.

Animal Thinking. Donald R. Griffin. 1984. 256p. pap. text 15.95 (*0-674-03713-8*) HUP.

Animal Virus Pathogenesis: A Practical Approach. Ed. by Michael B. Oldstone. 1990. (Practical Approach Ser.). (Illus.). 192p. pap. 45.00 (*0-19-963101-8*) OUP.

Animal Warden. Jack Rudman. 1994. (Career Examination Ser.: C-1844). pap. 23.95 (*0-8373-1844-0*) Nat Learn.

Animalcular & Cryptogamic Theories on the Origins of Fevers: An Original Anthology. Ed. by Barbara G. Rosenkrantz. 1977. LC 76-40658. (Public Health in America Ser.). reprint ed. 23.95 (*0-405-09839-1*) Ayer.

Animals & Alternatives in Toxicity Testing. Michael Balls et al. 1983. text 104.00 (*0-12-077480-1*) Acad Pr.

Animals & Disease: An Introduction to the History of Comparative Medicine. Lise Wilkinson. 1992. (Illus.). 282p. (C). text 80.00 (*0-521-37573-8*) Cambridge U Pr.

Animals Disease & Human Society: Human-Animal Relations & the Rise of Veterinary Science. Joanna Swabe. 1998. LC 98-25860. (Studies in Science, Technology, & Society: 2). 224p. (C). 90.00 (*0-415-18193-3*) Routledge.

Animals in Wildlife—Biology, Behavior, & Vectorisms for Disease: Index for New Information. Bruce J. McNally. 1995. LC 95-19213. 57.50 (*0-7883-0642-1*); pap. 47.50 (*0-7883-0643-X*) ABBE Pubs Assn.

Animals, Nature & Albert Schweitzer. Comment by Ann C. Free. rev. ed. 1989. LC 88-81164. (Illus.). 96p. 8.95 (*0-9617225-1-7*) Flying Fox Pr.

Animals, the Law & Veterinary Medicine: A Guide to Veterinary Law. Orland A. Soave. 1997. LC 97-19012. 195p. 75.00 (*1-57292-089-0*); 212p. pap. 56.95 (*1-57292-088-2*) Austin & Winfield.

Animals Without Backbones. Ralph Buchsbaum. 2nd rev. ed. 1972. LC 48-9508. (Illus.). 405p. pap. text 15.00 (*0-226-07870-1*) U Ch Pr.

Animus & Anima. Emma Jung. Tr. by Cary F. Baynes & Hildegard Nagel. 1985. LC 85-18299. 94p. reprint ed. pap. 11.00 (*0-88214-301-8*) Spring Pubns.

Anky Techua-Te: Classical Khamitic Afrikan Medicine. Cwolde Kyte. 1986. 181p. (Orig.). pap. 19.41 (*0-936901-00-4*) Ctr Sacred Healing.

Ann Arbor Learning Inventory: Skill Level C - Grades 5-8. Barbara M. Vitale & Waneta B. Bullock. 1992. stu. ed. 15.00 (*0-87879-852-8*); stu. ed. 8.00 (*0-87879-854-4*); (gr. 5-8). pap. 12.00 (*0-87879-853-6*, 853-6) Acad Therapy (Ann Arbor Div).

Anna Freud: A Biography. Elizabeth Y. Bruehl et al. 1994. pap. 14.95 (*0-393-31157-0*) Norton.

Anna Freud: A Life Dedicated to Children. Uwe H. Peters. 1985. LC 84-1278. (Illus.). 384p. 24.95 (*0-8052-3910-3*) Schocken.

Anna Freud: The Dream of Psychoanalysis. Robert Coles. 2000. pap. 10.95 (*0-201-62232-7*) Perseus Bks Grp.

Anna Freud's Letters to Eva Rosenfeld. Peter Heller. Tr. by Mary Weigand from GER. 1992. LC 91-51861. xiv, 210p. (C). 32.50 (*0-8236-0152-8*) Intl Univs Pr.

Annals of Child Development. Ed. by Ross Vasta. 1998. (Annals of Child Development Ser.: Vol. 13). 300p. (*1-85302-589-5*) Jessica Kingsley GBR. *Dist:* Taylor & Francis.

Annals of Child Development, Vol. 7. Ed. by Ross Vasta. 1990. 300p. 65.00 (*1-85302-081-8*) Taylor & Francis.

Annals of Clinical Research. Chris E. Stout. 1997. 131p. text 19.95 (*1-890056-07-3*, 1988-56081) Grayson Pub.

Annals of Insanity: Comprising a Selection of Curious & Interesting Cases in the Different Species of Lunacy, Melancholy, or Madness. William Perfect. 1976. LC 75-16726. (Classics in Psychiatry Ser.). reprint ed. 30.95 (*0-405-07449-2*) Ayer.

Annals of Internal Medicine: Time & Medicine. Ed. by Richard V. Lee & Frank Davidoff. 2000. (Illus.). 91p. pap. text 16.00 (*0-943126-96-7*, 330301890) Amer Coll Phys.

Annals of Life Insurance Medicine: Proceedings of the International Congress of Life Insurance, 13th, Madrid, 1979, Vol. 6. International Congress of Life Insurance Staff. Ed. by Eward W. Tanner & M. L. Hefti. 1980. (Illus.). 270p. 53.95 (*0-387-10050-4*) Spr-Verlag.

Annals of the Barber-Surgeons of London. Sidney Young. LC 75-23773. (Illus.). reprint ed. 72.00 (*0-404-13399-1*) AMS Pr.

Annals of the ICRP, Vol. 5, No. 1-6. Ed. by F. D. Sowby. 1980. (International Commission on Radiological Protection Ser.: No. 30, Supplement to Pt. 2). 751p. 142.00 (*0-08-026833-1*, Pergamon Pr) Elsevier.

Annals of Theoretical Psychology, Vol. 1. Ed. by Leendert P. Mos & Joseph R. Royce. 1984. LC 84-644088. 346p. 85.00 (*0-306-41327-2*, Plenum Trade) Perseus Pubng.

Annals of Theoretical Psychology, Vol. 4. Ed. by Leendert P. Mos et al. 1986. LC 84-644088. (Illus.). 420p. (C). 114.00 (*0-306-42327-8*, Plenum Trade) Perseus Pubng.

Annals of Theoretical Psychology, Vol. 5. Ed. by Leendert P. Mos & Arthur W. Staats. 1988. LC 84-644088. (Illus.). 382p. (C). 114.00 (*0-306-42652-8*, Plenum Trade) Perseus Pubng.

Annals of Theoretical Psychology, Vol. 6. Ed. by Leendert P. Mos & D. N. Robinson. 1990. LC 84-644088. (Illus.). 254p. (C). 95.00 (*0-306-43588-8*, Plenum Trade) Perseus Pubng.

Annals of Theoretical Psychology, Vol. 7. Ed. by Leendert P. Mos & P. Van Geert. 1991. (Illus.). 400p. (C). 95.00 (*0-306-44053-9*, Plenum Trade) Perseus Pubng.

Annals of Theoretical Psychology. Ed. by Leendert P. Mos et al. 1993. LC 84-644088. (Illus.). (C). Vol. 8. 306p. 95.00 (*0-306-44564-6*); Vol. 9. 280p. 95.00 (*0-306-44624-3*) Perseus Pubng (Plenum Trade).

Anniversary Issue, 50 Years of 'Cardiology' Ed. by J. J. Kellermann. 1987. (Journal: Vol. 74, No. 4, 1987). (Illus.). 88p. pap. 36.75 (*3-8055-4638-6*) S Karger.

Annotated Atlas of Electrocardiography: A Guide to Confident Interpretation. Thomas M. Blake. 1998. (Contemporary Cardiology Ser.: Vol. 3). 248p. LC 98-36685. 99.50 (*0-89603-762-2*); pap. 59.50 (*0-89603-768-1*) Humana.

Annotated Bibliography for Ethical Guidelines. Mary Silva. 1995. 45p. (Orig.). pap. 14.95 (*1-55810-110-1*, D-97) Am Nurses Pub.

***Annotated Bibliography for Managed Behavioral Health Care, 1989-1999.** Jane Kramer & Michael Freeman. 2001. 171p. (C). pap. text 35.00 (*0-7567-1106-1*) DIANE Pub.

Annotated Bibliography of Pediatric Cardiology. American Academy of Pediatrics Staff. 1994. 188p. pap. 29.95 (*0-910761-55-8*) Am Acad Pediat.

Annotated Bibliography of Scientific Articles on AIDS for Policymakers, Set. 1991. (AIDS Ser.). lib. bdg. 500.00 (*0-8490-4218-6*) Gordon Pr.

Annotated Bibliography of Teaching-Learning Materials for Schools of Nursing & Midwifery. 1975. (Offset Publications: No. 19). pap. text 51.00 (*92-4-052005-8*) World Health.

Annotated Bibliography on Leprosy. Corinne S. Wood. 1997. LC 97-42479. (Studies in Health & Human Services: Vol. 30). 208p. text 89.95 (*0-7734-8441-8*) E Mellen.

Annotated Listing of Resources for the Study of the History of Medicine & Health Care in Nevada. Ed. by Michael L. Ezell. 1991. (Great Basin History of Medicine Ser.). 84p. lib. bdg. 23.00 (*1-56475-004-3*) U NV Oral Hist.

Annotated Medical/legal Dict. Richard Sloane. 1987. (Paralegal). (Illus.). 787p. (C). mass mkt. 158.50 (*0-314-93512-6*) West Pub.

Annotated Syllabus of Geriatric References. Gail Sullivan et al. 1998. 50p. ring bd. 80.00 (*1-891509-00-4*) Univ CT Hlth.

Annuaire de la Recherche Biomedicale. 1995.Tr. of Directory of Biomedical Research in France. 656p. 109.00 (*2-906077-63-1*) Elsevier.

Annual Editions: Abnormal Psychology. Palladino. 1995. 256p. (C). per. (*1-56134-440-0*) Brown & Benchmark.

Annual Editions: Aging. Steven M. Cox. 12th ed. 1997. 240p. pap. 16.56 (*0-697-39296-1*) McGraw.

Annual Editions: Biopsychology, 95-96. Boyce Jubilan. 1995. (Illus.). 256p. (C). text 12.95 (*1-56134-336-6*, Dshkn McG-Hill) McGrw-H Hghr Educ.

Annual Editions: Human Development, 97-98. Freiberg. 25th ed. 1997. 256p. (C). text 12.25 net. (*0-697-37286-3*, WCB McGr Hill) McGrw-H Hghr Educ.

Annual Guide to Graduate Nursing Education 1997. National League for Nursing Staff. 1997. 210p. pap. 34.95 (*0-88737-749-1*, 19-7491, NLN Pr) Natl League Nurse.

Annual Handbook for Group Facilitators, 1981. Ed. by John E. Jones & J. William Pfeiffer. 10th ed. 1980. LC 73-92841. (Human Resource Development Ser.). (Illus.). 296p. pap. 49.00 (*0-88390-004-1*); ring bd. 99.00 (*0-88390-003-3*) Jossey-Bass (Pffr & Co).

Annual Index, 1989. Ed. by Jon C. Ransom. 1989. 472p. pap. text 29.95 (*0-914899-07-4*) Current Lit Pubns.

Annual Meeting of the Skin Pharmacology Society & of the 9th Meeting of the International Society for Bioengineering & the Skin - Abstracts: SPS Meeting, Cleveland, Ohio, October 1992; ISBS Meeting, Sendai, Japan, October 1992 - Journal: Skin Pharmacology, Vol. 5, No. 4, 1992. Ed. by H. Schaefer. 1992. 56p. pap. 47.00 (*3-8055-5692-6*) S Karger.

Annual 19, Side Effects Drugs, 1995. Ed. by J. K. Aronson & C. J. Van Boxtel. 1996. 532p. 190.50 (*0-444-82531-2*) Elsevier.

Annual of Psychoanalysis, Vol. I. Chicago Institute for Psychoanalysis Staff. 1973. LC 72-91376. 395p. (C). 70.00 (*0-8236-0361-X*) Intl Univs Pr.

Annual of Psychoanalysis. Ed. by Chicago Institute for Psychoanalysis Staff. Vol. IX. 1981. 70.00 (*0-8236-0370-9*); Vol. X. 1982. 70.00 (*0-8236-0371-7*) Intl Univs Pr.

Annual of Psychoanalysis, Vol. XIV. Chicago Institute for Psychoanalysis Staff. 1987. LC 72-91376. 375p. (C). 70.00 (*0-8236-0374-1*) Intl Univs Pr.

Annual of Psychoanalysis, Vol. XV. Ed. by Chicago Institute for Psychoanalysis Staff. 1987. (Chicago Institute for Psychoanalysis Ser.). 70.00 (*0-8236-0375-X*, BN00375) Intl Univs Pr.

Annual of Psychoanalysis, Vol. XVI. Ed. by Chicago Institute of Psychoanalysis Staff. 1988. 391p. 70.00 (*0-8236-0376-8*) Intl Univs Pr.

Annual of Psychoanalysis, Vol. 17. Ed. by Chicago Institute for Psychoanalysis Staff. 1989. 376p. text 36.00 (*0-88163-092-6*) Analytic Pr.

Annual of Psychoanalysis, Vol. 18. Ed. by Chicago Institute of Psychoanalysis Staff. 1990. (Annual Ser.). 272p. text 29.95 (*0-88163-093-4*) Analytic Pr.

Annual of Psychoanalysis, Vol. 19. Ed. by Chicago Inst. for Psychoanalysis Staff. 1991. 280p. text 32.50 (*0-88163-094-2*) Analytic Pr.

Annual of Psychoanalysis, Vol. 20. Ed. by Chicago Institute for Psychoanalysis Staff. 1992. 336p. 34.50 (*0-88163-133-7*) Analytic Pr.

Annual of Psychoanalysis. Ed. by Jerome A. Winer. Vol. 21. 1993. 336p. text 36.00 (*0-88163-134-5*); Vol. 22. 1994. 312p. text 36.00 (*0-88163-135-3*) Analytic Pr.

Annual of Psychoanalysis, 1974, Vol. II. Ed. by Chicago Institute for Psychoanalysis Staff. 1975. LC 72-91376. (Illus.). x, 420p. (C). 70.00 (*0-8236-0362-8*) Intl Univs Pr.

Annual of Psychoanalysis, 1975, Vol. III. Ed. by Chicago Institute for Psychoanalysis Staff. 1976. LC 72-91376. viii, 441p. (C). 70.00 (*0-8236-0363-6*) Intl Univs Pr.

Annual of Psychoanalysis, 1976, Vol. IV. Ed. by Chicago Institute for Psychoanalysis Staff. 1977. LC 72-91376. (Illus.). xi, 508p. (C). 70.00 (*0-8236-0364-4*) Intl Univs Pr.

Annual of Psychoanalysis, 1977, Vol. V. Ed. by Chicago Institute for Psychoanalysis Staff. 1978. LC 72-91376. (Illus.). ix, 443p. (C). 70.00 (*0-8236-0366-0*) Intl Univs Pr.

Annual of Psychoanalysis, 1978, Vol. VI. Ed. by Chicago Institute for Psychoanalysis Staff. 1979. LC 72-91376. (Illus.). x, 489p. (C). 70.00 (*0-8236-0367-9*) Intl Univs Pr.

Annual of Psychoanalysis, 1979, Vol. VII. Ed. by Chicago Institute for Psychoanalysis Staff. 1980. LC 72-91376. (Illus.). x, 416p. (C). 70.00 (*0-8236-0368-7*) Intl Univs Pr.

Annual of Psychoanalysis, 1980, Vol. VIII. Ed. by Chicago Institute for Psychoanalysis Staff. 1981. LC 72-91376. (Illus.). xiii, 359p. (C). 70.00 (*0-8236-0369-5*) Intl Univs Pr.

Annual of Psychoanalysis, 1983, Vol. XI. Ed. by Chicago Institute for Psychoanalysis Staff. 1984. LC 72-91376. xii, 365p. (C). 70.00 (*0-8236-0372-5*) Intl Univs Pr.

Annual of Psychoanalysis, 1985, Vol. XII-XIII. Ed. by Chicago Institute for Psychoanalysis Staff. 1985. LC 72-91376. 452p. 70.00 (*0-8236-0373-3*, 00373) Intl Univs Pr.

Annual of Psychoanalysis 1997, Vol. 25. Ed. by Jerome A. Winer. 25th ed. 1997. 288p. reprint ed. 39.95 (*0-88163-189-2*) Analytic Pr.

Annual Post-Graduate Course in Cardiothoracic Surgery: A State of the Art Review, 1999. 1999. spiral bd. 395.00 incl. cd-rom (*1-928852-08-4*) Amadeus Multi Tech.

Annual Progress in Child & Adolescent Psychiatry & Child Development, 1994. Ed. by Margaret E. Hertzig & Ellen A. Farber. 1994. LC 68-23452. 600p. text 66.95 (*0-87630-744-6*) Brunner-Routledge.

Annual Progress in Child Psychiatry & Child Development, 1980. Ed. by Stella Chess & Alexander Thomas. 1980. LC 68-23452. 624p. text 66.95 (*0-87630-248-7*) Brunner-Routledge.

Annual Progress in Child Psychiatry & Child Development, 1984. Ed. by Stella Chess & Alexander Thomas. 1984. LC 68-23452. 514p. text 66.95 (*0-87630-375-0*) Brunner-Routledge.

Annual Progress in Child Psychiatry & Child Development, 1985. Ed. by Stella Chess & Alexander Thomas. 1985. LC 68-23452. 664p. text 66.95 (*0-87630-402-1*) Brunner-Routledge.

Annual Progress in Child Psychiatry & Child Development, 1986. Ed. by Stella Chess et al. 1986. LC 68-23452. 704p. text 66.95 (*0-87630-437-4*) Brunner-Routledge.

Annual Progress in Child Psychiatry & Child Development, 1987. Ed. by Stella Chess et al. 1987. LC 68-23452. 650p. text 66.95 (*0-87630-476-5*) Brunner-Routledge.

Annual Progress in Child Psychiatry & Child Development, 1988. Ed. by Stella Chess et al. 1988. LC 68-23452. 704p. text 66.95 (*0-87630-538-9*) Brunner-Routledge.

Annual Progress in Child Psychiatry & Child Development, 1989. Ed. by Stella Chess & Margaret E. Hertzig. 1989. LC 68-23452. 576p. text 52.95 (*0-87630-569-9*) Brunner-Routledge.

Annual Progress in Child Psychiatry & Child Development, 1990. Ed. by Stella Chess & Margaret E. Hertzig. 1990. LC 68-23452. (Illus.). 624p. text 66.95 (*0-87630-602-4*) Brunner-Routledge.

Annual Progress in Child Psychiatry & Child Development, 1991. Ed. by Stella Chess & Margaret E. Hertzig. 1991. LC 68-23452. 656p. text 66.95 (*0-87630-651-2*) Brunner-Routledge.

Annual Progress in Child Psychiatry & Child Development, 1992. Ed. by Margaret E. Hertzig & Ellen A. Farber. 1992. LC 68-23452. 653p. text 66.95 (*0-87630-692-X*) Brunner-Routledge.

Annual Progress in Child Psychiatry & Child Development, 1995: A Selection of the Year's Outstanding Contributions to the Understanding & Treatment of the Normal & Disturbed Child. Ed. by Margaret E. Hertzig et al. 1995. 632p. text 66.95 (*0-87630-793-4*) Brunner-Routledge.

Annual Progress in Child Psychiatry & Child Development, 1996. Ed. by Margaret E. Hertzig & Ellen A. Farber. 1996. 608p. 69.95 (*0-87630-828-0*) Brunner-Routledge.

Annual Progress in Child Psychiatry & Child Development, 1998 Edition. Margaret E. Hertzig. 1999. 512p. 79.95 (*0-87630-992-9*) Brunner-Routledge.

Annual Progress in Child Psychiatry & Child Development, 1999. Margaret E. Hertzig & Ellen A. Farber. 2000. 400p. 79.95 (*1-58391-046-8*) Brunner-Routledge.

***Annual Register of Pharmaceutical Chemists, 2000.** Royal Pharmaceutical Society of Great Britain Staff. 2000. (*0-85369-453-2*) Pharmaceutical Pr GBR. *Dist:* Rittenhouse.

Annual Report of the Committees on Toxicity, Mutagenicity & Carcinogenicity of 1996. 1998. (*0-11-322115-0*, HM21150) Statnry Office GBR. *Dist:* Bernan Associates.

Annual Reports in Combinatorial Chemistry & Molecular Diversity. Ed. by Walter H. Moos et al. 1997. 300p. lib. bdg. (*90-72199-23-5*) ESCOM Sci Pubs NLD. *Dist:* Kluwer Academic.

Annual Reports in Medicinal Chemistry. Ed. by Annette M. Doherty. 2000. (Annual Reports in Medicinal Chemistry: Vol. 35). 500p. pap. 85.00 (*0-12-040535-0*) Acad Pr.

Annual Reports in Medicinal Chemistry. Ed. by James A. Bristol. (Illus.). Vol. 29. 1994. (Annual Reports in Medicinal Chemistry: Vol. 29). 397p. pap. text 78.00 (*0-12-040529-6*); Vol. 30. 1995. (Annual Reports in Medicinal Chemistry: Vol. 30). 400p. pap. text 74.00 (*0-12-040530-X*); Vol. 31. 1996. 413p. pap. text 70.00 (*0-12-040531-8*) Acad Pr.

Annual Reports in Medicinal Chemistry, Vol. 32. Ed. by James A. Bristol. 1997. (Illus.). 378p. pap. text 70.00 (*0-12-040532-6*) Morgan Kaufmann.

Annual Reports on NMR Spectroscopy. Ed. by Graham A. Webb. Vol. 21. 1989. 304p. text 157.00 (*0-12-505321-5*); Vol. 23. 1991. 425p. text 193.00 (*0-12-505323-1*); Vol. 28. 1994. 368p. text 139.00 (*0-12-505328-2*); Vol. 35. 1998. 350p. (*0-12-505335-5*) Acad Pr.

Annual Reports on NMR Spectroscopy, Vol. 34. Ed. by Graham A. Webb. 1997. (Illus.). 400p. text 125.00 (*0-12-505334-7*) Morgan Kaufmann.

Annual Review of Biochemistry. Ed. by Charles C. Richardson et al. LC 32-25093. (Illus.). Vol. 53. 1984. text 41.00 (*0-8243-0853-0*); Vol. 55. 1986. text 41.00 (*0-8243-0855-7*) Annual Reviews.

Annual Review of Biomedical Engineering, Vol. 2. 2000. 500p. text 131.00 (*0-8243-3502-3*) Annual Reviews.

Annual Review of Biophysics & Biophysical Chemistry, Vol. 14. Ed. by Donald M. Engelman et al. 1985. LC 79-188446. (Illus.). text 55.00 (*0-8243-1814-5*) Annual Reviews.

Annual Review of Cell Biology, Vol. 1. Ed. by George E. Palade et al. 1985. (Illus.). (C). text 41.00 (*0-8243-3101-X*) Annual Reviews.

Annual Review of Genetics. Ed. by Herschel L. Roman et al. LC 67-29891. (Illus.). Vol. 6. 1972. text 40.00 (*0-8243-1206-6*); Vol. 7. 1973. text 40.00 (*0-8243-1207-4*); Vol. 8. 1974. text 40.00 (*0-8243-1208-2*); Vol. 9. 1975. text 40.00 (*0-8243-1209-0*); Vol. 10. 1976. text 40.00 (*0-8243-1210-4*); Vol. 11. 1977. text 40.00 (*0-8243-1211-2*); Vol. 12. 1978. text 40.00 (*0-8243-1212-0*); Vol. 15. 1981. text 40.00 (*0-8243-1215-5*); Vol. 17. 1983. text 40.00 (*0-8243-1217-1*) Annual Reviews.

Annual Review of Gerontology & Geriatrics: Behavioral Science & Aging, Vol. 11. K. Warner Schaie. 1991. 284p. 46.00 (*0-8261-6493-5*) Springer Pub.

Annual Review of Gerontology & Geriatrics: Biological, Clinical, Behavioral & Social Issues. Ed. by Carl Eisdorfer. Vol. 1. 1980. 432p. 46.00 (*0-8261-3080-1*); Vol. 2. 1981. 432p. (C). 46.00 (*0-8261-3081-X*); Vol. 3. 1982. 448p. 46.00 (*0-8261-3082-8*) Springer Pub.

Annual Review of Gerontology & Geriatrics: Biological, Clinical, Behavioral Issues, Vol. 4. Carl Eisdorfer. 1984. 304p. 46.00 (*0-8261-3083-6*) Springer Pub.

Annual Review of Gerontology & Geriatrics: Biology of Aging, Vol. 10. Ed. by Vincent J. Cristofalo. 1990. 240p. (C). 46.00 (*0-8261-6492-7*) Springer Pub.

Annual Review of Gerontology & Geriatrics: Experimental & Applied Psychology, Vol. 7. Ed. by K. Warner Schaie. 1987. 352p. 46.00 (*0-8261-3086-0*) Springer Pub.

Annual Review of Gerontology & Geriatrics: Geriatric Health Care, Vol. 6. Carl Eisdorfer. 1987. 304p. 46.00 (*0-8261-3085-2*) Springer Pub.

Annual Review of Gerontology & Geriatrics: Geriatrics & Psychological Interventions, Vol. 9. Ed. by M. Powell Lawton. 1989. 416p. 46.00 (*0-8261-6491-9*) Springer Pub.

Annual Review of Gerontology & Geriatrics: Kinship, Aging, & Social Change. Ed. by George L. Maddox & M. Powell Lawton. 1993. (Annual Review of Gerontology Ser.: Vol. 13). 280p. text 46.00 (*0-8261-6495-1*) Springer Pub.

Annual Review of Gerontology & Geriatrics: Social & Psychological Aspects of Aging, Vol. 5. M. Powell Lawton & George L. Maddox. 1985. 352p. 46.00 (*0-8261-3084-4*) Springer Pub.

Annual Review of Gerontology & Geriatrics Vol. 8: Varieties of Aging. Ed. by George L. Maddox & M. Powell Lawton. 1988. 320p. 56.00 (*0-8261-6490-0*) Springer Pub.

Annual Review of Gerontology & Geriatrics Vol. 12: Medications & the Elderly. Ed. by John W. Rowe & Judith C. Ahronheim. 1992. 232p. 46.00 (*0-8261-6494-3*) Springer Pub.

Annual Review of Gerontology & Geriatrics Vol. 15: Focus on Nutrition. Ed. by John E. Morley. 1995. (Annual Review of Gerontology & Geriatrics Ser.). (Illus.). 280p. 54.00 (*0-8261-6497-8*) Springer Pub.

Annual Review of Gerontology & Geriatrics Vol. 16: Focus on Managed Care & Quality Assurance: Integrating Acute & Chronic Care, Vol. 16. Ed. by Robert J. Newcomer & Anne M. Wilkinson. 1996. (Illus.). 280p. 54.00 (*0-8261-6498-6*) Springer Pub.

Annual Review of Gerontology & Geriatrics Vol. 17: Focus on Emotion & Adult Development. Ed. by K. Warner Schaie & M. Powell Lawton. 1997. (Illus.). 384p. 56.00 (*0-8261-6499-4*) Springer Pub.

Annual Review of Hydrocephalus, 1988, Vol. 6. Ed. by Shoichi Matsumoto et al. 1990. (Illus.). 171p. 128.00 (*0-387-52204-2*) Spr-Verlag.

Annual Review of Hydrocephalus, 1990, Vol. 8. Ed. by Shoichi Matsumoto et al. 1992. (Illus.). 192p. 137.00 (*0-387-54846-7*) Spr-Verlag.

Annual Review of Immunology. Ed. by William E. Paul et al. Vol. 1. 1983. (Illus.). text 41.00 (*0-8243-3001-3*); Vol. 2. 1984. (Illus.). text 41.00 (*0-8243-3002-1*); Vol. 3. 1985. (Illus.). text 41.00 (*0-8243-3003-X*); Vol. 4. 1986. (Illus.). text 41.00 (*0-8243-3004-8*); Vol. 5. 1987. (Illus.). text 41.00 (*0-8243-3005-6*); Vol. 6. 1988. text 41.00 (*0-8243-3006-4*); Vol. 7. 1989. (Illus.). text 41.00 (*0-8243-3007-2*); Vol. 8. 1990. text 41.00 (*0-8243-3008-0*); Vol. 9. 1991. text 41.00 (*0-8243-3009-9*); Vol. 10. 1992. (Illus.). text 45.00 (*0-8243-3010-2*); Vol. 11. 1993. (Illus.). text 45.00 (*0-8243-3011-0*) Annual Reviews.

Annual Review of Immunology. Ed. by William E. Paul. Vol. 12. 1994. (Illus.). text 48.00 (*0-8243-3012-9*); Vol. 15. 1997. text 64.00 (*0-8243-3015-3*); Vol. 16. 1998. 714p. text 128.00 (*0-8243-3016-1*) Annual Reviews.

Annual Review of Immunology, Vol. 18. 2000. text 135.00 (*0-8243-3018-8*) Annual Reviews.

Annual Review of Immunology, 1995, Vol. 13. Ed. by William E. Paul. 1995. (Illus.). 825p. 48.00 (*0-8243-3013-7*) Annual Reviews.

Annual Review of Medicine. Ed. by Windsor C. Cutting. LC 51-1659. Vol. 2. 1951. 40.00 (*0-8243-0502-7*); Vol. 3. 1952. 40.00 (*0-8243-0503-5*) Annual Reviews.

Annual Review of Medicine, Vol. 6. Ed. by David A. Rytand. 1955. LC 51-1659. 40.00 (*0-8243-0506-X*) Annual Reviews.

Annual Review of Medicine. Ed. by Cecil H. Coggins. Vol. 45. 1994. LC 51-1659. (Illus.). text 47.00 (*0-8243-0545-0*); Vol. 46 (1996) 1995. (Illus.). 590p. text 47.00 (*0-8243-0546-9*); Vol. 47. 1996. LC 51-1659. (Illus.). text 52.00 (*0-8243-0547-7*); Vol. 49. 1998. LC 51-1659. text 60.00 (*0-8243-0549-3*); Vol. 51. 2000. 614p. text 127.00 (*0 8243 0551 5*) Annual Reviews.

Annual Review of Medicine: Selected Topics in the Clinical Sciences, Vol. 9. Ed. by William P. Creger et al. 1958. LC 51-1659. text 40.00 (*0-8243-0509-4*) Annual Reviews.

Annual Review of Medicine: Selected Topics in the Clinical Sciences. Ed. by David A. Rytand et al. LC 51-1659. Vol. 11. 1960. text 40.00 (*0-8243-0511-6*); Vol. 12. 1961. text 40.00 (*0-8243-0512-4*); Vol. 13. 1962. text 40.00 (*0-8243-0513-2*) Annual Reviews.

Annual Review of Medicine: Selected Topics in the Clinical Sciences. Ed. by Arthur C. Degraff et al. LC 51-1659. Vol. 14. 1963. text 40.00 (*0-8243-0514-0*); Vol. 15. 1964. text 40.00 (*0-8243-0515-9*); Vol. 17. 1966. text 40.00 (*0-8243-0517-5*) Annual Reviews.

Annual Review of Medicine: Selected Topics in the Clinical Sciences. Ed. by William P. Creger et al. Vol. 18. 1967. LC 51-1659. text 40.00 (*0-8243-0518-3*); Vol. 19. 1968. text 40.00 (*0-8243-0519-1*); Vol. 20. 1969. LC 51-1659. text 40.00 (*0-8243-0520-5*); Vol. 21. 1970. LC 51-1659. text 40.00 (*0-8243-0521-3*); Vol. 22. 1971. LC 51-1659. text 40.00 (*0-8243-0522-1*); Vol. 23. 1972. LC 51-1659. (Illus.). text 40.00 (*0-8243-0523-X*); Vol. 24. 1973. LC 51-1659. (Illus.). text 40.00 (*0-8243-0524-8*); Vol. 25. 1974. LC 51-1659. (Illus.). text 40.00 (*0-8243-0525-6*); Vol. 26. 1975. LC 51-1659. (Illus.). text 40.00 (*0-8243-0526-4*); Vol. 27. 1976. LC 51-1659. (Illus.). text 40.00 (*0-8243-0527-2*); Vol. 28. 1977. LC 51-1659. (Illus.). text 40.00 (*0-8243-0528-0*); Vol. 29. 1978. LC 51-1659. (Illus.). text 40.00 (*0-8243-0529-9*); Vol. 30. 1979. LC 51-1659. (Illus.). text 40.00 (*0-8243-0530-2*); Vol. 31. 1980. LC 51-1659. (Illus.). text 40.00 (*0-8243-0531-0*); Vol. 32. 1981. LC 51-1659. (Illus.). text 40.00 (*0-8243-0532-9*); Vol. 33. 1982. LC 51-1659. (Illus.). text 40.00 (*0-8243-0533-7*); Vol. 34. 1983. LC 51-1659. (Illus.). text 40.00 (*0-8243-0534-5*); Vol. 35. 1984. LC 51-1659. (Illus.). text 40.00 (*0-8243-0535-3*); Vol. 37. 1986. LC 51-1659. (Illus.). text 40.00 (*0-8243-0537-X*); Vol. 38. 1987. LC 51-1659. (Illus.). text 40.00 (*0-8243-0538-8*); Vol. 39. 1988. text 40.00 (*0-8243-0539-6*); Vol. 40. 1989. LC 51-1659. (Illus.). text 40.00 (*0-8243-0540-X*); Vol. 41. 1990. LC 51-1659. text 40.00 (*0-8243-0541-8*); Vol. 42. 1991. LC 51-1659. text 40.00 (*0-8243-0542-6*); Vol. 43. 1992. LC 51-1659. text 44.00 (*0-8243-0543-4*); Vol. 44. 1993. LC 51-1659. (Illus.). text 44.00 (*0-8243-0544-2*) Annual Reviews.

Annual Review of Medicine Vol. 50: Selected Topics in the Clinical Sciences 1999. Ed. by Cecil H. Coggins et al. 1999. 581p. 120.00 (*0-8243-0550-7*) Annual Reviews.

Annual Review of Microbiology, Vol. 26. Ed. by C. E. Clifton et al. 1972. LC 49-432. (Illus.). text 41.00 (*0-8243-1126-4*) Annual Reviews.

Annual Review of Microbiology. Ed. by Mortimer P. Starr et al. LC 49-432. (Illus.). Vol. 27. 1973. text 41.00 (*0-8243-1127-2*); Vol. 28. 1974. text 41.00 (*0-8243-1128-0*); Vol. 29. 1975. text 41.00 (*0-8243-1129-9*); Vol. 30. 1976. text 41.00 (*0-8243-1130-2*); Vol. 32. 1978. text 41.00 (*0-8243-1132-9*); Vol. 34. 1980. text 41.00 (*0-8243-1134-5*); Vol. 36. 1982. text 41.00 (*0-8243-1136-1*) Annual Reviews.

Annual Review of Microbiology, Vol. 37. Ed. by L. Nicholas Ornston et al. 1983. LC 49-432. (Illus.). text 41.00 (*0-8243-1137-X*) Annual Reviews.

Annual Review of Neuroscience. Ed. by W. Maxwell Cowan et al. (Illus.). Vol. 1. 1978. text 40.00 (*0-8243-2401-3*); Vol. 3. 1980. text 40.00 (*0-8243-2403-X*); Vol. 4. 1981. text 40.00 (*0-8243-2404-8*); Vol. 6. 1983. text 40.00 (*0-8243-2406-4*); Vol. 7. 1984. text 40.00 (*0-8243-2407-2*); Vol. 9. 1986. text 40.00 (*0-8243-2409-9*) Annual Reviews.

Annual Review of Neuroscience, Vol. 10. Ed. by W. Maxwell Cowan. 1987. (Illus.). text 40.00 (*0-8243-2410-2*) Annual Reviews.

Annual Review of Neuroscience. Ed. by W. Maxwell Cowan et al. Vol. 12. 1989. (Illus.). text 40.00 (*0-8243-2412-9*); Vol. 13. 1990. text 40.00 (*0-8243-2413-7*); Vol. 15. 1992. text 44.00 (*0-8243-2415-3*); Vol. 16. 1993. (Illus.). text 44.00 (*0-8243-2416-1*); Vol. 17. 1994. (Illus.). text 47.00 (*0-8243-2417-X*); Vol. 19. 1996. (Illus.). text 52.00 (*0-8243-2419-6*) Annual Reviews.

Annual Review of Neuroscience, Vol. 20. Ed. by W. Maxwell Cowan. 1997. text 60.00 (*0-8243-2420-X*) Annual Reviews.

Annual Review of Neuroscience, 1995, Vol. 18. Ed. by W. Maxwell Cowan. 1995. 550p. text 47.00 (*0-8243-2418-8*) Annual Reviews.

Annual Review of Nuclear & Particle Science, Vol. 28. Ed. by J. D. Jackson et al. 1978. LC 53-995. (Illus.). text 55.00 (*0-8243-1528-6*) Annual Reviews.

Annual Review of Nursing Research, Vol. 14. annuals Ed. by Joyce J. Fitzpatrick & Jane Norbeck. 1996. (Illus.). 320p. 45.00 (*0-8261-8233-X*) Springer Pub.

Annual Review of Nursing Research: Focus on Actual & Potential Health Problems, Vol. 5. Joyce J. Fitzpatrick & Roma L. Taunton. 1987. 272p. (C). 45.00 (*0-8261-4354-7*) Springer Pub.

Annual Review of Nursing Research: Focus on Chronic Illness & Long Term Care, Vol. 9. Ed. by Joyce J. Fitzpatrick et al. 1991. LC 94-183. 272p. 45.00 (*0-8261-4358-X*) Springer Pub.

Annual Review of Nursing Research: Focus on Community Nursing, Vol. 3. Harriet H. Werley & Joyce J. Fitzpatrick. 1985. 288p. 45.00 (*0-8261-4352-0*) Springer Pub.

Annual Review of Nursing Research: Focus on Current Critical Nursing Problems, Vol. 10. annuals Ed. by Joyce J. Fitzpatrick et al. 1992. 256p. 45.00 (*0-8261-4359-8*) Springer Pub.

Annual Review of Nursing Research: Focus on Family Nursing, Vol. 2. Harriet H. Werley & Joyce J. Fitzpatrick. 1984. 352p. 45.00 (*0-8261-4351-2*) Springer Pub.

Annual Review of Nursing Research: Focus on Human Development, Vol. 1. Harriet H. Werley & Joyce J. Fitzpatrick. 1984. 256p. 45.00 (*0-8261-4350-4*) Springer Pub.

Annual Review of Nursing Research: Focus on Human Development, Vol. 4. Harriet H. Werley et al. 1986. 304p. 45.00 (*0-8261-4353-9*) Springer Pub.

Annual Review of Nursing Research: Focus on Key Social & Health Issues, Vol. 13. annuals Ed. by Joyce J. Fitzpatrick & Joanne S. Stevenson. 1995. (Annual Review of Nursing Research Ser.). (Illus.). 360p. 48.00 (*0-8261-8232-1*) Springer Pub.

Annual Review of Nursing Research: Focus on Patient/Client Symptoms, Vol. 11. annuals Ed. by Joyce J. Fitzpatrick et al. 1993. 352p. 45.00 (*0-8261-8230-5*) Springer Pub.

Annual Review of Nursing Research: Focus on Physiological Aspects of Care. Ed. by Joyce J. Fitzpatrick et al. LC 84-649764. Vol. 7. 1989. 256p. 45.00 (*0-8261-4356-3*); Vol. 8. 1990. 272p. 45.00 (*0-8261-4357-1*) Springer Pub.

Annual Review of Nursing Research: Focus on Significant Clinical Issues, Vol. 12, 1994. annuals Ed. by Joanne S. Stevenson et al. 1994. 264p. 45.00 (*0-8261-8231-3*) Springer Pub.

Annual Review of Nursing Research: Focus on Specific Nursing Interventions, Vol. 6. Ed. by Joyce J. Fitzpatrick et al. 1988. 324p. (C). 45.00 (*0-8261-4355-5*) Springer Pub.

Annual Review of Nursing Research Vol. 15: Focus on "Significant Clinical Issues", Vol. 15. Joyce Fitzpatrick & Jane Norbeck. 1997. 328p. 45.00 (*0-8261-8234-8*) Springer Pub.

Annual Review of Nursing Research Vol. 17: Focus on Complementary Health & Pain Management. Ed. by Joyce J. Fitzpatrick. 1999. (Illus.). 360p. text 48.00 (*0-8261-8236-4*) Springer Pub.

Annual Review of Nursing Research Vol. 18: Focus on Chronic Illness. Ed. by Jean Goeppinger & Joyce J. Fitzpatrick. 2000. (Illus.). 352p. text 48.00 (*0-8261-1328-1*) Springer Pub.

A
B

Annual Review of Nutrition. Ed. by W. J. Darby et al. (Illus.). Vol. 1. 1981. text 43.00 (*0-8243-2801-9*); Vol. 2. 1982. text 43.00 (*0-8243-2802-7*); Vol. 3. 1983. text 43.00 (*0-8243-2803-5*); Vol. 4. 1984. text 43.00 (*0-8243-2804-3*) Annual Reviews.

Annual Review of Nutrition, Vol. 6. Ed. by Robert E. Olson et al. 1986. (Illus.). text 43.00 (*0-8243-2806-X*) Annual Reviews.

Annual Review of Nutrition, Vol. 7. Ed. by Robert E. Olson. 1987. (Illus.). text 43.00 (*0-8243-2807-8*) Annual Reviews.

Annual Review of Nutrition, Vol. 8. Ed. by Robert E. Olson et al. 1988. (Illus.). text 43.00 (*0-8243-2808-6*) Annual Reviews.

Annual Review of Nutrition, Vol. 13. Ed. by Robert E. Olson. 1993. (Illus.). text 45.00 (*0-8243-2813-2*) Annual Reviews.

Annual Review of Nutrition. Ed. by Donald B. McCormick. Vol. 15. 1995. text 48.00 (*0-8243-2815-9*); Vol. 18. 1998. text 60.00 (*0-8243-2818-3*) Annual Reviews.

Annual Review of Nutrition, Vol. 20. 2000. text 127.00 (*0-8243-2820-5*) Annual Reviews.

Annual Review of Pharmacology. Ed. by W. Cutting et al. LC 61-5649. Vol. 2. 1962. text 40.00 (*0-8243-0402-0*); Vol. 3. 1963. text 40.00 (*0-8243-0403-9*); Vol. 5. 1965. text 40.00 (*0-8243-0405-5*) Annual Reviews.

Annual Review of Pharmacology. Ed. by H. W. Elliott et al. LC 61-5649. Vol. 6. 1966. text 40.00 (*0-8243-0406-3*); Vol. 7. 1967. text 40.00 (*0-8243-0407-1*); Vol. 8. 1968. text 40.00 (*0-8243-0408-X*); Vol. 9. 1969. text 40.00 (*0-8243-0409-8*); Vol. 10. 1970. text 40.00 (*0-8243-0410-1*); Vol. 11. 1971. text 40.00 (*0-8243-0411-X*); Vol. 12. 1972. text 40.00 (*0-8243-0412-8*); Vol. 13. 1973. (Illus.). text 40.00 (*0-8243-0413-6*); Vol. 14. 1974. (Illus.). text 40.00 (*0-8243-0414-4*); Vol. 15. 1975. (Illus.). text 40.00 (*0-8243-0415-2*) Annual Reviews.

Annual Review of Pharmacology & Toxicology. Ed. by H. W. Elliott et al. LC 61-5649. (Illus.). Vol. 16. 1976. text 40.00 (*0-8243-0416-0*); Vol. 17. 1977. text 40.00 (*0-8243-0417-9*) Annual Reviews.

Annual Review of Pharmacology & Toxicology. Ed. by Robert George et al. Vol. 18. 1978. LC 61-5649. (Illus.). text 40.00 (*0-8243-0418-7*); Vol. 19. 1979. LC 61-5649. (Illus.). text 40.00 (*0-8243-0419-5*); Vol. 20. 1980. LC 61-5649. (Illus.). text 40.00 (*0-8243-0420-9*); Vol. 21. 1981. LC 61-5649. (Illus.). text 40.00 (*0-8243-0421-7*); Vol. 22. 1982. LC 61-5649. (Illus.). text 40.00 (*0-8243-0422-5*); Vol. 23. 1983. LC 61-5649. (Illus.). text 40.00 (*0-8243-0423-3*); Vol. 24. 1984. LC 61-5649. (Illus.). text 40.00 (*0-8243-0424-1*); Vol. 25. 1985. LC 61-5649. (Illus.). (C). text 40.00 (*0-8243-0425-X*); Vol. 26. 1986. LC 61-5649. text 40.00 (*0-8243-0426-8*); Vol. 27. 1987. LC 61-5649. (Illus.). text 40.00 (*0-8243-0427-6*); Vol. 28. 1988. LC 61-5649. (Illus.). text 40.00 (*0-8243-0428-4*); Vol. 29. 1989. (Illus.). text 40.00 (*0-8243-0429-2*); Vol. 30. 1990. LC 61-5649. text 40.00 (*0-8243-0430-6*) Annual Reviews.

Annual Review of Pharmacology & Toxicology. Ed. by Arthur K. Cho et al. LC 61-5649. Vol. 32. 1992. text 44.00 (*0-8243-0432-2*); Vol. 33. 1993. (Illus.). text 44.00 (*0-8243-0433-0*) Annual Reviews.

Annual Review of Pharmacology & Toxicology, Vol. 35. Ed. by Arthur K. Cho. 1995. LC 61-5649. (Illus.). 650p. text 47.00 (*0-8243-0435-7*) Annual Reviews.

Annual Review of Pharmacology & Toxicology, Vol. 36. Ed. by Arthur K. Cho et al. 1996. LC 61-5649. (Illus.). text 52.00 (*0-8243-0436-5*) Annual Reviews.

Annual Review of Pharmacology & Toxicology, Vol. 37. 1997. LC 61-5649. text 60.00 (*0-8243-0437-3*) Annual Reviews.

Annual Review of Pharmacology & Toxicology, Vol. 38. Ed. by Arthur K. Cho. 1998. LC 61-5649. 581p. text 60.00 (*0-8243-0438-1*) Annual Reviews.

Annual Review of Pharmacology & Toxicology, Vol. 40. 2000. text 127.00 (*0-8243-0440-3*) Annual Reviews.

Annual Review of Physical Chemistry, Vol. 36. Ed. by B. S. Rabinovitch et al. 1985. LC 51-1658. (Illus.). (C). text 44.00 (*0-8243-1036-5*) Annual Reviews.

Annual Review of Physiology. Ed. by J. H. Comroe, Jr. et al. LC 39-15404. (Illus.). Vol. 34. 1972. text 42.00 (*0-8243-0334-2*); Vol. 35. 1973. text 42.00 (*0-8243-0335-0*); Vol. 36. 1974. text 42.00 (*0-8243-0336-9*); Vol. 37. 1975. text 42.00 (*0-8243-0337-7*) Annual Reviews.

Annual Review of Physiology. Ed. by Ernst Knobil et al. LC 39-15404. (Illus.). Vol. 38. 1976. text 42.00 (*0-8243-0338-5*); Vol. 39. 1977. text 42.00 (*0-8243-0339-3*); Vol. 40. 1978. text 42.00 (*0-8243-0340-7*) Annual Reviews.

Annual Review of Physiology, Vol. 41. Ed. by I. S. Edelman et al. 1979. LC 39-15404. (Illus.). text 42.00 (*0-8243-0341-5*) Annual Reviews.

Annual Review of Physiology, Vol. 42. Ed. by Robert M. Berne & I. S. Edelman. 1980. LC 39-15404. (Illus.). 42.00 (*0-8243-0342-3*) Annual Reviews.

Annual Review of Physiology. Ed. by I. S. Edelman et al. LC 39-15404. (Illus.). Vol. 43. 1981. text 42.00 (*0-8243-0343-1*); Vol. 44. 1982. text 42.00 (*0-8243-0344-X*) Annual Reviews.

Annual Review of Physiology. Ed. by Robert M. Berne et al. LC 39-15404. (Illus.). Vol. 45. 1983. text 42.00 (*0-8243-0345-8*); Vol. 46. 1984. text 42.00 (*0-8243-0346-6*); Vol. 47. 1985. (C). text 42.00 (*0-8243-0347-4*); Vol. 48. 1986. text 42.00 (*0-8243-0348-2*); Vol. 49. 1987. text 42.00 (*0-8243-0349-0*) Annual Reviews.

Annual Review of Physiology. Ed. by Joseph F. Hoffman et al. LC 39-15404. Vol. 51. 1989. (Illus.). text 42.00 (*0-8243-0351-2*); Vol. 52. 1990. text 42.00 (*0-8243-0352-0*); Vol. 54. 1992. text 46.00 (*0-8243-0354-7*); Vol. 58. 1996. text 54.00 (*0-8243-0358-X*) Annual Reviews.

Annual Review of Physiology. Ed. by Joseph F. Hoffman. LC 39-15404. Vol. 60. 1998. 776p. text 62.00 (*0-8243-0360-1*); Vol. 61. 1999. 18p. 42.00 (*0-8243-0361-X*) Annual Reviews.

Annual Review of Physiology 1995 Vol. 57. Ed. by Joseph F. Hoffman. 1995. LC 63-8847. 800p. text 49.00 (*0-8243-0357-1*) Annual Reviews.

Annual Review of Psychology. Ed. by Calvin P. Stone et al. Vol. 4. 1953. text 40.00 (*0-8243-0204-4*); Vol. 5. 1954. text 40.00 (*0-8243-0205-2*) Annual Reviews.

Annual Review of Psychology, Vol. 8. Ed. by Paul R. Farnsworth et al. 1957. text 40.00 (*0-8243-0208-7*) Annual Reviews.

Annual Review of Psychology, Vol. 10. Ed. by Paul H. Mussen & Paul R. Farnsworth. 1959. LC 50-13143. 44.00 (*0-8243-0210-9*) Annual Reviews.

Annual Review of Psychology. Ed. by Paul H. Mussen. LC 50-13143. Vol. 22. 1971. text 40.00 (*0-8243-0222-2*); Vol. 23. 1972. text 40.00 (*0-8243-0223-0*); Vol. 24. 1973. (Illus.). text 40.00 (*0-8243-0224-9*) Annual Reviews.

Annual Review of Psychology. Ed. by Mark R. Rosenzweig. LC 50-13143. (Illus.). Vol. 26. 1975. text 40.00 (*0-8243-0226-5*); Vol. 27. 1976. text 40.00 (*0-8243-0227-3*); Vol. 28. 1977. text 40.00 (*0-8243-0228-1*); Vol. 29. 1978. text 40.00 (*0-8243-0229-X*); Vol. 30. 1979. text 40.00 (*0-8243-0230-3*); Vol. 32. 1981. text 40.00 (*0-8243-0233-8*); Vol. 34. 1983. text 40.00 (*0-8243-0234-6*) Annual Reviews.

Annual Review of Psychology, Vol. 35. Ed. by Mark R. Rosenzweig et al. 1984. LC 50-13143. (Illus.). text 40.00 (*0-8243-0235-4*) Annual Reviews.

Annual Review of Psychology. Ed. by Mark R. Rosenzweig. Vol. 36. 1985. LC 50-13143. (Illus.). text 40.00 (*0-8243-0236-2*); Vol. 37. 1986. LC 50-13143. (Illus.). text 40.00 (*0-8243-0237-0*); Vol. 39. 1988. LC 50-13143. (Illus.). text 40.00 (*0-8243-0239-7*); Vol. 40. 1989. LC 50-13143. (Illus.). text 40.00 (*0-8243-0240-0*); Vol. 41. 1990. LC 50-13143. text 40.00 (*0-8243-0241-9*); Vol. 42. 1991. LC 50-13143. text 40.00 (*0-8243-0242-7*); Vol. 43. 1992. text 43.00 (*0-8243-0243-5*) Annual Reviews.

Annual Review of Psychology, Vol. 44. Ed. by Lyman W. Porter. 1993. LC 50-13143. (Illus.). text 43.00 (*0-8243-0244-3*) Annual Reviews.

Annual Review of Psychology, Vol. 45. Ed. by Lyman W. Porter et al. 1994. LC 50-13143. (Illus.). text 46.00 (*0-8243-0245-1*) Annual Reviews.

Annual Review of Psychology, Vol. 47. Ed. by Janet T. Spense et al. 1996. (Illus.). text 48.00 (*0-8243-0247-8*) Annual Reviews.

Annual Review of Psychology, Vol. 49. Ed. by Janet T. Spence. 1998. LC 50-13143. text 55.00 (*0-8243-0249-4*) Annual Reviews.

Annual Review of Psychology Vol. 46: 1995. Ed. by Janet T. Spence. 1995. LC 50-13143. (Illus.). 650p. text 46.00 (*0-8243-0246-X*) Annual Reviews.

Annual Review of Pubic Health, Vol. 16. Ed. by Gilbert S. Omenn. 1995. text 52.00 (*0-8243-2716-0*) Annual Reviews.

Annual Review of Public Health. Ed. by Lester Breslow et al. Vol. 1. 1980. (Illus.). text 45.00 (*0-8243-2701-2*); Vol. 2. 1981. (Illus.). text 45.00 (*0-8243-2702-0*); Vol. 3. 1982. (Illus.). text 45.00 (*0-8243-2703-9*); Vol. 4. 1983. (Illus.). text 45.00 (*0-8243-2704-7*); Vol. 5. 1984. (Illus.). text 45.00 (*0-8243-2705-5*); Vol. 6. 1985. (Illus.). text 45.00 (*0-8243-2706-3*); Vol. 7. 1986. (Illus.). text 45.00 (*0-8243-2707-1*); Vol. 8. 1987. (Illus.). text 45.00 (*0-8243-2708-X*); Vol. 9. 1988. (Illus.). text 45.00 (*0-8243-2709-8*); Vol. 10. 1989. (Illus.). text 45.00 (*0-8243-2710-1*); Vol. 11. 1990. text 45.00 (*0-8243-2711-X*) Annual Reviews.

Annual Review of Public Health. Ed. by Gilbert S. Omenn et al. Vol. 12. 1991. text 45.00 (*0-8243-2712-8*); Vol. 13. 1992. text 49.00 (*0-8243-2713-6*); Vol. 14. 1993. (Illus.). text 49.00 (*0-8243-2714-4*); Vol. 15. 1994. (Illus.). text 52.00 (*0-8243-2715-2*); Vol. 17. 1996. (Illus.). text 57.00 (*0-8243-2717-9*) Annual Reviews.

Annual Review of Public Health, Vol. 19. Ed. by Jonathan E. Fielding. 1998. text 64.00 (*0-8243-2719-5*) Annual Reviews.

Annual Review of Sex Research. Ed. by John Bancroft. 1991. (C). text 45.00 (*0-9628266-0-X*) Soc Sci Study Sex.

Annual Review of Women's Health. Beverly J. McElmurry. Vol. I. 1993. 338p. pap. 38.95 (*0-88737-598-7*); Vol. II. 1995. 350p. pap. 38.95 (*0-88737-636-3*) Natl League Nurse.

Annual Review of Women's Health, Vol. III. Randy S. Parker & Beverly J. McElmurry. 1996. 350p. pap. 38.95 (*0-88737-672-X*) Natl League Nurse.

Annual Statement Diskette Filing Specifications - Health Maintenance Organizations. (Annual Ser.). (C). 1995. ring bd. 100.00 (*0-89382-344-9*); 1994. 136p. ring bd. 100.00 (*0-89382-286-8*) Nat Assn Insurance.

Annual Statement Diskette Filing Specifications - Hospital, Medical, Dental Service & Indemnity Corporation. 1994. 286p. (C). ring bd. 100.00 (*0-89382-287-6*) Nat Assn Insurance.

Annual Statement Diskette Filing Specifications for Health Maintenance Organization. 1992. 90p. (C). ring bd. 100.00 (*0-89382-207-8*) Nat Assn Insurance.

Annual Statement Diskette Filing Specifications for Life Insurers. 1992. 430p. (C). ring bd. 100.00 (*0-89382-204-3*) Nat Assn Insurance.

Annual Statement Instructions: Health for 2001. Ed. by Jean Buckley. 2000. 322p. ring bd. 175.00 (*0-89382-679-0*, ASI-HEA00) Nat Assn Insurance.

Annual Statement Instructions: Health Maintenance Organizations. Ed. by Jean Buckley. 1998. 210p. pap. 150.00 (*0-89382-553-0*, ASI-HU98) Nat Assn Insurance.

Annual Statement Instructions: Hospital, Medical, Dental & Indemnity Corporations. Ed. by Jean Buckley. rev. ed. 256p. 1999. ring bd. 150.00 (*0-89382-622-7*, ASI-MU99); 1998. ring bd. 150.00 (*0-89382-554-9*, ASI-MU98) Nat Assn Insurance.

Annual Statement Instructions - Health Maintenance Organizations. 1994. 77p. (C). ring bd. 150.00 (*0-89382-279-5*) Nat Assn Insurance.

Annual Statement Instructions - Hospital, Medical, Dental Service or Indemnity Corporations. 1994. 157p. (C). ring bd. 50.00 (*0-89382-280-9*) Nat Assn Insurance.

Annual Statement Instructions - Life, Accident & Health Insurance. 1994. 317p. (C). ring bd. 150.00 (*0-89382-276-0*) Nat Assn Insurance.

Annual Statement Instructions - Limited Health Services Organization. 1994. 58p. (C). ring bd. 50.00 (*0-89382-281-7*) Nat Assn Insurance.

Annual Statement Instructions Diskette Filing Specifications - Hospital, Medical & Dental Services & Indemnity Corporations. 1995. (Annual Ser.). (C). ring bd. 100.00 (*0-89382-345-7*) Nat Assn Insurance.

Annual Statement Instructions for Health Maintenance Organization. 1995. (Annual Ser.). 106p. (C). ring bd. 150.00 (*0-89382-334-1*) Nat Assn Insurance.

Annual Statement Instructions for Hospital, Medical & Dental Services & Indemnity Corporations. 1995. (Annual Ser.). 184p. (C). ring bd. 50.00 (*0-89382-335-X*) Nat Assn Insurance.

Annual Statement Instructions for Limited Health Services Organizations. (Annual Ser.). (C). 1995. 84p. ring bd. 50.00 (*0-89382-336-8*); 1994. ring bd. 50.00 (*0-89382-288-4*) Nat Assn Insurance.

Annual Statement Instructions Health Maintenance Organizations. 1993. 69p. ring bd. 150.00 (*0-89382-239-6*); 1992. 57p. (C). ring bd. 50.00 (*0-89382-195-0*) Nat Assn Insurance.

Annual Statement Instructions Limited Health Service Organizations. 1993. 58p. ring bd. 50.00 (*0-89382-241-8*); 1992. 53p. (C). ring bd. 50.00 (*0-89382-193-4*) Nat Assn Insurance.

Annual Statements Instructions: Limited Health Services Organizations. Ed. by Jean Buckley. rev. ed. 1999. 184p. ring bd. 150.00 (*0-89382-624-3*, ASI-SU99) Nat Assn Insurance.

Annual 20, Side Effects Drugs, 1997, Vol. 20. Ed. by J. K. Aronson. 1997. 524p. 204.50 (*0-444-82532-0*, North Holland) Elsevier.

Anomalies of Binocular Vision: Diagnosis & Management. Rutstein & Kent Michael Daum. 1997. LC 97-14847. (Illus.). 384p. (C). (gr. 13). text 64.95 (*0-8016-6916-2*, 06916) Mosby Inc.

Anomalies of the Fetal Head, Neck & Neural Axis: Ultrasound Diagnosis & Management. Frank A. Chervenak et al. 1988. (Illus.). 192p. text 98.00 (*0-7216-1957-6*) Saunders.

Anomalistic Psychology: A Study of Magical Thinking. Ed. by Leonard Zusne & Warren Jones. 2nd ed. 1989. 328p. (C). pap. 36.00 (*0-8058-0508-7*); text 69.95 (*0-8058-0507-9*) L Erlbaum Assocs.

Anomia: Neuroanatomical & Cognitive Correlates. Ed. by Harold Goodglass & Arthur Wingfield. 1997. LC 96-49185. (Foundations of Neuropsychology Ser.). (Illus.). 224p. text 59.95 (*0-12-289685-8*) Morgan Kaufmann.

Anonymi Medici: Edited with Translation & Introduction. Ivan Garofalo. Tr. by Brian Fuchs. 1996. LC 97-141934. (Studies in Ancient Medicine: No. 12). xxx, 375p. 155.50 (*90-04-10227-2*) Brill Academic Pubs.

Anorectal Disease in AIDS. 208p. (*0-340-54643-3*) E A GBR. *Dist:* Routldge.

Anorectal Malformations: A Surgeon's Experience. Subir K. Chatterjee. 1993. LC 93-5318. (Illus.). 228p. text 48.95 (*0-19-262453-9*) OUP.

Anorectal, Presacral & Sacral Tumors: Anatomy, Physiology, Pathogenesis & Management. S. Arthur Localio et al. 1987. (Illus.). 378p. text 135.00 (*0-7216-1982-7*) Saunders.

***Anorexia & Bulimia.** Alison Cotter. 2001. LC 00-12858. (Diseases & Disorders Ser.). (Illus.). (J). 27.45 (*1-56006-725-X*, Lucent Books) Gale.

Anorexia & Bulimia Nervosa: How to Help. Roger H. Slade. 1988. 256p. pap. (*0-335-09832-0*) OpUniv Pr.

Anorexia, Murder & Suicide. Malan. 2000. LC 97-29372. 224p. pap. (*0-7506-3003-5*) E A GBR. *Dist:* OUP.

Anorexia Nervosa. Ed. by H. Remschmidt & M. H. Schmidt. 1990. LC 90-4848. (Child & Youth Psychiatry: European Perspectives Ser.: Vol. 1). (Illus.). 200p. text 64.00 (*0-88937-041-9*) Hogrefe & Huber Pubs.

Anorexia Nervosa. Helmut Thoma. 1967. LC 67-27020. 342p. 55.00 (*0-8236-0360-1*) Intl Univs Pr.

Anorexia Nervosa: A Clinician's Guide to Treatment. Walter Vandereycken & Rolf Meermann. 1984. LC 84-72039. xiv, 252p. 79.25 (*3-11-009531-9*) De Gruyter.

Anorexia Nervosa: A Guide to Recovery. Lindsey Hall & Monika Ostroff. 1998. LC 98-29374. 187p. pap. 13.95 (*0-936077-32-8*) Gurze Bks.

Anorexia Nervosa: A Survival Guide for Families, Friends & Sufferers. Janet Treasure. 1997. LC 98-113586. 160p. pap. text 15.95 (*0-86377-760-0*) L Erlbaum Assocs.

Anorexia Nervosa: Starving for Attention. Dan Harmon. Ed. by Carol C. Nadelson. 1998. LC 98-25197. (Encyclopedia of Psychological Disorders Ser.). 144p. (gr. 7-12). 22.95 (*0-7910-4901-9*) Chelsea Hse.

Anorexia Nervosa: The Historical & Cultural Specificity. S. E. Van't Hof. 1994. 284p. pap. (*90-265-1424-7*) Swets.

Anorexia Nervosa: When Food Is the Enemy. Erica Smith. 1999. (Teen Eating Disorder Prevention Library). 64p. (YA). (gr. 3-10). pap. 6.95 (*1-56838-256-1*) Hazelden.

Anorexia Nervosa - Bulimia: A Source Guide. 1991. lib. bdg. 250.00 (*0-8490-4886-9*) Gordon Pr.

Anorexia Nervosa: A Guide to Recovery see Como Entender y Superar la Anorexia Nervosa

Anorexia Nervosa & Bulimia: An Annotated Bibliography. Izabella Taler. 1985. LC 85-14963. (CompuBibs Ser.: No. 13). 65p. pap. 15.00 (*0-914791-12-5*) Vantage Info.

Anorexia Nervosa & Recovery: A Hunger for Meaning. Karen Way. 1993. (Haworth Women's Studies). LC 91-22225. 146p. pap. 14.95 (*0-918393-95-7*, Harrington Park); LC 91-23995. 150p. lib. bdg. 39.95 (*1-56024-130-6*) Haworth Pr.

Anorexics on Anorexia. Ed. by Rosemary Shelley. 1997. LC 97-197988. 172p. pap. (*1-85302-471-6*) Jessica Kingsley GBR. *Dist:* Taylor & Francis.

Anorganisch-Chemische Praparate: Darstellung und Charakterisierung Ausgewahlter Vernindungen. Alfred Golloch et al. 1985. (GER., Illus.). xvi, 324p. 60.00 (*3-11-004821-3*) De Gruyter.

Another Day. Pat Seed. 1983. 100p. 9.95 (*0-434-67862-7*); pap. 8.50 (*0-434-68533-X*) Trafalgar.

Another Dimension to the Black Diaspora: Diet, Disease, & Racism. Kenneth F. Kiple & Virginia H. King. 1981. LC 81-7696. (Illus.). 314p. text 54.95 (*0-521-23664-9*) Cambridge U Pr.

Another Silenced Trauma: Twelve Feminist Therapists & Activists Respond to One Woman's Recovery from War. Ed. by Esther D. Rothblum & Ellen Cole. 1986. LC 86-9481. 124p. pap. 9.95 (*0-918393-29-9*, Harrington Park) Haworth Pr.

Ansiotensin in Receptors, Vol. 1. Ed. by Robert R. Ruffolo. 1994. 192p. 130.00 (*0-8493-8380-3*) CRC Pr.

Anson-Donaldson Surgical Anatomy of the Temporal Bone. James A. Donaldson et al. 4th ed. 1992. 576p. text 165.00 (*0-88167-915-1*, 2393) Lppncott W & W.

Answer in the Heart: Daily Meditations. Hazelden. 1995. (Hazelden Meditation Ser.). 400p. pap. text 11.00 (*0-89486-568-4*) Hazelden.

Answer Is at School: Bringing Health Care to Our Students. Illus. by Linda Bleck. 1993. 36p. (Orig.). pap. (*0-942054-07-5*) R W Johnson Found.

Answer to Job. Carl Gustav Jung. Tr. by R. F. C. Hull. 1973. (Bollingen Ser.: No. 283). 137p. pap. 12.95 (*0-691-01785-9*) Princeton U Pr.

Answer Within: A Clinical Framework of Ericksonian Hypnotherapy. Stephen R. Lankton & Carol H. Lankton. 1988. LC 82-20637. 392p. text 35.95 (*0-87630-320-3*) Brunner-Routledge.

Answering Your Questions about AIDS. Seth C. Kalichman. 1996. LC 96-4253. 273p. pap. 9.95 (*1-55798-339-9*, 4316680) Am Psychol.

Answers & Rationales for 1997 Assessment Test: Unsecured. Delores F. Saxton. 1996. 48p. (C). (gr. 13). pap. text (*0-8151-8677-0*, 28968) Mosby Inc.

Answers & Rationales for 1997 Assessment Test Secured. Delores F. Saxton. 1997. 48p. (C). (gr. 13). text (*0-8151-8676-2*, 28967) Mosby Inc.

Answers & Rationales for 1998 Assessment Test: Unsecured. Delores F. Saxton. 1997. 48p. (C). (gr. 13). pap. text (*0-8151-8678-9*, 28969) Mosby Inc.

Answers from the Family Doctor: Three Hundred Fifty Questions Patients Ask Most. Allan H. Bruckheim. 1994. LC 93-37715. 384p. pap. 12.95 (*1-56943-006-3*) NTC Contemp Pub Co.

Answers to Distraction. Edward M. Hallowell & John J. Ratey. 1996. LC 95-31278. 352p. pap. 13.95 (*0-553-37821-X*) Bantam.

Answers to Iridiagnosis Questions. Frederick W. Collins. 1993. 12p. reprint ed. spiral bd. (*0-7873-1180-4*) Hlth Research.

Answers to My Jehovah's Witness Friends. Thomas F. Heinze. 2000. 124p. pap. 5.95 (*0-937958-58-1*) Chick Pubns.

Answers to 10 Top Health Challenges: A Simple & Natural Approach to Prevention & Healing of High Blood Pressure, Heart Attacks & Strokes, Etc. Sheryl Simpson. Ed. by Carol Adler. unabr. ed. 1997. 230p. pap. 19.95 (*1-890243-07-8*) Trineurogenics.

Answers to the 50 Most Important Questions about Private Mental Health Practice. Bruce D. Forman & Wade H. Silverman. 1998. LC 98-8151. 94p. pap. text 16.95 (*0-398-06887-9*) C C Thomas.

Antacids & Anti-Reflux Agents. Ed. by Neena Washington. 1991. 320p. lib. bdg. 169.00 (*0-8493-5444-7*, RM365) CRC Pr.

Antecedent Control: Innovative Approaches to Behavioral Support. Ed. by James K. Luiselli & Michael J. Cameron. 1998. LC 98-19004. 416p. pap. 40.00 (*1-55766-334-3*, 3343) P H Brookes.

Antenatal Care. Ed. by Jo Alexander et al. 1994. 270p. pap. text 16.95 (*0-8020-7447-2*) U of Toronto Pr.

Antenatal Care Assessed: A Case Study of an Innovation in Aberdeen. M. Hall et al. 1985. (Illus.). 188p. text (*0-08-032427-4*) Aberdeen U Pr GBR. *Dist:* Macmillan.

Antenatal Fetal Assessment. Maureen Boyle. 1997. LC 97-178336. (Geological Society Miscellaneous Paper Ser.: Vol. 4). 80p. text 19.95 (*1-898507-25-2*) Buttrwrth-Heinemann.

Antenatal Investigations. Maureen Boyle. 1994. LC 94-219013. (Midwifery Practice Guides Ser.: No. 2). 61p. pap. text 12.50 (*1-898507-04-X*) Buttrwrth-Heinemann.

Antenatal Testing Handbook: The Complete Guide to Testing in Pregnancy. Vivienne Parry. 1998. 232p. pap. text 12.00 (*0-7881-5808-2*) DIANE Pub.

Antennas & Reaction Centers of Photosynthetic Bacteria: Structure, Interactions & Dynamics. Ed. by M. E. Michel-Beyerle. 1985. (Chemical Physics Ser.: Vol. 42). (Illus.). 367p. 74.95 (*0-387-16154-6*) Spr-Verlag.

Antepartal & Intrapartal Fetal Monitoring. Michelle L. Murray. 2nd rev. ed. 1996. (Illus.). 538p. otabind 78.00 (*0-942835-01-8*) Lrning Res Intl.

Anterior Approaches to the Spine. Ed. by Thomas A. Zdeblick. 1998. LC 98-36646. (Illus.). 291p. 145.00 (*1-57626-001-1*) Quality Med Pub.

Anterior Cervical Diskectomy. Oliver D. Grin & Dorothy L. Bouwman. 1990. (Patient Education Ser.). (Illus.). 18p. (Orig.). pap. text 3.50 (*0-929689-45-3*) Ludann Co.

Anterior Cruciate Ligament: Current & Future Concepts. Ed. by Douglas W. Jackson. 1993. LC 93-18586. 480p. text 149.00 (*0-7817-0039-6*) Lppncott W & W.

Anterior Ischemic Optic Neuropathy. S. S. Hayreh. 1975. LC 74-23702. (Illus.). 160p. 78.95 (*0-387-06916-X*) Spr-Verlag.

Anterior Segment & Strabismus Surgery: Proceedings of the 44th Annual Symposium, New Orleans, LA, U. S. A., February 9-12, 1995. Ed. by D. A. Long. 1996. LC 96-1883. (*90-6299-134-3*) Kugler NLD. *Dist:* Lib Res.

Anterior Segment Disease: Diagnostic Color Atlas. S. Arthur Boruchoff. 2000. LC 00-58663. (Illus.). 288p. text 125.00 (*0-7506-7181-5*) Buttrwrth-Heinemann.

Anterior Segment Repair & Reconstruction: Techniques & Medico-Legal Issues Techniques & Medico-Legal Issues. Bruce Noble & Ian Simmons. 2001. LC 2001-43646. (Illus.). 192p. 125.00 (*0-7506-4573-3*) Buttrwrth-Heinemann.

Anthology on Caring. Ed. by Peggy L. Chinn. 1991. 353p. pap. 34.95 (*0-88737-516-2*) Natl League Nurse.

Anthony: Anatomy & Physiology Lab Manual, No. 13 SE. Gary A. Thibodeau. 13th ed. 1989. 304p. pap. text 16.95 (*0-8016-6235-4*) Mosby Inc.

Anthony's Text of Anatomy & Physiology. Gary A. Thibodeau & Kevin T. Patton. 14th ed. 1993. (Illus.). 1008p. (C). (gr. 13). text 56.95 (*0-8016-7671-1*, 07671) Mosby Inc.

Anthony's Textbook of Anatomy & Physiology. Kevin T. Patton & Gary A. Thibodeau. 16th ed. 1999. (Illus.). 1200p. 57.00 (*0-323-00204-8*) Mosby Inc.

Anthracycline Antibiotics: New Analogues, Methods of Delivery & Mechanisms of Actions, Vol. 57. Ed. by Waldemar Priebe. 1995. LC 94-38929. (ACS Symposium Ser.: No. 574). (Illus.). 380p. 115.00 (*0-8412-3040-4*) Am Chemical.

Anthracycline Antibiotics in Cancer Therapy. Franco M. Muggia et al. 1982. text 226.00 (*90-247-2711-1*) Kluwer Academic.

Anthraquinone Laxatives: Proceedings of the Symposium, Bissone (Lugano), Switzerland, Sept. 1975. Symposium, Bissone Switzerland Staff. Ed. by J. W. Fairbairn. 1976. (Pharmacology Ser.: Vol. 14, Suppl. 1). (Illus.). pap. 39.25 (*3-8055-2426-9*) S Karger.

***Anthrax Immunization Program: Congressional Hearing.** Christopher Shays. 2001. 124p. reprint ed. pap. text 30.00 (*0-7567-1809-0*) DIANE Pub.

Anthropological Approaches to Diabetes: A Special Issue to the Journal of Medical Anthropology. Ed. by M. L. Urdaneta & R. Krehbiel. 1989. 130p. pap. text 44.00 (*2-88124-346-0*) Gordon & Breach.

Anthropological Approaches to the Study of Ethnomedicine, Vol. 2. Ed. by Mark Nichter. 1992. LC 92-20369. 260p. text 85.00 (*2-88124-530-7*); pap. text 36.00 (*2-88124-529-3*) Gordon & Breach.

Anthropological Legal, & Medical Studies on Pederasty in Europe. Veniamin M. Tarnovskii. LC 78-22239. (Gay Experience Ser.). reprint ed. 32.50 (*0-404-61530-9*) AMS Pr.

Anthropological Structure of Madness in Black Africa. I. Sow. Tr. by Joyce Diamonti from FRE. 1980. LC 80-13909. 248p. 37.50 (*0-8236-0385-7*) Intl Univs Pr.

Anthropological Studies in the Strange Sexual Practices of All Races in All Ages, Ancient & Modern, Oriental & Occidental, Primitive & Civilized. Iwan Bloch. Tr. by Keene Wallis from GER. LC 72-9615. reprint ed. 39.50 (*0-404-57410-6*) AMS Pr.

Anthropology & Epidemiology. Ed. by Craig R. Janes et al. 1986. pap. text 68.50 (*90-277-2249-8*); lib. bdg. 152.00 (*90-277-2248-X*) Kluwer Academic.

Anthropology & Homosexual Behavior. Evelyn Blackwood et al. 1986. LC 85-17758. (Journal of Homosexuality Ser.: Vol. 11, No. 3-4). 217p. 6.95 (*0-86656-328-8*); text 19.95 (*0-86656-420-9*) Haworth Pr.

Anthropology & Psychoanalysis: An Encounter Through Culture. Ed. by Suzette Heald & Ariane Deluz. 1994. LC 93-44324. 256p. (C). pap. 31.95 (*0-415-09743-6*, B3968) Routledge.

Anthropology in Public Health: Bridging Differences in Culture & Society. Ed. by Robert A. Hahn. 1999. LC 98-34571. (Illus.). 408p. text 65.00 (*0-19-512902-4*); pap. text 32.95 (*0-19-511955-X*) OUP.

Anthropology of Aging: A Partially Annotated Bibliography, 13. Ed. by Marjorie M. Schweitzer. 1991. LC 91-9707. (Bibliographies & Indexes in Gerontology Ser.: No. 13). 360p. lib. bdg. 78.50 (*0-313-26119-9*, SWZ/, Greenwood Pr) Greenwood.

Anthropology of Community Care. Ed. by Iain Edgar & Andrew Russell. 1998. LC 97-49568. (Illus.). 288p. (C). 90.00 (*0-415-16964-X*) Routledge.

Anthropology of Infectious Disease: International Health Perspectives. Marcia C. Inhorn & Peter J. Brown. 1998. 512p. pap. text (*90-5699-556-1*) GBSP NLD. *Dist:* Gordon & Breach.

Anthropology of Infectious Disease: International Health Perspectives. Ed. by Marcia C. Inhorn & Peter J. Brown. 1998. (Theory & Practice in Medical Anthropology & International Health Ser.). 512p. text (*90-5699-555-3*) GBSP NLD. *Dist:* Gordon & Breach.

Anthropology of Medicine: From Culture to Method. Daniel R. Moerman & Lola E. Romanucci-Ross. 1985. (Illus.). 416p. (C). text 44.95 (*0-03-062192-5*, Bergin & Garvey) Greenwood.

Anthropology of Medicine: From Culture to Method. Ed. by Lola E. Romanucci-Ross et al. 3rd ed. 1997. LC 96-53993. 416p. pap. 35.00 (*0-89789-516-9*, Bergin & Garvey) Greenwood.

Anthropology of Medicine: From Culture to Method. Ed. by Lola E. Romanucci-Ross & Daniel R. Moerman. 3rd ed. 1997. LC 96-53993. 416p. 90.00 (*0-89789-490-1*, Bergin & Garvey) Greenwood.

Anthropology of Minority Groups: Index of New Information with Authors & Subjects. American Health Research Institute Staff. rev. ed. 1994. LC 94-24771. 151p. 57.50 (*0-7883-0268-X*) ABBE Pubs Assn.

Anthropology of Pregnancy Loss: Comparative Studies in Miscarriage, Stillbirth & Neo-natal Death. Ed. by Rosanne Cecil. 1996. 226p. LC 96-9158. (*1-85973-120-1*); pap. (*1-85973-125-2*) Berg Pubs GBR. *Dist:* NYU Pr.

Anthropology of Self & Behavior. Gerald M. Erchak. 1992. LC 91-19666. 200p. (C). text 34.00 (*0-8135-1761-3*); pap. text 17.00 (*0-8135-1762-1*) Rutgers U Pr.

Anthropometric Facial Proportions in Medicine. Leslie G. Farkas & Ian R. Munro. 1987. (Illus.). 368p. (C). 98.95 (*0-398-05261-1*) C C Thomas.

Anthropometric Standards for the Assessment of Growth & Nutritional Status. A. Roberto Frisancho. 1990. LC 89-20695. 200p. text 85.00 (*0-472-10146-3*, 10146) U of Mich Pr.

Anthropometric Study of Hawaiians of Pure & Mixed Blood. L. C. Dunn. Ed. by Alfred M. Tozzer. 1928. (HU PMP Ser.). pap. 15.00 (*0-527-01220-3*) Periodicals Srv.

Anthropometry of the American Negro. Melville Jean Herskovits. LC 76-82369. (Columbia University. Contributions to Anthropology Ser.: No. 11). reprint ed. 32.50 (*0-404-50561-9*) AMS Pr.

Anthropometry of the American Negro. Melville Jean Herskovits. 1970. LC 73-121370. (Studies in Black History & Culture: No. 54). reprint ed. lib. bdg. 62.95 (*0-8383-1116-4*) M S G Haskell Hse.

Anthropometry of the Head & Face. Ed. by Leslie G. Farkas. 2nd ed. 1994. 432p. LC 94-991. 145.00 (*0-7817-0519-3*); text 159.00 (*0-7817-0159-7*) Lppncott W & W.

Anthropometry of the Natives of Arnhem Land & the Australian Race Problem. W. W. Howells. 1937. (HU PMP Ser.). pap. 25.00 (*0-527-01236-X*) Periodicals Srv.

Anthroposophic Medicine Today. Richard Leviton. 1988. 40p. pap. 5.95 (*0-88010-265-9*) Anthroposophic.

Anthroposophical Approach to Medicine, Vol. 1. Friedrich Husemann et al. 1983. (Illus.). 411p. 39.95 (*0-88010-031-1*) Anthroposophic.

Anthroposophical Approach to Medicine: An Outline of a Spiritual Scientifically Oriented Medicine, Vol. 2. Ed. by Otto Wolff. Tr. by G. Karnow from GER. 1987.Tr. of Bild des Menschen als Grundlage der Heilkunst. 39.95 (*0-88010-174-1*) Anthroposophic.

Anti-Aging for Dogs. Steve Duno. Ed. by John M. Simon. 1998. LC 98-22879. 224p. pap. 16.95 (*0-312-19060-3*) St Martin.

Anti-Aging Hormones: That Help You Beat the Clock. Ruth Winter. 1997. LC 97-12228. 304p. pap. 12.95 (*0-609-80015-9*, Chatham River Pr) Random Hse Value.

Anti-Aging Pills, I. Q. & Memory Boosters: Life Extension Innovations for a Healthier Longer Life. A. Glenn Braswell. 1993. 335p. 29.95 (*1-883201-00-4*) Hlth Quest.

Anti-Aging Plan: The Complete Guide to Natural Alternatives. Mario Kyriazis. 2000. (Illus.). 224p. pap. 16.95 (*1-86204-704-9*) Element MA.

Anti-Aging Secrets & Strategies. 1993. 176p. (Orig.). pap. 14.95 (*1-57327-015-6*, M Pr CA) Busn Concepts.

Anti-AIDS Drug Development: Challenges, Strategies & Prospects. Ed. by Prem Mohan. 1995. LC 96-139395. 304p. text 94.00 (*3-7186-5698-1*, Harwood Acad Pubs) Gordon & Breach.

Anti-Arthritis Diet: Increase Mobility & Reduce Your Pain with This 28-Day Life Changing Program. J. Kandel & D. Suddereth. 1998. LC 98-4604. 288p. pap. 16.00 (*0-7615-1260-8*, Prima Health) Prima Pub.

Anti-Cancer Cooking. 1992. lib. bdg. 88.00 (*0-8490-5361-7*) Gordon Pr.

***Anti-Cancer Drug Development.** Bruce C. Baguley. 2001. 397p. 99.95 (*0-12-072651-3*) Acad Pr.

Anti-Depressants in America - Therapeutic Use & Effects: Index of New Information. Jenette S. Pritchard. Date not set. 160p. 57.50 (*0-7883-1884-5*); pap. 47.50 (*0-7883-1885-3*) ABBE Pubs Assn.

Anti-Diabetic Agents, Vol. 27. Ed. by Urs Meyer et al. 1996. (Illus.). 240p. text 80.00 (*0-12-013327-X*) Acad Pr.

Anti-DNA Antibodies in SLE. Ed. by Edward W. Voss. 1987. 208p. 117.00 (*0-8493-6494-9*, RC924, CRC Reprint) Franklin.

Anti-Freud: Karl Kraus's Criticism of Psychoanalysis & Psychiatry. Thomas Szasz. 1990. Orig. Title: Karl Kraus & the Soul Doctors. 180p. reprint ed. pap. 17.95 (*0-8156-0247-2*) Syracuse U Pr.

Anti-Group: Destructive Forces in the Group & Their Creative Potential. Morris Nitsun. 2nd ed. 1996. LC 95-35988. (International Library of Philosophy, Psychology, & Scientific Method). 336p. (C). 89.95 (*0-415-10210-3*); pap. 31.95 (*0-415-10211-1*) Routledge.

Anti-Herpes Virus Chemotherapy: Experimental & Clinical Aspects. Ed. by K. K. Gauri. 1979. (Advances in Ophthalmology Ser.: Vol. 38). (Illus.). 129.75 (*3-8055-2991-0*) S Karger.

Anti-Idiotypic Antibodies As Vaccines. Kennedy. 1992. (*0-8493-5895-7*) CRC Pr.

Anti-Idiotypic Vaccines. Ed. by Gursaran P. Talwar. 1990. (Progress in Vaccinology Ser.: Vol. 3). (Illus.). 139p. 175.00 (*0-387-97142-4*) Spr-Verlag.

Anti-Infective Applications of Interferon-Gamma. Ed. by Bucalo S. Jaffe. 1992. (Illus.). 334p. text 189.00 (*0-8247-8688-2*) Dekker.

Anti-Infective Markets: Manufacturers Build Resistance Against Generic Competition & Evolving Microbials. Market Intelligence Staff. 1993. 229p. 1995.00 (*1-56753-494-5*) Frost & Sullivan.

Anti-Infectives: Recent Advances in Chemistry & Structure Activity Relationships. Ed. by P. H. Bentley & P. J. O'Hanlon. 1997. (Special Publications: No. 198). 350p. (C). (*0-85404-707-7*) Royal Soc Chem GBR. *Dist:* Spr-Verlag.

Anti-Inflammatory & Anti-Rheumatic Drugs: Anti-Rheumatic Drugs, Experimental Agents, & Clinical Aspects of Drug Use, Vol. III. Ed. by Kim D. Rainsford. 1985. 264p. 148.00 (*0-8493-6232-6*, RB405, CRC Reprint) Franklin.

Anti-Inflammatory & Anti-Rheumatic Drugs Vol. 1: Inflammation Mechanisms & Actions of Traditional Drugs. Ed. by Kim D. Rainsford. 1985. 208p. 119.00 (*0-8493-6230-X*, RM405, CRC Reprint) Franklin.

Anti-Inflammatory Drug Discovery: Novel Approaches for Therapeutic Development. Ed. by Ann Parkinson. 1997. (Biomedical Library). pap. (*1-57936-024-6*) Drug & Market Dev.

Anti-Inflammatory Drugs. Ed. by J. R. Vane & S. H. Ferreira. 1978. LC 78-1606. (Handbook of Experimental Pharmacology Ser.: Vol. 50, Pt. 2). (Illus.). 952p. 234.00 (*0-387-08640-4*) Spr-Verlag.

Anti-Inflammatory Drugs from Plant & Marine Sources. D. A. Lewis. 1989. (Agents & Actions Supplements Ser.: No. 27). 371p. 107.00 (*0-8176-2265-9*) Birkhauser.

Anti-Inflammatory Drugs in Asthma. Anthony P. Sampson & Martin K. Church. 1999. LC 99-10223. (Progress in Inflammation Research Ser.). viii, 276p. (*0-8176-5873-4*); 250p. 155.00 (*3-7643-5873-4*) Birkhauser.

Anti-Inflammatory Therapeutics: Development of New Therapeutic Approaches & Worldwide Market Opportunities. George B. Zavoico. Ed. by Susan C. DiClemente. 1997. (Illus.). 575p. spiral bd. (*1-57936-063-7*, 914) Drug & Market Dev.

Anti-Inflammatory Therapy, Bk. 3. John A. Mills. 1977. (Illus.). pap. text 16.50 (*0-89147-051-4*) CAS.

Anti-Judaism: A Psychohistory. Ernest A. Rappaport. 1976. LC 75-36297. 312p. 12.50 (*0-9603382-0-9*) Perspective Chicago.

Anti-Membrane Receptor Antibodies in Cardiac Disease. Leonar Sterin-Borda. 1997. (Medical Intelligence Unit Ser.). 250p. 89.95 (*0-412-13101-3*) Chapman & Hall.

Anti-Oxidants: Index of National & International Research Developments with Authors, Subjects & Bibliography. American Health Research Institute Staff. 1993. 180p. 47.50 (*1-55914-778-4*); pap. 44.50 (*1-55914-779-2*) ABBE Pubs Assn.

Anti-Oxidants & Effects on Longevity: Index of New Information with Authors, Subjects, & Bibliography. American Health Research Institute Staff. rev. ed. 1994. LC 94-35129. 171p. 57.50 (*0-7883-0266-3*); pap. 47.50 (*0-7883-0267-1*) ABBE Pubs Assn.

Anti-Oxidants & Toxicity Research Studies: Index of New Information with Authors, Subjects & Bibliography. American Health Research Institute Staff. 1993. 180p. 47.50 (*1-55914-782-2*); pap. 44.50 (*1-55914-783-0*) ABBE Pubs Assn.

Anti-Rheumatic Drugs, 3. E. C. Huskisson. 1983. (Clinical Pharmacology & Therapeutics Ser.). 776p. 132.50 (*0-275-91397-X*, C1397, Praeger Pubs) Greenwood.

Anti-Semitic Stereotypes: A Paradigm of Otherness in English Popular Culture, 1660-1830. Frank Felsenstein. 1999. (Johns Hopkins Jewish Studies). (Illus.). 374p. pap. text 19.95 (*0-8018-6179-9*) Johns Hopkins.

Anti-Stress Workbook. Barbara North & Penelope Crittenden. 1980. (Illus.). 79p. (Orig.). pap. 4.95 (*0-938480-00-6*) Healthworks.

Anti-Trust Law: A Guide for the Healthcare Professional. Jonathan P. Tomes. 1993. LC 92-35486. 90p. (Orig.). per. 24.95 (*1-882198-02-6*) Hlthcare Fin Mgmt.

***Anti-Tuberculosis Drug Resistance in the World.** World Health Organisation Staff. 2001. (*0-11-986243-3*) Statnry Office GBR. *Dist:* Balogh.

Anti-Viral Agents in Chronic Hepatitis B Virus Infection: Proceedings of an International Symposium, the Royal Society, London, UK, 11-12 Nov., 1985. Ed. by G. J. Alexander et al. 1987. 318p. 106.50 (*0-444-80901-5*) Elsevier.

Antiandrogen-Estrogen Therapy in Signs of Androgenization. Ed. by A. E. Schindler. 1987. (New Developments in Biosciences Ser.: No. 3). 244p. (C). pap. text 79.25 (*3-11-011402-X*) De Gruyter.

Antiandrogens in Prostate Cancer. Ed. by L. Denis & U. Veronesi. 1996. LC 95-45831. (ESO Monographs). (Illus.). 120p. 102.00 (*3-540-60599-1*) Spr-Verlag.

Antiangiogenic Agents in Cancer Therapy. Beverly A. Teicher. 1998. LC 98-45812. (Cancer Drug Discovery & Development Ser.: Vol. 3). (Illus.). 464p. 175.00 (*0-89603-641-3*) Humana.

Antiarrhythmic Agents Pocket Professor, No. 2. Henry J. Marriott. 1991. (YA). (gr. 13 up). text 16.95 (*0-944132-48-0*) Mosby Inc.

Antiarrhythmic Drugs. Ed. by E. M. Williams & T. J. Campbell. 1988. (Handbook of Experimental Pharmacology Ser.: Vol. 89). (Illus.). 650p. 377.00 (*0-387-19239-5*) Spr-Verlag.

Antiarrhythmic Drugs: A Practical Guide. Richard N. Fogoros. 1997. (Illus.). 168p. (Orig.). pap. 51.95 (*0-86542-532-9*) Blackwell Sci.

Antiarrhythmic Drugs: Mechanisms of Antiarrhythmic & Proarrhythmic Actions. Ed. by G. Breithardt et al. 1995. (*0-387-59254-7*); (Illus.). 410p. 99.00 (*3-540-59254-7*) Spr-Verlag.

Antiarrhythmic Therapy: A Pathophysiologic Approach. Sicilian Gambit Staff. 1994. LC 94-13905. (Illus.). 352p. 65.00 (*0-87993-596-0*) Futura Pub.

Antibacterial Therapy: Achievements, Problems & Future Perspectives. Ed. by W. D. Busse et al. 1997. LC 97-22632. (Illus.). 77p. pap. 64.95 (*3-540-62896-7*) Spr-Verlag.

Antibiosis & Host Immunity. Ed. by Andor Szentivanyi et al. 1987. LC 87-18514. (Illus.). 324p. 75.00 (*0-306-42600-5*, Plenum Trade) Perseus Pubng.

Antibiotic - Antimicrobial Use in Dental Practice. Michael G. Newman & Kenneth G. Kornman. 1990. LC 90-9099. (Illus.). 260p. pap. text 32.00 (*0-86715-172-2*) Quint Pub Co.

Antibiotic & Chemotherapy. Ed. by Harold P. Lambert & Francis O'Grady. 6th ed. 1991. (Illus.). 561p. text (*0-443-03203-3*) Church.

Antibiotic Associated Diarrhoea & Colitis. Ed. by S. P. Borriello. 1984. (Developments in Gastroenterology Ser.). 188p. text 122.00 (*0-89838-623-3*) Kluwer Academic.

Antibiotic Inhibitors of Bacterial Cell Wall Biosynthesis. D. J. Tipper. 2nd ed. 1988. LC 87-21572. (International Encyclopedia of Pharmacology & Therapeutics Ser.: No. 127). (Illus.). 277p. 203.00 (*0-08-036130-7*, Pergamon Pr) Elsevier.

Antibiotic Paradox: How the Misuse of Antibiotics Endangers Their Curative Power. Stuart B. Levy. 2nd ed. 2002. (Illus.). 376p. pap. text 17.50 (*0-7382-0440-4*) Perseus Bks Grp.

Antibiotic Resistance: From Molecular Basics to Therapeutic Options. Carlos F. Amabile-Cuevas. 1996. LC 96-47138. (Medical Intelligence Unit Ser.). 250p. pap. 89.95 (*0-412-13571-X*) Chapman & Hall.

Antibiotic Resistance: Origins, Evolution, Selection & Spread, Vol. 207. Derek J. Chadwick & Jamie Goode. 1997. LC 96-29697. (CIBA Foundation Symposia Ser.). 260p. 147.95 (*0-471-97105-7*) Wiley.

Antibiotic Resistance: Proceedings. Ed. by S. Mitsuhashi et al. 1981. (Illus.). 410p. 71.95 (*0-387-10322-8*) Spr-Verlag.

***Antibiotic Resistance & Infection Control.** Ed. by Helen F. Galley. 2001. (Critical Care Focus Ser.: Vol. 5). (Illus.). 54p. pap. text (*0-7279-1538-X*) BMJ Pub GBR. *Dist:* AIDC.

Antibiotic Resistance Methods & Protocols. Ed. by Stephen H. Gillespie. 2000. (Methods in Molecular Medicine Ser.: Vol. 48). 304p. 89.50 (*0-89603-777-0*) Humana.

Antibiotic Selection in Obstetrics & Gynecology. Gilles R. Monif. 1997. 140p. pap. 11.95 (*1-880906-07-4*) IDI Pub.

Antibiotics. Ed. by John H. Hash. 1975. (Methods in Enzymology Ser.: Vol. 43). text 199.00 (*0-12-181943-4*) Acad Pr.

Antibiotics: A Multidisciplinary Approach. Francesco Parenti et al. 1995. LC 95-11625. (Illus.). 288p. (C). text 69.50 (*0-306-44924-2*, Kluwer Plenum) Kluwer Academic.

Antibiotics: An Integrated View. Giancarlo L. Lancini & Francesco Parenti. 1982. (Microbiology Ser.). (Illus.). 253p. 124.00 (*0-387-90630-4*) Spr-Verlag.

Antibiotics & Chemotherapy. Lambert. 7th ed. 1997. text (*0-443-05255-7*, 00202) Church.

Antibiotics & Microbial Transformations. S. S. Lamba & C. A. Walker. 1987. LC 86-29908. 224p. 128.00 (*0-8493-6408-6*, QR88, CRC Reprint) Franklin.

Antibiotics & Milk. Harry Mol. 1975. 214p. 75.00 (*90-6191-010-2*) Ashgate Pub Co.

Antibiotics Containing the Beta-Lactam Structure One. Ed. by A. L. Demain & Nadine A. Solomon. 1983. (Handbook of Experimental Pharmacology Ser.: Vol. 67-I). (Illus.). 362p. 248.00 (*0-387-12107-2*) Spr-Verlag.

Antibiotics Containing the Beta-Lactam Structure Two. Ed. by A. L. Demain & Nadine A. Solomon. 1983. (Handbook of Experimental Pharmacology Ser.: Vol. 67, II). (Illus.). 479p. 312.00 (*0-387-12131-5*) Spr-Verlag.

Antibiotics, Hosts & Host Defences in Nosocomial Infections. Ed. by Thomas R. Beam. 35.00 (*0-915340-07-0*) PJD Pubns.

Antibiotics I: Beta-Lactams, Vol. 16 & 17. Ed. by E. Tomlinson & A. Regosz. 1985. 812p. 314.00 (*0-08-029235-6*, Pergamon Pr) Elsevier.

Antibiotics I: Lactams & Other Antimicrobial Agents, Vol. 2. Isao Kawamoto. 1992. 152p. pap. text 74.00 (*2-88124-855-1*) Gordon & Breach.

Antibiotics II: Antibiotics by Fermentation, Vol. 3. Sadao Teshiba. 1993. (Japanese Technology Reviews Ser.). 132p. pap. text 61.00 (*2-88124-889-6*) Gordon & Breach.

Antibiotics in Historical Perspective. David L. Cowen & Alvin B. Segelman. 1981. 238p. (*0-911910-71-9*) Merck-Sharp-Dohme.

Antibiotics in Laboratory Medicine. Victor Lorian. (Illus.). 3rd ed. 1991. 1268p. 190.00 (*0-683-05168-7*); 4th ed. 1996. 1008p. text 199.00 (*0-683-05169-5*) Lppncott W & W.

Antibiotics in Obstetrics & Gynecology: Developments in Perinatal Medicine, No. 2. William J. Ledger. 1982. 320p. text 171.00 (*90-247-2529-1*) Kluwer Academic.

Antibodies, Vol. 1. Maurizio Zanetti. 1995. 200p. text 94.00 (*3-7186-0602-X*); pap. text 66.00 (*3-7186-0610-0*) Gordon & Breach (Harwood Acad Pubs).

Antibodies, Vol. 4. Maurizio Zanetti & J. Donald Capra. 1998. 248p. pap. 85.00 (*90-5702-560-4*, Harwood Acad Pubs) Gordon & Breach.

Antibodies, Vol. 4. Ed. by Maurizio Zanetti & J. Donald Capra. 1997. 224p. text 85.00 (*90-5702-559-0*, Harwood Acad Pubs) Gordon & Breach.

Antibodies: A Laboratory Manual. Ed. by Ed Harlow & David Lane. 1988. (Illus.). 726p. pap. text 75.00 (*0-87969-314-2*) Cold Spring Harbor.

Antibodies: Protective, Destructive & Regulatory Role: International Convocation on Immunology, Amherst, N.Y., June 1984. Ed. by Felix Milgrom et al. 1985. (Illus.). xiv, 462p. 326.25 (*3-8055-3990-8*) S Karger.

Antibodies: Structure, Synthesis, Function, & Immunologic Intervention in Disease. Ed. by Andor Szentivanyi et al. 1987. LC 87-2457. (University of South Florida International Biomedical Symposia Ser.). 224p. 65.00 (*0-306-42559-9*, Plenum Trade) Perseus Pubng.

Antibodies: Their Structure & Function. M. W. Steward. 1984. (Outline Studies in Biology). 96p. pap. 9.95 (*0-412-25640-1*, NO. 6897) Chapman & Hall.

Antibodies, Antigens, & Molecular Mimicry. Ed. by John J. Langone et al. 1989. (Methods in Enzymology Ser.: Vol. 178). 835p. text 153.00 (*0-12-182079-3*) Acad Pr.

Antibodies As Carriers of Cytotoxicity. H. H. Sedlacek et al. Ed. by J. Czech et al. 1992. (Beitraege Zur Onkologie, Contributions to Oncology Ser.: Vol. 43). (Illus.). viii, 208p. 71.50 (*3-8055-5599-7*) S Karger.

Antibodies in Cytokines: The Concerted Action on the Antigenicity of rDNA Derived Pharmaceuticals. Ed. by Huub Schellekens. 1997. 98p. text 87.00 (*0-7923-4407-3*) Kluwer Academic.

Antibodies in Diagnosis & Therapy: Technologies Mechanisms & Clinical Data. Ed. by Siegfried Matzku & Rolf A. Stahel. 1999. (Studies in Medicinal Chemistry Ser.: Vol. 3). 328p. text 125.00 (*90-5702-310-5*, ECU113, Harwood Acad Pubs) Gordon & Breach.

Antibodies in Radiodiagnosis & Therapy. Ed. by Michael R. Zalutsky. 1988. 256p. 144.00 (*0-8493-6303-9*, RC271, CRC Reprint) Franklin.

***Antibodies in Viral Infection.** Ed. by D. R. Burton. 2001. (Current Topics in Microbiology & Immunology Ser.: Vol. 260). (Illus.). vi, 310p. 115.00 (*3-540-41611-0*) Spr-Verlag.

Antibodies to Endothelial Cells & Vascular Damage. Ricard Cervera. 1993. 208p. lib. bdg. 179.00 (*0-8493-4914-1*, RC694) CRC Pr.

Antibody Affinity: Thermodynamic Aspects & Biological Significance. Ed. by Michael W. Steward & Jens Steensgaard. 1983. 176p. 106.00 (*0-8493-5790-X*, QR187, CRC Reprint) Franklin.

Antibody Conjugates & Malignant Disease. Michael Magerstadt. 1991. (Illus.). 248p. lib. bdg. 190.00 (*0-8493-6089-7*, RC270) CRC Pr.

Antibody Engineering. Ed. by J. D. Capra. 1996. LC 96-34316. (Chemical Immunology Ser.: Vol. 65, 1996). (Illus.). xii, 212p. 195.75 (*3-8055-6356-6*) S Karger.

Antibody Engineering. Ed. by Carl A. Borrebaeck. 2nd ed. 1995. LC 94-25809. (Breakthroughs in Molecular Biology Ser.). (Illus.). 416p. pap. text 60.00 (*0-19-509150-7*) OUP.

Antibody Engineering: A Practical Approach. Ed. by John McCafferty et al. 1996. LC 95-49216. (Practical Approach Ser.: No. 169). (Illus.). 348p. text 95.00 (*0-19-963593-5*) OUP.

Antibody Engineering Vol. II: New Technology, Application & Commercialization. Ed. by Wendy Hori. 1997. (Biomedical Library). pap. (*1-57936-031-9*) Drug & Market Dev.

Antibody Fusion Proteins. Ed. by Steven M. Chamow & Avi Ashkenazi. 1999. LC 98-36471. (Illus.). 312p. 115.00 (*0-471-18358-X*) Wiley.

Antibody Techniques: A Guide for Nonimmunologists. Ed. by Vedpal S. Malik & Erik P. Lillehoj. 1994. LC 94-16438. (Illus.). 353p. pap. 53.00 (*0-12-466460-1*) Acad Pr.

Antibody Technology: A Comprehensive Overview. J. E. Liddell & I. Weeks. 1995. (Introduction to Biotechniques Ser.). 160p. (Orig.). pap. (*1-872748-87-2*) Bios Sci GBR. *Dist:* Coronet Bks.

Antibody Therapeutics. William J. Harris & John R. Adair. 1997. LC 96-27305. (Pharmacology & Toxicology Ser.). 384p. 119.95 (*0-8493-8547-4*) CRC Pr.

Antibody Therapy. E. J. Wawrzynczak. 1996. (Medical Perspectives Ser.). 160p. pap. (*1-872748-29-5*) Bios Sci GBR. *Dist:* Coronet Bks.

Antibody Usage in the Lab. Laura Caponi & Paola Migliorini. 1999. LC 99-11672. (Lab Manual Ser.). (Illus.). 160p. 62.00 (*3-540-65148-9*) Spr-Verlag.

***Anticancer Agents: Frontiers in Cancer Chemotherapy.** Ed. by Iwao Ojima et al. 2001. (ACS Symposium Ser.: Vol. No. 796). (Illus.). 272p. text 140.00 (*0-8412-3745-X*) Am Chemical.

Anticancer Chinese Drugs & Related Plants. Eric J. Lien & Wen Y. Li. Ed. by Don R. Bensen. 1996. 160p. pap. 10.95 (*0-941942-18-X*, Keats Pubng) McGraw-Hill Trade.

Anticancer Drug Development Guide: Preclinical Screening, Clinical Trials & Approval. Ed. by Beverly A. Teicher. 1997. LC 96-38113. (Cancer Drug Discovery & Development Ser.). (Illus.). 336p. 160.00 (*0-89603-461-5*) Humana.

Anticancer Drug Discovery & Development: Natural Products & New Molecular Models; Proceedings of the Second Drug Discovery & Development Symposium, Traverse City, Michigan, USA, June 27-29, 1991. Ed. by Frederick A. Valeriote et al. 1994. LC 94-11632. (Developments in Oncology Ser.: Vol. 74). 416p. (C). text 212.00 (*0-7923-2928-7*) Kluwer Academic.

Anticancer Drug Resistence: Advances in Molecular & Clinical Research. Ed. by Lori T. Goldstein & Robert F. Ozols. 1994. LC 94-10351. (Cancer Treatment & Research Ser.: Vol. 73). 294p. (C). text 268.00 (*0-7923-2836-1*) Kluwer Academic.

Anticancer Drugs. William B. Pratt et al. 2nd ed. 1994. (Illus.). 360p. pap. text 39.95 (*0-19-506739-8*); (C). text 69.95 (*0-19-506738-X*) OUP.

Anticancer Drugs: Antmetabolite Metabolism & Natural Anticancer Agents. Ed. by Garth Powis. 1994. 524p. 220.50 (*0-08-042334-5*, Pergamon Pr) Elsevier.

Anticancer Drugs: Reactive Metabolism & Drug Interactions. Ed. by Garth Powis. 1994. 460p. 220.50 (*0-08-042335-3*, Pergamon Pr) Elsevier.

Anticancer Drugs from Animals, Plants & Microorganisms. George R. Pettit et al. 1994. LC 93-46997. 688p. 145.00 (*0-471-03657-9*) Wiley.

Anticancer Pain: Potency & Mechanism of SPES. Xu H. Wang et al. 1994. (Illus.). (Orig.). pap. 85.00 (*0-9636432-3-1*) Int Med Res.

Anticancer Pain: Potency & Mechanism of SPES. Xu Hui Wang et al. 1994. (CHI., Illus.). (Orig.). pap. 85.00 (*0-9636432-2-3*) Int Med Res.

***Anticancer Therapy.** Patricia K. Anthony & Dal Yoo. 2001. (Illus.). 200p. pap. 25.00 (*1-56053-467-2*) Hanley & Belfus.

Anticarcinogenesis & Radiation Protection, No. 1. Ed. by Peter A. Cerutti et al. 1988. LC 87-36133. (Illus.). 524p. 135.00 (*0-306-42785-0*, Plenum Trade) Perseus Pubng.

Anticarcinogenesis & Radiation Protection 2. Ed. by Oddvar F. Nygaard & Arthur C. Upton. 1992. (Illus.). 488p. (C). text 174.00 (*0-306-44056-3*, Kluwer Plenum) Kluwer Academic.

Anticholinergic Agents in Upper & Lower Airways. Ed. by Sheldon L. Spector. 1999. LC 99-29626. (Lung Biology in Health & Disease Ser.). (Illus.). 240p. text 135.00 (*0-8247-1959-X*) Dekker.

Anticipating & Assessing Health Care, Vol. 4. Scenario Commission on Future Health Care Technolo & H. David Banta. 1988. (C). text 73.50 (*0-89838-410-9*) Kluwer Academic.

Anticipating & Assessing Health Care Technology, Vol. 2. Scenario Commission on Future Health Care Technolo. 1988. (C). pap. text 104.00 (*0-89838-379-X*) Kluwer Academic.

Anticipating & Assessing Health Care Technology. Scenario Commission on Future Health Care Technolo & H. David Banta. 1988. (C). Vol. 5. text 92.50 (*0-89838-411-7*); Vol. 6. text 92.50 (*0-89838-412-5*); Vol. 7. text 73.50 (*0-89838-413-3*); Vol. 8. text 92.50 (*0-89838-420-6*) Kluwer Academic.

Anticipating & Assessing Health Care Technology: A Report Commissioned by the Steering Committee on Future Health Scenarios, Vol. 3. Scenario Commission on Future Health Care Technolo & H. David Banta. 1988. (C). text 92.50 (*0-89838-419-2*) Kluwer Academic.

Anticipating & Assessing Health Care Technology: General Considerations & Policy Conclusions. a Report Commissioned by the Steering Committee on Future Health Scenarios, Vol. 1. H. David Banta. 1987. (C). pap. text 105.00 (*0-89838-897-X*) Kluwer Academic.

***Anticlote for Age? Seeking Novel Therapeutics for the Needs of an Aging Population.** Paul Evers et al. Ed. by Lynn M. Savage. 2001. (Illus.). 72p. spiral bd. 595.00 (*1-57936-198-6*, 9053, D&MD Reports) International Business.

Anticoagulant Rodenticides. 1995. (Environmental Health Criteria Ser.: Vol. 175). 121p. (C). pap. 28.00 (*92-4-157175-6*, 1160175) World Health.

Anticoagulants: Physiologic, Pathologic, Pharmacologic. Ed. by David Green. 1994. LC 93-47688. 288p. lib. bdg. 179.00 (*0-8493-4762-9*) CRC Pr.

Anticoagulation. Ed. by Christian Doutremepuich. 1994. LC 94-16729. (Illus.). 530p. 150.00 (*0-387-94318-8*) Spr-Verlag.

Anticoagulation, Hemostasis & Blood Preservation in Cardiovascular Surgery. Ed. by Roque Pifarre. 1993. (Illus.). 420p. 69.95 (*1-56053-098-7*) Hanley & Belfus.

Anticoagulation Therapy Management Manual. Jack E. Ansell. 1997. LC 97-6378. ring bd. 239.00 (*0-8342-0878-4*, S443) Aspen Pub.

Anticonvulsant Medicines: Medicines for People with Epilepsy. Michael G. Aman et al. 2000. (Project MED Ser.). pap. (*0-9658966-7-6*) OSU Nisonger.

Anticonvulsant Therapy: Pharmacological Basis & Practice. Mervyn J. Eadie. 3rd ed. 1989. (Illus.). 367p. text (*0-443-04010-9*) Church.

Anticonvulsants in Mood Disorders. Ed. by Russell T. Joffe & Joseph R. Calabrese. 1994. LC 94-21977. (Medical Psychiatry Ser.: 2). (Illus.). 264p. text 135.00 (*0-8247-9260-2*) Dekker.

Anticonvulsants in Psychiatry. Ed. by Kjell Modigh et al. 1994. LC 94-28069. 176p. (*1-871816-25-4*) Wrightson Biomed GBR. *Dist:* Taylor & Francis.

Antidepressant Era. David Healy. 1997. LC 97-23118. (Illus.). 352p. 41.50 (*0-674-03957-2*) HUP.

Antidepressant Fact Book: What Your Doctor Won't Tell You about Prozac, Zoloft, Paxil, Celexa & Luvox. Peter R. Breggin. 2001. 240p. pap. text 13.00 (*0-7382-0451-X*) Perseus Bks Grp.

Antidepressant Sourcebook: A User's Guide for Patients & Families. Andrew L. Morrison. 1999. LC 99-29949. 304p. pap. 12.95 (*0-385-49665-6*) Doubleday.

Antidepressant Survival Program: How to Enhance the Benefits & Beat the Side Effects of Your Medication. Robert J. Hedaya. 2001. LC 00-69081. (Illus.). 304p. reprint ed. pap. 12.95 (*0-609-80541-X*, Three Riv Pr) Crown Pub Group.

Antidepressants. Ed. by B. E. Leonard. 2000. (Milestones in Drug Therapy Ser.). (Illus.). 200p. 120.00 (*3-7643-5933-1*) Birkhauser.

Antidepressants: New Pharmacological Strategies. Ed. by Phil Skolnick. 1997. LC 97-16900. (Contemporary Neuroscience Ser.). (Illus.). 272p. 150.00 (*0-89603-469-0*) Humana.

Antidepressants & Receptor Function. CIBA Foundation Staff. 1986. (CIBA Foundation Symposia Ser.: No. 123). 304p. 128.00 (*0-471-91089-9*) Wiley.

Antidepressants for Elderly People. Ed. by Karabi Ghose. 1990. 296p. 80.00 (*0-412-32460-1*, A4453) Chapman & Hall.

Antidiabetic Drugs to Benzoquinone & Naphthoquinone Dyes, Vol. A3, Antidiabetic Drugs to Benzoquinone and Na. Wolfgang Gerhartz. 5th ed. 1985. LC 84-25829. (Illus.). 578p. 450.00 (*3-527-20103-3*, Wiley-VCH) Wiley.

Antidiscrimination in Health Care: Community Ratings & Preexisting Conditions. Richard A. Epstein. 1996. 36p. (Orig.). pap. 5.95 (*0-945999-45-3*) Independent Inst.

Antidotes for Poisoning by Cyanide. T. J. Meredith et al. 1994. LC 93-32558. (IPCS-CES Evaluation of Antidotes Ser.: No. 2). 203p. (C). pap. text 22.95 (*0-521-45458-1*) Cambridge U Pr.

Antidotes for Poisoning by Paracetamol. T. J. Meredith et al. 1995. (IPCS-CES Evaluation of Antidotes Ser.: No. 3). (Illus.). 109p. (C). text 49.95 (*0-521-49576-8*) Cambridge U Pr.

Antidromic Vasodilatation & Neurogenic Inflammation. L. A. Chahl et al. 1984. 352p. (C). (*963-05-3996-9*) Akade Kiado HUN. *Dist:* St Mut.

Antiemetics in the Supportive Care of Cancer Patients. M. Tonato. 1996. LC 96-33254. (Monographs of the European School of Oncology). (Illus.). 145p. 99.00 (*3-540-61201-7*) Spr-Verlag.

Antiepileptic Drug Monitoring. C. Gardner-Thorpe et al. 1977. pap. 70.00 (*0-8464-0138-X*) Beekman Pubs.

Antiepileptic Drug Trials, Vol. 76. Ed. by Jacqueline A. French et al. 1997. (Advances in Neurology Ser.). 304p. text 145.00 (*0-397-51848-X*) Lppncott W & W.

Antiepileptic Drugs. Ed. by Rene H. Levy et al. 4th ed. 1995. 1,150p. text 199.00 (*0-7817-0246-1*) Lppncott W & W.

Antiepileptic Drugs: Pharmacology & Therapeutics. Ed. by E. Ben-Menachem et al. 1999. LC 99-10225. (Handbook of Experimental Pharmacology Ser.: Vol. 138). (Illus.). 669p. 399.00 (*3-540-65374-0*) Spr-Verlag.

Antiepileptic Drugs in Psychiatry. Ed. by M. Berger et al. 1993. (Journal: Vol. 27, No. 3, 1993). (Illus.). 76p. pap. 58.50 (*3-8055-5839-2*) S Karger.

Antietam Hospitals. John W. Schildt. 1987. (Illus.). 64p. (Orig.). pap. 6.50 (*0-936772-04-2*) Antietam.

Antifolate Drugs in Cancer Therapy. Ed. by Ann L. Jackman. 1999. LC 00-501973. (Cancer Drug Discovery & Development Ser.: Vol. 4). 480p. 165.00 (*0-89603-596-4*) Humana.

Antifungal Drug Therapy: A Complete Guide for the Practitioner. Paul H. Jacobs & Lexie Nall. 1990. (Illus.). 352p. text 135.00 (*0-8247-8353-0*) Dekker.

Antifungals in Gynecology: Focus on Terconazole. Ed. by R. Y. Cartwright & H. A. Hirsch. 1985. (Journal: Vol. 25, Suppl. 1). (Illus.). iv, 120p. pap. 33.25 (*3-8055-4041-8*) S Karger.

Antigen & Antibody Molecular Engineering in Breast Cancer Diagnosis & Treatment: Diagnosis & Treatment. R. L. Ceriani. 1994. (Advances in Experimental Medicine & Biology Ser.: Vol. 353). (Illus.). 234p. (C). text 85.00 (*0-306-44720-7*, Kluwer Plenum) Kluwer Academic.

Antigen Depository of the Immune System: Follicular Dendritic Cells. Ed. by M. H. Kosco-Vilbois. 1995. LC 95-12910. (Current Topics in Microbiology & Immunology Ser.: Vol. 201). (Illus.). 224p. 150.00 (*3-540-59013-7*) Spr-Verlag.

Antigen Detection to Diagnose Bacterial Infections: Applications, I. R. B. Kohler. 1990. LC 86-12960. 118.00 (*0-8493-6698-4*, CRC Reprint) Franklin.

Antigen Detection to Diagnose Bacterial Infections: Applications. II. 1986. 280p. 159.00 (*0-8493-6699-2*); Set. 1987. 384.00 (*0-8493-6697-6*, QR186) Franklin.

Antigen Presentation by Intestinal Epithelial Cells. Dominique Kaiserlian. 1996. LC 96-553. 149p. 99.00 (*1-57059-337-X*) Landes Bioscience.

Antigen Processing - Recognition. Ed. by James McCluskey. 1991. 248p. lib. bdg. 195.00 (*0-8493-6932-0*, RB52) CRC Pr.

Antigen-Specific T-Cell Receptors. John J. Marchalonis. 1987. 168p. 163.00 (*0-8493-6167-2*);Vol. II. 144p. 86.00 (*0-8493-6168-0*) Franklin (CRC Reprint).

Antigenic Changes Associated with Complement Activation: Journal: Complement & Inflammation, Vol. 6, No. 3, 1989. Ed. by T. E. Mollnes. 1989. (Illus.). 120p. pap. 36.75 (*3-8055-5048-0*) S Karger.

Antigenic Determinants & Immune Regulation. Ed. by Eli E. Sercarz. 1989. (Chemical Immunology Ser.: Vol. 46). (Illus.). viii, 190p. 129.75 (*3-8055-4960-1*) S Karger.

Antigenic Variation: Molecular & Genetic Mechanisms of Relapsing Disease. Ed. by J. M. Cruse & R. E. Lewis. 1987. (Contributions to Microbiology & Immunology Ser.: Vol. 8). (Illus.). vi, 246p. 169.75 (*3-8055-4343-3*) S Karger.

Antigens & Antibodies 1, Vol. 10, Antigens and Antibodies 1. Ed. by Hans U. Bergmeyer. 3rd ed. 1986. LC 84-105641. 509p. 310.00 (*3-527-26050-1*, Wiley-VCH) Wiley.

Antiglobulins, Cryoglobulins & Glomerulonephritis. Ed. by C. Ponticelli et al. 1986. (Developments in Nephrology Ser.). lib. bdg. 188.00 (*0-89838-810-4*) Kluwer Academic.

Antihormones in Health & Disease. Ed. by M. K. Agarawal. 1991. (Frontiers of Hormone Research Ser.: Vol. 19). (Illus.). viii, 200p. 178.50 (*3-8055-5297-1*) S Karger.

Antihypertensive Drugs. Ed. by Peter A. Van Zwieten & William J. Greenlee. 1997. 704p. text 150.00 (*90-5702-122-6*, Harwood Acad Pubs) Gordon & Breach.

***Antihypertensive Treatment & Endothelial Vasodilatory Function.** Bengt Von Zur Muhlen. 2001. (Comprehensive Summaries of Uppsala Dissertatons from the Faculty of Medicine: No. 1027). (Illus.). 56p. pap. (*91-554-4999-9*) Uppsala Universitet SWE. *Dist:* Coronet Bks.

Antimalarial Chemotherapy: Mechanisms of Action, Resistance & New Directions in Drug Discovery. Ed. by Philip J. Rosenthal. 2001. LC 00-59762. (Infectious Disease Ser.). (Illus.). xi, 396p. 125.00 (*0-89603-670-7*) Humana.

Antimalarial Drugs. Ed. by W. Peters & W. H. Richards. 1984. (Handbook of Experimental Pharmacology Ser.: Vol. 68, Pt. 1). (Illus.). 484p. 295.00 (*0-387-12616-3*) Spr-Verlag.

Antimalarial Drugs II: Current Antimalarials & New Drug Developments. Ed. by W. Peters & W. H. Richards. 1984. (Handbook of Experimental Pharmacology Ser.: Vol. 68). (Illus.). 520p. 312.00 (*0-387-12617-1*) Spr-Verlag.

Antimicrobial Agents & Intracellular Pathogens. Didier Raoult. 1993. LC 93-2668. 400p. lib. bdg. 210.00 (*0-8493-4924-9*, RM409) CRC Pr.

Antimicrobial Drug Action: The Chemical Treatment of Infectious Diseases. R. A. Williams et al. 1996. (Medical Perspectives Ser.). 160p. (Orig.). pap. (*1-872748-81-3*) Bios Sci GBR. *Dist:* Bks Intl VA.

***Antimicrobial Pharmacodynamics in Theory & Clinical Practice.** Takeo Murakawa et al. Ed. by Charles H. Nightingdale. 2001. (Infectious Disease & Therapy Ser.). 416p. 175.00 (*0-8247-0561-0*) Dekker.

Antimicrobial Prophylaxis in Urology with Special Reference to the Quinolones. Ed. by T. C. Gasser. 1992. (Fortune West Ser.: Vol. 27). 88p. 29.00 (*0-387-91441-2*) Spr-Verlag.

Antimicrobial Resistance: A Crisis in Health Care. Ed. by Donald L. Jungkind et al. 1996. (Advances in Experimental Medicine & Biology Ser.: Vol. 390). (Illus.). 260p. 85.00 (*0-306-45207-3*, Kluwer Plenum) Kluwer Academic.

Antimicrobial Resistance: Issues & Options. Polly Harrison & Joshua Lederberg. 1998. LC 98-167581. 128p. pap. 25.00 (*0-309-06084-2*) Natl Acad Pr.

Antimicrobial Susceptibility Testing: Critical Issues for the 90s. Ed. by James Poupard et al. 1994. (Advances in Experimental Medicine & Biology Ser.: Vol. 349). (Illus.). 200p. (C). text 75.00 (*0-306-44673-1*, Kluwer Plenum) Kluwer Academic.

Antimicrobial Therapy - Abdominal Surgery: Precepts & Practices. Haragopal Thadepalli & Ashis K. Mandal. 1991. 120p. lib. bdg. 99.95 (*0-8493-4269-4*, RD540) CRC Pr.

Antimicrobial Therapy & Vaccines. Ed. by Victor L. Yu et al. 1998. LC 98-36941. (Illus.). 1,500p. text 189.00 (*0-683-30061-X*) Lppncott W & W.

Antimicrobial Therapy in the Elderly Patient. Ed. by Thomas T. Yoshikawa & Dean C. Norman. 1994. (Infectious Disease & Therapy Ser.: Vol. 9). (Illus.). 584p. text 199.00 (*0-8247-9163-0*) Dekker.

Antimicrobial Therapy in Veterinary Medicine. John F. Prescott et al. 3rd ed. 2000. LC 00-36967. (Illus.). xvi, 796p. text 99.95 (*0-8138-0779-4*) Iowa U Pr.

Antimutagenesis & Anticarcinogenesis Mechanisms. Ed. by Delbert M. Shankel et al. 1986. LC 86 15070. (Basic Life Sciences Ser.: Vol. 39). 618p. 125.00 (*0-306-42375-8*, Plenum Trade) Perseus Pubng.

Antimutagenesis & Anticarcinogenesis Mechanisms, No. II. Ed. by Y. Kuroda. 1990. (Basic Life Sciences Ser.: Vol. 52). (Illus.). 498p. 125.00 (*0-306-43403-2*, Plenum Trade) Perseus Pubng.

Antimutagenesis & Anticarcinogenesis Mechanisms 3. G. Bronzetti et al. 1993. (Basic Life Sciences Ser.: Vol. 61). (Illus.). 504p. (C). text 135.00 (*0-306-44577-8*, Kluwer Plenum) Kluwer Academic.

Antimutagens in Anticarcinogens. T. Hughes & B. Casto. 1993. 80p. pap. text 98.00 (*2-88124-605-2*) Gordon & Breach.

Antimycobacteria Susceptibility Testing for Myobacteriom Tuberculosis: Tentative Standard. 1995. 75.00 (*1-56238-270-5*, M24-T) NCCLS.

Antinuclear Antibodies. Ed. by F. Hiepe. 2000. (International Archives of Allergy & Immunology Ser.: Vol. 123, No. 1). (Illus.). 98p. 34.00 (*3-8055-7156-9*) S Karger.

Antioxidant. Lester Packer et al. 1999. LC 98-34992. (Illus.). 272p. 24.95 (*0-471-29768-2*) Wiley.

Antioxidant Methodology: In-Vivo & In-Vitro Concepts. Ed. by Susan L. Cuppett & Okezie I. Aruona. 1997. LC 97-3214. 85.00 (*0-935315-79-9*) Am Oil Chemists.

Antioxidant Miracle: Put Lipoic Acid, Pycogenol & Vitamins E & C to Work for You. Lester Packer. 1999. LC 99-52442. 272p. pap. 15.95 (*0-471-35311-6*) Wiley.

Antioxidant Nutrients & Immune Functions. A. Bendich et al. 1990. LC 89-26570. (Advances in Experimental Medicine & Biology Ser.: No. 262). (Illus.). 184p. (C). text 75.00 (*0-306-43396-6*, Kluwer Plenum) Kluwer Academic.

Antioxidants. Remi Cooper. 1997. (Woodland Health Ser.). 32p. pap. text 3.95 (*1-885670-52-4*) Woodland UT.

Antioxidants. Richard A. Passwater. 1985. (Good Health Guides). 30p. pap. 3.50 (*0-87983-404-8*, Keats Pubng) McGraw-Hill Trade.

Antioxidants: Free Radicals in Nutrition, Health & Disease. John M. Gutteridge & Barry Halliwell. 1995. LC 94-18907. (Illus.). 152p. text 39.95 (*0-19-854902-4*) OUP.

Antioxidants: In Science, Technology, Medicine & Nutrition. Gerald Scott. 1997. LC 97-198840. 350p. (*1-898563-31-4*) Horwood Pub GBR. *Dist:* Paul & Co Pubs.

Antioxidants Against Cancer. Ralph W. Moss. 2000. LC 99-57585. (Ralph Moss on Cancer Ser.). (Illus.). 128p. pap. 9.95 (*1-881025-28-4*) Equinox Pr.

Antioxidants & Disease Prevention. Ed. by Harinder S. Garewal. 1997. LC 96-45089. (Modern Nutrition Ser.). 208p. 129.95 (*0-8493-8509-1*) CRC Pr.

Antioxidants & Exercise. Jan Karlsson. 1997. LC 96-18843. (Illus.). 224p. text 40.00 (*0-87322-896-0*, BKAR0896) Human Kinetics.

Antioxidants for Life. Carolyn Reuben. 1998. LC 98-18105. pap. 14.00 (*0-7615-1446-5*) Prima Pub.

Antioxidants in Human Health & Disease. Tapan K. Basu et al. 1999. LC 98-33114. (CAB International Publication). (Illus.). 480p. text (*0-85199-334-6*) OUP.

Antioxidants in Therapy & Preventive Medicine. I. Emerit et al. 1990. (Advances in Experimental Medicine & Biology Ser.: Vol. 264). (Illus.). 608p. (C). text 145.00 (*0-306-43407-5*, Kluwer Plenum) Kluwer Academic.

Antiparasitic Chemotherapy. Ed. by H. Schoenfeld. 1981. (Antibiotics & Chemotherapy Ser.: Vol. 30). (Illus.). viii, 288p. 198.50 (*3-8055-2160-X*) S Karger.

AntiPatterns & Patterns in Software Configuration Management. William J. Brown et al. 1999. LC 99-10822. (Illus.). 336p. 44.99 (*0-471-32929-0*) Wiley.

Antiperspirants & Deodorants. Karl Laden. 2nd rev. ed. 1999. LC 98-50967. (Cosmetic Science & Technology Ser.). (Illus.). 408p. text 195.00 (*0-8247-1746-5*) Dekker.

Antiphospholipid Antibodies. Ed. by J. Monasterio et al. 1994. (Journal: Vol. 24, No. 3, 1994). (Illus.). iv, 56p. pap. 20.00 (*3-8055-6027-3*) S Karger.

***Antiplatelet Therapy - an Update: 20th Platelet Lake Ashi Conference, Hakone, Japan, October 1999.** Ed. by Y. Ikeda. 1999. iv, 52p. 25.25 (*3-8055-7201-8*) S Karger.

Antiprogestin Steroid RU 486 & Human Fertility Control. Ed. by Etienne-Emile Baulieu & Sheldon J. Segal. 1985. LC 85-19815. (Reproductive Biology Ser.). 364p. 95.00 (*0-306-42103-8*, Plenum Trade) Perseus Pubng.

Antipsychiatry Bibliography/Resource Guide. Frank. 2nd enl. rev. ed. 1979. 160p. pap. (*0-88974-006-2*) Press Gang Pubs CAN. *Dist:* LPC Group.

Antipsychotic Drugs & Their Side Effects. Ed. by T. R. Barnes. 1994. (Neuroscience Perspectives Ser.). (Illus.). 287p. text 78.00 (*0-12-079035-1*) Acad Pr.

Antipsychotics, No. 120. Ed. by J. G. Csernansky. 1996. (Handbook of Experimental Pharmacology Ser.: Vol. 120). (Illus.). 539p. 398.00 (*3-540-60118-X*) Spr-Verlag.

Antiquity of Disease. Roy L. Moodie. LC 75-23743. reprint ed. 29.50 (*0-404-13298-7*) AMS Pr.

Antiretroviral Therapy. Ed. by Erik D. DeClercq. 2001. LC 00-53111. (Illus.). x, 359p. 99.95 (*1-55581-156-6*) ASM Pr.

Antisense - From Technology to Therapy: Lab Manual & Textbook. R. Schlingensiepen et al. 1997. (Illus.). 365p. 120.00 (*0-86542-669-4*) Blackwell Sci.

Antisense Oligodeoxynucleotides & Antisense RNA: Novel Pharmacological & Therapeutic Agents. Benjamin Weiss. 1997. LC 97-183510. (Pharmacology & Toxicology Ser.). 272p. 179.95 (*0-8493-8552-0*) CRC Pr.

Antisense Research & Application. Ed. by Stanley T. Crooke & Sudhir Agrawal. 1998. LC 97-46586. (Handbook of Experimental Pharmacology Ser.). (Illus.). 656p. 399.00 (*3-540-63833-4*) Spr-Verlag.

Antisense Therapeutics. Ed. by Sudhir Agrawal. 1996. LC 96-3441. (Methods in Molecular Medicine Ser.: Vol. 1). (Illus.). 290p. 135.00 (*0-89603-305-8*) Humana.

Antisocial Behavior & Mental Health Problems: Explanatory Factors in Childhood & Adolescence. Rolf Loeber et al. 1998. LC 97-38123. 350p. (*0-8058-2956-3*) L Erlbaum Assocs.

Antisocial Behavior in Organizations. Robert A. Giacalone & Jerald Greenberg. 1997. LC 96-25241. 160p. 67.95 (*0-8039-7235-0*, 1105) Sage.

Antisocial Personalities. David T. Lykken. 1995. 272p. text 49.95 (*0-8058-1941-X*) L Erlbaum Assocs.

Antithrombotic Drugs in Thrombosis Models. Josef Hladovec. 1989. 240p. lib. bdg. 191.00 (*0-8493-5162-6*, RC694) CRC Pr.

Antithrombotics. William R. Bell. Ed. by Andrew C. Uprichard et al. 1998. LC 98-29079. (Handbook of Experimental Pharmacology Ser.: Vol. 132). (Illus.). 508p. 325.00 (*3-540-64691-4*) Spr-Verlag.

Antitrust: Challenge of the Health Care Field - Principles & Their Practical Application. Ed. by David Marx & James H. Sneed. 1990. 230p. 30.00 (*0-918945-08-9*) Am Hlth Lawyers.

Antitrust Health Care Handbook. 1993. LC 91-77251. 100p. pap. 35.00 (*0-89707-877-2*, 503-0229) Amer Bar Assn.

Antitrust Law. Douglas J. Colton. 1988. (Hospital Law in North Carolina Ser.: Chap. 12). 63p. (C). ring bd. 10.50 (*1-56011-084-8*, 85.03L) Institute Government.

Antitrust Problems & Solutions in a Changing Health Care System. 1994. LC 94-78409. 438p. pap. 50.00 (*0-89707-978-7*, 503-0250, ABA Antitrust) Amer Bar Assn.

Antitumor Compounds of Natural Origin Ed. by Adorjan Aszalos. 1981. Vol. 1. 256p. 148.00 (*0-8493-5520-6*, RC271); Vol. 2. 224p. 125.00 (*0-8493-5521-4*, RC271) Franklin (CRC Reprint).

Antitumor Drug-Radiation Interactions. Ed. by Bridget T. Hill & Angela S. Bellamy. 1989. 284p. 195.00 (*0-8493-4620-7*, RC271) CRC Pr.

Antiviral Agents: The Development & Assessment of Antiviral Chemotherapy, Set. H. J. Field. 1988. LC 87-9312. 183.00 (*0-8493-6683-6*, CRC Reprint) Franklin.

Antiviral Agents: The Development & Assessment of Antiviral Chemotherapy Ed. by H. J. Field. 1988. LC 87-9312. Vol. I: Successful Selective Inhibitors of Viruses. 192p. 100.00 (*0-8493-6684-4*, RM411); Vol. II: Chemotherapy of Herpes Simplex Encephalit. 160p. 84.00 (*0-8493-6685-2*, RM411) Franklin (CRC Reprint).

Antiviral Chemotherapy 5: New Directions for Clinical Application & Research. John Mills et al. 1999. LC 99-10159. (Advances in Experimental Medicine & Biology Ser.). (C). text (*0-306-46107-2*, Kluwer Plenum) Kluwer Academic.

Antiviral Chemotherapy. Richard Challand & Robert J. Young. 1996. LC 96-44658. (Biochemical & Medicinal Chemistry Ser.). (Illus.). 128p. (C). text (*0-935702-94-6*) Spektrum Acad GBR. *Dist:* Univ Sci Bks.

Antiviral Chemotherapy. Ed. by Hans W. Doerr et al. 1998. (Intervirology Ser.: Vol. 40, No. 5-6). (Illus.). 124p. pap. 51.50 (*3-8055-6725-1*) S Karger.

Antiviral Chemotherapy. Ed. by D. J. Jeffries & E. De Clercq. 1995. LC 94-30007. 604p. 270.00 (*0-471-93040-7*) Wiley.

Antiviral Chemotherapy 4: New Directions for Clinical Application & Research. Ed. by John Mills et al. 1996. (Advances in Experimental Medicine & Biology Ser.: Vol. 394). (Illus.). 454p. (C). text 144.00 (*0-306-45294-4*, Kluwer Plenum) Kluwer Academic.

Antiviral Chemotherapy, Interferons & Vaccines. D. O. White. 1984. (Monographs in Virology: Vol. 16). (Illus.). viii, 112p. 67.00 (*3-8055-3825-1*) S Karger.

Antiviral Drug Development: A Multidisciplinary Approach. Ed. by Erik De Clercq & R. T. Walker. 1988. (NATO ASI Series A, Life Sciences: Vol. 143). (Illus.). 314p. 85.00 (*0-306-42796-6*, Plenum Trade) Perseus Pubng.

Antiviral Drug Resistance. Ed. by Douglas D. Richman. 1996. LC 96-13385. 324p. 159.95 (*0-471-96120-5*) Wiley.

Antiviral Drugs. I. Becker. Ed. by Joseph L. Melnick. 1976. (Monographs in Virology: Vol. 11). (Illus.). 65.25 (*3-8055-2248-7*) S Karger.

Antiviral Drugs & Interferon: The Molecular Basis of Their Activity. Yechiel Becker. 1984. (Developments in Molecular Virology Ser.). 464p. text 159.00 (*0-89838-643-8*) Kluwer Academic.

Antiviral Methods & Protocols. Ed. by Derek Kinchington & Raymond F. Schinazi. 2000. LC 99-25099. (Methods in Molecular Medicine Ser.: Vol. 24). (Illus.). xiv, 404p. 110.00 (*0-89603-561-1*) Humana.

Antiviral Therapy. E. D. Blair et al. 1998. LC 97-41321. (Medical Perspectives Ser.). (Illus.). 161p. pap. 38.95 (*0-387-91510-9*) Spr-Verlag.

Antiviral Therapy. E. Littler et al. 1996. (Medical Perspectives Ser.). 160p. pap. text (*1-85996-070-7*) Bios Sci GBR. *Dist:* Bks Intl VA.

Antivirals. Ed. by Wendy Mori. 1997. (Illus.). (Orig.). pap. (*1-57936-042-4*) Drug & Market Dev.

Antivirals Against AIDS. Ed. by Ronald E. Unger et al. 2000. LC 00-31590. (Illus.). xii, 326p. text 150.00 (*0-8247-0358-8*) Dekker.

Antivirals in the Elderly. Ed. by James W. Cooper. LC 96-3445. (Journal of Geriatric Drug Therapy Ser.: Vol. 10, No. 2). 79p. (C). 1997. pap. 14.95 (*0-7890-0219-1*); 1996. 39.95 (*1-56024-820-3*) Haworth Pr (Pharmctl Prods).

Anutan Concepts of Disease: A Polynesian Study. Richard Feinberg. 1979. (Polynesian Studies: No. 3). 64p. (C). pap. text 6.95 (*0-939154-03-X*) Inst Polynesian.

Anxiety. Ed. by D. F. Klein. 1987. (Modern Problems of Pharmacopsychiatry Ser.: Vol. 22). (Illus.). viii, 196p. 85.25 (*3-8055-4488-X*) S Karger.

Anxiety: Psychobiological & Clinical Perspectives. Norman Sartorius et al. 1990. (Series in Health Psychology & Behavioral Medicine). 300p. 79.95 (*1-56032-064-8*) Hemisp Pub.

Anxiety: Psychological Perspectives on Panic & Agoraphobia. Richard S. Hallam. 1985. text 110.00 (*0-12-319620-5*) Acad Pr.

Anxiety - Prevention & Control: Index of New Information with Authors & Subjects. Dean A. Jobber. 1993. 180p. 47.50 (*1-55914-914-0*); pap. 44.50 (*1-55914-915-9*) ABBE Pubs Assn.

Anxiety & Cognition: A Unified Theory. Michael W. Eysenck. 1997. LC 97-198295. (Illus.). viii, 200p. (*0-86377-478-4*) Psychol Pr GBR. *Dist:* Taylor & Francis.

Anxiety & Defensive Strategies in Childhood & Adolescence. Gudmund J. Smith & Anna Danielsson. 1981. LC 81-23633. (Psychological Issues Monographs: No. 52, Vol. 13, No. 3). 212p. 32.00 (*0-8236-0389-X*) Intl Univs Pr.

Anxiety & Depression: A Natural Approach. Shirley Trickett. 1997. LC 97-60156. (Illus.). 144p. pap. 9.95 (*1-56975-118-8*) Ulysses Pr.

Anxiety & Depression: Your Questions Answered. Hallstrom. 1998. (C). pap. text (*0-443-04939-4*, H0576) Church.

Anxiety & Depression in Adults & Children. Ed. by Kenneth D. Craig & Keith S. Dobson. 1995. (Banff International Conference Ser.: Vol. 1). 296p. pap. 37.95 (*0-8039-7021-8*, 2852) Sage.

Anxiety & Ego Formation in Infancy. Sylvia Brody & Sidney Axelrad. 1993. 432p. (C). reprint ed. pap. 24.95 (*0-8236-8003-7*) Intl Univs Pr.

Anxiety & Its Treatment. John H. Greist et al. 1988. 304p. mass mkt. 6.99 (*0-446-35362-0*) Warner Bks.

Anxiety & Neurosis. Charles Rycroft. 1988. 166p. reprint ed. pap. text (*0-946439-52-4*) Karnac Bks GBR. *Dist:* Other Pr LLC.

***Anxiety & Panic Attacks.** Nancy R. Campbell. 2000. LC 00-12937. (Perspectives on Mental Health Ser.). (J). (gr. 5-12). lib. bdg. 23.93 (*0-7368-1030-7*, LifeMatters Bks) Capstone Pr.

Anxiety & Panic Attacks: Their Cause & Cure. Robert W. Handly. 1987. mass mkt. 6.99 (*0-449-21331-5*, Crest) Fawcett.

Anxiety & Related Disorders: A Handbook. Ed. by Benjamin B. Wolman & George Stricker. 1993. LC 93-925. (Personality Processes Ser.). 462p. 170.00 (*0-471-54773-5*) Wiley.

Anxiety & Ritual: The Theories of Malinowski & Radcliffe-Brown. George C. Homans. 1993. (Reprint Series in Social Sciences). (C). reprint ed. pap. text 1.00 (*0-8290-2725-4*, S-121) Irvington.

Anxiety & the Anxiety Disorders. Ed. by Hussain A. Tuma & Jack D. Maser. 1985. 1172p. text 160.00 (*0-89859-532-0*) L Erlbaum Assocs.

Anxiety & the Heart. Ed. by D. G. Byrne & Ray H. Rosenman. 1990. (Series in Health Psychology & Behavioral Medicine). 325p. 79.95 (*0-89116-860-5*) Hemisp Pub.

Anxiety as Symptom & Signal. Ed. by Steven P. Roose & Robert A. Glick. 1995. LC 94-44632. 192p. text 29.95 (*0-88163-118-3*) Analytic Pr.

Anxiety Cure: An Eight-Step Program for Getting Well. Robert L. DuPont et al. 1998. LC 97-44043. 256p. pap. 15.95 (*0-471-24701-4*) Wiley.

Anxiety, Depression, & Mania. Ed. by P. Soubrie. 1991. (Animal Models of Psychiatric Disorders Ser.: Vol. 3). (Illus.). 134p. 128.75 (*3-8055-5247-5*) S Karger.

Anxiety Disorders. Russell Noyes, Jr. & Rudolf Hoehn-Saric. 1998. LC 97-42566. (Illus.). 353p. (C). text 85.00 (*0-521-55207-9*) Cambridge U Pr.

Anxiety Disorders: A Rational-Emotive Perspective. R. Warren & George D. Zgourides. 1991. (Psychology Practitioner Guidebooks Ser.). 180p. text (*0-08-040623-8*); pap. text (*0-08-040622-X*) PPI GBR. *Dist:* Elsevier.

Anxiety Disorders: A Scientific Approach for Selecting the Most Effective Treatment. Samuel Knapp & Leon VandeCreek. 1994. LC 94-7201. (Practitioner's Resource Ser.). 114p. pap. 17.95 (*1-56887-000-0*, ADBP, Prof Resc Pr) Pro Resource.

Anxiety Disorders: Proceedings Medical Symposium on Buspirone, Dusseldorf, Germany, April 18-19, 1985. 1985. 99p. (Orig.). (*0-934205-01-9*) Academy Prof Inform.

Anxiety Disorders: Psychological & Biological Perspectives. Ed. by Brian F. Shaw et al. 1987. LC 87-6998. 268p. 79.50 (*0-306-42485-1*, Plenum Trade) Perseus Pubng.

Anxiety Disorders: Psychological Approaches to Theory & Treatment. Michelle Craske. 1998. LC 98-19027. (Perspectives in Clinical Psychology Ser.). 448p. text 70.00 (*0-8133-3250-8*) Westview.

Anxiety Disorders & Phobias: A Cognitive Perspective. Aaron T. Beck et al. 1990. 372p. pap. 22.00 (*0-465-00385-0*) Basic.

Anxiety Disorders in African Americans. Ed. by Steven Friedman. 1994. LC 94-17232. 248p. 41.95 (*0-8261-8540-1*) Springer Pub.

Anxiety Disorders in Children & Adolescents. John S. March. 1995. LC 94-30107. 448p. 48.00 (*0-89862-834-2*) Guilford Pubns.

***Anxiety Disorders in Children & Adolescents: Epidemiology, Risk Factors & Treatment.** Ed. by Cecilia Essau & Franz Petermann. 2001. 352p. 65.00 (*90-5823-213-1*, Harwood Acad Pubs) Gordon & Breach.

***Anxiety Disorders in Children & Adolescents: Epidemiology, Risk Factors, & Treatment.** Ed. by Cecilia Essau & Franz Petermann. 2001. LC 2001-43282. (Biobehavioural Perspectives on Health & Disease Prevention Ser.: Vol. 4). (*1-58391-232-0*) Brunner-Routledge.

Anxiety Disorders in Children & Adolescents: Research, Assessment & Intervention. Ed. by Wendy K. Silverman & Philip D. A. Treffers. 2001. LC 00-33696. (Child & Adolescent Psychiatry Ser.). (Illus.). 418p. (C). pap. text 64.95 (*0-521-78966-4*) Cambridge U Pr.

Anxiety Disorders in Youth: Cognitive-Behavioral Interventions. P. C. Kendall. 1991. (Psychology Practitioner Guidebooks Ser.). 248p. text (*0-08-040621-1*); pap. text (*0-08-040620-3*) PPI GBR. *Dist:* Elsevier.

Anxiety Disorders in Youth: Cognitive-Behavioral Interventions. P.C. Kendall. 1993. LC 94-124089. (Psychology Practitioner Guidebooks Ser.). 224p. (C). pap. text 48.00 (*0-205-14589-2*) Allyn.

Anxiety in Children. Ved P. Varma. 1984. 228p. (C). 35.00 (*0-416-01031-8*, 9206) Routledge.

Anxiety in Elementary School Children. Seymour B. Sarason et al. 1978. LC 77-26021. (Illus.). 351p. reprint ed. lib. bdg. 35.00 (*0-313-20075-0*, SAAE, Greenwood Pr) Greenwood.

Anxiety in Sports: An International Perspective. Ed. by Dieter Hackfort & Charles D. Spielberger. 1990. (Series in Health Psychology & Behavioral Medicine). 350p. pap. 34.95 (*1-56032-143-1*) Hemisp Pub.

Anxiety in the Elderly: Treatment & Research. Ed. by Carl Salzman & Barry D. Lebowitz. 1990. LC 90-10015. 336p. 41.95 (*0-8261-7090-0*) Springer Pub.

A B

Anxiety, Learning, & Instruction. J. E. Sieber et al. 1977. 272p. 49.95 (*0-89859-425-1*) L Erlbaum Assocs.

Anxiety Management Training: A Behavior Therapy. R. M. Suinn. 1990. LC 90-42069. (Behavior Therapy Ser.). (Illus.). 392p. (C). 59.50 (*0-306-43545-4*, Plenum Trade) Perseus Pubng.

Anxiety, Phobias, & Panic: Taking Charge & Conquering Fear. Reneau Z. Peurifoy. 1988. (Orig.). pap. 12.95 (*0-929437-11-X*) Warner Bks.

Anxiety Resolution, Relaxation & Systematic & Flexible Hierarchy Guides, Set-AH. Russell E. Mason. 1975. (Train-Ascendance Ser.). pap. 45.00 incl. audio (*0-89533-009-1*, 58.GT-AR) F I Comm.

Anxiety Sensitivity: Theory, Research, & Treatment of the Fear of Anxiety. Steven Taylor. 1999. LC 98-23956. (Personality & Clinical Psychology Ser.). xii, 370p. 49.95 (*0-8058-2865-6*) L Erlbaum Assocs.

Anxiolytic Beta-Carbolines: From Molecular Biology to the Clinic. Ed. by David N. Stephens. 1994. (Psychopharmacology Ser.: Vol. 11). (Illus.). 162p. 86.95 (*0-387-57144-2*) Spr-Verlag.

Anxiolytic Compounds: Perspectives in Drug Development. Neal R. Cutler et al. 1996. LC 95-39622. 176p. 99.95 (*0-471-95713-5*) Wiley.

***Anxious Parent's Guide to Pregnancy.** Gerard M. DiLeo. 2002. 256p. pap. 14.95 (*0-07-138307-7*, Contemporary) McGraw-Hill Trade.

Anxious Self: Diagnosis & Treatment of Fears & Phobias. Intro. by Ronald A. Kleinknecht. 1986. LC 85-14279. 236p. (C). 32.95 (*0-89885-264-1*); pap. 20.95 (*0-89885-266-8*) Kluwer Academic (Kluwer Acad Hman Sci).

Anyone Can Intubate. Christine E. Whitten. 4th rev. ed. 1997. LC 94-75815. (Illus.). 240p. (Orig.). (C). pap. text 19.95 (*0-929894-18-9*) K-W Pubns.

AO-ASIF Instruments & Implants: A Technical Manual. R. Texhammar & C. Colton. 2nd rev. ed. 1993. LC 93-21299. (Illus.). 585p. 145.00 (*0-387-56895-6*) Spr-Verlag.

AO-ASIF Principles in Spine Surgery: Techniques Recommended by the AOASIF Group, Spine Education Committee. M. Aebi et al. 1997. LC 97-30417. (Illus.). 249p. 199.00 (*3-540-62763-4*) Spr-Verlag.

AO Principles of Fracture Management. T. P. Ruedi & W. M. Murphy. 2000. LC 00-32598. (Illus.). xvii, 864p. pap. 369.00 (*0-86577-886-8*) Thieme Med Pubs.

AOFAS Foot & Ankle Manual. G. James Sammarco. 1991. LC 90-13349. (Illus.). 390p. text 49.50 (*0-8121-1368-3*) Lppncott W & W.

AORN Patient Classification Instrument for Perioperative Nursing. AORN Staff. Ed. by Carol Applegeet. rev. ed. 1993. 50p. (Orig.). pap. text 25.00 (*0-939583-83-6*) AORN.

Aortic Valve. Ed. by Robert W. Emery & Kit V. Arom. 1991. LC 90-83246. (Illus.). 332p. text 69.00 (*0-932883-97-4*) Hanley & Belfus.

Aortic Valve. Mano J. Thubrikar. 1989. 221p. 129.00 (*0-8493-4771-8*, QP114) CRC Pr.

AOTA Self Study Series: Neuroscience & Occupation: Links to Practice. Ed. by Charlotte B. Royeen. 1997. pap. text 290.00 (*0-910317-82-8*) Am Occup Therapy.

AOTCB Study Guide for the COTA Certification Examination. Ed. by Susan M. Lang & Martha S. O'Connor. rev. ed. 1996. 72p. (Orig.). (C). pap. text 20.00 (*0-9639373-0-8*) Am Occupat Ther.

AOTCB Study Guide for the OTR Certification Examination. Ed. by Susan M. Lang & Martha S. O'Connor. rev. ed. 1996. 76p. (Orig.). (C). pap. text 20.00 (*0-9639373-1-6*) Am Occupat Ther.

Ape, Primitive Man & Child: Essays in the History of Behavior. A. R. Luria & L. S. Vygotsky. Tr. by Evelyn Rossiter from RUS. 1992. LC 91-73523. (Classics in Soviet Psychology Ser.). (Illus.). 192p. (C). per. 31.95 (*1-878205-43-9*) St Lucie Pr.

Apes, Giants & Man. Franz Weidenreich. 1946. (Illus.). lib. bdg. 10.00 (*0-226-88147-4*) U Ch Pr.

Apes, Men & Morons. Earnest A. Hooton. 1977. LC 76-134095. (Essay Index Reprint Ser.). 25.95 (*0-8369-1956-4*) Ayer.

APG Handbook, 1998. 1998. pap. 245.00 (*1-57372-104-2*) Solucient.

APG Handbook, 1997. 1997. pap. 245.00 (*1-57372-067-4*) Solucient.

Apha Practical Guide to Natural Medicines: The First Authoritative Home Reference for Herbs & Natural Remedies, from the Nation's Largest. Andrea Peirce. 1999. LC 98-26810. (American Pharmaceutical Association Guide Ser.). (Illus.). xvi, 728p. 37.00 (*0-688-16151-0*, Wm Morrow) Morrow Avon.

Apha's Complete Math Review for Pharmacy Technician. William A. Hopkins, Jr. 2001. (Illus.). 150p. pap. 28.00 (*1-58212-012-9*) Am Pharm Assn.

Apha's Complete Review for the Pharmacy Technician. L. Michael Posey. 2001. LC 2001-22955. 200p. pap. 30.00 (*1-58212-009-9*) Am Pharm Assn.

Aphasia. Ed. by F. Clifford Rose et al. 1990. 578p. pap. 87.75 (*1-56593-578-0*, 0061) Singular Publishing.

Aphasia: A Clinical Approach. John C. Rosenbek et al. 1989. LC 90-52763. 311p. (C). pap. text 38.00 (*0-89079-270-4*, 1781) PRO-ED.

Aphasia: A Clinical Perspective. D. F. Benson & Alfredo Ardila. 1996. (Illus.). 456p. (C). text 52.50 (*0-19-508934-0*) OUP.

Aphasia: A Pathophysiological Key to Memory & Volitional Naming. Robert Cohn. 1995. 137p. lib. bdg. 125.00 (*1-56072-234-7*) Nova Sci Pubs.

Aphasia: Assessment & Treatment. Ed. by Ruben H. Douglas & Nancy R. Macciomei. 1986. (Special Education Ser.). 110p. (C). 24.95 (*0-582-28631-X*); pap. text 16.95 (*0-582-28617-4*) Longman.

Aphasia: What Is It? Barbara J. Lecomte. 1995. 16p. 14.95 (*0-937857-04-1*, 1550) Speech Bin.

Aphasia & Associated Disorders: Taxonomy, Localization & Recovery. Andrew Kertesz. 1979. 368p. text 58.00 (*0-8089-1193-7*, 792278, Grune & Strat) Harcrt Hlth Sci Grp.

Aphasia & Brain Organization. Ivar Reinvang. 1985. LC 85-9545. (Applied Psycholinguistics & Communication Disorders Ser.). 208p. 59.50 (*0-306-41975-0*, Plenum Trade) Perseus Pubng.

Aphasia & Related Neurogenic Language Disorders. Leonard L. LaPointe. 2nd rev. ed. 1996. LC 96-19737. (Illus.). 256p. (C). text 49.00 (*0-86577-622-9*) Thieme Med Pubs.

Aphasia & Sensory-Perceptual Deficits in Adults. Ralph M. Retian. 1984. 173p. (Orig.). pap. text 34.00 (*0-934515-00-X*) Neuropsych Pr.

Aphasia & Sensory-Perceptual Deficits in Children. Ralph M. Reitan. 1985. 208p. (Orig.). pap. text 32.00 (*0-934515-01-8*) Neuropsych Pr.

Aphasia, Apraxia of Speech, & Dysarthria Samples. David E. Hartman & James P. Dworkin. 1993. (Illus.). 12p. (Orig.). (C). pap., stu. ed. 24.50 (*1-56593-309-5*, 0601) Thomson Learn.

Aphasia in Atypical Populations. Ed. by Patrick Coppens et al. 1997. LC 97-41461. 300p. (*0-8058-1738-7*) L Erlbaum Assocs.

Aphasia, My World Alone. Helen H. Wulf. rev. ed. 1986. LC 79-11334. 144p. pap. 13.95 (*0-8143-1823-1*) Wayne St U Pr.

Aphasia Rehabilitation: An Auditory & Verbal Task Hierarchy. Deborah Ross & Sara H. Spencer. 1980. (Illus.). 272p. 48.95 (*0-398-04031-1*) C C Thomas.

Aphasia Therapy File. Sally Byng. 1999. LC 00-361735. ix, 164p. 39.95 (*0-86377-566-7*) L Erlbaum Assocs.

Aphasia Therapy Workbook, Vol. 1. Julie Guerrero. Ed. by Cindy Drolet. 1997. 325p. ring bd., wbk. ed. 49.00 (*1-883315-27-1*, 8521) Imaginart Intl.

Aphasia Treatment: World Perspectives. Ed. by Audrey L. Holland & Margaret M. Forbes. 1993. LC 93-18644. (Illus.). 392p. (Orig.). (C). pap. text 59.95 (*1-879105-64-0*, 0328) Thomson Learn.

Apheresis: Principles & Practice. Ed. by Bruce C. McLeod et al. 1997. LC 97-35728. text 169.00 (*1-56395-082-0*) Am Assn Blood.

APIC Infection Control & Applied Epidemiology: Principles & Practice. Association for Practitioners in Infection Control Staff. 1996. LC 96-14096. (Illus.). 1408p. (C). (gr. 13). text 165.00 (*0-8151-0243-7*, 24857) Mosby Inc.

APICE 1998: Anaesthesia, Pain, Intensive Care & Emergency Medicine. Ed. by A. Gullo. 1999. LC 99-16114. 1000p. pap. (*88-470-0051-3*) Spr-Verlag ITA. *Dist:* Spr-Verlag.

APICE 1995: Anaesthesia, Pain, Intensive Care & Emergency Medicine. Ed. by A. Gullo. 1995. (Illus.). 800p. pap. 139.00 (*3-540-75014-2*) Spr-Verlag.

APICE 1999: Anaesthesia, Pain, Intensive Care & Emergency Medicine. Ed. by A. Gullo. 2000. 120p. pap. text 99.00 (*88-470-0095-5*) Spr-Verlag.

***APICE 115: Anaesthesia, Pain, Intensive Care & Emergency Medicine.** Ed. by A. Gullo. 2001. 720p. (C). pap. (*88-470-0136-6*) Spr-Verlag ITA. *Dist:* Spr-Verlag.

Aplastic Anemia. Ed. by H. Heimpel et al. 1980. (Illus.). 292p. 51.00 (*0-387-09772-4*) Spr-Verlag.

Aplastic Anemia: Acquired & Inherited. Neal S. Young & Blanche P. Alter. 1993. (Illus.). 496p. text 142.00 (*0-7216-3702-7*) Saunders.

Aplastic Anemia: Pathophysiology & Treatment. Ed. by Hubert Schrezenmeier & Andrea Bacigalupo. 1999. LC 99-10964. (Illus.). 403p. text 110.00 (*0-521-64101-2*) Cambridge U Pr.

Aplastic Anemia & Other Bone Marrow Failure Syndromes. Ed. by N. T. Shahidi. 1989. (Illus.). 236p. 170.00 (*0-387-97030-4*, 2944) Spr-Verlag.

Apley's System of Orthopaedics & Fractures. A. Graham Apley & Louis Solomon. 7th ed. 1999. LC 92-48221. (Illus.). 805p. (*0-7506-0641-X*) E A GBR. *Dist:* OUP.

APLS: The Pediatric Emergency Medicine Course. American Academy of Pediatrics Staff & American College of Emergency Physicians Staff. 2nd ed. 1993. 280p. pap. 79.95 (*0-910761-45-0*) Am Acad Pediat.

Apnea Monitoring by Means of Thoracic Impedance Pneumography. 1989. 60p. pap. 90.00 (*0-910275-88-2*, TIR4-209) Assn Adv Med Instrn.

Apocalypse: Nuclear Catastrophe in World Politics. Louis R. Beres. LC 80-13541. (Illus.). (C). 1982. pap. text 9.95 (*0-226-04361-4*); 1980. lib. bdg. 24.00 (*0-226-04360-6*) U Ch Pr.

Apolipoprotein E & Alzheimer's Disease. Ed. by A. D. Roses et al. 1996. (Illus.). 216p. 81.95 (*3-540-60798-6*) Spr-Verlag.

Apolipoprotein E Genotyping in Alzheimer's Disease. Norman R. Relkin et al. 1997. LC 96-45654. (Annals of the New York Academy of Sciences Ser.). 225p. pap. 80.00 (*1-57331-049-2*) NY Acad Sci.

Apolipoprotein E Genotyping in Alzheimer's Disease: Proceedings of a Conference Sponsored by the National Institute on Aging & the Alzheimer's Association, October 21-22, 1995, Vol. 802. Ed. by Norman R. Relkin et al. 1996. 80.00 (*1-57331-048-4*) NY Acad Sci.

Apolipoprotein Immunoassays: Development & Recommended Performance Characteristics; Approved Guideline (1997) 1997. 95.00 (*1-56238-331-0*, I/LA15-A) NCCLS.

Apolipoprotein Immunoassays: Development & Recommended Performance Characteristics: Proposed Guideline. 1991. 95.00 (*1-56238-117-2*, I-LA15P) NCCLS.

Apollo Versus the Echomaker: A Langian Approach to Psychotherapy Dreams & Shamanism. Anthony Lunt. 1993. 120p. pap. 12.95 (*1-85230-153-8*) Element MA.

***Apoptosis.** A. H. Wyllie. (British Medical Bulletin Ser.: Vol. 53, No. 3). pap. (*1-85315-317-6*) Royal Soc of Medicine Pr Ltd GBR. *Dist:* Balogh.

Apoptosis: Practical Applications & Novel Therapies. 1997. (Biomedical Library). pap. (*1-57936-036-X*) Drug & Market Dev.

Apoptosis & Cancer. Seamus J. Martin. 1997. (Medical Intelligence Unit Ser.). 250p. 89.95 (*0-412-13511-6*) Chapman & Hall.

Apoptosis & Cancer. Seamus J. Martin. 1997. LC 97-10616. (Medical Ser.). 216p. 98.00 (*1-57059-452-X*) Landes Bioscience.

Apoptosis & Cancer. Seamus J. Martin. 1997. LC 97-10616. (Medical Ser.). (Illus.). 216p. 98.00 (*3-8055-6579-8*) S Karger.

Apoptosis & Cancer Chemotherapy. Ed. by John A. Hickman & Caroline Dive. 1999. LC 99-12556. (Cancer Drug Discovery & Development Ser.: Vol. 6). (Illus.). xv, 342p. 115.00 (*0-89603-743-6*) Humana.

Apoptosis & Cell Cycle Control in Cancer: Basic Mechanisms & Implications for Treating Malignant Disease. Ed. by N. S. Thomas. 1996. (UCL Molecular Pathology Ser.). 300p. (*1-872748-89-9*) Bios Sci GBR. *Dist:* Coronet Bks.

Apoptosis & It's Modulation by Drugs. Ed. by Ross G. Cameron & George Feuer. 2000. LC 99-52107. (Handbook of Experimental Pharmacology Ser.: Vol. 142). (Illus.). 512p. 350.00 (*3-540-66121-2*) Spr-Verlag.

Apoptosis & Programmed Cell Death (PCD) Protocols. Ed. by Graham J. Cowling. 1999. (Methods in Molecular Medicine Ser.: No. 22). 79.50 (*0-89603-557-3*) Humana.

Apoptosis & the Immune System. Ed. by Christopher D. Gregory. 1995. LC 94-41047. 432p. 152.00 (*0-471-01251-3*) Wiley.

Apoptosis in Cardiac Biology. Ed. by Heribert Schunkert. 2000. (Basic Science for the Cardiologist Ser.: Vol. 5). 353p. 179.00 (*0-7923-8648-5*, Kluwer Acad) Kluwer Academic.

Apoptosis in Hormone Dependent Cancers. Ed. by Martin Tenniswood & Horst Michna. 1995. LC 95-952. (Ernst Schering Research Foundation Ser.: Vol. 14). 264p. 61.95 (*3-540-58840-X*); (*0-387-58840-X*) Spr-Verlag.

Apoptosis in Immunology. Ed. by G. Kroemer & C. Martinez-A. 1996. LC 15-12910. (Current Topics in Microbiology & Immunology Ser.: Vol. 200). (Illus.). 272p. 137.00 (*3-540-58756-X*) Spr-Verlag.

Apoptosis in Normal Development & Cancer. Ed. by M. Sluyser. 1996. 275p. 126.00 (*0-7484-0444-9*) Taylor & Francis.

Apoptosis in Pharmacology & Toxicology: Approaches to Measurement & Quantification. Ed. by Myrtle A. Davis. 2002. (Methods in Pharmacology & Toxicology Ser.). 176p. 79.50 (*0-89603-890-4*) Humana.

Apoptosis Two: The Molecular Basis of Apoptosis in Disease. Ed. by L. David Tomei & Fred O. Cope. 1994. (Current Communications in Cell & Molecular Biology Ser.: No. 8). (Illus.). 300p. (C). pap. text 69.00 (*0-87969-395-9*) Cold Spring Harbor.

Apothecary in Eighteenth-Century Williamsburg. Colonial Williamsburg Foundation Staff. 1965. (Historic Trades Ser.). (Illus.). 37p. (Orig.). pap. 2.95 (*0-910412-16-2*) Colonial Williamsburg.

Apoyo Vital Basico Guia para Salvar Corazones (Spanish Basic Life Support Heartsaver Guide), 1997-99. 1997. (Emergency Cardiovascular Care Programs Ser.). (Illus.). 95p. pap. 3.50 (*0-87493-677-2*) Am Heart.

App Pathology Radiographers. Laudici. 1989. 625.00 (*0-7216-2988-1*) Harcourt.

Appelton & Lange Review of Internal Medicine. Robert E. Pieroni. 3rd ed. 1999. 200p. pap. text 19.95 (*0-8385-0216-4*, A0216-0) Appleton & Lange.

Appendicitis: The Etiology, Hygienic & Dietic Treatment (1909) with a Chapter on Diabetes. John H. Tilden. 1996. 180p. reprint ed. pap. 13.00 (*1-56459-773-3*) Kessinger Pub.

Appetite: Neural & Behavioural Bases. Ed. by Charles R. Legg & David A. Booth. 1995. LC 94-11806. (European Brain & Behavior Ser.). (Illus.). 346p. text 65.00 (*0-19-854787-0*) OUP.

Appetite & the Eye: Visual Aspects of Food & Its Presentation Within Their Historic Context. Ed. by C. Anne Wilson. 1991. (Food & Society in History Today Ser.). (Illus.). 162p. (*0-85224-640-4*) Edinburgh U Pr GBR. *Dist:* Col U Pr.

***Appetite Disturbances & Disorders - Early Behavior & Hyperphagia: Index of New Information & Guide-Book for Consumers, Reference & Research.** 2002. 180p. pap. 47.50 (*0-7883-2427-6*) ABBE Pubs Assn.

Apple a Day. Jo Petty. 1999. 9.95 (*0-7667-2978-8*) Gibson.

Apple Cider Vinegar: Miracle Health System. Paul C. Bragg & Patricia Bragg. 50th rev. ed. 1999. (Illus.). 128p. per. 6.95 (*0-87790-042-6*) Hlth Sci.

Appleton & Lange Quick Review: Pharmacy. Joyce A. Generali et al. 11th ed. 1997. LC 97-1372. 315p. pap. 34.95 (*0-8385-6342-2*, A6342-8) McGraw-Hill Prof.

Appleton & Lange Review of Pharmacology. Walter Singer et al. 3rd ed. 1999. 213p. (C). pap. text 15.50 (*0-8385-7839-X*, A7839-2) Appleton & Lange.

Appleton & Lange's Outline Review for the Physician Assistant Examination. Albert F. Simon & Anthony A. Miller. 2000. LC 00-37240. (Illus.). 504p. pap. 39.95 (*0-8385-0373-X*) McGraw-Hill Prof.

Appleton & Lange's Outline Review for the USMLE: Step 2. Joel S. Goldberg. 3rd ed. 1998. LC 98-33537. 680p. pap. 39.95 (*0-8385-0354-3*) McGraw-Hill Prof.

Appleton & Lange's Practice Test - Pediatrics. Hansbarger. 1998. (C). pap. text 19.95 (*0-8385-0359-4*) Appleton & Lange.

Appleton & Lange's Practice Test - Surgery. Metzler. 2nd ed. 1998. (C). pap. text 19.95 (*0-8385-0361-6*) Appleton & Lange.

Appleton & Lange's Practice Tests for the USMLE Step 1. Joseph Krzanowski, Jr. 1999. pap. 32.95 (*0-8385-6341-4*, Medical Exam) Appleton & Lange.

Appleton & Lange's Practice Tests for the USMLE Step 2. Samuel L. Jacobs. 2nd rev. ed. 1998. pap. 32.95 (*0-8385-0357-8*, Medical Exam) Appleton & Lange.

Appleton & Lange's Practice Tests for the USMLE Step 2: A Student to Student Guide. Joel S. Goldberg et al. rev. ed. 1999. (Illus.). 350p. (C). pap. 39.95 (*0-8385-0372-1*) McGraw-Hill Prof.

Appleton & Lange's Quick Review. Ed. by Richard R. Rahr et al. 4th ed. 2001. LC 00-68100. 429p. pap. 29.95 (*0-8385-0394-2*) McGraw-Hill Prof.

Appleton & Lange's Quick Review: Health Information Management. Susan P. Bailey. 7th ed. 1998. LC 98-13628. (& L's Quick Review Ser.). 320p. (C). pap. 32.95 (*0-8385-0353-5*) Appleton & Lange.

Appleton & Lange's Quick Review: Medical Assistant. Laverne Dreizen. 5th ed. 2000. 24.95 (*0-8385-0397-7*) Appleton & Lange.

Appleton & Lange's Quick Review: Therapeutic Massage & Bodywork. Jane S. Garofano. 2nd ed. 1999. LC 99-462641. (& L's Quick Review Ser.). 182p. (C). pap. 28.00 (*0-8385-0337-3*) P-H.

Appleton & Lange's Quick Review of Pharmacy. Joyce Generali & Michele A. Danish. 3rd ed. 2001. LC 00-60525. (Illus.). 478p. pap. 39.95 (*0-8385-0400-0*) McGraw-Hill Prof.

Appleton & Lange's Review for the Cardiovascular Interventional Technology Examination. Judy Vitanza. 1996. LC 94-49171. (& L's Review Ser.). 250p. (C). pap. text 39.95 (*0-8385-0248-2*, A0248-3, Apple Lange Med) McGraw.

Appleton & Lange's Review for the Chiropractic National Boards, Pt. I. Linda W. Shanks. rev. ed. 1992. (Illus.). 208p. (C). pap. text 42.95 (*0-8385-0224-5*, A0224-4, Apple Lange Med) McGraw.

Appleton & Lange's Review for the Radiography Examination. D. A. Saia. 4th ed. 2000. LC 00-267730. (Illus.). xxiv, 418p. (*0-07-135990-7*) Appleton & Lange.

Appleton & Lange's Review for the Radiography Examination. D. A. Saia. 4th ed. 2000. LC 00-267730. (Appleton & Lange's Review Ser.). (Illus.). 418p. pap. 39.95 (*0-8385-0389-6*) McGraw-Hill Prof.

Appleton & Lange's Review for the Surgical Technology Examination. Nancy M. Allmers. 4th rev. ed. 1998. LC 96-19661. 216p. (C). pap. 39.95 (*0-8385-0270-9*, A0270-7) McGraw-Hill Prof.

Appleton & Lange's Review for the Ultrasonography Examination. Charles S. Odwin et al. 2nd rev. ed. 1998. LC 92-49035. (& L's Review Ser.). (Illus.). 584p. (C). pap. text 65.00 (*0-8385-9073-X*, A9073-6, Apple Lange Med) McGraw.

***Appleton & Lange's Review for the USMLE**, Step 3. Samuel L. Jacobs. 3rd ed. 2000. (First Aid Ser.). (Illus.). 350p. pap. 36.95 (*0-8385-5039-8*, Apple Lange Med) McGraw.

Appleton & Lange's Review for the USMLE: Step 1. Thomas K. Barton. 3rd ed. 1999. LC 99-462606. (Illus.). 331p. pap. 39.95 incl. cd-rom (*0-8385-0375-6*) McGraw-Hill Prof.

Appleton & Lange's Review for the USMLE Step 1. Thomas K. Barton. 2nd rev. ed. 1997. LC 96-83674. (Review Ser.). 331p. (C). pap. 36.95 (*0-8385-0265-2*, A0265-7, Apple Lange Med) McGraw.

Appleton & Lange's Review of Anatomy USMLE, Step 1. Royce L. Montgomery et al. 5th ed. 1996. LC 94-31509. 331p. (C). pap. text 39.95 (*0-8385-0246-6*, A0246-7, Apple Lange Med) McGraw.

Appleton & Lange's Review of Epidemiology & Biostatistics for the USMLE. Edward J. Hanrahan & Gangadhur Madupu. 1994. LC 94-7416. (Appleton & Lange's Review Ser.). (Illus.). 109p. (C). pap. text 39.95 (*0-8385-0244-X*, A0244-2, Apple Lange Med) McGraw.

Appleton & Lange's Review of General Pathology. Martin G. Lewis et al. 3rd ed. 1995. LC 93-2667. (Appleton & Lewis's Review Ser.). (Illus.). 197p. (C). pap. text 34.95 (*0-8385-0161-3*, A0161-8, Apple Lange Med) McGraw.

Appleton & Lange's Review of Internal Medicine. Barry J. Goldlist. 1995. LC 95-33372. (C). pap. text 34.95 (*0-8385-0251-2*, A0251-7) Appleton & Lange.

Appleton & Lange's Review of Internal Medicine. Barry J. Goldlist. 2nd ed. 1998. LC 98-26247. (Appleton & Lange's Review Ser.). (Illus.). 189p. (C). pap. 39.95 (*0-8385-0355-1*) McGraw-Hill Prof.

Appleton & Lange's Review of Pediatrics. Martin I. Lorin. 6th ed. 2001. (Illus.). 222p. (C). pap. 34.95 (*0-8385-0303-9*, A-0303-6, Apple Lange Med) McGraw.

Appleton & Lange's Review of Pharmacy. Gary D. Hall & Barry S. Reiss. 7th ed. 2000. LC 00-41838. (Illus.). 384p. pap. 39.95 incl. cd-rom (*0-07-136088-3*) McGraw-Hill Prof.

Appleton & Lange's Review of Physiology - USMLE 1. Penney. 1997. LC 97-33321. (Illus.). 277p. (C). pap. 32.95 (*0-8385-0274-1*, A-0274-9, Apple Lange Med) McGraw.

Appleton & Lange's Review of Psychiatry. Ivan Oransky. 6th ed. 2000. LC 00-37252. (Illus.). 306p. pap. 39.95 (*0-8385-0370-5*) McGraw-Hill Prof.

Appleton & Lange's Review of Respiratory Care. Crystal Dunlevy. 2nd rev. ed. 1994. LC 94-23439. (Review Ser.). 320p. (C). pap. 39.95 (*0-8385-8414-4*, A8414-3) P-H.

Appleton & Lange's Review of Surgery. Simon Wapnick et al. 3rd ed. 1998. LC 97-17395. (Appleton & Lange's Review Ser.). 220p. (C). pap. 39.95 (*0-8385-0245-8*, A-0245-9) McGraw-Hill Prof.

Application & Dispersal of Pesticides. 1964. (Technical Report Ser.: No. 284). 27p. pap. text 3.00 (*92-4-120284-X*) World Health.

Application of Advances in Neurosciences for the Control of Neurological Disorders: Report of a WHO Study Group, 1978. 1978. (Technical Report Ser.: No. 629). 83p. pap. text 9.00 (*92-4-120629-2*, 1100629) World Health.

Application of Basic Neuroscience to Child Psychiatry. S. I. Deutsch et al. 1990. LC 90-7203. (Illus.). 420p. (C). text 69.50 (*0-306-43357-5*, Kluwer Plenum) Kluwer Academic.

Application of Biomarkers to Cancer Epidemiology. Ed. by P. Toniolo et al. 1998. (IARC Scientific Publications Ser.: No. 142). (Illus.). 342p. pap. text 95.00 (*92-832-2142-7*) OUP.

Application of Cancer Chemotherapy: Proceedings of the 10th International Congress, Zurich, September 1977. Anticancer-Symposium Staff et al. Ed. by H. Schoenfeld. 1978. (Antibiotics & Chemotherapy Ser.: Vol. 24). (Illus.). 64.50 (*3-8055-2831-0*) S Karger.

Application of Chaos Theory to Psychological Models. Rae F. Blackerby. 1998. LC 98-198230. 174p. (C). pap. text 22.00 (*0-9632885-3-9*) Perf Strategies.

Application of Cognitive Psychology: Problem Solving, Education & Computing. Ed. by Dale E. Berger et al. 1986. 264p. (C). text 49.95 (*0-89859-710-2*) L Erlbaum Assocs.

Application of Hyperthermia in the Treatment of Cancer. Ed. by R. D. Issels & W. Wilmanns. 1988. (Recent Results in Cancer Research Ser.: Vol. 107). (Illus.). 277p. 101.00 (*0-387-18486-4*) Spr-Verlag.

Application of Induced Sterility for Control of Lepidopterous Populations. International Atomic Energy Agency Staff. 1971. (Panel Proceedings Ser.). (Illus.). 169p. pap. (*92-0-111271-8*, ISP281) IAEA AUT. *Dist:* Bernan Associates.

Application of Learning Theory to ESP Performance. Charles T. Tart. 1975. LC 75-14709. (Parapsychological Monographs: No. 15). pap. 8.00 (*0-912328-25-8*) Parapsych Foun.

Application of Magnetic Resonance to the Study of Lung. Ed. by Antonio G. Cutillo. 1996. (Illus.). 624p. 98.00 (*0-87993-611-8*) Futura Pub.

Application of Mental Health Statistics: Uses in Mental Health Programmes of Statistics Derived from Psychiatric Service & Selected Vital & Morbidity Records. Matthew S. Kramer. 1969. (ENG, FRE & RUS., Illus.). 112p. pap. text 12.00 (*92-4-156013-4*, 1150003) World Health.

Application of NMR Techniques on the Body Composition of Live Animals: A Seminar Organized by the Commission of the European Communities in the Framework of the Community Programme for the Coordination of Agricultural Research & held at the Institut fur Tierzucht & Tierverhaven, Mariensee (FRG), 14-15 June 1988. Ed. by E. Kallweit et al. 1989. 176p. 39.75 (*1-85166-404-1*) Elsevier.

Application of Non-Animal Models to Biomedical & Behavioral Research. Micheal B. Kapis. 1993. 288p. lib. bdg. 89.95 (*0-87371-504-7*, L504) Lewis Pubs.

Application of Nonclonal Antibodies in Tumor Pathology. Ed. by Dirk J. Ruiter et al. 1987. (Developments in Oncology Ser.). lib. bdg. 225.50 (*0-89838-853-8*) Kluwer Academic.

*__Application of Noninvasive Vascular Techniques.__ Amil J. Gerlock, Jr. et al. 2nd ed. 2001. 540p. text (*0-7216-6876-3*) Saunders.

Application of Radioiodinated Rose Bengal & Colloidal Radiogold in the Detection of Hepatobiliary Disease. Leonard Rosenthall. 1969. LC 68-59353. (Illus.). 88p. 9.50 (*0-87527-068-9*) Green.

Application of Signal Processing Concepts to Hearing Aids. Ed. by Paul Yanick, Jr. & Stephen Freifield. 1978. 256p. text 37.50 (*0-8089-1106-6*, 794945, Grune & Strat) Harcrt Hlth Sci Grp.

Application of Systems Analysis to Health Management: Report of a WHO Expert Committee, 1976. 1976. (Technical Report Ser.: No. 596). 69p. pap. text 7.00 (*92-4-120596-2*, 1100596) World Health.

Application of the International Classification of Diseases to Dentistry & Stomatology (ICD-DA) 3rd ed. 1994. (CHI & FRE.). v, 238p. (C). pap. text 50.00 (*92-4-154467-8*, 1153086) World Health.

Application of the International Classification of Diseases to Neurology. WHO Staff. 2nd ed. 1996. LC 98-114235. 604p. 182.00 (*92-4-154502-X*) World Health.

Application of the International Classification of Diseases to Neurology ICD-NA. WHO Staff. 1987. 253p. 39.00 (*92-4-154205-5*) World Health.

Application of the Rorschach Test to Young Children, Vol. 23. Mary Ford. 1975. LC 70-141545. (University of Minnesota Institute of Child Welfare Monographs: No. 23). (Illus.). 114p. reprint ed. lib. bdg. 48.00 (*0-8371-5892-3*, CWFR, Greenwood Pr) Greenwood.

Application of Time Use Methodology in the Social Sciences. Ed. by W. E. Pentland et al. 1999. LC 98-47892. (Illus.). 281p. (C). 59.50 (*0-306-45951-5*, Plenum Trade) Perseus Pubng.

Applications & Engineering of Monoclonal Antibodies. D. J. King. 1998. LC 99-181593. x, 249p. 95.00 (*0-7484-0422-8*) Taylor & Francis.

Applications in Behavioral Medicine & Health Psychology: A Clinician's Source Book. Ed. by James A. Blumenthal & Daphne C. McKee. 1987. LC 86-62715. 616p. 39.95 (*0-943158-18-4*, ABMBP, Prof Resc Pr) Pro Resource.

Applications in Health Psychology. Ed. by Marie Johnston & Theresa Marteau. 1988. 220p. text 44.95 (*0-88738-254-1*) Transaction Pubs.

Applications in Medical Nutrition Therapy. Frances J. Zeman & Denise M. Ney. 2nd ed. 1995. LC 95-34138. 485p. pap. 62.00 (*0-13-375015-9*) P-H.

Applications Manual for Radiographic Anatomy & Positioning: An Integrated Approach. Diane H. Gronefeld et al. 1997. LC 96-48080. 450p. (C). pap., wbk. ed. 29.95 (*0-8385-8247-8*, A8247-7) McGraw-Hill Prof.

Applications of Antisense Therapies to Restenosis. Leroy E. Rabbani. 1999. LC 98-51825. (*0-7923-8423-7*) Kluwer Academic.

Applications of Behavior Analysis to Prevent Injuries from Vehicle Crashes. E. Scott Geller. Ed. by Sigrid S. Glenn. rev. ed. 1998. LC 98-20157. (Behavior Monographs). pap. 16.95 (*1-881317-08-0*) Cambdge Ctr Behav.

Applications of Biomaterials in Facial Plastic Surgery. Frederick H. Silver. Ed. by Alvin I. Glasgold. 1991. 360p. 199.00 (*0-8493-5251-7*, RD523, CRC Reprint) Franklin.

Applications of Biotechnology to Medicine. Edvotek Staff. 1997. (Illus.). 120p. text 99.95 (*1-58100-023-5*) Beckley Cardy.

Applications of Counseling in Speech-Language Pathology & Audiology. Thomas A. Crowe. 1997. LC 96-9331. 392p. pap. 33.95 (*0-683-02216-4*) Lppncott W & W.

Applications of Diffusion Theory to Cancer Care in the United States 1972-1981. Elinor R. Schoenfeld. 1990. (Studies in Historical Demography). 240p. reprint ed. text 15.00 (*0-8240-5198-X*) Garland.

Applications of Dynamic NMR Spectroscopy to Organic Chemistry. Michinori Oki. 1985. LC 84-20844. (Methods in Stereochemical Analysis Ser.: Vol. 4). 423p. lib. bdg. 140.00 (*0-89573-120-7*, Wiley-VCH) Wiley.

Applications of Environment-Behavior Research: Case Studies & Analysis. Paul D. Cherulnik. 1993. (Cambridge Series in Environment & Behavior: No. 9). 358p. (C). text 69.95 (*0-521-33189-7*) Cambridge U Pr.

Applications of Fluorescence in Immunoassays. Ilkka Hemmila et al. 1991. LC 90-27188. (Chemical Analysis Monographs: Vol. 117). 360p. 175.00 (*0-471-51091-2*) Wiley.

Applications of Genetic Engineering to Crop Improvement. Ed. by Glenn B. Collins & Joseph G. Petolino. 1984. (Advances in Agricultural Biotechnology Ser.). text 256.50 (*90-247-3084-8*) Kluwer Academic.

Applications of Glass Capillary Gas Chromatography. Jennings. 1981. (Chromatographic Science Ser.: Vol. 15). (Illus.). 648p. text 250.00 (*0-8247-1223-4*) Dekker.

Applications of Item Response Theory to Practical Testing Problems. Frederic M. Lord. 1980. LC 79-24186. (Illus.). 288p. text 69.95 (*0-89859-006-X*) L Erlbaum Assocs.

Applications of Molecular Biology to Blood Transfusion Medicine. Ed. by George Garratty. 1997. LC 97-38417. pap. text 79.00 (*1-56395-092-8*) Am Assn Blood.

Applications of Networking in Family & Community: A Special Issue of Journal of Family Therapy, Vol. 6, No. 2. Uri Rueveni. 1984. 80p. pap. 14.95 (*0-89885-246-3*, Kluwer Acad Hman Sci) Kluwer Academic.

Applications of Neuro Fuzzy Systems in Medicine & Bio-Medical Engineering. Horia-Nicolai Teodorescu et al. 1998. LC 98-36332. (International Series on Computational Intelligence Ser.). 432p. 94.95 (*0-8493-9806-1*, 9806) CRC Pr.

Applications of New Technology - External Dosimetry: 1996 Health Physics Society Summer School. Ed. by Jack F. Higginbotham. 1996. (Illus.). 464p. LC 96-76738. text 69.95 (*0-944838-68-5*); pap. text 35.95 (*0-944838-69-3*) Med Physics Pub.

Applications of NLP: '78-'84. Robert Dilts. 1983. LC 83-61049. 24.95 (*0-916990-13-3*) META Pubns.

Applications of Noninvasive Vascular Techniques. Amil J. Gerlock. 1988. (Illus.). 560p. text 103.00 (*0-7216-2335-2*) Saunders.

Applications of Nonlinear Dynamics to Developmental Process Modeling. Ed. by Karl M. Newell & Peter C. Molenaar. 1997. LC 97-3672. 275p. (*0-8058-2115-5*) L Erlbaum Assocs.

Applications of Nonverbal Behavioral Theories & Research. Ed. by Robert S. Feldman. 1992. 288p. pap. 32.50 (*0-8058-1033-1*); text 59.95 (*0-8058-1032-3*) L Erlbaum Assocs.

Applications of Pharmacokinetics to Patient Care. Charles A. Walker. Ed. by Charles A. Walker & Lambros Tterlikkis. 1982. LC 81-23377. 175p. 57.95 (*0-275-91383-X*, C1383, Praeger Pubs) Greenwood.

Applications of Physics to Medicine & Biology: Proceedings of the 2nd International Conference on the Applications of Physics to Medicine & Biology, Italy, November 1983. Ed. by Z. Bajzer et al. 1984. 664p. (C). 123.00 (*9971-966-81-6*) World Scientific Pub.

Applications of Social Science to Clinical Medicine & Health Policy. Ed. by Linda H. Aiken & David Mechanic. 1986. 500p. (C). pap. text 16.95 (*0-8135-1149-6*) Rutgers U Pr.

Applications of Traumatic Incident Reduction. Frank Gerbode. 1993. lib. bdg. 39.95 (*1-57444-108-6*) St Lucie Pr.

Applications of Ultrashort-Pulse Lasers in Medicine & Biology, Vol. 3255. Ed. by Joseph Neev. 1998. 130p. 59.00 (*0-8194-2694-6*) SPIE.

Applied Analysis of Variance in Behavioral Science. Lynne K. Edwards. 1993. (Statistics: Textbooks & Monographs: Vol. 137). (Illus.). 640p. text 225.00 (*0-8247-8896-6*) Dekker.

Applied Anatomy & Biomechanics in Sport. John Bloomfield et al. 1994. (Illus.). 304p. (Orig.). pap. text (*0-86793-305-4*, BBLO0305) Blckwell Science.

Applied Anatomy of the Back. A. M. Landolt et al. Tr. by R. R. Wilson & D. P. Winstanley from GER. 1985. LC 85-9937. (Illus.). 425p. 690.00 (*0-387-15132-X*) Spr-Verlag.

Applied Anatomy of the Pelvis. W. Lierse. 1987. (Illus.). 335p. 544.00 (*0-387-16750-1*) Spr-Verlag.

Applied Angiography for Radiographers. Paul Laudicina & Douglas Wean. 1994. LC 93-27002. text 52.50 (*0-7216-3283-1*) Saunders.

Applied Animal Ethics. Leland S. Shapiro. 1999. LC 99-14916. (Illus.). 512p. 52.95 (*0-8273-8494-7*) Delmar.

Applied Animal Reproduction. H. Joe Bearden & John W. Fuquay. 5th ed. 1999. LC 99-25858. (Illus.). 400p. 96.00 (*0-13-081976-X*) P-H.

Applied Aviation Psychology: Achievement Change & Challenge. Ed. by Andrew R. Low & Brent J. Hayward. 1996. LC 96-86206. 490p. 93.95 (*0-291-39840-5*) Ashgate Pub Co.

Applied Basic Science for Basic Surgical Training. Andrew T. Raftery. 2000. LC 99-38215. text (*0-443-06144-0*) Church.

Applied Bedside Cardiovascular Physiology. Michael R. Pinsky. 1997. LC 96-53123. (Update in Intensive Care & Emergency Medicine Ser.). (Illus.). 249p. 140.00 (*3-540-62411-2*) Spr-Verlag.

Applied Behavior Analysis. John O. Cooper et al. 1990. 672p. (C). 131.00 (*0-675-20223-X*, Merrill Coll) P-H.

Applied Behavior Analysis & School Psychology: A Research Guide to Principles & Procedures. H. A. Ninness & Sigrid S. Glenn. 1988. LC 87-29544. 298p. lib. bdg. 72.95 (*0-313-24267-4*, NBA/, Greenwood Pr) Greenwood.

Applied Behavior Analysis in Brain Injury Rehabilitation. Ed. by William H. Burke. 2nd ed. 1996. (Professional Series on Traumatic Brain Injury: Vol. 2). 68p. (Orig.). pap. 9.50 (*1-882855-43-4*) HDI Pubs.

Applied Behavior Analysis in the Classroom. Patrick Schloss & Maureen A. Smith. 2nd ed. 1997. LC 97-30862. 356p. pap. text 66.00 (*0-205-19683-7*) Allyn.

Applied Biochemistry of Clinical Disorders. Allan G. Gornall et al. 2nd ed. 1986. LC 65-9319. (Illus.). 598p. text 45.00 (*0-397-50768-2*, Lippnctt) Lppncott W & W.

Applied Bioelectricity: From Electrical Stimulation to Electropathology. J. Patrick Reilly. 1998. LC 97-48860. (Illus.). 582p. 92.00 (*0-387-98407-0*) Spr-Verlag.

Applied Biopharmaceutics & Pharmacokinetics. Leon Shargel & Andrew B. Yu. 3rd ed. 1996. (Illus.). 625p. (C). pap. 56.95 (*0-8385-0129-X*, A0129-5) McGraw-Hill Prof.

Applied Biopharmaceutics & Pharmacokinetics. Andrew B. Yu & Leon Shargel. 4th rev. ed. 1999. LC 98-49079. (Illus.). 792p. (C). text 55.00 (*0-8385-0278-4*) McGraw-Hill Prof.

Applied Blood Group Serology. Peter D. Issitt & David J. Anstee. 4th ed. 1998. LC 98-65364. xxiv, 1208p. text 125.00 (*0-935643-05-2*) Mont Sci Pubns.

Applied Body Composition Assessment. Vivian H. Heyward & Lisa M. Stolarczyk. 1996. LC 95-33160. (Illus.). 232p. (Orig.). pap. text 26.00 (*0-87322-653-4*, BHEY0653) Human Kinetics.

Applied Cardiovascular Biology, 1989. Ed. by P. P. Zilla et al. 1990. (International Society for Applied Cardiovascular Biology Ser.). (Illus.). x, 198p. 164.50 (*3-8055-5147-9*) S Karger.

Applied Cardiovascular Biology, 1990-91. Ed. by P. P. Zilla et al. 1992. (International Society for Applied Cardiovascular Biology Ser.: Vol. 2). (Illus.). x, 254p. 213.25 (*3-8055-5430-3*) S Karger.

Applied Clinical Pharmacokinetics. Larry A. Bauer. 2001. LC 00-45078. (Illus.). 759p. (C). pap. 44.95 (*0-8385-0388-8*) McGraw-Hill Prof.

Applied Cognitive Psychology: An Information Processing Approach. Paul J. Barber. 1988. (Illus.). 170p. pap. 15.95 (*0-416-08762-0*, 9181) Routledge.

Applied Computational Statistics Longitudinal Research. Michael J. Rovine & Alexander Von Eye. 1991. 237p. (C). pap. text 53.00 (*0-12-599450-8*) Acad Pr.

Applied Concepts in Vision Therapy with Accompanying Disk. Leonard J. Press. 1997. LC 96-21428. (Illus.). 416p. incl. disk (*0-8151-6729-6*, 24293) Mosby Inc.

Applied Cross-Cultural Psychology. Ed. by Richard W. Brislin. 14th ed. 1990. (Cross-Cultural Research & Methodology Ser.: Vol. 14). (Illus.). 368p. (C). pap. 36.95 (*0-8039-3786-5*, 7376) Sage.

Applied Developmental Psychology. Ed. by Celia B. Fisher & Richard M. Lerner. 1994. LC 93-43168. 512p. (C). text 61.25 (*0-07-021172-8*) McGrw-H Hghr Educ.

Applied Drug Information. Mirta Millares. 1998. LC 98-193486. pap. 40.00 (*0-915486-28-8*) Applied Therapeutics.

Applied Electro-Acupoint Therapy Workshop Manual. Carolyn W. Greenlee et al. rev. ed. 1982. (Illus.). 152p. 45.00 (*0-9607836-0-1*) See Do Pr.

Applied Epidemiology: Theory to Practice. Ed. by Ross C. Brownson & Diana B. Petitti. 1998. (Monographs in Epidemiology & Biostatistics). (Illus.). 416p. text 52.50 (*0-19-511190-7*) OUP.

Applied Field Research in Malaria in Africa. 1982. (Bulletin Supplement Ser.: No. 62). 128p. pap. text 22.00 (*92-4-068621-5*) World Health.

Applied Human Relations. Gary Dessler. 1983. (C). text 37.67 (*0-8359-0180-7*) P-H.

Applied Immunohematology. Kathy D. Blaney & Paula R. Howard. 1999. (Illus.). 464p. (C). text (*0-323-00165-3*) Mosby Inc.

Applied Immunohistochemistry for the Surgical Pathologist. Ed. by Anthony S. Leong. 1993. 448p. (*0-340-55148-8*) E A GBR. *Dist:* OUP.

Applied Industrial - Organizational Psychology. Michael G. Aamodt. 1990. 529p. (C). pap. 54.75 (*0-534-13770-9*); 2nd ed. 1995. mass mkt., suppl. ed. 15.75 (*0-534-33881-X*); 2nd ed. 1995. LC 95-17007. xviii, 568p. pap. 52.50 (*0-534-33880-1*) Brooks-Cole.

Applied Kinesiology: Muscle Response in Diagnosis, Therapy & Preventive Medicine. Tom Valentine & Carole Valentine. 1989. LC 92-43338. 144p. pap. 12.95 (*0-89281-328-8*, Heal Arts VT) Inner Tradit.

Applied Kinesiology: Synopsis. D. S. Walther. 1988. (Illus.). 584p. text 95.00 (*0-929721-00-4*) Systems DC.

Applied Laboratory Medicine. Ed. by Norbert W. Tietz et al. 1992. LC 92-13381. pap. text 34.95 (*0-7216-6474-1*) Saunders.

Applied Laparoscopic Anatomy of the Abdomen & Pelvis. Gary G. Wind & Moshe Dudai. 1997. LC 96-8433. (Illus.). 376p. text 139.00 (*0-683-09136-0*) Lppncott W & W.

Applied Management in Hospital Pharmacy. Ed. by C. Richard Talley. 1991. 200p. text 20.00 (*1-879907-03-8*) Am Soc Hlth-Syst.

*__Applied Math for Allied Health.__ McNicholas. 2001. 48p. 5.75 (*0-536-63451-3*) Pearson Custom.

Applied Medical Microbiology. J. G. Collee. 2nd ed. 1981. (Illus.). 158p. pap. text 21.00 (*0-632-00853-9*) Blackwell Sci.

Applied Neuromuscular Pharmacology. Ed. by B. J. Pollard. 1994. (Illus.). 450p. text 135.00 (*0-19-262148-3*) OUP.

Applied Nursing Research: Commonsense Strategies for Clinicians. Bradi B. Granger. 1999. LC 98-41363. 288p. spiral bd. 40.00 (*0-8385-1539-8*) P-H.

Applied Nutrition: Study Guide. Ed. by Deakin University Press Staff. 1988. (C). pap. text (*0-7300-0548-8*, SHN750) Deakin Univ AUS. *Dist:* St Mut.

Applied Nutrition 1: Study Guide. Ed. by Deakin University Press Staff. 1987. (C). pap. (*0-7300-0464-3*, SHN730) Deakin Univ AUS. *Dist:* St Mut.

Applied Nutrition & Diet Therapy for Nurses. Judi R. Davis & Kim Sherer. 2nd ed. (Illus.). 1994. tchr. ed. (*0-7216-5459-2*); 1993. LC 92-49079. 1178p. 62.95 (*0-7216-6785-6*) Saunders.

Applied Nutritional Principles in Health & Disease. Ed. by Geoffrey H. Bourne. 1987. (World Review of Nutrition & Dietetics Ser.: Vol. 53). (Illus.). x, 302p. 237.50 (*3-8055-4681-5*) S Karger.

Applied Pathology for Radiographies. Paul Laudicina. 1989. 308p. text 52.00 (*0-7216-2143-0*) Saunders.

Applied Pharmacokinetics: Principles of Therapeutic Drug Monitoring. Ed. by W. E. Evans et al. 3rd ed. 1992. LC 85-72244. 1202p. 70.00 (*0-915486-15-6*) Applied Therapeutics.

Applied Pharmacology for the Dental Hygienist. Barbara S. Requa-Clark. (Illus.). (C). (gr. 13). 3rd ed. 1994. LC 95-106202. 416p. pap. text 44.00 (*0-8151-7233-8*, 23812); 4th ed. 1999. LC 99-16182. 512p. pap. text 39.95 (*0-8151-3630-7*, 28851) Mosby Inc.

Applied Pharmacology for the Veterinary Technician. Boyce P. Wanamaker & Christy L. Pettes. 1995. LC 95-1003. (Illus.). 256p. pap. text 33.50 (*0-7216-4954-8*) Saunders.

Applied Pharmacology for Veterinary Technicians. Boyce P. Wanamaker & Christy L. Pettes. 2nd ed. 2000. LC 99-49766. (Illus.). 430p. pap. text 35.00 (*0-7216-8577-3*) Saunders.

Applied Pharmacology Nurses. Sylvia Prosser. 2000. 433p. pap. text 29.95 (*0-7234-2588-4*) Saunders.

Applied Physics for Radiation Oncology. Robert Stanton & Donna Stinson. 1996. LC 95-49184. (Illus.). 375p. 68.95 (*0-944838-61-8*); pap. text 53.95 (*0-944838-60-X*) Med Physics Pub.

Applied Physiology for Surgery & Critical Care. Michael A. Glasby & C. L. Huang. 1995. LC 94-10942. (Illus.). 756p. text 205.00 (*0-7506-1168-5*); Pt. 3. 1997. 784p. pap. text 115.00 (*0-7506-3593-2*) Buttrwrth-Heinemann.

Applied Physiology in Clinical Respiratory Care. O. Prakash. 1982. text 249.00 (*90-247-2662-X*) Kluwer Academic.

Applied Physiology in Respiratory Mechanics. J. Milic-Emili. 1997. LC 97-34796. 233p. 108.00 (*3-540-75041-X*) Spr-Verlag.

Applied Physiotherapy: Practical Clinical Applications with Emphasis on the Management of Pain & Related Symptoms. Paul A. Jaskoviak & R. C. Schafer. 1986. LC 85-71674. (Illus.). 413p. text 42.00 (*0-9606618-2-4*, K-17) Am Chiro Assn.

Applied Psychiatric: Mental Health Nursing Standards in Clinical Practice. Ed. by Mary J. Krebs & Kenneth H. Larson. 1989. LC 87-25311. 388p. text 30.95 (*0-8273-4274-8*) Delmar.

Applied Psychologist. Ed. by James Hartley & Alan Branthwaite. 2nd ed. 2000. LC 99-25143. 264p. (*0-335-20285-3*) OpUniv Pr GBR. *Dist:* Taylor & Francis.

Applied Psychology in Personnel Management. Wayne F. Cascio. 2nd ed. 1982. (Illus.). 496p. (C). (*0-8359-0283-8*); text (*0-8359-0282-X*) P-H.

Applied Quantitative Methods for Health Services Management. James Lewis et al. 1995. LC 95-3855. 272p. (C). 42.00 (*1-878812-24-6*) Hlth Prof Pr.

Applied Radiographic Calculations. Cynthia A. Dennis & Ronald L. Eisenberg. 1993. (Illus.). 190p. pap. (*0-7216-4885-1*); LC 92-28280. 192p. pap. text 35.95 (*0-7216-6596-9*) Saunders.

Applied Radiological Anatomy. Ed. by Paul Butler et al. 1999. LC 2001-266903. (Illus.). 453p. (C). text 200.00 (*0-521-48110-4*) Cambridge U Pr.

Applied Research in Gerontology. William J. McAuley. 1987. 258p. 120.00 (*0-471-29082-3*, VNR) Wiley.

Applied Research in Residential Treatment. Ed. by Gordon Northrup. 1995. LC 94-24683. 99p. 29.95 (*1-56024-687-1*) Haworth Pr.

Applied Scientific Inquiry in the Health Professions: An Epistemological Orientation. Anne C. Mosey. 2nd ed. 1996. (Illus.). 400p. (Orig.). pap. text 55.00 (*1-56900-032-8*) Am Occup Therapy.

Applied Screen Film Mammography. Gini Wentz. 1991. (Illus.). 192p. pap. text (*0-08-040687-4*); text (*0-08-040686-6*) PPI GBR. *Dist:* McGraw.

Applied Social Psychology & Organizational Settings. John Carroll. 1990. 240p. (C). text 49.95 (*0-8058-0541-9*) L Erlbaum Assocs.

Applied Social Psychology in India. Girishwar Misra. 1990. 320p. (C). 27.50 (*0-8039-9645-4*, 7937) Sage.

Applied Specialties in Psychology. Elizabeth M. Altmaier & Merle E. Meyer. 1985. 500p. text 39.95 (*0-89859-714-5*) L Erlbaum Assocs.

Applied Specialties in Psychology. Elizabeth M. Altmaier & Merle E. Meyer. 1985. 600p. (C). text 34.25 net. (*0-07-554880-1*) McGraw.

Applied Spectroscopy: A Compact Reference for Practitioners. Jerry Workman & Art Springsteen. 1998. LC 97-41175. (Illus.). 539p. 89.00 (*0-12-764070-3*) Acad Pr.

Applied Sport Psychology: Personal Growth to Peak Performance. Jean Williams. 4th ed. 2000. LC 00-64731. xxiii, 548p. pap. (*0-7674-1747-X*) Mayfield Pub.

Applied Supervision in Psychotherapy. Ed. by Michael Blumenfield. 1982. 240p. text 37.00 (*0-8089-1461-8*, 790627, Grune & Strat) Harcrt Hlth Sci Grp.

Applied Surgical Anatomy. M. A. Glasby et al. 1998. LC 98-10423. 320p. (*0-7506-0777-7*) E A GBR. *Dist:* OUP.

Applied Survival Analysis: Regression Modeling of Time to Event Data. David W. Hosmer, Jr. & Stanley Lemeshow. 1999. LC 98-27511. (Probability & Statistics Ser.). (Illus.). 408p. 94.50 (*0-471-15410-5*) Wiley.

Applied Techniques in Behavioral Medicine. Ed. by Charles Golden et al. 1981. 464p. text 51.00 (*0-8089-1404-9*, 791622, Grune & Strat) Harcrt Hlth Sci Grp.

Applied Therapeutics: The Clinical Use of Drugs. Ed. by Lloyd Y. Young & Mary A. Kimble. 6th ed. 1995. LC 95-75490. 2360p. (C). 117.00 (*0-915486-23-7*) Applied Therapeutics.

Applied Toxicology: Approaches Through Basic Science. Ed. by J. P. Seller & E. Vilanova. 1997. LC 96-46756. (Archives of Toxicology Ser.). (Illus.). 417p. 157.00 (*3-540-62211-X*) Spr-Verlag.

Applied Toxicology of Petroleum Hydrocarbons. Ed. by H. N. McFarland et al. 1984. LC 84-60312. (Advances in Modern Environmental Toxicology Ser.: Vol. 6). (Illus.). 287p. pap. text 65.00 (*0-911131-07-8*) Specialist Journals.

Applied Veterinary Anatomy. Alexander De Lahunta & Robert E. Habel. 1986. LC 85-8379. (Illus.). 330p. text 52.00 (*0-7216-1431-0*) Saunders.

Applied Veterinary Epidemiology. Ed. by T. Blaha. 1989. (Developments in Animal & Veterinary Science Ser.). 344p. 147.50 (*0-444-98854-8*) Elsevier.

Applied Veterinary Histology, Vol. 3. William J. Banks. 3rd ed. 1992. LC 92-10984. (Illus.). 512p. (C). (gr. 13). text 66.00 (*0-8016-6610-4*, 06610) Mosby Inc.

Applied Virology Research: New Vaccines & Chemotherapy, Vol. 1. E. Kurstak et al. 1988. LC 87-32835. (Illus.). 328p. (C). text 95.00 (*0-306-42659-5*, Kluwer Plenum) Kluwer Academic.

Applied Virology Research Vol. 2: Virus Variability, Epidemiology & Control. E. Kurstak et al. 1990. (Illus.). 353p. (C). text 114.00 (*0-306-43359-1*, Kluwer Plenum) Kluwer Academic.

Applied Virology Research Vol. 3: Diagnostic Procedures. E. Kurstak et al. 1994. (Applied Virology Research Ser.). (Illus.). 188p. (C). text 95.00 (*0-306-44668-5*, Kluwer Plenum) Kluwer Academic.

Applying Computers in Social Service & Mental Health Agencies: A Guide to Selecting Equipment Procedures & Strategies. Ed. by Simon Slavin. 1982. LC 81-20102. (Administration in Social Work Ser.: Vol. 5, Nos. 3 & 4). 184p. text 44.95 (*0-86656-102-1*) Haworth Pr.

Applying Health Services Research to Long Term Care. Ed. by James C. Romeis et al. 1996. LC 95-41301. (Illus.). 232p. 42.95 (*0-8261-9140-1*) Springer Pub.

Applying Inpatient Coding Skills under Prospective Payment. Vickie L. Rogers. rev. ed. 1998. 198p. pap. text 56.00 (*1-58426-015-7*, AC200398) Am Hlth Info.

Applying Medication Math Skills: A Dimensional Analysis Approach. Gary M. Lawler. 1998. LC 98-8415. (Illus.). 288p. pap. text 43.95 (*0-7668-0050-4*) Delmar.

Applying Nursing Process: A Step-by-Step Guide. Rosalinda A. Alfaro-Lefevre. 4th ed. 1997. LC 97-25194. 288p. pap. text 26.95 (*0-397-55453-2*) Lppncott W & W.

Applying Nursing Research: A Text & Workbook. James A. Fain. 1998. LC 97-50464. (Illus.). 371p. pap. 31.95 (*0-8036-0227-8*) Davis Co.

Applying Psychology. Virginia N. Quinn. 3rd ed. 1994. LC 94-33045. 546p. (C). pap. 70.00 (*0-07-051339-2*) McGrw-H Hghr Educ.

Applying Psychology IBM 5.25. Virginia N. Quinn. 3rd ed. 1994. (C). pap. text 51.50 net. incl. disk (*0-07-912025-3*) McGraw.

Applying Psychology in Business: The Manager's Handbook. John W. Jones et al. 1990. (Issues in Organization & Management Ser.). 878p. 160.00 (*0-669-15838-0*) Lxngtn Bks.

Applying Structured Learning Therapy. Arnold P. Goldstein et al. 1977. LC 76-16518. 46.00 (*0-08-021109-7*, Pergamon Pr) Elsevier.

Appraisal of the Longitudinal Approach to Studies of Growth & Development. D. Kodlin & D. J. Thompson. 1958. (SRCD M Ser.: Vol. 23, No. 1). pap. 25.00 (*0-527-01573-3*) Periodicals Srv.

Appreciating Dreams: A Group Approach. Montague Ullman. 1996. LC 95-50167. (C). 344p. 72.95 (*0-7619-0127-2*, 1841); pap. 34.95 (*0-7619-0128-0*, 1842) Sage.

Apprentice to Genius: The Making of a Scientific Dynasty. Robert Kanigel. 1993. LC 93-5669. 304p. (C). reprint ed. pap. text 16.95 (*0-8018-4757-5*) Johns Hopkins.

Approaches & Methods in Neurotoxicology. Louis W. Chang & William Slikker. 1994. text 149.00 (*981-02-1798-6*) World Scientific Pub.

Approaches in Neurosurgery: Central & Peripheral Nervous System. J. Fischer et al. 1994. LC 94-32117. (Illus.). 200p. 199.00 (*0-86577-541-9*) Thieme Med Pubs.

Approaches to Art Therapy: Theory & Technique. Ed. by Judith A. Rubin. 1987. LC 86-26376. 362p. text 35.95 (*0-87630-452-8*) Brunner-Routledge.

Approaches to Art Therapy with Children. Marcia Rosal. 1996. pap. text 23.95 (*1-885762-01-1*) Abbeygate Pr.

Approaches to Breast Cancer Prevention. Ed. by Basil A. Stoll. 1991. (Developments in Oncology Ser.). 256p. text 166.50 (*0-7923-0995-2*) Kluwer Academic.

Approaches to Case Study: A Handbook for Those Entering the Therapeutic Field. Robin Higgins. 1993. 250p. pap. 24.95 (*1-85302-182-2*) Taylor & Francis.

Approaches to Child Treatment: Introduction to Theory, Research & Practice. James H. Johnson & Lawrence J. Siegel. 1986. (General Psychology Ser.). 264p. 55.00 (*0-08-033630-2*, J115); pap. 19.95 (*0-08-033629-9*) Elsevier (Pergamon Pr).

Approaches to Child Treatment: Introduction to Theory, Research, & Practice. James H. Johnson et al. 2nd ed. 1997. LC 96-32666. 368p. (C). 74.00 (*0-205-15604-5*) Allyn.

Approaches to Cognition: Contrasts & Controversies. Ed. by Terry Knapp & Lynn C. Robertson. 1986. 344p. (C). text 69.95 (*0-89859-623-8*) L Erlbaum Assocs.

Approaches to Desgin & Synthesis of Antiparasitic Drugs, Vol. 25. Ed. by N. Anand. 1997. LC 97-16035. (Pharmacochemistry Library: 25). 524p. 222.00 (*0-444-89476-4*) Elsevier.

Approaches to Gene Mapping in Complex Human Diseases. Ed. by Jonathan L. Haines & Margaret Pericak-Vance. 1998. LC 97-42666. 464p. 84.95 (*0-471-17195-6*, Wiley-Liss) Wiley.

Approaches to Planning & Design of Health Care Facilities in Developing Areas. B. M. Kleczkowski & R. Pibouleau. (WHO Offset Publications: No. 45). Vol. 3. 1979. 149p. 18.00 (*92-4-170045-9*); Vol. 4. 1983. 322p. 25.00 (*92-4-170072-6*) World Health.

Approaches to Planning & Design of Health Care Facilities in Developing Areas, Vol. 5. Ed. by B. M. Kleczkowski et al. 1985. (WHO Offset Publications: No. 91). 106p. pap. text 9.90 (*92-4-170091-2*, 1120091) World Health.

Approaches to Psychology. William E. Glassman. 2nd ed. 1995. LC 95-1904. 400p. pap. (*0-335-19259-9*) OpUniv Pr.

Approaches to Research. Robin Higgins. 1995. 120p. pap. text (*1-85302-307-8*) Jessica Kingsley GBR. *Dist:* Taylor & Francis.

Approaches to Syntax. Jean-Pierre Paillet & Andre Dugas. 1982. (Lingvisticae Investigationes Supplementa Ser.: Vol. 5). viii, 282p. 78.00 (*90-272-3115-X*) J Benjamins Pubng Co.

Approaches to Teaching in the Health Sciences. Harry J. Knopke & Nancy L. Diekelmann. 1978. LC 78-52503. text (*0-201-01656-7*) Addison-Wesley.

Approaches to the Clivus: Approaches to No Man's Land. Madjid Samii & E. Knosp. 1992. (Illus.). 169p. 159.00 (*0-387-54015-6*) Spr-Verlag.

Approaches to the Mind: Movement of the Psychiatric Schools from Sects to Science. Leston L. Havens. 1987. LC 86-25827. 399p. 40.00 (*0-674-04184-4*); pap. 14.50 (*0-674-04185-2*) HUP.

Approaches to the Study of Motor Control & Learning. J. J. Summers. 1991. (Advances in Psychology Ser.: Vol. 84). 600p. 152.50 (*0-444-88455-6*, North Holland) Elsevier.

Approaches to the Treatment of Aphasia. Nancy Helm-Estabrooks & Audrey L. Holland. 1997. LC 97-29784. (Clinical Competence Ser.). 288p. spiral bd. 61.95 (*1-56593-841-0*, 1642) Thomson Learn.

Approaches to Traditional Chinese Medical Literature: Proceedings of an International Symposium on Translation Methodologies & Terminologies. Ed. by Paul U. Unschuld. 1989. (C). text 148.50 (*1-55608-041-7*) Kluwer Academic.

Approaching Death: Improving Care at the End of Life. Committee on Care at the End of Life, Institute of. Ed. by Marilyn J. Field & Christine K. Cassel. 1997. LC 97-21175. 375p. 34.95 (*0-309-06372-8*) Natl Acad Pr.

Approaching Hysteria: Disease & Its Interpretations. Mark S. Micale. 1994. LC 94-16596. 327p. 49.50 (*0-691-03717-5*) Princeton U Pr.

Appropriate Coding for Critical Care Services & Pulmonary Medicine. 2000. 116p. pap. 70.00 (*0-916609-19-7*) Am Chest Phys.

Appropriate Diagnostic Technology in the Management of Cardiovascular Diseases: Report of a WHO Expert Committee, 1988. 1988. (Technical Report Ser.: No. 772). 41p. pap. text 6.00 (*92-4-120772-8*, 1100772) World Health.

Appropriate Technology. 1985. (Illus.). 73p. pap. (*0-7279-0157-5*) BMJ Pub GBR. *Dist:* AIDC.

Appropriate Use of Fluorides for Human Health. 1986. 136p. pap. text 22.00 (*92-4-154203-9*, 1150241) World Health.

Appropriateness & Effectiveness of Vocational Rehabilitation in Florida: Costs, Referrals, Services, & Outcomes. John A. Gardner. 1988. 35.00 (*0-935149-12-0*, WC-88-2) Workers Comp Res Inst.

Appropriateness of Spinal Manipulation for Low-Back Pain: Data Collection Instruments & A Manual for Their Use. Paul G. Shekelle et al. 1995. 131p. pap. text 10.00 (*0-8330-1656-3*, R-4025/5) Rand Corp.

Approval Motive: Studies in Evaluative Dependence. Douglas P. Crowne & David Marlowe. 1980. LC 80-475. (Illus.). 233p. reprint ed. lib. bdg. 67.00 (*0-313-22365-3*, CRAM, Greenwood Pr) Greenwood.

Approved Drug Products with Therapeutic Equivalence Evaluations. 17th ed. 1997. 800p. pap. 35.00 (*0-8080-0225-2*, 5457) CCH INC.

Approved Drug Products with Therapeutic Equivalence Evaluations. 1997. (Illus.). (C). 16th ed. 753p. reprint ed. pap. text 95.00 (*0-7881-4627-0*); 17th ed. 760p. pap. text 95.00 (*0-7881-4628-9*) DIANE Pub.

Approved Drug Products with Therapeutic Equivalence Evaluations. Ed. by Barry Leonard. 18th ed. 1999. (Illus.). 770p. (C). pap. text 95.00 (*0-7881-7324-3*) DIANE Pub.

***Approved Drug Products with Therapeutic Equivalence Evaluations.** Ed. by Barry Leonard. 21st ed. 2001. 1000p. pap. 125.00 (*0-7567-1183-5*) DIANE Pub.

Approved Drug Products with Therapeutic Equivalence Evaluations, 1999. Ed. by Barry Leonard. 19th ed. 2000. 800p. (C). pap. text 95.00 (*0-7881-8679-5*) DIANE Pub.

Approved Drug Products with Therapeutic Evaluations. 1995. (Illus.). 780p. (Orig.). (C). (gr. 6-12). pap. text 95.00 (*0-7881-0405-5*) DIANE Pub.

Apraxia of Speech in Adults: The Disorder & Its Management. Robert T. Wertz et al. 1984. 336p. text 42.00 (*0-8089-1612-2*, 794798, Grune & Strat) Harcrt Hlth Sci Grp.

Apraxia of Speech in Adults: The Disorder & Its Management. Robert T. Wertz et al. 1991. (Illus.). 328p. (C). reprint ed. pap. text 39.95 (*1-879105-54-3*, 0239) Thomson Learn.

Apraxia Profile Kit. Hickman. 1997. 51.50 (*0-7616-3259-X*) Commun Skill.

Apraxia Treatment Manual. Beth A. Kaufman. Ed. by Cindy Drolet & C. Gilles Brown. 1997. 223p. spiral bd. 45.00 (*1-883315-26-3*, 8457) Imaginart Intl.

Aprendiendo a Promover la Salud: Un Libro de Metodos, Materiales e Ideas para Instructores que Trabajan en la Comunidad. Bill Bower & David B. Werner. Ed. by Lynn Gordon & Anna M. Briggs. 1985. LC 81-85010.Tr. of Helping Health Workers Learn: A Book of Methods, Aids & ideas for instructors at the Village Level. (SPA., Illus.). 640p. (C). pap. 20.00 (*0-942364-14-7*) Hesperian Found.

Apricot Power: How Laetrile Cured My Cancer. Helen M. Curran. 1994. 111p. (Orig.). pap. 12.00 (*0-9642185-0-X*) H M Curran.

Apricots & Oncogenes: On Vegetables & Cancer Prevention. Eileen Jennings. 1993. LC 93-77061. 309p. (Orig.). pap. 13.95 (*0-9635890-3-2*) McGuire & Beckley.

April Fool's Day. Bryce Courtenay. 1997. 674p. 24.95 (*0-433-39710-1*) Buttrwrth-Heinemann.

Aquacises: Terri Lee's Water Workout Book. Terri Lee. 1990. (Illus.). 240p. reprint ed. pap. text 15.00 (*0-9627703-0-2*) Lee Pub AZ.

Aquacises: Terri Lee's Water Workout Book. Terri Lee. 1984. 256p. spiral bd. 22.50 (*0-8359-0152-1*) P-H.

Aquactic Safety. American Red Cross Staff. 1992. (C). (gr. 13). 3.95 (*0-8016-7686-X*) Mosby Inc.

Aquaculture for Veterinarians. Peter Emily & Susanna Penman. 2nd ed. 1994. LC 93-33124. (Veterinary Handbook Ser.). text 88.00 (*0-08-042291-8*) Elsevier.

Aquaculture for Veterinarians: Fish Husbandry & Medicine. Ed. by Lydia Brown. 1993. LC 92-41237. 462p. text 155.00 (*0-08-040835-4*, Prgamon Press) Buttrwrth-Heinemann.

Aquarian Conspiracy: Personal & Social Transformation in Our Time. Marilyn Ferguson. rev. ed. 1987. LC 87-10188. 464p. pap. 16.95 (*0-87477-458-6*, Tarcher Putnam) Putnam Pub Group.

Aquatic Examiner Program Chapter Handbook. American Red Cross Staff. 1994. (gr. 13). 5.00 (*0-8151-0275-5*) Mosby Inc.

Aquatic Rehabilitation. Richard Ruoti. 1996. LC 96-2682. 432p. text 53.95 (*0-397-55152-5*) Lppncott W & W.

Aquatics: A Revived Approach to Pediatric Management. Ed. by Faye H. Dulcy. 1983. LC 83-85. (Physical & Occupational Therapy in Pediatrics Ser.: Vol. 3, No. 1). 92p. text 39.95 (*0-86656-215-X*) Haworth Pr.

Aqueous Polymeric Coatings for Pharmaceutical Dosage Forms. James W. McGinity. 2nd ed. 1996. LC 96-43038. (Drugs & the Pharmaceutical Sciences Ser.: Vol. 79). (Illus.). 600p. text 215.00 (*0-8247-9773-6*) Dekker.

Aquired Immune Deficiency Syndrome: Biological Medical Social & Legal Issues. Gerald J. Stine. 3rd ed. 1997. LC 97-42639. 600p. (C). 70.00 (*0-13-789991-2*) P-H.

Arab Medicine & Surgery: A Study of the Healing Art in Algeria. Melville W. Hilton-Simpson. LC 75-23721. reprint ed. 29.50 (*0-404-13279-0*) AMS Pr.

Arabian Medicine. Edward Brown. 1992. 19.95 (*0-935782-19-2*) Kazi Pubns.

Arabian Medicine & Its Influence on the Middle Ages, Set. Donald E. Campbell. LC 74-180330. reprint ed. 84.50 (*0-404-56235-3*) AMS Pr.

Arachidonate Metabolism in Immunologic Systems. Ed. by L. Levine. 1988. (Progress in Allergy Ser.: Vol. 44). (Illus.). viii, 216p. 128.75 (*3-8055-4773-0*) S Karger.

Arachidonic Acid Metabolism & Tumor Initiation. Lawrence J. Marnett. 1985. (Prostaglandins, Leukotrienes, & Cancer Ser.). text 113.50 (*0-89838-729-9*) Kluwer Academic.

Arachidonic Acid Metabolism & Tumor Promotion. Ed. by Susan M. Fischer & Thomas J. Slaga. 1985. (Prostaglandins, Leukotrienes, & Cancer Ser.). text 127.50 (*0-89838-724-8*) Kluwer Academic.

Arachidonic Acid Metabolism in Corneal Epithelial Cells: Identification of Lipoxygenase Isoforms. Maria Liminga. 2000. (Comprehensive Summaries of Uppsala Dissertations from the Faculty of Pharmacy Ser.: 222). (Illus.). 55p. pap. (*91-554-4666-3*) Uppsala Universitet SWE. *Dist:* Coronet Bks.

Arbeiterfrage: The Labor Question: with Particular Consideration of the Social Psychological Side of Modern Large-Scale Industry & Its Psycho-Physical Effect on Workers. Adolf Levenstein. 1975. LC 74-25767. (European Sociology Ser.). 410p. reprint ed. 34.95 (*0-405-06521-3*) Ayer.

Arbeitsdiagnose - Neue Wege der Chirurgischen Diagnose und Therapie. M. Hobsley. Tr. by Caroline Seemann from ENG. 1981. Orig. Title: Pathways in Surgical Management. (GER.). 480p. pap. 34.00 (*3-8055-0747-X*) S Karger.

Arboviruses & Human Disease: Report of a WHO Scientific Group, 1967. 1967. (Technical Report Ser.: No. 369). 84p. pap. text 5.00 (*92-4-120369-2*, 1100369) World Health.

ARC Foundations for Caregiving Textbook. American Red Cross Staff. 1993. 512p. (gr. 13). pap. text 22.50 (*0-8016-6515-9*) Mosby Inc.

Archaebacteria: Proceedings of the 1st International Workshop on Archebacteria, Munich 1981. O. Kandler. 1982. (Illus.). 366p. text 72.00 (*3-437-10797-6*) Lubrecht & Cramer.

Archeology of Disease. Charlotte Roberts & Keith Manchester. 2nd ed. 1997. LC 95-15961. (Illus.). 256p. pap. 23.95 (*0-8014-8448-0*) Cornell U Pr.

Archetypal Medicine. Alfred J. Ziegler. 2000. 169p. pap. 17.00 (*0-88214-374-3*) Spring Pubns.

Archetype of the Unconscious & the Transfiguration of Therapy: Reflections On Jungian Psychology. Charles Ponce. 1990. 120p. (Orig.). pap. 9.95 (*1-55643-070-1*) North Atlantic.

Architectural Design & Indoor Microbial Pollution. Ed. by Ruth B. Kundsin. 1988. (Illus.). 328p. text 55.00 (*0-19-504436-3*) OUP.

Architecture & Dynamics of Developing Mind: Experiential Structuralism As a Frame for Unifying Cognitive Developmental Theories. Andreas Demetriou et al. 1993. (Monographs of the Society for Research in Child Development). 216p. pap. text 19.50 (*0-226-14247-7*) U Ch Pr.

Architecture & Medicine: I. M. Pei Designs the Kirklin Clinic, University of Alabama at Birmingham Medical Center. Aaron Betsky. 1993. LC 92-28149. 144p. (C). lib. bdg. 40.00 (*0-8191-8878-6*) U Pr of Amer.

Architecture of Amnesia. Mary A. Staniszewski & Dennis Adams. Ed. by Susan Harris. 1990. (Illus.). 112p. pap. 30.00 (*1-878607-07-3*) Kent Gallery.

Architecture of Cognition. John R. Anderson. 1995. 352p. pap. text 39.95 (*0-8058-2233-X*) L Erlbaum Assocs.

Architecture of Fear. Ed. by Kathryn D. Cramer & Peter D. Pautz. 1989. 288p. pap. 3.95 (*0-380-70553-2*, Avon Bks) Morrow Avon.

Architecture of Imaging. Bill Rostenberg. 1995. LC 95-17090. pap. 120.00 (*1-55648-140-3*, 043183) AHPI.

Archive Fever: A Freudian Impression. Jacques Derrida. Tr. by Eric Prenowitz. 1996. LC 96-18568. (Religion & Postmodernism Ser.). 144p. 17.95 (*0-226-14336-8*) U Ch Pr.

Archives of the Foundation of Thanatology: Social Work & Terminal Care, Vol. 9. pap. 19.95 (*0-405-14207-2*) Ayer.

Archives of the Foundation of Thanatology, Vol. 8: Acute Grief III: Continuum of Anticipatory Grief; Dying & Death; Acute Grief; Bereavement; Recovery from Bereavement, or Pathological Bereavement; & Lifelong Bereavement, Vol. 4. pap. 18.95 (*0-405-13074-0*) Ayer.

Archives of the Foundation of Thanatology, Vol. 8: Urology & Psychosocial Aspects of Chronic, Critical & Terminal Illness: The Patient, the Family & the Staff, Vol. 3. 1980. pap. 18.95 (*0-405-13099-6*) Ayer.

Archives of the Foundation of Thanatology, Vol. 9: Psychosocial Aspects of Radiation Oncology: The Radiation Therapist & Supporting Staff, No. 1. pap. 19.95 (*0-405-13073-2*) Ayer.

Archives of the Foundation of Thanatology, Vol. 9: Veterinary Medical Practice: Pet Loss & Human Emotion, Vol. 2. pap. 18.95 (*0-405-13083-X*) Ayer.

Arctic Aeromedical Laboratory's Thyroid Function Study: A Radiological Risk & Ethical Analysis. NRC, Committee on Evaluation of 1950s Air Force Hu. 1996. 116p. (Orig.). pap. text 34.00 (*0-309-05428-1*) Natl Acad Pr.

Ardous Touch: Women's Voices in Health Care. Ed. by Amy M. Haddad & Kate H. Brown. 1999. LC 98-55266. 133p. pap. 15.95 (*1-55753-154-4*, NotaBell) Purdue U Pr.

ARDS: Acute Respiratory Distress in Adults. T. Evans & C. Haslett. 1996. LC 96-83464. (Illus.). 568p. (*0-412-56910-8*) E A GBR. *Dist:* OUP.

Are Existing Private Sector & State-Operated Health Care Alliances Working? Congressional Hearings. Ed. by Edolphus Towns. 1994. 138p. (C). pap. text 25.00 (*0-7881-8293-5*) DIANE Pub.

Are Existing Private Sector & State-operated Health Care Alliances Working? Hearing Before the Human Resources & Intergovernmental Relations Subcommittee of the Committee on Government Operations, House of Representatives, One Hundred Third Congress, Second Session, June 30, 1994. U. S. Government Printing Office Staff. 1997. LC 98-110191. iii, 138 p. (*0-16-055507-8*) USGPO.

Are the Medical Needs for the Treatment of Acute Pain Fulfilled? Istanbul, Turkey, October 5, 1996. Michael J. Parnham. 1997. LC 97-512. pap. (*0-8176-5679-0*) Birkhauser.

Are the Medical Needs for the Treatment of Acute Pain Fulfilled? Istanbul, Turkey, October 5th, 1996. Michael J. Parnham. 1997. LC 97-512. pap. 12.00 (*3-7643-5679-0*) Birkhauser.

Are There Alternate Therapies for Cancer & AIDS? Ernest W. Filberth & Juanita V. Cook. 1995. 112p. pap. 9.95 (*0-9649121-0-4*) J V Cook.

Are You a Genius? Ron Dalrymple. 1978. 15p. pap. 1.00 (*0-935882-00-6*) Celestial Gifts.

Are You Allergic? William G. Crook. rev. ed. 1978. pap. 6.95 (*0-933478-02-X*) Prof Bks Future Health.

Are You Confused? The Authoritative Answers to Controversial Questions. Paavo O. Airola. 1984. 224p. pap. 7.95 (*0-932090-04-4*) Health Plus.

Are You Considering Cosmetic Surgery? Arthur W. Perry. 1997. pap. 5.99 (*0-380-79159-5*, Avon Bks) Morrow Avon.

Are You Considering Psychoanalysis? Ed. by Karen Horney. 1962. pap. 9.95 (*0-393-00131-8*) Norton.

Are You Getting Enlightened or Losing Your Mind? A Spiritual Program for Mental Fitness. Dennis Gersten. 2000. 310p. reprint ed. text 25.00 (*0-7881-6868-1*) DIANE Pub.

Are You Radioactive? Linda Clark. 1973. LC 73-76155. 128p. pap. 9.95 (*0-8159-5013-6*) Devin.

Are You Ready for a Miracle?... With Chiropractic: A Practical Guide to Understanding Chiropractic Healing in Everyday Life. Angelica E. Wagner. Ed. by Murray Fisher. 2nd ed. 2000. 208p. reprint ed. pap. (*1-896375-02-2*) Mir1acleworks.

Are You Really Too Sensitive? How to Understand & Develop Your Sensitivity as the Strength It Is. Marcy Calhoun. 1987. LC 87-7983. 208p. pap. 12.95 (*0-931892-10-4*) B Dolphin Pub.

Are You Sad Too? Helping Children Deal with Loss & Death. Dinah Siebert et al. 1993. LC 92-21150. (*1-56071-117-5*) ETR Assocs.

Are You Sure It's Arthritis? A Guide to Soft-Tissue Rheumatism. Paul Davidson. 1985. LC 85-13668. 224p. 15.95 (*0-02-529770-8*) Macmillan.

Are You the Doctor, Doctor? Vol. IV: The Philosophy of Successful Practice. Frederick H. Barge. 3rd ed. 1993. 157p. pap. 24.95 (*1-885048-09-2*) Barge Chiropract.

Arena of Masculinity: Sports, Homosexuality, & the Meaning of Sex. Brian Pronger. 1992. LC 91-29264. (Stonewall Inn Editions Ser.). (Illus.). 320p. pap. 15.95 (*0-312-06293-1*) St Martin.

Arenaviridiae. M. S. Salvato. 1993. (Viruses Ser.). (Illus.). 426p. (C). text 110.00 (*0-306-44272-8*, Kluwer Plenum) Kluwer Academic.

Arginine Solution: The First Guide to America's New Cardio-Enhancing Supplement. Robert Fried et al. 2000. 304p. mass mkt. (*0-446-60784-3*) Warner.

Arhythmias. John A. Kastor. 2nd ed. 2000. LC 99-19076. (Illus.). viii, 603p. text 89.00 (*0-7216-7647-2*) Saunders.

Aristotle: The Power of Perception. Deborah K. Modrak. LC 86-19208. (C). 1995. x, 250p. 35.95 (*0-226-53338-7*); 1989. x, 260p. pap. text 17.00 (*0-226-53339-5*) U Ch Pr.

Arithmetical Word Problem Solving after Frontal Lobe Damage: A Cognitive Neuropsychological Approach. Luciano Fasotti. 1992. x, 134p. pap. (*90-265-1308-9*) Swets.

Arizona Health Care in Perspective 1999. Ed. by Kathleen O'Leary Morgan & Scott E. Morgan. 1999. 21p. spiral bd. 19.00 (*0-7401-0052-1*) Morgan Quitno Corp.

Arizona Health Care in Perspective 2000. Ed. by Kathleen O'Leary Morgan & Scott E. Morgan. 2000. 21p. spiral bd. 19.00 (*0-7401-0202-8*) Morgan Quitno Corp.

Arizona Health Care Perspective, 1998. Ed. by Kathleen O'Leary Morgan & Scott E. Morgan. 1998. 20p. pap. 19.00 (*1-56692-802-8*) Morgan Quitno Corp.

Arizona Law of Medical Malpractice. Robert Stephen, Jr. 1997. 320p. 88.00 (*0-916763-00-5*) Medilex Co.

Arizona Medical Association: The First Hundred Years. John W. Kenendy. Ed. by Kathy Bailey. 1993. (C). text 15.00 (*0-929690-19-2*) Herit Pubs AZ.

Arizona Territorial Hospital Records 1890-1910. Dora M. Whiteside. 1985. 61p. (Orig.). pap. 8.00 (*0-938353-04-7*) D M Whiteside.

Arkansas Health Care in Perspective 2000. Ed. by Kathleen O'Leary Morgan & Scott E. Morgan. 2000. 21p. spiral bd. 19.00 (*0-7401-0203-6*) Morgan Quitno Corp.

Arkansas Health Care Perspective, 1998. Ed. by Kathleen O'Leary Morgan & Scott E. Morgan. 1998. 20p. pap. 19.00 (*1-56692-803-6*) Morgan Quitno Corp.

Armchair Fitness. Manor Healthcare Corporation Staff & Betty Switkes. 1984. (Illus.). 64p. (*0-917025-00-8*) Manor Health.

Armfuls of Time: The Psychological Experience of the Child with a Life-Threatening Illness. Barbara M. Sourkes. 1996. LC 95-8667. 187p. pap. 19.95 (*0-8229-5565-2*); text 39.95 (*0-8229-3888-X*) U of Pittsburgh Pr.

Armica the Wonder Herb. Phyllis Speight. 1977. 103p. pap. (*0-85032-138-7*) C W Daniel GBR. *Dist:* Natl Bk Netwk.

Armies of Pestilence: The Effects of Pandemics on History. R. S. Bray. 1997. LC 97-156006. (Illus.). 258p. (*0-7188-2949-2*) Lutterwrth GBR. *Dist:* Parkwest Pubns.

Army Medical Department, 1818-1865. 1995. lib. bdg. 299.75 (*0-8490-7574-2*) Gordon Pr.

Army Medical Department, 1818-1865. Mary C. Gillett. 1987. LC 87-600095. (Army Historical Series, Center for Military History Publication: No. 330-5). (Illus.). 385p. (Orig.). per. 25.00 (*0-16-001954-0*, 008-029-00152-7) USGPO.

Army Medical Support to the Army after Next: Issues & Insights from the Medical Technology Workshop 1999. Gary Cecchine et al. 2001. LC 00-45831. (Illus.). pap. 15.00 (*0-8330-2914-2*) Rand Corp.

Army Surgeon's Manual. William Grace. 1992. (American Civil War Medical Ser.: No. 10). 200p. reprint ed. 45.00 (*0-930405-41-2*) Norman SF.

Arnica the Wonder Herb. Phyllis Speight. 1977. (C). pap. 7.95 (*0-8464-0992-5*) Beekman Pubs.

Arnold Gessell: Themes of His Work. Louise B. Ames. 1989. (Illus.). 288p. 45.95 (*0-89885-421-0*, Kluwer Acad Hman Sci) Kluwer Academic.

Aroma-Color-Plant-Sound Correlations for Healing: A Practical Reference Table. Jeanne Rose. 1990. (Illus.). stu. ed. 15.00 (*0-9620838-7-9*, J R Herb Pubns) Herb Studies Library.

Aroma Therapy Kit. Charla Devereux. 1993. 112p. 26.95 (*0-8048-1981-5*) Tuttle Pubng.

Aromatase Inhibition & Breast Cancer. William R. Miller & Richard J. Santen. 2000. LC 00-47464. (Illus.). 322p. text 150.00 (*0-8247-0412-6*) Dekker.

Aromaterapia Esencial. Kendra Grace. 2000. (SPA., Illus.). 264p. pap. 9.95 (*1-56718-289-5*) Llewellyn Pubns.

Aromatherapy. 2001. (Gem Ser.). (Illus.). 192p. pap. (*0-00-710146-5*) HarpC GBR. *Dist:* Trafalgar.

Aromatherapy. Viktor Blevi & Gretchen Sween. 1993. (Illus.). 176p. (Orig.). pap. 10.00 (*0-380-76429-6*, Avon Bks) Morrow Avon.

Aromatherapy. Ed. by Joanna Drew. 1997. (Select Pocket Library). 96p. 4.98 (*0-7858-0446-3*) Bk Sales Inc.

Aromatherapy. Clare Walters. 1998. LC 98-6664. (Illustrated Guides Ser.). (Illus.). 144p. pap. 19.95 (*1-86204-166-0*) Element MA.

Aromatherapy: A Lifetime Guide to Healing with Essential Oils. Valerie Gennari Cooksley. 1996. LC 95-53852. 220p. pap. 13.95 (*0-13-349432-2*) PH Pr.

Aromatherapy: An A-Z. Patricia Davis. enl. rev. ed. 1998. 368p. pap. (*0-85207-295-3*) C W Daniel GBR. *Dist:* Natl Bk Netwk.

Aromatherapy: For Health & Harmony. Evans. 2000. (Health & Well-Being Ser.). 64p. pap. (*1-84215-175-4*, Swater) Ann3ess GBR. *Dist:* AOL Time Warner, AOL Time Warner.

Aromatherapy: Principles & Practice. Carol Horrigan & Nicole Perez. 2002. 272p. pap. 37.50 (*0-7506-3807-9*) Buttrwrth-Heinemann.

Aromatherapy: The A-Z Guide to Healing with Essential Oils. Shelagh R. Masline & Barbara Close. 1997. LC 98-114031. (Essential Healing Arts Ser.). 240p. mass mkt. 5.99 (*0-440-22256-7*) Dell.

Aromatherapy: The Treatment of Illness with the Essences of Plants. Jean Valnet. 1980. 40.00 (*0-85027-141-X*) St Mut.

Aromatherapy: To Heal & Tend the Body. Robert B. Tisserand. 1988. (Illus.). 240p. pap. 10.95 (*0-941524-42-6*) Lotus Pr.

Aromatherapy A-Z. Connie Higley et al. 2001. (Illus.). 156p. pap. 11.95 (*1-56170-796-1*, 5527) Hay House.

Aromatherapy an A-Z. Patricia Davis. 1991. 382p. (Orig.). pap. 29.95 (*0-8464-1537-2*) Beekman Pubs.

Aromatherapy Chart. pap. (*0-86315-595-2*, 1742) Floris Bks GBR. *Dist:* Anthroposophic.

Aromatherapy During Your Pregnancy. Date not set. pap. 7.95 (*0-8464-4557-3*) Beekman Pubs.

Aromatherapy During Your Pregnancy. Frances R. Clifford. 1997. (Illus.). 96p. pap. (*0-85207-312-7*) C W Daniel GBR. *Dist:* Natl Bk Netwk.

Aromatherapy for Common Ailments: A Gaia Original. Shirley Price. 1991. LC 90-20746. (Illus.). 96p. pap. 14.95 (*0-671-73134-3*, Fireside) S&S Trade Pap.

Aromatherapy for Health Professionals. Shirley Price & Len Price. 1995. LC 95-20316. pap. text (*0-443-04975-0*) Church.

Aromatherapy for Horses. Caroline Ingraham. 1997. (Threshold Picture Guides Ser.). (Illus.). 24p. pap. 12.00 (*1-872082-98-X*) Half Halt Pr.

Aromatherapy for Midwives. Tiran. 1996. pap. text 30.00 (*0-7020-1978-X*) Saunders.

Aromatherapy for Women: A Practical Guide to Essential Oils for Health & Beauty. Maggie Tisserand. rev. ed. 1996. LC 95-43956. 176p. pap. 8.95 (*0-89281-628-7*, Heal Arts VT) Inner Tradit.

Aromatherapy for Women & Children: Pregnancy & Childbirth. Jane Dye. 1992. 103p. pap. (*0-85207-226-0*) C W Daniel GBR. *Dist:* Natl Bk Netwk.

Aromatherapy from Provence. Nelly Grosjean. 1993. 103p. (Orig.). pap. (*0-85207-266-X*) C W Daniel GBR. *Dist:* Natl Bk Netwk.

Aromatherapy Handbook: The Secret Healing Power of Essential Oils. Daniele Ryman. 1990. 196p. (Orig.). pap. 19.95 (*0-8464-1338-8*) Beekman Pubs.

Aromatherapy in Pregnancy & Childbirth. Jane Dye. 1991. 192p. (Orig.). pap. 23.95 (*0-8464-1536-4*) Beekman Pubs.

Aromatherapy Made Easy. Christine Wildwood. 1998. pap. (*0-7225-3452-3*) Thorsons GBR. *Dist:* Natl Bk Netwk.

Aronson's Neurosciences Pocket Lectures: Speech, Language, Voice. Arnold E. Aronson. 1999. LC 99-40696. 224p. pap. text 54.95 (*0-7693-0060-X*) Singular Publishing.

Arrhythmia Education Course. Competence Assurance Systems Staff. 1984. (Illus.). pap. text 40.00 (*0-89147-054-9*) CAS.

Arrhythmia Interpretation: ACLS Preparation & Clinical Approach. Ken Grauer & Dan Cavallaro. 1997. LC 96-40479. (Illus.). 392p. (C). (gr. 13). spiral bd. 24.00 (*0-8151-3624-2*, 28156) Mosby Inc.

Arrhythmia Management & Cardiac Arrest: A Pocket Brain Approach. Ken Grauer. 1998. (Illus.). iv, 64p. pap. text 10.00 (*0-9663389-1-X*) KG-EKG.

Arrhythmia Management in Chagas' Disease. Ed. by Maria Christina Tentori et al. 1999. LC 99-53035. (Illus.). 168p. 69.00 (*0-87993-450-6*) Futura Pub.

Arrhythmias. Ed. by John A. Kastor. 1993. LC 92-49316. (Illus.). 368p. text 103.00 (*0-7216-4228-4*) Saunders.

Arrhythmias. Mosby Staff. 1999. LC 98-47836. (Managing Major Diseases Ser.). 29.95 (*0-323-00854-2*) Mosby Inc.

Arrhythmias & Pacemakers. John L. Atlee. 1995. (Illus.). 469p. text 66.00 (*0-7216-5880-6*) Saunders.

Arrhythmogenic Right Ventricular Cardiomyopathy Dysplasia. Andrea Nava et al. 1997. LC 97-37685. (International Congress Ser.). 514p. 199.00 (*0-444-82447-2*) Elsevier.

ARRT Examination in Cardiovascular - Interventional Technology (CIT) Jack Rudman. (Admission Test Ser.). Date not set. 69.95 (*0-8373-5867-1*, ATS117); 1997. pap. 49.95 (*0-8373-5817-5*, ATS117) Nat Learn.

ARRT Examination in Computed Tomography (CT) Jack Rudman. (Admission Test Ser.: ATS-116). pap. 49.95 (*0-8373-5816-7*) Nat Learn.

ARRT Examination in Mammography (MAM) Jack Rudman. Date not set. (Admission Test Ser.). 69.95 (*0-8373-5868-X*, ATS118); pap. 49.95 (*0-8373-5818-3*, ATS118) Nat Learn.

Arsenic Exposure & Health Effects, Vol. 2. Ed. by Willard R. Chappell et al. 1997. LC 97-65629. (Illus.). xx, 416p. pap. 149.95 (*0-412-73470-2*, Chap & Hall NY) Chapman & Hall.

***Arsenic Exposure & Health Effects: Proceedings of the Fourth International Conference on Arsenic Exposure & Health Effects, July 18-22, 2000, San Diego, California.** Ed. by Willard R. Chappell et al. 2001. LC 2001-40631. 500p. 160.00 (*0-08-044067-3*) Elsevier.

Arsenic Exposure & Health Effects: Proceedings of the Third International Conference on Arsenic Exposure & Health Effects, July 12-15, 1998, San Diego, California. International Conference on Arsenic Exposure and Health Effects Staff et al. 1999. LC 99-54134. 440p. 136.50 (*0-08-043648-X*) Elsevier.

Arsrteagnga Htrdaya of Veagbharta: The Book of Eight Branches of Eayurveda : Text & English Translation. Veagbharta. 1999. LC 98-909519. (Indian Medical Science Ser.). (*81-7030-619-1*) Sri Satguru Pubns.

Art: Ideas for Elementary Classroom Teachers; Bulletin Board Suggestions; Patterns; Ideas for Holidays. Laura S. Crosby. 1985. (Illus.). spiral bd. 25.00 (*0-915114-04-6*) Lewis-Sloan.

Art & Aesthetics in Nursing. Peggy L. Chinn & Jean Watson. 1994. 363p. pap. 38.95 (*0-88737-609-6*, 14-2611, NLN Pr) Natl League Nurse.

Art & Practice of Children's Orthopaedics. Dennis R. Wenger & Mercer Rang. 1992. 768p. text 169.00 (*0-88167-867-8*) Lppncott W & W.

Art & Practice of Low Vision. Paul B. Freeman & Randall T. Jose. 1991. 139p. pap. 37.50 (*0-7506-9010-0*); 2nd ed. 1997. LC 97-12273. (Illus.). 320p. pap. text 34.99 (*0-7506-9685-0*) Buttrwrth-Heinemann.

Art & Practice of Plastic Surgery Set Ed. by Bruce M. Achauer. 2000. LC 00-38017. (Illus.). xl, 2887p. text 595.00 (*0-8151-0984-9*, 29441) Mosby Inc.

Art & Psyche: A Study in Psychoanalysis & Aesthetics. Ellen H. Spitz. 1989. 192p. (C). reprint ed. pap. 17.95 (*0-300-04620-0*) Yale U Pr.

Art & Psychoanalysis. Peter Fuller. 1981. (Art Ser.). (Illus.). 250p. 12.95 (*0-906495-24-5*); pap. 6.95 (*0-906495-32-6*) Writers & Readers.

Art & Science of 360 Degree Feedback. Richard Lepsinger & Antoinette D. Lucia. 1997. LC 96-39195. 304p. 46.00 (*0-7879-0855-X*) Jossey-Bass.

Art & Science of Assessment in Psychotherapy. Ed. by Chris J. Mace. 1995. LC 94-46785. 208p. (C). pap. 29.95 (*0-415-10539-0*, C0465) Routledge.

Art & Science of Cytopathology, Set. Richard M. DeMay. 1996. 1280p. 295.00 (*0-89189-322-9*) Am Soc Clinical.

Art & Science of Evaluation in the Arts Therapies: How Do You Know What's Working? Bernard Feder & Elaine Feder. 1998. LC 98-3547. (Illus.). 398p. 79.95 (*0-398-06873-9*) C C Thomas.

Art & Science of Massage. Walter. 1999. (Illus.). 352p. (gr. 13). pap. text 38.95 (*0-8151-9479-X*, 29268) Mosby Inc.

Art & Science of Massage. Jane Walter. 1998. tchr. ed. (*0-8151-9430-7*) Mosby Inc.

Art & Science of Medical Radiography. Jack C. Malott & Joseph Fodor, III. 7th ed. 1993. LC 92-49306. (Illus.). 320p. (gr. 13). pap. text 45.95 (*0-8016-6321-0*, 06321) Mosby Inc.

A
B

AB

Art & Science of Music Therapy: A Handbook. Ed. by Tony Wigram et al. 1995. xxi, 483p. text 88.00 (*3-7186-5634-5*); pap. text 29.00 (*3-7186-5635-3*) Gordon & Breach (Harwood Acad Pubs).

Art & Science of Operative Dentistry. Clifford M. Sturdevant et al. 3rd ed. 1994. (Illus.). 848p. (C). (gr. 13). text 84.00 (*0-8016-6366-0*, 06366) Mosby Inc.

Art & Science of Operative Dentistry. Clifford M. Sturdevant et al. 3rd ed. 1994. (Illus.). 848p. (*84-8174-187-6*) Mosby-Doyma Libros ESP. *Dist:* Mosby Inc.

Art & Science of Rational Eating. Albert Ellis et al. 1992. LC 92-17733. 342p. pap. 14.95 (*0-942637-60-7*) Barricade Bks.

Art & Science of Sclerology Certification Course, Incl. 4 videotapes & charting system. Jack Tips. 1996. (Illus.). 240p. 399.00 incl. VHS (*0-929167-08-2*) Apple-a-Day.

Art & Science of Wholeness. Herbert L. Beierle. 1975. 20.00 (*0-940480-00-X*) UNIPress.

Art & Soul. Howard McConeghy. 2000. (Illus.). 168p. pap. 18.50 (*0-88214-383-2*) Spring Pubns.

Art & Soul: Reflections on an Artistic Psychology. Bruce L. Moon. 1996. LC 96-32928. (Illus.). 156p. text 38.95 (*0-398-06676-0*); pap. text 27.95 (*0-398-06677-9*) C C Thomas.

Art & Technique of Analytic Group Therapy. Martin Grotjahn. LC 76-22916. 1977. 288p. 35.00 (*0-87668-252-2*); 1993. 232p. reprint ed. pap. (*0-87668-838-5*); 1993. 232p. reprint ed. pap. 35.00 (*1-56821-026-4*) Aronson.

***Art & the Human Blastocyst.** David K. Gardner & Michelle Lane. 2001. LC 00-67927. (Serono Symposia Ser.). (Illus.). xvi, 254p. 149.00 (*0-387-95245-4*) Spr-Verlag.

Art As Healing. Edward Adamson & John Timlin. 1991. pap. 18.95 (*0-904575-24-1*) Sigo Pr.

Art As Medicine: Creating a Therapy of the Imagination. Shaun McNiff. 1992. LC 92-50117. (Illus.). 224p. (Orig.). pap. 18.00 (*0-87773-658-8*) Shambhala Pubns.

Art As Therapy: An Introduction to the Use of Art As a Therapeutic Technique. Ed. by Tessa Dalley. 1984. 201p. pap. 16.95 (*0-422-78730-2*, NO. 9083) Routledge.

Art as Therapy with Children. Edith Kramer. 2nd ed. 1993. (Illus.). 238p. (C). reprint ed. pap. text 21.95 (*0-9613309-4-5*) Magnolia St Pub.

Art of Acupuncture Techniques. Robert Johns. 1996. LC 96-27949. 211p. 21.95 (*1-55643-230-5*) North Atlantic.

Art of Aromatherapy. Robert B. Tisserand. 1977. 320p. pap. 23.95 (*0-8464-0993-3*) Beekman Pubs.

Art of Aromatherapy: The Beautifying & Healing Properties of the Essential Oils of Flowers & Herbs. Robert B. Tisserand. 1987. LC 77-20493. (Illus.). 328p. pap. 14.95 (*0-89281-001-7*, Heal Arts VT) Inner Tradit.

Art of Art Therapy. Judith A. Rubin. 1986. LC 84-9344. 224p. text 35.95 (*0-87630-371-8*) Brunner-Routledge.

Art of Asylum-Keeping: Thomas Story Kirkbride & the Origins of American Psychiatry. Nancy Tomes. 1994. LC 93-49742. (Studies in Health, Illness, & Caregiving). Orig. Title: A Generous Confidence. (Illus.). 424p. (Orig.). reprint ed. pap. text 17.50 (*0-8122-1539-7*) U of Pa Pr.

Art of Balance in Health Policy: Maintaining Japan's Low-Cost, Egalitarian System. Naoki Ikegami. 1998. LC 97-23853. (Illus.). 240p. (C). text 54.95 (*0-521-57122-7*) Cambridge U Pr.

Art of Becoming Human. Mary E. Mercer. 1997. LC 96-47874. 146p. 23.00 (*1-57392-120-3*) Prometheus Bks.

Art of Breathing: Six Simple Lessons to Improve Performance, Health, & Well-Being. Nancy Zi. 4th rev. ed. 2000. LC 00-30864. (Illus.). 240p. pap. 15.95 (*1-58394-034-0*) Frog Ltd CA.

Art of Co-Therapy: How Therapists Work Together. Bill Roller & Vivian Nelson. 1991. LC 90-44744. 256p. 40.00 (*0-89862-557-2*) Guilford Pubns.

Art of Cooking for the Diabetic. Mary Abbot-Hess. 3rd ed. 1998. (Illus.). 496p. pap. 7.99 (*0-451-19533-7*, Sig) NAL.

Art of Cooking for the Diabetic. Mary Abbott Hess. 3rd rev. ed. 1997. 549p. pap. 16.95 (*0-8092-3087-9*, 308790, Contemporary) McGraw-Hill Trade.

Art of Effective Doctor-Patient Communication. David Singer. Ed. by Karen Hadley. 2nd rev. ed. 90p. pap. 19.95 (*0-9636712-0-0*) D Singer Ent.

Art of Examining & Interpreting Histologic Preparations: A Student Handbook. William J. Krause. 2001. LC 00-64991. (Illus.). 176p. pap., stu. ed. 29.95 (*1-85070-277-2*, Parthenon Pbng) CRC Pr.

Art of Getting Even. Gary Brodsky. 1995. 118p. 5.98 (*1-55521-663-3*) Bk Sales Inc.

Art of Getting Well. Anthony Di Fabio. 1997. LC 87-62790. (Illus.). 141p. pap. 7.00 (*0-9615437-1-X*) Arthritis Trust.

***Art of Getting Well: Maximizing Health & Well-Being When You Have a Chronic Illness.** David Spero. 2002. LC 2001-39722. 15.95 (*0-89793-357-5*) Hunter House.

Art of Hating. Gerald Schoenewolf. 1990. LC 90-45054. 224p. 40.00 (*0-87668-693-5*) Aronson.

Art of Healing. Lewis E. Mehl & Gayle Peterson. 350p. text (*0-8290-1804-2*) Irvington.

Art of Intervention in Dynamic Psychotherapy. Bert Kaplan. 1988. LC 88-6238. 263p. 50.00 (*0-87668-983-7*) Aronson.

Art of JAMA: One Hundred Covers & Essays from the Journal of the American Medical Association. M. Therese Southgate. 1996. LC 96-18876. (Illus.). 240p. (C). 59.95 (*0-8151-0994-6*, 29462) Mosby Inc.

Art of Laparoscopic Suturing. James A. Rosser. 1995. (*1-85775-022-5*) Radcliffe Med Pr GBR. *Dist:* Balogh.

Art of Lasik. Jeffery J. Machat et al. 2nd ed. 1999. (SPA., Illus.). 544p. 215.00 (*1-55642-421-3*) SLACK Inc.

Art of Lasik. Jeffery Machat et al. 2nd ed. 1998. LC 98-28025. (Illus.). xx, 520p. text 215.00 (*1-55642-386-1*, 63861) SLACK Inc.

Art of Letting Go. Slightly Off Center Writers Group Staff. 1995. (Orig.). pap. 9.95 (*1-56721-115-1*) Twenty-Fifth Cent Pr.

Art of Living: Erich Fromm's Life & Works. Gerhard P. Knapp. 1989. (American University Studies: Ser. VIII, Vol. 13). 270p. (C). text 49.95 (*0-8204-1034-9*) P Lang Pubng.

Art of Man: Faces of Plastic Surgery. Daniel Man & L. C. Faye. rev. ed. 1998. (Illus.). 247p. pap. 29.95 (*0-9666345-1-9*) BeautyArt Pr.

Art of Massage. John H. Kellogg. 1997. (Illus.). 293p. reprint ed. spiral bd. 29.50 (*0-7873-0489-1*) Hlth Research.

Art of Massage. John H. Kellogg. 1984. (Illus.). 293p. reprint ed. pap. text 25.00 (*0-87556-378-3*) Saifer.

Art of Massage. John H. Kellogg. fac. ed. 1997. LC 96-60567. 400p. reprint ed. per. 14.95 (*1-57258-116-6*) TEACH Servs.

Art of Massage: A Practical Manual for the Student, the Nurse & the Practitioner. John H. Kellogg. 1996. 294p. reprint ed. pap. 13.95 (*1-56459-936-1*) Kessinger Pub.

Art of Massage: A Practical Manual for the Student, the Nurse & the Practitioner. John H. Kellogg. 1991. lib. bdg. 250.00 (*0-87700-937-6*) Revisionist Pr.

Art of Medicine: Medical Teaching at the University of Paris, 1250-1400. Cornelius O'Boyle. 1998. LC 98-38400. (Education & Society in the Middle Ages & Renaissance Ser.: Vol. 9). (Illus.). 336p. 106.50 (*90-04-11124-7*) Brill Academic Pubs.

Art of Memory. Frances A. Yates. 2001. LC 66-22770. xvi, 448p. reprint ed. pap. text 22.00 (*0-226-95001-8*, P615) U Ch Pr.

Art of Midwifery. Ed. by Hilary Marland. 1994. (Wellcome Institute Series in the History of Medicine). (Illus.). 256p. (C). pap. 29.95 (*0-415-11675-9*) Routledge.

Art of Nursing. Wynona Bice-Stephens. 2nd ed. 1992. 64p. 9.95 (*0-8059-3254-2*) Dorrance.

Art of Psychotherapy. Anthony Storr. 2nd ed. 1990. 224p. pap. text (*0-7506-0428-X*) E A GBR. *Dist:* OUP.

Art of Psychotherapy. Anthony Storr. 1985. pap. 9.95 (*0-416-60321-1*); 2nd ed. 1990. LC 90-8067. 223p. (gr. 13). pap. 20.95 (*0-415-90302-5*, A4364) Routledge.

Art of Spiritual Healing. Joel S. Goldsmith. 1997. LC 97-5081. 213p. 18.95 (*1-889051-12-8*, I Lvl) Acrpls Bks GA.

Art of Spiritual Healing: Chakra & Energy Workbook. Keith Sherwood. 2nd ed. 2000. LC 85-10224. (New Age Ser.).Tr. of Kunst Spirituellen Heilens. (Illus.). 264p. pap. 9.95 (*0-87542-720-0*) Llewellyn Pubns.

Art of Surgery: Exceptional Cases - Unique Solutions. Michael Trede. 1999. LC 99-26557. (Illus.). 224p. 125.00 (*0-86577-845-0*) Thieme Med Pubs.

Art of Surgical Technique. Milton T. Edgerton. 1988. (Illus.). 218p. pap. text 59.95 (*0-683-02749-2*) Lppncott W & W.

Art of the Question: A Guide to Short-Term Question-Centered Therapy. Marilee C. Goldberg. 1997. LC 97-14144. (Couples & Family Dynamics & Treatment Ser.). 368p. 69.95 (*0-471-12387-0*) Wiley.

Art of True Healing: The Unlimited Power of Prayer & Visualization. Israel Regardie. Ed. by Marc Allen. 2nd ed. 1997. LC 96-43004. (Illus.). 112p. reprint ed. pap. 8.95 (*1-57731-012-8*) New Wrld Lib.

Art of Unknowing: Dimensions of Openness in Analytic Therapy. Stephen S. Kurtz. 1989. LC 88-39471. 280p. 45.00 (*0-87668-860-1*) Aronson.

Art of Veterinary Practice: A Guide to Client Communication. Myrna M. Milani. 1995. LC 94-40919. 294p. 29.95 (*0-8122-3260-7*) U of Pa Pr.

Art of Veterinary Practice Management. Mark Opperman. 1999. LC 98-61301. (Illus.). 240p. 49.95 (*0-935078-74-6*) Veterinary Hlthcare.

Art Projects for the Mentally Retarded Child. Ellen J. Sussman. 1976. (Illus.). 108p. 28.95 (*0-398-03535-0*) C C Thomas.

Art Psychotherapy. Harriet Wadeson. 1987. (Personality Processes Ser.). 384p. pap. 39.95 (*0-471-62904-9*) Wiley.

Art Psychotherapy & Psychosis. Ed. by Joy Schaverien & Katherine Killick. 1997. LC 97-160705. (Illus.). 280p. (C). 89.95 (*0-415-13841-8*); pap. 29.95 (*0-415-13842-6*) Routledge.

Art Psychotherapy in Groups. Sally Skaife & Valerie Huet. 1998. LC 97-42738. (Illus.). 224p. (C). 84.95 (*0-415-15072-8*); pap. 27.95 (*0-415-15073-6*) Routledge.

Art, Science & Technology of Pharmaceutical Compounding. Loyd V. Allen, Jr. 1998. LC 98-25173. (Illus.). 319p. text 70.00 (*0-917330-88-9*) Am Pharm Assn.

Art, Surgery, & Transplantation. Roy Calne. 1996. (Illus.). 227p. (*0-683-23094-8*) Lppncott W & W.

Art That Heals: The Image As Medicine in Ethiopia. Jacques Mercier. 1997. LC 96-80093. (Illus.). 128p. 49.95 (*3-7913-1606-0*) Prestel Pub NY.

Art Therapist: Artist, Teacher, Clinician, Healer. 1992. (Conference Proceedings Ser.). 147p. (Orig.). (C). 20.00 (*1-882147-14-6*) Am Art Therapy.

Art Therapy. Ed. by Cathy A. Malchiodi. (Journal of the American Art Therapy Association Ser.: Vol. 10, No. 4). (C). (Illus.). pap. 18.00 (*1-882147-45-6*); 1993. (Illus.). 55p. 16.00 (*1-882147-18-9*); 1993. (Illus.). 64p. 16.00 (*1-882147-17-0*); 1992. (Illus.). 56p. pap. 18.00 (*1-882147-15-4*); 1992. (Illus.). 52p. 16.00 (*1-882147-02-2*); 1992. 51p. 16.00 (*1-882147-01-4*); 1992. (Illus.). 60p. 16.00 (*1-882147-00-6*) Am Art Therapy.

Art Therapy. Ed. by Kathy A. Malchiodi. 1993. (Journal of the American Art Therapy Association Ser.: Vol. 10, No. 3). 66p. (C). pap. 18.00 (*1-882147-19-7*) Am Art Therapy.

Art Therapy: A Bridge Between Worlds. Ed. by Audrey E. Di Maria. 1981. (Conference Proceedings Ser.). 121p. (Orig.). pap. 7.00 (*1-882147-11-1*) Am Art Therapy.

Art Therapy: A Handbook. Ed. by Diane Waller & Andrea Gilroy. 1992. (Psychotherapy Handbooks Ser.). 256p. (*0-335-09886-X*); pap. (*0-335-09885-1*) OpUniv Pr.

Art Therapy: An Introduction. Judith A. Rubin. 1998. LC 98-35409. (Basic Principles into Practice Ser.). 29.95 (*0-87630-897-3*) Brunner-Routledge.

Art Therapy: European Perspect. Diane Waller. 1998. LC 98-5419. (*0-335-19448-6*); pap. (*0-335-19449-4*) OpUniv Pr.

Art Therapy: Expanding Horizons. Ed. by Linda Gantt et al. 1978. (Conference Proceedings Ser.). 142p. (Orig.). pap. 7.00 (*1-882147-05-7*) Am Art Therapy.

Art Therapy: New Directions in the Eighties. 1987. (Conference Proceedings Ser.). 110p. (Orig.). pap. 15.00 (*1-882147-13-8*) Am Art Therapy.

Art Therapy: Still Growing. Ed. by Audrey E. Di Maria. 1982. (Conference Proceedings Ser.). 171p. (Orig.). pap. 14.00 (*1-882147-06-5*) Am Art Therapy.

Art Therapy & Dramatherapy: Masks of the Soul. Sue Jennings & Ase Minde. 1993. (Illus.). 224p. (*1-85302-027-3*) Jessica Kingsley GBR. *Dist:* Taylor & Francis.

Art Therapy & Group Work: An Annotated Bibliography. Compiled by Kathleen M. Hanes. 1982. LC 81-13442. 191p. lib. bdg. 55.00 (*0-313-23172-9*, HAW/, Greenwood Pr) Greenwood.

Art Therapy & Psychotherapy: Blending Two Therapeutic Approaches. Victoria D. Coleman & Phoebe M. Farris-Dufrene. 1996. LC 95-26439. 144p. 39.95 (*1-56032-489-9*); pap. 19.95 (*1-56032-490-2*) Accel Devel.

Art Therapy for Groups: A Handbook of Themes, Games & Exercises. Marian Liebmann. 1986. (Illus.). 226p. (Orig.). pap. text 19.95 (*0-914797-24-7*) Brookline Bks.

Art Therapy in Palliative Care: The Creative Response. Amanda Pratt & Michele J. Wood. 1998. LC 97-51524. (Illus.). 208p. (C). pap. 27.95 (*0-415-16157-6*); 84.95 (*0-415-16156-8*) Routledge.

Art Therapy in Practice. Ed. by Marian Liebmann. 1990. 176p. pap. 24.00 (*1-85302-058-3*) Taylor & Francis.

Art Therapy in the United States. Elinor Ulman et al. 1977. (Illus.). 40p. pap. 3.95 (*0-8391-1164-9*) Art Therapy.

Art Therapy in Theory & Practice. Ed. by Elinor Ulman & Penny Dachinger. 1975. (Illus.). 404p. reprint ed. pap. 29.95 (*0-9613309-8-8*) Magnolia St Pub.

Art Therapy with Families in Crisis: Overcoming Resistance Through Nonverbal Expression. Ed. by Debra G. Linesch. 1993. LC 92-27839. (Illus.). 192p. text 29.95 (*0-87630-638-5*) Brunner-Routledge.

Art Therapy with Sexual Abuse Survivors. Stephanie L. Brooke. 1997. LC 97-22272. (Illus.). 188p. text 44.95 (*0-398-06805-4*); pap. text 28.95 (*0-398-06806-2*) C C Thomas.

Artemia Biology. Robert Browne et al. 1990. (Illus.). 384p. 259.00 (*0-8493-6729-8*, QL444) CRC Pr.

Artemis Speaks: V. B. A. C. Stories & Other Natural Childbirth Information. Nan U. Koehler. 2nd ed. 1985. LC 85-70586. (Illus.). 551p. pap. 12.95 (*0-9623851-0-7*) Freestone Pub Co.

Arteres des Muscles des Membres et du Tronc, Les Vois Anastomotiques Arterielles des Membres see Michel Salmon Anatomic Studies

Arterial Anatomy of Skin Flaps. George C. Cormack & B. George Lamberty. (Illus.). 1987. 484p. text (*0-443-03214-9*); 2nd ed. 1994. LC 94-5558. 538p. text (*0-443-04567-4*) Church.

Arterial & Venous Systems in Essential Hypertension. Ed. by Michel E. Safar. 1987. (Developments in Cardiovascular Medicine Ser.). text 247.50 (*0-89838-857-0*) Kluwer Academic.

Arterial Aneurysms: Diagnosis & Management. Ed. by Michael Horrocks. 1995. (Illus.). 256p. text 130.00 (*0-7506-1368-8*) Buttrwrth-Heinemann.

Arterial Behavior & Blood Circulation of the Brain. George I. Mchedlishvili. Tr. by John A. Bevan from RUS. 1986. (Illus.). 354p. (C). text 132.00 (*0-306-10985-9*, Kluwer Plenum) Kluwer Academic.

Arterial Blood Withdrawal: Direct & from Arterial-Lines. M. Wade Curl. 1991. LC 91-67113. (Illus.). 82p. (Orig.). (C). pap. 25.99 (*1-880610-13-2*) PRO-ACT Pub.

Arterial Chemoreception. Ed. by Carlos Eyzaguirre et al. 1990. (Illus.). 475p. 169.00 (*0-387-97225-0*) Spr-Verlag.

Arterial Chemoreceptors: Cell to System, 360. R. G. O'Regan et al. 1994. (Advances in Experimental Medicine & Biology Ser.). (Illus.). 416p. (C). text 115.00 (*0-306-44824-6*, Kluwer Plenum) Kluwer Academic.

Arterial Circulation: Physical Principles & Clinical Applications. John K. J. Li. 2000. LC 00-31955. 288p. 125.00 (*0-89603-633-2*) Humana.

Arterial Conduits in Myocardial Revascularisation. Gianni D. Angelini et al. 1996. 208p. (*0-340-61024-7*) E A GBR. *Dist:* OUP.

Arterial Grafting for Myocardial Revascularization: Indications, Surgical Techniques & Results. L. K. Von Segesser. 1990. (Illus.). 146p. 101.00 (*0-387-52596-3*) Spr-Verlag.

Arterial Grafts for Coronary Artery Bypass Surgery: A Textbook for Cardiovascular Clinicians. Guo-Wei He. 1999. LC 99-27971. (Illus.). 400p. 75.00 (*981-4021-06-7*) Spr-Verlag.

Arterial Hypertension: Pathogenisis, Diagnosis, & Therapy. Ed. by J. Rosenthal. Tr. by Terry C. Telger from GER. 1982. (Illus.). 576p. 248.00 (*0-387-90611-8*) Spr-Verlag.

Arterial Hypertension: Report of a WHO Expert Committee. 1978. (Technical Report Ser.: No. 628). 58p. pap. text 5.00 (*92-4-120628-4*, 1100628) World Health.

Arterial Lines. Springhouse Publishing Company Staff. 1992. (Procedures Video Ser.). 36.95 incl. VHS (*0-87434-428-X*) Springhouse Corp.

Arterial Occlusive Disease: Nursing Assessment & Patient Care. Mitzi A. Ekers. 1984. (Illus.). 58p. (Orig.). pap. text 9.50 (*0-932491-04-9*) Res Appl Inc.

Arterial Pulse. Michael O'Rourke et al. 1992. (Illus.). 276p. (*0-683-06641-2*) Lppncott W & W.

Arterial Remodeling: Critical Factor in Restenosis. Antoine Lafont & Eric J. Topol. 1997. LC 97-33314. (Developments in Cardiovascular Medicine Ser.). 600p. text 247.50 (*0-7923-8008-8*) Kluwer Academic.

Arterial Surgery. Ed. by H. H. Eastcott. 3rd ed. 1992. (Illus.). 670p. (Orig.). pap. text (*0-443-03674-8*) Church.

Arterial Surgery of the Lower Limb. P. R. Bell. 1991. (Illus.). 189p. text (*0-443-03541-5*) Church.

Arterial System in Hypertension. Ed. by Michel E. Safar. 1993. LC 93-1730. (Developments in Cardiovascular Medicine Ser.). 256p. (C). text 183.00 (*0-7923-2343-2*) Kluwer Academic.

Arterial Vasodilation. 256p. (*0-340-55398-7*) E A GBR. *Dist:* Routldge.

Arterial Vasodilation, Mechanisms & Therapy. Ed. by Michael O'Rourke et al. 1993. LC 92-49292. (Illus.). 231p. text 89.50 (*0-8121-1671-2*) Lppncott W & W.

Arterial Wall Disease & Stroke Prevention. Ed. by J. Bogousslavsky & F. Aichner. 2000. (Cerebrovascular Diseases Ser.: Vol. 10). (Illus.). iv, 48p. 25.25 (*3-8055-7150-X*) S Karger.

Arteries. Ed. by Wiley F. Barker. 1993. 503p. 89.95 (*1-879702-07-X*, LN0207) CRC Pr.

Arteriosclerosis. 1995. 61.00 (*0-387-00937-X*) Spr-Verlag.

Arteriosclerosis: New Insights into Pathogenetic Mechanisms & Prevention. Ed. by H. Just et al. 1995. (Illus.). 202p. 61.00 (*3-7985-0937-9*) Spr-Verlag.

Arteriosclerosis: New Insights into Pathogenetic Mechanisms & Prevention. A. M. Zeiher et al. 1993. 190p. 46.00 (*0-387-91433-1*) Spr-Verlag.

Arteriosclerosis & Herbal Chelation. Hanna Kroeger. 1984. 14p. (Orig.). pap. 1.00 (*1-883713-03-X*) Hanna Kroeger.

Artforus: A Visual Arts Curriculum to Develop Fine & Gross Motor Skills in Handicapped Students. Nigel Buss. 1986. 87p. tchr. ed. 10.00 (*1-878276-37-9*) Educ Systs Assocs Inc.

Artful Eye. Ed. by R. L. Gregory et al. 1995. (Illus.). 456p. 50.00 (*0-19-852195-2*) OUP.

Artherosclerosis: Clinical Evaluations & Therapy. Ed. by G. Descovisch & S. Lenzi. 1982. (Illus.). 500p. text 179.50 (*0-85200-449-4*) Kluwer Academic.

Arthritic, Realistic Fantastics & Artistic. B. Harlington Bratley. 1986. 130p. (*0-7223-1970-3*) A H S Ltd GBR. *Dist:* St Mut.

Arthritic's Cookbook. Collin H. Dong. 1995. pap. 8.95 (*0-8217-4883-1*, Zebra Kensgtn) Kensgtn Pub Corp.

Arthritic's Cookbook. H. Collin Dong. 1996. pap. 9.95 (*1-57566-158-6*) Kensgtn Pub Corp.

Arthritis. Lisa Newman. 1999. LC 99-37386. (Crossing Press Pocket Ser.). 96p. mass mkt. 6.95 (*1-58091-003-3*) Crossing Pr.

Arthritis. Joan Hustace Walker & Cal Orey. 1999. LC 99-22313. (Essential Guide to Natural Pet Care Ser.). (Illus.). xvi, 46p. pap. 6.95 (*1-889540-33-1*) Bowtie Press.

Arthritis: A Comprehensive Guide. James F. Fries. rev. ed. 1986. LC 86-8043. 272p. pap. 9.57 (*0-201-05408-6*) Addison-Wesley.

Arthritis: An Alternative Medicine Definitive Guide. Ellen Kamhi et al. 1999. LC 99-44153. (Illus.). 400p. pap. 18.95 (*1-887299-15-7*) AlternMed Bks.

Arthritis: An American Yoga Association Guide. Alice Christensen. 2001. (Illus.). 228p. pap. 12.00 (*1-57566-648-0*, Twin Streams) Kensgtn Pub Corp.

Arthritis: Diseases & Treatment, Set. 3rd ed. John A. Mills. Incl. Bk. 3. Anti-Inflammatory Therapy. (Illus.). 1977. pap. text 16.50 (*0-89147-051-4*); 1977. Set pap. text 48.00 (*0-89147-048-4*) CAS.

Arthritis: Everything You Need to Know. John Thompson. rev. ed. 1996. (Illus.). 294p. pap. 14.95 (1-55013-782-4) Firefly Bks Limited.

Arthritis: How You Can Benefit from Diet, Vitamins, Minerals, Herbs, Exercise & Other Natural Methods. Michael T. Murray. 1994. LC 93-50095. (Getting Well Naturally Ser.). 176p. pap. 12.95 (1-55958-491-2) Prima Pub.

Arthritis: Little Known Treatments. Anthony Di Fabio. 1995. LC 93-83495. (Orig.). pap. 7.00 (0-9615437-2-8) Arthritis Trust.

Arthritis: Osteoarthritis & Rheumatoid Disease Including Rheumatoid Arthritis. Anthony Di Fabio & Gus J. Prosch, Jr. 1997. LC 97-71310. (Illus.). 360p. (Orig.). pap. 10.00 (0-9615437-3-6) Arthritis Trust.

Arthritis: Questions You Have...Answers You Need. Ellen Moyer. rev. ed. 1997. LC 96-47270. 192p. pap. 12.95 (1-882606-52-3) Peoples Med Soc.

Arthritis: Stop Suffering, Start Moving. Darlene Cohen. 1995. LC 94-45682. (Illus.). 160p. pap. 14.95 (0-8027-7466-0) Walker & Co.

Arthritis: The Chinese Way of Healing & Prevention. Jwing-Ming Yang. Ed. by Alan Dougall. 2nd rev. ed. 1996. LC 96-60418. (Qigong Health & Healing Ser.). Orig. Title: Qigone for Arthritis. (Illus.). 160p. pap. 20.95 (1-886969-42-6, B015R/426) YMAA Pubn.

Arthritis: The Physical & Mental Connections. Michael Schwartz. 1994. 55p. (Orig.). pap. 3.50 (1-886722-03-X) Maps Pub.

Arthritis: What Exercises Work: Breakthrough Relief for the Rest of Your Life, Even after Drugs & Surgery Have Failed. Dava Sobel & Arthur C. Klein. 1995. LC 95-10962. pap. 11.95 (0-312-13025-2, St Martin Griffin) St Martin.

Arthritis: What Works. Dava Sobel & Arthur C. Klein. 1989. (Illus.). 512p. 22.95 (0-312-03289-7) St Martin.

Arthritis Action Plan: An Integrated Program of Traditional & Complementary Therapies. Michael E. Weinblatt. 2001. 352p. reprint ed. pap. 14.00 (0-684-86803-2, Fireside) S&S Trade Pap.

Arthritis Action Program: An Integrated Plan of Traditional & Complementary Therapies. Michael E. Weinblatt & Harvard Medical School Staff. 2000. LC 00-57340. (Illus.). 352p. 25.00 (0-684-86802-4) Free Pr.

Arthritis & Allied Conditions: A Textbook of Rheumatology. Daniel J. McCarty. 12th ed. 1992. LC 91-33513. (Illus.). 2151p. text 198.50 (0-8121-1430-2) Lppncott W & W.

Arthritis & Allied Conditions: A Textbook of Rheumatology. William J. Koopman. 14th ed. 2000. 2,848p. text 299.00 (0-7817-2240-3) Lppncott W & W.

Arthritis & Cetyl Myristoleate (CMO) Chuck Cochran. 1997. 24p. pap. 2.95 (0-9647080-8-6) Healing Wisdom.

Arthritis & Chinese Herbal Medicine. Pi-Kwang Tsung et al. 1987. (Educational Series on Chinese Medicine Ser.). 32p. pap. 4.95 (0-941942-25-2) Orient Heal Arts.

Arthritis & Common Sense. Dale Alexander. 1981. (Fireside Book Ser.). 256p. pap. 12.00 (0-671-42791-1) S&S Trade Pap.

Arthritis & Folk Medicine: An Almanac of Natural Health Care. D. C. Jarvis. 1997. 192p. 7.99 (0-88365-983-2) Galahad Bks.

Arthritis & Its Cure. 1994. lib. bdg. 250.95 (0-8490-5664-0) Gordon Pr.

Arthritis & Related Affections: Clinic, Pathology, & Treatment. Arnold Soren. 1993. LC 93-20236. (Illus.). 456p. 255.00 (0-387-55779-2) Spr-Verlag.

***Arthritis & Rheumatism.** Jill Wright. 2002. 128p. pap. (1-85703-723-5) How To Bks GBR. *Dist:* Midpt Trade.

Arthritis & Rheumatism: Your Questions Answered. Andrie Calin. 1996. pap. text (0-443-04988-2, C0826) Church.

Arthritis & Rheumatism in Practice. P. A. Dieppe et al. 1991. (Illus.). 128p. (gr. 13). text 39.95 (0-397-44588-1, GM0036) Mosby Inc.

Arthritis & Ulcer Disease: New Directions & Controversies. Patricia Leinen. 1994. (Audioconference Workbook Ser.). (Illus.). 12p. (0-944036-98-8) Medicine Grp USA.

Arthritis & Ulcer Disease: New Directions & Controversies NSAIDS in Arthritis. Ed. by Patricia Leinen. 1994. (Slide Resource Ser.: Pt. 1). (Illus.). (Orig.). (1-57130-001-5) Medicine Grp USA.

Arthritis & Ulcer Disease New Directions & Controversies: Approaches for the Prevention of NSAID-Induced GI Damage & Complications. Ed. by Patricia Leinen. 1994. (Slide Resource Ser.: Pt. 4). (Illus.). (Orig.). (1-57130-004-X) Medicine Grp USA.

Arthritis & Ulcer Disease New Directions & Controversies: Epidemiology of NSAID-Induced GI Damage. Ed. by Patricia Leinen. 1994. (Slide Resource Ser.: Pt. 3). (Illus.). (Orig.). (1-57130-003-1) Medicine Grp USA.

Arthritis & Ulcer Disease New Directions & Controversies: Pathophysiology of GI Injury: NSAIDS & H. Pylori. Ed. by Patricia Leinen. 1994. (Slide Resource Ser.: Pt. 2). (Illus.). (Orig.). (1-57130-002-3) Medicine Grp USA.

Arthritis Bible: A Comprehensive Guide to Alternative Therapies & Conventional Treatments for Arthritic Diseases Including Osteoarthrosis, Rheumatoid Arthritis, Gout, Fibromyalgia & More. Craig Weatherby & Leonid Gordin. 1999. LC 99-18474. 272p. pap. 14.95 (0-89281-825-5, Heal Arts VT) Inner Tradit.

Arthritis Breakthrough: The N. I. H. Trials of the New MIRA Therapy - How They Happened & What They Mean to You. Henry Scammell & Thomas M. Brown. 1993. LC 92-9712. 276p. pap. 11.95 (0-87131-690-0) M Evans.

Arthritis Breakthroughs. William L. Fischer & Ginny Brizzi. 1993. LC 92-73902. (Illus.). 242p. (Orig.). pap. 18.95 (0-915421-15-1) Fischer Pub.

Arthritis Cure. Jason Theodosakis et al. 1997. (Illus.). 228p. pap. 11.95 (0-312-19029-8, St Martin Griffin) St Martin.

Arthritis Cure: The Medical Miracle That Can Halt, Reverse & May Cure Osteoarthritis. Jason Theodosakis et al. 1999. (Illus.). 203p. text 23.00 (0-7881-5685-3) DIANE Pub.

Arthritis Cure: The Medical Miracle That Can Halt, Reverse, & May Even Cure Osteoarthritis. Jason Theodosakis et al. 1997. 282p. mass mkt. 6.99 (0-312-96453-6); 1996. LC 96-6579. 224p. 22.95 (0-312-15284-1) St Martin.

Arthritis Cure Fitness Solution. Brenda Adderly. 2000. 208p. reprint ed. pap. 12.95 (0-89526-244-4, LifeLine Press) Regnery Pub.

Arthritis Education Course. Competence Assurance Systems Staff. 1984. (Illus.). pap. text 75.00 (0-89147-067-0) CAS.

Arthritis Exercise Book. Gwen Ellert. 1990. (Illus.). 120p. spiral bd. 14.95 (0-8092-4094-7, 409470, Contemporary) McGraw-Hill Trade.

Arthritis Handbook. Arthritis Foundation of New South Wales Staff. 2nd ed. 1996. 187p. pap. 32.00 (0-8036-0376-2) Davis Co.

Arthritis Healthy Exchanges Cookbook. Joanna M. Lund. 1998. LC 97-32731. 320p. pap. 14.00 (0-399-52377-4, Perigee Bks) Berkley Pub.

Arthritis Helpbook see Como Convivir Con Su Artritis: Una Guia Para una Vida Activa y Saludable

Arthritis Helpbook. Kate Lorig. 3rd ed. 1990. pap. 12.95 (0-201-52403-1) Addison-Wesley.

Arthritis Helpbook: A Tested Self-Management Program for Coping with Your Arthritis & Fibromyalgia. Kate Lorig & James F. Fries. 4th ed. 2000. 288p. pap. 14.00 (0-201-40963-1) Perseus Bks Grp.

Arthritis Helpbook: HealthTrac Edition, Smart Version. 3rd ed. 1993. pap. (0-201-40683-7) Addison-Wesley.

Arthritis in Black & White Vol. 2. Anne C. Brower. Ed. by Lesteet Bralow. 2nd ed. 1996. 400p. text 83.00 (0-7216-5152-6) Saunders.

Arthritis Medicine A to Z: A Doctor's Guide to Today's Most Commonly Prescribed Arthritis Drugs. C. Michael Stein. 2001. LC 00-37432. 336p. pap. 14.00 (0-609-80507-X, Three Riv Pr) Harmony Bks.

Arthritis of the Bases of the Thumb. P. Saffar. Date not set. (Illus.). 225p. 175.00 (0-387-59586-4) Spr-Verlag.

Arthritis of the Hip & Knee: The Active Person's Guide to Taking Charge. Ronald J. Allen et al. 1997. LC 97-15388. (Illus.). 256p. pap. 14.95 (1-56145-149-5) Peachtree Pubs.

Arthritis of the Knee. Ed. by M. A. Freeman. 1980. (Clinical Features & Surgical Management Ser.). (Illus.). 320p. 135.00 (0-387-09699-X) Spr-Verlag.

Arthritis 101: Answers to Your Questions about Arthritis. Arthritis Foundation Staff. 1997. 176p. (Orig.). pap. 11.95 (1-56352-380-9) Longstreet.

Arthritis Relief: Breakthroughs in Natural Healing. Deborah L. Wilcox-Jamieson. 1998. LC 97-67979. (Illus.). 182p. (Orig.). pap. 14.95 (1-890394-04-1) Rhodes & Easton.

Arthritis Relief the Natural Way Vol. 1: Power Cutting Edge Nutritional & Mind/Body Programs to Combat Arthritis. Deborah L. Wilcox. rev. ed. 1997. (Illus.). 56p. pap. 9.95 (0-9633361-1-8) Hlth & Life.

Arthritis, Rheumatism & Allied Disorders: How's Your Liver? Why Die of Cancer? A. L. Allen. 1996. 120p. reprint ed. spiral bd. 12.00 (0-7873-0027-6) Hlth Research.

Arthritis, Rheumatism & Psoriasis. Jan De Vries. 1988. (By Appointment Only Ser.). 124p. pap. (1-85158-690-3) Mainstream Pubng GBR. *Dist:* Trafalgar.

Arthritis, Rheumatism & Sciatica. George S. Weger et al. 1993. 73p. reprint ed. spiral bd. 10.00 (0-7873-0943-5) Hlth Research.

Arthritis Solution. Joseph Kandel & David B. Sudderth. 1997. LC 97-13641. 224p. pap. 12.00 (0-7615-1172-5, Prima Health) Prima Pub.

Arthritis Sourcebook. Earl J. Brewer, Jr. & Kathy C. Angel. LC 92-39063. 1993. 252p. 21.95 (1-56565-036-0); 2nd ed. 1998. 240p. pap. 16.00 (1-56565-627-X) Lowell Hse.

Arthritis Sourcebook: Basic Consumer Health Information about Specific Forms of Arthritis & Related Disorders. Ed. by Allan R. Cook. 1998. (Health Reference Ser.). 650p. lib. bdg. 78.00 (0-7808-0201-2) Omnigraphics Inc.

Arthritis Surgery. Ed. by Clement B. Sledge et al. 1993. (Illus.). 976p. text 135.00 (0-7216-4912-2) Saunders.

Arthritis Survival: The Holistic Medical Treatment Program for Osteoarthritis. Robert S. Ivker & Todd Nelson. 2001. LC 00-53263. xxi, 336p. pap. 14.95 (1-58542-097-2, Tarcher Putnam) Putnam Pub Group.

Arthritis Therapy: A Clinician's Manual. Thomas Kantor. 1992. 243p. pap. 12.95 (0-929240-40-5) EMIS.

Arthrogryposis: A Text Atlas. Ed. by Lynn T. Staheli et al. 1998. (Illus.). 184p. (C). text 90.00 (0-521-57106-5) Cambridge U Pr.

Arthroplasty. Skinner. 1999. pap. text 175.00 (0-8385-0339-X) Appleton & Lange.

Arthropod-Borne & Rodent-Borne Viral Diseases. 1985. (Technical Reports: No. 719). 116p. pap. text 10.00 (92-4-120719-1, 1100719) World Health.

Arthropods & Human Skin. J. O'Donel Alexander. 1984. (Illus.). 430p. 210.00 (0-387-13235-X) Spr-Verlag.

Arthropods of Medical & Veterinary Importance: A Checklist of Preferred Names & Allied Terms. A. R. Pittaway. 1991. 192p. pap. 59.95 (0-8288-7365-8, 851987419) Fr & Eur.

Arthropods of Medical & Veterinary Importance: A Checklist of Preferred Names & Allied Terms. Compiled by A. R. Pittaway. 1991. 160p. pap. text 45.00 (0-85198-741-9) OUP.

Arthroscopic Atlas of the Temporomandibular Joint. David I. Blaustein & Leslie B. Heffez. 1989. LC 89-13158. (Illus.). 117p. 89.00 (0-8121-1242-3) Lppncott W & W.

Arthroscopic Laser Surgery: Clinical Implications. Allen T. Brillhart. 1994. LC 93-38570. (Illus.). 299p. 172.00 (0-387-94186-X) Spr-Verlag.

Arthroscopic Management of the Knee. David J. Dandy. 2nd ed. 1987. (Illus.). 236p. text (0-443-02958-X) Church.

Arthroscopic Surgery: The Foot & Ankle. Richard D. Ferkel. Ed. by Terry L. Whipple. 1995. (Arthroscopic Surgery Ser.). (Illus.). 360p. text 159.00 (0-397-51093-4) Lppncott W & W.

Arthroscopic Surgery: The Shoulder & Elbow. James C. Esch & Champ L. Baker. 1993. 336p. text 149.00 (0-397-51182-5) Lppncott W & W.

Arthroscopy of the Elbow. Ed. by Felix H. Savoie & Larry D. Field. 1995. LC 95-35650. 178p. (C). text (0-443-08923-X) Church.

Arthroscopy of the Knee. R. Aigner & J. Gillquist. 1991. (Flexibook Ser.). (Illus.). 228p. text 32.50 (0-86577-342-4) Thieme Med Pubs.

Arthroscopy of the Knee: A Guide for Patients. Marc J. Freidman. Ed. by David Seligson. 1996. (Orthopedic Ser.). (Illus.). (Orig.). pap. 2.95 (1-885274-15-7) Health InfoNet Inc.

Arthroscopy of the Knee: Diagnosis & Treatment. W. Norman Scott. 1990. (Illus.). 528p. text 145.00 (0-7216-8032-1) Saunders.

Arthroscopy of the Knee Joint. H. R. Henche. Tr. by P. A. Casey from GER. 1979. (Illus.). 86p. 81.00 (0-387-09314-1) Spr-Verlag.

Arthroscopy of the Shoulder: Diagnosis & Therapy. H. Resch & E. Beck. Tr. by M. L. Antoft & B. Marschall from GER. 1992. (Illus.). 190p. 169.00 (0-387-82339-5) Spr-Verlag.

Arthroscopy of the Temporomandibular Joint. Ed. by Mohan Thomas & Sidney L. Bronstein. 1991. (Illus.). 561p. text 190.00 (0-7216-3119-3) Saunders.

Arthroscopy of the Upper Extremities. Martti Vastamaki. 1996. LC 97-204553. text 162.00 (0-443-05001-5) Saunders.

Arthrosonography. H. Sattler & U. Harland. 1990. (Illus.). 164p. 117.00 (0-387-19482-7) Spr-Verlag.

***Arthur's Veterinary Reproduction & Obstetrics.** David E. Noakes et al. 8th ed. 2001. 868p. (0-7020-2556-9) W B Saunders GBR. *Dist:* Saunders.

Articles from the New England Journal of Medicine on Drug Therapy, Vol. 8. Ed. by Edwin W. Salzman. 1991. (NEJM Reprint Collection). (Illus.). 300p. reprint ed. text 49.00 (0-910133-33-6); pap. text 34.00 (0-910133-23-9) Mass Med Pub Div.

Articular Synovium. Ed. by P. Franchimont. 1982. (Illus.). viii, 184p. pap. 99.25 (3-8055-3461-2) S Karger.

Articulate Body. Pavel Machotka & John P. Spiegel. 1982. (Illus.). 250p. 32.50 (0-8290-0229-4) Irvington.

Articulation: A Physiological Approach. Samuel G. Fletcher. 1992. (Illus.). 316p. (Orig.). (C). pap. text 55.00 (1-879105-89-6, 0322) Singular Publishing.

Articulation & Phonological Disorders. John E. Bernthal & Nicholas W. Bankson. 4th ed. 1997. LC 97-13185. 432p. 80.00 (0-205-19693-4) P-H.

Articulation & Phonological Disorders: A Book of Exercises. Ken M. Bleile. 2nd ed. 1996. LC 96-23808. (Illus.). 306p. (C). pap. 49.95 (1-56593-688-4, 1350) Thomson Learn.

Articulation Therapy & Consonant Drill Book. Sidney Goda. 1970. LC 74-93566. 174p. text 36.50 (0-8089-0649-6, 791615, Grune & Strat) Harcrt Hlth Sci Grp.

Articulations: The Body & Illness in Poetry. Ed. by Jon Mukand. 1994. LC 94-16528. 452p. (Orig.). pap. 19.95 (0-87745-478-7) U of Iowa Pr.

Articulatory Organization: From Phonology to Speech Signals. Ed. by O. Fujimura. 1990. (Journal: Vol. 45, No. 2-4, 1988). (Illus.). iv, 122p. reprint ed. 50.50 (3-8055-5150-9) S Karger.

Articulatory Phonology. R. L. Diehl. 1992. (Journal Phonetica: Vol. 49, No. 3-4, 1992). (Illus.). 108p. pap. 47.00 (3-8055-5724-8) S Karger.

Artificial Auditory Stimulation Theories. Ed. by W. D. Keidel & P. Finkenzeller. 1984. (Advances in Audiology Ser.: Vol. 1). (Illus.). viii, 152p. 100.00 (3-8055-3720-4) S Karger.

Artificial Disc. M. Brock et al. 1991. (Illus.). 104p. 58.95 (0-387-51857-6) Spr-Verlag.

Artificial Heart. Yukiyasu Sezai. import ed. 1992. text 160.00 (0-7216-4299-3) Saunders.

Artificial Heart: Prototypes, Policies & Patients. Ed. by John R. Hogness et al. 1991. 312p. text 29.95 (0-309-04532-0) Natl Acad Pr.

Artificial Heart, No. 3: Proceedings of the 3rd International Symposium on Artificial Heart & Assist Devices February 16-17, 1990, Tokyo, Japan. Ed. by T. Akutsu & H. Koyanagi. 1992. (Illus.). 384p. 187.00 (0-387-70065-X) Spr-Verlag.

Artificial Insemination. Richard B. Bourne et al. 1972. LC 72-13433. (Illus.). 220p. (C). text 21.50 (0-8422-7077-9) Irvington.

Artificial Insemination & Embryo Transfer of Dairy & Beef Cattle. H. A. Herman & F. W. Madden. 8th ed. 1994. 416p. (gr. 12). pap. 49.95 (0-8134-2969-2, 2969) Interstate.

Artificial Intelligence in Medicine. Ed. by Peter Szolovits. 1982. (AAAS Selected Symposium Ser.: No. 51). 130p. pap. text 56.50 (0-89158-900-7) Westview.

Artificial Intelligence in Medicine: 5th Conference on Artificial Intelligence in Medicine, Europe, AIME '95, Pvia, Italy, June 1995. Ed. by Pedro Barahona et al. 1995. LC 95-30443. (Lecture Notes in Computer Science: Vol. 934). (0-387-60025-6) Spr-Verlag.

Artificial Intelligence in Medicine: 6th Conference on Artificial Intelligence Europe, AIME '97, Grenoble, France, March 1997, Proceedings. E. T. Keravnou. 1997. LC 97-6605. (Lecture Notes in Artificial Intelligence). 526p. pap. 84.95 (3-540-62709-X) Spr-Verlag.

Artificial Intelligence in Medicine: Interpreting Clinical Data: Papers from the 1994 Spring Symposium. Ed. by Isaac Kohane & Serdar Uckun. 1994. (Technical Reports). (Illus.). 168p. (Orig.). spiral bd. 25.00 (0-929280-57-1) AAAI Pr.

Artificial Intelligence in Medicine: Proceedings of the 5th Conference on Artificial Intelligence in Medicine Europe, AIME '95, Pavia, Italy, June 25-28, 1995. Ed. by Jeremy Wyatt et al. 1995. LC 95-30443. (Lecture Notes in Artificial Intelligence: Vol. 934). 449p. pap. 79.95 (3-540-60025-6) Spr-Verlag.

Artificial Intelligence Techniques in Breast Cancer Diagnosis & Prognosis. Ed. by Ashlesha Jain et al. 2000. (Series in Machine Perception & Artificial Intelligence: Vol. 39). 250p. 68.00 (981-02-4374-X) World Scientific Pub.

Artificial Kidney: Physiological Modeling & Tissue Engineering. John K. Leypoldt. 1999. LC 99-33005. (Tissue Engineering Intelligence Unit Ser.: Vol. 3). (Illus.). 151p. 89.00 (1-57059-602-6) Landes Bioscience.

Artificial Larynx. Y. Lebrun. 1973. (Neurolinguistics Ser.: Vol. 1). 90p. pap. (90-265-0173-0) Swets.

Artificial Larynx Handbook & Cassette Package. Shirley J. Salmon & Lewis P. Goldstein. 1978. 176p. text 63.00 (0-8089-1111-2, 793747, Grune & Strat) Harcrt Hlth Sci Grp.

Artificial Liver Support: Proceedings. F. W. Schmidt. Ed. by G. Brunner. 1981. (Illus.). 332p. 70.00 (0-387-10591-3) Spr-Verlag.

Artificial Minds. Stan Franklin. 1997. (Illus.). 464p. reprint ed. pap. 22.95 (0-262-56109-3, Bradford Bks) MIT Pr.

Artificial Neural Networks. Vanya Gant. 1997. (Medical Intelligence Unit Ser.). 200p. 89.95 (0-412-14151-5) Thomson Learn.

Artificial Neural Networks for Assessment of Patients with Suspected Acute Myocardial Infarction. Johan Ellenius. 2000. (Comprehensive Summaries of Uppsala Dissertations from the Faculty of Medicine Ser.: No. 937). (Illus.). 45p. pap. (91-554-4742-2) Uppsala Universitet SWE. *Dist:* Coronet Bks.

Artificial Nutrition Support in Clinical Practice. Ed. by Jason Payne-James et al. 2nd ed. 2001. (Greenwich Medical Media Ser.). (Illus.). 740p. text (1-900151-97-9) Greenwich Med GBR. *Dist:* JAMCO Dist.

Artificial Organs. W. J. Kolff. 1975. 180p. 3.5 hd 54.50 (0-7065-1525-0) Coronet Bks.

Artificial Reproduction & Reproductive Rights. Athena Nga Chee Liu. 1991. 223p. text (1-85521-022-3) Dartmth Pub GBR. *Dist:* Ashgate Pub Co.

Artificial Sweeteners: A Special Issue of the Journal Comments on Toxicology. Ed. by A. Wallace Hayes & William O. Berndt. 1989. 100p. pap. text 55.00 (2-88124-395-9) Gordon & Breach.

Artificial Urinary Sphincter, Incontinence, Impotence: Effects of a Prostatectomy, Pt. 1. Gene Washington. 2000. LC 00-191770. 229p. pap. 16.00 (0-7388-3249-9) Xlibris Corp.

Artist As Therapist. Arthur Robbins. 1987. LC 86-10466. 226p. 42.95 (0-89885-322-2); pap. 22.95 (0-89885-439-3) Kluwer Academic (Kluwer Acad Hman Sci).

Artistic Inquiry in Dance/Movement Therapy: Creative Research Alternatives. Lenore Wadsworth Hervey. 2000. LC 00-42305. xv, 174p. text 39.95 (0-398-07108-X); pap. text 24.95 (0-398-07109-8) C C Thomas.

Arts & Psychotherapy. Shaun McNiff. 1981. (Illus.). 260p. text 41.95 (0-398-04112-1) C C Thomas.

Arts Therapies & Eating Disorders. Ed. by Ditty Dokter. 1995. 250p. pap. 29.95 (1-85302-256-X) Taylor & Francis.

Aryan Medical Science: A Short History. H. H. Jee. 1993. (C). (81-85557-74-8) Low Price IND. *Dist:* S Asia.

A
B

Arzt und Heilkunde in den fruhmittelalterlichen Leges: Eine Wort- und Sachkundliche Untersuchung, Vol. 12. Annette Niederhellamnn. 1983. 3053p. 142.35 (*3-11-009607-2*) De Gruyter.

As Bill Sees It: Selected Writings of the A. A.'s Co-Founder. 1967. LC 87-402899. 332p. 3.35 (*0-916856-03-8*) AAWS.

As Boys Become Men: Learning New Male Roles. Doug Cooper Thompson. 1985. 81p. pap. 14.95 (*0-8290-1591-4*) Irvington.

As Dreams Are Made On: Previews of the Human Mind. David P. Pace & E. C. Barksdale. 1988. LC 87-91102. 18.95 (*0-87212-209-3*) Libra.

As I See It: Radial Keratotomy Before, During & After Surgery. Raymond J. Munna. 1986. (Illus.). 110p. pap. 9.95 (*0-935669-07-8*) A Granite Pubs.

As I Walked Out One Evening. Donald Wetzel. 1997. LC 96-27408. 141p. pap. 16.00 (*1-877946-94-X*) Permanent Pr.

As Perceived by the Patient: Introduction to the Literature of Patient Response. Jimmie R. Rankin. 1993. LC 93-26011. (Literature of Patient Response Ser.: Vol. I). 70p. pap., per. 12.95 (*1-883938-02-3*) Dry Bones Pr.

As They May Need: A History of the Addison Gilbert Hospital, 1889-1989. Laurence F. Brooks & W. Warren Babson. 1989. LC 89-16395. (Illus.). 360p. 18.00 (*0-914659-43-X*) Phoenix Pub.

As We Understood. Al-Anon Family Group Headquarters, Inc. Staff. 1985. LC 85-71379. 269p. 8.50 (*0-910034-56-7*) Al-Anon.

As You Eat, So Your Baby Grows: Prenatal Nutrition. Nikki Goldbeck. rev. ed. 2000. (Illus.). 16p. pap. 2.50 (*0-9606138-8-9*) Ceres Pr.

ASA 1999 Proceedings of the Section on Epidemiology & Section on Health Policy Statistics. 2000. 138p. pap. (*1-883276-91-8*) Amer Statist.

Asbestos: Medical & Legal Aspects. Barry I. Castleman. 3rd ed. 1995. 798p. 95.00 (*0-13-048414-8*) Aspen Law.

Asbestos: Medical & Legal Aspects. Barry I. Castleman. 4th ed. 1996. LC 95-47681. 1230p. 135.00 (*1-56706-275-X*) Panel Pubs.

Asbestos: The Unseen Peril in Our Environment. Edwin Flatto. 1983. pap. 7.95 (*0-935540-10-5*) Plymouth Pr.

Asbestos & Other Fibrous Materials: Mineralogy, Crystal Chemistry, & Health Effects. H. Catherine Skinner et al. 1988. (Illus.). 222p. text 65.00 (*0-19-503967-X*) OUP.

Asbestos & Other Natural Mineral Fibers. 1987. (Environmental Health Criteria Ser.: No. 53). 194p. pap. text 26.00 (*92-4-154193-8*, 1160053) World Health.

Asbestos Cancer: One Man's Experience. Myrna J. Grove. 1995. LC 93-74752. 12.95 (*0-8158-0498-9*) Chris Mass.

Asbestos Medicine on Trial—A Medical/Legal Outline. Norwood S. Wilner & Ilan A. Feingold. 1995. LC 95-36638. 115.00 (*0-9636246-6-0*) Andrews Pubns.

ASCA: National Profiles in Youth Psychopathology. Paul A. McDermott. 1993. 64p. pap. 34.95 (*0-9638072-3-4*) Ed & Psych.

Ascites & Renal Dysfunction in Liver Disease: Pathogenesis, Diagnosis & Treatment. Vicente Arroyo et al. 1999. LC 98-37812. (Illus.). xiii, 568p. 135.95 (*0-632-04342-3*) Blackwell Sci.

***Asclepius: The God of Medicine.** Gerald D. Hart. 2000. (History of Medicine Ser.). 284p. pap. (*1-85315-409-1*) Royal Soc of Medicine Pr Ltd GBR. *Dist:* Balogh.

Ascomycetes of Ohio, Pts. I & II. Bruce Fink. 1915. (Bulletin Ser.: No. 5). pap. text 3.00 (*0-86727-004-7*) Ohio Bio Survey.

Ascomycetes of Ohio, Pts. IV & V. Bruce Fink & Leafy J. Corrington. 1921. (Bulletin Ser.: No. 10). pap. text 3.00 (*0-86727-009-8*) Ohio Bio Survey.

Ascorbic Acid: Chemistry, Metabolism, & Uses. Bert M. Tolbert. Ed. by Paul A. Seib. 1982. LC 82-13795. (ACS Advances in Chemistry Ser.: No. 200). 69.95 (*0-8412-0632-5*) Am Chemical.

Aseptic Pharmaceutical Manufacturing: Technology for the 1990s. Ed. by Wayne Olson & M. Groves. 1987. 430p. 79.50 (*0-935184-06-6*) IHS Health Grp.

Aseptic Pharmaceutical Manufacturing II: Applications for the 1990s. Ed. by Michael J. Groves & Ram Murty. 1995. 520p. 179.00 (*0-935184-77-5*) IHS Health Grp.

***Ashgate Handbook of Chiral Drugs.** Ed. by Cynthia A. Challener. 2001. 800p. (*0-566-08411-2*) Ashgate Pub GBR. *Dist:* Ashgate Pub Co.

Asian - Pacific Islander American Health: Bibliography. January 1990 Through March 1995. Loretta D. Ulincy et al. 1995. 93p. (Orig.). (C). pap. text 30.00 (*0-7881-2023-9*) DIANE Pub.

Asian Americans: Personality Patterns, Identity, & Mental Health. Laura Uba. 1993. LC 93-41723. 302p. 37.00 (*0-89862-372-3*) Guilford Pubns.

Asian & Pacific Islander Task Force Report on the Year 2000: Health Promotion Objectives & Recommendations for California. 1993. 68p. (Orig.). (C). pap. text 30.00 (*0-7881-0089-0*) DIANE Pub.

Asian Contributions to Psychology. Ed. by Anand C. Paranjpe et al. 1988. LC 88-2334. 307p. 82.50 (*0-275-92524-2*, C2524, Praeger Pubs) Greenwood.

Asian Health Secrets: The Complete Guide to Asian Herbal Medicine. Letha Hadady. 1998. 512p. pap. 18.00 (*0-609-80105-8*) Random Hse Value.

Asian Nephrology: Proceedings of the Fifth Asian Pacific Congress of Nephrology, New Delhi, India, 9-13, December 1992. Ed. by K. S. Chugh et al. 1995. (Illus.). 796p. text 160.00 (*0-19-563401-2*) OUP.

Asian Pacific Congress on Antisepsis: Proceedings, 3rd Congress, Sydney, January 1997. Ed. by D. G. MacLellan & M. Ermini. 1997. (Dermatology Ser.: Vol. 195, Suppl. 2, 1997). (Illus.). iv, 160p. pap. 69.75 (*3-8055-6627-1*) S Karger.

Asian Perspectives on Psychology. Henry S. Kao & Durganand Sinha. 1997. LC 96-33402. (Cross-Cultural Research & Methodology Ser.). 284p. 49.95 (*0-8039-9293-9*, 80825) Sage.

Asian Perspectives on Psychology. Ed. by Henry S. Kao & Durganand Sinha. 1996. 284p. pap. 18.95 (*0-8039-9294-7*) Sage.

Asian Society for Stereotactic, Functional & Computer-Assisted Neurosurgery: 2nd Congress, Nagano Prefecture, November 1996 - Invited Papers & Abstracts. Ed. by Chihiro Ohye et al. 1998. (Stereotactic & Functional Neurosurgery Ser.: Vol. 70, Nos. 2-4). (Illus.). viii, 150p. pap. 99.25 (*3-8055-6797-9*) S Karger.

***Asian Society for Stereotactic, Functional & Computer-Assisted Neurosurgery: 3rd Congress, Seoul, June 1999 - Invited Papers & Abstracts.** Ed. by S. S. Chung et al. 2001. (Stereotactic & Functional Neurosurgery Ser.: Vol. 74, No. 3-4). (Illus.). xviii, 146p. 45.25 (*3-8055-7213-1*) S Karger.

***Asian Society for Stereotactic, Functional & Computer-Assisted Neurosurgery: 4th Congress, Beijing, October-November 2000: Selected Papers.** Ed. by Z. Liu et al. 2001. (Illus.). 106p. pap. 34.00 (*3-8055-7338-3*) S Karger.

Asian Voices: Asian & Asian American Health Educators Speak Out. Lin Zhan & National League for Nursing Staff. 1998. LC 97-34603. (*0-88737-741-6*) Natl League Nurse.

Asians in the United States: Abstracts of the Psychological & Behaviorial Literature, 1967-1991. Ed. by Frederick T. L. Leong & James R. Whitfield. 1992. LC 92-17379. (Bibliographies in Psychology Ser.: No. 11). 216p. pap. 19.95 (*1-55798-178-7*) Am Psychol.

***Ask a Nurse.** American Association of Colleges of Nursing Staff. 2002. (Illus.). 416p. pap. 15.00 (*0-7432-1940-6*, Fireside) S&S Trade Pap.

Ask a Nurse: From Home Remedies to Hospital Care. American Association of Colleges of Nursing Staff. Ed. by Polly Bednash. 2001. LC 00-47009. 415p. 25.00 (*0-684-85687-5*) Free Pr.

Ask Audrey: The Author's Personal & Professional Experience in the Day-to-Day Living with Inflammatory Bowel Disease. Audrey Kron. Date not set. 156p. pap. 12.00 (*0-9633877-0-7*) A Kron.

Ask Dr. Ian about Men's Health. Iain M. Banks et al. 1997. 206p. pap. (*0-85640-592-2*) Blackstaff Pr IRL. *Dist:* Dufour.

Ask Dr. Weil. Andrew Weil. 1999. pap. (*0-449-00311-6*) Fawcett.

Ask Dr. Weil. Andrew Weil. Ed. by Steven Petrow. 1998. LC 97-97188. 304p. pap. 12.95 (*0-449-00312-4*) Fawcett.

Ask Dr. Weil. Andrew Weil. Ed. by Steven Petrow. l.t. ed. 1998. LC 98-28573. 496p. pap. 18.95 (*0-375-70445-0*) Random Hse Lrg Prnt.

Ask Dr. Mike: Frequently Asked Questions about Psychology. Michael Atkinson. 2000. 188p. pap. 18.00 (*0-205-33109-2*) Allyn.

Ask the Children: Experiences of Physical Disability in the School Years. Nicola Madge & Meg Fassam. 1982. (Illus.). 160p. (Orig.). pap. 17.95 (*0-7134-1896-6*) Trafalgar.

Ask the Doctor: Herbs & Supplements for Better Health. Derrick DeSilva. 1997. LC 97-2748. (Illus.). 160p. pap. 12.95 (*1-883010-31-4*) Interweave.

Ask the Pharmacist: Drug & Health Information for the Consumer. Richard P. Hoffmann. 2000. LC 99-69147. 200p. pap. 9.95 (*1-884778-81-X*) Old Mountain.

Ask the Vet: Concise Answers to Common Questions. John H. Hunt. Ed. by Elizabeth Umphrey & Elizabeth Payne. 1994. (Useful Little Book Ser.: Vol. 1). (Illus.). 104p. pap. 7.95 (*0-9665422-0-7*) J H Hunt.

Ask Your Doctor, Ask Yourself. Annette Thornhill. Ed. by Emily McKeigue & Camilla Ayers. 1986. LC 84-62728. 160p. pap. 10.95 (*0-914918-67-2*, Whitford) Schiffer.

Ask Your Gynecologist. R. Scott Thornton & Kathleen Schramm. 1998. LC 98-17932. 256p. pap. 13.00 (*0-395-89262-7*) HM.

Ask Your Pharmacist: A Leading Pharmacist Answers Your Most Frequently Asked Questions. Lisa M. Chavis. 2001. LC 2001-19151. x, 399p. 29.95 (*0-312-26554-9*) St Martin.

Asking the Right Questions in Abnormal Psychology. Stuart M. Keeley. 1994. LC 94-30165. 160p. pap. text 21.80 (*0-13-291212-0*) P-H.

Asklepios: Cult of the Greek God of Medicine. A. Walton. 1979. 136p. pap. 15.00 (*0-89005-229-8*) Ares.

Asklepios at Athens: Epigraphic & Prosopographic Essays on Athenian Healing Cults. Sara B. Aleshire. 1992. (Illus.). xii, 256p. pap. (*90-5063-068-5*) Gieben NLD. *Dist:* J Benjamins Pubng Co.

***Aspartame Disease: An Ignored Epidemic.** H. S. Roberts. 2001. (Illus.). 1000p. lib. bdg. 75.00 (*1-884243-17-7*) Sunshine Sentinel.

Aspartame (NutraSweet) Is It Safe? H. J. Roberts. 1990. LC 89-81086. 328p. text 26.95 (*0-914783-37-8*) Charles.

Aspartic Proteinases: Physiology & Pathology. Ed. by Martin Fusek & Vaclav Vetvicka. 1995. LC 95-32355. 320p. 204.95 (*0-8493-7660-2*, 7660) CRC Pr.

Aspartic Proteinases: Structure, Function, Biology & Biomedical Implications, Vol. 362. Ed. by Kenji Takahashi. 1995. LC 94-43762. (Advances in Experimental Medicine & Biology Ser.: Vol. 362). (Illus.). 656p. (C). text 149.50 (*0-306-44830-0*, Kluwer Plenum) Kluwer Academic.

Aspartylglycosaminuria: Lysosomal Disease & Inborn Errors of Metabolism. Iikka Mononen. Ed. by Nathan N. Aronson, Jr. 1997. (Medical Intelligence Unit Ser.). 178p. 99.00 (*1-57059-443-0*) Landes Bioscience.

Aspects Actuels de la Contraception Hormonale. Ed. by P. J. Keller. 1991. (GER., Illus.). x, 88p. pap. 39.25 (*3-8055-5263-7*) S Karger.

Aspects & Treatments of Vulvar Cancer: Proceedings of the International Symposium, 1st, Madrid, 1971. International Symposium on Vulvar Cancer Staff. Ed. by L. Lopez De La Osa. 1972. (Illus.). 250p. 65.25 (*3-8055-1399-2*) S Karger.

Aspects for Treatment with Fosfomycin. Ed. by J. P. Guggenbichler. 1987. 150p. pap. 29.00 (*0-387-81986-X*) Spr-Verlag.

Aspects of Autonomy: The Autonomy Frustration Syndrome As Cause of Psychological Disorder & Autonomy Exercised As Precondition to Personal Well-Being & to the Good Society. Henry Stern. 1995. 270p. (Orig.). pap. 15.00 (*0-9646379-4-4*) H Stern.

Aspects of Avian Endocrinology: Practical & Theoretical Implications. Ed. by Colin G. Scanes. 1982. (Graduate Studies: No. 26). 411p. 59.95 (*0-89672-103-5*); pap. 29.95 (*0-89672-102-7*) Tex Tech Univ Pr.

Aspects of Childhood Nutrition. Ed. by Geoffrey H. Bourne. 1989. (World Review of Nutrition & Dietetics Ser.: Vol. 58). (Illus.). x, 166p. 128.75 (*3-8055-4918-0*) S Karger.

Aspects of Family Mental Health in Europe. D. Buckle et al. 1965. (Public Health Papers: No. 28). 123p. pap. text 5.00 (*92-4-130028-0*, 1110028) World Health.

Aspects of Food Production, Consumption & Energy Values. Ed. by Geoffrey H. Bourne. 1989. (World Review of Nutrition & Dietetics Ser.: Vol. 61). (Illus.). 212p. 172.25 (*3-8055-4993-8*) S Karger.

Aspects of Forensic Psychiatric Nursing. Ed. by Paul Morrison & Philip Burnard. 1992. 183p. (*1-85628-371-2*) Avebry GBR. *Dist:* Ashgate Pub Co.

Aspects of Greek Medicine. E. D. Phillips. 1987. LC 86-72186. 240p. text 32.95 (*0-914783-18-1*) Charles.

Aspects of Homogeneous Catalysis: A Series of Advances, Vol. 4. Ed. by Renato Ugo. 1981. 208p. text 155.50 (*90-277-1139-9*) Kluwer Academic.

Aspects of Human & National Nutrition. Ed. by Geoffrey H. Bourne. 1983. (World Review of Nutrition & Dietetics Ser.: Vol. 41). (Illus.). xii, 260p. 204.50 (*3-8055-3591-0*) S Karger.

Aspects of Human Nutrition. Ed. by Geoffrey H. Bourne. 1988. (World Review of Nutrition & Dietetics Ser.: Vol. 57). (Illus.). x, 334p. 258.50 (*3-8055-4810-9*) S Karger.

Aspects of Human Nutrition & Food Contaminants. Ed. by Geoffrey H. Bourne. 1979. (World Review of Nutrition & Dietetics Ser.: Vol. 34). (Illus.). 144.50 (*3-8055-3069-2*) S Karger.

Aspects of Hypertension Management. 120p. pap. text (*0-86471-057-7*) Adis Intl NZL. *Dist:* Lppncott W & W.

***Aspects of Illness.** Robert Dingwall. 2nd ed. 2001. 184p. text (*0-7546-1670-3*) Ashgate Pub GBR. *Dist:* Ashgate Pub Co.

Aspects of Leukemia Treatment with Special Reference to Drug Development Stuart Roath. 1990. 74p. text 141.00 (*3-7186-5077-0*) Gordon & Breach.

Aspects of Lyme Borreliosis. Ed. by K. Weber & William Burgdorfer. 1992. LC 92-48763. (Illus.). 392p. 194.00 (*0-387-55628-1*) Spr-Verlag.

Aspects of Manipulative Therapy. Ed. by E. F. Glasgow et al. 2nd ed. 1985. LC 84-5846. (Illus.). 208p. pap. (*0-443-03036-7*) Church.

Aspects of Microbial Metabolism & Ecology. Ed. by Geoffrey A. Codd. 1984. (Social Publication Society General Microbiology Ser.: No. 11). text 157.00 (*0-12-178050-3*) Acad Pr.

Aspects of Nutritional Physiology. Ed. by Geoffrey H. Bourne. 1988. (World Review of Nutrition & Dietetics Ser.: Vol. 56). (Illus.). x, 262p. 195.00 (*3-8055-4785-4*) S Karger.

Aspects of Oral Molecular Biology. Ed. by D. B. Ferguson. 1991. (Frontiers of Oral Physiology Ser.: Vol. 8). (Illus.). xii, 144p. 135.00 (*3-8055-5261-0*) S Karger.

Aspects of Public Health Nursing. Alcantara. Ed. by Ashurkov. 1961. (Public Health Papers: No. 4). 185p. 5.00 (*92-4-130004-3*) World Health.

Aspects of Slow & Persistent Virus Infections. Ed. by David A. Tyrrell. 1979. (New Perspectives in Clinical Microbiology Ser.: Vol. 2). 286p. text 126.50 (*90-247-2281-0*) Kluwer Academic.

Aspects of Some Vitamins, Minerals & Enzymes in Health & Disease. Ed. by Geoffrey H. Bourne. 1990. (World Review of Nutrition & Dietetics Ser.: Vol. 62). (Illus.). 216p. 188.00 (*3-8055-4994-6*) S Karger.

Aspects of Stroke Prevention. Ed. by J. D. Easton. 1992. (Journal: Vol. 2, Suppl. 1, 1992). (Illus.). iv, 48p. pap. 22.75 (*3-8055-5584-9*) S Karger.

***Aspects of Surgical Treatment of Morbid Obesity.** Agneta Westling. 2001. (Comprehensive Summaries of Uppsala Dissertations from the Faculty of Medicine Ser.: No. 1029). (Illus.). 46p. (*91-554-5003-2*) Uppsala Universitet SWE. *Dist:* Coronet Bks.

Aspects of Synaptic Transmission, Vol. 1: LTP, Galanin, Autonomic, Opioids & 5-HT. Ed. by Trevor W. Stone. 1991. 380p. (*0-85066-828-X*) Tay Francis Ltd GBR. *Dist:* Taylor & Francis.

Aspects of the Computer-Based Patient Record. Ed. by M. H. Ball et al. 1996. (Computers in Health Care Ser.). (Illus.). 316p. 59.95 (*0-387-97723-6*) Spr-Verlag.

Aspects of the Development of Competence Vol. 14: The Minnesota Symposium on Child Psychology. Ed. by W. Andrew Collins. 1981. LC 80-20568. 288p. 59.95 (*0-89859-070-1*) L Erlbaum Assocs.

Aspects of the Feminine. Carl Gustav Jung. 1983. LC 82-47629. (Jung Extracts Ser.). 189p. pap. 12.95 (*0-691-01845-6*) Princeton U Pr.

Aspects of the History of Psychology in America 1892-1992. Ed. by Helmut E. Adler & Robert W. Rieber. 1995. LC 94-42028. (Annals Ser.: Vol. 188). (Illus.). 147p. pap. 19.95 (*0-89766-867-7*) Am Psychol.

Aspects of the Introduction of Food Irradiation in Developing Countries. 1973. (Illus.). 113p. (Orig.). pap. (*92-0-111673-X*, ISP362) IAEA AUT. *Dist:* Bernan Associates.

Asperger Syndrome. Ed. by Ami Klin et al. 2000. LC 99-54492. 489p. 48.00 (*1-57230-534-7*, 8R0534) Guilford Pubns.

Asperger Syndrome: A Guide for Educators & Parents. Brenda Myles & Richard L. Simpson. 1997. LC 97-17269. 38.89 (*0-89079-727-7*, 8409) PRO-ED.

***Asperger Syndrome & Adolescence: Helping Preteens & Teens Get Ready for the Real World.** Theresa Bolick. 2001. 24.95 (*1-931412-69-3*) Fair Winds Pr.

Asperger Syndrome Employment Workbook: An Employment Workbook for Adults with Asperger Syndrome. Roger N. Meyer. 2001. LC 99-41650. 320p. pap., wbk. ed. (*1-85302-796-0*) Jessica Kingsley GBR. *Dist:* Taylor & Francis.

Asperger Syndrome or High Functioning Autism? E. Schopler et al. 1998. LC 98-3651. (Current Issues in Autism Ser.). (Illus.). 365p. (C). text 49.50 (*0-306-45746-6*, Kluwer Plenum) Kluwer Academic.

Asphyxia & Drowning. Jay D. Dix et al. 2000. LC 00-29735. (Causes of Death Atlas Ser.). (Illus.). ix, 110p. per. 34.95 (*0-8493-2369-X*) CRC Pr.

Asphyxia & Fetal Brain Damage. Ed. by Dev Maulik. 1998. LC 97-52695. 372p. 132.00 (*0-471-18427-6*, Wiley-Liss) Wiley.

Asphyxiation. Susan Black. 1996. LC 96-60922. 116p. 14.95 (*1-881636-08-9*) Windsor Hse Pub Grp.

Aspiration Biopsy. Leopold G. Koss et al. 2nd ed. 1992. LC 92-1467. (Illus.). 752p. 185.00 (*0-89640-212-6*) Igaku-Shoin.

Aspiration, Biopsy, Cytology, Part II: Cytology of Infradiaphragmatic Organs. J. Zajicek. 1979. (Monographs in Clinical Cytology Ser.: Vol. 7). (Illus.). 100.00 (*3-8055-2933-3*) S Karger.

Aspirin: Uses & Abuses. Jennifer James. rev. ed. 1999. pap. 0.50 (*0-89230-061-2*) Do It Now.

Aspirin - Reports of Harmful & Unfavorable Effects Including Illness & Wayward Behavior: Index of New Information with Authors & Subjects. Roy R. Zimmerman. 1993. 180p. 47.50 (*1-55914-838-1*); pap. 44.50 (*1-55914-839-X*) ABBE Pubs Assn.

Aspirin Alternative. Michael Loes. 1985. pap. 13.95 (*1-893910-04-0*) Freedom Pr Inc.

Aspirin & Other Salicylates. Ed. by John R. Vane & Regina M. Botting. 1993. (Illus.). 672p. (gr. 13). pap. 246.95 (*0-412-32370-2*) Chapman & Hall.

Aspirin, Platelets & Stroke: Background for a Clinical Trial. William S. Fields & William K. Hass. 1971. LC 74-153915. (Illus.). 178p. 15.00 (*0-87527-033-6*) Green.

Assault on Medical Freedom. P. Joseph Lisa. 1994. LC 95-130406. 336p. (Orig.). pap. 14.95 (*1-57174-003-1*) Hampton Roads Pub Co.

Assaults Within Psychiatric Facilities. John R. Lion & William H. Reid. 1985. 336p. (Orig.). pap. text 29.00 (*0-8089-1703-X*, 792567, Grune & Strat) Harcrt Hlth Sci Grp.

Assay for Ristocetin Cofactor: Proposed Guideline (1993) Contrib. by H. James Day. 1993. 75.00 (*1-56238-226-8*, H41-P) NCCLS.

Assay of Calcium Regulating Hormones. Ed. by D. D. Bikle. 1983. (Illus.). 290p. 135.00 (*0-387-90841-2*) Spr-Verlag.

Assays of the Heme Biosynthetic Enzymes. Ed. by D. F. Bishop & R. J. Desnick. 1982. (Enzyme Ser.: Vol. 28, No. 2-3). (Illus.). vi, 144p. pap. 84.50 (*3-8055-3573-2*) S Karger.

Assembly of Enveloped RNA Viruses. M. Dubois-Dalco et al. Ed. by D. W. Kingsbury. 1985. (Illus.). 250p. 111.00 (*0-387-81802-2*) Spr-Verlag.

Assert Yourself! How to Be Your Own Person. Merna D. Galassi & John P. Galassi. 1977. LC 76-57936. 256p. pap. 25.95 (*0-87705-299-9*, Kluwer Acad Hman Sci) Kluwer Academic.

Assertion Training Workshop. Laura G. Manis. 1998. LC 83-83316. 32p. pap., stu. ed. 7.45 (*1-55691-144-0*, 440) Learning Pubns.

Assertion Training Workshop: Leader Guide. Laura G. Manis. 2nd ed. 1998. LC 83-83316. 144p. pap., tchr. ed. 21.50 (*1-55691-140-8*, 408) Learning Pubns.

Assertive Communication: COPE Program for Depression. John H. Greist et al. 1999. (Illus.). 35p. pap. (*0-9702974-4-0*) Healthcare Sys.

Assertive Community Treatment of Persons with Severe Mental Illness. Leonard I. Stein. 1998. LC 97-38893. 224p. pap. 27.00 (*0-393-70258-8*) Norton.

Assertive Formula. A. D. Russo. 1982. (Human Resources Book Ser.). 95p. pap. 4.00 (*0-9610708-0-3*) Twenty Fst CT.

Assertive Option: Your Rights & Responsibilities. Patricia Jakubowski & Arthur J. Lange. 1978. LC 78-62904. 348p. (Orig.). pap. text 22.95 (*0-87822-192-1*, 1921) Res Press.

Assertiveness. Jeff Davidson. 1997. LC 97-73152. (Complete Idiot's Guides). 368p. pap. 16.95 (*0-02-861964-1*) Mac USA.

Assesment & Management of Central Auditory Processing Disorders in the Educational Setting: From Science to Practice. Teri J. Bellis. 1996. (Illus.). 364p. pap. text 57.95 (*1-56593-628-0*, 1302) Thomson Learn.

Assess for Success: Handbook on Transition Assessment. Patricia L. Sitlington et al. 1996. LC 96-8058. 136p. (Orig.). pap. text 30.00 (*0-86586-281-8*, P5155) Coun Exc Child.

Assess Your True Risk of Breast Cancer. Patricia T. Kelly. 2000. LC 00-44851. (Illus.). xiv, 253p. pap. 15.00 (*0-8050-6468-0*, Owl) H Holt & Co.

Assessing Adolescents: A Practitioner's Guide. G. D. Oster et al. 1988. (Psychology Practitioner Guidebooks). 192p. text 30.00 (*0-08-034941-2*); pap. text 15.95 (*0-08-034940-4*) Elsevier (Pergamon Pr).

Assessing Adolescents in Educational, Counseling & Forensic Settings. Robert D. Hoge. 1999. LC 98-41565. 328p. 39.95 (*0-8058-3094-4*) L Erlbaum Assocs.

Assessing Adolescents with the MACI: Using the Million Adolescent Clinical Inventory. Joseph T. McCann. 1999. LC 98-42307. (Illus.). 238p. 85.00 (*0-471-32619-4*) Wiley.

Assessing AIDS Prevention: Selected Papers Presented at the International Conference Held in Montreux (Switzerland), October 29-November 1, 1990. Ed. by F. Paccaud et al. 1992. x, 305p. 192.00 (*0-8176-2722-7*) Birkhauser.

Assessing Alcohol Problems: A Guide for Clinicians & Researchers. Ed. by John P. Allen & Megan Columbus. 1997. (Illus.). 575p. (Orig.). (C). pap. text 75.00 (*0-7881-3829-4*) DIANE Pub.

Assessing Allegations of Child Sexual Abuse. Kathryn Kuehnle. 1996. LC 95-31514. 400p. 65.45 (*1-56887-009-4*, AACBP, Prof Resc Pr) Pro Resource.

Assessing & Improving Billing & Collections. Ed. by Coker Group Staff. 2000. (Assessing & Improving Practice Operations Ser.). 75p. pap. 36.40 (*1-57947-078-5*) AMA.

Assessing & Improving Staffing & Organization. Ed. by Coker Group Staff. 2000. (Assessing & Improving Practice Operations Ser.). 75p. pap. 56.00 (*1-57947-080-7*) AMA.

Assessing & Improving the Patient Encounter Process. Ed. by Coker Group Staff. 2000. (Assessing & Improving Practice Operations Ser.). 75p. pap. 56.00 (*1-57947-079-3*) AMA.

Assessing & Managing Behavior Disabilities. Ed. by Norris G. Haring. 1987. LC 87-16008. 344p. 50.00 (*0-295-96563-0*) U of Wash Pr.

***Assessing & Modifying the Vulnerable Atherosclerotic Plaque.** Ed. by Valentin Fuster. 2001. LC 2001-55631. (American Heart Association Monographs). (Illus.). 208p. text (*0-87993-485-9*) Futura Pub.

Assessing & Screening Preschoolers: Psychological & Educational Dimensions. Ed. by Ena V. Nuttall et al. 2nd ed. 1998. LC 98-25701. 466p. (C). 86.00 (*0-205-26676-2*, Longwood Div) Allyn.

Assessing & Treating Culturally Diverse Clients: A Practical Guide. Freddy A. Paniagua. 2nd ed. 1998. LC 97-45260. (Multicultural Aspects of Counseling Ser.: Vol. 4). 161p. 89.95 (*0-7619-1049-2*, 81485); pap. 34.95 (*0-7619-1050-6*, 81486) Sage.

Assessing & Treating Victims of Violence. Vol. 64. Ed. by John Briere. 1994. LC 87-646993. (New Directions for Mental Health Services Ser.: No. MHS 64). Orig. Title: Violent Victimization. 104p. (Orig.). pap. 28.00 (*0-7879-9991-1*) Jossey-Bass.

Assessing Attention-Deficit/Hyperactivity Disorder. Arthur D. Anastopoulos & Terri L. Shelton. 2001. LC 00-49780. (Illus.). xvi, 349p. 45.00 (*0-306-46388-1*, Kluwer Plenum) Kluwer Academic.

Assessing Child & Adolescent Disorders: A Practice Manual. Masud Hoghughi. 2nd ed. 1992. (Illus.). 320p. (C). pap. 34.95 (*0-8039-8297-6*, 9178); text 69.95 (*0-8039-8296-8*) Sage.

Assessing Children's Vision: A Handbook. Carol A. Westall et al. 1998. LC 98-10424. 408p. pap. text 55.00 (*0-7506-0584-7*) Buttrwrth-Heinemann.

Assessing Chronic Pain. Ed. by P. M. Camic & F. D. Brown. 1989. (Contributions to Psychology & Medicine Ser.). (Illus.). 257p. 108.00 (*0-387-96942-X*) Spr-Verlag.

Assessing Clinical Reasoning: The Oral Examination & Alternative Methods. Ed. by Elliott L. Mancall & Philip G. Bashook. 1995. LC 95-79294. 224p. lib. bdg. 44.95 (*0-934277-21-4*) Am Bd Med Spec.

Assessing Community Health Needs & Coverage Module 2: Facilitator's Guide. Martine Hilton. 1993. (Primary Health Care Management Advancement Programme Modules Ser.). 59p. pap. text (*1-882839-09-9*) Aga Khan Fnd.

Assessing Community Health Needs & Coverage Module 2: User's Guide. Jack Reynolds. 1993. (Primary Health Care Management Advancement Programme Modules Ser.). 227p. pap. text (*1-882839-01-3*) Aga Khan Fnd.

***Assessing Competence: A Resource Manual.** 2001. (Illus.). pap. (*1-887759-99-9*) Am Phys Therapy Assn.

Assessing Competence to Consent to Treatment: A Guide for Physicians & Other Health Professionals. Thomas Grisso & Paul S. Appelbaum. 1998. LC 97-26915. (Illus.). 224p. text 29.95 (*0-19-510372-6*) OUP.

Assessing Development & Treating Disorders Within a Family, Vol. 1. (*0-89970-120-5*, OP-006) AMA.

Assessing E M F in the Workplace: A Guide for Industrial Hygienist. Robert M. Patterson et al. Ed. by American Conference of Governmental Industrial Hygenists Staff. 1998. LC 99-183495. (Illus.). 88p. pap. text 34.00 (*1-882417-28-3*, 9853) Am Conf Govt Indus Hygienist.

Assessing Educational Outcomes: Third National Conference on Measurement & Evaluation in Nursing. Ed. by Margery Garbin. 1991. 144p. (Orig.). (C). pap. text 29.95 (*0-88737-541-3*) Natl League Nurse.

Assessing Experience in Psychotherapy: Personal Construct Alternatives. A. J. Faidley & L. M. Leitner. 1993. LC 92-48993. 232p. 70.00 (*0-275-94260-0*, C4260, Praeger Pubs) Greenwood.

Assessing Exposure to Air Toxicants from Environmental Tobacco Smoke. Shelly L. Miller. 2000. (Illus.). 224p. reprint ed. pap. 40.00 (*0-7567-0386-7*) DIANE Pub.

Assessing for Special Educational Needs. Ed. by Sheila Wolfendale. 1993. LC 94-132789. (Special Needs in Ordinary Schools Ser.). (Illus.). 192p. pap. 31.95 (*0-304-32652-6*) Continuum.

Assessing for Special Educational Needs. Ed. by Sheila Wolfendale. 1993. LC 94-132789. (Special Needs in Ordinary Schools Ser.). (Illus.). 192p. 75.00 (*0-304-32654-2*) Weidner & Sons.

Assessing Genetic Risks: Implications for Health & Social Policy. Institute of Medicine Staff. Ed. by Lori B. Andrews et al. 1994. LC 93-47973. 352p. (C). text 44.95 (*0-309-04798-6*) Natl Acad Pr.

Assessing Health & Human Services Needs: Concepts, Methods & Applications. Ed. by Roger Bell et al. 1983. LC 81-20249. (Community Psychology Ser.: Vol. VIII). (Illus.). 352p. 45.95 (*0-89885-057-6*, Kluwer Acad Hman Sci) Kluwer Academic.

Assessing Health Care: A Study in Organizational Evaluation. Gilbert Smith & Caroline Cantly. 1985. LC 84-27215. 195p. (*0-335-15072-1*) OpUniv Pr.

Assessing Health Care Reform. Institute of Medicine Staff. Ed. by Marilyn J. Field et al. 1993. 88p. (C). pap. text 21.00 (*0-309-04926-1*) Natl Acad Pr.

Assessing Health Need Using the Life Cycle Framework. Chrissie Pickin & Selwyn St. Leger. 1992. LC 92-18760. 192p. (*0-335-15743-2*); pap. (*0-335-15742-4*) OpUniv Pr.

Assessing Health Risks from Contaminated Soil. B. D. Beck. 1987. text 77.00 (*2-88124-419-X*) Gordon & Breach.

Assessing Human Health Risks of Chemicals: Derivation of Guidance Values for Health-Based Exposure Limits. 1994. (Environmental Health Criteria Ser.: No. 170). (ENG, FRE & SPA.). 73p. pap. text 21.00 (*92-4-157170-5*, 1160170) World Health.

Assessing Hypertension Control & Management: Hypertension Management Audit Project: a WHO-WHL Study. Ed. by T. Strasser & L. Wilhelmsen. 1993. (WHO Regional Publications: No. 47). xiv, 181p. pap. text 39.00 (*92-890-1310-9*, 1310047) World Health.

Assessing Individual Differences in Human Behavior: New Concepts, Methods, & Findings. Ed. by David Lubinski & Rene V. Dawis. 1995. LC 95-11398. 780p. (C). text 49.95 (*0-89106-072-3*, 7220, Davies-Black Pub) Consulting Psychol.

Assessing Information Needs Module 1: Facilitator's Guide. Mary Millar. 1993. (Primary Health Care Management Advancement Programme Modules Ser.). 55p. pap. text (*1-882839-08-0*) Aga Khan Fnd.

Assessing Information Needs Module 1: User's Guide. Jack Reynolds. 1993. (Primary Health Care Management Advancement Programme Modules Ser.). 54p. pap. text (*1-882839-00-5*) Aga Khan Fnd.

Assessing Intelligence: Applying a Biocultural Model. Eleanor Armour-Thomas & Sharon-Ann Gopaul-McNicol. 1998. LC 97-45335. (Ethnic Minority Psychology Ser.). 264p. 74.95 (*0-7619-0520-0*, 80665); pap. 34.95 (*0-7619-0521-9*, 80666) Sage.

Assessing Interventions: Traditional & Innovative Methods. Fred Tudiver et al. Ed. by Moira A. Stewart. 1992. LC 92-19922. (Research Methods for Primary Care Ser.: Vol. 4). (Illus.). 260p. (C). 86.95 (*0-8039-4770-4*, 4781); pap. 37.95 (*0-8039-4771-2*, 4782) Sage.

Assessing Medical Technologies. Institute of Medicine Staff. 1985. 573p. text 49.95 (*0-309-03583-X*) Natl Acad Pr.

Assessing Object Relations Phenomena. Ed. by Morton Kissen. 1986. LC 86-10513. (Illus.). 400p. (C). 57.50 (*0-8236-0445-4*) Intl Univs Pr.

Assessing Organizational Readiness for Capitation. Ed. by Deborah M. Kolb. 1996. LC 96-4580. (Illus.). 90p. pap. 32.50 (*1-55648-154-3*, 131002) AHPI.

Assessing Outcome in Clinical Practice. Kevin S. Masters et al. 1996. LC 95-38901. 208p. (C). 56.00 (*0-205-19353-6*) Allyn.

Assessing Physical Fitness & Physical Activity in Population-Based Surveys 1994. lib. bdg. 600.75 (*0-8490-6432-5*); Set. 1995. lib. bdg. 602.99 (*0-8490-6729-4*) Gordon Pr.

Assessing Physically Disabled People at Home. Kathleen Maczka. Ed. by Jo Campling. 1992. (Therapy in Practice Ser.: No. 12). 128p. pap. 28.95 (*0-412-32480-6*, A4417) Chapman & Hall.

Assessing Problem Behaviors. MaryAnn Demchak & Karen W. Bossert. Ed. by Diane M. Browder. 1996. (Innovations Ser.). (Illus.). 44p. pap. 21.95 (*0-940898-39-X*) Am Assn Mental.

Assessing Psychological Trauma & PTSD. Ed. by John P. Wilson & Terence M. Keane. 1996. LC 96-30206. 577p. text 60.00 (*1-57230-162-7*, 0162) Guilford Pubns.

Assessing Psychopathology & Behavior Problems in Persons with Mental Retardation: A Review of Available Instruments. 1994. (Illus.). 239p. (Orig.). (C). pap. text 45.00 (*0-7881-0529-9*) DIANE Pub.

Assessing Quality of Life in Alzheimer's Disease. Steven M. Albert & Rebecca G. Logsdon. 2000. LC 99-88404. (Illus.). xiii, 191p. 41.95 (*0-8261-1333-8*) Springer Pub.

Assessing Risks to Health: Methodologic Approaches. Ed. by John C. Bailar, III et al. 1993. LC 88-6203. 344p. 72.50 (*0-86569-167-3*, T167, Auburn Hse) Greenwood.

Assessing Satisfaction in Health & Long-Term Care: Practical Approaches to Hearing the Voices of Consumers. Ed. by Robert A. Applebaum et al. 2000. LC 99-42882. (Illus.). 144p. pap. text 30.95 (*0-8261-1305-2*) Springer Pub.

Assessing Sexual Abuse: A Resource Guide for Practitioners. Ed. by Robert A. Prentky & Stacey B. Edmunds. 1997. 148p. (Orig.). pap. 25.00 (*1-884444-41-5*) Safer Soc.

Assessing Stress in Children. Louis A. Chandler. 1985. LC 85-12188. 240p. 55.00 (*0-275-90072-X*, C0072, Praeger Pubs) Greenwood.

Assessing the Economic Value of Anticancer Therapies. N. Neymark. 1998. LC 97-52408. (Recent Results in Cancer Research Ser.: Vol. 148). 296p. 109.00 (*3-540-64030-4*) Spr-Verlag.

Assessing the Handicaps & Needs of Mentally Retarded Children. Ed. by Brian Cooper. 1981. LC 81-66374. text 104.00 (*0-12-188020-6*) Acad Pr.

Assessing the Mentally Retarded. Ed. by Stephen Bruening & Johhny L. Matson. 1984. 480p. text 52.50 (*0-8089-1607-6*, 792809, Grune & Strat) Harcrt Hlth Sci Grp.

Assessing the Quality of Anthropometric Data: Background & Illustrated Guidelines for Survey Managers. Kees Kostermans. 1994. LC 93-47898. (Living Standards Measurement Study Papers: No. 101). (Illus.). 62p. pap. 22.00 (*0-8213-2755-0*, 12755) World Bank.

Assessing the Quality of Management Module 7: Facilitator's Guide. Mary Millar. 1993. (Primary Health Care Management Advancement Programme Modules Ser.). 47p. pap. text (*1-882839-13-7*) Aga Khan Fnd.

Assessing the Quality of Management Module 7: User's Guide. Lori D. Brown. 1993. (Primary Health Care Management Advancement Programme Modules Ser.). 90p. pap. text (*1-882839-05-6*) Aga Khan Fnd.

Assessing the Quality of Radioimmunoassay Systems: Approved Guideline, Vol. 5. National Committee for Clinical Laboratory Standards. 2nd ed. 1994. 75.00 (*1-56238-073-7*, LA1-A2) NCCLS.

Assessing the Quality of Services Module 6: Facilitator's Guide. Martine Hilton. 1993. (Primary Health Care Management Advancement Programme Modules Ser.). 45p. pap. text (*1-882839-12-9*) Aga Khan Fnd.

Assessing the Quality of Services Module 6: User's Guide. Lori D. Brown. 1993. (Primary Health Care Management Advancement Programme Modules Ser.). 190p. pap. text (*1-882839-04-8*) Aga Khan Fnd.

Assessing the Quality of Systems for Alpha-Fetoprotein (AFP) Assays Used in Prenatal Screening & Diagnosis of Neural Tube Defects: Approved Guideline (1997) 1997. 95.00 (*1-56238-322-1*, I/LA17-A) NCCLS.

Assessing the Quality of Systems for Alpha-Fetoprotein (AFP) Assays Used in Prenatal Screening & Diagnosis of Open Neural Tube Defects: Approved Guideline (1996) Contrib. by Robert F. Ritchie. 1996. 95.00 (*1-56238-202-0*, I/LA17-A) NCCLS.

Assessing the Skeletal Maturity of the Hand-Wrist: FELS Method. Alex F. Roche et al. 1988. (Illus.). 348p. (C). text 86.95 (*0-398-05452-5*) C C Thomas.

Assessing the Value of the Medical Practice: The Physician's Handbook for Measuring & Maximizing Practice Value. American Medical Association Staff. 1996. (Practice Success Ser.). pap. 54.00 (*0-89970-787-4*, OP315196WE) AMA.

Assessing the Youthful Offender: Issues & Techniques. Robert D. Hoge & D. A. Andrews. 1996. LC 96-39453. (Forensic Psychiatry & Psychology Library). (Illus.). 152p. (C). 42.00 (*0-306-45466-1*, Kluwer Plenum) Kluwer Academic.

Assessing Woman Battering in Mental Health Services. Edward W. Gondolf. 1997. LC 97-4882. 208p. 74.95 (*0-7619-1107-3*, 81643); pap. 34.95 (*0-7619-1108-1*, 81644) Sage.

Assessing Young Children with Special Needs: An Ecological Perspective. Susan M. Benner. 1992. 400p. (C). tchr. ed. (*0-8013-0489-X*, 78322) Longman.

Assessing Young Children's Development. Gayle Mindes. 1996. (C). pap. text, tchr. ed. 10.00 (*0-8273-6212-9*) Delmar.

Assessing Your Career Options. AMA Staff. 1998. (Career Development Ser.). 94p. 332.95 (*0-89970-887-0*) AMA.

Assessment Across Disorders: Perspectives, Practices & Procedures. Katharine G. Butler. 1993. LC 93-34702. (Topics in Language Disorders Ser.). 240p. pap. 44.00 (*0-8342-0593-9*) PRO-ED.

Assessment & Care Co-Ordination. NISW Staff. 1993. (*1-873153-13-9*) Natl Inst Soc Work GBR. *Dist:* St Mut.

Assessment & Care Fetus. Eden & Boehm. 2nd ed. 1999. pap. text 106.00 (*0-8385-0439-6*) Appleton & Lange.

Assessment & Care Management for Adults in Residential & Supported Accommodation: A Handbook for Care Manager & Social Care Staff. Philip Seed & Gillian Kaye. 1994. LC 93-41412. 200p. pap. 25.95 (*1-85302-227-6*) Taylor & Francis.

Assessment & Care of the Fetus: Physiological, Clinical & Medicolegal Principles. Robert D. Eden & Frank H. Boehm. 1992. (Illus.). 1043p. (C). pap. text 129.00 (*0-8385-0436-1*, A0436-4, Apple Lange Med) McGraw.

Assessment & Care of the Well Newborn. Patricia J. Thureen et al. Ed. by Maura Connor. 1998. LC 98-37948. (Illus.). 416p. (C). pap. text 39.00 (*0-7216-6142-4*) Saunders.

Assessment & Diagnosis of Personality Disorders: The International Personality Disorder Examination (IPDE) Ed. by Armand W. Loranger et al. 1997. LC 96-45992. (Illus.). 226p. (C). text 64.95 (*0-521-58043-9*) Cambridge U Pr.

Assessment & Evaluation Health: A Methods Text. Crispin Jenkinson. 1997. LC 97-2673. (Illus.). 208p. (*0-335-19706-X*); pap. (*0-335-19705-1*) OpUniv Pr.

Assessment & Intervention Issues across the Life Span. Ed. by Stephanie M. Dollinger & Lisabeth DiLalla. 1997. LC 96-27362. 320p. (C). text 79.95 (*0-8058-2164-3*) L Erlbaum Assocs.

Assessment & Protocols for Older Adults. Reynolds. 2000. (C). pap. text (*0-7216-6548-9*) Saunders.

Assessment & Remediation of Articulatory & Phonological Disorders. Nancy Creaghead et al. 2nd ed. 1990. 448p. (C). 93.00 (*0-675-20653-7*, Merrill Coll) P-H.

***Assessment & Therapy: Specialty Articles from the Encyclopedia of Mental Health.** Ed. by Howard S. Friedman. 2001. 392p. 99.95 (*0-12-267806-0*) Acad Pr.

Assessment & Treatment of Addictive Disorders. Ed. by Timothy B. Baker & Dale S. Cannon. 1988. LC 87-30537. 318p. 82.50 (*0-275-92388-6*, C2388, Praeger Pubs) Greenwood.

Assessment & Treatment of Adolescent Sex Offenders. Garry P. Perry & Janet Orchard. 1992. LC 92-14135. 160p. pap. 23.45 (*0-943158-75-3*, ATABP, Prof Resc Pr) Pro Resource.

Assessment & Treatment of Cancer Pain. Ed. by Richard Payne et al. 1998. LC 98-12346. (Progress in Pain Research & Management Ser.: Vol. 12). (Illus.). 331p. 71.00 (*0-931092-21-3*) Intl Assn Study Pain.

Assessment & Treatment of Childhood Problems: A Clinician's Guide. Carolyn S. Schroeder & Betty N. Gordon. 1991. LC 91-20201. 512p. 50.00 (*0-89862-565-3*) Guilford Pubns.

Assessment & Treatment of Depression in Children & Adolescents. Harvey F. Clarizio. 2nd ed. 1994. LC 89-90917. 250p. pap. 31.95 (*0-88422-103-2*) Clinical Psych.

Assessment & Treatment of Emotional or Behavioral Disorders. H. A. Ninness et al. 1993. LC 93-20502. 192p. 67.00 (*0-275-94098-5*, C4098, Praeger Pubs) Greenwood.

Assessment & Treatment of Multiple Personality & Dissociative Disorders. James P. Bloch. Ed. by Harold H. Smith, Jr. 1991. LC 91-52545. (Practitioner's Resource Ser.). 112p. pap. 17.95 (*0-943158-67-2*, ATMBP, Prof Resc Pr) Pro Resource.

Assessment & Treatment of Pancreatic Disease Vol. I, 1999: New Horizons & Aspects: Publication of the Educational Symposium Held During the 8th Meeting of the International Association of Pancreatology (IAP), Tokyo, Japan, July 1, 1998. Ed. by Katsusuke Satake et al. 1999. (Digestion Ser.: Vol. 60). (Illus.). iv, 140p. pap. 39.25 (*3-8055-6842-8*) S Karger.

Assessment & Treatment of Patients with Coexisting Mental Illness & Alcohol & Other Drug Abuse. Richard Ries. 1996. (Illus.). 114p. (C). reprint ed. pap. text 35.00 (*0-7881-3388-8*) DIANE Pub.

Assessment & Treatment of the Elderly Neuropsychiatric Patient, 4. Ed. by Gabe J. Maletta & Francis J. Pirozzolo. 1986. LC 86-9507. (Advances in Neurogerontology Ser.: Vol. 4). 291p. 68.50 (*0-275-92112-3*, C2112, Praeger Pubs) Greenwood.

Assessment, Evaluation, & Programming System for Infants & Children, Vol. 1: Measurement for Birth to Three Years. Ed. by Diane D. Bricker. 352p. (C). AEPS Child Progress Record, 02/1994, pkg. of 30. 1994. 18.00 (*1-55766-165-0*); Family Report, pkg. of 10. 1993. 17.00 (*1-55766-099-9*) P H Brookes.

Assessment for Decision, Vol. I. Ed. by Donald R. Peterson & Daniel B. Fishman. 1988. (Rutgers Symposia on Applied Psychology Ser.). 463p. (C). pap. text 20.00 (*0-8135-1247-6*) Rutgers U Pr.

Assessment for Reflexologists. Barbara Kunz & Kevin Kunz. 1999. (Illus.). 138p. pap. (*0-9606070-6-4*) Reflex Res Proj.

Assessment in Mental Handicap: A Guide to Assessment Practices, Tests & Checklists. Ed. by James Hogg & Norma V. Raynes. 1987. (Illus.). 289p. 19.95 (*0-914797-31-X*) Brookline Bks.

Assessment in Neuropsychology. Ed. by John R. Beech & Leonora Harding. 1996. LC 95-15757. (Assessment Library). 216p. (C). pap. 27.95 (*0-415-12953-2*) Routledge.

Assessment in Occupational Therapy & Physical Therapy. Julia Van Deusen & Denis Brunt. Ed. by Selma Kaszczuk. 1996. LC 96-6052. 432p. text 62.95 (*0-7216-4444-9*) Saunders.

Assessment in Speech-Language Pathology: A Resource Manual. Kenneth G. Shipley & Julie G. McAfee. 2nd ed. 1998. LC 97-42807. (Singular Textbook Ser.). (Illus.). 424p. spiral bd. 57.95 (*1-56593-870-4*) Thomson Learn.

Assessment Issues in Child Neuropsychology. M. G. Tramontana & S. R. Hooper. 1988. LC 88-22399. (Critical Issues in Neuropsychology Ser.). (Illus.). 408p. (C). 65.00 (*0-306-42898-9*, Plenum Trade) Perseus Pubng.

Assessment Made Incredibly Easy. Ed. by Patricia Schull. 1997. LC 97-7655. (Made Incredibly Easy Ser.). (Illus.). 328p. (Orig.). pap. 34.95 (*0-87434-888-9*) Springhouse Corp.

Assessment Manual for Medical Groups. Stephen J. Williams et al. 1995. 41.50 (*1-56829-008-X*) M G M A.

Assessment Measures in Medical School, Residency, & Practice: The Connections. Ed. by Joseph S. Gonnella et al. 1993. LC 93-35462. (Medical Education Ser.: Vol. 17). 240p. 37.95 (*0-8261-8350-6*) Springer Pub.

Assessment Methodology in Orthopaedics. A. Carr. Ed. by P. B. Pynsent et al. 1995. LC 96-37312. (Illus.). 273p. text (*0-7506-2214-8*) E A GBR. *Dist:* OUP.

Assessment Methods for Infants & Toddlers: Transdisciplinary Team Approaches. Doris Bergen. 1994. LC 94-12519. (Early Childhood Education Ser.). 336p. 52.00 (*0-8077-3380-6*); 490p. (C). pap. 25.95 (*0-8077-3379-2*) Tchrs Coll.

Assessment of Addictive Behaviors. Ed. by Dennis M. Donovan & G. Alan Marlatt. 1988. LC 87-19674. (Behavioral Assessment Ser.). 497p. 55.00 (*0-89862-144-5*) Guilford Pubns.

Assessment of Adolescent Alcohol & Drug Abuse. Ken C. Winters. 1994. 91p. 29.50 (*0-87424-291-6*, W-291) Western Psych.

Assessment of Adolescents with Special Needs: A Guide for Transition Planning. Margaret West. 1987. stu. ed. 50.00 (*0-295-96626-2*) U of Wash Pr.

Assessment of & Surgery for Impacted Third Molars: A Self-Instructional Guide, Bk. 6. James R. Hooley & Robert J. Whitacre. 3rd rev. ed. 1983. (Illus.). 104p. pap. 19.95 (*0-89939-061-7*) Stoma Pr.

Assessment of Antenatal & Obstetric Care Services in a Rural District of Nepal. Maureen D. Iang. 1999. xxi, 156p. (Medizin in Entwicklungslandern Ser.: Vol. 45). pap. 31.95 (*0-8204-4328-X*);Vol. 45. (Illus.). pap. 31.95 (*3-631-34718-9*) P Lang Pubng.

Assessment of Bilingual Aphasia. Michel Paradis & Gary Libben. 1990. 17.50 (*0-8058-0849-3*); 1990. 19.95 (*0-8058-0848-5*); 1987. 264p. text 45.00 (*0-89859-650-5*) L Erlbaum Assocs.

Assessment of Cell Proliferation in Clinical Practice. Ed. by P. A. Hall & Nicholas A. Wright. 1991. (Illus.). 210p. 118.00 (*0-387-19700-1*) Spr-Verlag.

Assessment of Child & Adolescent Personality. Ed. by Howard M. Knoff. 1986. LC 85-30585. 686p. 65.00 (*0-89862-668-4*) Guilford Pubns.

Assessment of Childhood Disorders. Ed. by Eric J. Mash & Leif G. Terdal. 3rd ed. 1997. LC 97-5159. 800p. text 75.00 (*1-57230-194-5*) Guilford Pubns.

Assessment of Children. Jerome M. Sattler. 3rd rev. ed. 1992. 1200p. (C). 58.00 (*0-9618209-2-6*) J M Sattler.

Assessment of Chronic Pain Patients with the MMPI-2. Laura S. Keller & James Neal Butcher. 1991. (MMPI-2 Monographs). (Illus.). 288p. (C). text 29.95 (*0-8166-1861-5*) U of Minn Pr.

Assessment of Cognitive Function in Epilepsy. W. Edwin Dodson et al. Ed. by Marcel Kinsbourne & Beat Hiltbrunner. 1991. 192p. 69.95 (*0-939957-45-0*) Demos Medical.

Assessment of Cognitive Processes: The PASS Theory of Intelligence. Jagannath P. Das et al. 1993. LC 93-13843. (Illus.). 256p. (C). 77.00 (*0-205-14164-1*, Longwood Div) Allyn.

Assessment of Diagnostic Technology in Health Care: Rationale, Methods, Problems, & Directions. Institute of Medicine Staff. 1989. 152p. pap. text 17.50 (*0-309-04099-X*) Natl Acad Pr.

Assessment of Early Child Development. Dorothy Flapan & Peter B. Neubauer. 1983. LC 84-450013. (Illus.). 184p. 20.00 (*0-87668-659-5*) Aronson.

Assessment of Eating Disorders: Obesity, Anorexia & Bulimia Nervosa. D. A. Williamson. Ed. by C. J. Davis et al. 1990. (Psychology Practitioner Guidebooks). 184p. text 32.50 (*0-08-036453-5*); pap. text 16.95 (*0-08-036452-7*) Elsevier (Pergamon Pr).

Assessment of Eating Disorders: Obesity, Anorexia, & Bulimia Nervosa. Donald A. Williamson. 1990. (Practitioner Guidebook Ser.). 216p. (C). pap. text 48.00 (*0-205-14507-8*, H4507, Longwood Div) Allyn.

Assessment of Fracture Risk & Its Application to Screening for Postmenopausal Osteoporosis: Report of a WHO Study Group. Ed. by World Health Organization Staff. 1994. LC 95-103031. (Technical Reports: No. 843). (CHI, ENG, FRE & SPA.). v, 129p. pap. text 22.00 (*92-4-120843-0*, 1100843) World Health.

Assessment of Future Scientific Needs for Live Variola Virus. Institute of Medicine Staff. 1999. LC 99-216014. (Illus.). xv, 108p. pap. 29.00 (*0-309-06441-4*) Natl Acad Pr.

Assessment of Health Care Technologies: Case Studies, Key Concepts, & Strategic Issues. Ed. by Ala Szczepura & Jari Kankaanpaa. 1996. LC 96-3533. 262p. 88.50 (*0-471-96571-5*) Wiley.

Assessment of Hearing Disability. King. 1992. 122p. pap. 47.75 (*1-56593-571-3*, 0317) Singular Publishing.

Assessment of Hormones & Drugs in Saliva in Biobehavioral Research. Ed. by C. Kirschbaum et al. 1993. (Illus.). 356p. 69.00 (*0-88937-050-8*) Hogrefe & Huber Pubs.

Assessment of Human Performance. Carrasco. 1998. (Standard Texts of Cosmetology Ser.). 39.95 (*0-8273-7522-0*) Delmar.

Assessment of Human Vertebral Strength: Relationships to Bone Mass & Trabecular Microstructure in Vitro. XiaoGuang Cheng. 1997. (Acta Biomedica Lovaniensia Ser.: Vol. 147). (Illus.). 154p. pap. (*90-6186-806-8*) Leuven Univ BEL. *Dist:* Coronet Bks.

Assessment of Hypertensive Organ Damage. Ed. by L. Hansson & William H. Birkenhager. 1997. (Handbooks of Hypertension: Vol. 18). 416p. 225.00 (*0-444-82217-8*) Elsevier.

Assessment of Immigration Status in Health Research. Sana Loue et al. 1999. LC 99-40419. (Vital Ser.). (*0-8406-0558-7*) Natl Ctr Health Stats.

Assessment of Individuals with Mental Retardation. Ed. by Ronald L. Taylor. 1997. LC 97-15243. (Illus.). 282p. (Orig.). pap. 39.95 (*1-56593-708-2*, 1396) Thomson Learn.

Assessment of Infants & Young Children. Libby G. Cohen & Loraine J. Spenciner. 1995. LC 92-35208. 528p. (C). tchr. ed. 24.00 (*0-8013-1248-5*, 79879) Longman.

Assessment of Intellectual Functioning. Lewis R. Aiken. 2nd ed. 1996. (Perspectives on Individual Differences Ser.). (Illus.). 424p. (C). 42.50 (*0-306-45152-2*, Kluwer Plenum) Kluwer Academic.

Assessment of Motor & Process Skills. Anne G. Fisher. 1995. pap. text 35.00 (*0-9645127-0-X*) Three Star Pr.

Assessment of Neuropsychological Functions in Psychiatric Disorders. Ed. by Avraham Calev. 1999. LC 98-29253. 608p. 74.95 (*0-88048-912-X*, 8912) Am Psychiatric.

Assessment of Nonorthopedic Sports Injuries: A Sideline Reference Manual. Jeff Lewandowski. 2000. LC 99-86957. (Illus.). 176p. pap. 24.00 (*1-55642-444-2*) SLACK Inc.

Assessment of Nutritional Status & Food Consumption Surveys: Proceedings of the European Nutritionists Group Symposium, 11th, Warsaw, April 1972. European Nutritionists Group Symposium Staff. Ed. by J. C. Somogyi. 1974. (Bibliotheca Nutritio et Dieta Ser.: No. 20). (Illus.). 224p. pap. 81.75 (*3-8055-1685-1*) S Karger.

Assessment of Object Relations Phenomena in Adolescents: TAT & Rorschach Measures. Francis D. Kelly. 1997. LC 96-38321. (Lea Series in Personality & Clinical Psychology Ser.). 272p. 34.50 (*0-8058-2235-6*) L Erlbaum Assocs.

Assessment of Oral health: Diagnostic Techniques & Validation Criteria. Ed. by R. V. Faller. 2000. LC 00-38432. (Monographs in Oral Science: Vol. 17). (Illus.). viii, 196p. 170.50 (*3-8055-7030-9*) S Karger.

Assessment of Personality & Behavior Problems: Infancy Through Adolescence. Roy P. Martin. LC 88-19030. 399p. 1988. 47.50 (*0-89862-727-3*); 1992. reprint ed. pap. 27.00 (*0-89862-026-0*) Guilford Pubns.

Assessment of Psychoses. T. R. Barnes. 1994. 256p. (gr. 13). 104.95 (*0-412-53590-4*) Chapman & Hall.

Assessment of Public Health & Social Problems Associated with the Use of Psychotropic Drugs. 1981. (Technical Report Ser.: No. 656). 54p. pap. text 4.00 (*92-4-120656-X*) World Health.

Assessment of Quality of Life & Childhood Asthma. Davina French & Margaret Christie. 1995. 209p. text 64.00 (*3-7186-5707-4*); pap. text 32.00 (*3-7186-5708-2*) Gordon & Breach (Harwood Acad Pubs).

Assessment of Reproductive & Tetragenic Hazards. Ed. by Myron A. Mehlman et al. 1983. LC 82-62165. (Advances in Modern Environmental Toxicology Ser.: Vol. 3). (Illus.). reprint ed. pap. text 58.00 (*0-911131-03-5*) Specialist Journals.

Assessment of Risk in the Term Newborn. Ed. by Susan Bakewell-Sachs et al. 1997. LC 97-8218. (*0-86525-074-X*) March of Dimes.

Assessment of Sexual Function: A Guide to Interviewing. Group for the Advancement of Psychiatry Staff. 1994. 100p. pap. 20.00 (*0-87668-128-3*) Aronson.

Assessment of Sexual Maturity Stages in Girls. American Academy of Pediatrics Staff. 1995. 15p. pap. 24.95 (*0-910761-95-7*) Am Acad Pediat.

***Assessment of Skeletal Maturity & Prediction of Adult Height (TW3) Method.** James M. Tanner et al. 2001. (Illus.). 125p. incl. cd-rom (*0-7020-2511-9*) W B Saunders GBR. *Dist:* Saunders.

Assessment of Stroke Outcome: Round Table. Ed. by J. M. Orgogozo & G. L. Lenzi. 1994. (Journal: Vol. 4, Suppl. 2, 1994). (Illus.). iv, 30p. pap. 15.00 (*3-8055-6064-8*) S Karger.

Assessment of Subjective Well-Being: The Subjective Well-Being Inventory (SUBI) R. Nagpal & H. Sell. 1993. (SEARO Regional Health Papers: No. 24). v, 37p. pap. text 6.30 (*92-9022-193-3*, 1580024) World Health.

Assessment of the Carcinogenicity & Mutagenicity of Chemicals: Proceedings of the WHO Scientific Group, Geneva, 1972. WHO Staff. 1974. (Technical Reports: No. 546). pap. text 4.00 (*92-4-120546-6*) World Health.

Assessment of the Clinical Accuracy of Laboratory Tests Using Receiver Operating Characteristic (ROC) Plots: Approval Guideline (1993) Contrib. by Mark H. Zweig. 1995. 75.00 (*1-56238-285-3*, GP10-A) NCCLS.

Assessment of the Human Stress Response. George S. Everly, Jr. & Steven A. Sobelman. 1987. LC 86-47604. (Stress in Modern Society Ser.: No. 4). 32.50 (*0-404-63254-8*) AMS Pr.

Assessment of the Lower Limb. Ed. by Linda M. Merriman & David R. Tollafield. 1995. LC 94-44955. text (*0-443-05030-9*) Church.

Assessment of the NIH Women's Health Initiative. Institute of Medicine Staff. Ed. by Susan Thaul & Dana Hoftra. 1993. LC 93-86833. 160p. (Orig.). pap. text 25.00 (*0-309-04989-X*) Natl Acad Pr.

Assessment of the Primary Health Care Needs of North & South Omaha. Genevieve Burch. 1981. 159p. (Orig.). pap. 10.50 (*1-55719-046-1*) U NE CPAR.

Assessment of the Use of Single Cytochrome P450 Enzymes in Drug Research. Ed. by M. R. Waterman & M. Hildebrand. 1994. LC 94-43228. (Ernst Schering Research Foundation Ser.: Vol. 13). (Illus.). 239p. 69.95 (*0-387-58343-2*) Spr-Verlag.

Assessment of Toxic Agents at the Workplace. Ed. by A. Berlin. 1983. 660p. text 376.50 (*0-89838-613-6*) Kluwer Academic.

Assessment of Tumor Response. B. W. Hancock. 1982. text 162.50 (*90-247-2712-X*) Kluwer Academic.

Assessment of Urinary Sediment by Electron Microscopy: Applications in Renal Disease. Anil K. Mandal. 1987. LC 87-14153. (Illus.). 284p. (C). text 90.00 (*0-306-42521-1*, Kluwer Plenum) Kluwer Academic.

Assessment of Ventricular Function. David H. Spodick. 1985. (Advances in Cardiology Ser.: Vol. 32). (Illus.). vi, 154p. 109.75 (*3-8055-3993-2*) S Karger.

Assessment of Young Children. Libby G. Cohen & Loraine J. Spenciner. 1994. LC 92-35208. 528p. (C). text 92.00 (*0-8013-0965-4*, 79247) Longman.

Assessment Strategies in Behavioral Medicine. Francis Keefe & James Blumental. 1982. 514p. text 55.00 (*0-8089-1442-1*, 792261, Grune & Strat) Harcrt Hlth Sci Grp.

Assessment Tool for the Roy Adaptation Model: Nursing Process Manual. Joan M. Seo-Cho. 1999. (Illus.). 88p. (C). pap. text 10.00 (*0-9669791-0-9*) Polaris Pub.

Assessment with Projective Techniques: A Concise Introduction. Albert I. Rabin. 1981. LC 80-26229. 352p. 46.95 (*0-8261-3550-1*) Springer Pub.

Assistant Bacteriologist. Jack Rudman. 1994. (Career Examination Ser.: C-25). pap. 27.95 (*0-8373-0025-8*) Nat Learn.

Assistant Director of Nursing Care. Jack Rudman. 1994. (Career Examination Ser.: C-2858). pap. 39.95 (*0-8373-2858-6*) Nat Learn.

Assistant Health Insurance Administrator. Jack Rudman. 1994. (Career Examination Ser.: C-358). pap. 34.95 (*0-8373-0358-3*) Nat Learn.

Assistant Hospital Administrator. Jack Rudman. 1994. (Career Examination Ser.: C-1107). pap. 34.95 (*0-8373-1107-1*) Nat Learn.

Assistant Microbiologist. Jack Rudman. 1994. (Career Examination Ser.: C-1811). pap. 29.95 (*0-8373-1811-4*) Nat Learn.

Assistant Public Health Engineer. Jack Rudman. 1994. (Career Examination Ser.: C-2232). pap. 29.95 (*0-8373-2232-4*) Nat Learn.

Assistant Radiologist. Jack Rudman. 1994. (Career Examination Ser.: C-1112). pap. 44.95 (*0-8373-1112-8*) Nat Learn.

Assisted Circulation, No. 3. Ed. by F. Unger. 1989. (Illus.). 621p. 256.00 (*0-387-50722-1*, 2642) Spr-Verlag.

Assisted Human Reproductive Technology. Ed. by E. S. Hafez. 1991. (Reproductive Health Technology Ser.). 248p. 132.00 (*1-56032-148-2*) Hemisp Pub.

Assisted Reproduction: Progress in Research & Practice. Robert W. Shaw. 1995. (Advances in Reproductive Endocrinology Ser.: Vol. 7). (Illus.). 156p. lib. bdg. 74.95 (*1-85070-679-4*, S1350, Parthenon Pbng) CRC Pr.

Assisted Reproductive Technologies. Ed. by Richard P. Marrs. 1993. LC 93-1410. (Illus.). 280p. 95.00 (*0-86542-203-6*) Blackwell Sci.

Assisted Reproductive Technology: What the Doctor Should Know. D. M. Saunders & L. J. Satchwell. 1995. (Illus.). 108p. lib. bdg. 27.95 (*1-85070-713-8*, Parthenon Pbng) CRC Pr.

Assisted Suicide - Legal, Medical, Ethical & Social Issues: Hearing Before the Committee on Commerce, U. S. House of Representatives. Ed. by Michael Bilirakis. 1998. 143p. (C). pap. text 30.00 (*0-7881-4971-7*) DIANE Pub.

Assisted Ventilation. J. Goldstone. 2nd ed. 1994. (Illus.). 124p. pap. (*0-7279-0843-X*) BMJ Pub GBR. *Dist:* AIDC.

Assisted Ventilation at Home: A Practical Guide. W. J. Kinnear. 1994. LC 93-33019. (Oxford Medical Publications). (Illus.). 110p. (C). text 37.95 (*0-19-262400-8*) OUP.

Assisted Ventilation of the Neonate. Jay P. Goldsmith & Edward H. Karotkin. Ed. by Judy Fletcher. 3rd ed. 1996. LC 95-20425. 512p. text 87.00 (*0-7216-5593-9*) Saunders.

Assisting in Long-Term Care. Barbara R. Hegner. 2nd ed. 1994. 454p. pap., stu. ed. 17.95 (*0-8273-5443-6*) Delmar.

Assisting in Long-Term Care. Barbara R. Hegner & Esther Caldwell. 2nd ed. 1994. 776p. pap., tchr. ed. 64.95 (*0-8273-5280-8*); 2nd ed. 1993. LC 92-22067. 688p. pap. 30.50 (*0-8273-5285-9*); 2nd ed. 1989. 776p. pap. text 10.95 (*0-8273-5258-1*); 3rd ed. 1997. 176p. text, tchr. ed. 19.95 (*0-8273-8260-X*); 3rd ed. 1997. 288p. text, wbk. ed. 18.95 (*0-8273-8261-8*) Delmar.

Assisting in Long-Term Care. Barbara R. Hegner et al. 3rd ed. 1997. LC 97-5158. (Illus.). 608p. (C). pap. text 48.95 (*0-8273-8259-6*) Delmar.

***Assisting in Long Term Care.** Barbara F. Hegner & Joan F. Needham. 4th ed. 2001. 704p. pap. 44.95 (*0-7668-3479-4*) Delmar.

Assisting in Long-Term Care. Barbara R. Hegner & Esther Caldwell. 4th ed. 1993. 776p. disk 49.95 (*0-8273-5476-2*) Delmar.

Assisting in Long Term Care - CTB. Barbara R. Hegner. 2nd ed. 1993. (Home Care Aide Ser.). 64.95 (*0-8273-5364-2*) Delmar.

***Assisting Survivors of Traumatic Brain Injury: The Role of Speech-Language Pathologists.** Karen Hux. 2002. LC 2001-48730. (*0-89079-895-8*) PRO-ED.

Assisting the Anaesthetist. N. S. Morton. 1997. (Illus.). 264p. text 79.50 (*0-19-262444-X*) OUP.

Assisting the Anaesthetist. Ed. by N. S. Morton. 1997. (Illus.). 264p. pap. text 39.95 (*0-19-262443-1*) OUP.

Assistive Devices for Persons with Hearing Impairment. Donald J. Schum. Ed. by Richard S. Tyler. 1994. LC 94-26290. 283p. (C). 78.00 (*0-205-15126-4*, Longwood Div) Allyn.

Assistive Products: An Illustrated Guide to Terminology. Gordon C. Krantz et al. 1998. (Illus.). 177p. pap. 37.00 (*1-56900-089-1*, 1130) Am Occup Therapy.

Assistive Technologies: Principles & Practice. Albert M. Cook et al. 1994. LC 94-30291. 736p. (C). (gr. 13). text 61.00 (*0-8016-1038-9*, 01038) Mosby Inc.

Assistive Technology: An Interdisciplinary Approach. Beverly K. Bain & Dawn Leger. 1997. LC 97-8215. pap. text (*0-443-07552-2*) Church.

Assistive Technology: Essential Human Factors. Thomas W. King. 1998. LC 98-8342. 305p. (C). pap. text 42.00 (*0-205-27326-2*) Allyn.

Assistive Technology & Occupational Therapy: A Link to Function, a Self-Study Course. Ed. by Joy Hammel. 1997. (Illus.). 600p. (Orig.). pap. 270.00 (*1-56900-039-5*, 3008A) Am Occup Therapy.

Assistive Technology for Persons with Disabilities: The Role of Occupational Therapy. William C. Mann & Joseph P. Lane. 2nd ed. 1995. 400p. (C). pap. text 58.00 (*1-56900-028-X*) Am Occup Therapy.

Assistive Technology for Rehabilitation Therapists. Jennifer Angelo et al. 1996. LC 96-19181. (Illus.). 254p. (C). pap. text 23.95 (*0-8036-0136-0*) Davis Co.

Assistive Technology in Traumatic Brain Injury Vocational Rehabilitation. C. Gerald Warren. Ed. by Robert Fraser & David Clemmons. 1991. LC 91-73659. (Traumatic Brain Injury Rehabilitation Training Ser.). 42p. spiral bd. 26.95 (*1-878205-07-2*) St Lucie Pr.

Associate Budget Analyst. Jack Rudman. 1994. (Career Examination Ser.: C-3172). pap. 39.95 (*0-8373-3172-2*) Nat Learn.

Associate Degree Nursing & the Nursing Home. 1988. 216p. pap. 22.95 (*0-88737-423-9*, 15-2241) Natl League Nurse.

Associate Degree Nursing Education: An Historical Annotated Bibliography, 1942-1988. Patricia T. Haase. 1990. LC 89-23713. 316p. (C). text 59.95 (*0-8223-0983-1*) Duke.

Associate Medical Examiner. Jack Rudman. 1994. (Career Examination Ser.: C-2722). pap. 44.95 (*0-8373-2722-9*) Nat Learn.

Associate Radiological Health Specialist. Jack Rudman. (Career Examination Ser.: C-3692). pap. 39.95 (*0-8373-3692-9*) Nat Learn.

Associated Systems Theory: A Systematic Approach to Cognitive Representations of Persons. Ed. by Robert S. Wyer, Jr. 1994. (Advances in Social Cognition Ser.). 256p. pap. 29.95 (*0-8058-1474-4*); text 55.00 (*0-8058-1473-6*) L Erlbaum Assocs.

Associateships: A Guide for Health Care Providers. Steven D. Chinn. 1995. LC 95-15484. 29.95 (*0-87814-446-3*) PennWell Corp.

***Associazione Urologi Italiani (AUROit) Selected Papers from the Congress.** Ed. by P. Puppo. 2001. (European Urology Ser.: Vol. 39, Suppl. 2). (Illus.). iv, 42p. 25.25 (*3-8055-7200-X*) S Karger.

Assumptions about Human Nature: A Social-Psychological Approach. Lawrence S. Wrightsman. 2nd ed. 1991. 368p. (C). 64.95 (*0-8039-2774-6*, 6622); pap. 32.95 (*0-8039-2775-4*, 6623) Sage.

Assumptions of Social Psychology: A Reexamination. Robert E. Lana. 1991. 160p. (C). pap. 19.95 (*0-8058-1023-4*); text 39.95 (*0-8058-1022-6*) L Erlbaum Assocs.

Assurance of Quality in Health Care. Best & Morey. 1994. (*0-08-042006-0*, Pergamon Pr) Elsevier.

Assyrian Medical Texts from the Originals in the British Museum. Ed. by Reginald C. Thompson. LC 78-72766. (Ancient Mesopotamian Texts & Studies). (Illus.). 120p. reprint ed. 47.50 (*0-404-18220-8*) AMS Pr.

Astha: Epidemiology, Anti-Inflammatory Therapy & Future Trends. Ed. by B. J. O'Connor & M. A. Giembycz. 2000. LC 99-57085. (Respiratory Pharmacology & Pharmacotherapy Ser.). 270p. 219.00 (*3-7643-5858-0*) Birkhauser.

Asthma Peter J. Barnes. 1997. LC 96-28935. 2,368p. text 299.00 (*0-397-51682-7*, Lippnctt) Lppncott W & W.

Asthma. Kristin Casler. 2000. 256p. pap. 5.99 (*0-380-73291-2*, HarpTorch) Morrow Avon.

Asthma. M. Eric Gershwin & E. L. Klingelhofer. 1986. pap. 10.53 (*0-201-11581-6*) Addison-Wesley.

Asthma. Kirk Hamilton. Ed. by Kristine Roberson et al. 1997. LC 99-176758. (Illus.). 67p. pap. 12.95 (*1-890302-02-3*) ITServices.

Asthma. Ed. by G. Jariwalla. 1988. (Practical Clinical Medicine Ser.). (C). pap. text 95.50 (*0-85200-672-1*) Kluwer Academic.

Asthma. Wendy B. Murphy. 1998. LC 97-52128. (Medical Library). (Illus.). 112p. (YA). (gr. 7-12). 24.90 (*0-7613-0364-2*) Millbrook Pr.

Asthma. Paul Thomas. 2001. (Questions & Answers Ser.). (Illus.). 100p. pap. 26.95 (*1-873413-90-4*) Merit Pub Intl.

Asthma. A. J. Wardlaw. 1993. (Medieval Mediterranean Ser.). (Illus.). 206p. (Orig.). pap. (*1-872748-26-0*) Bios Sci GBR. *Dist:* Coronet Bks.

Asthma. Ed. by T. J. H. Clark et al. 3rd ed. 1991. (Illus.). 640p. (C). (gr. 13). text 188.95 (*0-412-35900-6*) Chapman & Hall.

Asthma. Ed. by Tim Clark et al. 4th ed. 2000. LC 2001-268202. (Arnold Publication). (Illus.). viii, 476p. text 89.50 (*0-340-76123-7*) OUP.

Asthma. Ed. by Peter J. Barnes. 48th ed. 1993. (British Medical Bulletin Ser.: Vol. 48, 1). (Illus.). 320p. text (*0-443-04718-9*) Church.

Asthma: A Guide for Patients. Harold Nelson. Ed. by Archie Wilson. 1996. (Allergy Ser.). (Illus.). 32p. (Orig.). pap. 2.95 (*1-885274-34-3*) Health InfoNet Inc.

Asthma: A Link Between Environment, Immunology & the Airways. Ed. by Hugo E. Neffen et al. 1999. LC 99-65053. (Illus.). ix, 270p. 69.00 (*0-88937-220-9*) Hogrefe & Huber Pubs.

Asthma: An Epidemiological Overview. HMSO Staff. 1995. 61p. pap. (*0-11-321897-4*, HM18974) Statnry Office GBR. *Dist:* Bernan Associates, Balogh.

Asthma: Basic Mechanisms & Clinical Management. Ed. by Ian W. Rodger et al. 2nd ed. 1992. (Illus.). 782p. text 184.00 (*0-12-079026-2*) Acad Pr.

Asthma: Basic Mechanisms & Clinical Management. Ed. by Peter J. Barnes et al. 3rd ed. 1998. (Illus.). 864p. 150.00 (*0-12-079027-0*) Acad Pr.

Asthma: Current Studies in Therapy. Ed. by Vincent J. Fontana et al. 1978. 32.00 (*0-8422-7289-5*) Irvington.

Asthma: Immunopathology. 1996. (Illus.). 179p. text 43.95 (*3-211-82454-5*) Spr-Verlag.

Asthma: Immunopathology & Immunotherapy - Immunopathologie und Immunotherapie. Ed. by F. Kummer. 1996. (Illus.). 192p. 40.00 (*0-387-82454-5*) Spr-Verlag.

Asthma: Its Pathogenesis & Treatment. Peter J. Barnes et al. 1990. (Lung Biology in Health & Disease Ser.: Vol. 49). (Illus.). 808p. text 275.00 (*0-8247-8217-8*) Dekker.

Asthma: Materia Medica Relating to Asthma. 2000. LC 99-97767. 112p. pap. 6.95 (*1-929410-06-9*) dttm.

Asthma: Mechanisms & Protocols. Ed. by K. Fan Chung & Ian Adcock. 2000. LC 00-40930. (Methods in Molecular Medicine Ser.: Vol. 44). (Illus.). xi, 346p. 110.00 (*0-89603-626-X*) Humana.

Asthma: Practical & Easy-to-Follow Advice. Erika Harvey. 1998. LC 98-4680. (Your Child Ser.). 128p. pap. 9.95 (*1-86204-207-1*) Element MA.

Asthma: Questions You Have... Answers You Need. Kristin Casler. rev. ed. 1998. LC 98-20353. 192p. pap. 12.95 (*1-882606-42-6*) Peoples Med Soc.

***Asthma: Respiratory Symptoms, Atopy & Bronchial Hyperresponsiveness in Young Adults in Estonia & Sweden.** Rain Jogi. 2001. (Comprehensive Summaries of Uppsala Dissertations from the Faculty of Medicine Ser.: No. 1076). 56p. pap. (*91-554-5119-5*) Acta Univ SWE. *Dist:* Coronet Bks.

Asthma: Stop Suffering, Start Living. M. Eric Gershwin et al. 2nd ed. 1992. LC 92-15443. (Illus.). 240p. pap. 14.00 (*0-201-60847-2*) Addison-Wesley.

Asthma: Structural Body-Theophylline Today - Strukturelle Grundlagen - Theophyllin Heute. Friedrich Kummer. 1996. LC 95-18395. 43.95 (*3-211-82670-X*) Spr-Verlag.

Asthma: The Complete Guide for Sufferers & Careers. Deryk Williams et al. 1997. (Illus.). 192p. (Orig.). pap. text (*0-7499-1606-0*) Piatkus Bks GBR. *Dist:* London Brdge.

Asthma: The Complete Guide to Integrative Therapies. Jonathan Brostoff & Linda Gamlin. 2000. LC 00-40844. (Illus.). 512p. pap. 19.95 (*0-89281-932-4*, Heal Arts VT) Inner Tradit.

Asthma: The Facts. Donald J. Lane. 3rd ed. 1996. (Facts Ser.). (Illus.). 230p. pap. text 19.95 (*0-19-262151-3*) OUP.

Asthma: Theory, Treatment & Education. Louis-Philippe Boulet. 1998. (Illus.). 400p. text (*0-7735-1609-3*) McG-Queens Univ Pr CAN. *Dist:* CUP Services.

Asthma & Allergic Diseases: Physiology, Immunopharmacology & Treatment. Ed. by Gianni Marone et al. 1998. (Illus.). 439p. 95.00 (*0-12-473340-9*) Acad Pr.

Asthma & Allergies. Chris McLaughlin. 2000. (Illus.). 128p. pap. 16.95 (*1-56649-184-3*) Welcome Rain.

Asthma & Allergies: The Natural Way of Healing. Natural et al. 1995. LC 95-157963. (Natural Way of Healing Ser.). 400p. mass mkt. 5.99 (*0-440-21662-1*) Dell.

Asthma & Allergy: Advances in Understanding & Novel Therapeutic Approaches. Ed. by Wendy Hori. 1997. (Biomedical Library). pap. (*1-57936-028-9*) Drug & Market Dev.

Asthma & Chronic Obstructive Pulmonary Disease (COPD) Tim Peters. 1996. (Humanatomy Board Bks.). 10p. bds. 9.95 (*1-879874-49-0*) T Peters & Co.

Asthma & Emotion. Abraham Stern. 1980. 216p. 35.00 (*0-89876-002-X*) Gardner Pr.

Asthma & Hay Fever: Proven Drug-Free Methods to Combat the Causes. Leon Chaitow. 1990. 112p. pap. (*0-7225-1899-4*) Thorsons.

Asthma & Hayfever. Leon Chaitow. 1998. pap. (*0-7225-3591-0*) Thorsons GBR. *Dist:* Natl Bk Netwk.

Asthma & Immunological Diseases in Pregnancy & Early Infancy, Vol. 110. Michael Schwartz et al. 1997. LC 97-36791. (Lung Biology in Health & Disease Ser.). (Illus.). 1144p. text 275.00 (*0-8247-0095-3*) Dekker.

Asthma & Other Lung Disorders: The Physical & Mental Connections. Michael Schwartz. 1994. 62p. pap. 3.50 (*1-886722-02-1*) Maps Pub.

Asthma & Respiratory Infections. David P. Skoner. 2000. LC 00-50085. (Lung Biology in Health & Disease Ser.: Vol. 154). (Illus.). xv, 312p. text 150.00 (*0-8247-7710-7*) Dekker.

Asthma & Rhinitis. Stephen T. Holgate & W. Busse. 1994. (Illus.). 1520p. 250.00 (*0-86542-246-X*) Blackwell Sci.

Asthma & Rhinitis, Set. William W. Busse & Stephen T. Holgate. 2nd ed. 2000. LC 99-32708. (Illus.). 2176p. 399.95 (*0-632-04175-7*) Blackwell Sci.

Asthma As an Inflammatory Disease. Ed. by Paul M. O'Byrne. 1990. (Allergic Disease & Therapy Ser.: Vol. 2). (Illus.). 336p. text 175.00 (*0-8247-8220-8*) Dekker.

Asthma Breathe Again Naturally & Reclaim Your Life. Mimi Weisbord. 1997. LC 96-44531. 320p. pap. 14.95 (*0-312-14544-6*) St Martin.

Asthma Epidemic. John Mansfield. 1998. pap. 13.00 (*0-7225-3388-8*) General Distrib Services.

Asthma Epidemiology: Principles & Epidemiology. Neil Pearce et al. 1998. (Monographs in Epidemiology & Biostatistics). (Illus.). 288p. text 49.95 (*0-19-508016-5*) OUP.

***Asthma Free in 21 Days.** 2002. mass mkt. (*0-312-98141-4*) St Martin.

***Asthma Free in 21 Days: The Breakthroough Mindbody Healing Program.** Kathryn Shafer & Fran Greenfield. 2001. 246p. 22.00 (*0-7567-5133-0*) DIANE Pub.

Asthma Free in 21 Days: The Breakthrough Mind-Body Healing Program. Kathryn Shafer. 2000. LC 99-56136. (Illus.). 256p. 22.00 (*0-06-251597-7*) Harper SF.

Asthma in Children & Adolescents: Pediatrician Journal, Vol. 18, No. 4. Ed. by David W. Kaplan & E. F. Ellis. 1992. (Illus.). iv, 80p. pap. 51.50 (*3-8055-5523-7*) S Karger.

Asthma in Control. 1995. (*0-941549-11-9*) Creative Hlth.

***Asthma in History.** S. Cohen. 2001. ring bd. 89.95 (*1-84214-105-8*, Parthenon Pbng) CRC Pr.

Asthma in the Elderly. Robert A. Barbee & John W. Bloom. 1997. LC 97-22376. (Lung Biology in Health & Disease Ser.: Vol. 108). (Illus.). 312p. text 165.00 (*0-8247-9870-8*) Dekker.

Asthma in the Elderly: Considerations for Diagnosing & Managing Asthma in the Elderly. Claude Lenfant et al. 1997. (Illus.). 50p. (C). reprint ed. pap. text 25.00 (*0-7881-4229-1*) DIANE Pub.

Asthma in the Workplace. I. Leonard Bernstein et al. 1993. (Illus.). 688p. text 230.00 (*0-8247-8799-4*) Dekker.

Asthma in the Workplace. I. Leonard Bernstein. 2nd exp. rev. ed. 1999. LC 99-29230. (Illus.). xix, 742p. text 250.00 (*0-8247-1963-8*) Dekker.

Asthma Management: Clinical Pathways, Guidelines, & Patient Education. Health & Administration Development Group Aspen Publishers Staff. Ed. by Jo Gulledge & Shawn Beard. 1995. LC 99-31841. (Chronic Disease Management Ser.). 229p. pap. 76.00 (*0-8342-1705-8*) Aspen Pub.

Asthma Management for the New Millennium. 216p. pap. text (*0-86471-058-5*) Adis Intl NZL. *Dist:* Lppncott W & W.

Asthma Management in Minority Children: Practical Insights for Clinicians, Researchers & Public Health Planners. Ed. by Cynthia L. Arfken & David Evans. 1997. (Illus.). 60p. (C). reprint ed. pap. text 20.00 (*0-7881-4594-0*) DIANE Pub.

Asthma Prevention Management Guidelines: 1998, Japan (JGL 1998) Ed. by S. Makino et al. 2000. (International Archives of Allergy & Immunology Ser.: Vol. 121, Suppl. 1). (Illus.). viii, 78p. pap. 34.00 (*3-8055-7074-0*) S Karger.

Asthma Self-Care Book: How to Take Control of Your Asthma. G. Harrington. 1999. LC 99-211990. 368p. mass mkt. 6.50 (*0-06-109796-9*) HarperCollins Pubs.

Asthma Self-Help Book: A Comprehensive Guide to Management of Asthma in Children & Adults. Paul J. Hannaway. Ed. by Nancy Savles. 1991. LC 89-80071. (Illus.). 265p. (C). reprint ed. text 18.95 (*0-9621799-0-6*) Lighthse MA.

Asthma Self-Help Book: How to Live a Normal Life in Spite of Your Condition. Paul J. Hannaway. 2nd rev. ed. 1992. LC 91-40762. (Illus.). 250p. 19.95 (*1-55958-166-2*) Prima Pub.

Asthma Sourcebook. Francis V. Adams. 2nd rev. ed. 1998. LC 98-231451. (Illus.). 256p. pap. 17.00 (*0-7373-0016-7*, 00167W) NTC Contemp Pub Co.

Asthma Sourcebook: Basic Consumer Health Information about Asthma. Ed. by Annemarie S. Muth. 2000. LC 00-63716. (Health Reference Ser.). (Illus.). xiii, 627p. lib. bdg. 78.00 (*0-7808-0381-7*) Omnigraphics Inc.

Asthma Sourcebook: Everything You Need to Know. Francis V. Adams. 1996. (Illus.). 224p. pap. 16.00 (*1-56565-471-4*) Lowell Hse.

***Asthma Survival: The Holistic Medical Treatment for Asthma.** Robert S. Ivker & Todd H. Nelson. 2001. LC 2001-33210. (Illus.). 338p. pap. 14.95 (*1-58542-124-3*, Tarcher Putnam) Putnam Pub Group.

Asthma Treatment: A Multidisciplinary Approach. D. Olivieri et al. 1992. (NATO Advanced Science Institutes Ser.: Vol. 299). (Illus.). 306p. (C). text 105.00 (*0-306-44215-9*, Kluwer Plenum) Kluwer Academic.

Asthma Treatment Guide: Step-by-Step Instructions on Asthma Management. Elizabeth M. Lykins. Ed. by Gurline J. Baptiste. 1999. (Illus.). 51p. pap. 11.95 (*0-9701963-2-6*) B L Enter.

Asthma's Impact on Society: The Social & Economic Burden. Ed. by Kevin B. Weiss. 1999. LC 99-51987. (Lung Biology in Health & Disease Ser.: Vol. 138). (Illus.). 416p. text 125.00 (*0-8247-1942-5*) Dekker.

ASTM Standards on Electronic Data Interchange. American Society for Testing and Materials, Committee E-31 on Computerized Systems. 1995. LC 95-18101. 100p. pap. 51.00 (*0-8031-1808-2*, ELECDATA) ASTM.

ASTM Standards on Emergency Medical Services. Contrib. by American Society for Testing and Materials Staff. 2nd ed. 1998. LC 98-45636. 404p. pap. 49.00 (*0-8031-2593-3*) ASTM.

Aston Postural Assessment: Skills for Observing & Evaluating Body Patterns. Judith Aston. 1999. (Illus.). 208p. wbk. ed. 52.00 (*0-12-784593-3*) Acad Pr.

Astral Medicine: A Practical Treatise & Therapeutics Combining Astrology, Diet & Homeopathic Medicine. M. D. Duz. 1991. lib. bdg. 67.95 (*0-8490-4305-0*) Gordon Pr.

Astrocytes in Brain Aging & Neurodegeneration. Hyman M. Schipper. 1997. (Neuroscience Intelligence Unit Ser.). 200p. pap. 89.95 (*0-412-14181-7*) Thomson Learn.

Astrocytes in Brain Aging & Neurodegeneration. M. Hyman Schipper. 1998. LC 98-26335. 256p. 99.00 (*1-57059-489-9*) Landes Bioscience.

Astrocytes in Infectious & Immune-Related Diseases of the CNS. Lennart Mucke. 1997. (Neuroscience Intelligence Unit Ser.). 250p. 89.95 (*0-412-13451-9*) Chapman & Hall.

Astrocytomas: Diagnosis, Treatment, & Biology. Ed. by Peter Black et al. 1993. LC 92-10543. (Contemporary Issues in Neurological Surgery Ser.). (Illus.). 320p. 95.00 (*0-86542-217-6*) Blackwell Sci.

Astrologer's Handbook. Julia Parker. 1995. (Illus.). 256p. (Orig.). pap. 12.00 (*0-916360-59-8*) CRCS Pubns CA.

Astrology & Health: A Beginner's Guide. Dylan Warren-Davis. 1998. (Illus.). 96p. mass mkt. (*0-340-70518-3*) Hodder & Stought Ltd GBR. *Dist:* Lubrecht & Cramer, Trafalgar.

Asylum: The History of Friends Hospital & the Quaker Contribution to Psychiatry. Carol B. Perloff. 1994. LC 94-72152. (Illus.). 55p. (*0-9642252-0-4*) Frnds Hosp.

Asylum History: Buckinghamshire County Pauper Lunatic Asylum - St. John's. Ed. by John L. Crammer. 1990. 195p. pap. text (*0-902241-34-6*) Royal Coll Psych GBR. *Dist:* Parkwest Pubns, Balogh.

Asylum in the Community. Ed. by John Carrier & Dyland Tomlinson. 1996. LC 95-25158. 240p. (C). 80.00 (*0-415-10742-3*); pap. 29.95 (*0-415-10743-1*) Routledge.

Asylums: Essays on the Social Situation of Mental Patients & Other Inmates. Erving Goffman. 1961. LC 61-13812. 400p. pap. 13.95 (*0-385-00016-2*) Doubleday.

Asylums & After: A New History of the Mental Health Services. Kathleen Jones. rev. ed. 1993. LC 93-31413. 280p. (C). pap. (*0-485-12091-7*) Athlone Pr GBR. *Dist:* Transaction Pubs, Humanities.

Asymptotic Statistics: Proceedings of the Fifth Prague Symposium, Held from September 4-9, 1993. Ed. by P. Mandl & M. Huskova. 1994. (Contributions to Statistics Ser.). x, 474p. 93.95 (*0-387-91488-9*) Spr-Verlag.

Asyst 88 International Conference Proceedings: Connecting Users & Applications. Intro. by Kirsten Bartles. 1989. (Illus.). 300p. (Orig.). pap. 25.00 (*0-924729-00-7*) Keithley Instruments.

At-a-Glance Nutrition Counter. Patricia Hausman. 1984. 256p. mass mkt. 4.95 (*0-345-90191-6*) Ballantine Pub Grp.

At Home with Autism: Three Families' Stories. Danielle Morse et al. 1997. 40p. pap. 5.95 (*0-9650700-3-4*, PUP Bks) Potential Unltd.

At Home with Terminal Illness. Michael Appleton et al. 1994. LC 94-9604. 103p. pap. text 20.80 (*0-13-299843-2*) P-H.

At Odds with AIDS: Thinking & Talking about a Virus. Alexander G. Duttmann. Tr. by Peter Gilgen & Conrad Scott-Curtis from GER. 1996. LC 96-14817. (Meridian: Crossing Aesthetics Ser.). xv, 144p. 51.00 (*0-8047-2437-7*); 144p. pap. 15.95 (*0-8047-2438-5*) Stanford U Pr.

At Risk. Carlos Morton. 1997. LC 97-13870. (Carlos Morton Collection). 16p. (YA). (gr. 8-12). pap. 5.00 (*0-88734-442-9*) Players Pr.

At Risk: Can the Doctor Patient Relationship Survive in the High Tech World. Robert Charman. 1992. (Orig.). pap. 10.95 (*0-87233-094-X*) Bauhan.

At Risk in America: The Health & Health Care Needs of Vulnerable Populations in the United States. Lu Ann Aday. 2nd ed. 2001. LC 00-48758. (Jossey-Bass Health Ser.). 400p. 48.00 (*0-7879-4986-8*) Jossey-Bass.

At Risk Student in Our Schools: A Model Intervention Program for the At Risk Student's Most Common Learning & Behavior Problems. Stephen B. McCarney. 1994. 504p. pap. 36.00 (*1-878372-03-3*) Hawthorne Educ Servs.

At the Bedside: Innovations in Hospital Nursing. David A. Gould & Mathy D. Mezey. 1991. (Papers: No. 19). 32p. 10.00 (*0-934459-68-1*) United Hosp Fund.

At the Bench: A Laboratory Navigator. Kathy Barker. 1998. LC 98-15662. 49.00 (*0-87969-523-4*) Cold Spring Harbor.

At the Desert's Green Edge: An Ethnobotany of the Gila River Pima. Amadeo M. Rea. 1997. LC 97-4577. 480p. text 60.00 (*0-8165-1540-9*) U of Ariz Pr.

At the Edge of Development: Health Crises in a Transitional Society. Ed. by Richard L. Guerrant et al. 1996. LC 94-73847. (Illus.). 472p. 65.00 (*0-89089-788-3*) Carolina Acad Pr.

At the Extremity of Civilization: A Meticulously Descriptive Diary of an Illinois Physician's Journey in 1849 along the Oregon Trail to the Goldmines & Cholera of California, Thence in Two Years to Return by Boat Via Panama. Israel S. Lord. Ed. by Necia D. Liles. 1995. (Illus.). 451p. lib. bdg. 45.00 (*0-7864-0000-5*) McFarland & Co.

***At the Front Lines of Medicine: How the Health Care System Alienates Doctors & Mistreats Patients... And What We Can Do about It.** Howard Waitzkin. 2001. LC 2001-19739. (Illus.). 256p. 26.95 (*0-7425-0131-0*) Rowman.

At the Threshold: The Developing Adolescent. S. Shirley Feldman & Glen R. Elliott. 1990. LC 90-33784. (Illus.). 640p. 54.00 (*0-674-05035-5*) HUP.

At War Within: The Double-Edged Sword of Immunity. William R. Clark. 1997. (Illus.). 288p. pap. 13.95 (*0-19-511568-6*) OUP.

At Your Own Risk: A Saint's Testament. Derek Jarman. 1994. LC 92-24387. (Illus.). 144p. pap. 10.95 (*0-87951-538-4*) Overlook Pr.

Atals of Vascular Anatomy: An Angiographic Approach. Ranan Uflacker. 1996. LC 96-32248. 811p. text 225.00 (*0-683-18110-6*) Lppncott W & W.

Ataxia-Telangiectasia. Richard A. Gatti & Robert B. Painter. 1993. (NATO ASI Ser.: Vol. 77). (Illus.). 283p. (*3-540-56792-5*) Spr-Verlag.

Ataxia-Telangiectsia. Ed. by Richard A. Gatti & Robert B. Painter. 1993. LC 93-20625. (NATO ASI Ser.: Vol. 77). 283p. 159.00 (*0-387-56792-5*) Spr-Verlag.

ATCC Animal Viruses & Antisera, Chlamydiae, & Rickettsiae. Ed. by C. Buck et al. 7th ed. 1996. 256p. pap. text (*0-930009-58-4*) ATCC.

ATCC Bacteria & Bacteriophages. Ed. by P. Pienta et al. 19th ed. 1996. 804p. pap. text (*0-930009-59-2*) ATCC.

Atencao Pos - Aborto: Um Manual de Referencia para a Melhorar a Qualidade du Atencao. Ed. by Judith Winkler et al. 1996. (POR., Illus.). (Orig.). pap. text 15.00 (*0-929817-33-8*) JHPIEGO.

Atencion de las Enfermedades Prostaticas. Robert E. Weiss & William R. Fair. 2nd rev. ed. 1998.Tr. of Management of Prostate Diseases. (SPA.). 155p. per. 19.95 (*1-884735-34-7*) Prof Comms.

Atencion Posaborto: Manuel de Referencia par Mejorar la Calidad de la Atencion. Ed. by Judith Winkler et al. 1996. (SPA., Illus.). (Orig.). pap. text 15.00 (*0-929817-34-6*) JHPIEGO.

Atencion Primaria en Pediatria. Hoekelman. 3rd ed. 1998. (SPA.). (C). text 134.83 (*84-8174-316-X*) Harcourt.

Athabaskan Languages: Perspectives on a Native American Language Family. Ed. by Theodore B. Fernald & Paul Platero. 2000. LC 98-36532. (Oxford Studies in Anthropological Linguistics: No. 24). 344p. text 55.00 (*0-19-511947-9*) OUP.

Atherogenesis: Morphology, Metabolism & Function of the Arterial Wall, Proceedings of the 1st International Atherosclerosis Conference, Vienna, April 1977. International Atherosclerosis Conference Staff. Ed. by W. Auerswald et al. 1977. (Progress in Biochemical Pharmacology Ser.: Vol. 13). (Illus.). 103.50 (*3-8055-2761-6*) S Karger.

Atherogenesis & Aging. Ed. by S. R. Bates & E. Gangloff. 1987. (Illus.). 213p. 155.00 (*0-387-96393-6*) Spr-Verlag.

Atherosclerosis. I. V. Likar & R. W. Robinson. 1986. (Monographs on Atherosclerosis: Vol. 12). (Illus.). viii, 176p. 118.50 (*3-8055-4069-8*) S Karger.

Atherosclerosis: A Pediatric Perspective. Ed. by M. T. Subbiah. 1989. 304p. 164.00 (*0-8493-4773-4*, RJ426, CRC Reprint) Franklin.

Atherosclerosis: Cellular & Molecular Interactions in the Artery Wall. Ed. by Sergey Federoff et al. 1991. (Altschul Symposia Ser.: Vol. 1). (Illus.). 288p. (C). text 126.00 (*0-306-43923-9*, Kluwer Plenum) Kluwer Academic.

Atherosclerosis: Experimental Methods & Protocols. Ed. by Angela F. Drew. 2000. LC 00-38924. (Methods in Molecular Medicine Ser.: Vol. 52). (Illus.). 256p. 89.50 (*0-89603-751-7*) Humana.

Atherosclerosis: Gene Expresion, Cell Interactions, & Oxidation. Ed. by Roger Dean & David Kelly. 2000. (Illus.). 464p. text 130.00 (*0-19-850637-6*) OUP.

Atherosclerosis: Path Vascul Li. Jeffrey M. Isner. 1999. (C). text (*0-7020-1927-5*) Bailliere Tindall.

Atherosclerosis & Arteriosclerosis: Human Pathology & Experimental Animal Methods & Models. Ed. by Rodney A. White. 1989. 336p. 249.00 (*0-8493-6357-8*, RC692) CRC Pr.

Atherosclerosis & Atherectomy: Index of New Information & Medical Research Bible. Julius M. Hightower. 1994. 160p. 57.50 (*0-7883-0126-8*); pap. text 47.50 (*0-7883-0127-6*) ABBE Pubs Assn.

***Atherosclerosis & Autoimmununity.** Ed. by Yehuda Shoenfeld et al. 2001. LC 2001-18982. (Illus.). 396p. 113.50 (*0-444-50669-1*) Elsevier.

Atherosclerosis & Cardiovascular Disease. Ed. by S. Lenzi & G. C. Descovich. 1987. (C). text 288.00 (*0-85200-836-8*); 1984. text 225.00 (*0-85200-793-0*) Kluwer Academic.

Atherosclerosis & Cardiovascular Disease: 7th International Meeting. Ed. by G. C. Descovitch. 1990. (C). text 294.00 (*0-7923-8949-2*) Kluwer Academic.

Atherosclerosis & Thrombosis. A. Myasnikov. 1967. (Illus.). 229p. 25.00 (*0-8464-1078-8*) Beekman Pubs.

Atherosclerosis XI: Proceedings of the XXth International Symposium on Atherosclerosis, Held in Paris, France, on 5-9 October, 1997. B. Al Jacotot et al. 1998. LC 98-18211. 1228p. 262.50 (*0-444-82651-3*) Elsevier.

Atherosclerosis V: The 5th Saratoga International Conference. Fujio Numano et al. 2000. LC 00-36154. (Annals of the New York Academy of Sciences Ser.: Vol. 902). (Illus.). xv, 379p. (*1-57331-247-9*) NY Acad Sci.

Atherosclerosis V Vol. 902: The 5th Saratoga International Conference. Ed. by Fujio Numano & Michael A. Gimbrone, Jr. 2000. LC 00-36154. (Annals of the New York Academy of Sciences Ser.: Vol. 902). (Illus.). xv, 379p. 140.00 (*1-57331-246-0*) NY Acad Sci.

Atherosclerosis IV Vol. 811: Recent Advances in Atherosclerosis Research. Ed. by Fujio Numano & Russell Ross. 1997. LC 97-10469. 550p. 160.00 (*1-57331-022-0*) NY Acad Sci.

Atherosclerosis in Primates. Ed. by J. P. Strong. 1975. (Primates in Medicine Ser.: Vol. 9). (Illus.). 149.75 (*3-8055-2195-2*) S Karger.

Atherosclerosis IV: Recent Advances in Atherosclerosis Research. Numano, Fujio National Conference on Atheroscleros & Russell Ross. 1997. LC 97-10469. (Annals of the New York Academy of Sciences Ser.). pap. 160.00 (*1-57331-023-9*) NY Acad Sci.

Atherosclerosis Prevention: Identification & Treatment of the Child with High Cholesterol, Vol. 4. Ed. by Marc S. Jacobson. 1991. (Monographs in Clinical Pediatrics). xi, 164p. text 107.00 (*3-7186-5121-1*, Harwood Acad Pubs) Gordon & Breach.

Atherosclerosis X: Proceedings of the 10th International Symposium on Atherosclerosis, Montreal, October 9-14, 1994. Ed. by J. Davignon et al. 1995. LC 95-12158. (International Congress Ser.: No. 1066). 1106p. 357.00 (*0-444-82007-8*, Excerpta Medica) Elsevier.

Atherosclerosis III: Recent Advances in Atherosclerosis Research. Saratoga International Conference on Atheroscleros. Ed. by Robert W. Wissler & Fujio Numano. 1995. LC 94-46619. (Annals Ser.: Vol. 748). pap. 175.00 (*0-89766-812-X*) NY Acad Sci.

Atherosclerosis V: Proceedings of the Fifth International Symposium. Ed. by Antonio M. Gotto, Jr. et al. 1980. (Illus.). 843p. 200.00 (*0-387-90473-5*) Spr-Verlag.

Atherosclerosis VI: Proceedings. Ed. by F. Gotthard Schettler et al. 1982. (Illus.). 982p. 85.95 (*0-387-11450-5*) Spr-Verlag.

Atherosclerotic Plaques: Advances in Imaging for Sequential Quantitative Evaluation. R. W. Wissler et al. 1992. (ATO ASI Ser.: Vol. 219). (Illus.). 326p. (C). text 110.00 (*0-306-44083-0*, Kluwer Plenum) Kluwer Academic.

Athlete & Heart Disease: Diagnosis, Evaluation & Management. Richard A. Williams. 1998. LC 98-28127. (Illus.). 352p. pap. text 92.00 (*0-316-88001-9*) Lppncott W & W.

Athlete in You: A Sportsmedicine Self-Care Guide. William F. Bennett. 1997. LC 96-69341. 200p. (Orig.). pap. 12.95 (*0-9647700-3-2*) Capital Com Inc.

Athletes & Drugs: A No-Win Combination. Community Intervention, Inc. Staff. 1986. 36p. (Orig.). pap. 3.95 (*0-9613416-2-9*, 102P) Comm Intervention.

Athletes at Risk. Tricker. 1992. 15.00 net. (*0-697-20933-4*, WCB McGr Hill) McGrw-H Hghr Educ.

Athlete's Shoulder. Ed. by James R. Andrews & Kevin E. Wilk. 1993. (Illus.). 600p. text (*0-443-08847-0*) Church.

Athletic Ability & the Anatomy of Motion. Rolf Wirhed. 1988. text 22.95 (*0-7234-1540-4*) CRC Pr.

Athletic Drug Reference '94. Ed. by Robert J. Fuentes et al. rev. ed. 1994. (C). pap. 9.95 (*1-881011-00-3*) Clean Data.

Athletic Drug Reference '96. Ed. by Robert J. Fuentes et al. 1996. 400p. (Orig.). pap. 14.95 (*1-881011-07-0*) Clean Data.

Athletic Horse: Principles & Practice of Equine Sports Medicine. David R. Hodgson & Reuben J. Rose. 1994. LC 94-7652. (Illus.). 512p. text 99.00 (*0-7216-3759-0*) Saunders.

Athletic Injuries & Rehabilitation. David J. Magee et al. Ed. by Margaret Biblis. 1996. LC 95-23428. (Illus.). 992p. text 99.00 (*0-7216-4946-7*) Saunders.

Athletic Injuries of the Foot & Ankle. Ed. by Anunziato Amendola. Date not set. 432p. text 70.00 (*0-07-001219-9*) McGraw-Hill Med Pub.

***Athletic Injury Assessment with References.** James M. Booher & Gary A. Thibodeau. 4th ed. 1999. 67.50 (*0-07-239368-8*) McGrw-H Hghr Educ.

Athletic Injury Care: And Sports Conditioning. Gary Shankman. 1992. pap. 13.95 (*0-9630564-0-9*) Sports Hlth.

Athletic Protective Equipment: Care, Selection & Fitting. Scott A. Street & Debra Runkle. 1999. LC 99-18620. (Illus.). 320p. (C). pap. text 36.88 (*0-8151-8533-2*) McGrw-H Hghr Educ.

Athletic Taping: Canadian Version. Sports Medicine Council of British Columbia Staff. 1995. (Illus.). 128p. (C). pap. text 38.95 (*0-8036-0116-6*) Davis Co.

Athletic Taping & Bracing. David H. Perrin. 1995. LC 95-1519. 136p. spiral bd. 44.95 (*0-87322-502-3*, BPER0502) Human Kinetics.

Athletic Training: A Study & Laboratory. Daniel D. Arnheim. 2nd ed. 2000. (C). (gr. 13). text 13.12 (*0-8016-0331-5*, 00331) Mosby Inc.

Athletic Training & Sports Medicine. Ed. by Letha Y. Hunter-Griffin. 2nd ed. 1991. LC 91-70295. 1027p. 59.00 (*0-89203-044-5*) Amer Acad Ortho Surg.

Athletic Training & Sports Medicine. Ed. by Robert C. Schenck. 3rd ed. 2000. (Illus.). 925p. 95.00 (*0-89203-172-7*) Amer Acad Ortho Surg.

Athletic Training & Sports Medicine Instructor's Manual. Ed. by Letha Y. Hunter-Griffin. 1992. 515p. tchr. ed. 19.95 (*0-89203-067-4*) Amer Acad Ortho Surg.

Athletic Training Student Guide to Success. Lynn Van Ost & Karen Manfre. 2000. LC 00-30069. (Illus.). 240p. pap. 24.00 (*1-55642-379-9*, 43799) SLACK Inc.

Atkinson Morley's Hospital, 1869-1995. Terry Gould. 1996. LC 96-21899. x, 116p. (C). pap. 15.00 (*0-485-12125-5*); text 29.95 (*0-485-11505-0*) Brill Academic Pubs.

Atlas: The Biomechanics of the Normal & Diseased Hip. F. Pauwels. Tr. by R. J. Furlong & P. Maguet from GER. 1976. LC 75-31723. (Illus.). 276p. 287.00 (*0-387-07428-7*) Spr-Verlag.

Atlas & Dissection Guide for Comparative Anatomy. Saul Wischnitzer. 5th ed. 1993. LC 92-30800. (Illus.). 320p. (C). pap. text 37.95 (*0-7167-2374-3*) W H Freeman.

Atlas & Sourcebook of the Lesser Bushbaby, Galago Senegalensis. Haines Edgerton & James L. Stevens. 1982. 320p. 170.00 (*0-8493-6320-9*, QL737, CRC Reprint) Franklin.

Atlas & Textbook of Diagnostic Ultrasonography of the Dog & Cat. Cordula Poulsen Nautrup & Ralf Tobias. Ed. by Robert E. Cartee. 1999. (Illus.). 400p. (C). pap. text 149.00 (*1-884254-49-7*) Vet Lrn Syst.

Atlas & Textbook of Malignant Lymphomas: Cytology, Histopathology & Immunocytochemistry. P. Van Heerde. 1996. (Illus.). 288p. text 175.00 (*0-19-521269-X*) OUP.

Atlas Casebook of Primary Care. Ian Williams & Vivienne Ankrett. 1999. (Illus.). 68p. pap. text 24.95 (*1-873413-56-4*, 8291) Merit Pub Intl.

Atlas Clinical Ophthalmology 2. David J. Spalton. 2nd ed. 1993. (gr. 13). (*0-397-44632-2*) Gower-Mosby.

Atlas Clinical Anesthesia. Miller. 1999. text (*0-443-07907-2*) Church.

Atlas Cutaneous Manifestations. Tyring. 1997. text (*0-7216-4947-5*) Saunders.

Atlas de Anatomia. Victor Pauchet & S. Dupret. 6th ed. 1989. 520p. pap. 24.95 (*0-7859-5797-9*) Fr & Eur.

Atlas de Anatomia Seccional e Imagenes Radiologicas (Basic Atlas of Sectional Anatomy) With Correlated Imaging. Walter J. Bo et al. 3rd ed. 1998. (ENG & SPA., Illus.). 511p. (*84-8174-455-7*) Mosby-Doyma Libros ESP. *Dist:* Mosby Inc, Saunders.

***Atlas de Anestesia Regional (Atlas of Regional Anesthesia)** David L. Brown. (SPA.). (*84-8174-084-5*) Mosby-Doyma Libros ESP. *Dist:* Saunders.

Atlas de Histologia. Daniel B. Freeman & Bracegirdle. 2nd ed. 1981. (SPA., Illus.). 144p. pap. 24.95 (*0-7859-5100-8*) Fr & Eur.

Atlas de Histopatologia. R. C. Curran. 1979. (SPA.). 96p. 95.00 (*0-8288-4720-7*, S37588) Fr & Eur.

Atlas de las Enfermedades Cromosomicas. J. Grouchy & C. Turleau. 1978. (SPA.). 356p. 150.00 (*0-8288-4861-0*, S31931) Fr & Eur.

Atlas de Patologia Macroscopica. R. C. Curran & E. L. Jones. 1978. (SPA.). 148p. 85.00 (*0-8288-4862-9*, S37589) Fr & Eur.

Atlas der Chirurgischen Schnitt-und Nahttechnik. J. Zoltan. 2nd ed. 1980. (Illus.). 176p. 83.50 (*3-8055-0439-X*) S Karger.

Atlas der Dermatologie und Venerologie see Atlas of Dermatology

Atlas der Elektrokardiographie. O. Ritter & V. Fattorusso. 5th ed. 1976. 48.75 (*3-8055-2416-1*) S Karger.

Atlas der Topographischen und Angewamdten Anatomie Des Menschen see Atlas of Topographical & Applied Human Anatomy

Atlas der Topographischen und Angewnadten Anatomie Des Menschen see Atlas of Topographical & Applied Human Anatomy, Vol. 1, Head & Neck

Atlas d'Immuno-Allergologie see Atlas of Immuno-Allergology: An Illustrated Primer for Health Care Professionals

Atlas Diseases of Oral Mucosa. Jens Jrgen Pindborg. 5th ed. 1992. (C). text 160.00 (*0-7216-4988-2*) Harcourt.

Atlas Emergency Procedures. Susan M. Dunmire & Paul M. Paris. 1994. LC 93-25118. (Illus.). 240p. text 79.00 (*0-7216-3682-9*) Saunders.

Atlas Facial Aesthetic Skeletal Contouring. Ousterhout. 1997. (*0-7216-5460-6*) Saunders.

Atlas for Sterotaxy of the Human Brain: Anatomical, Physiological & Clinical Applications. Georges Schaltenbrand. Ed. by Earl A. Walker. 2nd ed. 1998. (Illus.). 32p. 499.00 (*0-86577-055-7*) Thieme Med Pubs.

Atlas for the Hutt Adaptation of the Bender-Gestalt Test. Max L. Hutt & Robert G. Gibby. 1970. LC 79-75147. (Illus.). 296p. text 55.00 (*0-8089-0213-X*, 792096, Grune & Strat) Harcrt Hlth Sci Grp.

Atlas Imaging Management Traum. Shaff & Morris. 1999. pap. text 85.00 (*0-8385-0125-7*, Medical Exam) Appleton & Lange.

Atlas Manual de Anatomia. Victor Pauchet & Garcia I. Rodrigo. 6th ed. 1978. (SPA.). 518p. pap. 29.95 (*0-8288-4863-7*, S12343) Fr & Eur.

Atlas Non-Neoplastic Orthopedic. Wold. 2001. (C). text (*0-7216-6111-4*) Harcrt Hlth Sci Grp.

Atlas of Abdominal Operations. Michael J. Zinner. 1999. 135.00 (*0-8385-0459-0*, Medical Exam) Appleton & Lange.

Atlas of Abdominal Surgery. Braasch et al. 1990. (Illus.). 480p. text 142.00 (*0-7216-5601-3*) Saunders.

Atlas of Acupuncture. Felix Mann. 1993. pap. text 72.50 (*0-7506-1678-4*) Buttrwrth-Heinemann.

Atlas of Adult Cardiac Surgery. William A. Gay, Jr. 1990. (Surgical Practice Illustrated Ser.). (Illus.). 189p. text (*0-443-08598-6*) Church.

Atlas of Adult EEG Rhythms. Bromfield & Nugent. 2000. 176p. pap. (*0-7506-9619-2*) Buttrwrth-Heinemann.

Atlas of Adult Foot & Ankle Surgery. Lowell D. Lutter. 1996. (Illus.). 368p. (C). (gr. 13). text 159.00 (*0-8016-6280-X*, 06280) Mosby Inc.

Atlas of Adult Orthodontics: Functional & Esthetic Enhancement. Ed. by Manuel H. Marks & Herman Corn. 1988. LC 86-21469. (Illus.). 645p. text 149.50 (*0-8121-1023-4*) Lppncott W & W.

Atlas of Advanced Gastric Surgery Techniques. Ed. by Nobura Sakakibara. 1997. (Illus.). 156p. text (*90-5702-073-4*) GBSP NLD. *Dist:* Gordon & Breach.

Atlas of Advanced Orthodontics: A Guide to Clinical Efficiency. Anthony D. Viazis. Ed. by Judy Fletcher. 1998. LC 97-29321. (Illus.). 240p. (C). text 159.00 (*0-7216-7637-5*) Saunders.

Atlas of Advanced Techni1ues in Laparoscopic Surgery: Solid Organ Procedures. Michel Gagner. 1998. (Illus.). 280p. (*0-683-03407-3*) Lppncott W & W.

***Atlas of Aesthetic Face & Neck Surgery.** Gregory LaTrenta. 2001. (Illus.). 285p. (*0-7216-8572-2*) Saunders.

Atlas of Aesthetic Plastic Surgery. John R. Lewis. 1973. (Illus.). 62.00 (*0-316-52335-6*, Little Brwn Med Div) Lppncott W & W.

Atlas of Aging. T. B. L. Kirkwood. 2001. (Encyclopedia of Visual Medicine Ser.). 120p. 88.00 (*1-84214-023-X*, Parthenon Pbng) CRC Pr.

Atlas of Alimentary Tract Pathology. LC 94-221500. (Illus.). 124.95 (*957-9069-15-8*) Global Pub NJ.

Atlas of Allergies. Philip Fireman. 2nd ed. 1995. 352p. 144.00 (*0-7234-2181-1*) Mosby Inc.

Atlas of Allergies. Philip Fireman & Raymond G. Slavin. 2nd ed. 1996. (Illus.). 352p. (*84-8174-278-3*) Mosby-Doyma Libros ESP. *Dist:* Mosby Inc.

Atlas of Allergy. P. Ewan. 2002. (Encyclopedia of Visual Medicine Ser.). (Illus.). 100p. 89.95 (*1-84214-018-3*, Parthenon Pbng) CRC Pr.

Atlas of Alzheimer's Disease. Ed. by M. J. De Leon. 1999. LC 99-32886. (Encyclopedia of Visual Medicine Ser.). (Illus.). 150p. 103.95 (*1-85070-912-2*, Parthenon Pbng) CRC Pr.

Atlas of Ambulatory Eeg. Shatcter. 1999. pap. text 59.95 (*0-12-621345-3*) Acad Pr.

Atlas of Ambulatory Surgery. Frank G. Moody. Ed. by Richard Lampert. 1999. LC 98-36267. (Illus.). xvi, 302p. text 125.00 (*0-7216-5517-3*) Saunders.

Atlas of Anatomic Correlations in CT & MRI. P. Gerhardt. 1988. (Illus.). 184p. 299.00 (*0-86577-227-4*) Thieme Med Pubs.

Atlas of Anatomy. Parramon Studios Staff. 1997. LC 96-79470. 19.95 (*0-7641-5000-6*) Barron.

Atlas of Anatomy: The Functional Systems of the Human Body. Elke Lutjen-Drecoll & Johannes W. Rohen. 1998. LC 98-23048. 159p. 19.95 (*0-683-30641-3*) Lppncott W & W.

Atlas of Anatomy Basic to Radiology. Isadore Meschan. 2nd ed. 1998. text (*0-7216-3533-4*) Saunders.

Atlas of Anatomy for Reconstruction Surgery. Khouri. 1999. text (*0-7216-5189-5*) Saunders.

Atlas of Angina. J. Abrams & G. Charlton. 2002. (Illus.). 120p. ring bd. 89.95 (*1-84214-048-5*, Parthenon Pbng) CRC Pr.

Atlas of Aortic Surgery. G. Melville Williams & Leon Schlossberg. 1997. LC 96-18087. (Illus.). 188p. 139.00 (*0-683-09102-6*) Lppncott W & W.

Atlas of Applied Internal Liver Anatomy. E. M. Gadzijev & D. Ravnik. 1996. LC 96-24183. 208p. 222.00 (*3-211-82793-5*) Spr-Verlag.

Atlas of Approaches for General Surgery of the Dog & Cat. Mark M. Smith & Don R. Waldron. 1993. LC 93-12637. (Illus.). 288p. text 73.00 (*0-7216-3515-6*) Saunders.

Atlas of Arterial Histology. Donald F. Bunce, 2nd. 1974. LC 72-13843. (Illus.). 250p. 37.50 (*0-87527-096-4*) Green.

Atlas of Asthma. R. Djukanovic & Stephen T. Holgate. 1999. LC 98-44810. (Encyclopedia of Visual Medicine Ser.). (Illus.). 100p. lib. bdg. 82.95 (*1-85070-908-4*, H2123, Parthenon Pbng) CRC Pr.

Atlas of Atherosclerosis: Progression & Regression. Herbert C. Stary. Ed. by Herbert C. Stary. 1999. LC 98-54979. (Encyclopedia of Visual Medicine Ser.). (Illus.). 132p. 88.95 (*1-85070-480-5*, Parthenon Pbng) CRC Pr.

Atlas of Automated Percutaneous Lumbar Discectomy (A.P.L.D.) According to the Onkik Method. A. Solini. 1990. (Illus.). 145p. 107.00 (*0-387-82172-4*, 3641) Spr-Verlag.

Atlas of Avian Radiographic Anatomy. Stephen A. Smith & Bonnie J. Smith. 1991. (Illus.). 238p. text 89.00 (*0-7216-3652-7*) Saunders.

Atlas of Back Pain. S. S. Haldeman & W. H. Kirkaldy-Willis. 2001. LC 2001-56029. (Encyclopedia of Visual Medicine Ser.). (Illus.). 150p. 87.95 (*1-84214-076-0*, Parthenon Pbng) CRC Pr.

Atlas of Bedside Procedures. Thomas J. Vander Salm. 2nd ed. 1988. pap. 55.00 (*0-316-89618-7*, Little Brwn Med Div) Lppncott W & W.

Atlas of Bedside Procedures. Thomas J. Vander Salm et al. 2nd ed. 1988. LC 79-65313. 80.00 (*0-316-89617-9*, Little Brwn Med Div) Lppncott W & W.

Atlas of Benign Gynecology/Obstetric Surgery, '95. Stovall. 1995. text 160.00 (*0-7234-2017-3*) Mosby Inc.

Atlas of Biliary Tract Surgery. Ed. by John L. Cameron. 1993. LC 93-9302. (Surgical Practice Illustrated Ser.). (Illus.). 240p. text (*0-443-08742-3*) Church.

Atlas of Blood Cells: Function & Pathology M. F. Greaves et al. 2nd ed. 1988. (Illus.). 789p. text 225.00 (*0-8121-1094-3*) Lppncott W & W.

Atlas of Blood Diseases: Cytology & Histology. Yoshihito Yawata. 1996. 224p. 104.00 (*1-85317-313-4*) Mosby Inc.

Atlas of Bone Marrow & Blood Pathology. Contrib. by Saunders, W.B., Publishing Staff. 2000. LC 00-32234. 220p. 195.00 (*0-7216-8735-0*) Saunders.

Atlas of Bone Marrow Pathology. B. Frisch & R. Bartl. 1990. (C). text 324.50 (*0-7923-8921-2*) Kluwer Academic.

Atlas of Bone Scintigraphy in the Developing Pediatric Skeleton: The Normal Skeleton, Its Variants & Pitfalls. Klaus Hahn et al. 1995. LC 93-5678. (Illus.). 316p. 139.00 (*0-387-56578-7*) Spr-Verlag.

Atlas of Bone Scintigraphy in the Pathological Pediatric Skeleton. Isky Gordon et al. 1996. LC 95-52577. (Illus.). 416p. 165.00 (*3-540-60471-5*) Spr-Verlag.

Atlas of Bovine Anatomy. Chris Pasquini. 1982. (Illus.). 340p. (Orig.). (C). pap. 24.95 (*0-9623114-0-5*) Sudz Pub.

Atlas of Brain Function. William W. Orrison. 1995. LC 94-46586. 176p. pap. 55.00 (*0-86577-528-1*) Thieme Med Pubs.

Atlas of Brain Mapping: Topographic Mapping of EEG & Evoked Potentials. Konrad Maurer & T. Dierks. 1991. (Illus.). 103p. 86.95 (*0-387-53090-8*) Spr-Verlag.

Atlas of Brain Tumors. K. Tabuchi & A. Nishimoto. 1988. (Illus.). 247p. 214.00 (*0-387-70024-2*) Spr-Verlag.

Atlas of Breast Cancer. R. Blamey et al. 1994. (Illus.). 100p. 29.95 (*1-873413-70-X*) Merit Pub Intl.

Atlas of Breast Cancer. Ed. by Daniel F. Hayes. 1993. LC 92-49328. (gr. 13). (*1-56375-010-4*) Gower-Mosby.

Atlas of Breast Cancer. Ed. by Daniel F. Hayes. 2nd ed. 2000. 150p. pap. text 95.00 (*0-7234-3176-0*) Saunders.

Atlas of Breast Disease. J. A. Hall & J. Knause. 2002. (Encyclopedia of Visual Medicine Ser.). (Illus.). 120p. lib. bdg. 89.95 (*1-85070-533-X*, Parthenon Pbng) CRC Pr.

Atlas of Breast Imaging. Marla K. Jones. 1997. xi, 250 p. 105.00 (*0-632-04303-2*) Blackwell Sci.

Atlas of Breast Imaging. Daniel B. Kopans. 1998. LC 98-43303. 208p. text 120.00 (*0-7817-1720-5*) Lppncott W & W.

Atlas of Breast Pathology. Merino. 1999. text (*0-7216-6116-5*) Saunders.

Atlas of Breast Pathology. R. M. Millis. 1983. (Current Histopathology Ser.). 144p. text 234.50 (*0-85200-329-3*) Kluwer Academic.

Atlas of Bullous Disease. Robert E. Jordon. 2000. (Illus.). 300p. text (*0-443-05863-6*) Church GBR. *Dist:* Saunders.

Atlas of Cancer Incidence in the Former German Democratic Republic, 1978-1982. W. H. Menhart et al. 1993. (IARC Scientific Publications Ser.: No. 106). (Illus.). 384p. pap. text 95.00 (*92-832-2106-0*) OUP.

Atlas of Cancer Mortality in Central Europe. Ed. by Peter Boyle et al. 1996. (IARC Scientific Publications Ser.: No. 134). (Illus.). 240p. text 89.50 (*92-832-2134-6*) OUP.

Atlas of Cancer Mortality in the European Economic Community. Ed. by Michael Smans et al. 1993. (IARC Scientific Publications Ser.: No. 107). (Illus.). 220p. text 70.00 (*92-832-2107-9*) OUP.

Atlas of Cancer of the Skin. Guenter Burg. Ed. by Judy Fletcher. 1999. LC 98-43444. (Illus.). x, 254p. text (*0-443-05821-0*) Church.

Atlas of Cancer Surgery. Norman Bloom & Edward J. Beattie. 2000. LC 99-59399. (Illus.). 510p. text (*0-7216-6199-8*) Saunders.

Atlas of Canine & Feline Anatomy. Chris Pasquini. 1990. (Illus.). 400p. (Orig.). (C). pap. 26.95 (*0-9623114-3-X*) Sudz Pub.

Atlas of Canine & Feline Dental Radiography. 1997. 248p. pap. text 89.00 (*1-884254-36-5*) Vet Lrn Syst.

***Atlas of Canine Opthamology.** 2001. (Illus.). 208p. (*0-7020-1997-6*) W B Saunders GBR. *Dist:* Saunders.

Atlas of Canine Surgical Techniques. P. G. C. Bedford. 1996. (Illus.). 194p. pap. (*0-632-01814-3*) Blackwell Sci.

Atlas of Cardiac Imaging. Ed. by Richard T. Lee & Eugene Braunwald. 1998. LC 97-36794. text (*0-443-07567-0*) Church.

Atlas of Cardiac NMR with Anatomical Correlations. C. Depre et al. 1991. (Series in Radiology). (C). text 208.50 (*0-7923-0941-3*) Kluwer Academic.

Atlas of Cardiothoracic Surgery. Ed. by L. Henry Edmunds, Jr. et al. 1989. LC 89-12294. (Illus.). 287p. text 142.50 (*0-8121-1224-5*) Lppncott W & W.

Atlas of Cardiothoracic Surgery. David C. Sabiston, Jr. 1995. LC 94-32213. (Illus.). 400p. text 189.00 (*0-7216-3498-2*) Saunders.

Atlas of Cardiovascular Monitoring. Jonathan B. Mark. 1997. LC 97-41359. text (*0-443-08891-8*) Church.

Atlas of Cardiovascular Pathology. E. G. Olsen. 1987. text 268.50 (*0-85200-866-X*) Kluwer Academic.

Atlas of Cardiovascular Pathology. Renu Virmani et al. Ed. by Lesley Day. 1996. LC 95-9479. (Atlases in Diagnostic Surgical Pathology Ser.). 272p. text 185.00 (*0-7216-4476-7*) Saunders.

Atlas of Cat Anatomy. Hazel E. Field & Mary E. Taylor. 2nd rev. ed. 1969. LC 69-16998. 134p. pap. text 32.50 (*0-226-24817-8*) U Ch Pr.

Atlas of Cataract Surgery. Ed. by Samuel Masket & Alan S. Crandall. 1999. 322p. (*1-85317-557-9*) Martin Dunitz GBR. *Dist:* Mosby Inc.

Atlas of Cerebrovascular Disease. Philip B. Gorelick. 2nd ed. 1995. LC 2001-53795. (Illus.). 384p. text 95.00 (*1-878132-16-4*) Current Med.

Atlas of Cervicofacial Rejuvenation. Bruce F. Connell & Timothy J. Marten. 2000. (Illus.). 500p. text 275.00 (*1-57626-123-9*) Quality Med Pub.

Atlas of Chest Infections. Margaret E. Hodson et al. 1992. LC 92-1568. (Illus.). 128p. (gr. 13). text (*1-56375-553-X*, GM0270) Gower-Mosby.

Atlas of Chinese Therapeutic Motion for Treatment & Health: A Guide to Traditional Chinese Massage & Exercise Therapy. Delta Staff. 1995. (Illus.). 173p. (*983-9808-31-1*) Delta Edits MYS. *Dist:* Weatherhill.

Atlas of Chinese Tongue Diagnosis. Barbara Kirschbaum. Tr. by Barbara Kirschbaum. 2000. LC 99-72892. (Illus.). xix, 260p. 75.00 (*0-939616-33-5*) Eastland.

Atlas of Chrysophycean Cysts. Katherine E. Duff et al. 1994. LC 94-30346. (Developments in Hydrobiology Ser.: 99). (Illus.). 200p. (C). text 213.00 (*0-7923-3039-0*) Kluwer Academic.

Atlas of Clinical & Surgical Orbital Anatomy. Jonathan J. Dutton. 1994. LC 93-11266. (Illus.). 256p. text 177.00 (*0-7216-5427-4*) Saunders.

***Atlas of Clinical Dermatology.** Anthony Du Vivier. 3rd ed. 2001. (Illus.). 625p. pap. (*0-7234-3173-6*) Mosby Inc.

Atlas of Clinical Dermatology. Anthony Du Vivier. 2nd ed. 1992. (*84-8086-109-6*) Mosby-Doyma Libros ESP. *Dist:* Mosby Inc.

Atlas of Clinical Diagnosis. M. A. Mir. 1995. text 45.00 (*0-7020-1846-5*) Saunders.

Atlas of Clinical Endocrinology, Set. Ed. by Stanley G. Korenman & Stanley G. Korenman. Incl. Human Nutrition & Obesity. Ed. by David Heber & David Heber. LC 99-33358. xiii, 226p. 125.00 (*0-632-04401-2*); Neuroendocrinology & Pituitary Disease. Ed. by Mark E. Molitch & Mark E. Molitch. LC 99-34471. 240p. 131.95 (*0-632-04405-5*); Osteoporosis. Ed. by Robert Marcus. LC 99-34891. 198p. 131.95 (*0-632-04403-9*); Thyroid Diseases. Ed. by Martin I. Surks. LC 98-35631. 201p. 125.00 (*0-632-04397-0*); sets. Diabetes. Ed. by C. Ronald Kahn. LC 98-35631. 212p. 125.00 (*0-632-04399-7*); 1999. (Illus.). 1999. 495.00 (*0-86542-588-4*) Blackwell Sci.

Atlas of Clinical Gastroenterology Two. J. J. Misiewicz. 2nd ed. 1993. (C). (gr. 13). (*0-397-44737-X*) Gower-Mosby.

Atlas of Clinical Gastrointestinal Endoscopy. C. Mel Wilcox. 1995. 256p. text 145.00 (*0-7216-5315-4*) Saunders.

Atlas of Clinical Hematology. Jan V. Hirschmann et al. 1999. LC 99-37692. (Illus.). 285p. text (*0-7216-7002-4*) Saunders.

Atlas of Clinical Hematology. Helmut Loeffler & Johann Rastetter. Tr. by T. C. Telger. 5th rev. ed. 1999. (Illus.). 352p. 199.00 (*3-540-65085-7*) Spr-Verlag.

Atlas of Clinical Hepatology. Norman Gitlin & Robert M. Strauss. 1995. 192p. text 135.00 (*0-7216-4356-6*) Saunders.

Atlas of Clinical Neonatology. Karen E. Bender. 1993. (*1-56375-090-2*) Gower-Mosby.

Atlas of Clinical Neurology. Ed. by Roger N. Rosenberg. 1997. LC 97-6024. 500p. text 155.00 (*0-7506-9922-1*) Buttrwrth-Heinemann.

Atlas of Clinical Neurology. John D. Spillane. 3rd ed. 1983. (Illus.). 550p. text 60.00 (*0-19-261286-7*) OUP.

Atlas of Clinical Nuclear Medicine. Ignac Fogelman et al. 2nd ed. 1993. LC 93-23372. (Illus.). 736p. (C). (gr. 13). text 247.00 (*0-8151-3341-3*, 24080) Mosby Inc.

Atlas of Clinical Nutrition. A. Shils. 2001. 150p. 98.00 (*1-84214-050-7*, Parthenon Pbng) CRC Pr.

Atlas of Clinical Ophthalmology. David J. Spalton. 2nd ed. 1993. (*84-8086-123-1*) Mosby-Doyma Libros ESP. *Dist:* Mosby Inc.

Atlas of Clinical Ophthalmology, Set. Daniel M. Albert & Frederick A. Jakobiec. 1995. LC 95-1015. (Illus.). 480p. text 235.00 (*0-7216-3417-6*) Saunders.

Atlas of Clinical Ophthalmology, '94. Spalton. 2nd ed. 1994. (*0-7234-1993-0*) Wolfe Publishing GBR. *Dist:* Mosby Inc.

Atlas of Clinical Pet. Maisey. 1998. 256p. pap. 184.00 (*0-412-78270-7*, Chap & Hall NY) Chapman & Hall.

Atlas of Clinical PET in Oncology: PET vs. CT& MRI. Ed. by H. G. Bender et al. 2000. LC 99-59592. (Illus.). 224p. 145.00 (*3-540-66726-1*) Spr-Verlag.

Atlas of Clinical Positron Emission Tomography. Michael N. Maisey et al. 1999. LC 00-500836. (An Arnold Publication). (Illus.). 360p. (*0-340-74098-1*) E A GBR. *Dist:* OUP.

Atlas of Clinical Skills. M. A. Mir. 1997. 282p. text 39.95 (*0-7020-1816-3*) Saunders.

Atlas of Clinical Vectorcardiography. Ljuba Bacharova. 1994. (Illus.). 121p. (Orig.). (C). pap. text 29.50 (*0-930329-59-7*) Kabel Pubs.

Atlas of Closed Nailing of the Tibia & Femur. C. M. Court-Brown. 1991. (Illus.). 240p. 130.00 (*0-387-91396-3*) Spr-Verlag.

Atlas of Color Coded Doppler Sonography: Vascular & Soft Tissue Structures of the Upper Extremity, Thoracic Outlet & Neck. Ed. by Franz X. Fruhwald & D. Eric Blackwell. Tr. by M. Lafortune & M. Dauzat. 1992. LC 92-2332. (ENG, FRE & GER., Illus.). 144p. 213.00 (*0-387-82325-5*) Spr-Verlag.

Atlas of Colorectal Surgery. M. R. Keighley. 1996. LC 96-16863. 395p. text (*0-443-07570-0*) Church.

Atlas of Colposcopy. Reid. 1996. text (*0-7216-3555-5*) Saunders.

Atlas of Common Diseases: A Guide to Their Visual Manifestations. M. R. Salkind. 1993. (Encyclopedia of Visual Medicine Ser.). (Illus.). 140p. (C). lib. bdg. 77.95 (*1-85070-291-8*) CRC Pr.

Atlas of Common Subluxations of the Human Spine. William J. Ruch. 1997. LC 96-46124. 256p. 119.95 (*0-8493-3117-X*) CRC Pr.

Atlas of Computerized Perimetry. Jorg Weber & Joseph Caprioli. Ed. by Richard Lampert. 1999. LC 99-16763. (Illus.). 255p. text (*0-7216-6737-6*) Saunders.

Atlas of Congenital Cardiac Surgery. Paul A. Ebert. 1989. (Surgical Practice Illustrated Ser.). (Illus.). 138p. text (*0-443-08532-3*) Church.

Atlas of Contraception. Malcolm Potts & Pramilla Senanayke. 1995. (Encyclopedia of Visual Medicine Ser.). (Illus.). 140p. lib. bdg. 85.95 (*1-85070-387-6*, Parthenon Pbng) CRC Pr.

Atlas of Contrast-Enhanced Angiography. R. Mohiaddin & N. Bunce. 2002. (Encyclopedia of Visual Medicine Ser.). (Illus.). 144p. lib. bdg. 89.95 (*1-84214-081-7*, Parthenon Pbng) CRC Pr.

Atlas of Corneal Disease. Eric R. Mandel & Michael D. Wagoner. 1989. 160p. text 189.00 (*0-7216-2160-0*) Saunders.

Atlas of Coronary Artery Disease. Michael Davies. 1998. LC 98-12094. 176p. text 139.00 (*0-397-58750-3*) Lppncott W & W.

Atlas of Correlative Imaging Anatomy of the Normal Dog. Feeney et al. 1990. (Illus.). 400p. text 197.00 (*0-7216-2744-7*) Saunders.

Atlas of Correlative Surgical Neuropathology & Imaging. G. Stuart Rutherfoord & R. H. Hewlett. 1994. LC 94-11237. (Current Histopathology Ser.: Vol. 24). 206p. (C). text 318.50 (*0-7923-8951-4*) Kluwer Academic.

Atlas of Cosmetic & Reconstructive Periodontal Surgery. Edward S. Cohen. 2nd ed. 1994. (Illus.). 424p. text 105.00 (*0-8121-1518-X*) Lppncott W & W.

Atlas of Cosmetic Dermatology. Zoe Diana Drelos. 2000. LC 00-25388. (Illus.). xiv, 190p. text (*0-443-06548-9*) Church.

Atlas of Cranial Base Surgery. Ed. by Madjid Samii et al. 1994. LC 94-4811. (Illus.). 264p. text 285.00 (*0-7216-3882-1*) Saunders.

Atlas of Craniofacial & Cleft Surgery. Janusz Bardach & Kenneth Sayler. 1998. LC 98-13316. (Illus.). 1,200p. text 399.00 (*0-397-51807-2*) Lppncott W & W.

Atlas of Craniofacial Growth. Riolo et al. 1979. (Craniofacial Growth Ser.: Vol. 2). (Illus.). 379p. reprint ed. 65.00 (*0-929921-01-1*) UM CHGD.

Atlas of Craniofacial Growth in Americans of African Descent. Elisha R. Richardson. 1991. (Craniofacial Growth Ser.: Vol. 26). (Illus.). 69.00 (*0-929921-22-4*) UM CHGD.

Atlas of Craniomaxillofacial Fixation. Robert M. Kellman & Lawrence Marentette. 1994. 352p. text 210.00 (*0-7817-0016-7*) Lppncott W & W.

Atlas of Critical Care Procedures. Ed. by Mitchell P. Fink & Alan Lisbon. 2001. (Illus.). 300p. text 79.00 (*0-07-020985-5*) McGraw-Hill Educ Grp.

Atlas of Cross Sectional Anatomy of Human 14 Meridians & Acupoints. Moxun Chen et al. 1996. (Illus.). 346p. pap. text 52.00 (*1-880132-21-4*) Sci Pr NY.

***Atlas of Cross-Sectional & Projective MR Cholangio-Pancreatography: A Teaching File.** L. Van Hoe et al. 2001. (Illus.). xxvii, 429p. pap. 99.00 (*3-540-41885-7*) Spr-Verlag.

***Atlas of Cryosurgery.** Ed. by N. N. Korpan. 2001. (Illus.). 520p. 189.00 (*3-211-83449-4*) Spr-Verlag.

Atlas of CT Pathology. Deborah L. Durham. Ed. by Lisa Biello. 1996. 192p. text 42.00 (*0-7216-6415-6*) Saunders.

***Atlas of Cutaneous Aesthetic Surgery.** Michael S. Kaminar et al. 2001. LC 2001-42967. (Illus.). 285p. (*0-7216-8413-0*) Saunders.

Atlas of Cutaneous Facial Flaps & Grafts: A Differential Diagnosis of Wound Closures. Ronald L. Moy. 1990. LC 89-13856. 224p. text 98.50 (*0-8121-1313-6*) Lppncott W & W.

Atlas of Cutaneous Surgery. Philip E. LeBoit et al. 1995. LC 94-25752. (Illus.). 432p. text 158.00 (*0-7216-5404-5*) Saunders.

Atlas of Cutaneous Surgery. Neil A. Swanson. 1986. (Illus.). 176p. 48.95 (*0-316-82474-7*, Little Brwn Med Div) Lppncott W & W.

Atlas of Cystic Neoplasms of the Pancreas. K. Yamaguchi & M. Tanaka. 2000. (Illus.). xiv, 130p. 213.25 (*3-8055-7055-4*) S Karger.

Atlas of Cytopathology of the Head & Neck: With Clinical & Histological Correlations. G. Warner-Learmonth. 1999. (Illus.). 164p. (*0-340-74103-1*) E A GBR. *Dist:* OUP.

Atlas of Dental & Maxillofacial Radiology. Gregory. 1994. (Illus.). 240p. (C). (gr. 13). text 108.00 (*0-8151-1284-X*, 22951) Mosby Inc.

Atlas of Dental Radiographic Anatomy. Myron J. Kasle. 4th ed. 1993. LC 93-2762. (Illus.). 336p. pap. text 46.00 (*0-7216-4858-4*) Saunders.

Atlas of Depression. D. Baldwin & J. Birtwistle. 2001. LC 2001-56028. (Encyclopedia of Visual Medicine Ser.). (Illus.). 112p. lib. bdg. 87.95 (*1-85070-942-4*, Parthenon Pbng) CRC Pr.

Atlas of Dermatology. Lionel Fry. 1997. LC 96-15108. (Encyclopedia of Visual Medicine Ser.). (Illus.). 222p. 107.95 (*1-85070-461-9*, Parthenon Pbng) CRC Pr.

Atlas of Dermatology. Gernot Rassner. 3rd ed. 1994.Tr. of Atlas der Dermatologie und Venerologie. (Illus.). 382p. text 89.00 (*0-8121-1601-1*) Lppncott W & W.

Atlas of Dermatopathology. Phillip H. McKee. 1992. (Illus.). 208p. (gr. 13). text (*1-56375-574-2*) Gower-Mosby.

Atlas of Dermatopathology. George F. Murphy & Arlene J. Herzberg. 1996. LC 95-1014. (Illus.). 382p. text 240.00 (*0-7216-4886-X*) Saunders.

Atlas of Descriptive Embryology. Mathews. 5th ed. 1997. LC 98-115859. 266p. (C). pap. 54.00 (*0-13-593740-X*, Prentice Hall) P-H.

Atlas of Developmental Embryology. Emil S. Szebenyi. 1976. LC 75-388. (Illus.). 338p. (C). 65.00 (*0-8386-1710-7*) Fairleigh Dickinson.

Atlas of Diabetes Mellitus. Ed. by I. N. Scobie. 1998. LC 96-19318. (Encyclopedia of Visual Medicine Ser.). (Illus.). 96p. lib. bdg. 85.95 (*1-85070-489-9*, Parthenon Pbng) CRC Pr.

Atlas of Diabetes Mellitus. I. N. Scobie. 2nd ed. 2002. LC 2001-50049. (Encyclopedia of Visual Medicine Ser.). (Illus.). 96p. lib. bdg. 87.95 (*1-84214-009-4*, Parthenon Pbng) CRC Pr.

Atlas of Diagnostic Cytopathology. Barbara F. Atkinson. 1992. (Illus.). 706p. text 240.00 (*0-7216-3528-8*) Saunders.

Atlas of Diagnostic Cytopathology. Gabrijela I. Kocjan. 2nd ed. 1997. pap. text (*0-443-05174-7*) Church.

Atlas of Diagnostic Oncology. Skarin. 2nd ed. 1995. text (*0-7234-2175-7*) Wolfe Publishing GBR. *Dist:* Mosby Inc.

Atlas of Diagnostic Radiology in Gastroenterology. Ramsay Vallance. 1998. LC 98-15826. (Illus.). 273.95 (*0-632-05022-5*, Blackwell Hlthcare) Blackwell Sci.

Atlas of Diagnostic Radiology of Exotic Pets. Rubel et al. 1991. text 182.00 (*0-7216-3493-1*) Saunders.

Atlas of Diagnostic Ultrasound & Pathology of Fetal Malformation. Heather S. Andrews & P. J. Berry. 1997. (Illus.). 250p. (*0-7020-1405-2*) W B Saunders GBR. *Dist:* Saunders.

Atlas of Differential Diagnosis in Dermatology. Klaus F. Helm & James G. Marks. 1997. LC 97-34014. 64p. text (*0-443-05605-6*) Church.

Atlas of Differential Diagnosis in HIV Disease. M. Lipman et al. 1994. LC 94-21470. (Encyclopedia of Visual Medicine Ser.). 140p. lib. bdg. 85.95 (*1-85070-474-0*, Parthenon Pbng) CRC Pr.

Atlas of Differential Diagnosis in HIV Disease. M. C. I. Lipman. 2nd ed. 2001. (Encyclopedia of Visual Medicine Ser.). (Illus.). 120p. 88.00 (*1-84214-026-4*, Parthenon Pbng) CRC Pr.

Atlas of Difficult Diagnoses in Cytopathology. Barbara F. Atkinson & Jan F. Silverman. Ed. by Alan Ross. 1998. LC 97-31213. 432p. (C). text 245.00 (*0-7216-4076-1*) Saunders.

Atlas of Digital Human Anatomy. Engineering Animation Incorporated Staff. 1998. LC 99-160755. (Illus.). 368p. (C). (gr. 13). text 59.00 (*0-8151-8656-8*, 28925) Mosby Inc.

Atlas of Disease Mortalities in Hong Kong for the Three Five-Year Periods in 1979-93. Owen L. Lloyd et al. 1997. (C). (*962-201-732-0*) Chinese Univ HKG. *Dist:* U of Mich Pr.

Atlas of Diseases of the Ear in Dog & Cat. Orsher. 1994. (*0-397-51199-X*) Lppncott W & W.

Atlas of Diseases of the Eye. E. S. Perkins et al. 3rd ed. 1986. (Illus.). 208p. (Orig.). pap. text (*0-443-02961-X*) Church.

Atlas of Diseases of the Kidney Ed. by Robert W. Schrier & Robert W. Schrier. Incl. Dialysis as Treatment of End-Stage Renal Disease/Transplantation as Treatment of End-Stage Renal Disease. Ed. by William L. Henrich & William M. Bennett. 1999. 131.95 (*0-632-04391-1*); Disorders of Water, Electrolytes & Acid Base/Acute Renal Failure. Ed. by Tomas Bert. 1998. 131.95 (*0-632-04385-7*); Glomerulonephritis & Vasculitis/Tubolointerstitial Disease. Ed. by Richard J. Glassock. 1998. 131.95 (*0-632-04387-3*); Hypertension & the Kidney. Ed. by Christopher S. Wilcox. 1999. 131.95 (*0-632-04389-X*); Systemic Diseases & the Kidney. Ed. by Saulo Klahr. 1998. 131.95 (*0-632-04437-3*); LC 98-29127. (Illus.). 1999. 519.95 (*0-86542-578-7*) Blackwell Sci.

Atlas of Diseases of the Nail. R. K. Scher & P. A. Rich. 2002. (Encyclopedia of Visual Medicine Ser.). (Illus.). 140p. 95.95 (*1-85070-595-X*, Parthenon Pbng) CRC Pr.

Atlas of Drosophila Development. Volker Hartenstein. 1995. (Illus.). 58p. pap. text 19.50 (*0-87969-472-6*) Cold Spring Harbor.

Atlas of Duplex Scanning: Extremities. John J. Cranley. 1992. (Illus.). 426p. text 185.00 (*0-7216-3466-4*) Saunders.

Atlas of Duplex Ultrasonography: Essential Images of the Vascular System. Sergio Salles-Cunha & George Andros. 1988. LC 87-30729. (Illus.). 200p. text 79.00 (*0-941022-08-0*) Davies Pubng.

Atlas of Dynamic Laryngeal Pathology: A Video-Text Package. C. Richard Stasney. 1996. (Illus.). 130p. 225.00 incl. VHS (*1-56593-622-1*, 1291) Singular Publishing.

Atlas of Ear, Nose & Throat Disorders. A. J. Gulya & W. R. Wilson. 1999. LC 99-40838. (Encyclopedia of Visual Medicine Ser.). (Illus.). 80p. 88.95 (*1-85070-937-8*, Parthenon Pbng) CRC Pr.

Atlas of Ear, Nose & Throat Disorders in Children. Steven D. Handler & Charles M. Myer, III. 1997. (Illus.). 195p. incl. cd-rom (*1-55009-042-9*) DEKR.

Atlas of Ear, Nose & Throat Pathology. L. Michaels. 1990. (C). text 287.50 (*0-7923-8934-4*) Kluwer Academic.

Atlas of Echocardiography. A. Greengart. 2001. (Encyclopedia of Visual Medicine Ser.). (Illus.). 100p. 85.00 (*1-85070-069-9*, Parthenon Pbng) CRC Pr.

Atlas of Echocardiography. Ernesto Salcedo. 2nd ed. 1985. (Illus.). 445p. text 99.00 (*0-7216-7899-8*) Saunders.

Atlas of EEG in the First Months of Life. A. W. De Weerd. 1995. LC 95-14334. (Illus.). 244p. 230.50 (0-444-89946-4) Elsevier.

Atlas of Elbow Surgery. R. Hotchkiss & T. G. Wadsworth. 1998. (Illus.). 320p. (0-443-08928-0) Church.

Atlas of Electro-Encephalography in the Dog & Cat. Richard W. Redding & Charles E. Knecht. 1984. LC 83-13693. (Illus.). 387p. 83.50 (0-275-91448-8, C1448, Praeger Pubs) Greenwood.

Atlas of Electroencephalography, 1. Robert R. Clancy et al. 1999. LC 93-27908. (Atlas of Electroencephalography Ser.: Vol. 1). 190p. pap. 94.00 (0-444-81239-3) Elsevier.

Atlas of Electroencephalography, Set. Sperling. 1999. 204.00 (0-444-81180-X) Elsevier.

Atlas of Emergency Medicine. Kevin Knoop et al. 1997. LC 97-1279. (Illus.). 544p. text 189.00 (0-07-035202-X) McGraw-Hill Prof.

***Atlas of Emergency Medicine.** Kevin J. Knoop et al. 2nd ed. 2001. (Illus.). 704p. 179.00 (0-07-135294-5, Apple Lange Med) McGraw.

Atlas of Emergency Procedures. Rosen & George L. Sternbach. 1999. LC 00-52538. (Illus.). xiv, 289p. (C). (gr. 13). text 125.00 (0-8151-7402-0, 23605) Mosby Inc.

Atlas of Emergency Radiology: Diagnosis & Treatment. Gary A. Johnson et al. 1999. LC 00-30111. (Illus.). 350p. text 60.00 (0-7216-7142-X) Saunders.

Atlas of Emergency Trauma Surgical Procedures. Norman E. McSwain & Drue N. Ware. 1994. LC 90-4546. (Illus.). 184p. 98.50 (0-89640-179-0) Igaku-Shoin.

Atlas of Endocrine Imaging. Michael Besser. 1993. 149p. (C). (gr. 13). (1-56375-583-1) Gower-Mosby.

Atlas of Endocrine Organs: Vertebrates & Invertebrates. Ed. by Akira Matsumoto & Susumu Ishii. Tr. by A. Urano from JPN. 1992. LC 92-28888. (Illus.). 307p. 273.00 (0-387-53158-0) Spr-Verlag.

Atlas of Endocrine Pathology. Bruce M. Wenig et al. Ed. by Lesley Day. 1997. LC 96-29338. 384p. text 205.00 (0-7216-5917-9) Saunders.

Atlas of Endodontic Surgery. Syngcuk Kim. 1998. 256p. text 140.00 (0-7216-4851-7) Saunders.

Atlas of Endometrial Histopathology. G. Dallenbach-Hellweg & Hemming Poulsen. 2nd exp. rev. ed. 1996. LC 96-16757. (Illus.). 240p. 208.00 (3-540-60908-3) Spr-Verlag.

Atlas of Endometriosis. R. W. Shaw. 1992. (Encyclopedia of Visual Medicine Ser.). (Illus.). 96p. lib. bdg. 77.95 (1-85070-390-6, Parthenon Pbng) CRC Pr.

Atlas of Endometriosis. C. Overton & M. Farrugia. 2nd ed. 2001. LC 2001-56112. (Encyclopedia of Visual Medicine Ser.). (Illus.). 140p. lib. bdg. 87.95 (1-84214-022-1, Parthenon Pbng) CRC Pr.

***Atlas of Endoscopic Anatomy for Endonasal Intracranial Surgery.** P. Cappablanca et al. 2001. (Illus.). 150p. 169.00 (3-211-83548-2) Spr-Verlag.

Atlas of Endoscopic Examination for Early Carcinoma of Esophagus & Gastric Cardia. Ed. by Wang Guoqing. 1996. (Illus.). 155p. (7-03-005004-5) Sci Pr CHN. *Dist:* Lubrecht & Cramer.

Atlas of Endoscopic Perforator Vein Surgery. Ed. by Peter Gloviczki & John J. Bergan. 1997. LC 97-16185. (Illus.). 352p. 350.00 (3-540-76171-3) Spr-Verlag.

Atlas of Endoscopic Sinonasal Surgery. Dinesh Mehta. 1992. (Illus.). 118p. text 95.00 (0-8121-1471-X) Lppncott W & W.

Atlas of Endoscopic Spine Surgery. Ed. by John J. Regan et al. 1995. (Illus.). 359p. 200.00 (0-942219-73-2) Quality Med Pub.

Atlas of Endoscopic Spine Surgery. John J. Regan et al. 1995. (Illus.). 359p. 225.00 (1-57626-046-1, QMP) Quality Med Pub.

Atlas of Endoscopic Techniques. Jeffrey M. Goldberg & Tommaso Falcone. 2000. 220p. text (0-7020-2435-X) W B Saunders GBR. *Dist:* Saunders.

Atlas of Endourology. Kurt Amplatz. 1991. (0-8151-0137-6) Mosby Inc.

Atlas of Enteroscopy. Ed. by Francesco P. Rossini & Nancy G. Gay. 1998. LC 98-20746. (Illus.). 187p. 149.00 (88-470-0025-4) Spr-Verlag.

Atlas of Epilepsy. David W. Smith et al. 1997. LC 97-987. (Encyclopedia of Visual Medicine Ser.). (Illus.). 158p. lib. bdg. 85.95 (1-85070-488-0, Parthenon Pbng) CRC Pr.

Atlas of Epilepsy. D. F. Smith. 2nd ed. 2001. (Encyclopedia of Visual Medicine Ser.). (Illus.). 120p. 88.00 (1-84214-027-2, Parthenon Pbng) CRC Pr.

Atlas of Equine Surgery. Stephen B. Adams & John F. Fessler. 1999. LC 99-42010. (Illus.). xi, 428p. text 115.00 (0-7216-4643-3) Saunders.

Atlas of Equine Ultrasonography. Reimer. 1997. LC 97-27369. (Illus.). 328p. (C). (gr. 13). text 84.95 (0-8151-2146-6, 30756) Mosby Inc.

Atlas of Esophageal Surgery. David B. Skinner. 1991. (Surgical Practice Illustrated Ser.). (Illus.). 186p. text (0-443-08610-9) Church.

Atlas of Exotic & Domestic Diseases of Animals. 1997. (Illus.). lib. bdg. 275.00 (0-8490-8146-7) Gordon Pr.

Atlas of Experimental Immunobiology & Immunopathology. Byron H. Waksman. 1970. LC 73-81434. (Illus.). 85.00 (0-300-01154-7) Yale U Pr.

Atlas of Experimental Toxicological Pathology, Vol. 13. C. Gopinath et al. 1987. (Current Histopathology Ser.). 176p. lib. bdg. 256.00 (0-85200-332-3) Kluwer Academic.

Atlas of Experimentally-Induced Neoplasia in the Beagle Dog. Stephen A. Benjamin. Ed. by Charles R. Watson & Gerald E. Dagle. 1997. LC 96-46999. viii, 172p. pap. 125.00 (1-57477-025-X) Battelle.

Atlas of Extraocular Muscle Surgery. John A. Dyer & David A. Lee. 2nd ed. 1984. LC 84-18090. 256p. 59.95 (0-275-91427-5, C1427, Praeger Pubs) Greenwood.

Atlas of Eyelid & Conjunctival Tumors. Jerry A. Shields & Carol L. Shields. 1999. LC 98-33790. 368p. text 169.00 (0-7817-1915-1) Lppncott W & W.

Atlas of Eyelid Surgery. Gary E. Borodic & Daniel J. Townsend. 1993. (Illus.). 160p. text 115.00 (0-7216-3640-3) Saunders.

Atlas of Feline Anatomy for Veterinarians. Lola C. Hudson & William P. Hamilton. 1993. LC 93-12640. (Illus.). 224p. text 104.00 (0-7216-4004-4) Saunders.

Atlas of Feline Ophthalmology. Barnett. 1997. text 150.00 (0-7020-1662-4) Saunders.

Atlas of Feline Ophthalmology. Kerry L. Ketring & Mary B. Glaze. 1994. LC 94-60003. 140p. pap. text 87.00 (1-884254-13-6) Vet Lrn Syst.

Atlas of Female Infertility Surgery. Robert B. Hunt. 2nd ed. 1992. (Illus.). 560p. (C). (gr. 13). text 136.00 (0-8151-4739-2, 22450) Mosby Inc.

Atlas of Female Urologic Surgery. Appell. 2001. 125.00 (0-397-51528-6, A0738) Lppncott W & W.

Atlas of Fetal Sectional Anatomy. G. Isaacson. 1986. (Illus.). 184p. 253.00 (0-387-96248-4) Spr-Verlag.

Atlas of Fetal Surgery. Michael Harrison. 1996. 272p. (0-412-99131-4) E A GBR. *Dist:* OUP.

Atlas of Film-Screen Mammography. Ellen S. De Paredes. 2nd enl. rev. ed. 1992. LC 88-20633. (Illus.). 628p. 150.00 (0-683-06758-3) Lppncott W & W.

Atlas of Fine Structure of Human Sperm Penetration, Eggs & Embryos Cultured In Vitro. Henry A. Sathananthan et al. 1985. LC 85-6400. 302p. 88.00 (0-275-91308-2, C1308, Praeger Pubs) Greenwood.

Atlas of Finger & Thumb Reconstruction. G. Loda. 1999. LC 99-12945. (Illus.). 240p. 179.00 (0-86577-585-0) Thieme Med Pubs.

Atlas of Fluorescein Angiography. Alexandre E. Jalkh & Jose M. Celorio. 1993. (Illus.). 272p. text 177.00 (0-7216-3641-1) Saunders.

Atlas of Foot & Ankle Surgery. Michael J. Shereff. 1993. LC 92-19403. (Illus.). 320p. text 110.00 (0-7216-3537-7) Saunders.

Atlas of Foot Radiology. Jacques Montagne. 1981. (C). (gr. 13). 81.50 (0-89352-097-7) Mosby Inc.

Atlas of Foot Surgery. Yu. 1999. text (0-443-08786-5) Saunders.

Atlas of Foot Surgery Vol. II: Rear Foot Surgery. O. A. Mercado. (Illus.). 75.00 (0-940542-04-8) Carolando.

Atlas of Forensic Pathology. Nancy L. Jones. 1996. LC 96-1929. (Illus.). 224p. 95.00 (0-89640-315-7) Igaku-Shoin.

Atlas of Forensic Pathology. Charles V. Wetli et al. 1998. LC 98-52752. 165.00 (0-89189-430-6) Am Soc Clinical.

Atlas of Fungal Pathology. Karlhanns Salfelder. 1990. (Current Histopathology Ser.). (C). text 287.50 (0-7923-8935-2) Kluwer Academic.

Atlas of Gastric Surgery. Michael J. Zinner. 1991. (Surgical Practice Illustrated Ser.). (Illus.). 242p. text (0-443-08770-9) Church.

Atlas of Gastroenterologic Endoscopy: By High-Resolution Video-Endoscope. Kou Nagasako et al. 1998. 164p. text 135.00 (4-260-14346-8) Lppncott W & W.

Atlas of Gastroenterology. C. R. Kapadia & C. Taylor. 2001. (Encyclopedia of Visual Medicine Ser.). (Illus.). 100p. lib. bdg. 89.95 (1-85070-581-X, Parthenon Pbng) CRC Pr.

Atlas of Gastroenterology. Tadataka Yamada. 2nd ed. 1998. LC 98-46289. 928p. text 229.00 (0-397-58767-8) Lppncott W & W.

Atlas of Gastrointestinal & Hepatobiliary Infections. W. Edmund Farrar & Martin J. Wood. 1992. (Illus.). 144p. (gr. 13). text (1-56375-555-6) Gower-Mosby.

Atlas of Gastrointestinal Cancer Staging by Endosonography. T. L. Tio. 1995. LC 94-21375. (Illus.). 216p. 149.50 (0-89640-267-3) Igaku-Shoin.

Atlas of Gastrointestinal Endoscopy. Emmet B. Keeffe et al. 1998. LC 97-45781. 232p. (C). text 129.00 (0-8385-0448-5) McGraw-Hill Prof.

Atlas of Gastrointestinal Endoscopy. Fred E. Silverstien & Guido N. Tytgat. 1987. (Illus.). 272p. text 209.00 (0-03-012792-0) Saunders.

***Atlas of Gastrointestinal Endoscopy & Related Pathology.** Klaus Schiller et al. 2001. (Illus.). 384p. 175.00 (0-632-05585-5) Blackwell Sci.

Atlas of Gastrointestinal Endosonography. Sivak. 1998. text (0-7216-3638-1) Saunders.

Atlas of Gastrointestinal Pathology. Frank A. Mitros. 1988. LC 65-40231. (Gower Bk.). (Illus.). 272p. (gr. 13). text (0-397-44651-9, GM0066) Gower-Mosby.

Atlas of Gastrointestinal Pathology. David A. Owen & James K. Kelly. 1994. LC 94-989. text 210.00 (0-7216-6730-9) Saunders.

Atlas of Gastrointestinal Surgery. Emilio Etala. Tr. by Alfred Axtmayer. 1997. LC 96-21197. (Illus.). 2,516p. text 325.00 (0-683-02837-5) Lppncott W & W.

Atlas of General Laparoscopic Surgery. Joseph Sanfilippo et al. 1995. (Illus.). 280p. (C). text 129.00 (0-397-51268-6, Lippnctt) Lppncott W & W.

Atlas of General Surgery. Niederhuber. 1999. pap. text 135.00 (0-8385-0060-9) Appleton & Lange.

Atlas of General Surgery. David C. Sabiston, Jr. 1993. LC 92-48756. (Illus.). 928p. text 175.00 (0-7216-7883-1) Saunders.

Atlas of General Surgery. Ed. by Hugh Dudley & David Carter. 2nd ed. 1993. (Illus.). 1000p. (gr. 13). pap. 138.95 (0-407-00377-0) Chapman & Hall.

Atlas of General Surgery. D. C. Carter et al. 3rd ed. 1996. (Illus.). 1208p. (0-412-72090-6) E A GBR. *Dist:* OUP.

Atlas of General Thoracic Surgery. Larry R. Kaiser. 1996. (Illus.). 256p. (C). (gr. 13). text 105.00 (0-8016-6380-6, 06380) Mosby Inc.

Atlas of General Thoracic Surgery. Mark M. Ravitch & Felician M. Steichen. 1988. (Illus.). 400p. text 220.00 (0-7216-7474-7) Saunders.

***Atlas of Genitourinary Oncology.** Movsas. 2001. (0-7216-8738-5) Saunders.

Atlas of Genitourinary Radiology. Rosalyn Kutcher & Everett M. Lautin. 1989. (Illus.). 300p. (gr. 13). text (0-397-44614-4) Gower-Mosby.

Atlas of Genitourinary Tract Infections. Martin J. Wood. 1992. (C). (gr. 13). text (1-56375-554-8) Gower-Mosby.

Atlas of Glomerular Histopathology. P. H. Schillings & H. J. Schuurmans Stekhoven. 1980. (Illus.). 85.25 (3-8055-0201-X) S Karger.

Atlas of Gross Neuropathology. Robert E. Slemmer. 1983. (Illus.). 320p. (C). 48.50 (0-87527-239-8) Green.

Atlas of Gross Pathology. Christopher D. Fletcher & Phillip H. McKee. 1988. (Illus.). 112p. pap. text (0-683-13024-2) E A GBR. *Dist:* Williams & Wilkins.

Atlas of Gross Pathology. Christopher D. Fletcher & Phillip H. McKee. 1987. (Illus.). 112p. pap. (0-397-44607-1, GM0058) Gower-Mosby.

Atlas of Growth in the Aging Craniofacial Skeleton. Behrents. 1986. (Craniofacial Growth Ser.: Vol. 18). (Illus.). 125p. 20.00 (0-929921-14-3) UM CHGD.

Atlas of Gynecolgic Pathology. Debra S. Heller. 1992. 85.00 (0-316-35501-1, Little Brwn Med Div) Lppncott W & W.

Atlas of Gynecologic & Peritoneal Surgical Pathology. Philip B. Clement & Robert H. Young. 2000. LC 99-59936. (Illus.). 360p. text (0-7216-2458-8) Saunders.

Atlas of Gynecologic Pathology. J. Donald Woodruff & Tim H. Parmley. 1988. LC 65-40256. (Gower Bk.). (Illus.). 240p. (0-397-44650-0, GM0065) Gower-Mosby.

Atlas of Gynecologic Pathology. J. Donald Woodruff et al. 2nd ed. 1993. LC 92-49463. (1-56375-074-0) Gower-Mosby.

Atlas of Gynecological Surgery: Including Breast Surgery & Related Urologic & Intestinal Surgical Procedures. Ed. by Hans A. Hirsch et al. Tr. by K. Tamussino & E. Kohron. 3rd ed. 1996. LC 96-8673. (Illus.). 616p. text 249.00 (0-86577-595-8) Thieme Med Pubs.

Atlas of Hair & Scalp Diseases. J. Powell & N. Stone. 2001. (Encyclopedia of Visual Medicine Ser.). (Illus.). 96p. lib. bdg. 87.95 (1-84214-013-2, Parthenon Pbng) CRC Pr.

Atlas of Hand Surgery. Bruce W. Conolly. 1997. LC 97-36173. text (0-443-05077-5) Church.

Atlas of Hand Surgery. S. Pechlaner. 2000. LC 99-48644. (Illus.). 567p. 229.00 (0-86577-865-5) Thieme Med Pubs.

Atlas of Head & Neck Pathology. Bruce M. Wenig. 1993. (Illus.). 448p. text 195.00 (0-7216-4032-X) Saunders.

Atlas of Head & Neck Surgery. Robert H. Ossoff. Date not set. text (0-7216-4922-X) Saunders.

Atlas of Head & Neck Surgery. Carl E. Silver. 2nd ed. 1999. LC 98-32247. viii, 348p. (C). text (0-443-05129-1) Church.

Atlas of Head & Neck Surgery. John M. Lore. 3rd ed. 1988. (Illus.). 1219p. text 199.00 (0-7216-5816-4) Saunders.

Atlas of Head & Neck Surgery, Vol. 2. Kenneth L. Mattox. 2nd ed. 1999. 350p. (C). text 125.00 (1-55664-254-7) Mosby Inc.

Atlas of Head & Neck Surgery - Otolaryngology. Ed. by Byron J. Bailey et al. 1996. (Illus.). 976p. text 259.00 (0-397-51315-1) Lppncott W & W.

Atlas of Headaches. Steven D. Silberstein & Todd D. Rozen. 2001. (Encyclopedia of Visual Medicine Ser.). (Illus.). 150p. lib. bdg. 89.95 (1-85070-547-X, Parthenon Pbng) CRC Pr.

Atlas of Hearing & Balance Organs. Andre LeBlanc. 1998. LC 98-29337. (Illus.). 68p. (C). pap. (2-287-59648-8) Spl France Editions FRA. *Dist:* Spr-Verlag.

Atlas of Hearing & Balance Organs. Andre LeBlanc. 1998. LC 98-29337. 55.00 (3-540-59648-8) Spr-Verlag.

Atlas of Heart & Vessel Pathology 1.0. Bruce McManus & Stanley J. Radio. 1997. 199.00 incl. cd-rom (0-412-09081-3) Chapman & Hall.

Atlas of Heart Disease. Eugene Braunwald. 1996. (C). (gr. 13). text 1625.00 (1-878132-21-0, 30366) Current Med.

Atlas of Heart Disease. Contrib. by Saunders, W.B., Publishing Staff. 6th ed. 2001. 230.00 incl. cd-rom (0-7216-8554-4); 245.00 incl. cd-rom (0-7216-8556-0) Saunders.

Atlas of Heart Disease: Heart Diseases in the Presence of Disorders of Other Organ Systems. Ed. by Michael H. Crawford. 1995. (Atlas of Heart Diseases Ser.: Vol. 6). (Illus.). 264p. text 134.00 (1-878132-28-8) Current Med.

Atlas of Heart Disease: Techniques in Interventional Cardiology, Vol. 13. Ed. by Eugene Braunwald & Mark A. Creager. 1997. LC 97-6325. (C). (gr. 13). 125.00 (1-878132-55-5, 26641) Current Med.

Atlas of Heart Disease Vol. 2: Cardiomyopathies, Myocarditis & Pericardial Disease. Ed. by Walter H. Abelmann. 1994. LC 94-31947. text 134.00 (1-878132-24-5) Current Med.

Atlas of Heart Disease Vol. 10: Atherosclerosis: Risk Factors & Treatment. Ed. by W. Virgil Brown & Eugene Braunwald. 1996. LC 95-50019. (Illus.). 248p. text 134.00 (1-878132-31-8) Current Med.

Atlas of Heart Disease Vol. 11: Valvular Heart Disease. Ed. by Eugene Braunwald & Shahbudin H. Rahimtoola. 1996. LC 95-42589. (Atlas of Heart Diseases Ser.: Vol. 11). (Illus.). 336p. 134.00 (1-878132-30-X) Current Med.

Atlas of Heart Disease Vol. 12: Congenital Heart Disease, Vol. 12. Ed. by Eugene Braunwald & Robert M. Freedom. 1996. LC 96-20464. (Atlas of Heart Diseases Ser.). (Illus.). 284p. (C). (gr. 13). text 130.00 (1-878132-33-4, 26645) Current Med.

Atlas of Heart Diseases: Arrhythmias: Electrophysiologic Principles, Vol. IX. Ed. by Melvin M. Scheinman & Eugene Braunwald. 1996. (Illus.). 240p. 134.00 (1-878132-22-9) Current Med.

Atlas of Heart Diseases: Cardiopulmonary Disease & Cardiac Tumors. Eugene Braunwald et al. 1995. LC 94-30333. (Atlas of Heart Diseases Ser.: 3). (Illus.). 312p. text 134.00 (1-878132-23-7) Current Med.

Atlas of Heart Diseases Vol. 8: Acute Myocardial Infarction & Other Acute Ischemic Syndromes. Ed. by Eugene Braunwald & Robert M. Califf. 1996. (Illus.). 320p. text 134.00 (1-878132-32-6) Current Med.

Atlas of Heart Failure. J. Cleland & M. Davis. 2002. (Encyclopedia of Visual Medicine Ser.). (Illus.). 120p. 95.95 (1-85070-041-9, Parthenon Pbng) CRC Pr.

Atlas of Heart Failure: Cardiac Function & Dysfunction. Ed. by Wilson S. Colucci & Eugene Braunwald. 2nd ed. 1998. LC 97-165613. (Atlas of Heart Diseases Ser.: Vol. 4). (Illus.). 250p. 136.95 (0-632-04381-4) Blackwell Sci.

***Atlas of Heart Failure: Cardiac Function & Dysfunction.** Ed. by Wilson S. Colucci. 3rd ed. 2002. LC 2001-53786. (1-57340-184-6) Current Med.

Atlas of Hematology. George A. McDonald et al. 5th ed. 1989. (Illus.). 296p. text (0-443-02560-6) Church.

Atlas of Hernia Surgery. George E. Wantz. 1990. (Illus.). 240p. text 139.00 (0-88167-724-8) Lppncott W & W.

Atlas of Hip Surgery. Ed. by R. Bauer et al. 1995. LC 96-130091. (Illus.). 334p. 229.00 (0-86577-601-6) Thieme Med Pubs.

Atlas of Histology. Shu-Xin Zhang. 1999. LC 97-47335. (Illus.). 448p. pap. 49.95 (0-387-94954-2) Spr-Verlag.

Atlas of Histopathology of Skin Diseases. D. T. Shum & L. C. Guenther. 1999. LC 98-30129. (Encyclopedia of Visual Medicine Ser.). (Illus.). 286p. lib. bdg. 93.95 (1-85070-929-7, Parthenon Pbng) CRC Pr.

Atlas of Histopathology of the Cervix Uteri. Ed. by Gisela Dallenbach-Hellweg & Hemming Poulsen. 1991. (Illus.). 180p. 182.00 (0-387-52295-6) Spr-Verlag.

Atlas of Histopathology of the Skin. David E. Elder. 1998. LC 98-27635. (Illus.). 464p. text 199.00 (0-397-58420-2) Lppncott W & W.

***Atlas of Human Anatomy.** Stanley Jacob. 2001. (Illus.). 250p. pap. (0-443-05364-2) Church GBR. *Dist:* Saunders.

Atlas of Human Anatomy Kiss. 1987. lib. bdg. (90-247-2264-0) M Nijhoff NLD. *Dist:* Kluwer Academic.

Atlas of Human Anatomy. Frank H. Netter. Ed. by Sharon Colacino. 1989. LC 89-60477. (Illus.). 592p. 79.95 (0-914168-18-5); pap. text 55.00 (0-914168-19-3) Icon Lrning Systs.

***Atlas of Human Anatomy.** Contrib. by Springhouse Corporation Staff. 2001. LC 2001-20027. (Illus.). 376p. 54.95 (1-58255-108-1) Springhouse Corp.

Atlas of Human Anatomy. J. A. Gosling et al. 3rd ed. 1996. (Illus.). 112p. pap. (84-8086-118-5) Mosby-Doyma Libros ESP. *Dist:* Mosby Inc.

Atlas of Human Anatomy. J. A. Gosling et al. 3rd ed. 1996. 112p. (0-7234-2657-0, QM23) Wolfe Publishing GBR. *Dist:* Mosby Inc.

Atlas of Human Anatomy, No. 614466. American Map Staff. 1997. (Illus.). pap. 2.95 (0-8416-1446-6) Am Map.

Atlas of Human Anatomy, English Vol. 1: Head, Neck, Upper Extremities. Johannes Sobotta. Ed. & Tr. by Anna N. Taylor from GER. 11th ed. 1990. (Illus.). 416p. text (0-683-07833-X) Urban & S DEU. *Dist:* Williams & Wilkins.

Atlas of Human Anatomy, English Vol. 3: Thorax, Abdomen, Pelvis, Lower Limbs, Skin. Johannes Sobotta. Ed. & Tr. by Anna N. Taylor from GER. 11th ed. 1990. (Illus.). 384p. text (0-683-07834-8) Urban & S DEU. *Dist:* Williams & Wilkins.

Atlas of Human Anatomy, Latin Vol. 2: Thorax, Abdomen, Pelvis, Lower Limbs. Johannes Sobotta. Ed. by Jochen Staubesand. Ed. & Tr. by Anna N. Taylor. 11th ed. 1989. (ENG & LAT., Illus.). 416p. text 79.00 (0-683-07840-2) Lppncott W & W.

Atlas of Human Anatomy, '95. McMinn. 3rd ed. 1994. (0-7234-1977-9) Wolfe Publishing GBR. *Dist:* Mosby Inc.

Atlas of Human Cross-Sectional Anatomy: With CT & MR Images. Donald R. Cahill et al. 3rd ed. 1995. LC 94-42877. 328p. 275.00 (0-471-59165-3) Wiley.

Atlas of Human Limb Joints. J. Guyot. (Illus.). 1980. 252p. 165.00 (*0-387-10380-5*); 2nd ed. 1989. 258p. 298.00 (*0-387-51709-X*, 3579) Spr-Verlag.

Atlas of Human Paleopathology. Michael R. Zimmerman & Marc A. Kelley. 1982. LC 81-19878. 220p. 59.95 (*0-275-91386-4*, C1386, Praeger Pubs) Greenwood.

Atlas of Human Parasitology. Lawrence R. Ash & Thomas C. Orihel. 1997. LC 89-17988. 300.00 (*0-89189-436-5*); 4th ed. LC 97-2149. 424p. text 155.00 (*0-89189-399-7*, 16-7-004-00) Am Soc Clinical.

Atlas of Human Prenatal Morphogenesis. Jan E. Jirasek. 1983. text 211.50 (*0-89838-558-X*) Kluwer Academic.

Atlas of Human Sex Anatomy. Robert L. Dickinson. 1971. LC 50-5564. (Illus.). 382p. reprint ed. 54.50 (*0-88275-014-3*) Krieger.

Atlas of Human Tumor Cell Lines. Ed. by Robert J. Hay et al. 1994. LC 93-25709. (Illus.). 486p. text 69.95 (*0-12-333530-2*) Acad Pr.

Atlas of Hypertension. Peter F. Semple & George B. Lindop. 1992. (Encyclopedia of Visual Medicine Ser.). (Illus.). 98p. (C). lib. bdg. 77.95 (*1-85070-354-X*, Parthenon Pbng) CRC Pr.

Atlas of Hypertension. Peter F. Semple & George B. Lindop. 2nd ed. 1998. LC 97-29563. (Encyclopedia of Visual Medicine Ser.). (Illus.). 96p. lib. bdg. 85.95 (*1-85070-949-1*, Parthenon Pbng) CRC Pr.

Atlas of Hysteroscopy: A Guide to Diagnosis. Herbert Guedj et al. 1997. LC 95-25335. (Encyclopedia of Visual Medicine Ser.). (Illus.). 72p. lib. bdg. 77.95 (*1-85070-506-2*, Parthenon Pbng) CRC Pr.

Atlas of Immuno-Allergology: An Illustrated Primer for Health Care Professionals. Jacques Centner et al. Tr. by Christine De Weck from FRE. 3rd ed. 1995. LC 95-9994.Tr. of Atlas d'Immuno-Allergologie. (Illus.). 200p. text 54.00 (*0-88937-142-3*); (FRE., text 54.00 (*0-88937-143-1*); (GER., text 54.00 (*0-88937-144-X*); (SPA., text 54.00 (*0-88937-145-8*) Hogrefe & Huber Pubs.

Atlas of Immunology. Julius M. Cruse. 1998. LC 98-25823. (Illus.). 464p. 99.95 (*0-8493-9489-9*) CRC Pr.

***Atlas of Immunology.** Julius M. Cruse & Robert E. Lewis. 1999. xii, 451p. 89.95 (*3-540-64807-0*) Spr-Verlag.

Atlas of Implant Surgery. Han. 1999. text (*0-7216-5883-0*) Saunders.

Atlas of In-Vitro Fertilization. P. R. Brinsden. 2001. (Encyclopedia of Visual Medicine Ser.). (Illus.). 140p. 120.00 (*1-84214-025-6*, Parthenon Pbng) CRC Pr.

Atlas of Indocyanine Green Angiography. Elias Reichel & Carmen A. Puliafito. 1996. LC 96-6149. (Illus.). 120p. 98.50 (*0-89640-310-6*) Igaku-Shoin.

Atlas of Infections of the Nervous System. W. Edmund Farrar. 1993. (C). (gr. 13). (*1-56375-615-3*) Gower-Mosby.

Atlas of Infections of the Skin. Raza Aly & Howard Maibach. Ed. by Judy Fletcher. 1999. LC 98-74079. (Illus.). 352p. (C). text (*0-443-05587-4*) Church.

Atlas of Infectious Diseases. Sherwood L. Gorbach & David R. Stone. 1999. LC 99-31874. (Illus.). vii, 211p. text 129.00 (*0-7216-7032-6*) Harcourt.

***Atlas of Infectious Diseases**, Set. Ed. by Gerald L. Mandell. 1998. (Illus.). 2806p. (*0-443-07880-7*) Church GBR. *Dist:* Saunders.

Atlas of Infective Endocarditis: Diagnosis & Management. C. Ward. 1996. LC 95-745. (Encyclopedia of Visual Medicine Ser.). (Illus.). 96p. lib. bdg. 85.95 (*1-85070-462-7*, Parthenon Pbng) CRC Pr.

Atlas of Infertility. Grant W. Patton, Jr. & Robert W. Kistner. 1984. 368p. 99.00 (*0-316-69387-1*, Little Brwn Med Div) Lppncott W & W.

Atlas of Infertility: Diagnostic & Therapeutic Imaging. Amy S. Thurmond. 1997. 128p. 95.00 (*0-632-04305-9*) Blackwell Sci.

Atlas of Internal Fixation: Fractures of Long Bones: Classification, Statistical Analysis, Technique, Radiology. R. Orozco et al. 2000. (Illus.). 368p. 199.00 (*3-540-65621-9*) Spr-Verlag.

Atlas of Internal Medicine. Eugene Braunwald. 1998. LC 98-21633. (Illus.). 125.00 (*1-57340-118-8*) Current Med.

Atlas of Interpretive Radiographic Anatomy of the Dog & Cat. Arlene Coulson & Noreen Lewis. 1998. LC 00-68009. (Illus.). 672p. (C). text (*0-632-04078-5*) Blckwell Science GBR. *Dist:* Iowa U Pr.

Atlas of Interventional Cardiology. Jeffrey J. Popma et al. 1994. LC 94-1694. (Illus.). 368p. text 110.00 (*0-7216-3569-5*) Saunders.

Atlas of Interventional Pain Management. Steven D. Waldman. Ed. by Allan Ross. 1998. LC 97-48245. (Illus.). 408p. (C). text 175.00 (*0-7216-7577-8*) Saunders.

Atlas of Interventional Radiology. Constantin Cope et al. 1990. LC 65-40421. (Gower Bk.). (Illus.). 264p. (gr. 13). text (*0-397-44656-X*, GM0034) Gower-Mosby.

Atlas of Intraocular Tumors. George E. Sanborn et al. 1993. LC 92-49183. (Illus.). 192p. text 195.00 (*0-7216-2452-9*) Saunders.

Atlas of Intraocular Tumors. Jerry A. Shields & Carol L. Shields. 1999. LC 98-33786. 384p. text 169.00 (*0-7817-1916-X*) Lppncott W & W.

Atlas of Ischemic Heart Disease: Clinical & Pathologic Aspects. James T. Willerson & Jay N. Cohn. 1996. LC 96-29163. text (*0-443-07924-2*) Church.

Atlas of Kidney Biopsies 1997. (Illus.). lib. bdg. 600.95 (*0-8490-8152-1*); 1995. lib. bdg. 259.99 (*0-8490-7573-4*) Gordon Pr.

Atlas of Laparoscopic & Pelvic Surgery. N. Kadar. 1994. (Illus.). 288p. 150.00 (*0-86542-417-9*) Blackwell Sci.

Atlas of Laparoscopic Colon Surgery. Moises Jacobs et al. 1996. LC 96-15262. (Illus.). 256p. 129.00 (*0-683-30032-6*) Lppncott W & W.

Atlas of Laparoscopic Retroperitoneal Surgery. Louis R. Kavoussi & Jay T. Bishoff. 2000. LC 00-24805. (Illus.). 330p. text (*0-7216-8451-3*) Saunders.

Atlas of Laparoscopic Surgery. Garth H. Ballantyne. 1999. LC 99-31883. (Illus.). xv, 537p. text 95.00 (*0-7216-6326-5*) Saunders.

Atlas of Laparoscopic Surgery. Darzi. 1997. text 110.00 (*0-7020-2011-7*) Saunders.

Atlas of Laparoscopic Surgery. Ed. by Theodore N. Pappas et al. 1996. (Illus.). 328p. text 149.00 (*1-878132-20-2*) Current Med.

Atlas of Laryngology. Mary Hawkshaw et al. 1999. LC 99-33587. 130p. pap. 154.50 net. (*0-7693-0026-X*) Thomson Learn.

Atlas of Laser Voice Surgery. Jean Abitbol. 1995. LC 94-6939. (Illus.). 480p. pap. 250.00 (*1-56593-190-4*, 0569) Thomson Learn.

Atlas of Liver, Biliary Tract & Pancreas Surgery. L.H. Blumgart & M. F. Brennan. 1998. (Illus.). 500p. (*0-443-07660-X*) Church.

Atlas of Liver Disease. A. Burroughs & D. Patch. 2002. (Encyclopedia of Visual Medicine Ser.). (Illus.). 140p. 95.95 (*1-84214-012-4*, Parthenon Pbng) CRC Pr.

Atlas of Liver, Pancreas & Kidney Transplantation. Ed. by B. Kremer et al. 1994. LC 93-44990. (Illus.). 161p. 209.00 (*0-86577-513-3*) Thieme Med Pubs.

Atlas of Liver Pathology. D. G. Wight. 2nd ed. 1993. LC 93-17187. (Current Histopathology Ser.: Vol. 23). (Illus.). 189p. text 264.50 (*0-7923-8819-4*) Kluwer Academic.

Atlas of Liver Surgery. Christoph E. Broelsch-Houssin. 1993. (Surgical Practice Illustrated Ser.). (Illus.). 248p. text (*0-443-08733-4*) Church.

Atlas of Lower Limb Orthotic Practice. David N. Condie & M. S. Turner. 1997. LC 96-84199. (Illus.). 104p. (*0-412-72770-6*) E A GBR. *Dist:* OUP.

Atlas of Lumphoid Hyperplasia & Lymphoma. Judith A. Ferry & Nancy L. Harris. Ed. by Lesley Day. 1997. LC 96-29401. (Atlases in Diagnostic Surgical Pathology Ser.). (Illus.). 264p. text 175.00 (*0-7216-5907-1*) Saunders.

Atlas of Lung Cancer. Raymond Yesner. 1997. LC 97-10918. (Illus.). 304p. text 199.00 (*0-397-51646-0*) Lppncott W & W.

Atlas of Lung Infections. J. F. Costello et al. 1996. (Encyclopedia of Visual Medicine Ser.). (Illus.). 112p. (C). lib. bdg. 93.95 (*1-85070-456-2*, Parthenon Pbng) CRC Pr.

Atlas of Macaca Mulatta. Emil S. Szebenyi. 1975. LC 79-78611. (Illus.). 307p. 65.00 (*0-8386-7347-3*) Fairleigh Dickinson.

Atlas of Macular Diseases. John Donald M. Gass. 4th ed. 1996. (Illus.). 1120p. (C). (gr. 13). text 310.00 (*0-8151-3416-9*, 25531) Mosby Inc.

Atlas of Male Reproductive System Pathological. I. D. Ansell. 1985. (Current Histopathology Ser.). text 274.00 (*0-85200-327-7*) Kluwer Academic.

Atlas of Malignant Haematology: Cytology, Histology & Cytogenetics. Ghulam J. Mufti et al. 1996. 432p. sl. (*0-397-51572-3*); LC 96-221254. (Illus.). text 225.00 (*0-397-51400-X*) Lppncott W & W.

Atlas of Mammalian Chromosomes. T. C. Hsu & Kurt Benirschke. (Illus.). 1. 1967. LC 67-19307. 100p. ring bd. 90.00 (*0-387-03878-7*); Vol. 8. 1974. xl, 252p. ring bd. 39.00 (*3-540-06755-8*) Spr-Verlag.

Atlas of Mammalian Viruses. Erskine L. Palmer & Mary L. Martin. 1982. 163p. 98.00 (*0-8493-6628-3*, QR363, CRC Reprint) Franklin.

Atlas of Mammographic Positioning. Lucinda K. Prue. 1993. LC 92-49800. (Illus.). 176p. text 43.00 (*0-7216-3683-7*) Saunders.

Atlas of Mammography. Michelin Travel Publications Staff. 1997. 368p. text (*0-412-56020-8*) Chapman & Hall.

Atlas of Mammography: New Early Signs in Breast Cancer. Parvis Gamagami. 1996. LC 96-44527. (Illus.). 364p. 204.95 (*0-86542-481-0*) Blackwell Sci.

Atlas of Manipulative Techniques for the Cranium & Face. Alain Gehin. 1985. LC 85-80135. (Illus.). 269p. (C). 40.00 (*0-939616-02-5*) Eastland.

Atlas of Measurements in Ultrasound. Goldberg. 1990. 480p. 79.95 (*0-8151-3862-8*) Mosby Inc.

Atlas of Medical Helminthology & Protozology. P. L. Chiodini et al. 4th ed. 2000. LC 00-46272. (Illus.). 95p. Price not set. (*0-443-06268-4*) Harcrt Hlth Sci Grp.

Atlas of Medical Helminthology & Protozoology. Hugh C. Jeffrey & R. M. Leach. 2nd ed. 1975. LC 74-81190. (Illus.). 126p. (C). (*0-443-01222-9*) Church.

Atlas of Medical Helminthology & Protozoology. Peter L. Chiodini et al. 4th ed. 2000. LC 00-46272. (Illus.). (*0-443-06267-6*) Harcrt Hlth Sci Grp.

Atlas of Medical Parasitology. Viqar Zaman. 3rd ed. 1992. (Illus.). 250p. (*9971-69-161-2*) Sngapore Univ Pr SGP. *Dist:* Coronet Bks.

Atlas of Medicinal Plants of Middle America: Bahamas to Yucatan Julia F. Morton. fac. ed. 1981. (Illus.). 1454p. 239.95 (*0-398-04036-2*) C C Thomas.

Atlas of Metabolic Diseases. William L. Nyhan & Pinar T. Ozand. 1999. LC 97-69678. (Illus.). 688p. (*0-412-47960-5*) E A GBR. *Dist:* OUP.

Atlas of Microbiology of the Skin. Ed. by J. L. Lesher. 2000. LC 98-50050. (Encyclopedia of Visual Medicine Ser.). (Illus.). 134p. 97.95 (*1-85070-904-1*, Parthenon Pbng) CRC Pr.

Atlas of Micropathology of the Temporal Bone. Fred H. Linthicum, Jr. & Jorge A. Schwartzman. 1994. (Illus.). 104p. (C). text 125.00 (*1-56593-377-X*, 0755) Thomson Learn.

Atlas of Microscopic Artifacts & Foreign Materials. John S. Brooks & Giuseppe G. Pietra. Ed. by I-Tien Yeh. 1997. LC 96-50067. (Illus.). 224p. text (*0-89640-331-9*) Igaku-Shoin.

Atlas of Microscopy of Medicinal Plants, Culinary Herbs, & Spices. Betty P. Jackson. 1990. 71.00 (*0-8493-7705-6*, SB) CRC Pr.

Atlas of Microscopy Techniques. H. Aebi. 1999. 260p. 115.00 (*0-12-044415-1*) Acad Pr.

Atlas of Microsurgical Composite Tissue Transplantation. Donald Serafin. 1995. LC 94-31118. (Illus.). 576p. text 285.00 (*0-7216-2870-2*) Saunders.

Atlas of Microvascular Surgery: Anatomy of Operative Techniques. Berish Strauch et al. 1993. LC 92-401. 560p. 199.00 (*0-86577-436-6*) Thieme Med Pubs.

Atlas of Microvascular Surgery in Head & Neck Reconstruction. Hayden. 1990. (Illus.). 350p. 85.00 (*0-8016-1682-4*) Mosby Inc.

Atlas of Migraine. Xavier Lataste. Date not set. (Encyclopedia of Visual Medicine Ser.). (Illus.). 96p. 85.00 (*1-85070-001-X*, Parthenon Pbng) CRC Pr.

Atlas of Mineralized Bone Histology. H. H. Malluche & Marie-Claude Faugere. 1986. (Illus.). xiii, 136p. 208.00 (*3-8055-4201-1*) S Karger.

Atlas of Minimal Access Surgical Anatomy. Alfred Cuschieri & Fiona Carter. 1997. LC 99-53181. (Illus.). 320p. text 149.00 (*0-397-51459-X*) Lppncott W & W.

Atlas of Minor Oral Surgery. Harry Dym & Orrett E. Ogle. 2000. 301p. text 88.75 (*0-7216-7977-3*) Saunders.

Atlas of Minor Surgery. Ian D. Cracknell & Michael Mead. 1998. LC 96-26057. (C). text (*0-443-05304-9*) Church.

Atlas of Mouse Development. Kaufman. 1992. (Illus.). 512p. 211.00 (*0-12-402035-6*) Acad Pr.

Atlas of MR Pathology. Deborah L. Durham. Ed. by Lisa Durham. 1996. LC 96-8867. 208p. text 42.00 (*0 7216 6416 4*) Saunders.

Atlas of Multiple Pregnancy: Biology & Pathology. Geoffrey A. Machin & Louis G. Keith. 1999. LC 97-20395. (Encyclopedia of Visual Medicine Ser.). (Illus.). 216p. lib. bdg. 147.95 (*1-85070-918-1*, Parthenon Pbng) CRC Pr.

Atlas of Musculoskeletal Imaging. Thomas L. Pope et al. 1999. LC 98-27858. (Illus.). 552p. 89.00 (*0-86577-695-4*) Thieme Med Pubs.

Atlas of Myocardial Infarction. D. S. Dymond. 2nd ed. 2002. (Encyclopedia of Visual Medicine Ser.). (Illus.). 140p. 95.95 (*1-84214-024-8*, Parthenon Pbng) CRC Pr.

Atlas of Myocardial Infraction: And Related Cardiovascular Complications. Duncan S. Dymond. 1994. LC 94-21976. (Encyclopedia of Visual Medicine Ser.). 136p. lib. bdg. 93.95 (*1-85070-505-4*, Parthenon Pbng) CRC Pr.

Atlas of Neonatal Anatomy. Jean-Pierre Lassau. 1982. (Illus.). 180p. (gr. 13). 73.00 (*0-89352-139-6*, MA139) Mosby Inc.

Atlas of Neonatal Brain Sonography. Paul Govaert & Linda S. De Vries. 1997. (Clinics in Developmental Medicine Ser.: Vol. 141). (Illus.). 300p. (C). (*1-898683-09-3*) Mc Keith Pr GBR. *Dist:* Cambridge U Pr.

***Atlas of Neonatal EEG Monitoring.** L. De Vries & L. Hellstrom-Westas. 2002. (Illus.). 150p. lib. bdg. 139.95 (*1-84214-111-2*, Parthenon Pbng) CRC Pr.

Atlas of Neonatal Electroencephalography. Janet E. Stockard-Pope et al. 2nd ed. 1991. 416p. text 129.00 (*0-88167-851-1*) Lppncott W & W.

Atlas of Neonatology. David A. Clark. 1999. LC 99-11887. (C). text (*0-7216-7636-7*) Saunders.

Atlas of Neuroanatomy: With Systems Organization & Case Correlations. Joseph J. Warner. 2000. (Illus.). 696p. text 145.00 (*0-7506-7250-1*) Buttrwrth-Heinemann.

Atlas of Neuroanatomy with Radiologic Correlation & Pathologic Illustration: Surface & Sectional, with CT Scanning Correlation. William B. Dublin & Arthur Dublin. 1982. LC 79-50199. (Illus.). 252p. (C). 62.50 (*0-87527-204-5*) Green.

Atlas of Neurofunctional Systems. H. J. Kretschmann. 1998. cd-rom 99.00 (*0-86577-812-4*) Thieme Med Pubs.

Atlas of Neuroradiologic Anatomy & Variants. J. Randy Jinkins. 1998. LC 99-40671. (Illus.). xvi, 732p. text 199.00 (*0-7817-1652-7*) Lppncott W & W.

Atlas of Neuroradiology. Matthew J. Kuhn. 1992. (Illus.). 256p. (gr. 13). text (*1-56375-008-2*) Gower-Mosby.

Atlas of Neuroradiology. Steven J. Willing. 1995. (Illus.). 560p. text 145.00 (*0-7216-4219-5*) Saunders.

Atlas of Neurosurgical Anatomy. J. L. Fox. 1989. (Illus.). 208p. 352.00 (*0-387-96838-5*) Spr-Verlag.

Atlas of Neurosurgical Techniques, Vol. 1. John M. Tew, Jr. & Harry R. Van Loveren. 1993. LC 92-49097. text 230.00 (*0-7216-3560-1*) Saunders.

Atlas of Normal & Variant Angiographic Anatomy. Saadoon Kadir. 1990. (Illus.). 544p. text 135.00 (*0-7216-2894-X*) Saunders.

Atlas of Normal Endourologic Appearances. David Albala. 1998. LC 97-42492. 224p. text 149.00 (*0-397-51676-2*) Lppncott W & W.

Atlas of Normal Human Skin. W. Montagna et al. 1994. (Illus.). 384p. 181.00 (*0-387-97769-4*) Spr-Verlag.

Atlas of Normal Radiographic Anatomy. Richard S. Snell & Alvin C. Wyman. 1976. LC 75-36765. 40.00 (*0-316-80207-7*, Little Brwn Med Div) Lppncott W & W.

Atlas of Normal Roentgen Variants That May Simulate Disease. Theodore E. Keats. 6th ed. 1995. LC 97-223793. (Illus.). 1040p. (C). (gr. 13). text 250.00 (*0-8151-4951-4*, 26574) Mosby Inc.

Atlas of Normal Roentgen Variants That May Simulate Disease. Theodore E. Keats. 6th ed. 1996. (Illus.). 1040p. (*84-8174-318-6*) Mosby-Doyma Libros ESP. *Dist:* Mosby Inc.

Atlas of Normal Roentgen Variants That May Simulate Disease. Theodore E. Keats & Mark W. Anderson. 7th ed. 2001. LC 00-51974. (Illus.). xx, 1207p. (*0-323-01322-8*) Mosby Inc.

Atlas of Nuclear Medicine. Marc Coel & Jimmy Leung. Ed. by Lisette Bralow. 1996. 720p. text 235.00 (*0-7216-3578-4*) Saunders.

Atlas of Nuclear Medicine. Douglas Van Nostrand & Sheldon Baum. 1988. LC 65-9541. (Illus.). text 95.00 (*0-397-50789-5*, Lippnctt) Lppncott W & W.

Atlas of Nuclear Medicine Imaging. Sheldon Baum. 2nd ed. 1994. (Illus.). 232p. (C). text 235.00 (*0-8385-0449-3*, A0449-7) McGraw-Hill Prof.

Atlas of Nursing: Atlas de la Enfermera. Ana M. Cimorra. 1987. (SPA., Illus.). 86p. pap. 19.95 (*0-7859-4943-7*) Fr & Eur.

Atlas of Nutritional Support Techniques. John L. Rombeau. 1989. 51.00 (*0-316-75575-3*, Little Brwn Med Div) Lppncott W & W.

Atlas of Obesity & Weight Control. G. A. Bray. 2001. (Illus.). 150p. lib. bdg. 87.95 (*1-84214-049-3*, Parthenon Pbng) CRC Pr.

Atlas of Obstetrical Ultrasonography. 304p. (*0-7131-4428-9*) E A GBR. *Dist:* Routldge.

Atlas of Oncology. Ronald W. Raven. 1994. (Encyclopedia of Visual Medicine Ser.). (Illus.). 238p. lib. bdg. 93.95 (*1 85070-363-9*, Parthenon Pbng) CRC Pr.

Atlas of Open Knee Surgery. D. G. Poitout. 1995. 200p. 381.95 (*0-412-58550-2*) Chapman & Hall.

Atlas of Operative Andrology: Selected Operations on Male Genitalia & Their Accessory Glands. Alpay Kelami. 1980. 202p. 142.35 (*3-11-008180-6*) De Gruyter.

Atlas of Operative Microneurosurgery Vol. 2: Tumors. John M. Tew, Jr. & Harry R. Van Loveren. 3rd ed. 2000. (Illus.). 335p. text 295.00 (*0-7216-5730-3*) Saunders.

Atlas of Operative Neurosurgery. Frederic B. Meyer. Ed. by Richard Zorab. 1998. LC 98-18407. (Illus.). 480p. (C). text (*0-443-08951-5*, M2039) Church.

Atlas of Ophthalmic Surgery: Cornea Gloucorna Lens, Vol. II. George I. Spaeth & Douglas D. Koch. Ed. by Klaus Heilmann & David Patton. 1987. (Illus.). 272p. text 179.00 (*0-86577-180-4*) Thieme Med Pubs.

Atlas of Ophthalmology. G. K. Krieglstein et al. 2000. (Illus.). 432p. 70.00 (*3-540-64454-7*) Spr-Verlag.

Atlas of Opthalmic Surgery. Jaffe. 2nd ed. 1995. text (*0-7234-2188-9*) Wolfe Publishing GBR. *Dist:* Mosby Inc.

Atlas of Oral & Maxillofacial Surgery. Ed. by David A. Keith. 1992. (Illus.). 346p. text 175.00 (*0-7216-2369-7*) Saunders.

Atlas of Oral & Maxillofacial Surgery. Wong. 1997. text (*0-7216-3392-7*) Saunders.

Atlas of Oral Implantology. Ed. by A. N. Cranin et al. 1993. LC 93-781. (Illus.). 342p. text 99.00 (*0-86577-449-8*) Thieme Med Pubs.

Atlas of Oral Implantology. A. Norman Cranin et al. 2nd ed. 1999. (Illus.). 416p. (C). text (*1-55664-552-X*) Mosby Inc.

Atlas of Oral Pathology. R. D. Lucas & John W. Eveson. 1985. (Current Histopathology Ser.). text 355.00 (*0-85200-328-5*) Kluwer Academic.

Atlas of Orbital Tumors. Jerry A. Shields & Carol L. Shields. 1999. LC 98-39677. 256p. text 169.00 (*0-7817-1917-8*) Lppncott W & W.

Atlas of Orbitocranial Surgery. Ed. by Bryant A. Toth et al. 1999. 351p. (*1-85317-376-2*) Martin Dunitz.

Atlas of Organ Transplantation. Ed. by M. Wayne Flye. 1994. LC 93-44256. text 165.00 (*0-7216-4611-5*) Saunders.

Atlas of Orthopaedic Pathololology. Peter G. Bullough. 3rd ed. 1996. text 189.00 (*0-7234-2236-2*) Mosby Inc.

Atlas of Orthopaedic Surgical Exposures. Christopher Jordan. 2000. LC 00-25384. 149.00 (*0-86577-776-4*) Thieme Med Pubs.

Atlas of Orthopedic Pathology. Wold et al. 1990. (Illus.). 320p. text 195.00 (*0-7216-2911-3*) Saunders.

Atlas of Orthotics Assistive Devices. American Academy of Orthopaedic Surgeons Staff. 3rd ed. 1996. (Illus.). 720p. (C). (gr. 13). text 134.00 (*0-8151-0052-3*, 25689) Mosby Inc.

Atlas of Osteoarthritis. Kenneth D. Brandt. 2001. LC 00-46482. (Encyclopedia of Visual Medicine Ser.). (Illus.). 160p. 87.95 (*1-85070-494-5*, Parthenon Pbng) CRC Pr.

Atlas of Osteoporosis. J. C. Stevenson & M. S. Marsh. 2nd ed. 1999. LC 99-35361. (Encyclopedia of Visual Medicine Ser.). (Illus.). 110p. lib. bdg. 88.95 (*1-85070-987-4*, Parthenon Pbng) CRC Pr.

Atlas of Otologic Surgery. Newton Coker & Herman A. Jenkins. 1999. LC 00-53800. (Illus.). xii, 679p. (C). text 175.00 (*0-7216-2216-X*) Saunders.

Atlas of Otology. Pulec. 2000. 226p. text 199.95 (*0-7693-0011-1*) Singular Publishing.

Atlas of Outpatient & Office Surgery. Robert B. Benjamin. 2nd ed. 1993. (Illus.). 290p. 89.50 (*0-8121-1540-6*) Lppncott W & W.

***Atlas of Pain Injection Techniques.** Therese O'Connor & Steven E. Abram. 2001. (Illus.). 251p. (*0-443-06380-X*) Church GBR. *Dist:* Saunders.

Atlas of Pain Management. D. B. Carr. 2001. (Encyclopedia of Visual Medicine Ser.). (Illus.). 120p. lib. bdg. 89.95 (*1-85070-564-X*, Parthenon Pbng) CRC Pr.

Atlas of Pain Management Injection Techniques. Steven D. Waldman. Date not set. LC 99-597401. (Illus.). 405p. text (*0-7216-8504-8*) Saunders.

Atlas of Palpatory Anatomy of the Lower Limbs: A Manual of the Surface. Serge Tixa. 1998. LC 98-55688. (Illus.). 220p. text 49.95 (*0-07-065357-7*) McGraw-Hill Prof.

Atlas of Pancreatic Exocrine Tumors: Morphology, Biology, & Diagnosis, with an International Guide for Tumor Classification. Ed. by P. M. Pour et al. 1994. LC 94-9950. 314p. 239.00 (*0-387-70129-X*) Spr-Verlag.

Atlas of Pancreatic Surgery. Ed. by Howard A. Reber. 2000. (Illus.). 300p. (C). (gr. 13). text 79.95 (*0-8151-7160-9*, 22453) Mosby Inc.

Atlas of Paramedic Skills. Bryan E. Bledsoe. 1987. (Illus.). 272p. pap. 66.67 (*0-89303-444-4*) P-H.

Atlas of Paranasal Sinus Surgery. Frank N. Ritter & Michael H. Fritsch. 1992. LC 91-7018. (Illus.). 296p. 115.00 (*0-89640-194-4*) Igaku-Shoin.

Atlas of Parasitic Pathology. Karlhanns Salfelder et al. 1992. LC 92-49790. (Current Histopathology Ser.: Vol. 20). 192p. (C). text 265.00 (*0-7923-8998-0*) Kluwer Academic.

Atlas of Parkinson's Disease & Related Disorders. G. D. Perkin. 1998. LC 97-37265. (Encyclopedia of Visual Medicine Ser.). (Illus.). 96p. lib. bdg. 85.95 (*1-85070-943-2*, Parthenon Pbng) CRC Pr.

Atlas of Pathological Computer Tomography: Computer Tomography of Neck, Chest, Spine & Limbs, Vol. 3. L. Jeanmart et al. 1983. (Illus.). 194p. 304.00 (*0-387-11439-4*) Spr-Verlag.

Atlas of Pathological Computer Tomography Vol. 1: Cranio-Cerebral Computed Tomography, Set. A. Wackenheim et al. 1980. (Illus.). 130p. 294.00 (*0-387-09879-8*) Spr-Verlag.

Atlas of Pediatric & Adolescent Gynecology. Morton A. Stenchever. 1998. LC 97-167386. 250p. (C). pap. text 129.00 (*0-8385-0318-7*, Apple Lange Med) McGraw.

Atlas of Pediatric & Fetal Ultrasound. Harris L. Cohen & Carlos J. Sivit. 2000. LC 99-88758. (Illus.). 656p. text 179.00 (*0-8385-8864-6*) McGraw-Hill Prof.

Atlas of Pediatric Clinical Diseases. Teresita A. Laude & Binita R. Shah. 1999. LC 99-19073. text 79.00 (*0-7216-7639-1*) Saunders.

Atlas of Pediatric Dermatology. S. B. Mallory. 2001. 150p. 95.00 (*1-84214-045-0*, Parthenon Pbng) CRC Pr.

Atlas of Pediatric Electroencephalography. Warren T. Blume & Masako Kaibara. 2nd ed. 1998. LC 98-29865. (Illus.). 416p. text 159.00 (*0-7817-1434-6*) Lppncott W & W.

Atlas of Pediatric Endoscopy. Winter. 1997. text (*0-7216-9489-6*) Saunders.

Atlas of Pediatric Gastrointestinal Disease. Ronald E. Kleinman et al. 1997. (Illus.). 238p. incl. cd-rom (*1-55009-038-0*) DEKR.

Atlas of Pediatric Infectious Diseases. Russell W. Steele et al. 1997. LC 97-8979. (Encyclopedia of Visual Medicine Ser.). 112p. 97.95 (*1-85070-914-9*, Parthenon Pbng) CRC Pr.

Atlas of Pediatric Neurosurgery. William R. Cheek. Ed. by Richard Zorab. 1996. 192p. text 165.00 (*0-7216-5138-0*) Saunders.

Atlas of Pediatric Neurosurgical Techniques: Atlas de Technicas Quirurgicas en Neurocirugia Infantil. F. J. Villarejo. Tr. by D. Applewhite from SPA. 1984. (Illus.). xii, 224p. 129.75 (*3-8055-3455-8*) S Karger.

Atlas of Pediatric Ophthalmic Surgery. Joseph H. Calhoun et al. 1987. (Illus.). 320p. text 115.00 (*0-7216-1104-4*) Saunders.

Atlas of Pediatric Ophthalmology & Strabismus Surgery. Monte A. Del Monte. 1992. (Illus.). 232p. text (*0-443-08708-3*) Church.

Atlas of Pediatric Orthopaedic Surgery Mihran O. Tachdjian. 1994. (Illus.). 1664p. text 335.00 (*0-7216-3733-7*) Saunders.

Atlas of Pediatric Orthopaedic Surgery. Raymond T. Morrissy & Stuart L. Weinstein. 3rd ed. 2000. LC 00-42045. 928p. text 225.00 (*0-7817-2095-8*) Lppncott W & W.

Atlas of Pediatric Otolaryngology. Charles D. Bluestone & Sylvan E. Stool. 1994. LC 93-40737. (Illus.). text 185.00 (*0-7216-3711-6*) Saunders.

Atlas of Pediatric Physical Diagnosis. Davis & Basil J. Zitelli. 3rd ed. 1997. LC 96-46308. (Illus.). 912p. (C). (gr. 13). text 110.00 (*0-8151-9930-9*, 27081) Mosby Inc.

Atlas of Pediatric Surgery. Keith W. Ashcraft & Thomas M. Holder. 1994. LC 93-1848. 336p. text 153.00 (*0-7216-3720-5*) Saunders.

Atlas of Pediatric Urologic Surgery. Frank Hinman, Jr. 1994. LC 94-4205. (Illus.). text 198.00 (*0-7216-4231-4*) Saunders.

Atlas of Pelvic Anatomy & Gynecologic Surgery. Michael S. Baggish & Mickey M. Karram. 2001. LC 2001-31120. (Illus.). 512p. (*0-7216-8318-5*) Saunders.

Atlas of Pelvic Surgery. Clifford R. Wheeless, Jr. 2nd ed. 1988. LC 87-3933. (Illus.). 475p. text 139.00 (*0-8121-1080-3*) Lppncott W & W.

Atlas of Perinatology. Silvio Aladjem & Dharmapuri Vidyasagar. 1982. (Illus.). 508p. text 180.00 (*0-7216-1080-3*) Saunders.

Atlas of Peripheral Nerve Disorders. Rosalind King. 1999. 232p. (*0-340-58666-4*) E A GBR. *Dist:* OUP.

Atlas of Peripheral Nerve Surgery. David G. Kline & Alan R. Hudson. 2000. LC 00-57417. (Illus.). 235p. text 235.00 (*0-7216-7988-9*) Harcrt Hlth Sci Grp.

Atlas of Phlebography of the Lower Limbs. Jacques Chermet. 1982. 256p. text 226.00 (*90-247-2525-9*) Kluwer Academic.

Atlas of Phonomicrosurgery & Other Endolaryngeal Procedures for Benign & Malignant Disease. Steven M. Zeitels. 2001. LC 00-30050. (Illus.). 274p. text 295.00 (*0-7693-0131-2*) Singular Publishing.

Atlas of Podiatric Anatomy see Mercado Atlas of Foot Anatomy

Atlas of Podiatric Surgery: Forefoot Surgery, Vol. 1. O. A. Mercado. 1980. (Illus.). 290p. 75.00 (*0-940542-03-X*) Carolando.

Atlas of Porcelain Restorations. H. Denissen et al. 1990. 94p. text (*1-57235-012-1*) Piccin Nuova.

Atlas of Posterior Fundus Changes in Pathologic Myopia. T. Tokoro. 1998. LC 98-3242. (Illus.). 218p. 180.00 (*4-431-70225-3*) Spr-Verlag.

Atlas of Practical Proctology. Alexander Neiger. 2nd enl. rev. ed. 1990. LC 89-71714. 170p. text 98.00 (*0-920887-76-7*) Hogrefe & Huber Pubs.

Atlas of Preimplantation Genetic Diagnosis: An Illustrated Textbook & Reference for Clinicians. Y. Verlinsky & A. Kuliev. 2000. LC 00-32387. (Encyclopedia of Visual Medicine Ser.). (Illus.). 174p. 149.95 (*1-85070-760-X*, Parthenon Pbng) CRC Pr.

Atlas of Prenatal Development in Conceptions with Chromosomal Anomalies. Dorothy Warburton et al. 1991. (Oxford Monographs on Medical Genetics: No. 27). (Illus.). 120p. 89.50 (*0-19-505145-9*) OUP.

Atlas of Prenatal Rat Brain Development. Joseph Altman & Shirley Bayer. 1994. (Illus.). 664p. 152.95 (*0-8493-8993-3*) CRC Pr.

Atlas of Preoperative Staging & Surgical Treatment Options for Rectal Cancer. Thomas M. Heimann & Arnold Szporn. LC 96-31454. 1997. (Illus.). 128p. 74.00 (*0-89640-326-2*); 1996. (*4-260-14326-3*) Igaku-Shoin.

Atlas of Primary Eyecare Procedures. Casser & Murray Fingeret. 2nd ed. 1997. LC 96-40178. (Illus.). 494p. (C). text 115.00 (*0-8385-0257-1*, A-0257-4) McGraw-Hill Prof.

Atlas of Primate Gross Anatomy. Daris R. Swindler & Charles D. Wood. 1982. LC 81-19350. 392p. reprint ed. lib. bdg. 52.00 (*0-89874-321-4*) Krieger.

Atlas of Procedures in Anesthesia & Critical Care. John F. Butterworth, IV. 1991. (Illus.). 251p. text 41.00 (*0-7216-2916-4*) Saunders.

Atlas of Procedures in Respiratory Medicine. Warren M. Gold et al. 2001. LC 2001-49543. (Illus.). 445p. (C). text (*0-7216-4086-9*) Saunders.

Atlas of Prostatic Diseases. R. S. Kirby. (EVM Ser.). (Illus.). 96p. 1997. LC 96-52992. lib. bdg. 93.95 (*1-85070-764-2*, K1078); 2nd ed. 1999. LC 99-21825. lib. bdg. 96.95 (*1-85070-096-6*) CRC Pr (Parthenon Pbng).

Atlas of Protein Sequence & Structure. Ed. by M. O. Dayhoff. LC 65-29342. Vol. 5, Suppl. No. 1. 1973. pap. 5.00 (*0-912466-04-9*); Vol. 5, Suppl. No. 3. 1979. pap. 25.00 (*0-912466-07-3*) Natl Biomedical.

Atlas of Psoriasis. L. Fry. 1992. (Encyclopedia of Visual Medicine Ser.). (Illus.). 111p. lib. bdg. 77.95 (*1-85070-410-4*, Parthenon Pbng) CRC Pr.

Atlas of Pulmonary Surgical Pathology. Howard D. Colby et al. 1990. (Illus.). 400p. text 205.00 (*0-7216-2893-1*) Saunders.

Atlas of Radiation Histopathology. David C. White. 1975. LC 75-17867. (AEC Technical Information Center Ser.). 236p. fiche 9.00 (*0-87079-235-0*, TID-26676) DOE.

Atlas of Radiographic Anatomy of the Dog & Cat. Horst Schebitz & Helmut Wilkins. 4th ed. 1987. (Illus.). 224p. text 180.00 (*0-03-012122-1*) Saunders.

Atlas of Radiography for Sports Injuries. Jock Anderson. 2000. (Illus.). 94p. pap. 39.95 (*0-07-470888-0*) McGraw-Hill Prof.

Atlas of Radiologic Anatomy. Lothar Wicke. 5th ed. 1993. (Illus.). 310p. pap. text 37.50 (*0-8121-1677-1*) Lppncott W & W.

Atlas of Radiologic Imaging. Ed. by E. George Kassner. 1989. (Illus.). 688p. (gr. 13). text (*0-397-44661-6*, GM0073) Gower-Mosby.

Atlas of Radiologic Imaging, Unit 4: Slide Atlas of Radiology of Adult Cardiac Disease. Lisa Diethelm & Benigno Soto. 1989. 54p. (gr. 13). (*0-397-46415-0*, GM0148) Gower-Mosby.

Atlas of Radiologic Measurement. Theodore E. Keats & Christopher Sistrom. 7th ed. 2001. LC 00-60938. (Illus.). 637p. 125.00 (*0-323-00161-0*) Mosby Inc.

Atlas of Rectal Endosonography. J. Beynon et al. 1991. (Illus.). 111p. 130.00 (*0-387-19690-0*) Spr-Verlag.

Atlas of Refractive Eye Surgery. Leo D. Bores. 1992. LC 92-21895. (Illus.). 624p. 250.00 (*0-86542-152-8*) Blackwell Sci.

Atlas of Regional Anatomy of the Brain Using MRI: With Functional Correlations. J. C. Tamraz & Y. G. Comair. 2000. LC 99-44535. (Illus.). 352p. 199.00 (*3-540-64099-1*) Spr-Verlag.

Atlas of Regional & Free Flaps for Head & Neck Reconstruction. Mark L. Urken. 1995. suppl. ed. 599.00 incl. sl. (*0-7817-0245-3*) Lppncott W & W.

Atlas of Regional & Free Flaps for Head & Neck Reconstruction. Mark L. Urken et al. 1994. LC 94-15911. (Illus.). 390p. text 299.00 (*0-7817-0197-X*) Lppncott W & W.

Atlas of Regional Anesthesia. David L. Brown. Ed. by Allan Ross. 2nd ed. 1998. LC 98-18198. (Illus.). 300p. (C). text 125.00 (*0-7216-7004-0*) Saunders.

Atlas of Regional Anesthesia. Jordan Katz. 2nd ed. 1994. (Illus.). 238p. (C). pap. text 135.00 (*0-8385-0452-3*, A0452-1, Apple Lange Med) McGraw.

Atlas of Removable Partial Denture Design. Russel J. Stratton & Frank J. Wiebelt. 1988. (Illus.). 336p. text 58.00 (*0-86715-190-0*) Quint Pub Co.

Atlas of Renal Pathology. William Kern et al. Ed. by Allan Ross. 1999. LC 98-18406. (Illus.). 285p. (C). text 179.00 (*0-7216-7067-9*) Saunders.

Atlas of Renal Ultrasonography. W. Charles O'Neill. 2000. LC 00-58857. (Illus.). 255p. text 112.25 (*0-7216-8913-2*) Saunders.

Atlas of Replantation & Transplantation of Teeth. Jens O. Andreasen. 1992. (Illus.). 304p. text 142.00 (*0-7216-6711-2*) Saunders.

Atlas of Reproductive Endocrinology. Daniel R. Mishell. 1998. LC 98-9640. (Atlas of Clinical Gynecology Ser.: Vol. 3). (Illus.). 250p. (C). text 129.00 (*0-8385-0319-5*) McGraw-Hill Prof.

***Atlas of Reproductive Function.** P. Motta. 2002. (Encyclopedia of Visual Medicine Ser.). (Illus.). 150p. 89.95 (*1-84214-121-X*, Parthenon Pbng) CRC Pr.

Atlas of Rheumatology. Gene G. Hunder. 1998. LC 97-43307. (Illus.). (*1-57340-116-1*) Appleton & Lange.

Atlas of Rheumatology. Gene G. Hunder. 1998. (Illus.). 146.95 (*0-632-04435-7*) Blackwell Sci.

Atlas of Rhinoplasty: Open & Endonasal Approaches. Gilbert Aiach. Tr. by Azita Madjiji et al. 1995. (Illus.). 206p. text 175.00 (*0-942219-64-3*) Quality Med Pub.

Atlas of Roentgenographic Measurement. Theodore E. Keats. 6th ed. 1990. (Illus.). 592p. (C). (gr. 13). text 115.00 (*0-8151-5657-X*, 20391) Mosby Inc.

Atlas of Roentgenographic Anatomy of the Newborn & Infant Skull. Charles N. Chasler. 1972. LC 76-96981. (Illus.). 228p. 25.00 (*0-87527-028-X*) Green.

Atlas of Schizophrenia. Ed. by M. D. Stefan & R. A. Murray. 2001. LC 2001-52033. (Encyclopedia of Visual Medicine Ser.). (Illus.). 100p. lib. bdg. 87.95 (*1-85070-074-5*, Parthenon Pbng) CRC Pr.

Atlas of Scrotal Ultrasound. B. Martin. 1993. (Illus.). 200p. 180.00 (*0-387-53309-5*) Spr-Verlag.

Atlas of Sectional Anatomy. Philomena McGrath & P. Mills. 2nd ed. 1985. (Illus.). viii, 238p. 71.50 (*3-8055-4060-4*) S Karger.

Atlas of Sectional Human Anatomy: Frontal, Sagittal, & Horizontal Planes. J. G. Koritke & H. Sick. 2nd ed. 1988. LC 88-20618. (Illus.). 346p. 175.00 (*0-683-04748-5*) Lppncott W & W.

Atlas of Serous Fluid Cytopathology. Arthur I. Spriggs & Michael M. Boddington. 1989. (C). text 304.50 (*0-7462-0091-9*) Kluwer Academic.

Atlas of Shoulder Surgery. Fu & Imhoff. 1997. 320p. (C). text 225.00 (*0-8385-0446-9*, A-0446-3) McGraw-Hill Prof.

Atlas of Shoulder Surgery. Richard J. Hawkins. 1995. (Illus.). 352p. (C). (gr. 13). text 130.00 (*0-8151-4196-3*, 20043) Mosby Inc.

Atlas of Sigmoidoscopy & Cytoscopy. Ed. by B. E. Miller & L. Chase. 2001. LC 00-68673. (Encyclopedia of Visual Medicine Ser.). (Illus.). 104p. lib. bdg. 87.95 (*1-85070-927-0*, Parthenon Pbng) CRC Pr.

Atlas of Skeletal Dysplasias. Ruth Wynne-Davies et al. 1985. (Illus.). 646p. text (*0-443-03047-2*) Church.

Atlas of Skeletal Muscle Pathology. Janice R. Anderson. 1985. LC 85-2956. text 309.00 (*0-85200-325-0*) Kluwer Academic.

Atlas of Skin Cancer. Anthony Du Vivier. 1991. (Illus.). 256p. (gr. 13). text (*0-397-44836-8*, GM0107) Gower-Mosby.

Atlas of Skin Pathology. R. M. Marks et al. 1986. (Current Histopathology Ser.). text 268.50 (*0-85200-324-2*) Kluwer Academic.

Atlas of Skin Repair. J. Zoltan. 1984. 304p. 139.25 (*3-8055-3511-2*) S Karger.

Atlas of Sleep Medicine. Ed. by John W. Shepard. 1991. (Illus.). 240p. 150.00 (*0-87993-509-X*) Futura Pub.

Atlas of Sleep Medicine in Infants & Children. Stephen H. Sheldon. 1998. LC 98-37769. 13p. 150.00 (*0-87993-423-9*) Futura Pub.

Atlas of Small Animal Reconstructive Surgery. Michael M. Pavletic. Ed. by Ray Kersey. 2nd ed. 1999. LC 98-37965. (Illus.). 380p. text 65.00 (*0-7216-7077-6*) Saunders.

Atlas of Small Animal Surgery. Robert T. DeHoff. 1999. text 75.00 (*0-7216-6787-2*) Saunders.

Atlas of Small Animal Surgery. Ira M. Gourley. 1992. (Illus.). 336p. (C). (gr. 13). text (*1-56375-015-5*) Gower-Mosby.

Atlas of Soft Tissue Tumors. Jeanne M. Meis & Franz M. Enzinger. 1993. (C). VHS, disk 500.00 (*1-56815-019-9*) Mosby Inc.

Atlas of Sperm Morphology. Marilyn M. Adelman & Eileen M. Cahill. 1989. LC 88-7867. (Illus.). 126p. 75.00 (*0-89189-275-3*) Am Soc Clinical.

Atlas of Spinal Operations. Ed. by R. Bauer et al. 1994. LC 93-37755. (Illus.). 229.00 (*0-86577-496-X*) Thieme Med Pubs.

Atlas of Spinal Surgery. Donlin M. Long & Paul C. McAfee. 1992. (Illus.). 464p. text 199.00 (*0-683-05149-0*) Lppncott W & W.

Atlas of Spinal Surgery. Robert B. Winter et al. 1995. LC 94-29593. (Illus.). 624p. text 165.00 (*0-7216-2958-X*) Saunders.

Atlas of Spine Imaging. Renfrew. 2002. text (*0-7216-9071-8*) Saunders.

***Atlas of Spontaneous & Chemically Induced Tumors in Nonhuman Primates.** Ed. by S. Takayama et al. 2000. viii, 154p. 298.25 (*3-8055-7159-3*) S Karger.

Atlas of Sputum Cytology. R. Djukanovic & P. Sterk. 2002. (Encyclopedia of Visual Medicine Ser.). (Illus.). 144p. lib. bdg. 89.95 (*1-84214-005-1*, Parthenon Pbng) CRC Pr.

Atlas of Steroid Structure, Vol. 2. Ed. by William L. Duax et al. 1983. LC 75-22419. 760p. 150.00 (*0-306-66102-0*, Kluwer Plenum) Kluwer Academic.

Atlas of Strabismus Surgery: Comprehensive Management of Motility Disorders. Helveston. 4th ed. 1992. (Illus.). 475p. text 79.00 (*0-8016-2144-5*) Mosby Inc.

Atlas of Stroke. P. F. Semple. 1998. LC 97-25927. (Encyclopedia of Visual Medicine Ser.). (Illus.). 96p. lib. bdg. 93.95 (*1-85070-738-3*, S2535, Parthenon Pbng) CRC Pr.

Atlas of Stroke. P. F. Semple & R. L. Sacco. 2nd ed. 1999. LC 99-14700. (Illus.). 108p. lib. bdg. 93.95 (*1-85070-082-6*, Parthenon Pbng) CRC Pr.

Atlas of Suction Assisted Lipectomy in Body Contouring. Frederick M. Grazer. 1991. (Illus.). 410p. text (*0-443-08625-7*) Church.

Atlas of Surgery: Soft Tissue, Endocrine Glands. Cameron. 1992. (gr. 13). 250.00 (*1-55664-253-9*) Mosby Inc.

Atlas of Surgery of the Spine. Howard S. Anderson & Lee H. Riley. 1998. 500p. text 249.00 (*0-7817-1219-X*) Lppncott W & W.

Atlas of Surgery of the Upper Urinary Tract. R. Hohenfellner & R. Wammack. 1998. (Illus.). 224p. (*0-443-05137-2*) Church.

Atlas of Surgical Anatomy & Surgical Approaches to the Hand. Yu Han-Liang & Strauch. 1999. 512p. (C). (gr. 13). text 200.00 (*0-8151-7927-8*, 24184) Mosby Inc.

Atlas of Surgical Anatomy for General Surgeons. Stephen W. Gray & John E. Skandalakis. 1988. LC 83-16883. (Illus.). 408p. 169.95 (*0-683-03733-1*) Lppncott W & W.

Atlas of Surgical Anatomy of the Hand. Eduardo A. Zancolli & Elbio P. Cozzi. 1991. (Illus.). 745p. text (*0-443-08176-X*) Church.

Atlas of Surgical Approaches to the Bones & Joints of the Dog & Cat. D. L. Piermattei. 3rd ed. 1992. LC 92-25778. (Illus.). 336p. text 61.00 (*0-7216-1012-9*) Saunders.

Atlas of Surgical Exposure of the Upper & Lower Extremity. Raoul Tubiana et al. 2000. (Illus.). 400p. (*1-85317-875-6*) Martin Dunitz GBR. *Dist:* Blackwell Sci.

Atlas of Surgical Exposures of the Lower Extremities. Alain C. Masquelet et al. 1993. 424p. text 269.00 (*0-397-58325-7*) Lppncott W & W.

Atlas of Surgical Exposures of the Upper Extremity. Raoul Tubiana et al. 1990. (Illus.). 360p. text 249.00 (*0-397-58316-8*) Lppncott W & W.

Atlas of Surgical Management of Anorectal Malformations. A. Pena. 1992. (Illus.). 104p. 120.00 (*0-387-97067-3*, 3064) Spr-Verlag.

Atlas of Surgical Management of Male Infertility. Anthony J. Thomas, Jr. & Harris M. Nagler. 1995. (Illus.). 152p. (*0-89640-282-7*) Lppncott W & W.

Atlas of Surgical Neurotology. Robert K. Jackler. 1995. (Illus.). 320p. (C). (gr. 13). text 221.00 (*0-8151-4920-4*, 24379) Mosby Inc.

Atlas of Surgical Oncology. Kirby I. Bland et al. 1995. LC 93-40050. (Illus.). 688p. text 165.00 (*0-7216-4223-3*) Saunders.

Atlas of Surgical Oncology. Ed. by John M. Daly & Blake Cady. 1992. LC 92-18763. text 129.00 (*0-8016-1272-1*) Mosby Inc.

Atlas of Surgical Oncology. Ed. by John H. Donohue et al. 1995. LC 94-18165. (Illus.). 336p. 135.00 (*0-86542-422-5*) Blackwell Sci.

Atlas of Surgical Oncology: Fundamental Procedures Ed. by Everette D. Sugarbaker. 1983. Vol. I. 200p. 112.00 (*0-8493-6365-9*, RD651); Vol. II. 320p. 176.00 (*0-8493-6366-7*, RD651) Franklin (CRC Reprint).

Atlas of Surgical Operations. Robert M. Zollinger, Jr. & Robert M. Zollinger. 6th ed. 1990. 473p. text 130.00 (*0-02-432070-6*, Macmillan Coll) P-H.

Atlas of Surgical Operations. Robert M. Zollinger. 7th ed. 1992. LC 92-49984. (Illus.). 484p. text 179.00 (*0-07-105417-0*) McGraw-Hill Prof.

Atlas of Surgical Orthodontic Corrective Dentistry. Bell. 1999. text (*0-7216-1487-6*) Saunders.

***Atlas of Surgical Pathology of the Brain.** L. Danaila et al. Ed. by Silvia Cinca. pap. text 39.99 (*1-930387-04-0*) Moonfall Pr VA.

Atlas of Surgical Pathology of the Colon, Rectum, & Anus. Jeremy R. Jass et al. 1989. (Illus.). 256p. text (*0-443-03738-8*) Church.

Atlas of Surgical Pathology of the Male Reproductive Tract. Jae Y. Ro et al. Ed. by Lesley Day. 1996. (Illus.). 240p. text 159.00 (*0-7216-5284-0*) Saunders.

Atlas of Surgical Techniques. Ed. by Marvin L. Gliedman. 1990. 548p. text 49.00 (*0-07-023491-4*) McGraw-Hill Prof.

Atlas of Surgical Techniques. Steven G. Economou & Tasia S. Economou. Ed. by Lisette Bralow. 2nd ed. 1996. (Illus.). 704p. 185.00 (*0-7216-1611-9*) Saunders.

Atlas of Surgical Techniques for the Hand & Wrist. Raoul Tubiana et al. 1998. 500p. text 259.00 (*0-397-51505-7*) Lppncott W & W.

Atlas of Synovial Fluid Cytopathology. A. J. Freemont & J. Denton. 1991. (C). text 276.50 (*0-7462-0090-0*) Kluwer Academic.

Atlas of Techniques in Breast Surgery. Susan M. Love et al. 1995. (Illus.). 176p. text 139.00 (*0-397-50946-4*) Lppncott W & W.

Atlas of Temporal Bone & Lateral Skull Base Surgery. Mario Sanna et al. 1995. LC 95-17700. 189p. 149.00 (*0-86577-591-5*) Thieme Med Pubs.

Atlas of the Canine Brain. O. S. Adrianov & T. A. Mering. Ed. by E. F. Domino. Tr. by E. Ignatieff. 1964. LC 64-63010. (Illus.). 349p. 95.00 (*0-916182-01-0*) NPP Bks.

Atlas of the Cellular Structure of the Human Nervous System. H. Hillman & D. Jarman. 1991. 228p. text 136.00 (*0-12-348770-6*) Acad Pr.

Atlas of the Cerebral Sulci. Michio Ono. 1990. (Illus.). 232p. text 199.00 (*0-86577-362-9*) Thieme Med Pubs.

Atlas of the Difficult Airway. Ed. by Martin L. Norton. 2nd ed. 1996. (Illus.). 256p. (C). (gr. 13). text 110.00 (*0-8151-6433-5*, 24216) Mosby Inc.

Atlas of the Diseases of the Mammary Gland: Atlas der Brustdruesenerkrankungen. I. Degrell. 1976. (Illus.). 186p. 121.75 (*3-8055-2219-3*) S Karger.

Atlas of the Dog & Cat Cytology. Ed. by Rose Raskin & Dennis J. Meyer. 1999. LC 00-49270. (Illus.). xiv, 430p. text (*0-7216-6335-4*) Saunders.

Atlas of the Hematology of the Laboratory Rat. Atsuhiko Hasegawa & Kazuhisa Furuhama. 1998. LC 98-9363. 186p. 169.50 (*0-444-82893-1*) Elsevier.

Atlas of the Human Body. Takeo J. Takahashi. 1994. LC 94-4162. (Illus.). 144p. pap. 25.00 (*0-06-273297-8*, Harper Ref) HarperCollins Pubs.

Atlas of the Human Brain. Ed. by Juergen K. Mai et al. 1997. LC 97-10171. (Illus.). 328p. pap. text 89.95 (*0-12-465361-8*) Morgan Kaufmann.

Atlas of the Human Brain. Ed. by Jurgen K. Mai et al. 1997. LC 97-10171. (Illus.). 328p. text 135.00 (*0-12-465360-X*) Morgan Kaufmann.

Atlas of the Human Brain. Jurgen K. Mai et al. deluxe ed. 1998. (Illus.). 328p. pap. text 109.95 incl. cd-rom (*0-12-465362-6*) Acad Pr.

Atlas of the Human Brain Stem & Spinal Cord. James D. Fix. 2nd ed. 1987. 180p. (C). spiral bd. 60.00 (*0-87189-858-6*) Aspen Pub.

Atlas of the Human Brainstem. Ed. by George T. Paxinos & Xu F. Huang. 1995. LC 95-15203. (Illus.). 149p. (C). spiral bd. 99.00 (*0-12-547615-9*) Acad Pr.

Atlas of the Human Embryo & Fetus: A Photographic Review of Human Prenatal Development. J. E. Jirasek. 2000. LC 00-33639. (Encyclopedia of Visual Medicine Ser.). (Illus.). 144p. lib. bdg. 108.95 (*1-85070-659-X*, Parthenon Pbng) CRC Pr.

***Atlas of the Human Skeleton.** Matt Hutchinson et al. 2001. LC 00-710320. v, 55p. (*0-8053-4988-X*) Benjamin-Cummings.

Atlas of the Human Skull. H Wayne Sampson et al. 1991. LC 90-11248. (Illus.). 216p. pap. 34.95 (*0-89096-488-2*) Tex A&M Univ Pr.

Atlas of the Liver. Ed. by Willis C. Maddrey. 2nd ed. 2000. LC 99-34180. (Gastroenterology & Hepatology Ser.: Vol. 1). (Illus.). 320p. text 124.95 (*1-57340-134-X*) Current Med.

Atlas of the Menopause. M. I. Whitehead et al. 1993. (Encyclopedia of Visual Medicine Ser.). (Illus.). 93p. (C). lib. bdg. 77.95 (*1-85070-388-4*, Parthenon Pbng) CRC Pr.

Atlas of the Menopause. M. I. Whitehead & A. Cooper. 2nd ed. 2001. (Encyclopedia of Visual Medicine Ser.). (Illus.). 120p. lib. bdg. 89.95 (*1-85070-948-3*, Parthenon Pbng) CRC Pr.

Atlas of the Neuropathology of HIV Infection. Ed. by Francoise Gray. 1993. LC 92-48766. (Illus.). 314p. (C). text 135.00 (*0-19-854776-5*) OUP.

Atlas of the Newborn. G. C. Di Renzo. 2001. 200p. 98.00 (*1-84214-044-2*, Parthenon Pbng) CRC Pr.

Atlas of the Newborn. N. O'Doherty. 1985. text 124.00 (*0-85200-924-0*) Kluwer Academic.

Atlas of the Newborn Arnold J. Rudolph. 1997. (Illus.). 1200p. incl. cd-rom (*1-55009-062-3*) DEKR.

Atlas of the Peripheral Ocular Fundus. William L. Jones & Robert W. Reidy. 1985. (Illus.). 214p. 100.00 (*0-7506-9450-5*) Buttrwrth-Heinemann.

Atlas of the Peripheral Ocular Fundus. William L. Jones. 2nd ed. 1998. LC 97-26003. (Illus.). 328p. text 115.00 (*0-7506-9050-X*) Buttrwrth-Heinemann.

Atlas of the Peripheral Retina. Frank C. Bell & William J. Stenstrom. 1983. (Illus.). 244p. text 170.00 (*0-7216-1669-0*) Saunders.

Atlas of the Prenatal Mouse Brain. Uta B. Schambra et al. 1991. LC 91-32888. (Illus.). 327p. text 99.00 (*0-12-622585-0*) Acad Pr.

Atlas of the Rabbit Brain & Spinal Cord. Judy W. Shek et al. 1985. (Illus.). xvi, 140p. 309.75 (*3-8055-3814-6*) S Karger.

***Atlas of the Skin & Systemic Disease.** Mark G. Lebwohl. 2nd ed. 2001. (Illus.). 255p. (*0-443-06539-X*) Church GBR. *Dist:* Saunders.

Atlas of the Surgical Techniques of Oliver H. Beahrs. Oliver H. Beahrs et al. 1985. LC 84-1231. (Illus.). 332p. text 110.00 (*0-7216-1602-X*) Saunders.

Atlas of the Ultrastructure of Human Oocytes: A Guide for Assisted Reproduction. Ed. by Mahmoud A. El-Shafie et al. 2000. (Encyclopedia of Visual Medicine Ser.). (Illus.). 188p. 115.95 (*1-85070-404-X*, Parthenon Pbng) CRC Pr.

Atlas of the Visible Human Female. Victor M. Spitzer & David G. Whitlock. 1998. (Illus.). 524p. (C). text 100.00 (*0-7637-0892-5*) Jones & Bartlett.

Atlas of Therapeutic Proctology. Emilio De Los Rios. 1984. 185p. text 165.00 (*0-7216-3036-7*) Saunders.

Atlas of Thoracic Surgery. Harold C. Urschel, Jr. & Joel D. Cooper. 1995. (Surgical Practice Illustrated Ser.). (Illus.). 240p. text (*0-443-08539-0*) Church.

Atlas of Thoracic Surgery. Harold C. Urschel, Jr. 2nd ed. 2000. (C). text (*0-443-06543-8*) Church.

Atlas of Thoracoscopic Surgery. Ed. by William T. Brown. 1994. LC 93-36925. text 167.00 (*0-7216-3793-0*) Saunders.

Atlas of Thoracoscopic Surgery. Mark J. Krasna & Michael J. Mack. 1993. (Illus.). LC 93-34146. 130.00 (*0-942219-45-7*); 216p. 175.00 (*1-57626-048-8*, QMP) Quality Med Pub.

***Atlas of Three-Dimensional Echocardiography.** Ed. by Navin C. Nanda & Vincent L. Sorrell. 2001. LC 2001-51142. (*0-87993-486-7*) Futura Pub.

Atlas of Thumb & Finger Reconstruction. Guillermo Loda. 1999. LC 99-12945. xi, 195p. (*3-13-101191-2*) Icon Lrning Systs.

Atlas of Tissue Doppler Echocardiography TDE. Ed. by H. J. Nesser et al. 1995. (Illus.). 178p. 155.00 (*3-7985-1020-2*) Spr-Verlag.

Atlas of Topographical Anatomy of the Brain & Surrounding Structures. Wolfgang Seeger. 1985. (Illus.). 544p. 95.00 (*0-387-81851-0*) Spr-Verlag.

Atlas of Topographical Anatomy of the Brain & Surrounding Structures: For Neurosurgeons, Neuroradiologists & Neuropathologists. Wolfgang Seeger. 1985. 544p. 80.00 (*3-211-81851-0*) Spr-Verlag.

Atlas of Topographical Anatomy of the Brain & Surrounding Structures for Neurosurgeons, Neuroradiologists, & Neuropathologists. Wolfgang Seeger. 1978. LC 77-16683. (Illus.). 544p. 179.00 (*0-387-81447-7*) Spr-Verlag.

Atlas of Topographical & Applied Human Anatomy, Set. Eduard Pernkopf. Ed. by Werner Platzer. Tr. by Harry Monsen from GER. 3rd enl. rev. ed. 1990.Tr. of Atlas der Topographischen und Angewamdten Anatomie Des Menschen. (Illus.). 804p. 295.00 (*0-683-06854-7*) Lppncott W & W.

Atlas of Topographical & Applied Human Anatomy Vol. 1: Head & Neck, 1. Eduard Pernkopf. Ed. by Werner Platzer. Tr. by Harry Monsen from GER. 3rd enl. rev. ed. 1989.Tr. of Atlas der Topographischen und Angewnadten Anatomie Des Menschen. (Illus.). 380p. 175.00 (*0-683-06852-0*) Lppncott W & W.

Atlas of Topographical & Applied Human Anatomy Vol. II: Thorax, Abdomen & Extremities, 2. Eduard Pernkopf. Ed. by Werner Platzer. Tr. by Harry Monson from GER. 3rd enl. rev. ed. 1989. (Illus.). 424p. text 175.00 (*0-683-06853-9*) Lppncott W & W.

Atlas of Total Hip Replacement. Douglas E. Padgett & Paul M. Pellicci. 1995. LC 95-9614. (Orthopaedic Surgical Skills Ser.). (Illus.). text (*0-443-08902-7*) Church.

Atlas of Total Knee Surgery. Windsor. 1998. (C). text (*0-443-08929-9*) Church.

Atlas of Transesophageal Color Doppler Echocardiography & Intraoperative Imaging. r. DeSimone et al. 1994. LC 94-31740. (Illus.). 204p. 155.00 (*0-387-57938-9*) Spr-Verlag.

Atlas of Transesophageal Echocardiography. Navin C. Nanda & Michael J. Domanski. 1998. LC 97-33648. 408p. text 189.00 (*0-683-06320-0*) Lppncott W & W.

Atlas of Transesophageal Echocardiography in Clinical Practice. Jos R. Roelandt et al. 1991. (Illus.). 224p. (gr. 13). (*0-397-44640-3*, GM0064) Gower-Mosby.

Atlas of Transvaginal Color Doppler. Ed. by Asim Kurjak & S. Kupesic. 2nd ed. 2000. LC 99-54490. (Encyclopedia of Visual Medicine Ser.). (Illus.). 472p. lib. bdg. 149.95 (*1-85070-093-1*, Parthenon Pbng) CRC Pr.

Atlas of Transvaginal Color Doppler: The Current State of the Art. Ed. by Asim Kurjak. 1994. LC 93-35739. (Encyclopedia of Visual Medicine Ser.). (Illus.). 370p. lib. bdg. 159.95 (*1-85070-459-7*, Parthenon Pbng) CRC Pr.

***Atlas of Transvaginal Surgery.** Shlomo Raz. 2nd ed. (Illus.). 300p. text (*0-7216-9113-7*) Saunders.

Atlas of Trauma Management: The First Hour. B. A. Landon & J. D. Goodall. 1994. (Encyclopedia of Visual Medicine Ser.). (Illus.). 151p. lib. bdg. 77.95 (*1-85070-411-2*, Parthenon Pbng) CRC Pr.

Atlas of Tumor Pathology of the Fischer Rat. Ed. by Sherman F. Stinson et al. 1990. 496p. lib. bdg. 299.00 (*0-8493-5462-5*, SF910) CRC Pr.

Atlas of Tumors of the Facial Skeleton. Ed. by J. Prein et al. 1986. (Illus.). 162p. 287.00 (*0-387-16167-8*) Spr-Verlag.

Atlas of Two-Dimensional Echocardiography in Congenital Cardiac Defects. G. J. Van Mill et al. 1986. pap. text 111.00 (*0-89838-783-3*) Kluwer Academic.

Atlas of Ultrasonography in Obstetrics & Gynecology. Ed. by Asim Kurjak. 1992. (Encyclopedia of Visual Medicine Ser.). (Illus.). 236p. (C). lib. bdg. 159.95 (*1-85070-362-0*, Parthenon Pbng) CRC Pr.

Atlas of Ultrasound & Ductal Echography of the Breast. Michael Halliwell & Michel Teboul. 1995. (Illus.). 336p. 357.95 (*0-632-03329-0*) Blackwell Sci.

Atlas of Ultrasound Color Flow Imaging. Barry B. Goldberg et al. 1997. 304p. (*1-85317-063-1*) Martin Dunitz GBR. *Dist:* Mosby Inc.

Atlas of Upper Respiratory & Head & Neck Infections. Itzhak Brook. 2nd ed. 2000. LC 99-462026. ix, 223p. (*1-57340-140-4*) Current Med.

Atlas of Uro-Oncology. Ed. by R. S. Kirby. 2001. (Encyclopedia of Visual Medicine Ser.). (Illus.). 120p. lib. bdg. 87.95 (*1-85070-614-X*, Parthenon Pbng) CRC Pr.

Atlas of Urodynamics. Ed. by Michael B. Chancellor & Jerry G. Blaivas. 1996. (Illus.). 336p. 129.00 (*0-683-01640-7*) Lppncott W & W.

Atlas of Urologic Imaging. Daniel Hoffman et al. 1995. LC 94-41745. 69.00 (*0-683-04084-7*) Lppncott W & W.

Atlas of Urologic Surgery. Frank Hinman, Jr. Ed. by Stephanie Donley. 2nd ed. 1998. LC 96-38015. 1008p. text 195.00 (*0-7216-6404-0*) Saunders.

Atlas of Urosurgical Anatomy. Frank Hinman, Jr. 1993. (Illus.). 560p. text 155.00 (*0-7216-3955-0*) Saunders.

Atlas of Valvular Heart Disease: Clinical & Pathologic Aspects. James T. Willerson et al. 1997. LC 97-26912. text (*0-443-07953-6*) Church.

Atlas of Vascular Anatomy of the Skeleton & Spinal Cord. Henry V. Crock. 9th ed. 1996. 328p. (*1-85317-302-9*) Martin Dunitz GBR. *Dist:* Mosby Inc.

Atlas of Vascular Surgery: Basic Techniques & Exposures. Robert B. Rutherford. 1993. (Illus.). 288p. text 91.00 (*0-7216-2956-3*) Saunders.

Atlas of Vascular Surgery: Operative Procedures. Kenneth Ouriel & Robert B. Rutherford. Ed. by Lisette Bralow. 1998. LC 97-22033. (Illus.). 384p. text 95.00 (*0-7216-6994-8*) Saunders.

Atlas of Veterinary Hematology: Blood & Marrow of Domestic Animals. John W. Harvey. 2001. LC 00-63569. (Illus.). 228p. (*0-7216-6334-6*) Saunders.

Atlas of Veterinary Surgery. J. Hickman et al. 3rd ed. 1992. (Illus.). 384p. (C). pap. 98.95 (*0-8464-4165-9*) Beekman Pubs.

Atlas of Visual Fields. Budenz. 1997. LC 96-47934. 368p. text 115.00 (*0-397-51741-6*) Lppncott W & W.

Atlas of Vitreo-Retinal Surgery. Travis Meredith. 1998. LC 98-22343. (Illus.). 256p. (C). text 175.00 (*0-8151-2834-7*, 30963) Mosby Inc.

Atlas of Vitreous Biomicroscopy. Charles L. Schepens et al. 1999. LC 99-20089. 168p. text 84.99 (*0-7506-7052-5*) Buttrwrth-Heinemann.

Atlas of Vulval Diseases: A Combined Dermatological, Gynecological & Venereological Approach. Michele Leibowitch et al. 1997. 208p. (*1-85317-431-9*) Martin Dunitz GBR. *Dist:* Mosby Inc.

Atlas of Whole Body MRI. R. H. Mohiaddin & D. B. Longmore. 1992. (Series in Radiology). (C). text 191.50 (*0-7923-8974-3*) Kluwer Academic.

Atlas of Whole Chromosome Paint Probes: Normal Patterns & Utility for Abnormal Cases. Syed M. Jalal et al. 1995. (Illus.). 150p. lab manual ed. 49.50 (*0-9627865-4-3*) Mayo Fndtn Med Ed & Res.

Atlas on the Surgical Anatomy of Laryngeal Cancer. John A. Kirchner. 1998. LC 97-45063. 200p. pap. 175.00 (*1-56593-776-7*, 1510) Thomson Learn.

Atlas Pediatric Oral & Maxillofacial Surgery. Kaban. 1999. text (*0-7216-5866-0*) Saunders.

Atlas Special. Wilcox. 1995. (Illus.). 192p. text 250.00 (*0-7216-6392-3*) Saunders.

Atlas/Text Clinical Imaging. Weir. 1997. text (*0-7234-2555-8*) Wolfe Publishing GBR. *Dist:* Mosby Inc.

Atman Project: A Transpersonal View of Human Development. Ken Wilber. 1980. (Illus.). 204p. pap. 14.00 (*0-8356-0730-5*, Quest) Theos Pub Hse.

Atmosphere-Surface Exchange of Particulate & Gaseous Pollutants (1974) Proceedings. Ed. by Rudolf J. Engelmann & George A. Sehmel. 1976. LC 75-38716. (ERDA Symposium Ser.). 1000p. pap. 33.00 (*0-87079-138-9*, CONF-740921); fiche 9.00 (*0-87079-139-7*, CONF-740921) DOE.

Atmospheric Aerosol: Source-Air Quality Relationships. Ed. by Edward S. Macias & Phillip K. Hopke. 1981. LC 81-10960. (ACS Symposium Ser.: No. 167). 359p. 43.95 (*0-8412-0646-5*) Am Chemical.

Atmospheric Nuclear Tests: Environmental & Human Consequences. NATO Staff. Ed. by Charles S. Shapiro. 1998. LC 97-38993. (NATO ASI Ser.: Vol. 35). (Illus.). 296p. 130.00 (*3-540-63804-0*) Spr-Verlag.

Atomic Absorption Spectrometry in Occupational & Environmental Health Practice: Determination of Individual Elements, Vol. II. Ed. by Dimiter L. Tsalev. 1984. 312p. 110.00 (*0-8493-5604-0*, QP534, CRC Reprint) Franklin.

Atomic Components of Thought. John R. Anderson & Christian J. Lebiere. 1998. 400p. (*0-8058-2816-8*); LC 97-51871. pap. 39.95 (*0-8058-2817-6*) L Erlbaum Assocs.

Atomic Spectroscopy in Japan. Ed. by K. Fuwa et al. 1981. (Journal Spectrochimica Acta Ser.: No. 36). 160p. pap. 19.25 (*0-08-028731-X*, Pergamon Pr) Elsevier.

Atoms, Radiation & Radiation Protection. James E. Turner. 1991. 346p. text 49.95 (*0-07-105320-4*) McGraw-Hill Med Pub.

Atoms Within Us. Ernest Borek. rev. ed. 1980. LC 80-19010. 272p. text 60.00 (*0-231-04386-4*); pap. text 21.00 (*0-231-04387-2*) Col U Pr.

Atopic Dermatitis: From Pathogenesis to Treatment. Ed. by Donald Leung. 1996. (Medical Intelligence Unit Ser.). (Illus.). 234p. (C). pap. 89.95 (*0-412-10191-2*) Chapman & Hall.

Atopic Palmoplantar Eczema. H. J. Schwanitz. 1988. (Illus.). 150p. 79.95 (*0-387-17863-5*) Spr-Verlag.

Atopy Syndrome in the Third Millennium. Ed. by Brunello Wuthrich. 1999. LC 99-14130. (Current Problems in Dermatology Ser.: Vol. 28). (Illus.). 200p. 174.00 (*3-8055-6655-7*) S Karger.

ATPases. Ed. by Thomas A. Pressley & Sandra Sabatini. 1996. (Journal: Vol. 22, No. 5-6). (Illus.). iv, 168p. pap. 92.25 (*3-8055-6398-1*) S Karger.

ATRA Annual in Therapeutic Recreation. Ed. by Cynthia Carruthers. (Orig.). Vol. 3. 1992. 95p. pap. 10.50 (*1-889435-01-5*); Vol. 4. 1993. 114p. pap. text 19.00 (*1-889435-04-X*); Vol. 5. 1994. 109p. pap. text 19.00 (*1-889435-06-6*); Vol. 6. 1996. 88p. pap. text 19.00 (*1-889435-08-2*) Am Therapeutic.

ATRA College & University Therapeutic Recreation Programs Directory. Ed. by Glenn Kastrinos. 1995. 24p. (Orig.). pap. text 10.00 (*1-889435-07-4*) Am Therapeutic.

Atrial & Ventricular Fibrillation: Mechanisms & Device Therapy. Ed. by Maurits A. Allessie & Martin Fromer. 1996. LC 96-29416. (Bakken Research Center Ser.: Vol. 9). (Illus.). 448p. 98.00 (*0-87993-650-9*) Futura Pub.

Atrial Arrhythmias: State of the Art. Ed. by John P. DiMarco & Eric N. Prystowsky. 1994. (American Heart Association Monographs). (Illus.). 448p. 70.00 (*0-87993-604-5*) Futura Pub.

Atrial Fibrillation. J. Rawles. 1991. (Illus.). 243p. 129.00 (*0-387-19699-4*) Spr-Verlag.

Atrial Fibrillation: A Treatable Disease? Ed. by J. H. Kingma et al. 1992. LC 92-49554. (Developments in Cardiovascular Medicine Ser.: Vol. 139). text 138.00 (*0-7923-2008-5*) Kluwer Academic.

Atrial Fibrillation: Facts from Yesterday - Ideas for Tomorrow. Ed. by Henri E. Kulbertus et al. 1994. (Bakken Research Center Ser.: Vol. 8). (Illus.). 176p. 55.00 (*0-87993-097-7*) Futura Pub.

Atrial Fibrillation: Mechanisms & Management. Rodney H. Falk. 2nd ed. 1997. LC 97-24977. 544p. text 115.00 (*0-397-51767-X*) Lppncott W & W.

Atrial Fibrillation after Cardiac Surgery. Ed. by Jonathan S. Steinberg. 2000. LC 99-47095. (Developments in Cardiovascular Medicine Ser.: Vol. 222). 169p. 125.00 (*0-7923-8655-8*) Kluwer Academic.

Atrial Fibrillation for the Clinician. Ed. by Francis D. Murgatroyd & A. John Camm. 1995. LC 95-176. (Clinical Approaches to Tachyarrhythmias Ser.: Vol. 4). (Illus.). 152p. 19.00 (*0-87993-614-2*) Futura Pub.

Atrial Flutter: Advances in Mechanisms & Management. Ed. by Albert L. Waldo & Paul Touboul. 1996. (Illus.). 496p. 109.00 (*0-87993-635-5*) Futura Pub.

Atrial Flutter & Fibrillation: From Basic to Clinical Applications. Ed. by Nadir Saoudi et al. 1998. LC 98-12981. (Illus.). 392p. 85.00 (*0-87993-661-4*) Futura Pub.

Atrial Tachycardia. Michael D. Lesh & Franz X. Roithinger. 1999. LC 99-40659. (Clinical Approaches to Tachyarrhythmias Ser.: Vol. 11). (Illus.). 80p. pap. 19.00 (*0-87993-442-5*) Futura Pub.

Atrioventricular Conduction in Congenital: Heart Disease - Surgical Anatomy. H. Kurosawa & Anton E. Becker. 1987. 272p. 349.00 (*0-387-70015-3*) Spr-Verlag.

ATSDR Public Health Assessment Guidance Manual. Edward J. Calabrese. 1992. 336p. lib. bdg. 75.00 (*0-87371-857-7*, L857) Lewis Pubs.

Attachment Across the Life Cycle. Ed. by Colin M. Parkes et al. 1993. 336p. (C). pap. 31.95 (*0-415-05651-9*, B0621) Routledge.

***Attachment & Family Systems: Conceptual, Empirical & Therapeutic Relatedness.** Phyllis Erdman & Tom Caffery. 2002. (C). text 39.95 (*1-58391-351-3*) Brunner-Routledge.

Attachment & Psychopathology. Ed. by Leslie Atkinson & Kenneth J. Zucker. 1997. LC 96-49001. 328p. text 40.00 (*1-57230-191-0*) Guilford Pubns.

Attachment & the Therapeutic Process: Essays in Honor of Otto Allen Will, Jr. M.D. Ed. by James L. Sacksteder et al. 1987. 500p. (C). 55.00 (*0-8236-0447-0*) Intl Univs Pr.

Attachment Disorganization. Ed. by Judith Y. Solomon & Carol George. 1999. LC 99-23365. 420p. text 45.00 (*1-57230-480-4*, CO480) Guilford Pubns.

Attachment in the Preschool Years: Theory, Research, & Intervention. Ed. by Mark T. Greenberg et al. 1993. LC 89-49657. (John D. & Catherine T. MacArthur Foundation Series on Mental Health & Development). (Illus.). 552p. 39.95 (*0-226-30629-1*); xx, 528p. (C). pap. text 23.95 (*0-226-30630-5*) U Ch Pr.

Attachment of Organisms to the Gut Mucosa. Ed. by Edgar C. Boedeker. 1984. Vol. I. 240p. 137.00 (*0-8493-5286-X*, QR171); Vol. II. 272p. 150.00 (*0-8493-5287-8*) Franklin (CRC Reprint).

Attachment Research & Psychoanalysis Pt. 1: Theoretical Considerations. Ed. by Diamond & Blatt. 1999. (Psychoanalytic Inquiry Ser.: Vol. 19, No. 4). pap. 20.00 (*0-88163-923-0*) Analytic Pr.

Attachment Research & Psychoanalysis Pt. 2: Clinical Implications. Ed. by Diamond & Blatt. 1999. (Psychoanalytic Inquiry Ser.: Vol. 19, No. 5). pap. 20.00 (*0-88163-922-2*) Analytic Pr.

Attachment Theory & Psychoanalysis. Peter Fonagy. 2001. LC 2001-32089. 261p. pap. 30.00 (*1-892746-70-0*) Other Pr LLC.

Attack Asthma: How to Conquer Environmental Illnesses & Allergies Without Drugs. William Vayda. 1995. 170p. (Orig.). pap. (*0-85091-626-7*) Lothian Pub AUS. *Dist:* Seven Hills Bk.

Attack on the Self: Adolescent Behavioral Disturbances & Their Treatment. Derek Miller. 1994. LC 93-74780. 352p. pap. 45.00 (*1-56821-214-3*); 1986. LC 86-17418. 340p. 55.00 (*0-87668-927-6*) Aronson.

***Attacked by Poison Ivy: A Psychological Understanding.** Ann Belford Ulanov. 2001. LC 2001-32606. (Jung on the Hudson Book Ser.). 224p. pap. 18.95 (*0-89254-058-3*) Nicolas-Hays.

Attempted Suicide: Its Social Significance & Effects, 4. Erwin Stengel et al. 1982. LC 82-6181. (Maudsley Monographs). 136p. reprint ed. lib. bdg. 55.00 (*0-313-23573-2*, STAT, Greenwood Pr) Greenwood.

Attempts to Understand Metastasis Formation Pt. 1, Vol. 213: Metastasis-Related Molecules. U. Gunthert & W. Birchmeier. 2nd ed. 1996. (Illus.). 304p. 149.50 (*3-540-60680-7*) Spr-Verlag.

Attempts to Understand Metastasis Formation Pt. 2: Regulatory Factors. U. Gunthert & W. Birchmeier. 1996. (Illus.). 330p. 149.50 (*3-540-60681-5*) Spr-Verlag.

Attempts to Understand Metastasis Formation Pt. 3: Therapeutic Approaches for Metastasis Treatment, Vol. 213/3. U. Gunthert & W. Birchmeier. 1996. (Illus.). 290p. 143.00 (*3-540-60682-3*) Spr-Verlag.

Attending to Children. (*0-340-52741-2*) E A GBR. *Dist:* Routldge.

Attention - Selection, Awareness, & Control: A Tribute to Donald Broadbent. Ed. by Alan D. Baddeley & Lawrence Weiskrantz. 1995. (Illus.). 454p. pap. text 50.00 (*0-19-852374-2*) OUP.

Attention & Avoidance: Strategies in Coping with Aversiveness. Ed. by Heinz W. Krohne. 1993. LC 92-48721. (Illus.). 380p. 56.00 (*0-88937-108-3*) Hogrefe & Huber Pubs.

Attention & Brain Function. Risto Naatanen. 1992. 494p. text 89.95 (*0-8058-0984-8*) L Erlbaum Assocs.

Attention & Interpretation. Wilfred R. Bion. 1995. LC 84-45115. 150p. pap. 30.00 (*1-56821-714-5*) Aronson.

Attention & Performance VIII. Ed. by Raymond S. Nickerson. 1980. LC 80-23850. (Attention & Performance Ser.). 864p. 180.00 (*0-89859-038-8*) L Erlbaum Assocs.

Attention & Performance XIII: Motor Representation & Control. Ed. by M. Jeannerod. 1990. 888p. 175.00 (*0-8058-0565-6*) L Erlbaum Assocs.

Attention & Performance XIV: Synergies in Experimental Psychology, Artificial Intelligence, & Cognitive Neuroscience a Silver Jubilee Volume. Ed. by David E. Meyer & Sylvan Kornblum. 1993. LC 93-211150. (Attention & Performance, Ser.: Vol. 14). (Illus.). 937p. 82.50 (*0-262-13284-2*, Bradford Bks) MIT Pr.

Attention & Self Regulation: A Control-Theory Approach to Human Behavior. Charles S. Carver & Michael F. Scheier. 1981. (Social Psychology Ser.). (Illus.). 403p. 80.00 (*0-387-90553-7*) Spr-Verlag.

***Attention Deficit: A Family Affair: The Latest Techniques, Tools & Tips for Managing ADD.** David Hall. 2001. 50p. pap. 8.30 (*1-878353-54-3*, 19105) Silent Partners.

Attention Deficit Disorder. David Sosin & Myra Sosin. 1997. (Professional's Guide Ser.). (Illus.). 80p. pap., tchr. ed. 9.95 (*1-55734-883-9*, TCA0883) Tchr Create Mat.

Attention Deficit Disorder, Vol. 4. Ed. by Lewis M. Bloomingdale & James Swanson. 1990. 360p. 114.50 (*0-08-036508-6*, Pergamon Pr) Elsevier.

Attention Deficit Disorder, Vol. 5. Ed. by Lewis M. Bloomingdale & Joseph A. Sergeant. 1988. 234p. 56.50 (*0-08-036509-4*, Pergamon Pr) Elsevier.

Attention Deficit Disorder: A Concise Source of Information for Parents & Teachers. H. Moghadam & Joel Fagan. 2nd rev. ed. 1994. (Illus.). 128p. pap. 12.95 (*1-55059-082-0*) Temeron Bks.

Attention Deficit Disorder: A Different Perception. Thom Hartmann. 2nd rev. ed. 1997. LC 97-23214. 227p. pap. text 12.00 (*1-887424-14-8*) Underwood Bks.

Attention Deficit Disorder: ADHD & ADD Syndromes. Dale R. Jordan. 3rd ed. 1998. LC 97-35479. 192p. pap. 19.00 (*0-89079-742-0*, 8544) PRO-ED.

Attention Deficit Disorder: Clinical & Basic Research. Ed. by Terje Sagvolden & Trevor Archer. 1988. (Attention & Performance Ser.). 424p. text 89.95 (*0-8058-0098-0*) L Erlbaum Assocs.

Attention Deficit Disorder: New Research in Attention, Treatment & Psychopharmacology, Vol. 3. Ed. by Lewis M. Bloomingdale. 1988. 220p. (*0-08-036466-7*) Pergamon Repr GBR. *Dist:* Franklin.

Attention Deficit Disorder: Practical Coping Methods. Barbara C. Fisher & Ross A. Beckley. 1998. LC 98-7960. 392p. 29.95 (*0-8493-1899-8*) CRC Pr.

Attention Deficit Disorder & Learning Disabilities: Reality, Myths & Controversial Treatments. Barbara D. Ingersoll & Sam Goldstein. 1993. LC 92-46645. 256p. pap. 12.95 (*0-385-46931-4*) Doubleday.

Attention Deficit Disorder in Adults. Lynn Weiss. 3rd rev. ed. 1997. LC 96-29579. 224p. pap. 12.95 (*0-87833-979-5*) Taylor Pub.

Attention Deficit Disorder Misdiagnosis: Approaching ADD from a Brain-Behavior - Neuropsychological Perspective for Assessment & Treatment. Barbara C. Fisher. 1997. LC 97-48340. 432p. 65.00 (*1-57444-097-7*) St Lucie Pr.

Attention Deficit Disorders: Assessment & Teaching. Janet W. Lerner et al. 1994. LC 94-20274. (Special Education Ser.). 258p. pap. text 39.95 (*0-534-25044-0*) Brooks-Cole.

Attention-Deficit Disorders & Comorbidities in Children, Adolescents & Adults. Ed. by Thomas E. Brown. 2000. LC 99-47756. 736p. 59.00 (*0-88048-711-9*, 8711) Am Psychiatric.

Attention Deficit Disorders & Hyperactivity in Children: Early Diagnosis & Intervention. Ed. by Pasquale J. Accardo et al. 1991. (Pediatric Habilitation Ser.: Vol. 7). (Illus.). 424p. text 65.00 (*0-8247-8429-4*) Dekker.

Attention Deficit Disorders, Hyperactivity & Associated Disorders: A Handbook for Parents & Professionals. Wendy S. Coleman. 6th rev. ed. 1996. 104p. pap. 12.95 (*0-9620187-2-4*) Calliope Bks.

Attention Deficit Disorders Intervention Manual. Stephen B. McCarney. 1989. 167p. pap. 22.00 (*1-878372-06-8*) Hawthorne Educ Servs.

Attention Deficit Hyperactivity & Learning Disorders: Questions & Answers. J. Gordon Millichap. 1998. LC 98-91663. (Illus.). xi, 253 p. pap. 14.95 (*0-9629115-4-2*) PNB Pub.

Attention Deficit Hyperactivity Disorder. 1996. lib. bdg. 250.95 (*0-8490-6043-5*) Gordon Pr.

Attention-Deficit Hyperactivity Disorder: A Clinical Guide to Diagnosis & Treatment for Health & Mental Health Professionals. Ed. by Larry B. Silver. 2nd ed. 1999. LC 98-27809. 320p. text 29.95 (*0-88048-940-5*, 8940) Am Psychiatric.

Attention-Deficit Hyperactivity Disorder: A Clinical Workbook. Russell A. Barkley & Kevin R. Murphy. 2nd ed. 1998. LC 98-193358. 134p. spiral bd., wbk. ed. 32.00 (*1-57230-301-8*, 0301) Guilford Pubns.

Attention-Deficit Hyperactivity Disorder: A Handbook for Diagnosis & Treatment. Russell A. Barkley. 2nd rev. ed. 1998. LC 97-52762. 628p. text 60.00 (*1-57230-275-5*, 0275) Guilford Pubns.

Attention Deficit Hyperactivity Disorder: Questions & Answers for Parents. Gregory S. Greenberg & Wade F. Horn. 1991. LC 91-61551. 144p. (Orig.). pap. text 12.95 (*0-87822-322-3*, 4516) Res Press.

Attention Deficit Hyperactivity Disorder in Adulthood: A Practitioner's Handbook. Santo J. Triolo. 1998. LC 98-24227. 34.95 (*0-87630-890-6*) Brunner-Routledge.

Attention-Deficit Hyperactivity Disorder in Adults. Paul H. Wender. (Illus.). 1995. LC 94-46139. 312p. 35.00 (*0-19-509227-9*); 1998. 304p. reprint ed. pap. 13.95 (*0-19-511922-3*) OUP.

Attention Deficit Hyperactivity Disorder Through the Lifespan. Michele West. 2nd rev. ed. 1999. (Illus.). 123p. pap. 24.95 (*1-57801-032-2*) Western Schls.

Attention-Deficit Scales for Adults (ADSA) Santo J. Triolo. 1995. Complete Kit. 50.00 (*0-87630-797-7*); Instrument/Scoring/Profile Sets (25) pap. text 25.00 (*0-87630-798-5*) Brunner-Routledge.

Attention-Deficit/Hyperactivity Disorder: Abstracts of the Psychological & Behavioral Literature, 1971-1994. Ed. by Robert J. Resnick & Kathleen McEvoy. 1994. (Bibliographies in Psychology Ser.: No. 14). 204p. pap. 19.95 (*1-55798-274-0*) Am Psychol.

Attention Deficits & Hyperactivity in Children. Stephen P. Hinshaw. 1994. LC 93-36735. (Developmental Clinical Psychology & Psychiatry Ser.: Vol. 29). 168p. (C). pap. 34.95 (*0-8039-5196-5*, 3402) Sage.

Attention Deficits, Learning Disabilities, & Ritalin: A Practical Guide. Robert B. Johnston. 2nd ed. 1991. (Illus.). 202p. (C). pap. text 32.95 (*1-879105-12-8*, A037) Singular Publishing.

Attention, Development & Psychopathology. Ed. by Jacob A. Burack & James T. Enns. 1997. LC 97-3395. 414p. text 50.00 (*1-57230-198-8*, 0198) Guilford Pubns.

***Attention, Genes & Attention Deficit Hyperactivity Disorder.** Florence Levy & David A. Hay. 2001. LC 00-65135. 272p. (*1-84169-193-3*) Psychol Pr GBR. *Dist:* Taylor & Francis.

Attention in Early Development: Themes & Variations. Holly A. Ruff & Mary K. Rothbart. 1996. LC 95-33048. (Illus.). 312p. text 45.00 (*0-19-507143-3*) OUP.

Attention, Memory, & Executive Function. G. Reid Lyon & Norman A. Krasnegor. 1995. LC 95-2540. 432p. 45.00 (*1-55766-198-7*) P H Brookes.

Attention, Please! A Comprehensive Guide for Successfully Parenting Children with Attention Disorders & Hyperactivity. Edna D. Copeland & Valerie L. Love. 2nd rev. ed. 1995. LC 91-62565. (Illus.). 352p. 25.00 (*1-886941-02-5*) Spec Pr FL.

Attention, Voluntary Contraction & Event-Related Cerebral Potentials. Ed. by J. E. Desmedt. 1977. (Progress in Clinical Neurophysiology Ser.: Vol. 1). 85.75 (*3-8055-2438-2*) S Karger.

Attention Without Tension: A Teacher's Handbook on Attention Deficit Disorders (ADHD & ADD) Edna D. Copeland & Valerie L. Love. 2nd rev. ed. 1995. (Illus.). 175p. pap. 28.00 (*1-886941-01-7*) Spec Pr FL.

Attention Zone: A Parent's Guide to Attention Deficit/Hyperactivity Disorder. Michael W. Cohen. 1997. LC 97-22972. 234p. 22.95 (*0-87630-860-4*) Brunner-Routledge.

Attentional Processing: The Brain's Art of Mindfulness. David LaBerge. 1995. LC 94-38071. (Perspectives in Cognitive Neuroscience Ser.). (Illus.). 256p. text 42.50 (*0-674-05268-4*, LABATT) HUP.

Attentive Brain. Ed. by Raja Parasuraman. (Bradford Book Ser.). (Illus.). 1998. LC 97-22985. 532p. 85.00 (*0-262-16172-9*); 2000. 604p. (C). reprint ed. pap. 39.95 (*0-262-66112-8*) MIT Pr (Bradford Bks).

Attitude & Attitude Change: The Social Judgment-Involvement Approach. Carolyn W. Sherif. 1982. LC 81-13265. (Illus.). 264p. reprint ed. lib. bdg. 68.50 (*0-313-23260-1*, SHAC, Greenwood Pr) Greenwood.

Attitude Organization & Change: An Analysis of Consistency among Attitude Components, Volume 3. Milton J. Rosenberg et al. 1980. LC 80-14704. (Yale Studies in Attitude & Communication: Vol. 3). (Illus.). 239p. reprint ed. lib. bdg. 72.50 (*0-313-22435-8*, ROAT) Greenwood.

Attitude Strength: Antecedents & Consequences. Richard E. Petty. Ed. by Jon A. Krosnick. 1995. 528p. pap. 49.95 (*0-8058-1087-0*) L Erlbaum Assocs.

Attitude Strength: Antecedents & Consequences. Ed. by Richard E. Petty & Jon A. Krosnick. 1995. 528p. text 110.00 (*0-8058-1086-2*) L Erlbaum Assocs.

Attitude Structure & Function. Ed. by Anthony R. Pratkanis et al. 1989. 472p. text 89.95 (*0-89859-991-1*); pap. text 49.95 (*0-8058-0323-8*) L Erlbaum Assocs.

Attitudes & Behavior: An Annotated Bibliography. David R. Siebold & Daniel J. Canary. 1984. LC 84-3389. 234p. 57.75 (*0-275-91137-3*, C1137, Praeger Pubs) Greenwood.

Attitudes & Behavioral Decisions. Ed. by A. Upmeyer. 1988. (Psychology Ser.). (Illus.). 268p. 107.00 (*0-387-96727-3*) Spr-Verlag.

Attitudes & Emotions. Compiled by Association for Research and Enlightenment, Readings Staff. (Library: Vol. 13). Pt. I. 1981. 445p. lib. bdg. 22.95 (*0-87604-138-1*, 1113); Pt. II. 1982. 393p. lib. bdg. 22.95 (*0-87604-140-3*, 1114) ARE Pr.

Attitudes, Personality, & Behavior. Icek Ajzen. 1988. 175p. (C). mass mkt. 20.75 (*0-534-10949-7*) Brooks-Cole.

Attitudes Toward Handicapped Students: Professional, Peer & Parent Reactions. Marcia D. Horne. 1985. (School Psychology Ser.). 288p. (C). text 59.95 (*0-89859-584-3*) L Erlbaum Assocs.

Attorney for the Damned: A Lawyer's Life with the Criminally Insane. Denis Woychuk. 1996. 288p. 23.00 (*0-02-935607-5*) Free Pr.

Attorneys' Dictionary of Medicine J. E. Schmidt. 16th ed. 1962. ring bd. 610.00 (*0-8205-1609-0*) Bender.

Attorney's Directory of Forensic Psychiatrists: 1996 Edition. 1996. 82p. (Orig.). pap. 20.00 (*0-935645-09-8*) AJFP.

Attorney's Master Guide to Courtroom Psychology: How to Apply Behavioral Science Techniques for New Trial Success. David L. Herbert & Roger K. Barrett. 1980. 69.50 (*0-13-050443-2*) Exec Reports.

Attorney's Medical Handbook. Samuel J. Faber & Stuart J. Faber. 1981. 256p. (Orig.). pap. text 32.50 (*0-89074-085-2*) Lega Bks.

Attorneys' Medical Reference. Barry Creighton et al. 4th ed. 1984. 270p. ring bd. 85.00 (*0-9614995-0-8*, 80163-10, MICHIE) LEXIS Pub.

Attorneys' Textbook of Medicine Roscoe N. Gray & Louise J. Gordy. 3rd ed. 1934. ring bd. 2953.00 (*0-8205-1300-8*) Bender.

Attorney's Textbook of Medicine: Manual of Traumatic Injuries, Set. 1989. ring bd. 439.00 (*0-8205-1009-2*) Bender.

Attractive Woman: A Physical Fitness Approach to Emotional & Spiritual Well-Being. Marvel Harrison-Davis & Catharine Stewart-Roache. 1989. (Illus.). 178p. pap. text 8.95 (*0-942421-07-8*, AW) BRAT Pub.

Attribution Theory: An Organizational Perspective. Ed. by Mark Martinko. 1995. LC 94-17213. (Illus.). 384p. 54.95 (*1-884015-19-0*) St Lucie Pr.

Attribution Theory: Applications to Achievement, Mental Health, & Interpersonal Conflict. Ed. by Sandra Graham & Valerie S. Folkes. 1990. (Applied Social Psychology Ser.). 232p. 69.95 (*0-8058-0531-1*) L Erlbaum Assocs.

Attributional Theory of Motivation & Emotion. B. Weiner. 1986. (Social Psychology Ser.). (Illus.). 340p. 65.00 (*0-387-96312-X*) Spr-Verlag.

Attributions & Psychological Change: Application of Attributional Theories to Clinical & Educational Practice. Ed. by Charles Antaki & Chris R. Brewin. 1982. LC 81-71575. (Illus.). text 103.00 (*0-12-058780-7*) Acad Pr.

Atypical Cognitive Deficits in Developmental Disorders: Implications for Brain Function. Ed. by Sarah H. Broman & Jordan Grafman. 1994. LC 93-12499. 352p. text 89.95 (*0-8058-1180-X*) L Erlbaum Assocs.

Atypical Infant Development. Ed. by Marci J. Hanson. 2nd ed. 1996. LC 83-14741. (Illus.). 529p. (C). text 43.00 (*0-89079-641-6*, 7636) PRO-ED.

Au Dela de la Psychologie Vol. 1: Introduction a la Metapsychologie, Set. Frank A. Gerbode. 1995. (FRE.). 252p. pap. 45.00 (*1-887927-01-8*) Inst Res Metapsychol.

Au Dela de la Psychologie Vol. 2: Introduction a la Metapsychologie. Frank A. Gerbode. 1995. (FRE.). 228p. pap. 45.00 (*1-887927-02-6*) Inst Res Metapsychol.

Au-Dela des Murs de la Clinique: Etudes de Cas sur la Distribution a Base Communautaire de Contraceptifs. James A. Wolff et al. Ed. by C. Elizabeth McCrory & Susanna C. Binzen. 1997.Tr. of Beyond the Clinic Walls: Case Studies in Community-Based Distribution. (FRE.). 163p. (Orig.). pap. 15.00 (*0-913723-42-8*) Mgmt Sci Health.

AUAA (American Urological Association Allied) Urologic Nursing: Principles & Practice. American Urological Association Staff. Ed. by Karen A. Karlowicz. 1994. LC 92-49388. (Illus.). 736p. text 91.50 (*0-7216-2731-5*) Saunders.

Audilogic Evaluation & Management & Speech Perception Assesment. Lisa Lucks Mendel & Jeffrey L. Danhauer. 1996. LC 96-29149. 290p. pap. 57.95 (*1-56593-692-2*, 1366) Thomson Learn.

Audio-Visual Aids in Health Biology: Index of Modern Information. Andy J. Cyrpinski. 1990. LC 88-47968. 150p. pap. 44.50 (*1-55914-211-1*) ABBE Pubs Assn.

Audiogram Workbook. Sharon Hepfner. 1997. (Illus.). 304p. pap., wbk. ed. 19.95 (*0-86577-719-5*) Thieme Med Pubs.

Audiologist. Jack Rudman. 1994. (Career Examination Ser.: C-1124). pap. 27.95 (*0-8373-1124-1*) Nat Learn.

Audiologist - Speech Pathologist. Jack Rudman. 1994. (Career Examination Ser.: C-59). pap. 27.95 (*0-8373-0059-2*) Nat Learn.

Audiologists' Desk Reference Volume I: Diagnostic Audiology Principles Procedures & Protocols, Vol. 1. James W. Hall, III & H. Gustav Mueller. 1996. LC 96-28454. (Singular Audiology Text Ser.). (Illus.). 914p. pap. text 99.95 (*1-56593-269-2*, 0591) Thomson Learn.

Audiology: The Fundamentals. Fred H. Bess & Larry E. Humes. 2nd ed. 1995. (Illus.). 352p. 57.95 (*0-683-00620-7*) Lppncott W & W.

Audiology & Auditory Dysfunction. George T. Mencher et al. 1996. LC 96-26053. (Illus.). 288p. (C). 66.00 (*0-205-16101-4*) Allyn.

Audiology Business & Practice Management. Holly Hosford-Dunn et al. 1995. (Illus.). 552p. (C). text 77.95 (*1-56593-345-1*, 0643) Thomson Learn.

Audiology Clinical Protocols. Robert H. Margolis et al. 1997. LC 97-1019. 224p. (C). pap. 61.00 (*0-205-26824-2*) Allyn.

Audiology Desk Reference: A Guide to the Practice of Audiology. Ed. by Ross J. Roeser. 1996. (Illus.). 400p. pap. 45.00 (*0-86577-574-5*) Thieme Med Pubs.

Audiology Diagnosis. Ross J. Roeser. 2000. LC 99-52571. (Illus.). 560p. 59.00 (*0-86577-857-4*) Thieme Med Pubs.

Audiology in Education. Ed. by Wendy McCracken & Siobhan Laoide-Kemp. 1997. 450p. 90.00 (*1-56593-911-5*, 1804) Singular Publishing.

Audiology Practice Management. Holly Hosford-Dunn et al. 2000. LC 99-50353. (Illus.). 496p. 59.00 (*0-86577-858-2*) Thieme Med Pubs.

Audiology Treatment. Michael Valente. 2000. LC 99-51912. (Illus.). 800p. 69.00 (*0-86577-859-0*) Thieme Med Pubs.

Audiometric Interpretation: A Manual of Basic Audiometry. Harriet Kaplan et al. 2nd ed. 1993. LC 92-46331. 352p. (C). pap. text 75.00 (*0-205-14753-4*, Longwood Div) Allyn.

Audiometry in Infancy. Sanford E. Gerber. 1977. 368p. text 45.00 (*0-8089-1038-8*, 791545, Grune & Strat) Harcrt Hlth Sci Grp.

Audiovestibular Toxicity of Drugs Jose A. De Oliviera. 1989. 256p. 152.00 (*0-8493-6959-2*, RF285, CRC Reprint) Franklin.

Audiovestibular Toxicity of Drugs, Vol. 2. Jose A. De Oliveira. 1989. 240p. 152.00 (*0-8493-6960-6*, RF285, CRC Reprint) Franklin.

Audit in Action. Richard Smith et al. 1993. (Illus.). 245p. pap. text (*0-7279-0317-9*) BMJ Pub GBR. *Dist:* AIDC.

Audit in Obstetrics & Gynecology. M. Maresh. 1994. (Illus.). 288p. 70.00 (*0-632-03352-5*) Blackwell Sci.

Auditing: Advances in Behavioral Research. Ed. by Lawrence A. Ponemon & D. R. Gadhart. 1991. (Recent Research in Psychology Ser.). (Illus.). 166p. 88.95 (*0-387-97619-1*) Spr-Verlag.

Audition. Pierre Buser & Michel Imbert. Tr. by Roy H. Kay. 1992. (Illus.). 280p. 55.00 (*0-262-02331-8*, Bradford Bks) MIT Pr.

Auditory & Speech Characteristics of Poor Readers. Guy L. Bond. LC 72-176578. (Columbia University. Teachers College. Contributions to Education Ser.: No. 657). reprint ed. 37.50 (*0-404-55657-4*) AMS Pr.

Auditory Brainstem, Vol. 7. D. R. Irvine. 1986. (Progress in Sensory Physiology Ser.). (Illus.). 279p. 85.95 (*0-387-16299-2*) Spr-Verlag.

***Auditory CNS Processing & Plasticity: A Series of Synopses Arising from the Auditory Function & Dysfunction Satellite Symposium of the 34th IUPS Congress.** Ed. by G. D. Housley et al. 2001. (Illus.). 76p. pap. 25.25 (*3-8055-7335-9*) S Karger.

Auditory Computation. Ed. by Harold L. Hawkins et al. 1995. LC 95-12906. (Springer Handbook of Auditory Research: Vol. 6). (Illus.). 517p. 101.00 (*0-387-97843-7*) Spr-Verlag.

Auditory Cortex. L. M. Aitkin. 1990. (Illus.). 160p. (C). (gr. 13). pap. text 125.95 (*0-412-32490-3*, A4949) Chapman & Hall.

Auditory Development in Infancy. Ed. by Sandra E. Trehub & Bruce Schneider. 1985. (Advances in the Study of Communication & Affect Ser.: Vol. 10). 258p. 65.00 (*0-306-41757-X*, Plenum Trade) Perseus Pubng.

Auditory Diagnosis: Principles & Applications. Schlomo Silman & Carol A. Silverman. 1997. (Illus.). 428p. (Orig.). pap. 64.95 (*1-56593-726-0*, 1410) Thomson Learn.

Auditory Disorders in Children. Helmer R. Myklebust. 1954. LC 54-7372. 367p. text 45.00 (*0-8089-0338-1*, 793025, Grune & Strat) Harcrt Hlth Sci Grp.

Auditory Disorders in School Children: The Law; Identification; Remediation. Ed. by Ross J. Roeser & Marion P. Downs. 3rd ed. 1995. (Illus.). 400p. text 45.00 (*0-86577-550-8*) Thieme Med Pubs.

Auditory Display: Sonification, Audification & Auditory Interfaces. Ed. by Gregory Kramer. 2000. 720p. (C). pap. 49.00 (*0-201-62604-7*) Perseus Bks Grp.

Auditory Evoked Magnetic Fields & Electric Potentials. Ed. by F. Grandon et al. 1990. (Advances in Audiology Ser.: Vol. 6). (Illus.). viii, 362p. 258.50 (*3-8055-5001-4*) S Karger.

Auditory Evoked Potentials in Man: Psychopharmacology Correlates of EPS. Ed. by J. E. Desmedt. 1977. (Progress in Clinical Neurophysiology Ser.: Vol. 2). 85.25 (*3-8055-2626-1*) S Karger.

Auditory Hallucinations. Robert Dunning. 3rd ed. 2000. (Illus.). 52p. 9.95 (*1-877633-57-7*) Luthers.

Auditory Imagery. Ed. by Daniel Reisberg. 1992. 288p. text 65.00 (*0-8058-0556-7*) L Erlbaum Assocs.

Auditory Neuropathy: Diagnosis, Management, & Prosthetic Devices. Linda J. Hood & Yvonne S. Sininger. 1998. 104p. 48.00 incl. audio (*1-58041-022-7*, 0112148) Am Speech Lang Hearing.

Auditory Perception Test for the Hearing Impaired. Susan G. Allen & Thomas S. Serwatka. 1994. 35p. pap. 13.95 (*0-931421-29-2*); pap. 26.95 (*0-931421-38-1*) Psychol Educ Pubns.

Auditory-Perceptual Development Remedial Activities: Auditory Discrimination. Karen G. Codding & Morrison F. Gardner. 1988. pap. 9.95 (*0-931421-31-4*) Psychol Educ Pubns.

Auditory-Perceptual Development Remedial Activities: Auditory Interpretation of Directions. Karen G. Codding & Morrison F. Gardner. 1988. pap. 9.95 (*0-931421-35-7*) Psychol Educ Pubns.

Auditory-Perceptual Development Remedial Activities: Auditory Processing. Karen G. Codding & Morrison F. Gardner. 1988. pap. 9.95 (*0-931421-36-5*) Psychol Educ Pubns.

Auditory-Perceptual Development Remedial Activities: Auditory Sentence Memory. Karen G. Codding & Morrison F. Gardner. 1988. pap. 9.95 (*0-931421-34-9*) Psychol Educ Pubns.

Auditory-Perceptual Development Remedial Activities: Auditory Sequential Memory. Karen G. Codding & Morrison F. Gardner. 1988. pap. 9.95 (*0-931421-32-2*) Psychol Educ Pubns.

Auditory-Perceptual Development Remedial Activities: Auditory Word Memory. Karen G. Codding & Morrison F. Gardner. 1988. pap. 9.95 (*0-931421-33-0*) Psychol Educ Pubns.

Auditory-Perceptual Development Remedial Activities: Remedial Activities. Karen G. Codding & Morrison F. Gardner. 1988. pap. 9.95 (*0-931421-30-6*) Psychol Educ Pubns.

Auditory Physiology & Perception: Proceedings of the Ninth International Symposium on Hearing, Carcens, France, 9-14 June 1991. Y. Cazals et al. 1992. (Advances in the Biosciences Ser.: No. 83). (Illus.). 590p. 210.50 (*0-08-041847-3*, Pergamon Pr) Elsevier.

Auditory Processes. Pamela Gillet. rev. ed. 1993. LC 74-80092. 96p. (gr. k-12). pap. 15.00 (*0-87879-094-2*) Acad Therapy.

Auditory Processing & Language: Clinical & Research Perspectives. Philip J. Levinson & Christine Sloan. 1980. 256p. text 36.50 (*0-8089-1305-0*, 792517, Grune & Strat) Harcrt Hlth Sci Grp.

Auditory Processing of Complex Sounds. Ed. by William A. Yost & Charles S. Watson. 1987. 344p. text 49.95 (*0-89859-981-4*) L Erlbaum Assocs.

Auditory Reasoning & Processing Remedial Activities. Morrison F. Gardner & Karen G. Codding. 1993. pap. 7.25 (*0-931421-80-2*) Psychol Educ Pubns.

Auditory Skills Curriculum: Preschool Supplement. Lexington School for the Deaf Staff. 1988. (Auditory Skills Instructional Planning System Ser.). 180p. ring bd. 35.00 (*0-943292-23-9*) Foreworks.

Auditory System: Proceedings of the Satellite Symposium of the Second Extraordinary International Symposium on Recent Advances in Otitis Media, Kyoto, Japan, April 5, 1993. Ed. by Iwao Honjo. 1994. LC 94-1074. (Illus.). viii, 90p. pap. text (*90-6299-104-1*) Kugler NLD. *Dist:* Lib Res.

Auditory System Plasticity & Regeneration. Ed. by Richard J. Salvi et al. 1996. LC 95-38677. 412p. 95.00 (*0-86577-580-X*) Thieme Med Pubs.

Auditory Training. Norman P. Erber. 1982. 208p. pap. text 23.95 (*0-88200-149-3*) Alexander Graham.

Audits of Voluntary Health & Welfare Organizations. annuals 2nd ed. (American Institute of CPAs Audit Guides Ser.). pap. 33.00 (*0-87051-027-4*) Am Inst CPA.

Audrey's Add No Salt Cookery. Audrey Greene. 1982. (Illus.). (*0-9608892-0-5*) Greene Pubns.

Augmentative & Alternative Communication. Howard C. Shane & Maggie Sauer. Ed. by Harvey Halpern. 1986. LC 86-16919. (PRO-ED Studies in Communicative Disorders). 88p. (Orig.). pap. text 9.00 (*0-89079-091-4*, 1381) PRO-ED.

Augmentative Communication Assessment for Children. Sharon L. Glennen & Denise C. Decoste. 1996. LC 96-28455. (Illus.). 920p. (Orig.). pap. text 83.95 (*1-56593-684-1*, 1360) Thomson Learn.

Augmented Breast: Radiologic & Clinical Perspectives. David P. Gorczyca & R. James Brenner. 1996. LC 96-44700. (Illus.). 300p. text 109.00 (*0-86577-612-1*) Thieme Med Pubs.

Aujeszky's Disease. G. Wittmann & S. A. Hall. 1982. text 141.50 (*90-247-2638-7*) Kluwer Academic.

Aunt Minnie's Atlas & Imaging-Specific Diagnosis. Kenneth L. Ford, III & Thomas L. Pope, Jr. 1997. LC 96-19736. (Illus.). 314p. 99.00 (*0-683-03309-3*) Lppncott W & W.

AUPHA Manual of Health Services Management. Robert J. Taylor & Susan B. Taylor. 1993. 680p. 96.00 (*0-8342-0363-4*, 20363) Aspen Pub.

Aural Habilitation: The Foundations of Verbal Learning in Hearing-Impaired Children. Daniel Ling & Agnes H. Ling. 1978. LC 78-56077. pap. text 26.95 (*0-88200-121-3*, C2441) Alexander Graham.

Aural Rehabilitation: Serving Children & Adults. Raymond H. Hull. 3rd ed. 1997. LC 96-25790. (Illus.). 530p. pap. text 55.00 (*1-56593-682-5*, 1378) Singular Publishing.

Aural Rehabilitation: Serving Children & Adults. Ed. by Raymond H. Hull. 4th ed. 2000. LC 00-49653. (Illus.). 543p. pap. text 60.95 (*0-7693-0127-4*) Singular Publishing.

Aural Rehabilitation for the Elderly. Ed. by Miriam A. Henoch. 1979. 240p. text 36.00 (*0-8089-1186-4*, 791968, Grune & Strat) Harcrt Hlth Sci Grp.

Aural Rehabilitation Hearing Aids & Assistive Listening Devices. Darius Kohan & Louise Levy. 1999. LC 99-52110. (Illus.). 67p. pap. text 25.00 (*1-56772-027-7*, 5506355) AAO-HNS.

Auranofin in Rheumatoid Arthritis. Ed. by Norman L. Gottlieb. 1987. LC 87-73225. 128p. 30.00 (*0-941741-00-1*) Adis Pr Intl.

Auricular Diagnosis, Treatment & Health Preservation. Shipei Liu. Tr. by Ren Gan & Zhining Tian. 1996. (Illus.). 307p. pap. 29.50 (*1-880132-23-0*) Sci Pr NY.

Auricular Therapy: Theory & Practice. Beatrice Bartnett. 1992. (Illus.). 146p. (Orig.). pap. 34.95 (*0-9622182-1-9*) Lifestyle Inst.

Aus den Lebenserinnerungen. Hans Herzfeld. Ed. by Willy Real. 1992. (Veroeffentlichungen der Historischen Kommission zu Berlin, Band 67, Beitraege zu Inflation und Wiederaufbau in Deutschland und Europa 1914-1924: Vol. 81). (GER.). x, 219p. (C). lib. bdg. 36.95 (*3-11-013520-5*, 102-92) De Gruyter.

Aus Der Reihe Frankfurter Beitrage Zur Geschichte, Theorie und Ethik der Medizin Vol. 15: Medizin in Frankfurt Am Main. Geburtstag Von Gert Preiser. 1994. (GER.). (*3-487-09894-6*) G Olms Pubs.

Aus Der Reihe Medizin der Antike Vol. 2: Der Sanitatsdienst Im Romischen Reich. Juliane C. Wilmanns. 1995. (GER.). (*3-487-07919-4*) G Olms Pubs.

Auscultation of the Heart: A Cardiophonetic Approach. T. Anthony Michael. 1997. LC 97-15124. (Illus.). 304p. pap. 49.95 (*0-07-018005-9*) McGraw-Hill Prof.

Auscultation Skills: Breath & Heart Sounds. Springhouse Publishing Company Staff. 1998. LC 98-11711. (Illus.). 288p. pap. 46.95 (*0-87434-962-1*) Springhouse Corp.

Australasian Radiology: A History. James F. Ryan et al. 1995. LC 97-179437. (Illus.). 150p. text (*0-07-470207-6*) McGraw-Hill Med Pub.

Australia Antigen & Viral Hepatitis: Proceedings of the International Symposium on Basic Progress in Blood Transfusion, 6th, Brussels, Feb., 1972. International Symposium on Basic Progress in Blood. Ed. by J. Desmyter & W. T. London. 1973. (Vox Sanguinis Ser.: Vol. 24). (Illus.). pap. 15.75 (*3-8055-1611-8*) S Karger.

Australian HIV - AIDS Legal Guide. John Godwin et al. 1991. 270p. pap. (*1-86287-058-6*) Federation Pr AUS. *Dist:* Gaunt.

***Australian Prescriber's Abnormal Laboratory Results.** Robert Dunstan. 2002. (Illus.). 120p. pap. 19.95 (*0-07-470926-7*) McGraw-Hill Prof.

Australian Women's Health: Innovations in Social Science & Community Research. Ed. by Lenore Manderson. 1998. LC 98-51297. 163p. 49.95 (*0-7890-0668-5*) Haworth Pr.

Auswertung und Deutung des EKG. A. H. Lemmerz & R. R. Schmidt. 12th ed. 1981. (Illus.). xii, 260p. pap. 41.75 (*3-8055-1932-X*) S Karger.

Autecology of the Copperhead. Henry S. Fitch. 2nd ed. 1980. (Museum Ser.: Vol. 13, No. 4). (Illus.). 203p. reprint ed. pap. 12.00 (*0-89338-016-4*) U KS Nat Hist Mus.

***Authentication of Chinese Medicinal Materials by DNA Technology.** Ed. by P. C. Shaw et al. 2001. 250p. 58.00 (*981-02-4621-8*) World Scientific Pub.

Author Catalog of the Library of the New York Academy of Medicine. New York Academy of Medicine Library Staff. 1983. 4910.00 (*0-8161-1388-2*, Macmillan Ref) Gale.

Author Index to Psychological Abstracts, 1964 to 1968. Columbia University Staff. 1982. 370.00 (*0-8161-1355-6*, Macmillan Ref) Gale.

Author-Title & Subject Catalogs of the Centers for Disease Control Library. Center for Disease Control Staff. 1983. 990.00 (*0-8161-0395-X*, Macmillan Ref) Gale.

Author Title Catalog of Francis & Countway Library of Medicine Imprints 1994. 2010.00 (*0-7838-2284-7*, Macmillan Ref) Gale.

Authoritative Guide to Books in Psychotherapy, Set. Aronson, Jason, Inc. Staff. 1996. 144p. pap. 2.00 (*0-7657-0112-X*) Aronson.

Authoritative Guide to Grapefruit Seed Extract: A Breakthrough in Alternative Treatment for Colds, Infectious, Candida, Allergies, Herpes, Parasites & Many Other Ailments. Allan Sachs. 1997. LC 96-44186. pap. 10.95 (*0-940795-17-5*) LifeRhythm.

Authoritative Guide to Self-Help Resources in Mental Health. John C. Norcross et al. 2000. (Clinician's Toolbox Ser.). 399p. 43.00 (*1-57230-506-1*, 8R0506); pap. 25.00 (*1-57230-580-0*, 8R0580) Guilford Pubns.

Authorized to Heal: Gender, Class & the Transformation of Medicine in Appalachia, 1880-1930. Sandra Lee Barney. 2000. LC 99-30433. (Illus.). xiii, 222p. lib. bdg. 39.95 (*0-8078-2522-0*) U of NC Pr.

Author's Guide to Biomedical Journals: Complete Manuscript Submission Instruction for 185 Leading Biomedical Periodicals. Ed. by Mary A. Liebert. 1994. 628p. 164.00 (*0-913113-61-1*) M Liebert.

Author's Guide to Journals in the Behavioral Sciences. Alvin Y. Wang. 1989. 496p. pap. 24.95 (*0-8058-0313-0*); 3.5 hd 49.95 (*1-56321-053-3*); 5.25 hd 49.95 (*1-56321-054-1*) L Erlbaum Assocs.

Author's Guide to Nursing Journals. Ed. by Susan C. Slaninka. 2nd ed. Date not set. (Orig.). pap. text 19.95 (*0-9628084-9-0*) Hlth Mngmnt Pubns.

Author's Handbook of Styles for Life Science Journals. Michel C. Atlas. 1995. LC 95-38010. 704p. 104.95 (*0-8493-2503-X*, 2503) CRC Pr.

Autism. Laura Schreibman. 1988. (Developmental Clinical Psychology & Psychiatry Ser.: Vol. 15). 160p. (C). pap. 34.95 (*0-8039-2810-6*, 6553) Sage.

Autism: A Reappraisal of Concepts & Treatment. Ed. by Michael Rutter & Eric Schopler. 1978. LC 77-26910. (Illus.). 552p. 49.50 (*0-306-31096-1*, Kluwer Plenum) Kluwer Academic.

Autism: A Sensorimotor Approach to Management. Ruth A. Huebner. 1991. LC 00-58298. (Illus.). xvii, 493p. 65.00 (*0-8342-1645-0*, 16450) PRO-ED.

Autism: An Introduction to Psychological Theory. Francesca Happe. 1998. (Illus.). 160p. pap. 14.50 (*0-674-05311-7*) HUP.

Autism: Behavior-Analytic Perspectives. Ed. by Patrick M. Ghezzi et al. 1999. LC 99-20586. 39.95 (*1-878978-32-2*) Context Pr.

Autism: Clinical & Research Issues. Ed. by Pasquale J. Accardo et al. 2000. (Illus.). (C). 45.00 (*0-912752-48-3*) York Pr.

Autism: Explaining the Enigma. Uta Frith. 1989. (Cognitive Development Ser.). pap. text 27.95 (*0-631-16824-9*) Blackwell Pubs.

***Autism: Explaining the Enigma.** Uta Frith. 2nd ed. 2001. (Cognitive Development Ser.). 288p. pap. 26.95 (*0-631-22901-9*) Blackwell Pubs.

Autism: Facts & Strategies for Parents. Janice E. Janzen. 1999. LC 99-32422. xiv, 169p. 45.00 (*0-7616-4550-0*, Thrpy Skill Bldrs) Commun Skill.

Autism: Identification, Education, & Treatment. Ed. by Dianne E. Berkell. 1992. 328p. pap. 34.50 (*0-8058-0897-3*); text 69.95 (*0-8058-0896-5*) L Erlbaum Assocs.

Autism: Identification, Education, & Treatment. Ed. by Dianne E. Zager. 2nd ed. 1999. LC 98-41273. 384p. 79.95 (*0-8058-2043-4*); pap. 36.00 (*0-8058-2044-2*) L Erlbaum Assocs.

Autism: Information & Resources for Parents, Families, & Professionals. Richard L. Simpson & Paul Zionts. 1992. LC 92-1. 188p. pap. text 26.00 (*0-89079-538-X*, 5192) PRO-ED.

Autism: Information & Resources for Professionals & Parents. Richard L. Simpson & Paul Zionts. 2nd ed. 1999. LC 99-13965. 40.28 (*0-89079-820-6*) PRO-ED.

Autism: Nature, Diagnosis & Treatment. Ed. by Geraldine Dawson. 1989. LC 88-16356. 417p. pap. 52.00 (*0-89862-724-9*, 2724) Guilford Pubns.

Autism: Nightmare Without End. Dorothy J. Beavers. Ed. by Debbie Hammond. 1982. LC 79-27669. 24.95 (*0-87949-167-1*) Ashley Bks.

Autism: Preparing for Adulthood. Patricia Howlin. 1996. LC 96-21556. (Illus.). 304p. (C). pap. 29.95 (*0-415-11532-9*) Routledge.

Autism: Strategies for Change. Gerald Groden & M. Grace Baron. 1991. LC 87-8682. 256p. (C). pap. text 23.95 (*0-89876-184-0*) Gardner Pr.

Autism: The Facts. Simon Baron-Cohen & Patrick Bolton. 1994. LC 92-49828. (Facts Ser.). (Illus.). 122p. pap. 19.95 (*0-19-262327-3*) OUP.

Autism: Understanding the Disorder. Gary B. Mesibov et al. 1998. LC 97-35645. (Clinical Child Psychology Library). (Illus.). (C). 136p. 45.00 (*0-306-45546-3*); 118p. pap. 25.00 (*0-306-45547-1*) Kluwer Academic (Kluwer Plenum).

Autism & Asperger Syndrome. Ed. by Uta Frith. 1992. 257p. (C). pap. text 27.95 (*0-521-38608-X*) Cambridge U Pr.

Autism & Austistic-Like Conditions in Mental Retardation. Dirk W. Draijer. 1997. LC 97-29573. 450p. (*90-265-1463-8*) Swets.

Autism & Childhood Psychosis. Francis Tustin. 1995. 224p. pap. text (*1-85575-110-0*) Karnac Bks GBR. *Dist:* Other Pr LLC.

Autism & Pervasive Developmental Disorders. Ed. by Fred R. Volkmar. 1998. LC 97-35997. (Monographs in Child & Adolescent Psychiatry). (Illus.). 294p. (C). text 80.00 (*0-521-55386-5*) Cambridge U Pr.

Autism & Post-Traumatic Stress Disorder: Ending Autistic Fixation. Ken Lenchitz. LC 00-32543. xi, 123p. 2001. text 36.95 (*0-398-07096-2*); 2000. pap. 19.95 (*0-398-07097-0*) C C Thomas.

Autism & the Family: Problems, Prospects & Coping with the Disorder. David E. Gray. 1998. LC 97-43533. 210p. text 47.95 (*0-398-06842-9*); pap. text 34.95 (*0-398-06843-7*) C C Thomas.

Autism as an Executive Disorder. James Russell. 1998. LC 97-37721. (Illus.). 328p. text 90.00 (*0-19-852349-1*) OUP.

Autism in Adolescents & Adults. E. Schopler & G. B. Mesibov. 1983. LC 82-22314. (Current Issues in Autism Ser.). (Illus.). 456p. (C). 63.00 (*0-306-41057-5*, Plenum Trade) Perseus Pubng.

Autism in Children & Adults: Etiology, Assessment & Intervention. Ed. by Johnny L. Matson. 1994. LC 93-2902. (Special Education Ser.). 275p. (C). 46.50 (*0-534-23826-2*) Thomson Learn.

***Autism Spectrum Disorders: A Communication Based Handbook.** Prelock. 1993. (*0-8342-1841-0*) PRO-ED.

Autism Spectrum Disorders: A Transactional Developmental Perspective. Amy M. Wetherby & Barry M. Prizant. 2000. LC 99-53060. (Communication & Language Intervention Ser.: Vol. 9). xvii, 422p. 39.95 (*1-55766-445-5*) P H Brookes.

Autism Treatment Guide. Elizabeth K. Gerlach. rev. ed. 1998. LC 93-91648. 133p. pap. 12.95 (*0-9637578-0-6*) Four Leaf Pr.

Autisme Infantile-Infantile Autism. F. Gremy et al. 1987. (Colloque de L'INSERM Ser.: No. 146). (ENG & FRE.). 360p. lib. bdg. 33.00 (*2-85598-316-9*) S M P F Inc.

Autistic Adults at Bittersweet Farms. Norman S. Giddan & Jane J. Giddan. LC 90-41945. (Haworth Series on Social & Community Horticulture). 219p. 1991. text 6.95 (*1-56024-042-3*); 1990. pap. text 17.95 (*1-56024-057-1*) Haworth Pr.

Autistic Child: Language Development Through Behavior Modification. O. Ivar Lovaas. LC 76-5890. (Illus.). 256p. 1984. pap. text 16.95 (*0-8290-1003-3*); 1986. (C). reprint ed. text 29.95 (*0-8290-0253-7*) Irvington.

Autistic Children: A Guide for Parents & Professionals. Lorna Wing. 2nd ed. 1985. LC 84-29276. 176p. text 28.95 (*0-87630-391-2*) Brunner-Routledge.

Autistic Spectrum: A Guide for Parents & Professionals. Lorna Wing. 1997. 239p. (*0-09-475160-9*) Constable & Co GBR. *Dist:* Trafalgar.

Autistic States in Children. Francis Tustin. rev. ed. 1992. 272p. (C). pap. 29.95 (*0-415-08129-7*, A7789) Routledge.

Autistic States in Children. Francis Tustin. rev. ed. 1992. 272p. (C). text (*0-415-08128-9*, A7785) Tavistock GBR. *Dist:* Routldge.

Autoantibodies. Ed. by James B. Peter & Yehuda Shoenfeld. 1996. LC 96-13604. 910p. 126.00 (*0-444-82383-2*) Elsevier.

Autoantibodies to Immunoglobulins. Ed. by Farouk Shakib. 1989. (Monographs in Allergy: Vol. 26). (Illus.). x, 274p. 208.75 (*3-8055-4913-X*) S Karger.

Autobiographical Consciousness of Aging. Edmund Sherman. 2000. 239p. pap. 14.95 (*0-9701446-0-1*) Ed Sherman.

Autobiographical Memory: Remembering What & Remembering When. Charles P. Thompson et al. 1955. 248p. text 55.00 (*0-8058-1514-7*) L Erlbaum Assocs.

Autobiographical Study. Sigmund Freud. Ed. & Tr. by James Strachey. 1989. reprint ed. pap. 8.95 (*0-393-00146-6*) Norton.

Autobiographies in Experimental Psychology. Ed. by Ronald Gandelman. 1985. LC 85-20585. 128p. (C). text 29.95 (*0-89859-544-4*) L Erlbaum Assocs.

Autobiography & Personal Philosophy of a Retired Physician. Cyril Hart. 1997. LC 97-48409. (Lives Ser.: Vol. 7). 240p. text 89.95 (*0-7734-8470-1*) E Mellen.

Autobiography of a Schizophrenic Girl: An Astonishing Memoir of Reality Lost & Regained. Frwd. by Frank Conroy. 1994. 192p. pap. 12.95 (*0-452-01133-7*, Mer) NAL.

Autobiography of an Androgyne. Earl Lind et al. 1975. LC 75-12333. (Homosexuality Ser.). reprint ed. 23.95 (*0-405-07400-X*) Ayer.

Autobiography of Andrew T. Still with a History of the Discovery & Development of the Science of Osteopathy. Andrew T. Still. 1972. LC 78-180591. (Medicine & Society in America Ser.). 508p. reprint ed. 30.95 (*0-405-03973-5*) Ayer.

Autobiography of Samuel D. Gross, M. D. with Sketches of His Contemporaries Samuel D. Gross. 1972. LC 71-180576. (Medicine & Society in America Ser.). 898p. reprint ed. Set. 56.95 (*0-405-03953-0*); Vol. 1. 28.95 (*0-405-03980-8*); Vol. 2. 28.95 (*0-405-03981-6*) Ayer.

Autocrine & Paracrine Mechanisms in Reproductive Endocrinology. Ed. by L. C. Krey et al. 1989. LC 90-6703. (Reproductive Biology Ser.). (Illus.). 214p. 69.50 (*0-306-43490-3*, Plenum Trade) Perseus Pubng.

Autoeval Medicine Interna. Farreras. 13th ed. 1996. (C). text 40.80 (*84-8174-110-8*) Mosby Inc.

Autogenes Training. 1987. text 24.95 (*3-540-15750-6*) Spr-Verlag.

Autogenic Training: The Effective Holistic Way to Better Health. Kai Kermani. 1996. 336p. pap. text (*0-285-63322-8*) Souvenir Pr Ltd GBR. *Dist:* IPG Chicago.

Autohemotherapy Reference Manual: The Definitive Guide to the Literature. S. H. Shakman. 1998. LC 98-96133. 278p. pap. text 29.95 (*1-892506-02-5*); 200p. pap. text 49.95 (*1-892506-09-2*) Inst of Science.

Autoimmune Aspects of Lung Disease. David A. Isenberg & Stephen G. Spiro. 1997. LC 97-48629. (Respiratory Pharmacology & Pharmacotherapy Ser.). 182.00 (*0-8176-5719-3*) Birkhauser.

Autoimmune Aspects of Lung Disease. Ed. by David A. Isenberg & Stephen G. Spiro. 1997. LC 97-48629. (Respiratory Pharmacology & Pharmacotherapy Ser.). 280p. text 182.00 (*3-7643-5719-3*) Birkhauser.

Autoimmune Disease: Aetiopathogenesis, Diagnosis, & Treatment. Ed. by Jonathon Brostoff & Peter M. Lydyard. 1994. LC 93-48904. (Illus.). 272p. (*0-632-03799-7*) Blckwell Science.

Autoimmune Disease: Focus on Sjogren's Syndrome. Ed. by David A. Isenberg & A. C. Horsfall. 1994. (University College, London, Molecular Pathology Ser.). 250p. (*1-872748-23-6*) Bios Sci GBR. *Dist:* Coronet Bks.

Autoimmune Disease Therapeutic Markets: New Therapies Target Causes, Not Symptoms. Market Intelligence Staff. 1992. 320p. 1895.00 (*1-56753-077-X*) Frost & Sullivan.

Autoimmune Diseases. Ed. by Noel R. Rose & Ian R. MacKay. 3rd ed. 1998. LC 98-84368. (Illus.). 895p. (C). 139.95 (*0-12-596923-6*) Acad Pr.

Autoimmune Diseases of the Endocrine System. Ed. by Robert Volpe. 1990. LC 96-21108. (Illus.). 376p. lib. bdg. 192.00 (*0-8493-6849-9*, RC649) CRC Pr.

***Autoimmune Diseases of the Skin.** Ed. by Michael Hertl. 2001. (Pathogenesis, Diagnosis, Management Ser.). (Illus.). 250p. 49.95 (*3-211-83598-9*) Spr-Verlag.

Autoimmune Diseases Two. Ed. by Noel R. Rose & Ian R. MacKay. 1992. (Illus.). 444p. text 105.00 (*0-12-596922-8*) Acad Pr.

Autoimmune Disorders of Blood. Ed. by Leslie E. Silberstein. 1996. (Illus.). 200p. pap. text 55.00 (*1-56395-067-7*, 960011) Am Assn Blood.

Autoimmune Endocrinopathies. Ed. by Robert Volpe. 1999. LC 99-10951. (Contemporary Endocrinology Ser.: Vol. 15). (Illus.). 433p. 175.00 (*0-89603-680-4*) Humana.

Autoimmune Hepatitis. Ed. by M. Nishioka et al. 1994. 358p. 201.25 (*0-444-88196-4*) Elsevier.

Autoimmune Liver Disease. Ed. by P. A. Berg et al. 1998. (Falk Symposium Ser.). 128p. text 80.00 (*0-7923-8730-9*) Kluwer Academic.

Autoimmune Liver Diseases. Edward L. Krawitt et al. 2nd ed. 1998. LC 98-28060. 674p. 246.50 (*0-444-82803-6*) Elsevier.

Autoimmune Neurological Disease. Michael P. Pender & Pamela A. McCombe. 1995. (Cambridge Reviews in Clinical Immunology Ser.). 385p. (C). text 95.00 (*0-521-46113-8*) Cambridge U Pr.

Autoimmune Reactions. Sudhir Paul. 1998. LC 98-28432. (Contemporary Immunology Ser.: Vol. 6). (Illus.). 448p. 145.00 (*0-89603-550-6*) Humana.

Autoimmune Rheumatic Disease. John Morrow et al. 2nd ed. 1999. LC 98-28029. (Illus.). 288p. text 75.00 (*0-19-262883-6*) OUP.

Autoimmune Thyroiditis: Approaches Towards Its Etiological Differentiation. Balthasar Weinheimer & W. A. Scherbaum. 1991. (Illus.). 340p. 95.00 (*0-387-53476-8*) Spr-Verlag.

***Autoimmunity.** Ed. by Andrzej Gorski et al. 2001. LC 2001-43409. 207p. 80.00 (*1-4020-0037-5*) Kluwer Academic.

Autoimmunity. Holborow. 1981. text 51.00 (*0-7216-4734-0*) Saunders.

Autoimmunity. W. Ollier & D. P. Symmons. 1992. (Medical Perspective Ser.). 152p. pap. (*1-872748-50-3*) Bios Sci GBR. *Dist:* Coronet Bks.

Autoimmunity: Basic Concepts & Systemic & Selected Organ-Specific Diseases. Ed. by J. M. Cruse & R. E. Lewis. 1985. (Concepts in Immunopathology Ser.: Vol. 1). (Illus.). viii, 362p. 172.25 (*3-8055-3908-8*) S Karger.

Autoimmunity: Experimental Aspects. Ed. by Moncef Zouali. 1994. LC 93-47074. (NATO ASI Ser.: Vol. 80). (Illus.). 302p. 175.00 (*0-387-57642-8*) Spr-Verlag.

Autoimmunity: Physiology & Disease. Ed. by Antonio Coutinho & Michel D. Kazatchkine. 1993. LC 93-12816. 474p. 160.00 (*0-471-59227-7*, Wiley-Interscience) Wiley.

Autoimmunity & Autoimmune Disease. CIBA Foundation Staff. 1987. LC 87-10493. (CIBA Foundation Symposia Ser.: No. 129). 288p. 128.00 (*0-471-91095-3*) Wiley.

Autoimmunity & Endocrine Diseases. Ed. by A. Pinchera & L. Vanhaelst. 1982. (Journal: Vol. 16, No. 5). (Illus.). 84p. pap. 35.75 (*3-8055-3658-5*) S Karger.

Autoimmunity & the Pathogenesis of Diabetes. Ed. by F. Ginsberg-Fellner & R. C. McEvoy. 1989. (Endocrinology & Metabolism Ser.: Vol. 4). (Illus.). 296p. 145.00 (*0-387-96645-5*, 2060) Spr-Verlag.

Autoimmunity in Nephritis. Ed. by Francis W. Ballardie. 1992. LC 91-35410. 130p. text 88.00 (*3-7186-5195-5*) Gordon & Breach.

Autoimmunity in Psoriasis. Ed. by Ernest H. Beutner. 1982. 328p. 182.00 (*0-8493-5473-0*, RL321, CRC Reprint) Franklin.

Autoimmunoregulation & Autoimmune Disease. Ed. by J. M. Cruse & R. E. Lewis. 1987. (Concepts in Immunopathology Ser.: Vol. 4). (Illus.). viii, 304p. 241.75 (*3-8055-4406-5*) S Karger.

Autologous Blood & Marrow Transplantation: Proceedings of the 9th International Symposium. Ed. by Karel A. Dicke & Armand Keating. 1999. (Illus.). pap. text 95.00 (*1-891524-04-6*) Carden Jennings.

***Autologous Blood & Marrow Transplantation: Proceedings of the Tenth International Symposium.** Ed. by Karel A. Dicke & Armand Keating. 2001. (Illus.). 744p. pap. 95.00 (*1-891524-08-9*) Carden Jennings.

***Autologous Fat Transplantation.** Ed. by Melvin A. Shiffman. 2001. LC 2001-17438. (Illus.). xii, 323p. text 150.00 (*0-8247-0484-3*) Dekker.

Autologous Marrow & Blood Transplantation: Proceedings of the 8th International Symposium. Ed. by Karel A. Dicke & Armand Keating. 1997. (Illus.). 744p. pap. text 65.00 (*1-891524-02-X*) Carden Jennings.

Autologous Stem Cell Transplantation: Biological & Clinical Results in Malignancies. Ed. by Angelo Carella. 1997. (Advances in Blood Disorders Ser.: Vol. 2). 600p. text 150.00 (*3-7186-5933-6*, Harwood Acad Pubs) Gordon & Breach.

Autologous Transfusion: Using Your Own Blood. B. G. Adhoute. 1992. (Illus.). 138p. 103.00 (*0-387-59554-6*) Spr-Verlag.

Autologous Transfusion Devices. 2nd ed. 1991. 13p. 70.00 (*0-910275-62-9*, AT6-209) Assn Adv Med Instrn.

Automated Blood Counts & Differentials: A Practical Guide. J. David Bessman. 1986. LC 85-24108. (Johns Hopkins Series in Contemporary Medicine & Public Health Ser.). (Illus.). 174p. pap. text 26.95 (*0-8018-3173-3*) Johns Hopkins.

Automated Cervical Cancer Screening. Ed. by Heinz K. Grohs & O. A. Husain. 1994. LC 94-2501. (Illus.). 400p. 115.00 (*0-89640-255-X*) Igaku-Shoin.

Automated Data Sources for Ambulatory Care Effectiveness Research. Ed. by Mary L. Grady & Harvey A. Schwartz. 1995. 74p. (Orig.). (C). pap. text 30.00 (*0-7881-2249-5*) DIANE Pub.

Automated Defibrillation. James Atkins & Taylor. 1991. pap. 15.25 (*0-13-514594-5*) P-H.

Automated Defibrillation for Professional & Lay Rescues. Jeffrey W. Myers. 1999. LC 98-31919. (Illus.). 144p. (C). pap. text 17.95 (*0-8036-0454-8*) Thomson Learn.

Automated External Defibrillation. American Red Cross Staff. 1998. LC 98-14957. 40.00 (*0-323-00439-3*) Mosby Inc.

Automated External Defibrillation. National Safety Council Staff. 1997. LC 98-140463. (Emergency Care Ser.). (Illus.). 64p. (C). pap. text 12.95 (*0-7637-0422-9*, 0422-9) Jones & Bartlett.

Automated Fabrication of Mobility Aids (AFMA) Below-Knee CASD-CAM Testing & Evaluation Program Results. 1993. (Illus.). 47p. (Orig.). (C). pap. text 20.00 (*1-56806-212-5*) DIANE Pub.

Automated Instrumentation for Radioimmunoassay. Lemuel J. Bowie. 1980. 224p. 119.00 (*0-8493-5747-0*, QP519, CRC Reprint) Franklin.

Automated Integration of Clinical Laboratories: A Reference. Ed. by Michael G. Bissell & John R. Petersen. 1998. 153p. pap. 53.00 (*1-890883-03-4*, 202028) Am Assn Clinical Chem.

Automated Perimetry in Glaucoma: Fluctuation Behavior & General & Local Reduction of Sensitivity. Christina T. Langerhorst. 1988. (Illus.). 172p. pap. text (*90-6299-025-8*) Kugler NLD. *Dist:* Lib Res.

Automated Peritoneal Dialysis. Ed. by C. Ronco et al. 1999. LC 99-40841. (Contributions to Nephrology Ser.: Vol. 129). (Illus.). x, 274p. 198.25 (*3-8055-6934-3*) S Karger.

Automated Static Perimetry. Douglas R. Anderson. 2nd ed. 1998. LC 98-29287. (Illus.). 377p. text 84.95 (*0-8151-4384-2*, 31269) Mosby Inc.

Automatic Analysis & Recognition of Speech. Ed. by Jean-Paul Haton. 1982. text 155.50 (*90-277-1443-6*) Kluwer Academic.

Automatic Control of Food Manufacturing Processes. Ian MacFarlane. 1983. (Illus.). 308p. 88.25 (*0-85334-200-8*, I-207-83) Elsevier.

Automatic Data Technology: Index of New Information with Authors, Subjects & References. Jerome C. Totter. 1995. LC 95-16103. 57.50 (*0-7883-0662-6*); pap. 47.50 (*0-7883-0663-4*) ABBE Pubs Assn.

Automatic External Defibrillators & Remote-Control Defibrillators. AAMI Staff. 1993. (Illus.). 29p. (Orig.). pap. 82.00 (*1-57020-000-9*, DF39-209) Assn Adv Med Instrn.

Automatic, General-Purpose EO Sterilizers & EO Sterilant Sources Intended for Use in Health Care Facilities. 2nd ed. 1992. pap. 70.00 (*1-57020-001-7*, ST24-209) Assn Adv Med Instrn.

Automatic Speech Recognition Research in the U. S. S. R. George Vysotsky. Ed. by Andrew A. Michta. 1986. (Illus.). 143p. (Orig.). pap. text 75.00 (*1-55831-055-X*) Delphic Associates.

Automating the Medical Record. Thomas Landholt. Ed. by Kay Stanley. 1998. (Practice Success Ser.). 96p. 54.00 (*0-89970-909-5*) AMA.

Automating the Physician's Office. Barry Wend. 1992. 60p. pap., stu. ed. 21.00 (*0-932223-14-1*) Churchill PC.

Automation & Validation of Information in Pharmaceutical Processing. Ed. by Joseph Despautz. 1998. LC 98-21356. (Drugs & the Pharmaceutical Sciences Ser.: 0). (Illus.). 464p. text 175.00 (*0-8247-0119-4*) Dekker.

Automation in Anesthesia: A Relief? A. P. Meijler. 1987. (Illus.). 181p. 66.95 (*0-387-18204-7*) Spr-Verlag.

Automation in Blood Transfusion: Proceedings of the Thirteenth Annual Symposium on Blood Transfusion, Groningen 1988. Ed. by Smith C. Sibinga et al. 1989. (Developments in Hematology & Immunology Ser.). (C). text 158.50 (*0-7923-0488-8*) Kluwer Academic.

Automation in the Clinical Lab. Ward. 1995. 345.00 (*0-7216-4764-2*) Saunders.

Automed - A to Z: The Automedical Index. S. H. Shakman. 1998. LC 98-96148. pap. text 19.95 (*1-892506-03-3*) Inst of Science.

Autonomic & Enteric Ganglia: Transmission & Its Pharmacology. Ed. by Alexander G. Karczmar et al. 1986. LC 85-19398. (Illus.). 532p. (C). text 162.00 (*0-306-42039-2*, Kluwer Plenum) Kluwer Academic.

Autonomic Control of the Respiratory System. Peter J. Barnes. 1997. (Autonomic Nervous System Ser). 352p. text 105.00 (*3-7186-5140-8*, Harwood Acad Pubs) Gordon & Breach.

Autonomic Functions in Human Physiology. G. E. Thews & P. Vaupel. Tr. by M. A. Biederman-Thorson from GER. 1984. (Springer Study Edition Ser.). (Illus.). 400p. 37.95 (*0-387-13217-1*) Spr-Verlag.

Autonomic Ganglia. Elspeth M. McLachlan. 1995. (Autonomic Nervous System Ser.). 529p. text 165.00 (*3-7186-5148-3*, Harwood Acad Pubs) Gordon & Breach.

Autonomic Innervation of the Skin. Judy L. Morris & Ian L. Gibbins. 1997. (Autonomic Nervous System Ser.). 432p. text 120.00 (*90-5702-235-4*, Harwood Acad Pubs) Gordon & Breach.

Autonomic Nervous System & Exercise. Hilary Green. 1990. 212p. (gr. 13). pap. 90.95 (*0-412-32500-4*, A4462) Chapman & Hall.

Autonomic Nervous System & Its Effectors. Alison S. Brading. 1999. LC 97-22696. (Illus.). viii, 370 p. 141.95 (*0-632-02624-3*) Blackwell Sci.

Autonomic Neuroeffector Mechanisms. Ed. by Geoffrey Burnstock. (Autonomic Nervous System Ser.). xii, 580p. 1995. pap. text 66.00 (*3-7186-5683-3*); 1992. text 198.00 (*3-7186-5135-1*) Gordon & Breach (Harwood Acad Pubs).

Autonomic Pharmacology. K. J. Broadley. 1996. 500p. text (*0-7484-0556-9*) Tay Francis Ltd GBR. *Dist:* Taylor & Francis.

***Autonomietraining: Gesundheit und Problemlosung Durch Anregung der Selbstregulation.** Ronald Grossarth-Maticek. 2000. (Illus.). 44.00 (*3-11-016881-2*) De Gruyter.

Autonomous Self: The Work of John D. Sutherland. Ed. by Jill S. Scharff. 1994. LC 93-22563. (Library of Object Relations). 480p. reprint ed. 65.00 (*1-56821-008-6*) Aronson.

Autopoiesis & Cognition: The Realization of the Living. Humberto Muturana & Francisco J. Varela. 1980. (Boston Studies in the Philosophy of Science: No. 42). 170p. (C). pap. text 45.00 (*90-277-1016-3*); lib. bdg. 94.00 (*90-277-1015-5*) Kluwer Academic.

Autopsy: A Manual & Atlas. Finkbeiner. 1999. text 90.00 (*0-443-07676-6*) Saunders.

Autopsy in Epidemiology & Medical Research. Ed. by E. Riboli & M. Delendi. 1991. (IARC Scientific Publications Ser.: No. 112). (Illus.). 298p. pap. text 57.50 (*92-832-2112-5*) OUP.

***Autopsy, Medicine & Mortality Statistics.** Randy Hanzlick. 2001. 50p. per. 6.50 (*0-16-050955-6*) USGPO.

Autoradiography & Correlative Imaging. Ed. by Howard Solomon & Walter E. Stumpf. 1995. (Illus.). 597p. text 158.00 (*0-12-675450-0*) Acad Pr.

Autosomal Dominant Polycystic Kidney Disease. Ed. by Adalberto Sessa. 1995. LC 95-24977. (Contributions to Nephrology Ser.: Vol. 115). (Illus.). x, 192p. 197.50 (*3-8055-6090-7*) S Karger.

Auxiliaries in Primary Health Care: An Annotated Bibliography. Ed. by Katherine Elliott. 1979. 126p. (Orig.). pap. (*0-903031-58-2*) Stylus Pub VA.

***Auxiliary Nurses Guide.** (Illus.). pap. (*0-7021-2883-X*) Juta & Co ZAF. *Dist:* Intl Spec Bk.

Auxiliary Personnel in Nursing: A Survey of Existing Legislation. WHO Staff. 1966. (International Digest of Health Legislation Offprints: Vol. 17, No. 2). 38p. 3.00 (*92-4-169172-7*) World Health.

Aversion, Avoidance & Anxiety: Perspectives on Aversively Motivated Behavior. Ed. by T. Archer & L. G. Nilsson. 1988. 512p. (C). text 99.95 (*0-8058-0132-4*) L Erlbaum Assocs.

Aversive Interpersonal Behaviors. Ed. by Robin M. Kowalski. 1997. LC 97-23743. (Series in Social/Clinical Psychology). 260p. (C). 49.50 (*0-306-45611-7*, Plenum Trade) Perseus Pubng.

Avery's Diseases of the Newborn. H. William Taeusch & Roberta A. Ballard. Ed. by Judy Fletcher. 7th ed. 1998. LC 97-42374. (Illus.). 1360p. (C). text 139.00 (*0-7216-5751-6*) Saunders.

Avery's Drug Treatment. Speight. 3rd ed. 1987. text 236.00 (*0-443-03923-2*) Saunders.

Avery's Drug Treatment. Trevor M. Speight. 4th ed. 1997. (Illus.). 1800p. (*0-86471-036-4*) Adis Intl NZL. *Dist:* Lppncott W & W.

Avian & Mammalian Wildlife Toxicology: Second Conference - STP 757. Ed. by Lamb & E. E. Kenaga. 1981. 170p. pap. 18.50 (*0-8031-0759-5*, STP757) ASTM.

Avian & Mammalian Wildlife Toxicology - STP 693. Ed. by E. E. Kenaga. 1979. 103p. pap. 16.25 (*0-8031-0287-9*, STP693) ASTM.

Avian Auditory-Vocal Motor Interfaces, No. 44, No. 4-5. Ed. by S. E. Brauth & W. S. Hall. 1994. (Journal: Vol. 44, No. 4-5). (Illus.). 100p. pap. 51.50 (*3-8055-6074-5*) S Karger.

Avian Cellular Immunology. Ed. by Sharma. 1990. 216p. 198.00 (*0-8493-6833-2*, SF995) CRC Pr.

Avian Endocrinology. Ed. by P. J. Sharp. 1993. 396p. 69.95 (*1-898099-01-4*) Blackwell Sci.

Avian-Exotic Animal Care Guides. R. W. Woerpel & W. J. Rosskopf, Jr. 1991. LC 88-83117. 85p. 39.95 (*0-939674-24-6*) Am Vet Pubns.

Avian Hematology & Cytology. Terry W. Campbell. 2nd ed. 1994. LC 94-36354. (Illus.). 112p. text 62.95 (*0-8138-2970-4*) Iowa U Pr.

Avian Immunology: Basis & Practice, Set. Ed. by Auli Toivanen & Paavo Toivanen. 1987. 420.00 (*0-8493-6767-0*, SF995) CRC Pr.

Avian Immunology: Basis & Practice, Vol. II: Cellular Cooperation in Immunity. Ed. by Auli Toivanen & Paavo Toivanen. 1987. 256p. 128.00 (*0-8493-6769-7*, CRC Reprint) Franklin.

Avian Immunology Basis & Practice, Vol. 1. Paavo Toivanen & Auli Toivanen. 1987. LC 86-14700. 141.00 (*0-8493-6768-9*, CRC Reprint) Franklin.

Avian Leukosis. Ed. by G. F. De Boer. 1987. (Developments in Veterinary Virology Ser.). (C). text 161.50 (*0-89838-872-4*) Kluwer Academic.

Avian Medicine. Ed. by Jaime Samour. 1999. (Illus.). 427p. text 99.95 (*0-7234-2960-X*) Mosby Inc.

Avian Medicine. Thomas Tully et al. 2000. LC 00-36020. (Illus.). 448p. text 95.00 (*0-7506-3598-3*) Buttrwrth-Heinemann.

Avian Medicine: Principles & Application. Ed. by Branson W. Ritchie et al. (Illus.). (C). 1994. LC 93-60501. 1384p. text 175.00 (*0-9636996-0-1*); 1997. 800p. pap. text 69.00 (*0-9636996-5-2*) Zoological Educ.

Avian Medicine & Surgery. Robert B. Altman et al. Ed. by Sandra Valkoff. 1996. LC 95-4641. (Illus.). 720p. text 99.00 (*0-7216-5446-0*) Saunders.

Avian Medicine & Surgery. B. H. Coles. 2nd ed. 1998. (Illus.). 416p. pap. text (*0-632-03356-8*) Blckwell Science GBR. *Dist:* Iowa U Pr.

Avian Reproductive Tactics: Female & Male Perspectives. Ed. by P. G. Parker & N. T. Burley. 1998. (Ornithological Monographs: Vol. 49). 20.00 (*0-935868-95-X*) Am Ornithologists.

Aviation Medicine. John Ernsting & Peter King. 2nd ed. 1988. (Illus.). 956p. pap. text 110.00 (*0-7506-2275-X*) Buttrwrth-Heinemann.

Aviation Medicine. John Ernstine et al. 3rd ed. 1999. LC 99-206430. (Illus.). 720p. (*0-7506-3252-6*) E A GBR. *Dist:* OUP.

Aviation Medicine. Richard M. Harding. Ed. by F. John Mills. 3rd ed. 1993. (Illus.). 228p. pap. text (*0-7279-0814-6*) BMJ Pub GBR. *Dist:* AIDC.

Aviation Psychology. Stanley N. Roscoe. 1982. LC 79-27539. (Illus.). 318p. reprint ed. pap. 29.95 (*0-8138-1927-X*) Iowa U Pr.

Aviation Psychology: A Science & a Profession. Klaus-Martin Goeters. 1998. LC 97-46524. 306p. text (*1-84014-325-8*, TL555.A94) Ashgate Pub GBR. *Dist:* Ashgate Pub Co.

Avicenna, His Life & Works. Soheil M. Afnan. 1980. LC 79-8705. 298p. reprint ed. lib. bdg. 38.50 (*0-313-22198-7*, AFAV, Greenwood Pr) Greenwood.

Avoiding Attendants from Hell: A Practical Guide to Finding, Hiring & Keeping Personal Care Attendants. June Price. l.t. ed. 1998. LC 98-89122. (Illus.). 120p. spiral bd. 16.95 (*1-888725-18-4*) Sci & Human Pr.

Avoiding Ethical Misconduct in Psychology Specialty Areas. Ed. by Robert M. Anderson, Jr. et al. 1998. LC 97-23109. 340p. text 72.95 (*0-398-06797-X*); pap. text 55.95 (*0-398-06798-8*) C C Thomas.

Avoiding Liability in Hospital Security. Ed. by Paul Leavitt & Jennifer Vaughan. 1998. 80p. pap. 97.00 (*1-887986-08-1*) Strafford Pubns.

Avoiding the Medicaid Trap. Armond D. Budish. 1991. 240p. pap. 15.00 (*0-380-71403-5*, Avon Bks) Morrow Avon.

Awaken Healing Energy Through the Tao Mantak Chia. Mantak Chia. 1983. 205p. pap. 14.00 (*0-943358-07-8*) Aurora Press.

Awaken the Genius in Your Child Through Positive Attitude Training. Nicola M. Tauraso & L. Richard Batzler. 1981. pap. 12.95 (*0-935710-01-9*) Hid Valley MD.

Awakening. Richard W. Heinberg. 1985. (Illus.). 10p. reprint ed. pap. 2.00 (*0-935427-25-2*) Foundation Hse.

Awakening Nature's Healing Intelligence: Expanding Ayurveda Through the Maharishi Vedic Approach to Health. Hari Sharma. 1998. LC 97-69848. (Illus.). 278p. pap. 17.95 (*0-914955-35-7*) Lotus Pr.

Awakening Nightmare. Albert M. Honig. 1972. LC 77-189003. 9.95 (*0-912834-00-5*) Am Faculty Pr.

***Awakening of a Surgeon: One Doctor's Journey to Fight the System & Empower Your Community.** David Janda. 2001. LC 2001-474. 192p. 18.95 (*1-886947-95-3*) Sleepng Bear.

Awakening Our Self-Healing Body: A Solution to the Health Care Crisis. Arthur M. Baker. 1994. LC 93-93516. 306p. (Orig.). pap. 12.95 (*1-883989-25-6*) Self Hlth Care.

Awakening the Heart: East-West Approaches to Psychotherapy & the Healing Relationship. Ed. by John Welwood. 1983. LC 83-42807. 219p. (Orig.). pap. 17.00 (*0-394-72182-9*) Shambhala Pubns.

Awakening to the Plant Kingdom. Robert Shapiro & Julie Rapkin. 1991. (Illus.). 140p. (Orig.). pap. 9.95 (*0-945946-12-0*) Cassandra Pr.

Awakenings. Oliver W. Sacks. 1999. LC 99-27880. (Illus.). 464p. pap. 14.00 (*0-375-70405-1*) Knopf.

Awareness: What It Is, What It Does. Chris Nunn. 1995. LC 95-13966. 176p. (C). pap. 22.95 (*0-415-13227-4*) Routledge.

Awareness, Dialogue & Process: Essays on Gestalt Therapy. Gary M. Yontef. 1993. 580p. pap. 35.00 (*0-939266-20-2*) Gestalt Journal.

Awareness During Anesthesia. Mohamed Ghoneim. 2000. LC 00-60810. (Illus.). 179p. text 64.99 (*0-7506-7201-3*) Buttrwrth-Heinemann.

Awareness of Deficit after Brain Injury: Clinical & Theoretical Issues. Ed. by George P. Prigatano & Daniel L. Schacter. 1991. (Illus.). 290p. text 52.50 (*0-19-505941-7*) OUP.

Awe & Trembling: Psychotherapy of Unusual States. E. Mark Stern & Robert B. Marchesani. 2000. LC 99-88149. (Illus.). xx, 203p. 39.95 (*0-7890-0973-0*); pap. text 24.95 (*0-7890-0991-9*) Haworth Pr.

Awesome Abs! The Gut-Busting Solution for Men & Women. Paul Chek. 1996. (Illus.). 47p. pap. (*1-55210-002-2*) MuscleMag Intl CAN. *Dist:* BookWorld.

Awhonn's Single Room Maternity Care for the 21st Century: The Phillips & Fenwick Model. Celeste R. Phillips & Loel Fenwick. 2000. LC 00-23780. (Illus.). 208p. pap. text 49.95 (*0-7817-2233-0*) Lppncott W & W.

Axon: Structure, Function & Pathophysiology. Ed. by Jeffery D. Kocsis et al. 1995. (Illus.). 714p. text 175.00 (*0-19-508293-1*) OUP.

Axonal Conduction Time & Human Cerebral Laterality: A Psychobiological Theory. Robert Miller. 1996. 304p. text 95.00 (*3-7186-5865-8*) Gordon & Breach.

Axonal Regeneration in the Mammalian Central Nervous System. D. E. Oorschot & D. G. Jones. 1990. (Advances in Anatomy, Embryology & Cell Biology Ser.: Vol. 119). (Illus.). 121p. 59.00 (*0-387-51757-X*) Spr-Verlag.

Axonal Transport in Neuronal Growth & Regeneration. Ed. by John S. Elam & Paul Cancalon. 1984. LC 84-16006. 300p. 79.50 (*0-306-41699-9*, Plenum Trade) Perseus Pubng.

Axoplasmic Transport. Zafar Igbal. 1986. 352p. 185.00 (*0-8493-6334-9*, QP363, CRC Reprint) Franklin.

Ayahuasca Analogues - Pangaean Entheogens. Jonathan Ott. 1994. 128p. 24.00 (*0-9614234-4-7*) Natural Prod.

AY's Neuroanatomy of C. Elegans for Computation. Theodore B. Acchacoso & William S. Yamamoto. 1991. 304p. 131.95 (*0-8493-4234-1*, QM451) CRC Pr.

Ayurveda: A Way of Life. Vinod Verma. 1995. LC 95-15228. (Illus.). 304p. (Orig.). pap. 14.95 (*0-87728-822-4*) Red Wheel ME.

Ayurveda: India's Art of Natural Medicine & Life Extension. Birgit Heyn. 1990. 176p. reprint ed. pap. 9.95 (*0-89281-333-4*, Heal Arts VT) Inner Tradit.

Ayurveda: The Complete Handbook. T. L. Devaraj. 2000. LC 99-949982. xi, 188p. pap. (*81-7476-287-6*) UBS Pubs IND. *Dist:* S Asia.

Ayurveda - A Life of Balance: The Complete Guide to Ayurvedic Nutrition & Body Types with Recipes. Maya Tiwari. 1994. LC 94-29178. 368p. pap. 24.95 (*0-89281-490-X*, Heal Arts VT) Inner Tradit.

Ayurveda & Aromatherapy: The Earth Essential Guide to Ancient Wisdom & Modern Healing. Light Miller & Bryan Miller. 1995. LC 95-80409. (Illus.). 368p. (Orig.). pap. 21.95 (*0-914955-20-9*) Lotus Pr.

Ayurveda & Life Impressions Bodywork: Seeking Our Healing Memories. Donald VanHowten. 1997. LC 96-79622. (Illus.). 296p. (Orig.). pap. 19.95 (*0-914955-24-1*) Lotus Pr.

Ayurveda & Panchakarma: The Science of Healing & Rejuvenation. Sunil V. Joshi. 1997. LC 96-79621. (Illus.). 316p. pap. 19.95 (*0-914955-37-3*) Lotus Pr.

Ayurveda Baby Massage. Samhita Enterprises Incorporated Staff. 1999. pap. text (*1-57582-039-0*) Samhita Enterprises.

Ayurveda Encyclopedia: Natural Secrets to Healing, Prevention, & Longevity. Sada Shiva Tirtha. 1998. (*81-7030-590-X*) Sri Satguru Pubns IND. *Dist:* S Asia.

Ayurveda Encyclopedia: Natural Secrets to Healing, Prevention & Longevity. Sada Shiva Tirtha. Ed. by Amrit Kaur Khalsa & Rob Paton. 1998. LC 97-77845. (Illus.). 686p. pap. 34.95 (*0-9658042-2-4*) Ayurveda Holistic.

Ayurveda for Health & Long Life. R. K. Garde. 1975. 120p. (Orig.). pap. text 11.95 (*0-89744-054-4*) Auromere.

Ayurveda for Women: A Guide to Vitality & Health. Robert E. Svoboda. 1999. (Illus.). 144p. pap. text (*0-7153-0855-6*) D & C Pub.

Ayurveda for Women: A Guide to Vitality & Health. Robert E. Svoboda. 2000. LC 00-57784. 192p. pap. 14.95 (*0-89281-939-1*, Inner Trad) Inner Tradit.

Ayurveda or Hindu System of Medical Science. 1998. 131p. (C). text (*81-7030-184-X*) Sri Satguru Pubns IND. *Dist:* S Asia.

Ayurveda Revisited. S. Dahanukar & U. Thatte. 1989. (*0-86132-223-1*) Popular Prakashan IND. *Dist:* S Asia.

Ayurveda, the Science of Self-Healing: A Practical Guide. Vasant Lad. 1984. LC 83-80620. (Illus.). 175p. (Orig.). pap. text 10.95 (*0-914955-00-4*) Lotus Pr.

***Ayurvedic Balancing.** Joyce Bueker. 2002. LC 2001-50442. pap. 14.95 (*0-7387-0188-2*) Llewellyn Pubns.

Ayurvedic Beauty Care: Ageless Techniques to Invoke Nature Beauty. Melanie A. Sachs. 1994. LC 93-80313. (Illus.). 285p. (Orig.). pap. 17.95 (*0-914955-11-X*) Lotus Pr.

Ayurvedic Drugs & Their Plant Sources. V. V. Sivarajan & Indira Balachandran. 1995. LC 94-900730. (C). (*81-204-0828-4*) Oxford IBH IND. *Dist:* S Asia.

Ayurvedic Healing. Frena Gray-Davidson. 2001. LC 2001-35784. (Healing Wisdom Ser.). 160p. pap. 11.95 (*0-658-01147-2*) McGraw-Hill Prof.

Ayurvedic Healing: A Comprehensive Guide. David Frawley. 2nd enl. rev. ed. 2000. LC 00-134620. (Illus.). x, 448p. pap. 22.95 (*0-914955-97-7*) Lotus Pr.

Ayurvedic Healing Cuisine. Harish Johari. 2000. LC 00-40914. 272p. pap. 19.95 (*0-89281-938-3*, Heal Arts VT) Inner Tradit.

Ayurvedic Healing for Women: Herbal Gynecology. Atreya. 1999. LC 99-11474. (Illus.). 304p. pap. 14.95 (*1-57863-116-5*) Red Wheel ME.

Ayurvedic Massage: Traditional Indian Techniques for Balancing Body & Mind. Harish Johari. 1996. LC 96-16436. (Illus.). 160p. pap. 19.95 (*0-89281-489-6*, Heal Arts VT) Inner Tradit.

Ayurvedic Secrets to Longevity & Total Health. Peter Anselmo. 1996. LC 96-2833. 320p. (C). pap. 13.95 (*0-13-156465-X*) PH Pr.

Azapropazone: Twenty Years of Clinical Use. Ed. by Kim D. Rainsford. 1990. 256p. text 141.50 (*0-7923-8911-5*) Kluwer Academic.

Azospirillum II: Genetics, Physiology, Ecology, Vol. 48. Ed. by W. Klingmuller. 1984. (Experientia Supplementa Ser.). 196p. 41.95 (*3-7643-1576-8*) Birkhauser.

B

B Cells & Autoantibody Production in Autoimmune Diseases. Christian Boitard. 1996. LC 95-22862. (Medical Intelligence Unit Ser.). 273p. pap. 89.95 (*0-412-10171-8*, 71207) Chapman & Hall.

B Cells & Autoantibody Production in Autoimmune Diseases. Christian Boitard. 1996. LC 95-22862. (Medical Intelligence Unit Ser.). 270p. 99.00 (*1-57059-209-8*) Landes Bioscience.

B. F. Skinner: A Life. Daniel W. Bjork. 2nd ed. 1997. LC 96-40385. (Illus.). 298p. reprint ed. pap. 19.95 (*1-55798-416-6*, 4316850) Am Psychol.

B. F. Skinner & Behaviorism in American Culture. Ed. by Laurence D. Smith & William R. Woodward. 1996. LC 95-42466. 352p. 47.50 (*0-934223-40-8*) Lehigh Univ Pr.

B-Lymphocytes & Autoimmunity, Vol. 815. Ed. by Nicholas Chiorazzi et al. 1997. LC 97-3680. 170.00 (*1-57331-076-X*) NY Acad Sci.

B. S. & Live Longer (Beat Stress) Jim Keelan. 1978. 6.00 (*0-9606554-2-5*) Comm Unltd.

***Babel's Shadow: Genetic Technologies in a Fracturing Society.** Pete Moore. 2001. LC 2001-2861. 14.95 (*1-893956-16-4*) Context Bks.

Babesiosis of Domestic Animals & Man, Vol. I. Ed. by Miodrag Ristic. 1988. 176p. 152.00 (*0-8493-4908-7*, QR201, CRC Reprint) Franklin.

Babies in Bottles: Twentieth-Century Visions of Reproductive Technology. Susan M. Squier. 1994. LC 94-10154. (Illus.). (C). 285p. text 48.00 (*0-8135-2116-5*); 270p. pap. text 17.00 (*0-8135-2117-3*) Rutgers U Pr.

Babies Remember Birth see Mind of Your Newborn Baby

Babies with Down Syndrome: A New Parents' Guide. Ed. by Karen Stray-Gundersen. 2nd ed. 1995. LC 95-34041. (Special Needs Collection). (Illus.). 340p. pap. 15.95 (*0-933149-64-6*) Woodbine House.

Baboon: Microbiology, Clinical Chemistry & Some Hematological Aspects. S. S. Kalter. 1973. (Primates in Medicine Ser.: Vol. 8). (Illus.). 62.75 (*3-8055-1442-5*) S Karger.

Baboon Mothers & Infants. Jeanne Altmann. LC 79-21568. (Illus.). 256p. 1981. pap. 15.95 (*0-674-05857-7*); 1980. 34.95 (*0-674-05856-9*) HUP.

Baby: He's a Doctor She's a Nurse Now They Must Decide If Their Own Baby Should Live or Die. Joseph A. Stirt. 1992. LC 92-60566. 314p. 22.95 (*0-88282-111-3*) New Horizon NJ.

Baby? ... Maybe: A Guide to Making the Most Fateful Decision of Your Life. Elizabeth M. Whelan. 1975. LC 75-6396. 256p. 10.95 (*0-672-52096-6*); pap. 6.95 (*0-672-52186-5*) Macmillan (Bobbs).

Baby & Child A to Z Medical Handbook: Parent's Easy Reference Guide to Children's Illnesses, Symptoms, & Treatment. Miriam Stoppard. 1996. 320p. pap. 15.95 (*0-399-51765-0*, Perigee Bks) Berkley Pub.

Baby & Child Emergency First-Aid Handbook. Ed. by Mitchell J. Einzig. 1992. LC 92-28339. (Illus.). 64p. 15.00 (*0-671-79204-0*) S&S Trade.

Baby & Child Emergency First Aid Handbook. Mitchell J. Einzig. rev. ed. 1995. (Illus.). 64p. pap. 8.00 (*0-671-51976-X*) S&S Trade.

Baby & Child Emergency First Aid Handbook: Simple Step-by-Step Instructions for the Most Common Childhood Emergencies. Ed. by Mitchell J. Einzig. 1992. LC 92-28339. (Illus.). 96p. 13.00 (*0-88166-195-3*) Meadowbrook.

Baby & Child Medical Care. Mitchell J. Einzig et al. 3rd ed. 1998. LC 97-36441. 9.00 (*0-88166-307-7*) Meadowbrook.

Baby & Infant Health Care: Index of New Information. Cathy L. Kauffman & Milton K. Kauffman. 1998. 160p. 57.50 (*0-7883-2018-1*); pap. 47.50 (*0-7883-2019-X*) ABBE Pubs Assn.

Baby & Me: The Essential Guide to Pregnancy see Mi Bebe y Yo: Una Guia Esencial para el Embarazo

Baby & the Bathwater. Nina Coltart. 1996. LC 96-28318. 35.00 (*0-8236-0535-3*) Intl Univs Pr.

Baby & Toddler Sleep Program. John Pearce. 2000. 144p. pap. 10.95 (*1-55561-279-2*) Fisher Bks.

Baby & Toddler Sleep Program: How to Get Your Child to Sleep Through the Night, Every Night. John Pearce. 1999. LC 98-51783. (Illus.). 144p. pap. 10.95 (*1-55561-175-3*) Fisher Bks.

Baby & Toddler Sleep Programme. John Pearce. pap. (*0-09-181571-1*) Ebury Pr GBR. *Dist:* Trafalgar.

Baby Books. Chris Hadden et al. 1982. pap. 7.90 (*0-941298-06-X*) M E Pinkham.

Baby Challenge: A Handbook on Pregnancy for Women with a Physical Disability. Mukti J. Campion. 1990. LC 89-39067. 219p. (C). pap. text 15.95 (*0-415-04859-1*, A4697) Routledge.

Baby ER: The Heroic Doctors & Nurses Who Perform Medicine's Tiniest Miracles. Edward Humes. 2000. LC 00-61870. 336p. 25.00 (*0-684-86410-X*) S&S Trade.

Baby Friendly/Mother Friendly. Susan F. Murray. 1996. mass mkt. 24.00 (*0-7234-2123-4*) Mosby Inc.

Baby Massage: Parent-Child Bonding Through Touch. Amelia Auckett. rev. ed. 1991. LC 82-2172. (Illus.). 128p. pap. 11.95 (*1-55704-022-2*) Newmarket.

Baby?...Maybe: A Guide to Making the Most Fateful Decision of Your Life. Elizabeth M. Whelan. rev. ed. 1980. LC 79-55437. 256p. pap. 8.95 (*0-672-52629-8*) Macmillan.

Baby Observation: Emotional Relationships During the First Year of Life. M. Perez-Sanchez. 1990. 219p. pap. (*0-902965-26-3*) Clunie Pr GBR. *Dist:* Other Pr LLC.

Baby Steps: A Parents' Guide to Understanding During the First Two Years. Claire B. Kopp & Donne L. Bean. 1993. LC 93-10365. 300p. (C). text 23.95 (*0-7167-2390-5*); pap. text 14.95 (*0-7167-2499-5*) W H Freeman.

Babyhood. Penelope Leach. 2nd enl. rev. ed. 1983. LC 82-48881. pap. 19.00 (*0-394-71436-9*) Knopf.

***Baby's First Year: Your Guide to a Happy & Healthy First Year with Baby.** Marion Finholm Jones et al. 2001. (Illus.). 28p. 8.00 (*0-9618935-9-1*, 20005) Linholm.

Bac-si: A Doctor Remembers Vietnam. Peter Caldwell. 1991. LC 90-90086. (Illus.). 144p. pap. 9.95 (*0-9626124-0-5*) Taote Pub.

Bach Flower Massage. Daniele L. Rito. Tr. by Tami Calliope from ITA. 1997. LC 97-26253. (Illus.). 208p. pap. 14.95 (*0-89281-736-4*, Heal Arts VT) Inner Tradit.

Bach Flower Remedies. Edward Bach & F. J. Wheeler. 2nd rev. ed. 1997. LC 97-29689. 248p. pap. 12.95 (*0-87983-869-8*, 38698K, Keats Pubng) McGraw-Hill Trade.

Bach Flower Remedies: Illustrations & Preparations. Nora Weeks & Victor Bullen. 1990. (Illus.). 104p. pap. (*0-85207-205-8*) C W Daniel GBR. *Dist:* Natl Bk Netwk.

Bach Flower Remedies & Other Flower Essences. Vivian Williamson & Andrew Tresider. 2001. (Illus.). 96p. 17.95 (*0-7548-0626-X*) Anness Pub.

Bach Flower Remedies for Animals. Gregory Vlamis & Helen Graham. 1999. 120p. pap. (*1-899171-72-X*) Findhorn Pr GBR. *Dist:* Lantern Books.

Bach Flower Remedies for Children: A Parents' Guide. Barbara Mazzarella. 1997. LC 97-302. 192p. pap. 14.95 (*0-89281-649-X*, Heal Arts VT) Inner Tradit.

Bach Flower Remedies for Men. 1996. pap. 13.95 (*0-8464-4558-1*) Beekman Pubs.

Bach Flower Remedies Illustrations & Preparations. Nora Weeks & Victor Bullen. (Illus.). 96p. (Orig.). pap. 14.95 (*0-8464-4209-4*) Beekman Pubs.

Bach Flower Remedies Repertory. F. J. Wheeler. 16th ed. 32p. pap. 7.95 (*0-8464-4207-8*) Beekman Pubs.

Bach Flower Remedies Step by Step. Judy Howard. 68p. (Orig.). pap. 8.95 (*0-8464-4208-6*) Beekman Pubs.

Bach Flower Remedies Step by Step. Judy Howard. 1990. 104p. pap. (*0-85207-223-6*) C W Daniel GBR. *Dist:* Natl Bk Netwk.

Bach Flower Remedies to the Rescue. Gregory Vlamis. 1990. (Illus.). 176p. pap. 10.95 (*0-89281-378-4*) Inner Tradit.

Bach Flower Remedies Workbook. 1998. pap., wbk. ed. 29.95 (*0-8464-4560-3*) Beekman Pubs.

Bach Flower Therapy: Theory & Practice. Mechthild Scheffer. 1987. LC 92-43337. 208p. pap. 12.95 (*0-89281-239-7*, Heal Arts VT) Inner Tradit.

Bach Remedies Repertory. F. J. Wheeler. 1996. pap. (*0-85207-300-3*) C W Daniel GBR. *Dist:* Natl Bk Netwk.

Bachelors: The Psychology of Men Who Haven't Married. Charles A. Waehler. 1996. LC 96-21323. 224p. 45.00 (*0-275-95668-7*, Praeger Pubs) Greenwood.

Back: Problems & Prevention, a Self-Help Guide. Vivian Grisogono. 1996. (Illus.). 230p. pap. (*0-7195-5531-0*) John Murray GBR. *Dist:* Trafalgar.

Back Almanac: The Best New Thinking on an Age-Old Problem. Lanier Publishing International Editors. 1992. LC 92-25976. 216p. pap. 14.95 (*0-89815-508-8*) Ten Speed Pr.

Back & Neck Disorders Sourcebook: Basic Information about Disorders & Injuries of the Spinal Cord & Vertebrae. Ed. by Karen Bellenir. 1997. LC 97-1006. (Health Reference Ser.: Vol. 24). 560p. 78.00 (*0-7808-0202-0*) Omnigraphics Inc.

Back Care: A Clinical Approach. Sheila Braggins. 2000. LC 99-50230. x, 265p. (*0-443-06488-1*) Church.

Back Care: An Illustrated Guide. Jean Oliver. (Illus.). 1994. LC 93-6254. 192p. pap. text 45.00 (*0-7506-0191-4*); 2nd ed. 2002. 224p. pap. 45.00 (*0-7506-4689-6*) Buttrwrth-Heinemann.

Back Care: How to Relieve & Prevent Pain from Low Back Problems. Ed. by Augustus A. White, III. 2nd ed. 1996. 24p. pap. 1.42 (*0-934230-43-9*) Medic Pub.

Back Care Basics: A Doctor's Gentle Yoga Program for Back & Neck Pain Relief. Mary P. Schatz. 1992. LC 91-78206. (Illus.). 248p. (Orig.). pap. 21.95 (*0-9627138-2-1*) Rodmell Pr.

Back Care Basics: A Doctor's Gentle Yoga Program for Back & Neck Pain Relief. Mary Pullig Schatz. 2000. (Illus.). 248p. reprint ed. text 27.00 (*0-7881-6987-4*) DIANE Pub.

Back Fitness the Yoga Way. Kareen Zebroff. 1989. (Illus.). 105p. pap. 14.95 (*0-88976-080-2*) Gordon Soules Bk.

Back from the Dead. Harry Hone. 1978. (Illus.). pap. text (*0-9601168-2-6*); pap. text (*0-9601168-3-4*) Am Biog Ctr.

Back in Action: Lumbar Laminectomy & Discectomy Surgery. Blynnsa Call. Ed. by Karen Hubbard. 2000. (Illus.). 24p. pap. text 4.50 (*0-939838-43-5*) Pritchett & Hull.

Back in Balance: A Chronic Pain Workbook. Barbara J. Headley. 1988. (Illus.). 174p. (Orig.). pap. 10.00 (*0-929538-02-1*) Innovat Systems.

Back in Balance - Back in Action: The Complete Guide to the Self-Treatment & Prevention of Back Pain. Tony Cardenas. 1994. (Illus.). 150p. (Orig.). 19.95 (*0-9641656-0-0*) T H I N K Pr.

Back in Shape: A Back Owner's Manual. Stephen H. Hochschuler. 1991. (Illus.). 208p. pap. 16.00 (*0-395-56273-2*) HM.

Back Injury & Litigation. R. W. Porter. 1995. 140p. pap. (*1-85996-110-X*) Bios Sci GBR. *Dist:* Coronet Bks.

A
B

Back Injury Prevention Handbook. David W. Apts. 1991. 208p. 83.95 (*0-87371-419-9*, L419) Lewis Pubs.

Back Labor No More! What Every Woman Should Know Before Labor. Janie M. King. Ed. by Becky Lormor. 1993. (Illus.). 136p. (Orig.). pap. 16.45 (*0-926218-00-X*) Plenary Systs.

Back Pack. Jane Hobden. 1999. 112p. pap. 22.95 (*0-312-24340-5*) St Martin.

Back Pain. Nachemson. 1993. (*0-397-51202-3*) Lppncott W & W.

Back Pain: A Guide for Patients. Mitchel Harris. Ed. by David Seligson. 1996. (Orthopedics Ser.). (Illus.). 32p. (Orig.). pap. 2.95 (*1-885274-14-9*) Health InfoNet Inc.

Back Pain: An International Review. Ed. by John K. Paterson & Loic Burn. 1990. (C). text 244.50 (*0-7923-8912-3*) Kluwer Academic.

Back Pain: Diagnosis & Treatment Using Manipulative Techniques. John M. Mennell. 1960. 226p. 46.95 (*0-316-56667-5*, Little Brwn Med Div) Lppncott W & W.

Back Pain - What Works: A Comprehensive Guide to Preventing & Overcoming Back Problems. Joseph Kandel. 1996. (Illus.). 224p. pap. 14.95 (*0-7615-0327-7*, Prima Health) Prima Pub.

Back Pain & Spinal Problems: Index of New Information with Authors, Subjects & References. Wilma V. Randoll. rev. ed. 1996. LC 96-185. 149p. 57.50 (*0-7883-1028-3*); pap. 47.50 (*0-7883-1029-1*) ABBE Pubs Assn.

Back Pain Book: A Self-Help Guide for the Daily Relief of Neck & Back Pain. Mike Hage. 1991. LC 92-2670. (Illus.). 256p. pap. 13.95 (*1-56145-042-1*) Peachtree Pubs.

***Back Pain Matters in Primary Care: Clinical Management of Back Pain in a Healthy & Safe Environment.** Ruth Chambers et al. 2001. 192p. pap. (*1-85775-418-2*) Radcliffe Med Pr GBR. *Dist:* Balogh.

Back Pain Rehabilitation. Brian D'Orazio. 1993. LC 93-11017. (Illus.). 282p. text 54.99 (*1-56372-029-9*) Buttrwrth-Heinemann.

Back Pain Revolution. Gordon Waddell. 1998. (C). text (*0-443-06039-8*) Church.

Back Pain Sourcebook. Stephanie Levin-Gervasi. 2nd rev. ed. 1998. (Illus.). 256p. pap. 17.00 (*0-7373-0015-9*, 00159W) NTC Contemp Pub Co.

***Back Sense: A Revolutionary Approach to Halting the Cycle of Chronic Back Pain.** Ronald D. Siegel et al. 2002. 256p. pap. 12.95 (*0-7679-0581-4*) Broadway BDD.

Back Sense: A Revolutionary Approach to Healing the Cycle of Chronic Back Pain. Ronald D. Siegel et al. 2001. LC 00-45466. (Illus.). 256p. 21.95 (*0-7679-0636-5*) Broadway BDD.

Back Talk: How to Diagnose & Treat Lower Back Pain & Sciatica. Loren Fishman & Carol Ardman. 1997. LC 97-426. (Illus.). 224p. 25.00 (*0-393-04129-8*) Norton.

Back to Balance: A Holistic Self-Help Guide to Eastern Remedies. Dylana Accolla & Peter Yates. 1996. LC 95-40330. (Illus.). 240p. pap. (*4-7700-1923-8*) Kodansha Intl JPN. *Dist:* Kodansha.

Back to Basics: Foundations of Healthcare Management. Health Administration Press Staff. 2000. LC 00-59692. (Illus.). vi, 415p. (*1-56793-140-5*) Health Admin Pr.

Back-to-Basics Management for Physicians: How to Reclaim Your Shrinking Profits. Paula Hartley. 1996. 320p. (Orig.). pap. 34.95 (*0-9647823-0-8*) Trisib Pubng.

Back to Basics with Herbs. Jim Jenks. 1984. 50p. pap. 3.95 (*0-913923-61-3*) Woodland UT.

Back to Bismarck: Eastern European Health Care in Systems Transition. Jorgen Marree & Peter Groenewegen. 1997. LC 96-79845. 144p. (*1-85972-617-8*) Avebry GBR. *Dist:* Ashgate Pub Co.

Back to Eden see Regreso al Eden

Back to Eden: The Classic Guide to Herbal Medicine, Natural Foods, & Home Remedies Since 1939. Jethro Kloss & Promise K. Moffet. 936p. reprint ed. rev. ed. 1989. 21.95 (*0-940985-13-6*); rev. ed. 1989. mass mkt. 9.95 (*0-940985-10-1*); 58th annot. exp. ed. 1997. pap. 14.95 (*0-940985-09-8*) Lotus Pr.

Back to Freud's Texts: Making Silent Documents Speak. Ilse Grubrich-Simitis. Tr. by Philip Slotkin. 1996. LC 96-8117. (Illus.). 352p. 45.00 (*0-300-06631-7*) Yale U Pr.

Back to Health see Health Sense: The Cancer Manual - Deal from Strength

Back to Health: A Comprehensive Medical & Nutritional Yeast Control Program. Dennis W. Remington & Barbara W. Higa. 1986. (Illus.). 256p. pap. 10.95 (*0-912547-03-0*, 801-224-9214) Vitality Hse Int Inc.

Back to One: A Practical Guide for Psychotherapists. Sheldon B. Kopp. 1977. LC 77-608269. 165p. pap. 11.95 (*0-8314-0055-2*) Sci & Behavior.

Back to Our Roots: Cooking for Control of Sickle Cell Anemia & Cancer Prevention. Dawud Ujamaa. 2nd rev. ed. 1995. LC 94-72181. (Illus.). 221p. pap. 18.95 (*1-884938-01-9*) Dawud Ujamma.

Back to Reality: A Critique of Postmodern Theory in Psychotherapy. Barbara S. Held. 1995. LC 95-13740. 272p. (C). 32.00 (*0-393-70192-1*) Norton.

Back to Reform: Values, Markets, & the Health Care System. Charles J. Dougherty. 1996. 192p. (C). 29.95 (*0-19-510397-1*) OUP.

Back to the Asylum: The Future of Mental Health Law in the United States. Mary L. Durham & John Q. La Fond. 1992. LC 91-42365. 280p. text 47.50 (*0-19-505520-9*) OUP.

Back to the Beanstalk: Enchantment & Reality for Couples. Judith R. Brown. 1980. LC 79-89476. (C). 9.95 (*0-930626-03-6*); pap. 6.95 (*0-930626-04-4*) Psych & Consul Assocs.

Back Trouble: A New Approach to Prevention & Recovery. Deborah Caplan. 1987. (Illus.). 224p. (Orig.). pap. 14.95 (*0-937404-26-8*) Triad Pub FL.

Backache. Ian Macnab & John A. McCulloch. 2nd ed. 1989. (Illus.). 448p. 62.00 (*0-683-05352-3*) Lppncott W & W.

Backache: 51 Ways to End the Agony. Charles B. Inlander & Porter Shimer. 1997. LC 97-991. 96p. (Orig.). 8.95 (*0-8027-7516-0*) Walker & Co.

Backache: What Exercises Work. Dava Sobel & Arthur C. Klein. 3rd ed. 1996. LC 96-5435. (Illus.). 208p. pap. 11.95 (*0-312-14281-1*, St Martin Griffin) St Martin.

Backcountry First Aid & Extended Care. Buck Tilton. 3rd ed. 1998. LC 92-47093. (Illus.). 80p. (Orig.). pap. 4.95 (*0-7627-0413-6*) Globe Pequot.

***Background & Current Practice of Fetal Tissue & Embryo Research in Canada.** 289p. pap. (*0-662-21389-0*) Can7 Govern Pub CAN. *Dist:* Intl Spec Bk.

BackHab: The Water Way to Mobility & Pain Free Living. Ruth Sova. Ed. by Susan Harpt & Mary Schmit. 2nd ed. 2001. (Illus.). 167p. (Orig.). pap. 23.95 (*1-889959-00-6*) D S L Ltd.

Backpower Program. David Imrie. 1990. LC 90-35741. 208p. pap. 15.95 (*0-471-52879-X*) Wiley.

Backwoods Surgery & Medicine. Charles S. Moody. 1974. (Shorey Lost Arts Ser.). reprint ed. pap. 10.00 (*0-8466-6034-2*, U 34) Shoreys Bkstore.

BackWorks: An Illustrated Guide to How Your Back Works & What to Do When It Doesn't. Timothy J. Gray. 2001. LC 92-63045. (Illus.). 208p. pap. 15.95 (*0-9622269-1-2*) BookPartners.

Backyard Medicine Chest: An Herbal Primer. Douglas Schar. 1995. LC 95-900. (Illus.). 160p. (Orig.). pap. 12.95 (*1-880216-28-0*, Elliott Clark) River City Pub.

Bacteria-Cytokine Interactions in Health & Disease. Ed. by Brian Henderson et al. 1998. (Illus.). 394p. text (*1-85578-114-X*) Portland Pr Ltd GBR. *Dist:* Ashgate Pub Co.

Bacteria, Germs, & Viruses Do Not Cause Disease: Discriminating Between Medical Myth & Biological Fact. Arthur M. Baker. 1994. LC 93-93558. 55p. (Orig.). pap. 8.95 (*1-883989-07-8*) Self Hlth Care.

Bacteria in Biology, Biotechnology & Medicine. Paul Singleton. 5th ed. 1999. LC 99-14378. 500p. 150.00 (*0-471-98877-4*) Wiley.

Bacteria in Nature Vol. 1: Bacterial Activities in Perspective, Vol. 1. E. R. Leadbetter & J. S. Poindexter. 1985. LC 85-3433. (Illus.). 282p. (C). text 85.00 (*0-306-41944-0*, Kluwer Plenum) Kluwer Academic.

Bacterial Adhesion: Mechanisms & Physiological Significance. D. C. Savage & M. Fletcher. 1985. LC 85-3434. (Illus.). 496p. (C). text 125.00 (*0-306-41941-6*, Kluwer Plenum) Kluwer Academic.

Bacterial Adhesion & Its Prevention in Dentistry. H. J. Busscher. 1991. 86p. pap. text 123.00 (*3-7186-5188-2*, Harwood Acad Pubs) Gordon & Breach.

Bacterial & Viral Zoonoses. 1982. (Technical Report Ser.: No. 682). 146p. pap. text 11.00 (*92-4-120682-9*) World Health.

Bacterial Conjugation. D. B. Clewell. 1993. (Illus.). 430p. (C). text 110.00 (*0-306-44376-7*, Kluwer Plenum) Kluwer Academic.

Bacterial Diarrheal Diseases. Yoshihiko Takeda & T. Miwatani. 1985. LC 84-1186. (New Perspectives in Clinical Microbiology Ser.). text 203.00 (*0-89838-681-0*) Kluwer Academic.

Bacterial Enzymes & Virulence. Ed. by Ian A. Holder. 1985. LC 84-16976. 208p. 121.00 (*0-8493-5296-7*, QR175, CRC Reprint) Franklin.

Bacterial Fish Pathogens: Diseases of Farmed & Wild Fish. B. Austin & D. Austin. 3rd rev. ed. 1999. LC 98-52790. 500p. (C). (*1-85233-120-8*) Spr-Verlag GBR. *Dist:* Spr-Verlag.

Bacterial Genetic Systems. Ed. by Jeffrey H. Miller et al. 1991. (Methods in Enzymology Ser.: Vol. 204). (Illus.). 706p. text 125.00 (*0-12-182105-6*) Acad Pr.

Bacterial Genetics in Natural Environments. J. C. Fry & M. J. Day. 1990. 192p. (C). (gr. 13). pap. text 167.95 (*0-412-35630-9*, A4385) Chapman & Hall.

Bacterial Growth & Division: Biochemistry & Regulation of Prokaryotic & Eukaryotic Division Cycles. Stephen Cooper. 1991. (Illus.). 501p. (C). text 77.00 (*0-12-187905-4*) Acad Pr.

Bacterial Infection: Close Encounters at the Host Pathogen Interface. Ed. by P. K. Vogt et al. 1997. (Current Topics in Microbiology & Immunology Ser.: Vol. 225). (Illus.). 169p. 139.00 (*3-540-63260-3*) Spr-Verlag.

Bacterial Infections. Ed. by Axel Dalhoff. 1999. (Chemotherapy Ser.: Vol. 45, No. 2 (1999)). (Illus.). 68p. pap. 25.25 (*3-8055-6841-X*) S Karger.

Bacterial Infections of Human: Epidemiology & Control. Ed. by Alfred S. Evans & Philip S. Brachman. 2nd ed. 1991. LC 90-14169. (Illus.). 840p. 95.00 (*0-306-43343-5*, Plenum Trade) Perseus Pubng.

Bacterial Infections of Humans: Epidemiology & Control. Alfred S. Evans & Philip S. Brachman. 3rd ed. 1998. LC 98-19429. (Illus.). 770p. (C). text 59.50 (*0-306-45323-1*, Kluwer Plenum) Kluwer Academic.

Bacterial Infections of Humans: Epidemiology & Control. Ed. by Alfred S. Evans & Philip S. Brachman. 3rd ed. 1998. LC 98-19429. (Illus.). 770p. (C). 125.00 (*0-306-45320-7*, Plenum Trade) Perseus Pubng.

Bacterial Interference. Raza Aly & Henry R. Shinefield. 1982. 192p. 102.95 (*0-8493-6285-7*, QR99, CRC Reprint) Franklin.

Bacterial Invasion into Eukarytic Cells. Ed. by Tobias A. Oelschlaeger & Jorg H. Hacker. 2000. LC 73-643479. (Subcellular Biochemistry Ser.: Vol. 33). 687p. 225.00 (*0-306-46290-7*, Kluwer Plenum) Kluwer Academic.

Bacterial Invasiveness, 209. Ed. by V.L. Miller. 1996. (Current Topics in Microbiology & Immunology Ser.: Vol. 209). (Illus.). 115p. 128.00 (*3-540-60065-5*) Spr-Verlag.

Bacterial Meningitis. Ed. by H. Schonfeld & H. Helwig. 1992. (Antibiotics & Chemotherapy Ser.: Vol. 45). (Illus.). viii, 276p. 205.25 (*3-8055-5484-2*) S Karger.

Bacterial Meningitis. Allan R. Tunkel. 2001. 288p. text 125.00 (*0-7817-1102-9*) Lppncott W & W.

Bacterial Pathogenesis. Ed. by John N. Abelson et al. 1997. LC 97-202919. (Selected Methods in Enzymology Ser.: Vols. 235 & 236). (Illus.). 827p. 79.95 (*0-12-175465-0*) Morgan Kaufmann.

Bacterial Pathogenesis: A Molecular Approach. Abigail A. Salyers & Dixie D. Whitt. 1994. LC 94-1468. (Illus.). 550p. pap. 49.95 (*1-55581-070-5*) ASM Pr.

***Bacterial Pathogenesis: A Molecular Approach.** Ed. by Abigail A. Salyers & Dixie D. Whitt. 2nd ed. 2002. 450p. pap. 56.95 (*1-55581-171-X*) ASM Pr.

Bacterial Pathogenesis Pt. B: Interaction of Pathogenic Bacteria with Host Cells. Ed. by Virginia L. Clark et al. 1994. (Methods in Enzymology Ser.: Vol. 236). 642p. text 115.00 (*0-12-182137-4*) Acad Pr.

Bacterial Protein Toxins. Ed. by J. E. Alouf et al. 1984. (Fems Symposia Ser.). text 83.00 (*0-12-053080-5*) Acad Pr.

Bacterial Resistance to Antimicrobial Agents. S. A. Lerner & G. W. Kaatz. Date not set. (Infectious Disease & Therapy Ser.). (*0-8247-9404-4*) Dekker.

Bacterial Skin Disease in the Dog: A Guide to Canine Pyoderma. Peter J. Ihrke. 1996. LC 95-62462. (Illus.). 98p. pap. text (*1-884254-30-6*) Vet Lrn Syst.

Bacterial Superantigens: Structure, Function & Therapeutic Potential. Jacques Thibodeau & Rafick Sekaly. 1995. LC 95-14947. (Molecular Biology Intelligence Unit Ser.). (Illus.). 245p. 99.00 (*1-57059-264-0*) Landes Bioscience.

Bacterial Toxins: Methods & Protocols. Ed. by Otto Holst. 2000. LC 99-41237. (Methods in Molecular Biology Ser.: Vol. 145). (Illus.). 392p. 89.50 (*0-89603-604-9*) Humana.

Bacterial Vaccines. Ed. by John B. Robbins et al. 1987. LC 86-9523. 589p. 125.00 (*0-275-92157-3*, C2157, Praeger Pubs) Greenwood.

Bacterial Wilt: The Disease & Its Causative Agent, Pseudomonas Solanacearum. G. L. Hartman & A. C. Hayward. 1992. 381p. pap. 186.00 (*1-86320-087-8*) St Mut.

Bacteriocins, Microcins, & Lantibiotics. Ed. by Richard James et al. 1993. LC 92-26374. (NATO ASI Ser.: Vol. 65). (Illus.). 519p. 341.00 (*0-387-54604-9*) Spr-Verlag.

Bacteriofagos. OAS General Secretariat, Department of Scientific Research Staff. 2nd rev. ed. 1980. (Serie de Biologia: No. 12). (SPA., Illus.). 102p. (C). pap. 2.00 (*0-8270-1301-9*) OAS.

Bacteriologist. Jack Rudman. 1994. (Career Examination Ser.: C-80). pap. 29.95 (*0-8373-0080-0*) Nat Learn.

Bacteriology. J. Spicer. 1998. (Illus.). 200p. pap. (*0-443-04365-5*) Church.

Bacteriology & Immunity for Nurses. Ronald Hare & E. Mary Cooke. 6th ed. 1984. (Churchill Livingstone Nursing Text Ser.). (Illus.). 232p. (Orig.). pap. text (*0-443-02878-8*) Church.

Bacteriophages, Vol. 1. R. Calendar. 1988. LC 88-9770. (Viruses Ser.). (Illus.). 614p. (C). text 135.00 (*0-306-42730-3*, Kluwer Plenum) Kluwer Academic.

Baculovirus Expression System: A Laboratory Guide. L. A. King & R. D. Possee. 1992. (Illus.). 192p. (C). (gr. 13). pap. 119.95 (*0-412-37150-2*, A6890) Chapman & Hall.

Baculovirus Expression Vectors: A Laboratory Manual. David O'Reilly et al. 1993. LC 93-43895. (Illus.). 364p. (C). spiral bd., lab manual ed. 65.00 (*0-19-509131-0*) OUP.

Baculovirus Expressions Systems & Biopesticides. Ed. by Michael L. Shuler et al. 1994. LC 94-17194. 259p. 130.00 (*0-471-06580-3*, Wiley-Liss) Wiley.

Baculoviruses. Ed. by Lois K. Miller. 1997. LC 97-17668. (Viruses Ser.). 468p. (C). text 110.00 (*0-306-45641-9*, Kluwer Plenum) Kluwer Academic.

Bad Back: Coping for Life. Lucy M. Dobkins. 1995. LC 94-41901. (Illus.). 208p. (Orig.). pap. 12.95 (*1-56554-062-X*) Pelican.

Bad Back Book. Jerry Wayne. 1983. LC 82-62473. reprint ed. pap. 12.95 (*0-918024-25-0*) Ox Bow.

Bad Blood: Crisis in the American Red Cross. Judith Reitman. 1998. (Illus.). 352p. pap. 6.99 (*0-7860-0508-4*, Pinncle Kensgtn) Kensgtn Pub Corp.

Bad Blood: The Tuskegee Syphilis Experiment. James H. Jones. exp. rev. ed. 1992. LC 92-34818. (Illus.). 304p. pap. 16.95 (*0-02-916676-4*) Free Pr.

Bad Breath Book: Your Complete Guide to Combating Halitosis. Fred Siemon. 1999. LC 99-71660. (Illus.). 187p. pap. 14.95 (*0-9670497-0-9*) Library Research Assocs.

Bad Medicine: How the American Medical Establishment Is Ruining Our Healthcare System. Lawrence J. O'Brien. 1999. LC 98-48718. 225p. 28.00 (*1-57392-260-9*) Prometheus Bks.

Bad Medicine: The Prescription Drug Industry in the Third World. Milton Silverman et al. 1992. LC 91-5085. 384p. (C). 51.00 (*0-8047-1669-2*) Stanford U Pr.

Bad Men Do What Good Men Dream: A Forensic Psychiatrist Illuminates the Darker Side of Human Behavior. Robert I. Simon. 1999. 362p. pap. 17.00 (*0-88048-995-2*, 8995); 1995. LC 95-10723. 368p. 23.95 (*0-88048-688-0*, 8688) Am Psychiatric.

Bad Object: Handling the Negative Therapeutic Reaction in Psychotherapy. Jeffrey Seinfeld. 1990. LC 89-15199. 336p. 50.00 (*0-87668-831-8*) Aronson.

Bag Balm & Duct Tape: Tales of a Vermont Doctor. Beach Conger. 1988. 224p. 16.95 (*0-316-15258-7*, Little Brwn Med Div) Lppncott W & W.

Bailey & Love's Short Practice of Surgery. C. V. Mann et al. 22nd ed. 1995. (Illus.). 1056p. (*0-412-49490-6*) E A GBR. *Dist:* OUP.

Bailey & Scott's Diagnostic Microbiology. Betty A. Forbes et al. 1998. (Illus.). 1072p. (*0-323-00492-X*); 10th ed. LC 97-46902. (C). (gr. 13). text 67.00 (*0-8151-2535-6*, 28830) Mosby Inc.

Bailliere's Comprehensive Veterinary Dictionary. D. C. Blood. 1988. 1312p. text 82.95 (*0-7020-1195-9*) Saunders.

Bailliere's Midwives' Dictionary. Tiran. 9th ed. 1998. (C). pap. text (*0-7020-2281-0*) Bailliere Tindall.

Bailliere's Nurse's Dictionary. Barbara F. Weller & Richard J. Wells. 21st ed. 1990. (Illus.). 619p. (*0-7020-1505-9*) W B Saunders GBR. *Dist:* Saunders.

Bailliere's Study Skills for Nurses. Maslin. 1997. pap. text (*0-7020-1979-8*) Bailliere Tindall.

***Bailliere's Study Skills for Nurses.** Sian Maslin-Prothero. 2001. (Illus.). 251p. pap. (*0-7020-2602-6*) W B Saunders GBR. *Dist:* Saunders.

Baker & Silverton's Introduction to Medical Laboratory Technology. Ed. by Chris Pallister et al. 7th ed. 2000. LC 97-48992. (Illus.). 464p. pap. (*0-7506-2190-7*) E A GBR. *Dist:* OUP.

Bakerman's ABC's of Adult & Pediatric Drug Therapy. Paul Bakerman & Seymour Bakerman. 1992. pap. text 28.50 (*0-945577-05-2*) Interpret Lab Data.

Baking Without Fat. George Mateljan. Ed. by Jim Burns. 1993. LC 93-77482. (Illus.). 175p. (Orig.). pap. 9.95 (*0-9633608-1-7*) Hlth Valley Foods.

Balance. Ed. by Richard Di Fabio. 1997. (Monograph Ser.). (Illus.). 261p. pap. 30.00 (*1-887759-17-4*, P-146) Am Phys Therapy Assn.

Balance: Your Personal Prescription for Supermetabolism, Renewed Vitality, Maximum Health & Instant Rejuvenation. Ozzie Garcia. 2000. LC 99-58685. 256p. pap. 13.00 (*0-06-098737-5*) HarperCollins Pubs.

Balance Disorders: A Case-Study Approach. Joseph M. Furman & Stephen P. Cass. 1996. LC 95-52576. (Illus.). 352p. (C). 74.00 (*0-8036-0166-2*) OUP.

Balance in Motion: Ivan Boszormenyi-Nagy & His Vision of Individual & Family Therapy. Ammy Van Heusden & ElseMarie Van den Eerenbeemt. 1992. LC 87-10379. 140p. pap. text 28.95 (*0-87630-693-8*) Brunner-Routledge.

Balance (Proceedings) Ed. by Pamela Duncan. 1990. 112p. pap. 25.00 (*0-912452-73-0*, P-66) Am Phys Therapy Assn.

Balance Within: The Science Connecting Health & Emotions. Esther M. Sternberg. 2000. LC 99-86775. (Illus.). xix, 288p. text 24.95 (*0-7167-3479-6*) W H Freeman.

Balance Your Act: A Book for Adults with Diabetes. Maria Alogna Ludi & Nancy Hull. Ed. by Karen Hubbard. l.t. ed. 2000. (Illus.). 96p. pap. 8.95 (*0-939838-55-9*) Pritchett & Hull.

Balance Your Body, Balance Your Life: Total Health Rejuvenation. Edward A. Taub. 2000. 480p. reprint ed. pap. 14.95 (*0-7434-1259-1*, PB Trade Paper) PB.

Balanced Food Medicine: A Comprehensive Guide for Your Health & Wellness. Timothy Yeh et al. 2000. (Illus.). 451p. pap. 49.95 (*0-9652967-6-8*) Yehs Ctr Nat Med.

Balancing Access, Costs, & Politics: The American Context for Health System Reform. John Holahan et al. 1991. (Reports: No. 91-6). (Illus.). 90p. (C). pap. text 18.50 (*0-87766-518-4*); lib. bdg. 38.50 (*0-87766-555-9*) Urban Inst.

Balancing Act. Cowley. 1998. 55.00 (*0-7616-6400-9*) Acad Pr.

Balancing Act: Getting & Keeping Your Life in Balance. Paul Heneks. 1995. LC 94-61885. 157p. (Orig.). pap. 15.95 (*0-87034-119-7*) Fraser Pub Co.

Balancing Act: Living with Spinal Cerebellar Ataxia. Patricia B. Hamilton. 1997. LC 96-92684. (Ataxia: A Lifestyle Change). 100p. (Orig.). spiral bd. 23.95 (*1-889826-00-6*) Scripts Pub.

Balancing Act: Memoir of a Southern Woman Doctor. Martha D. Yow. 1997. LC 97-7060. 205p. 19.95 (*1-57168-160-4*) Eakin Press.

Balancing Act: The New Medical Ethics of Medicine's New Economics. E. Haavi Morreim. 1995. LC 94-37058. (Clinical Medical Ethics Ser.). 224p. pap. 17.95 (*0-87840-584-4*) Georgetown U Pr.

Balancing Act: The New Medical Ethics of Medicine's New Economics. E. Haavi Morreim. 1991. 196p. (C). lib. bdg. (*0-7923-1170-1*) Kluwer Academic NLD. *Dist:* Kluwer Academic.

Balancing Heaven & Earth: A Memoir of Visions, Dreams, & Realizations. Robert A. Johnson & Jerry M. Ruhl. 1998. LC 97-22306. 320p. 24.00 (*0-06-251506-3*) Harper SF.

Balancing the Body's Energies. Wayne W. Topping. rev. ed. 1986. (Illus.). 128p. stu. ed. 16.00 (*0-935299-04-1*) Topping Inst.

Balancing the Request to Be Good: An Account of a Visit to the Outskirts of Child Psychotherapy. Sheila K. Cameron. 1995. (C). LC 97-194514. pap. (*1-85343-324-1*); 200p. (*1-85343-323-3*) Free Assoc Bks GBR. *Dist:* Intl Spec Bk, NYU Pr.

Balancing the Scales of Opportunity: Ensuring Racial & Ethnic Diversity in the Health Professions. Institute of Medicine Staff. Ed. by Marion E. Lewin & Barbara Rice. 1994. LC 94-66070. 100p. (Orig.). pap. text 23.00 (*0-309-05078-2*) Natl Acad Pr.

Balancing Your Emotions: For Women Who Want Consistency under Stress. Gayle G. Roper. 2000. LC 92-30983. 144p. pap. 7.99 (*0-87788-075-1*, H Shaw Pubs) Waterbrook Pr.

Bald No More. Morton Walker. 1998. LC 98-233152. 112p. mass mkt. 5.99 (*1-57566-308-2*) Kensgtn Pub Corp.

Balding: Hair Loss & Restoration. Gustavo J. Gomez. 1989. 160p. pap. 13.95 (*0-89697-299-2*) Intl Univ Pr.

Baldness (Alopecia) - Causes, Treatments & Chemotherapy: Index of New Information. Michael Y. Drake. 1998. 150p. 57.50 (*0-7883-2048-3*); pap. 47.50 (*0-7883-2049-1*) ABBE Pubs Assn.

Baldrige Assessor's Workbook: How to Perform the Examiner's Role for Internal & External Assessments. Kicab Castaneda-Mendez. 1997. LC 97-26526. 239p. spiral bd. 39.95 (*0-527-76325-X*) Product Pr.

Ballad, Bard & Bandage: Saga of Stillman Valley's Theatrical Physician. Anne B. Weyrauch. 1990. (Illus.). (Orig.). pap. 14.95 (*1-878924-90-7*) Beebe Bks.

Ballistic Trauma: Clinical Relevance in Peace & War. Ed. by James M. Ryan et al. 1997. LC 96-53122. (An Arnold Publication). (Illus.). 312p. (C). (*0-340-58114-X*) E A GBR. *Dist:* OUP.

Ballistocardiographic Methods & Cardiovascular Dynamics: Proceedings of the Ballistocardiography & Cardiovascular Dynamics Congress, 3rd World, 9th European Sofia, 1973. Ballistocardiography and Cardiovascular Dynamics Con. Ed. by A. Talakov. 1975. (Bibliotheca Cardiologica Ser.: No. 33). 300p. pap. 121.00 (*3-8055-1701-7*) S Karger.

Ballistocardiography - Research & Computer Diagnosis: Proceedings of the Ballistocardiograph Research Society, 16th Annual Meeting, Atlantic City, 1972. Ballistocardiograph Research Society Staff. Ed. by E. K. Franke. 1973. (Bibliotheca Cardiologica Ser.: No. 32). (Illus.). 160p. pap. 36.75 (*3-8055-1376-3*) S Karger.

Ballistocardiography & Cardiac Performance. Abraham Noordergraaf et al. 1967. LC 67-27246. 156p. 10.50 (*0-87527-062-X*) Green.

Ballistocardiography & Cardiovascular Therapy: Proceedings of the World Congress. World Congress on Ballistocardiography and Cardiovas. Ed. by A. Falcao De Freitas. 1970. (Bibliotheca Cardiologica Ser.: No. 26). pap. 82.75 (*3-8055-0033-5*) S Karger.

Ballistocardiography & Clinical Studies: Proceedings of the Ballistocardiograph Research Society, 14th Annual Meeting, Atlantic City, 1970. Ballistocardiograph Research Society Staff. Ed. by W. K. Harrison. 1971. (Bibliotheca Cardiologica Ser.: No. 27). pap. 21.75 (*3-8055-1188-4*) S Karger.

Bamboo Stone: The Evolution of a Chinese Medical Elite. Karen Minden. 1994. LC 94-205783. (Illus.). 490p. (C). text 45.00 (*0-8020-0550-0*) U of Toronto Pr.

Band of Brothers: Creators of Modern Vascular Surgery. W. Andrew Dale. Ed. by George Johnson, Jr. & James A. DeWeese. 1996. (Illus.). 528p. 50.00 (*0-9649826-1-7*) G Johnson.

Band Three Proteins: Anion Transporters, Binding Proteins, & Senescent Antigenes. Ed. by Ernst Bamberg & Hermann Passow. 1992. LC 92-22096. (Progress in Cell Research Ser.: Vol. 2). xvi,358p. 237.50 (*0-444-89547-7*) Elsevier.

Bandaging & Splinting. 1986. (Medical Ser.). lib. bdg. 79.95 (*0-8490-3568-6*) Gordon Pr.

Bangour Story: A History of Bangour Village & General Hospitals. William F. Hendrie & Donald A. Macleod. 1991. (Aberdeen University Press Bks.). (Illus.). 192p. text (*0-08-041402-8*); pap. text (*0-08-041401-X*) Aberdeen U Pr GBR. *Dist:* Macmillan.

***Banish Bloating.** Suzannah Olivier. 2001. 208p. pap. 10.00 (*0-7432-1864-7*) S&S Trade.

Banishing Tobacco. William U. Chandler. 1986. LC 85-52313. (Worldwatch Papers). pap. 5.00 (*0-916468-68-2*) Worldwatch Inst.

Bantam Medical Dictionary. Market House Books Ltd. Staff. 1990. 13.04 (*0-606-03045-X*) Turtleback.

Bantam Medical Dictionary. Laurence Urdang. 1996. mass mkt. 8.99 (*0-553-85103-9*); 1995. mass mkt. 8.99 (*0-553-85084-9*) Bantam.

Bantam Medical Dictionary. Ed. by Market House Books Ltd. Staff. 3rd rev. ed. 2000. LC 00-267332. (Illus.). 544p. mass mkt. 6.99 (*0-553-58189-9*) Bantam.

Baran & Dawber's Diseases of the Nails & their Management. R. Baran & R. P. R. Dawber. 3rd ed. 2001. LC 00-58490. (Illus.). 640p. 275.00 (*0-632-05358-5*) Blackwell Sci.

Barbers, Cars, & Cigars: Activity Programming for Older Men. Nancy Dezan. 1992. 52p. (Orig.). pap. 8.95 (*1-879633-12-4*) Eldersong.

Barbiturates: Sleeping Potions or Intoxicants? Jack E. Henningfield & Nancy Ator. 1992. LC 85-17432. (Encyclopedia of Psychoactive Drugs Ser.: No. 1). (Illus.). 124p. (YA). (gr. 7-11). lib. bdg. 19.95 (*0-87754-768-8*) Chelsea Hse.

Barbiturates & Other Depressants. Lawrence Clayton. 1998. (Drug Abuse Prevention Library). 64p. (YA). (gr. 7 up). reprint ed. pap. 6.95 (*1-56838-211-1*) Hazelden.

Barcena's Clinical Reference Pocket Guide to Abbreviations & Symbols Used in Hospitals. Theresa L. Barcena & William Donofrio. 1994. (Reference Pocket Guide Ser.). 116p. (C). pap. text 10.00 (*0-9643995-0-4*) Barcena & Co.

Barcode Medical Health Concerns 93. Saundersco. 1994. (C). pap. text 40.00 (*0-03-011217-6*) Harcourt Coll Pubs.

Barefoot Doctor's Manual. Tr. by Geographic Health Studies Staff. 1994. (Illus.). reprint ed. lib. bdg. 45.00 (*0-7808-0009-5*) Omnigraphics Inc.

Barefoot Doctor's Manual: Healing with Medicinal Herbs & Acupuncture. Set. 1984. lib. bdg. 600.00 (*0-87700-549-4*) Revisionist Pr.

Bargaining for Life: A Social History of Tuberculosis, 1876-1938. Barbara Bates. 1992. LC 91-40040. (Studies in Health, Illness, & Caregiving). (Illus.). 456p. (Orig.). (C). pap. text 20.95 (*0-8122-1367-X*) U of Pa Pr.

Bargaining with Uncertainty: Decision-Making in Public Health, Technological Safety, & Environmental Policy. Merrie G. Klapp. 1992. LC 91-32712. 168p. 58.00 (*0-86569-046-4*, T046, Auburn Hse) Greenwood.

Barium. 1990. (Environmental Health Criteria Ser.: No. 107). 148p. pap. text 28.00 (*92-4-157107-1*, 1160107) World Health.

Barksdale Stress Control Program Participant's Kit. Lilburn S. Barksdale. 1980. (Illus.). pap., stu. ed. 34.95 incl. audio (*0-918588-23-5*, 205) Barksdale Foun.

Barksdale Stress Control Program Script for Seminar Instructor. Lilburn S. Barksdale. 1980. 91p. pap., tchr. ed. 80.00 incl. audio (*0-918588-18-9*, 204) Barksdale Foun.

Barksdale Stress Control Seminar Instructor's Kit. Lilburn S. Barksdale. 1980. (Illus.). pap., vinyl bd. 80.00 incl. audio (*0-918588-21-9*, 204) Barksdale Foun.

***Barley Grass Juice: Rejuvenation Elixir & Natural, Healthy Power Drink Easy to Prepare & Totally Healthy, Barley Grass Juice Works True Wonders.** Barbara Simonsohn. 2001. (Illus.). 176p. pap. 14.95 (*0-914955-68-3*, Shangri-La) Lotus Pr.

Barnaby: The Struggle of a Word Blind Child. Mary L. Murphy. 1968. 74p. pap. 1.95 (*0-85225-535-7*) Ed Solutions.

***Barrett's Esophagus.** Ed. by H. W. Tilanus & A. E. Attwood. 2001. LC 2001-50222. 159.00 (*1-4020-0102-9*) Kluwer Academic.

***Barrett's Esophagus & Esophageal Adenocarcinoma.** Ed. by Prateek Sharma & Richard E. Sampliner. 2001. LC 00-67462. (Illus.). x, 230p. 99.95 (*0-632-04509-4*) Blackwell Sci.

Barrier Contraception & Breast Cancer. A. N. Gjorgov. 1980. (Contributions to Gynecology & Obstetrics Ser.: Vol. 8). (Illus.). pap. 42.75 (*3-8055-0330-X*) S Karger.

Barrier Contraceptives & Spermicides: Their Role in Family Planning Care. 1987. 81p. pap. 15.00 (*92-4-156101-7*) World Health.

Barriers Against Recovery. John O. Grimmett. 8p. reprint ed. pap. 1.50 (*0-89486-009-7*, 1180B) Hazelden.

Barriers & Fluids of the Eye & Brain. Segal. 1991. 110.00 (*0-8493-7707-2*, QP476) CRC Pr.

Barriers to Prenatal Care: An Examination of Use of Prenatal Care among Low-Income Women in New York City. Francis G. Caro et al. 1988. LC 89-170885. 122p. pap. 11.00 (*0-88156-069-3*) Comm Serv Soc NY.

Barron's Regents Exams & Answers: Biology. Ed. by Gabrielle I. Edwards. rev. ed. 1996. LC 58-19074. 300p. (YA). (gr. 9-12). pap. text 5.95 (*0-8120-3197-0*) Barron.

Bartonella & Afipia Species Emphasizing Bartonella Henselae. Ed. by Axel Schmidt. 1998. LC 98-22642. (Merged Book Ser.: Vol. 1). (Illus.). x, 218p. 127.00 (*3-8055-6649-2*) S Karger.

Basal & Squamous Cell Skin Cancers of the Head & Neck. Ed. by Randal S. Weber et al. 1996. LC 95-14204. (Illus.). 416p. 120.00 (*0-683-08888-2*) Lppncott W & W.

Basal Forebrain: Anatomy to Function. T. C. Napier et al. 1991. (Advances in Experimental Medicine & Biology Ser.: Vol. 295). (Illus.). 504p. (C). text 174.00 (*0-306-43932-8*, Kluwer Plenum) Kluwer Academic.

Basal Ganglia: Cellular & Functional Aspects. Ed. by R. Hassler & J. F. Christ. 1979. (Applied Neurophysiology Ser.: Vol. 42, No. 1-2). (Illus.). pap. 29.75 (*3-8055-3023-4*) S Karger.

Basal Ganglia Vol. 2: Structure & Function: Current Concepts. Ed. by M. B. Carpenter & A. Jayaraman. 1987. LC 87-15300. (Advances in Behavioral Biology Ser.: Vol. 32). (Illus.). 560p. 125.00 (*0-306-42616-1*, Plenum Trade) Perseus Pubng.

Basal Ganglia 3. Ed. by G. Bernardi. 1991. (Advances in Behavioral Biology Ser.: Vol. 39). (Illus.). 793p. (C). text 198.00 (*0-306-43720-1*, Kluwer Plenum) Kluwer Academic.

Basal Ganglia & Behavior: Sensory Aspects of Motor Functioning. Jay S. Schneider & Theodore I. Lidsky. 1987. LC 86-20893. 300p. (C). text 59.90 (*0-920887-13-9*) Hogrefe & Huber Pubs.

Basal Ganglia & Thalamus in Health & Movement Disorders. Ed. by Kristy Kultas-Llinsky & Igor A. Llinsky. 2001. LC 00-67119. (Illus.). 388p. 95.00 (*0-306-46543-4*, Kluwer Plenum) Kluwer Academic.

Basal Ganglia V: Proceedings of the Fifth Triennial Meeting of the International Basal Ganglia Society Held in Nemuno-Sato, Japan, May 23-26, 1995. International Basal Ganglia Society Staff. Ed. by Chihiro Ohye et al. 1997. LC 96-34816. (Advances in Behavioral Biology Ser.: Vol. 47). (Illus.). 534p. 167.00 (*0-306-45386-X*, Plenum Trade) Perseus Pubng.

Bascom Palmer Eye Institute's Atlas of Opthalmology. Richard K. Parrish, II. 1999. LC 99-14084. (Illus.). 500p. text 205.00 (*0-7506-7075-4*) Buttrwrth-Heinemann.

Base Excision Repair of DNA Damage. Ian D. Hickson. 1997. LC 97-13249. (Molecular Biology Intelligence Unit Ser.). 194p. 99.00 (*1-57059-449-X*) Landes Bioscience.

Baseline, 1997: A Survey of Medi-Cal Managed Care Plans in County Organized Health System & Two-Plan Counties. unabr. ed. 1999. (Illus.). 28p. pap. (*1-929008-14-7*) CA HlthCare Fnd.

Basic Accounting for Hospital Based Non-Financial Managers. Sandra H. Pelfrey. 1993. text 31.50 (*0-8273-4894-0*) Delmar.

Basic Adolescent Gynecology: An Office Guide. Ed. by Victor C. Strasburger. 1990. (Illus.). 270p. 48.00 (*0-683-07947-6*) Lppncott W & W.

Basic Aerohemodynamics. 1984. 17.95 (*0-930835-03-4*) Med Res Assocs.

Basic Allied Health Statistics & Analysis. Gerda Koch. 1995. LC 94-23929. 224p. (C). mass mkt. 31.00 (*0-8273-5525-4*) Delmar.

Basic Allied Health Statistics & Analysis. Gerda Koch & Frank Waterstraat. 2nd ed. 1999. LC 99-38063. 288p. 48.95 (*0-7668-1092-5*) Delmar.

Basic Analytical Toxicology. Ed. by R. J. Flanagan et al. 1995. LC 96-174836. (FRE., Illus.). 274p. (C). pap. 54.00 (*92-4-154458-9*, 1150437) World Health.

Basic Anatomical & Physiological Data for Use in Radiological Protection: The Skeleton. Ed. by H Smith. 1996. (International Commission on Radiological Protection Ser.: Vol. 70). 92p. pap. 57.00 (*0-08-042879-7*, Pergamon Pr) Elsevier.

Basic Anatomy of Movement. Carla Z. Hinkle. 1997. LC 98-233284. (Illus.). 288p. (gr. 13). pap. text, wbk. ed. 29.95 (*0-8151-2210-1*, 30824) Mosby Inc.

Basic & Advanced Colposcopy. Louis Burke. 2nd ed. 1999. 195.00 (*0-8385-0651-8*, Medical Exam) Appleton & Lange.

***Basic & Advanced Dermatology for Primary Care Physicians.** M. Joseph. 2002. 220p. 38.95 (*1-84214-126-0*, Parthenon Pbng) CRC Pr.

Basic & Advanced in Vitreous Surgery. Ed. by G. Blankenship et al. 1986. (FIDIA Research Ser.). 419p. 203.00 (*0-387-96330-8*) Spr-Verlag.

Basic & Advanced Laser Surgery in Gynecology. Michael S. Baggish. 2nd ed. 1999. 398p. (C). pap. text 85.00 (*0-8385-0521-X*, A0521-3) Appleton & Lange.

Basic & Applied Aspects of Vestibular Function. J. C. Hwang et al. 1988. 246p. (C). text (*962-209-214-4*) HK Univ Pr HKG. *Dist:* Intl Spec Bk, Coronet Bks.

Basic & Applied Concepts of Immunohematology. Kathy D. Blaney & Paula R. Howard. 2000. (Illus.). 376p. tchr. ed. (*0-323-00234-X*) Mosby Inc.

Basic & Applied Dental Biochemistry. R. A. Williams & J. C. Elliott. 2nd ed. 1989. (Dental Ser.). (Illus.). 536p. pap. text (*0-443-03144-4*) Church.

Basic & Applied Influenza Research & Progress Towards Epidemiological Control. Ed. by A. S. Beare. 1982. 288p. 119.95 (*0-8493-6250-4*, QR201) CRC Pr.

Basic & Applied Memory Research Vol. 1: Theory in Context. Ed. by Douglas Herrmann et al. 1996. 464p. pap. 45.00 (*0-8058-1543-0*); text 89.95 (*0-8058-1542-2*) L Erlbaum Assocs.

Basic & Applied Principles of Drug Actions. Ernst Mutschler & Hartmut Derendorf. 1994. LC 93-36069. 89.95 (*0-8493-7774-9*) CRC Pr.

Basic & Applied Science of Anesthesia. H. C. Hemmings. 2nd ed. 1999. text 129.50 (*0-7234-2787-9*) Mosby Inc.

Basic & Clinical Applications of Flow Cytometry: Proceedings of the 24th Annual Detroit Cancer Symposium Detroit, Michigan, April 30-May 2, 1992. Ed. by Frederick A. Valeriote et al. 1995. LC 95-39521. (Developments in Oncology Ser.). 336p. (C). text 133.00 (*0-7923-3809-X*) Kluwer Academic.

Basic & Clinical Applications of Vision Science the Professor Jay M. Enoch Festschrift. Lakshminarayanan. 1996. LC 96-49524. text 176.50 (*0-7923-4348-4*) Kluwer Academic.

Basic & Clinical Aspects of Chronic Abdominal Pain. Ed. by Emeran A. Mayer & Helen Raybould. 1993. LC 93-11488. (Pain Research & Clinical Management Ser.: Vol. 9). 356p. 258.00 (*0-444-89437-3*) Elsevier.

Basic & Clinical Aspects of Growth Hormone. Ed. by Barry B. Bercu. 1988. LC 88-12527. (Serono Symposia U. S. A. Ser.). (Illus.). 392p. 110.00 (*0-306-42921-7*, Plenum Trade) Perseus Pubng.

Basic & Clinical Aspects of Helicobacter Pylori Infection: Proceedings of the Fourth Workshop of the Helicobacter Pylori Study Group Held in Bologna, Italy, November 1991. Fourth Workshop of the Helicobacter Pylori Study G. Ed. by G. Gasbarrini & S. Pretolani. 1994. LC 93-43056. (Illus.). 326p. 136.00 (*0-387-56720-8*) Spr-Verlag.

Basic & Clinical Aspects of IGG Subclasses. Ed. by Farouk Shakib. 1986. (Monographs in Allergy: Vol. 19). (Illus.). 318p. 248.75 (*3-8055-4290-9*) S Karger.

Basic & Clinical Aspects of Intra-Uterine Devices. 1966. (Technical Report Ser.: No. 332). 25p. pap. text 3.00 (*92-4-120332-3*) World Health.

Basic & Clinical Aspects of Malignant Melanoma. Ed. by Larry Nathanson. 1987. 240p. (C). text 152.00 (*0-89838-856-2*) Kluwer Academic.

Basic & Clinical Aspects of Neuroscience Vol. 4: Somatostatin. Ed. by C. Weil et al. 1992. (Illus.). 66p. 25.95 (*0-387-54569-7*) Spr-Verlag.

Basic & Clinical Biostatistics. B. Dawson. 3rd ed. 2000. (Lange Medical Bks.). (Illus.). 399p. pap. 44.95 (*0-8385-0510-4*) McGraw-Hill Prof.

Basic & Clinical Concepts of Lung Cancer. Ed. by Heine H. Hansen & William L. McGuire. 1989. (Cancer Treatment & Research Ser.). (C). text 227.50 (*0-7923-0153-6*) Kluwer Academic.

Basic & Clinical Endocrinology. Ed. by Francis S. Greenspan & Gordon J. Strewler. 5th ed. 1997. 823p. (C). pap. 44.95 (*0-8385-0588-0*) McGraw-Hill Educ Grp.

Basic & Clinical Endocrinology. Strewler Greenspan. 6th ed. 2000. (Lange Medical Bks.). (Illus.). 900p. (C). 44.95 (*0-8385-0597-X*, Apple Lange Med) McGraw.

Basic & Clinical Hepatology. Ed. by P. M. Motta & L. J. Didio. 1981. 200p. text 191.50 (*90-247-2404-X*) Kluwer Academic.

Basic & Clinical Immunology. Mark Peakman & Diego Vergani. 1997. LC 97-1431. pap. (*0-443-04672-7*) Church.

Basic & Clinical Neuroscience. Sladek. 1998. text (*0-7216-6004-5*) Saunders.

Basic & Clinical Perspectives in Vision Research: A Celebration of the Career of Hisako Ikeda. Ed. by Jon G. Robbins et al. 1996. (Illus.). 244p. 85.00 (*0-306-45202-2*, Kluwer Plenum) Kluwer Academic.

Basic & Clinical Pharmacology for Podiatrists. Margaret Johnson & Rae Morgan. 2000. LC 00-33747. (Illus.). pap. 62.95 (*0-632-05445-X*) Blackwell Sci.

Basic & Clinical Pharmacology Made Memorable. J. Luty & P. Harrison. 1997. (Illus.). 116p. pap. (*0-443-05598-X*) Church.

Basic & Clinical Research on Renal Cell Carcinoma. Ed. by G. Staehler & S. Pomer. 1992. (Illus.). 237p. 112.00 (*0-387-54424-0*) Spr-Verlag.

Basic & Clinical Science of Mental & Addictive Disorders: Neuroscience & Neuropharmacology East & West at the Beginning of the European Decade of Brain Research CINP Regional Conference, Vienna/Prague, June 1995. Ed. by L. L. Judd et al. 1997. LC 97-1088. (Bibliotheca Psychiatrica Ser.: No. 167, 1997). (Illus.). xiv, 258p. 214.00 (*3-8055-6385-X*) S Karger.

Basic & Clinical Science of Substance Related Disorders: Congress, Basel, May, 1998. Ed. by D. Ladewig. 2nd ed. 1999. LC 99-32981. (Bibliotheca Psychiatrica Ser.: Vol. 168 (1999)). (Illus.). viii, 68p. 75.00 (*3-8055-6870-3*) S Karger.

Basic & Clinical Tumor Immunology. Ed. by Ronald B. Herberman. 1983. (Cancer Treatment & Research Ser.). text 192.00 (*0-89838-579-2*) Kluwer Academic.

Basic Animal Science. L. D. Wythe et al. 7th ed. 1985. (Illus.). 216p. reprint ed. stu. ed., spiral bd. 18.95 (*0-89641-154-0*) American Pr.

Basic Arrhythmia Reprint. Gail Walraven. 4th ed. 1998. 499p. pap. 49.00 (*0-13-084004-1*) P-H.

Basic Arrhythmias. Gail Walraven. 5th ed. 1998. LC 98-26272. 528p. pap. text 58.67 (*0-8359-5305-X*) P-H.

Basic Arrhythmias: A Practice Workbook. Louise Smith. 1984. 150p. (Orig.). 13.95 (*0-932491-02-2*); 159.00 (*0-932491-10-3*) Res Appl Inc.

Basic Aspects of Blood Trauma: A Workshop, Proceedings of the Symposium, Stolberg Near Aachen, Federal Rep. of Germany, Nov. 21-23, 1978. Basic Aspects of Blood Trauma in Extracorporeal Ox Staff. Ed. by H. Schmid Schonbein & P. Teitel. 1979. pap. text 191.50 (*90-247-2279-9*) Kluwer Academic.

Basic Aspects of the Eustachian Tube & Middle Ear Diseases. Ed. by Jacob Sade. 1991. LC 91-7088. (Illus.). 384p. lib. bdg. (*90-6299-076-2*) Kugler NLD. *Dist:* Lib Res.

Basic Atlas of Sectional Anatomy with Correlated Imaging. Walter J. Bo et al. 3rd ed. 1998. LC 97-26180. (Illus.). 560p. text 120.00 (*0-7216-3265-3*) Saunders.

Basic Attainments Programme for Young Handicapped Children. Bill Gillham. 1987. (Special Education Ser.). 96p. pap. text (*0-7099-3862-4*) C Helm GBR. *Dist:* Routldge.

Basic Background for Test Interpretation. Harley D. Christiansen. 1981. LC 81-7285. (Illus.). 96p. (Orig.). (C). pap. text 15.95 (*0-915456-04-4*) P Juul Pr.

Basic Behavioral Science Research for Mental Health: A National Investment. Gordon H. Bower & John F. Kihlstrom. 1998. 137p. (C). reprint ed. pap. text 40.00 (*0-7881-3301-2*) DIANE Pub.

Basic Behaviour Therapy. Murdoch. 1991. 200p. pap. 39.95 (*0-632-02322-8*) Blackwell Sci.

Basic Biomechanics of the Musculoskeletal System. Margareta Nordin & Victor H. Frankel. 3rd ed. 2001. LC 00-65519. 496p. pap. text 49.95 (*0-683-30247-7*) Lppncott W & W.

Basic Biostatistics: Concepts for the Health Sciences. Frank D. Bell. 1994. LC 93-73781. 192p. (C). pap. 31.25 (*0-697-14979-X*) McGrw-H Hghr Educ.

Basic Cancer Medicine. Maurie Markman. Ed. by Richard Zorab. 1997. LC 97-706. 128p. pap. text 35.00 (*0-7216-5824-5*) Saunders.

Basic Cancer Programs: Genes, Signals, Metabolites: Unified Holistic Theory of Evolution. Werner J. Schwemmler. 1998. LC 98-165536. (Illus.). x, 148p. pap. 41.75 (*3-8055-6667-0*) S Karger.

Basic Cardiac Electrophysiology for the Clinician. Jose Jalife et al. 1998. LC 98-33472. (Illus.). 320p. 55.00 (*0-87993-417-4*) Futura Pub.

Basic Cardiac Rhythms - Made Easy! Beverly Kempf. 1992. (Illus.). 80p. (C). pap. text 19.95 (*0-9635791-0-X*) Dimensions.

Basic Cardiac Rhythms - Made Easy! Beverly Teichgraeber & Martha Wright. 2nd ed. 1997. (Illus.). 72p. pap. text 19.95 (*0-9635791-1-8*) Dimensions.

Basic Causes of Modern Diseases: And How to Remedy Them. Hanna Kroeger. rev. ed. 1998. LC 98-9733. 224p. pap. 12.95 (*1-56170-527-6*, 558) Hay House.

Basic Chest Radiology. Robert D. Tarver. 1998. (Illus.). 512p. pap. 65.00 (*0-86577-702-0*) Thieme Med Pubs.

Basic Child Psychiatry. Philip Barker. 6th ed. 1994. LC 94-1898. (Illus.). 416p. pap. 52.95 (*0-632-03772-5*) Blackwell Sci.

Basic Childbirth Picture Book. Fran P. Hosken. 1981. (Childbirth Picture Bks.). (Illus.). 60p. pap. 7.00 (*0-942096-00-2*) WINNEWS.

Basic Chiropractic Paraprofessional Manual see Chiropractic Assistant

Basic Chiropractic Paraprofessional Manual. D. C. FICC Staff. Ed. by R. C. Schafer. 1978. LC 78-11974. 36.00 (*0-9606618-3-2*) Am Chiro Assn.

Basic Chiropractic Procedural Manual. D. C. FICC Staff. Ed. by R. C. Scafer. 4th ed. 1984. LC 83-73396. 42.00 (*0-9606618-4-0*) Am Chiro Assn.

Basic Clinic Lab: Complete Physical Therapy. John Eargle. 1998. (Physical Therapy Ser.). pap. 39.95 (*0-8273-6490-3*) Delmar.

Basic, Clinical & Surgical Nephrology. P. M. Motta. Ed. by L. J. DiDio. 1985. (Developments in Nephrology Ser.). text 186.00 (*0-89838-698-5*) Kluwer Academic.

Basic, Clinical & Therapeutic Aspects of Alzheimer's & Parkinson's Disease, Vol. 1. Ed. by T. Nagatsu et al. 1990. (Advances in Behavioral Biology Ser.: Vol. 38A). (Illus.). 830p. (C). text 210.00 (*0-306-43680-9*, Kluwer Plenum) Kluwer Academic.

Basic, Clinical & Therapeutic Aspects of Alzheimer's & Parkinson's Diseases, Vol. 2. Ed. by T. Nagatsu et al. 1990. (Advances in Behavioral Biology Ser.: Vol. 38B). (Illus.). 638p. (C). text 186.00 (*0-306-43681-7*, Kluwer Plenum) Kluwer Academic.

Basic Clinical Lab: Complete Respiratory Care. Gary C. White. 1987. (Respiratory Care Ser.). pap. 32.95 (*0-8273-2714-5*) Delmar.

Basic Clinical Lab Competencies For Respiratory Care. Gary C. White. 3rd ed. 1997. LC 97-27990. 480p. (C). pap. text 58.95 (*0-8273-7998-6*) Delmar.

Basic Clinical Lab Competencies for Respiratory Care: An Integrated Approach. Gary C. White. 2nd ed. 1993. LC 92-18591. 468p. (C). pap. 49.95 (*0-8273-5118-6*) Delmar.

Basic Clinical Neuroanatomy. Paul A. Young & Paul H. Young. 1997. LC 96-17643. (Illus.). 352p. 29.95 (*0-683-09351-7*) Lppncott W & W.

Basic Clinical Parasitology. Franklin A. Neva. 6th ed. 1996. (Illus.). 400p. text 49.95 (*0-8385-0624-0*, A0624-5) McGraw.

Basic Clinical Pharmacokinetics. Michael E. Winter. 3rd ed. 1994. LC 94-70212. 436p. (C). pap. 45.00 (*0-915486-22-9*) Applied Therapeutics.

Basic Clinical Pharmacokinetics Handbook. John White, Jr. & Mark W. Garrison. Ed. by Mary A. Koda-Kimble. 1994. LC 95-71941. (Illus.). 254p. (C). pap. 25.00 (*0-915486-21-0*) Applied Therapeutics.

Basic Clinical Radiobiology. Ed. by G. Gordon Steel. 2nd ed. 1997. LC 97-13980. (Arnold Publication). (Illus.). 266p. text 45.00 (*0-340-70020-3*) OUP.

Basic Clinical Ultrasound. Hylton B. Meire & Pat Farrant. 1982. (British Journal of Radiology Teaching Ser.: No. 4). (Illus.). 170p. pap. text (*0-905749-10-3*) Med Physics Pub.

Basic Community & Home Care Nursing. Mary K. Ringsven. 1988. (LPN/LVN Nursing Ser.). pap. 29.95 (*0-8273-2969-5*); pap., tchr. ed. 14.00 (*0-8273-2970-9*) Delmar.

Basic Complex Analysis. Marsden. 3rd ed. 1998. tchr. ed. 23.90 (*0-7167-2772-2*) W H Freeman.

Basic Concepts & Applications, Vol. 1. Robert W. Broyles & Colin Lay. 1980. LC 79-23280. 570p. 83.50 (*0-89443-153-6*) Aspen Pub.

Basic Concepts for Qualitative Research. Immy Holloway. 1997. LC 97-25880. (Illus.). 186p. pap. 38.95 (*0-632-04173-0*) Blackwell Sci.

Basic Concepts in Doppler Echocardiography. Ed. by James V. Chapman & A. Sgalambro. 1987. (Developments in Cardiovascular Medicine Ser.). text 184.00 (*0-89838-888-0*) Kluwer Academic.

Basic Concepts in Eidetic Psychotherapy. Akhter Ahsen. 1973. 434p. text 35.00 (*0-913412-12-0*) Brandon Hse.

Basic Concepts in Family Therapy: An Introductory Text. Linda Berg-Cross. 1987. LC 86-22774. 399p. text 29.95 (*0-86656-565-5*); 2nd ed. 2000. LC 99-54668. (Illus.). xvii, 616p. (C). 89.95 (*0-7890-0646-4*); 2nd ed. 1999. LC 99-54668. (Illus.). xvii, 616p. (C). pap. 59.95 (*0-7890-0941-2*) Haworth Pr.

Basic Concepts in Immunology: A Student's Survival Guide. John Clancy, Jr. 1997. LC 97-25668. (Basic Concepts Ser.). (Illus.). 216p. pap. 29.95 (*0-07-011371-8*) McGraw-Hill Prof.

Basic Concepts in Neuroscience: A Student's Survival Guide. Robert H. Thalmann. 1996. (Illus.). 320p. pap. text 24.95 (*0-07-064389-X*) McGraw.

Basic Concepts in Pathology: A Student's Survival Guide. Earl J. Brown. 1997. LC 97-35643. (Basic Concepts Ser.). (Illus.). 456p. pap. 29.95 (*0-07-008321-5*) McGraw-Hill Prof.

Basic Concepts in Pharmacology: A Student's Survial Guide. Janet L. Stringer. 1996. LC 95-40461. (Basic Concepts Ser.). (Illus.). 320p. pap. 29.95 (*0-07-063165-4*) McGraw-Hill Educ Grp.

Basic Concepts in Pharmacology: A Student's Survial Guide. Janet L. Stringer. 2nd ed. 2000. LC 00-55397. (Illus.). 285p. pap. 29.95 (*0-07-135699-1*) McGraw-Hill Prof.

Basic Concepts of Hemostasis & Thrombosis. Roger L. Bick. Ed. by Genesio Murano. 1980. 304p. 118.00 (*0-8493-5393-9*, RC633, CRC Reprint) Franklin.

Basic Concepts of Industrial Hygiene. Ronald M. Scott. 1997. LC 97-28597. 496p. (C). 84.95 (*1-56670-292-5*) Lewis Pubs.

Basic Concepts of Medical Terminology: Conceptos Basicos de Terminologia Medica. J. J. Reboiras. 1982. (SPA.). 157p. 27.95 (*0-8288-1876-2*, S12385) Fr & Eur.

Basic Concepts of Psychiatric-Mental Health Nursing. Louise Rebecca Shives. 2nd ed. 1989. (Illus.). 657p. text 27.95 (*0-397-54757-9*); 4th ed. 1997. LC 97-12761. 720p. pap. text 31.95 (*0-397-55457-5*) Lppncott W & W.

Basic Concepts of Psychopharmacology for People with Developmental Disabilities. Robert L. Sprague. 1996. pap. text 32.50 (*1-57654-011-1*, Creative Core) Creat Core.

Basic Concepts of the Digestive System. Glenn F. Bastian. 1997. LC 94-1897. (Illustrated Review of Anatomy of Physiology: Systems Ser.). 160p. (C). pap., wbk. ed. 14.20 (*0-06-501710-2*) Addson-Wesley Educ.

Basic Concepts of the Muscular & Skeletal Systems: The Muscular/Skeletal Systems. Glenn F. Bastian. 1997. LC 93-25475. (Illustrated Review of Anatomy of Physiology: Systems Ser.). (Illus.). 208p. (C). pap., wbk. ed. 14.20 (*0-06-501704-8*) Addson-Wesley Educ.

Basic Concepts of the Urinary System: The Urinary System. Glenn F. Bastian. 1997. (Illustrated Review of Anatomy of Physiology: Systems Ser.). 144p. (C). pap., wbk. ed. 14.20 (*0-06-501711-0*) Addson-Wesley Educ.

Basic Contact Lens Practice Update. Ian Davies. 2001. 160p. pap. 80.00 (*0-7506-4912-7*) Buttrwrth-Heinemann.

Basic CPT/HCPCS Coding. Rita Scichilone. rev. ed. 1999. (Illus.). 252p. pap. text 44.00 (*1-58426-018-1*, AC200699) Am Hlth Info.

Basic CPT/HCPCS Coding: 2000 Edition. Gail Smith & Sherri Mallett. rev. ed. 2000. 208p. pap. text 48.00 (*1-58426-034-3*, AC200600) Am Hlth Info.

Basic Cutaneous Surgery: A Primer in Technique. Christopher B. Zachary. 1990. (Practical Manuals in Dermatologic Surgery Ser.). (Illus.). 134p. pap. text (*0-443-08660-5*) Church.

Basic CV Science Review Book. J. Wesley Todd. 2nd rev. ed. 1996. (Illus.). 382p. spiral bd. 80.00 (*0-9653568-0-9*) Cardiac Self Assessmnt.

Basic Data Underlying Clinical Decision-Making in Vascular Surgery. Ed. by John M. Porter & Lloyd M. Taylor, Jr. 1994. 198p. 75.00 (*0-942219-71-6*) Quality Med Pub.

Basic Doppler Physics. Hans J. Smith & James A. Zagzebski. 1991. (Illus.). 136p. (C). pap. text 13.95 (*0-944838-15-4*) Med Physics Pub.

Basic Drug Calculations. Brown. 6th ed. 1999. pap. text 28.00 (*0-323-01004-0*) Mosby Inc.

Basic Drug Therapy & Arithmetic Review. Grace F. Bates et al. 5th ed. 1991. 419p. text 21.95 (*0-07-105244-5*) McGraw-Hill Med Pub.

Basic Dysrhythmias: Interpretation & Management. Robert J. Huszar. 2nd ed. 1994. (Illus.). 480p. (C). (gr. 13). pap. text 25.00 (*0-8016-7203-1*, 07203) Mosby Inc.

Basic ECG Interpretation. Methodist Hospital Staff. 1986. 256p. (C). (gr. 13). pap. text 29.95 (*0-8016-3401-6*, 03401) Mosby Inc.

Basic Electrocardiography. Stephen Scheidt. 1997. (Illus.). 19.95 (*0-914168-13-4*) Icon Lrning Systs.

Basic, Elementary Systematic Substitution Training, Set-ES. Russell E. Mason. 1973. pap. 35.00 incl. audio (*0-89533-015-6*) F I Comm.

Basic EMT. Norman E. McSwain. 1996. 1p. (gr. 13). text, wbk. ed. 45.95 (*0-8151-4580-2*, 30571) Mosby Inc.

Basic EMT: Comprehensive Pre-Hospital Patient Care. Norman E. McSwain. 1996. (Illus.). 864p. (C). (gr. 13). pap. text 37.95 (*0-8151-4647-7*, 29889) Mosby Inc.

Basic EMT: Comprehensive Pre-Hospital Patient Care. Norman E. McSwain et al. 1996. pap. text, tchr. ed. (*0-8151-4579-9*) Mosby Inc.

***Basic EMT: Comprehensive Pre-Hospital Patient Care.** Norman E. McSwain. 2nd ed. 2001. (Illus.). tchr. ed. (*0-323-01117-9*) Mosby Inc.

Basic EMT: Comprehensive Prehospital Patient Care. Norman E. McSwain et al. 1996. text, wbk. ed. (*0-8151-5979-X*) Mosby Inc.

Basic EMT: Comprehensive Prehospital Patient Care. McSwain. 2nd ed. 2001. LC 00-69943. (Illus.). xxix, 926p. text 41.95 (*0-323-01116-0*) Mosby Inc.

***Basic EMT: Comprehensive Prehospital Patient Care.** Norman E. McSwain. 2nd ed. 2001. (*0-323-01121-7*) Mosby Inc.

***Basic EMT: Comprehensive Prehospital Patient Care.** Norman E. McSwain & James L. Paturas. 2nd ed. 2001. (Illus.). wbk. ed. (*0-323-01118-7*) Mosby Inc.

Basic EMT: Comprehensive Prehospital Patient Care Text. Norman E. McSwain et al. 1996. text, wbk. ed. (*0-8151-4581-0*) Mosby Inc.

Basic EMT Prehospital Patient Care. Norman E. McSwain, Jr. et al. 1996. LC 96-8004. (Illus.). 928p. (C). (gr. 13). text 39.95 (*0-8151-5961-7*, 25287) Mosby Inc.

Basic Endocrinology: An Interactive Approach. J. Matthew Neal. 1999. LC 99-30331. (Illus.). 282p. pap. 29.95 (*0-632-04429-2*) Blackwell Sci.

Basic Endocrinology for Students of Pharmacy & Allied Health Sciences. Andrew Constanti et al. 1998. 156p. text 75.00 (*90-5702-250-8*); pap. text 24.00 (*90-5702-251-6*) Gordon & Breach (Harwood Acad Pubs).

Basic Environmental Toxicology. Ed. by Lorris G. Cockerham & Barbara S. Shane. 1993. 640p. 110.95 (*0-8493-8851-1*, QH545) CRC Pr.

Basic Epidemiological Methods & Biostatistics: A Practical Guidebook. Randy M. Page et al. 1995. (Life Science Ser.). (Illus.). 448p. (C). pap. text 48.95 (*0-86720-869-4*, 869-4) Jones & Bartlett.

Basic Epidemiology. R. Beaglehole et al. 1993. (CHI, ENG, FRE & SPA.). viii, 174p. pap. text 18.00 (*92-4-154446-5*, 1150395) World Health.

Basic Exercises in Immunochemistry: A Laboratory Manual. A. Nowotny. 2nd ed. 1979. LC 79-14029. (Illus.). 314p. 39.00 (*0-387-09453-9*) Spr-Verlag.

Basic Eye Care: Training Activities for Community Health Workers. Helen Keller International Staff. 1996. LC 96-36057. (*0-915173-36-0*) Helen Keller Intl.

Basic Facts in Orthopaedics. Patrick S. Browne. 2nd ed. 1985. (Illus.). 288p. (gr. 13). 23.95 (*0-86793-184-1*, B-0870-8) Mosby Inc.

Basic Family Therapy. Philip Barker. 4th ed. 1998. LC 98-11191. (Illus.). 320p. pap. 50.95 (*0-632-04259-1*) Blackwell Sci.

Basic Fault: Therapeutic Aspects of Regression. Michael Balint. 1992. 205p. reprint ed. pap. 21.00 (*0-8101-1025-3*) Northwestern U Pr.

Basic Filing for Health Information Management. Jan L. Johnson. 1994. 70p. tchr. ed. 16.00 (*0-8273-6284-6*); LC 93-13902. (C). mass mkt. 44.95 (*0-8273-5457-6*) Delmar.

Basic First Aid for Horses. Ed. by William E. Jones. 1973. (Horse Health & Care Ser.). (Illus.). pap. 6.95 (*0-912830-04-2*) Printed Horse.

Basic First Response. Grant B. Goold & Scott Vahradian. 1996. LC 96-22141. 448p. pap. text 53.00 (*0-8359-4914-1*) P-H.

Basic Flight Physiology. Richard O. Reinhart. 1992. 248p. 34.95 (*0-8306-3890-3*, 4141) McGraw-Hill Educ Grp.

Basic Flight Physiology. Richard O. Reinhart. 2nd ed. 1996. LC 95-50308. 285p. pap. 59.95 (*0-07-052223-5*) McGraw-Hill Prof.

Basic Formulary for General Practice. Grant B. Goold et al. 3rd ed. 1995. (Practical Guides for General Practice Ser.: No. 18). 108p. pap. text 25.00 (*0-19-262492-X*) OUP.

Basic Genetics. Daniel L. Hartl. 1991. (Illus.). sl. 195.00 (*0-86720-290-4*, 290-4) Jones & Bartlett.

Basic Genetics. Daniel L. Hartl & Davis. 1991. (Illus.). 544p. (C). pap. text, stu. ed. 13.75 (*0-86720-227-0*, 227-0) Jones & Bartlett.

Basic Genetics. Daniel L. Hartl. 2nd ed. 1991. (Illus.). 544p. text 48.75 (*0-86720-173-8*, 173-8) Jones & Bartlett.

Basic Genetics. Robert F. Weaver & Philip W. Hedrick. 2nd ed. 1994. 72p. (C). text, stu. ed. 16.50 net. (*0-697-24302-8*, WCB McGr Hill) McGrw-H Hghr Educ.

Basic Genetics: A Human Approach. BSCS Staff. 3rd ed. 1998. LC 97-76030. 144p. stu. ed., per. 18.99 (*0-7872-3023-5*) Kendall-Hunt.

Basic Geriatric Nursing. Gloria E. Wold. 2nd ed. 1998. LC 98-27917. (Illus.). 432p. (C). (gr. 13). pap. text 24.95 (*0-8151-8392-5*, 31692) Mosby Inc.

Basic Geriatric Nursing: Includes Testbank. Gloria E. Wold. 2nd ed. 1998. (Illus.). 432p. tchr. ed. (*0-8151-2823-1*) Mosby Inc.

Basic Groupwork. Tom Douglas. 1976. LC 76-1316. 208p. 30.00 (*0-8236-2245-2*) Intl Univs Pr.

Basic Guide to Pesticides: Their Characteristics & Hazards. Shirley Briggs. 1992. 320p. 52.95 (*1-56032-253-5*) Taylor & Francis.

Basic Guide to Understanding Clinical Laboratory Tests. Richard P. Murray. 1993. LC 93-77871. 110p. 14.95 (*1-882657-01-2*) Health Digest.

Basic Head & Neck Pathology. Karen H. Calhoun et al. 1996. LC 95-42455. (Monograph). (Illus.). 228p. (Orig.). pap. text 30.00 (*1-56772-020-X*) AAO-HNS.

Basic Health Physics: Problems & Solutions. Joseph J. Bevelacqua. 1999. LC 98-20472. (Illus.). 576p. 92.95 (*0-471-29711-9*, Wiley-Interscience) Wiley.

Basic Healthcare Statistics for Health Information Management Professionals. Karen G. Youmans. rev. ed. 2000. 182p. pap. text 50.00 (*1-58426-042-4*, AB120700) Am Hlth Info.

Basic Healthcare Statistics for HIM Professionals. Karen G. Youmans. 1996. (Illus.). 224p. pap. text 35.00 (*1-58426-019-X*, AB120796) Am Hlth Info.

Basic Healthcare Statistics for HIM Professionals: Instructor's Answer Guide. Karen G. Youmans. rev. ed. 1996. (Illus.). 48p. pap. text, tchr. ed. 15.00 (*1-58426-008-4*, AB101296) Am Hlth Info.

Basic Healthcare Terminology: With Anatomy Coloring Exercises. R. Whitney Williams. 1995. tchr. ed. (*0-8151-9346-7*); text, tchr. ed. (*0-323-00114-9*); 3rd ed. text (*0-8151-9307-6*) Mosby Inc.

Basic Healthcare Terminology, with Anatomy Coloring Exercises. R. Whitney Williams. 1995. LC 95-166754. (Illus.). 408p. (C). (gr. 13). spiral bd. 22.00 (*0-8151-9144-8*, 24687) Mosby Inc.

Basic Histology. L. Carlos Junqueira. 9th ed. 1998. (Illus.). 494p. (C). pap. 44.95 (*0-8385-0590-2*, A-0590-8) McGraw-Hill Prof.

Basic Histology: Examination & Board Review. Douglas F. Paulsen. 3rd ed. 1996. 368p. (C). pap. 32.95 (*0-8385-2282-3*, A2282-0, Apple Lange Med) McGraw.

Basic Histology & Atlas Value Pak. L. Carlos Junqueira. 8th ed. 1997. 65.00 (*0-8385-0581-3*) Appleton & Lange.

Basic Home Remedies: A Macrobiotic Guide to Special Drinks, Compresses, & Other Natural Applications. Michio Kushi. 1994. 64p. (Orig.). pap. 6.95 (*1-882984-08-0*) One Peaceful World.

Basic Homeopathy for Beast...& Man: Simple, Safe & Effective Treatments of Everyday Ailments... Ilse H. Garriss. 1997. LC 97-42476. (Illus.). spiral bd. 14.95 (*1-888994-06-1*) Howln Moon.

Basic Human Anatomy & Physiology: Clinical Implications for the Health Professionals. Paul D. Anderson. 1984. LC 83-23511. (C). pap., tchr. ed. 10.00 (*0-534-03090-4*); (Illus.). 450p. pap. text 35.00 (*0-534-03089-0*, 089-0) Jones & Bartlett.

Basic Human Anatomy As Seen in the Fetus. Hans Elias. 1971. LC 68-20944. (Illus.). 176p. 22.50 (*0-87527-031-X*) Green.

Basic Human Needs: An Interdisciplinary & International View. Ed. by IUBS-CBE Staff & Gerhard Schaefer. 1992. LC 92-40664. (Illus.). 243p. 48.00 (*3-631-45723-5*) P Lang Pubng.

Basic Human Neuroanatomy. Graig Watson. 2nd ed. 1985. 188p. 22.50 (*0-316-92470-9*, Little Brwn Med Div) Lppncott W & W.

Basic Human Neuroanatomy: An Introductory Atlas. Craig Watson. 5th ed. 1995. LC 94-32506. (Illus.). 256p. pap. text 29.95 (*0-316-92457-1*, Little Brwn Med Div) Lppncott W & W.

Basic Human Physiology. Richard G. Pflanzer. (C). Date not set. pap. text, tchr. ed., suppl. ed. 42.00 (*0-03-072773-1*); 2000. pap. text 31.00 (*0-03-072776-6*) Harcourt Coll Pubs.

Basic Humor Process: A Cognitive-Shift Theory & the Case Against Incongruity. Robert Latta. 1998. LC 98-30868. (Humor Research Ser.). 257p. 114.85 (*3-11-016103-6*) De Gruyter.

Basic ICD-9-CM Coding. Lou Ann Schraffenberger. rev. ed. 1999. (Illus.). 352p. pap. text 58.00 (*1-58426-017-3*, AC200599) Am Hlth Info.

Basic ICD-9-CM for Physician Office Coding. Anita C. Hazelwood & Carol A. Venable. 2000. 163p. (C). pap. text 60.00 (*1-58426-040-8*, AC400900) Am Hlth Info.

Basic ICD-9-CM for Physician Office Coding. Nancy R. Hirschl. rev. ed. 1999. (Illus.). 128p. pap. text 50.00 (*1-58426-024-6*, AC400999) Am Hlth Info.

Basic Ideas Reconsidered: Progress in Self Psychology. Ed. by Arnold Goldberg. 1996. (Progress in Self Psychology Ser.: Vol. 12). 336p. 45.00 (*0-88163-228-7*) Analytic Pr.

Basic Immunology: The Functions & Disorders of the Immune System. Abdul K. Abbas & Andrew H. Lichtman. 2001. (Illus.). 255p. text 39.95 (*0-7216-9316-4*) Saunders.

Basic Industrial Hearing Conservation. David F. Barr & Richard K. Miller. 26.95 (*0-915586-10-X*) Fairmont Pr.

Basic Interviewing: A Practical Guide for Counselors & Clinicians. Ed. by Michel Hersen & Vincent B. Van Hasselt. 1998. LC 97-30349. 250p. pap. (*0-8058-2369-7*) L Erlbaum Assocs.

Basic Introduction to Health Services Administration: Selected Readings. Ed. by William T. Hall. 1976. LC 76-26094. (Illus.). 331p. (C). pap. text 12.95 (*0-8422-0508-X*) Irvington.

Basic Introduction to Statistics for the Behavioral Sciences. Howard Tokunaga & Geoffrey Keppel. 2000. text (*0-7167-3320-X*) W H Freeman.

Basic Issues in Psychopathology. Ed. by Charles G. Costello. 1993. LC 92-48972. 465p. 58.00 (*0-89862-139-9*, 2139) Guilford Pubns.

Basic Keyboarding for Medical Office Assistant, IML. Edna J. Moss. 2nd ed. 1999. 100p. tchr. ed. 14.95 (*0-7668-0924-2*) Delmar.

Basic Keyboarding for the Medical Office Assistant. Edna J. Moss. 2nd ed. 1999. LC 98-53985. (Medical Assisting Ser.). 323p. (C). pap. text 35.95 (*0-7668-0923-4*) Delmar.

Basic Laboratory Methods in Medical Parasitology. 1991. (CHI, ENG, FRE & SPA.). viii, 114p. pap. text 21.00 (*92-4-154410-4*, 1150354) World Health.

Basic Laboratory Procedures in Clinical Bacteriology. Ed. by J. Vandepitte et al. 1991. (CHI, ENG, FRE & SPA.). vii, 121p. pap. text 21.00 (*92-4-154425-2*, 1150361) World Health.

Basic Law for Allied Health Professionals. Michael L. Cowdrey & Melinda Drew. 2nd ed. 1995. LC 94-38115. (Illus.). 336p. (C). pap. text 41.95 (*0-86720-710-8*, 710-8) Jones & Bartlett.

Basic Life Support: Skills Manual. Charles L. Phillips. 1977. LC 77-8351. pap. 14.95 (*0-87618-883-8*) P-H.

Basic Life Support for Healthcare Providers, 1997-99. 1997. (Emergency Cardiovascular Care Programs Ser.). (Illus.). 108p. pap. 10.00 (*0-87493-618-7*) Am Heart.

Basic Life Support Heartsaver Guide, 1997-99: A Student Handbook for Cardiopulmonary Resuscitation & First Aid Choking. 1997. (Emergency Cardiovascular Care Programs Ser.). (Illus.). 78p. pap. 3.50 (*0-87493-632-2*) Am Heart.

Basic Life Support Instructor's Manual, 1997-99. 1997. (Emergency Cardiovascular Care Programs Ser.). (Illus.). 129p. pap., tchr. ed. 25.00 (*0-87493-624-1*) Am Heart.

Basic Lifeguard Textbook. American Red Cross Staff. 1994. 336p. (C). (gr. 13). pap. text 20.00 (*0-8016-7555-3*) Mosby Inc.

Basic Malaria Microscopy Pt. 1: Learner's Guide. 1991. (ENG & FRE.). 72p. pap. text 14.00 (*92-4-154430-9*, 1151365) World Health.

Basic Malaria Microscopy Pt. 2: Tutor's Guide. 1991. (ENG & FRE.). 69p. pap. text 14.00 (*92-4-154431-7*, 1152365) World Health.

Basic Management for Staff Nurses: A Companion to Practice. Ed. by Nancy M. Nicol & Stanley Walker. 1991. 176p. (C). pap. text 28.00 (*0-412-35520-5*, A5239) Chapman & Hall.

Basic Masking: An Explanation & Procedure. Wayne J. Staab. 2nd ed. 1992. (Illus.). 24p. (C). pap. text 5.00 (*1-881148-07-6*) W J Staab.

Basic Maternal - Newborn Nursing. Barbara G. Anderson & Pamela J. Shapiro. 6th ed. 1994. LC 93-28313. 416p. (C). mass mkt. 46.95 (*0-8273-5747-8*) Delmar.

Basic Maternal - Pediatric Nursing. Shapiro. 1995. 256p. (C). stu. ed. 17.95 (*0-8273-6354-0*) Delmar.

Basic Maternal / Pediatric Nursing. Pamela J. Shapiro. 1994. LC 94-19097. 608p. (C). 63.95 (*0-8273-4993-9*) Delmar.

Basic Maternal Newborn Nursing: Instructor's Guide. Barbara G. Anderson & Pamela J. Shapiro. 6th ed. 1994. 27p. tchr. ed. 12.95 (*0-8273-5748-6*) Delmar.

Basic Maternity Nursing. Persis Mary Hamilton. 6th ed. 1988. (Illus.). 400p. (C). (gr. 13). pap. text 29.95 (*0-8016-2700-1*, 02700) Mosby Inc.

Basic Math & Medicines for Nurses. Delores F. Saxton. 1994. (Nursing Education Ser.). pap. 20.95 (*1-878060-02-3*) GW Medical.

Basic Mechanisms Controlling Term & Preterm Birth. Ed. by Kristof Schwalisz & Robert Garfield. 1993. LC 93-37409. (Schering Foundation Workshop Ser.: Vol. 7). (Illus.). 317p. 100.00 (*0-387-57191-4*) Spr-Verlag.

Basic Mechanisms in Mucosal Immunology: Journal: Immunologic Research, Vol. 10, Nos. 3-4, 1991. Ed. by M. Zeitz et al. 1991. (Illus.). vi, 370p. pap. 65.25 (*3-8055-5471-0*) S Karger.

Basic Mechanisms of Physiologic & Aberrant Lymphoproliferation in the Skin. W. C. Lambert et al. 1994. (NATO Advanced Science Institutes Ser.: 265). (Illus.). 664p. (C). text 145.00 (*0-306-44736-3*, Kluwer Plenum) Kluwer Academic.

Basic Mechanisms of the EEG. Ed. by Stephan Zschocke & Erwin-Joseph Speckmann. 1993. LC 92-48487. (Brain Dynamics Ser.). (Illus.). xv, 355p. 136.50 (*0-8176-3596-3*) Birkhauser.

Basic Medical Biochemistry: A Clinical Approach. Dawn B. Marks et al. 1996. (Illus.). 806p. pap. 42.00 (*0-683-05595-X*) Lppncott W & W.

Basic Medical Endocrinology. H. Maurice Goodman. 2nd ed. 1993. (Series in Physiology). 352p. text 69.00 (*0-7817-0106-6*) Lppncott W & W.

Basic Medical Histology: The Biology of Cells, Tissues & Organs. Richard G. Kessel. 1998. LC 97-6576. (Illus.). 672p. (C). text 54.50 (*0-19-509528-6*) OUP.

Basic Medical Laboratory Subjects. Patrick Cuviella & Hugh Woosley. 1975. LC 74-18675. (Allied Health Ser.). (gr. 11-12). pap. 7.20 (*0-672-61383-2*) Macmillan.

Basic Medical Laboratory Techniques. Norma J. Walters et al. 2nd ed. LC 85-12885. 412p. (gr. 12). 1991. pap., tchr. ed. 18.00 (*0-8273-3949-6*, 2512-6); 1990. pap. 34.95 (*0-8273-3948-8*, 2511-8) Delmar.

Basic Medical Laboratory Techniques. Norma J. Walters & Barbara H. Estridge. 3rd ed. 1996. LC 95-9991. 220p. text, tchr. ed. 18.00 (*0-8273-6228-5*) Delmar.

Basic Medical Laboratory Techniques, 4E. Barbara H. Estridge et al. 4th ed. 1999. LC 99-54759. (Medical Lab Technician Ser.). 576p. (C). pap. text 58.95 (*0-7668-1206-5*) Thomson Learn.

Basic Medical Microbiology. Robert F. Boyd & Bryan G. Hoerl. 3rd ed. 1985. 976p. 42.50 (*0-316-10441-8*, Little Brwn Med Div) Lppncott W & W.

Basic Medical Sciences for MRCP, Pt. 1. P. Easterbrook. 1994. (Illus.). 357p. text (*0-443-04035-4*); 2nd ed. 1999. LC 98-40968. (*0-443-06156-4*) Church.

Basic Medical-Surgical Nursing. Mildred A. Mason & Grace F. Bates. 5th ed. 1991. 915p. text 36.95 (*0-07-105295-X*) McGraw-Hill Med Pub.

Basic Medical Techniques & Patient Care in Imaging Technology. Lillian S. Torres et al. 5th ed. 1997. LC 96-38864. 368p. text 38.95 (*0-397-55398-6*) Lppncott W & W.

Basic Medical Terminology. J. Patrick Fisher. (Allied Health Ser.). 1975. LC 74-77820. (gr. 11-12). 115.50 incl. audio (*0-672-61387-5*, Bobbs); 1975. LC 74-77820. (gr. 11-12). pap. text 14.95 (*0-672-61385-9*, Bobbs); 2nd ed. 1983. 288p. incl. audio (*0-672-61575-4*); 2nd ed. 1983. 288p. tchr. ed. (*0-672-61574-6*); 2nd ed. 1983. 288p. pap. text (*0-672-61573-8*); 3rd ed. 1987. 36.51 net. (*0-02-685180-6*) Macmillan.

Basic Medical Terminology Concepts. Marilyn W. Wilson. 2nd ed. 1995. LC 94-45259. 208p. pap. 45.00 (*0-8359-4956-7*) P-H.

Basic Medical Terminology Instructors Guide. Meaus. 3rd ed. 1987. 11.10 net. (*0-02-685470-8*) Macmillan.

Basic Methods in Antibody Production & Characterization. Gary C. Howard & Delia R. Bethell. 2000. LC 00-33729. (Illus.). 288p. 99.95 (*0-8493-9445-7*) CRC Pr.

Basic Microbiology. Orten C. Skinner. 1975. LC 74-78590. (Allied Health Ser.). pap. 9.50 (*0-672-61390-5*, Bobbs) Macmillan.

Basic Microcomputer Models in Biology. James D. Spain. 1982. 368p. (C). text 35.50 (*0-201-10678-7*) Benjamin-Cummings.

Basic Microcurrent Therapy: Acupoint & Body Work Manual. Carolyn Wing Greenlee et al. 4th exp. rev. ed. 1998. LC 00-500758. (Illus.). 160p. spiral bd. 45.00 (*1-887400-19-2*, BK-1001) Earthen Vessel Prodns.

Basic Neurochemistry. George J. Siegel et al. 3rd ed. 1981. 39.00 (*0-316-79002-8*, Little Brwn Med Div) Lppncott W & W.

Basic Neurochemistry: Molecular, Cellular & Medical Aspects. George J. Siegel. 6th ed. 1998. LC 98-21392. 1,200p. text 72.00 (*0-397-51820-X*) Lppncott W & W.

Basic Neurochemistry: Molecular, Cellular & Medical Aspects. George J. Siegel & Bernard W. Agranoff. 6th ed. 1998. 1,200p. 125.00 (*0-7817-1746-9*) Lppncott W & W.

Basic Neurology. John Gilroy. 2nd ed. 1991. 384p. text 55.00 (*0-07-105271-2*); pap. text 42.00 (*0-07-105272-0*) McGraw-Hill Med Pub.

Basic Neurology. Ed. by John Gilroy. 3rd ed. 1999. LC 99-461903. (Illus.). 720p. pap. 49.95 (*0-07-105467-7*) McGraw-Hill Prof.

Basic Neurology. John Gilroy. 2nd ed. 1990. text (*0-08-040297-6*); pap. text (*0-08-040301-8*) PPI GBR. *Dist:* McGraw.

Basic Neuroradiology. Mohammad Sarwar et al. 1983. (Illus.). 863p. 95.00 (*0-87527-230-4*) Green.

Basic Neurosis: Oral Regression & Psychic Masochism. Edmund Bergler. rev. ed. 1978. 371p. text 21.95 (*0-8089-0054-4*, 790564, Grune & Strat) Harcrt Hlth Sci Grp.

Basic Notes in Psychopharmacology. M. Levi. 1993. 64p. (C). pap. text 14.00 (*0-7923-8806-2*) Kluwer Academic.

Basic Nursing: A Critical Thinking Approach. Patricia Castaldi. 4th ed. 1999. (Illus.). 432p. (C). pap., stu. ed. 18.95 (*0-323-00100-9*) Mosby Inc.

Basic Nursing: A Critical Thinking Approach. Patricia A. Potter & Anne G. Perry. 4th ed. 1998. tchr. ed. (*0-323-00103-3*); LC 98-23777. 1300p. (gr. 3). text 57.00 (*0-323-00099-1*); (Illus.). 1296p. (*0-323-00499-7*) Mosby Inc.

Basic Nursing: A Critical Thinking Approach. Patricia A. Potter & Anne G. Perry. 4th ed. 1999. (Illus.). 1290p. (*84-8174-094-2*) Mosby-Doyma Libros ESP. *Dist:* Mosby Inc.

Basic Nursing: Theory & Practice. Patricia A. Potter & Anne G. Perry. 3rd ed. (Illus.). tchr. ed., suppl. ed. (*0-8151-6756-3*) Mosby Inc.

Basic Nursing Education Programmes: A Guide to Their Planning. K. Lyman. 1961. (Public Health Papers: No. 7). 81p. 3.00 (*92-4-130007-8*) World Health.

Basic Nursing Procedures. Grace V. Hornemann. 3rd ed. LC 77-94835. (Illus.). 340p. 1980. tchr. ed. 11.00 (*0-8273-1321-7*); 1979. (C). (gr. 11-12). mass mkt. 37.95 (*0-8273-1320-9*) Delmar.

Basic Nursing Skills. Frances Britton. 1981. (Illus.). 272p. pap. text 7.95 (*0-87619-921-X*) P-H.

Basic Nursing Skills & Concepts Two. Ed. by Grace Cole. 2nd ed. 1995. (Illus.). 912p. (C). (gr. 13). text 41.95 (*0-8016-7884-6*, 07884) Mosby Inc.

Basic Nutrition. Sue R. Williams. 11th ed. 2000. (Illus.). 624p. pap. text 33.95 (*0-323-00569-1*) Mosby Inc.

Basic Nutrition & Diet Therapy. Sue R. Williams. 10th ed. 1994. (Illus.). text, tchr. ed., suppl. ed. 24.95 (*0-8151-9413-7*); 10th ed. 1994. LC 95-106110. (Illus.). 656p. (C). (gr. 13). pap. text 35.95 (*0-8151-9234-7*, 24135); 11th ed. 1999. tchr. ed. (*0-323-00619-1*) Mosby Inc.

***Basic Nutrition & Diet Therapy: Computerized Test Bank (IBM)** Sue Rodwell Williams. 2000. 500.00 (*0-323-00620-5*) Mosby Inc.

Basic Obstetrics & Gynecology. Norman Gant & F. Gary Cunningham. 1998. LC 93-218666. (Illus.). 472p. (C). pap. text 39.95 (*0-8385-9633-9*, A9633-7, Apple Lange Med) McGraw.

Basic Occupational Medicine: A Guide to Developing Delivery Systems. Robert R. Silver. 1991. 192p. 104.95 (*0-8493-4290-2*, RC963) CRC Pr.

Basic of Magnetic Resonance Imaging. William H. Oldendorf, Jr. 1988. (Topics in Neurology Ser.). (C). text 133.00 (*0-89838-964-X*) Kluwer Academic.

Basic Operative Surgery. Khatri. 2001. text (*0-7216-7864-5*) Saunders.

Basic Ophthalmic Investigative Techniques. Larry Benjamin & C. B. James. 2002. 112p. pap. 45.00 (*0-7506-4952-6*) Buttrwrth-Heinemann.

Basic Ophthalmology for Medical Students & Primary Care Residents. Cynthia A. Bradford. 7th ed. 1999. LC 98-27992. xv, 175 p. pap. 28.00 (*1-56055-098-8*) Am Acad Ophthal.

Basic Opthalmic Surgery. Alexander Foss. 2001. (Illus.). 336p. pap. text 55.00 (*0-7506-4197-5*) Buttrwrth-Heinemann.

Basic Orthopaedic Biomechanics. Ed. by Van C. Mow & Wilson C. Hayes. 2nd ed. 1997. LC 97-1336. 528p. text 110.00 (*0-397-51684-3*) Lppncott W & W.

Basic Pathology. Vinay Kumar. 6th ed. 1997. LC 96-46873. text 54.95 (*0-7216-5122-4*) Saunders.

Basic Pathology: An Introduction to the Mechanisms of Disease. Sunil Lakhani et al. 2nd ed. 1998. (Arnold Publication). (Illus.). 336p. pap. text 24.50 (*0-340-67787-2*) OUP.

Basic Patient Assessment. Mosby Staff. 1995. (Respiratory Care Workbook Ser.: No. 2). (C). wbk. ed. (*0-8151-6305-3*, 26023) Mosby Inc.

Basic Pediatric Nursing. Scipien. 1989. tchr. ed. 32.00 net. (*0-07-055566-4*) McGraw.

Basic Pediatric Nursing. Shapiro. 1997. (LPN/LVN Nursing Ser.). tchr. ed. 15.00 (*0-8273-7718-5*) Delmar.

Basic Pediatric Nursing. Persis M. Hamilton. 6th ed. 1990. (Illus.). 640p. (C). (gr. 13). pap. text 29.95 (*0-8016-5869-1*, 05869) Mosby Inc.

Basic Personal Counseling: A Training Manual for Counselors. David Geldard. 1989. (Illus.). 214p. (C). pap. text 42.95 (*0-398-05540-8*) C C Thomas.

Basic Pharmacology. Ed. by R. W. Foster. 4th ed. 1996. (Illus.). 569p. pap. text (*0-7506-2198-2*) E A GBR. *Dist:* OUP.

Basic Pharmacology. Henry Hitner & Barbara T. Nagle. 4th ed. 1999. LC 98-36021. (Illus.). 448p. (YA). (gr. 6-12). stu. ed. 33.00 (*0-02-804654-4*) Glencoe.

Basic Pharmacology & Clinical Drug Use in Dentistry. R. A. Clawson et al. 6th ed. 1995. LC 94-22240. 227p. pap. text (*0-443-05107-0*) Church.

Basic Pharmacology for Health Occupations. Henry Hitner & Barbara T. Nagle. 3rd ed. 1993. LC 93-13333. (Glencoe Seminar Ser.). (C). text 46.92 (*0-02-800679-8*); tchr. ed. (*0-02-800680-1*) Glencoe.

Basic Pharmacology for Health Occupations. Henry Hitner & Barbara T. Nagle. 1980. (Health Occupations Ser.). tchr. ed. (*0-672-61438-3*); pap. (*0-672-61437-5*) Macmillan.

Basic Pharmacology for Nurses. Bruce D. Clayton. (C). text (*981-4020-71-0*) Harcourt Coll Pubs.

Basic Pharmacology for Nurses. Bruce D. Clayton & Yvonne N. Stock. 11th ed. 1997. (C). 192p. pap. text, tchr. ed. (*0-8151-2147-4*, 30758); 208p. pap. text, stu. ed. (*0-8151-1508-3*, 28268) Mosby Inc.

Basic Pharmacology for Nurses. Bruce D. Clayton et al. 11th ed. 1996. LC 96-28659. (Illus.). 624p. (C). (gr. 13). pap. text 37.00 (*0-8151-1512-1*, 28266) Mosby Inc.

***Basic Pharmacology for Nurses: Instructor's Resource Manual.** Bruce D. Clayton & Yvonne N. Stock. 2001. (Illus.). (*0-323-00995-6*) Mosby Inc.

Basic Pharmacology for Nurses: Text & Student Learning Guide Package, Set. Bruce D. Clayton & Yvonne N. Stock. 11th ed. 1997. (Illus.). (C). text, stu. ed. (*0-8151-1513-X*) Mosby Inc.

Basic Pharmacology in Medicine: Pharmacology in Medicine. Ed. by M. D. DiPalma et al. 4th ed. 1994. (Illus.). 890p. pap. text 46.95 (*0-942447-04-2*) Med Surveill.

Basic Physical Therapy Techniques: A Manual for Use in Countries with Developing Physical Rehabilitation Programs. 1996. (*0-9650378-0-0*) MN-Commonwlth.

Basic Physics & Measurement in Anaesthesia. Gavin Kenny & Paul D. Davis. 2001. (Illus.). 384p. pap. (*0-7506-4828-7*) Buttrwrth-Heinemann.

Basic Physics & Measurement in Anesthesia. P. D. Davis et al. 4th ed. 2001. LC 95-184868. (Illus.). 360p. pap. text 55.00 (*0-7506-1713-6*) Buttrwrth-Heinemann.

Basic Physics of Radiation Therapy. Joseph Selman. 6th ed. 1990. (Illus.). 786p. (C). text 147.95 (*0-398-05685-4*) C C Thomas.

Basic Physiology. Ed. by P. D. Sturkie. 1984. (Illus.). 445p. 89.95 (*0-387-90485-9*) Spr-Verlag.

Basic Physiology for the Health Sciences. Ewald E. Selkurt. 2nd ed. 1982. 43.95 (*0-316-78048-0*, Little Brwn Med Div) Lppncott W & W.

Basic Prehospital Care. Rothenberg et al. 1991. (Illus.). 688p. stu. ed., wbk. ed. 12.95 (*0-8016-3418-0*) Mosby Inc.

Basic Principles, Pt. 2. R. Vance Hall. 1975. (Managing Behavior Ser.: Part 2). 71p. (C). pap. 11.00 (*0-89079-002-7*, 1046) PRO-ED.

Basic Principles for Control of Acute Respiratory Infections in Children in Developing Countries: A Joint WHO-UNICEF Statement. 1986. 18p. pap. text 2.70 (*92-4-156094-0*, 1150246) World Health.

***Basic Principles Gynaecological Obstetrics.** 1998. pap. (*1-919713-21-2*) U Cape Town.

Basic Principles in Transport. Ed. by R. K. Kinne. 1990. (Comparative Physiology Ser.: Vol. 3). (Illus.). viii, 160p. 127.00 (*3-8055-5078-2*) S Karger.

Basic Principles of Ayurveda. Bhagavan D. Dash & Lalitesh Kashyap. 1980. (Illus.). 628p. 70.00 (*0-940500-34-5*) Asia Bk Corp.

Basic Principles of Equine Massage-Muscle Therapy. Michael Scott. Ed. by Peter Tocci. 1997. (Illus.). 208p. pap. 27.95 (*0-9662677-0-2*) Massage-Muscle.

Basic Principles of Knee Arthroscopy: Normal & Pathological Findings Tips & Tricks. John M. Eichhorn et al. 1991. (Illus.). 253p. 140.00 (*0-387-53540-3*) Spr-Verlag.

Basic Principles of Nursing Care. Virginia Henderson. rev. ed. 1997. 96p. (C). text 29.95 (*0-9658360-0-2*) Intl Coun Nurses.

Basic Principles of Oral & Maxillofacial Radiology. Dale A. Miles et al. 1992. (Illus.). 240p. pap. text 42.00 (*0-7216-3471-0*) Saunders.

Basic Principles of Psychoanalysis. Abraham Arden Brill. 1985. LC 85-7407. 316p. reprint ed. pap. text 26.00 (*0-8191-4665-X*) U Pr of Amer.

Basic Principles of Radiographic Exposure. Diane C. De Vos. 2nd ed. 1995. LC 94-34821. (Illus.). 160p. pap. 29.00 (*0-683-02458-2*) Lppncott W & W.

Basic Principles of Rhinoplasty. J. Gregory Staffel & Nick Lang. 1996. 100p. pap. text 22.00 (*0-9651231-0-3*) Am Acad Facial.

Basic Principles of the Science of Mind. Frederick W. Bailes. Ed. by Frederick W. Bailes. 5th ed. 1987. 181p. reprint ed. pap. 20.95 (*0-87516-404-8*) DeVorss.

Basic Probability & Statistics for Nurses with Computer Applications. Archie W. Earl, Sr. 1999. 614p. lib. bdg. 69.95 (*1-884169-69-4*) Intl Educ Improve.

Basic Problems of Enthnopsychiatry. George Devereux. Tr. by Basia M. Gulati from FRE. 1980. LC 79-11104. 384p. reprint ed. lib. bdg. 37.50 (*0-226-14355-4*) U Ch Pr.

Basic Problems of Neurolinguistics. A. R. Luria. Tr. by Basil Haigh from RUS. 1976. (Janua Linguarum, Series Major: No. 73). text (*90-279-3205-0*) Mouton.

Basic Procedures. Lindy DuBois. 1998. LC 98-12042. (Basic Bookshelf for Eyecare Professionals Ser.). (Illus.). 128p. pap. text 30.00 (*1-55642-347-0*, 63470) SLACK Inc.

Basic Processes in Memory Development. Ed. by Charles J. Brainerd & M. Pressley. 1985. (Cognitive Development Ser.). (Illus.). 324p. 85.95 (*0-387-96064-3*) Spr-Verlag.

Basic Processes in Reading: Visual Word Recognition. Derek Besner & Glyn W. Humphreys. 1990. 352p. (C). pap. 55.00 (*0-8058-0994-5*); text 99.95 (*0-8058-0219-3*) L Erlbaum Assocs.

Basic Processes of Learning, Cognition & Motivation. Stephen M. Cormier. 1986. 472p. (C). text 89.95 (*0-89859-689-0*) L Erlbaum Assocs.

Basic Psychiatric Science & Treatment, Vol. 6, Basic Psychiatric Science and Treatment. Ed. by Joseph D. Noshpitz et al. 1998. (Handbook of Child & Adolescent Psychiatry Ser.: Vol. 6). 640p. 250.00 (*0-471-19331-3*) Wiley.

Basic Psychoanalytic Concepts on Metapsychology, Conflicts, Anxiety & Other Subjects. Ed. by Humberto Nagera. 1990. 232p. reprint ed. pap. text (*0-9507146-6-6*) Karnac Bks GBR. *Dist:* Other Pr LLC.

Basic Psychoanalytic Concepts on the Libido Theory. Ed. by Humberto Nagera. 1990. 194p. reprint ed. pap. text (*0-9507146-3-1*) Karnac Bks GBR. *Dist:* Other Pr LLC.

Basic Psychoanalytic Concepts on the Theory of Dreams, Vol. II. Ed. by Humberto Nagera. 1990. 124p. reprint ed. pap. text (*0-9507146-4-X*) Karnac Bks GBR. *Dist:* Other Pr LLC.

Basic Psychological Skills for Front-Line Staff of Residential Youth Facilities. Kenneth France. 1993. LC 92-37754. (Illus.). 212p. text 50.95 (*0-398-05840-7*) C C Thomas.

Basic Psychology. Henry Gleitman et al. 5th ed. 2000. (C). text 58.00 (*0-393-97609-2*) Norton.

Basic Psychology. Jonides. 5th ed. 1999. pap. text, stu. ed. 14.00 (*0-393-97361-1*) Norton.

Basic Psychology: Classroom Demos. J. Jonies. 4th ed. Date not set. (C). pap. (*0-393-96915-0*) Norton.

***Basic Psychology: Int Psy Crs Plat.** Henry Gleitman. 5th ed. 2001. (C). pap. text 23.25 (*0-393-94694-0*) Norton.

Basic Quality Assurance & Quality Control in the Clinical Laboratory. A. Wayne Bruce. 1984. 179p. 29.95 (*0-316-11252-6*, Little Brwn Med Div) Lppncott W & W.

Basic Questions on Addiction & Recovery. Gary P. Stewart. 2000. (Biobasics Ser.). 96p. pap. 4.99 (*0-8254-3076-3*) Kregel.

Basic Radiology. Michael Y. Chen et al. 1996. LC 95-19434. (Illus.). 461p. pap. 54.95 (*0-07-011148-0*) McGraw-Hill Educ Grp.

Basic Rehabilitation Techniques: A Self-Instructional Guide. Robert D. Sine et al. 4th ed. 1991. LC 99-59770. 339p. 43.00 (*0-8342-1732-5*) PRO-ED.

Basic Research & Clinical Aspects of Pseudomonas Aeruginosa. Ed. by G. Doering et al. 1987. (Antibiotics & Chemotherapy Ser.: Vol. 39). (Illus.). x, 314p. 221.00 (*3-8055-4541-X*) S Karger.

Basic Research in Urological Oncology. Ed. by Lucio Luciani et al. 1996. LC 95-25524. viii, 182p. 172.25 (*3-8055-6120-2*) S Karger.

Basic Respiratory Physiology. Norman C. Staub. 1991. (Illus.). 242p. pap. text (*0-443-08755-5*) Church.

Basic Science & Clinical Review: Study for Surgery Housestaff. Rittenhouse Book Staff. 1997. 39.00 (*0-01-570300-2*) Rittenhouse.

Basic Science in Obstetrics & Gynaecology Pt. 1: A Textbook for the MRCOG. Ed. by Michael De Swiet & Geoffrey V. Chamerlain. 2nd ed. 1992. (Illus.). 298p. pap. text (*0-443-04229-2*) Church.

Basic Science in Obstetrics & Gynaecology Pt. 1: A Textbook for the MRCOG. Michael De Swiet. 3rd ed. 2000. LC 2001-37989. Price not set. (*0-443-06150-5*) Harcrt Hlth Sci Grp.

Basic Science of Oncology. Ed. by Ian F. Tannock & R. P. Hill. 1987. (Illus.). 400p. 160.00 (*0-08-032389-8*); pap. 42.50 (*0-08-032388-X*) Elsevier (Pergamon Pr).

Basic Science of Oncology. Ian F. Tannock & Richard P. Hill. Ed. by Jim Morgan. 3rd ed. 1998. LC 98-2905. (Illus.). 488p. pap. 69.95 (*0-07-105484-7*) McGraw-Hill Prof.

Basic Science of Vascular Disease. Ed. by Anton N. Sidawy et al. 1997. LC 96-27629. (Illus.). 904p. 175.00 (*0-87993-627-4*) Futura Pub.

Basic Science Review for Otolaryngology. Thomas Van De Water & Hinrich Staecker. 2001. (Illus.). 612p. pap. 69.00 (*0-86577-901-5*) Thieme Med Pubs.

Basic Science Review for Surgeons. Ed. by Richard L. Simmons & David L. Steed. rev. ed. 1991. (Illus.). 460p. pap. text 55.00 (*0-7216-2984-9*) Saunders.

Basic Science Review for Surgery. Richard L. Simmons. 2nd ed. 1998. pap. text (*0-7216-5701-X*) Saunders.

Basic Science Review of Anesthesiology. Ed. by Guy L. Weinberg. 1996. LC 96-8665. (Illus.). 253p. pap. 45.00 (*0-07-069134-7*) McGraw-Hill Prof.

Basic Sciences. Wright & Michael Gleeson. 6th ed. 1996. (Scott Brown's Otolaryngology Ser.: Vol. 1). 804p. (*0-7506-0595-2*) E A GBR. *Dist:* OUP.

Basic Sciences: A Working Reference for Dental Laboratory Technicians. 1997. lib. bdg. 252.95 (*0-8490-8118-1*) Gordon Pr.

Basic Sciences for Obstetrics & Gynaecology. T. Chard & Richard Lilford. 5th ed. 1997. LC 97-17860. (Illus.). 216p. pap. text 39.00 (*3-540-76188-8*) Spr-Verlag.

Basic Sciences for Obstetrics & Gynaecology. Tim Chard & Richard J. Lilford. (Illus.). 2nd ed. 1986. 200p. 43.00 (*0-387-16214-3*); 3rd ed. 1990. 204p. 33.00 (*0-387-19591-2*) Spr-Verlag.

Basic Sciences for Obstetrics & Gynecology - MCQs. Tim Chard. 2nd ed. 1998. LC 97-46471. 128p. pap. 29.95 (*3-540-76206-X*) Spr-Verlag.

Basic Sciences for Sports Medicine. Ron J. Maughan. 1999. LC 99-17155. 368p. pap. text 45.00 (*0-7506-3466-9*) Buttrwrth-Heinemann.

Basic Sciences in Obstetrics & Gynecology. Tim Chard & Richard J. Lilford. 4th ed. 1996. LC 94-47954. 39.50 (*0-387-19903-9*); (Illus.). 203p. 42.95 (*3-540-19903-9*) Spr-Verlag.

Basic Shiatsu: How to Give an Energizing, Relaxing, Healthful Massage. Michio Kushi & Edward Esko. 1995. (Illus.). 96p. (Orig.). pap. 8.95 (*1-882984-10-2*) One Peaceful World.

Basic Sign Communication: Student Materials. William Newell. 1983. pap. 20.95 (*0-913072-56-7*, SL074) Natl Assn Deaf.

***Basic Skills for Living with Diabetes.** 2001. (Illus.). 96p. 14.95 (*1-931876-06-1*) Allina Health Pr.

Basic Skills for Ophthalmic Assistants. 1993. LC 93-21443. (*1-56055-100-3*) Am Acad Ophthal.

Basic Skills in Interpreting Laboratory Data. Ed. by Scott L. Traub. 1996. (Illus.). 400p. (Orig.). pap. text 55.00 (*1-879907-62-3*) Am Soc Hlth-Syst.

Basic Source Readings in the Psychology of Learning. Ed. by Edward Zamble. 1972. LC 72-6357. 296p. pap. text 19.95 (*0-8290-0652-4*) Irvington.

Basic Statistics. Chris Spatz. 3rd ed. 1984. (Psychology). tchr. ed. (*0-534-03211-7*) Wadsworth Pub.

Basic Statistics: Tales of Distribution. Chris Spatz. 6th ed. 1996. LC 96-20147. (Psychology Ser.). 496p. (C). pap. 88.95 (*0-534-26424-7*) Brooks-Cole.

Basic Statistics & Pharmaceutical Statistical Applications. James E. DeMuth. 1999. LC 99-30733. (Biostatistics Ser.). (Illus.). 624p. text 79.75 (*0-8247-1967-0*) Dekker.

Basic Statistics for Nurses. Rebecca G. Knapp. 2nd ed. 1989. LC 84-7274. 418p. (C). mass mkt. 47.95 (*0-8273-4271-3*) Delmar.

Basic Statistics for the Health Sciences. Jan W. Kuzma. 3rd ed. 1998. LC 97-34441. xvii, 344p. text 54.95 (*1-55934-951-4*, 1951) Mayfield Pub.

Basic Statistics for the Health Sciences. Stephen E. Bohnenblust. 4th ed. 2000. LC 00-38006. (Illus.). xvii, 364p. pap. (*0-7674-1752-6*) Mayfield Pub.

Basic Statistics Minitab Workbook. Jarrell. 1993. 192p. pap. 12.95 (*0-8016-2303-0*) Mosby Inc.

Basic Statistics Study Guide. Jarrell. 1993. 192p. pap. text 16.25 (*0-8016-7462-X*) Mosby Inc.

Basic Steps in Planning Nursing Research. Pamela J. Brink & Marilynn J. Wood. 2nd ed. 1983. LC 82-17426. (Illus.). 304p. (C). pap. text 22.50 (*0-534-01241-8*, 241-8) Jones & Bartlett.

Basic Steps in Planning Nursing Research: From Question to Proposal. Pamela J. Brink & Marilynn J. Wood. 4th ed. 1994. LC 93-41640. (Illus.). 400p. (C). text 47.95 (*0-86720-677-2*, 677-2); 5th ed. 1999. 416p. 47.95 (*0-7637-0538-1*) Jones & Bartlett.

Basic Structure & Evolution of Vertebrates, Vol. 2. E. Jarvik. 1981. LC 80-40244. text 209.00 (*0-12-380802-2*) Acad Pr.

Basic Structures of the Head & Neck: A Programmed Instruction in Clinical Anatomy for Dental Professionals. Gretchen M. Reed & Vincent F. Sheppard. 1976. (Illus.). 716p. pap., tchr. ed. (*0-7216-2035-3*); LC 75-298. pap. text 55.00 (*0-7216-7516-6*) Saunders.

Basic Surgery. Hiram C. Polk, Jr. et al. 5th ed. 1995. (Illus.). 1021p. pap. 48.00 (*0-942219-74-0*) Quality Med Pub.

Basic Surgical Exercises Using Swine. M. Michael Swindle. 1983. LC 82-24688. 237p. 77.00 (*0-275-91415-1*, C1415, Praeger Pubs) Greenwood.

Basic Surgical Instrumentation. Mary F. Smith & Joette Stehn. 1992. (Illus.). 256p. pap. text 36.00 (*0-7216-4211-X*) Saunders.

***Basic Surgical Operations.** M. E. Foster & Gareth Morris-Stiff. 2001. (Illus.). 135p. pap. (*0-443-06359-1*) Church GBR. *Dist:* Saunders.

Basic Surgical Skills Manual. Iain J. Skinner. 2000. (Illus.). 136p. 44.95 (*0-07-470608-X*) McGraw.

Basic Surgical Techniques. Raymond M. Kirk. 3rd ed. 1989. (Illus.). 304p. pap. text (*0-443-04004-4*) Church.

Basic Techniques for Metal Ceramics. Makoto Yamamoto. 1990. (Illus.). 117p. text 66.00 (*4-87417-280-6*) Quint Pub Co.

Basic Techniques in Clinical Laboratory Science. Jean J. Linne & Karen M. Ringsrud. 3rd ed. 1991. (Illus.). 600p. (gr. 13). text 39.95 (*0-8016-2864-4*, 02864) Mosby Inc.

Basic Techniques in Vascular Surgery. Bjorn F. Ericsson. 1988. LC 88-71787. (Illus.). 70p. (Orig.). (C). pap. text 14.95 (*0-9620916-0-X*) Davis & Geck.

Basic Techniques of Psychodynamic Psychotherapy. Michael P. Nichols & Thomas J. Paolino, Jr. 1998. 337p. (C). reprint ed. pap. text 22.00 (*0-7881-5610-1*) DIANE Pub.

Basic Terms of Anatomy & Physiology. Bruce P. Squires. 2nd ed. 1987. (Illus.). 184p. pap. 28.00 (*0-920513-00-X*) Saunders.

Basic Tests for Pharmaceutical Dosage Forms. 1991. v, 129p. pap. text 24.00 (*92-4-154418-X*, 1150359) World Health.

Basic Tests for Pharmaceutical Substances. 1986. (ARA, CHI, FRE & SPA.). 210p. pap. text, stu. ed. 34.00 (*92-4-154204-7*, 1150245) World Health.

Basic Textbook of Psychology. Charles A. Heidenreich. 1971. pap. 8.95 (*0-9600428-1-4*) Heidenreich.

Basic Theory of Psychoanalysis. Robert Waelder. 1964. LC 60-8304. 273p. 40.00 (*0-8236-0460-8*); pap. 24.95 (*0-8236-8008-8*, 20200) Intl Univs Pr.

Basic Transcription. Florence C. Maloney & Lois M. Burns. 1996. (Medical Assisting Ser.). 64p. pap., tchr. ed. 15.95 (*0-8273-6375-3*) Delmar.

Basic Transport Phenomena in Biomedical Engineering. Ronald L. Fournier. 1998. LC 98-18733. (Chemical Engineering Ser.). 312p. 85.00 (*1-56032-708-1*) Hemisp Pub.

Basic Trauma Life Support. Alabama ACEP Staff & John E. Campbell. 1985. (Illus.). 224p. (C). tchr. ed. 17.95 (*0-89303-363-4*) P-H.

Basic Trauma Life Support Access. James Gargan. 1995. 80p. pap. (*1-887321-00-4*) Emerg Trng Assocs.

Basic Trauma Life Support for Paramedics & Other Advanced EMS Providers. 4th ed. 2000. (C). (*0-13-086736-5*) S&S Trade.

Basic Trauma Life Support para Paramedicos y Proveedores Avanzados de SME: Primera Edicion en Espanol. John Emory Campbell. Tr. by Eduardo Romero Hicks from ENG. Date not set. (SPA.). (C). pap. text 12.00 (*0-9647418-2-2*) Basic Trauma.

Basic Ultrasound. Hylton B. Meire & Pat Farrant. 1995. LC 94-40651. 234p. pap. 95.00 (*0-471-91691-9*) Wiley.

Basic Urogynaecology. Linda Cardozo et al. 1993. LC 92-48233. 176p. 55.00 (*0-19-262360-5*) OUP.

Basic Virology. Edward K. Wagner & Martin J. Hewlett. 1999. LC 99-21382. (Illus.). 466p. pap. 69.95 (*0-632-04299-0*) Blackwell Sci.

Basic Vocabulary: American Sign Language for Parents & Children. Terrence J. O'Rourke. 1978. pap. 8.95 (*0-932666-00-0*) T J Pubs.

Basic Vocabulary & Language Thesaurus for Hearing-Impaired Children. Daniel Ling & Agnes H. Ling. 1977. LC 76-52826. 11.50 (*0-88200-078-0*, C1437) Alexander Graham.

Basic Water Rescue. American Red Cross Staff. 1997. 64p. (gr. 13). pap. text 4.75 (*0-8151-7955-3*) Mosby Inc.

Basic Writings in the History of Psychology. Robert I. Watson. 1979. (Illus.). 420p. pap. text 27.95 (*0-19-502444-3*) OUP.

Basic Writings of C. G. Jung. Carl Gustav Jung. Ed. & Intro. by Violet S. De Laszlo. 1993. LC 93-17801. (Modern Library Ser.). 736p. reprint ed. 21.00 (*0-679-60071-X*) Random.

Basic Writings of Sigmund Freud. Sigmund Freud. 1995. LC 95-13411. (Modern Library Ser.). 992p. 23.95 (*0-679-60166-X*) Random.

Basics: A Guide for Children's Emergencies. John Shufeldt. 1993. LC 93-9813. (Illus.). 96p. pap. 9.95 (*0-942963-35-0*) Distinctive Pub.

Basics Industrial Hygiene. 1998. (Occupational Health & Safety Ser.). (C). pap. 49.95 (*0-442-02601-3*, VNR) Wiley.

Basics of Acupuncture. Gabriel Stux & Bruce Pomeranz. 4th ed. 1997. LC 97-28726. (Illus.). 322p. pap. text 27.00 (*3-540-63235-2*) Spr-Verlag.

Basics of Anesthesia. Robert K. Stoelting & Ronald D. Miller. 3rd ed. 1994. LC 94-2905. text (*0-443-08962-0*) Church.

Basics of Anesthesia. Robert K. Stoelting & Ronald D. Miller. 4th ed. 2000. LC 99-53883. (Illus.). x, 507p. text (*0-443-06573-X*) Saunders.

Basics of Cancer Chemotherapy. Ellen Carr & Judith A. Killman. 3rd rev. ed. 1995. (Illus.). 115p. (C). pap. 39.95 (*1-878025-71-6*) Western Schls.

Basics of Chest Film Interpretation. Cynthia Umali. 1987. (Illus.). 190p. 45.95 (*0-316-88739-0*, Little Brwn Med Div) Lppncott W & W.

Basics of Computers & Nursing Informatics. Donna Gloe. Ed. by Pat Clutter. 2000. LC 13-3011. 232p. (YA). 22.95 (*1-880254-68-9*) Vista.

Basics of Film Processing in Medical Imaging. Arthur G. Haus & Susan M. Jaskulski. 1997. LC 97-18596. (Illus.). 340p. pap. text 69.95 (*0-944838-79-0*) Med Physics Pub.

Basics of Group Psychotherapy. Ed. by Harold S. Bernard & K. Roy MacKenzie. 1994. LC 94-16964. 224p. 32.00 (*0-89862-117-8*, 2117) Guilford Pubns.

Basics of Head & Neck Film Interpretation. G. V. Keller. 1989. 53.95 (*0-316-48649-3*, Little Brwn Med Div) Lppncott W & W.

Basics of Histotechnology: H & E Stain. Frieda L. Carson. 1992. 50.00 incl. VHS (*0-89189-351-2*) Am Soc Clinical.

Basics of Mistake Proofing. Robin E. McDermott et al. 1997. (Illus.). 66p. pap. 7.95 (*0-527-76327-6*) Product Pr.

Basics of Quality Assurance for Intermediate & Peripheral Laboratories. M. M. El-Nageh et al. 1992. (WHO Regional Publications: No. 2). xviii, 208p. pap. text 15.00 (*92-9021-160-1*, 1440002) World Health.

Basics of Radiology. William Erkonen. 1998. LC 98-2597. 416p. pap. text 59.95 (*0-397-51499-9*) Lppncott W & W.

Basics of Respiratory Therapy: A Laboratory Manual. Frank Sinsheimer. 1983. (C). pap. 20.00 (*0-316-79285-3*, Little Brwn Med Div) Lppncott W & W.

Basics of Transesophageal Echocardiography. Terence D. Rafferty. 1995. LC 95-2999. text (*0-443-08922-1*) Church.

Basics Toxicology. Kent. 1997. (Occupational Health & Safety Ser.). (C). pap. 49.95 (*0-442-02600-5*, VNR) Wiley.

Basis for Gene Therapy. Walter J. Burdette. 2001. LC 00-50784. (Illus.). xxv, 204p. 51.95 (*0-398-07158-6*); pap. 33.95 (*0-398-07159-4*) C C Thomas.

Basis for Sensorimotor Development-Normal & Abnormal: The Influence of Primitive, Postural Reflexes on the Development & Distribution of Tone. Mary R. Fiorentino. 1981. (Illus.). 184p. 40.95 (*0-398-04179-2*) C C Thomas.

Basis for the Application of Calcium Antagonists in Neurology. Ed. by J. M. Van Nuetem & A. Hartmann. 1990. (Journal: Vol. 30, Suppl. 2, 1989). vi, 42p. 21.00 (*3-8055-5173-8*) S Karger.

Basis for Variability of Response to Anti-Rheumatic Drugs. Ed. by P. M. Brooks et al. 1988. (AAS: Agents & Actions Supplements Ser.: Vol. 24). 300p. 82.50 (*0-8176-1959-3*) Birkhauser.

Basis of Toxicity Testing. Donald J. Ecobichon. 2nd ed. 1997. LC 97-204752. (Pharmacology & Toxicology: Basic & Clinical Aspects Ser.). 240p. 104.95 (*0-8493-8554-7*) CRC Pr.

Basis Research on Lung Surfactant. Ed. by P. Von Wichert. 1990. (Progress in Respiratory Research Ser.: Vol. 25). (Illus.). xii, 360p. 235.00 (*3-8055-5030-8*) S Karger.

Basiswissen-Ekg-Registrierung: 2., Erweiterte Auflage. A. H. Lemmerz. 1975. (Illus.). viii, 96p. 16.75 (*3-8055-2298-3*) S Karger.

Bates' Guide to Physical Examination & History Taking. Lynn S. Bickley et al. 7th ed. 1998. LC 98-21795. (Illus.). 816p. text 60.95 (*0-7817-1655-1*) Lppncott W & W.

Bates Method. Peter Mansfield. 1994. LC 95-143054. (Alternative Health Ser.). (Illus.). 166p. (Orig.). pap. 12.95 (*0-8048-3003-7*) Tuttle Pubng.

Bates Method: A Complete Guide to Improving Eyesight Naturally. Peter Mansfield. 1997. (Illus.). 178p. pap. (*0-09-181281-X*) Random GBR. *Dist:* Trafalgar.

Bates Method for Better Eyesight Without Glasses. William H. Bates. 1981. LC 80-39878. 208p. pap. 12.00 (*0-8050-0241-3*, Owl) H Holt & Co.

Bates' Pocket Guide to Physical Examination & History Taking. Lynn S. Bickley & Robert A. Hoekelman. 3rd ed. 2000. LC 99-38243. (Illus.). 288p. pap. text 27.95 (*0-7817-1869-4*) Lppncott W & W.

Battered Child. C. Henry Kempe & Ray E. Helfer. 3rd rev. ed. 1980. LC 80-14329. (Illus.). lib. bdg. 35.00 (*0-226-43038-3*) U Ch Pr.

Battered Children & Child Abuse: Proceedings of the CIOMS Round Table Conference, XIXth. Ed. by Z. Bankowski & M. Carballo. 1986. 187p. pap. text 20.00 (*92-9036-026-7*, 1830019) World Health.

Battered Rich. Steve Bassett. Ed. by Sylvia Ashton. 1980. LC 79-15043. 22.95 (*0-87949-159-0*) Ashley Bks.

Battered Wives. Del Martin. rev. ed. 1981. LC 81-12985. 281p. pap. 12.95 (*0-912078-70-7*) Volcano Pr.

Batteries for Implantable Biomedical Devices. B. B. Owens. 1986. LC 86-582. (Illus.). 380p. (C). text 107.00 (*0-306-42148-8*, Kluwer Plenum) Kluwer Academic.

Battering & Family Therapy: A Feminist Perspective. Marsali Hansen & Michele Harway. 1993. LC 92-42025. (Illus.). 332p. (C). pap. 34.95 (*0-8039-4321-0*, 3662) Sage.

Battle for Health: A Political History of the Socialist Medical Association, 1930-51. John Stewart. 1999. LC 98-34699. (History of Medicine in Context Ser.). 15p. text 86.95 (*1-85928-218-0*, RA413.5.G7S74) Ashgate Pub Co.

Battle of the WAC. Carolyn Bessey. 1999. (Illus.). 192p. per. 11.95 (*0-9670579-0-6*) C H Bessey.

Battle Station Sick Bay: Navy Medicine in World War II. Jan K. Herman. 1997. LC 96-44536. (Illus.). 312p. 36.95 (*1-55750-361-3*) Naval Inst Pr.

Battles of Life & Death. David Hellerstein. 1987. 288p. mass mkt. 6.95 (*0-446-38422-4*) Warner Bks.

Bay Area Baby: The Essential Guide to Local Resources for Pregnancy, Childbirth & Parenthood. Paula B. Reynolds & Jenny G. Andrus. 1991. LC 87-28445. (Illus.). 324p. (Orig.). pap. 14.95 (*0-944296-05-X*) Spirit Pr.

Bay Area Health Care Choices: The Families U. S. A. Guide to Quality & Cost. Ed. by Marc S. Miller. 1996. (Illus.). 240p. pap. 10.95 (*0-9617893-3-6*) Fam USA Found.

Bayerische Gesellschaft fuer Geburtshilfe und Frauenheilkunde, Tagung der Oesterreichischen Gesellschaft fuer Gynaekologie und Geburtshilfe und Jubilaeumstagung, Wuerzburg, May 1987. Ed. by Eduard Gitsch & E. Reinold. 1988. (Journal: Vol. 27, Suppl. 2, 1987). (Illus.). xii, 368p. pap. 87.00 (*3-8055-4743-9*) S Karger.

Bayerische Gesellschaft fuer Geburtshilfe und Frauenheilkunde und der Oesterreichischen Gesellschaft fuer Gynaekologie und Geburtshilfe, Jahrestagung, Innsbruck, May, 1989. Ed. by Eduard Gitsch & E. Reinold. 1989. (Journal: Vol. 29, Suppl. 2, 1989). (Illus.). xiv, 478p. pap. 148.00 (*3-8055-5104-5*) S Karger.

Bayesian Methods & Ethics in a Clinical Trial Design. Ed. by Joseph B. Kadane. 1996. LC 95-14352. (Probability & Statistics Ser.). 344p. 105.00 (*0-471-84680-5*, Wiley-Interscience) Wiley.

BCG - A New Standard for Superficial Bladder Cancer: Journal: European Urology, Vol. 21, Suppl. 2, 1992. Ed. by D. L. Lamm. 1992. (Illus.). iv, 48p. pap. 15.75 (*3-8055-5620-9*) S Karger.

BCG - The Optimal Approach in Superficial Bladder Cancer: Proceedings of the Symposium Held at the 14th European Association of Urology Congress, Stockholm, April, 1999. Ed. by A. Bohle. 1999. (European Urology Ser.: Vol. 37, Suppl. 1). (Illus.). iv, 40p. pap. 25.25 (*3-8055-7019-8*) S Karger.

BCG Vaccination Policies. 1980. (Technical Report Ser.: No. 652). 17p. pap. text 2.00 (*92-4-120652-7*) World Health.

BCG Vaccines & Tuberculins Part A & B. Ed. by L. Lugosi & W. Hennessen. 1987. (Developments in Biological Standardization Ser.: Vol. 58). (Illus.). xviii, 782p. pap. 61.00 (*3-8055-4279-8*) S Karger.

BDA Handbook for Non-Insulin Dependent Diabetes. John L. Day & British Diabetic Association Staff. 1998. LC 97-22984. 132p. pap. 40.00 (*0-471-97275-4*) Wiley.

Be a Natural Woman: Fitness for Teens. Judith Lessmann. Ed. by Harry Kaste. 1981. LC 81-80111. (Illus.). 184p. (Orig.). (gr. 7-12). pap. 5.95 (*0-939390-00-0*) Pizzazz Pr.

Be a Successful Resident. Woodson. 1999. 59.95 (*0-07-134159-5*) McGraw.

Be a Successful Resident. R. Dodge Woodson. 2000. LC 00-269781. (Complete Construction Ser.). (Illus.). 352p. pap. 39.95 (*0-07-134160-9*) McGraw-Hill Prof.

Be a Survivor: Your Guide to Breast Cancer Treatment. Vladimir Lange. 2nd ed. 2000. LC 98-84908. (Illus.). 158p. (C). pap. text 26.95 (*0-9663610-0-8*) Lange Prodns.

***Be Active, Feel Good.** Friga Dickwach & Eva Mainka. 2000. LC 95-932520. 160p. (*0-920905-46-3*) SPBP.

Be an Outrageous Older Man: Action Guide for Men 50 & Beyond. Bard Lindeman. 1998. LC 00-551035. 272p. pap. 14.95 (*1-879198-24-X*) Knwldg Ideas & Trnds.

Be Good to Your Back. William Evans. 1989. (*0-9619258-2-5*) Clearwtr Pools Pub Co.

Be Good to Your Gut: Recipes & Tips for People with Digestive Problems. Pat Baird. 1996. (Illus.). 160p. pap. 17.95 (*0-86542-472-1*) Blackwell Sci.

Be Good to Yourself. John MacKenzie. 1981. (Illus.). 150p. pap. 9.95 (*0-89496-026-1*); 12.95 (*0-89496-027-X*) Ross Bks.

Be Heart Smart: The HCF Way to a Healthy Heart. James W. Anderson. 1989. (Illus.). 120p. (Orig.). pap. 5.95 (*0-922859-00-0*) HCF NRF.

Be Sure Your Child Learns to Read. James Carroll & Barbara Overton. 1976. 160p. pap. 1.95 (*0-89826-000-0*) Natl Paperback.

Be Whole! Robert Conklin. 1997. LC 96-92796. ix, 229p. pap. 11.95 (*0-9654882-0-9*) CliffTop.

Be Your Own Boss: Starting Your Veterinary Practice. Shawn Messonnier. 1994. LC 94-71553. 196p. pap. text 29.95 (*0-939674-55-6*) Am Vet Pubns.

Be Your Own Doctor: How to Use Nature as a Healer & Builder of Health. Ann Wigmore. 2nd ed. 1982. 200p. pap. 3.95 (*0-89529-193-2*) Penguin Putnam.

Beard's Massage. Giovanni De Domenico & Elizabeth C. Wood. Ed. by Margaret Biblis. 4th ed. 1997. LC 96-14136. 256p. pap. text 34.00 (*0-7216-6234-X*) Saunders.

Bearing Meaning: The Language of Birth. Robbie P. Kahn. 1995. LC 94-42159. (Illus.). 456p. 32.95 (*0-252-02171-1*) U of Ill Pr.

Bearing of Basic Research on Clinical Otolaryngology. Ed. by C. R. Pfaltz et al. 1991. (Advances in OtoRhinoLaryngology Ser.: Vol. 46). (Illus.). x, 182p. 161.75 (*3-8055-5338-2*) S Karger.

Bearing of Certain Personality Factors Other Than Intelligence on Academic Success: Study of Tests Made at Teacher's College, Columbia University. Henry T. Tyler. LC 78-177693. (Columbia University. Teachers College. Contributions to Education Ser.: No. 468). reprint ed. 37.50 (*0-404-55468-7*) AMS Pr.

Bearing Unbearable States of Mind. Ruth Riesenberg-Malcolm. 1999. LC 98-39629. (New Library of Psychoanalysis : Vol. 34). ix, 201 p. pap. 29.99 (*0-415-20519-0*) Routledge.

Beast: A Reckoning with Depression. Tracy Thompson. 2000. 288p. reprint ed. 24.00 (*0-7881-9542-5*) DIANE Pub.

Beast: A Reckoning with Depression. Tracy Thompson. 1996. 304p. pap. 13.95 (*0-452-27695-0*, Plume) Dutton Plume.

Beast in the Temple. James G. Stuart. 1988. 199p. (*0-7855-0721-3*); pap. (*0-85335-254-2*) Stuart Titles Ltd GBR. *Dist:* St Mut.

Beast Within Me: Systemic Lupus Erythematosus. Dawn M. Grieshaber. 2000. LC 99-93678. pap. 9.95 (*0-533-13116-2*) Vantage.

Beat High Cost Health Care: A Resource & Guide to Quality Free & Low Cost Medical Treatment. David R. Hopfinger. Ed. by Thorn Bacon. 1994. LC 94-70325. (Illus.). 214p. (Orig.). pap. text 12.95 (*0-9637123-1-4*) Patient Med Progs.

Beat the Breathalyzer: A Survival Kit for Drinking Drivers. Christen A. Jamessen. 1979. pap. 8.95 (*0-9603918-0-0*) Poltergeist.

Beat the Fat...Cook Without It. 1993. (Illus.). 61p. (Orig.). reprint ed. text 8.95 (*0-9638671-0-5*) Beat the Fat.

Beat the Nursing Home Trap: A Consumer's Guide to Assisted Living & Long-Term Care. Joseph L. Matthews. 3rd ed. 2001. LC 98-51467. 336p. pap. 21.95 (*0-87337-515-7*) Nolo com.

***Beating Depression.** Maga E. Jackson-Triche et al. 2002. 256p. pap. 16.95 (*0-07-137627-5*) McGraw-Hill Trade.

Beating Menopause & Early Ovarian Failure with the Help of One Natural Ingredient. Julia Elliott. ltd. ed. 1996. 57p. 9.95 (*0-9658646-0-X*) SCB.

***Beating Sports Injuries Through Conventional & Alternative Methods.** Len Saputo. 2001. (Illus.). 144p. pap. 14.95 (*0-7641-1904-4*) Barron.

***Beating the Blood Sugar Blues: Guide to Low Blood Sugar Control.** Thomas A. Lincoln & John A. Eaddy. 2001. LC 2001-22773. 178p. pap. 14.95 (*1-58040-048-5*) Am Diabetes.

Beating the Food Giants. Paul A. Stitt. 1993. 288p. (Orig.). pap. 9.95 (*0-939956-06-3*) Natural Pr.

Beating Wife-Beating. Lee H. Bowker. 1983. LC 82-48603. 176p. text 35.00 (*0-669-06345-2*) Free Pr.

Beaumont: America's First Physiologist. Rodney B. Nelson, III. 1990. LC 89-82643. (Illus.). 400p. 42.00 (*0-9625624-0-8*) Grant Hse Pr.

Beautiful Again: Restoring Your Image & Enhancing Body Changes. Jan Willis. Ed. by Denise Anderson. 1994. LC 92-23698. (Illus.). 192p. pap. 20.00 (*0-929173-13-9*) Health Press.

Beauty & the Beam: Your Complete Guide to Cosmetic Laser Surgery. Deborah S. Sarnoff & Joan Swirsky. 1998. LC 97-48376. 318p. 23.50 (*1-57626-059-3*) Quality Med Pub.

Beauty & the Beam: Your Complete Guide to Cosmetic Laser Surgery. Deborah S. Sarnoff & Joan Swirsky. 3rd ed. 1998. LC 98-38504. (Illus.). 304p. pap. 19.95 (*0-312-19441-2*) St Martin.

Beauty & the East: Book of Oriental Body Care. Wendy Buonaventura. 1997. LC 99-203022. (Illus.). pap. (*0-86356-081-4*) Saqi GBR. *Dist:* Intl Spec Bk.

Beauty Born of Suffering: Journal of a Plague Year. Malachy Grange. 2000. 267p. pap. 10.00 (*0-9664016-1-1*) Fenix Pr.

Beauty Knows No Pain: The Anatomy of a Successful Facelift. Paula J. Lochmandy. 1994. LC 93-61905. (Illus.). 128p. (Orig.). pap. 20.00 (*0-9639890-7-3*) Tattersall Pr.

Beauty of Being: Psychological Tips for Holistic Wellness of the Person as a Whole - Mind, Body, Spirit & Soul. Fahmy Attallah. 1999. LC 99-14240. 264p. 18.95 (*0-929765-64-8*, Chapman Univ) Seven Locks Pr.

Beauty of Creation: Inspiration for Pregnancy & Childbirth. Elisa Roberson et al. 1998. LC 98-40575. (Illus.). 250p. pap. 14.95 (*0-9644932-3-3*) Kujichagulia Pr.

Because I Live Here: The Theory & Practice of Vita-Erg Ward Therapy with Deteriorated Psychotic Women. S. R. Slavson. 1970. LC 70-125477. 374p. 55.00 (*0-8236-0490-X*) Intl Univs Pr.

Because of Flowers & Dancers. Sandra S. Brackenridge. 1994. (Illus.). 14p. (Orig.). pap. 5.00 (*0-9603534-7-X*) Vet Practice.

Bech, Hamilton, & Zung Scales for Mood Disorders: Screening & Listening: A Twenty Years Update with References to DSM & ICD-10. Per Bech. 1995. LC 95-15491. (*0-387-59104-4*) Spr-Verlag.

Bech, Hamilton & Zung Scales for Moods Disorders Screening & Listening. Per Bech. 2nd rev. ed. 1996. (Illus.). 80p. pap. 89.95 (*3-540-61245-9*) Spr-Verlag.

Bechamp or Pasteur? The Myth of Pasteur's Germ Theory. E. Douglas Hume. 1991. lib. bdg. 250.00 (*0-87700-928-7*) Revisionist Pr.

Becker-Shaffer's Diagnosis & Therapy of the Glaucoma. Robert L. Stamper et al. 7th ed. 1999. LC 99-19994. (Illus.). 784p. (C). (gr. 13). text 195.00 (*0-8016-7726-2*, 07726) Mosby Inc.

Become the Dream: The Transforming Power of Hypnotic Dreamwork. Randal Churchill. Ed. by Cheryl Canfield. 1997. LC 97-60102. 279p. 29.95 (*0-9656218-0-4*) Transforming Pr.

Becoming: Basic Considerations for a Psychology of Personality. Gordon W. Allport. 1960. LC 55-5975. (Terry Lectures). (C). pap. 13.00 (*0-300-00002-2*, Y20) Yale U Pr.

Becoming a Care Supervisor. Clive Curtis & Jane Metcalf. 1992. LC 92-34226. (Skills for Caring Ser.). pap. text (*0-443-04621-2*) Church.

Becoming a Clinical Psychologist. Robert H. Woody & Malcolm H. Robertson. 1988. 343p. 49.50 (*0-8236-0491-8*, BN#00491) Intl Univs Pr.

Becoming a Clinician: A Primer for Students. Shirley M. Neitch & Maurice Mufson. 1998. LC 98-15024. (Illus.). 264p. pap. 29.95 (*0-07-046515-0*) McGraw-Hill Prof.

***Becoming a Complementary Therapist: How to Start a Career in the New Caring Professions.** Linda Wilson. 2001. 144p. pap. (*1-85703-628-X*) How To Bks GBR. *Dist:* Midpt Trade.

Becoming a Constant Object in Psychotherapy with the Borderline Patient. Charles Cohen & Vance R. Sherwood. 1991. LC 90-14556. 336p. 65.00 (*0-87668-613-7*) Aronson.

Becoming a Doctor: A Journey of Initiation in Medical School. Melvin Konner. 1988. LC 87-32832. 412p. pap. 15.00 (*0-14-011116-6*, Penguin Bks) Penguin Putnam.

Becoming a Family Physician. Ed. by M. Little et al. 1989. (Illus.). 286p. 59.00 (*0-387-96949-7*, 2588) Spr-Verlag.

Becoming a Good Doctor: The Place of Virtue & Character in Medical Ethics. James F. Drane. 2nd ed. 1988. LC 88-61721. 226p. (Orig.). pap. 12.95 (*1-55612-209-8*) Sheed & Ward WI.

Becoming a Mother: Research on Maternal Role Identity from Rubin to the Present. Ramona T. Mercer. 1995. LC 95-2601. (Focus on Women Ser.: Vol. 18). (Illus.). 408p. 58.95 (*0-8261-8970-9*) Springer Pub.

Becoming a Physician: What You Need to Know to Make the Decision & Go for It. Marita Danek & Jennifer Danek. 1997. LC 96-25092. 240p. (Orig.). pap. 15.95 (*0-471-12166-5*) Wiley.

Becoming a Practical & Vocational Nurse: A Complete Planning Guide. Linda L. Blair. 1998. LC 97-49685. (Illus.). 288p. (C). (gr. 13). text 23.00 (*0-8151-2620-4*, 31636) Mosby Inc.

Becoming a Psychoanalyst: A Study of Psychoanalytic Supervision. Pref. by Robert S. Wallerstein. 1981. LC 81-8337. (Monograph of the Supervision Study Group of the Committee on Psychoanalytic Education). xiii, 351p. (C). 52.50 (*0-8236-0492-6*) Intl Univs Pr.

Becoming a Psychotherapist: A Clinical Primer. Rosemary M. Balsam & Alan Balsam. 2nd ed. 1984. LC 83-24301. xxii, 370p. (C). pap. text 17.00 (*0-226-03636-7*) U Ch Pr.

Becoming an Adult Stepchild: Adjusting to a Parent's New Marriage. Pearl Ketover Prilik. 1998. LC 97-24487. 160p. 22.95 (*0-88048-870-0*, 8870) Am Psychiatric.

Becoming an Effective Supervisor: A Workbook for Counselors & Therapists. Jane Campbell. 2000. (Illus.). 128p. pap. 19.95 (*1-56032-847-9*) Taylor & Francis.

Becoming Doctors Vol. 2: The Professionalization of Medical Students. Jack Haas & William Shaffir. Ed. by Jaber F. Gubrium. 1987. LC 87-2858. (Contemporary Ethnographic Studies). 142p. 73.25 (*0-89232-718-9*) Jai Pr.

Becoming Kate. Theodore Jansma & Katherine St. Clair. 1990. LC 89-61782. 256p. 19.95 (*0-915677-46-6*) Roundtable Pub.

Becoming Men: The Development of Aspirations, Values, & Adaptational Styles. D. A. Hart. 1992. (Perspectives in Developmental Psychology Ser.). (Illus.). 234p. (C). 39.50 (*0-306-44274-4*, Plenum Trade) Perseus Pubng.

Becoming Miracle Workers: Language & Meaning in Brief Therapy. Gale Miller. 1997. LC 97-3300. (Social Problems & Social Issues Ser.). 250p. pap. text 22.95 (*0-202-30571-6*); lib. bdg. 43.95 (*0-202-30570-8*) Aldine de Gruyter.

Becoming Naturally Therapeutic: A Return to the True Essence of Helping. Jacquelyn Small. rev. ed. 1989. 176p. pap. 14.95 (*0-553-34800-0*) Bantam.

Becoming Solution-Focused in Brief Therapy. John L. Walter & Jane E. Peller. 1992. LC 91-43491. 288p. text 30.95 (*0-87630-653-9*) Brunner-Routledge.

Becoming Visible Bridenthal. 3rd ed. 1997. LC 97-72450. (C). pap. text 35.96 (*0-395-79625-3*) HM.

Bed Number Ten. Sue Baier & Mary Z. Schomaker. 1989. 304p. per. 29.95 (*0-8493-4270-8*, RC416) CRC Pr.

Bed Rest Survival Guide. Barbara E. Peterson. 1998. LC 98-9587. 176p. pap. 12.00 (*0-380-79506-X*, Avon Bks) Morrow Avon.

Bed Wetting: A Guide for Parents. Barbara H. Starfield & Frank A. Oski. 1999. (Pediatrics Ser.). (Illus.). pap. 2.95 (*1-885274-05-X*) Health InfoNet Inc.

Bed Wetting: Cause & Correction. Stanley M. Heston. 1987. 146p. text 29.95 (*0-9620473-0-9*); 2nd rev. ed. 1999. 226p. pap. 29.95 (*0-9620473-1-7*) Med Info Internatl.

Bedrest Before Baby: What's a Mother to Do? A Survival Handbook for High Risk Moms. Patricia D. Isennock. 1992. LC 92-80763. 104p. (Orig.). pap. 12.95 (*0-9632392-5-2*) Mustard Seed.

Bedside Approach to Clinical Neurology. Ed. by N. K. Gami. 1985. (C). (*0-89771-350-8*) Current Dist IND. *Dist:* St Mut.

Bedside Assessment of Swallowing Safety: The Clinician's Software User's Guide. T. Neil McKaig & Jim Thibodeau. 1997. 44p. pap. 59.99 incl. disk (*0-7506-7004-5*, RC815) Buttrwrth-Heinemann.

Bedside Cardiac Diagnosis. Henry J. L. Marriott. 1992. (Illus.). 320p. text 59.95 (*0-397-51085-3*) Lppncott W & W.

Bedside Cardiology. Contrib. by Jules Constant. 5th ed. 1999. LC 99-21282. (Illus.). ix, 342p. pap. text 59.95 (*0-7817-2168-7*) Lppncott W & W.

Bedside Critical Care Manual. Edward D. Chan. 1997. LC 97-31328. 29.95 (*1-56053-216-5*) Hanley & Belfus.

Bedside Diagnosis: An Annotated Bibliography of Literature on Physical Examination & Interviewing. Ed. by Henry Schneiderman & Aldo J. Peixoto. 3rd ed. 1997. LC 96-29487. 203p. (C). pap. text 27.00 (*0-943126-55-X*) Amer Coll Phys.

Bedside Logic in Diagnostic Gastroenterology. James Christensen. 1987. (Illus.). 174p. (Orig.). (C). pap. text (*0-443-08518-8*) Church.

Bedside Manner: Hospital & Health Care in Hong Kong. Robin Hutcheon. 1998. 260p. pap. (*962-201-798-3*) Chinese Univ HKG. *Dist:* U of Mich Pr.

Bedside Manners: An Anthology of Medical Wit & Wisdom. John Ballantyne. 1998. 266p. pap. text 16.00 (*0-7881-5650-0*) DIANE Pub.

Bedsides Approach to Clinical Neurology. G. Gami. 1985. (C). (*0-7855-4663-4*) Current Dist IND. *Dist:* St Mut.

Bedwetting: A Guide for Parents & Children. Arthur C. Houts & Robert M. Liebert. 1984. (Illus.). 110p. pap. 25.95 (*0-398-05074-0*) C C Thomas.

Bedwetting: A Treatment Manual for Professional Staff. J. Bollard & T. Nettelbeck. 1990. (Illus.). 208p. pap. 37.95 (*0-412-32520-9*, A4457) Chapman & Hall.

Bee in Balance: A Guide to Healing the Whole Person with Honeybees, Oriental Medicine & Common Sense. Amber Rose. Ed. by Alan Dumoff. 1994. (Illus.). 320p. (Orig.). pap. 34.95 (*0-9641810-0-2*) Starpoint Ent.

Bee Pollen & Your Health. Carlson Wade. 1978. LC 78-19928. (Pivot Original Health Bks.). 120p. pap. text 4.95 (*0-87983-184-7*, 31847K, Keats Pubng) McGraw-Hill Trade.

Bee Well Bee Wise: With Bee Pollen, Bee Propolis, Royal Jelly. Bernard Jensen. 1994. (Dr. Jensen's Health Handbooks Ser.: Vol. 5). (Illus.). 128p. pap. text 12.99 (*0-932615-30-9*, P-0295) B Jensen.

Before & After: Orthopedic Photography, Vol. 2. Horst Rieck. 1999. (Illus.). 120p. (*3-929078-87-2*) Kehayoff Verlag DEU. *Dist:* Prestel Pub NY.

Before & After: Spoliation of Evidence in Medical Negligence Litigation. Elliott B. Oppenheim. 5th ed. 1996. 200p. 180.00 (*1-930263-03-1*) Terra Firma NM.

Before Birth: Prenatal Testing for Genetic Disease. Elena O. Nightingale & Melissa Goodman. 1990. (Illus.). 128p. 31.00 (*0-674-06390-2*); pap. text 12.50 (*0-674-06391-0*) HUP.

***Before Birth: Understanding Prenatal Screening.** Ed. by Elizabeth Ettorre. 2001. 202p. text (*0-7546-1621-5*) Ashgate Pub GBR. *Dist:* Ashgate Pub Co.

Before Calling the Doctor. Phyllis Speight. 1976. (C). pap. 6.95 (*0-8464-0994-1*) Beekman Pubs.

Before Calling the Doctor. Phyllis Speight. 1976. 104p. pap. (*0-85032-137-9*) C W Daniel GBR. *Dist:* Natl Bk Netwk.

Before Freud: Neurasthenia & the American Medical Community, 1870-1910. F. G. Gosling. 1988. LC 87-6038. (Illus.). 214p. text 29.95 (*0-252-01406-5*) U of Ill Pr.

Before I Was I: Psychoanalysis & the Imagination. Ed. by Juliet Mitchell & Michael Parsons. 1998. 256p. reprint ed. 35.00 (*1-892746-10-7*) Other Pr LLC.

Before the Change: Taking Charge of Your Perimenopause. Ann L. Gittleman. LC 97-32146. 1999. (Illus.). 272p. pap. 14.00 (*0-06-251537-3*); 1998. 256p. 22.00 (*0-06-251539-X*) Harper SF.

Before the Change: Taking Charge of Your Perimenopause. Ann Louise Gittleman. 2000. 252p. reprint ed. text 22.00 (*0-7881-6811-8*) DIANE Pub.

Before Their Time: Adult Children's Experiences of Parental Suicide. Ed. by Mary Stimming & Maureen Stimming. 1999. LC 98-8173. 240p. pap. text 18.95 (*1-56639-655-7*) Temple U Pr.

Before Their Time: Fetuses & Infants at Risk. Libby G. Cohen. 1990. pap. 18.00 (*0-940898-26-8*) Am Assn Mental.

Before We Are Born: Essentials of Embryology & Birth Defects. Keith L. Moore & T. V. Persaud. Ed. by William Schmitt. 5th ed. 1998. LC 97-50318. (Illus.). 543p. (C). pap. text 40.00 (*0-7216-7377-5*) Saunders.

Before You Conceive: The Complete Pregnancy Guide. John R. Sussman & B. Blake Levitt. 1989. 464p. pap. 15.95 (*0-553-34718-7*) Bantam.

Before You See Your First Client: 55 Things Counselors & Human Service Providers Need to Know. Howard Rosenthal. 1998. LC 99-166422. 176p. pap. 15.95 (*1-55691-134-3*) Learning Pubns.

Beginner's Guide to Blood Cells. Barbara J. Bain. 1996. LC 95-53136. (Illus.). 120p. (Orig.). pap. 38.95 (*0-86542-717-8*) Blackwell Sci.

Beginner's Guide to Quantum Psychology. Stephen H. Wolinsky. 2000. pap. 14.95 (*0-9670362-3-2*) Quantum Inst Inc.

Beginner's Introduction to Ayurvedic Medicine. Vivek Shanbhag. 1994. 50p. (Orig.). pap. 3.95 (*0-87983-604-0*, 36040K, Keats Pubng) McGraw-Hill Trade.

Beginners Introduction to Homeopathy: Good Health Guide. Trevor Cook. 1987. 31p. pap. 3.95 (*0-87983-394-7*, 33947K, Keats Pubng) McGraw-Hill Trade.

Beginner's Introduction to Trace Minerals. Erwin DiCyan. Ed. by Richard A. Passwater & Earl R. Mindell. 1984. (Good Health Guides). 32p. pap. 3.95 (*0-87983-362-9*, 33629K, Keats Pubng) McGraw-Hill Trade.

Beginning an Academic Medical Career: Research, Writing, Speaking. Reginald C. Tsang & William Oh. 1993. LC 92-74264. (Illus.). 90p. 9.95 (*1-56053-064-2*) Hanley & Belfus.

Beginning Behavioral Research: A Conceptual Primer. Ralph L. Rosnow & Robert Rosenthal. 3rd ed. 1998. LC 98-20614. 475p. 86.00 (*0-13-791542-X*) P-H.

Beginning Bioethics: A Text with Integrated Readings. Ridley. 1997. LC 97-65376. 352p. pap. text 31.95 (*0-312-13291-3*) St Martin.

Beginning Child Psychiatry. Paul L. Adams & Ivan Fras. 1988. LC 87-32587. 624p. text 60.95 (*0-87630-493-5*) Brunner-Routledge.

Beginning Curricula A, B & Affixes Used in Signing Exact English. Gerilee Gustason. 1983. 124p. (Orig.). pap. text, stu. ed. 12.95 (*0-916708-09-8*) Modern Signs.

Beginning Life. Geraldine Lux Flanagan. 1996. LC 95-52790. (Illus.). 120p. 19.95 (*0-7894-0609-8*) DK Pub Inc.

Beginning Manual for Psychotherapists. Ernest Kramer. 2nd ed. 1978. LC 78-13510. 176p. text 32.95 (*0-8089-1120-1*, 792382, Grune & Strat) Harcrt Hlth Sci Grp.

Beginning of the School of Medicine at East Carolina University - 1964-1977, Vol. 1. Wayne C. Williams. 1998. LC 97-73944. 370p. 35.00 (*0-9626185-1-9*) Brookcliff Pubs.

Beginning with Awareness. Verena Tsuchudin. 1991. (Illus.). 164p. (*0-443-04290-X*); 132p. stu. ed. (*0-443-04292-6*) Church.

Beginning with Empathy. Tschudin. 1989. text 144.00 (*0-443-04244-6*) Saunders.

Beginning with the Handicapped. Verna Hart. 1978. (Illus.). 140p. spiral bd. 27.95 (*0-398-03179-7*) C C Thomas.

Beginnings: Egypt & Assyria. Warren R. Dawson. LC 75-23650. (Clio Medica Ser.: No. 1). reprint ed. 29.50 (*0-404-58901-4*) AMS Pr.

***Beginnings: Pregnancy, Birth & Beyond.** 2001. (Illus.). 242p. 29.95 (*1-931876-03-7*) Allina Health Pr.

Beginnings Count: American Values, Medical Technology & Health Care Policy. David J. Rothman. 1997. LC 96-46368. 208p. (C). text 24.95 (*0-19-511118-4*) OUP.

Beginnings of American Psychiatric Thought & Practice: Five Accounts, 1811-1830. 1978. LC 73-2384. (Mental Illness & Social Policy; the American Experience Ser.). 21.95 (*0-405-05192-1*) Ayer.

Beginnings of Cancer in the Cell: An Interdisciplinary Approach. Janos Ladik & Wolfgang Forner. 1994. LC 94-21255. (Illus.). 194p. 59.95 (*0-387-57962-1*) Spr-Verlag.

AB

Beginnings of Mental Hygiene in America: Three Selected Essays, 1833-1850. Amariah Brigham et al. 1973. (Mental Illness & Social Policy; the American Experience Ser.). 35.95 (*0-405-05193-X*) Ayer.

Behandlung von Herzrhythmusstoerungen bei Nierenkranken. J. Braun et al. 1984. (Illus.). viii, 248p. pap. 43.50 (*3-8055-3917-7*) S Karger.

Behandlungsprinzipien in der Rheumatologie. Ed. by G. Kaganas et al. 1979. (Fortbildungskurse fuer Rheumatologie Ser.: Vol. 5). (Illus.). 42.75 (*3-8055-2695-4*) S Karger.

Behaving Badly: Aversive Behaviors in Interpersonal Relationships. Ed. by Robin M. Kowalski. 2000. LC 00-41611. xiii, 333p. 49.95 (*1-55798-716-5*, 431-759A) Am Psychol.

Behavior: An Introduction to Psychology As a Biological Science. Geoffrey Hall. 1984. text 55.00 (*0-12-319580-2*) Acad Pr.

Behavior: The Control of Perception. William T. Powers. 1973. LC 73-75697. 309p. lib. bdg. 45.95 (*0-202-25113-6*) Aldine de Gruyter.

Behavior Analysis & Learning. W. David Pierce & W. Frank Epling. 2nd ed. 1998. LC 98-10083. 444p. (C). 68.00 (*0-13-080743-5*) P-H.

Behavior Analysis & Therapy in Nursing Homes. Duane A. Lundervold & Lewis M. Lewin. 1992. (Illus.). 178p. (C). text 49.95 (*0-398-05807-5*) C C Thomas.

Behavior Analysis & Treatment. Ed. by R. Van Houten & Saul Axelrod. 1993. (Applied Clinical Psychology Ser.). (Illus.). 406p. (C). 80.00 (*0-306-44371-6*, Plenum Trade) Perseus Pubng.

Behavior Analysis in Developmental Disabilities. Ed. by Brian A. Iwata. 3rd ed. 1997. (Illus.). 900p. (C). pap. 35.00 (*1-882018-03-6*) Jrnl Applied Behavior Analysis.

Behavior Analysis of Child Development. Sidney W. Bijou. 3rd ed. 1993. 160p. (C). pap. text 19.95 (*1-878978-03-9*) Context Pr.

Behavior Analysis of Language & Cognition: The Fourth International Institute on Verbal Relations. Ed. by Steven C. Hayes et al. 1994. (International Institute on Verbal Relations Ser.). (Illus.). 320p. (C). text 46.95 (*1-878978-18-7*) Context Pr.

Behavior Analytic View of Child Development. Henry D. Schlinger, Jr. 1995. LC 95-23848. (Applied Clinical Psychology Ser.). (Illus.). 280p. (C). 51.00 (*0-306-45059-3*, Plenum Trade) Perseus Pubng.

Behavior & Adaptation in Late Life. Ewald W. Busse & Eric Pfeiffer. 2nd ed. 1977. 24.50 (*0-316-11833-8*); pap. 18.50 (*0-316-11834-6*) Lppncott W & W (Little Brwn Med Div).

Behavior & Environment: Psychological & Geographical Approaches. Ed. by Tommy Garling & Reginald G. Golledge. 1993. LC 92-44318. (Advances in Psychology Ser.: Vol. 96). 484p. 153.00 (*0-444-89698-8*, North Holland) Elsevier.

Behavior & Evolution. Ed. by M. Hall et al. 1998. LC 98-36072. 314p. pap. 39.95 (*3-540-64752-X*) Spr-Verlag.

Behavior & Immunity. Alan J. Husband. 1991. 240p. 99.95 (*0-8493-0199-8*, QP56) CRC Pr.

Behavior & Its Causes: Philosophical Foundations of Operant Psychology. Terry L. Smith. 1994. LC 94-10400. (Studies in Cognitive Systems). 292p. (C). lib. bdg. (*0-7923-2815-9*) Kluwer Academic NLD. *Dist:* Kluwer Academic.

Behavior & Mood Disorders in Focal Brain Lesions. Ed. by Julien Bogousslavsky & Jeffrey L. Cummings. 2000. LC 99-46508. (*0-521-62342-1*) Cambridge U Pr.

Behavior Belongs in the Brain: Neuro Behavioral Syndromes. Ed. by Pasquale J. Accardo et al. 1997. LC 96-54476. (Illus.). (C). text 30.50 (*0-912752-41-6*) York Pr.

Behavior, Bias, & Handicaps: Labeling the Emotionally Disturbed Child. Judy Kugelmass. 1987. 260p. text 49.95 (*0-88738-114-6*) Transaction Pubs.

Behavior Change & Public Health in the Developing World. John P. Elder. 2000. LC 00-9852. (Behavioral Medicine & Health Psychology Ser.). (Illus.). xviii, 171p. pap. 29.95 (*0-7619-1779-9*, 83334) Sage.

Behavior Changes Resulting from a Study of Communicable Diseases: An Evaluation of the Effects of Learning on Certain Actions of High School Pupils. John Urban. LC 75-177687. (Columbia University. Teachers College. Contributions to Education Ser.: No. 896). reprint ed. 37.50 (*0-404-55896-8*) AMS Pr.

Behavior Cycle As a Framework for Dynamic Psychotherapy. Joseph Jacob. 1996. 312p. (C). text 29.95 (*0-89876-217-0*) Gardner Pr.

Behavior Description Interview. D. Janz. 1985. text 56.00 (*0-205-08597-0*) Allyn.

Behavior Development in Infants: A Survey of the Literature on Prenatal & Postnatal Activity 1920-1932. Evelyn Dewey. 1973. LC 72-343. (Body Movement Perspectives in Research Ser.). 334p. reprint ed. 26.95 (*0-405-03142-4*) Ayer.

Behavior Disorders of Adolescence: Research, Intervention, & Policy in Clinical & School Settings. Ed. by Robert J. McMahon & R. D. Peters. 1991. LC 91-1957. (Illus.). 242p. (C). 90.00 (*0-306-43813-5*, Plenum Trade) Perseus Pubng.

Behavior Disorders of Children & Adolescents: Assessment, Etiology, & Intervention. Marilyn T. Erickson. 3rd ed. 1997. LC 97-19787. 366p. (C). 87.00 (*0-13-649187-1*) P-H.

Behavior Genetic Approaches in Behavioral Medicine. Ed. by John K. Hewitt et al. 1995. LC 95-19341. (Perspectives on Individual Differences Ser.). (Illus.). 255p. (C). text 54.50 (*0-306-44969-2*, Kluwer Plenum) Kluwer Academic.

Behavior Guide. Stephen Rollnick. 11th ed. Date not set. 225p. (C). pap. text (*0-443-05850-4*) Church.

Behavior in Public Places: Notes on the Social Organization of Gatherings. Erving Goffman. 1966. LC 62-11850. 248p. pap. 17.95 (*0-02-911940-5*) Free Pr.

Behavior Modeling Training: Principles & Applications. Phillip J. Decker & Barry R. Nathan. 1985. LC 84-18155. 256p. 65.00 (*0-275-90084-3*, C0084, Praeger Pubs) Greenwood.

Behavior Modification: Behavioral Approaches to Human Problems. William H. Redd et al. 1978. text (*0-394-32134-0*) Random.

Behavior Modification: Contributions to Education. Ed. by Sidney W. Bijou & Roberto Ruiz. 1981. LC 80-278780. 352p. text 69.95 (*0-89859-051-5*) L Erlbaum Assocs.

Behavior Modification: Principles & Clinical Applications. Ed. by W. Stewart Agras. 2nd ed. 1978. 307p. 20.00 (*0-316-02031-1*, Little Brwn Med Div) Lppncott W & W.

Behavior Modification: Principles & Procedures. Raymond G. Miltenberger. 2nd ed. 2000. (Psychology Ser.). 608p. pap. text 72.95 (*0-534-36599-X*) Brooks-Cole.

Behavior Modification: The Scientific Way to Self Control. William C. Budd. 1973. LC 73-79774. 10.95 (*0-87212-027-9*) Libra.

Behavior Modification & the Child: An Annotated Bibliography, 3. Hazel B. Benson. 1979. LC 79-7358. (Contemporary Problems of Childhood Ser.: No. 3). 398p. lib. bdg. 80.00 (*0-313-21489-1*, BBM/, Greenwood Pr) Greenwood.

Behavior Modification & What It Is & How to Do It. Garry L. Martin & Joseph Pear. 3rd ed. 1988. (Illus.). 576p. pap. text 42.33 (*0-13-072315-0*) P-H.

Behavior Modification for Exceptional Children & Youth. Marcia D. Smith. 1993. LC 94-40045. 296p. text 37.00 (*1-56372-042-6*, 6940) PRO-ED.

Behavior Modification in Applied Settings. Alan E. Kazdin. 4th ed. 1989. 382p. (C). mass mkt. 29.00 (*0-534-11116-5*) Brooks-Cole.

Behavior Modification in Black Populations: Psychosocial Issues & Empirical Findings. Ed. by Samuel M. Turner & Russell T. Jones. 1982. LC 82-3746. 348p. 54.50 (*0-306-40867-8*, Plenum Trade) Perseus Pubng.

Behavior Modification in Business & Industry: A Selected Bibliography. Dolores Rescigno. 1984. (CPL Bibliographies Ser.: No. 140). 58p. 10.00 (*0-86602-140-X*, Sage Prdcls Pr) Sage.

Behavior Modification in Children & Adolescents: Dissertation for Ph.D. Degree. Geoffrey Wuzor. 1997. (Illus.). 252p. 29.00 (*0-9647631-1-7*) G O Wuzor.

Behavior Modification in the Human Services: A Systematic Introduction to Concepts & Applications. Sandra S. Sundel & Martin Sundel. 3rd ed. 1993. (Illus.). 428p. (C). 86.95 (*0-8039-3415-7*, 7155); pap. 46.95 (*0-8039-3416-5*, 7156, Sage Prdcls Pr) Sage.

Behavior Neurology. Orrin Devinsky. 1992. LC 92-49804. (One Hundred Maxims in Neurology Ser.). 35.95 (*0-8016-7280-5*) Mosby Inc.

Behavior of Adolescents: Health, Risks, Violence & Sex: Index of New Information. Vincent M. De La Fuente. 1998. 57.50 (*0-7883-1816-0*); pap. 47.50 (*0-7883-1817-9*) ABBE Pubs Assn.

Behavior of Industrial Work Groups: Prediction & Control. Leonard R. Sayles. Ed. by Leon Stein. 1977. LC 77-70530. reprint ed. lib. bdg. 19.95 (*0-405-10198-8*) Ayer.

Behavior of Marine Animals Vol. 4: Marine Birds. Ed. by Howard E. Winn et al. 1980. LC 79-167675. 532p. 95.00 (*0-306-37574-5*, Plenum Trade) Perseus Pubng.

Behavior of Marine Animals Vol. 5: Shorebirds: Breeding, Behavior & Populations. J. Burger & B. L. Olla. 1984. LC 79-167675. (Illus.). 452p. (C). text 115.00 (*0-306-41590-9*, Kluwer Plenum) Kluwer Academic.

Behavior of the Fetus. Ed. by William P. Smotherman & Scott R. Robinson. 1990. (Telford Press Ser.). (Illus.). 300p. 70.00 (*0-936923-13-X*) Telford Pr.

Behavior Problems in Children: And Their Aftermath in Adult Age. Ines S. Bustamante. Ed. & Tr. by Carlos De Varona from ENG. 1988. (SPA.). 268p. (Orig.). pap. 9.95 (*0-9619497-0-8*) ISB Edns.

Behavior Problems in Preschool Children: Clinical & Developmental Issues. Susan B. Campbell. 1990. LC 89-16838. 270p. 34.50 (*0-89862-395-2*) Guilford Pubns.

Behavior Problems in Small Animals: Practical Advice for the Veterinary Team. Sarah Heath. 2001. (Illus.). 192p. pap. 37.50 (*0-7506-4052-9*) Buttrwrth-Heinemann.

Behavior Recovery. Bill Rogers. (*0-86431-155-9*); pap. (*0-86431-154-0*) Aust Council Educ Res AUS. *Dist:* Stylus Pub VA.

Behavior Settings: A Revision & Extension of Roger G. Barker's 'Ecological Psychology' Phil Schoggen. 1989. LC 88-38736. 435p. 61.00 (*0-8047-1543-2*) Stanford U Pr.

Behavior Therapy: A Clinical Introduction. Richard I. Lanyon & Barbara P. Lanyon. 1978. LC 77-83022. (Topics in Clinical Psychology Ser.: 7). pap. text (*0-201-04100-6*) Addison-Wesley.

Behavior Therapy: Beyond the Conditioning Framework. O. Fontaine. Ed. by P. Eelen. 1986. 261p. (Orig.). pap. (*90-6186-197-7*) Leuven Univ BEL. *Dist:* Coronet Bks.

Behavior Therapy & Beyond. Arnold A. Lazarus. 1996. LC 96-16611. (Master Work Ser.). 320p. pap. 50.00 (*1-56821-839-7*, RA1) Aronson.

Behavior Therapy for Dev. & Physically Disabled. Johnny L. Matson. Ed. by Michel Hersen & Vincent B. Hasselt. 49.00 (*0-12-343050-X*) Acad Pr.

Behavior Therapy in Primary Care: A Practical Guide. R. France & M. Robson. 1986. LC 86-70732. 236p. pap. text 16.95 (*0-914783-12-2*) Charles.

Behavior Therapy with Children & Adolescents: A Clinical Approach. Ed. by Michel Hersen & Vincent B. Van Hasselt. 1991. 588p. (C). reprint ed. lib. bdg. 69.50 (*0-89464-606-0*) Krieger.

Behavioral & Biochemical Issues in Substance Abuse. Ed. by Frank R. George et al. 1991. LC 90-5325. (Advances in Alcohol & Substance Abuse Ser.). 266p. text 49.95 (*1-56024-088-1*) Haworth Pr.

Behavioral & Developmental Pediatrics: A Handbook for Primary Care. Ed. by Steven Parker & Barry S. Zuckerman. 1995. LC 94-17875. 480p. pap. text 49.95 (*0-316-69090-2*) Lppncott W & W.

Behavioral & Developmental Pediatrics: A Handbook for Primary Care. Steven Parker & Barry S. Zuckerman. 2nd ed. 2002. pap. text 49.95 (*0-7817-1683-7*) Lppncott W & W.

Behavioral & Metabolic Aspects of Breastfeeding: International Trends. A. P. Simopoulos. Ed. by I. D. Desai et al. 1995. (World Review of Nutrition & Dietetics Ser.: Vol. 78). (Illus.). xviii, 196p. 198.25 (*3-8055-6102-4*) S Karger.

Behavioral & Psychological Approaches to Breathing Disorders. Ed. by Beverly H. Timmons & Ronald Ley. 1994. LC 93-44087. (Illus.). 350p. (C). text 55.00 (*0-306-44446-1*, Kluwer Plenum) Kluwer Academic.

Behavioral & Social Contexts of HIV Infection Risk in Lesbians & Other Women Who Have Sex with Women: A Special Issue of "Women's Health", Vol. 2, No. 2, 1996. Mayes. 1996. pap. 20.00 (*0-8058-9885-9*) L Erlbaum Assocs.

Behavioral & Social Science: Fifty Years of Discovery. National Research Council Staff. 1986. 312p. text 29.50 (*0-309-03588-0*) Natl Acad Pr.

Behavioral Approach to Assessment of Youth with Emotional/Behavioral Disorders: A Handbook for School-Based Practitioners. Ed. by Michael J. Breen & Craig R. Fiedler. 1996. LC 95-22355. 729p. (C). pap. text 44.00 (*0-89079-625-4*, 7312) PRO-ED.

Behavioral Approaches to Alcoholism. Ed. by G. Alan Marlatt & P. E. Nathan. 1978. LC 77-620035. (NIAAA-RUCAS Alcoholism Treatment Ser.: No. 2). pap. 6.00 (*0-911290-48-6*) Rutgers Ctr Alcohol.

Behavioral Approaches to Brain Research. Terry E. Robinson. 1983. (Illus.). 352p. text 40.00 (*0-19-503258-6*) OUP.

Behavioral Approaches to Medical Treatment. Ed. by Redford B. Williams & W. Doyle Gentry. 1977. LC 76-30327. 288p. (C). 25.00 (*0-88410-136-3*, HarpBusn) HarpInfo.

Behavioral Approaches to Pattern Recognition & Concept Formation: Quantitative Analyses of Behavior, Vol. 8. Michael L. Commons et al. 1990. 240p. 69.95 (*0-8058-0398-X*) L Erlbaum Assocs.

Behavioral Aspects of AIDS. D. G. Ostrow. 1990. LC 90-7242. (Illus.). 430p. (C). 78.00 (*0-306-43452-0*, Plenum Trade) Perseus Pubng.

Behavioral Aspects of Cardiovascular Disease. Ed. by Andrew Baum & Alvin P. Shapiro. 1991. 368p. text 59.95 (*0-8058-0771-3*) L Erlbaum Assocs.

Behavioral Aspects of Neuroendocrinology. Ed. by D. Ganten & D. W. Pfaff. 1990. (Current Topics in Neuroendocrinology Ser.: Vol. 10). (Illus.). 295p. 131.00 (*0-387-52801-6*) Spr-Verlag.

Behavioral Aspects of Pediatric Burns. Ed. by K. J. Tarnowski. 1994. LC 94-30884. (Issues in Clinical Child Psychology Ser.). (Illus.). 302p. (C). 45.00 (*0-306-44840-8*, Plenum Trade) Perseus Pubng.

Behavioral Assessment: A Practical Handbook. Ed. by Michel Hersen & Alan S. Bellack. 1981. text 61.00 (*0-08-025956-1*); pap. text 21.00 (*0-08-025955-3*) Elsevier.

Behavioral Assessment: A Practical Handbook. Alan S. Bellack & Michael Hersen. 3rd ed. 1988. (General Psychology Ser.). 650p. text 70.00 (*0-08-032796-6*); pap. text 28.50 (*0-08-032795-8*) Elsevier (Pergamon Pr).

Behavioral Assessment & Management of Cardiovascular Disorders. Ed. by David S. Krantz & James A. Blumenthal. 1987. LC 87-42554. 192p. 24.45 (*0-943158-20-6*, BACBP, Prof Resc Pr) Pro Resource.

Behavioral Assessment & Rehabilitation of the Traumatically Brain Damaged. B. A. Edelstein & E. T. Couture. 1984. LC 83-22973. (Applied Clinical Psychology Ser.). (Illus.). 364p. (C). 80.00 (*0-306-41295-0*, Plenum Trade) Perseus Pubng.

Behavioral Assessment in School Psychology. Edward S. Shapiro. 1987. (School Psychology Ser.). 272p. text 59.95 (*0-89859-881-8*) L Erlbaum Assocs.

Behavioral Assessment in Schools: Conceptual Foundations & Practical Applications. Ed. by Edward S. Shapiro & Thomas R. Kratochwill. 1988. LC 87-11966. 555p. text 65.00 (*0-89862-711-7*, 2711) Guilford Pubns.

Behavioral Assessment of Childhood Disorders. Ed. by Eric J. Mash & Leif G. Terdal. 2nd ed. 1988. LC 88-26928. (Guilford Behavioral Assessment Ser.). 824p. text 85.00 (*0-89862-143-7*) Guilford Pubns.

Behavioral Assessment of Childhood Disorders: Selected Core Problems. Ed. by Eric J. Mash & Leif G. Terdal. 2nd ed. 1988. LC 88-24684. (Guilford Behavioral Assessment Ser.). 456p. (C). pap. 35.00 (*0-89862-512-2*) Guilford Pubns.

Behavioral Audiologic Evaluation of Infants & Young Children. Jane R. Madell. 1998. pap. 69.00 (*0-86577-804-3*); LC 98-4647. (Illus.). 300p. pap. 39.00 (*0-86577-692-X*) Thieme Med Pubs.

Behavioral Biology: Neuroendocrine Axis. Ed. by Trevor Archer & Stefan Hansen. 1991. 288p. text 69.95 (*0-8058-0790-X*) L Erlbaum Assocs.

***Behavioral Care Informatics.** Ed. by Naakesh A. Dewan et al. 2001. LC 2001-20192. (Health Informatics Ser.). (Illus.). 184p. 55.00 (*0-387-95265-9*, Copernicus) Spr-Verlag.

Behavioral Case Formulation. Ed. by Ira D. Turkat. 1985. LC 85-24463. (Illus.). 338p. (C). 84.00 (*0-306-42047-3*, Plenum Trade) Perseus Pubng.

Behavioral Cognitive Stuttering Therapy & Audiotape. Stanley A. Goldberg. 1981. 240p. spiral bd. 60.00 incl. audio (*1-56593-603-5*, 1238) Singular Publishing.

Behavioral Community Psychology: Progress & Prospects. Ed. by David Glenwick & Leonard Jason. 1980. LC 79-21457. 501p. 44.95 (*0-275-90488-1*, C0488, Praeger Pubs) Greenwood.

Behavioral Complications in Alzheimer's Disease. Ed. by Brian A. Lawlor. 1995. (Clinical Practice Ser.: No. 31). 272p. text 38.50 (*0-88048-477-2*, 8477) Am Psychiatric.

Behavioral Consequences of Antihypertensive Drugs. Jeffrey W. Elias et al. 1993. (*0-89116-058-2*) Hemisp Pub.

Behavioral Consultation & Therapy. J. R. Bergan & Thomas R. Kratochwill. 1989. (Applied Clinical Psychology Ser.). (Illus.). 526p. (C). 85.00 (*0-306-43345-1*, Plen Insight) Perseus Pubng.

Behavioral Consultation in Applied Settings: An Individual Guide. Thomas R. Kratochwill & J. R. Bergan. 1989. (Applied Clinical Psychology Ser.). (Illus.). 192p. (C). pap. 24.50 (*0-306-43346-X*, Plen Insight) Perseus Pubng.

Behavioral Counseling Model for Injection Drug Users, Intervention Manual. 1994. lib. bdg. 250.00 (*0-8490-8605-1*) Gordon Pr.

Behavioral Development: Concepts of Approach - Withdrawal & Integrative Levels. Ed. by Kathryn E. Hood et al. 1995. LC 94-24356. (Research in Developmental & Comparative Psychology Ser.: Vol. 1). 496p. text 87.00 (*0-8153-1709-3*, SS677) Garland.

Behavioral Development of Human Fetus & Neonates: Japanese Studies - Journal: Biology of the Neonate, Vol. 60, Suppl. 1, 1991. Ed. by N. Kobayashy & M. Ibuka. 1991. (Illus.). iv, 96p. pap. 30.50 (*3-8055-5454-0*) S Karger.

Behavioral Disease Management: Planning, Delivering, & Promoting a Successful Disease Management System. Ed. by Patrick E. Vega. 1999. 120p. pap. 137.00 (*1-884937-58-6*) Manisses Communs.

Behavioral Disorders: Understanding Clinical Psychopathology. Igor Grant. 1979. LC 78-15309. (Illus.). 318p. text 27.50 (*0-88331-114-3*) R B Luce.

Behavioral Disorders in Infants, Children, & Adolescents. Ed. by John Reisman. 1986. 416p. text 36.00 (*0-89859-887-7*) L Erlbaum Assocs.

Behavioral Effects of Nicotine: Proceedings of the International Workshop, Zurich, September 15-17, 1976. Ed. by K. Baettig. 1978. (Illus.). 42.75 (*3-8055-2763-2*) S Karger.

Behavioral Emergencies: A Field Guide for EMT's & Paramedics. Ellen L. Bassuk et al. 1983. tchr. ed. (*0-316-08331-3*, Little Brwn Med Div); pap. text 16.00 (*0-316-08330-5*) Lppncott W & W.

Behavioral Endocrinology. Ed. by Jill B. Becker et al. 1992. (Illus.). 688p. pap. 52.95 (*0-262-52171-7*, Bradford Bks) MIT Pr.

Behavioral Evolution & Integrative Levels. Ed. by Gary Greenberg & Ethel Tobach. 1984. (T. C. Schneirla Conference Ser.: Vol. 1). 320p. (C). text 89.95 (*0-89859-363-8*) L Erlbaum Assocs.

Behavioral Expression & Biosocial Bases of Sensation Seeking. Marvin Zuckerman. 1994. LC 93-40276. (Illus.). 479p. (C). text 90.00 (*0-521-43200-6*); pap. text 32.95 (*0-521-43770-9*) Cambridge U Pr.

Behavioral Family Intervention. M. R. Dadds & Matthew R. Sanders. 1991. (Psychology Practitioner Guidebooks Ser.). 192p. text (*0-08-037917-6*); pap. text (*0-08-037916-8*) PPI GBR. *Dist:* Elsevier.

Behavioral Family Therapy. Ed. by Bruce A. Thyer. 1989. (Illus.). 266p. text 60.95 (*0-398-05561-0*) C C Thomas.

Behavioral Family Therapy for Psychiatric Disorders. Kim T. Mueser & Shirley M. Glynn. 2nd ed. 1999. LC 98-68758. 399p. 49.95 (*1-57224-143-8*) New Harbinger.

Behavioral Foundations of Community Emergency Response Planning. Ronald W. Perry & Michael K. Lindell. 1992. (Illus.). 630p. 99.95 (*0-89116-620-3*) Hemisp Pub.

Behavioral Genetics: The Clash of Culture & Biology. Ronald A. Carson & Mark A. Rothstein. 1999. LC 98-43307. 224p. 44.95 (*0-8018-6069-5*) Johns Hopkins.

Behavioral Healthcare Quality & Accountability Tool Kit, Version I. Allen Daniels et al. 1997. 745.00 (*1-887452-14-1*) Manisses Communs.

Behavioral High-Risk Paradigm in Psychopathology. Ed. by Gregory A. Miller. 1995. LC 95-6678. (Series in Psychopathology). (Illus.). 303p. 137.00 (*0-387-94504-0*) Spr-Verlag.

Behavioral Intervention Techniques in Drug Abuse Treatment. 1986. lib. bdg. 79.95 (*0-8490-3521-X*) Gordon Pr.

Behavioral Interventions with Brain-Injured Children. A. MacNeill Horton, Jr. 1993. LC 93-41064. (Critical Issues in Neuropsychology Ser.). (Illus.). 230p. (C). 36.00 (*0-306-44438-0*, Plenum Trade) Perseus Pubng.

Behavioral Issues in Autism. Ed. by Eric Schopler & Gary B. Mesibov. 1994. (Current Issues in Autism Ser.). (Illus.). 314p. (C). 47.50 (*0-306-44600-6*, Plenum Trade) Perseus Pubng.

Behavioral Managed Care: Strategies for Integrating Behavioral Health Services. M. J. Werthman. 1997. LC 96-51529. 192p. text 45.00 (*0-7863-1092-8*, Irwn Prfssnl) McGraw-Hill Educ Grp.

*__Behavioral Management Guide: Essential Treatment Strategies for the Psychotherapy of Children, Their Parents & Families.__ Muriel Prince Warren. 2001. LC 2001-45699. pap. 50.00 (*0-7657-0354-8*) Aronson.

Behavioral Management of Stuttering. Mark Onslow. 1995. (Illus.). 232p. (C). reprint ed. pap. 45.00 (*1-56593-633-7*, 1312) Thomson Learn.

Behavioral Management of the Cardiac Patient. D. G. Byrne. Ed. by Glenn R. Caddy. 1987. LC 87-1324. (Developments in Clinical Psychology Ser.: Vol. 7). 224p. 77.00 (*0-89391-386-3*, Ablex) Greenwood.

Behavioral Measures of Neurotoxicity. National Research Council Staff. Ed. by Roger W. Russell et al. 1990. 452p. text 42.50 (*0-309-04047-7*) Natl Acad Pr.

Behavioral Mechanisms in Ecology. Douglass H. Morse. LC 80-12130. 391p. 1982. pap. 19.50 (*0-674-06461-5*); 1980. 48.50 (*0-674-06460-7*) HUP.

Behavioral Medicine. S. Araki. 1992. x382p. 164.50 (*0-444-89253-2*) Elsevier.

Behavioral Medicine: A Primary Care Approach. H. Russell Searight. 1998. LC 98-35106. 59.95 (*0-87630-981-3*); pap. 25.95 (*0-87630-982-1*) Brunner-Routledge.

Behavioral Medicine: Assessment & Treatment Strategies. Ed. by Daniel M. Doleys et al. 1982. LC 81-23376. 648p. (C). 90.00 (*0-306-40841-4*, Plenum Trade) Perseus Pubng.

Behavioral Medicine: Concepts & Procedures. E. Tunks & A. Bellissimo. 1991. (Psychology Practitioner Guidebooks Ser.). 272p. text (*0-08-036832-8*); pap. text (*0-08-036831-X*) PPI GBR. *Dist:* Elsevier.

Behavioral Medicine: Work, Stress & Health. Ed. by W. Doyle Gentry et al. 1986. (NATO Advanced Science Institutes Ser.). text 205.50 (*90-247-3264-6*) Kluwer Academic.

Behavioral Medicine Vol. 1: International Perspectives, 1. Don G. Byrne & Glenn R. Caddy. 1991. (Developments in Clinical Psychology Ser.). 430p. (C). 85.00 (*0-89391-620-X*, Ablex) Greenwood.

Behavioral Medicine Vol. 2: International Perspectives, 2. Don G. Byrne & Glenn R. Caddy. 1992. (Developments in Clinical Psychology Ser.). 432p. (C). 85.00 (*0-89391-680-3*, Ablex) Greenwood.

Behavioral Medicine Vol. 3: International Perspectives, 3. Paul R. Latimer et al. Ed. by Glenn R. Caddy et al. 1995. (Developments in Clinical Psychology Ser.: Vol. 3). (Illus.). 464p. (C). 85.00 (*0-89391-744-3*, Ablex) Greenwood.

Behavioral Medicine & Developmental Disabilities. Ed. by J. K. Luiselli. 1989. (Disorders of Human Learning, Behavior, & Communication Ser.). (Illus.). 242p. 82.95 (*0-387-96875-X*) Spr-Verlag.

Behavioral Medicine & Women: A Comprehensive Handbook. Ed. by Elaine A. Blechman & Kelly D. Brownell. 1997. LC 97-36130. 876p. 80.00 (*1-57230-218-6*, 0218) Guilford Pubns.

Behavioral Medicine Approaches to Cardiovascular Disease Prevention. Ed. by Kristina Orth-Gomer & Neil Schneiderman. 1995. LC 95-2986. 336p. text 69.95 (*0-8058-1820-0*) L Erlbaum Assocs.

Behavioral Medicine, Biofeedback, & Behavioral Approaches in Psychosomatic Medicine. Ed. by H. Leigh. 1982. (Journal: Vol. 36, No. 3-4, 1981). (Illus.). 122p. pap. 52.25 (*3-8055-3521-X*) S Karger.

Behavioral Medicine in Primary Care: A Practical Guide. W. Feldman. Ed. by John F. Christensen. 1998. 345p. (C). pap. 39.95 (*0-8385-0636-4*) McGraw-Hill Prof.

Behavioral Medicine Made Ridiculously Simple. Frank C. Seitz. 1997. LC 97-120731. (Orig.). pap. text 12.95 (*0-940780-29-1*) MedMaster.

Behavioral Medicine Treatment Planner. Arthur E. Jongsma, Jr. et al. 1999. LC 99-13574. (Practice Planners Ser.). 240p. pap. 44.95 (*0-471-31923-6*) Wiley.

Behavioral Medicine Treatment Planner. Arthur E. Jongsma, Jr. et al. 1999. LC 99-13574. (Practice Planners Ser.). 226p. pap. 175.00 incl. disk (*0-471-31926-0*) Wiley.

Behavioral Medicine with the Developmentally Disabled. D. C. Russo & J. H. Kedesdy. 1988. LC 88-17953. (Illus.). 308p. (C). 56.50 (*0-306-42884-9*, Plenum Trade) Perseus Pubng.

Behavioral Neurology. Jeffrey L. Cummings & Michael R. Trimble. 1996. 544p. text 95.00 (*0-7506-2360-8*) Buttrwrth-Heinemann.

Behavioral Neurology. Jonathan H. Pincus & Gary J. Tucker. 3rd ed. 1985. (Illus.). 320p. pap. text 21.95 (*0-19-503555-0*) OUP.

Behavioral Neurology: A Practical Approach. Howard S. Kirshner. 1985. (Clinical Neurology & Neurosurgery Monographs). (Illus.). 230p. text (*0-443-08410-6*) Church.

Behavioral Neurology & Neuropsychology. Ed. by Todd E. Feinberg & Martha Farah. 1996. (Illus.). 873p. text 79.00 (*0-07-020361-X*) McGraw-Hill Prof.

Behavioral Neurology & the Legacy of Norman Geschwind. Steven C. Schachter. 1996. LC 96-41088. 320p. text 129.00 (*0-397-51631-2*) Lppncott W & W.

*__Behavioral Neurology in the Elderly.__ Ed. by Jose Leon-Carrion & Margaret Joan Giannini. 2001. LC 2001-25749. (Illus.). 461p. 89.95 (*0-8493-2066-6*) CRC Pr.

*__Behavioral Neurology of White Matter.__ Christopher M. Filley. 2001. (Illus.). 304p. text 55.00 (*0-19-513561-X*) OUP.

Behavioral Neuroscience. Kolb & Whishaw. 2000. pap. text, stu. ed. 18.00 (*0-7167-5103-8*) W H Freeman.

Behavioral Objectives: Evaluation in Nursing. Dorothy E. Reilly & Marilyn H. Oermann. 3rd ed. 1990. 284p. pap. 27.95 (*0-88737-500-6*) Natl League Nurse.

Behavioral Observations in Cardiovascular Research. A. D. Appels. 1991. 130p. (*90-265-1036-5*) Swets.

Behavioral Pediatrics. Ed. by Donald E. Greydanus & Mark L. Wolraich. 1991. (Illus.). 471p. 139.00 (*0-387-97547-0*) Spr-Verlag.

Behavioral Pediatrics: Research & Practice. Dennis C. Russo et al. 1982. LC 82-3799. 432p. 65.00 (*0-306-40961-5*, Plenum Trade) Perseus Pubng.

Behavioral Pharmacology of 5-HT. P. Duphar et al. 1989. 528p. (C). text 89.95 (*0-8058-0135-9*) L Erlbaum Assocs.

Behavioral Phenotypes. Ed. by Gregory O'Brien & William Yule. 1996. (Clinics in Developmental Medicine Ser.: No. 138). 224p. (*1-898683-06-9*) Mc Keith Pr GBR. *Dist:* Cambridge U Pr.

Behavioral Primatology: Advances in Research & Theory, Vol. 1. Ed. by Allan M. Schrier. 1977. 208p. 39.95 (*0-89859-139-2*) L Erlbaum Assocs.

Behavioral Problems of Childhood. Ed. by Stewart Gabel. 1981. 464p. text 61.00 (*0-8089-1336-0*, 791475, Grune & Strat) Harcrt Hlth Sci Grp.

Behavioral Regulators of Behavior in Primates. Ed. by C. R. Carpenter. 1974. LC 72-3602. (Illus.). 303p. 40.00 (*0-8387-1099-9*) Bucknell U Pr.

Behavioral Relaxation Training & Assessment. R. Poppen. 1988. (General Psychology Ser.). 156p. text 28.00 (*0-08-035566-8*); pap. text 14.95 (*0-08-035565-X*) Elsevier (Pergamon Pr).

Behavioral Relaxation Training & Assessment. Roger Poppen. 2nd ed. 1998. LC 97-45278. 206p. 73.95 (*0-7619-1200-2*, 82069); pap. 36.95 (*0-7619-1201-0*, 82070) Sage.

Behavioral Risk Management: How to Avoid Preventable Losses from Mental Health Problems at Work. Rudy M. Yandrick. 1996. LC 95-26783. (Psychology Ser.). 410p. 47.00 (*0-7879-0220-9*) Jossey-Bass.

Behavioral Science. Sahler. 1999. pap. text (*0-7216-7093-8*) Harcourt.

Behavioral Science. Evan G. Pattishall. 8th ed. 1998. (Pretest Basic Sciences Ser.). (Illus.). 321p. pap. 24.95 (*0-07-052689-3*) McGraw-Hill Educ Grp.

Behavioral Science for Students. Frederick S. Sierles. 1993. (Illus.). 560p. 28.00 (*0-683-07730-9*) Lppncott W & W.

*__Behavioral Science for The Boards & Wards.__ Carlos Ayala. 2001. (Boards & Wards Ser.). (Illus.). 100p. pap. 14.95 (*0-632-04578-7*) Blackwell Sci.

Behavioral Science in Family Medicine. Compiled by STFM Task Force on Behavioral Science Staff. 1979. 118p. 5.00 (*0-942295-00-5*) Soc Tchrs Fam Med.

Behavioral Science in Family Medicine: A Program for Second & Third Year Family Medicine Residents Ser. Howard F. Stein. Ed. by Willam D. Grant. rev. ed. 1986. (Illus.). 94p. (C). pap. 15.00 (*0-9617230-1-7*) Univ Health Ctr.

Behavioral Science in HIV Prevention. Ed. by Anthony Robbins. 1996. (Illus.). 144p. (Orig.). (C). pap. text 35.00 (*0-7881-3721-2*) DIANE Pub.

Behavioral Science, 1996: Digging up the Bones, Vol. 5. Medical Review Staff. 1998. (Medical Review Ser.). (Illus.). 86p. pap. 19.95 (*0-07-038218-2*) McGraw-Hill Prof.

Behavioral Science Review. Sahler. 1999. pap. text (*0-7216-7095-4*) Harcourt.

Behavioral Science/Psychiatry: Review for New National Boards. Julia B. Frank. 1998. LC 97-70352. (Illus.). 229p. pap. text 25.00 (*1-888308-00-1*) J & S Pub VA.

Behavioral Sciences. Ronald S. Krug & Alvah R. Cass. (Oklahoma Notes). 1988. 271p. (C). 15.95 (*0-387-96333-2*); 2nd ed. 1991. 281p. 18.95 (*0-387-96967-5*) Spr-Verlag.

Behavioral Sciences. Robert E. Pieroni. 2nd ed. 1989. (Medical Examination Review Ser.). 248p. pap. 18.00 (*0-444-01049-1*) Elsevier.

Behavioral Sciences. Ronald S. Krug & Alvah R. Cass. 4th ed. 1995. LC 94-25309. (Oklahoma Notes). 311p. 24.95 (*0-387-94393-5*) Spr-Verlag.

Behavioral Sciences for Nurses. Jack Rudman. 1994. (College Level Examination Ser.: CLEP-39). pap. 27.95 (*0-8373-5339-4*) Nat Learn.

Behavioral Sciences in Psychiatry. Ed. by Jerry M. Wiener & Nancy Breslin. 3rd ed. 1996. LC 93-23682. (National Medical Series for Independent Study). (Illus.). 375p. pap. text 29.00 (*0-683-06203-4*) Lppncott W & W.

Behavioral Social Work: An Introduction. Barbara L. Hudson & Geraldine M. Macdonald. 1989. 289p. (C). reprint ed. pap. 28.95 (*0-534-11046-0*) Brooks-Cole.

Behavioral Social Work in Health Care Settings: Papers from the Seventh Doris Siegel Memorial Colloquium. Gary Rosenberg. 2000. LC 00-57553. (Illus.). xv, 112p. (*0-7890-1025-9*) Haworth Pr.

Behavioral Social Work in Health Care Settings: Papers from the Seventh Doris Siegel Memorial Colloquium. Gary Rosenberg & Andrew Weissman. 2000. LC 00-57553. (Illus.). xv, 112p. (*0-7890-1026-7*) Haworth Pr.

Behavioral Statistics. Richard B. Darlington. 1987. wbk. ed. 9.95 (*0-02-907861-X*) S&S Trade.

Behavioral Statistics: An Introduction. Sternberg. Date not set. (C). text 76.00 (*0-15-505203-9*) Harcourt Coll Pubs.

Behavioral Statistics: The Core. Richard P. Runyon et al. 1994. (C). pap., stu. ed. 25.00 (*0-07-054926-5*) McGraw.

Behavioral Statistics in Action. Mark V. Vernoy & Judith A. Vernoy. 2nd ed. 1996. LC 96-14983. (Psychology Ser.). 425p. (C). mass mkt. 89.95 (*0-534-23664-2*) Brooks-Cole.

Behavioral Statistics in Action. Mark W. Vernoy & Judith A. Vernoy. 2nd ed. 1996. (Psychology Ser.). (C). mass mkt., wbk. ed. 18.25 (*0-534-34281-7*) Brooks-Cole.

*__Behavioral Statistics in Action.__ Mark W. Vernoy. 3rd ed. 2001. LC 2001-18042. (*0-7674-2275-9*) Mayfield Pub.

Behavioral Systems. Robert L. Moraskey. 1982. LC 82-12334. 181p. 45.00 (*0-275-90863-1*, C0863, Praeger Pubs) Greenwood.

Behavioral Teratogenesis & Behavioral Mutagenesis: A Primer in Abnormal Development. Ernest L. Abel. 1989. (Illus.). 254p. (C). text 49.50 (*0-306-43053-3*, Kluwer Plenum) Kluwer Academic.

Behavioral Teratology: A Bibliography to the Study of Birth Defects of the Mind. Ernest L. Abel. 1985. LC 85-21946. 206p. lib. bdg. 62.50 (*0-313-25066-9*, ABT/, Greenwood Pr) Greenwood.

Behavioral Theories & Treatment of Anxiety. Ed. by Samuel M. Turner. 1984. 454p. 80.00 (*0-306-41593-3*, Plenum Trade) Perseus Pubng.

Behavioral Therapy for Rural Substance Abusers. Carl G. Leukefeld et al. 2000. LC 99-47768. (Illus.). 181p. (C). pap. 18.00 (*0-8131-0984-1*) U Pr of KY.

Behavioral Treatment for Asthma: Biofeedback-, Respondent-, & Relaxation-Based Approaches. Edward P. Sarafino. 1997. LC 97-28143. (Studies in Health & Human Services: Vol. 29). 100p. text 59.95 (*0-7734-8591-0*) E Mellen.

Behavioral Treatment for Persistent Insomnia. Patricia Lacks. 1987. (Psychology Practitioner Guidebooks). 192p. text 30.00 (*0-08-034318-X*); pap. text 15.95 (*0-08-034317-1*) Elsevier (Pergamon Pr).

Behavioral Treatments for Drug Abuse & Dependence. Ed. by Lisa S. Onken et al. 1995. (Illus.). 329p. (C). pap. text 35.00 (*0-7881-1871-4*) DIANE Pub.

Behavioral Treatments for Drug Abuse & Dependence, Set. 1994. lib. bdg. 350.00 (*0-8490-8606-X*) Gordon Pr.

Behavioral Types & the Art of Patient Management: Improving Quality of Care with Better Understanding of Physician-Patient Relationships. Stephen E. Prather et al. Ed. by Gregg Rogers. 1995. LC 95-16790. 212p. 44.95 (*1-57066-031-X*, ME018) Practice Mgmt Info.

Behaviorism. John E. Staddon. 1993. (Interpretations Ser.). 128p. pap. 14.95 (*0-7156-2488-1*) Focus Pub-R Pullins.

Behaviorism. John B. Watson. 1998. LC 97-27084. 262p. pap. text 21.95 (*1-56000-994-2*) Transaction Pubs.

Behaviorism & Phenomenology: Contrasting Bases for Modern Psychology. Ed. by T. W. Wann. 1993. LC 64-12257. pap. text 3.95 (*0-226-87283-1*, P192) U Ch Pr.

Behaviorism, Neobehaviorism & Cognitivism in Learning Theory: Historical & Contemporary Perspectives. Abram Amsel. 1988. 116p. 24.95 (*0-8058-0332-7*) L Erlbaum Assocs.

Behaviorism, Science, & Human Nature. Barry Schwartz & Hugh Lacey. 1982. (Illus.). 282p. (C). pap. text 19.00 (*0-393-95197-9*) Norton.

Behavioristic Study of the Activity of the Rat. Curt P. Richter. 1922. LC 24-2657. (Comparative Psychology Monographs: Vol. 1). pap. 40.00 (*0-527-24837-1*) Periodicals Srv.

Behaviors in Dementia: Best Practices for Successful Management. Ed. by Mary Kaplan & Stephanie B. Hoffman. 1998. LC 97-44288. 224p. pap. 29.95 (*1-878812-43-2*) Hlth Prof Pr.

Behaviour & Mind: Seven Pioneers of Psychology. Ed. by Ray Fuller. 1994. LC 94-9124. 176p. (C). (gr. 13). pap. 22.95 (*0-415-09980-3*, B3996) Routledge.

Behaviour & Pharmacology. 1977. (Modern Problems of Pharmacopsychiatry Ser.: Vol. 12). (Illus.). 41.00 (*3-8055-2691-1*) S Karger.

Behaviour Modification see Cognitive-Behavioural Therapy

Behaviour Problems in Horses. Susan McBane. 1987. (Illus.). 304p. 24.95 (*0-7153-8749-9*) Trafalgar.

Behaviour Problems in Mental Handicap: An Annotated Bibliography 1970-1985. Kenneth Day et al. 1988. 144p. (*0-902241-20-6*) Royal Coll Psych GBR. *Dist:* Parkwest Pubns.

Behaviour Studies in Psychiatry. S. J. Hutt & C. Hutt. 1970. (*0-08-015780-7*) Pergamon Repr GBR. *Dist:* Franklin.

Behavioural Models in Psychopharmacology: Theoretical, Industrial & Clinical Perspectives. Ed. by Paul Willner. 1991. (Illus.). 554p. (C). text 120.00 (*0-521-39192-X*) Cambridge U Pr.

Behavioural Sciences for Carers. 192p. pap. (*0-340-55436-3*) E A GBR. *Dist:* Routldge.

Behavioural Sciences for Dentistry. Gerry Humphris & Margaret S. Ling. 2000. LC 99-36939. (Illus.). ix, 149p. (*0-443-05190-9*) Church.

Behavioural Sciences for Health. Aitken. 1996. (C). pap. text 57.00 (*0-7020-1964-X*) Harcourt.

Behavioural Sciences for Nurses: Towards Project 2000. L. Fisher. 1992. pap. 14.95 (*0-7156-2336-2*) Focus Pub-R Pullins.

Behavioural Studies Related to Care of the Aged: Report on a WHO Working Group. 1982. (Euro Reports & Studies Ser.: No. 71). 39p. pap. text 4.00 (*92-890-1237-4*) World Health.

Behcet's Disease: A Guide to Its Clinical Understanding: Textbook & Atlas. Sungnack Lee et al. 2000. LC 00-30057. (Illus.). 221p. 150.00 (*3-540-66761-X*) Spr-Verlag.

Behcet's Disease: Basic & Clinical Aspects. Ed. by J. Desmond O'Duffy & Emre Kokmen. 1991. (Infectious Disease & Therapy Ser.: Vol. 8). (Illus.). 696p. text 275.00 (*0-8247-8476-6*) Dekker.

Behcet's Disease: Proceedings of the 6th International Conference on Behcet's Disease, Held in Paris, France, 30th June-1st July 1993. Ed. by Pierre Godeau & Bertrand Wechsler. 1993. LC 93-33060. (International Congress Ser.: No. 1037). 732p. 307.00 (*0-444-81615-1*, Excerpta Medica) Elsevier.

Behind Closed Doors: A Consumer's Guide to Psychiatric Hospitals. Sherer M. Murtiashaw. 1994. 128p. pap. text 9.95 (*0-9639267-9-9*) HRS.

Behind Closed Doors: Gender, Sexuality & Touch in the Doctor-Patient Relationship. Angelica Redleaf. 1998. LC 97-32947. 216p. 55.00 (*0-275-96146-X*, Praeger Pubs) Greenwood.

Behind Closed Doors: Gender, Sexuality & Touch in the Doctor/Patient Relationship. Susan Baird. 1998. LC 97-32947. 224p. 62.50 (*0-86569-285-8*, Auburn Hse) Greenwood.

Behind the Great Wall: A Post-Jungian Approach to Kafkaesque Literature. James Whitlark. 1992. LC 90-55830. 288p. 46.50 (*0-8386-3427-3*) Fairleigh Dickinson.

Behind the Masks: Personality Disorders in Religious Behavior. Wayne E. Oates. 1987. LC 87-8221. 140p. (Orig.). pap. 14.95 (*0-664-24028-3*) Westminster John Knox.

Behind the Playground Walls: Sexual Abuse in Preschools. Jill Waterman et al. 1993. LC 91-35420. 307p. 40.00 (*0-89862-523-8*, 2523) Guilford Pubns.

Behind the Poison Cloud: Union Carbide's Bhopal Massacre. Larry Everest. 1986. LC 85-26863. 192p. 21.95 (*0-916650-26-X*); pap. 8.95 (*0-916650-25-1*) Banner Pr Intl.

Behind the Screens: Nursing Somology & the Problem of the Body. Jocalyn Lawler. 1991. 264p. pap. (*0-443-04444-9*) Church.

Behind the Screens: Nursing, Somology, & the Problem of the Body. Jocalyn Lawler. 1993. LC 93-9933. (C). pap. text 24.50 (*0-8053-4090-4*) Benjamin-Cummings.

Behind the Therapists' Notes: Fears, Feelings & Hopes. Theodore C. Kent. 1993. LC 92-72426. 352p. pap. 12.95 (*0-87212-256-5*) Libra.

Behind the Wall of Respect: Experiments in Heroin Addiction Control in Chicago Neighborhoods. Patrick H. Hughes. 1997. LC 76-25640. 182p. 13.50 (*0-226-35930-1*) U Ch Pr.

Behinderte Kind. H. J. Roelli. Ed. by A. Anderhalden. 1982. (Paediatrische Fortbildungskurse fuer die Praxis Ser.: Vol. 56). (Illus.). vi, 110p. pap. 46.25 (*3-8055-3493-0*) S Karger.

Beilstein-Leitfaden: Eine Anleitung Zur Benutzung Von Beilsteins Handbuch der Organischen Chemie. Beilstein Institut fur Literatur der Organischen Chemie. 1975. 56p. 525.00 (*0-387-07431-7*) Spr-Verlag.

Being a Blessing: Fifty-Four Ways You Can Help People Living with AIDS. Harris R. Goldstein. 1994. LC 94-3620. 160p. (Orig.). pap. 13.95 (*1-881283-08-9*) Alef Design.

Being a Character: Psychoanalysis & Self-Experience. Christopher Bollas. 1994. 294p. pap. 11.00 (*0-8090-1569-2*) Hill & Wang.

Being a Counselor: Directions & Challenges. Jeannette A. Brown & Robert H. Pate, Jr. 1983. LC 82-20764. (Psychology Ser.). 450p. (C). text 43.95 (*0-534-01261-2*) Brooks-Cole.

Being a Food Service Worker. 1967. 276p. stu. ed. 13.95 Hosp Res & Educ.

***Being a Health Unit Coordinator.** Kay Cox-Stevens. 5th ed. 2001. 576p. pap. 49.27 (*0-13-091612-9*, Prentice Hall) P-H.

Being a Homemaker: Home Health Aide. Julie K. Wernig & Barbara Baranishyn. 1985. 192p. (C). pap., tchr. ed. 11.95 (*0-89303-460-6*) P-H.

Being a Homemaker: Home Health Aide. Elana Zucker. 1982. LC 81-21770. (Illus.). 320p. pap. text 18.95 (*0-89303-113-5*) P-H.

Being a Housekeeping Aide. 1967. 320p. stu. ed. 11.95 Hosp Res & Educ.

Being a Long-Term Care Nursing Assistant. Judith B. Eighmy & Connie Will-Black. 4th rev. ed. 1997. LC 97-36825. 432p. pap. text 49.00 (*0-8359-5169-3*) P-H.

***Being a Long-Term Care Nursing Assistant.** Connie Will-Black & Judith B. Eighmy. 5th ed. 2001. LC 2001-21467. 560p. pap. 48.00 (*0-13-089432-X*) P-H.

Being a Medical Clerical Worker: An Introductory Core Text. Jacquelyn R. Marshall & Kathleen S. Harris. 2nd ed. 1997. LC 97-31482. (Brady Medical Clerical Ser.). 288p. pap. text 46.00 (*0-8359-5147-2*) P-H.

Being a Medical Records Clerk. Kathryn McMiller. 1991. 224p. (C). 46.00 (*0-89303-807-5*, 740504); 2nd ed. 1999. LC 99-38985. (Illus.). 208p. pap. 46.00 (*0-13-086493-5*) P-H.

Being a Medical Transcriptionist. Norma L. Morrow. 1991. (Brady Medical Clerical Ser.). 208p. pap. text 42.00 (*0-89303-082-1*) P-H.

Being a Nursing Assistant. Rose Schniedman et al. 7th ed. 1996. pap., tchr. ed. 38.00 (*0-89303-020-1*) P-H.

***Being a Woman-Naturally: Dr. Jan McBarron's Guide to Natural Supplements Beyond 25.** Jan McBarron. 2001. 208p. pap. 15.95 (*1-893910-16-4*) Freedom Pr Inc.

***Being Alive: Building on the Work of Anne Alvarez.** Anne Alvarez. Ed. by Judith Edwards. 2001. LC 2001-35707. (*1-58391-130-8*); pap. (*1-58391-131-6*) Brunner-Routledge.

Being & Belonging: Group, Intergroup, & Gestalt. Gaie Houston. 1994. LC 93-3472. (Psychotherapy & Counselling Ser.). 234p. 269.95 (*0-471-93548-4*) Wiley.

Being & Loving: How to Achieve Intimacy with Another Person & Retain One's Own Identity. Althea J. Horner. rev. ed. 1986. LC 77-73972. 184p. 17.50 (*0-87668-931-4*) Aronson.

Being Called to Care. Mary E. Lashley et al. 1994. LC 93-7296. 215p. (C). text 23.50 (*0-7914-1839-1*); pap. text 22.95 (*0-7914-1840-5*) State U NY Pr.

Being Female: What Every Woman Should Know about Gynecological Health. Rita Baron-Faust. 1998. LC 97-37162. (Illus.). 384p. 25.00 (*0-688-12071-7*, Wm Morrow) Morrow Avon.

Being Ill: Personal & Social Meanings. Steven Mann. 1982. 204p. text 29.50 (*0-8290-0720-2*) Irvington.

Being Married Doing Gender: Critical Analysis of Gender Relationships in Marriage. Caroline Dryden. 1999. LC 98-29689. (Women & Psychology Ser.). 192p. (C). pap. 23.95 (*0-415-16559-8*) Routledge.

Being Married Doing Gender: Critical Analysis of Gender Relationships in Marriage. Ed. by Caroline Dryden. 1999. LC 98-29689. (Women & Psychology Ser.). 192p. (C). 75.00 (*0-415-16558-X*) Routledge.

Being Nice at a Price: Emotional Domination, Depression & the Search for Autonomy. Steven J. Russell. Ed. by Lisa McCoy. 1999. LC 99-60583. 160p. pap. 17.95 (*0-9660092-4-X*) Puget Sound.

Being Positive: The Lives of Men & Women with HIV. Robert Klitzman. 1997. LC 97-16116. 256p. 26.00 (*1-56663-164-5*) I R Dee.

Being Reasonable about the Economics of Health: Selected Essays by Alan Williams. Ed. by A. J. Culyer & Alan Maynard. 1997. LC 97-12051. 392p. 95.00 (*1-85898-648-6*) E Elgar.

Being Somebody: Spring the Mind-Traps That Keep You Fat & Frustrated With Your Life. Patricia Chamberlain. Ed. by Barbara Kyper. 1991. (Illus.). 19.99 (*1-880011-01-8*) Dundas-Devonhills Assoc.

Being There: Profiles of Mental Illness. Karlene K. Hale. 2nd ed. 1996. 109p. pap. 15.00 (*0-9639070-2-6*) ebooksonthe.

Being Vegetarian. American Dietetic Association Staff. 1996. (Nutrition Now Ser.). 88p. pap. 6.95 (*0-471-34661-6*) Wiley.

Being Who You Are. Stefan C. Nadzo. 1983. LC 82-84415. 140p. pap. 6.95 (*0-937226-02-5*) Laugh Cat.

Beitrage Zum Griechischen Liebesroman. Hans Gartner. 1984. (Olms GW Studien: Bd. 20). (GER.). xii, 478p. (*3-487-07497-4*) G Olms Pubs.

Beitrage zur Gestaltentwicklung Menschlicher Zahnanlagen der Ersten Dentition see Contributions to the Development of Human Deciduous Tooth Primordia

Bela Banerjee: Bringing Health to India's Villages. LaVonne G. Platt. 1988. LC 87-51688. (Illus.). xi, 178p. (Orig.). pap. 11.95 (*0-945530-00-5*) Wordsworth KS.

Belding H. Scribner Festschrift. Ed. by C. M. Kjellstrand. 1983. (Journal: Vol. 33, No. 2). (Illus.). 96p. pap. 69.75 (*3-8055-3675-5*) S Karger.

Belief & Imagination: Explorations in Psychoanalysis. Ronald Britton. LC 98-19593. 240p. 1999. pap. 31.95 (*0-415-19438-5*); 1998. (C). 90.00 (*0-415-19437-7*) Routledge.

Belief in a Just World: A Fundamental Delusion. M. J. Lerner. 1980. LC 80-16359. (Perspectives in Social Psychology Ser.). (Illus.). 224p. (C). 55.00 (*0-306-40495-8*, Plenum Trade) Perseus Pubng.

Belief in Psychology: A Study in the Ontology of Mind. Jay L. Garfield. 1988. 152p. 23.50 (*0-262-07108-8*, Bradford Bks) MIT Pr.

Beliefs & Self-Help: Cross-Cultural Perspectives & Approaches. George H. Weber & Lucy M. Cohen. 1982. LC 81-6706. (Illus.). 359p. (C). 45.95 (*0-89885-032-0*, Kluwer Acad Hman Sci) Kluwer Academic.

Beliefs, Behaviors, & Alcoholic Beverages: A Cross-Cultural Survey. Ed. by Mac Marshall. 1979. 504p. pap. text 32.50 (*0-472-08580-8*, 08580) U of Mich Pr.

Beliefs, Reasoning, & Decision Making: Psycho-Logic in Honor of Bob Abelson. Ed. by Roger C. Schank & Ellen J. Langer. 1994. LC 93-5714. 435p. text 89.95 (*0-8058-1456-6*) L Erlbaum Assocs.

Believe It or Not: True Emergency Room Stories. Kevin Pezzi. Ed. by Karla Lewk. 1998. (Illus.). 186p. pap. 12.95 (*0-9655606-2-7*) Transcope.

Believe the Heart: Our Dyslexic Days. Elizabeth Fleming. 1984. LC 84-75. (Illus.). 160p. pap. 7.95 (*0-89407-061-4*) LF Pub VA.

Bellagio Meeting on Vitamin A Deficiency & Childhood Mortality: Proceedings of "Public Health Significance of Vitamin A Deficiency & Its Control" Keith P. West, Jr. 1993. LC 93-10308. (Illus.). 74p. (Orig.). pap. 10.00 (*0-915173-21-2*) Helen Keller Intl.

Belle Epoque of Surgery: The Life & Times of Theodor Billroth. Set. Karel B. Absolon. enl. rev. ed. 1995. Orig. Title: The Surgeon's Surgeon. (Illus.). 312p. (Orig.). (C). text 59.50 (*0-930329-64-3*) Kabel Pubs.

***Bellevue Guide to Outpatient Medicine: An Evidence-Based Guide to Primary Care.** Ed. by Nathan Link et al. 2001. 402p. pap. text (*0-7279-1680-7*) BMJ Pub GBR. *Dist:* AIDC.

Bell's Orofacial Pains. Jeffrey P. Okeson. 5th ed. 1995. LC 95-1313. (Illus.). 400p. text 68.00 (*0-86715-293-1*) Quint Pub Co.

Belousov-Zhabotinskii Reaction. J. J. Tyson. Ed. by S. A. Levin. 1976. (Lecture Notes in Biomathematics: Vol. 10). (Illus.). 128p. 29.95 (*0-387-07792-8*) Spr-Verlag.

Beloved Son: Born with HIV. Therese Muamini. 1997. 192p. (*1-85375-205-3*) Prion GBR. *Dist:* Trafalgar.

Beloved Son: Born with HIV. Therese Muamini. 1997. 192p. pap. 9.95 (*1-85375-202-9*) Trafalgar.

Below Replacement Fertility in Industrial Societies: Causes, Consequences, Politics. Kingsley Davis et al. Ed. by Hoover Institute Staff. 1987. 380p. text 95.00 (*0-521-34324-0*) Cambridge U Pr.

Below-Replacement Fertility in Industrialized Societies: Causes, Consequences, Policies - Supplement to Population & Development Review, Vol. 12. Ed. by Kingsley Davis et al. 1987. LC 87-2458. pap. 14.00 (*0-87834-056-4*) Population Coun.

Beltway Baby: A Guide to Life in Washington's Baby Lanes. Evelyn Goldstein. 1994. LC 95-119598. (Illus.). 178p. (Orig.). pap. 10.95 (*0-915168-30-8*) Wash Bk Trad.

Bench Aids for the Diagnosis of Filarial Infections. 1997. (Illus.). 6p. pap. 36.00 (*92-4-154489-9*, 1150444) Am Soc Clinical.

Bench Aids for the Diagnosis of Intestinal Parasites. Lawrence R. Ash et al. 1994. (CHI, ENG, FRE & SPA.). 20p. pap. text 31.50 (*92-4-154476-7*, 1150417) World Health.

Bench Aids for the Diagnosis of Malaria: Plates No. 1-8. Illus. by Y. L. Fong. 1988. (FRE.). 8p. (C). 15.00 (*92-4-154232-2*, 1150294) World Health.

Bench & Me: Teaching & Learning Medicine. J. Willis Hurst. 1992. LC 92-1517. (Illus.). 112p. pap. 19.95 (*0-89640-223-1*) Igaku-Shoin.

Benchmark Study on Physicians' Use of the World Wide Web. American Medical Association Staff. 1999. 2800.00 (*0-89970-935-4*) AMA.

Benchmarking Strategies for Health Care Management. Mark T. Czarnecki. 1994. LC 94-18369. ring bd. 120.00 (*0-8342-0604-8*, S153) Aspen Pub.

Benchmarks: Alternative Methods in Toxicology. Ed. by Myron A. Mehlman. 1989. LC 88-63539. 219p. 50.00 (*0-911131-19-1*) Specialist Journals.

Benchmarks for Designing Workers' Compensation Medical Fee Schedules, 1994-1995. Philip L. Burstein. 1994. 50.00 (*0-935149-50-3*, WC-94-7) Workers Comp Res Inst.

Benchmarks for Designing Workers' Compensation Medical Fee Schedules, 1995-1996. Philip L. Burstein. 1996. LC 96-15349. 127p. (Orig.). pap. 50.00 (*0-935149-56-2*, WC-96-2) Workers Comp Res Inst.

Benchmarks of Fairness for Health Care Reform. Norman Daniels et al. 1996. LC 95-47820. (Illus.). 208p. text 36.50 (*0-19-510237-1*) OUP.

Bendectin & Birth Defects: The Challenges of Mass Toxic Substances Litigation. Michael D. Green. 1998. 384p. pap. 24.95 (*0-8122-1645-8*) U of Pa Pr.

Bender Gestalt Screening for Brain Dysfunction. 1. Patricia Lacks. 2nd ed. 1998. LC 98-7635. (Illus.). 288p. 80.00 (*0-471-24257-8*) Wiley.

Bender Gestalt Test: Its Qualification & Validity for Adults. Gerald R. Pascal & Barbara J. Suttell. 1953. LC 51-3749. (Illus.). 288p. text 40.00 (*0-8089-0358-6*, 793252, Grune & Strat) Harcrt Hlth Sci Grp.

Bender Gestalt Test for Young Children. Elizabeth M. Koppitz. LC 63-19130. 1963. (Illus.). 208p. text 30.00 (*0-8089-0239-3*, 792351); Vol. II. 1975. 224p. text 32.95 (*0-8089-0873-1*, 792352X) Harcrt Hlth Sci Grp (Grune & Strat).

Bender Visual Motor Gestalt Test for Children: A Manual. Aileen Clawson. 1962. LC 79-57294. (Illus.). 92p. pap. 42.50 (*0-87424-035-2*, W-35) Western Psych.

Beneath the Mask. Christopher F. Monte. 5th ed. 1994. (C). pap. text, tchr. ed., suppl. ed. 49.75 (*0-15-501856-6*) Harcourt Coll Pubs.

Beneficence & Health Care. Earl E. Shelp. 1982. 281p. text 112.50 (*90-277-1377-4*) Kluwer Academic.

Beneficial & Toxic Effects of Aspirin. Susan E. Feinman. 1993. LC 93-28097. (Pharmacology & Toxicology Ser.). 144p. 136.95 (*0-8493-7297-6*, RM666) CRC Pr.

Beneficial Effects of Endotoxins. Ed. by Alois Nowotny. 1983. LC 83-2256. 596p. 125.00 (*0-306-41147-4*, Plenum Trade) Perseus Pubng.

Beneficiary Beware: Inadequate Review of Medicare Managed Care Plans Results in Incomplete Information for Consumers: Ed. by Charles E. Grassley. 2000. (Illus.). 169p. (C). pap. text 30.00 (*0-7567-0150-3*) DIANE Pub.

Benefit Design: Clinical Preventive Services. 1994. lib. bdg. 250.00 (*0-8490-8544-6*) Gordon Pr.

Benefit Design: Patient Cost-Sharing, Background Paper. 1994. lib. bdg. 250.00 (*0-8490-8545-4*) Gordon Pr.

Benefit Risk Ratio: A Handbook for the Rational Use of Potentially Hazardous Drugs. Hans C. Korting & Monika Schafer-Korting. 1998. LC 98-10797. (Illus.). 400p. 134.95 (*0-8493-2791-1*) CRC Pr.

Benefit Your Business. James F. Schwoob. 1989. LC 89-90862. (Illus.). (Orig.). pap. 16.95 (*0-9622483-0-4*) Single-Knight.

Benefits & Risks of Oral Contraceptives Today. James O. Drife. 2nd ed. 1996. LC 96-6752. (Illus.). 48p. lib. bdg. 21.95 (*1-85070-707-3*, Parthenon Pbng) CRC Pr.

Benefits, Costs & Cycles in Workers Compensation. Ed. by Philip S. Borba & David Appel. 1990. (S. S. Huebner International Ser.: Vol. 9). (C). lib. bdg. 94.50 (*0-7923-9037-7*) Huebner Foun Insur.

Benefits in Medical Care Programs. Avedis Donabedian. 1990. (Illus.). 456p. 54.00 (*0-674-06580-8*) HUP.

Benefits of Marijuana: Physical, Psychological & Spiritual. Joan Bello. 2nd rev. unabr. ed. (Illus.). 160p. pap. 12.95 (*0-9660988-1-1*) Lifeservs Pr.

Benefits of Marijuana: Physical, Psychological & Spiritual. Joan Bello. Ed. by Guy Mount. 1996. 160p. per. 12.95 (*0-9604462-9-X*) Sweetlight.

Benefits of Recreation Research Update (1991-1994) Judy M. Sefton & W. Kerry Mummery. 1995. LC 95-60644. 40p. (C). pap. text 12.95 (*0-910251-75-4*, BRU80) Venture Pub PA.

Benefits of Valsartan. Ed. by Gordon McInnes. 1999. (Cardiology Ser.: Vol. 91). (Illus.). lv, 26p. 25.25 (*3-8055-6945-9*) S Karger.

Benefits Review Board Service: Longshore Reporter Bender's Editors. 1974. ring bd. 920.00 (*0-8205-1135-8*) Bender.

Benign & Malignant Bone Disease. Ed. by James H. McKillop & I. Fogelman. 1991. (Illus.). 160p. pap. text (*0-443-04436-8*) Church.

Benign & Malignant Lymphadenopathies: A Guide to Clinical & Laboratory Diagnosis. Ed. by Gerassimos A. Pangalis & Aaron Polliack. 1993. LC 92-49470. 338p. text 128.00 (*3-7186-5232-3*) Gordon & Breach.

Benign Breast Disease. 208p. (*0-7131-4579-X*) E A GBR. *Dist:* Routldge.

Benign Childhood Partial Seizures & Related Epileptic Syndromes. Panaiotopoulos. 1999. 416p. (*0-86196-577-9*) J Libbey Med GBR. *Dist:* Bks Intl VA, Buttrwrth-Heinemann.

Benign Diseases of the Vulva & Vagina. Raymond H. Kaufman. 4th ed. 1994. (Illus.). 415p. (C). (gr. 13). text 123.00 (*0-8016-6836-0*, 06836) Mosby Inc.

***Benign Diseases of the Vulva & Vagina: Enfermedades Benignas de la Vulva y Vagina.** Raymond H. Kaufman & Sebastian Faro. 4th ed. 1994. (ENG & SPA., Illus.). 415p. (*84-8174-118-3*) Mosby-Doyma Libros ESP. *Dist:* Mosby Inc.

Benign Disorders & Diseases of the Breast. Ed. by Les Hughes et al. 2nd ed. 1999. (Illus.). 275p. text (*0-7020-2069-9*) W B Saunders.

Benign Lesions of the Esophagus. 1989. (Illus.). 848p. 174.00 (*0-387-18446-5*) Spr-Verlag.

Benign Prostatic Hypeplasia. Kirby. 1992. (*1-56375-582-3*) Gower-Mosby.

Benign Prostatic Hyperplasia. 1995. lib. bdg. 251.95 (*0-8490-6847-9*) Gordon Pr.

Benign Prostatic Hyperplasia. Perinchery Narayan. 2000. 350p. text 149.00 (*0-443-05637-4*) Saunders.

Benign Prostatic Hyperplasia: Conservative & Operative Management. Ed. by G. Jakse et al. 1993. LC 92-49308. (Illus.). 240p. 107.00 (*0-387-55424-6*) Spr-Verlag.

Benign Prostatic Hyperplasia: Current Therapy. Christopher R. Chapple & John D. McConnell. 2000. (Illus.). 192p. (*1-85317-603-6*) Martin Dunitz GBR. *Dist:* Blackwell Sci.

Benign Prostatic Hyperplasia: Diagnosis & Treatment: Clinical Practice Guideline. 1995. (Illus.). 225p. (Orig.). (C). pap. text 50.00 (*0-7881-2094-8*) DIANE Pub.

Benign Prostatic Hyperplasia: Innovations in the Maanagement. Ed. by Z. Petrovich & L. Baert. 1994. LC 94-527. (Illus.). 384p. 174.00 (*0-387-56628-7*) Spr-Verlag.

Benign Prostatic Hyperplasia. Kirby. 2nd ed. 1997. text (*0-7234-2448-9*) Wolfe Publishing GBR. *Dist:* Mosby Inc.

Benign Prostatic Hypertrophy. Ed. by F. Hinman, Jr. 1983. (Illus.). 1097p. 260.00 (*0-387-90779-3*) Spr-Verlag.

Benign Prostatic Hypertrophy. David G. Williams. 1992. 26p. pap. 14.95 (*0-944649-11-4*) Mtn Home Pub.

Benign Structures of the Bile Ducts. Edward I. Galperin et al. 1987. 60.00 (*0-8236-0494-2*, BN#00494) Intl Univs Pr.

Benign to Malignant Progression in Cervical Squamous Epithelium. Robert L. Ehrmann. 1994. LC 93-31971. (Illus.). 280p. 98.50 (*0-89640-241-X*) Igaku-Shoin.

Benign Tumors in the Third Ventricle of the Brain: Diagnosis & Treatment. Walter O. Dandy. 1970. (Illus.). reprint ed. 25.00 (*0-87266-037-0*) Argosy.

Benign Tumors, Tumor-Like Conditions, & Pre-Neoplastic Lesions of the Adult Human Liver: Epidemiology & Pathogenesis in Medicolegal Autopsies & Clinical Patients. P. J. Karhunen. 1986. 70p. (Orig.). pap. 48.50 (*951-99803-0-X*) Coronet Bks.

Benigne & Maligne Gallenwegstenosen. 1999. 104p. 44.50 (*3-8055-6829-0*) S Karger.

Benjamin Rush: Revolutionary Gadfly. David F. Hawke. 1971. LC 70-145859. 27.50 (*0-672-51599-7*) Irvington.

Benjamin Silliman & His Circle: Studies on the Influence of Benjamin Silliman on Science in America. Ed. by Leonard G. Wilson. 1979. LC 77-21564. (Illus.). x, 227p. 10.00 (*0-88202-174-5*) Midewiwin.

Bennett & Rabbetts' Clinical Visual Optics. Arthur G. Bennett & Ronald B. Rabbetts. 3rd ed. 1998. LC 97-51177. 450p. text 120.00 (*0-7506-1817-5*) Buttrwrth-Heinemann.

Bennett's Opthalmic Prescription Work. Kelvin G. Wakefield. 4th ed. 2000. LC 00-41436. (Illus.). 366p. pap. text 69.99 (*0-7506-4669-1*) Buttrwrth-Heinemann.

Benomyl. 1993. (Environmental Health Criteria Ser.: No. 148). (ENG, FRE & SPA.). 135p. pap. text 29.00 (*92-4-157148-9*, 1160148) World Health.

Ben's Story: The Symptoms of Depression, ADHD, & Anxiety That Caused His Suicide. Trudy Carlson. 1998. LC 96-83889. (Illus.). 144p. (Orig.). pap. 9.95 (*0-9642443-6-5*) Benline Pr.

Benzene. 1993. (Environmental Health Criteria Ser.: No. 150). (ENG, FRE & SPA.). 156p. pap. text 30.00 (*92-4-157150-0*, 1160150) World Health.

Benzene—Index of New Information & Medical Research Bible. Duane J. DuBois. rev. ed. 1998. 149p. 57.50 (*0-7883-1964-7*); pap. 47.50 (*0-7883-1965-5*) ABBE Pubs Assn.

Benzene Carcinogenicity. Ed. by M. Aksoy. 1988. (Cancer Specialists & Hematologists Ser.). 192p. 100.00 (*0-8493-6670-4*, RC643, CRC Reprint) Franklin.

Benzodiazepine Dependence. Ed. by Cosmo Hallstrom. 1993. LC 93-20040. (Oxford Medical Publications). (Illus.). 392p. text 89.50 (*0-19-262094-0*) OUP.

Benzodiazepine Dependence, Toxicity, & Abuse. American Psychiatric Association Task Force Staff. 1990. LC 90-571. 116p. text 19.95 (*0-89042-228-1*, 2228) Am Psychiatric.

Benzodiazepines, No. II. H. Schutz. 1989. (Illus.). 623p. 214.00 (*0-387-50249-1*) Spr-Verlag.

Benzodiazepines: Current Standards for Clinical Practice. Ed. by D. E. Smith & Donald R. Wesson. 1985. text 193.50 (*0-85200-783-3*) Kluwer Academic.

Benzodiazepines & GHB: Detection & Pharmacology. Ed. by Salvatore J. Salamone. 2001. (Forensic Science & Medicine Ser.). 160p. 79.50 (*0-89603-981-1*) Humana.

Benzodiazepines, Use, Overuse, Misuse, & Abuse. J. Marks. 2nd ed. 1985. text 73.50 (*0-85200-870-8*) Kluwer Academic.

Benzopyrene. Martin R. Osborne & Neil T. Crosby. 1987. (Monographs on Cancer Research). 352p. text 90.00 (*0-521-30122-X*) Cambridge U Pr.

Bereaved Child: Analysis, Education, & Treatment - An Abstracted Bibliography. Gillian S. Mace et al. 1981. LC 81-8637. 292p. 95.00 (*0-306-65197-1*, Kluwer Plenum) Kluwer Academic.

Bereaved Parent. Harriet S. Schiff. 1978. LC 78-16098. 146p. pap. 11.95 (*0-14-005043-4*, Penguin Bks) Penguin Putnam.

Bereavement: Client Adaptation & Hospice Services. Ed. by Donna L. Infeld & Nadine R. Penner. 1997. LC 96-38929. (Hospice Journal: Vol. 11, No. 4). 136p. (C). 29.95 (*0-7890-0030-X*) Haworth Pr.

Bereavement: Its Psychological Aspects. Ed. by Bernard Schoenberg et al. 1975. LC 75-16422. 375p. text 66.50 (*0-231-03974-3*) Col U Pr.

Bereavement: Studies of Grief in Adult Life. Colin M. Parkes. 3rd ed. 1996. LC 95-47088. (*0-415-11033-5*) Routledge.

Bereavement & Adaptation: A Comparative Study of the Aftermath of Death. Marc Cleiren. 1992. LC 92-26136. 296p. 31.95 (*1-56032-279-9*) Hemisp Pub.

Bereavement & Health: The Psychological & Physical Consequences of Partner Loss. Wolfgang Stroebe & Margaret S. Stroebe. 1987. (Illus.). 304p. text 59.95 (*0-521-24470-6*); 302p. pap. text 21.95 (*0-521-28710-3*) Cambridge U Pr.

Bereavement & Support: Healing in a Group Environment. Marylou Hughes. 1995. 224p. 59.95 (*1-56032-370-1*); pap. 29.95 (*1-56032-371-X*) Taylor & Francis.

Bereavement Counseling: A Multidisciplinary Handbook. Ed. by B. Mark Schoenberg. 1980. LC 79-7471. (Illus.). 266p. lib. bdg. 65.00 (*0-313-21434-4*, SBR/, Greenwood Pr) Greenwood.

Bereavement of Physical Disability: Recommitment to Life, Health & Function. Ed. by John A. Downey et al. 1982. 20.95 (*0-405-14214-5*) Ayer.

Berengario da Carpi, on Fracture of the Skull or Cranium. L.R. Lind. 1990. LC 90-55267. (Transactions Ser.: Vol. 80, Pt. 4). (Illus.). 164p. (C). pap. 15.00 (*0-87169-804-8*, T804-LIL) Am Philos.

Bergey's Manual of Determinative Bacteriology. Ed. by John G. Holt et al. 9th rev. ed. 1993. LC 93-8438. (Illus.). 816p. pap. 79.95 (*0-683-00603-7*) Lppncott W & W.

Bergey's Manual of Systematic Bacteriology, Volume 2. Peter H. Sneath. 1986. (Illus.). 636p. text 139.00 (*0-683-07893-3*) Lppncott W & W.

Bergey's Manual of Systematic Bacteriology, Volume 3. Ed. by James T. Staley. 1989. (Illus.). 744p. text 139.00 (*0-683-07908-5*) Lppncott W & W.

Bergsma Doctors & Patients. Jurrit Bergsma. 1997. LC 96-53893. 200p. pap. text 37.00 (*0-7923-4395-6*) Kluwer Academic.

Bernheim's New Studies in Hypnotism. Hippolyte Bernheim. Tr. by Richard S. Sandor from GER. 1980. (Illus.). xix, 407p. (C). 60.00 (*0-8236-0496-9*) Intl Univs Pr.

Bernisches Mammasymposium: Festschrift fuer Max Berger Mammasymposium, Bern, September 1987. Ed. by E. Dreher. 1988. (Journal: Vol. 28, Suppl. 1, 1988). (Illus.). vi, 94p. pap. 30.50 (*3-8055-4832-X*) S Karger.

Berry & Kohn's Operating Room Technique. Lucy J. Atkinson & Nancymarie H. Fortunato. 8th ed. (Illus.). 1996. tchr. ed. (*0-8151-0826-5*); 1996. 320p. (C). (gr. 13). pap. text, stu. ed. (*0-8151-0827-3*, 27886); 1995. LC 95-41189. 1008p. (C). (gr. 13). text 53.00 (*0-8151-0103-1*, 24556) Mosby Inc.

Berry & Kohn's Operating Room Techniques. Nancymarie Fortunato. 9th ed. 2000. LC 99-46828. (Illus.). 955p. 56.00 (*0-323-00968-9*) Mosby Inc.

***Berry & Kohn's Operating Room Techniques: Resource Manual.** Nancymarie Fortunato. 9th ed. 2000. (Illus.). 250.00 (*0-323-01095-4*) Mosby Inc.

Berry & Kohn's Operating Room Techniques: Text & Resource Manual Package. Lucy J. Atkinson. 8th ed. 1996. (Illus.). (*0-8151-0828-1*) Mosby Inc.

Bert's Eye View: Coping with Macular Degeneration. Bert Silverman. l.t. ed. 1997. 48p. pap. 6.95 (*0-9659473-0-0*) Viewpt Pr.

Beryllium. 1990. (Environmental Health Criteria Ser.: No. 106). (ENG, FRE & SPA.). 210p. pap. text 37.00 (*92-4-157106-3*, 1160106) World Health.

Beryllium, Cadmium, Mercury, & Exposures in the Glass Manufacturing Industry. Ed. by World Health Organization Staff. 1993. (IARC Scientific Publications Ser.: Vol. 58). 444p. pap. text 75.00 (*92-832-1258-4*, 1720058) World Health.

Beryllium Health & Safety Guide. 1990. (Health & Safety Guides Ser.: No. 44). 30p. pap. text 5.00 (*92-4-151044-7*, 1860044) World Health.

Beside Ourselves: Our Hidden Personality in Everyday Life. Naomi L. Quenk. 1993. LC 93-4373. 465p. pap. text 17.95 (*0-89106-062-6*, 7378, Davies-Black Pub) Consulting Psychol.

***Best Alternative Medicine.** Kenneth Pelletier. 2002. 448p. pap. 15.00 (*0-7432-0027-6*, Fireside) S&S Trade Pap.

Best Alternatives: Sorting Fact from Fiction in Complementary & Alternative Medicine. Kenneth R. Pelletier. 2000. LC 99-26629. (Illus.). 448p. 26.00 (*0-684-84207-6*) S&S Trade.

Best & Promising Practices in Developmental Disabilities. Ed. by Alan Hilton & Ravic Ringlaben. 1998. LC 97-18844. 364p. pap. 38.00 (*0-89079-720-X*, 8381) Coun Exc Child.

Best & Worst Ideas for Health Care Reform. John C. Goodman. 1992. (Illus.). 28p. (C). pap. 5.00 (*0-943802-97-0*, BG118) Natl Ctr Pol.

Best Arthritis: The World Renowned Colgan Institute Reveals Its Programs for Nutritional Treatment. Michael Colgan. 2000. 168p. 14.95 (*1-896817-23-8*) Apple Pubg Co.

***Best Body Best Bones: Your Doctors Exercise Prescription for Life Long Fitness.** Raymond E. Cole. 2001. 180p. 24.95 (*0-917073-04-5*) Wellpower.

Best Guide to Allergy. Nathan D. Schultz et al. 3rd ed. 1994. LC 94-11376. (Illus.). 240p. reprint ed. 29.50 (*0-89603-283-3*) Humana.

Best Guide to Alternative Medicine. Paul Froemming. 1998. LC 98-7120. (Illus.). 304p. pap. 16.95 (*1-58063-017-0*) Renaissance.

Best Hospitals in America. Linda Sunshine & John W. Wright. 1989. 384p. reprint ed. pap. 9.95 (*0-380-70741-1*, Avon Bks) Morrow Avon.

Best in Medical Advertising & Graphics: Selections from the Rx Club Shows. 1989. (Illus.). 256p. 49.99 (*0-935603-20-4*, 30175) Rockport Pubs.

***Best Labour Possible.** Lesley Hobbs. 2001. 160p. pap. text 25.00 (*0-7506-5200-4*) Buttrwrth-Heinemann.

Best Labour Possible. Caroline M. Shepherd & Aileen Patton. 2000. 160p. pap. text 22.50 (*1-898507-24-4*) Buttrwrth-Heinemann.

Best Laid Schemes: The Psychology of the Emotions. Keith Oatley. 1992. (Studies in Emotion & Social Interaction). 543p. (C). pap. text 34.95 (*0-521-42387-2*) Cambridge U Pr.

Best Medical Advertising & Graphics 2: Selections from the RX Club. 2nd ed. 1992. (Illus.). 240p. 59.99 (*1-56496-025-0*, 30459) Rockport Pubs.

Best Medical Treatments for Women. Holly Atkinson & Pamela P. Novotny. 2000. LC 97-26409. 640p. 27.95 (*0-316-05636-7*) Little.

Best-Natured Man: Sir Samuel Garth, Physician & Poet. John F. Sena. 1986. LC 85-48009. (Studies in the Eighteenth Century: No. 9). 39.50 (*0-404-61475-2*) AMS Pr.

Best of Alert Diver. Peter B. Bennett et al. 1997. LC 97-73096. 19.95 (*0-941332-62-4*, D937) Best Pub Co.

Best of Behaviour Research & Therapy. Jack Rachman. 1997. LC 97-37215. 184p. 51.50 (*0-08-043078-3*, Pergamon Pr) Elsevier.

Best of Dental Humor. Ed. by Stephen T. Sonis & Gerald Shklar. 1996. LC 96-36809. (Illus.). 27.95 (*1-56053-067-7*) Hanley & Belfus.

Best of Everything for Your Baby. Krantz & Richard Exely. 1999. pap. 16.00 (*0-13-089271-8*) P-H.

Best of Jems: Timeless Essays from the First 15 Years. Ed. by Jim Page et al. 1996. LC 96-75305. (*0-8151-7342-3*) Jems Comm.

Best of Nursing Humor. Ed. by Colleen Kenefick & Amy Young. 1993. (Illus.). 170p. 29.95 (*1-56053-062-6*) Hanley & Belfus.

Best of Prevention. Mark Bricklin. 1997. LC 96-47050. (Illus.). 320p. pap. 12.95 (*0-87596-419-2*) Rodale Pr Inc.

Best of Psychology Today. Paul Chance. 1990. 350p. (C). pap. text (*0-07-010509-X*) McGraw.

Best of Psychology Today. Paul Chance & George T. Harris. 1990. 268p. (C). pap. 33.13 (*0-07-557138-2*) McGrw-H Hghr Educ.

Best of the Grapevine, Vol. I. 1985. (Illus.). 288p. 8.00 (*0-933685-00-9*) A A Grapevine.

Best Practice Occupational Therapy: In Community Service with Children & Families. Winnie W. Dunn. 2000. LC 00-27243. (Illus.). 373p. pap. text 42.00 (*1-55642-456-6*) SLACK Inc.

Best Practices for Comprehensive Tobacco: Control Programs. Terry F. Pechacek. 2001. 87p. (C). reprint ed. pap. 20.00 (*0-7881-8397-4*) DIANE Pub.

Best Practices for Health-System Pharmacy, 2000-2001: Positions & Practice Standards of ASHP. 2000. 560p. pap. 48.50 (*1-58528-019-4*) Am Soc Hlth-Syst.

Best Practices I: The Classroom As an Assessment Arena, Vol. 2. Ed. by Katharine G. Butler. 1992. LC 93-36264. (Topics in Language Disorders Ser.). 240p. pap. 44.00 (*0-8342-0586-6*, 20586) PRO-ED.

Best Practices II: The Classroom As an Intervention Context. Ed. by Katharine G. Butler. 1986. LC 93-36264. (Topics in Language Disorders Ser.). 240p. pap. 44.00 (*0-8342-0587-4*, 20587) PRO-ED.

Best Practices in Assessment for School & Clinical Settings. Ed. by Booney Vance. 1993. LC 91-75519. 555p. lib. bdg. 49.50 (*0-88422-114-8*) Clinical Psych.

Best Practices in Complementary & Alternative Medicine. Freeman. 2001. LC 00-63995. (Illus.). 604p. pap. 189.00 (*0-8342-1842-9*) Aspen Pub.

Best Practices in Medical Management. Peter R. Kongstvedt & David W. Plocher. 1998. LC 98-19519. (Managed Health Care Handbook Ser.). 800p. 92.00 (*0-8342-1090-8*, 10908) Aspen Pub.

Best Practices in School Psychology II. Ed. by Alex Thomas & Jeff Grimes. 1990. 1048p. pap. text 32.00 (*0-932955-11-8*) Natl Assn Schl Psych.

Best Practices in School Psychology III. Ed. by Alex Thomas & Jeff Grimes. rev. ed. 1995. 1296p. pap. text 90.00 (*0-932955-99-1*) Natl Assn Schl Psych.

Best Practics in Clinical Chirpractic. Robert D. Mootz & Howard T. Vernon. 1999. LC 99-29381. 200p. pap. 45.00 (*0-8342-1376-1*) Aspen Pub.

Best Self-Health Book & More: Your Shield from Stress, Illness, & Dis-ease, for Life! Jordan H. Jordann. 1993. 272p. 21.95 (*0-9639610-0-4*) Jordan Res.

Best Treatment. Isadore Rosenfeld. l.t. ed. 1993. LC 92-32815. (General Ser.). 600p. 24.95 (*0-8161-5657-3*, Macmillan Ref) Gale.

Best Year of My Life Bk. 1: Getting Diabetes. Jed Block. 1999. LC 99-90681. (Illus.). 28p. (J). (gr. 2-6). pap. 10.95 (*0-9672728-0-7*) J Block.

Beta-Adrenergic Pathway in the Failing Human Heart: Implications for Inotropic Therapy. Ed. by A. M. Feldman & M. R. Bristow. 1990. (Journal: Vol. 77, Suppl. 1). (Illus.). iv, 32p. pap. 15.75 (*3-8055-5195-9*) S Karger.

Beta-Adrenoceptors: Molecular Biology, Biochemistry & Pharmacology. Ed. by R. R. Ruffolo. 1991. (Progress in Basic & Clinical Pharmacology Ser.: Vol. 7). (Illus.). x, 240p. 213.25 (*3-8055-5366-8*) S Karger.

Beta Adrenoceptors in Asthma. Ed. by John Morley. 1984. (Perspectives in Asthma Ser.). text 83.00 (*0-12-506440-3*) Acad Pr.

Beta Agonists in the Treatment of Asthma. Ed. by J. F. Costello & R. D. Mann. 1992. LC 92-49662. 158p. lib. bdg. 74.95 (*1-85070-438-4*, Parthenon Pbng) CRC Pr.

Beta-Blockade & Cardiopreservation: Satellite Symposium American College of Cardiology. Ed. by Michael B. Fowler. 1999. 5p. pap. (*3-8055-7011-2*) S Karger.

Beta Blockers in Clinical Practice. J. M. Cruickshank. 2nd ed. 1994. text (*0-443-04522-4*) Church.

Beta-Blockers in Hypertension & Angina Pectoris: Different Compounds, Different Strategies. Ton M. Cleophas. 1995. LC 95-17076. 100p. (C). pap. text 44.50 (*0-7923-3516-3*) Kluwer Academic.

Beta-Blockers in the Elderly. Ed. by E. K. Lang. 1982. (Illus.). 107p. 32.00 (*0-387-11682-6*) Spr-Verlag.

Beta-Blockers in the Treatment of Hypertension in the 90s: Experience with Tertatolol. Ed. by K. Oenen & C. Diehm. 1993. (Journal: Vol. 83, Suppl. 1, 1993). (Illus.). iv, 72p. pap. 23.50 (*3-8055-5869-4*) S Karger.

Beta-Carotene. Richard A. Passwater. Ed. by Earl S. Mindell. 1984. (Good Health Guides). 32p. pap. 2.95 (*0-87983-363-7*, Keats Pubng) McGraw-Hill Trade.

Beta-Carotene & Other Carotenoids. Richard A. Passwater. 1996. (Good Health Guides). 48p. pap. 3.95 (*0-87983-705-5*, 37055K, Keats Pubng) McGraw-Hill Trade.

Beta-Lactam Antibiotics for Clinical Use. Webber et al. 1986. (Clinical Pharmacology Ser.). (Illus.). 680p. text 225.00 (*0-8247-7386-1*) Dekker.

Beta 3-Adrenergic Agonism: A New Concept in Human Pharmacotherapy. Ed. by Daniel E. Goldberg & William H. Frishman. 1994. (Illus.). 208p. 35.00 (*0-87993-601-0*) Futura Pub.

Beta Two-Microglobulin: Its Significance in Clinical Medicine. Ed. by M. D. Poulik. 1980. (Vox Sanguinis: Vol. 38, No. 6). (Illus.). pap. 28.75 (*3-8055-1560-X*) S Karger.

Beta Virus. Robert A. Kloner. unabr. ed. 1996. 251p. (Orig.). pap. 9.00 (*0-9626020-2-7*) Le Jacq Commns.

Betarezeptoren in der Kardiologie - Probleme aus klinischer Sicht: Proceedings of the Symposium, 1st, Bad Krozingen, October, 1977. Oberrheinisches Kardiologen Symposium Staff. Ed. by H. Roskamm. 1978. (Cardiology Ser.: Vol. 63, Suppl. 1). (FRE & GER., Illus.). 14.00 (*3-8055-2870-1*) S Karger.

Beta2-agonists in Asthma Treatment. Ed. by Romain Pauwels & Paul M. O'Byrne. 1997. LC 97-11742. (Lung Biology in Health & Disease Ser.). (Illus.). 472p. text 195.00 (*0-8247-9496-6*) Dekker.

Bethesda Cancer Manual. James Abraham. 2000. 688p. pap. text 45.00 (*0-7817-2300-0*) Lppncott W & W.

Bethesda System for Reporting Cervical Vaginal Cytologic Diagnoses: Definitions, Criteria & Explanatory Notes for Terminology & Specimen Adequacy. Robert Kurman et al. 1997. LC 93-31572. (Illus.). 96p. 32.00 (*0-387-94077-4*) Spr-Verlag.

Betrayal by the Brain: The Neurologic Basis of Chronic Fatigue Syndrome, Fibromyalgia Syndrome, & Related Neural Network Disorders. Jay A. Goldstein. 1996. LC 95-51124. 313p. (Illus.). 49.95 (*1-56024-977-3*); pap. 24.95 (*1-56024-981-1*) Haworth Pr (Hawrth Medical).

Betrayal in Psychotherapy & Its Antidotes: Challenges for Patient & Therapist. Intro. by E. Mark Stern. 1993. LC 92-45159. (Psychotherapy Patient Ser.: Vol. 8, Nos. 3-4). 186p. lib. bdg. 39.95 (*1-56024-448-8*) Haworth Pr.

Betrayal of Innocence: Incest & Its Devastation. Susan Forward & Craig Buck. rev. ed. 1988. LC 87-25776. 208p. pap. 12.95 (*0-14-011002-X*, Penguin Bks) Penguin Putnam.

Betrayal of the Soul in Psychotherapy. Robert Stein. 1998. 348p. pap. 19.00 (*1-882670-16-7*) Spring Pubns.

Betrayal of Trust: The Collapse of Global Public Health. Laurie Garrett. 2000. LC 00-33425. (Illus.). xiv, 754p. 30.00 (*0-7868-6522-9*) Hyperion.

Betrayal Trauma: The Logic of Forgetting Childhood Abuse. Jennifer J. Freyd. 1996. LC 96-9059. (Illus.). 288p. 26.95 (*0-674-06805-X*) HUP.

Betrayed. Gloria L. Bywalec & Anna M. Rzeppa. 1996. (Illus.). 200p. (Orig.). pap. 14.95 (*0-9652174-0-X*) JMJ Publng.

Better, Better Body Book. Marge Frank & Nancy Linton. 1985. LC 85-11851. pap. 10.95 (*0-310-42741-X*, 12736P) Zondervan.

***Better Birthing with Hypnosis.** Michelle Leclaire O'Neill. 2001. LC 2001-38351. 272p. pap. 16.95 (*0-658-01533-8*) McGraw-Hill Prof.

Better Breast Health Naturally with Chinese Medicine. Honora L. Wolfe & Bob Flaws. 1998. LC 97-78086. (Illus.). 175p. pap. 12.95 (*0-936185-90-2*) Blue Poppy Pr.

Better Buildings for Better Services: Innovative Developments in Primary Care. Jackie Bailey et al. 1997. LC 97-29165. (National Primary Care Research & Development Centre Ser.). (Illus.). 120p. pap. (*1-85775-287-2*) Radcliffe Med Pr GBR. *Dist:* Balogh.

***Better Communication & Cochlear Implants.** Donna S. Wayner et al. 1998. 81p. wbk. ed. 15.00 (*0-9664780-3-7*, 004) Hear Again.

Better Food for Patients: New Menus, Cooking, & Ward Service for Hospital Patients John Rice. 1975. (King Edward's Hospital Fund Ser.). pap. 25.00 (*0-8464-0191-6*) Beekman Pubs.

Better Health & the Reverse Effect. Walter A. Heiby. 1988. (Illus.). 112p. (Orig.). pap. 3.95 (*0-938869-03-5*) MediSci Pubs.

Better Health in Africa: Experience & Policy Issues. R. Paul Shaw & A. Edward Elmendorf. 1994. LC 94-18249. (Development in Practice Ser.). 260p. pap. 22.00 (*0-8213-2817-4*) World Bank.

Better Health with Foot Reflexology. Dwight C. Byers. rev. ed. (Illus.). 263p. (Orig.). 1987. 26.95 (*0-9611804-8-X*); 1983. pap. 26.95 (*0-9611804-2-0*); 1983. (FRE., pap. 18.95 (*0-9611804-4-7*) Ingham Pub.

Better Health with (Mostly) Chinese Herbs & Foods. Albert Y. Leung. 1984. (Illus.). 128p. pap. 9.95 (*0-9634979-1-X*) AYSL.

Better Iinformation, Better Outcomes? The Use of Health Technology Assessment & Clinical Effectiveness Data in Health Care Purchasing Decisions in the United Kingdom & the United States. Frwd. by Daniel M. Fox & Samuel L. Milbank. 2000. 36p. pap. (*1-887748-37-7*) Milbank Memorial.

Better Jobs, Better Care: Building the Home Care Work Force. Rick Surpin et al. 1994. LC 94-22797. (Papers). 56p. pap. 10.00 (*1-881277-03-8*) United Hosp Fund.

Better Living with Chronic Obstructive Pulmonary Disease: How Patients, Families & Care Givers Can Manage Emphysema & Asthmatic or Chronic Bronchitis. Rick Carter & Brooke Nicotra. 1998. (Illus.). 192p. (Orig.). pap. 29.95 (*1-882431-04-9*) New Technology.

Better Management - 100 Tips: Manager's Guide. Jack Reynolds et al. 1993. (Primary Health Care Management Advancement Programme Modules Ser.). 64p. pap. text (*1-882839-17-X*) Aga Khan Fnd.

Betty Ford Center Book of Answers. James W. West. 1997. LC 96-41485. 224p. pap. 12.00 (*0-671-00182-5*) PB.

Betty Neuman: The Neuman Systems Model. Karen S. Reed. 1993. LC 93-26131. (Notes on Nursing Theories Ser.: Vol. 11). (Illus.). 64p. (C). pap. 14.95 (*0-8039-4862-X*, 4684) Sage.

Between Analyst & Patient: New Dimensions in Countertransference & Transference. Ed. by Helen C. Meyers. 1986. 280p. text 45.00 (*0-88163-043-8*) Analytic Pr.

Between Bench & Bedside: Science, Healing, & Interleukin-2 in a Cancer Ward. Ilana Lowy. 1996. LC 96-25407. (Illus.). 384p. 44.50 (*0-674-06809-2*) HUP.

Between Biology & Medicine: The Formation of Intermediary Metabolism. Frederic L. Holmes. 1992. LC 91-62712. (Berkeley Papers in History of Science: No. 14). 115p. pap. text 18.00 (*0-918102-18-9*) U Cal Hist Sci Tech.

Between Doctors & Patients: The Changing Balance of Power. Lilian R. Furst. 1998. LC 97-17695. 292p. 37.50 (*0-8139-1755-7*) U Pr of Va.

Between Feminism & Psychoanalysis. Ed. by Teresa Brennan. 1989. 224p. 55.00 (*0-415-01489-1*, A3333) Routledge.

Between Freud & Klein: The Psychoanalytic Quest for Knowledge & Truth. Adam Limentani. 1989. LC 90-104872. xiv, 281 p. (*1-85343-063-3*) Free Assoc Bks.

Between Give & Take: A Clinical Guide to Contextual Therapy. Ivan Boszormenyi-Nagy & Barbara R. Krasner. 1986. LC 86-2219. 450p. text 48.95 (*0-87630-418-8*) Brunner-Routledge.

Between Heaven & Earth: A Guide to Chinese Medicine. Harriet Beinfield & Efrem Korngold. 1992. LC 92-90043. 448p. pap. 15.00 (*0-345-37974-8*) Ballantine Pub Grp.

Between Home & Nursing Home: The Board & Care Alternative. Ivy M. Down & Lorraine Schnurr. LC 91-21157. (Golden Age Bks.). 216p. (Orig.). (C). 1991. 34.00 (*0-87975-619-5*); 1990. pap. 21.00 (*0-87975-620-9*) Prometheus Bks.

Between Mind, Brain, & Managed Care: The Now & Future World of Academic Psychiatry. Roger E. Meyer & Christopher J. McLaughlin. 1998. LC 97-40588. 340p. pap. text 39.00 (*0-88048-815-8*, 8815) Am Psychiatric.

Between Person & Person: Toward a Dialogical Psychotherapy. Richard H. Hyncer. 1993. 186p. reprint ed. pap. 25.00 (*0-939266-23-7*) Gestalt Journal.

Between Philosophy & Psychoanalysis: Lacan's Reconstruction of Freud. Robert Samuels. 1993. LC 92-42806. 208p. (C). pap. 19.95 (*0-415-90676-8*) Routledge.

***Between Psyche & Soma: The Gerda Boyesen Methods of Biodynamic Psychology.** Gerda Boyesen. 2001. LC 2001-29287. (*0-940795-22-1*) LifeRhythm.

Between Psychology & Psychotherapy: A Poetics of Experience. Miller Mair. 1989. 272p. 49.95 (*0-415-00021-1*, A3317) Routledge.

Between Public & Private: The Lost Boundaries of the Self. Joseph Bensman & Robert Lilienfeld. 1979. LC 78-24751. pap. 12.95 (*0-02-902680-6*) Free Pr.

Between Reality & Fantasy. Simon A. Grolnik. 1995. LC 88-10517. 596p. pap. 50.00 (*1-56821-718-8*) Aronson.

Between Reality & Fantasy: Winnicott's Concepts of Transitional Objects & Phenomena. Ed. by Simon A. Grolnick & Leonard Barkin. 1988. LC 88-10517. 581p. reprint ed. 60.00 (*0-87668-884-9*) Aronson.

Between Safety Nets: Linking Distant Providers with Rural Community Care Systems. 1994. (Illus.). 51p. (Orig.). (C). pap. text 20.00 (*0-7881-1070-5*) DIANE Pub.

Between the Lines: (Reflections of a Family Physician) B. Lewis Barnett, Jr. 1989. (C). pap. 18.95 (*0-942295-17-X*) Soc Tchrs Fam Med.

Between Therapists: The Processing of Transference - Countertransference Material. Arthur Robbins. 1988. 227p. (C). 38.95 (*0-89885-373-7*, Kluwer Acad Hman Sci) Kluwer Academic.

Betwixt & Between: Patterns of Masculine & Feminine Initiation. Ed. by Louise C. Mahdi et al. 1987. LC 86-31271. (Reality of the Psyche Ser.). 528p. pap. 19.95 (*0-8126-9048-6*); (C). 39.95 (*0-8126-9047-8*) Open Court.

Beyond. Lori L. Yates. Ed. by Clare Redig et al. 1996. (Illus.). 168p. (Orig.). pap. 9.95 (*0-9656454-0-1*) Bum Prodns.

*__Beyond a Western Bioethics: Voices from the Developing World.__ Angeles Tan-Alora. Ed. by Josephine M. Lumitao. 2001. LC 2001-23502. (Clinical Medical Ethics Ser.). 176p. 59.95 (*0-87840-874-6*) Georgetown U Pr.

Beyond Addiction: A Step-by-Step Guide to the Spiritual Principles of Addiction & Recovery. Ray Geide. 1991. LC 90-85263. (Illus.). 232p. (Orig.). pap. 7.95 (*0-9628012-0-8*) Dexter KS.

Beyond Alcoholism: Alcohol & Public Health Policy. Dan E. Beauchamp. 1982. 240p. pap. 18.95 (*0-87722-286-X*) Temple U Pr.

Beyond Amalgam: The Hidden Health Hazard Posed by Jawbone Cavitations. Susan Stockton. 2000. (Illus.). 117p. pap. 12.95 (*0-9628770-2-6*) Power of One.

Beyond Anorexia: Narrative, Spirituality & Recovery. Catherine J. Garrett. 1998. LC 98-6161. 259p. (C). text 54.95 (*0-521-62015-5*); pap. text 19.95 (*0-521-62983-7*) Cambridge U Pr.

Beyond Antibiotics: Fifty (or So) Ways to Boost Immunity & Avoid Antibiotics. Lendon H. Smith et al. 2nd rev. ed. 1994. LC 93-42356. 328p. pap. 18.95 (*1-55643-180-5*) North Atlantic.

Beyond Baby M: Ethical Issues in New Reproductive Techniques. Ed. by Dianne M. Bartels et al. 1990. LC 89-49394. (Contemporary Issues in Biomedicine, Ethics, & Society Ser.). 296p. 49.50 (*0-89603-166-7*) Humana.

Beyond Backache: A Personal Guide to Back & Neck Pain Relief. Michael M. Livingston. 1988. LC 87-92101. 12.95 (*0-87212-212-3*) Libra.

Beyond Bedlam: Contemporary Women Psychiatric Survivors Speak Out. Ed. by Jeanine Grobe. LC 95-11003. 272p. 1996. 30.95 (*1-879427-23-0*); 1995. pap. 15.95 (*1-879427-22-2*) Third Side Pr.

Beyond Bedside Manner: 99 Ways to Show You Care. K. C. Warner. 1997. LC 97-74355. (Illus.). 99p. pap. 9.95 (*1-884926-80-0*, 99WAY) Amer Media.

Beyond Behavior Modification: A Cognitive-Behavioral Approach to Behavior Management in the School. Joseph S. Kaplan & Jane Carter. LC 89-77154. 2nd ed. 1991. 312p. pap. text 34.00 (*0-89079-224-0*, 1497); 3rd ed. 1995. 643p. pap. 39.00 (*0-89079-663-7*, 6964) PRO-ED.

Beyond Behaviorism. Vicki L. Lee. 1988. 216p. 39.95 (*0-8058-0115-4*) L Erlbaum Assocs.

Beyond Belief: Psychotherapy & Religion. Ed. by Samuel Stein. 2000. 232p. pap. (*1-85575-186-0*) Karnac Bks GBR. *Dist:* Other Pr LLC.

Beyond Biofeedback. Elmer Green & Alyce Green. 1989. (Illus.). 394p. pap. 14.95 (*0-940267-14-4*) Rinella Edit.

Beyond Biomechanics: Psychosocial Aspects of Musculoskeletal Disorders in Office Work. Ed. by Samuel D. Moon & Steven L. Sauter. 1995. 320p. (*0-7484-0321-3*); pap. (*0-7484-0322-1*) Tay Francis Ltd GBR. *Dist:* Taylor & Francis.

Beyond Blame: A New Way of Resolving Conflict in Relationships. Jeffrey A. Kottler. 1996. (Psychology Ser.). 256p. reprint ed. pap. 16.00 (*0-7879-0249-7*) Jossey-Bass.

Beyond Caring: Hospitals, Nurses, & the Social Organization of Ethics. Daniel F. Chambliss. 1996. LC 95-42835. (Morality & Society Ser.). 192p. pap. text 17.00 (*0-226-10102-9*) U Ch Pr.

Beyond Caring: Morality & Organization in Hospital Nursing. Daniel F. Chambliss. 1996. LC 95-42835. (Morality & Society Ser.). 201p. lib. bdg. 48.00 (*0-226-10071-5*) U Ch Pr.

Beyond Carl Rogers: Towards a Psychotherapy for the 21st Century. David Brazier. 1998. 287p. (Orig.). pap. (*0-09-472610-8*) Constable & Co GBR. *Dist:* Trafalgar.

Beyond Cholesterol: The Johns Hopkins Complete Guide for Avoiding Heart Disease. Peter O. Kwiterovich, Jr. 1989. LC 89-2548. (Illus.). 416p. 24.95 (*0-8018-3828-2*) Johns Hopkins.

Beyond Clinical Paths: Advanced Tools for Outcomes Management. Ed. by Patrice L. Spath. 1997. LC 97-16430. 267p. pap. 65.00 (*1-55648-201-9*) AHPI.

Beyond Codependency: And Getting Better All the Time. Melody Beattie. 1989. LC 88-45986. pap. 12.00 (*0-06-255418-2*) Harper SF.

Beyond Complementary Medicine: Legal & Ethical Perspectives on Health Care & Human Evolution. Michael H. Cohen. 2000. LC 99-50870. 224p. text 45.00 (*0-472-11135-3*, 11135) U of Mich Pr.

Beyond Consent: Seeking Justice in Research. Ed. by Jeffrey P. Kahn et al. 1998. LC 97-44169. 208p. text 39.95 (*0-19-511353-5*) OUP.

Beyond Control: Medical Power & Abortion Law. Sally Sheldon. 1997. (Law & Social Theory Ser.). LC 96-51823. (*0-7453-1168-7*); 208p. pap. (*0-7453-1167-9*) Pluto GBR GBR. *Dist:* Stylus Pub VA.

Beyond Countertransference: The Therapist's Subjectivity in the Therapeutic Process. Joseph M. Natterson. 1991. LC 90-14542. 256p. 50.00 (*0-87668-558-0*) Aronson.

Beyond Diagnosis: Case Formulation Approaches in CBT. Michael Bruch & Frank W. Bond. 1999. LC 98-2989. (Clinical Psychology & Personality Ser.). 238p. pap. 55.00 (*0-471-98222-9*) Wiley.

Beyond Dieting: Psychoeducational Interventions for Chronically Obese Women - A Non-Dieting Approach. Donna Ciliska. 1990. LC 90-1533. (Eating Disorders Monographs: No. 5). (Illus.). 192p. text 33.95 (*0-87630-583-4*) Brunner-Routledge.

Beyond Disengagement 2000. Ed. by Coker Group Staff. 2000. 144p. pap. 75.00 (*1-57947-076-9*) AMA.

Beyond Ego Psychology. Rubin Blanck & Gertrude Blanck. 1986. LC 85-21356. 248p. text 40.50 (*0-231-06266-4*) Col U Pr.

Beyond Empathy: A Therapy of Contact-in-Relationship. Janet Moursund et al. 1999. LC 99-20272. 380p. 44.95 (*0-87630-963-5*) Brunner-Routledge.

Beyond Evolution. Wilbur A. Jasson. 1986. LC 84-52700. (Illus.). 141p. 14.95 (*0-9614464-0-4*); pap. 8.95 (*0-9614464-1-2*) Sarasota Sci.

Beyond First Aid. Peter R. Hewett. 1992. (Illus.). 256p. (Orig.). pap. text (*0-443-04579-8*) Church.

Beyond Flexner: Medical Education in the Twentieth Century, 34. Ed. by Barbara M. Barzansky & Norman Gevitz. 1992. LC 91-24333. (Contributions in Medical Studies Ser.: No. 34). 264p. 68.00 (*0-313-25984-4*, BMU, Greenwood Pr) Greenwood.

Beyond Formal Operations: Late Adolescent & Adult Cognitive Development. Francis A. Richards & Cheryl Armon. Ed. by Michael L. Commons. 1984. LC 83-21142. 463p. 75.00 (*0-275-91139-X*, C1139, Praeger Pubs) Greenwood.

Beyond Gentle Teaching: A Nonaversive Approach to Helping Those in Need. J. J. McGee & F. J. Menolascino. 1991. (Illus.). 244p. (C). 42.00 (*0-306-43856-9*, Plenum Trade) Perseus Pubng.

Beyond Glasses! The Consumer's Guide to Laser Vision Correction. Franette Armstrong. 1997. LC 97-140161. (Illus.). 368p. pap. 19.95 (*0-9656505-0-2*) U C Books.

Beyond Grief: A Guide for Recovering from the Death of a Loved One. Carol Staudacher. 1987. 264p. pap. 14.95 (*0-934986-43-6*) New Harbinger.

Beyond Ideology: Philosophy, Public Policy, & Health Care Reform. Alan F. Kremen. 1994. LC 93-48682. (Essays in Public Policy Ser.: No. 46). 43p. pap. 5.00 (*0-8179-5512-7*) Hoover Inst Pr.

Beyond Infertility: The New Paths to Parenthood. Susan L. Cooper & Ellen S. Glazer. 1994. 376p. 19.95 (*0-02-911813-1*) Jossey-Bass.

Beyond Labeling. Gelman. 1998. 216p. pap. text 15.00 (*0-226-28707-6*) U Ch Pr.

Beyond M S: It's All in the Image. Nancy Bent. 1995. 281p. 25.00 (*0-913412-76-7*) Brandon Hse.

Beyond Managed Care: How Consumers & Technology Are Changing the Future of Health Care- Dean C. Coddington et al. 2000. LC 00-8789. (Jossey-Bass Health Care Ser.). (Illus.). 368p. 52.00 (*0-7879-5383-0*) Jossey-Bass.

Beyond Mind Games: The Marketing Power of Psychographics. Rebecca Piirto. 1991. LC 91-58121. 263p. (C). 34.50 (*0-936889-08-X*) Intertec Pub Bks.

Beyond Modularity: A Developmental Perspective on Cognitive Science. Annette Karmiloff-Smith. (Learning, Development, & Conceptual Change Ser.). (Illus.). 1992. LC 92-5006. 252p. 40.00 (*0-262-11169-1*); 1995. 256p. reprint ed. pap. text 20.00 (*0-262-61114-7*) MIT Pr (Bradford Bks).

*__Beyond Negative Thinking: Breaking the Cycle of Depressing & Anxious Thoughts.__ Martorano. 2001. 304p. pap. text 22.50 (*0-7382-0617-2*) Perseus Bks Grp.

Beyond Nutrition Counseling: Achieving Positive Outcomes Through Nutriton Therapy, a Publication of the Nutrition Entrepreneurs Dietetic Practice Group. Donna Israel & Susan Moores. 1996. LC 96-36493. 157p. pap. 19.95 (*0-88091-152-2*) Am Dietetic Assn.

Beyond Nutritional Recommendations: Imlementing Science for Healthier Populations. Ed. by Cutberto Garza et al. 1996. xi, 350p. (Orig.). pap. text 36.00 (*0-9655240-0-0*) Cornell U Div Nutrit Scis.

Beyond Obedience: Training with Awareness for You & Your Dog April Frost & Rondi Lightmark. 1999. (Illus.). 368p. reprint ed. pap. 13.00 (*0-609-80469-3*, Three Riv Pr) Crown Pub Group.

Beyond Operating Room Doors. Phyllis A. Roberts. 1997. (Illus.). (Orig.). pap. 15.95 (*0-9657819-0-9*) P Roberts.

Beyond Phen-fen: Healthier, Safer, Medically Proven Weight-Loss. Maher A. Abbas. 1998. (Illus.). 150p. (Orig.). pap. 12.95 (*0-9656065-2-X*) SYTAC Pub.

Beyond Prozac: Antidotes for Modern Times. Michael J. Norden. 1995. LC 95-16745. 272p. 23.00 (*0-06-039151-0*) HarperTrade.

Beyond Psychology. Otto Rank. 1958. 291p. pap. text 10.95 (*0-486-20485-5*) Dover.

Beyond Psychology: An Introduction to Methapsychology. Frank A. Gerbode. 3rd ed. 1995. 600p. 35.00 (*1-887927-00-X*) Inst Res Metapsychol.

Beyond Psychology: Letters & Journals, 1934-1939. Wilhelm Reich. Ed. & Intro. by Mary B. Higgins. 1994. LC 94-14721. 320p. 25.00 (*0-374-11247-9*) FS&G.

*__Beyond Psychotherapy: Programmed Writing & Structured Computer-Assisted Interventions.__ Luciano L'Abate. 2001. LC 2001-31648. (Developments in Clinical Psychology Ser.). 347p. 79.95 (*1-56750-654-2*) Greenwood.

Beyond Rage: Mastering Unavoidable Health Changes. JoAnn LeMaistre. rev. ed. 1993. LC 93-36467. 208p. 24.95 (*0-931712-11-4*) Alpine Guild.

Beyond Reason: The National Health Service & the Limits of Management. Ed. by J. Leopold et al. 1996. (Stirling School of Management Ser.). 288p. (*1-85972-031-5*) Avebry GBR. *Dist:* Ashgate Pub Co.

Beyond Regulations: Ethics in Human Subjects Research. Gail E. Henderson. Ed. by Nancy M. King et al. 1999. LC 98-29189. (Studies in Social Medicine). (Illus.). 296p. pap. 18.95 (*0-8078-4770-4*); lib. bdg. 39.95 (*0-8078-2468-2*) U of NC Pr.

Beyond Ritalin: Adults with Attention Deficit Disorders: Facts About Medication & Other Strategies for Helping Children, Adolescents, & Stephen W. Garber et al. 1997. 272p. pap. 13.50 (*0-06-097725-6*, Perennial) HarperTrade.

Beyond Second Opinions: Rethinking Questions about Fertility. Judith S. Turiel. LC 97-6044. (Illus.). 419p. 1998. pap. 18.95 (*0-520-20854-4*); 1996. text 45.00 (*0-520-08945-6*) U CA Pr.

Beyond Self Awareness. Wyatt Woodsmall. 1998. (Advanced Neuro Linguistic Programming Applications Ser.). 110p. spiral bd. 35.00 (*1-892876-07-8*) Next Step Pr.

Beyond Severe Disability: A Functional Bibliography. Lois S. Rood & Karen Faison. 1985. 32p. (Orig.). pap. 2.50 (*1-55719-014-3*) U NE CPAR.

Beyond Severe Disability: Models & Strategies for Change. Lois S. Rood. 1983. 43p. (Orig.). pap. 3.15 (*1-55719-006-2*) U NE CPAR.

Beyond Severe Disability: National Approaches & Networking Guide. Floyd T. Waterman et al. 1985. 305p. (Orig.). pap. 9.95 (*1-55719-018-6*) U NE CPAR.

Beyond Severe Disability: Nebraska Services Guide. Lois S. Rood. 1985. 38p. (Orig.). pap. 3.15 (*1-55719-013-5*) U NE CPAR.

Beyond Severe Disability: The Challenge of Private Enterprise. Lois S. Rood & Carole M. Davis. 1985. 38p. (Orig.). pap. 3.15 (*1-55719-015-1*) U NE CPAR.

Beyond Symptom Suppression: Improving Long-Term Outcomes of Schizophrenia. Committee on Psychopathology Staff. Ed. by Group for the Advancement of Psychiatry Staff. 1992. LC 91-26231. (Group for the Advancement of Psychiatry Ser.). 125p. 27.50 (*0-87318-202-2*) Grp Adv Psych.

Beyond Talk Therapy: Using Movement & Expressive Techniques in Clinical Practice. Ed. by Daniel J. Wiener. 1999. LC 99-13104. (Illus.). xix, 309p. 39.95 (*1-55798-585-5*, 431-618A) Am Psychol.

Beyond Teaching & Learning: Ways to Profoundly Improve the Experience & Results of Learning. Win Wenger. 2nd ed. 1992. (Compendium of Enhanced Learning Techniques Ser.). (Illus.). 315p. (Orig.). (C). pap. text 29.95 (*0-931865-04-2*) Proj Renaissance.

Beyond Technique: Psychotherapy for the 21st Century. Lawrence LeShan. 1996. LC 95-10750. 216p. 40.00 (*1-56821-550-9*) Aronson.

Beyond Technique: The Hidden Dimensions of Bodywork. Ronan M. Kisch. 1998. 376p. 34.95 (*0-9664761-0-7*) BLHY Growth Pubns.

Beyond the Boards: ECG Review. Brendan Phibbs. 1996. LC 96-18845. 280p. 34.95 (*0-316-70512-8*, Little Brwn Med Div) Lppncott W & W.

Beyond the Brain: Birth, Death, & Transcendence in Psychotherapy. Stanislav Grof. 1985. LC 85-14882. (Series in Transpersonal & Humanistic Psychology). 466p. (C). pap. text 20.95 (*0-87395-899-3*) State U NY Pr.

Beyond the Breast-Bottle Controversy. Penny Van Esterik. 1989. LC 88-18494. 220p. (C). text 35.00 (*0-8135-1382-0*); pap. text 16.00 (*0-8135-1383-9*) Rutgers U Pr.

Beyond the Call of Duty. David H. Sutton et al. 1990. 240p. (C). pap. (*0-86439-087-4*) Boolarong Pubns AUS. *Dist:* St Mut.

Beyond the Clinic Survival Skills for Opthalmologists. Merrick Murray & Philip Moseley. 2001. (Illus.). 256p. pap. 40.00 (*0-7506-4487-7*) Buttrwrth-Heinemann.

Beyond the Clinic Walls: Case Studies in Community-Based Distribution. James A. Wolff et al. 1990. LC 90-5281. (Library of Management for Development). (Illus.). 170p. pap. 14.95 (*0-931816-08-4*) Kumarian Pr.

Beyond the Clinic Walls: Case Studies in Community-Based Distribution see Au-Dela des Murs de la Clinique: Etudes de Cas sur la Distribution a Base Communautaire de Contraceptifs

Beyond the Crime Lab: The New Science of Investigation. Jon Zonderman. rev. ed. 1998. LC 98-14283. (Illus.). 272p. 29.95 (*0-471-25466-5*) Wiley.

Beyond the Crisis: Preserving the Capacity for Excellence in Health Care & Medical Science. Ed. by Henry M. Greenberg & Susan U. Raymond. 1994. LC 94-36768. (Annals of the New York Academy of Sciences Ser.: Vol. 729). pap. 30.00 (*0-89766-902-9*); (Illus.). 199p. 30.00 (*0-89766-901-0*) NY Acad Sci.

Beyond the Dark Cloud Vol. 1: Road to Recovery from Chronic Fatigue & Immune Dysfunction CFIDS Media Awareness. Thea Schlosser. 1996. (Illus.). 208p. (Orig.). 19.95 (*0-9653215-0-9*) T Schlosser.

Beyond the Dyad. Ed. by Michael Lewis. 1984. (Genesis of Behavior Ser.: Vol. 4). 346p. 65.00 (*0-306-41446-5*, Plenum Trade) Perseus Pubng.

Beyond the Germ Theory: The Story of Dr. Cooper Curice. Jeanne N. Logue. 1996. LC 95-21982. (Illus.). 168p. 33.95 (*0-89096-673-7*) Tex A&M Univ Pr.

Beyond the Inner & the Outer: Wittgenstein's Philosophy of Psychology. Michel Ter Hark. Tr. by Anthony P. Runia from DUT. 1990. (Synthese Library: No. 214). 356p. lib. bdg. (*0-7923-0850-6*) Kluwer Academic NLD. *Dist:* Kluwer Academic.

Beyond the Labels: "Creatively Gifted"... a Mother's Story. Elaine C. Gennari. 1995. 280p. (Orig.). pap. 12.95 (*0-9647794-0-4*) Karma Pubng.

Beyond the Mind. David Frawley. 1993. 180p. pap. 12.95 (*1-878423-14-2*) Morson Pub.

Beyond the Natural Body: An Archaeology of Sex Hormones. Nelly Oudshoorn. 1994. LC 94-4945. (Illus.). 224p. (C). pap. 27.95 (*0-415-09191-8*, A9982) Routledge.

Beyond the Nerves: The Effectiveness of Acupuncture. Robert Tien Huang. 1994. 176p. (Orig.). pap. (*0-9640207-0-X*) EO Acupuncture.

Beyond the Obvious: Bringing Intuition into Our Awakening Consciousness. Christine R. Page. 1998. pap. (*0-85207-322-4*) C W Daniel GBR. *Dist:* Natl Bk Netwk.

Beyond the Outsider. Colin Wilson. 1991. 256p. pap. 8.95 (*0-88184-704-6*) Carroll & Graf.

Beyond the Pain. Lecia J. Ritter. 2000. 65p. pap. 8.95 (*0-9701658-0-3*) Health Wealth Found.

Beyond the Pleasure Principle. Sigmund Freud. Ed. & Tr. by James Strachey. 1990. (Norton Library). 96p. reprint ed. pap. 8.95 (*0-393-00769-3*) Norton.

Beyond the Psychoanalytic Dyad: Developmental Semiotics in Freud, Peirce, & Lacan. John P. Muller. 1995. LC 95-14600. 256p. (C). 80.00 (*0-415-91068-4*); pap. 21.95 (*0-415-91069-2*) Routledge.

Beyond the Rule Book: Moral Issues & Dilemmas in the Practice of Psychotherapy. Ed. by Ellyn Kaschak & Marcia Hill. 1999. LC 99-33952. 153p. 29.95 (*0-7890-0772-X*); pap. 17.95 (*0-7890-0773-8*) Haworth Pr.

Beyond the Shame: Understanding & Treating the Child Molester. James A. Kitchens. 1991. 120p. (Orig.). (C). pap. 7.95 (*0-9624469-0-4*) Ads-Co.

Beyond the Smoke & Mirrors: Turmoil in the PPM Industry. William R. Dexheimer. 1999. LC 98-53529. 27.95 (*1-57359-018-5*, Starrhill Press) River City Pub.

Beyond the Successful Veterinary Practice: Succession Planning & Other Legal Issues. Thomas E. Catanzaro et al. 2000. LC 00-39679. (Illus.). xvii, 210p. 49.95 (*0-8138-1209-7*) Iowa U Pr.

Beyond the Unconscious: Essays of Henri F. Ellenberger in the History of Psychiatry. Ed. by Mark S. Micale. Tr. by Francoise Dubor. 1993. 488p. 65.00 (*0-691-08550-1*) Princeton U Pr.

Beyond the War on Drugs: Overcoming a Failed Public Policy. Steven Wisotsky. 1990. LC 89-70301. 319p. (C). reprint ed. pap. 25.00 (*0-87975-587-3*) Prometheus Bks.

Beyond Tomorrow: Trends & Prospects in Medical Science. 1977. LC 77-24824. 150p. pap. 2.95 (*0-87470-023-X*) Rockefeller.

Beyond Transference: When the Therapist's Real Life Intrudes. Ed. by Judith H. Gold & John C. Nemiah. 1993. LC 92-7053. 186p. text 14.95 (*0-88048-361-X*, 8361) Am Psychiatric.

Beyond Trauma: Cultural & Societal Dynamics. Ed. by Rolf J. Kleber et al. 1995. (Stress & Coping Ser.). (Illus.). 332p. (C). 49.50 (*0-306-45058-5*, Plenum Trade) Perseus Pubng.

Beyond Universals in Cognitive Development. David H. Feldman. 2nd ed. 1994. LC 94-16334. 232p. 73.25 (*1-56750-031-5*); pap. 39.50 (*1-56750-032-3*) Greenwood (Ablex).

Beyond Words: Interpretive Art Therapy. J. S. Bodtker. 1990. 158p. pap. (*0-902965-27-1*) Clunie Pr GBR. *Dist:* Other Pr LLC.

Beyond Words: The Story of Sensitivity Training & the Encounter Movement. Kurt W. Back. 1972. LC 73-182935. 266p. (Orig.). 45.00 (*0-87154-077-0*) Russell Sage.

*__Beyond Year 2000 Vol. 14, No. 3: Innovative Solutions for the Evolving Healthcare Information Management Environment,__ Vol. 14. 2000. pap. 26.00 (*0-7879-5453-5*) Jossey-Bass.

Beyond Yin & Yang. George P. Ulett. 1992. (Illus.). 172p. pap. 22.50 (*0-87527-490-0*) Green.

BH Mars Physiotherapy in Obstetrics & Gynaecology. Jill Mantle & Margaret Polden. 2002. (Illus.). 220.00 incl. disk (*0-7506-4291-2*) Buttrwrth-Heinemann.

Bharti Vyas' Two Day Treat: Perfect Wellbeing in a Weekend. Bharti Vyas. 2000. pap. (0-7225-4012-4) Thorsons GBR. *Dist:* Natl Bk Netwk.

Bias in Mental Testing. Arthur R. Jensen. 1980. LC 79-7583. (Illus.). 786p. 40.00 (0-02-916430-3) Free Pr.

Bias in Psychotherapy. Joan Murray & Paul R. Abramson. 1983. 398p. 72.95 (0-275-91050-4, C1050, Praeger Pubs) Greenwood.

Biased Selection in Health Care Markets, Vol. 6. Ed. by Richard M. Scheffler et al. 1985. (Advances in Health Economics & Health Services Research Ser.). 286p. 73.25 (0-89232-519-4) Jai Pr.

Biathanatos. John Donne. Ed. by Robert J. Kastenbaum. 1977. LC 76-19567. (Death & Dying Ser.). reprint ed. lib. bdg. 25.95 (0-405-09563-5) Ayer.

Bible & Healing: A Medical & Theological Commentary. John Wilkinson. 2000. 358p. pap. 20.00 (0-8028-4876-1) Eerdmans.

Bible for Stress Management? Maria Kuman. (Illus.). pap. 20.00 (1-893637-12-3) Hlth & Hap.

Bible Medicine with Healing Verses. George H. Brummel. 1984. LC 83-91263. 172p. (Orig.). pap. 9.95 (0-9613041-0-3) G Brummel Pub.

Bible Secret of Divine Health. Gordon Lindsay. 1960. 3.25 (0-89985-023-5) Christ for the Nations.

Bibliographic Guide to Psychology. New York Public Library Staff. 1996. 225.00 (0-7838-1339-2) Macmillan.

Bibliographic Guide to Psychology: 1987. New York Public Library Staff. 1988. 152p. 185.00 (0-8161-7094-0, Hall Reference) Macmillan.

Bibliographic Guide to Psychology: 1989. New York Public Library Staff. 1989. 150p. 200.00 (0-8161-7114-9, Macmillan Ref) Gale.

Bibliographic Guide to Psychology: 1998. 1999. 295.00 (0-7838-0228-5, Macmillan Ref) Gale.

Bibliographic Guide to Psychology 1988. Ed. by New York Public Library Staff. 1988. 190.00 (0-8161-7076-2, Macmillan Ref) Gale.

Bibliographic Guide to Psychology 1990. Ed. by New York Public Library Staff. 1991. 185.00 (0-8161-7147-5, Macmillan Ref) Gale.

Bibliographic Guide to Psychology, 1991. Research Libraries of the New York Public Library Staff & Library of Congress Staff. 1992. (Bibliographic Guides Ser.). 154p. 205.00 (0-8161-7168-8, Macmillan Ref) Gale.

Bibliographic Guide to Psychology 1992. New York Public Library Staff. 1993. 195.00 (0-8161-1681-4, Macmillan Ref) Gale.

Bibliographic Guide to Psychology 1994. New York Public Library Staff. 1995. 205.00 (0-7838-2195-6, Macmillan Ref) Gale.

Bibliographic Guide to Psychology 1996. 1997. 235.00 (0-7838-1774-6, Macmillan Ref) Gale.

Bibliographic Index of Health Education Periodicals (BIHEP) 1980 Cumulative Edition. William J. Bailey & Stephen J. Guynn. 1982. 428p. lib. bdg. 75.00 (0-941636-00-3) IN U Dept Health.

Bibliographic Management on Information in Health Science Libraries. Laurie Lynn Lightner Thompson. Ed. by Alison Bunting. 2000. LC 00-20426. (Current Practice in Health Sciences Librarianship Ser.: No. 6). (Illus.). 232p. 55.00 (0-8108-3783-8) Scarecrow.

Bibliographie Gastronomique. Georges Vicaire. 1996. (FRE.). 353p. reprint ed. 65.00 (1-888262-35-4) Martino Pubng.

Bibliographie Psychologie: Deutschsprachige Hochschulschriften & Veroffentlichungen Ausserhalb des Buchhandels 1966 bis 1980 Ed. by Monika Eichler & Margarethe Wolf. 1992. (GER.). Set. lib. bdg. (3-598-21927-X); Vol. 1. 416p. lib. bdg. (3-598-21928-8); Vol. 2. 416p. lib. bdg. (3-598-21929-6) K G Saur Verlag.

Bibliography & Resource Guide on Alcohol & Other Drugs for Social Work Educators. 1991. lib. bdg. 76.00 (0-8490-5047-2) Gordon Pr.

Bibliography for the Housing of Children with AIDS. Theresa Cameron. 1992. LC 92-10380. (CPL Bibliographies Ser.: No. 278). 10.00 (0-86602-278-3, Sage Prdcls Pr) Sage.

Bibliography of Bioethics. Ed. by LeRoy Walters & Tamar J. Kahn. Vol. 10. 1984. xi, 387p. 70.00 (0-9614448-0-0); Vol. 11. 1985. xi, 444p. 70.00 (0-9614448-1-9); Vol. 12. 1986. 475p. text 70.00 (0-9614448-2-7); Vol. 15. 1989. 601p. 70.00 (0-9614448-5-1); Vol. 16. 1990. 70.00 (0-9614448-6-X) Geo U Kennedy Inst.

Bibliography of Child Psychiatry & Child Mental Health: With a Selected List of Films. Ed. by Irving N. Berlin. 1976. LC 74-11813. 508p. 44.95 (0-87705-244-1, Kluwer Acad Hman Sci) Kluwer Academic.

Bibliography of Child Study. Louis N. Wilson. 1975. LC 74-21433. (Classics in Child Development Ser.). 360p. reprint ed. 33.95 (0-405-06482-9) Ayer.

Bibliography of Electrophoretic Studies of Biochemical Variation in Natural Vertebrate Populations. M. W. Smith et al. 1982. LC 82-62007. 105p. 19.95 (0-89672-106-X); pap. 8.00 (0-89672-105-1); ring bd. 5.00 (0-89672-104-3) Tex Tech Univ Pr.

Bibliography of Human Behavior, 7. Compiled by Hiram Caton. 1993. LC 93-3066. (Bibliographies & Indexes in Anthropology Ser.: No. 7). 600p. lib. bdg. 135.00 (0-313-27897-0, CBJ) Greenwood.

Bibliography of Lecithin: 683 References from 1793 to 1990, Extensively Annotated. Compiled by William Shurtleff & Akiko Aoyagi. 1990. (Bibliographies of Soya Ser.). 133p. spiral bd. 67.00 (0-933332-70-X) Soyfoods Center.

Bibliography of Medical & Biomedical Biography. Leslie T. Morton & Robert J. Moore. 2nd ed. 1994. LC 94-8284. 333p. (0-85967-981-0) Scolar Pr GBR. *Dist:* Ashgate Pub Co.

Bibliography of Medicine & Human Biology of Papua New Guinea. R. W. Hornabrook & G. H. Skeldon. 1989. 335p. 90.00 (0-7855-0599-7) St Mut.

Bibliography of Near Lenses & Vision Training Research. 1997. LC 97-12721. 100p. pap. 25.00 (0-943599-90-3) OEPF.

Bibliography of Noise for 1965-1970. Compiled by Mary K. Floyd. 1973. LC 72-87107. 403p. 17.00 (0-87875-029-0) Whitston Pub.

Bibliography of Noise for 1971. Compiled by Mary K. Floyd. 1973. LC 72-87107. 171p. 10.00 (0-87875-031-2) Whitston Pub.

Bibliography of Noise for 1972. Compiled by Mary K. Floyd. 1974. LC 72-87107. xvii, 126p. 10.00 (0-87875-054-1) Whitston Pub.

Bibliography of Noise for 1974. Compiled by Judith Kramer-Greene. 1976. LC 72-82107. 197p. 10.00 (0-87875-078-9) Whitston Pub.

Bibliography of Noise for 1973. Compiled by Mary K. Floyd. 1975. LC 72-87107. 164p. 10.00 (0-87875-055-X) Whitston Pub.

Bibliography of North American Indian Mental Health. Compiled by Dianne R. Kelso & Carolyn L. Attneave. 1981. LC 81-800. (Illus.). 411p. lib. bdg. 60.00 (0-313-22930-9, KEB/, Greenwood Pr) Greenwood.

Bibliography of Recent Works on Home Health Care. Ross M. Mullner & Mark Jewell. 2000. LC 00-32452. (Studies in Health & Human Services: Vol. 37). viii, 184p. 79.95 (0-7734-7763-2) E Mellen.

Bibliography of the History of Medicine. 1992. lib. bdg. 88.00 (0-8490-5256-4) Gordon Pr.

Bibliography of the History of Medicine of the United States & Canada, 1939-1960. Genevieve Miller. 1979. 37.95 (0-405-10616-5) Ayer.

Bibliography of the Writings of Harvey Cushing. Ed. by AANS Publications Committee. 3rd ed. 1993. 142p. 28.00 (1-879284-26-X) Am Assn Neuro.

Bibliography on Human Relations Training & Related Subjects. Compiled by Fred Massarik. 1985. pap. 8.00 (0-9610392-3-X) NTL Inst.

***Bibliography on Smoking & Health (1991)** Ed. by Barry Leonard. 2000. 734p. reprint ed. pap. text 65.00 (0-7567-0603-3) DIANE Pub.

***Bibliography on Smoking & Health (1992-1993) Selected Annotations.** Ed. by Barry Leonard. 2000. 505p. (C). reprint ed. pap. text 60.00 (0-7567-0604-1) DIANE Pub.

Bibliography on Smoking & Health (to 1990) Ed. by Barry Leonard. 2000. 343p. (C). reprint ed. pap. text 30.00 (0-7881-8966-2) DIANE Pub.

Bibliography on the Epidemiology of Cancer: Bibliography on the Epidemiology of Cancer: Nineteen Forty-Six to Nineteen Sixty. 1963. (ENG, FRE, RUS & SPA.). 168p. pap. text 12.00 (92-4-052000-7, 0150012) World Health.

Bibliography on Yaws. 1963. (ENG, FRE & RUS.). 106p. pap. text 9.00 (92-4-052003-1, 0150014) World Health.

Bibliotheca Chemica: A Catalogue of Alchemical & Pharmaceutical Books in the Collection of the Late James Young of Kelly & Durris, Set. John Ferguson. 1974. reprint ed. (3-487-05340-3) G Olms Pubs.

Bibliotheca Epidemiographica. Heinrich Haeser. 1971. xv, 230p. reprint ed. (3-487-04919-8) G Olms Pubs.

Bibliotheca Medicinae Practicae, Set. Albrecht V. Haller. 1987. reprint ed. (3-487-07334-X) G Olms Pubs.

Bibliotheca Medico-Historia. Johann L. Choulant. 1988. 279p. reprint ed. lib. bdg. 70.00 (3-487-00014-8) G Olms Pubs.

Bibliotheca Osleriana: A Catalogue of Books Illustrating the History of Medicine & Science. William Osler. Ed. by W. W. Francis et al. 1997. 822p. reprint ed. 95.00 (1-57898-015-1) Martino Pubng.

Bibliotherapy: A Guide to Using Books in Clinical Practice. John T. Pardeck. Ed. by Jean A. Pardeck. 1992. LC 92-49235. 168p. pap. text 59.95 (0-7734-1954-3) E Mellen.

Bibliotherapy & Its Widening Applications. Eleanor F. Brown. 1975. LC 74-28187. 414p. 37.00 (0-8108-0782-3) Scarecrow.

Bibliotherapy in Rehabilitation, Educational & Mental Health Settings. Joseph S. Zaccaria et al. 1978. pap. text 8.80 (0-87563-149-5) Stipes.

Biblisch-Talmudische Medizin: Beitraege zur Geschichte der Heilkunde und der Kultur Ueberhaupt. Julius Preuss. 1990. viii, 736p. reprint ed. 174.00 (3-8055-4976-8) S Karger.

Bicycle As a Factor in Genito Urinary Diseases, Prostratis, Prostatorrhea, or Prostatic Catarrh. H. H. Kane. 1983. 24p. pap. 10.00 (0-87556-575-1) Saifer.

Bicycle Fitness Book: Riding Your Bike for Health & Fitness. Rob Van der Plas. rev. ed. 1996. LC 89-61366. (Illus.). 143p. pap. 7.95 (0-933201-23-0) MBI Pubg.

Bien Salud: A Guide to Baja's Medical Services. Carlos Diez. Ed. by Sam Warren. Date not set. (Illus.). 200p. (Orig.). pap. 16.95 (0-945949-08-1) Warren Comns.

BIER-Steam Vessels. 1992. 7p. 62.00 (0-910275-74-2, ST45-209) Assn Adv Med Instrn.

Bifocals Without Tears. Les Swift. 1989. (C). (0-89771-745-7) Assn Brit Dispen Opticians GBR. *Dist:* St Mut.

Big Book of Health Tips. FC and A Publishing Staff. 2000. 387p. pap. 9.99 (0-915099-91-8) FC&A Pub.

Big Book Study Guide. Joe McQuany. 1986. 145p. pap. text 8.95 (1-883094-00-3) Kelly Fnd.

Big Deception. David W. Shave. 1989. LC 88-39726. 320p. (C). lib. bdg. 29.50 (0-89464-339-8) Krieger.

Big Five Personality Factors. Boele De Raad. 2000. LC 00-105124. (Illus.). vii, 128p. 24.50 (0-88937-236-5) Hogrefe & Huber Pubs.

Big Heart: Proceedings of the International School of Medical Sciences, Ettore Majorana Centre for Scientific Culture 1990, Italy. Ed. by R. D. Leachman & Angelo A. Raineri. 1994. LC 93-46071. (Ettore Majorana International Life Sciences Ser.: Vol. 14). (Illus.). 214p. text 61.00 (3-7186-5510-1) Gordon & Breach.

***Big Shot: Passion, Politics & the Struggle for an AIDS Vaccine.** Patricia Thomas. 2001. LC 2001-31959. 528p. text 27.50 (1-891620-88-6) PublicAffairs NY.

***Big Vitamin Dictionary: Unlocks the Door to Health, Nutrition & Longevity.** Michael LeVesque. 2001. 198p. pap. 9.95 (0-9706608-1-2) L Daro Prodns.

Bilateral Communication Between the Endocrine & Immune Systems. Charles J. Grossman. 1994. LC 93-26904. (Endocrinology & Metabolism Ser.: Vol. 7). 227p. 154.00 (0-387-94141-X) Spr-Verlag.

***Bilberry & Lutein: The Vision Enhancers.** Beth M. Ley. 2nd ed. 2001. LC 2001-53. (Health Learning Handbook Ser.). (Illus.). 40p. pap. 4.95 (1-890766-16-X) B L Pubns.

Bild des Menschen als Grundlage der Heilkunst see Anthroposophical Approach to Medicine: An Outline of a Spiritual Scientifically Oriented Medicine

Bildgebende Systeme in der Urologie. Ed. by H. Melchior. 1986. (Beitraege zur Urologie Ser.: Vol. 4). (GER., Illus.). xiv, 386p. 188.75 (3-8055-4335-2) S Karger.

Bile Acids: Chemistry, Physiology & Metabolism; Methods & Applications. K. D. Setchell et al. 1987. LC 71-138520. (Illus.). 604p. (C). text 155.00 (0-306-42622-6, Kluwer Plenum) Kluwer Academic.

Bile Acids & Cholesterol in Health & Disease. Ed. by G. Paumgartner et al. 1983. 350p. text 217.50 (0-85200-729-9) Kluwer Academic.

Bile Acids & Hepatobiliary Diseases - Basic Research & Clinical Application, Vol. 93. Ed. by G. Paumgartner et al. 1997. LC 97-188087. 352p. text 177.50 (0-7923-8725-2) Kluwer Academic.

Bile Acids & Immunology: Proceedings of the 86th Falk Symposium Held in Basel, Switzerland, October 17-18, 1995. Ed. by P. A. Berg & U. Leuschner. 1996. LC 96-17379. (Basel Liver Week Ser.: Pt. I). text 132.50 (0-7923-8700-7) Kluwer Academic.

Bile Acids & the Hepatobiliary System - From Basic Science to Clinical Practice: Proceedings of the 68th Falk Symposium Held in Basel, Switzerland, October 12-14, 1992. Falk Symposium Staff. Ed. by G. Paumgartner et al. 1993. LC 93-19224. text 147.00 (0-7923-8829-1) Kluwer Academic.

Bile Acids & the Liver. Ed. by G. Paumgartner et al. 1987. (Falk Symposium Ser.: No. 45). (C). text 227.50 (0-85200-675-6) Kluwer Academic.

Bile Acids As Therapeutic Agents from Basic Science to Clinical Practice. Ed. by G. Paumgartner et al. 1991. (Falk Symposium Ser.). (C). text 243.00 (0-7923-8954-9) Kluwer Academic.

Bile Acids, Cholestasis, Gallstones: Advances in Basic & Clinical Bile Acid Research: Proceedings of the Falk Symposium No. 84, Held in Berlin, Germany, June 9-10, 1995. Ed. by H. Fromm & U. Leuschner. 1996. text 206.00 (0-7923-8893-3) Kluwer Academic.

Bile Acids in Gastroenterology: Basic & Clinical Advances: Proceedings of the 80th Falk Symposium (XIII International Bile Acid Meeting), Held in San Diego, California, U. S. A. September 30-October 2, 1994. Falk Symposium 80 Staff. Ed. by A. F. Hofmann et al. 1995. LC 95-9443. text 169.00 (0-7923-8880-1) Kluwer Academic.

Bile Acids in Health & Disease. Ed. by T. C. Northfield. 1988. (C). text 156.00 (0-7462-0076-5) Kluwer Academic.

Bile Acids in Hepatobiliary Disease. Ed. by T. C. Northfield. 2000. (Falk Symposium Ser.). 368p. 190.00 (0-7923-8755-4) Kluwer Academic.

Bile Acids in Liver Diseases: Proceedings of the International Falk Workshop Held in Munich, Germany, January 26-27, 1995. Ed. by G. Paumgartner & U. Beuers. 1996. LC 95-24717. 176p. (C). text 73.50 (0-7923-8891-7) Kluwer Academic.

Bile Ducts & Bile Duct Stones. George Berci & Alfred Cuschieri. Ed. by Lisette Bralow. 1996. 320p. text 110.00 (0-7216-1488-4) Saunders.

Bilharzia: A History of Imperial Tropical Medicine. John Farley. 1991. (Cambridge History of Medicine Ser.). (Illus.). 371p. (C). text 69.95 (0-521-40086-4) Cambridge U Pr.

Biliary & Pancreatic Ductal Epithelia. Ed. by Longnecker & Alphonse E. Sirica. 1996. (Gastroenterology Ser.: Vol. 3). (Illus.). 592p. text 225.00 (0-8247-9414-1) Dekker.

Biliary Atresia: The Japanese Experience. Daniel M. Hays & Ken Kimura. 1980. LC 79-24677. (Commonwealth Fund Publications). (Illus.). 232p. 39.50 (0-674-07325-8) HUP.

Biliary Tract Radiology. Andy Adam & Plinio Rossi. 1996. LC 96-29096. (Medical Radiology Ser.). (Illus.). 504p. 259.00 (3-540-58776-4) Spr-Verlag.

Bilingual Dictionary of Dental Terms: Spanish-English & English-Spanish. Marcos Freiberg. 1990. (ENG & SPA.). 111p. 49.95 (0-7859-9284-7) Fr & Eur.

Bilingual Education, Health, & Manpower Programs. U. S. Senate Committee on Labor and Public Welfare. Ed. by Francesco Cordasco. 1978. LC 77-90563. (Bilingual-Bicultural Education in the U. S. Ser.). reprint ed. lib. bdg. 23.95 (0-405-11101-0) Ayer.

Bilingual Language, Speech, & Hearing Dictionary. Larry J. Mattes. 1985. 96p. (Orig.). pap. text 9.00 (0-930951-01-8) Acad Comm.

Bilingual Vocabulary for the Medical Profession. R. Escandon. 1982. (ENG & SPA.). 248p. pap. 17.95 (0-8288-0577-6, S 40307) Fr & Eur.

Bilingual Word Guides of the English & Spanish Language: Health & the Human Body. Armando B. Rico. (ENG & SPA.). spiral bd. (1-879219-13-1) Veracruz Pubs.

Billing Department Policy & Procedure Guideline Manual. Barbara Jenings. 1990. 55.00 (1-879575-06-X) Acad Med Sys.

***Billion-Dollar Bargain, Computer-Related Illness, Cause, Prevention & Treatment.** Anuthep Benja-Athon. 2001. (Health, Medicine & Science Ser.). (Illus.). 104p. pap. 30.00 (0-9706580-4-4) Muscle Joint.

Billion Dollar Battle: Merck vs. Glaxo. Matthew Lynn. 1993. pap. 13.95 (0-7493-1026-X) Trafalgar.

Billion Dollar Molecule: The Quest for the Perfect Drug. Barry Werth. 1995. 464p. pap. 15.00 (0-671-51057-6, Touchstone) S&S Trade Pap.

Bills of Health. Richard Lawson. 1996. LC 96-13782. (1-85775-101-9) Radcliffe Med Pr GBR. *Dist:* Balogh.

Binding & Linkage: Functional Chemistry of Biological Macromolecules. Jeffrey Wyman & Stanley Gill. 1990. (Illus.). 330p. (C). text 58.00 (0-935702-56-3) Univ Sci Bks.

Binding Proteins of Steroid Hormones. M. G. Forest & M. Pugeat. 1987. (Colloque de L'INSERM Ser.). (ENG & FRE.). 672p. pap. 85.00 (2-85598-310-X) S M P F Inc.

Bing & Haymaker's Neurological Diagnosis. Clifford B. Saper. 1995. 400p. 79.50 (0-8016-6937-5) Mosby Inc.

Binge Eating: Nature, Assessment & Treatment. Ed. by Christopher G. Fairburn & G. Terence Wilson. 1996. LC 92-48235. 419p. pap. 24.00 (0-89862-858-X, 2858) Guilford Pubns.

Binocular Anomalies: Diagnosis & Vision Therapy. John R. Griffin et al. 3rd rev. ed. 1995. LC 95-11233. (Illus.). 519p. (C). text 99.00 (0-7506-9410-6) Buttrwrth-Heinemann.

Binocular Vision: A Practical Guide. Michelle Rundstrom. 2001. 224p. pap. 63.00 (0-7506-5010-9) Buttrwrth-Heinemann.

Binocular Vision - Psychophysics. Ed. by Cronly. 1991. 137.00 (0-8493-7509-6, QP464) CRC Pr.

Binocular Vision & Ocular Motility. Gunter K. Von Noorden & Emilio C. Campos. 6th ed. Date not set. LC 2001-42586. (Illus.). 635p. text (0-323-01129-2) Mosby Inc.

Binocular Vision & Ocular Motility: Theory & Management of Strabismus. Gunter K. Von Noorden. 5th ed. 1995. (Illus.). 624p. (C). (gr. 13). text 138.00 (0-8151-9026-3, 25688) Mosby Inc.

Binocular Vision & Orthoptics Investigation & Management. Bruce Evans & Sandip Doshi. 2001. LC 2001-25320. (Illus.). 160p. pap. text 70.00 (0-7506-4713-2) Buttrwrth-Heinemann.

Binocular Vision & Stereopsis. Ian P. Howard & Brian J. Rogers. 1995. (Oxford Psychology Ser.: No. 29). (Illus.). 756p. text 145.00 (0-19-508476-4) OUP.

Bio Aerosols: Assessment & Control. Ed. by Janet Macher & American Conference of Governmental Industrial Hygenists Staff. 1998. 322p. text 89.00 (1-882417-29-1, 3180) Am Conf Govt Indus Hygienist.

Bio Behavioral Research & Psychosomatic Disorders. Ed. by D. H. Hellhammer. 1993. (Journal: Vol. 60, No. 1, 1993). (Illus.). 56p. pap. 43.50 (3-8055-5864-3) S Karger.

Bio-Etheric Healing: A Breakthrough in Alternative Therapies. Trudy Lanitis. 1999. LC 98-87550. (Illus.). 192p. pap. 14.95 (1-56184-139-0) New Falcon Pubns.

Bio-Ethics: Index of New Information & Current Research. Althea G. Skinner. 1996. LC 96-12515. 57.50 (0-7883-0940-4); pap. 47.50 (0-7883-0941-2) ABBE Pubs Assn.

Bio-Immobilization, No. C-066R. enl. rev. ed. 1994. LC 97-120149. 166p. 2850.00 (1-56965-010-1) BCC.

Bio-Incompatibility & Dialysis. Ed. by Marc E. De Broe et al. 1988. (Contributions to Nephrology Ser.: Vol. 62). (Illus.). viii, 152p. 111.50 (3-8055-4695-5) S Karger.

Bio-Informatics & Bio-Process Studies in the Physiology of Communication. Ed. by B. Rybak. 1978. (Health Communications & Informatics Biosciences Communications Ser.: Vol. 4, No. 3). (Illus.). 16.75 (3-8055-2856-6) S Karger.

Bio-Medical Fix: Human Dimensions of Bio-Medical Technologies. David L. Ellison. 1978. LC 77-91104. 171p. 58.00 (*0-313-20038-6*, ELB/, Greenwood Pr) Greenwood.

Bio-Medical Fluid Engineering. Ed. by R. A. Gerbsch & K. Ohba. 1995. LC 95-78828. (ASME/JSME Engineering Conference Ser.: FED-Vol. 212). 60p. 28.00 (*0-7918-1467-X*, G00962) ASME Pr.

Bio-Organization: Diagnosis & Theory. 3rd ed. 1992. LC 92-48847. (Regents - Prentice-Hall Medical Assistant Kit Ser.). 112p. pap. 27.13 (*0-13-225640-1*) P-H.

Bio-Organization: Diagnosis & Therapy. 1983. (Medical Ser.). (Illus.). 184p. pap. text 12.95 (*0-935920-13-7*, Ntl Pubs Blck) P-H.

Bioacoustics: A Comparative Approach. Ed. by B. Lewis. 1983. (Illus.). text 136.00 (*0-12-446550-1*) Acad Pr.

Bioactive Polymeric Systems: An Overview. Ed. by Charles G. Gebelein & Charles E. Carraher, Jr. 1985. LC 85-6399. 714p. 155.00 (*0-306-41855-X*, Plenum Trade) Perseus Pubng.

Bioadhesive Drug Delivery Systems. Ed. by Vincent M. Lenaerts & Robert Gurny. 1989. LC 96-21434. (Illus.). 272p. lib. bdg. 210.00 (*0-8493-5367-X*, RS201) CRC Pr.

Bioadhesive Drug Delivery Systems: Fundamentals, Novel Approaches & Development. Edith Mathiowitz et al. 1999. LC 99-32806. (Drugs & the Pharmaceutical Sciences Ser.: Vol. 98). (Illus.). xv, 670p. text 225.00 (*0-8247-1995-6*) Dekker.

Bioanalysis of Anticancer Drugs. Ernst A. Debruijn & Ubbo R. Tjaden. 1999. 120.00 (*0-8493-8977-1*) CRC Pr.

Bioanalysis of Drugs & Metabolites: Especially Anti-Inflammatory & Cardiovascular. Ed. by E. Reid et al. 1988. LC 88-22412. (Methodological Surveys in Biochemistry & Analysis Ser.: Vol. 18). (Illus.). 430p. 110.00 (*0-306-42996-9*, Plenum Trade) Perseus Pubng.

Bioartificial Organs Vol. 831: Science Medicine, & Technology. Ed. by Ales Prokop et al. 1997. LC 97-46923. 100.00 (*1-57331-098-0*) NY Acad Sci.

Bioartificial Organs Vol. 831: Science, Medicine, & Technology. Ales Prokop et al. 1997. (Annals of the New York Academy of Sciences Ser.). pap. 100.00 (*1-57331-099-9*) NY Acad Sci.

***Bioartificial Organs III: Tissue Sourcing, Immunoisolation & Clinical Trials.** David J. Hunkeler. 2001. 400p. 140.00 (*1-57331-342-4*) NY Acad Sci.

Bioartificial Organs II: Technology, Medicine & Materials. Ed. by David J. Hunkeler et al. 1999. LC 99-26595. (Annals of the New York Academy of Sciences Ser.: Vol. 875). (Illus.). xii, 415p. lib. bdg. 140.00 (*1-57331-194-4*) NY Acad Sci.

Bioavailability, Bioequivalence & Therapeutic Substitutions. Umesh V. Banakar. 1995. 300p. ring bd. 139.95 (*1-56676-350-9*) CRC Pr.

Bioavailability of Drugs: Proceedings. Conference on Bioavailability of Drugs, Washington. Ed. by B. B. Brodie & W. M. Heller. 1972. (Pharmacology Ser.: Vol. 8, Nos. 1-3). (Illus.). 56.75 (*3-8055-1456-5*) S Karger.

Bioavailability of Drugs - Principles & Problems: Proceedings of the WHO Scientific Group, Geneva, 1973. WHO Staff. 1974. (Technical Reports: No. 536). pap. text 4.00 (*92-4-120536-9*, 1100536) World Health.

Bioavailability of Nutrients for Animals: Amino Acids, Minerals, Vitamins. Ed. by Clarence B. Ammerman et al. 1995. LC 95-10078. (Illus.). 441p. text 69.00 (*0-12-056250-2*) Acad Pr.

***Biobased Economy of the Twenty-First Century: Agriculture Expanding into Health, Energy, Chemicals & Materials.** Ed. by Allan E. Aglesham et al. 2001. (Illus.). 196p. (C). pap. 25.00 (*0-7567-1033-2*) DIANE Pub.

***Biobehavioral Assessment of the Infant.** Ed. by Lynn T. Singer & Philip Sanford Zeskind. 2001. LC 2001-23247. (Illus.). xix, 476p. text 60.00 (*1-57230-669-6*) Guilford Pubns.

Biobehavioral Control of AIDS. Ed. by David G. Ostrow. 1987. (Illus.). 250p. (C). text 29.50 (*0-8290-2354-2*) Irvington.

Biobehavioral Measures of Dyslexia. Ed. by David Gray & James Kavanagh. 1985. LC 85-52392. 328p. text 33.00 (*0-912752-10-6*) York Pr.

Biobehavioral Self-Regulation: Eastern & Western Perspectives. Ed. by T. Kikuchi et al. 1995. (Illus.). 752p. 350.00 (*4-431-70153-2*) Spr-Verlag.

Bioceramics O. H. Andersson et al. 1996. pap. 469.00 (*0-08-042687-5*, Pergamon Pr) Elsevier.

Bioceramics. James F. Shackelford. 1999. 96p. text (*90-5699-612-6*) GBSP NLD. *Dist:* Gordon & Breach.

Bioceramics J. Wilson et al. 1996. 353.00 (*0-08-042686-7*, Pergamon Pr) Elsevier.

Bioceramics, Vol.6. P. Ducheyne & D. Christiansen. 1994. 528p. text 135.00 (*0-7506-1884-1*) Buttrwrth-Heinemann.

Bioceramics: Applications of Ceramic & Glass Materials in Medicine. Ed. by James F. Shackelford. 1998. (Materials Science Forum Ser.: Vol. 293). (Illus.). 120p. (C). text (*0-87849-822-2*) Trans T Pub CHE. *Dist:* Enfield Pubs NH.

Bioceramics: Materials & Applications. Ed. by Gary S. Fischman et al. 1995. (Ceramic Transactions Ser.: Vol. 48). 88.00 (*0-944904-82-3*, CT048) Am Ceramic.

Bioceramics: Materials & Applications II. Ed. by Richard P. Rusin & Gary S. Fischman. 1996. LC 96-295. (Ceramic Transactions Ser.: Vol. 63). 95.00 (*1-57498-006-8*, CT063) Am Ceramic.

Bioceramics: Proceedings of 10th International Symposium on Ceramics in Medicine, Paris, France, 5-8 October 1997, Vol. 10. Ed. by L. Sedel & C. Rey. 1997. 632p. 244.50 (*0-08-042692-1*, Pergamon Pr) Elsevier.

Bioceramics Vol. 8: Proceedings of the 8th International Symposium on Ceramics in Medicine, Florida, U.S.A. November, 1995. Ed. by J. Wilson et al. 1995. 552p. 199.50 (*0-08-042677-8*, Pergamon Pr) Elsevier.

Biochemic System of Medicine. George W. Carey. 26th ed. 1996. 535p. spiral bd. 38.50 (*0-7873-0144-2*) Hlth Research.

Biochemical & Clinical Aspects of Pteridines Vol. 2: Cancer, Immunology, Metabolic Diseases: Proceedings, Second Winter Workshop on Pterdines, March 6-9, 1983, St. Christoph, Arlberg, Austria. Ed. by H. Wachter et al. 1984. LC 83-24079. xv, 435p. 173.10 (*3-11-009813-X*) De Gruyter.

Biochemical & Immunologic Diagnosis of Cancer. Ed. by A. M. Neville. 1987. (Tumor Biology Ser.: Vol. 8, No. 2-3, 1987). (Illus.). 124p. pap. 71.50 (*3-8055-4665-3*) S Karger.

Biochemical & Molecular Aspects of Selected Cancers, Vol. 2. Ed. by Thomas G. Pretlow, II & Theresa P. Pretlow. 1994. (Illus.). 542p. text 136.00 (*0-12-564499-X*) Acad Pr.

***Biochemical & Physiological Aspects of Human Nutrition.** Martha H. Stipanuk. 2000. (Illus.). 1007p. tchr. ed. 75.00 (*0-7216-4453-8*) Saunders.

Biochemical Approach to Nutrition. R. A. Freedland & S. Briggs. 1977. pap. 13.95 (*0-412-13040-8*, NO.6113) Chapman & Hall.

Biochemical Aspects of Insect Development. P. S. Chen. 1971. (Monographs in Developmental Biology: Vol. 3). (Illus.). 62.75 (*3-8055-1265-1*) S Karger.

Biochemical Aspects of Renal Function: Journal: Renal Physiology & Biochemistry, Vol. 12, Nos. 5 & 6, 1989. Ed. by W. G. Guder. 1989. (Illus.). iv, 124p. pap. 102.75 (*3-8055-5119-3*) S Karger.

Biochemical Aspects of Renal Function: Proceedings of a Symposium Held in Honour of Professor Sir Hans Krebs FRS, at Merton College, Oxford, 16-19 September 1979. Ed. by D. B. Ross & W. G. Guder. 1980. (Illus.). 340p. pap. 67.00 (*0-08-025517-5*, Pergamon Pr) Elsevier.

Biochemical Bases of the Development of Physiological Functions. Ed. by Olga Greengard. 1974. (Enzyme Ser.: Vol. 15, Nos. 1-6). (Illus.). 386p. pap. 83.50 (*3-8055-1713-0*) S Karger.

Biochemical Basis of Inherited Human Disease. Shintaro Okada et al. 1973. 32.50 (*0-8422-7087-6*) Irvington.

Biochemical Basis of Neuropharmacology. Jack R. Cooper et al. 7th ed. 1996. (Illus.). 528p. (C). text 57.50 (*0-19-510398-X*); pap. text 32.50 (*0-19-510399-8*) OUP.

Biochemical Basis of Pediatric Disease. Steven J. Soldin et al. 3rd ed. 1998. LC 98-19476. 663p. pap. 85.00 (*1-890883-01-8*, AACC Pr) Am Assn Clinical Chem.

Biochemical Basis Plant Breeding: Carbon Metabolism, Vol. I. Carlos A. Neyra. 1985. 176p. 106.00 (*0-8493-5741-1*, SB123, CRC Reprint) Franklin.

Biochemical Mechanisms in Heart Function. Ed. by Ernst-Georg Krause. 1996. (Developments in Molecular & Cellular Biochemistry Ser.). 332p. (C). text 314.50 (*0-7923-4118-X*) Kluwer Academic.

Biochemical Messengers: Hormones, Neurotransmitters & Growth Factors. D. Grahame Hardie. 250p. 1991. (gr. 13). pap. 54.95 (*0-412-30350-7*, A5003); 1990. 65.00 (*0-412-30340-X*, A4999) Chapman & Hall.

Biochemical Methodology for the Assessment of Carotenes. Kenneth L. Simpson et al. 1987. (Illus.). 47p. (Orig.). pap. 9.00 (*0-944398-01-4*) ILSI.

Biochemical Methods for Monitoring Risk Pregnancies. Ed. by P. J. Keller. 1976. (Contributions to Gynecology & Obstetrics Ser.: Vol. 2). 136.75 (*3-8055-2386-6*) S Karger.

Biochemical Modulation: Its Pharmacological Basis & Clinical Applications Symposium, Singapore, October 1995. Ed. by Low Cheng Hock. 1996. (Journal: Vol. 54, Supplement 1, 1997). (Illus.). iv, 40p. pap. 24.50 (*3-8055-6450-3*) S Karger.

Biochemical Monitoring of the Fetus. Ed. by Molly S. Chatterjee. 1993. LC 93-1477. (Illus.). 89p. 49.95 (*0-387-97892-5*) Spr-Verlag.

Biochemical, Pharmacological & Clinical Aspects of Nitric Oxide: Proceedings of the 38th OHOLO Conference Held in Eilat, Israel, April 17-21, 1994. Ed. by Ben A. Weissman et al. 1995. 260p. 89.50 (*0-306-45113-1*, Kluwer Plenum) Kluwer Academic.

Biochemical Pharmacology As an Approach to Gastrointestinal Disorders Basic Science to Clinical Perspectives (1996) Ed. by Timothy S. Gaginella. 1997. LC 97-203803. 408p. text 227.50 (*0-7923-8719-8*) Kluwer Academic.

Biochemical Pharmacology of Blood & Blood-Forming Organs. Ed. by J. W. Fisher et al. 1992. (Handbook of Experimental Pharmacology Ser.: Vol. 101). (Illus.). 587p. 447.00 (*0-387-52844-X*) Spr-Verlag.

Biochemical Profiling in the Dog & Cat. A. H. Rebar et al. 1999. (Illus.). 108p. (*0-9678005-4-4*) Gloyd Grp Inc.

Biochemical Protozoology As a Basis for Drug Design. Ed. by Graham H. Coombs. 1991. 500p. (*0-7484-0000-1*); pap. (*0-7484-0001-X*) Tay Francis Ltd GBR. *Dist:* Taylor & Francis.

Biochemical Regulation of Myocardium. Ernst-Georg Krause. Ed. by Roland Vetter. 1996. LC 96-38430. (Developments in Molecular & Cellular Biochemistry Ser.). 336p. (C). text 314.50 (*0-7923-4259-3*) Kluwer Academic.

Biochemical Techniques: Theory & Practice. John F. Robyt & Bernard J. White. 1987. LC 86-26874. (Chemistry). 400p. 35.25 (*0-534-07944-X*) Brooks-Cole.

Biochemical Techniques in the Heart. Ed. by John H. McNeill. 1996. LC 96-2903. (Methods in the Life Sciences-Methods in Pharmacology Ser.). 144p. spiral bd. 74.95 (*0-8493-3333-4*) CRC Pr.

Biochemical Tests for Identification of Medical Bacteria. Jean F. MacFaddin. 3rd ed. 2000. 928p. spiral bd. 58.50 (*0-683-05318-3*) Lppncott W & W.

Biochemist. Jack Rudman. 1994. (Career Examination Ser.: C-85). pap. 29.95 (*0-8373-0085-1*) Nat Learn.

Biochemistry. Guttenplan. 1994. (Blond's Medical Guides Ser.). (Illus.). 264p. (C). pap. text 19.99 (*0-945819-49-8*) Sulzburger & Graham Pub.

Biochemistry. Alex F. Huang. 1993. (Licensing Examination Review Pop-up Book Series for Advanced Medical Study). 96p. (C). pap. text 35.95 (*1-884142-03-6*) AFH Softech.

Biochemistry. Olf. 1994. pap. text 36.00 (*0-443-05272-7*) Saunders.

Biochemistry. Michael S. Matta & Antony C. Wilbraham. 2nd ed. 1986. LC 85-15765. (Illus.). 800p. (C). pap. text, tchr. ed. 20.50 (*0-8053-9633-0*) Benjamin-Cummings.

Biochemistry: A Case-Oriented Approach. Rex Montgomery & Chappell. 6th ed. 1996. (Illus.). 704p. (C). (gr. 13). pap. text 57.00 (*0-8151-6483-1*, 26342) Mosby Inc.

Biochemistry: A Review with Questions. Paul J. Friedman. 3rd ed. 1987. 23.50 (*0-316-29374-1*, Little Brwn Med Div) Lppncott W & W.

Biochemistry: An Essential Slide Collection. David J. Williams. 1988. 121p. (gr. 13). text incl. sl. (*0-397-46424-X*, GM0096) Gower-Mosby.

Biochemistry: Mosby's USMLE Step 1 Reviews. John W. Pelley. 1996. LC 96-41726. (Ace the Boards Ser.). (Illus.). 400p. (C). (gr. 13). pap. text 29.95 (*0-8151-8652-5*, 28894); pap. text 29.95 (*0-8151-8668-1*, 28947) Mosby Inc.

Biochemistry: Review for USMLE, Step I. Ajit Kumar et al. 2nd ed. 2001. 260p. pap. 25.00 (*1-888308-10-9*) J & S Pub VA.

Biochemistry: The Molecular Basis of Cell Structure & Function. Albert L. Lehninger. 2nd ed. 1975. LC 75-11082. 1104p. text 84.95 (*0-87901-047-9*) Worth.

Biochemistry & Genetic Regulation of Commercially Important Antibiotics. Ed. by L. P. Vining. 1983. LC 83-2492. (Biotechnology Ser.: No. 2). (Illus.). 370p. (C). text (*0-201-10984-0*) Addison-Wesley.

***Biochemistry & Genetics: Self-Assessment & Review.** Golder Wilson. 2001. (Pretest Basic Sciences Ser.). (Illus.). 300p. pap. 24.95 (*0-07-137578-3*) McGraw-Hill Prof.

Biochemistry & Microbiology of the Female & Male Genital Tracts. 1965. (Technical Report Ser.: No. 313). 15p. pap. text 3.00 (*92-4-120313-7*) World Health.

Biochemistry & Molecular Biology. Ed. by R. Brambl & George A. Marzluf. 1996. (Mycota Ser.: Vol. 3). (Illus.). 456p. 229.00 (*3-540-58004-2*) Spr-Verlag.

Biochemistry & Molecular Genetics of Cancer Metastasis. Ed. by Karoly Lapis et al. 1986. (Developments in Oncology Ser.). text 127.00 (*0-89838-785-X*) Kluwer Academic.

Biochemistry & Pathology of Basement Membranes: Proceedings of the Colloquium, Paris, October 14-15, 1977. International Colloquium, Paris Staff. Ed. by L. Robert. 1979. (Frontiers of Matrix Biology Ser.: Vol. 7). (Illus.). 125.75 (*3-8055-2894-9*) S Karger.

Biochemistry & Pharmacology of Free Fatty Acids. Ed. by W. L. Holmes & W. M. Bortz. 1971. (Progress in Biochemical Pharmacology Ser.: Vol. 6). 84.50 (*3-8055-1211-2*) S Karger.

Biochemistry & Physiology of Bifidobacteria. Anatoly Bezkorovainy & Robin Miller-Catchpole. 1989. 192p. lib. bdg. 269.00 (*0-8493-4753-X*, QR82) CRC Pr.

Biochemistry & Physiology of Substance Abuse Ed. by Ronald R. Watson. Vol. 1. 1989. 264p. 199.95 (*0-8493-4461-1*, RC564); Vol. 2. 1990. 304p. 217.95 (*0-8493-4462-X*); Vol. 3. 1990. 304p. 219.00 (*0-8493-4463-8*, RC564) CRC Pr.

Biochemistry Collections: A Cross-Disciplinary Survey of the Literature. Ed. by Bernard S. Schlessinger. 1982. LC 81-13408. (Special Collections: Vol. 1, No. 2). 147p. 4.95 (*0-917724-48-8*) Haworth Pr.

Biochemistry for Medical Sciences. Isidore Danishefsky. 1980. text 34.00 (*0-316-17198-0*) Little.

Biochemistry for the Medical Sciences. Newsholme. 2nd ed. pap. (*0-471-93165-9*) Wiley.

Biochemistry Lab Manual. Mark C. Morvant. 1999. (C). pap. text 13.81 (*1-56870-364-3*) RonJon Pub.

Biochemistry of Alcohol & Alcoholism. P. M. Clark & Larry J. Kricka. 1979. LC 79-40252. (Chemical Science Ser.). 285p. 104.95 (*0-470-26712-7*) P-H.

Biochemistry of Arachidonic Acid Metabolism. Ed. by William E. Lands. 1985. LC 85-4853. (Prostaglandins, Leukotrienes, & Cancer Ser.). text 176.50 (*0-89838-717-5*) Kluwer Academic.

Biochemistry of Cellular Regulation Vol. I: Gene Expression. Michael J. Clemens. 1980. 288p. 157.00 (*0-8493-5454-4*, QH450, CRC Reprint) Franklin.

Biochemistry of Cellular Regulation Vol. III: Development & Differentiation. Margaret E. Buckingham. 1981. 272p. 151.00 (*0-8493-5456-0*, QH607, CRC Reprint) Franklin.

Biochemistry of Cellular Regulation Vol. IV: The Cell Surface. Ed. by Peter Knox. 1981. 336p. 184.00 (*0-8493-5457-9*, QH607, CRC Reprint) Franklin.

Biochemistry of Exercise & Training. Ron Maughan et al. 1997. LC 97-31837. (Illus.). 256p. text 95.00 (*0-19-262742-2*); pap. text 52.50 (*0-19-262741-4*) OUP.

Biochemistry of Exercise IX. Ed. by Ron J. Maughan & Susan M. Shirreffs. 1996. LC 96-10897. (International Series on Sport Sciences: Vol. 9). (Illus.). 608p. text 72.00 (*0-88011-486-X*, BMAU0486) Human Kinetics.

Biochemistry of Foreign Compounds. D. V. Parke. 1968. (*0-08-012202-7*) Pergamon Repr GBR. *Dist:* Franklin.

Biochemistry of Gene Expression in Higher Organisms: Proceedings. Ed. by J. K. Pollak & J. W. Lee. 1973. LC 72-97960. 656p. text 283.50 (*90-277-0289-6*) Kluwer Academic.

Biochemistry of Human Nutrition: A Desk Reference. Eva M. Hamilton & Sareen S. Gropper. 1987. (Illus.). 324p. (Orig.). (C). pap. 42.95 (*0-314-29520-8*) West Pub.

Biochemistry of Human Nutrition: A Desk Reference. Sareen S. Gropper. 2nd ed. 2000. LC 99-44550. (Health Sciences Ser.). 325p. pap. text 60.95 (*0-534-51543-6*) Wadsworth Pub.

Biochemistry of Hypertension. Ed. by J. Rosenthal et al. 1988. (Journal: Vol. 6, No. 3-4, 1988). (Illus.). 124p. pap. 58.50 (*3-8055-4849-4*) S Karger.

Biochemistry of Inflammation. Ed. by J. T. Wicher & S. W. Evansa. 1992. (Immunology & Medicine Ser.). (C). text 195.50 (*0-7923-8985-9*) Kluwer Academic.

Biochemistry of Mental Disorders: Proceedings of the WHO Scientific Group, Geneva, 1968. WHO Staff. 1969. (Technical Reports: No. 427). pap. text 5.00 (*92-4-120427-3*, 1100427) World Health.

Biochemistry of Migraine. Ed. by M. J. Eadie & J. H. Tyrer. 1985. text 171.00 (*0-85200-731-0*) Kluwer Academic.

Biochemistry of Neuroectodermal Tumors. Gerry Melino. 1994. 129p. pap. text 180.00 (*3-7186-5500-4*, Harwood Acad Pubs) Gordon & Breach.

Biochemistry of Neuroectodermal Tumors. Ed. by Gerry Melino et al. 1990. (Clinical Chemistry & Enzymology Communications Ser.). iv, 178p. pap. text 293.00 (*3-7186-5019-3*) Gordon & Breach.

Biochemistry of Neuroectodermal Tumors, Pt. I. Gerry Melino. 1994. 130p. pap. text 182.00 (*3-7186-5491-1*, Harwood Acad Pubs) Gordon & Breach.

Biochemistry of Non-Protein Amino Acids. Bell & Bruce Nash. 1998. (Biochemistry of Natural Products Ser.). (Illus.). 250p. pap. 99.95 (*0-412-58720-3*, Chap & Hall NY) Chapman & Hall.

Biochemistry of Normal & Abnormal Epidermal Differentiation. Ed. by I. A. Bernstein & M. Seiji. 1981. (Current Problems in Dermatology Ser.: Vol. 10). (Illus.). x, 442p. pap. 118.50 (*3-8055-1915-X*) S Karger.

Biochemistry of Peptide Antibiotics: Recent Advances in the Biotechnology of B-Lactams & Microbial Peptides. Ed. by Horst Kleinkauf & Hans Von Dohren. 1990. (Illus.). xiv, 522p. (C). lib. bdg. 238.50 (*3-11-011928-5*) De Gruyter.

Biochemistry of Pulmonary Emphysema. Ed. by C. Grassi et al. 1992. LC 92-2315. (Current Topics in Rehabilitation Ser.). (Illus.). 200p. 62.95 (*0-387-19775-3*) Spr-Verlag.

Biochemistry of Smooth Muscle. Ed. by Newman L. Stephens. 1983. Vol. I. 208p. 121.00 (*0-8493-6575-9*, QP321); Vol. II. 304p. 168.00 (*0-8493-6576-7*, QP321); Vol. III. 208p. 163.00 (*0-8493-6577-5*) Franklin (CRC Reprint).

Biochemistry of Smooth Muscle Contraction. Ed. by Michael Barany. 1995. LC 95-23967. (Illus.). 434p. text 115.00 (*0-12-078160-3*) Acad Pr.

Biochemistry of Steroidal Alkaloids. Roddick. 1999. (Illus.). 224p. pap. 99.95 (*0-412-58710-6*, Chap & Hall NY) Chapman & Hall.

Biochemistry of Sulfur. R. J. Huxtable. 1986. (Biochemistry of the Elements Ser.: Vol. 6). (Illus.). 460p. (C). text 120.00 (*0-306-42348-0*, Kluwer Plenum) Kluwer Academic.

Biochemistry of the Cardiac Glycosides. Malcolm. 1999. (Biochemistry of Natural Products Ser.). (Illus.). 250p. pap. 95.00 (*0-412-55540-9*, Chap & Hall NY) Chapman & Hall.

Biochemistry of the Eye. David R. Whikehart. (Illus.). 1994. LC 94-7076. 198p. pap. text 54.99 (*0-7506-9074-7*); 2nd ed. 2001. 224p. pap. 49.50 (*0-7506-7152-1*) Buttrwrth-Heinemann.

Biochemistry of the Human Body. Peter G. Markow. 1994. 80p. (C). 19.18 (*1-56870-030-X*) RonJon Pub.

Biochemistry of Vitamin A. Ed. by Jagannath Ganguly. 1989. 240p. 210.00 (*0-8493-6890-1*, QP772) CRC Pr.

Biochemistry of Vitamin B6 & PQQ. Ed. by G. Marino et al. 1994. LC 94-38750. (Advances in Life Sciences Ser.). (Illus.). 384p. 99.00 (*0-8176-5067-9*) Birkhauser.

Biochemistry Review for Windows. Alex F. Huang. 1998. (Licensing Examination Review Pop-Up Book Series for Advanced Medical Study). 128p. (C). pap. 69.95 (*1-884142-10-9*) AFH Softech.

Biologic Markers in Immunotoxicology. National Research Council Staff. 1992. 224p. (C). pap. text 37.95 (*0-309-04389-1*) Natl Acad Pr.

Biologic Markers in Urinary Toxicology. National Research Council Staff. Ed. by Subcommittee on Biologic Markers in Urinary Toxico. 1995. LC 94-69722. 210p. (Orig.). (C). pap. text 34.00 (*0-309-05228-9*) Natl Acad Pr.

Biologic Markers of Pulmonary Toxicology. National Research Council Staff. 1989. 196p. text 34.95 (*0-309-03992-4*); pap. text 24.95 (*0-309-03990-8*) Natl Acad Pr.

Biologic Rhythms in Clinical Laboratory & Medicine. Ed. by E. Haus & Yvan Touitou. 1994. (Illus.). 748p. 159.00 (*0-387-57592-8*) Spr-Verlag.

Biologic System Evaluation with Ultrasound. J. F. Greenleaf & C. M. Sehgal. 1992. (Illus.). 127p. 79.95 (*0-387-97851-8*) Spr-Verlag.

Biological Activities of Complement: Proceedings of the International Symposium of the Canadian Society for Immunology, 5th, Guleph, 1970. Canadian Society for Immunology Staff. Ed. by D. G. Ingram. 1972. (Illus.). 73.25 (*3-8055-1310-0*) S Karger.

Biological Aging Measurement: Clinical Applications. Ward Dean. Ed. by Hans U. Weber. 2nd ed. 1988. (Illus.). 472p. pap. text, per. 59.95 (*0-937777-00-5*) Ctr Bio-Gerontology.

Biological Aide. Jack Rudman. 1994. (Career Examination Ser.: C-86). pap. 27.95 (*0-8373-0086-X*) Nat Learn.

Biological & Behavioral Determinants of Language Development. Ed. by Richard L. Schiefelbusch et al. 1991. 544p. (C). text 145.00 (*0-8058-0635-0*); pap. 75.00 (*0-8058-0993-7*) L Erlbaum Assocs.

Biological & Clinical Aspects of Phagocyte Function: (International Congress, Pavia, Italy, Sept. 1986) C. Mauri. Ed. by M. Corn & Stuart Roath. 1986. (Hematology Reviews & Communications Ser.: Vol. 1). vii, 182p. pap. text 235.00 (*3-7186-0354-3*) Gordon & Breach.

Biological & Clinical Basis of Infectious Diseases. Stanford T. Shulman et al. Ed. by William Schmitt. 5th ed. 1996. 704p. pap. text 62.00 (*0-7216-5948-9*) Saunders.

Biological & Hormonal Therapies of Cancer. Ed. by Kenneth A. Foon & Hyman B. Muss. 1998. LC 97-28807. (Cancer Treatment & Research Ser.). 304p. 295.00 (*0-7923-9997-8*) Kluwer Academic.

Biological & Medical Research in Space: An Overview of Life Sciences Research in Microgravity. Ed. by David Moore et al. 1996. LC 95-49025. (Illus.). 569p. 148.00 (*3-540-60636-X*) Spr-Verlag.

Biological & Neurobehavioral Studies of Borderline Personality Disorder. Ed. by Kenneth R. Silk. 1994. LC 93-44846. (Progress in Psychiatry Ser.: Vol. 45). 288p. text 36.00 (*0-88048-480-2*, 8480) Am Psychiatric.

Biological & Neuropsychological Mechanisms: Life-Span Developmental Psychology. Ed. by Hayne W. Reese & Michael D. Franzen. 1997. LC 96-17641. (West Virginia Conference on Life-Span Developmental Psychology Ser.). 264p. 59.95 (*0-8058-1152-4*) L Erlbaum Assocs.

Biological & Psychological Aspects of Orofacial Pain. Sessle et al. Ed. by Christian S. Stohler & David S. Carlson. 1994. (Craniofacial Growth Ser.: Vol. 29). (Illus.). 195p. 55.00 (*0-929921-25-9*) UM CHGD.

Biological & Psychological Factors in Cardiovascular Disease. Ed. by T. F. Schmidt et al. 1986. (Illus.). 628p. 77.95 (*0-387-16577-0*) Spr-Verlag.

Biological Anomalies No. I: Humans I. William R. Corliss. 1992. LC 91-68541. (Catalog of Biological Anomalies Ser.). (Illus.). 304p. 19.95 (*0-915554-26-7*) Sourcebook.

Biological Anomalies No. II: Humans II. William R. Corliss. 1993. LC 91-68541. (Catalog of Biological Anomalies Ser.). (Illus.). 297p. (C). 19.95 (*0-915554-27-5*) Sourcebook.

Biological Anomalies No. III: Humans III. William R. Corliss. 1984. LC 91-68541. (Catalog of Biological Anomalies Ser.). (Illus.). 206p. 19.95 (*0-915554-29-1*) Sourcebook.

Biological Applications of Anti-Idiotypes Constantin A. Bona. 1988. 224p. Vol. I. 120.00 (*0-8493-6941-X*, QR186); Vol. II. 114.00 (*0-8493-6942-8*, QR186) Franklin (CRC Reprint).

Biological Approaches & Novel Applications for Molecular Nanotechnology. Ed. by Shelley Minden. 1997. (Biomedical Library). pap. (*1-57936-029-7*) Drug & Market Dev.

Biological Approaches to Rational Drug Design. Ed. by David B. Weiner & William V. Williams. 1994. LC 94-11157. (Pharmacology & Toxicology Ser.). 208p. 141.95 (*0-8493-9422-8*) CRC Pr.

Biological Aspects of Affective Disorders. Ed. by Roger Horton & Cornelius L. Katona. 1991. (Neuroscience Perspectives Ser.). (Illus.). 359p. text 74.00 (*0-12-356510-3*) Acad Pr.

Biological Aspects of Alcohol Consumption. O. Forsander & K. Eriksson. 1972. (Finnish Foundation for Alcohol Studies: Vol. 20). pap. 6.50 (*951-9192-09-3*) Rutgers Ctr Alcohol.

Biological Aspects of Alcoholism: Implications for Prevention, Treatment, & Policy, No. 4. Boris Tabakoff & Paula L. Hoffman. rev. ed. 1995. LC 94-19261. (WHO Expert Series on Neuroscience: Vol. 4). (Illus.). 312p. text 39.00 (*0-88937-130-X*) Hogrefe & Huber Pubs.

Biological Aspects of Alzheimer's Disease. Ed. by Robert Katzman. 1983. LC 82-19713. (Banbury Reports: No. 15). 495p. 55.00 (*0-87969-213-8*) Cold Spring Harbor.

Biological Aspects of Brain Tumors: Proceedings of the 8th Nikko Brain Tumor Conference Karatsu (Saga) 1990. Ed. by K. Tabuchi. 1991. (Illus.). 512p. 205.00 (*0-387-70078-1*) Spr-Verlag.

Biological Aspects of Disease: Contributions from Animal Models. Philip M. Iannaccone & Dante G. Scarpelli. 1997. 400p. text 60.00 (*3-7186-0612-7*); pap. text 34.95 (*3-7186-0613-5*) Gordon & Breach.

*__Biological Aspects of Mental Health Nursing.__ Shupi Rinomhota & Paul Marshall. 2001. (Illus.). 245p. pap. (*0-443-05990-X*) Church GBR. *Dist:* Saunders.

Biological Barriers in Behavioral Medicine. W. Linden. 1988. LC 87-36137. (Behavioral Psychophysiology Ser.). (Illus.). 348p. (C). 75.00 (*0-306-42651-X*, Plenum Trade) Perseus Pubng.

Biological Barriers to Protein Delivery. K. L. Audus & T. L. Raub. 1993. (Pharmaceutical Biotechnology Ser.: Vol. 4). (Illus.). 522p. (C). text 110.00 (*0-306-44368-6*, Kluwer Plenum) Kluwer Academic.

Biological Bases of Brain Function & Disease. Ed. by Alan Frazer. 1993. LC 93-16859. 464p. text 69.00 (*0-7817-0089-2*); pap. text 59.95 (*0-7817-0085-X*) Lppncott W & W.

Biological Basis & Therapy of Neuroses. Ed. by Ashoka J. Prasad. 1988. 208p. 119.00 (*0-8493-4899-4*, RC530, CRC Reprint) Franklin.

Biological Basis for Dose Limitation in the Skin. ICRP Staff. 1992. (International Commission on Radiological Protection Ser.: Vol. 59). 112p. pap. 62.50 (*0-08-041143-6*, Pergamon Pr) Elsevier.

Biological Basis for Mind Body Interactions. Ed. by E. Mayer & C. Saper. 2000. LC 99-59943. (Progress in Brain Research Ser.). 544p. 199.50 (*0-444-50049-9*, Excerpta Medica) Elsevier.

Biological Basis for Risk Assessment of Dioxins & Related Compounds. Ed. by Michael A. Gallo et al. 1991. (Banbury Reports: No. 35). (Illus.). 400p. (C). text 95.00 (*0-87969-235-9*) Cold Spring Harbor.

Biological Basis of Cancer. Robert G. McKinnell et al. 1998. LC 97-42369. (Illus.). 398p. (C). text 120.00 (*0-521-59298-4*); pap. text 47.95 (*0-521-59695-5*) Cambridge U Pr.

Biological Basis of Clinical Effect of Bleomycin. Ed. by A. Caputo. 1976. (Progress in Biochemical Pharmacology Ser.: Vol. 11). (Illus.). 200p. 110.50 (*3-8055-2338-6*) S Karger.

Biological Basis of Early Human Reproductive Failure: Applications to Medically-Assisted Conception. Ed. by Jonathan Van Blerkom. 1994. (Illus.). 464p. text 89.50 (*0-19-506036-9*) OUP.

Biological Basis of Human Behavior. Ed. by Robert W. Sussman. 2nd ed. 1998. LC 98-25995. 448p. (C). pap. text 46.00 (*0-13-799735-3*) P-H.

Biological Basis of Human Behavior. Ed. by Robert W. Sussman. 1997. 466p. (C). reprint ed. pap. text 69.00 (*0-536-59846-0*) Pearson Custom.

Biological Basis of Mental Activity. John I. Hubbard. 1975. 224p. (C). pap. (*0-201-03086-1*) Addison-Wesley.

Biological Basis of Oncologic Thermotherapy. C. Sterffer et al. 1990. (Clinical Thermology Ser.: Vol. 1). (Illus.). 169p. 118.00 (*0-387-51432-5*, 3612) Spr-Verlag.

Biological Basis of Psychiatric Treatment. Ed. by Samuel Gershon & R. Pohl. 1990. (Progress in Basic & Clinical Pharmacology Ser.: Vol. 3). (Illus.). x, 328p. 247.00 (*3-8055-5007-3*) S Karger.

Biological Basis of Substance Abuse. Ed. by Stanley G. Korenman & Jack D. Barchas. 1993. LC 92-49780. (Illus.). 536p. text 79.00 (*0-19-507154-9*) OUP.

Biological Basis of the Human Chondrodysplasias. Ed. by W. A. Horton. 1988. (Journal: Vol. 7, No. 1-2, 1988). (Illus.). 148p. pap. 82.75 (*3-8055-4855-9*) S Karger.

Biological Chemistry of Organelle Formation: Proceedings. Ed. by T. Buecher et al. 1981. (Colloquium der Gesellschaft fur Biologische Chemie in Mosbach Baden Ser.: Vol. 31). (Illus.). 254p. 61.95 (*0-387-10458-5*) Spr-Verlag.

Biological Components of Human Reproduction, Studies of Their Variations in Population Groups: Proceedings of the WHO Scientific Group, Geneva, 1968. WHO Staff. 1969. (Technical Reports: No. 435). pap. text 5.00 (*92-4-120435-4*, 1100435) World Health.

Biological Components of Substance Abuse & Addiction: Background Paper. 1994. lib. bdg. 250.00 (*0-8490-8607-8*) Gordon Pr.

Biological Consequences of Oxidative Stress: Implications for Carcinogenesis & Cardiovascular Disease. Ed. by Lawrence Spatz & Arthur D. Bloom. 1992. (Conte Institute Ser.: No. 1). (Illus.). 208p. text 39.95 (*0-19-507296-0*) OUP.

Biological Consequences of the European Expansion, 1450-1800. Ed. by Kenneth F. Kiple & Stephen V. Beck. 1997. LC 96-52045. (Expanding World Ser.: Vol. 26). 416p. text (*0-86078-518-1*) Variorum GBR. *Dist:* Ashgate Pub Co.

Biological Control of Vectors: Manual for Collecting, Field Determination & Handling of Biofactors for Control of Vectors of Diseases. Ed. by Jaroslav Weiser. 1991. LC 90-20612. 200p. 216.50 (*0-471-92864-X*) Wiley.

Biological Control of Vectors of Disease. 1982. (Technical Report Ser.: No. 679). 39p. pap. text 4.00 (*92-4-120679-9*) World Health.

Biological Determinants of Reinforcement: Quantitative Analyses of Behavior, Vol. 7. Ed. by Michael L. Commons et al. 1988. 312p. 69.95 (*0-89859-551-7*) L Erlbaum Assocs.

Biological Effects & Health Implications of Radiofrequency Radiation. S. M. Michaelson & J. C. Lin. 1987. (Illus.). 688p. (C). text 155.00 (*0-306-41580-1*, Kluwer Plenum) Kluwer Academic.

Biological Effects of Cholesterol Oxides. Peng Shi-Kaung & Robert J. Morin. 1991. (Illus.). 224p. lib. bdg. 189.00 (*0-8493-6776-X*, QP752) CRC Pr.

Biological Effects of Dietary Restriction. Ed. by L. Fishbein. 1991. (ILSI Monographs). (Illus.). 354p. 152.00 (*0-387-52294-8*) Spr-Verlag.

Biological Effects of Electropollution: Brain Tumors & Experimental Models. Ed. by Sisir K. Dutta & Richard M. Millis. 1986. LC 86-82834. (Illus.). x, 245p. (C). text 48.00 (*0-9617314-1-9*) Info Ventures Inc.

Biological Effects of External X & Gamma Radiation, Part 2. AEC Technical Information Center Staff. Ed. by Raymond E. Zirkle. 1956. (National Nuclear Energy Ser.: Vol. 22C). 487p. pap. 52.00 (*0-87079-146-X*, TID-5220); fiche 9.00 (*0-87079-147-8*, TID-5220) DOE.

Biological Effects of Low Level Exposures: Dose-Response Relationships. Ed. by Edward J. Calabrese. 1994. LC 93-50076. 320p. lib. bdg. 95.00 (*1-56670-093-0*, L1093) Lewis Pubs.

Biological Effects of Low Level Exposures to Chemicals. Edward J. Calabrese. 1992. 156p. lib. bdg. 71.95 (*0-87371-665-5*, L665) Lewis Pubs.

Biological Effects of Organolead Compounds. Ed. by Philippe Grandjean. 1984. 288p. 164.00 (*0-8493-5309-2*, RA1231, CRC Reprint) Franklin.

Biological Effects of Ultrasound: Mechanisms & Clinical Implications. 1983. LC 84-61833. (Report Ser.: No. 74). 268p. pap. text 55.00 (*0-913392-64-2*) NCRP Pubns.

Biological Evaluation of Medical Devices. AAMI Staff. 1996. (Illus.). 286p. (Orig.). pap. 210.00 (*1-57020-055-6*, BIOT3-209) Assn Adv Med Instrn.

Biological Evaluation of Medical Devices Pt. 1: Evaluation & Testing: ANSI/AAMI/ISO 10993-1: 1997. 2nd ed. 1998. (Illus.). 62p. pap. 100.00 (*1-57020-138-2*) Assn Adv Med Instrn.

Biological Evaluation of Medical Devices Pt. 5: Tests for Cytotoxicity, in Vitro Methods, ANSI/AAMI/ISO 10993-5:1999. 1999. (Illus.). pap. 100.00 (*1-57020-135-8*) Assn Adv Med Instrn.

Biological Evaluation of Medical Devices Pt. 9: Framework for Identification & Quantification of Potential Degradation Products, ANSI/AAMI/ISO 10993-9:1999. 1999. (Illus.). pap. 100.00 (*1-57020-136-6*) Assn Adv Med Instrn.

Biological Evaluation of Medical Devices Pt. 13: Identification & Quantification of Degradation Products from Polymeric Devices, ANSI/AAMI/ISO 10993-13:1999. 1999. (Illus.). pap. (*1-57020-137-4*) Assn Adv Med Instrn.

Biological Foundations of Behavior. Frederick Toates. 1986. LC 86-5158. (Guides to Psychology Ser.). 160p. (*0-335-15333-X*) OpUniv Pr.

Biological Foundations of Gesture: Motor & Semiotic Aspects. J. L. Nespoulous et al. 1986. 336p. (C). text 69.95 (*0-89859-645-9*) L Erlbaum Assocs.

Biological Foundations of Linguistic Communication: Towards a Biocybernetics of Language. Thomas T. Ballmer. 1983. (Pragmatics & Beyond Ser.: Vol. III, No. 7). x, 161p. (Orig.). pap. 57.00 (*90-272-2520-6*) J Benjamins Pubng Co.

Biological Function of Gangliosides: Proceedings of Novel Symposium 93. Ed. by Lars Svennerholm et al. 1994. LC 93-30538. (Progress in Brain Research Ser.: Vol. 101). 428p. 240.25 (*0-444-81658-5*) Elsevier.

Biological Functions of Proteinases. Ed. by H. Holzer & J. Tschesche. 1979. (Colloquium der Gesellschaft fur Biologische Chemie in Mosbach Baden Ser.: Vol. 30). (Illus.). 284p. 64.95 (*0-387-09683-3*) Spr-Verlag.

Biological Implications of the Nuclear Age: Proceedings. Ed. by Bernard Shore & Frederick Hatch. 1969. LC 74-603800. (AEC Symposium Ser.). 334p. pap. 16.25 (*0-87079-150-8*, CONF-690303); fiche 9.00 (*0-87079-151-6*, CONF-690303) DOE.

Biological Indicators for Ethylene Oxide Sterilization Processes in Health Care Facilities. 1986. 8p. pap. 62.00 (*0-910275-66-1*, ST21-209) Assn Adv Med Instrn.

Biological Indicators for Saturated Steam Sterilization Processes in Health Care Facilities. 1986. 8p. pap. 62.00 (*0-910275-58-0*, ST19-209) Assn Adv Med Instrn.

Biological Interrelations & Nutrition Biologische Wechselbeziehungen und Ernaehrung: Proceedings of the Institute of Nutrition Research Symposium, Zurich, 1969. Institute of Nutrition Research Symposium Staff. Ed. by J. C. Somogyi. 1971. (Bibliotheca Nutritio et Dieta Ser.: No. 15). (Illus.). pap. 55.75 (*3-8055-1155-8*) S Karger.

Biological Magnetic Resonance, Vol. 5. Ed. by Lawrence J. Berliner & Jacques Reuben. 1983. LC 78-16035. 322p. 85.00 (*0-306-41293-4*, Plenum Trade) Perseus Pubng.

Biological Manipulation of Life. Ed. by Harry Messel. 1981. (Illus.). 352p. text 44.00 (*0-08-024825-X*); pap. text 27.00 (*0-08-024824-1*) Elsevier (Pergamon Pr).

Biological Markers in Mental Disorders: Proceedings of the Symposium Held in Milan, Italy, June 1983. Ed. by Silvio Garattini & G. C. Tognoni. 1985. 200p. pap. 36.00 (*0-08-031848-7*, Pergamon Pr) Elsevier.

Biological Markers in Psychology. Usdin. 1982. 50.00 (*0-08-028874-X*, Pergamon Pr) Elsevier.

Biological Matrices & Tissue Reconstruction. Ed. by G. B. Stark et al. 1998. LC 97-32683. (Illus.). 312p. 119.00 (*3-540-63863-6*) Spr-Verlag.

Biological Membranes, Vol. 4. D. Chapman. 1982. text 199.00 (*0-12-168545-4*) Acad Pr.

Biological Membranes: Trigger Processes in Cell Biology, Vol. 5. David J. Chapman. 1985. (Biological Membranes Ser.). text 199.00 (*0-12-168546-2*) Acad Pr.

Biological Membranes in Toxicology. Ernest Foulkes. 1998. LC 98-17546. 153p. text 75.00 (*1-56032-762-6*) Hemisp Pub.

Biological Methylation & Drug Design: Experimental & Clinical Roles of S-Adenosylmethionine. Ed. by Ronald T. Borchardt et al. 1986. LC 86-7212. (Experimental Biology & Medicine Ser.: Vol. 12). (Illus.). 480p. 139.50 (*0-89603-102-0*) Humana.

Biological Mineralization & Demineralization: Report on the Dahlemn Workshop Berlin 1981. G. H. Nancollas et al. 1982. (Dahlem Workshop Reports Ser.: Vol. 23). (Illus.). 82p. 42.95 (*0-387-11521-8*) Spr-Verlag.

Biological Models in Radiopharmaceutical Development. Richard M. Lambrecht. 1996. LC 95-43931. (Developments in Nuclear Medicine Ser.: No. 27). 288p. (C). text 144.00 (*0-7923-3836-7*) Kluwer Academic.

Biological Modulation of Solid Tumours by Interferons. Ed. by K. Pummer. 1994. LC 94-5664. (European School of Oncology Monographs). (Illus.). 75p. 73.95 (*0-387-57764-5*) Spr-Verlag.

Biological Monitoring for Pesticide Exposure: Measurement, Estimation, & Risk Reduction. Ed. by Rhoda G. Wang et al. 1988. LC 88-39189. (ACS Symposium Ser.: No. 382). (Illus.). xi, 490p. 69.95 (*0-8412-1559-6*) Am Chemical.

Biological Monitoring of Toxic Metals. Ed. by T. W. Clarkson et al. 1988. LC 87-36128. (Rochester Series on Environmental Toxicity). (Illus.). 698p. (C). text 186.00 (*0-306-42809-1*, Kluwer Plenum) Kluwer Academic.

Biological Neural Networks: Hierarchical Concept of Brain Function. K. V. Baev. 1997. LC 97-30734. 273p. 95.00 (*0-8176-3859-8*) Birkhauser.

Biological Oxidants & Antioxidants: Molecular Mechanisms & Health Effects. Ed. by Lester Packer & Augustine S. Ong. 1998. LC 98-6432. (Illus.). 130.00 (*0-935315-91-8*, PC120) Am Oil Chemists.

Biological Oxidation of Nitrogen in Organic Molecules. Ed. by J. W. Gorrod & L. A. Damani. 1985. 445p. 105.00 (*3-527-26299-7*, Wiley-VCH) Wiley.

Biological, Physical & Clinical Aspects of Hyperthermia: Proceedings of the 1987 AAPM - NAHG Hyperthermia School Held at the Sheraton University Center, Durham, North Carolina, April 27-May 1, 1987. Ed. by Bhudatt R. Paliwal et al. 1988. (American Association of Physicists in Medicine Symposium Ser.: No. 16). 483p. 75.00 (*0-88318-558-X*) Am Inst Physics.

Biological Protection with Prostaglandins, Vol. I. Ed. by Max M. Cohen. 1985. 288p. 162.00 (*0-8493-5962-7*, QP801, CRC Reprint) Franklin.

Biological Protection with Prostaglandins, Vol. II. Max M. Cohen. 1986. 272p. 152.00 (*0-8493-5963-5*, QP801, CRC Reprint) Franklin.

Biological Psychiatry. Robert J. Hedaya. 1996. LC 96-2429. 192p. (C). 35.00 (*0-393-70191-3*) Norton.

*__Biological Psychiatry.__ E. C. Johnstone. 1996. (British Medical Bulletin Ser.: Vol. 52, No. 3). 269p. pap. (*1-85315-281-1*) Royal Soc of Medicine Pr Ltd GBR. *Dist:* Balogh.

Biological Psychiatry. Michael R. Trimble. 2nd ed. 1996. LC 95-24372. 480p. pap. 45.00 (*0-471-95374-1*); 211.50 (*0-471-96360-7*) Wiley.

Biological Psychiatry: Marching Backwards into the Future. Ed. by H. De Cuyper & G. Buyse. 1989. 152p. (Orig.). pap. (*90-6186-333-3*) Leuven Univ BEL. *Dist:* Coronet Bks.

Biological, Psychological, & Environmental Factors in Delinquency & Mental Disorder: An Interdisciplinary Bibliography, 4. Ed. by Deborah W. Denno & Ruth M. Schwarz. 1985. LC 85-5620. (Bibliographies & Indexes in Sociology Ser.: No. 4). 222p. lib. bdg. 62.95 (*0-313-24939-3*, DBP/) Greenwood.

Biological Psychology. James W. Kalat. 2nd ed. 1984. 524p. (C). mass mkt. 36.50 (*0-534-02982-5*) Brooks-Cole.

Biological Psychology. Kimble. 2nd ed. 1992. (C). pap. text, tchr. ed., suppl. ed. 35.00 (*0-03-040493-2*) Harcourt Coll Pubs.

Biological Psychology. Daniel P. Kimble. 2nd ed. 1992. (C). pap. text, stu. ed. 31.00 (*0-03-040494-0*); LC 91-32911. (Illus.). 482p. text 90.50 (*0-03-040487-8*) Harcourt Coll Pubs.

Biological Psychology. James W. Kalat. 3rd ed. 1987. 560p. (C). mass mkt. 46.00 (*0-534-08466-4*); 4th ed. 1992. 704p. (C). pap., stu. ed. 18.95 (*0-534-16255-X*); 4th ed. 1991. 704p. (C). text 57.95 (*0-534-16254-1*); 5th ed. 1994. LC 94-27415. 688p. mass mkt. 59.75 (*0-534-21108-9*); 5th ed. 1994. mass mkt., tchr. ed. (*0-534-21114-3*) Brooks-Cole.

Biological-Psychosocial Interactions in Early Adolescence: A Life-Span Perspective. Ed. by Richard M. Lerner & Terryl Foch. 1987. (Child Psychology Ser.). 408p. text 69.95 (*0-89859-787-0*) L Erlbaum Assocs.

Biological Reactions within the Extracorporeal Blood Circuit During Hemodialysis. Ed. by K. M. Koch & E. Streicher. 1988. (Contributions to Nephrology Ser.: Vol. 59). (Illus.). viii, 168p. 125.25 (*3-8055-4578-9*) S Karger.

Biological Reactive Intermediates 4: Molecular & Cellular Effects & Their Impact on Human Health. Ed. by Charlotte M. Witmer et al. 1991. LC 90-14326. (Advances in Experimental Medicine & Biology Ser.: Vol. 283). (Illus.). 912p. (C). text 234.00 (*0-306-43737-6*, Kluwer Plenum) Kluwer Academic.

Biological Reactive Intermediates 5: Basic Mechanistic Research in Toxicology & Human Risk Assessment, Vol. 387. Ed. by R. Snyder et al. 1996. LC 95-46530. (Advances in Experimental Medicine & Biology Ser.: No. 387). (Illus.). 476p. (C). text 150.00 (*0-306-45197-2*, Kluwer Plenum) Kluwer Academic.

Biological Reactive Intermediates III: Mechanisms of Action in Animal Model & Human Disease. Ed. by James J. Kocsis et al. 1986. LC 86-4973. (Advances in Experimental Medicine & Biology Ser.: Vol. 197). 1076p. 175.00 (*0-306-42264-6*, Plenum Trade) Perseus Pubng.

Biological Regulation & Development Vol. 3A: Hormone Action. Ed. by Robert F. Goldberger et al. 1982. LC 82-9841. 360p. 85.00 (*0-306-40925-9*, Plenum Trade) Perseus Pubng.

Biological Regulation of the Chondrocyte. Ed. by Monique Adolphe. 1992. 368p. lib. bdg. 219.00 (*0-8493-6733-6*, QP88) CRC Pr.

Biological Research in Schizophrenia: Proceedings of the WHO Scientific Group, Geneva, 1969. WHO Staff. 1970. (Technical Reports: No. 450). pap. 5.00 (*92-4-120450-8*, 1100450) World Health.

Biological Response Modifiers: A Self-Instruction Manual for Health Professionals. Kimberly A. Rumsey & Paula T. Rieger. 1992. LC 92-81530. 134p. 39.95 (*0-944496-30-X*) Precept Pr.

Biological Responses in Cancer: Progress Toward Potential Applications, Vol. 1. Ed. by Enrico Mihich. 1982. LC 82-18041. 322p. 85.00 (*0-306-41146-6*, Plenum Trade) Perseus Pubng.

Biological Responses in Cancer: Progress Toward Potential Applications, Vol. 3: Immunomodulation by Anticancer Drugs. Ed. by Enrico Mihich & Yoshio Sakurai. 1985. LC 84-18041. 230p. 85.00 (*0-306-41879-7*, Plenum Trade) Perseus Pubng.

Biological Responses in Cancer: Progress Toward Potential Applications; Vol. 4. Ed. by Enrico Mihich. 1985. LC 82-18041. 270p. 79.50 (*0-306-42044-9*, Plenum Trade) Perseus Pubng.

Biological Responses to Ultraviolet A Radiation: 2nd International Symposium. Ed. by Frederick Urback. 1992. (American Society for Photobiology Symposium Ser.). 433p. 80.00 (*0-9632105-0-5*); pap. 65.00 (*0-9632105-1-3*) Valdenmar.

Biological Rhythms. Ed. by Jurgen Aschoff. 1981. LC 80-21037. (Handbook of Behavioral Neurobiology Ser.: Vol. 4). 582p. 115.00 (*0-306-40585-7*, Plenum Trade) Perseus Pubng.

Biological Rhythms: Sleep & Shift Work. Ed. by L. C. Johnson et al. 1981. (Advances in Sleep Research Ser.: Vol. 7). 640p. text 65.00 (*0-88331-115-1*) R B Luce.

Biological Rhythms & Behavior. Herman M. Van Praag & Julien Mendlewicz. 1983. (Advances in Biological Psychiatry Ser.: Vol. 11). (Illus.). iv, 150p. pap. 86.25 (*3-8055-3672-0*) S Karger.

Biological Rhythms, Mood Disorders, Light Therapy & the Pineal Gland. Mohammad Shafii & Sharon L. Shafii. 1990. LC 89-18447. (Progress in Psychiatry Ser.: No. 24). 213p. text 11.95 (*0-88048-169-2*, 8169) Am Psychiatric.

Biological Risk Factors for Psychosocial Disorders. Ed. by Michael Rutter & Paul Casaer. 1991. (European Network on Longitudinal Studies on Individual Development). 364p. (C). text 90.00 (*0-521-40103-8*) Cambridge U Pr.

Biological Risks of Medical Irradiations: Proceedings of the AAPM Spring Symposium Held at the University of Texas Health Science Center, San Antonio, Texas, March 26-28, 1980. Ed. by Gary D. Fullerton et al. 1980. (American Association of Physicists in Medicine Symposium Ser.: No. 5). 340p. 42.00 (*0-88318-278-5*) Am Inst Physics.

Biological Role of Proteinases & Their Inhibitors in Skin. Ed. by H. Ogawa et al. 1986. 238p. 190.50 (*0-444-01086-6*) Elsevier.

Biological Role of Reactive Oxygen Species in Skin. Ed. by Osamu Hayaishi et al. 1987. 282p. 127.50 (*0-444-01247-8*) Elsevier.

Biological Science: Interaction of Experiments & Ideas (BSCS Second Course) Biological Sciences Curriculum Study Staff. 3rd ed. 1977. tchr. ed. 15.96 (*0-13-076919-3*, 07813-9-8); text 30.64 (*0-13-076562-7*) P-H.

Biological Sciences - Area Examination. Jack Rudman. 1994. (Graduate Record Examination Ser.: GRE-41). pap. 47.95 (*0-8373-5241-X*) Nat Learn.

Biological Signals Relevant to Sleep. Ed. by R. A. Velluti. 2000. (Biological Signals & Receptors Ser.: Vol. 9, No. 6 (2000)). iv, 68p. pap. 25.25 (*3-8055-7148-8*) S Karger.

Biological Significance of Superantigens. Ed. by B. Fleischer. 1992. (Chemical Immunology Ser.: Vol. 55). (Illus.). x, 200p. 170.50 (*3-8055-5587-3*) S Karger.

Biological Substances: International Standards & Reference Reagents 1990. 1991. (ENG & FRE.). 105p. pap. text 19.00 (*92-4-154429-5*, 1150362) World Health.

Biological Treatment in Psychiatry. Lothar B. Kalinowsky et al. 1982. 424p. text 71.00 (*0-8089-1423-5*, 792231, Grune & Strat) Harcrt Hlth Sci Grp.

Biological Treatment in Psychiatry. Rothschild. 1999. (C). text (*0-7216-7164-0*) Saunders.

Biological Treatments in Psychiarty. Reginald Herrington & Malcolm H. Lader. 2nd ed. 1996. (Illus.). 458p. (C). text 79.95 (*0-19-262652-3*) OUP.

Biological Unhappiness. Leland M. Heller. 1999. 438p. pap. 22.95 (*1-928947-00-X*) Dyslimbia Pr.

Biological Variation in Health & Illness: Race, Age, & Sex Differences. Theresa Overfield. 2nd ed. 1995. LC 94-42293. 220p. 149.95 (*0-8493-4577-4*, 4577) CRC Pr.

Biological Vulnerability to Drug Abuse. 1993. lib. bdg. 261.95 (*0-8490-8910-7*) Gordon Pr.

Biological Vulnerability to Drug Abuse: Genetics in the Etiology of Drug Abuse. 1991. lib. bdg. 250.00 (*0-8490-4344-1*) Gordon Pr.

Biological Woman: The Convenient Myth. Ruth Hubbard et al. 1982. LC 82-10781. 376p. pap. 18.95 (*0-87073-703-1*) Schenkman Bks Inc.

Biologically Active Products. Horace Culter & Stephen J. Cutler. 1999. LC 99-13027. (Illus.). 296p. 99.95 (*0-8493-1887-4*) CRC Pr.

Biologically-Based Methods for Cancer Risk Assessment. Ed. by Curtis C. Travis. 1989. (NATO ASI Series A, Life Sciences: Vol. 159). (Illus.). 340p. 95.00 (*0-306-43117-3*, Plenum Trade) Perseus Pubng.

Biologically Informed Psychotherapy for Depression. Stephen R. Shuchter et al. 1996. LC 96-4858. 224p. text 32.00 (*1-57230-069-8*, 0069) Guilford Pubns.

Biologie des Menschen. J. Wunderli. 4th ed. 1982. (Illus.). xiv, 194p. pap. 21.00 (*3-8055-2613-X*) S Karger.

Biologie des menschlichen Verhaltens: Grundriss der Humanethologie see Human Ethology

Biologist. Jack Rudman. 1994. (Career Examination Ser.: C-2013). pap. 29.95 (*0-8373-2013-5*) Nat Learn.

Biologists & Their World Series, Set. Ed. by Keir B. Sterling. 1978. (Illus.). lib. bdg. 3356.00 (*0-405-10641-6*) Ayer.

Biologos & Biopsychosocial Synthesis: The SAMA Foundation Lectures, Calabar, West Africa, 1982. Stacey B. Day. 1985. LC 84-82409. 130p. 35.00 (*0-934314-75-6*) Intl Found Biosocial Dev.

Biology. Eva M. Bushman. 1980. 205p. (J). 242.20 incl. audio (*0-89420-203-0*, 238000); (C). (gr. 9-12). pap. text 12.95 (*0-89420-110-7*, 238040) Natl Book.

Biology. Jack Rudman. 1994. (Regents College Proficiency Examination Ser.: CPEP-5). pap. 23.95 (*0-8373-5405-6*); (Graduate Record Examination Ser.: Vol. GRE-1). pap. 27.95 (*0-8373-5201-0*) Nat Learn.

Biology. John W. Kimball. 4th ed. 1978. (Life Sciences Ser.). LC 77-74322. (*0-201-03692-4*); LC 77-74322. stu. ed. (*0-201-03764-5*); LC 82-11636. text (*0-201-03761-0*) Addison-Wesley.

Biology. Sylvia S. Mader. 7th ed. 2000. LC 00-35477. (Illus.). 65.00 net. (*0-07-013657-2*) McGraw.

Biology: A Human Emphasis. Cecie Starr. 4th ed. 1999. (Biology Ser.). mass mkt. 46.75 (*0-534-56324-4*) Wadsworth Pub.

Biology: Study Guide & Workbook. Charles K. Levy. 3rd ed. 1983. LC 81-17556. (Biology Ser.). (Illus.). 620p. pap. text, stu. ed. 11.25 net. (*0-201-04566-4*) Addison-Wesley.

Biology & Biochemistry. Ed. by P. Shubik. 1974. (Physiopathology of Cancer Ser.: Vol. 1). (Illus.). 412p. 42.75 (*3-8055-1545-6*) S Karger.

Biology & Biochemistry of Normal & Cancer Cell Growth. Italo Nenci & L. Castagnetta. 1988. xiv, 274p. text 258.00 (*3-7186-4816-4*) Gordon & Breach.

Biology & Diseases of the Ferret. Ed. by James G. Fox. 1988. LC 87-26096. (Illus.). (C). text 49.50 (*0-8121-1139-7*) Lppncott W & W.

Biology & Diseases of the Ferret. Jame G. Fox. 2nd ed. 1998. LC 98-18196. (Illus.). 475p. 55.95 (*0-683-30034-2*) Lppncott W & W.

Biology & Emotion. Neil McNaughton. 1989. (Problems in the Behavioral Sciences Ser.). (Illus.). 256p. (C). pap. text 27.95 (*0-521-31938-2*) Cambridge U Pr.

Biology & Human Concerns. E. Peter Volpe & Claudia De Gruy. 3rd ed. 1983. 704p. (C). spiral bd. 42.19 (*0-697-04746-6*, WCB McGr Hill) McGrw-H Hghr Educ.

Biology & Human Progress. Charles Tanzer. 5th ed. 1977. text 28.52 (*0-13-076612-7*); (gr. 9-10). tchr. ed. 11.40 (*0-13-076638-0*, 07663-8); (gr. 9-10). wbk. ed. 9.92 (*0-13-076620-8*, 07662-0) P-H.

Biology & Knowledge: An Essay on the Relations Between Organic Regulations & Cognitive Processes. Jean Piaget. 1971. LC 70-157421. (C). lib. bdg. 19.00 (*0-226-66775-8*) U Ch Pr.

Biology & Management of Lung Cancer. Ed. by F. Anthony Greco. 1983. text 145.00 (*0-89838-554-7*) Kluwer Academic.

Biology & Management of Multiple Myeloma. Ed. by James R. Berenson. 2001. (Current Clinical Oncology Ser.). 400p. 125.00 (*0-89603-706-1*) Humana.

Biology & Medicine into the 21st Century. Ed. by M. A. Hardy & R. K. Kinne. 1991. (Issues in Biomedicine Ser.: Vol. 15). (Illus.). viii, 200p. 195.75 (*3-8055-5392-7*) S Karger.

Biology & Medicine of Rabbits & Rodents. John E. Harkness & Joseph E. Wagner. 1988. LC 88-13330. (Illus.). 230p. pap. text 28.50 (*0-8121-1176-1*) Lppncott W & W.

Biology & Molecular Genetics of Lung Cancer. Adi F. Gazdar & David P. Carbone. 1994. LC 94-2335. (Medical Intelligence Unit Ser.). 152p. 99.00 (*1-57059-008-7*) Landes Bioscience.

Biology & Pathology of Astrocyte-Neuron Interactions. S. Fedoroff et al. 1993. (Altschul Symposia Ser.: Vol. 2). (Illus.). 470p. (C). text 139.50 (*0-306-44565-4*, Kluwer Plenum) Kluwer Academic.

Biology & Pathology of Elastic Tissues. Ed. by A. M. Robert & L. Robert. 1980. (Frontiers of Matrix Biology Ser.: Vol. 8). (Illus.). viii, 232p. 108.00 (*3-8055-3078-1*) S Karger.

Biology & Physiology of the Blood-Brain Barrier: Transport, Cellular Interactions & Brain Pathologies. Ed. by Pierre-Olivier Couraud & Daniel Scherman. 1996. LC 96-34815. (Advances in Behavioral Biology Ser.: Vol. 46). (Illus.). 403p. (C). text 107.00 (*0-306-45362-2*, Kluwer Plenum) Kluwer Academic.

Biology & Physiology of the Osteoclast. Barry R. Rifkin. 1992. 512p. 199.00 (*0-8493-5437-4*, QP88) CRC Pr.

Biology & Prevention of Aerodigestive Tract Cancers. G. R. Newell & W. K. Hong. 1992. LC 92-21811. (Advances in Experimental Medicine & Biology Ser.: Vol. 320). (Illus.). 184p. (C). text 85.00 (*0-306-44244-2*, Kluwer Plenum) Kluwer Academic.

Biology & Social Behavior. Allan Mazur & Leon S. Robertson. 1972. LC 72-169236. (Illus.). 200p. 19.95 (*0-02-920450-X*) Free Pr.

Biology & the Social Crisis. John K. Brierley. 1975. LC 71-120071. (Illus.). 260p. 28.50 (*0-8386-7719-3*) Fairleigh Dickinson.

Biology & Therapy of Acute Leukemia. Lawrence H. Baker et al. 1985. (Developments in Oncology Ser.). text 120.00 (*0-89838-728-0*) Kluwer Academic.

Biology & Treatment of Colorectal Cancer Metastasis. Ed. by Anthony J. Mastromarino. 1986. (Developments in Oncology Ser.). text 120.50 (*0-89838-786-8*) Kluwer Academic.

Biology & Violence: From Birth to Adulthood. Deborah W. Denno. 1990. (Illus.). 232p. (C). text 49.95 (*0-521-36219-9*) Cambridge U Pr.

Biology in Human Affairs. Ed. by Edward M. East. 1977. LC 72-313. (Essay Index Reprint Ser.). reprint ed. 27.95 (*0-8369-2790-7*) Ayer.

Biology in the Health Sciences: Index of Modern Authors & Subjects with Guide for Rapid Research. J. H. Vickery. rev. ed. 1994. 57.50 (*0-7883-0174-8*); pap. 47.50 (*0-7883-0175-6*) ABBE Pubs Assn.

Biology in the Health Sciences: Index of Modern Authors & Subjects with Guide for Rapid Research. Joe H. Vickery. rev. ed. 1995. 143p. pap. 47.50 (*0-7883-0665-0*) ABBE Pubs Assn.

Biology in the Health Sciences: Index of Modern Authors & Subjects with Guide for Rapid Research. Joe H. Vickery. Ed. by J. H. Vickery. rev. ed. 1995. 143p. 57.50 (*0-7883-0664-2*) ABBE Pubs Assn.

Biology in the Nineteenth Century. W. Coleman. 1978. LC 77-83989. (Cambridge History of Science Ser.). (Illus.). 187p. pap. text 19.95 (*0-521-29293-X*) Cambridge U Pr.

Biology, Medicine & Surgery of South American Wild Animals. Ed. by Murray E. Fowler & Zalmir Cubas. 2001. LC 00-66967. (Illus.). x, 536p. 89.95 (*0-8138-2846-5*) Iowa U Pr.

Biology of Aging. Ed. by Richard L. Sprott et al. 1993. LC 93-31559. 144p. 26.95 (*0-8261-8370-0*) Springer Pub.

Biology of AIDS. Hong Y. Fan et al. 1989. (Illus.). 208p. (C). pap. text 22.50 (*0-86720-124-X*, 124-X) Jones & Bartlett.

Biology of AIDS. Hung Fan et al. 3rd ed. 1994. (Life Science Ser.). (Illus.). 192p. (C). pap. text 31.95 (*0-86720-346-3*, 346-3) Jones & Bartlett.

Biology of Alcohol Problems: Proceedings of the Seventh Congress of the International Society for Biomedical Research on Alcoholism, Australia, June 1994. Ed. by John S. Saunders & J. B. Whitfield. 1996. 586p. 130.50 (*0-08-042528-3*, Pergamon Pr) Elsevier.

Biology of Alcoholism Vol. 7: Pathogenesis of Alcoholism: Biological Factors. Ed. by Henri Begleiter & Benjamin Kissin. 1983. LC 82-22284. 666p. 120.00 (*0-306-41053-2*, Plenum Trade) Perseus Pubng.

Biology of & Novel Therapeutic Approaches for Epithelial Cancers of the Aerodigestive Tract. 1995. lib. bdg. 252.99 (*0-8490-6721-9*) Gordon Pr.

Biology of Animal Behavior. Grier-Burk. 2nd ed. 1994. tchr. ed. 8.75 (*0-697-23493-2*, WCB McGr Hill) McGrw-H Hghr Educ.

Biology of Anxiety Disorders. Ed. by Rudolf Hoehn-Saric & Daniel R. McLeod. 1993. LC 92-17631. (Progress in Psychiatry Ser.: No. 36). 259p. text 12.95 (*0-88048-476-4*, 8476) Am Psychiatric.

Biology of Baculoviruses, Set. Ed. by Robert R. Granados & Brian A. Federici. 1987. 358.00 (*0-8493-5986-4*, QR327) Franklin.

Biology of Baculoviruses, Vol. I. Brian A. Federici. 1987. 288p. 162.00 (*0-8493-5987-2*, CRC Reprint) Franklin.

Biology of Baculoviruses, Vol. 1: Practical Properties & Molecular Biology. Ed. by Robert R. Granados & Brian A. Federici. 1987. 288p. 163.00 (*0-8493-5988-0*, CRC Reprint) Franklin.

Biology of Brain Tumor. Ed. by Michael D. Walker & David G. Thomas. 1986. text 380.50 (*0-89838-775-2*) Kluwer Academic.

Biology of Carbohydrates, Vol. 3. Ed. by Victor Ginsberg & Phillips W. Robbins. 1991. 296p. 90.00 (*1-55938-014-4*) Jai Pr.

Biology of Carcinogenesis. Ed. by Michael J. Waring & B. A. Ponder. 1986. (Cancer Biology & Medicine Ser.). text 155.00 (*0-85200-935-6*) Kluwer Academic.

Biology of Change in Otolaryngology: Proceedings of the Third ARO Midwinter Research Meeting, Clearwater Beach, FL, February 2-6, 1986. Ed. by R. J. Ruben et al. 1987. 416p. 210.00 (*0-444-80844-2*) Elsevier.

Biology of Clinical Encounters: Psychoanalysis As a Science of Mind. John E. Gedo. 1991. 216p. 39.95 (*0-88163-126-4*) Analytic Pr.

Biology of Death: Series of Lectures Delivered at the Lowell Institute in Boston in Dec. 1920. Raymond Pearl. 1976. LC 75-38141. (Demography Ser.). (Illus.). reprint ed. 24.95 (*0-405-07994-X*) Ayer.

Biology of Depressive Disorders Pt. A: A Systems Perspective. J. J. Mann & D. J. Kupfer. 1993. (Depressive Illness Ser.: Vol. 3). (Illus.). 286p. (C). text 59.50 (*0-306-44295-7*, Kluwer Plenum) Kluwer Academic.

Biology of Depressive Disorders Pt. B: Subtypes of Depression & Comobid Disorders. J. J. Mann & D. J. Kupfer. 1993. (Depressive Illness Ser.: Vol. 4). (Illus.). 196p. (C). text 52.50 (*0-306-44296-5*, Kluwer Plenum) Kluwer Academic.

Biology of Disease. Ed. by Jonathon Phillips et al. 1995. LC 94-46340. 250p. 34.95 (*0-632-03855-1*) Blackwell Sci.

Biology of Disease. Jonathan Phillips et al. 2nd ed. 2001. LC 00-41405. (Illus.). xii, 323p. pap. 41.95 (*0-632-05404-2*) Blackwell Sci.

Biology of Drosophila. Ed. by Milislav Demerec. 1995. 632p. (C). reprint ed. text 39.00 (*0-87969-441-6*) Cold Spring Harbor.

Biology of Echinococcus & Hydatid Disease. Ed. by R.C. Thompson. 1985. LC 85-9066. (Illus.). 336p. (C). text 95.00 (*0-04-591020-0*) Routledge.

Biology of Elephantiasis, Lymphatic Filariasis & Albendazole: Index of New Information. John C. Bartonc. 1998. 150p. 57.50 (*0-7883-2036-X*); 1998. 150p. pap. 44.50 (*0-7883-2037-8*); 1999. 143p. pap. 47.50 (*0-7883-2201-X*) ABBE Pubs Assn.

Biology of Female Cancers. Ed. by Simon P. Langdon et al. 1997. LC 96-34494. 320p. 149.95 (*0-8493-9443-0*) CRC Pr.

Biology of Fertility Control by Periodic Abstinence: Report of a WHO Scientific Group, 1967. 1967. (Technical Report Ser.: No. 360). 20p. pap. text 3.00 (*92-4-120360-9*, 1100360) World Health.

Biology of Fungi. Cecil T. Ingold. 3rd rev. ed. (Hutchinson Biology Monographs). (Illus.). pap. text (*0-09-105120-7*) Brill Academic Pubs.

Biology of Germinal Centers in Lymphoid Tissue. G. Jeanette Thorbecke & Vincent K. Tsaigbe. 1998. LC 98-23745. (Biotechnology Intelligence Unit Ser.). 250p. 150.00 (*3-540-64559-4*) Spr-Verlag.

Biology of Germinal Centers in Lymphoid Tissue. G. Jeanette Thorbecke & Vincent K. Tsiagbe. 1998. LC 98-23745. (Biotechnology Intelligence Unit Ser.). 150.00 (*1-57059-533-X*) Landes Bioscience.

Biology of Heritable Skin Diseases. Ed. by K. D. Wuepper & Tobias Gedde-Dahl. 1987. (Current Problems in Dermatology Ser.: Vol. 17). (Illus.). viii, 256p. 212.25 (*3-8055-4398-0*) S Karger.

Biology of Human Aging. Alexander P. Spence. 2nd ed. 1994. LC 94-34128. 336p. 54.00 (*0-13-146267-9*) P-H.

Biology of Human Conflict: An Anatomy of Behavior, Individual & Social. Trigant Burrow. 1974. LC 73-14149. (Perspectives in Social Inquiry Ser.). 510p. reprint ed. 33.95 (*0-405-05495-5*) Ayer.

Biology of Hyaluronan. CIBA Foundation Staff. 1989. LC 89-30662. (CIBA Foundation Symposia Ser.: No. 143). 308p. 128.00 (*0-471-92305-2*) Wiley.

Biology of Idiotypes. Ed. by Mark I. Greene & Alfred Nisonoff. 1984. LC 83-13474. 520p. 125.00 (*0-306-41646-8*, Plenum Trade) Perseus Pubng.

Biology of Infections: Index of New Information. John C. Bartone. 1998. 160p. 57.50 (*0-7883-1766-0*); pap. 47.50 (*0-7883-1767-9*) ABBE Pubs Assn.

Biology of Inorganic Nitrogen & Sulfur Metabolism. Ed. by Hans-Werner Bothe & A. Trebst. 1981. (Proceedings in Life Sciences Ser.). (Illus.). 370p. 86.95 (*0-387-10486-0*) Spr-Verlag.

Biology of Insect Eggs, Set. H. E. Hinton. 1981. LC 77-30390. (Illus.). 1500p. (*0-08-021539-4*) Pergamon Repr GBR. *Dist:* Franklin.

Biology of Lung Cancer. Ed. by Madeleine A. Kane & Paul A. Bunn. 1998. LC 98-27854. (Lung Biology in Health & Disease Ser.). (Illus.). 632p. text 225.00 (*0-8247-0132-1*) Dekker.

Biology of Lung Cancer: Diagnosis & Treatment. Abrams. Ed. by Steven T. Rosen et al. 1988. (Lung Biology in Health & Disease Ser.: Vol. 37). (Illus.). 384p. text 175.00 (*0-8247-7642-9*) Dekker.

Biology of Malaria Parasites. 1987. (Technical Reports: No. 743). 229p. pap. text 32.00 (*92-4-120743-4*, 1100743) World Health.

Biology of Menopause: The Causes & Consequences of Ovarian Aging. R. C. Gosden. 1985. LC 84-14516. (Monograph Ser.). text 104.00 (*0-12-291850-9*) Acad Pr.

Biology of Mental Disorders. Research and Education Association Staff. 1995. LC 94-67652. 192p. pap. text 15.95 (*0-87891-960-0*) Res & Educ.

Biology of Moral Systems. Richard D. Alexander. 1987. (Evolutionary Foundations of Human Behavior Ser.). 323p. (C). pap. text 27.95 (*0-202-01174-7*) Aldine de Gruyter.

Biology of Music Making: Proceedings of the 1984 Denver Conference. Ed. by Frank P. Wilson & Frank L. Roehman. 1988. 316p. per. 14.95 (*0-918812-51-8*, ST 009) MMB Music.

Biology of Nicotine Dependence. CIBA Foundation Staff. 1990. LC 90-12213. (CIBA Foundation Symposia Ser.: No. 152). 274p. 147.95 (*0-471-92688-4*) Wiley.

Biology of Normal Proliferating Cells in Vitro Relevance for in Vivo Aging. A. Macieira-Coelho. 1987. (Interdisciplinary Topics in Gerontology Ser.: Vol. 23). (Illus.). vi, 218p. 148.00 (*3-8055-4660-2*) S Karger.

Biology of Organisms, Pt. 2. Helena Curtis & N. Sue Barnes. 5th ed. 1989. 668p. pap. text 32.95 (*0-87901-436-9*) Worth.

Biology of Personality Disorders. Ed. by Kenneth R. Silk. 1998. LC 98-10615. (Review of Psychiatry Ser.). 166p. pap. text 26.00 (*0-88048-835-2*, 8835) Am Psychiatric.

Biology of Phagocytes in Health & Disease: Proceedings of the International Congress on the Biological & Clinical Aspects of Phagocyte Function, 7-10 September, 1986, Pavia, Italy. Ed. by C. Mauri et al. 1988. 664p. 116.00 (*0-08-036133-1*, Pergamon Pr) Elsevier.

Biology of Poxviruses. S. Dales & Beatriz G. Pogo. 1981. (Virology Monographs: Vol. 18). (Illus.). 140p. 55.00 (*0-387-81643-7*) Spr-Verlag.

Biology of Rarity: Causes & Consequences of Rare-Common Differences. Ed. by W. Kunin & Kevin J. Gaston. 1996. LC 96-71014. (Population & Community Biology Ser.). (Illus.). 296p. (C). (gr. 13). (*0-412-63380-9*) Kluwer Academic.

Biology of Renal Cell Carcinoma. Ed. by Eric A. Klein et al. 1995. LC 95-16247. (Illus.). 275p. 217.00 (*0-387-94503-2*) Spr-Verlag.

Biology of Rickettsial Diseases David H. Walker. 1988. Vol. I. 160p. text 94.00 (*0-8493-4382-8*, RC114); Vol. II. 176p. text 103.00 (*0-8493-4383-6*, RC114) Franklin (CRC Reprint).

Biology of Schizophrenia: Proceedings of the 7th International Symposium of the Tokyo Institute of Psychiatry, Tokyo, Japan, October 19-20, 1992. Ed. by T. Moroji. 1994. LC 94-3420. (Developments in Psychiatry Ser.). 284p. 194.50 (*0-444-81772-7*) Elsevier.

Biology of Schizophrenia & Affective Disease. Ed. by Stanley J. Watson. 1995. LC 95-10715. 464p. text 61.50 (*0-88048-746-1*, 8746) Am Psychiatric.

Biology of Sleep Substances. Shojiro Inoue. 1989. 224p. lib. bdg. 166.00 (*0-8493-4822-6*, QP425) CRC Pr.

Biology of Spermatozoa: Proceedings of the Inserm Symposium at Nouzilly, Nov. 4-7, 1973. Inserm-International Symposium Staff. Ed. by E. S. Hafez & C. G. Thibault. 1975. (Illus.). vii, 256p. 95.75 (*3-8055-2104-9*) S Karger.

Biology of Stress in Farm Animals: An Integrative Approach. Ed. by P. R. Wiepkema & P. W. Van Adrichem. 1987. (Current Topics in Veterinary Medicine & Animal Science Ser.). (C). text 144.00 (*0-89838-895-3*) Kluwer Academic.

Biology of Taurine: Methods & Mechanisms. Ed. by Ryan J. Huxtable et al. 1987. LC 87-20335. (Advances in Experimental Medicine & Biology Ser.: Vol. 217). (Illus.). 418p. 95.00 (*0-306-42665-X*, Plenum Trade) Perseus Pubng.

Biology of the Arterial Wall. Bernard I. Levy & Alain Tedguin. 1999. LC 98-55059. (Basic Science for the Cardiologist Ser.). 278p. 155.00 (*0-7923-8458-X*) Kluwer Academic.

Biology of the Autistic Syndromes. Christopher Gillberg & Mary Coleman. 2nd ed. 1993. (Clinics in Developmental Medicine Ser.: No. 126). 300p. (C). text 74.95 (*0-521-43228-6*) Cambridge U Pr.

Biology of the Autistic Syndromes. Christopher Gillberg & Mary Coleman. 3rd ed. 2000. (Clinics in Developmental Medicine Ser.: No. 153/154). (Illus.). 352p. (C). (*1-898683-22-0*) Mc Keith Pr GBR. *Dist:* Cambridge U Pr.

Biology of the Chemotactic Response. Ed. by J. P. Armitage & J. M. Lackie. 1991. (Society for General Microbiology Symposia Ser.: No. 46). 420p. (C). text 130.00 (*0-521-40313-8*) Cambridge U Pr.

Biology of the General Adaptation Syndrome in Health & Disease: Index of New Information. Marshall E. Straus. 1997. 169p. 57.50 (*0-7883-1522-6*); pap. 47.50 (*0-7883-1523-4*) ABBE Pubs Assn.

Biology of the Integument: Vertebrates. Ed. by J. Bereiter-Hahn et al. 1986. (Biology of the Integument Ser.: Vol. 2). (Illus.). 870p. 362.00 (*0-387-13244-9*) Spr-Verlag.

Biology of the Intervertebral Disc. Peter Ghosh. 1988. LC 87-21781. Vol. 1. 256p. 146.00 (*0-8493-6711-5*, RD771); Vol. 2. 224p. 126.00 (*0-8493-6712-3*, RD771) Franklin.

Biology of the Joint. Hasselbach. 1981. text 60.00 (*0-7216-4569-0*) Saunders.

Biology of the Laboratory Rabbit. Ed. by Patrick J. Manning et al. 2nd ed. 1994. LC 93-39577. (American College of Laboratory Animal Medicine Ser.). (Illus.). 483p. text 132.00 (*0-12-469235-4*) Acad Pr.

Biology of the Mammal. A. G. Clegg & P. C. Clegg. 4th ed. 1975. (Illus.). (C). pap. 42.95 (*0-433-06122-7*) Coronet Bks.

Biology of the Mammary Gland. Ed. by Jan A. Mol & Roger A. Clegg. 2000. LC 00-33102. (Advances in Experimental Medicine & Biology Ser.: Vol. 480). (Illus.). xiv, 314p. 85.00 (*0-306-46414-4*) Plenum.

Biology of the Mycobacteria Vol. 2: Immunological & Environmental Aspects. Ed. by Colin Ratledge & John L. Stanford. 1983. text 209.00 (*0-12-582302-9*) Acad Pr.

Biology of the Ovary. Ed. by P. M. Motta & E. S. Hafez. 1980. (Developments in Obstetrics & Gynecology Ser.: No. 2). 345p. text 234.00 (*90-247-2316-7*) Kluwer Academic.

Biology of the Pancreas in Growing Animals. S. G. Pierzynowski & R. Zabielski. 1999. LC 99-34045. 476p. 171.00 (*0-444-50217-3*) Elsevier.

Biology of the Periodontal Connective Tissues. P. Mark Bartold & A. Sampath Narayanan. 1998. LC 98-17716. (Illus.). 278p. text 86.00 (*0-86715-340-7*) Quint Pub Co.

Biology of the Skin. R. K. Freinkel & D. T. Woodley. 2001. LC 00-29832. (Illus.). 432p. 97.95 (*1-85070-006-0*, Parthenon Pbng) CRC Pr.

Biology of the Species Porphyromonas Gingivalis. H. N. Shah & D. Myrand. 1993. LC 93-17936. 400p. 215.00 (*0-8493-6648-8*, QR201, CRC Reprint) Franklin.

Biology of the Sperm Cell. B. Bacetti & B. Afzelius. 1975. (Monographs in Developmental Biology: Vol. 10). (Illus.). 250p. 110.50 (*3-8055-2204-5*) S Karger.

Biology of the Uterus. R. M. Wynn & W. Jollie. 2nd rev. ed. 1989. (Illus.). 644p. (C). text 150.00 (*0-306-43057-6*, Kluwer Plenum) Kluwer Academic.

Biology of Tooth Movement. Ed. by Louis A. Norton & Charles J. Burstone. 1988. 384p. 259.00 (*0-8493-4733-5*, QP88) CRC Pr.

Biology of Trypanosoma & Leishmania, Parasites of Man & Domestic Animals. D. H. Molyneux & R. W. Ashford. 1983. 274p. (*0-85066-242-7*) Taylor & Francis.

Biology of Tubulo-Interstitial Cells, No. 6. Ed. by M. E. De Broe & M. J. F. Helbert. 1999. (Experimental Nephrology Ser.: Vol. 7, Nos. 5-6). (Illus.). iv, 146p. pap. 39.25 (*3-8055-6977-7*) S Karger.

Biology of Tumors: Proceedings of the 9th Annual Pezcoller Symposium Held in Rovereto, Italy, June 4-7, 1997. Ed. by Enrico Mihich & Carlo Croce. 1998. (Pezcoller Foundation Symposia Ser.: No. 9). (Illus.). 364p. 125.00 (*0-306-45932-9*, Kluwer Plenum) Kluwer Academic.

Biology of Vascular Disease. Ed. by Goran Holm & Magnus Bjorkholm. 1987. (Acta Medica Scandinavica Symposium Ser.: No. 3). (Illus.). 171p. 87.50 (*91-22-00866-7*) Coronet Bks.

Biology of Women. Ethel Sloane. 3rd ed. 1993. LC 92-48339. 760p. (C). pap. 63.95 (*0-8273-4938-6*) Delmar.

Biology of Women. Ethel Sloane & Patricia Sloane-White. 4th ed. 2001. LC 00-65690. (Illus.). 784p. text 72.95 (*0-7668-1142-5*) Delmar.

Biology Problem Solver. Research and Education Association Staff. rev. ed. 1999. LC 78-63610. (REA Problem Solvers Ser.). (Illus.). 1088p. pap. text 23.95 (*0-87891-514-1*) Res & Educ.

Biology Reviews Vol. 10, Pt. 3: Room Temperature & Low Temperature Magnetic Circular Dichroism of Hemoproteins & Related Compounds, Vol. 10. Yu. A. Sharonov. 1991. (Soviet Scientific Reviews Ser.: Section D). 118p. text 118.00 (*3-7186-5181-5*, Harwood Acad Pubs) Gordon & Breach.

Biology Reviews Vol. 11, Pt. 2: Enhancement of Macromolecule Penetration into Cells & Nontraditional Drug Delivery Systems, Vol. 11. A. Kabanov. 1992. (Soviet Scientific Reviews Ser.: Section D). 75p. pap. text 104.00 (*3-7186-5327-3*, Harwood Acad Pubs) Gordon & Breach.

Biology, Toxicology & Carcinogenesis of Respiratory Epithelium. David G. Thomassen & Paul Nettesheim. 1989. 94.95 (*0-89116-941-5*) Hemisp Pub.

Biology Two: Laboratory Manual. Darrell S. Vodopich & Moore. 1989. (Illus.). 320p. spiral bd., lab manual ed. 17.95 (*0-8016-5289-8*) Mosby Inc.

Biomagnetic & Herbal Therapy. Michael Tierra. 1997. LC 96-80512. (Illus.). 108p. pap. 10.95 (*0-914955-33-0*) Lotus Pr.

Biomarkers: Biochemical, Physiological, & Histological Markers of Anthropogenic Stress. Robert J. Huggett et al. 1992. 368p. 110.00 (*0-87371-505-5*, L505) Lewis Pubs.

Biomarkers: Medical & Workplace Applications. Mortimer L. Mendelsohn et al. 1998. LC 98-3882. 500p. (C). text 69.95 (*0-309-06422-8*) Natl Acad Pr.

Biomarkers: The Ten Keys to Prolonging Vitality. William Evans et al. 1992. LC 91-9133. (Illus.). 304p. per. 14.00 (*0-671-77898-6*) S&S Trade.

Biomarkers & Occupational Health: Progress & Perspectives. Ed. by Mortimer L. Mendelsohn et al. 1995. 350p. (C). text 54.95 (*0-309-05187-8*) Natl Acad Pr.

Biomarkers & Risk Assessment: Concepts & Principles. WHO Staff. 1993. (Environmental Health Criteria Ser.: No. 155). (FRE & SPA.). 92p. pap. text 24.00 (*92-4-157155-1*, 1160155) World Health.

Biomarkers for Agrochemicals & Toxic Substances: Applications & Risk Assessment, Vol. 643. Ed. by Jerry N. Blancato et al. 1996. LC 96-28772. (ACS Symposium Ser.: No. 643). (Illus.). 296p. text 110.00 (*0-8412-3449-3*) Am Chemical.

Biomaterial-Tissue Interfaces: Proceedings of the Ninth European Conference on Biomaterials, Chester, U. K., September 9-11, 1991. Ed. by P. J. Doherty et al. 1992. LC 92-49135. (Advances in Biomaterials Ser.: Vol. 10). xii,534p. 315.50 (*0-444-89065-3*) Elsevier.

Biomaterials: An Introduction. J. B. Park & R. S. Lakes. 2nd ed. 1992. (Illus.). 408p. (C). text 59.50 (*0-306-43992-1*, Kluwer Plenum) Kluwer Academic.

Biomaterials: Interfacial Phenomena & Applications. Ed. by Stuart L. Cooper & Nicholas A. Peppas. 1982. LC 82-6763. (ACS Advances in Chemistry Ser.: No. 199). 539p. lib. bdg. 76.95 (*0-8412-0631-7*) Am Chemical.

Biomaterials & Biodegradable Polymers & Macromolecules: Current Research & Industrial Applications: Proceedings of Symposium G on Biomaterials—perspectives for Research & Industry at the Century Change & Proceedings of Symposium H on Biodegradable Polymers & Macromolecules of the 1997 ICAM/E-MRS Spring Conference, Strasbourg, France, June 16-20, 1997. 1998. LC 99-183909. 320p. 344.00 (*0-444-20516-0*) Elsevier.

Biomaterials & Bioengineering Handbook. Donald L. Wise. 2000. LC 00-24962. (Illus.). 944p. pap. text 235.00 (*0-8247-0318-9*) Dekker.

Biomaterials Engineering & Devices - Human Applications Vol. 1: Fundamentals & Vascular & Carrier Applications Ed. by Donald L. Wise et al. 2000. LC 99-86203. (Illus.). 368p. 150.00 (*0-89603-858-0*) Humana.

Biomaterials Engineering & Devices - Human Applications Vol. 2: Orthopedic, Dental & Bone Graft Applications Ed. by Donald L. Wise et al. 2000. LC 99-86203. (Illus.). 368p. 149.50 (*0-89603-859-9*) Humana.

Biomaterials for Drug & Cell Delivery Vol. 331: Materials Research Society Symposium Proceedings. Ed. by Antonios G. Mikes et al. 1994. LC 94-9650. 289p. text 83.00 (*1-55899-230-8*) Materials Res.

Biomaterials in Otology. Ed. by J. J. Grote. 1983. 324p. text 199.50 (*0-89838-610-1*) Kluwer Academic.

Biomaterials in Surgery. Walenkamp. 1998. (Illus.). 141p. pap. 69.00 (*0-86577-805-1*) Thieme Med Pubs.

Biomaterials' Mechanical Properties. Ed. by Helen E. Kambic & A. Toshimitsu Yokobori, Jr. 1994. LC 93-48490. (STP Ser.: Vol. 1173). (Illus.). 312p. 89.00 (*0-8031-1894-5*, STP1173) ASTM.

Biomaterials, Medical Devices & Tissue Engineering: An Integrated Approach. F. H. Silver. 1993. (Illus.). 304p. (gr. 13). pap. 179.95 (*0-412-41260-8*) Chapman & Hall.

Biomaterials Science. Buddy D. Ratner & Jack E. Lemon. Ed. by Frederick J. Scheon et al. 1997. (Illus.). 484p. pap. text 79.95 (*0-12-582461-0*) Acad Pr.

Biomechanical Analysis of the Musculoskeletal Structure for Medicine & Sports. R. Arvikar & Ali A. Seireg. 1989. 700p. 120.00 (*0-89116-423-5*) Hemisp Pub.

Biomechanical & Morphological Analysis of Human Hand Joints. J. Koebke. 1983. (Advances in Anatomy, Embryology & Cell Biology Ser.: Vol. 80). (Illus.). 85p. 39.95 (*0-387-12438-1*) Spr-Verlag.

Biomechanical Basis of Human Movement. Joe Hamill & Kathleen Knutzen. 1995. LC 94-22325. (Illus.). 542p. 56.95 (*0-683-03863-X*) Lppncott W & W.

Biomechanical Measurement. Phillips. 1997. pap. text (*0-7216-4473-2*) Saunders.

Biomechanics: A Qualitative Approach for Studying Human Movement. Ellen Kreighbaum & Katharine Barthels. 4th ed. 1996. (C). tchr. ed. (*0-205-19145-2*, H9145-7) Allyn.

Biomechanics: An Approach to Vertebrate Biology. Carl Gans. 1980. LC 80-18705. 272p. (C). pap. text 22.95 (*0-472-08016-4*, 08016) U of Mich Pr.

Biomechanics: Mechanical Properties of Living Tissues. Yuan-Cheng Fung. 2nd ed. 1996. LC 92-33749. (Illus.). 568p. 69.95 (*0-387-97947-6*) Spr-Verlag.

Biomechanics: Principles & Applications. R. Huiskes. 1982. text 211.50 (*90-247-3047-3*) Kluwer Academic.

Biomechanics: Problem Solving for Functional Activity. Roberts. 1991. (Illus.). 216p. (gr. 13). pap. text 29.95 (*0-8016-4047-4*, 04047) Mosby Inc.

Biomechanics & Cells. Ed. by Fiona Lyall & A. J. El Haj. 1994. LC 93-42046. (Society for Experimental Biology Seminar Ser.: No. 54). (Illus.). 287p. (C). text 80.00 (*0-521-45454-9*) Cambridge U Pr.

Biomechanics & Medicine in Swimming, Vol. VII. J. Troup & D. Strass. 1996. LC 96-69459. 296p. (C). 110.00 (*0-419-20480-6*) Routledge.

Biomechanics & Motor Control of Human Movement. David A. Winter. 2nd ed. 1990. LC 89-70467. 296p. 110.00 (*0-471-50908-6*) Wiley.

Biomechanics-Functional Adaption & Remodeling. Ed. by K. Hayashi et al. 1996. (Illus.). 320p. 159.00 (*4-431-70173-7*) Spr-Verlag.

Biomechanics in Clinical Orthodontics. Ravindra Nanda. Ed. by Larry McGrew. 1996. 368p. text 130.00 (*0-7216-2784-6*) Saunders.

Biomechanics in Orthopedics. Ed. by S. Niwa et al. 1993. LC 92-49957. (*4-431-70108-7*); (*3-540-70108-7*); (Illus.). 340p. 181.00 (*0-387-70108-7*) Spr-Verlag.

Biomechanics in Sports: Performance Improvement & Injury Prevention. Ed. by Vladimir M. Zatsiorsky. 2000. LC 99-54566. (Encyclopedia of Sports Medicine Ser.: Vol. 9). (Illus.). 680p. 131.95 (*0-632-05392-5*) Blackwell Sci.

Biomechanics in the Musculoskeletal System. M. M. Panjabi & Augusta A. White. 2000. LC 00-64376. (Illus.). 255p. 59.00 (*0-443-06585-3*) Saunders.

Biomechanics of Diarthrodial Joints Ed. by V. C. Mow et al. 1990. (Illus.). Vol. I. 451p. 99.00 (*0-387-97378-8*); Vol. II. 464p. 99.00 (*0-387-97379-6*) Spr-Verlag.

Biomechanics Of Exercise Physiology. Arthur T. Johnson. 1991. LC 90-12842. 493p. 210.00 (*0-471-85398-4*) Wiley.

Biomechanics of Hearing. Ed. by John J. Rosowski & Albrecht Eiber. 1999. (Audiology & Neuro-Otology Ser.: Vol. 4, Nos. 3-4 (1999)). (Illus.). 90p. pap. 34.00 (*3-8055-6847-9*) S Karger.

Biomechanics of Human Movement. Marlene J. Adrian & John M. Cooper. 2nd ed. 1994. 592p. (C). text 80.31 (*0-697-16242-7*) McGrw-H Hghr Educ.

Biomechanics of Impact Injury & Injury Tolerances of the Abdomen, Lumbar Spine & Pelvic Complex. Ed. by Stanley H. Backaitis. 1995. 60p. pap. 149.00 (*1-56091-592-7*, PT47) Soc Auto Engineers.

Biomechanics of Impact Injury & Injury Tolerances of the Extremities. Ed. by Stanley H. Backaitis. 1996. LC 96-67656. (Progress in Technology Ser.). 896p. 149.00 (*1-56091-749-0*, PT-56) Soc Auto Engineers.

Biomechanics of Medical Devices. Dhanjoo N. Ghista. 1981. LC 80-15480. (Biomedical Engineering & Instrumentation Ser.: Vol. 7). (Illus.). 704p. text 275.00 (*0-8247-6848-5*) Dekker.

Biomechanics of Motion. Ed. by A. Morecki. 1981. (CISM Courses & Lectures: Vol. 263). (Illus.). 233p. 54.95 (*0-387-81611-9*) Spr-Verlag.

Biomechanics of Musculoskeletal Injury. William C. Whiting & Ronald F. Zernicke. 1998. LC 97-41020. (Illus.). 296p. text 49.00 (*0-87322-779-4*, BWHI0779) Human Kinetics.

Biomechanics of Normal & Pathological Human Articulating Joints. Ed. by Necip Berme et al. 1985. (NATO Advanced Science Institutes Ser.). text 184.00 (*90-247-3164-X*) Kluwer Academic.

Biomechanics of the Foot & Ankle. Robert A. Donatelli. 2nd ed. 1995. LC 95-24075. (Contemporary Perspectives in Rehabilitation Ser.). (Illus.). 391p. (C). 47.00 (*0-8036-0031-3*) Davis Co.

Biomechanics of the Hip. P. G. Maquet. 1984. (Illus.). 309p. 199.00 (*0-387-13257-0*) Spr-Verlag.

Biomechanics of the Knee. P. G. Maquet. 2nd ed. 1983. (Illus.). 306p. 217.00 (*0-387-12489-6*) Spr-Verlag.

Biomechanics of the Spine: Clinical & Surgical Perspective. Ed. by Vijay K. Goel & James N. Weinstein. 1989. 312p. 169.00 (*0-8493-6649-6*, RD768) CRC Pr.

Biomechanics of the Wrist Joint. Ed. by K. N. An et al. 1991. (Illus.). 174p. 84.95 (*0-387-97674-4*) Spr-Verlag.

Biomedical Advances in Aging. Ed. by Allan L. Goldstein. 1989. (GWUMC Department of Biochemistry & Molecular Biology Annual Spring Symposium Ser.). (Illus.). 598p. 135.00 (*0-306-43275-7*, Plenum Trade) Perseus Pubng.

Biomedical & Clinical Instrumentation: Fast Tracking from Concept Through Production in a Regulated Environment. Robert Meltzer. 1993. 274p. 135.00 (*0-935184-50-3*) IHS Health Grp.

Biomedical & Social Advances AIDS & Associated Tumors: Antibiotics & Chemotherapy, Vol. 43. 1991. (Illus.). viii, 284p. 215.75 (*3-8055-5303-X*) S Karger.

Biomedical Applications of Computer Modeling. Arthur Christopoulos. 2000. LC 00-44445. (Pharmacology & Toxicology Ser.). (Illus.). 264p. 99.95 (*0-8493-0100-9*) CRC Pr.

Biomedical Applications of Mass Spectrometry. Clarence H. Suelter. 1990. LC 54-7232. (Methods of Biochemical Analysis Ser.). 396p. 220.00 (*0-471-61303-7*) Wiley.

Biomedical Applications of Microencapsulation. Ed. by Franklin Lim. 1984. 192p. 101.00 (*0-8493-5440-4*, RS201, CRC Reprint) Franklin.

Biomedical Applications of Microprobe Analysis. Ingram Staff et al. 1999. LC 99-61699. (Illus.). xxv, 545p. 69.95 (*0-12-371020-0*) Acad Pr.

Biomedical Applications of Polymeric Materials. Ed. by Teiji Tsuruta et al. 1993. 512p. 225.00 (*0-8493-4519-7*, R857) CRC Pr.

Biomedical Applications of Spectroscopy. Ed. by R.J. Clark & R. E. Hester. 1996. LC 95-42360. (Advances in Spectroscopy Ser.: Vol. 25). 402p. 368.00 (*0-471-95918-9*) Wiley.

Biomedical Applications of Synthetic Biodegradable Polymers. Ed. by Jeffrey Hollinger. 1995. LC 95-8042. 256p. 199.95 (*0-8493-4896-X*, 4896) CRC Pr.

Biomedical Aspects of Drug Dependence: International Biomedical Research Symposium on Drug

Dependence, Tangier, Morocco, 11-15 October 1982. Ed. by A. A. Badawy. 1984. (Illus.). 120p. pap. 22.00 (0-08-030785-X, Pergamon Pr) Elsevier.

Biomedical Aspects of Intrauterine Devices. Ed. by H. Hasson et al. 1984. (Advances in Reproductive Health Care Ser.). text 225.00 (0-85200-806-6) Kluwer Academic.

***Biomedical Communications.** Jon D. Miller & Linda K. Kimmel. 2001. LC 2001-90864. (Illus.). 458p. pap. 29.95 (0-12-496751-5) Acad Pr.

Biomedical Desk Reference. Daniel J. Schneck. 1992. (C). text 65.00 (0-8147-7940-9) NYU Pr.

***Biomedical Diagnostic, Guidance, & Surgical-Assist Systems II: 25-25 January 2000, San Jose, California.** Ed. by Tuan Vo-Dinh et al. 2000. LC 00-710357. (Progress in Biomedical Optics & Imaging Ser.: No. 1). (Illus.). ix, 388p. (0-8194-3527-9) SPIE.

Biomedical Engineering: An International Symposium. Ed. by Wen-Jei Yang & Chun-Jean Lee. 1989. (Illus.). 375p. 94.95 (0-89116-827-3) Hemisp Pub.

Biomedical Engineering: Index of Modern Information. John C. Bartone, II. 1990. LC 88-48000. 150p. pap. 44.50 (1-55914-077-1) ABBE Pubs Assn.

Biomedical Engineering: Opening Doors, Set. Ed. by Donald C. Mikulecky & Alexander M. Clarke. 1990. (Monographs in Biomedical Engineering). 298p. (C). text 85.00 (0-8147-7908-5) NYU Pr.

Biomedical Engineering & Data Processing in Pneumonology: Proceedings of the International Titisee Conference, Titisee, October 19-21, 1978. International Titisee Conference Staff. Ed. by H. Matthys. 1979. (Progress in Respiratory Research Ser.: Vol. 11). (Illus.). 101.00 (3-8055-3012-9) S Karger.

Biomedical Engineering Dictionary. Coatrieux. 2001. (Biomedical Engineering Ser.). 400p. (C). 69.95 (0-12-177375-2) Acad Pr.

Biomedical Engineering Handbook. Joseph D. Bronzino. 2nd ed. 1999. (Electrical Engineering Handbook Ser.). 3168p. 139.95 (0-8493-8594-6) CRC Pr.

Biomedical Engineering Principles: An Introduction to Fluid, Heat & Mass Transport Processes. Ed. by David Cooney. 1976. (Biomedical Engineering & Instrumentation Ser.: Vol. 2). (Illus.). 464p. text 125.00 (0-8247-6347-5) Dekker.

Biomedical Equipment Vol. 2, Pt. 1: General Safety & Design, Equipment for Therapy & Surgery. 1996. (Illus.). 820p. (Orig.). pap. 260.00 (1-57020-046-7, BEBK6-1-209) Assn Adv Med Instrn.

Biomedical Equipment Vol. 2, Pt. 2: Monitoring & Diagnostic Equipment, 1995. 1995. (Illus.). pap. 235.00 (1-57020-047-5, BEBK5-2-209) Assn Adv Med Instrn.

Biomedical Ethics. Ed. by Terry O'Neil. 1998. LC 98-37239. (Opposing Viewpoints Digests Ser.). (Illus.). 144p. (J). (gr. 4-12). pap. 14.95 (1-56510-874-4, Greenhaven Pr) Gale.

Biomedical Ethics. Ed. by Thomas A. Mappes et al. 4th ed. 1995. LC 95-9348. 672p. (C). text 60.00 (0-07-040141-1) McGrw-H Hghr Educ.

Biomedical Ethics: Opposing Viewpoints. Ed. by Terry O'Neill. 1994. LC 93-7260. 312p. pap. 16.20 (1-56510-061-1); lib. bdg. 26.20 (1-56510-062-X) Gale (Greenhaven Pr).

Biomedical Ethics: Opposing Viewpoints. Ed. by Tamara L. Roleff. 1998. LC 97-51374. (Opposing Viewpoints Ser.). 252p. (YA). (gr. 5-12). pap. 16.20 (1-56510-792-6); lib. bdg. 26.20 (1-56510-793-4) Gale (Greenhaven Pr).

Biomedical Ethics & Fetal Therapy. Ed. by Carl Nimrod & Glenn Griener. 1988. (Calgary Institute for the Humanities Ser.). 122p. (C). pap. (0-88920-962-6) W Laurier U Pr.

Biomedical Ethics & the Law. Ed. by James M. Humber & Robert E. Almeder. 2nd ed. 1979. LC 79-17758. 672p. pap. 45.00 (0-306-40242-4, Plenum Trade) Perseus Pubng.

Biomedical Ethics in Canada. John Williams. 1986. LC 86-5453. 202p. lib. bdg. 89.95 (0-88946-149-X) E Mellen.

Biomedical Ethics in United States Public Policy. 1995. lib. bdg. 251.99 (0-8490-7567-X) Gordon Pr.

Biomedical Ethics Reviews - 1983. Ed. by James M. Humber & Robert F. Almeder. 1983. LC 83-74. (Biomedical Ethics Reviews Ser.). 220p. 59.50 (0-89603-041-5) Humana.

Biomedical Ethics Reviews - 1985. Ed. by James M. Humber & Robert F. Almeder. 1986. LC 84-640015. (Biomedical Ethics Reviews Ser.). 196p. 59.50 (0-89603-093-8) Humana.

Biomedical Ethics Reviews - 1987. Ed. by James M. Humber & Robert F. Almeder. 1988. LC 84-640015. (Biomedical Ethics Reviews Ser.). 195p. 55.50 (0-89603-136-5) Humana.

Biomedical Ethics Reviews - 1989. Ed. by James M. Humber & Robert F. Almeder. 1990. LC 84-640015. (Biomedical Ethics Reviews Ser.). 180p. 49.50 (0-89603-169-1) Humana.

Biomedical Ethics Reviews - 1990. Ed. by James M. Humber & Robert F. Almeder. 1991. LC 84-640015. (Biomedical Ethics Reviews Ser.). 257p. 49.50 (0-89603-203-5) Humana.

Biomedical Ethics Reviews - 1992. Ed. by James M. Humber & Robert F. Almeder. 1993. LC 84-640015. (Biomedical Ethics Reviews Ser.). 246p. 49.50 (0-89603-240-X) Humana.

Biomedical Functions & Biotechnology of Natural & Artificial Polymers, Self-assemblies, Hybrid Complexes & Biological Conjugates of Glycans, Liposomes, Polyethylene Glycols, Polyisopropylamides, & Polypeptides. Ed. by Manssur Yalpani. 1996. (Frontiers in Biomedicine & Biotechnology Ser.: Vol. 3). 296p. pap. 119.00 (1-882360-32-X) ATL Pr Sci.

Biomedical Functions & Biotechnology of Natural Artificial Polymers: Self-Assemblies, Hybrid Complexes & Biological Conjugates of Glycans, Liposomes, Polyethylene Glycols, Polyisoprpylacrylamides, & Polypeptides. Ed. by Manssur Yalpani. 1996. (Frontiers in Biomedicine & Biotechnology Ser.: Vol. 3). (Illus.). 296p. 220.00 (1-882360-02-8) ATL Pr Sci.

***Biomedical Globalization: The International Migration of Scientists.** Sergio Diaz-Briquets & Charles C. Cheney. 2001. 134p. 34.95 (0-7658-0104-3) Transaction Pubs.

Biomedical Image Analysis (WBIA '98) 1998 Workshop. Ed. by Baba C. Vemuri. 1998. LC 98-84706. pap. 120.00 (0-8186-8460-7) Inst Electrical.

Biomedical Image Processing & Three-Dimensional Microscopy. Ed. by R. S. Acharya et al. 1992. 126.00 (0-8194-0814-X, 1660) SPIE.

Biomedical Implications of Radiostrontium Exposure: Proceedings. Ed. by Marvin Goldman & Leo K. Bustad. 1972. LC 72-600049. (AEC Symposium Ser.). 412p. pap. 18.25 (0-87079-152-4, CONF-710201); fiche 9.00 (0-87079-153-2, CONF-710201) DOE.

Biomedical Information Technology: Global Social Responsibilities for the Democratic Information Age. Harold Sackman. 1997. LC 97-2836. (Library & Information Science Ser.). (Illus.). 316p. text 59.95 (0-12-613745-5) Morgan Kaufmann.

Biomedical Innovation. Ed. by Edward Roberts et al. 1981. (Illus.). 368p. 44.00 (0-262-18103-7) MIT Pr.

Biomedical Institutions, Biomedical Funding, & Public Policy. Ed. by H. Hugh Fudenberg. 1983. LC 83-11159. 236p. 45.00 (0-306-41231-4, Plenum Trade) Perseus Pubng.

Biomedical Issues in U. S. Public Policy. 1994. (Illus.). 92p. (Orig.). (C). pap. text 35.00 (0-7881-0448-9) DIANE Pub.

Biomedical Laser: Technology & Clinical Applications. Ed. by Leon Goldman. 1981. (Illus.). 350p. 159.00 (0-387-90571-5) Spr-Verlag.

Biomedical Light Microscopy. Ed. by J. James & H. J. Tanke. 1991. (C). text 146.50 (0-7923-0946-4) Kluwer Academic.

Biomedical Magnetic Resonance Technology. C. N. Chen & D. I. Hoult. 1989. (Medical Science Ser.). (Illus.). 362p. 163.00 (0-85274-118-9) Inst of Physics Pubng.

Biomedical Modeling & Simulation on a PC: A Workbench for Physiology & Biomedical Engineering. Ed. by R. P. Van Wijk van Brievingh et al. 1992. (Advances in Simulation Ser.: Vol. 6). (Illus.). 517p. 215.00 incl. 5.25 hd (0-387-97650-7) Spr-Verlag.

Biomedical Optics & Lasers: Diagnostics & Treatment. Ed. by Junheng Li & James A. Harrington. 1998. LC 98-233180. (Proceedings of SPIE Ser.: Vol. 3548). 250p. 80.00 (0-8194-3009-9) SPIE.

Biomedical Particle Accelerators. Waldemar H. Scharf. 1997. 480p. 107.00 (1-56396-089-3) Spr-Verlag.

Biomedical Physics & Biomaterials Science. Ed. by H. Eugene Stanley. 1972. LC 72-8855. (C). pap. text 20.00 (0-262-69038-1) MIT Pr.

Biomedical Policy & Mental Health. Donna R. Kempt. 1994. LC 93-43788. 240p. 70.00 (0-275-94812-9, Praeger Pubs) Greenwood.

Biomedical Politics. Institute of Medicine Staff. Ed. by Kathi E. Hanna. 1991. 360p. 29.95 (0-309-04486-3) Natl Acad Pr.

Biomedical Polymers: Designed-to-Degrade Systems. W. Shalaby. 1993. LC 93-50660. 352p. 128.00 (1-56990-159-7) Hanser-Gardner.

Biomedical Polymers: Molecular Design to Clinical Applications. Ed. by Daniel Cohn & Joseph Kost. 1993. LC 93-27080. 177p. pap. 228.50 (1-85861-043-5, Pergamon Pr) Elsevier.

Biomedical Polymers & Polymer Therapeutics. Ed. by Emo Chiellini. 2001. LC 00-52736. (Illus.). xviii, 451p. (J). 110.00 (0-306-46472-1, Kluwer Plenum) Kluwer Academic.

Biomedical Research: How to Plan, Publish & Present It. W. F. Whimster. 2nd ed. 1997. LC 96-42694. (Illus.). 276p. pap. 28.00 (3-540-19876-8) Spr-Verlag.

Biomedical Research Involving Animals: Proposed International Guiding Principles. Z. Bankowski & N. Howard-Jones. 1984. (CIOMS Round Table Proceedings Ser.: No. 17). pap. text 25.00 (92-9036-017-8) World Health.

Biomedical Research Using Radiochemicals: Current & Future Trends. Ed. by E. A. Evans & K. G. Oldham. 1988. LC 87-37182. (Critical Reports on Applied Chemistry). 162p. 618.95 (0-471-91878-4) Wiley.

Biomedical Science & Technology: Recent Developments in the Pharmaceutical & Medical Sciences. Ed. by A. Atilla Hincal & H. Suheyla Kas. 1998. LC 98-22345. (Illus.). 254p. (C). text 85.00 (0-306-45837-3, Kluwer Plenum) Kluwer Academic.

Biomedical Sciences. Margaret Dickenson. 1994. 165p. (C). 24.22 (1-56870-146-2) RonJon Pub.

Biomedical Sensing & Imaging Technologies, Vol. 3253. Ed. by Robert A. Lieberman & Tuan Vo-Dinh. 1998. 300p. 80.00 (0-8194-2692-X) SPIE.

Biomedical Sensing, Imaging & Tracking Technologies I: 29-31 January 1996, San Jose, California. Robert A. Lieberman et al. 1996. LC 95-72271. (Proceedings Ser.). vii, 384 p. 85.00 (0-8194-2050-6) SPIE.

Biomedical Sensing, Imaging & Tracking Technologies II, Vol. 2976. Ed. by Tuan Vo-Dinh et al. 1997. LC 98-103990. 390p. 107.00 (0-8194-2387-4) SPIE.

Biomedical Sensors, Fibers, & Optical Delivery Systems, Vol. 3570. Ed. by Nathan I. Croitoru et al. 1999. LC 99-225587. (Europto Ser.). (Illus.). ix, 304p. 80.00 (0-8194-3032-3) SPIE.

Biomedical Signal Processing. Metin Akay. 1994. LC 93-25710. 377p. text 58.00 (0-12-047145-0) Acad Pr.

Biomedical Signal Processing. Arnon Cohen. 2nd ed. 1994. 125.00 (0-8493-4238-4) CRC Pr.

Biomedical Significance of Peptide Research. F. A. Laszlo & F. Antoni. 1984. 278p. (C). (963-05-3886-5) Akade Kiado HUN. *Dist:* Intl Spec Bk, St Mut.

Biomedical Systems & Technologies. Ed. by Nathan I. Croitoru et al. 1996. (Europto Ser.: Vol. 2928). 292p. 76.00 (0-8194-2330-0) SPIE.

Biomedical Systems & Technologies II, Vol. 3199. Ed. by Francesco Baldini et al. 1998. LC 98-162135. (Europto Ser.). 316p. 80.00 (0-8194-2631-8) SPIE.

Biomedical Technician. Jack Rudman. (Career Examination Ser.: C-3695). pap. 29.95 (0-8373-3695-3) Nat Learn.

Biomedical Technologies & Health Policy. Ed. by Robert H. Blank & Miriam Mills. 1989. (Orig.). pap. 15.00 (0-944285-07-4) Pol Studies.

Biomedical Technology & Human Rights. Eugene B. Brody. 1993. LC 93-175. (Unesco Ser.). 326p. (1-85521-373-7) Dartmth Pub GBR. *Dist:* Ashgate Pub Co.

Biomedical Technology & Public Policy, 26. Ed. by Robert H. Blank & Miriam K. Mills. 1989. LC 89-16899. (Contributions in Medical Studies Ser.: No. 26). 250p. 68.00 (0-313-26629-8, BBH/, Greenwood Pr) Greenwood.

Biomedical Technology Resources: A Research Resources Directory. Ed. by Barry Leonard. 1998. 92p. reprint ed. pap. text 25.00 (0-7881-4187-2) DIANE Pub.

Biomedical Terminology: Greek-English & English-Greek Glossary. B. Samios. 1991. (ENG & GRE.). 733p. 250.00 (0-7859-9050-X) Fr & Eur.

Biomedical Transducers & Instruments. Tatsuo Togawa et al. 1997. LC 96-40279. 384p. 149.95 (0-8493-7671-8, 7671) CRC Pr.

Biomedical Uses of Radiation Pts. A & B Ed. by William R. Hendee. 1999. 1428p. 675.00 (3-527-29668-9) Wiley.

Biomedicine & Alternative Healing Systems in America: Issues of Class, Race & Gender. Hans A. Baer. 2001. LC 00-12733. xii, 222p. 55.00 (0-299-16690-2); pap. 21.95 (0-299-16694-5) U of Wis Pr.

Biomedicine Examined. Ed. by Margaret M. Lock & Deborah R. Gordon. 1988. (Culture, Illness & Healing Ser.: No. 13). 558p. pap. text 73.50 (1-55608-072-7) Kluwer Academic.

Biomembranes. Lester Packer. 1974. (Methods in Enzymology Ser.: Vol. 31). Pt. A. text 199.00 (0-12-181894-2); Pt. B. text 199.00 (0-12-181895-0) Acad Pr.

Biomembranes: Visual Pigments & Purple Membranes, II, Pt. I. Ed. by Sidney P. Colowick & Lester Packer. 1982. (Methods in Enzymology Ser.: Vol. 88). 750p. text 188.00 (0-12-181988-4) Acad Pr.

Biomembranes Pt. M: Transport in Bacteria, Mitochondria, & Chloroplasts: General Approaches & Transport Systems. Ed. by Sidney P. Colowick & Nathan O. Kaplan. 1986. (Methods in Enzymology Ser.: Vol. 125). text 178.00 (0-12-182025-4) Acad Pr.

Biomembranes Pt. K: Membrane Biogenesis: Assembly & Targeting (Prokaryotes, Mitochondria, & Chloroplasts) Ed. by Sidney Fleischer & Becca Fleischer. 1983. (Methods in Enzymology Ser.: Vol. 97). text 188.00 (0-12-181997-3) Acad Pr.

Biomembranes Pt. N: Transport in Bacteria, Mitochondria, & Chloroplasts: Protonmotive Force. Ed. by Sidney P. Colowick & Nathan O. Kaplan. 1986. (Methods in Enzymology Ser.: Vol. 126). text 178.00 (0-12-182026-2) Acad Pr.

Biomembranes Pt. R: Transport Theory: Cells & Model Membranes. Ed. by John N. Abelson et al. 1989. (Methods in Enzymology Ser.: Vol. 171). 900p. text 157.00 (0-12-182072-6) Acad Pr.

Biomembranes Vol. 11: Pathological Membranes. Ed. by Alois Nowotny. 1983. LC 82-22343. 494p. 110.00 (0-306-41065-6, Plenum Trade) Perseus Pubng.

Biomimetic Materials Chemistry. Ed. by Stephen Mann. 1995. 400p. 185.00 (0-471-18597-3) Wiley.

Biominerals. Ed. by F. C. M. Driessens. 1990. 440p. lib. bdg. 259.00 (0-8493-5280-0, QP88) CRC Pr.

Biomolecular Engineering in the European Community. Ed. by E. Magnien. 1986. text 445.50 (90-247-3400-2) Kluwer Academic.

Bion & Group Psychotherapy. Ed. by Malcolm Pines. 1985. (International Library of Philosophy, Psychology, & Scientific Method). 336p. 49.95 (0-7100-9949-5, 99495, Routledge Thoemms) Routledge.

Bion in New York & Sao Paulo. Wilfred R. Bion. Ed. by F. Bion. 1980. 128p. pap. (0-902965-13-1) Clunie Pr GBR. *Dist:* Other Pr LLC.

Bion's Legacy to Groups. Ed. by Parthenope Bion Talamo et al. 1998. 128p. pap. (1-85575-188-7) Karnac Bks GBR. *Dist:* Other Pr LLC.

Bioorganic Chemistry in Healthcare & Technology. Ed. by U. K. Pandit & F. C. Alderweireldt. 1991. (NATO Advanced Science Institutes Ser.: Vol. 207). (Illus.). 326p. (C). text 138.00 (0-306-44007-5, Kluwer Plenum) Kluwer Academic.

Biopathology of the Liver: An Ultrastructural Approach. Ed. by P. M. Motta. 1988. (C). text 254.00 (0-7462-0049-8) Kluwer Academic.

Biopharmaceutical Drug Design & Development. Ed. by Susanna Wu-Pong & Yongyut Rojanasakul. 1999. LC 98-53441. (Illus.). 448p. 99.50 (0-89603-691-X) Humana.

Biopharmaceutical Process Validation. Gail K. Sofer & Dane W. Zabriskie. 2000. LC 00-24958. (Biotechnology & Bioprocessing Ser.). (Illus.). 400p. text 150.00 (0-8247-0249-2) Dekker.

Biopharmaceutical Sequential Statistical Applications. Ed. by Karl A. Peace. 1992. (Statistics: Textbooks & Monographs: Vol. 128). (Illus.). 376p. text 165.00 (0-8247-8628-9) Dekker.

Biopharmaceuticals. Edwards. Date not set. (Pharmaceutical Engineering Ser.: No. 8). 170.00 (0-7506-5065-6) Buttrwrth-Heinemann.

Biopharmaceuticals: An Industrial Perspective. Gary Walsh & Brendan Murphy. 1999. LC 99-25678. (Illus.). x, 514p. (0-7923-5746-9) Kluwer Academic.

Biopharmaceuticals: Biochemistry & Biotechnology. Gary Walsh. 1998. LC 97-44167. 448p. 150.00 (0-471-97788-8); pap. 64.95 (0-471-97789-6) Wiley.

Biopharmaceuticals of Occular Drug Delivery. Edman. 1992. 224p. lib. bdg. 129.00 (0-8493-7296-8, RE994) CRC Pr.

Biopharmaceutics & Clinical Pharmacokinetics. Milo Gibaldi. 4th ed. 1990. LC 90-5614. (Illus.). 406p. text 47.95 (0-8121-1346-2) Lppncott W & W.

Biopharmaceutics & Clinical Pharmacokinetics: An Introduction. Robert E. Notari. 4th rev. ed. 1986. (Illus.). 440p. text 59.75 (0-8247-7523-6) Dekker.

Biophilosophy. Bernhard Rensch. Tr. by Cecilia Sym from GER. 1971. LC 72-132692. 61.00 (0-231-03299-4) Col U Pr.

Biophosphonates & Tumor-Osteolysis. Ed. by K. W. Brunner et al. 1989. (Recent Results in Cancer Research Ser.: Vol. 116). (Illus.). 95p. 43.00 (0-387-50560-1) Spr-Verlag.

Biophysical Approach to Excitable Systems: A Volume in Honor of Kenneth S. Cole on His 80th Birthday. Ed. by William J. Adelman, Jr. & David E. Goldman. 1981. LC 81-15759. 270p. 65.00 (0-306-40784-1, Plenum Trade) Perseus Pubng.

Biophysical Aspects of the Medical Use of Technetium-99m. James G. Kereiakes et al. 1976. (AAPM Monographs: No. 1). 126p. (Orig.). pap. text (1-888340-05-3) AAPM.

Biophysical Chemistry Part III: The Behavior of Biological Macromolecules. Charles R. Cantor & Paul R. Schimmel. 1980. LC 79-27860. (Illus.). 597p. (C). pap. text 64.95 (0-7167-1192-3) W H Freeman.

Biophysical Foundations of Human Movement. Ed. by Bruce Abernethy et al. 1997. LC 96-50009. (Illus.). 440p. pap. text 36.00 (0-88011-732-X, BABE0732) Human Kinetics.

Biophysical Models in Radiation Oncology. Ed. by Lionel Cohen. 1982. 192p. 110.00 (0-8493-6055-2, RC271, CRC Reprint) Franklin.

Biophysics & Cancer. Claudio Nicolini. 1986. LC 86-4926. (Illus.). 480p. (C). text 167.00 (0-306-42122-4, Kluwer Plenum) Kluwer Academic.

Biophysics & Physiology of Carbon Dioxide. Ed. by C Bauer et al. 1980. (Proceedings in Life Sciences Ser.). (Illus.). 453p. 71.95 (0-387-09892-5) Spr-Verlag.

Biophysics of Organ Cryopreservation. Ed. by Armand M. Karow, Jr. & David E. Pegg. 1988. LC 87-36059. (NATO ASI Series A, Life Sciences: Vol. 147). (Illus.). 496p. 135.00 (0-306-42812-1, Plenum Trade) Perseus Pubng.

Biophysics of the Pancreatic B-Cell. Ed. by Illani Atwater et al. 1987. LC 87-7713. (Advances in Experimental Medicine & Biology Ser.: Vol. 211). 506p. 125.00 (0-306-42555-6, Plenum Trade) Perseus Pubng.

Biophysics of the Skeletal Muscle Extracellular Potentials. Alexander Gydikov. 1992. (C). text 175.00 (0-7923-1468-9) Kluwer Academic.

Bioprosthesis in Cardiovascular Surgery: Problems & Perspectives. Irina Y. Zhouravliova. 1999. 243p. text 129.00 (1-56072-702-0) Nova Sci Pubs.

Biopsie und Operationspraeparat. U. E. Bonk. 1983. (Illus.). viii, 134p. pap. 19.25 (3-8055-3702-6) S Karger.

Biopsy Diagnosis in Rheumatic Diseases. J. T. Lie. 1997. LC 96-29142. (Illus.). 256p. 99.00 (0-89640-327-0) Igaku-Shoin.

Biopsy Diagnosis of Peripheral Neuropathy. Gyl Midroni et al. 1995. LC 95-6618. 477p. text 185.00 (0-7506-9552-8) Buttrwrth-Heinemann.

Biopsy Interpretation of Bone & Bone Marrow. B. Frisch & R. Bartl. 2nd ed. 1999. LC 99-18246. (Illus.). 384p. (0-340-74089-2) E A GBR. *Dist:* OUP.

Biopsy Interpretation of the Liver. Stephen Geller. 1998. text (0-397-51784-X) Lppncott W & W.

A B

Biopsy Interpretation of the Lung. Ed. by Yukio Shimosato & Roberta R. Miller. 1994. LC 94-954. (Biopsy Interpretation Ser.). 416p. text 109.00 (*0-7817-0168-6*) Lppncott W & W.

Biopsy of Bone in Internal Medicine: An Atlas & Sourcebook. R. Bartl & B. Frisch. 1993. LC 93-20357. (Current Histopathology Ser.: Vol. 21). 240p. (C). text 241.50 (*0-7923-8802-X*) Kluwer Academic.

Biopsy Pathology & Cytology of the Cervix. Dulcie V. Coleman. 2nd ed. 1999. LC 99-201835. (Illus.). 456p. (*0-340-74087-6*) E A GBR. *Dist:* OUP.

Biopsy Pathology of Melanocytic Disorders. W. J. Mooi & T. Krausz. 1992. LC 91-47890. (Biopsy Pathology Ser.: No. 17). (Illus.). 433p. (*0-412-32350-8*) E A GBR. *Dist:* OUP.

Biopsy Pathology of Muscle. Michael Swash & Martin S. Schwartz. 2nd ed. 1991. LC 91-70213. (Illus.). 247p. lib. bdg. 87.00 (*0-89089-449-3*) Carolina Acad Pr.

Biopsy Pathology of Oesophagus, Stomach & Duodenum. Day. 2nd ed. 1996. (Biopsy Pathology Ser.). 416p. (*0-412-63570-4*) E A GBR. *Dist:* OUP.

Biopsy Pathology of the Bronchi. Elizabeth M. McDowell & Theodore F. Beals. 1987. (Illus.). 410p. text 115.00 (*0-03-012119-1*) Saunders.

Biopsy Pathology of the Eye & Ocular Adnexa. N. A. Rao. 1996. (Biopsy Pathology Ser.). (Illus.). 416p. (*0-412-56720-2*) E A GBR. *Dist:* OUP.

Biopsy Pathology of the Oral Tissues. P. Morgan & Edward W. Odell. 1997. (Biopsy Pathology Ser.). 504p. (*0-412-54790-2*) E A GBR. *Dist:* OUP.

Biopsy Pathology of the Prostate. David G. Bostwick & P. Dundore. 1996. LC 96-86621. (Biopsy Pathology Ser.). (Illus.). 280p. (*0-412-75510-6*) E A GBR. *Dist:* OUP.

Biopsy Pathology of the Pulmonary Vasculature. C. A. Wagenvoort & W. J. Mooi. 1989. (Biopsy Pathology Ser.). (Illus.). 384p. (C). (gr. 13). pap. 169.95 (*0-412-27940-1*) Chapman & Hall.

Biopsy Pathology of the Skin. N. Kirkham. 1992. (Illus.). 408p. 99.95 (*0-442-31545-7*); 1991. 416p. (C). (gr. 13). 181.95 (*0-412-35080-7*) Chapman & Hall.

Biopsy Pathology of the Thyroid & Parathyroid. Otto Ljungberg. 1993. LC 92-49004. (Biopsy Pathology Ser.). 384p. (gr. 13). 181.95 (*0-412-34890-X*) Chapman & Hall.

Biopsych Notes. N. T. Late. 1994. 14p. (Orig.). pap. (*0-9641448-7-5*) N Late Pub.

Biopsychology. John P. Pinel. 1989. 608p. text 50.00 (*0-205-12052-0*, H20522) Allyn.

Biopsychology. Jubilan. 2nd annot. ed. 1996. tchr. ed. (*0-697-31662-9*, WCB McGr Hill) McGrw-H Hghr Educ.

Biopsychology. 4th ed. 1999. (C). text (*0-205-29815-X*, Longwood Div) Allyn.

Biopsychology. 4th ed. 1999. 608p. (C). (*0-205-31066-4*) S&S Trade.

Biopsychology. Mana. 4th ed. 1999. pap. text, stu. ed. 16.00 net. (*0-205-28993-2*) Allyn.

Biopsychology of Mood & Arousal. Robert E. Thayer. 1989. (Illus.). 256p. text 55.00 (*0-19-505162-9*) OUP.

Biopsychopathology. Hertzler. 2002. text (*0-7167-3088-X*) W H Freeman.

Biopsychosocial Approaches in Primary Care: State of the Art & Challenges for the 21st Century. Ed. by Hoyle Leigh. 1997. LC 97-3397. (Illus.). 252p. (C). text 89.50 (*0-306-45582-X*, Kluwer Plenum) Kluwer Academic.

Biopsychosocial Approach/Supershell Macintosh. Peterson. 2nd ed. 1996. text 49.69 (*0-673-54382-X*) Addison-Wesley.

Bioquest Curriculum Consortium. Contrib. by Bioquest Curriculum Consortium Staff. 2001. 197p. pap. 99.00 incl. cd-rom (*0-12-099473-9*) Acad Pr.

Bioradicals Detected by ESR Spectroscopy. Ed. by H. Ohya-Nishiguchi & Lester Packer. 1995. (Molecular & Cell Biology Updates Ser.). 337p. 139.00 (*3-7643-5077-6*) Birkhauser.

Bioregulators: Chemistry & Uses. Robert L. Ory & Falk R. Rittig. 1984. LC 84-10987. (ACS Symposium Ser.: No. 257). 296p. 49.95 (*0-8412-0853-0*) Am Chemical.

Biorelated Polymers & Gels: Controlled Release & Applications in Biomedical Engineering. Ed. by Teruo Okano. 1998. LC 97-50406. (Polymers, Interfaces & Biomaterials Ser.). (Illus.). 257p. text 95.00 (*0-12-525090-8*) Acad Pr.

Bioresonance & Multiresonance Therapy (BRT) New, Forward-Looking Forms of Therapy with Ultrafine Body Energies & Environmental Signals. Ed. by Hans Brugemann. Tr. by Robert E. Williams from GER. 1993. (Illus.). 277p. text (*2-8043-4010-4*) Edits Haug Intl BEL. *Dist:* Medicina Bio.

Biorhythm: A Personal Science. Bernard Gittelson. rev. ed. 1988. mass mkt. 4.95 (*0-446-34847-3*) Warner Bks.

Biorhythm for Life. Howard M. Thomson. 1997. LC 76-29578. (Illus.). 84p. (Orig.). pap. 11.12 (*0-9601070-1-0*) Evergreen MA.

Biosafety in Microbiological & Biomedical Laboratories. Ed. by John H. Richardson & W. Emmett Barkley. 2nd ed. 1993. (Illus.). 139p. (C). pap. text 35.00 (*1-56806-423-3*) DIANE Pub.

Biosafety in Microbiological & Biomedical Laboratories: Working with Infectious Agents in Laboratory Settings. 1992. lib. bdg. 250.00 (*0-8490-5539-3*) Gordon Pr.

Biosciences 2000: Current Aspects & Prospects for the Next Millennium. Charles A. Pasternak. 1999. LC 99-34736. (Series on Cell & Molecular Biology: Vol. 1). (Illus.). 275p. (*1-86094-195-8*) Imperial College GBR. *Dist:* World Scientific Pub.

Bioscientific Terminology. Donald M. Ayers. 1972. LC 74-163010. 325p. (C). pap. 15.95 (*0-8165-0305-2*) U of Ariz Pr.

Biosensors & Technical Medicine: Index of Modern Authors & Subjects with Guide for Rapid Research. Peter B. Zeiderhof. rev. ed. 1994. LC 94-32971. 171p. pap. 47.50 (*0-7883-0443-7*); text 57.50 (*0-7883-0442-9*) ABBE Pubs Assn.

Biosocial Bases of Violence: Proceedings of a NATO ASI Held in Rhodes, Greece, May 12-21, 1996. Ed. by Adrian Raine et al. 1997. LC 97-13920. (NATO ASI Series A: Vol. 292). 372p. 115.00 (*0-306-45601-X*) Plenum.

Biosocial Psychopathology: Epidemiologic Perspectives. Donald I. Templer et al. 1993. LC 93-25832. 344p. text 46.95 (*0-8261-8290-9*) Springer Pub.

***Biostatistical Genetics & Genetic Epidemiology.** Ed. by Robert C. Elston. 2002. 800p. 245.00 (*0-471-48631-0*) Wiley.

Biostatistician. Jack Rudman. 1994. (Career Examination Ser.: C-1135). pap. 29.95 (*0-8373-1135-7*) Nat Learn.

Biostatistics: A Foundation for Analysis in the Health Sciences. Wayne W. Daniel. 7th ed. 1998. LC 98-13102. (Illus.). 928p. text 96.95 (*0-471-16386-4*) Wiley.

Biostatistics: A Methodology for the Health Sciences. Lloyd Fisher. 1996. LC 92-24336. 1024p. pap. 94.95 (*0-471-16609-X*) Wiley.

Biostatistics: The Bare Essentials. Geoffrey R. Norman & David L. Streiner. 1998. (Illus.). 260p. pap. (*1-55009-085-2*) DEKR.

Biostatistics: The Bare Essentials. Geoffrey R. Norman & David L. Streiner. 1993. LC 92-48446. (*0-8016-2186-0*) Mosby Inc.

Biostatistics & Epidemiology: A Primer for Health Professionals. Sylvia Wassertheil-Smoller. 2nd ed. 1995. LC 94-44484. (Illus.). 185p. 42.95 (*0-387-94388-9*) Spr-Verlag.

Biostatistics & Epidemiology: Digging up the Bones, Vol. 9. Nikos M. Linardakis et al. 2nd ed. 1998. LC 98-2834. (Digging Up the Bones Ser.). (Illus.). 350p. pap. 19.95 (*0-07-038222-0*) McGraw-Hill Prof.

Biostatistics Cookbook: The Most User-Friendly Guide for the Bio/Medical Scientist. Seth Michelson & Timothy Schofield. 1996. LC 95-48001. 172p. lib. bdg. 87.00 (*0-7923-3884-7*) Kluwer Academic.

Biostatistics for Epidemiologists. Anders Ahlbom. 1993. 224p. lib. bdg. 79.95 (*0-87371-912-3*, L912) Lewis Pubs.

Biostatistics in Clinical Medicine. Joseph A. Ingelfinger et al. 3rd ed. 1994. LC 93-13482. (Illus.). 340p. pap. 39.95 (*0-07-105415-4*) McGraw-Hill Educ Grp.

Biostatistics in Pharmacology. Ed. by A. L. Delaunois. (International Encyclopedia of Pharmacology & Therapeutics Ser.). 1979. LC 78-40220. (*0-08-023168-3*); Set, Vols. 1 & 2. 1973. 1128p. (C). (*0-08-016556-7*) Pergamon Repr GBR. *Dist:* Franklin.

Biostats: A Primer for Health Care Professionals. Dennis B. Gillings & Chester W. Douglass. 2nd ed. 1985. LC 85-14927. (Illus.). 293p. 23.00 (*0-932137-02-4*) Cavco Pubns.

Biostats: Data Analysis for Dental Health Care Professionals. Jane A. Weintraub et al. 4th ed. 1985. (Illus.). 297p. (Orig.). (C). 23.00 (*0-932137-01-6*) Cavco Pubns.

Biosynthesis, Metabolism & Mode of Action of Inverterbrate Hormones. Ed. by J. Hoffmann & M. Porchet. 1984. (Proceedings in Life Sciences Ser.). (Illus.). 570p. 156.00 (*0-387-13667-3*) Spr-Verlag.

Biotechnological Innovations in Health Care. G. Turnock. 1991. (BIOTOL Ser.). 320p. pap. text 46.95 (*0-7506-1493-5*) Buttrwrth-Heinemann.

Biotechnology. Steve Prentis. 1984. LC 83-26571. (Illus.). 192p. 18.50 (*0-8076-1094-1*) Braziller.

Biotechnology: A Guide to Genetic Engineering. Pamela M. Peters. 1992. 272p. (C). pap. 64.38 (*0-697-12063-5*) McGrw-H Hghr Educ.

Biotechnology: Enzymes, Biomass, Food & Feed, Vol. 9, Enzymes, Biomass, Food and Feed. H. J. Rehm. 2nd ed. 1995. (Illus.). 804p. 425.00 (*3-527-28319-6*, Wiley-VCH) Wiley.

Biotechnology: Human Health & Nutrition: Bibliography January 1985-December 1992. Robert D. Warmbrodt & Daniel Cabirac. 1995. 26p. (Orig.). (C). pap. text 20.00 (*0-7881-2190-1*) DIANE Pub.

Biotechnology: Implications for Public Policy. Ed. by Sandra Panem. 1986. LC 85-48176. (Dialogues on Public Policy Ser.). 99p. text 10.95 (*0-8157-6903-2*) Brookings.

Biotechnology: Legal, Economic & Ethical Dimensions, Vol. 12, Modern Biotechnology. H. J. Rehm. 2nd ed. 1995. (Illus.). 695p. 425.00 (*3-527-28322-6*, Wiley-VCH) Wiley.

Biotechnology: Quality Assurance & Validation. Ed. by Kenneth Avis et al. 1998. LC 98-40953. (Drug Manufacturing Technology Ser.). 268p. 179.00 (*1-57491-089-2*) IHS Health Grp.

Biotechnology & Biopharmaceutical Manufacturing, Processing, & Preservation. Ed. by Kenneth E. Avis & Vincent Wu. 1996. (Drug Manufacturing Technology Ser.). (Illus.). 386p. 179.00 (*1-57491-016-7*) IHS Health Grp.

Biotechnology & Comparative Medicine. Ed. by R. Pandey. 1987. (Progress in Veterinary Microbiology & Immunology Ser.: Vol. 3). (Illus.). xvi, 268p. 182.75 (*3-8055-4399-9*) S Karger.

Biotechnology Business: A Strategic Analysis. Peter Daly. 1985. LC 85-10877. 150p. 44.50 (*0-8476-7460-6*) Rowman.

***Biotechnology in Agriculture, 1986-May 1992: Citations from Agricola Concerning Diseases & Other Environmental Considerations.** Ed. by Charles N. Beebee. 2001. 276p. (C). reprint ed. pap. text 40.00 (*0-7567-0816-8*) DIANE Pub.

Biotechnology in Blood Transfusion. Ed. by C. T. Sibinga. 1988. (Developments in Hematology & Immunology Ser.). (C). text 100.50 (*0-89838-404-4*) Kluwer Academic.

Biotechnology in Renal Replacement Therapy. Ed. by V. Bonomini et al. 1989. (Contributions to Nephrology Ser.: Vol. 70). (Illus.). xiv, 346p. 216.75 (*3-8055-4893-1*) S Karger.

Biotechnology Instrumentation & Software: Pharmaceutical Growth Expands Supplier Markets. Market Intelligence Staff. 1993. 293p. 1895.00 (*1-56753-468-6*) Frost & Sullivan.

Biotechnology International: International Developments in the Biotechnology Industry, Vol. 2. Ed. by Frederick Fox & Thomas Connor. 2nd unabr. ed. 1998. (Illus.). 350p. pap. text 145.00 (*1-890131-01-6*) Univ Med Pr.

Biotechnology International Vol. 3: The Biotech Millenium. Ed. by Babak N. Alizadeh et al. unabr. ed. 2001. (Illus.). 304p. pap. text 95.00 (*1-890131-02-4*) Univ Med Pr.

Biotechnology of Antibiotics. W. R. Strohl. 2nd ed. 1997. LC 97-20469. (Drugs & the Pharmaceutical Sciences Ser.: Vol. 82). (Illus.). 840p. text 230.00 (*0-8247-9867-8*) Dekker.

Biotechnology of Antibiotics & Other Bioactive Microbial Metabolites. G. Lancini & R. Lorenzetti. 1993. (Illus.). 244p. (C). text 69.50 (*0-306-44603-0*, Kluwer Plenum) Kluwer Academic.

Biotechnology of Insulin Therapy. J. C. Pickup. 1991. (Frontiers in Pharmacology & Therapeutics Ser.). (Illus.). 200p. 125.00 (*0-632-03038-0*) Blackwell Sci.

Biotechnology of Plasma Proteins: Haemostasis, Thrombosis & Iron Proteins. Ed. by Alberto Albertini et al. 1991. (Current Studies in Hematology & Blood Transfusion: No. 58). (Illus.). x, 216p. 182.75 (*3-8055-5250-5*) S Karger.

Biotechnology of Vitamins, Pigments & Growth Factors. Ed. by E. J. Vandamme. 1989. (Applied Biotechnology Ser.). 444p. pap. 234.95 (*1-85166-325-8*) Elsevier.

Biotelemetry International Symposium, 2nd, Davos, May 1974. Biotelemetry International Symposium. Ed. by P. A. Neukomm et al. 1974. 55.75 (*3-8055-2103-0*) S Karger.

***Bioterrorism & Biology of Botulism (Clostridium Boltlinum) Index of New Information & Guide-Book for Consumers, Reference & Research.** John C. Bartone. 2001. (Illus.). 200p. 57.50 (*0-7883-2710-0*); pap. 50.50 (*0-7883-2711-9*) ABBE Pubs Assn.

***Bioterrorism of Anthrax (Bacillus Anthracis) Index of New Information & Guide-Book for Consumers, Reference & Research.** John C. Bartone. 2001. (Illus.). 200p. 57.50 (*0-7883-2564-7*) ABBE Pubs Assn.

***Bioterrorism of Plague (Yersinia Infections) Index of New Information & Guide-Book for Consumers, Reference & Research.** John C. Bartone. 2001. (Illus.). 200p. 57.50 (*0-7883-2630-9*) ABBE Pubs Assn.

***Bioterrorism of Smallpox (Variola Virus) Index of New Information & Guide-Book for Consumers, Reference & Research.** John C. Bartone. 2001. (Illus.). 200p. pap. 50.50 (*0-7883-2589-2*) ABBE Pubs Assn.

***Bioterrorism, Threats & Biology of Toxins: Index of New Information & Guide-Book for Consumers, Reference & Research.** John C. Bartone. 2001. (Illus.). 200p. 57.50 (*0-7883-2698-8*); pap. 50.50 (*0-7883-2699-6*) ABBE Pubs Assn.

Biotherapeutic Agents & Infectious Diseases. Gary W. Elmer et al. 1999. LC 99-201903. (Illus.). 336p. 135.00 (*0-89603-647-2*) Humana.

Biotherapy: A Comprehensive Overview. Paula T. Rieger. (Nursing Ser.). (Illus.). 1995. 352p. text 52.95 (*0-86720-707-8*, 707-8); 2nd ed. 2000. LC 00-62679. 807p. (C). pap. text 54.95 (*0-7637-1428-3*, 1428-3) Jones & Bartlett.

Biothiols Pt. A: Monothiols & Dithiols, Protein Thiols & Thiyl Radicals. Melvin I. Simon. Ed. by Lester Packer et al. 1995. (Methods in Enzymology Ser.: Vol. 251). (Illus.). 529p. text 90.00 (*0-12-182152-8*) Acad Pr.

Biothiols in Health & Disease, No. 2. Ed. by Lester Packer & Enrique Cadenas. 1995. (Antioxidants in Health & Disease Ser.: Vol. 2). (Illus.). 552p. text 195.00 (*0-8247-9654-3*) Dekker.

BioWorld Biotechnology VC Directory, 2001: U. S. Venture Capital Companies & Contacts. Ed. by BioWorld Today Staff & Institute for Biotechnology Information Staff. 2001. pap. 299.00 (*1-931107-04-1*) Am Health Consults.

BioWorld 2000 Genomics Review. Ed. by BioWorld Today Staff. 2000. pap. 459.00 (*1-931107-07-6*) Am Health Consults.

BioWorld 2001 Genomics Review. Ed. by BioWorld Today Staff. 2001. pap. 459.00 (*1-931107-02-5*) Am Health Consults.

***Bipolar Child: The Definitive & Reassuring Guide to Childhood's Most Misunderstood Disorder.** Demitri Papolos & Janice Papolos. 2001. reprint ed. pap. 14.00 (*0-7679-0317-X*) Broadway BDD.

Bipolar Disorder. Judith Peacock. 2000. LC 99-56078. (Perspectives on Mental Health Ser.). 64p. (YA). (gr. 5-12). lib. bdg. 23.93 (*0-7368-0434-X*, LifeMatters Bks) Capstone Pr.

Bipolar Disorder: A Family-Focused Treatment Approach. David J. Miklowitz & Michael J. Goldstein. 1997. LC 97-26189. 318p. text 36.00 (*1-57230-283-6*, C0283) Guilford Pubns.

Bipolar Disorder: A Guide for Patients & Families. Francis Mark Mondimore. 1999. LC 98-41913. (Johns Hopkins Press Health Bks.). (Illus.). 312p. pap. 17.95 (*0-8018-6118-7*); 296p. 45.00 (*0-8018-6117-9*) Johns Hopkins.

Bipolar Disorder: Biological Models & Their Clinical Application. L. Trevor Young & Russell T. Joffe. 1997. LC 97-22826. (Medical Psychiatry Ser.: Vol. 7). (Illus.). 328p. text 140.00 (*0-8247-9872-4*) Dekker.

Bipolar Disorders: A Guide for Helping Children & Adolescents. Mitzi Waltz. Ed. by Linda Lamb. 2000. LC 99-56646. (Patient-Centered Guides). (Illus.). 460p. pap. 24.95 (*1-56592-656-0*, Patient-Centered) OReilly & Assocs.

Bipolar Disorders: Basic Mechanisms & Therapeutic Implications. Ed. by Jair C. Soares & Samuel Gershon. 2000. LC 00-703236. (Medical Psychiatry Ser.: Vol. 15). (Illus.). xv, 580p. 175.00 (*0-8247-0360-X*) Dekker.

Bipolar Disorders: CE Booklet. Beth Harris. 1999. 24p. pap. text 39.95 (*0-7817-1897-X*) Lppncott W & W.

Bipolar Puzzle Solution: A Mental Health Client's Perspective: 187 Answers to Questions Asked by Support Group Members about Living with Manic-Depressive Illness. Bryan L. Court & Gerald E. Nelson. 1996. LC 96-14284. (Psychological Disorders Ser.: Vol. 1). 160p. 19.95 (*1-56032-493-7*) Accel Devel.

Bipolar Theory of Living Processes: How to Treat Chronic Fatigue, Exhaustion & Death from an Electrical Energy Standpoint. G. W. Crile. 1991. lib. bdg. 88.95 (*0-8490-4933-4*) Gordon Pr.

Birational Theory of Degenerations. Ed. by Robert Friedman & David Morrison. 1982. (Progress in Mathematics Ser.: Vol. 29). 386p. (C). 60.50 (*0-8176-3111-9*) Birkhauser.

Bird Disease by Stroud. Robert Stroud. 1964. 483p. 19.95 (*0-86622-731-8*, AP-926) TFH Pubns.

Bird Respiration. T. J. Seller. 1987. LC 86-20700. Vol. 1. 103.00 (*0-8493-4691-6*, QL698); Vol. 2. 121.00 (*0-8493-4692-4*, QL698) Franklin (CRC Reprint).

Birdkeeping As a Source of Lung Cancer & Other Human Diseases: A Need for Higher Hygienic Standards. P. A. Holst. 1991. 136p. 32.00 (*0-387-53555-1*) Spr-Verlag.

Bird's Nest Fungi. Harold J. Brodie. 1975. LC 75-18476. pap. 12.95 (*0-8020-6766-2*) U of Toronto Pr.

Birds of Prey: Medicine & Management. Manfred Heidenreich. Tr. by Yvonne Oppenheim from GER. 1997. LC 97-136231. (Illus.). 284p. 250.00 (*0-632-04186-2*) Blackwell Sci.

Birkhauser Dictionary of Human Biology (Birkhauser Whorterbuch der Humanbiologie) English-German - German-English. Peter Reuter. 2000. LC 00-22420. (ENG & GER., Illus.). xiii, 973p. 120.00 (*3-7643-6198-0*) Birkhauser.

Birth after Cesarean: The Medical Facts. Bruce L. Flamm. 1992. 224p. per. 11.00 (*0-671-79218-0*, Fireside) S&S Trade Pap.

Birth & Death & Cybernation: Cybernetics of the Sacred. Paul Ryan. 1973. xiv, 176p. text 101.00 (*0-677-04320-1*) Gordon & Breach.

Birth & Fertility Rates for States, United States, 1990. Sally C. Clarke & Stephanie J. Ventura. Ed. by National Center for Health Statistics Staff. 1994. LC 94-24746. (Vital & Health Statistics Ser.: Series 21, Vol. 52). iv, 53p. (*0-8406-0502-1*) Natl Ctr Health Stats.

Birth & Fortune: The Impact of Numbers on Personal Welfare. Richard A. Easterlin. 2nd rev. ed. 1987. LC 86-30724. 242p. pap. text 24.00 (*0-226-18032-8*) U Ch Pr.

Birth & the Dialogue of Love. Marilyn A. Moran. 1981. LC 81-81200. (Illus.). 233p. (Orig.). (C). pap. 24.95 (*0-940128-01-2*) Terra Publng.

Birth As a Healing Experience: The Emotional Journey of Pregnancy Through Postpartum. Lois Hazel Freedman. 1999. LC 99-16075. 117p. 24.95 (*0-7890-0576-X*); pap. 14.95 (*1-56023-940-9*) Haworth Pr (Harrington Park).

Birth As an American Rite of Passage. Robbie E. Davis-Floyd. 1993. 382p. (C). pap. 18.95 (*0-520-08431-4*) U CA Pr.

Birth Atlas. Maternity Center Association Staff. 6th rev. ed. 1993. (Illus.). 19p. reprint ed. 55.00 (*0-912758-00-7*) Maternity Ctr.

Birth Book: Everything You Need to Know to Have a Safe & Satisfying Birth. William M. Sears & Martha Sears. 1994. LC 93-5748. (Sears Parenting Library). (Illus.). 280p. pap. 13.95 (*0-316-77907-5*, Back Bay) Little.

Birth By Design: Pregnancy, Maternity Care & Midwifery in North America & Europe. Ed. by Raymond Devries et al. 2000. LC 00-55327. (Illus.). xviii, 301p. 80.00 (*0-415-92337-9*); pap. 24.99 (*0-415-92338-7*) Routledge.

Birth Control. Maududi Abu-Ala. 1993. pap. 5.50 (*0-935782-52-4*) Kazi Pubns.

Birth Control & Controlling Birth: Women-Centered Perspectives. Betty B. Hoskins & Michael Gross. Ed. by Helen B. Holmes. 1981. LC 80-82173. (Contemporary Issues in Biomedicine, Ethics & Society Ser.). 338p. 59.95 (*0-89603-022-9*); pap. 39.95 (*0-89603-023-7*) Humana.

Birth Control & Family Planning in Nineteenth Century America. 1977. LC 73-20645. (Sex, Marriage & Society Ser.). (Illus.). 349p. reprint ed. 31.95 (*0-405-05795-4*) Ayer.

Birth Control Book. Philip A. Belcastro. 1986. (Illus.). 144p. (C). pap. text 38.95 (*0-86720-068-5*, 068-5) Jones & Bartlett.

Birth Control in Practice. Marie E. Kopp. 1974. LC 72-169390. (Family in America Ser.). 294p. reprint ed. 19.95 (*0-405-03867-4*) Ayer.

Birth Control Technologies: Prospects by the Year 2000. Michael J. Harper. 1983. LC 82-15940. 281p. pap. 10.95 (*0-292-70757-6*) U of Tex Pr.

Birth Control Vaccines. Ed. by Gursaran P. Talwar & Raj Raghupathy. 1995. LC 94-27362. (Medical Intelligence Unit Ser.). 165p. text 79.00 (*1-57059-126-1*) Landes Bioscience.

Birth Days: A Nurse-Midwife's Account. Frances Wirvin. 1994. 160p. pap. 17.95 (*1-55059-079-0*) Temeron Bks.

Birth Defects. Edward Edelson. 1993. LC 91-27448. (Encyclopedia of Health Ser.). (Illus.). 116p. (YA). (gr. 7-13). lib. bdg. 19.95 (*0-7910-0058-3*) Chelsea Hse.

Birth Defects - Including Drug, Diet & Chemical - Induced: Index of New Information for Reference & Research. American Health Research Institute Staff. 1997. (Illus.). 150p. 57.50 (*0-7883-1062-3*); pap. 47.50 (*0-7883-1063-1*) ABBE Pubs Assn.

Birth Defects & Infant Mortality: A National & Regional Profile 1996. Joann Petrini & March of Dimes Birth Defects Foundation Staff. 1996. LC 96-33556. (Statbook Technical Report Ser.). (*0-86525-072-3*) March of Dimes.

Birth Defects Encyclopedia, Set. M. Buyse. 1992. 275.00 (*0-86542-228-1*) Blackwell Sci.

Birth Environments: Emerging Trends & Implications for Design. Alice Lerman. 1991. (Publications in Architecture & Urban Planning: No. R91-3). (Illus.). 110p. (C). 15.00 (*0-938744-76-3*) U of Wis Ctr Arch-Urban.

Birth of Bioethics. Albert R. Jonsen. 1998. LC 97-41154. 448p. text 47.00 (*0-19-510325-4*) OUP.

Birth of Hatred: Developmental, Clinical & Technical Aspects of Intense Aggression. Ed. by Salman Akhtar et al. 1996. LC 94-23614. 172p. 35.00 (*1-56821-428-6*) Aronson.

Birth of the Hospital in the Byzantine Empire. Timothy S. Miller. 1997. LC 97-201618. 328p. reprint ed. pap. text 18.95 (*0-8018-5657-4*) Johns Hopkins.

Birth of the Other. Rosine Lefort. Tr. by Marc Du Ry et al. 1994. LC 93-40386. 344p. (C). text 49.95 (*0-252-01900-8*); pap. text 18.95 (*0-252-06393-7*) U of Ill Pr.

Birth Order: Its Influence on Personality. C. Ernst & J. Angst. 1985. (Illus.). 343p. 59.95 (*0-387-11248-0*) Spr-Verlag.

Birth Order & Life Roles. Lucille K. Forer. 1969. 184p. 29.95 (*0-398-00596-6*) C C Thomas.

Birth over Thirty-Five. Sheila Kitzinger. 1995. LC 94-21963. (Illus.). 192p. pap. 14.00 (*0-14-024141-8*, Penguin Bks) Penguin Putnam.

Birth Partner's Handbook: How to Help a Woman Through Childbirth. Penny Simkin. 1989. LC 87-31537. pap. 5.95 (*0-671-66403-4*) S&S Trade.

Birth Plan Guide. Jeanne Raycher. 1988. (Illus.). (Orig.). (C). pap. 9.95 (*0-944252-00-1*) CC Services.

Birth Power: The Case for Surrogacy. Carmel Shalev. 1989. 224p. (C). 30.00 (*0-300-04216-7*) Yale U Pr.

Birth Rates of the White Population in the United States, 1800-1860: An Economic Study. Yasukichi Yasuba. LC 78-64236. (Johns Hopkins University. Studies in the Social Sciences. Thirtieth Ser. 1912: 2). reprint ed. 37.50 (*0-404-61341-1*) AMS Pr.

Birth, Suffering, & Death: Catholic Perspectives at the Edges of Life. Ed. by Kevin W. Wildes. 1992. (Philosophy & Medicine Ser.). 248p. (C). lib. bdg. (*0-7923-1547-2*) Kluwer Academic NLD. *Dist:* Kluwer Academic.

Birth to Death: Science & Bioethics. Ed. by David C. Thomasma & Thomasine Kushner. 1996. (Illus.). 398p. (C). pap. text 27.95 (*0-521-55556-6*) Cambridge U Pr.

Birth to Old Age: Health in Transition. Ed. by Basiro Davey. 2nd ed. 1995. LC 94-27569. (Health & Disease Ser.: Bk. 5). 224p. (Orig.). pap. text (*0-335-19207-6*) OpUniv Pr.

***Birth to Old Age: Health in Transition.** Ed. by Basiro Davey. 2nd ed. 2001. LC 2001-21658. (Health & Disease Ser.: Bk. 5). 224p. (Orig.). pap. (*0-335-20836-3*) OpUniv Pr GBR. *Dist:* Taylor & Francis.

Birth Traditions & Modern Pregnancy Care. Jacqueline V. Priya. 1992. 149p. pap. 10.95 (*1-85230-321-2*) Element MA.

Birth Without Violence: The Book that Revolutionized the Way We Bring Our Children into the World. Frederick Leboyer. 1995. LC 95-13382.Tr. of Pour une Naissance sans Violence. (Illus.). 128p. pap. 14.95 (*0-89281-545-0*, Heal Arts VT) Inner Tradit.

Birthing from Within: An Extra-Ordinary Guide to Childbirth Preparation. Pam England & Rob Horowitz. 1998. LC 97-92447. (Illus.). 331p. (Orig.). pap. 19.95 (*0-9659873-0-2*) Partera Pr.

Birthing Normally: A Personal Growth Approach to Childbirth. Gayle Peterson. 2nd ed. 1991. (Illus.). 195p. reprint ed. pap. 17.95 (*0-9625231-1-9*) Shadow & Light.

Birthrate Plus: A Framework for Workforce Planning & Decision Making for Midwifery Services. Ball. 1997. LC 97-142349. 176p. pap. text 39.99 (*1-898507-41-4*) Buttrwrth-Heinemann.

Bisexualities: Theory & Research. Ed. by Fritz Klein et al. 1985. LC 85-7629. (Journal of Homosexuality Ser.: Vol. 11, Nos. 1-2). 255p. text 49.95 (*0-86656-336-9*) Haworth Pr.

Bisexualities: Theory & Research. Ed. by Fritz Klein & Timothy J. Wolf. 1985. LC 85-7629. (Journal of Homosexuality Ser.: Vol. 11, Nos. 1-2). (Illus.). 255p. pap. text 14.95 (*0-86656-423-3*) Haworth Pr.

Bisexuality & HIV-AIDS: A Global Perspective. Ed. by Rob Tielman et al. 1991. LC 91-16625. (New Concepts in Human Sexuality Ser.). 253p. 55.00 (*0-87975-666-7*) Prometheus Bks.

Bishay' New Illustrated Medical Dictionary: English-Arabic. Milad Bishay. 1991. (ARA & ENG.). 800p. 125.00 (*0-7859-7464-4*) Fr & Eur.

Bishop & the Future of Catholic Health Care: Challenges & Opportunities: Proceedings of the 16th Workshop for Bishops. Ed. by Daniel P. Maher. 1997. LC 97-36565. 230p. pap. 19.95 (*0-935372-41-5*) NCBC.

Bisphosphonates in Bone Disease: From the Laboratory to the Patient. Herbert A. Fleisch. 4th ed. 2000. LC 00-100337. 350p. 139.95 (*0-12-260371-0*); pap. 69.95 (*0-12-260370-2*) Acad Pr.

Bisphosphonates in Bone Disease: From the Laboratory to the Patient. Herbert A. Fleisch. 2nd ed. 1995. LC 95-37749. (Illus.). 176p. 42.95 (*1-85070-705-7*); 3rd ed. 1997. LC 96-47806. 184p. pap. text 45.00 (*1-85070-951-3*) CRC Pr (Parthenon Pbng).

Bisphosphonates in Clinical Oncology: The Development of Pamidronate. Beat Thuerlimann. 1998. LC 98-4053. (Recent Results in Cancer Research Ser.: Vol. 149). (Illus.). 127p. 119.00 (*3-540-63689-7*) Spr-Verlag.

Bite the Apple: Healthy Bites of Medical Knowledge. Mayer L. Horensten. Ed. by Jean Terra & Santha Swanson. 1997. LC 96-80260. (Illus.). 126p. pap. 7.95 (*1-887747-10-9*, 297-231-X) Legendary Pub.

Bites & Stings. Alvin Silverstein et al. 2001. LC 00-49989. (My Health Ser.). (Illus.). 48p. (J). (gr. 3-5). lib. bdg. 23.00 (*0-531-11861-4*) F Watts.

Biting off the Bracelet: A Study of Children in Hospitals. Ann H. Beuf. 2nd ed. 1988. LC 88-15329. 164p. (C). pap. text 17.95 (*0-8122-1278-9*) U of Pa Pr.

Bitter Blue: Tranquillisers, Drugs, Dependency. Jeremy Reed. 1996. LC 96-150111. 136p. (*0-7206-0892-9*) P Owen Ltd GBR. *Dist:* Dufour.

Bitter Grass: The Cruel Truth about Marijuana. Roy H. Hart. 1980. LC 79-91582. (Illus.). pap. 6.95 (*0-935688-00-5*) Menta Pubns.

Bitter Pills: Medicines & the Third World Poor. Dianna Melrose. 1982. (Illus.). 277p. (C). pap. (*0-85598-065-6*) Oxfam Pub GBR. *Dist:* Stylus Pub VA.

Bitter Sea: The Human Cost of Minamata Disease. Akio Mishima. 1992. LC 93-206173. 248p. pap. (*4-333-01479-4*) Kosei Pub Co JPN. *Dist:* Tuttle Pubng.

Bittersweet: The Recovery of an Adult Child of an Alcoholic. Mary Ann Haske. 1987. 183p. (Orig.). pap. 7.95 (*0-9619475-0-0*) M A Haske.

Bittersweet Notes from a Therapist. Dorothy Wagner. 1988. (Illus.). 240p. (Orig.). pap. 9.95 (*0-9621652-0-4*) Wagner Pub.

Bivad (David) For Parents of Learning Disabled Children. Anne Sheppard. 1983. 24p. (Orig.). pap. 1.95 (*0-8298-0650-4*) Pilgrim OH.

Black Adult Development & Aging. Ed. by Reginald L. Jones. 1989. 448p. text 27.95 (*0-943539-03-X*); pap. text 20.00 (*0-943539-04-8*) Cobb & Henry Pubs.

Black Alcohol Abuse & Alcoholism: A Bibliography. Thomas D. Watts & Roosevelt Wright, Jr. 1986. LC 85-28245. 284p. 72.50 (*0-275-92083-6*, C2083, Praeger Pubs) Greenwood.

Black American Health: An Annotated Bibliography, 17. Compiled by Mitchell F. Rice & Woodrow Jones, Jr. 1987. LC 86-25745. (Bibliographies & Indexes in Afro-American & African Studies: No. 17). 133p. lib. bdg. 57.75 (*0-313-24887-7*, RBH/, Greenwood Pr) Greenwood.

Black & Recovering. Peter Bell. 1993. 64p. pap., wbk. ed. 7.75 (*1-56246-079-X*, 6284, HazeldenJohnson Inst) Hazelden.

Black & White Identity Formation. Stuart T. Hauser & E. Kasendorf. 2nd ed. 1983. LC 82-16221. 252p. pap. 13.50 (*0-89874-055-X*) Krieger.

Black & White Skin Diseases. C. Archer. 1995. (Illus.). 320p. 165.00 (*0-632-02529-8*) Blackwell Sci.

Black Art of Cooking: How Cooked Food Produces Disease, an Introduction to the Unfired Diet. Carl Loeb. 1991. lib. bdg. 79.95 (*0-8490-4547-9*) Gordon Pr.

Black Death. J. F. C. Hecker. Tr. by B. G. Babington. 1972. 78p. pap. 5.00 (*0-87291-038-5*) Coronado Pr.

Black Death. Tr. by Rosemary Horrox. 1994. LC 93-50558. (Manchester Medieval Sources Ser.: Vol. 1). text (*0-7190-3498-1*) Manchester Univ Pr GBR. *Dist:* St Martin.

Black Death: The Impact of the Fourteenth-Century Plague. Ed. by Daniel Williman. 1989. LC 82-12435. (Medieval & Renaissance Texts & Studies: Vol. 13). (Illus.). 160p. reprint ed. 25.00 (*0-86698-050-4*, MR13) MRTS.

Black Death & Men of Learning. Anna M. Campbell. LC 31-29792. reprint ed. 37.50 (*0-404-01368-6*) AMS Pr.

Black Death of 1348 & 1349. Francis A. Gasquet. 2nd ed. LC 75-23713. reprint ed. 47.50 (*0-404-13264-2*) AMS Pr.

Black Hamlet. Wulf Sachs. Ed. by Saul Dubow & Jacqueline Rose. 1996. LC 95-39448. (Parallax Ser.). 328p. (C). pap. text 18.95 (*0-8018-5286-2*) Johns Hopkins.

Black Heart's Truth: The Early Career of W. D. Howells. John W. Crowley. 1985. LC 84-20908. xv, 192p. 34.95 (*0-8078-1632-9*) U of NC Pr.

Black Lung: Anatomy of a Public Disaster. Alan Derickson. 1998. LC 98-13612. (Illus.). 244p. 32.50 (*0-8014-3186-7*) Cornell U Pr.

Black Lung: The Human Cost of Industrialization. Alan Derickson. 1998. LC 98-13612. pap. (*0-8014-8286-0*) Cornell U Pr.

Black Male in America: Perspectives on His Status in Contemporary Society. Ed. by Doris Y. Wilkinson & Ronald L. Taylor. 1977. LC 76-44310. 384p. (C). text 42.95 (*0-88229-227-7*) Burnham Inc.

Black Medicine IV: The Equalizers. N. Mashiro. 1995. (Illus.). 96p. pap. 15.00 (*0-87364-815-3*) Paladin Pr.

Black Psychiatrists & American Psychiatry. Ed. by Jeanne Spurlock. 1999. LC 98-36902. 272p. 29.00 (*0-89042-411-X*, 2411) Am Psychiatric.

Black Skin: Structure & Function. Ed. by William Montagna et al. 1993. LC 93-14784. 158p. text 58.00 (*0-12-505260-X*) Acad Pr.

Black Stork: Eugenics & the Death of 'Defective' Babies in American Medicine & Motion Pictures Since 1945. Martin S. Pernick. 1996. LC 94-47668. (Illus.). 312p. text 29.95 (*0-19-507731-8*) OUP.

Black Sun: Depression & Melancholia. Julia Kristeva. Tr. by Leon S. Roudiez from FRE. 1992. 300p. pap. 18.00 (*0-231-06707-0*) Col U Pr.

Black Swan: The Twelve Lessons of Abandonment Recovery. Susan Anderson. 2000. LC 99-93501. (Illus.). 112p. pap. 16.99 (*0-9673755-1-7*) Rock Found.

Black Women in White: Racial Conflict & Cooperation in the Nursing Profession, 1890-1950. Darlene Clark Hine. 1989. LC 88-46023. (Blacks in the Diaspora Ser.). (Illus.). 288p. pap. 14.95 (*0-253-20529-8*, MB-529) Ind U Pr.

Black Women's Health: A Special Issue of Women's Health. Ed. by Hope Landrine & Elizabeth A. Klonoff. 1997. 210p. pap. 40.00 (*0-8058-9855-7*) L Erlbaum Assocs.

Black Women's Health Vol. 1: Research & Social Policy. Ed. by Erma Jean Lawson & LaFrancis Rodgers-Rose. unabr. ed. 1997. 262p. (Orig.). pap. text 15.95 (*0-934185-03-4*) Traces Inst.

Black Women's Health Book: Speaking for Ourselves. Ed. by Evelyn C. White. 2nd exp. ed. 1993. LC 93-28901. 396p. (Orig.). pap. 16.95 (*1-878067-40-0*) Seal Pr WA.

Blackburn's Introduction to Clinical Radiation Therapy Physics. Benjamin Blackburn. 1989. LC 88-13905. (Illus.). 220p. (Orig.). (C). text 31.95 (*0-944838-06-5*) Med Physics Pub.

Blacks - Their Psychology & Behavior: Index of Modern Information. Joseph F. Codipipoy. 1990. LC 90-30452. 143p. 47.50 (*1-55914-128-X*); pap. 44.50 (*1-55914-129-8*) ABBE Pubs Assn.

Blacks & Jews on the Couch: Psychoanalytic Reflections on Black-Jewish Conflict. Ed. by Alan Helmreich & Paul Marcus. 1998. LC 98-15620. 240p. 72.50 (*0-275-95666-0*, Praeger Pubs) Greenwood.

Blacks & Their Bio-Medical History: Index of Modern Authors & Subjects with Guide for Rapid Research. American Health Research Institute Staff. 1997. 155p. 57.50 (*0-7883-1570-6*); 1997. 155p. pap. 47.50 (*0-7883-1571-4*); 1991. LC 90-56302. 160p. 47.50 (*1-55914-404-1*); 1991. LC 90-56302. 160p. pap. 44.50 (*1-55914-405-X*) ABBE Pubs Assn.

Blacks in Science & Medicine. Vivian O. Sammons. 1989. 293p. 70.95 (*0-89116-665-3*) Hemisp Pub.

Black's Medical Dictionary. Ed. by C. W. Havard. 36th ed. 1990. (Illus.). (C). lib. bdg. 85.00 (*0-389-20901-5*) B&N Imports.

Black's Medical Dictionary. Ed. by Gordon Macpherson. 37th ed. 1992. 656p. (C). text 105.50 (*0-389-20989-9*) B&N Imports.

Blacks Medical Dictionary. Black. 38th ed. 1996. 109.50 (*0-389-21014-5*) B&N Imports.

Black's Medical Dictionary. Gordon MacPherson. 39th ed. 1999. (Black's Medical Dictionary Ser.). 640p. 39.95 (*1-56833-129-0*) Madison Bks UPA.

Black's Veterinary Dictionary. Ed. by Geoffrey West. 18th ed. 1994. (Illus.). 624p. (*0-7136-3946-6*) B T B GBR. *Dist:* Intl Spec Bk.

Black's Veterinary Dictionary. Geoffrey West. 17th ed. 1992. 672p. (C). text 120.50 (*0-389-20994-5*) B&N Imports.

Black's Veterinary Dictionary. Ed. by Edward Boden. 19th ed. 1998. (Black's Veterinary Dictionary Ser.). (Illus.). 608p. 109.50 (*0-389-21017-X*) B&N Imports.

Blackstone's Guide to the Human Fertilisation & Embryology Act, 1990: Abortion & Embryo Research, the New Law. Ed. by Derek Morgan & Robert G. Lee. 1991. 276p. (C). text (*1-85431-105-0*) Blackstone Pr GBR. *Dist:* Gaunt.

Blackstone's Statutes on Medical Law. Ed. by Michael Jones & Anne Morris. 1992. (C). (*1-85431-142-5*) Blackstone Pr GBR. *Dist:* Gaunt.

Blackwell Dictionary of Cognitive Psychology. Ed. by Michael W. Eysenck. 1994. (Illus.). 416p. (C). pap. 38.95 (*0-631-19257-3*) Blackwell Pubs.

Blackwell Dictionary of Neuropsychology. Ed. by J. Graham Beaumont et al. (Illus.). 1996. 928p. 110.95 (*0-631-17896-1*); 1999. 816p. reprint ed. pap. 39.95 (*0-631-21435-6*) Blackwell Pubs.

Blackwell Encyclopedia of Social Psychology. Ed. by Miles Hewstone & Anthony S. Manstead. 1995. (Illus.). 656p. (C). text 117.95 (*0-631-18146-6*) Blackwell Pubs.

Blackwell Reader in Developmental Psychology. Alan Slater & Darwin Muir. 1999. LC 98-29201. (Illus.). xxi, 558p. 76.95 (*0-631-20718-X*) Blackwell Pubs.

***Blackwell's Dictionary of Nursing.** (Illus.). pap. (*0-7021-3138-5*) Juta & Co ZAF. *Dist:* Intl Spec Bk.

***Blackwell's Primary Care Essentials.** Stanford I. Lamberg. 2nd ed. 2002. LC 2001-6469. (Blackwell's Primary Care Essentials Ser.). pap. (*0-632-04629-5*) Blackwell Sci.

***Blackwell's Primary Care Essentials.** David P. Moore. 2nd ed. 2001. LC 2001-5586. (Blackwell's Primary Care Essentials Ser.). pap. (*0-632-04631-7*) Blackwell Sci.

***Blackwell's Underground Clinical Vignettes: Anatomy.** Vikas Bhushan. 3rd ed. 2001. LC 2001-4887. (Underground Clinical Vignettes Ser.). pap. (*0-632-04541-8*) Blackwell Sci.

***Blackwell's Underground Clinical Vignettes: Behavioral Science.** Vikas Bhushan. 3rd ed. 2001. LC 2001-4886. (Underground Clinical Vignettes Ser.). pap. (*0-632-04543-4*) Blackwell Sci.

***Blackwell's Underground Clinical Vignettes: Biochemistry.** Vikas Bhushan. 3rd ed. 2001. LC 2001-4933. (Underground Clinical Vignettes Ser.). pap. (*0-632-04545-0*) Blackwell Sci.

***Blackwell's Underground Clinical Vignettes: Emergency Medicine.** Vikas Bhushan. 2nd ed. 2001. LC 2001-4874. (Underground Clinical Vignettes Ser.). pap. (*0-632-04561-2*) Blackwell Sci.

***Blackwell's Underground Clinical Vignettes: Internal Medicine.** Vikas Bhushan. 2nd ed. 2001. LC 2001-4893. (Underground Clinical Vignettes Ser.). pap. (*0-632-04563-9*) Blackwell Sci.

***Blackwell's Underground Clinical Vignettes: Microbiology.** Vikas Bhushan. 3rd ed. 2001. LC 2001-4932. (Underground Clinical Vignettes Ser.). (*0-632-04547-7*) Blackwell Sci.

***Blackwell's Underground Clinical Vignettes: Neurology.** Vikas Bhushan. 2nd ed. 2001. LC 2001-4892. (Underground Clinical Vignettes Ser.). pap. (*0-632-04567-1*) Blackwell Sci.

***Blackwell's Underground Clinical Vignettes: OB/GYN.** Vikas Bhushan. 2nd ed. 2001. LC 2001-4891. (Underground Clinical Vignettes Ser.). pap. (*0-632-04569-8*) Blackwell Sci.

***Blackwell's Underground Clinical Vignettes: Pathophysiology.** Vikas Bhushan. 3rd ed. 2001. LC 2001-4931. (Underground Clinical Vignettes Ser.). pap. (*0-632-04551-5*) Blackwell Sci.

***Blackwell's Underground Clinical Vignettes: Pediatrics.** Vikas Bhushan. 2nd ed. 2001. LC 2001-4890. (Underground Clinical Vignettes Ser.). pap. (*0-632-04571-X*) Blackwell Sci.

***Blackwell's Underground Clinical Vignettes: Pharmacology.** Vikas Bhushan. 3rd ed. 2001. LC 2001-4930. (Underground Clinical Vignettes Ser.). pap. (*0-632-04557-4*) Blackwell Sci.

***Blackwell's Underground Clinical Vignettes: Psychiatry.** Vikas Bhushan. 2nd ed. 2001. LC 2001-4889. (Underground Clinical Vignettes Ser.). pap. (*0-632-04573-6*) Blackwell Sci.

***Blackwell's Underground Clinical Vignettes: Surgery.** Vikas Bhushan. 2nd ed. 2001. LC 2001-4888. (Underground Clinical Vignettes Ser.). pap. (*0-632-04575-2*) Blackwell Sci.

Bladder. Ed. by Robert J. Krane & John M. Fitzpatrick. 1995. LC 95-9441. text (*0-443-04222-5*) Church.

Bladder Augmentation. Ed. by Paddy Dewan & Michael E. Mitchell. 2000. (An Arnold Publication). 160p. (*0-340-75957-7*) E A.

Bladder Cancer. Ed. by R. T. Oliver & M. J. Coptcoat. 1998. LC 97-78239. (Cancer Surveys Ser.). (Illus.). 170p. (C). text 93.00 (*0-87969-529-3*) Cold Spring Harbor.

A
B

Bladder Cancer. Ed. by Ismail Elsebai. 1983. Vol. I. 216p. 120.00 (*0-8493-5733-0*); Vol. II. 224p. 127.00 (*0-8493-5734-9*) Franklin (CRC Reprint).

Bladder Cancer: Biology, Diagnosis & Management. Ed. by Konstantinos N. Syrigos & Donald Skinner. 1999. LC 98-50047. (Oxford Medical Publications). (Illus.). x, 469p. text 129.50 (*0-19-263038-5*) OUP.

Bladder Cancer: Clinical Practice in Urology. Ed. by D. M. Wallace & Ernst J. Zingg. 1985. (Clinical Practice in Urology Ser.). (Illus.). 302p. 160.00 (*0-387-13239-2*) Spr-Verlag.

Bladder Cancer: Current Diagnosis & Treatment. Ed. by Michael J. Droller. 2001. LC 00-33523. (Current Clinical Urology Ser.). 445p. 135.00 (*0-89603-818-1*) Humana.

Blakiston's Gould Pocket Medical Dictionary. Blakiston. Ed. by Richard Stander et al. 4th ed. 1979. 992p. text 29.95 (*0-07-005715-X*) McGraw-Hill Med Pub.

Blakiston's Gould Pocket Medical Dictionary. Blakiston. Ed. by Leon Weiss et al. 4th ed. 1979. 992p. pap. text 27.50 (*0-07-005714-1*) McGraw-Hill Med Pub.

Blame It on Freud: A Guide to the Language of Psychology. F. K. Heussenstamm. 1993. 192p. pap. 12.95 (*1-880823-02-0*) N Star Pubns.

Blame It on the Brain? Distinguishing Chemical Imbalances, Brain Disorders, & Disobedience. Edward T. Welch. 1998. LC 98-7094. (Resources for Changing Lives Ser.). 204p. pap. 12.99 (*0-87552-602-0*) P & R Pubng.

Blaming the Brain: The Real Truth about Drugs & Mental Health. Elliott Valenstein. 1998. LC 98-27346. (Illus.). 336p. 25.00 (*0-684-84964-X*) Free Pr.

***Blanchard & Loeb Publishers Nurse's Choice for Better Care Drug Handbook 2002.** Ed. by Ross Blanchard & Stanley Loeb. 2001. (Illus.). 900p. pap. 26.95 (*1-930138-25-3*) Blanchard & Loeb.

Blanche Knott's Book of Truly Tasteless Anatomy Jokes, Vol. II. Blanche Knott. 1991. (Blanche Knott's Book of Truly Tasteless Anatomy Jokes Ser.: Vol. II). mass mkt. 4.50 (*0-312-92421-6*) St Martin.

Blastocyst-Endometrium Relationships. Ed. by F. Leroy. 1980. (Progress in Reproductive Biology & Medicine Ser.: Vol. 7). (Illus.). 338p. 172.25 (*3-8055-0988-X*) S Karger.

Blastocyst Implantation. Ed. by Koji Yoshinaga. 1989. (Illus.). 248p. (C). text 50.00 (*0-944903-04-5*) Adams Pub Group.

Blastomycosis. Y. Al-Doory & A. F. DiSalvo. 1991. (Current Topics in Infectious Disease Ser.). (Illus.). 288p. (C). text 75.00 (*0-306-43958-1*, Kluwer Plenum) Kluwer Academic.

Blaustein's Pathology of the Female Genital Tract. Ed. by Robert J. Kurman. 4th ed. 1997. LC 93-23252. (Illus.). 1280p. 217.00 (*0-387-94166-5*) Spr-Verlag.

Bleaching Techniques in Restorative Dentistry. Linda Greenwall. 2000. (Illus.). 224p. (*1-85317-772-5*) Martin Dunitz GBR. *Dist:* Thieme Med Pubs.

Bleeding Edge: The Business of Health Care in the New Century. J. D. Kleinke. 1998. LC 98-20691. 368p. 43.00 (*0-8342-1190-4*, 11904) Aspen Pub.

Blended Medicine: The Best Choices in Healing. Michael Castleman. 2000. LC 99-48384. (Illus.). xii, 708p. 29.95 (*0-87596-520-2*) Rodale Pr Inc.

Bleomycin: A Review. Stanley T. Crooke & W. T. Bradner. 35.00 (*0-915340-05-4*) PJD Pubns.

Blepharoplasty. Norman J. Pastorek. 3rd ed. 1994. LC 94-40392. (Self-Instructional Package Ser.). (Illus.). 137p. pap. text 25.00 (*1-56772-013-7*) AAO-HNS.

Bless Me Father for I Have Sinned: Perspectives on Sexual Abuse Committed by Roman Catholic Priests. Ed. by Thomas G. Plante. 1999. LC 98-56635. 200p. 62.50 (*0-275-96386-1*, C6386, Praeger Pubs) Greenwood.

Blessed by Illness. L. F. Mees. 1983. 248p. (Orig.). reprint ed. pap. 10.95 (*0-88010-054-0*) Anthroposophic.

Blessed Tragedy: Restoring New Life with Hope & Faith after a Head Injury. Karen Wells. 1997. LC 97-67343. (Illus.). 460p. 23.95 (*0-9649401-7-5*) Rhodes & Easton.

Blessings from the Fall: Turning a Fall from Grace into a New Beginning. Beverly Engel. 1997. LC 96-39728. 225p. pap. 10.95 (*1-55874-456-8*) Health Comm.

Blind. Jack Rudman. 1994. (Teachers License Examination Ser.: T-5). pap. 27.95 (*0-8373-8005-7*) Nat Learn.

Blind Eye: How the Medical Establishment Let a Doctor Get Away with Murder. James B. Stewart. 2000. LC 99-37044. (Illus.). 336p. pap. 14.00 (*0-684-86563-7*, Touchstone) S&S Trade Pap.

Blind in Society & Blindness, a New Seeing of the World. Jacques Lusseyran. Tr. by Dorothea Winkler from FRE. 1978. 32p. (gr. 7-12). pap. 1.50 (*0-913098-11-6*) Orion Society.

Blindfold on a Tightrope: Men's Myths & Men's Mysteries. Ramfls Firethorn. Date not set. (Illus.). 129p. (Orig.). pap. 14.95 (*1-885569-01-7*) Solar Crown.

Blindness & Children: An Individual Differences Approach. David H. Warren. 1994. LC 93-42678. (Illus.). 392p. (C). text 74.95 (*0-521-45109-4*); pap. text 27.95 (*0-521-45719-X*) Cambridge U Pr.

Blindness & Early Childhood Development. David Warren. rev. ed. 1984. LC 84-16796. 384p. pap. 34.95 (*0-89128-123-1*) Am Foun Blind.

Blindness & Visual Handicap: The Facts. John H. Dobree & Eric Boulter. 1982. (Facts Ser.). (Illus.). 200p. 13.95 (*0-19-261328-6*) OUP.

Blindness-Control, Preservation & Psychology: Index of New Information with Authors, Subjects & References. George J. Collins. 1998. 150p. 57.50 (*0-7883-1372-X*); pap. 47.50 (*0-7883-1373-8*) ABBE Pubs Assn.

Bliss Bibliographic Classification: Class H: Anthropology, Human Biology & Life Sciences. Ed. by Jack Mills & Vanda Broughton. 2nd ed. 1981. 326p. text (*0-408-70828-X*) Bowker.

Bliss Bibliographic Classification: Class I: Psychology & Psychiatry. Ed. by Jack Mills & Vanda Broughton. 1978. 62p. text (*0-408-70841-7*) Bowker.

Bliss of Becoming One! Integrating Feminine Feelings into the Male Psyche: Mainstreaming the Gender Community. Rachel Miller. 1995. LC 95-25566. (Illus.). 120p. (Orig.). pap. 12.95 (*1-56825-031-2*) Rainbow Books.

Bloat in Large Dogs. Siegfried Zahn. 1983. (Illus.). 24p. pap. 5.00 (*0-912183-00-4*) Univelt Inc.

Blocks & Freedoms in Sexual Life: A Handbook in Psychosexual Medicine. Ruth L. Skrine. 1995. LC 96-47139. 152p. pap. (*1-85775-159-0*) Radcliffe Med Pr GBR. *Dist:* Balogh.

Blood: An Epic History of Medicine & Commerce. Douglas Starr. 1998. LC 97-46815. (Illus.). 433p. 28.50 (*0-679-41875-X*) Knopf.

Blood: Atlas & Sourcebook of Hematology. Carola T. Kapff & James H. Jandl. 1981. 79.50 (*0-316-48276-5*, Little Brwn Med Div) Lppncott W & W.

Blood: Atlas & Sourcebook of Hematology. Carola T. Kapff. 2nd ed. 1991. 176p. text 139.00 (*0-316-48274-9*) Lppncott W & W.

Blood: Hemostasis, Transfusion, & Alternatives in the Perioperative Period. Ed. by Carol L. Lake & Roger A. Moore. 1995. LC 94-42192. (Illus.). 566p. text 154.00 (*0-7817-0267-4*) Lppncott W & W.

Blood: Physiology & Pathophysiology. Christopher J. Pallister. 1994. LC 95-103064. 384p. text (*0-7506-0581-2*) E A GBR. *Dist:* OUP.

Blood: Principles & Practice of Hematology. Ed. by Robert I. Handin et al. 1994. LC 94-27361. (Illus.). 2,328p. (C). text 199.00 (*0-397-50944-8*) Lppncott W & W.

Blood: Rheology, Hemolysis, Gas & Surface Interactions. Ed. by Dhanjoo N. Ghista et al. 1979. (Advances in Cardiovascular Physics Ser.: Vol. 3). (Illus.). 82.25 (*3-8055-2852-3*) S Karger.

Blood: Textbook of Hematology. James H. Jandl. 2nd ed. 1996. LC 96-4748. 1,900p. text 199.00 (*0-316-45731-0*) Lppncott W & W.

Blood: Textbook of Hematology + Kapff/Blood: Atlas & Sourcebook of Hematology James H. Jandl. 2nd ed. 1996. 96p. 175.95 (*0-316-48288-9*, J0436) Lppncott W & W.

Blood Alcohol Testing in the Clinical Laboratory. 1988. (Approved Guideline Ser.: Vol. 8). 75.00 (*1-56238-094-X*, TDM6-P) NCCLS.

Blood & Circulatory Disorders Sourcebook: Basic Information about Blood & Its Components, Anemias, Leukemias, Bleeding Disorders & Circulatory Disorders. Linda M. Ross. 1998. LC 98-33704. (Health Reference Ser.). 554p. lib. bdg. 78.00 (*0-7808-0203-9*) Omnigraphics Inc.

Blood & Its Third Anatomical Element. A. Bechamp. 1991. lib. bdg. 250.00 (*0-87700-927-9*) Revisionist Pr.

Blood & Marrow Stem Cell Transplantation. Marie Bakitas Whedon et al. 2nd ed. 1997. LC 97-2860. (Nursing Ser.). (Illus.). 608p. (C). text 71.95 (*0-7637-0356-7*, 0356-7) Jones & Bartlett.

Blood Bank GMPS. Ed. by Thomas G. Crouthamel. 1992. LC 92-81865. (Handi-Regs Ser.: No. 9206). 112p. (Orig.). pap. 21.95 (*0-940701-26-X*) Keystone Pr.

Blood Bank Regulations: A to Z. Kay McCurdy & Kay Gregory. 3rd ed. 2000. LC 00-50822. xi, 258p. pap. text (*1-56395-130-4*) Am Assn Blood.

Blood Bank Regulations: A-Z. American Association of Blood Banks Staff. Ed. by Kay Gregory & Kay McCurdy. 2nd ed. 1999. 160p. pap. (*3-8055-7058-9*) S Karger.

Blood Bank Regulations A-Z: A Handbook. Ed. by Kay McCurdy & Kay Gregory. 1997. LC 98-138828. pap. text 79.00 (*1-56395-085-5*) Am Assn Blood.

Blood Banking, Vol. 1. Ed. by Tibor J. Greenwalt et al. 1977. LC 76-27688. (Clinical Lab Science Ser.: Pt. D). 616p. 333.00 (*0-8493-7011-6*, RB37, CRC Reprint) Franklin.

Blood Banking. Ed. by Tibor J. Greenwalt & Edwin A. Steane. 1981. (Clinical Lab Science Ser.: Pt. D). Vol. 2. 400p. 211.00 (*0-8493-7012-4*, RB37); Vol. 3. 336p. 181.00 (*0-8493-7013-2*, RB37) Franklin (CRC Reprint).

Blood Banking & Regulation: Procedures, Problems, & Alternatives. Institute of Medicine, Forum on Blood Safety. Ed. by Edward A. Dauer. 1996. 136p. (Orig.). pap. text 27.00 (*0-309-05546-6*) Natl Acad Pr.

***Blood Banking & Transfusion Medicine.** Leslie E. Silberstein & Christopher D. Hillyer. 2001. (Illus.). 755p. (*0-443-06542-X*) Church GBR. *Dist:* Saunders.

Blood, Blood Products & HIV. R. Madhok et al. 2nd ed. 1993. LC 93-40109. 288p. (gr. 13). 150.95 (*0-412-40400-1*) Chapman & Hall.

Blood-Brain Barrier: Cellular & Molecular Biology. Ed. by William M. Pardridge. 1993. LC 92-48543. 496p. text 112.00 (*0-7817-0015-9*) Lppncott W & W.

Blood-Brain Barrier Amino Acids. M. B. Segal & B. V. Zlokovic. 1989. (C). text 146.00 (*0-7462-0122-2*) Kluwer Academic.

Blood Brothers: Siblings As Writers. Norman Kiell. 1982. LC 83-12677. xv, 434p. 65.00 (*0-8236-0545-0*) Intl Univs Pr.

Blood Cell Biochemistry, Vol. 8. Ed. by L.J. Fairbairn & N. G. Testa. 1999. (Illus.). 392p. (C). text 149.50 (*0-306-45962-0*, Kluwer Plenum) Kluwer Academic.

Blood Cell Biochemistry Vol. 1: Erythroid Cells. J. R. Harris. 1990. (Illus.). 537p. (C). text 120.00 (*0-306-43462-8*, Kluwer Plenum) Kluwer Academic.

Blood Cell Biochemistry Vol. 4: Basophil & Mast Cell Degranulation & Recovery. A. M. Dvorak. 1991. (Illus.). 415p. (C). text 105.00 (*0-306-43752-X*, Kluwer Plenum) Kluwer Academic.

Blood Cell Biochemistry Vol. 5: Macrophages & Related Cells. M. A. Horton. 1993. (Illus.). 454p. (C). text 115.00 (*0-306-44362-7*, Kluwer Plenum) Kluwer Academic.

Blood Cell Biochemistry Vol. 6: Molecular Basis of Human Blood Group Antigens. Ed. by J. P. Cartron & P. Rouger. 1995. (Illus.). 512p. (C). text 120.00 (*0-306-44853-X*, Kluwer Plenum) Kluwer Academic.

Blood Cell Biochemistry Vol. 7: Hematopoietic Cell Growth Factors & Their Receptors, Vol. 1. Ed. by Anthony D. Whetton & John Gordon. 1996. (Illus.). 413p. (C). text 110.00 (*0-306-45238-3*, Kluwer Plenum) Kluwer Academic.

Blood Cell Growth Factors: Their Present & Future Use in Hematology & Oncology. Ed. by Martin J. Murphy, Jr. 1991. 225p. (C). pap. text 49.00 (*1-880854-00-7*) AlphaMed Pr.

Blood Cell Morphology. Lynn Maedel & Sandra Sommer. 1993. sl. (*0-89189-329-6*) Am Soc Clinical.

Blood Cells: A Practical Guide. Barbara J. Bain. 2nd ed. (Illus.). 1996. 326p. pap. text 54.95 (*0-632-04155-2*); 1995. 368p. 95.00 (*0-86542-913-8*) Blackwell Sci.

***Blood Cells: A Practical Guide.** Barbara J. Bain. 3rd ed. 2001. LC 2001-37986. (*0-632-05734-3*) Blackwell Sci.

Blood Cells in Nuclear Medicine, Set, Pts. I & II. Ed. by M. R. Hardeman et al. LC 84-8100. (Developments in Nuclear Medicine Ser.). 1987. pap. text 124.50 (*0-89838-660-8*); 1984. lib. bdg. 209.00 (*0-89838-654-3*); 1984. text 252.50 (*0-89838-653-5*) Kluwer Academic.

Blood Chemistry & Clinical Nutrition. Jack Tips. 1993. 123p. 44.95 (*0-929167-07-4*) Apple-a-Day.

Blood Circulation in the Brain. B. N. Klosovskii. 1963. 320p. 3.5 hd 88.00 (*0-7065-0269-8*) Coronet Bks.

Blood Clots & Strokes: A Guide for Parents & Little Folks. Maureen Andrew. 1998. LC 99-180210. 40p. pap. (*1-55009-064-X*) DEKR.

Blood Coagulation & Hemostasis: A Practical Guide. Ed. by Jean M. Thomson. 4th ed. 1991. (Illus.). 300p. text (*0-443-04383-3*) Church.

Blood Coagulation, Fibrinolysis & Platelets. Ed. by E. W. Davie & E. Kakishita. 1996. (Illus.). 240p. pap. 89.00 (*4-431-70165-6*) Spr-Verlag.

Blood Collection: Special Procedures. Susan Phelan. 1991. 145.00 incl. VHS (*0-89189-309-1*, D47-9-055-VH) Am Soc Clinical.

Blood Collection: The Difficult Draw. Deanna Klosinski. 1992. 145.00 incl. VHS (*0-89189-350-4*) Am Soc Clinical.

Blood Collection: The Pediatric Patient. Susan Phelan. 1990. (NLM Ser.: No. WB382). 145.00 incl. VHS (*0-89189-302-4*, 47-9-052-VH) Am Soc Clinical.

Blood Collection: The Routine Venipuncture. Deanna Klosinski et al. 1989. 145.00 incl. VHS (*0-89189-291-5*, 47-9-051VH) Am Soc Clinical.

Blood Collection on Filter Paper for Neonatal Screening Programs: Approved Standard (1992) Contrib. by Robert M. Nakamura. 2nd ed. 1992. 75.00 (*1-56238-157-1*, LA4-A2) NCCLS.

Blood Collection on Filter Paper for Neonatal Screening Programs: Approved Standard (1997) 3rd ed. 1997. 75.00 (*1-56238-334-5*, LA4-A3) NCCLS.

Blood Compatibility, Set. Ed. by David F. Williams. 1987. 234.00 (*0-8493-6608-9*, R857, CRC Reprint) Franklin.

Blood Compatibility. D. Williams. 1987. LC 86-34337. reprint ed. Vol. 1. 240p. 135.00 (*0-8493-6604-6*); Vol. 2. 168p. 99.00 (*0-8493-6605-4*) Franklin (CRC Reprint).

Blood Compatible Materials & Devices. Ed. by Chandra P. Sharma & Michael Szycher. 1990. LC 90-71281. 303p. 39.95 (*0-87762-733-9*) CRC Pr.

Blood Compatible Materials & Their Testing. Ed. by Steen Dawids & A. Bantjes. 1986. (Developments in Hematology & Immunology Ser.). text 256.50 (*0-89838-813-9*) Kluwer Academic.

Blood Conservation in Cardiac Surgery. Ed. by Karl H. Krieger & O. W. Isom. 1997. LC 96-45492. (Illus.). 752p. 103.00 (*0-387-94908-9*) Spr-Verlag.

Blood Conservation in the Surgical Patient. Ed. by M. Ramez Salem. 1996. (Illus.). 446p. text 125.00 (*0-683-07531-4*) Lppncott W & W.

Blood Conservation with Aprotinin. Ed. & Intro. by Roque Pifarre. 1995. LC 95-6759. (Illus.). 407p. 55.00 (*1-56053-151-7*) Hanley & Belfus.

Blood Conspiracy: How to Avoid Getting AIDS & Hepatitis in a Transfusion. Joleen Ottosen. Ed. by Marilyn Ross. 1993. LC 92-71818. 326p. 24.95 (*0-9632963-3-7*) Aspen Leaf Pr.

Blood, Dirt & DNA: For Attorneys & Investigators. unabr. ed. 1998. (Illus.). viii, 106p. pap. 25.00 (*0-9666111-2-8*, BI-2) Baggetts.

Blood Donor Collection Practices. Ed. by Christina A. Kasprisin & Barbara Laird-Fryer. 1993. (Illus.). 203p. (C). text 40.00 (*1-56395-021-9*) Am Assn Blood.

Blood Feuds: AIDS, Blood & the Politics of Medical Disaster. Eric Feldman. 1999. LC 98-47064. 400p. pap. text 29.95 (*0-19-513160-6*) OUP.

Blood Feuds: AIDS, Blood, & the Politics of Medical Disaster. Eric Feldman. 1999. LC 98-47064. 400p. text 49.50 (*0-19-512929-6*) OUP.

Blood Filtration & Blood Cell Deformability. Ed. by John A. Dormandy. 1985. pap. text 73.00 (*0-89838-714-0*) Kluwer Academic.

Blood Flow in Large Arteries: Applications to Atherogenesis & Clinical Medicine. Ed. by Dieter W. Liepsch. 1989. (Monographs on Atherosclerosis: Vol. 15). (Illus.). viii, 288p. 235.00 (*3-8055-4983-0*) S Karger.

Blood Flow in the Heart & Large Vessels. Ed. by M. Sugawara et al. 1989. (Illus.). 226p. 211.00 (*0-387-70032-3*, 1524) Spr-Verlag.

***Blood Folate & Vitamin B12: United States, 1988-1994.** Jacqueline D. Wright. 2001. (Illus.). 78p. pap. 25.00 (*0-7567-1350-1*) DIANE Pub.

Blood Gas Preanalytical Considerations: Specimen Collection, Calibration, & Controls; Approved Guideline (1993) Contrib. by Sharon Ehrmeyer. 1993. 75.00 (*1-56238-190-3*, C27-A) NCCLS.

Blood Glucose Logbook. Charles E. Hugenberger. 2nd ed. 1998. 20p. pap. text 3.95 (*1-885057-11-3*) C E Hugenberger.

Blood Group Antigen Factsbook. Ed. by Marion E. Reid & Christine Lomas-Francis. 1996. LC 96-36684. (Factsbooks Ser.). (Illus.). 384p. pap. text 42.00 (*0-12-585965-1*) Morgan Kaufmann.

Blood Group Antigens & Antibodies. Marjory Stroup & Margaret Treacy. 1982. (Illus.). 255p. (Orig.). pap. text 35.00 (*0-910771-00-6*) Ortho Diag.

Blood Group Serology. Kathleen E. Boorman et al. 6th ed. 1987. (Illus.). 448p. text (*0-443-02636-X*) Church.

Blood Group Systems: Duffy, Kidd & Lutheran. Steven R. Pierce & Colin Macpherson. 1988. LC 88-19267. 151p. 25.00 (*0-915355-55-8*) Am Assn Blood.

Blood Group Systems: Kell. Ed. by Barbara Laird-Fryer. 1990. LC 90-949. 91p. (C). text 35.00 (*0-915355-80-9*) Am Assn Blood.

Blood Group Systems: MN & Gerbich. Phyllis Unger & Barbara Laird-Fryer. 1989. LC 89-17694. (Illus.). 107p. (C). text 25.00 (*0-915355-65-5*) Am Assn Blood.

Blood Group Systems: Rh. Ed. by Virginia Vengelen-Tyler & Steven R. Pierce. 1987. LC 87-14518. 103p. text 16.00 (*0-915355-41-8*) Am Assn Blood.

Blood Group Topics. Barbara E. Dodd. 1978. (Current Topics in Immunology Ser.: Vol. 3). (Illus.). pap. 21.25 (*0-8151-2710-3*) Mosby Inc.

Blood Grouping Reagents: Preparation & Application Methods. G. S. Nicholson et al. 1993. (WHO Regional Publications: No. 5). 87p. pap. text 9.00 (*92-9021-179-2*, 1440005) World Health.

Blood Groups: Ch-Rg, Kn-McC-Yk, Cromer. Ed. by JoAnn M. Moulds & Barbara Laird-Fryer. 1992. LC 92-49706. 66p. 43.00 (*1-56395-009-X*) Am Assn Blood.

Blood Groups: P, I, Sda & Pr. JoAnn M. Moulds & Laura L. Woods. 1991. LC 91-4870. (Illus.). 151p. (C). text 40.00 (*1-56395-002-2*) Am Assn Blood.

Blood Groups & Other Red Cell Surface Markers in Health & Disease. Ed. by Charles Salmon. 1984. LC 82-13096. (Illus.). 150p. (gr. 13). 47.50 (*0-89352-193-0*) Mosby Inc.

Blood Industry, No. C-071N. 1994. 2750.00 (*1-56965-017-9*) BCC.

Blood Industry (Update) Business Communications Co., Inc. Staff. 1991. 135p. 2250.00 (*0-89336-763-X*, C-071R) BCC.

Blood Irradiation: A User's Guide. Ed. by Suzanne H. Butch & Ann Tiehen. 1996. (Illus.). 124p. pap. 69.00 (*1-56395-057-X*, PC97-PR9605) Am Assn Blood.

Blood Lactate Response to Exercise. Arthur Weltman. 1995. LC 94-15638. (Current Issues in Exercise Science Ser.: Vol. 4). 128p. pap. text 24.00 (*0-87322-769-7*, BWEL0769) Human Kinetics.

Blood Leukocytes: Function & Use in Therapy. Ed. by C. F. Hogman et al. 1977. 88p. (Orig.). pap. text 18.50 (*91-506-0136-9*) Coronet Bks.

Blood Loss & Shock. Ed. by Niels H. Secher et al. 1994. 208p. (*0-340-56021-5*) E A GBR. *Dist:* OUP.

Blood Magic: The Anthropology of Menstruation. Ed. by Thomas Buckley & Alma Gottlieb. 1988. pap. text 19.95 (*0-520-06350-3*) U CA Pr.

Blood-Membrane Internation in Extracorporal Circuits. Ed. by L. W. Henderson & D. Chenoweth. 1987. (Journal: Vol. 5, No. 2-3, 1987). (Illus.). 96p. 60.00 (*3-8055-4580-0*) S Karger.

Blood Money: Modern Medicine's Abuse of Power. Surendra Kelwala. 1996. LC 96-67245. 322p. (Orig.). pap. 12.95 (*1-882792-20-3*) Proctor Pubns.

Blood Oxygenation. Ed. by Daniel Hershey. 1998. (Illus.). 374p. reprint ed. pap. text 50.00 (*0-916961-09-5*) Basal Books.

Blood Perfusion & Microenvironment of Human Tumors: Implications for Clinical Radiooncology. Ed. by M. Molls & P. Vaupel. 2000. (Medical Radiology Ser.). (Illus.). 238p. pap. 75.00 (*3-540-66994-9*) Spr-Verlag.

Blood Perfusion & Microenvironment of Human Tumors: Implications for Clinical Radiooncology. Ed. by M. Molls & Peter Vaupel. 1997. LC 97-20657. (Medical Radiology Ser.). (Illus.). 238p. (C). 139.00 (*3-540-58866-3*) Spr-Verlag.

Blood Plasma: The Promise & the Politics. Thomas Drees. 1983. LC 82-11617. (Illus.). 29.95 (*0-87949-225-2*) Ashley Bks.

Blood Plasma Safety: Plasma Product Risks Are Low If Good Manufacturing Practices Are Followed. Bernice Steinhardt. 1999. (Illus.). 56p. text 20.00 (*0-7881-7915-2*) DIANE Pub.

Blood Pressure. 1996. lib. bdg. 250.75 (*0-8490-5890-2*) Gordon Pr.

Blood Pressure. Andrew R. Nara et al. Ed. by Mary J. Pramik-Holdaway. 1989. (Biophysical Measurement Ser.). 109p. (Orig.). (C). 28.00 (*0-9627449-0-5*) SpaceLabs.

Blood Pressure: Questions You Have, Answers You Need. People's Medical Society Staff. 1996. LC 95-46873. 96p. pap. 9.95 (*1-882606-61-2*) Peoples Med Soc.

Blood Pressure & Heart Rate Variability: Computer Analysis, Methodology & Clinical Applications. Antonio Pedotti & Alberto Zanchetti. Ed. by M. Di Rienzo et al. 1993. LC 91-59040. (Studies in Health Technology & Informatics: Vol. 4). 277p. (YA). (gr. 12 up). 110.00 (*90-5199-077-4*) IOS Press.

Blood Pressure Book: How to Get It down & Keep It down. Stephen P. Fortmann & Prudence E. Breitrose. 1995. LC 95-11231. (Illus.). 144p. pap. 14.95 (*0-923521-32-1*) Bull Pub.

Blood Pressure Measurement. E. T. O'Brien & K. O'Malley. 1991. (Handbooks of Hypertension: Vol. 14). 460p. 225.00 (*0-444-81162-1*) Elsevier.

Blood Pressure Measurements. W. Meyer-Sabellek et al. 1990. 340p. 80.00 (*0-387-91332-7*, 1915) Spr-Verlag.

Blood Pressure Monitoring in Cardiovascular Medicine & Therapeutics. Ed. by William B. White. 2000. LC 00-33588. (Contemporary Cardiology Ser.). (Illus.). 328p. 99.00 (*0-89603-840-8*) Humana.

Blood Pressure Studies in Children: Report of a WHO Study Group, 1985. WHO Staff. 1985. (Technical Report Ser.: No. 715). 36p. 5.00 (*92-4-120715-9*) World Health.

***Blood Purification in Intensive Care: 2nd International Course on Critical Care Nephrology, Vicenza, May 2001 - Proceedings.** Ed. by C. Ronco et al. 2001. LC 2001-29339. (Contributions to Nephrology Ser.: No. 132). (Illus.). x, 433p. 248.75 (*3-8055-7207-7*) S Karger.

Blood Sacrifice Complex. Edwin M. Loeb. 1924. LC 24-4020. (American Anthropological Association Memoirs Ser.: No. 30). pap. 25.00 (*0-527-00529-0*) Periodicals Srv.

***Blood Safety & Availability: Congressional Hearing.** Ed. by Fred Upton. 2001. 149p. reprint ed. pap. 35.00 (*0-7567-1151-7*) DIANE Pub.

Blood Safety & Availability: Hearings Before the Subcommittee on Oversight & Investigations of the Committee on Commerce, House of Representatives, One Hundred Sixth Congress, First Session, September 23, October 6, & October 19, 1999. Ed. by U. S. Congress, House Committee on Commerce, Subcommittee on Oversight and Investigations. 1999. LC 00-325617. (*0-16-059934-2*) USGPO.

Blood Safety in the New Millennium. Ed. by Susan Linda Stramer. 2000. LC 2001-22052. (Illus.). xvi, 236p. pap. text (*1-56395-134-7*) Am Assn Blood.

Blood Safety, Minimizing Plasma Product Risks: Hearing Before the Subcommittee on Human Resources of the Committee on Government Reform & Oversight, House of Representatives, One Hundred Fifth Congress, Second Session, September 9, 1998. Contrib. by U. S. Congress, House Committee on Government Reform and Oversight, Subcommittee on Human Resources. 1999. LC 99-215635. (*0-16-058382-9*) USGPO.

Blood Saga: The Social History of the U. S. Hemophilia Community, 1948-1998. Susan Resnik. 1999. LC 98-14150. 294p. 29.95 (*0-520-21195-2*) U CA Pr.

Blood Specimen Collection for Healthcare Professionals: A Short Course. Marjorie Schaub Di Lorenzo & Susan King Strasinger. 2001. LC 2001-28564. (Illus.). 75p. per. 19.95 (*0-8036-0848-9*) Davis Co.

Blood Stem Cell Transplantation. Ed. by Jane N. Winter. 1997. LC 96-35387. (Cancer Treatment & Research Ser.). 432p. (C). text 407.00 (*0-7923-4260-7*) Kluwer Academic.

Blood Substitutes. Sarah Mangold. 1998. 45p. (C). 7.00 (*0-937013-77-3*) Potes Poets.

Blood Substitutes: New Challenges. Ed. by R. M. Winslow et al. 1996. LC 96-4628. 208p. (*3-7643-3878-4*); (Illus.). 224p. 79.95 (*0-8176-3878-4*) Birkhauser.

Blood Substitutes: Physiological Basis of Efficacy. Ed. by Robert M. Winslow et al. 1995. LC 95-2118. (Illus.). 205p. 69.95 (*0-8176-3804-0*) Birkhauser.

Blood Substitutes: Present & Future Perspectives. E. Tsuchida. 1998. LC 98-37069. 456p. 187.00 (*0-444-20524-1*) Elsevier.

Blood Substitutes: Principles, Methods, Products & Clinical Trials: Tissue Engineering. Thomas M. Chang. 1997. LC 97-36010. (Illus.). xiv, 142p. text 98.00 (*3-8055-6584-4*) S Karger.

Blood Substitutes - Principles, Methods, Products & Clinical Trials Vol. 2: A Karger Landes Systems Publication. Ed. by T. M. Chang. 1998. (Illus.). xviii, 236p. 98.00 (*3-8055-6633-6*) S Karger.

Blood Substitutes & Oxygen Carriers. Thomas M. Chang. 1992. (Illus.). 896p. text 250.00 (*0-8247-8810-9*) Dekker.

Blood Substitutes & Therapeutic Uses: Index of New Information with Authors, Subjects & Bibliography. Arthur T. Treadwell. 1993. 180p. 47.50 (*1-55914-762-8*); pap. 44.50 (*1-55914-763-6*) ABBE Pubs Assn.

Blood Sugar Blues: Overcoming the Hidden Dangers of Insulin Resistance & How You Can Detect & Overcome It. Miryam Ehrlich Williamson. 2001. LC 2001-26347. 252p. pap. 14.95 (*0-8027-7610-8*) Walker & Co.

Blood Supply: FDA Oversight & Remaining Issues of Safety. 1997. (Illus.). 158p. pap. text 35.00 (*1-57979-222-7*) DIANE Pub.

Blood Supply: Risks, Perceptions & Prospects for the Future. Ed. by Sandra T. Nance. 1994. (Illus.). 197p. (C). text 30.00 (*1-56395-033-2*) Am Assn Blood.

Blood Supply: Transfusion-Associated Risks. 1997. (Illus.). 92p. pap. text 35.00 (*1-57979-217-0*) DIANE Pub.

Blood Supply: Transfusion-Associated Risks. Marcia G. Crosse. 1999. (Illus.). 92p. (C). pap. text 20.00 (*0-7881-7636-6*) DIANE Pub.

Blood Supply of Bone: Scientific Aspects. Murray Brookes & William J. Revell. 1997. LC 97-31214. (Illus.). 300p. 125.00 (*3-540-76204-3*) Spr-Verlag.

Blood Thinner Cure: A Revolutionary Seven-Step Lifestyle Plan for Stopping Heart Disease & Stroke. Kenneth R. Kensey & Carol A. Turkington. 2001. LC 00-64481. (Illus.). 208p. pap. 14.95 (*0-8092-9841-4*, Contemporary) McGraw-Hill Trade.

Blood Transfusion: 2nd European Course (Madrid, 1990) Council of Europe Staff. 1992. (ENG & FRE.). (*92-871-2063-3*) Council of Europe FRA. *Dist:* Manhattan Pub Co.

Blood Transfusion: A Basic Text. Ed. by A. F. Britten et al. 1994. (WHO Regional Publications: No. 7). xi, 171p. pap. text 15.00 (*92-9021-181-4*, 1440007) World Health.

Blood Transfusion & Addendum 1978: A Guide to the Formation & Operation of a Transfusion Service. Ed. by C. C. Bowley et al. 1978. 147p. pap. text 14.00 (*92-4-154013-3*, 1150016) World Health.

Blood Transfusion & Blood Components. C. T. Sibinga. 1995. (WHO Regional Publications: No. 12). 54p. pap. text 9.00 (*92-9021-190-3*, 1440012) World Health.

Blood Transfusion & Problems of Bleeding. C. T. Sibinga & P. C. Das. 1982. text 126.50 (*90-247-3058-9*) Kluwer Academic.

Blood Transfusion ID Card & Book: For Safer Blood at the Time of AIDS, Hepatitis, VDs, etc. Antun Murkovic. 1989. (ENG & JPN.). 120p. (Orig.). pap. (*0-929602-00-5*) Mura Pub Co.

Blood Transfusion in Clinical Medicine. P. L. Mollison et al. 10th ed. 1997. LC 97-73. (Illus.). 754p. 225.00 (*0-86542-881-6*) Blackwell Sci.

Blood Transfusion Micro-Filters. 2nd ed. 1989. 10p. pap. 70.00 (*0-910275-93-9*, BF7-209) Assn Adv Med Instrn.

Blood Transfusion Services for the Developing World. Ed. by J. Leikola & M. Contreras. 1994. (Vox Sanguinis: Vol. 67, Supplement 5, 1994). (Illus.). iv, 66p. pap. 30.50 (*3-8055-6094-X*) S Karger.

Blood, Transfusion Therapy: A Physician's Handbook. Edward L. Snyder. 5th ed. 1996. LC 97-122522. (Illus.). 141p. pap. text 3.50 (*0-914404-97-0*, PC97-OP1762) Am Assn Blood.

Blood Transfusion Therapy: A Physician's Handbook. American Association of Blood Banks Staff. Ed. by Darrell J. Triulzi. 6th ed. 1999. (Illus.). 150p. pap. (*3-8055-7039-2*) S Karger.

Blood Transfusion Therapy: A Problem Oriented Approach. J. A. Napier. 1996. 498p. 275.00 (*0-471-95378-4*) Wiley.

Blood Transfusions: A History & Evaluation of the Religions, Biblical & Medical Objections. Jerry Bergman. 1994. 220p. (Orig.). (C). pap. 9.95 (*1-883858-27-5*) Witness CA.

Blood Transfusions & Infectious Diseases. E. G. Rondanelli. 1989. (Infectious Diseases Color Atlas Monographs: No. 2). 322p. text (*1-57235-029-6*) Piccin Nuova.

Blood Use in Cardiac Surgery. Ed. by N. Friedel et al. 1991. 320p. 87.00 (*0-387-91372-6*) Spr-Verlag.

Blood Vessel Changes in Hypertension, I. Ed. by Robert M. K. W. Lee. 1989. 216p. lib. bdg. 141.00 (*0-8493-4883-8*, RC685) CRC Pr.

Blood Vessel Changes in Hypertension, II. Ed. by R. Lee. 1989. 192p. lib. bdg. 149.00 (*0-8493-4884-6*, RC685) CRC Pr.

Blood Vessel Wall & Thrombosis: Hemostasis, Vol. 1. Ed. by Raymond Machovich. 1988. LC 87-24298. 320p. 145.00 (*0-8493-5626-1*, RC694, CRC Reprint) Franklin.

Blood Vessel Wall & Thrombosis: Thrombotic Processes in Atherogenesis, Vol. 2. Raymond Machovich. 1988. LC 87-24298. 280p. 112.00 (*0-8493-5627-X*, RC694, CRC Reprint) Franklin.

Blood Vessel Wall Interactions in Thrombogenesis. Ed. by A. Nordoy. 1979. (Haemostasis Ser.: Vol. 8, Nos. 3-5). pap. 68.00 (*3-8055-0117-X*) S Karger.

Blood Viscosity. Leopold Dintenfass. 1985. text 316.00 (*0-85200-413-3*) Kluwer Academic.

Blood Whispers: L. A. Writers on AIDS. Ed. by Terry Wolverton. 1991. LC 91-90365. 100p. pap. 7.95 (*0-9629528-0-X*) Silverton Bks.

Bloodborne Diseases - Reducing Your Risks at Work: Standard Precautions Review. Charles A. Illian. 1995. (In Service Sourcebook Ser.). 72p. pap. text 29.95 (*1-888343-01-X*) Hartman Pub.

Bloodborne Pathogens. National Safety Council Staff. 2nd ed. 1996. LC 96-47085. (Emergency Care Ser.). 80p. pap. 26.95 (*0-7637-0229-3*) Jones & Bartlett.

Bloodborne Pathogens: Four Color Edition. National Safety Council Staff. 1994. LC 93-26138. (Illus.). pap. text 26.95 (*0-86720-818-X*, 818-X) Jones & Bartlett.

Bloodborne Pathogens: Instructor's Resource Manual. National Safety Council Staff. 2nd ed. 1997. (Illus.). 92p. pap. text 15.00 (*0-7637-0732-5*, 0732-5) Jones & Bartlett.

Bloodborne Pathogens: Interactive Training. National Safety Council Staff. 1998. (Emergency Care Ser.). (Illus.). 32p. (C). pap. text, wbk. ed. 16.95 (*0-7637-0519-5*, 0519-5) Jones & Bartlett.

Bloodborne Pathogens - Academic. National Safety Council Staff. LC 92-49476. 1993. (Illus.). 80p. tchr. ed., ring bd. 395.00 (*0-86720-798-1*, 798-1); 1992. (Illus.). 64p. pap. text, tchr. ed. 15.00 (*0-86720-772-8*, 772-8); 1992. 80p. pap. text 15.00 (*0-86720-771-X*); 1992. (Illus.). 60p. sl. 195.00 (*0-86720-773-6*, 773-6) Jones & Bartlett.

Bloodborne Pathogens in the Workplace: Guidelines for Small Businesses. Erskine S. Walther. rev. ed. 1995. LC 95-79091. 92p. spiral bd. 50.00 (*1-885327-09-9*) Walther Cnslt.

Bloodborne Pathogens Initial Training Program for the School Setting. Jan Sanderson. 1997. 74p. stu. ed., ring bd. 60.00 incl. trans. (*1-880118-09-2*, 247-04) MESD Pr.

Bloodborne Pathogens Policy Manual. Victoria Wetle. 1994. LC 93-6416. (Illus.). 480p. (C). pap. text 103.95 (*0-86720-778-7*, 778-7) Jones & Bartlett.

Bloodborne Pathogens (Smithkline) National Safety Council Staff. 1993. pap. 12.50 (*0-86720-793-0*) Jones & Bartlett.

Bloodborne Pathogens Standard: A Pragmatic Approach. Jon T. O'Neal. 1996. 336p. text 60.95 (*0-442-01779-0*, VNR) Wiley.

Bloodborne Pathogens Update Training Program for the School Setting. Jan Sanderson. 1997. 38p. ring bd. 100.00 (*1-880118-16-5*, 247-05) MESD Pr.

Bloom & Fawcett: Concise Histology. Don W. Fawcett & Ronald P. Jensh. 1997. LC 96-19630. (An Arnold Publication). (Illus.). 320p. pap. (*0-412-07971-2*) E A GBR. *Dist:* OUP.

Blooming Bellany: Herbs & Herbal Healing. David Bellamy. 1994. (Illus.). 188p. (*0-563-36725-3*) BBC GBR. *Dist:* Parkwest Pubns.

BLR Encyclopedia of Safety & Health Training, Set. Ed. by John F. Brady. rev. ed. 1988. 1024p. 199.95 (*1-55645-591-7*, 591) Busn Legal Reports.

Blue Book: Suggested Procedures for the Detection & Identification of Certain Finfish & Shellfish Pathogens. Ed. by John C. Thoesen. 1994. LC 90-64152. (Illus.). stu. ed., ring bd. 91.00 (*0-9625505-2-3*, 530.19) Am Fisheries Soc.

Blue Collar Stress. Arthur B. Shostak. 1980. LC 79-16531. (A-W Occupational Stress Ser.). pap. 10.95 (*0-201-07688-8*) Addison-Wesley.

Blue Cross & Blue Shield: Experiences of Weak Plans & the Role of Effective State Oversight. 1994. (Illus.). 64p. (Orig.). (C). pap. text 40.00 (*0-7881-1149-3*) DIANE Pub.

Blue Fire: Selected Writings by James Hillman. James Hillman. 1997. LC 89-45043. 336p. reprint ed. pap. 14.00 (*0-06-092101-3*, Perennial) HarperTrade.

***Blue Print for Heart Failure: A Physician's Guide to Establishing a Heart Failure Center in the Private Practice Setting** Michael E. McIvor. 2001. (Illus.). 200p. pap. 99.95 (*1-928888-03-8*) Heart Gallery.

Blue Tongue, African Horse Sickness & Related Orbiviruses: International Symposium on Bluetongue, African Horse Sickness, & Related Orbiviruses, Second Conference, Paris, France, 1991. 1992. 1088p. 159.00 (*0-8493-5169-3*, SF809) CRC Pr.

***Blueprint for Action on Breastfeeding.** Ed. by Suzanne G. Haynes. 2001. 51p. (C). pap. text 15.00 (*0-7567-0793-5*) DIANE Pub.

Blueprint for Health. Mary A. Howard. 1985. 176p. (Orig.). pap. 4.70 (*0-310-42151-9*, 12776P) Zondervan.

Blueprint for Immortality. Harold S. Burr. 1972. 104p. pap. (*0-85435-281-3*) C W Daniel GBR. *Dist:* Natl Bk Netwk.

Blueprint for Use of Nursing Models: Education, Research, Practice & Administration. Patricia H. Walker & Betty M. Neuman. 1996. LC 96-19656. 360p. pap. 40.95 (*0-88737-656-8*) Natl League Nurse.

Blueprints for Managed Care: Mental Healthcare Concepts & Structure. Frank D. McGuirk et al. 1996. (Illus.). 79p. (C). reprint ed. pap. text 25.00 (*0-7881-3691-7*) DIANE Pub.

Blueprints for Thinking: The Role of Planning in Cognitive Development. Ed. by Sarah L. Friedman et al. 1987. (Illus.). 576p. text 130.00 (*0-521-25605-4*) Cambridge U Pr.

Blueprints in Medicine. Vincent Young. 2nd ed. 2000. LC 00-44409. (Blueprints Ser.). (Illus.). 250p. pap. 29.95 (*0-632-04484-5*) Blackwell Sci.

Blueprints in Medicine: Steps 2 & 3 Review Series. Allan H. Goroll et al. 1997. LC 97-6519. (Blueprints Ser.). (Illus.). 256p. pap. 28.95 (*0-86542-537-X*) Blackwell Sci.

Blueprints in Obstetrics & Gynecology. Tamara L. Callahan et al. 1997. LC 97-9851. (Blueprints Ser.). (Illus.). 224p. pap. 28.95 (*0-86542-505-1*) Blackwell Sci.

Blueprints in Obstetrics & Gynecology. Tamara Callahan et al. 2nd ed. 2000. LC 00-44415. (Blueprints Ser.). (Illus.). xii, 308p. pap. 29.95 (*0-632-04489-6*) Blackwell Sci.

Blueprints in Pediatrics. Bradley S. Marino et al. 1997. LC 97-9049. (Blueprints Ser.). (Illus.). 272p. pap. 28.95 (*0-86542-504-3*) Blackwell Sci.

Blueprints in Pediatrics. Bradley S. Marino & Katie Snead. 2nd ed. 2000. LC 00-44416. (Blueprints Ser.). (Illus.). xviii, 339p. pap. 31.95 (*0-632-04486-1*) Blackwell Sci.

Blueprints in Psychiatry. Michael J. Murphy et al. 1997. LC 97-7347. (Blueprints Ser.). (Illus.). 96p. pap. 25.95 (*0-86542-503-5*) Blackwell Sci.

Blueprints in Psychiatry. Michael J. Murphy. 2nd ed. 2000. LC 00-44411. (Blueprints Ser.). (Illus.). 128p. pap. 28.95 (*0-632-04488-8*) Blackwell Sci.

Blueprints in Surgery. Seth J. Karp et al. 1997. LC 97-7348. (Blueprints Ser.). (Illus.). 113p. pap. 25.95 (*0-86542-546-9*) Blackwell Sci.

Blueprints in Surgery. Seth Karp. 2nd ed. 2000. LC 00-44410. (Blueprints Ser.). (Illus.). 250p. pap. 28.95 (*0-632-04487-X*) Blackwell Sci.

***Blueprints Q&A Step 2: Medicine.** Michael S. Clement. 2001. LC 2001-2367. (Blueprint Q&A Ser.). (Illus.). 128p. pap. 10.00 (*0-632-04602-3*) Blackwell Sci.

***Blueprints Q&A Step 2: Obstetrics & Gynecology.** Michael S. Clement. 2001. LC 2001-3188. (Blueprints Q&A Ser.). (Illus.). 128p. pap. 10.00 (*0-632-04594-9*) Blackwell Sci.

***Blueprints Q&A Step 2: Pediatrics.** Michael S. Clement. 2001. LC 2001-2524. (Blueprint Q&A Ser.). (Illus.). 128p. pap. 10.00 (*0-632-04598-1*) Blackwell Sci.

***Blueprints Q&A Step 2: Psychiatry.** Michael S. Clement. 2001. LC 2001-2138. (Blueprint Q&A Ser.). (Illus.). 128p. pap. 10.00 (*0-632-04592-2*) Blackwell Sci.

***Blueprints Q&A Step 2: Surgery.** Michael S. Clement. 2001. LC 2001-3080. (Blueprint Q&A Ser.). (Illus.). 100p. pap. 10.00 (*0-632-04596-5*) Blackwell Sci.

Blueprints Series Bradley S. Marino. 2nd ed. 2000. (Blueprints Ser.). (Illus.). pap. 141.95 (*0-632-04512-4*) Blackwell Sci.

Bluetongue Viruses. Ed. by P. Roy & B. M. Gorman. 1990. (Current Topics in Microbiology & Immunology Ser.: Vol. 162). (Illus.). 192p. 114.00 (*0-387-51922-X*) Spr-Verlag.

Blunt Chest Trauma: General Principles of Management. Marvin M. Kirsh & Herbert Sloan. 1977. text 30.00 (*0-316-49501-8*, Little Brwn Med Div) Lppncott W & W.

Blunt Multiple Trauma: Pathophysiology & Comprehensive Therapy. John R. Border et al. 1990. (Illus.). 1024p. text 295.00 (*0-8247-8172-4*) Dekker.

Blurred Boundaries: My Therapist, My Friend. Marina C. Miller. 1993. (Orig.). pap. 14.95 (*0-9636710-5-7*) Shades of Gray.

BMA's General Practitioners Handbook. Norman Ellis & British Medical Association Staff. 1997. LC 97-11002. (*1-85775-241-4*) Radcliffe Med Pr GBR. *Dist:* Balogh.

BMDO Technologies for Biomedical Applications. Joan Zimmerman et al. 1999. (Illus.). 94p. (C). pap. text 25.00 (*0-7881-7600-5*) DIANE Pub.

BMT Data Book: A Manual for Bone Marrow & Blood Stem Cell Transplantation. Kerry Atkinson. 1997. LC 96-27079. (Illus.). 608p. (C). text 130.00 (*0-521-55615-5*) Cambridge U Pr.

Board Fund Raising Manual. Darla Struck & Sheri Campbell. 1992. 75p. 32.00 (*0-8342-0405-3*, 04053) Aspen Pub.

Board Member Manual, Vol. 1. 1995. 49.00 (*0-8342-0483-5*, 04835) Aspen Pub.

Board Member Manual Video, Vol. 2. 1995. 51.00 (*0-8342-0484-3*, 04843) Aspen Pub.

Board of Registry Study Guide - Histotechnology. Carson. 1994. 40.00 (*0-89189-375-X*) Am Soc Clinical.

Board of Registry Study Guide for Clinical Laboratory Certification Examinations. Barbara M. Castleberry et al. 4th ed. 1996. LC 96-2826. 40.00 (*0-89189-416-0*) Am Soc Clinical.

Board Self-Evaluation Manual. Barry S. Bader et al. 2nd ed. 1988. 141p. (Orig.). stu. ed. 59.00 (*0-915963-04-3*) Bader Assoc Inc.

Board Stiff Preparing for the Anaesthesia Orals. Christopher J. Gallagher & David Lebersky. 2nd ed. 2000. LC 00-41390. 368p. pap. text 49.99 (*0-7506-7157-2*) Buttrwrth-Heinemann.

***Board-Style Question & Answer Book.** 9th ed. 2001. 550p. stu. ed. 149.00 (*0-9640788-8-0*) MedStudy.

Boarding Time: A Psychiatry Candidate's Guide to Part II of the ABPN Examination. James Morrison & Rodrigo A. Munoz. 2nd ed. 1995. LC 95-34139. 256p. pap. text 29.95 (*0-88048-722-4*, 8722) Am Psychiatric.

Board's Role in Quality Care: A Practical Guide for Hospital Trustees. James E. Orlikoff & Mary K. Totten. 1991. LC 90-14512. 157p. (Orig.). pap. 32.95 (*1-55648-061-X*, 196126) AHPI.

Boater's Medical Companion. Robert S. Gould. 1990. LC 89-43018. (Cornell Boaters Library). (Illus.). 128p. pap. 6.95 (*0-87033-402-6*) Cornell Maritime.

Boating Safely Course. U. S. Coast Guard, Auxiliary Staff. 1997. LC 96-46739. 64p. (gr. 13). text 5.00 (*0-8151-4588-8*, 30069) Mosby Inc.

Bockus Gastroenterology. Ed. by William S. Haubrich et al. 5th ed. 1994. LC 93-2763. (Illus.). 3515p. text 625.00 (*0-7216-3687-X*) Saunders.

Bodies & Crimes: A Pathologist Speaks. F. D. Hocking. 1992. 300p. (C). (*0-86332-753-2*) St Mut.

Bodies & Souls: Politics & the Professionalization of Nursing in France, 1880-1922. Katrin Schultheiss. 2001. LC 00-61391. (Historical Studies: Vol. 139). (Illus.). vi, 248p. 49.95 (*0-674-00491-4*) HUP.

Bodies, Health & Consciousness: A Guide to Living Successfully in Your Body Through Rolfing & Yoga. Rosie Spiegel. 1994. (Illus.). 291p. (Orig.). pap. 24.95 (*0-9637824-0-1*) SRG Pubng.

Bodies in Glass: Genetics, Eugenics & Embryo Ethics. Steinberg. 1997. LC 96-8351. 192p. 59.95 (*0-7190-4667-X*) St Martin.

Bodies in Protest: Environmental Illness & the Struggle over Medical Knowledge. Steve Kroll-Smith. 2000. pap. text 17.50 (*0-8147-4752-3*) NYU Pr.

Bodies in Protest: Environmental Illness & the Struggle over Medical Knowledge. Steve Kroll-Smith et al. 1997. LC 97-4665. 240p. text 25.00 (*0-8147-4662-4*) NYU Pr.

Bodies of Evidence: The Fascinating World of Forensic Science & How It Helped Solved More Than 100 True Crimes. Brian Innes. 2000. LC 00-31084. (Illus.). 256p. 24.95 (*0-7621-0295-0*) RD Assn.

Bodies of Knowledge in Psychosocial Practice. Roann Barris et al. 1988. LC 88-43098. 172p. pap. 24.00 (*1-55642-071-4*) SLACK Inc.

Bodies under Siege: Self-Mutilation & Body Modification in Culture & Psychiatry. Armando R. Favazza. 2nd ed. 1996. LC 95-26098. (Illus.). 352p. (C). 52.95 (*0-8018-5299-4*); pap. text 18.95 (*0-8018-5300-1*) Johns Hopkins.

Bodily Alterations: An Introduction to a Sociology of the Body for Health Workers. Wendy Seymour. 1991. 176p. pap. text (*0-04-374009-X*) Allen & Unwin Pty AUS. *Dist:* Paul & Co Pubs.

Bodily Healing & the Atonement. T. J. McCrossan. 1982. pap. 5.95 (*0-89276-505-4*) Faith Lib Pubns.

Bodily Reflective Modes: A Phenomenological Approach for Psychology. Kenneth J. Shapiro. 1984. LC 84-26018. xxi, 230p. text 44.95 (*0-8223-0605-0*) Duke.

Body see Cuerpo

Body & Brain: A Trophic Theory of Neural Connections. Dale Purves. 1990. (Illus.). 272p. pap. 22.50 (*0-674-07716-4*) HUP.

Body & Emotion: The Aesthetics of Illness & Healing in the Nepal Himalayas. Robert R. Desjarlais. 1992. LC 92-23545. (Contemporary Ethnography Ser.). (Illus.). 320p. (Orig.). (C). text 45.00 (*0-8122-3166-X*); pap. text 18.95 (*0-8122-1434-X*) U of Pa Pr.

Body & Physical Difference: Discourses of Disability. Ed. by David T. Mitchell & Sharon L. Snyder. 1997. LC 97-20579. (Body, in Theory: Histories of Cultural Materialism Ser.). (Illus.). 320p. (C). text 55.00 (*0-472-09659-1*, 09659); pap. text 19.95 (*0-472-06659-5*, 06659) U of Mich Pr.

Body & Self: An Exploration of Early Female Development. Ed. by Dale Mendell. 1995. LC 94-32618. 276p. pap. text 50.00 (*1-56821-396-4*) Aronson.

Body & Social Psychology. Alan Radley. 1991. (Social Psychology Ser.). 213p. 107.00 (*0-387-97584-5*) Spr-Verlag.

Body & Soul: Children, Teenagers & Cancer. Mark Ragg. 1995. 350p. (Orig.). pap. (*0-85572-252-5*) Hill Content Pubng AUS. *Dist:* Seven Hills Bk.

Body & Soul: One Hundred Years at St. Vincent Hospital. David P. Kowal. 1993. (Illus.). 325p. 9.99 (*0-9636277-3-2*) Chandler Hse.

Body & Soul: The Black Woman's Guide to Physical Health & Emotional Well-Being. Ed. by Linda Villarosa. 1994. LC 94-13140. (Illus.). 608p. pap. 22.00 (*0-06-095085-4*) HarperCollins Pubs.

Body & the City: Psychoanalysis, Space, & Subjectivity. Steve Pile. 1996. LC 95-46814. (Illus.). 288p. (C). 90.00 (*0-415-06649-2*); pap. 29.95 (*0-415-14192-3*) Routledge.

Body Art - Human Physiology. Rhoades. 3rd ed. 1995. (C). pap. text, tchr. ed. 30.00 (*0-03-015862-1*) Harcourt Coll Pubs.

Body at War: The Story of Our Immune System. John Dwyer. 1994. (Illus.). 416p. pap. (*1-86373-484-8*) Allen & Unwin Pty AUS. *Dist:* IPG Chicago.

Body Awareness As Healing Therapy: The Case of Nora. Moshe Feldenkrais. 1993. LC 93-25025. 73p. (Orig.). pap. 12.95 (*1-883319-08-0*) Frog Ltd CA.

Body Basics for Life: Simple Steps to a Healthy, Painfree You! Karen Webb. 1998. (Illus.). 64p. pap. (*0-9682571-0-0*) Birchcliff CAN. *Dist:* Hushion Hse.

Body Bears the Burden: Trauma, Dissociation & Disease. Robert C. Scaer. 2001. LC 00-47213. (Illus.). 250p. (C). 59.95 (*0-7890-1245-6*); pap. text 32.95 (*0-7890-1246-4*) Haworth Pr (Hawrth Medical).

Body Betrayed: A Deeper Understanding of Women, Eating Disorders, & Treatment. Kathryn J. Zerbe. 1995. LC 93-5737. 447p. reprint ed. pap. 18.95 (*0-936077-23-9*) Gurze Bks.

Body Betrayed: Women, Eating Disorders, & Treatment. Kathryn J. Zerbe. 1993. LC 93-5737. 447p. 24.00 (*0-88048-522-1*, 8522) Am Psychiatric.

Body Build & Behavior in Young Children, Pt. 1. R. N. Walker. 1962. (SRCD M Ser.: Vol. 27, No. 3). pap. 25.00 (*0-527-01594-6*) Periodicals Srv.

Body-Centered Psychotherapy: The Hakomi Method. Ron Kurtz. 1997. 22.00 (*0-940795-18-3*) LifeRhythm.

Body Code: A Personalized Wellness & Weight Loss Plan Developed at the World Famous Green Valley Spa. Jay Cooper & Kathryn Lance. 1999. LC 99-18027. 320p. 24.00 (*0-671-02619-4*, PB Hardcover) PB.

Body Composition - Research Techniques & Nutritional Assessment. Ed. by Werner Overbeck & Dieter Bohm. 1990. (Internationale Zeitschrift fuer Infusionstherapie, Klinische Ernahrung und Transfusionsmedizin Ser.: Supplement 3 zu Band 17, April 1990). 18.50 (*3-8055-5228-9*) S Karger.

Body Composition Assessment in Children Adolescents. Ed. by T. Jurimae & A. P. Hills. 2001. LC 00-48745. (Medicine & Sport Science Ser.: Vol. 44). (Illus.). viii, 182p. 169.75 (*3-8055-7131-3*) S Karger.

Body Criticism: Imaging the Unseen in Enlightenment Art & Medicine. Barbara M. Stafford. 1993. (Illus.). 612p. pap. 39.95 (*0-262-69165-5*) MIT Pr.

Body CT: A Practical Approach. Dennis M. Balfe et al. 1999. LC 99-23503. (Illus.). 267p. text 79.00 (*0-07-058219-X*) McGraw-Hill Prof.

Body Ecology Diet: Recovering Your Health & Rebuilding Your Immunity. Donna Gates. Ed. by BED Publishing Staff. 4th ed. 1996. 260p. (Orig.). pap. 19.95 (*0-9638458-8-8*) Body Ecology.

Body Elite Gourmet. Wendi H. Schwartz. 1993. 123p. (Orig.). pap. (*0-9635503-0-6*) Bodyworks Pubs.

Body Experience in Fantasy & Behavior. Seymour Fisher. 1970. LC 71-111878. (Century Psychology Ser.). (C). 39.50 (*0-89197-046-0*); pap. text 12.95 (*0-89197-683-3*) Irvington.

Body Fat & Physical Fitness. Jana Parizkova. Tr. by K. Osancova from CZE. 1977. (Illus.). 280p. (*90-247-1925-9*) Kluwer Academic NLD. *Dist:* Kluwer Academic.

Body Fluid & Kidney Physiology. Stephen B. Hladky & Timothy J. Rink. 1988. (Physiology Principles in Medicine Ser.). 248p. (C). pap. text (*0-683-13037-4*) E A GBR. *Dist:* Williams & Wilkins.

Body Fluid Balance: Exercise & Sport. Ed. by Elsworth R. Buskirk & Susan M. Puhl. 1996. LC 95-53970. (Nutrition in Exercise & Sport Ser.). 352p. 104.95 (*0-8493-7918-0*) CRC Pr.

Body Fluid Homeostasis. Ed. by Barry M. Brenner & Jay H. Stein. 1986. (Contemporary Issues in Nephrology Ser.: Vol. 16). (Illus.). 454p. text (*0-443-08530-7*) Church.

Body Fluids: Laboratory Examination of Amniotic, Cerebrospinal, Seminal, Serous & Synovial Fluids. Carl R. Kjeldsberg & Joseph A. Knight. 3rd ed. 1993. LC 92-23968. (Illus.). 436p. 145.00 (*0-89189-344-X*) Am Soc Clinical.

Body Fluids & Electrolytes: A Programmed Presentation. Norma J. Weldy. 7th ed. 1995. LC 95-10053. (Illus.). 256p. (C). (gr. 13). spiral bd. 27.95 (*0-8151-9197-9*, 24780) Mosby Inc.

Body Fluids & Kidney Function. Ed. by Robert A. Brace et al. 1998. LC 97-13540. (Fetus & Neonate Ser.: No. 4). (Illus.). 340p. (C). text 110.00 (*0-521-59392-1*) Cambridge U Pr.

Body Image & Perceptual Dysfunction in Adults. Julia M. Van Deusen. 1992. (Illus.). 267p. pap. text 39.50 (*0-7216-3172-X*) Saunders.

Body Image & the Image of the Brain. Warren Gorman. 1969. LC 68-8293. (Illus.). 298p. 12.50 (*0-87527-037-9*) Green.

Body Image Disturbance: Assessment & Treatment. J. Kevin Thompson. 1990. (Psychology Practitioner Guidebooks Ser.). 160p. text (*0-08-036822-0*) PPI GBR. *Dist:* Elsevier.

Body Image Disturbance: Assessment & Treatment. J. Kevin Thompson. 1994. (Practitioner Guidebook Ser.). 156p. (C). pap. text 48.00 (*0-205-14482-9*, H4482, Longwood Div) Allyn.

Body Image, Eating Disorders & Obesity: An Integrative Guide for Assessment & Treatment. Ed. by J. Kevin Thompson. 1996. LC 95-36117. 517p. 49.95 (*1-55798-324-0*) Am Psychol.

Body in a Pocket. Richard M. Slone et al. 1998. LC 98-39686. 362p. pap. 35.00 (*0-07-134435-7*) McGraw-Hill Prof.

Body in Brief: Essentials for Health Care. Rebecca J. Rayman. 3rd ed. 1997. (Illus.). 400p. per. 38.95 (*1-56930-055-0*) Delmar.

Body in Everyday Life. Sarah Nettleton. 1998. LC 97-44695. 280p. (C). pap. 27.95 (*0-415-16201-7*) Routledge.

Body in Everyday Life. Ed. by Sarah Nettleton & Jonathan Watson. 1998. LC 97-44695. 320p. (C). 90.00 (*0-415-16200-9*) Routledge.

Body in Illness & Health: Themes & Images in Jane Austen. Anita G. Gorman. 1993. LC 92-36595. (American University Studies: Ser. IV, Vol. 154). XIV, 212p. 45.95 (*0-8204-1996-6*) P Lang Pubng.

Body in Medical Thought & Practice. Ed. by Drew Leder. 1992. LC 92-6258. (Philosophy & Medicine Ser.). 266p. (C). lib. bdg. (*0-7923-1657-6*) Kluwer Academic NLD. *Dist:* Kluwer Academic.

Body in Mind: Understanding Cognitive Processes. Mark Rowlands. 1999. LC 98-45620. (Cambridge Studies in Philosophy). 280p. text 74.95 (*0-521-65274-X*) Cambridge U Pr.

Body in Nursing: A Collection of Views. Ed. by J. Lawler. 1998. 240p. pap. (*0-443-05250-6*) Church.

Body in Psychotherapy: Inquiries in Somatic Psychology. Ed. by Don H. Johnson & Ian Grand. 1997. LC 97-21280. (IO Journals: no. 58). 275p. pap. 16.95 (*1-55643-251-8*) North Atlantic.

Body in Psychotherapy: International Congress, Geneva, February 1996. Ed. by Jose Gimon. 1997. LC 97-9894. (Illus.). x, 206p. 172.25 (*3-8055-6285-3*) S Karger.

Body in Recovery: Somatic Psychotherapy & the Self. John Conger. 1994. LC 93-37231. 277p. (Orig.). pap. 16.95 (*1-883319-06-4*) Frog Ltd CA.

Body, Land & Spirit: Health & Healing in Aboriginal Society. Janice Reid. 1985. (Illus.). 241p. reprint ed. pap. (*0-7022-1779-4*) Univ Queensland Pr AUS. *Dist:* Intl Spec Bk.

Body Mass Index: A Measure of Chronic Energy Deficiency in Adults. P. S. Shetty & W. P. James. 1994. (Food & Nutrition Ser.: 56). 68p. pap. (*92-5-103472-9*, F34729) FAO ITA. *Dist:* Bernan Associates.

Body Massage for the Beauty Therapist. Audrey G. Goldberg. 1972. (Illus.). pap. 22.95 (*0-434-90659-X*) Trafalgar.

Body Mechanics & Self Care Manual. Marian Wolfe Dixon. 2000. LC 00-35681. (Illus.). 290p. pap. 33.40 (*0-8385-0747-6*) P-H.

Body, Memory & Architecture. Kent C. Bloomer & Charles W. Moore. 1977. LC 77-76304. (Yale Paperbound Ser.). (Illus.). 147p. pap. 22.50 (*0-300-02142-9*) Yale U Pr.

Body Mind Connection in Human Movement Analysis. Susan Loman & Rose Brandt. 1992. LC 92-70393. 235p. (C). pap. text 12.00 (*1-881245-00-4*) Antioch New Eng.

Body Movement: Coping with the Environment. Irmgard Bartenieff & D. Lewis. 1980. xiv, 290p. text 60.00 (*0-677-05500-5*) Gordon & Breach.

Body Movement: Perspectives in Research Ed. by Martha Davis. 1975. (Illus.). 84.00 (*0-405-06197-8*) Ayer.

Body Movement & Speech in Medical Interaction. Christian Heath. 1986. (Cambridge Studies in Emotion & Social Interaction). (Illus.). 224p. text 64.95 (*0-521-25335-7*) Cambridge U Pr.

Body of Business: Is Your Business Fit? Ronald K. Law. 2001. (Illus.). 192p. 19.95 (*0-9706790-2-5*) Cor Bks.

***Body of Knowledge.** Steven Giegerich. 2002. pap. 13.00 (*0-684-86208-5*, Touchstone) S&S Trade Pap.

Body of Knowledge: An Introduction to Body/Mind Psychology. Robert Marrone. 1990. LC 89-28863. (Series in Transpersonal & Humanistic Psychology). 160p. (C). pap. text 19.95 (*0-7914-0388-2*) State U NY Pr.

Body of This Death: Historicity & Sociality in the Time of AIDS. William Haver. 1996. LC 96-856. xviii, 221p. 51.00 (*0-8047-2716-3*); 221p. pap. 18.95 (*0-8047-2728-7*) Stanford U Pr.

Body Parts: Property Rights & the Ownership of Human Biological Materials. E. Richard Gold. 1998. LC 96-11852. 236p. pap. 25.50 (*0-87840-661-1*) Georgetown U Pr.

Body Process: Working with the Body in Psychotherapy. James I. Kepner. 1993. 246p. 32.50 (*0-88163-283-X*) Analytic Pr.

Body Reflexology: Healing at Your Fingertips. Mildred Carter & Tammy Weber. 2nd rev. ed. 1994. LC 94-15863. 272p. (C). reprint ed. text 29.95 (*0-13-299728-2*, Parker Publishing Co) P-H.

Body Reflexology: Healing at Your Fingertips. Mildred Carter & Tammy Weber. 2nd rev. ed. 1994. LC 00-15863. (Illus.). xx, 343p. (C). reprint ed. pap. 13.00 (*0-13-299736-3*) PH Pr.

Body Remembers. Babette Rothschild. 2000. LC 00-62520. (Professional Book Ser.). (Illus.). 224p. 30.00 (*0-393-70327-4*) Norton.

Body Scripture: A Therapist's Journal of Recovery from Multiple Personality. Barbara Hope. 2000. 325p. pap. text 28.00 (*1-55605-297-9*) Wyndham Hall.

Body Sculpturing by Lipoplasty. Yves-Gerard Illouz & Yves T. De Villers. 1989. (Illus.). 496p. text (*0-443-03833-3*) Church.

Body Smart System: The Complete Guide to Cleansing & Rejuvenation. Helene Silver. rev. ed. 1995. (Illus.). 248p. pap. text 19.95 (*1-884334-60-1*) Hlthy Healing.

Body Snatching: The Robbing of Graves for the Education of Physicians in Early Nineteenth Century America. Suzanne M. Shultz. 1992. LC 90-53522. (Illus.). 144p. lib. bdg. 29.95 (*0-89950-587-2*) McFarland & Co.

Body, Soul, & Bioethics. Gilbert C. Meilaender. 1998. LC 95-17486. 144p. (C). reprint ed. pap. text 15.00 (*0-268-02153-8*) U of Notre Dame Pr.

Body, Soul & Blood: Recovering the Human in Medicine. William T. Sayers. 1980. LC 79-56194. 112p. pap. 7.95 (*0-935718-00-1*) Asclepiad.

Body Speaks: Therapeutic Dialogues for Mind-Body Problems. James Griffith & Melissa E. Griffith. 1994. LC 93-34330. (Illus.). 336p. 47.00 (*0-465-00716-3*) Basic.

Body Structures & Functions. Elizabeth Fong et al. 8th ed. 1993. LC 92-49599. 337p. pap. 62.95 (*0-8273-5903-9*); pap. 31.95 (*0-8273-5115-1*) Delmar.

Body Structures & Functions. Scott Fong. 9th ed. 1997. (C). 288p. mass mkt., wbk. ed. 13.75 (*0-8273-7898-X*); LC 97-21044. 384p. 51.95 (*0-8273-7897-1*) Delmar.

Body Structures & Functions. Ann S. Scott & Fong. 9th ed. 1998. 160p. (C). pap. text, tchr. ed. 14.00 (*0-8273-7899-8*) Delmar.

Body Surface Electrocardiographic Mapping. Ed. by David M. Mirvis. 1988. (Developments in Cardiovascular Medicine Ser.). (C). text 150.00 (*0-89838-983-6*) Kluwer Academic.

Body Surface Mapping of Cardiac Fields: Proceedings of the Symposium, Burlington, Vermont, 1972. Body Surface Mapping of Cardiac Fields Symposium. Ed. by E. Lepeschkin & S. Rush. 1974. (Advances in Cardiology Ser.: Vol. 10). (Illus.). 344p. 123.50 (*3-8055-1566-9*) S Karger.

Body Systems Review No. I: Hematopoietic/ Lymphoreticular, Respiratory, Cardiovascular: A Body Systems-Based Review for USMLE Step 1. National Medical School Review Staff. 2nd ed. 1997. LC 97-9560. (Board Simulator Ser.). 375p. pap. text 25.95 (*0-683-30298-1*) Lppncott W & W.

Body Systems Review No. II: Gastrointestinal, Renal, Reproductive, Endocrine: A Body Systems-Based Review for USMLE Step 1, No. II. National Medical School Review Staff. 2nd ed. 1997. LC 97-11572. (Board Simulator Ser.). (Illus.). 375p. pap. text 25.95 (*0-683-30299-X*) Lppncott W & W.

Body Systems Review No. III: Nervous, Skin/Connective Tissue, Musculoskeletal: A Body Systems-Based Review for USMLE Step 1. National Medical School Review Staff & Gerald D. Barry. 2nd ed. 1997. LC 97-8375. (Board Simulator Ser.). (Illus.). 375p. pap. text 25.95 (*0-683-30300-7*) Lppncott W & W.

Body Systems Review I: Hematopoietic Lymphoreticular, Respirataory, Cardiovascular. National Medical School Review Staff. 1996. LC 96-24459. (Board Simulator Ser.). 320p. pap. 24.95 (*0-683-06329-4*) Lppncott W & W.

Body Systems Review II: Gastrointestinal, Renal, Reproductive, Endocrine. National Medical School Review Staff. 1996. LC 96-24460. (Board Simulator Ser.). (*0-683-06332-4*) Lppncott W & W.

Body Systems Review III: Nervous, Skin Connective Tissue, Musculoskeletal. rev. ed. 1996. LC 96-24461. (Board Simulator Ser.). (*0-683-06328-6*) Lppncott W & W.

Body Talk: Looking & Being Looked at in Psychotherapy. Janice S. Lieberman. 2000. LC 99-88327. xiv, 305p. 45.00 (*0-7657-0258-4*) Aronson.

Body Talk: Rhetoric, Technology, Reproduction. Ed. by Mary M. Lay et al. 2000. LC 99-6903. (Samuel & Althea Stroum Book Ser.). xiii, 308p. pap. 24.95 (*0-299-16794-1*) U of Wis Pr.

Body Talk: Rhetoric, Technology, Reproduction. Mary M. Lay. 2000. LC 99-6903. (Rhetoric of the Human Sciences Ser.). xiii, 308p. 60.00 (*0-299-16790-9*) U of Wis Pr.

Body Talk: The Material & Discursive Regulation of Sexuality, Madness & Reproduction. Jane M. Ussher. 1997. LC 97-15836. 272p. (C). 84.95 (*0-415-15363-8*); pap. 27.95 (*0-415-15364-6*) Routledge.

Body Techniques. Joan G. Lafrentiere. 1984. (C). (gr. 13). 26.50 (*0-89352-205-8*) Mosby Inc.

Body Trauma: A Writer's Guide to Wounds & Injuries. David W. Page. 1996. LC 96-28627. (Howdunit Writing Ser.). (Illus.). 240p. pap. 16.99 (*0-89879-741-1*, 10488, Wrtrs Digest Bks) F & W Pubns Inc.

Body Voices: Using the Power of Breath, Sound & Movement to Heal & Create New Boundaries. Carolyn J. Braddock. 1995. LC 94-67842. (Illus.). 288p. pap. 19.95 (*1-879290-05-7*) PageMill Pr.

Body Wisdom: The Longevity Lifestyle. Ann Tyndall. 1997. 115p. (Orig.). pap. 14.95 (*0-9657027-0-7*) Healthy Wealthy & Wise.

Bodybuilding: The Weider Approach. Joe Weider. 1981. (Illus.). 232p. pap. 18.95 (*0-8092-5908-7*, 59087) NTC Contemp Pub Co.

Bodylink. Martin Sulway. Date not set. (Illus.). 96p. pap. text (*0-07-470002-2*) McGraw-Hill Med Pub.

Bodymind Energetics: Toward a Dynamic Model of Health. Mark D. Seem. 1989. LC 89-49072. 272p. pap. 18.95 (*0-89281-246-X*, Heal Arts VT) Inner Tradit.

Bodypower. Vernon Coleman. 1989. 128p. reprint ed. pap. 8.95 (*1-878290-00-2*) Intl Hlth MD.

Body's Battle Against Pollution. Radu Olinescu et al. 1997. LC 97-38186. 226p. lib. bdg. 65.00 (*1-56072-503-6*) Nova Sci Pubs.

BodySkills Manual. Judy K. Werder & Robert H. Bruininks. 1988. (gr. k-6). pap. text 49.95 (*0-88671-185-1*, 4901) Am Guidance.

Bodywise. Joseph Heller & William A. Henkin. 1991. LC 86-3757. (Illus.). 262p. pap. 17.95 (*0-914728-73-3*) Wingbow Pr.

Bodywise Woman. Judy M. Lutter & Lynn Jaffee. 2nd rev. ed. 1996. LC 96-13088. (Illus.). 328p. reprint ed. pap. 16.95 (*0-87322-606-2*, PLUT0606) Human Kinetics.

Bodywork: What Type of Massage to Get—& How to Make the Most of It. Thomas Claire. 1995. 25.00 (*0-688-12581-6*, Wm Morrow) Morrow Avon.

Bodywork Basics: A Guide to the Powers & Pleasures of Your Body. Anne Kent Rush & Greg Zelonka. 2000. LC 99-36563. (Omega Institute Mind, Body, Spirit Ser.). 256p. pap. 12.95 (*0-440-50870-3*, Dell Trade Pbks) Dell.

Bodywork Therapies for Women: A Guide. Delcia McNeil. 2001. pap. (*0-7043-4569-2*) Womens Press GBR. *Dist:* Trafalgar.

Boiling Energy: Community Healing among the Kalahari Kung. Richard Katz. 1984. LC 81-13383. (Illus.). 368p. pap. 18.95 (*0-674-07736-9*) HUP.

Bold Endeavors: Lessons from Polar & Space Exploration. Jack Stuster. 1996. LC 96-8131. (Illus.). 408p. 36.95 (*1-55750-749-X*) Naval Inst Pr.

Bolden & Tackle's Practice Nurse Handbook. Gillian Hampson. 3rd ed. 1994. (Illus.). 320p. pap. 26.95 (*0-632-03692-3*) Blackwell Sci.

Boletes of North America: A Compendium. Ernst E. Both. 1993. 431p. pap. 10.00 (*0-944032-54-0*) Buffalo SNS.

Boletin. Ed. by Blanca Vazquez. 1993. (Illus.). 240p. (Orig.). pap. (*1-878483-53-6*) Hunter Coll CEP.

Bolton's Handbook of Canine & Feline Electrocardiography. N. Joel Edwards. 2nd ed. 1987. (Illus.). 408p. pap. text 61.00 (*0-7216-1847-2*) Saunders.

Bomb in the Brain: A Heroic Tale of Science, Surgery & Survival. Steven J. Fishman. 1990. 336p. pap. 8.95 (*0-380-70898-1*, Avon Bks) Morrow Avon.

Bonded Ceramic Inlays. Jean-Francois Roulet & Stefan Herder. 1991. (Illus.). 103p. text 64.00 (*0-86715-244-3*) Quint Pub Co.

Bone: A Treatise. Brian K. Hall. (Telford Press Ser.). Vol. 5. 1991. (Illus.). 368p. 99.00 (*0-8493-8825-2*); Vol. 6. 1991. 304p. 99.00 (*0-8493-8826-0*); Vol. 7. 1992. (Illus.). 368p. 99.00 (*0-8493-8827-9*) CRC Pr.

Bone: Differentiation & Morphogenesis of Bone, Vol. 9. Ed. by Brian K. Hall. 1994. 208p. 141.95 (*0-8493-8994-1*, 8994) CRC Pr.

Bone: Mechanisms of Bone Development & Growth, Vol. 8. Ed. by Brian K. Hall. 1994. (Physiology of Substance Abuse Ser.). 240p. 167.95 (*0-8493-8903-8*, 8903) CRC Pr.

Bone: The Osteoclast, Vol. 4. Brian K. Hall. 1991. (Telford Press Ser.). (Illus.). 272p. 99.00 (*0-8493-8824-4*, QP88) CRC Pr.

Bone Vol. 2: The Osteoclast, Vol. 2. Brian K. Hall. 1991. LC 93-5671. (Telford Press Ser.). (Illus.). 288p. 110.00 (*0-8493-8822-8*, QP88) CRC Pr.

Bone: A Treatise: The Osteoclast, Vol. 3. Brian K. Hall. 1991. (Illus.). 344p. 99.00 (*0-8493-8823-6*, QP88) CRC Pr.

Bone & Bone Seeking Radionuclides: Physiology, Dosimetry, & Effects. Ed. by V. Volf. 1981. (European Applied Research Reports Special Topics Ser.). viii, 154p. text 220.00 (*3-7186-0061-7*) Gordon & Breach.

Bone & Joint Disorders: Conventional Radiologic Differential Diagnosis. Francis A. Burgener & Martti Kormano. 1996. LC 96-26197. (Illus.). 325p. 79.00 (*0-86577-673-3*) Thieme Med Pubs.

Bone & Joint Disorders of the Foot & Ankle. M. Bouysset & Pierre B. Cedex. 1998. (Illus.). 375p. 185.00 (*3-540-63992-6*) Spr-Verlag.

Bone & Joint Disorders of the Foot & Ankle. Maurice Bouysset & Andre Bardot. 1997. LC 97-42750. 144.00 (*3-540-59593-7*) Spr-Verlag.

***Bone & Joint Futures.** Woolf & Marinker. 2002. 192p. pap. (*0-7279-1548-7*) BMJ Pub GBR. *Dist:* AIDC.

Bone & Joint Imaging. Donald Resnick. Ed. by Lisette Bralow. 2nd ed. 1996. LC 95-37882. (Illus.). 944p. text 195.00 (*0-7216-6043-6*) Saunders.

Bone & Joint Infections. Shannon E. Perry. 1996. 200p. (*1-85317-132-8*) Mosby Inc.

Bone & Mineral Manual. Ed. by Michael Kleerekoper et al. 1999. LC 98-83212. 192p. (C). pap. text 39.95 (*0-12-412650-2*) Acad Pr.

Bone & Mineral Research Annual, No. 6. Ed. by William A. Peck. 1989. 350p. 226.50 (*0-444-81061-7*) Elsevier.

Bone & Renal Failure. Ed. by Marc E. De Broe & F. L. Van de Vyver. 1988. (Contributions to Nephrology Ser.: Vol. 64). (Illus.). vi, 182p. 29.75 (*3-8055-4738-2*) S Karger.

Bone & Soft Tissue Tumors: Clinical Features, Imaging, Pathology & Treatment. Mario Campanacci. 2nd rev. ed. 1999. (Illus.). 1300p. 379.00 (*3-211-83235-1*) Spr-Verlag.

Bone Biodynamics in Orthodontic & Orthopedic Treatment. Ed. by Steven A. Goldstein & David S. Carlson. 1992. LC 93-135645. (Craniofacial Growth Ser.: Vol. 27). (Illus.). 388p. 59.00 (*0-929921-23-2*) UM CHGD.

***Bone Biology & Skeletal Maturity in a Clinical Setting.** 2002. (Illus.). 100p. 87.00 (*3-8055-7313-8*) S Karger.

Bone-Biomaterial Interface. Ed. by J. E. Davies. 1991. 1040p. text 140.00 (*0-8020-5941-4*) U of Toronto Pr.

Bone, Breath, & Gesture: Practices of Embodiment, Vol. I. Ed. by Don H. Johnson. 1995. LC 95-3876. (Bone, Breath & Gesture Ser.: Vol. I). 200p. (Orig.). pap. 22.50 (*1-55643-201-1*) North Atlantic.

Bone Cement & Its Application. Saha. 1993. (*0-8493-4918-4*) CRC Pr.

Bone Cements: Up-to-Date Comparison of Physical & Chemical Properties of Commercial Materials. Klaus-Dieter Kuhn. 2000. LC 00-38825. (Illus.). 250p. 72.00 (*3-540-67207-9*) Spr-Verlag.

Bone Circulation & Vascularization in Normal & Pathological Conditions. A. Schoutens et al. 1993. (NATO Advanced Science Institutes Ser.: Vol. 247). (Illus.). 394p. (C). text 120.00 (*0-306-44523-9*, Kluwer Plenum) Kluwer Academic.

Bone Densitometry & Osteoporosis. Ed. by Harry K. Genant et al. 1997. LC 97-18415. (Illus.). 625p. 175.00 (*3-540-63149-6*) Spr-Verlag.

Bone Densitometry for Technologists: Application & Interpretation. Sydney Lou Bonnick & Lori A. Lawless. 2001. LC 2001-16675. (Illus.). 352p. 74.50 (*1-58829-020-4*) Humana.

Bone Densitometry in Clinical Practice: Application & Interpretation. Sydney Lou Bonnick. 1998. LC 98-12447. (Current Clinical Practice Ser.). (Illus.). 280p. 99.50 (*0-89603-513-1*) Humana.

Bone Density Program: Six Weeks to a Strong Mind & Body. George J. Kessler & Colleen Kapklein. 2001. LC 00-110317. (Illus.). 464p. pap. 14.95 (*0-345-43285-1*, Ballantine) Ballantine Pub Grp.

Bone Density Test: A Guide for Women of Every Age. Maggie Greenwood-Robinson. 2000. 224p. pap. 7.50 (*0-425-17782-3*) Berkley Pub.

Bone Disease in Renal Failure. Ed. by H. H. Malluche. 1992. (Mineral & Electrolyte Metabolism Ser.: Vol. 17, No. 4). (Illus.). 92p. pap. 59.25 (*3-8055-5506-7*) S Karger.

Bone Diseases: Macroscopic, Histological & Radiological Diagnosis of Structural Changes in the Skeleton. Claus-Peter Adler. Tr. by F. Steel & J. Steel. 2000. LC 99-58725. (Illus.). 624p. 159.00 (*3-540-65061-X*) Spr-Verlag.

Bone Formation & Repair: Proceedings of the International Symposium on Formation & Repair of Mineralized Extracellular Matrix, Hong Kong, 10-19 October, 1996. A. B. Rabie & Marshall R. Urist. 1997. LC 97-39183. (International Congress Ser.). 232p. 148.00 (*0-444-82652-1*) Elsevier.

Bone Grafts & Bone Substitutes. Mutaz B. Habal & A. Harri Reddi. 1992. (Illus.). 485p. text 142.00 (*0-7216-2809-5*) Saunders.

Bone Histomorphometry. Erik F. Eriksen et al. 1993. LC 93-24476. 88p. pap. text 22.95 (*0-7817-0122-8*) Lppncott W & W.

Bone Histomorphometry: Techniques & Interpretation. Ed. by Robert R. Recker. 1983. 312p. 179.00 (*0-8493-5373-4*, QM569, CRC Reprint) Franklin.

Bone Implant Grafting. Ed. by John Older. 1992. LC 92-2327. xviii, 226p. (*3-540-19720-6*); (Illus.). 226p. 247.00 (*0-387-19720-6*) Spr-Verlag.

Bone Ischaemia & Infarction in Sickle Cell Disease. Stanley P. Bohrer & Abass Alavi. 1981. LC 79-50182. (Illus.). 347p. (C). 44.50 (*0-87527-188-X*) Green.

Bone Marrow Biopsies Revisited. R. Bartl et al. 1984. (Illus.). xiv, 138p. 50.50 (*3-8055-3937-1*) S Karger.

Bone Marrow Biopsies Updated. Ed. by Bertha Frisch & R. Bartl. 1984. (Current Studies in Hematology & Blood Transfusion: No. 50). (Illus.). viii, 132p. 85.25 (*3-8055-3863-4*) S Karger.

Bone Marrow Disorders: The Biological Basis of Treatment. A. J. Barrett & M. Y. Gordon. 2nd ed. 1993. LC 92-22052. (Illus.). 432p. 165.00 (*0-632-03353-3*) Blackwell Sci.

Bone Marrow Failure Syndromes. Ed. by Neil S. Young. 2000. LC 00-23872. 223p. text 125.00 (*0-7216-7174-8*) Harcrt Hlth Sci Grp.

Bone Marrow Pathology. Kathryn Foucar. 1994. LC 94-16244. (Illus.). 564p. 175.00 (*0-89189-372-5*) Am Soc Clinical.

Bone Marrow Pathology. Barbara J. Bain et al. 2nd ed. 1996. LC 95-50024. 280p. text 195.00 (*0-86542-647-3*) Blackwell Sci.

Bone Marrow Pathology. Barbara J. Bain. 3rd ed. 2001. LC 00-51929. (Illus.). ix, 499p. 199.50 (*0-632-05578-2*) Blackwell Sci.

Bone Marrow Processing & Purging: A Practical Guide. Adrian P. Gee. 1991. (Illus.). 408p. 189.00 (*0-8493-6402-7*, RD123) CRC Pr.

Bone Marrow Transplant: Administrative Strategies & Clinical Concerns. Patricia C. Buchsel & Marie B. Whedon. 1995. (Nursing-Health Science Ser.). (Illus.). 528p. (C). text 68.95 (*0-86720-691-8*, 691-8) Jones & Bartlett.

Bone Marrow Transplantation. Richard K. Burt. 1999. LC 98-49747. 700p. spiral bd. 45.00 (*1-57059-560-7*) Landes Bioscience.

Bone Marrow Transplantation. Ed. by Richard E. Champlin. 1990. (Cancer Treatment & Research Ser.). (C). text 215.50 (*0-7923-0612-0*) Kluwer Academic.

Bone Marrow Transplantation. Ed. by S. J. Forman et al. 1993. LC 93-26102. (Illus.). 992p. 250.00 (*0-86542-253-2*) Blackwell Sci.

Bone Marrow Transplantation. S. Ikehara & F. Takaku. 1996. (Illus.). 364p. 82.95 (*4-431-70181-8*) Spr-Verlag.

Bone Marrow Transplantation. U. W. Schaefer & D. W. Beelen. 1991. (Illus.). 124p. pap. 28.75 (*3-8055-5518-0*) S Karger.

Bone Marrow Transplantation. Marie B. Whedon et al. 1991. (Illus.). 480p. (C). text 64.95 (*0-86720-440-0*, 440-0) Jones & Bartlett.

Bone Marrow Transplantation. U. W. Schaefer & D. W. Beelen. 2nd rev. ed. 1996. LC 96-20422. (Illus.). x, 126p. pap. 35.00 (*3-8055-6308-6*) S Karger.

Bone Marrow Transplantation: A Nursing Perspective. Ed. by Christina A. Kasprisin & Edward L. Snyder. 1990. 157p. (C). text 7.00 (*0-915355-86-8*) Am Assn Blood.

Bone Marrow Transplantation: Foundations for the 21st Century. Ed. by Robert Sackstein et al. 1995. LC 95-45313. (Annals of the New York Academy of Sciences Ser.: Vol. 770). 394p. pap. 90.00 (*0-89766-994-0*) NY Acad Sci.

Bone Marrow Transplantation & Other Treatment After Radiation Injury. H. Balner. 1977. pap. text 73.50 (*90-247-2056-7*) Kluwer Academic.

Bone Marrow Transplantation & Peripheral Blood Stem Cell Transplantation. rev. ed. 1996. (Illus.). 50p. (Orig.). pap. text 25.00 (*0-7881-3005-6*) DIANE Pub.

Bone Marrow Transplantation in Clinical Practice. Jennifer G. Treleaven & A. John Barrett. 1992. (Illus.). 400p. pap. text (*0-443-04413-9*) Church.

Bone Marrow Transplants: A Book of Basics for Patients. Susan K. Stewart. rev. ed. 1995. 170p. pap. 7.95 (*0-9647352-0-2*) Blood & Marrow.

Bone Marrow Transplants: A Guide for Cancer Patients & Their Families. Marianne Shaffer. 1994. LC 93-23704. 200p. 19.95 (*0-87833-855-1*) Taylor Pub.

Bone Mechanics. Ed. by Stephen C. Cowin. 1988. 320p. (C). 249.00 (*0-8493-4562-6*, QP303) CRC Pr.

Bone Mechanics Handbook. Ed. by Stephen C. Cowin. 2nd ed. 2001. LC 00-51909. 968p. 169.95 (*0-8493-9117-2*) CRC Pr.

Bone Medicine. Wolf Moondance. 1999. LC 99-12226. (Illus.). 192p. pap. 12.95 (*0-8069-9797-4*) Sterling.

Bone Metastasis. F. William Orr & Gurmit Singh. 1995. (Medical Intelligence Unit Ser.). 225p. 89.95 (*1-57059-319-1*) Landes Bioscience.

Bone Metastasis. William F. Orr. 1996. (Medicine Ser.). pap. 89.95 (*0-412-10341-9*, VNR) Wiley.

Bone Pathology. Ed. by E. Bonucci. 1987. (Journal: Vol. 5, No. 3, 1987). (Illus.). 56p. pap. 32.25 (*3-8055-4655-6*) S Karger.

Bone Regeneration & Repair: Biology & Clinical Applications. Ed. by Jay R. Lieberman & Gary E. Friedlaender. 2002. 400p. 125.00 (*0-89603-847-5*) Humana.

Bone Regulatory Factors: Morphology, Biochemistry, Physiology & Pharmacology. Ed. by A. Pecile & B. De Bernard. 1990. LC 90-6777. (NATO ASI Series A, Life Sciences: Vol. 184). (Illus.). 302p. 95.00 (*0-306-43500-4*, Plenum Trade) Perseus Pubng.

Bone Remodeling Orthodontics by Jaw Repositioning & Alveolar Growth. Leon Kussick. 1987. (Illus.). 225p. text 98.00 (*0-86715-158-7*) Quint Pub Co.

Bone Scintigraphy. E. K. Pauwels. 1981. 224p. text 154.00 (*90-6021-476-5*) Kluwer Academic.

Bone Structure & Remodeling. A. Odgaards & H. Weinans. 1995. (Recent Advances in Human Biology Ser.: Vol. 2). 268p. text 84.00 (*981-02-2190-8*) World Scientific Pub.

Bone Transplant. Ed. by M. Aebi & P. Regazzoni. 1989. (Illus.). 363p. 144.00 (*0-387-50165-7*) Spr-Verlag.

Bone Tumors see Dahlin's Bone Tumors: General Aspects & Data on 11,087 Cases

Bone Tumors. Dorfman & Czerniak. 1997. LC 97-36939. (Illus.). 1280p. (C). (gr. 13). text 225.00 (*0-8151-2746-4*, 24078) Mosby Inc.

Bone Tumors: Clinical, Radiologic & Pathologic Correlations, Vol. 1 & 2. Ed. by Joseph M. Mirra et al. 1989. LC 88-3019. (Illus.). 1857p. 295.00 (*0-8121-1156-7*) Lppncott W & W.

Bones & Joints. M. Runge. 1987. (Exercises in Radiological Diagnosis Ser.). (Illus.). 168p. 34.95 (*0-387-16544-4*) Spr-Verlag.

Bones & Joints. Ed. by W. S. Symmers et al. 3rd ed. 1998. (Systemic Pathology Ser.). (Illus.). 500p. text (*0-443-03428-1*) Church.

Bones & Joints: A Guide for Students. Christine Gunn. 2nd ed. 1996. LC 96-29143. text (*0-443-05422-3*) Church.

Bones & Joints in Diabetes Mellitus. S. Forgacs. 1982. text 94.00 (*90-247-2395-7*) Kluwer Academic.

Bone's Atlas of Pulmonary & Critical Care Medicine. Roger C. Bone et al. 1998. LC 98-4009. 250p. 85.00 (*0-683-30486-0*) Lppncott W & W.

Bones, Bodies, & Behavior: Essays in Behavioral Anthropology. Ed. by George W. Stocking, Jr. 1990. LC 87-40377. (History of Anthropology Ser.: No. 5). (Illus.). 272p. pap. 18.95 (*0-299-11254-3*) U of Wis Pr.

Bones in the Basement: Postmortem Racism in Nineteenth-Century Medical Training. Ed. by Robert L. Blakely & Judith M. Harrington. 1997. LC 96-53982. (Illus.). 464p. text 45.00 (*1-56098-750-2*) Smithsonian.

Bonica's Management of Pain John D. Loeser. 3rd ed. 2000. (Illus.). 2,208p. text 299.00 (*0-683-30462-3*) Lppncott W & W.

Bonne Pratique des Essais Cliniques des Medicaments. A. Spriet & Therese Dupin-Spriet. 1990. (Illus.). vi, 250p. 116.75 (*3-8055-5220-3*) S Karger.

Bonus Options in Health Insurance. Peter Zweifel & Otto Waser. 1992. LC 92-9931. (Developments in Health Economics & Public Policy Ser.: Vol. 2). 160p. (C). lib. bdg. 132.00 (*0-7923-1722-X*) Kluwer Academic.

Book for Midwives: A Manual for Traditional Birth Attendants & Community Midwives. Susan Klein. 1995. LC 94-7378. (Illus.). 519p. (Orig.). pap. 22.00 (*0-942364-22-8*) Hesperian Found.

Book of Acupuncture Points: Volume I of a Complete Course in Acupuncture. James Tin Yau So. Ed. by Robert L. Felt. 1993. (Illus.). 320p. text 32.00 (*0-912111-02-X*) Paradigm Publns.

Book of Ayurveda: A Holistic Approach to Health & Longevity. Judith Morrison. 1995. LC 94-44993. 192p. per. 16.00 (*0-684-80017-9*) S&S Trade.

Book of Children's Foods. Lorna Rhodes. 1992. (Illus.). 120p. pap. 12.00 (*1-55788-047-6*, HP Books) Berkley Pub.

Book of Family Therapy. Ed. by Andrew Ferber et al. 1990. LC 84-24171. 725p. reprint ed. 70.00 (*0-87668-671-4*) Aronson.

***Book of Healing Teas.** Sylvia Schneider. 2001. (Illus.). 160p. 22.95 (*1-55356-009-4*) Sarasota Press.

Book of Health. Susan Stockton. 2nd rev. ed. 1997. (Illus.). 316p. (Orig.). pap. 14.95 (*0-9628770-0-X*, 102) Natures Pubng.

Book of Heath. Ed. by Susan B. Silvester. 1985. LC 85-12421. (Illus.). 207p. 22.00 (*0-913993-02-6*) Paideia Pubs.

Book of Herbal Wisdom: Using Plants As Medicines. Matthew Wood. 1997. LC 96-49794. (Illus.). 250p. pap. 18.95 (*1-55643-232-1*) North Atlantic.

Book of Home Remedies. Betty Kirkpatrick. 1997. 188p. reprint ed. text 15.00 (*0-7881-5168-1*) DIANE Pub.

Book of Jook: Chinese Medicinal Porridges, a Healthy Alternative to the Typical Western Breakfast. Bob Flaws. 1998. 225p. (Orig.). pap. 16.95 (*0-936185-60-0*) Blue Poppy Pr.

Book of Life. Marsilio Ficino. Tr. by Charles Boer from LAT. 1980. LC 88-3073. (Dunquin Ser.: No. 12). xx, 218p. (Orig.). pap. 19.00 (*0-88214-212-7*) Spring Pubns.

Book of Macrobiotics. Michio Kushi & Alex Jack. enl. rev. ed. 1987. LC 85-81363. (Illus.). 216p. reprint ed. pap. 21.00 (*0-87040-667-1*) Japan Pubns USA.

Book of Man. Walter Bodmer. 1995. LC 94-38081. ix, 259p. 25.00 (*0-684-80102-7*) S&S Trade.

Book of Matthew: What Would You Do If Your Child Was Faced with a Serious Medical Problem? Betty J. Wylie. 1994. mass mkt. 5.95 (*1-56171-285-X*) SPI.

***Book of Meditation: Practical Ways to Health & Healing.** Chris Jarmey. 2001. (Illus.). 224p. pap. 22.95 (*1-58290-059-0*) Jrny Editions.

Book of Psychiatric Books. Ed. by Sidney Crown & Hugh Freeman. 1994. LC 92-49165. 440p. 50.00 (*0-87668-510-6*) Aronson.

Book of Ruth see Living with Alzheimer's: Ruth's Story

Book of Shiatsu. Paul Lundberg. 1992. (Illus.). 192p. (Orig.). pap. 14.95 (*0-671-74488-7*, Fireside) S&S Trade Pap.

Book of Stress Survival: Identifying & Reducing the Stress in Your Life. Alix Kirsta. 1987. (Illus.). 192p. pap. 16.00 (*0-671-63026-1*, Fireside) S&S Trade Pap.

Book of Tendons. Eleni Sikelianos. 1997. LC 97-22109. 33p. (Orig.). pap. 7.00 (*0-942996-29-1*) Post Apollo Pr.

Book of the Craft of Dying & Other Early English Tracts Concerning Death. Ed. by Frances M. Comper & Robert J. Kastenbaum. 1977. LC 76-19564. (Death & Dying Ser.). reprint ed. lib. bdg. 21.95 (*0-405-09560-0*) Ayer.

Book of Vision. Christopher Hills. 1995. 103p. (Orig.). pap. 4.95 (*0-916438-63-5*) Dr Hills Technol.

Book of Vitamins. Edmond B. Szekely. 1981. (Illus.). 48p. pap. 3.50 (*0-89564-045-7*) IBS Intl.

Book on Cataracts. G. Brock Magruder & Walter R. Gilbert, Jr. Ed. by Curley and Pynn Public Relations Management, Inc. St. 1988. (Illus.). (Orig.). (C). pap. text 4.95 (*0-9622095-2-X*) G B Magruder.

Book on Freud. H. Bloom. 1999. text (*0-670-80462-2*) Viking Penguin.

Booke Conteining...Experienced Medicines: The Fourth & Finall Booke of His Secretes. Piemontese Alessio. Tr. by R. Androse. 1977. LC 77-6846. (English Experience Ser.: No. 841). reprint ed. lib. bdg. 35.00 (*90-221-0841-4*) Walter J Johnson.

Books & Manuscripts of the Bakken. Judith A. Overmier & John E. Senior. 1992. LC 92-8512. (Illus.). 525p. 100.00 (*0-8108-2570-8*) Scarecrow.

Books, Manuscripts, & the History of Medicine: Essays on the Fiftieth Anniversary of the Osler Library. Ed. by Philip M. Teigen. 1982. 112p. 14.95 (*0-88202-199-0*, Sci Hist) Watson Pub Intl.

Boomerang: Health Care Reform & the Turn Against Government. Theda Skocpol. 1997. LC 97-179877. (Illus.). 256p. pap. 12.95 (*0-393-31572-X*) Norton.

Boost Your Brainpower. Ellen Michaud et al. 1993. 472p. 9.98 (*1-56731-026-5*, MJF Bks) Fine Comms.

Boost Your Health with Bovine Cartilage. Sally E. Osborne. 1998. 192p. pap. 14.95 (*0-87983-839-6*, Keats Pubng) McGraw-Hill Trade.

Boost Your Immune System Naturally: Your Essential Guide to Fighting Infection & Nurturing Your Health. Beth MacEoin. 2001. (Illus.). 128p. pap. (*1-84222-151-5*) Carlton Bks Ltd GBR. *Dist:* Natl Bk Netwk.

*__Boosting Digestive Health Through Conventional & Alternative Methods.__ Ed. by Len Saputo. 2001. (Illus.). 144p. pap. 14.95 (*0-7641-1903-6*) Barron.

Boosting Immunity with Power Plants. Linda R. Page. 2nd rev. ed. 1996. (Healthy Healing Library: Vol. 9). (Illus.). 32p. (Orig.). pap. 3.50 (*1-884334-34-2*) Hlthy Healing.

Boosting Your Brain Power: Stress, the Brain, Exercise & Nutrition. 1991. lib. bdg. 250.00 (*0-8490-4651-3*) Gordon Pr.

Boothe's Small Animal Formulary. Dawn Boothe. 5th ed. 2000. 208p. pap. (*1-58326-024-2*, AAHA Pr) Am Animal Hosp Assoc.

Booze: A Guide for Young People. Jim Parker. rev. ed. 1999. pap. 0.50 (*0-89230-139-2*) Do It Now.

Border Dispute: The Place of Logic in Psychology. John MacNamara. 1986. (Learning, Development & Conceptual Change Ser.). 230p. 27.50 (*0-262-13216-8*, Bradford Bks) MIT Pr.

*__Borderland Between Care & Self-Care.__ Anna Sarkadi. 2001. (Comprehensive Summaries of Uppsala Disertations from the Faculty of Medicine: No. 981). (Illus.). 108p. (Orig.). pap. (*91-554-4901-8*) Uppsala Universitet SWE. *Dist:* Coronet Bks.

Borderlands of Normal & Early Pathologic Findings in Skeletal Radiography. A. M. Koehler et al. Ed. & Tr. by Peter Winter from GER. 6th enl. rev. ed. 1993. LC 92-49475. (Illus.). 918p. 219.00 (*0-86577-461-7*) Thieme Med Pubs.

Borderline & Narcissistic Patients in Therapy. Ed. by Nonna Slavinska-Holy. 1988. 568p. (C). 80.00 (*0-8236-0572-8*) Intl Univs Pr.

Borderline & Other Self Disorders. Donald B. Rinsley. 1982. LC 81-20538. 336p. 50.00 (*0-87668-447-9*) Aronson.

Borderline Child: Etiology, Diagnosis & Treatment. Ed. by Kenneth S. Robson. 1997. LC 97-10432. (Master Works Ser.). 320p. pap. text 45.00 (*0-7657-0090-5*) Aronson.

Borderline Conditions & Pathological Narcissism. Otto F. Kernberg. 1990. LC 84-45864. 384p. reprint ed. 50.00 (*0-87668-762-1*) Aronson.

Borderline Disorders: Clinical Models & Techniques. Eda G. Goldstein. 1990. LC 90-3400. 240p. text 36.00 (*0-89862-442-8*, 2442) Guilford Pubns.

Borderline Patient. Roy R. Grinker, Sr. & Beatrice Werble. 1983. LC 84-45089. 240p. 25.00 (*0-87668-676-5*) Aronson.

Borderline Patient: Emerging Concepts in Diagnosis, Psychodynamics & Treatment. Ed. by James S. Grotstein et al. 1987. (Psychoanalytic Inquiry Book Ser.: Vol. 2). text 45.00 (*0-88163-055-1*) Analytic Pr.

Borderline Patients: Psychoanalytic Perspectives. Sander M. Abend et al. Ed. by Bernard D. Fine et al. 1983. LC 83-12750. (Kris Study Group Monographs: No. 7). viii, 255p. 37.50 (*0-8236-0576-0*) Intl Univs Pr.

Borderline Patients, the Psychosomatic Focus & the Therapeutic Process. Peter L. Giovacchini. 1993. LC 92-49191. 296p. 50.00 (*0-87668-295-6*) Aronson.

Borderline Personality: Vision & Healing. Nathan Schwartz-Salant. 1989. LC 88-25079. (Orig.). (C). 256p. 34.95 (*0-933029-30-6*); 362p. pap. 24.95 (*0-933029-31-4*) Chiron Pubns.

Borderline Personality Disorder. John G. Gunderson. 1984. LC 84-18411. 204p. text 38.00 (*0-88048-020-3*, 8020) Am Psychiatric.

Borderline Personality Disorder: A Clinical Guide. John G. Gunderson. 2001. LC 00-56945. (Illus.). xxii, 329p. 57.00 (*1-58562-016-5*, 62016) Am Psychiatric.

Borderline Personality Disorder: A Multidimensional Approach. Joel Paris. 1994. LC 93-48728. 288p. text 34.00 (*0-88048-655-4*, 8655) Am Psychiatric.

Borderline Personality Disorder: Clinical & Empirical Perspectives. Ed. by John F. Clarkin et al. 1991. LC 91-28304. (Guilford Personality Disorders Ser.). 352p. 47.00 (*0-89862-262-X*, 2262) Guilford Pubns.

Borderline Personality Disorder: Etiology & Treatment. Ed. by Joel Paris. 1992. 420p. text 52.00 (*0-88048-408-X*, 8408) Am Psychiatric.

Borderline Personality Disorder: Tailoring the Psychotherapy to the Patient. Leonard Horwitz et al. Ed. by Donald B. Colson. 1996. LC 95-36000. 269p. text 36.00 (*0-88048-689-9*, 8689) Am Psychiatric.

Borderline Personality Disorder: The Latest Assessment & Treatment Strategies. Melanie A. Dean. 2nd ed. 2001. LC 00-65754. (Condensed Reviews for Professionals Ser.). (Illus.). 84p. (C). reprint ed. pap. 14.95 (*1-887537-17-1*) Compact Clinicals.

Borderline Personality Disorders: The Concept, the Syndrome, the Patient. Ed. by Peter Hartocollis. 1977. LC 77-6152. 535p. 80.00 (*0-8236-0575-2*) Intl Univs Pr.

Borderline Phenomena & the Rorschach Test. Ed. by Jay S. Kwawer et al. 1980. LC 80-15693. 505p. 75.00 (*0-8236-0577-9*) Intl Univs Pr.

Borderline Psychotic Child: A Selective Integration. Trevor Lubbe. 2000. LC 99-48948. (Illus.). xv, 218p. pap. 29.95 (*0-415-22220-6*) Routledge.

Borg's Perceived Exertion & Pain Scales. Gunnar Borg. 1998. LC 97-46439. (Illus.). 120p. pap. text 26.00 (*0-88011-623-4*, BBOR0623) Human Kinetics.

Borish's Clinical Refraction. William J. Benjamin. Ed. by Richard Lampert. 1998. LC 96-49871. (Illus.). 960p. (C). text 150.00 (*0-7216-5688-9*) Saunders.

Born to Procreate: Women & Childbirth in France from the Middle Ages to the Eighteenth Century. Rolande J. Graves. 2001. LC 00-36395. (Studies in the Humanities: vol. 53). (Illus.). x, 162p. 49.95 (*0-8204-4907-5*) P Lang Pubng.

Born to Win. Lewis Timberlake & Marietta Reed. 1986. 224p. pap. 8.99 (*0-8423-0338-3*) Tyndale Hse.

Born to Win. Muriel James. 3rd ed. 1990. pap. 12.00 (*0-201-55016-4*) Addison-Wesley.

Boron Neutron Capture Therapy: Toward Clinical Trials of Glioma Treatment. Ed. by Detlaf Gabel & Ray Moss. 1993. LC 92-48775. (Illus.). 290p. (C). text 107.00 (*0-306-44350-3*, Kluwer Plenum) Kluwer Academic.

Borrowed Blood: Victory over Leukemia. Shawn S. Riley. 1991. 118p. (Orig.). pap. 5.00 (*0-936635-06-1*) Lion Pr & Vid.

Borrowed Time: A Surgeon's Struggle with Transfusion Induced AIDS. Orville J. Messenger & Dorothy Messenger. 1995. LC 95-197130. 160p. pap. 14.95 (*0-88962-582-4*) Mosaic.

Borrowed Time: An AIDS Memoir. Paul Monette. 1998. LC 98-219384. 352p. (gr. 1). pap. 13.00 (*0-15-600581-6*, Harvest Bks); 1988. LC 88-7215. 400p. 22.00 (*0-15-113598-3*) Harcourt.

Borrowed Time: An AIDS Memoir. Paul Monette. 1990. pap. 12.50 (*0-380-70779-9*, Avon Bks) Morrow Avon.

Bosquejos de Sermones para Bodas y Funerales: Sermon Outlines for Weddings & Funerals. Compiled by Jose L. Martinez. 1990. (SPA.). 112p. (Orig.). pap. 6.99 (*0-311-43042-2*) Casa Bautista.

Boston Colloquium on Cardiac Pacing. Ed. by J. Warren Harthorne & Hilbert J. Thalen. 1977. text 99.50 (*90-247-2006-0*) Kluwer Academic.

Boston Diagnostic Aphasia Examination. Harold Goodglass & Edith Kaplan. 3rd ed. 2000. 32p. 15.00 (*0-683-30561-1*) Lppncott W & W.

Boston Diagnostic Aphasia Examination: Boston Naming Test. Harold Goodglass & Edith Kaplan. 3rd ed. 2000. 30p. spiral bd. 35.00 (*0-683-30562-X*) Lppncott W & W.

Boston Diagnostic Aphasia Examination: Test Cards. Harold Goodglass & Edith Kaplan. 3rd ed. 2001. 30p. spiral bd. 50.00 (*0-683-30560-3*) Lppncott W & W.

Boston Diagnostic Aphasia Examination Set. Harold Goodglass & Edith Kaplan. 3rd ed. 2000. 140p. 150.00 (*0-683-30559-X*) Lppncott W & W.

Boswella: Herb for Pain. 1996. lib. bdg. 250.75 (*0-8490-5892-9*) Gordon Pr.

*__Botanical Dietary Supplements: Quality, Safety & Efficacy.__ Gail B. Mahady et al. 2001. LC 2001-31370. 276p. (*90-265-1855-2*) Swets NLD. *Dist:* Ashgate Pub Co.

Botanical Influences on Illness: A Sourcebook of Clinical Research. Melvyn R. Werbach & Michael T. Murray. 1994. LC 94-60010. 344p. text 39.95 (*0-9618550-4-5*); 2nd ed. 2000. LC 99-76898. (Illus.). xiii, 624p. text 59.95 (*1-891710-00-1*) Third Line Pr.

Botanical Medicine: A European Professional Perspective. Dan Kenner & Yves Requena. 1995. LC 96-45883. 350p. text 37.00 (*0-912111-48-8*) Paradigm Publns.

Botanical Pharmacy: The Pharmacology of Common Herbs. Heather Boon & Michael Smith. 1999. (Health Bks.). (Illus.). 320p. 39.95 (*1-55082-230-6*) Rockport Pubs.

Botany & Healing: Medicinal Plants of New Jersey & the Region. Cecil C. Still. 1998. LC 97-45725. (Illus.). (C). xi, 261p. text 59.00 (*0-8135-2507-1*); 304p. pap. text 22.00 (*0-8135-2508-X*) Rutgers U Pr.

Bottle in the Cupboard: Women & Alcohol. Yvonne Ward. 1993. 144p. pap. (*1-85594-066-3*) Attic Press.

Bottom Line Billing & Collections for the Medical Practice. Thomas Prince & Edward Mayberry. Date not set. 500p. (C). 169.00 (*1-56329-405-2*) Ingenix Inc.

Bottoms Up! A Pathologist's Essays on Medicine & the Humanities. William B. Ober. 1987. LC 87-13125. (Illus.). 356p. 21.95 (*0-8093-1419-3*) S Ill U Pr.

Botulinum & Tetanus Neurotoxins: Neurotransmission & Biomedical Aspects. B. R. DasGupta. 1993. LC 93-3845. (Illus.). 708p. (C). text 165.00 (*0-306-44412-7*, Kluwer Plenum) Kluwer Academic.

Botulinum Toxic Type A in Pain Management. Martin K. Childers. 2000. (Illus.). 136p. pap. text 29.95 (*0-9663422-2-4*) Acad Info Systs.

Botulinum Toxin Therapy. Dirk Dressler. 2000. (Illus.). 128p. pap. 39.00 (*0-86577-816-7*) Thieme Med Pubs.

Bound for Good Health: A Collection of Age Pages. 1993. 140p. (Orig.). (C). pap. text 35.00 (*0-7881-0060-2*) DIANE Pub.

Boundaries & Boundary Violations in Psychoanalysis. Glen O. Gabbard & Eva P. Lester. 1995. LC 95-30407. 223p. pap. 47.00 (*0-465-09577-1*) Basic.

Boundaries & Relationships: Knowing, Protecting & Enjoying the Self. Charles L. Whitfield. 1993. LC 92-40512. (Illus.). 288p. (Orig.). pap. 11.95 (*1-55874-259-X*, 259X) Health Comm.

Boundaries Between Promotion & Progression During Carcinogenesis. Ed. by O. Sudilovsky et al. 1991. (Basic Life Sciences Ser.: Vol. 57). (Illus.). 384p. (C). text 138.00 (*0-306-44031-8*, Kluwer Plenum) Kluwer Academic.

*__Boundaries in the Mind: A New Psychology of Personality.__ Ernest Hartmann. 2001. 274p. pap. 16.00 (*0-7881-9807-6*) DIANE Pub.

Boundaries of the Soul: The Practice of Jung's Psychology. June Singer. rev. ed. 1994. LC 94-9070. 528p. pap. 16.00 (*0-385-47529-2*) Doubleday.

Boundary & Space: An Introduction to the Work of D. W. Winnicott. Madeleine Davis & David Wallbridge. 1991. LC 90-48118. 240p. pap. 23.95 (*0-87630-641-5*) Brunner-Routledge.

Bounded Rationality: The Adaptive Toolbox. Gerd Gigerenzer & Reinhard Selten. 2001. LC 00-64589. (Illus.). xv, 377p. 39.95 (*0-262-07214-9*) MIT Pr.

Bourdillon's Spinal Manipulation. Edward R. Isaacs & Mark R. Bookhout. 6th ed. 2001. (Illus.). 392p. 75.00 (*0-7506-7239-0*) Buttrwrth-Heinemann.

Boutiquin Natural. Abel Delgado. 2000. LC 00-35287. (SPA.). 192p. pap. 12.95 (*1-57954-206-9*) Rodale Pr Inc.

Bovine Ephemeral Fever & Related Rhabdoviruses. Ed. by T. D. St. George et al. 1993. 141p. (Orig.). pap. 132.00 (*1-86320-088-6*) St Mut.

Bovine Practice. William E. Boden. 1991. pap. text 48.00 (*0-7020-1556-3*) Saunders.

Bovine Practice 2. William E. Boden. 2nd ed. 1997. (Illus.). 204p. pap. text 55.00 (*0-7020-2331-0*) Saunders.

Bovine Radiology. Uri Bargai et al. 1989. (Venture Series in Veterinary Medicine). (Illus.). 206p. (C). pap. text 49.95 (*0-8138-0185-0*) Iowa U Pr.

Bovine Respiratory Disease: A Symposium. Ed. by Raymond W. Loan. 1984. LC 83-40491. (Illus.). 544p. 39.95 (*0-89096-187-5*) Tex A&M Univ Pr.

Bovine Spongiform Encephalopathy. Richard H. Kimberlin. 1993. (Animal Production & Health Papers: No. 109). 76p. pap. (*92-5-103155-X*, F3155X) FAO ITA. *Dist:* Bernan Associates.

Bovine Spongiform Encephalopathy: The BSE Dilemma. Ed. by Clarence J. Gibbs. 1996. LC 96-13586. (Proceedings of the Serono Symposia Ser.). 413p. 154.00 (*0-387-94740-X*) Spr-Verlag.

Bowel Cancer: The Facts. John M. Northover & Joel D. Kettner. 1992. LC 92-12443. pap. 10.50 (*0-19-262207-2*) OUP.

Bowel Management: A Manual of Ideas & Techniques. Ed. by Raymond C. Cheever & Charles D. Elmer. 1975. 32p. pap. 3.50 (*0-915708-02-7*, #1420) Cheever Pub.

Bowel Obstruction: Differential Diagnosis & Clinical Management. John P. Welch. 1989. (Illus.). 711p. text 155.00 (*0-7216-1963-0*) Saunders.

Bowes & Church's Food Values of Portions Commonly Used. Jean A. T. Pennington. 17th ed. 1997. LC 97-24666. 512p. text 45.00 (*0-397-55435-4*) Lppncott W & W.

Box, the Amoeba, & the Egg: The Flow to Self-Discovery. Michael C. Giammatteo. rev. ed. 1999. (Illus.). pap. 8.95 (*0-918428-07-6*) Sylvan Inst.

Boxing & Medicine. Ed. by Robert C. Cantu. 1995. LC 94-33961. (Illus.). 224p. text 39.00 (*0-87322-797-2*, BCAN0797) Human Kinetics.

Boy Crazy: Analysing Adolescence, Memories, & Dreams. Janet Sayers. 1998. LC 98-10662. (Illus.). 192p. (C). pap. 24.99 (*0-415-19085-1*) Routledge.

Boy Crazy: Remembering Adolescence, Memories & Dreams. Janet Sayers. 1998. LC 98-10662. (Illus.). 185p. (C). 75.00 (*0-415-19084-3*) Routledge.

Boy or Girl? Elizabeth M. Whelan. 1977. LC 76-44667. (Illus.). 7.95 (*0-672-52276-4*, Bobbs) Macmillan.

Boy Sex Offender & His Later Career. Lewis J. Doshay. 1969. LC 69-14921. (Criminology, Law Enforcement, & Social Problems Ser.: No. 59). reprint ed. 20.00 (*0-87585-059-6*) Patterson Smith.

Boy Who Couldn't Stop Washing: The Experience & Treatment of Obesessive-Compulsive Disorder. Judith L. Rapoport. 1990. LC 89-14509. 272p. pap. 13.95 (*0-452-26365-4*, Plume) Dutton Plume.

Boyd's Introduction to the Study of Disease. Huntingdon Sheldon. 11th ed. 1992. (Illus.). 320p. text 49.00 (*0-8121-1561-9*) Lppncott W & W.

Boys in White: Student Culture in Medical School. Ed. by Howard S. Becker et al. rev. ed. 1976. LC 76-26951. 456p. reprint ed. pap. text 24.95 (*0-87855-622-2*) Transaction Pubs.

Boys into Men: Staying Healthy through the Teen Years. Mark A. Goldstein & Myrna Chandler Goldstein. 2000. LC 00-21045. (Illus.). 216p. (YA). (gr. 7 up). 45.00 (*0-313-30966-3*) Greenwood.

BPH Diseases Management: Proceedings of the Satellite Symposium Held at the XIVth Congress of the European Association of Urology, Stockholm, April 7, 1999. Ed. by C. R. Chapple. 1999. (European Urology Ser.: Vol. 36, Suppl. 3). (Illus.). iv, 64p. pap. 25.25 (*3-8055-6997-1*) S Karger.

BPPV: What You Need to Know. P. J. Haybach. Ed. by Jerry L. Underwood. 2000. (Illus.). 208p. 34.95 (*0-9632611-4-2*); pap. 24.95 (*0-9632611-3-4*) Vestibular.

Bracero Program in California: With Particular Reference to Health Status, Attitudes, & Practices. Henry P. Anderson. Ed. by Carlos E. Cortes. 1977. LC 76-1225. (Chicano Heritage Ser.). (Illus.). 28.95 (*0-405-09482-5*) Ayer.

Brachial Plexus. Boome. 1996. LC 97-204554. text 60.00 (*0-443-04838-X*) Saunders.

Brachial Plexus Injuries. Robert Leffert. 1986. LC 85-13319. (Illus.). 235p. text (*0-443-08026-7*) Church.

Brachial Plexus Lesions: Drawings of Explorations & Reconstructions by Algimantas Otonas Narakas. Ed. by Chantal Bonnard & Albert J. Slooff. 1998. LC 98-50980. (Illus.). 173p. 225.00 (*3-540-63428-2*) Spr-Verlag.

Brachial Plexus Palsy. Ed. by H. Kawai & H. Kawabata. 1997. 250p. text 33.00 (*981-02-3139-3*) World Scientific Pub.

Brachysira- Monographie der Gattung, Vol. 29. H. Lange-Bertalot & Gert Moser. 1994. (Bibliotheca Diatomologica Ser.: Band 29). (GER., Illus.). iv, 212p. lib. bdg. (*3-443-57020-8*) Gebruder Borntraeger DEU. *Dist:* Balogh.

Brachytherapy. Joslin. 1999. (Illus.). 576p. (C). pap. 184.00 (*0-412-63550-X*, Chap & Hall NY) Chapman & Hall.

Brachytherapy Physics: AAPM Summer School 1994. Ed. by Jeffrey F. Williamson et al. 1995. LC 95-80186. (Illus.). 715p. (Orig.). text 79.95 (*0-944838-50-2*) Med Physics Pub.

Bradford Hill's Principles of Medical Statistics. Austin B. Hill & I. D. Hill. 12th ed. 1991. 352p. pap. (*0-340-53739-6*) E A GBR. *Dist:* OUP.

Bradman Approach: Selected Topics. Leo H. Bradman. 1993. 150p. pap. (*1-883945-02-X*) UniPsych Pr.

Bradykinin, Kallidin & Kallikrein. Ed. by E. G. Erdoes. 1970. (Handbook of Experimental Pharmacology Ser.: Vol. 25). (Illus.). 768p. 219.00 (*0-387-04847-2*) Spr-Verlag.

Bradykinin, Kallidin & Kallikrein-Supplement. Ed. by E. G. Erdoes. 1979. (Handbook of Experimental Pharmacology Ser.: Vol. 25, Suppl.). (Illus.). 817p. 288.00 (*0-387-09356-7*) Spr-Verlag.

Brady's Introduction to Medical Terminology. Carol Lillis. 4th rev. ed. 1996. LC 96-8407. 275p. (C). pap. 30.20 (*0-8385-4321-9*, A-4321-4) P-H.

Bragg Healthy Heart: Keep Your Cardiovascular System Healthy & Fit at Any Age. Patricia Bragg & Paul C. Bragg. 14th rev. ed. 2000. LC 2001-268058. (Illus.). 230p. per. 8.95 (*0-87790-096-5*) Hlth Sci.

Brain. 1991. (Symposia on Quantitative Biology Ser.: Vol. LV). (Illus.). 1067p. text 200.00 (*0-87969-059-3*); pap. text 85.00 (*0-87969-060-7*) Cold Spring Harbor.

Brain: Aids to the Examination of the Peripheral Nervous System. 3rd ed. 1987. (Illus.). 68p. pap. text (*0-7020-1165-7*) Bailliere Tindall.

Brain: An Overview, a Source Guide. 1991. lib. bdg. 250.00 (*0-8490-4863-X*) Gordon Pr.

Brain: Biochemistry & Inherited Metabolic Disease. Ed. by N. R. Belton et al. 1983. 128p. text 107.50 (*0-85200-484-2*) Kluwer Academic.

Brain: Degeneration, Damage & Disorder. Ed. by Judith Metcalfe. 1998. LC 97-42430. (Biology Ser.). (Illus.). 270p. 39.95 (*3-540-63796-6*) Spr-Verlag.

Brain: Fetal & Infant. Samuel R. Berenberg. 1978. text 155.50 (*90-247-2022-2*) Kluwer Academic.

Brain: Introduction to Neuroscience 3. Thompson. 2000. 480p. pap. text 30.95 (*0-7167-3226-2*) W H Freeman.

Brain Activation. Pere E. Roland. (Professional Ser.). 600p. 1997. pap. 76.50 (*0-471-18441-1*); 1993. LC 92-49741. 179.00 (*0-471-50867-5*) Wiley.

Brain Aging: Molecular Neurobiology, the Aging Process & Neurodegenerative Disease. Ed. by H. Hendrie et al. 1990. LC 89-15337. (Neuronal Control of Bodily Function Ser.: Vol. 5). (Illus.). 320p. (C). text 69.00 (*0-920887-49-X*) Hogrefe & Huber Pubs.

Brain Allergies. William H. Philpott & Dwight K. Kalita. 1987. 235p. (Orig.). pap. 14.95 (*0-87983-426-9*, Keats Pubng) McGraw-Hill Trade.

Brain & Bannister's Clinical Neurology. Ed. by Roger Bannister. 7th ed. 1992. (Illus.). 634p. pap. text 52.50 (*0-19-261913-6*) OUP.

Brain & Behavior, Vol. 1. 1961. 10.00 (*0-934454-17-5*) Lubrecht & Cramer.

Brain & Behavior: An Introduction to Behavioral Neuroanatomy. David L. Clark & Nashaat N. Boutros. 1999. LC 99-21428. (Illus.). vii, 214p. 35.95 (*0-632-04295-8*) Blackwell Sci.

Brain & Behavior: Assessing Cortical Dysfunction Through ADL. Gudrun Arnadottir. 1990. (Illus.). 336p. (C). (gr. 13). text 47.95 (*0-8016-0334-X*, 00334) Mosby Inc.

Brain & Behavior: Mental Disorders & Substance Abuse. Contrib. by Marie Sosa. 1995. (Illus.). 60p. pap. 14.95 (*0-87168-559-0*, 95-33S) AAAS.

Brain & Behavior in Child Psychiatry. Ed. by A. Rothenberger. 1990. (Illus.). 414p. 112.00 (*0-387-52064-3*) Spr-Verlag.

Brain & Behavioural Development: Interdisciplinary Perspectives on Structure & Function. Ed. by John W. T. Dickerson & Harry McGurk. 1982. (Illus.). 266p. 69.95 (*0-903384-27-2*) Trans-Atl Phila.

Brain & Biodefence. Ed. by Yutaka Taniguchi & Tetsuro Hori. 1998. LC 99-159369. (Taniguchi Symposia on Brain Sciences Ser.: No. 21). (Illus.). x, 248p. 213.25 (*3-8055-6764-2*) S Karger.

Brain & Cardiac Surgery: Causes of Neurological Complications & Their Prevention. Stanton P. Newman & Michael J.G. Harrison. 2000. 416p. 112.00 (*90-5702-476-4*, Harwood Acad Pubs) Gordon & Breach.

Brain & Its Mind. H. Kuhlenbeck & J. Gerlach. 2nd ed. 1982. (Human Brain & Its Universe Ser.: Vol. 2). (Illus.). viii, 374p. 201.75 (*3-8055-2403-X*) S Karger.

Brain & Mind. Ed. by David A. Oakley. 1985. LC 84-29604. (Psychology in Progress Ser.). 320p. pap. 14.95 (*0-416-31630-1*, 9627) Routledge.

Brain & Oral Functions: Oral Motor Function & Dysfunction: Selected Papers from the Osaka International Oral Physiology Symposium on Brain & Oral Function, Osaka, 3-5 September 1994. Ed. by Toshifumi Morimoto et al. 1995. LC 95-8197. (International Congress Ser.: No. 1079). 662p. 240.00 (*0-444-81963-0*) Elsevier.

Brain & Personality. Graham Powell. 1979. LC 79-87638. 122p. 47.95 (*0-275-90408-3*, C0408, Praeger Pubs) Greenwood.

Brain & Pituitary Peptides II: Pulsatile Administration of Gn-Rh in Hypothalmic Failure-Basic & Clinical Aspects, Ferring Symposium on Brain & Pituitary Peptides, June 1982. H. Stock & L. Wildt. Ed. by G. Leyendecker et al. 1984. (Illus.). viii, 188p. 85.25 (*3-8055-3811-1*) S Karger.

Brain & Spinal Cord Tumors: Hope Through Research. 1995. lib. bdg. 251.99 (*0-8490-6717-0*); 1994. lib. bdg. 250.00 (*0-8490-8546-2*) Gordon Pr.

Brain & the Nervous System. Steve Parker. 1997. LC 96-36804. (Human Body Ser.). (*0-08-172480-2*) Elsevier.

Brain & Values. Ed. by Karl H. Pribaum. 1998. LC 98-17067. (INNS Series of Texts, Monographs, & Proceedings). 560p. pap. 95.00 (*0-8058-3154-1*) L Erlbaum Assocs.

Brain As an Endocrine Organ. Ed. by M. P. Cohen & Piero P. Foa. 1988. (Endocrinology & Metabolism Ser.: Vol. 3). (Illus.). 269p. 175.00 (*0-387-96644-7*) Spr-Verlag.

Brain Asymmetry. Ed. by Richard J. Davidson & Kenneth Hugdahl. 1994. 650p. 75.00 (*0-262-04144-8*, Bradford Bks) MIT Pr.

Brain Atlas & Functional Systems. Josephine C. Moore. 1993. (Illus.). 58p. (Orig.). (C). 26.00 (*1-56900-000-X*) Am Occup Therapy.

Brain Attack: Mapping Out Early Recovery from Stroke. Mary M. Castiglione & Cynthia C. Johnson. Ed. by Anna Hollingsworth. 1995. LC 95-3305. (Illus.). 48p. pap. text 8.95 (*0-939838-40-0*) Pritchett & Hull.

Brain Basics: An Integrated Biological Approach to Understanding & Assessing Human Behavior. Robert A. Williams. Ed. by Ellen Antill & Laura Lawrie. 1999. LC 00-500417. (Illus.). 320p. pap. 39.95 (*0-9668886-0-X*) Bio Psych.

Brain Biochemistry & Brain Disorders. Philip E. Strange. 1993. (Illus.). 354p. pap. text 39.95 (*0-19-854775-7*) OUP.

Brain Blood Supply. G. I. Mchedlishvili et al. 1977. 320p. (C). (*963-05-1130-4*) Akade Kiado HUN. *Dist:* St Mut.

Brain Book: Your Brain & Your Health. Contrib. by Marie Sosa. 1995. LC 98-105261. (Illus.). 60p. pap. 14.95 (*0-87168-561-2*, 95-07S) AAAS.

Brain Builders: A Lifelong Guide to Sharper Thinking, Better Memory, & an Age-Proof Mind. Richard Leviton. 1995. LC 95-32233. 432p. (C). pap. 14.95 (*0-13-303603-0*) PH Pr.

Brain-Building Nutrition: The Healing Power of Fats & Oils. Michael Schmidt. 2nd rev. ed. 2001. LC 2001-16176. 300p. pap. 16.95 (*1-58394-048-0*) Frog Ltd CA.

Brain Cancer. Michael Prados. 2000. (ACS Atlas of Clinical Oncology Ser.). 300p. incl. cd-rom (*1-55009-098-4*) DEKR.

***Brain Chemistry Diet: The Personalized Prescription for Balancing Mood, Relieving Stress, & Conquering Depression, Based on Your Personality Profile.** Michael Lesser & Colleen Kapklein. 2002. LC 2001-48358. 304p. text 24.95 (*0-399-14744-6*) Penguin Putnam.

Brain Cholinergic Systems. Ed. by Mircea Steriade & D. Biesold. 1991. (Illus.). 468p. text 150.00 (*0-19-854266-6*) OUP.

Brain Circuits & Functions of the Mind. Ed. by Colwyn Trevarthen. 1990. (Illus.). 448p. (C). pap. text 39.95 (*0-521-37874-5*) Cambridge U Pr.

Brain Code Mechanisms of Information Transfer & the Role of the Corpus Callosum. Norman D. Cook. 1986. 300p. 42.50 (*0-416-40840-0*, 9834) Routledge.

Brain-Compatible Science. Margaret A. Mangan. 1998. LC 98-60466. (Illus.). 256p. pap. 36.95 (*1-57517-081-7*, 1594) SkyLght Prof Dev.

Brain Control of Behaviour: An Analysis of Verbal Delayed Reactions & Their Impairment in Mental Disorders. P. Pinelli. 1997. LC 96-43505. (Illus.). xii, 342p. 299.25 (*3-8055-6305-1*) S Karger.

Brain Control of Responses to Trauma. Ed. by Nancy J. Rothwell & Frank Berkenbosch. 1994. (Illus.). 352p. (C). text 90.00 (*0-521-41939-5*) Cambridge U Pr.

Brain Control of the Reproductive System. Ed. by Akira Yokoyama. 1992. 88.00 (*0-8493-7754-4*, QP251) CRC Pr.

Brain, Culture & the Human Spirit: Essays from an Emergent Evolutionary Perspective. Ed. by James B. Ashbrook. 1992. (Illus.). 222p. (Orig.). (C). 65.50 (*0-8191-8853-0*); pap. 32.00 (*0-8191-8854-9*) U Pr of Amer.

***Brain-Damage: With a Cognitive Deficit & Pituitary Dysfunction: A Book about Overcoming Cognitive Deficit & Creating the New You.** Richard Edward Schmelzkopf. 2001. LC 2001-921. (*1-885373-35-X*) Emerald Ink.

Brain Damage Claims: Coping with Neuropsychological Evidence, Set. David Faust et al. 1991. LC 91-72274. 1000p. pap. 195.00 (*1-879689-00-6*) Law & Psych.

Brain Damage in the Preterm Infant. Nigel Paneth et al. 1995. (Clinics in Developmental Medicine Ser.: No. 131). (Illus.). 300p. (C). 69.95 (*0-521-68300-9*) Cambridge U Pr.

Brain Death. Douglas N. Walton. 1980. LC 80-80845. (Science & Society: Series in Science, Technology, & Human Values: Vol. 5). 102p. pap. 7.95 (*0-931682-12-6*) Purdue U Pubns.

Brain Death: Proceedings of the Second International Symposium on Brain Death, Havana, Cuba, February 27-March 1, 1996, No. 9. International Symposium on Brain Death Staff. Ed. by Calixto Machado. 1995. LC 95-34946. (Developments in Neurology Ser.: Vol. 9). 310p. 173.00 (*0-444-82267-4*) Elsevier.

Brain Death Criterion of Human Death. D. L. Stickel. 1982. (Illus.). 73p. pap. 23.00 (*0-08-025814-X*, Pergamon Pr) Elsevier.

Brain Development: Relationship to Dietary Lipid & Lipid Metabolism. Ed. by J. Jumpsen & M. T. Clandinin. 1995. 128p. 70.00 (*0-935315-65-9*) Am Oil Chemists.

Brain Development & Cognition: A Reader. Mark H. Johnson. 1993. LC 92-17620. 752p. pap. 33.95 (*0-631-18223-3*) Blackwell Pubs.

***Brain Development & Cognition: A Reader.** Ed. by Mark H. Johnson et al. 2nd ed. 2002. LC 2001-52407. (*0-631-21736-3*); pap. (*0-631-21737-1*) Blackwell Pubs.

Brain Development & Epilepsy. John W. Swann et al. 1995. LC 94-42513. (Illus.). 352p. text 59.95 (*0-19-507846-2*) OUP.

Brain-Disabling Treatments in Psychiatry: Drugs, Electroshock & the Role of the FDA. Peter Breggin. 1997. LC 97-3969. 320p. 43.95 (*0-8261-9490-7*) Springer Pub.

Brain Diseases & Disorders: Diagnostics & Treatment Products. 1991. 275p. 2650.00 (*0-89336-830-X*, C-139) BCC.

Brain Disorders Sourcebook. Roger S. Cicla. 1999. LC 99-15345. 432p. pap. 19.95 (*0-7373-0093-0*, 00930WW) NTC Contemp Pub Co.

Brain Disorders Sourcebook: Basic Consumer Health Information about Strokes, Epilepsy, Parkinson's Disease & More. Ed. by Karen Bellenir. 1999. LC 99-15539. (Health Reference Ser.). 600p. 78.00 (*0-7808-0229-2*) Omnigraphics Inc.

Brain Dissection & Surface Anatomy for Communication Sciences. Douglas B. Webster. 1997. 72p. pap. 24.95 (*1-56593-855-0*, 1670) Thomson Learn.

Brain Dissection & Surface Anatomy for the Communication Sciences. Douglas B. Webster. 1997. LC 96-52548. 100p. 190.00 (*1-56593-730-9*, 1420) Singular Publishing.

Brain Dopaminergic Imaging with Positron Tomography. Ed. by J. C. Baron et al. 1991. (Developments in Nuclear Medicine Ser.). 208p. text 118.00 (*0-7923-1476-X*) Kluwer Academic.

Brain Edema, No. VIII. Ed. by H. J. Reulen et al. 1991. (Acta Neurochirurgica Ser.: No. 51). (Illus.). 416p. 230.00 (*0-387-82240-2*) Spr-Verlag.

Brain Edema: A Pathogenetic Analysis. Ed. by G. I. Mchedlishvili et al. 1986. 365p. (C). (*963-05-4378-8*) Akade Kiado HUN. *Dist:* St Mut.

***Brain Edema XI.** A. D. Mendelow et al. 2001. (Acta Neurochirurgica Ser.: Vol. 76). 400p. 169.00 (*3-211-83561-X*) Spr-Verlag.

Brain Edema IX: Proceedings of the Ninth International Symposium, Tokyo, May 16-19, 1993. Ed. by Umeo Ito et al. 1994. LC 94-5220. (Acta Neurochirurgica Ser.: Vol. 60). 600p. 237.00 (*0-387-82532-0*) Spr-Verlag.

Brain Edema X: Proceedings of the 10th International Symposium, San Diego, California, October 20-23, 1996. Ed. by H. E. James et al. 1997. LC 97-39789. (Acta Neurochirurgica Ser.: Vol. 70). 314p. 189.00 (*3-211-82892-3*) Spr-Verlag.

Brain Encyclopedia. Carol Turkington. 1999. 320p. pap. 18.95 (*0-8160-3170-3*); 1996. LC 95-49503. 352p. 40.00 (*0-8160-3169-X*) Facts on File.

Brain-Endocrine Interaction I: Median Eminence-Structure & Function: Proceedings of the International Symposium, Munich, 1971. International Symposium on Brain-Endocrine Interac. Ed. by K. M. Knigge et al. 1971. (Illus.). xii, 368p. 104.50 (*3-8055-1257-0*) S Karger.

Brain Endocrine Interaction II: The Ventricular System in Neuroendocrine Mechanisms: Proceedings of the International Symposium, 2nd, Tokyo, October, 1974. International Symposium on Brain-Endocrine Interac. Ed. by K. M. Knigge & D. E. Scott. 1975. (Illus.). x, 406p. 123.50 (*3-8055-2176-6*) S Karger.

Brain Energy Metabolism: Molecules to Man: Congress, Blaubeuren, August 1995. Ed. by John Edmond & John B. Clark. 1996. (Journal: Vol. 18, No. 5-6). (Illus.). 232p. pap. 83.50 (*3-8055-6390-6*) S Karger.

Brain Energy Metabolism Fundamentals & Methodology. Avital Schurr & Benjamin M. Rigor. 1999. 99.95 (*0-8493-2689-3*) CRC Pr.

Brain Failure. Ed. by D. J. Bihari & J. W. Holaday. 1989. (Update in Intensive Care & Emergency Medicine Ser.: Vol. 9). (Illus.). 279p. 120.00 (*0-387-51655-7*, 3512) Spr-Verlag.

Brain Food Diet for Children. Ralph E. Minear & William Proctor. 1984. LC 83-3798. 228p. (*0-672-52755-3*) Macmillan.

Brain Function & Orthomolecular Nutrition. 1996. lib. bdg. 251.75 (*0-8490-5877-5*) Gordon Pr.

Brain Function & Oscillations Vol. II: Integrative Brain Function, Neurophysiology & Cognitive Processes. Erol Basar. 1998. (Series in Synergetics). (Illus.). 515p. 89.95 (*3-540-64345-1*) Spr-Verlag.

Brain Function in Hot Environment, Vol. 115. H. S. Sharma & Jan Westman. 1998. LC 97-49233. (Progress in Brain Research Ser.). 534p. 204.50 (*0-444-82377-8*) Elsevier.

Brain Functions of Neuropeptides: A Current View. Ed. by J. P. Burbach & D. De Wied. 1993. (Illus.). 142p. (C). lib. bdg. 53.95 (*1-85070-453-8*, Parthenon Pbng) CRC Pr.

Brain Gut Peptides & Reproductive Peptides. Charles D. Barnes. 1991. 304p. 106.00 (*0-8493-8848-1*, QP552) CRC Pr.

Brain, Head, Neck & Spine with Mr. Correlations: A Teaching File. Yock Myers. 2001. (Illus.). 608p. text 99.00 (*0-8151-9000-X*, 29915) Mosby Inc.

Brain, Heart & Tumor Imaging: Updated PET &: MRI: Proceedings of the 2nd International Osaka City University Symposium, Osaka, Japan, 2-4 October 1994. Ed. by Hironobu Ochi et al. 1995. LC 95-25119. (International Congress Ser.: No. 1090). 208p. 135.00 (*0-444-82155-4*) Elsevier.

Brain Hypothermia: Pathology, Pharmacology & Treatment of Severe Brain Injury. N. Hayashi. 2000. LC 00-41320. 240p. 80.00 (*4-431-70277-6*) Spr-Verlag.

Brain Imaging: Applications in Psychiatry. Ed. by Nancy C. Andreasen. 1989. LC 88-16775. 384p. 29.95 (*0-88048-229-X*, 8229) Am Psychiatric.

Brain Imaging: Case Review. Laurie A. Loevner. 1999. LC 99-10768. (Illus.). 224p. (C). text (*0-323-00430-X*) Mosby Inc.

Brain Imaging: Techniques & Applications. Ed. by N. A. Sharif & M. E. Lewis. 1989. 293p. 99.00 (*0-470-21471-6*) P-H.

Brain Imaging & Psychogeriatric Services in Geriatric Psychiatry: 23rd Symposium of the European Association of Geriatric Psychiatry, Lund, October 1995. Ed. by Lars Gustafson & Jarl Risberg. 1997. (Journal: Vol. 8, No. 2, 1997). (Illus.). 86p. pap. 34.00 (*3-8055-6454-6*) S Karger.

Brain Imaging in Clinical Psychiatry. Ed. by K. Ranga Rama Krishnan & Doraiswamy. 1997. LC 97-6337. (Medical Psychiatry Ser.). (Illus.). 672p. text 195.00 (*0-8247-9859-7*) Dekker.

***Brain Imaging in Epilepsy: Insights & Applications.** David Maudgil. 2001. 90p. pap. (*1-901346-24-2*) Remedica GBR. *Dist:* Gordon & Breach.

Brain Imaging in Psychiatry. Ed. by Shon Lewis & Nicholas Higgins. 1996. LC 96-6148. 312p. 157.95 (*0-632-03647-8*) Blackwell Sci.

Brain Imaging in Substance Abuse: Research, Clinical & Forensic Applications. Ed. by Marc J. Kaufman. 2000. LC 99-54063. (Forensic Science & Medicine Ser.). (Illus.). xxv, 425p. 135.00 (*0-89603-770-3*) Humana.

Brain Imaging of Nicotine & Tobacco Smoking. Ed. by E. F. Domino. 1995. LC 95-67172. (Illus.). 340p. 95.00 (*0-916182-10-X*) NPP Bks.

Brain Immune Axis & Substance Abuse: Proceedings of the Second Annual Symposium Held in Palm Beach, Florida, June 16-18, 1994. Ed. by Burt M. Sharp et al. 1995. LC 95-17727. (Advances in Experimental Medicine & Biology Ser.: Vol. 373). (Illus.). 356p. (C). text 95.00 (*0-306-45017-8*, Kluwer Plenum) Kluwer Academic.

Brain in Health & Disease Abstracts. IBRO Staff. 1982. (Neuroscience Ser.: No. 468). pap. 125.00 (*0-08-028896-0*, Pergamon Pr) Elsevier.

Brain in Human Aging. Gene D. Cohen. 1988. (Adulthood & Aging Ser.). 272p. (C). 37.95 (*0-8261-5830-7*) Springer Pub.

Brain in Pediatric AIDS. Ed. by P. B. Kozloski et al. 1990. (Illus.). xvi, 204p. 170.50 (*3-8055-5216-5*) S Karger.

Brain Injury: A Guide for Families. Tampa General Rehabilitation Center Staff. 2nd ed. 1995. (Coping Ser.: Vol. 1). 68p. (Orig.). pap. 9.50 (*1-882855-40-X*) HDI Pubs.

Brain Injury: A Home Based Cognitive Rehabilitation Program. Ed. by Tampa General Rehab Center Staff. 2nd rev. ed. 1997. (HDI Coping Ser.: Vol. 2). 84p. pap. 9.50 (*1-882855-58-2*) HDI Pubs.

Brain Injury & After: Towards Improved Outcome. Rose. 1996. 216p. pap. 55.00 (*0-471-96288-0*) Wiley.

Brain Injury & Gender Role Strain: Rebuilding Adult Lifestyles after Injury. Sharon A. Gutman. 2000. LC 00-58210. 155p. 49.95 (*0-7890-1186-7*); pap. 24.95 (*0-7890-1187-5*) Haworth Pr.

Brain Injury & Neuropsychological Trauma & Rehabilitation: International Perspectives. Ed. by Anne-Lise Christensen & Barbara P. Uzzell. 1994. (Institute for Research in Behavioral Neuroscience Ser.). 344p. pap. 36.00 (*0-8058-1448-5*) L Erlbaum Assocs.

Brain Injury & Pediatric Cardiac Surgery. Richard A. Jonas et al. 1995. LC 95-40257. 416p. text (*0-7506-9567-6*) E A GBR. *Dist:* OUP.

Brain Injury & Protection During Heart Surgery. Ed. by Mark Hilberman. 1987. (C). text 124.50 (*0-89838-952-6*) Kluwer Academic.

Brain Injury & Recovery: Theoretical & Controversial Issues. S. Finger et al. 1988. (Illus.). 362p. (C). 95.00 (*0-306-42756-7*, Kluwer Plenum) Kluwer Academic.

Brain Injury & the Family: A Life & Living Perspective. Arthur E. Dell Orto & Paul W. Power. 2nd ed. 2000. LC 99-89634. 256p. per. 44.95 (*0-8493-1325-2*) CRC Pr.

Brain Injury & the Family: An Aid for Better Understanding. Lesley A. Sitkin & Bruce E. Murdoch. 1987. (Illus.). (Orig.). (C). pap. text 9.47 (*0-943723-00-0*) Simmons & Hall Pub.

Brain Injury Case Management. Brooks. 1998. (Illus.). 224p. pap. 29.95 (*0-412-60910-X*, Chap & Hall NY) Chapman & Hall.

Brain Injury Glossary. Ed. by Don Lehmkuhl. 1993. 48p. reprint ed. pap. 9.50 (*1-882855-06-X*) HDI Pubs.

Brain Injury Neuropsychological Trauma & Rehabilitation: International Perspectives. Ed. by Anne-Lise Christensen & Barbara P. Uzzell. 1994. (Institute for Research in Behavioral Neuroscience Ser.). 344p. text 69.95 (*0-8058-1447-7*) L Erlbaum Assocs.

Brain Injury Pathway. McDermott. 1998. (C). pap. text 75.00 (*0-12-785065-1*) Acad Pr.

Brain Injury Rehabilitation: A Neuro-Functional Approach. Jo Clark-Wilson & Gordon M. Giles. 1992. LC 92-21407. (Therapy in Practice Ser.: Vol. 33). 458p. 55.00 (*1-56593-052-5*, 0300) Singular Publishing.

Brain Injury Rehabilitation: A Neurobehavioral Approach. Rodger L. Wood. 1987. 196p. 40.00 (*0-87189-314-2*) Aspen Pub.

Brain Injury Rehabilitation: Adaptive Driving after TBI. Ed. by William H. Burke. 2nd rev. ed. 1996. (Professional Series on Traumatic Brain Injury: Vol. 5). 40p. pap. 9.50 (*1-882855-52-3*) HDI Pubs.

Brain Injury Rehabilitation: Clinical Considerations. Ed. by M. Alan Finlayson & Scott H. Garner. 1993. LC 92-48433. (Rehabilitation Medicine Library). 332p. 79.00 (*0-683-03224-0*) Lppncott W & W.

Brain Injury Rehabilitation: Managing Anger & Aggression. Ed. by William H. Burke. 2nd rev. ed. 1996. (Professional Series on Traumatic Brain Injury: Vol. 6). 60p. pap. 9.50 (*1-882855-53-1*) HDI Pubs.

Brain Injury Rehabilitation Patient Education Manual. Aspen Reference Group Staff. 1996. ring bd. 189.00 (*0-8342-0744-3*, S304) Aspen Pub.

Brain Injury Rehabilitation with Children & Adolescents. Ed. by William H. Burke. 2nd rev. ed. 1996. (Professional Series on Traumatic Brain Injury: Vol. 12). 76p. pap. 9.50 (*1-882855-50-7*) HDI Pubs.

Brain Ischemia. 1995. (Illus.). 380p. 190.00 (*3-540-19850-4*) Spr-Verlag.

Brain Ischemia: Basic Concepts & Clinical Relevance. Ed. by Louis R. Caplan. 1995. LC 93-49746. (Illus.). 380p. 165.00 (*0-387-19850-4*) Spr-Verlag.

Brain Lateralization in Children: Developmental Implications. Ed. by Dennis L. Molfese & Sidney J. Segalowitz. 1988. LC 88-11269. 612p. 80.00 (*0-89862-719-2*, 2719) Guilford Pubns.

Brain Machine: The Development of Neurophysiological Thought. Marc Jeannerod. Tr. by David Urion from FRE. 1985. LC 85-7597. (Illus.). 192p. 31.00 (*0-674-08047-5*) HUP.

Brain Maturation & Cognitive Development: Comparative & Cross-Cultural Perspectives. Ed. by Kathleen R. Gibson & Anne C. Petersen. 1991. (Evolutionary Foundations of Human Behavior Ser.). (Illus.). 399p. lib. bdg. 72.95 (*0-202-01187-9*) Aldine de Gruyter.

Brain Mechanisms & Psychotropic Drugs. Ed. by Andrius Baskys & Gary Remington. 1996. LC 95-47545. (Pharmacology & Toxicology: Basic & Clinical Aspects Ser.). 288p. 139.95 (*0-8493-8386-2*) CRC Pr.

Brain Mechanisms & Spatial Vision. Ed. by David J. Ingle et al. 1984. lib. bdg. 225.00 (*90-247-3117-8*) Kluwer Academic.

Brain Mechanisms of Perception & Memory: From Neuron to Behavior. Ed. by Taketoshi Ono et al. 1993. LC 92-49789. (Illus.). 722p. text 125.00 (*0-19-507770-9*) OUP.

Brain Metallothionein in Neurological Disorders. Ed. by M. Ebadi. 1994. (Journal: Vol. 3, No. 4, 1994). (Illus.). 40p. pap. 30.50 (*3-8055-6057-5*) S Karger.

Brain, Mind & Behavior. Bloom. 2000. tchr. ed. (*0-7167-2758-7*) W H Freeman.

Brain, Mind & Behavior. H. J. G. Bloom & Larzen. 3rd ed. 2000. (C). pap. text (*0-7167-2389-1*) W H Freeman.

Brain, Mind & Behavior: A New Perspective on Human Nature. David L. Robinson. 1996. LC 95-43765. 192p. 58.00 (*0-275-95468-4*, Praeger Pubs) Greenwood.

Brain, Mind & Medicine: Charles Richet & the Origins of Physiological Psychology. Stewart G. Wolf. 1993. 302p. (C). text 49.95 (*1-56000-063-5*) Transaction Pubs.

Brain-Mind & Parapsychology: Proceedings of the International Conference, Aug. 24-25, 1978. International Conference, Montreal Canada Staff. Ed. by Betty Shapin & Lisette Coly. 1979. LC 79-84820. 17.00 (*0-912328-31-2*) Parapsych Foun.

Brain, Mind & the External Signs of Intelligence. Bernard Hollander. 1931. LC 78-72802. 32.50 (*0-404-60864-7*) AMS Pr.

Brain-Mind Problem: Philosophical & Neurophysiological Approaches. Ed. by B. Gulyas. 1987. (Louvain Philosophical Studies: No. 1). 125p. (Orig.). pap. (*90-6186-246-9*) Leuven Univ BEL. *Dist:* Coronet Bks.

A
B

Brain of the Common Marmoset (Callithrix Jacchus) Heinz Stephan et al. 1980. (Illus.). 91p. 135.00 (*0-387-09782-1*) Spr-Verlag.

Brain Oncology. Ed. by M. Chatel et al. 1987. (Developments in Oncology Ser.). (C). text 345.50 (*0-89838-954-2*) Kluwer Academic.

Brain Organization & Memory: Cells, Systems & Circuits. Ed. by James L. McGaugh et al. 1992. (Illus.). 432p. pap. text 60.00 (*0-19-507712-1*) OUP.

Brain Organization of Language & Cognitive Processes. A. Ardila & F. Ostrosky-Solis. 1989. LC 89-16051. (Critical Issues in Neuropsychology Ser.). (Illus.). 276p. (C). text 54.00 (*0-306-43169-6*, Kluwer Plenum) Kluwer Academic.

Brain-Pituitary-Adrenal Interrelationships: Proceedings of the International Symposium, Cincinnati, Ohio, June, 1973. International Symposium on Brain-Pituitary-Adrenal. Ed. by H. Brodish & S. Redgate. 1973. 127.00 (*3-8055-1457-3*) S Karger.

Brain Plasticity: Development & Aging: Proceedings of the Conference on Recent Advances in Neurobiology: Plasticity & Regeneration Held in St. Vincent, Italy, October 9-11, 1995. Ed. by Guido Filogamo et al. 1998. LC 97-35346. (Advances in Experimental Medicine & Biology Ser.: Vol. 429). 334p. 95.00 (*0-306-45765-2*, Kluwer Plenum) Kluwer Academic.

Brain Plasticity & Behavior. Bryan Kolb. 1995. (John M. MacEachran Memorial Lectures). 208p. text 45.00 (*0-8058-1520-1*) L Erlbaum Assocs.

Brain Policy: How the New Neuroscience Will Change Our Lives & Our Politics. Robert H. Blank. 1999. LC 98-46088. 224p. text 60.00 (*0-87840-712-X*) Georgetown U Pr.

Brain Policy: How the New Neuroscience Will Change Our Lives & Our Politics. Robert H. Blank. 1999. LC 98-46088. (Illus.). 208p. pap. 21.95 (*0-87840-713-8*) Georgetown U Pr.

Brain Power: A Neurosurgeon's Complete Program to Maintain & Enhance Brain Fitness Throughout Your Life. Vernon H. Mark & Jeffrey P. Mark. 1991. LC 89-7520. 256p. pap. 14.00 (*0-395-55001-7*) HM.

Brain Processes & Memory. Ed. by K. Ishikawa. 1996. LC 96-30634. (International Congress Ser.: Vol. 1108). 426p. 175.00 (*0-444-82303-4*, QP406) Elsevier.

Brain Protection in Aortic Surgery: Proceedings of the International Symposium on Current Techniques for Brain Protection in Aortic Surgery, Osaka, Japan, 15-16 September 1996. Ed. by Y. Kawashima & S. Takamoto. 1997. (International Congress Ser.: No. 1130). 274p. 148.00 (*0-444-82492-8*) Elsevier.

Brain Repair. Donald G. Stein & Simon Brailowsky. 1997. 176p. pap. 13.95 (*0-19-511918-5*) OUP.

Brain Scale of Dr. Brunler. Arthur M. Young. 1985. (Broadside Editions Ser.). 20p. reprint ed. pap. 3.95 (*0-931191-01-7*) Rob Briggs.

Brain Section Model: Including a Comprehensive Guide to Construction. E. M. Weber. 9th ed. 1996. (ENG & GER.). 11p. pap. 18.95 (*3-540-60474-X*) Spr-Verlag.

Brain Sex: The Real Difference Between Men & Women. Anne Moir. 1991. 17.95 (*0-8184-0543-0*, Delta Trade) Dell.

Brain Slices. Ed. by Raymond Dingledine. 1984. LC 83-22957. 460p. 89.50 (*0-306-41437-6*, Plenum Trade) Perseus Pubng.

Brain Slices: Fundamentals, Applications & Implications. Ed. by A. Schurr et al. 1987. (Illus.). vi, 194p. 148.00 (*3-8055-4490-1*) S Karger.

Brain Slices in Basic & Clinical Research. Ed. by Avital Schurr & Benjamin M. Rigor. 1995. LC 94-31343. 352p. 179.95 (*0-8493-4760-2*) CRC Pr.

Brain SPECT Imaging in Psychiatry. Ed. by F. Gruenwald et al. 1995. (Illus.). viii, 218p. (Orig.). (C). pap. text 152.30 (*3-11-014730-0*) De Gruyter.

Brain-Stem Localization & Function. Ed. by Louis R. Caplan et al. 1993. LC 93-5073. (Illus.). 279p. 95.00 (*0-387-56608-2*) Spr-Verlag.

Brain Structure & Aging. E. A. Wright et al. 1974. 297p. text 29.50 (*0-8422-7175-9*) Irvington.

Brain Surgery. Michael L. J. Apuzzo. 1998. incl. cd-rom (*0-443-07822-X*) Church.

Brain Surgery: Complication Avoidance & Management Ed. by Michael L. J. Apuzzo. 1992. (Illus.). 2616p. text (*0-443-08709-1*) Church.

Brain Surgery: What to Know & Ask. Elaine B. LePage. Ed. by Anna Hollingsworth. 1994. LC 93-23725. (Illus.). 36p. (Orig.). pap. text 7.75 (*0-939838-36-2*) Pritchett & Hull.

Brain Theory. Ed. by G. Shaw & G. Palm. 1988. (Advance Series on Neuroscience: Vol. 1). 800p. (C). reprint ed. pap. text 55.00 (*9971-5-0484-7*) World Scientific Pub.

Brain Theory: Spatio-Temporal Aspects of Brain Function. Ed. by A. M. Aertsen. 1993. LC 93-15872. (Illus.). 318p. 154.50 (*0-444-89839-5*) Elsevier.

Brain Tumor Biology. Ed. by M. L. Rosenblum & C. B. Wilson. 1984. (Progress in Experimental Tumor Research Ser.: Vol. 27). (Illus.). xvi, 260p. 136.75 (*3-8055-3698-4*) S Karger.

Brain Tumor Immunotherapy. Ed. by Linda M. Liau et al. 2001. LC 00-57512. (Illus.). xi, 373p. 135.00 (*0-89603-638-3*) Humana.

Brain Tumor Invasion: Biological, Clinical & Therapeutic Considerations. Ed. by Tom Mikkelsen et al. 1998. LC 97-29119. 464p. 132.00 (*0-471-15452-0*, Wiley-Liss) Wiley.

Brain Tumor Invasiveness. Ed. by Ronald H. Goldfarb. 1994. LC 94-8764. 90p. (C). text 176.50 (*0-7923-2791-8*) Kluwer Academic.

Brain Tumor Research & Therapy. Ed. by M. Nagai. 1996. (Illus.). 454p. 175.00 (*4-431-70164-8*) Spr-Verlag.

Brain Tumor Therapy. Ed. by M. L. Rosenblum & C. B. Wilson. 1984. (Progress in Experimental Tumor Research Ser.: Vol. 28). (Illus.). xvi, 288p. 136.75 (*3-8055-3699-2*) S Karger.

Brain Tumors. Harry S. Greenberg et al. 1999. LC 98-27811. (Contemporary Neurology Ser.: Vol. 54). (Illus.). 368p. text 110.00 (*0-19-512958-X*) OUP.

Brain Tumors. Ed. by Andrew H. Kaye & Edward R. Laws. 1997. LC 94-38014. text 230.00 (*0-443-04840-1*) Saunders.

Brain Tumors: A Comprehensive Text. Ed. by Robert A. Morantz & John W. Walsh. 1993. (Neurological Disease & Therapy Ser.: Vol. 20). (Illus.). 864p. text 275.00 (*0-8247-8826-5*) Dekker.

***Brain Tumors: An Encyclopedic Approach.** Andrew H. Kaye & Edward Laws, Jr. 2nd rev. ed. 2001. (Illus.). 1215p. (*0-443-06426-1*) Church GBR. *Dist:* Saunders.

Brain Tumors: Pathology & Biological Correlates. Davide Schiffer. 1993. LC 92-49398. (*3-540-55864-0*) Spr-Verlag.

Brain Tumors: Pathology & Its Biological Correlates. Davide Schiffer. 2nd ed. 1996. LC 96-41506. (Illus.). 695p. 249.00 (*3-540-61622-5*) Spr-Verlag.

Brain Tumors - Biopathology & Therapy: Proceedings of the Brain Tumor Workshop - Verona 1 Held in Verona, Italy, 13-14 June 1985. Ed. by M. A. Gerosa et al. 1986. LC 86-785. (Advances in the Biosciences Ser.: No. 58). (Illus.). 254p. 96.00 (*0-08-032013-9*, Pergamon Pr) Elsevier.

Brain Tumors Completely. K. J. Zulch. 3rd rev. ed. 1986. (Illus.). 704p. 327.00 (*0-387-10933-1*) Spr-Verlag.

Brain Tumors in Children: Principles of Diagnosis & Treatment. Michael E. Cohen & Patricia K. Duffner. 2nd ed. 1993. LC 93-34357. (International Review of Child Neurology Ser.). 512p. text 115.00 (*0-7817-0064-7*) Lppncott W & W.

Brain Waves through Time: 12 Principles for Understanding the Evolution of the Human Brain & Man's Behav. R. T. DeMoss. 2000. LC 99-17252. (Illus.). 300p. (C). 26.95 (*0-306-46010-6*) Perseus Bks Grp.

Brain Wellness Plan: Breakthrough Medical, Nutritional & Immune-Boosting Therapies to Prevent. Jay Lombard & Carl Germano. LC 97-72050. 1997. 240p. 20.00 (*1-57566-230-2*); 1998. 304p. pap. 14.00 (*1-57566-293-0*, Knsington) Kensgtn Pub Corp.

Brain Without Oxygen. Peter Lutz. 1997. (Neuroscience Intelligence Unit Ser.). 250p. pap. 89.95 (*0-412-13061-0*) Chapman & Hall.

Brain Without Oxygen: Causes of Failure & Mechanisms for Survival. Peter L. Lutz & Goran E. Nilsson. 2nd ed. 1997. LC 97-20847. (Neuroscience Intelligence Unit Ser.). 99.00 (*1-57059-458-9*) Landes Bioscience.

Brainedness, Handedness & Mental Abilities: The Foundations of Neuropsychology (*0-404-60850-7*) AMS Pr.

Brainlash: Maximize Your Recovery from Mild Brain Injury. Gail L. Denton. Ed. by Fagan & Gerard. 1996. LC 95-94718. (Illus.). 383p. pap. 39.95 (*0-9646653-5-2*) Attention Span Bks.

Brainlash: Maximize Your Recovery from Mild Brain Injury. Gail L. Denton. 2nd ed. 1999. (Illus.). 256p. pap. 24.95 (*1-888799-37-4*) Demos Medical.

***Brain's Diseases of the Nervous System.** Michael Donaghy. Ed. by Michael Donaghy. 11th ed. 2001. (Illus.). 1104p. text 229.95 (*0-19-262618-3*) OUP.

Brain's Mind: A Neuroscience Perspective on the Mind-Body Problem. Ed. by Dalbir Bindra. 1980. LC 80-13998. (Illus.). 128p. text 23.95 (*0-89876-003-8*) Gardner Pr.

Brainstem (PRE) Motor Mechanisms & the Stereotypy of Motor Patterns: 5th International Congress of Vertebrate Morphology, Bristol, July 1997. Ed. by J. L. Dubbeldam. 5th ed. 1999. (Acta Anatomica Ser.: Vol. 163, No. 3). (Illus.). 52p. pap. 75.75 (*3-8055-6848-7*) S Karger.

Brainstorming: The Science & Politics of Opiate Research. Solomon H. Snyder. 1989. LC 89-11096. (Illus.). 208p. text 24.95 (*0-674-08048-3*) HUP.

Brainstorms: Philosophical Essays on Mind & Psychology. Daniel Clement Dennett. 1981. LC 78-13723. (Bradford Bks.). 353p. pap. text 19.00 (*0-262-54037-1*) MIT Pr.

Brainstorms - Epilepsy in Our Words: Personal Accounts of Living with Seizures. Ed. by Steven C. Schachter. 1993. LC 92-36754. 128p. pap. text 35.00 (*0-88167-997-6*) Lppncott W & W.

Brainstorms Healer: Epilepsy in Our Experience. Steven C. Schachter & A. James Rowan. 1998. LC 98-200025. 198p. pap. text 35.00 (*0-7817-1688-8*) Lppncott W & W.

Brainstorms Woman: Epilepsy in Our Lives. Steven C. Schachter et al. 2000. 144p. pap. text 35.00 (*0-7817-2749-9*) Lppncott W & W.

Brainwashing-Deprogramming Controversy: Sociological, Psychological, Legal & Historical Perspectives. Ed. by David G. Bromley & James T. Richardson. 1983. LC 83-4346. (Studies in Religion & Society: Vol. 5). 376p. lib. bdg. 99.95 (*0-88946-868-0*) E Mellen.

Branch Chain Amino Acids for Health. 1996. lib. bdg. 250.75 (*0-8490-5905-4*) Gordon Pr.

Branched Chain Amino & Keto Acids in Health & Disease. S. A. Adibi. Ed. by S. A. Adibi et al. 1985. (Illus.). xiv, 572p. 129.75 (*3-8055-3996-7*) S Karger.

Branching Processes Applied to Cell Surface Aggregation Phenomena. C. A. Macken & Alan S. Perelson. 1985. (Lecture Notes in Biomathematics: Vol. 58). 122p. 31.95 (*0-387-15656-9*) Spr-Verlag.

Branding Health Services: Defining Yourself in the Marketplace. Gilbert G. Bashe & Nancy J. Hicks. 2000. LC 99-88085. (Illus.). 304p. 54.00 (*0-8342-1175-0*) Aspen Pub.

Branemark Osseointegrated Implant. Ed. by Thomas Albrektsson & George A. Zarb. 1989. LC 89-3685. (Illus.). 262p. text 132.00 (*0-86715-208-7*) Quint Pub Co.

Brass Errings: A Case Study of a Mental Patient. Sarah A. Edwards. 1999. LC 99-95042. pap. 10.95 (*0-533-13274-6*) Vantage.

Brass Tacks: Oral Biography of a Twentieth Century Physician. Adelaide Suits. 1985. LC 84-81444. 144p. pap. text 10.00 (*0-916717-00-3*) Halyburton.

Brassinosteroids: A New Class of Plant Hormones. V. A. Khripach et al. 1998. LC 98-87079. (Illus.). 456p. (C). 85.00 (*0-12-406360-8*) Acad Pr.

Braunwald's Heart Disease: Review & Assessment. Michael Mendelsohn. 3rd ed. 1997. (Illus.). 300p. pap. text 52.00 (*0-7216-6631-0*) Saunders.

Braving the Void: Journeys into Healing. Michael Greenwood. Ed. by Susan Clark. 2000. 318p. pap. (*0-9695822-1-8*) Prdox Pubng CAN. *Dist:* New Centry Pr.

Brazilian Medical Contributions. Leonidio Ribeiro. 1976. lib. bdg. 69.95 (*0-8490-1548-0*) Gordon Pr.

Brazil's National Alcohol Program: Technology & Development in an Authoritarian Regime. F. Joseph Demetrius. 1990. LC 89-16243. 181p. 60.00 (*0-275-93183-8*, C3183, Praeger Pubs) Greenwood.

Brazos Vacios: Como Vivir con el Aborto la Muerte Prenatala y la Muerte Infantil. Sherokee Ilse. 1999.Tr. of Empty Arms - Coping with Miscarriage, Stillbirth & Infant Loss. (SPA.). 96p. reprint ed. pap. 9.50 (*0-9609456-7-9*) Wntergrn.

Break in Your Cycle: The Medical & Emotional Causes & Effects of Amenorrhea. Theresa Francis-Cheung. 1998. 176p. pap. 14.95 (*0-471-34663-2*); LC 98-230252. pap. 14.95 (*1-56561-164-0*) Wiley.

Break the Anger Trap. Betty Doty. 1985. LC 85-71508. (Illus.). 90p. (Orig.). pap. 8.95 (*0-930822-06-4*) Bookery.

Break the Stress Cycle! 10 Steps to Reducing Stress for Women. Judith Sachs. 1998. LC 97-45179. 256p. pap. 9.95 (*1-58062-007-8*) Adams Media.

Breakdown: A Personal Crisis & a Medical Dilemma. Stuart Sutherland. 2nd ed. 1998. 320p. (C). 35.00 (*0-19-852380-7*) OUP.

Breakdown & Breakthrough: Psychotherapy in a New Dimension. Nathan Field. 1996. LC 96-5997. 168p. (C). 84.95 (*0-415-10957-4*); pap. 27.95 (*0-415-10958-2*) Routledge.

Breakdown in Human Adaptation to 'Stress' Towards a Multidisciplinary Approach Ed. by J. Cullen et al. 1983. lib. bdg. 144.00 (*0-89838-607-1*) Kluwer Academic.

Breakdown of Speech: Causes & Remediation. Nancy R. Milloy. (Therapy in Practice Ser.: No. 20). pap. 32.50 (*0-412-31550-5*) Chapman & Hall.

Breaking Addictions. 1996. lib. bdg. 252.99 (*0-8490-5904-6*) Gordon Pr.

Breaking Destructive Patterns: Multiple Strategies for Treating Partner Abuse. Janet A. Geller. 1992. LC 91-47754. 182p. 35.00 (*0-02-911605-8*) Free Pr.

Breaking Free from Compulsive Eating. Geneen Roth. 1993. LC 93-13034. 242p. reprint ed. pap. 12.95 (*0-452-27084-7*, Plume) Dutton Plume.

Breaking Free of Managed Care: A Step-by-Step Guide to Regaining Control of Your Practice. Dana C. Ackley. 1997. LC 96-48406. (Clinician's Toolbox Ser.). 317p. text 42.00 (*1-57230-105-8*, 0105) Guilford Pubns.

Breaking New Ground: Developing Innovative AIDS Care Residences. Betsy Lieberman & Donald Chamberlain. 1993. 311p. pap. 39.95 (*0-9639595-0-6*); LC 93-71111. 250p. pap. text 39.95 (*0-9636595-0-2*) AIDS Hse WA.

Breaking Out of Environmental Illness: Essential Reading for Anyone with Chronic Fatigue Syndrome, Allergies, & Chemical Sensitivities. Robert Sampson & Patricia Hughes. 1997. LC 97-7512. 272p. (Orig.). pap. 14.00 (*1-879181-41-X*) Bear & Co.

Breaking the Bonds of Irritable Bowel Syndrome: A Psychological Approach to Regaining Control of Your Life. Barbara Bradley Bolen. 2000. (Illus.). 177p. pap. 14.95 (*1-57224-188-8*) New Harbinger.

Breaking the Fine Rain of Death: African American Health Issues & a Womanist Ethic of Care. Emilie M. Townes. 1998. LC 92-36883. 224p. 24.95 (*0-8264-1121-5*) Continuum.

Breaking the Impasse in the War on Drugs, 159. Steven Wisotsky. 1986. LC 86-7574. (Contributions in Political Science Ser.: No. 159). 293p. 66.00 (*0-313-24266-6*, WLW/, Greenwood Pr) Greenwood.

Breaking the Patterns of Depression. Michael D. Yapko. 1998. 384p. pap. 12.95 (*0-385-48370-8*) Doubleday.

Breaking the Rules: Counseling Ethnic Minorities. Celina Pagani-Tousignant. 1992. 40p. pap. 5.95 (*1-56246-031-5*, 3274, HazeldenJohnson Inst) Hazelden.

Breaking the Rules: Women in Prison & Feminist Therapy. Ed. by Judy Harden & Marcia Hill. 1998. LC 97-45550. 194p. pap. 19.95 (*1-56023-107-6*, Harrington Park); (Women & Therapy Monograph Ser.: Vol. 20, No. 4 & Vol. 21, No. 1). 49.95 (*0-7890-0365-1*) Haworth Pr.

Breaking the Silence: A Guide to Help Children with Complicated Grief: Suicide, Homicide, AIDS, Violence, & Abuse. Linda Goldman. 1996. LC 96-13029. 256p. pap. text 31.95 (*1-56032-434-1*) Taylor & Francis.

Breaking the Silence: Art Therapy with Children from Violent Homes. Cathy A. Malchiodi. 1990. LC 90-1466. (Illus.). 230p. text 30.95 (*0-87630-578-8*) Brunner-Routledge.

Breaking the Silence: Group Therapy for Childhood Sexual Abuse - A Practitioner's Manual. Judith A. Margolin. 1998. LC 98-39343. (Illus.). 152p. lib. bdg. 29.95 (*0-7890-0200-0*) Haworth Pr.

Breaking the Stress Habit: A Modern Guide to One Minute Stress Management. Andrew Goliszek. 1987. 266p. 16.95 (*0-9616475-2-3*); pap. 9.95 (*0-9616475-3-1*) Healthnet Pr.

Breaking the Vicious Cycle: Intestinal Health Through Diet. Elaine Gottschall. 2nd rev. ed. 1994. (Illus.). 170p. pap. (*0-9692768-1-8*) Kirkton Pr.

Breaking the Walls of Silence: AIDS & Women in a New York State Maximum Security Prison. A. C. E. Program of the Bedford Hills Correctional Staff. 1998. LC 92-35997. (Illus.). 336p. 29.95 (*0-87951-500-7*, Elephants Eye) Overlook Pr.

Breaking Through... Alternative Pathways to Healing. Polly A. Petersen. Ed. by Frank J. Thomason. 1997. (Illus.). 184p. pap. 18.95 (*0-9655549-1-0*) Table Top.

Breaking Your Prescribed Addiction: A Guide to Coming off Tranquilizers, Antidepressants, Pain Pills & More, Using Amino Acids & Nutrients. Billie Jay Sahley & Katherine M. Birkner. 3rd ed. 1998. LC 98-65759. (Illus.). 132p. pap. 9.95 (*1-889391-09-3*) Pain & Stress.

Breakthrough: The Race to Find the Breast Cancer Gene. Kevin Davies & Michael James Denham White. 1996. LC 95-30911. 310p. 24.95 (*0-471-12025-1*) Wiley.

Breakthrough for Back Pain! William V. Zucker & Brian W. Nelson. 1992. (Illus.). 213p. (Orig.). pap. 15.00 (*0-9634440-0-X*) Lester St Pub.

Breakthrough Leadership: Achieving Organizational Alignment Through Hoshin Planning. Mara M. Melum & Casey Collett. 1995. LC 94-48029. 344p. 69.00 (*1-55648-133-0*) AHPI.

Breakthroughs in Antipsychotic Medications. Peter J. Weidenbeck, Jr. 1999. LC 99-17205. 240p. pap. 22.95 (*0-393-70303-7*) Norton.

Breakthroughs in Family Therapy with Drug Abusing & Problem Youth. Jose Szapocznik & William M. Kurtines. 1989. 208p. 29.95 (*0-8261-6850-7*) Springer Pub.

Breakthroughs in Medicine: From Superstition to Empirical & Scientific Medicine. David Erlik. 1992. 208p. (*965-229-078-5*) Gefen Pub Hse ISR. *Dist:* Gefen Bks.

Breakthroughs in Natural Healing. David G. Williams. 1992. 25p. pap. 9.95 (*0-944649-09-2*) Mtn Home Pub.

Breast: Comprehensive Management of Benign & Malignant Diseases. Kirby I. Bland & Edward M. Copeland, III. 2nd ed. 1998. LC 97-135. (Illus.). 1824p. (C). text 225.00 (*0-7216-6656-6*) Saunders.

Breast: Guides to Clinical Aspiration Biopsy. Tilde S. Kline. 1989. LC 89-1938. (Illus.). 272p. 87.50 (*0-89640-159-6*) Igaku-Shoin.

Breast: Science & Surgery. P. Forrest. 1998. (Illus.). 300p. (*0-443-04997-1*) Church.

Breast & Gynecologic Cancer Epidemiology. J. L. Kelsey & N. G. Hildreth. 1983. LC 82-9629. 101.00 (*0-8493-6385-3*, CRC Reprint) Franklin.

Breast Awareness: Breast Lumps & Cancer. S. Eva Singletary. 1994. (OB-GYN Ser.). 32p. pap. text 2.95 (*1-885274-04-1*) Health InfoNet Inc.

Breast Book. Miriam Stoppard. 1996. LC 95-44848. (Illus.). 208p. pap. 24.95 (*0-7894-0420-6*) DK Pub Inc.

***Breast Cancer.** 1997. pap. (*1-85343-369-1*) Free Assoc Bks GBR. *Dist:* Intl Spec Bk.

Breast Cancer. Patrick I. Borgen & Arnold Hill. 2000. spiral bd. 45.00 (*1-57059-578-X*) Landes Bioscience.

Breast Cancer. Leah Cartabruno. 1992. 21p. pap. (*1-58703-005-5*, CRB-92-004) CA Res Bureau.

Breast Cancer. Lesley Fallowfield & Andrew Clark. Ed. by Psychology Staff. 1993. (Experience of Illness Ser.). 160p. (C). (gr. 13). pap. 24.99 (*0-415-03841-3*, A7633) Routledge.

Breast Cancer. Ed. by Barth Hoogstraten & Robert W. McDivitt. 1981. 304p. 172.00 (*0-8493-5731-4*, RC280, CRC Reprint) Franklin.

***Breast Cancer.** Ed. by Kelly K. Hunt. 2001. LC 2001-20191. (Cancer Care Ser.). (Illus.). 504p. pap. 59.95 (*0-387-95190-3*) Spr-Verlag.

Breast Cancer. John J. Kavanagh et al. 1998. LC 99-167587. (Illus.). viii, 187p. 99.95 (*0-632-04431-4*) Blackwell Sci.

Breast Cancer. Judith Peacock. 2000. LC 00-12364. (Perspectives on Disease & Illness Ser.). (Illus.). (J). (gr. 5-12). lib. bdg. 23.93 (*0-7368-1028-5*, LifeMatters Bks) Capstone Pr.

Breast Cancer. Ed. by S. E. Singletary. 1998. LC 98-4702. (M. D. Anderson Solid Tumor Oncology Ser.: Vol. 2). (Illus.). 296p. 95.00 (*0-387-98369-4*) Spr-Verlag.

Breast Cancer. David J. Winchester & David P. Winchester. 1999. LC 00-421468. (ACS Atlas of Clinical Oncology Ser.). (Illus.). viii, 294p. incl. cd-rom (*1-55009-112-3*) DEKR.

Breast Cancer, Vol. 1. Ed. by Edwin W. Salzman. 1990. (NEJM Reprint Collection). (Illus.). 420p. pap. 39.00 (*0-910133-18-2*); text 65.00 (*0-910133-24-7*) Mass Med Pub Div.

Breast Cancer: A Family Survival Guide. Lucille M. Pederson & Janet M. Trigg. 1995. LC 94-37836. 304p. pap. 24.00 (*0-89789-438-3*); 72.50 (*0-89789-293-3*) Greenwood (Bergin & Garvey).

Breast Cancer: A Guide for Fellows. Ed. by Orlando E. Silva & Stefano Zurrida. 1999. 324p. pap. 70.00 (*0-444-50117-7*) Elsevier.

Breast Cancer: A Guide to Detection & Multidisciplinary Therapy. Ed. by Michael H. Torosian. 2002. (Current Clinical Oncology Ser.). 425p. 125.00 (*0-89603-839-4*) Humana.

Breast Cancer: A Practical Guide to Diagnosis, Vol. 1. Wende W. Logan-Young & Nancy Yanes-Hoffman. 1994. (Illus.). 500p. 110.00 (*0-9640886-1-4*) Mount Hope Pub.

Breast Cancer: A Practical Guide to Diagnosis & Treatment. Ed. by Lewis Venet. 1979. text 30.00 (*0-88331-116-X*) R B Luce.

Breast Cancer: A Psychological Treatment Manual. Sandra Haber. 1994. LC 94-35284. (Illus.). 160p. 27.95 (*0-8261-8790-0*) Springer Pub.

Breast Cancer: An Annotated Guide to the Current Literature. Ed. by N. G. Arashvili. annot. ed. 1995. 202p. pap. text 95.00 (*1-56072-112-X*) Nova Sci Pubs.

Breast Cancer: Can You Prevent It? James S. Lawson & Amelia Lawson. 1999. (Illus.). 224p. pap. 24.95 (*0-07-470723-X*) McGraw-Hill Prof.

Breast Cancer: Causes, Prevention & Treatment. Agatha Thrash & Calvin L. Thrash. 1999. (Illus.). 126p. pap. 12.95 (*0-942658-14-0*) NLB.

Breast Cancer: Diagnosis & Management. J. M. Dixon. 2000. LC 00-49024. (Illus.). 436p. 109.00 (*0-444-50011-1*) Elsevier.

Breast Cancer: Diagnosis & Treatment: A Special Report from the Editors of Women's Health Advisor. Marianne Doran. Ed. by Orli Etingin & Gabrielle Weiner. 2000. (Illus.). 59p. pap. 19.95 (*1-929942-06-0*) Torstar.

Breast Cancer: Health Care Needs Assessment; the Epidemiologically Based Needs Assessment Reviews, No. 2. Andrew Stevens et al. 1997. LC 97-13351. (*1-85775-216-3*) Radcliffe Med Pr GBR. *Dist:* Balogh.

Breast Cancer: Journey to Recovery. Carroll N. Hoskins et al. 2001. LC 00-46388. (Illus.). viii, 128p. pap. (*0-8261-1392-3*) Springer Pub.

Breast Cancer? Let Me Check My Schedule! Peggy McCarthy & John Loren. 1997. LC 97-16378. 288p. pap. 14.00 (*0-465-00763-5*) Basic.

***Breast Cancer: Market Opportunities for Novel Diagnostic & Therapeutic Approaches.** Kate Sheldon. Ed. by Susan C. DiClemente & Sarah L. Young. 2001. (Illus.). 233p. spiral bd. 4950.00 (*1-57936-172-2*, 9027, D&MD Reports) International Business.

Breast Cancer: Molecular Genetics, Pathogenesis & Therapeutics. Anne M. Bowcock. 1999. LC 98-21525. (Contemporary Cancer Research Ser.). 608p. 145.00 (*0-89603-560-3*) Humana.

Breast Cancer: Myths & Facts, What You Need to Know. Alice F. Judkins & S. Eva Singletary. 1997. (Illus.). 56p. (Orig.). pap. (*0-9641823-3-5*) PRR.

Breast Cancer: Myths & Facts: What You Need to Know. S. Eva Singletary & Alice F. Judkins. (Illus.). 56p. (Orig.). 1998. (SPA.). pap. 9.95 (*1-891483-03-X*); 1997. pap. 9.95 (*0-9641823-7-8*) PRR.

Breast Cancer: Origins, Detection & Treatment. Ed. by Marvin A. Rich et al. 1986. (Developments in Oncology Ser.). text 120.50 (*0-89838-792-2*) Kluwer Academic.

Breast Cancer: Physician's Volume. Daniel F. Roses. 1999. LC 98-12904. 688p. (C). text (*0-443-05581-5*) Church.

Breast Cancer: Poisons, Profits & Prevention. Liane Clorfene-Casten. 1996. LC 96-29233. 342p. pap. 18.95 (*1-56751-094-9*); 350p. lib. bdg. 29.95 (*1-56751-095-7*) Common Courage.

Breast Cancer: Progress in Biology, Clinical Management & Prevention. Ed. by Marvin A. Rich et al. 1989. (Developments in Oncology Ser.). (C). text 118.50 (*0-7923-0507-8*) Kluwer Academic.

Breast Cancer: Questions & Answers for Young Women. Carole Garbuny Vogel. 2001. LC 00-32569. (Single Titles Ser.). (Illus.). 176p. (J). (gr. 7-12). lib. bdg. 25.90 (*0-7613-1855-0*) TFC Bks NY.

Breast Cancer: Scientific & Clinical Progress. Ed. by Marvin A. Rich et al. 1988. (C). text 190.00 (*0-89838-387-0*) Kluwer Academic.

Breast Cancer: Strategies for Husbands to Support Their Wives. James K. Eckmann. 1995. LC 94-69145. (Illus.). 102p. (Orig.). pap. 9.95 (*0-9644135-0-7*) Nehemiah Pubng.

Breast Cancer: Textbook for General Practitioners. Ed. by Europe Against Cancer Staff & U. Veronesi. 1990. (EC Series for General Practitioners). (Illus.). 67p. 47.95 (*0-387-53102-5*) Spr-Verlag.

Breast Cancer: The Complete Guide. Yashar Hirshaut et al. 3rd rev. ed. 2000. LC 00-39279. (Illus.). 256p. pap. 15.95 (*0-553-38081-8*, Delta Trade) Dell.

Breast Cancer: The Psychological Effects of the Disease & Its Treatment. Karin Gyllenskold. Tr. by Patricia Crampton. 1982. (*0-422-76820-0*, NO. 3623) Tavistock GBR. *Dist:* Routldge.

Breast Cancer: The Social Construction of an Illness. Susan J. Ferguson & Anne S. Kasper. 2000. 400p. 27.50 (*0-312-21710-2*) St Martin.

Breast Cancer: Twenty Women's Stories. Susan D. Moch & Allan Graubard. 1995. 162p. pap. 19.95 (*0-88737-654-1*) Natl League Nurse.

Breast Cancer: Twenty Women's Stories: Becoming More Alive Through the Experience. Susan D. Moch & Allan Graubard. 1995. 12.95 (*0-88737-669-X*) Natl League Nurse.

Breast Cancer: What Every Woman Should Know. Paul Rodriguez. 1988. (Illus.). 138p. (Orig.). pap. text 11.45 (*0-9622118-0-X*) Aurora KS.

Breast Cancer: What You Should Know (But May Not Be Told) about Prevention, Diagnosis & Treatment. Steve Austin & Cathy Hitchcock. 1994. LC 93-49716. (Illus.). 336p. pap. 16.00 (*1-55958-362-2*) Prima Pub.

Breast Cancer: What You Should Know (but May Not Have Been Told) about Prevention, Diagnosis & Treatment. Steve Austin & Cathy Hitchcock. 2nd rev. ed. 2000. 336p. pap. 16.00 (*0-7615-1258-6*) Prima Pub.

***Breast Cancer - Beyond Convention: The World's Foremost Authorities on Complementary & Alternative Medicine Offer Advice on Healing.** Ed. by Mary Tagliaferri et al. 2002. (Illus.). 384p. 26.00 (*0-7434-1011-4*, PB Hardcover) PB.

Breast Cancer - Biological & Clinical Progress: Proceedings of the Conference of the International Association for Breast Cancer Research, St. Vincent, Aosta Valley, Italy, May 26-29, 1991. Ed. by L. Dogliotti. 1992. (Developments in Oncology Ser.). 336p. (C). text 163.50 (*0-7923-1655-X*) Kluwer Academic.

Breast Cancer - Black Woman. Edwin T. Johnson. 2nd rev. ed. 2000. LC 98-86265. (Illus.). xxi, 240p. 24.75 (*0-9635435-1-2*) Van Slyke Bray.

Breast Cancer - Patient Volume. D. F. Roses. 1998. (Illus.). 200p. pap. (*0-443-05582-3*) Church.

Breast Cancer - Physician & Patient Volumes D. F. Roses. 1998. (*0-443-05613-7*) Church.

Breast Cancer - Treatments & Therapy Including Drugs: Index of New Information. Audrey M. Anson. 1996. 150p. pap. 47.50 (*0-7883-0905-6*) ABBE Pubs Assn.

Breast Cancer? Breast Health! The Wise Woman Way. Susun S. Weed. 1996. LC 94-71323. (Wise Woman Herbal Ser.: No. 4). (Illus.). 380p. (Orig.). pap. 14.95 (*0-9614620-7-8*) Ash Tree.

Breast Cancer? Let Me Check My Schedule! Donna Cederberg et al. 1994. 250p. pap. 12.95 (*0-9641386-0-3*) Innovat Med.

Breast Cancer & You: Bettering the Odds. Martha L. Grigg. Ed. by Adolph Caso. 1995. (Illus.). 195p. pap. 14.95 (*0-8283-2010-1*) Branden Bks.

Breast Cancer & You: International Breast Cancer Treatments. Michael L. Holcomb. 1998. 300p. pap. 34.95 (*0-9644990-3-7*) Intl Toxicol.

***Breast Cancer Case Studies.** Harnett. 2001. (Illus.). 148p. (*1-84110-054-4*) Greenwich Med GBR. *Dist:* JAMCO Dist.

Breast Cancer Collaborative Management. Ed. by Jay K. Harness et al. 1988. (Illus.). 390p. lib. bdg. 97.00 (*0-87371-106-8*, L106) Lewis Pubs.

Breast Cancer, Fat & Adipose Tissue with Toxic & Non-Toxic Chemicals & Residues: Index of New Information. John C. Bartone. 1997. 160p. 57.50 (*0-7883-1714-8*); pap. 47.50 (*0-7883-1715-6*) ABBE Pubs Assn.

Breast Cancer Handbook: Taking Control after You've Found a Lump. Joan Swirsky. 2nd ed. 1998. pap. text 12.95 (*1-888315-05-9*) Power NY.

Breast Cancer Immunodiagnosis & Immunotherapy. Ed. by Roberto L. Ceriani. 1989. (Illus.). 272p. 85.00 (*0-306-43338-9*, Plenum Trade) Perseus Pubng.

***Breast Cancer in African-American Women.** Ed. by Lovell Allan Jones. 2001. 500p. 95.00 (*1-57331-356-4*) NY Acad Sci.

Breast Cancer in the Life Course: Women's Experiences. Ed. by Julianne S. Oktay & Carolyn Walter. 1991. (Social Work Ser.: Vol. 20). 232p. 28.95 (*0-8261-7110-9*) Springer Pub.

Breast Cancer in Younger Women. 1997. lib. bdg. 250.99 (*0-8490-8154-8*) Gordon Pr.

Breast Cancer-Its Impact on the Patient, Family, & Community: Proceedings of the San Francisco Cancer Symposium, 11th, San Francisco, California, November, 1975. San Francisco Cancer Symposium Staff. Ed. by J. M. Vaeth. 1976. (Frontiers of Radiation Therapy & Oncology Ser.: Vol. 11). (Illus.). 200p. 76.75 (*3-8055-2340-8*) S Karger.

Breast Cancer Journal: A Century of Petals. Juliet Wittman. 1993. LC 92-54765. 304p. 21.95 (*1-55591-136-6*) Fulcrum Pub.

Breast Cancer: Myths & Facts: What You Need to Know. S. Eva Singletary & Alice F. Judkins. rev. ed. 2001. (Myths & Facts Series). (Illus.). 49p. pap. 9.95 (*1-891483-10-2*) PRR.

***Breast Cancer New Medical Therapies.** 2000. 14.99 (*0-9673029-7-8*) CenterWatch.

Breast Cancer, 1971-91: Prevention, Treatment, & Research. 1995. (Illus.). 48p. (Orig.). (C). pap. text 25.00 (*0-7881-2354-8*) DIANE Pub.

***Breast Cancer Nursing.** 1995. pap. 35.95 (*0-412-41200-4*) Chapman & Hall.

Breast Cancer Nursing. S. Denton. 1995. (Illus.). 256p. pap. text 57.50 (*1-56593-033-9*, 0281) Thomson Learn.

Breast Cancer Prevention Diet: The Powerful Foods, Supplements & Drugs That Can Save Your Life. Bob Arnot. l.t. ed. 1999. (Nonfiction Ser.). 303p. 30.95 (*0-7838-8563-6*, Thorndike) Gale.

Breast Cancer Prevention Program. Samuel S. Epstein & David Steinman. 2000. 416p. (C). reprint ed. text 25.00 (*0-7881-6910-6*) DIANE Pub.

Breast Cancer Prevention Program: The First Complete Survey of the Causes of Breast Cancer. Samuel S. Epstein et al. 1997. LC 97-22253. 416p. 24.95 (*0-02-536192-9*) Hungry Minds.

Breast Cancer Research Stamp: Millions Raised for Research, but Better Cost Recovery Criteria Needed. Ed. by Bernard L. Ungar. 2000. 51p. pap. text 20.00 (*0-7567-0327-1*) DIANE Pub.

Breast Cancer Screening. Ismail Jatoi. 1997. LC 97-15077. (Medical Intelligence Unit Ser.). 187p. 99.00 (*1-57059-457-0*) Landes Bioscience.

Breast Cancer Screening. Ismail Jatoi. 1997. (Medical Intelligence Unit Ser.). 200p. pap. 89.95 (*0-412-14161-2*) Thomson Learn.

Breast Cancer Screening in Europe. Ed. by A. Gad & M. Rosselli Del Turco. 1993. LC 93-13231. (Monographs of the European School of Oncology). (Illus.). 148p. 128.00 (*0-387-56577-9*) Spr-Verlag.

Breast Cancer Survival Manual: A Step-by-Step Guide for the Woman with Newly Diagnosed Breast Cancer. John Link. 2nd rev. ed. 2000. LC 99-47515. (Illus.). 224p. pap. 15.00 (*0-8050-6400-1*, Owl) H Holt & Co.

Breast Cancer Survival Rates & Health Plan Services. Joel Cohen. 2000. 23p. pap. (*1-58703-118-3*, CRB-00-001) CA Res Bureau.

Breast Cancer Survivors' Club: A Nurse's Experience. Lillie Shockney. rev. ed. 1996. LC 96-44260. 269p. pap. 12.95 (*1-881636-22-4*) Windsor Hse Pub Grp.

***Breast Cancer, There & Back: A Woman-to-Woman Guide.** Jami Bernard. 2001. LC 2001-17943. 272p. pap. (*0-446-67753-1*) Warner.

Breast Cancer Treatment Options. Robert P. Lenk. 1998. (Illus.). 279p. lib. bdg. 37.00 (*1-56072-396-3*) Nova Sci Pubs.

Breast Cancer Wars: Hope, Fear & the Pursuit of a Cure in Twentieth-Century America. Barron H. Lerner & Barron Lerner. 2001. LC 00-6391. (Illus.). 400p. 30.00 (*0-19-514261-6*) OUP.

Breast Cancers: Index of New Information - Chemically Induced. John C. Bartone. 1995. (Illus.). 160p. 57.50 (*0-7883-0698-7*); pap. 47.50 (*0-7883-0699-5*) ABBE Pubs Assn.

Breast Carcinoma: Risk & Detection. Cushman D. Haagensen et al. 3rd ed. 1981. LC 80-53370. 542p. text 140.00 (*0-7216-4438-4*) Saunders.

Breast Care. Deni Bown et al. 1997. LC 97-17384. (101 Essential Tips Ser.). (Illus.). 72p. pap. 3.95 (*0-7894-1975-0*) DK Pub Inc.

Breast Care: A Clinical Guidebook for Women's Primary Health Care Providers. Ed. by William H. Hindle. 1998. LC 97-49307. (Illus.). 484p. 79.00 (*0-387-98348-1*) Spr-Verlag.

Breast Care Options. Paul Kuehn. 1986. LC 86-61100. (Illus.). 178p. 17.95 (*0-938539-00-0*) Newmark Pub.

Breast Care Options for the 1990's. Paul Kuehn. 1991. LC 91-60345. 255p. 19.95 (*0-938539-04-3*) Newmark Pub.

Breast Conservation vs. Mastectomy: Patient Survival in Day-to-Day Medical Practice & in Randomized Studies. 1995. (Illus.). 48p. (Orig.). (C). pap. text 35.00 (*0-7881-1691-6*) DIANE Pub.

Breast Cytopathology: A Diagnostic Atlas. Peter A. Trott. 1995. (Illus.). 168p. (*0-412-28280-1*) E A GBR. *Dist:* OUP.

Breast Disease. Douglas J. Marchant. Ed. by William Schmitt. 1997. LC 96-51068. (Illus.). 288p. text 52.00 (*0-7216-6429-6*) Saunders.

Breast Disease. Ed. by H. J. Stewart et al. 1991. (British Medical Bulletin Ser.: Vol. 47, No. 2). (Illus.). 264p. text (*0-443-04492-9*) Church.

***Breast Disease: A Problem-Based Approach.** J. Michael Dixon & Monica Morrow. 1999. (Illus.). 228p. pap. (*0-7020-2325-6*) W B Saunders GBR. *Dist:* Saunders.

Breast Disease for Clinicians. Barbara B. Bennett et al. 2001. LC 00-140210. (Illus.). 238p. text 65.00 (*0-8385-0514-7*) McGraw-Hill Prof.

Breast Disease for Primary Care Physicians. B. A. Eskin et al. 1998. LC 98-22292. (Illus.). 184p. lib. bdg. 64.95 (*1-85070-744-8*, Parthenon Pbng) CRC Pr.

Breast Disease in Women & Men: A Clinician's Handbook. Pam Shuler. 1993. (Illus.). pap. text 12.95 (*0-929240-54-5*) EMIS.

Breast Disease Test & Syllabus. Edward A. Sickles et al. 1993. LC 93-41764. (Professional Self-Evaluation & Continuing Education Program: Vol. 36). (Illus.). 470p. 220.00 (*1-55903-037-2*) Am Coll Radiology.

Breast Diseases. Jay R. Harris et al. 1987. LC 65-9244. (Illus.). 751p. text 99.00 (*0-397-50760-7*, Lippnctt) Lppncott W & W.

Breast Epithelial Antigens. Ed. by Roberto L. Ceriani. 1991. (Illus.). 256p. (C). text 114.00 (*0-306-44009-1*, Kluwer Plenum) Kluwer Academic.

Breast Feeding: A Guide for Midwives. Dora Henschell. 1995. LC 96-115857. 136p. pap. text 25.00 (*1-898507-12-0*) Buttrwrth-Heinemann.

Breast Feeding & Child Development. B. K. Mishra. 1993. viii, 178p. (*81-7024-567-2*) Ashish Pub Hse IND. *Dist:* Nataraj Bks.

Breast-Feeding & Fertility. Ed. by G. Hafez & K. Bagchi. 1995. (Regional Publications, Eastern Mediterranean Ser.: Vol. 13). 55p. (C). pap. 9.00 (*92-9021-171-7*, 1440013) World Health.

Breast-Feeding Patterns: A Review of Studies in the Eastern Mediterranean Region. Contrib. by A. O. Musaiger & J. K. Harfouche. 2nd rev. ed. 1993. (EMRO Technical Publications: No. 4). ix, 231p. pap. text 9.00 (*92-9021-156-3*, 1452004) World Health.

Breast Fitness: An Optimal Exercise & Health An Optimal Exercise & Health Plan for Reducing Your Risk of Breast Cancer. Anne Mctiernan et al. 2000. LC 00-31817. (Illus.). xii, 333p. 25.95 (*0-312-25312-5*) St Martin.

***Breast Fitness: An Optimal Exercise & Health Plan for Reducing Your Risk of Breast Cancer.** Anne Mctiernan et al. 2001. (Illus.). 352p. pap. 14.95 (*0-312-26298-1*, St Martin Griffin) St Martin.

Breast Health. Miriam Stoppard. 1998. LC 97-46128. (DK Healthcare Ser.). (Illus.). 96p. pap. 7.95 (*0-7894-3096-7*) DK Pub Inc.

Breast Health: A Guide for Women. Eva Singletary. Ed. by William Spellacey. 2000. (Gyn Ser.). (Illus.). 13p. (Orig.). pap. text 1.95 (*1-885274-63-7*) Health InfoNet Inc.

Breast Health Vol. 4: Women's Health Discourses. Jack Tips. 1996. 26p. 7.95 (*0-929167-17-1*) Apple-a-Day.

Breast Health Cookbook: Fast & Simple Recipes to Reduce the Risk of Breast Cancer. Robert Arnot et al. 2001. LC 00-46942. 272p. 25.95 (*0-316-05133-0*) Little.

Breast Health Medical Information Delivery System: 230 Breast Health Patient Teaching Topics. Judy C. Kneece. 1995. 300p. pap. (*1-886665-03-6*) EduCare Pub.

Breast Health the Natural Way: Six Step Natural Program to Optimal Breast Wellness with Nutrition, Herbal Medicine, Exercise & Mind-Body Techniques. Deborah Gordon et al. 2001. LC 00-66252. (Women's Natural Health Ser.). (Illus.). 288p. pap. 14.95 (*0-471-37958-1*) Wiley.

***Breast Health with Nutribionics: The Mysteries of Eastern Medicine & Nutrition Are Unlocked to Fight Breast Diseases.** Romi Roy. 2000. pap. 22.95 (*1-56492-348-7*) Laredo.

Breast Imaging. Daniel B. Kopans. 2nd ed. 1997. 896p. 375.00 (*0-7817-2027-3*); 299.00 (*0-7817-1953-4*); LC 97-34814. text 225.00 (*0-397-51302-X*) Lppncott W & W.

Breast Imaging: A Teaching File. Gilda Cardenosa. 1998. (Teaching File Ser.). (Illus.). (*0-683-30218-3*) Lppncott W & W.

Breast Imaging: Diagnosis & Morphology of Breast Diseases. Robert L. Egan. 1988. (Illus.). 656p. text 152.00 (*0-7216-2320-4*) Saunders.

Breast Imaging Companion. Gilda Cardenosa. 2nd ed. 2000. LC 00-60600. (Illus.). 512p. pap. text 65.00 (*0-7817-2891-6*) Lppncott W & W.

Breast Implant Story: Communication & Uncertainty. Marsha L. Vanderford & David H. Smith. 1996. LC 96-13566. (LEA's Communication Ser.). 312p. text 49.95 (*0-8058-1706-9*); pap. text 22.50 (*0-8058-1707-7*) L Erlbaum Assocs.

Breast Implants: An Informative Update, 1998. Ed. by Sharon S. Holston. rev. ed. 2000. 62p. pap. text 20.00 (*0-7881-8865-8*) DIANE Pub.

Breast Implants: Everything You Need to Know. Nancy Pauline Bruning. 2nd ed. 1995. LC 94-46995. (Illus.). 224p. 21.95 (*0-89793-176-9*); pap. 12.95 (*0-89793-175-0*) Hunter Hse.

Breast Implants - Harmful, Hostile & Sometimes Dangerous: Index of New Information. Ruby D. Kinkel. 1997. 177p. 57.50 (*0-7883-1584-6*); 1997. 177p. pap. text 47.50 (*0-7883-1585-4*); 1996. 150p. 57.50 (*0-7883-0906-4*); 1996. 150p. pap. 47.50 (*0-7883-0907-2*) ABBE Pubs Assn.

Breast Implants or Aspartame (Nutrasweet) Disease? The Suppressed Opinion about a Perceived Medicolegal Travesty. H. J. Roberts. 1999. LC 98-91122. 62p. pap. 12.00 (*1-884243-10-X*) Sunshine Sentinel.

Breast Pathology. Robert E. Fechner & Stacey E. Mills. 1990. LC 90-647. (Illus.). 182p. text 50.00 (*0-89189-298-2*, 16-1-049-00) Am Soc Clinical.

Breast Pathology: Diagnosis by Needle Core Biopsy. Paul P. Rosen. 1998. LC 98-31090. 336p. text 199.00 (*0-397-58790-2*) Lppncott W & W.

Breast Reconstruction. W. W. Shaw. 1998. (Illus.). 448p. text (*0-443-05684-6*) Church.

Breast Reconstruction Following Mastectomy for Carcinoma. William M. Cocke, Jr. 1977. text 27.50 (*0-316-14920-9*, Little Brwn Med Div) Lppncott W & W.

Breast Reconstruction with Autologous Tissue: Art & Artistry. Stephen S. Kroll. 1999. LC 98-51594. (Illus.). 400p. 280.00 (*0-387-98670-7*) Spr-Verlag.

A
B

Breast Self-Examination. Albert R. Milan. 1980. LC 79-56529. (Illus.). 128p. pap. 3.50 (*0-89480-124-4*, 419) Workman Pub.

Breast Sourcebook: Everything You Need to Know about Cancer Detection, Treatment, & Prevention. M Sara Rosenthal. 2nd ed. 1999. LC 99-54494. (Illus.). xvi, 360p. pap. 18.95 (*0-7373-0249-6*, 02496W) NTC Contemp Pub Co.

Breast Sourcebook: Everything You Need to Know about Cancer Detection, Treatment, & Prevention. M Sara Rosenthal. 2nd ed. 1997. 352p. reprint ed. pap. 16.00 (*1-56565-819-1*, Anodyne) Lowell Hse.

Breast Specimen Radiography. Eva Rubin & Jean F. Simpson. 1997. LC 98-114593. (Illus.). 224p. text 105.00 (*0-397-51667-3*) Lppncott W & W.

Breast Surgery. N. Bricout. Tr. by D. LeVay. 1996. (Illus.). 445p. pap. 185.00 (*2-287-59632-1*) Spr-Verlag.

***Breast Surgery.** John R. Farndon. 2nd ed. 2001. 220p. (*0-7020-2595-X*) W B Saunders GBR. *Dist:* Saunders.

Breast Ultrasound. C. Sohn. 1998. LC 98-38151. (Illus.). 174p. 59.00 (*0-86577-722-5*) Thieme Med Pubs.

Breast Ultrasound. A. Thomas Stavros. 1998. (Illus.). text 159.00 (*0-397-51624-X*) Lppncott W & W.

Breast Ultrasound Update. Ed. by H. Madjar et al. 1995. (Illus.). x, 376p. 100.00 (*3-8055-5860-0*) S Karger.

Breastfeed Book. Maire Messenger Davies. 1998. 128p. pap. (*0-7112-0677-5*) F Lincoln GBR. *Dist:* St Mut.

Breastfeeding. Karen Salt. 1999. LC 99-12294. (Baby Tips Ser.). (Illus.). 144p. pap. 6.95 (*1-55561-191-5*) Fisher Bks.

Breastfeeding: A Guide to the Medical Profession. Ruth A. Lawrence. 5th ed. 1998. LC 98-42918. (Illus.). 981p. (C). (gr. 13). text 54.95 (*0-8151-2615-8*, 31637) Mosby Inc.

Breastfeeding: A Mother's Gift. Pamela K. Wiggins. 1996. LC 96-94363. (Illus.). 176p. (Orig.). pap. 9.95 (*0-9623529-9-3*, 005) Lactation Assocs Pub.

Breastfeeding: A Problem-Solving Manual. Stephen Saunders et al. 4th ed. 1995. pap. 14.95 (*0-929240-68-5*) EMIS.

Breastfeeding: Something Special for Mother & Baby. Toni Berg. rev. ed. 1992. (Illus.). 26p. reprint ed. pap. 2.95 (*0-945886-10-1*) New Futures.

Breastfeeding: The Art of Mothering. Maurice Teitel et al. rev. ed. 1988. (Illus.). 48p. pap. 5.95 (*0-9618860-1-3*) Alive Prodns.

Breastfeeding & Human Lactation. Kathleen G. Auerbach & Janice Riordan. 1993. (Nursing-Health Science Ser.). (Illus.). 720p. (C). text 88.75 (*0-86720-343-9*, 343-9) Jones & Bartlett.

Breastfeeding & Human Lactation. Jan Riordan & Kathleen Auerbach. 2nd ed. 1998. LC 98-3502. (Nursing Ser.). (Illus.). 704p. (C). text 93.95 (*0-7637-0545-4*, 0545-4) Jones & Bartlett.

Breastfeeding & Human Lactation. Jan Riordan & Kathleen G. Auerbach. 2nd ed. 1999. (Illus.). (C). pap. text, stu. ed. 24.95 (*0-7637-0829-1*, 0829-1) Jones & Bartlett.

Breastfeeding Care: Setting the Environment, Supporting the Process. Ruth A. Lawrence et al. 1994. LC 94-29660. (*0-86525-058-8*) March of Dimes.

Breastfeeding Promotion Through the Women, Infants & Children (WIC) Program. 1994. (Illus.). 122p. (Orig.). (C). pap. text 35.00 (*0-7881-0568-X*) DIANE Pub.

Breastfeeding Pure & Simple. Gwen Gotsch. 2000. LC 93-80164. (Illus.). 117p. pap. 9.95 (*0-912500-42-5*) La Leche.

Breastfeeding Secrets & Solutions. Janis Graham. Ed. by Claire Zion. 1993. 256p. (Orig.). pap. 10.00 (*0-671-74963-3*) PB.

Breastfeeding Source Book: Where to Get What You Need to Breastfeed Successfully. Marilyn Grams. 1988. LC 88-6191. (Illus.). 220p. (Orig.). pap. 9.95 (*0-932707-17-3*) Achievement Pr.

Breastfeeding Sourcebook. M Sara Rosenthal. 2nd rev. ed. 1998. (Illus.). 336p. pap. 18.00 (*0-7373-0019-1*, 00191W) NTC Contemp Pub Co.

Breastfeeding Sourcebook: Everything You Need to Know. M Sara Rosenthal. 1996. 320p. pap. 16.00 (*1-56565-478-1*) Lowell Hse.

Breastfeeding Success for Working Mothers. Marilyn Grams. 1985. LC 85-71326. (Illus.). 160p. pap. 15.00 (*0-932707-14-9*) Achievement Pr.

Breastfeeding the Healthy Newborn: A Nursing Perspective. Marie Biancuzzo & Margaret Comberford Freda. Ed. by Karla Damus. 1994. (*0-86525-064-2*) March of Dimes.

Breastfeeding Triage Tool. Sandra Jolley & Ellen Phillips-Angeles. 4th rev. ed. 1998. (Illus.). 116p. pap., spiral bd. 10.00 (*1-893234-00-2*) Seattle-King Cty Dept.

Breath of Life: Mastering the Breathing Techniques of Pranayama & Qi Gong. George Ellis. Ed. by Gina R. Gross. 1993. (Illus.). 192p. (Orig.). pap. 12.95 (*0-87877-183-2*, New Page Bks) Career Pr Inc.

Breath Sounds Methodology. Noam Gavriely. 1995. LC 94-25914. 219p. 204.95 (*0-8493-5500-1*) CRC Pr.

Breathe! An Anti-Smoking Anthology. Ed. by Shel Horowitz. 1981. (Illus.). 62p. pap. 5.00 (*0-942292-08-1*) Warthog Pr.

Breathe Again Naturally. Bernard Jensen. 1983. pap. 12.99 (*0-932615-08-2*) B Jensen.

Breathe Better, Feel Better: Learn to Increase Your Energy, Control Anxiety & Anger, Relieve Health Problems & Just Relax with Simple Breathing Techniques. Howard Kent. 1997. LC 96-48544. (Illus.). 128p. pap. 27.95 (*1-882606-73-6*) Peoples Med Soc.

Breathe Free: Nutritional & Herbal Care for Your Respiratory System. Daniel Gagnon & Amadea Morningstar. 1991. LC 90-24413. (Illus.). 179p. (Orig.). pap. 14.95 (*0-914955-07-1*) Lotus Pr.

Breathe! You Are Alive: Sutra on the Full Awareness of Breathing. Thich Nhat Hanh. rev. ed. 1996. LC 88-15894. 103p. pap. 11.00 (*0-938077-93-7*) Parallax Pr.

Breathing & Mechanical Support. A. Oczenski. 1997. 65.00 (*0-632-04859-X*) Blackwell Sci.

Breathing Apparatus Guide: Leader's Guide. Shirley Ayers. 1992. 60p. (Orig.). pap. 20.00 (*0-945790-03-1*) Detrick Lawrence.

Breathing Disorders of Sleep. Ed. by Norman H. Edelman & Teodoro Santiago. 1986. (Contemporary Issues in Pulmonary Disease Ser.: Vol. 5). (Illus.). 274p. text (*0-443-08398-3*) Church.

Breathing Disorders Sourcebook. Francis V. Adams. 1998. LC 98-27806. 256p. pap. 17.00 (*0-7373-0006-X*, 0006XW) NTC Contemp Pub Co.

Breathing Easy: Your Guide to Living with Asthma & Allergies. Elizabeth M. Lykins. Ed. by Gurline J. Baptiste. 1999. (Illus.). 117p. pap. 18.95 (*0-9701963-0-X*) B L Enter.

Breathing Exercises for Asthma. Karen R. Butts. 3rd ed. 1999. LC 87-71059. (Illus.). 57p. (Orig.). pap. text, tchr. ed. 12.95 (*0-9618671-0-8*) CKRB Pub.

***Breathing Pattern & Lung Mechanics During Assisted Ventilation.** Richard Sindelar. 2001. (Comprehensive Summaries of Uppsala Dissertations from the Faculty of Medicine Ser.: No. 1043). (Illus.). 51p. (*91-554-5039-3*) Uppsala Universitet SWE. *Dist:* Coronet Bks.

Breathing the ABC's see Ways to Better Breathing

Breathless: An Asthma Journal. Louise A. DeSalvo. 1998. LC 96-46405. 168p. pap. 12.00 (*0-8070-7097-1*) Beacon Pr.

Breathwork Experience: Exploration & Healing in Nonordinary States of Consciousness. Kylea Taylor. 1994. 192p. per. 16.95 (*0-9643158-0-7*) Hanford Mead.

Breathworks for Your Back: Strengthening Your Back from the Inside Out. Nancy L. Swayzee. 1998. LC 97-36517. (Illus.). pap. 12.00 (*0-380-79044-0*, Avon Bks) Morrow Avon.

Breeding Primates: Proceedings of the International Symposium on Breeding Non-Human Primates for Laboratory Use, Berne, 1971. International Symposium on Breeding Non-Human Prim. Ed. by W. I. Beveridge. 1972. (Illus.). 300p. 55.75 (*3-8055-1369-0*) S Karger.

Breeding, Whelping & Natal Care of Dogs. Louis L. Vine. 1977. LC 77-1817. pap. 2.50 (*0-668-04160-9*, Arc) Hungry Minds.

Breezing Through the Change: Managing Menopause Naturally. Ellen Hodgson Brown & Lynne P. Walker. 1994. LC 93-26662. 197p. pap. 14.95 (*1-883319-12-9*) Frog Ltd CA.

Brenner & Rector's the Kidney Ed. by Barry M. Brenner & Floyd C. Rector. 6th ed. 2000. LC 99-11888. (Illus.). xix, 2653p. (*0-7216-7999-4*); (*0-7216-8000-3*) Saunders.

Breuiary of Helthe, for All Maner of Syckenesses & Diseases, the Whiche May Be in Man, or Woman Deth Folowe, Set. Andrew Borde. 1971. LC 71-38106. (English Experience Ser.: No. 362). 356p. reprint ed. 50.00 (*90-221-0362-5*) Walter J Johnson.

Breuss Cancer Cure: Advice for the Prevention & Natural Treatment of Cancer, Leukemia & Other Seemingly Incurable Diseases. Rudolf Breuss. 1995. LC 95-910587. 130p. pap. 11.95 (*0-920470-56-4*) Alive Bks.

Brewer Medical Diet for Normal & High-Risk Pregnancy: A Leading Obstetrician's Guide to Every Stage of Pregnancy. Gail S. Brewer & Thomas H. Brewer. 1983. 8.95 (*0-671-42635-4*, Fireside) S&S Trade Pap.

Brewer's Yeast, Wheat Germ, Lecithin & Other High Power Foods. Beatrice T. Hunter. 1982. (Good Health Guides). 31p. pap. 3.95 (*0-87983-278-9*, 32789K, Keats Pubng) McGraw-Hill Trade.

Bridge Between Acupuncture & Modern Bio-Energetic Medicine. Stuart J. Zoll. 1993. (Illus.). 184p. pap. text (*2-8043-4001-5*) Edits Haug Intl BEL. *Dist:* Medicina Bio.

Bridge to Recovery: An Introduction to 12-Step Programs. Robert L. DuPont & John P. McGovern. 1994. LC 93-26758. 159p. 24.50 (*0-88048-669-4*, 8669) Am Psychiatric.

Bridges: Psychic Structures, Functions, & Processes. Rosemary Gordon. 1995. LC 94-44022. pap. text 39.95 (*1-56000-819-9*) Transaction Pubs.

Bridges Between Psychology & Linguistics: A Swarthmore Festschrift for Lila Gleitman. Ed. by Donna J. Napoli & J. Kegl. 1991. 312p. (C). text 59.95 (*0-8058-0783-7*) L Erlbaum Assocs.

Bridges Not Walls: A Book about Interpersonal Communication. John Stewart. 3rd ed. 1982. (Illus.). 368p. (C). pap. text 10.00 (*0-394-34986-5*) McGraw.

Bridges of Compassion: Insights & Interventions in Developmental Disabilities. Alex R. Campbell & Lorne Ladner. 1998. LC 97-40101. (Illus.). 248p. 35.00 (*0-7657-0131-6*) Aronson.

Bridges to Tomorrow: The Best of ACLD, Vol. 2. Ed. by William M. Cruickshank & Archie A. Silver. 1981. pap. 22.50 (*0-8156-2237-6*) Syracuse U Pr.

Bridging Paradigms: Positive Development in Adulthood & Cognitive Aging. Ed. by Jan D. Sinnott & John C. Cavanaugh. 1991. LC 90-49073. 288p. 67.00 (*0-275-93617-1*, C3617, Praeger Pubs) Greenwood.

***Bridging Science & Service: A Report by the National Advisory Mental Health Council's Clinical Treatment & Services Research Workgroup.** Pref. by Steven E. Hyman. 2001. 64p. reprint ed. pap. 25.00 (*0-7567-1163-0*) DIANE Pub.

Bridging Separate Gender Worlds: Why Men & Women Clash & How Therapists Can Bring Them Together. Carol L. Philpot et al. 1997. LC 96-41554. 410p. text 29.95 (*1-55798-381-X*) Am Psychol.

Bridging the Gap: A Training Module in Personal & Professional Development. J. Hildebrand. 1998. LC 00-361736. (Systemic Thinking & Practice Ser.). 136p. pap. (*1-85575-181-X*) Karnac Bks GBR. *Dist:* Other Pr LLC.

Bridging the Gap Between Theory & Practice: Exploring Clinical Practice Guidelines. Ed. by Hospital Research and Educational Trust Staff. 1993. (Illus.). 194p. (Orig.). pap. 19.95 (*0-87258-652-9*, 169511) Am Hospital.

Bridging the Gap Between Theory & Practice: Exploring Continuous Quality Improvement. Ed. by Hospital Research and Educational Trust Staff. 1992. (Illus.). 130p. (Orig.). pap. 19.95 (*0-87258-587-5*, 169510) Am Hospital.

Bridging the Gap Between Theory & Practice: Exploring Outcomes Management. Ed. by Hospital Research and Educational Trust Staff. 1994. (Illus.). 122p. (Orig.). pap. 19.95 (*0-87258-664-2*, 169512) Am Hospital.

Bridging Worlds: Understanding & Facilitating Adolescent Recovery from the Trauma of Abuse. Joycee Kennedy & Carol J. McCarthy. 1998. LC 97-37274. (Illus.). 215p. 39.95 (*0-7890-0089-X*); pap. 24.95 (*0-7890-0227-2*) Haworth Pr (Maltreatment & Trauma Pr).

Brief But Comprehensive Psychotherapy: The Multimodal Way. Arnold A. Lazarus. 1997. LC 96-39552. (Behavior Therapy & Behavioral Medicine Ser.). (Illus.). 192p. 35.95 (*0-8261-9640-3*) Springer Pub.

Brief Collaborative Therapy: A Practical Guide for Practitioners. Bonnie A. Rudolph. 1999. 184p. pap. 18.95 (*0-275-96745-X*, Praeger Pubs) Greenwood.

Brief Collabortive Therapy: A Practical Guide for Practitioners. Bonnie A. Rudolph. 1996. LC 96-2202. 184p. 60.00 (*0-275-95469-2*, Praeger Pubs) Greenwood.

Brief Counseling in Action. John M. Littrell. 1998. LC 97-39263. (Professional Book Ser.). (Illus.). 256p. 32.00 (*0-393-70265-0*) Norton.

Brief Counseling That Works: A Solution-Focused Approach for School Counselors. Gerald B. Sklare. 1997. LC 96-45867. (Counseling Techniques Ser.). (Illus.). 136p. 45.95 (*0-8039-6466-8*, 80063); 122p. pap. 19.95 (*0-8039-6467-6*, 80064) Corwin Pr.

Brief Counselling: A Practical Guide for Beginning Practitioners. Windy Dryden & Colin Feltham. 1992. LC 92-8610. pap. (*0-335-09972-6*) OpUniv Pr.

Brief Encounters (Brief Psychotherapy) Karl K. Lewin. 1970. LC 78-96987. 288p. 15.00 (*0-87527-048-4*) Green.

Brief Epidemiology of Crime: With Particular Reference to the Relationship Between Caffeine & Alcohol Use & Crime. Peter D. Hays. rev. ed. 2000. 44p. pap. text 13.95 (*1-885554-09-5*) P D Hays.

Brief Field of View & Elderly Drivers: A Research Study. A. Thompson Perry, 2nd. 1995. (Illus.). 109p. (Orig.). (C). pap. text 40.00 (*0-7881-1615-0*) DIANE Pub.

Brief Group Counselling: Integrating Individual & Group Cognitive-Behavioral Approaches. Michael J. Scott & Stephen G. Stradling. 1998. LC 97-45638. (Brief Therapy & Counselling Ser.). 218p. pap. 49.95 (*0-471-97838-8*) Wiley.

Brief Guide to Brief Therapy. Brian Cade & William H. O'Hanlon. 1993. LC 92-48864. 224p. (C). 25.00 (*0-393-70143-3*) Norton.

Brief Guide to Current Methods of Assessing Vitamin A Status. International Vitamin A Consultative Group Staff. 1993. (Illus.). 37p. pap. 3.50 (*0-944398-10-3*) ILSI.

Brief History of Chinese Medicine. 1997. 130p. lib. bdg. 34.00 (*981-02-2717-5*); 2nd ed. pap. text 15.00 (*981-02-2803-1*) World Scientific Pub.

Brief History of Medicine in the Spartanburg Region & of the Spartanburg County Medical Society 1700-1990: To Which Are Added Biographies of the Spartanburg Physicians. William C. Herbert, Jr. 1992. LC 92-49376. 25.00 (*0-87152-461-9*) Reprint.

***Brief History of Surgery.** Harold Ellis. 2001. (Greenwich Medical Media Ser.). (Illus.). 264p. pap. (*1-84110-023-4*) Greenwich Med GBR. *Dist:* JAMCO Dist.

Brief History of Systems Approaches in Counseling & Psychotherapy. Joseph M. Bauserman & Warren R. Rule. 74p. (C). 2002. pap. text 20.50 (*0-8191-9997-4*); 1995. lib. bdg. 34.50 (*0-8191-9996-6*) U Pr of Amer.

Brief History of Wound Care. Frwd. by I. Kelman Cohen. 1997. (Illus.). 52p. text (*0-9660389-0-8*) OCC.

Brief Interventions & Therapies for Substance Abuse. Ed. by Kristen Lawton Barry & Sandra Clunies. 2000. (Illus.). 234p. (C). pap. text 35.00 (*0-7567-0167-8*) DIANE Pub.

Brief Introduction to Health Occupations. Shirley A. Badasch & Doreen S. Chesebro. 1999. LC 93-24610. 304p. 45.00 (*0-89303-170-4*) P-H.

Brief Psychotherapy: CMT. Francis Macnab. 1993. LC 93-17761. 342p. pap. 100.00 (*0-471-94078-X*) Wiley.

Brief Psychotherapy with the Latino Immigrant Client. Marlene D. De Rios. 2001. LC 00-33531. (Illus.). 192p. pap. 24.95 (*0-7890-1090-9*) Haworth Pr.

Brief Psychotherapy with the Latino Immigrant Client. Ed. by Marlene D. De Rios. 2001. LC 00-33531. (Illus.). 191p. 49.95 (*0-7890-1089-5*) Haworth Pr.

Brief Rational Emotive Behaviour Therapy. Windy Dryden. 1995. LC 95-223794. (Brief Therapy & Counselling Ser.). 244p. pap. 70.00 (*0-471-95786-0*) Wiley.

Brief Separations. Christoph M. Heinicke & Ilse Westheimer. 1966. LC 65-25911. 355p. 52.50 (*0-8236-0600-7*) Intl Univs Pr.

Brief Strategic Problem-Solving Group Therapy: Making Group Therapy Work for You. Terence T. Gorski. 1996. 84p. (Orig.). pap. text 6.25 (*0-8309-0733-5*, Indep Pr) Herald Pub Hse.

Brief Strategic Problem-Solving Group Therapy: Making Group Therapy Work in the Managed Care Environment. Terence T. Gorski. 1995. 84p. (Orig.). pap. text 9.00 (*0-8309-0716-5*, Indep Pr) Herald Pub Hse.

Brief Strategic Solution-Oriented Therapy of Phobic & Obsessive Disorders. Giorgio Nardone. 1996. LC 95-52096. xxviii, 188p. 45.00 (*1-56821-804-4*) Aronson.

Brief Study Course in Homoeopathy. Elizabeth Wright-Hubbard. Ed. by Alain Naude. 1977. pap. 4.95 (*0-89378-071-5*) Formur Intl.

Brief Therapeutic Consultations: An Approach to Systemic Counselling. Eddy Street & Jim Downey. 1996. LC 96-21695. (Brief Therapy & Counselling Ser.). 174p. pap. 60.00 (*0-471-96343-7*) Wiley.

Brief Therapy: Myths, Methods, & Metaphors. Jeffrey K. Zeig. Ed. by Stephen G. Gilligan. 1990. LC 90-1498. 492p. text 57.95 (*0-87630-577-X*) Brunner-Routledge.

Brief Therapy: Short-Term Psychodynamic Intervention. Gregory P. Bauer & Joseph C. Kobos. 1987. LC 87-1487. 312p. 50.00 (*0-87668-940-3*) Aronson.

Brief Therapy & Eating Disorders: A Practical Guide to Solution-Focused Work with Clients. Barbara McFarland. 1995. LC 94-38947. (Jossey-Bass Social & Behavioral Science Ser.). 284p. 40.00 (*0-7879-0053-2*) Jossey-Bass.

Brief Therapy & Managed Care: Readings for Contemporary Practice. Michael F. Hoyt. 1995. LC 94-44548. (Social & Behavioral Sciences-Health Ser.). 444p. 45.00 (*0-7879-0077-X*) Jossey-Bass.

Brief Therapy Approaches to Treating Anxiety & Depression. Ed. by Michael D. Yapko. 1989. LC 89-15746. 384p. text 47.95 (*0-87630-508-7*) Brunner-Routledge.

Brief Therapy for Adolescent Depression. Scott Temple. 1997. LC 97-20410. (Practitioner's Resource Ser.). 112p. pap. 17.95 (*1-56887-028-0*, BTABP, Prof Resc Pr) Pro Resource.

Brief Therapy for PTSD: Traumatic Incident Reduction & Related Techniques. Stephen Bisbey & Lori B. Bisbey. 1998. LC 97-45185. 192p. pap. 65.00 (*0-471-97567-2*) Wiley.

Brief Therapy Homework Planner. Gary M. Schultheis. 1998. LC 97-41088. (Psychotherapy Treatment Planners Ser.). (Illus.). 256p. pap. text 49.95 incl. disk (*0-471-24611-5*) Wiley.

Brief Therapy with Couples: An Integrative Approach. Maria Gilbert & Diana Shmukler. 1996. LC 96-33200. 218p. pap. 54.95 (*0-471-96206-6*) Wiley.

Brief Therapy with Individuals & Couples. Jon Carlson & Len Sperry. 2000. LC 00-28969. xvii, 571p. 59.95 (*1-891944-43-6*) Zeig Tucker Theisen.

Brief Therapy with Intimidating Cases: Changing the Unchangeable. Richard Fisch & Karin Schlanger. 1998. LC 98-36779. 192p. 40.00 (*0-7879-4364-9*) Jossey-Bass.

Brief Therapy with Single-Parent Families. Anita Morawetz & Gillian Walker. 1985. LC 83-21367. 294p. text 41.95 (*0-87630-350-5*) Brunner-Routledge.

Brief vs. Long Psychotherapy: When, Why & How. James P. Gustafson. 1995. LC 94-49234. 400p. 55.00 (*1-56821-470-7*) Aronson.

BriefBook: Biotechnology & Genetic Diversity. Steven C. Witt. 1985. LC 88-606951. (Illus.). 145p. (Orig.). pap. 14.50 (*0-912005-03-3*) Ctr Sci Info.

Briefe Discourse of a Disease Called the Suffocation of the Mother. Edward Jorden. 1971. LC 77-171768. (English Experience Ser.: No. 392). 58p. reprint ed. 25.00 (*90-221-0392-7*) Walter J Johnson.

Brigden's Operating Department. Clarke. 1998. LC 98-3309. (C). text 153.00 (*0-443-05188-7*) Saunders.

Briggs' Information-Processing Model of the Binary Classification Task. Samuel Mudd. 1983. 152p. (C). text 29.95 (*0-89859-291-7*) L Erlbaum Assocs.

Brigham & Women's Hospital Handbook of Diagnostic Imaging. Barbara J. McNeil & Herbert L. Abrams. 1985. 342p. 21.00 (*0-316-56322-6*, Little Brwn Med Div) Lppncott W & W.

Bright Air, Brilliant Fire: On the Matter of the Mind. Gerald M. Edelman. 1993. LC 91-55454. 304p. reprint ed. pap. 18.00 (*0-465-00764-3*) Basic.

Bright Colors Falsely Seen: Synaesthesia & the Search for Transcendental Knowledge. Kevin Dann. 1998. LC 98-15990. 240p. 35.00 (*0-300-06619-8*) Yale U Pr.

***Bright Red Scream: Self-Mutilation & the Language of Pain.** Marilee Strong. 2001. 232p. reprint ed. 25.00 (*0-7881-9917-X*) DIANE Pub.

Bright Red Scream: Self-Mutilation & the Language of Pain. Marilee Strong. 1999. 256p. pap. 14.00 (*0-14-028053-7*, Penguin Bks) Penguin Putnam.

Bring Out Your Dead: The Great Plague of Yellow Fever in Philadelphia in 1793. John H. Powell. 1976. LC 77-112567. (Rise of Urban America Ser.). (Illus.). reprint ed. 23.95 (*0-405-02471-1*) Ayer.

Bringing AID from HIV. Grady L. Etheridge & Myrna L. Etheridge. 1992. 90p. (Orig.). pap. 6.95 (*0-937417-11-4*) Etheridge Minist.

Bringing Cultural Diversity to Feminist Psychology: Theory, Research & Practice. Ed. by Hope Landrine. 1995. LC 95-18570. (Psychology of Women Bks.). (Illus.). 465p. text 39.95 (*1-55798-292-9*) Am Psychol.

Bringing Ethics Alive: Feminist Ethics in Psychotherapy Practice. Intro. by Nanette K. Gartrell. 1994. LC 93-44928. (Women & Therapy Ser.: Vol. 15, No. 1). (Illus.). 113p. pap. 9.95 (*1-56023-051-7*, Harrington Park); 39.95 (*1-56024-511-5*) Haworth Pr.

Bringing Grandy Home: For End-of-Life Care with Family with Year 2000 Update Form. N. Laurie Clark. l.t. rev. ed. 1994. LC 94-94607. (Illus.). 250p. pap. 18.95 (*0-9641197-0-6*) Clark Pubs.

Bringing Health Care Online. 1996. lib. bdg. 255.99 (*0-8490-6373-6*) Gordon Pr.

Bringing Health Care Online: The Role of Information Technologies. 1997. lib. bdg. 250.95 (*0-8490-6223-3*) Gordon Pr.

Bringing Health to Work. Ilise L. Feitshans. Date not set. (Illus.). 163p. 25.00 (*0-9662216-0-5*) Emalyn Pr.

***Bringing Heart Health Tolatinos: A Guide for Building Community Programs.** Ed. by Claude Lenfant. 2001. (Illus.). 86p. (C). pap. text 20.00 (*0-7567-1295-5*) DIANE Pub.

Bringing Out the Best in People: How to Apply the Astonishing Power of Positive Reinforcement. Aubrey Daniels. 2000. 245p. pap. 16.95 (*0-07-136409-9*) McGraw-Hill Educ Grp.

Bringing the Hospital Home: Ethical & Social Implications of High-Tech Home Care. Ed. by John D. Arras. 1995. LC 95-11547. 256p. 44.00 (*0-8018-4990-X*) Johns Hopkins.

Bringing Your Practice into Focus. John A. Wilde. 1994. (Illus.). 276p. 44.95 (*0-87814-410-2*) PennWell Corp.

Bristol Detox Diet for Cancer Patients. Alec Forbes. 1985. LC 84-52563. 196p. reprint ed. pap. 3.95 (*0-87983-419-6*, Keats Pubng) McGraw-Hill Trade.

Bristol-Myers Squibb: World's Largest Pharmaceutical Sales Force in Action. Market Intelligence Staff. 1992. 210p. (Orig.). 995.00 (*1-56753-047-8*) Frost & Sullivan.

***British Contributions to Medicine.** A. Banerjee. 2001. (Illus.). 370p. 87.95 (*1-84214-104-X*, Parthenon Pbng) CRC Pr.

British Masters of Medicine. Ed. by D'Arcy Power. 1977. LC 79-99721. (Essay Index Reprint Ser.). 28.95 (*0-8369-1375-2*) Ayer.

British Medical Journal 1994-1996. A and L New Media Staff. 1997. cd-rom 295.00 (*0-8385-0828-6*, Apple Lange Med) McGraw.

***British National Formulary.** Mehta. 2001. No. 41. (*0-85369-478-8*); No. 42. (*0-85369-479-6*) Pharmaceutical Pr GBR. *Dist:* Rittenhouse.

British National Health Service: State Intervention in the Medical Marketplace, 1911-1948. Sharon Grimes. Ed. by Peter Stansky. 1991. LC 91-13278. (Modern European History Ser.). 256p. text 20.00 (*0-8240-2547-4*) Garland.

British Pediatric Association Manual on Infections & Immunizations in Children. Ed. by Peter Rudd & Angus Nicoll. 2nd ed. 1991. (Illus.). 320p. pap. 27.50 (*0-19-262118-1*) OUP.

British Pharmacopoeia, Set. 1999. (Illus.). 150p. incl. audio compact disk (*0-11-322258-0*, HM22580) Statnry Office GBR. *Dist:* Balogh, Bernan Associates.

***British Pharmacopoeia 2001,** Set. British Pharmacopoeia Commission Staff. 2001. 3200p. incl. cd-rom (*0-11-322446-X*) Statnry Office GBR. *Dist:* Balogh, Bernan Associates.

Broad Scope of Psychoanalysis: Selected Papers of Leopold Bellak. Donald P. Spence. 1967. (Illus.). 400p. text 80.00 (*0-8089-0447-7*, 794230, Grune & Strat) Harcrt Hlth Sci Grp.

Broad Spectrum Psychotherapist. Wyn Bramley. 1996. 275p. (C). pap. (*1-85343-327-6*); (*1-85343-328-4*) Free Assoc Bks GBR. *Dist:* Intl Spec Bk, NYU Pr.

Broader Implications of Ericksonian Therapy. Ed. by Stephen R. Lankton. 1990. LC 89-71310. (Ericksonian Monographs: No. 7). 128p. 28.95 (*0-87630-582-6*) Brunner-Routledge.

Broadribb's Introductory Pediatric Nursing. Margaret G. Marks. 5th ed. 1998. LC 97-24540. 544p. pap. text 31.95 (*0-397-55450-8*) Lppncott W & W.

Broca's Brain. Carl Sagan. 1986. 416p. mass mkt. 6.99 (*0-345-33689-5*) Ballantine Pub Grp.

Brocklehurst's Pocket Book of Geriatrics & Gerontology. Ed. by R. C. Tallis et al. 5th ed. 1998. (Illus.). 400p. pap. (*0-443-05371-5*) Church.

Brocklehurst's Textbook of Geriatric Medicine & Gerontology. R. C. Tallis. 5th ed. 1998. text (*0-443-05370-7*, T0890) Church.

Brodifacoum. 1995. (Health & Safety Guides Ser.: No. 93). 25p. (C). pap. text 4.50 (*92-4-151093-5*, 1860093) Am Soc Clinical.

Broken Bones: Anthropological Analysis of Blunt Force Trauma. Alison Galloway. 1999. LC 99-34122. (Illus.). 392p. text 69.95 (*0-398-06992-1*) C C Thomas.

Broken Bottles, Broken Dreams: Understanding & Helping the Children of Alcoholics. Charles Deutsch. 1982. LC 81-5729. 318p. pap. 18.95 (*0-8077-2663-X*) Tchrs Coll.

Broken Boys - Men: Recovery from Childhood Sexual Abuse. Stephen D. Grubman-Black. 1990. pap. 12.95 (*0-8306-3562-9*) McGraw-Hill Educ Grp.

Broken Brain. Nancy C. Andreasen. 1985. LC 83-48782. (Illus.). 288p. pap. 15.00 (*0-06-091272-3*, PL 1272, Perennial) HarperTrade.

Broken Brains or Wounded Hearts: What Causes Mental Illness? Ty C. Colbert. 1996. LC 96-76762. (Illus.). 316p. 23.95 (*0-9643635-4-2*) Kevco Pubg.

Broken Connection: On Death & the Continuity of Life. Robert J. Lifton. 1996. 474p. pap. text 39.00 (*0-88048-874-3*, 8874) Am Psychiatric.

Broken Connections: Alzheimer's Disease. Liduin E. Souren & Emile H. Franssen. 1994. LC 93-25579.Tr. of Verbroken Verbindigen. (DUT.). Pt. I. 172p. pap. (*90-265-1334-8*); Pt. II. 330p. pap. text (*90-265-1371-2*) Swets.

Broken Images, Broken Selves: Dissociative Narratives in Clinical Practice. Stanley Krippner & Susan M. Powers. 1997. LC 97-26048. 450p. 26.95 (*0-87630-851-5*) Brunner-Routledge.

Broken Memories: Case Studies in Memory Impairment. Ed. by Ruth Campbell & Martin Conway. 1995. (Illus.). 496p. pap. 39.95 (*0-631-18723-5*); 68.95 (*0-631-18722-7*) Blackwell Pubs.

Broken Structures: Severe Personality Disorder & Their Treatment. Salman Akhtar. 2000. pap. 50.00 (*0-7657-0255-X*) Aronson.

Broken Taboo: Sex in the Family. Blair Justice & Rita Justice. 1979. LC 78-23720. 304p. 42.95 (*0-87705-389-8*); pap. 20.95 (*0-87705-482-7*) Kluwer Academic (Kluwer Acad Hman Sci).

Broken Toys Broken Dreams: Understanding & Healing Boundaries, Codependence, Compulsion & Family Relationships. Terry Kellogg. 1990. 242p. pap. 10.95 (*1-56073-001-3*, BTBD) BRAT Pub.

Bromadiolone. 1995. (Health & Safety Guides Ser.: No. 94). 25p. (C). pap. text 4.50 (*92-4-151094-3*, 1860094) Am Soc Clinical.

Brominated Diphenyl Ethers. 1994. (Environmental Health Criteria Ser.: No. 162). 347p. pap. text 62.00 (*92-4-157162-4*, 1160162) World Health.

Bronchial Asthma: Its Etiology & Control with Traditional Herbal Extracts. Muhammed Majeed. 1998. pap. text 2.00 (*0-9647856-5-X*) Nutrisci Pubs.

Bronchial Asthma: Principles of Diagnosis & Treatment. Ed. by M. Eric Gershwin & Georges M. Halpern. 3rd ed. 1994. LC 93-38240. (Illus.). 792p. text 149.00 (*0-89603-253-1*) Humana.

Bronchial Asthma: Principles of Diagnosis & Treatment. Ed. by M. Eric Gershwin & Timothy E. Albertson. 4th ed. 2001. LC 00-54101. 400p. 125.00 (*0-89603-861-0*) Humana.

Bronchial Carcinoma: An Integrated Approach to Diagnosis & Management. Ed. by M. Bates. 1985. (Illus.). 240p. 125.00 (*0-387-13234-1*) Spr-Verlag.

Bronchial Circulation. Ed. by John Butler. 1992. (Lung Biology in Health & Disease Ser.: Vol. 57). (Illus.). 832p. text 285.00 (*0-8247-8443-X*) Dekker.

Bronchial Hygiene. Lonny J. Ashworth. 1998. (CPG Mentor - Patient Cases in Respiratory Care Ser.: Unit 4). (*0-8151-2286-1*) Mosby Inc.

Bronchial Hyperresponsiveness. Ed. by Hartmut Zwick. 1992. LC 92-49734. 100p. (*3-211-82375-1*); (Illus.). 33.95 (*0-387-82375-1*) Spr-Verlag.

Bronchial Hyperresponsiveness & Structural Changes in the Asthmic Airway. Alistair G. Stewart. 1997. (Medical Intelligence Unit Ser.). 250p. 89.95 (*0-412-13111-0*) Chapman & Hall.

Bronchitis: Materia Medica Relating to Bronchitis. 1999. LC 99-93311. 83p. pap. 5.95 (*1-929410-00-X*) dttm.

Bronchogenic Carcinoma. Omar M. Salazar et al. 1981. (Oncologic Division of Radiation Oncology Ser.: Vol. 13). (Illus.). 384p. pap. 135.00 (*0-08-027464-1*, Pergamon Pr) Elsevier.

Brookings Institution: A Fifty-Year History. Charles B. Saunders, Jr. 1966. LC 66-27855. 118p. 4.50 (*0-8157-7714-0*); pap. 2.00 (*0-8157-7713-2*) Brookings.

Brother Animal: The Story of Freud & Tausk. Paul Roazen. 1990. 224p. (C). pap. text 24.95 (*0-88738-851-5*) Transaction Pubs.

Brother to Brother: You Don't Have to Die with Prostate Cancer. Thomas L. Walker. 1998. (Illus.). xv, 182p. pap. 15.95 (*0-9665465-0-4*, 2001) Eternal Gold.

Brothers & Sisters: A Guide for Families of Children with Epilepsy. Epilepsy Foundation of America Staff. 1992. 95p. pap. 10.95 (*0-916570-03-7*) Epilepsy Foundation of America.

Brothers Beyond Blood: A Battalion Surgeon in the South Pacific. George Sharpe. Ed. by Melissa Roberts. 1989. (Illus.). 240p. 18.95 (*0-89015-689-1*) Eakin Press.

Browning Outcomes Survey Scale: For Brief Therapy Charles H. Browning & Beverley J. Browning. 1996. (Illus.). (Orig.). pap. text, wbk. ed. 75.00 (*0-911663-11-8*) Duncliffs Intl.

BRS Obstetrics & Gynecology. Elmar P. Sakala. 2nd ed. 2000. LC 99-40829. 448p. pap. text 29.95 (*0-683-30743-6*) Lppncott W & W.

***BRS Pediatrics.** Lloyd G. Brown. 2001. (Board Review Ser.). (Illus.). 525p. pap. (*0-7817-2129-6*) Lppncott W & W.

BRS Surgical Specialties. Traves D. Crabtree. 2000. LC 00-25010. 288p. pap. text 29.95 (*0-7817-2771-5*) Lppncott W & W.

Bruce-Chwatt's Essential Malariology. Leonard J. Bruce-Chwatt. Ed. by Herbert M. Gilles & David A. Warrell. 3rd ed. 1993. 368p. (*0-340-57190-X*) E A GBR. *Dist:* OUP.

Brucellosis. Ed. by Lyon Valette & W. Hennessen. 1984. (Developments in Biological Standardization Ser.: Vol. 56). (Illus.). xiv, 782p. pap. 61.00 (*3-8055-3944-4*) S Karger.

Brucellosis: Clinical & Laboratory Aspects. Ed. by Edward J. Young & Michael J. Corbel. 1989. 192p. 210.00 (*0-8493-6661-5*, RC123) CRC Pr.

Brucellosis: Proceedings of the International Symposium on Standardization & Control of Vaccines & Reagents, 24, Tunise & Bourse du Travail, 1968. Ed. by Microbiological Standardization, Permanent Section. 1970. (Immunobiological Standardization Symposia Ser.: Vol. 12). 26.25 (*3-8055-0634-1*) S Karger.

Brugada Syndrome. Ed. by Charles Antzelevitch et al. 1999. LC 99-19225. (Clinical Approaches to Tachyarrhythmias Ser.: Vol. 10). (Illus.). 112p. pap. 21.00 (*0-87993-434-4*) Futura Pub.

Bruising Apothecary: Images of Pharmacy & Medicine in Health Care. Arnold. 1989. pap. (*0-85369-223-8*) Pharmaceutical Pr GBR. *Dist:* Rittenhouse.

Brunner & Suddarth's Textbook of Medical-Surgical Nursing. Lillian Sholtis Brunner et al. 9th ed. 1999. LC 99-16398. (Illus.). 2096p. 87.95 (*0-7817-1575-X*) Lppncott W & W.

Brunner & Suddarth's Textbook of Medical-Surgical Nursing. Suzanne C. Smeltzer & Brenda G. Bare. 9th ed. 2000. LC 99-47902. 832p. pap. text 24.95 (*0-7817-2091-5*) Lppncott W & W.

Brunnstrom's Clinical Kinesiology. Laura K. Smith et al. 5th ed. 1995. LC 95-4491. (Illus.). 468p. (C). text 39.95 (*0-8036-7916-5*) Davis Co.

Brunnstrom's Movement Therapy in Hemiplegia: A Neurophysiologic Approach. Kathryn A. Sawner & Jeanne M. LaVigne. 2nd ed. 1992. (Illus.). 288p. text 50.95 (*0-397-54808-7*) Lppncott W & W.

Brush Foundation Study of Child Growth & Development I: Psychometric Tests. Elizabeth Ebert & Katherine Simmons. 1972. (SRCD M Ser.: Vol. 8, No. 2). reprint ed. 25.00 (*0-527-01527-X*, SRCD.M 35) Periodicals Srv.

Brush Foundation Study of Child Growth & Development II: Physical Growth & Development. Katherine Simmons. 1972. (SRCD M Ser.: Vol. 9, No. 1). reprint ed. 25.00 (*0-527-01530-X*, SRCD.M 37) Periodicals Srv.

BSAVA Manual of Small Animal Clinical Pathology. Ed. by Malcolm Davidson et al. 1998. (Illus.). 230p. pap. text (*0-905214-41-2*) BSAVA GBR. *Dist:* Iowa U Pr.

BSAVA Manual of Small Animal Fracture Repair & Management. Ed. by Andrew Coughlan & Andrew Miller. 1997. (Illus.). 200p. pap. (*0-8138-2794-9*) BSAVA GBR. *Dist:* Iowa U Pr.

BSAVA Manual of Small Animal Fracture Repair & Management. Ed. by Andrew R. Coughlan & Andrew Miller. 1998. LC 98-167590. 348p. 94.95 (*0-905214-37-4*) Brynwood Publishing Co.

B3 Adrenoreceptor. A. D. Strosberg. 2000. LC 00-23999. (Taylor & Francis Series in Pharmaceutical Sciences Ser.). (Illus.). 192p. (gr. 13). text 110.00 (*0-7484-0804-5*) Taylor & Francis.

BTLS: Basic Trauma Life Support for the EMT-B & First Responder. Contrib. by John E. Campbell. 3rd ed. 1999. LC 99-35610. 336p. pap. 50.00 (*0-13-084581-7*) P-H.

Bucket Diagrams: A Problem-Solving Approach to Renal Physiology. Herbert F. Janssen. 1993. (Illus.). 144p. (C). pap. text 17.50 (*0-89672-323-2*) Tex Tech Univ Pr.

Buddha's Art of Healing: Tibetan Paintings Rediscovered. Frwd. by Dalai Lama XIV, pseud. 1998. LC 97-51770. (Illus.). 208p. pap. 35.00 (*0-8478-2090-4*); 65.00 (*0-8478-2089-0*) Rizzoli Intl.

Buddhism & Jungian Psychology. J. Marvin Spiegelman & Mokusen Miyuki. 2nd ed. 1987. LC 85-70850. 224p. (Orig.). pap. 12.95 (*1-56184-111-0*) New Falcon Pubns.

Buddhism & the Art of Psychotherapy. Hayao Kawai. 1996. LC 95-43421. (Carolyn & Ernest Fay Series in Analytical Psychology: Vol. 5). (Illus.). 156p. (C). 22.95 (*0-89096-698-2*) Tex A&M Univ Pr.

Buddhist & Freudian Psychology. Padmasiri De Silva. 3rd ed. 1992. 230p. (*9971-69-167-1*) Sngapore Univ Pr SGP. *Dist:* Coronet Bks.

Budget Reconciliation Recommendations of the Committee on Finance (spending Provisions) As Submitted to the Committee on the Budget Pursuant to H. Con. Res. 84. Contrib. by U. S. Congress, Senate Committee on Finance. 1997. LC 97-186980. (*0-16-055188-9*) USGPO.

Budgeting & Financial Management Nurse Managers. Russell C. Swansburg. 1997. LC 96-50949. (Nursing Ser.). (Illus.). 336p. (C). text 48.95 (*0-7637-0232-3*, 0232-3) Jones & Bartlett.

Budgeting Concepts for Nurse Managers. Steven A. Finkler. 2nd ed. (Illus.). 392p. 1992. pap., tchr. ed. (*0-7216-4348-5*); 1991. pap. text 44.00 (*0-7216-3279-3*) Saunders.

Bufotenin (Dimethylserotonin - Mappine) Index of New Information & Medical Research Bible. Patrick M. Pfeifer. 1994. 160p. 57.50 (*0-7883-0218-3*); pap. 47.50 (*0-7883-0219-1*) ABBE Pubs Assn.

Bugcards: The Complete Microbiology Review for Class, the Boards & the Wards. Jason Levine & Sarah Bhalla. 1998. (Illus.). 154p. (C). 26.50 (*0-9671655-0-4*) B L Publishing.

Build a Better Staff: Hiring, Evaluating, & Firing Staff Members. Ed. by Darla Struck & Jeff Stratton. 1992. 194p. ring bd. 163.00 (*0-8342-0403-7*, 04037) Aspen Pub.

Build Bone Health: Prevent & Treat Osteoporosis. Freedolph Anderson. 1999. LC 99-61964. pap. 7.95 (*1-890694-22-3*) IMPAKT Communs.

Building a Cancer Information Network in Texas: A Demonstration in the Heart of Texas Region. Lonna Milburn. 1989. (Special Project Reports: Vol. SP-BC). 277p. pap. 10.00 (*0-89940-864-8*) LBJ Sch Pub Aff.

Building a Career: The Effect of Initial Job Experiences & Related Work Attitudes on Later Employment. Joseph A. Raelin. 1980. LC 80-24848. 178p. pap. 5.00 (*0-911558-73-X*) W E Upjohn.

Building a Database for Nursing Education Enrollment Management. American Association of Colleges of Nursing Staff. 1989. 175p. 18.00 (*0-922148-03-1*) AACN.

Building a Dynamic Vision Therapy Practice. Ed. by Willard B. Bleything. 1998. (Illus.). 152p. pap. 25.00 (*0-943599-27-X*) OEPF.

Building a Group Practice: Creating a Shared Vision for Success. American Psychological Association Staff & Coopers and Lybrand Staff. 1995. (APA Practitioner's Toolbox Ser.). pap. 29.95 (*1-55798-318-6*) Am Psychol.

Building a Healthy America: Conquering Disease & Disability. Ed. by Terry Lierman. 2nd rev. ed. 1987. 248p. 49.00 (*0-913113-12-3*) M Liebert.

Building a Healthy Heart. Eric F. Powell. 1961. pap. 8.95 (*0-8464-0997-6*) Beekman Pubs.

Building a Healthy Heart. Eric F. Powell. 1980. 19.50 (*0-85032-177-8*) St Mut.

Building a Legacy: Voices of Oncology Nurses. Brenda Nevidjon. 1995. LC 95-4063. (Nursing Ser.). (Illus.). 464p. (C). text 52.95 (*0-86720-727-2*, 727-2) Jones & Bartlett.

Building a Medical Vocabulary. Peggy C. Leonard. (Illus.). 3rd ed. 1993. pap., tchr. ed. (*0-7216-4739-1*); 4th ed. 1997. 555p. pap., tchr. ed. (*0-7216-9643-0*); 4th ed. 1997. LC 96-15373. 555p. pap. text 38.00 (*0-7216-9642-2*) Saunders.

***Building a Medical Vocabulary.** Peggy Leonard. 5th ed. 2001. (Illus.). pap., tchr. ed. (*0-7216-9462-4*) Saunders.

***Building a Medical Vocabulary: ExaMaster.** Peggy Leonard. 5th ed. 2001. (Illus.). pap. (*0-7216-9461-6*) Saunders.

Building a National Immunization System: A Guide to Immunization Services & Resources. Children's Defense Fund Staff. 1994. 136p. pap. 9.95 (*1-881985-06-7*) Childrens Defense.

Building a National Policy Agenda: Ten Principles for Woman-Focused HIV/AIDS Prevention. Belinda Rochelle et al. 1996. 28p. pap. 8.00 (*1-877966-28-2*) Ctr Women Policy.

Building a Neuropsychology Practice: A Guide to Respecialization. Marvin H. Podd & Donald P. Seelig. 1998. LC 97-34797. (Developments in Clinical Psychiatry Ser.). 192p. 50.00 (*0-7657-0146-4*) Aronson.

Building a New Dream: A Family Guide to Coping with Chronic Illness & Disability. Janet R. Maurer. 1990. pap. 9.57 (*0-201-55098-9*) Addison-Wesley.

Building a New Stomach. Victor G. Rocine. 1991. (Nutrition Ser.). lib. bdg. 75.00 (*0-8490-4260-7*) Gordon Pr.

Building a Pharmacist's Patient Data Base. Nancy A. Mason & Leslie A. Shimp. 1993. (Clinical Skills Program, Advancing Pharmaceutical Care Ser.). 96p. ring bd. 50.00 (*1-879907-32-1*) Am Soc Hlth-Syst.

Building a Practice with Patterns of Excellence: For Counseling Practitioners, Therapists, & All Mental Health Practitioners. C. Rex Heisler. 1987. 357p. 39.95 (*0-929564-00-6*) Pneumatikos Counsel Inst.

Building a Solid Foundation for Health: A Report on Public Health System Development. 1995. (Illus.). 45p. (Orig.). (C). pap. text 25.00 (*0-7881-2476-5*) DIANE Pub.

Building A Successful Health Outcomes Program Vol. 1: Collecting, Analyzing & Using Clinical Data. Chris Arslanian. 2001. LC 00-133508. (Illus.). 112p. pap. 59.95 (*0-9703224-0-2*) Symphonic Lion.

Building a Successful Medical Transcription Business. 1993. 196p. pap. 495.00 incl. VHS (*0-934385-57-2*) Hlth Prof Inst.

Building a Successful Practice: A Step by Step Guide to Building Your Own Profitable Business. Jason Liles & Shiroko Sokitch. 3rd rev. ed. 1997. 60p. pap. text 19.95 (*0-9660950-0-6*) Hrt to Hrt Med.

Building America's Health: A Report President's Commission on Health Needs. 1976. LC 75-17239. (Social Problems & Social Policy Ser.). (Illus.). reprint ed. Set. 134.95 (*0-405-07508-1*); Vol. 1. 66.95 (*0-405-07509-X*); Vol. 4. 66.95 (*0-405-07510-3*) Ayer.

Building & Managing Effective Physician Organizations under Capitation. Douglas E. Goldstein. 1996. 384p. 128.00 (*0-8342-0809-1*, 20809) Aspen Pub.

Building & Managing Your Private Practice. Daniel L. Richards. 1990. 268p. pap. text 32.95 (*1-55620-071-4*, 72031) Am Coun Assn.

Building & Sustaining Systems of Care for Substance-Using Pregnant Women & Their Infants. M. Poland Laken & E. Hutchins. 1995. LC 95-71705. 68p. pap. text (*1-57285-021-3*) Nat Ctr Educ.

Building & Using a Model of Nursing. 2nd ed. (*0-340-52627-0*) E A GBR. *Dist:* Routldge.

Building Basic Therapeutic Skills: A Practical Guide for Current Mental Health Practice. Jeanne Heaton. 1998. LC 97-45300. 288p. 38.00 (*0-7879-3984-6*) Jossey-Bass.

Building Blocks of APGs: Preparing for Change in the Outpatient Arena. 1996. 104p. (Orig.). pap. 99.00 (*1-889115-13-4*) Med Learn.

Building Bright Futures: An Annotated Bibliography on Substance Abuse Prevention for Families with Young Children. Carole J. Oshinsky et al. 1996. LC 96-15063. 52p. pap. 8.00 (*0-926582-19-4*) NCCP.

Building Communicative Competence with Individuals Who Use Augmentative & Alternative Communication. Janice B. Light & Cathy Binger. 1998. LC 97-33599. 304p. 37.95 (*1-55766-324-6*) P H Brookes.

Building Community: A Manual Exploring Issues of Women & Disability. Women and Disability Awareness Project Staff. 1984. tchr. ed. 15.00 (*0-931629-01-2*) Educ Equity Con.

Building Community Services - The Mental Illness Specific Grant - A Review. 1995. 118p. pap. (*0-11-321900-8*, HM19008) Statnry Office GBR. *Dist:* Bernan Associates.

Building Endurance. 1999. (Fitness, Health & Nutrition Ser.). (Illus.). 144p. (YA). (gr. 7). 17.95 (*0-8094-6154-4*) Time-Life.

***Building Hospital Palliative Care Programs: Lessons from the Field.** Susan Shampaine Hopper. 2001. LC 00-54504. (Special Report Ser.). pap. (*1-881277-57-7*) United Hosp Fund.

Building Muscle Mass, Performance & Health with HMB. Richard A. Passwater & John C. Fuller. 1997. (Good Health Guides). 48p. pap. 3.95 (*0-87983-867-1*, 38671K, Keats Pubng) McGraw-Hill Trade.

Building New Nursing Organizations: Visions & Realities. Cathleen K. Wilson. 1991. LC 91-22412. 240p. 72.00 (*0-8342-0307-3*, 20307) Aspen Pub.

Building Outdoor Playthings for Kids, with Project Plans. Bill Barnes. 1988. (Illus.). 240p. (Orig.). 21.95 (*0-8306-0971-7*, 1971); pap. 14.95 (*0-8306-1971-2*) McGraw-Hill Educ Grp.

Building Partnerships: Educating Health Professionals for the Communities They Serve. Ronald W. Richards et al. 1995. LC 95-9652. (Health Ser.). 216p. 43.00 (*0-7879-0150-4*) Jossey-Bass.

Building Partnerships in Hospital Care: Empowering Patients, Families & Professionals. Mary D. Scheller. 1990. 148p. pap. 16.95 (*0-923521-07-0*) Bull Pub.

Building Pathology: Principles & Practice. David Watt. 1999. LC 98-51354. (Building Pathology Ser.). pap. 80.00 (*0-632-04875-1*) Blackwell Sci.

Building People, Building Programs: A Practitioner's Guide for Introducing the Myers-Briggs Type Indicator to Individuals & Organizations. Gordon D. Lawrence & Charles R. Martin. 2000. LC 00-26200. (Illus.). v, 274p. pap. 24.95 (*0-935652-54-X*) Ctr Applications Psych.

Building Primary Health Care in New York City's Low-Income Communities. Anjean B. Carter & Christel Brellochs. 1990. LC 90-198029. 80p. pap. 9.00 (*0-88156-107-X*) Comm Serv Soc NY.

Building Productive Organizations Through Health & Wellness Programs. Douglas B. Gutknecht & David M. Gutknecht. 1990. LC 89-22491. 252p. (C). pap. text 70.50 (*0-8191-7580-3*); lib. bdg. 111.00 (*0-8191-7579-X*) U Pr of Amer.

Building Regional Health Care Networks in Europe. Ed. by John Oates & Benrik Bjerregarrd Jensen. 2000. (Studies in Health Technology & Informatics: Vol. 67). 240p. (*90-5199-506-7*) IOS Press.

Building Rural Hospital Networks: Lessons in Providing Care to Underserved Populations. William Manning et al. 1995. LC 95-174. 244p. pap. 19.50 (*1-56793-028-X*, 0958) Health Admin Pr.

Building Safe Communities: State & Local Strategies for Preventing Injury & Violence Within Our Communities. Prod. by National Center for Education in Maternal and Child Health Staff. 1994. LC 94-69180. 232p. pap. (*1-57285-006-X*) Nat Ctr Educ.

Building Sight. 1995. 180p. pap. (*0-11-701993-3*, HM19933) Statnry Office GBR. *Dist:* Bernan Associates.

Building Supportive Communities for At-Risk Adolescents: It Takes More Than Services. Martha R. Burt et al. 1997. LC 97-32411. 314p. pap. 24.95 (*1-55798-466-2*, 431-703A) Am Psychol.

Building the Healing Partnership: Parents, Professionals & Children with Chronic Illnesses & Disabilities. Patricia Taner-Leff & Elaine Walizer. 1993. 312p. (C). text 34.95 (*0-914797-63-8*); pap. text 24.95 (*0-914797-60-3*) Brookline Bks.

Building the Successful Veterinary Practice: Leadership Tools, Vol. 1. Thomas E. Catanzaro. 1997. LC 97-374. (Building the Successful Veterinary Practice Ser.: Vol. 1). (Illus.). 180p. (Orig.). (C). pap. text 24.95 (*0-8138-2819-8*) Iowa U Pr.

Building the Successful Veterinary Practice Vol. 2: Programs & Procedures, Vol. 2. Thomas E. Catanzaro. 1997. LC 97-374. (Building the Successful Veterinary Practice Ser.: Vol. 2). (Illus.). 368p. pap. 44.95 (*0-8138-2399-4*) Iowa U Pr.

Building the Successful Veterinary Practice Vol. 3: Innovation & Creativity, Vol. 3. Thomas E. Catanzaro. 1998. LC 97-374. (Building the Successful Beterinary Practice Ser.: Vol. 3). (Illus.). 200p. pap. text 34.95 (*0-8138-2984-4*) Iowa U Pr.

Building up to Financial Freedom: Financial & Retirement Planning for Dentists. James B. Jackson. 1986. 296p. 10.00 (*0-87814-302-5*) PennWell Corp.

Building Your Ideal Private Practice: How to Love What You Do & Be Highly Profitable Too. Contrib. by Lynn Grodzki. 2000. LC 99-58069. (Professional Bks. for Psychotherapists). 224p. 29.00 (*0-393-70331-2*) Norton.

Building Your Million Dollar Solo Practice. Edward L. Silker. 1995. 416p. 59.95 (*0-9645815-0-7*) Silk Pages Pub.

Building Your Rheumatology Practice. Joseph J. Weiss. 1984. 140p. pap. 18.75 (*0-9613906-0-3*) Belleraphon.

Built to Survive: A Comprehensive Guide to the Use of Anabolic Steroids, Nutrition, & Exercise for HIV Therapy. Nelson R. Vergel & Michael Mooney. 1999. (Illus.). 190p. pap. 24.95 (*0-9662231-0-1*) Prog Wellness Res.

Bulimarexia: The Binge Purge Cycle. Marlene Boskind-White. 2nd ed. 1991. LC 86-23733. pap. 13.95 (*0-393-30117-6*) Norton.

Bulimia: A Guide for Family & Friends. Roberta T. Sherman & Ron A. Thompson. 1996. LC 96-45095. (Jossey-Bass Psychology Ser.). 176p. pap. 15.16 (*0-7879-0361-2*) Jossey-Bass.

Bulimia: A Guide for Sufferers & Their Families. David Haslam. 1996. pap. 9.99 (*0-7493-2456-2*) Buttrwrth-Heinemann.

Bulimia: A Guide to Recovery. Lindsey Hall & Leigh Cohn. 5th rev. ed. 1999. LC 98-34618. (Illus.). 192p. pap. 14.95 (*0-936077-31-X*) Gurze Bks.

Bulimia: Book for Therapist & Client. Barbara G. Bauer et al. 1986. LC 85-72774. 210p. (Orig.). pap. text 23.95 (*0-915202-56-5*) Accel Devel.

Bulimia: Disease of Addiction. 1993. 12p. (Orig.). pap. 2.00 (*0-9638074-1-2*) Food Addicts.

Bulimia: Psychoanalytic Treatment & Theory. Ed. by Harvey J. Schwartz. 1988. 564p. 80.00 (*0-8236-0605-8*, BN 00605) Intl Univs Pr.

Bulimia Anorexia. Boskind-White. 3rd ed. 2001. 228p. pap. 14.95 (*0-393-31923-7*) Norton.

Bulimia Nervosa. James Mitchell. 1990. 188p. (C). 27.95 (*0-8166-1626-4*) U of Minn Pr.

Bulimia Nervosa & Binge-Eating: A Guide to Recovery. Peter J. Cooper. 1995. LC 95-8359. (Illus.). 160p. (C). text 35.00 (*0-8147-1522-2*); pap. 13.95 (*0-8147-1523-0*) NYU Pr.

Bulimic College Student: Evaluation, Treatment, & Prevention. Ed. by Leighton C. Whitaker & William N. Davis. 1989. LC 88-34725. (Journal of College Student Psychotherapy Ser.: Vol. 3, Nos. 2-4). 340p. pap. 19.95 (*0-86656-832-8*); 49.95 (*0-86656-874-3*) Haworth Pr.

Bulleins Bulwarke of Defence Againste All Sickness, Sorness & Woundes. William Bullein. 1971. LC 73-37139. (English Experience Ser.: No. 350). (Illus.). 488p. reprint ed. 125.00 (*90-221-0350-1*) Walter J Johnson.

Bullein's Dialogue Against the Fever Pestilence. Mark W. Bullen. Ed. by Arthur H. Bullen. 1972. (EETS, ES Ser.: No. 52). reprint ed. 40.00 (*0-527-00258-5*) Periodicals Srv.

Bullet Penetration: Modeling the Dynamics & the Incapacitation Resulting from Wound Trauma. Duncan MacPherson. 1994. LC 94-79577. (Illus.). 303p. 39.95 (*0-9643577-0-4*) Ballistic Pubns.

Bullough & Vigorita's Atlas of Orthopaedic Pathology. Peter G. Bullough. 2nd ed. 1991. (Illus.). 448p. (gr. 13). (*0-397-44621-7*, GM0241) Gower-Mosby.

Bunyaviridae. Ed. by Richard M. Elliott. 1996. LC 96-4224. (Viruses Ser.). (Illus.). 360p. 95.00 (*0-306-45178-6*, Kluwer Plenum) Kluwer Academic.

Buprenorphine: An Alternative Treatment for Opioid Dependence. 1995. lib. bdg. 251.95 (*0-8490-6837-1*) Gordon Pr.

Buprenorphine: Combatting Drug Abuse with a Unique Opioid. Ed. by Alan Cowan & John W. Lewis. 1995. LC 94-28470. (Illus.). 342p. 137.00 (*0-471-56198-3*, Wiley-Liss) Wiley.

Burdens of Disease: Epidemics & Human Response in Western History. J. N. Hays. 1998. LC 97-39328. (Illus.). (C). 361p. 50.00 (*0-8135-2527-6*); 440p. pap. text 24.00 (*0-8135-2528-4*) Rutgers U Pr.

Bureau of Biological Survey: Its History, Activities, & Organization. Jenks Cameron. 1974. LC 73-17805. (Natural Sciences in America Ser.). 354p. reprint ed. 26.95 (*0-405-05722-9*) Ayer.

Bureaucratic Malpractice: Hospital Regulation in N. J. 1974. 120p. 17.00 (*0-943136-03-2*) Ctr Analysis Public Issues.

Burford NDU Model: Caring in Practice. Ed. by Christopher Johns. 1994. LC 94-12532. 240p. pap. 39.95 (*0-632-03886-1*) Blackwell Sci.

Burger's Medicinal Chemistry & Drug Discovery Ed. by Manfred E. Wolff. 5th ed. Set. 1997. 3992p. 1425.00 (*0-471-57561-5*); Vol. 1. 1994. LC 94-12687. (Burger's Medicinal Chemistry & Drug Discovery Ser.: Vol. 1). 1088p. 325.00 (*0-471-57556-9*); Vol. 4. 1997. LC 94-12687. (Burger's Medicinal Chemistry & Drug Discovery Ser.: Vol. 4). 656p. 325.00 (*0-471-57559-3*) Wiley.

Burger's Medicinal Chemistry & Drug Discovery Vol. 2: Therapeutic Agents, Vol. 2. Ed. by Manfred E. Wolff. 5th ed. 1996. 680p. 325.00 (*0-471-57557-7*) Wiley.

Burger's Medicinal Chemistry & Drug Discovery Vol. 3: Therapeutic Agents, Vol. 3. Ed. by Manfred E. Wolff. 5th ed. 1996. LC 94-12687. 664p. 325.00 (*0-471-57558-5*) Wiley.

Burger's Medicinal Chemistry & Drug Discovery Vol. 5: Therapeutic Agents, Vol. 5. Ed. by Manfred E. Wolff. 5th ed. 1997. LC 94-12687. (Burger's Medicinal Chemistry & Drug Discovery Ser.: Vol. 5). 879p. 325.00 (*0-471-57560-7*) Wiley.

Burket's Oral Medicine. Ed. by Malcolm A. Lynch. 8th ed. 1983. (Illus.). 875p. text 55.00 (*0-397-52106-5*, 65-07131, Lippnctt) Lppncott W & W.

Burkitt Lymphoma, Hemostasis & Intercellular Matrix: Barbara Robert Memorial. Ed. by L. Robert et al. 1976. (Frontiers of Matrix Biology Ser.: Vol. 3). (Illus.). 155.75 (*3-8055-2326-2*) S Karger.

Burn Care. Steven E. Wolf & David N. Herndon. 1999. LC 99-24714. (Vademecum Ser.). spiral bd. 45.00 (*1-57059-526-7*) Landes Bioscience.

Burn Care & Therapy. Gretchen Carrougher. 1998. LC 98-10872. (Illus.). 496p. (C). (gr. 13). text 59.95 (*0-8151-1396-X*, 29559) Mosby Inc.

Burn Wound Coverings. Ed. by Donald L. Wise. 1984. Vol. I. 192p. 109.00 (*0-8493-5706-3*, RD96); Vol. II. 176p. 103.00 (*0-8493-5707-1*, RD96) Franklin (CRC Reprint).

Burning Within. RaNelle Wallace. 1994. LC 94-260. 16.95 (*1-882723-05-8*) Phoenix Soc.

Burnout & Stress Management Handbook: Professional Handbook Ser. Pref. by James J. Messina. 1982. 78p. (Orig.). pap. text 11.00 (*0-931975-14-X*) Advanced Dev Sys.

Burnout in HIV/AIDS Health Care & Support: Impact for Professionals & Volunteers. Ed. by Huib Van Dis & Emma Van Dongen. 1994. 79p. (Orig.). (C). pap. text (*90-5356-042-4*) Amsterdam U Pr NLD. *Dist:* U of Mich Pr.

Burnout Syndrome: Current Research, Theory, Interventions. John W. Jones. 1981. LC 81-84967. 179p. (Orig.). pap. 12.95 (*0-930171-00-4*) London Hse.

Burns: Therapy & Psychology with Subject Analysis & Research Bibliography. Lynn P. Chenn. rev. ed. 1997. 149p. 57.50 (*0-7883-1626-5*); pap. 47.50 (*0-7883-1627-3*) ABBE Pubs Assn.

Burns: Treatment & Research. Ed. by Peter C. Leung et al. 1991. 324p. (C). text 104.00 (*9971-5-0674-2*) World Scientific Pub.

Burns Sourcebook: Basic Consumer Health Information about Various Types of Burns & Scalds. Ed. by Allan R. Cook. 1999. LC 99-24510. (Health Reference Ser.). (Illus.). 595p. lib. bdg. 78.00 (*0-7808-0204-7*) Omnigraphics Inc.

***Burns Trauma: Management & Nursing Care.** Chrissie Bosworth. 2nd ed. 2001. 280p. (C). pap. (*1-86156-240-3*) Whurr Pub GBR. *Dist:* Taylor & Francis.

Burnt - A Teenage Addict's Road to Recovery see High School, Vol. 1, A Teenager's Drug Addiction, Treatment & Lasting Recovery

Burt Affair. R. B. Joynson. 1989. (General Psychology Ser.). 400p. 35.00 (*0-415-01039-X*, A3371) Routledge.

Burwell & Metcalfe's Heart Disease & Pregnancy: Physiology & Management. James Metcalfe et al. 2nd ed. 1986. 408p. 125.00 (*0-316-56797-3*, Little Brwn Med Div) Lppncott W & W.

Business Administration for the Dental Assistant. Ann Ehrlich. 4th ed. 1991. (Illus.). 185p. pap. text 23.95 (*0-940012-33-2*) Colwell Syst.

Business Administration for the Medical Assistant. Ann Ehrlich et al. 4th ed. 1991. LC 81-67045. (Illus.). pap. text 23.95 (*0-940012-32-4*) Colwell Syst.

Business Applications of Neuro Linguistic Programming. Wyatt Woodsmall. 1998. (Advanced Neuro Linguistic Programming Applications Ser.). 154p. spiral bd. 40.00 (*1-892876-02-7*) Next Step Pr.

Business Aspects of Medical Practice. Hoyt W. Torras & James R. Lyle. 1992. rev. ed. pap. 49.95 (*1-879249-05-7*); 2nd ed. pap. 49.95 (*1-879249-10-3*) HlthCare Consult.

Business Aspects of Optometry. John G. Classe. 1997. LC 96-50465. (Illus.). 384p. text 84.99 (*0-7506-9614-1*) Buttrwrth-Heinemann.

Business Awareness for Optometrists: A Primer. Nizar K. Hirji. 1999. LC 99-22338. 128p. pap. text 55.00 (*0-7506-3961-X*) Buttrwrth-Heinemann.

Business, Education, Health, Information Studies, Law & Social Work, 1999, Bk. 6. Peterson's Guides Staff. 1998. (Peterson's Graduate & Professional Program Ser.). 1999p. (*1-56079-986-2*) Intl School Servs.

Business English for the Pharmaceutical Industry: English-German, German-English. Reinhard Rychlik. 1993. (ENG & GER.). 407p. 150.00 (*0-7859-9982-5*) Fr & Eur.

Business Genetics. Charles Fine. 1998. (*0-201-31142-9*) Addison-Wesley.

Business, Legal, & Tax Planning for Dental Practices. William P. Prescott. 1994. LC 94-30140. 79.95 (*0-87814-424-2*) PennWell Corp.

Business Management for the Veterinary Practitioner. James F. Wilson et al. Ed. & Pref. by David A. Chubb. 1995. (Illus.). 368p. 59.95 (*1-888026-25-1*) Chubb Commun.

Business of Critical Care: A Textbook. William J. Sibbald et al. Ed. by Thomas A. Massaro. 2nd ed. 1996. (Illus.). 472p. 75.00 (*0-87993-623-1*) Futura Pub.

Business of Hypnotherapy: Establishing & Maintaining a Successful Practice. Katherine Zimmerman. 2nd ed. 1996. 137p. pap. 28.00 (*1-929957-00-9*) TranceTime.

Business of Medical Practice: Profit Maximizing Skill for Savvy Doctors. David Edward Marcinko. 2000. LC 99-54299. (Illus.). 368p. 55.95 (*0-8261-1311-7*) Springer Pub.

Business of Medicine. Julie K. Silver. 1998. LC 98-12942. 387p. 29.95 (*1-56053-254-8*) Hanley & Belfus.

Business of Nursing. American Organization of Nurse Executives Staff. 1996. LC 95-47785. 86p. pap. 45.00 (*1-55648-151-9*, 154153) AHPI.

Business of Opticianry, Vol. IV. William A. Borover. 1984. per. 48.00 (*0-9606398-4-5*) Gracie Ent.

Business of Orthodontics: Management & Administration of Your Orthodontic Practice. Karen Moawad et al. 1991. 550p. pap. (*0-9631446-0-X*) Hummingbrd WA.

Business of Psychotherapy. Robert L. Barker. 1982. LC 82-1307. (Illus.). 376p. text 57.50 (*0-231-05438-6*) Col U Pr.

Business of Veterinary Practice. Ed. by John Sheridan & Owen McCafferty. 1993. LC 92-41236. (Veterinary Handbook Ser.). pap. text 45.00 (*0-08-040846-X*, Pergamon Pr) Elsevier.

Business Perspective on Industry & Health Care. W. B. Goldbeck. 1978. LC 77-7982. (Springer Series in Industry & Health Care: Vol. 2). 70p. 57.00 (*0-387-90298-8*) Spr-Verlag.

Business Side of Medicine: A Survival Guide for Medical Students & Residents. Ronald P. Kaufman. 1999. LC 99-62644. 160p. (C). pap. 25.00 (*0-924674-72-5*) Am Coll Phys Execs.

Business Skills for Nurse Managers. Rundio. 1997. (Nursing Education Ser.). (C). pap. text 19.95 (*0-8273-5681-1*) Delmar.

Business Skills for Young Dentists: A Hands-on Guide for the Young Professional. John P. Sullivan. rev. ed. 1993. 125p. pap. 29.95 (*0-9638856-0-X*) Pronet Pr.

Business Strategies for a Caring Profession: A Practitioner's Guidebook. Sharon L. Yenney & American Psychological Association Staff. 1994. LC 94-13771. 159p. pap. 19.95 (*1-55798-254-6*) Am Psychol.

Business Yardsticks: An Introduction to Financial Ratios. 1991. 97p. pap. 41.00 (*1-883066-07-7*) Natl Comm Mental.

***But First Do No Harm.** George L. Druger. 2001. pap. 15.95 (*0-533-13846-9*) Vantage.

But I Didn't Say Goodbye: For Parents & Professionals Helping Child Suicide Survivors. Barbara Rubel. 2000. LC 99-96975. 112p. pap. (*1-892906-00-7*) Griefwork Ctr.

But Is It True: A Citizen's Guide to Environmental Health & Safety Issues. Aaron Wildavsky. 1997. (Illus.). 584p. pap. text 22.95 (*0-674-08923-5*) HUP.

But Westward Look: Nursing in Western Australia 1829-1979. Victoria Hobbs. 1981. (*0-85564-179-7*) Univ of West Aust Pr AUS. *Dist:* Intl Spec Bk.

But Where Is God? Psychotherapy & the Religious Search. John C. Robinson. 1999. 246p. pap. 18.95 (*1-56072-504-4*, Nova Troitsa Bks) Nova Sci Pubs.

Butadiene & Styrene: Assessment of Health Hazard. Ed. by K. Peltonen et al. 1994. (IARC Scientific Publications Ser.: No. 127). (Illus.). 424p. pap. text 95.00 (*92-832-2127-3*) OUP.

Butorphanol Tartrate: Research Advances in Multiple Clinical Settings. Ed. by C. E. Rosow. 1988. (Journal: Vol. 12, Suppl. 1, 1986). (Illus.). iv, 80p. pap. 26.25 (*3-8055-4752-8*) S Karger.

Butterfly & Life Span Nutrition. Majid Ali. 1995. 419p. (Orig.). pap. 16.99 (*1-879131-01-3*) Inst of Prev Med.

Butterfly Caste: A Social History of Pellagra in the South, 17. Elizabeth W. Etheridge. 1972. LC 70-176431. (Contributions in American History Ser.: No. 17). 278p. 68.50 (*0-8371-6276-9*, EHP/, Greenwood Pr) Greenwood.

Butterworth-Heinemann Handbook of Ophthalmic Diagnosis & Treatment. Ed. by Myron Yanoff. 1998. LC 98-11384. 320p. pap. text 49.99 (*0-7506-7014-2*) Buttrwrth-Heinemann.

Butterworth-Heinemann Pocket Book of Ophthalmology. Philip I. Murray & Alistair R. Fielder. 1997. LC 96-51444. (Illus.). 128p. pap. text 22.00 (*0-7506-2371-3*) Buttrwrth-Heinemann.

Butterworths Medico-Legal Reports. Ed. by Cardiff Law School Staff. 1992. 160p. 58.00 (*0-406-44001-8*, UK, MICHIE) LEXIS Pub.

Butterworths Medico-Legal Reports, Set. (*0-406-44000-X*, U.K., MICHIE) LEXIS Pub.

Buyer Be Wise! The Consumer's Guide to Buying Quality Nutritional Supplements. Karolyn A. Gazella. 1998. (Illus.). 93p. pap. 7.95 (*1-890694-04-5*) IMPAKT Communs.

Buyer's Guide to Choosing the Best Healthcare. Intro. by John J. Connolly. 2000. Orig. Title: How to Find the Best Doctors, Hospitals & HMOs for You & Your Family. 312p. pap. 12.95 (*1-883769-61-2*) Castle Connolly Med.

Buyer's Guide to Dentistry. Gordon J. Christensen. 1994. 256p. (C). (gr. 13). text 56.95 (*0-8016-6776-3*, 06776) Mosby Inc.

Buying Equipment & Programs for Home or Office. Ed. by C. J. McDonald. 1987. (M. D. Computing Benchmark Papers). (Illus.). 216p. 54.00 (*0-387-96455-X*) Spr-Verlag.

Buying, Selling & Merging a Medical Practice. Kenneth M. Hekman. 1996. text 50.00 (*0-7863-1155-X*, Irwn Prfssnl) McGraw-Hill Educ Grp.

Buying, Selling, & Merging Medical Practices: How to Structure, Negotiate, & Implement Transactions for Long-Term Success. Kenneth M. Hekman. 1996. LC 96-17364. 204p. text 50.00 (*0-7863-0815-X*, Irwn Prfssnl) McGraw-Hill Educ Grp.

Buying, Selling, & Owning the Medical Practice: The Physician's Handbook to Ownership Options. American Medical Association Staff. 1996. (Practice Success Ser.). pap. 54.00 (*0-89970-788-2*, OP315396WE) AMA.

By Accident, Not Design: The Case for Comprehensive Injury Reparations. Eli P. Bernzweig. 1980. LC 80-20815. 221p. 65.00 (*0-275-91686-3*, C1686, Praeger Pubs) Greenwood.

By No Extraordinary Means: The Choice to Forgo Life-Sustaining Food & Water. Ed. by Joanne Lynn. exp. ed. 1989. LC 85-45781. (Medical Ethics Ser.: Vol. 517). 323p. pap. 6.75 (*0-253-20517-4*, MB-517) Ind U Pr.

By Reason of Insanity: Essays on Psychiatry & the Law. Ed. by Lawrence Z. Freedman. 1983. LC 83-3314. 256p. lib. bdg. 45.00 (*0-8420-2203-1*) Scholarly Res Inc.

By The Ages: Behavior & Development of Children Prebirth through 8. K. Eileen Allen. 2000. LC 00-694635. (Illus.). 244p. pap. text 16.95 (*0-7668-2048-3*) Delmar.

By the London Post. John Lister. Ed. by Arnold S. Relman. 1985. 248p. (Orig.). pap. text 13.95 (*0-910133-13-1*) Mass Med Pub Div.

By the Patient & Not by the Book: Constancy & Change in Small Town Doctoring, 1893-1987. Paul I. Crellin & John K. Crellin. 1988. (Illus.). xi, 76p. (Orig.). pap. 12.95 (*0-89386-021-2*) Acorn NC.

Bye Bye Backache. David C. Lindsey. 1981. LC 81-67080. (Illus.). 256p. 17.95 (*0-939342-00-6*); pap. 10.95 (*0-939342-01-4*) DCarlin Pub.

Bye-Bye Bypass: The Truth about Chelation Therapy. Arline Brecher. 1989. (Illus.). 296p. (Orig.). pap. 5.95 (*0-927839-58-X*) HlthSavers Pr.

Byers Neurotherapy Reference Library. Ed. by Alvah P. Byers. 2nd ed. 1998. 515p. pap. text 75.00 (*1-887114-04-1*) AAPB.

Byssinosis-Causative Agent & Clinical Aspects. Shirley Inst. Staff. 1982. (C). (*0-7855-4570-0*) British Textile Tech GBR. *Dist:* St Mut.

C

C. G. Jung: His Myth in Our Time. Marie-Louise Von Franz. 1998. LC 98-155493. (Studies in Jungian Psychology by Jungian Analysts: Vol. 77). (Illus.). 384p. pap. (*0-919123-78-3*) Inner City Bks CAN. *Dist:* BookWorld.

C. G. Jung: Word & Image. Carl Gustav Jung & Wystan Hugh Auden. Ed. by Aniela Jaffe. 1983. LC 78-17319. (Princeton/Bollingen Paperbacks Ser.: Vol. XCVII, No. 2). (Illus.). 252p. pap. 29.95 (*0-691-01847-2*) Princeton U Pr.

C. G. Jung Letters Vol. 1: 1906-1950. Carl Gustav Jung. Ed. by Gerhard Adler & Aniela Jaffe. Tr. by R. F. C. Hull. 1992. LC 74-166378. (Bollingen Ser.: No. 95). (Illus.). 2p. 99.50 (*0-691-09895-6*) Princeton U Pr.

C. G. Jung Speaking: Interviews & Encounters. Carl Gustav Jung. Ed. by William McGuire. Tr. by R. F. C. Hull & Ralph Manheim. 1987. LC 77-71985. (Bollingen Ser.: No. 97). 520p. pap. 24.95 (*0-691-01871-5*) Princeton U Pr.

C. G. Jung's Psychology of Religion & Synchronicity. Robert Aziz. 1990. LC 89-30039. (Series in Transpersonal & Humanistic Psychology). 269p. (C). text 64.50 (*0-7914-0166-9*); pap. text 24.95 (*0-7914-0167-7*) State U NY Pr.

C. I. C. D. Collegium Internationale Chirurgiae Digestive: Abstracts-9th World Congress, Jerusalem, Aug.-Sept. 1986. Ed. by M. M. Feuchtwanger. 1986. (Journal: Vol. 3, No. 2). 140p. pap. 63.50 (*3-8055-4466-9*) S Karger.

C-Myc Function in Neoplasia. Chi V. Dang. 1996. (Medicine Ser.). 196p. pap. 89.95 (*0-412-10231-5*) Chapman & Hall.

C-Myc in B-Cell Neoplasia: 14th Workshop on Mechanics in B-Cell Neoplasia - The Workshop "Mechanisms in B-Cell Neoplasia" Ed. by M. Potter. 1997. (Current Topics in Microbiology & Immunology Ser.: Vol. 224). (Illus.). 291p. 119.00 (*3-540-62892-4*) Spr-Verlag.

C-Reactive Proteins in Health, Disease, Injuries & Diagnostics: Index of New Information. Jerry U. Simmons. 1997. 160p. 57.50 (*0-7883-1764-4*); pap. 47.50 (*0-7883-1765-2*) ABBE Pubs Assn.

CA Advisor Training Manual. Cindy Rondberg. 1998. (Illus.). 120p. lib. bdg. 50.00 (*0-9647168-5-2*) Chiropractic Jrnl.

CA Clinical Hematology. A. Victor Hoffbrand. 2nd ed. 1994. 344p. (*1-56375-592-0*) Gower-Mosby.

CA 2 Plus Plus Antagonists in CNS: Proceedings of Investigators' Meeting. Ed. by R. A. Janis & D. J. Triggle. 1994. (Drugs in Development Ser.). (Illus.). 520p. (Orig.). pap. text 75.00 (*0-9637603-1-9*) Neva Pr.

CA 2 Plus Pump of Plasma Membrane. Alcides F. Rega. Ed. by Patricio J. Garrahan. 1986. 184p. 108.00 (*0-8493-6253-9*, QH601, CRC Reprint) Franklin.

Cabinet of Medical Curiosities. Jan Bondeson. 1997. LC 97-20749. (Illus.). 320p. (gr. 10-12). 35.00 (*0-8014-3431-9*) Cornell U Pr.

Cabinet of Medical Curiosities. Jan Bondeson. 1999. LC 97-20749. (Illus.). 250p. pap. 14.00 (*0-393-31892-3*) Norton.

Cada Dia Un Nuevo Comienzo: Reflexiones Para Mujeres. Hazelden Publishing Staff. abr. ed. 1994. (SPA.). 400p. pap. 16.95 (*968-39-0794-6*, 6293) Hazelden.

Cadmium. 1992. (Environmental Health Criteria Ser.: No. 134). (ENG, FRE & SPA.). 280p. pap. text 50.00 (*92-4-157134-9*, 1160134) World Health.

Cadmium. Ed. by E. C. Foulkes. 1986. (Handbook of Experimental Pharmacology Ser.: Vol. 80). (Illus.). 450p. 327.00 (*0-387-16025-6*) Spr-Verlag.

Cadmium - Environmental Aspects. 1992. (Environmental Health Criteria Ser.: No. 135). 156p. pap. text 30.00 (*92-4-157135-7*, 1160135) World Health.

Cadmium & Health: A Toxicological & Epidemiological Appraisal, Vol. I. Ed. by Lars F. Friberg et al. 1985. 224p. 127.00 (*0-8493-6690-9*, RA1231, CRC Reprint) Franklin.

Cadmium & Health: A Toxicological & Epidemiological Appraisal Effects Response, Vol. II. Ed. by Lars Friberg et al. 1986. 320p. 179.00 (*0-8493-6691-7*, RA1231, CRC Reprint) Franklin.

Cadmium in the Human Environment: Toxicity & Carcinogenicity. Ed. by G. F. Nordberg et al. 1993. (IARC Scientific Publications Ser.: No. 118). (Illus.). 482p. pap. text 125.00 (*92-832-2118-4*) OUP.

Caesarean Birth: Experience, Practice & History. Helen Churchill. 1997. LC 97-204566. 120p. pap. text 34.99 (*1-898507-51-1*, RG761) Buttrwrth-Heinemann.

Caffeine: The Most Popular Stimulant. Richard Gilbert. 1986. LC 85-25970. (Encyclopedia of Psychoactive Drugs Ser.: No. 1). (Illus.). 124p. (YA). (gr. 7-11). lib. bdg. 19.95 (*0-87754-756-4*) Chelsea Hse.

Caffeine & Nicotine. Richard S. Lee & Mary Price Lee. 1998. LC 94-2279. (Drug Abuse Prevention Library). (Illus.). 64p. (YA). (gr. 7-12). lib. bdg. 17.95 (*0-8239-2745-8*, DRCANI) Rosen Group.

Caffey's Pediatric X-ray Diagnosis: An Integrated Imaging Approach. Ed. by Frederic N. Silverman. 9th ed. 1992. LC 92-18838. (Illus.). 2304p. text 360.00 (*0-8151-1462-1*, 22134) Mosby Inc.

Cahoon's Formulating X-Ray Techniques. Thomas T. Thompson. 9th ed. 1979. LC 79-87805. xii, 322p. text 32.95 (*0-8223-0431-7*) Duke.

CAI Network Evaluation Criteria & Methodology (Seattle, Wash. Nov., 1973) 2nd ed. 1976. 76p. 6.00 (*0-917054-10-5*) Med Communications.

***Cailliet's Soft Tissue Pain Syndromes.** Gary W. Jay. 4th ed. 2001. (Pain Ser.). (Illus.). 352p. pap. 29.95 (*0-8036-0773-3*) Davis Co.

Cajal on the Cerebral Cortex: An Annotated Translation of the Complete Writings. Santiago R. Cajal & FIDIA Research Foundation Staff. Ed. & Tr. by Javier DeFelipe & Edward G. Jones. 1988. (History of Neuroscience Ser.: No. 1). (Illus.). 672p. text 79.50 (*0-19-505280-3*) OUP.

Cajal's Degeneration & Regeneration of the Nervous System. Ed. by Javier DeFelipe & Edward G. Jones. Tr. by Raoul M. May. 1991. (History of Neuroscience Ser.: No. 5). (Illus.). 976p. text 79.50 (*0-19-506516-6*, 11153) OUP.

Cajal's Histology of the Nervous System S. Ramon y Cajal. Ed. by Larry W. Swanson. Tr. by Neely Swanson from FRE. 1995. LC 93-35437. (History of Neuroscience Ser.: No. 6). (Illus.). 1672p. text 195.00 (*0-19-507401-7*) OUP.

Calcification in Biological Systems. Ed. by Ermanno Bonucci. 1992. 432p. lib. bdg. 249.00 (*0-8493-5735-7*, QP535) CRC Pr.

Calcified Tissue. David W. Hukins. 1989. 88.00 (*0-8493-7115-5*, QP88) CRC Pr.

Calcitonine: Fisiologia e Farmacologia. M. Azria. 1990. (Illus.). x, 152p. 85.25 (*3-8055-5088-X*) S Karger.

Calcitonins: Physiology & Pharmacology. M. Azria. 1989. (Illus.). x, 152p. 85.25 (*3-8055-4851-6*) S Karger.

Calcium: Proliferator, Differentiator, & Killer. James F. Whitfield. 1997. (Molecular Biology Intelligence Unit Ser.). 200p. pap. 89.95 (*0-412-14061-6*) Thomson Learn.

Calcium & Hypertension. Ed. by Carlo Gennari & Shaul G. Massry. 1987. (American Journal of Nephrology: Vol. 6, Suppl. 1, 1986). (Illus.). vi, 166p. pap. 50.50 (*3-8055-4370-0*) S Karger.

Calcium & Magnesium in Early Life. Ed. by Reginald C. Tsang. 1995. LC 94-21058. 176p. 149.95 (*0-8493-4613-4*) CRC Pr.

Calcium & Phosphorus in Health & Disease. Ed. by John J. Anderson & Sanford C. Garner. 1995. (Modern Nutrition Ser.). 416p. 179.95 (*0-8493-7845-1*, 7845) CRC Pr.

Calcium & Your Health. Takuo Fujita. 1987. LC 87-80495. (Illus.). 144p. pap. 9.95 (*0-87040-691-4*) Japan Pubns USA.

Calcium Antagonists: Mechanisms of Action on Cardiac Muscle & Vascular Smooth Muscle. Ed. by Nicholas Sperelakis & James Caulfield. 1984. (Developments in Cardiovascular Medicine Ser.). text 131.50 (*0-89838-655-1*) Kluwer Academic.

Calcium Antagonists in Clinical Medicine. Murray Epstein. 2nd ed. 1997. LC 97-25775. 590p. 65.00 (*1-56053-223-8*) Hanley & Belfus.

Calcium Antagonists in the Treatment of Hypertension in Pregnancy. A. L. Tranquilli & C. Romanini. 1999. LC 98-11883. (Illus.). 170p. lib. bdg. 52.95 (*1-85070-468-6*, Parthenon Pbng) CRC Pr.

Calcium Antagonists Pharmacology & Clinical Research. Ed. by Theophile Godfraind et al. 1993. LC 93-15059. (Medical Science Symposia Ser.: Vol. 3). 404p. (C). text 200.50 (*0-7923-2259-2*) Kluwer Academic.

Calcium Antogonista & the Kidney: Journal: American Journal of Nephrology Vol. 7, Suppl. 1, 1987. Ed. by M. Epstein. 1988. (Illus.). iv, 68p. pap. 24.50 (*3-8055-4648-3*) S Karger.

Calcium As an Intracellular Messenger in Eucaryotic Microbes. Ed. by Danton H. O'Day. 1990. (Illus.). 418p. 99.95 (*1-55581-023-3*) ASM Pr.

Calcium As Cell Signal: Proceedings of the Yamada Conference XXXIX on Calcium As Cell Signal, April 26-28, 1994, Tokyo, Japan. Ed. by Koscak Maruyama et al. Date not set. LC 95-47710. (*4-260-14309-3*) Igaku-Shoin.

Calcium Bible: How to Have Better Bones All Your Life. Patricia Hausman. 1985. LC 84-42932. 224p. 13.95 (*0-89256-284-6*, Rawson Assocs) Macmillan.

Calcium-Binding Protein Protocols Vol. 1: Reviews & Case Histories. Ed. by Hans J. Vogel. 2001. LC 00-63354. (Methods in Molecular Biology Ser.: Vol. 172). (Illus.). 352p. 125.00 (*0-89603-688-X*) Humana.

Calcium-Binding Protein Protocols Vol. 2: Methods & Techniques. Ed. by Hans J. Vogel. 2002. (Methods in Molecular Biology Ser.: Vol. 173). 434p. 99.50 (*0-89603-689-8*) Humana.

Calcium-Binding Proteins: Biological Functions, Vol. II: Biological Functions. Marvin P. Thompson. 1988. LC 87-18375. 160p. 92.00 (*0-8493-4859-5*, QP552, CRC Reprint) Franklin.

Calcium-Binding Proteins: Characterization & Properties, Vol. I: Characterization & Properties. Marvin P. Thompson. 1988. LC 87-18375. 176p. 95.00 (*0-8493-4858-7*, QP552, CRC Reprint) Franklin.

Calcium Binding Proteins in Normal & Transformed Cells. Ed. by R. Pochet et al. 1990. LC 90-6704. (Advances in Experimental Medicine & Biology Ser.: Vol. 269). (Illus.). 224p. (C). text 102.00 (*0-306-43491-1*, Kluwer Plenum) Kluwer Academic.

Calcium, Cell Cycles, & Cancer. Ed. by James F. Whitfield. 1990. 280p. lib. bdg. 228.00 (*0-8493-6233-4*, QP535) CRC Pr.

Calcium-Dependent Processes in the Liver. Ed. by C. Heilmann et al. 1988. (Falk Symposium Ser.). (C). text 209.50 (*0-7462-0075-7*) Kluwer Academic.

Calcium Entry in Endothelium & in Mast Cells: Mechanisms & Modulation. Marion Gericke. 1996. (Acta Biomedica Lovaniensia Ser.: No. 124). (Illus.). 137p. (Orig.). pap. (*90-6186-729-0*) Leuven Univ BEL. *Dist:* Coronet Bks.

Calcium Factor: The Scientific Secret of Health & Youth. Robert R. Barefoot & Carl M. Reich. 1992. 110p. (Orig.). pap. 14.95 (*0-9633703-2-4*) Bokar Cnslts.

Calcium Homeostasis: Hypercal & Hypocalcaemia. Mundy. 1989. 122.00 (*0-948269-67-7*) CRC Pr.

Calcium Homeostasis: Hypercalcemia & Hypocalcemia. Gregory R. Mundy. 2nd ed. 1990. (Illus.). 284p. text 80.00 (*0-19-520894-3*) OUP.

Calcium Hunger: Behavioral & Biological Regulation. Jay Schulkin. 2000. LC 00-34212. (Illus.). 220p. text 80.00 (*0-521-79170-7*) Cambridge U Pr.

Calcium Hypothesis of Aging & Dementia. Ed. by John F. Disterhoft et al. 1995. LC 94-41979. (Annals Ser.: No. 747). 130.00 (*0-89766-878-2*) NY Acad Sci.

Calcium in Biological Systems. Ed. by Ronald P. Rubin et al. 1985. LC 84-18246. 760p. 145.00 (*0-306-41747-2*, Plenum Trade) Perseus Pubng.

Calcium in Cell Cycles & Cancer. James F. Whitfield. 2nd ed. 1995. LC 94-41530. 242p. 239.95 (*0-8493-4420-4*) CRC Pr.

Calcium in Muscle Activation. Johann C. Ruegg. 1988. (Zoophysiology & Ecology Ser.: Vol. 19). (Illus.). 300p. reprint ed. 69.00 (*0-387-18278-0*) Spr-Verlag.

Calcium in Your Life. American Dietetic Association Staff. 1997. 168p. (Orig.). pap. 5.95 (*0-471-34667-5*) Wiley.

Calcium in Your Life. American Dietetic Association Staff & Colleen Pierre. 1997. LC 98-231828. 168p. (Orig.). pap. 5.95 (*1-56561-117-9*) Wiley.

Calcium Ion Antagonists in Cardiovascular Disease: Proceedings of an International Conference, 12-13 October 1979, Toronto, Canada. Ed. by J. Morch. 1981. 200p. pap. 48.00 (*0-08-027376-9*, Pergamon Pr) Elsevier.

Calcium Ion Modulators: The New Wave of Psychotropic Drugs. Ed. by Kazuhide Inoue & Yasuo Watanabe. 1998. 208p. pap. text (*90-5702-080-7*, ECU63) GBSP NLD. *Dist:* Gordon & Breach.

Calcium Ions in Nerve Cell Function. Platon G. Kostyuk. 1992. (Illus.). 228p. text 69.50 (*0-19-854672-6*) OUP.

Calcium Metabolism. John A. Kanis. 1990. (Progress in Basic & Clinical Pharmacology Ser.: Vol. 4). (Illus.). viii, 188p. 146.25 (*3-8055-5146-0*) S Karger.

Calcium Neuronal Function & Transmitter Release. Ed. by Rami Rahamimoff & Bernard Katz. 1986. text 183.50 (*0-89838-791-4*) Kluwer Academic.

Calcium Oxalate in Biological Systems. Ed. by Saeed R. Khan. 1995. LC 95-36917. 400p. 129.95 (*0-8493-7673-4*, 7673) CRC Pr.

Calcium, Oxygen Radicals & Cellular Damage. Ed. by C. J. Duncan. 1991. (Society for Experimental Biology Seminar Ser.: No. 46). (Illus.). 234p. (C). text 69.95 (*0-521-38068-5*) Cambridge U Pr.

Calcium-Regulating Hormones, Set: Vol. 90-91. 1991. (Contributions to Nephrology Ser.). (Illus.). xxii, 382p. 269.75 (*3-8055-5451-6*) S Karger.

Calcium-Regulating Hormones Vol. 1: Role in Disease & Aging. Ed. by H. Morii. 1991. (Contributions to Nephrology Ser.: Vol. 90). (Illus.). xiv, 230p. 49.75 (*3-8055-5371-4*) S Karger.

Calcium-Regulating Hormones Vol. II: Calcium Transport, Bone Metabolism & New Drugs. Ed. by H. Morii. 1991. (Contributions to Nephrology Ser.: Vol. 91). (Illus.). viii, 152p. 49.75 (*3-8055-5372-2*) S Karger.

Calcium Regulating Hormones & Cardiovascular Function. M. F. Crass. 1994. 352p. 168.95 (*0-8493-8661-6*) CRC Pr.

Calcium Regulating Hormones, Vitamin D Metabolites, & Cyclic AMP Assays & Their Clinical Application. Ed. by H. Schmidt-Gayk et al. 1990. (Illus.). 370p. 125.00 (*0-387-52229-8*) Spr-Verlag.

Calcium Requirements. 1962. (Technical Report Ser.: No. 230). 54p. pap. text 4.00 (*92-4-120230-0*) World Health.

Calcium Signaling Protocols. David Lambert. 1999. LC 98-44482. (Methods in Molecular Biology Ser.: Vol. 114). (Illus.). 376p. 99.50 (*0-89603-597-2*) Humana.

Calcium-Signalling in Smooth Muscle: Recent Development. Ed. by C. Kwan. 1994. (Journal: Vol. 2, No. 5, 1993). (Illus.). 76p. pap. 28.75 (*3-8055-5968-2*) S Karger.

Calcium Signalling in the Nervous System. Ed. by Platon G. Kostyuk & A. Verkhratsky. 1996. 220p. 200.00 (*0-471-95941-3*) Wiley.

Calcium, Vitamin D, & Prevention of Colon Cancer. Martin Lipkin et al. 1991. (Illus.). 416p. lib. bdg. 129.00 (*0-8493-4264-3*, RC280) CRC Pr.

Calculate with Confidence. Deborah Gray. 2nd ed. 1997. LC 97-21619. (Illus.). 432p. (C). (gr. 13). pap. text 29.00 (*0-8151-2607-7*, 31077) Mosby Inc.

Calculated Risk: A Provider's Guide to Assessing & Controlling the Financial Risk of Managed Care. Ed. by Bruce S. Pyenson. 1995. 77p. pap. 32.00 (*1-55648-131-4*, 131001) AHPI.

Calculated Risks: The Toxicity & Human Health Hazards of Chemicals in Our Environment. Joseph V. Rodricks. 1994. (Illus.). 282p. (C). pap. text 19.95 (*0-521-42331-7*) Cambridge U Pr.

Calculation Methods for Industrial Hygiene. Salvatore R. DiNardi. 1995. (Illus.). 304p. text 54.95 (*0-442-01821-5*, VNR) Wiley.

Calculation of Drug Dosages. Caroline Janney & Jane Flahive. 5th ed. 1996. 256p. (C). reprint ed. pap. text 24.95 (*0-939287-11-0*); 6th ed. 2000. (Illus.). pap. text, wbk. ed. 35.95 (*0-939287-12-9*) T J Designs.

Calculation of Drug Dosages. Sheila J. Ogden & Ruth K. Radcliff. 6th ed. 1999. LC 98-54874. (Illus.). xviii, 508p. pap. text 36.00 (*0-323-00698-1*) Mosby Inc.

Calculation of Genetic Risks: Worked Examples in DNA Diagnostics. Peter J. Bridge. 2nd ed. 1997. LC 97-20471. (Illus.). 248p. 59.95 (*0-8018-5744-9*) Johns Hopkins.

Calculations for Veterinary Nurses. Margaret Moore & Norman Palmer. 2000. LC 00-46797. (Illus.). ix, 157p. pap. (*0-632-05498-0*) Blckwell Science GBR. *Dist:* Iowa U Pr.

Calculations for Veterinary Professionals. Vicki C. Mcconnell & Branson W. Ritchie. 2000. LC 99-47112. 204p. pap. 24.95 (*0-8138-0879-0*) Iowa U Pr.

Calculus: A Genetic Approach. Otto Toeplitz. Ed. by Gottfried Kothe. Tr. by Louise Lange. 1996. LC 63-9731. 208p. pap. text 16.50 (*0-226-80667-7*) U Ch Pr.

Calculus Disease. Ed. by Graeme R. Catto. 1988. (New Clinical Applications in Nephrology Ser.). (C). text 95.50 (*0-7462-0074-9*) Kluwer Academic.

C
D

Calculus for Biology & Medicine: Companion Website. 1999. *(0-13-085880-3)* P-H.

Calendar of Congresses of Medical Sciences, 1989: Bilingual English/French. 1989. (CIOMS Publication Ser.: No. 50). pap. text 10.00 *(92-9036-035-6)* World Health.

California Art Therapy Trends. Evelyn Virshup. 1993. (Illus.). 428p. (C). pap. text 29.95 *(0-9613309-3-7)* Magnolia St Pub.

California Consumers Talk about Health Care Quality: Findings from Focus Group Discussions. Peter D. Hart. unabr. ed. 1999. 44p. pap. *(1-929008-21-X)* CA HlthCare Fnd.

California Health Care in Perspective 2000. Ed. by Kathleen O'Leary Morgan & Scott E. Morgan. 2000. 21p. spiral bd. 19.00 *(0-7401-0204-4)* Morgan Quitno Corp.

California Health Care Perspective, 1998. Ed. by Kathleen O'Leary Morgan & Scott E. Morgan. 1998. 20p. pap. 19.00 *(1-56692-804-4)* Morgan Quitno Corp.

California Herbal Remedies: The History & Uses of Native Medicinal Plants. Lolo Westrich. 1989. (Illus.). 180p. pap. 14.95 *(0-87201-457-6,* 1457) Lone Star Bks.

California Indian Shamanism. Ed. by Lowell J. Bean & Sylvia B. Vane. 1992. LC 92-6167. (Anthropological Papers: No. 39). (Illus.). 274p. text 34.00 *(0-87919-125-2)*; pap. text 28.50 *(0-87919-124-4)* Ballena Pr.

California Institute of Psychology Modern Guide to Psychotherapy. John F. Fielder et al. 1991. pap. 13.95 *(0-9631938-5-6)* CIP Comms.

California Law for California Pharmacists. William L. Marcus & Marsha Cohen. Ed. by Mary A. Koda-Kimble. 1997. 235p. pap. text 27.50 *(0-915486-27-X)* Applied Therapeutics.

California Mental Health: The Struggle for Turf. Harold E. Simmons. 1978. pap. 10.00 *(0-87312-008-6)* Gen Welfare Pubns.

California Telemedicine: A Reimbursement Dilemma. Feedback Research Services Staff. 1998. 56p. spiral bd. 195.00 *(1-889713-19-8)* Feedback Rsch.

California Toxic Fungi. Thomas J. Duffy & Paul P. Vergeer. 1977. LC 77-76180. (Toxicology Monograph: No. 1). (Illus.). 2.00 *(0-918942-00-4)* Mycological.

California's Disproportionate Share Hospital Program: Background Paper. William Huen. 1999. (Illus.). 12p. pap. *(1-929008-24-4)* CA HlthCare Fnd.

Californium - 252: Isotope for 21st Century Radiotherapy: Proceedings of the NATO Advanced Research Workshop on Californium - 252, Isotope for 21st Century Radiotherapy, Detroit, U. S. A. April 24-27, 1996. Jacek G. Wierzbicki & North Atlantic Treaty Organization Staff. 1997. LC 97-8452. (NATO Advanced Science Institutes Ser.). 324p. text 184.00 *(0-7923-4543-6)* Kluwer Academic.

Call a Doctor, Please: Memoirs of a Surgeon. Edgar W. Barber & Patricia A. Paton. 1988. (Illus.). 326p. 24.95 *(0-9620899-0-7)*; pap. 14.95 *(0-9620899-1-5)* Whitaker Pub.

Call from Home: Armenia & Karabagh - My Journal. Carolann S. Najarian. 1999. LC 99-476349. (Illus.). xiv, 306p. 22.95 *(0-9664985-0-X)* Arpen Pr.

Call Me a Doctor: Tales of Six Medical Men Who Went Elsewhere & Did Other Things. Jack Griffitts. 1991. (Illus.). 244p. 15.95 *(0-9629072-0-0)* Amer Spectator.

Called to Care: A Christian Theology of Nursing. Judith A. Shelly & Arlene B. Miller. 1999. LC 99-10868. 288p. pap. 19.99 *(0-8308-1598-8,* 1598) InterVarsity.

***Callifornia Patient's Guide: Your Health Care Rights & Remedies.** Ed. by Barry Leonard. 2001. 79p. (C). pap. text 20.00 *(0-7567-1843-0)* DIANE Pub.

Callous Problem. G. Kuntscher. 1974. (Illus.). 160p. 9.50 *(0-87527-133-2)* Green.

Calories & Weight. 1991. lib. bdg. 150.00 *(0-8490-5139-8)* Gordon Pr.

Calorimetry: Fundamentals & Practice. Wolfgang Hemminger & Guenther Hohne. 1984. (Illus.). 310p. 105.00 *(0-89573-056-1,* Wiley-VCH) Wiley.

Calvary Hospital: A Model for Pallitaive Care in Advanced Cancer. Ed. by James E. Cimino & Michael Brescia. 1998. LC 98-71723. 180p. text 49.95 *(0-930194-98-5)* Ctr Thanatology.

Calving Problems & Early Viability of the Calf. Ed. by B. Hoffmann & I. L. Mason. 1979. (Current Topics in Veterinary Medicine & Animal Science Ser.: No. 4). text 206.50 *(90-247-2195-4)* Kluwer Academic.

Cambridge Companion to Freud. Ed. by Jerome Neu. 1991. (Cambridge Companions to Philosophy Ser.). 368p. (C). text 74.95 *(0-521-37424-3)*; pap. text 27.95 *(0-521-37779-X)* Cambridge U Pr.

Cambridge Companion to Jung. Ed. by Polly Young-Eisendrath & Terence Dawson. 1997. (Illus.). 366p. (C). text 59.95 *(0-521-47309-8)*; pap. text 21.95 *(0-521-47889-8)* Cambridge U Pr.

Cambridge Dictionary of Statistics in the Medical Sciences. B. S. Everitt. 1995. (Illus.). 287p. (C). text 69.95 *(0-521-47382-9)*; pap. text 24.95 *(0-521-47928-2)* Cambridge U Pr.

Cambridge Encyclopedia of Human Growth & Development. Ed. by Stanley J. Ulijaszek. 1998. LC 97-14707. (Illus.). 509p. (C). text 100.00 *(0-521-56046-2)* Cambridge U Pr.

Cambridge Encyclopedia of Human Paleopathology. Arthur C. Aufderheide & Conrado Rodriguez-Martin. 1998. LC 97-16223. (Illus.). 496p. (C). text 100.00 *(0-521-55203-6)* Cambridge U Pr.

Cambridge Handbook of Psychology, Health & Medicine. Ed. by Andrew Baum et al. 1997. (Illus.). 678p. (C). pap. text 74.95 *(0-521-43686-9)* Cambridge U Pr.

Cambridge Illustrated History of Medicine. Ed. by Roy Porter. 1996. (Illustrated Histories Ser.). (Illus.). 400p. (C). text 54.95 *(0-521-44211-7)* Cambridge U Pr.

Cambridge Medical Ethics Workbook: Case Studies, Commentaries & Activities. Michael Parker & Donna Dickenson. 2001. LC 00-42939. 374p. text 130.00 *(0-521-78301-1)*; (Illus.). pap. text 47.95 *(0-521-78863-3)* Cambridge U Pr.

Cambridge Medical Reviews: Haematological Oncology, Vol. 3. Ed. by Alan Burnett et al. 1994. (Illus.). 258p. (C). text 95.00 *(0-521-44208-7)* Cambridge U Pr.

Cambridge Medical Reviews Vol. 1: Neurobiology & Psychiatry. Ed. by Robert Kerwin et al. 1992. (Illus.). 200p. (C). text 85.00 *(0-521-39542-9)* Cambridge U Pr.

Cambridge Medical Reviews Vol. 2: Neurobiology & Psychiatry. Ed. by Robert Kerwin. 1993. (Illus.). 235p. (C). text 85.00 *(0-521-43483-1)* Cambridge U Pr.

Cambridge Textbook of Accident & Emergency Medicine. Ed. by Andrew Swain et al. 1997. LC 96-50952. (Illus.). 1285p. (C). text 260.00 *(0-521-43379-7)* Cambridge U Pr.

Cambridge World History of Human Disease. Ed. by Kenneth F. Kiple. 1993. (Illus.). 1200p. (C). text 175.00 *(0-521-33286-9)* Cambridge U Pr.

Camdex-R: The Cambridge Examination for Mental Disorders of the Elderly. Felicia A. Huppert et al. Ed. by Martin Roth. 2nd rev. ed. 1999. LC 97-16498. (Illus.). 114p. (C). text 160.00 *(0-521-46261-4)* Cambridge U Pr.

Came to Believe. 1973. LC 73-164457. 121p. pap. 1.20 *(0-916856-05-4)* AAWS.

Cameral Analysis: A Method of Treating the Psychoneuroses Using Hypnosis. David L. Pedersen. 1994. LC 93-37852. (Illus.). (C). 240p. 78.95 *(0-415-10424-6,* B3806); 224p. pap. 26.95 *(0-415-10425-4,* B3910) Routledge.

Cameras for Image Intensifier Fluorography, No. 15. International Commission on Radiation Units and Measurements Staff. 1969. LC 73-97641. 25.00 *(0-913394-08-4)* Intl Comm Rad Meas.

Camilla, Montana Prairie Pioneer. Camilla M. Anderson. 1996. LC 96-83562. *(1-888875-01-1)* P Diamond.

Campaign Safe & Sober. Mary Jagin et al. Ed. by Laurie Flaherty & Susan MacLean. unabr. ed. 1996. (Illus.). 233p. (Orig.). pap. 15.00 *(0-935890-05-X)* Emerg Nurses IL.

Campath-1H: Emerging Frontline Therapy in Chronic Lymphocytic Leukemia. Kanti R. Rai & Janet Stephenson. 2001. (Illus.). 128p. lib. bdg. 64.95 *(1-84214-060-4,* Parthenon Pbng) CRC Pr.

***Campbell's Operative Orthopaedics.** S. Terry Canale. 9th ed. 1999. 475.00 *(0-323-00494-6)*; 675.00 incl. cd-rom *(0-323-00493-8)* Mosby Inc.

Campbell's Operative Orthopaedics. S. Terry Canale. 9th ed. 1997. LC 97-33348. (Illus.). 4656p. (C). (gr. 13). text 450.00 *(0-8151-2087-7,* 28867) Mosby Inc.

Campbell's Operative Orthopaedics S. Terry Canale. 1998. (Illus.). 9th ed. 4656p. *(84-8174-328-3)*; Vol. 1. *(84-8174-353-4)*; Vol. 2. *(84-8174-354-2)*; Vol. 3. *(84-8174-355-0)*; Vol. 4. *(84-8174-356-9)* Mosby-Doyma Libros ESP. *Dist:* Mosby Inc.

Campbell's Urology Patrick C. Walsh. 7th ed. 1997. LC 96-40836. (Illus.). 3432p. text 395.00 *(0-7216-4461-9)* Saunders.

Campbell's Urology Study Guide. Patrick C. Walsh et al. Ed. by Richard Zorab. 1997. 432p. pap. text, stu. ed. 49.95 *(0-7216-6020-7)* Saunders.

Camptotheca Acuminata Decaisne, Xi Shu, a Promising Anti-Tumor & Anti-Viral Tree for the Twenty-First Century. Shiyou Li & Kent T. Adair. (Illus.). 268p. 45.00 *(0-938361-11-2)* Austin Univ Forestry.

Camptothecins: From Discovery to the Patient. Panayotis Pantazis et al. 1996. LC 96-39276. (Annals of the New York Academy of Sciences Ser.). 100.00 *(1-57331-056-5)*; pap. 100.00 *(1-57331-057-3)* NY Acad Sci.

Camptothecins: New Anti-Cancer Agents. Milan Potmesil & Herbert M. Pinedo. 1994. 160p. lib. bdg. 149.00 *(0-8493-4764-5,* 4764) CRC Pr.

Camptothecins: Unfolding Their Anticancer Potential. Ed. by Joachim G. Liehr et al. 2000. LC 00-51567. (Annals of the New York Academy of Sciences Ser.: Vol. 922). (Illus.). xii, 363p. *(1-57331-291-6)* NY Acad Sci.

Campus Community Confronts Sexual Assault: Institutional Issues & Campus Awareness. Juneau M. Gary. 1994. pap. 21.95 *(1-55691-113-0,* 130) Learning Pubns.

Campus Health Guide: The College Student's Handbook for Healthy Living. Carol L. Otis & Roger Goldingay. 1989. 460p. (C). pap. 14.95 *(0-87447-317-9)* College Bd.

Campus Mental Health Issues, Best Practices: A Guide for Colleges. Meg Mackenhaupt. 2000. 36p. pap. text 15.00 *(0-89292-256-7)* Educ Dev Ctr.

Campylobacter: Progress in Research. Ed. by D. G. Newell. 1982. (Illus.). 400p. text 183.00 *(0-85200-455-9)* Kluwer Academic.

Campylobacter Infection in Man & Animals. Ed. by Jean-Paul Butzler. 1984. 256p. 147.00 *(0-8493-5446-3,* QR201, CRC Reprint) Franklin.

CAMS Expressive Language Program. Vonda Douglass & Richard Baer. Ed. by Glendon Casto. 1979. LC 79-88181. (Curriculum & Monitoring System Ser.). 80p. pap. text 11.90 *(0-8027-9063-1)* Walker & Co.

CAMS Motor Program. Adrienne Peterson & Karen Sedjo. Ed. by Glendon Casto. 1979. LC 79-64724. (Curriculum & Monitoring System Ser.). 192p. pap. text 17.20 *(0-8027-9064-X)* Walker & Co.

CAMS Self-Help Program. Karen Sedjo & Richard Baer. Ed. by Glendon Casto. 1979. LC 79-64892. (Curriculum & Monitoring System Ser.). 180p. pap. text 16.80 *(0-8027-9065-8)* Walker & Co.

CAMS Training Manual. Ed. by Glendon Casto. 1979. LC 79-64723. (Curriculum & Monitoring System Ser.). 102p. 9.70 *(0-8027-9061-5)* Walker & Co.

Can a Woman Over Forty? Lynne Norris. 1979. LC 79-12587. 204p. 10.95 *(0-933380-41-0)*; pap. 5.95 *(0-933380-47-X)* Olive Pr Pubns.

Can Anyone Help my Child? Therapies & Treatment for Attention Deficit & Other Learning & Behavioral Disorders in Children, Adolescents, & Adults. Guy D. Ogan. rev. ed. 1991. 186p. (Orig.). pap. 9.95 *(0-9631880-1-1)* Faith Pub & Media.

Can Bacteria Cause Cancer? Alternative Medicine Confronts Big Science. David J. Hess. 1997. LC 97-4910. 234p. text 27.50 *(0-8147-3561-4)*; pap. text 18.50 *(0-8147-3562-2)* NYU Pr.

Can Health Care Costs Be Controlled? A Study in Production & Development in Health Care. Ingemar Stahl. 1986. (Illus.). 164p. (Orig.). pap. text 55.00 *(91-7504-048-4)* Coronet Bks.

Can Mandatory Treatment Be Therapeutic?, Vol. 75. Ed. by Mark R. Munetz. 1997. pap. 28.00 *(0-7879-9877-X)* Jossey-Bass.

Can Psychotherapists Hurt You? Judi Striano. 1989. LC 88-32208. 140p. (Orig.). (C). pap. 7.95 *(0-943659-03-5)* J Striano Bks.

Can Stress Heal? Converting a Major Health Hazard into a Surprising Health Benefit. Kenneth H. Cooper. 1998. LC 97-33082. 288p. 19.99 *(0-7852-8315-3)* Nelson.

Can Survive: Reclaiming Your Life after Cancer. Susan Nessim & Judith Ellis. rev. ed. 2000. LC 99-58373. xvi, 255p. pap. 15.00 *(0-618-00417-3)* HM.

Can You Avoid Cancer: An Investigation. Peter Goodwin. 1986. 166p. pap. *(0-563-21062-1)* BBC GBR. *Dist:* Parkwest Pubns.

Canada Nursing Job Guide, 1989. Ed. by Martha J. Denney. 1989. 166p. pap. 50.00 *(0-932834-06-X)* Prime Natl Pub.

Canadian Drug Identification Code. Health Protection Branch, National Health and Welfare Staff. 19th ed. 1993. 1023p. (Orig.). pap. *(0-660-57987-1)* Can7 Govern Pub.

Canadian Fundamentals of Nursing: Includes Testbank. Patricia A. Potter et al. 1997. tchr. ed. *(0-8151-2788-X)* Mosby Inc.

Canadian Guidelines for the Prevention, Diagnosis, Management & Treatment of Sexually Transmitted Diseases in Neonates, Children, Adolescents & Adults, April 1992, Vol. 18S1. Health and Welfare Canada Staff. 1992. 213p. (Orig.). pap. *(0-660-14767-X)* Can7 Govern Pub.

Canadian Health Care System: Lessons for the United States. Ed. by Susan Brown Eve et al. 1995. (Illus.). 304p. (C). reprint ed. pap. text 46.00 *(0-7618-0006-9)*; LC 97-4015. lib. bdg. 64.00 *(0-7618-0005-0)* U Pr of Amer.

Canadian Nurses & the Law. Morris. 1991. 205p. 50.00 *(0-409-80190-9,* MICHIE) LEXIS Pub.

Canadian Nurses & the Law. John J. Morris et al. 2nd ed. 1999. 330p. pap. text *(0-433-41609-2)* Butterwrth CAN Ltd CAN. *Dist:* Gaunt.

Canadian Nursing: Issues & Perspectives. Janet Ross Kerr. 1990. *(0-8016-2632-3)*; 2nd ed. (Illus.). 416p. (C). (gr. 13). pap. text 32.50 *(0-8016-6274-5,* 06274) Mosby Inc.

Canadian Nursing: Issues & Perspectives. Janet Ross Kerr & Jannetta Macphail. 3rd ed. 1995. (Illus.). 448p. (C). (gr. 13). pap. text 37.00 *(0-8151-5225-6,* 24348) Mosby Inc.

Canadian Nursing Faces the Future: Development & Change. Alice J. Baumgart & Jenniece Larson. 2nd ed. 1992. (Illus.). 680p. (C). (gr. 13). pap. text 30.00 *(0-8016-6330-X,* 06330) Mosby Inc.

Canadian Patient's Book of Rights. Lorne E. Rozovsky & Fay Rozovsky. 1994. LC 94-227688. 256p. pap. 18.95 *(0-385-25449-0)* Doubleday.

Canadian Transcultural Nursing: Assessment & Intervention. Joyce Newman Giger & Ruth Elaine Davidhizar. 1998. LC 98-20114. (Illus.). 416p. (C). (gr. 13). pap. text 37.00 *(0-8151-4389-3,* 31683) Mosby Inc.

Canakkale Bebek Dostu Hastane: Canakkale State Hospital BFHI Experience. UNICEF Turkey Staff. 1994. 40p. *(92-806-3076-8)* U N I C E F.

Canary & Chronic Fatigue. Majid Ali. 1995. 580p. pap. 20.00 *(1-879131-04-8)* Inst of Prev Med.

Cancer. Cal Orey & Joan Hustace Walker. 1999. LC 98-43387. (Essential Guide to Natural Pet Care Ser.: Vol. 2). (Illus.). 64p. pap. 6.95 *(1-889540-35-8)* Bowtie Press.

Cancer. Lisa Yount. 2000. LC 99-11431. (Contemporary Issues Companion Ser.). 190p. (YA). (gr. 9-12). lib. bdg. 27.45 *(0-7377-0161-7,* Greenhaven Pr) Gale.

Cancer, Vol. IV. Ingrid Naiman. 2nd ed. 1997. (Astrology of Healing Ser.). (Illus.). 216p. reprint ed. 35.00 *(1-882834-04-6)* Seventh Ray.

Cancer, Vols. 13, 13a & 13b. Arthur Frank et al. 1978. (Courtroom Medicine Ser.). ring bd. 674.00 *(0-8205-1259-1)* Bender.

Cancer: A Beginner's Guidebook of Hope. Jane Peters. rev. ed. 1991. 96p. pap. 6.95 *(0-9628806-1-2)* Encouraging Words.

Cancer: A Comprehensive Clinical Guide. Ed. by David Morris et al. 1998. 321p. pap. text 38.00 *(90-5702-216-8,* ECU32, Harwood Acad Pubs) Gordon & Breach.

Cancer: A Comprehensive Clinical Guide. Ed. by David Morris & John Kearsley. 1998. 321p. text 75.00 *(90-5702-215-X,* ECU83, Harwood Acad Pubs) Gordon & Breach.

***Cancer: A Modern Overview.** I. Edward Alcamo & Aronson. 2002. (Illus.). (C). pap. text 32.95 *(0-7637-1770-3,* 1770-3) Jones & Bartlett.

Cancer: A Natural Approach. Ed. by Christine Murphy. 2001. 96p. pap. 10.00 *(1-930051-31-X)* Lantern Books.

Cancer: Acute & Chronic Deleterious Effects of the Present Conventional Medical Therapy to Cancer Patients. Jacques Melek. 1984. 600p. (Orig.). pap. text 19.95 *(0-942330-04-8,* Sunbright Bks) J Melek.

Cancer: Affinity & Pool of Iron from the Red Blood Cells by the Highly Acidic Chromosomal Nucleic Acid of Cancer Cell As the Source of Energy of Cancer Cell & Loss of Weight by Cancer Patient. Jacques Melek. 1984. 400p. (Orig.). pap. text 8.95 *(0-942330-07-2,* Sunbright Bks) J Melek.

Cancer: Can Alternative Therapies Really Help? Linda R. Page. 2nd rev. ed. 1998. (Dr. Linda Page's Guides: Vol. 12). 96p. per. 8.95 *(1-884334-36-9)* Hlthy Healing.

Cancer: Cause - Prevention - Treatment. Lew Strogat, pseud. Ed. by Boris P. Berest. Tr. by Jack E. Evans. 1991. (Illus.). 272p. (Orig.). 20.00 *(0-939636-07-7)* Literary Frontiers Pubs.

Cancer: Causes, Occurrence & Control. L. Tomatis. 1990. (IARC Scientific Publications Ser.: No. 100). (Illus.). 368p. pap. text 50.00 *(92-832-0110-8)* OUP.

Cancer: Causes, Prevention & Treatment-the Total Approach. Paavo O. Airola. 1984. 48p. pap. 3.95 *(0-932090-05-2)* Health Plus.

Cancer: Egg-Shell Formation on Cancer Cell. Jacques Melek. 1984. (Illus.). 500p. (Orig.). pap. text 19.95 *(0-942330-05-6,* Sunbright Bks) J Melek.

Cancer: Epidemiology & Prevention in Public Health Practice. Phillip C. Nasca. Date not set. 350p. 65.00 *(0-8342-0769-9)* Aspen Pub.

Cancer: Etiology, Diagnosis & Treatment. Walter Burdette. 1997. LC 97-25674. (Illus.). 576p. text 39.00 *(0-07-008992-2)* McGraw-Hill Med Pub.

Cancer: Experiments & Concepts. R. Suess et al. 1977. LC 70-189962. (Springer Study Edition Ser.). (Illus.). xxii, 290p. 94.00 *(0-387-90042-X)* Spr-Verlag.

Cancer: Genetics & the Environment. Ed. by H. Leon Bradlow et al. 1997. LC 97-32681. (Annals of the New York Academy of Sciences Ser.: No. 833). 220p. 60.00 *(1-57331-114-6)* NY Acad Sci.

Cancer: Herencia y Ambiente. Cristina Cortinas. (Ciencia para Todos Ser.). (SPA.). pap. 6.99 *(968-16-3572-8)* Fondo CA.

Cancer: How Worthwhile Is Non-Curative Treatment? Ed. by M. L. Slevin et al. 1998. LC 97-18096. (Focus on Cancer Ser.). (Illus.). 327p. pap. 39.95 *(3-540-76083-0)* Spr-Verlag.

Cancer: Inherited Tumors. David Malkin. 1997. pap. text 39.00 *(3-540-19975-6)* Spr-Verlag.

Cancer: Materia Medica Relating to Cancer. 1999. LC 99-96160. 68p. pap. 6.95 *(1-929410-02-6)* dttm.

Cancer: Nursing Assessment & Care: A Self-Learning Text. Carol Smith. 1980. (Illus.). text 19.95 *(0-07-059106-7)* McGraw.

Cancer: Oral & Cutaneous Signs of Malignancy. Ed. by Dido Franceschi et al. 5th rev. ed. 1995. (Illus.). 105p. (Orig.). pap. text 34.00 *(1-879772-07-8)* Health Studies.

Cancer: Palliative Care. R. Dunlop. Ed. by R. Rubens. 1997. LC 97-36628. (Focus on Cancer Ser.). 181p. pap. 45.00 *(3-540-19974-8)* Spr-Verlag.

Cancer: Prevention, Detection, Causes, Treatment. Ed. by Clifford T. Stewart. 1987. (Orig.). 24.95 *(0-9617667-0-0)*; pap. 12.95 *(0-9617667-1-9)* Hamp Court Pr.

Cancer: Principles & Practice of Oncology. Ed. by Vincent T. DeVita, Jr. et al. 5th ed. 1996. (Illus.). 3456p. 325.00 incl. cd-rom *(0-397-58425-3)*; 355.00 incl. cd-rom *(0-397-58426-1)* Lppncott W & W.

Cancer: Principles & Practice of Oncology. Vincent T. DeVita, Jr. et al. 6th ed. 3,504p. 2001. 299.00 *(0-7817-2387-6)*; 2000. text 259.00 *(0-7817-2229-2)* Lppncott W & W.

Cancer: Rates & Risks. Ed. by Angela Harras. 4th ed. 1998. (Illus.). 205p. (C). pap. text 35.00 *(0-7881-7411-8)* DIANE Pub.

Cancer: The Outlaw Cell. Ed. by Richard E. LaFond. 2nd ed. 1988. LC 88-14517. (Illus.). 289p. text 35.00 *(0-8412-1419-0)*; pap. text 25.00 *(0-8412-1420-4)* Am Chemical.

Cancer: The Positive Approach: A No-Nonsense Prevention &Treatment Guide. Deborah Lee. 1999. 256p. pap. text 14.95 (*1-58054-045-7*) Woodland UT.

Cancer: Through the Eyes of Ten Women. Ed. by Patricia Duncker & Vicky Wilson. 1996. LC 98-211628. 256p. (*0-04-440980-X*) Pandora GBR. *Dist:* NYU Pr.

Cancer: What It Means: A Guide for People Who Have Just Learned They Have Cancer. 1998. (Illus.). 36p. pap. 5.30 (*0-939838-41-9*) Pritchett & Hull.

Cancer: What to Do about It. Ray Lowenthal. 1997. pap. text (*0-85091-644-5*) Lothian Pub AUS. *Dist:* Seven Hills Bk.

Cancer: What's It Doing in My Life? Mary A. Geier. 2nd ed. 1997. LC 85-17559. 128p. (Orig.). pap. 9.95 (*0-932727-05-0*) Hope Pub Hse.

Cancer Vol. 1: A Comprehensive Treatise, Etiology: Chemical & Physical Carcinogenesis. Ed. by Frederick F. Becker et al. 2nd ed. 1982. LC 81-21050. 736p. 125.00 (*0-306-40701-9*, Plenum Trade) Perseus Pubng.

Cancer, AIDS & Quality of Life: Proceedings of the Second International Conference of the International Council for Global Health Progress (ICGHP) Held in Paris, France, January 15-17, 1996. Ed. by Jay A. Levy et al. 1997. LC 97-5782. (Illus.). 211p. 85.00 (*0-306-45517-X*, Kluwer Plenum) Kluwer Academic.

Cancer-Anaphylactic: The Jacques Melek Cytokinetic Induced Respond Immune Response & Molecular Theory Effect on Cancer Cells. Jacques Melek. 1984. 600p. (Orig.). pap. 24.95 (*0-942330-03-X*, Sunbright Bks) J Melek.

Cancer & Aging. Ed. by Alvaro Macieira-Coelho. 1990. 304p. lib. bdg. 149.00 (*0-8493-6878-2*, RC262) CRC Pr.

Cancer & AIDS. Ed. by J. M. Vaeth. 1985. (Frontiers of Radiation Therapy & Oncology Ser.: Vol. 19). (Illus.). x, 186p. 142.75 (*3-8055-3923-1*) S Karger.

Cancer & Anti-Oxidants: Index of New Information & Bibliography. Jonas E. Webster. 1996. 150p. 57.50 (*0-7883-1004-6*); 1996. 150p. pap. 47.50 (*0-7883-1005-4*); 1998. 167p. 57.50 (*0-7883-1882-9*); 1998. 167p. pap. 47.50 (*0-7883-1883-7*) ABBE Pubs Assn.

Cancer & Autoimmunity. Yehuda Shoenfeld & M. Eric Gershwin. 2000. LC 99-37344. (Autoantibody Library). 468p. 170.00 (*0-444-50331-5*) Elsevier.

Cancer & Carcinogens in Your Environment at Home, Work & Recreation. American Health Research Institute Staff. 1995. LC 95-17724. 150p. 57.50 (*0-7883-0748-7*); pap. 47.50 (*0-7883-0749-5*) ABBE Pubs Assn.

***Cancer & Chromosome Aberrations: Index of New Information & Guide-Book for Consumers, Reference & Research.** John C. Bartone. 2002. 180p. pap. 47.50 (*0-7883-2421-7*) ABBE Pubs Assn.

Cancer & Chronic Lung Disease in the Workplace. 1991. lib. bdg. 250.00 (*0-8490-4342-5*) Gordon Pr.

Cancer & Common Sense: Combining Science & Nature to Control Cancer. Douglas S. Brodie & Michael Culbert. Ed. by Paul L. Engstrom. 1997. pap. 12.95 (*1-884367-03-8*) Winning St Paul.

Cancer & Consciousness. Barry Bryant. 1990. 277p. pap. 18.95 (*0-938434-74-8*) Sigo Pr.

Cancer & Emotion: A Practical Guide to Psycho-Oncology. Jennifer Barraclough. 3rd ed. 1999. LC 98-37039. 236p. (C). pap. 49.95 (*0-471-98597-X*) Wiley.

Cancer & Faith: Reflections on Living with a Terminal Illness. John Carmody. 1994. LC 94-60080. 160p. (Orig.). pap. 9.95 (*0-89622-594-1*) Twenty-Third.

Cancer & Genetics: Answering Your Patients' Questions. Randi L. Gould et al. 1997. (Illus.). 150p. (Orig.). pap. 14.95 (*0-9641823-6-X*) PRR.

Cancer & HIV Clinical Nutrition. Gail Wilkes. 2nd ed. 1999. (Illus.). 272p. (C). pap. text (*0-7637-1128-4*) Jones & Bartlett.

Cancer & HIV Nutrition Pocket Guide. Gail M. Wilkes. 1995. LC 95-1041. (Nursing Ser.). (Illus.). 224p. (C). spiral bd. 35.00 (*0-86720-726-4*, 726-4) Jones & Bartlett.

Cancer & Its Causes: Index of Modern Authors & Subjects with Guide for Rapid Research. John C. Bartone. 1991. LC 90-56234. (Illus.). 205p. 47.50 (*1-55914-244-8*); pap. 44.50 (*1-55914-245-6*) ABBE Pubs Assn.

Cancer & Its Management. Jeffrey S. Tobias & Robert L. Souhami. 2nd ed. 1995. LC 94-21772. (Illus.). 592p. pap. 59.95 (*0-632-03371-1*) Blackwell Sci.

Cancer & Its Management. Robert L. Souhami & Jeffrey S. Tobias. 3rd ed. 1998. LC 97-26658. 524p. pap. 78.95 (*0-86542-774-7*) Blackwell Sci.

***Cancer & Its Palliative Care: Index of New Information & Guide-Book for Consumers, References & Research.** Ed. by Research and Development Division Staff & John C. Bartone. 2001. (Illus.). 190p. 47.50 (*0-7883-2478-0*); pap. 44.50 (*0-7883-2479-9*) ABBE Pubs Assn.

Cancer & Its Psychological Influences: Index of Modern Authors & Subjects with Guide for Rapid Research. John C. Bartone. 1991. 180p. 47.50 (*1-55914-246-4*); pap. 44.50 (*1-55914-247-2*) ABBE Pubs Assn.

Cancer & Natural Medicine: A Textbook of Basic Science & Clinical Research. John C. Boik. 1996. LC 95-69639. (Illus.). 332p. (Orig.). pap. 28.00 (*0-9648280-0-6*) OR Med Pr.

Cancer & Nutrition. Ed. by K. N. Prasad & W. C. Cole. 1997. LC 97-75197. 251p. 86.00 (*90-5199-377-3*) IOS Press.

Cancer & Nutrition: Prevention & Treatment. Ed. by J. Mason & G. Nitenberg. 2000. LC 00-37108. (Nestle Nutrition Workshop Ser.: Vol. 4). (Illus.). xvi, 300p. 198.25 (*3-8055-7081-3*) S Karger.

Cancer & Nutrition Vol. 7. R. B. Alfin-Slater & D. Kritchevsky. 1991. (Human Nutrition Ser.). (Illus.). 508p. (C). text 110.00 (*0-306-43425-3*, Kluwer Plenum) Kluwer Academic.

Cancer & Pre-Cancer of the Cervix. Ed. by David Luesley & R. Barrasso. 1999. LC 98-70533. (Illus.). 472p. (*0-412-56600-1*) E A GBR. *Dist:* OUP.

***Cancer & Pregnancy.** Ed. by E. R. Barnea et al. 2001. LC 00-49240. x, 310p. 139.00 (*1-85233-374-X*) Spr-Verlag.

Cancer & the Adolescent. Peter Selby & Clifford Bailey. 1996. 256p. pap. text (*0-7279-0893-6*) BMJ Pub GBR. *Dist:* AIDC.

Cancer & the Elderly. Ed. by J. L. Meyer & J. M. Vaeth. 1986. (Frontiers of Radiation Therapy & Oncology Ser.: Vol. 20). (Illus.). viii, 202p. 161.00 (*3-8055-4145-7*) S Karger.

Cancer & the Family. Lea Baider et al. 2nd ed. 2000. LC 99-56524. (Illus.). 572p. 149.95 (*0-471-80300-6*) Wiley.

Cancer & the Heart. Ed. by A. S. Kapoor. 1986. (Illus.). xvii, 318p. 126.00 (*0-387-96245-X*) Spr-Verlag.

Cancer & the Law: A Medical Negligence Guide. Jonathan Waxman & Daniel Simons. 1999. LC 99-35052. 110.95 (*0-632-04852-2*) Blackwell Sci.

Cancer & the Search for Selective Biochemical Inhibitors. E. J. Hoffman. 1999. LC 98-49306. 584p. 139.95 (*0-8493-9118-0*) CRC Pr.

Cancer & Vitamin C: A Discussion of the Nature, Causes, Prevention, & Treatment of Cancer, with Special Reference to the Value of Vitamin C. Ewan Cameron & Linus Pauling. rev. ed. 1993. LC 93-12150. (Illus.). 278p. pap. 13.95 (*0-940159-21-X*) Camino Bks.

Cancer Answer. Albert E. Carter. 252p. (*0-9619041-1-9*) ALM Pubs.

Cancer Answers: Encouraging Answers to 25 Questions You Were Always Afraid to Ask. Errol C. Friedberg. 1992. LC 92-13491. 191p. pap. text 10.95 (*0-7167-7023-7*) W H Freeman.

Cancer As Initiation: Surviving the Fire. Barbara Stone. 1994. LC 94-36451. (Dreamcatcher Ser.: Vol. 2). 284p. 38.95 (*0-8126-9273-X*); pap. 17.95 (*0-8126-9274-8*) Open Court.

Cancer Battle Plan: Six Strategies for Beating Cancer from a Recovered "Hopeless Case" Anne E. Frahm & David J. Frahm. 1997. LC 97-25467. 172p. 12.95 (*0-87477-893-X*, Tarcher Putnam) Putnam Pub Group.

Cancer Battle Plan: Six Strategies for Beating Cancer, from a Recovered "Hopeless Case" David J. Frahm & Anne E. Frahm. 1992. LC 92-39675. 171p. (Orig.). pap. 14.00 (*0-89109-690-6*) Pinon Press.

Cancer Biology. Roger J. King. 2nd ed. 2000. LC 99-42884. xv, 308p. (*0-582-40432-0*) P-H.

Cancer Biology. Raymond W. Ruddon. 3rd ed. 1995. (Illus.). 544p. pap. text 52.50 (*0-19-509691-6*) OUP.

Cancer Biology & Biosynthesis. Samuel H. Wilson. 1991. 192p. 111.00 (*0-936923-50-4*, RC261) CRC Pr.

Cancer Book: A Guide to Understanding the Causes, Prevention & Treatment of Cancer. Geoffrey M. Cooper. 1993. LC 93-16282. (Illus.). 248p. (C). pap. text 24.95 (*0-86720-770-1*, 770-1) Jones & Bartlett.

***Cancer Breakthrough You've Never Heard Of: Your Guide to Limited Surgery in the Treatment of Cancer.** Richard A. Evans. 2001. Orig. Title: Making the Right Choice - Treatment Options in Cancer Surgery. (Illus.). 375p. pap. 16.95 (*0-9668865-3-4*) Murdock Pubng.

***Cancer Care.** David. 1994. pap. 35.95 (*0-412-55430-5*) Chapman & Hall.

Cancer Care: A Nurses' Guide. Brenda M. Nevidjon & Kevin W. Sowers. 2000. LC 99-55266. 528p. pap. text 39.95 (*0-7817-1587-3*) Lppncott W & W.

Cancer Care - Aid & Facilities: Index of New Information & Resources. Helen N. Bloggett. 1997. 160p. 57.50 (*0-7883-1532-3*); pap. 47.50 (*0-7883-1533-1*) ABBE Pubs Assn.

Cancer Care in the Hospital. Ed. by Barry W. Hancock. 1995. (*1-85775-120-5*) Radcliffe Med Pr GBR. *Dist:* Balogh.

***Cancer Caregivers a Resource Guide: Hundreds of Essential Tips.** Karen Kirzner Adler & Rozlyn Forman Kleiman. 2001. 250p. pap. 17.95 (*0-9701058-5-1*) Upstream Pr TX.

Cancer, Cause, Cure & Cover-Up. Ron Gdanski. 2000. 479p. pap. (*0-9685665-0-2*) Nadex Pub CAN. *Dist:* New Centry Pr.

Cancer Causes & Natural Controls. Lynn Dallin. 1984. LC 82-13765. 374p. 24.95 (*0-87949-224-4*) Ashley Bks.

Cancer Causes & Prevention. Ed. by Swedish Cancer Committee Staff. 1992. 500p. 220.00 (*0-85066-344-X*) Taylor & Francis.

Cancer Cell. Ed. by K. Sikora et al. 1991. (British Medical Bulletin Ser.: Vol. 47, No. 1). (Illus.). 1991p. text (*0-443-04489-9*) Church.

Cancer Chemo-& Immunopharmacology Part 1: Chemopharmacology. Ed. by G. Mathe & Franco M. Muggia. 1980. (Recent Results in Cancer Research Ser.: Vol. 74). (Illus.). 315p. 86.00 (*0-387-10162-4*) Spr-Verlag.

Cancer Chemoprevention. Lee W. Wattenberg. 1992. 656p. lib. bdg. 189.00 (*0-8493-4715-7*, RC268) CRC Pr.

Cancer Chemotherapeutic Agents. Ed. by William O. Foye. 1995. LC 94-39366. (ACS Professional Reference Bk.). 718p. 175.00 (*0-8412-2920-1*) Am Chemical.

Cancer Chemotherapy. Margaret Barton-Burke. 1991. 480p. 50.00 (*0-86720-434-6*) Jones & Bartlett.

Cancer Chemotherapy. Ed. by John A. Hickman & Thomas R. Tritton. 1993. LC 92-49872. (Frontiers in Pharmacology & Therapeutics Ser.). (Illus.). 384p. 145.00 (*0-632-03441-6*) Blackwell Sci.

Cancer Chemotherapy. Ed. by F. Homburger. 1979. (Oncology One Ser.). (Illus.). pap. 13.25 (*3-8055-3026-9*) S Karger.

Cancer Chemotherapy. T. J. Priestman. 3rd ed. 1989. 224p. 45.00 (*0-387-19551-3*) Spr-Verlag.

Cancer Chemotherapy: A Nursing Process Approach. Margaret B. Burke et al. 2nd ed. 1996. (Nursing Ser.). (Illus.). 752p. (C). text 65.95 (*0-86720-718-3*, 718-3) Jones & Bartlett.

Cancer Chemotherapy: A Veterinary Handbook. Ed. by Kevin A. Hahn & Ralph C. Richardson. 1994. LC 94-4930. (*0-8121-1693-3*) Lppncott W & W.

Cancer Chemotherapy: Challenges for the Future, Vol. 9. Ed. by K. Kimura et al. (International Congress Ser.: No. 1078). 252p. 162.50 (*0-444-81966-5*, Excerpta Medica) Elsevier.

Cancer Chemotherapy: Concepts, Clinical Investigations & Therapeutic Advances. Ed. by Franco M. Muggia. 1988. (Cancer Treatment & Research Ser.). (C). text 160.50 (*0-89838-381-1*) Kluwer Academic.

Cancer Chemotherapy: Reprinted Selected Top Articles Published 1976-1978. Ed. by F. Homburger. 1979. (Oncology Two Ser.). (Illus.). pap. 13.75 (*3-8055-3029-3*) S Karger.

Cancer Chemotherapy Vol. 10: Challenges for the Future. Ed. by K. Kimura et al. 1995. (International Congress Ser.). 326p. 191.50 (*0-444-82320-4*, Excerpta Medica) Elsevier.

Cancer Chemotherapy & Biological Response Modifiers. Ed. by H. M. Pinedo et al. 1997. (Cancer Chemotherapy Annual Ser.: Vol. 17). 768p. 190.50 (*0-444-82671-8*, North Holland); 1994. 732p. 324.25 (*0-444-82056-6*) Elsevier.

Cancer Chemotherapy & Biological Response Modifiers: Annual 14, Vol. 14. Ed. by H. M. Pinedo et al. 1993. 698p. 320.50 (*0-444-81509-0*) Elsevier.

Cancer Chemotherapy & Biological Response Modifiers: Annual 16, Vol. 16. Ed. by H. M. Pinedo et al. 1995. 704p. 305.75 (*0-444-82326-3*) Elsevier.

***Cancer Chemotherapy & Biological Response Modifiers: Annual 19**, Annual 19. Ed. by G. Giaccone et al. 2001. (Cancer Chemotherapy Annual 19 Ser.). 746p. 181.50 (*0-444-50561-X*) Elsevier.

Cancer Chemotherapy & Biotherapy: Principles & Practice. Ed. by Bruce A. Chabner & Dan L. Longo. 2nd ed. 1995. 848p. text 129.00 (*0-397-51418-2*) Lppncott W & W.

Cancer Chemotherapy & Biotherapy: Principles & Practice. Bruce A. Chabner. 3rd ed. 2001. text 179.00 (*0-7817-2269-1*) Lppncott W & W.

Cancer Chemotherapy & Biotherapy: The Reference Guide. Linda Tenenbaum. 2nd ed. 1994. LC 94-6844. (Illus.). 634p. pap. text 47.00 (*0-7216-6720-1*) Saunders.

Cancer Chemotherapy & Selective Drug Development: Proceedings of the Tenth Anniversary Meeting of the Coordination Committee for Human Tumor Investigations, Brighton, England (24-28 October, 1983) K. R. Harrap et al. 1984. (Developments in Oncology Ser.). 615p. text 141.00 (*0-89838-673-X*) Kluwer Academic.

Cancer Chemotherapy by Infusion. Ed. by Jacob J. Lokich. 2nd ed. 1990. LC 90-61367. 659p. 129.00 (*0-944496-14-8*) Precept Pr.

***Cancer Chemotherapy Care Plans Handbook.** Margaret Barton Burke et al. 3rd ed. 2001. LC 2001-38541. (Illus.). 416p. (C). text 31.95 (*0-7637-1481-X*, 1481-X, N L N Bart) Jones & Bartlett.

Cancer Chemotherapy Guidelines & Recommendations for Practice. Ed. by Maryanne Fishman & Mary Mrozek-Orlowski. 2nd rev. ed. 1999. LC 99-62505. (Illus.). 146p. pap. text 45.00 (*1-890504-11-4*) Oncology Nursing.

Cancer Chemotherapy Handbook. Dorr. 2nd ed. 1994. text 90.00 (*0-8385-1068-X*) McGraw-Hill Educ Grp.

Cancer Chemotherapy Handbook. Robert T. Dorr & Daniel D. Von Hoff. 2nd ed. 1996. 1020p. (C). pap. text 115.00 (*0-8385-1036-1*, A1036-1, Apple Lange Med) McGraw.

Cancer Chemotherapy Handbook. Robert T. Dorr. 3rd ed. 1999. 80.00 (*0-8385-1534-7*, Medical Exam) Appleton & Lange.

Cancer Chemotherapy Handbook. David S. Fischer & M. Tish Knobf. 5th ed. 1997. LC 97-5017. (Illus.). 640p. (C). (gr. 13). pap. text 39.95 (*0-8151-3314-6*, 29158) Mosby Inc.

Cancer Chemotherapy I. Franco M. Muggia. 1983. text 187.00 (*90-247-2713-8*) Kluwer Academic.

Cancer Chemotherapy in Small Animal Practice. Jane M. Dobson & Neil T. Gorman. 1993. LC 93-3434. (Library of Veterinary Practice). (Illus.). 224p. pap. 41.95 (*0-632-03694-X*) Blackwell Sci.

Cancer Chemotherapy Order. Sather. 1979. pap. text (*90-247-2170-9*) M Nijhoff NLD. *Dist:* Kluwer Academic.

Cancer Chemotherapy Pocket Guide. Robert Ignoffo. 1997. LC 96-50069. 480p. pap. text 55.00 (*0-397-51521-9*) Lppncott W & W.

Cancer Chemotherapy Treatment Protocols. David Khayat et al. 1998. LC 97-6107. (Illus.). 145p. pap. 75.00 (*0-86542-693-7*) Blackwell Sci.

***Cancer Chronicles.** Ann H. Milam. 2001. pap. 7.95 (*0-533-13572-9*) Vantage.

Cancer Clinical Trials: Experimental Treatments & How They Can Help You. Robert Finn. Ed. by Linda Lamb. 1999. LC 99-38927. (Patient-Centered Guides Ser.). (Illus.). 226p. pap. 14.95 (*1-56592-566-1*, Patient-Centered) OReilly & Assocs.

Cancer Combat: Cancer Survivors Share Their Guerrilla Tactics to Help You Win the Fight of Your Life. Dean King et al. 1998. LC 97-44801. 432p. pap. 12.95 (*0-553-37845-7*) Bantam.

Cancer Control. 1963. (Technical Report Ser.: No. 251). 27p. pap. text 3.00 (*92-4-120251-3*) World Health.

Cancer Control in Children: Report on a Study. O. Hrodek. 1983. (Euro Reports & Studies Ser.: No. 75). 37p. pap. text 5.00 (*92-890-1241-2*) World Health.

Cancer Control in the Countries of the Council of Mutual Economic Assistance. N. P. Napalkov & S. Eckhardt. 1982. 741p. (C). (*963-05-3036-8*) Akade Kiado HUN. *Dist:* St Mut.

Cancer Control in the Countries of the Council of Mutual Economic Assistance. N. P. Napalkov & S. Eckhardt. 1982. 742p. 177.00 (*0-569-08718-X*) St Mut.

Cancer Control in the Eastern Mediterranean Region. 1995. (EMRO Technical Publications: No. 20). iii, 52p. (C). pap. text 7.20 (*92-9021-194-6*, 1450020) World Health.

Cancer Culture. Colditz. 1995. 24.95 (*0-226-11321-3*) U Ch Pr.

Cancer Cure: The Complete Guide to Finding. Gary L. Schine. 1996. LC 96-166037. 183p. pap. 13.00 (*1-57566-024-5*) Kensgtn Pub Corp.

Cancer Cure That Worked! The Rife Report Fifty Years of Suppression. Barry Lynes. 1987. 167p. (Orig.). pap. 10.95 (*0-919951-30-9*) New Leaf Dist.

Cancer Curers - Or Quacks? The Story of a Secret Herbal Remedy. T. Llew Jones & Dafydd W. Jones. 1998. 128p. pap. 13.95 (*0-8464-4700-2*) Beekman Pubs.

Cancer Curing the Incurable Without Surgery, Chemotherapy & Radiation. William D. Kelley. 200p. mass mkt. 29.95 (*0-9669422-9-9*) Metabolic Medicine.

Cancer Cytogenetics. Sverre Heim & Felix Mitelman. 2nd ed. 1995. LC 95-7451. 552p. 99.95 (*0-471-12052-9*) Wiley.

Cancer de la Prostata. Sheldon Marks. 1997. LC 97-9313. (SPA.). 320p. pap. 18.50 (*1-55561-136-2*) Fisher Bks.

Cancer Diagnosis: Early Detection. Ed. by P. Bannasch. 1992. (Illus.). 272p. 74.95 (*0-387-54503-4*) Spr-Verlag.

Cancer Diagnosis in Children. L. D. Samuels. 1972. (CRC Uniscience Ser). 46.00 (*0-87819-009-0*, R) CRC Pr.

Cancer Diagnostic Imaging Markets. Market Intelligence Staff. 1994. LC 97-197198. 410p. 2295.00 (*0-7889-0139-7*) Frost & Sullivan.

Cancer, Diagnostics, & Chemotherapy: A Reference Manual. Cynthia C. Chernecky. 1991. pap. text 34.00 (*0-7216-3187-8*) Saunders.

Cancer Dictionary. Roberta Altman & Michael J. Sarg. 1994. (Illus.). 360p. reprint ed. pap. 16.95 (*0-8160-3027-8*) Facts on File.

Cancer Dictionary. Roberta Altman & Michael J. Sarg. rev. ed. 1999. LC 99-21201. (Illus.). xi, 387p. text 40.00 (*0-8160-3953-4*); pap. text 19.95 (*0-8160-3954-2*) Facts on File (Checkmark).

Cancer Disarmed: Healing Benefits of a Natural Plant Formula. Nina Anderson & Howard Peiper. 2000. 40p. mass mkt. 4.95 (*0-9701110-6-1*) New Cent Pub CT.

Cancer Disease & Patients: Emotional Feelings, Fears & Future: Index of New Information. John C. Bartone. 1997. 160p. 57.50 (*0-7883-1756-3*); pap. 47.50 (*0-7883-1757-1*) ABBE Pubs Assn.

Cancer Doesn't Have to Hurt: How to Conquer Pain Caused by Cancer & Cancer Treatment. Pamela J. Haylock & Carol P. Curtiss. 1997. LC 96-18194. (Illus.). 192p. pap. 14.95 (*0-89793-213-7*) Hunter Hse.

Cancer Doesn't Have to Hurt: How to Conquer the Pain Caused by Cancer & Cancer Treatment. Pamela J. Haylock & Carol P. Curtiss. 1997. LC 96-18194. (Illus.). 192p. 24.95 (*0-89793-214-5*) Hunter Hse.

Cancer Education Resources for American Indians & Alaska Natives. Linda Burhan-Stipanov & Kathleen C. Barry. 1996. (Illus.). 73p. (Orig.). (C). pap. text 20.00 (*0-7881-3001-3*) DIANE Pub.

***Cancer Encyclopedia - Collections of Anti-Cancer & Anti-Carcinogenic Agents, Chemicals, Drugs & Substances: Index of New Information & Guide-Book for Consumers, Reference & Research** John C. Bartone. 2002. 180p. Set. (Illus.). 1310.00 (*0-7883-2650-3*); Set. (Illus.). pap. 1110.00 (*0-7883-2651-1*); Vol. 1 (1966-1979) (Illus.). 65.50 (*0-7883-2652-X*); Vol. 1 (1966-1979) (Illus.). pap. 55.50 (*0-7883-2653-8*); Vol. 2 (1980-1985) (Illus.). 65.50 (*0-7883-2654-6*); Vol. 2 (1980-1985) (Illus.). pap. 55.50 (*0-7883-2655-4*); Vol. 3 (1986-1988) (Illus.). 65.50 (*0-7883-2656-2*); Vol. 3 (1986-1988) (Illus.). pap. 55.50 (*0-7883-2657-0*); Vol. 4 (1989-1991) (Illus.). 65.50 (*0-7883-2658-9*); Vol. 4 (1989-1991) (Illus.). pap. 55.50 (*0-7883-2659-7*); Vol. 5 (1992) (Illus.). 65.50 (*0-7883-2660-0*); Vol. 5 (1992) (Illus.). pap. 55.50

(0-7883-2661-9); Vol. 6 (1993) (Illus.). 65.50 (0-7883-2662-7); Vol. 6 (1993) (Illus.). pap. 55.50 (0-7883-2663-5); Vol. 7 (1994) (Illus.). 65.50 (0-7883-2664-3); Vol. 7 (1994) (Illus.). pap. 55.50 (0-7883-2665-1); Vol. 8 (1995A) (Illus.). 65.50 (0-7883-2666-X); Vol. 8 (1995A) (Illus.). pap. 55.50 (0-7883-2667-8); Vol. 9 (1995B) (Illus.). 65.50 (0-7883-2668-6); Vol. 9 (1995B) (Illus.). pap. 55.50 (0-7883-2669-4); Vol. 10 (1996A) (Illus.). 65.50 (0-7883-2670-8); Vol. 10 (1996A) (Illus.). pap. 55.50 (0-7883-2671-6); Vol. 11 (1996B) (Illus.). 65.50 (0-7883-2672-4); Vol. 11 (1996B) (Illus.). pap. 55.50 (0-7883-2673-2); Vol. 12 (1997A) (Illus.). 65.50 (0-7883-2674-0); Vol. 12 (1997A) (Illus.). pap. 55.50 (0-7883-2675-9); Vol. 13 (1997B) 65.50 (0-7883-2676-7); Vol. 13 (1997B) (Illus.). pap. 55.50 (0-7883-2677-5); Vol. 14 (1998A) (Illus.). 65.50 (0-7883-2678-3); Vol. 14 (1998A) (Illus.). pap. 55.50 (0-7883-2679-1); Vol. 15 (1998B) (Illus.). 65.50 (0-7883-2680-5); Vol. 15 (1998B) (Illus.). pap. 55.50 (0-7883-2681-3); Vol. 16 (1999A) (Illus.). 65.50 (0-7883-2682-1); Vol. 16 (1999A) (Illus.). pap. 55.50 (0-7883-2683-X); Vol. 17 (1999B) (Illus.). 65.50 (0-7883-2684-8); Vol. 17 (1999B) (Illus.). pap. 55.50 (0-7883-2685-6); Vol. 18 (2000A) (Illus.). 65.50 (0-7883-2686-4); Vol. 18 (2000A) (Illus.). pap. 55.50 (0-7883-2687-2); Vol. 19 (2000B) (Illus.). 65.50 (0-7883-2688-0); Vol. 19 (2000B) (Illus.). pap. 55.50 (0-7883-2689-9); Vol. 20 (2000C) (Illus.). 65.50 (0-7883-2690-2); Vol. 20 (2000C) (Illus.). pap. 55.50 (0-7883-2691-0) ABBE Pubs Assn.

Cancer Epidemic: Shadow of the Conquest of Nature. Gotthard Booth. 1980. LC 59-7362. (Illus.). 277p. 89.95 (0-88946-625-4) E Mellen.

***Cancer Epidemics Are World-Wide & Affecting All Parts of the Human Body: Index of New Information of Neoplasms Ranging the Human Body.** John C. Bartone. 2002. (Illus.). 250p. 67.50 (0-7883-2404-7) ABBE Pubs Assn.

Cancer Epidemiology & Prevention. Ed. by David Schottenfeld & Joseph F. Fraumeni, Jr. 2nd ed. 1996. (Illus.). 1544p. text 225.00 (0-19-505354-0) OUP.

Cancer-Free: 30 Who Triumphed over Cancer Naturally. East West Foundation Staff & Ann Fawcett. 1991. LC 81-60393. (Illus.). 256p. (Orig.). pap. 18.00 (0-87040-794-5) Japan Pubns USA.

Cancer Free: The Comprehensive Cancer Prevention Program. Sidney J. Winawer & Moshe Shike. 1996. (Illus.). 416p. per. 14.00 (0-684-81512-5, Fireside) S&S Trade Pap.

Cancer Free: The Comprehensive Prevention Program Developed by Physicians at Memorial Sloan-Kettering Cancer Center. Sidney J. Winawer et al. 1995. LC 94-37680. 448p. 25.00 (0-671-79967-3) S&S Trade.

***Cancer from Cure to Cure: Palliative Care Dilemmas in General Practice.** David Jeffrey. 2000. 145p. pap. (1-898507-83-X) Books For Midwives Pr GBR. *Dist:* Balogh.

Cancer Gene Therapy: Past Achievements & Future Challenges. Ed. by Nagy A. Habib. 2000. LC 99-44529. (Advances in Experimental Medicine & Biology Ser.: Vol. 465). (Illus.). 508p. 165.00 (0-306-46191-9, Kluwer Plenum) Kluwer Academic.

Cancer Genes: Functional Aspects; Proceedings of the Seventh Pezcoller Symposium Held in Trento, Italy, June 14-16, 1995. Ed. by Enrico Mihich & David Housman. 1997. LC 96-41755. (Pezcoller Foundation Symposia Ser.: Vol. 7). 300p. 95.00 (0-306-45482-3, Kluwer Plenum) Kluwer Academic.

Cancer Genetics: A Guide for Counseling Families. Gwendolyn M. Reiser & G. Bradley Schaefer. 1996. (Illus.). 63p. ring bd. 45.00 (1-889843-00-8) Munroe-Meyer Inst.

Cancer Genetics for the Clinician. Ed. by Gail L. Shaw. 1999. LC 99-37279. (0-306-46194-3, Kluwer Plenum) Kluwer Academic.

Cancer Genetics in Women, Set. S. Kullander. Ed. by H. T. Lynch. 1987. 220.00 (0-8493-5180-4, RC281, CRC Reprint) Franklin.

Cancer Genetics in Women. Ed. by Henry T. Lynch. 1987. Vol. I. 184p. 107.00 (0-8493-5183-9); Vol. II. 192p. 113.00 (0-8493-5184-7) Franklin (CRC Reprint).

***Cancer Handbook,** Set. Ed. by Malcolm R. Alison. 2001. 1500p. 375.00 (1-56159-289-7) Nature Pubg Grp.

Cancer Handbook: A Guide for the Nonspecialist. Darrell E. Ward. 1995. LC 95-8318. (Illus.). 130p. pap. 15.00 (0-8142-0675-1) Ohio St U Pr.

Cancer Imaging with Radiolabeled Antibodies. Ed. by David M. Goldenberg. 1990. (Cancer Treatment & Research Ser.). (C). text 277.00 (0-7923-0631-7) Kluwer Academic.

Cancer Immunoembryotherapy: A New Weapon Against Cancer. F. Columbus. 1994. 72p. (Orig.). pap. 35.00 (1-56072-107-3) Nova Sci Pubs.

Cancer Immunology. Houghton. 208p. pap. (0-471-16404-6) Wiley.

Cancer Immunology: Innovative Approaches to Therapy. Ed. by Ronald B. Herberman. 1986. (Cancer Treatment & Research Ser.). text 141.00 (0-89838-757-4) Kluwer Academic.

Cancer Immunotherapy Protocols. Ed. by Luc Michiels & Kris Motmans. 2000. (Methods in Molecular Medicine Ser.). 375p. 99.50 (0-89603-829-7) Humana.

Cancer in Atomic Bomb Survivors. Ed. by Itsuzo Shigematsu & Abraham Kagan. 1986. (Gann Monographs on Cancer Research: No. 32). (Illus.). 204p. (C). text 102.00 (0-306-42501-7) Plenum.

***Cancer in Children.** J. S. Malpas. 1996. (British Medical Bulletin Ser.: Vol. 52, No. 4). 263p. pap. (1-85315-282-X) Royal Soc of Medicine Pr Ltd GBR. *Dist:* Balogh.

Cancer in Children. Ed. by P. A. Voute et al. 2nd enl. rev. ed. 1986. (Current Treatment of Cancer Ser.). (Illus.). 400p. 64.00 (0-387-15342-X) Spr-Verlag.

Cancer in Children: Clinical Management. Ed. by P. A. Voute et al. 4th ed. 1998. (Illus.). 372p. text 110.00 (0-19-262897-6) OUP.

Cancer in Children: Clinical Management. Ed. by P. A. Voute et al. 3rd rev. ed. 1992. (Current Treatment of Cancer Ser.). (Illus.). 365p. 100.00 (0-387-55186-7) Spr-Verlag.

Cancer in Costa Rica. R. Sierra & R. Barrantes. 1988. (IARC Scientific Publications Ser.: No. 1). 95p. text 30.00 (92-832-1412-9) World Health.

Cancer in Italian Migrant Populations. Ed. by M. Geddes et al. 1993. (IARC Scientific Publications Ser.: No. 123). (Illus.). 302p. (C). pap. text 75.00 (92-832-2123-0) OUP.

Cancer in Organ Transplant Recipients. Ed. by Dietrich Schmahl & I. Penn. 1991. (Illus.). 183p. 98.00 (0-387-53020-7) Spr-Verlag.

Cancer in Pregnancy: Maternal & Fetal Risks. Ed. by Gideon Koren et al. 1996. (Illus.). 233p. (C). text 69.95 (0-521-47176-1) Cambridge U Pr.

***Cancer in Primary Care.** Gore & Russell. 2001. (Illus.). 300p. (1-901865-26-6) Isis Med GBR. *Dist:* Bks Intl VA.

Cancer in Thailand 1988-1991. D. M. Parkin & S. Sontipong. 1993. (IARC Scientific Publications Ser.: No. 16). xiv, 164p. pap. text 30.00 (92-832-1430-7, 1770016) World Health.

Cancer in the African Population of Bulawayo, Zimbabwe, 1963-1977: Incidence, Time Trends, & Risk Factors. D. M. Parkin et al. 1993. (IARC Scientific Publications Ser.: No. 15). vi, 123p. pap. text 27.00 (92-832-1429-3, 1770015) World Health.

Cancer in the Community: Class & Medical Authority. Martha Balshem. 1993. LC 92-48963. (Series in Ethnographic Inquiry). (Illus.). 192p. text 42.00 (1-56098-250-0); pap. text 16.95 (1-56098-251-9) Smithsonian.

Cancer in the Elderly. Ed. by F. I. Caird & T. B. Brewin. 1990. (Illus.). 295p. text 185.00 (0-7236-0972-1) Buttrwrth-Heinemann.

Cancer in the Elderly: A Nursing & Medical Perspective. Ed. by K. Redmond & M. S. Aapro. 1997. 110p. 83.50 (0-444-82858-3) Elsevier.

Cancer in the Elderly: Approaches to Early Detection & Treatment. Ed. by Jerome W. Yates. 1989. LC 89-21664. 272p. 44.95 (0-8261-6930-9) Springer Pub.

Cancer in the Elderly: Directions for Research. Ed. by Ian S. Fentiman & Silvio Monfardini. 1994. LC 94-24864. (Illus.). 184p. text 95.00 (0-19-262200-5) OUP.

Cancer in the Family: Helping Children Cope with a Parents Illness. Sue P. Heiney. 2001. LC 2001-22090. (Illus.). 288p. pap. 18.95 (0-944235-34-4) Am Cancer NY.

Cancer in the First Year of Life: Leukemia, Neuroblastomas, Soft Tissue Sarcomas. Ed. by F. Lampert et al. 1991. (Beitraege Zur Onkologie, Contributions to Oncology Ser.: Vol. 41). (Illus.). viii, 174p. 61.75 (3-8055-5233-5) S Karger.

Cancer in the Nervous System. Ed. by Victor A. Levin. 1995. LC 95-35116. 474p. text (0-443-08880-2) Church.

Cancer in the Netherlands, Set. Ed. by F. J. Cleton & J. W. Coebergh. 1988. (C). pap. text 86.00 (0-89838-400-1) Kluwer Academic.

Cancer in the United States. Abraham M. Lilienfeld et al. 1972. LC 72-80658. (American Public Health Association. Vital & Health Statistics Monographs). (Illus.). 572p. 57.50 (0-674-09425-5) HUP.

Cancer in Transplantation, Prevention & Treatment: Proceedings of the 27th Conference on Transplantation & Clinical Immunology 22-24 May 1995. Ed. by J. L. Touraine. 1996. (Transplantation & Clinical Immunology Ser.). 400p. (C). text 166.00 (0-7923-3863-4) Kluwer Academic.

Cancer in Women. John J. Kavanagh et al. 1998. LC 97-43312. (Illus.). 666p. 209.95 (0-86542-465-9) Blackwell Sci.

***Cancer in Women.** John Kavanagh et al. 2nd ed. 2002. (Illus.). (C). text 224.95 (0-7637-1854-8, 1854-8) Jones & Bartlett.

Cancer Incidence by Occupation & Industry in Tianjin, China, 1981-1987. Manolis Kogevinas et al. 1994. (IARC Scientific Publications Ser.: No. 22). vi, 95p. pap. text 27.00 (92-832-1433-1, 1770022) World Health.

Cancer Incidence in Five Continents, Vol. VII. Ed. by D. M. Parkin et al. 1999. (IARC Scientific Publications Ser.: No. 143). (Illus.). 1286p. text 250.00 (92-832-2143-5) OUP.

Cancer Incidence in Jewish Migrants to Israel, 1961-1981. Ruth Steinitz et al. 1990. (IARC Scientific Publications Ser.: No. 98). (Illus.). 328p. pap. 65.00 (92-832-1198-7) OUP.

Cancer-Increasing Your Odds for Survival: A Resource Guide for Integrating Mainstream, Alternative & Complementary Therapies. David Bognar. 1998. LC 98-34440. (Illus.). 352p. 25.95 (0-89793-248-X); pap. 15.95 (0-89793-247-1) Hunter Hse.

Cancer Industry: The Classic Expose on the Cancer Establishment. Ralph W. Moss. pap. 14.95 (1-55778-439-6); 1996. LC 96-84574. 41p. pap. 16.95 (1-881025-09-8) Equinox Pr.

Cancer Information Service: A 15-Year History of Service & Research. 1995. lib. bdg. 251.95 (0-8490-6728-6) Gordon Pr.

Cancer, Its Cause, Prevention & Cure. Edward H. Smalpage. 1996. 127p. reprint ed. spiral bd. 13.00 (0-7873-0800-5) Hlth Research.

Cancer Journals. Audre Geraldine Lorde. 2nd ed. 1980. LC 80-53110. 77p. pap. 7.00 (1-879960-26-5) Aunt Lute Bks.

Cancer Journals: Special Edition. Audre Geraldine Lorde. 1997. LC 97-10954. (Illus.). 112p. 12.95 (1-879960-51-6) Aunt Lute Bks.

Cancer Journals & Serials: An Analytical Guide, 11. Ed. by Pauline M. Vaillancourt. 1988. LC 87-29580. (Annotated Bibliographies of Serials: A Subject Approach Ser.: No. 11). 281p. lib. bdg. 70.00 (0-313-24055-8, VCC/, Greenwood Pr) Greenwood.

***Cancer Management: A Multidisciplinary Approach.** Ed. by Richard Pazdur et al. 6th rev. ed. 2002. (Illus.). 1000p. pap. text 49.95 (1-891483-13-7) PRR.

Cancer Management: A Multidisciplinary Approach: Medical, Surgical, & Radiation Oncology. Ed. by Richard Pazdur, MD et al. 5th rev. ed. 2001. (Illus.). 982p. per. 49.95 (1-891483-08-0) PRR.

Cancer Management in Man: Biological Response Modifiers, Chemotherapy, Antibiotics, Hyperthermia Supporting Measures. Paul V. Woolley. 1989. (C). text 207.50 (0-89838-999-2) Kluwer Academic.

Cancer Management in Man: Detection, Diagnosis, Surgery, Radiology, Chronobiology, Endocrine Therapy. Ed. by Alfred L. Goldson. 1989. (C). text 207.50 (0-89838-998-4) Kluwer Academic.

Cancer Medicine, No. 5. Robert C. Bast, Jr. et al. 5th ed. 2000. LC 2001-265836. (ACS Atlas of Clinical Oncology Ser.). (Illus.). 2546p. incl. cd-rom (1-55009-113-1) DEKR.

Cancer Medicine, Vol. 2. James F. Holland & Emil Frei. 3rd ed. 1993. (Illus.). 2600p. text 198.50 (0-8121-1422-1) Lppncott W & W.

Cancer Medicine Review. James F. Holland & Emil Frei, III. 2000. (ACS Atlas of Clinical Oncology Ser.). 300p. incl. cd-rom (1-55009-115-8) DEKR.

Cancer Medicine Review. Richard M. Stone et al. 1997. LC 96-48209. 230p. pap. 35.00 (0-683-30059-8) Lppncott W & W.

Cancer Metastasis. Ed. by V. Schirrmacher & R. Schwartz-Albiez. 1989. (Illus.). 268p. 69.95 (0-387-50471-0, 2962) Spr-Verlag.

Cancer Metastasis: Biological & Biochemical Mechanisms & Clinical Aspects. Ed. by G. Prodi et al. 1988. (Advances in Experimental Medicine & Biology Ser.: Vol. 233). (Illus.). 504p. 125.00 (0-306-42907-1, Plenum Trade) Perseus Pubng.

Cancer Metastasis: From Mechanisms to Therapies. Ed. by Richard G. Vile. 1995. LC 94-5291. (Molecular Medical Science Ser.). 220p. 155.00 (0-471-95266-4) Wiley.

Cancer Metastasis: In Vitro & In Vivo Experimental Approaches, Vol. 29. D. Rusciano et al. 2000. LC 99-53890. (Laboratory Techniques in Biochemistry & Molecular Biology Ser.: Vol. 29). (Illus.). 372p. 147.50 (0-444-82372-7); pap. 68.00 (0-444-82358-1) Elsevier.

Cancer Metastasis, Molecular & Cellular Mechanisms. Wen G. Jiang & Robert E. Mansel. 2000. (Cancer Metastasis Ser.). 444p. 183.00 (0-7923-6395-7) Kluwer Academic.

Cancer Microbe. Alan Cantwell, Jr. Ed. by Suzanne Henig. 1990. (Illus.). 281p. pap. 19.95 (0-917211-01-4) Aries Rising.

Cancer Modeling. James R. Thompson & Brown. 1987. (Statistics: Textbooks & Monographs: Vol. 83). (Illus.). 440p. text 175.00 (0-8247-7773-5) Dekker.

Cancer Mortality & Morbidity Statistics: Japan & the World, 1993. Ed. by Suketami Tominaga et al. 1994. LC 93-35677. (Gann Monographs on Cancer Research: No. 41). 94.95 (0-8493-7748-X, RC271) CRC Pr.

Cancer Mortality by Occupation & Social Class. 1997. (Studies on Medical & Population Subjects: No. 81020271). (0-11-690776-2, HM07762) Statnry Office GBR. *Dist:* Bernan Associates.

Cancer Neutron Capture Therapy: Proceedings of the Sixth International Symposium Held in Kobe, Japan, October 31-November 4, 1994. Ed. by Yutaka Mishima. 1996. (Illus.). 947p. 210.00 (0-306-45307-X, Kluwer Plenum) Kluwer Academic.

***Cancer Nursing.** Ed. by Sylvia Denton. pap. (0-7487-3300-0) Nelson Thornes GBR. *Dist:* Intl Spec Bk.

Cancer Nursing. Susan L. Groenwald. (C). 1988. 75.00 (0-86720-403-6); 1987. (Illus.). text 110.00 (0-86720-351-X, 351-X) Jones & Bartlett.

Cancer Nursing. Susan L. Groenwald et al. 2nd ed. 1990. 1376p. 125.00 (0-86720-435-4) Jones & Bartlett.

Cancer Nursing. Susan L. Groenwald. 3rd ed. (Illus.). 1994. 1600p. (C). pap. text 100.00 (0-86720-722-1, 722-1); 1993. 1724p. text 125.00 (0-86720-640-3, 640-3) Jones & Bartlett.

Cancer Nursing: A Comprehensive Textbook. Ruth McCorkle et al. 2nd ed. 1996. (Illus.). 1487p. text 150.00 (0-7216-5668-4) Saunders.

Cancer Nursing: Care in Context. Contrib. by Jessica Corner & Christopher Bailey. 2001. LC 99-47592. 592p. pap. 69.95 (0-632-03998-1) Blackwell Sci.

Cancer Nursing: Principles & Practice. Susan L. Groenwald et al. 4th ed. 1997. LC 96-48548. (Nursing Ser.). (Illus.). 1920p. text 139.95 (0-7637-0219-6, 0219-6) Jones & Bartlett.

Cancer Nursing: Principles & Practice. Connie H. Yarbro et al. 5th ed. 2000. (Illus.). 1952p. (C). pap. text 138.95 (0-7637-1164-0, 1164-0) Jones & Bartlett.

Cancer Obstetrics & Gynecology. Edward L. Trimble & Cornelia Liu Trimble. 1999. LC 99-21823. (Illus.). 288p. text 92.00 (0-7817-1410-9) Lppncott W & W.

Cancer Occurrence in Developing Countries. D. M. Parkin. 1986. (IARC Scientific Publications Ser.: No. 75). (Illus.). 350p. text 40.00 (92-832-1175-8) OUP.

Cancer of the Bile Ducts & Pancreas. Preece et al. 1989. 320p. text 135.00 (0-7216-2631-9) Saunders.

Cancer of the Breast. William L. Donegan & John S. Spratt. 4th ed. 1995. LC 94-12235. (Illus.). 720p. text 173.00 (0-7216-4694-8) Saunders.

Cancer of the Cervix. Stephen G. Brown & Philip J. Disaia. 1981. (Oncologic Ser.: Vol. 14). (Illus.). 308p. pap. 135.00 (0-08-027465-X, Pergamon Pr) Elsevier.

Cancer of the Colon, Rectum & Anus. Ed. by Alfred M. Cohen & Sidney J. Winawer. 1994. (Illus.). 1154p. text 135.00 (0-07-011601-6) McGraw-Hill Med Pub.

Cancer of the Esophagus. Ed. by Tom R. DeMeester & Bernard Levin. 1985. 320p. text 99.00 (0-8089-1665-3, 791023, Grune & Strat) Harcrt Hlth Sci Grp.

Cancer of the Esophagus. Carl J. Pfeiffer. 1982. Vol. I. 176p. 100.00 (0-8493-6213-X, RC280); Vol. II. 280p. 155.00 (0-8493-6214-8, RC280) Franklin (CRC Reprint).

Cancer of the Esophagus: Approaches to the Etiology. Valda M. Craddock. 1993. (Cambridge Monographs on Cancer Research). (Illus.). 296p. (C). text 110.00 (0-521-37393-X) Cambridge U Pr.

Cancer of the Exocrine Pancreas: From Oncogenes to Unresectable Tumors. Ed. by J. Delmont & A. G. Harris. 1986. (Frontiers of Gastrointestinal Research Ser.: Vol. 12). (Illus.). x, 306p. 216.75 (3-8055-4329-8) S Karger.

Cancer of the Face & Mouth: Pathology & Management for Surgeons. Ian A. McGregor & Frances M. McGregor. 1986. (Illus.). 624p. text (0-443-02455-3) Church.

Cancer of the Head & Neck. Louis Harrison. 1998. LC 98-36344. 1,120p. text 199.00 (0-397-51777-7) Lppncott W & W.

Cancer of the Head & Neck. Schantz. 1996. (0-7216-5287-5) Saunders.

Cancer of the Head & Neck. Ed. by Eugene N. Myers & James Y. Suen. 2nd ed. 1989. (Illus.). 1132p. text (0-443-08597-8) Church.

Cancer of the Head & Neck. James Y. Suen & Eugene N. Myers. Ed. by Larry McGrew. 3rd ed. 1996. LC 95-35682. 736p. text 190.00 (0-7216-5550-5) Saunders.

Cancer of the Larynx Ed. by A. Ferlito. 1985. Vol. I. 216p. 126.00 (0-8493-6587-2, RC280); Vol. II. 248p. pap. text 141.00 (0-8493-6588-0, RC280); Vol. 3. LC 84-9509. 216p. 123.00 (0-8493-6589-9) Franklin (CRC Reprint).

Cancer of the Larynx: Current Concepts in the Treatment of the Neck. Ed. by A. Ferlito & W. Arnold. 2000. (ORL Ser.: Vol. 62). (Illus.). 62p. pap. 25.25 (3-8055-7126-7) S Karger.

***Cancer of the Larynx & Hypopharynx.** Ed. by William I. Wei & Jonathan S. T. Shem. 2000. (Illus.). 272p. (1-899066-64-0) Isis Med GBR. *Dist:* Bks Intl VA.

Cancer of the Lung: From Molecular Biology to Treatment Guidelines. Ed. by Alan B. Weitberg. 2001. (Current Clinical Oncology Ser.). 354p. 125.00 (0-89603-830-0) Humana.

Cancer of the Nervous System. Peter M. Black & Jay S. Loeffler. 1997. LC 96-33386. (Illus.). 935p. 295.00 (0-86542-384-9) Blackwell Sci.

Cancer of the Pharynx & Larynx. Nick Stafford. 1998. 288p. (0-632-03515-3) Blckwell Science.

Cancer of the Prostate. Sakti Das & Crawford. 1993. LC 92-48552. (Basic & Clinical Oncology Ser.: Vol. 3). (Illus.). 480p. text 195.00 (0-8247-8863-X) Dekker.

Cancer of the Prostate, 18. Malcolm A. Bagshaw. 1984. (Oncologic Ser.: Vol. 18). (Illus.). 260p. pap. 120.00 (0-08-027471-4, Pergamon Pr) Elsevier.

Cancer of the Skin. Friedman et al. 1990. (Illus.). 640p. text 225.00 (0-7216-2328-X) Saunders.

Cancer of the Urinary Bladder: With Emphasis on Treatment by Irradiation. William L. Caldwell. 1970. LC 72-96980. (Illus.). 128p. 12.50 (0-87527-003-4) Green.

Cancer of the Vulva, Vagina, & Cervix. Patricia J. Eifel & Charles Levenback. 2000. (ACS Atlas of Clinical Oncology Ser.). 300p. incl. cd-rom (1-55009-107-7) DEKR.

Cancer Oncogenes & Tumor Suppressor Genes in Human Malignancies. Ed. by Christopher C. Benz & Edison T. Liu. 1993. LC 92-49212. (Cancer Treatment & Research Ser.: Vol. CTAR 63). (C). text 254.00 (*0-7923-1960-5*) Kluwer Academic.

Cancer Overcome by Diet: An Alternative to Surgery. Louise Greenfield. 1987. LC 86-61770. (Illus.). 133p. (Orig.). pap. 7.95 (*0-9617947-0-4*) L Greenfield.

Cancer Pain. Ed. by M. Swerdlow & V. Ventafridda. 1987. lib. bdg. 80.50 (*0-85200-858-9*) Kluwer Academic.

Cancer Pain Handbook. Cynthia King. 2002. (Illus.). 320p. (C). pap. text 36.95 (*0-7637-1477-1*, 1477-1) Jones & Bartlett.

Cancer Pain Management. Deborah McGuire et al. 2nd ed. 1995. (Nursing Ser.). (Illus.). 400p. (C). text 52.95 (*0-86720-725-6*, 725-6) Jones & Bartlett.

Cancer Pain Management: A Comprehensive Approach. Ed. by Karen H. Simpson & Keith Budd. 2000. LC 00-32389. (Illus.). 286p. text 59.95 (*0-19-262877-1*) OUP.

Cancer Pain Management: Principles & Practice. Winston C. Parris. 1996. LC 96-28928. 596p. text 145.00 (*0-7506-9491-2*) Buttrwrth-Heinemann.

Cancer Pain Relief: With a Guide to Opioid Availability. 2nd ed. 1996. (FRE & SPA.). vi, 63p. (C). pap. text 15.30 (*92-4-154482-1*, 1152247) World Health.

Cancer Pain Relief & Palliative Care: Report of a WHO Expert Committee. 1990. (Technical Reports: No. 804). (CHI, ENG, FRE & SPA.). 75p. pap. text 9.00 (*92-4-120804-X*, 1100804) World Health.

Cancer Pain Sourcebook. Roger Cicala. 2001. LC 00-53478. 320p. pap. 17.95 (*0-7373-0423-5*) McGraw-Hill Prof.

Cancer Patient & Supportive Care. Ed. by Donald J. Higby. 1985. (Cancer Treatment & Research Ser.). text 141.00 (*0-89838-690-X*) Kluwer Academic.

Cancer Patient Folllow-Up. Ed. by Frank E. Johnson & Katherine S. Virgo. 1997. LC 96-50270. (Illus.). 576p. (C). (gr. 13). text 69.00 (*0-8151-4925-5*, 26019) Mosby Inc.

Cancer Patient's Guide to Radiation Therapy. Richard Steeves. 1992. LC 92-1624. (Focus on Health Ser.). (Illus.). 94p. pap. 11.95 (*0-944838-26-X*) Med Physics Pub.

Cancer Patient's Handbook. Margaret Greeley. 1978. LC 78-70591. (Illus.). pap. 6.95 (*0-932904-01-7*) Magoos Umbrella.

Cancer Policy: Research & Methods. Charles L. Bennett & Tammy S. Pajeau. 1998. LC 98-22296. (Cancer Treatment & Research Ser.). 200p. 165.00 (*0-7923-8203-X*) Kluwer Academic.

Cancer Policy Framework. Ed. by Christopher DeRosa. 2000. 57p. (C). reprint ed. pap. text 20.00 (*0-7881-8864-X*) DIANE Pub.

Cancer Prevention: From the Laboratory to the Clinic: Implications of Genetic, Molecular, & Preventive Research. Ed. by Umberto Veronesi et al. 1995. LC 95-21867. (Annals of the New York Academy of Sciences Ser.: Vol. 768). 342p. 95.00 (*0-89766-947-9*) NY Acad Sci.

***Cancer Prevention: Molecular Mechanisms to Clinical Applications.** Ed. by Michael P. Osborne. 2001. LC 2001-54674. (Annals of the New York Academy of Sciences Ser.: Vol. 952). (*1-57331-350-5*); pap. (*1-57331-351-3*) NY Acad Sci.

Cancer Prevention: Novel Nutrient & Pharmaceutical Developments. H. L. Bradlow. 2000. (Annals of the New York Academy of Science Ser.). (Illus.). 264p. pap. text 21.50 (*0-8018-6544-1*) Johns Hopkins.

Cancer Prevention: Novel Nutrient & Pharmaceutical Developments. Contrib. by H. Leon Bradlow et al. 1999. LC 99-51355. (Annals of the New York Academy of Sciences Ser.: Vol. 889). (Illus.). ix, 264p. (*1-57331-198-7*) NY Acad Sci.

Cancer Prevention: Novel Nutrient & Pharmaceutical Developments. H. Leon Bradlow et al. 1999. LC 99-51355. (Annals of the New York Academy of Sciences Ser.: Vol. 889). (Illus.). ix, 264p. pap. (*1-57331-199-5*) NY Acad Sci.

Cancer Prevention & Control. Ed. by Peter Greenwald et al. 1994. LC 94-35430. (Basic & Clinical Oncology Ser.: Vol. 6). (Illus.). 824p. text 225.00 (*0-8247-9258-0*) Dekker.

Cancer Prevention & Control: Index of Modern Information. Mary R. Bartone. 1990. LC 88-47856. 150p. 47.50 (*1-55914-176-X*); pap. 44.50 (*1-55914-177-8*) ABBE Pubs Assn.

***Cancer Prevention Book: Holistic Guidelines from the World-Famous Bristol Cancer Help Centre.** Rosy Daniel & Rachel Ellis. 2002. LC 2001-39723. 15.95 (*0-89793-360-5*) Hunter House.

***Cancer Prevention Book: Holistic Guidelines from the World-Famous Bristol Cancer Help Centre.** Rosy Daniel & Rachel Ellis. 2002. LC 2001-39723. pap. 15.95 (*0-89793-361-3*) Hunter Hse.

Cancer Prevention Diet: Michio Kushi's Nutritional Blueprint for the Relief & Prevention of Disease. Michio Kushi & Alex Jack. rev. ed. 1993. 544p. 24.95 (*0-312-09257-1*) St Martin.

Cancer Prevention Good Health Diet. Martin Katahn. 2000. LC 00-31882. (Illus.). 288p. pap. 14.95 (*0-393-32058-8*) Norton.

Cancer Prevention in Primary Care. Ed. by Joan Austoker. 1995. 150p. (Orig.). pap. text (*0-7279-0825-1*) BMJ Pub GBR. *Dist:* AIDC.

Cancer Radiotherapy Protocols. Ed. by Robert A. Huddart. 2001. (Methods in Molecular Medicine Ser.). 400p. 99.50 (*0-89603-831-9*) Humana.

Cancer Recovery Eating Plan: The Right Foods to Help Fuel Your Recovery. Daniel W. Nixon. 1996. LC 97-188693. pap. 15.00 (*0-8129-2590-4*, Crown) Crown Pub Group.

Cancer Registration in the European Economic Community. M. P. Coleman & E. Domaret. 1988. (IARC Scientific Publications Ser.: No. 3). 172p. text 30.00 (*92-832-1414-5*) World Health.

Cancer Rehabilitation Continuing Care. Blunk & J. P. Gudas. 1999. (*0-7506-9538-2*) Buttrwrth-Heinemann.

Cancer Related Information Seeking. David J. Johnson. Ed. by Gary Kreps. 1997. LC 97-13365. (Communication Ser.). 256p. text 52.50 (*1-57273-138-9*); pap. text 21.95 (*1-57273-139-7*) Hampton Pr NJ.

Cancer Research: Cell Biology, Molecular Biology & Tumor Virology. Ed. by Robert G. Gallo. 1977. (Uniscience Ser.). Vol. 1. 280p. 137.00 (*0-8493-5138-3*, RC268); Vol. 2. 240p. 137.00 (*0-8493-5139-1*, RC268) Franklin (CRC Reprint).

Cancer Research at the European Level. S. S. Baig. 1995. LC 95-7527. (Biomedical & Health Research Ser.: Vol. 11). 60.00 (*90-5199-215-7*) IOS Press.

Cancer Research Campaign Atlas of Cancer Incidence in England & Wales, 1968-1985. Anthony Swerdlow & Isabel Dos Santos Silva. 1994. (Illus.). 294p. text 250.00 (*0-19-261993-4*) OUP.

Cancer Research in Hispanic Populations in the United States. 1997. lib. bdg. 250.00 (*0-8490-6087-7*) Gordon Pr.

Cancer Resources on the Internet. Ed. by M. Sandra Wood & Eric P. Delozier. 1997. LC 97-19030. 110p. 29.95 (*0-7890-0344-9*); pap. 14.95 (*0-7890-0345-7*) Haworth Pr.

Cancer Risk Assessment: A Quantitative Approach. Samuel C. Morris. 1990. (Occupational Safety & Health Ser.: Vol. 20). (Illus.). 416p. text 160.00 (*0-8247-8239-9*) Dekker.

Cancer Risk by Social Class & Occupation: A Survey of 109,000 Cancer Cases among Finns of Working Age. Eero Pukkala. 1995. LC 95 1186. (Contributions to Epidemiology & Biostatistics Ser.: Vol. 7). (Illus.). x, 278p. 104.50 (*3-8055-6152-0*) S Karger.

Cancer Risks: Strategies for Elimination. Ed. by P. Bannasch. 1987. (Illus.). 199p. 34.95 (*0-387-17465-6*) Spr-Verlag.

Cancer Risks & Incidence Trends: The Connecticut Perspective. George Roush et al. 1987. (Illus.). 435p. 176.00 (*0-89116-412-X*) Hemisp Pub.

Cancer S. O. S. Strategies of Survival. Rose Welsh & Shirley Grandahl. Ed. & Illus. by Susan Ross. 1998. 184p. pap. 29.95 (*0-9660057-5-9*) Alba Pub.

Cancer Salves: A Botanical Approach to Treatment. Ingrid Naiman. 3rd rev. ed. (Illus.). 1999. 272p. 45.00 (*1-882834-16-X*); 1999. 272p. pap. text 27.50 (*1-882834-15-1*); 1997. 220p. 30.00 (*1-882834-11-9*) Seventh Ray.

Cancer Screening. Ed. by A. B. Miller et al. 1991. 456p. (C). text 105.00 (*0-521-41041-X*) Cambridge U Pr.

Cancer Screening. Ed. by Douglas Reintgen & Robert A. Clark. 1996. LC 95-33562. (Illus.). 304p. (C). (gr. 13). text 74.00 (*0-8151-7142-0*, 24303) Mosby Inc.

Cancer Screening. Mary E. Wheat & Ernest H. Rosenbaum. Ed. by Sheila Mahoney & Nancy Wiltsek. 1984. (Illus.). 29p. pap. 2.50 (*0-933161-03-4*) Better H Prog.

Cancer Screening: A Practical Guide for Physicians. Ed. by Khalid Aziz & George Y. Wu. 2001. (Current Clinical Practice Ser.). 328p. 89.00 (*0-89603-865-3*) Humana.

Cancer Selection: The New Theory of Evolution. James Graham. 1992. LC 91-73759. (Illus.). xvi, 213p. 35.00 (*0-9630242-0-5*) Aculeus Pr.

Cancer Self-Help Groups: A Guide. Pat Kelly. 2000. (Your Personal Health Ser.). (Illus.). 176p. pap. 15.95 (*1-55209-478-2*) Firefly Bks Limited.

Cancer Solution. Robert E. Willner. 1994. 323p. 23.95 (*0-9642316-0-3*) Peltec Pubng.

Cancer Solutions for Dogs. Shawn Messonnier. 2001. LC 2001-41419. pap. 14.00 (*0-7615-2583-1*) Prima Pub.

Cancer Source Book for Nurses. American Cancer Society Staff. 7th ed. 1996. LC 96-29088. (Nursing Ser.). (Illus.). 496p. (C). pap. text 41.95 (*0-7637-0242-0*, 0242-0) Jones & Bartlett.

Cancer Sourcebook: Basic Consumer Health Information about Major Forms & Stages of Cancer. Ed. by Edward J. Prucha. 3rd ed. 2000. LC 00-36307. (Health Reference Ser.). (Illus.). xii, 1069p. lib. bdg. 78.00 (*0-7808-0227-6*) Omnigraphics Inc.

Cancer Sourcebook: Basic Information on Cancer Types, Symptoms, Diagnostic Methods, & Treatments, Including Statistics on Cancer Occurrences Worldwide & the Risks Associated with Known Carcinogens & Activities. Ed. by Frank E. Bair. 1990. (Health Reference Ser.: Vol. 1). (Illus.). viii, 932p. lib. bdg. 78.00 (*1-55888-888-8*) Omnigraphics Inc.

Cancer Sourcebook for Women: Basic Consumer Health Information about Specific Forms of Cancer That Affect Women. Ed. by Karen Bellenir. 2nd ed. 2002. (Health Reference Ser.). 600p. lib. bdg. 78.00 (*0-7808-0226-8*) Omnigraphics Inc.

Cancer Sourcebook for Women: Basic Information about Specific Forms of Cancer That Affect Women, Vol. 10. Ed. by Allan R. Cook & Peter D. Dresser. 1995. LC 95-36875. (Health Reference Ser.). 524p. lib. bdg. 78.00 (*0-7808-0076-1*) Omnigraphics Inc.

Cancer Statistics. Office for National Statistics Staff. Date not set. iv, 72p. (*0-11-621247-0*) Statnry Office GBR. *Dist:* Balogh.

Cancer Statistics: Report of a WHO/IARC Expert Committee. 1979. (Technical Report Ser.: No. 623). 47p. pap. text 5.00 (*92-4-120632-2*, 1100632) World Health.

Cancer Statistics No. 24, 1991. HMSO Staff. 1997. 120p. pap. 50.00 (*0-11-620967-4*, HM09674) Bernan Associates.

Cancer Stories: Creativity & Self-Repair. Esther Dreifuss-Kattan. 1994. (Psychoanalytic Inquiry Book Ser.: Vol. 11). 288p. reprint ed. pap. 29.95 (*0-88163-204-X*) Analytic Pr.

Cancer, Stress & Death. S. B. Day. 2nd ed. 1986. LC 86-570. 392p. (C). text 59.50 (*0-306-42187-9*, Kluwer Plenum) Kluwer Academic.

Cancer Surgery. James C. Harvey & Edward J. Beattie. 1995. LC 95-4090. 528p. text 126.00 (*0-7216-5173-9*) Saunders.

Cancer Surgery for General Surgeons. Ed. by David Winchester et al. 1998. LC 98-27799. 352p. text 139.00 (*0-397-58470-9*) Lppncott W & W.

Cancer Survival: An International Comparison of Outcomes. 1994. (Illus.). 48p. (Orig.). (C). pap. text 35.00 (*0-7881-1066-7*) DIANE Pub.

Cancer Survival Cookbook: 200 Quick & Easy Recipes with Helpful Eating Hints. Donna L. Weihofen. 1997. LC 00-127499. 304p. pap. 16.95 (*0-471-34668-3*) Wiley.

Cancer Survival in Developing Countries. R. Sankaranarayanan et al. 1999. LC 99-228703. (IARC Scientific Publications Ser.: 145). (Illus.). 184p. pap. text 69.00 (*92-832-2145-1*) OUP.

Cancer Survival Trends in England & Wales, 1971-1995: Deprivation & NHS Region. Office for National Statistics Staff & Michel P. Coleman. 1999. 695p. (*0-11-621031-1*) Statnry Office GBR. *Dist:* Balogh, Bernan Associates.

Cancer Survivor's Almanac: Charting Your Journey. National Coalition for Cancer Survivorship Staff. 1996. 352p. pap. 18.95 (*0-471-34669-1*) Wiley.

Cancer Survivor's Almanac: Charting Your Journey. National Coalition for Cancer Survivorship Staff. Ed. by Barbara Hoffman. 2nd rev. ed. 1996. 354p. pap. 18.95 (*1-56561-104-7*) Wiley.

Cancer Survivor's Nutrition & Health Guide: Eating Well & Getting Better During & after Cancer Treatment. Gene F. Spiller & Bonnie Bruce. 1996. LC 96-32749. 256p. pap. 15.95 (*0-7615-0581-4*, Prima Health) Prima Pub.

Cancer Symptom Management. Margaret Frogge et al. Ed. by Susan L. Groenwald. 1996. LC 96-2452. (Nursing Ser.). (Illus.). 624p. (C). text 90.00 (*0-86720-732-9*, 732-9) Jones & Bartlett.

Cancer Symptom Management. Connie Henke Yarbro et al. 2nd ed. 1999. LC 98-43134. (Series in Oncology). (Illus.). 672p. (C). text 98.95 (*0-7637-0864-X*, 0864-X) Jones & Bartlett.

Cancer Symptom Management: Patient Self Care Guides. Susan L. Groenwald et al. 1997. LC 97-33689. (Nursing Ser.). (Illus.). 264p. (C). ring bd. 153.95 (*0-7637-0210-2*, 0210-2) Jones & Bartlett.

Cancer Symptom Managment: Rhone Version. Susan L. Groenwald et al. 1996. (Illus.). 624p. (C). pap. text 20.00 (*0-7637-0688-4*, 0688-4) Jones & Bartlett.

Cancer... Then Healing! 15 Decisions to Make When You or a Loved One Are Told You Have Cancer or Any Life Threatening Disease. Micki Voisard. 1998. v, 230p. pap. 14.95 (*0-9664082-0-9*) Stray Dog.

Cancer Therapeutics: Experimental & Clinical Agents. Ed. by Beverly A. Teicher. 1996. LC 96-38113. (Cancer Drug Discovery & Development Ser.: Vol. 1). (Illus.). 464p. 170.00 (*0-89603-460-7*) Humana.

Cancer Therapies: Awesome New Advances. Anna R. Spickler. 1998. (Awesome Science of Biology Ser.). (Illus.). 304p. pap. 19.95 (*1-880319-22-5*) Biotech.

Cancer Therapy. Ed. by P. Bannasch. 1989. (Illus.). 256p. 51.95 (*0-387-51034-6*, 2833) Spr-Verlag.

Cancer Therapy. Ed. by H. G. Beger et al. 1988. 308p. 103.00 (*0-387-19293-X*) Spr-Verlag.

Cancer Therapy: Differentiation, Immunomodulation, & Angiogenesis. Ed. by Natale D'Alessandro et al. 1993. LC 93-10491. (NATO ASI Ser.: Vol. 75). 288p. 227.00 (*0-387-54603-0*) Spr-Verlag.

Cancer Therapy: Radiolabeled Antibodies. David M. Goldenberg. 1994. 336p. lib. bdg. 249.00 (*0-8493-5112-X*) CRC Pr.

Cancer Therapy: The Independent Consumer's Guide to Non-Toxic Treatment & Prevention. Ralph W. Moss. 1992. 41p. pap. 19.95 (*1-881025-06-3*) Equinox Pr.

Cancer Therapy—Methods, Treatment, Trials & Drug Use: Index of New Information. Judy T. Gilahan. 1995. LC 95-15403. 57.50 (*0-7883-0738-X*); pap. 47.50 (*0-7883-0739-8*) ABBE Pubs Assn.

Cancer Therapy Sourcebook. Barry Tepperman. 2001. 272p. pap. text 25.95 (*0-7373-0185-6*) Lowell Hse.

Cancer Treatment. Charles M. Haskell. (Illus.). 4th ed. 1995. LC 94-29906. 1056p. text 175.00 (*0-7216-4907-6*); 5th ed. 2000. 1275p. text 195.00 (*0-7216-7833-5*) Saunders.

Cancer Treatment: Proceedings of the WHO Expert Committee, Geneva, 1965. WHO Staff. 1966. (Technical Reports: No. 322). (ENG, FRE, RUS & SPA.). 55p. pap. text 5.00 (*92-4-120322-6*, 1100322) World Health.

Cancer Treatment & Diagnostic Products. Crull & Park. 1995. LC 96-143455. 185p. 2650.00 (*1-56965-043-8*, C-047N) BCC.

Cancer Treatment & Marijuana Therapy: Marijuana's Use in the Reduction of Nausea & Vomiting & for Appetite Stimulation in Cancer Patients. Testimony from Historic Federal Hearings. Ed. by Robert C. Randall. 1990. LC 90-81972. (Marijuana, Medicine & the Law Ser.). 365p. (Orig.). pap. 23.95 (*0-936485-05-1*, Galen Pr DC) Lkng Glass Pubns.

Cancer Treatment & Survival Rates: Site-Specific Registries in Japan, Vol. 43. Ed. by Shaw Wantanabe et al. 1995. LC 95-33187. (Gann Monographs on Cancer Research). 120.00 (*0-8493-7778-1*) CRC Pr.

Cancer Treatment by Hyperthermia, Radiation & Drugs. Ed. by Tadayoshi Matsuda. 1993. 380p. (*0-85066-837-9*) Tay Francis Ltd GBR. *Dist:* Taylor & Francis.

Cancer Treatment Mob. Spiegel. 1999. (*0-465-09547-X*) HarperCollins Pubs.

Cancer Treatment Modalities. Susan L. Groenwald. 1991. (Illus.). (C). pap. text 32.50 (*0-86720-302-1*, 302-1) Jones & Bartlett.

Cancer Treatment Research. Paul Chang. Ed. by Joseph Aisner. 1980. (Developments in Oncology Ser.: Vol. 2). (Illus.). xvi, 272p. text 131.50 (*90-247-2358-2*) Kluwer Academic.

***Cancer Trends in England & Wales, 1950-1999 No. 66: Studies on Medical & Population Subjects.** Mike Quinn et al. 2001. (Illus.). 250p. pap. (*0-11-621393-0*) Statnry Office GBR. *Dist:* Balogh, Bernan Associates.

Cancer Vaccines: Index of New Information for Reference & Research. John C. Bartone. 1997. 160p. 57.50 (*0-7883-1668-0*); pap. 47.50 (*0-7883-1669-9*) ABBE Pubs Assn.

Cancer Vaccines & Immunotherapy. Ed. by Peter L. Stern et al. 2000. LC 99-48963. (Illus.). 296p. text 90.00 (*0-521-62263-8*) Cambridge U Pr.

Cancer Variations & Mortality: Index of Modern Information. Erwin D. Frazier. 1990. LC 88-47855. 150p. 47.50 (*1-55914-190-5*); pap. 44.50 (*1-55914-191-3*) ABBE Pubs Assn.

Cancer Virology, Immunology & Biology. 1991. lib. bdg. 75.00 (*0-8490-4338-7*) Gordon Pr.

Cancer Wars: How Politics Shape What We Know & Don't Know about Cancer. Robert N. Proctor. 1996. (Illus.). 368p. pap. 17.50 (*0-465-00859-3*) Basic.

Cancerproof Your Body. Ross Horne. 1998. (Illus.). 192p. pap. 13.95 (*0-207-18900-5*) HarperCollins Pubs.

Cancers - By Diverse Experiments & Chemically Produced: Index of New Information Including Authors, Methods & Results. John C. Bartone. 1995. (Illus.). 210p. 57.50 (*0-7883-0440-2*); pap. 47.50 (*0-7883-0441-0*) ABBE Pubs Assn.

Cancers - Research on Causes of the Disease: Index of New Information Including Theories & Sources in Life, Work, Hobbies & Environmental Types of Recreation. John C. Bartone. 1995. LC 95-15408. (Illus.). 185p. 57.50 (*0-7883-0436-4*); pap. 47.50 (*0-7883-0437-2*) ABBE Pubs Assn.

Cancers of the Mouth & Throat: A Patient's Guide to Treatment. William Lydiatt & Perry Johnson. 2000. LC 00-11134. (Illus.). viii, 172p. pap. 14.95 (*1-886039-44-5*) Addicus Bks.

Cancers Produced by Radiation: Index of New Information Including Human Risks & Results. John C. Bartone, Sr. 1995. (Illus.). 185p. 57.50 (*0-7883-0624-3*); pap. 47.50 (*0-7883-0625-1*) ABBE Pubs Assn.

Cancers Produced by Radiation: Index of New Information Including Human Risks & Results. John C. Bartone. rev. ed. 1996. LC 96-187. 135p. 57.50 (*0-7883-1016-X*); pap. 47.50 (*0-7883-1017-8*) ABBE Pubs Assn.

CancerScam: Diversion of Federal Cancer Funds to Politics. James T. Bennett & Thomas J. DiLorenzo. 1997. LC 97-26547. 189p. 32.95 (*1-56000-334-0*) Transaction Pubs.

Candid Camera in General Psychology. Allen Funt. 1993. text (*0-07-022801-9*) McGraw.

Candida: A Natural Approach. Karen Brody & Shirley Trickett. 1999. LC 98-85069. (Illus.). 208p. reprint ed. pap. 11.95 (*1-56975-153-6*) Ulysses Pr.

Candida: A Nutritional Approach. Louise Tenney. 1988. (Woodland Health Ser.: No. 1). 32p. pap. 3.95 (*0-913923-28-1*) Woodland UT.

Candida: A Twentieth Century Disease. Shirley Lorenzani. 1986. LC 85-81549. (Pivot Original Health Bks.). 176p. (Orig.). pap. 4.95 (*0-87983-375-0*, Keats Pubng) McGraw-Hill Trade.

Candida: Your Guide to Complementary Therapies, Alternative Techniques & Conventional Treatments. Simon Martin. 1998. LC 98-12757. (Natural Way Ser.). 128p. pap. 5.95 (*1-86204-193-8*) Element MA.

Candida Adherence to Epithelial Cells. Ed. by Mahmoud A. Ghannoum. 1990. 280p. lib. bdg. 230.00 (*0-8493-5979-1*, QR201) CRC Pr.

Candida Albicans. Sarah Brewer. 1997. pap. (*0-7225-3391-8*) Thorsons GBR. *Dist:* Natl Bk Netwk.

Candida Albicans: Cellular & Molecular Biology. Ed. by R. Prasad. 1991. (Illus.). 296p. 183.00 (*0-387-51926-2*) Spr-Verlag.

Candida Albicans Epidemic. 1992. lib. bdg. 75.00 (*0-8490-8706-6*) Gordon Pr.

Candida & Candidamycosis. Ed. by E. Tumbay et al. 1991. (FEMS Symposium Ser.: No. 50). (Illus.). 320p. (C). text 126.00 (*0-306-43829-1*, Kluwer Plenum) Kluwer Academic.

***Candida & Candidiasis.** Ed. by Richard A. Calderone. 2001. LC 2001-53525. 472p. 99.95 (*1-55581-212-0*) ASM Pr.

Candida & Candidosis. Odds. 2nd ed. 1988. 448p. text 126.00 (*0-7020-1265-3*) Saunders.

Candida Diet Against It: What You Eat Can Help Direct Your Immune System to Help You. Luc De Schepper. 1994. pap. (*0-572-01501-1*) W Foulsham GBR. *Dist:* Trans-Atl Phila.

Candida Directory: The Comprehensive Guidebook to Yeast-Free Living. Helen Gustafson & Maureen O'Shea. 1995. LC 93-50920. (Illus.). 192p. pap. 13.95 (*0-89087-714-9*) Celestial Arts.

Candida, The Silent Epidemic: Vital Information to Detect, Combat & Prevent Yeast Infections. Gail Burton. 1999. ix, 63p. (*0-9703256-0-6*) G Burton.

Candida Yeast & Other Parasites: The Battle in Your Body. Jonathon D. Miller. rev. ed. Date not set. (Orig.). pap. 4.98 (*0-935815-03-1*) Lifecircle.

Candidate Reference Method for Serum Digoxin: A Model for Radioimmunoassay Reference Methods; Tentative Guideline (1996) Contrib. by David D. Bayse. 1996. 75.00 (*1-56238-298-5*, I/LA9-T) NCCLS.

Candle & Darkness: Current Research in Alzheimer's Disease. Joseph Rogers. 1998. LC 98-9280. (Illus.). 166p. pap. 13.95 (*1-56625-095-1*) Bonus Books.

Candle Therapy. Catherine Riggs-Bergesen. 1992. (Illus.). 153p. (Orig.). pap. 16.95 (*0-9640440-1-3*) Other Worldly.

Cando Medical et Pharmaceutique. J. Chevalier. 4th ed. 1984. 1016p. 99.95 (*0-8288-1796-0*, M6069) Fr & Eur.

Canine Acupressure: A Treatment Workbook. Nancy A. Zidonis & Marie K. Soderberg. Ed. by Mickey Rubin. 1995. (Illus.). 117p. (Orig.). pap., stu. ed. 20.00 (*0-9645982-0-5*) Tallgrass Pubs.

Canine Anatomy. Bonnie J. Smith. 1999. LC 98-52915. (National Veterinary Medical Series for Independent Study). 640p. 34.95 (*0-683-30080-6*) Lppncott W & W.

Canine & Feline Cardiac Arrhythmias: Self Assessment. Larry P. Tilley. 1993. (Illus.). 212p. pap. 36.00 (*0-8121-1517-1*) Lppncott W & W.

Canine & Feline Dermatology: Diagnosis & Treatment. Gene Nesbitt & Lowell J. Ackerman. 1998. LC 98-175581. 300p. pap. text 99.00 (*1-884254-39-X*) Vet Lrn Syst.

Canine & Feline Endocrinology & Reproduction. Edward C. Feldman & Richard W. Nelson. Ed. by Ray Kersey. 2nd ed. 1996. (Illus.). 672p. text 96.00 (*0-7216-3634-9*) Saunders.

Canine & Feline Geriatrics. Mike Davies. 1994. LC 96-20438. (Library of Veterinary Practice). (Illus.). 166p. pap. 49.95 (*0-632-03479-3*) Blackwell Sci.

Canine & Feline Nephrology & Urology. Ed. by Carl A. Osborne & Delmar R. Finco. 1995. LC 94-34694. (Illus.). 960p. 79.00 (*0-683-06666-8*) Lppncott W & W.

Canine & Feline Nutrition. Linda P. Case & Diane L. Carey. 1994. LC 95-119829. (Illus.). 432p. (C). (gr. 13). text 65.00 (*0-8151-1536-9*, 25123) Mosby Inc.

Canine & Feline Nutrition. Linda P. Case et al. 1995. (Illus.). 432p. (*84-8174-246-5*) Mosby-Doyma Libros ESP. *Dist:* Mosby Inc.

Canine & Feline Reproduction. Shirley D. Johnson et al. 1999. LC 00-49229. (Illus.). 592p. text 69.00 (*0-7216-5607-2*) Saunders.

Canine As a Biomedical Research Model: Immunological, Hematological & Oncological Aspects. DOE Technical Information Center Staff. Ed. by Moshe Shifrine & Floyd D. Wilson. 1980. LC 80-24174. 436p. 19.00 (*0-87079-122-2*, DOE/TIC-10191); 9.00 incl. fiche (*0-87079-457-4*, DOE/TIC-10191) DOE.

Canine Behavior: A Guide for Veterinarians. Bonnie V. Beaver. Ed. by Ray Kersey. 1998. LC 98-17176. (Illus.). 368p. (C). pap. 29.95 (*0-7216-5965-9*) Saunders.

Canine Behavior: A History of Domestication; Behavioral Development & Adult Behavior Patterns; Neurophysiology; Psychobiology; Training, Inheritance, Early Experience & Psycho Social Relationships; Experimental Neuroses & Sports Behavioral Anomalities, Congenital Anomalies & Differential Diagnosis of Neurologic Disease. M. W. Fox. fac. ed. 1978. (Illus.). 152p. 29.95 (*0-398-00599-0*) C C Thomas.

Canine Clinical Parasitology. Jay R. Georgi & M. E. Georgi. 1992. LC 91-14154. (Illus.). 227p. text 55.00 (*0-8121-1469-8*) Lppncott W & W.

Canine Dentistry Including a Section on Felines. Patricia Frost. 5th ed. 1995. 76p. (C). pap. text 14.95 (*0-9648369-0-4*) J H D Communs.

Canine Distemper Virus. M. J. Appel & J. H. Gillespie. 1972. (Virology Monographs: Vol. 11). (Illus.). 153p. 45.00 (*0-387-81059-5*) Spr-Verlag.

Canine Medicine & Therapeutics. Ed. by E. A. Chandler. 3rd ed. 1990. (Illus.). 896p. pap. 72.95 (*0-86542-824-7*) Blackwell Sci.

Canine Medicine & Therapeutics. Neil T. Gorman & British Small Animal Veterinary Association Staff. 4th ed. 1998. LC 97-27105. 1086p. 124.95 (*0-632-04045-9*) Blackwell Sci.

Canine Orthopedics. W. G. Whittick. 2nd ed. 1990. LC 88-2999. (Illus.). 936p. text 135.00 (*0-8121-1086-2*) Lppncott W & W.

Canine Parvovirus: A New Pathogen. C. Vella & S. W. Ketteridge. 1991. (Illus.). 58p. 32.00 (*0-387-54314-7*) Spr-Verlag.

Canine Practice. William E. Boden. 1991. pap. text 44.95 (*0-7020-1522-9*) Saunders.

Canine Practice No. 2. Edward Boden. 2nd ed. 1996. (Illus.). 217p. pap. text 49.00 (*0-7020-2082-6*) Saunders.

Canine Sports Medicine & Surgery. Mark S. Bloomberg et al. 1998. LC 96-24186. (Illus.). 496p. (C). text 95.00 (*0-7216-5022-8*) Saunders.

Cannabinoids As Therapeutic Agents. Raphael Mechoulam. 1986. 200p. 115.00 (*0-8493-5772-1*, RM666, CRC Reprint) Franklin.

Cannabis: Physiopathology, Epidemiology, Detection, Proceedings of the Second International Symposium, Paris, April 8-9, 1992. Gabriel G. Nahas. Ed. by Colette Latour. 1992. 432p. 156.95 (*0-8493-8310-2*, QP801) CRC Pr.

Cannabis & Cognitive Functioning. Nadia Solowij. 1998. LC 97-38655. (International Research Monographs in the Addictions). (Illus.). 306p. (C). text 85.00 (*0-521-59114-7*) Cambridge U Pr.

Cannabis in Medical Practice: A Legal, Historical & Pharmacological Overview of the Therapeutic Use of Marijuana. Ed. by Mary L. Mathre. 1997. LC 97-10944. (Illus.). 247p. per. 29.95 (*0-7864-0361-6*) McFarland & Co.

***Cannabis Therapeutics in HIV/AIDS.** Ed. by Ethan Russo. 2001. LC 2001-51488. (Journal of Cannabis Therapeutics Ser.: No. 1). (*0-7890-1698-2*); pap. (*0-7890-1699-0*) Haworth Pr (Integrative Healing Pr).

Canon of Medicine. Ibn S. Avicenna. 1997. 500p. (C). 59.95 (*1-871031-67-2*) Kazi Pubns.

Canonical Status of Catholic Health Care Facilities in the Province of New Brunswick in Light of Recent Provincial Government Legislation. Michael McGowan. 2000. LC 00-32874. (Canadian Studies: Vol. 26). xxiii, 351p. 99.95 (*0-7734-7683-0*) E Mellen.

Cansell Controversy: Why Is a Possible Cure for Cancer Being Suppressed? Louise B. Trull. 1993. 140p. pap. 9.95 (*1-878901-76-1*) Hampton Roads Pub Co.

Can't Live Without It! The Story of Hemoglobin in Sickness & in Health. Loren F. Hazelwood. 1997. LC 98-170262. (Illus.). xi, 265p. pap. 15.95 (*0-9660784-0-3*) Autodidactics.

Can't Wait to Communicate! Fun Activities That Shape Nonverbal Communication. Robbie Wise. Ed. by Cindy Drolet. 1989. (Illus.). 76p. spiral bd. 31.00 (*0-9609464-2-X*, 8501) Imaginart Intl.

Can't Your Child See? A Guide for Parents & Professionals about Young Children Who Are Visually Impaired. Eileen P. Scott et al. 3rd ed. 1995. LC 94-9262. (Illus.). 279p. (C). pap. text 26.00 (*0-89079-604-1*, 6801) PRO-ED.

Cantaneous Medicine & Surgery: Self Assessment & Review, Vol. 1. Philip E. LeBoit et al. 1995. LC 94-21584. (Illus.). 304p. pap. text 42.00 (*0-7216-5408-8*) Saunders.

CAOS - Computer-Assisted Orthopedic Surgery. Ed. by L. P. Nolte. 1999. LC 98-3828. (Illus.). 290p. text 49.00 (*0-88937-168-7*) Hogrefe & Huber Pubs.

Capacity, Capital, & Calories. Beryl Levinger & National Council for International Health. 1996. LC 96-45936. (Martin J. Forman Memorial Lectures). (*0-915173-04-2*) Helen Keller Intl.

Capacity for Emotional Growth. Elizabeth R. Zetzel. 1971. LC 71-126355. 316p. 47.50 (*0-8236-0650-3*) Intl Univs Pr.

CAPD CCPD in Children. Richard N. Fine et al. 2nd ed. 1998. LC 98-42542. 250.00 (*0-7923-8236-6*) Kluwer Academic.

Capillarity Today: Proceedings of an Advanced Workshop on Capillarity Held In Memoriam Raymond Defay at Brussels, Belgium, 7-10 May 1990. Ed. by G. Petre et al. 1991. (Lecture Notes in Physics: Vol. 386). 384p. 59.95 (*0-387-54367-8*) Spr-Verlag.

Capillary Electrophoresis: Theory & Practice. Patrick Camilleri. 1993. LC 93-10058. (New Directions in Organic & Biological Chemistry Ser.). 512p. 136.95 (*0-8493-7862-1*, QP519) CRC Pr.

Capillary Electrophoresis Methods for Pharmaceutical Analysis. George Lunn. 2000. LC 98-48818. 1544p. 295.00 (*0-471-33188-0*) Wiley.

Capillary Electrophoresis of Carbohydrates. Ed. by Pierre Thibault & Susumu Honda. 2000. (Methods in Molecular Biology Ser.). 350p. 84.50 (*0-89603-826-2*) Humana.

Capillary Electrophretic Separations of Drugs, Vol. 735. A. S. Cohen et al. 1996. LC 96-33181. 458p. 272.00 (*0-444-82519-3*) Elsevier.

Capillary Functions & White Cell Interaction. Ed. by K. Messmer. 1991. (Progress in Applied Microcirculation Ser.: Vol. 18). (Illus.). x, 138p. 124.50 (*3-8055-5397-8*) S Karger.

Capital Health's 1997 Managed Care Glossary. 1996. 16p. (Orig.). pap. 4.65 (*1-890074-00-4*) CapitalHlth Pub.

Capital Health's 1997 Managed Care Glossary: Including Insurance Terminology. 1996. 40p. (Orig.). pap. 7.25 (*1-890074-01-2*) CapitalHlth Pub.

Capital Health's 1997 Medicare Glossary Including Managed Care Terminology: Consumer Edition. 1997. (*1-890074-03-9*) CapitalHlth Pub.

Capital Medicine: A Tradition of Excellence. Nancy B. Paull. 1994. (Illus.). 128p. 29.95 (*1-882933-02-8*) Cherbo Pub Grp.

Capitalizing Medical Groups: Positioning Physicians for the Future. Dean C. Coddington et al. 1997. LC 97-48342. 300p. 75.00 (*0-07-012023-4*) McGraw.

Capitation: New Opportunities & Risks in Managing Healthcare. David I. Samuels. 1995. LC 95-44282. 250p. (C). text 45.00 (*1-55738-640-4*, Irwn Prfssnl) McGraw-Hill Educ Grp.

Capitation: Tools, Trends, Traps & Techniques. Ed. by Steve Venable. 1998. LC 97-39422. 200p. (Orig.). pap. text 49.95 (*1-57066-072-7*, ME102) Practice Mgmt Info.

Capitation & Other Managed Care Payment Systems for Orthopaedic Surgeons. Ed. by AAOS Staff. 1996. 100p. pap. 45.00 (*0-89203-154-9*) Amer Acad Ortho Surg.

Capitation & Risk Sharing: A Guidebook for Physicians & Alternate Site Providers. Alison Cherney. 1995. LC 95-36379. 300p. (C). text 60.00 (*1-55738-643-9*, Irwn Prfssnl) McGraw-Hill Educ Grp.

Capitation for Physicians: Understanding & Negotiating Contracts to Maximize Reimbursement & Manage Financial Risk. John F. McCally. 1996. text 40.00 (*0-7863-1149-5*); LC 96-6446. (Illus.). 240p. text 45.00 (*0-7863-1006-5*) McGraw-Hill Educ Grp (Irwn Prfssnl).

Capitation in California: A Study of Physician Organizations Managing Risk. Maurice J. Penner. 1997. LC 96-39279. 281p. pap. 44.00 (*1-56793-051-4*) Health Admin Pr.

Capitation Rates in the Medi-Cal Managed Care Program. unabr. ed. 1999. (Illus.). 32p. pap. (*1-929008-13-9*) CA HlthCare Fnd.

Capped Langur in Bangladesh: Behavioral Ecology & Reproductive Tactics. C. B. Stanford. 1991. (Contributions to Primatology Ser.: Vol. 26). (Illus.). xviii, 180p. 107.00 (*3-8055-5396-X*) S Karger.

Capsaicin: The Anti-Arthritic Phytochemical. Muhammed Majeed. 1997. (Illus.). 84p. pap. (*0-9647856-2-5*) Nutrisci Pubs.

Capsaicin in the Study of Pain. Ed. by John N. Wood. 1993. (Neuroscience Perspectives Ser.). (Illus.). 304p. text 78.00 (*0-12-762855-X*) Acad Pr.

Capsaicin-Sensitive Afferent Nerves in Gastric Mucosal Damage & Protection. Gy Mozsik et al. 1997. 124p. pap. (*963-05-7437-3*) Akade Kiado HUN. *Dist:* Intl Spec Bk, St Mut.

Capsicum: The Woodland Health Series. Rita Elkins. 1997. (Woodland Health Ser.). 32p. pap. text 3.95 (*1-885670-41-9*) Woodland UT.

Capture Gamma-Ray Spectroscopy & Related Topics 1984. S. Raman. 1984. LC 84-73303. (Conference Proceedings Ser.: No. 125). 984p. (C). 65.00 (*0-88318-324-2*) Am Inst Physics.

Cara: Growing with a Retarded Child. Martha M. Jablow. 1982. LC 82-3283. 250p. pap. 12.95 (*0-87722-269-X*) Temple U Pr.

Caraka-Samhita Tr. by A. Chandra Kaviratna & P. Sharma from SAN. 2nd rev. ed. 1996. LC 96-902820. (*81-7030-471-7*) Sri Satguru Pubns IND. *Dist:* S Asia.

Carbaryl. Ed. by World Health Organization Staff. 1994. (Environmental Health Criteria Ser.: No. 153). (ENG, FRE & SPA.). 358p. pap. text 67.00 (*92-4-157153-5*, 1160153) World Health.

Carbendazim. 1993. (Environmental Health Criteria Ser.: No. 149). (ENG, FRE & SPA.). 132p. pap. text 29.00 (*92-4-157149-7*, 1160149) World Health.

Carbohydrate Addict's Gram Counter. Rachael F. Heller & Richard F. Heller. 1993. 96p. (Orig.). pap. 4.99 (*0-451-17717-7*, Sig) NAL.

Carbohydrate Addict's Healthy Heart Program: Break Your Carbo-Insulin Connection to Heart Disease. Richard F. Heller et al. 2000. 368p. pap. 14.95 (*0-345-42612-6*, Ballantine); 1999. LC 99-26067. (Illus.). xi, 352p. 24.95 (*0-345-42610-X*) Ballantine Pub Grp.

Carbohydrate Building Blocks. Mikael Bols. 1995. LC 95-16543. 182p. 80.00 (*0-471-13339-6*) Wiley.

Carbohydrate Metabolism. Ed. by W. A. Wood et al. 1967. (Methods in Enzymology Ser.: Vol. 9). text 209.00 (*0-12-181809-8*) Acad Pr.

Carbohydrate Metabolism, Pt. C. Ed. by W. A. Wood. 1975. (Methods in Enzymology Ser.: Vol. 42). text 199.00 (*0-12-181942-6*) Acad Pr.

Carbohydrate Metabolism, Pt. D. Ed. by Sidney P. Colowick & Willis A. Wood. 1982. (Methods in Enzymology Ser.: Vol. 89). 656p. text 188.00 (*0-12-181989-2*) Acad Pr.

Carbohydrate Metabolism, Pt. B. Ed. by W. A. Wood. 1975. (Methods in Enzymology Ser.: Vol. 41). text 199.00 (*0-12-181941-8*) Acad Pr.

Carbohydrate Metabolism, Pt. E. Ed. by Sidney P. Colowick & Willis A. Wood. 1982. (Methods in Enzymology Ser.: Vol. 90). 559p. text 188.00 (*0-12-181990-6*) Acad Pr.

Carbohydrate Metabolism in Cultured Cells. Ed. by Michael J. Morgan. 1986. LC 86-12170. (Illus.). 536p. (C). text 174.00 (*0-306-42240-9*, Kluwer Plenum) Kluwer Academic.

Carbohydrate Metabolism in Pregnancy & the Newborn IV. Ed. by H. W. Sutherland et al. 1989. (Illus.). 377p. 182.00 (*0-387-19547-5*, 2660) Spr-Verlag.

Carbohydrate-Protein Interaction. Ed. by Irwin J. Goldstein. 1979. LC 78-25788. (ACS Symposium Ser.: No. 88). 223p. 29.95 (*0-8412-0466-7*) Am Chemical.

Carbohydrates: Structure & Biology. Lehmann. 1998. 98.00 (*0-86577-790-X*) Thieme Med Pubs.

Carbohydrates: Structures & Biology. Lehmann. 1998. pap. 59.00 (*0-86577-795-0*) Thieme Med Pubs.

Carbohydrates: What You Need to Know American Dietetic Association Staff. 1998. pap. 41.70 (*1-56561-144-6*) Wiley.

Carbohydrates & Energy Metabolism. Ed. by Alan A. Boulton et al. 1989. LC 88-26609. (Neuromethods Ser.: Vol. 11). (Illus.). 403p. 159.00 (*0-89603-143-8*) Humana.

Carbohydrates in Drug Design. Zbigniew J. Witczak & Karl A. Nieforth. 1997. LC 97-12543. (Illus.). 720p. text 215.00 (*0-8247-9982-8*) Dekker.

Carbohydrates in Infant Nutrition. 1997. text 19.00 (*3-540-99540-4*) Spr-Verlag.

Carbohydrates in Solution. Ed. by Horace S. Isbell. 1973. LC 73-81038. (Advances in Chemistry Ser.: No. 117). 421p. 36.95 (*0-8412-0178-1*) Am Chemical.

Carbohydrates, Lipids & Accessory Growth Factors. Ed. by Miloslav Rechcigl, Jr. 1976. (Comparative Animal Nutrition Ser.: Vol. 1). (Illus.). 85.25 (*3-8055-2268-1*) S Karger.

Carbon-13 Nuclear Magnetic Resonance Spectroscopy. George C. Levy et al. 2nd ed. 1992. 352p. (C). reprint ed. lib. bdg. 59.95 (*0-89464-796-2*) Krieger.

Carbon Dioxide & Climate: Dedicated to Williard F. Libby & Hans E. Suss. L. M. Libby. 1980. (Illus.). 270p. pap. 48.00 (*0-08-026240-6*, Pergamon Pr) Elsevier.

Carbon Disulfide. 1979. (Environmental Health Criteria Ser.: No. 10). 100p. pap. text 16.00 (*92-4-154070-2*, 1160010) World Health.

Carbon Monoxide. 1979. (Environmental Health Criteria Ser.: No. 13). 125p. pap. text 19.00 (*92-4-154073-7*, 1160013) World Health.

Carbon Monoxide. Ed. by J. Descotes et al. 1999. (Indoor & Build Environment Ser.: Vol. 8, No. 3, 1999). (Illus.). 64p. pap. 25.25 (*3-8055-6994-7*) S Karger.

Carbon Monoxide. Ed. by David G. Penney. 1996. LC 95-53854. 304p. 119.95 (*0-8493-4796-3*) CRC Pr.

Carbon Monoxide—Accidents, Poisoning & Suicide Attempts Via Car Exhaust: Index of New Information for Reference & Research. Jose T. Bardoza. rev. ed. 1998. 167p. pap. 47.50 (*0-7883-2119-6*) ABBE Pubs Assn.

Carbon Monoxide & Human Lethality: Fire & Non-Fire Studies. Ed. by Marcelo M. Hirschler et al. 1993. LC 93-3411. vi, 424p. mass mkt. 184.95 (*1-85861-015-X*) Elsevier.

Carbon Monoxide Poisoning. K. K. Jain. 1990. 200p. pap. 37.50 (*0-87527-258-4*) Green.

***Carbon Monoxideand Cardiovascular Functions.** Contrib. by Nader G. Abraham et al. 2001. 336p. 129.95 (*0-8493-1041-5*) CRC Pr.

Carbon-13 NMR Spectral Problems. Robert B. Bates & William A. Beavers. 1981. LC 79-92216. (Organic Chemistry Ser.). 259p. text 99.50 (*0-89603-010-5*) Humana.

Carbonic Anhydrases: New Horizons. Ed. by R. W. Chegwidden. 2000. LC 00-27796. (Experientia Supplementa Ser.: Vol. 90). (Illus.). 350p. 249.00 (*3-7643-5670-7*) Birkhauser.

Carboplatin: Present Status & Future Directions. Ed. by D. Khayat. 1993. (Journal: Vol. 50, Suppl. 2, 1993). (Illus.). iv, 54p. pap. 25.25 (*3-8055-5891-0*) S Karger.

Carcinogen Risk Assessment. C. C. Travis. 1988. LC 87-37403. (Contemporary Issues in Risk Analysis Ser.: Vol. 3). (Illus.). 220p. (C). text 85.00 (*0-306-42848-2*, Kluwer Plenum) Kluwer Academic.

Carcinogen Risk Assessment: New Directions in the Qualitative & Quantitative Aspects. Ed. by Ronald W. Hart & Fred D. Hoerger. 1988. (Banbury Reports: No. 31). (Illus.). 356p. 85.00 (*0-87969-231-6*) Cold Spring Harbor.

Carcinogenesis: Fundamental Mechanisms & Environmental Effects. Ed. by Bernard Pullman et al. 1980. (Jerusalem Symposia on Quantum Chemistry & Biochemistry Ser.: No. 13). 560p. text 191.50 (*90-277-1171-2*) Kluwer Academic.

Carcinogenesis & Adducts in Animals & Humans. Ed. by Miriam C. Poirier & F. A. Beland. 1987. (Progress in Experimental Tumor Research Ser.: Vol. 31). (Illus.). viii, 116p. 103.50 (*3-8055-4457-X*) S Karger.

Carcinogenesis & Aging. V. N. Anisimov. 1987. 176p. 105.00 (*0-8493-6278-4*, CRC Reprint) Franklin.

Carcinogenesis & Aging, Set. Ed. by V. N. Anisimov. 1987. LC 86-18778. 199.00 (*0-8493-6277-6*, RC268, CRC Reprint) Franklin.

Carcinogenesis & Aging, Vol. 2. V. N. Anisimov. 1987. LC 86-18778. 94.00 (*0-8493-6279-2*, RC268, CRC Reprint) Franklin.

Carcinogenesis & Dietary Fat. Ed. by S. Abraham. 1989. (Prostaglandins, Leukotrienes, & Cancer Ser.). (C). text 258.00 (*0-7923-0117-X*) Kluwer Academic.

Carcinogenesis & Mutagenesis. 1977. LC 77-91833. 388p. 39.00 (*0-930376-02-1*) Chem-Orbital.

Carcinogenesis & Mutagenesis Testing. Ed. by J. Fielding Douglas. 1984. LC 84-12820. (Contemporary Biomedicine Ser.: Vol. 4). 355p. 119.50 (*0-89603-042-3*) Humana.

Carcinogenesis in Animals & Humans. A. R. Gregory. 1988. 125p. text 173.00 (*2-88124-412-2*) Gordon & Breach.

Carcinogenic & Mutagenic Metal Compounds, Vol. 14. Ed. by Ernest Merian. 1991. (Current Topics in Environmental & Toxicology Ser.). xvi, 638p. text 303.00 (*2-88124-781-4*) Gordon & Breach.

Carcinogenic & Mutagenic Metal Compounds: Environmental & Analytical Chemistry & Biological Effects. R. W. Frei et al. 1985. (Current Topics In Environmental & Toxicological Chemistry Ser.: Vol. 8). xii, 550p. text 318.00 (*2-88124-022-4*) Gordon & Breach.

Carcinogenic & Mutagenic Metal Compounds 2, Vol. 11. Ernest Merian et al. 1988. xiv, 544p. text 203.00 (*2-88124-663-X*) Gordon & Breach.

Carcinogenic Potency Database & President's Cancer Panel Conference on Avoidable Causes of Cancer. Ed. by Thomas J. Goehl & Michael P. Dieter. 1997. (Illus.). 320p. (Orig.). (C). pap. text 50.00 (*0-7881-4492-8*) DIANE Pub.

Carcinogenic Potency Database; Endocrine Disruptors. Ed. by Lois Swirsky Gola. 2000. (Illus.). 129p. (C). pap. text 25.00 (*0-7881-8536-5*) DIANE Pub.

Carcinogenicity & Pesticides: Principles, Issues, & Relationships. Ed. by Nancy N. Ragsdale & Robert E. Menzer. 1989. LC 89-18052. (ACS Symposium Ser.: No. 414). (Illus.). 237p. text 65.00 (*0-8412-1703-3*) Am Chemical.

Carcinogens: Index of Modern Information. American Health Research Institute Staff. 1990. LC 88-47988. 150p. 47.50 (*1-55914-196-4*); pap. 44.50 (*1-55914-197-2*) ABBE Pubs Assn.

Carcinogens & Anti-Carcinogens in the Human Diet: A Comparison of Naturally Occurring & Synthetic Substances... National Research Council Staff. 1996. LC 95-73149. 436p. (Orig.). pap. text 44.95 (*0-309-05391-9*) Natl Acad Pr.

Carcinogens & Mutagens in the Environment: Food Products, Vol. 1. Ed. by Hans F. Stich. 1982. 320p. 181.00 (*0-8493-5881-7*, RC268, CRC Reprint) Franklin.

Carcinogens & Mutagens in the Environment: The Workplace, Vol. V. Hans F. Stich. 1985. 192p. 110.00 (*0-8493-5885-X*, RC268, CRC Reprint) Franklin.

Carcinoid Tumors. Ed. by M. Rothmund et al. 1995. (Journal: Vol. 55, Suppl. 3, 1994). (Illus.). iv, 116p. pap. 49.75 (*3-8055-6121-0*) S Karger.

Carcinological Fauna of India. A. Alcock. 1968. 700p. pap. (*0-7855-2720-6*) Intl Bks & Periodicals IND. *Dist:* St Mut.

Carcinoma Corporis Uteri. E. Held et al. Ed. by A. Reist. 1973. (Fortschritte der Geburtshilfe & Gynaekologie Ser.: Vol. 49). (Illus.). 150p. 41.75 (*3-8055-1564-2*) S Karger.

Carcinoma of the Bladder: Innovations in Management. Ed. by Zbigniew Petrovich et al. 1997. LC 97-11285. (Medical Radiology Ser.). (Illus.). 325p. 170.00 (*3-540-60885-0*) Spr-Verlag.

Carcinoma of the Breast. I. K. Dhawan & V. K. Kapoor. 1987. (C). (*81-85017-37-9*) Interprint IND. *Dist:* St Mut.

Carcinoma of the Cervix. E. S. Hafez. 1982. text 289.50 (*90-247-2574-7*) Kluwer Academic.

Carcinoma of the Esophagus & Gastric Cardia. Ed. by Guo J. Huang & Ying K'Ai Wu. 1984. (Illus.). 395p. 273.00 (*0-387-12535-3*) Spr-Verlag.

Carcinoma of the Kidney & Testis & Rare Urologic Malignancies: Innovations in Management. Ed. by Zbigniew Petrovich et al. 1998. LC 98-21388. (Medical Radiology Ser.). (Illus.). 400p. 189.00 (*3-540-63215-8*) Spr-Verlag.

Carcinoma of the Lip. Robert P. Zitsch, 3rd & Gregory J. Renner. 1996. LC 96-22954. (Self-Instructional Package Ser.). (Illus.). 73p. (Orig.). pap. text 25.00 (*1-56772-023-4*) AAO-HNS.

Carcinoma of the Oesophagus: Proceedings of the First South African Conference, Cape Town, 26-28 January 1977. Ed. by W. Silber. 1978. 476p. 99.00 (*0-86961-098-8*) Ashgate Pub Co.

Carcinoma of the Oral Cavity & Oropharynx, No. 134. Ed. by H. D. Pape et al. 1994. LC 93-30355. (Recent Results in Cancer Research Ser.: Vol. 134). 98.00 (*0-387-56819-0*) Spr-Verlag.

Carcinoma of the Prostate: Innovations in Management. Ed. by Z. Petrovich et al. 1996. LC 95-52110. (Medical Radiology Ser.). (Illus.). 400p. 198.00 (*3-540-58749-7*) Spr-Verlag.

Carcinoma of the Supraglottic Larynx. James H. Boyd et al. 1993. (Self-Instructional Package Ser.). (Illus.). 77p. pap. text 25.00 (*1-56772-008-0*) AAO-HNS.

***Carcinoma of the Supraglottic Larynx.** Jonas T. Johnson & Hugh Curtin. 2nd ed. 2001. LC 00-68941. (Self-Instructional Package Ser.). (Illus.). 77p. 30.00 (*1-56772-033-1*, 5506535) AAO-HNS.

Carcinomas of Esophagus & Colon. M. Webber & Lea I. Sekely. 1984. LC 84-1838. (In Vitro Models Cancer Research Ser.). 256p. 142.00 (*0-8493-5581-8*, CRC Reprint) Franklin.

Carcinomas of Liver & Pancreas. M. Webber & Lea I. Sekely. 1985. LC 84-1838. (In Vitro Models Cancer Research Ser.: Vol. 2). 264p. 147.00 (*0-8493-5582-6*, CRC Reprint) Franklin.

Carcinomas of the Head & Neck. Ed. by Charlotte Jacobs. 1990. (C). text 215.50 (*0-7923-0668-6*) Kluwer Academic.

Cardiac Adaptation & Failure. 1995. 214.00 (*4-431-70133-8*) Spr-Verlag.

Cardiac Adaptation & Failure. Ed. by Yosh Maruyama et al. 1995. LC 94-40505. 195.00 (*0-387-70133-8*) Spr-Verlag.

Cardiac Anaesthesia: A Practical Handbook. Nian C. Hwang & Michael Sinclair. 1997. LC 97-158393. (Illus.). 170p. (C). text 85.00 (*0-19-262836-4*) OUP.

Cardiac Anaesthesia: Problems & Innovations. Ed. by S. De Lange et al. 1986. (Developments in Critical Care, Medicine, & Anesthesiology Ser.). text 140.00 (*0-89838-794-9*) Kluwer Academic.

Cardiac & Pulmonary Management. M. Gabriel Khan et al. 1992. LC 92-11602. (Illus.). 977p. pap. text 49.50 (*0-8121-1494-9*) Lppncott W & W.

Cardiac & Vascular Diseases. 1989. (International Nomenclature of Diseases Ser.: No. 5). pap. text 20.00 (*92-9036-037-2*) World Health.

Cardiac Anesthesia. Clutton-Brock. 2000. (Illus.). 256p. pap. 64.95 (*0-412-71710-7*, Chap & Hall NY) Chapman & Hall.

Cardiac Anesthesia. Ed. by Joel A. Kaplan. 3rd ed. 1993. LC 92-24342. (Illus.). 1376p. text 210.00 (*0-7216-6707-4*) Saunders.

Cardiac Anesthesia. Joel A. Kaplan. Ed. by Allan Ross. 4th ed. 1998. LC 97-43985. (Illus.). 1260p. text 279.00 (*0-7216-7509-3*) Saunders.

Cardiac Anesthesia: Principles & Clinical Practice. F. G. Estafanous et al. 2nd ed. 2001. LC 00-67813. (Illus.). 1,056p. text 199.00 (*0-7817-2195-4*) Lppncott W & W.

Cardiac Angiography. Stephen W. Miller. 1984. 430p. 105.00 (*0-316-57367-1*, Little Brwn Med Div) Lppncott W & W.

Cardiac Arrest: Practice in Running a Code. 1999. (Illus.). 50p. pap. 10.00 (*0-9663389-5-2*) KG-EKG.

Cardiac Arrhythmia. Philip J. Podrid & Peter R. Kowey. 2nd ed. 2001. text 159.00 (*0-7817-2486-4*) Lppncott W & W.

Cardiac Arrhythmia: Mechanisms, Diagnosis, & Management. Ed. by Philip J. Podrid & Peter R. Kowey. 1994. (Illus.). 1,472p. text 169.00 (*0-683-06905-5*) Lppncott W & W.

Cardiac Arrhythmias. William J. Mandel. 3rd ed. 1995. 1,296p. text 199.00 (*0-397-51185-X*) Lppncott W & W.

Cardiac Arrhythmias. David H. Bennett. 4th ed. 1993. LC 93-15125. (Illus.). 224p. pap. text 55.00 (*0-7506-1638-5*) Buttrwrth-Heinemann.

Cardiac Arrhythmias: A Practical Guide for the Clinician. Ed. by Robert A. Waugh et al. 2nd ed. 1994. (Illus.). 480p. (C). 75.00 (*0-8036-9114-9*) OUP.

Cardiac Arrhythmias: An Approach to Their Electrocardiographic Recognition. Alan E. Lindsay & Alberto Budkin. 2nd ed. 1975. (Illus.). 178p. pap. 26.50 (*0-8151-5428-3*) Mosby Inc.

Cardiac Arrhythmias: An Integrated Approach for the Clinician. Eric N. Prystowsky & George Klein. 1994. (Illus.). 452p. text 67.00 (*0-07-050984-0*) McGraw-Hill Prof.

Cardiac Arrhythmias: New Therapeutic Drugs & Devices. Ed. by Joel Morganroth & E. Neil Moore. 1985. (Developments in Cardiovascular Medicine Ser.). text 132.00 (*0-89838-716-7*) Kluwer Academic.

Cardiac Arrhythmias: Practical Notes on Interpretation & Treatment. David H. Bennett. 5th ed. 1997. LC 96-53898. (An Arnold Publication). (Illus.). 264p. pap. (*0-7506-3369-7*) E A GBR. *Dist:* OUP.

Cardiac Arrhythmias: The Management of Atrial Fibrillation. Ed. by Ronald W. Campbell & Michiel J. Janse. 1992. LC 92-49869. (*3-540-55588-9*) Spr-Verlag.

Cardiac Arrhythmias 1997: Proceedings of the 5th International Workshop on Cardiac Arrhythmias, Venice, 7-10 October, 1997. Antonio Raviele. 1997. LC 97-36011. 562p. 98.00 (*88-470-0002-5*) Spr-Verlag.

Cardiac Arrhythmias-Electrophy. Grace. 2001. text (*0-7020-1880-5*) W B Saunders GBR. *Dist:* Saunders.

Cardiac Arrhythmias in the Pediatric Patient. Edward Walsh. 1997. LC 2001-29376. text 159.00 (*0-397-58744-9*) Lppncott W & W.

Cardiac Arrhythmias 1999: Proceedings of the 6th International Workshop on Cardiac Arrhythmias, Venice, 5-8 October 1999. International Workshop on Cardiac Arrhythmias Staff & Antonio Raviele. 1999. LC 99-44747. (Illus.). 600p. (C). (*88-470-0071-8*) Spr-Verlag ITA. *Dist:* Spr-Verlag.

Cardiac Arrhythmias, Pacing & Electrophysiology: The Expert View. Ed. by Panos E. Vardas. 1998. LC 97-49833. (Developments in Cardiovascular Medicine Ser.). 496p. 199.00 (*0-7923-4908-3*) Kluwer Academic.

***Cardiac Arrythmias: Practical Notes on Interpretation & Treatment.** David H. Bennett. 6th ed. 2001. (Arnold Publication). 288p. (Orig.). pap. text (*0-340-80731-8*) E A GBR. *Dist:* OUP.

***Cardiac Arrythmias after Surgery for Congenital Heart Disease.** Ed. by Seshadri Balaji et al. 2001. (Arnold Publication). 354p. text 98.50 (*0-340-76207-1*) OUP.

Cardiac Assist Devices. Ed. by Daniel J. Goldstein & Mehmet Oz. 1999. LC 99-48126. (Illus.). 464p. 115.00 (*0-87993-449-2*) Futura Pub.

Cardiac Auscultation. Antonio C. deLeon. 29p. 9.75 (*1-886128-00-6*) Laennec Pub.

Cardiac Bioassist. Ed. by Alain Carpentier et al. 1997. LC 96-41246. (Bakken Research Center Ser.: Vol. 11). (Illus.). 656p. 125.00 (*0-87993-647-9*) Futura Pub.

Cardiac Catheterization. Kirk L. Peterson & Pascal Nicod. Ed. by Richard Zorab. 1996. LC 95-3944. (Illus.). 560p. text 99.00 (*0-7216-3064-2*) Saunders.

Cardiac Catheterization: And Other Cardiac Diagnostic Tests & Radiological Procedures. Julia A. Purcell. Ed. by Nancy R. Hull. rev. ed. 1995. LC 82-10133. (Illus.). 32p. pap. 5.95 (*0-939838-10-9*) Pritchett & Hull.

Cardiac Catheterization, Angiography & Intervention. William Grossman & Donald S. Baim. 4th ed. 1990. LC 90-5835. (Illus.). 698p. text 82.00 (*0-8121-1342-X*) Lppncott W & W.

Cardiac Catheterization, Angiography & Intervention. William Grossman & Donald S. Balm. 5th ed. 1995. LC 95-13453. (*0-683-03645-9*) Lppncott W & W.

Cardiac Catheterization Handbook, Vol. 3. Ed. by Morton J. Kern. 3rd ed. 1998. LC 98-13814. (Illus.). 672p. (C). (gr. 13). spiral bd. 44.95 (*0-8151-2614-X*, 31638) Mosby Inc.

Cardiac Catheterization Policy & Procedure Guidelines. Judith Smith. 1995. 508p. spiral bd. 135.00 (*1-879575-40-X*) Acad Med Sys.

Cardiac Catheters: Forecasts for 22 Products in an Evolving Market. Market Intelligence Staff. 1993. 413p. 1995.00 (*1-56753-426-0*) Frost & Sullivan.

***Cardiac Cellular Electrophysiology.** Edward Carmeliet & J. Vereecke. 2001. LC 2001-38980. (Basic Science for the Cardiologist Ser.: Vol. 9). (Illus.). 432p. 205.00 (*0-7923-7544-0*) Kluwer Academic.

Cardiac Colloquy: The First Comprehensive Video Textbook of Cardiac Surgery Technique. Ed. by Ann S. Adams & Arthur J. Roberts. 1988. (Illus.). 205p. 595.00 (*0-944903-00-2*) Adams Pub Group.

Cardiac Conduction System in Unexplained Sudden Death. Saroja Bharati & Maurice Lev. 1990. (Illus.). 416p. 115.00 (*0-87993-362-3*) Futura Pub.

Cardiac Contraction & the Pressure-Volume Relationship. Kiichi Sagawa et al. 1988. (Illus.). 496p. (C). text 75.00 (*0-19-504320-0*) OUP.

Cardiac Cuisine: A Guide to Healthy Eating. Gail Underbakke. 1988. LC 88-6087. 114p. (Orig.). pap. 9.95 (*0-299-97064-7*) U of Wis Pr.

Cardiac Diagnostic Tests: A Guide for Nurses. Sharon VanRipper & John VanRipper. Ed. by Barbara Nelson-Cullen. 1996. LC 96-18816. (Illus.). 365p. pap. text 35.00 (*0-7216-2493-6*) Saunders.

Cardiac Disease in the Dog & Cat: A Diagnostic Handbook. American Animal Hospital Association Staff. 1986. 220p. 17.95 (*0-9616498-0-1*) Am Animal Hosp Assoc.

***Cardiac Disease in the Elderly: Interventions, Ethics, Economics.** Ed. by M. Preiss et al. 2001. 140p. pap. (*3-7985-1286-8*) D Steinkopff DEU. *Dist:* Spr-Verlag.

Cardiac Disorders. Mosby, C. V., Company Staff. 1999. LC 98-40594. (Managing Major Diseases Ser.). (*0-323-00741-4*) Mosby Inc.

Cardiac Doppler Diagnosis. Ed. by Merrill P. Spenser. 1983. (Developments in Cardiovascular Medicine Ser.). lib. bdg. 175.00 (*0-89838-591-1*) Kluwer Academic.

Cardiac Doppler Diagnosis, Vol. II. Ed. by Merrill P. Spencer. 1986. lib. bdg. 173.50 (*0-89838-767-1*) Kluwer Academic.

Cardiac Drug Therapy. Khan. 4th ed. 1995. pap. text 43.00 (*0-7020-1996-8*) Saunders.

Cardiac Drug Therapy. Gabriel M. Khan. 5th ed. 1999. 446p. (*0-7020-2479-1*) W B Saunders.

Cardiac Dynamics: A Selection of Papers Presented at the Third International Conference on Cardiovascular System Dynamics Held at the University of Leiden, the Netherlands, August 1978. Ed. by Jan Baan et al. 1980. (Developments in Cardiovascular Medicine Ser.: No. 2). 545p. text 239.50 (*90-247-2212-8*) Kluwer Academic.

Cardiac Dysfunction in Chronic Uremia. Ed. by Patrick S. Parfrey & John D. Harnett. 1991. (Topics in Renal Medicine Ser.). (C). text 237.00 (*0-7923-1351-8*) Kluwer Academic.

Cardiac Electrophysiology: From Cell to Bedside. Ed. by Douglas P. Zipes & Jose Jalife. 2nd ed. 1994. LC 94-2557. (Illus.). 1612p. text 255.00 (*0-7216-4941-6*) Saunders.

Cardiac Electrophysiology: From Cell to Bedside. Douglas P. Zipes & Jose Jalife. Ed. by Richard Zorab. 3rd ed. 1999. LC 98-31649. (Illus.). xxiii, 1111p. (C). text 230.00 (*0-7216-7811-4*) Saunders.

Cardiac Electrophysiology, Circulation & Transport. Ed. by Samuel Sideman et al. 1991. (Developments in Cardiovascular Medicine Ser.). (C). text 179.50 (*0-7923-1145-0*) Kluwer Academic.

Cardiac Emergencies. Alan Mackintosh & Nolan. 1998. 208p. pap. (*0-7506-3833-8*) E A GBR. *Dist:* OUP.

Cardiac Emergencies. Melvin M. Scheinman. 2nd ed. 1984. (Illus.). 416p. text 75.00 (*0-7216-7958-7*) Saunders.

Cardiac Energetics: From Emax to Pressure-Volume Area. Ed. by Martin M. Lewinter et al. 1995. LC 95-25025. (Developments in Cardiovascular Medicine Ser.: Vol. 177). 256p. (C). text 141.50 (*0-7923-3721-2*) Kluwer Academic.

Cardiac Gap Junctions: Physiology, Regulation, Pathophysiology & Pharmacology. Stefan Dhein. 1998. LC 97-48990. (Illus.). xii, 148p. 112.25 (*3-8055-6567-4*) S Karger.

Cardiac Glycosides, Pt. 1: Experimental Pharmacology of Cardiac Glycosides. Ed. by K. Creeff. 1981. (Handbook of Experimental Pharmacology Ser.: Vol. 56-1). (Illus.). 682p. 287.00 (*0-387-10917-X*) Spr-Verlag.

Cardiac Growth & Regeneration. Ed. by William C. Claycomb & Paolo Di Nardo. 1995. LC 95-2609. (Annals of the New York Academy of Sciences Ser.: No. 752). 135.00 (*0-89766-929-0*) NY Acad Sci.

Cardiac Health - Rehab & Graded Exercise Testing. Jody C. Heggestad. 1999. 444p. per. 150.00 (*1-879575-02-7*) Acad Med Sys.

Cardiac Imaging: An Atlas & Teaching File. Pamela Woodard. 2001. (Illus.). 304p. 99.00 (*0-86577-867-1*) Thieme Med Pubs.

Cardiac Imaging: Case Review. Steiner. 2000. pap. text (*0-323-01176-4*) Mosby Inc.

Cardiac Intensive Care. David L. Brown. 1998. LC 96-28909. (Illus.). 860p. 125.00 (*0-7216-6006-1*) Saunders.

Cardiac Involvement in Systemic Diseases. J. David Talley. 1996. LC 96-45182. (Topics in Clinical Cardiology Ser.). (Illus.). 192p. 59.95 (*0-89640-317-3*) Igaku-Shoin.

Cardiac Ion Channels. Ed. by A. E. Busch. 1999. (Cellular Physiology & Biochemistry Ser.: Vol. 9, No. 4-5, 1999). (Illus.). 112p. pap. 34.00 (*3-8055-7012-0*) S Karger.

Cardiac Ischemia: From Injury to Protection. Bohuslav Ostadal & Frantisek Kolar. 1999. LC 99-40853. (*0-7923-8642-6*) Kluwer Academic.

Cardiac Left Ventricular Hypertrophy. Ed. by H. E. Ter Keurs & J. J. Schipperheyn. 1983. text 162.50 (*0-89838-612-8*) Kluwer Academic.

Cardiac Lymph Circulation & Cardiac Disorders. Ed. by F. Solti & H. Jellinek. 1989. (Illus.). 177p. (*963-05-4863-1*) Akade Kiado HUN. *Dist:* St Mut.

Cardiac Mapping. Ed. by Mohammad Shenasa et al. 2nd ed. 2002. (Illus.). (*0-87993-404-2*, Futura Media) Futura Pub.

Cardiac Markers. Alan H.B. Wu. 1998. LC 97-37500. (Pathology & Laboratory Medicine Ser.: Vol. 3). (Illus.). 312p. 135.00 (*0-89603-434-8*) Humana.

Cardiac Mechanical Assistance Beyond Balloon Pumping. Ed. by Susan J. Quaal. 1992. LC 92-25096. (Illus.). 395p. (C). (gr. 13). pap. text 43.95 (*0-8016-6442-X*, 06442) Mosby Inc.

Cardiac Mechanics & Function in the Normal & Diseased Heart. Ed. by Motoo Hori et al. 1990. (Illus.). 368p. 189.00 (*0-387-70043-9*, 2857) Spr-Verlag.

Cardiac Metabolism in Health & Disease. Ed. by Salah Abdel-Aleem & James E. Lowe. 1998. LC 97-42768. (Developments in Molecular & Cellular Biochemistry Ser.). 202p. 225.00 (*0-7923-8104-1*) Kluwer Academic.

Cardiac Monitoring in a Complex Patient Care Environment. Association for the Advancement of Medical Instruments Staff & Alan S. Berson. 1982. 89p. (Orig.). pap. text 30.00 (*0-910275-09-2*, TAR3-209) Assn Adv Med Instrn.

Cardiac Monitors, Heart Rate Meters & Alarms. 2nd ed. 1992. 44p. pap. 90.00 (*0-910275-03-3*, EC13-209) Assn Adv Med Instrn.

Cardiac Myocyte - Connective Tissue Interactions in Health & Disease. Ed. by T. F. Robinson & R. K. Kinnel. 1990. (Issues in Biomedicine Ser.: Vol. 13). (Illus.). x, 150p. 128.75 (*3-8055-5028-6*) S Karger.

Cardiac Nuclear Medicine. Ed. by Myron C. Gerson. 2nd ed. 1992. 608p. text 97.00 (*0-07-023443-4*) McGraw-Hill Educ Grp.

Cardiac Nuclear Medicine. Ed. by Myron C. Gerson. 3rd ed. 1996. LC 96-46198. (Illus.). 830p. text 155.00 (*0-07-032848-X*) McGraw-Hill Prof.

Cardiac Output: Biophysical Measurements. T. Andrew Bowdle et al. 1990. 65p. (C). 28.00 (*0-9627449-2-1*) SpaceLabs.

Cardiac Output & Regional Flow in Health & Disease. Ed. by Abdul-Majeed Salmasi & Abdulmassih S. Iskandrian. 1993. LC 92-49733. (Developments in Cardiovascular Medicine Ser.: Vol. 138). text 339.00 (*0-7923-1911-7*) Kluwer Academic.

Cardiac Pacemakers & Implantable Defibrillators Vol. 3: A Workbook in 3 Volumes: Transtelephonic, Electrocardiography, & Troubleshooting: A Case Approach Janet R. Christiansen. Ed. by David L. Hayes et al. 1997. (Illus.). 98p. wbk. ed. 25.00 (*0-87993-697-5*) Futura Pub.

Cardiac Pacemakers & Implantable Defibrillators Vol. 4: A Multi-Volume Workbook: ICDs & Pacemakers. Ed. by David L. Hayes & Paul J. Wang. 2000. (Illus.). 120p. pap., wbk. ed. 29.00 (*0-87993-451-4*) Futura Pub.

Cardiac Pacemakers & Implantable Defibrillators - A Workbook in 3 Volumes Vol. 1: Cardiac Pacing: A Case Approach David L. Hayes et al. Ed. by David L. Hayes & Paul J. Wang. 1997. (Illus.). 102p. pap. 25.00 (*0-87993-695-9*) Futura Pub.

Cardiac Pacemakers & Implantable Defibrillators - A Workbook in 3 Volumes Vol. 2: Implantable Defibrillators: A Case Approach Paul J. Wang et al. Ed. by Paul J. Wang & David L. Hayes. 1997. (Illus.). 72p. pap. 25.00 (*0-87993-696-7*) Futura Pub.

Cardiac Pacing. Cooper. 1988. 188p. (gr. 13). text 26.95 (*0-944132-17-0*) Mosby Inc.

Cardiac Pacing. Fred M. Kusumoto & Nora F. Goldschlager. 2000. LC 00-63997. 512p. text 99.00 (*0-683-30704-5*) Lppncott W & W.

Cardiac Pacing. Charles J. Love. 1998. LC 98-26333. (Vademecum Ser.). (Illus.). 145p. spiral bd. 45.00 (*1-57059-492-9*) Landes Bioscience.

Cardiac Pacing. Kenneth A. Ellenbogen. 2nd ed. 1996. LC 96-19016. (Practical Cardiac Diagnosis Ser.). (Illus.). 480p. pap. text 52.95 (*0-86542-471-3*) Blackwell Sci.

***Cardiac Pacing.** Kenneth A. Ellenbogen. 3rd ed. 2001. LC 2001-1216. (Illus.). xi, 530p. pap. 49.95 (*0-86542-586-8*) Blackwell Sci.

Cardiac Pacing: Electrophysiology & Pacemaker Technology. G. A. Feruglio. 1983. 1146p. text (*1-57235-047-4*) Piccin Nuova.

Cardiac Pacing: New Advances. Rosenqvist. 1998. text (*0-7020-2215-2*) Bailliere Tindall.

Cardiac Pacing & Defibrillation: A Clinical Approach. David L. Hayes et al. 2000. LC 00-34098. (Illus.). vii, 600p. 89.00 (*0-87993-462-X*) Futura Pub.

Cardiac Pacing & Electrophysiology: A Bridge to the 21st Century. Ed. by A. E. Aubert et al. 1994. LC 93-38818. text 148.50 (*0-7923-2627-X*) Kluwer Academic.

Cardiac Pacing in Clinical Practice. Wilhelm Fischer & P. Ritter. Tr. by Rodolphe Ruffy from ENG. 1998. LC 98-12136. (*0-387-63595-5*); 2nd ed. (Illus.). 480p. 68.00 (*3-540-63595-5*) Spr-Verlag.

Cardiac Pearls. W. Proctor Harvey. 1993. 345p. 74.00 (*1-886128-03-0*) Laennec Pub.

Cardiac Positron Emission Tomography. Ed. by Markus Schwaiger. 1996. LC 95-4109. (Developments in Cardiovascular Medicine Ser.: Vol. 165). 416p. (C). text 302.50 (*0-7923-3417-5*) Kluwer Academic.

Cardiac Positron Emission Tomography: Viability, Perfusion, Receptors & Cardiomyopathy. Ernst E. Van der Wall et al. 1995. LC 95-14245. (Developments in Cardiovascular Medicine Ser.: Vol. 166). 276p. text 125.00 (*0-7923-3472-8*) Kluwer Academic.

Cardiac Preexcitation Syndromes. Ed. by David G. Benditt & D. Woodrow Benson. 1986. text 242.00 (*0-89838-771-X*) Kluwer Academic.

Cardiac Problems in Pregnancy: Diagnosis & Management of Maternal & Fetal Disease. Uri Elkayam & Norbert Gleicher. 3rd ed. 1998. LC 97-18625. 773p. 279.00 (*0-471-16358-9*) Wiley.

Cardiac Puzzles. J. Willis Hurst. 1995. LC 95-32144. (C). 36.00 (*0-7234-2469-1*) Mosby Inc.

Cardiac Radiology - The Requisites. Stephen W. Miller. 1996. (Illus.). 466p. (C). (gr. 13). text 85.00 (*0-8016-6478-0*, 06478) Mosby Inc.

Cardiac Rate & Rhythm. L. N. Bouman & H. J. Jongsma. 1982. text 268.50 (*90-247-2626-3*) Kluwer Academic.

Cardiac Reconstructions with Allograft Valves. Ed. by R. A. Hopkins. 1989. (Illus.). 194p. 152.00 (*0-387-96855-5*) Spr-Verlag.

Cardiac Rehabilitation. 1997. lib. bdg. 250.95 (*0-8490-8156-4*) Gordon Pr.

Cardiac Rehabilitation. Ed. by Dee Jones & Robert West. 1995. 264p. (Orig.). pap. text (*0-7279-0852-9*) BMJ Pub GBR. *Dist:* AIDC.

Cardiac Rehabilitation. Michael A. Lojek & Patricia Bement. Ed. by Oliver D. Grin & Dorothy L. Bouwman. 1992. (Patient Education Ser.). (Illus.). 26p. (Orig.). pap. text 4.00 (*0-929689-48-8*) Ludann Co.

Cardiac Rehabilitation: A Guide for Patients. Robert De Busk. Ed. by Elliott Rapaport. 1996. (Cardiology Ser.). (Illus.). 32p. (Orig.). pap. 2.95 (*1-885274-39-4*) Health InfoNet Inc.

Cardiac Rehabilitation: A Guide to Practice in the 21st Century. Nanette K. Wenger. 1999. LC 99-29625. (Fundamental & Clinical Cardiology Ser.). (Illus.). 630p. text 185.00 (*0-8247-6092-1*) Dekker.

Cardiac Rehabilitation: Proceedings of the International Congress, 1st, Hamburg, Sept., 1977. International Congress on Cardiac Rehabilitation Staff. Ed. by H. Denolin & K. G. Koenig. 1978. (Advances in Cardiology Ser.: Vol. 24). (Illus.). 85.25 (*3-8055-2827-2*) S Karger.

Cardiac Rehabilitation: Proceedings of the International Congress on Cardiac Rehabilitation, 1st, Hamburg, Sept. 12-14, 1977. International Congress on Cardiac Rehabilitation Staff. Ed. by K. G. Koenig. 1977. (Journal: Vol. 62, No. 2). 26.25 (*3-8055-2774-8*) S Karger.

Cardiac Rehabilitation, Adult Fitness, & Exercise Testing. Paul S. Fardy & Frank G. Yanowitz. 3rd ed. 1996. LC 94-37793. (Illus.). 520p. 49.95 (*0-683-03031-0*) Lppncott W & W.

Cardiac Rehabilitation & Graded Exercise Testing. Jody C. Heggestad. rev. ed. 1995. 252p. stu. ed. 60.00 (*1-879575-04-3*) Acad Med Sys.

Cardiac Rhythms: A Systematic Approach to Interpretation. Raymond E. Phillips & Mary K. Feeney. 3rd ed. 1990. (Illus.). 608p. pap. text 42.00 (*0-7216-2427-8*) Saunders.

Cardiac Risk Assessment Before Vascular Surgery. Ed. by Andris Kazmers. 1994. LC 93-43088. (Illus.). 364p. 52.00 (*0-87993-578-2*) Futura Pub.

Cardiac Sarcoplasmic Reticulum Function & Regulation of Contractility. Ed. by Robert G. Johnson & Evangelia G. Kranias. 1998. LC 98-23010. (Annals of the New York Academy of Sciences Ser.). 395p. pap. 140.00 (*1-57331-130-8*); 140.00 (*1-57331-129-4*) NY Acad Sci.

Cardiac Spect Imaging. E. Gordon DePuey et al. 2nd ed. 2000. LC 00-60557. 368p. text 169.00 (*0-7817-2007-9*) Lppncott W & W.

Cardiac Stress Testing & Imaging: A Clinician's Guide. Ed. by Thomas H. Marwick. 1996. LC 96-24943. 638p. text (*0-443-07652-9*) Church.

Cardiac Surgery. Patricia C. Seifert. 1994. LC 93-42494. (Perioperative Nursing Ser.). (Illus.). 512p. (C). (gr. 13). text 54.95 (*0-8016-6542-6*, 06542) Mosby Inc.

Cardiac Surgery John W. Kirklin & Brian G. Barratt-Boyes. 2nd ed. 1992. (Illus.). 1976p. (C). text (*0-443-08845-4*) Church.

Cardiac Surgery. Kouchoukos. 3rd ed. 1998. (C). text (*0-443-07526-3*) Church.

Cardiac Surgery: Biological & Psychological Implications. Herman C. Denber. 1994. LC 94-29707. 272p. 35.00 (*0-87993-599-5*) Futura Pub.

Cardiac Surgery: Current Issues, Vol. 2. A. C. Cernaianu & A. J. DelRossi. 1994. (Illus.). 262p. (C). text 95.00 (*0-306-44671-5*, Kluwer Plenum) Kluwer Academic.

Cardiac Surgery: Operative Technique. Donald B. Doty. 1996. LC 96-2567. (Illus.). 448p. (C). (gr. 13). text 195.00 (*0-8151-2761-8*, 24295) Mosby Inc.

Cardiac Surgery: Proceedings of the Fifth Annual Meeting Held in St. Thomas, Virgin Islands, November 18-20, 1993. Ed. by Aurel C. Cernaianu & Anthony J. DelRossi. 1995. (Current Issues in Autism Ser.: Vol. 3). 206p. 79.50 (*0-306-45015-1*, Kluwer Plenum) Kluwer Academic.

Cardiac Surgery: Safeguards & Pitfalls in Operative Technique. Siavosh Khonsari. 2nd ed. 1996. LC 96-2753. 352p. text 229.00 (*0-397-51626-6*) Lppncott W & W.

Cardiac Surgery Vol. 1: Current Issues, Vol. 1. A. C. Cernaianu & A. J. DelRossi. 1992. (Illus.). 222p. (C). text 95.00 (*0-306-44319-8*, Kluwer Plenum) Kluwer Academic.

Cardiac Surgery & Concomitant Disease. Ed. by J. Ennker. 1999. (Illus.). 337p. 69.00 (*3-7985-1130-6*) Spr-Verlag.

Cardiac Surgery & Current Issues Vol. 4: Proceedings of the Seventh Annual Symposium Held in St. Thomas, Virgin Islands, November 9-12, 1994, Vol. 4. Ed. by Aurel C. Cernaianu & Anthony J. DelRossi. 1996. (Illus.). 225p. 79.50 (*0-306-45188-3*, Kluwer Plenum) Kluwer Academic.

Cardiac Surgery & the Brain. Ed. by Peter L. Smith & K. M. Taylor. 1993. (Illus.). 296p. (*0-340-55315-4*) E A GBR. *Dist:* OUP.

Cardiac Surgery & the Conduction System. Saroja Bharati et al. 2nd rev. ed. 1991. (Illus.). 176p. 75.00 (*0-87993-522-7*) Futura Pub.

Cardiac Surgery in the Adult. Ed. by Louis H. Edmunds, Jr. 1997. LC 96-37119. (Illus.). 1632p. text 225.00 (*0-07-018963-5*) McGraw-Hill Prof.

Cardiac Surgery of the Neonate & Infant. Aldo R. Castaneda et al. 1994. LC 93-22880. (Illus.). 528p. text 205.00 (*0-7216-4301-9*) Saunders.

Cardiac Surgery Secrets. Ed. by Paulo R. Soltoski et al. 2000. LC 99-88126. (Secrets Ser.). (Illus.). 350p. pap. 39.95 (*1-56053-361-7*) Hanley & Belfus.

Cardiac Therapy. Ed. by Michael R. Rosen & Brian F. Hoffman. 1983. text 290.50 (*0-89838-564-4*) Kluwer Academic.

Cardiac, Thoracic & Vascular Anesthesia. J. A. Youngberg. 1998. LC 98-20111. 1360p. (*0-443-08920-5*) Church.

Cardiac Toxicology. Tibor Balazs. 1981. Vol. I. 240p. 134.00 (*0-8493-5555-9*, RC682); Vol. II. 240p. 138.00 (*0-8493-5556-7*, RC682); Vol. III. 232p. 133.00 (*0-8493-5558-3*, RC682) Franklin (CRC Reprint).

Cardiac Transplantation. Kirklin. 1999. (C). text (*0-443-07655-3*) Church.

Cardiac Transplantation: A Manual for Health Care Professionals. Ed. by Jeffrey D. Hosenpud et al. 1990. (Illus.). 265p. 83.00 (*0-387-97304-4*) Spr-Verlag.

Cardiac Ultrasound. Ed. by John P. Panidis. 1995. LC 95-40944. (Practical Cardiac Diagnosis Ser.). (Illus.). 354p. pap. 59.95 (*0-86542-275-3*) Blackwell Sci.

Cardiac Value Replacement: Current Status. Ed. by Jack M. Matloff. 1985. text 160.50 (*0-89838-722-1*) Kluwer Academic.

Cardiac Valve Allografts 1962-1987. Ed. by A. C. Yankah et al. 1988. 400p. 116.00 (*0-387-91313-0*) Spr-Verlag.

Cardiac Valve Allografts II: Science & Practice. Ed. by A. C. Yankah & M. H. Yacoub. 1998. 385p. 99.00 (*3-7985-1064-4*) Spr-Verlag.

Cardiac Valve Disease in Children. J. Dunn. 1987. (Illus.). 370p. (C). (gr. 13). pap. 105.95 (*0-412-04471-4*) Chapman & Hall.

Cardiac-Vascular Remodeling & Functional Interaction, Vol. XII. Y. Maruyama et al. 1997. (Illus.). 416p. 207.00 (*4-431-70188-5*) Spr-Verlag.

Cardio Assessement for Physical Therapy. Loveridge. 1998. text (*0-7216-3276-9*) Saunders.

***Cardio Cures: Alternative Strategies for a Healthy Heart.** Gary Bushkin & Estitta Bushkin. 2001. LC 2001-38352. 288p. pap. 16.95 (*0-658-01531-1*) McGraw-Hill Prof.

Cardio-Pulmonary Technician. Jack Rudman. 1994. (Career Examination Ser.: C-1159). pap. 39.95 (*0-8373-1159-4*) Nat Learn.

***Cardioangioscopy.** Yasumi Uchida. 2001. (Illus.). (*0-87993-487-5*) Futura Pub.

Cardiocirculatory Function in Renal Disease. Shaul G. Massry & Eberhard Ritz. 1985. (Contributions to Nephrology Ser.: Vol. 41). (Illus.). xii, 460p. 29.75 (*3-8055-3914-2*) S Karger.

CardioFax. Dennis A. Tighe et al. 2000. LC 00-31250. (ClinicoFax Ser.). (Illus.). xii, 239p. 29.95 (*0-86542-563-9*) Blackwell Sci.

Cardiogenic Embolism. Ed. by Werner G. Daniel et al. 1996. LC 95-12357. (Illus.). 320p. 75.00 (*0-683-02359-4*) Lppncott W & W.

***Cardiogenic Shock: Diagnosis & Treatment.** Ed. by David Hasdai et al. 2002. LC 2001-39902. 400p. 135.00 (*1-58829-025-5*) Humana.

Cardiograms: Theory & Applications. Ed. by Dhanjoo N. Ghista et al. 1979. (Advances in Cardiovascular Physics Ser.: Vol. 2). (Illus.). 85.25 (*3-8055-2851-5*) S Karger.

Cardiolipin Antigens. M. Pangborn & J. Almeida. 1951. (WHO Monograph Ser.: No. 6). 63p. 5.00 (*92-4-140006-4*) World Health.

Cardiological Dilemmas. R. A. Blackwood & B. N. J. Daily. 1995. viii,87p. (*0-906584-40-X*) Beaconsfield GBR. *Dist:* Medicina Bio.

Cardiologist's Managed Care Manual. Ed. by David B. Nash. 1997. (Illus.). 250p. (Orig.). spiral bd. 54.95 (*1-890045-03-9*) T L C Med Pub.

Cardiologist's Painless Prescription for a Healthy Heart & a Longer Life. Joe D. Goldstrich. 1994. LC 93-92831. 416p. 19.95 (*0-9639877-0-4*) Nine-Heart-Nine.

Cardiology. Michael H. Crawford & John P. DiMarco. 2000. (Illus.). 1795p. 139.00 (*0-7234-3138-8*) Mosby Inc.

Cardiology. Sergio Dalla Volta et al. 1999. (Clinical Medicine Ser.). (Illus.). 891p. pap. text 79.95 (*0-07-709518-9*) McGraw-Hill Med Pub.

Cardiology. 2nd ed. 1984. (Medical Ser.). (Illus.). 72p. (C). pap. text 12.95 (*0-935920-22-6*, Ntl Pubs Blck) P-H.

Cardiology. Martin D. Lowe et al. 2nd ed. 1998. LC 97-22076. (Colour Guide Ser.). (C). pap. text 16.95 (*0-443-05912-8*) Harcrt Hlth Sci Grp.

Cardiology. Joel W. Heger et al. 3rd ed. 1992. LC 92-48965. (House Officer Ser.). 416p. pap. 21.95 (*0-683-03949-0*) Lppncott W & W.

Cardiology. Ed. by Cindy Jennings. 3rd ed. 1997. LC 92-48257. (Regents - Prentice-Hall Medical Assistant Kit Ser.). 112p. pap. 12.40 (*0-13-146598-8*) P-H.

Cardiology. Joel W. Heger et al. 4th ed. 1998. LC 97-51976. (House Officer Ser.). 450p. 29.95 (*0-683-30204-3*) Lppncott W & W.

Cardiology. Desmond G. Julian et al. 7th ed. 1998. (C). pap. text 36.00 (*0-7020-2211-X*) Saunders.

Cardiology: An Essential Slide Collection. Adam D. Timmis. 2nd ed. 148p. incl. sl. (*0-397-46497-5*, GM0091) Gower-Mosby.

Cardiology: Crash Course. Anjana Siva & Mark Noble. 2000. 227p. text (*0-7234-3152-3*) Mosby Inc.

Cardiology: Evolution of Ideas. Richard J. Bing. 1992. LC 92-1542. 319p. text 74.00 (*3-7186-0549-X*) Gordon & Breach.

Cardiology: Peterborough Symposium. Ed. by F. J. Fawcett. 1975. 19.95 (*0-8464-1081-8*) Beekman Pubs.

Cardiology: The Evolution of the Science & the Art. Ed. by Richard J. Bing. 2nd ed. 1999. LC 98-44410. (Illus.). 368p. (C). text 55.00 (*0-8135-2627-2*); pap. text 24.00 (*0-8135-2628-0*) Rutgers U Pr.

Cardiology & Co-Existing Disease. Ed. by Elliott Rapaport. 1993. (Illus.). 352p. text (*0-443-08887-X*) Church.

Cardiology Board Certification Review Guide - Interventional Cardiology. Ed. by Jeffrey J. Popma & Ross Prpic. 1999. LC 99-64879. (Illus.). 350p. ring bd. 195.00 (*1-58397-005-3*, CBCRG) Am Coll Cardiology.

Cardiology Color Guide. John J. Hunter et al. 2nd ed. 1999. LC 98-46713. (Illus.). (C). pap. text (*0-443-06113-0*) Church.

Cardiology Explained. William Drake et al. 1996. LC 97-131372. 218p. pap. 24.95 (*0-412-73680-2*) Chapman & Hall.

***Cardiology for the MRCP.** de Belder & Chin. 2002. (Illus.). 208p. pap. (*1-84110-010-2*) Greenwich Med GBR. *Dist:* JAMCO Dist.

Cardiology for the Primary Care. George W. Vetrovec. 1999. text (*0-7216-6519-5*) Saunders.

Cardiology for the Primary Care Physician. Ed. by Joseph S. Alpert. 1996. (Illus.). 384p. text 95.00 (*1-57340-024-6*) Current Med.

Cardiology for the Primary Care Physician. Joseph S. Alpert. 2nd ed. 1997. LC 97-41983. (*1-57340-115-3*) Current Med.

***Cardiology Futures.** Poole-Wilson & Marinker. 2001. 120p. pap. (*0-7279-1588-6*) BMJ Pub GBR. *Dist:* AIDC.

Cardiology Handbook. Diana Holdright et al. 1998. (Illus.). 96p. pap. 19.95 (*1-873413-71-8*, 8289) Merit Pub Intl.

Cardiology Handbook for Health Professionals. M. Wayne Cooper. 1988. (Illus.). 186p. pap. 22.50 (*0-87527-366-1*) Green.

Cardiology in AIDS. Steven E. Lipshultz. 1998. LC 97-42609. (Current Topics in Cardiology Ser.). (Illus.). 256p. (*0-412-08861-4*) E A GBR. *Dist:* OUP.

***Cardiology in Critical Illness.** Helen F. Galley. 6th ed. 2001. (Critical Care Focus Ser.: No. 6). (Illus.). 60p. pap. (*0-7279-1543-6*) BMJ Pub GBR. *Dist:* AIDC.

Cardiology in Primary Care. Ed. by William Branch et al. 2000. LC 00-699799. (Illus.). 940p. text 79.95 (*0-07-007162-4*) McGraw-Hill Prof.

Cardiology in Transition. John O. Goodman & Conrad Vernon. 1989. 175p. 9.95 (*0-9625207-0-5*) J Goodman & Assocs.

Cardiology Medical Transcription. S. Turley. 1993. 176p. (C). ring bd. (*0-933195-59-1*) CA College Health Sci.

Cardiology, 1998. James T. Willerson. Ed. by William C. Roberts et al. 1998. (Illus.). 611p. 98.00 (*0-87993-405-0*) Futura Pub.

Cardiology 1994. William C. Roberts. 1994. 504p. text 115.00 (*0-7506-9591-9*) Buttrwrth-Heinemann.

Cardiology of the Horse. Ed. by Celia Marr. 1997. (Illus.). 260p. (*0-7020-2240-3*) W B Saunders GBR. *Dist:* Saunders.

Cardiology Pearls. Blase A. Carabello. 1993. 223p. pap. (*84-8086-143-6*) Mosby-Doyma Libros ESP. *Dist:* Mosby Inc.

Cardiology Pearls. Ed. by Blase Carabello. 2nd ed. 2001. LC 00-23117. (Illus.). 250p. pap. 45.00 (*1-56053-403-6*) Hanley & Belfus.

Cardiology Pearls of Wisdom: Over 3000 Questions. Michael Zevitz. 1999. (Pearls of Wisdom Ser.). pap. (*1-890369-15-2*) Boston Medical.

Cardiology Pocket Consultant. R. H. Swanton. 4th ed. 1998. LC 97-29781. (Pocket Consultant Ser.). 559p. pap. 62.95 (*0-632-04839-5*) Blackwell Sci.

Cardiology Reviews: Regulation of Myocardial Contractile Function & Metabolism, Vol. 2. Ed. by Eugene I. Chazov. 1989. (Soviet Medical Reviews Ser.: Vol. 2, Pt. A). xii, 388p. pap. text 582.00 (*3-7186-4893-8*, Harwood Acad Pubs) Gordon & Breach.

Cardiology Reviews Vol. 3, Pt. 1: The Role of Endogenous Epinephrine in the Development of Experimental Hypertension, Vol. 3. O. S. Medvedev. 1991. (Soviet Medical Reviews Ser.: Section A). 128p. pap. text 184.00 (*3-7186-5234-X*, Harwood Acad Pubs) Gordon & Breach.

Cardiology Reviews Vol. 3, Pt. 2: Profiles & Pharmacological Aspects of Selected Cardiovascular Drugs, Vol. 3. L. Lukoshkova. 1992. (Soviet Medical Reviews Ser.: Section A). 196p. pap. text 143.00 (*3-7186-5312-5*, Harwood Acad Pubs) Gordon & Breach.

Cardiology Reviews 1: Human Atherosclerosis, Vol. 1. Ed. by Eugene I. Chazov & V. N. Smirnov. 1987. (Soviet Medical Reviews Ser., Section A). xviii, 406p. text 544.00 (*3-7186-0349-7*) Gordon & Breach.

***Cardiology Rotation.** George J. Taylor. 2001. LC 00-68002. (Illus.). 320p. pap. 19.95 (*0-632-04352-0*) Blackwell Sci.

Cardiology Secrets: Questions You Will Be Asked on Rounds, in the Clinic, on Oral Exams. Ed. by Olivia Adair & Edward P. Havranek. 1994. (Secrets Ser.). (Illus.). 275p. (Orig.). pap. 39.95 (*1-56053-104-5*) Hanley & Belfus.

Cardiology Today. Ed. by B. Guggenheim. 1984. (Illus.). xii, 396p. 142.75 (*3-8055-3761-1*) S Karger.

Cardiology 2000: An Internet Resource Guide. Ed. by Dan Goldenson. 2000. 450p. pap. 24.95 (*0-9676811-8-9*) eMedguides.

Cardiology Words & Phrases. 2nd ed. 1995. 575p. pap. text 41.00 (*0-934385-63-7*) Hlth Prof Inst.

Cardiomyopathies. 1984. (Technical Report Ser.: No. 697). 68p. pap. text 7.00 (*92-4-120697-7*) World Health.

Cardiomyopathies. Ed. by J. F. Goodwin & E. G. Olsen. 1993. LC 92-49589. (*3-540-55608-7*); (Illus.). 315p. 132.00 (*0-387-55608-7*) Spr-Verlag.

Cardiopathies Valvulaires Acquises. J. Acar et al. 1985. (FRE., Illus.). 656p. 130.00 (*2-257-10441-2*) S M P F Inc.

Cardioprotective Role of HRT: A Clinical Update. P. Collins & C. Beale. 1996. (Illus.). 60p. (C). lib. bdg. 27.95 (*1-85070-740-5*, C1864, Parthenon Pbng) CRC Pr.

Cardiopulmonary. 1997. LC 99-173212. 200p. pap. 30.00 (*1-887759-12-3*, P-137) Am Phys Therapy Assn.

Cardiopulmonary Anatomy & Physiology. DesJardins. 1988. (Respiratory Care Ser.). tchr. ed. 16.00 (*0-8273-2837-0*) Delmar.

Cardiopulmonary Anatomy & Physiology. Terry R. Desjardins. 1988. (C). pap. text 12.95 (*0-8273-2840-0*); pap. 29.95 (*0-8273-2836-2*) Delmar.

***Cardiopulmonary Anatomy & Physiology.** George H. Hicks. 2000. (Illus.). pap. 21.95 (*0-7216-9191-9*) Saunders.

Cardiopulmonary Anatomy & Physiology. George H. Hicks. 1999. (Illus.). 315p. pap. text (*0-7216-5199-2*) Saunders.

Cardiopulmonary Anatomy & Physiology. DesJardins. 4th ed. 2001. (C). pap., wbk. ed. 16.75 net. (*0-7668-2535-3*) Delmar.

Cardiopulmonary Anatomy & Physiology. Terry R. Desjardins. 4th ed. 2001. LC 2001-47593. 448p. (C). pap. text 47.95 (*0-7668-2533-7*) Delmar.

Cardiopulmonary Anatomy & Physiology: Essentials for Respiratory Care. DesJardins. 3rd ed. 1998. 240p. pap. text, tchr. ed. 18.00 (*0-8273-8257-X*) Delmar.

Cardiopulmonary Anatomy And Physiology 3E: Essentials of Respiratory Care. Terry R. Des Jardins. 3rd ed. 1997. LC 97-8797. 416p. (C). pap. text 53.95 (*0-8273-8256-1*) Delmar.

Cardiopulmonary Bypass: Current Concepts & Controversies. Tinker. 1989. 160p. text 75.00 (*0-7216-8831-4*) Saunders.

Cardiopulmonary Bypass: Principles & Management. Kenneth M. Taylor. 1987. (Illus.). 440p. 74.00 (*0-683-08105-5*) Lppncott W & W.

Cardiopulmonary Bypass: Principles & Techniques of Extracorporeal Circulation. Ed. by Christina T. Mora et al. 1997. LC 94-29083. (Illus.). 504p. 184.00 (*0-387-94242-4*) Spr-Verlag.

Cardiopulmonary Bypass Bibliography. Howard D. Johnson & Marc S. Morgan. Ed. by Joe R. Utley et al. 1990. LC 89-80769. (Cardiothoracic Surgery Monographs). 610p. text 50.00 (*0-9623617-8-X*) Cardiothoracic Rsch.

***Cardiopulmonary Critical Care.** Ed. by T. Higgins et al. 2001. (Critical Care Ser.). 304p. pap. (*1-85996-237-8*) Bios Sci GBR. *Dist:* Spr-Verlag.

Cardiopulmonary Critical Care. David R. Dantzer & Steven M. Scharf. Ed. by Judy Fletcher. 3rd ed. 1997. LC 96-36901. (Illus.). 800p. text 125.00 (*0-7216-6543-8*) Saunders.

Cardiopulmonary Interactions in Acute Respiratory Failure. J. L. Vincent & P. M. Suter. 1987. (Update in Intensive Care & Emergency Medicine Ser.: Vol. 2). (Illus.). 265p. 79.95 (*0-387-17474-5*) Spr-Verlag.

Cardiopulmonary Pharmacology Handbook: A Handbook for Cardiopulmonary Practitioners & Other Allied Health Personnel. Cynthia L. Howder. 2nd ed. 1996. LC 96-686. (Illus.). 632p. pap. text 32.00 (*0-683-16313-2*) Lppncott W & W.

Cardiopulmonary Physical Therapy. Scot Irwin. 3rd ed. 1995. text, stu. ed. (*0-8151-4887-9*) Mosby Inc.

Cardiopulmonary Physical Therapy. Scot Irwin & Jan S. Tecklin. 3rd ed. 1995. (Illus.). 640p. (C). (gr. 13). stu. ed. (*0-8016-7926-5*, 07926) Mosby Inc.

Cardiopulmonary Physical Therapy: A Clinical Manual. Joanne Watchie. 1995. 368p. pap. text 30.00 (*0-7216-6709-0*) Saunders.

Cardiopulmonary Physiology in Anesthesiology. Michael G. Levitzky et al. 1996. LC 94-2822. (Illus.). 322p. text 49.00 (*0-07-037534-8*) McGraw-Hill Prof.

Cardiopulmonary Physiology in Critical Care. Ed. by Steven M. Scharf. 1992. (Fundamental & Clinical Cardiology Ser.: Vol. 7). (Illus.). 464p. text 135.00 (*0-8247-8649-1*) Dekker.

Cardiopulmonary Rehabilitation. Ed. by Ciro Rampulla et al. 1995. LC 93-13742. (Current Topics in Rehabilitation Ser.). 69.00 (*0-387-19836-9*) Spr-Verlag.

Cardiopulmonary Rehabilitation: Basic Theory & Application. Frances J. Brannon et al. 3rd ed. 1997. LC 97-24298. (Contemporary Perspectives in Rehabilitation Ser.). (Illus.). 486p. 55.95 (*0-8036-0318-5*) Davis Co.

Cardiopulmonary Resuscitation. David V. Skinner & Richard I. Vincent. 2nd ed. 1996. (Oxford Handbooks in Emergency Medicine Ser.: No. 16). (Illus.). 232p. pap. text 49.50 (*0-19-262693-0*) OUP.

Cardiopulmonary System. D. Richardson et al. 1997. (Integrated Medical Sciences Ser.). (C). pap. 29.95 (*1-889325-30-9*) Blackwell Sci.

Cardiorenal Disease. Ed. by M. Timio & V. Wizemann. 1994. LC 93-38201. (Contributions to Nephrology Ser.: Vol. 106). (Illus.). x, 206p. 49.75 (*3-8055-5830-9*) S Karger.

Cardiorespiratory & Cardiosomatic Psychophysiology. Ed. by P. Grossman et al. 1986. LC 86-21252. (NATO ASI Series A, Life Sciences: Vol. 114). 376p. 95.00 (*0-306-42395-2*, Plenum Trade) Perseus Pubng.

Cardiorespiratory & Motor Coordination. Ed. by H. P. Koepchen & T. Huopaniemi. 1991. (Illus.). 352p. 135.00 (*0-387-52279-4*) Spr-Verlag.

Cardiorespiratory Disease. Alex Habel & Rod Scott. 1998. LC 98-23207. (Illus.). 160p. pap. (*0-7506-2444-2*) E A GBR. *Dist:* OUP.

Cardiorespiratory Diseases of the Dog & Cat. Mike Martin & Brendan Corcoran. 1996. LC 96-15365. (Library of Veterinary Practice). (Illus.). 416p. (Orig.). (C). pap. text (*0-632-03298-7*) Blckwell Science GBR. *Dist:* Iowa U Pr.

Cardiorespiratory Nursing. Ed. by Caroline Shuldham. 1998. (Illus.). 596p. pap. (*0-7487-3301-9*) Nelson Thornes GBR. *Dist:* Intl Spec Bk, Trans-Atl Phila.

Cardiothoracic Interrelationships in Clinical Practice. Ed. by Anthony M. Cosentino & Richard J. Martin. 1997. LC 96-38646. (Illus.). 232p. 47.00 (*0-87993-655-X*) Futura Pub.

Cardiothoracic Surgery. Fritz J. Baumgartner. 2nd ed. 1999. LC 99-31800. (Vademecum Ser.). spiral bd. 45.00 (*1-57059-559-3*) Landes Bioscience.

Cardiothoracic Trauma. P. Symbas. 1989. 448p. text 145.00 (*0-7216-2827-3*) Saunders.

Cardiovascular Actions of Anesthetics & Drugs Used in Anesthesia, Set: Vols. 1 & 2. Ed. by B. M. Altura & S. Halevy. 1987. (Illus.). xx, 570p. 352.75 (*3-8055-4159-7*) S Karger.

Cardiovascular Actions of Anesthetics & Drugs Used in Anesthesia: Basic Aspects, Vol. 1. Ed. by B. M. Altura & S. Halevy. 1986. (Illus.). viii, 268p. 169.75 (*3-8055-4157-0*) S Karger.

Cardiovascular & Musculoskeletal Systems. Ed. by Thomas C. Jones et al. 1991. (Monographs in Pathology of Laboratory Animals). (Illus.). 312p. 383.00 (*0-387-53876-3*) Spr-Verlag.

Cardiovascular & Renal Actions of Dopamine. Ed. by P. Soares-de-Silva. 1993. (Advances in the Biosciences Ser.: Vol. 88). 270p. 190.25 (*0-08-042209-8*, Pergamon Pr) Elsevier.

Cardiovascular & Respitory Physiotherapy. Mandy Smith & Valerie Ball. 1998. (Illus.). 264p. pap. 29.95 (*0-7234-2595-7*) Mosby Inc.

Cardiovascular & Vascular Disease of the Aorta. Lars G. Svensson & E. Stanley Crawford. Ed. by Lisette Bralow. 1996. 512p. text 149.00 (*0-7216-5426-6*) Saunders.

Cardiovascular Anesthesia. Carol L. Lake. 1984. (Illus.). 467p. 98.00 (*0-387-96028-7*) Spr-Verlag.

Cardiovascular Applications of Doppler Ultrasound. Ed. by Abdul-Majeed Salmasi & Andrew N. Nicolaides. 1989. (Illus.). 388p. text (*0-443-03592-X*) Church.

Cardiovascular Applications of Magnetic Resonance. Ed. by Gerald M. Pohost. 1993. LC 92-48279. (American Heart Association Monograph Ser.). (Illus.). 480p. 86.00 (*0-87993-548-0*) Futura Pub.

Cardiovascular Biology of Purines Geoffrey Burnstock. 1998. LC 98-37372. (Developments in Cardiovascular Medicine Ser.). 374p. 210.00 (*0-7923-8334-6*) Kluwer Academic.

Cardiovascular Biomaterials. Ed. by Garth W. Hastings. 1991. (Illus.). 198p. 150.00 (*0-387-19666-8*) Spr-Verlag.

Cardiovascular Biomechanics. K. B. Chandran. 1992. (Biomedical Engineering Ser.). (Illus.). 300p. (C). text 80.00 (*0-8147-1471-4*) NYU Pr.

Cardiovascular Care of the Elderly. Ed. by T. Strasser. 1987. 174p. pap. text 29.00 (*92-4-156098-3*, 1150265) World Health.

Cardiovascular Complications of Liver Disease. Ed. by Arieh Bomzon & Laurence M. Blendis. 1990. 384p. lib. bdg. 202.00 (*0-8493-4735-1*, RC848) CRC Pr.

Cardiovascular Diagnosis by Ultrasound. P. Hanrath. 1982. text 126.50 (*90-247-2692-1*) Kluwer Academic.

Cardiovascular Disease. A. R. Lorimer & W. S. Hillis. 1985. (Treatment in Clinical Medicine Ser.). (Illus.). 289p. 47.95 (*0-387-15426-4*) Spr-Verlag.

Cardiovascular Disease: Assessment & Intervention. Mary Stein & Kathy Templin. Ed. by Barbara Halliburton. 4th ed. 1996. 198p. (C). reprint ed. pap. text 49.95 (*1-878025-93-7*) Western Schls.

Cardiovascular Disease: Cellular & Molecular Mechanisms, Prevention, & Treatment: Proceedings of the Fourteenth Washington International Spring Symposium at the George Washington University Held in Washington, DC, June 6-10, 1994. Ed. by Linda L. Gallo. 1995. (GWUMC Department of Biochemistry & Molecular Biology Annual Spring Symposium Ser.: Vol. 2). (Illus.). 378p. (C). text 120.00 (*0-306-44992-7*, Kluwer Plenum) Kluwer Academic.

Cardiovascular Disease: Molecular & Cellular Mechanisms, Prevention & Treatment. L. L. Gallo. 1987. LC 87-20224. (GWUMC Department of Biochemistry & Molecular Biology Annual Spring Symposium Ser.). (Illus.). 608p. (C). text 186.00 (*0-306-42537-8*, Kluwer Plenum) Kluwer Academic.

Cardiovascular Disease: Nutrition for Prevention & Treatment. American Dietetic Association Staff. Ed. by Penny M. Kris-Etherton. 1990. LC 90-1031. (Illus.). 349p. (Orig.). pap. text 42.00 (*0-88091-078-X*, 0104) Am Dietetic Assn.

Cardiovascular Disease, Aging & Behavior. Ed. by Jeffrey W. Elias & Philip H. Marshall. 1987. (Series in Health Psychology & Behavioral Medicine). 196p. 73.95 (*0-89116-401-4*) Hemisp Pub.

Cardiovascular Disease in Diabetes. Ed. by Makoto Nagano et al. 1992. (Developments in Cardiovascular Medicine Ser.). 416p. (C). text 187.00 (*0-7923-1554-5*) Kluwer Academic.

Cardiovascular Disease in Older People. Ed. by Fran E. Kaiser et al. 1997. LC 97-4380. (Illus.). 280p. 42.95 (*0-8261-9850-3*) Springer Pub.

Cardiovascular Disease in the Elderly. Ed. by Franz H. Messerli. 1984. (Developments in Cardiovascular Medicine Ser.). text 141.00 (*0-89838-596-2*) Kluwer Academic.

Cardiovascular Disease in Women. Ed. by R. C. Becker & J. S. Alpert. 1990. (Journal: Vol. 77, Suppl. 2). (Illus.). iv, 140p. pap. 43.50 (*3-8055-5222-X*) S Karger.

Cardiovascular Disease in Women: Journal: Cardiology, 1995. Ed. by R. C. Becker & J. S. Alpert. 1995. (Journal: Vol. 86, No. 4, 1995). (Illus.). 98p. pap. 22.75 (*3-8055-6197-0*) S Karger.

***Cardiovascular Disease Matters in Primary Care.** Ruth Chambers et al. 2001. 216p. pap. (*1-85775-419-0*) Radcliffe Med Pr GBR. *Dist:* Balogh.

Cardiovascular Disease Programme of WHO in Europe. G. Lamm. 1981. (Public Health in Europe Ser.: No. 15). 139p. pap. text 11.00 (*92-890-1151-3*) World Health.

Cardiovascular Disease Risk Factors: New Areas for Research: Report of a WHO Scientific Group. Ed. by World Health Organization Staff. 1994. LC 95-103036. (Technical Reports: No. 841). (CHI, FRE & SPA.). vi, 53p. pap. text 10.00 (*92-4-120841-4*, 1100841) World Health.

Cardiovascular Diseases. Ed. by H. S. Rosenberg & J. Bernstein. 1988. (Perspectives in Pediatric Pathology Ser.: Vol. 12). (Illus.). x, 162p. 172.25 (*3-8055-4716-1*) S Karger.

Cardiovascular Diseases: Genetics, Epidemiology & Prevention. James J. Nora et al. 1991. (Oxford Monographs on Medical Genetics: No. 22). (Illus.). 208p. text 39.95 (*0-19-506032-6*, 2924) OUP.

Cardiovascular Diseases & Disorders Sourcebook: Basic Information about Cardiovascular Diseases & Disorders. Ed. by Karen Bellenir & Peter D. Dresser. 1995. LC 95-10583. (Health Reference Ser.: Vol. 5). 683p. lib. bdg. 78.00 (*0-7808-0032-X*) Omnigraphics Inc.

Cardiovascular Diseases & Pregnancy. O. M. Eliseev. 1988. 190p. 83.00 (*0-387-19174-7*) Spr-Verlag.

Cardiovascular Diseases in the United States. Iwao Moriyama et al. 1971. LC 73-154498. (Vital & Health Statistics Monographs, American Public Health Association). (Illus.). 524p. 45.00 (*0-674-09640-1*) HUP.

Cardiovascular Disorders & Behavior Vol. 3: Handbook of Psychology & Health. David S. Krantz et al. 1981. 400p. text 79.95 (*0-89859-185-6*) L Erlbaum Assocs.

Cardiovascular Drug Therapy. Springhouse Publishing Company Staff. 1994. LC 94-3076. (Professional Quick Reference Ser.). (Illus.). 384p. 29.95 (*0-87434-714-9*) Springhouse Corp.

Cardiovascular Drug Therapy - Current Concepts: Journal: Cardiology, Vol. 72, Nos. 5 & 6. Ed. by Ezra A. Amsterdam. 1985. (Illus.). 164p. pap. 62.75 (*3-8055-4081-7*) S Karger.

Cardiovascular Drug Therapy in the Elderly. Adam Schneeweiss & F. Gotthard Schettler. 1988. (Developments in Cardiovascular Medicine Ser.). 400p. (C). text 175.50 (*0-89838-883-X*) Kluwer Academic.

Cardiovascular Dynamics: A Psycholphysiological Study Behavioral Control, Type A, Task Performance, Test Anxiety, & Cardiovascular Responses. M. W. Van Schijndel. 1987. x, 166p. pap. (*90-265-0793-3*) Swets.

Cardiovascular Education Course. Competence Assurance Systems Staff. 1984. (Illus.). pap. text 60.00 (*0-89147-055-7*) CAS.

Cardiovascular Education Course: Acute Care. Competence Assurance Systems Staff. (Illus.). 195p. pap. text 75.00 (*0-89147-112-X*) CAS.

Cardiovascular Effects of Dihydropyridine Type Calcium Antagonists & Agonists. Ed. by Albrect Fleckenstein et al. 1986. (Bayer Symposium Ser.: No. 9). (Illus.). 511p. 99.00 (*0-387-15455-8*) Spr-Verlag.

Cardiovascular Effects of Histamine & H2-Receptor Antagonists. W. Kirch. 1994. (Clinical Pharmacology Ser.: Vol. 10). (Illus.). 74p. text (*3-88603-516-6*) W Zuckschwerdt DEU. *Dist:* Scholium Intl.

Cardiovascular Effects of Verapamin. 1979. (Landmark Ser.). 34.00 (*0-8422-4112-4*) Irvington.

***Cardiovascular Emergencies.** Crispin Davies et al. 2001. (Illus.). 408p. pap. text (*0-7279-1484-7*) BMJ Pub GBR. *Dist:* AIDC.

Cardiovascular Emergencies: Current Therapy. Edward K. Chung. 1985. (Illus.). xii, 244p. 147.00 (*3-8055-3679-8*) S Karger.

Cardiovascular Engineering. Ed. by D. N. Ghista et al. 1983. (Advances in Cardiovascular Physics Ser.: Pt. I-IV). (Illus.). xxxxviii, 960p. 377.50 (*3-8055-3613-5*) S Karger.

Cardiovascular Engineering: Prostheses, Assist & Artificial Organs, Pt. IV. Ed. by D. N. Ghista et al. 1983. (Advances in Cardiovascular Physics Ser.: Vol. 5). (Illus.). viii, 292p. 124.50 (*3-8055-3612-7*) S Karger.

Cardiovascular Engineering Part III: Diagnosis. Ed. by D. N. Ghista et al. 1983. (Advances in Cardiovascular Physics Ser.: Vol. 5). (Illus.). x, 158p. 99.25 (*3-8055-3611-9*) S Karger.

Cardiovascular Engineering, Part I: Modelling. Ed. by D. N. Ghista et al. 1983. (Advances in Cardiovascular Physics Ser.: Vol. 5). (Illus.). xiv, 230p. 124.50 (*3-8055-3609-7*) S Karger.

Cardiovascular Engineering, Part II: Monitoring. Ed. by D. N. Ghista et al. 1983. (Advances in Cardiovascular Physics Ser.: Vol. 5). (Illus.). viii, 280p. 124.50 (*3-8055-3610-0*) S Karger.

Cardiovascular Evaluation of Athletes. Bruce F. Waller & W. Proctor Harvey. 213p. 74.00 (*1-886128-02-2*) Laennec Pub.

Cardiovascular Fluid Dynamics. Uri Dinnar. 1981. 264p. 150.00 (*0-8493-5573-7*, QP105, CRC Reprint) Franklin.

Cardiovascular Function of Peripheral Dopamine Receptors. Ed. by J. Paul Hieble. 1989. (Clinical Pharmacology Ser.: Vol. 15). (Illus.). 384p. text 195.00 (*0-8247-8100-7*) Dekker.

***Cardiovascular Genetics for Clinicians.** Ed. by Pieter A. Doevendans & A. A. M. Wilde. 2001. LC 2001-50227. (Developments in Cardiovascular Medicine Ser.: Vol. 239). 244p. 87.00 (*1-4020-0097-9*) Kluwer Academic.

***Cardiovascular Haemodynamics & Doppler Waveforms Explained.** Ed. by Crispian Oates. 2001. (Illus.). 178p. pap. (*1-84110-021-8*) Greenwich Med GBR. *Dist:* JAMCO Dist.

Cardiovascular Health & Disease in Women. Pamela S. Douglas. 1993. LC 92-48884. (Illus.). 388p. text 90.00 (*0-7216-4567-4*) Saunders.

Cardiovascular Health & Risk Management: The Role of Nutrition & Medication in Clinical Practice. Sylvia Wassertheil-Smoller et al. 1988. (Illus.). 228p. pap. 44.95 (*0-8151-9179-0*) Mosby Inc.

Cardiovascular Imaging by Ultrasound. Ed. by P. Hanrath et al. 1992. LC 92-13423. (Developments in Cardiovascular Medicine Ser.: Vol. 134). 500p. text 340.50 (*0-7923-1755-6*) Kluwer Academic.

Cardiovascular Implants - Cardiac Valve Prostheses. 1991. 9p. pap. 65.00 (*0-910275-06-8*, CV5840-209) Assn Adv Med Instrn.

Cardiovascular Infections. Ed. by Gerald L. Mandell & Oksana M. Korzeniowski. 1998. LC 97-15076. (Atlas of Infectious Diseases Ser.: Vol. 10). (Illus.). 202p. text (*0-443-07750-9*) Church GBR. *Dist:* Saunders.

Cardiovascular Involvement in Systemic Diseases. Ed. by J. David Talley. 1996. LC 96-45182. (Topics in Clinical Cardiology Ser.). (*4-260-14317-4*) Igaku-Shoin.

Cardiovascular Magnetic Resonance Spectroscopy. Ed. by Saul Schaefer & Robert S. Balaban. 1992. (C). text 171.50 (*0-7923-1686-X*) Kluwer Academic.

Cardiovascular Medicine. James T. Willerson. 2nd ed. 1999. LC 00-22728. 100p. text (*0-443-07000-8*) Saunders.

***Cardiovascular Medicine: Practice & Management.** Ed. by Richard C. Becker & Joseph S. Alpert. 2001. (Arnold Publication). 832p. 125.00 (*0-340-76286-1*) OUP.

***Cardiovascular Mega Trends: The 21st Century.** John O. Goodman & Conrad Vernon. 2001. 69.95 (*0-9625207-4-8*) J Goodman & Assocs.

***Cardiovascular Morbidity & Mortality among Swedish Farmers & Non-Farmers: A Population-Based Study.** Eva-Lena Stiernstrom. 2000. (Comprehensive Summaries of Uppsala Dissertations from the Faculty of Medicine Ser.: No. 968). (Illus.). 76p. (Orig.). pap. (*91-554-4839-9*) Uppsala Universitet SWE. *Dist:* Coronet Bks.

Cardiovascular Nuclear Medicine. Ed. by A. Donath & A. Righetti. 1980. (Progress in Nuclear Medicine Ser.: Vol. 6). (Illus.). viii, 228p. 128.75 (*3-8055-0618-X*) S Karger.

Cardiovascular Nuclear Medicine. Kenneth P. Lyons. 1992. (Illus.). 334p. (C). pap. text 120.00 (*0-8385-1052-3*, A1052-8, Apple Lange Med) McGraw.

Cardiovascular Nuclear Medicine & MRI. Ed. by Johan H. Reiber & Ernst E. Van der Wall. 1992. (Developments in Cardiovascular Medicine Ser.). 384p. (C). text 247.50 (*0-7923-1467-0*) Kluwer Academic.

Cardiovascular Nursing. Jeanne Holland. 1977. pap. text 10.95 (*0-316-36998-5*, Little Brwn Med Div) Lppncott W & W.

Cardiovascular Nursing: Holistic Practice, Vol. 1. Cathie E. Guzzetta. 1992. (Illus.). 816p. (C). (gr. 13). text 52.95 (*0-8016-2784-2*, 02784) Mosby Inc.

Cardiovascular Nutrition: Strategies & Tools for Disease Management & Prevention. Penny Kris-Etherton & Julie Burns. 1998. (Illus.). 307p. 35.00 (*0-88091-159-X*) Am Dietetic Assn.

Cardiovascular Outcomes: Collaborative, Path-Based Approaches. Suzanne Smith Blancett & Dominick L. Flarey. 1998. LC 98-13313. 350p. pap. 72.00 (*0-8342-1138-6*, 11386) Aspen Pub.

Cardiovascular Pathology Ed. by Malcolm D. Silver. 2nd ed. 1991. (Illus.). 2043p. text (*0-443-08664-8*) Church.

Cardiovascular Pathology Ed. by Malcolm D. Silver & Avrum Il Gotlieb. 3rd ed. 1998. (*0-443-07576-X*) Church.

Cardiovascular Pathology. Malcolm D. Silver & Avrum Il Gotlieb. 3rd ed. 2000. LC 2001-25319. (Illus.). viii, 808p. text 260.00 (*0-443-06535-7*) Saunders.

Cardiovascular Pathology, Vol. 23. Virmani & Cecilia M. Fenoglio-Preiser. 1990. (Illus.). 480p. text 92.00 (*0-7216-3232-7*) Saunders.

Cardiovascular Pathology in Infants & Children. James B. Arey. 1984. (Illus.). 392p. text 145.00 (*0-7216-1395-0*) Saunders.

Cardiovascular Pathophysiology. F. Kusumoto. 1998. (Pathophysiology Ser.). pap. 30.95 (*1-889325-00-7*) Blackwell Sci.

Cardiovascular Pharmacology. Ed. by William W. Parmley & Kanu Chatterjee. 1994. LC 93-7862. (gr. 13). (*1-56375-160-7*) Gower-Mosby.

Cardiovascular Pharmacology 1987. J. Gy Papp. 1986. 649p. (C). (*963-05-4651-5*) Akade Kiado HUN. *Dist:* St Mut.

Cardiovascular Pharmacology & Therapeutics. Ed. by Bramah N. Singh et al. 1993. (Illus.). 1264p. text (*0-443-08814-4*) Church.

Cardiovascular Pharmacology of 5-Hydroxytryptamine: Prospective Therapeutic Applications. Ed. by P. R. Saxena et al. 1990. (Developments in Cardiovascular Medicine Ser.). (C). text 309.50 (*0-7923-0502-7*) Kluwer Academic.

Cardiovascular Pharmacotherapeutics. William H. Frishman & Edmund H. Sonnenblick. 1997. LC 96-43577. (Illus.). 1722p. text 125.00 (*0-07-022481-1*) McGraw-Hill Prof.

Cardiovascular Pharmacotherapeutics: Companion Handbook. Ed. by William H. Frishman & Edmund H. Sonnenblick. 1998. LC 98-9637. (Illus.). 550p. pap. 39.95 (*0-07-022488-9*) McGraw-Hill Prof.

Cardiovascular Physiology. H. S. Badeer. 1984. (Continuing Education Ser.: Vol. 6). (Illus.). xvi, 276p. 50.50 (*3-8055-3796-4*) S Karger.

Cardiovascular Physiology. Jon Goerke & Allan H. Mines. 1988. (Physiology Ser.). (Illus.). 232p. text 50.00 (*0-88167-413-3*) Lppncott W & W.

Cardiovascular Physiology. William R. Milnor. 1990. (Illus.). 520p. text 39.95 (*0-19-505884-4*) OUP.

Cardiovascular Physiology. Ed. by H. J. Priebe & K. Skarvan. 1995. 200p. (Orig.). (C). pap. text (*0-7279-0781-6*) BMJ Pub GBR. *Dist:* AIDC.

Cardiovascular Physiology. David E. Mohrman & Lois J. Heller. 4th ed. 1996. LC 96-35519. (Illus.). 254p. pap. 34.95 (*0-07-028025-8*) McGraw-Hill Prof.

Cardiovascular Physiology. Robert M. Berne & Mathew N. Levy. 7th ed. 1996. LC 96-28899. (Illus.). 336p. (C). (gr. 13). pap. text 35.95 (*0-8151-0901-6*, 28159) Mosby Inc.

Cardiovascular Physiology. Robert M. Berne & Matthew N. Levy. 8th ed. 2000. LC 00-32430. (Mosby Physiology Monograph Ser.). (Illus.). xiv, 312p. 32.95 (*0-323-01127-6*) Mosby Inc.

Cardiovascular Physiology in the Genetically Engineered Mouse. Brian D. Hoit & Richard A. Walsh. 1998. LC 98-45055. (Developments in Cardiovascular Medicine Ser.). x, 286p. (*0-7923-8356-7*) Kluwer Academic.

Cardiovascular Psychophysiology: A Perspective. Paul A. Obrist. 1981. LC 80-28582. 246p. 45.00 (*0-306-40599-7*, Plenum Trade) Perseus Pubng.

Cardiovascular Radiology. Eugene Gedgaudas et al. 1985. (Illus.). 269p. text 115.00 (*0-7216-1084-6*) Saunders.

Cardiovascular Reactivity & Stress: Patterns of Physiological Response. J. R. Turner. 1994. (Series in Behavioral Psychophysiology & Medicine). (Illus.). 256p. (C). 39.50 (*0-306-44612-X*, Plenum Trade) Perseus Pubng.

Cardiovascular Reactivity to Psychological Stress & Disease. Ed. by Jim Blascovich & Edward S. Katkin. 1993. (Illus.). 242p. pap. text 19.95 (*1-55798-337-2*) Am Psychol.

Cardiovascular Regulation. Ed. by D. Jordan & J. M. Marshall. 1995. (Studies in Physiology: Vol. 2). (Illus.). 172p. (Orig.). (C). pap. text (*1-85578-024-0*) Portland Pr Ltd GBR. *Dist:* Ashgate Pub Co.

Cardiovascular Response to Exercise. Gerald F. Fletcher. 1993. LC 93-22393. (American Heart Association Monograph Ser.). (Illus.). 416p. 75.00 (*0-87993-559-6*) Futura Pub.

Cardiovascular Review Book for Invasive CV Technology, Set. J. Wesley Todd. 2nd rev. ed. 1996. (Illus.). 1540p. spiral bd. 190.00 (*0-9653568-1-7*) Cardiac Self Assessmnt.

Cardiovascular Review Book for Invasive CV Technology Vol. I: Anatomy, Physiology & Pathology. J. Wesley Todd. 2nd rev. ed. 1996. (Cardiovascular Review Bk.). (Illus.). 490p. (Orig.). spiral bd. 80.00 (*0-9653568-2-5*) Cardiac Self Assessmnt.

Cardiovascular Review Book for Invasive CV Technology Vol. II: Diagnostic Techniques. J. Wesley Todd. 2nd rev. ed. 1996. (Cardiovascular Review Bk.). (Illus.). 445p. (Orig.). spiral bd. 80.00 (*0-9653568-3-3*) Cardiac Self Assessmnt.

Cardiovascular Risk Factors. John D. Swales & David P. De Bono. 1992. LC 92-49565. (gr. 13). text (*1-56375-551-3*) Gower-Mosby.

Cardiovascular Sciences: Recent Advances. Ed. by Y. S. Chan et al. 1995. (Journal: Vol. 4, No. 3, 1995). (Illus.). 90p. pap. 31.50 (*3-8055-6264-0*) S Karger.

***Cardiovascular Solid Mechanics: Cells, Tissues & Organs.** Jay D. Humphrey. 2001. LC 00-69244. (Illus.). 768p. 79.95 (*0-387-95168-7*) Spr-Verlag.

Cardiovascular Specialty Manual. Association of Surgical Technologists. 2001. (Allied Health Ser.). (C). pap. 40.00 net. (*0-7668-1210-3*) Delmar.

Cardiovascular Specific Gene Expression. Peter A. Doevendans et al. 1999. LC 99-13442. (Developments in Cardiovascular Medicine Ser.: Vol. 214). (*0-7923-5633-0*) Kluwer Academic.

Cardiovascular Surgery: Thoracic Surgery. Ed. by E. Wolner et al. 1994. LC 94-36670. (Fibrin Sealing in Surgical & Nonsurgical Fields Ser.: 6). (*0-387-58381-5*) Spr-Verlag.

Cardiovascular Survey Methods. G. A. Rose & H. Blackburn. 1982. (Monographs: No. 56). (ENG, FRE, RUS & SPA.). 178p. pap. text 22.00 (*92-4-140056-0*, 1140056) World Health.

Cardiovascular System. Thomas Braem. 1993. (The Organs of the Human Anatomy: Vol. 1). 48p. (C). spiral bd. 15.95 (*1-878576-25-9*) Flash Anatomy Inc.

Cardiovascular System: General Considerations & Congenital Malformations, Pt. A. Ed. by William B. Robertson. 3rd ed. 1993. LC 92-20957. (Systemic Pathology Ser.: Vol. 10, Pt. A). text (*0-443-03096-0*) Church.

Cardiovascular System Pt. B: Acquired Diseases of the Heart. Ed. by W. S. Symmers et al. 3rd ed. 1995. (Systemic Pathology Ser.: No. 10). (Illus.). 600p. (*0-443-04930-0*) Church.

Cardiovascular System & Physical Exercise. Victor L. Karpman. 1987. 208p. 189.00 (*0-8493-6528-7*, QP114) CRC Pr.

Cardiovascular System at a Glance. P. I. Aaronson et al. 1999. LC 98-54927. (At a Glance Ser.). (Illus.). 125p. pap. 26.95 (*0-632-04971-5*) Blackwell Sci.

Cardiovascular Therapeutics. Thomas W. Smith. Ed. by Richard Zorab. 1996. LC 95-30947. (Illus.). 720p. text 99.00 (*0-7216-5660-9*) Saunders.

Cardiovascular Therapeutics: A Companion to Braunwald's Heart Disease. Elliott M. Antman. 2nd ed. 2001. LC 2001-49606. (Illus.). 435p. text (*0-7216-8733-4*) Saunders.

Cardiovascular Therapy & Drug Market. Ed. by Peter Allen. 1988. 300p. pap. 1495.00 (*0-941285-38-3*) FIND-SVP.

Cardiovascular Thrombosis. Marc Verstraete. 2nd ed. 1998. LC 97-42477. 896p. text 159.00 (*0-397-58772-4*) Lppncott W & W.

Cardiovascular Toxicity of Cocaine. 1993. lib. bdg. 265.95 (*0-8490-8911-5*) Gordon Pr.

Cardiovascular Transformation: A Business Guide for Successful Growth. John O. Goodman & Conrad Vernon. 1994. 170p. ring bd. 219.00 (*0-8342-0611-0*) Aspen Pub.

Cardiovascular Trials Review. Robert A. Kloner & Yochai Birnbaum. unabr. ed. 1996. 312p. (Orig.). pap. text 22.00 (*0-9626020-3-5*) Le Jacq Commns.

Cardiovascular Trials Review. Ed. by Robert Kloner & Yochai Birnbaum. 3rd ed. 1998. 640p. pap. 58.00 (*0-9626020-7-8*) Le Jacq Commns.

Care: Discovery & Uses in Clinical & Community Nursing. Ed. by Madeleine M. Leininger. 1988. LC 88-10804. (Human Care & Health Ser.). 202p. pap. 22.95 (*0-8143-1997-1*) Wayne St U Pr.

Care: The Essence of Nursing & Health. Ed. by Madeleine M. Leininger. 1988. LC 87-30043. (Human Care & Health Ser.). 278p. (C). reprint ed. pap. 22.95 (*0-8143-1995-5*) Wayne St U Pr.

Care & Cure of Crippled Children. Gathrone R. Giralestone. Ed. by William R. Phillips & Janet Rosenberg. 1980. LC 79-6900. (Physically Handicapped in Society Ser.). (Illus.). reprint ed. lib. bdg. 16.95 (*0-405-13111-9*) Ayer.

Care & Education of Crippled Children in the United States. Edith R. Sollenberger. 1974. LC 74-1706. (Children & Youth Ser.: Vol. 21). (Illus.). 270p. reprint ed. 30.95 (*0-405-05983-3*) Ayer.

Care & Feeding of the Chronologically Gifted Brain. Joanne McClellan Egnor. 2000. pap. 6.95 (*0-533-13372-6*) Vantage.

Care & Feeding of the Prostate. Arnold Perrin. 1980. pap. 1.00 (*0-939736-49-7*) Wings ME.

Care & Management of People with Sickle Cell & Thalassaemia. Lola Oni et al. 2002. (Illus.). 288p. pap. 55.00 (*0-7506-3000-0*) Buttrwrth-Heinemann.

Care, Concern & Cure in Perinatal Medicine: Recent Advances & Developments. J. G. Koppe. 1993. (Illus.). 613p. ring bd. (*1-85070-398-1*, Parthenon Pbng) CRC Pr.

Care, Cure, & Education of the Crippled Child: A Study of American Social & Professional Facilities to Care for, Cure, & Educate Crippled Children. Henry E. Abt. 1974. LC 74-1659. (Children & Youth Ser.). (Illus.). 240p. reprint ed. 26.95 (*0-405-05941-8*) Ayer.

Care for Frail Elders: Developing Community Solutions. Walter N. Leutz et al. 1992. LC 92-11506. 315p. 68.00 (*0-86569-029-4*, T029, Auburn Hse) Greenwood.

Care for the Caregiver: A Guide for Staff in the Helping Professions. Terrance P. McGuire & Kathleen McGowan. 1991. LC 90-62085. (Illus.). 54p. (Orig.). (C). pap. 8.95 (*1-55612-400-7*) Sheed & Ward WI.

Care Gaps. W. Halamandaris. 1992. LC 92-6438. (Illus.). 114p. (Orig.). (C). 49.50 (*0-8191-8658-9*); pap. 23.00 (*0-8191-8659-7*) U Pr of Amer.

Care in Labour. D. Gibb & C. Warwick. 1995. (Illus.). 192p. pap. 24.95 (*0-86542-922-7*) Blackwell Sci.

Care in the Community: Illusion or Reality. Julian P. Leff. LC 96-3425. 230p. 1998. pap. 65.00 (*0-471-96982-6*); 1997. 150.00 (*0-471-96981-8*) Wiley.

Care Management & Health Care of Older People: The Darlington Community Care Project. David Challis et al. 384p. 1996. pap. (*1-85742-190-6*); 1995. (*1-85742-184-1*) Arena GBR. *Dist:* Ashgate Pub Co.

Care Management of Skin Diseases: Life Quality & Economic Impact. Rukmini Rajagopalan et al. 1998. LC 97-42815. (Illus.). 485p. text 175.00 (*0-8247-0128-3*) Dekker.

Care Matters: Concepts, Practice & Research in Health & Social Care. Ann Brechin et al. 1998. LC 98-75102. (Social Work Ser.). (Illus.). 193p. 74.00 (*0-7619-5565-8*, 81441) Sage.

Care of Children in Hospital: A Study. Else Stenbak. 1986. (Illus.). 68p. pap. text 12.00 (*92-890-1033-9*, 1340027) World Health.

Care of Children with Long-Term Tracheostomies. Ed. by Ken M. Bleile. 1993. LC 93-3951. (Illus.). 300p. (Orig.). (C). pap. text 55.00 (*1-56593-094-0*, 0398) Thomson Learn.

Care of Chronically & Severely Ill: Comparative Social Policies. Ed. by J. Rogers Hollingsworth & Ellen J. Hollingsworth. 1994. LC 93-38398. (Social Institutions & Social Change Ser.). 256p. pap. text 26.95 (*0-202-30486-8*); lib. bdg. 49.95 (*0-202-30485-X*) Aldine de Gruyter.

Care of Congenital Hand Anomalies. Adrian E. Flatt. 2nd ed. 1993. LC 94-20707. (Illus.). 466p. text 89.00 (*0-942219-35-X*) Quality Med Pub.

Care of Drug Users in General Practice: A Harm-Minimization Approach. Berry Beaumont. 1997. LC 97-20285. (*1-85775-236-8*) Radcliffe Med Pr GBR. *Dist:* Balogh.

Care of Frail Elderly People in the United Kingdom. A. Tinker et al. 1994. 114p. pap. (*0-11-321610-6*, HM16106) Statnry Office GBR. *Dist:* Bernan Associates.

Care of Handicapped Children, Vol. 7. Ed. by Robert H. Bremner. 1978. LC 74-1671. (Children & Youth Ser.). 22.95 (*0-405-05951-5*) Ayer.

Care of Individuals with Cancer. Susan L. Groenwald. 1991. (Illus.). (C). pap. text 49.95 (*0-86720-305-6*, 305-6) Jones & Bartlett.

Care of Mind/Care of Spirit: A Psychiatrist Explores Spiritual Direction. Gerald G. May. 1992. LC 91-58190. 256p. reprint ed. pap. 14.00 (*0-06-065567-4*) Harper SF.

Care of Neuropathic Limbs: A Practical Manual. Grace Warren & Sydney Nade. 1999. LC 98-50051. (Illus.). 178p. lib. bdg. 78.95 (*1-85070-048-6*) CRC Pr.

Care of Patients: Examples of Compliance. Joint Commission on Accreditation of Healthcare Organizations. 1999. (Illus.). 359p. pap. 50.00 (*0-86688-611-7*, TX-100) Joint Comm Hlthcare.

Care of Patients with Urologic Problems. Edwina A. McConnell & Mary F. Zimmerman. 1982. (Illus.). 309p. text 22.50 (*0-397-54402-2*, 64-03430, Lippnctt) Lppncott W & W.

Care of People with Diabetes: A Manual of Nursing Practice. Trisha Dunning. 1994. LC 93-46697. 188p. pap. 39.95 (*0-632-03876-4*) Blackwell Sci.

Care of Strangers: The Rise of America's Hospital System. Charles E. Rosenberg. 1995. LC 94-36036. (Illus.). 456p. pap. text 17.95 (*0-8018-5082-7*) Johns Hopkins.

Care of the Aged Persons in the United States. Florence E. Parker & Estelle M. Stewart. 1976. LC 75-17235. (Social Problems & Social Policy Ser.). reprint ed. 25.95 (*0-405-07504-9*) Ayer.

Care of the Aged, the Dying, & the Dead. Ed. by Robert J. Kastenbaum. 2nd ed. 1977. LC 76-19596. (Death & Dying Ser.). reprint ed. lib. bdg. 16.95 (*0-405-09590-2*) Ayer.

Care of the Alzheimer's Patient. Fuzy. 1996. (C). pap. text, tchr. ed. 12.00 (*0-8273-7934-X*) Delmar.

Care of the Arthritic Hand. Adrian E. Flatt. 5th ed. 1995. LC 95-21359. (Illus.). 454p. text 99.00 (*0-942219-83-X*) Quality Med Pub.

Care of the Burn Wound. Ed. by S. R. May & G. Dogo. 1985. (Illus.). xiv, 246p. 191.50 (*3-8055-3991-6*) S Karger.

Care of the Critically Ill Child. MacNab. 1999. text 79.00 (*0-443-05394-4*) Saunders.

Care of the Critically Ill Patient. Ed. by Jack Tinker & Warren M. Zapol. 1986. (Illus.). 1150p. 129.00 (*0-387-11289-8*) Spr-Verlag.

Care of the Critically Ill Patient. Jack Tinker & Warren M. Zapol. 2nd ed. 1991. (Illus.). 1504p. 179.00 (*3-540-19617-X*) Spr-Verlag.

Care of the Critically Ill Patient. Ed. by Warren M. Zapol & Jack Tinker. 2nd ed. 1991. (Illus.). 1504p. 198.00 (*0-387-19617-X*) Spr-Verlag.

Care of the Critically Ill Surgical Patient. Ed. by Iain D. Anderson. 1999. (Illus.). 192p. pap. (*0-340-70092-0*) E A GBR. *Dist:* OUP.

Care of the Dying Child. Ed. by Ann Goldman. 1994. (Illus.). 224p. pap. text 29.95 (*0-19-261983-7*) OUP.

Care of the Elderly: A Family Approach. Elsie M. Pinkston & Nathan L. Linsk. 1984. (Psychology Practitioner Guidebooks). (Illus.). 128p. text 28.00 (*0-08-030978-X*); pap. text 14.95 (*0-08-030977-1*) Elsevier (Pergamon Pr).

Care of the Elderly: Clinical Aspects of Aging. Ed. by William Reichel et al. 4th ed. 1995. LC 94-26125. (Illus.). 672p. 65.00 (*0-683-07209-9*) Lppncott W & W.

Care of the Elderly Patient: Policy Issues & Research Opportunities. Institute of Medicine Staff. 1989. 152p. pap. text 18.00 (*0-309-04097-3*) Natl Acad Pr.

Care of the High-Risk Neonate. Ed. by Marshall H. Klaus & Avroy A. Fanaroff. 4th ed. 1993. LC 92-20397. (Illus.). 558p. text 58.00 (*0-7216-3709-4*) Saunders.

Care of the Mentally Retarded. Marian Blackwell. 1979. 19.50 (*0-316-09890-6*, Little Brwn Med Div) Lppncott W & W.

Care of the Newborn & Mother. Fuzy. (C). 1998. 19.95 (*0-8273-7929-3*); 1996. pap. text, tchr. ed. 12.00 (*0-8273-7930-7*) Delmar.

Care of the Older Person. Christine A. McMahon et al. 1996. LC 96-27717. 256p. (Orig.). pap. 38.95 (*0-632-03985-X*) Blackwell Sci.

***Care of the Ophthalmic Patient.** Perry. 2nd ed. 1997. pap. 28.95 (*0-412-59290-8*) Chapman & Hall.

Care of the Ophthalmic Patient. Perry. 2nd ed. 1995. 480p. pap. 79.75 (*1-56593-334-6*, 0664) Singular Publishing.

Care of the Pregnant Woman & Her Baby. Norman A. Beischer et al. 2nd ed. 1990. (Illus.). 424p. text (*0-7295-0297-X*) Bailliere Tindall.

Care of the Professional Voice. D. Garfield Davies & Anthony J. Jahn. 1999. LC 98-22187. (Illus.). 176p. pap. (*0-7506-3640-8*) E A GBR. *Dist:* OUP.

Care of the Psyche: A History of Psychological Healing. Stanley W. Jackson. 1999. LC 98-37512. 480p. 45.00 (*0-300-07671-1*) Yale U Pr.

Care of the Renal Patient: A Family Medicine Guide. David Z. Levine. Ed. by Ray Kersey. 3rd ed. 1997. LC 96-26583. 315p. text 52.00 (*0-7216-6243-9*) Saunders.

Care of the Skin. Audrey G. Goldberg. 1975. (Illus.). pap. 22.95 (*0-434-90673-5*) Trafalgar.

Care of the Teeth: A Natural Approach. Ed. by Christine Murphy. 2000. 96p. pap. 15.00 (*1-930051-07-7*) Lantern Books.

Care of the Wild: Family First Aid & Care for All Wild Creatures. W. J. Jordan & John Hughes. 1983. LC 82-42699. (Illus.). 228p. 13.95 (*0-89256-226-9*); pap. 8.95 (*0-89256-240-4*) Macmillan (Rawson Assocs).

Care of the Wild: First Aid for Wild Creatures. William J. Jordan et al. 1991. (Illus.). 240p. reprint ed. pap. 14.95 (*0-299-13184-X*) U of Wis Pr.

Care of the Wild Feathered & Furred: Treating & Feeding Injured Birds & Animals, 25th Anniversary Edition. Mae Hickman & Maxine Guy. 25th anniv. ed. 1998. LC 93-78383. (Illus.). 143p. reprint ed. pap. 15.95 (*0-935576-53-3*) Kesend Pub Ltd.

Care of the Wounded in Vietnam. Robert M. Hardaway. 1988. (Illus.). 244p. pap. 15.00 (*0-89745-106-6*) Sunflower U Pr.

Care of Well Children in Day-Care Centers & Institutions. 1963. (Technical Report Ser.: No. 256). 34p. pap. text 3.00 (*92-4-120256-4*) World Health.

Care of Wounds. Carol Dealey. 2nd ed. 1999. LC 99-37337. pap. 49.95 (*0-632-05237-6*) Blackwell Sci.

Care of Wounds: A Guide for Nurses. Carol Dealey. 1994. LC 93-47189. (Advanced Nursing Ser.). 256p. pap. (*0-632-03864-0*) Blckwell Science.

Care Pack. (*0-340-52521-5*) E A GBR. *Dist:* Routldge.

Care Planning for the Older Adult: Nursing Diagnosis in Long-Term Care. Richard S. Ferri. 1994. (Illus.). 381p. pap. text 31.00 (*0-7216-2132-5*) Saunders.

Care Planning Pocket Guide. Janet R. Lederer. 4th ed. 1991. 288p. (C). pap. text 19.95 (*0-8053-4103-X*) Addison-Wesley.

Care Planning Pocket Guide: A Nursing Diagnosis Approach. Janet R. Lederer. 22nd ed. 1988. LC 87-28987. pap. 17.50 (*0-201-16399-3*) Addison-Wesley.

Care Planning with the MDS+ for the Geriatric Nurse. Mattie Locke. 1995. 258p. (Orig.). (C). 49.50 (*1-877735-46-9*, 2268PP) Prof Prnting & Pub.

Care Plans That Work with MDS. Mattie Locke et al. 3rd ed. 1996. 214p. (C). 49.50 (*1-877735-03-5*, 2104PP) Prof Prnting & Pub.

Carebook: A Workbook for Caregiver Peace of Mind. Joyce Beedle. Ed. by Louise Dunn. 1991. 51p. ring bd., wbk. ed. 24.50 (*0-9630730-5-2*) Lady Bug.

Career Choices for Veterinarians: Beyond Private Practice. Carin A. Smith. 1998. LC 97-91960. 256p. (Orig.). pap. 27.95 (*1-885780-08-7*) Smith Vet Srvs.

Career Connections: Great Careers for People Interested in the Human Body, Vol. 2. Lois Edwards. 1993. LC 93-78078. (Career Connections Ser.: Series 1). (Illus.). 48p. (J). (gr. 6-9). text 30.00 (*0-8103-9386-7*, GML14099-102104, UXL) Gale.

Career Counseling: Applied Concepts of Life Planning. Vernon G. Zunker. 2nd ed. 1985. LC 85-21353. (Psychology-Counseling Ser.). 432p. (C). pap. 36.00 (*0-534-05508-7*) Brooks-Cole.

Career Decision Making. Ed. by W. Bruce Walsh & Samuel H. Osipow. 1988. 280p. text 39.95 (*0-89859-756-0*) L Erlbaum Assocs.

Career Guide for the Health Services Manager. Anthony R. Kovner & Alan H. Channing. 3rd ed. 1999. LC 99-28565. xii, 201p. pap. 38.00 (*1-56793-111-1*) Health Admin Pr.

Career Guide in Pathology. Ellis S. Benson et al. 1997. LC 97-42841. 20.00 (*0-89189-428-4*) Am Soc Clinical.

Career in Clinical Psychology: From Training to Employment. Robert H. Woody & Malcolm H. Robertson. 1996. LC 96-25086. 242p. 37.50 (*0-8236-0652-X*) Intl Univs Pr.

***Career in Medicine.** R. M. Kirk. 1998. 120p. pap. text (*1-900151-68-5*) Greenwich Med GBR. *Dist:* JAMCO Dist.

***Career in Medicine: Do You Have What It Takes?** Ed. by Harvey White. 2000. 75p. pap. (*1-85315-462-8*) Royal Soc of Medicine Pr Ltd GBR. *Dist:* Balogh.

Career Inventories for the Learning Disabled (CAI) Carol Weller & Mary Buchanan. 1983. stu. ed. 55.00 (*0-87879-350-X*); 20.00 (*0-87879-351-8*) Acad Therapy.

Career Inventories for the Learning Disabled (CAI) Interest Inventories. Carol Weller & Mary Buchanan. 1983. 10.00 (*0-87879-352-6*) Acad Therapy.

Career of William Beaumont & the Reception of His Discovery: An Original Anthology. William Beaumont. Ed. by I. Bernard Cohen. 1980. LC 79-7949. (Three Centuries of Science in America Ser.). (Illus.). lib. bdg. 25.95 (*0-405-12530-5*) Ayer.

Career Opportunities in Health Care. Shelly Field. 1997. (Career Opportunities Ser.). LC 96-48138. 240p. 29.95 (*0-8160-3381-1*); 320p. reprint ed. pap. text 18.95 (*0-8160-3382-X*) Facts on File.

Career Options in Health Care. Edward J. Hopkins. 1998. 224p. pap. 25.00 (*0-8342-0891-1*, 20891) Aspen Pub.

Career Pathways in Psychiatry: Transition in Changing Times. Ed. by Arthur Lazarus. 1996. LC 95-48245. 216p. 36.00 (*0-88163-217-1*) Analytic Pr.

Career Perspectives: Interviews with Blind & Visually Impaired Professionals. Compiled by Marie Attmore. l.t. ed. 1990. LC 90-430. 96p. pap. 19.95 (*0-89128-170-3*) Am Foun Blind.

Career Planning: A Nurse's Guide to Career Advancement. Patricia Winstead-Fry. 1990. 256p. 29.95 (*0-88737-462-X*) Natl League Nurse.

Career Planning for Nurses. Bette Case. 1996. LC 96-21218. (Professional Reference-Nursing Ser.). 352p. (C). pap. text 44.95 (*0-8273-7165-9*) Delmar.

Career Planning for Psychiatrists. Ed. by Kathleen M. Mogul & Leah J. Dickstein. 1995. LC 95-1384. (Issues in Psychiatry Ser.). 288p. pap. text 19.95 (*0-88048-197-8*, 8197) Am Psychiatric.

Career Planning Guide for the Allied Health Professions. Zubie W. Metcalf, Jr. 1998. 192p. pap. 15.95 (*0-683-30166-7*) Lppncott W & W.

Career Recovery: Best Practices in the Vocational Rehabilitation of Persons with Serious Mental Illness. Michael S. Shafer et al. unabr. ed. 1998. LC 98-2512. 109p. pap. 29.00 (*1-883302-24-2*) Trning Res.

Careers & Identities. Michael A. Banks et al. 1991. 224p. (*0-335-09715-4*); pap. (*0-335-09714-6*) OpUniv Pr.

Careers for Caring People: And Other Sensitive Types. Adrian R. Paradis. 1995. LC 95-542. (Illus.). 205p. pap. 9.95 (*0-8442-4476-7*, 44767, VGM Career Bks) McGraw-Hill Trade.

Careers in Anesthesiology Vol. I: Autobiographical Memoirs. William Hamilton et al. Ed. by B. Raymond Fink. 1997. LC 97-60921. (Illus.). 217p. pap. 25.00 (*0-9614932-9-1*) Wood Lib-Mus.

Careers in Clinical Research: Obstacles & Opportunities. Institute of Medicine Staff. Ed. by William N. Kelley & Mark A. Randolph. 1994. LC 94-13014. 344p. (C). text 39.95 (*0-309-04890-7*) Natl Acad Pr.

Careers in Health Care. Barbara M. Swanson. 1984. LC 83-73721. 350p. text 14.95 (*0-87094-443-6*, Irwn Prfssnl) McGraw-Hill Educ Grp.

Careers in Health Care. Barbara M. Swanson. (Professional Careers Ser.). 1994. (Illus.). 320p. 17.95 (*0-8442-4198-9*, 41989); 2nd ed. 1991. 304p. 16.95 (*0-8442-8698-2*) McGraw-Hill Trade (VGM Career Bks).

Careers in Health Care & Medicine. Mark A. Taylor. 1998. (Illus.). 86p. (Orig.). pap. 10.95 (*0-9664171-0-0*) M A Taylor.

Careers in Medicine. Terence J. Sacks. 1994. LC 92-15866. (Professional Careers Ser.). 160p. 16.95 (*0-8442-4178-4*); 2nd ed. pap. 12.95 (*0-8442-4179-2*) McGraw-Hill Trade (VGM Career Bks).

Careers in Medicine. Terence J. Sacks. 2nd ed. 1996. LC 96-26670. (VGM Professional Careers Ser.). (Illus.). 144p. 17.95 (*0-8442-4448-1*, 44481); 340p. pap. 13.95 (*0-8442-4449-X*, 4449X) NTC Contemp Pub Co.

Careers in Nursing. Terence J. Sacks. 1998. LC 98-10328. (VGM Professional Careers Ser.). (Illus.). 278p. pap. 13.95 (*0-8442-4555-0*, 45550, VGM Career Bks) McGraw-Hill Trade.

Careers in Social & Rehabilitation Services. Geraldine O. Garner. 1994. LC 93-14049. (Professional Careers Ser.). (Illus.). 245p. pap. 13.95 (*0-8442-4190-3*, 41903); 152p. 17.95 (*0-8442-4188-1*, 41881) McGraw-Hill Trade (VGM Career Bks).

Careers Inside the World of Health Care. Beth Wilkinson. rev. ed. 1999. LC 2001-268659. (Careers & Opportunities Ser.). (Illus.). 64p. (J). (gr. 7-12). lib. bdg. 17.95 (*0-8239-2886-1*, CIHECA) Rosen Group.

Careers of Care: Survivors of Traumatic Brain Injury & the Response of Health & Social Care. P. E. Higham & Kay Phelps. 1998. LC 97-49933. 289p. text (*1-85742-425-5*, RD594.H53) Ashgate Pub GBR. *Dist:* Ashgate Pub Co.

Caregiver Connection: Training Manual. 1994. (Illus.). 165p. (Orig.). (C). pap. text 35.00 (*0-7881-1371-2*) DIANE Pub.

Caregiver Sourcebook: Central New York. Jane J. White. Ed. by Sherry L. Fleckenstein. 1998. Orig. Title: Thompson's Resource Guide for Aging. ring bd. 29.95 (*0-9645965-6-3*) Res for Aging.

Caregiver Sourcebook: Finger Lakes. Jane J. White. Ed. by Sherry L. Fleckenstein. 1998. Orig. Title: Thompson's Resource Guide for Aging. ring bd. 29.95 (*0-9645965-5-5*) Res for Aging.

Caregiver Sourcebook: National. Jane J. White. Ed. by Sherry L. Fleckenstein. 1998. Orig. Title: Thompson's Resource Guide for Aging. ring bd. 69.95 (*0-9645965-3-9*) Res for Aging.

Caregiver Sourcebook: Western New York. Jane J. White. Ed. by Sherry L. Fleckenstein. 1998. Orig. Title: Thompson's Resource Guide for Aging. ring bd. 29.95 (*0-9645965-4-7*) Res for Aging.

Caregiver Therapy. Julie Kuebelbeck & Victoria O'Connor. 1995. LC 96-77810. (Elf-Help Bks.). 88p. pap. 4.95 (*0-87029-285-4*) Abbey.

Caregiver's Book: Caring for a Loved One, Caring for Yourself. James E. Miller. 1996. LC 96-23938. 64p. pap. 14.99 (*0-8066-2985-1*, 9-2985, Augsburg) Augsburg Fortress.

Caregivers Guide: Giving Medicines. 1999. 48p. text, tchr. ed. 42.60 (*0-13-085293-7*) P-H.

Caregiver's Guide: Helping Older Friends & Relatives with Health & Safety Concerns. Caroline Rob & Janet Reynolds. 1992. 320p. pap. 15.00 (*0-395-58780-8*) HM.

Caregiver's Guide to Giving Medicines. Carol Heerema. 1999. LC 99-19490. (Illus.). x, 182p. spiral bd. 19.93 (*0-8359-5388-2*, Prentice Hall) P-H.

Caregiver's Handbook: A Complete Guide to Home Health Care. Deni Bown. 1998. LC 97-35911. (Illus.). 192p. pap. 14.95 (*0-7894-1969-6*) DK Pub Inc.

Caregiving: A Step-by-Step Resource for Caring for the Cancer Patient at Home. Peter S. Houts et al. 2000. LC 00-32789. (Illus.). xv, 314p. pap. 18.95 (*0-944235-20-4*) Am Cancer NY.

Caregiving: Readings in Knowledge, Practice, Ethics, & Politics. Ed. by Suzanne Gordon et al. 1996. LC 96-19693. (Studies in Health, Illness, & Caregiving). 328p. (Orig.). pap. text 22.95 (*0-8122-1582-6*) U of Pa Pr.

Caregiving Across Cultures: Working with Dementing Illness & Ethnically Diverse Populations. Ramon Valle & Helen Cook-Gait. 1997. LC 97-30918. pap. 27.95 (*1-56032-530-5*) Taylor & Francis.

Caregiving & Loss: Family Needs, Professional Responses. Ed. by Kenneth J. Doka & Joyce D. Davidson. 2001. LC 00-134618. 336p. pap. (*1-893349-02-0*) Hospice Fndt Amer.

Caregiving at a Glance: Finger Tip Help for Families Taking Care of People with Alzheimers. Lin E. Noyes. rev. ed. 2000. 28p. pap. (*0-9678646-0-7*) Family Respte.

Caregiving Dilemma: Work in an American Nursing Home. Nancy Foner. LC 93-27426. 190p. 1995. pap. text 15.95 (*0-520-20337-2*); 1994. (C). text 45.00 (*0-520-08359-8*) U CA Pr.

Caregiving in Dementia, Vol. 2. Ed. by Gemma M. Jones & M. Bere Miesen. 1997. 392p. (C). 90.00 (*0-415-13844-2*); pap. 34.95 (*0-415-13845-0*) Routledge.

Caregiving Sourcebook: Basic Consumer Health Information for Caregivers, Including a Profile of Caregivers. Ed. by Joyce Brennfleck Shannon. 2001. LC 2001-33129. (Health Reference Ser.). (Illus.). xiii, 602p. lib. bdg. 78.00 (*0-7808-0331-0*) Omnigraphics Inc.

Caregiving Systems: Informal & Formal Helpers. Ed. by K. Warner Schaie et al. 1993. (Social Structure & Aging Ser.). 416p. text 79.95 (*0-8058-1094-3*) L Erlbaum Assocs.

Carence En Fer Chez la Femme. Thomas H. Bothwell & Robert W. Carlton. Ed. by James D. Cook et al. Tr. by Marc Vicent. 1983. (FRE., Illus.). 136p. (Orig.). pap. text 3.50 (*0-935368-37-X*) ILSI.

Carence En Fer Chez le Nourrisson Et Che L'Enfant. Peter R. Dallman et al. Ed. by Thomas H. Bothwell et al. 1985. (FRE., Illus.). 57p. (Orig.). pap. text 3.50 (*0-935368-45-0*) ILSI.

CarePooling: How to Get the Help You Need to Care for the Ones You Love. Paula C. Lowe. 1993. LC 93-26746. 300p. pap. 14.95 (*1-881052-16-8*) Berrett-Koehler.

Carer's Guide to Good Health. Sheryl Navin et al. 1994. 61p. (Orig.). pap. (*0-85572-207-X*) Hill Content Pubng AUS. *Dist:* Seven Hills Bk.

***Carer's Guide to Schizophrenia.** G. Wilkinson et al. 2nd ed. 2000. 72p. pap. (*1-85315-408-3*) Royal Soc of Medicine Pr Ltd GBR. *Dist:* Balogh.

Carewise for Older Adults: Self-Care for Lifelong Health. 1996. (Illus.). 448p. (Orig.). pap. (*1-886444-02-1*) CareWise.

Carewise Guide: Self-Care from Head to Toe. Acamedica Press Staff. 1995. LC 94-72787. 448p. pap. 19.95 (*1-886444-00-5*) CareWise.

CareWise Guide: Self-Care from Head to Toe. Ed. by Reliance Medical Information, Inc. Staff et al. 2nd rev. ed. 1996. LC 96-83132. (Illus.). 448p. pap. 19.95 (*1-886444-01-3*) CareWise.

Caribbean Contraceptive Prevalence Surveys. St. Kitts Nevis & Tirbani P. Jagdeo. 1985. (*0-916683-16-8*) Intl Plan Parent.

Caribbean Contraceptive Prevalence Surveys-2 Moutserrat. Tirbani P. Jagdeo. 1985. (*0-916683-12-5*) Intl Plan Parent.

Caribbean Medicine Forward to Eden: A Source Book on the Healing Modalities of Guyana, The Caribbean & The Americas. Cwolde Kyte. 1988. (Illus.). 190p. (Orig.). 28.90 (*0-936901-07-1*); pap. 14.90 (*0-936901-06-3*) Ctr Sacred Healing.

Caries Prevention by Domestic Salt Fluoridation. K. Toth. 1984. 248p. (C). (*963-05-3476-2*) Akade Kiado HUN. *Dist:* St Mut.

Caring. Ed. by Gosia M. Brykczynska & Moya Jolley. 1997. LC 97-122198. 224p. pap. (*0-340-66196-8*) E A GBR. *Dist:* Routldge.

Caring: Compassion & Wisdom. Ed. by Gosia M. Brykczynska. 1996. 224p. pap. 38.25 (*1-56593-769-4*, 1496) Thomson Learn.

Caring: The Compassionate Healer. Ed. by Delores A. Gaut & Madeleine M. Leininger. 1991. 16.50 (*0-88737-518-9*) Natl League Nurse.

Caring - An Essential Human Need: Proceedings of the Three National Caring Conferences. Ed. by Madeleine M. Leininger. 1988. LC 87-29577. (Human Care & Health Ser.). 178p. (C). reprint ed. pap. 22.95 (*0-8143-1993-9*) Wayne St U Pr.

Caring & Community: Concepts & Models for Service-Learning in Nursing. Ed. by Jane S. Norbeck et al. 1998. (Service-Learning in the Disciplines Ser.). 208p. pap. 28.50 (*1-56377-009-1*, SLIODS) Am Assn Higher Ed.

Caring & Compassion in Clinical Practice: Issues in the Selection, Training, & Behavior of Helping Professionals. Seymour B. Sarason. 1995. LC 95-3544. (Master Work Ser.). 244p. pap. 40.00 (*1-56821-528-2*) Aronson.

Caring & Curing: Health & Medicine in the Western Religious Traditions. Ed. by Ronald L. Numbers & Darrel W. Amundsen. 1997. LC 97-28500. 622p. reprint ed. pap. text 22.50 (*0-8018-5796-1*) Johns Hopkins.

Caring & Nursing: Explorations in Feminist Perspectives. Ed. by R. Neil & R. Watts. 1990. 275p. pap. 29.95 (*0-88737-501-4*) Natl League Nurse.

Caring & Responsibility: The Crossroads of Holistic Practice & Traditional Medicine. June S. Lowenberg. 1989. LC 88-15067. (Studies in Health, Illness, & Caregiving). (Illus.). 306p. (C). pap. 18.95 (*0-8122-1408-0*); text 42.50 (*0-8122-8174-8*) U of Pa Pr.

Caring Approach in Nursing Administration. Jan J. Nyberg. 1998. LC 97-49688. (Illus.). 288p. 34.95 (*0-87081-478-8*) Univ Pr Colo.

Caring as Healing: Renewal Through Hope. Ed. by Delores A. Gaut & Anne Boykin. 1994. LC 94-5923. 350p. pap. 36.95 (*0-88737-607-X*) Natl League Nurse.

Caring Families: Food Choices. Ed. by Sue N. Butkus. 1997. (Illus.). 206p. reprint ed. pap. text 35.00 (*0-7881-4584-3*) DIANE Pub.

Caring Families: Supports & Interventions. Deborah S. Bass. 1990. LC 90-6277. 281p. pap. text 23.95 (*0-87101-185-9*) Natl Assn Soc Wkrs.

Caring for a Loved One with AIDS: The Experiences of Families, Lovers, & Friends. Marie A. Brown & Gail M. Powell-Cope. 1992. LC 92-2695. (Illus.). 76p. pap. 5.95 (*0-295-97183-5*) U of Wash Pr.

Caring for a Person with Memory Loss & Confusion. Ed. by Mardi Richmond. 1995. (Illus.). 32p. 3.95 (*1-56885-059-X*) Journeyworks Pub.

Caring for America: The Story of Family Practice. John R. Stanard. 1997. LC 97-1850. (*0-89865-992-2*) Donning Co.

Caring for an Alzheimer's Patient: A Family Guide. 1994. (Illus.). 36p. pap. 2.00 (*1-930181-05-1*) A H A F.

Caring for Cambodian Americans: A Mutlidisciplinary Resource for the Helping Professions. Sharon K. Ratliff. 1997. LC 97-33180. (Asian Americans Ser.). 408p. text 89.00 (*0-8153-2989-X*) Garland.

Caring for Cancer Patients: A Handbook for the Home Care Aide. Janet Zhun Nassif. 3rd rev. ed. 1999. iii, 120p. pap. (*1-930304-01-3*) Home Care Univ.

Caring for Children. (*0-340-51840-5*) E A GBR. *Dist:* Routldge.

Caring for Children. Mary Wanda Draper. 2nd ed. 1979. (gr. 9-12). tchr. ed. 33.48 (*0-02-662840-6*); text 45.00 (*0-02-662810-4*); stu. ed. 10.20 (*0-02-662820-1*) Glencoe.

Caring for Children with HIV & AIDS. (*0-340-55256-5*) E A GBR. *Dist:* Routldge.

Caring for Depression. Kenneth B. Wells et al. 1999. 264p. pap. text 19.95 (*0-674-09730-0*); 1996. LC 96-4951. (Illus.). 256p. 44.50 (*0-674-09729-7*) HUP.

Caring for Elderly Parents: Juggling Work, Family & Caregiving in Middle & Working Class Families. Deborah M. Merrill. 1997. LC 96-45347. 248p. 60.00 (*0-86569-269-6*, Auburn Hse) Greenwood.

Caring for Elderly People. Jim Marr. Ed. by Betty Kershaw. 1998. (Illus.). 304p. (Orig.). pap. 32.95 (*1-56593-764-3*, 1486) Singular Publishing.

Caring for Elderly People: A Workbook in Tswana. Francie Lund & Nozizwe Madlala. 1993. (TSW., Illus.). 92p. pap. (*0-86980-899-0*) Univ Natal Pr ZAF. *Dist:* Intl Spec Bk.

Caring for Elderly People: A Workbook in Xhosa. Francie Lund & Nozizwe Madlala. 1993. (XHO., Illus.). 92p. pap. (*0-86980-900-8*) Univ Natal Pr ZAF. *Dist:* Intl Spec Bk.

Caring for Elderly People: A Workbook in Zulu. Francie Lund & Nozizwe Madlala. 1993. (ZUL., Illus.). 92p. pap. (*0-86980-901-6*) Univ Natal Pr ZAF. *Dist:* Intl Spec Bk.

Caring for Frail Elderly People: New Directions in Care. OECD Staff. 1994. LC 94-234147. 143p. (Orig.). pap. 27.00 (*92-64-14160-X*) OECD.

Caring for Health: From Childhood. Derek Fatchett. 1995. pap. text 27.95 (*0-7020-1792-2*) Saunders.

Caring for Health: History & Diversity. Ed. by Charles Webster. 1993. LC 92-45734. (Health & Disease Ser.: Bk. 6). 224p. pap. (*0-335-19118-5*) OpUniv Pr.

Caring for Infants & Toddlers with Disabilities in Family Child Care: Annotated Resource Directory. Children's Foundation Staff. 1995. 44p. pap. text 8.00 (*1-884093-06-X*) Chldrns Fnd.

Caring for Life & Death. Nelda Samarel. 1991. (Death Education, Aging & Health Care Ser.). (Illus.). 160p. 38.95 (*1-56032-124-5*) Hemisp Pub.

Caring for Maria: An Experience of Successfully Coping with Alzheimer's Disease. B. Heywood. 1994. LC 94-25494. 192p. pap. 11.95 (*1-85230-502-9*) Element MA.

Caring for Mental Health in the Future. Scenario Committee on Mental Health and Mental Healt. 1992. (C). pap. text 180.50 (*0-7923-1565-0*) Kluwer Academic.

Caring for Mothers & Newborns. Jetta Fuzy & Kathlene Benson. 1998. (Illus.). 106p. pap. 29.95 (*1-888343-16-8*) Hartman Pub.

***Caring for Muslim Patients.** Ed. by Aziz Sheikh & Abdul Rashid Gatrad. 2000. LC 00-340767. 160p. pap. (*1-85775-372-0*) Radcliffe Med Pr GBR. *Dist:* Balogh.

Caring for Neighbors: An Examination of Non-Resident Use of New York City Hospitals. Melvin I. Krasner. 1993. LC 92-44742. (Papers). 10.00 (*0-934459-67-3*) United Hosp Fund.

Caring for Older Adults: Basic Skills & Concepts. Joan C. Breitung. 1987. (Illus.). 400p. text 32.00 (*0-7216-1576-7*) Saunders.

Caring for Older People. 1998. 352p. pap. 29.00 net. (*0-340-61374-2*) Thomson Learn.

Caring for Older People. Malcolm Geeves & Terry Smith. 1996. LC 97-187339. 180p. pap. (*0-7329-3125-8*) Macmill Educ AUS. *Dist:* Paul & Co Pubs.

Caring for Older People. Smyth. 1997. pap. (*0-333-57053-7*) Macmillan GBR. *Dist:* Trans-Atl Phila, St Martin.

Caring for Older People in a Mixed Economy. Open Learning Foundation Staff. 1996. 146p. pap. (*0-443-05734-6*) Church.

Caring for Older People in the Community. Idris Williams. 3rd ed. 1995. pap. (*1-85775-025-X*) Radcliffe Med Pr GBR. *Dist:* Balogh.

Caring for Our Special Children: Early Intervention Services. Josefina M. Vallarta. 1996. LC 96-92458. (Illus.). x, 276p. (Orig.). pap. 16.95 (*0-9653591-0-7*) Puget Snd.

Caring for Patients: A Critique of the Medical Model. Allen Barbour. 418p. 1997. pap. 25.95 (*0-8047-3153-5*); 1995. LC 94-27113. 66.00 (*0-8047-2389-3*) Stanford U Pr.

Caring for Patients, Caring of Student Nurses. Annette M. Jinks. 1997. LC 97-71716. (Developments in Nursing & Health Care Ser.). (Illus.). 221p. text (*1-85972-549-X*) Ashgate Pub GBR. *Dist:* Ashgate Pub Co.

Caring for Patients from Different Cultures: Case Studies from American Hospitals. Geri-Ann Galanti. 2nd ed. 1997. LC 96-35530. 184p. pap. text 16.95 (*0-8122-1608-3*) U of Pa Pr.

Caring for Patients with the 25 Most Serious, Most Common Disorders: Diabetes Millitus. 1998. LC 98-27919. (Illus.). 224p. (C). (gr. 13). spiral bd. 29.95 (*0-8151-2040-0*, 32017) Mosby Inc.

Caring for People. Jenny Rogers. 1990. 192p. pap. (*0-335-09429-5*) OpUniv Pr.

Caring for People from Birth to Death. James E. Hightower, Jr. enl. rev. ed. 1999. LC 98-47910. (Illus.). xi, 204p. lib. bdg. 39.95 (*0-7890-0571-9*, Haworth Pastrl) Haworth Pr.

Caring for People in Pain. Bryn D. Davis. 2000. LC 99-36130. (Essentials for Nurses Ser.). (Illus.). vi, 256p. pap. 24.99 (*0-415-18891-1*) Routledge.

Caring for People with Alzheimer's Disease: A Training Manual for Direct Care Providers. Gayle Andresen. 1995. LC 94-31057. 208p. pap. 26.95 (*1-878812-22-X*) Hlth Prof Pr.

Caring for People with HIV: A Community Perspective. Surinder Singh & Sara Madge. 1998. LC 98-70993. xii, 204p. pap. text (*1-85742-398-4*); (Illus.). 300p. text (*1-85742-397-6*) Ashgate Pub GBR. *Dist:* Ashgate Pub Co.

Caring for People with Multiple Disabilities: An Interdisciplinary Guide for Caregivers. Cindy French. 1998. 145p. pap. text 36.00 (*0-12-784555-0*) Acad Pr.

Caring for People with Physical Impairment: The Journey Back. Group for the Advancement of Psychiatry Staff. 1993. LC 92-22055. (GAP Reports: No. 135). 178p. text 14.95 (*0-87318-203-0*, 7203) Am Psychiatric.

Caring for People with Severe Mental Disorders: A National Plan of Research to Improve Services. 1993. 80p. (Orig.). (C). pap. text 35.00 (*1-56806-885-9*) DIANE Pub.

Caring for School Age Children. Click. 1992. (Teaching Methods Ser.). pap., tchr. ed. 14.00 (*0-8273-5412-6*) Delmar.

Caring for School Age Children. Phyllis Click. 1992. 213p. pap. 21.00 (*0-8273-5411-8*) Delmar.

Caring for Someone in Your Home. K. N. Tigges et al. 1992. LC 92-81466. (Illus.). 172p. (Orig.). pap. 11.95 (*0-9633017-0-5*) Mast Hlth Grp.

Caring for the Cardiac Patient. Whitman. 1999. text 85.00 (*0-7216-6036-3*) Harcourt.

Caring for the Chronic Mentally Ill. Ursula C. Gerhart. 1990. LC 89-61482. 319p. (C). pap. text 44.00 (*0-87581-333-X*, CMI) F E Peacock Pubs.

Caring for the Coronary Patient. David R. Thompson & Webster. 2nd ed. 2000. 256p. pap. 50.00 (*0-7506-4315-3*) Buttrwrth-Heinemann.

Caring for the Country: A History & Celebration of the First 150 Years of the American Medical Association. American Medical Association Staff. 1997. (Illus.). 192p. 49.95 (*0-375-50000-6*) Random.

Caring for the Developing Child. Patricia E. Marhoefer & Lisa A. Vadnais. 2nd ed. 1992. (C). mass mkt., tchr. ed. 13.00 (*0-8273-4682-4*); pap. 36.95 (*0-8273-4681-6*) Delmar.

Caring for the Developing Child Workbook. Patricia E. Marhoefer. 2nd ed. 1992. (C). pap. 13.00 (*0-8273-4902-5*) Delmar.

Caring for the Diabetic Soul: Restoring Emotional Balance for Yourself & Your Family. Hope Warshaw. 1997. LC 97-7990. (Diabetes Forecast Book Ser.). 213p. pap. 9.95 (*0-945448-81-3*, 4815-01) Am Diabetes.

Caring for the Disabled Elderly: Who Will Pay? Alice M. Rivlin & Joshua M. Wiener. 1988. LC 88-10528. 318p. pap. text 16.95 (*0-8157-7497-4*) Brookings.

Caring for the Dying Patient & the Family. J. Robbins & J. E. Moscrop. 3rd ed. 1995. 304p. pap. 49.95 (*1-56593-328-1*, 0658) Singular Publishing.

***Caring for the Dying Patient & Their Family.** Robbins. 1995. pap. 35.95 (*0-412-57840-9*) Chapman & Hall.

Caring for the Elderly at Home: A Policy Perspective on Consumer Experiences with Publicly-Funded Home Care Programs in New York City. Francis G. Caro & Arthur E. Blank. 1987. LC 89-105204. 143p. pap. text 12.00 (*0-88156-052-9*) Comm Serv Soc NY.

Caring for the Exercising Woman. R. Hale. 1991. (Current Topics in Obstetrics & Gynecology Ser.). (Illus.). 160p. (C). (gr. 13). text 71.95 (*0-412-04581-8*) Chapman & Hall.

Caring for the Healing Heart: An Eating Plan for Recovery from Heart Attack. Eleanor Cousins. 1989. pap. 3.95 (*0-380-70744-6*, Avon Bks) Morrow Avon.

Caring for the HIV/AIDS Caregiver. Ed. by Vincent J. Lynch & Paul A. Wilson. 1996. LC 96-15503. 176p. 57.95 (*0-86569-239-4*, Auburn Hse) Greenwood.

Caring for the Mind: The Comprehensive Guide to Mental Health. Dianne Hales et al. 1996. 896p. pap. 26.95 (*0-553-37511-3*) Bantam.

Caring for the Parkinson Patient: A Practical Guide. Ed. by Raye L. Dippel & J. Thomas Hutton. 1989. LC 89-10658. (Golden Age Bks.). (Illus.). 196p. pap. 18.00 (*0-87975-562-8*) Prometheus Bks.

Caring for the Person Recovering from Stroke. Ann Summers. 1999. (Illus.). 81p. pap. 29.95 (*1-888343-27-3*) Hartman Pub.

Caring for the Person with Alzheimer's or Other Dementias. Paula Siciliano. 1995. (In Service Sourcebook Ser.). 72p. pap. text 29.95 (*1-888343-02-8*) Hartman Pub.

Caring for the Person with Alzheimer's or Other Dementias. Paula Siciliano & Charles A. Illian. 2nd rev. ed. 1999. (Illus.). 87p. pap. 29.95 (*1-888343-34-6*) Hartman Pub.

Caring for the Psychogeriatric Client. Priscilla Ebersole. 1990. LC 89-11516. 304p. 35.95 (*0-8261-6420-X*) Springer Pub.

Caring for the Retarded in America: A History. 15. Peter L. Tyor & Leland V. Bell. 1984. LC 84-6575. (Contributions in Medical History Ser.: No. 15). (Illus.). 215p. 60.00 (*0-313-20977-4*, TVS/, Greenwood Pr) Greenwood.

Caring for the Rural Community: An Interdisciplinary Curriculum. Ed. by American Psychological Association Staff. 1995. LC 94-49194. 76p. pap. 14.95 (*1-55798-288-0*) Am Psychol.

Caring for the Sick at Home. Tieneke Van Bentheim et al. 1987. 160p. pap. 12.95 (*0-88010-254-3*) Anthroposophic.

Caring for the Vascular Patient. Lynda M. Herbert. 1997. LC 97-22823. text (*0-443-05423-1*) Church.

Caring for the Working Man: The Rise & Fall of the Dispensary. Ed. by Charles E. Rosenberg. 1989. (Medical Care in the United States Ser.). 250p. reprint ed. text 20.00 (*0-8240-8341-5*) Garland.

Caring for Victims of Torture. Ed. by James M. Jaranson & Michael K. Popkin. 1998. LC 97-50112. 296p. text 24.95 (*0-88048-774-7*, 8774) Am Psychiatric.

Caring for Women through the Life Cycle. Elaine Weil. 1999. Orig. Title: Nursing for Women's Health. (Illus.). 246p. pap. (*1-57801-030-6*) Western Schls.

Caring for Women with Circumcision: A Technical Manual for Health Care Providers. Nahid Toubia. 1999. (Illus.). 96p. pap. (*1-893136-01-9*) RAINBO.

Caring for Your Aging Parents: When Love Is Not Enough. Barbara Deane. 1989. LC 89-62760. 276p. pap. 12.00 (*0-89109-578-0*) NavPress.

Caring for Your Dog. Gary Nowell. (Illus.). 224p. (*0-85493-164-3*) V Gollancz GBR. *Dist:* Trafalgar.

Caring for Your Geriatric Resident: In-Services Based on HCFA's RAI MDS 2.0 Manual. Katherine Vaughn. 2000. (Illus.). 118p. pap. 34.95 (*1-888343-35-4*) Hartman Pub.

Caring for Your Older Cat. Christopher C. Pinney. 1996. LC 95-25360. (Barron's Educational Ser.). pap. 10.95 (*0-8120-9148-5*) Barron.

Caring for Your Sick Cat. Carol A. Himsel. 1994. 192p. pap. 11.95 (*0-8120-1726-9*) Barron.

Caring for Your Wife in Sickness & in Health: A Husband's Guide to Understanding the Special Health Needs of a Woman. Richard H. Dominguez. 1995. LC 94-43736. 224p. 14.99 (*0-929239-68-7*) Discovery Hse Pubs.

Caring from the Heart: AIDS & the Caregiver. Charles A. Illian. 1999. (Illus.). 260p. pap. 29.95 (*1-888343-18-4*) Hartman Pub.

Caring Hands: Planning & Implementing a Caregiver Retreat. Joyce Bryan & Thomas F. Edson. 1995. 63p. (Orig.). pap. 25.00 (*0-9644874-0-3*) Orange Caregiver.

Caring in Crisis: A Handbook of Intervention Skills for Nurses. Bob Wright. 2nd ed. 1993. LC 92-49335. (Orig.). pap. text (*0-443-04599-2*) Church.

Caring in Crisis: An Oral History of Critical Care Nursing. Jacqueline Zalumas. 1994. (Studies in Health, Illness, & Caregiving). 240p. (Orig.). (C). text 39.95 (*0-8122-3255-0*) U of Pa Pr.

Caring in Emergencies. Sandra Mallan. 1992. (Skills for Caring Ser.). (Illus.). 48p. (Orig.). pap. text (*0-443-04622-0*) Church.

Caring Jurisprudence: Listening to Patients at the Supreme Court. Susan M. Behuniak. 1999. LC 99-16198. 224p. pap. 24.95 (*0-8476-9455-0*); 208p. text 65.00 (*0-8476-9454-2*) Rowman.

Caring Physician: The Life of Dr. Francis W. Peabody. Paul Oglesby. 1991. (Illus.). 220p. (C). text 24.95 (*0-674-09738-6*) HUP.

Caring Prescriptions: Comprehensive Health Care Strategies for Young Children in Poverty. Karen N. Bell & Linda S. Simkin. 1993. LC 92-48194. (Illus.). 96p. (Orig.). pap. 8.00 (*0-926582-09-7*) NCCP.

Caring Relationship: Elderly People & Their Families. Alan Walker & Hazel Qureshi. 1989. LC 89-8344. (Health, Society, & Policy Ser.). (C). 37.95 (*0-87722-663-6*) Temple U Pr.

Caring Relationships: The Dying & the Bereaved. Ed. by Richard A. Kalish. 1981. (Perspectives on Death & Dying Ser.: Vol. 2). 160p. (C). pap. 21.95 (*0-89503-010-1*) Baywood Pub.

Caring Services. Bill Clarke. 1992. (Skills for Caring Ser.). (Illus.). 48p. (Orig.). pap. text (*0-443-04527-5*) Church.

Cariology. Ernest Newbrun. 3rd ed. 1989. (Illus.). 389p. text 60.00 (*0-86715-205-2*) Quint Pub Co.

Cariology for the Nineties. Ed. by William H. Bowen & Lawrence A. Tabak. 1993. LC 92-48515. (Illus.). 475p. (C). 90.00 (*1-878822-17-9*) Univ Rochester Pr.

Carl Gustav Jung. Frank McLynn. 1998. 340p. pap. 18.95 (*0-312-19445-5*); 1997. LC 97-12830. 640p. 29.95 (*0-312-15491-7*) St Martin.

Carl Gustav Jung: Critical Assessments, Set. Ed. by Renos Papadopoulos. 1992. LC 92-1044. 1875p. (C). 693.00 (*0-415-04830-3*, A7769) Routledge.

Carl Jung & Soul Psychology. Karen Gibson & Donald Lathrop. 1991.Tr. of Voices: The Art & Science of Psychotherapy. (Orig.). pap. 19.95 (*1-56023-001-0*, Harrington Park) Haworth Pr.

Carl Jung & Soul Psychology. Ed. by Karen Gibson. 1987. LC 86-29497.Tr. of Voices: The Art & Science of Psychotherapy. 192p. (Orig.). reprint ed. text 49.95 (*0-86656-632-5*) Haworth Pr.

Carl Rogers. Brian Thorne. 1992. (Key Figures in Counselling & Psychotherapy Ser.). (Illus.). 160p. (C). pap. 25.95 (*0-8039-8463-4*, 9808) Sage.

Carl Rogers Reader. Ed. by Howard Kirschenbaum & Valerie L. Henderson. 1989. 512p. pap. 17.00 (*0-395-48357-3*) HM.

Carlson Wade's Amino Acids Book. Carlson Wade. 1985. LC 84-80809. (Pivot Original Health Bks.). 144p. pap. 4.50 (*0-87983-372-6*, 33726K, Keats Pubng) McGraw-Hill Trade.

CAR'97 Computer Assisted Radiology & Surgery: Proceedings of the 11th International Symposium & Exhibition, Berlin, Germany, 25-28 June 1997. Ed. by H. U. Lemke et al. 1997. (International Congress Ser.: No. 1134). 1108p. 272.50 (*0-444-82756-0*) Elsevier.

Carnitine: Its Role in Lung & Heart Disorders. Ed. by E. Kaiser. 1987. (Illus.). x, 140p. 58.50 (*3-8055-4438-3*) S Karger.

Carnitine & Its Uses. 1996. lib. bdg. 251.99 (*0-8490-5909-7*) Gordon Pr.

Carnitine Connection. Winifred Conkling. 2000. LC 00-698946. (Illus.). xi, 223p. mass mkt. 5.99 (*0-312-97458-2*, St Martins Paperbacks) St Martin.

Carnitine Defense: A Nutraceutical Formula to Prevent & Treat Heart Disease, the Nation's #1 Killer. Stephen L. DeFelice. 2000. (Illus.). 240p. pap. 14.95 (*1-57954-339-1*, Rodale Reach) Rodale Pr Inc.

Carnitine, Enzymes & Isoenzymes in Disease. Ed. by D. M. Goldberg et al. 1986. (Advances in Clinical Enzymology Ser.: Vol. 4). viii, 190p. 155.75 (*3-8055-4322-0*) S Karger.

Carnitine System: A New Therapeutical Approach to Cardiovascular Diseases, No. 162. Ed. by J. W. De Jong & R. Ferrari. 1995. LC 94-46324. (Developments in Cardiovascular Medicine Ser.: Vol. 162). 400p. text 184.00 (*0-7923-3318-7*) Kluwer Academic.

Carotenoid As Colorants & Vitamin A Precursors: Technological & Nutritional Applications. Ed. by Jack C. Bauerfeind. 1981. LC 80-984. (Food Science & Technology Ser.). text 194.00 (*0-12-082850-2*) Acad Pr.

Carotenoids: Chemistry & Biology. N. I. Krinsky et al. 1989. (Illus.). 390p. (C). text 120.00 (*0-306-43607-8*, Kluwer Plenum) Kluwer Academic.

Carotenoids Vols. 1A & 1B: Isolation & Analysis; Spectroscopy. Ed. by G. Britton et al. 1994. LC 94-40358. (Illus.). 368p. 129.00 (*0-8176-2908-4*) Birkhauser.

Carotic Body Chemoreceptors. Constancio Gonzalez. 1997. (Medical Intelligence Unit Ser.). 250p. pap. 89.95 (*0-412-11501-8*) Chapman & Hall.

Carotid & the Eye. Ed. by Ramon Berguer & Harold Weiss. 1985. LC 85-6336. 223p. 49.95 (*0-275-91332-5*, C1332, Praeger Pubs) Greenwood.

Carotid Artery Disease. Larry J. Robson & Dorothy L. Bouwman. Ed. by Dorothy L. Bouwman & Oliver D. Grin. 1990. (Patient Education Ser.). (Illus.). 26p. (Orig.). pap. text 4.00 (*0-929689-39-9*) Ludann Co.

Carotid Artery Plaques. Ed. by M. Hennerici et al. 1988. viii, 200p. 68.75 (*3-8055-4715-3*) S Karger.

Carotid Artery Surgery. Ed. by Christopher M. Loftus & Timothy F. Kresowik. 1999. LC 99-30338. (Illus.). 379p. 159.00 (*0-86577-769-1*) Thieme Med Pubs.

Carotid Body Chemoreceptors. Constancio Gonzalez. 1997. LC 97-19788. (Medical Intelligence Unit Ser.). 236p. 99.00 (*1-57059-465-1*) Landes Bioscience.

Carotid Endarterectomy: A Practical Guide. Norman L. Browse et al. 1997. LC 97-206421. 144p. text (*0-7506-0530-8*) E A.

Carotid Endarterectomy: Principles & Techniques. Christopher M. Loftus. 1995. 242p. text 130.00 (*0-942219-69-4*) Quality Med Pub.

Carpal Injuries: Anatomy, Radiology, Current Treatment. P. Saffar. 1991. (Illus.). 202p. 227.00 (*0-387-59534-1*) Spr-Verlag.

Carpal Tunnel Syndrome: A Guide for Patients. Robert Belsole. Ed. by David Seligson. 1995. (Orthopedic Ser.). (Illus.). 24p. (Orig.). pap. 2.95 (*1-885274-08-4*) Health InfoNet Inc.

Carpal Tunnel Syndrome: Prevention & Treatment. Kate Montgomery. Ed. by Diane Gage. (Illus.). 1992. 80p. stu. ed. 14.95 (*1-878069-03-9*); 3rd rev. ed. 1994. LC 95-161098. 41p. pap. 16.95 (*1-878069-35-7*) Sports Touch.

Carpal Tunnel Syndrome: Prevention & Treatment. Kate Montgomery. Ed. by Diane Gage. 4th ed. 1996. (Illus.). 117p. (Orig.). pap., wbk. ed. 19.95 (*1-878069-05-5*) Sports Touch.

Carpal Tunnel Syndrome: Prevention, Treatment & Hand Exercises. 1992. lib. bdg. 250.95 (*0-8490-5610-1*) Gordon Pr.

Carpal Tunnel Syndrome: Selected References. 1996. (Illus.). 110p. reprint ed. pap. text 20.00 (*0-7881-2789-6*) DIANE Pub.

Carpal Tunnel Syndrome - Causes, Symptoms, Diagnosis, Treatments & Surgery: Index of New Information Including Complications. American Health Research Institute Staff. 1995. (Illus.). 170p. 57.50 (*0-7883-0350-3*); 1995. (Illus.). 170p. pap. 47.50 (*0-7883-0351-1*); 1996. LC 96-3127. 131p. 57.50 (*0-7883-1102-6*); 1996. LC 96-3127. 131p. pap. 47.50 (*0-7883-1103-4*) ABBE Pubs Assn.

Carpal Tunnel Syndrome & Other Disorders of the Median Nerve. Ochoa. 2001. 415p. 95.00 (*0-7506-7314-1*) Buttrwrth-Heinemann.

Carpal Tunnel Syndrome & Other Disorders of the Median Nerve. Richard B. Rosenbaum & Jose L. Ochoa. 1992. LC 92-49623. 358p. text 115.00 (*0-7506-9229-4*) Buttrwrth-Heinemann.

Carpal Tunnel Syndrome & Repetitive Stress Injuries: The Comprehensive Guide to Prevention, Treatment & Recovery. Tammy Crouch. 2nd ed. 1996. LC 96-8576. (Illus.). 164p. (Orig.). pap. 14.95 (*1-883319-50-1*) Frog Ltd CA.

Carpe Diem: Enjoying Every Day with a Terminal Illness. Edward F. Madden. 1993. (Illus.). 128p. (C). pap. text 19.95 (*0-86720-782-5*, 782-5) Jones & Bartlett.

Carpentier-Edwards Pericardial Bioprosthesis Mini-Symposium. Ed. & Illus. by Silent Partners, Inc. Staff. 1989. 133p. (Orig.). pap. (*1-878353-00-4*) Silent Partners.

Carrier & Bioreactor Red Blood Cells for Drug Delivery & Targeting. DeLoach & Way. 1994. (Advances in the Biosciences Ser.: No. 92). (Illus.). 210p. 165.00 (*0-08-042496-1*, Pergamon Pr) Elsevier.

Carrier State: An Original Anthology. Ed. by Barbara G. Rosenkrantz. 1977. LC 76-40660. (Public Health in America Ser.). (Illus.). reprint ed. 19.95 (*0-405-09870-7*) Ayer.

Carroll County Physicians of the Nineteenth & Early Twentieth Century. Theodore E. Woodward. 1989. (Illus.). 16.00 (*0-9614125-8-5*) Hist Soc Carroll.

Carry on Osteopathy. Susan G. Royle. 1992. 14.95 (*0-533-10176-X*) Vantage.

Cars '99: Computer Assisted Radiology & Surgery: Proceedings of the 13th International Congress & Exhibition, Paris, 23-26 June 1999. Ed. by Heinz U. Lemke. 1999. LC 99-35458. (International Congress Ser.). 1158p. 247.50 (*0-444-50290-4*, Excerpta Medica) Elsevier.

Cars 2000: Computer Assisted Radiology & Surgery: Proceedings of the 14th International Congress & Exhibition, San Francisco, June 28-July 1, 2000. H. U. Lemke. 2000. LC 00-34105. (International Congress Ser.: No. 1214). (Illus.). 1124p. 215.50 (*0-444-50536-9*) Elsevier.

***CARS 2001: Computer Assisted Radiology & Surgery.** Ed. by H. U. Lemke et al. 2001. (International Congress Ser.: Vol. 1230). 1264p. 265.50 (*0-444-50866-X*, Excerpta Medica) Elsevier.

Carvedilol - A Wide Therapeutic Potential in Cardiovascular Syndromes. Ed. by S. H. Taylor & L. Storstein. 1993. (Journal: Vol. 82, Suppl. 3, 1993). (Illus.). iv, 60p. pap. 20.00 (*3-8055-5874-0*) S Karger.

***Casarett & Doull's Toxicology: The Basic Science of Poisons.** Curtis D. Klaassen. 6th ed. 2001. LC 2001-276259. (Illus.). 1275p. text 79.00 (*0-07-134721-6*) McGraw-Hill Prof.

Case Analyses for Abnormal Psychology. Randall E. Osborne et al. 1999. LC 99-39603. 192p. pap. text 24.95 (*0-86377-584-5*) L Erlbaum Assocs.

Case Analyses for Abnormal Psychology: Learning to Look Beyond the Symptoms. Randall E. Osborne et al. 2000. LC 99-39603. 200p. (*0-86377-583-7*) Psychol Pr GBR. *Dist:* Taylor & Francis.

Case Approach to Counseling & Psychotherapy. Gerald Corey. (Psychology-Counseling Ser.). 2nd ed. 1985. LC 85-9683. 320p. (C). pap. 19.50 (*0-534-05262-2*); 4th ed. 1995. LC 95-15146. 364p. pap. 41.95 (*0-534-26580-4*) Brooks-Cole.

Case Approach to Medical-Psychiatric Practice. Antoinette A. Wyszynski & Bernard Wyszynski. 1996. LC 95-24976. 452p. spiral bd. 58.00 (*0-88048-530-2*, 8530) Am Psychiatric.

Case Atlas of Gastroenterology. J. Thomas Danzi & Silviu Landman. 1995. (Illus.). 335p. 129.00 (*0-683-02366-7*) Lppncott W & W.

Case-Based Telematic Systems: Equity in Health Care. Ed. by Roger France et al. 1994. LC 94-7752. (Studies in Health Technology & Informatics: Vol. 14). 207p. 93.00 (*90-5199-182-7*) IOS Press.

***Case-Book of John Hunter FRS.** Elizabeth Allen et al. 1993. (History of Medicine Ser.). 700p. (*1-85315-203-X*) Royal Soc of Medicine Pr Ltd GBR. *Dist:* Balogh.

Case Books of John Hunter, FRS. Ed. by Elizabeth Allen et al. 1993. (Illus.). 699p. 148.00 (*1-85070-542-9*, Parthenon Pbng) CRC Pr.

Case Commentaries in Obstetrics & Gynecology. P. N. Baker et al. 1997. (Illus.). 265p. pap. text (*0-7020-2235-7*) W B Saunders GBR. *Dist:* Saunders.

Case Conceptualization & Treatment Planning: Exercises for Integrating Theory with Clinical Practice. Pearl S. Berman. 1997. LC 96-51275. 272p. 81.95 (*0-7619-0214-7*, 2091); pap. 39.95 (*0-7619-0215-5*, 2092) Sage.

Case Control Studies: Design, Conduct, Analysis. James J. Schlesselman & Paul D. Stolley. 1982. (Monographs in Epidemiology & Biostatistics: No. 2). (Illus.). 350p. (C). text 39.95 (*0-19-502933-X*) OUP.

Case Development Problems in Hematology: Ser. 1, the Red Cell, Problems 1-8. John W. Harris & Daniel L. Horrigan. 1963. LC 63-6774. (Commonwealth Fund Publications). (Illus.). 204p. pap. 7.95 (*0-674-09850-1*) HUP.

Case Files in Anesthesia: Medical-Legal Issues. RiskCare Staff. 2000. 70p. pap. 150.00 (*1-893929-12-4*) RiskCare.

Case for Intravenous EDTA Chelation Therapy. Martin Dayton. 1995. pap. 12.00 (*0-9664838-0-4*) Martin Dayton.

Case for Legalizing Drugs. Richard L. Miller. 1991. LC 90-7379. 264p. 35.00 (*0-275-93459-4*, C3459, Praeger Pubs) Greenwood.

Case for New Paradigms in Cell Biology & in Neurobiology. Harold Hillman. 1991. LC 91-29811. (Illus.). 356p. lib. bdg. 99.95 (*0-7734-9690-4*) E Mellen.

Case for Physician-Assisted Suicide. Sheila Mclean & Alison Britton. 1997. LC 98-212243. (Pandora Soap Box Ser.). 128p. pap. (*0-04-440983-4*) Rivers Oram GBR. *Dist:* NYU Pr.

Case Histories: How One-Hundred People Lost Twenty-Five or More Pounds. Charles F. Sexauer. Ed. by Health Services Group Staff. 1981. pap. 8.95 (*0-9607148-1-2*) C F Sexauer.

Case Histories in Human Physiology. Donna M. Van Wynsberghe & Gregory M. Cooley. 2nd ed. 1995. 144p. (C). spiral bd. 27.81 (*0-697-13791-0*) McGrw-H Hghr Educ.

***Case Histories in Human Physiology.** Donna M. Van Wynsberghe & Gregory M. Cooley. 3rd ed. 1997. (C). 25.00 (*0-07-303865-2*) McGrw-H Hghr Educ.

Case Histories in Infectious Diseases. Nick J. Beeching & J. Cheesbrough. 1993. (Illus.). 35.00 (*0-7234-1799-7*) Mosby Inc.

Case Histories in Rheumatology. Lesley Hordon & A. Isdale. 1994. 23.00 (*0-7234-1962-0*) Mosby Inc.

Case Histories of Professional Liability Losses. John P. Bachner. 1996. (Orig.). pap. (*1-58074-055-3*) ASFE.

Case Law in Health Care Administration. George D. Pozgar & Nina Santuzzi Pozgar. 2nd ed. 1998. LC 98-44120. 228p. pap. 46.00 (*0-8342-1204-8*, 12048) Aspen Pub.

Case Management: A Dynamic Process. Ed. by Debbie K. Kozeny et al. unabr. ed. 1996. (Illus.). 134p. (Orig.). pap. text 35.00 (*0-935890-02-5*, P27) Emerg Nurses IL.

Case Management: A Guide to Strategic Evaluation. Gerri Lamb et al. 1998. 256p. (C). ring bd. 59.95 (*0-323-00086-X*) Mosby Inc.

Case Management: Meeting the Needs of Women with HIV/AIDS. Leslie R. Wolfe et al. 1996. 12p. (Orig.). pap. 5.00 (*1-877966-31-2*) Ctr Women Policy.

Case Management by Nurses. Kathleen A. Bower. 1992. 80p. pap. 17.95 (*1-55810-073-3*, NS-32) Am Nurses Pub.

Case Management for Healthcare Professionals. Ed. by Rufus S. Howe. 1994. LC 93-83247. 211p. pap. 44.95 (*0-944496-37-7*) Precept Pr.

Case Management for Mentally Ill Patients: Theory & Practice. Ed. by Maxine Harris & Helen Bergman. 1993. LC 92-42246. 296p. text 48.00 (*3-7186-0565-1*) Gordon & Breach.

Case Management for Straight Chiropractors. Joseph B. Strauss. 2nd ed. 1993. 246p. (C). text 26.00 (*1-890419-05-2*) Fnd Chiropractic Educ.

Case Management Handbook. Cindy Ling. 1999. 250p. (C). ring bd. 97.95 (*1-56930-080-1*) Delmar.

Case Management in Community Care. David Challis & Bleddyn Davies. 1989. 289p. pap. text (*0-566-05816-2*) Arena GBR. *Dist:* Ashgate Pub Co.

Case Management in Healthcare: A Practical Guide. Peggy G. Rossi. Ed. by Tim Eoyang. 1998. LC 98-9757. (Illus.). 416p. (C). pap. text 39.95 (*0-7216-7175-6*) Saunders.

Case Management in Mental Health Services. Ed. by Charlotte J. Sanborn. 1983. LC 82-15495. 198p. text 49.95 (*0-86656-109-9*) Haworth Pr.

Case Management Practice Guidelines. Margaret St. Coeur. 1998. (Illus.). 160p. (C). text, suppl. ed. (*0-323-00225-0*) Mosby Inc.

Case Management Resource Guide, Set. Ed. by Kevin F. O'Grady et al. 1999. 4147p. pap. 225.00 (*1-880874-33-4*) Dorland Hlthcare.

Case Management Resource Guide Vol. 1: Eastern U. S. Ed. by Kevin F. O'Grady et al. 1998. 986p. pap. 60.00 (*1-880874-34-2*) Dorland Hlthcare.

Case Management Resource Guide Vol. 2: Southern U. S. Ed. by Kevin F. O'Grady et al. 1998. 1180p. pap. 60.00 (*1-880874-35-0*) Dorland Hlthcare.

Case Management Resource Guide Vol. 3: Midwestern U. S. Ed. by Kevin F. O'Grady et al. 1998. 1123p. pap. 60.00 (*1-880874-36-9*) Dorland Hlthcare.

Case Management Resource Guide Vol. 4: Western U. S. Ed. by Kevin F. O'Grady et al. 1998. 858p. pap. 60.00 (*1-880874-37-7*) Dorland Hlthcare.

***Case Manager's Desk Reference.** Aspen Health and Science Staff & Fran Snowden. 2nd ed. 2001. LC 2001-22444. (Illus.). 400p. pap. 75.00 (*0-8342-2042-3*, 9111124996) Aspen Pub.

Case Manager's Guide: Acquiring the Skills for Success. Alice Easterling et al. 1995. 203p. pap. 56.00 (*1-55648-148-9*, 027104) AHPI.

Case Manager's Handbook. Catherine M. Mullahy. 2nd ed. 1998. LC 98-5033. 448p. 59.00 (*0-8342-1073-8*, 10738) Aspen Pub.

Case Manager's Sourcebook: A Guide to Designing & Implementing a Centralized Case Management Sourcebook. Cherilyn G. Murer. 1997. LC 97-12459. (HFMA Healthcare Financial Management Ser.). 280p. 60.00 (*0-7863-1221-1*, Irwn Prfssnl) McGraw-Hill Educ Grp.

Case Manager's Survival Guide: Winning Strategies for Clinical Practice. Toni G. Cesta et al. 1997. LC 99-208413. (Illus.). 288p. (C). (gr. 13). pap. text 32.95 (*0-8151-1771-X*, 30312) Mosby Inc.

***Case of Chronic Neglect: Education & Training of Health Professionals on Family Violence.** Ed. by Institute of Medicine Staff. 2001. 300p. 39.95 (*0-309-07431-2*) Natl Acad Pr.

Case of Sigmund Freud: Medicine & Identity at the Fin de Siecle. Sander L. Gilman. 1994. 320p. reprint ed. pap. text 18.95 (*0-8018-4974-8*) Johns Hopkins.

Case Presentation in Clinical Tuberculosis. Peter D. O. Davies & Peter Ormerod. 1999. LC 99-22798. (An Arnold Publication). (Illus.). 328p. pap. (*0-340-74159-7*) E A GBR. *Dist:* OUP.

Case Presentations for the MRCS & AFRCS, Vol. 2. Philip Hornick et al. 1997. 176p. pap. text (*0-7506-3258-5*) E A GBR. *Dist:* OUP.

Case Presentations for the MRCS & the AFRCS, Vol. 1. Philip Hornick et al. 1997. LC 97-187323. 192p. pap. text (*0-7506-3257-7*) E A GBR. *Dist:* OUP.

Case Presentations for the MRCS & the AFRCS, Vol. 3. Ed. by Philip Hornick et al. 1997. (Case Presentations for the Mrcs & the Afrcs Ser.: Vol. 3). 208p. pap. text (*0-7506-3259-3*) E A GBR. *Dist:* OUP.

Case Presentations in Accident & Emergency Medicine. Francis Morris et al. 1992. LC 92-49711. 192p. pap. text (*0-7506-1378-5*) E A GBR. *Dist:* OUP.

Case Problems in Management & Organizational Behavior. Randall S. Schuler et al. Ed. by Fenton. 4th ed. 1991. (SWC-Management). 437p. (C). mass mkt. 33.75 (*0-314-66805-5*) West Pub.

Case Profiles in Respiratory Care. William A. French. 1995. LC 95-9196. (Health & Life Science Ser.). 288p. (C). mass mkt. 34.95 (*0-8273-6684-1*) Delmar.

Case Records of the Massachusetts General Hospital. Andrew E. Rosenberg. 1995. 700.00 (*1-56815-028-8*) Mosby Inc.

Case Reports I: Clinical Studies in Extracorporeal Circulation. Ed. by J. M. Toomasian et al. 1994. (Orig.). pap. text 50.00 (*0-9643233-0-3*) Perfusion Res.

Case Studies for Family Nurse Practitioners. Joyce D. Cappiello & Jeffrey A. Eaton. 1998. LC 98-11267. (Illus.). 360p. (C). (gr. 13). pap. text 39.95 (*0-8151-1559-8*, 31762) Mosby Inc.

Case Studies for Interpreting the MMPI-A. Yossef S. Ben-Porath & Daniel L. Davis. 1996. LC 96-30416. 230p. pap. 25.95 (*0-8166-2729-0*) U of Minn Pr.

Case Studies from Primary Health Care Settings. Ed. by Marie L. Talashek et al. 1998. LC 97-52764. (Illus.). 312p. pap. 32.00 (*0-07-105487-1*) McGraw-Hill Prof.

Case Studies in Abnormal Psychology. Thomas F. Oltmanns et al. 5th ed. 1998. LC 98-35239. 416p. pap. 38.95 (*0-471-25216-6*) Wiley.

Case Studies in Autism: A Young Child & Two Adolescents. Cheryl D. Seifert. 1990. 130p. (C). lib. bdg. 45.50 (*0-8191-7722-9*) U Pr of Amer.

***Case Studies in Benign Prostatic Hyperplasia.** Jerry G. Blaivas. 2001. (Illus.). 144p. pap. (*1-901865-62-2*) Isis Med GBR. *Dist:* Bks Intl VA.

Case Studies in Child & Adolescent Counseling. Larry Golden. 2nd ed. 1997. LC 97-35617. 176p. (C). pap. text 34.00 (*0-13-716291-X*) P-H.

Case Studies in Child & Adolescent Psychopathology. Robin K. Morgan. 1998. LC 98-27727. xii, 123p. pap. text 25.40 (*0-13-079604-2*) P-H.

Case Studies in Clinical Anatomy. Stuart W. McDonald. 1995. 74p. (gr. 13). 20.00 (*0-7234-2202-8*, QM23) Mosby Inc.

Case Studies in Clinical Examination. Owen Epstein et al. 2nd ed. 1998. text 14.95 (*0-7234-2579-5*) Mosby Inc.

Case Studies in Communication & Disenfranchisement: Social Health Issues & Implications. Ed. by Eileen B. Ray. 1996. (LEA's Communication Ser.). 294p. text 59.95 (*0-8058-1674-7*); pap. text 29.95 (*0-8058-1675-5*) L Erlbaum Assocs.

Case Studies in Community Health Nursing: A Problem-Based Learning Approach. Juliann G. Sebastian & Marcia Stanhope. 1998. 224p. tchr. ed. (*0-323-00574-8*); LC 98-37371. x, 214p. text 29.95 (*0-323-00260-9*) Mosby Inc.

Case Studies in Couple & Family Therapy: Systemic & Cognitive Perspectives. Ed. by Frank M. Dattilio. 1998. LC 97-40877. (Guilford Family Therapy Ser.). 486p. 50.00 (*1-57230-297-6*, C0297) Guilford Pubns.

Case Studies in Cultural Diversity: A Workbook. Vernice D. Ferguson. 1997. LC 97-46651. 15.95 (*0-88737-728-9*, 14-7289, NLN Pr) Natl League Nurse.

Case Studies in Depression: Based on the Edgar Cayce Health Methods. David McMillin. 1997. LC 97-11151. (Edgar Cayce Health Ser.). 152p. (Orig.). pap. 14.95 (*0-87604-385-6*, 497) ARE Pr.

Case Studies in Emergency Medicine & the Health of the Public. Edward Bernstein & Judith Bernstein. 1996. LC 96-1930. (Medical Ser.). (Illus.). 352p. (C). pap. text 56.95 (*0-7637-0029-0*, 0029-0) Jones & Bartlett.

Case Studies in Emergency Medicine for the House Officer. Lidia Pousada et al. 1993. LC 92-48917. (Illus.). 244p. 20.00 (*0-683-06966-7*) Lppncott W & W.

Case Studies in Endocrinology, Diabetes, & Metabolism: A Problem-Oriented Approach. Matthew J. Neal. 1996. LC 95-32574. (Illus.). 248p. 39.50 (*0-89640-297-5*) Igaku-Shoin.

Case Studies in Environmental Health & Safety. 1990. 106p. pap. 35.00 (*0-913359-54-8*) APPA VA.

Case Studies in General & Systematic Pathology. J. C. Underwood et al. 1996. (Illus.). 178p. pap. (*0-443-05096-1*) Church.

Case Studies in General Surgery: Problem-Oriented Learning. John B. Herrmann & Michael D. Wertheimer. 1988. 288p. pap. text 20.00 (*0-683-03967-9*) Lppncott W & W.

Case Studies in Health Care Supervision. Charles R. McConnell. 1998. LC 98-20876. 288p. pap. 35.00 (*0-8342-1133-5*, 11335) Aspen Pub.

Case Studies in Health Communication. Ed. by Eileen B. Ray. 1993. (Communication Textbooks, Applied Communication Subseries). 328p. (C). pap. 29.95 (*0-8058-1109-5*); text 79.95 (*0-8058-1108-7*) L Erlbaum Assocs.

Case Studies in Immunology. Rosen. 1998. pap. text 23.00 (*0-443-05725-7*) Saunders.

Case Studies in Immunology: A Clinical Companion. Fred S. Rosen & Raif Geha. 2nd ed. 1996. LC 98-46006. (Illus.). 134p. pap. text 24.95 (*0-8153-2174-0*) Garland.

***Case Studies in Incontinence.** Jerry G. Blaivas. 2001. (Illus.). 144p. pap. (*1-901865-61-4*) Isis Med GBR. *Dist:* Bks Intl VA.

Case Studies in Insomnia. Peter J. Hauri. 1991. (Critical Issues in Psychiatry Ser.). (Illus.). 268p. (C). text 49.50 (*0-306-43791-0*, Kluwer Plenum) Kluwer Academic.

Case Studies in Law & Nursing: A Course Book for Project 2000 Training. Young. 1992. 278p. pap. 47.75 (*1-56593-034-7*, 0282) Thomson Learn.

Case Studies in Medical Ethics. Robert M. Veatch. 1980. 437p. pap. 22.50 (*0-674-09932-X*) HUP.

Case Studies in Medicine for the Elderly. S. C. Allen et al. 1987. pap. text 73.50 (*0-85200-698-5*) Kluwer Academic.

Case Studies in Music Therapy. Ed. by Kenneth E. Bruscia. 1991. 656p. (C). pap. text 40.00 (*0-9624080-1-8*) Barcelona Pubs.

***Case Studies in Natural Medicine.** Melvyn R. Werbach. 2002. 350p. text 49.95 (*1-891710-02-8*); cd-rom 49.95 (*1-891710-03-6*) Third Line Pr.

Case Studies in Neuropsychological Rehabilitation. Barbara A. Wilson. 1998. LC 98-23697. (Illus.). 400p. text 39.50 (*0-19-506598-0*) OUP.

Case Studies in Neuroscience. Ralph F. Jozefowicz & Robert G. Holloway. 1999. LC 98-48503. (Illus.). 230p. (C). pap. text 26.95 (*0-8036-0304-5*) Davis Co.

Case Studies in Neurosurgery for the House Officer. Ed. by Robert Solomon. 1989. (House Officer Ser.). 250p. pap. text 20.00 (*0-683-07858-5*) Lppncott W & W.

Case Studies in Non-Directive Play Therapy. Virginia Ryan & Kate Wilson. 1996. 258p. pap. text (*0-7020-1830-9*) W B Saunders GBR. *Dist:* Saunders.

***Case Studies in Nursing Ethics.** Veatch & Fry. 2nd ed. 1995. (Illus.). 336p. (C). pap. text 42.95 (*0-86720-481-8*, 481.8) Jones & Bartlett.

Case Studies in Nursing Ethics. Sara T. Fry & Robert M. Veatch. 3rd ed. 2000. LC 00-22091. (Illus.). 416p. (C). pap. text 42.95 (*0-7637-1333-3*, 1333-3) Jones & Bartlett.

Case Studies in Occupational Epidemiology. Ed. by Kyle Steenland. 1992. LC 92-6175. (Illus.). 224p. text 38.50 (*0-19-506831-9*) OUP.

Case Studies in Occupational Health Practice. C. Elding & H. A. Waldron. 2000. (Illus.). 160p. pap. text (*0-7506-4470-2*) E A GBR. *Dist:* OUP.

Case Studies in Pathology. Stevens. 1994. text (*0-7234-2196-X*) Wolfe Publishing GBR. *Dist:* Mosby Inc.

Case Studies in Pediatric Surgery. R. Lawrence Moss et al. 2000. 416p. (C). pap. 75.00 (*0-8385-1548-7*) McGraw-Hill Prof.

Case Studies in Psychology. Ed. by Robert M. Berne & Matthew N. Levy. 1994. (Illus.). 224p. (C). (gr. 13). pap. text 20.00 (*0-8151-0544-4*, 24349) Mosby Inc.

Case Studies in Psychotherapies. Ed. by Danny Wedding & Raymond J. Corsini. 3rd ed. 2000. LC 00-134166. xii, 246p. (C). pap. text 32.00 (*0-87581-437-9*) F E Peacock Pubs.

Case Studies in Public & Community Health. Jo Fairbanks & Judith Candelaria. 1998. LC 98-8878. viii, 79p. pap. 26.95 (*0-7619-1405-6*, 82368) Sage.

Case Studies in Public Health Ethics. Ed. by Steven S. Coughlin et al. 1997. LC 97-76770. 182p. (Orig.). pap., tchr. ed. 37.00 (*0-87553-232-2*) Am Pub Health.

Case Studies in Rehabilitation. Patricia A. Ghikas & Michele Clopper. 2000. LC 00-49691. (Illus.). 113p. pap. text 29.00 (*1-55642-425-6*) SLACK Inc.

Case Studies in Rehabilitation Instructor's Manual. Patricia A. Ghikas & Michele Clopper. 2000. LC 00-49691. 80p. pap., tchr. ed. (*1-55642-438-8*) SLACK Inc.

Case Studies in Reproductive Endocrinology. Shahla Nader. 2000. (Arnold Publication). 240p. pap. 35.00 (*0-340-75963-1*) OUP.

Case Studies in Schizophrenia. David McMillin. 1997. LC 97-3237. (Edgar Cayce Health Ser.). 292p. (Orig.). pap. 14.95 (*0-87604-382-1*, 494) ARE Pr.

Case Studies in Sex Therapy. Raymond C. Rosen & Sandra R. Leiblum. 1995. LC 94-49590. 400p. 47.00 (*0-89862-848-2*, C2848) Guilford Pubns.

Case Studies in Sport Psychology. Bob Rotella et al. 1997. LC 97-9654. (Health Science Ser.). (Illus.). 224p. (C). pap. text 31.95 (*0-7637-0355-9*, 0355-9) Jones & Bartlett.

Case Studies in the Neuropsychology of Reading. Elaine Funnell. 2000. 240p. 44.95 (*0-86377-558-6*) L Erlbaum Assocs.

***Case Studies in the Neuropsychology of Vision.** Glyn W. Humphreys. 2001. 336p. pap. (*0-86377-896-8*) Psychol Pr GBR. *Dist:* Taylor & Francis.

Case Studies in Transfusion Medicine. Lynn Hoffstadter et al. 1992. 35.00 (*0-89189-311-3*, 35-6-001-00) Am Soc Clinical.

Case Studies Through the Health Care Continuum: A Workbook for the Occupational Therapy Student. Patricia Halloran & Nancy Lowenstein. 2000. LC 00-26537. (Illus.). 323p. (C). pap. text 30.00 (*1-55642-405-1*) SLACK Inc.

Case Study & Computing: Advanced Qualitative Methods in the Study of Human Behavior. Robert W. Lawler & Kathleen Carley. 1996. (Illus.). 290p. pap. 65.00 (*1-56750-132-X*, Ablex) Greenwood.

Case Study Workbook. 1995. pap., wbk. ed. 34.95 (*0-923369-26-0*) MedBooks.

Case Workbook in Personality. Robert W. White et al. 1982. 259p. (C). pap. text, wbk. ed. 19.95 (*0-917974-80-8*) Waveland Pr.

Casebase in Pediatric Radiology: "The Baby Minnie of Pediatric Radiology" Joanna J. Seibert & Charles A. James. 1997. LC 97-25643. (*3-13-107891-X*) G Thieme DEU. *Dist:* Thieme Med Pubs.

Casebase in Pediatric Radiology Casebase. Joanna J. Seibert. 1998. LC 97-25643. (Illus.). 633p. pap. 69.00 (*0-86577-697-0*) Thieme Med Pubs.

Casebook for Herfindal & Gourley's Textbook of Therapeutics: Drug & Disease Management. Donna Schroeder. 6th ed. 1996. 173p. pap., tchr. ed. (*0-683-18089-4*) Lppncott W & W.

Casebook for Herfindal & Gourley's Textbook of Therapeutics: Drug & Disease Management. Dick R. Gourley & Greta Gourley. 7th ed. 2000. LC 00-42813. xviii, 428p. pap. text 35.00 (*0-7817-2415-5*) Lppncott W & W.

Casebook in Abnormal Psychology. John Vitkus. 2nd ed. 1992. LC 92-49349. (C). pap. text 19.50 net. (*0-07-006546-2*) McGraw.

Casebook in Abnormal Psychology. Timothy A. Brown & David H. Barlow. 2nd rev. ed. 2000. LC 00-49402. (Psychology Ser.). (Illus.). 352p. pap. text 43.95 (*0-534-36316-4*) Brooks-Cole.

Casebook in Abnormal Psychology: An Integrative Approach. Timothy A. Brown & David H. Barlow. 1996. LC 96-28116. (Psychology Ser.). 334p. (C). mass mkt. 25.95 (*0-534-34247-7*) Brooks-Cole.

Casebook in Abnormal Psychology: From the Files of Experts. Ed. by Richard P. Halgin & Susan K. Whitbourne. 1998. LC 97-9227. 304p. (C). pap. text 29.95 (*0-19-509298-8*) OUP.

Casebook in Child Behavior Disorders. Kearney. 1998. LC 98-29815. (Psychology Ser.). 331p. pap. text 31.95 (*0-534-34643-X*) Brooks-Cole.

Casebook in Social & Behavioral Pharmacy. Ed. by Mickey C. Smith et al. 1987. LC 86-51242. ix, 187p. pap. text 2.00 (*0-9606488-6-0*) H W Bks.

Casebook of Child & Pediatric Psychology. Ed. by Michael C. Roberts & C. Eugene Walker. 1989. LC 88-37197. 468p. 55.00 (*0-89862-739-7*, 2739) Guilford Pubns.

Casebook of Child Psychotherapy: Strategies & Techniques. Shirley Cooper & Leon R. Wanerman. 1993. LC 93-31139. (Master Work Ser.). 272p. pap. 40.00 (*1-56821-116-3*) Aronson.

Casebook of Clinical Hypnosis. Ed. by Steven J. Lynn et al. 1996. LC 96-11150. 429p. 49.95 (*1-55798-365-8*) Am Psychol.

***Casebook of Cognitive Therapy for Psychosis.** Ed. by Tony Morrison. 2001. LC 2001-35706. (*1-58391-205-3*) Brunner-Routledge.

Casebook of Forensic Detection: How Science Solved 100 of the World's Most Baffling Crimes. Colin Evans. 1996. LC 95-26002. 320p. 24.95 (*0-471-07650-3*) Wiley.

Casebook of Marital Therapy. Ed. by Alan S. Gurman. 1991. LC 85-9778. (Guilford Family Therapy Ser.). 392p. pap. 21.95 (*0-89862-466-5*) Guilford Pubns.

Casebook of Medical Ethics. Terrence F. Ackerman & Carson Strong. 1989. 264p. pap. text 27.50 (*0-19-503917-3*) OUP.

Casebook of Systemic Family Therapy. Michael E. Kerr. (*1-56821-010-8*) Aronson.

Casebook of the Brief Psychotherapies. Ed. by R. A. Wells & V. J. Giannetti. 1993. (Applied Clinical Psychology Ser.). (Illus.). 410p. (C). pap. 42.50 (*0-306-44393-7*); 75.00 (*0-306-44392-9*) Perseus Pubng (Plenum Trade).

Casebook on the Termination of Life-Sustaining Treatment & the Care of the Dying. Ed. by Cynthia B. Cohen. 1988. LC 88-45101. (Medical Ethics Ser.). 176p. (Orig.). 25.00 (*0-253-31321-X*); pap. 4.25 (*0-253-21207-3*) Ind U Pr.

Cases & Select Readings in Health Care Marketing. Ed. by Robert Sweeney et al. 1989. LC 88-16033. (Series in Marketing & Health Services Administration: No. 2). 351p. text 59.95 (*0-86656-429-2*) Haworth Pr.

Cases in Cardiology. Buckley & Gimple. 1997. audio compact disk 99.00 (*0-7872-4549-6*) Kendall-Hunt.

Cases in Chemical Pathology: A Diagnostic Approach. R. N. Walmsley et al. 1994. 464p. pap. text 28.00 (*981-02-1068-X*); 3rd ed. 1994. 464p. text 78.00 (*981-02-1067-1*); 4th ed. 1999. 300p. 68.00 (*981-02-4034-1*); 4th ed. 1999. 300p. pap. 32.00 (*981-02-4035-X*) World Scientific Pub.

Cases in Developmental Psychology & Psychopathology. Robert G. Meyer. 1989. 410p. pap. text 28.00 (*0-205-11907-7*, H19078) Allyn.

Cases in Healthcare Finance. Louis C. Gapenski. 1999. LC 99-41176. 200p. pap. 75.00 (*1-56793-113-8*) Health Admin Pr.

Cases in Long-Term Care Management Vol. II: Leadership Challenges in Managing Change. Ed. by Donna L. Infeld & John R. Kress. 1995. 310p. (C). pap. text 44.00 (*1-56793-033-6*, 0965) Health Admin Pr.

Cases in Medical Microbiology & Infectious Diseases. Peter H. Gilligan et al. 2nd ed. 1997. LC 96-40181. (Illus.). 350p. 39.95 (*1-55581-106-X*) ASM Pr.

Cases in Neurogenic Communicative Disorders: A Workbook. James P. Dworkin & David E. Hartman. 2nd ed. 1993. LC 93-30762. (Illus.). 416p. (Orig.). (C). pap. text, wbk. ed. 55.00 (*1-56593-264-1*, 0586) Thomson Learn.

Cases in Neurogenic Communicative Disorders: A Workbook & Audio Tape Set: & Aphasia, Apraxia of Speech, & Dysarthria Samples: Audiotape, Manual & Test Stimuli. James P. Dworkin & David E. Hartman. 2nd ed. 1993. (Illus.). 428p. (Orig.). (C). pap., wbk. ed. 65.00 (*1-56593-310-9*, 0602) Thomson Learn.

Cases in Pathology: A Clinical Approach for Students. Nancy Standler & Bernard Klionsky. 1991. (Illus.). 242p. (Orig.). pap. text (*0-443-08759-8*) Church.

Cases, Materials & Problems on Bioethics & Law. Michael H. Shapiro & Roy G. Spece, Jr. 1981. LC 80-28699. (American Casebook Ser.). 892p. (C). 65.00 (*0-8299-2134-6*) West Pub.

Casework: A Psychosocial Therapy. M. E. Woods & Florence Hollis. 4th ed. 1990. 550p. (C). text 79.06 (*0-07-557294-X*) McGrw-H Hghr Educ.

Casework: A Psychosocial Therapy. Florence Hollis & Mary E. Woods. 5th ed. 1999. LC 99-28076. 696p. text 80.94 (*0-07-290179-9*) McGrw-H Hghr Educ.

Cash's Textbook of Orthopaedics & Rheumatology for Physiotherapists. Patricia A. Downie. 1984. LC 65-73208. text 19.75 (*0-397-58293-5*, Lippnctt) Lppncott W & W.

Cast Manual for Adults & Children. F. Freuler et al. Tr. by P. A. Casey from GER. 1979. (Illus.). 38.95 (*0-387-09590-X*) Spr-Verlag.

Cast the First Stone: Ethics in Analytic Practice. Ed. by Lena B. Ross & Manisha Roy. 1995. LC 94-40573. 168p. (Orig.). pap. 16.95 (*0-933029-89-6*) Chiron Pubns.

Casting Nets & Testing Specimens: Two Grand Methods of Psychology. Philip J. Runkel. 1990. LC 89-48665. 208p. 60.00 (*0-275-93533-7*, C3533, Greenwood Pr) Greenwood.

Castle Connolly Guide: How to Find the Best Doctors for You & Your Family in the New York Metro Area. John J. Connolly. Ed. by Sue Berkman & Sandra Beach. 1993. LC 93-72954. (Illus.). 608p. pap. 21.95 (*1-883769-59-0*) Castle Connolly Med.

C D

Castration of Oedipus: Psychoanalysis, Postmodernism, & Feminism. J.C. Smith & Carla J. Ferstman. 1996. LC 95-41726. (Illus.). 336p. (C). pap. text 19.50 (*0-8147-8019-9*) NYU Pr.

Casualties of Progress: Personal Histories from the Chemically Sensitive. Ed. by Alison Johnson. 2000. 276p. pap. 14.00 (*0-9675619-0-6*) M C S ME.

Cat: Diseases & Clinical Management Ed. by Robert G. Sherding. 2nd ed. 1994. (Illus.). 2159p. text 279.00 (*0-7216-5936-5*) Saunders.

CAT: Facts about Fantasy. Mary R. Haworth. 1966. LC 65-24643. (Illus.). 322p. text 47.00 (*0-8089-0180-X*, 791940, Grune & Strat) Harcrt Hlth Sci Grp.

Cat Anatomy Slides: A Visual Guide to Dissection. rev. ed. 1990. (C). tchr. ed. 179.00 incl. sl. (*0-9627559-1-5*) Spyglass Pubns.

Cat Care Book. Sheldon L. Gerstenfeld. 2nd rev. ed. 2000. LC 88-39579. 280p. pap. 16.00 (*0-201-09569-6*) Perseus Bks Grp.

Cat Care, Naturally: Celeste Yarnall's Complete Guide to Holistic Health Care for Cats. Celeste Yarnall. 1995. LC 94-39373. (Illus.). 256p. 24.95 (*0-8048-3025-8*) Tuttle Pubng.

Cat First Aid: A Guide to Emergency Treatment & General Health Care. George E. Boyle & Charles L. Blood. Ed. by Ben Watson. 1990. LC 90-50019. (Illus.). 128p. (Orig.). pap. 9.95 (*0-88266-626-6*) Storey Bks.

Cat Musculature: A Photographic Atlas. Gordon M. Greenblatt. 2nd ed. 1981. LC 80-25610. (Illus.). 32p. pap. text 10.00 (*0-226-30656-9*) U Ch Pr.

***Cat Primary Visual Cortex.** Ed. by Alan Peters & Bertram Payne. 2001. LC 2001-93294. (Illus.). 725p. 199.95 (*0-12-552104-9*) Acad Pr.

Cat Repair Book: A Do-It-Yourself Guide for the Cat Owner. Ruth B. James. 1996. (Illus.). 288p. (Orig.). pap. 19.95 (*0-9615114-2-7*) Alpine Pr.

Cataclysms, Crises, & Catastrophes: Psychology in Action. Ed. by Gary R. VandenBos & Brenda K. Bryant. 1987. LC 87-19134. (Master Lectures: Vol. 6). 235p. (Orig.). pap. 24.95 (*0-912704-77-2*) Am Psychol.

Catalog of Chromosome Aberrations in Cancer Felix Mitelman. Ed. by Bertil Johansson & Fredrik Mertens. 5th ed. 1994. LC 94-30796. 4252p. 675.00 (*0-471-11183-X*) Wiley.

Catalog of Human Cancer Genes: Mckusick's Mendelian Inheritance in Man for Clinical & Research Oncologists (ONCO-MIM) John J. Mulvihill. 1999. LC 98-54978. 670p. 150.00 (*0-8018-4799-0*) Johns Hopkins.

Catalog of Prenatally Diagnosed Conditions. David D. Weaver & Ira K. Brandt. 3rd ed. 1999. LC 98-17788. 711p. 130.00 (*0-8018-6044-X*) Johns Hopkins.

***Catalog of Teratogenic Agents.** Thomas H. Shepard. 10th ed. 2001. LC 2001-29349. 680p. 160.00 (*0-8018-6722-3*) Johns Hopkins.

Catalog of the Dental School Library, Set. Ed. by Northwest U Staff & Minnie Organos. 1978. 950.00 (*0-8161-0239-2*, Macmillan Ref) Gale.

Catalog of the Library of the American Hospital Association, Asa S. Bacon Memorial Library, Chicago, Set. American Hospital Association Staff. 1976. 610.00 (*0-8161-1210-X*, Macmillan Ref) Gale.

Catalog of the Menninger Clinic Library Menninger Foundation Staff. 1972. 455.00 (*0-8161-0961-3*, Macmillan Ref) Gale.

Catalogue of Chromosome Aberrations in Cancer. Felix Mitelman. 1983. (Journal: Vol. 36, No. 1-2). (Illus.). 516p. pap. 115.00 (*3-8055-3813-8*) S Karger.

Catalogue of Printed Books in the Wellcome Historical Medical Library, Vol. 1 & 2. rev. ed. 1996. 944p. 200.00 (*1-888262-04-4*) Martino Pubng.

Catalogue of Salmonella First Isolations, 1965-1984. E. Kelterborn. 1987. text 201.00 (*0-89838-832-5*) Kluwer Academic.

Catalogue of Seventeenth Century Printed Books in the National Library of Medicine. Peter Krivatsky. 1999. 1315p. reprint ed. 110.00 (*1-57898-125-5*) Martino Pubng.

Catalogue of Sixteenth Century Printed Books in the National Library of Medicine. Richard J. Durling. 1999. 698p. reprint ed. 75.00 (*1-57898-137-9*) Martino Pubng.

Catalogue of the Printed Books in the Wellcome Historical Medical Library Vol. 1: Books Printed Before 1641, Vol. 1. Frwd. by Henry H. Dale. rev. ed. 1996. 422p. 100.00 (*1-888262-02-8*) Martino Pubng.

Catalogue of the Printed Books in the Wellcome Historical Medical Library Vol. 2: 1641-1850 rev. ed. 1996. 551p. 100.00 (*1-888262-03-6*) Martino Pubng.

Catalyst Deactivation. Eugene E. Petersen & Alexis T. Bell. 1987. (Chemical Industries Ser.: Vol. 30). (Illus.). 376p. text 210.00 (*0-8247-7741-7*) Dekker.

Catalyst of Power: The Assemblage Point of Man. Jon Whale. 2001. 250p. pap. (*1-899171-73-8*) Findhorn Pr GBR. *Dist:* Lantern Books.

Catalytic Activation of Carbon Monoxide. Ed. by Peter Ford. 1981. LC 81-1885. (ACS Symposium Ser.: No. 152). 358p. 43.95 (*0-8412-0620-1*) Am Chemical.

Catalytic Antibodies. Ed. by P. Sudhir. 2000. (Chemical Immunology Ser.: Vol. 77). (Illus.). xii, 162p. 171.50 (*3-8055-7099-6*) S Karger.

Catalytic Naphtha Reforming: Science & Technology. Ed. by George J. Antos et al. 1994. LC 94-29127. (Chemical Industries Ser.: Vol. 61). (Illus.). 528p. text 215.00 (*0-8247-9236-X*) Dekker.

Catalytical & Radical Polymerization. 1986. (Advances in Polymer Science Ser.: Vol. 81). (Illus.). 249p. 99.00 (*0-387-16754-4*) Spr-Verlag.

Cataract: Biochemistry, Epidemiology & Pharmacology. John Harding. 1991. 382p. (C). (gr. 13). pap. text 239.95 (*0-412-36050-0*, A5562) Chapman & Hall.

Cataract 1993. Ed. by Otto Hockwin & K. Sasaki. 1994. (Journal: Vol. 26, Suppl. 1, 1994). (Illus.). iv, 90p. pap. 28.75 (*3-8055-5986-0*) S Karger.

Cataract & Posterior Capsule Opacification, 1997: Joint Conference with the 8th Scheimpflug Club Meeting, Amsterdam, September-October 1997. Ed. by G. F. Vrensen et al. 1999. (Opthalmologica Ser.: Vol. 31, No. 2). (Illus.). 94p. pap. 55.75 (*3-8055-6825-8*) S Karger.

Cataract Breakthrough: The Booklet. Alex Duarte. 1994. 60p. pap. text 8.00 (*1-891036-00-9*) Nutri Tapes.

Cataract Epidemiology. Ed. by K. Sasaki et al. 1987. (Developments in Ophthalmology Ser.: Vol. 15). (Illus.). vi, 106p. 76.75 (*3-8055-4597-5*) S Karger.

Cataract Epidemiology: International Forum on Advanced Techniques in Lens & Cataract Research, Kanazawa, June 1995. Ed. by K. Sasaki & Otto Hockwin. 1996. LC 96-41777. (Developments in Ophthalmology Ser.: Vol. 27). (Illus.). viii, 120p. 95.75 (*3-8055-6360-4*) S Karger.

Cataract in Adults: Management of Functional Impairment. 1994. (Illus.). 226p. (Orig.). (C). pap. text 50.00 (*0-7881-0294-X*) DIANE Pub.

Cataract in Adults: Management of Functional Impairment. 1995. (Orig.). lib. bdg. 255.75 (*0-8490-6804-5*) Gordon Pr.

Cataract Pathogenesis: Results of Epidemiological Studies & Experimental Models. Ed. by Otto Hockwin & K. Sasaki. 1994. (Developments in Ophthalmology Ser.: Vol. 26). (Illus.). viii, 100p. 102.75 (*3-8055-5987-9*) S Karger.

***Cataract Surgery.** Dartry. 2002. (Fundamentals in Clinical Ophthalmology Ser.). 200p. (*0-7279-1201-1*) BMJ Pub GBR. *Dist:* AIDC.

Cataract Surgery. Dodick. 1994. 39.00 (*0-316-18829-8*, Little Brwn Med Div) Lppncott W & W.

Cataract Surgery: A Literature Review & Ratings of Appropriateness & Cruciality. Paul P. Lee et al. 1993. LC 93-25076. pap. text 20.00 (*0-8330-1405-6*, JRA-06) Rand Corp.

Cataract Surgery: Technique, Complications & Management. Roger F. Steinert. 1995. (Illus.). 448p. text 199.00 (*0-7216-5044-9*) Saunders.

Cataract Surgery: The State of the Art. James P. Gills. 1997. LC 97-31712. (Illus.). 272p. text 125.00 (*1-55642-362-4*, 63624) SLACK Inc.

Cataract Surgery & Its Complications. Norman S. Jaffe. 6th ed. 1997. LC 97-20149. (Illus.). 528p. (C). (gr. 13). text 160.00 (*0-8151-4865-8*, 29486) Mosby Inc.

Cataract Surgery in Complicated Cases. Lucio Buratto et al. 2000. LC 2001-267419. (Illus.). xi, 466p. (C). text 165.00 (*1-55642-467-1*) SLACK Inc.

Cataracts: A Guide for Patients. Walter J. Stark. Ed. by Morton Goldberg. 1997. (Ophthalmology Ser.: Vol. O802). 32p. (Orig.). pap. 2.95 (*1-885274-49-1*) Health InfoNet Inc.

Cataracts: The Complete Guide from Diagnosis to Recovery, for Patients & Families. Julius Shulman. rev. ed. 1995. LC 95-17388. pap. 11.95 (*0-312-13039-2*, St Martin Griffin) St Martin.

Catastrophe Ahead: AIDS & the Case for a New Public Policy. William B. Johnston & Kevin R. Hopkins. 1990. LC 89-72139. 256p. 68.00 (*0-275-93589-2*, C3589, Praeger Pubs) Greenwood.

Catastrophic Brain Injury. Ed. by Harvey S. Levin et al. 1996. LC 95-11592. (Illus.). 282p. text 42.50 (*0-19-508533-7*) OUP.

Catastrophic Diseases: Who Decides What?: A Psychosocial & Legal Analysis of the Problems Posed by Hemodialysis & Organ Transplantation. Jay Katz & Alexander M. Capron. 1975. LC 75-7175. 280p. 34.95 (*0-87154-439-3*) Russell Sage.

Catastrophic Diseases: Who Decides What? A Psychosocial & Legal Analysis of the Problems posed by Hemodialysis & Organ Transplantation. Jay Katz & Alexander M. Capron. 1982. LC 80-21899. 275p. reprint ed. pap. text 24.95 (*0-87855-686-9*) Transaction Pubs.

Catastrophic Illness & the Family. Bert E. Park. 1992. LC 91-70967. 19.95 (*0-8158-0471-7*) Chris Mass.

Catastrophic Injuries in High School & College Sports. Frederick O. Mueller et al. 1995. LC 95-31210. (Sport Science Monographs: Vol. 8). (Illus.). 120p. pap. text 19.00 (*0-87322-674-7*, BMUE0674) Human Kinetics.

Catch a Falling Star: Living with Alzheimer's Disease. Betty B. Spohr & Jean V. Bullard. 1995. LC 95-15655. (Illus.). 214p. (Orig.). pap. 9.95 (*0-9641357-1-X*) Storm Peak.

Catching Babies: The Professionalization of Childbirth, 1870-1920. Charlotte G. Borst. 1995. LC 95-5261. (Illus.). 288p. (C). 45.00 (*0-674-10262-2*) HUP.

Catching Cold. Pete Davies. 320p. text (*0-7181-4349-3*) M Joseph GBR. *Dist:* Trafalgar.

Catching My Breath: An Asthmatic Explores His Illness. Tim Brookes. 1998. 291p. text 22.00 (*0-7881-5713-2*) DIANE Pub.

Catching Ourselves in the Act: Situated Activity, Interactive Emergence, Evolution, & Human Thought. Horst Hendriks-Jansen. 1996. LC 96-972. (Complex Adaptive Systems Ser.). (Illus.). 379p. (C). 52.00 (*0-262-08246-2*, Bradford Bks) MIT Pr.

Catching the Thread: Sufism, Dreamwork, & Jungian Psychology. Llewellyn Vaughan-Lee. rev. ed. 1998. LC 97-38191. 304p. pap. 14.95 (*1-890350-00-1*) Golden Sufi Ctr.

Catechism of Health. Bernhard C. Faust. Tr. by J. H. Basse from GER. 1972. LC 74-180574. (Medicine & Society in America Ser.). 116p. reprint ed. 18.95 (*0-405-03951-4*) Ayer.

Catecholamines & Behaviour. Stephen T. Mason. 1984. LC 83-7722. 480p. text 85.00 (*0-521-24930-9*); pap. text 39.95 (*0-521-27082-0*) Cambridge U Pr.

Catecholamines & Heart Disease. Pallab K. Ganguly. 1991. 304p. 210.00 (*0-8493-5810-8*, RC682) CRC Pr.

Catecholamines & Stress. Ed. by Earl Usdin et al. 1976. 644p. (*0-08-020588-7*) Pergamon Repr GBR. *Dist:* Franklin.

Catecholamines & Their Enzymes in the Neuropathology of Schizophrenia. Steven Matthysse & Seymour S. Kety. 1975. LC 75-4093. (Illus.). 382p. (*0-08-018242-9*) Pergamon Repr GBR. *Dist:* Franklin.

Catecholamines II. Ed. by U. Trendelenburg & Neal O. Weiner. 1988. (Handbook of Experimental Pharmacology Ser.: Vol. 90). (Illus.). 487p. 357.00 (*0-387-19117-8*) Spr-Verlag.

Catecholamines in Normal & Abnormal Cardiac Function. William M. Manger. 1982. (Advances in Cardiology Ser.: Vol. 30). (Illus.). xxiv, 152p. 85.25 (*3-8055-3516-3*) S Karger.

Catecholamines One. Ed. by U. Trendelenburg & Neal O. Weiner. 1988. (Handbook of Experimental Pharmacology Ser.: Vol. 90-1). (Illus.). 571p. 357.00 (*0-387-18904-1*) Spr-Verlag.

Categorical Perceptions. Ed. by Stevan R. Harnad. 1987. (Illus.). 616p. text 110.00 (*0-521-26758-7*) Cambridge U Pr.

Catharsis & Cognition in Psychotherapy. B. J. Guinagh. 1987. (Illus.). 131p. 76.95 (*0-387-96530-0*) Spr-Verlag.

Catheter Ablation of Cardiac Arrhythmias: Basic Bio-Electrical Effects & Clinical Indications. Ed. by Melvin M. Scheinman. 1988. (Developments in Cardiovascular Medicine Ser.). (C). text 140.50 (*0-89838-967-4*) Kluwer Academic.

Catheter Introducers. Les Geddes & LaNelle Geddes. Ed. by Michael Boo et al. 1993. (Illus.). (*0-916371-13-1*) Mobium Pr.

Catheter-Related Infections. Ed. by Harold Seifert et al. 1997. LC 97-2630. (Infectious Disease & Therapy Ser.: Vol. 20). (Illus.). 480p. text 150.00 (*0-8247-9848-1*) Dekker.

Catheter Sleeve: A Morphological Study in Experimental Animals. Da Zhen Xiang. 1999. (Illus.). 144p. (*90-5867-007-4*) Leuven Univ BEL. *Dist:* Coronet Bks.

Catholic Ethicists on HIV/AIDS Prevention. James F. Keenan. 2000. 50.00 (*0-8264-1251-3*) Continuum.

***Catholic Health Care Ethics: A Manual for Ethics Committees.** Ed. by Peter J. Cataldo & Albert S. Moraczewski. 2001. LC 2001-44175. (*0-935372-44-X*) NCBC.

Catholic Identity in Health Care: Principles & Practice. Orville N. Griese. 1987. LC 87-2270. 537p. (Orig.). pap. 17.95 (*0-935372-19-9*) NCBC.

Catholic Perspectives on Medical Morals: Foundational Issues. Ed. by Edmund D. Pellegrino et al. 1989. 314p. (C). lib. bdg. (*1-55608-083-2*) Kluwer Academic NLD. *Dist:* Kluwer Academic.

***Catholicism & Health-Care Justice: Problems, Potential & Solutions.** S. S. Keane. 2002. LC 2001-54567. pap. 26.95 (*0-8091-4059-4*) Paulist Pr.

Cation Ordering & Electron Transfer. Ed. by J. B. Goodenough & C. K. Jorgensen. 1985. (Structure & Bonding Ser.: Vol. 61). (Illus.). 167p. 79.95 (*0-387-15446-9*) Spr-Verlag.

Cato Major. Marcus Tullius Cicero. Ed. by Robert J. Kastenbaum. 1979. LC 78-22193. (Aging & Old Age Ser.). reprint ed. lib. bdg. 18.95 (*0-405-11810-4*) Ayer.

Catologoe de Especialidades Farmaceuticas 1996. 1996. 1997p. 295.00 (*0-7859-9485-8*) Fr & Eur.

Cats: Homoeopathic Remedies. George MacLeod. 1990. 156p. pap. 19.95 (*0-8464-1335-3*) Beekman Pubs.

Cats: Homoeopathic Remedies. George MacLeod. 1990. 128p. pap. (*0-85207-190-6*) C W Daniel GBR. *Dist:* Natl Bk Netwk.

Cats Claw: Healing Vine of Peru. Kenneth Jones. 1995. 52p. pap. 9.95 (*0-9625638-3-8*) Sylvan Pr WA.

Cat's Claw: The Wondrous Herb from the Peruvian Rain Forest. Phillip Steinberg. 1996. 20p. (Orig.). pap. 2.95 (*0-9647080-4-3*) Healing Wisdom.

Cattle Ailments: Recognition & Treatment. Ed Straiton. 6th ed. 1993. (Illus.). 192p. (*0-85236-250-1*) Farming Pr GBR. *Dist:* Diamond Farm Bk.

Cattle Embryo Transfer Procedure. John L. Curtis. 1990. (Orig.). (C). pap. text 39.50 (*0-9627130-0-7*) J Curtis KS.

Cattle Footcare & Claw Trimming. E. Toussaint Raven. 1985. (Illus.). 128p. (Orig.). pap. (*0-85236-149-1*) Farming Pr GBR. *Dist:* Diamond Farm Bk.

Caught in the Middle: Protecting the Children of High-Conflict Divorce. Carla B. Garrity & Mitchell A. Baris. 1997. LC 97-15535. 192p. pap. 19.00 (*0-7879-3879-3*) Jossey-Bass.

Caught-in-the-Middle Management. Clyde Jackson et al. 1996. (Illus.). 168p. (Orig.). pap. 22.00 (*1-56829-075-6*, 4892) M G M A.

***Causal Analysis in Biomedicine & Epidemiology: Based on Minimal Sufficient Causation.** Mikel Aickin. 2001. LC 2001-52772. (*0-8247-0748-6*) Dekker.

Causal Cognition: A Multidisciplinary Approach. Ed. by David Premack et al. 1996. (Fyssen Foundation Symposium Ser.). (Illus.). 690p. reprint ed. pap. text 45.00 (*0-19-852402-1*) OUP.

Causal Inference. Ed. & Intro. by Kenneth J. Rothman. 1988. LC 87-22227. 207p. (Orig.). pap. text 25.00 (*0-917227-03-4*) Epidemiology.

Causal Mechanisms of Behavioural Development. Ed. by Jerry A. Hogan & Johan J. Bolhuis. 1994. (Illus.). 436p. (C). text 110.00 (*0-521-43241-3*) Cambridge U Pr.

Causal Thinking in the Child. Monique Laurendeau & Adrien Pinard. 1963. LC 62-21895. 309p. 42.50 (*0-8236-0680-5*) Intl Univs Pr.

Causation & Clinical Management of Pelvic Radiation Disease. Ed. by Philip F. Schofield & E. Lupton. 1989. (Illus.). 153p. 129.00 (*0-387-19561-0*, 3098) Spr-Verlag.

Causation & Disease: A Chronological Journal. A. S. Evans. 1993. (Illus.). 254p. (C). 36.50 (*0-306-44283-3*, Plenum Trade) Perseus Pubng.

Causation & Prevention of Human Cancer. Ed. by M. J. Hill & A. Giacosa. 1991. (Developments in Oncology Ser.). (C). text 89.00 (*0-7923-1084-5*) Kluwer Academic.

Causation, Course & Treatment of Reflex Insanity in Women. Horatio R. Storer. 1979. LC 71-180592. (Medicine & Society in America Ser.). 240p. reprint ed. 23.95 (*0-405-03974-3*) Ayer.

Causation of Rheumatoid Disease & Many Human Cancers: A Precis & Addenda Including the Nature of Multiple Sclerosis. Roger Wyburn-Mason. 1983. LC 83-71522. 32p. 10.00 (*0-931150-13-2*) Arthritis Trust.

***Cause & Cure of Human Illness: Kranke Menschen.** Tr. by Ludwig Max Fischer. 2001. (Illus.). 160p. pap. 14.95 (*1-884772-02-1*) Ehret Lit.

Cause & Defect: Drinking, Drugs & Pregnancy. Danielle Hain. rev. ed. 2000. pap. 0.50 (*0-89230-219-4*) Do It Now.

Causes & Consequences of Chromosomal Aberrations. Ed. by Ilan R. Kirsch. 1992. 544p. 199.00 (*0-8493-8893-7*, RB155) CRC Pr.

Causes & Control of Colorectal Cancer: A Model for Cancer Prevention. Ed. by Gabriel A. Kune. 1996. (Developments in Oncology Ser.). 400p. (C). text 175.50 (*0-7923-4059-0*) Kluwer Academic.

Causes & Cures of Criminality. Hans J. Eysenck & Gisli H. Gudjonsson. 1989. (Perspectives on Individual Differences Ser.). (Illus.). 326p. (C). 49.50 (*0-306-42968-3*, Plenum Trade) Perseus Pubng.

Causes, Controls & Organization of Behavior in the Neonate. Peter H. Wolff. 1966. LC 66-22207. (Psychological Issues Monographs: No. 17, Vol. 5, No. 1). 105p. pap. 27.50 (*0-8236-0700-3*) Intl Univs Pr.

Causes Du Suicide. Maurice Halbwachs. 1975. LC 74-25757. (European Sociology Ser.).Tr. of Causes of Suicide. (FRE.). 530p. reprint ed. 42.95 (*0-405-06511-6*) Ayer.

Causes of Crime. Arthur E. Fink. 1985. LC 84-22493. 309p. reprint ed. lib. bdg. 72.50 (*0-313-24746-3*, FICA, Greenwood Pr) Greenwood.

Causes of Death Contributing to Changes in Life Expectancy: United States, 1984-1989. Kenneth D. Kochanek et al. 1994. LC 94-671. (Vital & Health Statistics Ser. 20: Data from the National Vital Statistics System: No. 23). (*0-8406-0488-2*) Natl Ctr Health Stats.

Causes of Death in the Workplace. J. Paul Leigh. 1995. LC 94-36796. 328p. 67.95 (*0-89930-951-8*, Quorum Bks) Greenwood.

Causes of Development: Interdisciplinary Perspectives. Ed. by George Butterworth & Peter Bryant. 1990. 288p. 59.95 (*0-8058-0796-9*) L Erlbaum Assocs.

Causes of Diabetes: Genetic & Environmental Factors. Ed. by R. D. Leslie. 1993. LC 93-11222. 376p. 314.00 (*0-471-94040-2*) Wiley.

Causes of Suicide see Causes Du Suicide

Cautionary Tales: Authentic Case Histories from Medical Practice. John Murtagh. 1992. 220p. text 39.00 (*0-07-452806-8*) McGraw-Hill Med Pub.

***Caveolins & Lipid Rafts: New Elements in the Modulation of Volume-Regulated Anion Channels.** Dominique Trouet. 2000. (Acta Biomedica Lovanuensia Ser.: No. 222). (Illus.). 121p. pap. (*90-5867-077-5*) Leuven Univ BEL. *Dist:* Coronet Bks.

Cavernous Sinus. Ed. by V. V. Dolenc. 1987. (Illus.). 419p. 205.00 (*0-387-82000-0*) Spr-Verlag.

Cavernous Sinus: A Comprehensive Text. Mark Eisenberg & Ossama Al-Mefty. 1999. LC 99-33747. 416p. text 189.00 (*0-397-51844-7*) Lppncott W & W.

CBS Course of Mycology. W. Gams et al. 3rd ed. 1987. (Illus.). 136p. text (*90-70351-12-9*) Ctrl Bur voor Schimmel NLD. *Dist:* Lubrecht & Cramer.

CCL Home Study Course for Natural Family Planning. John F. Kippley & Sheila K. Kippley. 1987. stu. ed. 59.95 (*0-9601036-0-0*) Couple to Couple.

CCTA/WHO African Conference on Ancylostomiasis. 1963. (Technical Report Ser.: No. 255). 30p. pap. text 3.00 (*92-4-120255-6*) World Health.

CCU Intern Pocket Survival Guide. Thomas M. Masterson & Todd C. Rothenhaus. 2nd ed. 1992. 78p. pap. text 7.50 (*0-9634063-1-0*) Intl Med Pub.

CCU Pocket Professor. Jonni Cooper. 1991. (C). (gr. 13). text 16.95 (*0-944132-46-4*) Mosby Inc.

CD-ROM Atlas of Pathology: Gynecologic Cytopathology: Cervix. C. Marsan et al. 1998. (ENG & FRE.). 149.00 incl. cd-rom (*3-540-14655-5*) Spr-Verlag.

CD-ROM Atlas of Pathology: Leukemias. G. Flandrin. 1998. (ENG & FRE.). 149.00 incl. cd-rom (*3-540-14656-3*) Spr-Verlag.

CD-ROM Atlas of Pathology: Stomatology - ENT. C. Brocheriou et al. 1998. (ENG & FRE.). 149.00 incl. cd-rom (*3-540-14654-7*) Spr-Verlag.

CD-ROM Atlas of Pathology: Urological Pathology. A. Vieillefond et al. 1998. (ENG & FRE.). 149.00 incl. cd-rom (*3-540-14657-1*) Spr-Verlag.

CD-ROM Implementation & Networking in Health Sciences Libraries. Ed. by M. Sandra Wood. 1993. LC 92-44603. (Illus.). 165p. lib. bdg. 29.95 (*1-56024-381-3*) Haworth Pr.

CD-Rom Internal Medicine: Version 2.0. Jay H. Stein. 1998. 199.00 incl. cd-rom (*0-323-00373-7*) Mosby Inc.

CD23: A Novel Multifunctional Regulator of the Immune System That Binds IgE. Ed. by J Gordon. 1991. (Monographs in Allergy: Vol. 29). (Illus.). viii, 208p. 214.00 (*3-8055-5358-7*) S Karger.

CDC Prevention Guidelines: A Guide to Action. Andrew Friede et al. 1,000p. 1997. LC 96-20767. (Illus.). pap. 55.00 (*0-683-30005-9*); 1996. pap. 75.00 incl. cd-rom (*0-683-03360-3*) Lppncott W & W.

CD14 in the Inflammatory Response. Ed. by R. S. Jack. 1999. (Chemical Immunology Ser.: Vol. 74). (Illus.). viii, 182p. 172.25 (*3-8055-6917-3*) S Karger.

CDIA Training & Test Preparation Guide. Richard Harrison. Ed. by Susan Schmidt. 1998. LC 98-224184. (Illus.). 197p. pap. text (*0-9663920-2-7*) Specialized Solns.

CDT-2: Current Dental Terminology. Contrib. by James B. Davis. 1996. LC 97-30411. 250p. pap. text 39.95 (*1-57066-071-9*, 9718) Practice Mgmt Info.

CE Marking for Medical Devices: A Handbook to the Medical Devices Directives: Medical Devices Directive 93 42 EEC: The Active Implantable Medical Devices Directive 90 396 EEC. C. C. Schoenmakers. 1997. LC 97-41283. (*1-55937-946-4*) IEEE Standards.

Ce Qui ne va Pas Dans le Systeme de la Sante Mentale et Comment y Remedier. 1999.Tr. of What's Wrong with the Mental Health System & What Can Be Done About It. (FRE.). pap. 3.00 (*1-58429-049-8*) Rational Isl.

Cecil Essentials of Medicine. Thomas E. Andreoli et al. Ed. by Lisette Bralow. 4th ed. 1997. LC 96-18701. (Illus.). 780p. pap. text 45.00 (*0-7216-6697-3*) Saunders.

Cecil Essentials of Medicine. Thomas E. Andreoli et al. 5th ed. 2000. LC 99-89413. (Illus.). xxiii, 1070p. pap. text 49.00 (*0-7216-8179-4*) Saunders.

Cecil Review of General Internal Medicine. J. Allen D. Cooper, Jr. et al. Ed. by Ray Kersey. 6th ed. 1996. 288p. pap. text 39.95 (*0-7216-6264-1*) Saunders.

Cecil Review of General Internal Medicine. J. Allen D. Cooper, Jr. & Peter G. Pappas. 7th ed. 2000. (Illus.). 255p. pap. text 55.00 (*0-7216-7789-4*) Saunders.

Cecil Textbook of Medicine. Bennett. 20th ed. (C). text (*0-8089-2155-X*, Grune & Strat) Harcrt Hlth Sci Grp.

Cecil Textbook of Medicine. Ed. by Lee Goldman & J. Claude Bennett. 21st ed. 2000. LC 98-52751. (Illus.). xli, 2308p. (C). 110.00 (*0-7216-7996-X*) Harcrt Hlth Sci Grp.

Cecil Textbook of Medicine, Set. Russell L. Cecil. Ed. by Lee Goldman & J. Claude Bennett. 21st ed. 2000. LC 98-52751. (Illus.). 2525p. (C). text 125.00 (*0-7216-7995-1*) Saunders.

Cecil Textbook of Medicine Ed. by Russell L. Cecil et al. 20th ed. 1996. LC 94-43773. Vol. 1. (*0-7216-3574-1*); Vol. 2. (*0-7216-3575-X*) Saunders.

Celebrating Life: African American Women Speak Out about Breast Cancer. Sylvia Dunnavant. Ed. by Sharon Egiebor. 1995. LC 95-60852. (Illus.). 256p. pap. 19.95 (*0-9643211-4-9*) USFI.

Celebrating Small Victories: A Primer of Approaches & Attitudes for Helping Clients with Dual Disorders. Ken Montrose & Dennis Daley. 1995. LC 95-18958. 177p. 19.95 (*1-56838-092-5*) Hazelden.

Celebrating the Second Year of Life: A Parent's Guide for a Happy Child. Lucie W. Barber. 1979. LC 78-21484. 148p. (Orig.). pap. 10.95 (*0-89135-015-2*) Religious Educ.

Celebration of Birth. Sheila Kitzinger. 1986. LC 86-62953. 29p. (Orig.). pap. 7.95 (*0-937604-08-9*, Pennypr) Intl Childbirth.

Celebration of Chiropractic. Mosby Staff. 1995. 24p. (gr. 13). text 17.95 (*0-8151-6556-0*) Mosby Inc.

Celebration of Medical History. Ed. by Lloyd G. Stevenson. 1982. LC 81-17168. (Illus.). 236p. (C). 34.00 (*0-8018-2733-7*) Johns Hopkins.

Celiac Disease: Methods & Protocols. Ed. by Michael N. Marsh. 2000. (Methods in Molecular Medicine Ser.: Vol. 41). 304p. 99.50 (*0-89603-650-2*) Humana.

Celioscopy & Ancillary Techniques in the Study of Gynecological Pathology. E. Cittadini & T. Rossi. 1974. 96p. text (*1-57235-058-X*) Piccin Nuova.

Cell Activation & Apoptosis in HIV Infection: Implications for Pathogenesis & Therapy. Ed. by Jean-Marie Andrieu & Wei Lu. 1995. LC 95-17728. (Advances in Experimental Medicine & Biology Ser.: Vol. 374). 258p. 89.50 (*0-306-45063-1*, Kluwer Plenum) Kluwer Academic.

Cell Adhesion & Human Disease: Symposium No. 189. CIBA Foundation Staff. 1995. LC 94-39499. (CIBA Foundation Symposia Ser.: Vol. 189). 254p. 128.00 (*0-471-95279-6*) Wiley.

Cell Adhesion & Invasion in Cancer Metastasis. Ed. by Pnina Brodt. 1996. LC 95-46850. (Medical Intelligence Unit Ser.). 245p. (gr. 13). pap. 89.95 (*0-412-10151-3*) Chapman & Hall.

Cell Adhesion & Invasion Mechanisms in Cancer Metastasis. Pnina Brodt. 1996. LC 95-12647. (Medical Intelligence Unit Ser.). 258p. 99.00 (*1-57059-263-2*) Landes Bioscience.

Cell Adhesion Molecules in Cancer & Inflammation. Agamemnon A. Epenetos. 1995. (Cell Adhesion & Communication Ser.). 250p. text 121.00 (*3-7186-5516-0*, Harwood Acad Pubs) Gordon & Breach.

Cell Adhesion Molecules in Human Organ Transplants. Gustav Steinhoff. 1997. (Medical Intelligence Unit Ser.). 250p. 89.95 (*0-412-13091-2*) Chapman & Hall.

Cell Adhesion Molecules in Organ Transplantation. Gustav Steinhoff. 2nd ed. 1999. LC 98-10904. (Medical Intelligence Unit Ser.). 216p. 99.00 (*1-57059-517-8*) Landes Bioscience.

Cell & Animal Models in Aging & Dementia Research. Ed. by S. Hoyer et al. 1995. 96.00 (*0-387-82549-5*) Spr-Verlag.

Cell & Molecular Biology. E. D. De Robertis & E. M. De Robertis, Jr. 8th ed. 1987. LC 86-123. (Illus.). 734p. text 48.00 (*0-8121-1012-9*) Lppncott W & W.

Cell & Molecular Biology of Colon Cancer. Ed. by Leonard H. Augenlicht. 1989. LC 88-7589. 224p. 125.00 (*0-8493-4710-6*, RC280, CRC Reprint) Franklin.

Cell & Molecular Biology of Pancreatic Carcinoma: Recent Developments in Research & Experimental Therapy. J. Matthias Lohr. 1999. LC 99-34747. (Annals of the New York Academy of Sciences Ser.: Vol. 880). (Illus.). xii, 380p. (*1-57331-219-3*) NY Acad Sci.

Cell & Molecular Biology of Pancreatic Carcinoma: Recent Developments in Research & Experimental Therapy. J. Matthias Lohr & New York Academy of Sciences Staff. 1999. LC 99-34747. (Annals of the New York Academy of Sciences Ser.: Vol. 880). (Illus.). xii, 380p. (*1-57331-220-7*) NY Acad Sci.

Cell & Molecular Biology of Pancreatic Carcinoma Vol. 880: Recent Developments in Research & Experimental Therapy. J. Matthias Lohr et al. 1999. 350p. 140.00 (*1-57331-206-1*) NY Acad Sci.

Cell & Molecular Biology of the Cytoskelton. Ed. by Jerry W. Shay. 1986. LC 86-4912. (Illus.). 356p. (C). text 114.00 (*0-306-42175-5*, Kluwer Plenum) Kluwer Academic.

Cell & Molecular Biology of the Ear. Janet Stoeckert. Ed. by David J. Lim. 2000. LC 00-36371. (Illus.). xviii, 267p. 145.00 (*0-306-46374-1*) Plenum.

Cell & Molecular Biology of the Testis. Ed. by Claude Desjardins & Larry L. Ewing. 1993. (Illus.). 512p. (C). text 125.00 (*0-19-506269-8*) OUP.

Cell & Molecular Biology of the Uterus. Ed. by W. W. Leavitt. 1988. LC 88-5793. (Advances in Experimental Medicine & Biology Ser.: Vol. 230). (Illus.). 254p. 75.00 (*0-306-42836-9*, Plenum Trade) Perseus Pubng.

Cell & Muscle Motility. Ed. by Jerry W. Shay & Robert M. Dowden. LC 81-13827. Vol. 1. 1981. 414p. 85.00 (*0-306-40703-5*); Vol. 2. 1982. 328p. 85.00 (*0-306-40798-1*); Vol. 3. 1983. 324p. 89.50 (*0-306-41157-1*); Vol. 4. 1983. 348p. 89.50 (*0-306-41227-6*) Perseus Pubng (Plenum Trade).

Cell & Muscle Motility Vol. 5: The Cytoskeleton. Ed. by Jerry W. Shay. 1984. LC 81-13827. 434p. 85.00 (*0-306-41443-0*, Plenum Trade) Perseus Pubng.

Cell & Tissue Culture for Medical Research. Alan Doyle & Bryan Griffiths. 2000. LC 99-89625. (Illus.). 468p. pap. 105.00 (*0-471-85213-9*) Wiley.

Cell & Tissue Culture Models in Dermatological Research. A. Bernd et al. 1993. LC 92-36359. (Illus.). 363p. 172.00 (*0-387-55972-8*) Spr-Verlag.

Cell Biological Aspects of Disease: The Plasma Membrane & Lysosomes. Ed. by W. T. Daems et al. 1981. (Boerhaave Series for Postgraduate Medical Education: No. 19). 330p. text 184.00 (*90-6021-466-8*) Kluwer Academic.

Cell Biology: Review for New National Boards. Mark R. Adelman & Kurt E. Johnson. 1995. LC 95-75532. (Illus.). 203p. pap. 25.00 (*0-9632873-8-9*) J & S Pub VA.

Cell Biology & Histology. Leslie P. Gartner et al. 3rd ed. 1997. LC 97-18242. (Board Review Ser.). 390p. pap. text 27.95 (*0-683-30103-9*) Lppncott W & W.

Cell Biology & Pathology of Myelin: Evolving Biological Concepts & Therapeutic Approaches. Ed. by Bernhard H. Juurlink et al. 1997. LC 97-8136. (AS Ser.: Vol. 4). 408p. (C). text 125.00 (*0-306-45595-1*, Kluwer Plenum) Kluwer Academic.

Cell Biology Course. Competence Assurance Systems Staff. 1978. (Illus.). pap. text 45.00 (*0-89147-057-3*) CAS.

Cell Biology of the Secretory Process. Ed. by M. Cantin. 1983. (Illus.). viii, 624p. 259.25 (*3-8055-3619-4*) S Karger.

Cell Biology of Tooth Enamel Formation. T. Sasaki et al. 1990. (Monographs in Oral Science: Vol. 14). (Illus.). x, 204p. 200.00 (*3-8055-5045-6*) S Karger.

Cell Biology of Trauma. Ed. by Constance Oliver. 1995. LC 94-30688. 384p. 149.95 (*0-8493-2453-X*) CRC Pr.

Cell Biology of Triggers in Coagulation. Ed. by H. Prydz. 1985. (Journal: Vol. 14, No. 5). (Illus.). 68p. pap. 48.75 (*3-8055-4046-9*) S Karger.

Cell Calcium Metabolism: Physiology, Biochemistry, Pharmacology & Clinical Implications. Gary Fiskum. 1989. (GWUMC Department of Biochemistry & Molecular Biology Annual Spring Symposium Ser.). (Illus.). 638p. (C). text 155.00 (*0-306-43069-X*, Kluwer Plenum) Kluwer Academic.

Cell-Cell Interactions in the Release of Inflammatory Mediators: Eicosanoids, Cytokines & Adhesion. P. Y. Wong & C. N. Serhan. 1992. (Illus.). 400p. (C). text 120.00 (*0-306-44108-X*, Kluwer Plenum) Kluwer Academic.

Cell Communication in Health & Disease: Readings from Scientific American. Howard Rasmussen. 1991. (Scientific American Reader Ser.). (Illus.). 144p. (C). text 16.95 (*0-7167-2224-0*) W H Freeman.

Cell Culture. Ed. by William B. Jacoby & Ira H. Pastan. 1979. (Methods in Enzymology Ser.: Vol. 58). text 134.00 (*0-12-181958-2*) Acad Pr.

Cell Culture. Ed. by William B. Jakoby & Ira H. Pastan. 1988. (Methods in Enzymology Ser.: Vol. 58). 642p. reprint ed. spiral bd. 50.00 (*0-12-181776-8*) Acad Pr.

Cell Culture in Pharmaceutical Research, 11. Ed. by N. E. Fusenig et al. 1994. (Ernst Schering Research Foundation Ser.: Vol. 11). (Illus.). 300p. 69.95 (*0-387-58141-3*) Spr-Verlag.

Cell Culture in the Neurosciences. Ed. by Jane E. Bottenstein & Gordon H. Sato. 1985. LC 85-3435. (Current Topics in Neurobiology Ser.). 402p. 99.50 (*0-306-41942-4*, Plenum Trade) Perseus Pubng.

Cell Culture Techniques in Heart & Vessel Research. Ed. by Hans M. Piper. 1990. (Illus.). 362p. 115.00 (*0-387-51934-3*) Spr-Verlag.

Cell Cycle: Regulators, Targets & Clinical Applications. V. W. Hu. 1994. (Illus.). 442p. (C). text 125.00 (*0-306-44672-3*, Kluwer Plenum) Kluwer Academic.

Cell Cycle & Oncogenes. Ed. by W. Tanner & D. Gallwitz. 1987. (Colloquium der Gesellschaft fur Biologische Chemie in Mosbach Baden Ser.: Vol. 37). (Illus.). 171p. 94.00 (*0-387-17251-3*) Spr-Verlag.

Cell Cycle Effects of Drugs. Ed. by L. A. Dethlefsen. 1986. (International Encyclopedia of Pharmacology & Therapeutics Ser.: Section 121). (Illus.). 351p. 240.00 (*0-08-032015-5*, Pergamon Pr) Elsevier.

Cell Cycle in Malignancy & Immunity: Proceedings. Ed. by James C. Hampton. 1975. LC 74-600181. (ERDA Symposium Ser.). 617p. fiche 9.00 (*0-87079-158-3*, CONF-731005) DOE.

Cell Cycle Regulation. Ed. by Robert R. Ruffolo, Jr. et al. 1997. (New Horizons in Therapeutics Ser.). 192p. text 80.00 (*90-5702-204-4*, Harwood Acad Pubs) Gordon & Breach.

Cell Cycle Regulators in Cancer. Phillip Hinds. 1997. (Molecular Biology Intelligence Unit Ser.). 200p. 89.95 (*0-412-13151-X*) Chapman & Hall.

Cell Cycle Regulators in Cancer. K. Musunuru & P. W. Hinds. 1997. LC 97-22377. (Illus.). x, 162p. 98.00 (*3-8055-6561-5*) S Karger.

Cell Death. W. J. Mergner. 1990. 110.00 (*0-938607-39-1*) Field & Wood Inc Medical.

Cell Death & Diseases of the Nervous System. Vassilis E. Koliatsos & Rajiv R. Ratan. 1998. LC 98-22462. (Contemporary Neuroscience Ser.). (Illus.). 698p. 175.00 (*0-89603-413-5*) Humana.

Cell Death in Biology & Pathology. I. D. Bowen & R. Lockshin. 1981. (Illus.). 450p. 85.00 (*0-412-16010-2*, NO.6491) Chapman & Hall.

Cell Death in Reproductive Physiology. U. S. A. Serono Symposia Staff. Ed. by Jonathan L. Tilly et al. 1997. LC 97-36129. (Serono Symposia Ser.). (Illus.). 305p. 154.00 (*0-387-98344-9*) Spr-Verlag.

Cell Differentiation & Cancer. Schwartz. 1992. 14.95 (*0-8493-6324-1*) CRC Pr.

Cell Differentiation, Genes & Cancer. Ed. by T. Kakunaga et al. 1989. (IARC Scientific Publications Ser.: No. 92). (Illus.). 222p. pap. 60.00 (*92-832-1192-8*) OUP.

Cell Function & Disease. Ed. by L. Canedo et al. 1988. (Illus.). 534p. 125.00 (*0-306-43201-3*, Plenum Trade) Perseus Pubng.

Cell Fusion. A. E. Sowers. 1987. LC 86-30392. (Illus.). 560p. (C). text 130.00 (*0-306-42351-0*, Kluwer Plenum) Kluwer Academic.

Cell Growth & Oncogenesis. Peter Bannasch. 1998. LC 97-40596. (Molecular & Cell Biology Updates Ser.). (*0-8176-5727-4*) Birkhauser.

Cell Growth & Oncogenesis. Ed. by Peter Bannasch et al. 3rd ed. 1998. (Molecular & Cell Biology Updates Ser.). (Illus.). 350p. text 125.00 (*3-7643-5727-4*) Birkhauser.

Cell Injury & Protection in the Gastrointestinal Tract from Basic Sciences to Clinical Perspectives 1996. Ed. by G. Y. Mozsik. 1997. LC 97-212611. x, 358p. text 227.50 (*0-7923-8720-1*) Kluwer Academic.

Cell Interactions in Visual Development. Ed. by S. R. Hilfer & J. B. Sheffield. 1988. (Cell & Developmental Biology of the Eye Ser.). (Illus.). 175p. 175.00 (*0-387-96829-6*) Spr-Verlag.

Cell Kinetic Modelling & the Chemotherapy of Cancer. H. Knolle. 1988. (Lecture Notes in Biomathematics: Vol. 75). 157p. 41.95 (*0-387-50153-3*) Spr-Verlag.

Cell Markers. Ed. by G. Jasmin. 1981. (Methods & Achievements in Experimental Pathology Ser.: Vol. 10). (Illus.). xii, 296p. 144.50 (*3-8055-1736-X*) S Karger.

Cell-Mediated Effects of Immunoglobulins. Wolf H. Fridman & Catherine Sautes. 1996. LC 96-33465. (Molecular Biology Intelligence Unit Ser.). 206p. 99.00 (*1-57059-396-5*) Landes Bioscience.

Cell-Mediated Immune Responses: Proceedings of the WHO Scientific Group, Geneva, 1968. WHO Staff. 1969. (Technical Reports: No. 423). 61p. pap. text 5.00 (*92-4-120423-0*, 1100423) World Health.

Cell-Mediated Immunity in Ruminants. Bruno M. L. Goddeeris. 1994. 256p. lib. bdg. 189.00 (*0-8493-4952-4*, SF757) CRC Pr.

Cell Mediated Reactions, Miscellaneous Topics Vol. 3: PAR, Pseudo-Allergic Reactions. Involvement of Drugs & Chemicals. Ed. by P. Dukor et al. 1982. (Illus.). viii, 160p. 68.75 (*3-8055-0960-X*) S Karger.

Cell Membranes: Methods & Reviews. Ed. by Elliot Elson et al. Vol. 1. 1983. 212p. 65.00 (*0-306-41298-5*); Vol. 2. 1984. 396p. 95.00 (*0-306-41761-8*) Perseus Pubng (Plenum Trade).

Cell Motility Factors. Ed. by Irving D. Goldberg. 1991. (Experientia Supplementa Ser.: Vol. 59). xii, 224p. 161.50 (*0-8176-2569-0*) Birkhauser.

Cell Movements. Dennis Bray. 1992. LC 91-24911. (Illus.). 450p. text 49.00 (*0-8153-0404-8*, 3-0404-8); pap. text 31.00 (*0-8153-0717-9*) Garland.

Cell Physiology of Blood. Ed. by Robert Gunn & John L. Parker. 1988. 450p. 50.00 (*0-87470-044-2*) Rockefeller.

Cell Proliferation & Cytogenesis in the Mouse Hippocampus. K. Y. Reznikov. Ed. by F. Beck et al. 1991. (Advances in Anatomy, Embryology & Cell Biology Ser.: Vol. 122). (Illus.). 83p. 72.00 (*0-387-53689-2*) Spr-Verlag.

Cell Proliferation in Cancer: Regulatory Mechanisms of Neoplastic Cell Growth. Ed. by Claire E. Lewis et al. 1996. LC 94-24053. (Illus.). 418p. text 145.00 (*0-19-854791-9*) OUP.

Cell Proliferation in Lymphomas. J. Crocker. 1993. (Illus.). 224p. 145.00 (*0-632-02925-0*) Blackwell Sci.

Cell Signalling. Ed. by P. Parker & T. Pawson. 1996. LC 96-226674. (Cancer Surveys Ser.: Vol. 27). (Illus.). 450p. (C). text 90.00 (*0-87969-484-X*) Cold Spring Harbor.

Cell Surface Carbohydrates & Cell Development. Minoru Fukuda. 1991. 352p. lib. bdg. 210.00 (*0-8493-6435-3*, QH545) CRC Pr.

Cell Surface in Development & Cancer, Vol. 3. M. Steinberg. 1986. LC 85-3406. (Developmental Biology Ser.). (Illus.). 380p. (C). text 114.00 (*0-306-42165-8*, Kluwer Plenum) Kluwer Academic.

Cell Surface Labeling. Robert P. Becker & Om Johari. 1979. (Illus.). 100p. pap. text 10.00 (*0-931288-07-X*) Scanning Microscopy.

Cell Surface Peptidases in Health & Disease. Ed. by J. Kenny & C. M. Boustead. 1997. (Illus.). 400p. (*1-85996-275-0*) Bios Sci GBR. *Dist:* Bks Intl VA.

Cell, the Human Organism & Cancer. A. Leroi. 1973. lib. bdg. 79.95 (*0-87968-538-7*) Krishna Pr.

Cell Therapy. Ed. by Y. Ikeda et al. 2000. LC 00-25437. (Keio University Symposia for Life Science & Medicine Ser.: Vol. 5). (Illus.). 260p. 169.00 (*4-431-70253-9*) Spr-Verlag.

Cell Therapy: Stem Cell Transplantation, Gene Therapy, & Cellular Immunotherapy. Ed. by George Morstyn & William Sheridan. 1996. (Cancer Ser.). (Illus.). 647p. (C). text 130.00 (*0-521-47315-2*) Cambridge U Pr.

Cell-to-Cell Communication. W. C. De Mello. 1987. LC 87-18573. (Illus.). 388p. (C). text 105.00 (*0-306-42623-4*, Kluwer Plenum) Kluwer Academic.

Cell Transplantation for Neurological Disorders: Toward Reconstruction of the Human Central Nervous System. Thomas B. Freeman & Hakan Widner. 1998. LC 98-18085. (Contemporary Neuroscience Ser.). (Illus.). 368p. 175.00 (*0-89603-449-6*) Humana.

Cell Types in the Adenohypophysis of the Primitive Actinopterygians: With Special Reference to Immunocytochemical Identification of Pituitary Hormone Producing Cells in the Distal Lobe. G. N. Hansen. 1983. (Illus.). 88p. pap. 29.00 (*0-08-029827-3*, Pergamon Pr) Elsevier.

***Cell Volume: Sensors, Regulators & Functional Significance.** Ed. by F. Wehner. 2001. (Cellular Physiology & Biochemistry Ser.: Vol. 10, No. 5-6). (Illus.). 192p. 85.00 (*3-8055-7216-6*) S Karger.

Cell Volume Regulation: The Molecular Mechanism & Volume Sening Machinery: Proceedings of the 23rd Taniguichi Foundation Biophysics Symposium Held in Okazaki, Japan, 17-21 November, 1997. Okada Yasunobu Tion. 1998. LC 98-8800. (International Congress Ser.). 230p. 129.00 (*0-444-82951-2*) Elsevier.

Cellars at Marcelcave: A Yank Doctor in the BEF. Christopher J. Gallagher. 1998. LC 98-2974. (Illus.). 266p. 24.95 (*1-57249-110-8*, Burd St Pr) White Mane Pub.

Cells: Principles of Molecular Structure & Function. David Prescott. 1988. 640p. (C). 51.25 (*0-86720-092-8*); (Illus.). pap. text, stu. ed. 16.95 (*0-86720-098-7*, 098-7) Jones & Bartlett.

Cells & Cytokines in Lung Inflammation. Ed. by Michel Chignard et al. 1994. LC 94-18939. (Annals Ser.: Vol. 725). pap. 110.00 (*0-89766-856-1*) NY Acad Sci.

Cells & Tissues. Ed. by Andy W. Rogers. 1983. pap. text 52.00 (*0-12-593120-4*) Acad Pr.

Cells, Development & the Biology of Cancer. Harold E. Varmus & Robert A. Weinberg. 1992. LC 92-20554. vii, 214p. text 32.95 (*0-7167-5037-6*) W H Freeman.

Cells, Embryos & Evolution. John Gerhart & Marc Kirschner. 1997. LC 96-51650. (Illus.). 500p. pap. 77.95 (*0-86542-574-4*) Blackwell Sci.

Cells in the Liver. 1995. (Illus.). 156p. 121.00 (*3-540-59099-4*) Spr-Verlag.

Cells, Membranes & Disease: Including Renal. Ed. by E. Reid et al. 1987. LC 87-22060. (Methodological Surveys in Biochemistry & Analysis Ser.: Vol. 17). (Illus.). 506p. (C). text 174.00 (*0-306-42678-1*, Kluwer Plenum) Kluwer Academic.

Cells, Tissues & Disease. Guido Majno & Isabelle Joris. 1996. LC 94-44912. (Illus.). 832p. 68.95 (*0-86542-372-5*) Blackwell Sci.

Cellular Adhesion: Molecular Definition to Therapeutic Potential. B. W. Metcalf et al. 1994. (New Horizons in Therapeutics Ser.). (Illus.). 339p. (C). text 89.50 (*0-306-44685-5*, Kluwer Plenum) Kluwer Academic.

Cellular Ageing. Ed. by H. W. Sauer. 1984. (Monographs in Developmental Biology: Vol. 17). (Illus.). x, 278p. 128.75 (*3-8055-3860-X*) S Karger.

Cellular Ageing Pt. 1: Concepts & Mechanisms: General Concepts. Mechanisms I: Fidelity of Information Flow Ed. by R. G. Cutler. 1976. (Interdisciplinary Topics in Gerontology Ser.: Vol. 9). (Illus.). 150p. pap. 99.25 (*3-8055-2283-5*) S Karger.

Cellular Ageing Pt. 2: Concepts & Mechanisms: Mechanisms II: Translation, Transcription & Structural Properties Ed. by R. G. Cutler. 1976. (Interdisciplinary Topics in Gerontology Ser.: Vol. 10). (Illus.). 150p. pap. 65.25 (*3-8055-2284-3*) S Karger.

Cellular & Humoral Components of Cerebrospinal Fluid in Multiple Sclerosis. Ed. by A. Lowenthal & J. Raus. 1987. (NATO ASI Series A, Life Sciences: Vol. 129). (Illus.). 538p. 135.00 (*0-306-42578-5*, Plenum Trade) Perseus Pubng.

Cellular & Humoral Defense against Disease. Ed. by Max E. Rafelson. 1983. (Journal: Vol. 1, No. 2-5, 1983). (Illus.). 228p. pap. 113.25 (*3-8055-3693-3*) S Karger.

Cellular & Molecular Alterations in the Failing Human Heart. Ed. by G. Hasenfuss et al. 1992. 368p. 87.00 (*0-387-91419-6*) Spr-Verlag.

Cellular & Molecular Aspects of Fiber Carcinogenesis. Ed. by B. R. Brinkley et al. 1991. (Current Communications in Cell & Molecular Biology Ser.: No. 2). (Illus.). 260p. (C). text 36.00 (*0-87969-361-4*) Cold Spring Harbor.

Cellular & Molecular Aspects of Implantation. Ed. by Stanley R. Glasser & David W. Bullock. 1981. LC 80-20471. 518p. 115.00 (*0-306-40581-4*, Plenum Trade) Perseus Pubng.

Cellular & Molecular Aspects of Inflammation. G. Poste & S. T. Crooke. 1988. LC 87-37400. (New Horizons in Therapeutics Ser.). (Illus.). 496p. (C). text 125.00 (*0-306-42852-0*, Kluwer Plenum) Kluwer Academic.

Cellular & Molecular Bases of Neuroendocrine Processes: Symposium of the International Society of Psychoneuro-Endocrinology, Visegrad, Hungary, 17-20 Dec. 1975. Elemer Endroczi. 1976. 622p. (C). (*963-05-1073-1*) Akade Kiado HUN. *Dist:* St Mut.

Cellular & Molecular Basis of Cystic Fibrosis. Ed. by G. Mastella & P. M. Quinton. 1988. (Illus.). 20.00 (*0-911302-63-8*) San Francisco Pr.

Cellular & Molecular Biology: Proceedings of the "Takahashi Memorial Forum," Held in Tokyo, Japan on 5 November 1994. Ed. by Masami Y. Yamanaka et al. 1995. LC 95-39978. (International Congress Ser.: Vol. 1086, No. 1). (Illus.). 154p. 165.50 (*0-444-82099-X*) Elsevier.

Cellular & Molecular Biology of Airway Chemoreceptors. E. Cutz. 1997. (Medical Intelligence Unit Ser.). 200p. (C). pap. 89.95 (*0-412-10801-1*) Chapman & Hall.

Cellular & Molecular Biology of Airway Chemoreceptors. Ernest Cutz. 1997. LC 97-24582. (Medical Intelligence Unit Ser.). 132p. text 99.00 (*1-57059-473-2*) Landes Bioscience.

Cellular & Molecular Biology of Atherosclerosis. Ed. by A. J. Gotto, Jr. 1992. (Illus.). 180p. 118.00 (*0-387-19704-4*) Spr-Verlag.

Cellular & Molecular Biology of Bone. Ed. by Masaki Noda. 1993. LC 93-14783. (Illus.). 567p. text 121.00 (*0-12-520225-3*) Acad Pr.

Cellular & Molecular Biology of Invertebrate Development: The Belle W. Baruch Library in Marine Science. Roger H. Sawyer & Richard M. Showman. 1985. LC 85-22695. (Belle W. Baruch Library in Marine Science: No. 15). 346p. text 42.95 (*0-87249-464-0*) U of SC Pr.

Cellular & Molecular Biology of Mammary Cancer. D. Medina et al. 1988. LC 87-25756. (Illus.). 528p. (C). text 139.50 (*0-306-42761-3*, Kluwer Plenum) Kluwer Academic.

Cellular & Molecular Biology of the Kidney. Ed. by H. Koide et al. 1992. (Contributions to Nephrology Ser.: Vol. 95). (Illus.). x, 288p. 49.75 (*3-8055-5424-9*) S Karger.

Cellular & Molecular Events in Spermiogenesis As Targets for Fertility. D. W. Hamilton & G. M. Waites. 1990. (Basic Science Topics in Fertility Regulation Research Ser.). (Illus.). 352p. (C). text 115.00 (*0-521-37265-8*) Cambridge U Pr.

Cellular & Molecular Mechanisms: Report of the Dahlem Workshop on Cellular & Molecular Mechanisms Underlying Higher Neural Functions, Berlin, 1993, February 28-March 5. Ed. by P. Ascher & Allen I. Selverston. 1994. LC 93-46293. (Life Sciences Research Reports: Vol. 54). 344p. 290.00 (*0-471-94304-5*) Wiley.

Cellular & Molecular Mechanisms in Hypertension. R. H. Cox. 1992. (Advances in Experimental Medicine & Biology Ser.: Vol. 308). (Illus.). 264p. (C). text 95.00 (*0-306-44084-9*, Kluwer Plenum) Kluwer Academic.

Cellular & Molecular Mechanisms of Cell-Mediated Allergic Reactions, Chemistry of Allergens & Transactions: Proceedings of the Collegium Internationale Allergologicum, 8th Symposium, Montreux, 1970. Collegium Internationale Allergologicum Staff. Ed. by P. Kallos et al. 1971. (International Archives of Allergy & Immunology Ser.: Vol. 41, No. 1). pap. 47.00 (*3-8055-1191-4*) S Karger.

Cellular & Molecular Mechanisms of Drugs of Abuse: Cocaine, Ibogaine, & Substituted Amphetamines. Syed F. Ali & Yasuo Takahashi. 1996. LC 96-36646. (Annals of the New York Academy of Sciences Ser.: Vol. 801). 125.00 (*1-57331-036-0*) NY Acad Sci.

Cellular & Molecular Mechanisms of Drugs of Abuse: Cocaine, Ibogaine & Substituted Amphetamines. Syed F. Ali & Yasuo Takahashi. 1996. LC 96-36646. (Annals of the New York Academy of Sciences Ser.). pap. 125.00 (*1-57331-037-9*) NY Acad Sci.

Cellular & Molecular Networks in Clinical Immunology & Allergy. Ed. by Stephen T. Holgate. 1991. (Journal: Vol. 94, No. 1-4, 1991). (Illus.). 380p. pap. 358.50 (*3-8055-5507-5*) S Karger.

Cellular & Molecular Neurobiology. Ed. by Constance Hammond. 1996. (Illus.). 488p. pap. text 65.00 (*0-12-322040-8*) Acad Pr.

Cellular & Molecular Neurobiology of Renin-Angiotensin System. Ed. by Mohan K. Raizada et al. 1993. 592p. 240.00 (*0-8493-4622-3*, QP572) CRC Pr.

Cellular & Molecular Pathogenesis. Ed. by Alphonse E. Sirica. 1995. LC 95-20665. (Illus.). 576p. text 125.00 (*0-7817-0301-8*) Lppncott W & W.

Cellular & Molecular Regulation of Testicular Cells. Ed. by Claude Desjardins. 1996. LC 95-46670. (Illus.). 371p. 152.00 (*0-387-94648-9*) Spr-Verlag.

Cellular & Molecular Targets Cancer Chemoprevention. Ed. by Vernon E. Steele. 1992. 400p. 110.00 (*0-8493-4530-8*, RC268) CRC Pr.

Cellular & Viral FOS Genes. Peter A. Herrlich. 1994. 322p. 199.95 (*0-8493-4573-1*) CRC Pr.

Cellular Aspects of Autoimmunity. Ed. by J. M. Cruse & R. E. Lewis, Jr. 1988. (Concepts in Immunopathology Ser.: Vol. 6). (Illus.). vi, 202p. 148.00 (*3-8055-4728-5*) S Karger.

Cellular Aspects of Hypertension. Ed. by G. Bruschi & A. Borghetti. 1991. (Illus.). 271p. 94.00 (*0-387-53987-5*) Spr-Verlag.

Cellular Basis of Cardiovascular Function in Health & Disease. Ed. by Pawan K. Singal et al. 1998. LC 97-21934. (Developments in Molecular & Cellular Biochemistry Ser.). 352p. text 291.50 (*0-7923-9974-9*) Kluwer Academic.

Cellular Basis of Central Nervous System HIV-1 Infection & the AIDS Dementia Complex. Ed. by Richard W. Price & John J. Sidtis. 1996. 49.95 (*1-56024-774-6*, Hawrth Medical) Haworth Pr.

Cellular Basis of Renal Function: Journal: Renal Physiology & Biochemistry. Ed. by N. G. De Santo. 1993. (Journal: Vol. 16, Nos. 1 & 2, 1993). (Illus.). 92p. pap. 88.75 (*3-8055-5770-1*) S Karger.

Cellular Cancer Markers. Ed. by Carleton T. Garrett & Stewart Sell. 1995. LC 95-1286. (Contemporary Biomedicine Ser.: Vol. 12). (Illus.). 496p. 145.00 (*0-89603-210-8*) Humana.

Cellular Cardiomyoplasty: Myocardial Repair with Cell Implantation. Race L. Kao & Ray C. Chiu. 1997. (Medical Intelligence Unit Ser.). 201p. 99.00 (*1-57059-451-1*) Landes Bioscience.

Cellular Characteristics of Cord Blood & Cord Blood Transplantation. American Association of Blood Banks Staff. Ed. by Hal E. Broxmeyer. 1998. (Illus.). 150p. (*3-8055-6749-9*) S Karger.

Cellular Characteristics of Cord Blood & Cord Blood Transplantation. Ed. by Hal E. Broxmeyer. 1998. LC 98-9427. 227p. text 149.00 (*1-56395-084-7*) Am Assn Blood.

Cellular Cloud. Frederick W. Barnes. 1995. (Illus.). xiii, 221p. 35.00 (*0-9653311-0-5*) F W Barnes.

Cellular Communication During Ocular Development. Ed. by J. B. Sheffield & S. R. Hilfer. 1982. (Cell & Developmental Biology of the Eye Ser.). (Illus.). 196p. 136.00 (*0-387-90773-4*) Spr-Verlag.

Cellular Communication in Reproduction. Ed. by F. Facchinetti et al. 1993. 228p. 55.00 (*1-898099-00-6*) Blackwell Sci.

Cellular Energy Metabolism & Its Regulation. Daniel E. Atkinson. 1977. text 79.00 (*0-12-066150-0*) Acad Pr.

Cellular Immune Mechanisms & Tumor Dormancy. Stewart. 1992. 384p. 121.00 (*0-8493-4520-0*, RC268) CRC Pr.

Cellular Inter-Relationships in the Pancreas: Implications for Islet Transplantation. William P. Duguid & Lawrence M. Rosenberg. 1996. LC 96-34373. (Medical Intelligence Unit Ser.). (Illus.). 219p. 99.00 (*1-57059-403-1*) Landes Bioscience.

Cellular Inter-Relationships in the Pancreas: Implications for Islet Transplantation. Lawrence Rosenberg & William P. Duguid. 1996. LC 96-34373. (Medical Intelligence Unit Ser.). 216p. pap. 79.95 (*0-412-12591-9*) Chapman & Hall.

Cellular Interactions in Allergy. Ed. by F. Kristensen et al. 1981. (Journal: Vol 66, Supp. 1). (Illus.). vi, 298p. pap. 64.50 (*3-8055-3439-6*) S Karger.

Cellular Interactions in Cardiac Pathophysiology. Ed. by Jan Slezak. 1995. (Developments in Molecular & Cellular Biochemistry Ser.). 172p. (C). text 224.00 (*0-7923-3573-2*) Kluwer Academic.

Cellular Interactions in the Immune Response: Proceedings of the International Convocation in Immunology, 2nd, Buffalo, New York, 1970. International Convocation in Immunology Staff. Ed. by S. Cohen et al. 1971. 86.00 (*3-8055-1202-3*) S Karger.

Cellular Metabolism of the Arterial Wall & Central Nervous System: Selected Aspects. Ed. by F. Gotthard Schettler et al. 1993. LC 93-19198. (Ver Offentlichungen Aus der Geomedizinischen Forschungstelle der Heidelberg Akademie der Wissenschaften Ser.). (Illus.). 312p. 64.95 (*0-387-56603-1*) Spr-Verlag.

Cellular Methods in Immunology. Rafael Fernandez-Botran & Vaclav Vetvicka. 2000. 192p. spiral bd. 79.95 (*0-8493-2125-5*) CRC Pr.

Cellular Microbiology: Bacteria-Host Interactions in Health & Disease. Brian Henderson. 1999. LC 98-46842. (Illus.). 478p. 149.95 (*0-471-98678-X*) Wiley.

Cellular, Molecular & Genetic Approaches to Immunodiagnosis & Immunotherapy. Ed. by Motomichi Torisu et al. 1987. (Illus.). xvi, 510p. 243.50 (*3-8055-4649-1*) S Karger.

Cellular Neurophysiology & Integration: An Interpretive Introduction. W. R. Uttal. 1975. 310p. 39.95 (*0-89859-429-4*) L Erlbaum Assocs.

Cellular Oncology: New Approaches in Biology, Diagnosis & Treatment, 1. Ed. by Peter Moloy & Garth, L. Nicolson. 1983. LC 83-11222. (Cancer Research Monographs). 305p. 72.95 (*0-275-91405-4*, C1405, Praeger Pubs) Greenwood.

Cellular Pathology. D. J. Cook. 1998. LC 98-28024. 384p. pap. (*0-7506-3111-2*) E A GBR. *Dist:* OUP.

Cellular Pathophysiology. Ed. by Mohammed M. Sayeed. 1989. 176p. lib. bdg. 153.00 (*0-8493-4061-6*, RB112) CRC Pr.

Cellular Peptidases in Immune Functions & Diseases: Proceedings of an International Conference Held in Magdeburg, Germany, November 3-5, 1996. Ed. by Siegfried Ansorge et al. 1997. LC 97-21524. (Advances in Experimental Medicine & Biology Ser.: Vol. 421). 350p. (C). text 95.00 (*0-306-45616-8*, Kluwer Plenum) Kluwer Academic.

Cellular Physiology of Nerve & Muscle. Gary G. Matthews. 3rd ed. 1997. LC 97-14314. (Illus.). 240p. pap. 57.95 (*0-632-04354-7*) Blackwell Sci.

Cellular Recognition. M. F. Greaves. 1975. pap. 6.95 (*0-412-13110-2*, NO.6129) Chapman & Hall.

Cellular Structure of the Mammalian Nervous System. H. Hillman. 1986. text 288.00 (*0-85200-916-X*) Kluwer Academic.

Cellular Therapy. Ed. by H. Wekerle et al. 1997. LC 97-26852. (Ernst Schering Research Foundation Ser.: Vol. 20). (Illus.). 178p. 49.00 (*3-540-63049-X*) Spr-Verlag.

Cellulite Solution: A Wholistic Guide for a Beautiful Body. Laura Simms. Ed. by Wilhelmine Hartnack. 1990. (Illus.). 192p. (Orig.). pap. 12.95 (*0-9625499-0-8*) Natural CA.

CEN Examination Review. Renebe S. Holleran. 3rd ed. 2000. LC 00-41574. (Illus.). xv, 293p. 39.95 (*0-323-01234-5*) Mosby Inc.

CEN Review Manual. Ed. by Lorene Newberry et al. 2nd rev. ed. 1996. (Illus.). 362p. (Orig.). pap. text 40.00 (*0-935890-00-9*, C2) Emerg Nurses IL.

Centenarians in Hungary. Ed. by Edit Beregi. 1990. (Interdisciplinary Topics in Gerontology Ser.: Vol. 27). (Illus.). xii, 210p. 146.25 (*3-8055-5204-1*) S Karger.

Centennial History of African Americans in Radiology. Alan E. Oestreich et al. unabr. ed. 1996. (Illus.). 100p. 40.00 (*0-9651714-0-X*) Nat Med Assn.

Centennial History of Sheltering Arms Hospital. Anne R. Lower. 1989. (Illus.). 96p. pap. (*0-9623370-1-3*); lib. bdg. 20.00 (*0-9623370-0-5*) Sheltering Arms.

Centennial of Surgical Anesthesia. John F. Fulton. 1999. 102p. reprint ed. 55.00 (*1-57898-122-0*) Martino Pubng.

Center, the Group under Observation, Sources of Information & Studies in Progress. Harold C. Stuart. 1939. (SRCD M Ser.: Vol. 4, No. 1). 28.00 (*0-527-01508-3*) Periodicals Srv.

***CenterWatch Compilation Reports: Report on Academic Medical Centers.** Ken Getz. 2001. (Illus.). 70p. pap. 399.00 (*1-930624-20-4*) CenterWatch.

***CenterWatch Compilation Reports: Report on Contract Research Organizations.** Ken Getz. 2001. (Illus.). 70p. pap. 399.00 (*1-930624-21-2*) CenterWatch.

Central & Peripheral 5-HT3 Receptors. Ed. by Michel Hamon. 1992. (Neuroscience Perspectives Ser.). (Illus.). 314p. text 78.00 (*0-12-322370-9*) Acad Pr.

Central & Peripheral Dopamine Receptors: Biochemistry & Pharmacology. Ed. by Giovanni Biggio et al. 1988. (FIDIA Research Ser.: Vol. 5). 283p. 130.00 (*0-387-96736-2*) Spr-Verlag.

Central Auditory Dysfunction. Ed. by Robert W. Keith. 1977. LC 77-10777. 400p. text 42.00 (*0-8089-1061-2*, 792270, Grune & Strat) Harcrt Hlth Sci Grp.

Central Auditory Processing & Neural Modeling: Proceedings of an International Workshop Held in Kaohsiung, Taiwan, January 26-29, 1997. Ed. by Paul W. Poon & John F. Brugge. 1998. LC 98-4100. (Illus.). 292p. 95.00 (*0-306-45836-5*, Kluwer Plenum) Kluwer Academic.

Central Auditory Processing Disorders: Mostly Management. M. Gay Masters et al. 1998. LC 98-11753. 288p. (C). 57.00 (*0-205-27361-0*) Allyn.

Central Auditory Processing Disorders: New Perspectives. Gail D. Chermak & Frank E. Musiek. 1997. LC 97-4466. 392p. pap. 55.00 (*1-56593-697-3*, 1354) Thomson Learn.

Central Auditory System. Gunter Ehret & Raymond Romand. 1996. LC 96-2376. (Illus.). 416p. text 59.50 (*0-19-509684-3*) OUP.

Central Autonomic Network: Functional Organization & Clinical Correlations. Eduardo E. Benarroch. 1997. LC 97-17397. (Illus.). 698p. 125.00 (*0-87993-673-8*) Futura Pub.

Central Cancer Registries: Design, Management, & Use. Ed. by Herman Menck & Charles Smart. 1994. LC 94-1853. 312p. text 55.00 (*3-7186-0579-1*) Gordon & Breach.

Central Cancer Registries: Design, Management & Use. Ed. by Herman Menck & Charles Smart. 1994. 312p. pap. text 25.00 (*3-7186-0587-2*) Gordon & Breach.

Central Cholinergic Mechanism & Adaptive Dysfunctions. Ed. by Man M. Singh et al. 1985. LC 84-18125. 418p. 110.00 (*0-306-41835-5*, Plenum Trade) Perseus Pubng.

Central Nervous Control of Autonomic Function. Ed. by David Jordan. 1997. (Autonomic Nervous System Book Ser.: Vol. 11). 304p. text 105.00 (*3-7186-5141-6*, Harwood Acad Pubs) Gordon & Breach.

Central Nervous System: Structure & Function. Per Brodal. 2nd ed. 1997. LC 96-40369. (Illus.). 688p. text 54.50 (*0-19-511741-7*) OUP.

Central Nervous System & Eye Infections. Ed. by Gerald L. Mandell & Thomas P. Bleck. 1995. LC 94-41262. (Atlas of Infectious Diseases Ser.: Vol. 3). (Illus.). 258p. text 135.00 (*0-443-07700-2*) Current Med.

Central Nervous System Angitis. James W. Schmidley. 2000. LC 99-53888. (Illus.). 240p. text 84.99 (*0-7506-7153-X*) Buttrwrth-Heinemann.

Central Nervous System, Autonomic Nervous System, Sense Organs & Skin, Peripheral Nerves & Vessels, Vol. 3. Johannes Sobotta. Ed. by Frank H. Figge & Walter J. Hild. 1978. 366p. text 45.00 (*0-8067-1739-4*) Lppncott W & W.

Central Nervous System Control of the Heart. Ed. by T. Stober et al. 1986. (Topics in the Neurosciences Ser.). text 139.50 (*0-89838-820-1*) Kluwer Academic.

Central Nervous System Diseases. Ed. by H. S. Rosenberg & J. Bernstein. 1987. (Perspectives in Pediatric Pathology Ser.: Vol. 10). viii, 264p. 229.75 (*3-8055-4403-0*) S Karger.

Central Nervous System Diseases: Innovative Animal Models from Lab to Clinic. Ed. by Dwaine F. Emerich et al. 2000. LC 99-25833. (Contemporary Neuroscience Ser.). (Illus.). 532p. 135.00 (*0-89603-724-X*) Humana.

Central Nervous System; Heart; Eye; Mesothelium. Ed. by Ulrich Mohr. 1994. (Illus.). 92p. pap. text 30.00 (*92-832-0127-2*) OUP.

Central Nervous System in AIDS. Ed. by J. Artigas et al. 1993. (Illus.). 250p. (*3-540-55839-X*) Spr-Verlag.

Central Nervous System in AIDS: Neurology, Radiology, Pathology, Ophthalmology. Ed. by Artigas G. Grosses et al. 1993. LC 93-22713. 246p. 239.00 (*0-387-55839-X*) Spr-Verlag.

Central Nervous System Infectious Diseases & Therapy. Ed. by Karen L. Roos. 1997. LC 97-7153. (Neurological Disease & Therapy Ser.: Vol. 44). (Illus.). 784p. text 235.00 (*0-8247-9811-2*) Dekker.

Central Nervous System Leukemia Prevention & Treatment. Ed. by R. Mastrangelo. 1983. (Developments in Oncology Ser.). text 126.50 (*0-89838-570-9*) Kluwer Academic.

Central Nervous System Monitoring in Anesthesia & Intensive Care. Ed. by J. Schulte Am Esch & E. Kochs. 1993. LC 94-2610. (Illus.). 354p. 106.00 (*0-387-57134-5*) Spr-Verlag.

Central Nervous System Pathology: A New Approach. G. N. Kryzhanovsky. Tr. by Nicholas Bobrov from RUS. 1986. (Illus.). 444p. 155.00 (*0-306-10982-4*, Kluwer Plenum) Kluwer Academic.

Central Nervous System Trauma Research Techniques, Vol. 4. Ed. by S. Tsuyoshi Ohnishi et al. 1995. LC 94-41529. (Membrane-Linked Diseases Ser.). 592p. 199.95 (*0-8493-8094-4*, 8094) CRC Pr.

Central Neural Mechanisms of Cardiovascular Regulation. Ed. by George Kunos & John Ciriello. 1991. (Illus.). xv, 282p. 140.50 (*0-8176-3545-9*) Birkhauser.

Central Pain: A Neurosurgical Survey. Valentino Cassinari & Carlo A. Pagni. 1969. LC 68-54017. (Illus.). 102p. 21.50 (*0-674-10540-0*) HUP.

Central Regulation of Autonomic Functions. Ed. by Arthur D. Loewy & K. Michael Spyer. 1990. (Illus.). 416p. text 85.00 (*0-19-505106-8*) OUP.

Central Regulation of Energy Metabolism. Katsuya Nagai. 1992. 208p. lib. bdg. 129.00 (*0-8493-6657-7*, QP356) CRC Pr.

Central Serotonin Receptors & Psychotropic Drugs. C. A. Marsden & D. J. Heal. 1992. (Frontiers in Pharmacology & Therapeutics Ser.). (Illus.). 336p. 145.00 (*0-632-02883-1*) Blackwell Sci.

Centrifugal Analysers in Clinical Chemistry. Ed. by Christopher/P. Price & Kevin C. Spencer. 1980. LC 80-81330. (Illus.). 520p. 132.50 (*0-275-91339-2*, C1339, Praeger Pubs) Greenwood.

Centural Neural Mechanisms in Cardiovascular Regulation, Vol. 2. Ed. by George Kunos & John Ciriello. 1992. (Illus.). x, 480p. 140.50 (*0-8176-3569-6*) Birkhauser.

Century for Psychiatry. Freeman. 1999. pap. text (*0-7234-3174-4*) Mosby Inc.

Century of Arterial Hypertension, 1896-1996. Nicolas Postel-Vinay & International Society of Hypertension Staff. 1997. LC 96-8699. (Illus.). 224p. 79.95 (*0-471-96788-2*) Wiley.

Century of Biological Research. Harlow B. Mills et al. Ed. by Frank N. Egerton, 3rd. 1978. LC 77-74240. (History of Ecology Ser.). (Illus.). reprint ed. lib. bdg. 18.95 (*0-405-10409-X*) Ayer.

Century of Black Surgeons: The U. S. A. Experience. Ed. by Margaret M. Kosiba. 1991. 973p. reprint ed. 75.00 (*0-9617380-0-6*) C H Organ.

Century of Caring. Ohio Veterinary Medical Association Staff. Ed. by Flournoy and Gibbs, Inc. Staff. 1984. (Illus.). 132p. 30.00 (*0-9613273-0-8*) Ohio Vet.

Century of Concern: A History of the American Association on Mental Deficiency 1876-1976. W. Sloan. 1976. pap. 10.00 (*0-940898-01-2*) Am Assn Mental.

Century of Darwin. Ed. by Samuel A. Barnett. 1977. LC 71-76891. (Essay Index Reprint Ser.). 25.95 (*0-8369-1019-2*) Ayer.

Century of Developmental Psychology. Ed. by Ross D. Parke et al. 1994. LC 94-4484. 684p. pap. text 34.95 (*1-55798-238-4*, 431-6411) Am Psychol.

Century of Excellence: A 100th Anniversary History of the American Academy of Otolaryngology-Head Neck Surgery & Its Predecessor Organizations. Loring W. Pratt et al. Ed. by T. Susan Hill. 1996. (Illus.). 546p. (Orig.). 50.00 (*1-56772-051-X*); pap. 40.00 (*1-56772-052-8*) AAO-HNS.

Century of Psychology: Progress, Paradigms, & Prospects for the New Millennium. Ray Fuller et al. 1997. LC 97-3892. (Illus.). 352p. (C). 85.00 (*0-415-16219-X*); pap. 25.99 (*0-415-16220-3*) Routledge.

Century of Psychology As Science. Ed. by Sigmund Koch & David E. Leary. 1992. 1008p. reprint ed. text 29.95 (*1-55798-171-X*) Am Psychol.

Century of X-Rays & Radioactivity in Medicine with Emphasis on Photographic Records of the Early Years. R. F. Mould. 1993. LC 93-19005. (Illus.). 236p. 105.00 (*0-7503-0224-0*) Inst of Physics Pubng.

CEO's Guide to Health Care Information Systems. Joseph M. DeLuca & Rebecca E. Cagan. 1996. LC 96-16758. 128p. pap. 40.95 (*1-55648-158-6*, 093105) AHPI.

Cephalometrics: Contemporary. Anthony D. Viazis. 1998. text (*0-7216-5916-0*) Saunders.

Cephalopod Behaviour. Rodney Lee Johnson, Sr. & John B. Messenger. 1998. 248p. pap. text 35.95 (*0-521-64583-2*) Cambridge U Pr.

Cephalosporin-Therapie der Gonorrhoe. H. C. Korting. 1987. (Illus.). xii, 110p. 36.75 (*3-8055-4586-X*) S Karger.

Cephalosporins in the Treatment of Severe Infections, 3rd Generation. Ed. by W. Michael Scheld et al. 1990. (Journal: Vol. 35, Suppl. 2, 1989). (Illus.). 44p. pap. 21.75 (*3-8055-5149-5*) S Karger.

Ceramic Microstructures '86: Role of Interfaces. Ed. by Joseph A. Pask & A. G. Evans. 1987. LC 87-22758. (Materials Science Research Ser.: Vol. 21). 1002p. 175.00 (*0-306-42681-1*, Plenum Trade) Perseus Pubng.

***Cerbral Palsy Handbook: A Practical Guide for Parents & Carers.** Marion Stanton. 2002. 256p. pap. (*0-09-187676-1*) Random GBR. *Dist:* Trafalgar.

Cerebellar Functions. Ed. by J. Dichgans et al. 1984. (Proceedings in Life Sciences Ser.). (Illus.). 335p. 128.00 (*0-387-13728-9*) Spr-Verlag.

Cerebellar Infarct: Minimal Invasive Endoscopy Neurosurgery - Midline Tumors. Ed. by B. L. Bauer et al. 1994. LC 94-196067. (Illus.). 332p. 84.95 (*0-387-57668-1*) Spr-Verlag.

Cerebellar Tumors: Clinical Analysis & Physiopathologic Correlations. R. Amici et al. 1976. (Monographs in Neural Sciences: Vol. 4). pap. 55.75 (*3-8055-2358-0*) S Karger.

Cerebellum: From Structure to Control. D. I. Zeeuw et al. 1997. LC 97-4339. (Progress in Brain Research Ser.). 626p. 214.50 (*0-444-82313-1*) Elsevier.

Cerebellum & Neuronal Plasticity. Ed. by Mitchell Glickstein et al. 1988. LC 88-2409. (NATO ASI Series A, Life Sciences: Vol. 148). (Illus.). 368p. 95.00 (*0-306-42822-9*, Plenum Trade) Perseus Pubng.

Cerebellum in Health & Disease. William S. Fields et al. 1970. LC 78-78016. (Illus.). 588p. 37.50 (*0-87527-009-3*) Green.

Cerebellum Revisited. Ed. by Rodolfo R. Llinas & C. Sotelo. 1992. (Illus.). 339p. 148.00 (*0-387-97693-0*) Spr-Verlag.

Cerebral & Spinal Computed Tomography. Thomas H. Grumme. 3rd ed. 1998. LC 98-35432. 280p. 195.00 (*0-632-04855-7*) Blackwell Sci.

Cerebral Aneurysms: Microvascular & Endovascular Management. R. R. Smith et al. 1994. LC 93-23192. (Illus.). 216p. 236.00 (*0-387-94132-0*) Spr-Verlag.

Cerebral Aneurysms: Perioperative Management, Vol. 6. Fremont P. Wirth & Robert A. Ratcheson. 1994. (Illus.). 208p. 75.00 (*0-683-09199-9*) Lppncott W & W.

Cerebral Angiography. H. Krayenbuehl & M. G. Yasargil. 2nd ed. 1982. (Illus.). 597p. 169.00 (*0-86577-067-0*) Thieme Med Pubs.

Cerebral Angiography. Anne G. Osborn. 2nd ed. 1998. LC 98-39295. 480p. text 159.00 (*0-397-58404-0*) Lppncott W & W.

Cerebral Asymmetries in Sensory & Perceptual Processing. Stephen Christman. 1997. LC 97-43233. (Advances in Psychology Ser.: Vol. 123). 580p. 129.50 (*0-444-82510-X*, North Holland) Elsevier.

Cerebral Blood Flow: Mathematical Models, Instrumentation, & Imaging Techniques. Ed. by A. Rescigno & A. Boicelli. 1988. LC 88-25519. (NATO ASI Series A, Life Sciences: Vol. 153). (Illus.). 272p. 95.00 (*0-306-43019-3*, Plenum Trade) Perseus Pubng.

Cerebral Blood Flow & Intracranial Pressure: Proceedings of the International Symposium on Cerebral Blood Flow Regulation, Acid-Base & Engergy Metabolism Acute Brain Injuries, 5th, Roma Siena, 1971 International Symposium on Cerebral Blood Flow Regulation Staff. Ed. by C. Fieschi. 1972. 139.25 (*3-8055-1440-9*) S Karger.

Cerebral Blood Flow in Acute Head Injury: The Regulation of Cerebral Blood Flow & Metabolism During the Acute Phase of Head Injury, & Its Significance for Therapy. G. E. Cold. 1990. (Acta Neurochirurgica Ser.: Supplementum No. 49). (Illus.). 100p. 79.95 (*0-387-82224-0*) Spr-Verlag.

Cerebral Blood Flow, Metabolism & Epilepsy. Baldy-Moulinier. 1983. (Current Problems in Epilepsy Ser.: Vol. 1). (Illus.). (*0-86196-038-6*) J Libbey Med GBR. *Dist:* Bks Intl VA.

Cerebral Computer. Robert Baron. 1987. 552p. pap. 55.00 (*0-8058-0037-9*) L Erlbaum Assocs.

Cerebral Contusions, Lacerations & Hematomas. Ed. by R. A. Frowein. 1991. (Advances in Neurotraumatology Ser.: Vol. 3). (Illus.). 259p. 128.00 (*0-387-81982-7*) Spr-Verlag.

Cerebral Cortex: Association & Auditory Cortices, Vol. 4. A. Peters & E. G. Jones. 1985. LC 84-1982. (Illus.). 376p. (C). text 105.00 (*0-306-42040-6*, Kluwer Plenum) Kluwer Academic.

Cerebral Cortex: Cellular Components of the Cerebral Cortex, Vol. 1. A. Peters & E. G. Jones. 1984. LC 84-1982. (Illus.). 580p. (C). text 120.00 (*0-306-41544-5*, Kluwer Plenum) Kluwer Academic.

Cerebral Cortex: Visual Cortex, Vol. 3. A. Peters & E. G. Jones. 1985. LC 84-1982. (Illus.). 438p. (C). text 105.00 (*0-306-42025-2*, Kluwer Plenum) Kluwer Academic.

Cerebral Cortex Vol. 2: Functional Properties of Cortical Cells. E. G. Jones & A. Peters. 1984. LC 84-1982. (Illus.). 354p. 95.00 (*0-306-41755-3*, Kluwer Plenum) Kluwer Academic.

Cerebral Cortex Vol. 5: Sensory-Motor Areas & Aspects of Cortical Connectivity. E. G. Jones & A. Peters. 1986. LC 84-1982. (Illus.). 528p. 120.00 (*0-306-42174-7*, Kluwer Plenum) Kluwer Academic.

Cerebral Cortex Vol. 7: Development & Maturation of Cerebral Cortex. A. Peters & E. G. Jones. 1988. LC 84-1982. (Illus.). 536p. (C). text 120.00 (*0-306-42881-4*, Kluwer Plenum) Kluwer Academic.

Cerebral Cortex Vol. 8A: Comparative Structure & Evolution of Cerebral Cortex, Pt. I. Edward G. Jones & Alan A. Peters. 1990. LC 84-1982. (Illus.). 388p. (C). text 105.00 (*0-306-43477-6*, Kluwer Plenum) Kluwer Academic.

Cerebral Cortex Vol. 8B: Comparative Structure & Evolution of Cerebral Cortex, Pt. 2. E. G. Jones & A. Peters. 1990. LC 84-1982. (Illus.). 512p. (C). text 120.00 (*0-306-43635-3*, Kluwer Plenum) Kluwer Academic.

Cerebral Cortex Vol. 9: Normal & Altered States of Function. A. Peters & E. G. Jones. 1991. LC 84-1982. (Illus.). 552p. (C). text 120.00 (*0-306-43648-5*, Kluwer Plenum) Kluwer Academic.

Cerebral Cortex Vol. 10: Primary Visual Cortex in Primates. A. Peters & K. S. Rockland. 1994. (Illus.). 576p. (C). text 125.00 (*0-306-44605-7*, Kluwer Plenum) Kluwer Academic.

Cerebral Cortex Vol. 11: The Barrel Cortex of Rodents, Vol. 11. Ed. by E. G. Jones & I. T. Diamond. 1995. (Illus.). 462p. (C). text 120.00 (*0-306-44847-5*, Kluwer Plenum) Kluwer Academic.

Cerebral Cortex Vol. 12: Extrastriate Cortex in Primates, Vol. 12. Ed. by Kathleen S. Rockland et al. 1998. (Illus.). 870p. (C). text 191.00 (*0-306-45530-7*, Kluwer Plenum) Kluwer Academic.

Cerebral Cortex Vol. 13: Models of Cortical Circuits, Vol. 13. P. S. Ulinski et al. 1999. (Illus.). 590p. (C). text 165.00 (*0-306-45727-X*, Kluwer Plenum) Kluwer Academic.

Cerebral Damage Before & after Cardiac Surgery. Ed. by Allen Willner. 1993. (Developments in Critical Care, Medicine, & Anesthesiology Ser.). 280p. (C). text 200.50 (*0-7923-1928-1*) Kluwer Academic.

Cerebral Dominance: The Biological Foundations. Ed. by Norman Geschwind & Albert M. Galaburda. 1984. (Illus.). 240p. 52.50 (*0-674-10658-X*) HUP.

Cerebral Dominance & Its Relation to Psychological Function. Oliver L. Zangwill. LC 78-72831. (Brainedness, Handedness, & Mental Abilities Ser.). reprint ed. 28.00 (*0-404-60899-X*) AMS Pr.

Cerebral Dysfunction: Pathophysiology & Management of Mental Decline. Kewal K. Jain et al. 1990. (Illus.). 600p. 94.95 (*0-88416-608-2*) Mosby Inc.

Cerebral Dysgenesis: Embryology & Clinical Expression. Harvey B. Sarnat. 1992. (Illus.). 496p. (C). text 79.50 (*0-19-506442-9*) OUP.

Cerebral Embolism. Ed. by Michael Hennerici. 1995. (Journal: Vol. 5, No. 2, 1995). (Illus.). 94p. (Orig.). pap. 31.50 (*3-8055-6153-9*) S Karger.

Cerebral Energy Metabolism & Metabolic Encephalopathy. Ed. by D. W. McCandless. 1985. 478p. 125.00 (*0-306-41797-9*, Plenum Trade) Perseus Pubng.

Cerebral Ischemia. G. W. Kramer et al. 1991. (Illus.). 238p. 83.00 (*0-387-52341-3*) Spr-Verlag.

Cerebral Ischemia: Clinical Implications & Therapeutics. Ed. by Robert H. Rosenwasser et al. 1994. (Illus.). 179p. (C). lib. bdg. 145.00 (*1-56072-137-5*) Nova Sci Pubs.

Cerebral Ischemia: From Pathophysiology to Treatment - Journal: Cerebrovascular Diseases, Vol. 1, Suppl. 1, 1991. Ed. by Jose Biller et al. 1991. (Illus.). iv, 140p. pap. 62.75 (*3-8055-5448-6*) S Karger.

Cerebral Ischemia: From Pharmacology to Modern Techniques & Clinical Implications. Value of Almitrine-Raubasine: International Symposium, Hangzhou, People's Republic of China, May 14, 1994. Ed. by J. Bogousslavsky & X. D. Wang. 1995. (Journal: Vol. 35, Suppl. 1, 1995). (Illus.). iv, 48p. pap. 22.75 (*3-8055-6232-2*) S Karger.

Cerebral Ischemia: Molecular & Cellular Pathophysiology. Wolfgang Walz. 1999. LC 98-32443. (Contemporary Neuroscience Ser.). (Illus.). ix, 278p. 125.00 (*0-89603-540-9*) Humana.

Cerebral Ischemia & Basic Mechanisms. Ed. by A. Hartman et al. 1994. LC 93-24247. (Illus.). 443p. 280.00 (*0-387-56573-6*) Spr-Verlag.

Cerebral Ischemia & Dementia. Ed. by A. Hartmann et al. 1991. (Illus.). 472p. 198.00 (*0-387-53331-1*) Spr-Verlag.

Cerebral Ischemia Resuscitation. Ed. by Schurr. 1990. 456p. lib. bdg. 139.00 (*0-8493-6715-8*, RC171) CRC Pr.

Cerebral Laterality: Theory & Research. Ed. by Frederick L. Kitterle. 1991. 248p. (C). text 49.95 (*0-8058-0471-4*) L Erlbaum Assocs.

Cerebral Metabolism in Aging & Neurological Disorders, Second Joint Meeting. A. Agnoli et al. Ed. by H. Lechner et al. 1987. (Journal: Vol. 33, No. 3-4, 1987). (Illus.). 164p. pap. 95.75 (*3-8055-4640-8*) S Karger.

Cerebral Microcirculation. Ed. by F. Hammersen & K. Messmer. 1990. (Progress in Applied Microcirculation Ser.: Vol. 16). (Illus.). x, 102p. 76.75 (*3-8055-5054-5*) S Karger.

Cerebral Monitoring in the Operating Room & the Intensive Care Unit: Development in Critical Care Medicine & Anaesthesiology. Enno Freye. 1990. 196p. (C). text 166.50 (*0-7923-0439-X*) Kluwer Academic.

Cerebral Motor Control in Man: Cerebral Event-Related Potentials. Ed. by J. E. Desmedt. 1978. (Progress in Clinical Neurophysiology Ser.: Vol. 4). (Illus.). 102.75 (*3-8055-2712-8*) S Karger.

Cerebral Palsies: Causes, Consequences, & Management. Geoffrey Miller & Gary Clark. 1998. LC 97-52631. (Illus.). 384p. text 79.99 incl. audio (*0-7506-9964-7*) Buttrwrth-Heinemann.

Cerebral Palsies: Epidemiology & Causal Pathways. Fiona J. Stanley et al. 2000. LC 00-421463. (Clinics in Developmental Medicine Ser.: No. 151). (Illus.). xx, 251p. (C). (*1-898683-20-4*) Mc Keith Pr GBR. *Dist:* Cambridge U Pr.

Cerebral Palsies of Children: A Clinical Study from the Infirmary for Nervous Diseases, Philadelphia. William Osler. 1991. (Classics in Developmental Medicine Ser.: No. 1). (Illus.). 92p. (C). text (*0-521-41326-5*) Mc Keith Pr GBR. *Dist:* Cambridge U Pr.

Cerebral Palsy. Daniel Boone. 1972. LC 76-190708. (Studies in Communicative Disorders). (C). pap. text (*0-672-61290-9*, Bobbs) Macmillan.

Cerebral Palsy. Ed. by Lesley Cogher et al. 1992. (Management of Disability Ser.: No. 1). (Illus.). 240p. text (*0-412-30900-9*) E A GBR. *Dist:* OUP.

Cerebral Palsy. Eugene T. McDonald & B. Chance, Jr. 1964. pap. text 25.67 (*0-13-122812-9*) P-H.

Cerebral Palsy. Merlin J. Mecham. Ed. by Harvey Halpern. 2nd ed. 1996. LC 86-3271. (PRO-ED Studies in Communicative Disorders). (Illus.). 180p. (Orig.). pap. text 26.00 (*0-89079-627-0*, 7318) PRO-ED.

Cerebral Palsy: A Complete Guide for Caregiving. Freeman Miller & Steven J. Bachrach. 2nd ed. 1998. (Johns Hopkins Press Health Bks.). 488p. reprint ed. pap. 19.95 (*0-8018-5949-2*) Johns Hopkins.

Cerebral Palsy Vol. 1: Discussion & Reviews. 1995. 413p. pap. 47.00 (*1-887759-04-2*, P-123) Am Phys Therapy Assn.

Cerebral Palsy Vol. 2: Research. 1995. 346p. pap. 47.00 (*1-887759-05-0*, P-124) Am Phys Therapy Assn.

Cerebral Palsy Vol. 3: Case Reports, Orthotics & Devices, Measurement & Assessment & Schools & Education. 1995. 312p. pap. 47.00 (*1-887759-07-7*, P-125) Am Phys Therapy Assn.

Cerebral Palsy Not Necessary: No Cause for Life Long Handicap. Hildegard Winky-Lotz. 1989. (Illus.). 85p. spiral bd. 30.00 (*0-936112-04-2*) Willyshe Pub.

Cerebral Perivascular Cells. D. N. Angelov et al. Ed. by F. Beck et al. 1998. LC 98-25894. (Advances in Anatomy, Embryology & Cell Biology Ser.: Vol. 147). (Illus.). 92p. pap. 69.95 (*3-540-64638-8*) Spr-Verlag.

Cerebral Reorganization of Function after Brain Damage. Ed. by Harvey S. Levin & Jordan Grafman. 2000. LC 99-47749. (Illus.). 412p. text 55.00 (*0-19-512026-4*) OUP.

Cerebral Revascularization by Microneurosurgical Bypass. P. Conforti et al. 1984. 240p. text (*1-57235-042-3*) Piccin Nuova.

Cerebral Sinus Thrombosis: Experimental & Clinical Aspects. Ed. by K. Einhupl et al. 1990. LC 91-2456. (Illus.). 242p. (C). text 102.00 (*0-306-43832-1*, Kluwer Plenum) Kluwer Academic.

Cerebral Vascular Spasm: A New Diagnostic & Neurosurgical Approach Based on Advances in Neuropharmacology & Neurosciences. Ed. by Paul Glees & Dieter Voth. 1985. LC 84-22983. (Illus.). xii, 515p. 113.85 (*3-11-010029-0*) De Gruyter.

Cerebral Veins. Ed. by L. M. Auer & F. Loew. 1984. (Illus.). 381p. 148.00 (*0-387-81767-0*) Spr-Verlag.

Cerebral Visual Disturbance in Infantile Encephalogathy. O. Van Nieuwenhuizen. 1987. (Monographs in Ophthalmology). text 161.50 (*0-89838-860-0*) Kluwer Academic.

Cerebrospinal Fluid. Ed. by Robert M. Herndon & Roger A. Brumback. 1989. (C). text 199.50 (*0-7923-0121-8*) Kluwer Academic.

Cerebrospinal Fluid & the Brain Edemas. Thomas H. Milhorat. 1987. (Illus.). 172p. (C). 45.00 (*0-944809-00-6*) NeuroSci Soc NY.

Cerebrospinal Fluid Collections. Ed. by Howard H. Kaufman. 216p. 95.00 (*1-879284-48-0*) Am Assn Neuro.

Cerebrospinal Fluid (CSF) & Peptide Hormones. Ed. by E. M. Rodriguez & T. Van Wimersma Greidanus. 1981. (Frontiers of Hormone Research Ser.: Vol. 9). (Illus.). viii, 220p. 115.00 (*3-8055-2823-X*) S Karger.

Cerebrospinal Fluid in Diseases of the Nervous System. Robert A. Fishman. 2nd ed. 1992. (Illus.). 416p. text 77.00 (*0-7216-3557-1*) Saunders.

Cerebrospinal Fluid in Neurology & Psychiatry. Ed. by Joseph Bianchine & H. McConnell. 1994. LC 94-70978. (Illus.). 336p. (C). (gr. 13). 127.95 (*0-412-53570-X*, Chap & Hall NY) Chapman & Hall.

Cerebrospinal Meningitis in West Africa & the Sudan in the Twentieth Century. K. David Patterson & Gerald W. Hartwig. 1984. pap. 15.00 (*0-918456-55-X*) African Studies Assn.

Cerebrovascular Disease. Ed. by H. Hunt Batjer et al. 1996. LC 96-13565. 1,310p. text 299.00 (*0-397-51661-4*) Lppncott W & W.

***Cerebrovascular Disease.** Ed. by Pak H. Chan. 2001. LC 2001-25936. text 90.00 (*0-521-80254-7*) Cambridge U Pr.

Cerebrovascular Disease: Imaging & International Treatment Options. Ed. by Calvin L. Rumbaugh et al. 1995. LC 94-27327. (Illus.). 544p. 225.00 (*0-89640-259-2*) Igaku-Shoin.

***Cerebrovascular Disease: Momentum at the Turn of the Millennium.** Ed. by Dennis W. Choi et al. 2001. (American Heart Association Monographs). (Illus.). 384p. text (*0-87993-484-0*) Futura Pub.

Cerebrovascular Disease: Pathology, Diagnosis & Management Myron D. Ginsberg & Julien Bogousslavsky. Incl. Vol. 1. 185.00 (*0-632-04423-3*); Vol. 2. 260.00 (*0-632-04424-1*); 1998. LC 97-2036. (Illus.). 418.95 (*0-86542-425-X*);Vol. 1. 1998. 185.00 (*0-632-04423-3*);Vol. 2. 1998. 260.00 (*0-632-04424-1*) Blackwell Sci.

Cerebrovascular Disease in Childhood & Adolescence. Michael Edwards & Harold Hoffman. 1988. (Illus.). 512p. 115.00 (*0-683-02747-6*) Lppncott W & W.

Cerebrovascular Diseases: Nineteenth Princeton Stroke Conference. Ed. by Michael A. Moskowitz & Louis R. Caplan. 1995. 552p. text 195.00 (*0-7506-9603-6*) Buttrwrth-Heinemann.

Cerebrovascular Diseases: Proceedings of the WHO Expert Committee, Monaco, 1970. WHO Staff. 1971. (Technical Reports: No. 469). 57p. pap. text 5.00 (*92-4-120469-9*, 1100469) World Health.

Cerebrovascular Diseases in Children. Ed. by Anthony J. Raimondi et al. 1992. (Principles of Pediatric Neurosurgery Ser.). (Illus.). 256p. 138.00 (*0-387-97626-4*) Spr-Verlag.

Cerebrovascular Disorders. James F. Toole. 5th ed. 1998. LC 98-35963. 560p. text 105.00 (*0-397-51834-X*) Lppncott W & W.

Cerebrovascular Disorders: A Clinical & Research Classification. WHO Staff. 1978. (WHO Offset Publications: No. 43). 82p. 12.00 (*92-4-170043-2*) World Health.

Cerebrovascular Evaluation with Dopler Ultrasound. Merrill P. Spencer & John M. Reid. 1981. text 126.50 (*90-247-2384-1*) Kluwer Academic.

Cerebrovascular Pathology in Alzheimer's Disease. Ed. by Jack C. De La Torre & Vladimir Hachinski. 1997. LC 97-213174. (Annals of the New York Academy of Sciences Ser.: No. 826). 523p. 160.00 (*1-57331-086-7*); pap. 160.00 (*1-57331-087-5*) NY Acad Sci.

Cerebrovascular Pathology in Alzheimer's Disease. Jack C. De La Torre. 1999. (Annals of the New York Academy of Sciences Ser.). 544p. pap. text 29.95 (*0-8018-6214-0*) Johns Hopkins.

Cerebrovascular Surgery. Ed. by J. M. Fein & E. S. Flamm. 1985. (Illus.). Vol. 1. 300p. 275.00 (*0-387-90995-8*); Vol. 2. 300p. 275.00 (*0-387-90996-6*); Vol. 3. 465p. 324.00 (*0-387-96041-4*); Vol. 4. 350p. 275.00 (*0-387-96026-0*) Spr-Verlag.

Ceremonial Chemistry: The Ritual Persecution of Drugs, Addicts, & Pushers. Thomas S. Szasz. rev. ed. 1987. 272p. pap. 25.95 (*1-55691-019-3*, 193) Learning Pubns.

Cerenex Family Health Counselor. Hippocrates Magazine Editors. 1994. 256p. stu. ed. (*0-9644119-0-3*) Time Inc Health.

Ceres SV System - Endoscopic Saphenous Vein Harvesting Training Manual. 1998. (Illus.). vii, 49p. (*1-878353-44-6*) Silent Partners.

Certain Necessary Directions As well for the Cure of the Plague As for Preventing the Infection: Also Certaine Select Statutes. London College of Physicians Staff. 1979. LC 79-84120. (English Experience Ser.: No. 939). 148p. reprint ed. lib. bdg. 14.00 (*90-221-0939-9*) Walter J Johnson.

Certaine Workes of Chirurgerie. Thomas Gale. 1971. LC 79-38108. (English Experience Ser.: No. 420). (Illus.). 200p. reprint ed. 90.00 (*90-221-0420-6*) Walter J Johnson.

Certifiably Bulimic. Susan L. Merkel. 1991. LC 91-14993. 136p. pap. 12.95 (*0-942963-15-6*) Distinctive Pub.

Certification Completion for Basic First Response. Brady Games Staff. 1996. pap. text (*0-8359-5125-1*) Brady Pub.

Certification Examination for Medical Assistants. Jack Rudman. 1994. (Admission Test Ser.: ATS-93). pap. 29.95 (*0-8373-5093-X*) Nat Learn.

Certification Examination for Medical Assistants (CMA) Jack Rudman. (Admission Test Ser.: Vol. 93). 49.95 (*0-8373-5193-6*) Nat Learn.

Certification Examination for Occupational Therapy Assistant (OTA) Jack Rudman. (Admission Test Ser.: Vol. 69). 49.95 (*0-8373-5169-3*); 1994. pap. 29.95 (*0-8373-5069-7*) Nat Learn.

Certification for Home Care/Hospice Executives Study Guide. Home Care University Staff. 1999. (Illus.). iv, 175p. pap. (*1-930304-02-1*) Home Care Univ.

Certification for Home/Hospice Executives Resource Manual: Content References. Ed. by Home Care University Staff. 1999. (Illus.). v, 600p. pap. (*1-930304-03-X*) Home Care Univ.

Certification, Recertification, & Lifetime Learning in Psychiatry. Ed. by James H. Shore & Stephen C. Scheiber. 1994. LC 93-4217. (Issues in Psychiatry Ser.). 220p. text 10.95 (*0-88048-465-9*, 8465) Am Psychiatric.

Certification Review for Perianesthesia Nursing. American Society of Post Anesthesia Nurses Staff. Ed. by Kathy Carlson. 3rd ed. 1995. LC 95-36450. (Illus.). 379p. pap. text 33.00 (*0-7216-4492-9*) Saunders.

Certification Review for Pharmacy Technicians. Noah Reifman. 1996. pap. text 32.95 (*0-914373-34-X*) Wieser & Wieser.

Certification Review to Accompany Health Unit Coordinating. Myrna LaFleur Brooks & Elaine T. Gillingham. Ed. by Selma Kaszczuk. 4th ed. 1998. LC 97-36631. 192p. (C). pap. 22.50 (*0-7216-7283-3*) Saunders.

Certified Clinical Microbiologist Database. Stewart. 1992. 225.00 (*0-87371-579-9*, L579) Lewis Pubs.

Certified Complete Emergency 1st. Poliafico. 1996. 10p. pap. text (*0-8359-5053-0*) Brady Pub.

Certified Dental Technician (CDT) Jack Rudman. (Admission Test Ser.: Vol. 106). 69.95 (*0-8373-5856-6*); 1994. pap. 49.95 (*0-8373-5806-X*) Nat Learn.

Certified Laboratory Assistant. Jack Rudman. 1994. (Career Examination Ser.: C-179). pap. 27.95 (*0-8373-0179-3*) Nat Learn.

Certified Manager of Patient Accounts Examination Study Guide. Healthcare Financial Management Association Staff. 136p. (Orig.). pap. text, stu. ed. 35.00 (*0-930228-38-3*) Hlthcare Fin Mgmt.

Certified Mental Health Counselor. Jack Rudman. 1994. (Career Examination Ser.: C-3560). pap. 39.95 (*0-8373-3560-4*) Nat Learn.

Certified Nurse Examination Series. Jack Rudman. 1994. pap. (*0-8373-6100-1*) Nat Learn.

Certified Occupational Therapy Assistant: Principles, Concepts & Techniques. Ed. by Sally E. Ryan. 2nd ed. 1992. LC 92-50395. (Illus.). 304p. (C). pap. 30.00 (*1-55642-178-8*, 31788) SLACK Inc.

Certified Ophthalmic Assistant Exam Review Manual. Janice K. Ledford. 1996. LC 96-44190. (Basic Bookshelf for Eyecare Professionals Ser.). (Illus.). 240p. pap. text 33.00 (*1-55642-333-0*, 63330) SLACK Inc.

Certified Ophthalmic Technician Exam Review Manual. Janice K. Ledford. 1997. LC 97-10166. (Basic Bookshelf for Eyecare Professionals Ser.). (Illus.). 256p. (Orig.). pap. text 33.00 (*1-55642-324-1*, 63241) SLACK Inc.

Certified Opthalmic Medical Technologist Exam Review Manual. Janice K. Ledford. 1999. (Illus.). 240p. pap. text 36.00 (*1-55642-422-1*) SLACK Inc.

Cervical & Thoracic Spine: Mechanical Diagnosis & Therapy. Robin A. McKenzie. 1990. (Illus.). 320p. (C). text (*0-9597746-7-X*) Spinal Pubns Ltd NZL. *Dist:* Orthopedic Phys.

Cervical Cancer: Current Bibliographies in Medicine: January 1993 Through March 1996. Lori J. Klein & Edward L. Trimble. 1996. 47p. (Orig.). pap. text 20.00 (*0-7881-3342-X*) DIANE Pub.

Cervical Cancer & Preinvasive Neoplasia. Ed. by Stephen C. Rubin & William J. Hoskins. 1996. LC 95-26460. 512p. text 160.00 (*0-397-51645-2*) Lppncott W & W.

Cervical Cancer Screening Programmes: Managerial Guidelines. A. B. Miller. 1992. (FRE & SPA., Illus.). viii, 50p. pap. text 12.00 (*92-4-154447-3*, 1150390) World Health.

Cervical Laminectomy. Oliver D. Grin & Dorothy L. Bouwman. 1993. (Patient Education Ser.). (Illus.). 24p. (Orig.). pap. text 4.00 (*0-929689-59-3*) Ludann Co.

Cervical Neoplasia. Ed. by Franco Rilke. 1987. (Journal: Vol. 5, No. 1). (Illus.). 76p. pap. 41.75 (*3-8055-4605-X*) S Karger.

Cervical Spinal Disorders: A Textbook for Rehabilitation Sciences Students. Ed. by S. W. Lee. 1999. LC 99-10460. (Illus.). 400p. pap. (*981-4021-29-6*) U Auckland NZL. *Dist:* Spr-Verlag.

Cervical Spine. Ed. by Charles R. Clark & Thomas B. Ducker. 3rd ed. 1997. LC 97-4392. 1,024p. text 189.00 (*0-397-51535-9*) Lppncott W & W.

Cervical Spine, No. II. Ed. by R. Louis & A. Weidner. 1990. (Illus.). 304p. 112.00 (*0-387-82151-1*, 3624) Spr-Verlag.

Cervical Spine: A Surgical Atlas. Henry H. Sherk. 3rd ed. 1994. 352p. text 159.00 (*0-397-51203-1*) Lppncott W & W.

Cervical Spine I. Ed. by P. Kehr & A. Weidner. 1987. (Illus.). 330p. 126.00 (*0-387-81953-3*) Spr-Verlag.

Cervical Spondylosis & Similar Disorders in the Cervical Spine. Ed. by K. Ono et al. 1997. LC 98-9990. 763p. lib. bdg. 58.00 (*981-02-2744-2*) World Scientific Pub.

Cervical Spondylotic Myelopathy. R. L. Saunders & P. M. Bernini. 1992. (Contemporary Issues in Neurological Surgery Ser.). (Illus.). 240p. 95.00 (*0-86542-193-5*) Blackwell Sci.

Cervical Syndrome. Ruth Jackson. 4th ed. 1978. (Illus.). 416p. 65.95 (*0-398-03696-9*) C C Thomas.

Cervix Cancer. Ed. by Earl A. Surwit & David S. Alberts. 1987. (Cancer Treatment & Research Ser.). text 150.00 (*0-89838-822-8*) Kluwer Academic.

Cesarean Delivery in the United States, 1990. S. M. Tafel. 1994. LC 94-10794. (Vital & Health Statistics. Series 21, Data on Natality, Marriage, & Divorce: No. 51). (*0-8406-0490-4*) Natl Ctr Health Stats.

Cesarean Section: Guidelines for Appropriate Utilization. Ed. by Bruce L. Flamm & Edward J. Quilligan. 1995. LC 94-29533. (Clinical Perspectives in Obstetrics & Gynecology Ser.). (Illus.). 278p. 89.00 (*0-387-94238-6*); (*3-540-94238-6*) Spr-Verlag.

Cesium-137 from the Environment to Man: Metabolism & Dose. 1977. LC 77-77789. (Report Ser.: No. 52). 48p. pap. text 20.00 (*0-913392-34-0*) NCRP Pubns.

CFIDs, Fibromyalgia & the Virus-Allergy Link: New Therapy for Chronic Functional Illnesses. R. Bruce Duncan. 2000. LC 00-22098. (Illus.). xxxv, 330p. pap. 39.95 (*0-7890-1073-9*); lib. bdg. 79.95 (*0-7890-1072-0*) Haworth Pr (Hawrth Medical).

CFIDS Resource Directory: A Comprehensive Guide to Chronic-Fatigue Related Services. Ed. by Taia Butterworth & Maritza O. Dunn. 1997. 242p. (Orig.). pap. 34.90 (*0-925133-48-5*) Volt Directory.

CFRN Study Guide. Contrib. by Lura Donnelly et al. 2nd ed. 1996. 217p. (Orig.). pap. text, stu. ed. 26.00 (*0-935890-01-7*) Emerg Nurses IL.

CFS: Conquering the Crippler: Nature & Management of Chronic Fatigue Syndrome. 1993. pap. (*0-9636487-0-5*) C&C Communs.

CFTR & the Molecular Basis for Cystic Fibrosis. Jeffrey Wine. 1997. (Medical Intelligence Unit Ser.). 250p. 89.95 (*0-412-13481-0*) Chapman & Hall.

CGFNS Qualifying Exam: Practice English Test Audio Tape. Commission on Graduates of Foreign Nursing Schools. (C). No. 1. 1992. 20p. incl. audio (*0-9630592-1-1*); No. 2. 1995. 28p. incl. audio (*0-9630592-3-8*) Grads of For Nursing.

CGRP Family: CGRP, Amylin & Adrenomedullin. David Poyner & Ian Marshall. 2000. LC 99-34620. (Medical Intelligence Unit Ser.). (Illus.). 261p. 89.00 (*1-57059-592-5*) Landes Bioscience.

Chagas' Disease & the Nervous System. 1999. (Scientific Publications: No. 547). 362p. text 30.00 (*92-75-11547-8*) PAHO.

Chaga's Disease Vectors, Vol. III. Brenner & Stoka. 1987. 168p. 99.00 (*0-8493-4349-6*, CRC Reprint) Franklin.

Chagas' Disease Vectors: Anatomic & Physiological Aspects. R. Brenner & Stoka A. Merced. 1987. LC 87-13209. reprint ed. 88.00 (*0-8493-4348-8*, CRC Reprint) Franklin.

Chagas' Disease Vectors: Taxonomic Ecological & Epidemiological Aspects. R. Brenner & Stoka A. Merced. 1987. LC 87-13209. 168p. reprint ed. 99.00 (*0-8493-4347-X*, CRC Reprint) Franklin.

Chaim - To Good Health & Life: A History of Montefiore Hospital Pittsburgh, PA, 1898-1990. Carol S. Bleier et al. 1997. LC 97-71894. (Illus.). viii, 286p. pap. 35.00 (*0-945704-05-4*) Genesis Comns.

Chain of Friendship: Selected Letters of Dr. John Fothergill of London, 1735-1780. John Fothergill. Ed. by Betsy C. Corner & Christopher C. Booth. 1971. LC 75-127877. (Illus.). 566p. 47.50 (*0-674-10660-1*, Belknap) HUP.

Chained to the Desk: A Guidebook for Workaholics, Their Partners & Children, & the Clinicians Who Treat Them. Bryan E. Robinson. 1998. LC 97-45349. 280p. 24.95 (*0-8147-7480-6*) NYU Pr.

Chairman, Nursing. Jack Rudman. 1994. (Teachers License Examination Ser.: CH-31). pap. 39.95 (*0-8373-8181-9*) Nat Learn.

Chalk Talks on Alcohol. Joseph Martin. 1989. LC 82-47750. 192p. pap. 13.00 (*0-06-250593-9*) Harper SF.

***Challenge & Change: A History of the Dalhousie School of Nursing, 1949-1989.** Peter Twohig. 1998. 128p. pap. (*1-895686-95-4*) Fer1nwd Publ Co CAN. *Dist:* Eiron.

Challenge & Crisis in Missionary Medicine. David J. Seel. 1979. LC 79-16015. (Illus.). 149p. pap. 4.99 (*0-87808-172-0*) William Carey Lib.

Challenge & Innovation: Methodological Advances in Social Research on HIV-AIDS. Ed. by Mary Boulton. 1994. LC 94-4131. (Social Aspects of AIDS Ser.). 240p. (*0-7484-0197-0*); pap. (*0-7484-0198-9*) Tay Francis Ltd GBR. *Dist:* Taylor & Francis.

Challenge for Psychoanalysis & Psychotherapy: Solutions for the Future. Stefan De Schill. 1998. LC 99-231336. (International Library of Group Analysis). 250p. pap. (*1-85302-477-5*) Jessica Kingsley GBR. *Dist:* Taylor & Francis.

Challenge for Science, Medicine & Public Health System. Ed. by H. F. Rabenau et al. 2001. LC 00-50676. (Contributions to Microbiology Ser.: 7). (Illus.). viii, 164p. 155.00 (*3-8055-7124-0*) S Karger.

Challenge of Adolescent Health: Views from Catholic Social Teaching & the Social & Medical Sciences. Brenda W. Donnelly et al. 1996. LC 96-35135. 242p. pap. text 33.00 (*0-7618-0561-3*); lib. bdg. 63.00 (*0-7618-0560-5*) U Pr of Amer.

Challenge of Aging: A Multidisciplinary Approach to Extended Care. Ed. by Marion W. Shaw. 2nd ed. 1991. (Illus.). 192p. (Orig.). pap. text (*0-443-04357-4*) Church.

Challenge of AIDS in the Workplace: An IDI Report. Gilles R. Monif et al. 2nd ed. 1995. (Illus.). 56p. text 149.00 (*1-880906-24-4*) IDI Pub.

Challenge of Attachment for Caregiving. Dorothy Heard & Brian Lake. 1997. LC 96-29387. 240p. (C). 84.95 (*0-415-14017-X*); pap. 27.95 (*0-415-14018-8*) Routledge.

Challenge of Cognitive Therapy: Applications to Nontraditional Populations. T. M. Vallis et al. 1991. LC 90-14306. (Applied Clinical Psychology Ser.). (Illus.). 198p. (C). 52.50 (*0-306-43629-9*, Plenum Trade) Perseus Pubng.

Challenge of Dermato-Epidemiology. Ed. by Hywel C. Williams & David P. Strachan. 1997. LC 96-9820. 384p. 139.95 (*0-8493-7689-0*) CRC Pr.

Challenge of Environmental Management in Urban Areas. Ed. by Adrian Atkinson et al. 1999. LC 99-72605. (Studies in Environmental Policy & Practice). 302p. text (*1-84014-525-0*) Ashgate Pub GBR. *Dist:* Ashgate Pub Co.

Challenge of Epidemiology: Issues & Selected Readings. C. Buck & A. Llopis. 1988. (PAHO Scientific Publication Ser.: No. 505). 1003p. text 60.00 (*92-75-11505-2*) World Health.

Challenge of Epilepsy. Sally Fletcher. rev. ed. 1986. LC 85-90992. (Illus.). 128p. pap. 9.95 (*0-9615513-9-9*) Aura Pub Co.

Challenge of Epilepsy: New Antiepileptic Drugs. H. Stefan et al. 1998. (Illus.). 272p. 83.95 (*3-89412-385-0*) Blackwell Sci.

Challenge of Ethics in Pharmacy Practice: A Symposium. David A. Knapp. 1985. 68p. 6.00 (*0-931292-15-8*) Am Inst Hist Pharm.

Challenge of Geriatric Medicine. Bernard Isaacs. 1992. (Illus.). 254p. 79.50 (*0-19-262022-3*); pap. text 34.50 (*0-19-262021-5*) OUP.

Challenge of Health Care Leadership: Executive Strategies for Managing Responsible Change. Earl A. Simendinger. 1997. LC 97-14540. 206p. pap. 44.00 (*1-55648-205-1*) AHPI.

Challenge of Maturity: A Comprehensive Guide to Understand & Achieve Psychological & Social Self-Actualization As We Grow Older. William D. Eldridge. 1991. 342p. (C). pap. text 32.00 (*0-8191-8178-1*) U Pr of Amer.

Challenge of Overpopulation, 1955 edition see Standing Room Only: The World's Exploding Population

***Challenge of Rising PSA. Can We Delay Prostate Cancer Progression? AstraZeneca-Sponsored Satellite Symposium, EAU, Geneva, April 2001.** Ed. by R. Kirby. 2001. (Illus.). 32p. pap. 25.25 (*3-8055-7324-3*) S Karger.

Challenge of Severe Mental Handicap: A Behavior Analytic Approach. Ed. by Bob Remington. 1991. LC 90-13162. (Clinical Psychology & Personality Ser.: No. 1837). 416p. 425.00 (*0-471-92503-9*) Wiley.

Challenge of the Aged. Abraham Epstein. 1976. LC 75-17219. (Social Problems & Social Policy Ser.). reprint ed. 35.95 (*0-405-07490-5*) Ayer.

Challenge of the Borderline Patient: Competency in Diagnosis & Treatment. Jerome Kroll. 1988. (Professional Bks.). 237p. 32.00 (*0-393-70047-X*) Norton.

Challenge the Wilderness: A Family Saga of Robert & Alice Tomlinson - Pioneer Medical Missionaries. George D. Tomlinson & Judith Young. 1993. (Illus.). 503p. reprint ed. 22.95 (*1-883183-01-4*); pap. 16.95 (*1-883183-02-2*) NW Wilderness.

Challenge to the NHS. David G. Green. 1986. (Hobart Paperback Ser.: No. 23). 116p. (Orig.). (C). pap. text (*0-255-36194-7*) Transatl Arts.

Challenges. Serge Lang. 1997. LC 94-7180. (Illus.). 832p. pap. 34.95 (*0-387-94861-9*) Spr-Verlag.

Challenges & Innovations in Homecare. Ed. by Joanne Handy & Charlotte K. Scheurman. 1994. (Critical Debates in an Aging Society Ser.). 101p. (Orig.). pap. 19.95 (*0-9640387-1-4*) Am Soc Aging.

Challenges & Opportunities in Pediatric Oncology. Frederick F. Holmes. 1999. (Annals of the New York Academy of Sciences Ser.). 256p. pap. text 24.95 (*0-8018-6211-6*) Johns Hopkins.

Challenges & Perspectives in Neuroscience. Ed. by David Ottoson et al. 1995. LC 95-22622. (Wenner-Gren International Ser.: Vol. 66). 312p. 188.00 (*0-08-042515-1*, Pergamon Pr) Elsevier.

Challenges Facing Dwarf Parents: Preparing for a New Baby. Ellen H. Fernandez. 1990. LC 90-80575. 64p. pap. 7.95 (*0-942963-03-2*) Distinctive Pub.

Challenges for Neuroscience in the 21st Century. Ed. by O. Hayaishi. 2000. (Taniguchi Symposia on Brain Sciences Ser.: Vol. 22). (Illus.). x, 306p. 243.50 (*3-8055-7034-1*) S Karger.

Challenges in Acute Coronary Syndromes. David P. De Bono & Burton Sobel. 2001. LC 00-60891. (Blackwell Science Challenges Ser.). (Illus.). 320p. 103.95 (*0-632-05579-0*) Blackwell Sci.

Challenges in Aging. Ed. by Manfred Bergener et al. 1991. (Sandoz Lectures in Gerontology). (Illus.). 304p. text 99.95 (*0-12-090163-3*) Acad Pr.

Challenges in Breast Cancer. Ian S. Fentiman. 1999. LC 99-15250. (Illus.). 268p. 152.95 (*0-632-05242-2*) Blackwell Sci.

***Challenges in Chronic Obstructive Pulmonary Disease.** Pearson. 2001. (Illus.). 99.00 (*0-632-05972-9*) Blackwell Sci.

Challenges in Clinical Practice: Pharmacologic & Psychosocial Strategies. Ed. by Mark H. Pollack et al. 1996. LC 96-7348. 504p. text 60.00 (*1-57230-067-1*, 0067) Guilford Pubns.

Challenges in Colorectal Cancer. John Scholefield. 2000. LC 99-57131. (Illus.). 230p. 152.95 (*0-632-05116-7*) Blackwell Sci.

Challenges in Colorectal Surgery. Ed. by Paul B. Boulos & Steven D. Wexner. 2000. 228p. text (*0-7020-2559-3*) W B Saunders GBR. *Dist:* Saunders.

Challenges in Emergency Nursing: A Self-Study Certification Review. Judy Selfridge-Thomas et al. Ed. by Robin Carter. 2nd ed. 1998. LC 98-21737. (Illus.). 352p. (C). pap. text 32.00 (*0-7216-7746-0*) Saunders.

Challenges in Growth Hormone Therapy. John P. Monson. 1999. LC 99-17635. (Illus.). xiv, 305p. 152.95 (*0-632-05164-7*) Blackwell Sci.

Challenges in Inflammatory Bowel Disease. D. P. Jewell et al. 2001. (Illus.). 320p. 139.00 (*0-632-05169-8*) Blackwell Sci.

Challenges in Medical Care. Ed. by Andrew Grubb. 1992. LC 91-27615. 206p. 159.95 (*0-471-93102-0*, Wiley-Liss) Wiley.

***Challenges in Melanoma.** Julia Newton-Bishop. 2001. LC 2001-35202. (Illus.). 320p. 139.95 (*0-632-05772-6*) Blackwell Sci.

Challenges in Military Health Care: Perspectives on Health Status & the Provision of Care. Jay Stanley & John D. Blair. 1993. 192p. (C). text 34.95 (*1-56000-650-1*) Transaction Pubs.

Challenges in Prostate Cancer. Winsor Bowsher. 2000. LC 00-36192. (Illus.). xi, 236p. 104.95 (*0-632-05422-0*) Blackwell Sci.

Challenges in Reproductive Health Research: UNDP-UNFPA-WHO-World Bank Special Programme of Research, Development, & Research Training in Human Reproduction: Biennial Report 1992-1993. Ed. by J. Khanna et al. 1994. (ENG & FRE.). 202p. pap. text 39.00 (*92-4-156170-X*, 1150414) World Health.

Challenges in Rheumatoid Arthritis. Howard A. Bird & Michael L. Snaith. 1999. LC 98-42399. (Illus.). xi, 319p. 115.95 (*0-632-04939-1*) Blackwell Sci.

Challenges in Studying the Socioeconomic Dimensions in Cancer Therapy. Ed. by Maureen O'Reilly. 1995. 88p. (Orig.). (*1-57130-013-9*) Medicine Grp USA.

Challenges in Studying the Socioeconomic Dimensions in Cancer Therapy: Proceedings of a Symposium held in Cologne, Germany. Ed. by Maureen O'Reilly. 1995. (Illus.). 124p. (Orig.). (*1-57130-016-3*) Medicine Grp USA.

Challenges in Women's Health: Menopause. Elaine Weil. 2000. (Illus.). 80p. pap. (*1-57801-049-7*) Western Schls.

Challenges in Women's Health: PMS. Elaine Weil. 2000. (Illus.). 35p. pap. (*1-57801-053-5*) Western Schls.

Challenges in Women's Health: Reproductive Choices. Elaine Weil. 2000. (Illus.). 80p. pap. (*1-57801-051-9*) Western Schls.

Challenges of Medical Practice Variations. Ed. by Tavs F. Andersen & Gavin H. Mooney. 1990. text 60.00 (*0-333-47508-9*) Intl Spec Bk.

Challenging Behavior: Analysis & Intervention in People with Learning Disabilities. Eric Emerson. 1996. (Illus.). 243p. (C). pap. text 39.95 (*0-521-40665-X*) Cambridge U Pr.

Challenging Behavior of Persons with Mental Health Disorders & Severe Disabilities. Norman A. Wieseler et al. 1999. LC 99-33488. (Illus.). x, 278p. 39.95 (*0-940898-66-7*) Am Assn Mental.

Challenging Behaviour & Intellectual Disability: A Psychological Perspective. Ed. by Robert S. Jones & Caroline B. Eayrs. 1993. 375p. 105.00 (*1-873791-20-8*) Taylor & Francis.

Challenging Cases in Endocrinology. Ed. by Mark E. Molitch. 2002. (Contemporary Endocrinology Ser.). 436p. 145.00 (*0-89603-914-5*) Humana.

Challenging Diagnoses in the Academy Collection: Quick Reference Guides for Family Physicians. Margaret E. McCahill & Erik Lindbloom. 1998. LC 98-22561. (Academy Collection). 200p. pap. 29.95 (*0-683-30423-2*) Lppncott W & W.

Challenging Dream of Heart Surgery: From the Pampas to Cleveland. Rene G. Favaloro. Tr. by Peter Willshaw from SPA. 1993. LC 93-36345.Tr. of De/La Pampa a los Estados Unidos. 24.95 (*0-316-26026-6*, Little Brwn Med Div) Lppncott W & W.

Challenging Family Therapy Situations: Perspectives in Social Constructionism. Ed. by Joan D. Atwood. 1997. LC 97-23148. (Illus.). 296p. 43.95 (*0-8261-9820-1*) Springer Pub.

Challenging Ideas in Psychiatric Nursing. Liam Clarke. 1999. LC 98-32451. 208p. text 90.00 (*0-415-18696-X*) Routledge.

Challenging Medicine. Ed. by Jonathan Gabe et al. 1994. LC 93-46699. 240p. (C). pap. 27.99 (*0 415 08817 8*, B3450) Routledge.

Challenging Medicine. Ed. by Jonathon Gabe et al. 1994. LC 93-46699. 240p. (C). 80.00 (*0-415-08816-X*, B3446) Routledge.

Challenging the Therapeutic State: Critical Perspectives on Psychiatry & the Mental Health System. David Cohen. 1990. 350p. pap. 25.00 (*0-930195-05-1*) Inst Mind Behavior.

Challenging the Therapeutic State Pt. 2: Further Disquisitions on the Mental Health System. David Cohen. 1994. LC 82-642121. (Special Issue of the Journal of Mind & Behavior Ser.). 212p. pap. text 20.00 (*0-930195-07-8*) Inst Mind Behavior.

Challenging Women: Psychology's Exclusions, Feminist Possibilities. Erica Burman et al. 1995. LC 95-30473. 224p. pap. (*0-335-19510-5*) OpUniv Pr.

Challenging Your Preconceptions: Thinking Critically about Psychology. Randolph A. Smith. 2nd ed. 1994. LC 94-35321. mass mkt. 11.25 (*0-534-19972-0*) Brooks-Cole.

Chamberlain's Symptoms & Signs in Clinical Medicine: An Introduction to Medical Diagnosis. Colin Ogilvie et al. 12th ed. 1997. LC 97-5699. 392 p. (*0-7506-3683-1*) Buttrwrth-Heinemann.

Chamberlain's Symptoms & Signs in Clinical Medicine: An Introduction to Medical Diagnosis. Colin Ogilvie et al. 12th ed. 1997. LC 97-5699. (Illus.). 408p. pap. (*0-7506-2030-7*) E A GBR. *Dist:* OUP.

Chamberlens & the Midwifery Forceps. James H. Aveling. LC 75-23677. reprint ed. 41.50 (*0-404-13230-8*) AMS Pr.

Champignons Filamenteux d'Interet Medical. Guy St. Germain & Richard Summerbell. 1996. (FRE., Illus.). 320p. lib. bdg. 59.95 (*0-89863-179-3*, 179-3) Star Pub CA.

Champignons "Opportunistes" Ed. by D. Grigoriu. 1979. (Dermatologica Ser.: Vol. 159, Suppl. 1, 1979). (Illus.). pap. 67.00 (*3-8055-0084-X*) S Karger.

Championship Care. John R. Griffith. 1999. LC 99-47683. (Self-Study Ser.). (*1-56793-118-9*) Health Admin Pr.

Championship Clinical Organization. John R. Griffith. 1999. LC 99-48026. (Self-Study Ser.). (*1-56793-119-7*) Health Admin Pr.

Championship Cost & Quality Management. John R. Griffith. 1999. LC 99-47685. (Self-Study Ser.). (*1-56793-120-0*) Health Admin Pr.

Championship Governance. John R. Griffith. 1999. LC 99-47722. (Self-Study Ser.). (*1-56793-117-0*) Health Admin Pr.

Championship Performance Improvement. John R. Griffith. 1999. LC 99-51567. (Self-Study Ser.). (*1-56793-121-9*) Health Admin Pr.

Chance & Design: Reminiscences of Science in Peace & War. Alan Hodgkin. 1992. (Illus.). 424p. (C). text 100.00 (*0-521-40099-6*) Cambridge U Pr.

Chance of a Lifetime: The Birth of a New Medical School in Hong Kong. Arthur E. Starling. 1989. 214p. (Orig.). pap. 27.50 (*962-201-424-0*) Coronet Bks.

Chance to Live: The Heroic Story of the Global Campaign to Immunize the World's Children. June Goodfield. 1991. 288p. text 22.95 (*0-02-544655-X*) Macmillan.

Chandler & Grant's Glaucoma. Ed. by David L. Epstein et al. 4th ed. 1997. LC 96-11484. (Illus.). 688p. text 139.00 (*0-683-02808-1*) Lppncott W & W.

Change: Principles of Problem Formation & Problem Resolution. Paul Watzlawick et al. 1974. LC 73-17485. (Illus.). 172p. 22.50 (*0-393-01104-6*) Norton.

Change, Adaptation & Learning: A Science Masters Series Book. Mary C. Bateson. 176p. 1998. pap. (*0-465-00915-8*); 1997. 25.00 (*0-465-00914-X*) Basic.

Change Before the Change: Everything You Need to Know to Stay Healthy in the Decade Before Menopause. Laura E. Corio & Linda G. Kahn. 2000. LC 00-31205. (Illus.). 448p. 24.95 (*0-553-10876-X*) Bantam.

***Change Before the Change: Everything You Need to Know to Stay Healthy in the Decade Before Menopause.** Laura E. Corio & Linda G. Kahn. 2002. 448p. reprint ed. pap. 14.95 (*0-553-38031-1*) Bantam Dell.

Change Drivers: Information Systems for Managed Care. Ed. by Roy Ziegler. 1998. LC 97-20670. 220p. 50.00 (*1-55648-209-4*) AHPI.

Change in the Context of Group Therapy. Mary W. Nicholas. 1987. LC 84-1718. 272p. text 40.95 (*0-87630-358-0*) Brunner-Routledge.

Change of Heart: The Bypass Experience. Nancy Y. Hoffman. 1985. LC 85-8759. (Illus.). 384p. 17.95 (*0-15-116641-2*) Harcourt.

Change of Sight: Classical German Surgery & Pathology As Mirrored in the Fine Arts. F. Oelschlegel. 1994. (Illus.). 215p. (C). pap. 29.50 (*0-930329-42-2*) Kabel Pubs.

Change Processes in Child Psychotherapy: Revitalizing Treatment & Research. Steven R. Shirk & Robert L. Russell. 1996. LC 96-15603. 395p. text 45.00 (*1-57230-095-7*, 0095) Guilford Pubns.

Change Your Smile. Ronald E. Goldstein et al. 3rd ed. 1996. LC 96-9359. (Illus.). 328p. 38.00 (*0-86715-291-5*, B2915) Quint Pub Co.

Change Your Thinking, Change Your Life: A Practical Course in Successful Living, Vol. II. Ernest Holmes. 1984. 240p. pap. 24.95 (*0-911336-93-1*) Sci of Mind.

Change'll Do You Good: The Baby Boomers Guide to Menopause. Carol Schulen. 2000. LC 99-62714. 128p. pap. 14.95 (*0-9672352-0-0*) D C S Pubg.

Changemakers: A Jungian Perspective on Sibling Positions & the Family Atmosphere. Louis H. Stewart. 1993. LC 92-1050. (Illus.). 176p. (C). (gr. 13). pap. 27.99 (*0-415-07444-4*, B0218) Routledge.

Changes: You & Your Body. 1988. 3.00 (*0-930659-01-5*) CHOICE.

Changes in Sensory Motor Behavior in Aging. Ed. by Anne-Marie Ferrandez & Normand Teasdale. 1995. LC 95-46144. (Advances in Psychology Ser.: No. 114). 406p. 123.00 (*0-444-82101-5*, North Holland) Elsevier.

Changes Workbook: A Woman's Journal for Self-Awareness & Personal Planning. Judy Edmondson et al. 1993. LC 87-14383. (Illus.). 104p. (Orig.). pap., stu. ed. 6.95 (*0-911655-41-7*) Advocacy Pr.

Changing & Learning in the Lives of Physicians. Robert D. Fox & Paul E. Maxmanian. 1989. LC 89-3886. 201p. 67.00 (*0-275-93338-5*, C3338, Praeger Pubs) Greenwood.

Changing Assessments: Alternative Views of Aptitude, Achievement & Instruction. Ed. by Bernard R. Gifford. 1991. 352p. (C). lib. bdg. 101.00 (*0-7923-9177-2*) Kluwer Academic.

Changing Attitudes: Student Booklet. American Psychological Association Staff. 1981. (Human Behavior Curriculum Project Ser.). 64p. (Orig.). (gr. 9-12). pap. text 3.95 (*0-8077-2621-4*) Tchrs Coll.

Changing Attitudes: Teachers Handbook & Duplication Masters. American Psychological Association Staff. 1981. (Human Behavior Curriculum Project Ser.). 50p. 9.95 (*0-8077-2622-2*) Tchrs Coll.

Changing Attitudes in the Treatment of BPH: Journal: European Urology, Vol. 20, Suppl. 2, 1991. Ed. by F. H. Schroeder & A. Steg. 1991. (Illus.). iv, 92p. pap. 29.75 (*3-8055-5516-4*) S Karger.

Changing Behavior in Individuals, Couples & Groups: Identifying, Analyzing & Manipulating the Elements Involved in Change in Order to Promote or Inhibit Alteration of Behavior. Leonard Blank. 1996. (Illus.). 202p. 46.95 (*0-398-06656-6*); pap. 30.95 (*0-398-06657-4*) C C Thomas.

Changing Behaviour: Teaching Children with Emotional & Behavioural Difficulties in Primary & Secondary Classrooms (Resource Materials for Teachers) Sylvie McNamara & Gill Moreton. 1995. 96p. pap. (*1-85346-350-7*) David Fulton GBR. *Dist:* Taylor & Francis.

Changing Bodies, Changing Lives. Ruth Bell. Date not set. (*0-679-45221-4*) McKay.

Changing Bodies, Changing Lives: A Handbook for Teenagers. Ruth Bell et al. 1981. (Illus.). 17.95 (*0-394-50304-X*) Random.

Changing Cancer Patterns & Topics in Cancer Epidemiology. Ed. by Minoru Kurihara et al. 1987. LC 87-61140. (Gann Monographs on Cancer Research: No. 33). (Illus.). 240p. (C). text 114.00 (*0-306-42704-4*) Plenum.

Changing Character of the Medical Profession: An International Perspective. Ed. by Fredric W. Hafferty & John B. McKinlay. 1993. LC 92-48382. (Illus.). 272p. (C). text 49.95 (*0-19-507592-7*) OUP.

Changing Childbirth: Family Birth in the Hospital. Diony Young. 1982. LC 82-9492. (Illus.). 536p. (Orig.). pap. 20.00 (*0-943114-00-4*) Childbirth Graphics.

Changing Childhood. Ed. by Martin Hoyles. 1981. (Education Ser.). (Illus.). 304p. (C). 14.00 (*0-904613-91-7*); pap. 5.95 (*0-904613-79-8*) Writers & Readers.

Changing Complexion of DNA Viruses. Ed. by T. Albrecht. 1990. (Journal: Vol. 31, Nos. 1-2, 1990). (Illus.). 184p. pap. 161.75 (*3-8055-5103-7*) S Karger.

Changing Conceptions of Crowd Mind & Behavior. Carl F. Graumann & S. Moscovici. 1985. (Social Psychology Ser.). (Illus.). 241p. 79.95 (*0-387-96187-9*) Spr-Verlag.

Changing Conceptions of Psychoanalysis: The Legacy of Merton M. Gill. Ed. by Doris K. Silverman & David L. Wolitzky. 2000. LC 00-46903. 336p. pap. 36.00 (*0-88163-235-X*) Analytic Pr.

***Changing Consumers & Changing Technology in Health Care & Health Care Delivery.** Ed. by J. J. Kronenfeld. 2001. (Research in the Sociology of Health Care Volume 19 Ser.: Vol. 19). 250p. 89.00 (*0-7623-0808-7*) Jai Pr.

Changing Context of Social Health Care: Its Implications for Providers & Consumers. Ed. by Helen Rehr & Gary Rosenberg. 1991. 143p. pap. 2.95 (*1-56024-144-6*) Haworth Pr.

Changing Definition of Masculinity. Clyde W. Franklin, II. 1984. (Perspectives in Sexuality Ser.). (Illus.). 246p. (C). 57.00 (*0-306-41554-2*, Plenum Trade) Perseus Pubng.

Changing Disciplines: Lectures on the History, Method & Motives of Social Pathology. John A. Ryle. 1994. 123p. (C). pap. text 21.95 (*1-56000-746-X*) Transaction Pubs.

Changing Eating & Exercise Behavior: A Handbook for Professionals. Paula Hunt & Melvyn Hillsdon. 1996. LC 96-16809. (Illus.). 192p. pap. 38.95 (*0-632-03927-2*) Blackwell Sci.

Changing Economics of Medical Technology, Vol. 2. Institute of Medicine Staff. Ed. by Annetine C. Gelijns & Ethan A. Halm. 1991. (Medical Innovation at the Crossroads Ser.). 224p. text 24.95 (*0-309-04491-X*) Natl Acad Pr.

Changing Employment Relations: Behavioral & Social Perspectives. Ed. by Lois Tetrick & Julian Barling. 1995. LC 95-20863. (APA Science Volumes Ser.). 385p. text 29.95 (*1-55798-315-1*) Am Psychol.

Changing Expectations: A Key to Effective Psychotherapy. Irving Kirsch. 1990. 304p. (C). text 71.95 (*0-534-12648-0*) Brooks-Cole.

Changing Face of Health Care: A Christian Appraisal of Managed Care, Resource Allocation, & Patient-Caregiver Relationships. Center for Bioethics and Human Dignity Staff. Ed. by John F. Kilner et al. 1997. LC 98-22481. (Horizons in Bioethics Ser.). 328p. pap. 19.00 (*0-8028-4533-9*) Eerdmans.

Changing Face of Health Care Social Work: A Guide for Professional Empirical Practice. Sophia F. Dziegielewski. 1998. LC 97-52604. (Illus.). 320p. 59.95 (*0-8261-1196-3*) Springer Pub.

Changing Faces: The Challenge of Facial Disfigurement. James Partridge. 1990. pap. 11.95 (*0-14-011597-8*) Phoenix Soc.

Changing Families: A Family Therapy Reader. Ed. by Jay Haley. 1971. LC 72-118654. 366p. text 40.95 (*0-8089-0681-X*, 791829, Grune & Strat) Harcrt Hlth Sci Grp.

Changing Families: A Group Activities Manual for Middle & High School Students from Separated, Divorced, or Single-Parent Families or Stepfamilies. Teresa M. Schmidt. 1994. LC 93-45455. 206p. pap. 65.95 (*1-56246-087-0*, 3122, HazeldenJohnson Inst) Hazelden.

Changing Federal Role in U. S. Health Care Policy. Jennie J. Kronenfeld. 1997. LC 97-19036. 200p. 60.00 (*0-275-95023-9*); pap. 23.95 (*0-275-95024-7*) Greenwood (Praeger Pubs).

Changing Health & Changing Culture: The Yemenite Jews in Israel. Michael A. Weingarten. 1992. LC 91-38329. 208p. 62.50 (*0-275-94230-9*, C4230, Praeger Pubs) Greenwood.

Changing Health Care: Creating Tomorrow's Winning Health Enterprises Today. Kenneth R. Jennings et al. 1997. 336p. 24.95 (*1-888232-18-8*) Spurge ink.

Changing Health Care Market. Employee Benefit Research Institute Staff. 1987. LC 87-619. (Orig.). 39.95 (*0-86643-055-5*); pap. 19.95 (*0-86643-053-9*) Empl Benefit Res Inst.

Changing Health Care Market. Ed. by Frank B. McArdle. 1987. LC 87-619. (EBRI-ERF Policy Forum Ser.). 292p. (Orig.). (C). 71.00 (*0-8191-6510-7*); 37.00 (*0-8191-6511-5*) U Pr of Amer.

Changing Health Care Systems: Trends in Spending, Coverage & Delivery. Ed. by Linda F. Wolf. 2000. (Illus.). 81p. (C). reprint ed. pap. text 20.00 (*0-7881-8530-6*) DIANE Pub.

Changing Health Care Systems & Rheumatic Disease. Ed. by Frederick J. Manning et al. 1997. LC 97-116822. 256p. (Orig.). pap. 30.00 (*0-309-05683-7*, Joseph Henry Pr) Natl Acad Pr.

Changing Health Care Team-Improving Effectiveness: Proceedings of the Hawaii Conference on Advances in Patient Care, 3rd Annual. Hawaii Conference on Advances in Patient Care Staff. Ed. by Stephen R. Yarnall & Spring Zoog. 1976. 19.00 (*0-917054-11-3*) Med Communications.

Changing Ideas in Health Care. Ed. by David Seedhouse & Alan Cribb. 1990. 252p. pap. 69.95 (*0-471-92068-1*) Wiley.

Changing Lives Through Redecision Therapy. Mary M. Goulding & Robert L. Goulding. rev. ed. 1997. LC 97-1141. 288p. reprint ed. pap. 13.00 (*0-8021-3511-0*, Grove) Grove-Atltic.

Changing Men: New Directions in Research on Men & Masculinity. Michael S. Kimmel. 1988. (Focus Editions Ser.: Vol. 88). 320p. pap. 38.95 (*0-8039-2997-8*, 68063) Sage.

Changing Mental Health Services: The Politics & Policy. Tom Butler. 1992. LC 92-30606. 206p. pap. 41.50 (*1-56593-035-5*, 0283) Thomson Learn.

Changing Minds: The History of Psychotherapy As an Answer to Human Suffering. Frank Tallis. 1998. LC 99-218089. 171p. 59.95 (*0-304-70362-1*) Continuum.

Changing Minds: The History of Psychotherapy as an Answer to Human Suffering. Frank Tallis. 1998. LC 99-218089. 160p. pap. 19.95 (*0-304-70363-X*) Continuum.

Changing Mindsets: The Potential Unconscious. Maria C. Gear et al. 1993. 320p. (C). pap. text 17.50 (*0-8147-3061-2*) NYU Pr.

Changing Moods: The Psychology of Mood & Mood Regulation. Brian Parkinson. 1996. LC 96-17192. 250p. (C). pap. text 30.13 (*0-582-27814-7*) Addison-Wesley.

Changing Nature of Nursing in a Managerial Age. Sarah Cowley. 1999. LC 99-17633. 192p. pap. 47.95 (*0-632-04252-4*) Blackwell Sci.

Changing Nature of Pain Complaints over the Lifespan. M. R. Thomas & R. Roy. 1999. LC 98-41541. (Adult Development & Aging Ser.). (Illus.). 234p. (C). 55.00 (*0-306-45954-X*, Kluwer Plenum) Kluwer Academic.

Changing Nervous System: Neurobehavioral Consequences of Early Brain Disorders. Ed. by Sarah H. Broman & Jack M. Fletcher. 1999. LC 98-45750. (Illus.). 428p. text 65.00 (*0-19-512193-7*) OUP.

Changing Nursing Practice. (*0-7131-4581-1*); 2nd ed. 208p. pap. (*0-340-63181-3*) E A GBR. *Dist:* Routldge.

Changing Nursing Practice. Stephen G. Wright. 2nd ed. 1997. (Illus.). 160p. pap. 29.95 (*1-56593-758-9*, 1474) Singular Publishing.

Changing Patient Behavior: Improving Outcomes in Health & Disease Management. Patterson. 1999. 75.00 (*1-55648-246-9*) AHPI.

Changing Patient Behavior: Improving Outcomes in Health & Disease Management. Ed. by Richard Patterson. 2000. LC 00-10153. (Jossey-Bass/AHA Press Ser.). 272p. 75.00 (*0-7879-5279-6*) Jossey-Bass.

Changing Patterns in Suicide Behaviour: Report on a WHO Working Group. 1982. (Euro Reports & Studies Ser.: No. 74). 45p. pap. text 4.00 (*92-890-1240-4*) World Health.

Changing Patterns of Law: The Courts & the Handicapped: An Original Anthology. Ed. by William R. Phillips & Janet Rosenberg. 1980. LC 79-6009. (Physically Handicapped in Society Ser.). lib. bdg. 44.95 (*0-405-13101-1*) Ayer.

Changing People: The Law & Ethics of Behavior Modification. Alexander M. Smith. 1994. (*1-85521-031-2*) Dartmth Pub GBR. *Dist:* Ashgate Pub Co.

Changing Perspectives: Multi-Viewing Model. Frances K. Wiggins. 1986. (Illus.). 18p. (Orig.). pap. 4.00 (*0-942937-00-7*) Rivijon Pr.

Changing Perspectives on Menopause. Ed. by Ann M. Voda et al. 1982. (Illus.). 424p. text 45.00 (*0-292-71069-0*) U of Tex Pr.

Changing Physician Behavior Through Practice Guidelines: The Zitter Group's 1996 Implementing Practice Guidelines Seminar Proceedings. Ed. by Dean H. Anderson. 1996. 131p. (Orig.). pap. text 247.00 (*0-9645360-3-X*) Cor Hlthcare.

Changing Physician Practice Patterns: Strategies for Success in a Capitated Health Care System. Elaine Zablocki. 1995. 212p. ring bd. 226.00 (*0-8342-0688-9*) Aspen Pub.

Changing Primary Health Care: The Teamcare Valleys Experience. Rosamund Bryar & Bill Blytheway. 1996. (Illus.). 256p. (Orig.). pap. 39.95 (*0-632-03938-8*) Blackwell Sci.

Changing Problem Behavior in Schools. Alex Molnar & Barbara Lindquist. 1989. LC 88-31388. 224p. 33.00 (*1-55542-134-2*) Jossey-Bass.

Changing Role of Volunteerism. Ed. by Susan Wyant & Phyllis Brooks. 1993. LC 93-9491. (Papers). 32p. pap. 10.00 (*1-881277-05-4*) United Hosp Fund.

Changing Roles & Relationships in Nursing & Health Care. Mary B. Williams. 1999. LC 00-500426. 183p. (C). pap. 19.95 (*0-87527-527-3*) Green.

Changing Roles of Occupational Therapists in the 1980s. Ed. by Florence S. Cromwell. 1984. LC 83-22818. (Occupational Therapy in Health Care Ser.: Vol. 1, No. 1). 99p. text 29.95 (*0-86656-294-X*) Haworth Pr.

Changing Scene of Health Care & Technology. Ed. by R. G. Kensett. 1990. 220p. pap. 78.95 (*0-442-31287-3*) Chapman & Hall.

Changing Scene of Health Care & Technology: Proceedings of the 11th International Congress of Hospital Engineering, June 1990, London, U. K. Ed. by R. G. Kensett. 1990. (Illus.). 240p. (C). pap. 120.00 (*0-419-16740-4*, Spon) Routledge.

Changing Shape of Nursing Practice: The Role of Nurses in the Hospital Division of Labour. Davina Allen. 2000. LC 00-30822. 224p. pap. 25.95 (*0-415-21649-4*) Routledge.

Changing Shape of Nursing Practice: The Role of Nurses in the Hospital Divison of Labour. Davina Allen. 2000. LC 00-30822. 224p. 85.00 (*0-415-21648-6*) Routledge.

Changing the Odds: Cancer Prevention Through Personal Choice & Public Policy. R. Grant Sheen. 1995. LC 94-25291. 400p. 35.00 (*0-8160-3167-3*) Facts on File.

Changing the Patterns Vol. II: Participants Manual - from the "A Path to Responsibility" Treatment Program. G. Richard Kishur. 1994. 168p. pap. text, stu. ed. 19.95 (*1-885473-02-8*) Wood N Barnes.

Changing the Rules: A Client-Directed Approach to Therapy. Barry L. Duncan et al. 1992. LC 92-1550. (Family Therapy Ser.). 284p. 38.00 (*0-89862-108-9*, 2108) Guilford Pubns.

Changing the Rules: Psychology in the Netherlands, 1900-1985. Trudy Dehue. 1995. (Cambridge Studies in the History of Psychology). (Illus.). 216p. (C). text 64.95 (*0-521-47522-8*) Cambridge U Pr.

Changing the Self: Philosophies, Techniques, & Experiences. Ed. by Thomas M. Brinthaupt & Richard P. Lipka. 1994. LC 93-10522. (SUNY Series, Studying the Self). 373p. (C). pap. text 21.95 (*0-7914-1868-5*) State U NY Pr.

Changing the Subject: Psychology Social Regulation & Subjectivity. Julian Henriques et al. 2nd ed. 1998. LC 97-30854. 360p. (C). pap. 27.95 (*0-415-15138-4*) Routledge.

Changing the U. S. Health Care System: Key Issues in Health Services, Policy & Management. Ed. by Ronald M. Andersen et al. 1996. LC 96-22517. (Health Ser.). 480p. 46.95 (*0-7879-0224-1*) Jossey-Bass.

Changing the U. S. Health Care System: Key Issues in Health Services, Policy & Management. Ronald Andersen et al. 2nd ed. 2001. LC 00-50675. (Health Ser.). (Illus.). 608p. 49.00 (*0-7879-5404-7*) Jossey-Bass.

Changing Tides Training System: A Child-Parent Bereavement Program. Estelle D'Costa & Grace Zambelli. 1998. (Illus.). 235p. (J). (ps up). pap. 125.00 incl. VHS (*0-9622089-2-2*) Ctr Hospice Care.

Changing Trends in Coronary Heart Disease: Journal: Cardiology, Vol. 72, Nos. 1 & 2. Ed. by K. Pyorala et al. 1985. (Illus.). 104p. pap. 61.00 (*3-8055-4015-9*) S Karger.

Changing Values in Medical & Healthcare Decision-Making. Ed. by Gavin H. Mooney & Uffe J. Jensen. 1990. LC 89-70700. 206p. 239.95 (*0-471-92634-5*) Wiley.

Changing Values in Medicine. Ed. by Eric J. Cassell & Mark Siegler. 1979. LC 85-10033. 221p. pap. 24.95 (*0-313-27060-0*, P7060); lib. bdg. 62.95 (*0-313-27050-3*, U7050) Greenwood (Greenwood Pr).

Changing Visions: Human Cognitive Maps: Past, Present & Future. Ervin Laszlo et al. 1996. LC 96-15309. (Praeger Studies on the 21st Century). 144p. 62.50 (*0-275-95676-8*); pap. 18.95 (*0-275-95677-6*) Greenwood (Praeger Pubs).

Changing Visual System: From Early to Late Stages of Life. Ed. by P. Bagnoli & William Hodos. 1992. (NATO Advanced Science Institutes Ser.: Vol. 222). (Illus.). 432p. (C). text 156.00 (*0-306-44090-3*, Kluwer Plenum) Kluwer Academic.

Changing Woman & Her Sisters. Sheila Moon. 1985. LC 84-27901. 233p. (Orig.). 14.00 (*0-917479-02-5*); pap. 11.50 (*0-917479-03-3*) Guild Psy.

Changing Youth in a Changing Society: Patterns of Adolescent Development & Disorder. Michael Rutter. 1980. LC 82-242973. (Illus.). 333p. 39.50 (*0-674-10875-2*) HUP.

Channel Divergences: Deeper Pathways of the Web. Miki Shima & Charles Chace. 2000. (Illus.). 300p. 39.95 (*1-891845-15-2*) Blue Poppy Pr.

Channelling in Intermediary Metabolism. Ed. by L. Agius. 1996. (Research Monographs: Vol. 9). 352p. (C). text (*1-85578-075-5*) Portland Pr Ltd GBR. *Dist:* Ashgate Pub Co.

Channelopathies of the Nervous System. Ed. by Michael R. Rose & Robert Griggs. 2001. LC 2001-25590. (Illus.). 368p. text 95.00 (*0-7506-4507-5*) Buttrwrth-Heinemann.

Chaos & Complexity: Implications for Psychological Theory & Practice. Michael R. Butz. 1997. LC 97-19038. pap. 27.95 (*1-56032-419-8*) Taylor & Francis.

Chaos & the Changing Nature of Science & Medicine: An Introduction: Proceedings (1995: Mobile, AL) Ed. by Donald E. Herbert et al. 1996. LC 96-85220. (Conference Proceedings Ser.: No. 376). 203p. (C). 60.00 (*1-56396-442-2*, Q172) Am Inst Physics.

Chaos in Medicine. Sataloff. 2000. 620p. 59.95 (*1-56593-953-0*) Singular Publishing.

Chaos Theory in Psychology. Frederick D. Abraham & Albert R. Gilgen. 1995. LC 94-29848. 400p. pap. 31.95 (*0-275-95140-5*, Praeger Pubs);27. 75.00 (*0-313-28961-1*, Greenwood Pr) Greenwood.

Chaos Theory in Psychology & the Life Sciences. Ed. by Robin Robertson & Allan Combs. 1995. 408p. LC 95-17298. text 79.95 (*0-8058-1736-0*); pap. text 39.95 (*0-8058-1737-9*) L Erlbaum Assocs.

Chaperonin Protocols. Ed. by Christine Schneider. 2000. LC 99-41622. (Methods in Molecular Biology Ser.: Vol. 140). 224p. 79.50 (*0-89603-739-8*) Humana.

Chaplain-Physician Relationship. Ed. by Laurel A. Burton. 1991. LC 90-19258. (Journal of Health Care Chaplaincy Ser.). 78p. text 39.95 (*1-56024-108-X*) Haworth Pr.

Chapman's Orthopaedic Surgery. Michael W. Chapman et al. 3rd ed. 2000. 5,152p. text 475.00 (*0-7817-1487-7*) Lppncott W & W.

Chapter One: The Socialization of an Adolescent Alcoholic, Vol. 1. Joseph B. Whitty, II. 1980. 14p. pap. 2.50 (*0-9607254-0-7*) Newspaper Agcy.

Chapters from Dim. Human Sex. Byer & Shainberg. 4th ed. 1993. 30.25 net. (*0-697-24650-7*, WCB McGr Hill) McGrw-H Hghr Educ.

Character Analysis. Wilhelm Reich. Tr. by Vincent R. Carfagno from GER. 3rd rev. ed. 1980. 576p. pap. 22.00 (*0-374-50980-8*) FS&G.

Character & Health. Yves Requena. Ed. by Robert L. Felt. Tr. by Carol Bell from FRE. 1995. (Illus.). 224p. (Orig.). pap. text 25.00 (*0-912111-23-2*) Paradigm Publns.

Character & Neurosis: An Integrative View. Claudio Naranjo. 2001. LC 94-21263. 352p. (Orig.). reprint ed. pap. 24.95 (*0-89556-066-6*) Gateways Bks & Tapes.

Character & Personality of Children from Broken Homes. Nehemiah Wallenstein. LC 70-177664. (Columbia University. Teachers College. Contributions to Education Ser.: No. 721). reprint ed. 37.50 (*0-404-55721-X*) AMS Pr.

Character & Self-Experience: Working with Obsessive-Compulsive, Depressive-Masochistic, Narcissistic, & Other Character Styles. Lawrence Josephs. 1995. 344p. pap. 40.00 (*1-56821-580-0*) Aronson.

Character Disorders & Adaptive Mechanisms. Peter L. Giovacchini. rev. ed. 1984. LC 83-11957. 552p. 60.00 (*0-87668-641-2*) Aronson.

Character of Mind: An Introduction to the Philosophy of Mind. Colin McGinn. 2nd ed. 1997. LC 96-35172. 186p. pap. text 16.95 (*0-19-875208-3*); (C). text 65.00 (*0-19-875209-1*) OUP.

Character Styles. Stephen M. Johnson. 1994. LC 93-42540. 320p. (C). 32.00 (*0-393-70171-9*) Norton.

***Characterisation of CtBP: A Co-Repressor of Transcription That Interacts with the Adenovirus E1A Protein.** Anders Sundqvist. 2001. (Comprehensive Summaries of Uppsala Dissertations from the Faculty of Medicine Ser.: No. 1089). (Illus.). 50p. pap. (*91-554-5144-6*) Acta Univ SWE. *Dist:* Coronet Bks.

Characteristics & Potentials of Blood Stem Cells, Vol. 16, Supplement 1. T. M. Fliedner & D. Hoelzer. 1998. 305p. text 69.00 (*1-880854-21-X*); pap. text 49.00 (*1-880854-25-2*) AlphaMed Pr.

Characteristics of the Present Age, 2. Johann G. Fichte. Tr. by W. Smith. 1977. LC 77-72191. (Contributions to the History of Psychology Ser.: Pt. A, Orientations). 495p. reprint ed. lib. bdg. 85.00 (*0-313-26926-2*, U6926, Greenwood Pr) Greenwood.

Characteristics of Work-Related Injuries & Illnesses in Maine. Janet A. Callahan. 1993. (Illus.). 67p. (Orig.). (C). pap. text 20.00 (*1-56806-343-1*) DIANE Pub.

Characterization & Performance of Calcium Phosphate Coatings for Implants. Ed. by Emanual Horowitz & Jack E. Parr. 1994. LC 94-4736. (Special Technical Publications: No. 1196). (Illus.). 220p. pap. 59.00 (*0-8031-1854-6*, STP1196) ASTM.

Characters & Probable History of the Hawaiian Rat. G. S. Miller, Jr. 1972. (BMB Ser.). reprint ed. pap. 25.00 (*0-527-02117-2*) Periodicals Srv.

Charcot - Marie - Tooth Disorders. Ed. by Robert E. Lovelace et al. 1999. LC 99-43216. (Annals of the New York Academy of Sciences Ser.: Vol. 883). (Illus.). xviii, 544p. lib. bdg. 150.00 (*1-57331-182-0*) NY Acad Sci.

Charge Master: Review Strategies for Improved Billing & Reimbursement. Duane C. Abbey. 1997. LC 97-16895. (HFMA Healthcare Financial Management Ser.). 282p. 175.00 (*0-7863-0997-0*, Irwn Prfssnl) McGraw-Hill Educ Grp.

Charge Nurse Survival Skills: Long Term Care. 1997. wbk. ed. 49.95 incl. VHS (*0-8151-1312-9*) Mosby Inc.

Charge Nurse Survival Skills: OB. 1997. wbk. ed. 49.95 incl. VHS (*0-8151-1301-3*) Mosby Inc.

Charge Nurse Survival Skills: Perioperative Nursing. 1997. wbk. ed. 49.95 incl. VHS (*0-8151-1311-0*) Mosby Inc.

Charge Nurse Survival Skills: Taking Charge Core. Vivian Biggers. 1997. (Illus.). 30p. pap., wbk. ed. (*0-8151-2459-7*) Mosby Inc.

Charge Nurse Survival Skills: Taking Charge LTC. Vivian Biggers. 1997. (Illus.). 30p. pap., wbk. ed. (*0-8151-1315-3*) Mosby Inc.

Charge Nurse Survival Skills: Taking Charge OB. Vivian Biggers. 1997. (Illus.). 30p. pap., wbk. ed. (*0-8151-1313-7*) Mosby Inc.

Charge Nurse Survival Skills: Taking Charge OR. Vivian Biggers. 1997. (Illus.). 30p. pap., wbk. ed. (*0-8151-1314-5*) Mosby Inc.

Charge of the Parasols: Women's Entry to the Medical Profession. Catriona Blake. 1994. pap. 16.99 (*0-7043-4239-1*) Interlink Pub.

Chargemaster Coding & Reimbursement. 1997. 243p. pap. 149.00 (*1-889115-14-2*) Med Learn.

Charitable Knowledge: Hospital Pupils & Practitioners in Eighteenth-Century London. Susan C. Lawrence. 1996. (History of Medicine Ser.). (Illus.). 407p. (C). text 80.00 (*0-521-36355-1*) Cambridge U Pr.

Charles Bragg on Medicine. Charles Bragg. 1984. (Illus.). 80p. (Orig.). mass mkt. 7.95 (*0-446-38059-8*) Warner Bks.

Charles Press Handbook of Current Medical Abbreviations. Charles Press Publishers Staff. 5th ed. 1997. LC 97-12402. 472p. pap. text 16.95 (*0-914783-81-5*) Charles.

Charles R. Kleeman Festschrift. Ed. by Shaul G. Massry. 1987. (Journal: Vol. 12, Nos. 5-6, 1986). (Illus.). lv, 124p. pap. 61.00 (*3-8055-4454-5*) S Karger.

Charlie: An Unwanted Child? Ed. by Michael Jacobs. 1995. LC 94-29010. (In Search of a Therapist Ser.). 160p. (*0-335-19199-1*) OpUniv Pr.

Chart of Accounts for Hospitals: An Accounting & Reporting Reference Guide. L. Vann Seawell. 1994. 200p. per. 65.00 (*1-55738-619-6*, Irwn Prfssnl) McGraw-Hill Educ Grp.

Chartbook on Health Data on Older Americans: United States. 1994. lib. bdg. 250.00 (*0-8490-8547-0*) Gordon Pr.

Chartbook on Health Data on Older Americans: United States, 1992. Ed. by Robin A. Cohen et al. 1992. LC 92-48231. (Vital & Health Statistics Ser.: Series 3, No. 29). (Illus.). (*0-8406-0475-0*) Natl Ctr Health Stats.

Charter for Health Care Workers. Pontifcal Council for Pastoral Assistance to Health. 142p. pap. 3.95 (*0-8198-1538-1*) Pauline Bks.

Charting: The Systematic Approach to Achieving Control. Janice L. Roth. 1994. 38p. pap. 6.95 (*0-9631701-0-4*) R A Rapaport.

Charting a Course for the Future of Women's & Perinatal Health: Concepts, Findings & Recommendations Women's and Perinatal Health Policy Group Staff. Ed. by Holly A. Grason et al. 1999. (Illus.). 90p. pap. (*1-893692-02-7*); pap. (*1-893692-04-3*) Wom & Child Hlth.

Charting a Course for the Future of Women's & Perinatal Health Vol. II: Reviews of Key Issues. Women's and Perinatal Health Policy Group Staff. Ed. by Holly Allen Grason et al. 1999. (Illus.). 279p. pap. (*1-893692-03-5*) Wom & Child Hlth.

Charting by Exception: Cost Effective in Nursing Documentation. Ed. by Laura Burke & Judy Murphy. 1989. (Orig.). pap. text 41.95 (*0-8273-4216-0*) Delmar.

Charting Made Incredibly Easy. Springhouse Publishing Company Staff. 1997. LC 97-36360. (Made Incredibly Easy Ser.). 288p. pap. 34.95 (*0-87434-934-6*) Springhouse Corp.

Charting Your Course: A Life-Long Guide to Health & Compassion. Ed. by Sally Coleman & David S. Anderson. 1998. LC 98-3010. 400p. pap. 16.00 (*0-268-00827-2*) U of Notre Dame Pr.

Chasdei Aurahom: Hacoloh B'Halacha. Abraham Friedlander. 1994. 620p. 17.50 (*0-9643008-1-8*) A Friedlander.

Chase, Chance, & Creativity. James H. Austin. 1985. LC 77-23011. 236p. pap. text 23.00 (*0-231-04295-7*) Col U Pr.

Chasing Dirt: The American Pursuit of Cleanliness. Suellen Hoy. 1994. 22.95 (*0-02-915295-X*) S&S Trade.

Chasing Grace: Reflections of a Catholic Girl, Grown Up. Martha Manning. 1997. LC 96-6773. 240p. pap. 11.00 (*0-06-251312-5*) Harper SF.

Chasing the Dragon's Tail: Theory & Practice of Acupuncture in the Work of Yoshio Manaka. Yoshio Manaka et al. 1996. 453p. text 60.00 (*0-912111-53-4*) Paradigm Publns.

***Chassin's Operative Strategy in General Surgery: An Expositive Atlas.** Carol E. H. Scott-Conner. 3rd ed. 2001. LC 2001-20044. (Illus.). 888p. 179.00 (*0-387-95204-7*) Spr-Verlag.

Chasteen's Essentials of Clinical Dental Assisting. Cara Miyasaki-Ching. 5th ed. 1997. 480p. tchr. ed. (*0-8151-4489-X*) Mosby Inc.

Cheater's Diet. Daniel Tremblay. 1984. LC 84-13299. 162p. 16.95 (*0-13-128307-3*); pap. 7.95 (*0-13-128299-9*) P-H (Busn).

Check-Up: English Through Medical Readings. B. Sturgeon. 1994. (Illus.). 353p. pap. (*0-86577-732-2*) Thieme Med Pubs.

Checkbook's Guide to 1998 Health Insurance Plans for Federal Employees. Walton Francis & Washington Consumers' Checkbook Magazine Editors. rev. ed. 1997. 125p. pap. 8.95 (*1-888124-02-4*) Ctr Study Serv.

Checkbook's Guide to 1999 Health Insurance Plans for Federal Employees. Walton Francis & Washington Consumer's Checkbook Editors Staff. 20th rev. ed. 1998. 120p. pap. 8.95 (*1-888124-04-0*) Ctr Study Serv.

Checklist in Clinical Methods. Michael Swash. 1998. pap. text 9.50 (*0-7020-1724-8*) Harcourt.

Checklist Intensive Care Medicine: Including Poisoning. H. P. Schuster et al. Ed. by A. Sturm et al. 1993. (Flexibook Ser.). 362p. text 32.00 (*0-86577-320-3*) Thieme Med Pubs.

Checklist Manual Medicine. J. Dvorak & V. Dvorak. Ed. by A. Sturm et al. Tr. by Wolfgang G. Gilliar from GER. 1991. (Flexibook Ser.). (Illus.). 180p. pap. text 22.00 (*0-86577-386-6*) Thieme Med Pubs.

Checklist of the Newberry Library's Printed Books in Science, Medicine, Technology, & the Pseudosciences. Jean S. Gottlieb. 1992. LC 92-17941. (Illus.). 328p. text 25.00 (*0-8240-5171-8*, H01195) Garland.

Checklists & Illustrative Financial Statements for Health Care Organizations. AICPA Staff. 1998. 120p. pap. 33.75 (*0-87051-236-6*, 008722) Am Inst CPA.

Checklists for Skills Demonstration & Guidelines for Their Administration. Ed. by Carrie Lenberg. 2nd ed. 1999. 26p. pap. (*1-930304-06-4*) Home Care Univ.

CheckMate Classic. Angela G. Clarkson & Anne M. Larson. 3rd rev. ed. 2000. (Critical Care CheckMate Ser.). 210p. vinyl bd. (*0-9700484-9-1*) NNCC.

Chefs Creating Lean: A Nutrition Course for Food Professionals. Carolyn Leontos & Jeanne Palmer. 1994. LC 94-38126. ring bd. 95.00 (*0-88091-136-0*) Am Dietetic Assn.

Cheirolumbar Dysostosis. A. Wackenheim. 1980. (Illus.). 102p. 53.95 (*0-387-10371-6*) Spr-Verlag.

Chekhov's Lie. Harold L. Klawans. 1997. LC 97-25498. 278p. 24.95 (*1-888799-12-9*) Demos Medical.

Chelates & Clathrates: Markets & Opportunities. 1997. (Report Ser.: No. C-173R). 263p. 2850.00 (*1-56965-380-1*) BCC.

Chelates in Nutrition. Frank H. Kratzer & Pran N. Vohra. 1986. 184p. 106.00 (*0-8493-6544-9*, QP141, CRC Reprint) Franklin.

Chelation Can Cure: How to Reverse Heart Disease, Diabetes, Stroke, High Blood Pressure & Poor Circulation Without Drugs or Surgery. Edward W. McDonagh. 1983. 225p. (Orig.). pap. 9.95 (*0-912815-00-0*) Platinum Pen Pubs.

Chelation Therapies. Woodland Publishing Staff. 1997. (Woodland Health Ser.). 30p. pap. text 3.95 (*1-885670-95-8*) Woodland UT.

Chelation Therapy: The Key to Unclogging Your Arteries, Improving Oxygenation, Treating Vision Problems, Etc. John P. Trowbridge & Morton Walker. 3rd rev. ed. 1990. (Dr. Morton Walker Better Health Booklets Ser.). 64p. pap. 4.95 (*0-8159-5228-7*) Devin.

Chelation Therapy, Vol. 2, No. 1 - 2: Special Issue of Journal of Advancement in Medicine. Ed. by Elmer M. Cranton. 1989. (Illus.). 280p. pap. 21.95 (*0-89885-480-6*, Kluwer Acad Hman Sci) Kluwer Academic.

Chelation Therapy & Your Health. Michael Janson. 1998. (Keats Good Health Guides). 48p. pap. 3.95 (*0-87983-899-X*, 3899XK, Keats Pubng) McGraw-Hill Trade.

Chemical & Biochemical Methodology for the Assessment of Hazards of Pesticides for Man: Proceedings of the WHO Scientific Group, Geneva, 1974. WHO Staff. 1975. (Technical Reports: No. 560). pap. text 6.00 (*92-4-120560-1*, 1100560) World Health.

Chemical & Biological Aspects of Drug Dependence. S. J. Mule & Henry Brill. 1972. LC 72-191695. (Drug Dependence Ser.). 576p. 55.00 (*0-87819-011-2*, CRC Reprint) Franklin.

***Chemical & Biological Respiratory Protection Workshop Report.** John M. Dower. Ed. by Linda Rosenstock. 2001. 76p. (C). pap. text 25.00 (*0-7567-1139-8*) DIANE Pub.

Chemical & Radionuclide Food Contamination. M. E. Alpert et al. 1973. (Illus.). 220p. (C). text 29.50 (*0-8422-7091-4*) Irvington.

Chemical & Structural Approaches to Rational Drug Design. David B. Weiner & William V. Williams. 1994. 288p. 167.95 (*0-8493-7818-4*, 7818) CRC Pr.

Chemical Brain Injury. Kaye H. Kilburn. 1997. LC 97-24105. (Biology Ser.). (Illus.). 848p. 89.95 (*0-442-02427-4*, VNR) Wiley.

Chemical Carcinogenesis: Models & Mechanisms. Ed. by F. Feo et al. 1988. LC 88-29013. (Illus.). 696p. 135.00 (*0-306-43085-1*, Plenum Trade) Perseus Pubng.

Chemical Carcinogenesis & Mutagenesis I. Ed. by C. S. Cooper & P. L. Grover. 1989. (Handbook of Experimental Pharmacology Ser.: Vol. 94-I). (Illus.). 604p. 422.00 (*0-387-51182-2*, 3138) Spr-Verlag.

Chemical Carcinogenesis & Mutagenesis II. Ed. by C. S. Cooper & P. L. Grover. 1990. (Handbook of Experimental Pharmacology Ser.: Vol. 94, Pt. 2). (Illus.). 467p. 349.00 (*0-387-51183-0*, 3316) Spr-Verlag.

Chemical Carcinogenesis 2: Modulating Factors. Ed. by A. Columbano et al. 1991. (Illus.). 666p. (C). text 186.00 (*0-306-43896-8*, Kluwer Plenum) Kluwer Academic.

Chemical Carcinogens. M. Castegnaro & Eric B. Sansone. 1986. 97p. 24.95 (*0-387-16719-6*) Spr-Verlag.

Chemical Carcinogens & DNA Philip L. Grover. 1979. Vol. 1. 256p. 141.00 (*0-8493-5303-3*, RC268); Vol. 2. 224p. 128.00 (*0-8493-5304-1*, RC268) Franklin (CRC Reprint).

Chemical Changes in Food During Processing. Thomas J. Richardson & John W. Finley. 1995. LC 85-18638. (IFT Symposium Ser.). (Illus.). 167.00 (*0-87055-504-9*) Aspen Pub.

Chemical Concepts of Psychosis. Max Rinkle & H. C. Denber. 1958. (Illus.). 24.95 (*0-8392-1012-4*) Astor-Honor.

Chemical Contaminants in Human Milk. Allan A. Jensen & Stuart A. Slorach. 1990. (Illus.). 640p. 239.00 (*0-8493-6607-0*, RJ216) CRC Pr.

Chemical Contamination & Its Victims: Medical Remedies, Legal Redress, & Public Policy. Ed. by David Schnare & Martin T. Katzman. 1989. LC 88-37436. 186p. 59.95 (*0-89930-428-1*, KCV, Quorum Bks) Greenwood.

Chemical Control of the Human Environment: Plenary Lectures Presented at the International Symposium on the Chemical Control of the Human Environment held in Johannesburg, South Africa, 14-18 July 1969. International Symposium on the Chemical Control of the Human Environment et al. 1970. LC 73-166794. (*0-408-70086-6*) Buttrwrth-Heinemann.

Chemical Dependence: Diagnosis, Treatment & Prevention. H. T. Milhorn, Jr. 1990. (Illus.). 370p. 154.00 (*0-387-97292-7*) Spr-Verlag.

Chemical Dependence: Yes, You Can Do Something. Carole Remboldt. 1987. 20p. pap. 2.95 (*0-935908-35-8*, 3222, HazeldenJohnson Inst) Hazelden.

Chemical Dependence Treatment Documentation Sourcebook: A Comprehensive Collection of Program Management Tools, Clinical Documentation, & Psychoeducational Materials for Substance Abuse Treatment Professionals. James R. Finley & Brenda S. Lenz. 1998. LC 98-22930. 320p. pap. text 49.95 incl. disk (*0-471-31285-1*) Wiley.

Chemical Dependence Treatment Homework Planner. James R. Finley & Brenda S. Lenz. 1999. LC 99-17989. (Practice Planners Ser.). 320p. pap. 49.95 incl. disk, cd-rom (*0-471-32452-3*) Wiley.

Chemical Dependence Treatment Planner. Robert R. Perkinson & Arthur E. Jongsma, Jr. 1997. LC 97-35792. 256p. pap. 49.95 (*0-471-23795-7*); pap. text 175.00 incl. disk (*0-471-23794-9*) Wiley.

Chemical Dependency: A Family Affair. Olivia Curtis. 1998. LC 98-21058. 200p. pap. text 24.95 (*0-534-35583-8*) Brooks-Cole.

Chemical Dependency: A Systems Approach. C. Aaron McNeece & Diana M. DiNitto. 2nd ed. 1998. LC 97-35141. 462p. pap. text 51.00 (*0-205-26485-9*) P-H.

Chemical Dependency: Theoretical Approaches & Strategies Working with Individuals & Families. Ed. by Eileen B. Isaacson. 1991. LC 91-20793. (Illus.). 178p. lib. bdg. 39.95 (*1-56024-148-9*) Haworth Pr.

Chemical Dependency: Women at Risk. Ed. by Brenda L. Underhill & Dana G. Finnegan. 1996. LC 96-33337. 179p. (C). 34.95 (*0-7890-0001-6*, Haworth Pastrl); (Journal of Chemical Dependency Treatment Ser.: Vol. 6, Nos. 1/2). pap. 14.95 (*1-56023-088-6*, Harrington Park) Haworth Pr.

Chemical Dependency Aftercare (in Minnesota) A Status Report. 1995. (Illus.). 310p. (C). pap. text 40.00 (*0-7881-2457-9*) DIANE Pub.

Chemical Dependency & Antisocial Personality Disorder: Psychotherapy & Assessment Strategies. Gary G. Forrest. 1994. LC 92-924. (Original Book Ser.). (Illus.). 366p. lib. bdg. 59.95 (*1-56024-308-2*) Haworth Pr.

Chemical Dependency Counseling: A Practical Guide. Robert R. Perkinson. 1997. LC 96-51207. 464p. (C). pap. 49.95 (*0-7619-0859-5*, 08595) Sage.

Chemical Dependency in Nursing: The Deadly Diversion. Eleanor J. Sullivan. 1988. LC 87-31887. 228p. (C). pap. text 26.95 net. (*0-201-07581-4*) Addison-Wesley.

Chemical Dependency Treatment: Innovative Group Approaches. L. Donald McVinney. 1997. LC 97-37554. 125p. 39.95 (*0-7890-0354-6*) Haworth Pr.

Chemical Dependency Treatment Accountability Plan. Patricia A. Harrison. 1993. 50p. (Orig.). (C). pap. text 30.00 (*0-7881-0155-2*) DIANE Pub.

Chemical Dependency Treatment Planning Handbook. Richard J. Laban. 1997. LC 97-8006. 174p. spiral bd. 31.95 (*0-398-06776-7*) C C Thomas.

Chemical Deterioration of Proteins. Ed. by John R. Whitaker & Maseo Fujimaki. 1980. LC 79-27212. (ACS Symposium Ser.: No. 123). 38.95 (*0-8412-0543-4*) Am Chemical.

Chemical Engineering & the Pharmaceutical Industry. ICHEM Engineers Staff. 1983. (Institute of Chemical Engineers Symposia Ser.). pap. 14.00 (*0-08-031410-4*, Pergamon Pr) Elsevier.

Chemical Equilibrium & Analysis. Richard W. Ramette. 1981. (Chemistry Ser.). (Illus.). 672p. (C). text (*0-201-06107-4*) Addison-Wesley.

Chemical Exposure & Human Health: A Reference to 314 Chemicals, with a Guide to Symptoms & a Directory of Organizations. Cynthia Wilson. 1993. LC 92-51010. 351p. lib. bdg. 55.00 (*0-89950-810-3*) McFarland & Co.

Chemical Exposure & Toxic Responses. Stephen K. Hall et al. 1996. LC 96-20459. 304p. lib. bdg. 59.95 (*1-56670-239-9*) Lewis Pubs.

Chemical Factors in Neural Growth, Degeneration & Repair. Ed. by Christopher Bell. 1996. LC 97-132250. 528p. 259.00 (*0-444-82529-0*) Elsevier.

Chemical Formulary, Vol. 23. Ed. by H. Bennett. 1981. 70.00 (*0-8206-0282-5*) Chem Pub.

Chemical Formulary, Vol. 26. H. Bennett. 1985. 70.00 (*0-8206-0313-9*) Chem Pub.

Chemical Hazards in the Workplace. Ronald M. Scott. 1989. (Industrial Toxicology Ser.). (Illus.). 208p. lib. bdg. 79.95 (*0-87371-134-3*, L134) Lewis Pubs.

Chemical Illnesses. 1996. lib. bdg. 250.99 (*0-8490-5874-0*) Gordon Pr.

Chemical Indicators - Guidance for the Selection, Use & Interpretation of Results in Health Care Facilities: AAMI TIR25:1999. 2000. (Illus.). pap. 100.00 (*1-57020-127-7*) Assn Adv Med Instrn.

Chemical Induction of Cancer: Modulation & Combination Effects: An Inventory of the Many Factors Which Influence Carcinogenesis. Ed. by Joseph C. Arcos et al. LC 94-29782. 1995. 725p. 145.50 (*0-8176-3766-4*); 1994. (*3-7643-3766-4*) Birkhauser.

Chemical Induction of New Tumors & Cancers: Index of New Information Including Human Risks & Results. John C. Bartone. 1995. (Illus.). 190p. 57.50 (*0-7883-0482-8*); pap. 47.50 (*0-7883-0483-6*) ABBE Pubs Assn.

Chemical Information. Ed. by H. R. Collier. 1990. (Illus.). 311p. 113.00 (*0-387-51804-5*, 3720) Spr-Verlag.

Chemical Information Manual. OSHA Staff. 3rd ed. 1995. 341p. pap. text 115.00 (*0-86587-469-7*) Gov Insts.

Chemical Mechanisms in Bioenergetics. Ed. by D. Rao Sanadi. 1976. LC 76-26707. (ACS Monograph: No. 172). 272p. 37.95 (*0-8412-0274-5*) Am Chemical.

Chemical Mediators & Cellular Interactions in Clinical Immunology. Ed. by Gianni Marone. 1993. (Illus.). (Journal: Vol. 99 Nos. 2-4). 348p. 314.00 (*3-8055-5723-X*); (International Archives of Allergy & Immunology Ser.: Vol. 99, Nos. 2-4, 1992). 346p. reprint ed. 213.25 (*3-8055-5757-4*) S Karger.

Chemical Methods in Bacterial Systematics. Ed. by Michael Goodfellow & David E. Minnikin. 1985. LC 84-11032. (Society for Applied Bacteriology Technical Ser.). text 104.00 (*0-12-289675-0*) Acad Pr.

Chemical, Microbiological, Health & Comfort Aspects of Indoor Air Quality - State of the Art in SBS: Based on the Lectures Given During the Eurocourse on Chemical, Microbiological, Health & Comfort Aspects of Indoor Air Quality - State of the Art in SBS Held at the Joint Research Centre, Ispra, Italy, March 23-27, 1992. Ed. by Kelmut Knoppel. 1992. 388p. (C). text 185.00 (*0-7923-1703-3*) Kluwer Academic.

Chemical Modification of Proteins. Ed. by Alexander N. Glazer et al. 1975. LC 74-84210. (Laboratory Techniques in Biochemistry & Molecular Biology Ser.: Vol. 4, Pt. 1). 205p. pap. 41.25 (*0-444-10811-4*, North Holland) Elsevier.

Chemical Mutagens: Principles & Methods for Their Detection, Vol. 7. Ed. by Frederick J. De Serres & Alexander Hollaender. 1982. LC 79-640909. 524p. 95.00 (*0-306-40771-X*, Plenum Trade) Perseus Pubng.

Chemical Mutagens: Principles & Methods for Their Detection, Vol. 10. Ed. by Frederick J. De Serres. 1986. LC 79-640909. (Illus.). 572p. (C). text 174.00 (*0-306-42171-2*, Kluwer Plenum) Kluwer Academic.

Chemical Pathology Interpretative Pocket Book. R. N. Walmsley & H. J. Cain. 1996. LC 96-32476. (*981-02-2802-3*); pap. (*981-02-2849-X*) World Scientific Pub.

Chemical Peeling. Harold J. Brody. 2nd ed. 1997. LC 97-120805. (Illus.). 256p. (C). (gr. 13). text 99.00 (*0-8151-1261-0*, 26992) Mosby Inc.

Chemical Pharmacy Enters the University: Johannes Hartmann & the Didactic Care of Chymiatria. Bruce T. Moran. 1991. 90p. 16.00 (*0-931292-24-7*); (C). pap. 8.50 (*0-931292-23-9*) Am Inst Hist Pharm.

Chemical Reactivity & Modification of Keratin Fibres. N. H. Leon. 1975. 81p. 120.00 (*0-7855-7186-8*) St Mut.

Chemical Recognition in Biology. Ed. by F. Chapeville & A. O. Haenni. 1980. (Molecular Biology, Biochemistry & Biophysics Ser.: Vol. 32). (Illus.). 430p. 91.00 (*0-387-10205-1*) Spr-Verlag.

Chemical Risks: Fears, Facts, & the Media. Media Institute Media Institute Staff. 1985. LC 85-60247. (Illus.). 72p. (Orig.). (C). pap. 12.95 (*0-937790-28-1*) Media Institute.

Chemical Sensitivity: A Guide to Coping with Hypersensitivity Syndrome, Sick Building Syndrome & Other Environmental Illnesses. Bonnye L. Matthews. 1992. LC 92-54089. 291p. lib. bdg. 39.95 (*0-89950-731-X*) McFarland & Co.

Chemical Sensitivity: The Truth about Environmental Illness. Stephen J. Barrett. 1998. LC 97-53181. (Consumer Health Library). 220p. 30.00 (*1-57392-195-5*) Prometheus Bks.

Chemical Sensitivity: Tools for Diagnosis & Methods of Treatment, Vol. 4. William J. Rea. 1996. 928p. 114.95 (*0-87371-965-4*, L965) Lewis Pubs.

Chemical Sensitivity Vol. 1: Principles & Mechanisms, Vol. 1. William J. Rea. 1992. 560p. 99.95 (*0-87371-541-1*, L541) Lewis Pubs.

Chemical Sensitivity Vol. 2: Sources of Total Body Load. William J. Rea. 1994. 592p. lib. bdg. 95.00 (*0-87371-963-8*, L963) Lewis Pubs.

Chemical Sensitivity Vol. 3: Clinical Manifestations of Pollutant Overload, Vol. 3. William J. Rea. 1995. 928p. 114.95 (*0-87371-964-6*, L964) Lewis Pubs.

Chemical Sensitivity of the Mammalian Genome. James L. Hargrove & Carolyn D. Berdanier. 1999. 90.00 (*0-8493-2762-8*) CRC Pr.

Chemical Signals in Vertebrates, Vol. 3. Ed. by Robert M. Silverstein & Dietland Muller-Schwarze. 1983. LC 83-2151. 378p. 79.50 (*0-306-41254-3*, Plenum Trade) Perseus Pubng.

Chemical Stability of Pharmaceutricals: A Handbook for Pharmacists. Kenneth A. Connors et al. 2nd ed. 1986. LC 85-31455. 864p. 200.00 (*0-471-87955-X*) Wiley.

Chemical Sterilants & Sterilization Methods: A Guide to Selection & Use. 1990. 42p. pap. 90.00 (*0-910275-98-X*, TIR7-209) Assn Adv Med Instrn.

Chemical Synthesis of Ether Lipids, Vol. 12. G. A. Serebrennikova & R. P. Evstigneeva. 1989. (Soviet Scientific Reviews Ser.: Vol. 12, Pt. 4). iv, 66p. pap. text 69.00 (*3-7186-4900-4*) Gordon & Breach.

Chemical Transmission of Nerve Impulses: A Historical Sketch. Z. M. Bacq. 1975. (*0-08-020512-7*) Pergamon Repr GBR. *Dist:* Franklin.

Chemical Transport in Metasomatic Processes. Ed. by Harold C. Helgeson. 1987. (C). text 374.50 (*90-277-2618-3*) Kluwer Academic.

Chemical Villains: A Biology of Pollution. James W. Berry et al. 1974. LC 73-11099. vii, 189p. (*0-8016-0663-2*) Mosby Inc.

Chemical Warfare Medicine: Aspects & Perspectives from the Persian Gulf War. Ed. by Yehuda L. Danon & Joshua Shemer. 1994. (Illus.). 228p. (C). text (*965-229-103-X*) Gefen Pub Hse ISR. *Dist:* Gefen Bks.

Chemically Induced Alterations in Sexual & Functional Development: The Wildlife-Human Connection, Vol. 8, No. 4. Ed. by T. Colburn & C. Clement. 1992. (Advances in Modern Environmental Toxicology Ser.: Vol. 21). (Illus.). 403p. (Orig.). 68.00 (*0-911131-35-3*) Specialist Journals.

Chemically Induced Birth Defects. Jame L. Schardein. 2nd exp. rev. ed. 1993. (Illus.). 920p. text 295.00 (*0-8247-8775-7*) Dekker.

Chemicals, Cancer & Choices: Risk Reduction Through Markets. Peter VanDoren. 1999. LC 99-26599. 99p. 16.95 (*1-882577-78-7*); pap. text 8.95 (*1-882577-79-5*) Cato Inst.

Chemie im Laboratorium. K. Lauber. 4th ed. 1983. (Illus.). viii, 376p. pap. 68.00 (*3-8055-3547-3*) S Karger.

Chemistry & Application of Green Tea. Ed. by T. Yamamoto et al. 1997. LC 97-11614. 176p. 74.95 (*0-8493-4006-3*, 4006) CRC Pr.

Chemistry & Biology of Serpins: Proceedings of the International Symposium Held in Chapel Hill, North Carolina, April 13-16, 1996. Ed. by Frank C. Church et al. 1998. LC 97-31140. (Advances in Experimental Medicine & Biology Ser.: Vol. 425). (Illus.). 384p. 95.00 (*0-306-45698-2*, Kluwer Plenum) Kluwer Academic.

Chemistry & Medicine: Papers Presented at the Fiftieth Anniversary of the Founding of the Medical School of the University of Minnesota. Ed. by Maurice B. Visscher. 1977. LC 67-30234. (Essay Index Reprint Ser.). 25.95 (*0-8369-0962-3*) Ayer.

Chemistry & Metabolism of the Vitamin B6 Antagonist, 4' Deoxypyridoxine. Stephen P. Coburn. 1981. 224p. 79.00 (*0-8493-5783-7*, QP772, CRC Reprint) Franklin.

Chemistry & Physiology of Bile Acids & Their Influence on Atherosclerosis. W. T. Beher. 1976. (Monographs on Atherosclerosis: Vol. 6). (Illus.). 85.25 (*3-8055-2242-8*) S Karger.

Chemistry & Physiology of the Gametes. 1966. (Technical Report Ser.: No. 333). 23p. pap. text 3.00 (*92-4-120333-1*) World Health.

Chemistry & Specifications of Pesticides: Thirteenth Report of the WHO Expert Committee on Vector Biology & Control. 1990. (Technical Reports: No. 798). (ENG, FRE & SPA.). 77p. pap. text 9.00 (*92-4-120798-1*, 1100798) World Health.

Chemistry & the Food System. American Chemical Society, Committee on Chemistry and Public Affairs. 1980. LC 80-11194. 138p. 14.95 (*0-8412-0557-4*); pap. 14.95 (*0-8412-0563-9*) Am Chemical.

Chemistry & Toxicology of Diverse Classes of Alkaloids. Ed. by Murray S. Blum. 1996. LC 95-80642. (Illus.). 386p. (C). text 99.50 (*1-880293-06-4*) Alaken.

Chemistry, Ecology & Health. Ed. by K. G. Ione. 1996. 452p. lib. bdg. 145.00 (*1-56072-236-3*) Nova Sci Pubs.

Chemistry for Health Science. George I. Sackheim & Dennis D. Lehman. 8th ed. 1997. LC 97-23061. 643p. 88.00 (*0-13-744319-6*) P-H.

Chemistry, Health Physics, & Nuclear Instrumentation. Ed. by Robert W. Deutsch & J. W. Whitney. 1972. (Academic Program for Nuclear Power Plant Personnel Ser., BWR Version: Vol. IV). (Illus.). 454p. tchr. ed. 195.00 (*0-87683-157-9*); stu. ed. 25.00 (*0-87683-164-1*); stu. ed. 35.00 (*0-87683-171-4*); ring bd. 39.50 (*0-87683-150-1*, A 373977) GP Courseware.

Chemistry, Matter, & Life. Stephen Miall & Laurence M. Miall. 1977. LC 70-39099. (Essay Index Reprint Ser.). reprint ed. 25.95 (*0-8369-2703-6*) Ayer.

Chemistry of Antitumor Antibiotics, Vol. 2. William A. Remers. 1988. 290p. 210.00 (*0-471-08180-9*) Wiley.

Chemistry of Antitumour Agents. Ed. by D. E. Wilman. 1990. 352p. 160.00 (*0-412-02031-9*, A3602, Chap & Hall NY) Chapman & Hall.

Chemistry of Atopic Allergens. L. Berrens. 1971. (Monographs in Allergy: Vol. 7). 81.00 (*3-8055-1150-7*) S Karger.

Chemistry of Behavior: A Molecular Approach to Neuronal Plasticity. Stanislav Reinis & Jerome M. Goldman. 1982. LC 82-13294. 622p. 110.00 (*0-306-41161-X*, Plenum Trade) Perseus Pubng.

Chemistry of Linear Oligopyrroles & Bile Pigments. H. Falk. 1989. (Illus.). 621p. 199.95 (*0-387-82112-0*, 2795) Spr-Verlag.

Chemistry of Mind-Altering Drugs: History, Pharmacology, & Cultural Context. Daniel M. Perrine. 1996. LC 96-28908. (American Chemical Society Publication). (Illus.). 500p. pap. text 45.00 (*0-8412-3253-9*) Am Chemical.

Chemistry of N-Thiosulfinylamines. Yoshio Inagaki & Renji Okazaki. 1982. (Sulfur Reports: Vol. 2, No. 4). 40p. pap. text 135.00 (*3-7186-0126-5*) Gordon & Breach.

Chemistry of Nucleosides & Nucleotides, Vol. 2. L. B. Townsend. 1991. LC 88-22359. (Illus.). 478p. (C). text 135.00 (*0-306-43646-9*, Kluwer Plenum) Kluwer Academic.

Chemistry of over the Counter Drugs. Carol Eby & Tatum. 1989. (Illus.). (Orig.). pap. text 15.95 (*1-877991-06-6*, AP4277) Flinn Scientific.

Chemistry of Silica: Solubility, Polymerization, Colloid & Surface Properties & Biochemistry of Silica. Ralph K. Iler. 1979. LC 78-23960. 896p. 285.00 (*0-471-02404-X*) Wiley.

Chemistry of Structure-Function Relationships in Cheese: Proceedings of ACS Symposium Held in Chicago, Illinois, August 23-25, 1993. Ed. by Edyth L. Malin & Michael H. Tunick. 1995. (Advances in Experimental Medicine & Biology Ser.: Vol. 367). (Illus.). 408p. 120.00 (*0-306-44982-X*, Kluwer Plenum) Kluwer Academic.

Chemists' Views of Imaging Centers: Proceedings of an ACS Symposium Held in Chicago, Illinois, August 22-27, 1993. Ed. by Ali M. Emran. 1995. (Illus.). 552p. (C). text 139.50 (*0-306-44912-9*, Kluwer Plenum) Kluwer Academic.

Chemo & Lunch. Susan Winn. 1990. LC 90-2784. 128p. (Orig.). pap. 8.95 (*0-931832-53-5*) Fithian Pr.

Chemoarchitechture of the Brain. R. Nieuwenhuys. 1985. (Illus.). 246p. 115.00 (*0-387-15349-7*) Spr-Verlag.

Chemoarchitectonic Atlas of the Developing Mouse Brain. David M. Jacobowitz & Louise C. Abbott. 1997. LC 97-42895. 304p. lib. bdg. 195.00 (*0-8493-2667-2*) CRC Pr.

Chemoarchitecture of the Brain. Rudolf Nieuwenhuys. 1985. 246p. pap. 110.00 (*3-540-15349-7*) Spr-Verlag.

Chemokine Protocols. Ed. by Amanda E. I. Proudfoot et al. 2000. (Methods in Molecular Biology Ser.: Vol. 138). (Illus.). 332p. 99.50 (*0-89603-722-3*) Humana.

Chemokine Receptors. Ed. by John N. Abelson et al. 1997. (Methods in Enzymology Ser.: Vol. 288). (Illus.). 480p. text 99.95 (*0-12-182189-7*) Morgan Kaufmann.

Chemokines & Cancer. Barrett J. Rollins. 1999. LC 98-48424. (Contemporary Cancer Research Ser.). (Illus.). 336p. 125.00 (*0-89603-562-X*) Humana.

Chemokines & Skin. Ed. by E. Kownatzki & J. Norgauer. 1998. (Progress in Inflammation Research Ser.: Vol. 1). 151p. 109.00 (*3-7643-5818-1*) Spr-Verlag.

Chemokines & Skin. Eckhard Kownatzki & Johannes Norgauer. 1998. LC 98-18186. (PIR - Progress in Inflammation Research Ser.). (*0-8176-5818-1*) Birkhauser.

Chemokines in Allergic Disease. Ed. by Marc E. Rothenberg. 1999. LC 99-49547. (Illus.). 592p. text 235.00 (*0-8247-0286-7*) Dekker.

Chemokines in Disease. Alisa E. Koch & Robert Strieter. 1996. LC 96-22712. (Medical Intelligence Unit Ser.). 218p. 99.00 (*1-57059-365-5*) Landes Bioscience.

Chemokines in Disease: Biology & Clinical Research. Ed. by Caroline A. Hebert. 1999. LC 98-55169. (Contemporary Immunology Ser.: Vol. 8). (Illus.). 352p. 135.00 (*0-89603-703-7*) Humana.

Chemometrics: A Textbook. D. L. Massart et al. 1988. 488p. 144.50 (*0-444-42660-4*) Elsevier.

Chemopotentiation by Hyperthermia. Ed. by M. Urano & E. Douple. 1994. (Hyperthermia & Oncology Ser.: Vol. 4). 360p. 215.00 (*90-6764-166-9*) Coronet Bks.

Chemoprevention in Cancer Control. Ed. by M. Hakema et al. 1996. LC 96-183921. (IARC Scientific Publications Ser.: No. 136). (Illus.). 174p. pap. text 86.00 (*92-832-2136-2*) OUP.

Chemoprevention of Cancer. Daniel W. Nixon. 1994. 156p. 110.00 (*0-8493-6850-2*, 6850) CRC Pr.

Chemoprevention of Cancer: A Clinical Update. International Society of Cancer Chemoprevention Staff. Ed. by H. J. Senn et al. 1999. LC 98-36643. (Recent Results in Cancer Research Ser.: Vol. 151). (Illus.). 144p. 119.00 (*3-540-64710-4*) Spr-Verlag.

Chemoprevention of Disease, Anti-Cancer Attempts, Strategy for Health Protection & Chemical Therapies: Index of New Information. John C. Bartone. 1999. 147p. rev. ed. pap. 47.50 (*0-7883-2153-6*); 2nd rev. ed. 57.50 (*0-7883-2152-8*) ABBE Pubs Assn.

Chemoprevention of Disease, Anti-Cancer Attempts, Strategy for Health Protection & Clinical Therapies: Index of New Information. John C. Bartone. 1998. 150p. 57.50 (*0-7883-1368-1*); pap. 47.50 (*0-7883-1369-X*) ABBE Pubs Assn.

C D

Chemoprophylaxis & Virus Infections of the Respiratory Tract. Ed. by John S. Oxford. 1977. (Uniscience Ser.). 1. 133.00 (*0-8493-5136-7*, RC732); 2. 139.00 (*0-8493-5137-5*, RC732) Franklin (CRC Reprint).

Chemoradiation: An Integrated Approach to Cancer Treatment. Madhu J. John et al. 1993. LC 92-48953. (Illus.). 824p. text 110.00 (*0-8121-1482-5*) Lppncott W & W.

Chemosensitivity Testing in Gynecologic Malignancies & Breast Cancer. Ed. by O. R. Koechli et al. 1994. (Contributions to Gynecology & Obstetrics Ser.: Vol. 19). (Illus.). x, 200p. 186.25 (*3-8055-5949-6*) S Karger.

Chemosensory Information Processing. Ed. by D. Schild. 1990. (NATO ASI Ser.: Vol. 39). (Illus.). 403p. 146.00 (*0-387-51769-3*, 3800) Spr-Verlag.

Chemotaxis: Its Biology & Biochemistry. Ed. by E. Sorkin et al. 1974. (Antibiotics & Chemotherapy Ser.: Vol. 19). (Illus.). 300p. 143.50 (*3-8055-1688-6*) S Karger.

Chemotherapeutic Antibacterial Agents. Scott L. Dax. 1995. LC 94-47608. 59.95 (*0-412-04161-8*) Chapman & Hall.

Chemotherapeutics & Disease Control. Ed. by Mary Howe-Grant. 1993. (Encyclopedia Reprints Ser.). 1008p. 225.00 (*0-471-59633-7*) Wiley.

Chemotherapie - Kompendium fuer das Pflegepersonal. Angela Loeser et al. 1990. (Illus.). viii, 48p. pap. 14.00 (*3-8055-5295-5*) S Karger.

Chemotherapie bei Soliden Tumoren und Malignen Systemerkrankungen. Harry J. Sauer. 1990. (Illus.). viii, 36p. pap. 13.25 (*3-8055-5296-3*) S Karger.

Chemotherapie Urologischer Malignome. Ed. by G. H. Jacobi & J. E. Altwein. 1979. (Beitraege Zur Onkologie, Contributions to Oncology Ser.: Vol. 1). pap. 25.25 (*3-8055-0313-X*) S Karger.

Chemotherapy & Cancer: The Patient, Family & Staff. Ed. by Michael A. Zevon et al. 1993. LC 88-183830. (Current Thanatology Ser.). 120p. pap. 17.95 (*0-930194-45-4*) Ctr Thanatology.

Chemotherapy & Drug Resistance in Malaria W. Peters. 2nd ed. 1987. Vol. 1. 542p. text 209.00 (*0-12-552721-7*); Vol. 2. 650p. text 209.00 (*0-12-552722-5*) Acad Pr.

Chemotherapy & Radiation Therapy Survival Guide: Information, Suggestions & Support to Help You Get Through Treatment. Judith McKay & Nancee Hirano. 2nd rev. ed. 1998. LC 97-69490. Orig. Title: The Chemotherapy Survival Guide. 192p. pap. 14.95 (*1-57224-070-9*) New Harbinger.

Chemotherapy & Radiotherapy of Gastrointestinal Tumors. Ed. by H. O. Klein. 1981. (Recent Results in Cancer Research Ser.: Vol. 79). (Illus.). 118p. 45.00 (*0-387-10938-2*) Spr-Verlag.

Chemotherapy & Urological Malignancy. Ed. by Alexander S. Spiers. 1982. (Clinical Practice in Urology Ser.). (Illus.). 163p. 117.00 (*0-387-11543-9*) Spr-Verlag.

Chemotherapy & You: A Guide to Self-help During Cancer Treament. Ed. by Barry Leonard. rev. ed. 2000. (Illus.). 66p. pap. text 20.00 (*0-7567-0515-0*) DIANE Pub.

Chemotherapy & You: A Guide to Self-Help During Treatment. 1992. (Illus.). 56p. (Orig.). (C). pap. text 20.00 (*1-56806-102-1*) DIANE Pub.

Chemotherapy & You: A Guide to Self-Help During Treatment. Ed. by Barry Leonard. 2000. (Illus.). 56p. (C). pap. text 15.00 (*0-7881-7518-1*) DIANE Pub.

Chemotherapy Care Plans: Designs for Nursing Care. Margaret Barton-Burke. 1992. (Nursing-Health Science Ser.). (Illus.). 432p. (C). spiral bd. 34.95 (*0-86720-339-0*, 339-0) Jones & Bartlett.

Chemotherapy Care Plans Handbook. Margaret B. Burke et al. 2nd ed. 1997. LC 97-41987. (Nursing Ser.). (Illus.). 608p. (C). spiral bd. 38.95 (*0-7637-0424-5*, 0424-5) Jones & Bartlett.

Chemotherapy Certification Program: Self-Learning Module. Nancy J. Bush. 1993. 220p. pap. 500.00 (*0-9638351-0-6*) Valentine & Assocs.

Chemotherapy Gives New Meaning to a Bad Hair Day: A Healing Book. Eileen Marin. 1996. (Illus.). 120p. 11.50 (*1-885676-08-5*) On A Shoestring.

Chemotherapy in Psychiatry. Ross J. Baldessarini. enl. rev. ed. 1985. (Illus.). 416p. 45.95 (*0-674-11383-7*) HUP.

Chemotherapy Memory Bank. Fredrica A. Preston & Cecila Wilfinger. 2nd ed. 1992. (Nursing-Health Science Ser.). (Illus.). 264p. (C). spiral bd. 31.25 (*0-86720-629-2*, 629-2) Jones & Bartlett.

Chemotherapy of Bilharziasis. 1966. (Technical Report Ser.: No. 317). 71p. pap. text 5.00 (*92-4-120317-X*) World Health.

Chemotherapy of Cancer: Proceedings of the WHO Expert Committee, 1st, Geneva, 1961. WHO Staff. 1962. (Technical Reports: No. 232). (ENG, FRE, RUS & SPA.). 52p. pap. text 3.00 (*92-4-120232-7*, 1100232) World Health.

Chemotherapy of Fungal Diseases. Ed. by J. F. Ryley. 1990. (Handbook of Experimental Pharmacology Ser.: Vol. 96). (Illus.). 558p. 348.00 (*0-387-52232-8*) Spr-Verlag.

Chemotherapy of Gliomas: Basic Research, Experiences & Results. Ed. by P. Krauseneck & Dieter Voth. 1984. LC 84-22980. (Illus.). xii, 440p. 113.85 (*3-11-009990-X*) De Gruyter.

Chemotherapy of Gynecologic Cancers: Society of Gynecologic Oncologists Handbook. Ed. by Stephen C. Rubin. 1996. LC 95-50021. 240p. pap. text 34.95 (*0-397-51736-X*) Lppncott W & W.

Chemotherapy of Gynecological & Breast Cancer. M. Kaufmann et al. 2nd rev. ed. 1990. (Illus.). xiii, 94p. pap. 28.00 (*3-8055-5074-X*) S Karger.

Chemotherapy of Leprosy: Report of a WHO Study Group. 1994. LC 95-187524. (Technical Reports: No. 847). (ENG, FRE & SPA.). v, 24p. pap. text 6.00 (*92-4-120847-3*, 1100847) World Health.

Chemotherapy of Malaria. 1961. (Technical Report Ser.: No. 226). 92p. pap. text 5.00 (*92-4-120226-2*) World Health.

Chemotherapy of Malaria. W. Peters et al. 2nd ed. 1986. (Monographs: No. 27). 261p. pap. text 39.60 (*92-4-140127-3*, 1142027) World Health.

Chemotherapy of Malaria: Report of a WHO Scientific Group, 1967. 1967. (Technical Report Ser.: No. 375). 91p. pap. text 5.00 (*92-4-120375-7*, 1100375) World Health.

Chemotherapy of Malaria & Resistance to Antimalarials: Proceedings of the WHO Scientific Group, Geneva, 1972. WHO Staff. 1973. (Technical Reports: No. 529). pap. text 7.00 (*92-4-120529-6*, 1100529) World Health.

Chemotherapy of Parasitic Diseases. Ed. by William C. Campbell & Robert S. Rew. 1986. LC 85-19377. (Illus.). 684p. (C). text 174.00 (*0-306-42029-5*, Kluwer Plenum) Kluwer Academic.

Chemotherapy of Psoriasis. H. P. Baden. 1984. (International Encyclopedia of Pharmacology & Therapeutics Ser.: 110). 325p. 122.50 (*0-08-029823-0*, Pergamon Pr) Elsevier.

Chemotherapy of Solid Tumours: Report of a WHO Expert Committee, 1977. 1977. (Technical Report Ser.: No. 605). 106p. pap. text 10.00 (*92-4-120605-5*, 1100605) World Health.

Chemotherapy Quick Reference. Shirley Otto. 2nd ed. 1996. (Illus.). 64p. (C). (gr. 13). pap. text 8.95 (*0-8151-8956-7*, 29033) Mosby Inc.

Chemotherapy Scenarios. Ed. by Sara Parkerson & Mervianna Thompson. 1997. 56p. pap. 15.00 (*1-890504-08-4*) Oncology Nursing.

Chemotherapy Source Book. Michael C. Perry. (Illus.). 1991. 1192p. 140.00 (*0-683-06859-8*); 2nd ed. 1996. LC 96-685. 1,184p. text 110.00 (*0-683-06868-7*) Lppncott W & W.

Chemotherapy Survival Guide see Chemotherapy & Radiation Therapy Survival Guide: Information, Suggestions & Support to Help You Get Through Treatment

Chemotherapy under Special Conditions. Ed. by H. Schoenfeld et al. 1973. (Antibiotics & Chemotherapy Ser.: Vol. 18). (Illus.). 210p. 85.25 (*3-8055-1646-0*) S Karger.

Chernobyl: A Decade: Proceedings of the 5th Chernobyl Sasakawa Medical Cooperation Symposium, Kiev, Ukraine, 14-15 October, 1996. Shunichi Yamashita et al. 1997. LC 97-41262. (International Congress Ser.). 634p. 210.00 (*0-444-82800-1*) Elsevier.

Chernobyl Update & in the Future. Ed. by Shigenobu Nagataki. 1994. LC 94-35040. (International Congress Ser.: No. 1074). 292p. 151.50 (*0-444-81953-3*) Elsevier.

Cherry & Merkatz's Complications of Pregnancy. Wayne R. Cohen et al. 5th ed. 1999. LC 98-32438. (Illus.). 928p. text 169.00 (*0-683-01673-3*) Lppncott W & W.

Cheshire Cat Syndrome: My Adventures with Arthritis. Ethel E. Radmer. 1996. (Illus.). 240p. (Orig.). pap. 14.95 (*0-9651182-0-7*) Euphonia Pub.

Chesney's Care of the Patient in Diagnostic Radiography. Pauline J. Chesney & D. Noreen Chesney. 7th ed. 1995. LC 94-30883. (Illus.). 416p. pap. 40.95 (*0-632-03762-8*) Blackwell Sci.

Chest Atlas: Correlated Thin-Section Anatomy in Five Planes. J. T. Littleton & M. L. Durizch. 1993. LC 92-49474. 321p. 324.00 (*0-387-97928-X*); 336p. (*3-540-97928-X*) Spr-Verlag.

Chest Disease (Fifth Series) Test & Syllabus, Vol. 40. Heber MacMahon et al. Ed. by Robert H. Choplin. 1996. (Professional Self-Evaluation Ser.). (Illus.). 660p. 220.00 (*1-55903-040-2*) Am Coll Radiology.

Chest Disease (Fourth Series) Test & Syllabus. Anthony V. Proto et al. 1989. (Professional Self-Evaluation & Continuing Education Program Ser.: Vol. 27). (Illus.). 814p. 165.00 (*1-55903-027-5*) Am Coll Radiology.

Chest Drainage. Springhouse Publishing Company Staff. 1992. (Procedures Video Ser.). 36.95 incl. VHS (*0-87434-372-0*) Springhouse Corp.

Chest, Heart & Lungs, Vols. 11 & 11a. Jules R. Kalisch & Harold Williams. 1975. (Courtroom Medicine Ser.). ring bd. 535.00 (*0-8205-1254-0*, 254) Bender.

Chest Imaging. Godwin. 1998. text (*0-7216-5038-4*) Saunders.

Chest Imaging Companion. Eric Stern. 1998. 448p. pap. text 65.00 (*0-397-51732-7*) Lppncott W & W.

Chest Medicine. P. S. Shankar. 1990. (*81-204-0502-1*) Oxford IBH IND. *Dist:* S Asia.

Chest Medicine: Essentials of Pulmonary & Critical Care Medicine. Ronald B. George. 2nd ed. 1990. (Illus.). 512p. pap. 72.00 (*0-683-03453-7*) Lppncott W & W.

Chest Medicine: Essentials of Pulmonary & Critical Care Medicine. Ed. by Ronald B. George. 3rd ed. 1995. LC 94-38017. (Illus.). 736p. 79.00 (*0-683-03458-8*) Lppncott W & W.

Chest Medicine: Essentials of Pulmonary & Critical Care Medicine. Ronald B. George et al. 4th ed. 2000. LC 00-20038. 704p. text 99.00 (*0-683-30667-7*) Lppncott W & W.

***Chest Pain.** Ed. by J. Willis Hurst & Douglas C. Morris. 2001. (Illus.). 528p. 79.00 (*0-87993-482-4*) Futura Pub.

Chest Pain: Most Common Complaints. Richard C. Becker. 2000. LC 99-87184. (Most Common Complaints Ser.). (Illus.). 136p. pap. text 24.99 (*0-7506-7141-6*) Buttrwrth-Heinemann.

Chest Pain - Is It Your Heart? David Andres. Ed. by Rhonda L. Shemtov & Janet Andres. 1987. LC 87-70554. (Illus.). 140p. (Orig.). pap. 9.95 (*0-9618345-0-1*) Colco Pub.

Chest Pain with Normal Coronary Angiograms: Pathogenesis, Diagnosis & Management. Juan C. Kaski. 1999. LC 98-54994. (Developments in Cardiovascular Medicine Ser.). (*0-7923-8421-0*) Kluwer Academic.

Chest Radiographic Analysis. Norman Blank. 1989. (Illus.). 670p. text (*0-443-08658-3*) Church.

Chest Radiology: Plain Film Patterns & Differential Diagnoses. James C. Reed. 4th ed. 1996. (Illus.). 496p. (C). (gr. 13). text 95.00 (*0-8151-7122-6*, 27076) Mosby Inc.

Chest Radiology: Pre-Test Self Assessment & Review. Juzar Ali et al. 2001. LC 00-52713. (Pretest Clinical Science Ser.). (Illus.). 350p. pap. 24.95 (*0-07-135959-1*) McGraw-Hill Prof.

Chest Radiology: The Essentials. Jannette Collins & Eric J. Stern. 2000. LC 99-31263. 304p. text 99.00 (*0-7817-1582-2*) Lppncott W & W.

Chest Roentgenology. Benjamin Felson. 1973. LC 73-188387. (Illus.). 574p. text 78.00 (*0-7216-3591-1*) Saunders.

Chest (Thorax) Injuries: Index of New Information for Reference & Research. Roy D. Galacter. 1997. 160p. 57.50 (*0-7883-1782-2*); pap. 47.50 (*0-7883-1783-0*) ABBE Pubs Assn.

Chest Trauma: Diagnosis & Management. W. Glinz. 1981. (Illus.). 303p. 80.00 (*0-387-10409-7*) Spr-Verlag.

***Chest X-Ray in Practice.** Jonathan Corne et al. 2001. (Illus.). 175p. pap. (*0-443-07010-5*) Church GBR. *Dist:* Saunders.

Chest X-Ray Interp. Primary Care. A and L New Media Staff. 1998. cd-rom 155.00 (*0-8385-1073-6*, Apple Lange Med) McGraw.

Chest X-Ray Made Easy. Jonathan Corne. 1997. LC 96-24944. 115p. pap. text (*0-443-05194-1*) Church.

***Chest X-Ray Made Easy.** Jonathan Corne et al. 2nd ed. 2001. (Illus.). 125p. pap. (*0-443-07008-3*) Church GBR. *Dist:* Saunders.

Chewa Medical Botany Part 1: A Study of Herbalism in Southern Malawi. Brian Morris & Jerome Msonthi. 1995. 568p. text 84.95 (*3-8258-2637-6*) Transaction Pubs.

Chi Gung: Chinese Healing, Energy, & Natural Magick. L. V. Carnie. 1999. LC 97-32002. (Illus.). 288p. pap. 17.50 (*1-56718-113-9*) Llewellyn Pubns.

Chicago Area Health Care Choices: The Families U. S. A. Guide to Quality & Cost. Ed. by Marc S. Miller. 1996. (Illus.). 240p. (Orig.). pap. 10.95 (*0-9617893-2-8*) Fam USA Found.

Chicago Institute Lectures. Heinz Kohut. Ed. by Paul Tolpin & Marian Tolpin. 1996. LC 96-6374. 432p. 55.00 (*0-88163-116-7*) Analytic Pr.

Chicago 1992. Mary A. Mattoon. 1995. 550p. pap. 35.00 (*3-85630-538-6*); text 25.00 (*3-85630-537-8*) Continuum.

Chicago Review Press NCLEX-PN. Berta Roland & Linda Waide. rev. ed. 1998. LC 98-20596. (Illus.). 252p. pap. 17.95 (*1-55652-329-7*) Chicago Review.

Chicago Review Press NCLEX-RN. Berta Roland & Linda Waide. 2nd rev. ed. 1998. LC 98-29573. 252p. pap. 17.95 (*1-55652-328-9*) Chicago Review.

Chicken Egg Yolk Antibodies, Production & Application: IgY-Technology. Ed. by Ruediger Schade et al. 2000. LC 00-41914. (Lab Manual Ser.). (Illus.). 250p. spiral bd., lab manual ed. 74.00 (*3-540-66679-6*) Spr-Verlag.

Chicken Soup & Other Folk Remedies. Joan Wilen & Lydia Wilen. rev. ed. 2000. LC 00-702856. (Illus.). 272p. pap. 14.00 (*0-345-44061-7*, Ballantine) Ballantine Pub Grp.

***Chickenpox.** Alvin Silverstein & Laura Silverstein Nunn. 2001. (My Health Ser.). 48p. (gr. 3-5). pap. 6.95 (*0-531-13970-0*) F Watts.

Chicorel Abstracts to Reading & Learning Disabilities. Ed. by Robert E. Lynn. 1983rd ed. 1984. (Chicorel Index Ser.: Vol. 19). 325p. text 125.00 (*0-934598-85-1*) Am Lib Pub Co.

Chicorel Abstracts to Reading & Learning Disabilities: 1977 Annual. Ed. by Marietta S. Chicorel. 1977. (Chicorel Index Ser.: Vol. 19). text 125.00 (*0-934598-17-7*) Am Lib Pub Co.

Chicorel Abstracts to Reading & Learning Disabilities: Periodicals, 1978 Annual. 1979. (Chicorel Index Ser.: Vol. 19). 584p. lib. bdg. 125.00 (*0-934598-16-9*) Am Lib Pub Co.

Chicorel Abstracts to Reading & Learning Disabilities: Periodicals, 1979 Annual. 1980. (Chicorel Index Ser.: Vol. 19). 414p. lib. bdg. 125.00 (*0-934598-10-X*) Am Lib Pub Co.

Chicorel Abstracts to Reading & Learning Disabilities, 1976 Annual. Marietta S. Chicorel. 1976. (Chicorel Index Ser.: Vol. 19). 384p. text 125.00 (*0-934598-15-0*) Am Lib Pub Co.

Chicorel Abstracts to Reading & Learning Disabilities, 1981. Ed. by Robert E. Lynn. 1983. (Chicorel Index Ser.: Vol. 19). 490p. 125.00 (*0-934598-83-5*) Am Lib Pub Co.

Chicorel Abstracts to Reading & Learning Disabilities, 1982. Ed. by Robert E. Lynn. 1984. (Chicorel Index Ser.: Vol. 19). 424p. 125.00 (*0-934598-84-3*) Am Lib Pub Co.

Chicorel Abstracts to Reading & Learning Disabilities, Periodicals, 1980 Annual. Ed. by Marietta S. Chicorel. 1982. (Chicorel Index Ser.: Vol. 19). 380p. 125.00 (*0-934598-80-0*) Am Lib Pub Co.

Chicorel Index to Learning Disorders Ed. by Marietta S. Chicorel. 1975. LC 75-9713. (Chicorel Index Ser.: Vols. 18 & 18A). 1000p. 18. lib. bdg. (*0-934598-30-4*); 18A. lib. bdg. (*0-934598-31-2*); Set. 250.00 (*0-934598-32-0*) Am Lib Pub Co.

Chicorel Index to Mental Health Book Reviews, 1974 Annual. Ed. by Marietta S. Chicorel. 1982. (Chicorel Index Ser.: Vol. 26). 322p. text 125.00 (*0-934598-81-9*) Am Lib Pub Co.

Chicorel Index to Mental Health Book Reviews, 1975 Annual. Ed. by Marietta S. Chicorel. 1982. (Chicorel Index Ser.: Vol. 26). 287p. 125.00 (*0-934598-82-7*) Am Lib Pub Co.

Chicorel Index to Mental Health Book Reviews, 1978 Annual. 1980. (Chicorel Index Ser.: Vol. 26). 400p. text 125.00 (*0-934598-08-8*) Am Lib Pub Co.

Chicorel Index to Mental Health Book Reviews, 1979 Annual. 1980. (Chicorel Index Ser.: Vol. 26). 400p. lib. bdg. 125.00 (*0-934598-79-7*) Am Lib Pub Co.

Chicorel Index to Mental Health Book Reviews, 1980-84 Ed. by Marietta S. Chicorel. 1986. (Chicorel Index Ser.: Vol. 26). text 375.00 (*0-934598-93-2*) Am Lib Pub Co.

Chicorel Index to Mental Health Book Reviews, 1997 Annual. 1978. (Chicorel Index Ser.: Vol. 26). 400p. 125.00 (*0-934598-77-0*) Am Lib Pub Co.

Chicorel Index to Reading & Learning Disabilities: An Annotated Guide, 1976. Ed. by Marietta S. Chicorel. 1976. (Chicorel Index Ser.: Vol. 14A). text 125.00 (*0-934598-49-5*) Am Lib Pub Co.

Chicorel Index to Reading & Learning Disabilities: Books, 1977 Annual. Ed. by Marietta S. Chicorel. 1977. LC 76-14381. (Chicorel Index Ser.: Vol. 14A). text 125.00 (*0-934598-50-9*) Am Lib Pub Co.

Chicorel Index to Reading & Learning Disabilities: Books, 1978 Annual. 1980. (Chicorel Index Ser.: Vol. 14A). 400p. text 125.00 (*0-934598-09-6*) Am Lib Pub Co.

Chicorel Index to Reading Disabilities: An Annotated Guide. Ed. by Marietta S. Chicorel. 1974. (Chicorel Index Ser.: Vol. 14). 500p. 125.00 (*0-934598-51-7*) Am Lib Pub Co.

Chid Development. Nora Newcombe. 8th ed. 1996. (C). pap. text, stu. ed. 26.25 (*0-673-99332-9*) Addson-Wesley Educ.

Chief Medical Examiner. Jack Rudman. 1994. (Career Examination Ser.: C-1180). pap. 59.95 (*0-8373-1180-2*) Nat Learn.

Chief Occupational Therapist. Jack Rudman. (Career Examination Ser.: C-3699). pap. 39.95 (*0-8373-3699-6*) Nat Learn.

Chief Physical Therapist. Jack Rudman. 1994. (Career Examination Ser.: C-3384). pap. 39.95 (*0-8373-3384-9*) Nat Learn.

Chief Police Surgeon. Jack Rudman. 1994. (Career Examination Ser.: C-1181). pap. 49.95 (*0-8373-1181-0*) Nat Learn.

Chief Psychologist. Jack Rudman. 1994. (Career Examination Ser.: C-2194). pap. 44.95 (*0-8373-2194-8*) Nat Learn.

Chief Public Health Nutritionist. Jack Rudman. 1994. (Career Examination Ser.: C-1567). pap. 34.95 (*0-8373-1567-0*) Nat Learn.

Chief Recreation Therapist. Jack Rudman. 1994. (Career Examination Ser.: C-3279). pap. 39.95 (*0-8373-3279-6*) Nat Learn.

Chief Resident As Manager. Neal A. Whitman et al. 1988. 143p. (Orig.). pap. text 20.00 (*0-940193-05-1*) Univ UT Sch Med.

Chikitsa Nyaya Shastra: (Medical Jurisprudence) B. L. Babel. 1988. (HIN.). (C). 40.00 (*0-7855-5116-6*) St Mut.

Child. Eli Siegel. 1970. pap. (*0-911492-16-X*) Aesthetic Realism.

Child: His Nature & His Needs. Ed. by M. V. O'Shea. 1975. LC 74-21424. (Classics in Child Development Ser.). (Illus.). 576p. reprint ed. 56.95 (*0-405-06473-X*) Ayer.

Child: His Thinking, Feeling, & Doing. Amy E. Tanner. enl. rev. ed. LC 78-72826. (Brainedness, Handedness, & Mental Abilities Ser.). reprint ed. 40.00 (*0-404-60894-9*) AMS Pr.

Child Abuse. Eli H. Newberger. 1982. 52.95 (*0-316-60410-0*, Little Brwn Med Div) Lppncott W & W.

Child Abuse. Peggy Murray & Mary Stein. 4th rev. ed. 1997. (Illus.). 231p. pap. 44.95 (*1-57801-008-X*) Western Schls.

Child Abuse: A Handbook for Health Care Practitioners. Ivan Blumenthal. 1994. LC 96-126567. 160p. pap. (*0-340-60141-8*) E A GBR. *Dist:* OUP.

Child Abuse: A Medical Reference. Ed. by Stephen Ludwig & Allan E. Kornberg. 2nd ed. 1991. (Illus.). 563p. text (*0-443-08722-9*) Church.

Child Abuse: Abstracts of the Psychological & Behavioral Literature. Ed. by Diane J. Willis et al. 1991. LC

91-18149. (Bibliographies in Psychology Ser.: No. 9). Vol. 1, 1967-1985. 225p. pap. 19.95 (*1-55798-163-9*); Vol. 2, 1986-1990. 280p. pap. 19.95 (*1-55798-147-7*) Am Psychol.

Child Abuse: Abstracts of the Psychological & Behavioral Literature 1990-1995. Ed. by Seth C. Kalichman & Anthony T. Gary. 1996. LC 96-30460. (Bibliographies in Psychology Ser.: Vol. 3). 403p. pap. text 19.95 (*1-55798-394-1*) Am Psychol.

Child Abuse: An Interactional Event. Alfred Kadushin & Judith A. Martin. 1981. LC 80-39654. (Illus.). 360p. text 57.50 (*0-231-04774-6*) Col U Pr.

Child Abuse: Implications for Child Development & Psychopathology. David A. Wolfe. 1987. (Developmental Clinical Psychology & Psychiatry Ser.: Vol. 10). 160p. 74.95 (*0-8039-2832-7*, 5939); pap. 34.95 (*0-8039-2833-5*, 5940) Sage.

Child Abuse: Medical Diagnosis & Management. Robert M. Reece & Stephen Ludwig. 2nd ed. 2001. 608p. text 99.00 (*0-7817-2444-9*) Lppncott W & W.

Child Abuse: Quick Reference for Healthcare Professionals, Social Services & Law Enforcement. Ed. by James A. Monteleone. 2000. LC 97-40035. (Illus.). 350p. (Orig.). pap. 39.95 (*1-878060-28-7*, 31142) GW Medical.

Child Abuse: Recognition & Management. Debbie Warley & Julie Pettet. 1997. 125p. (*0-7020-2238-1*) W B Saunders GBR. *Dist:* Saunders.

Child Abuse: The Legal Approach to Medical Evidence. R. Ough & Alan M. McClelland. Ed. by Duncan Matheson et al. 1995. 258p. pap. (*0-406-04980-7*, OCAL, MICHIE) LEXIS Pub.

***Child Abuse & Neglect.** Connie Burrows Horton & Tracy K. Cruise. 2001. LC 2001-23132. (Guilford School Practitioner Ser.). 200p. text 30.00 (*1-57230-673-4*) Guilford Pubns.

Child Abuse & Neglect: A Clinician's Handbook. Christopher J. Hobbs et al. 1993. LC 92-48782. 384p. text (*0-443-04146-6*) Church.

Child Abuse & Neglect: A Clinician's Handbook. C. J. Hobbs et al. 2nd ed. 1998. (Illus.). 368p. text (*0-443-05896-2*) Church.

Child Abuse & Neglect: An Annotated Bibliography, 2. Beatrice J. Kalisch. 1978. LC 78-3123. (Contemporary Problems of Childhood Ser.: No. 2). 535p. lib. bdg. 80.00 (*0-313-20376-8*, KBA/, Greenwood Pr) Greenwood.

Child Abuse & Neglect: An Information & Reference Guide. Timothy J. Iverson & Marilyn Segal. LC 89-71495. 232p. 1991. pap. text 19.95 (*0-8153-0468-4*, SS423); 1990. text 44.00 (*0-8240-7776-8*, SS423) Garland.

Child Abuse & Neglect: Facing the Challenge. Ed. by Wendy S. Rogers et al. 1989. (Illus.). 288p. 29.95 (*0-7134-6216-7*) Trafalgar.

Child Abuse & Neglect Prevention Strategies: Milwaukee County. Shirley R. Berry. 1990. 176p. (Orig.). (C). pap., tchr. ed. 27.50 (*0-9627724-0-2*) Blckbrry Crtns.

Child Abuse & Violence. Intro. by David G. Gil. 1979. LC 77-91865. (Studies in Modern Society: Political & Social Issues: No. 13). 34.50 (*0-404-16044-1*); pap. 14.00 (*0-404-16045-X*) AMS Pr.

Child Abuse in the Classroom. Phyllis Schlafly. 1984. LC 84-61629. 4.95 (*0-934640-10-6*) Pere Marquette.

Child Abuse Man. James McGovern. 1989. LC 88-50592. 215p. (Orig.). pap. 10.00 (*0-916383-70-9*, Univ Edtns) Aegina Pr.

Child Abuse Trauma: Theory & Treatment of the Lasting Effects. John N. Briere. 1992. (Interpersonal Violence Ser.: Vol. 2). 200p. (C). 79.95 (*0-8039-3712-1*, 3431); pap. 31.95 (*0-8039-3713-X*, 3432) Sage.

Child Advocacy for the Clinician: An Approach to Child Abuse & Neglect. Lawrence S. Wissow. 1989. (Illus.). 250p. 37.00 (*0-683-09204-9*) Lppncott W & W.

Child Analysis & Therapy. Ed. by Jules Glenn. 1992. LC 78-65122. 776p. reprint ed. 60.00 (*0-87668-356-1*) Aronson.

Child Analysis with Anna Freud. Peter Heller. 1990. LC 89-2146. (Illus.). 400p. 57.50 (*0-8236-0835-2*) Intl Univs Pr.

Child Analyst at Work. Ed. by Elisabeth R. Geleerd. 1967. LC 67-20281. 310p. 45.00 (*0-8236-0740-2*) Intl Univs Pr.

Child & Adolescent Analysis: Its Significance for Clinical Work with Adults. Ed. by Scott Dowling. 1990. LC 90-5089. (Workshop Series of the American Psychoanalytic Association: Monograph 6). 243p. 35.00 (*0-8236-0750-X*) Intl Univs Pr.

Child & Adolescent Athlete. Ed. by Oded Bar-Or et al. 1995. LC 95-182. (Encyclopedia of Sports Medicine Ser.: Vol. 6). 672p. 162.95 (*0-86542-904-9*) Blackwell Sci.

Child & Adolescent Clinical Psychopharmacology. Wayne H. Green. 1991. (Illus.). 256p. pap. 33.00 (*0-683-03766-8*); 2nd ed. 1995. LC 95-10273. 288p. pap. 44.95 (*0-683-03767-6*) Lppncott W & W.

Child & Adolescent Development. Edward P. Sarafino & James W. Armstrong. 2nd ed. 1986. (Illus.). 624p. (C). mass mkt. 49.25 (*0-314-93411-1*); mass mkt., stu. ed. 28.25 (*0-314-93412-X*) West Pub.

Child & Adolescent Disorders: Developmental & Health Psychology Perspectives. Ed. by Sam B. Morgan & Theresa M. Okwumabua. 1990. 480p. 99.95 (*0-8058-0514-1*) L Erlbaum Assocs.

Child & Adolescent Mental Health: Health Care Needs Assessment: The Epidemiologically Based Needs Assessment Reviews, Second Series. Andrew Stevens et al. 1997. LC 97-13347. (*1-85775-295-3*) Radcliffe Med Pr GBR. *Dist:* Balogh.

Child & Adolescent Mental Health Consultation in Hospitals, Schools, & Courts. Gregory K. Fritz et al. 1993. LC 92-48975. 316p. text 39.50 (*0-88048-418-7*, 8418) Am Psychiatric.

Child & Adolescent Neurology. Ronald B. David. 3rd ed. 1997. LC 96-49799. (Neurology Psychiatry Access Ser.). (Illus.). 656p. (C). (gr. 13). text 64.95 (*0-8151-2320-5*, 26884) Mosby Inc.

Child & Adolescent Nurse. Jack Rudman. 1994. (Certified Nurse Examination Ser.: CN-7). pap. 27.95 (*0-8373-6107-9*) Nat Learn.

Child & Adolescent Preventive Care: Access, Quality, & Outcomes. Ed. by Linda F. Wolf. 2000. (Illus.). 147p. reprint ed. pap. text 30.00 (*0-7881-8529-2*) DIANE Pub.

Child & Adolescent Psychiatry. Ed. by Dean X. Parmelee. 1996. LC 95-52516. (Access Ser.). (Illus.). 360p. (C). (gr. 13). text 66.95 (*0-8151-6809-8*, 25198) Mosby Inc.

Child & Adolescent Psychiatry: A Comprehensive Textbook. Melvin Lewis. (Illus.). 1991. 1318p. 139.00 (*0-683-04954-2*); 2nd ed. 1996. LC 95-23168. 1,538p. text 179.00 (*0-683-04955-0*) Lppncott W & W.

Child & Adolescent Psychiatry for the Specialty Board Review. Robert L. Hendren. 2nd rev. ed. 1997. (Continuing Education in Psychiatry & Psychology Ser.: Vol. 6). 128p. 69.95 incl. disk (*0-87630-849-3*); LC 96-54815. xvi, 157p. pap. 24.95 (*0-87630-840-X*) Brunner-Routledge.

Child & Adolescent Psychiatry in Europe. Ed. by H. Remschmidt. 1999. 420p. (C). (*3-7985-1170-5*) D Steinkopff DEU. *Dist:* Spr-Verlag.

Child & Adolescent Psychological Disorders: A Comprehensive Textbook. Ed. by Sandra D. Netherton et al. 1999. LC 98-7279. (Oxford Textbooks in Clinical Psychology Ser.). (Illus.). 624p. (C). text 69.95 (*0-19-509961-3*) OUP.

Child & Adolescent Psychology. M. Rutter. 3rd ed. 1995. pap. 141.95 (*0-632-02821-1*) Blackwell Sci.

Child & Adolescent Psychopharmacology. Stanley P. Kutcher. Ed. by Judy Fletcher. 1997. LC 96-43068. 480p. pap. text 58.00 (*0-7216-5749-4*) Saunders.

Child & Adolescent Therapy. Margaret Semrud-Clikeman. 1995. LC 95-2154. 224p. (C). 59.00 (*0-205-15026-8*, Longwood Div) Allyn.

Child & Adolescent Therapy: A Handbook. Ed. by David A. Lane & Andrew Miller. 1993. LC 92-18914. (Psychotherapy Handbooks Ser.). 256p. pap. (*0-335-09890-8*) OpUniv Pr.

Child & Adolescent Therapy: Cognitive-Behavioral Procedures. Philip C. Kendall. 2nd ed. 2000. LC 00-25796. (Illus.). 432p. text 46.00 (*1-57230-556-8*) Guilford Pubns.

Child & Adult Development: A Psychoanalytic Introduction for Clinicians. Calvin A. Colarusso. 1992. (Critical Issues in Psychiatry Ser.). (Illus.). 240p. (C). 45.00 (*0-306-44285-X*, Plenum Trade) Perseus Pubng.

Child & Family: Concepts of Nursing Practice. Marjorie Smith. 1991. 46.95 (*0-8016-6050-5*) Mosby Inc.

Child & Family Assessment: Clinical Guidelines for Practitioners. Ian Wilkinson. 2nd ed. 1998. LC 97-26566. (Illus.). 280p. (C). 78.95 (*0-415-16806-6*); pap. 26.95 (*0-415-16807-4*) Routledge.

Child & Family Development. Debra P. Hymovich & Robert Chamberlin. 1980. (Illus.). text 31.95 (*0-07-031650-3*) McGraw.

Child Art Therapy: Understanding & Helping Children Grow Through Art. Judith A. Rubin. 2nd ed. 1984. (Illus.). 320p. pap. 85.00 (*0-471-28951-5*, VNR) Wiley.

Child Art Therapy: Understanding & Helping Children Through Art. Judith A. Rubin. 2nd ed. 1984. (Illus.). 336p. pap. 48.95 (*0-442-27767-9*, VNR) Wiley.

Child Behavior Analysis & Therapy. Donna M. Gelfand & Donald P. Hartmann. 2nd ed. 1984. LC 74-14707. (General Psychology Ser.: No. 50). 304p. text 70.00 (*0-08-028054-4*); pap. text 24.50 (*0-08-028053-6*) Elsevier (Pergamon Pr).

Child Behavior Modification: A Manual for Teachers, Nurses & Parents. Leslie Watson & A. Goldstein. 1973. LC 72-83403. (Pergamon General Psychology Ser.: Vol. 24). (*0-08-016823-X*) Pergamon Repr GBR. *Dist:* Franklin.

Child Behavior Ri. Frances L. Ilg et al. 1992. LC 91-50503. 368p. reprint ed. pap. 14.00 (*0-06-092276-1*, Perennial) HarperTrade.

Child Behavior Therapy. Alan O. Ross. 1987. LC 87-3517. 444p. (C). reprint ed. lib. bdg. 46.50 (*0-89464-229-4*) Krieger.

Child Behavior Therapy Casebook. M. Hersen & C. G. Last. 1988. LC 88-15125. (Illus.). 424p. (C). 59.50 (*0-306-42868-7*, Plenum Trade) Perseus Pubng.

Child Behavioral Assessment: Principles & Procedures. Ed. by Michel Hersen & Thomas H. Ollendick. 1984. (General Psychology Ser.: No. 129). (Illus.). 280p. text 60.00 (*0-08-029370-0*); pap. text 24.50 (*0-08-029369-7*) Elsevier (Pergamon Pr).

Child Care Aide Skills. Flora S. Conger & Irene B. Rose. 1978. (Careers in Home Economics Ser.). (Illus.). text 25.84 (*0-07-012420-5*) McGraw.

Child Care Alternatives & Emotional Well-Being. Judith D. Schiller. 1980. LC 80-409. 204p. 38.50 (*0-275-90546-2*, C0546, Praeger Pubs) Greenwood.

Child Care & Health for Nursery Nurses. Jean Brain & Molly D. Martin. 3rd ed. 1995. pap. 21.00 (*0-7175-1196-0*) Dufour.

Child Care & Health for Nursery Nurses. Jean Brain et al. 3rd ed. 1989. 288p. (C). pap. (*1-871402-13-1*) Nelson Thornes GBR. *Dist:* Trans-Atl Phila.

Child Care Crisis: A Reference Handbook. Diane L. Reeves. 1992. LC 92-38144. (Contemporary World Issues Ser.). 173p. lib. bdg. 39.50 (*0-87436-645-3*) ABC-CLIO.

***Child Care Health Handbook.** Ed. by Iris Graville. 2001. (Illus.). 220p. ring bd. 18.00 (*1-893234-01-0*) Seattle-King Cty Dept.

Child Care in General Practice. Cyril Hart & John Bain. 3rd ed. 1989. (Illus.). 486p. pap. text (*0-443-03943-7*) Church.

Child Care in Rural America. 1977. LC 70-169360. (Family in America Ser.). (Illus.). 462p. 33.95 (*0-405-03884-4*) Ayer.

Child Care in the 1990s: Trends & Consequences. Ed. by Alan Booth. 1992. 264p. text 69.95 (*0-8058-1060-9*); pap. 29.95 (*0-8058-1061-7*) L Erlbaum Assocs.

***Child Care Law for Health Professionals.** Judith Hendrick. 1993. 176p. pap. (*1-870905-29-6*) Radcliffe Med Pr GBR. *Dist:* Balogh.

Child-Centerd Family Therapy. Lucille L. Andreozzi. 1996. LC 95-52822. (Couples & Family Dynamics & Treatment Ser.). 374p. 100.00 (*0-471-14858-X*) Wiley.

Child-Centered Group Guidance of Parents. S. R. Slavson. 1958. LC 58-11380. pap. 24.95 (*0-8236-8016-9*, 20760) Intl Univs Pr.

Child Centered Play Therapy. Janet West. 2nd ed. 1996. 256p. 29.95 (*1-56593-872-0*, 1704) Singular Publishing.

Child Clinical Documentation Sourcebook: A Comprehensive Collection of Forms & Guidelines for Efficient Record-Keeping in Child Mental Health Practice. Donald K. Freedheim & Jeremy P. Shapiro. 2nd ed. 1999. LC 98-44173. (Practice Planners Ser.). (Illus.). 256p. 49.95 incl. disk (*0-471-29111-0*) Wiley.

Child Custody Litigation: A Guide for Parents & Mental Health Professionals. Richard A. Gardner. 1986. LC 85-28029. xii, 385p. 35.00 (*0-933812-12-4*) Creative Therapeutics.

Child Development. Greta Fein. 1978. (Illus.). stu. ed. 8.95 (*0-13-132555-8*) P-H.

Child Development. Robert S. Feldman. 1997. 320p. (C). pap. text, stu. ed. 20.80 (*0-13-757642-0*) P-H.

Child Development. Fergus P. Hughes et al. 1988. 533p. (C). mass mkt. 48.00 (*0-314-64017-7*) West Pub.

Child Development. Neil J. Salkind. (Illus.). 864p. (C). pap. text 23.95 (*0-15-501031-X*) Harcourt Coll Pubs.

Child Development. Morrison. 2nd ed. 1995. (Early Childhood Education Ser.). pap., tchr. ed. 12.00 (*0-8273-4585-2*) Delmar.

Child Development. Dworetzky. 5th ed. Date not set. pap. text, tchr. ed. (*0-314-02169-8*); 1993. mass mkt., stu. ed. 14.75 (*0-314-02170-1*) West Pub.

Child Development. Nora Newcombe. 8th ed. 1998. (C). pap. text 22.00 (*0-673-97491-X*) Addson-Wesley Educ.

Child Development. Nora Newcombe. 8th ed. 1997. stu. ed. 92.00 (*0-201-34982-5*) Allyn.

Child Development. John W. Santrock. 9th ed. 2000. LC 00-28271. (Illus.). xxvii, 585p. text 45.74 net. (*0-697-36215-9*) McGraw.

Child Development: An Introduction. John W. Santrock. 6th ed. 1993. 640p. (C). text 58.00 (*0-697-14511-5*) Brown & Benchmark.

Child Development: Change over Time. Nora Newcombe. 8th rev. ed. 1997. LC 95-12721. 736p. (C). 92.00 (*0-673-99311-6*) Addson-Wesley Educ.

Child Development: Risk & Opportunities. Krantz. 1994. (Education Ser.). stu. ed. 18.00 (*0-534-13171-9*) Wadsworth Pub.

Child Development & Behavioral Pediatrics: Toward Understanding Children & Health. Ed. by Marc H. Bornstein & Janice L. Genevro. 1996. (Crosscurrents in Contemporary Psychology Ser.). 200p. text 39.95 (*0-8058-2364-6*) L Erlbaum Assocs.

Child Development & Education: A Piagetian Perspective. David Elkind. 1976. 304p. (C). pap. text 24.95 (*0-19-502069-3*) OUP.

Child Development & Learning. Ed. by William C. Johnson. 1973. LC 73-655. 193p. pap. text 12.95 (*0-8422-0294-3*) Irvington.

Child Development & Parenting. Herr. 1995. (C). text 21.95 (*0-8273-5594-7*) Delmar.

Child Development, Health, & Safety: Educational Materials for Home Visitors & Parents. Luanne G. Gardner Sheaffer et al. 1996. LC 96-21527. spiral bd. 70.00 (*0-8342-0845-8*) PRO-ED.

Child Development in Cultural Context. Ed. by Jaan Valsiner. 1989. LC 87-8799. (Illus.). 320p. (C). 38.00 (*0-88937-015-X*) Hogrefe & Huber Pubs.

Child Development in India: Health, Welfare & Management, Set. R. Kumar. 1988. (C). (*81-7024-189-8*) Ashish Pub Hse IND. *Dist:* S Asia.

Child Development in Life-Span Perspective. Ed. by E. Mavis Hetherington et al. 1988. 336p. text 69.95 (*0-8058-0189-8*); pap. text 36.50 (*0-8058-0190-1*) L Erlbaum Assocs.

Child Eyewitness Testimony: Ecological Sexual Abuse Investigations. Bruce E. Mapes. 1995. LC 94-41029. (*0-88422-154-7*) Clinical Psych.

Child Group Psychotherapy: Future Tense. Ed. by Albert E. Riester & Irvin A. Kraft. 1986. LC 86-10486. (American Group Psychotherapy Association Monographs). 45.00 (*0-8236-0765-8*, BN#00765) Intl Univs Pr.

Child Growth & Development. Elizabeth B. Hurlock. 5th ed. 1977. (American Home & Family Ser.). (Illus.). (gr. 10-12). text 30.56 (*0-07-031437-3*) McGraw.

Child Growth & Nutrition in Developing Countries: Priorities for Action. Ed. by Harold Alderman et al. 1994. LC 94-31497. (Food Systems & Agrarian Change Ser.). (Illus.). 496p. pap. 32.50 (*0-8014-8189-9*) Cornell U Pr.

Child Guidance & Education: Collected Papers. Rudolf Dreikurs. pap. 6.50 (*0-918560-11-X*) Adler Sch Prof Psy.

Child Health. Ed. by David Harvey & Ilya Kovar. 2nd ed. 1991. (Illus.). 460p. pap. text (*0-443-04026-5*) Church.

Child Health: The Screening Tests. Aidan MacFarlane et al. 1989. (Practical Guides for General Practice Ser.: No. 11). (Illus.). 64p. pap. 12.95 (*0-19-261768-0*) OUP.

Child Health & Disease. B. K. Chakraborty. 1989. (C). (*0-89771-378-8*) Current Dist IND. *Dist:* St Mut.

Child Health Care & the Working Mother: The Juggling Act. Jenny Hewison & Therese Dowswell. 1993. LC 93-36300. 192p. pap. 41.50 (*1-56593-235-8*, 0555) Singular Publishing.

Child Health Care Communication. Ed. by William K. Frankenburg & Susan M. Thornton. 1984. LC 84-13270. 385p. 78.75 (*0-275-91430-5*, C1430, Praeger Pubs) Greenwood.

Child Health Care Communications. Ed. by Susan M. Thornton. 1983. (Pediatric Round Table Ser.: No. 8). 217p. 10.00 (*0-931562-08-2*) J & J Consumer Prods.

Child Health Care in Ayurveda. Abhimanya Kuman. 1994. LC 94-900263. (C). (*81-7030-389-3*) Sri Satguru Pubns IND. *Dist:* S Asia.

Child Health Care Nursing: Concepts, Theory & Practice. Bernadette Carter et al. 1995. LC 95-22040. (Illus.). 800p. pap. 44.95 (*0-632-03689-3*) Blackwell Sci.

Child Health Guide: Put Prevention into Practice. 1995. (Illus.). 40p. (Orig.). (C). pap. text 20.00 (*0-7881-2184-7*) DIANE Pub.

Child Health in the Tropics. Ed. by R. E. Eeckels. 1985. text 226.00 (*0-89838-719-1*) Kluwer Academic.

Child Health Nursing: Care of the Child & Family Adele Pillitteri. 1999. LC 98-51353. 1,232p. text 59.95 (*0-7817-1624-1*) Lppncott W & W.

Child Health Nursing: Essential Care of Children & Families. James & Sandra R. Mott. Ed. by Debra Hunter. 1988. 1315p. (C). stu. ed. 12.76 (*0-201-14056-X*) Addison-Wesley.

Child Health Nursing: Essential Care of Children & Families. Susan R. James & Sandra R. Mott. Ed. by Debra Hunter. 1988. 1315p. (C). text 55.95 (*0-201-14178-7*) Addison-Wesley.

***Child Health Nursing: Review & Rationales.** Mary A. Hogan & Judy White. 2001. 384p. pap. 19.46 (*0-13-030452-2*) P-H.

Child Health, Nutrition, & Physical Activity. Ed. by Lilian W. Cheung & Julius B. Richmond. 1995. LC 94-43674. (Illus.). 392p. text 40.00 (*0-87322-774-3*, BCHE0774) Human Kinetics.

Child Health Psychology. Paul Karoly. 1982. (C). 55.95 (*0-205-14384-9*, H4384) Allyn.

Child Health Psychology. Neil Schneiderman & Barbara G. Melamed. 1987. 360p. pap. text 29.95 (*0-8058-0085-9*) L Erlbaum Assocs.

Child Health Psychology: Concepts & Issues. Ed. by Paul Karoly et al. 1982. (General Psychology Ser.: No. 113). (Illus.). 288p. 55.00 (*0-08-029368-9*, J115, Pergamon Pr) Elsevier.

Child Health Services & Pediatric Education: Report of the Committee for the Study of Child Health Services. American Academy of Pediatrics Staff. 1974. LC 74-1661. (Children & Youth Ser.). 304p. reprint ed. 28.95 (*0-405-05943-4*) Ayer.

Child Health Supervision: Analytical Studies in the Financing, Delivery, & Cost-Effectiveness of Preventive. Ed. by M. R. Solloway & P. P. Budetti. 1995. 420p. pap. (*1-57285-014-0*) Nat Ctr Educ.

Child in Latin America: Health, Development & Rights. Ed. by Ernest J. Bartell & Alejandro O'Donnell. 2000. LC 00-62894. (From the Helen Kellogg Institute for International Studies Ser.). (Illus.). xxxi, 378p. 50.00 (*0-268-02257-7*) U of Notre Dame Pr.

Child in the Family. Jay Belsky et al. 1984. LC 83-12255. (Illus.). 288p. (C). pap. text 33.50 net. (*0-07-554803-8*) McGraw.

Child Is Being Killed: On Primary Narcissism & the Death Drive. Serge LeClaire. 1998. LC 97-23343. (Meridian: Crossing Aesthetics Ser.). 37.00 (*0-8047-3140-3*) Stanford U Pr.

Child Is Being Killed: On Primary Narcissism & the Death Drive. Serge LeClaire. Tr. by Marie-Claude Hays. 1998. LC 97-23343. (Meridian: Crossing Aesthetics Ser.). 85p. pap. 13.95 (*0-8047-3141-1*) Stanford U Pr.

C D

Child Is Born. Lennart Nilsson. 1986. (Illus.). 216p. pap. 19.95 (*0-440-50691-3*) Dell.

Child Language & Developmental Dysphasia: Linguistic Studies of the Acquisition of German. Harald Clahsen. Tr. by Karin Richman from GER. 1991. LC 91-22437. (Studies in Speech Pathology & Clinical Linguistics: Vol. 2). x, 350p. 110.00 (*1-55619-388-2*) J Benjamins Pubng Co.

Child Language Aphasia & Phonological Universals. Roman Jakobson. 1968. (Janua Linguarum, Ser. Minor: No. 72). (Orig.). pap. text (*90-279-2103-2*) Mouton.

Child Language Development. Sandra Bochner et al. 1997. 150p. 39.95 (*1-56593-885-2*, 1734) Singular Publishing.

Child Language Disability Vol. 2: Semantic & Pragmatic Difficulties. Ed. by Kay Mogford-Bevan & Jane Sadler. 1991. 114p. (*1-85359-128-9*); pap. (*1-85359-127-0*) Multilingual Matters GBR. *Dist:* Taylor & Francis.

Child Language Disability Vol. 3: Hearing Impairment. Ed. by Kay Mogford-Bevan & Jane Sadler. 1992. 120p. pap. (*1-85359-168-8*); text (*1-85359-169-6*) Multilingual Matters GBR. *Dist:* Taylor & Francis.

Child Life in Hospitals: Theory & Practice. Richard H. Thompson & Gene Stanford. 1981. 286p. pap. 41.95 (*0-398-04456-2*) C C Thomas.

Child-Lovers: A Study of Pedophiles in Society. Glenn D. Wilson & David N. Cox. 1983. 132p. (*0-7206-0603-9*) P Owen Ltd GBR. *Dist:* Dufour.

Child Maltreatment: A Clinical Guide & Photographic Reference 2nd rev. ed. James A. Monteleone. Incl. Vol. 1. Child Maltreatment: A Clinical Guide & Reference. 698p. 2000. 110.00 (*1-878060-22-8*, 30958); Vol. 2. Child Maltreatment: A Comprehensive Photographic Reference Identifying Potential Child Abuse. 357p. 1998. 115.00 (*1-878060-23-6*, 30959); LC 97-41395. (Illus.). 1055p. 1998. 195.00 (*1-878060-26-0*) GW Medical.

Child Maltreatment: A Clinical Guide & Reference, Vol. 1. James A. Monteleone. 2nd rev. ed. 2000. LC 97-41395. (Illus.). 698p. 110.00 (*1-878060-22-8*, 30958) GW Medical.

Child Maltreatment: A Comprehensive Photographic Reference Identifying Potential Child Abuse, Vol. 2. James A. Monteleone. 2nd rev. ed. 1998. LC 97-41395. (Illus.). 357p. 115.00 (*1-878060-23-6*, 30959) GW Medical.

Child Maltreatment: Expanded Concepts of Helping. Ed. by M. Rothery & G. Cameron. 1990. 336p. text 69.95 (*0-8058-0455-2*) L Erlbaum Assocs.

Child Maltreatment: Theory & Research on the Causes & Consequences of Child Abuse & Neglect. Ed. by Dante Cicchetti & Vicki K. Carlson. 1989. (Illus.). 816p. (C). pap. text 53.95 (*0-521-37969-5*) Cambridge U Pr.

Child Maltreatment & the Family: Background Briefing Report with Seminar Presentations. M. Anne Powell. 1994. 94p. pap. 10.00 (*0-929722-80-9*) CA State Library Fndtn.

Child Maltreatment in the United States: A Challenge to Social Institutions. Saad Z. Nagi. 1977. LC 77-22121. text 52.50 (*0-231-04394-5*) Col U Pr.

Child Mental Health & Psychosocial Development: Report of a WHO Expert Committee, 1977. 1977. (Technical Report Ser.: No. 613). 71p. pap. text 7.00 (*92-4-120613-6*, 1100613) World Health.

Child Mental Health & the Law. Barry Nurcombe & David F. Partlett. 1994. LC 93-50557. 628p. 39.95 (*0-02-923245-7*) Free Pr.

***Child Mental Health in Primary Care.** Quentin Spender et al. 2001. 392p. pap. (*1-85775-262-7*) Radcliffe Med Pr GBR. *Dist:* Balogh.

Child Mental Health in the 1990s: Curricula for Graduate & Undergraduate Professional Education. 1994. lib. bdg. 250.00 (*0-8490-5751-5*) Gordon Pr.

Child Mental Health Practice from the Ecological Perspective. Richard L. Munger. 1991. 426p. (C). pap. 46.00 (*0-8191-8319-9*); lib. bdg. 75.50 (*0-8191-8318-0*) U Pr of Amer.

Child Mental Status Examination. Jerome D. Goodman & John A. Sours. 1994. LC 93-74193. (Master Work Ser.). 148p. pap. 22.50 (*1-56821-187-2*) Aronson.

Child Multimodal Therapy. Donald B. Keat, II. Ed. by Glenn Caddy. 1990. LC 89-6835. (Developments in Clinical Psychology Ser.: Vol. 12). 184p. (C). 77.00 (*0-89391-420-7*, Ablex) Greenwood.

Child Neurology. John H. Menkes & Harvey B. Sarnat. 6th ed. 2000. LC 99-46285. 1,296p. text 139.00 (*0-7817-2385-X*) Lppncott W & W.

Child Neurology: A Clinical Manual. Bruce O. Berg. 1986. LC 84-80920. (Illus.). 316p. pap. text 19.95 (*0-930010-05-1*) Jones Med.

Child Neurology: A Clinical Manual. Bruce O. Berg. 2nd ed. 1994. (Illus.). 400p. text 64.95 (*0-397-51328-3*) Lppncott W & W.

Child Neuropsychology, Vol. 1. John E. Obrzut & George W. Hynd. 1986. (Perspectives in Neurolinguistics, Neuropsychology & Psycholinguistics Ser.). pap. text 55.00 (*0-12-524043-0*) Acad Pr.

Child Neuropsychology: An Introduction to Theory, Research & Clinical Practice. Byron P. Rourke et al. 1991. LC 83-1657. 389p. reprint ed. pap. 30.00 (*0-89862-468-1*, 2468) Guilford Pubns.

Child Neuropsychology: Assessment & Interventions for Neurodevelopmental Disorders. Phyllis A. Teeter & Margaret Semrud-Clikeman. 1997. LC 96-54722. 330p. (C). 74.00 (*0-205-16331-9*) Allyn.

Child Nurturance Vol. 1: Philosophy, Children, & the Family. Ed. by Albert C. Cafagna et al. 1982. LC 82-3701. 392p. 75.00 (*0-306-41003-6*, Plenum Trade) Perseus Pubng.

Child Nutrition: An International Perspective. Noel W. Solomons. 1999. (Modern Nutrition Ser.). 69.95 (*0-8493-8507-5*) CRC Pr.

Child Nutrition & Health. Bobbie Hutchins. 1979. (Careers in Home Economics Ser.). (Illus.). text 18.12 (*0-07-031527-2*) McGraw.

Child Nutrition in South East Asia: Eighth Nutricia - Cow & Gate Symposium. Ed. by H. K. Viser & J. G. Bindels. 1990. (Nutricia Symposium Ser.). (C). text 191.50 (*0-7923-0690-2*) Kluwer Academic.

Child Observation Skills. Phillip Slee. 1987. 192p. lib. bdg. (*0-7099-5408-5*) C Helm GBR. *Dist:* Routldge.

Child of Your Dreams: Approaching Conception & Pregnancy with Inner Peace & Reverence for Life. Laura A. Huxley & Piero Ferrucci. 1992. (Illus.). 112p. pap. 12.95 (*0-89281-365-2*, Heal Arts VT) Inner Tradit.

Child Offenders: A Study in Diagnosis & Treatment. Harriet L. Goldberg. 1969. LC 69-14928. (Criminology, Law Enforcement, & Social Problems Ser.: No. 75). reprint ed. 22.00 (*0-87585-075-8*) Patterson Smith.

Child Patient & the Therapeutic Process: A Psychoanalytic, Developmental, Object Relations Approach. Diana Siskind. 1992. LC 91-47068. 328p. 45.00 (*0-87668-494-0*) Aronson.

Child Phonology: Vol. II, Perception. Ed. by Grace H. Yeni-Komshian et al. 1980. LC 80-981. (Perspectives in Neurolinguistics & Psycholinguistics Ser.). text 65.00 (*0-12-770602-X*) Acad Pr.

Child Protection Clinical Practice & the Law. Mattie Blackburn & Liz Davies. 2000. 256p. pap. 32.00 (*0-7506-4319-6*) Buttrwrth-Heinemann.

Child Protection Handbook. Wilson. 1995. pap. text 38.95 (*0-7020-1743-4*) Saunders.

***Child Protection Handbook.** Kate Wilson & Adrian James. 2nd ed. 2001. (Illus.). 555p. (*0-7020-2584-4*) W B Saunders GBR. *Dist:* Saunders.

Child Protection in Early Childhood Services. Ed. by Gillian Pugh & Anne Hollows. 1995. 108p. (*1-874579-19-9*) Natl Childrens Bur GBR. *Dist:* Paul & Co Pubs.

***Child Protection in Primary Care.** Ed. by Janet C. Polnay. 2001. 192p. pap. (*1-85775-224-4*) Radcliffe Med Pr GBR. *Dist:* Balogh.

Child Psychiatric Epidemiology: Concepts, Methods & Findings. Frank C. Verhulst & Hans M. Koot. 1991. (Developmental Clinical Psychology & Psychiatry Ser.: Vol. 23). 152p. (C). 74.95 (*0-8039-3996-5*, 7565); pap. 34.95 (*0-8039-3997-3*, 7566) Sage.

Child Psychiatric Units: At the Crossroads. Ed. by Rosemary Chesson & Douglas Chisholm. 1995. LC 95-36660. 278p. pap. text (*1-85302-329-9*) Jessica Kingsley GBR. *Dist:* Taylor & Francis.

Child Psychiatry. R. Goodman & S. Scott. 1997. LC 97-7393. (Illus.). 256p. pap. 57.95 (*0-632-03885-3*) Blackwell Sci.

Child Psychiatry. Leo Kanner. 4th ed. 1979. (Illus.). 768p. 101.95 (*0-398-02199-6*) C C Thomas.

Child Psychiatry: A Primer for Those Who Work with Children. Ed. by R. Dean Coddington & Mollie M. Wallack. abr. ed. 1990. (Illus.). 266p. pap., tchr. ed. 37.50 (*0-87527-361-0*) Green.

***Child Psychiatry & Child Protection Litigation.** Julia Brophy. 2001. 134p. (*1-901242-66-8*) Royal Coll Psych GBR. *Dist:* Balogh.

Child Psychiatry & the Law. Ed. by Dora Black et al. 2nd ed. 1991. 200p. text (*0-88048-608-2*, 8608) Royal Coll Psych GBR. *Dist:* Parkwest Pubns.

Child Psychiatry in the Soviet Union: Preliminary Observations. Nancy Rollins. 1972. LC 72-76560. (Illus.). 315p. 43.00 (*0-674-11475-2*) HUP.

Child Psychology. Contrib. by Gale Group Staff. 2001. LC 2001-37062. (Macmillan Psychology Ser.: Vol. 1). (Illus.). 130.00 net. (*0-02-865618-0*, Macmillan Ref) Gale.

Child Psychology. Ross Vasta et al. 3rd ed. 1998. 1062p. text, stu. ed. 124.90 (*0-471-34557-1*) Wiley.

Child Psychology. E. Mavis Hetherington et al. 5th ed. 1998. LC 98-15013. 784p. text 83.75 (*0-07-028469-5*) McGrw-H Hghr Educ.

Child Psychology: A Contemporary Viewpoint. E. Mavis Hetherington & Ross D. Parke. 4th ed. 1993. LC 92-21106. (C). text 60.25 net. (*0-07-028444-X*) McGraw.

Child Psychology: A Contemporary Viewpoint. Janis Jacobs. 4th ed. 1993. (C). pap., stu. ed. 24.69 (*0-07-028445-8*) McGrw-H Hghr Educ.

Child Psychology in Action: Linking Research & Practice. Ed. by John Harris. 1986. 273p. text 24.95 (*0-914797-19-0*) Brookline Bks.

Child Psychopathology. Ed. by Eric J. Mash & Russell A. Barkley. 1996. LC 96-4857. 650p. 66.00 (*1-57230-065-5*, 0065) Guilford Pubns.

Child Psychopathology: A Social Work Perspective. Ed. by Francis J. Turner. 1989. 576p. 39.95 (*0-02-933101-3*) Free Pr.

Child Psychopathology Developmental Disorders: Diagnostic Criteria & Clinical Assessment Richard E. Mattison & George W. Hynd. 1991. (C). Set. text 120.00 (*0-8058-0330-0*); Vol. 1: Diagnostic Criteria. 504p. text 89.95 (*0-8058-0328-9*); Vol. 2: Developmental Disorders. 336p. pap. 59.95 (*0-8058-0329-7*) L Erlbaum Assocs.

Child Psychopharmacology. Ed. by B. Timothy Walsh. 1998. LC 97-52694. (Review Ser.). 181p. pap. text 27.00 (*0-88048-833-6*, 8833) Am Psychiatric.

Child Psychotherapy: A Report from the Tavistock Clinic. Daws & Loose. 1999. (Psychoanalytic Inquiry Ser.: Vol. 19, No. 2). pap. 20.00 (*0-88163-925-7*) Analytic Pr.

Child Psychotherapy: Developing & Identifying Effective Treatments. Alan E. Kazdin. 1988. (General Psychology Ser.). 176p. 30.00 (*0-08-034961-7*); pap. 15.95 (*0-08-034960-9*) Elsevier (Pergamon Pr).

Child Psychotherapy: From Initial Therapeutic Contact to Termination. Sophie L. Lovinger & Robert L. Lovinger. 1998. LC 97-10296. 232p. 45.00 (*0-7657-0084-0*) Aronson.

Child Psychotherapy: Practice & Theory. Ed. by Mary R. Haworth. 1994. LC 94-71315. (Master Work Ser.). 475p. pap. 45.00 (*1-56821-265-8*) Aronson.

Child Psychotherapy Primer: Suggestions for the Beginning Therapist. Josiah Dodds. 1985. 166p. pap. 20.95 (*0-89885-310-9*, Kluwer Acad Hman Sci) Kluwer Academic.

Child Psychotherapy Progress Notes Planner. Arthur E. Jongsma et al. 2001. LC 00-43466. (Practice Planners Ser.). 432p. pap. 44.95 (*0-471-38102-0*) Wiley.

Child Psychotherapy Treatment Planner. Arthur E. Jongsma, Jr. et al. 2nd ed. 2000. LC 99-47916. (Practice Planners Ser.). 336p. pap. 44.95 (*0-471-34764-7*) Wiley.

Child Rearing: Influence on Prosocial & Moral Development. Ed. by J. M. Janssens & J. R. Gerris. 1992. iv, 196p. (*90-265-1181-7*) Swets.

Child Rearing & Psycho-Social Development. Motilal Lidhoo. 1991. (C). (*81-7024-300-9*) Ashish Pub Hse IND. *Dist:* S Asia.

Child Rorschach Responses: Developmental Trends from Two to Ten Years. Louise B. Ames & Ruth W. Metraux. rev. ed. 1995. LC 94-44161. (Master Work Ser.). (Illus.). 150p. pap. 60.00 (*1-56821-454-5*) Aronson.

Child Sacrificed to the Deaf Culture. Tom Bertling. 1994. 112p. pap. 18.95 (*0-9637813-4-0*) Kodiak Media.

Child Safety Is No Accident: A Parents' Handbook of Emergencies. Jay M. Arena & Miriam Bachar. 1978. LC 77-80346. xi, 296p. text 24.95 (*0-8223-0390-6*) Duke.

Child Sexual Abuse: A Guide for Health Professionals. Celia Doyle. 1994. 304p. 40.99 (*1-56593-136-X*, 0448) Singular Publishing.

Child Sexual Abuse: A Handbook for Health Care & Legal Professionals. Diane H. Schetky & Arthur H. Green. 1988. LC 87-31987. 264p. text 36.95 (*0-87630-495-1*) Brunner-Routledge.

Child Sexual Abuse: An Interdisciplinary Manual for Diagnosis, Case Management, & Treatment. Kathleen C. Faller. 1989. (Illus.). 428p. pap. text 29.00 (*0-231-06471-3*) Col U Pr.

Child Sexual Abuse: Impact & Aftershocks. Project Impact Staff. Ed. by Sue Freese. 1989. 272p. (Orig.). pap. 7.00 (*0-9622478-0-4*) Project Impact.

Child Sexual Abuse: Informing Practice from Research. David Phillip Jones et al. 1999. LC 99-495118. (Illus.). 136p. pap. (*1-85775-362-3*) Radcliffe Med Pr GBR. *Dist:* Balogh.

Child Sexual Abuse: The Initial Effects. Beverly Gomes-Schwartz et al. 1990. (Library of Social Research: Vol. 179). (Illus.). 203p. (C). 86.95 (*0-8039-3610-9*, 7711); pap. 37.95 (*0-8039-3611-7*, 7712) Sage.

Child Sexual Abuse & False Memory Syndrome. Robert A. Baker. 1998. LC 97-40899. 479p. 38.00 (*1-57392-182-3*) Prometheus Bks.

Child Stress & the School Experience. Edward W. Schultz & Charles M. Huechert. 1983. 160p. (C). 40.95 (*0-89885-132-7*); pap. 20.95 (*0-89885-151-3*) Kluwer Academic (Kluwer Acad Hman Sci).

Child Survival. Ed. by Nancy Scheper-Hughes. 1987. (C). lib. bdg. 158.50 (*1-55608-028-X*) Kluwer Academic.

Child Survival, Health & Social Work. Sandhya Joshi. 1996. (*81-7022-576-0*) Concept IND. *Dist:* S Asia.

Child Survivors & Perpetrators of Sexual Abuse: Treatment Innovations. Mic Hunter. 1995. LC 94-42211. 152p. 61.95 (*0-8039-7194-X*, 1061); pap. 31.95 (*0-8039-7195-8*, 1062) Sage.

Child Therapy: Concepts, Strategies & Decision Making. Jerry M. Lewis, 3rd & Mark J. Blotcky. 1997. LC 97-22378. (Basic Principles into Practice Ser.: No. 15). 270p. 37.95 (*0-87630-822-1*) Brunner-Routledge.

Child Therapy Today. Ed. by Laura Slap-Shelton. 1994. (Child Therapy News Ser.: Vol. 1). 279p. text 36.95 (*1-882732-12-X*) Childswork.

Child Therapy Today, Vol. 2. Ed. by Roger Phillips et al. 1996. 277p. 36.95 (*1-882732-50-2*) Childswork.

Child Training & Personality: A Cross-Cultural Study. John W. Whiting & Irvin L. Child. 1984. LC 84-10794. 353p. reprint ed. lib. bdg. 68.00 (*0-313-24387-5*, WHCT, Greenwood Pr) Greenwood.

Child Welfare in the United Kingdom, 1948-1998. Olive Stevenson. 1998. LC 98-25920. (Working Together for Children, Young People, & Their Families Ser.). pap. 52.95 (*0-632-04993-6*) Blackwell Sci.

Child with a Limb Deficiency. Shriners Hospitals for Crippled Children Staff et al. Ed. by John A. Herring & John G. Birch. 1998. LC 98-11882. (Symposium Ser.). (Illus.). 480p. 95.00 (*0-89203-175-1*) Amer Acad Ortho Surg.

Child with a Spinal Cord Injury. Ed. by Randal R. Betz & American Academy of Orthopaedic Surgeons Staff. 1996. 888p. pap. 80.00 (*0-89203-146-8*) Amer Acad Ortho Surg.

Child with Cancer: A Textbook of Complete Family-centred Care. Contrib. by Helen Langton. 2000. LC 99-29466. xvi, 404p. text (*0-7020-2300-0*) W B Saunders.

***Child with Headache: Diagnosis & Treatment.** Ed. by Patricia A. McGrath & Loretta M. Hillier. 2001. LC 00-47140. (Progress in Pain Research & Management Ser.: Vol. 19). (Illus.). xii, 292p. 82.00 (*0-931092-30-2*) Intl Assn Study Pain.

Child with Multiple Birth Defects. M. Michael Cohen, Jr. 2nd ed. 1996. (Oxford Monographs on Medical Genetics: No. 31). (Illus.). 288p. text 72.50 (*0-19-509926-5*) OUP.

Childbearing Family, No. 2. Mary Ann Miller. 1983. 30.50 (*0-316-57338-8*, Little Brwn Med Div) Lppncott W & W.

Childbed Fever: A Documentary History. Irvine Loudon. 1995. LC 94-33390. (Disease, Epidemics & Medicine Ser.: Vol. 2). (Illus.). 288p. text 61.00 (*0-8153-1079-X*, SS868) Garland.

Childbed Fever: A Scientific Biography of Ignaz Semmelweis, 39. K. Codell Carter & Barbara R. Carter. 1994. LC 93-32618. (Contributions in Medical Studies Ser.: No. 39). 144p. 45.00 (*0-313-29146-2*, Greenwood Pr) Greenwood.

Childbirth. Deni Bown. 1997. (101 Essential Tips Ser.). (Illus.). 72p. pap. 4.95 (*0-7894-1079-6*) DK Pub Inc.

Childbirth. Miriam Stoppard. 1998. LC 97-46130. (DK Healthcare Ser.). (Illus.). 96p. pap. 7.95 (*0-7894-3095-9*) DK Pub Inc.

Childbirth: Changing Ideas & Practices in Britain & America, 1600 to the Present. Set. Ed. & Intro. by Philip K. Wilson. 1996. 377.00 (*0-8153-2235-6*) Garland.

Childbirth & Obstetric Techniques. Farook Al-Azzawi. 2nd ed. 1998. (Illus.). 174p. 34.95 (*0-7234-3099-3*) Mosby Inc.

Childbirth & Pain Relief: An Anesthesiologist Explains Your Options. Sanjay Datta. 2001. LC 00-48985. (Illus.). 90p. pap. 16.95 (*0-9626003-9-3*) Next Decade.

Childbirth Education: Practice, Research & Theory. Francine H. Nichols & Sharron S. Humenick. 1988. (Illus.). 544p. text 61.95 (*0-7216-2052-3*) Saunders.

Childbirth in America: Anthropological Perspectives. Karen L. Michaelson et al. 1988. LC 87-37490. 313p. 55.00 (*0-89789-136-8*, Bergin & Garvey) Greenwood.

Childbirth Kit: Ideas & Images to Help You Through Labor. M. Fellenstein Hale & Liz Chalmers. 1995. LC 94-92447. (Illus.). 96p. pap. 22.95 (*0-9643530-0-8*) Swanstone Pr.

Childbirth with Hypnosis. William S. Kroger. 1975. (Illus.). pap. 5.00 (*0-87980-021-6*) Wilshire.

Childbirth Without Fear. Grantly Dick-Read. 1979. mass mkt. 3.95 (*0-06-080490-4*, Perennial) HarperTrade.

Childcare: Development. American Red Cross Staff. 1995. pap. text, wbk. ed. 5.95 (*0-86536-184-3*) Mosby Inc.

Childcare: Health & Safety Units. American Red Cross Staff. 1995. pap. text, wbk. ed. 8.25 (*0-86536-183-5*) Mosby Inc.

Childers' Diet to Stop Arthritis: Nightshades, Aging & Ill Health. Ed. by Norman F. Childers. 5th rev. ed. 1995. (Illus.). 246p. pap. 18.00 (*0-938378-05-8*) N F Childers.

Childes - Bib: An Annotated Bibliography of Child Language & Language Disorders. Roy Higginson & Brian MacWhinney. 1991. 1176p. (C). 200.00 (*0-8058-0859-0*) L Erlbaum Assocs.

Childes/Bib: An Annotated Bibliography of Child Language & Language Disorders, 1994 Supplement. Roy Higginson & Brian MacWhinney. 1994. 700p. text 125.00 (*0-8058-1478-7*) L Erlbaum Assocs.

Childhood. Steinberg. 1994. (C). pap., stu. ed. 23.44 (*0-07-061235-8*) McGrw-H Hghr Educ.

Childhood Abuse: Effects on Clinicians' Personal & Professional Lives. Helene Jackson & Ronald Nuttall. 1997. LC 96-45839. (C). 265p. 86.95 (*0-8039-4780-1*, 4927); 276p. pap. 39.95 (*0-8039-4781-X*, 4928) Sage.

Childhood Aggression & Violence: Sources of Influence, Prevention, & Control. D. H. Crowell et al. 1987. LC 86-30359. (Applied Clinical Psychology Ser.). (Illus.). 318p. (C). 65.00 (*0-306-42355-3*, Plenum Trade) Perseus Pubng.

Childhood & Adolescence: Counseling Theory & Technique. Ed. by William M. Walsh. rev. ed. 1985. LC 84-61506. 424p. (C). 37.25 (*0-8211-2262-2*) McCutchan.

Childhood & Adolescent Diabetes. S. Court & B. Lamb. 1997. LC 97-3042. 384p. 130.00 (*0-471-97003-4*) Wiley.

Childhood & Adolescent Diabetes. Ed. by Christopher J. Kelnar. 1994. (Illus.). 656p. (*0-412-48610-5*) E A GBR. *Dist:* OUP.

Childhood & Adolescent Drug Abuse: A Physicians Guide to Office Practice. Robert C. Petersen. rev. ed. 1991. LC 87-70131. 55p. pap. 3.00 (*0-942348-20-6*) Am Council Drug Ed.

Childhood & Human Nature: The Development of Personality. Sula Wolff. 1989. 256p. pap. 16.95 (*0-415-01129-9*, A3353) Routledge.

Childhood & Medicine Use in a Cross-Cultural Perspective: A European Concerted. Deanna J. Trakas & E. Sanz. 1996. 366p. pap. (*92-827-4978-9*, CGNA-16646-ENC) Comm Europ Commun BEL. *Dist:* Bernan Associates.

Childhood & Society. Erik H. Erikson. 1993. LC 93-11229. 448p. pap. 13.95 (*0-393-31068-X*) Norton.

Childhood Antecedents of Multiple Personality Disorder. Ed. by Richard P. Kluft. 1985. LC 85-5986. 258p. pap. text 22.50 (*0-88048-082-3*, 8082) Am Psychiatric.

Childhood Asthma: A Guide for Parents. Eggleston. 2000. (Illus.). pap. 2.95 (*1-885274-00-9*) Health InfoNet Inc.

Childhood Asthma: Pathophysiology & Treatment. Ed. by David G. Tinkelman & Charles K. Naspitz. 2nd exp. rev. ed. 1992. LC 92-29092. (Allergic Disease & Therapy Ser.: Vol. 6). (Illus.). 640p. text 195.00 (*0-8247-8751-X*) Dekker.

Childhood Asthma & Other Wheezing Disorders. Ed. by Micheal Silverman. 1995. (Illus.). 534p. (*0-412-56900-0*) E A GBR. *Dist:* OUP.

Childhood Bereavement & Its Aftermath. Ed. by Sol Altschul. 1988. (Chicago Institute for Psychoanalysis Emotions & Behavior Monograph Ser.: No. 8). 67.50 (*0-8236-0772-0*) Intl Univs Pr.

***Childhood Brain & Spinal Cord Tumors: A Guide for Families, Friends & Caregivers.** Tania Shiminski-Maher et al. 2001. LC 2001-52057. (Patient-Centered Guides Ser.). (*0-596-50009-2*) OReilly & Assocs.

Childhood Cancer: A Nursing Overview. Susan K. Maul & Jeanette N. Adams. 1987. (Illus.). (C). text 65.95 (*0-86720-381-1*, 381-1) Jones & Bartlett.

Childhood Cancer: A Parent's Guide to Solid Tumor Cancers. Honna Janes-Hodder & Nancy Keene. Ed. by Linda Lamb. 1999. LC 99-33120. (Patient-Centered Guides Ser.). (Illus.). 540p. pap. 24.95 (*1-56592-531-9*) OReilly & Assocs.

Childhood Cancer: The Challenge to Hawaii's Healthcare System. Jean P. Creadick & Nell Cammack. 1994. 55p. (Orig.). (C). pap. text 25.00 (*0-7881-0663-5*) DIANE Pub.

Childhood Cancer: Triumph Over Tragedy. Ed. by J. M. Vaeth. 1982. (Frontiers of Radiation Therapy & Oncology Ser.: Vol. 16). (Illus.). viii, 192p. 126.25 (*3-8055-3020-X*) S Karger.

Childhood Cancer: Understanding & Coping. H. Ekert. 1989. xviii, 186p. pap. text 38.00 (*2-88124-356-8*) Gordon & Breach.

Childhood Cancer & Nuclear Installations. Ed. by Valerie Beral et al. 1993. 496p. pap. text (*0-7279-0815-4*) BMJ Pub GBR. *Dist:* AIDC.

Childhood Cancer Management. C. R. Pinkerton et al. 1993. (Illus.). 288p. pap. 75.95 (*0-412-41080-X*) Chapman & Hall.

Childhood Cancer Survivors: A Practical Guide to Your Future. Nancy Keene et al. Ed. by Linda Lamb. 2000. LC 99-98177. (Patient-Centered Guides Ser.). (Illus.). xxviii, 482p. pap. 27.95 (*1-56592-460-6*, Patient-Centered) OReilly & Assocs.

Childhood Deafness: Causation, Assessment & Management. Ed. by Fred H. Bess. 1977. 368p. text 68.00 (*0-8089-1043-4*, 790575, Grune & Strat) Harcrt Hlth Sci Grp.

Childhood Depression. Ed. by Theodore A. Petti. 1983. LC 83-58. (Journal of Children in Contemporary Society: Vol. 15, No. 2). 95p. text 39.95 (*0-917724-95-X*) Haworth Pr.

Childhood Depression: School-Based Intervention. Kevin D. Stark. 1990. LC 90-3085. (Guilford School Practitioner Ser.). 234p. pap. 25.00 (*0-89862-236-0*, 2236) Guilford Pubns.

Childhood Depression Sourcebook. Jeffrey A. Miller. 1998. LC 98-45345. 288p. pap. 16.00 (*0-7373-0001-9*, 00019W) NTC Contemp Pub Co.

Childhood Diabetes: The Facts. Oman Craig. 1982. (Facts Ser.). (Illus.). 178p. 17.50 (*0-19-261330-8*) OUP.

Childhood Dialogues & the Lifting of Repression: Character Structure & Psychoanalytic Technique. Paul G. Myerson. 1991. 192p. (C). 32.00 (*0-300-04928-5*) Yale U Pr.

Childhood Disability & Family Systems. Ed. by Michael Ferrari & Marvin B. Sussman. 1987. LC 87-11839. (Marriage & the Family Ser.: Vol. 11, Nos. 1-2). 246p. text 49.95 (*0-86656-671-6*) Haworth Pr.

Childhood Disorder: A Psychosomatic Approach. Philip Pinkerton. 1975. LC 74-18488. (Illus.). 192p. text 46.00 (*0-231-03955-7*) Col U Pr.

Childhood Ear Infections see Healing Childhood Ear Infections: Prevention, Home Care, & Alternative Treatment

Childhood Encopresis & Enuresis: Causes & Therapy. Charles E. Schaefer. 1993. LC 93-3999. 192p. pap. 40.00 (*1-56821-073-6*) Aronson.

Childhood Environment & Adult Disease. CIBA Foundation Staff. 1991. LC 90-13144. (CIBA Foundation Symposia Ser.: No. 156). 252p. 128.00 (*0-471-92957-3*) Wiley.

Childhood Epilepsies & Brain Development. Ed. by Astrid Nehlig. 1999. 320p. (*0-86196-578-7*) J Libbey Med GBR. *Dist:* Buttrwrth-Heinemann.

Childhood Epilepsy: A Pediatric-Psychiatric Approach. R. Bouchard et al. 1977. LC 76-46814. 136p. 27.50 (*0-8236-0774-7*) Intl Univs Pr.

Childhood Feeding Disorders: Biobehavioral Assessment & Intervention. Jurgen H. Kedesdy & Karen S. Budd. 1998. LC 97-52164. 416p. 34.95 (*1-55766-316-5*) P H Brookes.

Childhood Hand That Disturbs Projective Test: A Diagnostic & Therapeutic Drawing Test. Roseline d. Davido. 1994. LC 93-23677. 200p. 62.50 (*0-275-94417-4*, Praeger Pubs) Greenwood.

Childhood Illness: Knowing When to Call the Doctor. Paul L. McCarthy. 1997. (Pediatrics Ser.). 32p. pap. text 2.95 (*1-885274-29-7*) Health InfoNet Inc.

***Childhood Illness: Meaning.** Evelyn K. Oremland. 2001. 96p. pap. 24.95 (*1-887841-50-4*, Psychosocial) Intl Univs Pr.

Childhood Illnesses. Miriam Stoppard. 1998. LC 97-46129. pap. text 7.95 (*0-7894-3094-0*) DK Pub Inc.

Childhood Immunization: Opportunities to Improve Immunization Rates at Lower Cost. 1993. (Illus.). 59p. (Orig.). (C). pap. text 25.00 (*0-7881-0087-4*) DIANE Pub.

Childhood in Contemporary Cultures. Ed. by Margaret Mead & Martha Wolfenstein. 1994. LC 55-10248. pap. text 6.50 (*0-226-51507-9*, P124) U Ch Pr.

Childhood Language Disorders in Context: Infancy through Adolescence. Nickola W. Nelson. 2nd ed. 1998. LC 97-32508. 594p. 71.00 (*0-205-19787-6*) Allyn.

Childhood Learning Disabilities & Prenatal Risk. Ed. by Catherine C. Brown. 1983. (Pediatric Round Table Ser.: No. 9). 109p. 10.00 (*0-931562-11-2*) J & J Consumer Prods.

Childhood Leukemia: A Guide for Families, Friends & Caregivers. Nancy Keene. Ed. by Linda Lamb. 2nd ed. 1999. LC 99-39059. (Patient-Centered Guides Ser.). (Illus.). 516p. pap. 24.95 (*1-56592-632-3*, Patient-Centered) OReilly & Assocs.

Childhood Leukemia: Present Problems & Future Prospects. Ed. by Noboru Kobayashi et al. 1991. (Developments in Oncology Ser.). (C). text 114.50 (*0-7923-1138-8*) Kluwer Academic.

Childhood Leukemias. Ed. by Ching-Hon Pui. 1999. LC 98-46407. (Illus.). 580p. (C). text 190.00 (*0-521-58176-1*) Cambridge U Pr.

Childhood Lymphoblastic Leukemia. Ed. by Carl Pochedly. 1985. LC 85-9331. 237p. 70.00 (*0-275-90048-7*, C0048, Praeger Pubs) Greenwood.

Childhood Nutrition. Ed. by Fima Lifshitz. 1994. LC 94-14377. (Modern Nutrition Ser.). 288p. 104.95 (*0-8493-2764-4*, 2764) CRC Pr.

***Childhood Nutrition & Disease Prevention.** Lucas & Stanley H. Zlotkin. 2002. (Fast Facts Ser.). (Illus.). 60p. pap. (*1-899541-93-4*) Health Pr GBR. *Dist:* JAMCO Dist.

Childhood Obsessive Compulsive Disorder. Greta Francis & Rod A. Gragg. 1996. LC 96-10084. (Developmental Clinical Psychology & Psychiatry Ser.: Vol. 35). 118p. 74.95 (*0-8039-5921-4*, 2923); (Illus.). pap. 34.95 (*0-8039-5922-2*, 29222) Sage.

Childhood Phases of Maturity: Sexual Developmental Psychology. Ernest Borneman. Tr. by Michael A. Lombardi-Nash from GER. 1994. LC 94-18036. 325p. (C). 65.00 (*0-87975-895-3*) Prometheus Bks.

Childhood Psychopathology & Adult Psychoses. Thomas Freeman. 1976. LC 75-31854. 45.00 (*0-8236-0775-5*) Intl Univs Pr.

Childhood Psychopharmacology: Current Concepts. Ed. by Julien Mendlewicz & H. M. Van Praag. 1978. (Advances in Biological Psychiatry Ser.: Vol. 2). (Illus.). pap. 34.00 (*3-8055-2901-5*) S Karger.

Childhood Psychotherapy: A Bioenergetic Approach. Ed. by C. D. Ventling. 2001. LC 00-48124. x, 88p. 49.75 (*3-8055-7149-6*) S Karger.

Childhood Rhinitis & Sinusitis: Pathophysiology & Treatment. Charles K. Nespitz. Ed. by David G. Tinkelman. 1990. (Allergic Disease & Therapy Ser.: Vol. 3). (Illus.). 304p. text 145.00 (*0-8247-8228-3*) Dekker.

Childhood Schizophrenia. Sheila Cantor. 1988. LC 88-5180. 193p. 34.00 (*0-89862-713-3*) Guilford Pubns.

Childhood Seizures. Ed. by S. Shinnar et al. 1994. (Pediatric & Adolescent Medicine Ser.: Vol. 6). (Illus.). viii, 200p. 203.50 (*3-8055-6009-5*) S Karger.

Childhood Sexual Learning: The Unwritten Curriculum. Ed. by Elizabeth Roberts. 1980. 304p. text 29.95 (*0-88410-374-9*, HarpBusn) HarpInfo.

Childhood Sexuality: Normal Sexual Behavior & Development. Ed. by Theo G. Sandfort & Jany Rademakers. 2000. LC 00-61353. (Journal of Psychology & Human Sexuality Monograph: Vol. 12, Nos. 1-2). 157p. 49.95 (*0-7890-1198-0*) Haworth Pr.

Childhood Socialization. Ed. by Gerald Handel. 1988. 423p. (C). pap. text 31.95 (*0-202-30336-5*); lib. bdg. 59.95 (*0-202-30335-7*) Aldine de Gruyter.

Childhood Stress. Ed. by L. Eugene Arnold. 1990. LC 90-30510. (Child & Adolescent Mental Health Ser.). 624p. 235.00 (*0-471-50868-3*) Wiley.

Childhood Trauma & HIV: Women at Risk. Laura E. Whitmire. 1999. LC 98-35611. 200p. text 59.95 (*0-87630-947-3*) Brunner-Routledge.

Childhood Traumatic Brain Injury: Diagnosis, Assessment, & Intervention. Ed. by Erin D. Bigler et al. 1997. LC 97-7468. 312p. pap. text 34.00 (*0-89079-718-8*, 8379) PRO-ED.

Childhood Tuberculosis: Modern Imaging & Clinical Concepts. Bryan J. Cremin. Ed. by Douglas H. Jamieson. 1995. LC 95-7046. (Illus.). 122p. 115.00 (*3-540-19925-X*) Spr-Verlag.

Childhood, Welfare & Justice in Britain. Michael King. 1981. 160p. (C). pap. 16.95 (*0-7134-3713-8*) Trafalgar.

Childhood's Deadly Scourge: The Campaign to Control Diphtheria in New York City, 1880-1930. Evelynn M. Hammonds. 1999. LC 98-38209. 312p. 42.95 (*0-8018-5978-6*) Johns Hopkins.

Childhood's Thief: One Woman's Journey of Healing from Sexual Abuse. Rose M. Evans. 1994. LC 93-44913. 336p. 22.00 (*0-02-536610-6*, Lisa Drew) Scribner.

Children. John W. Santrock. 4th ed. 1994. 496p. (C). text, stu. ed. 22.50 (*0-697-15043-7*) Brown & Benchmark.

Children. John W. Santrock. 5th ed. 1996. LC 95-83693. 648p. (C). pap. 67.81 (*0-697-23592-0*) McGrw-H Hghr Educ.

Children. John W. Santrock et al. 5th ed. 1996. (C). pap., stu. ed. 21.25 (*0-697-23594-7*) McGrw-H Hghr Educ.

Children: Their Growth & Development. Sheila G. Terry et al. 1979. (Careers in Home Economics Ser.). (Illus.). text 19.96 (*0-07-063731-8*) McGraw.

Children above One Hundred Eighty IQ Stanford-Binet: Origins & Development. Leta S. Hollingworth. 1997. LC 74-21417. (Classics in Child Development Ser.). (Illus.). 356p. reprint ed. 35.95 (*0-405-06467-5*) Ayer.

Children Act 1989 & Medical Practice. Barbara Mitchels. Ed. by Alister Prince. 1992. 120p. (C). (*0-85308-142-5*) Jordan Pubng GBR. *Dist:* U Toronto Pr.

Children Adapt: A Theory of Sensorimotor-Sensory Development. Elnora M. Gilfoyle et al. 2nd ed. 1990. LC 86-43125. 312p. pap. 36.00 (*1-55642-187-7*) SLACK Inc.

Children, Adolescents, & AIDS. Ed. by Jeffrey M. Seibert & Roberta A. Olson. 1989. LC 89-4866. (Children & the Law Ser.). 243p. text 27.50 (*0-8032-4186-0*) U of Nebr Pr.

Children & Adolescents. Scott W. Henggeler et al. 1998. LC 98-10618. (Treatment Manuals for Practitioners Ser.). 287p. text 35.00 (*1-57230-106-6*, C0106) Guilford Pubns.

Children & Adolescents. David Elkind. 3rd ed. 1981. 265p. (C). text 34.95 (*0-19-502820-1*) OUP.

Children & Adolescents with Mental Health Problems. Wendy Sharman. 1997. (Illus.). 285p. pap. (*0-7020-1920-8*) Bailliere Tindall.

Children & Counselling. (*0-340-55435-5*) E A GBR. *Dist:* Routldge.

Children & Death. Ed. by Costa Papadatos & Danai Papadatou. 1991. (Death Education, Aging & Health Care Ser.). 280p. 72.95 (*1-56032-043-5*) Hemisp Pub.

Children & Disasters. N. Gordon et al. 1999. LC 98-50828. (Series in Trauma & Loss, Ser.). 192p. text 29.95 (*0-87630-932-5*) Brunner-Routledge.

Children & Disasters. C. F. Saylor. 1993. (Issues in Clinical Child Psychology Ser.). (Illus.). 260p. (C). 47.00 (*0-306-44431-3*, Plenum Trade) Perseus Pubng.

Children & Emotion: The Development of Psychological Understanding. Paul Harris. 1989. (Dunn: Understanding Childrens' Worlds Ser.). 224p. pap. text 28.95 (*0-631-16753-6*) Blackwell Pubs.

Children & Families: Studies in Prevention & Intervention. Ed. by Euthymia D. Hibbs. 1988. 570p. (C). 80.00 (*0-8236-0790-9*) Intl Univs Pr.

Children & Families in Health & Illness. Marion Broome et al. 1998. LC 97-45403. 97.95 (*0-8039-5902-8*, 2951); pap. 53.95 (*0-8039-5903-6*, 2950) Sage.

Children & Family Breakdown. 1986. (EURO Reports & Studies: No. 101). 56p. pap. text 7.00 (*92-890-1267-6*, 1330101) World Health.

Children & Health Care: Moral & Social Issues. Ed. by Loretta M. Kopelman & John C. Moskop. 1989. 364p. (C). lib. bdg. (*1-55608-078-6*) Kluwer Academic NLD. *Dist:* Kluwer Academic.

Children & HIV/AIDS. Ed. by Gary Anderson et al. 1999. LC 98-29901. 271p. pap. 22.95 (*0-7658-0488-3*) Transaction Pubs.

Children & Mental Health: Group Rejection & Self-Rejection. Ed. by James R. Greenley & Morris Rosenberg. 1979. (Research in Community & Mental Health Ser.: Vol. 1). 386p. 73.25 (*0-89232-063-X*) Jai Pr.

Children & Nonviolence. Bob Aldridge et al. 1987. LC 87-4126. 136p. (Orig.). lib. bdg. 16.95 (*0-932727-18-2*) Hope Pub Hse.

Children & Other Strangers. Ruth S. Ginzberg. 1991. LC 91-17362. ix, 108p. (C). text 29.95 (*0-88738-445-5*) Transaction Pubs.

Children & Parents in Hospitals. Ed. by J. Lind et al. 1980. (Journal: Vol. 9, No. 3-4). (Illus.). 120p. pap. 17.25 (*3-8055-1476-X*) S Karger.

Children & Sexuality: Perspectives in Health Care. Tony Harrison. 1998. (Illus.). 190p. pap. (*0-7020-2208-X*) Bailliere Tindall.

Children & Solitude. Elise Boulding. 1962. LC 62-22235. (C). pap. 4.00 (*0-87574-125-8*) Pendle Hill.

Children & Stress: Theoretical Perspectives & Recent Research. James H. Humphrey. 1987. LC 87-45804. (Stress in Modern Society Ser.: No. 18). 32.50 (*0-404-63269-6*) AMS Pr.

***Children & Stress: Understanding & Helping.** Ed. by Beverly Hardcastle Stanford & Kaoru Yamamoto. 2001. LC 2001-41234. pap. (*0-87173-153-3*) ACEI.

Children & the HIV/AIDS Crisis: Youth Who Are Infected & Affected. Carrie McVicker. Ed. by Laura A. Barnitz. 1999. 38p. pap. 6.00 (*0-9663709-6-1*) Youth Advocate.

Children & the Threat of Nuclear War: An Annotated Bibliography. Nancy A. Guenther. 1985. (CompuBibs Ser.: No. 7). 42p. pap. 11.50 (*0-914791-06-0*) Vantage Info.

Children & Their Development: Knowledge Base, Research Agenda, & Social Policy Application, Vol. 44. Ed. by Frances D. Horowitz & Marion O'Brien. 1989. (Special Issue American Psychologist Ser.: Vol. 44, No. 2). 395p. pap. 20.00 (*1-55798-054-3*) Am Psychol.

Children & Their Families: The Continuum of Care. Vicky R. Bowden et al. Ed. by Kevin Law. 1998. LC 97-11069. (Illus.). 1824p. text 69.95 (*0-7216-5179-8*) Saunders.

***Children & Their Families: The Continuum of Care, ExaMaster.** Vicky R. Bowden et al. 1998. (*0-7216-5184-4*) Saunders.

***Children & Their Families: The Continuum of Care, Test Manual.** Vicky R. Bowden et al. 1998. (*0-7216-8051-8*) Saunders.

Children & Trauma: A Guide for Parents & Professionals. Cynthia Monahon. 1997. LC 97-15328. 240p. pap. 19.95 (*0-7879-1071-6*) Jossey-Bass.

Children & Traumatic Stress: Understanding & Training PTSD in Children & Adolescents. William Yule. 2001. 200p. pap. 30.00 (*0-471-97667-9*) Wiley.

Children & Young Adults with Sex Chromosome Aneuploidy: Follow-up, Clinical, & Molecular Studies. J. Evans et al. 1991. LC 90-12715. (Birth Defects Original Article Ser.). 328p. 415.00 (*0-471-56846-5*) Wiley.

Children As Research Subjects: Science, Ethics & Law. Ed. by Michael A. Grodin & Leonard E. Glantz. 1994. LC 93-3589. 272p. (C). text 43.95 (*0-19-507103-4*) OUP.

Children at Birth. Marjie Hathaway & Jay Hathaway. 1978. (Illus.). pap. 12.95 (*0-931560-00-4*) Academy Pubns.

Children at Play: Clinical & Developmental Approaches to Meaning & Representation. Ed. by Arietta Slade & Dennie P. Wolf. 1994. LC 93-606. (Illus.). 328p. (C). text 55.00 (*0-19-504414-2*) OUP.

Children at Risk: An Evaluation of Factors Contributing to Child Abuse & Neglect. R. T. Ammerman & M. Hersen. 1990. LC 90-7228. (Illus.). 332p. (C). 57.50 (*0-306-43437-7*, Kluwer Plenum) Kluwer Academic.

Children at Risk: Assessment, Longitudinal Research, & Intervention. Ed. by Michael Brambring et al. 1989. (Prevention & Intervention in Childhood & Adolescence Ser.: Vol. 7). xiv, 490p. (C). lib. bdg. 69.95 (*3-11-012134-4*) De Gruyter.

Children at Risk: In the Web of Parental Mental Illness. Ronald Feldman et al. 1987. 285p. text 40.00 (*0-8135-1192-5*) Rutgers U Pr.

Children Changed by Trauma: A Healing Guide. Debra Whiting Alexander. 1999. LC 99-74369. xvii, 204p. pap. 13.95 (*1-57224-166-7*) New Harbinger.

Children Communicating: The First Five Years (& a Little Bit Beyond...) Beth Haslett & Wendy Samter. 1997. LC 96-37758. (LEA's Communication Ser.). 320p. 69.95 (*0-8058-0066-2*); pap. (*0-8058-2668-8*) L Erlbaum Assocs.

Children Exposed to Domestic Violence: Current Issues in Research, Intervention, Prevention & Policy Development. Ed. by Robert Geffner et al. 1999. 373p. (C). LC 00-35034. 69.95 (*0-7890-0785-1*); pap. 34.95 (*0-7890-0820-3*) Haworth Pr (Maltreatment & Trauma Pr).

Children, Families, & Chronic Disease: Psychological Models & Methods of Care. Roger Bradford. 1996. LC 95-50973. 232p. (C). pap. 27.95 (*0-415-13147-2*); (Illus.). 84.95 (*0-415-13146-4*) Routledge.

Children, Families & Health Care Decision-Making. Lainie Friedman Ross. 1999. LC 98-27581. (Issues in Biomedical Ethics Ser.). 210p. text 45.00 (*0-19-823763-4*) OUP.

Children in Care: The Medical Contribution. Ed. by M. Oxtoby. 1989. (C). (*0-903534-81-9*) Brit Ag for Adopt & Fost GBR. *Dist:* St Mut.

Children in Difficulty: A Guide to Understanding & Helping. Julian Elliott & Maurice Place. 1998. LC 97-42582. (C). 240p. 80.00 (*0-415-14458-2*); 232p. pap. 26.95 (*0-415-14459-0*) Routledge.

Children in Exile: Therapeutic Work in the Community & the Clinic with Child Survivors of Political Violence & War. Sheila Melzak. 1999. LC 99-41645. 300p. (*1-85302-585-2*) Jessica Kingsley.

Children in Families at Risk: Maintaining the Connections. Lee Combrinck-Graham. 1995. LC 95-8793. 429p. 50.00 (*0-89862-852-0*, 2852) Guilford Pubns.

Children in Family Contexts: Perspectives on Treatment. Ed. by Lee Combrinck-Graham. 1988. LC 88-5108. 537p. 55.00 (*0-89862-732-X*, 2732) Guilford Pubns.

Children in Foster Care & Adoption: A Guide to Bibliotherapy. John T. Pardeck & Jean A. Pardeck. 1998. LC 98-15323. 120p. lib. bdg. 55.00 (*0-313-30775-X*, Greenwood Pr) Greenwood.

*__Children in Intensive Care: A Nurse's Survival Guide.__ Joanna Davies & Lynda Hassell. 2000. (Illus.). 155p. pap. (*0-443-06178-5*) Church GBR. *Dist:* Saunders.

Children in Pain: Clinical & Research Issues from a Developmental Perspective. Ed. by J. P. Bush & S. W. Harkins. 1991. (Illus.). 476p. 115.00 (*0-387-97501-2*) Spr-Verlag.

Children in Pain: Helping Chronically Addicted Adolescents. C. C. Nuckols. 1992. 224p. pap. 12.95 (*0-8306-3768-0*, 4096) McGraw-Hill Educ Grp.

Children in Recovery. Rosalie C. Jesse. 1989. 276p. (C). 24.95 (*0-393-70074-7*) Norton.

Children in the Crossfire: The Tragedy of Parental Kidnapping. Sally Abrahms. 1983. LC 82-73030. 320p. 14.95 (*0-689-11339-0*) Atheneum Yung Read.

Children in the Hospital. Thesi Bergmann & Anna Freud. LC 65-28803. 162p. 1974. pap. 24.95 (*0-8236-8017-7*, 020800); 1966. 27.50 (*0-8236-0800-X*) Intl Univs Pr.

Children in the Hospital: A Guide for Family & Care Givers. Richard Lansdown. 1996. (Illus.). 276p. pap. 29.95 (*0-19-262357-5*) OUP.

Children in Treatment: A Primer for Beginning Therapists. M. S. Cooper & Leon R. Wanerman. 1988. LC 77-7637. 191p. pap. text 19.95 (*0-87630-333-5*) Brunner-Routledge.

Children, Medicines, & Culture. Ed. by Alan Prout et al. 1997. LC 95-17497. 420p. (C). pap. 19.95 (*0-7890-0210-8*, Pharmctl Prods) Haworth Pr.

Children, Medicines, & Culture. Emilio J. Sanz. 1996. LC 95-17497. (Illus.). 420p. (C). 49.95 (*1-56024-937-4*, Pharmctl Prods) Haworth Pr.

Children Mourning, Mourning Children. Ed. by Kenneth J. Doka. 1995. LC 95-12114. 180p. pap. 19.95 (*1-56032-447-3*) Taylor & Francis.

Children Need Groups: A Practical Manual for Group Work with Young Children. R. Silveira et al. 1989. 170p. text 29.00 (*0-08-036413-6*); pap. text 17.00 (*0-08-036414-4*) Elsevier (Pergamon Pr).

Children of a Toxic Harvest: An Environmental Autobiography. Eve Hillary. 1997. 192p. pap. (*0-85091-850-2*) Lothian Pub AUS. *Dist:* Seven Hills Bk.

Children of Alcoholics: A Critical Appraisal of Theory & Research. Kenneth J. Sher. 1991. LC 91-2414. (John D. & Catherine T. MacArthur Foundation Series on Mental Health & Development). (Illus.). 236p. 28.95 (*0-226-75271-2*) U Ch Pr.

Children of Alcoholics: Critical Perspectives. Ed. by Michael Windle & John S. Searles. LC 89-23468. (Substance Abuse Ser.). 244p. 1990. 42.00 (*0-89862-168-2*); 1992. reprint ed. pap. 20.95 (*0-89862-035-X*) Guilford Pubns.

Children of Alcoholics-Addicts. Richard L. Towers. 1989. 80p. pap. 9.95 (*0-8106-0242-3*) NEA.

Children of Battered Women. Peter G. Jaffe & David A. Wolfe. Ed. by Susan K. Wilson. 1990. (Developmental Clinical Psychology & Psychiatry Ser.: Vol. 21). 136p. (C). pap. 34.95 (*0-8039-3384-3*) Sage.

Children of Choice: Freedom & the New Reproductive Technologies. John A. Robertson. 1994. LC 93-35880. 296p. 52.50 (*0-691-03353-6*) Princeton U Pr.

Children of Depressed Mothers: From Early Childhood to Maturity. Marian Radke-Yarrow et al. Ed. by Donna Ronsaville. 1998. LC 98-17213. (Illus.). 240p. (C). text 42.95 (*0-521-55131-5*) Cambridge U Pr.

Children of Depressed Parents: Risk Identification & Intervention. Ed. by Helen L. Morrison. 1983. 296p. text 40.00 (*0-8089-1545-2*, 792982, Grune & Strat) Harcrt Hlth Sci Grp.

Children of Different Worlds: The Formation of Social Behavior. Beatrice B. Whiting & Carolyn P. Edwards. 1992. (Illus.). 352p. pap. 20.45 (*0-674-11617-8*) HUP.

Children of Divorce: Developmental & Clinical Issues. Intro. by Craig A. Everett. 1989. LC 88-35622. (Journal of Divorce: Vol. 12, Nos. 2-3). (Illus.). 348p. text 69.95 (*0-86656-886-7*) Haworth Pr.

Children of Exceptional Parents. Ed. by Mary Frank. 1983. LC 82-25481. (Journal of Children in Contemporary Society: Vol. 15, No. 1). 99p. text 39.95 (*0-917724-96-8*) Haworth Pr.

Children of Heroin Addicts: An Assessment of Health, Learning, Behavioral, & Adjustment Problems. Barbara J. Sowder & Marvin R. Burt. 1980. LC 80-24408. 151p. 55.00 (*0-275-90555-1*, C0555, Praeger Pubs) Greenwood.

Children of Maria: Adolescent Substance Abusers, Their Families & Schooling. Christina Andersson. 1993. (Studies in Education: No. 46). 136p. (Orig.). pap. (*91-554-3086-4*) Uppsala Universitet SWE. *Dist:* Coronet Bks.

Children of Oedipus: Brother & Sister Incest in Psychiatry, Literature, History & Mythology. Luciano P. Santiago. 1973. LC 73-79773. 12.95 (*0-87212-028-7*) Libra.

Children of Parting Parents. Lora Heims Tessman. 1978. LC 77-94094. 624p. 40.00 (*0-87668-307-3*); 2nd ed. (*1-56821-055-8*) Aronson.

Children of Poverty: Research, Health, & Policy Issues. Ed. by Barry S. Zuckerman et al. 1995. LC 94-11694. (Reference Books on Family Issues: Vol. 23). (Illus.). 392p. text 65.00 (*0-8153-1738-7*, SS968) Garland.

Children of Prenatal Substance Abuse. Shirley N. Sparks. 1992. LC 92-28621. (School-Age Children Ser.). (Illus.). 204p. (C). pap. text 42.00 (*1-56593-071-1*, 0375) Thomson Learn.

Children of Silence: Or, the Story of the Deaf. Joseph A. Seiss. 1972. 69.95 (*0-87968-849-1*) Gordon Pr.

Children of the Atomic Bomb: An American Physician's Memoir of Nagasaki, Hiroshima, & the Marshall Islands. James N. Yamazaki & Louis B. Fleming. 1995. LC 95-6683. (Asia-Pacific, Culture, Politics, & Society Ser.). (Illus.). 182p. 18.95 (*0-8223-1658-7*) Duke.

Children of the Kibbutz: A Study in Child Training & Personality. Melford E. Spiro & Audrey G. Spiro. 1975. LC 74-21689. 534p. pap. 19.50 (*0-674-11606-2*) HUP.

Children of Trauma: Stressful Life Events & Their Effects on Children & Adolescents, No. 8. Ed. by Thomas W. Miller. 1997. LC 97-15597. (International Universities Press Stress & Health Ser.: Monograph 8). 267p. 42.50 (*0-8236-0810-7*) Intl Univs Pr.

Children, Parents, Lollipops: Tales of Pediatrics. Vladimir A. Tsesis. 1995. LC 95-5801. 296p. 24.95 (*0-89876-214-6*) Gardner Pr.

Children, Parents, Lollipops: Tales of Pediatrics. Vladimir A. Tsesis. 1996. 297p. 24.95 (*0-9657336-0-2*) Golden Meridian.

Children Solving Problems. Stephanie Thornton. 1995. LC 95-1114. (Developing Child Ser.). (Illus.). 160p. (C). 25.95 (*0-674-11623-2*) HUP.

Children Speak for Themselves: Using the Kempe Interactional Assessment to Evaluate Allegations of Parent-Child Sexual Abuse. Clare Haynes-Seman & David Baumgarten. 1994. LC 94-10231. 224p. text 27.95 (*0-87630-745-4*) Brunner-Routledge.

Children Surviving Persecution: An International Study of Trauma & Healing. Ed. by Judith Kestenberg & Charlotte Kahn. 1998. LC 98-11124. 264p. 72.50 (*0-275-96261-X*, Praeger Pubs) Greenwood.

Children Talk about the Mind. Karen Bartsch & Henry M. Wellman. 1997. (Illus.). 248p. reprint ed. pap. text 24.95 (*0-19-511566-X*) OUP.

Children, Teenagers & Health: The Key Data. Caroline Woodroffe et al. 1993. LC 93-16795. xiii, 193p. (C). pap. (*0-335-19125-8*) OpUniv Pr.

Children, What Are They? Understanding Child Development. E. C. Frijling-Schreuder. Tr. by Katherine Stechmann from DUT. 1975. LC 74-19889. 154p. pap. 24.95 (*0-8236-8020-7*, 20830) Intl Univs Pr.

Children Who Abuse Chemicals. 1993. 87p. (Orig.). (C). pap. text 25.00 (*0-7881-0156-0*) DIANE Pub.

Children Who Don't Want to Live: Understanding & Treating the Suicidal Child. Israel Orbach. 1988. LC 87-46338. (Social & Behavioral Science Ser.). 267p. 43.00 (*1-55542-076-1*) Jossey-Bass.

Children Who Murder: A Psychological Perspective. Robert V. Heckel & David M. Shumaker. 2001. LC 00-42776. (Illus.). 200p. 64.95 (*0-275-96618-6*, Praeger Pubs) Greenwood.

Children with Asthma: A Manual for Parents. Thomas F. Plaut. 2nd rev. ed. 1998. LC 98-19135. (Illus.). xxi, 276p. pap. 10.00 (*0-914625-21-7*) Pedipress.

Children with Autism: A Developmental Perspective. Marian Sigman. 1997. LC 96-53484. (Developing Child Ser.). 288p. pap. text 15.95 (*0-674-05313-3*) HUP.

Children with Autism: A Developmental Perspective. Marian Sigman & Lisa Capps. 1997. LC 96-53484. (Developing Child Ser.). 288p. 32.50 (*0-674-05314-1*); pap. 14.00 (*0-674-05315-X*) HUP.

Children with Autism: Diagnosis & Interventions to Meet Their Needs. Colwyn Trevarthen et al. 2nd ed. 1997. LC 98-178203. 280p. pap. (*1-85302-555-0*) Jessica Kingsley GBR. *Dist:* Taylor & Francis.

Children with Cancer. B. F. Last & VanVeldhuizn. 1991. viii, 280p. (*90-265-1038-1*) Swets.

Children with Conduct Disorders: A Psychotherapy Manual. Paulina F. Kernberg & Saralea Chazen. 1991. LC 90-55665. 320p. pap. 47.50 (*0-465-01055-5*) Basic.

Children with Disabilities. Mark L. Batshaw. 4th ed. 1997. LC 97-6941. 960p. 58.00 (*1-55766-293-2*) P H Brookes.

Children with Downs Syndrome: A Developmental Perspective. Ed. by Dante Cicchetti & Marjorie Beeghly. 1990. (Illus.). 486p. (C). text 90.00 (*0-521-37458-8*); pap. text 32.95 (*0-521-38667-5*) Cambridge U Pr.

Children with Down's Syndrome: A Guide for Teachers & Learning Support Assistants in Mainstream Society. Stephanie Lorenz. 1998. LC 99-200425. pap. (*1-85346-506-2*) David Fulton GBR. *Dist:* Taylor & Francis.

Children with Emotional Disorders & Developmental Disabilities: Assessment & Treatment. Ed. by Marian D. Sigman. 1985. LC 85-958. 400p. text 42.00 (*0-8089-1700-5*, 794072, Grune & Strat) Harcrt Hlth Sci Grp.

Children with Language Impairments: An Introduction. Morag L. Donaldson. 1995. 144p. pap. (*1-85302-313-2*) Jessica Kingsley GBR. *Dist:* Taylor & Francis.

Children with Learning Difficulties. Diana Montgomery. 1990. 224p. pap. 29.95 (*0-89397-351-3*) Nichols Pub.

Children with Learning Disabilities: A Five Year Follow-up Study. Elizabeth M. Koppitz. 1971. LC 70-167977. 218p. text 42.00 (*0-8089-0726-3*, 792365, Grune & Strat) Harcrt Hlth Sci Grp.

Children with Mental Handicaps: A Guide for Parents & Carers. Fred Heddell. 1989. 256p. pap. (*1-85223-069-X*) Crowood Pr GBR. *Dist:* Trafalgar.

Children with Physical Handicaps: A Guide for Parents & Carers. Fred Heddell. 1989. 320p. pap. (*1-85223-074-6*) Crowood Pr GBR. *Dist:* Trafalgar.

Children with Prenatal Alcohol &/Or Other Drug Exposure: Weighing the Risks of Adoption. Susan B. Edelstein. 1995. LC 95-237744. (Orig.). pap. text 12.95 (*0-87868-630-4*) Child Welfare.

Children with Prenatal Drug Exposure. Ed. by Lynette S. Chandler & Shelly J. Lane. LC 96-19136. (Physical & Occupational Therapy in Pediatrics Ser.: Vol. 16, Nos. 1/2). 199p. (C). 1997. pap. 19.95 (*0-7890-0221-3*); 1996. 39.95 (*1-56024-837-8*) Haworth Pr.

Children with Specific Language Impairment. Laurence Leonard. 1997. LC 96-37594. (Language, Speech, & Communication Ser.). 347p. 60.00 (*0-262-12206-5*, Bradford Bks) MIT Pr.

Children with Specific Speech & Language Impairment. Corinne Haynes & Sandhya Naidoo. 1991. (Clinics in Developmental Medicine Ser.: No. 119). (Illus.). 289p. (C). text 80.00 (*0-521-41275-7*) Cambridge U Pr.

Children with Speech & Language Difficulties. Alec Webster & Christine McConnell. 1987. 192p. pap. text 33.95 (*0-304-31378-5*) Continuum.

Children with Tourette Syndrome: A Parents' Guide. Ed. by Tracy Haerle. 1992. LC 90-50766. (Special Needs Collection). (Illus.). 340p. (Orig.). pap. 14.95 (*0-933149-44-1*) Woodbine House.

Children with Tracheostomies Resource Guide. Kertoy. 2001. LC 2001-47701. (Singular Resource Guide Ser.). pap. 40.00 net. (*0-7693-0157-6*) Singular Publishing.

Children with Visual Impairments: A Parent's Guide. Ed. by M. Cay Holbrook. 1996. LC 95-25645. (Special Needs Collection). (Illus.). 395p. pap. 16.95 (*0-933149-36-0*) Woodbine House.

Children Without Childhood: A Study of Childhood Schizophrenia. Benjamin B. Wolman. 1970. LC 71-100072. 248p. text 52.00 (*0-8089-0544-9*, 794900, Grune & Strat) Harcrt Hlth Sci Grp.

Children's Access to Health Coverage: Congressional Hearing. Ed. by Bill Thomas. 2000. (Illus.). 108p. (C). reprint ed. pap. text 25.00 (*0-7567-0229-1*) DIANE Pub.

Children's Adaptive Behavior Scale Cards: Administrator's Stimulus Manual. Bert O. Richmond & Richard H. Kicklighter. rev. ed. 1983. 42p. (Orig.). (C). pap. 14.95 (*0-89334-040-5*) Humanics Pub Grp.

Children's Adaptive Behavior Scale Manual. Bert O. Richmond & Richard H. Kicklighter. 1982. 16p. (Orig.). pap. 10.95 (*0-89334-030-8*) Humanics Pub Grp.

Children's Adjustment to Adoption: Developmental & Clinical Issues. David Brodzinsky et al. 1998. LC 97-45404. (Developmental Clinical Psychology & Psychiatry Ser.). 150p. 74.95 (*0-7619-0515-4*, 80643); pap. 34.95 (*0-7619-0516-2*, 80644) Sage.

Children's Bureau Studies. Ed. by Robert H. Bremner. 1974. LC 74-1676. (Children & Youth Ser.: Vol. 3). 386p. 36.95 (*0-405-05955-8*) Ayer.

Children's Conceptions of Death. Richard Lonetto. 1980. LC 79-24334. (Death & Suicide Ser.: Vol. 3). (Illus.). 238p. 34.95 (*0-8261-2550-6*) Springer Pub.

Children's Consent to Surgery. Priscilla Alderson. 1993. LC 93-1413. 224p. (C). (*0-335-15733-5*); pap. (*0-335-15732-7*) OpUniv Pr.

Children's Difficulties in Reading, Spelling & Writing: Challenges & Responses. Ed. by Peter D. Pumfrey & Colin D. Elliot. 1990. 260p. pap. 39.95 (*1-85000-691-1*) Taylor & Francis.

Children's Drawings As Diagnostic Aids. Joseph H. DiLeo. 1988. LC 73-79882. (Illus.). 240p. reprint ed. pap. text 23.95 (*0-87630-249-5*) Brunner-Routledge.

Children's Dreaming & the Development of Consciousness. David Foulkes. 1998. LC 98-26307. 208p. 29.00 (*0-674-11620-8*) HUP.

Children's Dreams in Clinical Practice. S. Catalano. 1990. LC 89-28470. (Illus.). 240p. (C). 45.00 (*0-306-43308-7*, Plenum Trade) Perseus Pubng.

Children's Early Text Construction. Ed. by Clotilde Pontecorvo et al. 1996. 384p. text 79.95 (*0-8058-1504-X*) L Erlbaum Assocs.

*__Children's Environmental Health & Cancer in Children.__ Ed. by Joy E. Carlson & Steven K. Galson. 2001. 160p. (C). pap. 30.00 (*0-7567-1043-X*) DIANE Pub.

Children's Environmental Health Research: Indoor Mold & Children's Health. Ed. by Allen Dearry & Gwen Collman. 2000. (Illus.). 133p. (C). pap. text 35.00 (*0-7881-8535-7*) DIANE Pub.

Children's Fractures: Radiological Diagnosis & Radiographic Technique. A. Thornton & C. Gyll. 1998. (Illus.). 260p. pap. text (*0-7020-2164-4*) W B Saunders GBR. *Dist:* Saunders.

Children's Friendship. Zick Rubin. 1980. (Developing Child Ser.). (Illus.). 165p. pap. text 11.95 (*0-674-11619-4*) HUP.

Children's Head Injury: Who Cares? David Johnson et al. 1989. 254p. pap. 27.50 (*0-86377-188-2*) L Erlbaum Assocs.

Children's Health: Quick Reference Guides for Family Physicians. Jeanne P. Spencer. 2000. LC 00-39132. (Academy Collection). 272p. pap. text 29.95 (*0-7817-2052-4*) Lppncott W & W.

Children's Health & Achievement in School. Jere R. Behrman & Victor Lavy. 1994. LC 94-12591. (LSMS Working Papers: No. 104). 56p. pap. 22.00 (*0-8213-2853-0*, 12853) World Bank.

Children's Health Care: Issues for the Year 2000 & Beyond. Thomas P. Gullotta et al. 1999. LC 98-58079. 79.95 (*0-7619-1931-7*, 85035) Sage.

Children's Health Care: Issues for the Year 2000 & Beyond. Thomas Gullotta et al. 1999. LC 98-58079. pap. 34.95 (*0-7619-1932-5*, 85036) Sage.

Children's Health Care Policy Issues in Texas: Options for Financing Coverage & Data Book Policy Research Project on Health Policy Issues in TX. 1995. (Working Papers Ser.: Vol. 84). 89p. pap. 7.50 (*0-89940-562-2*) LBJ Sch Pub Aff.

Children's Health in America: A History. Charles King. 1993. LC 93-6756. 240p. 26.95 (*0-8057-4101-1*); pap. 14.95 (*0-8057-4111-9*) Gale (Macmillan Ref).

Children's Health in Primary Schools. Berry Mayall et al. 1996. 240p. 79.95 (*0-7507-0544-2*); pap. 27.95 (*0-7507-0545-0*) Taylor & Francis (Falmer Pr).

Children's Health Insurance Program: State Implementation Approaches Are Evolving. Carolyn Yocom. 2000. (Illus.). 108p. pap. text 25.00 (*0-7881-8808-9*) DIANE Pub.

Children's Hospital of Boston. Clement A. Smith. 1983. 284p. 22.50 (*0-316-80170-4*, Little Brwn Med Div) Lppncott W & W.

Children's Hospital of Philadelphia 1974-1994: An Informal Report. Shirley Bonnem. 1995. (Illus.). (*0-9617370-3-4*); pap. (*0-9617370-2-6*); text (*0-9617370-1-8*) Childrens Hospital of Philadelphia.

Children's Hospital of Philadelphia Guide to Common Childhood Infections. Lou Bell et al. 1998. LC 98-18546. (Illus.). 336p. pap. 22.95 (*0-02-860435-0*) Hungry Minds.

Children's Interpersonal Trust: Sensitivity to Lying, Deception & Promise Violations. Ed. by K. J. Rotenberg. 1991. (Illus.). 172p. 59.95 (*0-387-97511-X*) Spr-Verlag.

Children's Interview for Psychiatric Syndromes (ChIPS) Report Forms for ChIPS. Elizabeth B. Weller et al. 1999. pap. 19.95 (*0-88048-899-9*) Am Psychiatric.

Children's Interview for Psychiatric Syndromes (ChIPS) Scoring Forms. Ed. by Elizabeth B. Weller et al. 1999. 24.95 (*0-88048-846-8*, 8846) Am Psychiatric.

Children's Language. Ed. by Keith E. Nelson. Vol. 4. 1983. 496p. text 89.95 (*0-89859-272-0*); Vol. 5. 1985. 472p. (C). text 89.95 (*0-89859-346-8*) L Erlbaum Assocs.

Children's Language & Communication Vol. 12: The Minnesota Symposium on Child Psychology. Ed. by W. Andrew Collins. 1979. LC 79-364. (Illus.). 256p. text 49.95 (*0-89859-000-0*) L Erlbaum Assocs.

Children's Medical Record. Consumer Guide Editors. 1997. 128p. pap. 2.99 (*0-451-19270-2*, Sig) NAL.

Children's Medications: A Guide to Schools & Day Care Centers. Richard D. Bates & Milap C. Nahata. 1995. LC 95-8554. viii, 360p. pap. text 29.95 (*0-929375-15-7*) H W Bks.

Children's Medications: A Parent's Guide. Richard D. Bates & Milap C. Nahata. 1995. LC 95-8561. (Illus.). viii, 360p. (Orig.). pap. 19.95 (*0-929375-16-5*) H W Bks.

Children's Medicine & Surgery. Forrester Cockburn et al. 1996. (Illus.). 556p. pap. text (*0-340-55143-7*) E A GBR. *Dist:* OUP.

Children's Mental Health: Problems & Services. Ed. by Technology Assessment Office Staff & Leonard M. Saxe. 1987. LC 86-600539. (Illus.). viii, 184p. (C). text 45.95 (*0-8223-0796-0*); pap. text 18.95 (*0-8223-0815-0*) Duke.

Children's Minds. Margaret Donaldson. 1979. (Illus.). (C). pap. text 10.50 (*0-393-95101-4*) Norton.

Children's National Medical Center A to Z Guide to Your Child's Behavior. Children's National Medical Center Staff et al. 1993. LC 92-40260. 384p. pap. 14.95 (*0-399-51796-0*, Perigee Bks) Berkley Pub.

Children's Needs II: Development, Problems & Alternatives. Ed. by George Bear et al. 3rd exp. ed. 1997. LC 97-3781. 930p. pap. text 80.00 (*0-932955-96-7*) Natl Assn Schl Psych.

Children's Nursing. Linda McQuaid et al. 1996. LC 96-25830. text (*0-443-05087-2*) Church.

Children's Nursing & Reflective Thinking. Ian Guy. 2000. (Illus.). 256p. pap. 30.00 (*0-7506-4320-X*) Buttrwrth-Heinemann.

Children's Nursing in Practice: The Nottingham Model. Fiona Smith. 1995. LC 94-23687. 256p. pap. 36.95 (*0-632-03909-4*) Blackwell Sci.

Children's Orthopaedics & Fractures. Michael K. Benson. 1994. text (*0-443-04372-8*) Church.

*__Children's Orthopaedics & Fractures.__ Michael K. D. Benson et al. 2nd ed. 2001. (Illus.). 700p. (*0-443-06459-8*) Church GBR. *Dist:* Saunders.

Children's Phantasies: The Shaping of Relationships. Otto Weininger. 1989. 314p. pap. text (*0-946439-54-0*) Karnac Bks GBR. *Dist:* Other Pr LLC.

Children's Prescription Drugs: A Parent's Guide to the Most Commonly Recommended Drugs for Children. Contrib. by Consumer Guide Editors. 1997. LC 96-70997. (Illus.). 400p. (*0-7853-2163-2*) Pubns Intl Ltd.

Children's Psychological Testing: A Guide for Nonpsychologists. David L. Wodrich. 3rd rev. ed. 1997. LC 96-38720. 416p. text 38.95 (*1-55766-277-0*) P H Brookes.

Children's Reasoning & the Mind. Peter Mitchell. 1999. 336p. 59.95 (*0-86377-854-2*) L Erlbaum Assocs.

***Children's Reasoning & the Mind.** Peter Mitchell & Kevin Riggs. 2001. 480p. pap. (*0-86377-855-0*) Psychol Pr GBR. *Dist:* Taylor & Francis.

Children's Rights & the Wheel of Life. Elise Boulding. 1980. LC 78-62890. 179p. text 34.95 (*0-87855-295-2*) Transaction Pubs.

Children's Rights, Therapists' Responsibilities: Feminist Commentaries. Ed. by Gail Anderson & Marcia Hill. 1997. LC 97-5226. 141p. 34.95 (*0-7890-0326-0*); pap. 19.95 (*1-56023-100-9*, Harrington Park) Haworth Pr.

Children's Sleep: A Series of Studies on the Influence of Motion Pictures. Samuel Renshaw et al. 1970. LC 76-124031. (Literature of Cinema Ser.). reprint ed. 21.95 (*0-405-01631-X*) Ayer.

Children's Social Networks & Social Supports. Deborah Belle. 1989. LC 88-18704. (Personality Processes Ser.). 384p. 195.00 (*0-471-62879-4*) Wiley.

Children's Strategies: Contemporary Views of Child Development. Ed. by David F. Bjorklund. 1990. 348p. text 69.95 (*0-8058-0315-7*) L Erlbaum Assocs.

Children's Theories of Mind: The Development of the Social Understanding of Self & Others. D. Frye & C. Moore. 1991. 224p. (C). pap. 27.50 (*0-8058-0418-8*); text 49.95 (*0-8058-0417-X*) L Erlbaum Assocs.

Children's Thinking: Developmental Function & Individual Differences. David F. Bjorklund. 1988. LC 88-22241. 357p. (C). text 44.95 (*0-534-09384-1*) Brooks-Cole.

Children's Understanding: The Development of Mental Models. Graeme Halford. 1993. 528p. pap. 45.00 (*0-8058-1233-4*); text 99.95 (*0-89859-970-9*) L Erlbaum Assocs.

Children's Vaccine Initiative: Achieving the Vision. Institute of Medicine Staff. Ed. by Violaine S. Mitchell et al. 1993. LC 93-84552. 240p. (Orig.). (C). pap. text 24.95 (*0-309-04940-7*) Natl Acad Pr.

Children's Views of Foreign People: A Cross-National Study. Wallace E. Lambert & Otto Klineberg. 1967. LC 66-24057. (Century Psychology Ser.). (Illus.). 31.00 (*0-89197-076-2*) Irvington.

Child's Conception of Physical Causality. Jean Piaget & Jane Valsiner. 2000. LC 99 462314. xxii, 309p. pap. text 29.95 (*0-7658-0641-X*) Transaction Pubs.

Child's Conception of the World. Jean Piaget. 1975. (Quality Paperback Ser.: No. 213). 398p. reprint ed. pap. 17.95 (*0-8226-0213-X*) Littlefield.

Child's Construction of Knowledge: Piaget for Teaching Children. George E. Forman & David S. Kuschner. 1983. LC 77-8676. 244p. reprint ed. pap. text 6.00 (*0-912674-92-X*, NAEYC #116) Natl Assn Child Ed.

Child's Eye. Baljean Dhillon & Geoffrey T. Millar. 1995. LC 92-48410. (Oxford Medical Publications). 144p. 85.00 (*0-19-262303-6*); (Illus.). 142p. pap. text 46.00 (*0-19-262302-8*) OUP.

Child's Eyes: A Guide for Pediatric Primary Care. John W. Simon & Joseph H. Calhoun. 1998. LC 97-48979. (Illus.). 224p. (Orig.). pap. text 39.95 (*0-937404-52-7*) Triad Pub FL.

Child's Foot & Ankle. Ed. by James C. Drennan. 1992. 576p. text 169.00 (*0-88167-879-1*) Lppncott W & W.

Child's Health Record: Two Years & Up. Sandy Abrams et al. Ed. by Jack Caravella. 1995. (Illus.). 120p. (Orig.). pap. 9.95 (*0-9641332-5-3*) Jormax Pubng.

***Child's Medical Encyclopedia**, Vol. 1. Betty Zed. 2000. (Illus.). 144p. pap. (*1-55068-048-X*) Vanwell Publ.

Child's Medical Record Book. Anne Seymour Odden. 1999. LC 99-90240. 64p. pap. 12.95 (*0-9670221-1-8*) Minot Pubg.

Child's Parent Dies: Studies in Childhood Bereavement. Erna Furman. 1981. LC 73-86894. pap. 22.00 (*0-300-02645-5*) Yale U Pr.

Child's Path to Spoken Language. John L. Locke. 1993. LC 92-34661. (Illus.). 480p. (Orig.). text 51.95 (*0-674-11640-2*) HUP.

Child's Play Life: An Ethnographic Study. Diana Kelly-Byrne. 1989. (Early Childhood Education Ser.: No. 20). 304p. (C). pap. 19.95 (*0-8077-2941-8*) Tchrs Coll.

Child's Reality: Three Developmental Themes. David Elkind. 1978. 180p. 36.00 (*0-89859-224-0*) L Erlbaum Assocs.

Child's Talk: Learning to Use Language. Jerome S. Bruner. 1985. LC 83-42676. (Illus.). 144p. (C). pap. 9.50 (*0-393-95345-9*) Norton.

Child's Therapy: Hour by Hour. Mary R. Haworth. 1990. LC 89-15374. 240p. 37.50 (*0-8236-0838-7*) Intl Univs Pr.

Child's World: Infancy Through Adolescence. Diane E. Papalia et al. 8th ed. 1998. LC 98-5943. 68.06 (*0-07-048785-5*); (*0-07-115828-6*) McGraw.

Child's World of Illness: The Development of Health & Illness Behaviour. Simon Wilkinson. 1988. (Illus.). 304p. text 85.00 (*0-521-32873-X*) Cambridge U Pr.

Chile: The Adult Health Policy Challenge. 1995. LC 95-8630. (Country Study). 246p. pap. 22.00 (*0-8213-3224-4*, 13224) World Bank.

Chile Health Insurance Issues: Old Age & Catastrophic Health Costs. Contrib. by World Bank Staff. 2001. LC 00-53381. (World Bank Country Study Ser.). (Illus.). viii, 43p. pap. 22.00 (*0-8213-4878-7*) Wrld Bank.

Chimaeras in Development Biology. Ed. by Nicole Le Douarin & Anne McLaren. 1984. text 104.00 (*0-12-440580-0*) Acad Pr.

Chimeric Virus-Like Particles as Vaccines. Ed. by Wolfram H. Gerlich et al. 1996. (Journal: Vol. 39, No. 1-2). (Illus.). 134p. pap. 75.00 (*3-8055-6431-7*) S Karger.

Chimpanzee: Immunological Specificities of Blood. Ed. by C. Kratochvil. 1972. (Primates in Medicine Ser.: Vol. 6). 150p. 51.50 (*3-8055-1389-5*) S Karger.

Chimpanzee Conservation & Public Health: Environments for the Future. Ed. by J. Erwin & John C. Landon. 1992. 171p. pap. 40.00 (*0-9632658-0-6*) Diagnon Bioqual.

Chin. Ed. by Jacque Levignac & S. Anthony Wolfe. 1990. (Illus.). 174p. text (*0-443-04221-7*) Church.

China's Sports Medicine. Ed. by Q. Mianyu & Y. Changlong. 1989. (Medicine & Sport Science Ser.: Vol. 28). (Illus.). viii, 120p. 86.25 (*3-8055-4806-0*) S Karger.

China's Strategic Demographic Initiative. H. Yuan Tien. 1991. LC 90-20614. 336p. 72.50 (*0-275-93824-7*, C3824, Praeger Pubs) Greenwood.

Chinese - English Medical Dictionary. Commercial Press Staff. (CHI & ENG.). 150.00 (*0-8288-2483-5*, F45700) Fr & Eur.

Chinese Acupuncture. George Soulie de Morant. Ed. by Paul Zmiewski. Tr. by Dhruva Grinnell et al from FRE. 1993. (ENG.). 916p. text 108.00 (*0-912111-31-3*) Paradigm Publns.

Chinese Acupuncture & Moxibustion. Ed. by Lian-yu Li et al. 1993. LC 92-49859. text (*0-443-04223-3*) Church.

Chinese Acupuncture & Moxibustion. Cheng Xinnong. 2000. (Illus.). (*7-119-01758-6*) Beijing Foreign Lang.

Chinese Acupuncture & Moxibustion. Ed. by Cheng Xinnong. 1987. (Illus.). 544p. (*7-119-00378-X*) Beijing Foreign Lang CHN. *Dist:* China Bks.

Chinese Acupuncture & Moxibustion. Ed. by Cheng Xinnong. rev. ed. 1987. (Illus.). 544p. 65.00 (*0-8351-2109-7*) China Bks.

Chinese American Family Therapy: A New Model for Clinicians. Marshall Jung. 1998. LC 97-51420. xiii, 265p. 42.00 (*0-7879-4045-3*) Jossey-Bass.

Chinese Americans in Loss & Separation: Social, Medical & Psychiatric Perspectives. Ed. by Clarence Chen et al. 1996. LC 92-74036. 110p. pap. 16.95 (*0-930194-48-9*) Ctr Thanatology.

Chinese & Western Daily Practical Health Guide. Betty Yulin Ho. 1982. LC 81-20848. (System of Government in the Living Body Ser.). (Illus.). 122p. pap. 15.00 (*0-9600148-4-5*) Juvenescent.

Chinese & Western Guide to Better Health & Longer Life. Betty Yulin Ho. 1974. LC 74-12332. 50p. pap. 10.00 (*0-87576-046-5*) Juvenescent.

Chinese Bodywork: A Complete Manual of Chinese Theapeutic Massage. Ed. by Sun Chengnan. Tr. by Wang Qiliang. 1993. LC 93-85293. (Illus.). 320p. pap. text 50.00 (*1-881896-23-4*) Pacific View Pr.

Chinese Bodywork: A Complete Manual of Chinese Therapeutic Massage. Ed. by Sun Chengnan. Tr. by Wang Qiliang. 1993. LC 93-85293. (Illus.). 320p. text 50.00 (*1-881896-06-4*) Pacific View Pr.

Chinese Drugs of Plant Origin: Chemistry, Pharmacology, & Use in Traditional & Modern Medicine. Gerhard Eisenbrand & W. Tang. 1992. (Illus.). 1056p. 171.00 (*0-387-19309-X*) Spr-Verlag.

Chinese-English Classified Dictionary of Traditional Chinese Medicine & Pharmacology: Standard Book of Computer Dictionary Base. 1996. (CHI & ENG.). 1974p. (*7-03-003606-9*) Sci Pr CHN. *Dist:* Lubrecht & Cramer.

Chinese-English Dictionary of Traditional Chinese Medicine. Ed. by Ou Ming. 1988. 640p. (*962-04-0207-3*) Joint Pub HKG. *Dist:* Cheng & Tsui.

Chinese Exercise Book see Chinese Exercises & Massage for Health & Longevity: Everyday Exercises for Harmony of Mind, Body & Spirit

Chinese Exercises & Massage for Health & Longevity: Everyday Exercises for Harmony of Mind, Body & Spirit. Dahong Zhuo. rev. ed. 1997. LC 97-49115. Orig. Title: Chinese Exercise Book. (Illus.). 316p. pap. 19.95 (*0-88179-158-X*) Hartley & Marks.

***Chinese Family Acupoint Massage.** Wang Chuangui. 2001. (Illus.). 232p. reprint ed. 30.00 (*0-7567-5151-9*) DIANE Pub.

Chinese Family Acupoint Massage. Wang Chuangui. 1995. (Illus.). (*983-9808-21-4*) Delta Edits MYS. *Dist:* Weatherhill.

Chinese Healing Foods & Herbs. Albert Y. Leung. Orig. Title: Chinese Herbal Remedies. (Illus.). 192p. reprint ed. pap. 10.95 (*0-9634979-0-1*) AYSL.

Chinese Healing Secrets. Bill Schoenbart & Ellen Shefi. 1997. LC 97-67522. 256 p. (*0-7853-2517-4*) Pubns Intl Ltd.

Chinese Healing Secrets. Ed. by Signet Staff. 1998. 256p. mass mkt. 5.99 (*0-451-19418-7*, Sig) NAL.

Chinese Health Care Secrets: A Natural Lifestyle Approach. Henry B. Lin. 2000. LC 99-45849. (Illus.). 528p. pap. 24.95 (*1-56718-434-0*) Llewellyn Pubns.

Chinese Herb Medicine & Therapy. Hong-yen Hsu. rev. ed. 1993. 15.00 (*0-941942-12-0*) Orient Heal Arts.

Chinese Herb Selection Guide: A Traditional & Modern Clinical Repertory with a Summary Materia Medica for the Health Care Practitioner. Charles A. Belanger. 1997. LC 97-91745. xxiv, 892p. (Orig.). pap. 59.95 (*0-9657310-3-0*) Phytotech Database.

Chinese Herbal Cures. Henry C. Lu. 1993. LC 93-43376. (Illus.). 160p. pap. 10.95 (*0-8069-0762-2*) Sterling.

Chinese Herbal Medicine. Daniel P. Reid. 1987. LC 86-17814. (Illus.). 180p. reprint ed. pap. 29.95 (*0-87773-398-8*) Shambhala Pubns.

Chinese Herbal Medicine: A Step-by-Step Guide. Helen Thomas. 1997. LC 97-18371. (In a Nutshell Ser.). (Illus.). 64p. 7.95 (*1-86204-105-9*) Element MA.

Chinese Herbal Medicine: Comprehensive Guide. Ze-lin Chen. 1999. 492p. pap. text 9.99 (*0-7858-1076-5*) Bk Sales Inc.

Chinese Herbal Medicine: Formulas & Strategies. Dan Bensky & Randall Barolet. 1990. LC 89-81674. (Illus.). 592p. (C). text 85.00 (*0-939616-10-6*) Eastland.

Chinese Herbal Medicine: Materia Medica. Ed. by Dan Bensky & Ted J. Kaptchuk. Tr. by Dan Bensky & Andrew Gamble from CHI. rev. ed. 1993. LC 92-74516. (Illus.). 556p. (C). 75.00 (*0-939616-15-7*) Eastland.

Chinese Herbal Medicine & the Problems of Aging. Bokuso Terashi. 1993. pap. 12.00 (*0-941942-17-1*) Orient Heal Arts.

Chinese Herbal Medicine Made Easy: Effective & Natural Remedies for Common Illnesses. Thomas R. Joiner. 2000. LC 99-58835. (Illus.). xvi, 416p. 34.95 (*0-89793-276-5*); pap. 24.95 (*0-89793-275-7*) Hunter Hse.

Chinese Herbal Medicine Materia Medica Study Guide. Mark Saltzman & Marisa Saltzman. 2000. LC 00-47584. 80p. reprint ed. pap. 9.95 (*0-9673034-2-7*) Complmtry Medcne.

Chinese Herbal Remedies see Chinese Healing Foods & Herbs

Chinese Herbs: Their Botany, Chemistry & Pharmacodynamics. John D. Keys. 1989. (Illus.). 346p. pap. 24.95 (*0-8048-1667-0*) Tuttle Pubng.

Chinese Herbs in the Western Clinic: A Guide to Prepared Herbal Formulas Indexed by Western Disorders & Supported by Case Studies. Andrew Gaeddart. 255p. pap. 15.95 (*0-9638285-0-9*) Get Well Fnd.

Chinese Herbs Made Easy. Frank Miesse. Date not set. 20p. pap. 2.95 (*0-913923-64-8*) Woodland UT.

Chinese Learner: Cultural, Psychological & Contextual Influences. Ed. by John Watkins & John B. Biggs. 1997. LC 97-161362. 288p. pap. (*0-86431-182-6*) Aust Council Educ Res AUS. *Dist:* Stylus Pub VA.

Chinese Massage for Infants & Children: Traditional Techniques for Alleviating Colic, Colds, Earaches & Other Common Childhood Conditions. Kyle Cline. 1999. LC 99-18421. (Illus.). 160p. pap. 19.95 (*0-89281-797-6*, Heal Arts VT) Inner Tradit.

Chinese Materia Medica: Chemistry, Pharmacology & Applications. You-Ping Zhu. 1998. (Illus.). 528p. text 95.00 (*90-5702-285-0*, ECU79, Harwood Acad Pubs) Gordon & Breach.

Chinese Materia Medica: Dragon & Snake Drugs. Bernard E. Read. 1979. lib. bdg. 300.00 (*0-8490-3063-3*) Krishna Pr.

Chinese Materia Medica: Vegetable Kingdom. F. P. Smith. 1980. 300.00 (*0-87968-469-0*) Krishna Pr.

Chinese Materia Medica: Vegetable Kingdom. G. A. Stuart. 1985. 570p. (C). reprint ed. (*81-7089-022-5*) Intl Bk Distr IND. *Dist:* St Mut.

Chinese Materia Medica: Vegetable Kingdom. G. A. Stuart. 1990. 570p. pap. 325.00 (*0-7855-2745-1*) St Mut.

Chinese Medical Modernization: Comparative Policy Continuities 1930's-1980's. Anelissa Lucas. 1982. LC 81-23361. 188p. 55.00 (*0-275-90851-8*, C0851, Praeger Pubs) Greenwood.

Chinese Medical Palmistry: Your Health in Your Hand. Zong Xiao-Fan & Gary Liscam. Ed. & Intro. by Bob Flaws. Tr. by Zong Xiao-Fan. 1995. LC 95-77408. (Illus.). 205p. pap. 17.95 (*0-936185-64-3*) Blue Poppy Pr.

Chinese Medical Terminology: English to Chinese. F. C. Liu & L. Y. Mau. 1980. (CHI & ENG.). 262p. 39.95 (*0-8288-0559-8*, M9399) Fr & Eur.

Chinese Medicinal Teas: Simple, Proven, Folk Formulas for Common Diseases & Promoting Health. Gary Liscum et al. Ed. by Bob Flaws. 1996. LC 96-85056. 190p. pap. 19.95 (*0-936185-76-7*) Blue Poppy Pr.

Chinese Medicinal Wines & Elixirs. Bob Flaws. 1994. 240p. (Orig.). pap. 19.95 (*0-936185-58-9*) Blue Poppy Pr.

Chinese Medicine. Giovanni Maciocia. 1996. (C). pap. 229.00 incl. cd-rom (*0-443-07821-1*) Harcourt.

Chinese Medicine. Paul U. Unschuld. Tr. by Nigel Wiseman from GER. 1998. LC 98-15490. 144p. pap. 14.95 (*0-912111-55-0*) Paradigm Publns.

Chinese Medicine. William R. Morse. LC 75-23661. (Clio Medica Ser.: 11). (Illus.). reprint ed. 36.00 (*0-404-58911-1*) AMS Pr.

Chinese Medicine: Acupuncture, Herbal Remedies, Nutrition, Qigong & Meditation for Total Health. Tom Williams. 1997. (Health Essentials Ser.). 128p. pap. 9.95 (*1-86204-065-6*) Element MA.

Chinese Medicine: The Complete Guide to Acupuncture, Chinese Herbal Medicine, Food Cures, & Preventive Care. Barbara Bernie. Ed. by Duo Gao. 1998. LC 98-156070. (Illus.). 256p. pap. 22.95 (*1-56025-176-X*, Thunders Mouth) Avalon NY.

Chinese Medicine: The Treatment of Disease with Acupuncture & Chinese Herbs. Giovanni Macviocia. 1994. LC 93-10311. text (*0-443-04305-1*) Church.

Chinese Patent Medicine: A Beginner's Guide. Mark Taylor. 1998. LC 98-204959. (Illus.). 304p. pap. (*0-9662973-0-X*) Global Eyes.

Chinese Patterns of Behavior: A Sourcebook of Psychological & Psychiatric Studies. Ed. by David Yau-Fai Ho et al. 1989. LC 88-32335. 512p. 175.00 (*0-275-93270-2*, C3270, Praeger Pubs) Greenwood.

Chinese Pediatric Massage: A Practitioner's Guide. Kyle Cline. 2000. LC 99-49254. (Illus.). 304p. 45.00 (*0-89281-842-5*, Heal Arts VT) Inner Tradit.

Chinese Pediatric Massage Therapy: A Parent & Practitioner's Guide to the Treatment & Prevention of Childhood Diseases. Fan Ya-li. Ed. & Intro. by Bob Flaws. 1994. LC 93-74981. (Illus.). 150p. pap. 12.95 (*0-936185-54-6*) Blue Poppy Pr.

Chinese Pulse Diagnosis: A Contemporary Approach. Leon Hammer. 2001. 812p. (C). 85.00 (*0-939616-25-4*) Eastland.

Chinese Qigong & the Science of Energy: Improving Mental & Physical Health & Increasing Longevity. 1992. (Alternative Medicine Ser.). lib. bdg. 93.95 (*0-8490-5391-9*) Gordon Pr.

Chinese Qigong Massage: General Massage. Jwing-Ming Yang. Ed. by Alan Dougall. 1992. (Illus.). 336p. pap. 29.95 (*0-940871-25-4*, B016/254) YMAA Pubn.

Chinese Self-Massage Therapy: The Easy Way to Health. Fan Ya-Li. Ed. by Bob Flaws. 1997. LC 96-86693. (Illus.). 155p. pap. 15.95 (*0-936185-74-0*) Blue Poppy Pr.

Chinese System of Natural Cures. Henry C. Lu. 1994. LC 94-13706. 160p. pap. 10.95 (*0-8069-0616-2*) Sterling.

Chinese Therapeutical Methods of Acupuncture & Moxibustion. Research Institute of Acupuncture and Moxibustion, China Staff. 1994. 18p. reprint ed. spiral bd. 8.00 (*0-7873-1023-9*) Hlth Research.

Chinese to English Dictionary Traditional Chinese Medicine, Pharmacology. 1994. (CHI & ENG.). 1974p. 125.00 (*0-320-00582-8*) Fr & Eur.

Chinese to English Dictionary Traditional Chinese Veterinary Medicine. 1991. (CHI & ENG.). 426p. 79.95 (*0-320-00603-4*) Fr & Eur.

Chinese Tonic Herbs. 1992. (Alternative Medicine Ser.). lib. bdg. 88.95 (*0-8490-5396-X*) Gordon Pr.

Chinese Way to Healing: Many Paths to Wholeness. Misha R. Cohen & Kalia Doner. 1996. LC 96-1390. 272p. pap. 15.95 (*0-399-52232-8*, Perigee Bks) Berkley Pub.

Chinese Way to Health: A Self-Help Guide to Traditional Chinese Medicine. Stephen Gascoigne. 1997. LC 96-27183. 160p. pap. 22.95 (*0-8048-3120-3*) Tuttle Pubng.

Chiral Separations by Hplc. Ed. by Ante M. Krstulovic. 1989. 548p. 119.00 (*0-470-21299-3*) P-H.

Chirality & Biological Activity of Drugs. Roger Crossley. 1995. LC 95-21285. 208p. 179.95 (*0-8493-9140-7*, 9140) CRC Pr.

Chiropractic. R. C. Schafer & Louis Sportelli. 1995. LC 95-149404. (VGM Careers for You Ser.). 160p. 13.95 (*0-8442-4131-8*) NTC Contemp Pub Co.

Chiropractic: A Philosophy for Alternative Health Care. Douglass Coulter. 1999. LC 99-27299. 117p. pap. text 39.95 (*0-7506-4006-5*) Buttrwrth-Heinemann.

Chiropractic: An Illustrated History. Dennis Peterson. 1994. (Illus.). 528p. (C). (gr. 13). text 73.00 (*0-8016-7735-1*, 07735) Mosby Inc.

Chiropractic: Early Concepts in Their Historical Setting. Pierre-Louis Gaucher-Peslherbe. Ed. by Dana J. Lawrence. Tr. by Elizabeth Weeks from FRE. 1993. (Illus.). 261p. (C). text 59.95 (*0-9615849-1-2*) Natl Coll Chiro.

Chiropractic: The Victim's Perspective. George Magner. Ed. by Stephen Barrett. 1995. LC 95-21978. (Illus.). 252p. 30.00 (*1-57392-041-X*) Prometheus Bks.

Chiropractic - The Superior Alternative. William H. Koch. 1995. (Illus.). 192p. pap. (*1-896209-22-X*) Bayeux Arts.

Chiropractic Analysis Through Palpation. F. P. DeGiacomo. Ed. by James McDonnell. 1980. (Illus.). 192p. (C). 20.00 (*0-938470-00-0*) NY Chiro Coll.

Chiropractic Assistant. R. C. Schafer. 2nd ed. 1992. Orig. Title: Basic Chiropractic Paraprofessional Manual. (Illus.). 583p. text 60.00 (*0-9606618-6-7*) Am Chiro Assn.

Chiropractic Business Management Guide. 2000. 256p. (C). 19.20 (*0-536-02161-9*) Pearson Custom.

Chiropractic Care for Special Populations. Robert D. Mootz & Linda J. Bowers. 1999. LC 99-31809. 200p. pap. 45.00 (*0-8342-1374-5*) Aspen Pub.

Chiropractic Care of the Older Patient. Ed. by Brian J. Gleberson. 2001. LC 2001-281214. (Butterworth-Heinemann Professional Complementary Medicine Ser.). (Illus.). 496p. 99.00 (*0-7506-4729-9*) Buttrwrth-Heinemann.

Chiropractic College Directory. Kevin P. McNamee et al. 6th ed. 1999. (Illus.). 236p. pap. 19.95 (*0-945947-05-4*) KM Enterprises.

Chiropractic Concepts in Healing. Frank Zolli & A. E. Cianciulli. 1984. 39p. 5.50 (*0-938470-01-9*) NY Chiro Coll.

Chiropractic Diagnosis & Management. 2nd ed. 2000. (Illus.). 608p. text 84.95 (*0-8151-4373-7*, 31171) Mosby Inc.

Chiropractic First: The Fastest Growing Healthcare Choice Before Drugs or Surgery. Terry A. Rondberg. 1996. LC 95-92445. (Illus.). 160p. pap. 12.95 (*0-9647168-2-8*) Chiropractic Jrnl.

Chiropractic for Natural Health & Wellness Care. Donald A. Dahlin. 1993. 136p. pap. 10.95 (*1-883243-00-9*) D A Dahlin.

Chiropractic History. 1992. 55p. (Orig.). pap. 14.50 (*0-9614296-8-2*) Wrld-Wide Bks.

Chiropractic Insights: A Handbook on Natural Health-Care. Jerrold J. Simon. 1987. LC 87-90728. (Illus.). 70p. (Orig.). (C). pap. 5.75 (*0-9619896-0-2*) Amer Hlth Heritage.

Chiropractic Management of Spine Related Disorders. Meridel I. Gatterman. 1990. 437p. 89.00 (*0-683-03438-3*); 2nd ed. 1998. (Illus.). 89.00 (*0-683-30240-X*) Lppncott W & W.

Chiropractic Manipulative Skills: The Fundamentals of Clinical Practice. David Byfield. 1995. LC 95-30545. (Illus.). 336p. pap. text 65.00 (*0-7506-0968-0*) Buttrwrth-Heinemann.

Chiropractic Name Techniques. Brian J Gleberzon. 2001. 256p. pap. 70.00 (*0-7506-4728-0*) Buttrwrth-Heinemann.

Chiropractic Office Manual. Steven C. Eggleston. 1996. (Office Manual Ser.). 191p. 89.00 (*1-890018-09-0*) Anadem Pubng.

Chiropractic Peripheral Joint Technique. Raymond T. Broome. 2000. LC 99-17378. 320p. pap. text 75.00 (*0-7506-3289-5*) Buttrwrth-Heinemann.

Chiropractic Philosophy. Joseph B. Strauss. 2nd ed. 1991. 213p. (C). text 25.00 (*1-890419-03-6*) Fnd Chiropractic Educ.

Chiropractic Physiology: A Review of Scientific Principles As Related to the Chiropractic Adjustment with Emphasis on the Bio Energetic Synchronization Technique. M. T. Morter, Jr. 1988. LC 88-70369. 120p. 32.00 (*0-944994-01-6*) BEST Research.

Chiropractic Practice, Methods & Trends: Index of New Information with Authors & Subjects. Billy J. Sweeney. 1994. LC 94-32483. 57.50 (*0-7883-0374-0*); pap. 47.50 (*0-7883-0375-9*) ABBE Pubs Assn.

Chiropractic Research Abstracts Collection (CRAC) 1990, Vol. 4. John P. Mrozek & Marilyn E. Schafer. 1991. 130p. 38.00 (*0-683-01420-X*) Lppncott W & W.

Chiropractic Secrets. Ed. by Seth Gardner & John S. Mosby. 1999. (Secrets Ser.). (Illus.). 325p. pap. 36.95 (*1-56053-318-8*) Hanley & Belfus.

Chiropractic Standards of Practice & Quality of Care. Herbert J. Vear. 1995. LC 91-22234. 324p. 87.00 (*0-8342-0242-5*) Aspen Pub.

Chiropractic Technique. Hooper & Curl. 1998. text 70.00 (*0-8385-6130-6*) Appleton & Lange.

Chiropractic Technique: Principles & Procedures. Thomas F. Bergmann et al. 1993. (Illus.). 816p. text (*0-443-08752-0*) Church.

Chiropractic Techniques. Bergmann. 2nd ed. 1998. text 125.00 (*0-443-07633-2*) Saunders.

Chiropractic Technologies. Robert D. Mootz & Daniel T. Hansen. 1999. LC 99-31808. (Topics in Clinical Chiropractic Ser.). (Illus.). xxvi, 198p. pap. 45.00 (*0-8342-1373-7*) Aspen Pub.

Chiropractic Theories. Robert A. Leach. 3rd ed. 1983. LC 93-17891. (Illus.). 426p. 54.00 (*0-683-04904-6*) Lppncott W & W.

Chiropractic Two Thousand. Lawrence. 2000. (Illus.). 350p. text 73.00 (*0-8151-2860-6*, 31806) Mosby Inc.

Chiropractic Two Thousand & One. Lawrence. 2001. text 73.00 (*0-8151-2871-1*, 31807) Mosby Inc.

Chiropractic Two Thousand & Three. Lawrence. 2002. text 73.00 (*0-8151-2880-0*, 31808) Mosby Inc.

Chiropractor. D. D. Palmer. 1996. 115p. reprint ed. pap. 13.00 (*0-7873-0652-5*) Hlth Research.

Chiropractor: The Quest for Professional Respect. Kent Boyer. 1994. LC 93-28885. 188p. pap. text 24.95 (*1-879904-12-8*) Halo Bks.

Chiropractor (1914) D. D. Palmer. 1996. 117p. reprint ed. pap. 12.95 (*1-56459-775-X*) Kessinger Pub.

Chiropractors: History & Evolution of a Profession. Walter I. Wardwell. 1992. LC 92-8436. (Illus.). 368p. (gr. 13). text 52.95 (*0-8016-6883-2*, 06883) Mosby Inc.

Chiropractor's Health Book. Leonard Mcgill. 1997. LC 96-23966. 208p. pap. 16.00 (*0-517-88818-1*, Crown) Crown Pub Group.

***Chiroptractic Pediatrics: A Clinical Handbook.** Neil J. Davies. 2001. (Illus.). 475p. pap. (*0-443-06253-6*) Church GBR. *Dist:* Saunders.

Chirotherapy: A Text on Joint Movements for Masseurs, Chiropractors & Laymen. 1991. lib. bdg. 250.00 (*0-8490-4538-X*) Gordon Pr.

Chirurgie dans l'Egypte Greco-Romaine d'apres les Papyrus Litteraires Grecs. Marie-Helene Marganne. 1998. (Studies in Ancient Medicine: Vol. 17). (Illus.). 256p. 75.50 (*90-04-11134-4*) Brill Academic Pubs.

Chirurgische Therapie des Mammakarzinoms. Ed. by F. Judmaier. 1980. (Beitraege Zur Onkologie, Contributions to Oncology Ser.: Band 2). (Illus.). viii, 60p. pap. 18.50 (*3-8055-1350-X*) S Karger.

Chirurgische Traumatologie & Rehabiltation. Ed. by U. Laffer & M. Duerig. 1990. (Basler Beitraege zur Chirurgie Ser.: Vol. 3). (Illus.). vi, 118p. 71.50 (*3-8055-5164-9*) S Karger.

***Chirurgisches Forum '99 fur Experimentelle und Klinische Forschung: 116. Kongress der Deutschen Gesellschaft fur Chirurgie, Munchen, 06.04.-10.04.1999.** Ed. by D. Ruehland et al. 1999. (Deutsche Gesellschaft fur Chirurgie Ser.). (ENG & GER., Illus.). xxiv, 773p. pap. 141.00 (*3-540-65669-3*) Spr-Verlag.

Chlamydia. P. A. Mardh et al. 1989. (Illus.). 388p. (C). text 85.00 (*0-306-42965-9*, Kluwer Plenum) Kluwer Academic.

Chlamydia Pneumoniae & Chronic Diseases: Proceedings of the State-of-the-Art Workshop, Held at the Robert Koch-Institut Berlin, on 19 & 20 March 1999. Johanna L'age-Stehr. 2000. LC 00-49222. (Illus.). x, 203p. (C). pap. 64.95 (*3-540-41136-4*) Spr-Verlag.

Chlamydia Pneumoniae Infection: The Lung & the Heart. Luigi Allegra & F. Blasi. 1999. LC 98-54981. 213p. (C). pap. (*88-470-0047-5*) Spr-Verlag ITA. *Dist:* Spr-Verlag.

Chlamydia Research: Proceedings of the European Society. 1988. 320p. (Orig.). pap. 87.50 (*91-22-01220-6*) Coronet Bks.

Chlamydial Infections. Ed. by R. Reeve. 1987. (Illus.). 126p. 55.95 (*0-387-16552-5*) Spr-Verlag.

Chlamydial Infections: Proceedings of the 9th International Symposium on Human Chlamydial Infection. Ed. by R. S. Stephens et al. 1998. (Illus.). 661p. 50.00 (*0-9664383-0-2*) Intl Chlamydia.

Chlamydial Infections: Proceedings of the Seventh International Symposium on Human Chlamydial Infections. Ed. by R. Jones et al. 1990. 623p. (C). text 130.00 (*0-521-39082-6*) Cambridge U Pr.

Chloride Channels & Carriers in Nerve, Muscle & Glial Cells. F. J. Alvarez-Leefmans & J. M. Russell. 1990. (Illus.). 444p. (C). text 125.00 (*0-306-43426-1*, Kluwer Plenum) Kluwer Academic.

Chlorinated Drinking-Water: Chlorination By-Products; Some Other Halogenated Compounds; Cobalt & Cobalt Compounds. 1991. (IARC Scientific Publications Ser.: Vol. 52). 544p. pap. text 88.00 (*92-832-1252-5*, 1720052) World Health.

Chlorobenzenes Other Than Hexachlorobenzene. 1991. (Environmental Health Criteria Ser.: No. 128). 252p. pap. text 45.00 (*92-4-157128-4*, 1160128) World Health.

Chloroform. 1994. (Environmental Health Criteria Ser.: No. 163). (ENG, FRE & SPA.). 174p. pap. text 36.00 (*92-4-157163-2*, 1160163) World Health.

Chloroplasts. Ed. by J. Reinert. 1980. (Results & Problems in Cell Differentiation Ser.: Vol. 10). (Illus.). 240p. 64.95 (*0-387-10082-2*) Spr-Verlag.

Chlorothalonil. 1995. (Health & Safety Guides Ser.: No. 98). 30p. (C). pap. text 4.50 (*92-4-151098-6*, 1860098) Am Soc Clinical.

Chocolate Is My Kryptonite: Feeding Your Feelings: How to Survive the Forces of Food. Matthew S. Keene. 1998. LC 97-69389. (Illus.). 208p. pap. 12.95 (*0-9659847-2-9*) Saguaro Pub AZ.

Choe Notes: A Handbook of Pharmacology. Jae Y. Choe. 2nd rev. ed. 1996. LC 96-14950. (Illus.). xii, 411p. pap. 34.95 (*0-940473-34-8*) Wm Caxton.

Choice: The Essential Element in Human Action. Alan Donagan. 1987. (Studies in Philosophical Psychology). 192p. lib. bdg. 35.00 (*0-7102-1168-6*, Routledge Thoemms) Routledge.

Choice Awareness: Systematic, Eclectic Counseling Theory. Richard C. Nelson. 1990. LC 90-81967. 420p. (Orig.). (C). pap. 17.95 (*0-932796-30-3*) Ed Media Corp.

Choice, Decision, & Measurement: Essays in Honor of R. Duncan Luce. Ed. by A. A. Marley. 1996. LC 96-41621. 400p. 80.00 (*0-8058-2234-8*) L Erlbaum Assocs.

Choice in Healing: Integrating the Best of Conventional & Alternative Approaches to Cancer. Michael Lerner. 1994. LC 93-39913. (Illus.). 693p. 38.50 (*0-262-12180-8*) MIT Pr.

Choice in Human Affairs: An Application to Aging-Accident-Illness Problems. Elmer Luchterhand & Daniel Sydiaha. 1966. pap. 15.95 (*0-8084-0075-4*) NCUP.

Choice of Foods: How It Can Protect Against Depression, Stroke & Alzheimer's Disease. 1991. lib. bdg. 79.95 (*0-8490-4642-4*) Gordon Pr.

Choice over Time. Ed. by George Loewestein & Jon Elster. 1992. LC 91-42816. (Illus.). 352p. 39.95 (*0-87154-558-6*) Russell Sage.

Choice Theory: A New Psychology of Personal Freedom. William Glasser. 1998. LC 97-36025. (Illus.). 352p. 24.00 (*0-06-019109-0*) HarperCollins Pubs.

Choice Theory: A New Psychology of Personal Freedom. William Glasser. 2000. 340p. reprint ed. 23.00 (*0-7881-9316-3*) DIANE Pub.

Choices: A Guide to Sex Counseling with Physically Disabled Adults. Maureen E. Neistadt & Maureen Freda. 1987. LC 86-2888. 132p. pap. 9.95 (*0-89464-201-4*); text 15.50 (*0-89874-903-4*) Krieger.

Choices: Realistic Alternatives in Cancer Treatment. Marion Morra & Eve Potts. rev. ed. 1980. 976p. pap. 12.95 (*0-380-75308-1*, Avon Bks) Morrow Avon.

Choices? The Whole-Person Health Profile. Raymond E. Cole. 2nd ed. 1986. LC 86-50257. 52p. reprint ed. pap. 4.95 (*0-917073-02-9*) Wellpower.

Choices & Conflict: Explorations in Health Care Ethics. Ed. by Emily Friedman. 1992. LC 92-816. 209p. pap. 45.00 (*1-55648-082-2*, 025105) AHPI.

Choices & Consequences: What to Do When a Teenager Uses Alcohol-Drugs, A Step-By-Step System That Really Works. Dick Schaefer. rev. ed. 1996. LC 87-22717. 156p. (Orig.). pap. 14.25 (*0-935908-42-0*, 3124, HazeldenJohnson Inst) Hazelden.

Choices & Decisions in Health Care. Andrew Grubb. 1993. 258p. 215.00 (*0-471-93621-9*) Wiley.

Choices for Terminally Ill Parents: A Guide for State Law Makers. Yolande M. Samerson. 1997. LC 97-25086. (*1-57073-465-8*) Amer Bar Assn.

Choices in Healing: Integrating the Best of Conventional & Alternative Approaches to Cancer. Michael Lerner. 1996. LC 93-39913. 696p. reprint ed. pap. text 20.00 (*0-262-62104-5*) MIT Pr.

Choices in Health Policy: An Agenda for the European Union. Brian Able-Smith et al. 1995. (Illus.). 200p. text (*1-85521-755-4*); pap. text (*1-85521-762-7*) Dartmth Pub GBR. *Dist:* Ashgate Pub Co.

***Choking & Air-Way Obstructions: Index of New Information & Guide-Book for Consumers.** Joanne C. Silvester. 2002. 180p. pap. 47.50 (*0-7883-2547-7*) ABBE Pubs Assn.

Cholangiography after Orthotopic Liver Transplantation. G. Noldge et al. 1995. LC 95-46876. 104p. pap. 75.00 (*3-540-60491-X*) Spr-Verlag.

Cholecystokinin. Ed. by Joseph R. Reeve, Jr. 1994. LC 94-4554. (Annals Ser.: Vol. 713). pap. 130.00 (*0-89766-858-8*) NY Acad Sci.

Cholecystokinin & Anxiety: From Neuron to Behavior. Jacques Bradwejn & Eero Vasar. 1995. LC 95-548. (Neuroscience Intelligence Unit Ser.). 173p. 79.00 (*1-57059-293-4*) Landes Bioscience.

Cholecystokinin Antagonists in Gastroenterology: Basic & Clinical Status. Ed. by G. Adler & C. Beglinger. 1991. (Illus.). 233p. 131.00 (*0-387-53582-9*) Spr-Verlag.

Cholelithiasis: Causes & Treatment. Fumio Nakayama. 1996. LC 96-42979. (*4-260-14334-4*) Igaku-Shoin.

Cholelithiasis: Causes & Treatment. Fumio Nakayama. 1996. LC 96-42979. 312p. 121.95 (*0-89640-334-3*) Igaku-Shoin.

Cholera. D. Barua & W. B. Greenough. 1992. (Current Topics in Infectious Disease Ser.). (Illus.). 392p. (C). text 69.50 (*0-306-44077-6*, Kluwer Plenum) Kluwer Academic.

Cholera & Related Diarrheas: Molecular Aspects of a Global Health Problem. WHO, 43rd Nobel Symposium. Ed. by O. Ouchterlony & J. Holmgren. 1980. (Illus.). 100.00 (*3-8055-3060-9*) S Karger.

Cholera Bulletin. Association of Physicians Staff. 1972. LC 77-180564. (Medicine & Society in America Ser.). 198p. reprint ed. 21.95 (*0-405-03942-5*) Ayer.

Cholera Immunology: Proceedings of the WHO Scientific Group, Teheran, 1968. WHO Staff. 1969. (Technical Reports: No. 414). pap. text 3.00 (*92-4-120414-1*, 1100414) World Health.

Cholera in Postrevolutionary Paris: A Cultural History. Catherine J. Kudlick. 1996. LC 95-25418. (Studies on the History of Society & Culture: Vol. 25). (Illus.). 319p. (C). text 50.00 (*0-520-20273-2*) U CA Pr.

Cholera on the American Continents. Ed. by A. F. De Castro & W. F. Almeida. 1993. LC 93-61303. (Illus.). 196p. pap. 37.50 (*0-944398-12-X*) ILSI.

Cholera Problem. Oscar Felsenfeld. 1967. LC 67-26004. (Illus.). 180p. 10.00 (*0-87527-008-5*) Green.

Cholera Years: The United States in 1832, 1849, & 1866. Charles E. Rosenberg. 1997. LC 62-18121. pap. text 8.00 (*0-226-72679-7*, P320) U Ch Pr.

Cholera Years: The United States in 1832, 1849, & 1866. Charles E. Rosenberg. 1987. LC 62-18121. (Illus.). x, 276p. (C). pap. text 12.00 (*0-226-72677-0*) U Ch Pr.

Cholescintigraphy: Developments in Nuclear Medicine, No. 1. Peter H. Cox. 1981. 250p. text 149.50 (*90-247-2524-0*) Kluwer Academic.

Cholestatic Liver Diseases. Ed. by M. P. Manns et al. 1998. (Falk Symposium Ser.). 320p. 173.00 (*0-7923-8746-5*) Kluwer Academic.

Cholestatic Liver Diseases: New Strategies for Prevention & Treatment of Hepatobiliary & Cholestatic Liver Diseases. Ed. by G. P. Van Berge Henegouwen. 1994. LC 94-23373. 352p. (C). text 115.00 (*0-7923-8867-4*) Kluwer Academic.

Cholestatic Liver Diseases in Children & Adults. Ed. by Christoph E. Broelsch-Houssin. 1997. (Falk Symposium Ser.). 128p. (C). text 60.00 (*0-7923-8710-4*) Kluwer Academic.

Cholesteatoma & Anterior Tympanotomy. Tamotsu Morimitsu. 1997. LC 97-20738. (Illus.). 128p. 85.00 (*4-431-70197-4*) Spr-Verlag.

Cholesteatoma & Mastoid Surgery. Ed. by Mirkos Tos et al. 1989. LC 89-19867. (Illus.). 1248p. lib. bdg. (*90-6299-056-8*) Kugler NLD. *Dist:* Lib Res.

Cholesteatoma & Mastoid Surgery: Proceedings of the Fourth International Conference, Nigata, Japan, September 8-12, 1993. Ed. by Yuichi Nakano. 1993. LC 93-41769. (Illus.). lib. bdg. (*90-6299-102-5*) Kugler NLD. *Dist:* Lib Res.

Cholesterol: Friend or Foe? David G. Williams. 1988. 76p. pap. 6.95 (*0-944649-03-3*) Mtn Home Pub.

Cholesterol 7 Alpha & Hydroxylase (7 Alpha Monooxygenase) Robin Fears & John R. Sabine. 1986. 256p. 125.00 (*0-8493-6553-8*, QP603, CRC Reprint) Franklin.

Cholesterol & Atherosclerosis: Diagnosis & Treatment. Scott M. Grundy. 1990. (Illus.). 176p. (gr. 13). text (*0-397-44674-8*, GM0082) Gower-Mosby.

Cholesterol & Your Health - the Great American Rip-Off!, Pt. 1. Chris Mudd. 1990. (Illus.). 170p. pap. (*0-9624515-1-7*) Am Lite Co.

Cholesterol Connections. Joan Bissen et al. 1990. 56p. stu. ed. (*1-884153-02-X*) Prk Nicollet.

Cholesterol Conspiracy. Russell Smith. 1991. 400p. (Orig.). pap. text 27.75 (*0-87527-476-5*) Green.

Cholesterol Cures: From Almonds & Antioxidants to Garlic, Golf, Wine & Yogurt - 325 Quick & Easy Ways to Lower Cholesterol & Live Longer. Richard Turbo. Ed. by Prevention Magazine Editors. 1996. LC 95-39324. 336p. pap. 15.95 (*0-87596-399-4*) Rodale Pr Inc.

Cholesterol Hoax: 101 + Lies. Sheldon Zerden. 1997. LC 97-40599. (Illus.). 130p. (C). pap. 9.95 (*0-9640104-2-9*) Bridger Hse.

Cholesterol in Children: Healthy Eating Is a Family Affair. 1994. (Illus.). 52p. (Orig.). (C). pap. text 15.00 (*0-7881-0329-6*) DIANE Pub.

Cholesterol in Membrane Models. Martin-Scott Finegold. 1992. 304p. lib. bdg. 110.00 (*0-8493-4207-4*, QP752) CRC Pr.

Cholesterol in School Age Children: A Program to Develop Awareness. Johanna C. Burani. 1990. (Illus.). 88p. spiral bd. 39.95 (*1-879339-12-9*) Infinity Impress.

Cholesterol-Lowering Therapy: Evaluation of Clinical Trial Evidence. Marcel Dekker. 1999. 352p. text 150.00 (*0-8247-8216-X*) Dekker.

Cholesterol Measurement: Test Accuracy & Factors That Influence Cholesterol Levels. 1995. (Illus.). 69p. (Orig.). (C). pap. text 30.00 (*0-7881-1822-6*) DIANE Pub.

Cholesterol Systems in Insects & Animals. Jacqueline Dupont. 1982. 160p. 79.95 (*0-8493-5315-7*, QL495) CRC Pr.

Cholesterol Treatment: A Review of the Clinical Trials Evidence. 1996. 107p. (Orig.). (C). pap. text 30.00 (*0-7881-3357-8*) DIANE Pub.

Cholesterosis - Membrane Cholesterol: Theoretical & Clinical Aspects, Vol. 4. Ed. by Yu. M. Lopukhin et al. 1984. (Physicochemical Biology Reviews Supplement Ser.: Soviet Scientific Reviews, Sect. D). xxii, 382p. text 515.00 (*3-7186-0159-1*) Gordon & Breach.

Choline, Lecithin, Inositol, Vol. 1. Jeffrey Bland. Ed. by Richard A. Passwater. 1983. (Good Health Guides). 30p. pap. 2.95 (*0-87983-277-0*, 32770K, Keats Pubng) McGraw-Hill Trade.

Choline, Phospholipids, Health, & Disease. Ed. by Steven H. Zeisel & Bernard F. Seuhaj. 1998. LC 98-39864. (Illus.). 160p. lib. bdg. 95.00 (*0-935315-86-1*) Am Oil Chemists.

Cholinergic Basis for Alzheimer Therapy. Ed. by Robert E. Becker & Ezio Giacobini. 1991. (Advances in Alzheimer's Disease Therapy Ser.). (Illus.). x, 480p. 96.50 (*0-8176-3566-1*) Birkhauser.

Cholinergic Function & Dysfunction. Ed. by A. Claudio Cuello. 1993. LC 93-2319. (Progress in Brain Research Ser.: Vol. 98). 484p. 273.50 (*0-444-89717-8*) Elsevier.

Cholinergic Synapse. Ed. by V. P. Whittaker. 1988. (Handbook of Experimental Pharmacology Ser.: Vol. 86). (Illus.). 762p. 537.00 (*0-387-18613-1*) Spr-Verlag.

Cholinesterase. 1986. (Monographs in Human Genetics: Vol. 11). x, 134p. 113.25 (*3-8055-4257-7*) S Karger.

Cholinesterase Genes: Multileveled Regulation. Hermona Soreq. Ed. by Haim Zakut. 1990. (Monographs in Human Genetics: Vol. 13). (Illus.). viii, 108p. 85.25 (*3-8055-5137-1*) S Karger.

Cholinesterase Inhibitors in Alzheimer's Disease. 120p. pap. text (*0-86471-066-6*) Adis Intl NZL. *Dist:* Lppncott W & W.

Cholinesterases: Fundamental & Applied Aspects. Ed. by M. Brzin et al. 1984. LC 84-12062. xiv, 527p. 152.35 (*3-11-009873-3*) De Gruyter.

Choose Health, Choose Lean: A Guide for a Supermarket Lean Meat Nutrition Education Program. California Project Lean Staff. Ed. by Prudence Breitrose. 1992. 84p. (Orig.). pap. 19.50 (*1-879552-09-4*) SCRDP.

Choose Life. James J. Mulligan. 1991. LC 91-31394. 383p. pap. text 17.95 (*0-935372-31-8*) NCBC.

Choose Life & Not Death: A Primer on Abortion, Euthanasia, & Suicide. William F. Maestri. 1986. LC 85-28687. pap. 9.95 (*0-8189-0490-9*) Alba.

***Choose Life Diets: Patients Teaching Manual.** Vinola Fowler. 2001. text (*0-9704354-0-1*) SHE.

Choose to Be Healthy. Susan S. Jones. 1995. LC 86-26842. 264p. pap. 11.95 (*0-89087-482-4*) Celestial Arts.

Choose to Live: An AIDS Healing Companion. Laurence E. Badgley. 1993. LC 87-81624. 70p. pap. 13.95 (*0-941523-01-2*) Human Energy Pr.

Choosing: A Better Way to Live. Richard C. Nelson. 1978. LC 78-67188. (Illus.). pap. 5.95 (*0-932570-00-3*) Guidelines Pr.

Choosing a Health Plan: Providing Medicare Beneficiaries with the Right Tools: Congressional Hearing. Ed. by Charles E. Grassley. 2000. (Illus.). 135p. reprint ed. pap. text 25.00 (*0-7881-8685-X*) DIANE Pub.

Choosing a Nurse-Midwife: Your Guide to Safe, Sensitive Care During Pregnancy & the Birth of Your Child. Catherine Poole & Elizabeth Parr. 1994. LC 93-33105. 200p. pap. 12.95 (*0-471-58452-5*) Wiley.

Choosing a Practice. Kronhaus. 1993. 161p. 48.95 (*0-387-97164-5*) Spr-Verlag.

Choosing a Wheelchair System. Ed. by Seldon P. Todd, Jr. 1993. (Illus.). 118p. (Orig.). (C). pap. text 30.00 (*1-56806-213-3*) DIANE Pub.

Choosing & Using an HMO. Ellyn Spragins. 1998. LC 97-33612. (Bloomberg Personal Bookshelf Ser.). (Illus.). 272p. 19.95 (*1-57660-010-6*) Bloomberg NJ.

Choosing Assisted Reproduction: Social, Emotional & Ethical Considerations. Susan L. Cooper & Ellen S. Glazer. 1998. LC 97-36563. 400p. 24.95 (*0-944934-19-6*) Perspect Indiana.

Choosing Life: Guidelines to Avoiding Extinction. 1997. (Illus.). 176p. (Orig.). pap. text 24.95 (*0-9659224-0-5*) LifeWays Pr.

Choosing Medical Care in Old Age: What Kind, How Much, When to Stop. Muriel R. Gillick. 1994. LC 94-11333. 208p. text 19.95 (*0-674-12812-5*, GILCHO) HUP.

Choosing Unsafe Sex: AIDS-Risk Denial among Disadvantaged Women. Elisa J. Sobo. 1995. (Illus.). 256p. pap. text 14.95 (*0-8122-1553-2*) U of Pa Pr.

Choosing Waterbirth: Reclaiming the Sacred Power of Birth. Lakshmi Bertram. 2000. (Illus.). 160p. pap. 14.95 (*1-57174-152-6*) Hampton Roads Pub Co.

Choosing Who's to Live: Ethics & Aging. Ed. by James W. Walters. 1996. LC 95-41785. 224p. pap. text 16.95 (*0-252-06541-7*) U of Ill Pr.

Chopra Center Herbal Handbook: Forty Natrual Prescriptions for Natural Health. David Simon & Deepak Chopra. 2000. LC 00-24451. (Illus.). xi, 260p. pap. 14.95 (*0-609-80390-5*, Three Riv Pr) Crown Pub Group.

Choreocapillaries & Pigment Epithelium Involvements in Macular Diseases: Proceedings of the Jules Gonin Club, 12th Meeting, Crans, Montana, March 1980. Gonin, Jules, Club Staff. Ed. by A. Wessing. 1981. (Journal: Vol. 183, No. 1). (Illus.). ii, 52p. pap. 38.50 (*3-8055-3457-4*) S Karger.

Choreography of Object Relations. Penny Lewis & David L. Singer. 1982. LC 82-73067. 196p. (C). pap. text 9.95 (*1-881245-06-3*) Antioch New Eng.

Chorionic Villi Sampling (CVS) Ed. by G. Pescia & H. Nguyen The. 1986. (Contributions to Gynecology & Obstetrics Ser.: Vol. 15). (Illus.). viii, 116p. 69.75 (*3-8055-4326-3*) S Karger.

***Christ-Centered Therapy: Empowering the Self.** Ed. by Russ Harris. 2001. LC 2001-24394. (Illus.). 275p. text 49.95 (*0-7890-1227-8*); pap. text 24.95 (*0-7890-1228-6*) Haworth Pr (Haworth Pastrl).

***Christal - Coping with Spina Bifida.** Karen Snyder Travis. Ed. by Adolph Caso. 2001. LC 2001-18411. (Illus.). 92p. pap. 9.95 (*0-8283-2062-4*) Branden Bks.

Christensen's Physics of Diagnostic Radiology. Thomas S. Curry, III et al. 4th ed. 1990. LC 90-5586. (Illus.). 522p. text 59.00 (*0-8121-1310-1*) Lppncott W & W.

Christian Ethics in Health Care. John Wilkinson. 1990. (C). pap. (*0-905312-35-X*) Arthur James GBR. *Dist:* St Mut.

Christian Family Guide to Healing. Merle E. Koepke. 1994. 176p. reprint ed. 24.00 (*1-891125-02-8*) Hands Jesus.

Christian Healing. Charles Fillmore. 1993. reprint ed. pap. (*1-872736-44-0*) Mandrake Pr GBR. *Dist:* Holmes Pub.

Christian Healing Ministry. Morris Maddocks. 1989. pap. 14.95 (*0-281-04462-7*) Intl Pubs Mktg.

Christian Parenting & Child Care see Parenting & Child Care

Christian Physician Looks at Stress & Healing. Michael F. Elmore & Gary Johnson. 1997. pap. 10.00 (*0-9660594-7-6*) MCK.

Christian Theology & Medical Ethics: Four Contemporary Approaches, Vol. 7. James B. Tubbs, Jr. 1995. LC 95-31705. (Theology & Medicine Ser.). x, 206p. lib. bdg. (*0-7923-3657-7*) Kluwer Academic NLD. *Dist:* Kluwer Academic.

Christian Virtues in Medical Practice. Edmund D. Pellegrino & David C. Thomasma. 1996. LC 94-11007. 176p. 27.95 (*0-87840-566-6*) Georgetown U Pr.

Christianity & Bioethics: Confronting Clinical Issues. Mark W. Foreman. 1999. LC 99-24048. 299p. pap. text 19.99 (*0-89900-755-4*) College Pr Pub.

Christianity & the Environmental Ethos. Ed. by Robert A. Brungs & Marianne Postiglione. 1996. LC 96-222430. (Illus.). 213p. (Orig.). pap. 15.95 (*1-885583-04-4*) ITEST Faith.

Christmas in Purgatory: A Photographic Essay on Mental Retardation. Burton Blatt & Fred Kaplan. 1974. (Illus.). 12.25 (*0-937540-00-5*, HPP-3) Human Policy Pr.

Chrohn's Disease & Ulcerative Colitis. Fred Saibil. 1997. (Your Personal Health Ser.). (Illus.). 176p. (Orig.). pap. 14.95 (*1-55209-114-7*) Firefly Bks Limited.

Chromatin, Vol. 304. Ed. & Pref. by Paul M. Wassarman. 1999. (Methods in Enzymology Ser.: Vol. 304). (Illus.). 815p. 115.00 (*0-12-182205-2*) Acad Pr.

Chromatographic Chiral Separations. Crane & Morris Zief. 1987. (Chromatographic Science Ser.: Vol. 40). (Illus.). 432p. text 210.00 (*0-8247-7786-7*) Dekker.

Chromatographic (Microcolumn) Determination of Hemoglobin A2-2. 1989. (Approved Standard Ser.: Vol. 9). 75.00 (*1-56238-040-0*, H9-A) NCCLS.

Chromatographic Separations of Stereoisomers. Rex W. Souter. 1985. LC 85-7850. 256p. 210.00 (*0-8493-6127-3*, QP519) CRC Pr.

Chromatography & Modification of Nucleosides Pt. C: Modified Nucleosides in Cancer & Normal Metabolism - Methods & Applications. Ed. by C. W. Gehrke & K. C. Kuo. 1990. (Journal of Chromatography Ser.: No. 45C). 452p. 255.75 (*0-444-88598-6*) Elsevier.

Chromium Connection: A Lesson in Nutrition. Betty Kamen. 4th rev. ed. 1994. 202p. pap. 12.95 (*0-944501-08-7*) Nutrition Encounter.

Chromium in Health, Disease & Industry: Index of New Information & Research Bible. Aron R. Sichler. 1994. 150p. 57.50 (*0-7883-0062-8*); pap. 47.50 (*0-7883-0063-6*) ABBE Pubs Assn.

Chromium, Nickel, & Welding. 1990. (IARC Scientific Publications Ser.: Vol. 49). 677p. pap. text 105.00 (*92-832-1249-5*, 1720049) World Health.

Chromosomal Aberrations: Basic & Applied Aspects. Ed. by G. Obe & A. T. Natarajan. 1990. (Illus.). 319p. 159.00 (*0-387-52540-8*) Spr-Verlag.

Chromosomal Alterations: Origin & Significance. Ed. by G. Obe & A. T. Natarajan. 1994. LC 94-8275. (Illus.). 402p. 203.00 (*0-387-57812-9*) Spr-Verlag.

Chromosomal Aspects of the Male Sterility in Mammals: Workshops on Abstracts. Ed. by A. G. Searle & P. De Boer. 1980. (Journal: Vol. 27; No. 4). (Illus.). 84p. pap. 9.75 (*3-8055-1610-X*) S Karger.

Chromosomal Nonhistone Proteins Vol. 4: Structural Association. Ed. by Lubomir S. Hnilica. 1984. 320p. 179.00 (*0-8493-5514-1*, QP625, CRC Reprint) Franklin.

Chromosomal Translocations & Oncogenic Transcription Factors. Ed. by P. K. Vogt & F. J. Rauscher, III. 1997. (Current Topics in Microbiology & Immunology Ser.: Vol. 220). (Illus.). 180p. 134.00 (*3-540-61402-8*) Spr-Verlag.

Chromosomal Variation in Man: A Catalog of Chromosomal Variants & Anomailies. Digamber S. Borgaonkar. 8th ed. 1997. LC 97-37684. 1175p. 200.00 (*0-471-24332-9*, Wiley-Liss) Wiley.

Chromosome. Ed. by J. S. Heslop-Harrison & R. Flavell. 1993. (Illus.). 302p. (*1-872748-32-5*) Bios Sci GBR. *Dist:* Coronet Bks.

Chromosome Abnormalities & Genetic Counseling. R. J. M. Gardner & G. R. Sutherland. 2nd ed. 1996. (Oxford Monographs on Medical Genetics: No. 29). (Illus.). 496p. (C). text 59.50 (*0-19-510615-6*) OUP.

Chromosome Analysis Protocols. Ed. by John R. Gosden. 1994. LC 93-34459. (Methods in Molecular Biology Ser.: Vol. 29). 508p. 109.50 (*0-89603-289-2*) Humana.

Chromosome Analysis Protocols. Ed. by Ernst-Jan Speel & A. H. N. Hopman. 2nd ed. 2001. (Methods in Molecular Biology Ser.). 425p. 89.50 (*0-89603-792-4*) Humana.

Chromosome Structure & Function: Impact of New Concepts. J. P. Gustafson & R. Appels. 1988. LC 88-17814. (Stadler Genetics Symposia Ser.). (Illus.). 342p. (C). text 105.00 (*0-306-42933-0*) Plenum.

Chromosomes & Genes in Acute Lumphoblastic Leukemia. Lorna M. Secker-Walker. 1997. (Medical Intelligence Unit Ser.). 250p. (C). pap. 89.95 (*0-412-10761-9*) Chapman & Hall.

Chromosomes & Genes in Acute Lymphoblastic Leukemia. Lorna M. Secker-Walker. 1997. LC 96-43702. (Medical Intelligence Unit Ser.). 179p. 99.00 (*1-57059-411-2*, 0-412-10761-9) Landes Bioscience.

Chromosomes in Evolution of Eukaryotic Groups, Vol. I. Arun K. Sharma. 1983. 304p. 151.00 (*0-8493-6496-5*, QH371, CRC Reprint) Franklin.

Chromosomes in Evolution of Eukaryotic Groups, Vol. II. Ed. by Arun K. Sharma & Archana Sharma. 1984. 208p. 159.00 (*0-8493-6497-3*, QH371, CRC Reprint) Franklin.

Chromosomes in Mitosis & Interphase. Ed. by H. G. Schwarzacher. 1976. (Handbuch der Mikroskopischen Anatomie Des Menschen Ser.: Vol. 1, Pt 3). (Illus.). 182p. 108.00 (*0-387-07456-2*) Spr-Verlag.

Chromosomes Today, Vol. 13. Ed. by E. Olmo & C. A. Redi. 2000. (Illus.). 350p. 139.00 (*3-7643-5799-1*) Birkhauser.

Chronic Ambulatory Peritoneal Dialysis (CAPD) And Chronic Cycling Peritoneal Dialysis (CCPD) in Children. Ed. by Richard N. Fine. 1987. (Topics in Renal Medicine Ser.). (C). text 174.00 (*0-89838-859-7*) Kluwer Academic.

Chronic & Acute Leukemias in Adults. Ed. by Clara D. Bloomfield. 1985. (Cancer Treatment & Research Ser.). text 186.00 (*0-89838-702-7*) Kluwer Academic.

Chronic & Recurrent Pain in Children & Adolescents. Ed. by Patrick J. McGrath & G. Allen Finley. 1999. LC 99-23564. (Progress in Pain Research & Management Ser.: Vol. 13). (Illus.). ix, 275p. 67.00 (*0-931092-27-2*) Intl Assn Study Pain.

***Chronic & Terminal Illness: New Perspectives on Caring & Carers.** Ed. by Sheila Payne & Caroline Ellis-Hill. 2001. LC 2001-21774. (Illus.). 170p. (Orig.). pap. 35.00 (*0-19-263167-5*) OUP.

Chronic Anxiety: Generalized Anxiety Disorder & Mixed Anxiety-Depression. Ed. by Ronald M. Rapee & David H. Barlow. 1991. LC 91-24737. 214p. 35.00 (*0-89862-771-0*) Guilford Pubns.

Chronic Aortic Regurgitation. Ed. by William H. Gaasch & Herbert J. Levine. 1988. (Developments in Cardiovascular Medicine Ser.). (C). text 179.50 (*0-89838-364-1*) Kluwer Academic.

Chronic Atrophic Gastritis. F. Di Mario et al. 1991. (Advances in Gastroenterology Ser.: No. 4). 132p. text (*1-57235-020-2*) Piccin Nuova.

Chronic Back Pain: Moving On. Julie Zimmerman. 1991. LC 90-85648. (Illus.). 120p. (Orig.). pap. 9.95 (*1-879418-04-5*) Biddle Pub.

Chronic Bronchitis & Emphysema Handbook. Francois Haas & Shelia S. Haas. 1990. (Science Editions Ser.). 272p. pap. 15.95 (*0-471-62263-X*) Wiley.

Chronic Bronchitis in the 90's Vol. 58, Supp. 1: Journal: Respiration. Ed. by D. Olivieri & Jay A. Nadel. 1991. (Illus.). vi, 58p. pap. 28.00 (*3-8055-5452-4*) S Karger.

Chronic Care Management, a Toolbox for Action. Mary J. Osmick & Linnea Smith Varner. 1999. (Illus.). xiv, 528p. pap. 130.00 (*0-9677724-0-0*) Natl Resource Ctr.

Chronic Childhood Disease: An Introduction to Psychological Theory & Research. Christine Eiser. 1990. 184p. (C). text 59.95 (*0-521-38519-9*); pap. text 19.95 (*0-521-38682-9*) Cambridge U Pr.

Chronic Complications of Diabetes. Ed. by John C. Pickup et al. 1994. LC 93-29976. (Illus.). 336p. 115.00 (*0-632-03795-4*) Blackwell Sci.

Chronic Condition: Why Health Reform Fails. Sherry Glied. 1998. LC 97-23827. (Illus.). 288p. 46.95 (*0-674-12893-1*) HUP.

Chronic Constipation. 1991. lib. bdg. 250.00 (*0-8490-5120-7*) Gordon Pr.

Chronic Disease & Disability: A Contemporary Rehabilitation Approach to the Practice of Medicine. Ed. by Ross M. Hays et al. 1994. LC 94-38226. (Illus.). 296p. pap. text 34.95 (*0-939957-46-9*) Demos Medical.

Chronic Disease Epidemiology & Control. Ed. by Ross C. Brownson et al. 358p. 1993. pap. 35.00 (*0-87553-214-4*, 072); 2nd ed. 1998. LC 98-74062. pap. 45.00 (*0-87553-237-3*) Am Pub Health.

***Chronic Disease Management.** Aspen Health and Administration Development Group. 1995. pap. 252.00 (*0-8342-1749-X*) Aspen Pub.

***Chronic Disease Management.** Health and Science Development Staff. 1997. cd-rom 200.00 (*0-8342-0996-9*) Aspen Pub.

***Chronic Disease Management: Asthma.** Health and Science Development Staff. 1997. disk 50.00 (*0-8342-1001-0*) Aspen Pub.

***Chronic Disease Management: Hypertension.** Health and Science Development Staff. 1997. disk 50.00 (*0-8342-0998-5*) Aspen Pub.

Chronic Disease Management Manual. Aspen Reference Group Staff. 1997. LC 97-2652. ring bd. 179.00 (*0-8342-0872-5*, S315) Aspen Pub.

Chronic Disease Modelling: Measurement & Evaluation of the Risks of Chronic Disease Processes. Kenneth G. Manton & Eric Stallard. 1988. (Charles Griffin Ser.: No. 2). (Illus.). 288p. text 69.00 (*0-19-520617-7*) OUP.

Chronic Disease (1907) W. H. Burgess. 1998. 320p. reprint ed. pap. 24.95 (*0-7661-0516-4*) Kessinger Pub.

Chronic Disease Patient Education Manual. Suzanne Niemeyer & Sara N. Dilima. 1997. LC 97-11530. ring bd. 179.00 (*0-8342-0941-1*, 5459) Aspen Pub.

Chronic Diseases. 1973. (Public Health in Europe Ser.: No. 2). 198p. 20.00 (*92-9020-121-5*, 1320002) World Health.

Chronic Diseases: Perspectives on Behavioral Medicine. Ed. by Marvin Stein & Andrew S. Baum. 1995. (Perspectives on Behavioral Medicine Ser.). 344p. text 69.95 (*0-8058-1855-3*) L Erlbaum Assocs.

Chronic Diseases in the Year 2005, Vol. 1. Chronic Diseases Scenario Committee Staff & A. F. Casparie. 1991. (C). pap. text 97.50 (*0-7923-1377-1*) Kluwer Academic.

Chronic Diseases in the Year Two Thousand Five Vol. 2: Scenarios on Chronic Non-Specific Lung Diseases 1990-2005 Scenario Report Commissioned by the Steering Committee on Future Health Scenarios. Chronic Diseases Scenario Committee Staff. 1993. 245p. (C). pap. text 102.50 (*0-7923-2354-8*) Kluwer Academic.

Chronic Disorders & the Family. Ed. by Froma Walsh & Carol Anderson. 1988. LC 87-31196. (Journal of Psychotherapy & the Family Ser.: Vol. 3, No. 3). (Illus.). 183p. pap. text 19.95 (*0-86656-926-X*); text 49.95 (*0-86656-700-3*) Haworth Pr.

Chronic Fatigue: A Resource Guide to Chronic Fatigue Syndrome, Infectious Diseases Syndrome & Musculoskeletal Diseases. 1991. lib. bdg. 250.00 (*0-8490-5109-6*) Gordon Pr.

Chronic Fatigue: Poisoned by the Mercury in Your Mouth? Annika Jeppsson-McClintock & Christer Malmstrom. rev. ed. 1997. 80p. pap. 6.95 (*0-941011-16-X*) Bio-Probe.

Chronic Fatigue: Self Help Book. Susan M. Lark. 3rd ed. 1995. LC 95-10916. 240p. pap. 16.95 (*0-89087-772-6*) Celestial Arts.

Chronic Fatigue & Its Syndromes. Simon Wessely. 1999. (Illus.). 448p. pap. text 59.95 (*0-19-263046-6*) OUP.

Chronic Fatigue & Related Immune Deficiency Syndromes. Ed. by Paul J. Goodnick & Nancy G. Klimas. 1993. LC 93-9228. (Progress in Psychiatry Ser.: No. 40). 168p. text 31.00 (*0-88048-468-3*, 8468) Am Psychiatric.

Chronic Fatigue Epidemic. 1992. lib. bdg. 250.00 (*0-8490-5240-8*) Gordon Pr.

Chronic Fatigue Syndrome. Jesse A. Stoff & Charles R. Pellegrino. 304th ed. 1992. LC 91-50504. 384p. reprint ed. pap. 14.00 (*0-06-092260-5*, Perennial) HarperTrade.

Chronic Fatigue Syndrome. 1992. lib. bdg. 250.00 (*0-8490-8784-8*) Gordon Pr.

Chronic Fatigue Syndrome. Ed. by David M. Dawson & Thomas D. Sabin. 1993. LC 92-49249. 300p. 74.95 (*0-316-17748-2*, Little Brwn Med Div) Lppncott W & W.

Chronic Fatigue Syndrome. Rona Moss-Morris & Keith J. Petrie. 2001. LC 00-62727. (Experience of Illness Ser.). (Illus.). 168p. pap. 25.95 (*0-415-20240-X*); lib. bdg. 85.00 (*0-415-20239-6*) Routledge.

Chronic Fatigue Syndrome. Ed. by Stephen E. Straus. 1994. LC 94-14914. (Infectious Disease & Therapy Ser.: Vol. 14). (Illus.). 488p. text 165.00 (*0-8247-9187-8*) Dekker.

Chronic Fatigue Syndrome: A Treatment Guide. Erica F. Verrillo & Lauren M. Gellman. 1998. LC 97-39912. 381p. 15.95 (*1-57626-053-4*) Quality Med Pub.

Chronic Fatigue Syndrome: A Victim's Guide to Understanding, Treating & Coping with This Debilitating Illness. Gregg C. Fisher et al. 1989. 224p. pap. 10.99 (*0-446-39004-6*) Warner Bks.

Chronic Fatigue Syndrome: Advances in Epidemiologic, Clinical & Basic Science Research. Ed. by Roberto Patarca-Montero. 1999. LC 99-48701. (Journal of Chronic Fatigue Syndrome Ser.: Vol. 5, Nos. 3/4). 338p. 69.95 (*0-7890-0697-9*); pap. text 29.95 (*0-7890-0821-1*) Haworth Pr.

Chronic Fatigue Syndrome: Charting Your Course to Recovery. Mary E. O'Brien. 1997. LC 97-199925. (Illus.). 100p. pap. 14.25 (*0-9646891-9-7*) Anadem Pubng.

Chronic Fatigue Syndrome: Critical Reviews & Clinical Advances. Ed. by Kenny De Meirleir & Roberto Patarca-Montero. 2000. LC 00-56714. 176p. 49.95 (*0-7890-0998-6*, Hawrth Medical) Haworth Pr.

Chronic Fatigue Syndrome: Proceedings of the Second Farber Center International Conference Held at Bar-Ilan University, Ramat Gan, Israel, December 12-13, 1995. Ed. by Shlomo Yehuda & David I. Mostofsky. 1997. LC 97-7774. (Illus.). 200p. 79.50 (*0-306-45587-0*, Kluwer Plenum) Kluwer Academic.

Chronic Fatigue Syndrome - Symposium No. 173. CIBA Foundation Staff. 1993. LC 00-92. (CIBA Foundation Symposia Ser.: No. 173). 376p. 128.00 (*0-471-93618-9*) Wiley.

Chronic Fatigue Syndrome, AIDS, & Immune Dysfunction Disease: The Cause & the Cure. Suzann M. Angelus. 1994. (Illus.). 240p. (Orig.). pap. 15.95 (*0-9640559-9-6*) Symbolic Prods.

Chronic Fatigue Syndrome & the Yeast Connection: A Get-Well Guide for People with this Often Misunderstood Illness & Those Who Care for Them. William C. Crook. 1992. (Illus.). 400p. (Orig.). pap. 14.95 (*0-933478-20-8*) Prof Bks Future Health.

Chronic Fatigue Syndrome, Fibromyalgia & Other Invisible Illnesses: A Comprehensive & Compassionate Guide. Katrina Berne. 3rd rev. ed. 2000. LC 2001-39721. (Illus.). 352p. pap. 15.95 (*0-89793-280-3*) Hunter Hse.

Chronic Fatigue Syndrome Treatment. Erica F. Verrillo & Lauren M. Gellman. 2nd ed. 1998. LC 97-50214. 404p. pap. 16.95 (*0-312-18066-7*) St Martin.

Chronic Fatigue Syndromes: The Limbic Hypothesis. Jay A. Goldstein. 1993. LC 92-48706. 234p. 49.95 (*1-56024-433-X*); pap. 19.95 (*1-56024-904-8*) Haworth Pr.

Chronic Fatiques Syndrome: Information for Physicians. Ed. by Barry Leonard. 1998. 60p. (C). pap. text 20.00 (*0-7881-4378-6*) DIANE Pub.

Chronic Gastritis-Achlorhydria in the Elderly. Peter R. Holt. 1993. 240p. 189.00 (*0-8493-6970-3*, RC840) CRC Pr.

Chronic Granulocytic Leukemia. Ed. by Michael T. Shaw. 1982. LC 81-23356. 261p. 78.00 (*0-275-91379-1*, C1379, Praeger Pubs) Greenwood.

Chronic Heart Failure. M. Bohm & Erland Erdmann. Ed. by G. Riecker et al. 1997. LC 97-41344. (Illus.). 256p. pap. 66.00 (*3-540-63579-3*) Spr-Verlag.

Chronic Hepatitis: New Concepts of Pathogenesis, Diagnosis & Treatment. H. P. Dienes et al. 2000. (Falk Symposium Ser.: Vol. 116b). 296p. 142.00 (*0-7923-8763-5*) Kluwer Academic.

Chronic Hepatitis: Proceedings of the International Symposium on Problems of Chronic Hepatitis, Montecatini, 1975. International Symposium on Problems of Chronic Hepatitis Staff. Ed. by Paolo Gentilini. 1976. (Illus.). 208p. 85.25 (*3-8055-2321-1*) S Karger.

Chronic Hyperandrogenic Anovulation. Ed. by H. J. Coelingh-Bennink et al. 1990. (Illus.). 192p. (C). lib. bdg. 85.95 (*1-85070-322-1*, Parthenon Pbng) CRC Pr.

Chronic Illness. Ilene Lubkin & Pamela Larsen. 4th ed. 1998. LC 98-14256. (Nursing Ser.). (Illus.). 608p. (C). text 60.95 (*0-7637-0549-7*, 0549-7) Jones & Bartlett.

***Chronic Illness.** Ilene Morof Lubkin & Pamala D. Larsen. 5th ed. 2001. (Illus.). 608p. (C). text 58.95 (*0-7637-1570-0*, 1570-0) Jones & Bartlett.

Chronic Illness: From Experience to Policy. Ed. by S. Kay Toombs et al. 1995. LC 94-30389. (Medical Ethics Ser.). 224p. 29.95 (*0-253-36011-0*) Ind U Pr.

Chronic Illness: Impact & Interventions. Ilene M. Lubkin. 3rd ed. 1995. LC 94-37265. (Series in Nursing). (Illus.). 592p. text 49.95 (*0-86720-712-4*, 712-4) Jones & Bartlett.

*__Chronic Illness: Living with a Thorn.__ Karlton Douglas. 2001. 100p. pap. 16.00 (*0-7388-6506-0*) Xlibris Corp.

Chronic Illness: Research & Theory for Nursing Practice. Ruth Bernstein Hyman & Juliet M. Corbin. 2000. LC 00-22099. x, 316p. (*0-8261-1353-2*) Springer Pub.

Chronic Illness & Disabilities in Childhood & Adolescence. Ed. by Robert Blum. 1984. 496p. text 63.00 (*0-8089-1635-1*, 790624, Grune & Strat) Harcrt Hlth Sci Grp.

Chronic Illness & Disability Through the Life Span: Effects on Self & Family, No. 7. Ed. by Myron G. Eisenberg et al. 1984. (Series on Rehabilitation: Vol. 4). 304p. (C). 42.95 (*0-8261-4180-3*) Springer Pub.

Chronic Illness & Retirement in Jamaica. Sudhanshu Handa & Monica Neitzert. 1998. LC 97-38752. (Living Standards Measurement Study Working Papers: No. 131). 64p. pap. 22.00 (*0-8213-4087-5*, 14087) World Bank.

Chronic Illness & the Older Adult Vol. II: Advances in Gerontological Nurses. Ed. by Elizabeth A. Swanson & Toni Trip-Reimer. 1997. (Illus.). 234p. 41.95 (*0-8261-9111-8*) Springer Pub.

Chronic Illness & Uncertainty: A Personal & Professional Guide to Poorly Understood Syndromes. Don L. Goldenberg. 1996. LC 96-92858. (Illus.). (Orig.). pap. 16.50 (*0-9656102-0-9*) Dorset Pr MA.

Chronic Illness in Children & Adults: A Psychosocial Approach. Ed. by Debra P. Hymovich & Gloria A. Hagopian. 1991. (Illus.). 344p. pap. text 44.00 (*0-7216-2355-7*) Saunders.

Chronic Illness in Young Children. Ed. by David W. Kaplan. 1988. (Journal: Vol. 15, No. 1-2). (Illus.). 108p. 63.50 (*3-8055-4813-3*) S Karger.

Chronic Illness Trajectory Frameworks: The Corbin & Strauss Nursing Model. Ed. by Pierre Woog. 1992. LC 91-5198. 112p. 25.95 (*0-8261-8000-0*) Springer Pub.

Chronic Infection, Chlamydia & Coronary Heart Disease. Sandeep Gupta. 1999. LC 99-29127. (Cardiovascular Medicine Developments Ser.). xiv, 144p. (*0-7923-5797-3*) Kluwer Academic.

Chronic Inflammation in Hemodialysis. Ed. by J. Botella et al. 2000. (Blood Purification Ser.: Vol. 18, No. 3). (Illus.). vi, 78p. 98.00 (*3-8055-7083-X*) S Karger.

Chronic Inflammation of the Bronchi: Proceedings of the Gesellschaft fuer Lungen und Atmungsforschung, Bochum, 1969. Societas Europaea Physiologiae Clinicae Respirator. Ed. by W. T. Ulmer. 1971. (Progress in Respiratory Research Ser.: Vol. 6). 139.25 (*3-8055-1189-2*) S Karger.

Chronic Inflammatory Bowel Disease: Proceedings of the Falk Symposium Held in Lubeck, Germany, 4-5, March 1994. Ed. by E. F. Stange. 1995. LC 94-39943. 224p. (C). text 99.50 (*0-7923-8876-3*) Kluwer Academic.

Chronic Ischemic Heart Disease. George A. Beller. 1995. LC 95-1751. (Atlas of Heart Diseases Ser.: Vol. 5). (Illus.). 264p. text 134.00 (*1-878132-29-6*) Current Med.

Chronic Ischemic Heart Disease (Atlas of Heart Disease), Vol. 5. Ed. by Eugene Braunwald. 1996. 210.00 (*1-57340-060-2*) Current Med.

Chronic Kids, Constant Hope: Help & Encouragement for Parents of Kids with Chronic Conditions. Elizabeth M. Hoekstra & Mary M. Bradford. 2000. LC 00-9201. 240p. pap. 12.99 (*1-58134-184-9*) Crossway Bks.

Chronic Leukemia: Approach to Diagnosis. Harold R. Schumacher & James D. Cotelingam. 1993. LC 94-27327. (Illus.). 392p. 82.00 (*0-89640-220-7*) Igaku-Shoin.

Chronic Leukemias & Lymphomas: Clinical Management. Ed. by Gary J. Schiller. 2001. (Current Clinical Oncology Ser.). 300p. 135.00 (*0-89603-907-2*) Humana.

Chronic Liver Disease. Ed. by M. U. Dianzani & Paolo Gentilini. 1986. (Frontiers of Gastrointestinal Research Ser.: Vol. 9). (Illus.). x, 282p. 170.50 (*3-8055-4205-4*) S Karger.

Chronic Low Back Pain: Assessment & Treatment from a Behavioral Rehabilitation Perspective. J. W. Vlaeyen. 1991. (Series in Rehabilitation Research: Vol. 1). xvi, 264p. pap. (*90-265-1173-6*) Swets.

Chronic Lung Disease in Early Infancy. R. D. Bland & J. J. Coalson. 1999. LC 99-37342. (Lung Biology in Health & Disease Ser.: Vol. 137). (Illus.). 1096p. text 250.00 (*0-8247-9871-6*) Dekker.

Chronic Lymphocytic Leukemia Aaron Polliack & D. Catovsky. 1988. xii, 390p. text 240.00 (*3-7186-4802-4*) Gordon & Breach.

Chronic Lymphocytic Leukemia: Scientific Advances & Clinical Development. Ed. by Bruce D. Cheson. 1992. LC 92-49857. (Basic & Clinical Oncology Ser.: Vol. 1). (Illus.). 440p. text 165.00 (*0-8247-8736-6*) Dekker.

Chronic Mental Illness in Children & Adolescents. Ed. by John G. Looney. 1988. LC 87-1472. 267p. text 14.95 (*0-88048-236-2*, 8236) Am Psychiatric.

Chronic Mental Patient. Ed. by John A. Talbott. 1984. 368p. text 44.00 (*0-8089-1649-1*, 794502, Grune & Strat) Harcrt Hlth Sci Grp.

Chronic Mentally Ill: Treatment, Programs, Systems. Ed. by John Talbott. 1981. LC 80-24874. 374p. 45.95 (*0-87705-086-4*, Kluwer Acad Hman Sci) Kluwer Academic.

Chronic Mercury Toxicity: New Hope Against an Endemic Disease. H.L. Sam Queen. 1988. (Doctor's Guide for Lifestyle Counseling Ser.: Vol. 1). (Illus.). 302p. (C). text 45.00 (*0-9620479-1-0*) Inst for Health Real.

Chronic Muscle Pain Syndrome. Paul Davidson. 1991. 272p. pap. 6.50 (*0-425-12775-3*) Berkley Pub.

Chronic Muscle Pain Syndrome: How to Recognize & Treat It & Feel Better All Over! Paul Davidson. 2001. LC 00-65191. 272p. reprint ed. pap. 14.00 (*0-425-18180-4*) Berkley Pub.

Chronic Musculoskeletal Injuries in the Workplace. Don Ranney. Ed. by Richard Lampert. 1996. 400p. pap. text 54.00 (*0-7216-6841-0*) Saunders.

Chronic Myelogenous Leukemia: Molecular Approaches. Deisseroth & Ralph B. Arlinghaus. 1990. (Hematology Ser.: Vol. 13). (Illus.). 504p. text 215.00 (*0-8247-8352-2*) Dekker.

Chronic Non-Cancer Pain: Assessment & Practical Management. Ed. by S. Andersson et al. 1987. pap. text 55.50 (*0-7462-0047-1*) Kluwer Academic.

Chronic Obstructive Pulmonary Disease. Ed. by P. M. Calverley & N. B. Pride. 1994. LC 93-71830. (An Arnold Publication). (Illus.). 600p. (*0-412-46450-0*) E A GBR. *Dist:* OUP.

Chronic Obstructive Pulmonary Disease. Ed. by Thomas L. Petty. 2nd ed. 1985. (Lung Biology in Health & Disease Ser.: Vol. 28). (Illus.). 512p. text 215.00 (*0-8247-7385-3*) Dekker.

Chronic Obstructive Pulmonary Disease: A Behavioral Perspective. McSweeny & Grant Staff. 1988. (Lung Biology in Health & Disease Ser.: Vol. 36). (Illus.). 336p. text 175.00 (*0-8247-7693-3*) Dekker.

Chronic Obstructive Pulmonary Disease: Current Concepts. John E. Hodgkin & Thomas L. Petty. 1987. (Illus.). 334p. pap. text 52.00 (*0-7216-1897-9*) Saunders.

Chronic Obstructive Pulmonary Disease No. 234: Pathogenesis to Treatment. William MacNee & Novartis Foundation Symposium Staff. 234th ed. 2001. LC 00-63291. (Novartis Foundation Symposium Ser.: Vol. 234). (Illus.). 296p. 125.00 (*0-471-49437-2*) Wiley.

*__Chronic Obstructive Pulonary Disease.__ William MacNee & Rennard. 2002. (Fast Facts Ser.). (Illus.). pap. (*1-899541-99-3*) Health Pr GBR. *Dist:* JAMCO Dist.

Chronic Pain. 1984. lib. bdg. 79.95 (*0-87700-540-0*) Revisionist Pr.

Chronic Pain. Rowbotham. 2000. (*1-85317-878-0*) Martin Dunitz GBR. *Dist:* Blackwell Sci.

Chronic Pain. Ed. by Thomas W. Miller. 1990. Vol. I. 400p. 57.50 (*0-8236-0850-6*); Vol. II. 550p. 77.50 (*0-8236-0851-4*) Intl Univs Pr.

Chronic Pain: A Family Matter. Barbara J. Headley. Ed. by J. David Haddox. 1988. (Illus.). 40p. (Orig.). pap. text 5.00 (*0-929538-01-3*) Innovat Systems.

Chronic Pain: A Handbook for Nurses. Marcus Munafo. 2000. LC 00-23641. (Illus.). 192p. pap. text 35.00 (*0-7506-4120-7*) Buttrwrth-Heinemann.

Chronic Pain: Diagnosis, Assessment, & Management. Michael Margoles & Richard Weiner. 1998. LC 99-174421. 528p. 79.95 (*1-57444-103-5*, SL1035) St Lucie Pr.

Chronic Pain: Taking Command of Our Healing: Understanding the Emotional Trauma Underlying Chronic Pain. William R. B. Anderson & Jesse F. Taylor. 1995. (Illus.). 130p. (Orig.). pap. 10.95 (*0-9642979-0-6*) New Energy Pr.

Chronic Pain: The Complete Guide to Relief. Arthur C. Klein. 2001. 320p. pap. 14.00 (*0-7867-0834-4*) Carroll & Graf.

Chronic Pain: The Natural Way of Healing. Natural et al. 1995. LC 95-157965. (Natural Way of Healing Ser.). 352p. mass mkt. 5.99 (*0-440-21658-3*) Dell.

Chronic Pain: The Psychotherapeutic Spectrum. Anthony Bellissimo & Eldon Tunks. 1984. LC 84-9909. 384p. 93.95 (*0-275-91422-4*, C1422, Praeger Pubs) Greenwood.

Chronic Pain & Old Age: An Integrated Biopsychosocial Perspective. Ed. by Ranjan Roy. 1995. LC 95-166830. 380p. pap. 19.95 (*0-8020-7359-X*) U of Toronto Pr.

Chronic Pain & the Family: A Problem-Centered Perspective. R. Roy. 1989. (Illus.). 256p. 32.95 (*0-89885-443-1*, Kluwer Acad Hman Sci) Kluwer Academic.

Chronic Pain Control Workbook: A Step-by-Step Guide for Coping with & Overcoming Pain. Ellen M. Catalano & Kimeron N. Hardin. 2nd rev. ed. 1996. LC 96-67938. (Illus.). 252p. pap. 18.95 (*1-57224-050-4*) New Harbinger.

Chronic Pain Evaluation: A Valid, Standardized Assessment Instrument. Karen S. Rucker. 2000. LC 00-25645. (Illus.). 176p. pap. text 44.99 (*0-7506-7121-1*) Buttrwrth-Heinemann.

Chronic Pain in Old Age: An Integrated Biopsychosocial Perspective. Ed. by Ranjan Roy. 1995. LC 95-166830. 500p. text 50.00 (*0-8020-2859-4*) U of Toronto Pr.

Chronic Pain Management for Physical Therapists. Ed. by Harriet Wittink & Theresa H. Michel. 1997. LC 97-4332. 282p. pap. text 49.99 (*0-7506-9740-7*) Buttrwrth-Heinemann.

Chronic Pain Management Sourcebook. David Drum. 1999. LC 99-21948. xiv, 349p. pap. 18.95 (*0-7373-0101-5*, 01015W) NTC Contemp Pub Co.

Chronic Pain Patient. Philip L. Gildenberg. Ed. by R. A. DeVaul. 1984. (Pain & Headache Ser.: Vol. 7). (Illus.). viii, 148p. 55.00 (*3-8055-3911-8*) S Karger.

Chronic Pancreatitis: Erice, Italy, 14-15 October 1996. Ed. by Eugene P. DiMagno. 1998. (Science & Culture Ser.). 600p. 110.00 (*981-02-3440-6*) World Scientific Pub.

Chronic Pancreatitis: Research & Clinical Management. Ed. by H. G. Beger et al. 1990. (Illus.). 574p. 139.00 (*0-387-52034-1*) Spr-Verlag.

Chronic Pelvic Pain: An Integrated Approach. John F. Steege et al. Ed. by William Schmitt. 1997. LC 97-7203. (Illus.). 352p. text 60.00 (*0-7216-6529-2*) Saunders.

Chronic Pelvic Pain: Evaluation & Management. Ed. by Richard E. Blackwell & David L. Olive. 1997. LC 97-9562. (Illus.). 225p. 69.00 (*0-387-98207-8*) Spr-Verlag.

Chronic Physical Illness & Depression among Ethnic Minority Elderly. Janet L. Bell. 1992. LC 91-37482. (Studies on the Elderly in America). 168p. text 25.00 (*0-8153-0513-3*) Garland.

Chronic Psychiatric Patient in the Community: Principles of Treatment. Ed. by I. Barofsky & R. D. Budson. 1983. LC 82-7338. 570p. text 57.95 (*0-88331-117-8*) R B Luce.

Chronic Pulmonary Conditions in Children: Case Studies for Nutrition Management. Sherie Sondel. 1999. LC 99-51563. ix, 91p. pap. (*0-88091-182-4*) Am Dietetic Assn.

Chronic Pulmonary Hyperinflation. Ed. by A. Grassino et al. 1991. (Current Topics in Rehabilitation Ser.). (Illus.). 175p. 64.95 (*0-387-19662-5*) Spr-Verlag.

Chronic Renal Failure. Ed. by Graeme R. Catto. 1988. (New Clinical Applications in Nephrology Ser.). (C). text 134.50 (*0-7462-0048-X*) Kluwer Academic.

Chronic Renal Failure. Ed. by F. Santos & S. Malaga. 1991. (Journal of Child Nephrology & Urology: Vol. 11, No. 3, 1991). (Illus.). 68p. pap. 53.25 (*3-8055-5527-X*) S Karger.

Chronic Respiratory Illness. Simon Williams. 1993. LC 92-39592. (Experience of Illness Ser.). x, 145p. (*0-415-09697-9*) Tavistock GBR. *Dist:* Routldge.

Chronic Reversible Myocardial Dysfunction: Clinical & Experimental Studies. Bharati Shivalkar. 1998. (Acta Biomedica Lovaniensia Ser.). (Illus.). 135p. pap. (*90-6186-884-X*) Leuven Univ BEL. *Dist:* Coronet Bks.

Chronic Schizophrenia. Thomas Freeman et al. 1966. 25.00 (*0-8236-0860-3*) Intl Univs Pr.

Chronic Venous Insufficiency: Diagnosis & Treatment. Ed. by J. J. Bergan & J. Ballard. 2000. LC 99-22604. xii, 204p. (C). (*1-85233-172-0*) Spr-Verlag GBR. *Dist:* Spr-Verlag.

Chronic Viral Hepatitis: Diagnosis & Therapeutics. Ed. by Raymond S. Koff & George Y. Wu. 2001. (Clinical Gastroenterology Ser.). 352p. 99.50 (*0-89603-880-7*) Humana.

Chronic Wound Care: A Clinical Source Book for Healthcare Professionals. Ed. by Diane Krasner & Dean Kane. 2nd ed. 1997. (Illus.). 500p. 69.95 (*0-9628084-4-X*) Hlth Mngmnt Pubns.

*__Chronic Wound Healing: The Evidence for Change.__ R. Mani. 2002. (Illus.). 450p. 88.95 (*1-84214-084-1*, Parthenon Pbng) CRC Pr.

Chronically Evolving Viral Hepatitis. Ed. by C. De Bac et al. 1992. LC 92-2366. (Archives of Virology Ser.: Suppl. 4). (Illus.). 250p. 189.00 (*0-387-82350-6*) Spr-Verlag.

Chronically Mentally Ill: Assessing Community Support Programs. Richard Tessler & Howard H. Goldman. 1982. LC 82-3884. 240p. text 34.95 (*0-88410-379-X*, HarpBusn) HarpInfo.

Chronicle: The Human Side of AIDS. Mike Greenly. 1986. LC 86-10643. 422p. 20.95 (*0-8290-1800-X*) Irvington.

Chronicle Health Occupations Guidebook. Ed. by Paul Downes. rev. ed. 1994. (Illus.). 100.65 (*1-55631-017-X*) Chron Guide.

Chronicles of Drug Discovery, Vol. 3. Ed. by Daniel Lednicer. 1993. LC 81-11471. (ACS Professional Reference Bk.). (Illus.). 350p. 95.00 (*0-8412-2523-0*); pap. text 45.00 (*0-8412-2733-0*) Am Chemical.

Chronicles of the Christmas Reindeer. Wayne Bomar. Ed. by Isabel Anders. 1996. (Illus.). 250p. (Orig.). pap. 14.95 (*1-886371-51-2*) Dragonfire.

Chronisch Kranke Kind. Ed. by S. Fink. 1982. (Paediatrische Fortbildungskurse fuer die Praxis Ser.: Vol. 54). (Illus.). 90p. pap. 28.75 (*3-8055-3422-1*) S Karger.

Chronobiology: Principles & Applications to Shifts in Schedules. Lawrence E. Scheving & Franz Halberg. 1981. (NATO Advanced Study Institutes Ser.: Behavioral Social Sciences, No. 3). 597p. text 184.00 (*90-286-0940-7*) Kluwer Academic.

Chronobiology & Chronomedicine: Basic Research & Applications: Proceedings of the 6th Annual Meeting of the European Society for Chronobiology, Barcelona, 1990. Ed. by Antoni Diez-Noguera & Trinitat Cambras. 1992. LC 92-15665. (Illus.). VIII, 415p. 63.00 (*3-631-44960-7*) P Lang Pubng.

Chronobiology & Chronomedicine: Basic Research & Applications, Proceedings of the 7th Annual Meeting of the European Society for Chronobiology, Marburg, 1991. Ed. by Christoph Gutenbrunner et al. 1993. LC 93-3998. (Illus.). VIII, 708p. 93.00 (*3-631-45239-X*) P Lang Pubng.

Chronology of Medicine & Related Sciences. Leslie T. Morton & Robert J. Moore. 1997. LC 96-42257. 800p. text (*1-85928-215-6*) Scolar Pr GBR. *Dist:* Ashgate Pub Co.

Chronology of Noteworthy Events in American Psychology. Warren R. Street. 1994. LC 94-29690. 425p. 39.95 (*1-55798-267-8*) Am Psychol.

Chronology of Nuclear Medicine. Marshall Brucer. Ed. by Robert R. Buntaine. 1990. (Illus.). 514p. (C). lib. bdg. 55.00 (*0-9625674-0-X*) Heritage MO.

Chumash Healing. Phillip L. Walker & Travis Hudson. 1993. LC 92-62437. 16.95 (*0-939046-33-4*); pap. 12.95 (*0-939046-34-2*) Malki Mus Pr.

Churches & Health Care in the Third World. Ed. by Jean Pirotte & Henri Derroitte. 1991. LC 91-9389. (SCM Ser.: No. 5). (ENG & FRE.). xxvi, 176p. 75.00 (*90-04-09470-9*) Brill Academic Pubs.

Churchill Livingstone Nurse's Dictionary. Churchill Livingstone Staff. 16th ed. 1989. 480p. pap. text (*0-443-02242-9*) Church.

*__Churchill Livingstone's Dictionary of Nursing.__ Ed. by Christine Brooker. 18th ed. 2001. LC 2001-37183. (*0-443-06483-0*) Church.

Churchill Livingstone's International Dictionary of Homeopathy. Jeremy Swayne. 2000. LC 99-89779. 288p. (*0-443-06009-6*) Church.

Churchill Livingstone's Medical Word Guide. 1991. 340p. pap. text (*0-443-08833-0*) Church.

Churchill Pocketbook of Oncology. Barr. 1997. pap. text 23.95 (*0-443-05102-X*) Saunders.

Churchill's Clinical Microbiology. Inglis. 1998. (C). pap. text (*0-443-05913-6*) Church.

Churchill's Clinical Pharmacology. Walker. 1998. (C). pap. text (*0-443-05536-X*) Church.

Churchill's Doctor: A Biography of Lord Moran. Richard Lovell. 1993. (Illus.). 457p. 49.00 (*1-85070-485-6*, Parthenon Pbng) CRC Pr.

*__Churchill's Doctor: A Biography of Lord Moran.__ Richard Lovell. 1992. (History of Medicine Ser.). 457p. pap. (*1-85315-183-1*) Royal Soc of Medicine Pr Ltd GBR. *Dist:* Balogh.

Churchill's House Physician's Survival Guide. Roger A. Fisken. 1995. LC 94-26803. 271p. pap. text (*0-443-04895-9*) Church.

Churchill's House Surgeon's Survival Guide. Henry K. Gompertz et al. 1992. LC 92-22883. 338p. pap. text (*0-443-04342-6*) Church.

Churchill's House Surgeon's Survival Guide. G. Henry K. Gompertz & Michael Rhodes. 2nd ed. 2000. LC 92-22883. 350p. Price not set. (*0-443-06223-4*) Harcrt Hlth Sci Grp.

*__Churchill's Mastery of Dentistry Vol. 1: Oral Pathology, Surgery & Medicine.__ P. Coulthard. 2001. (Illus.). 220p. pap. (*0-443-06192-0*) Church GBR. *Dist:* Saunders.

Churchill's Medical Dictionary. 1989. (Illus.). 2121p. text (*0-443-08691-5*) Church.

Churchill's Pocketbook of Cardiology. Neil R. Grubb & David E. Newby. 2000. LC 99-89463. (*0-443-06221-8*) Harcrt Hlth Sci Grp.

Churchill's Pocketbook of Clinical Dentistry. I. G. Chestnutt & J. Gibson. 1997. LC 97-6335. 478p. pap. text (*0-443-05375-8*) Church.

Churchill's Pocketbook of Clinical Microbiology. T. J. Inglis. 1998. LC 97-42804. (*0-443-05914-4*) Church.

Churchill's Pocketbook of Diabetes. Andrew J. Krentz. 2000. 155p. pap. text 24.95 (*0-443-06118-1*) Saunders.

*__Churchill's Pocketbook of Differential Diagnosis.__ Andrew T. Raftery. 2000. 501p. (*0-443-06260-9*) Church GBR. *Dist:* Saunders.

Churchill's Pocketbook of General Practice. Stephen Cartwright & C. J. Godlee. 1998. 296p. pap. (*0-443-04863-0*) Church.

Churchill's Pocketbook of Intensive Care. Simon M. Whiteley et al. 1998. LC 97-28647. (C). pap. text (*0-443-05363-4*) Church.

*__Churchill's Pocketbook of Medicine.__ P. Hayes et al. 2001. 445p. (*0-443-06498-9*) Church GBR. *Dist:* Saunders.

Churchill's Pocketbook of Medicine. Peter C. Hayes. 1997. LC 96-26059. 417p. pap. text (*0-443-05365-0*) Church.

Churchill's Pocketbook of Medicine. Peter C. Hayes et al. 2nd ed. 1996. LC 96-6479. (*0-443-05325-1*) Church.

Churchill's Pocketbook of Obstetrics & Gynaecology. B. Magowan. 1996. (Illus.). 241p. pap. (*0-443-05483-5*) Church.

Churchill's Pocketbook of Obstetrics & Gynaecology. Brian Magowan. 1996. LC 96-5330. (*0-463-05483-0*) Church.

Churchill's Pocketbook of Obstetrics & Gynaecology. Brian Magowan. 2nd ed. 2000. LC 99-89414. (Illus.). xv, 278p. (*0-443-06424-5*); (*0-443-06423-7*) Harcrt Hlth Sci Grp.

Churchill's Pocketbook of Pain. Catherine F. Stannard & Sara Booth. 1998. LC 97-43466. (C). pap. text (*0-443-05322-7*) Church.

Churchill's Pocketbook of Surgery. A. T. Raftery. 1996. pap. text 28.00 (*0-443-05057-0*) Saunders.

*__Churchill's Pocketbook of Surgery.__ Andrew Raftery. 2001. (Illus.). 523p. (*0-443-07042-3*) Church GBR. *Dist:* Saunders.

*__Churchill's Pocketbook of Toxicology.__ Alison Jones & Paul Dargan. 2001. (Illus.). 251p. pap. (*0-443-06476-8*) Church GBR. *Dist:* Saunders.

Chyrology for the Deaf: Reading, Spelling & Ciphering by the Fingers. T. M. Lucas. 1972. 250.00 (*0-87968-054-7*) Gordon Pr.

CIBA Collection of Medical Illustrations, Set. Illus. by Frank H. Netter. Incl. Ciba Collection of Medical Illustrations Pt. I: Nervous System: Anatomy & Physiology. 1997. 50.00 (*0-914168-10-X*); Vol. 1, Pt. 2. Ciba Collection of Medical Illustrations Vol. 1, Pt. II: Nervous System: Neurologic & Neuromuscular Disorders. 1997. 52.00 (*0-914168-11-8*); Vol. 3. Ciba Collection of Medical Illustrations Vol. 3, Pt. I: Digestive System; Upper Digestive Tract. 1997. 39.00 (*0-914168-03-7*); Vol. 3, Pt. 2. Ciba Collection of Medical Illustrations Vol. 3, Pt. II: Digestive System: Lower Digestive Tract. 1997. 41.00 (*0-914168-04-5*); Vol. 3, Pt. 3. Digestive System Vol. 3, Pt. III: Liver, Biliary Tract & Pancreas. 1957. 38.00 (*0-914168-05-3*); Vol. 4. Ciba Collection of Medical Illustrations Endocrine System & Selected Metabolic Diseases: Endocrine System & Selected Metabolic Diseases. 1997. 47.50 (*0-914168-06-1*); Vol. 5. Ciba Collection of Medical Illustrations. 1997. lib. bdg. 55.00 (*0-914168-07-X*); Vol. 6. Ciba Collection of Medical Illustrations: Kidneys, Ureters & Urinary Bladder. 1997. 55.00 (*0-914168-08-8*); Vol. 7. Ciba Collection of Medical Illustrations: Respiratory System. 1997. 55.00 (*0-914168-09-6*); Vol. 8, Pt. 1. Ciba Collection of Medical Illustrations Vol. 8, Pt. I: Musculoskeletal System: Anatomy, Physiology & Metabolic Disorders. 1997. 55.00 (*0-914168-14-2*); Vol. 8, Pt. II. Ciba Collection of Medical Illustrations: Musculoskeletal System: Developmental Disorders, Tumors, Rheumatic Diseases & Joint Replacement. 1997. 58.50 (*0-914168-15-0*); LC 53-2151. (Illus.). 1997. 425.00 (*0-914168-00-2*) Icon Lrning Systs.

Ciba Collection of Medical Illustrations, Vol. 5. Illus. by Frank H. Netter. 1997. LC 53-2151. lib. bdg. 55.00 (*0-914168-07-X*) Icon Lrning Systs.

Ciba Collection of Medical Illustrations: Kidneys, Ureters & Urinary Bladder, Vol. 6. Illus. by Frank H. Netter. 1997. LC 53-2151. 55.00 (*0-914168-08-8*) Icon Lrning Systs.

Ciba Collection of Medical Illustrations: Musculoskeletal System: Developmental Disorders, Tumors, Rheumatic Diseases & Joint Replacement, Vol. 8, Pt. II. Illus. by Frank H. Netter. 1997. LC 53-2151. 58.50 (*0-914168-15-0*) Icon Lrning Systs.

Ciba Collection of Medical Illustrations: Respiratory System, Vol. 7. Illus. by Frank H. Netter. 1997. LC 53-2151. 55.00 (*0-914168-09-6*) Icon Lrning Systs.

Ciba Collection of Medical Illustrations Pt. I: Nervous System: Anatomy & Physiology. Illus. by Frank H. Netter. 1997. LC 53-2151. 50.00 (*0-914168-10-X*) Icon Lrning Systs.

Ciba Collection of Medical Illustrations Vol. 1, Pt. II: Nervous System: Neurologic & Neuromuscular Disorders, Vol. 1, Pt. 2. Illus. by Frank H. Netter. 1997. LC 53-2151. 52.00 (*0-914168-11-8*) Icon Lrning Systs.

Ciba Collection of Medical Illustrations Vol. 3, Pt. I: Digestive System; Upper Digestive Tract, Vol. 3. Illus. by Frank H. Netter. 1997. LC 53-2151. 39.00 (*0-914168-03-7*) Icon Lrning Systs.

Ciba Collection of Medical Illustrations Vol. 3, Pt. II: Digestive System: Lower Digestive Tract, Vol. 3, Pt. 2. Illus. by Frank H. Netter. 1997. LC 53-2151. 41.00 (*0-914168-04-5*) Icon Lrning Systs.

Ciba Collection of Medical Illustrations Vol. 8, Pt. I: Musculoskeletal System: Anatomy, Physiology & Metabolic Disorders, Vol. 8, Pt. 1. Illus. by Frank H. Netter. 1997. LC 53-2151. 55.00 (*0-914168-14-2*) Icon Lrning Systs.

Ciba Collection of Medical Illustrations Endocrine System & Selected Metabolic Diseases: Endocrine System & Selected Metabolic Diseases, Vol. 4. Illus. by Frank H. Netter. 1997. LC 53-2151. 47.50 (*0-914168-06-1*) Icon Lrning Systs.

CIBA Vision Symposium: 12th Symposium, Osaka/Tokyo, November 1999: Proceedings. Ed. by Y. Oguchi & Y. Honda. 2001. (Opthalmologica Ser.: Vol. 215, Suppl. 1, 2001). (Illus.). iv, 54p. 25.25 (*3-8055-7204-2*) S Karger.

*__Ciba Vision Symposium: 13th Symposium, Tokyo/osaka, November-december 2000: Proceedings.__ Ed. by Y. Honda & Y. Oguchi. 2001. (Illus.). 44p. pap. 25.25 (*3-8055-7368-5*) S Karger.

CIC Handbook. Ed. by Marshall Chasin. 1997. LC 97-11451. (Illus.). 240p. (Orig.). pap. 39.95 (*1-56593-829-1*, 1596) Thomson Learn.

Cicatrising Conjunctivitis. Ed. by Wolfgang Bernauer et al. 1997. LC 97-28508. (Developments in Ophthalmology Ser.: Vol. 28, 1997). (Illus.). xvi, 266p. 248.00 (*3-8055-6443-0*) S Karger.

Ciclopidine. Ed. by J. R. O'Brien & Marc Verstraete. 1983. (Journal: Vol. 13, Suppl. 1). (Illus.). ii, 54p. pap. 41.75 (*3-8055-3816-2*) S Karger.

Ciclosporin. Ed. by J. F. Borel. 1986. (Progress in Allergy Ser.: Vol. 38). (Illus.). vi, 474p. 169.75 (*3-8055-4221-6*) S Karger.

Ciclosporin in Pediatric Renal Transplantation. Ed. by Wolff & Provoost. 1986. (Clinical Research Ser.: No. 4). ix, 122p. (Orig.). (C). pap. text (*3-11-013367-9*) Mouton.

Ciclosporin in Renal Transplantation. Ed. by C. Ponticelli & A. De Vecchi. 1987. (Contributions to Nephrology Ser.: Vol. 51). (Illus.). viii, 168p. 29.75 (*3-8055-4357-3*) S Karger.

CIDI Researchers' Manual, Version 1.1. World Health Organization: CIDI Editorial Committe. 1994. pap. text 19.95 (*0-88048-982-0*, 8982) Am Psychiatric.

Cigarette Smoking & the Kidney: Seminar on Cigarette Smoking & Kidney Involvement, Milan, October 1999. Ed. by A. Sessa et al. 2000. LC 00-27362. (Contributions to Nephrology Ser.: Vol. 130). (Illus.). viii, 140p. 147.00 (*3-8055-7064-3*) S Karger.

Ciguatera Poisoning - Traditional Remedies in the South Pacific. see Gratte ou Ciguatera (Ciguatera Poisoning): Ses Remedes Traditionnels dans le Pacifique Sud (Traditional Remedies in the South Pacific)

52 Maneras de Prevenir la Enfermedad Cadriaca. Terry Shintani & J. M. Miller. 1996. (Serie "52 Maneras" Ser.). (SPA.). 150p. pap. 7.99 (*0-88113-353-1*) Caribe Betania.

52 Maneras de Protegerse del Cancer. Terry Shintani & J. M. Miller. 1996. (Serie "52 Maneras" Ser.). (SPA.). 150p. pap. 7.99 (*0-88113-356-6*) Caribe Betania.

CINDI, Countrywide Integrated Noncommunicable Diseases Intervention Programme: Baseline Evaluation. Ed. by F. Gotthard Schettler et al. 1991. (Supplement zu den Sitzungsberichten der Mathematisch-Naturwissenschaftlichen Klasse Ser.). (Illus.). 70p. 15.95 (*0-387-54646-4*) Spr-Verlag.

Cinq Lecons sur la Psychanalyse. Sigmund Freud. 1989. (FRE.). pap. (*0-7859-3037-X*, 2228881260) Fr & Eur.

CIOMS Calendar of Congresses: Bilingual English/French. 1991. pap. text 10.00 (*92-9036-047-X*) World Health.

CIOMS Calendar of Congresses of Medical Sciences 1996. 1996. (FRE.). iv, 67p. (C). pap. text 9.00 (*92-9036-063-1*, 0810057) World Health.

CIOMS Calendar of Congresses of Medical Sciences, 1997. 1997. 62p. pap. 9.00 (*92-9036-065-8*, 0810058) Am Soc Clinical.

Ciprofloxacin: Defining its Role in Serious Infections. C. Garrard. 1995. LC 94-31566. 160p. 32.00 (*0-387-58174-X*) Spr-Verlag.

Circadian Cancer Therapy. Ed. by William J. Krushesky. 1994. LC 93-48014. 298p. lib. bdg. 180.95 (*0-8493-4989-3*) CRC Pr.

Circadian Rhythms in Psychiatry. Ed. by T. A. Wehr & F. K. Goodwin. (Illus.). (Orig.). 28.50 (*0-910286-89-2*) Boxwood.

Circadian Rhythms of Cardiovascular Disoders. Ed. by Prakash C. Deedwania. 1996. LC 96-44295. (Illus.). 240p. 55.00 (*0-87993-632-0*) Futura Pub.

Circadian Variation in Cardiovascular Disease: The Need for Compliance - Journal: Cardiology, Vol. 80, Suppl. 1, 1992. Ed. by F. R. Buehler. 1992. (Illus.). iv, 60p. pap. 20.00 (*3-8055-5613-6*) S Karger.

Circle of Poison: Pesticides & People in a Hungry World. David Weir & Mark Schapiro. 1981. LC 81-13384. 118p. pap. 7.95 (*0-935028-09-9*) Inst Food & Develop.

*__Circulating Nucleic Acids in Plasma or Serum II.__ Ed. by Y. M. Dennis Lo et al. 2001. LC 2001-45285. (Annals of the New York Academy of Sciences Ser.: Vol. 945). (*1-57331-378-5*); pap. (*1-57331-379-3*) NY Acad Sci.

Circulating Regulatory Factors & Neuroendocrine Function. Ed. by J. C. Porter & D. Jezova. 1990. LC 90-7365. (AEMB Ser.). (Illus.). 520p. (C). text 174.00 (*0-306-43609-4*, Kluwer Plenum) Kluwer Academic.

Circulation in Native & Artificial Kidneys: 3rd Annual Symposium on Applied Physiology of the Peripheral Circulation, Barcelona, September 1996. Ed. by Claudio Ronco et al. 1997. (Reprint of Blood Purification Ser.: Vol. 15, Nos. 4-6, 1997). (Illus.). iv, 172p. 78.25 (*3-8055-6599-2*) S Karger.

Circulation in the Female: From the Cradle to the Grave. Ed. by J. Ginsburg. 1989. (Illus.). 174p. 78.00 (*1-85070-210-1*, Parthenon Pbng) CRC Pr.

Circulation of the Blood: Men & Ideas. Ed. by Alfred P. Fishman & Dickinson W. Richards. 1988. (American Physiological Society Book). (Illus.). 879p. text 56.00 (*0-19-520699-1*) OUP.

Circulation Physiology & Medical Chemistry in England, 1650-1680. Audrey B. Davis. 1973. (Illus.). 263p. 17.50 (*0-87291-059-8*) Coronado Pr.

Circulatory Assist & Ballistocardiographic Studies: Proceedings of the Ballistocardiograph Research Society Annual Meeting, 15th, Atlantic City, 1971. Ballistocardiograph Research Society Staff. Ed. by D. H. Jackson. 1972. (Bibliotheca Cardiologica Ser.: No. 29). pap. 34.00 (*3-8055-1323-2*) S Karger.

Circulatory Response to the Upright Posture. Ed. by Smith. 1990. 200p. 99.50 (*0-8493-6518-X*, RC685) CRC Pr.

Circulatory Support Devices in Interventional Cardiology, International Symposium, Goettingen, May 1993: Journal: Reprint of Cardiology 1994, Vol. 84, No. 3. Ed. by H. R. Figulla & K. H. Scholz. 1994. (Illus.). iv, 98p. reprint ed. 49.75 (*3-8055-5977-1*) S Karger.

Circulatory System Course. Competence Assurance Systems Staff. 1981. (Illus.). pap. text 50.00 (*0-89147-053-0*) CAS.

Circumacreolar Techniques for Breast Surgery. Tolbert S. Wilkinson et al. 1995. LC 94-32696. (Illus.). 212p. 191.00 (*0-387-94378-1*) Spr-Verlag.

Circumcision: What Every Parent Should Know. Anne Briggs. 1985. (Illus.). 183p. pap. 4.95 (*0-9615484-0-1*) Birth & Parenting.

Circumcision - the Pros & Cons: Index of New Information. Janice D. Gibbons. 1995. LC 95-16983. 57.50 (*0-7883-0726-6*); pap. 47.50 (*0-7883-0727-4*) ABBE Pubs Assn.

Circumcision in Man & Woman: Its History, Psychology & Ethnology. Felix Bryk. LC 72-9625. reprint ed. 37.50 (*0-404-57420-3*) AMS Pr.

Circumcision-the Pros & Cons: Index of New Information. Janice D. Gibbons. 1994. 150p. 57.50 (*0-7883-0024-5*); pap. 47.50 (*0-7883-0025-3*) ABBE Pubs Assn.

Circumplex Model: Systemic Assessment & Treatment of Families. Ed. by David H. Olson et al. 1989. LC 88-30151. (Journal of Psychotherapy & the Family Ser.: Vol. 4, Nos. 1 & 2). (Illus.). 296p. text 49.95 (*0-86656-776-3*) Haworth Pr.

Circumvaginal Musculature & Sexual Function. Ed. by B. Graber. 1982. (Illus.). x, 126p. 42.75 (*3-8055-3017-X*) S Karger.

Circumventricular Organs & Body Fluids. P. Gross. 1987. LC 87-10356. 224p. reprint ed. Vol. 1. 124.00 (*0-8493-6797-2*); Vol. 3. 125.00 (*0-8493-6799-9*) Franklin (CRC Reprint).

Circumventricular Organs & Brain Fluid Environment: Molecular & Functional Aspects. Ed. by Armin Ermisch et al. 1992. LC 92-18263. (Progress in Brain Research Ser.: Vol. 91). xxiv,486p. 304.00 (*0-444-81419-1*) Elsevier.

Cirrhosis, Hepatic Encephalopathy & Ammonium Toxicity, Vol. 272. Ed. by Santiago Grisolia et al. 1990. (Advances in Experimental Medicine & Biology Ser.). (Illus.). 284p. (C). text 114.00 (*0-306-43666-3*, Kluwer Plenum) Kluwer Academic.

Cirrhosis, Hyperammonemia & Hepatic Encephalopathy. S. Grisolia & V. Felipo. 1993. (Advances in Experimental Medicine & Biology Ser.: Vol. 341). (Illus.). 156p. (C). text 75.00 (*0-306-44595-6*, Kluwer Plenum) Kluwer Academic.

Cisplatin derzeitiger Stand und neue Entwicklungen in der Chemotherapie maligner Neoplasien. Ed. by S. Seeber et al. 1980. (Beitraege Zur Onkologie, Contributions to Oncology Ser.: Band 3). (Illus.). 184p. pap. 25.25 (*3-8055-1364-X*) S Karger.

CISS Grantees Meeting Proceedings, Pt. II. Prod. by National Center for Education in Maternal and Child Health Staff. 1995. LC 95-69808. 96p. pap. (*1-57285-016-7*) Nat Ctr Educ.

Citizen's Alcohol & Other Drug Prevention Directory: Resources. 1991. lib. bdg. 75.00 (*0-8490-4351-4*) Gordon Pr.

Citizen's Alcohol & Other Drug Prevention Directory: Resources for Getting Involved. 1992. lib. bdg. 288.95 (*0-8490-8826-7*) Gordon Pr.

Citizens Alert! Alternatives for Low-Profile Survival. Virgil A. Postlethwaite. Ed. by Paul M. Clemens. 1981. (Orig.). pap. text 7.95 (*0-931892-02-3*) B Dolphin Pub.

Citric Acid Cycle. Ed. by J. M. Lowenstein et al. 1969. (Methods in Enzymology Ser.: Vol. 13). text 209.00 (*0-12-181870-5*) Acad Pr.

City Crime Rankings Vol. II: Crime in Metropolitan America. Ed. by Kathleen O'Leary Morgan et al. 1996. 400p. (Orig.). lib. bdg. 34.95 (*1-56692-309-3*) Morgan Quitno Corp.

City Hospitals: The Undercare of the Underprivileged. Harry F. Dowling. 1982. (Illus.). 256p. 42.00 (*0-674-13197-5*) HUP.

City of Columbus & Franklin County, Ohio, 1995-96 Community Health Risk Assessment. Columbus Health Department Staff & Franklin County Board of Health Staff. 1997. (Columbus Community Health Assessment Ser.: Vol. 6). (Illus.). vii, 102p. pap. (*1-888492-52-X*) Columbus Hlth.

Civil Rights: HIV Testing, Contact Tracing, & Quarantine. Neal A. Dickerson. 1993. LC 93-2598. (Politics of AIDS Ser.: Vol. 2). (Illus.). xii, 230p. pap. 15.00 (*0-930383-34-6*) Monument Pr.

Civil War Letters of Dr. Harvey Black: A Surgeon with Stonewall. Ed. by Glenn L. McMullen. 1995. LC 95-223100. (Army of Northern Virginia Ser.: Vol. 3). 249p. 30.00 (*0-935523-45-6*) Butternut & Blue.

Civil War Medicine. Alfred Jay. Bollett. 2001. (Illus.). 375p. pap. (*1-883620-03-1*) Galen AZ.

Civil War Medicine. Richard Hephner. 1998. (Illus.). 12p. pap. 3.00 (*1-890327-03-4*) Longwood Ctr.

Civil War Medicine. C. Keith Wilbur. 1999. LC 98-44799. (Illustrated Living History Ser.). (Illus.). 119p. (J). (gr. 5-9). 19.95 (*0-7910-5207-9*) Chelsea Hse.

Civil War Medicine. C. Keith Wilbur. 1998. LC 98-30569. (Illustrated Living History Ser.). (Illus.). 288p. pap. 14.95 (*0-7627-0341-5*) Globe Pequot.

Civil War Medicine: Care & Comfort of the Wounded. Robert E. Denney. 1995. (Illus.). 422p. (Orig.). pap. 19.95 (*0-8069-0880-7*) Sterling.

Civil War Nurse: The Diary & Letters of Hannah Ropes. John R. Brumgardt. 1980. LC 79-28372. 164p. (C). pap. 13.95 (*0-87049-790-1*) U of Tenn Pr.

Civilian Vascular Trauma. D. Preston Flanigan. 1992. (Illus.). 490p. text 98.50 (*0-8121-1426-4*) Lppncott W & W.

Civilization & Its Discontents. Sigmund Freud. Ed. by James Strachey. 1989. 128p. reprint ed. pap. 8.95 (*0-393-30158-3*) Norton.

Civilization & the Cripple. Frederick Watson. Ed. by William R. Phillips & Janet Rosenberg. 1980. LC 79-6927. (Physically Handicapped in Society Ser.). (Illus.). reprint ed. lib. bdg. 18.95 (*0-405-13134-8*) Ayer.

*__Claim for Compensation Form CA-7 & Attending Physician's Report Form CA-20.__ 2001. 6p. per. 32.00 (*0-16-061795-2*, Labor Dept) USGPO.

*__Claim for Compensation on Account of Traumatic Injury or Occupational Disease Form CA-7, & Attending Physician's Report Form CA-20.__ 2001. 6p. per. 12.00 (*0-16-061789-8*, Labor Dept) USGPO.

Claiming Power in Doctor-Patient Talk. Nancy Ainsworth-Vaughn. 1998. LC 97-36258. (Oxford Studies in Sociolinguistics). (Illus.). 224p. pap. 19.95 (*0-19-509607-X*) OUP.

Claims Medical Manual. Packard Thurber & Packard Thurber, Jr. 4th rev. ed. 1991. LC 90-7652. (Illus.). 128p. pap. 12.95 (*0-87015-257-2*) Pacific Bks.

CLAO-Allergan. Dabezies. 1989. 130.00 (*0-316-17061-5*, Little Brwn Med Div) Lppncott W & W.

CLAO Guide to Spectacles & Optical Dispensing: A Primer for Ophthalmologists. Harold A. Stein et al. 1999. (Illus.). viii, 160p. pap. text (*1-929652-02-X*) CLAO Inc.

CLAO LL Set. Dabezies. 2nd ed. 1989. 85.00 (*0-316-17060-7*, Little Brwn Med Div) Lppncott W & W.

CLAO Pocket Guide to Contact Lens Fitting. CLAO, Inc. Staff. 2nd rev. ed. (Illus.). viii, 126p. pap. text 38.00 (*1-929652-00-3*) CLAO Inc.

CLAO Residents Contact Lens Curriculum Manual. Harold A. Stein et al. Ed. by Lynn Maund. 1999. (Illus.). ix, 220p. pap. text 125.00 (*1-929652-01-1*) CLAO Inc.

CLAO Set. Dabezies. 2nd ed. 1989. 295.00 (*0-316-17055-0*, Little Brwn Med Div) Lppncott W & W.

CLAO Update LL. Dabezies. No. 4. 1989. 45.00 (*0-316-17054-2*); No. 5. 1989. 45.00 (*0-316-17062-3*); No. 6. 1990. 45.00 (*0-316-17063-1*); No. 7. 1990. 45.00 (*0-316-17065-8*); No. 8. 1991. 45.00 (*0-316-17066-6*) Lppncott W & W (Little Brwn Med Div).

Clarifying & Summarizing the Fundamentals of Counseling: Hebrew Translation. Harvey Jackins. 1987. pap. 1.00 (*0-913937-22-3*) Rational Isl.

Clarifying Concepts in Nursing Research. Audrey G. Gift. 1997. LC 97-9521. 24.95 (*0-8261-9980-1*) Springer Pub.

Clarke's Isolation & Identification of Drugs. Moffat. 2nd ed. 1992. (*0-85369-166-5*) Pharmaceutical Pr GBR. *Dist:* Rittenhouse.

Clark's Clinical Dentistry, 3. Jefferson F. Hardin. 1996. (C). (gr. 13). spiral bd. 99.95 (*0-8151-2003-6*, 31765) Mosby Inc.

Clark's Clinical Dentistry: 1998 Update. Jefferson F. Hardin. 1998. (Illus.). 860p. pap. text 110.00 (*0-8151-2540-2*, 30736) Mosby Inc.

Clark's Clinical Dentistry-1996. Jefferson F. Hardin. rev. ed. 1996. (Illus.). 534p. (C). (gr. 13). pap. text 89.00 (*0-8151-2224-1*, 30576) Mosby Inc.

Clark's Clinical Dentistry, 1997. Jefferson F. Hardin. rev. ed. 1997. (Illus.). 550p. (C). (gr. 13). 99.95 (*0-8151-2541-0*, 30715) Mosby Inc.

Clark's Clinical Dentistry, 2000. Jefferson F. Hardin. rev. ed. 2000. (Illus.). 550p. pap. text 99.95 (*0-8151-4351-6*, 31024) Mosby Inc.

Clark's Positioning in Radiography. R. A. Swallow et al. 11th ed. 1996. 400p. (*0-7506-0340-2*) E A GBR. *Dist:* OUP.

Clark's Special Procedures in Diagnostic Imaging. Stewart Whitley et al. 1999. LC 98-20552. (Illus.). 432p. (*0-7506-1715-2*) E A GBR. *Dist:* OUP.

Clashing Views on Controversial Issues in Abnormal Psychology. Richard Halgin. 2000. (Taking Sides Ser.). 400p. (C). pap. 20.31 (*0-07-237193-5*) McGrw-H Hghr Educ.

Clashing Views on Controversial Psychological Issues. Brent Slife. 11th ed. 2000. (Taking Sides Ser.). 416p. (C). pap. 19.38 (*0-07-237142-0*) McGrw-H Hghr Educ.

Clasificacion Diagnostica en Puerto Rico. Guillermo Bernal & Wanda C. Rodriguez. 1992. (SPA.). 68p. pap. (*0-929441-26-5*) Pubns Puertorriquenas.

Class Mammalia: The Animal Kingdom Arranged in Conformity with Its Organization by the Baron Cuvier. Georges Cuvier. Ed. by Keir B. Sterling. 1978. LC 77-81117. (Biologists & Their World Ser.). (Illus.). reprint ed. Set, Vols 1-5. lib. bdg. 237.95 (*0-405-10746-3*); Vol. 1-5. lib. bdg. 49.95 (*0-405-10765-X*); Vol. 2. lib. bdg. 49.95 (*0-405-10766-8*); Vol. 3. lib. bdg. 49.95 (*0-405-10767-6*); Vol. 4. lib. bdg. 49.95 (*0-405-10768-4*); Vol. 5. lib. bdg. 49.95 (*0-405-10769-2*) Ayer.

Classic & Innovative Treatment for Superficial Bladder Tumors: International Symposium: KLH: An Innovative Immunomodulator for Installation Prophylaxis in Superficial Bladder Carcinoma. Ed. by K. H. Kurth. 2000. (European Urology Ser.: Vol. 37, Suppl. 3 (2000)). (Illus.). iv, 56p. pap. 25.25 (*3-8055-7092-9*) S Karger.

Classic Cases in Medical Ethics: Accounts of Cases that Have Shaped Medical Ethics. Gregory E. Pence. 3rd ed. 1999. LC 99-24647. 528p. (C). pap. 31.25 (*0-07-303986-1*) McGrw-H Hghr Educ.

Classic Descriptions of Disease: With Biographical Sketches of the Authors. Ralph H. Major. 3rd ed. 1978. (Illus.). 712p. 115.95 (*0-398-01202-4*) C C Thomas.

Classic Discoveries of Neuroendocrine Syndromes of the Pancreas & Gut. Ed. by Stanley R. Friesen. 1993. 281p. 89.95 (*1-879702-63-0*, LN0263) CRC Pr.

Classic of Difficulties: A Translation of the Nan Jing. Bob Flaws. 1999. LC 98-74994. x, 140p. pap. text 15.95 (*1-891845-07-1*) Blue Poppy Pr.

***Classic Papers in Breast Disease.** Baum & Henderson. 2001. (Illus.). 256p. (*1-901865-83-5*) Isis Med GBR. *Dist:* Bks Intl VA.

Classic Presentations & Rapid Reviews for USMLE, Step 2. Theodore X. O'Connell et al. 1999. LC 98-66122. pap. 25.00 (*1-888308-05-2*) J & S Pub VA.

Classic Radiologic Signs: An Atlas & History. Michael E. Mulligan. 1996. LC 96-13052. (Illus.). 208p. 54.95 (*1-85070-664-6*, Parthenon Pbng) CRC Pr.

Classic Readings in Psychology. Ed. by James V. McConnell & Daniel W. Gorenflo. 1989. LC 89-7620. (C). 13.00 (*0-03-027614-4*) Harcourt Coll Pubs.

Classic Studies in Abnormal Psychology. Steven Schwartz. 1993. LC 92-49375. 254p. (C). pap. text 26.95 (*0-87484-866-0*, 866) Mayfield Pub.

Classic Studies in Psychology. Steven Schwartz. 1986. LC 86-62208. (Illus.). x, 196p. (C). (gr. 12). pap. text 23.95 (*0-87484-796-6*, 796) Mayfield Pub.

Classic Teachings in Clinical Cardiology: A Tribute to W. Proctor Harvey Ed. by Michael A. Chizner. 1996. 145.00 (*1-886128-06-5*) Laennec Pub.

Classic Texts: Health, the Professionals & the NHS. Lesley Mackay et al. 1998. LC 98-15950. 352p. pap. text 35.00 (*0-7506-2738-7*) Buttrwrth-Heinemann.

Classic Vision Vol. 2: The Retreat from Extremity. Murray Kreiger. 1973. LC 77-167984. 390p. pap. text 20.95 (*0-8018-1551-7*) Johns Hopkins.

Classic Works in Medical Ethics: Core Philosophical Readings. Gregory E. Pence. 1997. LC 97-1300. 384p. pap. 31.25 (*0-07-038115-1*) McGrw-H Hghr Educ.

Classical Anesthesia Files. David M. Little, Jr. 1985. LC 85-12088. 335p. 35.00 (*0-9614932-0-8*) Wood Lib-Mus.

Classical Conditioning. Ed. by William F. Prokasy. 1965. LC 65-16466. (Century Psychology Ser.). (Illus.). 32.50 (*0-89197-082-7*) Irvington.

Classical Conditioning. Ed. by I. Gormezano et al. 3rd ed. 1986. 424p. (C). text 89.95 (*0-89859-507-X*) L Erlbaum Assocs.

***Classical Homeopathy.** Michael Carlston. 2001. (Illus.). 315p. (*0-443-06565-9*) Church GBR. *Dist:* Saunders.

Classical Psychoanalysis Vol. 1: Unconscious Mental Life & Reality. Ed. by Ricard Ekins. 2001. 176p. pap. (*1-85575-197-6*) Karnac Bks GBR. *Dist:* Other Pr LLC.

Classical Swine Fever & Related Viral Infections. Ed. by B. Liese. 1987. (Developments in Veterinary Virology Ser.). (C). text 159.00 (*0-89838-969-0*) Kluwer Academic.

Classical Transmitters in the CNS, Pt. I. Ed. by Anders T. Bjorklund et al. 1985. (Handbooks of Chemical Neuroanatomy: Vol. 2, pt. I). 464p. 280.00 (*0-444-90330-5*, Excerpta Medica) Elsevier.

Classical Transmitters in the CNS, Pt. II. Anders T. Bjorklund et al. 1984. (Handbooks of Chemical Neuroanatomy: Vol. 3, pt. II). 436p. 267.00 (*0-444-90352-6*) Elsevier.

Classics in Ophthalmology, Set. Paul Henkind. 1979. 150.00 (*0-88275-933-7*); lthr. 199.50 (*0-88275-934-5*) Krieger.

Classics in Psychiatry Ser. Ed. by Eric T. Carlson. 1976. 1985.00 (*0-405-07410-7*) Ayer.

Classics in Psychology, Set. Ed. by Howard Gardner & Judith K. Gardner. 1047.00 (*0-405-05130-1*) Ayer.

Classics of American Psychiatry Eighteen-Ten to Nineteen Thirty-Four. John P. Brady. 1975. LC 72-85641. (Illus.). 336p. 17.50 (*0-87527-093-X*) Green.

Classics of Cardiology. John A. Callahan et al. 1988. LC 82-7830. Pt. 1, Vol. 4. 600p. lib. bdg. 80.00 (*0-89874-872-0*); Pt. 2, Vol. 4. 514p. lib. bdg. 75.00 (*0-89464-265-0*) Krieger.

Classics of Cardiology Ed. by Thomas E. Keys & Fredrick A. Willius. 1983. LC 82-7830. Set. 1536p. 235.00 (*0-89874-513-6*); Vol. 1: Repr. of 1941 Ed. 424p. 49.50 (*0-89874-514-4*); Vol. 2: Repr. of 1941 Ed. 472p. 56.50 (*0-89874-515-2*) Krieger.

Classics of Cardiology, Vol. 3. Ed. by John A. Callahan et al. 1983. LC 82-7830. 640p. 80.00 (*0-89874-516-0*) Krieger.

Classics of Neurology. Ed. by Emerson C. Kelly. deluxe ed. 1971. LC 78-158127. 384p. lthr. 39.50 (*0-88275-029-1*) Krieger.

Classification & Diagnosis of Alzheimer Disease: An International Perspective. Ed. by T. Hovaguimian et al. 1989. LC 88-13716. (Illus.). 200p. (C). text 68.00 (*0-920887-31-7*) Hogrefe & Huber Pubs.

Classification & Nomenclature of Viruses. Ed. by R. E. Matthews. 1982. (Journal: Vol. 17, No. 1-3, 1982). (Illus.). 200p. 31.50 (*3-8055-3557-0*) S Karger.

Classification in Mental Retardation. Ed. by Herbert J. Grossman. 1983. LC 83-8779. 228p. text 5.00 (*0-940898-12-8*) Am Assn Mental.

Classification, Monitoring & Evaluation of Cataracts: 4th Scheimpflug Club Meeting 1989 Gamagori, Japan, April 1989. Ed. by K. Sasaki. 1990. (Journal: Vol. 22, Suppl. 1, 1990). vi, 102p. pap. 33.25 (*3-8055-5224-6*) S Karger.

Classification of Child & Adolescent Mental Diagnoses in Primary Care. American Academy of Pediatrics Staff. Ed. by Mark L. Wolrarch. 1996. LC 95-75817. 368p. pap. 39.95 (*0-910761-71-X*) Am Acad Pediat.

Classification of Chronic Pain: Descriptions of Chronic Pain Syndromes & Definitions of Pain Terms. International Assn. for the Study of Pain, Task Fo. Ed. by Harold Merskey & Nikolai Bogduk. 2nd ed. 1994. LC 94-8062. 240p. pap. 12.00 (*0-931092-05-1*) Intl Assn Study Pain.

Classification of Endogenous Psychoses & Their Differentiated Etiology. Karl Leonhard. Ed. by Helmut Beckmann. Tr. by C. H. Cahn from GER. 2nd enl. rev. ed. 1999. LC 99-35446. 450p. 62.00 (*3-211-83259-9*) Spr-Verlag.

Classification of Musculoskeletal Trauma. J. Fairbank et al. 1999. LC 98-30092. (Illus.). 320p. (*0-7506-2722-0*) E A GBR. *Dist:* OUP.

Classification of Natural Communities. Robert H. Whittaker. Ed. by Frank N. Egerton, 3rd. 1978. LC 77-74257. (History of Ecology Ser.). reprint ed. lib. bdg. 21.95 (*0-405-10426-X*) Ayer.

Classification of Nursing Diagnoses: Proceedings of the Eleventh Conference. North American Nursing Diagnosis Association Staff. Ed. by Priscilla LeMone & Marilyn J. Rantz. 1995. LC 95-25622. 30.00 (*0-910478-54-6*) Cum Index Nursing.

Classification of Nursing Diagnoses: Proceedings of the Third & Fourth National Conferences. Ed. by Mija Kim & Derry A. Moritz. 1982. (Illus.). 448p. text 24.95 (*0-07-034547-3*) McGraw.

Classification of Nursing Diagnoses: Proceedings of the Twelfth Conference. North American Nursing Diagnosis Association Staff et al. Ed. by Marilyn J. Rantz & Priscilla Lemone. 1997. LC 97-19692. 45.00 (*0-910478-58-9*) Cum Index Nursing.

Classification of Psychopathology: Neokraepelinian & Quantitative Approaches. R. K. Blashfield. 1984. LC 83-26871. (Illus.). 354p. (C). 80.00 (*0-306-41405-8*, Plenum Trade) Perseus Pubng.

Classification of the Tumors of the Glioma Group on a Histogenetic Basis with a Correlated Study of Prognosis. Percival Bailey & Harvey Cushing. 1970. (Illus.). reprint ed. 20.00 (*0-87266-049-4*) Argosy.

Classified Dictionary of Traditional Chinese Medicine. Zhu-Fan Xie et al. 1994. LC 97-210513. (CHI, ENG & LAT.). 726p. (*7-80005-226-5*) New World Pr CHN. *Dist:* China Bks.

Classroom Management Through Curricular Adaptations: Educating Minority Handicapped Students. John J. Hoover & Catherine Collier. 1986. LC 86-82580. 80p. pap. text 8.50 (*0-940059-00-2*) Hamilton Pubns.

Classroom Manager to Accompany Health Assessment: Instructor's Resource Kit. Estes. 1998. (Nursing Education Ser.). 368p. tchr. ed. 250.00 (*0-8273-7148-9*) Delmar.

Classroom Manager to Accompany Psychiatric Mental Health Nursing: Instructor's Resource Kit. Frisch. 1998. (Nursing Education Ser.). 464p. tchr. ed. 250.00 (*0-8273-7234-5*) Delmar.

Claude Bernard & Animal Chemistry. Frederick L. Holmes. 1974. LC 73-88497. (Commonwealth Fund Publications). 640p. 62.00 (*0-674-13485-0*) HUP.

Claude M. Sing Around: Fighting Against Multiple Sclerosis. John Mythen. 1990. pap. 14.95 (*0-9694457-0-9*) Gordon Soules Bk.

Clays Handbook of Environmental Health. Bassett. 1991. (Mechanical Engineering Ser.). text 121.95 (*0-412-39480-4*) Chapman & Hall.

Clay's Handbook of Environmental Health. W. H. Bassett. 16th ed. 1992. 752p. 99.95 (*0-442-31488-4*) Chapman & Hall.

Clayton's Electrotherapy. Kitchen. 10th ed. 1995. pap. text 49.95 (*0-7020-1762-0*) Saunders.

***Clean Living Movements: American Cycles of Health Reform.** Ruth Clifford Engs. 2001. 328p. pap. 24.95 (*0-275-97541-X*, Praeger Pubs) Greenwood.

Clean Needle Technique Manual for Acupuncturists: Guidelines & Standards for the Clean & Safe Clinical Practice. Ed. by June Brazil et al. 4th rev. ed. 1997. 58p. 15.00 (*0-9670262-1-0*) Natl Acup Fndt.

Clean Room Design: Minimizing Contamination Through Proper Design. Bengt Ljungqvist & Berit Reinmuller. 1996. (Illus.). 124p. 89.00 (*1-57491-032-9*) IHS Health Grp.

Clean Water & the Health of the Cities: An Original Anthology. Ed. by Barbara G. Rosenkrantz. 1977. LC 76-40661. (Public Health in America Ser.). (Illus.). reprint ed. lib. bdg. 23.95 (*0-405-09871-5*) Ayer.

Cleaning Yourself Up. Jennifer James. rev. ed. 2000. pap. 0.50 (*0-89230-058-2*) Do It Now.

Clear Body, Clear Mind. L. Ron Hubbard. 1990. 306p. 35.00 (*0-88404-549-8*) Bridge Pubns Inc.

Clear Body Clear Mind: The Effective Purification Program. L. Ron Hubbard. 1990. 306p. 17.95 (*0-88404-588-9*) Bridge Pubns Inc.

Clear Corneal Lens Surgery. I. Howard Fine. 1998. LC 98-37810. (Illus.). 384p. text 125.00 (*1-55642-381-0*, 63810) SLACK Inc.

Clearing in the Crowd: Innovations in Emergency Services. Janette Cooke & Kathleen Finneran. 1994. LC 94-2739. (Papers). 48p. 10.00 (*1-881277-11-9*) United Hosp Fund.

Clearing the Air: An Assessment of Asthma & Indoor Allergens. Committee on the Assessment of Asthma and Indoor Air et al. 2000. LC 00-25801. (Illus.). xvi, 438p. 54.00 (*0-309-06496-1*) Natl Acad Pr.

Cleavage Lines of the Skin. A. Namikawa. 1986. (Bibliotheca Anatomica Ser.: No. 27). (Illus.). viii, 140p. 77.50 (*3-8055-4202-X*) S Karger.

Cleft, Set. D. Ralph Millard, Jr. 1980. 2,964p. text 662.00 (*0-316-57148-2*) Lppncott W & W.

Cleft Craft: Alveolar & Palatal Deformities, Vol. III. D. Ralph Millard, Jr. 1980. text 235.00 (*0-316-57139-3*, Little Brwn Med Div) Lppncott W & W.

Cleft Craft: Bilateral & Rare Deformities, Vol. 2. D. Ralph Millard, Jr. 1976. text 235.00 (*0-316-57138-5*, Little Brwn Med Div) Lppncott W & W.

Cleft Craft - The Evolution of Its Surgery Vol. 1: The Unilateral Deformity, Vol. 1. D. Ralph Millard, Jr. 1976. text 235.00 (*0-316-57137-7*) Lppncott W & W.

Cleft Lip & Palate: A System of Management. Desmond A. Kernahan & Sheldon Rosenstein. 1989. (Illus.). 352p. 72.00 (*0-683-04599-7*) Lppncott W & W.

Cleft Lip & Palate: Examination, Surgery & Rehabilitation. Rene Malek. 2000. (Illus.). 360p. (*1-85317-491-2*) Martin Dunitz GBR. *Dist:* Thieme Med Pubs.

Cleft Lip & Palate: Perspectives in Management with an Introduction to Craniofacial Anomalies, Vols. 1 & 2. Samuel Berkowitz. 1996. (Illus.). 904p. pap. 390.00 (*1-56593-590-X*, 1206) Thomson Learn.

Cleft Management. Helfrick. 1998. text (*0-7216-6505-5*) Saunders.

Cleft Palate. Gene R. Powers. 1973. LC 72-86554. (Studies in Communicative Disorders). 37p. pap. text 4.50 (*0-672-61288-7*, Bobbs) Macmillan.

Cleft Palate. Gene R. Powers. Ed. by Harvey Halpern. 1986. LC 86-3062. (PRO-ED Studies in Communicative Disorders). (Illus.). 52p. pap. text 9.00 (*0-89079-094-9*, 1384) PRO-ED.

Cleft Palate: Interdisciplinary Issues & Treatment. Ed. by Karlind T. Moller & Clark D. Starr. 1993. LC 92-12022. (For Clinicians by Clinicians Ser.). 409p. pap. text 36.00 (*0-89079-567-3*, 4046) PRO-ED.

Cleft Palate & Craniofacial Anomalies. Ruscello. 1995. (Dental Assisting Procedures Ser.). text 34.95 (*0-8273-5688-9*) Delmar.

Cleft Palate & Related Disorders. Grace F. Middleton & Mary Pannbacker. Ed. by Kirsteen Anderson. 1997. LC 97-74552. (Illus.). 301p. ring bd. 59.50 (*1-883315-25-5*, 7431) Imaginart Intl.

Cleft Palate & Velopharyngeal Insufficiency. Ed. by Jeno Hirschberg. 1997. (Journal: Vol. 49, Nos. 3-4, 1997). (Illus.). 108p. pap. 50.50 (*3-8055-6494-5*) S Karger.

Cleft Palate Children & Intelligence. J. A. Heineman-De Boer. 1984. xiv, 150p. pap. (*90-265-0605-8*) Swets.

Cleft Palate Speech. McWilliams et al. 2nd ed. 1989. (Illus.). 400p. (C). text 65.95 (*1-55664-238-5*) Mosby Inc.

Cleft Palate Speech. Sally J. Peterson-Falzone et al. 3rd ed. 1999. LC 00-55908. (Illus.). 432p. (gr. 13). text 58.00 (*0-8151-3153-4*, 29901) Mosby Inc.

Cleft Palate Speech Management: A Multidiscipline. Robert J. Sprintzen & Janusz Bardach. 1994. (Illus.). 400p. (C). (gr. 13). text 69.00 (*0-8016-6447-0*, 06447) Mosby Inc.

Cleft Palate Story. Samuel Berkowitz. 1994. 240p. 29.95 (*1-56593-745-7*, 1448) Singular Publishing.

***Clemente Dissector: A Guide to Individual Dissections in Human Anatomy.** Carmine D. Clemente. 2002. LC 2001-29950. (Illus.). xii, 379p. spiral bd. 39.95 (*0-7817-3290-5*) Lppncott W & W.

Cleveland Clinic Home Care Services: Home Therapy Standards, Policies, & Procedures. Ed. by Charlene L. Szunyog. 1995. LC 92-10859. ring bd. 195.00 (*0-8342-0330-8*, S55) Aspen Pub.

Cleveland Symposium on Behavioral Research in Rehabilitation. Ed. by William R. Phillips & Janet Rosenberg. rev. ed. 1980. LC 79-6898. (Physically Handicapped in Society Ser.). reprint ed. lib. bdg. 25.95 (*0-405-13110-0*) Ayer.

CLIA & Transfusion Medicine: A Guide to Total Compliance. Ed. by Kay McCurdy & Susan L. Wilkenson. 1996. ring bd. 109.00 (*1-56395-053-7*, PC97-PR9603) Am Assn Blood.

Client Access to Records: Participation in Social Work. David Shemmings. 1991. 123p. text (*1-85628-107-8*) Avebry GBR. *Dist:* Ashgate Pub Co.

Client-Centered & Experiential Psychotherapy: A Paradigm in Motion. Robert Hutterer. 1996. 97.93 (*0-8204-2985-6*) P Lang Pubng.

Client-Centered & Experiential Psychotherapy in the Nineties. Ed. by G. Lietaer et al. 1990. 863p. (Orig.). pap. (*90-6186-364-3*) Leuven Univ BEL. *Dist:* Coronet Bks.

Client-Centered Therapy: Its Current Practice, Implications & Theory. Carl Ransom Rogers. 1995. 560p. reprint ed. pap. 33.50 (*0-09-453990-1*) Trans-Atl Phila.

Client-Centered Therapy & the Person-Centered Approach: New Directions in Theory, Research & Practice. Ed. by Ronald F. Levant & John M. Shlien. 1984. LC 84-6832. 480p. 69.50 (*0-275-91215-9*, C1215, Praeger Pubs) Greenwood.

Client-Centered Therapy & the Person-Centered Approach: New Directions in Theory, Research, & Practice. Ed. by Ronald F. Levant & John M. Shlien. 1987. LC 84-6832. 480p. pap. 24.00 (*0-275-92821-7*, B2821, Praeger Pubs) Greenwood.

Client-Centred Practice in Occupational Therapy: A Guide to Implementation. Thelma Sumsion. 1999. LC 98-43689. xi, 123p. (*0-443-06127-0*) Church.

Client Education: Theory & Practice. Dorothy E. Babcock. 1993. LC 93-12114. (Illus.). 344p. (C). (gr. 13). pap. text 35.00 (*0-8016-6942-1*, 06942) Mosby Inc.

Client-Oriented, Provider-Efficient Services (COPE) AVSC International Staff. Ed. by Joanne Tzanis. 1995. pap. text 15.00 (*1-885063-01-6*) EngenderHlth.

***Client Profiles in Nursing - Child Health 1.** G. Campbell & Sadik. 2001. (Illus.). 208p. pap. (*1-84110-013-7*) Greenwich Med GBR. *Dist:* JAMCO Dist.

Client Teaching Guides for Home Health Care. Donna Meyers. 2nd ed. 225p. 1995. 109.00 incl. disk (*0-8342-1054-1*, 10541); 1997. LC 97-18555. pap. text 72.00 incl. disk (*0-8342-0968-3*, 20968) Aspen Pub.

Clients As Individuals. Ken Messenger. 1992. (Skills for Caring Ser.). (Illus.). 48p. (Orig.). pap. text (*0-443-04530-5*) Church.

Clifford W. Beers: Advocate for the Insane. Norman Dain. 1980. LC 79-24290. (Contemporary Community Health Ser.). (Illus.). 424p. text 49.95 (*0-8229-3419-1*) U of Pittsburgh Pr.

Climacteric: An Update. Ed. by H. B. Van Herendael et al. 1984. 180p. lib. bdg. 45.00 (*0-85200-852-X*) Kluwer Academic.

Climacteric & Its Treatment. Ed. by Nils-Otto Sjoberg et al. 1997. (Swedish Consensus of Obstetrics & Gynecology Ser.: Vol. 1). (Illus.). 126p. lib. bdg. 38.95 (*1-85070-997-1*, Parthenon Pbng) CRC Pr.

Climacteric Hot Flush. Ed. by E. Schoenbaum. 1991. (Progress in Basic & Clinical Pharmacology Ser.: Vol. 6). (Illus.). x, 166p. 138.50 (*3-8055-5260-2*) S Karger.

Climacteric in Perspective. Ed. by M. Notevitz & P. A. Van Keep. 1986. text 392.50 (*0-85200-919-4*) Kluwer Academic.

Climate & Human Ecology. Jim Norwine. 1978. LC 78-52975. (Illus.). pap. 9.95 (*0-918464-19-6*) D Armstrong.

Climate for Learning. Mike Torbe & Peter Medway. 1982. LC 82-14768. 149p. (C). pap. text 19.00 (*0-86709-041-3*, 0041) Boynton Cook Pubs.

Climb of My Life: A Miraculous Journey from the Edge of Death to the Victory of a Lifetime. Laura Evans. 1996. LC 96-9497. 288p. 22.00 (*0-06-258658-0*) Harper SF.

Climbing Back: A Journey with Cancer. Mark H. Gerner. 1998. LC 97-41658. 165p. pap. 18.95 (*1-56072-512-5*, Nova Kroshka Bks) Nova Sci Pubs.

Climbing Toward the Light: A Journey of Growth, Understanding & Love. Ardath Rodale. 1989. LC 89-32896. (Illus.). 240p. 17.95 (*0-87857-834-X*, 05-406-0) Rodale Pr Inc.

Clincal Disorders of Erythropoieses. Stephen A. Feig. 1993. 192p. 169.00 (*0-8493-6678-X*, R) CRC Pr.

Clincial Practice with Adolescents. DGM Consulting Inc. Staff. 2001. 39.00 net. (*0-534-52382-X*) Wadsworth Pub.

Clinic Administrator. Jack Rudman. 1994. (Career Examination Ser.: C-915). pap. 39.95 (*0-8373-0915-8*) Nat Learn.

Clinic Habit. Camille Lambert, Jr. & Howard E. Freeman. 1967. pap. 17.95 (*0-8084-0083-5*) NCUP.

Clinic Supervisor (Drug Abuse) Jack Rudman. 1994. (Career Examination Ser.: C-3007). pap. 39.95 (*0-8373-3007-6*) Nat Learn.

***Clinica de Pequenos Animales (Handbook of Small Animal Practice)** Rhea V. Morgan. 3rd ed. 1997. (ENG & SPA., Illus.). 1463p. (*84-8174-351-8*) Mosby-Doyma Libros ESP. *Dist:* Saunders.

***Clinica Mayo: Guia de Autocuidades.** Philip T. Hagen. 1999.Tr. of Mayo Clinic Guide to Self Care. (SPA., Illus.). 244p. (*968-11-0354-8*) Bertelsmann MEX. *Dist:* Libros Fronteras.

Clinica Mayo Guia de Autocuidados. Philip T. Hagen. 1999.Tr. of Mayo Clinic Guide to Self-Care. (SPA.). 272p. pap. (*0-9627865-9-4*) Mayo Fndtn Med Ed & Res.

Clinical Acid-Base Balance. Ed. by William S. Thomson & James F. Adams. 1997. LC 98-121486. (Illus.). 260p. pap. text 48.50 (*0-19-262769-4*) OUP.

Clinical Acupuncture: Scientific Basis. Ed. by Gabriel Stux & Richard Hammerschlag. 2000. LC 00-39485. (Illus.). 248p. pap. 25.00 (*3-540-64054-1*) Spr-Verlag.

Clinical Administration in Audiology & Speech-Language Pathology. Ed. by Stephen R. Rizzo, Jr. & Michael D. Trudeau. 1993. LC 93-25798. (Illus.). 306p. (Orig.). (C). pap. text 59.95 (*1-56593-088-6*, 0393) Thomson Learn.

Clinical Advances in Physical Medicine & Rehabilitation. Ed. by Frederic J. Kottke & E. A. Amate. 1991. (PAHO Scientific Publications: No. 533). (ENG & SPA.). xii, 450p. pap. text 68.00 (*92-75-11533-8*, 1610533) World Health.

Clinical Advisor: 2000 Edition. Fred F. Ferri. 1999. LC 00-269154. (Illus.). xxviii, 1278p. 54.95 (*0-323-00971-9*) Mosby Inc.

Clinical Ambulatory Monitoring. William A. Littler. 1981. (Illus.). 174p. 60.00 (*0-8151-5482-8*, ACT-1) Mosby Inc.

***Clinical Anatomy.** W. S. Monkhouse. 2001. (Master Medicine Ser.). (Illus.). 295p. pap. (*0-443-06395-8*) Church GBR. *Dist:* Saunders.

Clinical Anatomy. Ernest W. April. 3rd ed. 1997. LC 96-1552. (National Medical Series for Independent Study). (Illus.). 670p. pap. text 29.00 (*0-683-06199-2*) Lppncott W & W.

Clinical Anatomy. Richard S. Snell. 3rd ed. 1986. 45.00 (*0-316-80217-4*, Little Brwn Med Div) Lppncott W & W.

Clinical Anatomy: A Revision & Applied Anatomy for Clinical Students. Harold Ellis. 9th ed. 1997. LC 96-33109. (Illus.). 512p. pap. 73.95 (*0-86542-882-4*) Blackwell Sci.

Clinical Anatomy: An Illustrated Review with Questions & Explanations. Richard S. Snell. 3rd ed. 2000. LC 99-57554. 288p. pap. text 28.95 (*0-7817-1827-9*) Lppncott W & W.

Clinical Anatomy & Management for Thoracic Spine Pain. Lynton Giles & Kevin P. Singer. 2000. LC 99-56627. (Illus.). 320p. pap. text 69.99 (*0-7506-4789-2*) Buttrwrth-Heinemann.

Clinical Anatomy & Management of Cervical Spine Pain. L. G. F. Giles. Ed. by K. P. Singer. 2001. LC 97-25513. 192p. pap. text 65.00 (*0-7506-2397-7*) Buttrwrth-Heinemann.

Clinical Anatomy & Management of Low Back Pain. L. G. Giles & K. P. Singer. 1997. LC 97-175759. 411p. pap. text 80.00 (*0-7506-2395-0*) Buttrwrth-Heinemann.

Clinical Anatomy & Management of Thoracic Spine Pain. Ed. by Lynton Giles & Kevin P. Singer. 1999. (Clinical Anatomy & Management of Back Pain Ser.). pap. text 55.00 (*0-7506-2396-9*) Buttrwrth-Heinemann.

***Clinical Anatomy & Physiology for Veterinary Technicians.** Thomas P. Colville. 2001. (Illus.). 512p. pap. (*0-323-00819-4*) Mosby Inc.

Clinical Anatomy Atlas. Class et al. 1995. LC 95-10658. (Illus.). 608p. (C). (gr. 13). spiral bd. 58.00 (*0-8151-4012-6*, 24426) Mosby Inc.

Clinical Anatomy for Emergency Medicine. Richard S. Snell & Mark S. Smith. 1993. LC 92-49973. (Illus.). 862p. (C). (gr. 13). text 160.00 (*0-8016-6549-3*, 06549) Mosby Inc.

Clinical Anatomy for Laparoscopic & Thoracoscopic Surgery. Ed. by Harold Ellis & Raghu Savalgi. 1995. (*1-85775-070-5*) Radcliffe Med Pr GBR. *Dist:* Balogh.

Clinical Anatomy for Medical Students. Richard S. Snell. 6th ed. 2000. LC 99-53905. 912p. pap. text 56.95 (*0-7817-1574-1*) Lppncott W & W.

Clinical Anatomy Made Ridiculously Simple. Stephen Goldberg. 1991. (Illus.). 175p. pap. text 19.95 (*0-940780-02-X*) MedMaster.

***Clinical Anatomy Made Ridiculously Simple.** Stephen Goldberg. 2nd rev. ed. 2001. (Illus.). 175p. pap. 19.95 (*0-940780-53-4*) MedMaster.

Clinical Anatomy of the Cervical Spine. Johannes Lang. 1993. (Illus.). 188p. text 149.00 (*0-86577-486-2*) Thieme Med Pubs.

Clinical Anatomy of the Eye. Richard S. Snell et al. 2nd ed. 1997. LC 97-39908. (Illus.). 423p. pap. 73.00 (*0-632-04344-X*) Blackwell Sci.

Clinical Anatomy of the Lumbar Spine & Sacrum. N. Bogduk. 3rd ed. 1997. (Illus.). 261p. pap. (*0-443-06014-2*) Church.

Clinical Anatomy of the Masticatory Apparatus & the Peripharyngeal Spaces. Johannes Lang. 1995. (Illus.). 220p. 169.00 (*0-86577-551-6*) Thieme Med Pubs.

Clinical Anatomy of the Nose, Nasal Cavity & Paranasal Sinuses. J. Lang. 1989. (Illus.). 144p. text 139.00 (*0-86577-330-0*) Thieme Med Pubs.

Clinical Anatomy of the Visual System. Lee A. Remington. 1997. LC 97-16054. 272p. text 74.99 (*0-7506-9558-7*) Buttrwrth-Heinemann.

Clinical & Biological Basis of Lung Cancer Prevention. Y. Martinet. 1997. LC 97-29086. (Respiratory Pharmacology & Pharmacotherapy Ser.). (*0-8176-5778-9*) Birkhauser.

Clinical & Biological Basis of Lung Cancer Prevention. Ed. by Y. Martinet et al. 1997. (Respiratory Pharmacology & Pharmacotherapy Ser.). (Illus.). 350p. 135.00 (*3-7643-5778-9*) Spr-Verlag.

Clinical & Diagnostic Interviewing. Ed. by Robert J. Craig. LC 89-29. 1989. 355p. 55.00 (*0-87668-848-2*); 1995. 380p. reprint ed. pap. 40.00 (*1-56821-526-6*) Aronson.

Clinical & Educational Applications of Temperament Research. Ed. by W. B. Carey & S. C. McDevitt. 1989. 208p. (*90-265-0971-5*) Swets.

Clinical & Educational Interventions with Fathers. Ed. by Jay Fagan & Alan J. Hawkins. 2000. LC 00-40775. (Haworth Marriage & the Family Ser.). xxiii, 313p. 69.95 (*0-7890-0645-6*); pap. 34.95 (*0-7890-1238-3*) Haworth Pr (Haworth Clinical).

Clinical & Event Sports Massage: Developing a Multidisciplinary Approach to Athletic Injuries & Sports Enhancement. James Waslaski. 2nd ed. 1996. (Illus.). pap. 24.95 (*0-9647865-9-1*) Other Stuff.

Clinical & Experimental Dermatology: Festschrift to Professor Kint. Ed. by J. De Bersaques. 1994. (Journal: Vol. 189, Supplement 2, 1994). (Illus.). iv, 72p. pap. 33.25 (*3-8055-6099-0*) S Karger.

Clinical & Experimental Hypnosis: In Medicine, Dentistry & Psychology. William S. Kroger. 2nd ed. 1977. LC 77-10320. 406p. text 89.00 (*0-397-50377-6*, 65-02678, Lippncott) Lppncott W & W.

Clinical & Experimental Pathology of Lung Cancer. Ed. by J. G. McVie et al. 1985. (Developments in Oncology Ser.). text 160.00 (*0-89838-764-7*) Kluwer Academic.

Clinical & Experimental Pheochromocytoma. William M. Manger & Ray Gifford. 2nd ed. 1996. LC 95-12314. (Illus.). 400p. 152.95 (*0-86542-494-2*) Blackwell Sci.

Clinical & Experimental Studies in Personality. Morton Prince. rev. ed. 1970. LC 72-100197. (Illus.). 671p. reprint ed. lib. bdg. 100.00 (*0-8371-3995-3*, PRPE, Greenwood Pr) Greenwood.

***Clinical & Experimental Studies of Organ-Specific Autoimmune Diseases: With Special References to Addison Disease & Autoimmune Hepatitus.** Gennet Gebre-Medhin. 2001. (Comprehensive Summaries of Uppsala Dissertations from the Faculty of Medicine Ser.: Vol. 1045). (Illus.). 70p. (*91-554-5043-1*) Uppsala Universitet SWE. *Dist:* Coronet Bks.

Clinical & Forensic Applications of Capillary Electrophoresis. Ed. by John R. Petersen & Amin A. Mohammad. 2001. LC 2001-16677. (Pathology & Laboratory Medicine Ser.). (Illus.). x, 453p. 125.00 (*0-89603-645-6*) Humana.

Clinical & Forensic Interviewing of Children & Families: Guidelines for the Mental Health, Education, Pediatric, & Child Maltreatment Fields. 1997. LC 97-67148. (Illus.). 1135p. (C). text 70.00 (*0-9618209-4-2*) J M Sattler.

Clinical & Functional Histology for Medical Students. Richard S. Snell. 1983. 856p. 60.00 (*0-316-80216-6*, Little Brwn Med Div) Lppncott W & W.

Clinical & Laborataory Performance of Bone Plates. Ed. by J. Paul Harvey, Jr. & Robert F. Games. 1994. LC 93-49642. (Special Technical Publications: Vol. 1217). (Illus.). 125p. pap. 39.00 (*0-8031-1897-X*, STP1217) ASTM.

Clinical & Molecular Aspects of Autoimmune Diseases. Ed. by J. M. Cruse & R. E. Lewis, Jr. 1991. (Concepts in Immunopathology Ser.: Vol. 8). (Illus.). x, 258p. 215.75 (*3-8055-5402-8*) S Karger.

Clinical & Molecular Aspects of Neurotropic Virus Infection. Ed. by Donald H. Gilden & Howard L. Lipton. 1989. (Developments in Medical Virology Ser.). (C). text 227.50 (*0-7923-0027-0*) Kluwer Academic.

Clinical & Nursing Implications of Laboratory Tests. Sarko M. Tilkian et al. 5th ed. 1995. LC 95-223101. (Illus.). 688p. (C). (gr. 13). pap. text 36.95 (*0-8151-8807-2*, 25867) Mosby Inc.

Clinical & Nursing Staff Development: Current Competence, Future Focus. Karen J. Kelly. 2nd ed. 1998. LC 98-10655. (Illus.). 432p. pap. text 49.50 (*0-397-55416-8*) Lppncott W & W.

Clinical & Observational Psychoanalytic Research: Roots of a Controversy. Joseph Sandler et al. 2000. LC 00-59732. (Psychoanalytic Monographs: Vol. 5). xix, 163p. 32.50 (*0-8236-0945-6*) Intl Univs Pr.

Clinical & Pathogenic Microbiology. Howard. 2nd ed. 1993. (Illus.). 1008p. (gr. 13). text 73.00 (*0-8016-6426-8*, 06426) Mosby Inc.

Clinical & Practice Issues in Adoption: Bridging the Gap Between Adoptees Placed As Infants & As Older Children. Ed. by Victor F. Groza & Karen Rosenberg. 1998. LC 98-11122. 192p. 60.00 (*0-275-95816-7*, Praeger Pubs) Greenwood.

Clinical & Projective Use of the Bender-Gestalt Test. Eugene X. Perticone. 1998. LC 97-43203. (Illus.). 150p. text 38.95 (*0-398-06834-8*); pap. text 24.95 (*0-398-06835-6*) C C Thomas.

Clinical & Radiographic Interpretation of Facial Fractures. Amil J. Gerlock & Douglas P. Sinn. 1981. (Illus.). 75.00 (*0-316-30836-6*, Little Brwn Med Div) Lppncott W & W.

Clinical & Research Uses of Ambulatory Monitoring. Ed. by Nancy K. Jacobsen. 1977. pap. 17.50 (*0-917054-13-X*) Med Communications.

Clinical & Resuscitative Data: A Compendium of Intensive, Medical, & Anaesthetic Resuscitative Data. R. P. Dunnill & M. P. Colvin. 5th ed. 1998. LC 97-18409. pap. 52.95 (*0-86542-788-7*) Blackwell Sci.

Clinical & Social Realities. Ed. by Donald M. Kaplan & Louise J. Kaplan. 1995. LC 95-1285. 512p. 50.00 (*1-56821-472-3*) Aronson.

Clinical Anesthesia. Paul G. Barash et al. 4th ed. 2000. 1,600p. text 169.00 (*0-7817-2268-3*) Lppncott W & W.

Clinical Anesthesia in Neurosurgery. Frost. 2001. 704p. 135.00 (*0-7506-7083-5*) Buttrwrth-Heinemann.

Clinical Anesthesia in Neurosurgery. Elizabeth A. M. Frost. 2nd ed. 1990. (Illus.). 608p. text 125.00 (*0-409-90171-7*) Buttrwrth-Heinemann.

Clinical Anesthesia Procedures of the Massachusetts General Hospital. Massachusetts General Hospital, Dept. of Anesthesi & Harvard Medical School Staff. Ed. by J. Kenneth Davison et al. 4th ed. 1993. LC 92-48517. (Handbook Ser.). (Illus.). 728p. pap. text 38.95 (*0-316-17714-8*) Lppncott W & W.

Clinical Anesthesia Procedures of the Massachusetts General Hospital. William E. Hurford & Michael T. Bailin. 5th ed. 1997. LC 97-17479. 816p. pap. text 39.95 (*0-7817-1523-7*) Lppncott W & W.

Clinical Anesthesiology. G. Edward Morgan. 2nd ed. 1996. 1005p. (C). pap. text 54.95 (*0-8385-1381-6*, A1381-1, Apple Lange Med) McGraw.

Clinical Anesthesiology. Morgan. 3rd ed. 2001. 1042p. (C). pap. 64.95 (*0-8385-1553-3*) McGraw-Hill Prof.

Clinical Answer Book. Springhouse Publishing Company Staff. 1995. (Illus.). 552p. 36.95 (*0-87434-825-0*) Springhouse Corp.

Clinical Aphasiology. Ed. by Thomas E. Prescott. Vol. 18. 1989. 531p. (C). pap. text 49.00 (*0-89079-322-0*, 1774); Vol. 19. 1991. (Illus.). 331p. pap. text 45.00 (*0-89079-407-3*, 1587); Vol. 20. 1992. 369p. text 49.00 (*0-89079-466-9*, 1803) PRO-ED.

Clinical Aphasiology. Ed. by Margaret L. Lemme. Vol. 21. 1992. LC 86-647891. 364p. (C). text 49.00 (*0-89079-564-9*, 1808); Vol. 22. 1994. 363p. (C). text 49.00 (*0-89079-595-9*, 1809); Vol. 24. 1996. 277p. text 49.00 (*0-89079-695-5*, 6901) PRO-ED.

Clinical Application of Blood Gases. Paul Mathew & Barbara Ludwig. 5th ed. 1994. 128p. pap. text, wbk. ed. 15.95 (*0-8151-7586-8*, 23839) Mosby Inc.

Clinical Application of Blood Gases. Barry A. Shapiro. 5th ed. 1993. (Illus.). 427p. (C). (gr. 13). text 54.00 (*0-8016-7839-0*, 07839) Mosby Inc.

Clinical Application of Current Techniques & Treatment in Cardiology: Proceedings of the Cardiovascular Disease Conference, 6th, Snowmass at Aspen, Colorado, 1975. Cardiovascular Disease Conference Staff. Ed. by H. K. Vogel. 1976. (Advances in Cardiology Ser.: Vol. 17). 109.75 (*3-8055-2267-3*) S Karger.

Clinical Application of Mechanical Ventilation. David W. Chang. abr. rev. ed. 1996. LC 96-8592. (Respiratory Care Ser.). 544p. (C). mass mkt. 56.95 (*0-8273-7320-1*) Delmar.

Clinical Application of Mechanical Ventilation - IML. Chang. 2nd abr. rev. ed. 1996. 160p. tchr. ed. 14.95 (*0-8273-8287-1*) Delmar.

Clinical Application of Mechanical Ventilation Workbook. Chang. abr. rev. ed. 1996. 224p. (C). pap. 20.25 net. (*0-8273-8285-5*) Delmar.

Clinical Application of Mifepristone (RU 486) & Other Antiprogestins: Assessing the Science & Recommending a Research Agenda. Institute of Medicine Staff. Ed. by Molla S. Donaldson et al. 1993. LC 93-85360. 304p. (Orig.). (C). pap. text 33.00 (*0-309-04949-0*) Natl Acad Pr.

Clinical Application of MMPI Special Scales. Eugene E. Levitt. 1989. 136p. 29.95 (*0-8058-0047-6*) L Erlbaum Assocs.

Clinical Application of MMPI Special Scales. Eugene E. Levitt & Edward E. Gotts. 2nd ed. 1995. 200p. text 39.95 (*0-8058-1770-0*) L Erlbaum Assocs.

Clinical Application of Neuropsychological Test Batteries. Ed. by Theresa Incagnoli et al. 1986. LC 85-25674. (Illus.). 424p. (C). text 90.00 (*0-306-42045-7*, Kluwer Plenum) Kluwer Academic.

Clinical Application of Outcomes Assessment. Steven G. Yeomans. 1999. LC 99-73500. (Illus.). 696p. pap. 79.95 (*0-8385-1528-2*) McGraw-Hill Prof.

Clinical Application of Projective Drawings. Emanuel F. Hammer. 1980. (Illus.). 688p. 68.95 (*0-398-00768-3*) C C Thomas.

Clinical Application of 3D Sonography. Ed. by A. Kurjak. 2000. LC 00-39998. (Illus.). 272p. 97.95 (*1-84214-006-X*, Parthenon Pbng) CRC Pr.

***Clinical Applications in Neurosurgical Monitoring.** Cheri A. Sulek. 2001. (Illus.). 395p. (*0-7216-7691-X*) Saunders.

Clinical Applications of Bowen Family Systems Theory. Ed. by Peter Titelman. 1998. LC 98-6169. (Illus.). 423p. 69.95 (*0-7890-0468-2*); pap. 39.95 (*0-7890-0469-0*) Haworth Pr.

Clinical Applications of Capillary Electrophoresis. Ed. by Stephen M. Palfrey. 1999. (Methods in Molecular Medicine Ser.: Vol. 27). (Illus.). 208p. 99.50 (*0-89603-639-1*) Humana.

Clinical Applications of Cardiovascular Drugs. Ed. by Leonard S. Dreifus & Albert N. Brest. 1980. (Developments in Cardiovascular Medicine Ser.: No. 5). (Illus.). 275p. pap. text 85.50 (*90-247-2369-8*); lib. bdg. 123.50 (*90-247-2295-0*) Kluwer Academic.

Clinical Applications of Cognitive Therapy. Arthur Freeman et al. 1990. LC 90-6706. (Illus.). 388p. (C). 54.50 (*0-306-43311-7*, Plenum Trade) Perseus Pubng.

Clinical Applications of Continuous Infusion Chemotherapy & Concomitant Radiation Therapy. Ed. by C. J. Rosenthal & M. Rotman. 1986. LC 86-4890. 262p. 75.00 (*0-306-42260-3*, Plenum Trade) Perseus Pubng.

Clinical Applications of Cryobiology. Barry J. Fuller & Brian W. Grout. 1991. 256p. 189.95 (*0-8493-5429-3*, QH324) CRC Pr.

Clinical Applications of Cytokines: Role in Pathogenesis, Diagnosis, & Therapy. Ed. by Joost J. Oppenheim et al. 1993. LC 92-49062. (Illus.). 400p. text 150.00 (*0-19-507129-8*) OUP.

Clinical Applications of Cytokines & Growth Factors. John R. Wingard & George D. Demetri. 1999. LC 99-22740. (Developments in Oncology Ser.: Vol. 80). (Illus.). xii, 407p. (*0-7923-8486-5*) Kluwer Academic.

Clinical Applications of Doppler Ultrasound. Ed. by Kenneth J. Taylor et al. 2nd ed. 1995. (Illus.). 416p. text 159.00 (*0-7817-0184-8*) Lppncott W & W.

Clinical Applications of Flow Cytometry: Immunophenotyping of Leukemic Cells; Proposed Guideline (1993) Contrib. by Michael Borowitz. 1993. 85.00 (*1-56238-219-5*, H43-P) NCCLS.

Clinical Applications of Flow Cytometry: Quality Assurance & Immunophenotyping of Peripheral Blood Lymphocytes; Tentative Guideline (1992) Contrib. by Alan L. Landay. 1992. 85.00 (*1-56238-155-5*, H42-T) NCCLS.

Clinical Applications of Herbal Medicine. D. Paul Barney. 1996. 200p. 10.95 (*1-885670-23-0*) Woodland UT.

Clinical Applications of Herbal Medicine, Vol. 2. Paul Barney. 1997. pap. text 11.95 (*1-885670-66-4*) Woodland UT.

Clinical Applications of Immunophenotypic Analysis. Katalin Paloczi. 1994. LC 94-32881. (Medical Intelligence Unit Ser.). 99.00 (*1-57059-194-6*) Landes Bioscience.

Clinical Applications of Immunotoxins. Ed. by A. Frankel et al. 1998. (Current Topics in Microbiology & Immunology Ser.: Vol. 234). (Illus.). 122p. 129.00 (*3-540-64097-5*) Spr-Verlag.

Clinical Applications of Intravenous Immunoglobulin Therapy. Ed. by Peng L. Yap. 1992. (Illus.). 256p. (Orig.). pap. text (*0-443-04588-7*) Church.

Clinical Applications of Medical Imaging. Jeffrey Bisker. 1986. LC 86-15093. (Illus.). 242p. (C). text 78.00 (*0-306-42199-2*, Kluwer Plenum) Kluwer Academic.

Clinical Applications of Monoclonal Antibodies. Ed. by R. Hubbard & V. Marks. 1988. (Illus.). 268p. 75.00 (*0-306-43142-4*, Plenum Trade) Perseus Pubng.

Clinical Applications of MR Spectroscopy. Suresh K. Mukherji & Mauricio Castillo. 1998. LC 97-26486. (Illus.). 317p. 115.00 (*0-471-16178-0*, Wiley-Liss) Wiley.

Clinical Applications of Nursing Diagnosis: Adult, Child, Women's, Psychiatric, Gerontic, & Home Health Considerations. Helen C. Cox et al. 3rd ed. 1997. LC 96-34957. (Illus.). 800p. (C). pap. text 36.95 (*0-8036-0177-8*) Davis Co.

***Clinical Applications of Nursing Diagnosis: Adult, Child, Women's, Psychiatric, Gerontic, & Home Health Considerations.** Helen C. Cox. 4th ed. 2001. LC 2001-47231. 768p. per. 39.95 (*0-8036-0913-2*) Davis Co.

Clinical Applications of Pathophysiology. Valentina L. Brashers. 1998. (Illus.). 432p. (C). text (*0-323-00149-1*) Mosby Inc.

Clinical Applications of PCR. Ed. by Y. M. Dennis Lo. 1998. LC 97-51264. (Methods in Molecular Medicine Ser.: Vol. 16). (Illus.). 364p. 129.50 (*0-89603-499-2*) Humana.

Clinical Applications of PCR. Ed. by Y. M. Dennis Lo & J. S. Wainscoat. 1998. LC 97-51264. (Methods in Molecular Medicine Ser.: Vol. 16). (Illus.). 364p. spiral bd. 99.50 (*0-89603-359-7*) Humana.

Clinical Applications of Radioimmunoassay. Ferenc A. Laszlo & Tibor Janaky. 1992. 230p. pap. (*963-05-6219-7*) Akade Kiado HUN. *Dist:* Intl Spec Bk, St Mut.

Clinical Applications of Radiolabelled Platelets. Ed. by C. Kessler et al. 1990. (C). text 155.00 (*0-7923-0729-1*) Kluwer Academic.

Clinical Applications of Rational-Emotive Therapy. A. Ellis & M. E. Bernard. 1985. LC 85-3709. (Illus.). 372p. (C). 65.00 (*0-306-41971-8*, Plenum Trade) Perseus Pubng.

Clinical Applications of Respiratory Care. Barry A. Shapiro. 4th ed. 1990. 560p. (C). (gr. 13). text 64.95 (*0-8151-7670-8*, 20393) Mosby Inc.

Clinical Applications of the Interferons. Ed. by Charles H. Stuart-Harris & R. Penny. 1997. LC 96-86292. (Illus.). 448p. (*0-412-60250-4*) E A GBR. *Dist:* OUP.

Clinical Applications of the Intra-Aortic Balloon Pump. Ed. by Hooshang Bolooki. 3rd rev. ed. 1998. LC 98-6276. (Illus.). 484p. 98.00 (*0-87993-401-8*) Futura Pub.

Clinical Applications of the Physics of Radiology & Nuclear Medicine. Carl R. Bogardus, Jr. 1969. LC 67-26010. (Illus.). 248p. 15.00 (*0-87527-002-6*) Green.

Clinical Applications of the Scanning Electron Microscope. H. W. Carter et al. Ed. by Om Johari & R. P. Becker. 1980. (Illus.). pap. 10.00 (*0-931288-16-9*) Scanning Microscopy.

Clinical Applications of Ultrasonic Fetal Measurements. Evans. 1991. pap. (*0-905749-24-3*) Med Physics Pub.

Clinical Applications of Ventilatory Support. Ed. by Robert R. Kirby et al. 1990. (Illus.). 546p. text (*0-443-08613-3*) Church.

Clinical Applied Psychophysiology. Ed. by J. G. Carlson et al. 1994. (Behavioral Psychophysiology Ser.). (Illus.). 292p. (C). 49.50 (*0-306-44555-7*, Plenum Trade) Perseus Pubng.

Clinical Approach: A Companion for the Practising Doctor. R. D. Lele. 1997. LC 97-164935. (Illus.). 372p. 49.50 (*0-19-563729-1*) OUP.

Clinical Approach to Antiphospholipid Antibodies. Steven R. Levine & Robin L. Brey. 2000. LC 99-53901. (Illus.). 168p. text 59.99 (*0-7506-7177-7*) Buttrwrth-Heinemann.

Clinical Approach to Children's Rorschachs. Florence Halpern. 1953. LC 53-11013. 288p. text 44.00 (*0-8089-0170-2*, 791850, Grune & Strat) Harcrt Hlth Sci Grp.

C
D

Clinical Approach to Infection in the Compromised Host. Ed. by R. H. Rubin & L. S. Young. 3rd ed. 1994. (Illus.). 780p. (C). text 145.00 (*0-306-44617-0*, Kluwer Plenum) Kluwer Academic.

Clinical Approach to Medicine. Ed. by Ong Yong Yau et al. 2001. LC 00-48103. 850p. pap. 75.00 (*981-02-4455-X*) World Scientific Pub.

Clinical Approaches to the Erotic Transference & Countertransference. David Mann. 1999. LC 98-30535. 85.00 (*0-415-18452-5*); 192p. pap. 29.95 (*0-415-18453-3*) Routledge.

Clinical Approaches to the Mentally Disordered Offender. Ed. by Kevin Howells & Clive R. Hollin. 1993. LC 92-48423. (Clinical Approaches to Criminal Behavior Ser.). 274p. 225.00 (*0-471-93908-0*) Wiley.

Clinical Aromatherapy in Nursing. Jane Buckle. 1997. LC 97-205859. (Illus.). 304p. (Orig.). pap. 39.95 (*1-56593-876-3*, 1716) Singular Publishing.

Clinical Art Therapy: A Comprehensive Guide. Helen B. Landgarten. 1987. LC 80-22564. 416p. text 34.95 (*0-87630-237-1*) Brunner-Routledge.

Clinical Aspects of Cardiac Arrhythmias. Ed. by A. John Camm & David E. Ward. 1988. (Current Status of Clinical Cardiology Ser.). (C). text 235.50 (*0-85200-972-0*) Kluwer Academic.

Clinical Aspects of Compliance. Ed. by Levine & Reed. 1999. (Psychoanalytic Inquiry Ser.: Vol. 19, No. 1). pap. 20.00 (*0-88163-926-5*) Analytic Pr.

Clinical Aspects of Dental Materials. Contrib. by Michael D. Bagby & Marcia A. Gladwin. 1999. LC 99-29257. 296p. pap. text 37.95 (*0-683-30291-4*) Lppncott W & W.

Clinical Aspects of Fibrinolysis. T. K. Nilsson et al. 1991. (Illus.). 187p. 158.00 (*91-22-01436-5*) Coronet Bks.

Clinical Aspects of Hearing. Ed. by T. R. Van De Water et al. 1995. LC 95-9347. (Springer Handbook of Auditory Research: Vol. 13). (Illus.). 317p. 98.00 (*0-387-97842-9*) Spr-Verlag.

Clinical Aspects of IgG Subclasses & Therapeutic Implications. Ed. by F. Skavril et al. 1988. (Monographs in Allergy: Vol. 23). (Illus.). x, 294p. 172.25 (*3-8055-4671-8*) S Karger.

Clinical Aspects of Immunology. Ed. by P. J. Lachmann et al. 5th ed. 1993. LC 92-48808. (Illus.). 2328p. 299.95 (*0-86542-297-4*) Blackwell Sci.

Clinical Aspects of Implantable Cardioverter-Defibrillator Therapy. Martin Fromer. 1998. (Clinical Approaches to Tachyarrhythmias Ser.: Vol. 9). (Illus.). 126p. 19.00 (*0-87993-411-5*, Futura Media) Futura Pub.

Clinical Aspects of Microcirculation: Proceedings of the European Conference on Microcirculation, 7th, Aberdeen, 1972 Part II. European Conference on Microcirculation Staff. 1974. (Bibliotheca Anatomica Ser.: No. 12). (Illus.). 563p. 248.75 (*3-8055-1572-3*) S Karger.

Clinical Aspects of Microdialysis. A. Mendelowitsch. 1996. LC 96-18565. (Acta Neurochirurgica Ser.). (Illus.). 75p. 95.00 (*3-211-82834-6*) Spr-Verlag.

Clinical Aspects of Neutron Capture Therapy. Ed. by R. G. Fairchild et al. 1989. (Illus.). 384p. 89.50 (*0-306-43114-9*, Plenum Trade) Perseus Pubng.

Clinical Aspects of O2-Transport & Tissue Oxygenation. Ed. by K. Reinhart & K. Eyrich. 1989. (Illus.). 511p. 146.00 (*0-387-51470-8*, 3312) Spr-Verlag.

Clinical Aspects of Oral Gestogens. 1966. (Technical Report Ser.: No. 326). 24p. pap. text 3.00 (*92-4-120326-9*) World Health.

Clinical Aspects of Renovascular Hypertension. Ed. by R. Van Schilfgaarde & J. C. Stanley. 1983. text 148.50 (*0-89838-574-1*) Kluwer Academic.

Clinical Aspects of Sensory Motor Integration. Ed. by A. Struppler & A. Weindl. 1987. (Advances in Applied Neurological Sciences Ser.: Vol. 4). (Illus.). 353p. 108.00 (*0-387-17012-X*) Spr-Verlag.

Clinical Aspiration Cytology. Joseph A. Linsk et al. Ed. by Sixten Franzen. 2nd ed. 1989. LC 65-9913. (Illus.). 432p. text 125.00 (*0-397-50826-3*, Lippnctt) Lppncott W & W.

Clinical Assessment & Intervention Planning, Vol. 5, Clinical Assessment and Intervention Plann. Ed. by Joseph D. Noshpitz et al. 1998. (Handbook of Child & Adolescent Psychiatry Ser.: Vol. 5). 848p. 250.00 (*0-471-19330-5*) Wiley.

Clinical Assessment & Management of Severe Personality Disorders. Ed. by Paul S. Links. 1995. (Clinical Practice Ser.: No. 35). 256p. text 35.00 (*0-88048-488-8*, 8488) Am Psychiatric.

Clinical Assessment & Treatment of HIV: Rehabilitation of a Chronic Illness. Ed. by Mary L. Galantino. 1991. LC 90-53246. (Illus.). 280p. pap. 36.00 (*1-55642-181-8*) SLACK Inc.

Clinical Assessment in Respiratory Care. Robert L. Wilkins et al. (Illus.). 3rd ed. 1994. LC 94-35037. 400p. (C). (gr. 13). pap. text 43.00 (*0-8151-9334-3*, 24152); 4th ed. 2000. 450p. pap. 44.00 (*0-323-00909-3*) Mosby Inc.

*__Clinical Assessment in Respiratory Care.__ Robert L. Wilkins et al. 4th ed. 2000. (Illus.). pap., tchr. ed. 750.00 (*0-323-00910-7*) Mosby Inc.

Clinical Assessment in Respiratory Care: Quick Reference Guide. A. Wilkins. 1994. (Illus.). 64p. (gr. 13). pap. text 9.95 (*0-8151-9288-6*, 25895) Mosby Inc.

*__Clinical Assessment in Respiratory Care: Testbank.__ Robert L. Wilkins et al. 4th ed. 2000. pap. (*0-323-00997-2*) Mosby Inc.

Clinical Assessment of Child & Adolescent Behavior. H. Booney Vance & Andres J. Pumariega. 2001. LC 00-61965. (Illus.). 576p. 55.00 (*0-471-38046-6*, J874-Y3H) Wiley.

*__Clinical Assessment of Child & Adolescent Personality & Behavior.__ Randy W. Kamphaus & Paul J. Frick. 2nd ed. 2001. 496p. 100.00 (*0-205-33459-8*) Allyn.

Clinical Assessment of Children's Intelligence. Randy W. Kamphaus. 1992. LC 92-18063. 544p. 110.00 (*0-205-13934-5*) Allyn.

Clinical Assessment of Dangerousness: Empirical Contributions. Ed. by Georges-Franck Pinard & Linda Pagani. 2000. LC 00-23779. (Illus.). 336p. (C). text 59.95 (*0-521-64123-3*) Cambridge U Pr.

Clinical Assessment of Language Comprehension. Jon F. Miller & Rhea Paul. 1994. LC 94-35065. 208p. spiral bd. 34.95 (*1-55766-176-6*) P H Brookes.

Clinical Assessment of Malingering & Deception. Ed. by Richard Rogers. 2nd ed. 1997. LC 96-43033. 525p. text 52.00 (*1-57230-173-2*, 0173) Guilford Pubns.

Clinical Assessment of Nutritional Status. Alan H. Pressman & Alan H. Adams. 2nd ed. 1990. 220p. 40.00 (*0-683-06970-5*) Lppncott W & W.

Clinical Athletic Training. Jeff Konin. 1996. LC 96-42296. 320p. 35.00 (*1-55642-315-2*, 43152) SLACK Inc.

Clinical Atlas of Chinese Infants. Anita M. Li & Chap-Yung Yeung. 1996. LC 97-178884. (Illus.). 97p. (Orig.). pap. (*962-209-390-6*) HK Univ Pr HKG. *Dist:* Intl Spec Bk, Coronet Bks.

Clinical Atlas of Endodontic Surgery. Ralph Bellizzi & Robert Loushine. 1991. (Illus.). 135p. text 59.00 (*0-86715-234-6*) Quint Pub Co.

Clinical Atlas of Muscle & Musculocutaneous Flaps. Stephen J. Mathes & Foad Nahai. 1979. LC 79-10739. (Illus.). 520p. (C). (gr. 13). text 90.95 (*0-8016-3141-6*, 03141) Mosby Inc.

Clinical Atlas of Peripheral Retinal Disorders. Keith M. Zinn. 1988. (Illus.). 156p. 361.00 (*0-387-96459-2*) Spr-Verlag.

Clinical Atlas of Respiratory Diseases. Margaret E. Turner-Warwick et al. 1989. (Illus.). 550p. (gr. 13). text (*0-397-44590-3*, GM0052) Gower-Mosby.

Clinical Atlas of Surgical Oncology. Mark Roh. 2001. (Illus.). 600p. text 125.00 (*1-57626-014-3*) Quality Med Pub.

Clinical Atlas of Transesophageal Echocardiography. Martin E. Goldman. 1993. LC 93-3794. (Illus.). 392p. 149.00 (*0-87993-539-1*) Futura Pub.

Clinical Atlas of Uveitis. Spalton. 2001. 176p. 125.00 (*0-7506-9795-4*) Buttrwrth-Heinemann.

Clinical Atlas of Vascular Disorders. Ed. by J. Latorre & M. Monreal. 1988. 128p. 24.95 (*0-8151-5325-2*, CDA-1) Mosby Inc.

Clinical Audiology: An Introduction. Brad Stach. 1998. LC 97-51972. (Illus.). 604p. pap. text 59.95 (*1-56593-346-X*, 0644) Thomson Learn.

Clinical Audiometry & Masking. Frederick N. Martin. 1972. LC 74-183115. (Studies in Communicative Disorders). (C). pap. 3.25 (*0-672-61282-8*, Bobbs) Macmillan.

Clinical Audit in Mental Health: Toward a Multidisciplinary Approach. John Riordan. 1997. LC 96-48521. 182p. pap. 47.00 (*0-471-96332-1*) Wiley.

Clinical Audit in Pharmaceutical Development. Michael R. Hamrell. 1999. LC 99-47751. (Drugs & the Pharmaceutical Sciences Ser.: Vol. 104). (Illus.). 224p. text 135.00 (*0-8247-0309-X*) Dekker.

Clinical Audit in Physiotherapy: From Theory into Practice. Sue Barnard & Gayle Hartigan. 1998. LC 98-20594. 144p. pap. text 45.00 (*0-7506-3779-X*) Buttrwrth-Heinemann.

Clinical Auscultation of the Cardiovascular System. W. Proctor Harvey & David C. Canfield. 1989. 95.00 incl. audio (*1-886128-01-4*); 1996. (Illus.). 95.00 incl. audio (*1-886128-08-1*) Laennec Pub.

Clinical Autonomic Disorders. Ed. by Philip A. Low. 2nd ed. 1997. LC 97-11278. (Illus.). 849p. text 199.00 (*0-316-53281-9*) Lppncott W & W.

Clinical Avian Medicine & Surgery: Including Aviculture. Greg J. Harrison & Linda R. Harrison. 1986. (Illus.). 717p. text 126.00 (*0-7216-1241-5*) Saunders.

Clinical Aviation Medicine. Russell B. Rayman et al. 3rd rev. ed. 2000. LC 00-111788. xiii, 346p. 99.95 (*0-9707305-0-0*); xiii,346p. pap. 99.95 (*1-883769-86-8*) Cas Con Grad Med.

Clinical Behavior Analysis. Mike Dougher. 1999. LC 99-43532. 304p. 42.95 (*1-878978-38-1*) Context Pr.

Clinical Behavior Therapy. Marvin R. Goldfried & Gerald C. Davison. expurg. ed. 1994. LC 94-16335. (Clinical Psychology & Personality Ser.). 352p. pap. 54.95 (*0-471-07633-3*) Wiley.

Clinical Behavior Therapy with Children. Thomas H. Ollendick & Jerome A. Cerny. 1981. LC 81-17891. (Applied Clinical Psychology Ser.). (Illus.). 364p. (C). text 71.00 (*0-306-40774-4*, Kluwer Plenum) Kluwer Academic.

Clinical Behavioral Medicine: Some Concepts & Procedures. I. E. Wickramasekera. 1988. LC 88-1055. (Illus.). 334p. (C). 49.50 (*0-306-42734-6*, Plenum Trade) Perseus Pubng.

Clinical Behavioral Pediatrics: An Interdisciplinary Biobehavioral Approach. James W. Varni. 1983. (General Psychology Ser.: No. 125). 275p. 45.00 (*0-08-027172-3*, Pergamon Pr) Elsevier.

Clinical Benefits of Leukodepleted Blood Products. Ed. by Joseph Sweeney & Andrew Heaton. 1995. LC 94-39668. (Medical Intelligence Unit Ser.). 190p. text 99.00 (*1-57059-122-9*) Landes Bioscience.

Clinical Biochemical & Hematological Reference Values in Normal Experimental Animals & Normal Humans. Brij M. Mitruka & Howard M. Rawnsley. 2nd expurg. ed. 1981. LC 81-17157. (Illus.). 432p. (gr. 13). 68.50 (*0-89352-163-9*) Mosby Inc.

Clinical Biochemistry. Marshall. 3rd ed. 1995. 31.00 (*0-7234-2190-0*) Mosby Inc.

Clinical Biochemistry: An Illustrated Colour Text. Allan Gaw. 2nd ed. 1999. LC 99-10541. (Illus.). viii, 165p. (*0-443-06183-1*) Church.

Clinical Biochemistry Vol. 2: Principals, Methods, Applications: Data Presentation-Interpretation. Ed. by H. Keller & C. Trendelenburg. 1989. LC 89-11959. (Clinical Biochemistry Ser.: Vol. 2). xxii, 479p. (C). lib. bdg. 211.55 (*3-11-010735-X*) De Gruyter.

Clinical Biochemistry & the Sick Child. Barbara E. Clayton & Joan M. Round. 2nd ed. 1994. LC 93-38329. (Illus.). 576p. 208.95 (*0-632-03681-8*) Blackwell Sci.

Clinical Biochemistry for Medicine. Laker. 1995. pap. text 33.00 (*0-7020-1690-X*) Saunders.

Clinical Biochemistry in Hepatobiliary Diseases. 1989. (Progress in Clinical Biochemistry & Medicine Ser.: Vol. 8). (Illus.). 196p. 115.00 (*0-387-50705-1*, 2622) Spr-Verlag.

Clinical Biochemistry Made Ridiculously Simple. Stephen Goldberg. 2nd ed. 1999. (Illus.). 95p. (Orig.). pap. text 22.95 (*0-940780-30-5*) MedMaster.

Clinical Biochemistry of Lipids. A. Dubin. Ed. by Max E. Rafelson. 1984. (Journal: Vol. 2, No. 2-3). (Illus.). 80p. pap. 69.75 (*3-8055-3859-6*) S Karger.

Clinical Bioethics: Theory & Practice in Medical-Ethical Decision Making. James F. Drane. 1994. LC 93-46600. 300p. (Orig.). pap. 24.95 (*1-55612-612-3*) Sheed & Ward WI.

Clinical Biomechanics. Zeevi Dvir. 2000. LC 99-37691. viii, 275p. (C). text (*0-443-07945-5*) Harcrt Hlth Sci Grp.

Clinical Biomechanics. Ed. by Gary M. Greenstein. 1996. (Illus.). 304p. (C). (gr. 13). text 49.00 (*0-8151-3948-9*, 23706) Mosby Inc.

Clinical Biomechanics of Spinal Manipulation. Walter Herzog. 1998. (Illus.). 295p. pap. text (*0-443-07808-4*) Church.

Clinical Biomechanics of the Foot. Shavelson. 1998. text (*0-7216-3999-2*) Harcourt.

Clinical Biomechanics of the Lower Extremities. Ed. by Ronald L. Valmassy. 1995. LC 95-35679. (Illus.). 528p. (C). (gr. 13). text 89.95 (*0-8016-7986-9*, 07986) Mosby Inc.

Clinical Biomechanics of the Spine. Augustus A. White. 2nd ed. 1990. (Illus.). 752p. text 159.00 (*0-397-50720-8*) Lppncott W & W.

Clinical Biophysics. Michael Anbar. Ed. by Alvin F. Gardner. 1985. (Allied Health Professions Monograph). (Illus.). 772p. 75.00 (*0-87527-316-5*) Green.

Clinical Biostatistics: An Introduction to Evidence-Based Medicine. Graham Dunn & Brian S. Everitt. 1999. LC 95-171090. (An Arnold Publication). 160p. pap. (*0-340-59531-0*) E A GBR. *Dist:* OUP.

Clinical Blood Gases, Vol. 7. Karen Milikowski. 1995. (Respiratory Care Workbook Ser.). 24p. (C). (gr. 13). text, wbk. ed. 8.95 (*0-8151-6310-X*, 26028) Mosby Inc.

Clinical Blood Gases: Invasive & Noninvasive Techniques & Applications. Malley. 1990. (Illus.). 400p. text 52.00 (*0-7216-5861-X*) Saunders.

Clinical Blood Rheology. Ed. by Gordon D. O. Lowe. 1988. Vol. I. 224p. 137.00 (*0-8493-4598-7*, RB45); Vol. II. 240p. 146.00 (*0-8493-4599-5*, RB45) Franklin (CRC Reprint).

Clinical Briefs in Infectious Disease & HIV/AIDS. 2000. 200p. pap. 99.00 (*0-9603332-4-X*) Am Health Consults.

Clinical Briefs in Neurology. 2000. 200p. pap. 99.00 (*0-9603332-5-8*) Am Health Consults.

Clinical Briefs in Obstetrics & Gynecology. 2000. 200p. pap. 99.00 (*0-9603332-6-6*) Am Health Consults.

Clinical Briefs in Oncology. 2000. 200p. pap. 99.00 (*0-9603332-7-4*) Am Health Consults.

Clinical Briefs in Pharmacology. 2000. 200p. pap. 99.00 (*0-9603332-8-2*) Am Health Consults.

Clinical Briefs in Primary Care, Vol. 5. 2000. 200p. pap. 99.00 (*0-9603332-9-0*) Am Health Consults.

Clinical Calculations. Daniels. 1986. (Education Ser.). pap., tchr. ed. 9.95 (*0-8273-2518-5*) Delmar.

Clinical Calculations. Joyce LeFever Kee & Sally M. Marshall. 4th ed. 1999. LC 99-35200. (C). pap. text (*0-7216-8304-5*) Saunders.

Clinical Calculations: A Unified Approach. Joanne M. Daniels & Loretta M. Smith. 1986. LC 86-2131. 272p. (C). Apple II 49.95 (*0-8273-2516-9*); pap. 24.95 (*0-8273-2517-7*) Delmar.

Clinical Calculations: A Unified Approach. Joanne Daniels & Loretta Smith. 4th ed. 1998. LC 98-15353. 400p. (C). pap. text 49.95 (*0-7668-0167-5*) Delmar.

Clinical Calculations: A Unified Approach - Instructor's Guide. Joanne M. Daniels & Loretta M. Smith. 3rd ed. 1994. 132p. 14.95 (*0-8273-5946-2*) Delmar.

Clinical Calculations: With Applications to General & Specialty Areas. Joyce L. Kee & Sally M. Marshall. 3rd ed. 1996. (Illus.). 317p. pap., tchr. ed. (*0-7216-5451-7*) Saunders.

Clinical Calculations: With Applications to General & Specialty Areas. Joyce L. Kee & Sally M. Marshall. Ed. by Dan Ruth. 3rd ed. 1995. LC 95-14150. (Illus.). 320p. pap. text 28.00 (*0-7216-5444-4*) Saunders.

*__Clinical Calculations: With Applications to General & Specialty Areas.__ Joyce LeFever Kee & Sally M. Marshall. 4th ed. 2000. (Illus.). 384p. pap., tchr. ed. 75.00 (*0-7216-8306-1*) Saunders.

Clinical Calculations 3e. Joanne M. Daniels & Loretta M. Smith. 3rd ed. 1993. LC 93-19225. (Student Material TV). 375p. (C). mass mkt. 41.95 (*0-8273-5945-4*) Delmar.

Clinical Calculations Test Booklet. Daniels. 1986. (Education Ser.). pap. 24.95 (*0-8273-2540-1*) Delmar.

Clinical Cancer Genetics: Risk Counseling & Management. Kenneth Offitt. 1997. LC 97-14958. (Illus.). 448p. 84.95 (*0-471-14655-2*) Wiley.

Clinical Capillaroscopy: A Guide to Its Use in Clinical Research & Practice. Ed. by Alfred Bollinger & Bengt Fagrell. 1990. LC 90-5052. (Illus.). 168p. text 64.00 (*0-88937-048-6*) Hogrefe & Huber Pubs.

Clinical Cardiac Assessment, Interventions, & Assist-Technology. Ed. by Dhanjoo N. Ghista. 1990. (Advances in Cardiovascular Physics Ser.: Vol. 7). (Illus.). xii, 178p. 189.75 (*3-8055-5024-3*) S Karger.

Clinical Cardiac Magnetic Resonance. Warren J. Manning & Dudley J. Pennell. 1999. (Illus.). 300p. (C). 99.00 (*0-443-07519-0*) Saunders.

Clinical Cardiac Pacing. Ellen Bogen et al. 1994. (Illus.). 736p. text 188.00 (*0-7216-5462-2*) Saunders.

Clinical Cardiac Pacing & Defibrillation. Ellen Bogen. 2nd ed. 1999. LC 98-53093. xv, 1007p. text (*0-7216-7683-9*) Saunders.

Clinical Cardiac Rehabilitation: A Cardiologist's Guide. Ed. by Fredric J. Pashkow & William A. DaFoe. 2nd ed. 1998. LC 98-15106. 394p. 115.00 (*0-683-30224-8*) Lppncott W & W.

Clinical Cardiac Roentgen Diagnosis. Alphons Jacob. 1971. LC 70-96985. (Illus.). 322p. 24.50 (*0-87527-044-1*) Green.

Clinical Cardiology. Peter C. Gazes. 3rd ed. 1989. LC 89-12512. (Illus.). 594p. text 69.95 (*0-8121-1235-0*) Lppncott W & W.

Clinical Cardiology. Elliot Chesler. 5th ed. 1992. (Illus.). 451p. 163.00 (*0-387-97712-0*) Spr-Verlag.

Clinical Cardiology. Melvin D. Cheitlin & Maurice Sokolow. 6th ed. 1996. LC 93-239139. 741p. (C). pap. text 54.95 (*0-8385-1093-0*, A1093-2, Apple Lange Med) McGraw.

Clinical Cardiology. Melvin D. Cheitlin. 7th ed. 1999. (C). pap. text 43.95 (*0-8385-1385-9*) Appleton & Lange.

Clinical Cardiology: A Cost Effective Approach. Peter C. Gazes. 4th ed. 1997. LC 96-36033. 688p. pap. (*0-412-11281-7*) E A GBR. *Dist:* OUP.

Clinical Cardiology: An Illustrated Text. Ed. by K. Chaterjee & G. Sutton. 2nd ed. 1999. (Illus.). 440p. (*0-412-78310-X*) E A GBR. *Dist:* OUP.

Clinical Cardiology in the Elderly. Ed. by Elliot Chesler. 2nd ed. 1999. LC 98-42493. (Illus.). 840p. 165.00 (*0-87993-421-2*) Futura Pub.

Clinical Cardiovascular Medicine in Anaesthesia. Ed. by Pierre Coriat et al. 1997. 300p. pap. text (*0-7279-1127-9*) BMJ Pub GBR. *Dist:* AIDC.

Clinical Care in the Rheumatic Diseases. Ed. by Stephen T. Wegener et al. 1996. LC 96-41776. (Illus.). 224p. (Orig.). pap. 35.00 (*0-9654316-0-6*) Am College Rheum.

Clinical Care of the Aged Person: An Interdisciplinary Perspective. David G. Satin. 1994. LC 93-38279. (Illus.). 512p. text 69.50 (*0-19-505290-0*) OUP.

Clinical Care Plans for Medical-Surgical Nursing. Ed. by Marlene G. Mayers & Carol Pankratz. 2nd ed. 1994. LC 95-155433. (Clinical Care Plans Ser.). 362p. text 29.95 (*0-07-105464-2*) McGraw-Hill Med Pub.

Clinical Care Plans for Perinatal-Neonatal Nursing. Ed. by Marlene G. Mayers & Annette L. Jacobson. 2nd ed. 1994. (McGraw-Hill Clinical Care Plans Ser.). 320p. pap. 26.00 (*0-07-105463-4*) McGraw-Hill Educ Grp.

Clinical Case Management: An Approach to Comprehensive Treatment of Serious Mental Illness. Ed. by Robert W. Surber. 1994. LC 93-34552. (Sage Focus Editions Ser.: Vol. 167). 275p. (C). pap. 38.95 (*0-8039-4387-3*, 8076) Sage.

Clinical Case Management with Persons Having Mental Illness: A Relationship-Based Perspective. Joseph Walsh. 1999. LC 99-36796. 320p. pap. text 43.95 (*0-534-34852-1*) Wadsworth Pub.

Clinical Case Reporting in Evidence-Based Medicine. Milos Jenicek. 1999. LC 99-35353. 176p. (Orig.). pap. (*0-7506-4592-X*) E A GBR. *Dist:* OUP.

*__Clinical Case Reporting in Evidence-Based Medicine.__ Milos Jenicek. 2nd ed. 2001. (Arnold Publication). 256p. (Orig.). pap. text 27.50 (*0-340-76399-X*) OUP.

Clinical Case Studies - Concepts of Human Anatomy. Kent M. Van De Graaff & Stuart Ira Fox. 4th ed. 1995. 28p. (C). text 11.00 net. (*0-697-29202-9*, WCB McGr Hill) McGrw-H Hghr Educ.

Clinical Case Studies in the Behavioral Treatment of Alcoholism. Ed. by William H. Hay & Peter E. Nathan. 1982. LC 82-18048. 324p. 55.00 (*0-306-40940-2*, Plenum Trade) Perseus Pubng.

Clinical Cases for Learning Pediatric Occupational Therapy: A Problem-Based Approach. Diane E. Watson. 1998. pap. text 43.00 (*0-12-784590-9*) Acad Pr.

Clinical Cases for the MRCs & AFRCs. Gareth J. Morris-Stiff. 1998. LC 98-2837. (Illus.). 200p. pap. text (*0-340-69268-5*) E A GBR. *Dist:* St Martin.

Clinical Cases in Anesthesia. Ed. by Allan P. Reed. 2nd ed. 1995. LC 94-23730. text (*0-443-08899-3*) Church.

Clinical Cases in Contact Lenses. Ronald K. Watanabe. 2001. 240p. pap. 44.99 (*0-7506-9044-5*) Buttrwrth-Heinemann.

Clinical Cases in Neurology. L. P. Rouland & A. V. H. Schapira. 2001. LC 00-68888. (Illus.). 288p. pap. text 45.00 (*0-7506-4304-8*) Buttrwrth-Heinemann.

Clinical Cases in Ophthalmology. Hon Bing Hoh & David L. Easty. 1995. LC 94-44574. (Illus.). 224p. pap. text 55.00 (*0-7506-2102-8*) Buttrwrth-Heinemann.

Clinical Cases in Physical Therapy. Mark A. Brimer & Michael L. Moran. 1995. LC 95-13055. 103p. pap. text 29.99 (*0-7506-9637-0*) Buttrwrth-Heinemann.

Clinical Challenges in Gastroenterology. Ed. by Michael J. G. Farthing. 1996. 224p. (*1-85317-252-9*) Martin Dunitz GBR. *Dist:* Mosby Inc.

Clinical Challenges in Inflammatory Bowel Diseases: Diagnosis, Prognosis & Treatment. Ed. by G. Bianchi-Porro et al. 1998. (Falk Symposium Ser.). 288p. 125.00 (*0-7923-8733-3*) Kluwer Academic.

***Clinical Challenges in Orthopaedics: The Hip.** Northmore-Ball & Bannister. 2001. (Illus.). 256p. (*1-899066-83-7*) Isis Med GBR. *Dist:* Bks Intl VA.

***Clinical Challenges in Orthopaedics: The Knee.** Colin M. Fergusson et al. Ed. by Robin L. Allum. 2001. (Illus.). 240p. (*1-899066-63-2*) Isis Med GBR. *Dist:* Bks Intl VA.

Clinical Chaos: A Therapist's Guide to Nonlinear Dynamics & Therapeutic Change. Michael R. Butz & Linda L. Chamberlain. 1998. LC 98-25958. (*0-87630-925-2*) Brunner-Routledge.

Clinical Chemistry. Ed. by Donald T. Forman & Richard W. Mattoon. 1976. LC 76-49983. (ACS Symposium Ser.: No. 36). 29.95 (*0-8412-0345-8*) Am Chemical.

Clinical Chemistry. Muriel Kanter. 1975. LC 75-4050. (Allied Health Ser.). pap. 12.04 (*0-672-61380-8*, Bobbs) Macmillan.

Clinical Chemistry. Jack Rudman. 1994. (College Level Examination Ser.: CLEP-32). pap. 27.95 (*0-8373-5332-7*) Nat Learn.

Clinical Chemistry. William J. Marshall. 4th ed. 2001. LC 99 56728. 362p. pap. text 39.95 (*0 7234 3159 0*) Mosby Inc.

Clinical Chemistry: A Fundamental Textbook. Donald F. Calbreath. 1992. (Illus.). 490p. tchr. ed. (*0-7216-2622-X*) Saunders.

Clinical Chemistry: Concepts & Applications. Shauna C. Anderson & Susan Cockayne. 1992. (Illus.). 768p. text 65.00 (*0-7216-3372-2*) Saunders.

Clinical Chemistry: Principles, Procedures, Correlations. Michael Bishop et al. 4th ed. 2000. LC 99-36820. 720p. text 60.95 (*0-7817-1776-0*) Lppncott W & W.

Clinical Chemistry: Theory, Analysis, & Correlation. Ed. by Lawrence A. Kaplan & Amadeo J. Pesce. 3rd ed. 1996. LC 95-47197. (Illus.). 1232p. (C). (gr. 13). text 75.00 (*0-8151-5243-4*, 24163) Mosby Inc.

Clinical Chemistry in Diagnosis & Treatment. Philip Mayne. 6th ed. 1994. (Illus.). 478p. pap. text (*0-340-57647-2*) E A GBR. *Dist:* OUP.

Clinical Chemistry Laboratory Manual. Najih Naser & Saleh A. Naser. 1998. (Illus.). 380p. (C). pap., wbk. ed. (*0-8151-2581-X*) Mosby Inc.

Clinical Chemistry Profile Data for Hispanics, 1982-84. Matthew F. Najjar. 1992. LC 92-48934. (Vital & Health Statistics Ser.: Series 11, No. 241). (*0-8406-0467-X*) Natl Ctr Health Stats.

Clinical Child Interview. Jan N. Hughes & David B. Baker. 1991. LC 91-6501. (Guilford School Practitioner Ser.). 230p. pap. 25.00 (*0-89862-240-9*, 2240) Guilford Pubns.

Clinical Child Neuropsychiatry. Christopher Gillberg. 1995. (Illus.). 384p. (C). text 100.00 (*0-521-43388-6*) Cambridge U Pr.

Clinical Child Psychiatry. William M. Kylkylo et al. Ed. by Judy Fletcher. 1998. LC 97-72380. (Illus.). 560p. (C). text 50.00 (*0-7216-3840-6*) Saunders.

Clinical Child Psychology. Ed. by Steven I. Pfeiffer. 1985. 480p. text 44.00 (*0-8089-1680-7*, 793298, Grune & Strat) Harcrt Hlth Sci Grp.

Clinical Child Psychology. Martin Herbert. 2nd ed. 1999. (Stanford Series on Methods & Technique). 438p. pap. 75.00 (*0-471-97663-6*) Wiley.

Clinical Chiropractic: The Management of Pain & Disability: Upper Body Complaints. R. C. Schafer. 1990. LC 90-61201. (Illus.). 528p. (C). 59.00 (*0-924889-01-2*) Motion Palpat Inst.

Clinical Chiropractic Care No. 1: Clinical Care. Phillips et al. 1994. 400p. pap. 45.00 (*0-8016-6822-0*) Mosby Inc.

Clinical Chronopharmacology. Ed. by B. Lemmer & H. Huller. 1990. (Clinical Pharmacology Ser.: Vol. 6). (Illus.). 208p. text (*3-88603-374-0*) W Zuckschwerdt DEU. *Dist:* Scholium Intl.

Clinical Chronopharmacology. Alain Reinberg. 1990. 260p. 109.00 (*0-89116-943-1*) Hemisp Pub.

Clinical Clerking: A Short Introduction to Clinical Skills. Carol A. Seymour & Paul Siklos. 2nd ed. 1994. LC 93-46628. (Illus.). 211p. (C). text 27.95 (*0-521-46235-5*) Cambridge U Pr.

Clinical Clerkship Manual. Ed. by Larry E. Boh. 1993. LC 92-71899. 416p. (Orig.). (C). pap. 39.50 (*0-915486-17-2*) Applied Therapeutics.

Clinical Clerkship Manual. Larry E. Boh. 2nd ed. 2001. LC 00-67322. 832p. (Orig.). pap. text 40.00 (*0-7817-2541-0*) Lppncott W & W.

Clinical Clerkships: Real Medicine at Last. Peter Ways et al. 2000. LC 00-8075. (Surviving Medical School Ser.). (Illus.). xii, 204p. pap. 21.95 (*0-7619-1831-0*, 83610) Sage.

Clinical Coding Compendium. Deborah Day-Oliver. rev. ed. 1994. 415p. (C). pap. text 54.00 (*1-884103-00-6*) Hlth Data Concepts.

Clinical Communication Skills: The Importance of Good Patient Care. Richard Fielding. 1996. LC 98-105648. 352p. (Orig.). pap. (*962-209-371-X*) HK Univ Pr HKG. *Dist:* Intl Spec Bk, Coronet Bks.

Clinical Companion for Health Assessment & Physical Examination. Tamera Cauthorne-Burnette & Mary E. Estes. 1998. LC 97-24664. 384p. (C). pap. text 32.95 (*0-8273-8243-X*) Delmar.

Clinical Companion to Medical-Surgical Nursing. Shannon R. Dirksen et al. 1996. (Illus.). 768p. (C). (gr. 13). text 19.95 (*0-8151-5420-8*, 28204) Mosby Inc.

Clinical Companion to Medical-Surgical Nursing: Assessment & Management of Clinical Problems. Shannon Ruff Dirksen et al. 5th ed. 2000. LC 99-29383. (Illus.). (C). 24.95 (*0-323-00404-0*) Mosby Inc.

Clinical Companion to Nursing Care of Children: Principles & Practice. Jean W. Ashwill & Susan C. Droske. 1997. LC 97-188443. (Illus.). 240p. pap. text 19.95 (*0-7216-6489-X*) Saunders.

Clinical Companion to Sleep Disorders Medicine. Sudhansu Chokroverty. 2nd ed. 2000. LC 99-53900. 232p. pap. text 34.99 (*0-7506-9687-7*) Buttrwrth-Heinemann.

Clinical Competencies for Occupational Therapy: Instructors Manual. 2001. (C). 23.33 (*0-8385-1556-8*) Appleton & Lange.

Clinical Competencies in Occupational Therapy. Cindy A. Kief. 2000. 668p. pap. 53.00 (*0-8385-1248-8*) P-H.

Clinical Computers in Nuclear Medicine. Ed. by Katherine L. Rowell. 1992. LC 91-5207. (Illus.). 86p. 49.00 (*0-932004-40-7*) Soc Nuclear Med.

Clinical Concepts for COTAs. Ed. by Vicki Smith. 1998. 147p. pap. text 27.00 (*1-56900-093-X*, 1172) Am Occup Therapy.

Clinical Considerations in Perioperative Nursing. Edwina A. McConnell. 1987. LC 64-4347. text 24.95 (*0-397-54494-4*, Lippnctt) Lppncott W & W.

Clinical Consultation & Letters by Ippolito Francesco Albertini, Francesco Torti, & Other Physicians. Francesco Albertini et al. 1989. (Illus.). lxix, 356p. 24.95 (*0-88135-089-3*, Sci Hist) Watson Pub Intl.

Clinical Consultations of Giambattista Morgagni: The Edition of Enrico Benassi, 1935. Giambattista Morgani. Tr. & Intro. by Saul Jarcho. 1984. c, 450p. 25.00 (*0-88135-103-2*, Sci Hist) Watson Pub Intl.

Clinical Contact Lens Practice. Elisabeth A. W. Millis. 2001. (Illus.). 256p. 85.00 (*0-7506-4327-7*) Buttrwrth-Heinemann.

***Clinical Core Text for Integrated Curricula with Self Assessment: Master Medicine.** Peter Winstanley & Tom Walley. 2001. 229p. pap. text (*0-443-07055-5*) Church GBR. *Dist:* Saunders.

Clinical Cosmetology: A Medical Approach to Esthetics Procedures. Victoria Rayner. 1993. LC 92-22650. (Skin Ser.). (Illus.). 440p. (C). pap. 41.95 (*1-56253-056-9*) Thomson Learn.

Clinical Cosmetology: A Medical Approach to Esthetics Procedures. Victoria Raynor. 1993. 41.95 (*1-56293-056-7*) Phoenix Soc.

Clinical Counselling in Context: An Introduction. John Lees. 1999. LC 98-29006. (Clinical Counselling in Context Ser.). 75.00 (*0-415-17955-6*); pap. 26.95 (*0-415-17956-4*) Routledge.

***Clinical Counselling in Medical Settings.** Ed. by Peter Thomas et al. 2001. (Illus.). 184p. (C). pap. 27.95 (*0-415-21718-0*); text 59.95 (*0-415-21717-2*) Routledge.

Clinical Counselling in Primary Care. John Lees. 1999. LC 98-29005. (Clinical Counselling in Context Ser.). 75.00 (*0-415-17953-X*); x, 201p. pap. 26.95 (*0-415-17954-8*) Routledge.

Clinical Covernance in Healthcare Practice. Thoreya Swage. 2000. (Illus.). 272p. pap. text 36.00 (*0-7506-4453-2*) Buttrwrth-Heinemann.

Clinical Criteria & Indicators for Nutrition Services in Developmental Disabilities, Psychiatric Disorders, & Substance Abuse. 1993. LC 93-31212. 33.00 (*0-88091-127-1*) Am Dietetic Assn.

Clinical Cytopathology & Aspir Biology. Ibrahim Ramzy. 2nd ed. 2000. LC 2001-265919. (Illus.). 619p. text 199.00 (*0-8385-1069-8*) McGraw-Hill Prof.

***Clinical Cytopathology of the Head & Neck: A Text & Atlas.** Ed. by Gabrijela I. Kocjan. 2001. (Illus.). 210p. (*1-900151-76-6*) Greenwich Med GBR. *Dist:* JAMCO Dist.

***Clinical Data Interpretation in Anaesthesia & Intensive Care.** Christopher Dodds & Steven Bonner. 2001. (Illus.). 350p. pap. (*0-443-06453-9*) Church GBR. *Dist:* Saunders.

***Clinical Data Management.** Ed. by Florian Leiner. 2001. (*0-387-95159-8*) Spr-Verlag.

Clinical Data Management. R. K. Rondell & S. A. Varley. 2nd ed. 2000. LC 99-31926. (Illus.). 366p. 120.00 (*0-471-98329-2*) Wiley.

Clinical Decision Analysis. Milton C. Weinstein & Harvey V. Fineberg. 1980. (Illus.). 400p. text 52.00 (*0-7216-9166-8*) Saunders.

Clinical Decision for Respiratory Care. Patricia F. Carroll. 1996. wbk. ed. (*0-8151-1474-5*) Mosby Inc.

Clinical Decision for Respiratory Care: Evaluator's Guide. Patricia F. Carroll. 1996. (*0-8151-1475-3*) Mosby Inc.

Clinical Decision Making & Treatment Planning in Osseointegration. Michael J. Engelman. 1996. LC 96-24841. (Illus.). 219p. ring bd. 82.00 (*0-86715-318-0*) Quint Pub Co.

Clinical Decision Making for Nurse Practitioners: A Case Study Approach. Denise L. Robinson. 1997. LC 97-17251. (Illus.). 528p. pap. text 39.95 (*0-397-55459-1*) Lppncott W & W.

Clinical Decision Making for Nurses & Health Professionals. Shane A. Thomas et al. 1991. (Illus.). 144p. pap. text (*0-7295-0339-9*) Bailliere Tindall.

Clinical Decision Making from Theory to Practice: A Collection of Essays from the Journal of the American Medical Association. David M. Eddy. 1996. LC 96-4705. (Illus.). 457p. (C). pap. text 46.95 (*0-7637-0143-2*, 0143-2) Jones & Bartlett.

Clinical Decision Making in Colorectal Surgery. Verava & Steven D. Wexner. Ed. by Anthony M. Vernava. 1995. LC 95-3242. (Illus.). 544p. 89.00 (*0-89640-262-2*) Igaku-Shoin.

Clinical Decision Making in Optometry. Michael W. Rouse & Ellen R. Ettinger. 1996. 440p. pap. text 54.99 (*0-7506-9571-4*) Buttrwrth-Heinemann.

Clinical Decision-Making in Psychiatry: Pocketbook Edition. Siegfried Kasper & Joseph Zohar. 2000. 106p. pap. (*1-85317-594-3*) Martin Dunitz GBR. *Dist:* Blackwell Sci.

Clinical Decision Making in Rehabilitation: Efficacy & Outcomes. Ed. by John V. Basmajian & Sikhar N. Banerjee. 1996. LC 96-2745. 240p. text (*0-443-08993-0*) Church.

Clinical Decision Making in the Diagnosis & Treatment of Fluency Disorders. Walter H. Manning. 1996. LC 95-43920. (Health & Life Science Ser.). 316p. (C). mass mkt. 55.95 (*0-8273-6396-6*) Delmar.

Clinical Decision Making in Therapeutic Exercise. Markos Sullivan. 1994. LC 94-20009. 429p. (C). 66.00 (*0-8385-4045-7*, A-4045-9) P-H.

Clinical Decision Making (Proceedings) Ed. by Rose & Myers. 1989. 95p. pap. 21.00 (*0-912452-71-4*, P-68) Am Phys Therapy Assn.

Clinical Decision Manual. Kim A. Eagle. 2000. 160p. pap. text 24.95 (*0-7817-2222-5*) Lppncott W & W.

Clinical Decision Support Systems: Theory & Practice. Ed. by E. S. Berner et al. 1998. LC 98-21883. (Health Informatics Ser.). (Illus.). 264p. 54.95 (*0-387-98575-1*) Spr-Verlag.

Clinical Decisions in Glaucoma. Anderson et al. 1993. (Illus.). 216p. (C). (gr. 13). text 93.00 (*0-8016-6799-2*, 06799) Mosby Inc.

Clinical Decisions in Platelet Therapy. Ed. by Sanford R. Kurtz & Daniel B. Brubaker. 1992. LC 92-49648. 127p. 45.00 (*1-56395-013-8*) Am Assn Blood.

Clinical Delegation in the Emergency Care Setting. Sherri-Lynne A. Almeida et al. Date not set. (Regional Conference Ser.). (Illus.). ring bd. 475.00 (*0-935890-23-8*) Emerg Nurses IL.

Clinical Delegation Skills: A Handbook for Professional Practice. Ruth I. Hansten & Marilynn J. Washburn. 2nd ed. 1998. LC 98-9984. 350p. pap. 55.00 (*0-8342-1129-7*, 11297) Aspen Pub.

Clinical Dentistry Loose Leaf Reference Services Staff. Ed. by Garrett Hardin. 1988. ring bd. 395.00 (*0-06-148003-7*) Lppncott W & W.

Clinical Depression During Addiction Recovery. Martin D. Kantor. 1996. (Illus.). 256p. text 125.00 (*0-8247-9622-5*) Dekker.

Clinical Dermatology Loose Leaf Reference Services Staff. Ed. by D. Joseph Demis et al. ring bd. 450.00 (*0-06-148004-5*) Lppncott W & W.

Clinical Dermatology. Baker. 4th ed. 1989. (Illus.). 320p. text 40.95 (*0-7020-1359-5*) Saunders.

Clinical Dermatology. Rona M. MacKie. 4th ed. 1996. (Illus.). 334p. pap. text 39.95 (*0-19-262761-9*) OUP.

Clinical Dermatology: A Color Guide to Diagnosis & Therapy. Thomas P. Habif. 3rd ed. 1995. LC 95-35912. (Illus.). 912p. (C). (gr. 13). text 140.00 (*0-8151-4242-0*, 24205) Mosby Inc.

Clinical Dermatology: Diagnosis & Therapy. Thomas P. Habif. 1996. 500p. (C). (gr. 13). pap. text 299.00 incl. cd-rom (*0-8151-4189-0*, 28281) Mosby Inc.

Clinical Dermatology 2000 Satellite Symposia, Vancouver, May 1996: Topical Lamiail - New Indications & Dosage Forms/Proceedings of Oral Lamiail - 1996 Worldwide Experience Update. Ed. by G. Evans et al. 1997. (Journal: Vol. 194, Suppl. 1, 1997). (Illus.). ii, 50p. pap. 22.75 (*3-8055-6516-X*) S Karger.

Clinical Dermatology Illustrated: A Regional Approach. John R. Reeves & Howard I. Maibach. 3rd ed. 1997. LC 97-13921. (Illus.). 431p. (C). spiral bd. 54.95 (*0-8036-0279-0*) Davis Co.

Clinical Dermatology of Dogs & Cats: A Guide to Diagnosis & Therapy. Tom Willemse. 1991. (Illus.). 141p. 105.00 (*0-8121-1460-4*) Lppncott W & W.

Clinical Dermatopathology: A Text & Colour Atlas. Alan Stevens et al. 1989. (Illus.). 208p. text (*0-443-02583-5*) Church.

Clinical Detective: Techniques in the Evaluation of Sexual Abuse. Aaron N. Hoorwitz. 1992. LC 91-27039. 240p. 34.95 (*0-393-70124-7*) Norton.

Clinical Detective Stories: A Problem-Based Approach to Clinical Cases in Energy & Acid-Base. M. L. Halperin & F. S. Rolleston. 1993. (Illus.). 300p. (Orig.). (C). (*1-85578-999-X*) Portland Pr Ltd GBR. *Dist:* Ashgate Pub Co.

Clinical Development: Strategic, Pre-Clinical, Clinical, & Regulatory Issues. Janice Steiner. 1996. LC 96-41276. (Illus.). 250p. 149.00 (*1-57491-028-0*) IHS Health Grp.

Clinical Diabetes: An Illustrated Text. G. Michael Besser et al. 1988. LC 65-40116. (Gower Bk.). (Illus.). 304p. (C). (gr. 13). text (*0-397-44565-2*, GM0014) Gower-Mosby.

Clinical Diabetes Mellitus. George P. Kozak. 1982. (Illus.). 541p. text 140.00 (*0-7216-5502-5*) Saunders.

Clinical Diabetes Mellitus: A Problem Oriented Approach. John K. Davidson. 3rd ed. 2000. LC 99-42914. (Illus.). 928p. 189.00 (*0-86577-840-X*) Thieme Med Pubs.

Clinical Diagnosis: A Companion to Hutchinson's Clinical Methods. Ed. by Michael Swash. 1998. 250p. pap. text (*0-7020-1513-X*) W B Saunders GBR. *Dist:* Saunders.

Clinical Diagnosis: A Physiologic Approach. Richard D. Judge & George D. Zuidema. 5th ed. 1988. 607p. 44.95 (*0-316-47585-8*, Little Brwn Med Div) Lppncott W & W.

Clinical Diagnosis & Management by Lab Methods. Henry. 19th ed. 1998. (C). pap. text 11.25 (*0-8089-2091-X*) Harcourt.

Clinical Diagnosis & Management by Laboratory Methods. John B. Henry. Ed. by Lesley Day. 19th ed. 1996. (Illus.). 1440p. text 86.95 (*0-7216-6030-4*) Saunders.

Clinical Diagnosis & Management by Laboratory Methods. John Bernard Henry. 20th ed. 2001. LC 00-58856. (Illus.). xxiv, 1512p. text 99.00 (*0-7216-8864-0*) Saunders.

Clinical Diagnosis & Management of Alzheimer's Disease. Ed. by Serge Gauthier. 1996. LC 96-191682. 400p. text 75.00 (*0-7506-9845-4*) Buttrwrth-Heinemann.

Clinical Diagnosis & Management of Alzheimer's Disease. Ed. by Serge Gauthier. 2nd ed. 1999. 386p. (*1-85317-655-9*) Martin Dunitz.

Clinical Diagnosis & Management of Eating Disorders. Robert Anding et al. Ed. by Richard C. Hall. 1990. LC 89-64482. 334p. text 50.00 (*0-9625272-0-3*) Ryandic Pub.

Clinical Diagnosis of Atherosclerosis: Quantitative Methods of Evaluation. Ed. by M. G. Bond et al. 1983. (Illus.). 585p. 65.00 (*0-387-90780-7*) Spr-Verlag.

Clinical Diagnostic Immunology: Protocols in Quality Assurance & Standardization. Robert M. Nakamura & James D. Folds. 1998. LC 98-21394. (Illus.). 512p. 115.95 (*0-86542-518-3*) Blackwell Sci.

Clinical Diagnostic Ultrasound. E. Barnett & P. Morley. 1986. (C). (gr. 13). 350.00 (*0-632-00897-0*, B-0482-6) Mosby Inc.

Clinical Diagnostic Ultrasound. Grant M. Baxter et al. 2nd ed. 1999. LC 98-25578. (Illus.). 687p. 341.95 (*0-632-03744-X*) Blackwell Sci.

Clinical Dialysis. Allen Nissenson. 3rd ed. 1996. LC 95-11757. 1005p. (C). pap. text 250.00 (*0-8385-1379-4*, A1379-5, Apple Lange Med) McGraw.

Clinical Diary of Sandor Ferenczi. Sandor Ferenczi. Tr. by Michael Balint & Nicola Z. Jackson from GER. 1988. LC 88-16244. (Illus.). 256p. 42.50 (*0-674-13526-1*) HUP.

Clinical Dictionary: Klinisches Woerterbuch. Willibald Pschyrembel. 1993. (GER.). 1876p. 95.00 (*0-8288-1839-8*, 3110126923) Fr & Eur.

Clinical Dictionary of Chinese Medicine. Nigel A. Wiseman. 1997. 1100p. (C). text 125.00 (*0-912111-45-3*) Paradigm Publns.

Clinical Dietetics & Nutrition. F. P. Antia & Philip Abraham. 4th ed. 1998. LC 97-914015. 540p. text 65.00 (*0-19-564165-5*) OUP.

Clinical Director's Handbook 1. Hirst. 95th ed. 1995. (C). pap. text 157.00 (*0-443-05038-4*) Harcourt.

Clinical Disorders & Stressful Life Events, No. 7. Ed. by Thomas W. Miller. 1997. LC 96-39360. (International Universities Press Stress & Health Ser.: Monograph 7). xxx, 416p. 62.50 (*0-8236-0910-3*) Intl Univs Pr.

Clinical Disorders of Balance, Posture & Gait. Ed. by Thomas Brandt et al. 1996. LC 96-4706. (An Arnold Publication). 360p. (*0-340-60145-0*) E A GBR. *Dist:* OUP.

Clinical Disorders of Bone & Mineral Metabolism. Ed. by Michael Kleerekoper & Stephen M. Krane. 1989. 660p. 305.00 (*0-913113-21-2*) M Liebert.

Clinical Disorders of Memory. Aman U. Khan. 1986. (Critical Issues in Psychiatry Ser.). (Illus.). 284p. (C). text 78.00 (*0-306-42259-X*, Kluwer Plenum) Kluwer Academic.

Clinical Disorders of the Endometrium & Menstrual Cycle. Ed. by I. T. Cameron et al. 1998. (Illus.). 462p. text 149.50 (*0-19-262724-4*) OUP.

Clinical Documentation Sourcebook: A Comprehensive Collection of Mental Health Practice Forms,

Handouts, & Records. Donald E. Wiger. 2nd ed. 1999. LC 98-38798. (Practice Planners Ser.). (Illus.). 304p. pap. 49.95 incl. disk (*0-471-32692-5*) Wiley.

Clinical Doppler Echocardiography. Jose C. Missri. 1990. 316p. text 89.00 (*0-07-042436-5*) McGraw-Hill Educ Grp.

Clinical Doppler Ultrasound. Paul L. P. Allan. 2000. 293p. text 50.00 (*0-443-05549-1*) Saunders.

Clinical Drug Therapy: Rationales for Nursing Practice. Anne Collins Abrams. 6th ed. 2001. 1,104p. pap. text 52.95 (*0-7817-2121-0*) Lppncott W & W.

*__Clinical Drug Therapy: Rationales for Nursing Practice.__ Anne Collins Abrams. 6th ed. 2001. 272p. pap. text, stu. ed. 19.95 (*0-7817-2401-5*) Lppncott W & W.

Clinical Echocardiography. Ed. by John B. Chambers. 1995. 260p. text (*0-7279-0810-3*) BMJ Pub GBR. *Dist:* AIDC.

Clinical Echocardiography. Masatsugu Iwase & Iwao Sotobata. 1989. (Developments in Cardiovascular Medicine Ser.). (C). text 255.50 (*0-7923-0004-1*) Kluwer Academic.

Clinical Echocardiography. Catherine M. Otto. Ed. by Ricahrd Zorab. 1996. (Illus.). 832p. text 173.00 (*0-7216-6019-3*) Saunders.

Clinical Economics in Gastroenterology. Keith Bodger et al. 1999. LC 99-26447. (Illus.). x, 269p. 157.95 (*0-632-05033-0*) Blackwell Sci.

Clinical Education Vol. 1: An Anthology. 1992. 470p. pap. 82.50 (*0-912452-82-X*, E-25) Am Phys Therapy Assn.

Clinical Education & Supervision: An Instructional Guide. AOTA Staff. 1991. 350p. (C). ring bd. 225.00 incl. VHS (*0-910317-65-8*) Am Occup Therapy.

Clinical Educator Role. Moore. 1996. pap. text 60.00 (*0-443-05300-6*) Saunders.

Clinical Effectiveness & Primary Care. Mark R. Baker et al. 1997. LC 97-6232. (*1-85775-129-9*) Radcliffe Med Pr GBR. *Dist:* Balogh.

Clinical Effectiveness in Allied Health Practices: Critical Literature Review. Ed. by Judith T. Barr. 1996. 179p. (Orig.). (C). pap. text 45.00 (*0-7881-2639-3*) DIANE Pub.

Clinical Effects of Environmental Chemicals: A Guide to Etiologic Diagnosis. Renate D. Kimbrough et al. 1989. 200p. 79.95 (*0-89116-921-0*) Hemisp Pub.

Clinical Efficacy of Position Emission Tomography. Ed. by W. D. Heiss et al. 1987. (Developments in Nuclear Medicine Ser.). (C). text 261.50 (*0-89838-898-8*) Kluwer Academic.

Clinical Electro-Cardiography. Maiti & G. Goswami. 1989. (C). (*0-89771-373-7*) Current Dist IND. *Dist:* St Mut.

Clinical Electrocardiographic Diagnosis: A Problem-Based Approach. Noble O. Fowler. 2000. LC 99-45306. 256p. pap. text 59.95 (*0-7817-1957-7*) Lppncott W & W.

Clinical Electrocardiography: A Simplified Approach. Ary L. Goldberger. 6th ed. 1998. LC 98-4102. pap. text 39.95 (*0-323-00252-8*) Mosby Inc.

Clinical Electrocardiography: A Textbook. Antonio Bayes de Luna. 2nd ed. 1998. LC 97-22254. (Illus.). 416p. 125.00 (*0-87993-682-7*) Futura Pub.

Clinical Electrocardiography: PreTest Self-Assessment & Review. Franklin H. Zimmerman. 1993. LC 93-13548. (Pretest Specialty Level Ser.). (Illus.). 416p. pap. 49.95 (*0-07-052008-9*) McGraw-Hill Prof.

Clinical Electrocardiography: Self-Assessment & Review. Donald A. Underwood. 1993. (Illus.). 320p. pap. text 60.00 (*0-7216-6692-2*) Saunders.

Clinical Electroencephalography & Topographic Brain Mapping. F. H. Duffy et al. 1989. (Illus.). 304p. 137.00 (*0-387-96856-3*) Spr-Verlag.

Clinical Electromyography. William F. Brown & Charles F. Bolton. 2nd ed. 1993. (Illus.). 810p. text 180.00 (*0-7506-9204-9*) Buttrwrth-Heinemann.

Clinical Electromyography: A Case Study Approach. Bashar Katirji. 1998. LC 98-13762. (Illus.). 302p. (C). (gr. 13). pap. text 54.95 (*0-8151-4971-9*, 26882) Mosby Inc.

Clinical Electrophysiology. Lynn Snyder-Mackler & Andrew J. Robinson. 2nd ed. 1995. (Illus.). 400p. pap. 49.00 (*0-683-07817-8*) Lppncott W & W.

Clinical Electrophysiology of the Heart. David E. Ward & A. John Camm. 1988. (Current Topics in Cardiovascular Medicine Ser.). (Illus.). 400p. (C). (*0-683-13096-X*) E A GBR. *Dist:* Williams & Wilkins.

Clinical Electrophysiology of the Somatosensory Cortex: A Combined Study Using Electrocortigraphy, Scalp-EEG, & Magnetoencephalography. C. Baumgartner. 1993. (Illus.). 220p. 103.00 (*0-387-82391-3*) Spr-Verlag.

Clinical Electrophysiology Review. George J. Klein & Eric N. Prystowsky. 1996. LC 96-43397. (Illus.). 270p. pap. 45.00 (*0-07-035169-4*) McGraw-Hill Prof.

Clinical Electrotherapy. Roger M. Nelson & Dean P. Currier. 2nd ed. 1998. (Illus.). 432p. (C). 53.28 (*0-8385-1334-4*, A1334-0) Appleton & Lange.

Clinical Electrotherapy. Roger M. Nelson et al. 3rd rev. ed. 1999. LC 98-50864. (Illus.). 480p. (C). 63.00 (*0-8385-1491-X*) P-H.

Clinical Embryology Color Atlas & Text. Murray Brookes & Anthony L. Zietman. 1998. LC 98-22967. (Illus.). 341p. lib. bdg. 39.95 (*0-8493-1255-8*) CRC Pr.

Clinical Encounter: A Guide to the Medical Interview & Case Presentation. J. Andrew Billings & John D. Stoeckle. 2nd ed. 1998. LC 98-21886. (Illus.). 368p. (C). (gr. 13). pap. text 29.95 (*0-8151-1374-9*, 29932) Mosby Inc.

Clinical Endocrine Oncology. Richard Sheaves et al. 1997. LC 96-5659. (Illus.). 600p. 230.00 (*0-86542-862-X*) Blackwell Sci.

Clinical Endocrinology. Ed. by Ashley B. Grossman. 1992. (Illus.). 1080p. 235.00 (*0-632-02548-4*) Blackwell Sci.

Clinical Endocrinology. Ashley Grossman. 2nd ed. 1997. LC 97-7266. (Illus.). 1120p. 523.95 (*0-86542-629-5*) Blackwell Sci.

Clinical Endocrinology: Theory & Practice. A. Labhart. 1976. LC 75-11535. 60.00 (*0-387-90175-2*) Spr-Verlag.

Clinical Endocrinology of Dogs & Cats: An Illustrated Text. H. A. Hazewinkel et al. Ed. by Adam Rijnberk. 1995. LC 95-7371. (Illus.). 256p. (C). lib. bdg. 195.00 (*0-7923-3415-9*) Kluwer Academic.

Clinical Endocrinology of Dogs & Cats: An Illustrated Text. Ed. by Adam Rijnberk. 1995. 256p. (C). pap. text 102.50 (*0-7923-3416-7*) Kluwer Academic.

Clinical Endocrinology Two. Michael Besser. 2nd ed. 1994. (C). (gr. 13). (*1-56375-552-1*) Gower-Mosby.

Clinical Endocrinology Update Syllabus, 1997. Leonard Wartofsky. 1997. (Illus.). 408p. (C). 75.00 (*1-879225-28-X*) Endocrine Soc.

Clinical Endodontics: A Textbook. L. Tronstad. 1991. (Illus.). 256p. pap. 32.00 (*0-86577-411-0*) Thieme Med Pubs.

Clinical ENT: An Illustrated Textbook. Gerard O'Donoghue et al. 1992. (Illus.). 234p. text 49.95 (*0-19-262226-9*) OUP.

Clinical Enzymology, Vol. 3. George Kaldor. 1983. LC 82-19115. (Methods in Laboratory Medicine Ser.: Vol. 3). 222p. 68.50 (*0-275-91399-6*, C1399, Praeger Pubs) Greenwood.

Clinical Enzymology Symposia Vl. 4: Proceedings of the 10th International Symposium 1984. A. Burlina & L. Galzigna. 1984. 212p. text (*1-57235-051-2*) Piccin Nuova.

Clinical Enzymology Symposia Vol. 1: Proceedings of the 7th International Symposium, April 1976. A. Burlina & L. Galzigna. 1977. 382p. text (*1-57235-048-2*) Piccin Nuova.

Clinical Enzymology Symposia Vol. 2: Proceedings of the 8th International Symposium, April 1978. A. Burlina & L. Galzigna. 1980. 646p. text (*1-57235-049-0*) Piccin Nuova.

Clinical Enzymology Symposia Vol. 3: Proceedings of the 9th International Symposium, April 1980. A. Burlina & L. Galzigna. 1980. 222p. text (*1-57235-050-4*) Piccin Nuova.

Clinical Enzymology Symposia Vol. 5: Proceedings of the 11th International Symposium 1984. A. Burlina & L. Galzigna. 1986. 212p. pap. text (*1-57235-052-0*) Piccin Nuova.

Clinical Epidemiology. Robert Fletcher. 2nd ed. 1987. (Illus.). 260p. pap. 32.00 (*0-683-03251-8*) Lppncott W & W.

Clinical Epidemiology: A Basic Science for Clinical Medicine. David Sackett et al. 1985. LC 96-960076. (Illus.). 380p. 31.50 (*0-316-76595-3*); 2nd ed. 1991. 442p. pap. text 39.95 (*0-316-76599-6*) Lppncott W & W (Little Brwn Med Div).

Clinical Epidemiology: The Architecture of Clinical Research. Alvan R. Feinstein. 1985. 450p. text 133.00 (*0-7216-1308-X*) Saunders.

Clinical Epidemiology: The Essentials. Robert H. Fletcher et al. 3rd ed. 1996. LC 95-8382. (Illus.). 304p. pap. 29.95 (*0-683-03269-0*) Lppncott W & W.

Clinical Epidemiology: The Study of the Outcome of Illness. Noel S. Weiss. 2nd ed. 1996. LC 96-24639. (Monographs in Epidemiology & Biostatistics: No. 27). (Illus.). 176p. text 34.50 (*0-19-511026-9*) OUP.

Clinical Epidemiology & Biostatistics: A Primer for Clinical Investigators & Decision-Makers. Matthew S. Kramer. 1991. (Illus.). 286p. reprint ed. 62.00 (*0-387-18874-6*) Spr-Verlag.

*__Clinical Epidemiology & Evidence-based Medicine: Fundamental Principles of Clinical Reasoning & Research.__ David L. Katz. 2001. LC 2001-1275. (Illus.). 280p. pap. 32.95 (*0-7619-1939-2*) Sage.

Clinical Epidemiology for Nurses. Chavigny. 1993. text (*0-397-54657-2*) Lppncott W & W.

Clinical Epidemiology of Chronic Obstructive Pulmonary Disease. Michael J. Hensley. Ed. by Nicholas A. Saunders. 1989. (Lung Biology in Health & Disease Ser.: Vol. 43). (Illus.). 408p. text 199.00 (*0-8247-8087-6*) Dekker.

Clinical Ethics: A Practical Approach to Ethical Decisions in Clinical Medicine. Albert R. Jonsen et al. 4th ed. 1997. LC 97-219072. (Illus.). 224p. pap. 29.95 (*0-07-033120-0*) McGraw-Hill Prof.

Clinical Ethics: An Invitation to Healing Professionals. William Depender & Wanda Ikeda-Chandler. 1990. LC 89-16224. 152p. 58.00 (*0-275-93437-3*, C3437, Praeger Pubs) Greenwood.

Clinical Ethics: Theory & Practice. Ed. by Barry Hoffmaster et al. 1989. LC 88-13579. (Contemporary Issues in Biomedicine, Ethics, & Society Ser.). 258p. 55.50 (*0-89603-138-1*) Humana.

Clinical Ethics & Values, Issues & Insights in a Changing Healthcare Environment. Diann B. Uustal. 1995. LC 93-73395. 203p. (Orig.). reprint ed. pap. text 24.95 (*0-9638759-0-6*) Educ Res Hlth.

Clinical Ethics Casebook. Peter Horn. 1998. LC 98-34610. 208p. pap. text 27.95 (*0-534-55151-3*) Thomson Learn.

Clinical Evaluation & Management of Spasticity. Ed. by David A. Gelber & Douglas R. Jeffery. 2000. (Current Clinical Neurology Ser.). 335p. 125.00 (*0-89603-636-7*) Humana.

Clinical Evaluation of a Food Additive: Assessment of Aspartame. Ed. by Christian Tschanz et al. 1996. LC 95-26438. 320p. 144.95 (*0-8493-4973-7*) CRC Pr.

Clinical Evaluation of Amoxycillin. J. P. Van Waardhuizen. 1973. (Journal: Vol. 18, Suppl.). (Illus.). 120p. pap. 25.25 (*3-8055-1538-3*) S Karger.

Clinical Evaluation of Antitumor Therapy. Ed. by Franco M. Muggia & Marcel Rozencweig. 1986. (Developments in Oncology Ser.). text 139.50 (*0-89838-803-1*) Kluwer Academic.

Clinical Evaluation of Medical Devices: Principles & Case Studies. Ed. by Karen Becker Witkin. 1997. LC 97-23205. (Illus.). 288p. 145.00 (*0-89603-446-1*) Humana.

Clinical Evaluation of Psychotropic Drugs for Psychiatric Disorders: Principles & Proposed Guidelines. Ed. by P. Grof. 1993. LC 91-7039. (WHO Expert Series on Neuroscience: Vol. 2). (Illus.). 210p. text 38.00 (*0-88937-063-X*) Hogrefe & Huber Pubs.

Clinical Evaluation of the Nervous System. John F. Simpson & Kenneth R. Magee. 1973. (Illus.). 13.50 (*0-316-79184-9*, Little Brwn Med Div) Lppncott W & W.

Clinical Evaluation of Young Children with the McCarthy Scales. Ed. by Alan S. Kaufman & Nadeen L. Kaufman. 1977. LC 77-8969. 320p. text 40.95 (*0-8089-1013-2*, 792255, Grune & Strat) Harcrt Hlth Sci Grp.

Clinical Evaluations of School-Aged Children: A Structured Approach to the Diagnosis of Child & Adolescent Mental Disorders. Susan K. Samuels & Susana A. Sikorsky. 2nd ed. 1998. LC 98-11269. 384p. 44.95 (*1-56887-027-2*, CES2BP, Prof Resc Pr) Pro Resource.

Clinical Examination. Owen Epstein et al. 2nd ed. 1998. text 44.95 (*0-7234-2576-0*) Mosby Inc.

Clinical Examination. Nicholas J. Talley. 3rd ed. 1996. pap. text 36.95 (*0-86542-689-9*) Blackwell Sci.

Clinical Examination Cases in Ophthalmology. David Broadway et al. 1999. LC 99-25521. (Illus.). 336p. pap. text 85.00 (*0-7506-2500-7*) Buttrwrth-Heinemann.

Clinical Examination for Medical Students. Wai-Ching Leung. LC 97-171541. 192p. pap. (*0-340-66192-5*) E A GBR. *Dist:* OUP, Routldge.

Clinical Examination Manual for Nurses. Saltman. 1988. pap. text 31.00 (*0-7295-0284-8*) Saunders.

Clinical Examination of Horses. Victor C. Speirs. 1997. LC 96-72080. (Illus.). 358p. text 52.50 (*0-7216-6506-3*) Saunders.

Clinical Examination of the Nervous System. Sid Gilman. 1999. LC 99-19468. (Illus.). ix, 321p. text 69.95 (*0-07-024252-6*) McGraw-Hill Educ Grp.

Clinical Examination of the Patient: A Pocket Atlas. J. S. Lumley & Pierre-Marc G. Bouloux. 1994. LC 95-102576. (Illus.). 312p. pap. (*0-7506-1671-7*) E A GBR. *Dist:* OUP.

Clinical Examination of the Spine: A Multidisciplinary Approach. Swartz. 2000. (Illus.). 350p. (C). (gr. 13). text 39.95 (*0-8151-7949-9*, 24902) Mosby Inc.

Clinical Examination of Voice. Minoru Hirano. 1982. (Disorders of Human Communication Ser.: Vol. 5). (Illus.). 100p. 49.00 (*0-387-81659-3*) Spr-Verlag.

Clinical Exchange: Techniques Derived from Self & Motivational Systems. Joseph D. Lichtenberg et al. 1996. LC 96-28332. (Psychoanalytic Inquiry Book Ser.: Vol. 16). 272p. 45.00 (*0-88163-220-1*) Analytic Pr.

Clinical Exercise Physiology. Ed. by Scott M. Hasson. 1993. (Illus.). 288p. (C). (gr. 13). text 48.00 (*0-8151-4210-2*, 22146) Mosby Inc.

Clinical Exercise Testing. Norman L. Jones. Ed. by Judy Fletcher. 4th ed. 1997. LC 96-9821. 320p. text 52.00 (*0-7216-6511-X*) Saunders.

Clinical Exercise Testing & Prescription: Theory & Application. Ed. by Scott O. Roberts et al. 1997. LC 96-24940. 336p. 94.95 (*0-8493-4593-6*) CRC Pr.

Clinical Experience: The Construction & Reconstruction of Medical Reality. Paul A. Atkinson. 2nd ed. 1997. LC 97-73874. (Cardiff Papers in Qualitative Research). 224p. text (*1-85628-577-4*) Ashgate Pub GBR. *Dist:* Ashgate Pub Co.

Clinical Experiences in Athletic Training: A Modular Approach. Kenneth L. Knight. 2nd rev. ed. 1998. LC 98-15280. 160p. spiral bd. 25.00 (*0-87322-950-9*, BKNI0950) Human Kinetics.

Clinical Experiences with Platinum & Etoposide Therapy in Lung Cancer. Ed. by Paul A. Bunn et al. 1992. (Journal: Vol. 49, Suppl. 1, 1992). (Illus.). iv, 76p. pap. 24.50 (*3-8055-5639-X*) S Karger.

Clinical Faces of Childhood Volume I: The Oppositional Child, The Inhibited Child, The Depressed Child. Ed. by E. James Anthony & Doris C. Gilpin. 1994. LC 94-72350. 272p. pap. text 25.00 (*1-56821-334-4*) Aronson.

Clinical Faces of Childhood Volume II: The Hysterical Child, The Anxious Child, The Borderline Child. Ed. by E. James Anthony & Doris C. Gilpin. 1994. LC 94-72350. (Master Work Ser.). 336p. pap. text 25.00 (*1-56821-335-2*) Aronson.

Clinical Facts & Curios: A Compendium of Unique Insights from the Medical Literature. James A. Stockton, III. 1994. LC 94-11041. (*1-885046-00-6*) Am Bd Pediatrics.

Clinical Facts & Curios: A Compendium of Unique Insights from the Medical Literature, Vol. 1. James A. Stockman, III. 1994. (Illus.). 458p. incl. cd-rom (*1-885046-02-2*) Am Bd Pediatrics.

Clinical Fetal Assessment. Johnson. 1995. (C). text (*0-7216-5583-1*) Saunders.

Clinical Finals & How to Pass Them. K. P. Hanretty et al. 1998. 303p. pap. (*0-443-05923-3*) Church.

Clinical Foot Roentgenology. Felton O. Gamble & Irving Yale. 2nd ed. 1976. LC 74-15632. (Illus.). 448p. reprint ed. 52.50 (*0-88275-102-6*) Krieger.

Clinical Forensic Medicine. Ed. by W. D. McLay. 1991. 376p. pap. text 39.50 (*0-86187-155-3*) St Martin.

Clinical Gastroenterology. Edgar Achkar et al. 2nd ed. 1992. (Illus.). text 115.00 (*0-8121-1363-2*) Lppncott W & W.

Clinical Gastroenterology. Howard M. Spiro et al. 4th ed. 1993. LC 93-21707. (Illus.). 1232p. text 159.00 (*0-07-105434-0*) McGraw-Hill Educ Grp.

Clinical Gastroenterology: A Practical Problem-Based Approach. Nicholas J. Talley & Christopher J. Martin. 1996. 448p. pap. 63.00 (*0-8036-0374-6*) Davis Co.

Clinical Gastroenterology: Companion Handbook. Basil Rigas & Howard M. Spiro. 4th ed. 1995. LC 95-15756. (Illus.). 665p. pap. 36.00 (*0-07-003341-2*) McGraw-Hill Prof.

Clinical Gastroenterology in the Dog & Cat. Murdoch. 1991. (*0-632-01402-4*) Mosby Inc.

Clinical Gastroenterology in the Elderly. Ed. by Alvin M. Gelb. 1996. (Gastroenterology Ser.: Vol. 2). (Illus.). 320p. text 145.00 (*0-8247-9398-6*) Dekker.

Clinical Gastrointestinal Physiology. D. Neil Granger et al. 1985. (Monographs in Physiology Ser.). (Illus.). 255p. text 48.00 (*0-7216-1283-0*) Saunders.

Clinical Gated Cardiac SPECT. Daniel S. Berman. Ed. by Guido Germano. 1999. LC 99-19070. (Illus.). 387p. 125.00 (*0-87993-432-8*) Futura Pub.

Clinical Gene Analysis & Manipulation: Tools, Techniques & Troubleshooting. Ed. by J. A. Jankowski & J. M. Polak. 1996. (Postgraduate Medical Science Ser.). (Illus.). 475p. (C). pap. text 39.95 (*0-521-47896-0*) Cambridge U Pr.

Clinical Genetics. Bonthron. 1997. pap. text (*0-7020-2351-5*) Bailliere Tindall.

Clinical Genetics. Golder N. Wilson. 2000. LC 99-40663. 496p. pap. 49.95 (*0-471-29806-9*, Wiley-Liss) Wiley.

Clinical Genetics Handbook. Arthur Robinson. 2nd ed. 1993. 624p. pap. 44.95 (*0-86542-194-3*, 93-010567) Blackwell Sci.

Clinical Genetics in Nursing Practice. Felissa R. Lashley. 2nd ed. 1998. LC 98-12409. (Illus.). 543p. 79.95 (*0-8261-1177-7*) Springer Pub.

Clinical Geriatric Neurology. Ed. by Laurie Barclay. 1993. LC 92-20248. (Illus.). 513p. text 98.00 (*0-8121-1610-0*) Lppncott W & W.

Clinical Geriatric Psychopharmacology. Carl Salzman. (Illus.). 2nd ed. 1992. 392p. 65.00 (*0-683-07495-4*); 3rd ed. 1997. LC 97-12801. 614p. 120.00 (*0-683-30021-0*) Lppncott W & W.

Clinical Gerontological Nursing: A Guide to Advanced Practice. Joyce T. Stone et al. Ed. by Terri Wood. 2nd ed. 1998. LC 98-12903. (Illus.). 672p. (C). text 55.00 (*0-7216-5918-7*) Saunders.

Clinical Gerontology: A Guide to Assessment & Intervention. Ed. by T. L. Brink. 1986. LC 86-240. (Clinical Gerontologist Ser.: Vol. 5, Nos. 1-4). 517p. 79.95 (*0-86656-536-1*) Haworth Pr.

Clinical Geropsychology. Ed. by Inger Hilde Nordhus et al. 1998. LC 98-14132. 371p. 39.95 (*1-55798-519-7*) Am Psychol.

Clinical GI Physiology for the Exam Taker. Eugene D. Jacobson & Joel S. Levine. 1993. LC 93-8348. (Illus.). 128p. pap. text 29.00 (*0-7216-3701-9*) Saunders.

Clinical Glaucoma Management: Critical Signs in Diagnosis & Therapy. Ronald L. Gross. 1999. LC 99-48219. 510p. text 159.00 (*0-7216-7272-8*) Saunders.

*__Clinical Governance: Making It Happen.__ Myriam Lugon & Jonathan Secker-Walker. 1999. 222p. pap. (*1-85315-383-4*) Royal Soc of Medicine Pr Ltd GBR. *Dist:* Balogh.

*__Clinical Guide for Contraception.__ Leon Speroff. 3rd ed. 2001. LC 00-63972. (Illus.). xi, 448p. pap. text 34.95 (*0-7817-2984-X*) Lppncott W & W.

Clinical Guide for the Care of Older Women. Richard L. Byyny & Leon Speroff. 1990. (Illus.). 384p. 68.00 (*0-683-01150-2*) Lppncott W & W.

Clinical Guide for the Care of Older Women: Primary & Preventive Care. Richard L. Byyny & Leon Speroff. 2nd ed. 1996. LC 95-49918. (Illus.). 560p. 79.00 (*0-683-01151-0*) Lppncott W & W.

Clinical Guide for the Treatment of Schizophrenia. A. S. Bellack. 1989. LC 88-32137. (Illus.). 344p. (C). text 59.50 (*0-306-43064-9*, Kluwer Plenum) Kluwer Academic.

Clinical Guide to Alcohol Treatment: The Community Reinforcement Approach. Robert J. Meyers & Jane Ellen Smith. 1995. LC 95-546. (Substance Abuse Ser.). 211p. 32.00 (*0-89862-857-1*, 2857) Guilford Pubns.

Clinical Guide to Anaerobic Infections. Sydney M. Finegold et al. 1991. (Illus.). 160p. 34.95 (*0-89863-162-9*) Star Pub CA.

Clinical Guide to Cancer Nursing. Susan L. Groenwald et al. 4th ed. (Nursing Ser.). (Illus.). (C). 1998. LC 97-46106. 720p. pap. text 39.95 (*0-7637-0540-3*, 0540-3); 1997. pap. text 37.50 (*0-7637-0771-6*) Jones & Bartlett.

***Clinical Guide to Cancer Nursing.** Connie Henke Yarbro et al. 5th ed. 2001. (Illus.). (C). pap. text 38.95 (*0-7637-1809-2*, 1809-2, N L N Bart) Jones & Bartlett.

Clinical Guide to Cancer Nursing: A Companion to Cancer Nursing. Susan L. Groenwald et al. 3rd ed. 1995. LC 95-180. (Nursing Ser.). 632p. spiral bd. 37.50 (*0-86720-708-6*) Jones & Bartlett.

Clinical Guide to Cardiac Autonomic Tests. Marek Malik. 1998. LC 98-27478. (Developments in Cardiovascular Medicine Ser.). 423p. (*0-7923-5178-9*) Kluwer Academic.

Clinical Guide to Child Psychiatry. Ed. by David Shaffer et al. 1984. LC 84-57887. 624p. (C). 60.00 (*0-02-929020-1*) Free Pr.

Clinical Guide to Chinese Herbs & Formulae. Chen Songyu & Li Fei. Ed. by Francesca Diebschlag. Tr. by Jin Huide. 1993. LC 92-22810. text (*0-443-04680-8*) Church.

Clinical Guide to Comprehensive Ophthalmology. David A. Lee & Eve J. Higginbotham. 1998. LC 98-30784. (Illus.). 744p. 159.00 (*0-86577-766-7*) Thieme Med Pubs.

Clinical Guide to Depression in Children & Adolescents. Ed. by Mohammad Shafii & Sharon L. Shafii. 1991. LC 91-22112. 304p. text 41.50 (*0-88048-356-3*, 8356) Am Psychiatric.

Clinical Guide to Drug & Alcohol Problems. Joseph Westermeyer. 1986. LC 86-530. 336p. 72.50 (*0-275-92162-X*, C2162, Praeger Pubs) Greenwood.

Clinical Guide to Glaucoma Management. Higginbotham & Lee. 2001. 544p. pap. 80.00 (*0-7506-7310-9*) Buttrwrth-Heinemann.

Clinical Guide to Inherited Metabolic Diseases. Joe T. Clarke. 1996. LC 96-36666. (Illus.). 300p. (C). text 110.00 (*0-521-48064-7*); pap. text 41.95 (*0-521-48524-X*) Cambridge U Pr.

Clinical Guide to Laboratory Tests. Ed. by Norbert W. Tietz. 3rd ed. 1995. LC 94-33795. (C). pap. text (*0-7216-5052-X*); (Illus.). 1136p. pap. text 46.00 (*0-7216-5035-X*) Saunders.

Clinical Guide to Neonatal Seizures. Eli Mizrahi. 1997. LC 97-28764. (Illus.). 192p. text 99.00 (*0-7817-0296-8*) Lppncott W & W.

Clinical Guide to Periodontics. Murray Schwartz et al. 1994. LC 94-4810. pap. text 35.00 (*0-7216-4823-1*) Saunders.

Clinical Guide to Primary Bone Tumors. Jerome Levesque et al. 1998. LC 97-34657. 301p. text 125.00 (*0-683-30255-8*) Lppncott W & W.

Clinical Guide to Proper Selection of Acupoints. Wenfu Li. Tr. by Chengnian Huang & Junxuan Zhou. 1996. (Illus.). 211p. pap. 27.50 (*1-880132-25-7*) Sci Pr NY.

Clinical Guide to Prosthodontics. Hoffman. 1998. (Illus.). 260p. pap. text (*0-7216-6627-2*) Saunders.

Clinical Guide to Prosthodontics: A Compendium of Prosthodontic Procedures by Jules M. Hoffman, DDS. Jules M. Hoffman et al. 1999. (Illus.). 285p. 64.00 (*1-929475-00-4*) Delphi Pub.

Clinical Guide to Reproductive & Developmental Toxicology. Anthony R. Scialli. 1991. 304p. 129.00 (*0-8493-6737-9*) CRC Pr.

Clinical Guide to Soft Contact Lenses. Michael R. Spinell. 1979. LC 78-14621. 18.50 (*0-8019-6786-4*) NP-Chilton.

Clinical Guide to Stem Cell & Bone Marrow Transplantation. Terry W. Shapiro et al. 1997. LC 97-9563. (Nursing Ser.). (Illus.). 464p. (C). pap. text 39.95 (*0-7637-0217-X*, 0217-X) Jones & Bartlett.

Clinical Guide to the Treatment of the Human Stress Response. G. S. Everly, Jr. 1989. (Stress & Coping Ser.). (Illus.). 406p. (C). 42.50 (*0-306-43068-1*, Plenum Trade) Perseus Pubng.

Clinical Guideline Development: An Algorithm Approach. James P. Mozena et al. 1996. LC 95-39261. 176p. pap. 101.00 (*0-8342-0734-6*, 20734) Aspen Pub.

Clinical Guidelines: Diagnostic & Treatment Manual. Ed. by J. C. Desenclos. 3rd ed. 1993. (Medecins Sans Frontieres - Hatier Ser.). 283p. vinyl bd. 27.95 (*2-218-03480-8*) Hatier Pub.

Clinical Guidelines & the Law: Negligence, Discretion & Judgement. Brian Hurwitz. 1998. LC 98-17986. 132p. pap. (*1-85775-044-6*) Radcliffe Med Pr GBR. *Dist:* Balogh.

Clinical Guidelines for Involuntary Outpatient Treatment. J. Reid Meloy et al. Ed. by Harold H. Smith, Jr. 1990. LC 89-43652. (Practitioner's Resource Ser.). 78p. pap. 16.95 (*0-943158-45-1*, CGIBP, Prof Resc Pr) Pro Resource.

Clinical Guidelines for Managed Home Care. Donna J. Behrendt. 1996. LC 96-44666. ring bd. 99.00 (*0-8342-0815-6*) Aspen Pub.

Clinical Guidelines in Adult Health. Mary V. Graham & Constance R. Uphold. 1994. (Illus.). 729p. (Orig.). (C). pap. text 45.00 (*0-9646151-2-6*) Barmarrae Bks.

Clinical Guidelines in Adult Health. Constance R. Uphold & Mary V. Graham. 2nd ed. 1998. (Illus.). 720p. pap. 55.00 (*0-9646151-5-0*) Barmarrae Bks.

Clinical Guidelines in Child Health. Mary V. Graham & Constance R. Uphold. (Illus.). 2nd ed. 1994. 660p. (C). pap. text 45.00 (*0-9646151-1-8*); 3rd ed. 1998. 720p. pap. 55.00 (*0-9646151-4-2*) Barmarrae Bks.

Clinical Guidelines in Family Practice. Mary V. Graham & Constance R. Uphold. 2nd ed. 1994. (Illus.). 852p. (C). pap. text 50.00 (*0-9646151-0-X*) Barmarrae Bks.

Clinical Guidelines in Family Practice. Constance R. Uphold & Mary V. Graham. 3rd ed. 1998. (Illus.). 912p. pap. 60.00 (*0-9646151-3-4*) Barmarrae Bks.

Clinical Gynecologic Imaging. Arthur C. Fleischer. 1996. LC 96-8780. 448p. text 169.00 (*0-397-51706-8*) Lppncott W & W.

Clinical Gynecologic Oncology. Philip J. Disaia. 5th ed. 1997. LC 97-11272. (Illus.). 720p. (C). (gr. 13). text 119.00 (*0-8151-2506-2*, 28279) Mosby Inc.

Clinical Gynecologic Oncology. Philip J. Disaia & William T. Creasman. 5th ed. 1997. (Illus.). 720p. (*84-8174-339-9*) Mosby-Doyma Libros ESP. *Dist:* Mosby Inc.

Clinical Gynecologic Oncology, No. 5. Philip J. Disaia et al. 1997. (Illus.). 750p. (C). (gr. 13). text 139.95 (*0-8151-2387-6*, 31039) Mosby Inc.

Clinical Gynecologic Oncology Review. Tung Van Dinh & Edward V. Hannigan. 2nd ed. 1997. LC 99-222782. 160p. (C). (gr. 13). pap. text 24.95 (*0-8151-2501-1*, 29173) Mosby Inc.

Clinical Gynecologic Pathology. Enrique Hernandez & Barbara Atkinson. 1995. (Illus.). 416p. text 145.00 (*0-7216-5170-4*) Saunders.

Clinical Gynecology. Varma. 1991. 150.00 (*0-7131-4574-9*) Routledge.

Clinical Haematology. Ed. by Christopher A. Ludlam. 1990. (Illus.). 496p. pap. text (*0-443-03834-1*) Church.

Clinical Haematology: A Postgraduate Exam Companion. Drew Provan et al. 1997. LC 96-53901. 336p. pap. (*0-7506-2920-7*) E A GBR. *Dist:* OUP.

Clinical Handbook for Biotherapy. Paula T. Rieger. 1999. LC 98-42753. (Nursing Ser.). (Illus.). 416p. (C). pap. text 35.95 (*0-7637-0649-3*, 0649-3) Jones & Bartlett.

Clinical Handbook for Biotherapy - Genentech. Paula T. Rieger. 1999. (Illus.). 416p. (C). pap. text 35.95 (*0-7637-1152-7*, 1152-7) Jones & Bartlett.

Clinical Handbook for Maternal Newborn Nursing. Sally B. Olds. 1992. (C). pap. text 25.31 (*0-8053-5588-X*) Addison-Wesley.

Clinical Handbook for Surgical Critical Care. K. W. Burchard & D. S. Gann. 2001. LC 98-22291. (Clinical Handbook Ser.). (Illus.). 360p. pap. 38.95 (*1-85070-633-6*, Parthenon Pbng) CRC Pr.

Clinical Handbook Medical Surgical Nuring: Critical Thinking in Client Care. Priscilla LeMone. 2nd ed. 1999. LC 99-34472. (C). pap. text 22.00 (*0-8053-8126-0*) Benjamin-Cummings.

Clinical Handbook of Anxiety Disorders in Children & Adolescents. Ed. by Andrew R. Eisen et al. 1995. LC 94-18064. 624p. 60.00 (*1-56821-294-1*) Aronson.

Clinical Handbook of Child Abuse & Neglect. Lane J. Veltkamp & Thomas W. Miller. 1994. LC 93-15721. 188p. 27.50 (*0-8236-0950-2*) Intl Univs Pr.

Clinical Handbook of Child Psychiatry & the Law. Diane H. Schetky & Elissa P. Benedek. 1991. 352p. 58.00 (*0-683-07589-6*) Lppncott W & W.

Clinical Handbook of Chinese Prepared Medicine. Chun-Han Zhu. Ed. by Richard Feit. 1995. 368p. pap. text 27.00 (*0-912111-43-7*) Paradigm Publns.

Clinical Handbook of Couple Therapy. Neil S. Jacobson & Alan S. Gurman. 1995. LC 95-17655. 510p. 60.00 (*0-89862-855-5*, C2855) Guilford Pubns.

Clinical Handbook of Depression. 1991. 386p. (C). pap. text 32.50 (*0-89876-174-3*) Gardner Pr.

Clinical Handbook of Ear, Nose & Throat Disorders. W. R. Wilson & Joseph B. Nadol, Jr. 2001. (Clinical Handbook Ser.). (Illus.). 450p. lib. bdg. 38.95 (*1-85070-605-0*, Parthenon Pbng) CRC Pr.

Clinical Handbook of Endocrinology & Metabolic Disease. Noel I. Robin. 1996. LC 95-30949. (Clinical Handbook Ser.). 506p. 29.95 (*1-85070-637-9*, Parthenon Pbng) CRC Pr.

Clinical Handbook of Family Nursing. Judith M. McFarlane. 1989. LC 85-31446. 562p. pap. text 34.95 (*0-8273-4304-3*) Delmar.

Clinical Handbook of Health Psychology. Ed. by P. Camic & S. Knight. 1998. LC 97-77702. (Illus.). 658p. text 49.50 (*0-88937-177-6*) Hogrefe & Huber Pubs.

Clinical Handbook of Marriage & Couples Interventions. W. Kim Halford et al. 1997. LC 96-24024. (Clinical Psychology & Personality Ser.). 748p. 225.00 (*0-471-95519-1*) Wiley.

Clinical Handbook of Ophthalmology. Robert G. Small. 1994. LC 94-10570. (Clinical Handbook Ser.). (Illus.). 160p. lib. bdg. 26.95 (*1-85070-584-4*, Parthenon Pbng) CRC Pr.

Clinical Handbook of Pediatric Infectious Disease. Russell W. Steele. (Clinical Handbook Ser.). (Illus.). 1994. LC 94-8896. 422p. lib. bdg. 29.95 (*1-85070-575-5*); 2nd ed. 2000. LC 00-22210. 280p. lib. bdg. 42.95 (*1-85070-342-6*) CRC Pr (Parthenon Pbng).

Clinical Handbook of Pediatrics. M. William Schwartz. Ed. by Louis M. Bell et al. 2nd ed. 1998. LC 98-7539. 800p. pap. 34.00 (*0-683-30448-8*) Lppncott W & W.

Clinical Handbook of Perinatal & Pediatric Respiratory Care. Ed. by Sherry L. Barnhart & Michael P. Czervinske. 1995. (Illus.). 731p. spiral bd. 34.95 (*0-7216-6740-6*) Saunders.

Clinical Handbook of Psychiatry & the Law. Thomas G. Gutheil & Paul S. Appelbaum. 3rd ed. 2000. LC 99-59487. 432p. text 85.00 (*0-7817-2031-1*) Lppncott W & W.

Clinical Handbook of Psychotropic Drugs: CD-ROM Version 1.0. Kalyna Z. Bezchlibnyk-Butler & J. Joel Jeffries. 9th ed. 2000. 75.00 (*0-88937-228-4*, 5685448) Hogrefe & Huber Pubs.

Clinical Handbook of Sleep Disorders: Diagnosis & Management. Antonio Culebras. 1996. LC 96-23960. 524p. pap. text 59.99 (*0-7506-9644-3*) Buttrwrth-Heinemann.

Clinical Handbook of Sleep Disorders in Children. Charles E. Schaefer. Ed. by Charles E. Schaefer. 1995. LC 94-19702. (Child Therapy Ser.). 360p. 65.00 (*1-56821-324-7*) Aronson.

Clinical Handbook of Small Animals. Moriello. 2000. pap. text (*0-7216-6092-4*) Saunders.

Clinical Handbook to Accompany Essentials of Maternal Newborn Nursing. Patricia W. Ladewig. 4th ed. 1997. LC 97-41302. 368p. (C). pap. text 27.19 (*0-8053-5629-0*) Addison-Wesley.

Clinical Handbook to Accompany Fundamentals of Nursing: Concepts, Process& Practices. Barbara Kozier. 6th ed. 2001. LC 99-461893. 294p. (C). pap. text 18.67 (*0-8053-8353-0*) Benjamin-Cummings.

Clinical Handling of Dental Materials. Smith et al. 1995. 272p. pap. text 85.00 (*0-7236-1023-1*) Buttrwrth-Heinemann.

Clinical Health Issues Handbook. Karil Bellah. 2nd ed. 1997. LC 98-192974. 208p. pap. text 30.95 (*0-534-53707-3*) Brooks-Cole.

Clinical Health Psychology in Medical Settings: A Practitioner's Handbook. Cynthia D. Belar & William W. Deardorff. 2nd rev. ed. 1995. LC 94-49604. 296p. text 29.95 (*1-55798-277-5*); 277p. pap. text 24.95 (*1-55798-287-2*) Am Psychol.

Clinical Hematology. A. Victor Hoffbrand. 3rd ed. 1999. 346p. 179.00 (*0-7234-3115-9*) Mosby Inc.

Clinical Hematology: A Problem-Oriented Approach. James Isbister & D. Harmening Pittiglio. 1988. (Illus.). 264p. pap. 35.00 (*0-683-04349-8*) Lppncott W & W.

Clinical Hematology: Principles, Procedures & Correlations. Cheryl A. Lotspeich-Steininger et al. 1991. LC 65-9558. (Illus.). 720p. 49.95 (*0-397-50790-9*, Lippnctt) Lppncott W & W.

Clinical Hematology: Principles, Procedures & Correlations. E. Anne Stiene-Martin et al. 2nd ed. 1997. LC 97-17765. (Illus.). 848p. text 62.95 (*0-397-55321-8*) Lppncott W & W.

Clinical Hematology: Theory & Procedures. Mary L. Turgeon. 3rd ed. 1998. LC 98-38545. 480p. text 55.00 (*0-316-85623-1*, Little Brwn Med Div) Lppncott W & W.

Clinical Hematology & Fundamentals of Hemostasis. Denise M. Harmening. 3rd ed. 1996. (Illus.). 743p. 69.00 (*0-8036-0135-2*) Davis Co.

***Clinical Hematology & Fundamentals of Hemostasis.** Ed. by Denise Harmening. 4th ed. 2001. LC 2001-47699. 784p. kivar 75.00 (*0-8036-0783-0*) Davis Co.

Clinical Hematology Atlas. Jacqueline H. Carr & Bernadette F. Rodak. Ed. by Adrianne Williams. 1998. LC 98-5824. (Illus.). 224p. (C). pap. text 39.00 (*0-7216-4174-1*) Saunders.

Clinical Hemorheology. Ed. by S. Chein et al. 1987. lib. bdg. 184.00 (*0-89838-807-4*) Kluwer Academic.

Clinical Hemostasis. Sommer. 1997. (Medical Lab Technician Ser.). pap. 21.75 (*0-8273-6263-3*) Delmar.

Clinical Hepatology. O. Grady. 1999. 688p. 179.95 (*0-7234-3106-X*) Mosby Inc.

***Clinical History Taking & Examination: An Illustrated Color Text.** Philip Welsby. 2nd ed. 2001. (Illus.). 163p. pap. (*0-443-07088-1*) Church GBR. *Dist:* Saunders.

Clinical History Taking & Examination: An Illustrated Colour Text. Philip D. Welsby. 1996. LC 95-33680. (Illus.). 161p. pap. text (*0-443-04328-0*) Church.

Clinical Hypertension. J. I. Robertson. 1992. (Handbooks of Hypertension: Vol. 15). 812p. 225.00 (*0-444-81294-6*) Elsevier.

Clinical Hypertension. Norman M. Kaplan & Ellin Lieberman. 7th ed. 1998. LC 97-14181. (Illus.). 500p. 110.00 (*0-683-30132-2*) Lppncott W & W.

Clinical Hyperthermia. Ed. by F. N. Gilly et al. 1993. (Journal: Vol. 50, No. 5, 1993). (Illus.). 64p. pap. 88.75 (*3-8055-5854-6*) S Karger.

Clinical Hypnosis: A Multidisciplinary Approach. William C. Wester, II & Alexander H. Smith, Jr. 1991. (Illus.). 660p. (C). reprint ed. pap. 25.00 (*0-938837-06-0*) Behav Sci Ctr Pubs.

Clinical Hypnosis: Principles & Applications. Harold B. Crasilneck & James A. Hall. 2nd ed. 1985. 496p. text 39.00 (*0-8089-1681-5*, 790934, Grune & Strat) Harcrt Hlth Sci Grp.

Clinical Hypnosis & Memory: Guidelines for Clinicians & for Forensic Hypnosis. D. Corydon Hammond et al. 1995. LC 95-6572. (*1-886610-01-0*) Am Soc Clin Hyp Pr.

Clinical Hypnosis & Self-Regulation: Cognitive - Behavioral Perspectives. Ed. by Irving Kirsch et al. 1999. LC 98-29427. (Dissociation, Trauma, Memory, & Hypnosis Ser.). (Illus.). 370p. text 39.95 (*1-55798-535-9*) Am Psychol.

Clinical Hypnosis & Therapeutic Suggestion in Patient Care. Ed. by Rothlyn P. Zahourek. 1990. LC 90-2235. 270p. text 28.95 (*0-87630-606-7*) Brunner-Routledge.

Clinical Hypnosis Primer. George J. Pratt et al. 1984. LC 79-92665. (C). 36.00 (*0-930626-07-9*) Psych & Consul Assocs.

Clinical Hypnosis Primer: Updated & Expanded. George J. Pratt et al. enl. rev. ed. 1988. LC 88-5566. 407p. 215.00 (*0-471-61384-3*) Wiley.

Clinical Hypnosis with Children. Ed. by William C. Wester & Donald J. O'Grady. 1991. LC 90-15157. 288p. text 37.95 (*0-87630-605-9*) Brunner-Routledge.

Clinical Hypnotherapy. David B. Cheek & Leslie M. LeCron. 1968. LC 68-16304. 256p. text 44.95 (*0-8089-0097-8*, 790825, Grune & Strat) Harcrt Hlth Sci Grp.

Clinical Hypnotherapy: A Transpersonal Approach. Allen S. Chips. 1999. LC 00-699667. (Illus.). xi, 300p. text 27.95 (*1-929661-00-2*) EIH Pubng.

Clinical Hypnotherapy: The Application of Ideometer Technicians. David B. Cheek. 2nd ed. 320p. (*0-205-18595-9*) Allyn.

Clinical Imaging: An Atlas of Differential Diagnosis. Ronald L. Eisenberg. 2nd ed. 1991. 1152p. 173.50 (*0-7817-0208-9*); 3rd ed. 1996. 1,264p. text 225.00 (*0-397-51679-7*) Lppncott W & W.

Clinical Imaging: With Skeletal, Chest & Abdomen Pattern Differentials. Dennis M. Marchiori. 1999. (Illus.). 1200p. (*84-8174-469-7*) Mosby-Doyma Libros ESP. *Dist:* Mosby Inc.

Clinical Imaging in Non-Pulmonary Tuberculosis. Francis McGuinness et al. 1999. LC 99-35196. (Illus.). 176p. 99.00 (*3-540-65940-4*) Spr-Verlag.

Clinical Imaging of the Small Intestine. Ed. by Hans Herlinger et al. 2nd ed. 1998. LC 98-16317. (Illus.). 591p. 165.00 (*0-387-98516-6*) Spr-Verlag.

Clinical Immunodermatology. Mark V. Dahl. 3rd ed. 1995. LC 95-43751. (Illus.). 448p. (C). (gr. 13). text 96.00 (*0-8151-2312-4*, 25101) Mosby Inc.

Clinical Immunology. Williams. 1998. (Allied Health Ser.). text 37.95 (*0-8273-5690-0*) Delmar.

Clinical Immunology: An Introductory Text. Reginald M. Gorczynski & Jacqueline Stanley. 2000. LC 99-34618. (Vademecum Ser.). (Illus.). 403p. spiral bd. 45.00 (*1-57059-625-5*) Landes Bioscience.

Clinical Immunology: Principles & Laboratory Diagnosis. Sheehan. 1990. (Illus.). 480p. text 29.95 (*0-397-50890-5*) Lppncott W & W.

Clinical Immunology: Principles & Laboratory Diagnosis. Catherine Sheehan. 2nd ed. 1997. LC 96-37572. 416p. text 43.00 (*0-397-55313-7*) Lppncott W & W.

Clinical Immunology: Principles & Practice. Ed. by Robert R. Rich. 1995. (Illus.). 2912p. (C). (gr. 13). text 320.00 (*0-8016-7636-3*, 07636) Mosby Inc.

***Clinical Immunology: Principles & Practice.** Robert R. Rich et al. 2nd ed. 2001. (Illus.). (*0-7234-3161-2*) Mosby Inc.

***Clinical Immunology & Allergy: Color Guide.** Unsworth. 2001. (Illus.). 125p. pap. (*0-443-06248-X*) Church GBR. *Dist:* Saunders.

Clinical Immunology & Serology: A Laboratory Perspective. Christine Stevens. 1995. LC 95-22305. (Illus.). 343p. (C). pap. text 39.95 (*0-8036-0050-X*) Davis Co.

Clinical Immunology & Transplantation. Guillou. 1998. (Illus.). 650p. (C). pap. 124.50 (*0-412-63490-2*); (gr. 13). pap. 39.95 (*0-412-63500-3*) Chapman & Hall (Chap & Hall NY).

Clinical Immunology Outline. J. Brostoff. 1994. (*1-56375-664-1*) Gower-Mosby.

Clinical Impact of Bone & Connective Tissue Markers. Ed. by E. Lindh & Jan Thorell. 1989. 350p. text 104.00 (*0-12-450740-9*) Acad Pr.

Clinical Impact of H Plus, K Plus-ATP-ase Inhibitors: Journal: Digestion, Vol. 44, Suppl. 1, 1989. Ed. by C. B. Lamers. 1989. 98p. pap. 32.25 (*3-8055-5111-8*) S Karger.

Clinical Impact of the Monitoring of Allergic Inflammation. Ed. by Per Matsson et al. 1991. (Illus.). 272p. text 83.00 (*0-12-480265-6*) Acad Pr.

Clinical Implications of Drug Use, Vol. 1. T. K. Basu. 1980. 160p. 46.95 (*0-8493-5391-2*, RM300) CRC Pr.

Clinical Implications of Drug Use, Vol. 2. T. K. Basu. 1980. 144p. 86.00 (*0-8493-5392-0*, RM300, CRC Reprint) Franklin.

Clinical Implications of Irritable Bowel Syndrome. Ed. by Philippe Denis. 1997. 56p. pap. 38.70 (*3-11-015860-4*) De Gruyter.

Clinical Importance of Surfactant Defects. Ed. by P. Von Wichert. 1981. (Progress in Respiratory Research Ser.: Vol. 15). (Illus.). 320p. 142.75 (*3-8055-1011-X*) S Karger.

Clinical Improvement Action Guide. Ed. by Eugene C. Nelson et al. 1998. LC 97-76552. 210p. 45.00 (*0-86688-553-6*, AG-100) Joint Comm Hlthcare.

Clinical in Vitro Fertilization. Ed. by Carl Wood & Alan O. Trounson. (Illus.). 1984. 225p. 52.00 (*0-387-12812-3*); 2nd ed. 1989. 166p. 104.00 (*0-387-19534-3*) Spr-Verlag.

C
D

Clinical Infectious Disease: Diagnosis-Management. Cunha. 1998. text (*0-7216-4672-7*) Saunders.

Clinical Infectious Diseases: A Practical Approach. Ed. by Richard K. Root et al. 1998. LC 98-14548. (Illus.). 1040p. text 149.50 (*0-19-508103-X*) OUP.

Clinical Inference: How to Draw Meaningful Conclusions from Psychological Tests. Audrey M. O'Neill. 1992. LC 92-52846. pap. 24.95 (*0-88422-117-2*) Clinical Psych.

Clinical Information System for Oncology. Ed. by J. P. Enterline et al. 1989. (Computers & Medicine Ser.). (Illus.). 268p. 84.00 (*0-387-96956-X*, 2614) Spr-Verlag.

Clinical Information Technology: A Practical Guide to Personal Computing for Healthcare Clinicians & Managers. Harry Purser & David Rowley. 1987. 220p. 59.25 (*1-56593-580-2*, 0064) Singular Publishing.

Clinical Instruction in Blood Banking. Betty L. Theriot & Elizabeth Williams. 3rd ed. 1995. (Illus.). 200p. (C). stu. ed. 29.95 (*0-9641523-1-2*) Creative Educ.

Clinical Integration: Strategies & Practices for Organized Delivery Systems. Mary Tonges. 1998. LC 98-2503. 239p. 48.00 (*0-7879-4039-9*) Jossey-Bass.

Clinical Intensive Care. Ken Hillman & Gillian Bishop. 1996. (Illus.). 855p. (C). pap. text 69.95 (*0-521-47812-X*) Cambridge U Pr.

Clinical Interaction & the Analysis of Meaning: A New Psychoanalytic Theory. Theodore L. Dorpat & Michael L. Miller. 1992. 344p. text 49.95 (*0-88163-146-9*) Analytic Pr.

Clinical Internal Medicine. L. Barth Reller et al. 1979. 28.50 (*0-316-73970-7*, Little Brwn Med Div) Lppncott W & W.

Clinical Interpretation of Objective Psychological Tests. Charles J. Golden. 1979. 272p. text 26.00 (*0-8089-1163-5*, 791620, Grune & Strat) Harcrt Hlth Sci Grp.

Clinical Interpretation of the Wechsler Adult Intelligence Scale. Irla L. Zimmerman et al. 1973. LC 72-11825. 232p. text 26.95 (*0-8089-0780-8*, 794975, Grune & Strat) Harcrt Hlth Sci Grp.

Clinical Interpretation of the Woodcock-Johnson Test of Cognitive Ability. Ed. by Kevin S. McGrew. 1986. 320p. text 26.95 (*0-8089-1827-3*, 792939, Grune & Strat) Harcrt Hlth Sci Grp.

Clinical Interpretation of the Woodcock-Johnson Tests of Cognitive Ability. Kevin S. McGrew. rev. ed. 1994. LC 93-31670. (C). (*0-205-14701-1*) Allyn.

Clinical Interview Vol. 1: Diagnosis, Vol. 1. Felix Deutsch & William F. Murphy. 1997. 613p. text 70.00 (*0-8236-0920-0*) Intl Univs Pr.

Clinical Interview Vol. 2: Therapy. Felix Deutsch & William F. Murphy. 1967. LC 54-12140. 355p. text 52.50 (*0-8236-0940-5*) Intl Univs Pr.

Clinical Interview of the Adolescent: From Assessment & Formulation to Treatment Planning. Francis D. Kelly. 1997. LC 97-12042. 234p. text 62.95 (*0-398-06779-1*); pap. text 47.95 (*0-398-06780-5*) C C Thomas.

Clinical Interview of the Child. Stanley I. Greenspan & Nancy T. Greenspan. 2nd ed. 1991. LC 90-14571. 245p. text 44.95 (*0-88048-420-9*, 8420) Am Psychiatric.

Clinical Interview Using DSM-IV: Fundamentals, Vol. 1. Ekkehard Othmer & Sieglinde C. Othmer. 2nd ed. 1998. (Clinical Interview Using Dsm-IV Ser.: Vol. 1). 544p. pap. text 36.00 (*0-88048-825-5*, 8825) Am Psychiatric.

Clinical Interview Using DSM-IV: The Difficult Patient, Vol. 2. Ekkehard Othmer & Sieglinde C. Othmer. 1994. LC 94-2525. (Clinical Interview Using Dsm-IV Vol. 2 Ser.: Vol. 2). 576p. text 51.95 (*0-88048-520-5*, 8520) Am Psychiatric.

Clinical Interviewing. John Sommers-Flanagan & Rita Sommers-Flanagan. 2nd ed. 1999. LC 98-30786. (Illus.). 436p. 91.75 (*0-471-29567-1*) Wiley.

Clinical Introduction to Lacanian Psychoanalysis: Theory & Technique. Bruce Fink. 1997. LC 96-52127. (Illus.). 352p. 37.95 (*0-674-13535-0*) HUP.

Clinical Investigation in Gastroenterology. M. C. Bateson. 1988. (C). text 88.00 (*0-7462-0103-6*) Kluwer Academic.

Clinical Investigation of Gastric Function. Ed. by Porro G. Bianchi & C. Scarpignato. 1990. (Frontiers of Gastrointestinal Research Ser.: Vol. 17). (Illus.). viii, 300p. 233.25 (*3-8055-5100-2*) S Karger.

Clinical Investigation of Skin Disorders. Ed. by Rino Cerio & C. Archer. 1997. (Illus.). 168p. (*0-412-59230-4*) E A GBR. *Dist:* OUP.

Clinical Investigations in Gastroenterology. Malcolm C. Bateson & Ian A. Bouchier. 2nd ed. 1997. LC 96-6551. 256p. text 110.50 (*0-7923-4391-3*) Kluwer Academic.

Clinical Judgement: Evidence in Practice. Robin S. Downie & Jane MacNaughton. 2000. LC 99-59423. (Illus.). 224p. pap. text 27.50 (*0-19-263216-7*) OUP.

Clinical Judgement & Decision Making: The Future with Nursing Diagnosis. Kathryn J. Hannah. 1989. text 31.50 (*0-8273-4254-3*) Delmar.

Clinical Judgment: A Critical Appraisal. Ed. by H. Tristram Engelhardt et al. 1979. (Philosophy & Medicine Ser.). 304p. text 97.50 (*90-277-0952-1*) Kluwer Academic.

Clinical Kidney Transplants 1985. Ed. by Paul I. Terasaki. 1985. 15.00 (*0-9604606-1-6*) UCLA Tissue.

Clinical Kinesiology for Physical Therapist Assistants. Lynn S. Lippert. 3rd ed. 2000. LC 00-20083. (Illus.). xvi, 475p. pap. text 36.95 (*0-8036-0453-X*) Davis Co.

***Clinical Knowledge & Practice in the Information Age: A Toolkit for Clinicians.** Jeremy C. Wyatt. 2001. 100p. pap. (*1-85315-483-0*) Royal Soc of Medicine Pr Ltd GBR. *Dist:* Balogh.

Clinical Lab Computer/Mechanical Ventilation. Treanor. 1997. (Respiratory Care Ser.). tchr. ed. 12.00 (*0-8273-7297-3*) Delmar.

Clinical Lab Computer/Mechanical Ventilation. Treanor. 1997. (Respiratory Care Ser.). pap. 29.95 (*0-8273-7296-5*, VNR) Wiley.

Clinical Lab Science: Toxicology, Vol. 1. Ed. by Irving Sunshine & David Seligson. 1978. 432p. 236.00 (*0-8493-7051-5*, RB37, CRC Reprint) Franklin.

Clinical Lab Science: Virology & Rickettsiology Gueh-Djen Hsiung & Robert H. Green. 1979. (Illus.). 448p. Pt. 1, Vol. 1. 245.00 (*0-8493-7061-2*, RB37); Pt. 2, Vol.1. 243.00 (*0-8493-7062-0*) Franklin (CRC Reprint).

Clinical Lab Science Ser., Vol. 1. Ed. by Richard Spencer & David Seligson. 1977. (Nuclear Medicine Ser.). 632p. 339.00 (*0-8493-7071-X*, RB37, CRC Reprint) Franklin.

Clinical Lab Science Ser., Vol. 1. Ed. by Raymond Yesner & Byron H. Waksman. 1978. (Pathology Ser.). 368p. 202.00 (*0-8493-7041-8*, RB37, CRC Reprint) Franklin.

Clinical Lab Techniques. Pettit. (Nursing Education Ser.). 2001. (C). pap. 54.00 (*0-8273-7671-5*); 1998. tchr. ed. 12.00 (*0-8273-7672-3*) Delmar.

Clinical Laboratory Animal Medicine: An Introduction. Karen Hrapkiewicz et al. 2nd ed. 1998. LC 97-34537. (Illus.). 304p. pap. 34.95 (*0-8138-2555-5*) Iowa U Pr.

Clinical Laboratory Assistant/Phlebotomist. Jacquelyn R. Marshall. Ed. by Kay Cox-Stevens. 1999. LC 98-70063. (Clinical Allied Healthcare Ser.). (Illus.). 500p. pap. text 44.95 (*0-89262-434-5*) Career Pub.

Clinical Laboratory Assistant/Phlebotomist: Instructor's Guide. Jacquelyn R. Marshall. Ed. by Kay Cox-Stevens. 1999. (Clinical Allied Healthcare Ser.). (Illus.). 448p. tchr. ed., ring bd. 99.95 (*0-89262-442-6*) Career Pub.

Clinical Laboratory Automation, Robotics & Knowledge Optimization. Gerald J. Kost. 1996. LC 95-38368. 952p. 130.00 (*0-471-03179-8*) Wiley.

Clinical Laboratory Disposable Markets: Chemistry Tests & Reagents, Toxicology & Pathology Supplies. Market Intelligence Staff. 1993. 416p. 1895.00 (*1-56753-520-8*) Frost & Sullivan.

Clinical Laboratory Disposable Markets: Microbiology, Hematology & Immunology. Market Intelligence Staff. 1993. 413p. 1695.00 (*1-56753-521-6*) Frost & Sullivan.

Clinical Laboratory Instrumentation & Automation: Principles, Applications, & Selection. Ed. by Kory M. Ward et al. 1993. LC 92-48469. (Illus.). 496p. pap. text 41.95 (*0-7216-4218-7*) Saunders.

Clinical Laboratory Investigator. Jack Rudman. 1994. (Career Examination Ser.: C-2098). pap. 39.95 (*0-8373-2098-4*) Nat Learn.

Clinical Laboratory Management. Eleanor M. Travers. 1997. LC 96-5093. (Illus.). 840p. 99.00 (*0-683-08376-7*) Lppncott W & W.

Clinical Laboratory Medicine. Kenneth D. McClatchey. 1994. (Illus.). 1,920p. text 109.00 (*0-683-05755-3*) Lppncott W & W.

Clinical Laboratory Medicine: Clinical Application of Laboratory Data. Richard Ravel. 6th ed. 1994. LC 94-30386. (Illus.). 736p. (C). (gr. 13). pap. text 47.00 (*0-8151-7148-X*, 23833) Mosby Inc.

Clinical Laboratory Medicine: Self-Assessment & Review. Kenneth D. McClatchey et al. 1997. LC 96-47824. 360p. pap. 32.00 (*0-683-05757-X*) Lppncott W & W.

Clinical Laboratory Pearls. Steven L. Jones. 2000. LC 00-61818. (Illus.). 656p. pap. text 45.00 (*0-7817-2579-8*) Lppncott W & W.

Clinical Laboratory Safety: Approved Guideline (1996) Contrib. by Robert P. Buchwald. 1996. 95.00 (*1-56238-300-0*, GP17-A) NCCLS.

Clinical Laboratory Science: Basic & Routine Laboratory Techniques. Jean J. Linne & Karen M. Ringsrud. 4th ed. 1999. (Illus.). 812p. (C). pap. 49.00 (*1-55664-505-8*) Mosby Inc.

Clinical Laboratory Science: Exam Review. Leclair. 1999. (C). pap. text 31.95 (*0-7216-4957-2*) Saunders.

Clinical Laboratory Science: Strategies for Practice. Brenta G. Davis et al. 1988. (Illus.). 1024p. text 57.50 (*0-397-50860-3*) Lppncott W & W.

Clinical Laboratory Science Education & Management. M. Ann Wallace et al. Ed. by Selma Kaszczuk. 1997. LC 96-49581. (Illus.). 368p. pap. text 34.95 (*0-7216-4543-7*) Saunders.

Clinical Laboratory Science in the Changing Scene of Health Care. Ed. by John P. Ashby. 1987. text 114.50 (*0-85200-685-3*) Kluwer Academic.

Clinical Laboratory Science Review. Ed. by Robert R. Harr. 2nd ed. 1999. LC 99-23448. (Illus.). 412p. pap. text 36.95 (*0-8036-0443-2*) Davis Co.

Clinical Laboratory Science Review: A Bottom Line Approach. Betty L. Theriot et al. 1995. (Illus.). 238p. (C). pap. text 39.95 (*0-9641523-0-4*) Creative Educ.

Clinical Laboratory Science Series, CRC: Section F, Immunology Alexander Baumgarten & Frank F. Richards. Pt. 1, Vol 1. 1978. 251.00 (*0-8493-7021-3*, RB37); Pt. 2, Vol. 1. 1979. 480p. 257.00 (*0-8493-7022-1*) Franklin (CRC Reprint).

Clinical Laboratory Technical Procedure Manuals: Approved Guideline (1992) Contrib. by Gerald A. Hoeltge. 2nd ed. 1992. 95.00 (*1-56238-156-3*, GP2-A2) NCCLS.

Clinical Laboratory Tests: Values & Implications. Lippincott, Williams and Wilkins Staff. 3rd ed. 2001. LC 00-66123. (Illus.). xii, 692p. pap. 39.95 (*1-58255-081-6*) Springhouse Corp.

Clinical Laboratory Waste Management: Approved Guideline (1993) Contrib. by Gerald A. Hoeltge. 1993. 85.00 (*1-56238-218-7*, GP5-A) NCCLS.

Clinical Laparoscopy. G. Dagnini. 1980. 308p. text (*1-57235-056-3*) Piccin Nuova.

Clinical Lasers: Expert Strategies for Practical & Profitable Management. Ed. by Byron Breedlove & David M. Schwartz. 1985. LC 85-70926. (Illus.). 356p. text 78.00 (*0-9603332-3-1*) Am Health Consults.

Clinical Leadership in Nursing. Judith T. Rocchiccioli & Mary S. Tilbury. Ed. by Thomas Eoyang. 1998. LC 97-34010. (Illus.). 320p. pap. text 29.95 (*0-7216-5442-8*) Saunders.

Clinical Lectures on Klein & Bion. Ed. by Robin Anderson. 1991. (New Library of Psychoanalysis : No. 14). 156p. (C). pap. 25.99 (*0-415-06993-9*, A6481) Routledge.

Clinical Lectures on Senile & Chronic Diseases. Jean M. Charcot. Ed. by Robert J. Kastenbaum. Tr. by William S. Tuke. 1979. LC 78-22189. (Aging & Old Age Ser.). reprint ed. lib. bdg. 27.95 (*0-405-11807-4*) Ayer.

Clinical Leprosy. V. N. Sehgal. 1979. 100p. 14.95 (*0-7069-0866-X*) Asia Bk Corp.

Clinical Light Damage to the Eye. Ed. by D. Miller. 1987. (Illus.). 225p. 242.00 (*0-387-96451-7*) Spr-Verlag.

Clinical Linguistics. David Crystal. 1981. 240p. 39.95 (*1-56593-521-7*, 0021) Singular Publishing.

Clinical Low Vision. Eleanor E. Faye. 2nd ed. 1984. 505p. 49.95 (*0-316-27621-9*, Little Brwn Med Div) Lppncott W & W.

Clinical Magnetic Resonance Imaging, Set. Robert R. Edelman et al. 2nd ed. 1996. LC 95-20424. 2336p. text 325.00 (*0-7216-5221-2*) Saunders.

Clinical Management of Acute Malaria. 2nd ed. 1986. (Regional Publications, South-East Asia Ser.: No. 9). 118p. pap. text 7.00 (*92-9022-109-7*, 1560009) World Health.

Clinical Management of Anxiety Disorders. Ed. by William Coryell & George Winokur. 1991. (Illus.). 176p. text 32.50 (*0-19-505953-0*) OUP.

Clinical Management of Articulatory & Phonologic Disorders. Curtis Weiss et al. 2nd ed. 1987. (Illus.). 372p. 54.95 (*0-683-08926-9*) Lppncott W & W.

Clinical Management of Basic Maxillofacial Orthopedic Appliances: Diagnostics. John W. Witzig & Terrance J. Spahl. 1989. 99.95 (*0-8151-9245-2*) Mosby Inc.

Clinical Management of Bereavement: A Handbook for Health Care Professionals. George M. Burnell & Adrienne L. Burnell. 1989. 192p. 38.95 (*0-89885-424-5*, Kluwer Acad Hman Sci) Kluwer Academic.

Clinical Management of Bladder Cancer. Ed. by Reginald Hall. 1998. LC 99-204517. (Illus.). 400p. (*0-340-74092-2*) E A GBR. *Dist:* OUP.

Clinical Management of Childhood Stuttering. Meryl J. Wall & Florence L. Myers. 2nd ed. 1995. LC 94-6972. 336p. 38.00 (*0-89079-602-5*, 6780) PRO-ED.

Clinical Management of Chronic Fatigue Syndrome: Clinical Conference, American Association of Chronic Fatigue Syndrome. Paul H. Levine & Roberto Patarca. Ed. by Nancy G. Klimas et al. 1996. LC 95-47749. (Journal of Chronic Fatigue Syndrome Ser.: Vol. 1, Nos. 3/4). 244p. (C). 39.95 (*1-56024-792-4*, Hawrth Medical) Haworth Pr.

Clinical Management of Communication Problems in Adults with Traumatic Brain Injury. Anita S. Halper et al. 1997. LC 91-22270. 183p. 79.00 (*0-8342-0279-4*) PRO-ED.

Clinical Management of Diabetic Neuropathy. Aristidis Veves. 1998. (Contemporary Endocrinology Ser.: Vol. 7). (Illus.). 360p. 145.00 (*0-89603-528-X*) Humana.

Clinical Management of Dysarthric Speakers. Kathryn M. Yorkston et al. 1988. LC 87-3380. (Illus.). 386p. (C). pap. text 39.00 (*0-89079-316-6*, 1575) PRO-ED.

Clinical Management of Dysphagia in Adults & Children. Ed. by Leora R. Cherney et al. 2nd ed. 1995. 246p. spiral bd. 79.00 (*0-8342-0376-6*, 20376) PRO-ED.

Clinical Management of Early Pregnancy. Ed. by Prendiville & J. Scott. 1998. (Illus.). 304p. pap. 138.95 (*0-412-58960-5*, Chap & Hall NY) Chapman & Hall.

Clinical Management of Early Pregnancy. W. Prendiville. 1999. LC 98-73728. (Illus.). 208p. text (*0-340-74100-7*) E A GBR. *Dist:* OUP.

Clinical Management of Electrolyte Disorders. Mary G. McGeown. 1983. text 135.00 (*0-89838-559-8*) Kluwer Academic.

Clinical Management of Feeding Disorders: Case Studies. Florence L. Yossem. 1997. LC 97-27402. 203p. pap. text 39.99 (*0-7506-9854-3*) Buttrwrth-Heinemann.

Clinical Management of Gastrointestinal Cancer. Ed. by Jerome J. DeCosse & Paul Sherlock. 1984. (Cancer Treatment & Research Ser.). 386p. text 192.50 (*0-89838-601-2*) Kluwer Academic.

Clinical Management of Herpes Viruses. Ed. by S. L. Sacks. 1995. LC 95-7667. 120.00 (*90-5199-227-0*) IOS Press.

Clinical Management of Infections in Immunocompromised Infants & Children. Christian C. Patrick. 2000. LC 00-60888. (Illus.). 672p. text 139.00 (*0-7817-1718-3*) Lppncott W & W.

Clinical Management of Infectious Diseases: A Guide to Diagnosis & Therapy. Seymour I. Schlager. 1998. LC 97-50109. 937p. pap. 39.95 (*0-683-30568-9*) Lppncott W & W.

Clinical Management of Itching. Arthur B. Fleischer, Jr. 2000. LC 97-25928. (Illus.). 210p. 85.95 (*1-85070-779-0*, Parthenon Pbng) CRC Pr.

Clinical Management of Malignant Melanoma. Ed. by John J. Costanzi. 1984. (Cancer Treatment & Research Ser.). text 103.50 (*0-89838-656-X*) Kluwer Academic.

Clinical Management of Melanoma. Hilliard F. Seigler. 1982. text 268.50 (*90-247-2584-4*) Kluwer Academic.

Clinical Management of Memory Problems. Wilson. 2nd ed. 1992. 338p. pap. 55.00 (*1-879105-90-X*, 0277) Singular Publishing.

Clinical Management of Motor Speech Disorders in Children. Anthony J. Caruso & Edythe A. Strand. 1999. LC 99-17630. (*3-13-111381-2*) Icon Lrning Systs.

Clinical Management of Myopia. Theodore Grosvenor & David A. Goss. 1998. LC 98-46246. 248p. text 64.99 (*0-7506-7060-6*) Buttrwrth-Heinemann.

Clinical Management of Neuromotor Based Feeding & Swallowing Problems. Janice Flegle & Paul Laikko. 1997. (Illus.). 100p. 25.00 (*1-889843-06-7*) Munroe-Meyer Inst.

Clinical Management of Nicotine Dependence. Ed. by J. A. Cocores. 1991. (Illus.). 336p. 144.00 (*0-387-97464-4*) Spr-Verlag.

Clinical Management of Perimenopause. Shawky Z. Badawy. 1998. LC 97-42808. 300p. pap. 79.95 (*0-412-12851-9*) Chapman & Hall.

Clinical Management of Poisoning & Drug Overdose. Lester M. Haddad et al. Ed. by Judy Fletcher. 3rd ed. 1997. LC 96-43968. (Illus.). 1056p. text 150.00 (*0-7216-6409-1*) Saunders.

Clinical Management of Renal Transplantation. Ed. by Mary G. McGeown. 1992. (Developments in Nephrology Ser.). 400p. (C). text 255.50 (*0-7923-1604-5*) Kluwer Academic.

Clinical Management of Right Hemisphere Dysfunction. Anita S. Halper et al. 2nd ed. 1990. LC 96-2715. (Rehabilitation Institute of Chicago Procedure Manual Ser.). spiral bd. 69.00 (*0-8342-0810-5*, 20845) PRO-ED.

Clinical Management of Sensorimotor Speech Disorders. Ed. by Malcolm R. McNeil & William H. Perkins. 1996. (Current Therapy of Communication Disorders Ser.). (Illus.). 352p. text 49.00 (*0-86577-527-3*) Thieme Med Pubs.

Clinical Management of Strabismus. Elizabeth Caloroso et al. 1993. LC 92-49704. 367p. pap. text 69.99 (*0-7506-9047-X*) Buttrwrth-Heinemann.

***Clinical Management of Stuttering in Older Children & Adults.** Richard E. Ham. tchr. ed. (*0-8342-1691-4*) PRO-ED.

Clinical Management of Systemic Lupus Erythematosus. Peter H. Schur. 2nd ed. 1996. LC 96-23364. 272p. text 79.00 (*0-397-51473-5*) Lppncott W & W.

Clinical Management of the Airway. Ed. by James T. Roberts. 1994. LC 93-12115. (Illus.). 512p. text 84.00 (*0-7216-3670-5*) Saunders.

Clinical Management of the Child & Teenager with Diabetes. Leslie Plotnick & Randi Henderson. 1998. LC 98-16878. (Series in Ambulatory Pediatric Medicine). 280p. 57.00 (*0-8018-5908-5*); (Illus.). pap. text 26.00 (*0-8018-5909-3*) Johns Hopkins.

Clinical Management of the Disabled Dental Patient: A Working Manual for Dental Professionals, Vol. 1. Leslie B. Levine. Ed. by Leslie C. Mason. 1989. (Illus.). 65p. (Orig.). (C). pap. text 10.95 (*0-9622139-0-X*) Denta Pr.

Clinical Management of the Perimenopause. Ed. by Shawky ZA Badawy. 1999. (Arnold Publication). 208p. 49.95 (*0-340-74150-3*) OUP.

***Clinical Management of the Transplant Patient.** Ed. by Rebecca A. Schroeder et al. 2001. (Arnold Publication). 296p. (Orig.). pap. text 55.00 (*0-340-76127-X*) OUP.

Clinical Management of Urticaria & Anaphylaxis. Ed. by Alan L. Schocket. 1992. LC 92-49730. (Allergic Disease & Therapy Ser.: Vol. 5). (Illus.). 264p. text 135.00 (*0-8247-8632-7*) Dekker.

Clinical Management of Voice Disorders. James L. Case. 3rd ed. 1995. LC 90-14313. 417p. text 41.00 (*0-89079-674-2*, 7311) PRO-ED.

Clinical Management Seizures. Robert C. Solomon. 2nd ed. 1983. (C). pap. text 58.00 (*0-7216-8493-9*) Harcourt.

Clinical Manifestations of Respiratory Disease. Terry R. Des Jardins. 3rd ed. 1995. (Illus.). 584p. (C). (gr. 13). pap. text 53.00 (*0-8016-7988-5*, 07988) Mosby Inc.

Clinical Manual. John Bradley et al. 1994. LC 93-34267. (Illus.). 384p. pap. 36.95 (*0-632-03312-6*) Blackwell Sci.

Clinical Manual for Binocular Vision. Mitchell M. Scheiman. 1993. 544p. spiral bd. 69.95 (*0-397-51133-7*) Lppncott W & W.

Clinical Manual for Laryngectomy & Head & Neck Cancer Rehabilitation. Janina K. Casper & Raymond H. Colton. 1992. (Clinical Competence Ser.). (Illus.). 214p. (Orig.). (C). pap. text 34.95 (*1-879105-61-6*, 0326) Thomson Learn.

Clinical Manual For Laryngectomy And Head/Neck Cancer Rehabilitation. Janina K. Casper & Raymond H. Colton. 2nd ed. 1998. LC 98-17724. (Illus.). 290p. spiral bd. 51.95 (*1-56593-959-X*, 1892) Thomson Learn.

Clinical Manual for Nursing. McClelland. 1985. 18.75 (*0-534-03993-6*) Jones & Bartlett.

Clinical Manual for Nursing Assistants. Sharon McClelland. 1985. LC 84-11985. (Illus.). 440p. (C). pap. text 39.95 (*0-86720-365-X*, 365-X) Jones & Bartlett.

Clinical Manual for Pain Management. Christine Miaskowski. 1999. pap. text 29.95 (*0-7216-6073-8*) Saunders.

Clinical Manual for Swallowing Disorders. Thomas Murry. 2000. LC 00-34507. (Illus.). viii, 184p. pap. 49.95 (*0-7693-0065-0*) Singular Publishing.

Clinical Manual Fundamental Anatomy & Physiology. Frederic H. Martini. 2nd ed. 1992. pap. text 22.00 (*0-13-335357-5*) P-H.

Clinical Manual of Chinese Herbal Medicine & Acupuncture. Zhong Y. Zhou & Jin H. De. 1996. (Illus.). 585p. (*0-443-05128-3*) Church.

Clinical Manual of Electrophysiology. Igor Singer & Joel Kupersmith. 1992. (Illus.). 496p. 70.00 (*0-683-07735-X*) Lppncott W & W.

Clinical Manual of Emergency Pediatrics. Ellen Crain & Jeffrey C. Gershel. 3rd ed. 1996. LC 96-23809. (Illus.). 731p. pap. 39.95 (*0-07-013429-4*) McGraw-Hill Prof.

Clinical Manual of Geriatric Medicine. Edmund Lonergan. 1996. 632p. (C). pap. text 44.95 (*0-8385-1094-9*, A1094-0, Apple Lange Med) McGraw.

Clinical Manual of Gerontological Nursing. Mildred O. Hogstel. 1992. (Illus.). 301p. spiral bd. 32.95 (*0-8016-2814-8*) Mosby Inc.

Clinical Manual of Health Assessment. Arden C. Bowers. 4th ed. 1991. (Illus.). 657p. (C). (gr. 13). pap. text 47.95 (*0-8016-0826-0*, 00826) Mosby Inc.

Clinical Manual of Medical-Surgical Nursing: Concepts & Clinical Practice. Judith K. Sands et al. 3rd ed. 1995. LC 95-1131. (Illus.). 464p. (C). (gr. 13). text 36.95 (*0-8016-7889-7*, 07889) Mosby Inc.

Clinical Manual of Otolaryngology. Ed. by Terence M. Davidson. 2nd ed. 1992. LC 91-3857. (Clinical Manual Ser.). (Illus.). 267p. pap. 29.50 (*0-07-105399-9*, RF56) McGraw-Hill Educ Grp.

Clinical Manual of Pediatric Anesthesia. Ed. by Deborah K. Rasch & Dawn E. Webster. 1993. (Clinical Manual Ser.). (Illus.). 624p. pap. text 39.00 (*0-07-051119-5*) McGraw-Hill Med Pub.

Clinical Manual of Pediatric Nursing Procedure. Bowden. 2001. 2259p. pap. text (*0-7216-5178-X*) Saunders.

Clinical Manual of Psychiatric Diagnosis & Treatment: A Biopsychosocial Approach. Ronald W. Pies. 1994. LC 93-48517. 544p. spiral bd. 51.95 (*0-88048-534-5*, 8534) Am Psychiatric.

Clinical Manual of Psychiatric Nursing. Ruth P. Rawlins & Patricia E. Heacock. 2nd ed. 1992. LC 92-12910. (Illus.). 416p. (C). (gr. 13). spiral bd. 35.00 (*0-8016-6333-4*, 06333) Mosby Inc.

Clinical Manual of Specialized Contact Lens Prescribing. Nieves Fernandes & Terry Scheid. 2001. (Illus.). 232p. pap. 44.99 (*0-7506-9924-8*) Buttrwrth-Heinemann.

Clinical Manual of Substance Abuse. Jean Kinney. 2nd ed. 1996. (Illus.). 480p. (C). text 39.95 (*0-8151-5092-X*, 24428) Mosby Inc.

Clinical Manual of Supportive Psychotherapy. Peter N. Novalis et al. 1993. LC 92-18064. 362p. spiral bd. 48.50 (*0-88048-403-9*, 8403) Am Psychiatric.

Clinical Manual of Urology. Ed. by Philip M. Hanno & Alan J. Wein. 2nd ed. 1994. (Illus.). 672p. pap. text 39.95 (*0-07-105435-9*, Apple Lange Med) McGraw.

Clinical Manual of Urology. Philip M. Hanno et al. 3rd ed. 2001. (Illus.). 924p. pap. 54.95 (*0-07-136201-0*) McGraw-Hill Prof.

Clinical Manual: Photodynamic Therapy of Malignancies. James S. McCaughan. 1993. (Medical Intelligence Unit Ser.). 250p. 189.00 (*1-879702-31-2*) CRC Pr.

Clinical Maps for Acute Care: Managing Care Through Collaborative Practice, Sup. 1. Clyde E. Wesp, Jr. & Donna E. Hartman. 1996. LC 95-30025. ring bd. 159.00 (*0-8342-0808-3*) Aspen Pub.

Clinical Marker hCG. Robert O. Hussa. 1987. LC 87-2434. 290p. 95.00 (*0-275-92365-7*, C2365, Praeger Pubs) Greenwood.

Clinical Masking Procedures. William S. Yacullo. 1995. LC 95-35670. 384p. pap. text 71.00 (*0-205-17352-7*) Allyn.

Clinical Maternal-Fetal Medicine. H. N. Winn & J. C. Hobbins. 2000. LC 99-27094. (Illus.). 976p. 138.95 (*1-85070-798-7*, Parthenon Pbng) CRC Pr.

Clinical Maternal-Fetal Medicine. Ed. by H. Winn & R. H. Petrie. 1998. 400p. 125.00 (*0-86542-213-3*) Blackwell Sci.

Clinical Maternal-Fetal Nutrition. Barbara Luke et al. 1993. LC 92-48905. (Illus.). 368p. 79.95 (*0-316-53614-8*, Little Brwn Med Div) Lppncott W & W.

Clinical Measurement in Coloproctology. Ed. by Devinder Kumar et al. 1991. (Illus.). 216p. 144.00 (*0-387-19643-9*) Spr-Verlag.

Clinical Measurement in Drug Evaluation. Ed. by Walter S. Nimmo & Gregory T. Tucker. 1995. LC 94-40650. 344p. 235.95 (*0-471-94391-6*) Wiley.

Clinical Measurement in Gastroenterology Vol. 1: The Oesophagus. Ed. by David F. Evans & Graham K. Buckton. 1997. LC 97-2122. (Illus.). 227p. 130.00 (*0-86542-662-7*) Blackwell Sci.

Clinical Measurement of Joint Motion. Ed. by Walter B. Greene & James D. Heckman. 1994. 152p. 22.00 (*0-89203-090-9*) Amer Acad Ortho Surg.

Clinical Measurement of Speech & Voice. Ronald J. Baken. 1996. (Illus.). 528p. (Orig.). reprint ed. pap. text 59.95 (*1-56593-809-7*, 1582) Thomson Learn.

Clinical Measurement of Speech & Voice. Ronald J. Baken & Robert F. Orlikoff. 2nd ed. 1999. LC 99-24709. (Illus.). 864p. (Orig.). pap. text 93.95 (*1-56593-869-0*, 1698) Thomson Learn.

Clinical Mechanics of the Hand. Paul W. Brand & Anne Hollister. 2nd ed. 1992. (Illus.). 386p. (C). (gr. 13). text 85.00 (*0-8016-6978-2*, 06978) Mosby Inc.

Clinical Mechanics of the Hand. Paul W. Brand. 3rd ed. 1999. LC 98-42919. (Illus.). 388p. text 79.00 (*0-8151-2786-3*, 31248) Mosby Inc.

Clinical Medical Assistant. Mary A. Woods. (Illus.). 1994. 546p. tchr. ed. (*0-7216-5236-0*); 1993. 512p. text 33.00 (*0-7216-5235-2*) Saunders.

Clinical Medical Assisting: Professional Practice. Stiles. 1991. (Education Ser.). 27.95 (*0-8273-3443-5*); tchr. ed. 8.00 (*0-8273-3444-3*) Delmar.

Clinical Medical Asst Training Prog Wrkbk. Boston Reed Company Staff. 1998. (Medical Assisting Ser.). (C). pap., wbk. ed. 16.00 (*0-7668-0933-1*) Delmar.

Clinical Medical Ethics. Ed. by Edwin Salzman. 1986. (Medical Ethics Ser.). (Illus.). 109p. pap. text 15.00 (*0-910133-17-4*) Mass Med Pub Div.

Clinical Medical Ethics: Cases & Readings. David C. Thomasma & Patricia A. Marshall. 1995. LC 94-22890. 636p. (Orig.). (C). pap. 64.00 (*0-8191-9725-4*) U Pr of Amer.

Clinical Medical Ethics: Cases in Practice. Terry M. Perlin. 1992. LC 92-12544. 33.95 (*0-316-69959-4*, Little Brwn Med Div) Lppncott W & W.

Clinical Medicine. Bhattacharyya. 1989. (C). (*0-89771-372-9*) Current Dist IND. *Dist:* St Mut.

Clinical Medicine. Peter C. Hayes & Niall D. Finlayson. 1994. LC 94-4031. (Colour Guide, Picture Tests Ser.). pap. text (*0-443-04957-2*) Church.

Clinical Medicine. Ed. by Harry L. Greene et al. 2nd ed. 1995. (Illus.). 992p. (C). (gr. 13). pap. text 49.00 (*0-8151-4026-6*, 24427) Mosby Inc.

Clinical Medicine. Kumar. 4th ed. 1998. text 53.00 (*0-7020-2019-2*) Saunders.

Clinical Medicine: Key Questions Answered. Wai-Ching Leung. 1998. LC 98-15855. (Key Questions Answered Ser.). 300p. (Orig.). pap. text 32.50 (*0-19-262891-7*) OUP.

Clinical Medicine: Self-Assessment Questions in Colour. Pierre-Marc G. Bouloux. 1993. pap. (*1-56375-613-7*) Wolfe Publishing GBR. *Dist:* Mosby Inc.

Clinical Medicine for the Occupational Physician. M. K. Alderman & Hanley. 1982. (Occupational Safety & Health Ser.: Vol. 7). (Illus.). 552p. text 210.00 (*0-8247-7957-6*) Dekker.

Clinical Medicine in Optometric Practice. Bruce G. Muchnick. 1994. (Illus.). 480p. (C). (gr. 13). text 64.00 (*0-8016-6306-7*, 06306) Mosby Inc.

Clinical Medicine of the Dog & Cat. Ed. by Michael Schaer. 2000. (Illus.). 352p. 64.95 (*0-8138-0332-2*) Iowa U Pr.

Clinical Mental Health Counselor Crossword Puzzle. Maurice Ptito & AMHCA Staff. 1998. 32p. pap. text 18.00 (*0-7872-5301-4*) Kendall-Hunt.

Clinical Meta-Analysis. George Davey-Smith. 2001. 150p. 54.95 (*0-471-96706-8*) Wiley.

Clinical Method: A General Practice Approach. Robin C. Fraser. 1999. LC 99-13001. 199p. pap. text 35.00 (*0-7506-4005-7*) Buttrwrth-Heinemann.

Clinical Methods & Practicum in Speech-Language Pathology. Ben R. Kelly et al. 1993. LC 93-28364. (Illus.). 368p. (C). pap. text 39.95 (*1-56593-161-0*, 0471) Thomson Learn.

Clinical Methods in Communication Disorders. William R. Leith. 2nd ed. 1993. LC 92-17022. 288p. pap. text 31.00 (*0-89079-568-1*, 4047) PRO-ED.

Clinical Methods in Study of Cholesterol Metabolism. H. S. Sodhi et al. 1979. (Monographs on Atherosclerosis: Vol. 9). (Illus.). pap. 71.50 (*3-8055-2986-4*) S Karger.

Clinical Methods in Transcultural Psychiatry. Ed. by Samuel O. Okpaku. 1998. LC 97-47207. 496p. text 67.00 (*0-88048-710-0*, 8710) Am Psychiatric.

Clinical Microbiology. Roger Silletti & Victor Lorian. 1994. (Illus.). 512p. 65.00 (*0-683-07712-0*) Lppncott W & W.

Clinical Microbiology. Jennie Wilson. 2000. 410p. pap. text (*0-7020-2316-7*) W B Saunders GBR. *Dist:* Saunders.

Clinical Microbiology. E. Joan Stokes & G. L. Ridgeway. 6th ed. 1988. (Illus.). 352p. (C). pap. (*0-683-13078-1*) E A GBR. *Dist:* Williams & Wilkins.

Clinical Microbiology. Ed. by D. E. Stokes et al. 7th ed. 1993. (Illus.). 416p. pap. text (*0-340-55423-1*) E A GBR. *Dist:* OUP.

Clinical Microbiology in the ICU. Van Saene. 1997. (Illus.). 176p. (C). text (*0-412-61780-3*, Chap & Hall NY) Chapman & Hall.

Clinical Microbiology Made Ridiculously Simple. Mark Gladwin & Bill Trattler. 2nd rev. ed. 1999. 272p. (Orig.). (C). pap. text 23.95 (*0-940780-32-1*) MedMaster.

***Clinical Microbiology Made Ridiculously Simple.** Mark Gladwin & Bill Trattler. 3rd rev. ed. 2001. (Illus.). 288p. (Orig.). pap. 24.95 (*0-940780-49-6*) MedMaster.

Clinical Microbiology Procedures Handbook, Set. Ed. by Henry D. Isenberg et al. 1992. (Illus.). 2468p. 159.95 (*1-55581-038-1*) ASM Pr.

***Clinical Microbiology Review.** Peter Q. Warinner. 3rd ed. 2001. 150p. pap. 35.95 (*0-9677839-3-3*) Wysteria Ltd.

Clinical Monitoring for Anesthesia & Critical Care. Ed. by Carole L. Lake. 2nd ed. 1994. LC 93-41600. (Illus.). 590p. text 145.00 (*0-7216-5269-7*) Saunders.

Clinical MR Imaging: A Practical Approach. Ed. by Peter Reimer et al. 1999. LC 98-53094. (Illus.). 558p. pap. 129.00 (*3-540-64098-3*) Spr-Verlag.

Clinical MR Spectroscopy: First Principles. Nouha Salibi & Mark A. Brown. 1997. LC 97-13903. (Illus.). 236p. pap. 66.50 (*0-471-18280-X*) Wiley.

Clinical Musculoskeletal Anatomy. Neal E. Pratt. 1991. (Illus.). 333p. text 48.00 (*0-397-54825-7*, Lippnctt) Lppncott W & W.

Clinical Musculoskeletal Pathology. William F. Enneking. 3rd rev. ed. 1990. 508p. (C). 59.95 (*0-8130-1016-0*) U Press Fla.

Clinical Nephrology. Woo K. Thye. 1998. LC 98-6430. 340p. (C). pap. 13.00 (*981-02-3484-8*) World Scientific Pub.

Clinical Nephrology: Immunologic Considerations, Invasive Techniques & Dialytic Strategies. Ed. by G. Colasanti & G. D'Amico. 1989. (Contributions to Nephrology Ser.: Vol. 69). (Illus.). 29.75 (*3-8055-4857-5*) S Karger.

Clinical Nephrology in Medical Practice. Gavin J. Becker et al. 1992. (Essentials Ser.). (Illus.). 400p. 100.00 (*0-632-03167-0*) Blackwell Sci.

Clinical Nephrotoxins: Renal Injury from Drugs & Chemical. M. E. De Broe. 1997. LC 97-11284. 528p. lib. bdg. 265.00 (*0-7923-3611-9*) Kluwer Academic.

Clinical Neuro-Urology. Robert J. Krane. 2nd ed. 1991. 120.00 (*0-316-50332-0*, Little Brwn Med Div) Lppncott W & W.

Clinical Neuroanatomy for Medical Students. Richard S. Snell. 2nd ed. 1986. 35.50 (*0-316-80198-4*, Little Brwn Med Div) Lppncott W & W.

Clinical Neuroanatomy Made Ridiculously Simple. Stephen Goldberg. 2nd rev. ed. 2000. LC 00-266198. (Illus.). 97p. pap. text 13.95 (*0-940780-46-1*) MedMaster.

Clinical Neuroanesthesia. Armin Schubert. 1996. LC 96-33435. 406p. spiral bd. 74.99 (*0-7506-9502-1*) Buttrwrth-Heinemann.

Clinical Neuroanesthesia. Roy F. Cucchiara et al. 2nd ed. 1997. LC 97-41358. (Illus.). 704p. text (*0-443-07928-5*, C9409) Church.

Clinical Neurocardiology. Louis R. Caplan et al. 1999. LC 99-26885. (Fundamental & Clinical Cardiology Ser.). (Illus.). 520p. text 195.00 (*0-8247-1991-3*) Dekker.

Clinical Neuroimmunology. Jack P. Antel et al. 1997. LC 97-2678. (Illus.). 204.95 (*0-86542-411-X*) Blackwell Sci.

Clinical Neurology Ed. by Robert J. Joynt. (Annual Revision Service Ser.). ring bd. 450.00 (*0-06-148006-1*) Lppncott W & W.

Clinical Neurology. C. D. Marsden. 480p. pap. text (*0-7131-4432-7*) E A GBR. *Dist:* Routldge.

Clinical Neurology. C. David Marsden & Timothy J. Fowler. 2nd ed. 1998. LC 97-33688. (Arnold Publication). (Illus.). 466p. pap. 49.95 (*0-340-64611-X*) OUP.

Clinical Neurology: A Lange Medical Book. Roger P. Simon et al. 4th rev. ed. 1999. LC 00-265520. (Illus.). 344p. (C). pap. 44.95 (*0-8385-0515-5*) McGraw-Hill Prof.

Clinical Neurology: A Modern Approach. Anthony Hopkins. 1993. (Illus.). 494p. pap. text 49.50 (*0-19-262262-5*) OUP.

Clinical Neurology: Essential Concepts. Simon J. Ellis. 1997. LC 97-31681. 208p. pap. text 45.00 (*0-7506-3343-3*) Buttrwrth-Heinemann.

Clinical Neurology & Neuropsychiatry. Jeffrey Cummings. 1985. 272p. text 56.00 (*0-8089-1722-6*, 790955, Grune & Strat) Harcrt Hlth Sci Grp.

Clinical Neurology Casebook. Thomas M. Walshe & Richard Schwartz. 1999. (*0-7506-9563-3*) Buttrwrth-Heinemann.

Clinical Neurology for Psychiatrists. David M. Kaufman. 5th ed. 2001. LC 00-63722. (Illus.). xvii, 727p. 89.00 (*0-7216-8995-7*) Harcrt Hlth Sci Grp.

Clinical Neurology for Psychiatrists. David M. Kaufman. 4th ed. 1995. LC 94-46917. (Illus.). 592p. text 86.00 (*0-7216-5829-6*) Saunders.

Clinical Neurology in Rheumatic Diseases. Richard R. Rosenbaum et al. 1996. LC 96-28925. 436p. pap. text 99.00 (*0-7506-9613-3*) Buttrwrth-Heinemann.

Clinical Neurology of Aging. Ed. by Martin L. Albert & Janice E. Knoefel. 2nd rev. ed. 1994. (Illus.). 728p. reprint ed. text 145.00 (*0-19-507167-0*) OUP.

Clinical Neurology of Old Age. R. C. Tallis. 1989. 602p. 522.00 (*0-471-91108-9*) Wiley.

Clinical Neuromythology & Other Arguments & Essays, Pertinent & Impertinent. Ed. by William Landau. 1998. LC 97-46589. (Illus.). 556p. 70.00 (*0-87993-698-3*) Futura Pub.

Clinical Neurooncology Berger. 2000. text (*0-7216-8148-4*) Saunders.

Clinical Neuropathology. James S. Nelson & Paul E. McKeever. 1994. (C). 600.00 incl. disk (*1-56815-020-2*) Mosby Inc.

Clinical Neurophysiological Aspects of Psychopathological Coniditions. Ed. by C. Perris. 1980. (Advances in Biological Psychiatry Ser.: Vol. 4). (Illus.). viii, 192p. pap. 53.25 (*3-8055-0604-X*) S Karger.

Clinical Neurophysiology: Electroencephalography, Paediatric Neurophysiology, Special Techniques & Applications. John W. Osselton et al. 2001. (Illus.). 448p. 140.00 (*0-7506-1663-6*) Buttrwrth-Heinemann.

Clinical Neurophysiology: Electromyography, Nerve Conduction & Evoked Potentials, Vol. 1. Colin D. Binnie et al. Ed. by John W. Osselton. 1995. (Illus.). 592p. text 175.00 (*0-7506-1183-9*) Buttrwrth-Heinemann.

Clinical Neurophysiology: From Receptors to Perception. International Congress of Electroencephalography and Clinical Neurophysiology Staff & G. Comi. 1999. LC 99-36444. (Electroencephalography & Clinical Neurophysiology Ser.). 672p. 234.50 (*0-444-50048-0*) Elsevier.

Clinical Neurophysiology of Epilepsy: Handbook of Electroencephalography & Clinical Neurophysiology, No. 4. Ed. by J. A. Wada & R. J. Ellingson. 1990. 508p. 266.50 (*0-444-81241-5*) Elsevier.

Clinical Neurophysiology of Infancy & Childhood. Jones. 2001. 800p. 175.00 (*0-7506-7251-X*) Buttrwrth-Heinemann.

***Clinical Neurophysiology of the Vestibular System.** Robert W. Baloh. 3rd ed. 2001. LC 00-140077. (Contemporary Neurology Ser.). (Illus.). 432p. text 98.50 (*0-19-513982-8*) OUP.

Clinical Neuropsychiatry. Thomas Jobe & Moises Gaviria. 1997. LC 96-45558. (Illus.). 500p. (Orig.). 155.00 (*0-86542-528-0*) Blackwell Sci.

Clinical Neuropsychiatry of Stroke: Cognitive, Behavioral & Emotional Disorders Following Vascular Brain Injury. Robert G. Robinson. 1998. LC 97-26484. (Illus.). 503p. (C). text 95.00 (*0-521-44234-6*) Cambridge U Pr.

Clinical Neuropsychological Assessment: A Cognitive Approach. Ed. by Robert L. Mapou & Jack Spector. 1995. (Critical Issues in Neuropsychology Ser.: Vol. 1). (Illus.). 380p. (C). text 75.00 (*0-306-44869-6*, Kluwer Plenum) Kluwer Academic.

Clinical Neuropsychology. Pierre J. Vinken et al. 1985. (Handbooks of Clinical Neurology: Vol. 45(1)). 570p. 323.00 (*0-444-90356-9*) Elsevier.

Clinical Neuropsychology. Ed. by Kenneth M. Heilman & Edward Valenstein. 3rd ed. 1993. LC 92-49919. (Illus.). 752p. text 72.50 (*0-19-508123-4*) OUP.

Clinical Neuropsychology: Behavioral & Brain Science. John L. Bradshaw & Jason B. Mattingley. 1995. LC 94-49187. (Illus.). 458p. pap. text 39.95 (*0-12-124545-4*) Acad Pr.

Clinical Neuropsychology: Interface with Neurological & Psychiatric Disorders. Ed. by Charles J. Golden et al. 1983. text 32.95 (*0-8089-1541-X*, 791623, Grune & Strat) Harcrt Hlth Sci Grp.

Clinical Neuropsychology: Theoretical Foundations for Practitioners. Ed. by Mark E. Maruish & James A. Moses. 1996. 400p. 79.95 (*0-8058-1343-8*) L Erlbaum Assocs.

Clinical Neuropsychology & Brain Function: Research, Measurement, & Practice. Ed. by Thomas J. Boll & Brenda K. Bryant. 1988. LC 88-14558. (Master Lectures: Vol. 7). 202p. pap. 24.95 (*1-55798-038-1*) Am Psychol.

Clinical Neuropsychology of Attention. Adriaan H. Van Zomeren & Wiebo H. Brouwer. 1994. LC 93-17824. (Illus.). 264p. text 38.00 (*0-19-506373-2*) OUP.

Clinical Neuropsychopharmacology. Dornan. 2000. pap. text 37.00 net. (*0-534-25698-8*) Thomson Learn.

Clinical Neuroradiology: A Textbook. Ed. by Eberhard Lohr et al. 1995. LC 94-35189. (Illus.). 336p. text 135.00 (*0-88937-132-6*) Hogrefe & Huber Pubs.

Clinical Neuroscience. Lambert et al. 2002. text (*0-7167-5227-1*) Worth.

Clinical Neuroscience: Brain, Mind, Sex, Emotion, Development, Language, Cognition. Rhawn Joseph. 3rd ed. 2002. (Illus.). 1400p. (C). 150.00 (*0-9700733-3-X*) Univ Pr CA.

Clinical Neuroscience: From Neuroanatomy to Psychodynamics. Jay E. Harris. 1985. 304p. 45.95 (*0-89885-238-2*, Kluwer Acad Hman Sci) Kluwer Academic.

Clinical Neuroscience, Neuropsychology & Neuropsychiatry: Development, Sexuality, Emotion. Rhawn Joseph. 3rd ed. 2000. 109.95 (*0-12-390125-1*) Acad Pr.

Clinical Neurosis. Philip Snaith. 2nd ed. 1991. (Illus.). 256p. pap. 32.50 (*0-19-262067-3*) OUP.

Clinical Neurosurgery, Vol. 34. John Little. 1987. (Illus.). 718p. 64.95 (*0-683-02029-3*) Lppncott W & W.

Clinical Neurosurgery, Vol. 35. Ed. by Peter E. Black. 1988. (Proceedings of the Congress of Neurological Surgeons Ser.). (Illus.). 576p. 65.00 (*0-683-02032-3*) Lppncott W & W.

Clinical Neurosurgery, Vol. 39. Warren R. Selman. 1992. (Illus.). 602p. 85.00 (*0-683-02036-6*) Lppncott W & W.

Clinical Neurosurgery, Volume 44. CNS Staff. 1997. 603p. text 105.00 (*0-683-18313-3*) Lppncott W & W.

Clinical Neurosurgery, Volume 46. M. Sean Grady. 2000. 650p. text 115.00 (*0-7817-2533-X*) Lppncott W & W.

Clinical Neurosurgery: Proceedings of the Congress of Neurological Surgeons, Vol. 32. Ed. by John R. Little. 1985. (Illus.). 680p. 54.00 (0-683-02027-7) Lppncott W & W.

Clinical Neurosurgery: Proceedings of the Congress of Neurological Surgeons, Vol. 33. John R. Little. 1986. (Illus.). 702p. (0-683-02028-5) Lppncott W & W.

Clinical Neurosurgery: Proceedings of the Congress of Neurological Surgeons, Vol. 36. Peter M. Black. 1989. (Illus.). 512p. 65.00 (0-683-02033-1) Lppncott W & W.

Clinical Neurosurgery: Proceedings of the Congress of Neurological Surgeons, Vol. 40. Warren R. Selman. 1993. (Illus.). 561p. 85.00 (0-683-02037-4) Lppncott W & W.

Clinical Neurosurgery Vol. 37: Proceedings of the Congress of Neurological Surgeons. Peter M. Black. 1990. (Illus.). 844p. 66.00 (0-683-02034-X) Lppncott W & W.

Clinical Neurosurgery Vol. 42: Proceedings of the Congress of Neurological Surgeons, 42. Congress of Neurological Surgeons Staff. 1996. (Illus.). 538p. (0-683-02039-0) Lppncott W & W.

Clinical Neurosurgery Vol. 43: Proceedings of the Congress of Neurological Surgeons, Vol. 43. Christopher M. Loftus. 1997. (Illus.). 458p. (0-683-18300-1) Lppncott W & W.

Clinical Neutron Dosimetry Pt. 1: Determination of Absorbed Dose in a Patient Treated by External Beams of Fast Neutrons. ICRU Staff. 1989. LC 88-25113. (ICRU Report Ser.: No. 45). pap. text 50.00 (0-913394-39-4) Intl Comm Rad Meas.

Clinical Notes for the FRCA. Charles D. Deakin. 1997. LC 96-5332. 308p. pap. text (0-443-05386-3); 2nd ed. 1999. LC 99-53893. (Illus.). xii, 432p. (0-443-06403-2) Church.

Clinical Nuclear Cardiology. George A. Beller. 1995. LC 94-25345. (Illus.). 336p. text 110.00 (0-7216-3332-3); 2nd ed. 1999. 495p. text 120.00 (0-7216-7715-0) Saunders.

Clinical Nuclear Medicine. Michael N. Maisey. 1983. 97.50 (0-7020-1243-2) Saunders.

Clinical Nuclear Medicine. Michael N. Maisey et al. 1983. (Illus.). 525p. text 142.00 (0-7216-1087-0) Saunders.

Clinical Nuclear Medicine. Ed. by M. N. Maisey et al. 3rd ed. 1999. LC 97-76965. (Illus.). 784p. (0-412-75180-1) E A GBR. *Dist:* OUP.

Clinical Nurse. Jack Rudman. 1994. (Career Examination Ser.: C-947). pap. 29.95 (0-8373-0947-6) Nat Learn.

Clinical Nurse Specialist: Perspectives on Practice. Ed. by Shirley W. Menard. 1989. pap. text 33.50 (0-8273-4311-6) Delmar.

Clinical Nurse Specialist in Theory & Practice. Ann B. Hamric & Judith A. Spross. 2nd ed. 1989. (Illus.). 466p. text 47.00 (0-7216-4486-4) Saunders.

Clinical Nurse Specialist Role in Critical Care. American Association of Critical-Care Nurses Staff. Ed. by Anna Gawlinski & Leslie S. Kern. 1994. LC 93-30391. (Illus.). 335p. text 55.00 (0-7216-3715-9) Saunders.

Clinical Nursing. June M. Thompson et al. 4th ed. 1997. LC 97-4331. (Illus.). 1848p. (C). (gr. 13). text 49.95 (0-8151-8893-5, 29632) Mosby Inc.

Clinical Nursing. Rolf Wirhed. 4th ed. 1997. text (0-7234-2643-0) Wolfe Publishing GBR. *Dist:* Mosby Inc.

Clinical Nursing Interventions with Critical Elements. Mary A. Riley & Mary J. Beltran. 1989. LC 85-20360. 385p. pap. text 28.50 (0-8273-4338-8) Delmar.

***Clinical Nursing Practices: Guidelines for Evidence-Based Practice.** Elizabeth Jamieson et al. 4th ed. 2001. (Illus.). 491p. pap. (0-443-07020-2) Church GBR. *Dist:* Saunders.

Clinical Nursing Procedures. Ed. by Kathleen H. Belland & Mary A. Wells. 1984. LC 83-25982. (Illus.). 400p. (C). pap. text 43.95 (0-86720-374-9, 374-9) Jones & Bartlett.

Clinical Nursing Procedures. Kathleen Hoerth Belland. 1984. 27.95 (0-534-03154-4) Jones & Bartlett.

Clinical Nursing Procedures. Leahy. 1998. pap. text 42.50 (0-7216-5004-X) Harcourt.

Clinical Nursing Research - ONS. Frank Stromberg. 1991. (Illus.). (C). text, tchr. ed. 44.95 (0-86720-340-4, 340-4) Jones & Bartlett.

Clinical Nursing Skills. Carol B. Lammon et al. 1995. LC 93-44872. (Illus.). 784p. pap. text 47.00 (0-7216-6680-9) Saunders.

Clinical Nursing Skills. Smith. 4th ed. 1997. 1152p. (C). 69.33 (0-8385-1527-4) P-H.

Clinical Nursing Skills: Basic to Advanced Skills. Smith et al. 5th ed. 1999. 1199p. pap. 72.00 (0-8385-1566-5) P-H.

Clinical Nursing Skills: Textbook/Checklist Package. Textbook/Checklist Package. Carol B. Lammon et al. 1995. (Illus.). 811p. text 58.00 (0-7216-6217-X) Saunders.

Clinical Nursing Skills & Techniques. Anne G. Perry & Patricia A. Potter. 4th ed. 1998. 1392p. (0-8151-4308-7); tchr. ed. (0-8151-4307-9) Mosby Inc.

Clinical Nursing Skills & Techniques. Anne G. Perry & Patricia A. Potter. 4th ed. 1998. (Illus.). 1392p. pap. (84-8174-342-9) Mosby-Doyma Libros ESP. *Dist:* Mosby Inc.

Clinical Nursing Skills & Techniques. Patricia A. Potter & Anne G. Perry. 4th ed. 1997. (Illus.). 1392p. (C). (gr. 13). pap. text 52.00 (0-8151-4305-2, 29659) Mosby Inc.

Clinical Nursing Skills & Techniques: Checklists. Patricia A. Potter & Anne G. Perry. 4th ed. 1997. 490p. (C). (gr. 13). pap. text 14.95 (0-8151-4306-0) Mosby Inc.

Clinical Nutrition. Ed. by Bennion. 1978. (C). text (0-321-01537-1) Addson-Wesley Educ.

Clinical Nutrition: A Functional Approach. 1999. (Illus.). xxvi, 324p. pap. 85.00 (0-9624859-1-8) HealthComm Intl.

Clinical Nutrition: Enteral & Tube Feeding. John L. Rombeau & Rolando H. Rolandelli. Ed. by Ray Kersey. 3rd ed. 1996. (Illus.). 670p. text 99.00 (0-7216-2155-4) Saunders.

Clinical Nutrition: Parenteral Nutrition. John L. Rombeau & Michael D. Caldwell. 2nd ed. 1993. (Illus.). 912p. text 130.00 (0-7216-3600-4) Saunders.

Clinical Nutrition: Parenteral Nutrition. John L. Rombeau & Rolando H. Rolandelli. 2nd ed. 2000. LC 99-50227. (Illus.). xvi, 623p. text 134.50 (0-7216-8120-4) Saunders.

Clinical Nutrition: Proceedings of the European Nutritionists Group Symposium, Saltsjoebaden, June 10, 1971. European Nutritionists Group Symposium Staff. Ed. by J. C. Somogyi. 1973. (Bibliotheca Nutritio et Dieta Ser.: No. 19). (Illus.). 165p. pap. 56.75 (3-8055-1500-6) S Karger.

Clinical Nutrition & Metabolic Research. Ed. by G. Dietze & G. Kleinberger. 1986. (Illus.). 400p. pap. 108.00 (3-8055-4388-3) S Karger.

Clinical Nutrition Case Studies. Wayne E. Billon. 2nd ed. 1996. 293p. 25.25 (0-314-07169-5) West Pub.

Clinical Nutrition for Pain, Inflammmation & Tissue Healing. David R. Seaman. 1998. LC 98-88132. x, 282p. pap. 64.95 (0-9667211-0-1) NutrAnalysis Inc.

Clinical Nutrition for the Balanced Body. John A. Allocca. 1997. (Illus.). 398p. pap. text 60.00 (0-9659987-1-1) Allocca Biotech.

Clinical Nutrition for the Health Scientist. Daphne A. Roe. 1980. 144p. 83.00 (0-8493-5417-X, QP141, CRC Reprint) Franklin.

Clinical Nutrition of the Dog & Cat. J. W. Simpson et al. 1993. LC 92-36752. (Library of Veterinary Practice). (Illus.). 160p. pap. 47.95 (0-632-03363-0) Blackwell Sci.

Clinical Nutrition of the Essential Trace Elements & Minerals: The Guide for Health Professionals. Ed. by John D. Bogden & Leslie M. Klevay. 2000. LC 00-4979. (Nutrition & Health Ser.). (Illus.). 416p. 125.00 (0-89603-598-0) Humana.

Clinical Nutrition Using the Seven Lines of Defense Against Disease. Robert J. Peshek. 1980. 10.00 (0-9605902-3-4) Color Coded Charting.

Clinical Obesity. Peter G. Kopelman & Michael Stock. 1998. LC 97-46120. (Illus.). 631p. 208.95 (0-632-04198-6) Blackwell Sci.

Clinical Obstetrical Ultrasound, Vol. 1. William J. Ott. 1999. LC 98-32454. (Illus.). 416p. 167.00 incl. cd-rom (0-471-32927-4) Wiley.

Clinical Obstetrics & Gynaecology. Isabel Stabile et al. 2nd ed. 2000. LC 99-56572. 232p. pap. 45.00 (1-85233-615-3) Spr-Verlag.

Clinical Obstetrics & Gynecology. Alexander F. Burnett. 2000. LC 00-39760. (Illus.). x, 462p. (C). pap. 36.95 (0-632-04353-9) Blackwell Sci.

Clinical Obstetrics & Gynecology. Drife. 2000. (Illus.). 410p. text 46.50 (0-7020-1775-2) Saunders.

Clinical Occupational Medicine. Linda Rosenstock & Mark R. Cullen. 1986. (Illus.). 305p. text 38.00 (0-7216-1145-1) Saunders.

Clinical Ocular Oncology. Devron H. Char. 1988. (Illus.). 402p. text (0-443-08569-2) Church.

Clinical Ocular Pathology: Test Yourself. Gary P. Misson. 2001. 256p. pap. 40.00 (0-7506-2264-4) Buttrwrth-Heinemann.

Clinical Ocular Pharmacology. David W. Lamberts & David E. Potter. 1987. 560p. 89.95 (0-316-51286-9, Little Brwn Med Div) Lppncott W & W.

Clinical Ocular Pharmacology. Jimmy D. Bartlett & Siret D. Jaanus. 4th ed. 2001. LC 00-62170. (Illus.). 1100p. text 110.00 (0-7506-7039-8) Buttrwrth-Heinemann.

Clinical Ocular Pharmacology: Pocket Handbook. Jimmy D. Bartlett et al. 3rd ed. 1996. LC 96-42981. 512p. pap. text 45.00 (0-7506-9641-9) Buttrwrth-Heinemann.

Clinical Ocular Photography. Denise Cunningham. 1998. LC 98-13365. (Basic Bookshelf for Eyecare Professionals Ser.). (Illus.). 160p. pap. text 30.00 (1-55642-377-2, 63772) SLACK Inc.

Clinical Ocular Physiology: An Introductory Text. N. Victor Chong. 1997. LC 96-20041. 192p. pap. text 36.50 (0-7506-2718-2) Buttrwrth-Heinemann.

Clinical Oncology. Ed. by Martin D. Abeloff et al. 1995. LC 95-744. 2,350p. text (0-443-08941-8) Church.

Clinical Oncology. Ed. by Raymond E. Lenhard, Jr. et al. 2000. LC 00-32290. (Illus.). 800p. 60.95 incl. cd-rom (0-944235-15-8) Blackwell Sci.

Clinical Oncology. Anthony J. Neal & Peter J. Hoskin. 1994. 328p. pap. (0-340-59436-5) E A GBR. *Dist:* OUP.

Clinical Oncology. Geoffrey R. Weiss. 1993. LC 93-218387. (Illus.). 416p. (C). pap. text 39.95 (0-8385-1325-5, A1325-8, Apple Lange Med) McGraw.

Clinical Oncology. Martin D. Abeloff. 2nd ed. 1999. LC 99-26164. (Illus.). xxix, 2963p. (C). text (0-443-07545-X) Church.

Clinical Oncology. Philip F. Rubin. 8th ed. 1999. LC 00-58852. 971p. text incl. cd-rom (0-7216-7496-8) Saunders.

Clinical Oncology: A Quantitative Approach. N. M. Emmanuel & L. S. Evseenko. 1973. 280p. 3.5 hd 71.00 (0-7065-1337-1) Coronet Bks.

Clinical Oncology: Basic Principles & Practice. Anthony J. Neal & Peter J. Hoskin. 2nd ed. 1997. LC 96-39632. (Illus.). 256p. pap. text (0-340-67748-1) E A GBR. *Dist:* OUP.

Clinical Oncology for Physicians & Students: A Multidisciplinary Approach. Philip F. Rubin. 7th ed. 1993. (Illus.). 804p. pap. text 25.00 (0-7216-3761-2) Saunders.

Clinical Oncology for Students of Radiation Therapy Technology. John A. Stryker. 1992. (Illus.). 400p. (Orig.). (C). pap. 42.50 (0-87527-488-9) Green.

Clinical Ophthalmic Pathology. John Harry & Gary Misson. 2001. (Illus.). 376p. 195.00 (0-7506-2171-0) Buttrwrth-Heinemann.

Clinical Ophthalmology. Jack J. Kanski. 4th ed. 1999. LC 99-15484. 560p. pap. text (0-7506-4009-X) Buttrwrth-Heinemann.

Clinical Ophthalmology: A Systematic Approach. Jack J. Kanski. 1999. 3rd ed. LC 94-11863. (Illus.). 514p. text 130.00 (0-7506-1886-8); 4th ed. LC 99-15484. 673p. text 160.00 (0-7506-4014-6) Buttrwrth-Heinemann.

Clinical Ophthalmology: A Test Yourself Atlas. Jack J. Kanski. 2002. 192p. pap. 54.99 (0-7506-4938-0) Buttrwrth-Heinemann.

Clinical Ophthalmology: A Test Yourself Atlas. Jack J. Kanski et al. 1995. LC 95-6471. (Illus.). 410p. pap. text 45.00 (0-7506-2189-3) Buttrwrth-Heinemann.

Clinical Ophthalmology Pt. 3: Self-Assessment for the MRCOPHTH/FRCOPHTH. S. James Talks & Daniel Byles. 1998. (Arnold Publication). (Illus.). 112p. (Orig.). pap. text 27.50 (0-340-70577-9) OUP.

Clinical Ophthalmology the Essentials. Jack J. Kanski. 2001. (Illus.). 320p. pap. 63.00 (0-7506-4545-8) Buttrwrth-Heinemann.

Clinical Optics. Troy E. Fannin et al. 2nd ed. 1996. LC 96-191. 420p. text 99.00 (0-7506-9670-2) Buttrwrth-Heinemann.

Clinical Optics. A. R. Elkington et al. 3rd ed. 1999. LC 99-20296. (Illus.). pap. 57.95 (0-632-04989-8) Blackwell Sci.

Clinical Optics & Refraction. Ed. by O. J. Lehmann et al. 1998. LC 97-51984. 160p. pap. text 36.50 (0-7506-2188-5) Buttrwrth-Heinemann.

Clinical Optometric Pharmacology & Therapeutics: Clinical Text, Annual New. Bruce Onofrey. 1992. (Illus.). 170p. ring bd. 115.00 (0-397-52133-2) Lppncott W & W.

Clinical Oral Science. Ed. by Malcolm Harris et al. 1998. LC 97-42624. 347p. (0-7236-1059-2, QP146) John Wright GBR. *Dist:* Buttrwrth-Heinemann.

Clinical Orthopaedic Physical Therapy. Janice K. Richardson & Z. Annette Iglarsh. 1993. LC 93-7209. (Illus.). 816p. text 75.00 (0-7216-3257-2) Saunders.

Clinical Orthopaedic Rehabilitation. Ed. by S. Brent Brotzman. 1995. LC 95-42300. (Illus.). 416p. (C). (gr. 13). text 89.95 (0-8151-1034-0, 24183) Mosby Inc.

***Clinical Orthopaedic Rehabilitation.** Steven B. Brotzman. 2nd ed. 2001. (0-323-01186-1) Mosby Inc.

Clinical Orthopedic & Neurology. Talmage. 1999. pap. text 75.00 (0-8385-1533-9, Medical Exam) Appleton & Lange.

Clinical Orthopedic Anesthesia. John E. Tetzlaff. 1995. LC 95-32956. 406p. spiral bd. 74.99 (0-7506-9478-5) Buttrwrth-Heinemann.

Clinical Orthopedic Assessment Guide. Janice Loudon et al. 1998. LC 97-49234. (Illus.). 248p. pap. text 34.00 (0-88011-507-6, BLOU0507) Human Kinetics.

Clinical Orthopedic Examination. Ronald McRae. 4th ed. LC 97-10029. 1998. (0-443-05812-1); 1997. pap. text (0-443-05602-1) Church.

Clinical Orthopedic Tests. Gogia. 1998. (C). pap. text 74.00 (0-12-784592-5) Acad Pr.

Clinical Orthopedics for the Physical Therapist Assistant. Steven G. Lesh. 2000. LC 99-45181. (Illus.). 538p. (C). pap. text 39.95 (0-8036-0449-1) Davis Co.

Clinical Orthoptics. Fiona J. Rowe. 1997. (Illus.). 336p. (Orig.). pap. 89.95 (0-632-04274-5) Blackwell Sci.

Clinical Otology. Gordon B. Hughes & Myles L. Pensak. rev. ed. 1996. (Illus.). 528p. text 135.00 (0-86577-616-4) Thieme Med Pubs.

Clinical Otology & Audiology. G. G. Browning. 2nd ed. 1998. LC 98-20406. (Illus.). 224p. pap. (0-7506-3373-5) E A GBR. *Dist:* OUP.

Clinical Otoscopy: An Introduction to Ear Diseases. Michael Hawke et al. 2nd ed. 1990. (Illus.). 144p. pap. text (0-443-04044-3) Church.

Clinical Outcomes in Home Health Care: A Guide to Performance Measurement & Oryx Implementation. Leonard C. Rogers et al. 1998. LC 98-24895. 352p. ring bd. 159.00 (0-8342-0979-9, S477) Aspen Pub.

Clinical Outline of Oral Pathology: Diagnosis & Treatment. Lewis R. Eversole. 3rd ed. 1992. LC 91-17379. (Illus.). 488p. text 56.00 (0-8121-1425-6) Lppncott W & W.

Clinical Outlines for Health Assessment. June M. Thompson. 1997. LC 97-27471. (Illus.). 168p. (C). (gr. 13). pap. text 12.95 (0-8151-2578-X, 31365) Mosby Inc.

Clinical Overview & Pathogenesis of the Fibromyalgia Syndrome, Myofascial Pain Syndrome, & Other Pain Syndromes. Ed. by I. Jon Russell. 1996. LC 96-7347. (Journal of Musculoskeletal Pain Ser.: Vol. 4, No. 1/2). 254p. (C). 39.95 (1-56024-833-5, Hawrth Medical) Haworth Pr.

Clinical Paediatric Endocrinology. C. Brook. 3rd ed. 1995. (Illus.). 864p. 295.00 (0-632-03632-X) Blackwell Sci.

Clinical Paediatric Endocrinology. C. G. D. Brook & P. C. Hindmarsh. 4th ed. 2000. LC 00-58501. 528p. 350.00 (0-632-05148-5) Blackwell Sci.

Clinical Paediatric Endocrinology: 3rd Serono Symposia Workshop, Verona, September 1999. Ed. by K. Albertsson-Wikland et al. 2000. (Hormone Research Ser.: Vol. 53, Suppl. 1, 2000). iv, 98p. pap. 34.00 (3-8055-7097-X) S Karger.

Clinical Paediatrics. Ed. by E. M. Ross et al. 1997. (Illus.). 420p. (0-7020-1726-4) W B Saunders GBR. *Dist:* Saunders.

Clinical Paediatrics for Postgraduate Examinations. T. Stephenson & H. Wallace. 2nd ed. 1995. (Illus.). 212p. pap. (0-443-05226-3) Church.

Clinical Paediatrics for Postgraduate Examinations: A Guide to Success in the MRCP & DCH Examinations. Terence Stephenson & Hamish Wallace. 1990. 170p. pap. text (0-443-04172-5) Church.

***Clinical Paediatric Endocrinology: 4th Serono Symposia Workshop, Salamaca, Spain, September 2000.** Ed. by K. Albertsson-Wikland et al. 2001. (Hormone Research Ser.: Vol. 55). (Illus.). iv, 46p. pap., suppl. ed. 25.25 (3-8055-7238-7) S Karger.

Clinical Parasitology: A Practical Approach. Elizabeth A. Zeibig. Ed. by Selma Kaszczuk. 1997. LC 96-41184. (Illus.). 304p. pap. text 37.00 (0-7216-5187-9) Saunders.

Clinical Pathology. Alan Remaley et al. 1997. (0-89189-315-6) Am Soc Clinical.

Clinical Pathology in the Elderly: A Textbook of Laboratory Interpretations. Hazel Rochman. 1988. (Illus.). xiv, 222p. 77.50 (3-8055-4694-7) S Karger.

Clinical Pathology of Fibro-Osteo-Cemental Lesions in the Cranio-Facial & Jaw Bones. M. Makek. 1983. (Illus.). x, 230p. 138.50 (3-8055-3704-2) S Karger.

Clinical Pathology of Pancreatic Disorders. Ed. by John A. Lott. 1997. LC 97-14956. (Pathology & Laboratory Medicine Ser.: Vol. 2). (Illus.). 232p. 135.00 (0-89603-475-5) Humana.

Clinical Paths: Tools for Outcomes Management. Ed. by Patrice L. Spath. 1994. LC 94-13825. 265p. pap. 65.00 (1-55648-120-9, 027101) AHPI.

Clinical Paths in Medical-Surgical Nursing. Carole Birdsall & Sandra Sperry. 1996. LC 96-7476. (Illus.). 448p. (C). (gr. 13). text 59.95 (0-8151-0484-7, 27084) Mosby Inc.

Clinical Pathways for Ambulatory Care Case Management. Ed. by Rufus Howe. 1996. LC 95-53083. 400p. ring bd. 189.00 (0-8342-0780-X) Aspen Pub.

Clinical Pathways for Collaborative Practice. Donna D. Ignatavicius & Kathy A. Hausman. 1995. (Illus.). 378p. pap. text 40.95 (0-7216-4741-3) Saunders.

Clinical Pathways for Medical Rehabilitation. Aspen Reference Group Staff. 1998. LC 98-21821. ring bd. 179.00 (0-8342-1080-0, S519) Aspen Pub.

Clinical Pathways for Multidisciplinary Home Care Teams. Ed. by Barbara Stover Gingerich & Deborah Anne Ondeck. 2nd ed. 2000. LC 00-51061. (Illus.). 288p. ring bd. 249.00 incl. cd-rom (0-8342-1915-8) Aspen Pub.

Clinical Pathways in Glaucoma. Thomas J. Zimmerman & Karanjit Kooner. 2001. LC 00-55190. (Illus.). 448p. 99.00 (0-86577-919-8) Thieme Med Pubs.

Clinical Pathways in Neuro-Ophthalmology: An Evidence Based Approach. Andrew G. Lee & Paul W. Brazis. 1998. LC 97-51525. 398p. 79.00 (0-86577-755-1) Thieme Med Pubs.

Clinical Pathways in Nursing: A Guide to Managing Care from Hospital to Home. Poirrier & Oberleitner. 1998. LC 98-38636. 312p. pap. 39.95 (0-87434-930-3) Springhouse Corp.

Clinical Pearls, 1990: In Nutrition & Preventive Medicines. Kirkham R. Hamilton. 1991. 453p. 34.95 (0-9628840-0-6) ITServices.

Clinical Pearls, 1991: In Nutrition & Preventive Medicine. Kirkham R. Hamilton. Ed. by Joan Howell. 1992. 543p. spiral bd. 98.00 (0-9628840-2-2); 471p. spiral bd. 29.95 (0-9628840-1-4) ITServices.

Clinical Pearls, 1992: In Nutrition & Preventive Medicine. Kirkham R. Hamilton. Ed. by Joan Howell. 1993. 573p. 59.95 (0-9628840-4-9) ITServices.

Clinical Pediatric Anesthesia. J. Michael Badgwell & Steven C. Hall. 1997. LC 97-18627. (Illus.). 512p. text 129.00 (0-397-51476-X) Lppncott W & W.

Clinical Pediatric Arrhythmias. Paul C. Gillette & Arthur Garson. Ed. by Richard Zorab. 2nd ed. 1999. LC 98-40585. (Illus.). 300p. text (0-7216-6629-9) Saunders.

Clinical Pediatric Dermatology: A Textbook of Skin Disorders of Childhood & Adolescence. Sidney Hurwitz. (Illus.). 2nd ed. 1993. LC 92-20398. 704p. text 135.00 (0-7216-1515-5); Vol. 181. 1981. 656p. text 138.00 (0-7216-4872-X) Saunders.

Clinical Pediatric Endocrinology. Joel A. Kaplan. 2nd ed. 1989. (Illus.). 480p. text 99.00 (0-7216-5283-2) Saunders.

Clinical Pediatric Endocrinology: Serono Symposia Workshop, Arles, France, September 8-9, 1997. Ed. by Kerstin Albertsson-Wikland et al. 1998. (Hormone Research Ser.: Vol. 49, Supplement 2, 1998). (Illus.). iv, 82p. 37.50 (*3-8055-6700-6*) S Karger.

Clinical Pediatric Gastroenterology. Steven M. Altschuler & Christopher A. Liacouras. 1998. LC 97-47601. (Illus.). 704p. (C). text (*0-443-05542-4*) Church.

Clinical Pediatric Nephrology. Ed. by Kanwal K. Kher & Sudesh P. Makker. 1990. 416p. text 85.00 (*0-07-034543-0*) McGraw-Hill Educ Grp.

Clinical Pediatric Neurology: A Signs & Symptoms Approach. Gerald M. Fenichel. Ed. by Bill Schmitt. 3rd ed. 1996. 480p. text 72.00 (*0-7216-6852-6*) Saunders.

Clinical Pediatric Optometry. Leonard J. Press & Bruce D. Moore. 1992. (Illus.). 400p. text 84.99 (*0-7506-9080-1*) Buttrwrth-Heinemann.

Clinical Pediatric Orthopedics: The Art of Diagnosis & Principles Management. Mihran O. Tachdjian. 1996. LC 96-8406. 1248p. (C). pap. text 139.00 (*0-8385-1106-6*, A1106-2, Apple Lange Med) McGraw.

Clinical Pediatric Urology Panayotis P. Kelalis. 3rd ed. 1992. (C). text 320.00 (*0-7216-3233-5*) Harcourt.

*__Clinical Pediatric Urology.__ King et al. 4th ed. 2001. (Illus.). 700p. (*1-901865-63-0*) Isis Med GBR. *Dist:* Bks Intl VA.

Clinical Pediatrics, Vols. 1-4. N. J. Shaw et al. 1999. (Illus.). audio compact disk (*0-412-82170-2*) E A GBR. *Dist:* OUP.

Clinical Performance in Nursing Examination Study Guide. 1997. (Illus.). 205p. (Orig.). pap. text, stu. ed. (*1-889403-08-3*) Regnts College.

Clinical Periodontology. Carranza. 8th ed. 1998. text 14.29 (*0-8089-2156-8*, Grune & Strat) Harcrt Hlth Sci Grp.

Clinical Periodontology. Fermin A. Carranza, Jr. et al. 8th ed. 1995. (Illus.). 816p. text 85.00 (*0-7216-6728-7*) Saunders.

Clinical Periodontology for the Dental Hygienist. Fermin A. Carranza, Jr. & Dorothy A. Perry. 1986. (Illus.). 301p. pap. text 39.95 (*0-7216-1352-7*) Saunders.

Clinical Personality Assessment: Practical Approaches. Ed. by James Neal Butcher. 1995. LC 94-12405. (Illus.). 576p. (C). text 67.95 (*0-19-508569-8*) OUP.

Clinical Perspectives in the Management of Down Syndrome. Ed. by D. C. Van Dyke et al. 1989. (Disorders of Human Learning, Behavior, & Communication Ser.). (Illus.). 246p. 103.00 (*0-387-96987-X*, 2748) Spr-Verlag.

Clinical Perspectives on a New Gestodene Oral Contraceptive Containing 20jg of Ethinylestradiol. Ed. by S. O. Skouby. 1997. LC 97-12869. (Illus.). 80p. lib. bdg. 35.95 (*1-85070-786-3*, Parthenon Pbng) CRC Pr.

Clinical Perspectives on Multiple Personality Disorder. Ed. by Richard P. Kluft & Catherine G. Fine. 1993. LC 92-48949. 398p. text 54.00 (*0-88048-365-2*, 8365) Am Psychiatric.

Clinical Perspectives on Psychotherapy Supervision. Ed. by Stanley E. Greben & Ronald Ruskin. 1994. 273p. text 38.00 (*0-88048-552-3*, 8552) Am Psychiatric.

Clinical Perspectives on the Supervision of Psychoanalysis & Psychotherapy. L. Caligor et al. 1984. (Critical Issues in Psychiatry Ser.). (Illus.). 302p. (C). text 75.00 (*0-306-41403-1*, Kluwer Plenum) Kluwer Academic.

Clinical Pet on Oncology: Proceedings of the Second International Symposium. T. Matsuzawa. 1994. 452p. text 109.00 (*981-02-1825-7*) World Scientific Pub.

Clinical Pharmacokinetics. Intro. by John E. Murphy. 1993. (Illus.). 383p. (Orig.). pap. 48.00 (*1-879907-31-3*) Am Soc Hlth-Syst.

Clinical Pharmacokinetics: A Modern Approach to Individualized Drug Therapy, 2. Joseph Wartak. 1983. LC 82-18577. (Clinical Pharmacology & Therapeutics Ser.: Vol. 2). 216p. 68.50 (*0-275-91417-8*, C1417, Praeger Pubs) Greenwood.

Clinical Pharmacokinetics: A Short Introduction. D. R. Krishna & U. Klotz. 1990. (Illus.). 149p. 45.95 (*0-387-52458-4*) Spr-Verlag.

Clinical Pharmacokinetics: Concepts & Applications. Malcolm Rowland & Thomas N. Tozer. 3rd ed. 1995. LC 94-26305. (Illus.). 608p. 55.95 (*0-683-07404-0*) Lppncott W & W.

Clinical Pharmacokinetics: The MCQ Approach. Stephen H. Curry. 1988. (Telford Press Ser.). (Illus.). 184p. (C). lib. bdg. 59.95 (*0-936923-03-2*); lib. bdg. 39.95 (*0-936923-02-4*) Telford Pr.

Clinical Pharmacokinetics of Sulfonamides & Their Metabolites. T. B. Vree & Y. A. Heckster. 1987. (Antibiotics & Chemotherapy Ser.: Vol. 37). (Illus.). viii, 216p. 153.25 (*3-8055-4511-8*) S Karger.

Clinical Pharmacology. Ed. by Cesare Sirtori et al. 2001. (Clinical Medicine Ser.). (Illus.). 700p. pap. 79.95 (*0-07-709522-7*) McGraw-Hill Prof.

Clinical Pharmacology. Ed. by Kenneth L. Melmon et al. 3rd ed. 1991. (*0-08-040305-0*); pap. (*0-08-040644-0*) PPI GBR. *Dist:* McGraw.

Clinical Pharmacology. Paul Turner et al. 5th ed. 1986. LC 85-24295. (Churchill Livingstone Medical Text Ser.). (Illus.). 320p. text (*0-443-03237-8*) Church.

Clinical Pharmacology. D. R. Laurence et al. 8th ed. 1998. LC 96-26060. x, 710p. (C). pap. text (*0-443-04990-4*) Church.

Clinical Pharmacology, No. 1. Shepherd. 1991. (*0-933755-24-4*) Mosby Inc.

Clinical Pharmacology: Flavonoids & Vascular Wall, Proceedings of the Symposia Angiologica Santoriana, 4th International Symposium, Fribourg-Nyon, 1972. Symposia Angiologica Santoriana Staff. Ed. by M. Comel & L. Laszt. 1973. (Illus.). 55.75 (*3-8055-1587-1*) S Karger.

Clinical Pharmacology: The European Challenge. 1991. (WHO Regional Publications: No. 39). viii, 84p. pap. text 14.85 (*92-890-1302-8*, 1310039) World Health.

Clinical Pharmacology & Nursing. Harold L. Baer & Bradley R. Williams. 3rd ed. 1995. LC 95-21515. (Illus.). 1408p. 54.95 incl. disk (*0-87434-772-6*) Springhouse Corp.

Clinical Pharmacology & Nursing Management. Roberta T. Spencer et al. 2nd ed. 1986. LC 64-4453. (Illus.). 1168p. stu. ed. 14.95 (*0-397-54550-9*, Lippnctt) Lppncott W & W.

Clinical Pharmacology & Nursing Management. Laurel Eisenhauer et al. 5th ed. 1997. LC 97-8454. 1,216p. text 58.95 (*0-397-55329-3*) Lppncott W & W.

Clinical Pharmacology & Therapeutics. Eric Toby Herfindal et al. 5th ed. 1992. (Illus.). 1648p. stu. ed. 95.00 (*0-683-03966-0*) Lppncott W & W.

Clinical Pharmacology Course. Competence Assurance Systems Staff. 1985. (Illus.). pap. text 35.00 (*0-89147-071-9*) CAS.

Clinical Pharmacology for Nurses. John R. Trounce. 14th ed. 1993. LC 93-323. 336p. pap. (*0-443-04888-6*) Church.

Clinical Pharmacology for Nurses. Trounce. 15th ed. 1997. pap. text 24.95 (*0-443-05457-6*) Saunders.

Clinical Pharmacology for Nurses. J. R. Trounce. 16th ed. 2000. LC 99-29503. (Illus.). 382p. (*0-443-06244-7*) Church.

Clinical Pharmacology in Dental Practice. Clark et al. 4th ed. 1987. (Illus.). 624p. (C). (gr. 13). pap. text 43.95 (*0-8016-2260-3*, 02260) Mosby Inc.

Clinical Pharmacology in Dentistry. R. A. Cawson & R. G. Spector. 5th ed. 1989. (Illus.). 250p. pap. text (*0-443-04043-5*) Church.

Clinical Pharmacology in Elderly Subjects: Reference Ranges & Biological Variations after Repeated Measurements. H. P. Breuel. 1995. (Illus.). 270p. pap. 145.00 (*3-540-59495-7*) Spr-Verlag.

Clinical Pharmacology in Psychiatry. Ed. by S. G. Dahl & L. F. Gram. 1989. (Psychopharmacology Ser.: Vol. 7). (Illus.). 329p. 66.00 (*0-387-50770-1*, 3077) Spr-Verlag.

Clinical Pharmacology in Psychiatry: Strategies in Psychotropic Drug Development. Ed. by S. G. Dahl et al. 1993. (Psychopharmacology Ser.: Vol. 10). (Illus.). 268p. 132.00 (*0-387-56329-6*) Spr-Verlag.

Clinical Pharmacology in the Elderly. Ed. by Cameron G. Swift. 1987. (Clinical Pharmacology Ser.: Vol. 8). (Illus.). 680p. text 250.00 (*0-8247-7628-3*) Dekker.

Clinical Pharmacology Made Incrediby Easy. Springhouse Publishing Company Staff. 2001. LC 00-41972. (Made Incredibly Easy Ser.). (Illus.). vi, 376p. pap. 32.95 (*1-58255-042-5*) Springhouse Corp.

Clinical Pharmacology Made Ridiculously Simple. James Olson. 1998. (Illus.). 162p. (C). pap. text 19.95 (*0-940780-17-8*) MedMaster.

*__Clinical Pharmacology Made Ridiculously Simple.__ James Olson. 2nd rev. ed. 2001. (Illus.). 164p. pap. 19.95 (*0-940780-50-X*) MedMaster.

Clinical Pharmacology of Antihypertensive Drugs. Ed. by A. E. Doyle. 1984. (Handbooks of Hypertension: Vol. 5). 418p. 230.50 (*0-444-90354-2*) Elsevier.

Clinical Pharmacology of Cerebral Ischemia. Ed. by Gert J. Ter Horst & Jakob Korf. 1996. LC 96-43894. (Contemporary Neuroscience Ser.). (Illus.). 320p. 145.00 (*0-89603-378-3*) Humana.

Clinical Pharmacology of Drug Dependence. P. F. Mannaioni. 1984. 282p. pap. text (*1-57235-060-1*) Piccin Nuova.

Clinical Pharmacology of Drug Interactions. R. Rondanelli. 1988. 864p. text (*1-57235-032-6*) Piccin Nuova.

Clinical Pharmacology of Learning & Memory. Walter B. Essman. 1983. LC 82-3321. (Illus.). 202p. text 39.50 (*0-88331-119-4*) R B Luce.

Clinical Pharmacology of Local Anesthetics. John E. Tetzlaff. 1999. LC 99-37383. 272p. pap. text 50.00 (*0-7506-9797-0*) Buttrwrth-Heinemann.

Clinical Pharmacology of Psychotherapeutic Drugs. Ed. by Leo E. Holister & John Csernansky. 3rd ed. 1989. (Illus.). 204p. text (*0-443-08670-2*) Church.

Clinical Pharmacology of Serotonin: Proceedings of the Symposium, Satellite, Helsinki, July, 1975. Clinical Pharmacology of Serotonin Symposium Staff. Ed. by F. Sicuteri & E. Schoenbaum. 1976. (Monographs in Neural Sciences: Vol. 3). (Illus.). 180p. 55.75 (*3-8055-2328-9*) S Karger.

Clinical Pharmacology of Sport & Exercise: Proceedings of the Esteve Foundation Symposium VII, Sitges, Spain, 2-5 October 1996. Antonio Esteve Fundacion et al. 1997. LC 97-11696. (International Congress Ser.). 324p. 152.50 (*0-444-82454-5*) Elsevier.

Clinical Pharmacology, Scope, Organization, Training: Proceedings of the WHO Scientific Group, Geneva, 1969. WHO Staff. 1970. (Technical Reports: No. 446). pap. text 3.00 (*92-4-120446-X*, 1100446) World Health.

Clinical Pharmacy & Therapeutics. Roger Walker & Clive Edwards. 2nd ed. 1998. LC 98-15065. (C). text (*0-443-05816-4*) Church.

Clinical Phonetics. Lawrence D. Shriberg & Ray Kent. 2nd ed. 1994. LC 81-15988. 512p. (C). pap. 86.67 (*0-02-410213-X*, Macmillan Coll) P-H.

Clinical Phonetics & Linguistics. Ed. by Wolfram Ziegler & Karin Deger. 1998. 320p. 65.00 (*1-56593-919-0*, 1820) Singular Publishing.

Clinical Phonology: Assesment & Treatment of Articulation Disorders in Children & Adults. Edward S. Klein. 1995. (Illus.). 408p. (Orig.). pap. text 62.95 (*1-56593-602-7*, 1236) Thomson Learn.

Clinical Photography in Plastic Surgery. Gerald D. Nelson & John L. Krause. 1987. (Illus.). 176p. 79.95 (*0-316-60315-5*, Little Brwn Med Div) Lppncott W & W.

Clinical Photomedicine. Lim & Nicholas A. Soter. 1993. (Basic & Clinical Dermatology Ser.: Vol. 6). (Illus.). 428p. text 185.00 (*0-8247-8862-1*) Dekker.

Clinical Physiology in Obstetrics. Geoffrey Chamberlain & Fiona Broughton-Pipkin. 3rd ed. 1998. LC 97-42723. (Illus.). 510p. 208.95 (*0-86542-948-0*) Blackwell Sci.

Clinical Physiology Made Ridiculously Simple. Stephen Goldberg. 1999. 160p. (Orig.). (C). pap. text 19.95 (*0-940780-21-6*) MedMaster.

Clinical Physiology of Acid-Base & Electrolyte Disorders. Burton D. Rose. 4th ed. 1993. LC 93-20532. (Illus.). 915p. pap. 45.00 (*0-07-053663-5*) McGraw-Hill Educ Grp.

Clinical Physiology of Acid-Base & Electrolyte Disorders. Bud Rose et al. 5th ed. 2000. LC 2001-265857. (Illus.). 992p. pap. 44.95 (*0-07-134682-1*) McGraw-Hill Prof.

Clinical Physiology of Sleep. Ed. by Ralph Lydic & Julian F. Biebuyck. 1988. (Clinical Physiology Ser.). (Illus.). 254p. text 49.00 (*0-19-520780-7*) OUP.

Clinical Policies & Procedures for Home Health Care Organizations. Barbara Stover Gingerich & Deborah Anne Ondeck. 1997. LC 97-1073. ring bd. 169.00 (*0-8342-0939-X*, 5458) Aspen Pub.

Clinical Postreproductive Gynecology. Samir Hajj & Wendy Evans. 1993. (Illus.). 1135p. (C). pap. text 95.00 (*0-8385-8038-6*, A8038-0, Apple Lange Med) McGraw.

Clinical Practice & Cost Containment: A Physician's Perspective. Henry A. Shenkin. 1985. LC 85-25589. 160p. 57.95 (*0-275-92045-3*, C2045, Praeger Pubs) Greenwood.

*__Clinical Practice Cardiac Anesthesia.__ Troiano. 2002. LC 2001-55836. text (*0-323-00874-7*) EHS.

Clinical Practice Examination. Howard S. Barrows et al. 1992. (Illus.). 192p. (Orig.). (C). pap. 20.95 (*0-931369-24-X*) Southern IL Univ Sch.

Clinical Practice Gastroenterology Brandt. 1998. LC 98-22058. (Illus.). xxv, 1647p. (C). text (*0-443-06520-9*) Church.

Clinical Practice Guideline on Depression in Primary Care, Set. 1994. lib. bdg. 499.75 (*0-8490-9058-X*) Gordon Pr.

Clinical Practice Guidelines. Warren Todd et al. 48p. pap. text (*0-86471-042-9*) Adis Intl NZL. *Dist:* Lppncott W & W.

Clinical Practice Guidelines. Bonnie Wesorick & Diane Hanson. 2000. LC 00-134114. 400p. (C). spiral bd. 50.00 (*0-9648264-8-8*) Pract Field.

Clinical Practice Guidelines: Directions for a New Program. Institute of Medicine Staff. Ed. by Marilyn J. Field & Kathleen N. Lohr. 1990. 168p. (C). pap. text 30.00 (*0-309-04346-8*) Natl Acad Pr.

Clinical Practice Guidelines: Examination & Intervention for Rehabilitation. Carol Schunk & Kelly Reed. 1995. LC 00-26641. 493p. spiral bd. 99.00 (*0-8342-1774-0*) PRO-ED.

Clinical Practice Guidelines Directory. 1998. 200p. pap. 179.95 (*0-89970-955-9*) AMA.

Clinical Practice Guidelines Directory 2000. Naomi Kuznets. 2000. 320p. pap. 179.95 (*1-57947-008-4*) AMA.

Clinical Practice Guidelines of the American Academy of Pediatrics: A Compendium of Evidence-Based Research for Pediatric Practice. 3rd ed. 2000. 600p. pap. 49.95 (*1-58110-063-9*) Am Acad Pediat.

Clinical Practice Improvement Methodology: Implementation & Evaluation. Susan D. Horn. 1997. LC 98-142462. (Medical Outcomes & Practice Guidelines Library). xviii, 363 p. (*1-57987-026-0*) Faulkner & Gray.

Clinical Practice in Adoption. R. C. Winkler et al. 1988. (General Psychology Ser.). 160p. text 30.00 (*0-08-034222-1*); pap. text 15.95 (*0-08-034221-3*) Elsevier (Pergamon Pr).

Clinical Practice in Correctional Medicine. Michael Puisis. 1998. LC 98-34369. (Illus.). 450p. (C). (gr. 13). text 86.00 (*0-8151-2704-9*, 31339) Mosby Inc.

Clinical Practice in Respiratory Care. James B. Fink & Gerald E. Hunt. 1998. LC 98-21741. (Illus.). 516p. text 55.00 (*0-397-55093-6*) Lppncott W & W.

*__Clinical Practice in Sexually Transmissable Infections: An Atlas & Text.__ A. McMillan & F. Judson. 2001. (Illus.). 508p. (*0-7020-2538-0*) W B Saunders GBR. *Dist:* Saunders.

Clinical Practice Management for Speech-Language Pathologists. Becky Sutherland Cornett. 1995. LC 99-21827. 266p. pap. 41.00 (*0-8342-1094-0*, 21094) PRO-ED.

Clinical Practice of Critical Care Neurology. Ed. by Eelco F. M. Wijdicks. 1997. LC 97-9850. (Illus.). 432p. text 125.00 (*0-316-94759-8*) Lppncott W & W.

Clinical Practice of Emergency Medicine. Ann L. Harwood-Nuss et al. 3rd ed. 2000. 1,872p. text 199.00 (*0-7817-1680-2*) Lppncott W & W.

Clinical Practice of Gastroenterology Lawrence J. Brandt & Fredric Daum. 1999. LC 98-22058. (Illus.). xxv, 1647, 84 p. (*0-443-06522-5*) Church.

Clinical Practice of Hypnotherapy. M. Erik Wright & Beatrice A. Wright. 1987. LC 86-18473. (Clinical & Experimental Hypnosis Ser.). 292p. 40.00 (*0-89862-337-5*, 2337) Guilford Pubns.

Clinical Practice of Nephrology, Vol. 3. Harry Preuss. 1989. 69.00 (*0-938607-26-X*) Field & Wood Inc Medical.

Clinical Practice of Neurological & Neuroscience Nursing. Joanne V. Hickey. 4th ed. 1996. LC 96-24963. (Illus.). 768p. text 73.00 (*0-397-55319-6*) Lppncott W & W.

Clinical Practice of Nuclear Medicine. Ed. by Andrew Taylor, Jr. & Frederick L. Datz. 1991. (Illus.). 471p. text (*0-443-08384-3*) Church.

Clinical Practice of Pediatric Anesthesia. Ed. by W. S. Schecter & R. S. Holzman. 1998. (Illus.). 600p. pap. (*0-443-07675-8*) Church.

Clinical Practice of Psychology: A Practical Guide for Mental Health Professionals. Ed. by C. Eugene Walker. 1981. (General Psychology Ser.). 96.00 (*0-08-025591-4*); pap. 40.00 (*0-08-025590-6*) Elsevier (Pergamon Pr).

Clinical Practice of the Dental Hygienist. Esther M. Wilkins. 7th ed. 1994. LC 93-39743. (Illus.). 893p. 56.00 (*0-683-09078-X*); 8th ed. 1999. 1,032p. 84.50 (*0-7817-2178-4*) Lppncott W & W.

Clinical Practice of Transfusion Medicine. Ed. by Lawrence D. Petz et al. 3rd ed. 1995. LC 95-32421. 1115p. text (*0-443-08981-7*) Church.

Clinical Practice with Caregivers of Dementia Patients. Mary Kaplan. 1996. LC 96-22382. 200p. 69.95 (*1-56032-471-6*); pap. 29.95 (*1-56032-472-4*) Taylor & Francis.

Clinical Practice with Families: Supporting Creativity & Competence. M. A. Rothery & George Enns. 2000. LC 00-40783. xvi, 253p. pap. 29.95 (*0-7890-1085-2*) Haworth Pr.

Clinical Practice with Families: Supporting Creativity & Competence. Ed. by Michael Rothery & George Enns. 2000. LC 00-40783. xvi, 253p. lib. bdg. 69.95 (*0-7890-1084-4*) Haworth Pr.

Clinical Practice with Individuals. Mark A. Mattaini. 1996. LC 96-42938. (Illus.). 360p. (Orig.). (C). pap. text 28.95 (*0-87101-270-7*) Natl Assn Soc Wkrs.

Clinical Practitioners Pocket Guide to Respiratory Care. Dana Oakes. 4th ed. 1996. (Illus.). 320p. ring bd. 19.95 (*0-932887-12-0*) Health Ed Pubns.

Clinical Pre-Computer Proforma for the International Computer Database for Radiation Exposure Case Histories. A. E. Baranov et al. 1994. LC 94-211290. (Illus.). 128p. 62.95 (*0-387-57596-0*) Spr-Verlag.

Clinical Prediction of Violent Behavior. John Monahan. 1995. LC 95-42845. 152p. pap. 30.00 (*1-56821-489-8*) Aronson.

Clinical Preventive Medicine. Richard N. Matzen. 1993. (Illus.). 1263p. (C). (gr. 13). text 105.00 (*0-8016-3176-9*, 03176) Mosby Inc.

Clinical Preventive Medicine: Health Promotion & Disease Prevention. T. Warner Hudson. 1988. 768p. 56.95 (*0-316-37909-3*, Little Brwn Med Div) Lppncott W & W.

Clinical Preventive Services. 1995. (Medical Ser.). lib. bdg. 250.99 (*0-8490-7576-9*) Gordon Pr.

Clinical Problem Solving in Dentistry. E. W. Odell. 2000. LC 99-48086. 193p. text (*0-443-05631-5*) Church.

Clinical Problems in Gastroenterology. Johnathan M. Rhodes. 1995. 280p. (C). (gr. 13). pap. text 47.95 (*0-8151-7334-2*, 23042) Mosby Inc.

Clinical Problems in Gastroenterology. Jonathan M. Rhodes & Her Hsin Tsai. 1995. 280p. pap. (*84-8174-164-7*) Mosby-Doyma Libros ESP. *Dist:* Mosby Inc.

Clinical Problems in General Medicine & Surgery: A Problem-Solving Approach to Medicine & Surgery. Peter Devitt & Juliet Barker. 1993. (Illus.). 533p. text (*0-7295-1409-9*) Bailliere Tindall.

Clinical Problems in Obstetric Anaesthesia. Ed. by G. Lyons & I. F. Russell. 1997. (Illus.). 304p. (*0-412-71600-3*) E A GBR. *Dist:* OUP.

Clinical Problems in Oncology. Carol S. Portlock. 1986. 10.95 (*0-316-71427-5*, Little Brwn Med Div) Lppncott W & W.

Clinical Problems In Pediatric & Adolescent Gynecology. Alvin Goldfarb. 1996. (Illus.). 144p. (gr. 13). (*0-412-07201-7*) E A GBR. *Dist:* OUP.

Clinical Problems in Pediatric & Adolescent Gynecology, Vol. II. Alvin Goldfarb. rev. ed. 1998. 176p. pap. 54.95 (*0-412-13011-4*) Thomson Learn.

Clinical Problems in Sexually Transmitted Diseases. D. Taylor-Robinson. 1985. LC 85-4924. (New Perspectives in Clinical Microbiology Ser.). text 247.50 (*0-89838-720-5*) Kluwer Academic.

Clinical Problems in Vascular Surgery. Ed. by Robert B. Galland & C. A. C. Clyne. 1994. (Illus.). 280p. (*0-340-56437-7*) E A GBR. *Dist:* OUP.

Clinical Problems, Injuries & Complications of Gynecologic & Obstetric Surgery. Ed. by David H. Nichols & John O. L. Delancey. rev. ed. 1995. LC 94-44911. 400p. text 129.00 (*0-683-06497-5*) Lppncott W & W.

Clinical Procedures for Medical Assistants. Sharron M. Zakus. 3rd ed. 1995. (Illus.). 736p. (C). (gr. 13). pap. text 42.00 (*0-8016-6983-9*, 27775) Mosby Inc.

Clinical Procedures for Medical Assistants. Kathy Bonewit-West. (Illus.). 4th ed. 1995. tchr. ed. (*0-7216-5414-2*); 4th ed. 1995. 708p. text, stu. ed. 48.00 (*0-7216-6104-1*); 4th ed. 1995. pap. text, stu. ed. 17.95 (*0-7216-5337-5*); 5th ed. LC 99-48210. 735p. text (*0-7216-8406-8*) Saunders.

*__Clinical Procedures for Medical Assistants.__ Kathy Bonewit-West. 5th ed. 2000. (Illus.). 735p. 66.95 (*0-7216-9202-8*) Saunders.

*__Clinical Procedures for Medical Assistants: ExaMaster.__ Kathy Bonewit-West. 5th ed. 2000. 500.00 (*0-7216-8408-4*) Saunders.

Clinical Procedures for Medical Assisting. Mary A. Frew & David R. Frew. 1990. LC 90-2929. (Illus.). 535p. pap. 33.95 (*0-8036-3851-5*) Davis Co.

Clinical Procedures for Medical Assisting: A Patient-Centered Approach. 1999. (Illus.). (gr. 6-12). stu. ed., wbk. ed. 17.44 (*0-02-802435-4*) Glencoe.

Clinical Procedures for Ocular Examination. Nancy B. Carlson et al. 2nd ed. 1996. LC 95-49332. 493p. (C). pap. 44.95 (*0-8385-1319-0*, A1319-1) McGraw-Hill Prof.

Clinical Procedures for the Medical Assistant. Kathy Bonewit-West. 4th ed. 1995. LC 94-10991. (Illus.). 708p. text 36.50 (*0-7216-5413-4*) Saunders.

Clinical Procedures for Third Molar Surgery. Karl Koerner. 1986. 214p. 49.95 (*0-87814-311-4*, D4249) PennWell Corp.

Clinical Procedures in Anesthesia & Intensive Care. Jonathan L. Benumof. 1992. (Illus.). 992p. text 175.00 (*0-397-50950-2*) Lppncott W & W.

Clinical Procedures in Emergency Medicine. James R. Roberts & Jerrie R. Hedges. Ed. by Judy Fletcher. 3rd ed. 1997. LC 96-37054. (Illus.). 1184p. text 150.00 (*0-7216-6055-X*) Saunders.

Clinical Procedures in Optometry. J. Boyd Eskridge et al. 1991. (Illus.). 808p. text 139.00 (*0-397-50984-7*) Lppncott W & W.

Clinical Procedures in Primary Eye Care. David B. Elliott et al. 1997. LC 97-25703. 240p. pap. text 55.00 (*0-7506-3213-5*) Buttrwrth-Heinemann.

Clinical Procedures in Therapeutic Exercise. Patricia Sullivan & Prudence Markos. 2nd ed. 1996. LC 95-24975. 288p. (C). pap. 47.00 (*0-8385-1339-5*, 1339-9) P-H.

Clinical Process One Outcomes Measurement Directory. 1998. 200p. pap. 149.95 (*0-89970-954-0*) AMA.

Clinical Process Redesign: A Facilitator's Guide. Steven L. Strongwater & Vincent P. Pelote. 1996. LC 96-20523. spiral bd. 61.00 (*0-8342-0857-1*, 20857) Aspen Pub.

Clinical Processes. 1983. (Medical Ser.). (Illus.). 144p. pap. text 12.95 (*0-935920-08-0*, Ntl Pubs Blck) P-H.

Clinical Processes for Medical Assisting. 3rd ed. 1993. LC 92-48262. (Regents - Prentice-Hall Medical Assistant Kit Ser.). 240p. pap. 28.40 (*0-13-722885-6*) P-H.

Clinical Progress in Nutrition Research. Ed. by A. Sitges-Serra et al. 1988. (Illus.). viii, 282p. 101.75 (*3-8055-4683-1*) S Karger.

Clinical Protocols in Obstetrics & Gynecology: The "TAN" Book. John E. Turrentine & Martin Aviles. 2000. LC 99-40821. (Illus.). 220p. 46.95 (*1-85070-308-6*, Parthenon Pbng) CRC Pr.

Clinical Proton Dosimetry. International Commission on Radiation Units and Measurements Staff. 1998. LC 97-52065. (ICRU Report Ser.: Vol. 59). 50.00 (*0-913394-58-0*) Intl Comm Rad Meas.

Clinical Psychiatry. Emil Kraepelin. 1981. LC 80-25289. (History of Psychology Ser.). 624p. 75.00 (*0-8201-1352-2*) Schol Facsimiles.

Clinical Psychiatry. Howard S. Sudak. 1985. 512p. 55.00 (*0-87527-333-5*) Green.

Clinical Psychiatry for Medical Students. Alan Stoudemire. 3rd ed. 1998. LC 98-12186. 864p. pap. text 41.95 (*0-397-58460-1*) Lppncott W & W.

Clinical Psychoanalysis. Ed. by Shelly Orgel & Bernard D. Fine. 1979. LC 79-51910. (Downstate Psychoanalytic Institute Twenty-Fifth Anniversary Ser.: Vol. III). 360p. 60.00 (*0-87668-368-5*) Aronson.

Clinical Psychologist. Jack Rudman. 1994. (Career Examination Ser.: C-149). pap. 34.95 (*0-8373-0149-1*) Nat Learn.

Clinical Psychologist Intern. Jack Rudman. 1994. (Career Examination Ser.: C-1196). pap. 29.95 (*0-8373-1196-9*) Nat Learn.

Clinical Psychologist's Handbook of Epilepsy: Assessment & Management. Christine Cull & Laura H. Goldstein. 1997. LC 96-52980. (Illus.). 248p. (C). 84.95 (*0-415-13050-6*); pap. 27.95 (*0-415-13051-4*) Routledge.

Clinical Psychology. Kendall. text (*0-471-13740-5*) Wiley.

Clinical Psychology. Dennis P. Saccuzzo. 1984. LC 83-15800. (C). text 92.00 (*0-205-08075-8*, H80757) Allyn.

Clinical Psychology. E. Jerry Phares. 4th ed. 1992. 640p. (C). text 45.00 (*0-534-16830-2*) Brooks-Cole.

Clinical Psychology: Concepts, Methods & Professions. E. Jerry Phares. 3rd ed. 1988. 596p. (C). mass mkt. 42.50 (*0-534-10762-1*) Brooks-Cole.

Clinical Psychology: Historical & Research Foundations. C. E. Walker. 1991. (Applied Clinical Psychology Ser.). (Illus.). 552p. (C). 90.00 (*0-306-43757-0*, Plenum Trade) Perseus Pubng.

Clinical Psychology: Research & Developments. Ed. by Helen Dent. 1987. 368p. lib. bdg. (*0-7099-4544-2*) C Helm GBR. *Dist:* Routldge.

Clinical Psychology: Scientific & Professional Dimensions. Philip C. Kendall & Julian D. Norton-Ford. 1982. LC 81-16035. 699p. (C). 89.95 (*0-471-04350-8*) Wiley.

Clinical Psychology: Theory & Practice. R. M. Verma. 1985. xii, 212p. (*81-208-0025-7*) Motilal Bnarsidass IND. *Dist:* S Asia.

Clinical Psychology & Medicine: A Behavioral Perspective. Ed. by Chris J. Main et al. 1981. LC 81-19978. 384p. 65.00 (*0-306-40900-3*, Plenum Trade) Perseus Pubng.

Clinical Psychology Handbook. Ed. by Michel Hersen et al. 1983. (General Psychology Ser.: No. 120). 864p. 150.00 (*0-08-028058-7*, Pergamon Pr) Elsevier.

Clinical Psychology Handbook. Ed. by M. Hersen et al. 2nd ed. 1991. (General Psychology Ser.). 896p. (*0-08-036441-1*); (*0-08-040640-8*) PPI GBR. *Dist:* Elsevier.

Clinical Psychology Intellectual Disabilities. Eric Emerson. 1999. LC 98-33515. (Clinical Psychology & Personality Ser.). 360p. pap. 55.00 (*0-471-97662-8*) Wiley.

Clinical Psychology since 1917: Science, Practice, & Organization. D. K. Routh. 1994. LC 93-50551. (Applied Clinical Psychology Ser.). (Illus.). 300p. (C). 59.50 (*0-306-44452-6*, Kluwer Plenum) Kluwer Academic.

Clinical Psychopharmacology. Lawson. 2nd ed. 1994. 432p. 59.00 (*0-8342-1836-4*) PRO-ED.

Clinical Psychopharmacology: A Practical Reference for Nonmedical Psychotherapists. Gary W. Lawson & Craig C. Cooperrider. 2000. LC 87-33480. 398p. (C). 79.00 (*0-87189-751-2*) PRO-ED.

Clinical Psychopharmacology for the Busy Practitioner. Hugo Rosen. Ed. by Susan E. Wills. 2nd rev. ed. 1993. LC 93-76875. (Illus.). 362p. lib. bdg. 39.00 (*1-883122-01-5*) Pearce Pub.

Clinical Psychopharmacology Made Ridiculously Simple. John Preston. 4th ed. 2000. LC 00-266197. (Rapid Learning & Retention Through the Medmaster Ser.). (Illus.). 74p. pap. text 13.95 (*0-940780-44-5*) MedMaster.

Clinical Pulmonary Hypertension. Ed. by A. K. Morice. 1995. (Portland Press Research Monographs: Vol. 8). (Illus.). 292p. text (*1-85578-074-7*) Portland Pr Ltd GBR. *Dist:* Ashgate Pub Co.

Clinical Radiation Oncology. Leonard L. Gunderson & Joel E. Tepper. 2000. LC 99-31877. (Illus.). xxii, 1296p. (C). text (*0-443-07609-X*) Saunders.

Clinical Radiobiology. A. H. Nias. 2nd ed. 1989. (Illus.). 304p. text (*0-443-03340-4*) Church.

Clinical Radiology. Richard H. Daffner. 1993. LC 92-12314. (Illus.). 408p. 35.00 (*0-683-02330-6*) Lppncott W & W.

Clinical Radiology: The Essentials. Richard H. Daffner. 2nd ed. 1998. LC 98-27066. 420p. pap. 40.95 (*0-683-30517-4*) Lppncott W & W.

Clinical Radiology & Endoscopy of the Colon. Jacques W. Reeders & Gerd Rosenbusch. Ed. by Peter Winter. Tr. by Clifford Bergman et al. 1993. LC 93-30486. (Illus.). 199.00 (*0-86577-508-7*) Thieme Med Pubs.

Clinical Radiology for Medical Students. K. T. Evans et al. 2nd ed. 1995. LC 87-6373. 140p. pap. text 42.00 (*0-7506-1659-8*) Buttrwrth-Heinemann.

Clinical Radiology for Medical Students. G. M. Roberts et al. 3rd ed. 1998. LC 98-2712. 160p. pap. (*0-7506-1408-0*) E A GBR. *Dist:* OUP.

Clinical Radiology of the Horse. Janet A. Butler et al. 1992. (Illus.). 560p. (C). 268.95 (*0-8464-4162-4*) Beekman Pubs.

Clinical Radiology of the Horse. Janet A. Butler et al. 1993. (Illus.). 560p. 160.95 (*0-632-03271-5*) Blackwell Sci.

Clinical Radiology of the Small Intestine. Herlinger & Maglinte. 1989. 544p. text 199.00 (*0-7216-4608-5*) Saunders.

Clinical Reasoning: Forms of Inquiry in Occupational Therapy. Cheryl Mattingly & Maureen H. Fleming. 1993. LC 93-31102. (Illus.). 378p. (C). text 35.95 (*0-8036-5937-7*) Davis Co.

Clinical Reasoning: The Art & Science of Critical & Creative Thinking. Herman Pesut. 2nd ed. 1999. LC 98-37445. (Professional Reference - Nursing Ser.). 224p. (C). pap. text 33.95 (*0-8273-7869-6*) Delmar.

Clinical Reasoning for Physiotherapists. Mark Jones & Darren Rivett. 2001. (Illus.). 288p. pap. 45.00 (*0-7506-3906-7*) Buttrwrth-Heinemann.

Clinical Reasoning in Physical Disabilities. Rebecca Dutton. 1995. LC 94-24714. (Illus.). 352p. 37.00 (*0-683-02740-9*) Lppncott W & W.

Clinical Reasoning in the Health Professions. Ed. by Mark Jones & Joy Higgs. 2nd ed. 2000. LC 99-51959. 336p. pap. text 57.50 (*0-7506-3907-5*) Buttrwrth-Heinemann.

Clinical Recognition of Congenital Heart Disease. Joseph K. Perloff. 4th ed. 1994. LC 93-32195. text 135.00 (*0-7216-5504-1*) Saunders.

Clinical Relaxation Strategies. Kenneth L. Lichstein. 1988. LC 87-25296. (Personality Processes Ser.). 426p. 215.00 (*0-471-81592-6*) Wiley.

Clinical Relevance of Hemostaseological Findings: Abstracts. Ed. by E. Wenzel & P. Hellstern. 1985. (Journal: Vol. 15). 88p. pap. 35.00 (*3-8055-4068-X*) S Karger.

Clinical Repertory. John Henrik Clarke. 1980. 40.00 (*0-85032-179-4*) St Mut.

Clinical Repertory to the Dictionary of Materia Medica. John Henrik Clarke. 1995. 360p. (*0-85032-061-5*) C W Daniel GBR. *Dist:* Natl Bk Netwk.

Clinical Reports 1995 Vol. 7: In Nutrition & Preventive Medicine. Kirkham R. Hamilton. Ed. by Kristine Simpson & Karen R. Hamilton. Date not set. pap. 49.95 (*0-9628840-7-3*) ITServices.

Clinical Reproductive Endocrinology. Ed. by Rodney P. Shearman. 1985. LC 84-12156. (Illus.). 776p. text (*0-443-02645-9*) Church.

Clinical Reproductive Neuroendocrinology: Proceedings of the International Seminar on Reproductive Physiology & Sexual Endocrinology, 6th, Brussels, May-June, 1976. International Seminar on Reproductive Physiology &. Ed. by P. O. Hubinont. 1977. (Progress in Reproductive Biology & Medicine Ser.: Vol. 2). (Illus.). 101.00 (*3-8055-2382-3*) S Karger.

Clinical Research: Hearing Before the Committee on Appropriations, United States Senate. Composed by Diane Publishing Staff. 1998. 59p. pap. text 25.00 (*0-7881-4882-6*) DIANE Pub.

Clinical Research & Documentation: Single-Subject Research Designs & Documentation for the Neurologically Impaired Adult. M. Ann Karas & Janis J. Daly. 1997. (C). pap. 34.95 (*0-9621991-2-5*) NDTA.

Clinical Research As the Basis of Clinical Practice. Antczak-Bouckoms et al. Ed. by Katherine D. Vig & Peter S. Vig. 1991. (Craniofacial Growth Ser.: Vol. 25). (Illus.). 222p. 55.00 (*0-929921-21-6*) UM CHGD.

Clinical Research Coordinator Handbook. Deborah Norris. 2nd ed. 2000. LC 00-36695. (Illus.). ix, 82p. pap. 34.95 (*0-937548-43-X*) Plexus Pub.

*__Clinical Research for Complimentary Therapy.__ George Lewith et al. 2001. (Illus.). 275p. pap. (*0-443-06367-2*) Church GBR. *Dist:* Saunders.

Clinical Research for Health Professionals: A User-Friendly Guide. Mitch Batavia. 2000. LC 00-31219. (Illus.). 216p. pap. text 29.99 (*0-7506-7193-9*) Buttrwrth-Heinemann.

Clinical Research in Allied Health & Special Education. Franklin Stein & Susan K. Cutler. 3rd ed. 1996. LC 95-46566. 464p. pap. text 61.95 (*1-56593-631-0*, 1308) Thomson Learn.

Clinical Research in Communicative Disorders: Principles & Strategies. M. N. Hegde. 2nd ed. 1994. LC 93-41146. (Illus.). 467p. (C). text 41.00 (*0-89079-594-0*, 6691) PRO-ED.

Clinical Research in Diabetes amd Obesity Vol. 1: Methods, Assessment & Metabolic Regulation. Ed. by Boris Draznin & Robert Rizza. 1997. LC 97-5726. (Contemporary Biomedicine Ser.: Vol. 14). (Illus.). 408p. 160.00 (*0-89603-350-3*) Humana.

Clinical Research in Diabetes & Obesity Vol. 2: Diabetes & Obesity. Ed. by Boris Draznin & Robert Rizza. 1997. LC 97-5726. (Contemporary Biomedicine Ser.: Vol. 15). (Illus.). 408p. 160.00 (*0-89603-492-5*) Humana.

Clinical Research in Gastroenterology. Ed. by S. Matern. (C). 2nd ed. 1989. text 90.50 (*0-7923-8906-9*); Vol. I. 1987. text 119.00 (*0-85200-696-9*) Kluwer Academic.

Clinical Research in Occupational Therapy. Franklin Stein & Susan K. Cutler. 4th ed. 2000. LC 99-86956. 574p. pap. text 59.95 (*0-7693-0047-2*) Singular Publishing.

Clinical Research in Pharmaceutical Development. Barry Bleidt & Michael Montagne. 1996. LC 96-26648. (Drugs & the Pharmaceutical Sciences Ser.: Vol. 75). (Illus.). 368p. text 155.00 (*0-8247-9745-0*) Dekker.

Clinical Research in Psychiatry. Williams & Curran. 1998. 200p. pap. (*0-7506-4073-1*) E A GBR. *Dist:* OUP.

Clinical Research Monitor Handbook: GCP Tools & Techniques. Deborah Rosenbaum & Fred O. Smith. 1997. (Practical Clinical Trials Ser.: Vol. 3). (Illus.). 428p. 145.00 (*1-57491-048-5*) IHS Health Grp.

*__Clinical Research Monitor Handbook: GCP Tools & Techniques.__ Deborah Rosenbaum & Fred Smith. 2nd ed. 2002. LC 2001-39555. (Practical Clinical Trials Ser.). (*1-57491-125-2*) IHS Health Grp.

Clinical Research Opportunities: A Physician's Guide to Participating in Clinical Research Studies. Anthony Boyle. Ed. by Maureen Lynch & Kathryn Swanson. 1996. LC 95-14125. 175p. pap. 49.95 (*1-57066-030-1*, ME072) Practice Mgmt Info.

Clinical Research Process in the Pharmaceutical Industry. Gary M. Matoren. 1983. (Drugs & the Pharmaceutical Sciences Ser.: Vol. 19). (Illus.). 576p. text 75.00 (*0-8247-1914-X*) Dekker.

Clinical Resource & Quality Management. Ed. by Scott B. Ransom & William Pinsky. 1999. LC 98-86857. xi, 447p. (*0-924674-67-9*) Am Coll Phys Execs.

Clinical Respiratory Physiology. Taylor et al. 1989. 272p. pap. text 33.00 (*0-7216-2484-7*) Saunders.

Clinical Retinopathies. J. M. Gibson et al. 1994. (Illus.). 184p. (*0-412-35930-8*) E A GBR. *Dist:* OUP.

Clinical Rheumatology. Gene V. Ball & William J. Koopman. 1986. (Illus.). 367p. text 79.00 (*0-7216-1451-5*) Saunders.

Clinical Risk Management. Ed. by Charles Vincent. Date not set. 588p. (Orig.). (C). pap. text (*0-7279-0947-9*) BMJ Pub GBR. *Dist:* AIDC.

Clinical Risk Management & Modification. Ed. by John Tingle & Jo Wilson. 1999. LC 99-191728. (Illus.). 208p. pap. text 35.00 (*0-7506-2939-8*) Buttrwrth-Heinemann.

Clinical Risk Management in Midwifery: The Right to a Perfect Baby? John Tingle. Date not set. 256p. pap. 27.00 (*0-7506-2851-0*) Buttrwrth-Heinemann.

Clinical Rotation Handbook: The Practicum Guide for Nurses. Marlene Audrey Reimer et al. 1998. 240p. (C). pap. text 28.95 (*0-7668-0540-9*) Delmar.

Clinical Rotations. Thomson. 1997. (Health Occupations Ser.). 258p. (C). pap. text 30.95 (*0-8273-6290-0*) Delmar.

Clinical Safety & Efficacy Testing of Cosmetics. Ed. by William C. Waggoner. 1989. (Cosmetic Science & Technology Ser.: Vol. 8). (Illus.). 352p. text 165.00 (*0-8247-7941-X*) Dekker.

Clinical Scenarios in Pain. W. A. Chambers & W. A. McRae. 2000. (Greenwich Medical Media Ser.). 140p. pap. 34.95 (*1-900151-70-7*) OUP.

Clinical Science of Electroconvulsive Therapy. Ed. by C. Edward Coffey. 1993. (Progress in Psychiatry Ser.: No. 38). 259p. text 12.95 (*0-88048-470-5*, 8470) Am Psychiatric.

Clinical Science Question Bank. Stanley Zaslau. Ed. & Illus. by Paul L. McGrath. 1997. 136p. spiral bd., wbk. ed. 19.00 (*1-886468-16-8*) FMSG.

Clinical Self-Hypnosis: The Power of Words & Images. Shirley Sanders. 1990. LC 90-3407. (Guilford Clinical & Experimental Hypnosis Ser.). 244p. 40.00 (*0-89862-342-1*) Guilford Pubns.

Clinical Signs. Peter C. Hayes & Derek Bell. 1990. (Colour Aids Ser.). (Illus.). 112p. pap. text (*0-443-04051-6*) Church.

Clinical Signs. Peter C. Hayes & Derek Bell. 1996. LC 96-6472. (Colour Guide Ser.). 108p. pap. text 16.95 (*0-443-05193-3*) Harcrt Hlth Sci Grp.

Clinical Signs & Diagnosis. Ford. 1988. text 116.00 (*0-7216-5928-4*) Saunders.

Clinical Simulations - The Right Way! The Complete Guide to Respiratory Care. C. J. Peters. 1990. 370p. pap. text 49.95 (*0-931657-20-2*) Learning Proc Ctr.

Clinical Simulations in Laboratory Medicine. Shauna C. Anderson et al. 1986. LC 65-9095. (Illus.). 224p. text 28.50 (*0-397-50746-1*, Lippnctt) Lppncott W & W.

Clinical Simulations in Respiratory Care. Thomas A. Barnes. 1999. (C). cd-rom 52.95 (*0-8036-0246-4*) Davis Co.

Clinical Skills: The Medical Interview, Physical Examination & Assessment of the Patient's Problems. R. G. Larkins & R. A. Smallwood. 1994. 396p. pap. (*0-522-84467-7*) Melbourne Univ Pr AUS. *Dist:* Paul & Co Pubs.

Clinical Skills & Assessment Techniques in Nursing. Vicki V. Earnest. 2nd ed. 1992. LC 92-19632. (Illus.). 1,232p. pap. text 52.95 (*0-397-54926-1*) Lppncott W & W.

Clinical Skills for Assistive Personnel. Sheila A. Sorrentino. 1998. (Illus.). 208p. (*0-323-00074-6*); tchr. ed. (*0-323-00169-6*) Mosby Inc.

Clinical Skills for Assistive Personnel: Textbook for Nursing Assistants & Clinical Skills Package. Sheila A. Sorrentino. 1998. (Illus.). (*0-8151-1567-9*) Mosby Inc.

Clinical Skills for Pharmacists. Karen J. Tietze & Janice A. Gaska. 1997. LC 97-11635. (Illus.). 256p. (C). (gr. 13). pap. text 29.00 (*0-8016-6484-5*, 06484) Mosby Inc.

Clinical Skills For Speech-Language Pathologists: Practical Applications. Stanley A. Goldberg. 1996. LC 96-3306. 427p. pap. text 62.95 (*1-56593-686-8*, 1362) Thomson Learn.

Clinical Skills in Neurology. Michael J. Harrison. 1996. 153p. pap. text 37.50 (*0-7506-2520-1*) Buttrwrth-Heinemann.

Clinical Skills in Treating the Foot. David R. Tollafield & Linda M. Merriman. 1997. LC 96-39915. text (*0-443-05033-3*) Church.

Clinical Skills Matrix. Jane Dacre & Maggie Nicol. 1996. (*1-85775-195-7*) Radcliffe Med Pr GBR. *Dist:* Balogh.

Clinical Skills Performance Evaluation Tools for Physical Therapists: Cardiopulmonary. 2001. 28p. pap. 20.00 (*1-887759-89-1*) Am Phys Therapy Assn.

Clinical Skills Performance Evaluation Tools for Physical Therapists: Geriatric. 2001. 25p. pap. 20.00 (*1-887759-91-3*) Am Phys Therapy Assn.

Clinical Skills Performance Evaluation Tools for Physical Therapists: Pediatric. 2001. 37p. pap. 20.00 (*1-887759-94-8*) Am Phys Therapy Assn.

Clinical Skills Performance Evaluation Tools for Physical Therapists: Sports Physical Therapy. 2001. 19p. pap. 20.00 (*1-887759-95-6*) Am Phys Therapy Assn.

Clinical Skills Program: Advancing Pharmaceutical Care - Module 1. Reviewing Patient Medical Charts. Michele F. Shepherd. 1992. 64p. (C). pap. text 45.00 (*1-879907-26-7*) Am Soc Hlth-Syst.

Clinical Skills Program: Advancing Pharmaceutical Care, Module LN: Designing & Recommending a Pharmacist's Care Plan. William N. Jones & Suzanne Campbell. 1994. 112p. (C). pap. text 63.00 (*1-879907-43-7*) Am Soc Hlth-Syst.

Clinical Small Animal Behavior. Karen L. Overall. 1997. LC 96-18753. (Illus.). 560p. (C). (gr. 13). text 52.95 (*0-8016-6820-4*, 06820) Mosby Inc.

Clinical Small Animal Behavior: Case Study. Victoria L. Voith. 1999. text (*0-7216-5024-4*) Saunders.

Clinical Social Work: Definition, Practice, & Vision. Rachelle A. Dorfman. 1996. LC 96-15973. (Basic Principles into Practice Ser.: Vol. 9). 224p. pap. text 24.95 (*0-87630-808-6*) Brunner-Routledge.

Clinical Social Work: Research & Practice. Mary N. Russell. 1991. (Sourcebooks for the Human Services: Vol. 14). (Illus.). 192p. (C). 89.95 (*0-8039-3782-2*); pap. 39.95 (*0-8039-3783-0*, 8204) Sage.

Clinical Social Workers as Psychotherapists. Florence Lieberman. 1982. LC 82-3109. 29.95 (*0-89876-037-2*) Gardner Pr.

Clinical Society of London: Report on Myxoedema, 1888. Intro. by Clark T. Sawin. 1992. (Illus.). 215p. reprint ed. lib. bdg. 19.95 (*0-88135-063-X*, Sci Hist) Watson Pub Intl.

Clinical Sonography. Ed. by Roger C. Sanders. 3rd ed. 1997. 575p. pap. text 55.00 (*0-316-77105-8*) Lppncott W & W.

Clinical Sonography: A Practical Guide. Roger C. Sanders. 1984. 396p. 37.00 (*0-316-77010-8*, Little Brwn Med Div) Lppncott W & W.

Clinical Sonography: A Practical Guide. Roger C. Sanders & Nancy Smith Miner. 3rd ed. 1997. LC 97-33686. 640p. pap. text 64.00 (*0-7817-1556-3*) Lppncott W & W.

Clinical Specialist in Adult Psychiatric & Mental Health Nursing. Jack Rudman. 1994. (Certified Nurse Examination Ser.: CN-14). pap. 27.95 (*0-8373-6114-1*) Nat Learn.

Clinical Specialist in Child & Adolescent Psychiatric & Mental Health Nursing. Jack Rudman. 1994. (Certified Nurse Examination Ser.: CN-15). pap. 27.95 (*0-8373-6115-X*) Nat Learn.

Clinical Specialist in Medical-Surgical Nursing. Jack Rudman. 1994. (Certified Nurse Examination Ser.: CN-13). pap. 27.95 (*0-8373-6113-3*) Nat Learn.

Clinical Speech & Voice Measurement: Laboratory Exercises. Robert F. Orlikoff & Ronald J. Baken. 1993. LC 93-14930. (Illus.). 488p. (Orig.). (C). pap. text 55.00 (*1-879105-91-8*, 0354) Thomson Learn.

Clinical Speech & Voice Measurement Laboratory Exercises: Instructor's Manual. Robert F. Orlikoff & Ronald J. Baken. 1993. (Illus.). 150p. (Orig.). (C). pap. text 24.95 (*1-56593-215-3*, 0576) Singular Publishing.

Clinical Sports Medicine. William A. Grana & Kalenak. 1990. (Illus.). 656p. text 90.00 (*0-7216-2604-1*) Saunders.

Clinical Sports Nutrition. Ed. by Louise Burke & Vicki Deakin. 2nd ed. 2000. LC 2001-274246. (Illus.). 759p. pap. 54.95 (*0-07-470828-7*) McGraw-Hill Prof.

Clinical Stories & Their Translations. Howard F. Stein & Maurice Apprey. 1990. LC 89-16615. (Ethnicity, Medicine, & Psychoanalysis Ser.). text 40.00 (*0-8139-1241-5*) U Pr of Va.

Clinical Strabismus Management. Arthur L. Rosenbaum & Alvina P. Santiago. Ed. by Richard Lambert. 1999. LC 98-48475. (Illus.). 575p. (C). text 185.00 (*0-7216-7673-1*) Saunders.

Clinical Studies Vol. 2-1: International Journal of Psychoanalysis. Ed. by Laura C. Szichman. 1996. 100p. (C). pap. 9.00 (*1-883831-04-0*) Critical Pr.

Clinical Studies Vol. 2-2: International Journal of Psychoanalysis. Ed. by Laura C. Szichman. 1996. 100p. (C). 9.00 (*1-883831-06-7*) Critical Pr.

Clinical Studies in Medical Biochemistry. Ed. by Robert H. Glew & Yoshifumi Ninoyama. 2nd ed. 1997. (Illus.). 398p. pap. text 39.95 (*0-19-509929-X*) OUP.

Clinical Studies in Psychiatry. Harry Stack Sullivan. 1973. (Norton Library: No. N688). 400p. reprint ed. pap. 14.95 (*0-393-00688-3*) Norton.

Clinical Studies in Transpersonal Psychotherapy. Seymour Boorstein. 1997. LC 96-23228. (SUNY Series in the Philosophy of Psychology). 191p. (C). text 49.50 (*0-7914-3333-1*); pap. text 17.95 (*0-7914-3334-X*) State U NY Pr.

Clinical Supervision: A Systems Approach. Elizabeth L. Holloway. 1995. LC 95-7711. (Illus.). 213p. 74.95 (*0-8039-4223-0*, 3719); 266p. pap. 39.95 (*0-8039-4224-9*, 3720) Sage.

Clinical Supervision: Skills for Substance Abuse Counselors. David J. Powell. 1980. LC 79-20586. stu. ed. 20.95 (*0-87705-407-X*); 240p. pap., stu. ed. 30.95 (*0-89885-442-3*) Kluwer Academic (Kluwer Acad Hman Sci).

Clinical Supervision & Mentorship in Nursing. Tony Butterworth et al. 1998. pap. (*0-7487-3304-3*) Nelson Thornes GBR. *Dist:* Intl Spec Bk, Trans-Atl Phila.

Clinical Supervision in Alcohol & Drug Abuse Counseling: Principles, Models, Methods. David J. Powell & Archie Brodsky. 1993. LC 93-14505. 344p. 47.95 (*0-02-925055-2*) Jossey-Bass.

Clinical Supervision in Alcohol & Drug Abuse Counseling Vol. 1: Principles, Models, Methods. David J. Powell. 1997. LC 97-42941. 352p. pap. 28.00 (*0-7879-4074-7*) Jossey-Bass.

Clinical Supervision in Speech Pathology & Audiology. George W. Schubert. 1978. LC 77-81799. 256p. 12.75 (*0-87527-162-6*) Green.

Clinical Surgery. Alfred Cuschieri et al. 1996. LC 96-13646. (Illus.). 450p. (Orig.). pap. text 64.95 (*0-632-03146-8*) Blackwell Sci.

Clinical Surgery. Ed. by Michael M. Henry & Jeremy N. Thompson. 1998. (Illus.). 750p. text 37.50 (*0-7020-1588-1*) Saunders.

Clinical Surgery. D. Das. 3rd ed. 1989. (C). (*0-7855-4650-2*) Current Dist IND. *Dist:* St Mut.

Clinical Surgery in General. Ed. by R. M. Kirk et al. 1993. LC 93-6785. (*0-443-04574-7*) Church.

Clinical Surgery in General: RCS Course Manual. Kirk. 2nd ed. 1996. text (*0-443-05461-4*, C1660) Church.

Clinical Surgery in General: RCS Course Manual. R. M. Kirk et al. 3rd ed. 1999. LC 99-10536. xii, 453p. (*0-443-06219-6*) Church.

Clinical Symposium on the Recognition & Management of Immunodeficient Disorders, Proceedings of. 1986. (Vox Sanguinis: Vol. 51, Suppl. 2, 1986). iv, 104p. pap. 38.50 (*3-8055-4366-2*) S Karger.

Clinical Syndromes. Wiedema. 3rd ed. 1997. text 150.00 (*0-7234-2950-2*) Mosby Inc.

Clinical Syndromes in Adult Neuropsychology. R. F. White. 1992. 498p. 303.25 (*0-444-81271-7*) Elsevier.

Clinical Syndromes in Veterinary Neurology. Kyle G. Braund. 2nd ed. 1993. LC 93-12662. (Illus.). 477p. (gr. 13). text 70.00 (*0-8016-7354-2*, 07354) Mosby Inc.

Clinical Synopsis of Moss & Adams' Heart Disease in Infants, Children, & Adolescents: Including the Fetus & Young Adult. George C. Emmanouilides et al. 5th ed. 1997. LC 97-42673. 600p. pap. 59.95 (*0-683-18003-7*) Lppncott W & W.

Clinical Teaching & Evaluation for Manual for Respiratory Care. D. Graham & J. Yestingsmeir. Ed. by Beth Smith. 1992. LC 85-4154. (Illus.). 336p. pap. text 39.95 (*0-933195-01-X*) CA College Health Sci.

Clinical Teaching for Medical Residents: Roles, Techniques & Programs. Ed. by Janine C. Edwards & Robert L. Marier. 1987. (Medical Education Ser.). 288p. (C). 39.95 (*0-8261-5600-2*) Springer Pub.

Clinical Teaching in Nursing Education. Dorothy E. Reilly & Marilyn H. Oermann. 2nd ed. 1992. 528p. (C). pap. text 36.95 (*0-88737-549-9*) Natl League Nurse.

Clinical Teaching Strategies in Nursing. Kathleen B. Gaberson & Marilyn H. Oermann. 1999. LC 99-24713. (Series on the Teaching of Nursing). (Illus.). 256p. text 39.95 (*0-8261-1278-1*) Springer Pub.

***Clinical Team Advantage.** McEachern. 2001. 250p. 41.95 (*0-7879-4156-5*) Wiley.

Clinical Telemedicine Payment Models: Analysis of Current Services & Revenue Potential. Feedback Research Services Staff. 1998. 113p. spiral bd. 495.00 (*1-889713-18-X*) Feedback Rsch.

Clinical Tests in Ophthalmology. M. J. E. Huber. 1991. (Illus.). 176p. (C). (gr. 13). pap. text 46.00 (*0-8016-6291-5*, 06291) Mosby Inc.

Clinical Tests of Respiratory Function. G. J. Gibson. 2nd ed. 1995. (Illus.). 392p. (*0-412-56890-X*) E A GBR. *Dist:* OUP.

Clinical Textbook for Veterinary Technicians. Dennis M. McCurnin. Ed. by Selma Kaszczuk. 4th ed. 1998. LC 97-17014. (Illus.). 928p. text 62.50 (*0-7216-2196-1*) Saunders.

Clinical Textbook for Veterinary Technicians. Dennis M. McCurnin & Joanna Bassert. 5th ed. 2001. LC 2001-20898. (Illus.). 830p. text (*0-7216-9164-1*) Saunders.

Clinical Textbook of Addictive Disorders. Ed. by Richard J. Frances & Sheldon I. Miller. 2nd ed. 1998. LC 98-28510. 637p. pap. 66.00 (*1-57230-383-2*, C0383) Guilford Pubns.

Clinical Therapy in Breastfeeding Patients. Thomas W. Hale. 1999. 190p. pap. text 19.95 (*0-9636219-2-0*) Pharmasft Pub.

Clinical Thinking of Wilfred Bion. Joan Symington & Neville Symington. 1996. LC 95-31603. (Makers of Modern Psychotherapy Ser.). 216p. (C). 84.95 (*0-415-09352-X*); pap. 29.95 (*0-415-09353-8*) Routledge.

Clinical Thrombosis. Ed. by Hau C. Kwaan & Meyer M. Samama. 1989. 576p. 139.00 (*0-8493-6327-6*, RC694) CRC Pr.

Clinical Toxicology. Marsha Ford et al. 1999. 815p. text 156.25 (*0-7216-5485-1*) Saunders.

Clinical Toxicology of Commercial Products: Acute Poisoning. Robert E. Gosselin et al. 5th ed. 1984. (Illus.). 2012p. 160.00 (*0-683-03632-7*) Lppncott W & W.

Clinical Training & Health Care Costs: A Basic Curriculum for Medical Education. Mohan L. Garg & Warren M. Kleinberg. 1985. LC 84-15152. 170p. 55.00 (*0-275-91313-9*, C1313, Praeger Pubs) Greenwood.

Clinical Training in Psychotherapy. Ed. by Tom H. Peake et al. 1985. LC 84-15873. (Clinical Supervisor Ser.: Vol. 2, No. 4). 129p. text 4.95 (*0-86656-334-2*); pap. text 19.95 (*0-86656-335-0*) Haworth Pr.

Clinical Training Skills for Reproductive Health Professionals see Competences en Formation Clinique pour les Professionels en Sante de la Reproduction

Clinical Training Skills for Reproductive Health Professionals. Rick Sullivan et al. 1997. (RUS., Illus.). 200p. pap. text 15.00 (*0-929817-52-4*); 1995. pap. text 15.00 (*0-929817-06-0*) JHPIEGO.

Clinical Training Skills for Reproductive Health Professionals. Rick Sullivan. 2nd rev. ed. 1998. (Illus.). pap. 15.00 (*0-929817-55-9*) JHPIEGO.

Clinical Transesophageal Echocardiography: A Problem-Oriented Approach. Ed. by Yasu Oka et al. 1995. LC 95-35651. (Illus.). 400p. text 199.00 (*0-397-51426-3*) Lppncott W & W.

Clinical Transplantation: Current Practice & Future Prospects. Ed. by G. D. Catto. 1987. (Immunology & Medicine Ser.). 296p. (C). text 176.50 (*0-85200-960-7*) Kluwer Academic.

Clinical Transplants, 1986. Ed. by Paul I. Terasaki. 1986. 15.00 (*0-9604606-2-4*) UCLA Tissue.

Clinical Transplants, 1987. Ed. by Paul I. Terasaki. 1987. 15.00 (*0-9604606-3-2*) UCLA Tissue.

Clinical Transplants, 1988. Ed. by Paul I. Terasaki. 1988. 15.00 (*0-9604606-4-0*) UCLA Tissue.

Clinical Transplants, 1989. Ed. by Paul I. Terasaki. 1990. 15.00 (*0-9604606-5-9*) UCLA Tissue.

Clinical Transplants, 1991. Ed. by Paul I. Terasaki & J. Michael Cecka. 1992. 20.00 (*0-9604606-8-3*) UCLA Tissue.

Clinical Transplants, 1992. Ed. by Paul I. Terasaki & J. M. Cecka. 1993. 40.00 (*0-9604606-9-1*) UCLA Tissue.

Clinical Transplants, 1994. Ed. by Paul I. Terasaki & J. M. Cecka. 1995. 90.00 (*1-880318-02-4*) UCLA Tissue.

Clinical Transplants, 1997. J. Michael Cecka & Paul I. Terasaki. 1998. (Illus.). 650p. 90.00 (*1-880318-06-7*) UCLA Tissue.

Clinical Treatment of the Criminal Offender in Outpatient Mental Health Settings: The New & Emerging Perspectives. Ed. by Sol Chaneles & Nathaniel J. Pallone. 1990. LC 90-4008. (Journal of Offender Counseling, Services & Rehabilitation: Vol. 15, No. 1). 175p. text 39.95 (*0-86656-982-0*) Haworth Pr.

Clinical Treatment of the Violent Person. Ed. by Loren H. Roth. 1987. LC 86-19543. 270p. pap. 25.00 (*0-89862-914-4*) Guilford Pubns.

Clinical Trial Methodology in Pediatric RTI. Ed. by R. Dagan & G. Syrogiannopoulos. 1992. (Journal: Vol. 38, Suppl. 2, 1992). (Illus.). iv, 40p. pap. 12.25 (*3-8055-5651-9*) S Karger.

***Clinical Trials.** Lelia Duley & Barbara Farrell. 2001. 144p. pap. text (*0-7279-1599-1*) BMJ Pub.

Clinical Trials. Daniel Schwartz et al. 1981. LC 80-40684.Tr. of L'Essai Therapeutiques Chez L'Homme. text 136.00 (*0-12-632440-9*) Acad Pr.

Clinical Trials: A Practical Approach. Ed. by Stuart J. Pocock. 1984. LC 83-1316. (Medical Publications). 278p. 170.00 (*0-471-90155-5*, Wiley-Liss) Wiley.

Clinical Trials: Decision Tools for Measuring & Improving Performance. Bryan Beck. 1996. (Illus.). 152p. 169.00 (*1-57491-019-1*) IHS Health Grp.

Clinical Trials: Design, Conduct & Analysis. Curtis L. Meinert. 1986. (Monographs in Epidemiology & Biostatistics: No. 8). (Illus.). 512p. (C). text 89.50 (*0-19-503568-2*) OUP.

Clinical Trials: Issues & Approaches. Louis. Ed. by Stanley H. Shapiro. 1983. (Statistics: Textbooks & Monographs: Vol. 46). (Illus.). 224p. text 115.00 (*0-8247-1741-4*) Dekker.

Clinical Trials: What You Should Know Before Volunteering to Be a Research Subject. J. Joseph Giffels. 1996. LC 96-5309. 48p. pap. 9.95 (*1-888799-02-1*) Demos Medical.

Clinical Trials & Tribulations. Allen E. Cato. 1988. (Drugs & the Pharmaceutical Sciences Ser.: Vol. 34). (Illus.). 432p. text 65.00 (*0-8247-7854-5*) Dekker.

Clinical Trials Dictionary: Terminology & Usage Recommendations. Curtis L. Meinert. Date not set. LC 95-94294. 480p. text 95.00 (*0-9646424-0-9*) C L Meinert.

Clinical Trials for the Treatment of Sepsis, 19. Ed. by J. L. Vincent & William J. Sibbald. 1994. LC 94-23238. (Update in Intensive Care & Emergency Medicine Ser.). (Illus.). 593p. 130.00 (*3-540-58380-7*) Spr-Verlag.

Clinical Trials in Cardiology. Bertram Pitt. 1997. 386p. text (*0-7020-2156-3*) Bailliere Tindall.

Clinical Trials in Cardiovascular Medicine: A Companion to Braunwald's Heart Disease. Charles H. Hennekens. Ed. by Richard Zorab. 1998. (Illus.). 475p. (C). text 130.00 (*0-7216-6867-4*) Saunders.

Clinical Trials in Multiple Sclerosis. Ed. by F. Clifford Rose. 1987. (Journal: Vol. 6, No. 1-2, 1987). (Illus.). 92p. pap. 59.25 (*3-8055-4577-0*) S Karger.

Clinical Trials in Neurologic Practice. Jose Biller & Julien Bogousslavasky. 2000. LC 00-56441. (Illus.). 448p. text 99.00 (*0-7506-7140-8*) Buttrwrth-Heinemann.

Clinical Trials in Ophthalmology: A Summary & Practice Guide. Peter J. Kertes & Mandi D. Conway. 1998. LC 97-42620. 344p. pap. 59.95 (*0-683-30205-1*) Lppncott W & W.

***Clinical Trials in the Pharmacologic Management of Hypertension.** Ed. by Henry R. Black. 2001. LC 2001-28065. (Illus.). xi, 659p. text 225.00 (*0-8247-0270-0*) Dekker.

Clinical Trials in the Rheumatic Diseases: A Selected Critical Review. David Rosenbloom et al. 1985. LC 84-9911. 386p. 93.95 (*0-275-91323-6*, C1323, Praeger Pubs) Greenwood.

Clinical Trials of Genetic Therapy with Antisense DNA & DNA Vectors. Ed. by Eric Wickstrom. 1998. LC 98-13317. (Illus.). 448p. text 185.00 (*0-8247-0085-6*) Dekker.

Clinical Tropical Medicine. G. O. Cowan & B. J. Heap. 1993. LC 92-49006. 328p. (gr. 13). pap. 56.95 (*0-412-43330-3*) Chapman & Hall.

Clinical Tuberculosis. Ed. by P. D. Davies. 1994. LC 93-26568. 426p. (gr. 13). pap. 115.95 (*0-412-48630-X*, Chap & Hall NY) Chapman & Hall.

Clinical Tuberculosis. Ed. by P. D. O. Davies. 2nd ed. 1999. (An Arnold Publication). (Illus.). 744p. text (*0-412-80340-2*) E A GBR. *Dist:* OUP.

Clinical Tumor Immunology. Ed. by Joseph Wybran & Maurice J. Staquet. 1976. 230p. 65.00 (*0-08-020570-4*); pap. 53.00 (*0-08-021101-1*) Elsevier (Pergamon Pr).

Clinical Ultrasound: A Comprehensive Text, Set. Ed. by Peter Wilde et al. 1993. (Illus.). 3072p. text (*0-443-04846-0*) Church.

Clinical Ultrasound: Abdominal & General Ultrasound: A Comprehensive Text Ed. by Keith Dewbury et al. 1993. (Illus.). 2048p. text (*0-443-04277-2*) Church.

Clinical Ultrasound: Cardiac Ultrasound: A Comprehensive Text. Ed. by Peter Wilde. 1993. (Illus.). 550p. text (*0-443-04280-2*) Church.

Clinical Ultrasound: Ultrasound in Obstetrics & Gynecology: A Comprehensive Text. Ed. by Keith Dewbury et al. 1993. (Illus.). 600p. text (*0-443-04279-9*) Church.

***Clinical Ultrasound Vol. 3: A Comprehensive Text.** Hylton Meire et al. 2001. (Illus.). (*0-443-06154-8*) Church GBR. *Dist:* Saunders.

Clinical Urography: An Atlas & Textbook of Urological Imaging Howard M. Pollack. Incl. Vol. 1. text 198.00 (*0-7216-1556-2*); Vol. 2. text 198.00 (*0-7216-1557-0*); Vol. 3. text 198.00 (*0-7216-1558-9*); 3168p. 1989. 525.00 (*0-7216-1555-4*);Vol. 1. text 198.00 (*0-7216-1556-2*);Vol. 2. text 198.00 (*0-7216-1557-0*);Vol. 3. text 198.00 (*0-7216-1558-9*) Saunders.

Clinical Urogynecology. Scotti. 2000. 85.00 (*0-07-105440-5*) McGraw.

Clinical Urogynecology & Reconstructive Pelvic Surgery, Vol. 2. Ed. by Mark D. Walters & Mickey M. Karram. 2nd ed. 1999. LC 99-10976. (Illus.). 432p. text 98.00 (*0-8151-3671-4*, 31392) Mosby Inc.

Clinical Urology. John Fitzpatrick et al. 1994. (Illus.). 1,392p. (C). text 210.00 (*0-397-51161-2*, Lippnctt) Lppncott W & W.

Clinical Urology Howard M. Pollack et al. 2nd ed. 2000. LC 99-15252. (Illus.). xxxi, 3434p. text (*0-7216-6935-2*) Saunders.

Clinical Use & Interpretation of the Wechsler Intelligence Scale for Children. Shawn Cooper. 1995. LC 95-14202. (Illus.). 466p. (C). rev. ed. text 82.95 (*0-398-06523-3*); 3rd rev. ed. pap. text 59.95 (*0-398-06524-1*) C C Thomas.

Clinical Use of Antibodies: Tumors, Infection, Infarction, Rejection in the Diagnosis of AIDS. Ed. by R. P. Baum et al. 1991. (C). text 122.00 (*0-7923-1424-7*) Kluwer Academic.

Clinical Use of Antiviral Drugs. Ed. by Erik D. DeClercq. 1988. (Developments in Medical Virology Ser.). 416p. text 190.00 (*0-89838-357-9*) Kluwer Academic.

Clinical Use of Calcium Antagonist Drugs. Lionel H. Opie. 1989. (C). text 145.00 (*0-7923-0155-2*) Kluwer Academic.

Clinical Use of Emission Tomography in Focal Epilepsy. M. Baldy-Moulinier et al. 1989. (Current Problems in Epilepsy Ser.: Vol. 7). 192p. (*0-86196-206-0*) J Libbey Med GBR. *Dist:* Bks Intl VA.

Clinical Use of Intravenous Immunoglobulins. U. E. Nydegger & A. Morell. 1986. text 121.00 (*0-12-523282-9*) Acad Pr.

Clinical Use of Laboratory Data: A Practical Guide. D. Robert Dufour. 1997. LC 97-12909. 613p. pap. 59.95 (*0-683-18017-7*) Lppncott W & W.

Clinical Use of Mitoxantrone for Injection Concentrate: Clinical Use in Advanced Breast Cancer. Ed. by Chris Fellner. 1994. (Orig.). (*1-57130-009-0*) Medicine Grp USA.

Clinical Use of Mitoxantrone for Injection Concentrate: Clinical Use in Lymphoma. Ed. by Chris Fellner. 1994. (Orig.). pap. (*1-57130-012-0*) Medicine Grp USA.

Clinical Uses of Cerebral, Brainstem & Spinal Somatosensory Evoked Potentials. Ed. by John E. Desmedt. 1979. (Progress in Clinical Neurophysiology Ser.: Vol. 7). (Illus.). 120.00 (*3-8055-2936-8*) S Karger.

Clinical Uses of Prism: A Spectrum of Applications. Ed. by Susan Cotter. 1995. (Illus.). 320p. (C). (gr. 13). pap. text 39.95 (*0-8151-1810-4*, 24310) Mosby Inc.

Clinical Uses of Radionuclides: Critical Comparison with Other Techniques: Proceedings. Ed. by Francis A. Goswitz et al. 1972. LC 72-660271. (AEC Symposium Ser.). 718p. 26.00 (*0-87079-002-1*, CONF-711101); fiche 9.00 (*0-87079-164-8*, CONF-711101) DOE.

Clinical Utilization of Microcomputer Technology. Raymond G. Romanczyk. 1985. (Psychology Practitioner Guidebooks). 128p. text 30.00 (*0-08-031946-7*); pap. text 15.95 (*0-08-031945-9*) Elsevier (Pergamon Pr).

Clinical Vademecum of the Medical Practice: Vademecum Clinico del Medico Practico, del Sintoma a la Receta. 5th ed. 1982. 1398p. 95.00 (*0-8288-1861-4*, S25225) Fr & Eur.

Clinical Vademecum of the Medical Practice (Vademecum Clinique du Medecin Practicien) V. Fattorusso & Otto Ritter. 13th ed. 1990. (FRE.). 1760p. 125.00 (*0-7859-4631-4*, F137430) Fr & Eur.

Clinical Veterinary Dentistry. Ed. by Robert B. Wiggs. 1997. LC 96-43290. 762p. pap. text 49.95 (*0-397-51385-2*) Lppncott W & W.

C D

***Clinical Vignettes for the USMLE Step 1: Self-Assessment & Review.** McGraw-Hill Staff. 2nd ed. 2001. (Pretest Self-Assessment & Review Ser.). (Illus.). 300p. pap. 24.95 (*0-07-137376-4*, Apple Lange Med) McGraw.

Clinical Vignettes for the USMLE Step 2. McGraw-Hill Editors. 2nd ed. 2000. (Pretest Clinical Science Ser.). (Illus.). 309p. pap. 24.95 (*0-07-136453-6*) McGraw-Hill Prof.

Clinical Vignettes for USMLE. Ed. by McGraw-Hill Editors. 1999. (Illus.). 287p. pap. 24.95 (*0-07-135558-8*) McGraw-Hill Educ Grp.

Clinical Virology. Douglas D. Richman et al. 1996. LC 96-48084. text (*0-443-07653-7*) Church.

Clinical Virology in Oral Medicine & Dentistry. Crispian Scully & Laksham P. Samaranayake. 1992. (Illus.). 499p. (C). text 185.00 (*0-521-40102-X*) Cambridge U Pr.

Clinical Visual Optics. A. G. Bennett & Ronald B. Rabbetts. 2nd ed. 1990. (Illus.). 529p. 115.00 (*0-7506-0454-9*) Buttrwrth-Heinemann.

***Clinical Vivas for the FRCA Final.** Mills et al. 2001. (Illus.). 256p. pap. (*1-84110-070-6*) Greenwich Med GBR. *Dist:* JAMCO Dist.

Clinical Voice Disorders: An Interdisciplinary Approach. Arnold E. Aronson. 3rd ed. 1990. (Illus.). 398p. text 49.00 (*0-86577-337-8*) Thieme Med Pubs.

Clinical Voice Pathology. Bernice K. Gerdeman et al. 3rd ed. 2000. LC 99-57053. 544p. pap. text 70.95 (*0-7693-0005-7*) Singular Publishing.

Clinical Voice Pathology: Theory & Management. Joseph Stemple et al. 2nd ed. 1994. LC 94-27024. (Illus.). 342p. (C). 55.00 (*1-56593-342-7*, 0640) Thomson Learn.

Clinical vs. Statistical Prediction: A Theoretical Analysis & a Review of the Evidence. Paul E. Meehl. 1996. LC 96-5094. reprint ed. 40.00 (*1-56821-831-1*) Aronson.

Clinical Wisdom & Interventions in Critical Care: A Thinking-in-Action Approach. Patricia Benner et al. Ed. by Thomas Eoyang. 1998. cd-rom 699.00 (*0-7216-7512-3*); LC 98-12040. xx, 588p. (C). pap. text 25.00 (*0-7216-7511-5*) Saunders.

Clinical Work with Adolescents. Judith M. Mishne. 1986. LC 86-148222. 320p. 32.95 (*0-02-921260-X*) Free Pr.

Clinical Work with Children. Judith M. Mishne. 1983. LC 82-70990. 365p. 32.95 (*0-02-921630-3*) Free Pr.

Clinical Workbook for Psychotherapists. Robert J. Langs. 1992. 528p. pap. text (*1-85575-004-X*) Karnac Bks GBR. *Dist:* Other Pr LLC.

Clinical Worksheet. Jane A. Sennett. 1999. 250p. pap. 9.95 (*0-9670164-1-X*) Jalor Med.

Clinical Wound Management. Prem P. Gogia. 1995. 264p. pap. 35.00 (*1-55642-234-2*, 42342) SLACK Inc.

Clinically Applied Microcirculation Research. Ed. by John H. Barker et al. 1995. LC 95-1029. 512p. 289.95 (*0-8493-4870-6*, 4870) CRC Pr.

***Clinically Based Long-Term Care Survey Prep Guide.** Janie L. Krechting. 2001. LC 2001-22199. 440p. spiral bd. 199.00 (*0-8342-1966-2*) Aspen Pub.

Clinically Integrated Histology. David H. Cormack. 1997. LC 97-26178. 336p. pap. text 42.95 (*0-7817-1211-4*) Lppncott W & W.

Clinically Organ-Confined Adenocarcinoma of the Prostate: Natural History, Selection Criteria for Radical Prostatectomy & Prognostic Factors Based on Long-Term Follow-Up. Ed. by H. P. Schmid. 1996. (Illus.). 74p. pap. 29.00 (*3-7985-0998-0*) Spr-Verlag.

Clinically Oriented Anatomy. Keith L. Moore. (Illus.). 3rd ed. 1992. 930p. 53.00 (*0-683-06133-X*); 4th ed. 1998. LC 98-48704. 1,164p. (C). pap. text 65.00 (*0-683-06141-0*) Lppncott W & W.

Clinically Speaking: The Authentic Language of Clinical Medicine. Jones Staff. 1994. 144p. text 155.00 incl. cd-rom (*0-471-94417-3*) Wiley.

Clinician Pocket Reference. Leonard G. Gomella. 8th ed. 1996. 720p. (C). pap. 34.95 (*0-8385-1476-6*) McGraw-Hill Educ Grp.

Clinician to Academician: A Handbook for Those Who Aspire to Become Faculty Members. Caroline R. Brayley. 1996. 65p. (Orig.). pap. 20.00 (*1-56900-031-X*, 1141) Am Occup Therapy.

Clinician's Companion: A Study Guide for Effective & Humane Patient Care. David H. Alpers & Stephen M. Wittenberg. 1986. (Illus.). 224p. 29.95 (*0-316-03511-4*, Little Brwn Med Div) Lppncott W & W.

Clinician's Complete Reference to Complementary Medicine. Donald W. Novey. 1999. 855p. 39.95 (*0-323-00755-4*) Mosby Inc.

***Clinician's Drug Reference 2002.** Leonard G. Gomella. 2001. 224p. pap. 14.95 (*0-07-137934-7*) McGraw-Hill Prof.

Clinician's Electronic Thesaurus, Version 5.0: Software to Streamline Psychological Report Writing. Edward L. Zuckerman. 2000. (Clinician's Toolbox Ser.). 64p. pap. 49.95 incl. cd-rom (*1-57230-586-X*, 8R0586) Guilford Pubns.

Clinician's Guide to Ace Inhibition. Ed. by John Cleland. 1993. (Illus.). 224p. text (*0-443-04855-X*) Church.

Clinician's Guide to Alaryngeal Speech Therapy. Minnie S. Graham. 1997. LC 97-21510. 395p. pap. text 49.99 (*0-7506-9862-4*) Buttrwrth-Heinemann.

Clinician's Guide to Alternative Medicine. Rosenberg. 1999. 7p. (*0-7506-9639-7*) Buttrwrth-Heinemann.

Clinicians Guide to Aspirin. A. Bayer. 1999. (Illus.). 192p. text (*0-412-81900-7*) E A GBR. *Dist:* OUP.

Clinician's Guide to Chemotherapy Pharmacokinetics & Pharmacodynamics. Ed. by Louise B. Grochow & Matthew M. Ames. 1997. LC 97-30019. 504p. 85.00 (*0-683-18111-4*) Lppncott W & W.

Clinician's Guide to Cocaine Addiction: Theory, Research, & Treatment. Ed. by Thomas R. Kosten & Herbert D. Kleber. 1992. LC 92-1521. (Substance Abuse Ser.). 405p. 45.00 (*0-89862-192-5*) Guilford Pubns.

***Clinician's Guide to Controversial Illnesses: Chronic Fatigue Syndrome, Fibromyalgia & Multiple Chemical Sensitivities.** Renee R. Taylor et al. 2001. LC 00-47837. 182p. 34.45 (*1-56887-068-X*, Prof Resc Pr) Pro Resource.

***Clinician's Guide to Diagnosing Lung Cancer.** Pamela Calarese et al. 2001. (Illus.). (C). pap. text 29.95 (*0-7637-1861-0*, 1861-0) Jones & Bartlett.

***Clinicians' Guide to Epilepsy.** P. E. M. Smith & S. J. Wallace. 2001. (Arnold Publication). 240p. text (*0-340-76293-4*) E A GBR. *Dist:* OUP.

Clinician's Guide to Fungal Disease. Stephen O. B. Roberts et al. 1984. LC 84-14932. (Infectious Disease & Therapy Ser.: Vol. 5). (Illus.). 264p. text 135.00 (*0-8247-7190-7*) Dekker.

Clinician's Guide to Getting Better Bit(e) By Bit(e) Janet Treasure & Ulrike Schmidt. 1997. LC 97-197624. 240p. (*0-86377-730-9*) Psychol Pr GBR. *Dist:* Taylor & Francis.

***Clinicians Guide to Headache.** Silberstein et al. 2001. 96p. pap. (*1-901865-89-4*) Isis Med GBR. *Dist:* Bks Intl VA.

Clinicians' Guide to Helicobacter Pylori. J. Calam. 1995. (Clinicians' Guide Ser.). (Illus.). 192p. (*0-412-74000-1*) E A GBR. *Dist:* OUP.

Clinician's Guide to Inflamatory Bowel Disease. Alastair Forbes. 1997. (Clinicians' Guide Ser.). 280p. (*0-412-78850-0*) E A GBR. *Dist:* OUP.

Clinician's Guide to Legal Issues in Psychotherapy: Or Proceed with Caution. William H. Reid. 1999. LC 99-19558. 198p. pap. 22.95 (*1-891944-08-8*) Zeig Tucker Theisen.

Clinicians' Guide to Lipids & Coronary Heart Disease. D. Betteridge & J. M. Morrell. 1997. (Illus.). 292p. pap. (*0-412-75720-6*) E A GBR. *Dist:* OUP.

Clinician's Guide to Managed Behavioral Care. Norman Winegar. 2nd ed. 1996. LC 95-45916. (Illus.). 324p. 49.95 (*0-7890-6012-4*); pap. 24.95 (*0-7890-6013-2*) Haworth Pr.

Clinician's Guide to Managed Mental Health Care. Norman Winegar. 1992. LC 91-22226. 342p. lib. bdg. 49.95 (*1-56024-204-3*); 2nd ed. 310p. pap. 19.95 (*1-56024-205-1*) Haworth Pr.

Clinician's Guide to Medical & Surgical Abortion. Maureen Paul et al. Ed. by William Schmitt. 1999. LC 98-43931. (Illus.). 395p. text (*0-443-07529-8*) Church.

Clinician's Guide to Medical Informatics, the Internet & Telemedicine. E. Coiera. 1997. LC 97-199098. 408p. pap. (*0-412-75710-9*) E A GBR. *Dist:* OUP.

Clinician's Guide to Menopause. Ed. by Donna E. Stewart & Gail E. Robinson. 1997. LC 97-3185. (Clinical Practice Ser.). 272p. text 39.00 (*0-88048-754-2*, 8754) Am Psychiatric.

Clinician's Guide to Neuro-Psychological Assessment. Ed. by Rodney D. Vanderploeg. 1994. 320p. text 69.95 (*0-8058-1253-9*); 1994. 320p. pap. text 34.50 (*0-8058-1254-7*); 2nd ed. 1999. LC 99-31882. 551p. pap. (*0-8058-2834-6*) L Erlbaum Assocs.

Clinician's Guide to Nutrition in HIV & AIDS. Cade Fields-Gardner et al. 1997. 180p. 26.00 (*0-88091-147-6*); 1996. LC 96-36494. (*0-88091-148-4*) Am Dietetic Assn.

Clinician's Guide to Obesity. Finer. 1999. 192p. pap. 72.95 (*0-412-75480-0*, Chap & Hall NY) Chapman & Hall.

Clinicians' Guide to Oesophageal Disease. Stephen P. Wilkinson. 1999. LC 98-71761. (An Arnold Publication). (Illus.). 186p. text (*0-412-80910-9*) E A GBR. *Dist:* OUP.

Clinicians' Guide to Pain. T. W. I. Lovel & W. U. Hassan. 1999. (Clinicians' Guide Ser.). (Illus.). 214p. pap. (*0-340-74097-3*) E A GBR. *Dist:* OUP.

***Clinician's Guide to PPS.** Charles W. Tidd et al. 2001. (Illus.). 185p. pap. (*1-930304-15-3*) Home Care Univ.

Clinician's Guide to Psychodrama. Eva Leveton. 2nd ed. 1991. LC 91-4823. Orig. Title: Psychodrama for the Timid Clinician. (Illus.). 192p. pap. 29.95 (*0-8261-2262-0*) Springer Pub.

***Clinician's Guide to Psychodrama.** Eva Leveton. 3rd ed. 2001. LC 00-67913. Orig. Title: Psychodrama for the Timid Clinician. 224p. (*0-8261-2263-9*) Springer Pub.

***Clinicians' Guide to Sleep Medicine.** Neil J. Douglas. 2002. (Arnold Publication). 224p. pap. text 39.95 (*0-340-74205-4*) OUP.

Clinician's Guide to Successful Treatment Planning for Managed Care. Alex D'Alessandro. 1995. LC 95-21475. 79.00 (*0-935255-43-5*) Of Course Pubns.

Clinician's Guide to the Expanded Evaluation of Dysphagia in Adults. Russell H. Mills. 2000. LC 99-39484. (For Clinicians by Clinicians Ser.). (Illus.). xiv, 349p. pap. (*0-89079-836-2*) PRO-ED.

Clinician's Guide to the Personality Profiles of Alcohol & Drug Abusers: Typological Descriptions Using the MMPI. Donald J. Tosi et al. 1993. LC 93-24274. (Illus.). 156p. (C). text 41.95 (*0-398-05885-7*) C C Thomas.

Clinician's Guide to Ulcerative Colitis & Crohn's Disease. P. P. Jewell et al. 1992. (Illus.). 80p. (Orig.). pap. text (*0-443-04803-7*) Church.

Clinicians' Guide to Viral Hepatitis. Tibbs. 1999. 192p. pap. 74.95 (*0-412-79120-X*, Chap & Hall NY) Chapman & Hall.

Clinician's Guidebook to ADHD: Helping Parents Help Their Children. Edward H. Jacobs. 2000. LC 00-20328. xx, 247p. 35.00 (*0-7657-0273-8*) Aronson.

Clinician's Handbook: Integrated Diagnostics, Assessment & Intervention in Adult & Adolescent Psychopathology. Robert G. Meyer & Sarah E. Deitsch. 4th ed. 1995. LC 95-4215. 528p. (C). 105.00 (*0-205-17181-8*) Allyn.

Clinician's Handbook of Natural Healing: The First Comprehensive Guide to Scientific Peer Review. Gary Null. 1998. LC 97-75439. 880p. 60.00 (*1-57566-284-1*) Kensgtn Pub Corp.

Clinician's Handbook of Natural Healing: The First Scientific Guide to the Treatment Benefits of Herbs & Supplements. Gary Null. 2000. 880p. reprint ed. pap. 25.00 (*1-57566-720-7*, Knsington) Kensgtn Pub Corp.

***Clinician's Handbook of Natural Medicine.** Joseph E. Pizzorno et al. 2001. 335p. (*0-443-07080-6*) Church GBR. *Dist:* Saunders.

Clinician's Handbook of Prescription Drugs. Seymour Ehrenpreis & Eli Ehrenpreis. 2001. LC 2001-30501. 979p. pap. 34.95 (*0-07-134385-7*) McGraw-Hill Prof.

Clinician's Handbook of Preventive Services, Set. 1995. (Medical Ser.). lib. bdg. 627.95 (*0-8490-7514-9*) Gordon Pr.

Clinician's Handbook of Preventive Services: Put Prevention into Practice. 1995. (Illus.). 342p. (Orig.). (C). pap. text 40.00 (*0-7881-2294-0*) DIANE Pub.

Clinician's Handbook of Preventive Services: Put Prevention into Practice. Larry L. Dickey. 2nd ed. 1998. (Illus.). 524p. (C). pap. text 60.00 (*0-7881-7246-8*) DIANE Pub.

Clinician's Handbook of Preventive Services: Put Prevention into Practice. U. S. Public Health Service Staff et al. 2nd ed. 1998. (Illus.). 498p. (C). pap. 20.00 (*1-883205-32-8*) Intl Med Pub.

Clinician's Management Handbook. Ed. by David M. Hansell & Brian Salter. 1995. (Illus.). 195p. pap. text 42.00 (*0-7020-1915-1*) Saunders.

Clinician's Pocket Guide to Home Parenteral Medications. Roger S. Klotz & Kathryn T. Andrusko-Furphy. 2nd ed. 1993. 233p. pap. text 8.95 (*1-883202-00-0*) Spec Clin Srvs.

Clinician's Pocket Guide to Home Parenteral Medications. 3rd ed. 1994. pap. text 12.95 (*1-883202-01-9*); 4th ed. 1995. pap. text 19.95 (*1-883202-02-7*) Spec Clin Srvs.

Clinician's Pocket Reference. 9th ed. 2001. 720p. (C). pap. 34.95 (*0-8385-1552-5*, Apple Lange Med) McGraw.

***Clinician's Pocket Reference: And Drug Reference 2002.** Leonard G. Gomella. 9th ed. 2002. (Illus.). pap. 39.95 (*0-07-139232-7*) McGraw-Hill Prof.

Clinician's Practical Guide to Attention-Deficit Hyperactivity Disorder. Marianne Mercugliano et al. 1998. LC 98-35194. 39.95 (*1-55766-358-0*) P H Brookes.

Clinician's Reading List on Alcohol & Other Drug Dependencies. 1992. lib. bdg. 88.95 (*0-8490-8746-5*) Gordon Pr.

Clinician's Thesaurus: A Guidebook to Wording Psychological Reports & Other Evaluations. Edward L. Zuckerman. 2nd ed. 1992. (Clinician's Toolbox Ser.). 174p. reprint ed. pap. text 19.95 (*0-9622281-2-5*) Three Wishes.

Clinician's Thesaurus: The Guidebook for Writing Psychological Reports Edward L. Zuckerman. 5th ed. 2000. LC 00-699878. (Clinician's Toolbox Ser.). 385p. pap. 37.00 (*1-57230-569-X*, 8R0569) Guilford Pubns.

Clinico-Pathological Atlas of Congenital Fundus Disorders. Juan Orellana & Alan H. Friedman. 1993. LC 92-49529. (Illus.). 268p. 236.00 (*0-387-97936-0*) Spr-Verlag.

Clinico-Pharmacological Models for the Assay of Topical Corticoids. H. Wendt & P. J. Frosch. 1982. (Illus.). 64p. pap. 28.75 (*3-8055-3538-4*) S Karger.

Clinicopathologic Correlations in Dermatopathology. Clay J. Cockerell. 1995. LC 95-3181. (Illus.). 144p. 59.50 (*0-89640-270-3*) Igaku-Shoin.

Clinicopathologic Principles for Veterinary Medicine. Ed. by Wayne F. Robinson & Clive R. Huxtable. 1988. (Illus.). 448p. text 100.00 (*0-521-30883-6*) Cambridge U Pr.

Clinics, Contraception & Communication: Evaluation Studies of Family Planning Programs in Four Latin American Countries. Ed. by J. Mayone Stycos. 1973. LC 79-184865. (Illus.). 29.00 (*0-89197-625-6*) Irvington.

ClintonCare: Putting Government in Charge of Your Health. Barry Asmus. 1994. 101p. (Orig.). pap. 9.95 (*0-9640421-0-X*) Amerpress.

Clinton's Specialist Quota: Shaky Premises, Questionable Consequences. David Dranove & William D. White. 1994. (Special Studies in Health Reform). 32p. (Orig.). pap. 9.95 (*0-8447-7024-8*, AEI Pr) Am Enterprise.

Clio Medica: A Series of Primers on the History of Medicine Ed. by Edward B. Krumbhaar. reprint ed. (*0-404-58900-6*) AMS Pr.

Clitoris. Thomas P. Lowry. 1976. LC 73-704. (Illus.). 304p. 22.50 (*0-87527-112-X*) Green.

CLMA Guide to Managing a Clinical Laboratory. Ed. by Bettina G. Martin. 1991. (Illus.). 95p. (Orig.). pap. text 35.00 (*0-9625414-1-9*) Clinical Lab Mgmnt Assn.

CLMA Guide to Managing a Clinical Laboratory. Ed. by Anthony S. Kuree et al. 2nd rev. ed. 1996. (Illus.). 134p. (Orig.). pap. text 35.00 (*0-9625414-3-5*) Clinical Lab Mgmnt Assn.

CLMA Guide to Managing a Clinical Laboratory. Ed. by Anthony S. Kurec et al. 3rd rev. ed. 2000. (Illus.). pap. text (*1-892942-02-X*) Clinical Lab Mgmnt Assn.

CLMA Guide to Medicare Compliance for the Laboratory. Jeffrey Boothe & Julie Gayken. 1997. 332p. ring bd. 399.00 (*0-9625414-8-6*) Clinical Lab Mgmnt Assn.

Cloak of Competence: Stigma in the Lives of the Mentally Retarded. Robert B. Edgerton. rev. ed. 1993. LC 93-5292. 276p. (C). text 48.00 (*0-520-08225-7*); pap. text 17.95 (*0-520-08226-5*) U CA Pr.

Clock & the Mirror: Girolamo Cardano & Renaissance Medicine. Nancy G. Siraisi. 1997. LC 96-46354. xiv, 361p. 57.50 (*0-691-01189-3*) Princeton U Pr.

Clock Drawing: A Neuropsychological Analysis. Morris Freedman et al. 1994. LC 93-13481. (Illus.). 192p. (C). text 39.95 (*0-19-505906-9*, 9427) OUP.

Cloning Systems: A Laboratory Manual. Ed. by Bruce Birren et al. 1998. (Genome Analysis Ser.: No. 3). (Illus.). 650p. (C). text 230.00 (*0-87969-512-9*); pap. text 145.00 (*0-87969-513-7*) Cold Spring Harbor.

Cloning Vectors. P. H. Pouwels et al. 1986. 296p. ring bd., suppl. ed. 58.00 (*0-444-90452-2*) Elsevier.

Close Encounters: A Relational View of the Therapeutic Process. Robert Winer. 1994. LC 93-5090. (Library of Object Relations). 296p. 40.00 (*0-87668-165-8*) Aronson.

Close Relationship Loss: Theoretical Approaches. Ed. by Terri L. Orbuch. 1992. (Illus.). 233p. 148.00 (*0-387-97727-9*) Spr-Verlag.

Close Relationships: Perspectives on the Meaning of Intimacy. Ed. by George Levinger & Harold L. Raush. 1977. LC 77-900. (Illus.). 208p. 30.00 (*0-87023-238-X*) U of Mass Pr.

Close Relationships: The Study of Love & Friendship. Duncan Cramer. 1998. LC 98-13915. (Arnold Publication). (Illus.). 224p. text 75.00 (*0-340-62533-3*); pap. text 24.95 (*0-340-62534-1*) OUP.

Close Relationships & Socioemotional Development, 7. Jay Belsky et al. Ed. by Shmuel Shulman. 1995. (Human Development Ser.: Vol. 7). (Illus.). 248p. 77.00 (*1-56750-114-1*, Ablex) Greenwood.

Close to the Bone: Life-Threatening Illness & the Search for Meaning. Jean S. Bolen. 1998. 224p. per. 12.00 (*0-684-83530-4*, Touchstone) S&S Trade Pap.

Close to the Knives: A Memoir of Disintegration. David Wojnarowicz. 1991. LC 90-50210. 288p. (Orig.). pap. 14.00 (*0-679-73227-6*) Vin Bks.

Close up on Psychology: Supplemental Readings from the APA Monitor. Ed. by Jill N. Reich et al. 1997. LC 97-10904. 168p. pap. 9.95 (*1-55798-427-1*) Am Psychol.

Closed Functional Treatment of Fractures. Augusto Sarmiento & Loren L. Latta. 1981. (Illus.). 608p. 231.00 (*0-387-10384-8*) Spr-Verlag.

Closed Head Injury. D. Eugene Wiley & Carol E. Roberts. Ed. by Oliver D. Grin & Dorothy L. Bouwman. 1992. (Patient Education Ser.). (Illus.). 26p. (Orig.). pap. text 4.00 (*0-929689-46-1*) Ludann Co.

Closed-Head Injury: A Clinical Source Book. Peter G. Bernad. 2nd ed. 1998. LC 98-86445. 475p. 100.00 (*0-327-00276-X*, 6057311) LEXIS Pub.

Closed-Head Injury: A Clinical Source Book, 1999 Supplement, Pocketpart. Peter G. Bernad. 1999. 63p. (*0-327-01667-1*, 6057412) LEXIS Pub.

Closed Head Injury: Its Pathology & Legal Medicine. Rufus Crompton. 1988. 100p. (*0-683-13012-9*) E A GBR. *Dist:* Williams & Wilkins.

Closet: A Therapeutic Workbook for Adult Survivors of Childhood Abuse. Susan Wolf. 1995. (Illus.). 187p. ring bd., wbk. ed. 49.95 (*1-888474-00-9*); 40p. ring bd., wbk. ed. 14.95 (*1-888474-01-7*) Little Tree Pr.

Closing & Opening of a Millennium: A Journey from Old to New Relationships in the Work Setting. Bonnie Wesorick. 1996. LC 96-70090. (Wisdom from the Field Nursing Ser.: Bk. 2). (Illus.). 153p. (Orig.). (C). pap. 15.00 (*0-9648264-1-0*) Pract Field.

Closing & Opening of a Millennium: A Journey from Old to New Thinking. Bonnie Wesorick. 1995. LC 95-71362. (Wisdom from the Field Nursing Ser.: Bk. 1). (Illus.). 170p. (Orig.). (C). pap. 15.00 (*0-9648264-0-2*) Pract Field.

Closing the Gap: Symbolic vs. Subsymbolic Processing. Ed. by John Dinsmore. 1992. (Technical Monographs & Edited Collections in Cognitive Science). 280p. (C). text 59.95 (*0-8058-1079-X*) L Erlbaum Assocs.

Closing the Theory-Practice Gap: A New Paradigm for Nursing. Gary Rolfe. 1996. LC 96-15969. 224p. pap. text 40.00 (*0-7506-2616-X*) Buttrwrth-Heinemann.

Closing Your Practice. AMA Staff. 1998. (Career Development Ser.). 80p. 27.95 (*0-89970-889-7*) AMA.

***Clostridia: Biotechnology & Medical Applications.** Hubert Bahl & Peter Durre. 2001. 292p. 115.00 (*3-527-30175-5*) Wiley.

Clostridia: Molecular Biology & Pathogenesis. Ed. by Julian Rood et al. 1997. LC 96-37807. (Illus.). 480p. text 129.95 (*0-12-595020-9*) Morgan Kaufmann.

Clostridia in Gastrointestinal Disease. Ed. by S. Peter Borriello. 1985. 248p. 143.00 (0-8493-5656-3, RC862, CRC Reprint) Franklin.

Clostridial Neurotoxins: The Molecular Pathogenesis of Tetanus & Botulism. Ed. by C. Montecucco. 1995. LC 15-12910. (Current Topics in Microbiology & Immunology Ser.: Vol. 195). (Illus.). 278p. 166.00 (3-540-58452-8) Spr-Verlag.

Clostridium Botulinum: Ecology & Control in Foods. Ed. by Andreas H. Hauschild & Karen L. Dodds. 1992. LC 92-29096. (Food Science & Technology Ser.: No. 54). (Illus.). 440p. text 185.00 (0-8247-8748-X) Dekker.

Clostridium Difficile. Ed. by K. Aktories et al. 2000. (Current Topics in Microbiology & Immunology Ser.: Vol. 250). (Illus.). 170p. 94.00 (3-540-67291-5) Spr-Verlag.

Clostridium Difficile. Ed. by Rial D. Rolfe & Sydney M. Finegold. 1988. (Role in Intestinal Disease Ser.). 384p. text 146.00 (0-12-593410-6) Acad Pr.

Clothing—Healthful, Hazardous, Styles & Image Psychology: Index of New Information & Medical Research Bible. American Health Research Institute Staff. 1994. 150p. 57.50 (0-7883-0144-6); pap. 47.50 (0-7883-0145-4) ABBE Pubs Assn.

Clothing for the Handicapped, the Aged & Other People with Special Needs. Adeline M. Hoffman. 1979. (Illus.). 212p. 41.95 (0-398-03860-0) C C Thomas.

Clown Ambassador of Health Vol. 2: Your Habits Are Knocking at Your Door. Steven L. Doernberg. 1996. 9p. (Orig.). pap. (0-9648663-1-5) Clown Natural Hlth.

Club & Coral Mushrooms (Clavarias) of the United States & Canada. William C. Coker. 1974. LC 74-82202. (Illus.). 320p. reprint ed. pap. 7.95 (0-486-23101-1) Dover.

Clubfoot: The Present & a View of the Future. Ed. by George W. Simons. 1993. (Illus.). 587p. 244.00 (0-387-97876-3) Spr-Verlag.

Clues: Investigating Solutions in Brief Therapy. Steve De Shazer. 1988. LC 87-34799. (Professional Bks.). 202p. 23.95 (0-393-70054-2) Norton.

Clues to Diagnosis in Dermatopathology, Vol. I. A. Bernard Ackerman et al. 1991. LC 89-18029. (Illus.). 432p. text 160.00 (0-89189-296-6, 16-1-048-00) Am Soc Clinical.

Clues to Diagnosis in Dermatopathology. A. Bernard Ackerman. Vol. II. 1992. 436p. text 50.00 (0-89189-339-3, D16-1-051-00); Vol. III. 1993. (Illus.). 427p. 50.00 (0-89189-354-7) Am Soc Clinical.

Clumsy Child Syndromes: Descriptions, Evaluation, & Remediation. Bryant J. Cratty. 1993. LC 92-34999. 649p. text 81.00 (3-7186-0548-1); pap. text 57.00 (3-7186-0575-9) Gordon & Breach.

Clusterin: Role in Vertebrate Development, Function, & Adaptation. Judith A. Harmony. 1996. (Molecular Biology Intelligence Unit Ser.). 188p. pap. 89.95 (0-412-09921-7, VNR) Wiley.

Clusterin in Normal Brain Functions & During Degeneration. Caleb E. Finch. 1999. LC 98-50223. (Neuroscience Intelligence Unit Ser.: Vol. 2). (Illus.). 123p. 99.00 (1-57059-583-6) Landes Bioscience.

Cluttering: A Clinical Perspective. Myers. 1995. 148p. reprint ed. pap. 29.95 (1-56593-543-8, 0488) Thomson Learn.

CMA Review Manual. Cody. 1998. (Medical Assisting Ser.). tchr. ed. 14.95 (0-8273-7184-5) Delmar.

CMEA Chemotherapy Symposium, 1984. S. Kerpel Eckhardt & E. Fronius. 1985. 646p. (C). (963-05-4188-2) Akade Kiado HUN. *Dist:* St Mut.

CMO: A Natural Treatment for Arthritis & Other Joint-Related Diseases. Rita Elkins. 1997. (Woodland Health Ser.). pap. text 3.95 (1-58054-010-4) Woodland UT.

CMV-Related Immunopathology: 1st International Consensus Round Table Meeting, Frankfurt, August 1997. Ed. by Martin Scholz et al. 1997. LC 97-42392. (Monographs in Virology: Vol. 21, 1998). (Illus.). xii, 308p. 236.50 (3-8055-6602-6) S Karger.

CNOR Study Guide. Linda Groah. 4th rev. ed. 1999. 364p. pap., stu. ed. 40.00 (0-9670222-0-7) Certi Board.

CNRH Analogues in Cancer & Human Reproduction: Benign & Malignant Tumors. Ed. by B. H. Vickery & Bruno Lunenfeld. 1990. (C). lib. bdg. 135.00 (0-7923-8930-1) Kluwer Academic.

CNRH Analogues in Cancer & Human Reproduction: Precocious Puberty, Contraception & Safety Issues, Vol. 4. Ed. by B. H. Vickery & Bruno Lunenfeld. 1990. (C). text 129.00 (0-7923-8931-X) Kluwer Academic.

CNS Aging & Its Neuropharmacology: Experimental & Clinical Aspects. Ed. by W. Meier-Ruge. 1979. (Interdisciplinary Topics in Gerontology Ser.: Vol. 15). (Illus.). pap. 76.75 (3-8055-2980-5) S Karger.

CNS Control Mechanisms on Glucose Metabolism. E. H. Grote. 1981. (Acta Neurochirurgica Ser.: No. 31). (Illus.). 160p. pap. 47.00 (0-387-81619-4) Spr-Verlag.

CNS Injuries: Cellular Responses & Pharmacological Strategies. M. Berry & Ann Logan. 1998. LC 97-52407. (Pharmacology & Toxicology: Basic & Clinical Aspects Ser.). 226p. lib. bdg. 129.95 (0-8493-8309-9) CRC Pr.

CNS Neurotransmitters & Neuromodulators: Acetylcholine. Trevor E. Stone. 1994. LC 94-26310. 272p. 178.95 (0-8493-7630-0) CRC Pr.

CNS Neurotransmitters & Neuromodulators: Dopamine. Ed. by Trevor E. Stone. 1996. LC 95-45931. (CNS Neurotransmitters & Neuromodulators Ser.). 272p. 159.95 (0-8493-7632-7) CRC Pr.

CNS Neurotransmitters & Neuromodulators: Neuroactive Steroids. Trevor W. Stone. 1996. LC 95-46396. (CNS Neurotransmitters & Neuromodulators Ser.). 256p. 189.95 (0-8493-7633-5) CRC Pr.

CNS Protection During Hypothermic Circulatory Arrest. W. Baumgartner. 1997. (Medical Intelligence Unit Ser.). 200p. (C). 89.95 (0-412-10791-0) Chapman & Hall.

CNS Regeneration: Basic Science & Clinical Advances. Ed. by Mark H. Tuszynski & Jeffrey Kordower. 1998. LC 98-87916. (Illus.). 678p. (C). 89.95 (0-12-705070-1) Acad Pr.

Co-Constructing Therapeutic Consultations: A Consultation of Restraint. Ivan Inger & Jeri Inger. 1992. 112p. pap. text (1-85575-023-6) Karnac Bks GBR. *Dist:* Other Pr LLC.

Co-Counseling for Married Couples. Harvey Jackins. 1965. pap. 2.00 (0-911214-13-5) Rational Isl.

Co-Op Home Care: A Win-Win for Client & Caregiver. Rick Surpin. 1991. 35p. pap. text 10.00 (1-55516-643-1, 6126) Natl Conf State Legis.

Co-Operative Enterprise in the Health & Social Care Sectors. United Nations, Department for Policy Coordination Staff. 1997. LC 97-193676. 20.00 (92-1-130179-3) UN.

Co-Planar Stereotaxic Atlas of the Human Brain: 3-D Proportional System: An Approach to Cerebral Imaging. J. Talairach & P. Tournoux. 1988. (Illus.). 132p. 199.00 (0-86577-293-2) Thieme Med Pubs.

Coach: How to Make the Human Connection with Your Doctor. Carol L. Fernow. 1995. 116p. (Orig.). pap. 16.95 (0-9643160-5-6) Hlth Care Systs.

Coaches Guide to Drugs & Sport. Kevin R. Ringhofer & Martha E. Harding. 1995. LC 95-16965. (Illus.). 208p. pap. 21.95 (0-87322-715-8, PRIN0715) Human Kinetics.

Coaches Guide to Sport Psychology. Rainer Martens. 1987. LC 87-16814. (Illus.). 208p. pap. text 25.00 (0-87322-022-6, BMAR0022) Human Kinetics.

Coaches Guide to Sport Rehabilitation. Steven R. Tippett. 1990. LC 90-5659. (Illus.). 168p. pap. text 25.00 (0-88011-399-5, PTIP0399) Human Kinetics.

Coaching to Win: Building Your Business by Building Your Team. W. Bradford Swift. 1997. LC 97-60330. 106p. pap. 19.95 (0-935078-64-9, 97-060330) Veterinary Hlthcare.

Coagulase-Negative Staphylococci. Ed. by K. H. Schleifer & Peter-Anders Mardh. 1986. (Illus.). 222p. (Orig.). 78.50 (91-22-00783-0) Coronet Bks.

Coagulation. ring bd. 250.00 (1-56238-236-5, SC12-L) NCCLS.

Coagulation & Bleeding Disorders: The Role of Factor VIII & Von Willebrand Factor. Zimmerman & Zaverio Ruggeri. 1988. (Hematology Ser.: Vol. 9). (Illus.). 392p. text 210.00 (0-8247-8013-2) Dekker.

Coagulation & Blood Transfusion. Ed. by C. Th. Smit Sibinga. 1991. (Developments in Hematology & Immunology Ser.). (C). text 91.00 (0-7923-1331-3) Kluwer Academic.

Coagulation & Cancer. Ed. by Maria B. Donati. 1988. (Journal: Vol. 18, No. 1, 1988). (Illus.). 72p. pap. 30.50 (3-8055-4768-4) S Karger.

Coagulation & Lipids. Ed. by Robert F. Zwaal. 1988. 208p. 135.00 (0-8493-6762-X, QP93, CRC Reprint) Franklin.

Coagulation-Inflammation Interface: Coagulation Assembly on Leukocytes. Dario C. Altieri. 1997. (Molecular Biology Intelligence Unit Ser.). 203p. pap. 89.95 (0-412-13991-X) Chapman & Hall.

Coalescent Argumentation. Michael A. Gilbert. 1997. LC 96-32875. 176p. 36.00 (0-8058-2519-3); pap. 18.00 (0-8058-2520-7) L Erlbaum Assocs.

Coalition Formation. Ed. by A. A. Wilke. 1985. (Advances in Psychology Ser.: Vol. 24). 294p. 87.00 (0-444-87702-9) Elsevier.

Coated Pharmaceutical Dosage Forms: Fundamentals, Manufacturing Techniques, Biopharmaceutical Aspects, Test Methods, & Raw Materials. Kurt H. Bauer. Tr. by Erdmute Stanienda from GER. 1998. LC 97-52405. 119.95 (0-8493-7518-5) CRC Pr.

Coblentz Vigilanc Performance. Coblentz A. Asid. 1989. lib. bdg. 171.00 (0-7923-0302-4) Kluwer Academic.

Cocaine. M. S. Gold. 1993. LC 92-45165. (Drugs of Abuse: Vol. 3). (Illus.). 248p. (C). text 47.00 (0-306-44386-4, Kluwer Plenum) Kluwer Academic.

Cocaine. Roger D. Weiss et al. 2nd ed. 1993. LC 93-15802. 204p. 22.50 (0-88048-549-3, 8549) Am Psychiatric.

Cocaine: A Clinician's Handbook. Ed. by Arnold M. Washton & Mark S. Gold. 1987. LC 87-12015. 262p. 40.00 (0-89862-725-7, 2725) Guilford Pubns.

Cocaine: A New Epidemic. Chris-Ellyn Johanson. 1987. LC 85-25969. (Encyclopedia of Psychoactive Drugs Ser.: No. 1). (Illus.). 124p. (YA). (gr. 7-12). lib. bdg. 19.95 (0-87754-765-3) Chelsea Hse.

Cocaine: A Symposium. Ed. by Carla J. Brink. 1985. LC 85-17797. (Illus.). 69p. (Orig.). pap. text 10.00 (0-9615363-0-6) Wis Inst Drug Abuse.

Cocaine: A Treatment Guide for Counselors. Alan Meyers. 1988. 120p. (Orig.). pap. 9.95 (0-937119-01-6) Meyers Pub.

Cocaine: An Annotated Bibliography Carlton E. Turner et al. 1988. LC 88-29584. 1500p. text 125.00 (0-87805-382-4);Set. 5.25 hd 150.00 (0-87805-577-0) U Pr of Miss.

Cocaine: Effects on the Developing Brain, Vol. 846. Ed. by John A. Harvey & Barry E. Kosofsky. 1998. LC 98-6824. (Annals of the New York Academy of Sciences Ser.). 436p. 140.00 (1-57331-127-8); pap. 140.00 (1-57331-128-6) NY Acad Sci.

Cocaine: Impressions & Opinions. Aleister Crowley. Ed. by Edward Arliss. 1995. pap. 4.95 (1-55818-320-5) Holmes Pub.

Cocaine: Pharmacology, Addiction & Therapy. Ed. by Mark S. Gold & Marc Galanter. 1987. LC 86-29392. (Advances in Alcohol & Substance Abuse Ser.: Vol. 6, No. 2). 184p. text 49.95 (0-86656-615-5) Haworth Pr.

Cocaine: Pharmacology, Effects & Treatment of Abuse. 1986. lib. bdg. 250.00 (0-8490-3509-0) Gordon Pr.

Cocaine: Pharmacology, Effects, & Treatment of Abuse. Ed. by John Grabowski. 1994. 135p. (Orig.). (C). pap. text 40.00 (0-7881-0743-7) DIANE Pub.

Cocaine: Pharmacology, Physiology & Clinical Strategies. Joan M. Lakoski et al. 1991. 464p. 149.00 (0-8493-8813-9, QP801) CRC Pr.

Cocaine: Physiological & Physiopathological Effects. Ed. by Alfonso Paredes et al. 1993. LC 92-19390. (Journal of Addictive Diseases Ser.: Vol. 11, No. 4). (Illus.). 120p. 39.95 (1-56024-311-2) Haworth Pr.

Cocaine: Physiological & Physiopathological Effects. Ed. by Alfonso Paredes & David A. Gorlick. 1992. 130p. pap. 10.95 (1-56024-385-6) Haworth Pr.

Cocaine: Scientific & Social Dimensions. CIBA Foundation Staff. Ed. by Griffith Edwards. 1992. LC 92-230348. (CIBA Foundation Symposia Ser.: No. 166). 316p. 128.00 (0-471-93179-9, Wiley-Interscience) Wiley.

Cocaine: The Great White Plague. Gabriel G. Nahas. 1989. 320p. 19.95 (0-8397-1700-8) Eriksson.

Cocaine: The Users Guide to Self-Help Treatment. H. Alan Meyers. rev. ed. 1985. pap. 9.95 (0-937119-00-8) Meyers Pub.

Cocaine: Waking up to a Nightmare. Christina Dye. rev. ed. 2000. pap. 0.50 (0-89230-102-3) Do It Now.

Cocaine Abuse: Behavior, Pharmacology & Clinical Applications. Stephen T. Higgins & Jonathon L. Katz. 1998. LC 98-84982. (Illus.). 445p. (C). 79.95 (0-12-347360-8) Acad Pr.

Cocaine Abuse: New Directions in Treatment & Research. Ed. by Henry I. Spitz & Jeffrey S. Rosecan. 1988. LC 86-32676. 352p. text 46.95 (0-87630-461-7) Brunner-Routledge.

Cocaine Addiction. Arnold M. Washton. 2nd ed. Date not set. (0-393-70302-9) Norton.

Cocaine Addiction: Theory, Research & Treatment. Jerome J. Platt. 1997. LC 96-37435. 448p. 54.00 (0-674-13632-2) HUP.

Cocaine Affected Babies: A Bibliography. 1994. 49p. (Orig.). (C). pap. text 20.00 (0-7881-0566-3) DIANE Pub.

Cocaine AIDS & Intravenous Drugs. Samuel Friedman. 1991. pap. 10.95 (1-56023-004-5, Harrington Park) Haworth Pr.

Cocaine & Its Damaging Influences: Index of Modern Authors & Subjects with Guide for Rapid Research. American Health Research Institute Staff. 1994. LC 94-34580. 57.50 (0-7883-0256-6); pap. 47.50 (0-7883-0257-4) ABBE Pubs Assn.

Cocaine & Pregnancy: A Bibliography. 1994. 58p. (Orig.). (C). pap. text 20.00 (0-7881-0567-1) DIANE Pub.

Cocaine Changes: The Experience of Using & Quitting. Dan Waldorf et al. 1992. (Health, Society, & Policy Ser.). pap. 22.95 (1-56639-013-3) Temple U Pr.

Cocaine Crisis. Ed. by David F. Allen. 1987. LC 86-30518. 270p. 65.00 (0-306-42482-7, Plenum Trade) Perseus Pubng.

Cocaine-Exposed Infants: Social, Legal & Public Health Issues. James A. Inciardi et al. 1997. LC 97-4589. 116p. 64.95 (0-8039-7086-2, 2727); pap. 31.95 (0-8039-7087-0, 2726) Sage.

Cocaine in the Brain. Ed. by Nora D. Volkow & Alan C. Swann. 1990. LC 89-70177. (Mind & Medicine Ser.). (Illus.). 250p. (C). text 40.00 (0-8135-1564-5) Rutgers U Pr.

Cocaine, Marijuana, Designer Drugs: Chemistry, Pharmacology, & Behavior. Ed. by Kinfe K. Redda et al. 1989. 248p. 208.95 (0-8493-6853-7, RM316) CRC Pr.

Cocaine Solutions: Help for Cocaine Abusers & Their Families. Jennifer Rice-Licare & Katharine Delaney-McLoughlin. 1990. LC 90-4843. 150p. (Haworth Series in Addictions Treatment Ser.: Vol. 4). 39.95 (1-56024-035-0); (Addiction Treatment Ser.). pap. text 14.95 (0-918393-82-5) Haworth Pr.

Cocaine Treatment: Early Results from Various Approaches. 1996. (Illus.). 34p. (Orig.). (C). pap. text 20.00 (0-7881-3392-6) DIANE Pub.

Cocaine Treatment: Research & Clinical Perspectives. 1994. lib. bdg. 250.00 (0-8490-8608-6) Gordon Pr.

Cocaine Use in America: Epidemiological & Clinical Perspectives. 1986. lib. bdg. 250.00 (0-87700-876-0) Revisionist Pr.

Cocaine Use in America: Epidemmiologic & Clinical Perspectives. Ed. by Nicholas J. Kozel & Edgar H. Adams. 1996. 235p. (Orig.). (C). reprint ed. pap. text 30.00 (0-7881-2968-6) DIANE Pub.

Coccidian Parasites of Rodents. Ed. by Norman D. Levine & Virginia R. Ivens. 1989. 150p. lib. bdg. 139.00 (0-8493-4898-6, QL368) CRC Pr.

Coccidioidomycosis: Proceedings of the 5th International Conference. Ed. by Hans E. Einstein & Antonio Catanzaro. 1996. LC 96-72110. (Illus.). 431p. text 40.00 (0-9614520-3-X) NFID.

Coccidiosis of Man & Domestic Animals. Ed. by Peter L. Long. 1990. 352p. 205.00 (0-8493-6269-5, QR201) CRC Pr.

COCHE, Curriculum for Outreach Centered Health Education: A Vehicle for Implementing Health Education with Farmworkers. Farmworker Health Service Staff. 2000. (Illus.). 156p. pap. (0-9702892-0-0) Farmworker Hlth.

Cochlea. Ed. by Peter Dallos et al. 1996. (Springer Handbook of Auditory Research: Vol. 8). (Illus.). 551p. 99.00 (0-387-94449-4) Spr-Verlag.

Cochlear Implant & Related Sciences Update, 1st Asia Pacific Symposium, Kyoto, April 1996: 1st Asia Pacific Symposium, Kyoto, April 1996. Ed. by Iwao Honjo & Haruo Takahashi. 1992. LC 96-48816. (Advances in OtoRhinoLaryngology Ser.: Vol. 52, 1997). (Illus.). xii, 340p. 216.50 (3-8055-6369-8) S Karger.

Cochlear Implant Rehabilitation in Children & Adults. Ed. by Dianne J. Allum. 1996. LC 96-218443. (Illus.). 342p. (Orig.). pap. 55.00 (1-56593-794-5, 1550) Singular Publishing.

Cochlear Implantation. Jack M. Kartush et al. 1994. LC 94-16224. (Self-Instructional Package Ser.). (Illus.). 103p. pap. text 25.00 (1-56772-012-9) AAO-HNS.

Cochlear Implantation for Infants & Children. Ed. by Graeme R. Clark et al. 1997. LC 96-49000. (Singular Audiology Text Ser.). 288p. text 88.95 (1-56593-727-9, 1412) Thomson Learn.

Cochlear Implants. Ed. by J. M. Miller & F. A. Spelman. 1989. (Illus.). 422p. 169.00 (0-387-97033-9, 2956) Spr-Verlag.

Cochlear Implants. Susan Waltzman. 1999. (Illus.). 416p. 89.00 (0-86577-882-5) Thieme Med Pubs.

Cochlear Implants: A Handbook. Bonnie Tucker. 1998. LC 98-67679. (Illus.). 215p. lib. bdg. 34.50 (0-7864-0534-1) McFarland & Co.

Cochlear Implants: A Practical Guide. Ed. by Huw Cooper. 1991. (Illus.). 400p. (Orig.). (C). pap. text 75.00 (1-879105-32-2, 0014) Thomson Learn.

Cochlear Implants: Audiological Foundations. Ed. by Richard S. Tyler. 1992. LC 92-19404. (Illus.). 411p. (Orig.). (C). pap. text 59.95 (1-879105-81-0, 0344) Thomson Learn.

Cochlear Implants: New Perspectives. Ed. by B. Fraysse & O. Deguine. 1993. (Advances in OtoRhinoLaryngology Ser.: Vol. 48). (Illus.). x, 282p. 248.75 (3-8055-5767-1) S Karger.

Cochlear Implants & Children: A Handbook for Parents, Teachers & Speech & Hearing Professionals. Nancy Tye-Murray. 1993. (Illus.). 206p. (Orig.). (C). pap. text 28.95 (0-88200-173-6) Alexander Graham.

Cochlear Implants for Kids. Ed. by Warren Estabrooks. 1998. LC 98-71880. 404p. pap. text 39.95 (0-88200-208-2) Alexander Graham.

Cochlear Implants for Young Children: The Nottingham Approach to Assessment & Habilitation. Barry McCormick et al. 1994. (Illus.). 302p. (Orig.). (C). pap. text 59.95 (1-56593-372-9, 0720) Singular Publishing.

Cochlear Implants in Children. M. Mondain. 1995. LC 95-10372. (Advances in OtoRhinoLaryngology Ser.: Vol. 50). (Illus.). x, 210p. 173.25 (3-8055-6095-8) S Karger.

***Cochlear Implants in Children: Ethics & Choices.** Ed. by John B. Christiansen & Irene W. Leigh. 2001. LC 2001-56888. (Illus.). 340p. 49.95 (1-56368-116-1) Gallaudet Univ Pr.

Cochlear Implants in Clinical Use. Ed. by W. D. Keidel & P. Finkenzeller. 1984. (Advances in Audiology Ser.: Vol. 2). (Illus.). viii, 176p. 121.75 (3-8055-3721-2) S Karger.

Cochlear Mechanisms: Structure, Function, & Models. Ed. by J. P. Wilson & D. T. Kemp. 1989. (NATO ASI Series A, Life Sciences: Vol. 164). (Illus.). 518p. 135.00 (0-306-43152-1, Plenum Trade) Perseus Pubng.

Cochlear Mechanisms & Otoacoustic Emissions. Ed. by F. Grandori & D. T. Kemp. 1990. (Advances in Audiology Ser.: Vol. 7). (Illus.). x, 180p. 172.25 (3-8055-5082-0) S Karger.

Cochlear Nucleus: Structure & Function in Relation to Modeling, Vol. 3. Ed. by W. A. Ainsworth. 1996. 616p. 157.00 (1-55938-430-1) Jai Pr.

Cochlear Prostheses. Ed. by Graeme M. Clark et al. 1990. (Illus.). 288p. text (0-443-03582-2) Church.

***Cocina de Medico de Familia.** Ed. by Javier Rodriguez. 1997.Tr. of Kitchen of the Family Doctor. (SPA.). 191p. (84-922423-9-6) Jaguar Ed ESP. *Dist:* Libros Fronteras.

Cockroaches As Models for Neurobiology, I. Ed. by Ivan Huber. 1990. 280p. lib. bdg. 210.00 (0-8493-4838-2, QP357) CRC Pr.

Cockroaches As Models for Neurobiology, II. Ed. by Huber. 1990. 344p. lib. bdg. 210.00 (0-8493-4839-0, QP357) CRC Pr.

Code Blue: Cardiac Arrest & Resuscitation. Mickey S. Eisenberg et al. 1987. (Blue Bk.). 272p. pap. text 32.00 (0-7216-1822-7) Saunders.

Code Blue: Health Care in Crisis. Edward R. Annis. 1993. LC 92-44875. 288p. 21.95 (0-89526-515-X) Regnery Pub.

***Code It Right 2001.** Ingenix, Inc. Staff. pap. 64.95 (1-56337-321-1) Ingenix Inc.

Code It Right 2000. Ingenix, Inc. Staff. 1999. (Illus.). ii, 420p. (C). pap. 59.95 (1-56337-333-5) Thomson Learn.

Code Medical Ethics: Current Opinions with Annotations. American Medical Association Staff. 1998. 34.95 (0-89970-960-5) AMA.

C
D

***Code of Federal Regulations, Title 21: Food & Drugs.** rev. ed. 2001. per. 44.00 (*0-16-065086-0*); 203p. per. 15.00 (*0-16-065087-9*) USGPO.

Code of Medical Ethics: Current Opinions with Annotations 2000-2001. Ed. by AMA Counsel on Ethics Staff. 2000. (Illus.). 228p. pap. 38.00 (*1-57947-077-7*) AMA.

Code of Practice for Brachtherapy Physics: Report of the Radiation Therapy Committee Task Group #56. 1998. (Report Ser.: No. 59). 42p. pap. text 10.00 (*1-888340-14-2*) AAPM.

Code-Som: Composite Diagnostic Evaluation of Somatoform Disorders. Donald G. Catron. 1995. 192p. pap. text 30.00 (*0-9651214-3-7*) Somnos Programs.

Code Trainer DX. Patricia T. Aalseth. 2000. 59.00 (*0-8342-1757-0*) Aspen Pub.

***Code Warrior Compiler.** Metrowerks, Inc. Staff. 2001. (Illus.). (C). audio compact disk 12.95 (*0-7637-1889-0*, 1889-0) Jones & Bartlett.

CodeBusters: A Quick Guide to Coding & Billing Compliance for Medical Practices. Patricia T. Aalseth. 1998. LC 98-43607. 48p. pap. 28.00 (*0-8342-1317-6*, 13176) Aspen Pub.

Codelink Ophthalmology 1999. Ed. by Leslie Garvey. 1999. 300p. pap. 99.95 (*1-57066-137-5*, 9951) Practice Mgmt Info.

Codelink - Anesthesiology. ADP Context Software Staff. 1997. 1200p. (Orig.). pap. text 129.95 (*1-57066-106-5*, 9750) Practice Mgmt Info.

Codelink - Obstetrics & Gynecology. ADP Context Software Staff. 3rd rev. ed. 1998. 210p. pap. text 99.95 (*1-57066-107-3*, 9756) Practice Mgmt Info.

Codelink - Ophthalmology. ADP Context Software Staff. 3rd rev. ed. 1998. 260p. pap. text 99.95 (*1-57066-108-1*, 9751) Practice Mgmt Info.

Codelink - Oral & Maxillary Surgery. ADP Context Software Staff. 3rd ed. 1997. 315p. pap. text 99.95 (*1-57066-109-X*, 9752) Practice Mgmt Info.

Codelink - Otolaryngology. ADP Context Software Staff. 3rd rev. ed. 1998. 450p. pap. text 99.95 (*1-57066-111-1*, 9754) Practice Mgmt Info.

Codelink - Plastic Surgery. Context Software Staff. 3rd ed. 1997. 850p. pap. text 79.95 (*1-57066-112-X*, 9755) Practice Mgmt Info.

Codelink for Anesthesia, 2000. ADP Context Staff. 4th rev. ed. 2000. pap. text (*1-57066-169-3*) Practice Mgmt Info.

***Codelink for Anesthesiology 2001.** annuals ADP Context Staff. Ed. by Leslie Garvey. 2001. pap. text 129.95 (*1-57066-200-2*, 21050) Practice Mgmt Info.

Codelink for Maxillofacial Surgery, 2000. ADP Context Staff. 3rd rev. ed. 2000. 340p. pap. text 99.95 (*1-57066-172-3*, 20052) Practice Mgmt Info.

Codelink for OB/GYN, 2000. ADP Context Staff. 3rd rev. ed. 2000. 250p. pap. text 99.95 (*1-57066-170-7*, 20056) Practice Mgmt Info.

***Codelink for Ob/Gyn 2001.** annuals ADP Context Staff. Ed. by Leslie Garvey. 2001. pap. text 99.95 (*1-57066-201-0*, 21056) Practice Mgmt Info.

***Codelink for Ophthalmology 2001.** annuals ADP Context Staff. Ed. by Leslie Garvey. 2001. pap. text 99.95 (*1-57066-202-9*, 21051) Practice Mgmt Info.

Codelink for Ophthalmology, 2000. ADP Context Staff. 4th rev. ed. 2000. 300p. pap. text 99.95 (*1-57066-171-5*, 20051) Practice Mgmt Info.

***Codelink for Oral Maxillofacial Surgery 2001.** annuals ADP Context Staff. Ed. by Leslie Garvey. 2001. pap. text 99.95 (*1-57066-203-7*, 21052) Practice Mgmt Info.

Codelink for Orthopaedics, 2000. ADP Context Staff. 3rd rev. ed. 2000. 800p. pap. text 129.95 (*1-57066-173-1*, 20053) Practice Mgmt Info.

***Codelink for Orthopaedics 2001.** annuals ADP Context Staff. Ed. by Leslie Garvey. 2001. pap. text 129.95 (*1-57066-204-5*, 21053) Practice Mgmt Info.

***Codelink for Otolaryngology 2001.** annuals ADP Context Staff. Ed. by Leslie Garvey. 2001. pap. text 99.95 (*1-57066-205-3*, 21054) Practice Mgmt Info.

Codelink for Otolaryngology, 2000. ADP Context Staff. 4th rev. ed. 2000. 475p. pap. text 99.95 (*1-57066-174-X*, 20054) Practice Mgmt Info.

***Codelink for Plastic Surgery 2001.** annuals ADP Context Staff. Ed. by Leslie Garvey. 2001. pap. text 99.95 (*1-57066-206-1*, 21055) Practice Mgmt Info.

Codelink for Plastic Surgery, 2000. ADP Context Staff. 4th rev. ed. 2000. pap. text 99.95 (*1-57066-175-8*, 20055) Practice Mgmt Info.

Codelink Oral & Maxillofacial Surgery 1999. Ed. by Leslie Garvey. 1999. 300p. pap. 99.95 (*1-57066-138-3*, 9952) Practice Mgmt Info.

Codelink Orthopedics, 1999. Ed. by Leslie Garvey. 3rd rev. ed. 1999. 400p. pap. text 129.95 (*1-57066-110-3*, 9953) Practice Mgmt Info.

Codependency: A Christian Perspective Small Group Leader's Guide. Pat Springle. 1990. 51p. pap. 5.00 (*0-945276-08-7*) Rapha Pub.

Codependency: A Second-Hand Life. Stephanie Abbott. 1985. 11p. (Orig.). pap. 1.55 (*0-89486-317-7*, 5450B) Hazelden.

Codependency Issues in Treatment. Bruce Carruth et al. 1994. LC 89-1998. 167p. pap. 14.95 (*0-86656-942-1*); 1991. 39.95 (*0-86656-920-0*) Haworth Pr.

Codependent Counselor: Guidelines for Self-Assessment & Change. Philip J. Beebe. 1990. 178p. pap. 13.00 (*0-8309-0560-X*) Herald Pub Hse.

Codependent No More see Ya No Seas Codependiente

***Coders' Desk Reference 2001.** Ingenix, Inc. Staff. (Illus.). per. 99.95 (*1-56337-315-7*) Ingenix Inc.

***Coders' Desk Reference for Pathology & Laboratory 2001.** Ingenix, Inc. Staff. pap. 99.95 (*1-56337-317-3*) Ingenix Inc.

Coder's Handbook 2000. James B. Davis. Ed. by Kathryn Swanson. Date not set. text 99.95 (*1-57066-164-2*, 20045) Practice Mgmt Info.

***Coder's Handbook 2001.** James B. Davis & Marilyn DeLong. 2001. (Illus.). 1100p. pap. text 99.95 (*1-57066-211-8*, 21045) Practice Mgmt Info.

Codes of Professional Responsibility. Ed. by Rena A. Gorlin. 4th ed. 1999. 304p. 95.00 (*0-87179-489-6*, 0489) BNA Books.

Codes of Professional Responsibility: Ethics Standards in Business, Health, & Law. Rena A. Gorlin. 4th ed. 1998. LC 98-31152. 1166p. 95.00 (*1-57018-148-9*, 1148-PR9) BNA Books.

Codice de la Cruz Badiano (Codez de la Cruz Badiano) (Book of Indigenous Medicinal Herbs), Set. Martin De la Cruz. 2nd ed. 1991. (SPA., Illus.). 260p. pap. 99.99 (*968-16-3607-4*) Fondo CA.

Codification of Medical Morality Vol. 1: Historical & Philosophical Studies of the Formalization of Western Medical Morality in the Eighteenth & Nineteenth Centuries, No. 45. Ed. by Robert Baker et al. 1993. LC 92-49845. 238p. (C). lib. bdg. (*0-7923-1921-4*) Kluwer Academic NLD. *Dist:* Kluwer Academic.

***Coding Companion for Cardiology 2001.** Ingenix, Inc. Staff. (Illus.). spiral bd. 179.95 (*1-56329-717-5*) Ingenix Inc.

***Coding Companion for General Surgery 2001.** Ingenix, Inc. Staff. (Illus.). spiral bd. 179.95 (*1-56329-745-0*) Ingenix Inc.

***Coding Companion for OB/GYN 2001.** Ingenix, Inc. Staff. (Illus.). spiral bd. 179.95 (*1-56329-719-1*) Ingenix Inc.

***Coding Companion for Ophthalmology 2001.** Ingenix, Inc. Staff. (Illus.). spiral bd. 179.95 (*1-56329-718-3*) Ingenix Inc.

***Coding Companion for Orthopaedics 2001.** Ingenix, Inc. Staff. (Illus.). spiral bd. 179.95 (*1-56329-720-5*) Ingenix Inc.

Coding for Ambulatory Surgery Procedures. 1997. 536p. 149.00 (*1-889115-19-3*) Med Learn.

Coding for Pediatrics: A Manual for Documentation & Reimbursement. American Academy of Pediatrics Staff. Ed. by A. D. Jacobsen et al. 4th ed. 1998. LC 98-71822. 163 p. (*1-58110-012-4*) Am Acad Pediat.

Coding Guide for Surgeries & Procedures of the Breast. Sharon M. Mikolanis. 2000. LC 00-20167. 150p. ring bd. 89.00 (*0-8342-1722-8*) Aspen Pub.

***Coding Illustrated Cardiovascular & Respiratory 2001.** Ingenix, Inc. Staff. (Illus.). pap. 149.95 (*1-56337-358-0*) Ingenix Inc.

***Coding Illustrated Gastrointestinal System 2001.** Ingenix, Inc. Staff. (Illus.). pap. 149.95 (*1-56337-359-9*) Ingenix Inc.

***Coding Illustrated Genitourinary System 2001.** Ingenix, Inc. Staff. (Illus.). pap. 149.95 (*1-56337-360-2*) Ingenix Inc.

***Coding Illustrated Head & Neck 2001.** Ingenix, Inc. Staff. (Illus.). pap. 149.95 (*1-56337-361-0*) Ingenix Inc.

***Coding Illustrated Lower Extremity 2001.** Ingenix, Inc. Staff. (Illus.). pap. 149.95 (*1-56337-363-7*) Ingenix Inc.

***Coding Illustrated Nervous System & Spine 2001.** Ingenix, Inc. Staff. (Illus.). pap. 149.95 (*1-56337-375-0*) Ingenix Inc.

***Coding Illustrated Upper Extremity 2001.** Ingenix, Inc. Staff. (Illus.). pap. 149.95 (*1-56337-362-9*) Ingenix Inc.

Coding the Therapeutic Process: Emblems of Encounter, A Manual for Counsellors & Therapists. Murray Cox. 1978. pap. 21.00 (*1-85302-029-X*) Taylor & Francis.

Coding Workbook for the Physician's Office. Alice Covell. 1996. (Medical Assisting Ser.). 96p. (C). wbk. ed. 19.95 (*0-8273-8074-7*) Delmar.

Coding Workbook for the Physician's Office - IML, 1998. Covell. 1998. 10p. tchr. ed. 4.95 (*0-7668-0082-2*) Delmar.

Coeliac Disease. W. T. Hekkens & A. S. Pena. 1974. text 148.50 (*90-207-0463-X*) Kluwer Academic.

Coeliac Disease. M. N. Marsh. 1992. (Illus.). 384p. 190.00 (*0-632-03097-6*) Blackwell Sci.

Coeliac Disease: Forty Years Gluten-Free. Ed. by M. L. Mearin & Chris J. Mulder. 1991. (Developments in Gastroenterology Ser.). (C). text 146.50 (*0-7923-1160-4*) Kluwer Academic.

Coenzyme Contents of Arterial Tissue. J. E. Kirk. 1974. (Monographs on Atherosclerosis: Vol. 4). (Illus.). 130p. 47.00 (*3-8055-1670-3*) S Karger.

***Coenzyme Q - Qbiquinone: Index of New Information & Guide-Book for Consumers, Reference & Research.** Adolph A. Smithson. 2002. 180p. pap. 57.50 (*0-7883-2499-3*) ABBE Pubs Assn.

CoEnzyme Q 10 & Its Uses. 1996. lib. bdg. 250.75 (*0-8490-5906-2*) Gordon Pr.

Coenzyme Q10 & the Heart. Stephen T. Sinatra & Judi Quilici-Timmcke. 1998. LC 99-207053. (Good Health Guides). 48p. pap. 3.95 (*0-87983-808-6*, 38086K, Keats Pubng) McGraw-Hill Trade.

Coercion & Aggressive Community Treatment: A New Frontier in Mental Health Law. Ed. by Deborah L. Dennis & John Monahan. 1996. (Plenum Series in Social-Clinical Psychology). (Illus.). 236p. (C). 47.00 (*0-306-45167-0*, Plenum Trade) Perseus Pubng.

Coercion & Punishment in Long-Term Perspectives. Ed. by Joan McCord. 1995. (Illus.). 408p. (C). text 69.95 (*0-521-45069-1*) Cambridge U Pr.

Coercive Care: The Ethics of Choice in Health & Medicine. Torbjorn Tannsjo. 1999. LC 98-47880. x, 163p. 80.00 (*0-415-20849-1*) Routledge.

Coevolution. Ed. by Matthew H. Nitecki. LC 83-47773. 382p. 2000. lib. bdg. 30.00 (*0-226-58686-3*); 1994. pap. text 18.95 (*0-226-58687-1*) U Ch Pr.

Cofactors in HIV-1 Infection & AIDS. Ed. by Ronald R. Watson. 1989. 256p. 210.00 (*0-8493-5845-0*, QD431) CRC Pr.

Coffee & Health. Ed. by Brian MacMahon & Takashi Sugimura. 1984. LC 84-14199. (Banbury Reports: Vol.17). 259p. 47.50 (*0-87969-217-0*) Cold Spring Harbor.

Coffee Rust: Epidemiology, Resistance, & Management. Ed. by A. C. Kushalappa & A. B. Eskes. 1989. 336p. lib. bdg. 259.00 (*0-8493-6899-5*, SB608) CRC Pr.

Coffee, Tea, Mate, Methylxanthines, & Methylglyoxal. 1991. (IARC Scientific Publications Ser.: Vol. 51). 513p. pap. text 88.00 (*92-832-1251-7*, 1720051) World Health.

Cogito & the Unconscious. Slavoj Zi Zek. 1998. LC 97-35189. (Sic Ser.). (*0-8223-2083-5*) Duke.

Cogito & the Unconscious. Ed. by Slavoj Zizek. 1998. LC 97-35189. (Sic Ser.: Vol. 2). 279p. pap. 17.95 (*0-8223-2097-5*) Duke.

Cognative Processes. Malim. 1997. pap. 14.95 (*0-333-58811-8*) St Martin.

Cognition. John C. Jahnke & Ronald H. Nowaczyk. 1997. LC 97-11919. 520p. 81.00 (*0-13-140286-2*) P-H.

Cognition. Arnold L. Glass et al. 2nd ed. 1985. 522p. (C). pap. text 51.00 net. (*0-07-554878-X*) McGraw.

Cognition. Daniel Reisberg. 2nd ed. 2001. LC 00-46293. (Illus.). xii, 502p. 59.00 (*0-393-97622-X*, Norton Paperbks) Norton.

Cognition. Margaret W. Matlin. 4th ed. 1997. LC 96-79969. 594p. (C). text 107.00 (*0-15-504081-2*) Harcourt Coll Pubs.

Cognition: An Epistemological Inquiry. Joseph Owens. 1992. LC 92-70254. (C). text 34.50 (*0-268-00792-6*); pap. text 17.50 (*0-268-00791-8*) U of Notre Dame Pr.

Cognition: Conceptual & Methodological Issues. Ed. by Herbert L. Pick, Jr. et al. 1992. (Illus.). 374p. text 39.95 (*1-55798-165-5*) Am Psychol.

Cognition: Testbank, Testbank. Sternberg. 1995. (C). pap. text, tchr. ed., suppl. ed. 44.50 (*0-03-047163-X*) Harcourt Coll Pubs.

Cognition: Theory & Applications. Stephen K. Reed. (Experimental Psychology Ser.). 2nd ed. 1987. LC 87-11785. 348p. (C). mass mkt. 40.50 (*0-534-08172-X*); 3rd ed. 1992. LC 91-14250. 400p. (C). text 41.80 (*0-534-14760-7*); 4th ed. 1995. LC 95-15683. xix, 488p. mass mkt. 54.25 (*0-534-21954-3*) Brooks-Cole.

Cognition & Affect: A Developmental Psychology. Laurence R. Simon. 1986. LC 86-18659. (Psychology Ser.). 280p. 38.00 (*0-87975-340-4*) Prometheus Bks.

Cognition & Communication: Judgmental Biases, Research Methods & the Logic of Conversation. Norbert Schwarz. 1996. LC 96-31266. (MacEachran Lectures). 150p. 22.50 (*0-8058-2314-X*) L Erlbaum Assocs.

Cognition & Culture: A Cross-Cultural Approach to Cognitive Psychology. Ed. by Jeanette Altarriba. 1993. LC 93-36251. (Advances in Psychology Ser.: Vol. 103). 420p. 138.00 (*0-444-89639-2*, North Holland) Elsevier.

Cognition & Emotion: From Order to Disorder. Ed. by Erich Eichman. 2000. LC 99-34377. (Counterpoints Ser.). (Illus.). 272p. text 49.95 (*0-19-511333-0*) OUP.

Cognition & Emotion: From Order to Disorder. Michael J. Power & Tim Dalgleish. 1997. LC 97-202012. (Illus.). xii, 496p. pap. (*0-86377-739-2*) Psychol Pr GBR. *Dist:* Taylor & Francis.

Cognition & Fact: Materials on Ludwik Fleck. Ed. by Robert S. Cohen & Thomas Schnelle. 1986. 480p. text 201.00 (*90-277-1902-0*) Kluwer Academic.

Cognition & Motor Processes. Ed. by W. Prinz & A. F. Sanders. 1984. (Illus.). 385p. 89.95 (*0-387-12855-7*) Spr-Verlag.

Cognition & Occupation in Rehabilitation: Cognitive Models for Intervention in Occupational Therapy. Ed. by Noomi Katz. 1998. LC 98-204990. 343p. pap. text 45.00 (*1-56900-085-9*, 1173) Am Occup Therapy.

Cognition & Perception in the Stroke Patient: A Guide to Functional Outcomes in Occupational Therapy. Kathleen Okkema. 1996. LC 92-48191. (Rehabilitation Institute of Chicago Publication Ser.). 75.00 (*0-8342-0362-6*, 20362) PRO-ED.

Cognition & Psychotherapy. M. J. Mahoney & A. Freeman. 1985. LC 85-3370. (Illus.). 370p. (C). 84.00 (*0-306-41858-4*, Plenum Trade) Perseus Pubng.

Cognition & Social Behavior. John S. Carroll & John W. Payne. 1976. LC 76-48939. 290p. text 59.95 (*0-89859-111-2*) L Erlbaum Assocs.

Cognition & the Menstrual Cycle. Ed. by J. T. Richardson. 1991. (Contributions to Psychology & Medicine Ser.). (Illus.). 216p. 108.00 (*0-387-97612-4*) Spr-Verlag.

Cognition & the Symbolic Processes, Vol. 2. Ed. by Walter B. Weimer & David S. Palermo. 1982. 416p. 99.95 (*0-89859-066-3*) L Erlbaum Assocs.

Cognition & the Visual Arts. Robert L. Solso. 1996. (Cognitive Psychology Ser.). (Illus.). 312p. reprint ed. pap. 22.95 (*0-262-69186-8*, Bradford Bks) MIT Pr.

Cognition, Convention, & Communication. Mark H. Bickhard. 1980. LC 80-20799. 270p. 72.95 (*0-275-90455-5*, C0455, Praeger Pubs) Greenwood.

Cognition, Creativity, & Behavior: Selected Essays. Robert Epstein. 1996. LC 95-30657. 376p. 82.50 (*0-275-94452-2*, Praeger Pubs) Greenwood.

Cognition, Culture & Language in Bilingual Children: Conceptual & Semantic Development. Virginia Gonzalez. 1996. LC 95-23776. 265p. (C). text 69.95 (*1-57292-013-0*); pap. text 53.00 (*1-57292-012-2*) Austin & Winfield.

Cognition, Education, & Deafness: Directions for Research & Instruction. Ed. by David S. Martin. 1985. LC 85-12992. 248p. text 21.95 (*0-930323-12-2*) Gallaudet Univ Pr.

Cognition in Early Childhood. Janie D. Osborn & D. Keith Osborn. 1983. LC 83-71727. (Illus.). 237p. (C). pap. text 9.95 (*0-918772-12-5*) Daye Pr.

Cognition in Human Motivation & Learning. Ed. by G. D'Ydewalle & W. Lens. 1981. 304p. (Orig.). pap. (*90-6186-099-7*) Leuven Univ BEL. *Dist:* Coronet Bks.

Cognition in Human Motivation & Learning. Ed. by Gery D'Ydewalle & Willy Lens. 1981. LC 80-23715. 304p. text 59.95 (*0-89859-067-1*) L Erlbaum Assocs.

Cognition in Schizophrenia & Paranoia: The Integration of Cognitive Processes. Peter A. Magaro. 1980. LC 80-13870. 351p. text 69.95 (*0-89859-028-0*) L Erlbaum Assocs.

Cognition, Information Processing, & Psychophysics: Basic Issues. Hans-Georg Geissler et al. 1992. 334p. text 69.95 (*0-8058-0995-3*) L Erlbaum Assocs.

Cognition, Language, & Consciousness: Integrative Levels. Ed. by Gary Greenberg & Ethel Tobach. 1987. (T. C. Schneirla Conference Ser.: Vol. 2). 312p. 79.95 (*0-89859-722-6*) L Erlbaum Assocs.

Cognitive-Affective Processes: New Ways of Psychoanalytic Modeling. Ed. by U. Moser & I. Von Zeppelia. 1991. (Monographien der Breuninger-Stiffung Stuttgart Ser.). (Illus.). 183p. 62.95 (*0-387-53993-X*) Spr-Verlag.

Cognitive Analysis of Social Behavior. J. P. Codol & J. P. Leyens. 1982. lib. bdg. 141.50 (*90-247-2701-4*) Kluwer Academic.

Cognitive Analytic Therapy: Developments in Theory & Practice. Ed. by Anthony Ryle. 1995. LC 94-45112. (Psychotherapy & Counselling Ser.). 210p. pap. 75.00 (*0-471-94355-X*) Wiley.

Cognitive Analytical Therapy & Borderline Personality Disorder: The Model & the Method. Anthony Ryle. 1997. LC 97-8657. 206p. 98.95 (*0-471-97617-2*); pap. 60.00 (*0-471-97618-0*) Wiley.

Cognitive & Behavioral Interventions: An Empirical Approach to Mental Health Problems. Ed. by Linda Craighead et al. 1993. LC 93-31930. 464p. (C). 78.00 (*0-205-14586-8*) Allyn.

Cognitive & Behavioral Performance Factors in Atypical Aging. Ed. by M. L. Howe et al. 1990. (Illus.). 258p. 72.95 (*0-387-97129-7*, 3321) Spr-Verlag.

Cognitive & Behavioral Treatment: Methods & Application. Ed. by Donald K. Granvold. 1993. LC 93-24064. 370p. 53.04 (*0-534-19194-0*) Brooks-Cole.

Cognitive & Constructive Psychotherapies: Theory, Research, & Practice. Ed. by Michael J. Mahoney. 1994. (Illus.). 232p. 38.95 (*0-8261-8610-6*) Springer Pub.

Cognitive & Linguistic: Analyses of Test Performance, 22. Ed. by Roy O. Freedle & Richard Duran. 1987. LC 86-10888. (Advances in Discourse Processes Ser.: Vol. 22). 416p. 85.00 (*0-89391-295-6*, Ablex) Greenwood.

Cognitive & Linguistic Analyses of Test Performance. Ed. by Roy O. Freedle & Richard Duran. 1987. LC 86-10888. (Advances in Discourse Processes Ser.: Vol. 22). 416p. pap. 42.50 (*0-89391-366-9*, Ablex) Greenwood.

Cognitive & Neurological Approaches to Mental Imagery. Ed. by Michel Denis et al. 1988. text 211.50 (*90-247-3659-5*) Kluwer Academic.

Cognitive & Perceptual Dysfunction. Carolyn Unsworth. 1999. LC 99-19072. (Illus.). 524p. (C). pap. text 32.95 (*0-8036-0399-1*) Davis Co.

Cognitive Appraisal, Emotion, & Empathy. Becky Omdahl. 1995. 274p. text 59.95 (*0-8058-1479-5*) L Erlbaum Assocs.

Cognitive Approaches in Neuropsychological Rehabilitation. Ed. by X. Seron & G. Deloche. 1989. (Neuropsychology & Neurolinguistics Ser.). 416p. 79.95 (*0-89859-615-7*) L Erlbaum Assocs.

Cognitive Approaches to Human Perception. Ed. by Soledad Ballesteros. 1994. LC 93-6805. 304p. 69.95 (*0-8058-1043-9*) L Erlbaum Assocs.

Cognitive Approaches to Learning Disabilities. D. Kim Reid et al. 3rd ed. 1996. LC 90-19787. 686p. text 43.00 (*0-89079-685-8*, 7820) PRO-ED.

Cognitive Approaches to Neuropsychology. Ed. by J. Mark Williams & C. J. Long. 1988. LC 88-25178. (Human Neuropsychology Ser.). (Illus.). 374p. 95.00 (*0-306-43024-X*, Plenum Trade) Perseus Pubng.

Cognitive Aspects of Reporting Cancer Prevention Examinations & Tests. Seymour Sudman et al. 1994. LC 94-35224. (Vital & Health Statistics Ser.: Series 6, No. 7). 12.00 (*0-8406-0499-8*) Natl Ctr Health Stats.

Cognitive Assessment. Carol R. Glass & Myles Genest. Ed. by Thomas V. Merluzzi et al. 1976. LC 85-32041. 532p. (C). pap. text 25.00 (*0-8147-5425-2*) NYU Pr.

Cognitive Bases of Mental Disorders. Peter A. Magaro. 1991. (Annual Review of Psychopathology Ser.: Vol. 1). 352p. (C). 64.95 (*0-8039-4009-2*, 3927); pap. 36.95 (*0-8039-4010-6*, 3928) Sage.

Cognitive-Behavior Therapy: A Restructuring Approach. Rian E. McMullin & Thomas Giles. 1981. (Current Issues in Behavioral Psychology Ser.). 132p. text 24.00 (*0-8089-1362-X*, 792848, Grune & Strat) Harcrt Hlth Sci Grp.

Cognitive Behavior Therapy for Chronic Medical Problems - A Guide to Assessment & Treatment in Practice. Craig A. White. 2001. LC 00-47748. (Clinical Psychology & Personality Ser.). (Illus.). 320p. 64.95 (*0-471-49480-1*) Wiley.

Cognitive Behavior Therapy of DSM-IV Personality Disorders: Highly Effective Interventions for the Most Common Personality Disorders. Len Sperry. 1999. LC 98-54187. (Tree of Liberty Ser.: Vol. 2). 360p. 37.95 (*0-87630-900-7*) Brunner-Routledge.

Cognitive Behavior Therapy with Children. A. W. Meyers & W. E. Craighead. 1984. LC 83-16116. (Applied Clinical Psychology Ser.). (Illus.). 514p. (C). 85.00 (*0-306-41291-8*, Plenum Trade) Perseus Pubng.

Cognitive Behavior Therapy with Children in Schools. Jan N. Huges. 1988. (General Psychology Ser.). 296p. 40.00 (*0-08-034326-0*); pap. 18.95 (*0-08-034325-2*) Elsevier (Pergamon Pr).

Cognitive-Behavior Therapy with Women: A Special Issue of Journal of Rational-Emotive & Cognitive-Behavior Therapy. Ed. by Susan N. Walen & Russell M. Grieger. 1987. 120p. pap. 16.95 (*0-89885-384-2*, Kluwer Acad Hman Sci) Kluwer Academic.

Cognitive-Behavioral Approach to Counseling Psychology: Implications for Practice, Research, & Training. Gerald L. Stone. 1980. LC 80-21344. 185p. 59.95 (*0-275-90557-8*, C0557, Praeger Pubs) Greenwood.

Cognitive-Behavioral Coping Skills Therapy Manual: A Clinical Research Guide for Therapists Treating Individuals with Alcohol Abuse & Dependence. Ed. by Ronald Kadden et al. 1994. (Illus.). 101p. (Orig.). (C). pap. text 35.00 (*0-7881-0899-9*) DIANE Pub.

Cognitive-Behavioral Interventions. Clive R. Hollin. 1992. 200p. (C). pap. text 54.95 (*0-205-14369-5*, H4369); pap. text 48.00 (*0-205-14368-7*, H4368, Longwood Div) Allyn.

Cognitive Behavioral Interventions for Treating Abused Children: Treatment Manual. Esther Deblinger & Anne H. Heflin. 1996. LC 96-9963. (Interpersonal Violence Ser.: Vol. 16). 208p. 79.95 (*0-8039-5928-1*, 1915); pap. 31.95 (*0-8039-5929-X*, 1916) Sage.

Cognitive Behavioral Interventions with Young Offenders. Clive R. Hollin. 1990. (Psychology Practitioner Guidebooks). 192p. text 30.00 (*0-08-035870-5*); pap. text 15.95 (*0-08-035871-3*) Elsevier (Pergamon Pr).

Cognitive-Behavioral Marital Therapy. Donald H. Baucom & Norman B. Epstein. 1990. LC 89-7279. 448p. text 59.95 (*0-87630-558-3*) Brunner-Routledge.

Cognitive Behavioral Play Therapy. Susan M. Knell. 1995. 304p. pap. text 45.00 (*1-56821-719-6*) Aronson.

Cognitive-Behavioral Psychology in the Schools: A Comprehensive Handbook. Ed. by Jan N. Hughes & Robert J. Hall. 1989. LC 88-23598. 581p. 68.00 (*0-89862-736-2*, 2736) Guilford Pubns.

Cognitive-Behavioral Relaxation Training: A New System of Strategies for Treatment & Assessment. Jonathan Smith. 1990. 176p. 34.95 (*0-8261-7070-6*) Springer Pub.

Cognitive-Behavioral Strategies in Crisis Intervention. Ed. by Frank M. Dattilio & Arthur Freeman. 2nd rev. ed. 2000. LC 00-24985. 470p. 48.00 (*1-57230-579-7*, 8R0579) Guilford Pubns.

Cognitive-Behavioral Therapies for Trauma. Ed. by Victoria M. Follette et al. 1998. LC 98-37114. 431p. text 45.00 (*1-57230-400-6*, C0400) Guilford Pubns.

Cognitive Behavioral Therapy: An Introduction. Robert L. Leahy. 1996. 30.00 (*1-56821-367-0*) Aronson.

Cognitive-Behavioral Therapy for Bipolar Disorder. Monica R. Basco & A. John Rush. 1996. LC 96-13739. 291p. text 36.00 (*1-57230-090-6*, 0090) Guilford Pubns.

Cognitive-Behavioral Therapy for Impulsive Children. Philip C. Kendall & Lauren Braswell. 2nd ed. 1993. LC 92-49966. 239p. 31.00 (*0-89862-013-9*, 2013) Guilford Pubns.

Cognitive Behavioral Therapy with Schizophrenia: A Practice Manual. Hazel Nelson. 1997. 224p. 39.95 (*1-56593-934-4*, 1854) Singular Publishing.

Cognitive Behavioral Treatment for Adult Survivors of Childhood Trauma: Imagery, Rescripting & Reprocessing. Mervin Smucker. 1999. LC 98-53686. (New Directions in Cognitive-Behavior Therapy Ser.). (Illus.). xxiii, 256p. 40.00 (*0-7657-0213-4*) Aronson.

Cognitive-Behavioral Treatment of Borderline Personality Disorder. Marsha M. Linehan. 1993. LC 93-20483. (Diagnosis & Treatment of Mental Disorders Ser.). 558p. text 52.00 (*0-89862-183-6*, 2183) Guilford Pubns.

Cognitive Behaviour Therapy for Children & Families. Ed. by Philip Graham. 1998. LC 97-29374. (Monographs on Child & Adolescent Psychiatry). (Illus.). 310p. (C). text 110.00 (*0-521-57252-5*); pap. text 44.95 (*0-521-57626-1*) Cambridge U Pr.

Cognitive Behaviour Therapy for Psychiatric Problems: A Practical Guide. Ed. by Keith E. Hawton et al. 1989. (Illus.). 470p. pap. text 44.50 (*0-19-261587-4*) OUP.

Cognitive Behaviour Therapy in Primary Care. Richard France & Meredith Robson. 1997. LC 97-197680. 300p. pap. (*1-85302-410-4*) Jessica Kingsley GBR. *Dist:* Taylor & Francis.

Cognitive-Behavioural Interventions with Psychotic Disorders. Ed. by Gillian Haddock & Peter D. Slade. 1996. LC 95-16043. (Illus.). 304p. (C). 84.95 (*0-415-10289-8*); pap. 31.95 (*0-415-10290-1*) Routledge.

Cognitive-Behavioural Therapy. Brian Sheldon. enl. rev. ed. 1995. LC 94-18585. Orig. Title: Behaviour Modification. 296p. (C). pap. 29.95 (*0-415-09374-0*, B3997) Routledge.

Cognitive Behavioural Therapy for Chronic Medical Problems: A Guide to Assesment & Treatment in Practice. Craig A. White. 2000. LC 00-47748. (Clinical Psychology & Personality Ser.). (Illus.). 320p. pap. 55.00 (*0-471-49482-8*) Wiley.

Cognitive Behavioural Therapy with Schizophrenia: A Practice Manual. Hazel E. Nelson. 1997. (Illus.). 262p. (Orig.). pap. (*0-7487-3305-1*) Nelson Thornes GBR. *Dist:* Intl Spec Bk, Trans-Atl Phila.

Cognitive-Behavorial Therapies for Persons with Disabilities. Ed. by Cynthia Radnitz. 2000. LC 99-41432. (New Directions in Cognitive-Behavior Therapy Ser.). (Illus.). 359p. pap. 50.00 (*0-7657-0238-X*) Aronson.

Cognitive Biases. Ed. by Jean-Paul Caverni et al. 1990. (Advances in Psychology Ser.: No. 68). iv,576p. 201.50 (*0-444-88413-0*, North Holland) Elsevier.

Cognitive Case Conceptualization: A Guidebook for Practitioners. Lawrence D. Needleman. 1999. LC 98-31852. (Personality & Clinical Psychology Ser.). 352p. 39.95 (*0-8058-1908-8*) L Erlbaum Assocs.

Cognitive-Communication Disorders Following Traumatic Brain Injury: A Practical Guide. Jane Freund. 1998. pap. text 44.00 (*0-12-784584-4*) Acad Pr.

Cognitive-Communicative Abilities Following Brain Injury: A Functional Approach. Leila L. Hartley. 1994. LC 94-28243. (Neurogenic Communication Disorders Ser.). (Illus.). 304p. (Orig.). (C). pap. text 56.95 (*1 56593 102 5*, 0405) Thomson Learn.

Cognitive Components in Cerebral Event Related Potentials & Selective Attention. Ed. by J. E. Desmedt. 1979. (Progress in Clinical Neurophysiology Ser.: Vol. 6). (Illus.). 102.75 (*3-8055-2760-8*) S Karger.

Cognitive Control: A Study of Individual Consistencies in Cognitive Behavior. Riley W. Gardner et al. 1959. (Psychological Issues Monographs: No. 4, Vol. 1, No. 4). 85p. (Orig.). 27.50 (*0-8236-1000-4*) Intl Univs Pr.

Cognitive Control Therapy with Children & Adolescents. Sebastino Santostefano. 1985. (Psychology Practitioner Guidebooks). 200p. text 35.00 (*0-08-031581-X*); pap. text 17.95 (*0-08-031580-1*) Elsevier (Pergamon Pr).

Cognitive Counseling & Persons with Special Needs: Adapting Behavioral Approaches to the Social Context. Herbert Lovett. 1985. LC 85-3495. 160p. pap. 20.95 (*0-275-91651-0*, B1651, Praeger Pubs) Greenwood.

Cognitive Development. Thomas F. Gross. 1984. LC 84-14982. (Psychology Ser.). 255p. (C). mass mkt. 26.75 (*0-534-03363-6*) Brooks-Cole.

Cognitive Development. John H. Flavell et al. 3rd ed. 1992. LC 92-24487. 416p. pap. text 49.33 (*0-13-140039-8*) P-H.

Cognitive Development, Vol. 3. Ed. by Paul H. Mussen et al. 4th ed. 1983. LC 83-3468. 942p. 94.95 (*0-471-09064-6*) Wiley.

Cognitive Development: A Functional Approach. Peter J. Valletutti & Leonie Dummett. 1992. LC 92-10903. (Illus.). 224p. (Orig.). (C). pap. 39.95 (*1-879105-63-2*, 0327) Thomson Learn.

Cognitive Development: The Child's Acquisition of Diagonality. David R. Olson. 1996. 240p. pap. 29.95 (*0-8058-2302-6*) L Erlbaum Assocs.

Cognitive Development & Child Psychotherapy. S. R. Shirk. 1988. LC 88-17854. (Perspectives in Developmental Psychology Ser.). (Illus.). 360p. (C). 70.00 (*0-306-42880-6*, Plenum Trade) Perseus Pubng.

Cognitive Development in Adulthood. Ed. by M. L. Howe & Charles J. Brainerd. 1988. (Cognitive Development Ser.). (Illus.). 334p. 207.00 (*0-387-96697-8*) Spr-Verlag.

Cognitive Development in Atypical Children: Progress in Cognitive Development Research. Ed. by L. S. Siegel & F. J. Morrison. 1984. (Cognitive Development Ser.). (Illus.). 184p. 71.95 (*0-387-96008-2*) Spr-Verlag.

Cognitive Development in Children: Five Monographs of the SRCD. Society for Research in Child Development Staff. 1992. LC 78-103136. lib. bdg. 30.00 (*0-226-76755-8*) U Ch Pr.

Cognitive-Development Psychology of James Mark Baldwin: Current Theory & Research in Genetic Epistemology. John M. Broughton & John D. Freeman-Moir. 1982. LC 81-7885. (Publications for the Advancement of Theory & History in Psychology, the PATH Ser.). 386p. 73.25 (*0-89391-043-0*, Ablex) Greenwood.

Cognitive Development Today: Piaget & His Critics. Peter Sutherland. 1992. (Education Ser.). 192p. pap. (*1-85396-133-7*, 83904) P Chapman GBR. *Dist:* Sage.

Cognitive Developmental Therapy with Children. Tammie Ronen. 1997. LC 97-9107. 202p. pap. 49.95 (*0-471-97007-7*) Wiley.

Cognitive Disorders: Pathophysiology & Treatment. Ed. by Leon J. Thal et al. 1992. (Neurological Disease & Therapy Ser.: Vol. 11). (Illus.). 400p. text 195.00 (*0-8247-8601-7*) Dekker.

Cognitive Dissonance: Progress on a Pivotal Theory in Social Psychology. Ed. by Judson Mills & Eddie Herman-Jones. 1999. LC 98-49316. (Science Conference Ser.). 411p. Not sold separately (*1-55798-565-0*) Am Psychol.

Cognitive Dysfunctions in Chronic Cannabis Users Observed During Treatment: An Integrative Approach. Thomas Lundqvist. 1995. (Studia Psychologica et Paedagogica). 282p. (Orig.). pap. 58.00 (*91-22-01699-6*) Coronet Bks.

Cognitive Ecology. Ed. by Morton P. Friedman & Edward C. Carterette. 2nd ed. 1996. LC 95-20313. (Handbook of Perception & Cognition Ser.). (Illus.). 416p. text 65.00 (*0-12-161966-4*) Acad Pr.

Cognitive Effects of Early Brain Injury. Casey Dorman & Bilha Katzir. 1994. LC 94-6782. (Johns Hopkins Series in Psychiatry & Neuroscience Ser.). 336p. 57.95 (*0-8018-4856-3*) Johns Hopkins.

Cognitive Ergonomics. G. C. Van der Veer et al. 1992. 338p. 118.00 (*0-444-89504-3*, North Holland) Elsevier.

Cognitive Foundations of Calculated Speech: Controlling Understandings in Conversation & Persuasion. Robert Sanders. 1986. LC 86-5869. (SUNY Series in Human Communication Processes). 273p. (C). pap. text 24.95 (*0-88706-351-9*) State U NY Pr.

Cognitive Foundations of Personality Traits. S. Kreitler & H. Kreitler. 1990. LC 89-38261. (Emotions, Personality, & Psychotherapy Ser.). (Illus.). 422p. (C). 70.00 (*0-306-43179-3*, Plenum Trade) Perseus Pubng.

Cognitive Hypnotherapy. E. Thomas Dowd. 2000. LC 99-14701. (Illus.). xii, 240p. 40.00 (*0-7657-0228-2*) Aronson.

Cognitive Learning & Memory in Children. Ed. by M. Pressley & Charles J. Brainerd. 1985. (Cognitive Development Ser.). (Illus.). 250p. 83.95 (*0-387-96076-7*) Spr-Verlag.

Cognitive-Linguistic Improvement Program CLIP: A Program for Speech-Language Pathologists Treating Neuropathologies of Speech & Language & Learning Disabilities. Deborah G. Ross-Swain. 1992. (Illus.). 264p. (Orig.). (C). pap. text 49.95 (*1-879105-62-4*, 0276) Thomson Learn.

Cognitive Microgenesis: A Neuropsychological Perspective. Ed. by R. E. Hanlon. 1991. (Illus.). 323p. 151.00 (*0-387-97407-5*) Spr-Verlag.

***Cognitive Models & Spiritual Maps: Interdisciplinary Explorations of Religious Experience.** Jensine Andresen & Robert K. C. Forman. 2001. 288p. pap. (*0-907845-13-4*) Imprint Acad.

Cognitive Models of Memory. Ed. by Martin A. Conway. 1997. LC 96-43748. (Studies in Cognition). (Illus.). 320p. pap. 32.00 (*0-262-53148-8*); 55.00 (*0-262-03245-7*) MIT Pr.

Cognitive Motor Learning. Kenneth W. Adolph. 1997. LC 98-111048. 240p. pap. text 15.00 (*0-226-00766-9*) U Ch Pr.

Cognitive Neuropsychology. Alan J. Parkin. 1996. (Illus.). 256p. (C). 72.95 (*0-631-19472-X*) Blackwell Pubs.

Cognitive Neuropsychology: A Clinical Introduction. Rosaleen A. McCarthy & Elizabeth K. Warrington. 1990. 428p. text 89.95 (*0-12-481845-5*); pap. text 45.00 (*0-12-481846-3*) Acad Pr.

Cognitive Neuropsychology & Neurolinguistics: Advances in Models of Cognitive Function & Impairment. Ed. by Alfonso Caramazza. 1990. 312p. 89.95 (*0-89859-892-3*) L Erlbaum Assocs.

Cognitive Neuropsychology in Clinical Practice. Ed. by David I. Margolin. 1992. LC 91-24105. (Illus.). 560p. text 75.00 (*0-19-506422-4*) OUP.

Cognitive Neuropsychology of Alzheimer-Type Dementia. Ed. by Robin G. Morris. 1997. LC 96-22542. (Illus.). 370p. text 89.50 (*0-19-852343-2*) OUP.

Cognitive Neuroscience. Ed. by Michael D. Rugg. 1997. LC 96-39229. (Studies in Cognition). 402p. pap. 32.95 (*0-262-68094-7*); (Illus.). 75.00 (*0-262-18181-9*) MIT Pr.

Cognitive Neuroscience: The Biology of the Mind. Michael S. Gazzaniga et al. 1998. LC 97-36771. (Illus.). 600p. (C). text 65.00 (*0-393-97219-4*) Norton.

***Cognitive Neuroscience: The Biology of the Mind.** Michael S. Gazzaniga et al. 2nd ed. 2002. LC 2001-44542. (*0-393-97777-3*) Norton.

Cognitive Neuroscience of Attention: A Developmental Perspective. Ed. by John E. Richards. 1998. LC 97-35558. 374p. (*0-8058-2409-X*) L Erlbaum Assocs.

Cognitive Neuroscience of Memory. Hans J. Markowitsch & Lars-Goran Nilsson. 1999. LC 99-71722. (Illus.). 312p. 59.00 (*0-88937-213-6*) Hogrefe & Huber Pubs.

***Cognitive Neuroscience of Memory: An Introduction.** Howard Eichenbaum. 2002. (Illus.). 480p. pap. text 39.50 (*0-19-514175-X*) OUP.

Cognitive Organization & Change: An Information-Processing Approach. Robert S. Wyer, Jr. 1974. LC 74-12312. 502p. (C). text 89.95 (*0-89859-200-3*) L Erlbaum Assocs.

Cognitive Paradigm. Marc De Mey. 1982. lib. bdg. 117.50 (*90-277-1382-0*) Kluwer Academic.

Cognitive Practices: Human Language & Human Knowledge. Rita Nolan. 1994. 200p. pap. 26.95 (*0-631-18974-2*) Blackwell Pubs.

Cognitive Process Instruction: Research on Teaching Thinking Skills. Ed. by Jack Lochhead & John Clement. 1979. LC 78-22122. (Illus.). 339p. pap. 59.95 (*0-89859-729-3*) L Erlbaum Assocs.

Cognitive Processes & Emotional Disorders: A Structural Approach to Psychotherapy. Vittorio F. Guidano & G. Liotti. LC 83-13188. (Guilford Clinical Psychology & Psychotherapy Ser.). 347p. reprint ed. 1986. pap. 35.00 (*0-89862-907-1*, 2907); 1983. text 40.00 (*0-89862-006-6*) Guilford Pubns.

Cognitive Processes in Choice & Decision Behavior. Ed. by Thomas S. Wallsten. 1990. LC 79-27553. (Illus.). 304p. text 59.95 (*0-89859-054-X*) L Erlbaum Assocs.

Cognitive Processes in Comprehension. Ed. by M. A. Just & P. A. Carpenter. 1977. 352p. text 79.95 (*0-89859-127-9*) L Erlbaum Assocs.

Cognitive Processes in Translation & Interpreting. Joseph H. Danks et al. 1997. LC 96-45778. (Applied Psychology Ser.: Vol. 3). 276p. (C). 79.95 (*0-7619-0054-3*, 1673) Sage.

Cognitive Processing in Bilinguals. R. J. Harris. 1992. (Advances in Psychology Ser.: Vol. 83). 592p. 157.00 (*0-444-88922-1*, North Holland) Elsevier.

Cognitive Processing Therapy for Rape Victims: A Treatment Manual. Patricia A. Resick & Monica K. Schnicke. 1993. (Interpersonal Violence Ser.: Vol. 4). (Illus.). 174p. (C). pap. 31.95 (*0-8039-4902-2*, 4301) Sage.

Cognitive Psychoanalysis: Cognitive Processes in Psychopathology. Irving Bieber. 1996. LC 96-104217. 411p. pap. 50.00 (*1-56821-760-9*) Aronson.

Cognitive Psychodynamics: From Conflict to Character. Mardi J. Horowitz. 1998. LC 98-5925. 240p. 100.00 (*0-471-11772-2*) Wiley.

Cognitive Psychology. Ronald T. Kellogg. 1995. LC 95-11732. (Advanced Psychology Texts Ser.: Vol. 2). (Illus.). 544p. (C). 76.95 (*0-8039-5329-1*, 4811) Sage.

Cognitive Psychology. Payne. (C). Date not set. pap., tchr. ed. 11.96 (*0-395-68574-5*); 1998. text 65.96 (*0-395-68573-7*) HM.

Cognitive Psychology. Robert J. Sternberg. 1996. 576p. (C). text 81.50 (*0-03-037947-4*) Harcourt Coll Pubs.

Cognitive Psychology. Medin. 2nd ed. 1997. (C). pap. text 44.50 (*0-15-504006-5*) Harcourt Coll Pubs.

Cognitive Psychology. Douglas L. Medin & Brian H. Ross. 2nd ed. 1996. LC 96-78285. 626p. (C). text 98.50 (*0-15-502843-X*) Harcourt Coll Pubs.

Cognitive Psychology. Robert J. Sternberg. 2nd ed. 1998. LC 98-72574. (Illus.). 608p. (C). text 107.00 (*0-15-508354-6*) Harcourt Coll Pubs.

Cognitive Psychology. John B. Best. Ed. by Baxter Staff & Crochiere. 3rd ed. 1992. 550p. (C). text 48.75 (*0-314-90894-3*) West Pub.

Cognitive Psychology. John B. Best. 4th ed. 1994. LC 94-31727. 508p. (C). mass mkt. 54.50 (*0-314-04445-0*) West Pub.

Cognitive Psychology. Best. 5th ed. 1998. LC 98-40566. (Psychology Ser.). 632p. (C). spiral bd. 84.95 (*0-534-35417-3*) Wadsworth Pub.

Cognitive Psychology. Robert L. Solso. 6th ed. 2000. LC 00-46880. (Illus.). 602p. 83.00 (*0-205-30937-2*) Allyn.

Cognitive Psychology: An Essay in Cognitive Science. George Mandler. 1985. 144p. (C). pap. 6.95 (*0-89859-659-9*); text 29.95 (*0-89859-537-1*) L Erlbaum Assocs.

Cognitive Psychology: Current Issues & Debates. Freedman. 1919. (Psychology Ser.). (C). pap. 57.95 (*0-534-34943-9*) Brooks-Cole.

Cognitive Psychology & Emotional Disorders. Colin MacLeod et al. 2nd ed. 1997. LC 96-32464. (Clinical Psychology & Personality Ser.). 416p. pap. 80.00 (*0-471-94430-0*) Wiley.

Cognitive Psychology & Information Processing: An Introduction. Roy Lachman et al. 1979. 592p. (C). text 99.95 (*0-89859-131-7*) L Erlbaum Assocs.

Cognitive Psychology & Instruction. Ed. by Alan M. Lesgold et al. 1978. LC 77-27133. (NATO Conference Series III, Human Factors: Vol. 5). 540p. 75.00 (*0-306-32886-0*, Plenum Trade) Perseus Pubng.

Cognitive Psychology & Instruction. Roger H. Bruning et al. 3rd ed. 1998. LC 98-7091. 433p. pap. text 54.00 (*0-13-716606-0*, Merrill Coll) P-H.

Cognitive Psychology & Its Implications. John R. Anderson. 4th ed. 1995. LC 94-39006. 544p. (C). text 66.95 (*0-7167-2385-9*) W H Freeman.

Cognitive Psychology Applied: A Symposium at the 22nd International Congress of Applied Psychology. Ed. by Chizuko Izawa. 1993. 256p. text 59.95 (*0-8058-0830-2*) L Erlbaum Assocs.

Cognitive Psychology In & Out of the Laboratory. Galotti. 2nd ed. 1998. LC 98-25622. (Psychology Ser.). 556p. spiral bd. 79.95 (*0-534-34650-2*) Brooks-Cole.

Cognitive Psychology in the Middle Ages, 33. Simon Kemp. 1996. LC 96-10765. (Contributions in Psychology Ser.). 152p. 55.00 (*0-313-30051-8*, Greenwood Pr) Greenwood.

Cognitive Psychology of Knowledge. Ed. by Gerhard Strube & Karl F. Wender. 1993. LC 93-29886. (Advances in Psychology Ser.: Vol. 101). 470p. 169.25 (*0-444-89942-1*, North Holland) Elsevier.

Cognitive Psychology of Mass Communication. Richard J. Harris. 2nd ed. 1993. (Mass Communication Ser.). 328p. text 34.50 (*0-8058-1264-4*) L Erlbaum Assocs.

Cognitive Psychology of Planning. Ed. by Jean-Michel Hoc. 1988. (Computers & People Ser.). 200p. text 79.95 (*0-12-350770-7*) Acad Pr.

Cognitive Psychology of School Learning. Ellen D. Gagne. 1985. (C). text 27.95 (*0-316-30165-5*, Little Brwn Med Div) Lppncott W & W.

Cognitive Psychophysiology: Event-Related Potentials & the Study of Cognition, the Carmel Conferences, Vol. 1. Ed. by E. Donchin. 1984. (Illus.). 448p. (C). text 89.95 (*0-89859-150-3*) L Erlbaum Assocs.

Cognitive Psychophysiology: Principles of Covert Behavior. Frank J. McGuigan. 1978. LC 78-18542. (Century Psychology Ser.). 34.95 (*0-13-139519-X*) P-H.

Cognitive Psychotherapy. Ed. by C. Perris et al. 1988. (Illus.). 422p. 137.00 (*0-387-18870-3*) Spr-Verlag.

Cognitive Psychotherapy of Psychotic Disorders: Handbook of Theory & Practice. Carlo Perris & Patrick D. McGorry. 1999. LC 98-3825. 468p. 160.00 (*0-471-98221-0*) Wiley.

Cognitive Rehabilitation. Toglia. 1998. (Illus.). 383p. (C). pap. text 44.00 (*0-12-784583-6*) Acad Pr.

Cognitive Rehabilitation: An Integrative Neuropsychological Approach. McKay Moore Sohlberg & Catherine A. Mateer. 2001. LC 00-65445. (Illus.). 492p. 55.00 (*1-57230-613-0*) Guilford Pubns.

Cognitive Rehabilitation: Conceptualization & Intervention. Ed. by Lance Trexler. 1982. LC 82-7619. 292p. 65.00 (*0-306-41016-8*, Plenum Trade) Perseus Pubng.

Cognitive Rehabilitation for Neuropsychiatric Disorders. Ed. by Patrick W. Corrigan & Stuart C. Yudofsky. 1996. LC 96-13648. 477p. text 72.95 (*0-88048-551-5*, 8551) Am Psychiatric.

Cognitive Rehabilitation for Persons with Traumatic Brain Injury. Jeffrey S. Kreutzer & Paul H. Wehman. 1996. LC 95-45066. 310p. pap. 29.00 (*1-883315-15-8*, 7214) Imaginart Intl.

Cognitive Rehabilitation of Closed Head Injured Patients: A Dynamic Approach. Brenda B. Adamovich et al. 1985. LC 90-50381. 160p. (Orig.). (C). pap. text 31.00 (*0-89079-389-1*, 1600) PRO-ED.

Cognitive Rehabilitation of Memory: A Practical Guide. Minnie Harrell et al. 1991. LC 91-31706. 261p. 71.00 (*0-8342-0285-9*) PRO-ED.

Cognitive Rehabilitation Workbook. Pamela M. Dougherty & Radoms. 1987. 336p. pap. 89.00 (*0-8342-1193-9*) PRO-ED.

Cognitive Research on Response Error in Survey Questions on Smoking. 1993. 97p. (Orig.). (C). pap. text 30.00 (*1-56806-502-7*) DIANE Pub.

Cognitive Revolution in Psychology. Bernard J. Baars. 1986. LC 84-25311. 443p. pap. 33.00 (*0-89862-912-8*, 2912) Guilford Pubns.

Cognitive Science: An Introduction. David W. Green. 1996. (Illus.). 432p. 76.95 (*0-631-19859-8*) Blackwell Pubs.

Cognitive Science & Clinical Disorders. Ed. by Daniel L. Stein & Jeffrey Young. 1992. LC 92-11148. (Illus.). 399p. text 79.95 (*0-12-664720-8*) Acad Pr.

Cognitive Science & Genetic Epistemology: A Case Study of Understanding. D. Leiser & C. Gilleron. 1990. LC 89-22970. (PATH in Psychology Ser.). (Illus.). 216p. (C). 55.00 (*0-306-43193-9*, Plenum Trade) Perseus Pubng.

Cognitive Science & Psychoanalysis. Kenneth M. Colby & R. J. Stoller. 1988. 176p. 39.95 (*0-8058-0177-4*) L Erlbaum Assocs.

Cognitive Science & Psychoanalysis. R. J. Stoller. 1988. 176p. pap. 19.95 (*0-88163-076-4*) L Erlbaum Assocs.

Cognitive Science & the Mind-Body Problem: From Philosphy to Psychology to Artificial Intelligence to Imaging of the Brain. Morton Wagman. 1998. LC 97-26183. 168p. 62.50 (*0-275-96031-5*, Praeger Pubs) Greenwood.

Cognitive Science & the Unconscious. Ed. by Dan J. Stein. 1997. LC 96-30885. (Progress in Psychiatry Ser.: Vol. 53). 232p. text 35.00 (*0-88048-498-5*, 8498) Am Psychiatric.

Cognitive Science Foundations of Instruction. Ed. by Mitchell Rabinowitz. 1993. 248p. text 59.95 (*0-8058-1279-2*) L Erlbaum Assocs.

Cognitive Science in Europe. Ed. by M. Imbert et al. 1987. (Recent Research in Psychology Ser.). 236p. 54.95 (*0-387-96595-5*) Spr-Verlag.

Cognitive Science in Medicine: Biomedical Modeling. Ed. by David A. Evans & Vilma Patel. 1989. 350p. 46.50 (*0-262-05037-4*, Bradford Bks) MIT Pr.

Cognitive Science Perspectives on Personality & Emotion, Vol. 124. Gerald Matthews. 1997. LC 97-45697. (Advances in Psychology Ser.). 574p. 129.50 (*0-444-82450-2*) Elsevier.

Cognitive Skills & Their Acquisition. Ed. by John R. Anderson. 1981. (Carnegie Mellon Symposia on Cognition Ser.). 384p. text 79.95 (*0-89859-093-0*) L Erlbaum Assocs.

Cognitive Social Factors in Early Deception. Ed. by S. J. Ceci et al. 1992. 192p. text 39.95 (*0-8058-0953-8*) L Erlbaum Assocs.

Cognitive Strategies Special Education. Adrian F. Ashman & Robert N. Conway. 250p. 1997. LC 96-27652. text 49.95 (*0-415-00594-9*, A1690); 1988. pap. text 15.95 (*0-415-00595-7*, A1694) Routledge.

Cognitive Strategy Research: Psychological Foundations, 1. Ed. by M. Presley & J. R. Levin. 1983. (Cognitive Development Ser.). (Illus.). 350p. 88.95 (*0-387-90818-8*) Spr-Verlag.

Cognitive Structure & Development in Nonhuman Primates. Francesco Antinucci. 1989. 272p. (C). pap. 36.50 (*0-8058-0544-3*); text 69.95 (*0-8058-0242-8*) L Erlbaum Assocs.

Cognitive Structure of Emotions. Andrew Ortony et al. 1990. (Illus.). 221p. (C). pap. text 21.95 (*0-521-38664-0*) Cambridge U Pr.

Cognitive Styles: Essence & Origins- Field Dependence & Field Independence. Herman A. Witkin & Donald R. Goodenough. 1981. LC 80-39995. (Psychological Issues Monographs: No. 51). (Illus.). 153p. 27.50 (*0-8236-1003-9*) Intl Univs Pr.

Cognitive Technology in Psychiatric Rehabilitation. Ed. by William D. Spaulding. 1994. LC 93-23685. 246p. text 45.00 (*0-8032-4224-7*) U of Nebr Pr.

Cognitive Theory, Vol. 1. Ed. by H. R. Lindman et al. 1975. LC 74-14293. 320p. text 69.95 (*0-89859-436-7*) L Erlbaum Assocs.

Cognitive Theory, Vol. 3. Ed. by Frank Restle & N. J. Castellan, Jr. 1978. 336p. 69.95 (*0-89859-438-3*) L Erlbaum Assocs.

Cognitive Theory of Cultural Meaning. Claudia Strauss & Naomi Quinn. 1998. LC 97-14944. (Publications of the Society for Psychological Anthropology: Vol. 9). 335p. (C). text 74.95 (*0-521-59409-X*) Cambridge U Pr.

Cognitive Therapy. Mark McMinn. (Resources for Christian Counseling Ser.: Vol. 27). 22.99 (*0-8499-0876-0*) Nelson Ref & Elec Pub.

Cognitive Therapy: Applications in Psychiatric & Medical Settings. Ed. by Arthur Freeman & Vincent Greenwood. 1986. (Illus.). 234p. 42.95 (*0-89885-285-4*); 20.95 (*0-89885-311-7*) Kluwer Academic (Kluwer Acad Hman Sci).

Cognitive Therapy & Emotional Disorders. Aaron T. Beck. 1976. LC 75-33518. 365p. (Orig.). 52.50 (*0-8236-1005-5*) Intl Univs Pr.

Cognitive Therapy & the Emotional Disorders. Aaron T. Beck. 1979. pap. 15.95 (*0-452-00928-6*) NAL.

Cognitive Therapy for Anxiety & Depression: A Practitioner's Guide. Ivy-Marie Blackburn & Kate M. Davidson. 2nd ed. 1995. LC 95-22027. 228p. pap. 54.95 (*0-632-03986-8*) Blackwell Sci.

Cognitive Therapy for Bipolar Disorder: A Therapist's Guide to Concepts, Methods & Practice. Dominic H. Lam. 1999. LC 99-20568. (Wiley Series in Clinical Psychology). (Illus.). 320p. 85.00 (*0-471-97939-2*) Wiley.

Cognitive Therapy for Delusions, Voices & Paranoia. Paul Chadwick et al. LC 96-1475. (Clinical Psychology & Personality Ser.). 230p. 1999. pap. 65.00 (*0-471-96173-6*); 1996. 225.00 (*0-471-93888-2*) Wiley.

Cognitive Therapy for Depressed Adolescents. T. C. R. Wilkes et al. 1994. LC 94-13340. (Mental Health & Psychopathology Ser.). 396p. 44.00 (*0-89862-119-4*, C2119) Guilford Pubns.

Cognitive Therapy for Personality Disorders. Kate Davidson. 2000. 161p. pap. (*0-7506-4488-5*) E A GBR. *Dist:* OUP.

Cognitive Therapy for Personality Disorders: A Schema-Focused Approach. Jeffrey E. Young. 3rd ed. 1999. LC 98-50869. (Practitioner's Resource Ser.). 96p. pap. 17.95 (*1-56887-047-7*, CTPDBP, Prof Resc Pr) Pro Resource.

Cognitive Therapy in Action: A Practitioner's Casebook. Ivy-Marie Blackburn & Vivien Twaddle. 1996. 320p. pap. text (*0-285-63282-5*) Souvenir Pr Ltd GBR. *Dist:* IPG Chicago.

Cognitive Therapy in Clinical Practice. Ed. by Jan Scott et al. 1989. 256p. (C). lib. bdg. 39.95 (*0-415-00518-3*, A2736) Routledge.

Cognitive Therapy in Practice: A Case Formulation Approach. Jacqueline B. Persons. 1989. 227p. (C). 29.00 (*0-393-70077-1*) Norton.

Cognitive Therapy of Anxiety Disorders: A Practice Manual & Conceptual Guide. Adrian Wells. 1997. LC 96-46488. 328p. pap. 65.00 (*0-471-96476-X*) Wiley.

Cognitive Therapy of Borderline Personality Disorder. Mary A. Layden et al. 1993. LC 93-16298. (Practitioner Guidebook Ser.). 256p. (C). 56.00 (*0-205-14807-7*, 48077, Longwood Div) Allyn.

Cognitive Therapy of Depression. Aaron T. Beck et al. LC 79-19967. (Clinical Psychology & Psychotherapy Ser.). 425p. 1987. 27.00 incl. audio compact disk (*0-89862-919-5*, 2919); 1979. pap. 46.95 (*0-89862-000-7*) Guilford Pubns.

Cognitive Therapy of Personality Disorders. Aaron T. Beck & Arthur Freeman. 1990. LC 90-33575. 396p. 45.00 (*0-89862-434-7*, 2434) Guilford Pubns.

Cognitive Therapy of Substance Abuse. Aaron T. Beck et al. 1993. LC 93-5208. 354p. 45.00 (*0-89862-115-1*, 2115) Guilford Pubns.

Cognitive Therapy of Suicidal Behavior: A Manual for Treatment. Arthur Freeman & Mark A. Reinecke. 1993. LC 92-48342. (Death & Suicide Ser.: Vol. 12). 256p. 37.95 (*0-8261-6500-1*) Springer Pub.

Cognitive Therapy with Children & Adolescents: A Casebook for Clinical Practice. Ed. by Mark A. Reinecke et al. 1995. LC 95-36991. 416p. text 46.00 (*1-57230-022-1*, 0022) Guilford Pubns.

Cognitive Therapy with Couples. Frank M. Dattilio & Christine A. Padesky. 1990. LC 90-52991. 150p. pap. 22.45 (*0-943158-49-4*, CTCBP, Prof Resc Pr) Pro Resource.

Cognitive Therapy with Couples & Groups. A. Freeman. 1983. LC 83-13210. (Illus.). 358p. (C). 75.00 (*0-306-41149-0*, Plenum Trade) Perseus Pubng.

Cognitive Therapy with Schizophrenic Patients. C. Perris. 1989. LC 88-24467. 240p. 34.95 (*0-89862-737-0*) Guilford Pubns.

Cognitive Unconscious: A Piagetian Approach to Psychotherapy. Melvin L. Weiner. 1975. LC 75-12937. (Illus.). 202p. 35.00 (*0-915662-01-9*) Intl Psych Pr.

Cognitive Vulnerability to Depression. Rick E. Ingram et al. 1997. LC 97-48997. 330p. text 40.00 (*1-57230-304-2*, C304) Guilford Pubns.

Cognitively Diagnostic Assessment. Ed. by Paul D. Nichols et al. 1995. 480p. 89.95 (*0-8058-1588-0*); pap. 49.95 (*0-8058-1589-9*) L Erlbaum Assocs.

Cohen Diabetic Rat. Ed. by A. M. Cohen & E. Rosenmann. 1991. (Illus.). xii, 200p. pap. 58.50 (*3-8055-5025-1*) S Karger.

Coherence Domain Optical Methods in Biomedical Science & Clinical Applications, Vol. 2981. Ed. by Valery V. Tuchin et al. 1997. LC 97-200958. 262p. 69.00 (*0-8194-2392-0*) SPIE.

Coherence Domain Optical Methods in Biomedical Science & Clinical Applications II, Vol. 3251. Ed. by Valery V. Tuchin & Joseph A. Izatt. 1998. LC 98-227301. 290p. 80.00 (*0-8194-2690-3*) SPIE.

Coherence in Psychotic Discourse. Branca T. Ribeiro. 1994. LC 92-49156. (Oxford Studies in Sociolinguistics). (Illus.). 336p. text 75.00 (*0-19-506597-2*) OUP.

Colbert's Medico English - Spanish Instant Communication for the Medical Profession. Roman Colbert. 1991. 322p. pap. (*0-9630253-0-9*) R Colbert.

Cold & Flu Fighter see Jane Brody's Cold & Flu Fighter

Cold Knife Surgery. Suzette Bishop. 1998. 36p. pap. 5.00 (*1-891387-00-6*) Red Dragon VA.

Cold Sheet Treatment. John R. Christopher. 1991. pap. 2.00 (*1-879436-07-8*, 99107) Christopher Pubns.

Cold Spring Harbor Symposia on Quantitative Biology: Chromatin, Vol. 42. Cold Spring Harbor Symposia on Quantitative Biolog. 1978. (Illus.). 1260p. 139.00 (*0-87969-041-0*) Cold Spring Harbor.

Cold Spring Harbor Symposia on Quantitative Biology: Origins of Lymphocyte Diversity, Set, Vol. 41. Cold Spring Harbor Symposia on Quantitative Biolog. 1977. (Illus.). 1024p. 107.50 (*0-87969-040-2*) Cold Spring Harbor.

Cold Spring Harbor Symposia on Quantitative Biology: Sensory Receptors, Vol. 30. Cold Spring Harbor Symposia on Quantitative Biolog. 1966. (Illus.). 663p. 38.00 (*0-87969-029-1*) Cold Spring Harbor.

Cold Water Cure. Vincent Priessnitz. 1996. 48p. reprint ed. spiral bd. 12.50 (*0-7873-0677-0*) Hlth Research.

Cold Weather Emergencies: Principles of Patient Management. Ed. by James L. Paturas et al. 1990. 64p. pap. text 15.00 (*1-887272-00-3*) Amer Med Pub.

Colds: Materia Medica Relating to Colds. 2000. LC 99-96051. 95p. pap. 6.95 (*1-929410-01-8*) dttm.

Colds (Acute Coryza) & Related Subjects. Herbert M. Shelton et al. 1996. 65p. reprint ed. spiral bd. 10.00 (*0-7873-1017-4*) Hlth Research.

Colds & Flu: The Physical & Mental Connections. Michael Schwartz. 1994. 65p. pap. 3.50 (*1-886722-04-8*) Maps Pub.

Colds, Flu & You: Building Optimum Immunity. Linda R. Page. 3rd rev. ed. 1996. (Healthy Healing Library). (Illus.). 32p. pap. 3.50 (*1-884334-47-4*) Hlthy Healing.

Coliform Index & Waterborne Disease: Problems of Microbial Drinking Water Assessment. Cara Gleesoon & Nick F. Gray. 1996. LC 96-70578. (Illus.). 208p. (C). 65.00 (*0-419-21870-X*, Spon) Routledge.

Colitis Diet. 1991. lib. bdg. 75.00 (*0-8490-5137-1*) Gordon Pr.

Collaboration: A Health Care Imperative. Toni J. Sullivan. 1997. LC 98-124561. (Illus.). 672p. pap. 49.95 (*0-07-063350-9*) McGraw-Hill Prof.

Collaboration among Competing Managed Care Organizations for Quality Improvement. 1999. 62p. 18.00 (*0-309-06386-8*) Natl Acad Pr.

Collaboration in Care. Ed. by Jenny Wright et al. 1989. (C). (*0-86242-067-9*) Age Concern Eng GBR. *Dist:* St Mut.

Collaboration in Health Care: Hartford Hospital's Experience in Changing Management & Practice. Ed. by Cheryl B. Stetler et al. 1995. LC 95-14079. 307p. pap. 69.00 (*1-55648-139-X*) AHPI.

***Collaboration in Primary Mental Health.** 2001. pap. (*0-7487-5874-7*) Nelson Thornes GBR. *Dist:* Intl Spec Bk.

Collaborative Brain Injury Intervention: Positive Everyday Routines. Mark Ylvisaker & Timothy Feeney. 1998. LC 98-30364. (Illus.). 300p. pap. text 72.95 (*1-56593-733-3*, 1426) Thomson Learn.

Collaborative Clinical Education: The Foundation of Effective Health Care. Jane Westberg & Hilliard Jason. 1992. LC 92-49817. (Medical Education Ser.: Vol. 16). 432p. 49.95 (*0-8261-8030-2*) Springer Pub.

Collaborative Community Mental Health Care. 384p. pap. text (*0-340-54241-1*) E A GBR. *Dist:* Routldge.

***Collaborative Design Planning.** 112p. ring bd. 30.00 (*0-9677733-0-X*) Inst Fmly Ctr.

Collaborative Health Care: A Family-Oriented Model. Michael M. Glenn. 1987. LC 87-2420. 235p. 77.00 (*0-275-92319-3*, C2319, Praeger Pubs) Greenwood.

Collaborative Nursing Case Management: A Handbook for Development & Implementation. Virginia Del Togno-Armanasco et al. 1993. LC 93-14984. 200p. 29.95 (*0-8261-8110-4*, 93-14984) Springer Pub.

Collaborative Psychoanalysis: Anxiety, Depression, Dreams & Personality Change. Walter Bonime. 1989. LC 86-46161. 416p. 55.00 (*0-8386-3298-X*) Fairleigh Dickinson.

Collaborative Research in Developmental Therapy: A Model with Studies of Learning Disabled Children. Ed. by Kenneth J. Ottenbacher & Margaret A. Short-DeGraff. 1986. LC 86-11978. 157p. text 49.95 (*0-86656-570-1*) Haworth Pr.

***Collagen Revolution: Living Pain Free.** Marc Darrow. 2002. (Illus.). 192p. pap. 25.00 (*0-9714503-0-7*) Protex Pr.

Collagenases. Warren Hoeffler. 1999. LC 98-50414. (Medical Intelligence Unit Ser.: Vol. 10). (Illus.). 259p. 99.00 (*1-57059-562-3*) Landes Bioscience.

Collateral Circulation: Heart, Brain, Kidney, Limbs. Ed. by Wolfgang Schaper & Jutta Schaper. 1992. text 194.50 (*0-7923-2012-3*) Kluwer Academic.

Collect What You Produce. Cathy Jameson. 1996. LC 96-15336. xv, 231p. 44.95 (*0-87814-588-5*) PennWell Corp.

Collected Essays in Drama Therapy: The Double Life. Robert J. Landy. 1995. 268p. pap. text (*1-85302-322-1*) Jessica Kingsley GBR. *Dist:* Taylor & Francis.

Collected Essays on Public Health & Epidemiology Rudolf Virchow. 1985. LC 85-2042. (Illus.). 1. (*0-88135-076-1*); 2. (*0-88135-077-X*) Watson Pub Intl.

Collected Letters of Antoni Van Leeuwenhoek, Vol. 13. Antoni Van Leeuwenhoek. 1994. xviii, 344p. text (*90-265-1239-2*) Swets.

Collected Papers of David Rapaport. David Rapaport. 1996. (Master Work Ser.). 95.00 (*1-56821-473-1*) Aronson.

Collected Papers of Paul Ehrlich: Complete Bibliography, Set. F. Himmelweit & M. Marquardt. 1957. (*0-08-013123-9*) Pergamon Repr GBR. *Dist:* Franklin.

Collected Papers on Schizophrenia & Related Subjects. Harold F. Searles. 1966. LC 65-21320. 798p. 80.00 (*0-8236-0980-4*) Intl Univs Pr.

***Collected Questions & Answers.** Mark E. Brecher. 2001. (*1-56395-147-9*) Am Assn Blood.

Collected Questions & Answers. Ed. by Richard J. Davey & Ann McMican. 4th ed. 1994. 79p. (C). pap. text 28.00 (*1-56395-036-7*) Am Assn Blood.

Collected Studies on the Dionne Quintuplets. William E. Blatz. 1975. LC 74-21401. (Classics in Child Development Ser.). (Illus.). 294p. reprint ed. 44.95 (*0-405-06454-3*) Ayer.

Collected Works of C. G. Jung Supplementary Vol. A: The Zofingia Lectures. Carl Gustav Jung. Ed. by William McGuire. Tr. by Jan van Heurck. 1983. LC 83-42592. (Bollingen Ser.: No. 20). (Illus.). 160p. 47.50 (*0-691-09899-9*) Princeton U Pr.

Collected Works of C. G. Jung Vol. 1: Psychiatric Studies. Carl Gustav Jung. Ed. by G. Adler & R. F. C. Hull. 1970. (Bollingen Ser.: No. 20). 238p. 59.50 (*0-691-09768-2*) Princeton U Pr.

Collected Works of C. G. Jung Vol. 2: Experimental Researches. Carl Gustav Jung et al. Ed. by Gerhard Adler et al. Tr. by Leopold Stein & Diana Riviere. 1973. LC 73-159406. (Bollingen Ser.: No. 20). (Illus.). 664p. 85.00 (*0-691-09764-X*) Princeton U Pr.

Collected Works of C. G. Jung Vol. 3: The Psychogenesis of Mental Disease. Carl Gustav Jung et al. Ed. by G. Adler et al. (Bollingen Ser.: No. 20). 316p. 1984. pap. 19.95 (*0-691-01859-6*); 1960. 65.00 (*0-691-09769-0*) Princeton U Pr.

Collected Works of C. G. Jung Vol. 4: Freud & Psychoanalysis. Carl Gustav Jung. Ed. by G. Adler. Tr. by R. F. C. Hull. 1961. LC 52-8757. (Bollingen Ser.: No. 20). 392p. 65.00 (*0-691-09765-8*) Princeton U Pr.

Collected Works of C. G. Jung Vol. 5: Symbols of Transformation. Carl Gustav Jung et al. Ed. by G. Adler et al. 2nd ed. (Bollingen Ser.: No. 20). 597p. 1977. (Illus.). pap. 24.95 (*0-691-01815-4*); 1967. 85.00 (*0-691-09775-5*) Princeton U Pr (Bollingen).

Collected Works of C. G. Jung Vol. 7: Two Essays on Analytical Psychology. Carl Gustav Jung et al. Ed. by Gerhard Adler et al. Tr. by R. F. C. Hull. 2nd ed. (Bollingen Ser.: No. 20). 396p. 1972. pap. 19.95 (*0-691-01782-4*); 1967. 65.00 (*0-691-09776-3*) Princeton U Pr.

Collected Works of C. G. Jung Vol. 8: The Structure & Dynamics of the Psyche. Carl Gustav Jung. Ed. by Gerhard Adler et al. Tr. by R. F. C. Hull. 2nd ed. 1970. (Bollingen Ser.: No. 20). 606p. 79.50 (*0-691-09774-7*) Princeton U Pr.

Collected Works of C. G. Jung Vol. 9, Pt. 1: Archetypes & the Collective Unconscious. Carl Gustav Jung et al. Ed. by Gerhard Adler et al. Tr. by R. F. C. Hull. 2nd ed. (Bollingen Ser.: No. 20). 474p. 1981. pap. 29.95 (*0-691-01833-2*); 1969. LC 82-182882. 95.00 (*0-691-09761-5*) Princeton U Pr.

Collected Works of C. G. Jung Vol. 9, Pt. 2: Aion - Researches into the Phenomenology of the Self. Ed. by Gerhard Adler et al. Tr. by R. F. C. Hull. 2nd ed. (Collected Works of C. G. Jung No. 9: No. 20). 353p. 1979. pap. 18.95 (*0-691-01826-X*); 1969. 59.50 (*0-691-09759-3*) Princeton U Pr.

Collected Works of C. G. Jung Vol. 10: Civilization in Transition. Carl Gustav Jung et al. Ed. by Gerhard Adler et al. Tr. by R. F. C. Hull. 2nd ed. 1970. LC 81-160172. (Bollingen Ser.: No. 20). (Illus.). 630p. 79.50 (*0-691-09762-3*) Princeton U Pr.

Collected Works of C. G. Jung Vol. 11: Psychology & Religion: West & East. Carl Gustav Jung et al. Ed. by Gerhard Adler et al. Tr. by R. F. C. Hull. 2nd ed. 1970. LC 74-13858. (Bollingen Ser.: No. 20). (Illus.). 712p. 85.00 (*0-691-09772-0*) Princeton U Pr.

Collected Works of C. G. Jung Vol. 12: Psychology & Alchemy. Carl Gustav Jung et al. Ed. by Gerhard Adler et al. Tr. by R. F. C. Hull. 2nd ed. (Bollingen Ser.: No. 20). 617p. 1980. pap. 21.95 (*0-691-01831-6*); 1968. 85.00 (*0-691-09771-2*) Princeton U Pr.

Collected Works of C. G. Jung Vol. 13: Alchemical Studies. Carl Gustav Jung et al. Ed. by Gerhard Adler et al. Tr. by R. F. C. Hull. (Bollingen Ser.: No. 20). 617p. 1983. (Illus.). pap. 35.00 (*0-691-01849-9*); 1968. 85.00 (*0-691-09760-7*) Princeton U Pr.

Collected Works of C. G. Jung Vol. 14: Mysterium Coniunctionis: An Inquiry into the Separation & Synthesis of Psychic Opposites in Alchemy. Carl Gustav Jung et al. Ed. by Gerhard Adler et al. Tr. by R. F. C. Hull. 2nd ed. (Collected Works of C.G. Jung: No. 20). (Illus.). 714p. 1977. LC 78-314608. pap. 24.95 (*0-691-01816-2*); 1970. LC 75-302998. 85.00 (*0-691-09766-6*) Princeton U Pr.

Collected Works of C. G. Jung Vol. 15: The Spirit in Man, Art & Literature, Carl Gustav Jung et al. Ed. by Gerhard Adler et al. Tr. by R. F. C. Hull. 1966. LC 96-149588. (Bollingen Ser.: No. 20). 176p. 35.00 (*0-691-09773-9*) Princeton U Pr.

Collected Works of C. G. Jung Vol. 15: The Spirit in Man, Art, & Literature. Carl Gustav Jung et al. Ed. by Gerhard Adler et al. Tr. by R. F. C. Hull. 1971. LC 77-373351. (Bollingen Ser.: No. 20). 176p. pap. 14.95 (*0-691-01775-1*) Princeton U Pr.

Collected Works of C. G. Jung Vol. 16: The Practice of Psychotherapy. Carl Gustav Jung. 1985. (Bollingen Ser.: No. 20). 416p. pap. 21.95 (*0-691-01870-7*) Princeton U Pr.

Collected Works of C. G. Jung Vol. 16: The Practice of Psychotherapy. Ed. by Gerhard Adler et al. Tr. by R. F. C. Hull. 2nd ed. 1966. (Bollingen Ser.: No. 20). 416p. 70.00 (*0-691-09767-4*) Princeton U Pr.

Collected Works of C. G. Jung Vol. 18: The Symbolic Life: Miscellaneous Writings. Carl Gustav Jung et al. Ed. by Gerhard Adler et al. Tr. by R. F. C. Hull. 1977. LC 81-160155. (Collected Works of C.G. Jung: No. 20). 1024p. 125.00 (*0-691-09892-1*) Princeton U Pr.

Collected Works of C. G. Jung Vol. 19: General Bibliography of C. G. Jung's Writings. Ed. by Gerhard Adler et al. Tr. by R. F. C. Hull. rev. ed. 1979. LC 91-32917. (Bollingen Ser.: No. 20). 366p. 55.00 (*0-691-09893-X*) Princeton U Pr.

Collected Works of C. G. Jung Vol. 20: General Index. Ed. by Gerhard Adler et al. Tr. by R. F. C. Hull. 1979. LC 80-453172. (Bollingen Ser.: No. 20). 751p. 95.00 (*0-691-09867-0*) Princeton U Pr.

Collected Works of L. S. Vygotsky Vol. 1: Problems of General Psychology, Including the Volume "Thinking & Speech" L. S. Vygotsky. 1988. (Cognition & Language Ser.). (Illus.). 406p. (C). 71.00 (*0-306-42441-X*, Plenum Trade) Perseus Pubng.

Collected Works of L. S. Vygotsky Vol. 2: Fundamentals of Defectology (Abnormal Psychology & Learning Disabilities) L. S. Vygotsky. 1993. (Cognition & Language). (Illus.). 362p. (C). 71.00 (*0-306-42442-8*, Plenum Trade) Perseus Pubng.

Collected Works of L. S. Vygotsky Vol. 3: Problems of the Theory & History of Psychology, Vol. 3. Ed. by Robert W. Rieber & Jeffrey Wollock. 1997. (Cognition & Language). (Illus.). 438p. (C). 59.50 (*0-306-45488-2*, Plenum Trade) Perseus Pubng.

Collected Works of L. S. Vygotsky Vol. 5: Child Psychology. Ed. by Robert W. Rieber. 1998. (Cognition & Language Ser.). (Illus.). 380p. (C). 59.50 (*0-306-45707-5*, Kluwer Plenum) Kluwer Academic.

Collected Works of Lawrence W. Macdonald, Vol. 1. Lawrence W. Macdonald. Ed. by Abraham Shapiro. 1992. (Illus.). 299p. (C). lib. bdg. 18.00 (*0-943599-56-3*) OEPF.

Collected Works of Lawrence W. Macdonald, Vol. 2. Lawrence W. Macdonald. Ed. by Ira Schwartz & Abraham Shapiro. 1992. (Illus.). 350p. (C). lib. bdg. 18.00 (*0-943599-58-X*) OEPF.

Collected Works of Lydia Sicher: An Adlerian Perspective. Lydia Sicher. Ed. by Adele K. Davidson. 1991. LC 90-26254. (Illus.). 608p. (Orig.). pap. 24.95 (*0-936609-22-2*) QED Ft Bragg.

Collected Works of Peter G. Ossorio Vol. I: Persons. Peter G. Ossorio. 1995. 289p. text 70.00 (*0-9625661-8-7*) Descriptive Psych Pr.

Collected Works of Peter G. Ossorio Vol. II: Essays on Clinical Topics. Peter G. Ossorio. 1997. 70.00 (*0-9625661-9-5*) Descriptive Psych Pr.

Collected Works of Peter G. Ossorio Vol. III: Place. Peter G. Ossorio. 1998. 70.00 (*1-891700-00-6*) Descriptive Psych Pr.

Collected Writings. Paul R. Harrington. 1992. (Illus.). 376p. 100.00 (*0-932845-56-8*) Lowell Pr.

Collecting Information from Health Care Consumers: A Resource Manual of Tested Questionnaires & Practical Advice. Norbert Goldfield et al. 1996. ring bd. 189.00 (*0-8342-0676-5*, S177) Aspen Pub.

Collection & Processing of Drug Information. 1986. lib. bdg. 79.95 (*0-8490-3513-9*) Gordon Pr.

Collection & Use of Human Blood & Plasma in Europe: Report Prepared by Prof. Dr. W. G. Van Aken. 1993. (*92-871-2240-7*) Council of Europe FRA. *Dist:* Manhattan Pub Co.

Collection Containers for Specimens for Toxicological Analysis. 1986. (Proposed Guideline Ser.: Vol. 6). 75.00 (*1-56238-058-3*, H31-P) NCCLS.

Collection Development & Assessment in Health Sciences Libraries. Daniel T. Richards & Dottie Eakin. Ed. by Alison Bunting. 1997. LC 96-31662. (Current Practice in Health Sciences Librarianship Ser.: Vol. 4). 360p. 55.00 (*0-8108-3201-1*) Scarecrow.

Collection Manual for Healthcare Providers. Noelle Floreen. 1998. 55.00 (*0-07-134831-X*) McGraw.

Collection of Ceramic Works: A Communication of Tool for the Dental Office & Laboratory. Hitoshi Oshima. 1992. (Illus.). 92p. text 64.00 (*4-87417-386-1*) Quint Pub Co.

Collection of Recipes for the Use of Special Diet Kitchens in Military Hospitals. Helen Wittenmyer. 13.95 (*0-8488-0006-0*, J M C & Co) Amereon Ltd.

Collection, Transport, & Processing of Blood Specimens for Coagulation Testing & Performance of Coagulation Assays. 2nd ed. 1991. (Approved Guideline Ser.: Vol. 6). 85.00 (*1-56238-129-6*, H21-A2) NCCLS.

Collections Made Easy! Michael J. Berry. Ed. by Kathryn Swanson. 2nd ed. 1999. pap. text 44.95 (*1-57066-146-4*, ME124) Practice Mgmt Info.

Collective Behavior & Social Movements: Process & Structure. Gary T. Marx & Douglas McAdam. 1993. LC 92-29657. (Prentice Hall Foundations of Modern Sociology Ser.). 160p. (C). pap. text 30.40 (*0-13-142100-X*) P-H.

College Level Program for Learning Disabled Students. John R. Moss et al. 1980. (C). pap. 15.95 (*0-937660-01-9*) PIP.

College Outline: Introduction to Psychology. King. 1999. (C). pap. text (*0-15-601686-9*) Harcourt Coll Pubs.

College Peer Groups: Problems & Prospects for Research. Ed. by Theodore M. Newcomb & Everett K. Wilson. 1966. LC 65-29033. (Monographs in Social Research: No. 8). 15.00 (*0-202-09002-7*) Natl Opinion Res.

College Physics: Student Study Guide. Vincent P. Coletta. 1993. 240p. 18.95 (*0-8016-7723-8*) Mosby Inc.

College Student Development. Ed. by Richard E. Slimak. 1993. LC 92-42183. (Journal of College Student Psychotherapy Ser.: Vol. 6, Nos. 3-4). (Illus.). 240p. pap. text 19.95 (*1-56024-314-7*); lib. bdg. 49.95 (*1-56024-313-9*) Haworth Pr.

Colleges of Podiatry Admission Test (CPAT) Jack Rudman. (Admission Test Ser.: Vol. 37). 49.95 (*0-8373-5137-5*); 1994. reprint ed. pap. 29.95 (*0-8373-5037-9*) Nat Learn.

Colleges That Enable: A Guide to Support Services Offered to Physically Disabled Students on 40 U. S. Campuses. Prudence K. Tweed & Jason C. Tweed. 1989. (Illus.). 106p. (Orig.). pap. text 10.95 (*0-922466-12-2*) JIST Pubng.

Collegium Internationale Neuro-Psychopharmacologicum, 10th Congress: Proceedings, Set. Ed. by P. Deniker. 1978. (*0-08-021506-8*) Pergamon Repr GBR. *Dist:* Franklin.

Collision Sports: Injury & Repair. David Fevre. 1998. LC 98-28064. 288p. pap. text 45.00 (*0-7506-3142-2*) Buttrwrth-Heinemann.

Colloid Science, Vols. 1-2. D. H. Everett. 1973. LC 72-95096. 36.00 (*0-85186-508-9*) Am Chemical.

Colloidal Carriers/Controlled Drug Delivery & Targeting. Rainer H. Muller. 1991. 110.00 (*0-8493-7714-5*) CRC Pr.

Colloidal Drug Delivery Systems. Ed. by Jorg Kreuter. 1994. LC 94-14913. (Drugs & the Pharmaceutical Sciences Ser.: Vol. 66). (Illus.). 368p. text 150.00 (*0-8247-9214-9*) Dekker.

Colloque International sur la Thrombolyse Paris, Mars 1985. Ed. by A. Serradimigni. 1986. (Journal: Vol. 16, Suppl. 4, 1986). (Illus.). 160p. pap. 50.50 (*3-8055-4375-1*) S Karger.

Colloquies on the Simples & Drugs of India. G. D. Orta. 509p. (C). 1985. text (*0-89771-616-7*); 1979. reprint ed. (*0-7855-3127-0*) Intl Bk Distr IND. *Dist:* St Mut.

Colloquium on the Use of Embryonic Cell Transplantation for Correction of CNS Disorders. Ed. by V. H. Mark et al. 1984. (Journal: Vol 47, No. 1-2). (Illus.). 96p. pap. 30.50 (*3-8055-3952-5*) S Karger.

Colo-Proctology. Ed. by J. C. Givel & F. Saegesser. 1984. (Illus.). 182p. 51.95 (*0-387-12557-4*) Spr-Verlag.

Cologne Atherosclerosis Conference No. 2: Lipids. Michael J. Parnham. 1984. (Agents & Actions Supplements Ser.: No. 16). 75.00 (*0-8176-1645-4*) Birkhauser.

Cologne Atherosclerosis Conference Three: Platelets. Ed. by Michael J. Parnham & G. Prop. 1986. (Agents & Actions Supplements Ser.: No. 20). 278p. 85.00 (*0-8176-1805-8*) Birkhauser.

Colon & Rectal Cancer. Peter S. Edelstein. 2000. LC 99-462081. 480p. 137.00 (*0-471-35145-8*) Wiley.

Colon & Rectal Cancer. John M. MacKeigan & Kathleen M. Hillary. Ed. by Oliver D. Grin & Dorothy L. Bouwman. 1990. (Patient Education Ser.). (Illus.). 30p. pap. text 4.00 (*0-929689-44-5*) Ludann Co.

Colon & Rectal Cancer. Christopher Willett. 2000. (ACS Atlas of Clinical Oncology Ser.). 320p. incl. cd-rom (*1-55009-110-7*) DEKR.

Colon & Rectal Cancer: A Comprehensive Guide for Patients & Families. Lorraine Johnston. Ed. by Linda Lamb. 1999. LC 99-53773. (Patient-Centered Guides Ser.). (Illus.). 552p. pap. 24.95 (*1-56592-633-1*, Patient-Centered) OReilly & Assocs.

Colon & Rectal Cancer: A Patient's Guide to Treatment. Paul Ruggieri. 2001. LC 2001-177. (Illus.). 160p. pap. 14.95 (*1-886039-51-8*) Addicus Bks.

Colon & Rectal Cancer: All You Need to Know to Take an Active Part in Your Treatment. Michael E. Pezim. 1992. (Illus.). 214p. pap. (*0-9696125-0-8*) ITPG.

Colon & Rectal Surgery. Marvin L. Corman. 4th ed. 1998. LC 98-3238. 1,440p. text 269.00 (*0-7817-1013-8*) Lppncott W & W.

***Colon Cancer: Greater Use of Screening Would Save Lives: Congressional Hearing.** Charles E. Grassley. 2001. 80p. pap. text 20.00 (*0-7567-1573-3*) DIANE Pub.

Colon Cancer & the Polyps Connection. Stephen Fisher. 2000. LC 95-17811. (Illus.). 288p. pap. 16.95 (*1-55561-080-3*) Fisher Bks.

Colon Handbook: A Guide to Health. 1991. lib. bdg. 75.00 (*0-8490-5119-3*) Gordon Pr.

Colon Health: Key to a Vibrant Life. N. W. Walker. rev. ed. 1995. 132p. pap. 7.95 (*0-89019-069-0*) Norwalk Pr.

Colon Health Handbook. Robert Gray. 12th rev. ed. 1991. 80p. pap. 7.95 (*0-9615757-2-7*) Emerald NV.

Colon, Rectum & Anus. Ed. by C. Richard Boland. 1996. LC 95-32010. (Gastroenterology & Hepatology Ser.: Vol. 2). (Illus.). 241p. text 85.00 (*1-878132-79-2*) Current Med.

Colon, Rectum & Anus. L. P. Fielding & S. M. Goldberg. 5th ed. Date not set. (Operative Surgery Ser.). Vol. 1. text (*0-7506-1234-7*); Vol. 2. (*0-7506-1244-4*) Chapman & Hall.

Colonial American Medicine. Susan N. Terkel. 1993. LC 92-43988. (Colonial America Ser.). (Illus.). 112p. (J). (gr. 5-8). lib. bdg. 24.00 (*0-531-12539-4*) F Watts.

Colonial Disease: A Social History of Sleeping Sickness in Northern Zaire, 1900-1940. Maryinez Lyons. 1992. (History of Medicine Ser.). (Illus.). 351p. (C). text 90.00 (*0-521-40350-2*) Cambridge U Pr.

Colonial Physician & Other Essays. Whitfield J. Bell, Jr. 1975. LC 75-6652. (Illus.). 236p. text 16.00 (*0-88202-024-2*, Sci Hist) Watson Pub Intl.

Colonial Psychiatry & 'The African Mind' Jock McCulloch. 1995. 195p. (C). text 59.95 (*0-521-45330-5*) Cambridge U Pr.

Colonialism, Health, & Illness in French Equatorial Africa, 1885-1935. Rita Headrick. Ed. by Daniel R. Headrick. 1995. LC 94-29444. 48.00 (*0-918456-71-1*) African Studies Assn.

Colonialism, Tropical Disease & Imperial Medicine: Rockefeller Philanthropy in Sri Lanka. Soma Hewa. 1995. LC 95-13578. 222p. (C). lib. bdg. 49.00 (*0-8191-9939-7*) U Pr of Amer.

Colonic Drug Absorption & Metabolism. Ed. by Peter R. Bieck. 1993. LC 93-17265. (Drugs & the Pharmaceutical Sciences Ser.: Vol. 60). (Illus.). 240p. text 155.00 (*0-8247-9013-8*) Dekker.

Colonic Microbiota, Nutrition & Health. Contrib. by Glenn R. Gibson & M. B. Roberfroid. 1999. LC 99-40946. 312p. 149.00 (*0-412-79880-8*, Kluwer Plenum) Kluwer Academic.

Colonizing the Body: State Medicine & Epidemic Disease in Nineteenth-Century India. David Arnold. 1993. LC 92-25623. (C). text 55.00 (*0-520-08124-2*); pap. text 24.95 (*0-520-08295-8*) U CA Pr.

***Colonoscopy: Introduction & Development, Completion Rates, Complications & Cancer Detection.** George Dafnis. 2001. (Comprehensive Summaries of Uppsala Dissertatons from the Faculty of Medicine: No. 1039). (Illus.). 82p. pap. (*91-554-5030-X*) Uppsala Universitet SWE. *Dist:* Coronet Bks.

Colonoscopy: Principles & Techniques. Nord Raskin. Ed. by Jeffrey B. Raskin & H. Juergen Nord. 1995. LC 95-3481. (Illus.). 384p. 89.50 (*0-89640-277-0*) Igaku-Shoin.

Coloproctology. J. Nicholls & Richard Glass. 1985. (Illus.). 236p. 61.95 (*0-387-15140-0*) Spr-Verlag.

Color & Human Response. Faber Birren. 1978. LC 77-12505. (Illus.). 120p. pap. 29.95 (*0-442-20961-4*, VNR) Wiley.

Color & Power Doppler Teaching File. R. Jeffrey, Jr. 1997. LC 97-21997. 320p. text 149.00 (*0-397-51779-3*) Lppncott W & W.

Color & Spectral Doppler Ultrasound of the Carotid Artery & Peripheral Vessels. E. Meredith James et al. 1991. (C). 700.00 incl. disk (*1-56815-006-7*) Mosby Inc.

Color & the Edgar Cayce Readings. Roger Lewis. 1973. 48p. pap. 4.95 (*0-87604-068-7*, 264) ARE Pr.

Color Atlas: Test of Flow Cytometric Analysis of Hematologic Neoplasms. Tsieh Sun. 1993. LC 93-3103. (Illus.). 232p. 148.50 (*0-89640-232-0*) Igaku-Shoin.

Color Atlas: Text of Ureteroscopy. Lawrence B. Kandel. 1993. LC 92-48832. (Illus.). 336p. 159.95 (*0-89640-210-X*) Igaku-Shoin.

Color Atlas - Text of Advanced Laparoscopy for Surgeons. Barry A. Salky. 1995. LC 94-9399. (Illus.). 168p. 98.50 (*0-89640-224-X*) Igaku-Shoin.

Color Atlas - Text of Excimer Laser Surgery: The Cornea. Frank B. Thompson & Peter J. McDonnell. 1993. LC 92-1551. (Illus.). 176p. 125.00 (*0-89640-225-8*) Igaku-Shoin.

Color Atlas & Identification Manual of Gram Stain Images. Linda M. Marler et al. 2000. LC 00-64291. 320p. spiral bd. 45.95 (*0-7817-2663-8*) Lppncott W & W.

Color Atlas & Instruction Manual of Peripheral Blood Morphology. Barbara H. O'Connor. 1984. (Illus.). 316p. (C). pap. text 49.95 (*0-683-06624-2*) Lppncott W & W.

Color Atlas & Synopsis of Clinical Dermatology. Thomas B. Fitzpatrick et al. 2nd ed. 1991. 824p. text 49.00 (*0-07-021209-0*) McGraw-Hill Med Pub.

Color Atlas & Synopsis of Clinical Dermatology. Thomas B. Fitzpatrick et al. 4th ed. 2000. LC 00-56632. (Illus.). 1041p. pap. 55.00 (*0-07-136038-7*) McGraw-Hill Prof.

***Color Atlas & Synopsis of Pediatric Dermatology.** Kay S. Kane et al. 2001. (Illus.). 750p. pap. 79.00 (*0-07-006294-3*) McGraw-Hill Prof.

Color Atlas & Synopsis of Pigmented Lesions. Raymond L. Barnhill et al. 1995. (Illus.). 250p. text 59.95 (*0-07-005110-0*) McGraw-Hill Med Pub.

Color Atlas & Synopsis of Sexually Transmitted Diseases. H. Hunter Handsfield. 2nd ed. 2000. LC 00-41552. (Illus.). 216p. pap. 59.95 (*0-07-026033-8*) McGraw-Hill Prof.

Color Atlas & Test Neurology. G. David Perkin. 1997. text (*0-7234-2497-7*) Wolfe Publishing GBR. *Dist:* Mosby Inc.

Color Atlas & Text of Adult Dementias. David M. Mann et al. 1994. LC 94-43604. (*0-7234-1784-9*) Wolfe Publishing.

Color Atlas & Text of Bone Marrow Transplantation. Ed. by Peter Wiernik & Jennifer G. Treleaven. 1994. (Illus.). 240p. (C). (gr. 13). text 93.00 (*0-8151-8848-X*, 22742) Mosby Inc.

Color Atlas & Text of Clinical Medicine. Charles D. Forbes & William F. Jackson. 2nd ed. 1997. 534p. pap. 46.00 (*0-7234-2198-6*) Mosby Inc.

Color Atlas & Text of Clinical Medicine. Charles D. Forbes & William F. Jackson. 2nd ed. 1997. (Illus.). 576p. pap. (*84-8174-333-X*) Mosby-Doyma Libros ESP. *Dist:* Mosby Inc.

Color Atlas & Text of Complete Prosthodontics. Grant Staff. 1993. (Illus.). 144p. (C). (gr. 13). 56.95 (*0-8151-3546-7*, 22954) Mosby Inc.

Color Atlas & Text of Dental & Maxillo-Facial Implantology. John A. Hobkirk & Peter G. Watson. 1994. LC 94-23608. text 145.00 (*0-7234-1786-5*) Mosby Inc.

Color Atlas & Text of Dental Care for the Elderly. Yemm. 1994. (Illus.). 216p. (C). (gr. 13). text 99.95 (*0-8151-9751-9*, 22890) Mosby Inc.

Color Atlas & Text of Endodontics. Christopher Stock & Gulabiuaza. 2nd ed. 1995. 352p. text 148.50 (*0-7234-1890-X*) Mosby Inc.

Color Atlas & Text of Endodontics. Christopher J. R. Stock et al. 2nd ed. 1995. (Illus.). 352p. (*84-8174-137-X*) Mosby-Doyma Libros ESP. *Dist:* Mosby Inc.

Color Atlas & Text of Equine Ophthalmology. K. C. Barnett et al. 1994. text (*0-7234-1925-6*) Wolfe Publishing.

Color Atlas & Text of Neuro-Ophthalmology, '97. Cumming. 1998. text 199.00 (*0-7234-1964-7*) Mosby Inc.

Color Atlas & Text of Obstetric & Gynecologic Dermatology. Martin M. Black et al. 1996. (Illus.). 192p. text (*0-7234-2009-2*) Martin Dunitz GBR. *Dist:* Mosby Inc.

Color Atlas & Text of Osteoarthritis. M. Doherty et al. 1993. 105.00 (*0-8151-2752-9*, 22853) Mosby Inc.

Color Atlas & Text of Surgical Pathology of the Dog & Cat, 1. Julie A. Yager. 1994. LC 93-2094. text (*0-7234-1827-6*) Wolfe Publishing GBR. *Dist:* Mosby Inc.

Color Atlas & Textbook of Diagnostic Parasitology. Tsieh Sun. 1988. LC 87-29308. (Illus.). 328p. 125.00 (*0-89640-135-9*) Igaku-Shoin.

Color Atlas & Textbook of Equine Ophthalmology. K. C. Barnett. 1994. (C). (gr. 13). text 110.00 (*0-8151-0420-0*, 23000) Mosby Inc.

Color Atlas & Textbook of Human Anatomy: Locomotor System, Vol. I. Werner Platzer et al. 4th ed. 1992. (Illus.). 440p. pap. 29.90 (*0-86577-423-4*) Thieme Med Pubs.

Color Atlas & Textbook of Human Anatomy Vol. 2: Internal Organs, No. 2. Kahle. 4th ed. 1993. pap. 29.90 (*0-86577-484-6*) Thieme Med Pubs.

Color Atlas & Textbook of Oral Anatomy, Histology, & Embryology. B. K. Berkovitz et al. 2nd rev. ed. 1992. LC 92-12712. (Illus.). 328p. (C). (gr. 13). text 73.00 (*0-8151-0697-1*, 21901) Mosby Inc.

Color Atlas & Textbook of the Histopathology of Mycotic Diseases. Robin S. Chapman. 1981. (Illus.). 333p. (C). (gr. 13). 142.00 (*0-8151-1637-3*, 09846) Mosby Inc.

Color Atlas Dermatology. Callen. 1994. 1100.00 (*0-7216-3757-4*) Harcourt.

Color Atlas Histology. Dennis Strete. 1997. LC 95-181. (Illus.). 448p. (C). pap. 28.40 (*0-673-99190-3*) Addson-Wesley Educ.

Color Atlas of Acoustic Neuroma Microsurgery. Mario Sanna. 1998. LC 97-34732. (Illus.). 200p. 139.00 (*0-86577-726-8*) Thieme Med Pubs.

Color Atlas of Aesthetic Surgery of the Abdomen. Jorge Psillakis et al. 1991. (Illus.). 96p. text 119.00 (*0-86577-343-2*) Thieme Med Pubs.

Color Atlas of AIDS. Alvin E. Friedman-Kien. Ed. by Lisette Bralow & Judy Fletcher. 2nd ed. 1996. LC 95-20377. 224p. text 62.00 (*0-7216-4949-1*) Saunders.

Color Atlas of AIDS in the Tropics. Ansary. 1989. (Illus.). text 85.00 (*0-7234-1567-6*) CRC Pr.

Color Atlas of Anatomy: A Photographic Study of the Human Body. Johannes W. Rohen et al. 4th ed. 1998. LC 97-42744. (Illus.). 486p. 67.95 (*0-683-30492-5*) Lppncott W & W.

Color Atlas of Arthropods in Clinical Medicine. Wallac Peters. 1992. (Illus.). 256p. (C). (gr. 13). text 165.00 (*0-8151-6679-6*, 21938) Mosby Inc.

Color Atlas of Basic Histology. Irwin Berman. 2nd rev. ed. 1997. LC 97-223478. (Illus.). 356p. (C). spiral bd. 54.95 (*0-8385-1435-9*, A-1435-5) McGraw-Hill Prof.

Color Atlas of Basic Histopathology. Clara Milikowski & Irwin Berman. 1996. (Illus.). 615p. (C). text 59.95 (*0-8385-1382-4*, A1382-9) McGraw-Hill Prof.

Color Atlas of Bone & Joint Disease in the Elderly. Chakravorty. 160p. 60.00 (*0-8151-1613-6*) Mosby Inc.

Color Atlas of Brain Disorders in the Newborn. Devries. 1990. (Illus.). (C). (gr. 13). 105.00 (*0-8151-2964-5*, 20267) Mosby Inc.

Color Atlas of Breast Diseases. Robert E. Mansel. 1994. (Illus.). 128p. (C). (gr. 13). text 29.95 (*0-8151-5756-8*, 21951) Mosby Inc.

Color Atlas of Breast Diseases. Robert E. Mansel & Nigel J. Bundred. 1994. LC 94-44123. (Illus.). text 37.50 (*0-7234-1721-0*) Mosby Inc.

Color Atlas of Cancer Cytology. Masayoshi Takahashi. 2nd ed. 1981. LC 80-85297. (Illus.). 580p. 160.00 (*0-89640-050-6*) Igaku-Shoin.

Color Atlas of Chinese Traditional Drugs, Vol. I. Zhichen. 1989. 109.00 (*7-03-001616-5*) CRC Pr.

Color Atlas of Clinical Anatomy of Dogs & Cats. J. S. Boyd. 1991. 65.95 (*0-7234-2047-5*) Mosby Inc.

Color Atlas of Clinical Anatomy of the Dog & Cat. J. S. Boyd & Callum Paterson. 2nd ed. 2000. (Illus.). 220p. 69.00 (*0-7234-3169-8*) Mosby Inc.

Color Atlas of Clinical Embryology. Keith L. Moore et al. 1994. LC 93-26435. text 105.00 (*0-7216-4663-8*); 2nd ed. 2000. (Illus.). 270p. text (*0-7216-8263-4*) Saunders.

Color Atlas of Clinical Hematology. Bong H. Hyun et al. 1986. LC 84-25275. (Illus.). 285p. 120.00 (*0-89640-110-3*) Igaku-Shoin.

Color Atlas of Clinical Neurology. Malcolm L. Parsons. 2nd ed. 1993. (Illus.). 320p. (C). (gr. 13). text 113.00 (*0-8151-6613-3*, 22762) Mosby Inc.

Color Atlas of Clinical Operative Dentistry: Crowns & Bridges. J. Ralph Grundy. 2nd ed. 1992. (Illus.). 192p. (C). (gr. 13). text 75.95 (*0-8151-3622-6*, 21949) Mosby Inc.

Color Atlas of Clinical Oral Pathology. Brad W. Neville et al. (Illus.). 1990. LC 89-13980. 385p. text 99.50 (*0-8121-1311-X*); 2nd ed. 1998. LC 98-3616. 482p. text 99.95 (*0-683-30208-6*) Lppncott W & W.

Color Atlas of Common Oral Diseases. Robert P. Langlais & Craig S. Miller. (Illus.). 1992. LC 89-12561. 182p. text 38.00 (*0-8121-1249-0*); 2nd ed. 1997. LC 97-2654. 224p. pap. 45.95 (*0-683-30173-X*) Lppncott W & W.

Color Atlas of Congenital Heart Disease. Ho & Baker. 1994. 128p. 123.00 (*0-7234-1712-1*) Mosby Inc.

Color Atlas of Congenital Malformation Syndromes. Baraitser. 1995. 81.95 (*0-7234-2073-4*) Mosby Inc.

Color Atlas of Corneal Dystrophies & Degenerations. Thomas A. Casey. 1991. (Illus.). 126p. (C). (gr. 13). text 90.00 (*0-8151-1445-1*, 21948) Mosby Inc.

Color Atlas of Corneal Topography: Interpreting Videokeratography. Yaron S. Rabinowitz et al. 1993. LC 93-208. (Illus.). 96p. 125.00 (*0-89640-235-5*) Igaku-Shoin.

Color Atlas of Critical & Intensive Care: Diagnosis & Investigation. G. Park & D. W. Ryan. 1995. 64.95 (*0-7234-1956-6*) Mosby Inc.

Color Atlas of Cutaneous Disorders of the Lower Extremities. Joseph A. Witkowski & Harvey Lemont. 1993. LC 92-48718. (Illus.). 144p. 98.50 (*0-89640-233-9*) Igaku-Shoin.

Color Atlas of Cutaneous Infections. Lawrence C. Parish et al. 1995. (Illus.). 200p. 99.95 (*0-86542-435-7*) Blackwell Sci.

Color Atlas of Cytology for the Dog & Cat. Rebecca Baker & John H. Lumsden. 1999. LC 99-37111. (Illus.). ix, 288p. (C). (gr. 13). text 99.00 (*0-8151-0402-2*, 23968) Mosby Inc.

Color Atlas of Dermato-Immuno Histocytology. Ueki & Yadita. 1989. (Illus.). text 145.00 (*0-7234-1584-6*) CRC Pr.

Color Atlas of Dermatology. Jeffrey P. Callen et al. 1993. LC 93-10914. (Illus.). 368p. text 175.00 (*0-7216-3756-6*) Saunders.

Color Atlas of Dermatology. Jeffrey P. Callen. 2nd ed. 1999. LC 99-42915. (Illus.). 395p. (C). text 145.00 (*0-7216-8256-1*) Saunders.

Color Atlas of Dermatopathology. David A. Mehregan & Darius R. Mehregan. 1997. (Illus.). 500p. text 129.00 (*0-07-041330-4*) McGraw.

Color Atlas of Diagnostic Endoscopy in Otorhinolaryngology. Eiji Yanagisawa. 1997. LC 96-15369. (Illus.). 208p. 168.50 (*0-89640-316-5*) Igaku-Shoin.

Color Atlas of Diagnostic Microbiology. Luis M. De la Maza & Ellen Jo Baron. 1997. LC 98-130864. (Illus.). 224p. (C). (gr. 13). text 71.00 (*0-8151-0621-1*, 24752) Mosby Inc.

Color Atlas of Differential Diagnosis in Exfoliative & Aspiration Cytopathology. Sudha R. Kini. 1998. LC 98-22558. 352p. text 169.00 (*0-683-30675-8*) Lppncott W & W.

Color Atlas of Differential Diagnosis of Hair Loss. David A. Whiting & F. Fester Howsden. 1995. (Illus.). 96p. (*0-9647749-0-9*) Canfield Pubng.

Color Atlas of Difficult Diagnoses in Dermatology. Lawrence C. Parish et al. 1993. LC 92-1573. (Illus.). 184p. 135.00 (*0-89640-226-6*) Igaku-Shoin.

Color Atlas of Diseases & Disorders in the Horse. Derek C. Knottenbelt. 1994. (Illus.). 224p. (C). (gr. 13). text 145.00 (*0-8151-5117-9*, 22880) Mosby Inc.

Color Atlas of Diseases & Disorders of Cattle. R. W. Blowey & A. D. Weaver. 1990. LC 90-85771. (Illus.). 224p. (C). text 92.95 (*0-7234-1597-8*) Iowa U Pr.

Color Atlas of Diseases & Disorders of Sheep. Linklater. 1993. (Illus.). 256p. (gr. 13). text 115.00 (*0-8151-5438-0*, 22882) Mosby Inc.

Color Atlas of Diseases & Disorders of the Horse. Derek C. Knottenbelt & Reg R. Pascoe. 1993. LC 93-2092. text 159.00 (*0-7234-1702-4*) Mosby Inc.

Color Atlas of Diseases & Disorders of the Pig. W. J. Smith et al. 1989. (Illus.). 192p. text (*0-7234-0996-X*) Wolfe Publishing GBR. *Dist:* Mosby Inc.

Color Atlas of Ear, Nose, & Throat Diagnosis. T. R. Bull. 2nd ed. 1987. (Illus.). 368p. (C). (gr. 13). 53.00 (*0-8151-1317-X*, 09834) Mosby Inc.

Color Atlas of Embryology. Ulrich Drews. Tr. by David B. Meyer. 1995. LC 95-298. (Illus.). 384p. 32.00 (*0-86577-544-3*) Thieme Med Pubs.

Color Atlas of Endocrinology. Reginald Hall. 2nd ed. 1990. (Illus.). (C). (gr. 13). 100.00 (*0-8151-4249-8*, 20282) Mosby Inc.

Color Atlas of Endoscopic Diagnosis in Early Stage Lung Cancer. Harubumikato. 1992. (Illus.). 176p. (C). (gr. 13). text 145.00 (*0-8151-4982-4*, 21908) Mosby Inc.

Color Atlas of ENT Diagnosis. Bull. 1989. (*0-7234-1506-4*) Wolfe Publishing.

Color Atlas of ENT Diagnosis. T. R. Bull. 3rd ed. 1995. pap. text (*0-7234-2271-0*) Wolfe Publishing GBR. *Dist:* Mosby Inc.

Color Atlas of Fiberoptic Endoscopy of the Upper Respiratory Tract. John D. Shaw. 1987. (Illus.). 96p. (C). (gr. 13). 76.00 (*0-8151-7720-8*, 09472) Mosby Inc.

Color Atlas of Flourescein Angiography. Barbara A. Harney. 1993. (Illus.). 160p. (C). (gr. 13). text 98.00 (*0-8151-4155-6*, 22879) Mosby Inc.

Color Atlas of Foot & Ankle Anatomy. Hutchings & Robert M. McMinn. 2nd ed. 1995. text 35.00 (*0-7234-1995-7*) Mosby Inc.

Color Atlas of Foot & Ankle Dermatology. Gary L. Dockery & Mary E. Crawford. 1998. LC 98-12982. 416p. text 179.00 (*0-397-51519-7*) Lppncott W & W.

Color Atlas of Foot Conditions. M. A. Zatouroff & Lillian Bouffler. 1992. (Illus.). 264p. (C). 99.00 (*0-8151-9878-7*, 22473) Mosby Inc.

Color Atlas of Forefoot Surgery. Roger Butterworth. 1992. (Illus.). 264p. (gr. 13). text 108.00 (*0-8151-1387-0*, 21710) Mosby Inc.

Color Atlas of Gastrointestinal Surgery, Set. C. Cordiano & G. L. Nardi. 1989. 896p. text (*1-57235-039-3*) Piccin Nuova.

Color Atlas of General Pathology. G. Austin Gresham. 2nd ed. 1992. 160p. (C). (gr. 13). 39.00 (*0-8151-3989-6*, 22822) Mosby Inc.

Color Atlas of General Surgical Diagnosis. Garden. 1995. mass mkt. (*0-7234-2057-2*) Wolfe Publishing GBR. *Dist:* Mosby Inc.

Color Atlas of Genetics. Eberhard Passarge. 2nd ed. 2001.Tr. of Taschenatlas der Genetik. (Illus.). 370p. pap. 32.00 (*0-86577-958-9*) Thieme Med Pubs.

Color Atlas of Glaucoma. M. Bruce Shields. 4th ed. 1997. LC 96-48757. (Illus.). 250p. text 169.00 (*0-683-07696-5*) Lppncott W & W.

Color Atlas of Gross Placental Pathology. Cynthia G. Kaplan. 1994. LC 93-33096. (Illus.). 128p. 99.50 (*0-89640-249-5*) Igaku-Shoin.

Color Atlas of Hair & Nail Diagnosis. Levene. 1991. (Illus.). (*0-8151-5437-2*) Mosby Inc.

Color Atlas of Hair Restoration Surgery. James M. Swinehart. 1996. 411p. (C). pap. text 225.00 (*0-8385-3567-4*, 3567-3, Apple Lange Med) McGraw.

Color Atlas of Heart Failure. Leonard M. Shapiro. 2nd ed. 1995. text (*0-7234-2023-8*) Martin Dunitz GBR. *Dist:* Mosby Inc.

Color Atlas of Hematological Cytology. Frank G. Hayhoe & R. J. Flemans. 3rd ed. 1992. 384p. (C). (gr. 13). text 140.00 (*0-8151-4218-8*, 21892) Mosby Inc.

Color Atlas of Histology. Leslie Gartner & James Hiatt. 3rd ed. 2000. LC 99-86179. (Illus.). xv, 444p. 45.00 (*0-683-30642-1*) Lppncott W & W.

Color Atlas of Human Anatomy. Thompson. 1993. (Illus.). 32p. (C). (gr. 13). pap. text (*0-8016-7772-6*, 07772) Mosby Inc.

Color Atlas of Human Anatomy. Ed. by Vanio Vannini & Giuliano Pogliani. 1981. LC 81-47550. 112p. pap. 12.00 (*0-517-54514-4*) Harmony Bks.

Color Atlas of Hysteroscopy. Osamu Sugimoto. 1999. LC 98-37346. (Illus.). 188p. 165.00 (*4-431-70244-X*) Spr-Verlag.

Color Atlas of Immunology. G. R. Burmester & A. Pezzuto. 2001. (Illus.). 293p. pap. 29.00 (*0-86577-964-3*) Thieme Med Pubs.

Color Atlas of Infectious & Inflammatory Diseases of the External Eye. H. Bruce Ostler et al. 1987. LC 86-15941. (Illus.). 166p. 145.00 (*0-683-06650-1*) Lppncott W & W.

Color Atlas of Infectious Diseases. Ronald T. Emond. 1984. (Year Book Color Atlas Ser.). (Illus.). 384p. pap. 36.75 (*0-8151-3121-6*) Mosby Inc.

Color Atlas of Infectious Diseases. Ronald T. Emond et al. 3rd ed. 1995. (Illus.). pap. 29.95 (*0-7234-2127-7*) Mosby Inc.

Color Atlas of Intestinal Parasites. Francis M. Spencer & Lee S. Monroe. 2nd ed. 1982. (Illus.). 176p. (C). 58.95 (*0-398-04557-7*) C C Thomas.

Color Atlas of Lacrimal Surgery. Jane Olver. 2001. LC 2001-43712. (Illus.). 208p. 130.00 (*0-7506-4486-9*) Buttrwrth-Heinemann.

Color Atlas of Medical Microbiology. Tony Hart & Paul Shears. 1996. LC 89-13294. (Illus.). 314p. pap. (*0-7234-2322-9*) Wolfe Publishing GBR. *Dist:* Mosby Inc.

Color Atlas of Microneurosurgery: Intracranial Tumors, Vol. 1. Wolfgang T. Koos et al. 2nd enl. rev. ed. 1993. LC 93-20014. (Illus.). 704p. text 349.00 (*0-86577-477-3*) Thieme Med Pubs.

Color Atlas of Microneurosurgery Vol. 2: Cerebrovascular Lesions. J. Lang. Ed. by Wolfgang T. Koos & Robert F. Spetzler. 2nd ed. 1996. (Illus.). 415p. text 349.00 (*0-86577-478-1*) Thieme Med Pubs.

Color Atlas of Microneurosurgery Microanatomy, Approaches & Techniques Vol. III: Intra- & Extracranial Revascularization & Intraspinal Pathology. W. T. Koos et al. 2nd ed. 1999. (Illus.). 496p. 299.00 (*0-86577-780-2*) Thieme Med Pubs.

Color Atlas of Microneurosurgical Approaches: Cranial Base & Intracranial Midline. J. D. Day et al. 1997. LC 97-199400. (Illus.). 320p. text 199.00 (*0-86577-630-X*) Thieme Med Pubs.

Color Atlas of Microscopic Anatomy. P. Motta. 1990. 268p. text (*1-57235-011-3*) Piccin Nuova ITA. *Dist:* Gordon & Breach.

Color Atlas of Multiple Sclerosis. C. W. M. Adams. 1991. (Illus.). (*0-8151-0095-7*) Mosby Inc.

Color Atlas of Muscle Pathology. W. J. Cumming. 1994. LC 94-42133. (Illus.). (*0-7234-2016-5*) Wolfe Publishing.

Color Atlas of Neonatology. Abraham M. Rudolph. 1997. (*0-7216-6716-3*) Saunders.

Color Atlas of Neuropathology. David Graham. 2nd ed. 1995. (Illus.). 224p. (C). (gr. 13). text 86.95 (*0-8151-3855-5*, 23093) Mosby Inc.

Color Atlas of Neuroscience. B. Greenstein. 2000. LC 99-37655. (Flexibook Ser.). (Illus.). 400p. pap. text 29.90 (*0-86577-710-1*) Thieme Med Pubs.

Color Atlas of Nonhuman Primate Histology. Ed. by Shozo Takayama et al. 3rd ed. 1999. LC 00-265185. (Illus.). viii, 235p. 426.25 (*3-8055-6879-7*) S Karger.

Color Atlas of Normal Cytology. Arlene J. Herzberg et al. Ed. by Marc Strauss. 1999. LC 98-4057. (Illus.). 464p. (C). text (*0-443-07547-6*) Church.

Color Atlas of Obstetric & Gynecologic Pathology. Richard L. Voet. 1997. LC 96-36128. (Illus.). 256p. (C). (gr. 13). text 155.00 (*0-8151-9048-4*, 24381) Mosby Inc.

Color Atlas of Occlusion & Malocclusion. Alison P. Howat. 1992. (SPA.). (C). (gr. 13). text 76.50 (*0-7234-1764-4*) Mosby Inc.

Color Atlas of Ocular Manifestations of AIDS: Diagnosis & Management. Juan Orellana et al. 1995. LC 94-33155. 120p. 98.50 (*0-89640-273-8*) Igaku-Shoin.

Color Atlas of Office Skin Surgery. Moy & Richard P. Usatine. 1998. LC 97-42561. (Illus.). 336p. (C). (gr. 13). text 69.95 (*0-8151-7362-8*, 28047) Mosby Inc.

Color Atlas of Ophthalmology: The Manhattan Eye, Ear & Throat Hospital Pocket Guide. Suresh Mandava et al. 1998. LC 98-25048. (Illus.). 640p. pap. 59.00 (*0-86577-685-7*) Thieme Med Pubs.

Color Atlas of Oral Diseases in Children & Adolescents. George Laskaris. 1999. LC 99-36035. xii, 338p. (*3-13-111511-4*) Icon Lrning Systs.

Color Atlas of Oral Diseases in Children & Adolescents. George Laskaris. 1999. LC 99-36035. (Illus.). 352p. 129.00 (*0-86577-789-6*, L2371) Thieme Med Pubs.

Color Atlas of Oral Manifestations of AIDS. Sol Silverman. 2nd ed. 1995. 176p. (C). (gr. 13). text 59.95 (*0-8151-7897-2*, 25546) Mosby Inc.

Color Atlas of Oral Medicine. William R. Tyldesley. 2nd ed. 1994. 128p. text 69.00 (*0-7234-1918-3*) Mosby Inc.

Color Atlas of Oral Pathology. Crispian Scully. 1995. (Illus.). 137p. (C). (gr. 13). text 71.95 (*0-8151-7590-6*, 21954) Mosby Inc.

Color Atlas of Oral Pathology. Peter A. Reichart & Hans Peter Philipsen. 2000. (Illus.). 304p. 199.00 (*0-86577-932-5*) Thieme Med Pubs.

Color Atlas of Oro-Facial Diseases. William R. Tyldesley. 2nd ed. 1991. (Illus.). 286p. (C). (gr. 13). text 29.95 (*0-8151-4999-9*, 09298) Mosby Inc.

Color Atlas of Orthopaedics. L. Kessel. 1980. (C). (gr. 13). 89.95 (*0-8151-5021-0*, 09438) Mosby Inc.

Color Atlas of Osteochondrosis in the Dog. Carmichael. 1993. (Illus.). (*0-8151-1438-9*) Mosby Inc.

Color Atlas of Otorhinolaryngology. Bruce Benjamin et al. 1994. (Illus.). 352p. text 225.00 (*0-397-51422-0*) Lppncott W & W.

Color Atlas of Otoscopy: From Diagnosis to Surgery. Mario Sanna. 1998. (Illus.). 160p. 79.00 (*0-86577-721-7*) Thieme Med Pubs.

Color Atlas of Paediatric. Bill Chaudry & David Harvey. 2001. 414p. text (*0-7234-2436-5*) Wolfe Publishing GBR. *Dist:* Mosby Inc.

Color Atlas of Parasitology. John T. Sullivan. 1998. (Illus.). 120p. (C). spiral bd. 30.00 (*0-9665807-0-2*) Parasitology.

Color Atlas of Pathology. Ivan Damjanov & James Linder. 1999. 544p. (C). (gr. 13). text 179.00 (*0-8151-2248-9*, 24114) Mosby Inc.

Color Atlas of Pathology of the Nervous System. Asao Hirano et al. 2nd ed. 1988. LC 88-12812. (Illus.). 248p. 165.00 (*0-89640-148-0*) Igaku-Shoin.

Color Atlas of Pathophysiology. S. Silbernagl. 2000. LC 99-59262. (Illus.). 380p. pap. 35.00 (*0-86577-866-3*) Thieme Med Pubs.

Color Atlas of Pediatric Dermatology. Samuel Weinberg et al. 3rd ed. 1997. LC 97-42667. (Illus.). 304p. text 89.95 (*0-07-069249-1*) McGraw-Hill Prof.

Color Atlas of Pediatric Diseases with Differential Diagnosis. Ed. by R. Soll. 4th ed. 1999. LC 97-3047. 420p. (C). (gr. 13). 135.00 (*0-412-08131-8*) OUP.

Color Atlas of Pediatric Emergencies. Thomas F. Beattie. 1997. (Illus.). 160p. (C). (gr. 13). text 64.95 (*0-8151-0550-9*, 21952) Mosby Inc.

Color Atlas of Pediatric Gastroenterology & Hepatology. Kelly. 1996. 79.95 (*0-7234-1966-3*) Mosby Inc.

Color Atlas of Pediatric Infectious Disease. C. A. Hart & R. L. Broadhead. 1992. (Illus.). 208p. (C). text 79.95 (*0-8151-4143-2*, 21947) Mosby Inc.

Color Atlas of Pediatric Neurology. Ed. by Richard W. Newton. 1995. LC 94-42132. (Illus.). 256p. (gr. 13). 86.95 (*0-7234-1879-9*) Mosby Inc.

Color Atlas of Pediatric Surgery. Peter S. Liebert. Ed. by Larry McGrew. 2nd ed. 1996. LC 95-33478. 268p. text 239.00 (*0-7216-5885-7*) Saunders.

Color Atlas of Periodontal Surgery. Ito. 1994. text (*0-7234-2039-4*) Wolfe Publishing GBR. *Dist:* Mosby Inc.

Color Atlas of Peripheral Nerve Pathology. Shin J. Oh. 2001. (Illus.). 296p. otabind 159.95 (*0-8493-1676-6*) CRC Pr.

Color Atlas of Peripheral Vascular Diseases. J. J. Belch et al. 2nd ed. 1996. text 76.95 (*0-7234-2074-2*) Mosby Inc.

Color Atlas of Preprosthetic Oral Surgery. Russell Hopkins. 1987. (Illus.). 193p. text 85.00 (*0-8121-1097-8*) Lppncott W & W.

Color Atlas of Radical Hysterectomy with Pelvic Lymph Node Dissection. Ed. by Heung-Tat Ng. 1993. (Illus.). 120p. (C). (*1-899015-01-9*) Euromed Communs GBR. *Dist:* St Mut.

Color Atlas of Removable Partial Dentures. Davenport. 1988. (C). (gr. 13). 55.00 (*0-7234-1620-6*) Mosby Inc.

Color Atlas of Renal Diseases. George Williams. 2nd ed. 1994. (Illus.). 160p. (C). (gr. 13). text 99.00 (*0-8151-9337-8*, 22968) Mosby Inc.

Color Atlas of Reproductive Pathology of Domestic Animals. Claus D. Buergelt. 1996. LC 96-25861. (Illus.). 240p. (C). (gr. 13). text 110.00 (*0-8151-1305-6*, 28149) Mosby Inc.

Color Atlas of Respiratory Disease. D. Geraint James. 2nd ed. 1992. (Illus.). 366p. (C). (gr. 13). 115.00 (*0-7234-1695-8*) Mosby Inc.

Color Atlas of Rheumatology. Michael Shipley. 3rd ed. 1992. 176p. text 35.00 (*0-8151-7660-0*) Mosby Inc.

Color Atlas of Scleritis. Peter G. Watson. 1995. (C). (gr. 13). 76.00 (*0-8151-9185-5*, 22888) Mosby Inc.

Color Atlas of Sexual Assault. Ed. by Barbara Girardin. 1997. LC 97-14866. (Illus.). 224p. (C). (gr. 13). text 49.95 (*0-8151-3842-3*, 30729) Mosby Inc.

Color Atlas of Small Animal Dermatology. Linda Medleau & Keith A. Hnilica. 2001. LC 2001-20139. (Illus.). xi, 356p. text (*0-7216-8152-2*) Saunders.

Color Atlas of Small Animal Dermatology. George T. Wilkinson & Richard Harvey. 2nd ed. 1994. (Illus.). 304p. (*84-8174-145-0*) Mosby-Doyma Libros ESP. *Dist:* Mosby Inc.

Color Atlas of Small Animal Dermatology: A Guide to Diagnosis. George T. Wilkinson & Richard G. Harvey. 2nd ed. 1994. LC 93-2093. 288p. (gr. 13). text 119.00 (*0-7234-1898-5*) Mosby Inc.

Color Atlas of Small Animal Disorders. Simon J. Wheeler. 1994. 128p. text 127.50 (*0-7234-1897-7*) Mosby Inc.

Color Atlas of Small Animal Endoscopy. Malcom J. Brearly. 1991. (Illus.). 128p. (C). (gr. 13). text 78.95 (*0-8151-1195-9*, 21728) Mosby Inc.

Color Atlas of Soft Tissue Tumors. Jeanne M. Meis-Kindblom et al. 1995. LC 95-9592. (Illus.). 320p. (C). (gr. 13). text 129.00 (*0-8151-5895-5*, 24079) Mosby Inc.

Color Atlas of Stabismus Surgery: Strategies & Techniques. 2nd rev. ed. 1999. (Illus.). 265p. (C). 145.00 (*0-9675536-0-1*) Wright Pubg.

Color Atlas of Surface Anatomy: Clinical & Applied. Kenneth M. Backhouse & Ralph T. Hutchings. 1986. (Illus.). 350p. (C). pap. text 35.00 (*0-683-00307-0*) Lppncott W & W.

Color Atlas of Surface Anatomy. Backhou. 2nd ed. 1997. mass mkt. (*0-7234-2495-0*) Wolfe Publishing GBR. *Dist:* Mosby Inc.

Color Atlas of Surgery for the Removal of Melanoma, Vol. 40. McCarthy. 1991. (Illus.). (*0-8151-5859-9*) Mosby Inc.

Color Atlas of Surgical Anatomy for Esophageal Cancer. Ed. by T. Sato & T. Iizuka. 1993. LC 92-49824. (Illus.). 156p. 225.00 (*0-387-70100-1*) Spr-Verlag.

Color Atlas of Temporomandibular Joint Surgery. Hoffman & Quinn. 1997. (Illus.). 288p. (C). (gr. 13). text 138.00 (*0-8151-4540-3*, 26900) Mosby Inc.

Color Atlas of the Blood & Systemic Disease. Greaves. 1996. 49.95 (*0-7234-1905-1*) Mosby Inc.

Color Atlas of the Eye in Systemic Disease. Daniel Gold. 1996. LC 00-44370. (Illus.). xviii, 652p. text 189.00 (*0-397-51525-1*) Lppncott W & W.

Color Atlas of the Hair, Scalp & Nails. R. Baran. 1991. (Illus.). 192p. (C). (gr. 13). text 69.00 (*0-8151-0417-0*, 21727) Mosby Inc.

Color Atlas of the Horse's Foot. Christopher C. Pollitt. 1995. (C). (gr. 13). text 115.00 (*0-8151-6743-1*, 22965) Mosby Inc.

Color Atlas of the Horse's Foot. Christopher C. Pollitt. 1995. (SPA.). (*84-8174-397-6*) Mosby-Doyma Libros ESP. *Dist:* Mosby Inc.

Color Atlas of the Human Anatomy. P. H. Abrahams. 4th ed. 1998. text (*0-7234-2641-4*) Wolfe Publishing GBR. *Dist:* Mosby Inc.

Color Atlas of the Nail in Clinical Diagnosis. Donald W. Beaven. 2nd ed. 1994. 256p. 39.95 (*0-7234-1991-4*) Mosby Inc.

Color Atlas of the Nail in Clinical Diagnosis. Donald W. Beaven & E. Brooks. 2nd ed. 1994. pap. 32.00 (*0-7234-2026-2*) Mosby Inc.

Color Atlas of the Surgery & Management of Intestinal Stomas. L. R. Celestin. 1987. (Illus.). 96p. (C). (gr. 13). 89.95 (*0-8151-1484-2*, 09093) Mosby Inc.

Color Atlas of Tropical Medicine & Parasitology. Wallace Peters & Herbert M. Gilles. 3rd ed. 1989. (Illus.). 104.00 (*0-7234-1535-8*) CRC Pr.

Color Atlas of Tropical Medicine & Parasitology. Wallace Peters & Herbert M. Gilles. 4th ed. 1996. pap. 49.95 (*0-7234-2069-6*) Mosby Inc.

Color Atlas of Urine Microscopy. D. F. Birch et al. 1994. LC 93-14519. 160p. (gr. 13). 207.95 (*0-412-47950-8*) Chapman & Hall.

Color Atlas of Urology. R. W. Lloyd-Davies. 2nd ed. 1993. 288p. (C). (gr. 13). (*0-7234-1912-4*) Wolfe Publishing GBR. *Dist:* Mosby Inc.

Color Atlas of Urology. W. Lloyd-Davies et al. 2nd ed. 1994. (Illus.). 288p. (*84-8174-266-X*) Mosby-Doyma Libros ESP. *Dist:* Mosby Inc.

Color Atlas of Urology of the Dog & Cat: Diagnosis, Indications, Techniques. Peter E. Holt. 1994. LC 94-44185. text (*0-7234-1817-9*) Wolfe Publishing GBR. *Dist:* Mosby Inc.

Color Atlas of Uterine Cancer Cytology. Ed. by Franz A. Ikle & Yi-Jing Shu. 1992. (Illus.). 480p. text 105.00 (*0-07-057212-7*) McGraw-Hill Med Pub.

Color Atlas of Uveitis Diagnosis. Michelson. 2nd ed. 1992. (Illus.). 158p. (C). (gr. 13). text 83.00 (*0-8151-5872-6*, 21944) Mosby Inc.

Color Atlas of Vascular Diseases. C. Diehm et al. Tr. by W. H. C. Burgdorf from GER. 2000. LC 99-43213. (Illus.). 416p. 189.00 (*3-540-62619-0*) Spr-Verlag.

Color Atlas of Veterinary Anatomy: Ruminants. Ashdown. 2nd ed. 1996. pap. (*0-7234-2662-7*) Wolfe Publishing GBR. *Dist:* Mosby Inc.

Color Atlas of Veterinary Anatomy Vol. 1: The Ruminants. Raymond R. Ashdown & Stan Done. 1983. LC 65-40637. (Illus.). 230p. text (*0-397-44679-9*, GM0002) Gower-Mosby.

Color Atlas of Veterinary Anatomy Vol. 2: Horse. Ashdown. 2nd ed. 1996. pap. (*0-7234-2574-4*) Wolfe Publishing GBR. *Dist:* Mosby Inc.

Color Atlas of Veterinary Anatomy Vol. 3: The Dog & Cat. Stanley H. Done et al. 1996. (Illus.). 464p. pap. (*84-8174-200-7*) Mosby-Doyma Libros ESP. *Dist:* Mosby Inc.

Color Atlas of Veterinary Cardiology. Peter G. G. Darke & Bonogura. 1995. 71.00 (*0-7234-1907-8*) Mosby Inc.

Color Atlas of Veterinary Forensic Medicine. Chapman. 1993. (Illus.). 116p. 65.00 (*0-8151-1618-7*) Mosby Inc.

Color Atlas of Veterinary Histology. Contrib. by William J. Bacha & Linda M. Bacha. 2nd ed. 2000. LC 99-46388. (Illus.). 336p. text 49.95 (*0-683-30618-9*) Lppncott W & W.

***Color Atlas of Veterinary Ophthalmology.** Kirk N. Gelatt. 2001. LC 2001-23444. (Illus.). xviii, 420p. pap. text 95.00 (*0-7817-2998-X*) Lppncott W & W.

Color Atlas/Text of Salivary Gland Tumor Pathology. Irving Dardick. 1996. LC 95-26461. (Illus.). 288p. 129.50 (*0-89640-308-4*) Igaku-Shoin.

Color Blood Flow Imaging of the Heart. D. Redel. 1988. (Illus.). 130p. 217.00 (*0-387-16521-5*) Spr-Verlag.

Color-Coded Allergy Cookbook. Gloria D. Autry & T. Diener Allen. 1983. LC 82-17826. 400p. 19.95 (*0-672-52746-4*) Macmillan.

Color Coding EKGs. Tim Carrick. 1994. (Illus.). 29p. (C). text 14.95 (*0-943202-45-0*) H & H Pub.

Color Doppler Flow Imaging. W. Dennis Foley. 1991. 192p. text (*0-9626521-2-1*) E A GBR. *Dist:* OUP.

Color Doppler Flow Imaging. Ed. by Jos R. Roelandt. 1986. (Developments in Cardiovascular Medicine Ser.). lib. bdg. 184.00 (*0-89838-806-6*) Kluwer Academic.

Color Doppler Imaging in Obstetrics & Gynecology. Ed. by Richard Jaffe & Steven L. Warsof. 1992. (Illus.). 320p. text 98.00 (*0-07-105420-0*) McGraw-Hill Educ Grp.

Color Doppler in Clinical Cardiology. Walter J. Duncan. 1988. (Illus.). 176p. (C). text 170.00 (*0-03-014267-9*) SCP.

Color Doppler Sonography in Obstetrics & Gynecology: With Related Applications. Arthur C. Fleischer & Donald S. Emerson. 1993. (Illus.). 366p. text (*0-443-08864-0*) Church.

Color Duplex Sonography: Principles & Clinical Applications. Ed. by K. J. Wolf & F. Fobbe. 1995. (Illus.). 308p. 159.00 (*0-86577-542-7*) Thieme Med Pubs.

Color for Philosophers: Unweaving the Rainbow. C. L. Hardin. 1988. LC 87-15160. 268p. (C). pap. text 16.95 (*0-87220-039-6*); lib. bdg. 37.95 (*0-87220-040-X*) Hackett Pub.

***Color Guide: Forensic Medicine.** John Gall et al. 2001. (Color Guide Ser.). 120p. pap. (*0-443-06499-7*) Church GBR. *Dist:* Saunders.

Color Guide to the Nursing Management of Wounds. Moya Morison. 2nd ed. 1997. 335p. pap. text (*0-7234-2557-4*) Wolfe Publishing GBR. *Dist:* Mosby Inc.

Color Handbook of Ear Diseases of the Dog & Cat. Richard G. Harvey et al. 2001. (Illus.). 320p. 79.95 (*0-8138-0302-0*) Iowa U Pr.

Color Handbook of Occupational Dermatology. John S. English. 1998. pap. 69.95 (*0-8385-1074-4*, Apple Lange Med) McGraw.

Color Handbook of Skin Diseases in the Dog & Cat: A Problem-Oriented Approach to Diagnosis & Treatment. Patrick J. McKeever. 1998. LC 99-172752. (Illus.). 288p. 59.95 (*0-8138-2983-6*) Iowa U Pr.

Color Handbook of Veterinary Histology & Correlates. Elizabeth Aughey & Fredric Frye. 2001. (Illus.). 320p. 99.95 (*0-8138-2874-0*) Iowa U Pr.

Color Medicine: The Secrets of Color Vibrational Healing. Charles Klotsche. 1993. LC 94-181642. 114p. (Orig.). pap. 11.95 (*0-929385-27-6*) Light Tech Pubng.

Color of Angels: Cosmology, Gender & the Aesthetic Imagination. Constance Classen. 1998. LC 98-21837. (Illus.). 288p. (C). (gr. 13). 80.00 (*0-415-18073-2*, D6056) Routledge.

Color Synopsis of Refractive Surgery. Louis E. Probst & John F. Doane. 2000. (Illus.). 275p. 89.00 (*0-86577-914-7*) Thieme Med Pubs.

Color Text of Contact Dermatitis. Ed. by Walter G. Larsen et al. 1991. (Illus.). 252p. text 135.00 (*0-7216-3518-0*) Saunders.

Color Textbook of Histology. Leslie P. Gartner & James L. Hiatt. Ed. by Bill Schmitt. 1996. LC 96-16721. 512p. text 41.95 (*0-7216-5124-0*) Saunders.

Color Textbook of Pediatric Dermatology. William L. Weston et al. 2nd ed. 1996. (Illus.). 416p. (C). (gr. 13). text 99.95 (*0-8151-9201-0*, 24434) Mosby Inc.

Color Therapy: An Introductory Guide to the Healing Power of Color. Pauline Wills. 2000. (New Perspectives Ser.). (Illus.). 128p. pap. (*1-86204-766-9*) Oneworld.

Color Therapy Workbook: The Use of Color for Health & Healing. Theo Gimbel. 1993. LC 93-6133. 112p. pap., stu. ed. 16.95 (*1-85230-388-3*) Element MA.

Color Vision. Dain. Date not set. text (*0-7506-1446-3*) Buttrwrth-Heinemann.

Color Vision: Perspectives from Different Disciplines. Ed. by Werner G. Backhaus et al. 1998. LC 97-46863. 430p. 89.95 (*3-11-016100-1*); pap. 49.95 (*3-11-015431-5*) De Gruyter.

Color Vision Deficiencies. Ed. by Y. Ohta. 1990. LC 90-5233. (Illus.). 267p. lib. bdg. (*90-6299-063-0*) Kugler NLD. *Dist:* Lib Res.

Color Vision Deficiencies VIII. Ed. by Guy Verriest. 1987. (Documenta Ophthalmologica Proceedings Ser.). text 306.50 (*0-89838-801-5*) Kluwer Academic.

Color Vision Deficiency & Color Blindness. Mary M. Olsen & Kenneth R. Harris. 1988. 62p. (Orig.). pap. 8.50 (*0-9615332-2-6*) Fern Ridge Pr.

Colorado Health Care in Perspective 2000. Ed. by Kathleen O'Leary Morgan & Scott E. Morgan. 2000. 21p. spiral bd. 19.00 (*0-7401-0205-2*) Morgan Quitno Corp.

Colorado Health Care Perspective, 1998. Ed. by Kathleen O'Leary Morgan & Scott E. Morgan. 1998. 20p. pap. 19.00 (*1-56692-805-2*) Morgan Quitno Corp.

ColorCards: Inner Guidance Made Simple Through the Vibration of Color. Arlene Arnold. 2nd enl. rev. ed. 2000. 160p. pap. 29.95 (*0-9649990-1-3*) Transform WA.

Colorectal Cancer. Ed. by Jonathan Cebon. 1995. (Journal: Vol. 4, No. 2-3, 1995). (Illus.). 84p. pap. 47.00 (*3-8055-6150-4*) S Karger.

Colorectal Cancer. Jack D. Hardcastle. 1993. LC 93-23750. (EC Series for General Practitioners). (Illus.). 30p. pap. (*3-540-56702-X*) Spr-Verlag.

***Colorectal Cancer.** Ed. by Colin S. McArdle et al. 2000. (Illus.). 160p. (*1-899066-72-1*) Isis Med GBR. *Dist:* Bks Intl VA.

Colorectal Cancer. Ed. by Kees Welvaart et al. 1980. (Boerhaave Series for Postgraduate Medical Education: No. 18). (Illus.). 290p. text 171.00 (*90-6021-465-X*) Kluwer Academic.

***Colorectal Cancer.** Taylor et al. 2nd ed. 2002. (Fast Facts Ser.). (Illus.). 96p. pap. (*1-903734-08-8*) Health Pr GBR. *Dist:* JAMCO Dist.

Colorectal Cancer: A Guide for Patients. Jorge Marcet. Ed. by Larry C. Carey. 1996. (Surgery Ser.). (Illus.). 32p. (Orig.). pap. 2.95 (*1-885274-25-4*) Health InfoNet Inc.

Colorectal Cancer: Methods & Protocols. Ed. by Steven M. Powell. 2001. LC 00-22073. (Methods in Molecular Medicine Ser.: Vol. 50). (Illus.). 294p. 119.50 (*0-89603-767-3*) Humana.

Colorectal Cancer: Multimodality Management. Ed. by Leonard Saltz. 2001. (Current Clinical Oncology Ser.). 850p. 150.00 (*0-89603-935-8*) Humana.

Colorectal Cancer: New Aspects of Molecular Biology & Immunology & Their Clinical Applications. C. Hanski et al. 2000. LC 00-39443. (Annals of the New York Academy of Sciences Ser.: Vol. 910). (Illus.). ix, 272p. pap. (*1-57331-278-9*) NY Acad Sci.

***Colorectal Cancer: New Aspects of Molecular Biology & Immunology, & Their Clinical Applications.** Ed. by Christoph Hanski et al. 2001. (Annals of the New York Academy of Sciences Ser.). 350p. pap. 30.00 (*0-8018-6698-7*) NY Acad Sci.

Colorectal Cancer: Textbook for General Practitioners. Ed. by Jack D. Hardcastle. 1993. LC 93-23750. 48p. 51.95 (*0-387-56702-X*) Spr-Verlag.

Colorectal Cancer Vol. 910: New Aspects of Molecular Biology & Immunology & Their Clinical Applications. Ed. by Christoph Hanski et al. 2000. LC 00-39443. (Annals of the New York Academy of Sciences Ser.: Vol. 910). (Illus.). ix, 272p. 95.00 (*1-57331-277-0*) NY Acad Sci.

Colorectal Cancer - Questions & Answers. Mario Dicato. 2001. (Questions & Answers Ser.). (Illus.). 124p. pap. text 26.95 (*1-873413-18-1*) Merit Pub Intl.

Colorectal Cancer Screening: Early Detection. Jorge E. Marcet. Ed. by Larry Carey. abr. ed. 1996. (Surgery Ser.). (Illus.). 16p. pap. 1.95 (*1-885274-62-9*) Health InfoNet Inc.

Colorectal Cancer Screening: Technical Review. Ed. by Barry Leonard. 2000. 154p. reprint ed. pap. text 30.00 (*0-7567-0052-3*) DIANE Pub.

Colorectal Disease. Gordon Deans et al. 1998. (Illus.). 328p. text 169.50 (*0-19-262704-X*) OUP.

Colorectal Physiology: Fecal Incontinence. Han C. Kuijpers. 1994. 304p. 189.00 (*0-8493-4565-0*) CRC Pr.

Colorectal Surgery. Ed. by Robin Phillips. 1997. (Companion Guide to Specialist Surgical Practice Ser.: Vol. 4). (Illus.). 380p. text (*0-7020-2143-1*) W B Saunders GBR. *Dist:* Saunders.

***Colorectal Surgery: A Companion to Specialist Surgical Practice.** Robin K. S. Phillips. 2nd ed. 2001. (Illus.). 403p. (*0-7020-2590-9*) W B Saunders GBR. *Dist:* Saunders.

Colorectal Tumors. Oliver H. Beahrs et al. 1986. LC 65-8436. (Illus.). 334p. text 69.50 (*0-397-50677-5*, Lippnctt) Lppncott W & W.

Colorful Introduction to the Anatomy of the Human Brain: A Brain & Psychology Coloring Book. John P. Pinel. 1997. 226p. pap. text 19.00 (*0-205-16299-1*) P-H.

Coloring Atlas of Human Anatomy. Stephen W. Langjahr & Robert D. Brister. 2nd ed. 1992. 202p. (C). (*0-8053-4021-1*) Benjamin-Cummings.

***Coloring Guide to Regional Human Anatomy.** Alan Twietmeyer & Thomas McCracken. 3rd ed. 2001. LC 2001-29396. (Illus.). 220p. pap. text 25.95 (*0-7817-3042-2*) Lppncott W & W.

Coloring Review Guide of Human Anatomy & Physiology. Robert J. Stone & Judith A. Stone. 1995. (Illus.). 344p. (C). spiral bd. 38.13 (*0-697-17109-4*, WCB McGr Hill) McGrw-H Hghr Educ.

Coloring Review Guide to Human Anatomy. W. Hogin McMurtrie & James E. Rikel. 1990. 448p. (C). spiral bd. 50.94 (*0-697-03150-0*, WCB McGr Hill) McGrw-H Hghr Educ.

Colour Atlas & Text of Infectious Diseases. Christopher Conlon & Geoff Pasvol. 1999. (Illus.). 320p. mass mkt. (*0-7234-2434-9*) Wolfe Publishing GBR. *Dist:* Mosby Inc.

Colour Atlas & Text of Obstetrics. I. A. Greer. 2000. (Illus.). 352p. text (*0-7234-2435-7*) Wolfe Publishing GBR. *Dist:* Mosby Inc.

Colour Atlas & Text of Ocular Plastic Surgery. Van Der Meulen & Joseph Gruss. 1995. 215.00 (*0-7234-1924-8*) Mosby Inc.

Colour Atlas of Anatomical Pathology. Robin A. Cooke & Brian Stewart. 2nd ed. 1995. LC 95-7285. pap. text (*0-443-05062-7*) Church.

Colour Atlas of Anatomy of Small Laboratory Animals, 1. Peter Popesko. 1992. (Illus.). text 165.00 (*0-7234-1822-5*) CRC Pr.

Colour Atlas of Anatomy of Small Laboratory Animals, 2. Peter Popesko. 1992. (Illus.). text 165.00 (*0-7234-1823-3*) CRC Pr.

Colour Atlas of Burn Care. Contrib. by Saunders, W.B., Publishing Staff. 2000. (Illus.). 256p. 135.00 (*0-7020-2508-9*) Saunders.

Colour Atlas of Burn Injuries. John A. Clarke. 1992. LC 92-49022. (Medical Atlas Ser.: No. 9). (Illus.). 128p. (*0-412-34840-3*) E A GBR. *Dist:* OUP.

Colour Atlas of Cardio-Pulmonary Resuscitation Techniques. Kenneth Mills et al. 1986. (Illus.). 96p. text (*0-7234-1029-1*) Wolfe Publishing.

Colour Atlas of Chinese Traditional Drugs, Vol. 1. Ed. by National Institute for the Control of Pharmaceuticals. 1987. (Illus.). 300p. text (*0-945345-09-7*) Sci Pr CHN. *Dist:* Lubrecht & Cramer.

Colour Atlas of Clinical Genetics. Francis Baraitser & Robin Winter. 1988. (Illus.). 159p. text (*0-7234-1547-1*) Wolfe Publishing.

Colour Atlas of Clinical Rheumatology. Nicholas Bellamy. 1985. text 236.50 (*0-85200-761-2*) Kluwer Academic.

Colour Atlas of Developing Embryos. Jonathan B.L. Bard. 1993. LC 92-48738. 24.95 (*0-8151-0412-X*) Mosby Inc.

Colour Atlas of Diseases of the Vulva. C. M. Ridley et al. 1993. (Medical Atlas Ser.: No. 8). (Illus.). 128p. (gr. 13). text 188.95 (*0-412-36520-0*) Chapman & Hall.

Colour Atlas of Doppler Ultrasonography in Obstetrics. Ed. by Kevin P. Harrington & Stuart Campbell. 1995. (Illus.). 160p. text (*0-340-56952-2*) E A GBR. *Dist:* OUP.

Colour Atlas of First Pass Functional Imaging of the Heart. Ed. by N. Schadd et al. 1985. text 449.00 (*0-85200-798-1*) Kluwer Academic.

Colour Atlas of Gastrointestinal Endoscopy. K. F. Schiller et al. 1987. (Illus.). 240p. text 195.00 (*0-7216-2150-3*) Saunders.

Colour Atlas of Hand Disorders. Geoffrey Hooper. 1989. (Illus.). 192p. pap. text (*0-443-04064-8*) Church.

Colour Atlas of Head & Neck Anatomy. Robert M. McMinn et al. 2nd ed. 1994. LC 93-43540. (Illus.). 256p. (C). (gr. 13). reprint ed. (*0-7234-1994-9*) Wolfe Publishing GBR. *Dist:* Mosby Inc.

Colour Atlas of Histology. Paul R. Wheater et al. 1992. (Illus.). 159p. (Orig.). pap. text (*0-582-35269-X*) Church.

Colour Atlas of Inflammatory Bowel Disease. Pounder & Allison. 1998. 75.00 (*0-7234-1888-8*) Mosby Inc.

Colour Atlas of Medical Entomology. N. R. Burgess & G. O. Cowan. 1993. LC 92-49003. (Medical Atlas Ser.: Vol. 10). 152p. (C). (gr. 13). pap. text 179.95 (*0-412-32340-0*) Chapman & Hall.

Colour Atlas of Mouth, Throat & Ear Disorders in Children. John Bain et al. 1985. text 124.00 (*0-85200-767-1*) Kluwer Academic.

Colour Atlas of Neuropathology. R. O. Weller. 1984. (Oxford Color Atlases of Pathology Ser.). (Illus.). 208p. text 85.00 (*0-19-921044-6*) OUP.

Colour Atlas of Nuclear Cardiology. M. Goris & J. Bretille. 1992. (Illus.). 336p. 124.95 (*0-442-31620-8*) Chapman & Hall.

Colour Atlas of Nuclear Cardiology. Michael Goris & Josiane Bretille. 1992. (Medical Atlas Ser.). (Illus.). 336p. (C). (gr. 13). text 151.95 (*0-412-38950-9*, Chap & Hall NY) Chapman & Hall.

Colour Atlas of Ophthalmic Plastic Surgery. J. R. O. Collin & A. G. Tyers. 2001. 368p. text 160.00 (*0-7506-4254-8*) Buttrwrth-Heinemann.

Colour Atlas of Ophthalmology. Arthur S. Lim & Ian Constable. 3rd ed. 1995. 170p. text 38.00 (*981-02-2286-6*) World Scientific Pub.

Colour Atlas of Opthalmology. Arthur S. Lim & Ian Constable. 3rd ed. 1995. 170p. pap. text 25.00 (*981-02-2339-0*) World Scientific Pub.

Colour Atlas of Oral Disease. William H. Binnie. 2nd ed. 1993. 356p. (C). (gr. 13). (*1-56375-594-7*) Gower-Mosby.

Colour Atlas of Paediatric Haematology. Ian M. Hann et al. 3rd ed. 1996. (Illus.). 202p. (C). text 165.00 (*0-19-262696-5*) OUP.

Colour Atlas of Poisonous Fungi: Handbook for Pharmacists, Doctors, & Biologists. A. Bresinsky. 1990. (Illus.). (C). (gr. 13). 102.00 (*0-7234-1576-5*) Mosby Inc.

Colour Atlas of Posterior Chamber Implants. Arthur S. Lim. 1985. (Illus.). 692p. text 142.00 (*0-7216-1573-2*) Saunders.

Colour Atlas of Respiratory Diseases. D. Geraint James & Peter R. Studdy. 2nd ed. 1992. LC 92-24902. (*0-8151-4845-3*) Mosby Inc.

Colour Atlas of Respiratory Infections. J. T. Macfarlane et al. 1993. (Medical Atlas Ser.: No. 12). (Illus.). 144p. (gr. 13). 188.95 (*0-412-38960-6*) Chapman & Hall.

Colour Atlas of Salmonid Diseases. Ed. by David W. Bruno & Trygve T. Poppe. 1996. (Illus.). 208p. text 120.00 (*0-12-137810-1*) Acad Pr.

Colour Atlas of Sexually Transmitted Diseases. L. K. Bhutani. 1990. 208p. (C). (*81-85017-23-9*) Interprint IND. *Dist:* St Mut.

Colour Atlas of Trauma Pathology. Fischer. 1991. (Illus.). 136p. (C). (gr. 13). text 99.00 (*0-8016-6294-X*, 06294) Mosby Inc.

Colour Atlas of Tropical Dermatology & Venerology. K. F. Schaller. Ed. by F. A. Bahmer. 1994. (Illus.). 320p. 165.00 (*0-387-53327-3*) Spr-Verlag.

Colour Atlas of Tropical Dermatology & Venerology. K. F. Schaller. 1993. (Illus.). 320p. (*3-540-53327-3*) Spr-Verlag.

Colour Atlas of Vertebrate Anatomy: An Integrated Text & Color Dissection Guide. Gillian M. King & David R. Custance. 1982. (Illus.). 136p. (C). text 49.95 (*0-632-01007-X*) Blackwell Sci.

Colour Atlas of Wounds & Wounding. G. A. Gresham. 1986. text 248.00 (*0-85200-156-8*) Kluwer Academic.

Colour Atlas Ophthalmic Plastic Surgery. A. G. Tyers & J. R. Collin. 1995. LC 94-17532. (Illus.). 338p. text (*0-443-04452-X*) Church.

Colour Guide: Picture Tests in Neonatology & Paediatrics. Warren Hyer et al. 1997. LC 97-12425. pap. text (*0-443-04956-4*) Church.

Colour Me Healing: Colorpuncture: A New Medicine of Light. Jack Allanach. 1998. LC 97-25596. (Illus.). 192p. pap. 15.95 (*1-86204-143-1*) Element MA.

Colour Vision: Physiology & Psychophysics. Ed. by John Mollon & L. Ted Sharpe. 1983. text 135.00 (*0-12-504280-9*) Acad Pr.

Colour Vision Deficiencies, IX. Ed. by B. Drum & Guy Verriest. 1988. (Documenta Ophthalmologica Proceedings Ser.). (C). text 380.00 (*0-89838-403-6*) Kluwer Academic.

Colour Vision Deficiencies: Proceedings of the Seventh Symposium of the International Research Group on Color Vision Deficiencies, Geneva 1983, No. VII. Guy Verriest. 1984. (Documenta Ophthalmologica Proceedings Ser.). (Illus.). 434p. text 256.50 (*90-6193-735-3*) Kluwer Academic.

Colour Vision Deficiencies Vol. XIII: Proceedings of the International Symposium, Pau 1995. Ed. by C. R. Cavonius. 1997. (Documenta Ophthalmologica Proceedings Ser.). 544p. (C). text 234.00 (*0-7923-4224-0*) Kluwer Academic.

Colour Vision Deficiencies Four: Proceedings of the Symposium, Parma, June 1977. International Research Group on Colour Vision Deficiencies. Ed. by E. B. Streiff & Guy Verriest. 1978. (Modern Problems in Ophthalmology Ser.: Vol. 19). (Illus.). 172.25 (*3-8055-2800-0*) S Karger.

Colour Vision Deficiencies, No. 11: Proceedings of the Eleventh International Symposium, Sydney, Australia, 21-23 June 1991. Ed. by B. Drum. 1993. LC 92-23627. (Documenta Ophthalmologica Proceedings Ser.: Vol. 56). (C). text 313.00 (*0-7923-1864-1*) Kluwer Academic.

Colour Vision Deficiencies Six. Guy Verriest. 1982. text 332.00 (*90-6193-729-9*) Kluwer Academic.

Colour Vision Deficiencies Ten. Ed. by B. Drum et al. 1991. (Documenta Ophthalmologica Proceedings Ser.). (C). text 375.00 (*0-7923-0948-0*) Kluwer Academic.

Colour Vision Deficiencies Three: Proceedings of the Symposium, 3rd. International Research Group on Colour Vision Deficiencies. Ed. by Guy Verriest. 1976. (Modern Problems in Ophthalmology Ser.: Vol. 17). 300p. 155.00 (*3-8055-2297-5*) S Karger.

Colour Vision Deficiencies Twelve: Proceedings of the Twelfth Symposium of the International Research Group on Colour Vision Deficiencies, Vol. XII, No. 57. Ed. by B. Drum et al. 1995. LC 94-13946. (Documenta Ophthalmologica Proceedings Ser.: Vol. 57). 572p. (C). text 257.50 (*0-7923-2889-2*) Kluwer Academic.

Colour Vision Deficiencies Two: Proceedings of the Symposium, 2nd, Edinburgh, June 1973. International Research Group on Colour Vision Deficiencies. Ed. by Guy Verriest. 1974. (Modern Problems in Ophthalmology Ser.: Vol. 13). 300p. 138.50 (*3-8055-1698-3*) S Karger.

Colour Your Life: Discovering Your True Personality Through the Colour Reflection Reading. Howard Sun & Dorthy Sun. 1996. (Illus.). 182p. (Orig.). pap. text (*0-7499-1149-2*) Piatkus Bks GBR. *Dist:* London Brdge.

Colpopoliesis from the Colon. M. Kun. 1975. 172p. (C). (*963-05-0161-9*) Akade Kiado HUN. *Dist:* St Mut.

Colposcopy: A Scientific & Practical Approach to the Cervix, Vagina & Vulva in Health & Disease. Malcolm Coppleson et al. 3rd ed. 1986. (Illus.). 624p. (C). 107.95 (*0-398-05153-4*) C C Thomas.

***Colposcopy: Principles & Practice.** Barbara S. Apgar et al. 2002. LC 2001-57596. (Illus.). 510p. text (*0-7216-8494-7*) Saunders.

Colposcopy, Cervical Pathology: Textbook & Atlas. E. Burghardt et al. Tr. by Andrew G. Ostor & Karl Tamussino from GER. 3rd ed. 1998. LC 98-6919. ix, 323p. 139.00 (*0-86577-634-2*) Thieme Med Pubs.

Colposcopy in Diagnosis & Treatment of Preneoplastic Lesions. Ed. by H. E. Stegner & M. Coppleson. 1987. (Illus.). 90p. 31.50 (*0-387-17947-X*) Spr-Verlag.

***Colposcopy Management Options.** Walter Prendiville et al. 2001. (Illus.). 155p. (*0-7020-2491-0*) W B Saunders GBR. *Dist:* Saunders.

Columbia HCA: Healthcare on Overdrive. Sandy Lutz & E. Preston Gee. 1997. LC 97-44835. (Illus.). 232p. 21.95 (*0-07-024804-4*) McGraw.

Columbia Review Intensive Preparation for the MCAT. Stephen Bresnick. 1997. LC 95-25627. 825p. pap. 46.95 (*0-683-01027-1*) Lppncott W & W.

Columbia Review MCAT Practice Tests. Stephen D. Bresnick & William H. Bresnick. 1997. LC 97-6524. (Illus.). 208p. pap. 26.95 (*0-683-18099-1*) Lppncott W & W.

Columbia University Department of Pediatrics Children's Medical Guide: The Quick Reference Guide to Children's Symptoms. H. B. Valman. 1997. LC 96-35924. (Illus.). 216p. 29.95 (*0-7894-1443-0*) DK Pub Inc.

Columbia University School of Public Health 40 Plus Guide to Good Health. Robert J. Weiss et al. rev. ed. 1993. LC 92-43953. (*0-89043-541-3*) Consumers Union.

Columbus & the New World: Medical Implications. Ed. by Guy A. Settipane. 1995. LC 94-69156. (Illus.). 148p. (C). 49.50 (*0-936587-07-5*) OceanSide Pubns.

Colyer's Variations & Diseases of the Teeth of Animals. Ed. by A. E. Miles & C. Grigson. 2nd ed. 1990. (Illus.). 686p. text 140.00 (*0-521-25273-3*) Cambridge U Pr.

Coma, a Healing Journey: A Guide for Family, Friends & Helpers. Amy Mindell. 1998. LC 98-88184. (Illus.). 330p. 21.00 (*1-887078-05-3*) Lao Tse Pr.

Coma & Impaired Consciousness: A Clinical Perspective. Ed. by G. Bryan Young et al. 1997. LC 98-122136. (Illus.). 672p. pap. 69.00 (*0-07-072371-0*) McGraw-Hill Prof.

Coma Work & Palliative Care. Stan Tomandl. 2nd ed. 1991. LC 96-27296. (Illus.). 80p. (*0-9696200-0-4*) WBB CAN. *Dist:* Interact Media.

Combat Medic. Isadore L. Valenti. 1998. LC 98-61564. pap. 19.95 (*1-891231-01-4*) Word Assn.

Combat Sports Injuries. G. McLatchie. 1982. 192p. 50.00 (*0-9506989-2-X*) St Mut.

Combating Destructive Thought Processes: Voice Therapy & Separation Theory. Robert W. Firestone. 1997. LC 96-35618. 400p. 81.95 (*0-7619-0550-2*, 81013); pap. 39.95 (*0-7619-0551-0*, 81014) Sage.

Combating HIV-AIDS in Developing Countries. 1992. (Illus.). 35p. (Orig.). (C). pap. text 20.00 (*1-56806-009-2*) DIANE Pub.

Combating Infectious Diseases. U. S. Government Printing Office Staff. 1998. LC 98-217067. (S. Hrg. Ser.). iii, 52p. (*0-16-057141-3*) USGPO.

Combating Iron Deficiency in Chile: A Case Study. Vivian Beyda et al. Ed. by Catherine E. Adams et al. 1986. (Illus.). 58p. (Orig.). pap. text 3.50 (*0-935368-48-5*) ILSI.

***Combating Methampetamine Proliferation in America: Congressional Hearing.** Ed. by Orrin G. Hatch. 2001. 61p. reprint ed. pap. text 20.00 (*0-7567-1727-2*) DIANE Pub.

Combating Nutritional Blindness in Children: A Case Study of Technical Assistance in Indonesia. Carl Fritz. 1980. (Policy Studies). 74.00 (*0-08-024636-2*, Pergamon Pr) Elsevier.

Combination Drug Therapy for Hypertension. Lionel H. Opie & Franz H. Messerli. 1997. 190p. pap. text 59.95 (*1-881063-05-4*) Lppncott W & W.

Combination Therapies Vol. 1: Biological Response Modifiers in the Treatment of Cancer & Infectious Diseases. A. L. Goldstein & E. Garaci. 1992. (Illus.). 346p. (C). text 95.00 (*0-306-44115-2*, Kluwer Plenum) Kluwer Academic.

Combination Therapies Vol. 2: Biological Response Modifiers in the Treatment of Cancer & Infectious Diseases. A. L. Goldstein & E. Garaci. 1993. (Illus.). 266p. (C). text 95.00 (*0-306-44589-1*, Kluwer Plenum) Kluwer Academic.

***Combination Therapy for Asthma & Chronic Obstructive Pulmonary Disease.** Monica Kraft. Ed. by Richard J. Martin. 2000. LC 00-698406. (Lung Biology in Health & Disease Ser.: Vol. 145). (Illus.). 336p. text 150.00 (*0-8247-0371-5*) Dekker.

Combination Therapy in Urological Malignancy. Ed. by P. H. Smith. 1989. (Clinical Practice in Urology Ser.). (Illus.). 278p. 139.00 (*0-387-19528-9*, 2549) Spr-Verlag.

Combination Vaccines: Development, Clinical Research & Approval. Ronald W. Ellis. 1999. LC 98-55262. (Illus.). 292p. 125.00 (*0-89603-717-7*) Humana.

***Combinatorial Chemistry: A Practical Approach.** Ed. by Willie Bannwarth & Eduard Felder. 2000. LC 2001-278179. (Methods & Principles in Medicinal Chemistry Ser.: Vol. 9). (Illus.). 450p. 145.00 (*3-527-30186-0*) Wiley.

Combinatorial Chemistry & Molecular Diversity in Drug Discovery. Ed. by Eric M. Gordon & James F. Kerwin. 1998. LC 97-38036. 544p. 99.95 (*0-471-15518-7*, Wiley-Liss) Wiley.

Combinatorial Chemistry in Drug Design. Nielsen. 1998. (Illus.). 320p. text (*0-7514-0387-3*) B Acad & Prof GBR. *Dist:* Routldge.

Combined Analyses of Cancer Mortality among Nuclear Industry Workers in Canada, the United Kingdom & the United States of America. E. Cardis & E. Gilbert. 1995. (IARC Scientific Publications Ser.: No. 25). 147p. text 30.00 (*92-832-1440-4*) World Health.

Combined Antimicrobial Therapy. Ed. by William Brumfitt et al. 1980. (New Perspectives in Clinical Microbiology Ser.: No. 3). text 141.50 (*90-247-2280-2*) Kluwer Academic.

Combined Care of the Rheumatic Patient. A. Bird et al. 1985. (Illus.). 320p. 73.95 (*0-387-13557-X*) Spr-Verlag.

Combined Effects of Chemotherapy & Radiotherapy on Normal Tissue Tolerance: Proceedings of the Annual West Coast Cancer Symposium, 13th, San Francisco, CA, March 1978. Annual West Coast Cancer Symposium. Ed. by J. M. Vaeth. 1979. (Frontiers of Radiation Therapy & Oncology Ser.: Vol. 13). (Illus.). 126.75 (*3-8055-2932-5*) S Karger.

Combined Effects of Drugs & Toxic Agents: Modern Evaluation in Theorie & Practice. Gerald Poch. 1993. LC 92-43470. (*3-211-82434-0*); (Illus.). 178p. 62.95 (*0-387-82434-0*) Spr-Verlag.

Combined Modality Cancer Therapy: Radiation & Infusional Chemotherapy. Ed. by Jacob J. Lokich & John E. Byfield. 1991. LC 91-61357. 264p. 99.00 (*0-944496-22-9*) Precept Pr.

Combined Modality Therapy of Central Nervous System Tumors. Ed. by Zbigniew Petrovich et al. 2000. LC 00-55628. (Medical Radiology Ser.). (Illus.). 600p. 250.00 (*3-540-66053-4*) Spr-Verlag.

Combined Modality Therapy of Gastrointestinal Tract Cancer. Ed. by P. M. Schlag & P. Hohenberger. 1988. (Recent Results in Cancer Research Ser.: Vol. 110). (Illus.). 301p. 113.00 (*0-387-18610-7*) Spr-Verlag.

Combined Radiotherapy & Chemotherapy in Clinical Oncology. Horwich. 1992. 272p. 89.50 (*0-340-55159-3*) Trafalgar.

Combined Scintigraphic & Radiographic Diagnosis of Bone & Joint Diseases. Yong-Whee Bahk. 2nd enl. rev. ed. 2000. LC 99-52113. (Illus.). 304p. 189.00 (*3-540-66424-6*) Spr-Verlag.

***Combined Treatments for Mental Disorders: A Guide to Psychological & Pharmacological Interventions.** Ed. by Morgan T. Sammons & Norman B. Schmidt. 2001. 345p. 39.95 (*1-55798-780-7*, 431-775A) Am Psychol.

Combined Volume: COTA & Practice Issues in Occupational Therapy. Sally E. Ryan. 2nd ed. 1995. (Illus.). 770p. pap. 50.00 (*1-55642-290-3*, 32903) SLACK Inc.

Combining Medication & Psychosocial Treatments for Addictions. Joseph R. Volpicelli et al. 2001. LC 00-69163. 208p. text 30.00 (*1-57230-618-1*) Guilford Pubns.

Combining Neuro-Developmental Treatment & Sensory Integration Principles: An Approach to Pediatr. Erna I. Blanche et al. 1998. 175p. pap. text 58.00 (*0-12-784570-4*) Acad Pr.

Combining Psychotherapy & Drug Therapy in Clinical Practice. Ed. by Bernard D. Beitman & Gerald L. Klerman. 1984. LC 84-14144. 288p. text 39.95 (*0-88331-120-8*) R B Luce.

Come See About Nutrition & Exercise: Teacher's Guide. Jeanne M. Scott. 1996. (Foundations in Health Ser.: Vol. 5). (Illus.). 33p. (Orig.). (J). (gr. 3-8). pap. text, tchr. ed., wbk. ed. (*1-886728-09-7*) Visual Mentor.

Come See How We Fight Infection: Teacher's Guide. Jeanne M. Scott. 1996. (Foundations in Health Ser.: Vol. 3). (Illus.). 46p. (Orig.). (J). (gr. 3-8). pap. text, tchr. ed., wbk. ed. (*1-886728-05-4*) Visual Mentor.

Come See What First Aid You Can Do: Teacher's Guide. Jeanne M. Scott. 1996. (Foundations in Health Ser.: Vol. 4). (Illus.). 33p. (Orig.). (J). (gr. 3-8). pap. text, tchr. ed., wbk. ed. (*1-886728-07-0*) Visual Mentor.

Comfort & Care in a Final Illness: Support for the Patient & Caregiver. June C. Kolf. 1999. LC 98-32312. 176p. pap. 12.95 (*1-55561-188-5*) Fisher Bks.

Comforting the Confused: Strategies for Managing Dementia. Stephanie B. Hoffman & Constance A. Platt. 1991. 224p. reprint ed. pap. 33.95 (*0-8261-7850-2*); 2nd ed. 2000. LC 99-51495. (Illus.). 256p. pap. text (*0-8261-1261-7*) Springer Pub.

Comforts of Unreason: A Study of the Motives Behind Irrational Thought. Rupert Crawshay-William. 1970. LC 71-98217. 206p. reprint ed. lib. bdg. 67.00 (*0-8371-3398-X*, CRUN, Greenwood Pr) Greenwood.

Coming Health Crisis: How to Finance Care for the Aged in the Twenty-First Century. John R. Wolfe. 1993. LC 92-17098. (Illus.). 172p. (C). 24.95 (*0-226-90515-2*) U Ch Pr.

Coming Home: A Discharge Manual for Families of Persons with a Brain Injury. Dana S. DeBoskey. 1995. (Illus.). 80p. (Orig.). pap. 12.50 (*1-882855-34-5*) HDI Pubs.

Coming Home: A Guide to Home Care for the Terminally Ill. Deborah Duda. rev. ed. 1984. (Illus.). 275p. pap. (*0-912528-39-7*) Avalon Travel.

Coming Home to Preschool: The Sociocultural Context of Early Education, 7. Irving E. Sigel et al. 1993. (Advances in Applied Developmental Psychology Ser.: Vol. 7). 310p. 87.50 (*0-89391-875-X*, Ablex) Greenwood.

Coming of Age. Duncan Neuhauser. 2nd ed. 1995. LC 93-81268. 361p. 25.00 (*1-56793-009-3*, 0519) Health Admin Pr.

Coming Physician Surplus: In Search of a Public Policy. Eli Ginzberg & Miriam Ostow. 1984. LC 84-4894. (Conservation of Human Resources Ser.: Vol. 23). 144p. 55.50 (*0-8476-7364-2*) Rowman.

Coming Plague: Newly Emerging Diseases in a World Out of Balance. Laurie Garrett. 1995. 768p. pap. 15.95 (*0-14-025091-3*, Penguin Bks) Penguin Putnam.

Coming Through the Whirlwind: Case Studies in Psychotherapy. Michael Eigen. 1991. LC 91-623. 252p. (Orig.). pap. 5.95 (*0-933029-53-5*) Chiron Pubns.

Coming to Life. Leston L. Havens. 1993. LC 92-23563. 208p. text 22.50 (*0-674-14432-5*) HUP.

Commandments & Virtues: Moral Methodology & Duties of a Physician. Thomas G. Hooyman. 1998. LC 97-35587. 360p. 79.00 (*1-57309-215-0*) Intl Scholars.

Commemorative Volume in Honour of Prof. Streiff. Ed. by Michael J. Roper-hall et al. 1978. (Advances in Ophthalmology Ser.: Vol. 36). (FRE & GER., Illus.). 163.50 (*3-8055-2828-0*) S Karger.

Comment Debuter "La Re-Evaluation par la Co-Ecoute" 1999.Tr. of How to Begin "Re-Evaluation Counseling". (FRE.). 20p. pap. 1.00 (*1-58429-045-5*) Rational Isl.

Commentaries on Abend, Porder & Willicks "Borderline Patients - Psychoanalytic Perspectives" Ed. by Bornstein. 1988. (Psychoanalytic Inquiry Ser.: Vol. 8, No. 3). 20.00 (*0-88163-961-3*) Analytic Pr.

Commentaries on Narcotic Drugs & Psychotropic Substances Act, 1985 with Allied State & Central Rules & Noti. K. Kumar. 2nd ed. 1993. (C). (*81-7012-511-1*) Eastern Book IND. *Dist:* St Mut.

Commentaries on the Causes, Forms, Symptoms & Treatment, Moral & Medical, of Insanity. George M. Burrows. 1976. LC 75-16693. (Classics of Psychiatry Ser.). reprint ed. 59.95 (*0-405-07422-0*) Ayer.

Commentary on the Medical Writings of Rudolf Virchow: Based on Schwalbe's Virchow-Bibliographie, 1843-1901. Lelland J. Rather. 1990. (Bibliography Ser.: No. 3). (Illus.). 236p. 125.00 (*0-930405-19-6*) Norman SF.

Commerce & the Spread of Pests & Disease Vectors. Ed. by Marshall Laird. 1984. LC 83-16627. (Illus.). 354p. 70.00 (*0-275-91208-6*, C1208, Praeger Pubs) Greenwood.

Commercial Opportunities in Pharmacogenomics. Ed. by CTB Emerging Pharmaceutical Group Staff. 1998. spiral bd. 857.00 (*1-887566-11-2*, RPC-01) CTB Intl.

Commission on Chronic Illness, Vol. 2: Care of the Long-Term Patient, Vol. 2. Commission on Chronic Illness Staff. 1956. (Illus.). 620p. 61.50 (*0-674-09650-9*) HUP.

Commission on Chronic Illness, Vol. 3: Chronic Illness in a Rural Area: The Hunterdon Study, Vol. 3. Commission on Chronic Illness Staff. 1956. 454p. 50.00 (*0-674-12901-6*) HUP.

Commission on Chronic Illness, Vol. 4: Chronic Illness in a Large City: The Baltimore Study, Vol. 4. Commission on Chronic Illness Staff. 1957. (Commission on Chronic Illness Ser.: Vol. 4). (Illus.). 642p. 56.00 (*0-674-12900-8*) HUP.

Commission on Graduates of Foreign Nursing Schools Qualifying Examinations (CGFNS) Jack Rudman. 1994. (Admission Test Ser.: ATS-90). pap. 39.95 (*0-8373-5090-5*) Nat Learn.

Commissioned Papers on Historical, Institutional & Economic Contexts of Drug Treatment. 1994. lib. bdg. 250.95 (*0-8490-6422-8*) Gordon Pr.

Commissioned Reviews of 250 Psychological Tests Ed. by John Maltby et al. 2000. LC 00-52519. (Studies in Psychology: Vol. 2A). 476p. 109.95 (*0-7734-7452-8*); (Mellon Studies in Psychology: Vol. 2B). 484p. 109.95 (*0-7734-7454-4*) E Mellen.

Commitment to Caring: Enthusiasm Lithograph. 1993. 29.00 (*1-56066-089-9*, 35162) Mosby Inc.

Commitment to Deviance: The Nonprofessional Criminal in the Community, 5. Robert A. Stebbins. 1971. LC 75-95504. (Contributions in Sociology Ser.: No. 5). 201p. 27.50 (*0-8371-2339-9*, STDPB, Greenwood Pr) Greenwood.

***Commitment to Improving Quality in Mental Helath Care: Concepts & Case Studies.** Barbara Dickey & Lloyd Sederer. 2001. 400p. (*0-88048-963-4*, 8963) Am Psychiatric.

Commitment to Sobriety: A Relapse Prevention Guide for Adults in Recovery. Martin Fleming. 1981. 40p. pap. 5.50 (*1-56246-023-4*, 3226, HazeldenJohnson Inst) Hazelden.

Commitment to the Committed. J. T. Feldbrugge. 1986. xvi, 276p. pap. (*90-265-0678-3*) Swets.

***Committed to Memory: How We Remember & Why We Forget.** Rebecca Rupp. 2002. 331p. reprint ed. 23.00 (*0-7567-5373-2*) DIANE Pub.

Committee on Medical Aspects Report - Nutritional Aspects of Development of Cancer. 1998. (Health & Social Subjects Reports: No. 48). (*0-11-322089-8*, HM20898) Statnry Office GBR. *Dist:* Bernan Associates.

Common Ailments & Their Natural Remedies. Rudolf Steiner. 1973. lib. bdg. 250.00 (*0-87968-557-3*) Krishna Pr.

Common & Chronic Symptoms in Pediatrics: A Companion to the Atlas of Pediatric Physical Diagnosis. J. Carlton Gartner & Basil J. Zitelli. 2nd ed. 1997. LC 97-10508. (Illus.). 560p. (C). (gr. 13). pap. text 64.95 (*0-8151-3407-X*, 24724) Mosby Inc.

Common & Uncommon Sense of Social Behavior. Francis C. Dane. 1987. LC 87-15833. 182p. (C). mass mkt. 17.00 (*0-534-08406-0*) Brooks-Cole.

Common Beliefs about the Rural Elderly: What Do National Data Tell Us? 1993. LC 93-3076. (Vital & Health Statistics Ser. 3: Analytical & Epidemiological Studies: No. 28). (*0-8406-0477-7*) Natl Ctr Health Stats.

Common Bile Duct Exploration. A. Cushieri. 1984. (Developments in Surgery Ser.). lib. bdg. 212.50 (*0-89838-639-X*) Kluwer Academic.

Common Blood Tests: What Every Patient Must Know about Lab Tests. Ed. by N. L. Gifford. 3rd ed. 1996. LC 96-9498. 200p. (C). pap. 15.00 (*1-881818-08-X*) TBL.

Common Bonds: Reflections of a Cancer Doctor. E. Roy Berger & Linda Mittiga. 1994. LC 94-24684. 246p. 24.95 (*1-883257-07-7*) Hlth Edu Lit.

Common Conditions. Michael Mead. 1999. LC 98-40970. 122p. (C). (*0-443-06021-5*) Church.

Common Conditions in Gynecology: A Problem Solving Approach. Ed. by David Luesley. 1997. LC 97-66879. (Illus.). 312p. pap. (*0-412-72380-8*) E A GBR. *Dist:* OUP.

Common Contact Lens Complications, Their Recognition & Man: Diagnosis & Management. Lyndon Jones et al. 2000. LC 99-44549. (Illus.). 114p. pap. text 45.00 (*0-7506-3542-8*) Buttrwrth-Heinemann.

Common Cures for Common Ailments: A Doctor's Guide to Nonprescription, Over-the-Counter Medicines & His Recommendations for Their Use. Albert Marchetti. 1981. LC 77-16114. 368p. pap. 8.95 (*0-8128-6107-8*, Scrbrough Hse) Madison Bks UPA.

Common Diagnostic Procedures: Orthopedics & Neurology. 1993. ring bd. 166.00 (*0-8205-1039-4*) Bender.

Common Dilemmas in Family Medicine. Ed. by J. Fry. 1983. lib. bdg. 35.00 (*0-85200-565-2*) Kluwer Academic.

Common Diseases: Their Nature, Incidence & Care. John Fry. 3rd ed. 1983. lib. bdg. 29.00 (*0-85200-454-0*); 4th ed. 1985. text 74.00 (*0-85200-918-6*) Kluwer Academic.

***Common Disorders Natural Remedies.** N. D. Renders. 2001. 275p. pap. 22.95 (*0-9711551-1-9*) Rndrs Wllns.

Common Disorders of the Hip. Mary C. Singleton & Eleanor F. Branch. 1986. LC 86-3074. (Physical Therapy in Health Care Ser.: Vol. 1, No. 1). 116p. 39.95 (*0-86656-557-4*) Haworth Pr.

Common Disorders of the Nasal Cavity. Tim Peters. 1994. (Humanatomy Board Bks.). (Illus.). 12p. bds. 9.95 (*1-879874-02-4*) T Peters & Co.

Common Factors in Psychotherapy. Ed. by A. M. Van Kalmthout et al. 1985. xii, 194p. pap. (*90-265-0639-2*) Swets.

Common Food Intolerances One: Epidemiology of Coeliac Disease. Ed. by S. Auricchio & J. Visakorpi. 1993. (Dynamic Nutrition Research Ser.: Vol. 2). (Illus.). x, 192p. 161.75 (*3-8055-5616-0*) S Karger.

Common Food Intolerances Two: Milk in Human Nutrition & Adult-Type Hypolactasia. Ed. by S. Auricchio & R. Troncone. 1993. (Dynamic Nutrition Research Ser.: Vol. 3). (Illus.). x, 212p. 170.50 (*3-8055-5741-8*) S Karger.

Common Foot Problems in Primary Care. Richard B. Birrer et al. 2nd ed. 1998. LC 97-41961. 236p. 59.95 (*1-56053-222-X*) Hanley & Belfus.

Common Foundation Studies in Nursing. Ed. by Neil Kenworthy et al. 1992. LC 92-15511. (Illus.). 400p. (Orig.). pap. text (*0-443-04401-5*) Church.

Common Foundation Studies in Nursing. Neil Kenworthy et al. 2nd ed. 1996. LC 96-25831. (Orig.). pap. text (*0-443-05280-8*) Church.

Common Ground: The Arts, Therapy, & Spirituality. 1993. (Conference Proceedings Ser.). 168p. (Orig.). pap. 25.00 (*1-882147-21-9*) Am Art Therapy.

Common Ground of Psychoanalysis. Ed. by Robert S. Wallerstein. 1992. LC 91-18035. 336p. 60.00 (*0-87668-555-6*) Aronson.

Common Gynaecological Emergencies. Patricia Wilson. 1999. LC 98-46285. (Illus.). xi, 308p. pap. 52.95 (*0-632-05174-4*) Blackwell Sci.

Common Hand Problems in Primary Care. Ed. by Matthew J. Concannon. 1999. LC 98-37041. (Illus.). 184p. 39.95 (*1-56053-209-2*) Hanley & Belfus.

Common Head, Neck, & Back Injuries. Jacob Green. 1988. LC 85-24220. 160p. lib. bdg. 25.00 (*0-89874-912-3*) Krieger.

Common Health Complaints. Ken Fujihara et al. 1995. 54p. 4.95 (*0-941942-07-4*) Orient Heal Arts.

Common Herbs for Natural Health. Juliette De Bairacli Levy. exp. ed. 1997. LC 96-84261. (Herbals by Our Foremothers Ser.). (Illus.). 236p. reprint ed. pap. 11.95 (*0-9614620-9-4*) Ash Tree.

Common Heroes: Facing a Life Threatening Illness. Eric Blau. 1989. (Illus.). 96p. pap. 15.95 (*0-939165-12-0*) NewSage Press.

Common Illnesses. Andrew Weil. Ed. by Steven Petrow. 1997. LC 97-93712. (Ask Dr. Weil Ser.). mass mkt. 2.99 (*0-8041-1676-8*) Ivy Books.

Common Infections. Ed. by Louis G. Keith. 1985. (Infectious Agents & Pathogenesis Ser.). text 248.00 (*0-85200-733-7*) Kluwer Academic.

***Common Mechanism for Teratogenicity of Antiepileptic Drugs: Drug-Induced Embryonic Arrhythmia & Hypoxia-Reoxygenation Damage.** Faranak Azarbayjani. 2001. (Comprehensive Summaries of Uppsala Dissertations from the Faculty of Pharmacy Ser.: No. 253). (Illus.). 54p. pap. (*91-554-5065-2*) Uppsala Universitet SWE. *Dist:* Coronet Bks.

Common Mechanisms of Transformation by Small DNA Tumor Viruses. Ed. by Luis P. Villarreal. 1989. (Illus.). 276p. text 89.95 (*1-55581-013-6*) ASM Pr.

Common Medical Abbreviations. Luis DeSousa et al. 1994. LC 94-26241. 272p. (C). pap. text 34.95 (*0-8273-6643-4*) Delmar.

Common Medical Diagnosis. Patricia M. Healey. 3rd ed. 1999. LC 99-37694. (Illus.). xii, 235p. pap. text 35.00 (*0-7216-7732-0*) Saunders.

Common Medical Diagnosis: An Algorithmic Approach. Patrice M. Healey & Edwin J. Jacobson. 2nd ed. 1994. LC 93-38502. (Illus.). 240p. pap. text 44.00 (*0-7216-5401-0*) Saunders.

Common Mental Disorders. David Goldberg & Peter J. Huxley. 1991. 224p. (C). pap. 27.99 (*0-415-05987-9*, A6592); text 52.95 (*0-415-06100-8*, A6588) Routledge.

Common Mental Disorders in Primary Care: Essays in Honour of Professor Sir David Goldberg. Michele Tansella et al. 1999. LC 99-24250. xxvii, 244p. text (*0-415-20572-7*) Routledge.

Common Musculoskeletal Problems. Ed. by Arun B. Mehta. 1996. LC 96-20354. (Illus.). 369p. (Orig.). pap. 36.95 (*1-56053-173-8*) Hanley & Belfus.

Common Neuroses of Children & Adults. Oliver S. English & Gerald H. Pearson. 1937. (C). 6.00 (*0-393-01005-8*) Norton.

Common Pediatric Emergencies. David Crosley. 1999. (Illus.). 55p. pap. (*1-57801-042-X*) Western Schls.

Common Perioperative Problems & the Anesthetist. Gerald M. Woerlee. 1988. (Developments in Critical Care, Medicine, & Anesthesiology Ser.). (C). text 245.00 (*0-89838-402-8*) Kluwer Academic.

Common Principles in the Neuroethology of Acoustic & Electric Communication. Ed. by W. Wilczynski et al. 1987. (Journal: Vol. 28, NO. 13). (Illus.). 156p. pap. 100.00 (*3-8055-4462-6*) S Karger.

Common Principles of Psychotherapy. Chris L. Kleinke. 1993. LC 93-30265. (Counseling Ser.). 301p. 47.94 (*0-534-19998-4*) Brooks-Cole.

Common Problems in Neuroophthalmology. Acheson. 1996. text (*0-7020-1879-1*) Bailliere Tindall.

Common Problems in Pediatric Pathology. Vijay V. Joshi. 1994. LC 93-38969. (Illus.). 536p. 125.00 (*0-89640-242-8*) Igaku-Shoin.

Common Reptile Diseases & Treatments. Shawn Messonnier. 1996. LC 96-32365. (Illus.). 160p. (Orig.). pap. text 29.95 (*0-86542-553-1*) Blackwell Sci.

Common Sense about Dyslexia. Anne M. Huston. 1987. (Illus.). 300p. (Orig.). (C). pap. 18.00 (*0-8191-5666-3*); lib. bdg. 26.50 (*0-8191-6323-6*) U Pr of Amer.

Common Sense Approach to a Healthy Lifestyle. Thom Slagle. 1993. LC 93-84106. (Illus.). 86p. (Orig.). pap. 15.95 (*0-9636421-7-0*) Pacific Word.

Common-Sense Guide to Weight Loss. Barbara Hansen & Shauna S. Roberts. 1998. LC 97-45833. (Illus.). 288p. pap. 19.95 (*0-945448-85-6*, 00856Q) Am Diabetes.

Common Sense Psychology for Everyday Living. Brian M. Scully. 2000. 151p. pap. (*0-9703594-0-3*) Psychgy Srce.

Common Sense Toxics in the Workplace. Ilene R. Danse. 1991. 272p. text 55.95 (*0-442-00154-1*, VNR) Wiley.

Common Skin Diseases. Thomas F. Poyner. 2000. LC 99-21441. (Illus.). vii, 176p. pap. 36.95 (*0-632-05134-5*) Blackwell Sci.

Common Skin Disorders. Ernst Epstein. 5th ed. 2000. LC 00-41275. (Illus.). 335p. text 65.00 (*0-7216-8898-5*) Harcrt Hlth Sci Grp.

Common Skin Disorders. Ernst Epstein. 4th ed. 1994. (Illus.). 384p. pap. text 60.00 (*0-7216-6751-1*) Saunders.

***Common Small Animal Medical Diagnosis.** Linda Shell & Charlotte Davies. 2001. LC 2001-49545. (Illus.). 235p. (*0-7216-8478-5*) Saunders.

Common Surgical Diseases: An Algorithmic Approach to Problem Solving. Ed. by Theodore J. Saclarides & Keith W. Millikan. 1997. LC 97-33655. (Illus.). 534p. pap. 39.95 (*0-387-94983-6*) Spr-Verlag.

Common Symptom Guide: A Guide to the Evaluation of Common Adult & Pediatric Symptoms. Ed. by John H. Wasson. 4th ed. 1996. LC 96-230246. (Illus.). 400p. pap. 29.95 (*0-07-068469-3*) McGraw-Hill Prof.

Common Symptoms Described for Nurses. John Gibson. 1976. LC 77-356698. 195 p. (*0-632-00428-2*) Blackwell Sci.

Common Symptoms of Disease in Children. Ronald S. Illingworth. 3rd ed. 1971. LC 76-501769. 320 p. (*0-632-07980-0*); 5th ed. 1975. LC 76-675857. 375 p. (*0-632-00367-7*) Blackwell Sci.

Common Symptoms of Disease in the Elderly. H. M. Hodkinson. 1976. LC 77-352736. 147 p. (*0-632-00199-2*) Blackwell Sci.

Common Symptons of Disease in Children. Ronald S. Illingworth. 4th ed. 1973. LC 73-595434. 323 p. (*0-632-09710-8*) Blackwell Sci.

Common Vertebral Joint Problems. Gregory P. Grieve. 2nd ed. 1989. (Illus.). 804p. text (*0-443-03365-X*) Church.

Common Whiplash Injury: A Modern Epidemic. Michael Livingston. 1999. LC 98-38332. (Illus.). 224p. text 47.95 (*0-398-06911-5*); pap. text 36.95 (*0-398-06912-3*) C C Thomas.

***Commonalities in Nursing Area A.** Tiffany D. Dickinson. 2000. 144p. (C). pap. text 325.00 (*0-9700638-0-6*) Distance Learning.

Commonalities in Nursing Care: Area A. Jack Rudman. (Regents External Degree Ser.: Vol. 17). 43.95 (*0-8373-5667-9*); 1994. pap. 23.95 (*0-8373-5617-2*) Nat Learn.

Commonalities in Nursing Care: Area B. Jack Rudman. (Regents External Degree Ser.: Vol. 18). 43.95 (*0-8373-5668-7*); 1994. pap. 23.95 (*0-8373-5618-0*) Nat Learn.

Commonalities in Nursing Care, Area A. Jack Rudman. (ACT Proficiency Examination Program Ser.: Vol. 41). 43.95 (*0-8373-5591-5*); 1994. pap. 23.95 (*0-8373-5541-9*) Nat Learn.

Commonalities in Nursing Care, Area B. Jack Rudman. (ACT Proficiency Examination Program Ser.: Vol. 42). 43.95 (*0-8373-5592-3*); 1994. pap. 23.95 (*0-8373-5542-7*) Nat Learn.

Commonalities in Psychosomatic Medicine. Harold Geist. 1991. 119p. pap. 19.75 (*0-87527-485-4*) Green.

Commonly Used Chinese Herb Formulas with Illustrations. Hong-Yen Hsu & Chau S. Hsu. rev. ed. 1993. LC 93-2033. (*0-941942-41-4*) Orient Heal Arts.

Commonsense Approach to Coronary Care. Marielle Vinsant-Crawford. 6th ed. 1994. (Illus.). 560p. (C). (gr. 13). pap. text 42.95 (*0-8016-6949-9*, 06949) Mosby Inc.

Commonsense Cardiology. Gillian Strube & George Strube. 1989. (Commonsense Ser.). (C). text 68.50 (*0-7462-0078-1*) Kluwer Academic.

Commonsense Paediatrics. M. Pollak & J. Fry. 1986. text 144.00 (*0-85200-945-3*) Kluwer Academic.

Commonsense Psychiatry of Dr. Adolf Meyer: Fifty-Two Selected Papers. Adolf Meyer. Ed. by Alfred Lief. 1973. LC 73-2406. (Mental Illness & Social Policy; the American Experience Ser.). reprint ed. 46.95 (*0-405-05216-2*) Ayer.

***Commonsense Rebellion: Debunking Psychiatry, Confronting Society: An A to Z Guide to Rehumanizing Our Lives.** Bruce E. Levine. 2001. LC 00-65828. x, 331p. text 27.95 (*0-8264-1315-3*) Continuum.

Commonsense Use of Medicines. J. Fry et al. 1987. (Commonsense Ser.). 208p. (C). text 102.00 (*0-85200-996-8*) Kluwer Academic.

Commotion in the Blood: Life, Death, & the Immune System. Stephen S. Hall. 1999. 544p. text 30.00 (*0-7881-6043-5*) DIANE Pub.

Commotion in the Blood: Life, Death & the Immune System. Stephen S. Hall. 1998. (Sloan Technology Ser.). (Illus.). 560p. pap. 16.95 (*0-8050-5841-9*, Owl) H Holt & Co.

Communicable & Non-Communicable Disease Basics: A Primer. Madeline M. Hurster. 1997. LC 97-12667. 168p. 52.95 (*0-89789-507-X*); pap. 17.95 (*0-89789-508-8*) Greenwood (Bergin & Garvey).

Communicable Disease: Epidemiology & Control. N. D. Noah. 1998. LC 97-26054. 274p. 137.50 (*0-471-97273-8*) Wiley.

Communicable Disease Control Plan for School District Employees. Jan Sanderson & Dee K. Bauer. rev. ed. 1997. 85p. spiral bd. 27.50 (*1-880118-08-4*, 247-03) MESD Pr.

Communicable Disease Statistics. Office of Population Censuses and Surveys Staff. 1997. (OPCS Series MB2: No. 22, 1995). 66p. pap. (*0-11-691557-9*, HM09194) Statnry Office GBR. *Dist:* Bernan Associates.

Communicable Disease Statistics (OPCS Series MB2) 1992, No. 19. Office of Population Censuses and Surveys Staff. 1994. 66p. pap. (*0-11-691572-2*, HM15722) Statnry Office GBR. *Dist:* Bernan Associates.

Communicable Diseases: Policies & Procedures. Marguerite A. Bouvette. 3rd ed. 1996. 238p. (C). ring bd. 28.50 (*1-877735-23-X*, 2139PP) Prof Prnting & Pub.

Communicable Diseases 1998 Edition: Policies & Procedures. Marguerite A. Bouvette. 1998. 52.00 (*0-929442-34-2*, 2143PP) Prof Prnting & Pub.

Communicable Diseases & Infection Control for EMS. Robert G. Nixon. 1999. LC 99-44939. 118p. pap. text 30.60 (*0-13-084384-9*) P-H.

Communicating Care: Nursing Language in Action. Paul Crawford et al. 1998. (Illus.). pap. (*0-7487-3306-X*) Nelson Thornes GBR. *Dist:* Intl Spec Bk, Trans-Atl Phila.

Communicating Effectively in Multicultural Health Care Settings. Gary L. Kreps & Elizabeth N. Kunimoto. 1994. (Communicating Effectively in Multicultural Contexts Ser.: Vol. 3). 160p. (C). pap. 24.95 (*0-8039-4714-3*, 4504) Sage.

Communicating Effectively with Hispanic Patients: The Complete Guide to Key Vocabulary Words & Essential & Functional Phrases in Spanish for Direct Patient Contact. Set. Miriam Diaz-Gilbert. unabr. ed. 1991. (ENG & SPA.). 96p. (Orig.). pap., pap. text 175.00 incl. audio (*0-9628364-0-0*) ICPC.

Communicating for Better Health: A Guide through the Medical Mazes. Ed. by Allyn and Bacon Editorial Staff. 2000. LC 00-58272. 350p. 42.00 (*0-205-30777-9*, Longwood Div) Allyn.

Communicating for Learning: Classroom Observation & Collaboration. Elaine R. Silliman & Louise C. Wilkinson. 1991. LC 90-23748. 384p. 70.00 (*0-8342-0203-4*) Aspen Pub.

***Communicating Health: Personal, Cultural, & Political Complexities.** Patricia Geist-Martin et al. 2002. 448p. pap. text 48.95 (*0-534-53102-4*) Wadsworth Pub.

***Communicating Health & Illness.** Richard Gwyn. 2001. 182p. 83.00 (*0-7619-6474-6*); pap. 25.95 (*0-7619-6475-4*) Sage.

Communicating Issues in Thanatology. Thomas P. Fleming. 1979. 20.95 (*0-405-12512-7*) Ayer.

Communicating Issues in Thanatology. Thomas P. Fleming et al. 1976. text 37.50 (*0-8422-7272-0*) Irvington.

Communicating Risk in a Changing World. Ed. by Tim L. Tinker et al. 1998. LC 99-178794. 198p. pap. text 42.50 (*1-883595-20-7*, 23046, OEM Pr) OEM Health.

Communicating Therapeutic Risks. L. A. Morris. 1989. (Recent Research in Psychology Ser.). 186p. 64.95 (*0-387-97192-0*, 3675) Spr-Verlag.

Communicating with Patients: Improving Communication, Satisfaction & Compliance. Philip Ley. 1989. 240p. 49.95 (*0-7099-4161-7*); pap. 17.95 (*0-7099-4174-9*) Routledge.

Communicating with Your Doctor: Getting the Most Out of Health Care. J. Alfred Jones et al. Ed. by Gerald M. Phillips. 1995. (Communication Series). 256p. LC 95-37595. text 52.50 (*1-57273-022-6*); LC 95-37895. pap. text 21.95 (*1-57273-023-4*) Hampton Pr NJ.

Communicating Women's Health Messages: A Resource Book. Roxanne L. Parrott & Celeste M. Condit. 1996. 445p. 97.95 (*0-7619-0056-X*, 1693); pap. 49.95 (*0-7619-0057-8*, 1694) Sage.

Communication. 1995. 17.00 (*0-8342-0719-2*); VHS 94.00 (*0-8342-0720-6*) Aspen Pub.

Communication: Key to Effective Nursing. Ernestine Wiedenbach & Caroline E. Falls. 1978. LC 78-50063. (Illus.). 128p. pap. text 9.00 (*0-913292-23-0*) Tiresias Pr.

Communication: The Key to the Therapeutic Relationship. Pamela Schuster. 1999. LC 99-38640. (Illus.). xvi, 267p. pap. text 31.95 (*0-8036-0469-6*) Davis Co.

Communication Access for Persons with Hearing Loss: Compliance with the Americans with Disabilities Act. Ed. by Mark Ross. 1994. LC 94-2594. (Illus.). 306p. (C). pap. text 37.50 (*0-912752-35-1*) York Pr.

Communication, Aging, & Health: A Special Issue of Health Communication. Vol. 8, No. 3, 1996. Ed. by Ellen B. Ryan. 1996. 112p. pap. 20.00 (*0-8058-9909-X*) L Erlbaum Assocs.

Communication & Assertion Skills for Older Persons. Leilani Doty. 1987. (Death Education, Aging & Health Care Ser.). 110p. 46.95 (*0-89116-400-6*) Hemisp Pub.

Communication & Cognition in Normal Aging & Dementia. Kathryn A. Bayles et al. 1987. LC 90-21692. 400p. (Orig.). (C). pap. text 36.00 (*0-89079-330-1*, 1606) PRO-ED.

Communication & Communication Disorders: A Clinical Introduction. Plante & Beeson. 1998. LC 98-28923. 321p. pap. 62.67 (*0-205-28320-9*) Allyn.

Communication & Disenfranchisement: Social Health Issues & Implications. Ed. by Eileen B. Ray. 1996. (LEA's Communication Ser.). 504p. text 89.95 (*0-8058-1530-9*); 472p. pap. text 39.95 (*0-8058-1531-7*) L Erlbaum Assocs.

Communication & Education Skills for Dietetics Professionals. Betsy B. Holli & Richard J. Calabrese. 3rd ed. 1997. LC 97-6053. 243p. pap. 42.00 (*0-683-30015-6*) Lppncott W & W.

Communication & Health: Systems & Applications. Ed. by Eileen B. Ray & L. Donohew. 1989. 224p. 49.95 (*0-8058-0154-5*); pap. 22.50 (*0-8058-0697-0*) L Erlbaum Assocs.

Communication & Health Outcomes. Ed. by Gary L. Kreps & Dan O'Hair. 1995. LC 95-31622. (Speech Communication Association Applied Communication Ser.). 256p. text 59.50 (*1-881303-52-7*); pap. text 26.50 (*1-881303-53-5*) Hampton Pr NJ.

Communication & Interpersonal Relations: Text & Cases. William V. Haney. 6th ed. 1991. 608p. (C). text 64.95 (*0-256-06974-3*, 11-0283-06, Irwn McGrw-H) McGrw-H Hghr Educ.

Communication & Language Acquisition: Discoveries from Atypical Development. Lauren Adamson & Mary A. Romski. 1997. LC 96-37329. 352p. text 44.00 (*1-55766-279-7*) P H Brookes.

Communication & Medical Practice: Social Relations in the Clinic. David Silverman. 1987. 288p. (C). pap. 26.50 (*0-8039-8109-0*, 7001) Sage.

Communication & Parapsychology: Proceedings of an International Conference Held in Vancouver, Canada; August 9-10, 1979. Ed. by Betty Shapin & Lisette Coly. 1980. LC 80-80486. 17.00 (*0-912328-32-0*) Parapsych Foun.

Communication & Persuasion. R. E. Petty & John T. Cacioppo. 1986. (Social Psychology Ser.). (Illus.). 262p. 58.00 (*0-387-96344-8*) Spr-Verlag.

Communication & Persuasion: Psychological Studies of Opinion Change. Carl I. Hovland et al. 1982. LC 81-20104. 315p. reprint ed. lib. bdg. 49.75 (*0-313-23348-9*, HOVC, Greenwood Pr) Greenwood.

Communication & Swallowing Management Of Tracheostomized & Ventilator Dependent Adults. Karen J. Dikeman & Marta S. Kazandjian. 1995. (Illus.). 384p. (C). pap. text 73.95 (*1-56593-347-8*, 0645) Thomson Learn.

Communication & Swallowing Solutions for the ALS/MND Community: A CINI Manual. Communication Independence for the Neurologically Impaired Staff. Ed. by Marta S. Kazandjian. 1996. LC 96-32631. (Illus.). 100p. (Orig.). pap. 39.95 (*1-56593-808-9*, 1580) Thomson Learn.

Communication & the Mentally Ill Patient: Developmental & Linguistic Approaches to Schizophrenia. Ed. by Jenny France & Niki Muir. 1997. LC 97-108394. 208p. pap. (*1-85302-414-7*) Jessica Kingsley GBR. *Dist:* Taylor & Francis.

C
D

Communication Development: Foundations, Processes & Clinical Applications. William O. Haynes & Brian B. Shulman. 2nd ed. 1998. LC 97-33647. (Illus.). 405p. 50.00 (*0-683-30278-7*) Lppncott W & W.

Communication Difficulties in Childhood: A Practical Guide. Frances P. Glascoe & Geoff Thorley. Ed. by Rashmin C. Tamhne et al. 1999. LC 2001-347046. (Illus.). 264p. pap. (*1-85775-098-5*) Radcliffe Med Pr GBR. *Dist:* Balogh.

Communication Disorders. Ed. by Robert W. Rieber. 1981. LC 80-18394. (Applied Psycholinguistics & Communication Disorders Ser.). 366p. 65.00 (*0-306-40527-X*, Plenum Trade) Perseus Pubng.

Communication Disorders: An Introduction for Community-Based Rehabilitation Workers. Gillian Clezy et al. 1996. LC 97-143638. (Illus.). 172p. (Orig.). pap. (*962-209-389-2*) HK Univ Pr HKG. *Dist:* Intl Spec Bk, Coronet Bks.

Communication Disorders & Children with Psychiatric & Behavioral Disorders. Diana L. Rogers-Adkinson & Penny L. Griffith. 1998. LC 98-23248. (School-Age Children Ser.). (Illus.). 420p. pap. 49.95 (*1-56593-746-5*, 1454) Thomson Learn.

Communication Disorders & Interventions in Low Incidence Pediatric Populations. Lisa Schoenbrodt et al. 1995. 262p. (Orig.). (C). pap. 45.00 (*1-56593-220-X*, 0580) Thomson Learn.

Communication Disorders Following Traumatic Brain Injury: Management of Cognitive, Language, & Motor Impairments. Ed. by David R. Beukelman & Kathryn M. Yorkston. 1991. LC 89-14560. (Illus.). 439p. (C). pap. text 37.00 (*0-89079-295-X*, 1586) PRO-ED.

Communication Disorders Following Traumatic Brain Injury: Management of Cognitive, Language & Motor Impairments. Sky E. Mcdonald. 1999. LC 00-361287. (Brain Damage, Behaviour & Cognition Ser.). xiv, 338p. 59.95 (*0-86377-724-4*) L Erlbaum Assocs.

Communication Disorders in Infants & Toddlers: Assessment & Intervention. Frances P. Billeaud. 2nd ed. 1998. LC 97-43983. 304p. text 44.99 (*0-7506-9952-3*) Buttrwrth-Heinemann.

***Communication Disorders in Multilingual Populations: Second International Symposium, Kwa Maritane, South Africa, July 2000.** Ed. by M. Fredman & N. Miller. 2000. (Special Issue Ser.: Vol. 53, No. 3). (Illus.). 70p. 25.25 (*3-8055-7237-9*) S Karger.

Communication Disorders Sourcebook: Basic Information about Deafness & Hearing Loss, Speech, & Language Disorders, Voice Disorders, Balance, & Vestibular Disorders, & Disorders of Smell, Taste, & Touch. Ed. by Linda M. Ross. 1996. (Health Reference Ser.: Vol. 11). lib. bdg. 78.00 (*0-7808-0077-X*) Omnigraphics Inc.

Communication for Health Professionals: A Relational Perspective. Teresa L. Thompson. 1988. 176p. (C). reprint ed. pap. text 23.50 (*0-8191-6994-3*) U Pr of Amer.

Communication for Nursing Practice: A Skills Based Approach. Henry Minardi & Martin Riley. 1997. LC 96-53895. 224p. pap. text 34.50 (*0-7506-1579-6*) Buttrwrth-Heinemann.

Communication in Cancer Care. Ivan Lichter. 1987. LC 86-20764. (Illus.). 209p. text (*0-443-03698-5*) Church.

Communication in Medicine. McManus. 1999. (Illus.). 160p. (C). pap. 23.95 (*0-412-61820-6*, Chap & Hall NY) Chapman & Hall.

Communication in Medicine: A Challenge to the Profession. O. K. Harlem. 1977. (Illus.). 15.75 (*3-8055-2387-4*) S Karger.

Communication in Nursing: Communicating Assertively & Responsibly in Nursing. Julia Blazer-Riley. 4th ed. 2000. LC 99-33660. (Illus.). 454p. pap. 34.95 (*0-323-00872-0*) Mosby Inc.

Communication in Nursing Practice. Eleanor C. Hein. 2nd ed. 1980. 280p. 14.00 (*0-316-35453-8*, Little Brwn Med Div) Lppncott W & W.

Communication in the Counseling Relationship. Bonnie J. Headington. 1979. LC 78-9026. pap. 11.00 (*0-910328-24-2*); text 16.50 (*0-910328-23-4*) Sulzburger & Graham Pub.

Communication in the Nursing Context. Jean C. Bradley & Mark A. Edinberg. 3rd ed. 1990. (Illus.). 276p. (C). pap. 38.80 (*0-8385-1327-1*, A1327-4) P-H.

Communication Intervention: Birth to Three. Louis M. Rossetti. 1996. (Illus.). 272p. (C). pap. text 53.95 (*1-56593-101-7*, 0404) Thomson Learn.

Communication of Caring in Nursing. Virginia Knowlden. 1999. (Monographs). (Illus.). 76p. (C). pap. text 20.00 (*0-9656391-7-7*, 1061) Sigma Theta Tau.

Communication of Emotion: Current Research from Diverse Perspectives, Vol. 77. K. Barrett. 1997. pap. 28.00 (*0-7879-9895-8*) Jossey-Bass.

Communication of Language-Impaired Children. H. Van Balkom. 1991. xiv, 266p. pap. (*90-265-1183-3*) Swets.

Communication Options in the Education of Deaf Children. Wendy Lynas. 1994. LC 95-108460. 126p. (Orig.). (C). pap. text 34.95 (*1-56593-373-7*, 0750) Singular Publishing.

Communication Policy & Planning in the American Cancer Society Public Education Program. Gerald E. Klonglan & Chun-Nan Lo. 1984. (Institute of Culture & Communication Case Studies: No. 8). xii, 61p. (Orig.). pap. text 5.00 (*0-86638-044-2*) EW Ctr HI.

Communication Problems: After a Brain Injury or Stroke. Judith L. McKrell. Ed. by Richard Sweetman. 1996. LC 96-48516. (Illus.). 24p. (Orig.). pap. 5.95 (*0-939838-44-3*) Pritchett & Hull.

Communication Problems in Autism. E. Schopler & G. B. Mesibov. 1985. LC 85-3416. (Current Issues in Autism Ser.). (Illus.). 350p. (C). 59.00 (*0-306-41859-2*, Plenum Trade) Perseus Pubng.

Communication Skills for Doctors. Peter Maguire. 2001. (Arnold Publication). 192p. (Orig.). pap. 19.95 (*0-340-66309-X*) OUP.

Communication Skills for Medicine. Lloyd. 1996. pap. text 17.95 (*0-443-05168-2*) Saunders.

Communication Skills for the Health Care Professional: Concepts & Techniques. Gwen Van Servellen. 1996. LC 96-26915. 416p. pap. 52.00 (*0-8342-0766-4*, 20766) Aspen Pub.

Communication Skills in Hearing-Impaired Children: An Overview. R. John Bench. 1992. LC 92-18568. 340p. 50.00 (*1-56593-075-4*, 0381) Singular Publishing.

Communication Skills in Helping Relationships: A Framework for Facilitating Personal Growth. Vonda O. Long. 1995. LC 95-23584. 290p. stu. ed., wbk. ed. 23.07 (*0-534-33870-4*) Brooks-Cole.

Communication Skills in Medicine. Charles R. Hind. 1997. 161p. (Orig.). pap. (*0-7279-1152-X*) BMJ Pub GBR. *Dist:* AIDC.

Communication Skills in Pharmacy Practice. William N. Tindall et al. 3rd ed. 1994. (Illus.). 218p. pap. text 29.95 (*0-8121-1633-X*) Lppncott W & W.

Communication Skills in Practice: A Practical Guide for Health Professionals. Diana Williams. 1996. 382p. pap. (*1-85302-232-2*) Jessica Kingsley GBR. *Dist:* Taylor & Francis.

Communication Skills Training for Health Professionals. D. A. Dickson et al. 1996. (Illus.). 368p. pap. 45.00 (*1-56593-766-X*, 1490) Singular Publishing.

Communication Therapy for Adults with Sensory Loss. Erber. 1996. 32.00 net. (*1-56593-889-5*) Singular Publishing.

Communication Unbound: How Facilitated Communication Is Challenging Traditional Views of Autism & Ability-Disability. Douglas P. Biklen. 1993. LC 92-34555. (Special Education Ser.: No. 13). (C). 335p. pap. 17.95 (*0-8077-3221-4*); 240p. text 39.00 (*0-8077-3222-2*) Tchrs Coll.

Communication with the Cancer Patient: Information & Truth. Ed. by Antonella Surbone & Matjaz Zwitter. 1997. LC 96-29490. 540p. 90.00 (*0-89766-985-1*) NY Acad Sci.

Communication with the Cancer Patient: Information & Truth, Vol. 809. Antonella Surbone & Matjaz Zwitter. 1997. LC 96-29490. (Annals of the New York Academy of Sciences Ser.). pap. 90.00 (*0-89766-986-X*) NY Acad Sci.

Communications Examples for Child Health. Susan M. Thorton. 1983. (Johnson & Johnson Pediatric Round Table Ser.). 66p. (Orig.). pap. text 6.00 (*0-931562-10-4*) J & J Consumer Prods.

Communications for Responders. 1998. (Training in a Box Ser.). 56p. ring bd. 49.00 (*1-57927-036-0*) APCO Inst.

Communications in Nursing: Communicating Assertively & Responsibly in Nursing. Julia Balzer-Riley. 3rd ed. 1995. (Illus.). 496p. (C). (gr. 13). pap. text 35.00 (*0-8151-0562-2*, 25467) Mosby Inc.

Communicative Alternatives to Challenging Behavior: Integrating Functional Assessment & Intervention Strategies. Ed. by Joe Reichle & David Wacker. 1993. LC 93-14787. 496p. 45.00 (*1-55766-082-4*) P H Brookes.

Communicative Competence of Young Children. Susan H. Foster. 1990. (Studies in Language & Linguistics). (Illus.). 272p. (Orig.). (C). pap. text 33.55 (*0-582-55271-0*, 78583) Longman.

Communicative Disorders Related to Cleft Lip & Palate. Kenneth R. Bzoch & Janet Givens-Ackerman. 4th ed. 1997. LC 96-22641. (Illus.). 690p. pap. text 42.00 (*0-89079-701-3*, 7956) PRO-ED.

Communimed: Multilingual Patient Assessment Manual. Brent Kelland. 3rd ed. 1994. LC 94-231854. (Illus.). 352p. (C). (gr. 13). text 9.95 (*0-8151-5241-8*, 24307) Mosby Inc.

Communism: Medical Subject Index of Current Progress with Bibliography. Stanley M. Thompson. 1990. LC 88-47552. 150p. 47.50 (*1-55914-170-0*); pap. 44.50 (*1-55914-171-9*) ABBE Pubs Assn.

Communities at Risk: Collective Responses to Technical Hazards. Stephen R. Couch & J. Stephen Kroll-Smith. 1991. LC 89-13557. (Worcester Polytechnic Institute Studies in Science, Technology, & Culture: Vol. 3). (Illus.). VI, 320p. (C). text 50.95 (*0-8204-0712-7*) P Lang Pubng.

Communities That Care: Action for Drug Abuse Prevention. J. David Hawkins et al. 1992. LC 92-11010. (Joint Publication of the Jossey-Bass Social & Behavioral S Ser.). 272p. pap. 38.00 (*1-55542-471-6*) Jossey-Bass.

Community-Acquired Infections & Diseases: Index of New Information with Authors, Subjects & References. Ellen M. Majors. 1996. 150p. 57.50 (*0-7883-1262-6*); pap. 47.50 (*0-7883-1263-4*) ABBE Pubs Assn.

Community-Acquired Pneumonia. Thomas J. Marrie. 2001. LC 00-34931. (Illus.). 930p. 165.00 (*0-306-46432-2*, Kluwer Plenum) Kluwer Academic.

Community & Contagion: A Neighborhood's Reception to a Nursing Home for People with AIDS. Jane Balin. 1999. LC 98-36506. (Anthropology of Contemporary Issues Ser.). 200p. pap. 15.95 (*0-8014-8579-7*) Cornell U Pr.

Community & Home Health Nursing. Judith Ann Allender. 1997. LC 97-19138. (Lippincott's Review Ser.). 316p. pap. text 25.95 (*0-397-55456-7*) Lppncott W & W.

Community & Home Health Nursing. Ida Androwich et al. 1996. LC 95-36419. (Plans of Care for Specialty Practice Ser.). 408p. (C). pap. 33.50 (*0-8273-6227-7*) Delmar.

Community & Municipal Action on Alcohol. 1995. LC 96-145878. (WHO Regional Publications, European Ser.: No. 63). 102p. (Orig.). pap. text 23.00 (*92-890-1327-3*, 1310063) World Health.

Community & Nursing Home Practice Drug Therapy OBRA Monitoring & Patient Education Guidelines, 1993. James W. Cooper, Jr. 1993. LC 93-70156. 350p. (C). pap. text 42.50 (*0-9635702-4-2*) J W Cooper Cnslt.

Community & Public Health Dentistry. Schnuth. 1995. (Dental Assisting Procedures Ser.). text 37.95 (*0-8273-5677-3*) Delmar.

Community & Public Health Nursing. Marcia Stanhope & Jeanette Lancaster. 5th ed. 2000. LC 99-47288. (Illus.). 1243p. text 58.00 (*0-323-00749-X*) Mosby Inc.

***Community & Public Health Nursing: Instructor's Resource Kit.** Marcia Stanhope & Jeanette Lancaster. 5th ed. 2000. (Illus.). (*0-323-00750-3*) Mosby Inc.

Community Approach to AIDS Intervention: Exploring the Miami Outreach Project for Injecting Drug Users & Other High Risk Groups, 33. Dale D. Chitwood et al. 1991. LC 91-19872. (Contributions in Medical Studies Ser.: No. 33). 248p. 67.00 (*0-313-27319-7*, ICP, Greenwood Pr) Greenwood.

Community Approaches to the Prevention & Cessation of Smoking: A Manual for Community Health Professionals. Health Promotion Resource Center Staff. Ed. by John McManus et al. 2nd ed. 1991. 130p. reprint ed. pap. 19.50 (*1-879552-15-9*) SCRDP.

Community As Doctor. Robert N. Rapopart et al. Ed. by Gerald N. Grob. 1980. LC 78-22587. (Historical Issues in Mental Health Ser.). (Illus.). reprint ed. lib. bdg. 25.95 (*0-405-11938-0*) Ayer.

Community As Method: Therapeutic Communities for Special Populations & Special Settings. George De Leon. 1997. LC 96-26292. 328p. 72.95 (*0-275-94818-8*) Greenwood.

Community As Partner: Theory & Practice in Nursing. Elizabeth T. Anderson & Judith M. McFarlane. 3rd ed. 2000. LC 00-21600. 464p. pap. text 35.00 (*0-7817-2125-3*) Lppncott W & W.

Community Assessment: Guidelines for Developing Countries. Douglas Stockman. 1994. 144p. pap. (*1-85339-224-3*) Intermed Tech GBR. *Dist:* Stylus Pub VA.

***Community-Based Animal Healthcare: A Practical Guide to Improving Primary Veterinary Services.** Ed. by Andy Catley et al. 2001. 250p. pap. (*1-85339-485-8*) Intermed Tech GBR. *Dist:* Stylus Pub VA.

Community-Based Drug Demand Reduction & HIV-AIDS Prevention: A Manual for Planners, Practitioners, Trainer & Evaluators. Economic and Social Commission for Asia and the Pacific Staff. 1995. 152p. pap. 20.00 (*92-1-119708-2*, RA644) UN.

Community-Based Education of Health Personnel. 1987. (Technical Reports: No. 746). 89p. pap. text 12.00 (*92-4-120746-9*, 1100746) World Health.

Community-Based Long Term Care: Agenda for the 21st Century. Rita M. Gallagher. 1995. 80p. pap. text 22.95 (*1-55810-116-0*, CH-43) Am Nurses Pub.

Community-Based Medical Education. Ann Boaden. 1999. LC 99-224373. (Illus.). 160p. pap. text (*0-340-70012-2*) E A GBR. *Dist:* OUP.

Community Based Nursing: An Introduction. Melanie McEwen. Ed. by Thomas Eoyang. 1998. LC 97-41326. 608p. (C). pap. 27.95 (*0-7216-6109-2*) Saunders.

Community Based Nursing: Foundation for Practice. Ginger Armentrout. 1998. LC 97-45780. 250p. (C). pap. 36.60 (*0-8385-1522-3*, A-1522-0) P-H.

Community-Based Nursing Care: Making the Transition. Martha Ayers et al. 1999. LC 98-50554. (Illus.). 431p. (C). (gr. 13). pap. text 29.00 (*0-8151-1339-0*, 29954);Includes Testbank. tchr. ed. (*0-323-00747-3*) Mosby Inc.

Community Based Nursing Practice: Integrating Concepts & Skills. Roberta Hunt. 1997. 752p. pap. text 24.95 (*0-397-55188-6*) Lppncott W & W.

Community-Based Nursing Practice: Learning Through Students' Stories. Jeanne Sorrell & Georgine Redmond. 2001. LC 2001-28654. (Illus.). 464p. per. 30.95 (*0-8036-0067-9*) Davis Co.

Community-Based Prevention: Programs That Work. Ross C. Brownson et al. 1998. LC 98-43313. 320p. pap. 41.00 (*0-8342-1241-2*, 12412) Aspen Pub.

Community Based Rehabilitation. Peat. 1997. pap. text 50.00 (*0-7020-1941-0*) Saunders.

Community-Based Systems of Long-Term Care. Ed. by Rick Zawadski. 1984. LC 83-22703. (Home Health Care Services Quarterly Ser.: Vol. 4, Nos. 3-4). 247p. text 49.95 (*0-86656-255-9*) Haworth Pr.

Community-Based Teaching: A Guide to Developing & Implementing Education Programs for Medical Students & Residents in the Practitioner's Office. Ed. by Susan L. Deutsch. 1997. LC 97-6376. 284p. (Orig.). (C). pap. text 34.00 (*0-943126-59-2*) Amer Coll Phys.

Community Benefit & Tax-Exempt Status: A Self-Assessment Guide for Hospitals. American Hospital Association Staff. 1988. 100p. (Orig.). 40.00 (*0-87258-498-4*, 001800) Am Hospital.

Community Care. 320p. pap. (*0-340-61390-4*) E A GBR. *Dist:* Routldge.

Community Care: Asking the Users. Ed. by Gail Wilson. 1995. 278p. 39.95 (*1-56593-419-9*, 1085) Singular Publishing.

Community Care: Initial Training & Beyond. Ed. by David Skidmore. 1996. 180p. (Orig.). pap. 34.95 (*1-56593-772-4*) Singular Publishing.

Community Care: New Agendas & Challenges from the U. K. & Overseas. Ed. by David Challis et al. 1994. 336p. (*1-85742-208-2*) Arena GBR. *Dist:* Ashgate Pub Co.

Community Care: The Provision of Mental Health Services in North Wales. Ed. by Charles Crosby & Margaret Barry. 1995. 288p. (*1-85628-531-6*) Avebry GBR. *Dist:* Ashgate Pub Co.

Community Care for Health Professionals. Ann Compton & Mary Ashwin. 1992. 288p. pap. text 52.50 (*0-7506-0185-X*); 2nd ed. 2000. LC 00-36081. (Illus.). 223p. pap. text 45.00 (*0-7506-3290-9*) Buttrwrth-Heinemann.

Community Care for Older People: A Comparative Perspective. Susan Tester. 1996. LC 96-14143. 232p. text 59.95 (*0-312-15912-9*) St Martin.

Community Care in Context. NISW Staff. 1992. (*0-7855-2688-9*) Natl Inst Soc Work GBR. *Dist:* St Mut.

Community Care in England & France: Reforms & the Improvement of Equity & Efficiency. Bleddyn Davies et al. 1998. LC 98-71404. 250p. text (*1-84014-584-6*) Ashgate Pub GBR. *Dist:* Ashgate Pub Co.

Community Care Nurses & Caring. N. Malin. 1999. LC 98-40515. (Social Science for Nurses & the Caring Professions Ser.). 192p. pap. (*0-335-19670-5*) OpUniv Pr.

Community Care Nurses & Caring. N. Malin et al. 1999. LC 98-40515. (Social Science for Nurses & the Caring Professions Ser.). (Illus.). 206p. pap. (*0-335-19671-3*) OpUniv Pr.

Community Child Health: An Action Plan for Today. Judith S. Palfrey. LC 94-8641. 328p. 1995. pap. 26.95 (*0-275-95472-2*); 1994. 62.95 (*0-275-94696-7*) Greenwood (Praeger Pubs).

Community Child Health & Paediatrics. David Harvey et al. Ed. by Diane Smyth. 1995. LC 94-11861. (Illus.). 720p. text (*0-7506-1323-8*) E A GBR. *Dist:* OUP.

Community Genetics Services in Europe: Report on a Survey. B. Modell et al. 1991. (WHO Regional Publications: No. 38). (ENG, FRE & GER.). x, 137p. pap. text 24.00 (*92-890-1301-X*, 1310038) World Health.

Community Health. Gold. 2001. pap. text 25.00 (*0-697-00707-3*) McGraw.

Community Health. Richard H. Grimmett. 1999. LC 99-54062. (Rypins' Intensive Reviews Ser.). 176p. pap. text 23.00 (*0-397-51558-8*) Lppncott W & W.

Community Health. Wilkerson. 2000. pap. text 11.97 net. (*0-395-97322-8*) HM.

Community Health Analysis: A Global Awareness at the Local Level. G. E.Alan Dever. 2nd rev. ed. 1991. (Health Care Administration Ser.). (Illus.). 416p. (C). pap. 65.00 (*0-8342-0191-7*) Aspen Pub.

Community Health & Mental Health Care Delivery for North American Indians. E. Fuller Torrey et al. 1975. (Health Problems of N. A. Indians Ser.: Vol. 3). 22.00 (*0-8422-7218-6*) Irvington.

Community Health & Sanitation. Ed. by Charles Kerr. 1990. (Illus.). 300p. pap. (*1-85339-018-6*) Intermed Tech GBR. *Dist:* Stylus Pub VA.

Community Health Care Nursing. Ed. by David Sines. 1995. LC 95-1289. (Illus.). 224p. pap. 32.95 (*0-632-03856-X*) Blackwell Sci.

Community Health Care Nursing: Principles for Practice. Sheila Twinn et al. 1996. LC 96-210726. (Illus.). 544p. pap. text 62.50 (*0-7506-1590-7*) Buttrwrth-Heinemann.

Community Health Care Nursing, Second Edition. David Sines et al. 2nd ed. 2001. LC 00-50773. (Illus.). 400p. pap. 37.95 (*0-632-05657-6*) Blackwell Sci.

Community Health Centers: Adapting to Changing Health Care Environment Key to Continued Success. Helene Toiv & Anne Dievler. 2001. 51p. (C). pap. text 25.00 (*0-7567-0585-1*) DIANE Pub.

Community Health Centers: Changes in Transitioning to Prepaid Managed Care. 1996. 42p. (Orig.). (C). pap. text 20.00 (*0-7881-2932-5*) DIANE Pub.

Community Health Education. Breckon. 4th ed. 1998. tchr. ed. 49.00 (*0-8342-1153-X*) Aspen Pub.

Community Health Education & Promotion: A Guide to Program Design & Evaluation. Aspen Reference Group Staff et al. 1997. LC 97-75. 428p. pap. 62.00 (*0-8342-0953-5*, 20953) Aspen Pub.

Community Health Education & Promotion Manual. Aspen Reference Group Staff. 1996. LC 96-17242. 428p. ring bd. 199.00 (*0-8342-0774-5*, S195) Aspen Pub.

*Community Health Education Methods. Robert Bensley. 2nd ed. 2002. (Illus.). (C). pap. text 37.95 (0-7637-1801-7, 1801-7) Jones & Bartlett.
Community Health in the 21st Century. Patricia A. Reagan & Jodi Brookins-Fisher. 1997. (C). pap., tchr. ed. (0-205-26492-1, T6492-7); 1996. LC 96-24914. 532p. pap. text 73.00 (0-205-19749-3) Allyn.
Community Health Information Systems: Lessons for the Future. K. A. Duncan. 1998. LC 97-39549. xx, 165p. 44.00 (1-56793-071-9) Health Admin Pr.
Community Health Need Assessment. Timothy W. Bosworth. 1995. LC 95-36932. 256p. (C). text 45.00 (1-55738-647-1, Irwn Prfssnl) McGraw-Hill Educ Grp.
Community Health NSG/Public Health. Paula Brabec. 2001. (Nursing Education Ser.). 44.00 (0-8273-5691-9) Delmar.
Community Health Nurse. Jack Rudman. 1994. (Certified Nurse Examination Ser.: CN-4). pap. 27.95 (0-8373-6104-4) Nat Learn.
Community Health Nursing. Brabec. 1997. (Nursing Education Ser.). tchr. ed. 12.50 (0-8273-5692-7) Delmar.
Community Health Nursing. Gastrell. 1996. (C). pap. text 42.00 (0-7020-1890-2) Harcourt.
Community Health Nursing. Vec Staff & Delmar Publishing Staff. Ed. by Cecilia Mulvey. 1995. LC 95-4727. (NSNA Review Ser.). 224p. mass mkt. 21.50 (0-8273-7074-1) Delmar.
Community Health Nursing. McMurray. 2nd ed. 1993. pap. 29.00 (0-443-04865-7) Saunders.
Community Health Nursing. Ed. by Mary A. Nies & Melanie McEwen. 3rd ed. 2001. LC 00-54788. text 58.00 (0-7216-9161-7) Harcrt Hlth Sci Grp.
Community Health Nursing. Kathleen M. Leahy et al. 4th ed. 1982. 432p. text 25.95 (0-07-036834-1) McGraw.
Community Health Nursing. Judith Ann Allender & Barbara W. Spradley. 5th ed. 2000. LC 00-61819. (Illus.). 832p. text 56.95 (0-7817-2122-9) Lppncott W & W.
Community Health Nursing. Brabec. 5th ed. 1997. (Nursing Education Ser.). (0-8273-5693-5, VNR) Wiley.
Community Health Nursing: A Case Study Approach. Tamara Hertenstein-McKinnon. 1997. LC 96-41028. 336p. pap. text 28.95 (0-397-55460-5, Lippnctt) Lppncott W & W.
Community Health Nursing: An Alliance for Health. Marilyn B. Klainberg et al. 1997. LC 97-227580. (McGraw-Hill Nursing Core Ser.). (Illus.). 504p. pap. 39.95 (0-07-105478-2) McGraw-Hill Prof.
Community Health Nursing: Caring for the Public's Health. Kay Saucier Lundy et al. 2001. (Illus.). 832p. (C). text 68.95 (0-7637-0706-6, 0706-6) Jones & Bartlett.
Community Health Nursing: Caring in Practice to Community Health Nursing. Janice E. Hitchcock et al. 1999. LC 98-46716. (Nursing Education Ser.). 968p. (C). 68.95 (0-8273-6485-7) Delmar.
Community Health Nursing: Proceedings of the WHO Expert Committee, Geneva, 1974. WHO Staff. 1974. (Technical Reports: No. 558). pap. text 4.00 (92-4-120558-X, 1100558) World Health.
Community Health Nursing: Process & Practice for Promoting Health. Marcia Stanhope & Jeanette Lancaster. 4th ed. 1996. (Illus.). tchr. ed. (0-8151-8513-8) Mosby Inc.
Community Health Nursing: Process & Practice for Promoting Health. Ed. by Marcia Stanhope & Jeanette Lancaster. 4th ed. 1995. LC 95-39516. (Illus.). 1184p. (C). (gr. 13). text 58.00 (0-8151-8142-6, 25908) Mosby Inc.
Community Health Nursing: Promoting the Health of Aggregates. Ed. by Janice M. Swanson & Mary Nies. 1993. (Illus.). tchr. ed. (0-7216-4921-1) Saunders.
Community Health Nursing: Promoting the Health of Aggregates. Janice M. Swanson & Mary Nies. Ed. by Ilde Rader. 2nd ed. 1997. LC 96-31896. (Illus.). 895p. text 52.00 (0-7216-6167-X) Saunders.
Community Health Nursing: Promoting the Health of Aggregates. Ed. by Janice M. Swanson & Mary Nies. 2nd ed. 1997. (Illus.). 965p. tchr. ed. (0-7216-6168-8) Saunders.
Community Health Nursing: Theory & Practice. Ed. by Claudia M. Smith & Frances A. Maurer. 1995. (Illus.). tchr. ed. (0-7216-5892-X) Saunders.
Community Health Nursing: Theory & Practice. Claudia M. Smith & Frances A. Maurer. 1995. LC 94-13122. (Illus.). 872p. text 52.50 (0-7216-2742-0) Saunders.
Community Health Nursing: Theory & Practice. Claudia Smith. 2nd ed. 2000. 933p. pap. Price not set. (0-7216-7470-4) Saunders.
Community Health Nursing Care Plans. Susan L. Scherman. 2nd ed. 1990. (Nursing Education Ser.). pap. 32.20 (0-8273-4357-4) Delmar.
Community Health Nursing Care Plans: A Guide for Home Health Care Professionals. Susan L. Scherman. 1989. LC 84-17274. 564p. pap. text 32.20 (0-8273-4356-6) Delmar.
Community Health Nursing Handbook. Mary Jo Clark. 1998. LC 98-37952. (Illus.). 272p. (C). pap. 18.67 (0-8385-1070-1) P-H.
Community Health Nursing Supervisor: A Handbook for Community-Home Care Managers. Ruth N. Knollmueller. 1986. 216p. (Orig.). pap. 22.95 (0-88737-249-X, 21-1999) Natl League Nurse.
Community Health Promotion Ideas That Work: A Field Book for Practitioners. Marshall W. Kreuter et al. 1997. LC 97-3555. (Health Science Ser.). (Illus.). 224p. (C). pap. text 38.95 (0-7637-0408-3, 0408-3) Jones & Bartlett.
Community Health Psychology: Empowerment for Diverse Communities. Victor De La'Cancela et al. 1998. LC 97-21660. 288p. (C). 90.00 (0-415-91426-4); pap. 26.95 (0-415-91427-2) Routledge.
Community Health Services: Index of New Information with Authors, Subjects & References. Ellen M. Majors. 2nd ed. 1996. 150p. 57.50 (0-7883-1260-X); pap. 47.50 (0-7883-1261-8) ABBE Pubs Assn.
Community Health Worker: Working Guide, Guidelines for Training, Guidelines for Adaptation. rev. ed. 1987. (CHI, FRE & SPA.). 463p. pap. text 22.00 (92-4-156097-5, 1150262) World Health.
Community Health Workers. G. Walt. 1990. 192p. (0-335-15433-6) OpUniv Pr.
Community Healthcare Nursing. Blackie. 1998. LC 98-10211. (C). pap. text 29.95 (0-443-05291-3) Saunders.
Community Hospitals of Kansas City, Missouri, 1870-1915. Joan E. Lynaugh. 1989. (Medical Care in the United States Ser.). 200p. text 15.00 (0-8240-8337-7) Garland.
Community in African Primary Health Care: Strengthening Participation & a Proposed Strategy. Charles M. Good. 1988. LC 88-12828. (Studies in African Health & Medicine: Vol. 2). 175p. lib. bdg. 79.95 (0-88946-138-4) E Mellen.
Community Integrated Service Systems & Home Visiting for At-Risk Families Grant Programs: Abstracts of Active Projects, FY 1995. Prod. by National Center for Education in Maternal and Child Health Staff. 1995. LC 95-70485. 108p. pap. (1-57285-018-3) Nat Ctr Educ.
Community Integration Following Traumatic Brain Injury. 352p. (0-340-53709-4) E A GBR. *Dist:* Routldge.
Community Integration for People with Severe Disabilities. Ed. by Steven J. Taylor et al. 1987. (Special Education Ser.). 256p. 31.95 (0-8077-2847-0); pap. text 18.95 (0-8077-2846-2) Tchrs Coll.
Community Integration Program. Missy Armstrong & Sara Lauzen. 2nd ed. 1994. 321p. ring bd. 50.00 (1-882883-03-9, B245) Idyll Arbor.
Community Involvement in Health: From Passive Recipients to Active Participants. Jan Smithies & Georgina Webster. 1998. LC 98-12737. 313p. text 84.95 (1-85742-428-X, RA485.S59) Ashgate Pub Co.
Community Living Skills Development: Teaching Methods. Ed. by William H. Burke. 2nd rev. ed. 1996. (Professional Series on Traumatic Brain Injury: Vol. 3). 76p. (Orig.). pap. 9.50 (1-882855-44-2) HDI Pubs.
Community Living Skills Workbook for the Head-Injured Adult. Deborah K. Angle & Julie M. Buxton. 1991. LC 91-4532. 384p. spiral bd. 120.00 (0-8342-0210-7) PRO-ED.
Community Mental Health: A Practical Guide. Loren R. Mosher & Lorenzo Burti. abr. ed. 1994. LC 93-28408. 224p. (C). pap. 17.00 (0-393-70165-4) Norton.
Community Mental Health: A Sourcebook for Professionals & Advisory, Boards Members. Ed. by Wade H. Silverman. 1981. LC 80-25984. 499p. 78.75 (0-275-90718-X, C0718, Praeger Pubs) Greenwood.
Community Mental Health: Practical Approaches to Long-Term Problems. Morgan. 1993. 268p. pap. 44.75 (1-56593-138-6, 0450) Singular Publishing.
Community Mental Health: Practical Approaches to Long Term Problems - Therapy in Practice. S. Morgan. 1993. 272p. pap. (0-412-46940-5) Chapman & Hall.
Community Mental Health & Behavioral-Ecology: A Handbook of Theory, Research, & Practice. A. M. Jeger & R. S. Slotnick. 1982. LC 82-13122. (Illus.). 540p. (C). 95.00 (0-306-40850-3, Plenum Trade) Perseus Pubng.
Community Mental Health & Social Psychiatry: A Reference Guide. Harvard University, Medical School Staff. 1990. LC 62-9425. 161p. pap. 4.50 (0-674-15100-3) HUP.
Community Mental Health & the Law. Steven J. Schwartz & Stephen F. Ferrarone. 1981. LC 80-18872. 256p. 31.50 (0-8290-0239-1) Irvington.
Community Mental Health in Texas: Four Case Studies. David C. Warner et al. 1990. (Special Project Reports: Vol. SP-CM). 250p. pap. 10.50 (0-89940-869-9) LBJ Sch Pub Aff.
Community Mental Health Nurse. Jack Rudman. 1994. (Career Examination Ser.: C-3223). pap. 34.95 (0-8373-3223-0) Nat Learn.
Community Nursing. 224p. pap. (0-340-59799-2) E A GBR. *Dist:* Routldge.
Community Nursing: Dimensions & Dilemmas. Ed. by Paul Cain et al. 1995. 192p. pap. 34.95 (1-56593-612-4, 1270) Singular Publishing.
Community Nursing: Research & Recent Developments. G. Baker et al. 1986. 240p. (Orig.). pap. (0-7099-4415-2) C Helm GBR. *Dist:* Routldge.
Community Nutrition. Boyle & Morris. 3rd ed. 2001. (Health Sciences Ser.). 52.50 net. (0-534-55188-2) Wadsworth Pub.
Community Nutrition: Applying Epidemiology to Contemporary Practice. Gail C. Frank-Spohrer. 1996. 450p. 62.00 (0-8342-0784-2); 2nd ed. 2001. 600p. 80.00 (0-8342-1869-0) Aspen Pub.
Community Nutrition: Challenges & Opportunities. annuals Jeannette B. Endres. 1998. LC 98-14509. 398p. 81.00 (0-13-509191-8) P-H.
Community Nutrition: People, Policies & Programs. Compiled by Helen S. Wright. 1982. (Illus.). 583p. (C). pap. text 43.95 (0-86720-382-X, 382-X) Jones & Bartlett.
Community Nutrition in Action: An Entrepreneurial Approach. Mari Boyle & Diane H. Morris. 1994. LC 94-8255. 500p. (C). 48.50 (0-314-02819-6) West Pub.
Community Nutrition in Action: An Entrepreneurial Approach. Boyle & Morris. 2nd ed. 1998. LC 98-38212. (Health Sciences Ser.). 650p. spiral bd. 79.95 (0-534-53829-0) Wadsworth Pub.
Community Occupational Therapy with Mentally Handicapped Adults. D. Isaac. Ed. by Jo Campling. 1990. (Therapy in Practice Ser.). 200p. pap. 23.00 (0-412-32720-1, A4416) Chapman & Hall.
Community Oral Health. Cynthia M. Pine. 1996. LC 97-108396. 288p. pap. text (0-7236-1095-9, RK52) John Wright GBR. *Dist:* Buttrwrth-Heinemann.
Community Organizing & Community Building for Health. Ed. by Meredith Minkler. 1997. LC 96-49716. 416p. (C). text 60.00 (0-8135-2435-0) Rutgers U Pr.
Community-Oriented Primary Care: From Principle to Practice. Paul A. Nutting. 1990. LC 90-12627. 572p. reprint ed. pap. 22.50 (0-8263-1230-6) U of NM Pr.
Community-Oriented Primary Care: Health Care for the 21st Century. Ed. by Robert RhyneRhyne et al. 1998. LC 98-74064. 228p. pap. 39.00 (0-87553-236-5) Am Pub Health.
Community Oriented Primary Care: Training for Urban Practice. Jo I. Boufford & Pat A. Shonubi. 1985. LC 85-6495. 187p. 45.00 (0-275-91307-4, C1307, Praeger Pubs) Greenwood.
Community Paediatrics. Ed. by L. Polnay & D. Hull. 2nd ed. 1993. (Illus.). 479p. pap. (0-443-04250-0) Church.
Community Participation in Health: The Politics of Primary Care in Costa Rica. Lynn M. Morgan. 1993. LC 92-9575. (Cambridge Studies in Medical Anthropology). (Illus.). 195p. (C). text 54.95 (0-521-41898-4) Cambridge U Pr.
Community Participation in Maternal & Child Health - Family Planning Programmes: An Analysis Based on Case Study Materials. Susan B. Rifkin. 1990. (CHI, ENG, FRE & SPA.). ix, 38p. pap. text 9.50 (92-4-156135-1, 1150338) World Health.
Community Prevention & Control of Cardiovascular Disease. 1986. (Technical Reports: No. 732). 62p. (Orig.). pap. text 9.00 (92-4-120732-9, 1100732) World Health.
Community Prevention Trials for Alcohol Problems: Methodological Issues. Ed. by Harold D. Holder & Jan M. Howard. 1992. LC 92-9804. 336p. 65.00 (0-275-94196-5, C4196, Praeger Pubs) Greenwood.
Community Programs for Mental Health: Theory, Practice, Evaluation. Ruth Kotinsky & Helen L. Witmer. 1955. LC 55-11030. (Commonwealth Fund Publications). 381p. 39.50 (0-674-15151-8) HUP.
Community Programs for the Depressed Elderly: A Rehabilitation Approach. Ed. by Ellen D. Taira. 1987. LC 86-31956. (Physical & Occupational Therapy in Geriatrics Ser.: Vol. 5, No. 1). 89p. text 29.95 (0-86656-644-9) Haworth Pr.
Community Programs for the Health- Impaired Elderly. Ed. by Ellen D. Taira. 1989. LC 88-2084. (Physical & Occupational Therapy in Geriatrics Ser.: Vol. 6, No. 1). (Illus.). 87p. text 29.95 (0-86656-760-7) Haworth Pr.
Community Psychiatric Nursing: A Research Perspective. Ed. by Charles Brooker. 1990. 320p. 40.50 (0-412-34790-3, A4880) Chapman & Hall.
Community Psychiatric Nursing: A Research Perspective, Vol. 2. Charles Brooker & Edward White. 1992. LC 92-49002. pap. 54.95 (1-56593-002-9, 0243) Thomson Learn.
Community Psychiatric Nursing, Vol. 2: A Research Perspective. Ed. by Charles Brooker & Edward White. 1992. LC 92-49002. (0-412-43600-0) Chapman & Hall.
Community Psychiatry in Action: Analysis & Prospects. Ed. by Peter Tyrer & Francis Creed. 1995. (Illus.). 175p. (C). text 54.95 (0-521-47427-2) Cambridge U Pr.
Community Psychology: Perspectives in Training & Research. Ed. by Ira Iscoe & Charles D. Spielberger. 1970. LC 76-102038. (Century Psychology Ser.). (C). 32.00 (0-89197-095-9) Irvington.
Community Psychology: Theory & Practice. Jim Orford. 1992. LC 91-30651. 302p. pap. 90.00 (0-471-93810-6) Wiley.
Community Psychology & Mental Health. Margaret S. Gibbs. 1992. pap. text 34.95 (0-89876-136-0) Gardner Pr.
Community Re-Entry for Head-Injured Adults. Ed. by Mark Ylvisaker & Eva M. Gobble. 1987. LC 90-21329. (Illus.). 444p. (C). text 40.00 (0-89079-337-9, 1574) PRO-ED.
Community Reinforcement Approach to Addiction Treatment. Ed. by Robert J. Meyers & William R. Miller. 2001. LC 00-46747. (International Research Monographs in the Addictions). (Illus.). 224p. (C). text 74.95 (0-521-77107-2) Cambridge U Pr.
Community Resources for the Older Adult. Ed. by Mildred O. Hogstel. 1998. LC 98-127838. (Illus.). 384p. spiral bd. 57.95 (0-8151-4493-8, 30689) Mosby Inc.
Community Response to AIDS: Report of the Dallas Aids Planning Commission. Dallas Aids Planning Commission Staff. Ed. by Halcyon Press Staff. 1988. (Illus.). 260p. (Orig.). pap. 7.00 (0-9621114-0-6) Halcyon TX.
Community Risk Profiles: A Tool to Improve Environment & Community Health. Iddo K. Wernick et al. 1995. (Illus.). 96p. (Orig.). (0-9646419-0-9) Prog Human Environ.
Community Substance Abuse Indicators Handbook. 1995. (Illus.). 86p. (Orig.). (C). pap. text 35.00 (0-7881-2447-1) DIANE Pub.
Community Support System for Mentally Handicapped Adults: An Alternative to Spatially Distributed Human Service Facilities. Amiram Gonen. 1977. (Discussion Papers: No. 96). pap. 10.00 (1-55869-014-X) Regional Sci Res Inst.
Community Surveys in Psychiatric Disorders. Ed. by Myrna M. Weissman et al. 1986. (Psychosocial Epidemiology Ser.: Vol. 4). (Illus.). 544p. (C). pap. text 25.00 (0-8135-1055-4) Rutgers U Pr.
Community Toxicity Testing, STP 920. John Cairns. 1986. LC 86-20568. (Special Technical Publications). (Illus.). 345p. text 48.00 (0-8031-0488-X, STP920) ASTM.
Community Wastewater Collection & Disposal. Daniel A. Okun & G. Ponghis. 1975. pap. text 37.80 (92-4-156045-2, 1150026) World Health.
Community Water Safety. American Red Cross Staff. (C). 1996. pap. text 10.00 (0-8151-0925-3); 1994. 96p. (gr. 13). pap. text 10.00 (0-8016-7550-2) Mosby Inc.
Community Water Supply: Proceedings of the WHO Expert Committee, Geneva, 1968. WHO Staff. 1969. (Technical Reports: No. 420). pap. text 3.00 (92-4-120420-6, 1100420) World Health.
Como Conocer y Resolver los Problemas Emocionales De Sus Hijos. Maria E. Del Real. 1990. (SPA., Illus.). 240p. (Orig.). pap. 3.50 (0-944499-47-3) Editorial Amer.
Como Convivir Con Su Artritis: Una Guia Para una Vida Activa y Saludable. Virginia M. Gonzalez et al. 2001. LC 96-49424.Tr. of Arthritis Helpbook. (SPA., Illus.). 324p. pap. 16.95 (0-923521-37-2) Bull Pub.
*Como Entender y Superar la Anorexia Nervosa. Lindsey Hall & Leigh Cohn. 2001.Tr. of Anorexia Nervosa: A Guide to Recovery. (SPA.). 192p. pap. 13.95 (0-936077-39-5) Gurze Bks.
Como Mejorar la Salud Con al Reflexologia. Mildred Carter & Tammy Weber. 2nd ed. 1997. LC 97-15496. (SPA., Illus.). 400p. (C). text 24.95 (0-13-858044-8) P-H.
Como Mejorar la Salud Con la Reflexologia. Mildred Carter. 2000. (SPA., Illus.). 383p. pap. 14.00 (0-7352-0192-7) PH Pr.
Como Mejorar la Salud Usando La Reflexologia. Mildred Carter & Tammy Weber. 2nd ed. 1997. LC 97-15496. (SPA., Illus.). 400p. pap. text 12.95 (0-13-848730-8) P-H.
Comorbidity & Developmental Neurocognitive Disorders. Ed. by Heikki Lyytinen. 1995. 104p. pap. 20.00 (0-8058-9941-3) L Erlbaum Assocs.
Comorbidity in Affective Disorders. Ed. by Mauricio Tohen. 1998. LC 98-45749. (Medical Psychiatry Ser.). (Illus.). 337p. text 145.00 (0-8247-0212-3) Dekker.
Comorbidity of Addictive & Psychiatric Disorders. Ed. by Barry Stimmel. 1993. LC 93-24682. (Journal of Addictive Diseases Ser.: Vol. 12, No. 3). (Illus.). 185p. lib. bdg. 49.95 (1-56024-457-7) Haworth Pr.
Comorbidity of Mood & Anxiety Disorders. Ed. by Jack D. Maser & C. Robert Cloninger. 1990. 867p. text 78.00 (0-88048-324-5, 8324) Am Psychiatric.
Comp Cancer Nursing Review. Susan L. Groenwald et al. 2nd ed. 1995. (Nursing Ser.). 680p. pap. 42.50 (0-86720-720-5) Jones & Bartlett.
Comp Obstetrics Review. Saade. 2000. text (0-323-00878-X) Mosby Inc.
Comp Package for Fundamentals of Nursing. Potter. 3rd ed. 1993. (0-8016-7299-6) Mosby Inc.
Comp Package of Rawlins Mental Health-Psychiatric. Ruth P. Rawlins. 3rd ed. 1993. (0-8016-7359-3) Mosby Inc.
Compact American Medical Dictionary: A Concise & Up-To-Date Guide to Medical Terms. Ed. by American Heritage Dictionary Editors. 1998. LC 98-20456. (Illus.). 506p. pap. text 12.00 (0-395-88409-8, AHD & Ref) HM.
Compact Encyclopedia of Psychological Problems. Clyde M. Narramore. 1984. LC 83-12265. 400p. 11.95 (0-310-29880-6, 12265) Zondervan.
Compact Euro-Woerterbuch/Medicine/Pharmacy: English, French, German, Italian, Spanish. Date not set. (ENG, FRE, GER, ITA & SPA.). 95.00 (0-7859-9592-7) Fr & Eur.
Compact Physician ICD9-CM, 1999-2000, Vol. 1-2. Medicode, Med-Index Division Staff. 1999. (C). pap. 48.00 (1-56337-313-0) Thomson Learn.
Companion Animal Death: A Practical & Comprehensive Guide for Veterinary Practice. Mary F. Stewart. 1999. LC 99-25565. 188p. pap. text 30.00 (0-7506-4076-6) Buttrwrth-Heinemann.

C D

Companion Animal Therapeutic Markets: Profiting from Human Pharmaceutical Research. Market Intelligence Staff. 1992. 276p. (Orig.). 1895.00 (*1-56753-381-7*) Frost & Sullivan.

Companion Animals in Human Health. Ed. by Cindy C. Wilson & Dennis C. Turner. 1997. LC 97-21077. 256p. 81.95 (*0-7619-1061-1*, 81487); pap. 39.95 (*0-7619-1062-X*, 81488) Sage.

Companion Encyclopedia of Psychology, Set. Ed. by Andrew M. Colman. 1994. LC 94-177554. (Companion Encyclopedia Ser.). 1356p. (C). 320.00 (*0-415-06446-5*) Routledge.

Companion Encyclopedia of the History of Medicine Ed. by W. F. Bynum & Roy Porter. 1997. (Routledge Companion Encyclopedias Ser.). (Illus.). 1864p. (C). pap. 120.00 (*0-415-16418-4*) Routledge.

Companion Encyclopedia of the History of Medicine Ed. by William F. Bynum & Roy Porter. LC 92-26013. (Companion Encyclopedia Ser.). 1. 1994. 1400p. (*0-415-09242-6*); 2. 1994. 1400p. (*0-415-09243-4*); Set. 1993. 1792p. (C). 305.00 (*0-415-04771-4*, B0377) Routledge.

Companion Guide to Infectious Diseases of Mice & Rats. National Research Council Staff. 1991. 108p. pap. text 16.00 (*0-309-04283-6*) Natl Acad Pr.

Companion Handbook. 13th ed. 1994. 79.95 (*1-56712-181-0*, F0301) Franklin Elect.

Companion Handbook of Pediatric Symptoms. Bruno Bissonnette & Bernard J. Dalens. 2001. (Illus.). 512p. Price not set. (*0-07-135455-7*) McGraw-Hill Med Pub.

Companion Handbook to the Chemotherapy Sourcebook. Michael C. Perry et al. 1998. LC 98-42010. 512p. pap. 49.95 (*0-683-30248-5*) Lppncott W & W.

Companion Manual to Ethical Practices in Pharmacy: A Guidebook for Pharmacy Technicians. Robert A. Buerki & Louis D. Vottero. 1997. 28p. pap. text, tchr. ed. 5.00 (*0-931292-29-8*) Am Inst Hist Pharm.

Companion to Bioethics. Peter Albert David Singer & Helga Kuhse. 1998. LC 97-50242. (Companions to Philosophy Ser.). 512p. 110.95 (*0-631-19737-0*) Blackwell Pubs.

Companion to Clinical Anaesthesia Exams. C. F. Corke & I. J. Jackson. 1994. LC 94-1429. text (*0-443-04962-9*) Church.

Companion to Clinical Neurology. William Pryce-Phillips. 1995. LC 94-19605. 1,024p. text 120.00 (*0-316-72041-0*, Little Brwn Med Div) Lppncott W & W.

Companion to Gynaecology. C. L. Huang & V. G. Daniels. 1985. text 132.00 (*0-85200-378-1*) Kluwer Academic.

Companion to Neonatal Medicine. Ed. by C. L. Huang & V. G. Daniels. 1982. (Companion Ser.). (Illus.). 120p. text 59.00 (*0-85200-380-3*) Kluwer Academic.

Companion to Pharmacology: A Study Guide for Self Assessment & Revision. M. M. Dale & A. H. Dickenson. 1993. LC 92-19270. (Illus.). 206p. pap. text (*0-443-04178-4*) Church.

Companion to Psychiatric Studies. Ed. by R. E. Kendell & A. K. Zealley. 5th ed. 1993. LC 92-49324. text (*0-443-04668-9*) Church.

Companion Volume to Dr. Jay A. Goldstein's Betrayal by the Brain: A Guide for Patients & Their Physicians. Katie Courmel & Jay A. Goldstein. 1996. LC 96-20456. 98p. pap. 14.95 (*0-7890-0119-5*) Haworth Pr.

Companionship Preference & Dominance in the Social Interaction of Young Chimpanzees. Vincent Nowlis. 1941. (Comparative Psychology Monographs). pap. 25.00 (*0-527-24920-3*) Periodicals Srv.

Company They Keep: Friendships in Childhood & Adolescence. Ed. by William M. Bukowski et al. 1998. (Cambridge Studies in Social & Emotional Development). (Illus.). 438p. (C). reprint ed. pap. text 24.95 (*0-521-62725-7*) Cambridge U Pr.

Comparability of Statistics of Causes of Death According to the Fifth & Sixth Revisions of the International List. 1952. pap. text 2.00 (*92-4-156007-X*, 1150023) World Health.

Comparability of the Birth Certificate & the 1988 National Maternal & Infant Health Survey Questionnaire. Kenneth C. Schoendorf et al. 1992. LC 92-49066. (Vital & Health Statistics Ser.: Series 2, No. 116). (*0-8406-0473-4*) Natl Ctr Health Stats.

Comparative Abdominal & Pelvic Anatomy by Computed Tomography & Ultrasound. Michael M. Raskin. 1979. 304p. 130.00 (*0-8493-5369-6*, RC944, CRC Reprint) Franklin.

Comparative Analysis of Amino-Acid Sequences of Key Enzymes of Replication & Expression of Positive-strand Rna Viruses, Vol. 11. A. Gorbalenya & Steven E. Koonin. 1993. (Soviet Scientific Reviews Series, Section D: Biology Reviews: Vol. 11, Pt. 3). 109p. pap. text 135.00 (*3-7186-5396-6*) Gordon & Breach.

Comparative Anatomy: Manual of Vertebrate Dissection. Dale W. Fishbeck & Aurora Sebastiani. 2000. (Illus.). 368p. (Orig.). (C). ring bd. 49.95 (*0-89582-517-1*) Morton Pub.

Comparative Anatomy of the Vertebrates. George C. Kent & Larry Miller. 8th ed. 1996. LC 96-86791. 528p. (C). text 57.00 net. (*0-697-24378-8*, WCB McGr Hill) McGrw-H Hghr Educ.

Comparative Animal Physiology. Philip C. Withers. 1992. LC 91-50762. 900p. (C). text 95.50 (*0-03-012847-1*) SCP.

Comparative Animal Physiology, Set. Ed. by C. Ladd Prosser. 4th ed. 1991. 1378p. 260.00 (*0-471-56093-6*) Wiley.

Comparative Animal Physiology: Environmental & Metabolic Animal Pysiology, Pt. A, Set. C. Ladd Prosser. 4th ed. 1991. LC 90-27165. (Comparative Animal Physiology Ser.: Vol. A). 592p. 195.00 (*0-471-85767-X*) Wiley.

Comparative Animal Physiology Pt. B: Neural & Integrative Animal Physiology, Vol. 2. Ed. by C. Ladd Prosser. 4th ed. 1991. LC 90-27164. 786p. 162.00 (*0-471-56071-5*) Wiley.

Comparative Approaches in Brief Dynamic Psychotherapy. Ed. by William Borden. 1999. LC 99-43056. (Psychoanalytic Social Work Monograph Ser.: Vol. 6, Nos. 3-4). 245p. (C). (Illus.). 49.95 (*0-7890-0833-5*); pap. text 24.95 (*0-7890-0844-0*) Haworth Pr.

Comparative Approaches in Medical Reasoning. Ed. by M. E. Cohen & D. L. Hudson. 1995. LC 94-48854. (Advances in Fuzzy Systems Ser.: Vol. 3). 328p. text 86.00 (*981-02-2162-2*) World Scientific Pub.

Comparative Aspects of Neuroendocrine Control of Behavior. Ed. by C. Valverde-Rodriguez & H. Arechiga. 1980. (Frontiers of Hormone Research Ser.: Vol. 6). (Illus.). 85.75 (*3-8055-0571-X*) S Karger.

Comparative Aspects of Neuropeptide Function. Ed. by Ernst Florey & George B. Stefano. 1992. LC 92-23207. (Studies in Neurosciences: No. 2). 362p. 193.00 (*0-08-041984-4*, Pergamon Pr) Elsevier.

Comparative Aspects of Nutritional & Metabolic Diseases. Ed. by James C. Woodard & Michael Bruss. 1983. 160p. 91.00 (*0-8493-5697-0*, RC620, CRC Reprint) Franklin.

Comparative Aspects of Tumor Development. Ed. by Hans E. Kaiser. 1988. (Cancer Growth & Progression Ser.). (C). text 211.50 (*0-89838-994-1*) Kluwer Academic.

Comparative Biochemistry of Parasitic Helminths. Ed. by Eva Bennett et al. 1989. 256p. 65.00 (*0-412-32730-9*) Chapman & Hall.

Comparative Biology of Cancer. Mulcahy. 1997. 240p. pap. 64.95 (*0-412-57160-9*) Chapman & Hall.

Comparative Biology of the Normal Lung, Vol. 1. Andre Parent. 1992. 848p. 195.00 (*0-8493-8839-2*, RC732) CRC Pr.

Comparative Brain Research in Mammals, Vol. 1: Insectivora. Heinz Stephan et al. 1991. (Illus.). 573p. 169.00 (*0-387-97505-5*) Spr-Verlag.

Comparative Carcinogenicity of Ionizing Radiation & Chemicals. 1989. LC 88-15200. (Report Ser.: No. 96). 179p. (Orig.). pap. text 40.00 (*0-913392-96-0*) NCRP Pubns.

Comparative Cardiovascular Dynamics of Mammals. John K. Li. 1995. LC 95-45491. 176p. 149.95 (*0-8493-0169-6*, 169) CRC Pr.

Comparative Coachability of Certain Types of Intelligence Tests. Hsuan-Shan Chen. (Columbia University. Teachers College. Contributions to Education Ser.: No. 338). reprint ed. 32.50 (*0-404-55338-9*) AMS Pr.

Comparative Development of Adaptive Skills: Evolutionary Implications. Ed. by Eugene S. Gollin. 1985. 288p. text 49.95 (*0-89859-519-3*) L Erlbaum Assocs.

Comparative Ecology of Gorilla & Pan Troglodytes in Rio Muni, West Africa. C. Jones & J. Sabater Pi. 1971. (Bibliotheca Primatologica Ser.: No. 13). pap. 21.75 (*3-8055-0293-1*) S Karger.

Comparative Endocrinology of Calcium Regulations. C. Dacke et al. 1996. 238p. 89.95 (*1-898099-08-1*) Blackwell Sci.

Comparative Health Systems: Descriptive Analyses of Fourteen National Health Systems. Ed. by Marshall M. Raffel. 1984. LC 83-43032. (Illus.). 480p. 49.50 (*0-271-00363-4*) Pa St U Pr.

Comparative Health Systems No. 1: The Future of National Health Care Systems & Economic Analysis. Ed. by Richard M. Scheffler et al. 1990. (Advances in Health Economics & Health Services Research Ser.). 256p. suppl. ed. 73.25 (*1-55938-006-3*) Jai Pr.

Comparative Immunology: Proceedings of the Verona Workshop, 16-17 July 1980, Verona, Italy. Ed. by L. S. Azzolina. 1982. (Illus.). 180p. pap. 45.00 (*0-08-028019-6*, Pergamon Pr) Elsevier.

Comparative Leukemia Research, 1969: Proceedings of the International Symposium, 4th, Cherry Hill, New Jersey, 1969. International Symposium on Comparative Leukemia Research Staff. Ed. by R. M. Dutcher. 1971. (Bibliotheca Haemotologica Ser.: No. 36). 135.75 (*3-8055-1160-4*) S Karger.

Comparative Leukemia Research, 1975: Proceedings of the Symposium, 7th International, Copenhagen, October 1975. Comparative Leukemia Research Symposium Staff. Ed. by J. Clemmesen et al. 1976. (Bibliotheca Haemotologica Ser.: Vol. 43). (Illus.). 600p. 185.25 (*3-8055-2316-5*) S Karger.

Comparative Mental Health: From Institutional to Community Care. Simon Goodwin. 1997. LC 97-217907. 183p. 69.95 (*0-8039-7728-X*, 81983); pap. 27.95 (*0-8039-7729-8*, 81984) Sage.

Comparative Methods in Psychology. Ed. by Marc H. Bornstein. 1980. LC 79-27558. (Crosscurrents in Contemporary Psychology Ser.). (Illus.). 320p. text 69.95 (*0-89859-037-X*) L Erlbaum Assocs.

Comparative Morphology of the Inner Ear in Salamanders: Caudata-Amphibia. R. E. Lombard. 1977. (Contributions to Vertebrate Evolution Ser.: Vol. 2). 65.25 (*3-8055-2408-0*) S Karger.

Comparative Musculoskeletal Examination. Ed. by George H. Thompson. 1998. (Illus.). 304p. text (*0-443-08787-3*) Church.

Comparative Neurobiology: Problems for a New Decade: 1st Annual Karger Workshop - Journal: Brain, Behavior & Evolution, Vol. 36, Nos. 2 & 3, 1990. Ed. by R. G. Northcutt. 1990. 104p. pap. 130.50 (*3-8055-5319-6*) S Karger.

Comparative Neurology of the Optic Tectum. Ed. by Horacio Vanegas. 1984. LC 84-3372. 870p. 145.00 (*0-306-41236-5*, Plenum Trade) Perseus Pubng.

Comparative Overview of Mammalian Fertilization. Bonnie S. Dunbar & M. G. O'Rand. 1991. (Illus.). 480p. (C). text 115.00 (*0-306-43841-0*, Kluwer Plenum) Kluwer Academic.

Comparative Pathobiology of Viral Diseases. Ed. by Richard G. Olsen et al. 1985. 232p. 134.00 (*0-8493-5946-5*, SF780); 130.00 (*0-8493-5945-7*, SF780) Franklin (CRC Reprint).

Comparative Pathology of the Heart: Proceedings of the Symposium, Boston, Sept. 1973. Comparative Pathology of the Heart Symposium Staff. Ed. by F. Homburger & I. Lucas. 1974. (Advances in Cardiology Ser.: Vol. 13). 250p. 226.25 (*3-8055-1697-5*) S Karger.

Comparative Pathology of Zoo Animals. Ed. by Richard J. Montali & George Migaki. 1980. LC 79-24354. (Research Symposia of the National Zoological Park Ser.: No. 6). (Illus.). 684p. pap. text 29.95 (*0-87474-643-4*, MOCCP) Smithsonian.

Comparative Pathophysiology of Regulatory Reptides. Ed. by Adam Rijnberk & Wimersma Greidanus. 1987. (Frontiers of Hormone Research Ser.: Vol. 17). (Illus.). viii, 236p. 185.25 (*3-8055-4621-1*) S Karger.

Comparative Performance of U. S. Hospitals: The Sourcebook, 1997. 1996. pap. 399.00 (*1-57372-064-X*) Solucient.

Comparative Performance of U. S. Hospitals: The Sourcebook, 1998. 1997. pap. 399.00 (*1-57372-102-6*) Solucient.

Comparative Perinatal & Pediatric Respiratory Care. Whitaker. 2nd ed. 1996. (Respiratory Care Ser.). lab manual ed. 15.50 (*0-8273-7393-7*) Delmar.

Comparative Perspectives on the Development of Memory. Ed. by Robert V. Kail, Jr. & Norman E. Spear. 1984. 384p. text 89.95 (*0-89859-317-4*) L Erlbaum Assocs.

Comparative Pharmacokinetics: Principles, Techniques & Applications. Jim Riviere. 1999. LC 98-31926. (Illus.). 338p. text 94.95 (*0-8138-2931-3*) Iowa U Pr.

Comparative Pharmacology, Set. Ed. by M. J. Michelson. 1973. 1008p. (C). (*0-08-016389-0*) Pergamon Repr GBR. *Dist:* Franklin.

Comparative Physical Biology. N. R. Joseph. 1973. (Illus.). 260p. 75.75 (*3-8055-1485-9*) S Karger.

Comparative Physiology of Environmental Adaptations, Set, Vols. 1-3. 1987. (Illus.). xx, 580p. 417.50 (*3-8055-4473-1*) S Karger.

Comparative Physiology of Regulatory Peptides. Ed. by Susanne Holmgren. 1989. 360p. 85.00 (*0-412-32740-6*, A3703) Chapman & Hall.

Comparative Physiology of Temperature Regulation in Laboratory Rodents. Christopher J. Gordon. 1993. (Illus.). 292p. (C). text 80.00 (*0-521-41426-1*) Cambridge U Pr.

Comparative Physiology of the Brain & Comparative Psychology. Jacques Loeb. 1978. LC 73-2973. (Classics in Psychology Ser.). reprint ed. 26.95 (*0-405-05146-8*) Ayer.

Comparative Psychology & Hygiene of the Overweight Child. Kathryn McHale. LC 72-177027. (Columbia University. Teachers College. Contributions to Education Ser.: No. 221). reprint ed. 37.50 (*0-404-55221-8*) AMS Pr.

Comparative Psychology of Audition: Perceiving Complex Sounds. Ed. by R. J. Dooling & S. H. Hulse. 1989. 496p. 99.95 (*0-8058-0020-4*); pap. 55.00 (*0-8058-0384-X*) L Erlbaum Assocs.

Comparative Psychology of Mental Development. Heinz Werner. 1970. 564p. pap. 24.95 (*0-8236-8024-X*, 021020) Intl Univs Pr.

Comparative Records for Health Information Management. Peden. 1998. (Home Care Aide Ser.). tchr. ed. 14.00 (*0-8273-7521-2*) Delmar.

Comparative Records for Health Information Management. Ann Peden. 1997. LC 97-28555. (Health Services Administration Ser.). 512p. (C). pap. text 55.95 (*0-8273-7520-4*) Delmar.

Comparative Renal Handling of Solutes & Water. Ed. by William H. Dantzler. 1985. (Journal: Vol. 8, No. 4-5, 1985). (Illus.). 112p. pap. 54.00 (*3-8055-4147-3*) S Karger.

Comparative Respiratory Tract Carcinogenesis Hildegard M. Reznik-Schuller. 1983. 272p. 148.00 (*0-8493-5421-8*, RC280); 224p. 128.00 (*0-8493-5422-6*, RC280) Franklin (CRC Reprint).

Comparative Socioecology. Ed. by Valerie Standen & R. A. Foley. 1989. (Special Publication of the British Ecological Society Ser.: No. 8). (Illus.). 528p. (C). text 110.00 (*0-632-02361-9*) Blackwell Sci.

Comparative Studies in Hypertension: Journal: Nephron, Vol. 47, suppl. 1. Ed. by J. Ian Robertson et al. 1987. (Illus.). vi, 152p. pap. 48.00 (*3-8055-4710-2*) S Karger.

Comparative Studies of American & African Trypanosomiasis: Proceedings of the WHO Scientific Group, Washington, 1967. WHO Staff. 1969. (Technical Reports: No. 411). pap. text 5.00 (*92-4-120411-7*, 1100411) World Health.

Comparative Studies of Hearing in Invertebrates. Ed. by Arthur N. Popper & Richard R. Fay. 1980. (Proceedings in Life Sciences Ser.). (Illus.). 457p. 175.00 (*0-387-90460-3*) Spr-Verlag.

Comparative Study of Ayurveda & Treatment by Indian Drugs. P. K. Chitale. 1998. (C). (*81-7030-555-1*) Sri Satguru Pubns IND. *Dist:* S Asia.

Comparative Study of Responses of Children of Different Nationalities & Environments on Intelligence & Achievement Tests. Adelin Scott. LC 73-177807. (Columbia University. Teachers College. Contributions to Education Ser.: No. 367). reprint ed. 37.50 (*0-404-55367-2*) AMS Pr.

Comparative Study of the Organisation & Functioning of Emergency Medical Assistance Services. Council of Europe Staff. 1990. (*92-871-1727-6*) Council of Europe FRA. *Dist:* Manhattan Pub Co.

Comparative Study of the Organization & Performance of Hospital Emergency Services. Basil S. Georgopoulos & Robert A. Cooke. 1980. 512p. (Orig.). pap. 20.00 (*0-87944-253-0*) Inst Soc Res.

Comparative Treatments for Relationship Dysfunction. Frank M. Dattilio & Louis Bevilacqua. 2000. LC 99-88867. (Series on Comparative Treatments for Psychological Disorders). (Illus.). xvii, 414p. text 43.95 (*0-8261-1324-9*) Springer Pub.

Comparative Treatments of Eating Disorders. Katherine J. Miller & J. Scott Mizes. 2000. LC 00-27400. (Springer Series on Comparative Treatments for Psychological Disorders). xxi, 365p. (*0-8261-1358-3*) Springer Pub.

Comparative Ultrsonographic Imaging of Equine Lameness. K. J. Dik. 1997. (Illus.). 116p. text (*3-87706-523-6*) Schlutersche Verlags DEU. *Dist:* Iowa U Pr.

Compare Ultrastructural Path: Selected Tumors in Man & Animals. Hildegard M. Reznick-Schuller. 1989. 208p. 179.00 (*0-8493-5662-8*, RC269) CRC Pr.

Comparing Behavior: Studying Man Studying Animals. D. W. Rajecki. 1983. 304p. (C). 69.95 (*0-89859-259-3*) L Erlbaum Assocs.

Comparing Psychoanalytic Psychotherapies: Developmental, Self, & Object Relations; Self Psychology; Short-Term Dynamic. James F. Masterson et al. 1991. LC 91-8288. 312p. text 39.95 (*0-87630-640-7*) Brunner-Routledge.

Comparing Theories of Child Development. R. Murray Thomas. 4th ed. 1995. LC 95-15016. 592p. mass mkt. 47.25 (*0-534-33903-4*) Brooks-Cole.

Comparing Theories of Child Development. R. Murray Thomas. 3rd ed. 1991. 575p. (C). mass mkt. 42.75 (*0-534-16302-5*) Wadsworth Pub.

Comparison & Harmonization of Denominator Data for Primary Health Care Research: The European Denominator Project. Ed. by Martin Schlaud. 1999. LC 99-64856. (Biomedical & Health Research Ser.: Vol. 35). (Illus.). 129p. 71.00 (*0-9673355-2-3*) IOS Press.

Comparison of an Eight-Hour Plant & a Ten-Hour Plant: U. S. Public Health Bulletin, No. 106. Josephine Goldmark & Mary D. Hopkins. Ed. by Leon Stein. 1977. LC 77-70495. reprint ed. lib. bdg. 23.95 (*0-405-10168-6*) Ayer.

Comparison of Brain-Injured & Non-Brain-Injured Mentally Retarded Children on Several Psychological Variables. J. J. Gallagher. 1957. (SRCD M Ser.: Vol. 22, No. 2). pap. 25.00 (*0-527-01570-9*) Periodicals Srv.

Comparison of Probabilistic Unfolding Theories for Paired Comparisons Data. P. Bossuyt. 1990. (Recent Research in Psychology Ser.). 186p. 28.00 (*0-387-52491-6*) Spr-Verlag.

Comparison of the Intellectual & Educational Status of Neurotic & Normal Children in Public Schools. Esther K. Rosen. LC 78-177208. (Columbia University. Teachers College. Contributions to Education Ser.: No. 188). reprint ed. 37.50 (*0-404-55188-2*) AMS Pr.

Comparison of Urinalysis Technologies for Drug Testing in Criminal Justice. Christy Visher. 1995. (Illus.). 44p. (Orig.). (C). pap. text 30.00 (*0-7881-2097-2*) DIANE Pub.

Comparisons in Human Development: Understanding Time & Context. Ed. by Jonathan Tudge et al. 1996. (Cambridge Studies in Social & Emotional Development). (Illus.). 377p. (C). text 49.95 (*0-521-48202-X*) Cambridge U Pr.

Compartmental Analysis. Ed. by F. Kajiya et al. 1985. x, 190p. 115.00 (*3-8055-3696-8*) S Karger.

Compartmental Distribution of Radiotracers. Ed. by James S. Robertson. 1983. 208p. 118.00 (*0-8493-6010-2*, R895, CRC Reprint) Franklin.

Compartments, Pools & Spaces in Medical Physiology: Proceedings. Ed. by Erik E. Bergner et al. 1967. LC 67-61865. (AEC Symposium Ser.). 600p. pap. 21.00 (*0-87079-167-2*, CONF-661010); fiche 9.00 (*0-87079-168-0*, CONF-661010) DOE.

Compass Vol. 1: Your Roadmap Through Menopause. Ranny Riley & Linda Bark. Ed. by Tracy A. Howard. 1998. (Illus.). 136p. pap. 29.95 (*0-9666839-4-3*) Lifeline Inst.

Compass of Health: Using the Ancient Art of Sasang Medicine to Maximize Your Health. Kihyon Kim. 2001. LC 00-54889. (Illus.). 255p. pap. 14.99 (*1-56414-559-X*, New Page Bks) Career Pr Inc.

Compass of the Heart: Embodying Medicine Wheel Teachings. Loren Cruden. 1996. LC 95-48807. 192p. pap. 14.95 (*0-89281-600-7*, Destiny Bks) Inner Tradit.

Compassion: The Core Value That Animates Psychotherapy. Roger A. Lewin. 1996. LC 95-23012. 360p. 50.00 (*1-56821-678-5*) Aronson.

Compassion Fatigue: Coping with Secondary Traumatic Stress Disorder in Those Who Treat the Traumatized. Ed. by Charles R. Figley. 1995. LC 94-49230. (Psychosocial Stress Ser.: No. 23). 296p. text 37.95 (*0-87630-759-4*) Brunner-Routledge.

Compassionate Care, Practical Love for Your Aging Parents. Marilyn Fanning. 1994. LC 94-173392. 196p. reprint ed. pap. 5.50 (*1-56616-003-0*, 535013) Aglow Communs.

Compassionate Living for Personal Healing. Joanne Stepaniak. 2001. LC 00-67854. 192p. pap. 11.95 (*0-658-01088-3*) McGraw-Hill Prof.

Compassionate Therapy: Working with Difficult Clients. Jeffrey A. Kottler. 1992. LC 91-30554. (Jossey-Bass Social & Behavioral Science Ser.). 272p. 35.00 (*1-55542-422-8*) Jossey-Bass.

Compassionate Touch: Hands-On Caregiving for the Elderly, the Ill & the Dying. Dawn Nelson. 1993. LC 93-48423. 160p. pap. 17.95 (*0-88268-149-4*) Station Hill Pr.

***Compassion's Way: A Doctor's Quest into the Soul of Medicine.** Ralph Crawshaw. 2002. LC 2001-44469. (*0-936741-15-5*) Medi-Ed Pr.

Compatible & Incompatible Relationships. Ed. by W. Ickes. 1985. (Social Psychology Ser.). (Illus.). 615p. 71.95 (*0-387-96024-4*) Spr-Verlag.

Compelled Compassion: Government Intervention in the Treatment of Critically Ill Newborns. Ed. by Arthur L. Caplan et al. 1992. LC 91-44190. (Contemporary Issues in Biomedicine, Ethics & Society Ser.). 352p. 59.50 (*0-89603-224-8*) Humana.

Compend of the Principles of Homeopathy. William Boericke. 1996. 160p. reprint ed. spiral bd. 14.00 (*0-7873-0114-0*) Hlth Research.

Compendio de Anatomia Descriptiva. J. A. Fort. (SPA.). 546p. pap. 19.95 (*0-7859-0869-2*, S-50272) Fr & Eur.

Compendio de la Humana Salud: Biblioteca Nacional, Madrid I-51. Ed. by Maria T. Herrera. 1987. (Medieval Spanish Medical Texts Ser.: No. 9). (SPA.). 4p. 10.00 incl. fiche (*0-940639-05-X*) Hispanic Seminary.

Compendio de Medicina, Biblioteca Universitaria, Salamanca, 2262. Gomez De Salamanca. Ed. by M. Jesus Mancho. 1987. (Medieval Spanish Medical Texts Ser.: No. 12). (SPA.). 8p. 10.00 incl. fiche (*0-940639-08-4*) Hispanic Seminary.

Compendium for the Study of Christian Science No. 4: Mind Max Kappeler. 1951.Tr. of Leitfaden fur das Studium der Christlichen Wissenschaft, Gemut. 36p. 4.50 (*0-85241-058-1*) Kappeler Inst Pub.

Compendium of Abnormal Psychology. Henry H. Reiter. 2nd ed. 1980. 110p. pap. text 5.00 (*0-9606044-0-5*) Psychometric.

Compendium of Beet Diseases & Insects. Ed. by E. D. Whitney & J. E. Duffus. 1986. LC 86-71222. (Compendium of Plant Disease Ser.). 116p. 49.00 (*0-89054-070-5*) Am Phytopathol Soc.

Compendium of Bone Pathology. Jasvir S. Khurana et al. 1999. (Illus.). v, 276p. (*1-893941-00-0*) United Path Pr.

Compendium of Dr. Vodder's Manual Lymph Drainage. Renato Kasseroller. Ed. by Kathryn McKillip Thrift. Tr. by David M. Fogg. 1998. (Illus.). 211p. (C). text (*3-7760-1729-5*) K F Haug Pubs DEU. *Dist:* Medicina Bio.

Compendium of Facilities for Drugs of Abuse Testing & General Analytical Toxic Eur 15980 (Health & Safety) R. Zeeuw et al. 1995. 608p. pap. text (*92-826-9127-6*) Comm Europ Commun BEL. *Dist:* Bernan Associates.

Compendium of Informal Antitrust Enforcement Agency Advice in Health Care. 1991. LC 91-55451. 188p. pap. 50.00 (*0-89707-688-5*, 503-0207, ABA Antitrust) Amer Bar Assn.

Compendium of International AIDS Programs & Policies. George M. Worthington. 1989. 310p. (C). 29.50 (*0-9623474-2-6*) G M Worthington.

Compendium of Methods for the Microbiological Examination of Foods. Ed. by Carl Vanderzant & Don Splittstoesser. 3rd ed. 1992. 1264p. 90.00 (*0-87553-173-3*, 032) Am Pub Health.

Compendium of Neuropsychological Tests: Adminstration, Norms & Commentary. Otfried Spreen & Esther Strauss. 2nd ed. 1998. LC 96-34724. (Illus.). 752p. text 68.50 (*0-19-510019-0*) OUP.

Compendium of Oriental Healing. W. Craig Dodd. 1997. LC 97-171680. (Gift of Health Ser.). (Illus.). 96p. pap. text (*1-85368-669-7*) New Holland Pubs GBR. *Dist:* Sterling.

Compendium of Postpartum Care. Ed. by Patricia O. Beachy et al. 1996. (Illus.). 150p. pap., wbk. ed. (*0-931562-18-X*) J & J Consumer Prods.

Compendium of Quality of Life Instruments, Set. Ed. by Sam Salek. 1999. LC 97-42714. 1626p. pap. text 1495.00 incl. cd-rom (*0-471-98145-1*) Wiley.

Compendium of Terminology & Nomenclature of Properties in Clinical Laboratory Sciences: The Silver Book. J. C. Rigg et al. 1995. LC 95-19173. 304p. pap. 28.50 (*0-86542-612-0*) Blackwell Sci.

Compendium of Turfgrass Diseases. Richard W. Smiley et al. 2nd ed. 1992. LC 91-77313. (Compendium of Plant Disease Ser.). (Illus.). 128p. pap. 49.00 (*0-89054-124-8*) Am Phytopathol Soc.

Compendium of Veterinary Products. Ed. by Aurora Arrioja-Dechert. 4th ed. 1997. 1452p. pap. 85.00 (*1-889750-00-X*) Nrth Amer Compendiums.

Compensating Key Personnel in the Health Care Industry. Jay R. Schuster. 1985. LC 85-14166. 176p. text 24.95 (*0-88331-121-6*) R B Luce.

Compensation for Personal Injury in Sweden & 17 Other Countries. Ed. by Carl Oldertz & Eva Tidefelt. 1988. 408p. 87.50 (*91-7598-197-1*) Coronet Bks.

Compensation for Psychological Deficits & Declines: Managing Losses & Promoting Gains. Ed. by Roger A. Dixon & Lars Backman. 1995. 360p. text 59.95 (*0-8058-1559-7*) L Erlbaum Assocs.

Compensation Report on Management Employees in Hospital & Nursing Home Management Companies 1989. Zabka, John R., Associates Inc. Staff. 1989. 50p. pap. 250.00 (*0-939326-58-2*) Hosp & Hlthcare.

Compensation Report on Management Employees in Hospital & Nursing Home Management Companies, 1993. pap. 250.00 (*0-939326-74-4*) Hosp & Hlthcare.

Competence Assessment Tools for Health-System Pharmacies. Lee B. Murdaugh. 1998. 346p. spiral bd. 249.00 (*1-879907-85-2*) Am Soc Hlth-Syst.

Competence, Courage, & Change: An Approach to Family Therapy. David B. Waters & Edith C. Lawrence. 1993. LC 93-718. 180p. (C). 22.95 (*0-393-70139-5*) Norton.

Competence to Consent. Becky C. White. 1994. LC 94-9917. (Clinical Medical Ethics Ser.: No. 1). 240p. 45.00 (*0-87840-559-3*); pap. 17.95 (*0-87840-560-7*) Georgetown U Pr.

Competences Avancees en Formation pour les Professionnels en Sante de la Reproduction. Lois Schaefer et al. 2000.Tr. of Advanced Training Skills for Reproductive Health Professionals. (FRE., Illus.). 235p. pap. text 15.00 (*0-929817-73-7*) JHPIEGO.

Competences en Conception de Programmes Pedagogiques pour les Professionnels en Sante de la Reproduction. Rick Sullivan & Lynne Gaffikin. Ed. by Ann Blouse & Dana Lewison. 1998.Tr. of Instructional Design Skills for Reproductive Health Professionals. (FRE., Illus.). 220p. pap. text 15.00 (*0-929817-50-8*) JHPIEGO.

Competences en Formation Clinique pour les Professionnels en Sante de la Reproduction. Rick Sullivan et al. 2nd ed. 1999.Tr. of Clinical Training Skills for Reproductive Health Professionals. (FRE., Illus.). 270p. pap. text 15.00 (*0-929817-70-2*) JHPIEGO.

Competences en Formation Clinique pour les Professionnels en Sante de la Reproduction. Rick Sullivan et al. 1996. (FRE.). pap. text 15.00 (*0-929817-26-5*) JHPIEGO.

Competencies & Issues in Community Health Nursing. Schroeder. 1993. text (*0-397-54698-X*) Lppncott W & W.

Competencies of the Associate Degree Nurse: Valid Definers of Entry-Level Practice. Verle Waters & Sharlene Limon. 1987. (Orig.). pap. 12.95 (*0-88737-342-9*, 23-2172) Natl League Nurse.

Competency: A Study of Informal Competency Determinations in Primary Care. Ed. by Mary A. Cutter & Earl E. Shelp. 1991. (Philosophy & Medicine Ser.). 308p. lib. bdg. (*0-7923-1304-6*) Kluwer Academic NLD. *Dist:* Kluwer Academic.

Competency Assessment: Allied Health. American Society for Healthcare Education and Training Staff. Ed. by Francis L. Ulschak & Barbara A. Hayman. 1994. (Illus.). 208p. (Orig.). pap. 125.00 (*0-87258-661-8*, 049855) Am Hospital.

Competency Assessment: Challenges & Opportunities for Health Care Educators. American Society for Healthcare Education and Training Staff. 1992. 258p. (Orig.). pap. 130.00 (*0-87258-582-4*, 049906) Am Hospital.

Competency-Based Curriculum Development in Medical Education: An Introduction. W. McGaghie et al. 1978. (Public Health Papers: No. 68). 91p. pap. text 9.00 (*92-4-130068-X*, 1110068) World Health.

Competency-Based Education & Training in Psychology: A Primer. Scott Sumerall & Shane J. Lopez. Ed. by Mary E. Oehlert. 2000. LC 99-57927. xi, 118p. 19.95 (*0-398-07041-5*) C C Thomas.

Competency Based Orientation Manual for Hemodialysis Nursing. Roberta A. Stokes. 1991. 70p. pap. (*0-08-040696-3*) PPI GBR. *Dist:* McGraw.

Competency-Based Rad Tech Workbook. Mary Anne Kiser. 1991. 422p. pap. text 28.95 (*0-7216-3972-0*) Saunders.

Competency Exam Preparation & Review for Nursing Assistant. Barbara Kast & Barbara Acello. 2nd ed. 1996. LC 96-26238. (Illus.). 352p. (C). pap. text 36.95 (*0-8273-7996-X*) Delmar.

Competency Exam Preparation & Review for Nursing Assistants. Barbara Kast. 3rd ed. 2000. (Illus.). 400p. pap. text 36.95 (*0-7668-1429-7*) Delmar.

Competency Exam Preparation for Nurse Assistant. Barbara Kast. (Home Care Aide Ser.). 1990. 20.95 (*0-8273-4139-3*); 1989. pap., tchr. ed. 12.75 (*0-8273-4140-7*) Delmar.

Competency Exam Preparation Review for the Nursing Assistant. Barbara Kast. 2nd ed. 1997. (C). pap. text, tchr. ed. 13.00 (*0-8273-7997-8*) Delmar.

Competency in Home Care. Tarasa M. Astaritta et al. 1998. LC 98-15036. 288p. pap. 61.00 (*0-8342-1050-9*, 10509) Aspen Pub.

Competency Manual: Radiographic Anatomy & Positioning. Andrea G. Cornuelle. 1997. 200p. (C). pap. 29.95 (*0-8385-8239-7*, A-8239-4) McGraw-Hill Prof.

Competency Skills for the Dental Assistant. Charline M. Dofka. 1995. LC 94-24642. (Health & Life Science Ser.). (Illus.). 576p. (C). pap. text 43.95 (*0-8273-6685-X*) Delmar.

Competency to Stand Trial Evaluations: A Manual for Practice. Thomas Grisso. 1988. LC 88-42897. 136p. pap. 21.45 (*0-943158-51-6*, CSTBP, Prof Resc Pr) Pro Resource.

Competing Realities: Issues in Mental Health Advocacy. Susan M. Chandler. 1990. LC 89-22815. 208p. 60.00 (*0-275-93356-3*, C3356, Greenwood Pr) Greenwood.

Competing Solutions: American Health Care Proposals & International Experience. Joseph White. 1995. LC 95-7675. 392p. (C). text 44.95 (*0-8157-9364-2*); pap. text 19.95 (*0-8157-9363-4*) Brookings.

Competition & Efficiency in Education & Health: The Professional's Response. Mike Bottery. 1998. LC 99-231564. ix, 181p. 89.50 (*0-304-70156-4*); pap. 32.50 (*0-304-70157-2*) Continuum.

Competition & Monopoly in Medical Care. H. E. Frech, III. 1996. LC 96-11636. 200p. 37.95 (*0-8447-3884-0*) Am Enterprise.

Competition & Planning in the NHS: The Danger of Unplanned Markets. C. R. Paton. 1992. 174p. pap. 57.50 (*1-56593-058-4*, 0364) Singular Publishing.

Competition in the Health Care Sector: Ten Years Later. Ed. by Warren Greenberg. 1988. LC 88-21920. 153p. text 32.95 (*0-8223-0893-2*) Duke.

Competition in the Provision of Health Care. Allan Bruce & Ernest Jonsson. 1996. LC 96-85813. 212p. text (*1-85742-305-4*) Arena GBR. *Dist:* Ashgate Pub Co.

Competitive Advantage through Diversity: Organizational Learning from Difference. Peter Herriot & Carole Pemberton. 1994. 272p. 74.50 (*0-8039-8884-2*, 9487) Sage.

Competitive Approaches to Health Care Reform. Ed. by Richard J. Arnould et al. 1993. LC 93-1603. 384p. pap. text 36.00 (*0-87766-604-0*) Urban Inst.

Competitive Edge for Audiologists Negotiating with Managed Care Organizations. Ann C. Napp & Kenneth E. Wolf. 1997. LC 98-176669. 38.00 incl. audio (*1-58041-005-7*, 0112072) Am Speech Lang Hearing.

Competitive Ethos & Democratic Education. John G. Nicholls. 1989. LC 88-16303. (Illus.). 280p. 51.95 (*0-674-15417-7*) HUP.

Competitive Health Care in Europe: Future Prospects. A. F. Casparie et al. 1990. 429p. text (*1-85521-186-6*) Dartmth Pub GBR. *Dist:* Ashgate Pub Co.

Competitive Managed Care: The Emerging Health Care System. John D. Wilkerson et al. 1996. LC 96-24679. (Jossey-Bass Health Ser.). 405p. 45.00 (*0-7879-0309-4*) Jossey-Bass.

Competitive Market Strategies in Healthcare: Meeting the Marketing Challenges in an Integrated Delivery System. Terrence J. Rynne. 1995. 225p. (C). text 45.00 (*1-55738-635-8*, Irwn Prfssnl) McGraw-Hill Educ Grp.

Competitive Pricing for Medicare. Bryan E. Dowd et al. 1996. 180p. pap. 9.95 (*0-8447-7034-5*) Am Enterprise.

Competitive Status of the U. S. Pharmaceutical Industry. National Academy of Engineering Staff. 1983. LC 83-50568. 102p. pap. text 12.95 (*0-309-03396-9*) Natl Acad Pr.

Competitive Strategies in the Pharmaceutical Industry. Robert B. Helms. 1996. LC 95-18401. 200p. 35.95 (*0-8447-3882-4*) Am Enterprise.

Compilation of Odor & Taste Threshold Values Data-DS 48A: Compilations Parens. 1978. 508p. 55.00 (*0-8031-0306-9*, DS48A) ASTM.

Compilation of Principles & Practices Board Statements, Nos. 1-13. HFMA P and P Board Staff. 1991. 99p. 15.00 (*0-930228-56-1*) Hlthcare Fin Mgmt.

Compilation on Sex. Alice A. Bailey. 1980. pap. 10.00 (*0-85330-136-0*) Lucis.

Complaint Behavior: Beyond Obedience to Authority. Ed. by Max Rosenbaum. 1983. 254p. 35.95 (*0-89885-115-7*, Kluwer Acad Hman Sci) Kluwer Academic.

Complaint Handling: Worldwide Regulations for Healthcare Manufacturers. Ed. by Amy Davis & Michael H. Anisfeld. 1996. LC 97-143866. 66p. pap. 119.00 (*1-57491-033-7*) IHS Health Grp.

Complaints & Disorders: The Sexual Politics of Sickness. Barbara Ehrenreich & Deirdre English. 1973. LC 73-18356. (Glass Mountain Pamphlet Ser.: Vol. 2). (Illus.). 96p. pap. 6.95 (*0-912670-20-7*) Feminist Pr.

Complaints & Grievances in Psychotherapy: A Handbook of Ethical Practice. Fiona Palmer Barnes. 1998. LC 98-18079. 208p. (C). 78.95 (*0-415-15250-X*); pap. 26.95 (*0-415-15251-8*) Routledge.

Compleat Cardiologist: Heart Attack Handbook. Mark Lambert. 1997. 200p. pap. 21.95 (*0-9641170-0-2*) Gosport Pubng.

Complement. Ed. by H. J. Muller-Eberhard & Peter A. Miescher. 1985. (Illus.). 474p. 111.00 (*0-387-15075-7*) Spr-Verlag.

Complement: Clinical Aspects & Relevance to Disease. Paul Morgan. 1991. 215p. text 62.00 (*0-12-506955-3*) Acad Pr.

Complement & Infectious Diseases. Ed. by Douglas P. Fine. 1981. 176p. 100.00 (*0-8493-6075-7*, RC112, CRC Reprint) Franklin.

Complement in Health & Disease. Ed. by K. Whaley. (Immunology & Medicine Ser.). 1987. text 195.50 (*0-85200-954-2*); 2nd ed. 1993. 400p. (C). text 155.50 (*0-7923-8823-2*) Kluwer Academic.

Complement in Human Disease, Third European Meeting, Bratislava, Abstracts, September 1990: Journal: Complement & Inflammation, Vol. 7, No. 3. Ed. by Z. Starsia & U. E. Nydegger. 1990. 60p. pap. 37.50 (*3-8055-5282-3*) S Karger.

Complement in Laboratory Medicine. Ed. by A. P. Dalmasso. 1988. (Journal: Vol. 6, No. 1, 1989). (Illus.). 72p. pap. 51.50 (*3-8055-4914-8*) S Karger.

Complement Methods & Protocols. Ed. by B. Paul Morgan. 2000. LC 99-58849. (Methods in Molecular Biology Ser.: Vol. 150). (Illus.). ix, 268p. 89.50 (*0-89603-654-5*) Humana.

Complement System. D. R. Schultz. 1971. (Monographs in Allergy: Vol. 6). 38.00 (*3-8055-1086-1*) S Karger.

Complement System. K. Rother et al. 2nd rev. ed. 1997. LC 97-1035. (Illus.). 564p. 170.00 (*3-540-61894-5*) Spr-Verlag.

Complement Today. Ed. by J. M. Cruse & R. E. Lewis, Jr. 1993. (Complement Profiles Ser.: Vol. 1). (Illus.). x, 156p. 106.25 (*3-8055-5673-X*) S Karger.

***Complementary & Alternative Medicine.** Edzard Ernst & David Eisenberg. 2001. 444p. (*0-7234-3207-4*) Mosby Inc.

Complementary & Alternative Medicine: Challenge & Change. Ed. by Merrijoy Kelner & Beverly Wellman. 2000. 256p. 57.00 (*90-5823-098-8*); pap. 23.99 (*90-5823-099-6*) Gordon & Breach (Harwood Acad Pubs).

Complementary & Alternative Medicine: Legal Boundaries & Regulatory Perspectives. Michael H. Cohen. 1998. LC 97-21874. 190p. pap. text 18.95 (*0-8018-5689-2*) Johns Hopkins.

Complementary & Alternative Medicine & Psychiatry. Ed. by Philip R. Muskin. 2000. (Review of Psychiatry Ser.: Vol. 19, No. 1). 320p. pap. 28.50 (*0-88048-174-9*, 8174) Am Psychiatric.

***Complementary & Alternative Medicine Management.** Bowman & Lawlis. 2001. 418p. ring bd. 249.00 (*0-8342-1763-5*) Aspen Pub.

Complementary & Alternative Therapies: An Implementation Guide to Integrative Health Care. Doris Milton & Samuel G. Benjamin. 1999. LC 98-45876. 184p. pap. 38.00 (*1-55648-252-3*) AHPI.

***Complementary Formulary: A Guide for Prescribers.** Colin Lessell. 2001. 280p. pap. 24.99 (*0-7506-5389-2*) Buttrwrth-Heinemann.

Complementary Medicine. Ed. by John W. Spencer & Joseph J. Jacobs. 1998. LC 98-36023. (Illus.). 464p. (C). (gr. 13). pap. text 39.95 (*0-8151-2989-0*, 31792) Mosby Inc.

Complementary Medicine: A Practical Guide. Jamil. 1997. 272p. pap. text 37.50 (*0-7506-2881-2*) Buttrwrth-Heinemann.

Complementary Medicine: A Research Perspective. Charles Vincent et al. 1997. LC 97-4321. 312p. pap. 59.95 (*0-471-96645-2*) Wiley.

Complementary Medicine: An Objective Appraisal. Edzard Ernst. 1996. LC 96-16044. 176p. pap. text 47.50 (*0-7506-3141-4*) Buttrwrth-Heinemann.

Complementary Medicine: Knowledge in Practice. Ed. by Sarah Cant & Ursula Sharma. 1997. 220p. pap. (*1-85343-352-7*); (C). (*1-85343-351-9*) Free Assoc Bks GBR. *Dist:* Intl Spec Bk.

Complementary Medicine & Disability: Alternatives for People with Disabling Conditions. Andrew Vickers. 1993. 310p. pap. 44.75 (*1-56593-232-3*, 0551) Singular Publishing.

Complementary Medicine & the Law. Julie Stone & Joan Matthews. 1996. 328p. text 65.00 (*0-19-825970-0*); pap. text 26.00 (*0-19-825971-9*) OUP.

***Complementary Medicine in Acute Care: A Western Approach.** Steven Rosenzweig. 2001. (Illus.). 315p. (*0-443-06568-3*) Church GBR. *Dist:* Saunders.

Complementary Medicine Today: Practitioners & Patients. Ursula Sharma. 1991. LC 91-617. 256p. (C). pap. 27.99 (*0-415-04794-3*, A5934) Routledge.

Complementary Sports Medicine: Balancing Traditional & Nontraditional Treatments. Phillip Maffetone. 1999. LC 98-52399. (Illus.). 440p. text 99.95 (*0-88011-869-5*) Human Kinetics.

Complementary Therapies. 2001. (Gem Ser.). (Illus.). 192p. pap. (*0-00-710149-X*) HarpC GBR. *Dist:* Trafalgar.

Complementary Therapies for Healthcare Providers. Merrily A. Kuhn. 1999. LC 99-10977. (Illus.). 398p. pap. text 24.95 (*0-7817-1919-4*) Lppncott W & W.

***Complementary Therapies for Pharmacists.** Kayne. 2002. 224p. (*0-85369-430-3*) Pharmaceutical Pr GBR. *Dist:* Rittenhouse.

Complementary Therapies for Physical Therapists: A Theoretical & Clinical Exploration. Robert A. Charman. 2000. LC 00-23620. (Illus.). 320p. pap. text 52.50 (*0-7506-4079-0*) Buttrwrth-Heinemann.

Complementary Therapies for Pregnancy & Childbirth. Denise Tiran & Sue Mack. 2000. LC 99-53489. (Illus.). 29.00 (*0-443-06427-X*) Harcrt Hlth Sci Grp.

Complementary Therapies for Pregnancy & Childbirth. Ed. by Denise Tiran & Sue Mack. 1995. (Illus.). 317p. pap. text (*0-7020-1795-7*) W B Saunders GBR. *Dist:* Saunders.

***Complementary Therapies for Pregnancy & Childbirth.** Denise Tiran & Sue Mack. 2nd ed. 2000. (Illus.). 319p. pap. (*0-7020-2328-0*) W B Saunders GBR. *Dist:* Saunders.

Complementary Therapies in Childhood & Adolescence: A Practical Guide for Healthcare Professionals. 2002. 192p. pap. 29.95 (*0-7506-5175-X*) Buttrwrth-Heinemann.

Complementary Therapies in Dental Practice. Varley. 1998. LC 97-42650. 304p. pap. text 50.00 (*0-7236-1033-9*) Buttrwrth-Heinemann.

Complementary Therapies in Dental Practice. Ed. by Peter Varley. 1997. (Illus.). pap. (*0-7236-0248-4*) John Wright GBR. *Dist:* Macmillan.

Complementary Therapies in Rehabilitation: Holistic Approaches for Prevention & Wellness. Carol M. Davis. 1996. LC 96-44699. 352p. pap. 35.00 (*1-55642-281-4*, 42814) SLACK Inc.

Complementary/Alternative Therapies in Nursing. Mariah Snyder & Ruth Lindquist. 3rd ed. 1998. LC 97-37261. 14p. 48.95 (*0-8261-1169-6*) Springer Pub.

***Complementary/Alternative Therapies in Nursing.** Ed. by Mariah Snyder & Ruth Lindquist. 4th ed. 2001. LC 2001-49710. (Illus.). 352p. 49.95 (*0-8261-1446-6*) Springer Pub.

Complete A-Z Common Ailments & Their Natural Remedies. Judy Jacka. 1996. 352p. pap. (*0-572-02152-6*) W Foulsham GBR. *Dist:* Trans-Atl Phila.

Complete Adult Psychotherapy Treatment Planner. Arthur E. Jongsma, Jr. & Mark L. Peterson. 2nd ed. 1999. (Practice Planners Ser.). 288p. LC 98-39258. pap. 44.95 (*0-471-31924-4*); pap. text 175.00 incl. disk, 3.5 hd (*0-471-31957-0*) Wiley.

Complete Allergy Book. June Engel. 1998. LC 97-932379. (Illus.). 318p. pap. 14.95 (*1-55209-203-8*) Firefly Bks Limited.

Complete Appreciation of Oneself. Harvey Jackins. 1964. pap. 2.00 (*0-911214-08-9*) Rational Isl.

Complete Aromatherapy Gift Set: Essential Oils for Radiant Health. Cassandra Eason. deluxe ed. 1992. LC 90-24305. (Illus.). 240p. 29.95 (*0-8069-5687-9*) Sterling.

Complete Aromatherapy Handbook: Essential Oils for Radiant Health. Susanne Fischer-Rizzi. 1991. LC 90-24305. (Illus.). 240p. pap. 16.95 (*0-8069-8222-5*) Sterling.

Complete BBC Diet. Barry Lynch. 1994. pap. (*0-14-023722-4*) Pnguin Bks Ltd GBR. *Dist:* Trafalgar.

Complete Bedside Companion: No-Nonsense Advice on Caring for the Seriously Ill. Rodger McFarlane & Phillip Bashe. 1998. LC 97-43746. 544p. 27.00 (*0-684-80143-4*) S&S Trade.

Complete Bedside Companion: No-Nonsense Advice on Caring for the Seriously Ill. Rodger McFarlane & Phillip Bashe. 1999. (Illus.). 544p. pap. 16.00 (*0-684-84319-6*, Fireside) S&S Trade Pap.

Complete Body, Mind & Spirit. Ed. by Nancy Allison. 2001. LC 00-53477. 432p. pap. 24.95 (*0-658-00704-1*) McGraw-Hill Prof.

Complete Book of Acupuncture. Stephen Chang. 1995. LC 75-28762. (Illus.). 264p. text 12.95 (*0-89087-124-8*) Celestial Arts.

Complete Book of Alternative Nutrition: Powerful New Ways to Use Foods, Herbs, Supplements & Special Diets to Prevent & Cure Disease. Selene Craig et al. 1997. LC 96-27098. 464p. text 27.95 (*0-87596-322-6*) Rodale Pr Inc.

Complete Book of Ayurvedic Home Remedies: Based on the Timeless Wisdom of India's 5,000 Year Old Medical System. Vasant Lad. 1999. (Illus.). 336p. pap. 15.00 (*0-609-80286-0*) Crown Pub Group.

Complete Book of Breast Care. Niels Lauersen. 1998. LC 98-96299. 464p. pap. 14.95 (*0-449-91241-8*) Fawcett.

Complete Book of Breastfeeding. Marvin S. Eiger & Sally W. Olds. rev. ed. 1986. LC 86-40201. (Illus.). 320p. pap. 8.95 (*0-89480-153-8*, 1153) Workman Pub.

Complete Book of Children's Allergies. B. Robert Feldman & David Carroll. 1989. 320p. pap. 10.95 (*0-446-38765-7*) Warner Bks.

Complete Book of Complementary Therapies. Peter Albright. 1997. LC 96-39297. (Illus.). 176p. pap. 29.95 (*1-882606-72-8*) Peoples Med Soc.

Complete Book of Dog Care. Leon F. Whitney & George D. Whitney. rev. ed. 1985. LC 84-28763. (Illus.). 480p. pap. 13.95 (*0-385-15547-6*) Doubleday.

Complete Book of Dog Health. Animal Medical Center Staff et al. 1990. (Illus.). 272p. pap. 15.00 (*0-87605-455-6*, Howell) Hungry Minds.

Complete Book of Forms for the School Health Professional: Ready-to-Use Forms for the School Health Professional. Jerry Newton. 1987. 480p. text 34.95 (*0-13-156498-6*) P-H.

Complete Book of Homeopathy. Michael Weiner. 1997. 320p. 7.98 (*1-56731-181-4*, MJF Bks) Fine Comms.

***Complete Book of Laser Eye Surgery.** Stephen G. Slade et al. 2002. 336p. mass mkt. 6.99 (*0-553-58422-7*) Bantam.

Complete Book of Laser Eye Surgery. Stephen G. Slade et al. 2000. LC 00-44043. (Illus.). xiii, 311p. pap. 19.95 (*1-57071-633-1*) Sourcebks.

Complete Book of Medical Symptoms in Children. Martin Edwards. 1994. pap. (*0-572-01922-X*) W Foulsham GBR. *Dist:* Trans-Atl Phila.

Complete Book of Menopause. Carol Landau et al. 1995. 368p. pap. 15.95 (*0-399-51906-8*, Perigee Bks) Berkley Pub.

Complete Book of Men's Health: The Definitive, Illustrated Guide to Healthy Living, Exercise, & Sex. Ed. by Men's Health Book Editors. 2000. (Illus.). 288p. pap. 19.95 (*1-57954-298-0*) Rodale Pr Inc.

Complete Book of Men's Health: The Definitive, Illustrated Guide to Healthy Living, Exercise, & Sex. Men's Health Books Editors. 1998. LC 98-8658. (Illus.). 288p. 31.95 (*0-87596-528-8*) Rodale Pr Inc.

Complete Book of Natural Pain Relief: Safe & Effective Self-Help for Everyday Aches & Pains. Richard Thomas. 1998. (Illus.). 160p. pap. 19.95 (*1-55209-168-6*) Firefly Bks Limited.

Complete Book of Pregnancy & Childbirth. Sheila Kitzinger. 2nd exp. rev. ed. 1996. LC 96-17649. 432p. 25.00 (*0-679-45028-9*) Knopf.

Complete Book of Reiki Healing: Heal Yourself, Others, & the World Around You. Brigitte Muller & Horst H. Gunther. 1995. LC 94-47299. pap. 15.95 (*0-940795-16-7*) LifeRhythm.

Complete Book of Self-Hypnosis. John M. Yates. 1994. mass mkt. 4.95 (*0-8041-9817-9*) Ivy Books.

Complete Book of Sports Medicine. Dominguez. 1979. 2.95 (*0-684-16384-5*, Macmillan Ref) Gale.

Complete Book of Symptoms & Treatments. Roland Bettschart et al. 1998. LC 98-3697. 992p. pap. 24.95 (*1-86204-424-4*) Element MA.

Complete Book of Vitamins & Minerals. Consumer Guide Editors. 1989. 288p. (Orig.). 7.98 (*0-88176-497-3*) Pubns Intl Ltd.

Complete Book of Walking. Charles T. Kuntzleman. 1989. mass mkt. 6.50 (*0-671-70074-X*) PB.

Complete Breast Book: Everything You Need to Know about Breast Disease. June Engel. 1996. (Illus.). 276p. pap. 19.95 (*1-55013-748-4*) Firefly Bks Limited.

Complete Cancer Nursing Review. Susan L. Groenwald et al. 4th ed. 1997. (Illus.). (C). pap. text 10.00 (*0-7637-0768-6*) Jones & Bartlett.

Complete Cancer Survival Guide: Everything You Must Know & Where to Go for State-of-the-Art Treatment of the 25 Most Common Forms of Cancer. Peter Teeley & Philip Bashe. 2000. LC 98-28588. (Illus.). 992p. pap. 19.95 (*0-385-48605-7*, Main St Bks) Doubleday.

Complete Care Manual for Long-Term Care. Connie March. rev. ed. 1997. LC 96-40182. (Illus.). 103p. 40.95 (*1-55648-184-5*, 130106) AHPI.

Complete Care Plan Manual for Long-Term Care. Connie March. rev. ed. 1997. 124p. 45.00 (*0-7879-5525-6*) Jossey-Bass.

Complete Cat Health Manual. Race Foster. 1997. LC 97-2777. 288p. 19.95 (*0-87605-675-3*, Howell) Hungry Minds.

Complete Child Care in Body & Mind. I. Newton Kugelmass. 1959. 25.95 (*0-8084-0367-2*) NCUP.

Complete Coding Tutor: ICD-9-CM,CPT,HCPCS Level II. St. Anthony's Publishing Staff. 1999. (Medical Assisting Ser.). (C). pap. text 72.00 (*1-56329-624-1*) Delmar.

***Complete Coding Tutor 2001.** Ingenix, Inc. Staff. per. 99.95 (*1-56329-741-8*) Ingenix Inc.

Complete Coding Tutor/ICD9, CPT, HCPCS Level II. Ed. by Anita Hart & Julia Palmer. 1999. (Medical Assisting Ser.). 550p. (C). pap. 189.00 (*1-56329-512-1*) Ingenix Inc.

Complete Correspondence of Sigmund Freud & Ernest Jones, 1908-1939. Ed. by R. Andrew Paskauskas. 1993. LC 92-23913. (Illus.). 888p. 48.00 (*0-674-15423-1*, Belknap) HUP.

Complete Dental Assistant. 1994. text 75.00 (*0-8151-3361-8*) Mosby Inc.

Complete Dental Bleaching. Ronald E. Goldstein & David A. Garber. 1995. LC 95-14260. 176p. text 68.00 (*0-86715-290-7*) Quint Pub Co.

Complete Dental Hygiene. Daniel. 2001. text (*0-323-00993-X*) Mosby Inc.

Complete Diabetic Cookbook. Mary J. Finsand. 1990. LC 79-91382. (Illus.). 192p. pap. 10.95 (*0-8069-8908-4*) Sterling.

Complete Directory for Pediatric Disorders 2000. Ed. by Joy Bartnett et al. 2000. (Illus.). 993p. 165.00 (*1-891482-60-2*, Sedgwick Pr) Grey Hse Pub.

Complete Drug Reference, 2001. Micromedex Staff et al. 2000. LC 91-37304. (Complete Drug Reference Ser.). (Illus.). 1728p. 44.95 (*0-89043-942-7*) Consumer Reports.

Complete Eldercare Planner: Where to Start, Questions to Ask & How to Find Help. Joy Loverde. 1997. LC 96-43370. 288p. (J). pap. 14.95 (*0-7868-8229-8*) Hyperion.

Complete Electrocardiology I. G. MacFarlane. 1988. 395.00 (*0-08-035567-6*, Pergamon Pr) Elsevier.

Complete Encyclopedia of Natural Healing: A Comprehensive A-Z Listing of Common & Chronic Illnesses & Their Proven Natural Treatments. Gary Null. 1998. LC 97-73471. 612p. 35.00 (*1-57566-258-2*, Knsington) Kensgtn Pub Corp.

Complete Encyclopedia of Natural Healing: A Comprehensive A-Z Listing of Common & Chronic Illnesses & Their Proven Natural Treatments. Gary Null. 2000. 612p. reprint ed. pap. 20.00 (*1-57566-719-3*, Knsington) Kensgtn Pub Corp.

Complete Encyclopedia of the History of Medicine. Date not set. (C). Vol. 1. 808p. (*0-415-16419-2*); Vol. 2. 1040p. (*0-415-16420-6*) Routledge.

Complete Equine Veterinary Manual. Tony Pavord & Marcy Pavord. 1998. LC 98-133359. (Illus.). 288p. (*0-7153-0330-9*) D & C Pub GBR. *Dist:* F & W Pubns Inc.

Complete Family Guide to Alternative Medicine: An Illustrated Encyclopedia of Natural Healing. Richard Thomas. 1996. LC 96-34077. (Illus.). 288p. pap. 24.95 (*1-85230-901-6*) Element MA.

Complete Family Guide to Homeopathy. Christopher Hammond. 1996. LC 95-44025. (Illustrated Health Ser.). (Illus.). 256p. (*1-85230-748-X*) Element MA.

Complete Family Health Book. American Medical Women's Association Staff. 2000. 40.00 (*1-58238-019-8*, Whitman Coin) St Martin.

Complete Family Health Book. Roselyn P. Epps & Donna Shelly. 2001. (American Medical Women's Association Ser.). (Illus.). 768p. 40.00 (*0-312-25308-7*) St Martin.

Complete Feng Shui Health Handbook: How You Can Protect Yourself Against Harmful Energies & Create Positive Forces for Health & Prosperity. Wilhelm Gerstung & Jens Mehlhase. 2000. (Illus.). 248p. pap. 16.95 (*0-914955-60-8*) Lotus Pr.

Complete Foaling Manual. Theresa Jones. Ed. by Christine King & Don M. Wagoner. 1996. (Illus.). 332p. 48.00 (*0-935842-11-X*) Equine Res.

Complete German Commission E Monographs: Therapeutic Guide to Herbal Medicines. Ed. by Mark Blumenthal et al. Tr. by R. Rister & S. Klein from GER. 1998. LC 96-78896. 8500p. 165.00 (*0-9655555-0-X*, B181) Amer Botanical.

Complete German Commission E Monographs: Therapeutic Guide to Herbal Medicines. Mark Blumenthal. 1999. 199.00 (*0-9670772-7-3*) Integratv Med Commn.

Complete Guide to Acupressure. Iona M. Teeguarden. 1995. LC 92-70447. (Illus.). 364p. (Orig.). pap. 29.00 (*0-87040-880-1*) Japan Pubns USA.

Complete Guide to Better Dental Care. Jerry F. Taintor & Mary J. Taintor. 1999. 288p. pap. 12.95 (*0-8160-4005-2*, Checkmark); 2nd rev. ed. 1997. LC 96-51103. (Illus.). 256p. 25.95 (*0-8160-3383-8*) Facts on File.

Complete Guide to Children's Dental Care from Prenatal Through Teens. Karen B. Greenberg. 1993. 136p. pap. 14.95 (*0-9635998-0-1*) Hlth Monitor.

Complete Guide to Christian Videos. Anne Zanko. 1995. LC 95-60926. 381p. pap. 16.95 (*0-9646611-0-1*) Venture NJ.

Complete Guide to Experiential Psychotherapy. Alvin R. Mahrer. 1995. LC 95-7302. 412p. 150.00 (*0-471-12438-9*) Wiley.

Complete Guide to Fertility & Family Planning. Sarah Freeman & Vern L. Bullough. 1993. LC 93-10850. (Illus.). 129p. 36.00 (*0-87975-785-X*); pap. 22.00 (*0-87975-798-1*) Prometheus Bks.

Complete Guide to Foot Reflexology. Kevin Kunz & Barbara Kunz. rev. ed. 1991. LC 89-23112. 168p. pap. 10.95 (*0-13-155342-9*) P-H.

Complete Guide to Foreign Medical Schools. Nilanjan Sen. Ed. by Ilana Sparrow. 1997. (In Plain English Ser.). (Illus.). 150p. (Orig.). (C). pap. 12.95 (*1-890838-00-4*) Indus Pub.

Complete Guide to Graduate School Admission: Psychology & Related Programs. Ed. by Patricia C. Keith-Spiegel. 1990. 296p. (C). text 49.95 (*0-8058-0637-7*) L Erlbaum Assocs.

Complete Guide to Healing Foods. Amanda Ursell. 2000. LC 99-86947. (Illus.). 256p. 29.95 (*0-7894-5163-8*) DK Pub Inc.

Complete Guide to Health Claims Examining Insurance Career Development Center Staff & Caitlind L. Alexander. Ed. by Caitlind L. Alexander & Sharon E. Brown. 2nd ed. 1999. (Illus.). 875p. (C). reprint ed. pap. text 57.00 (*1-881159-24-8*, 24408) ICDC Pubng.

Complete Guide to Health Insurance: How to Beat the High Cost of Being Sick. Kathleen Hogue et al. 1990. 384p. mass mkt. 4.95 (*0-380-70785-3*, Avon Bks) Morrow Avon.

Complete Guide to Health Insurance: How to Beat the High Cost of Being Sick. Kathleen Hogue et al. 1988. 336p. 24.95 (*0-8027-1024-7*) Walker & Co.

Complete Guide to Homeopathy: The Principles & Practice of Treatment with a Comprehensive Range of Self-Help Remedies for Common Ailments. Andrew Lockie & Nicola Geddes. 1997. LC 95-6746. (Illus.). 240p. 29.95 (*0-7894-0148-7*, 6-70479) DK Pub Inc.

Complete Guide to Informed Consent in Clinical Trials. Terry Hartnett. 2000. 164p. 99.00 (*0-9701533-0-9*) Pharmsource.

Complete Guide to Integrative Healing. David Peters, pseud & Anne Woodham. 2000. LC 99-50060. (Illus.). 192p. 29.95 (*0-7894-5177-8*) DK Pub Inc.

Complete Guide to Managed Behavioral Health Care. Ed. by Chris E. Stout et al. 1997. 320p. pap. 225.00 (*0-471-14680-3*) Wiley.

Complete Guide to Mercury Toxicity from Dental Fillings: How to Find Out If Your Dental Fillings Are Poisoning You & What You Can Do about It. Joyal Taylor. 1988. LC 88-90719. (Illus.). 208p. (Orig.). pap. 14.95 (*0-944796-36-2*) EDA Pubg.

Complete Guide to Natural Healing. 1998. (Illus.). ring bd. (*1-886614-96-2*) Intl Masters Pub.

Complete Guide to Natural Healing. Tom Monte. 1997. LC 97-3527. 608p. pap. 16.95 (*0-399-52312-X*, Perigee Bks) Berkley Pub.

Complete Guide to Natural Healing. Tom Monte. 2000. 613p. reprint ed. text 35.00 (*0-7881-9121-7*) DIANE Pub.

Complete Guide to Nutritional Supplements. Brenda D. Adderly. 1998. pap. 108.00 (*0-7871-1782-X*, Dove Audio) NewStar Media.

Complete Guide to Nutritional Supplements: Everything You Need to Make Informed Choices For Optimum Health. Brenda D. Adderly. 1998. 464p. pap. 18.00 (*0-7871-1769-2*, Dove Audio) NewStar Media.

Complete Guide to Ocular History Taking. Janice K. Ledford. 1998. LC 98-36725. (Illus.). 144p. pap. text 30.00 (*1-55642-369-1*, 63691) SLACK Inc.

Complete Guide to OSHA Compliance. Joel M. Cohen. 1995. LC 95-42176. 416p. 75.00 (*0-87371-681-7*, L681) Lewis Pubs.

Complete Guide to Part B Billing & Compliance (BCP) Ed. by Sheila Parvis & Karen Kachur. 1999. 400p. (C). pap. 279.00 (*1-56329-604-7*) Thomson Learn.

Complete Guide to Pediatric Symptoms, Illness, & Medications. H. Winter Griffith. 1989. pap. 15.95 (*0-89586-816-4*, Body Pr-Perigee) Berkley Pub.

Complete Guide to Premedical Success: Achieving the Doctor Dream. Gregory A. Andrews. 1998. LC 98-204564. 317p. per. 20.00 (*0-9660525-0-1*) MedLaw Bks Inc.

Complete Guide to Prescription & Non-Prescription Drugs. H. Winter Griffith. Ed. by Douglas Morrison. 1987. LC 87-25596. 1056p. (Orig.). 25.00 (*0-89586-594-7*, HP Books) Penguin Putnam.

Complete Guide to Prescription & Non-Prescription Drugs. H. Winter Griffith. rev. ed. 1992. (*0-399-51714-6*, Body Pr-Perigee) Penguin Putnam.

***Complete Guide to Prescription & Nonprescription Drugs 2002.** Stephen Moore. 2001. 1104p. pap. 17.95 (*0-399-52716-8*, Perigee Bks) Berkley Pub.

Complete Guide to Preventing Cancer: How You Can Reduce Your Risks. Elizabeth Whelan. rev. ed. 1994. LC 94-11606. 385p. (C). 34.00 (*0-87975-890-2*) Prometheus Bks.

Complete Guide to Psychiatric Drugs: Straight Talk for Best Results. Edward H. Drummond. 2000. LC 99-50236. 320p. pap. 17.95 (*0-471-35370-1*) Wiley.

Complete Guide to Refractive Surgery: Nearsightedness, Farsightedness, & Astigmatism. Stanley C. Grandon et al. Ed. by Susan Giffin. 2nd rev. ed. 1999. Orig. Title: Good-Bye, Glasses. (Illus.). 240p. (Orig.). pap. 10.95 (*0-9628886-2-1*) Patton Pub.

Complete Guide to Safe Sex. Ted McIlvenna et al. 1987. 200p. (Orig.). pap. text 6.95 (*0-930846-05-2*) Specific Pr.

Complete Guide to Sensible Eating. Gary Null. 3rd ed. 1998. LC 97-22206. (Illus.). 352p. pap. 16.95 (*1-888363-61-4*) Seven Stories.

Complete Guide to Sports Injuries. H. Winter Griffith. rev. ed. 1997. LC 97-33690. 528p. pap. 16.95 (*0-399-52305-7*, Perigee Bks) Berkley Pub.

Complete Guide to Sports Nutrition. Anita Bean. 3rd ed. 2000. 256p. pap. (*0-7136-5389-2*) A & C Blk GBR. *Dist:* Lubrecht & Cramer, Midpt Trade.

Complete Guide to Symptoms, Illness & Surgery. H. Winter Griffith. 2nd ed. 1992. (Illus.). (*0-89586-830-X*, Body Pr-Perigree) Berkley Pub.

Complete Guide to Symptoms, Illness, & Surgery. H. Winter Griffith. 3rd rev. ed. 1995. LC 96-222733. 1104p. pap. 17.95 (*0-399-51942-4*, Perigee Bks) Berkley Pub.

Complete Guide to Symptoms, Illness & Surgery for People over Fifty. H. Winter Griffith. 1992. (Illus.). 896p. pap. 19.95 (*0-399-51749-9*, Body Pr-Perigree) Berkley Pub.

Complete Guide to Symptoms over Fifty. H. Winter Griffith. 1992. pap. 29.95 (*0-399-51760-X*) Berkley Pub.

Complete Guide to Women's Health. Bruce Shepard et al. 3rd rev. ed. 1997. LC 96-26960. (Illus.). 528p. pap. 23.95 (*0-452-27792-2*, Plume) Dutton Plume.

Complete Guide to Your Children's Health. American Medical Association Staff et al. 1998. LC 98-6970. (Illus.). 710p. 39.95 (*0-679-45776-3*) Random.

Complete Handbook for Medical Secretaries & Assistants. Jean M. Doyle & Robert L. Dennis. 2nd ed. 1978. pap. text 18.95 (*0-316-18082-3*, Little Brwn Med Div) Lppncott W & W.

Complete Handbook of Children's Reading Disorders: You Can Prevent or Correct Learning Disorders. Hilda L. Mosse. 2nd ed. 1987. (Illus.). 714p. (Orig.). pap. text 34.95 (*0-942311-00-0*) Riggs Inst Pr.

Complete Handbook of Health Tips. R. Emil Neuman. rev. ed. 1995. 256p. pap. 12.95 (*0-9614924-1-4*) United Res CA.

Complete Healing: Regaining Your Health Through Anthroposophical Medicine. Michael Evans & Iain Rodger. 2000. 192p. pap. 14.95 (*0-88010-489-9*) Anthroposophic.

Complete Herbal Handbook for Farm & Stable. Juliette D. Levy. 4th ed. 1991. LC 91-192224. 384p. (Orig.). pap. 21.95 (*0-571-16116-2*) Faber & Faber.

Complete Herbal Handbook for the Dog & Cat. Juliette D. Levy. rev. ed. 1991. (Orig.). pap. 16.00 (*0-571-16115-4*) Faber & Faber.

Complete Herbalist: The People Their Own Physicians. O. Phelps Brown. 1996. 504p. reprint ed. pap. 30.00 (*0-7873-0121-3*) Hlth Research.

Complete Herbalist: The People Their Own Physicians. O. Phelps Brown. 1992. 504p. pap. 35.00 (*0-89540-118-5*, SB-118) Sun Pub.

Complete Home Healer: Your Guide to Every Treatment Available for 300 of the Most Common Problems. Angela Smyth. LC 93-40025. pap. 12.00 (*0-06-251259-5*) HarperCollins Pubs.

Complete Home Health Advisor. Rita Elkins. 1994. 388p. pap. 17.95 (*0-913923-96-6*) Woodland UT.

***Complete Home Health Advisor: Instant Access to: Leading Cures, Reliable Remedies, Self-Help Strategies & Life-Saving Facts.** Compiled by Deborah Mitchell. 2001. LC 2001-36467. 500p. pap. 16.00 (*0-7352-0288-5*) PH Pr.

Complete Home-Study Course for Training in Cognitive-Behavioral Exposure Based Psychotherapy for the Treatment of PTSD & Other Anxiety Disorders, Vol. 1. Larry D. Smyth. 1999. pap., stu. ed. 400.00 incl. VHS (*1-889287-98-9*) Red Toad Rd.

***Complete Home Wellness Handbook: Home Remedies, Prevention, Self Care.** John Swartzberg & Sheldon Margen. 2001. LC 2001-19197. 672p. 34.95 (*0-929661-64-8*) Rebus.

Complete Homeopathy Handbook: Safe & Effective Ways to Treat Fevers, Coughs, Colds & Sore Throats, Childhood Ailments, Food Poisoning, Flu, & a Wide Range of Everyday Complaints. Miranda Castro. 1991. (Illus.). 272p. pap. 15.95 (*0-312-06320-2*) St Martin.

Complete Idiot's Guide to Acupuncture & Acupressure. David W. Sollars. 2000. LC 2001-266805. (Complete Idiot's Guides Ser.). (Illus.). 312p. pap. 16.95 (*0-02-863942-1*) Mac USA.

Complete Idiot's Guide to Alternative Medicine. 1999. pap. text 17.95 (*0-02-865450-1*) S&S Trade.

Complete Idiot's Guide to Back Pain. Deborah S. Romaine & Dawn E. DeWitt. 1999. LC 98-5121. (Complete Idiot's Guides Ser.). (Illus.). 368p. pap. 16.95 (*0-02-863115-3*) Mac USA.

Complete Idiot's Guide to Conquering Allergies & Asthma. Bill Shields. 2000. (Complete Idiot's Guides Ser.). 352p. 16.95 (*0-02-863931-6*) Macmillan.

Complete Idiot's Guide to First Aid. Karla Dougherty & Stephen J. Rosenberg. 1996. LC 95-83358. 352p. 16.95 (*0-02-861099-7*) Macmillan.

Complete Idiot's Guide to Homeopathy. David W. Sollars. 2001. (Complete Idiot's Guides Ser.). 336p. pap. 16.95 (*0-02-864003-9*) Mac USA.

Complete Idiot's Guide to Living with Breast Cancer. Sharon Sorenson & Suzanne Metzger. 2000. (Complete Idiot's Guides Ser.). (Illus.). 400p. pap. 18.95 (*0-02-863938-3*) Mac USA.

Complete Idiot's Guide to Managed Health Care. Macmillan General Reference Staff. 1998. 17.95 (*0-02-865115-4*) Macmillan.

Complete Idiot's Guide to Online Medical Resources. Joan Price. 2000. LC 99-67315. (Complete Idiot's Guides Ser.). (Illus.). 352p. pap. 18.95 (*0-7897-2297-6*) Que.

Complete Idiot's Guide to Total Nutrition. Prentice-Hall Staff. 2000. pap. 25.95 (*0-13-086722-5*, Prentice Hall) P-H.

Complete Idiot's Guide to Walking for Health. Erika Peters. 2001. (Complete Idiot's Guides Ser.). (Illus.). 312p. pap. 16.95 (*0-02-864002-0*) Mac USA.

Complete Illustrated Guide to Ayurveda: The Ancient Indian Healing Tradition. Gopi Warrier & Deepika Gunawant. 1997. LC 97-14115. (Complete Illustrated Guide to Ser.). (Illus.). 192p. pap. 24.95 (*1-85230-953-9*) Element MA.

Complete Illustrated Guide to Chinese Medicine: A Comprehensive System for Health & Fitness. Tom Williams. 1996. LC 96-32554. (Complete Illustrated Guide to Ser.). (Illus.). 256p. pap. 24.95 (*1-85230-904-0*) Element MA.

Complete Illustrated Guide to Flower Remedies: A Practical Approach to Healing with 400 Essences from Around the World. Carol Rudd. 2000. (Illus.). 224p. pap. 24.95 (*1-86204-366-3*) Element MA.

Complete Illustrated Guide to Nutritional Healing. Denise Mortimore. 1998. LC 98-21697. (Illus.). 224p. pap. text 24.95 (*1-86204-176-8*) Element MA.

Complete Illustrated Guide to Shiatsu: The Japanese Healing Art of Touch for Health & Fitness. Elaine Liechti. 1998. LC 98-6450. (Complete Illustrated Guide to Ser.). (Illus.). 224p. pap. 24.95 (*1-86204-177-6*) Element MA.

Complete Illustrated Guide to Vitamins & Minerals: A Practical Approach to a Healthy Diet & Safe Supplements. Denise Mortimore. 2000. (Illus.). 192p. pap. 24.95 (*1-86204-453-8*) Element MA.

Complete Illustrated Holistic Herbal: A Safe & Practical Guide to Making & Using Herbal Remedies. David Hoffman. 1996. LC 96-1804. (Illus.). 256p. pap. 24.95 (*1-85230-758-7*) Element MA.

Complete in All Its Parts: Nursing Education at the University of Iowa, 1898-1998. Lee Anderson & Kathy Penningroth. 1998. LC 98-13929. (Illus.). 320p. text 50.00 (*0-472-10966-9*, 10966) U of Mich Pr.

Complete Learning Disabilities Handbook: Ready-to-Use Techniques for Teaching Learning Handicapped Students. Joan Harwell. 1989. 224p. pap. 29.95 (*0-87628-239-7*) Ctr Appl Res.

Complete Letters of Sigmund Freud to Wilhelm Fliess: 1887-1904. Sigmund Freud. Ed. & Tr. by Jeffrey M. Masson. 1986. (Illus.). 544p. pap. text 18.95 (*0-674-15421-5*, Belknap) HUP.

Complete Letters of Sigmund Freud to Wilhelm Fliess: 1887-1904. Sigmund Freud. Tr. by Jeffrey M. Masson from GER. 1985. (Illus.). 544p. 39.95 (*0-674-15420-7*, Belknap) HUP.

Complete Manual of Natural Allergy Control. David Williams. 2nd ed. 1987. 92p. pap. 6.95 (*0-944649-00-9*) Mtn Home Pub.

Complete MCQs in Psychiatry: Self-Assessment for Parts 1 & 2 of the MRCpsych. Basant K. Puri & Anne D. Hall. 1999. LC 00-502201. (Arnold's Self-Assessment Ser.). 528p. pap. (*0-340-74035-3*) E A GBR. *Dist:* OUP.

Complete Medical Marketing Handbook: A Guide for Physicians & Managers. Maryann Szotstak-Ricardo. 1994. 112p. stu. ed., ring bd. 49.95 (*1-57066-028-X*, ME061) Practice Mgmt Info.

Complete Medical School Preparation & Admissions Guide. Andrew Goliszek. 1986. LC 86-70723. 184p. pap. 8.95 (*0-9616475-0-7*); 2nd ed. 1990. LC 89-82535. 224p. pap. text 14.95 (*0-9616475-5-8*) Healthnet Pr.

Complete Medicinal Herbal. Penelope Ody. (Illus.). 1997. LC 92-53415. 192p. 29.95 (*1-56458-187-X*); 2nd ed. 2000. LC 00-25779. 240p. 29.95 (*0-7894-6785-2*) DK Pub Inc.

***Complete Mental Health Directory, 2002.** Ed. by Laura Mars. 3rd ed. 2002. 750p. pap. 165.00 (*1-930956-06-1*, Sedgwick Pr) Grey Hse Pub.

Complete Micropsychology. Ashok G. Patel et al. 1995. pap. text 32.50 (*0-7020-2067-2*) Saunders.

Complete Mothercare Manual: An Illustrated Guide to Pregnancy, Birth & Childcare Through Age Five. Rosalind Y. Ting et al. rev. ed. 1992. (Illus.). 304p. pap. 15.00 (*0-671-78978-3*, Fireside) S&S Trade Pap.

Complete MRCP3. Beynon. 2nd ed. 1998. (C). pap. text (*0-443-05690-0*) Church.

Complete MRCPsych. Ed. by Ashok G. Patel. 1994. 255p. pap. text (*0-7020-1808-2*) W B Saunders GBR. *Dist:* Saunders.

Complete Natural Health Encyclopedia: Natural Treatments for the World's 350 Most Common Ailments. David H. Nyholt. 2nd ed. (Illus.). 398p. pap. (*0-921202-07-5*) Gloh CAN. *Dist:* BookWorld.

Complete Neuroticist. Robert L. McKinley. 1969. 125p. 12.50 (*0-9609644-1-X*) Candle Bks.

Complete Nutrition Counter. Lynn Sonberg. 1993. LC 93-218253. 400p. (Orig.). pap. 7.99 (*0-425-13859-3*) Berkley Pub.

Complete Patient History. Maurice Kraytman. 2nd ed. 1990. (Illus.). 504p. pap. 34.95 (*0-07-035614-9*) McGraw-Hill Prof.

Complete Preparation for Childbirth: A Self Help Manual for Expectant Parents. Janice Morton. 1990. 240p. (C). pap. text (*962-209-220-9*) HK Univ Pr HKG. *Dist:* Intl Spec Bk, Coronet Bks.

Complete Preparation for the AHPAT, 1999: Allied Health Professions Admission Test. Betz. 1998. pap. 27.95 (*0-683-30554-9*) Lppncott W & W.

Complete Preparation for the DAT, 2001: Dental Admission Test. Lippincott, Williams and Wilkins Staff. 2000. 256p. pap. text 29.95 (*0-7817-2838-X*) Lppncott W & W.

Complete Preparation for the MCAT. Aftab Hassan & Dorothy H. Air. 7th ed. 1996. LC 96-33436. 49.50 (*0-683-30078-4*) Lppncott W & W.

Complete Preparation for the MCAT: Betz Guide. Williams and Wilkins Staff. 1997. pap. text 49.50 (*0-683-30521-2*) Lppncott W & W.

Complete Preparation for the MCAT, 2001: Medical College Admission Test. Lippincott, Williams and Wilkins Staff. 2000. 676p. pap. text 49.95 (*0-7817-2839-8*) Lppncott W & W.

Complete Preparation for the OAT, 2001: Optometry Admission Test. Lippincott, Williams and Wilkins Staff. 2000. 248p. pap. text 29.95 (*0-7817-2840-1*) Lppncott W & W.

Complete Preparation for the PCAT, 2001: Pharmacy College Admission Test. Lippincott, Williams and Wilkins Staff. 2000. 320p. pap. text 29.95 (*0-7817-2841-X*) Lppncott W & W.

Complete Preparation for the VETS, 2001: Veterinary Entrance Tests. Lippincott, Williams and Wilkins Staff. 2000. 280p. pap. text 29.95 (*0-7817-2842-8*) Lppncott W & W.

Complete Preparation for the VETs, 1999: Vet Entrance Tests. Betz. 1998. pap. 27.95 (*0-683-30553-0*) Lppncott W & W.

Complete Preschool Program. Arlene L. Martin. 1987. 143p. pap. text 19.95 (*1-55691-008-8*, 088) Learning Pubns.

Complete Problem Solving for Wellness & Mental Health. Kime. 1995. 15.00 net. (*0-697-34846-6*) McGraw.

Complete Psychological Works of Sigmund Freud: Standard Edition, Set. Sigmund Freud. Ed. & Tr. by James Strachey from GER. 1976. (C). 995.00 (*0-393-01128-3*) Norton.

Complete Q & A for the NCLEX-PN. Patricia A. Hoefler. rev. ed. 1998. 424p. (C). pap. text 34.95 incl. cd-rom (*1-56533-028-5*) M E D S Inc.

Complete Quick & Hearty Diabetic Cookbook. American Diabetes Association. 1998. LC 97-46530. (Illus.). 256p. pap. 12.95 (*1-58040-002-7*, 00027Q) Am Diabetes.

Complete RBRVS (RBRC) Ed. by Mark Painter & Cathy Hopkins. rev. ed. 1998. 500p. pap. 109.95 (*1-56329-501-6*) Ingenix Inc.

Complete RBRVS (RBRC) Print. Mark Painter et al. Date not set. 400p. 89.95 (*1-56329-331-5*) Ingenix Inc.

Complete Recovery: An Expanded Model of Community Healing. Michael Picucci. 1996. 23.95 (*0-9650380-1-7*) Mombaccus Pubng.

Complete Recovery Room Book. Anthea Hatfield & Michael Tronson. 2nd ed. 1996. (Illus.). 494p. pap. text 49.50 (*0-19-262715-5*) OUP.

***Complete Reiki Course.** Master Naharo & Gail Radford. 2001. (Quality of Life Ser.). (Illus.). 244p. pap. (*965-494-119-8*) Astrolog Pub ISR. *Dist:* IPG Chicago.

Complete Reiki Handbook. Walter Lubeck. 1994. (Shangri-La Ser.). 191p. pap. 14.95 (*0-941524-87-6*) Lotus Pr.

Complete Review of Radiography. Kathryn M. Marzano & Pauline D. Lyons. 1989. LC 86-9117. (Red Bks.). 252p. pap. text 29.95 (*0-8273-4233-0*) Delmar.

Complete Scarsdale Medical Diet: Plus Dr. Tarnower's Lifetime Keep-Slim Program. Herman Tarnower & Samm S. Baker. 1982. 240p. mass mkt. 7.50 (*0-553-26886-4*) Bantam.

Complete Set. Ed. by A. P. Simopoulos et al. 1994. (World Review of Nutrition & Dietetics Ser.: Vols. 75 - 76). (Illus.). xxxii, 350p. 326.25 (*3-8055-6089-3*) S Karger.

Complete Set MRCP H. L. Beynon et al. 1992. (Complete MRCP Ser.). (Illus.). (Orig.). pap. text (*0-443-04311-6*) Church.

Complete Spleen: Structure, Function & Clinical Disorders. Ed. by Anthony J. Bowdler. 2nd ed. 2001. (Illus.). 328p. 195.00 (*0-89603-555-7*) Humana.

Complete Step-By-Step Diabetic Cookbook. Oxmoor House Staff. 1995. LC 94-74028. 368p. 17.95 (*0-8487-1431-8*) Oxmoor Hse.

Complete Textbook of Phlebotomy. Lynn B. Hoeltke. 1993. LC 93-5846. 216p. (C). mass mkt. 38.95 (*0-8273-6231-5*) Delmar.

Complete Textbook of Phlebotomy, 2E. Lynn B. Hoeltke. 2nd ed. 1999. LC 99-36290. (Medical Lab Technician Ser.). 96p. (C). pap. text 45.95 (*0-7668-0927-7*) Delmar.

Complete Therapist. Jeffrey A. Kottler. 1991. LC 90-5197. (Social & Behavioral Science Ser.). 240p. 33.00 (*1-55542-302-7*) Jossey-Bass.

Complete Woman's Herbal: A Manual of Healing Herbs & Nutrition for Personal Well-Being & Family Care. Anne McIntyre. 1995. LC 94-29291. (Reference Bks.). 287p. pap. 25.00 (*0-8050-3537-0*) H Holt & Co.

Complete Women's Health Directory 2001. Ed. by Laura Mars. 2002. 800p. 165.00 (*1-891482-45-9*) Grey Hse Pub.

Complete Womens Health Directory 2001. Ed. by Laura Mars. 2002. 800p. 190.00 (*1-891482-46-7*) Grey Hse Pub.

Complete Workers' Compensation Guide for Texas Physicians. Barbara A. Langham. 2nd rev. ed. 1997. LC 97-217475. (C). 169.00 (*0-9640262-8-7*) TX Med Assn.

***Complete Worker's Compensation Manual for Texas Physicians.** Julie Shank. 3rd rev. ed. 2001. (C). 169.00 (*1-893621-03-0*) TX Med Assn.

Completing a Qualitative Project: Details & Dialogue. Janice M. Morse. 1997. LC 97-4679. 432p. 81.95 (*0-7619-0600-2*, 80989); pap. 39.95 (*0-7619-0601-0*, 80990) Sage.

Complex & Revision Problems in Shoulder Surgery. Jon Warner. 1997. LC 96-39277. 448p. text 179.00 (*0-397-51657-6*) Lppncott W & W.

Complex Archetype Symbol in the Psychology of C. J. Jung. Jolande Jacobi. Tr. by R. Manheim. 1971. (Bollingen Ser.: Vol. 57). (Illus.). 248p. pap. 17.95 (*0-691-01774-3*, 241) Princeton U Pr.

Complex Arrhythmias: Self Assessment. E. K. Chung. 1985. (Illus.). xiv, 310p. 71.50 (*3-8055-3639-9*) S Karger.

Complex Carbohydrates. Ed. by Elizabeth F. Neufeld et al. 1966. (Methods in Enzymology Ser.: Vol. 8). text 209.00 (*0-12-181808-X*) Acad Pr.

Complex Carbohydrates, Pt. D. Ed. by Sidney P. Colowick & Victor Ginsburg. 1982. (Methods in Enzymology Ser.: Vol. 83). text 188.00 (*0-12-181983-3*) Acad Pr.

Complex Carbohydrates, Pt. B. Ed. by Victor Ginsburg. 1972. (Methods in Enzymology Ser.: Vol. 28). text 209.00 (*0-12-181891-8*) Acad Pr.

Complex Cases with LASIK: Advanced Techniques & Complication Management. Louis Probst. 1999. LC 99-40823. (Illus.). xii, 517p. text 175.00 (*1-55642-404-3*, 64043) SLACK Inc.

Complex Craniofacial Problems. Ed. by Craig R. Dufresne et al. 1992. (Illus.). 556p. text (*0-443-08624-9*) Church.

Complex Foot & Ankle Trauma. Ed. by Robert S. Adelaar. 1999. LC 98-7630. (Illus.). 304p. text 139.00 (*0-397-51374-7*) Lppncott W & W.

Complex Information Processing: The Impact of Herbert A. Simon. Ed. by David Klahr & K. Kotovsky. 1989. (Carnegie-Mellon Symposium on Cognition Ser.). 480p. 99.95 (*0-8058-0178-2*); pap. 45.00 (*0-8058-0179-0*) L Erlbaum Assocs.

Complex Interpersonal Conflict Behaviour: Theorectical Frontiers. Evert Van de Vliert. 1997. LC 98-113616. (Essays in Social Psychology Ser.). 208p. 37.50 (*0-86377-716-3*) L Erlbaum Assocs.

Complex Mixtures: Methods for In Vivo Toxicity Testing. National Research Council Staff. 1988. 240p. text 35.00 (*0-309-03778-6*) Natl Acad Pr.

Complex Mixtures & Cancer Risk. Ed. by Harri Vainio et al. 1990. (IARC Scientific Publications Ser.: No. 104). (Illus.). 450p. pap. text 95.00 (*92-832-2104-4*) OUP.

Complex Operations at Massachusetts General Hospital. Ronald A. Malt et al. 1983. (Illus.). 272p. text 135.00 (*0-7216-6008-8*) Saunders.

Complex Policy Planning: The Governance Strategic Management of the Social Care Market. Philip Haynes. 1999. LC 99-72606. (Illus.). xix, 258p. text (*1-84014-818-7*) Ashgate Pub GBR. *Dist:* Ashgate Pub Co.

Complex Problem Solving: Principles & Mechanisms. Ed. by R. J. Sternberg & P. Frensch. 1991. 424p. (C). pap. 49.95 (*0-8058-0651-2*); text 89.95 (*0-8058-0650-4*) L Erlbaum Assocs.

Complex Secret of Brief Psychotherapy: A Panorama of Approaches. James P. Gustafson. 1997. LC 96-52287. 472p. pap. text 50.00 (*0-7657-0063-8*) Aronson.

Complex Socket Deformities. Stephen L. Bosniak & Byron C. Smith. 1991. (Advances in Ophthalmic Plastic & Reconstructive Surgery Ser.: No. 9). (Illus.). 272p. (*0-08-040293-3*) PPI GBR. *Dist:* McGraw.

Complex Treatment for Stutterers. Laszlo Vekassy. 1994. 172p. (*963-05-6603-6*) Akade Kiado HUN. *Dist:* Intl Spec Bk.

Complexity in Structure & Function of the Lung. Ed. by Michael P. Hlastala & H. Thomas Robertson. 1998. LC 98-27993. (Lung Biology in Health & Disease Ser.). (Illus.). 680p. text 215.00 (*0-8247-9879-1*) Dekker.

Complexity of Creativity. Ake E. Andersson & Nils-Eric Sahlin. 1996. LC 96-50128. (Synthese Library). 151p. lib. bdg. 77.00 (*0-7923-4346-8*) Kluwer Academic.

Compliance Across the Continuum: A Comprehensive Look at Healthcare Corporate Compliance. Ed. by Corporate Compliance Resource Center Staff. 1998. LC 98-214672. 200p. pap. text 89.00 (*1-57839-024-9*) Opus Communs.

Compliance Auditing for Pharmaceutical Manufacturers: A Practical Guide to In-Depth Systems Auditing. Karen Ginsbury & Gil Bismuth. 1994. 402p. ring bd. 249.00 (*0-935184-60-0*) IHS Health Grp.

Compliance Guide to Electronic Health Records. Jonathan P. Tomes. 1994. 200p. pap. 149.95 (*1-881393-23-2*) Faulkner & Gray.

Compliance Guide to the Medical Staff Standards: Winning Strategies for Your JCAHO Survey. Richard E. Thompson. 2nd ed. 1998. (Illus.). 156p. (Orig.). pap. text 87.00 (*1-57839-025-7*) Opus Communs.

Compliance in Healthcare & Research. Lora E. Burke & Ira S. Ockene. 2001. LC 00-51414. (American Heart Association Monograph Ser.). (Illus.). xiii, 368p. 49.00 (*0-87993-474-3*) Futura Pub.

Compliance Manual for Healthcare Providers. W. H. Heaton. 1994. 200p. ring bd. 99.00 (*1-881057-75-5*) Heaton Pubns.

Compliance Manual for OSHA's Bloodborne Pathogens Standard 29 CFR 1910.1030. James Testo. Ed. by Failsafe Risk Management Alternatives Staff. 1993. (Illus.). 370p. (Orig.). ring bd. 99.00 (*0-931690-47-1*) Genium Pub.

Compliance Manual for OSHA's Hazard Communication Standard. 1992. 222p. pap. text 99.00 (*0-931690-43-9*) Genium Pub.

Compliance Programs: A Resource Guide. Robert J. Saner et al. 1998. 33p. spiral bd. (*1-56829-087-X*) M G M A.

Complicated Medical Patient: New Approaches to Psychomedical Syndromes. John I. Walker et al. 1987. LC 86-20808. 290p. 45.95 (*0-89885-331-1*, Kluwer Acad Hman Sci) Kluwer Academic.

Complications in Anesthesia. John L. Atlee. Ed. by Allan Ross. 1998. LC 98-5821. 928p. (C). text 95.00 (*0-7216-7161-6*) Saunders.

Complications in Anesthesiology. Ed. by Nikolaus Gravenstein & Robert R. Kirby. 2nd ed. 1995. 864p. text 169.00 (*0-397-51299-6*) Lppncott W & W.

Complications in Arterial Surgery. W. B. Campbell. 1996. LC 96-162886. 224p. text 125.00 (*0-7506-0568-5*) Buttrwrth-Heinemann.

Complications in Diagnostic Interventional Radiology. Michael A. Bettmann et al. 3rd rev. ed. 1996. (Illus.). 704p. 265.00 (*0-86542-243-5*) Blackwell Sci.

Complications in Foot & Ankle Surgery: Prevention & Management. Jeffrey M. Carrel & Howard M. Sokoloff. 3rd ed. 1992. (Illus.). 486p. 80.00 (*0-683-01465-X*) Lppncott W & W.

Complications in Gynecologic Surgery: Prevention, Recognition & Management. James W. Orr, Jr. et al. Ed. by J. Marion Sims. 1994. LC 93-41475. (Illus.). 320p. text 99.00 (*0-397-51269-4*, Lippnctt) Lppncott W & W.

Complications in Hand Surgery. John Boswick, Jr. 1986. (Illus.). 401p. text 155.00 (*0-7216-1877-4*) Saunders.

Complications in Head & Neck Surgery. Yosef P. Krespi & Robert H. Ossoff. 1992. (Illus.). 600p. text 105.00 (*0-7216-2980-6*) Saunders.

Complications in Laparoscopic Surgery. Robert W. Bailey et al. 1996. 416p. (*0-683-30053-9*) Lppncott W & W.

Complications in Modern Ophthalmic Surgery. Ed. by Ilse Strempel. 1987. (Developments in Ophthalmology Ser.: Vol. 13). (Illus.). xii, 160p. 111.50 (*3-8055-4413-8*) S Karger.

Complications in Neurosurgery I. Ed. by A. M. Landolt. 1984. (Progress in Neurological Surgery Ser.: Vol. 11). (Illus.). x, 174p. 85.25 (*3-8055-3691-7*) S Karger.

Complications in Ophthalmic Surgery. Ed. by Theodore Krupin et al. 2nd ed. 1999. LC 98-41938. (Illus.). xi, 387p. 195.00 (*0-7234-3109-4*) Mosby Inc.

Complications in Ophthalmic Surgery. Theodore Krupin et al. 2nd ed. 1999. (Illus.). 398p. (*84-8174-474-3*) Mosby-Doyma Libros ESP. *Dist:* Mosby Inc.

Complications in Orthopaedic Surgery, In Two Volumes. Ed. by Charles H. Epps, Jr. 3rd ed. 1994. LC 93-40983. 1,536p. text 279.00 (*0-397-51216-3*) Lppncott W & W.

Complications in Orthopaedic Surgery, In Two Volumes. Charles H. Epps. 3rd ed. 1994. LC 93-40983. 1,536p. text 379.00 (*0-397-51452-2*) Lppncott W & W.

Complications in Orthopaedics. Neil Citron. 2000. (Illus.). 192p. (*0-7506-2922-3*) E A GBR. *Dist:* OUP.

Complications in Pediatric Ophthalmology. Ed. by Charles H. Epps, Jr. & J. Richard Bowen. 1994. (Illus.). 912p. text 179.00 (*0-397-51217-1*) Lppncott W & W.

Complications in Pediatric Otolaryngology. Wohl. 2001. pap. 80.00 net. (*0-7693-0111-8*) Singular Publishing.

Complications in Phacoemulsification. William J. Fishkind. 2001. (Illus.). 352p. 99.00 (*0-86577-959-7*) Thieme Med Pubs.

Complications in Small Animal Surgery: Diagnosis, Management, Prevention. Ed. by Alan J. Lipowitz et al. 1996. (Illus.). 500p. 49.00 (*0-683-05047-8*) Lppncott W & W.

Complications in Spinal Surgery. Richard A. Balderston & Howard S. An. 1990. (Illus.). 208p. text 70.00 (*0-7216-3522-9*) Saunders.

Complications in Urologic Surgery: Prevention & Management. Samir S. Taneja et al. 3rd ed. 1999. (Illus.). (C). text 180.00 (*0-7216-7688-X*) Saunders.

Complications in Vascular Surgery. Ed. by Victor M. Bernhard & Jonathan B. Towne. 1991. 522p. 89.00 (*0-942219-20-1*) Quality Med Pub.

Complications of Abortion: Technical & Managerial Guidelines for Prevention & Treatment. 1995. (CHI, FRE & SPA.). 147p. (C). pap. text 35.00 (*92-4-154469-4*, 1150418) World Health.

***Complications of Cardiothoracic Surgery: Avoidance & Treatment.** Ed. by Alex G. Little & Kevin D. Murray. 2001. (Illus.). (*0-87993-427-1*) Futura Pub.

Complications of Cataract Surgery: A Primer. Bruce Noble & Ian Simmons. 2001. (Illus.). 108p. text 80.00 (*0-7506-4799-X*) Buttrwrth-Heinemann.

Complications of Colon & Rectal Surgery. Ed. by Terry C. Hicks et al. 1996. LC 96-15263. (Illus.). 512p. 129.00 (*0-683-30033-4*) Lppncott W & W.

Complications of Colon & Rectal Surgery: Prevention & Management. Bernard T. Ferrari et al. 1985. (Illus.). 450p. text 105.00 (*0-7216-3622-5*) Saunders.

Complications of Coronary Angioplasty. Ed. by Alexander J. Black. 1991. (Fundamental & Clinical Cardiology Ser.: Vol. 3). (Illus.). 280p. text 150.00 (*0-8247-8440-5*) Dekker.

Complications of Dermatologic Surgery: Prevention & Treatment. Ed. by Marwali Harahap. 1992. LC 92-48955. (Illus.). 272p. 126.00 (*0-387-55337-1*) Spr-Verlag.

Complications of Endoscopic & Laparoscopic Surgery: Prevention & Management. Ed. by Jeffrey L. Ponsky. 1997. LC 97-10755. 304p. text 139.00 (*0-316-98927-4*) Lppncott W & W.

Complications of Interventional Procedures. Ed. by Jerre Lutz. 1995. LC 94-46842. (Topics in Clinical Cardiology Ser.). (Illus.). 264p. 73.95 (*0-89640-260-6*) Igaku-Shoin.

Complications of Interventional Techniques. Ed. by Culley C. Carson, 3rd. 1995. LC 95-24468. (Topics in Clinical Urology Ser.). (Illus.). 256p. 69.50 (*0-89640-285-1*) Igaku-Shoin.

Complications of Laparoscopic Surgery. Ed. by Robert W. Bailey & John L. Flowers. 1995. LC 94-32028. (Illus.). 416p. 175.00 incl. VHS (*0-942219-47-3*) Quality Med Pub.

Complications of Laparoscopy & Hysteroscopy. Alan H. DeCherney et al. Ed. by R. S. Corfman & M. Diamond. 1992. (Illus.). 288p. 85.00 (*0-86542-201-X*) Blackwell Sci.

Complications of Laparoscopy & Hysteroscopy. Randle S. Corfman et al. 2nd ed. 1997. LC 97-15481. (Illus.). 304p. 105.00 (*0-86542-507-8*) Blackwell Sci.

Complications of Liver Cirrhosis: Internationaler Falk-Workshop, Bonn, February, 1998. Ed. by T. Sauerbruch et al. 1998. (Digestion Ser.: Vol. 59). (Illus.). iv, 98p. pap. 44.50 (*3-8055-6715-4*) S Karger.

Complications of Long-Term Dialysis. Ed. by Edwina Brown & Patrick Parfrey. 1999. LC 98-22503. (Oxford Clinical Nephrology Ser.). (Illus.). 354p. text 139.50 (*0-19-262829-1*) OUP.

Complications of Orthopedic Surgery, Set. Charles H. Epps, Jr. et al. 2nd ed. 1986. (Illus.). 1584p. text 175.00 (*0-397-50638-4*, Lippnctt) Lppncott W & W.

Complications of Pregnancy: Medical, Surgical, Gynecologic, Psychosocial & Perinatal. Sheldon H. Cherry et al. 4th ed. 1991. (Illus.). 1352p. 155.00 (*0-683-01672-5*) Lppncott W & W.

Complications of Regional Anesthesia. Brendan T. Finucane. Ed. by Allan Ross. 1999. LC 98-27027. 270p. text (*0-443-07536-0*) Church.

Complications of Shoulder Surgery. Louis U. Bigliani. 1993. LC 92-49883. (Illus.). 296p. 99.00 (*0-683-00751-3*) Lppncott W & W.

Complications of Spine Surgery. Steven R. Garfin. 1989. (Illus.). 500p. 80.00 (*0-683-03435-9*) Lppncott W & W.

Complications of Total Hip Arthroplasty. Richard H. Rothman & William J. Hozak. 1988. 256p. text 115.00 (*0-7216-2447-2*) Saunders.

Complications of Trauma. Ed. by Kenneth L. Mattox. 1994. (Illus.). 616p. text (*0-443-08851-9*) Church.

Complications of Trauma & Critical Care. Kimball I. Maull et al. 135th ed. 1996. LC 95-15497. (Illus.). 528p. text 120.00 (*0-7216-4940-8*) Saunders.

Complications of Urologic Surgery: Prevention & Management. Robert B. Smith & Erlich. 2nd ed. 1990. 544p. text 135.00 (*0-7216-8414-9*) Saunders.

Complications of Viral & Mycoplasmal Infections in Rodents to Toxicology Research & Testing. Ed. by Thomas E. Hamm, Jr. 1986. LC 84-12789. (Chemical Industry Institute of Toxicology Ser.). (Illus.). 300p. 115.00 (*0-89116-388-3*) Hemisp Pub.

Complying with OBRA: Managing Restraint Reduction Programs in Nursing Home & Healthcare Centers. Joseph K. Egbebike. Ed. by Jeff Gollin. 1994. LC 95-87071. (Illus.). 98p. (Orig.). pap. 36.95 (*0-9639841-0-1*) PTS Pubng.

Complying with the Bloodborne Pathogen Standard: A Step-by-Step Guide. Jane M. Whitehouse. 1992. 102p. pap. text 65.00 (*0-86587-327-5*) Gov Insts.

Component Selection: Polemics & Politics. Ed. by Joy L. Fridey & Marcus B. Simpson, Jr. 1996. LC 97-140511. (Illus.). 94p. pap. text 55.00 (*1-56395-065-0*, PC97-960012) Am Assn Blood.

Composite Materials for Implant Applications in the Human Body: Characterization & Testing. Ed. by Russel D. Jamison & Leslie N. Gilbertson. 1993. LC 92-44626. (Special Technical Publications: No. STP 1178). (Illus.). 165p. text 45.00 (*0-8031-1852-X*, STP1178) ASTM.

Composite Rhytidectomy. Sam T. Hamra. 1992. (Illus.). 252p. 245.00 incl. VHS (*1-57626-045-3*, QMP); LC 92-49030. (C). 200.00 (*0-942219-30-9*) Quality Med Pub.

Composite Tissue Transplantation. Charles W. Hewitt & Kirby S. Black. 1999. LC 98-8851. (Tissue Engineering Intelligence Unit Ser.: Vol. 2). (Illus.). 292p. 99.00 (*1-57059-554-2*) Landes Bioscience.

Comprehending Behavioral Statistics. Russell T. Hurlburt. (Psychology Ser.). 1995. 16.50 (*0-534-17424-8*); 1993. 25.50 (*0-534-17419-1*); 1993. pap., stu. ed. 18.50 (*0-534-17420-5*); 2nd ed. 1997. pap. 17.25 (*0-534-35043-7*); 2nd ed. 1997. LC 97-26026. 571p. spiral bd. 88.95 (*0-534-34889-0*) Brooks-Cole.

Comprehensive Adolescent Health Care. Ed. by Friedman. 2nd ed. 1997. LC 95-296. (Illus.). 1376p. (C). (gr. 13). text 150.00 (*0-8151-3386-3*, 27146) Mosby Inc.

Comprehensive, Annotated Bibliography of Selected Psychological Tests: Interpersonal Checklist, MMPI Short Forms, the Blacky Pictures. Earl S. Taulbee & Thomas L. Clark. 1982. LC 81-52806. x, 248p. 39.50 (*0-87875-231-5*) Whitston Pub.

Comprehensive Approach to Stereotactic Breast Biopsy. Laurie L. Fajardo et al. 1996. LC 95-44397. 250p. 95.00 (*0-86542-467-5*) Blackwell Sci.

Comprehensive Bibliography for Hyperemesis: Gravidarum &/or Morning Sickness. Ed. by Miriam Erick. rev. ed. 1993. 55p. 17.00 (*0-9613063-6-X*) Grinnen-Barrett Pub Co.

Comprehensive Bibliography of the Thanatology Literature. Martin L. Kutscher. 1979. 18.95 (*0-405-12510-0*) Ayer.

Comprehensive Bibliography of the Thanatology Literature. Ed. by Martin L. Kutscher et al. 1976. LC 75-5627. 285p. 14.00 (*0-8422-7274-7*) Irvington.

Comprehensive Bibliography on American Sign Language: A Resource Manual. Tom Federlin. 1979. LC 79-54021. pap. 15.00 (*0-9603136-0-5*) Federlin.

Comprehensive Biotechnology: The Principles, Applications & Regulations of Biotechnology in Industry, Agriculture & Medicine Ed. by M. Moo-Young. 1985. (Illus.). 3764p. 1562.00 (*0-08-026204-X*); 632p. 314.50 (*0-08-032510-6*) Elsevier (Pergamon Pr).

Comprehensive Breast Care: Surviving Breast Cancer. Joel A. Berman. Ed. by Adolph Caso. 2000. LC 00-42943. (Illus.). 308p. pap. 19.95 (*0-8283-2057-8*) Branden Bks.

Comprehensive Cancer Cytopathology of the Cervix Uteri. Ed. by Yi-Jing Shu et al. 1995. (Illus.). 496p. pap. 105.00 (*0-07-057219-4*) McGraw-Hill Educ Grp.

Comprehensive Cancer Nursing Review. Susan L. Groenwald. 1992. (Nursing-Health Science Ser.). (Illus.). 576p. (C). pap. text 34.95 (*0-86720-335-8*, 335-8) Jones & Bartlett.

Comprehensive Cancer Nursing Review. Susan L. Groenwald et al. 4th ed. 1997. LC 97-42396. (Nursing Ser.). (Illus.). 800p. (C). pap. text 44.95 (*0-7637-0541-1*, 0541-1) Jones & Bartlett.

Comprehensive Cancer Nursing Review. Connie H. Yarbro et al. 5th ed. 2001. (Illus.). 704p. (C). pap. text 42.95 (*0-7637-1473-9*, 1473-9) Jones & Bartlett.

Comprehensive Cardiac Rehabilitation, 2nd World Congress, Jerusalem, 1981. Ed. by J. J. Kellermann. 1982. (Advances in Cardiology Ser.: Vol. 31). (Illus.). x, 246p. 104.50 (*3-8055-3539-2*) S Karger.

Comprehensive Cardiovascular Community Control Programmes in Europe. P. Puska & E. Leparski. 1988. (Euro Reports & Studies Ser.: No. 106). 91p. pap. text 6.00 (*92-890-1272-2*) World Health.

Comprehensive Cardiovascular Medicine. Eric J. Topol. 1998. 3376p. 374.95 (*0-7817-1864-3*) Lppncott W & W.

Comprehensive Care for People with Epilepsy. Margarete Pfafflin et al. 2001. 350p. (*0-86196-610-4*) John Libby GBR. *Dist:* Buttrwrth-Heinemann.

Comprehensive Care of the Pediatric Patient: Prehospital Through Rehabilitation. Anne C. Albers et al. Ed. by Marion E. Broome. Date not set. 249p. pap. text 16.00 (*0-935890-25-4*) Emerg Nurses IL.

Comprehensive Case Management for Substance Abuse Treatment. Ed. by Sandra Clunies. 2000. 121p. reprint ed. pap. text 25.00 (*0-7567-0255-0*) DIANE Pub.

Comprehensive Casebook of Cognitive Therapy. Ed. by Arthur Freeman & F. M. Dattilio. 1992. (Illus.). 410p. (C). 75.00 (*0-306-44069-5*); pap. 42.50 (*0-306-44070-9*) Perseus Pubng (Plenum Trade).

Comprehensive Chemical Kinetics: Complex Catalytic Processes, Vol. 20. Ed. by C. H. Bamford & C. F. Tipper. 1978. xii,414p. 333.00 (*0-444-41651-X*) Elsevier.

Comprehensive Chemical Kinetics Vol. 30: Electron Tunneling in Chemistry. Ed. by R. G. Compton. 1989. 360p. 323.50 (*0-444-87364-3*) Elsevier.

Comprehensive Classification of Fractures. M. E. Miller. 1994. 300p. 145.00 incl. audio compact disk (*0-387-14150-2*) Spr-Verlag.

Comprehensive Classification of Fractures of Long Bones. M. E. Muller et al. 1994. (Illus.). 224p. 95.00 (*0-387-18165-2*) Spr-Verlag.

Comprehensive Clinical Management of the Epilepsies. Epilepsy Foundation of America Staff. 1992. 32p. pap. 2.95 (*0-916570-19-3*) Epilepsy Foundation of America.

Comprehensive Clinical Nephrology. Ed. by Richard J. Johnson & John Feehally. 1999. 179.95 (*0-7234-3117-5*) Mosby Inc.

Comprehensive Clinical Neurophysiology. Ed. by Kerry H. Levin & Hans O. Luders. Date not set. LC 99-59398. (Illus.). 605p. text (*0-7216-7656-1*) Saunders.

Comprehensive Clinical Psychology Ed. by Michel Hersen & Alan S. Bellack. 1998. LC 97-50185. (Illus.). 7000p. 3495.00 (*0-08-042707-3*, Pergamon Pr) Elsevier.

Comprehensive Community Health Nursing. Susan Clemen-Stone et al. 5th ed. 1997. LC 97-35023. (Illus.). 888p. (C). (gr. 13). text 51.00 (*0-8151-1324-2*, 29597) Mosby Inc.

Comprehensive Community Health Nursing: Includes Testbank. Susan Clemen-Stone et al. 5th ed. 1998. (Illus.). 888p. tchr. ed. (*1-55664-432-9*) Mosby Inc.

Comprehensive Curriculum for Trauma Nursing. Elizabeth W. Bayley & Turcke. 1992. (Nursing Ser.). (Illus.). (C). pap. text 49.95 (*0-86720-331-5*, 331-5) Jones & Bartlett.

Comprehensive Curriculum for Trauma Nursing. Elizabeth W. Bayley & Susan A. Turcke. 2nd rev. ed. Date not set. (Illus.). 696p. pap. text 55.00 (*0-935890-19-X*) Emerg Nurses IL.

Comprehensive Cytopathology. Marluse Bibbo. Ed. by Lesley Day. 2nd ed. 1996. LC 95-48273. (Illus.). 1216p. text 205.00 (*0-7216-5752-4*) Saunders.

Comprehensive Dental Assisting. Betty Ladley Finkbeiner & Claudia S. Johnson. 1995. (Illus.). 256p. (C). (gr. 13). pap. text, stu. ed. (*0-8151-3203-4*, 25102) Mosby Inc.

Comprehensive Dental Assisting. Patt Finkbeiner. 1993. (Illus.). text (*0-397-54870-2*) Lppncott W & W.

Comprehensive Dental Assisting. Gabriel. 1990. (Education Ser.). pap., tchr. ed. 8.00 (*0-8273-3939-9*); pap., wbk. ed. 14.95 (*0-8273-3940-2*) Delmar.

Comprehensive Dental Assisting: A Clinical Approach. Ed. by Betty Ladley Finkbeiner & Claudia S. Johnson. 1994. LC 94-31991. (Illus.). 1200p. (C). (gr. 13). text 46.00 (*0-8151-3239-5*, 24181) Mosby Inc.

Comprehensive Dental Hygiene Care. Irene R. Woodall. 4th ed. 1993. (Illus.). 896p. (C). (gr. 13). text 67.00 (*0-8016-7019-5*, 07019) Mosby Inc.

Comprehensive Diagnosis, Ethics & Quality of Life. Ed. by J. E. Mezzich & M. Schmolke. 1999. (Psychopathology Ser.: Vol. 32, No. 3 (1999)). (Illus.). 56p. pap. 25.25 (*3-8055-6839-8*) S Karger.

Comprehensive Diagnostic Test to Evaluate Motor & Cognitive Ability for the Ambulatory Severely Mentally Retarded. George Redey & Eugene Spatz. 1976. LC 76-23718. 100p. 5.00 (*0-935484-00-0*) Universe Pub Co.

Comprehensive Electrocardiology: Theory & Practice in Health & Disease, Set. Ed. by Peter W. Macfarlane & T. D. Lawrie. 1988. LC 88-17891. (Illus.). 1900p. 715.00 (*0-08-035568-4*, Pergamon Pr) Elsevier.

Comprehensive Evaluation & Treatment of Epilepsy: A Practical Guide. Ed. by Steven C. Schachter & Donald L. Schomer. (Illus.). 1997. LC 97-10913. 300p. text 34.95 (*0-12-621355-0*); 1998. 268p. (C). reprint ed. pap. text 34.95 (*0-12-621356-9*) Morgan Kaufmann.

Comprehensive Exit Examination for Undergraduate (B.Sc) Degree Program in Health Care Administration. Edward Khiwa-Kiwuwa. 1994. 5p. (C). text, stu. ed. 25.95 (*0-9643899-2-4*) E K Kiwuwa.

Comprehensive Fertility Awareness & Natural Family Planning see Couple's Guide to Fertility: The Complete Sympto-Thermal Method

Comprehensive Forensic Services Manual: The Essential Resources for All Experts. James Mangraviti, Jr. et al. 2000. 621p. 124.99 (*1-892904-07-1*) SEAK.

Comprehensive Geriatric Oncology. Ed. by Lodovico Balducci et al. 1997. 824p. text 185.00 (*90-5702-225-7*, Harwood Acad Pubs) Gordon & Breach.

Comprehensive Glossary of Psychiatry & Psychology. Harold I. Kaplan & Benjamin J. Sadock. 1991. 224p. 34.95 (*0-683-04527-X*) Lppncott W & W.

Comprehensive Glossary of Recreational Therapy. David R. Austin. 1994. 54p. (Orig.). pap. text 12.50 (*1-889435-05-8*) Am Therapeutic.

Comprehensive Guide to Arthritis. James F. Fries. 3rd ed. 1990. pap. 12.95 (*0-201-52402-3*) Addison-Wesley.

Comprehensive Guide to Attention Deficit Disorder in Adults: Research, Diagnosis, & Treatment. Ed. by Kathleen G. Nadeau. 1995. LC 94-44015. 432p. 39.95 (*0-87630-760-8*) Brunner-Routledge.

Comprehensive Guide to Child Psychotherapy. Christiane Brems. 1993. LC 92-24692. 416p. 107.00 (*0-205-14708-9*) Allyn.

Comprehensive Guide to Malpractice Risk Management in Psychiatry. Ed. by Frederic F. Flach. 1998. LC 97-36799. (CME Bks.). 384p. pap. 39.95 (*1-57826-013-2*, Five Star Pub) Hatherleigh.

Comprehensive Guide to Medical Halachah. Abraham S. Abraham. 1990. Orig. Title: Medical Halacha for Everyone. 25.95 (*0-87306-529-8*) Feldheim.

Comprehensive Guide to the Cannabis Literature. Compiled by Ernest L. Abel. 1979. LC 78-20014. 699p. lib. bdg. 115.00 (*0-313-20721-6*, ACG/, Greenwood Pr) Greenwood.

Comprehensive Guide to the Hazardous Properties of Chemical Substances. Pradyot Patnaik. 1992. 800p. text 119.95 (*0-442-00191-6*, VNR) Wiley.

Comprehensive Guide to the Therapeutic Use of Aminoglutethimide. Ed. by R. J. Santen et al. 2nd rev. ed. 1981. (Pharmanual Ser.: Vol. 2). (Illus.). vi, 162p. pap. 37.50 (*3-8055-3452-3*) S Karger.

Comprehensive Guide to the Therapeutic Use of Cefsulodin. Ed. by L. D. Sabath & M. Finland. 1980. (Pharmanual Ser.: Vol. 1). (Illus.). vi, 94p. pap. 21.00 (*3-8055-1042-X*) S Karger.

Comprehensive Guide to the Therapeutic Use of Trasicor. Ed. by J. Stevo. 1984. (Pharmanual Ser.: Vol. 4). (Illus.). viii, 116p. pap. 33.25 (*3-8055-3836-7*) S Karger.

Comprehensive Guide to Work Injury Management. Ed. by Susan J. Isernhagen. 2000. 854p. 99.00 (*0-8342-0558-0*, 20558) PRO-ED.

Comprehensive Gynecology. Morton A. Stenchever & Daniel R. Mishell. 3rd ed. 1997. LC 96-35516. (Illus.). 1296p. (C). (gr. 13). text 119.95 (*0-8151-6955-8*, 27227) Mosby Inc.

***Comprehensive Gynecology: Tratado de Ginecologia.** Daniel R. Mishell et al. 3rd ed. 1997. (ENG & SPA., Illus.). 1296p. (*84-8174-324-0*) Mosby-Doyma Libros ESP. *Dist:* Mosby Inc.

Comprehensive Gynecology Package Review. Daniel R. Mishell & Frank W. Ling. 1997. 139.95 (*0-8151-6342-8*) Mosby Inc.

Comprehensive Gynecology Review. Frank W. Ling & Laube. 3rd ed. 1997. LC 97-163936. (Illus.). 288p. (C). (gr. 13). pap. text 33.95 (*0-8151-5512-3*, 28451) Mosby Inc.

Comprehensive Handbook for the Practitioner. K. Majumdar. 1984. (C). (*0-89771-354-0*) Current Dist IND. *Dist:* St Mut.

Comprehensive Handbook of Cognitive Therapy. Ed. by Arthur Freeman et al. 1989. (Illus.). 640p. (C). 95.00 (*0-306-43052-5*, Plenum Trade) Perseus Pubng.

Comprehensive Handbook of Drug & Alcohol Addiction. Ed. by Norman S. Miller. 1991. (Illus.). 1360p. text 75.00 (*0-8247-8474-X*) Dekker.

Comprehensive Handbook of Psychopathology. Ed. by Henry E. Adams & Patricia B. Sutker. (Illus.). 2nd ed. 1993. 930p. (C). text 114.00 (*0-306-44169-1*); 3rd ed. 2000. LC 00-46622. xviii, 970p. 125.00 (*0-306-46490-X*) Kluwer Academic (Kluwer Plenum).

Comprehensive Handbook of Psychotherapy Integration. Ed. by George Stricker & J. R. Gold. 1993. (Illus.). 576p. (C). 85.00 (*0-306-44280-9*, Plenum Trade) Perseus Pubng.

Comprehensive Health Care for Everyone: A Guide for Body, Mind & Spirit. Thomas Collins. 1995. LC 95-18693. (Illus.). 418p. (Orig.). pap. 19.95 (0-931892-97-X) B Dolphin Pub.

Comprehensive Human Physiology Ed. by R. Greger & U. Windhorst. 1996. (Illus.). 2551p. 138.00 (0-387-58109-X) Spr-Verlag.

Comprehensive Human Physiology: From Cellular Mechanisms to Integration. Ed. by R. Greger & U. Windhorst. 1995. LC 95-34793. (Illus.). 2527p. (3-540-58109-X) Spr-Verlag.

Comprehensive Index of Group Psychotherapy Writings. Bernard Lubin. 1987. (American Group Psychotherapy Association Monographs: No. 2). (C). 85.00 (0-8236-1045-4) Intl Univs Pr.

Comprehensive Index to the Journal of Forensic Sciences, 1972-1986. Ed. by Abel M. Dominguez. 1987. LC 87-17453. 35.00 (0-8031-0984-9, JOFSINDX87) ASTM.

Comprehensive Insect Physiology, Biochemistry & Pharmacology, Set. Ed. by G. A. Kerkut. 1985. (Illus.). 8536p. 3717.50 (0-08-026850-1, Pergamon Pr) Elsevier.

Comprehensive Intraaortic Balloon Counterpulsation. Susan J. Quaal. 2nd ed. 1993. LC 92-48411. (Illus.). 581p. (C). (gr. 13). pap. text 38.95 (0-8016-6656-2, 06656) Mosby Inc.

Comprehensive Management of Head & Neck Tumors. Stanley E. Thawley. 2nd ed. 1999. LC 96-46194. xxix, 1981 p. (0-7216-5599-8) Saunders.

Comprehensive Management of Head & Neck Tumors. Stanley E. Thawley et al. Ed. by Stephanie Donley. 2nd ed. 1998. LC 96-46194. (Illus.). 1792p. (C). text 295.00 (0-7216-5582-3) Saunders.

Comprehensive Management of Parkinson's Disease. Andrea M. Cohen & William J. Weiner. 1994. LC 94-26984. (Comprehension Neurologic Rehabilitation Ser.: Vol. 8). 288p. text 44.95 (0-939957-74-4) Demos Medical.

Comprehensive Management of Spina Bifida. Ed. by Harold L. Rekate. 1990. 264p. 139.00 (0-8493-0151-3, RJ496) CRC Pr.

Comprehensive Management of Spinal Cord Injury. Lorraine Buchanan. 1987. 288p. 45.00 (0-683-01128-6) Lppncott W & W.

Comprehensive Management of Spine Trauma. Ed. by Daniel A. Capen & Willi Haye. 1998. LC 97-42383. (Illus.). 512p. text 125.00 (0-8151-1463-X, 29184) Mosby Inc.

Comprehensive Management of the Menopause. Ed. by Jacques Lorrain et al. 1994. LC 93-3255. (Clinical Perspectives in Obstetrics & Gynecology Ser.). (Illus.). 455p. 115.00 (0-387-97972-7) Spr-Verlag.

Comprehensive Management of the Upper Limb Amputee. Ed. by D. J. Atkins & R. H. Meier, III. 1988. (Illus.). 260p. 119.00 (0-387-96779-6) Spr-Verlag.

Comprehensive Manual of Taping & Wrapping Techniques. Kenneth E. Wright & William R. Whitehill. 2nd rev. ed. 1996. (Illus.). 177p. pap. text 24.95 (1-889366-00-5) Cramer Prods.

Comprehensive Maternity Nursing. Martha Auvenshine & Martha Enriquez. 2nd ed. 1989. 1000p. 58.75 (0-86720-421-4) Jones & Bartlett.

Comprehensive Medical. Chesebro. 1995. pap. text, wbk. ed. (0-89303-153-4) Brady Pub.

Comprehensive Medical Assisting. Shirley A. Badasch & Doreen Chesebro. 1995. (C). (0-89303-154-2) Appleton & Lange.

Comprehensive Medical Assisting. Lindh. 1997. (Medical Assisting Ser). (C). pap., wbk. ed. 19.25 (0-8273-6765-1) Thomson Learn.

Comprehensive Medical Assisting. Lindh. 1997. (Medical Assisting Ser.). tchr. ed. 19.95 (0-8273-6763-5, VNR) Wiley.

Comprehensive Medical Assisting: Competencies for Administrative & Clinical Practice. Mary A. Frew et al. 3rd ed. 1994. (Illus.). 930p. (C). text 43.95 (0-8036-3871-X) Davis Co.

Comprehensive Medical Codes. Carol J. Buck. Ed. by Adrianne Williams. 1999. LC 98-38028. (Illus.). xxiv, 1357p. text 60.00 (0-7216-7787-8) Saunders.

Comprehensive Medical Handbook. M. Majumdar. 1984. (C). (0-7855-4665-0) Current Dist IND. *Dist:* St Mut.

Comprehensive Medical Terminology - IML. Jones Staff. 1998. 240p. tchr. ed. 21.95 (0-7668-0495-X) Delmar.

Comprehensive Medical Thesaurus with Concise Etymological Analysis. John Ohno. 1999. 304p. pap. 29.95 (1-58244-012-3) Rutledge Bks.

Comprehensive Medicinal Chemistry Ed. by Corwin Hansch. 1990. (Rational Design, Mechanistic Study & Therapeutic Application of Chemical Compounds Ser.). (Illus.). 6000p. 1750.00 (0-08-030700-0, Pergamon Pr) Elsevier.

Comprehensive Medicine: An Oriental & Occidental Overview of Biopsychosocial Medicine. Katsutaro Nagata et al. 1998. LC 98-71383. (Illus.). 205p. lib. bdg. 52.00 (0-934314-02-0) Intl Found Biosocial Dev.

Comprehensive Multimedia Pharmacology Course. Anne Nichols & Michael Gibbs. 2000. 80p. 99.95 incl. cd-rom (0-9679170-2-6) NPeducationcom.

Comprehensive NCLEX PN Review 2000. Patricia A. Hoefler. 4th ed. 1999. 368p. (C). pap. text 34.95 incl. cd-rom (1-56533-036-6) M E D S Inc.

Comprehensive NCLEX-RN Review 2000. Patricia A. Hoefler. 9th ed. 1998. (Illus.). 374p. (C). pap. text 34.95 incl. cd-rom (1-56533-307-1) M E D S Inc.

Comprehensive Neonatal Nursing: A Physiologic Perspective. Carole A. Kenner et al. Ed. by Ilze Rader. 2nd ed. 1997. LC 97-703. (Illus.). 1104p. text 99.00 (0-7216-6535-7) Saunders.

Comprehensive Neurology. Ed. by Roger N. Rosenberg & David E. Pleasure. 2nd ed. 1998. LC 97-40569. 948p. 257.00 (0-471-16958-7, Wiley-Liss) Wiley.

Comprehensive Neurosurgery Board Review. Jonathan S. Citow. 2000. LC 99-59264. 392p. pap. 79.00 (0-86577-889-2) Thieme Med Pubs.

Comprehensive Nursing Care in Multiple Sclerosis. Ed. by June Halper & Nancy J. Holland. 1996. LC 96-46912. 286p. pap. text 39.95 (1-888799-05-6) Demos Medical.

Comprehensive Perinatal & Pediatric Respiratory Care. Kent Whitaker. 1993. pap. 39.95 (0-8273-3850-3); 1992. pap., stu. ed. 17.95 (0-8273-3855-4) Delmar.

Comprehensive Perinatal & Pediatric Respiratory Care. Kent B. Whitaker. 2nd ed. 1997. 720p. pap. (0-8273-8286-3); 1996. LC 96-9269. 768p. (C). mass mkt. 53.95 (0-8273-7392-9) Delmar.

Comprehensive Periodontics for the Dental Hygienist. Ed. by Mea A. Weinberg. 2000. LC 00-63717. 627p. (C). pap. text 46.00 (0-8385-1554-1) P-H.

Comprehensive Perioperative Nursing Barbara J. Gruendemann & Billie Fernsebner. 1995. (Nursing Ser.). Set. text 80.95 (0-86720-731-0); Vol. 1. (Illus.). 576p. (C). text 52.95 (0-86720-647-0, 647-0); Vol. 2. (Illus.). 592p. (C). text 52.95 (0-86720-719-1, 719-1) Jones & Bartlett.

Comprehensive Perioperative Nursing Review. Susan Fairchild. 1993. (Illus.). 350p. (C). pap. text 47.95 (0-86720-644-6, 644-6) Jones & Bartlett.

Comprehensive Pharmacy Review. Shargel. 2nd ed. 1993. (National Medical Series for Independent Study). 30.00 (0-683-06253-0) Lppncott W & W.

Comprehensive Pharmacy Review. Leon Shargel et al. 4th ed. 2001. 1,248p. pap. text 38.00 (0-7817-2147-4) Lppncott W & W.

Comprehensive Pharmacy Review: Practice Exams. Alan H. Mutnick et al. 1997. (National Medical Series for Independent Study). 175p. (0-683-23137-5) Lppncott W & W.

Comprehensive Pharmacy Review Practice Exams. Ed. by Alan H. Mutnick et al. 2nd rev. ed. 1994. LC 93-47687. 19.95 (0-683-06255-7) Lppncott W & W.

Comprehensive Physical Therapy Assistant Board Review. Shirley J. Brister. 1995. LC 95-31273. (Illus.). 304p. (C). (gr. 13). pap. text 39.95 (0-8151-1010-3, 26358) Mosby Inc.

Comprehensive Podiatric Medicine & Surgery. Tessler. Ed. by Stephen J. Kominsky. 1997. 1480p. (C). (gr. 13). text 189.95 (0-8151-5250-7) Mosby Inc.

Comprehensive Postanesthesia Care. Ed. by Morris Brown & Eli M. Brown. 1997. LC 96-14627. (Illus.). 586p. 89.00 (0-683-01116-2) Lppncott W & W.

Comprehensive Primer on Medical Genetics. T. F. Thurmon. 1999. LC 99-10581. (Illus.). 484p. 43.95 (1-85070-066-4) CRC Pr.

Comprehensive Psychiatric Nursing. Ed. by Judith Haber et al. 5th ed. 1996. LC 96-46940. (Illus.). 960p. (C). (gr. 13). text 52.00 (0-8151-4179-3, 27651) Mosby Inc.

Comprehensive Psychiatric Nursing: Includes Testbank. Judith Haber et al. 5th ed. 1997. (Illus.). tchr. ed. (0-8151-4272-2) Mosby Inc.

Comprehensive Psychotherapy, Vol. 3. Paul T. Olsen. 1984. 183p. pap. 109.00 (0-677-16369-X) Gordon & Breach.

Comprehensive Radiographic Pathology. Ronald L. Eisenberg & Cynthia A. Dennis. 2nd ed. 1995. (Illus.). 416p. (C). (gr. 13). text 54.00 (0-8151-3144-5, 24084) Mosby Inc.

Comprehensive Rehabilitation Nursing. Jill B. Derstine & Shirlee Drayton-Hargrove. 2000. LC 99-40815. (Illus.). viii, 631p. text 69.00 (0-7216-6977-8) Saunders.

Comprehensive Respiratory Care. David R. Dantzker et al. 1995. (Illus.). 1104p. text 66.00 (0-7216-2844-3) Saunders.

Comprehensive Respiratory Care. Eubanks et al. 2nd ed. 1990. (Illus.). 1040p. (C). (gr. 13). text 59.95 (0-8016-2932-2, 02932) Mosby Inc.

Comprehensive Respiratory Home. Minderman. 1999. text (0-7216-6546-2) Saunders.

Comprehensive Review. Linda Anne Silvestri. 1999. LC 98-3399. (C). pap. text 32.95 (0-7216-7795-9) Saunders.

Comprehensive Review for the Certification & Recertification Examinations. American Academy of Physician Assitants Staff et al. Ed. by Sarah Zarbock Goltzer & Rebeca Lovell Scott. 1999. LC 98-32027. 293p. 37.95 (0-683-30367-8) Lppncott W & W.

Comprehensive Review for the Radiology Registry: A Centralized Resource. Mark F. Pierce & Richard L. Carnovale. 1998. LC 97-42655. (Illus.). 250p. pap. 29.95 (0-683-30145-4) Lppncott W & W.

Comprehensive Review for Veterinary Technicians. Tighe & Brown. 1998. (Illus.). 441p. (C). (gr. 13). pap. text 29.95 (0-8151-9044-1, 29175) Mosby Inc.

Comprehensive Review in Respiratory Care. Vijay M. Deshpande et al. 1988. LC 88-14495. (Illus.). 398p. (C). pap. 52.21 (0-8385-1295-X, A1295-3) P-H.

Comprehensive Review in Toxicology for Emergency Clinicians. Peter D. Bryson. 3rd ed. 1996. LC 96-9209. 960p. 125.00 (1-56032-612-3) Hemisp Pub.

Comprehensive Review of Canadian Nursing. Delores F. Saxton. 1996. (Illus.). 1024p. (C). (gr. 13). pap. text 32.90 (0-8151-8673-8, 28965) Mosby Inc.

Comprehensive Review of Dental Assisting. Patt Finkbeiner et al. 1997. LC 96-45090. (Illus.). 560p. (C). (gr. 13). pap. text 34.95 (0-8151-3303-0, 26957) Mosby Inc.

Comprehensive Review of Geriatric Psychiatry II. Ed. by Joel Sadavoy et al. 2nd ed. 1996. LC 90-1203. 1152p. text 99.00 (0-88048-723-2, 8723) Am Psychiatric.

Comprehensive Review of Nursing for Canada. Delores F. Saxton. 1996. 25.80 (0-8151-4606-X) Mosby Inc.

Comprehensive Review of Radiography. Callaway. 2nd rev. ed. 2000. 315p. text 39.95 (0-323-01191-8) Mosby Inc.

***Comprehensive Russian - English Medical Dictionary.** Ed. by Russo, Moscow Staff. 2nd ed. 2001. (ENG & RUS.). 694p. (5-88721-184-9) Russo RUS. *Dist:* Coronet Bks.

Comprehensive School Health Challenge: Promoting Health Through Education. Ed. by Peter Cortese & Kathleen Middleton. 1993. LC 93-24711. 62.95 (1-56071-344-5) ETR Assocs.

Comprehensive Sourcebook of Bacterial Protein Toxins. Joseph E. Alouf. 2nd ed. 1999. LC 99-62163. (Illus.). 704p. 159.95 (0-12-053075-9) Acad Pr.

Comprehensive Sports Injury Management. Jim Taylor et al. 2001. 300p. pap. 55.00 (0-8342-1643-4) PRO-ED.

Comprehensive Stress Management. Greenberg. 5th ed. 1995. tchr. ed. 12.81 (0-697-22307-8) McGraw.

Comprehensive Study Questions for the EMI-A: Basic Life Support. Jim Murray. 1982. (C). pap. text 22.00 (0-8359-0895-X) P-H.

Comprehensive Textbook of Ethics & Law in the Practice of Psychology. Ed. by Steven F. Bucky et al. 2000. LC 00-22848. (Issues in the Practice of Psychology Ser.). (0-306-46236-2, Kluwer Plenum) Kluwer Academic.

Comprehensive Textbook of Foot Surgery, Set, Vols. 1 & 2. E. Dalton McGlamry et al. 2nd ed. 1992. (Illus.). 1840p. text 325.00 (0-683-05857-6) Lppncott W & W.

Comprehensive Textbook of Oncology A. R. Moossa et al. 2nd ed. 1990. 1918p. 199.00 (0-683-06147-X) Lppncott W & W.

Comprehensive Textbook of Psychiatry Harold I. Kaplan & Benjamin J. Sadock. 5th ed. 1989. (Illus.). 2360p. 229.00 (0-683-04517-2) Lppncott W & W.

Comprehensive Textbook of Suicidology. Ronald W. Maris et al. 2000. LC 00-37640. 650p. 75.00 (1-57230-541-X, 8R0541) Guilford Pubns.

Comprehensive Textbook of Thoracic Oncology. Ed. by Joseph Aisner et al. 1996. LC 95-2030. (Illus.). 992p. text 165.00 (0-683-00062-4) Lppncott W & W.

Comprehensive Textbook of Vascular Access. Ed. by Scott Berman et al. 2000. (Illus.). 300p. text 85.00 (1-57626-000-3) Quality Med Pub.

Comprehensive Toxicology, Set. Sipes et al. 1997. 3161.00 incl. cd-rom (0-08-042981-5) Elsevier.

Comprehensive Training: Relaxation, Feeling & Value Solutions, Set Russell E. Mason. 1975. pap. 145.00 incl. audio (0-89533-021-0, 69.ST-CT) F I Comm.

Comprehensive Treatise of Electrochemistry Vol. 6: Electrodics-Transport. Ed. by John O. Bockris et al. 1982. LC 82-13144. (Illus.). 546p. (C). text 156.00 (0-306-40942-9, Kluwer Plenum) Kluwer Academic.

Comprehensive Treatise of Electrochemistry Vol. 10: Bioelectrochemistry. J. O. Bockris et al. 1985. (Illus.). 566p. (C). text 156.00 (0-306-41541-0, Kluwer Plenum) Kluwer Academic.

Comprehensive Urology. Robert M. Weiss et al. 2000. 225.00 (0-7234-2949-9) Mosby Inc.

Comprehensive Vascular Exposures. Ronald J. Stoney & David J. Effeney. 1998. LC 97-31576. (Illus.). 208p. text 139.00 (0-397-51342-9) Lppncott W & W.

Comprehensive Vet Dictionary. Baillieres. 1990. pap. text 40.95 (0-7020-1395-1) Saunders.

Comprehensive Virology Vol. 17: Methods Used in the Study of Viruses. Ed. by Heinz Fraenkel-Conrat & Robert R. Wagner. 1981. LC 80-21841. 480p. 89.50 (0-306-40418-4, Plenum Trade) Perseus Pubng.

Comprehensive Virology Vol. 19: Viral Cytopathology: Cellular Macromolecular Synthesis & Cytocidal Viruses. Ed. by Heinz Fraenkel-Conrat & Robert R. Wagner. 1984. LC 84-16081. (Illus.). 556p. (C). text 156.00 (0-306-41698-0, Kluwer Plenum) Kluwer Academic.

Comprehensive Wellness for Firefighters: Fitness & Health Guide for Fire & Rescue Workers. Jon Pearson et al. 1995. (Industrial Health & Safety Ser.). 368p. pap. 74.95 (0-471-28709-1, VNR) Wiley.

Comprehensive Wound Management. Glenn Irion. 2001. 350p. (C). pap. text 35.00 (1-55642-477-9) SLACK Inc.

Compression Anastomosis by Biofragmentable Rings: Proceedings of the Second European Workshop. Ed. by R. Engemann & A. Thiede. LC 94-33288. (Illus.). 184p. 1995. 114.00 (3-540-58418-8); 1994. 107.00 (0-387-58418-8) Spr-Verlag.

Compression for Clinicians. Theodore Venema. 1998. LC 98-28845. (Illus.). 161p. pap. text 49.95 (1-56593-973-5, 1926) Thomson Learn.

Comprogram: Hospital Space Allocation Ed. by Clifford D. Stewart et al. 1972. LC 73-158290. 58.00 (0-915250-02-0) Environ Design.

Compromised Scientist: William James in the Development of American Psychology. Daniel W. Bjork. 1983. LC 82-14690. (Illus.). 221p. text 61.50 (0-231-05500-5) Col U Pr.

Compulsion & Doubt, Set. Wilhelm Stekel. Ed. by Emil A. Guthiel. rev. ed. 1949. (C). 14.40 (0-87140-845-7) Liveright.

Compulsions to Confess: On the Psycho Analysis of Crime & Punishment. Theodor Reik. 1977. LC 72-1146. (Essay Index Reprint Ser.). reprint ed. 38.95 (0-8369-2856-3) Ayer.

Compulsory Health Insurance: The Continuing American Debate, 11. Ed. by Ronald L. Numbers. 1982. LC 82-6145. (Contributions in Medical History Ser.: No. 11). 172p. 55.00 (0-313-23436-1, NHI/, Greenwood Pr) Greenwood.

Compulsory Treatment of Drug Abuse: Research & Clinical Practice. 1991. lib. bdg. 75.00 (0-8490-4347-6) Gordon Pr.

Computation & Cognition: Toward A Foundation for Cognitive Science. Zenon W. Pylyshyn. 1986. 320p. (C). pap. 21.95 (0-262-66058-X, Bradford Bks) MIT Pr.

Computation, Dynamics, & Cognition. Marco Giunti. 1997. LC 96-12616. (Illus.). 192p. text 45.00 (0-19-509009-8) OUP.

Computational & Clinical Approaches to Pattern Recognition & Concept Formation: Quantitative Analyses of Behavior, Vol. 9. Michael L. Commons et al. 1990. 176p. 59.95 (0-8058-0399-8) L Erlbaum Assocs.

Computational Approaches in Molecular Radiation Biology: Monte Carlo Methods. M. N. Varma & A. Chatterjee. 1995. (Basic Life Sciences Ser.: Vol. 63). (Illus.). 274p. (C). text 89.50 (0-306-44995-1, Kluwer Plenum) Kluwer Academic.

Computational Approaches to Enzyme Structure & Function: Reprinted from the Journal, Enzyme, Vol. 36, No. 1-2, 1986. Ed. by H. Weinstein. 1986. (Illus.). 164p. pap. 69.75 (3-8055-4492-8) S Karger.

Computational Biology of the Heart. Ed. by Alexander Panfilov & Arun V. Holden. 1997. LC 97-139642. 428p. 220.00 (0-471-96020-9) Wiley.

Computational Biomedicine. Carlos A. Brebbia et al. Ed. by K. D. Held et al. 1993. LC 93-71017. (BIOMED Ser.: Vol. 2). 366p. (1-56252-162-4, 2386) WIT Pr GBR. *Dist:* Computational Mech MA.

Computational Brain. Patricia S. Churchland et al. 1994. (Computational Neuroscience Ser.). (Illus.). 576p. pap. 27.95 (0-262-53120-8, Bradford Bks) MIT Pr.

Computational Explorations in Cognitive Neuroscience: Understanding the Mind by Stimulating the Brain. Randall C. O'Reilly & Yuko Munakata. 2000. LC 99-86066. (Illus.). xxvii, 504p. pap. 50.00 (0-262-65054-1, Bradford Bks) MIT Pr.

Computational Medicine, Public Health & Biotechnology: Building a Man in the Machine. 1996. LC 96-210905. 2250p. 353.00 (981-02-2500-8); lib. bdg. 131.00 (981-02-2968-2); lib. bdg. 131.00 (981-02-2969-0); lib. bdg. 131.00 (981-02-2970-4) World Scientific Pub.

***Computational Models for the Prediction of Intestinal Membrane Permeability.** Patric Stenberg. 2001. (Comprehensive Summaries of Uppsala Dissertations from the Faculty of Pharmacy Ser.: No. 247). (Illus.). 66p. pap. (91-554-4934-4) Uppsala Universitet SWE. *Dist:* Coronet Bks.

Computational Neuroscience. Ed. by Eric L. Schwartz. (System Development Foundation, Benchmark Ser.). 456p. 1993. pap. 40.00 (0-262-69164-7, Bradford Bks); 1990. (Illus.). 55.00 (0-262-19291-8) MIT Pr.

Computational Neuroscience: Trends in Research. Ed. by James M. Bower. 1996. LC 96-207956. (International Review of Neurobiology Ser.: No. 1). (Illus.). 489p. pap. text, suppl. ed. 59.95 (0-12-121041-3) Acad Pr.

Computational Neuroscience: Trends in Research, 1997: Proceedings of the Annual Computational Neuroscience Conference Held in Boston, Massachusetts, July 14-17, 1996. Ed. by James M. Bower. 1997. LC 97-23178. 982p. 195.00 (0-306-45699-0, Kluwer Plenum) Kluwer Academic.

Computational Neuroscience: Trends in Research, 1998. Ed. by J. M. Bower. 1998. LC 98-25793. (Illus.). 658p. (C). text 175.00 (0-306-45919-1, Kluwer Plenum) Kluwer Academic.

Computational Psycholinguistics: AI & Connectionist Models of Human Language Processing. Ed. by Ton Dijkstra & Koenrad De Smedt. 1996. 288p. 89.95 (0-7484-0465-1); pap. 34.95 (0-7484-0466-X) Taylor & Francis.

Computational Psycholinguistics: An Interdisciplinary Approach to the Study of Language. Matthew W. Crocker. 1996. LC 95-43997. (Studies in Theoretical Psycholinguistics: Vol. 20). 260p. (C). lib. bdg. 112.00 (0-7923-3802-2) Kluwer Academic.

Computed Body Tomography with MRI Correlation. Ed. by Joseph K. Lee et al. 3rd ed. 1997. LC 96-17612. 1,664p. text 325.00 (0-7817-0291-7) Lppncott W & W.

Computed Tomography of the Lung. S. Galluzzi et al. 1988. 194p. text (1-57235-033-4) Piccin Nuova.

Computed Tomography of the Trunk: Normal & Pathological Anatomy. J. Hureau & J. Pradel. 1990. 488p. text (1-57235-034-2) Piccin Nuova.

Computed Tomographic Atlas of the Head & Neck. Wilma Maue-Dickson et al. 1983. 453p. 145.00 (0-316-55081-7, Little Brwn Med Div) Lppncott W & W.

C D

***Computed Tomography: Fundamentals, System Technology, Image Quality & Applications.** Willie A. Kalender. 2nd ed. 2000. (Illus.). 220p. 55.00 (*3-89578-081-2*) Wiley.

Computed Tomography & Magnetic Resonance Imaging. John R. Haaga et al. 3rd ed. 1994. (Illus.). 1826p. (C). (gr. 13). text 314.00 (*0-8016-7057-8*, 07057) Mosby Inc.

Computed Tomography & Magnetic Resonance Imaging. John R. Haaga et al. 3rd ed. 1995. (Illus.). 1826p. (*84-8174-171-X*) Mosby-Doyma Libros ESP. *Dist:* Mosby Inc.

Computed Tomography & Magnetic Resonance Imaging of the Head & Neck. Anthony Mancuso et al. 2nd ed. 1985. (Illus.). 504p. 102.00 (*0-683-05476-7*) Lppncott W & W.

Computed Tomography & Magnetic Resonance of the Thorax. David P. Naidich & Elias A. Zerhouni. 3rd ed. 1998. LC 98-36942. 784p. text 169.00 (*0-7817-1660-8*) Lppncott W & W.

Computed Tomography & Magnetic Resonance Tomography of Intracranial Tumors. Ed. by E. Kazner et al. 2nd ed. 1989. (Illus.). 685p. 600.00 (*0-387-50576-8*, 1954) Spr-Verlag.

***Computed Tomography & MRI of the Whole Body.** John R. Haaga & Charles Lanzieri. 4th ed. 2001. LC 2001-42808. (Illus.). 1995p. (*0-323-01133-0*) Mosby Inc.

Computed Tomography in Intracranial Tumors: Differential Diagnosis & Clinical Aspects. Ed. by E. Kazner et al. Tr. by F. C. Dougherty from GER. 1982. (Illus.). 548p. 267.00 (*0-387-10815-7*) Spr-Verlag.

Computed Tomography of CNS Disease. Douglas H. Yock. 2nd ed. 1990. (Illus.). 526p. (C). (gr. 13). pap. text 105.00 (*0-8151-9778-0*, 20394) Mosby Inc.

Computed Tomography of the Body: With Magnetic Resonance Imaging Ed. by Albert A. Moss et al. 2nd ed. 1991. (Illus.). 1477p. text 299.00 (*0-7216-2415-4*) Saunders.

Computed Tomography of the Body Vol. 1: With Magnetic Resonance Imaging: Thorax & Neck. Ed. by Albert A. Moss et al. 2nd ed. 1991. (Illus.). 492p. text 155.00 (*0-7216-4358-2*) Saunders.

Computed Tomography of the Body Vol. 2: With Magnetic Resonance Imaging: Bone & Joint, Vol. 2. Ed. by Albert A. Moss et al. 2nd ed. 1991. (Illus.). 492p. text 75.00 (*0-7216-4359-0*) Saunders.

Computed Tomography of the Body Vol. 3: With Magnetic Resonance Imaging: Abdomen, Vol. 3. Ed. by Albert A. Moss et al. 2nd ed. 1991. (Illus.). 493p. text 199.00 (*0-7216-4503-8*) Saunders.

Computed Tomography of the Cranial Skeleton: Face & Skull. M. Megret. Tr. by M. T. Wackenheim from FRE. 1986. (Exercises in Radiological Diagnosis Ser.). (Illus.). 168p. 35.95 (*0-387-15389-6*) Spr-Verlag.

Computed Tomography of the Gastrointestinal Tract. Ed. by M. A. Meyers. 1986. (Illus.). 279p. 200.00 (*0-387-96232-8*) Spr-Verlag.

Computed Tomography of the Pituitary Gland. J. F. Bonneville et al. 1986. (Illus.). 256p. 301.00 (*0-387-15324-1*) Spr-Verlag.

Computed Tomography of the Retroperitoneum. M. A. Feldberg. 1983. (Radiology Ser.). text 206.50 (*0-89838-573-3*) Kluwer Academic.

Computer Advancements in the Health Sciences: Index of New Information with Authors & Subjects. Richard L. Hasborough. 1992. LC 92-54220. 180p. pap. 44.50 (*1-55914-001-1*) ABBE Pubs Assn.

Computer Aid in Gastroenterology. Ed. by P. Rozen & F. T. De Dombal. 1984. (Frontiers of Gastrointestinal Research Ser.: Vol. 7). (Illus.). viii, 196p. 71.50 (*3-8055-3770-0*) S Karger.

Computer-Aided Diagnosis in Medical Imaging: Proceedings of the First International Workshop on Computer-Aided Diagnosis, Chicago, U.S.A., 20-23 September 1998. Ed. by Kunio Doi. 1999. LC 99-35907. (International Congress Ser.). 580p. 186.00 (*0-444-50058-8*) Elsevier.

Computer-Aided Drug Design: Methods & Applications. C. Propst & Thomas Perun. 1989. (Illus.). 516p. text 175.00 (*0-8247-8037-X*) Dekker.

Computer-Aided Electromyography. Ed. by J. E. Desmedt. 1983. (Progress in Clinical Neurophysiology Ser.: Vol. 10). (Illus.). x, 334p. 143.50 (*3-8055-3748-4*) S Karger.

Computer Aids to Clinical Decisions Ed. by Ben T. Williams. 1982. 168p. 99.00 (*0-8493-5575-3*, R858); 216p. 123.00 (*0-8493-5576-1*, R858) Franklin (CRC Reprint).

Computer Analysis of Electrophysiological Signals. John Dempster. 1993. (Biological Techniques Ser.). (Illus.). 228p. 73.00 (*0-12-208940-5*) Acad Pr.

Computer & the Brain. John Von Neumann. 1979. LC 58-6542. (Silliman Lectures Ser.). pap. 10.00 (*0-300-02415-0*) Yale U Pr.

Computer & the Brain. John Von Neumann et al. 2nd ed. 2000. LC 00-26937. (Mrs. Hepsa Ely Silliman Memorial Lectures). xxviii, 82p. pap. 9.95 (*0-300-08473-0*) Yale U Pr.

Computer & the Mind: An Introduction to Cognitive Science. P. N. Johnson-Laird. 1988. LC 87-29841. (Illus.). 448p. 40.00 (*0-674-15615-3*) HUP.

Computer Applications for Augmenting the Management of Speech, Language & Hearing Disorders. Franklin H. Silverman. 1996. LC 96-9411. 324p. 70.00 (*0-13-124140-0*) P-H.

Computer Applications in Biotechnology: The 6th International Conference, Garmisch-Partenkirchen, Germany, May 14-17, 1995. Ed. by A. Munack & K. Schugerl. 1995. (IFAC Ser.). 378p. pap. 79.50 (*0-08-042377-9*, Pergamon Pr) Elsevier.

Computer Applications in Dermatology. William V. Stoecker. 1993. LC 93-9621. (Illus.). 272p. pap. 85.00 (*0-89640-238-X*) Igaku-Shoin.

Computer Applications in Diagnostic Radiology Study. Ritenour. 1985. 64p. (C). (gr. 13). text, wbk. ed. 20.95 (*0-8016-1351-5*, 01351) Mosby Inc.

Computer Applications in Engineering & Medicine (CAIME-95), 8th International Conference, March 15-17, 1995, Indianapolis, Indiana, U.S.A: March 15-17, 1995, Indianapolis, IN. Ed. by M. El-Sharkaway & E. Berbari. 1995. (Conference Proceedings Ser.). 316p. (C). (*1-880843-11-0*) Int Soc Comp App.

Computer Applications in Nursing Education & Practice. Ed. by J. Arnold & G. Pearson. 1992. 400p. (C). pap. 36.95 (*0-88737-522-7*) Natl League Nurse.

Computer Applications in Nutrition & Dietetics: An Annotated Bibliography. John Orta. 1988. LC 87-30450. 256p. text 15.00 (*0-8240-6621-9*) Garland.

Computer Applications in the Evaluation of Physician Competence. Ed. by John S. Lloyd & Donald G. Langsley. 1984. 241p. lib. bdg. 29.95 (*0-934277-04-4*) Am Bd Med Spec.

Computer Applications Mental Health, 1991: Education & Evaluation. Intro. by Marvin J. Miller. 1992. LC 92-1541. (Computers in Human Services Ser.: Vol. 8, Nos. 3-4). (Illus.). 200p. pap. text 19.95 (*1-56024-353-8*); text 49.95 (*1-56024-279-5*) Haworth Pr.

Computer Assisted Analyses of Cell Locomotion & Chemotaxis. P. B. Noble & M. D. Levine. 1986. 152p. 92.00 (*0-8493-6342-X*, QH647, CRC Reprint) Franklin.

Computer-Assisted Bacterial Systematics. Ed. by Michael Goodfellow et al. 1985. (Society for General Microbiology Special Publications: No. 15). text 104.00 (*0-12-289665-3*) Acad Pr.

Computer-Assisted Cardiac Nuclear Medicine. B. Leonard Holman & J. Anthony Parker. 1981. 546p. 64.00 (*0-316-37054-1*, Little Brwn Med Div) Lppncott W & W.

Computer-Assisted Drug Design. Ed. by Ralph E. Christoffersen & Edward C. Olson. 1979. LC 79-21038. (ACS Symposium Ser.: No. 112). 65.95 (*0-8412-0521-3*) Am Chemical.

Computer-Assisted Eye Examination. Elwyn Marg. 1980. (Illus.). 20.00 (*0-911302-40-9*) San Francisco Pr.

Computer-Assisted Image Analysis Cytology. Ed. by S. D. Greenberg. 1984. (Monographs in Clinical Cytology Ser.: Vol. 9). (Illus.). x, 202p. 85.25 (*3-8055-3902-9*) S Karger.

Computer Assisted Instruction in the Health Sciences: Index of New Information with Authors & Subjects. Mary R. Bartone. 1992. LC 92-54230. 180p. 47.50 (*1-55914-608-7*); pap. 44.50 (*1-55914-609-5*) ABBE Pubs Assn.

Computer-Assisted Instruction in the Health Sciences: Index of New Information with Authors & Subjects. Mary R. Bartone. 1997. 159p. 57.50 (*0-7883-1566-8*); pap. 47.50 (*0-7883-1567-6*) ABBE Pubs Assn.

Computer-Assisted Medical Decision Making, Vol. 2. Ed. by J. A. Reggia & S. Tuhrim. 1985. (Computers & Medicine Ser.). (Illus.). 296p. 79.00 (*0-387-96136-4*) Spr-Verlag.

Computer-Assisted Medical Decision Making I. Ed. by J. A. Reggia & S. Tuhrim. 1985. (Computers & Medicine Ser.). (Illus.). 275p. 54.00 (*0-387-96104-6*) Spr-Verlag.

Computer-Assisted Neurosurgery. Japanese Society of Computers in Neurosurgery Staf. Ed. by Norihiko Tamaki & K. Ehara. 1998. LC 97-43643. (Illus.). 200p. 129.00 (*4-431-70211-3*) Spr-Verlag.

Computer Assisted New Drug Application (CANDA) Guidance Manual (1994) 2nd ed. 1995. 320p. (C). pap. text 60.00 (*0-7881-2120-0*) DIANE Pub.

Computer Assisted Physicians Offices: Journal: Health Communications & Informatics, Vol. 5, No. 2, 1979. Ed. by J. F. Brandejs. 1979. (Illus.). pap. 16.75 (*3-8055-3063-3*) S Karger.

Computer Assisted Radiology - Computergestutze Radiologie: Proceedings of the International Symposium. Ed. by H. U. Lemke et al. 1993. (Illus.). 836p. 180.00 (*0-387-56595-7*) Spr-Verlag.

Computer Assisted Radiology Computergestutzte Radiologie: Proceedings of the International Symposium Vortrage des Internationalen Symposiums, CAR '91 Computer Assisted Radiology. Ed. by H. U. Lemke et al. 1991. (Illus.). 944p. 208.00 (*0-387-54143-8*) Spr-Verlag.

Computer Based Diagnostic Systems. Eta Berner. 1997. (Medical Intelligence Unit Ser.). 200p. 89.95 (*0-412-13021-1*) Chapman & Hall.

Computer-Based Examinations for Board Certification. Ed. by Elliott L. Mancall et al. 1996. LC 96-86080. (Illus.). 212p. 44.95 (*0-934277-22-2*) Am Bd Med Spec.

Computer-Based Medical Systems: Proceedings of the Tenth IEEE Symposium on Computer-Based Medical Systems, Maribor, Slovenia, 1997. 1997. LC 10-637125. 250p. pap. 110.00 (*0-8186-7928-X*) IEEE Comp Soc.

Computer-Based Medical Systems, 9th IEEE Symposium. 1996. LC 10-637125. 350p. 70.00 (*0-8186-7439-3*, PRO7439) IEEE Comp Soc.

Computer-Based Oral Health Record: A New Foundation for Oral Health Information Systems. John Eisner et al. 1993. 270p. (Orig.). pap. 50.00 (*0-9639893-0-8*) U Buffalo Sch Dental.

Computer-Based Patient Record: An Essential Technology for Health Care. Ed. by Richard S. Dick et al. rev. ed. 1997. LC 97-31030. 270p. 34.95 (*0-309-05532-6*) Natl Acad Pr.

Computer-Based Patient Record: Its Role in the Healthcare Enterprise, Vol. 12, No. 4. Julie Forema. 1998. pap. 28.00 (*0-7879-4245-6*) Jossey-Bass.

***Computer-Based Patient Records.** Lucy Mancini Newell. 2001. (HIMSS Guidebook Ser.). 148p. pap. 35.00 (*0-9704287-5-8*) Healthcare Info.

Computer Buying Guide: 2001 Edition. annuals Consumer Guide Editors. 2000. LC 85-645006. (Consumer Guide Computer Buying Guide Ser.). 160p. pap. 9.99 (*0-7853-4042-4*) NAL.

Computer Communication Networks in Science & Medicine: Index of New Information. Shoog D. Sewell. 1994. 150p. 57.50 (*0-7883-0132-2*); 1994. 150p. pap. 47.50 (*0-7883-0133-0*); 1997. 143p. 57.50 (*0-7883-1506-4*); 1997. pap. 47.50 (*0-7883-1507-2*) ABBE Pubs Assn.

Computer Concepts & Applications for the Medical Office. Kathy Bonewit-West. 1993. 296p. pap. text 34.00 (*0-7216-4945-9*) Saunders.

Computer Experience & Cognitive Development: A Child's Learning in a Computer Culture. Robert W. Lawler. 1985. LC 85-5534. (Cognitive Science Ser.). 275p. pap. 31.95 (*0-470-20194-0*) P-H.

Computer Health Hazards. Marija M. Hughes. LC 90-93371. 1990. 67p. 42.45 (*0-912560-05-3*); Vol. 2. 1993. (Illus.). 132p. pap. 55.45 (*0-912560-00-2*) Hughes Pr.

Computer in Clinical Dentistry: Proceedings of the First International Conference, Houston, Texas, September 26-29, 1991. Ed. by Jack D. Preston. 1993. LC 92-49188. (Illus.). 228p. pap. text 52.00 (*0-86715-229-X*) Quint Pub Co.

Computer in der Medizin. Dimitris N. Chorafas. 1973. (Illus.). 127p. (C). 43.10 (*3-11-004031-X*) De Gruyter.

Computer in Experimental Psychology. R. Bird. 1981. LC 80-41610. (Computers & People Ser.). 256p. text 147.00 (*0-12-099760-6*) Acad Pr.

Computer-Integrated Surgery: Technology & Clinical Applications. Ed. by Russell Taylor et al. 1995. LC 94-27743. (Illus.). 736p. (C). 125.00 (*0-262-20097-X*) MIT Pr.

Computer Literacy for Health Care Professionals. Sandra Anderson. 1992. (C). mass mkt. 44.95 (*0-8273-4171-7*) Delmar.

Computer Literacy for Health Care Professions Instructors Guide. Sandra Anderson. 1992. pap., tchr. ed. 13.00 (*0-8273-4172-5*) Delmar.

Computer Models of Mind: Computational Approaches in Theoretical Psychology. Margaret A. Boden. 1988. (Problems in the Behavioral Sciences Ser.: No. 6). (Illus.). 304p. pap. text 29.95 (*0-521-27033-2*) Cambridge U Pr.

***Computer Programs for Epidemiologists: PEPI v. 4.0.** J. H. Abramson & Paul M. Gahlinger. 4th ed. 2001. (Illus.). 308p. pap. 59.95 incl. cd-rom (*0-9703130-2-0*) Sagebrush UT.

Computer Programs in Clinical & Laboratory Medicine. D. J. Doyle. 1989. (Illus.). 189p. 57.00 (*0-387-96879-2*) Spr-Verlag.

Computer Psychotherapy Systems: Theory & Research Foundations. Morton Wagman. 1988. LC 87-25111. xviii, 262p. text 119.00 (*2-88124-207-3*) Gordon & Breach.

Computer Science in Health Sciences: Index of Information with Authors, Subjects & References. Anna R. Goodrich. 1994. LC 95-15950. 150p. 47.50 (*1-55914-524-2*); pap. 44.50 (*1-55914-525-0*) ABBE Pubs Assn.

Computer Simulation of Carcinogenic Processes. Ed. by B. D. Silverman. 1987. (Cancer Researchers & Biomedical Engineers Ser.). 208p. 110.00 (*0-8493-6539-2*, RC268, CRC Reprint) Franklin.

Computer Simulations for Clinical Nursing, Vol. 2. Nancy Ann Sickles Corbett & Phyllis Beveridge. 1986. 783.00 (*0-7216-1368-3*); text 783.00 (*0-7216-1343-8*) Saunders.

Computer Simulations in Biomedicine. Ed. by H. Power & R. T. Hart. 1995. LC 95-67479. (BIOMED Ser.: Vol. 3). 668p. (*1-56252-245-0*, 3218) WIT Pr GBR. *Dist:* Computational Mech MA.

Computer Simulations in Clinical Nursing, Vol. 1. Nancy Ann Sickles Corbett & Phyllis Beveridge. 1983. 665.00 (*0-7216-1023-4*); pap. text, stu. ed. 16.00 (*0-7216-1154-0*) Saunders.

Computer Systems Validation for the Pharmaceutical & Medical Device Industries. R. L. Chamberlain. 1994. 216p. 235.00 (*0-9631489-0-7*); 2nd ed. 350p. 247.00 incl. disk (*0-9631489-5-8*) Alaren Pr.

Computer Techniques in Neuroanatomy. J. J. Capowski. 1989. (Illus.). 502p. (C). text 115.00 (*0-306-43263-3*, Kluwer Plenum) Kluwer Academic.

Computer Techniques in Preclinical & Clinical Drug Development. Robert C. Jackson. 1996. LC 96-4704. 256p. 139.95 (*0-8493-7682-3*) CRC Pr.

Computer Tomographic Imaging & Anatomic Correlation of the Human Brain. C. Plets et al. 1987. (Series in Radiology). text 184.00 (*0-89838-811-2*) Kluwer Academic.

Computer Tomography: Physical Principles, Clinical Applications & Quality Control. Euclid Seeram. 1994. LC 94-2598. (Illus.). 352p. text 55.00 (*0-7216-6710-4*) Saunders.

Computer Tomography: State of the Art & Future Applications. Ed. by T. J. Vogl & W. Claus. 1995. (Illus.). 281p. 71.95 (*3-540-60050-7*) Spr-Verlag.

Computer Tutorial Guide for Medical Terminology: For Stenotypists. George P. Andrews. 1993. (Realtime Machine Shorthand Ser.). 67p. (C). pap. text 8.00 (*0-938643-28-2*, 452) Stenotype Educ.

Computer Vision, Virtual Reality, & Robotics in Medicine: First International Conference, CVRMed '95, Nice, France, April 3-6, 1995, Proceedings. Ed. by Nicholas Ayache. 1995. LC 95-7442. (Lecture Notes in Computer Science: Vol. 905). (*0-387-59120-6*) Spr-Verlag.

Computerisation of Medical Data in Hospital Services Including University Hospitals. Council of Europe Staff. 1989. (*92-871-1602-4*) Council of Europe FRA. *Dist:* Manhattan Pub Co.

Computerised Monitoring & Evaluation in Cardiovascular Pathophysiology & Pharmacology. D. W. Harron. 1991. 178p. pap. text 444.00 (*2-88124-801-2*) Gordon & Breach.

Computerization & Automation in Health Facilities: Computerization & Automation. Ed. by Martin Rubin. 1984. 296p. 167.00 (*0-8493-5143-X*, RC268, CRC Reprint) Franklin.

Computerization of Behavioral Healthcare: How to Enhance Clinical Practice, Management, & Communications. Ed. by Tom Trabin & Michael A. Freeman. 1996. LC 95-26784. (Psychology Ser.). 284p. 37.00 (*0-7879-0221-7*) Jossey-Bass.

Computerization of French Hospital Institutions: Social & Technical Implications for System Development. Karin J. Schneider. 1999. LC 99-26068. (Koinon: Vol. 1). (Illus.). 128p. pap. text 28.95 (*0-8204-3561-9*) P Lang Pubng.

Computerized Adaptive Testing: From Inquiry to Operation. Ed. by William A. Sands et al. 1997. LC 97-25695. 292p. pap. 34.95 (*1-55798-442-5*) Am Psychol.

Computerized CardioPulmonary Exercise Testing (CPX) Ed. by U. J. Winter et al. 1991. 185p. 65.00 (*0-387-91404-8*) Spr-Verlag.

Computerized Medical Office Management. Joan M. Johnson & Marcus W. Johnson. 1993. LC 92-48214. 347p. (C). pap. 52.95 (*0-8273-5112-7*) Delmar.

Computerized Medical Office Management: Instructor's Guide. Joan M. Johnson & Marcus W. Johnson. 1993. 82p. pap. 16.00 (*0-8273-5113-5*) Delmar.

Computerized Testbank for Nursing in the Community: IBM Version. Mary J. Clark. 2nd ed. 1995. (C). (*0-8385-7106-9*, A7106) Appleton & Lange.

Computerized Tomography-Brain Metabolism-Spinal Injuries. Ed. by W. Driesen et al. 1982. (Advances in Neurosurgery Ser.: Vol. 10). (Illus.). 408p. 75.00 (*0-387-11115-8*) Spr-Verlag.

Computerizing Healthcare Records: Developing Electronic Patient & Medical Records. Michael W. Davis. 1994. LC 94-171540. 200p. (C). text 60.00 (*1-55738-609-9*, Irwn Prfssnl) McGraw-Hill Educ Grp.

Computers: Manager's Guide. Paul Richardson. 1993. (Primary Health Care Management Advancement Programme Modules Ser.). 76p. pap. text (*1-882839-20-X*) Aga Khan Fnd.

Computers & Clinical Audit: An Introduction for Doctors & Healthcare Professionals. Sue Kinn & Tanya Siann. 1993. (Illus.). 200p. (Orig.). (C). (gr. 13). pap. 54.95 (*0-412-49280-6*, Chap & Hall NY) Chapman & Hall.

Computers & Control in Clinical Medicine. Ed. by Ewart R. Carson & D. G. Cramp. 1985. 272p. 79.50 (*0-306-41892-4*, Plenum Trade) Perseus Pubng.

Computers in Activation Analysis & Gamma-Ray Spectroscopy: Proceedings. Ed. by B. Stephen Carpenter et al. 1979. LC 79-19600. (DOE Symposium Ser.). 905p. pap. 30.50 (*0-87079-117-6*, CONF-780421); fiche 9.00 (*0-87079-169-9*, CONF-780421) DOE.

Computers in Biomedicine. Ed. by K. D. Held et al. 1991. LC 91-75140. (BIOMED Ser.: Vol. 1). 456p. (*1-56252-075-X*, 1487) WIT Pr GBR. *Dist:* Computational Mech MA.

***Computers in Cardiology 2001.** 2001. LC 80-641097. 860p. pap. (*0-7803-7266-2*) IEEE Standards.

Computers in Diagnostic Radiology: A Book of Selected Readings. Euclid Seeram. 1989. (Illus.). 402p. (C). text 81.95 (*0-398-05559-9*) C C Thomas.

Computers in Health & Safety. Ed. by Greg Rawls. 1990. 255p. 40.00 (*0-932627-39-0*) Am Indus Hygiene.

Computers in Human Services: An Overview for Clinical & Welfare Services. Ed. by J. W. Murphy & John T. Pardech. 1990. x, 150p. text 84.00 (*3-7186-5009-6*); pap. text 43.00 (*3-7186-5005-3*) Gordon & Breach.

Computers in Medical Physics. Ed. by A. R. Benedetto et al. 1990. (American Association of Physicists in Medicine Symposium Ser.: No. 17). 417p. 75.00 (*0-88318-802-3*) Am Inst Physics.

Computers in Medicine: Applications & Possibilities. Jonathan Javitt. 1986. (Illus.). 317p. pap. text 28.00 (*0-7216-1578-3*) Saunders.

Computers in Nuclear Medicine: A Practical Approach. Kai Lee. 1992. LC 91-4859. (Illus.). 290p. (Orig.). 42.00 (*0-932004-36-9*) Soc Nuclear Med.

Computers in Nursing: Concepts & Issues. Linda Q. Thede. 1998. LC 98-25817. 432p. pap. text 33.95 (*0-7817-1557-1*) Lppncott W & W.

Computers in Nursings: Nurses' Guide to the Internet. Leslie H. Nicoll. 3rd ed. 2000. 256p. pap. text 31.95 (*0-7817-2459-7*) Lppncott W & W.

Computers in Nutrition Education. 1984. 117p. pap. 12.00 (*0-910869-21-9*) Soc Nutrition Ed.

Computers in Private Practice Management. B. B. Oberst & J. L. Long. 1987. (Illus.). 240p. 110.00 (*0-387-96502-5*) Spr-Verlag.

Computers in Psychology: Application in Education, Research & Psychodiagnostics. Ed. by L. J. Mulder et al. 1991. 240p. (*90-265-1170-1*) Swets.

Computers in Psychology: Applications, Methods & Instrumentation. Ed. by F. J. Maarse et al. 1994. (Computers in Psychology Ser.: Vol. 5). 286p. (*90-265-1415-8*) Swets.

Computers in Psychology: Methods, Instrumentation, & Psychodiagnostics. F. J. Maarse et al. 1988. 220p. (*90-265-0896-4*) Swets.

Computers in Psychology: Tools for Experimental & Applied Psychology. Ed. by F. J. Maarse et al. 1992. LC 92-49200. 246p. (*90-265-1268-6*) Swets.

Computers in Radiology: Proceedings. International Meeting on the Use of Computers in R. Ed. by A. Wambersie & R. De Haene. 1971. 102.75 (*3-8055-0805-0*) S Karger.

Computers in Small Bytes: The Computer Workbook. Irene Joos et al. 2nd ed. 1996. 258p. pap., wbk. ed. 33.95 (*0-88737-680-0*) Natl League Nurse.

Computers in Stereotactic Neurosurgery. Ed. by P. J. Kelly & B. Kall. 1992. (Contemporary Issues in Neurological Surgery Ser.). (Illus.). 384p. 94.95 (*0-86542-145-5*) Blackwell Sci.

Computers in the Dental Office: How to Evaluate, Select & Get the Most Out of Your System. Frank J. Sapienza. 1992. LC 92-80574. 128p. ring bd. 39.95 (*0-9632212-6-4*) Mare Pub Dist.

Computers in the Doctor's Office. Stephen Radin & Harold Greenberg. 1984. LC 84-8378. 151p. 55.00 (*0-275-91245-0*, C1245, Praeger Pubs) Greenwood.

Computers in the Medical Office: Using MediSoft. Ed. by Claire Baptist et al. 1995. LC 94-20025. 281p. 55.96 (*0-02-803042-7*) Glencoe.

Computers in the Medical Office: Using Medisoft for Windows. Susan M. Sanderson. 2nd ed. 1998. LC 97-43098. pap. 33.00 (*0-02-801990-3*) Glencoe.

Computers in the Medical Office: Using Medisoft for Windows. Susan M. Sanderson. 3rd ed. 2001. LC 00-52536. (Illus.). xii, 301p. pap., stu. ed. incl. disk (*0-07-823134-5*) McGraw.

Computers in the Primary Care Office. American Academy of Pediatrics Staff. 3rd ed. 1995. LC 95-75174. 248p. spiral bd. 54.95 (*0-910761-70-1*) Am Acad Pediat.

Computers, the Patient, & the Psychiatrist. Ed. by Zebulon Taintor. 1997. (Review of Psychiatry Ser.: Vol. 16, Sect. VI). 96p. (Orig.). pap. text 19.95 (*0-88048-435-7*, 8435) Am Psychiatric.

Computing & Monitoring Anesthesia & Intensive Care: Recent Technological Advances. Ed. by K. Ikeda et al. 1992. (Illus.). 518p. 149.00 (*0-387-70101-X*) Spr-Verlag.

Computing for Clinicians. Tim Chard. 1992. LC 92-2228. (*0-387-19721-4*) Spr-Verlag.

Computing in Psychology: An Introduction to Programming Methods & Concepts. James H. Reynolds. 1987. (Illus.). 320p. pap. text 36.40 (*0-13-165812-3*) P-H.

Comtemporary Nutrition. Wardlaw. 5th ed. 2002. 47.00 net. (*0-07-231616-0*) McGraw.

Comunidad y la Salud. Ed. by Maria Sosa & Edward Gonzalez. 1996. LC 96-164193. (Illus.). 102p. pap. (*0-87168-577-9*, 96-035) AAAS.

Con Heart Disease. Liberthson. 1989. 85.00 (*0-316-52413-1*, Little Brwn Med Div) Lppncott W & W.

Conan Doyle's Tales of Medical Humanism & Values: Round the Red Lamp. Ed. by Jack D. Key. 1992. 496p. (C). lib. bdg. 52.50 (*0-89464-571-4*) Krieger.

Conations: On Striving, Willing & Wishing & Their Relationship with Cognition, Emotions, & Motives. Henrik Poulsen. 1991. 160p. (C). pap. (*87-7288-358-8*) Aarhus Univ Pr DNK. *Dist:* David Brown.

Conceiving Sexuality: Approaches to Sex Research in a Postmodern World. Ed. by Richard G. Parker & John H. Gagnon. 1994. LC 94-17761. 320p. (C). pap. 27.95 (*0-415-90928-7*, B3848) Routledge.

Conceiving the Embryo: Ethics, Law, & Practice in Human Embryology. Ed. by Donald Evans & Neil Pickering. 1996. LC 96-5362. lib. bdg. (*90-411-0208-6*) M Nijhoff NLD. *Dist:* Kluwer Academic.

Conceiving the Self: Presence & Absence in Psychoanalytic Theory. Barbara J. Socor. 1997. LC 96-29441. xiv, 310p. 47.50 (*0-8236-1030-6*, BN 01030) Intl Univs Pr.

Concentrate on What You Can Do: Bottom Line to Getting Healthy. Toni Fain. Date not set. (Orig.). pap. 5.00 (*0-9656189-0-0*) Healing Arts Therapies.

***Concentration & Choice in Healthcare.** Ed. by Brian Ferguson et al. 1997. 150p. pap. (*0-443-05939-X*) Royal Soc of Medicine Pr Ltd GBR. *Dist:* Balogh.

Concentration Cockpit: Explaining Attention Deficits to Children. Melvin D. Levine. 2nd rev. ed. 1995. 15.00 (*0-8388-1991-5*) Ed Pub Serv.

Concept & Case Studies In Nursing: A Life Cycle Approach. Gertrude T. Redmond & Frances Ouellette. 1983. pap. (*0-201-06207-0*, Health Sci) Addison-Wesley.

Concept & Measurement of Quality of Life in the Frail Elderly. Ed. by James E. Birren et al. 1991. LC 91-13951. (Illus.). 385p. (C). text 64.95 (*0-12-101275-1*) Acad Pr.

Concept Development in Nursing: Foundations, Techniques, & Applications. Beth L. Rodgers & Kathleen A. Knafl. 2000. LC 99-31082. (Illus.). 405p. pap. text (*0-7216-8243-X*) Saunders.

Concept Development in Nursing: Foundations, Techniques, & Applications. Ed. by Beth L. Rodgers & Kathleen A. Knafl. 1993. (Illus.). 270p. pap. text 43.00 (*0-7216-3674-8*) Saunders.

Concept of Anxiety. Soren Kierkegaard. Ed. by Howard V. Hong & Edna H. Hong. Tr. by Reider Thomte. LC 79-3217. (Kierkegaard's Writings: VIII). 304p. 1981. pap. 18.95 (*0-691-02011-6*); 1980. 57.50 (*0-691-07244-2*) Princeton U Pr.

Concept of Defense Mechanisms in Contemporary Psychology: Theoretical, Research, & Clinical Perspectives. Ed. by Uwe Hentschel et al. 1993. LC 92-48254. (Illus.). 439p. 83.95 (*0-387-94003-0*) Spr-Verlag.

Concept of Development Vol. 15: The Minnesota Symposium on Child Psychology. Ed. by W. Andrew Collins. 1982. 192p. 49.95 (*0-89859-159-7*) L Erlbaum Assocs.

Concept of Heart Failure: From Avicenna to Albertini. Saul Jarcho. 1980. (Commonwealth Fund Publications). 416p. 58.00 (*0-674-15635-8*) HUP.

Concept of Mind. Gilbert Ryle. 1984. LC 83-24147. 334p. (C). pap. text 15.00 (*0-226-73295-9*) U Ch Pr.

Concept of Moral Consensus: The Case of Technological Interventions into Human Reproduction. Ed. by Kurt Bayertz. 1994. LC 93-40700. (Philosophy & Medicine Ser.: Vol. 46). 256p. (C). lib. bdg. (*0-7923-2615-6*) Kluwer Academic NLD. *Dist:* Kluwer Academic.

Concept of Probability in Psychological Experiments. Carl-Axel S. Stael Von Holstein. 1974. LC 74-83873. (Theory & Decision Library: No. 8). lib. bdg. 96.00 (*90-277-0523-2*) Kluwer Academic.

Concept of Research in Psychoanalysis. Anna Ursula Dreher. 2000. (UCL/AFC Ser.). 256p. pap. (*1-85575-244-1*) Karnac Bks GBR. *Dist:* Other Pr LLC.

Concept of Structure in Psychoanalysis. Ed. by Theodore Shapiro. 1991. LC 90-36624. 390p. 57.50 (*0-8236-1041-1*) Intl Univs Pr.

Conception, Pregnancy, & Birth. Miriam Stoppard. 1993. LC 92-34181. (Illus.). 352p. (*1-56458-182-9*) DK Pub Inc.

Conceptions & Misconceptions: A Guide Through the Maze of In Vitro Fertilization & Other Assisted Reproduction Techniques. Arthur L. Wisot & David R. Meldrum. 1997. LC 97-10710. 224p. (Orig.). pap. 19.95 (*0-88179-147-4*) Hartley & Marks.

Conceptions of Modern Psychiatry. Harry Stack Sullivan. 1966. pap. 10.95 (*0-393-00740-5*) Norton.

Concepts & Issues in Nursing Practice. Erb Kozier et al. 2nd ed. 1992. 672p. (C). pap. text 50.63 (*0-8053-3520-X*) Benjamin-Cummings.

Concepts & Strategies in New Drug Development, 4. Ed. by Peter Nwangu. 1983. LC 83-19248. (Clinical Pharmacology & Therapeutics Ser.). 265p. 72.50 (*0-275-91406-2*, C1406, Praeger Pubs) Greenwood.

Concepts & Theories of Human Development. Richard M. Lerner. 1976. LC 75-12098. (Illus.). (C). text 22.00 (*0-394-34773-0*) Random.

Concepts & Theories of Human Development. Richard A. Lerner. 2nd ed. 1985. 512p. text 34.50 (*0-89859-886-9*) L Erlbaum Assocs.

Concepts & Theories of Human Development. Richard M. Lerner. 2nd ed. 1986. 512p. (C). text 33.25 net. (*0-07-554899-2*) McGraw.

Concepts & Theories of Parapsychology: Proceedings of the International Conference, Dec. 6, 1980. International Conference, New York Staff. Ed. by Betty Shapin & Lisette Coly. 1981. LC 81-83135. 112p. (C). 16.00 (*0-912328-35-5*) Parapsych Foun.

Concepts & Theories of Traditional Chinese Medicine. Ed. by L. Yubin & L. Chengcai. LC 95-8084. (Traditional Chinese Medicine Ser.: Vol. 2). 265p. 70.00 (*90-5199-243-2*, 243-2) IOS Press.

Concepts Basic to Nursing. P. Mitchell. 3rd ed. 1981. (Illus.). 720p. text 36.95 (*0-07-042582-5*) McGraw.

Concepts for Healthy Living with InfoTrac. Sandra M. Alters-Gottfried. 1998. (Health Sciences Ser.). 39.50 incl. cd-rom (*0-534-36329-6*) Brooks-Cole.

Concepts for Professional Nursing. Grant Staff. (Illus.). 750p. (*0-8016-2590-4*) Mosby Inc.

Concepts for the Ideal Diabetes Clinic. Ed. by C. E. Mogensen & E. Standl. 1993. LC 92-49365. xiv, 402p. (C). pap. text 113.85 (*3-11-013231-1*) De Gruyter.

Concepts Human Physiology. Richard L. Malvin et al. 1997. LC 96-32232. 450p. (C). 90.00 (*0-673-98562-8*) Addison-Wesley Educ.

Concepts in Athletic Training: Instructor's Manual. Ronald P. Pfeiffer & Brent Mangus. 1995. (Physical Education Ser.). (Illus.). 96p. (C). pap. text, tchr. ed. 10.00 (*0-86720-949-6*, 949-6) Jones & Bartlett.

Concepts in Canadian Nursing. Janet R. Kerr & Jannetta MacPhail. 1996. LC 95-36946. (Illus.). 136p. (C). (gr. 13). pap. text 20.00 (*0-8016-8107-3*, 08107) Mosby Inc.

Concepts in Clinical Pharmacokinetics. Joseph T. DiPiro et al. 1991. (Orig.). pap. text 69.00 (*0-930530-86-1*) Am Soc Hlth-Syst.

Concepts in Community Health Nursing: A Canadian Perspective. Janet Ross Kerr & Jannetta Mcphail. 1996. (Illus.). 192p. (C). (gr. 13). pap. text 24.00 (*0-8151-4930-1*, 29137) Mosby Inc.

Concepts in Drug Metabolism, Pt. A. Jenner & Bernard Testa. 1980. (Drugs & the Pharmaceutical Sciences Ser.: Vol. 10). (Illus.). 424p. text 170.00 (*0-8247-6906-6*) Dekker.

Concepts in Fetal Movement Research. Intro. by Joyce W. Sparling. 1993. LC 92-48442. (Physical & Occupational Therapy in Pediatrics Ser.: Vol. 12, Nos. 2 & 3). (Illus.). 207p. lib. bdg. 49.95 (*1-56024-449-6*) Haworth Pr.

Concepts in Gene Therapy. Ed. by Michael Strauss & John A. Barranger. 1997. LC 97-31282. 570p. text 99.95 (*3-11-014984-2*) De Gruyter.

Concepts in Gross Anatomy: A Review for the USMLE, Step 1. William T. Mosenthal. 1997. LC 96-47926. (USMLE Concepts Ser.). 260p. 29.95 (*1-85070-928-9*, M3762, Parthenon Pbng) CRC Pr.

Concepts in Hand Rehabilitation. Barbara G. Stanley et al. 1992. (Contemporary Perspectives in Rehabilitation Ser.: Vol. 9). (Illus.). 582p. text 48.95 (*0-8036-8092-9*) Davis Co.

Concepts in Immunology & Immunotherapeutics. Ed. by Jim Koeller & Joseph Tanci. 2nd rev. ed. 1992. (Illus.). 500p. (C). reprint ed. pap. text (*1-879907-06-2*) Am Soc Hlth-Syst.

Concepts in Immunology & Immunotherapeutics. 3rd rev. ed. 1997. LC 97-225251. 250p. pap. text 55.00 (*1-879907-71-2*) Am Soc Hlth-Syst.

Concepts in Inhalation Toxicology. Roger O. McClellan & Rogene F. Henderson. 2nd ed. 1995. LC 95-13914. 648p. 136.00 (*1-56032-368-X*) Hemisp Pub.

Concepts in Learning Disabilities: Selected Writings, Vol. 2. William M. Cruickshank. 1981. LC 80-29024. 296p. text 45.00 (*0-8156-2239-2*) Syracuse U Pr.

Concepts in Medical Radiog. Imaging. Tortori. 1992. 420.00 (*0-7216-6743-0*) Harcourt.

Concepts in Medical Radiographic Imaging: Circuitry, Exposure & Quality Control. Ed. by Marianne Tortorici. 1992. (Illus.). tchr. ed. (*0-7216-3118-5*); 377p. pap. text, lab manual ed. 27.95 (*0-7216-3497-4*); 377p. text 55.00 (*0-7216-3117-7*) Saunders.

Concepts in Microbiology, Immunology, & Infectious Disease: A Review for the USMLE Step 1. Kapil Gupta & Lynn Pulliam. 1997. LC 97-16254. (USMLE Concepts Ser.). (Illus.). 168p. lib. bdg. 19.95 (*1-85070-797-9*, Parthenon Pbng) CRC Pr.

Concepts in Nonsurgical Periodontal Therapy. Kathleen Hodges. 1997. LC 96-48459. (Rp-Dental Assisting Procedures Ser.). 560p. (C). pap. text 58.95 (*0-8273-6274-9*) Delmar.

Concepts in Oncology Therapeutics. Ed. by Rebecca S. Finley. 1991. (Illus.). 500p. (Orig.). (C). pap. text (*1-879907-08-9*) Am Soc Hlth-Syst.

Concepts in Oncology Therapeutics. Ed. by Rebecca S. Finley & Carol Balmer. 2nd rev. ed. 1998. LC 00-265334. (Orig.). pap. text (*1-879907-78-X*) Am Soc Hlth-Syst.

Concepts in Oncology Therapeutics: A Self-Instructional Course. Ed. by Rebecca S. Finley & Carol Balmer. 2nd rev. ed. 1998. (Illus.). 432p. (C). 75.00 (*1-879907-68-2*) Am Soc Hlth-Syst.

Concepts in Pediatric Neurosurgery. P. H. Chapman. 1985. (Concepts in Pediatric Neurosurgery Ser.: Vol. 6). (Illus.). xii, 244p. 151.50 (*3-8055-4136-8*) S Karger.

Concepts in Pediatric Neurosurgery. Ed. by R. P. Humphreys. 1983. (Concepts in Pediatric Neurosurgery Ser.: No. 4). (Illus.). xiv, 394p. 201.75 (*3-8055-3734-4*) S Karger.

Concepts in Pediatric Neurosurgery. Ed. by A. E. Marlin. 1989. (Concepts in Pediatric Neurosurgery Ser.: Vol. 9). (Illus.). viii, 236p. 184.50 (*3-8055-4835-4*) S Karger.

Concepts in Pediatric Neurosurgery. Ed. by American Society of Pediatric Neurosurgery Staff. 1982. (Illus.). No. 1. x, 238p. 165.25 (*3-8055-2904-X*); No. 2. x, 222p. 165.25 (*3-8055-3454-X*) S Karger.

Concepts in Pediatric Neurosurgery, No. 3. Ed. by Anthony J. Raimondi. 1983. (Illus.). xxii, 226p. 172.25 (*3-8055-3580-5*) S Karger.

Concepts in Pediatric Neurosurgery, Vol. 5. Ed. by Robin P. Humphreys. 1985. (Illus.). xii, 244p. 142.75 (*3-8055-3915-0*) S Karger.

Concepts in Pediatric Neurosurgery. Ed. by A. E. Marlin. (Illus.). Vol. 7. 1987. viii, 240p. 182.75 (*3-8055-4396-4*); Vol. 8. 1988. viii, 224p. 161.75 (*3-8055-4622-X*); Vol. 11. 1991. viii, 164p. 187.00 (*3-8055-5328-5*) S Karger.

Concepts in Pediatric Neurosurgery Series, Vol. 10. Ed. by A. E. Marlin. 1990. (Illus.). 262p. 220.00 (*3-8055-5022-7*) S Karger.

Concepts in Physiology: A Review for the USMLE, Step 1. Kapil Gupta & James W. Pasley. 1996. LC 96-6754. (USMLE Concepts Ser.). (Illus.). 148p. lib. bdg. 19.95 (*1-85070-730-8*, G0939, Parthenon Pbng) CRC Pr.

Concepts in Vaccine Development. Ed. by Stefan H. Kaufmann. 1996. LC 96-11977. (Illus.). xxi, 583p. (C). text 119.00 (*3-11-014815-3*, 129/96) De Gruyter.

Concepts in Viral Pathogenesis. Ed. by Michael B. Oldstone & A. L. Notkins. 1984. (Illus.). 390p. 87.00 (*0-387-90982-6*) Spr-Verlag.

Concepts in Viral Pathogenesis II. Ed. by Michael B. Oldstone & A. L. Notkins. 1986. (Illus.). 450p. 104.00 (*0-387-96322-7*) Spr-Verlag.

Concepts in Viral Pathogenesis III. Ed. by M. B. Oldstone & A. L. Notkins. 1989. (Illus.). 389p. 109.00 (*0-387-96974-8*, 2692) Spr-Verlag.

Concepts, Kinds, & Cognitive Development. Frank C. Keil. 1989. (Learning, Development & Conceptual Change Ser.). 344p. 40.00 (*0-262-11131-4*, Bradford Bks) MIT Pr.

Concepts, Mechanisms, & New Targets for Chemotherapy. Ed. by Franco M. Muggia. 1995. LC 95-17716. (Cancer Treatment & Research Ser.: Vol. 78). 256p. (C). text 212.00 (*0-7923-3525-2*) Kluwer Academic.

Concepts of Alzheimer Disease: Biological, Clinical, & Cultural Perspectives. Peter J. Whitehouse. 2000. LC 99-27293. (Illus.). 312p. 57.00 (*0-8018-6233-7*) Johns Hopkins.

Concepts of Athletic Training. Ronald P. Pfeiffer & Brent C. Mangus. (Illus.). (C). 1995. LC 95-1456. 400p. pap. text 43.75 (*0-86720-839-2*, 839-2); 2nd ed. 1997. LC 97-20506. 384p. pap. text 48.95 (*0-7637-0235-8*, 0235-8) Jones & Bartlett.

Concepts of Care: Developments in Health & Social Welfare. Richard Hugman et al. 1997. LC 98-161052. 216p. pap. (*0-340-65254-3*) E A.

Concepts of Chemical Dependency. Harold E. Doweiko. 1990. 384p. (C). pap. 28.00 (*0-534-12834-3*); 3rd ed. 1995. LC 95-19833. 608p. pap. 37.00 (*0-534-33904-2*); 4th ed. 1998. LC 97-51593. 510p. pap. text 55.95 (*0-534-35755-5*) Brooks-Cole.

Concepts of Chinese Science & Traditional Healing Arts. P. Y. Ho & P. Lisowski. 1993. 116p. text 48.00 (*981-02-1495-2*); pap. text 21.00 (*981-02-1496-0*) World Scientific Pub.

***Concepts of Fitness & Wellness with HealthQuest 3.0.** Corbin. 4th ed. 2001. 526p. 37.50 incl. cd-rom (*0-07-248599-X*) McGrw-H Hghr Educ.

Concepts of Fitness & Wellness with Laboratories. Charles B. Corbin & Ruth Lindsey. 2nd ed. 1996. LC 95-83958. 464p. (C). text 24.50 net. (*0-697-25877-7*) Brown & Benchmark.

Concepts of Health & Disease: Interdisciplinary Perspectives. Arthur L. Caplan et al. 1981. 608p. (C). pap. text (*0-201-00973-0*, Health Sci) Addison-Wesley.

Concepts of Health, Illness & Disease: A Comparative Perspective. Ed. by Caroline Currer & Meg Stacey. 1987. LC 85-20759. 324p. 49.50 (*0-907582-18-4*); pap. 19.50 (*0-907582-19-2*) Berg Pubs.

Concepts of Human Anatomy & Physiology: Survey of Infectious & Parasitic Diseases. Kent M. Van De Graaff & Ira S. Fox. 4th ed. 1994. LC 95-166649. 108p. (C). text, suppl. ed. 8.00 net. (*0-697-27535-3*, WCB McGr Hill) McGrw-H Hghr Educ.

Concepts of Occupational Therapy. Kathlyn L. Reed & Sharon R. Nelson. 3rd ed. 1992. (Illus.). 410p. 36.00 (*0-683-07207-2*) Lppncott W & W.

Concepts of Person: An Analysis of Concepts of Person, Self & Human Being. Catherine McCall. 1990. 210p. text (*1-85628-039-X*) Avebry GBR. *Dist:* Ashgate Pub Co.

Concepts of Physical Fitness. Charles B. Corbin & Ruth Lindsey. 9th ed. 1996. LC 95-83959. 408p. (C). text 20.50 net. (*0-697-25890-4*, WCB McGr Hill) McGrw-H Hghr Educ.

Concepts Physical Fitness. Charles B. Corbin et al. 10th ed. 1999. LC 99-14989. (Illus.). xvi, 422p. pap. text 20.50 net. (*0-697-29567-2*) McGraw.

Conceptual & Methodological Issues in Cancer Psychotherapy Intervention Studies. Ed. by H. Balner & Y. Van Rood. 1990. (Publications of the Helen Dowling Institute for Biopsychosocial Medicine). 100p. pap. (*90-265-1138-8*) Swets.

Conceptual Bases of Professional Nursing. Susan Leddy & Mae J. Pepper. 4th ed. 1998. LC 97-42746. 496p. pap. text 38.95 (*0-397-55277-7*) Lppncott W & W.

Conceptual Basis for Rural Nursing. Helen J. Lee. 1998. LC 98-18898. (Illus.). 520p. 48.95 (*0-8261-1189-0*) Springer Pub.

Conceptual Basis for the Determination of Dose Equivalent, No. 25. International Commission on Radiation Units and Measurements Staff. 1976. LC 76-24373. 25.00 (*0-913394-44-0*) Intl Comm Rad Meas.

Conceptual Change - Japanese Perspectives. Ed. by G. Hatano. 1994. (Journal: Vol. 37, No. 4). (Illus.). 70p. pap. 20.00 (*3-8055-6039-7*) S Karger.

Conceptual Foundation of Occupational Therapy. Gary Kielhofner. 2nd ed. 1997. LC 97-4078. (Illus.). 358p. (C). text 47.95 (*0-8036-0256-1*) Davis Co.

***Conceptual Foundations: The Bridge to Professional Nursing Practice.** Joan L. Creasia & Barbara Parker. 3rd ed. 2001. (Illus.). pap., tchr. ed. (*0-323-01228-0*) Mosby Inc.

Conceptual Foundations of Professional Nursing Practice. Ed. by Joan L. Creasia & Barbara J. Parker. 2nd ed. 1996. (Illus.). 528p. (C). (gr. 13). pap. text 37.00 (*0-8151-1406-0*, 24506) Mosby Inc.

Conceptual Framework of the International Classification of Impairments, Disabilities & Handicaps (ICIDH) Council of Europe Staff. 1992. (*92-871-1972-4*) Council of Europe FRA. *Dist:* Manhattan Pub Co.

Conceptual History of Modern Embryology. Ed. by Scott F. Gilbert. 1994. LC 93-31904. 280p. pap. text 26.95 (*0-8018-4737-0*) Johns Hopkins.

Conceptual History of Modern Embryology Vol. 7. S. F. Gilbert. 1991. (Developmental Biology Ser.). (Illus.). 280p. (C). text 85.00 (*0-306-43842-9*, Kluwer Plenum) Kluwer Academic.

Conceptual Issues in Psychoanalysis: Essays in History & Method. John E. Gedo. 1986. 256p. text 37.50 (*0-88163-050-0*) Analytic Pr.

Conceptual Issues in Psychological Medicine. Michael Shepherd. 2nd ed. 1998. LC 97-18007. (Illus.). 264p. (C). pap. 31.95 (*0-415-16530-X*) Routledge.

Conceptual Issues in Psychology. Elizabeth Valentine. 2nd ed. 1991. (Illus.). 208p. (C). pap. 26.95 (*0-415-03925-8*, A6699) Routledge.

Conceptual Models of Nursing: Analysis & Application. Fitzpatrick et al. 3rd ed. 1996. LC 96-4864. 389p. (C). pap. 59.00 (*0-8385-1064-7*, A1064-3) P-H.

Conceptual Nursing in Practice. M. Fraser. 2nd ed. 1996. LC 96-68956. (Illus.). 280p. (C). pap. text 39.95 (*1-56593-418-0*, 1084) Singular Publishing.

Conceptual Self in Context: Culture, Experience, Self Understanding. Ed. by Ulriv Neisser & David Jopling. 1997. (Emory Symposia in Cognition Ser.: Vol. 7). (Illus.). 295p. (C). text 59.95 (*0-521-48203-8*) Cambridge U Pr.

Conceptual Structure in Childhood & Adolescence: The Case of Everyday Physics. Christine Howe. 1998. LC 97-27800. (International Library of Philosophy, Psychology, & Scientific Method). 208p. (C). 84.95 (*0-415-14729-8*) Routledge.

Conceptualization & Measurement of Organism-Environment Interaction. Ed. by Theodore D. Wachs & Robert Plomin. 1991. 191p. pap. text 19.95 (*1-55798-264-3*) Am Psychol.

Conceptualization & Mental Processing in Language: Including a Selection of Papers from the First International Cognitive Linguistics Conference, Duisburg, Germany, March-April 1989. Ed. by Richard A. Geiger & Brygida Rudzka-Ostyn. 1993. LC 93-19401. (Cognitive Linguistics Research Ser.: Vol. 3). (Illus.). xiv, 825p. (C). lib. bdg. (*3-11-012714-8*) Mouton.

Conceptualization in Psychotherapy: The Models Approach. Frederic M. Levine & Evelyn Sandeen. 1985. 232p. (C). text 49.95 (*0-89859-549-5*) L Erlbaum Assocs.

Conceptualizing the Evaluation of Clinical Counseling. William D. Eldridge. 1993. LC 93-2284. 544p. (C). reprint ed. pap. 69.00 (*0-8191-9192-2*); 2001. LC 96-50978. 660p. 70.50 (*0-7618-0679-2*) U Pr of Amer.

Concern for Europe's Tomorrow: Health & Environment in the WHO European Region. 1994. LC 94-240283. (WHO Regional Publications, European Ser.: No. 53). (ENG, FRE, GER & RUS.). viii, 88p. pap. text 12.60 (*92-890-1317-6*, 1310053) World Health.

Concerning Our Girls & What They Tell Us: A Study of Some Phases of the Confidential Relationship of Mothers & Adolescent Daughters. Eugenie Leonard. LC 75-176986. (Columbia University. Teachers College. Contributions to Education Ser.: No. 430). reprint ed. 37.50 (*0-404-55430-X*) AMS Pr.

Concerning the Biosynthesis of Vitamin B12. A. I. Scott. 1976. pap. 15.50 (*0-08-020478-3*, Pergamon Pr) Elsevier.

***Concise Anatomy for Anaesthesia.** Erdman. 2001. (Illus.). 142p. (*1-84110-069-2*) Greenwich Med GBR. *Dist:* JAMCO Dist.

Concise Cardiology. 1991. 28.00 (*0-387-91394-7*) Spr-Verlag.

Concise Dental Anatomy & Morphology. James L. Fuller et al. 2nd ed. 1999. LC 99-10445. (*0-87414-114-1*) U IA Pubns Dept.

***Concise Dental Anatomy & Morphology.** James L. Fuller et al. 4th ed. 2001. (Illus.). 218p. (C). pap. 45.00 (*0-87414-125-7*) U IA Pubns Dept.

Concise Dictionary of Biomedicine & Molecular Biology. Ed. by Pei S. Juo. 1996. LC 95-38363. 992p. 94.95 (*0-8493-2460-2*, 2460) CRC Pr.

Concise Dictionary of Medical-Legal Terms: A General Guide to Interpretation & Usage. Joseph A. Bailey. 1998. LC 97-8985. 164p. 32.95 (*1-85070-680-8*, Parthenon Pbng) CRC Pr.

Concise Dictionary of Psychology. David A. Statt. 3rd ed. 1998. LC 97-30856. (Illus.). 160p. (C). 68.95 (*0-415-17939-4*); pap. 19.95 (*0-415-17940-8*) Routledge.

Concise Dictionary of the System of Psychological Understanding. K. K. Platanov. 2nd ed. 1984. (RUS.). 174p. 12.95 (*0-8288-2212-3*, M15380) Fr & Eur.

Concise Encyclopedia of Biological & Biomedical Measurement Systems. Peter A. Payne. 1991. (Advances in Systems Control & Information Engineering Ser.: No. 3). 504p. 223.00 (*0-08-036188-9*, Pergamon Pr) Elsevier.

Concise Encyclopedia of Chronic Fatigue Syndrome. Ed. by Roberto Patarca-Montero. 2000. LC 99-56033. 200p. 69.95 (*0-7890-0922-6*); pap. text 24.95 (*0-7890-0923-4*) Haworth Pr (Hawrth Medical).

Concise Encyclopedia of Foods & Nutrition. A. H. Ensminger et al. 1986. 1184p. 49.95 (*0-941218-07-4*) Pegus Pr.

Concise Encyclopedia of Medical & Dental Materials. Ed. by David Williams. 1990. (Advances in Materials Science & Engineering Ser.: No. 5). 432p. 161.00 (*0-08-036194-3*, Pergamon Pr) Elsevier.

Concise Encyclopedia of Medical & Dental Materials. David F. Williams. 1990. 150.00 (*0-262-23149-2*) MIT Pr.

Concise Encyclopedia of Psychology. Ed. by Raymond J. Corsini & Alan Auerbach. 1996. LC 95-26497. 1035p. 375.00 (*0-471-13159-8*) Wiley.

Concise Encyclopedia of Psychology. Raymond J. Corsini & Alan Auerbach. 2nd abr. ed. 1998. LC 98-14293. 952p. pap. 70.00 (*0-471-19282-1*) Wiley.

Concise Gray's Anatomy. H. Gray. 1997. (Reference Library). 304p. pap. (*1-85326-394-X*, 394XWW) Wrdsworth Edits GBR. *Dist:* Combined Pub.

Concise Guide to Alternative Therapies in the Horse. David W. Ramey. 1999. LC 00-501017. (Equestrian Library). (Illus.). 224p. pap. 16.95 (*1-58245-062-5*, Howell) Hungry Minds.

Concise Guide to Arthritis in the Horse. David W. Ramey. 1998. LC 97-52816. (Concise Guides). (Illus.). 128p. pap. 16.95 (*0-87605-091-7*, Howell) Hungry Minds.

Concise Guide to Assessment & Management of Violent Patients. Kenneth Tardiff. 2nd ed. 1996. LC 96-12775. (Concise Guides Ser.). 180p. pap. text 22.95 (*0-88048-344-X*, 8344) Am Psychiatric.

Concise Guide to Brief Dynamic Psychotherapy. Hanna Levenson et al. 1997. LC 97-17250. (Concise Guides/American Psychiatric Press Ser.). 224p. pap. text 22.95 (*0-88048-346-6*, 8346) Am Psychiatric.

Concise Guide to Child & Adolescent Psychiatry. Mina K. Dulcan & D. Richard Martini. 2nd ed. 1998. LC 98-22463. (Concise Guides / American Psychiatric Press). 400p. pap. text 22.95 (*0-88048-905-7*, 8905) Am Psychiatric.

Concise Guide to Colic in the Horse. David W. Ramey. 1996. (Concise Guide Ser.). 128p. pap. 14.95 (*0-87605-911-6*, Howell) Hungry Minds.

Concise Guide to Consultation Psychiatry. James R. Rundell & Michael G. Wise. 3rd ed. 2000. LC 99-52943. (Concise Guides / American Psychiatric Press). (Illus.). xxi, 350p. pap. 22.95 (*0-88048-394-6*, 8394) Am Psychiatric.

Concise Guide to Evaluation & Management of Sleep Disorders. Martin L. Reite et al. 2nd ed. 1997. LC 96-29956. (Concise Guides/American Psychiatric Press Ser.). 304p. pap. text 22.95 (*0-88048-906-5*, 8906) Am Psychiatric.

Concise Guide to Geriatric Psychiatry. James E. Spar & Asenath La Rue. 2nd rev. ed. 1997. LC 96-29957. (Concise Guides). 350p. pap. text 22.95 (*0-88048-796-8*, 8796) Am Psychiatric.

Concise Guide to Group Psychotherapy. Ed. by Sophia Vinogradov & Irvin D. Yalom. 1989. LC 88-38281. (Concise Guides / American Psychiatric Press). 169p. pap. text 22.95 (*0-88048-327-X*, 8327) Am Psychiatric.

Concise Guide to Laboratory & Diagnostic Testing in Psychiatry. Richard B. Rosse et al. 1989. LC 89-3. (Concise Guides Ser.). 151p. pap. text 22.95 (*0-88048-333-4*, 8333) Am Psychiatric.

Concise Guide to Marital & Family Therapy. Leslie B. Kadis & Ruth McClendon. 1998. LC 97-41044. (Concise Guide Ser.). 320p. pap. text 22.95 (*0-88048-775-5*, 8775) Am Psychiatric.

Concise Guide to Navicular Syndrome in the Horse. David W. Ramey. 1996. LC 96-8496. 112p. 14.95 (*0-87605-913-2*, Howell) Hungry Minds.

Concise Guide to Neuropsychiatry & Behavioral Neurology. Jeffrey L. Cummings & Michael R. Trimble. 1995. LC 95-1386. (Concise Guides Ser.). 368p. pap. text 22.95 (*0-88048-493-4*, 8493) Am Psychiatric.

Concise Guide to Proper Nutrition Natural Remedies & Therapies to Prevent Dis-ease Balance & Maintain Body Mind & Spirit. Kay Hornsby. 1998. 105p. spiral bd. 14.95 (*0-9666622-0-2*) Healing Connect.

Concise Guide to Psychiatry & Law for Clinicians. Robert I. Simon. 2nd ed. 1998. LC 97-51794. (Concise Guides Ser.). 296p. pap. text 22.95 (*0-88048-329-6*, 8329) Am Psychiatric.

Concise Guide to Psychiatry for Law & Clinicians. Robert I. Simon. 3rd ed. 2001. LC 00-47538. 320p. pap. 27.95 (*1-58562-024-6*, 62024) Am Psychiatric.

Concise Guide to Psychiatry for Primary Care Practitioners. Ed. by Michael F. Gliatto et al. 1999. LC 98-32241. (Concise Guides / American Psychiatric Press). 248p. pap. text 22.95 (*0-88048-345-8*, 8345) Am Psychiatric.

Concise Guide to Psychodynamic Psychotherapy: Principles & Techniques in the Era of Managed Care. Robert J. Ursano et al. 2nd ed. 1998. LC 97-25925. (Concise Guides/American Psychiatric Press Ser.). 251p. 22.95 (*0-88048-347-4*, 8347) Am Psychiatric.

Concise Guide to Psychopharmacology & Electroconvulsive Therapy. Laurence B. Guttmacher. 2nd rev. ed. 1994. LC 93-5676. (Concise Guides Ser.). 224p. pap. text 22.95 (*0-88048-340-7*, 8340) Am Psychiatric.

Concise Guide to Tendon & Ligament Injuries in the Horse. David W. Ramey. 1996. LC 95-25005. (Concise Guide Ser.). (Illus.). 128p. pap. 14.95 (*0-87605-912-4*, Howell) Hungry Minds.

Concise Guide to the Cytochrome P450 System for Psychiatrists: Drug Interaction Principles for Medical Practice. Kelly L. Cozza & Scott C. Armstrong. 2001. LC 00-46471. 272p. pap. 29.95 (*1-58562-000-9*, 62000) Am Psychiatric.

Concise Guide to Treatment of Alcoholism & Addictions. Richard J. Frances & John E. Franklin. 1989. LC 89-413. (Concise Guides Ser.). 172p. pap. text 22.95 (*0-88048-326-1*, 8326) Am Psychiatric.

***Concise Guide to Women's Mental Health.** Vivien K. Burt & Victoria C. Hendrick. 2nd ed. 2001. LC 00-67406. 208p. pap. 27.95 (*1-58562-030-0*, 62030) Am Psychiatric.

Concise Handbook of Human Anatomy. McMinn. 1998. 192p. (C). pap. 34.95 (*0-8385-1564-9*) McGraw-Hill Educ Grp.

Concise Handbook of Respiratory Diseases. Satter Farzan et al. 1978. (Illus.). pap. text 25.95 (*0-87909-180-0*) P-H.

Concise Handbook of Respiratory Disorders. Sattar Farzan & Doris A. Farzan. 4th ed. 1997. LC 96-40177. 492p. (C). 64.00 (*0-8385-1493-6*, A-1493-4) P-H.

Concise Human Physiology. M. Y. Sukkar et al. (Illus.). 1993. 516p. pap. 34.95 (*0-632-03383-5*); 2nd ed. 2000. LC 99-53652. 552p. (C). pap. 41.95 (*0-632-05586-3*) Blackwell Sci.

Concise Illustrated Dental Dictionary. F. J. Harty. 2nd ed. 1994. LC 95-168346. (Illus.). 304p. text 49.99 (*0-7236-1014-2*) Buttrwrth-Heinemann.

Concise Introduction to Modern Chemistry. Vijaya Korlipara. 1999. pap. 39.95 (*0-8385-1523-1*, Medical Exam) Appleton & Lange.

Concise Korner Coding Book for General Surgery & Urology. Compiled by R. Earlam. 2nd ed. 1991. 112p. pap. 23.95 (*0-412-43230-7*) Chapman & Hall.

Concise Medical Dictionary. 5th ed. 1998. LC 97-45023. pap. (*0-19-262916-6*) OUP.

Concise Medical Physiology. C. Chaudhuri. 1988. (C). (*0-7855-6120-X*) Current Dist IND. *Dist:* St Mut.

Concise Medical Physiology. S. Chowdhury. 1989. (C). (*0-89771-376-1*) Current Dist IND. *Dist:* St Mut.

Concise Neurosurgery. E. Pasztor. 1980. (Illus.). 292p. 81.75 (*3-8055-1431-X*) S Karger.

***Concise Paediatrics.** Mike Thomson. Ed. by Rachel U. Sidwell. 2000. (Greenwich Medical Media Ser.). (Illus.). 546p. pap. (*1-84110-027-7*) Greenwich Med GBR. *Dist:* JAMCO Dist.

Concise Pathology. Parakrama Chandrasoma & Clive R. Taylor. 3rd ed. 1997. (Illus.). 990p. (C). pap. text 43.95 (*0-8385-1499-5*, A-1499-1, Apple Lange Med) McGraw.

Concise Pediatric Surgery. Lewis Spitz & Arnold G. Coran. 1997. LC 97-69056. (Rob & Smith's Operative Surgery Ser.). (Illus.). 360p. text (*0-412-82780-8*) E A GBR. *Dist:* OUP.

Concise Psychological Dictionary. Ed. by A. Petrovsky. 1987. 358p. (C). 60.00 (*0-7855-3895-X*) St Mut.

Concise Psychological Dictionary. Ed. by A. V. Petrovsky & Petr N. Shikhirev. 1988. LC 87-4167. 358p. 10.95 (*0-7178-0657-X*) Intl Pubs Co.

Concise Review of Clinical Laboratory Science. Joel D. Hubbard. 1997. LC 96-47287. (Illus.). 545p. pap. 37.00 (*0-683-04219-X*) Lppncott W & W.

Concise Reviews in Clinical & Experimental Hematology. Ed. by Martin J. Murphy, Jr. 1992. LC 92-17634. 385p. 69.00 (*1-880854-01-5*) AlphaMed Pr.

Concise Surgery: An Illustrated Introduction. Ed. by Kevin Lafferty & John A. Rennie. 1998. (Arnold Publication). (Illus.). 512p. pap. 32.95 (*0-340-70611-2*) OUP.

Concise System of Orthopaedics & Fractures. A. Graham Apley & Louis Solomon. 2nd ed. 1994. (Illus.). 360p. pap. (*0-7506-1767-5*) E A GBR. *Dist:* OUP.

Concise Text of Neuroscience. Robert E. Kingsley. 1996. LC 95-37148. (Illus.). 456p. (*0-683-04621-7*); 2nd ed. 1999. LC 99-20294. 696p. pap. text 45.00 (*0-683-30460-7*) Lppncott W & W.

Concise Textbook of Clinical Psychiatry. Harold I. Kaplan & Benjamin J. Sadock. 1996. LC 96-3941. (Illus.). 736p. pap. text 49.95 (*0-683-30009-1*) Lppncott W & W.

Concise Vascular Surgery. Ed. by C. W. Jamieson Staff. 1997. (Illus.). 352p. text (*0-412-82450-7*) E A GBR. *Dist:* OUP.

Concomitant Continuous Infusion Chemotherapy & Radiation. Ed. by M. Rotman et al. 1991. (Medical Radiology Ser.). (Illus.). 304p. 186.00 (*0-387-52545-9*) Spr-Verlag.

Concordance to the Science of Mind. Martha A. Stewart & Albert G. Lowe. 1980. 312p. pap. 21.95 (*0-911336-82-6*) Sci of Mind.

Concordance to the Standard Edition of the Complete Works of Sigmund Freud. Samuel A. Guttman et al. 1984. lxiii, 5512p. Vol. 1. LC 83-22874. 140.00 (*0-8236-1071-3*); Vol. 2. LC 83-22874. 140.00 (*0-8236-1072-1*); Vol. 3. LC 83-22874. 140.00 (*0-8236-1073-X*); Vol. 4. 140.00 (*0-8236-1074-8*); Vol. 5. 140.00 (*0-8236-1075-6*); Vol. 6. LC 83-22874. 140.00 (*0-8236-1076-4*) Intl Univs Pr.

Concordantia in Mulomedicinam Chironis. Contrib. by Deane R. Blackman & Gavin G. Betts. 1998. (Alpha-Omega, Reihe A Ser..: Vol. LXXXVI). (GER.). vi, 974p. (*3-487-10641-8*) G Olms Pubs.

Conditioning & Learning: Student Booklet. American Psychological Association Staff. 1981. (Human Behavior Curriculum Project Ser.). 64p. (gr. 9-12). pap. text 3.95 (*0-8077-2623-0*) Tchrs Coll.

Conditioning & Learning: Teachers Handbook & Duplication Masters. American Psychological Association Staff. 1981. (Human Behavior Curriculum Project Ser.). 64p. 9.95 (*0-8077-2624-9*) Tchrs Coll.

Conditioning, Cognition & Methodology: Contemporary Issues in Experimental Psychology. Ed. by Joseph B. Sidowski. 1989. 286p. 53.00 (*0-8191-7496-3*) U Pr of Amer.

Conditioning with Physical Disabilities. Kevin F. Lockette & Ann M. Keyes. 1994. LC 93-47606. 288p. pap. 23.95 (*0-87322-614-3*, PLOC0614) Human Kinetics.

Conditions in Occupational Therapy: Effect on Occupational Performance. Ruth Hansen & Ben Atchison. 1993. (Illus.). 386p. pap. 37.00 (*0-683-03878-8*) Lppncott W & W.

Conditions of Aging in the Academy Collection: Quick Reference Guides for Family Physicians. Lanyard K. Dial & American Academy of Family Physicians Staff. 1998. LC 98-22643. (Academy Collection). 150p. pap. 29.95 (*0-683-30421-6*) Lppncott W & W.

Conditions of Awareness: Subjective Factors in the Social Adaptations of Man & Other Primates. Anthony Shafton. 1976. LC 76-26201. pap. 20.00 (*0-9601130-1-0*) Riverstone.

Conditions of Life in the Sea: Short Account of Quantitative Marine Biological Research. James Johnstone. Ed. by Frank N. Egerton, 3rd. 1978. LC 77-74232. (History of Ecology Ser.). (Illus.). reprint ed. lib. bdg. 30.95 (*0-405-10401-4*) Ayer.

Condom: Increasing Utilization in United States. 1985. (AIDS & Venereal Disease Ser.). lib. bdg. 90.00 (*0-8490-3960-6*) Gordon Pr.

Condoms. Adrian Mindel. 2000. (Illus.). 230p. pap. text (*0-7279-1267-4*) BMJ Pub GBR. *Dist:* AIDC.

Condoms & Sexually Transmitted Diseases Including AIDS. 1991. lib. bdg. 75.00 (*0-8490-5147-9*) Gordon Pr.

Condrau, Gion, Festschrift: Depression - Medizinische, Kulturelle und Anthropologische Aspekte, Zuerich, 10.-11. Juni 1988. Ed. by A. Hicklin. 1989. (Journal: Vol. 6, No. 1-2). 148p. pap. 43.50 (*3-8055-4964-4*) S Karger.

Conduct Disorder & Underachievement: Risk Factors, Assessment, Treatment & Prevention. Harvey P. Mandel. 1997. LC 96-23333. 304p. 105.00 (*0-471-13147-4*) Wiley.

Conduct Disorders & Severe Antisocial Behavior. P. J. Frick. 1998. LC 98-15094. (Clinical Child Psychology Library). (Illus.). 160p. (C). pap. text 23.50 (*0-306-45841-1*, Kluwer Plenum) Kluwer Academic.

Conduct Disorders & Severe Antisocial Behavior. P. J. Frick. 1998. LC 98-15094. (Clinical Child Psychology Library). (Illus.). 140p. (C). 39.50 (*0-306-45840-3*, Plenum Trade) Perseus Pubng.

Conduct Disorders in Childhood & Adolescence, Vol. 9. Alan E. Kazdin. 2nd ed. 1995. LC 95-5295. (Developmental Clinical Psychology & Psychiatry Ser.: No. 9). (Illus.). 200p. (Orig.). pap. 34.95 (*0-8039-7181-8*, 1042) Sage.

Conduct Disorders in Children & Adolescents. Ed. by G. Pirooz Sholevar. 1994. LC 94-26150. 448p. text 54.00 (*0-88048-517-5*, 8517) Am Psychiatric.

Conduct Disorders of Childhood: Psychodynamics & Psychotherapy. Richard A. Gardner. 1994. LC 94-6855. 550p. pap. 40.00 (*0-933812-32-9*) Creative Therapeutics.

Conduct of Care: Understanding Nursing Practice. Joanna Latimer. 2000. LC 00-36012. pap. 41.95 (*0-632-05575-8*) Blackwell Sci.

Conduct Unbecoming a Woman: Medicine on Trial in Turn of the Century Brooklyn. Regina Morantz-Sanchez. 1999. LC 98-29764. (Illus.). 304p. 30.00 (*0-19-512624-6*) OUP.

Conducting a Qualitative Assessment of Vitamin A Deficiency: A Field Guide for Program Managers. Helen Keller International Staff & David S. Rosen. 1993. LC 93-16646. (Illus.). 53p. (Orig.). pap. text 10.00 (*0-915173-22-0*) Helen Keller Intl.

Conducting & Reading Research in Health & Human Performance. Ted A. Baumgartner & Clinton H. Strong. 1994. 352p. (C). text 41.00 net. (*0-697-11169-5*) Brown & Benchmark.

***Conducting & Reading Research in Health & Human Performance.** Ted A. Baumgartner et al. 3rd ed. 2001. LC 2001-30403. xvi, 432p. (*0-07-235388-0*) McGraw.

Conducting Clinical Trials. Frank L. Iber et al. 1987. LC 87-15273. (Illus.). 366p. (C). text 85.00 (*0-306-42626-9*, Kluwer Plenum) Kluwer Academic.

Conducting Epidemiological Research. Harris Pastides. 1999. 74.95 (*0-87371-558-6*, L558) Lewis Pubs.

Conducting Experiments in Psychology: Measuring the Weight of Smoke. Pelham. 1998. LC 98-27537. (Psychology Ser.). pap. 29.50 (*0-534-35718-0*) Brooks-Cole.

Conducting GCP Compliant Clinical Research: A Practical Guide. Wendy Bohaychuk & Graham Ball. 1999. LC 98-54676. 226p. 145.00 (*0-471-98824-3*) Wiley.

Conducting Group Therapy with Addicts: A Guidebook for Professionals. Ivan R. Elder. rev. ed. 1995. 172p. pap. 19.99 (*0-945819-86-2*) Sulzburger & Graham Pub.
Conducting Group Therapy with Addicts: A Handbook for Professionals. Ivan R. Elder. 1990. pap. 17.95 (*0-8306-3567-X*) McGraw-Hill Educ Grp.
Conducting Insanity Evaluations. Richard Rogers & Daniel W. Shuman. 2nd ed. 2000. LC 99-52484. 371p. 42.00 (*1-57230-521-5*, C0521) Guilford Pubns.
Conducting On-Farm Animal Research: Procedures & Economic Analysis. Pervaiz Amir & Hendrik C. Knipscheer. 1989. 244p. 12.50 (*1-57360-010-5*) Winrock Intl.
Conducting Research & Evaluation in Gifted Education: A Handbook of Methods & Applications. Ed. by Nina K. Buchanan & John F. Feldhusen. 1991. (Education & Psychology of the Gifted Ser.: No. 6). 360p. (C). text 50.00 (*0-8077-3083-1*); pap. text 25.95 (*0-8077-3082-3*) Tchrs Coll.
***Conducting Research in Anaesthesia & Intensive Care Medicine.** Alex M. Zbinden & Dick Thomson. 2001. LC 00-46765. 568p. pap. text 69.95 (*0-7506-4544-X*) Buttrwrth-Heinemann.
Conducting Research in Psychology: Measuring the Weight of Smoke (International Version) Brett W. Pelham. 1998. LC 98-27537. 380p. spiral bd. 48.95 (*0-534-36358-X*) Brooks-Cole.
Conducting Research in the Practice Setting. Ed. by Fred Tudiver et al. 1993. (Research Methods for Primary Care Ser.: Vol. 5). (Illus.). 272p. LC 93-973. 86.95 (*0-8039-5126-4*, 4307); pap. 37.95 (*0-8039-5127-2*, 4308) Sage.
Conducting School-Based Assessments of Child & Adolescent Behavior. Ed. by Edward S. Shapiro & Thomas R. Kratochwill. 2000. (Guilford School Practitioner Ser.). 318p. text 35.00 (*1-57230-567-3*, C0567) Guilford Pubns.
Conducting Scientifically Crafted Child Custody Evalutations. Jonathan W. Gould. 1998. LC 98-19718. 387p. 79.95 (*0-7619-1100-6*, 81873); pap. 39.95 (*0-7619-1101-4*, 81874) Sage.
Conduction Aphasia. Ed. by Susan E. Kohn. 1992. LC 92-18219. 184p. 45.00 (*0-8058-0681-4*) L Erlbaum Assocs.
Conduction Blockade for Postoperative Analgesia. McClure. 1991. 256p. pap. (*0-340-55041-4*) E A GBR. *Dist:* Routldge.
Conduction Heart Order. Hein J. Wellens. 1978. pap. text (*90-247-2080-X*) M Nijhoff NLD. *Dist:* Kluwer Academic.
Conduction System of the Mammalian Heart: An Anatomico-Histological Study of the Atrioventricular Bundle & the Purkinje Fibers. S. Tawara. Tr. by Kozo Suma & Munehiro Shimada from GER. 1998. (Cardiopulmonary Medicine Ser.). 250p. 48.00 (*981-02-3502-X*) World Scientific Pub.
Conexion Salud-Desarrollo. Rosalia Rodriguez-Garcia et al. 1996. (ENG & SPA., Illus.). xv, 207p. (Orig.). pap. text (*0-9636369-1-X*) PAHO.
Confederate Nurse: The Diary of Ada W. Bacot 1860-1863. Ed. by Jean V. Berlin. 1994. LC 93-30098. (Women's Diaries & Letters of the Nineteenth-Century South). 220p. 24.95 (*0-87249-970-7*) U of SC Pr.
Confederate States Medical & Surgical Journal. Samuel P. Moore. 1992. (American Civil War Medical Ser.: No. 12). 272p. reprint ed. 95.00 (*0-930405-40-4*) Norman SF.
Confederate Surgeon. 1985. (Illus.). 152p. 25.00 (*0-9619508-1-1*) W R Scaife.
Conference of Directors of Schools of Public Health: Report of a WHO Inter-Regional Conference, 1967. 1967. (Technical Report Ser.). 24p. pap. text 3.00 (*92-4-120351-X*, 1100351) World Health.
Conference on Malaria in Africa - Proceedings: Practical Considerations on Malaria Vaccines & Clinical Trials. Intro. by Alfred A. Buck. 1988. 328p. (Orig.). pap. (*0-936829-02-8*) Am Inst Bio Sci.
Conference on Medicine & Public Health in the Arctic & Antarctic. 1963. (Technical Report Ser.: No. 253). 29p. pap. text 3.00 (*92-4-120253-X*) World Health.
Conferences on Cellular Dynamics: Proceedings of the 5th Interdisciplinary Conference Interdisciplinary Conference Staff. Ed. by L. D. Peachey. 1969. 446p. 173.00 (*0-677-65010-8*) Gordon & Breach.
Conferencia Internacional Sober la Hiperplasia Prostatica Benigna, Paris, June 26-27, 1991. A. T. Cockett. 1991. (SPA.). 272p. pap. (*84-7978-064-9*) Ediciones Diaz ESP. *Dist:* IBD Ltd.
Confessing Excess: Women & the Politics of Body Reduction. Carole Spitzack. 1990. LC 89-36513. (SUNY Series in Gender & Society). 200p. (C). text 64.50 (*0-7914-0271-1*); pap. text 22.95 (*0-7914-0272-X*) State U NY Pr.
***Confession of an Estrogen Evangelist: Setting the Record Straight on Estrogen Replacement Therapy.** Joyce A. Kakkis. 2001. (Illus.). 254p. pap. 19.95 (*0-9709399-0-6*, 01) J Kakkis.
Confessions in Psychotherapy. Sharon Hymer. 1988. LC 87-19623. text 29.95 (*0-89876-134-4*) Gardner Pr.
Confessions of a Medical Heretic. Robert S. Mendelsohn. 1990. 208p. reprint ed. pap. 16.95 (*0-8092-4131-5*, 413150, Contemporary) McGraw-Hill Trade.
Confessions of a Medicine Man: An Essay in Popular Philosophy. Alfred I. Tauber. 1999. LC 98-27288. (Bradford Book Ser.). (Illus.). 160p. 25.00 (*0-262-20114-3*, Bradford Bks) MIT Pr.
Confessions of an English Opium Eater. Thomas de Quincey. Tr. by Aileen Ward. 1985. 336p. mass mkt. 4.95 (*0-88184-130-7*) Carroll & Graf.
Confessions of an Estrogen Evangelist: Setting the Record Straight on Estrogen Replacement Therapy. Joyce A. Kakkis & David Paul Green. 2001. 288p. pap. 15.00 (*1-57566-618-9*, Knsington) Kensgtn Pub Corp.
Confident Childbirth: Your Guide Through Pregnancy, Labor, Birth & Early Parenthood. Mary J. Smith. 1991. (Illus.). 100p. (Orig.). pap. 12.95 (*0-9630874-0-1*) A P P L E Fam.
Confidentiality of Health Records: The Meeting of Law, Ethics, & Clinical Issues. Herman Schuchman et al. 1982. LC 82-990. text 30.00 (*0-89876-024-0*) Gardner Pr.
Confidentiality Versus the Duty to Protect: Foreseeable Harm in the Practice of Psychiatry. Ed. by James C. Beck. 1990. LC 90-13. (Issues in Psychiatry Ser.). 212p. text 16.95 (*0-88048-170-6*, 8170) Am Psychiatric.
Configuration Management & Document Control: Fundamentals for Medical Device & Quality Certified Manufacturing. Daniel P. Brennand & David P. Tondreau. 1997. LC 96-93026. x, 284 p. (*0-9656032-0-2*) CMDC Systs.
Confined Space Emergency: Leader's Guide. Shirley Ayers. 1995. 56p. pap. 20.00 (*0-945790-10-4*) Detrick Lawrence.
Confirmation Learning Theory. Raymond E. Hartley & Carl D. Williams. 1988. (American University Studies: Ser. VIII). 419p. (C). text 50.50 (*0-8204-0713-5*) P Lang Pubng.
Conflict & Cohesion in Families: Causes & Consequences. Ed. by Martha J. Cox & Jeanne Brooks-Gunn. 1999. LC 98-28381. (Advances in Family Research Ser.). 372p. 79.95 (*0-8058-2410-3*) L Erlbaum Assocs.
Conflict & Compromise: Therapeutic Implications. Ed. by Scott Dowling. 1991. LC 91-30989. (Workshop Series of the American Psychoanalytic Association: Monograph 7). 248p. (C). 37.50 (*0-8236-1038-1*) Intl Univs Pr.
Conflict & Confrontation: A Training Program. Peter Muniz & Robert Chasnoff. 1981. 26p. (C). pap. text 7.00 (*0-943300-01-0*) LABS.
Conflict & Continuity: A History of Ideas in Social Equality & Human Development. Ed. by John R. Snarey et al. 1981. LC 80-83476. (Reprint Ser.: No. 15). 471p. pap. 16.95 (*0-916690-17-2*) Harvard Educ Rev.
Conflict & Harmony: A Source-Book of Man in His Environment. Ed. by Grace E. King. 1972. 450p. pap. 25.00 (*0-8464-0274-2*) Beekman Pubs.
Conflict & Social Psychology. Ed. by Knud S. Larsen. 1993. 272p. (C). text 65.00 (*0-8039-8745-5*) Sage.
Conflict in Child & Adolescent Development. Ed. by Carolyn U. Shantz & Willard W. Hartup. 1992. (Cambridge Studies in Social & Emotional Development). (Illus.). 463p. (C). text 90.00 (*0-521-40416-9*) Cambridge U Pr.
Conflict in General Practice. Hobden. 1998. (C). pap. text (*0-443-05936-5*) Church.
Conflict in Intimate Relationships. Dudley D. Cahn. 1992. LC 92-1556. (Series on Intimate Relationships). 148p. 45.00 (*0-89862-975-6*); pap. 21.00 (*0-89862-982-9*, 2982) Guilford Pubns.
Conflict of the Faculties. Immanuel Kant. Tr. & Intro. by Mary J. Gregor. 1992. LC 92-16151. 217p. pap. text 18.00 (*0-8032-7775-X*) U of Nebr Pr.
***Conflicts in Care: Medicine & Nursing.** MacKay. 1992. pap. 26.95 (*0-412-47860-9*) Chapman & Hall.
Conflicts of Interest in Clinical Practice & Research. Ed. by Roy G. Spece, Jr. et al. 1996. 472p. text 49.95 (*0-19-508024-6*) OUP.
Confocal Laser Scanning Microscopy. C. Sheppard & D. Shotton. 1997. LC 97-24717. (Microscopy Handbooks: No. 38). (Illus.). 106p. pap. 37.95 (*0-387-91514-1*) Spr-Verlag.
Confocal Microscopy. Sidney P. Colowick. 1999. (Methods in Enzymology Ser.: Vol. 307). 602p. 105.00 (*0-12-182208-7*) Acad Pr.
Confocal Microscopy: Methods & Protocols. Stephen W. Paddock. 1998. LC 98-38205. (Methods in Molecular Biology Ser.: Vol. 122). (Illus.). 464p. 99.50 (*0-89603-526-3*) Humana.
Confrontation Analysis: Theory & Practice. Abraham Cohen. 1981. 528p. text 56.00 (*0-8089-1417-0*, 790876, Grune & Strat) Harcrt Hlth Sci Grp.
Confrontation Between the Young Deaf-Blind Child & the Outer World. M. R. Jurgens. 1977. vi, 58p. pap. (*90-265-0261-3*) Swets.
Confronting Abuse: An LDS Perspective on Understanding & Healing Emotional, Physical, Sexual, Psychological, & Spiritual Abuse. Ed. by Anne L. Horton et al. 1993. LC 92-42824. xv, 389p. 16.95 (*0-87579-637-0*) Deseret Bk.
Confronting Abusive Beliefs: Group Treatment for Abusive Men. Mary N. Russell. 1995. (Interpersonal Violence Ser.: Vol. 12). 12p. LC 96-35124. 79.95 (*0-8039-5807-2*, 9747); pap. 31.95 (*0-8039-5808-0*, 9748) Sage.
Confronting AIDS: Directions for Public Health, Health Care, & Research. Ed. by Institute of Medicine Staff. 1986. LC 86-23779. 374p. pap. text 29.95 (*0-309-03699-2*) Natl Acad Pr.
Confronting AIDS: Public Priorities in a Global Epidemic. World Bank, Policy Research Department Staff. rev. ed. 1999. LC 99-48248. (World Bank Publications). (Illus.). 300p. pap. text 30.00 (*0-19-521591-5*) OUP.
Confronting AIDS: Public Priorities in a Global Epidemic. World Bank, Policy Research Department Staff. 1997. LC 97-17434. (World Bank Policy Research Reports). (Illus.). 300p. pap. text 30.00 (*0-19-521117-0*, 61117) World Bank.
Confronting AIDS: Update 1988. Institute of Medicine Staff. 1988. 256p. pap. 24.95 (*0-309-03879-0*) Natl Acad Pr.
Confronting Autism: The Aurora on the Dark Side of Venus: A Practical Guide to Hope, Knowledge, & Empowerment. Victoria A. Beck. 1999. LC 00-500203. xxv, 162p. pap. 18.00 (*0-9674969-0-X*) New Destiny Ed.
Confronting Cancer: How to Care for Today & Tomorrow. M. M. Sherry. 1994. LC 94-2301. (Illus.). 400p. (C). pap. 16.95 (*0-306-44644-8*) Perseus Bks Grp.
Confronting Cancer, Constructing Change: New Perspectives on Women & Cancer. Ed. by Midge Stocker. 1993. LC 92-16998. (Women - Cancer - Fear - Power Ser.: Vol. 2). 304p. (Orig.). 30.95 (*1-879427-17-6*) Third Side Pr.
Confronting Cholera: The Development of a Hemispheric Response to the Epidemic. Ed. by Henry Hamman. 1991. 74p. (C). pap. text 11.95 (*0-935501-39-8*) U Miami N-S Ctr.
Confronting Critical Health Issues of Asian & Pacific Islander Americans. Ed. by Nolan Zane et al. 1994. LC 93-34623. (Illus.). 452p. (C). 86.95 (*0-8039-5113-2*, 4991) Sage.
Confronting Death. Richard W. Momeyer. 1988. LC 87-45439. (Medical Ethics Ser.). 204p. 27.50 (*0-253-31403-8*) Ind U Pr.
Confronting Life-Threatening Illness: Maintaining Control & Establishing Positive Objectives. Ed. by John D. Whitacre. 1992. 96p. pap. 12.95 (*0-87650-304-0*) Pierian.
Confronting Life-Threatening Illness: Mind - Body Approaches. Ed. by Suzanne R. Engelman. 1993. pap. 19.95 (*0-8290-2473-5*) Irvington.
Confronting Mitral Valve Prolapse Syndrome. Lyn Frederickson. 1992. LC 92-9871. (Illus.). 182p. reprint ed. pap. 13.99 (*0-446-39407-6*) Warner Bks.
Confronting Public Health Risks: A Decision Maker's Guide. Laura C. Leviton et al. 1998. LC 97-33795. 78.95 (*0-8039-5356-9*, 4581); pap. 36.95 (*0-8039-5357-7*, 4582) Sage.
Confronting Substance Abuse: An Action Plan for Change. 1993. 250p. (Orig.). (C). pap. text 50.00 (*1-56806-767-4*) DIANE Pub.
Confronting the AIDS Epidemic: Cross-Cultural Perspectives on HIV/AIDS Education. Ed. by Davidson C. Umeh. 1996. LC 97-550. 560p. 79.95 (*0-86543-526-X*); pap. 21.95 (*0-86543-527-8*) Africa World.
Confronting Traumatic Brain Injury: Devastation, Hope & Healing. William J. Winslade. 1998. LC 97-32406. (Illus.). 220p. 40.00 (*0-300-07026-8*) Yale U Pr.
Confused Consumer's Guide to Choosing a Health Care Plan: Everything You Need to Know. Martin Gottlieb. 1998. LC 98-24775. 272p. (J). pap. 12.95 (*0-7868-8233-6*) Hyperion.
Confused Professionals: Exploring the Myth of Dementia. Nancy H. Harding & Colin Palfrey. 1996. 200p. pap. (*1-85302-257-8*) Jessica Kingsley GBR. *Dist:* Taylor & Francis.
Confusional States in Older People. Eleanor J. Byrne. 1994. 112p. pap. text (*0-340-56298-6*) E A GBR. *Dist:* OUP.
Congenital Adrenal Hyperplasia. M. I. News & L. S. Levine. 1984. (Monographs in Endocrinology: Vol. 26). (Illus.). 88p. 62.95 (*0-387-12259-1*) Spr-Verlag.
Congenital & Perinatal Infections: Prevention, Diagnosis & Treatment. Ed. by James McIntyre & Marie-Louise Newell. 2000. LC 00-708630. (Illus.). 356p. (C). pap. text 59.95 (*0-521-78979-6*) Cambridge U Pr.
Congenital Cardiac Surgery. Ed. by Bruce A. Reitz & David D. Yuh. 2001. 350p. (C). 195.00 (*0-8385-1542-8*) Appleton & Lange.
Congenital Chromosome Aberrations & Tumour Predisposition. Gy. Fekete. 1990. (Illus.). 161p. (C). (*963-05-5753-3*) Akade Kiado HUN. *Dist:* Intl Spec Bk, St Mut.
Congenital Clubfoot: Fundamentals for Treatment. Ignacio Ponseti. 1996. (Illus.). 150p. (C). text 125.00 (*0-19-262765-1*) OUP.
Congenital Diaphragmatic Hernia. Ed. by P. Puri. 1989. (Modern Problems in Pediatrics Ser.: Vol. 24). (Illus.). 164p. 104.50 (*3-8055-4807-9*) S Karger.
Congenital Disorders Sourcebook: Basic Information about Disorders Acquired During Gestation. Ed. by Karen Bellenir. 1997. LC 97-17092. (Health Reference Ser.: Vol. 29). xi, 607p. lib. bdg. 78.00 (*0-7808-0205-5*) Omnigraphics Inc.
Congenital Displacement of the Hip Joint. J. A. Wilkinson. 1985. (Illus.). 153p. 257.00 (*0-387-13947-8*) Spr-Verlag.
Congenital Dysplasia & Dislocation of the Hip in Children & Adults. D. Tonis. Tr. by Terry C. Telger from GER. 1987. (Illus.). 536p. 366.00 (*0-387-16286-0*) Spr-Verlag.
Congenital External & Middle Ear Malformations: Management. Ed. by B. Ars. 1992. LC 92-49672. (Illus.). 80p. (*90-6299-086-X*) Kugler NLD. *Dist:* Lib Res.
Congenital Heart Disease. Burton W. Fink. 1975. (Illus.). 183p. pap. 29.95 (*0-8151-3222-0*) Mosby Inc.
Congenital Heart Disease. Ed. by F. J. Macartney. 1985. (Current Status of Clinical Cardiology Ser.). text 155.50 (*0-85200-719-1*) Kluwer Academic.
Congenital Heart Disease: A Diagrammatic Atlas. Charles E. Mullins & David C. Mayer. 1991. (Illus.). 394p. pap. 160.00 (*0-471-58817-2*, Wiley-Liss) Wiley.
Congenital Heart Disease: Textbook of Angiocardiography Robert M. Freedom et al. 1997. LC 96-42295. (Illus.). 1552p. 275.00 (*0-87993-656-8*) Futura Pub.
Congenital Heart Disease in Adolescents & Adults. Ed. by John Hess & George R. Sutherland. 1992. LC 92-49625. (Developments in Cardiovascular Medicine Ser.: Vol. 136). 216p. (C). text 185.00 (*0-7923-1862-5*) Kluwer Academic.
Congenital Heart Disease in Adults. Joseph K. Perloff & John S. Child. 2nd ed. 1997. LC 96-50089. (Illus.). 352p. text 110.00 (*0-7216-2998-9*) Saunders.
Congenital Heart Disease in Adults: A Practical Guide. Andrew Redington et al. 1994. (Illus.). 270p. text (*0-7020-1913-5*) W B Saunders GBR. *Dist:* Saunders.
Congenital Heart Disease with Cyanosis Symposium, Amsterdam 1968. Congenital Heart Disease with Cyanosis Symposium S. Ed. by A. C. Klinkhammer. 1970. (Radiologia Clinica et Biologica Ser.: Vol. 39, No. 2). reprint ed. pap. 28.00 (*3-8055-0802-6*) S Karger.
***Congenital Heart Diseases in the Adult.** Welton Gersony & Marlon Rosenbaum. 2001. (Illus.). 300p. text 99.00 (*0-07-032909-5*) McGraw-Hill Prof.
Congenital Heart Surgery: Current Techniques & Controversies. Ed. by Anthony L. Moulton. 1984. LC 83-21342. (Illus.). 347p. text 97.50 (*0-941022-00-5*) Davies Pubng.
Congenital Hemiplegia. Ed. by Brian Neville & Robert Goodman. 2001. (Clinics in Developmental Medicine Ser.: No. 150). 200p. (C). text (*1-898683-19-0*) Mc Keith Pr GBR. *Dist:* Cambridge U Pr.
Congenital Limb Deficiencies in Hungary: Genetic & Teratologic Epidemiological Studies. E. Czeizel et al. 1994. LC 95-177096. 420p. pap. (*963-05-6631-1*) Akade Kiado HUN. *Dist:* Intl Spec Bk, St Mut.
Congenital Malformation Syndromes. Ed. by D. Donnai & R. Winter. 1995. (Illus.). 640p. (gr. 13). (*0-412-56590-0*) E A GBR. *Dist:* OUP.
Congenital Malformations of the Brain: Pathological, Embryological, Clinical, Radiological & Genetic Aspects. Margaret G. Norman et al. 1995. (Illus.). 472p. text 98.50 (*0-19-506245-0*) OUP.
Congenital Malformations of the Female Genital Tract: Diagnosis & Management. Gita P. Gidwani. 1999. LC 98-52913. 272p. text 85.00 (*0-7817-1725-6*) Lppncott W & W.
Congenital Malformations of the Female Reproductive Tract & Their Treatment. Barry S. Verkauf. 1993. (Illus.). 240p. (C). pap. text 75.00 (*0-8385-1377-8*, A1377-9, Apple Lange Med) McGraw.
Congenital Malformations of the Hand & Upper Extremity. D. Buck-Gramcko. 1997. (Illus.). 704p. (*0-443-03560-1*) Church.
Congenital Malformations of the Urinary Tract. F. Douglas Stephens. 1983. LC 83-11207. (Illus.). 577p. 53.95 (*0-275-91414-3*, C1414, Praeger Pubs) Greenwood.
Congenital Malformations Worldwide: A Report from the International Clearing House for Birth Defects Monitoring Systems. Ed. by P. W. Peters. 1991. 220p. 143.25 (*0-444-89137-4*) Elsevier.
Congenital Muscular Dystrophies, Vol. 13. Ed. by Yukio Fukuyama et al. 1997. LC 97-17026. (Developments in Neurology Ser.: 13). (Illus.). 458p. 219.50 (*0-444-82487-1*) Elsevier.
Congenital, Perinatal & Neonatal Infections. Ed. by Ann Greenhough et al. 1992. (Illus.). 245p. text (*0-443-04508-9*) Church.
Congenital Toxoplasmosis: Scientific Background, Clinical Management & Control. P. Ambroise-Thomas & E. L. Petersen. 2000. LC 99-52109. (Illus.). 300p. pap. (*2-287-59664-X*) Spl France Editions FRA. *Dist:* Spr-Verlag.
Congestive Cardiac Failure: Pathophysiology & Treatment. Ed. by David B. Barnett et al. 1993. LC 93-7106. (Fundamental & Clinical Cardiology Ser.: Vol. 14). (Illus.). 408p. text 185.00 (*0-8247-8821-4*) Dekker.
Congestive Heart Failure. David McCall & Shahbudin Rahimtoola. 1995. (Illus.). 448p. (*0-412-04441-2*) E A GBR. *Dist:* OUP.
Congestive Heart Failure. Douglas Wetherill & Dean J. Kereiakes. 2000. LC 00-22111. (What You Should Know Ser.). (Illus.). viii, 136p. pap. 6.99 (*1-55870-551-1*, Betrwy Bks) F & W Pubns Inc.
***Congestive Heart Failure.** Douglas L. Wetherill & Dean J. Kereiakes. 2nd ed. 2001. (What You Should Know Ser.). (Illus.). 136p. pap. 8.99 (*0-632-04527-2*) Blackwell Sci.

***Congestive Heart Failure: Advances in Treatment & Their Market Potential.** Gerry Harnisch. Ed. by Susan C. DiClemente & Sarah L. Young. 2001. (Illus.). 237p. spiral bd. 4950.00 (*1-57936-138-2*) Drug & Market Dev.

Congestive Heart Failure: Current Clinical Issues. Ed. by Gemma T. Kennedy & Michael H. Crawford. 1994. LC 93-40981. (American Heart Association Monograph Ser.). (Illus.). 183p. pap. 27.00 (*0-87993-586-3*) Futura Pub.

Congestive Heart Failure: Pathophysiology, Diagnosis & Comprehensive Approach to Management. Ed. by Jeffrey D. Hosenpud & B. Greenberg. 1993. (Illus.). 810p. (*3-540-94017-0*) Spr-Verlag.

Congestive Heart Failure: Pathophysiology, Diagnosis & Comprehensive Approach To Management. Jeffrey D. Hosenpud & Barry Greenberg. 2nd ed. 1999. LC 99-36855. (Illus.). xix, 858p. text 169.00 (*0-683-30437-2*) Lppncott W & W.

Congestive Heart Failure: Pathophysiology, Diagnosis & Treatment. Jon D. Blumenfeld & John H. Laragh. 1994. 215p. per. 19.95 (*0-9632400-6-4*) Prof Comms.

Congestive Heart Failure: Proceedings of Symposium on New Drugs & Devices, October 30-31, 1986, Philadelphia, PA. Ed. by Joel Morganroth. 1987. (Developments in Cardiovascular Medicine Ser.). (C). text 138.00 (*0-89838-955-0*) Kluwer Academic.

Congress of Nephrology 1998: Joint Scientific Meeting Gesellschaft fur Nephrologie Deutsche Arbeitsgemeinschaft fur Klinische Nephrologie, Erlangen, September 1998. Ed. by R. Bernd Sterzel & Walter Schulz. 1998. (Kidney & Blood Pressure Research Ser.: Vol. 21, Nos. 2-4 (1998)). 216p. pap. 68.00 (*3-8055-6763-4*) S Karger.

Congress of Nephrology 2000: Joint Scientific Meeting: Gesellschaft fur Nephrologie, Deutsche Arbeitsgemeinschaft fur Klinische Nephrologie, Osterreichische Gesellschaft fur Nephrologie, Vienna, September 2000: Abstracts. Ed. by W. H. Horl et al. 2000. (Kidney & Blood Pressure Research Ser.: Vol. 23, No. 3-5). (Illus.). 212p. pap. 48.75 (*3-8055-7153-4*) S Karger.

Congress of Neurological Surgeons. CNS Clinical Neurosurgery Staff & Warren R. Selman. (Illus.). Vol. 38. 1992. 736p. 67.00 (*0-683-02035-8*); Vol. 41. 1994. 586p. (*0-683-02038-2*) Lppncott W & W.

Congress on Electrocardiology, 1st, Wiesbaden, Oct. 1974. Congress on Electrocardiology, 1st, Wiesbaden, Oct. Ed. by H. Abel. 1976. (Advances in Cardiology Ser.: Vol. 16). 111.50 (*3-8055-2197-9*) S Karger.

Conjoint Behavioral Consultation: A Procedural Manual. Susan M. Sheridan et al. 1996. LC 95-46987. (Applied Clinical Psychology Ser.). (Illus.). 208p. (C). 23.50 (*0-306-45155-7*, Plenum Trade) Perseus Pubng.

Conjoint Family Therapy. Virginia M. Satir. 3rd rev. ed. 1982. LC 82-61781. pap. 17.95 (*0-8314-0063-3*) Sci & Behavior.

Conjoint Marital Therapy. R. V. Fitzgerald. 1990. LC 73-81208. (Conjoint Marital Therapy CL Ser.). 256p. reprint ed. 40.00 (*0-87668-091-0*) Aronson.

Conjugate Vaccines. Ed. by J. M. Cruse & R. F. Lewis, Jr. 1989. (Contributions to Microbiology & Immunology Ser.: Vol. 10). (Illus.). vi, 198p. 143.50 (*3-8055-4932-6*) S Karger.

Conjugation-Deconjugation Reactions in Drug Metabolism & Toxicity. Ed. by Frederick C. Kauffman. 1994. LC 93-43134. (Handbook of Experimental Pharmacology Ser.: Vol. 112). (Illus.). 530p. 435.00 (*0-387-57122-1*) Spr-Verlag.

Conjugation Reactions in Drug Metabolism: An Integral Approach. Ed. by Gerard J. Mulder. 1990. 300p. 148.00 (*0-85066-738-0*) Taylor & Francis.

Conjunctivitis of the Newborn: Prevention & Treatment at the Primary Health Care Level. 1986. (Illus.). 35p. pap. text 13.00 (*92-4-156088-6*, 1150244) World Health.

Connecticut Health Care in Perspective 2000. Ed. by Kathleen O'Leary Morgan & Scott E. Morgan. 2000. 21p. spiral bd. 19.00 (*0-7401-0206-0*) Morgan Quitno Corp.

Connecticut Health Care Perspective, 1998. Ed. by Kathleen O'Leary Morgan & Scott E. Morgan. 1998. 20p. pap. 19.00 (*1-56692-806-0*) Morgan Quitno Corp.

Connecting with the New Healthcare Consumer: Defining Your Strategy. David B. Nash. 1999. LC 99-59088. xxiv, 544p. 60.00 (*0-07-134672-4*) McGraw.

Connectionist-Symbolic Integration: From Unified to Hybrid Approaches. Ed. by Ron Sun & Frederic Alexandre. 1996. LC 97-30217. 400p. 60.00 (*0-8058-2348-4*); pap. 30.00 (*0-8058-2349-2*) L Erlbaum Assocs.

Connections: A Self-Help & Resource Guide for Individuals with Mental Illness, Their Families & Social Service Professionals. Eleanor Owen. 9th rev. ed. 1996. 225p. (C). pap. text 33.00 (*0-926980-00-9*) WA Advocates.

Connections & Symbols. Ed. by Steven Pinker & Jacques A. Mehler. 1988. LC 88-6774. (Cognitive Special Issues Ser.). 255p. (Orig.). pap. 22.00 (*0-262-66064-4*, Bradford Bks) MIT Pr.

Connections Between Sex & Aggression. Dolf Zillmann. 1984. LC 83-20633. 272p. 29.95 (*0-89859-333-6*) L Erlbaum Assocs.

Connections, Cognition & Alzheimer's Disease. B. T. Hyman et al. 1997. LC 96-40405. (Research & Perspectives in Alzheimer's Disease Ser.). (Illus.). 245p. 119.00 (*3-540-62205-5*) Spr-Verlag.

Connections for Health. Kathleen D. Mullen et al. 3rd ed. 1993. 624p. (C). (*0-697-17345-3*) Brown & Benchmark.

***Connections for Health.** Kathleen M. Conley. 4th ed. 1996. stu. ed., wbk. ed. 64.38 (*0-697-33556-9*) McGrw-H Hghr Educ.

Connections for Health. Mullen. 4th ed. 1996. 79.06 (*0-697-21569-5*, WCB McGr Hill) McGrw-H Hghr Educ.

Connections for Health. Mullen et al. 5th ed. 1999. 34.74 net. (*0-697-29421-8*, WCB McGr Hill) McGrw-H Hghr Educ.

Connections for Health: Ancillary Binder. Mullen et al. 3rd ed. 1996. 31.74 net. (*0-697-21570-9*, WCB McGr Hill) McGrw-H Hghr Educ.

Connective Tissue: Biological & Clinical Aspects. Ed. by K. Kuehn & T. Krieg. 1986. (Rheumatology Ser.: Vol. 10). (Illus.). x, 490p. 304.50 (*3-8055-4225-9*) S Karger.

Connective Tissue & Its Disorders: Molecular, Genetic, & Medical Aspects. Ed. by Peter M. Royce & Beat Steinmann. 1992. LC 00-92. 724p. 489.00 (*0-471-58819-9*, Wiley-Liss) Wiley.

Connective Tissue Disease: Molecular Pathology of the Extracellular Matrix. Jouni Uitto. Ed. by Andrew Perejda. 1986. (Biochemistry of Disease Ser.: Vol. 12). (Illus.). 568p. text 250.00 (*0-8247-7533-3*) Dekker.

Connective Tissue Diseases. Ed. by Jill J. F. Belch & Robert B. Zurier. 1995. (Illus.). 412p. (*0-412-48620-2*) E A GBR. *Dist:* OUP.

Connective Tissue Diseases. Tuffanelli. 1991. (*0-8151-8862-5*) Mosby Inc.

Connective Tissue Diseases. Graham R. Hughes. 4th ed. 1994. LC 93-38328. (Illus.). 328p. 95.00 (*0-632-03752-0*) Blackwell Sci.

Connective Tissue Diseases of the Skin. Ed. by Charles M. Lapiere & Thomas Krieg. 1993. (Basic & Clinical Dermatology Ser.: Vol. 9). (Illus.). 408p. text 199.00 (*0-8247-9133-9*) Dekker.

Connective Tissue in Health & Disease. Ed. by Marcos Rojkind. 1989. 224p. lib. bdg. 35.00 (*0-8493-4161-2*, RC924) CRC Pr.

Connective Tissue Manipulations. Maria Ebner. 1985. LC 84-9636. 288p. (C). lib. bdg. 31.50 (*0-89874-763-5*) Krieger.

Connective Tissues in Arterial & Pulmonary Disease. T. F. McDonald. Ed. by A. B. Chandler. 1981. (Illus.). 355p. 106.00 (*0-387-90623-1*) Spr-Verlag.

Connexin Methods & Protocols. Ed. by Roberto Bruzzone & Christian Giaume. 2000. LC 99-87338. (Methods in Molecular Biology Ser.: Vol. 154). (Illus.). xiv, 491p. 125.00 (*0-89603-658-8*) Humana.

Conn's Current Therapy, 1998: Latest Approved Methods of Treatment for the Practicing Physician. Robert E. Rakel. Ed. by Ray Kersey. 98th ed. 1998. (Illus.). 1312p. text 59.00 (*0-7216-7223-X*) Saunders.

Conn's Current Therapy 1999. Robert E. Rakel. Ed. by Ray Kersey. 99th ed. 1998. 1310p. (C). text 59.00 (*0-7216-7224-8*) Saunders.

Conquer Candida: And Restore Your Immune System. Jack Tips. 1987. 163p. pap. 14.95 (*0-929167-00-7*) Apple-a-Day.

Conquer Depression Now: From Sad to Glad at Home, School & Work. David S. Wiesenberg. 1996. LC 95-94635. (Illus.). 320p. pap. 14.95 (*0-9647692-5-5*) Meadow Mtn Pr.

Conquer Fatigue in 30 Days! A Wellness Program to Increase Your Energy Vitality & Productivity. Elizabeth A. Walker. 2001. 238p. pap. 19.95 (*0-9704348-0-4*) Vitality Dr.

Conquer Odds. Charlotte Libov. 1999. text 23.95 (*0-525-94166-5*) Viking Penguin.

Conquer Your Headaches: How to Get Rid of Your Headaches & on with Your Life. Robert G. Ford & Kay T. Ford. 1994. LC 94-75614. 100p. pap. 15.95 (*0-9636292-5-5*) Intl Headache.

Conquering Asthma: An Illustrated Guide to Understanding & Care for Adults. Michael T. Newhouse & Peter J. Barnes. 1995. (Illus.). 124p. (Orig.). pap. 12.95 (*0-9695171-1-4*) Login Pubs Consort.

Conquering Bladder & Prostate Problems: The Authoritative Guide for Men & Women. Jerry G. Blaivas. 1998. LC 98-12045. (Illus.). 340p. (C). 26.95 (*0-306-45864-0*) Perseus Bks Grp.

Conquering Cancer: An Invitation to Hope. Paul Johnson. 1991. 256p. pap. 12.99 (*0-310-53781-9*) Zondervan.

Conquering Carpal Tunnel Syndrome: And Other Repetitive Strain Injuries. Sharon J. Butler. 1996. LC 94-96893. 160p. pap. text 17.95 (*1-57224-039-3*) New Harbinger.

Conquering Childhood Asthma. Bruce K. Rubin. 1995. 12.95 (*0-9697781-7-1*) Login Pubs Consort.

Conquering Childhood Asthma: An Illustrated Guide to Understanding the Treatment & Control of Childhood Asthma. Bruce K. Rubin et al. 1998. LC 98-206940. (Illus.). iv, 114p. (*1-896998-02-X*) Decker Art.

Conquering Chronic Disease: Through Maharishi Vedic Medicine. Kumuda Reddy & Linda Egenes. 2000. (Illus.). 350p. pap. 18.95 (*1-929297-00-9*) Samhita Prodns.

Conquering Chronic Disease Through Maharishi Vedic Medicine. Kumuda Reddy et al. 2001. (Illus.). 350p. pap. 18.95 (*1-930051-55-7*) Lantern Books.

***Conquering Diabetes: Are We Taking Full Advantage of the Scientific Opportunities for Research? - Congressional Hearing.** Ed. by Susan M. Collins. 2001. (Illus.). 156p. (C). pap. 35.00 (*0-7567-1294-7*) DIANE Pub.

Conquering Diabetes: Are We Taking Full Advantage of the Scientific Opportunities for Research? : Hearing Before the Permanent Subcommittee on Investigations of the Committee on Governmental Affairs, United States Senate, One Hundred Sixth Congress, First Session, October 14, 1999. Ed. by U. S. Congress, Senate Committee on Governmental Affairs, Permanent Subcommittee on Investigations. 2000. LC 00-325539. (Illus.). iv, 156p. (*0-16-060070-7*) USGPO.

Conquering Hair Loss: A Complete Medical Guide to Hair Loss Assessment, Prevention & Restoration. Nasser Razack. unabr. ed. 1997. LC 96-92990. (Illus.). iv, 270p. (Orig.). pap. 29.95 (*0-9656921-0-8*) Raztec Entrprises.

Conquering Hepatitis. Willis C. Maddrey. 2000. LC 2001-411067. (Illus.). 100p. pap. (*1-896998-06-2*, Empowering Pr) Decker.

Conquering High Blood Pressure: The Complete Guide to Managing Hypertension. Stephen Wood & Bert Griffith. 1997. LC 97-33320. (Illus.). 296p. (C). pap. 20.00 (*0-306-45632-X*) Perseus Bks Grp.

Conquering Hypertension: An Illustrated Guide to Understanding Treatment & Control of High Blood Pressure. R. Bryan Haynes & Frans H. H. Leenen. 1995. (Illus.). 168p. (Orig.). pap. 12.95 (*0-9697781-2-0*) Login Pubs Consort.

Conquering Kids Cancer: Triumphs & Tragedies of a Children's Cancer Doctor. Ken Lazarus. 1999. LC 98-40258. 240p. pap. 19.95 (*1-885373-22-8*) Emerald Ink.

***Conquering Lymphatic Disease: Setting the Research Agenda: Proceedings of an NIH Think Tank Conference, May 11-13, 2000.** Marlys H. Witte. Ed. by Marlys H. Witte. 2001. (Illus.). 287p. pap. text 60.00 (*0-9711731-0-9*) Univ AZ Surg.

Conquering Otitis Media. Charles D. Bluestone. 1999. LC 00-690016. (Illus.). vii, 111p. (*1-896998-05-4*, Empowering Pr) Decker.

Conquering Pain: An Illustrated Guide to Pain Relief & Pain Management. Jay B. Forrest. 1995. (Illus.). 88p. (Orig.). pap. text 12.95 (*0-9697781-0-4*) Login Pubs Consort.

Conquering Psoriasis. Eugene M. Farber & Lexie Nall. 1997. LC 98-206292. (Illus.). 160p. 12.95 (*0-9697781-5-5*) Login Pubs Consort.

Conquering Rheumatoid Arthritis. William Bensen & Wynn Bensen. 1996. LC 98-206414. 90 p. pap. (*0-9697781-8-X*, Empowering Pr) Decker.

Conquering Rheumatoid Arthritis: The Latest Breakthroughs & Treatments. Thomas F. Lee. 2001. LC 2001-16111. (Illus.). 255p. pap. 20.00 (*1-57392-886-0*) Prometheus Bks.

Conquering Senility. Arthur C. Walsh. 1985. 96p. (Orig.). pap. 5.95 (*0-939332-15-9*) J Pohl Assocs.

Conquering the Darkness: One Woman's Story of Recovering from Brain Injury. Deborah A. Quinn. 1998. LC 98-14373. 420p. pap. 15.95 (*1-55778-763-8*) Paragon Hse.

Conquering Your Migraine: The Essential Guide to Understanding & Treating Migraines for All Sufferers & Their Families. Seymour Diamond et al. 2001. LC 00-66178. 223p. pap. 13.00 (*0-684-87310-9*, Fireside) S&S Trade Pap.

Conquest of Bacteria, from Salvarsan to Sulphapyridine. Frank S. Taylor. 1977. LC 78-142705. (Essay Index Reprint Ser.). reprint ed. 19.95 (*0-8369-2375-8*) Ayer.

Conquest of Cancer: Vaccines & Diet. Virginia Livingston-Wheeler & Edmond G. Addeo. 1993. pap. 9.95 (*0-9627145-1-8*, Cyrus Pr) Waterside Prodns.

Conquest of Deficiency Diseases: Achievements & Prospects. W. R. Aykroyd. 1970. (Freedom from Hunger Campaign Basic Study Ser.: No. 24). 98p. pap. text 9.00 (*92-4-156018-5*, 1150024) World Health.

Conquest of Disease: The Psychology of Mental & Spiritual Healing. Eugene Del Mar. 1997. 250p. reprint ed. pap. 24.95 (*0-7661-0025-1*) Kessinger Pub.

Conquest of Epidemic Disease: A Chapter in the History of Ideas. Charles-Edward A. Winslow. 1980. LC 79-48055. 424p. reprint ed. pap. 16.95 (*0-299-08244-X*) U of Wis Pr.

Conquest of Pollution. Morris Goran. 1982. LC 81-184272. 281p. (C). 30.00 (*0-915250-37-3*) Environ Design.

Conrad Ferdinand Meyer & Freud: The Beginnings of Applied Psychoanalysis. Alexander Grinstein. 1992. 424p. (C). 60.00 (*0-8236-1046-2*) Intl Univs Pr.

Conscious & Unconscious: Freud's Dynamic Distinction Reconsidered. Patricia S. Herzog. 1991. (Psychological Issues Monographs: No. 58). 124p. 30.00 (*0-8236-1042-X*) Intl Univs Pr.

Conscious & Unconscious Processes: Psychodynamic, Cognitive & Neurophysiological Convergences. Howard Shevrin et al. 1996. LC 96-1714. 302p. text 47.00 (*1-57230-091-4*, 0091) Guilford Pubns.

Conscious & Unconscious Programs in the Brain. B. Kissin. 1986. LC 86-12310. (Psychology of Human Behavior Ser.: Vol. 1). (Illus.). 406p. (C). text 80.00 (*0-306-42243-3*, Kluwer Plenum) Kluwer Academic.

Conscious Conception: Elemental Journey Through the Labyrinth of Sexuality. Jeannine Baker et al. 1986. LC 86-26994. (Illus.). 411p. lib. bdg. 20.00 (*0-938190-83-0*) North Atlantic.

Conscious Ear: My Life of Transformation Through Listening. Alfred A. Tomatis. 1992. (Illus.). 352p. pap. 19.95 (*0-88268-108-7*) Station Hill Pr.

Conscious Mind, Sleeping Brain: Perspectives in Lucid Dreaming. J. Gackenbach & S. LaBarge. 1988. LC 88-6034. (Illus.). 468p. (C). 70.00 (*0-306-42849-0*, Plenum Trade) Perseus Pubng.

Conscious Sedation, Anesthesia & the JCAHO. Dean F. Smith. Ed. by David Beardsley. 1999. LC 00-268201. (Illus.). v, 180p. pap. text 87.00 (*1-57839-061-3*) Opus Communs.

Consciousness. Colin McGinn. 2001. (Illus.). 288p. pap. 17.00 (*0-465-01377-5*) HarperCollins Pubs.

Consciousness: Natural & Artificial. James T. Culbertson. 1983. LC 81-81617. 13.95 (*0-87212-152-6*) Libra.

Consciousness & Behavior. Benjamin Wallace & Leslie E. Fisher. 4th ed. 1998. LC 98-23669. 295p. (gr. 12). pap. text 63.00 (*0-205-27701-2*) Allyn.

Consciousness & Human Identity. Ed. by John Cornwell. 1998. LC 98-18360. (Illus.). 248p. 24.95 (*0-19-850323-7*) OUP.

Consciousness & Self-Consciousness: A Defense of the Higher-Order Thought Theory of Consciousness. Rocco J. Gennaro. 1995. LC 95-39111. (Advances in Consciousness Research Ser.: Vol. 6). x, 220p. pap. 38.95 (*1-55619-186-3*) J Benjamins Pubng Co.

Consciousness & Self-Regulation: Advances in Research & Theory, Vol. 3. Ed. by Gary E. Schwartz et al. 1983. 240p. 45.00 (*0-306-41214-4*, Plenum Trade) Perseus Pubng.

Consciousness & the Brain: A Scientific & Philosophical Inquiry. Ed. by Gordon G. Globus et al. 1976. LC 75-44478. (Illus.). 378p. 69.50 (*0-306-30878-9*, Plenum Trade) Perseus Pubng.

Consciousness, Dreams, & Self: A Transdisciplinary Approach. John B. Arden. 1996. LC 96-16622. 204p. 28.50 (*1-887841-01-6*, BN 61043, Psychosocial) Intl Univs Pr.

Consciousness in Philosophy & Cognitive Neuroscience. Ed. by Antti Revonsuo & Matti Kamppinen. 1994. 312p. text 59.95 (*0-8058-1509-0*) L Erlbaum Assocs.

Consciousness Lost & Found: A Neuropsychological Exploration. Lawrence Weiskrantz. 1997. (Illus.). 302p. 30.00 (*0-19-852301-7*) OUP.

Consciousness Redux: Waking, Sleeping, Dreaming, & States In-Between: Collected Papers of Martin H. Stein, M. D. Ed. by Barbara Stimmel. 1998. LC 97-24498. 288p. 60.00 (*0-7657-0119-7*) Aronson.

Consecratio Medici & Other Papers. Harvey W. Cushing. 1977. LC 70-99688. (Essay Index Reprint Ser.). 25.95 (*0-8369-1565-8*) Ayer.

Consensus Development at the NIH: Improving the Program. Institute of Medicine Staff. 1990. 96p. (C). pap. text 15.00 (*0-309-04242-9*) Natl Acad Pr.

Consensus Formation in Healthcare Ethics. Ed. by Henk A. Ten Have & Hans-Martin Sass. 1998. LC 97-50308. (Philosophy & Medicine Ser.). 272p. text 110.00 (*0-7923-4944-X*) Kluwer Academic.

Consensus in Clinical Nutrition. Richard V. Heatley et al. 1994. LC 93-42563. (Illus.). 520p. (C). text 110.00 (*0-521-44134-X*) Cambridge U Pr.

Consensus on Hyperthermia for the 1990's: Clinical Practice in Cancer Treatment. Ed. by Haim I. Bicher et al. 1990. LC 90-7312. (Advances in Experimental Medicine & Biology Ser.: Vol. 267). (Illus.). 572p. (C). text 174.00 (*0-306-43533-0*, Kluwer Plenum) Kluwer Academic.

***Consent, Rights & Choices in Health Care for Children & Young People.** British Medical Association Staff. 2001. 296p. pap. text (*0-7279-1228-3*) BMJ Pub GBR. *Dist:* AIDC.

Consent to Treatment. Nancy M. King. 1990. (Hospital Law in North Carolina Ser.: Chap. 14). 67p. (C). ring bd. 10.50 (*1-56011-178-X*, 85.03N) Institute Government.

Consent to Treatment: A Practical Guide. Fay Rozovsky. 1984. LC 83-81948. 669p. 80.00 (*0-316-76073-0*) Aspen Law.

Consent to Treatment: A Practical Guide. Fay Rozovsky. 2nd ed. 1998. (Illus.). 670p. 149.00 (*0-8342-1105-X*, S676) Aspen Pub.

***Consent to Treatment: A Practical Guide.** Fay Rozovsky. 3rd ed. 2000. 2120p. 199.00 (*0-8342-1875-5*) Aspen Pub.

Consentimiento Informado y Esterilizacion Voluntaria: Guia Practica para Administradores de Programas. AVSC International Staff. 1995. (SPA.). 26p. reprint ed. pap. text 5.00 (*1-885063-14-8*) EngenderHlth.

Consequences & Prevention of Unsafe Abortion. Merrill Wolf. Ed. by Katie E. McLaurin & Laszlo G. Lampe. 1994. (Issues in Abortion Care Ser.: Vol. 3). 21p. (Orig.). pap. 6.00 (*1-882220-05-6*) IPAS.

Consequences of European Competition Law for National Health Policies. Ed. by Danny Pieters & Stefaan Van den Bogaert. 1997. LC 98-166102. (*90-6215-547-2*) Maklu Uitgev BEL. *Dist:* Gaunt.

Consequences of Maternal Morbidity & Maternal: Report of a Workshop. Committee on Population, National Research Council et al. 2000. 44p. pap. 12.00 (*0-309-06943-2*) Natl Acad Pr.

Consequences of Programme Changes in Antenatal Care. Anna Berglund. 1999. (Comprehensive Summaries of Uppsala Dissertations from the Faculty of Medicine Ser.: No. 888). (Illus.). 74p. (Orig.). pap. (*91-554-4538-1*) Uppsala Universitet SWE. *Dist:* Coronet Bks.

Conservation in Thoracic Surgery. Lo Cicero. 2000. text (*0-7216-4842-8*) Harcrt Hlth Sci Grp.

Conservation of Nonhuman Primates in Nineteen Seventy. Barbara Harrisson. 1971. (Primates in Medicine Ser.: Vol. 5). 24.50 (*3-8055-1243-0*) S Karger.

Conservation Surgery & Radiation Therapy in the Treatment of Operable Breast Cancer. J. M. Vaeth. 1982. (Frontiers of Radiation Therapy & Oncology Ser.: Vol. 17). (Illus.). viii, 156p. 123.50 (*3-8055-3560-0*) S Karger.

Conservative Dentistry: An Integrated Approach. Ed. by P. H. Jacobsen. 1990. (Illus.). 224p. pap. text (*0-443-03958-5*) Church.

Conservative Management of Sports Injuries. Thomas E. Hyde, Jr. & Marianne S. Gengenbach. 1996. LC 96-5025. (Illus.). 768p. 99.00 (*0-683-03944-X*) Lppncott W & W.

Conservative Management of Squint. W. Aust. Tr. by C. H. Bedwell & H. Obstfeld. 1970. (Illus.). 152p. 24.50 (*3-8055-0752-6*) S Karger.

Conserving Human Life. Orville N. Griese et al. Ed. by Russell E. Smith. 1989. LC 89-16155. 336p. pap. 17.95 (*0-935372-26-1*) NCBC.

Conserving Nutrients in Dietetic Services. Rita Jackson. 1988. (Illus.). 206p. pap. text 24.50 (*0-9624150-1-4*) Amer Nutri-Tech.

Consider This... Recovering Harmony & Balance Naturally. Ayn W. Cates. 1995. (Illus.). (Orig.). pap. (*1-899171-40-1*) Findhorn Pr GBR. *Dist:* Words Distrib.

Consideration of Some Learning Variables in the Context of Psychoanalytic Theory: Toward a Psychoanalytic Learning Perspective. Stanley I. Greenspan. 1975. LC 74-19890. (Psychological Issues Monographs: No. 33, Vol. 9, No. 1). pap. 27.50 (*0-8236-1050-0*) Intl Univs Pr.

Considerations in Contact Lens Use under Adverse Conditions: Proceedings of a Symposium. National Research Council Staff. Ed. by Pamela E. Flattau. 1991. 178p. (C). pap. text 23.00 (*0-309-04438-3*) Natl Acad Pr.

Considerations in the Simultaneous Measurement of Blood Gases, Electrolytes, & Related Analytes in Whole Blood: Proposed Guideline (1993) Contrib. by Robert F. Moran. 1993. 75.00 (*1-56238-206-3*, C32-P) NCCLS.

Considerations Regarding the Unintended Radiation Exposure of the Embryo, Fetus or Nursing Child. Intro. by Charles B. Meinhold. 1994. LC 94-18566. (Commentary Ser.: No. 9). 21p. (Orig.). pap. text 20.00 (*0-929600-36-3*) NCRP Pubns.

Considering Plastic Surgery? John M. Finley. 1991. LC 90-22163. (Illus.). 176p. (Orig.). 20.95 (*0-88289-803-5*) Pelican.

Consistency & Cognition: A Theory of Causal Attribution. Shelley Duval et al. 1983. 176p. (C). text 29.95 (*0-89859-220-8*) L Erlbaum Assocs.

Consistency in Personality. D. J. Ozer. 1986. (Recent Research in Psychology Ser.). (Illus.). 78p. 51.95 (*0-387-96299-9*) Spr-Verlag.

Consistency, Scalability, & Personality Measurement. K. Lanning. 1990. (Recent Research in Psychology Ser.). (Illus.). 157p. 54.95 (*0-387-97438-5*) Spr-Verlag.

Consolidating & Restructuring Health Care: A Resource Guide. Keith M. Korenchuk. 1998. 404p. pap. 95.00 (*1-56829-090-X*) M G M A.

Conspiracy of Silence: The Trauma of Incest. Sandra Butler. 1996. LC 78-1975. 215p. pap. 13.95 (*1-884244-12-2*) Volcano Pr.

Conspiracy of Silence - Alcoholism. Leo P. Hennigan. 1991. (Illus.). 170p. pap. 17.95 (*0-9626382-2-6*) Gannel Pubns.

Constancy & Change in Human Development. Ed. by Orville G. Brim, Jr. & Jerome Kagan. 1980. LC 80-13457. (Illus.). 760p. 61.00 (*0-674-16625-6*) HUP.

Constant Ferment: A History of the Thyroid Clinic & Laboratory at the Massachusetts General Hospital: 1913-1990. John B. Stanbury. 1991. (Illus.). 238p. 20.00 (*0-938864-14-9*) Ipswich Pr.

Constantine the African & Ali ibn al-Abbas al-Magusi: The Pantegni & Related Texts. Ed. by Charles Burnett & Danielle Jacquart. 1994. LC 94-33854. (Studies in Ancient Medicine: Vol. 10). ix, 364p. 107.50 (*90-04-10014-8*) Brill Academic Pubs.

Constipation. Ed. by Michael A. Kamm & John E. Lennard-Jones. 1994. 560p. (*1-871816-24-6*) Wrightson Biomed GBR. *Dist:* Taylor & Francis.

Constipation: A New Reading on the Subject. J. H. Tilden. 1996. 66p. reprint ed. pap. 9.00 (*1-56459-810-1*) Kessinger Pub.

Constipation: Etiology, Evaluation & Management. Ed. by Steven D. Wexner & David C. Bartolo. 1995. LC 94-27778. (Illus.). 272p. text (*0-7506-0776-9*) E A GBR. *Dist:* OUP.

Constipation & Ano-Rectal Insufficiency. Ed. by K. Ewe et al. 1997. (Falk Symposium Ser.: No. 95). 256p. text 167.00 (*0-7923-8727-9*) Kluwer Academic.

Constipation & Fecal Incontinence & Mobility Disturbances of the Gut. Ed. by J. Yokoyama & T. A. Angerpointner. 1989. (Progress in Pediatric Surgery Ser.: Vol. 24). (Illus.). 235p. 175.00 (*0-387-50813-9*, 3096) Spr-Verlag.

Constitution of Man Considered in Relation to External Objects. George Combe. 2nd ed. 1974. LC 74-16109. (History of Psychology Ser.). 313p. reprint ed. 50.00 (*0-8201-1136-8*) Schol Facsimiles.

Constraining Cognitive Theories: Issues & Options. Zenon W. Pylyshyn. 1998. LC 96-32728. (Tutorial Monographs in Cognitive Science Ser.). 230p. 77.00 (*1-56750-299-7*); pap. 39.50 (*1-56750-300-4*) Greenwood (Ablex).

Constraints on Language Acquisition: Studies of Atypical Children. Ed. by Helen Tager-Flusberg. 1994. 248p. text 49.95 (*0-8058-0667-9*) L Erlbaum Assocs.

Construct of Language Proficiency: Applications of Psychological Models to Language Assessment. Ed. by Ludo T. Verhoeven & John H. A. L. De Jong. 1992. LC 92-23643. viii, 212p. 58.00 (*1-55619-461-7*) J Benjamins Pubng Co.

Constructed Body: AIDS, Reproductive Technology, & Ethics. Julien S. Murphy. 1995. LC 94-30815. 185p. (C). text 44.50 (*0-7914-2517-7*); pap. text 14.95 (*0-7914-2518-5*) State U NY Pr.

Constructing a Patient's Drug Therapy Problem List. Leslie A. Shimp & Nancy A. Mason. 1993. (Clinical Skills Program: Advancing Pharmaceutical Care Ser.). 126p. ring bd. 50.00 (*1-879907-36-4*) Am Soc Hlth-Syst.

Constructing a Psychology of Teaching & Learning. Kelvin Seifert. 1999. LC 98-72084. xxxii, 505 p. (*0-395-70808-7*) HM.

Constructing (In)Competence: Disabling Evaluations in Clinical & Social Interaction. Ed. by Dana Kovarsky et al. 1998. LC 98-24197. 384p. 79.95 (*0-8058-2590-8*) L Erlbaum Assocs.

Constructing Realities: Meaning-Making Perspectives for Psychotherapists. Ed. by Hugh Rosen & Kevin T. Kuehlwein. 1996. LC 95-37811. (Jossey-Bass Social & Behavioral Science Ser.). 532p. 50.00 (*0-7879-0195-4*) Jossey-Bass.

Constructing the Self in a Mediated World. Debra Grodin & Thomas R. Lindlof. 1996. LC 95-32497. (Inquiries in Social Construction Ser.: Vol. 18). 240p. 76.95 (*0-8039-7011-0*, 2847); pap. 37.95 (*0-8039-7012-9*, 2846) Sage.

Constructing the Subject: Historical Origins of Psychological Research. Kurt Danziger. 1994. (Cambridge Studies in the History of Psychology). (Illus.). 263p. (C). pap. text 21.95 (*0-521-46785-3*) Cambridge U Pr.

Constructing Therapeutic Narratives. Haim Omer & Nahi Alon. 1997. LC 96-13384. 280p. 50.00 (*1-56821-856-7*) Aronson.

Construction & Operation of Clandestine Drug Laboratories. Jack B. Nimble. 2nd rev. ed. 1994. LC 93-80258. (Illus.). 132p. (C). pap. 17.95 (*1-55950-108-1*, 85178) Loompanics.

Construction & Understanding of Psychotherapeutic Change: Conversations, Memories, & Theories. Jack Martin. 1994. LC 93-44505. (Counseling & Development Ser.). 160p. (C). text 35.00 (*0-8077-3337-7*) Tchrs Coll.

Construction & Understanding of Psychotherapeutic Change: Conversations, Memories & Theories. Jack Martin. 1994. LC 93-44505. (Counseling & Development Ser.). 235p. (C). pap. 16.95 (*0-8077-3336-9*) Tchrs Coll.

Construction of Objectivity: A New Look at the First Months of Life. Ed. by R. Melkman. 1988. (Contributions to Human Development Ser.: Vol. 19). (Illus.). xiv, 130p. 86.25 (*3-8055-4746-3*) S Karger.

Construction of Psychological Processes in Interpersonal Communication. Maria C. Lyra & Jaan Valsiner. 1998. LC 97-20464. (Child Development Within Culturally Structured Environments Ser.: Vol. 4). pap. 39.50 (*1-56750-415-9*, Ablex) Greenwood.

Construction Versus Choice in Cognitive Measurement: Issues in Constructed Response, Performance Testing, & Portfolio Assessment. Ed. by Randy Bennett & William C. Ward. 1993. 344p. text 69.95 (*0-8058-0964-3*) L Erlbaum Assocs.

Constructional Morphology & Evolution. Ed. by N. Schmidt-Kittler & K. Vogel. 1991. (Illus.). 424p. 217.00 (*0-387-53279-X*) Spr-Verlag.

Constructions of Deviance. Frederick R. Adler. Date not set. (Adaptable Courseware-Softside Ser.). pap. 33.00 (*0-534-56600-6*) Wadsworth Pub.

Constructions of Deviance: Social Power, Context, & Interaction. Patricia A. Adler & Peter Adler. 1993. 588p. mass mkt. 30.75 net. (*0-534-21342-1*) Wadsworth Pub.

Constructions of Personality. Sarah E. Hampson. rev. ed. 1988. (Introduction to Modern Psychology Ser.). 320p. text 49.95 (*0-415-00255-9*) Routledge.

Constructive Therapies. Ed. by Michael F. Hoyt. (Constructive Therapies Ser.: Vol. 1). Vol. 1. 1997. 340p. 23.00 (*1-57230-281-X*, C0281); Vol. 2. 1998. LC 94-14220. 388p. (C). 24.00 (*1-57230-424-3*, C0424) Guilford Pubns.

Constructive Thinking: COPE Program for Depression. John H. Greist et al. 1999. (Illus.). 97p. pap. (*0-9702974-2-4*) Healthcare Sys.

Constructive Thinking: The Key to Emotional Intelligence. Seymour Epstein. 1998. LC 97-37560. 304p. pap. 24.95 (*0-275-95885-X*, Praeger Pubs) Greenwood.

Constructivism in Practice: Methods & Challenges. Cynthia Franklin & Paula S. Nurius. 1998. LC 97-36573. 440p. 29.95 (*0-87304-303-0*) Manticore Pubs.

Constructivism in Psychotherapy. Ed. by Robert A. Neimeyer & Michael J. Mahoney. 1999. LC 94-23952. 436p. pap. 29.95 (*1-55798-645-2*) Am Psychol.

Constructivist Perspectives on Developmental Psychopathology & Atypical Development. Ed. by D. Keating & H. Rosen. 1990. 280p. (C). text 69.95 (*0-8058-0437-4*) L Erlbaum Assocs.

Constructual Marital Therapy: Theory & Practice. Marshall Jung. 1993. LC 92-34219. 256p. (C). pap. text 24.95 (*0-89876-191-3*) Gardner Pr.

Construing Person. Jack R. Adams-Webber. Ed. by James C. Mancuso. 1982. LC 81-12101. 309p. 40.95 (*0-275-90853-4*, C0853, Praeger Pubs) Greenwood.

Consultant in Audiology. Jack Rudman. 1994. (Career Examination Ser.: C-1213). pap. 34.95 (*0-8373-1213-2*) Nat Learn.

Consultation. A. Michael Dougherty. 2nd ed. 1994. (Counseling Ser.). pap., tchr. ed. (*0-534-25129-3*) Brooks-Cole.

Consultation: Practice & Perspectives. A. Michael Dougherty. 1989. LC 89-9724. 352p. (C). text 43.95 (*0-534-10362-6*) Brooks-Cole.

Consultation: Practice & Perspectives in School & Community Settings. A. Michael Dougherty. 2nd ed. 1994. LC 94-18259. 392p. pap. 52.25 (*0-534-25128-5*) Brooks-Cole.

Consultation: School Mental Health Professionals as Consultants. Don C. Dinkmeyer, Jr. et al. LC 93-13252. 294p. (C). pap. text 28.95 (*1-55959-036-X*) Accel Devel.

Consultation: School Mental Health Professionals as Consultants. Don C. Dinkmeyer, Jr. 2nd ed. 2001. LC 00-50800. (Accelerated Development Ser.). (Illus.). xiii, 202p. pap. 36.95 (*1-56032-849-5*) Hemisp Pub.

Consultation Guide. Paul W. Ladenson. 1998. LC 98-23835. 600p. pap. text 49.00 (*0-683-30525-5*) Lppncott W & W.

Consultation in Community, School, & Organizational Practice: Gerald Caplan's Contributions to Professional Psychology. Ed. by William P. Erchul. 1993. (Clinical & Community Psychology Ser.). 250p. 54.95 (*1-56032-264-0*) Hemisp Pub.

Consultation in Gastroenterology. William J. Snape, Jr. 1995. LC 95-11486. (Illus.). 784p. text 135.00 (*0-7216-4670-0*) Saunders.

Consultation in Internal Medicine. John T. Harrington. 2nd ed. 1996. LC 96-19077. (Illus.). 624p. (C). (gr. 13). spiral bd. 43.95 (*0-8151-4164-5*, 26062) Mosby Inc.

Consultation in Residential Care. Ed. by W. Raza Silveira. 1991. (Aberdeen University Press Bks.). 192p. pap. text (*0-08-040908-3*) Aberdeen U Pr GBR. *Dist:* Macmillan.

Consultation-Liaison Psychiatry. Ed. by Robert O. Pasnau. 1975. (Seminars in Psychiatry Ser.). 352p. text 64.00 (*0-8089-0901-0*, 793265, Grune & Strat) Harcrt Hlth Sci Grp.

Consultation-Liaison Psychiatry: 1990 & Beyond. H. Leigh. 1994. (Illus.). 250p. (C). 75.00 (*0-306-44725-8*, Plenum Trade) Perseus Pubng.

Consultation-Liaison Psychiatry: Current Trends & New Perspectives. Finkel. 1983. 352p. text 53.00 (*0-8089-1585-1*, 791263, Grune & Strat) Harcrt Hlth Sci Grp.

***Consultation-Liaison Psychiatry in Japan.** I. Fukunishi. 2001. (Advances in Psychosomatic Medicine Ser.: Vol. 23). (Illus.). viii, 130p. 98.25 (*3-8055-7243-3*) S Karger.

Consultation Liaison Throughout the World. Ed. by T. N. Wise & H. Freyberger. 1983. (Advances in Psychosomatic Medicine Ser.: Vol. 11). (Illus.). xvi, 216p. 111.50 (*3-8055-3667-4*) S Karger.

Consultation with Your Sports Doctor. Gabe Mirkin. 1985. (Orig.). pap. 6.95 (*0-671-50491-6*) PB.

Consultations in Feline Internal Medicine. John R. August. 4th ed. 2001. LC 00-53796. (Illus.). xx, 650p. text 95.00 (*0-7216-8003-8*) Harcrt Hlth Sci Grp.

Consultations in Feline Internal Medicine, Vol. 1. John R. August. 1990. (Illus.). 672p. text 105.00 (*0-7216-2226-7*) Saunders.

Consultations in Feline Internal Medicine, Vol. 2. Ed. by John R. August. 2nd ed. 1993. LC 93-1499. (Illus.). 608p. text 90.00 (*0-7216-4674-3*) Saunders.

Consultations in Feline Internal Medicine No. 3, Vol. III. John R. August. Ed. by Ray Kersey. 3rd ed. 1996. LC 96-18814. text 90.00 (*0-7216-5814-8*) Saunders.

***Consultative Thrombosis & Hemostasis.** Ed. by Craig S. Kitchens et al. 2001. (Illus.). 795p. (*0-7216-8264-2*) Saunders.

Consulting for Success: Professional Forms for the Consultant Dietitian & Dietary Manager. Rosemary Behrens & Anne K. Blocker. 1994. LC 94-31597. 110p. pap. text 41.95 (*0-8138-2478-8*) Iowa U Pr.

Consulting Therapist: A Guide for OTs & PTs in Schools. Barbara E. Hanft & Patricia A. Place. 1998. 154p. (C). pap. text 47.50 (*0-12-784557-7*) Acad Pr.

Consulting with Children. Ian C. Lewis et al. 1993. (Illus.). 144p. text (*0-7295-0337-2*) Bailliere Tindall.

Consulting with Pediatricians: Psychological Perspectives. Dennis Drotar. 1995. (Issues in Clinical Child Psychology Ser.). (Illus.). 270p. (C). text 39.50 (*0-306-44935-8*, Kluwer Plenum) Kluwer Academic.

Consumer & Patient Satisfaction: Index of Modern Information. Rosetta R. Hardine. rev. ed. 1994. 157p. LC 88-47549. 57.50 (*0-7883-0396-1*); pap. 47.50 (*0-7883-0397-X*) ABBE Pubs Assn.

Consumer & Public Disclosures of Condoms: Index of New Information. Corine S. Wayne. 1994. 150p. pap. 47.50 (*0-7883-0013-X*) ABBE Pubs Assn.

Consumer Attitudes & Wishes about Health Care: Index of New Information with Authors, Subjects & Bibliography. Lucille W. Quarles. rev. ed. 1995. 149p. 57.50 (*0-7883-0701-0*); pap. 47.50 (*0-7883-0702-9*) ABBE Pubs Assn.

Consumer Guide to Modern Cataract Surgery. William Maloney et al. 1986. LC 85-80392. (Illus.). pap. 12.95 (*0-918916-05-4*) Lasenda.

Consumer Health & Medical Information on the Internet. Michael S. Brown & FIND/SVP Staff. 1996. LC 98-207835. iv, 126p. (*1-56241-402-X*) FIND-SVP.

Consumer Health & Safety Activities. Patricia R. Toner. 1993. LC 93-8219. (Just for the Health of It!: Unit 1). 144p. (YA). (gr. 7-12). pap., tchr. ed. 19.95 (*0-87628-263-X*) Ctr Appl Res.

Consumer Health Informatics: Emerging Issues. 1998. 56p. (C). reprint ed. pap. text 20.00 (*0-7881-3470-1*) DIANE Pub.

Consumer Health Information: Managing Hospital-Based Centers. Salvinija G. Kernaghan & Barbara E. Giloth. 1991. 99p. (Orig.). pap. 8.00 (*0-87258-605-7*, 070200) Am Hospital.

Consumer Health Information Service, 1985-1987 Index. Ed. by Alan M. Rees. 1987. 120p. pap. 25.00 (*0-8357-0721-0*) Univ Microfilms.

Consumer Health Information Service, 1987-1989 Index. Ed. by Alan M. Rees. 1989. 143p. pap. 25.00 (*0-8357-0808-X*) Univ Microfilms.

Consumer Health Information Service, 1985 Index. Ed. by Alan M. Rees. 1985. 58p. pap. 25.00 (*0-8357-0700-8*) Univ Microfilms.

Consumer Health Information Source Book. Alan M. Rees. 6th ed. 2000. LC 99-52937. (Illus.). 232p. 59.50 (*1-57356-123-1*, Oryx) Greenwood.

Consumer Health Resource Centers: A Guide to Successful Planning & Implementation. Mary E. Longe & Karen Thomas. 1998. LC 97-53188. 180p. pap. 28.00 (*1-55648-231-0*) AHPI.

Consumer Health U. S. A., Vol. 2. Alan M. Rees. 2nd ed. 1997. LC 94-37594. (Consumer Health U. S. A. Ser.: Vol. 2). (Illus.). 608p. 65.00 (*1-57356-068-5*, Oryx) Greenwood.

Consumer Health USA: Essential Information from the Federal Health Network. Ed. by Alan M. Rees. 1994. LC 94-37594. 552p. 55.00 (*0-89774-889-1*, Oryx) Greenwood.

Consumer Information in a Changing Health Care System. Ed. by Linda P. Wolf et al. 1998. (Illus.). 295p. reprint ed. pap. text 50.00 (*0-7881-4214-3*) DIANE Pub.

Consumer Protection Issues Involving in Vitro Fertilization Clinics. 1990. lib. bdg. 74.00 (*0-8490-4015-9*) Gordon Pr.

Consumer Reference Book & Index about HIV, AIDS & Treatments. John C. Bartone. 1994. 90p. pap. 47.50 (*0-7883-0299-X*) ABBE Pubs Assn.

Consumer Reference Book & Index about HIV, AIDS, & Treatments. John C. Bartone. rev. ed. 1996. LC 96-188. 125p. pap. 47.50 (*0-7883-1025-9*) ABBE Pubs Assn.

Consumer Reference Book & Index about Informed Consent. John C. Bartone. 1994. 150p. pap. 47.50 (*0-7883-0285-X*) ABBE Pubs Assn.

Consumer Reports' Complete Guide to Health Services for Seniors: What Your Family Needs to Know about Finding & Financing Medicare, Assisted Living, Nursing Home, Adult Day Care with Ratings of Medic HMO's & Supplemental Policies. Trudy Lieberman & Consumer Reports Books Editors. 2000. LC 00-23453. 592p. pap. 19.95 (*0-8129-3147-5*, Three Riv Pr) Harmony Bks.

Consumer Satisfaction in Medical Practice. Paul A. Sommers. 1999. LC 98-54478. (Illus.). 197p. 49.95 (*0-7890-0713-4*) Haworth Pr.

Consumer Update on Asthma. Nancy J. Sander. 2nd ed. (Illus.). 49p. pap. (*1-885543-00-X*) Allergy & Asthma.

Consumers as Providers in Psychiatric Rehabilitation. Ed. by Carol T. Mowbray. 1997. LC 98-226152. xvii, 525p. (*0-9655843-1-3*) Intl Assn Psych.

Consumer's Attitudes to Health Care: Index of Modern of Information. Lucille W. Quarles. rev. ed. 1994. 155p. LC 88-47542. 57.50 (*0-7883-0692-8*); pap. 47.50 (*0-7883-0693-6*) ABBE Pubs Assn.

Consumer's Good Chemical Guide: A Jargon-Free Guide to Controversial Chemicals. John Emsley. 1994. LC 94-8286. (Illus.). 320p. text 20.00 (*0-7167-4505-4*) W H Freeman.

Consumer's Guide to Alternative Medicine: A Close Look at Homeopathy, Acupuncture, Faith-Healing & Other Unconventional Treatments. Kurt Butler. 1992. LC 92-19859. 299p. (Orig.). (C). pap. 24.00 (*0-87975-733-7*) Prometheus Bks.

Consumer's Guide to Art Therapy: For Prospective Employers, Clients & Students. Susan R. Makin. 1994. 112p. (C). text 33.95 (*0-398-05917-9*) C C Thomas.

Consumer's Guide to Colorado Nursing Homes: 1995-1996. Nancy Schwalm & Maria Arellano. 1995. 200p. pap. text 19.95 (*0-9649636-3-9*) Action Health.

Consumer's Guide to Doctoral Degree Programs in Nursing. Ed. by Judith C. Allen. 1990. 165p. 15.95 (*0-88737-455-7*) Natl League Nurse.

Consumer's Guide to Emergency Medical Services. Greg H. Williams. 1983. LC 83-62132. (Illus.). 129p. (Orig.). pap. 10.95 (*0-911223-00-2*) Star Valley.

Consumer's Guide to Homeopathy: The Definitive Resource for Understanding Homeopathic Medicine & Making It Work for You. Dana Ullman. 1996. LC 95-18442. 336p. 13.95 (*0-87477-813-1*, Tarcher Putnam) Putnam Pub Group.

Consumers' Guide to Long Term Health Care Facilities, Set. BGA Staff & Bryan Doyle. 2nd ed. 1994. (Illus.). 200p. pap. 25.00 (*0-9641280-0-4*) Better Government.

Consumer's Guide to Managed Health Care. Sophie M. Korczyk. 1997. 19.95 (*0-02-862042-9*) Macmillan.

***Consumer's Guide to Mental Health.** Susan Waggoner & Michael Aronoff. pap. 15.95 (*0-14-023708-9*) Penguin Putnam.

Consumer's Guide to Psychiatric Drugs. John D. Preston et al. 1998. LC 97-75482. 340p. pap. 16.95 (*1-57224-111-X*) New Harbinger.

Consumers' Reference & Index of What's Going on in Life, Health & Stress Research. Thelma F. Harrison. 1994. 150p. 47.50 (*1-55914-528-5*); pap. 44.50 (*1-55914-529-3*) ABBE Pubs Assn.

Consumers' Reference Book & Index about Food, Diet & Cancer. John C. Bartone. 1994. 160p. pap. 47.50 (*0-7883-0279-5*) ABBE Pubs Assn.

Consumers' Reference Book & Index about Relaxation & Its Methods. John C. Bartone. rev. ed. 1997. 149p. pap. 47.50 (*0-7883-1472-6*) ABBE Pubs Assn.

Consumers' Reference Book & Index about Rights to Medical Treatment. John C. Bartone. 1994. 155p. pap. 47.50 (*0-7883-0311-2*) ABBE Pubs Assn.

Consumer's Reference Book & Index Concerning Diagnostic Errors in Medicine. John C. Bartone. 1994. 150p. pap. 47.50 (*0-7883-0303-1*) ABBE Pubs Assn.

Consumers' Reference Book & Index Concerning Medical Malpractice. John C. Bartone. 1994. 160p. pap. 47.50 (*0-7883-0301-5*) ABBE Pubs Assn.

Consumption Coagulpathies. Ed. by A. Larcan et al. 1987. 176p. (gr. 13). 73.50 (*2-225-80981-X*, MA981) Mosby Inc.

Consumption in New England: Locality, One of Its Chief Causes & Is Consumption Contagious, or Communicated by One Person to Another in Any Manner? Henry I. Bowditch. Ed. by Barbara G. Rosenkrantz. 1977. LC 76-25653. (Public Health in America Ser.). (Illus.). reprint ed. lib. bdg. 18.95 (*0-405-09806-5*) Ayer.

Contact Allergy Predictive Test in Guinea Pigs. Ed. by K. E. Andersen & Howard I. Maibach. 1985. (Current Problems in Dermatology Ser.: Vol. 14). (Illus.). viii, 300p. 141.00 (*3-8055-4053-1*) S Karger.

Contact & Occupational Dermatology. James C. Marks & Deleo. 2nd ed. 1997. LC 96-47750. (Illus.). 416p. (C). (gr. 13). text 89.95 (*0-8151-6954-X*, 27226) Mosby Inc.

Contact Hypersensitivity in Experimental Animals. Ed. by D. Parker & J. L. Turk. 1974. (Monographs in Allergy: Vol. 8). (Illus.). 182p. 73.25 (*3-8055-1666-5*) S Karger.

Contact Lens & Ocular Disease. Ed. by Michael G. Harris. 1996. LC 96-182394. (Illus.). 176p. (C). (gr. 13). pap. text 37.95 (*0-8151-4645-0*, 24878) Mosby Inc.

Contact Lens Design & Fitting. MacDonald. 1995. (Home Care Aide Ser.). pap. 29.95 (*0-8273-6376-1*) Delmar.

Contact Lens Manual: A Practical Fitting Guide. Andrew Gasson & Judith Morris. 2nd ed. 1998. LC 98-9509. (Manual Ser.). (Illus.). 416p. pap. 65.00 incl. cd-rom (*0-7506-3187-2*) Buttrwrth-Heinemann.

Contact Lens Practice. Robert Fletcher et al. 1994. (Modern Optometry Ser.). (Illus.). 264p. 110.00 (*0-632-03287-1*) Blackwell Sci.

Contact Lens Practice. Robert B. Mandell. 4th ed. 1988. (Illus.). 1040p. (C). text 95.95 (*0-398-05509-2*) C C Thomas.

Contact Lens Practice: Clinical & Scientific Aspects. M. Guillon. Ed. by Montague Ruben. 1994. (Illus.). 1176p. (gr. 13). 649.95 (*0-412-35120-X*) Chapman & Hall.

Contact Lens Problem Solving. Edward S. Bennett. 1994. LC 94-19441. (Illus.). 199p. (C). (gr. 13). pap. text 39.95 (*0-8151-0424-3*, 24262) Mosby Inc.

Contact Lens Yearbook. Efron. 1995. text 30.40 net. (*0-7020-1926-7*) Saunders.

Contact Lenses: Fundamentals & Clinical Use. Harold A. Stein et al. 1996. LC 96-44189. (Illus.). 304p. pap. text 59.00 (*1-55642-340-3*, 63403) SLACK Inc.

Contact Lenses: International Ophthalmology Clinics, Vol. 31, No. 2. 1991. 39.00 (*0-316-80240-9*) Little.

Contact Lenses: Procedures & Techniques. Gerald E. Lowther & Christopher Snyder. 2nd ed. 1992. 432p. text 84.99 (*0-7506-9187-5*) Buttrwrth-Heinemann.

Contact Lenses: The CLAO Guide to Basic Science & Clinical Practice. Ed. by Oliver H. Dabezies, Jr. et al. 1984. 848p. text 225.00 (*0-8089-1642-4*, 790957, Grune & Strat) Harcrt Hlth Sci Grp.

Contact Lenses: The CIAO Guide to Basic Sciences & Clinical Practice, 1987. Oliver Dabezies, Jr. 1987. LC 79-959. 152p. text 63.00 (*0-8089-1869-9*, Grune & Strat) Harcrt Hlth Sci Grp.

Contact Lenses: Update No. 1, Nineteen Eighty-Six. Oliver Dabezies, Jr. et al. 1986. 104p. text 56.00 (*0-8089-1799-4*, 790958, Grune & Strat) Harcrt Hlth Sci Grp.

Contact Lenses Fitting: A Clinical Text. Frank J. Weinstock et al. 1989. LC 65-40520. (Illus.). 150p. (gr. 13). text (*0-397-44671-3*, GM0081) Gower-Mosby.

Contact Lenses for Pre & Post Surgery. Ed. by Michael G. Harris. 1996. (Illus.). 192p. (C). (gr. 13). pap. text 36.95 (*0-8151-1400-1*, 24370) Mosby Inc.

Contact Urticaria Syndrome. Ed. by Arto Lahti. 1997. LC 97-12227. (Illus.). 384p. lib. bdg. 99.95 (*0-8493-7352-2*) CRC Pr.

Contacts: Communicating Interpersonally. Teri K. Gamble & Michael W. Gamble. 1997. LC 97-2297. 440p. pap. text 57.00 (*0-205-16634-2*) P-H.

Contagion: Disease, Government & the 'Social Question' in Nineteenth-Century France. Andrew R. Aisenberg. 1999. LC 98-36505. 294p. 46.00 (*0-8047-3395-3*) Stanford U Pr.

Contagion & Confinement: Controlling Tuberculosis along the Skid Road. Barron H. Lerner. 1998. LC 98-5700. (Illus.). 264p. 44.50 (*0-8018-5898-4*) Johns Hopkins.

Contagion & the State in Europe, 1830-1930. Peter Baldwin. 1999. LC 98-39337. 596p. (C). text 74.95 (*0-521-64288-4*) Cambridge U Pr.

Contagious & Non-Contagious Infectious Diseases Sourcebook: Basic Information about Contagious Diseases & Non-Contagious Infectious Diseases. Ed. by Karen Bellenir & Peter D. Dresser. 1995. (Health Reference Ser.: Vol. 8). lib. bdg. 78.00 (*0-7808-0075-3*) Omnigraphics Inc.

Contagious Emotions: Staying Well When Your Loved One Is Depressed. Ronald M. Podell. Ed. by Claire Zion. 1993. reprint ed. pap. 10.00 (*0-671-70240-8*) PB.

Containing Costs in Japanese Health Care. Ed. by Naoki Ikegami & John C. Campbell. 1996. LC 96-26049. 376p. text 55.00 (*0-472-10538-8*, 10538) U of Mich Pr.

Containing Costs in Minnesota's Health Care System: A Report to Governor Arne H. Carlson & the Minnesota Legislature. Ed. by Gerald Brost. 1999. 177p. (C). reprint ed. pap. text 30.00 (*0-7881-8320-6*) DIANE Pub.

Containing Health Benefit Costs: The Self-Insurance Option. Ed. by R. H. Egdahl & Diana C. Walsh. 1979. (Springer Series in Industry & Health Care: Vol. 6). (Illus.). 181p. 38.00 (*0-387-90385-2*) Spr-Verlag.

Containing Rage, Terror & Despair: An Object Relations Approach to Psychotherapy. Jeffrey Seinfeld. 2000. LC 95-408. 256p. pap. 50.00 (*1-56821-578-9*); pap. 35.00 (*0-7657-0298-3*) Aronson.

Contaminating Theatre: Intersections of Theatre, Therapy, & Public Health. Ed. by Jill R. MacDougall & P. Stanley Yoder. 1998. LC 98-7121. (Psychosocial Issues Ser.). (Illus.). 256p. 102.00 (*0-8101-1534-4*); pap. 24.00 (*0-8101-1535-2*) Northwestern U Pr.

Contamination Control, 1981 Vol. III: Proceedings of the 27th Annual Technical Meeting of the Institute of Environmental Sciences, Los Angeles - Contamination Control, 1981. LC 62-38584. 85p. pap. 40.00 (*0-915414-64-3*) IEST.

Contemplation & Action: The Spiritual Autobiography of a Muslim. Seyyed H. Badakhchani. 1999. pap. (*1-86064-523-2*) I B T GBR. *Dist:* St Martin.

Contemporary Adolescence: A Social Psychological Approach. Patrick C. Heaven. 1994. LC 95-122796. 280p. (*0-7329-2620-3*); pap. (*0-7329-2619-X*) Macmill Educ AUS. *Dist:* Paul & Co Pubs.

Contemporary Adulthood. Munson. 5th ed. 1994. (C). pap. text, tchr. ed. 33.75 (*0-15-501157-X*) Harcourt Coll Pubs.

Contemporary Approaches to Neuropsychological Assessment. Ed. by Gerald Goldstein & Theresa M. Incagnoli. 1997. LC 97-16600. (Critical Issues in Neuropsychology Ser.). 430p. (C). text 65.00 (*0-306-45521-8*, Kluwer Plenum) Kluwer Academic.

Contemporary Approaches to Psychotherapy & Counseling: The Self-Regulation & Maturity Model. Joseph F. Burke. 1989. LC 88-39587. 427p. (C). text 57.95 (*0-534-10146-1*) Brooks-Cole.

Contemporary Ayurveda: Medicine & Research in Maharishi Ayur-Veda. Hari M. Sharma & Christopher Clark. 1997. LC 97-21470. (Complementary & Alternative Medicine Ser.). pap. text (*0-443-05594-7*) Church.

Contemporary Behavior Therapy. Michael D. Spiegler & David Guevremont. 2nd ed. 1992. 515p. (C). mass mkt. 54.25 (*0-534-12990-0*) Brooks-Cole.

Contemporary Behavior Therapy. Michael D. Spiegler. 3rd ed. 1997. LC 97-28203. (Counseling Ser.). 632p. spiral bd. 88.95 (*0-534-33893-3*) Brooks-Cole.

Contemporary Behavior Therapy: Conceptual & Empirical Foundations. Ed. by G. Terence Wilson & Cyril M. Franks. 1982. LC 82-949. 597p. pap. 79.95 (*0-89862-614-5*) Guilford Pubns.

Contemporary Behavioral Neurology. Michael R. Trimble & Jeffrey L. Cummings. 1996. LC 96-28926. (Blue Books of Practical Neurology). 348p. text 95.00 (*0-7506-9839-X*) Buttrwrth-Heinemann.

Contemporary Cephalometric Radiography. Kunihiko Miyashita. 1996. (Illus.). 292p. text 195.00 (*4-87417-517-1*) Quint Pub Co.

Contemporary Chiropractic. Daniel Redwood. 1997. LC 97-18583. 354p. text (*0-443-07809-2*) Church.

Contemporary Clinical Management of Gynecology Malignancies. Benjamin Greer. 1999. LC 98-26948. (Atlas of Clinical Gynecology Ser.: Vol. 4). (Illus.). 377p. text 129.00 (*0-8385-0316-0*) McGraw-Hill Prof.

Contemporary Clinical Psychology. Thomas G. Plante. 1998. LC 98-20474. (Illus.). 440p. 77.95 (*0-471-31626-1*) Wiley.

Contemporary Community Nursing. S. Burley. Ed. by S. Chilton et al. 1997. 256p. (Orig.). pap. 32.50 (*1-56593-822-4*, 1616) Singular Publishing.

Contemporary Conservative Care for Painful Spinal Disorders. Tom G. Mayer et al. 1991. LC 91-9298. (Illus.). 588p. text 105.00 (*0-8121-1344-6*) Lppncott W & W.

Contemporary Constructions of the Child: Essays in Honor of William Kessen. F. Kessel et al. 1991. 344p. (C). text 69.95 (*0-8058-0607-5*) L Erlbaum Assocs.

***Contemporary Dental Assisting.** Darlene Novak. 2001. (Illus.). pap., tchr. ed. 250.00 (*0-323-01394-5*) Mosby Inc.

Contemporary Diagnosis & Management in Primary Care Gynecology. William L. Frangipane. 2000. (Illus.). 275p. pap. 32.95 (*1-884065-52-X*, Hndbks Hlth Care) Assocs in Med.

Contemporary Diagnosis & Management of Allergic Diseases & Asthma. James E. Gern & W. W. Busse. 3rd ed. 1999. LC 98-74078. 271p. 29.95 (*1-884065-47-3*, Hndbks Hlth Care) Assocs in Med.

Contemporary Diagnosis & Management of Alzheimer's Disease. David S. Geldmacher. 2000. (Illus.). 200p. (C). pap. 29.95 (*1-884065-39-2*) Assocs in Med.

Contemporary Diagnosis & Management of Arthritis. Sergio Schwartzman. 2000. LC 98-70187. (Illus.). 144p. pap. 27.95 (*1-884065-29-5*, Hndbks Hlth Care) Assocs in Med.

Contemporary Diagnosis & Management of Attention Deficit/Hyperactivity Disorder. L. Eugene Arnold. 2000. LC 99-66879. (Illus.). 188p. pap. 29.95 (*1-884065-53-8*, Hndbks Hlth Care) Assocs in Med.

Contemporary Diagnosis & Management of Bronchitis. Antonio Anzueto. (Illus.). 1999. 135p. (C). pap. 28.95 (*1-884065-33-3*, Hndbks Hlth Care); 3rd ed. 2000. LC 00-105247. 128p. (*1-884065-88-0*) Assocs in Med.

Contemporary Diagnosis & Management of Common Psychiatric Disorders. Eric Hollander & Cheryl M. Wong. 2000. LC 98-71700. (Illus.). 188p. (C). pap. 29.95 (*1-884065-42-2*) Assocs in Med.

Contemporary Diagnosis & Management of Erectile Dysfunction. Tom F. Lue. 1999. LC 98-70695. (Illus.). 139p. pap. text 29.95 (*1-884065-27-9*) Assocs in Med.

Contemporary Diagnosis & Management of Gynecologic Infections. Sebastian Faro. 1997. (Illus.). 172p. (Orig.). (C). pap. text 28.95 (*1-884065-15-5*) Assocs in Med.

Contemporary Diagnosis & Management of Headache & Migraine. Seymour Diamond. 1998. LC 98-70181. (Illus.). 145p. (Orig.). (C). pap. text 29.95 (*1-884065-28-7*) Assocs in Med.

Contemporary Diagnosis & Management of Heart Failure. Barry Greenberg & Denise Hermann. 2001. (Illus.). 200p. pap. 29.50 (*1-884065-46-5*, Hndbks Hlth Care) Assocs in Med.

Contemporary Diagnosis & Management of HIV/AIDS Infections. John P. Phair & Robert L. Murphy. 1997. (Illus.). 175p. (Orig.). (C). pap. text 29.95 (*1-884065-18-X*) Assocs in Med.

Contemporary Diagnosis & Management of Hpylori-Associated GI Diseases. David Y. Graham. 1998. LC 98-71695. pap. text 27.95 (*1-884065-26-0*) Assocs in Med.

Contemporary Diagnosis & Management of Hypertension. Myron H. Weinberger. 1999. LC 96-79872. (Illus.). 155p. (C). pap. text 29.95 (*1-884065-14-7*) Assocs in Med.

Contemporary Diagnosis & Management of Ischemic Heart Disease. Spencer B. King. 2000. (Illus.). 200p. pap. 29.95 (*1-884065-49-X*) Assocs in Med.

Contemporary Diagnosis & Management of Lipid Disorders. Antonio M. Gotto, Jr. 1999. LC 98-70186. (Illus.). (C). pap. text 29.95 (*1-884065-25-2*) Assocs in Med.

Contemporary Diagnosis & Management of Male Impotence. John P. Mulhall & Irwin Goldstein. 2000. (Illus.). 150p. pap. 29.95 (*1-884065-32-5*) Assocs in Med.

Contemporary Diagnosis & Management of Neonatal Respiratory Diseases. Thomas N. Hansen & Leonard E. Weisman. 2nd ed. 1998. 336p. pap. 39.95 (*1-884065-23-6*, Hndbks Hlth Care) Assocs in Med.

Contemporary Diagnosis & Management of Obesity. George A. Bray. 1998. LC 98-70972. (Illus.). 298p. pap. 29.95 (*1-884065-30-9*) Assocs in Med.

Contemporary Diagnosis & Management of Osteoporosis. Daniel T. Baran. 2000. LC 98-75544. (Illus.). 128p. (C). pap. 29.95 (*1-884065-48-1*) Assocs in Med.

Contemporary Diagnosis & Management of Otitis Media. Russell W. Steele & Dana L. Suskind-Liu. 2000. LC 98-74011. (Illus.). 256p. (C). pap. 29.95 (*1-884065-45-7*) Assocs in Med.

Contemporary Diagnosis & Management of Pain. Donlin M. Long. (Illus.). 1997. 206p. pap. 29.95 (*1-884065-13-9*); 2nd ed. 2000. LC 98-70971. 224p. pap. (*1-884065-37-6*) Assocs in Med.

Contemporary Diagnosis & Management of Pain in Oncological & AIDS Patients. Russell K. Portenoy. 2nd ed. 1998. (Illus.). 206p. (Orig.). (C). pap. 28.95 (*1-884065-40-6*) Assocs in Med.

Contemporary Diagnosis & Management of Sinusitis. George A. Pankey et al. 3rd ed. 2000. LC 99-66841. (Illus.). 174p. (*1-884065-69-4*) Assocs in Med.

Contemporary Diagnosis & Management of Stroke. Jesse Weinberger. 2nd ed. 2000. LC 99-68884. (Illus.). 176p. (Orig.). pap. text (*1-884065-85-6*) Assocs in Med.

Contemporary Diagnosis & Management of Thyroid Disorders. John F. Wilber. 2000. LC 98-70975. (Illus.). 110p. pap. 28.50 (*1-884065-31-7*) Assocs in Med.

Contemporary Diagnosis & Management of Ulcerative Colitis & Proctitis. Mark A. Peppercorn. 1995. LC 94-74425. pap. 39.95 (*1-884065-08-2*) Assocs in Med.

Contemporary Diagnosis & Management of Urologic Emergencies. Ed. by John P. Mulhall. 2000. (Illus.). 230p. (C). pap. 29.50 (*1-884065-38-4*) Assocs in Med.

Contemporary Directions in Human Resource Management: A Sourcebook for Human Service Organizations. 1990. 300p. pap. 19.50 (*1-883066-01-8*) Natl Comm Mental.

Contemporary Fixed Prosthodontics. Stephen F. Rosenstiel et al. 2nd ed. 1994. LC 93-40196. (Illus.). 688p. (C). (gr. 13). text 74.00 (*0-8016-6528-0*, 06528) Mosby Inc.

Contemporary Fixed Prosthodontics. Stephen Rosenstiel et al. 3rd ed. 2000. LC 2001-268271. (Illus.). xi, 868p. (C). (gr. 13). text 69.95 (*0-8151-5559-X*, 30603) Mosby Inc.

Contemporary Geriatric Medicine. Ed. by Steven R. Gambert. Vol. 1. 1983. LC 83-10978. 436p. 110.00 (*0-306-41301-9*); Vol. 3. 1988. LC 84-643208. (Illus.). 502p. (C). text 156.00 (*0-306-42736-2*) Kluwer Academic (Kluwer Plenum).

Contemporary Geriatric Medicine Vol. 2. Ed. by Steven R. Gambert. 1986. LC 84-643208. (Illus.). 566p. (C). text 156.00 (*0-306-42055-4*, Kluwer Plenum) Kluwer Academic.

Contemporary Hair Transplant Surgery. Kenneth A. Buchwach & Raymond J. Konior. 1997. LC 96-44701. (Illus.). 176p. text 79.00 (*0-86577-577-X*) Thieme Med Pubs.

Contemporary Health. Sandra M. Alters-Gottfried. Date not set. (Health Sciences Ser.). 39.50 (*0-314-12517-5*) Brooks-Cole.

Contemporary Health Issues. Eric Banister et al. 1987. (Orig.). (C). pap. text 40.00 (*0-86720-077-4*) Jones & Bartlett.

Contemporary Health Issues. Corporation for Com. Col. TV Staff. 3rd ed. 1984. (C). pap. text, stu. ed. 17.50 net. (*0-07-554753-8*) McGraw.

Contemporary Health Policy. Beaufort B. Longest. 2000. LC 00-58102. (Illus.). xi, 579p. (*1-56793-139-1*) Health Admin Pr.

Contemporary Hematology - Oncology. Ed. by Albert S. Gordon et al. (Illus.). Vol. 2. 1981. 568p. 110.00 (*0-306-40683-7*); Vol. 3. 1984. 288p. 85.00 (*0-306-41535-6*) Kluwer Academic (Kluwer Plenum).

Contemporary Hypnosis Research. Ed. by Erika Fromm & Michael R. Nash. 1992. LC 92-1570. 591p. 68.00 (*0-89862-893-8*, 2893) Guilford Pubns.

Contemporary Implant Dentistry. Carl E. Misch. 2nd ed. 1998. LC 98-27520. (Illus.). 702p. (C). (gr. 13). text 125.00 (*0-8151-7059-9*, 27496) Mosby Inc.

Contemporary Industrial - Organizational Psychology. Linda N. Jewell & Marc Siegall. Ed. by Marshall. 2nd ed. 1990. 568p. (C). mass mkt. 49.75 (*0-314-58409-9*) West Pub.

Contemporary Internal Medicine: Clinical Case Studies. J. Bowen & E. L. Mazzaferri. (Illus.). (C). Vol. 1. 1988. LC 88-22379. 336p. text 95.00 (*0-306-43000-2*); Vol. 2. 1989. 296p. text 95.00 (*0-306-43329-X*); Vol. 3. 1991. 304p. text 95.00 (*0-306-43684-1*) Kluwer Academic (Kluwer Plenum).

Contemporary International Hypnosis: Proceedings of the XIIIth International Congress on Hypnosis, Melbourne, Australia, August 6-12, 1994. Ed. by Graham D. Burrows & Robb Stanley. 1995. LC 95-6640. 410p. 260.00 (*0-471-95829-8*) Wiley.

Contemporary Interpersonal Theory & Research: Personality, Psychopathology, & Psychotherapy. Donald J. Kiesler. 1996. LC 95-39129. (Clinical Psychology & Personality Ser.). 398p. 110.00 (*0-471-14847-4*) Wiley.

Contemporary Issues in Behavior Therapy: Improving the Human Condition. Ed. by Joseph R. Cautela & Waris Ishaq. 1996. (Applied Clinical Psychology Ser.). (Illus.). 432p. (C). 69.50 (*0-306-45168-9*, Plenum Trade) Perseus Pubng.

Contemporary Issues in Bioethics. Ed. by Thomas L. Beauchamp & LeRoy Walters. 2nd ed. 1982. 614p. (C). pap. 28.00 net. (*0-534-01102-0*) Wadsworth Pub.

Contemporary Issues in Bioethics. Thomas L. Beauchamp & LeRoy Walters. 4th ed. 1994. 752p. 49.25 (*0-534-22314-1*) Wadsworth Pub.

Contemporary Issues in Biomedical Ethics. Ed. by John W. Davis et al. 1979. LC 78-71406. (Contemporary Issues in Biomedicine, Ethics & Society Ser.). 336p. 59.50 (*0-89603-002-4*) Humana.

Contemporary Issues in Breast Cancer. Karen Hassey-Dow. 1996. (Nursing Ser.). (Illus.). 320p. (C). text 58.95 (*0-86720-713-2*, 713-2) Jones & Bartlett.

Contemporary Issues in Breast Cancer - Custom. Karen Hassey Dow. 1997. (Nursing Ser.). 336p. 15.00 (*0-7637-0618-3*) Jones & Bartlett.

Contemporary Issues in Chronic Pain Management. Ed. by Winston C. Parris. 1991. (Current Management of Pain Ser.). 311p. (C). text 188.00 (*0-7923-1182-5*) Kluwer Academic.

***Contemporary Issues in Colorectal Cancer: A Nursing Perspective.** Ed. by Deborah T. Berg. 2001. (Series in Oncology). (Illus.). 296p. (C). text 51.95 (*0-7637-1475-5*, 1475-5) Jones & Bartlett.

Contemporary Issues in Cross-Cultural Psychology. Ed. by N. Bleichrodt & Pieter J. D. Drenth. 1991. viii, 464p. pap. (*90-265-1117-5*) Swets.

Contemporary Issues in Law, Medicine & Ethics. Sheila A. McLean. 1995. (Medico-Legal Ser.). (Illus.). 288p. text (*1-85521-586-1*) Dartmth Pub GBR. *Dist:* Ashgate Pub Co.

***Contemporary Issues in Lung Cancer.** Marilyn L. Haas. 2002. (Illus.). (C). pap. text 52.95 (*0-7637-1914-5*, 1914-5) Jones & Bartlett.

Contemporary Issues in Maternal Health Care in Africa. J. K. Mati et al. 1995. LC 00-500198. 448p. text 132.00 (*3-7186-5560-8*, Harwood Acad Pubs) Gordon & Breach.

Contemporary Issues in Nursing. Biley. 1996. pap. text 17.95 (*0-443-05351-0*) Saunders.

Contemporary Issues in Pediatric Ethics. Ed. by Michael M. Burgess & Brian E. Woodrow. 1991. LC 91-31141. 124p. lib. bdg. 59.95 (*0-7734-9673-4*) E Mellen.

Contemporary Issues in Perimenopause & Menopause. Frances R. Batzer. 1999. LC 97-71114. (Illus.). 297p. (C). pap. text 29.95 (*1-884065-16-3*) Assocs in Med.

Contemporary Issues in Prostate Cancer: A Nursing Perspective. Ed. by Jeanne Held-Warmkessel. 2000. LC 99-44509. (Series in Oncology). (Illus.). 336p. (C). pap. text 51.95 (*0-7637-1081-4*, 1081-4) Jones & Bartlett.

Contemporary Issues in Public Health: A Special Issue of Journal of Community Health. Ed. by James E. Banta. 1987. 132p. pap. 16.95 (*0-89885-375-3*, Kluwer Acad Hman Sci) Kluwer Academic.

Contemporary Issues in the Treatment of Schizophrenia. Ed. by Christian L. Shriqui & Henry A. Nasrallan. 1995. 960p. text 99.95 (*0-88048-681-3*, 8681) Am Psychiatric.

Contemporary Jungian Analysis: Post Jungian Perspectives from the Sap. Ed. by Ian Alister & Christopher Hauke. 1998. LC 97-41078. (Illus.). 328p. (C). 84.95 (*0-415-14165-6*) Routledge.

Contemporary Jungian Analysis: Postjungian Perspectives from the Sap. Ed. by Ian Alister & Christopher Hauke. 1998. LC 97-41078. 272p. (C). pap. 27.95 (*0-415-14166-4*) Routledge.

Contemporary Kleinians of London. Ed. by Roy Schafer. 1997. LC 96-39138. 461p. 65.00 (*0-8236-1055-1*, BN01055) Intl Univs Pr.

Contemporary Learning Theories. Ed. by Stephen B. Klein & Robert R. Mowrer. 1989. (C). 336p. text 79.95 (*0-89859-915-6*);Set. text 125.00 (*0-8058-0526-5*);Vol. II. 304p. text 69.95 (*0-8058-0318-1*) L Erlbaum Assocs.

Contemporary Learning Theory & Research. Roger M. Tarpy. 1997. LC 96-36652. (*0-07-063118-2*) McGraw.

Contemporary Learning Theory & Research. Roger M. Tarpy. 1997. LC 96-36652. 608p. (C). text 85.00 (*0-07-063117-4*) McGrw-H Hghr Educ.

Contemporary Managed Care. Marsha R. Gold. 1998. LC 98-2665. vii, 369 p. 48.00 (*1-56793-078-6*) Health Admin Pr.

Contemporary Management of Motor Control Problems: Proceedings of the II Step Conference. 1991. 279p. 39.95 (*0-9628807-0-1*) FPT VA.

Contemporary Management of Spinal Cord Injuries: From Impact to Rehabilitation. Ed. by Charles H. Tator & Edward C. Benzel. 2000. 365p. 95.00 (*1-879284-72-3*) Am Assn Neuro.

***Contemporary Maternal-Newborn Nursing Care.** Patricia W. Ladewig et al. 5th ed. 2001. 912p. 63.33 (*0-8053-8051-5*) Addison-Wesley.

Contemporary Maternity Nursing. Gloria H. Wold. 1997. (Illus.). 256p. (C). (gr. 13). pap. text, stu. ed. (*0-8151-9372-6*); LC 96-51996. 528p. (C). (gr. 13). pap. text 31.95 (*0-8151-9373-4*, 27247); stu. ed. (*0-8151-9371-8*) Mosby Inc.

Contemporary Medical Office Procedures. Doris Humphrey. 1990. 576p. (C). pap. 32.95 (*0-538-70015-7*, RL43AB) S-W Thomson.

Contemporary Medical Office Procedures. Humphrey. 2nd ed. 1996. (Medical Assisting Ser.). 204p. text, tchr. ed. 16.00 (*0-8273-7421-6*) Delmar.

Contemporary Medical Office Procedures. Humphrey. 2nd ed. 1996. (Medical Assisting Ser.). pap. 32.95 (*0-538-71223-6*) S-W Thomson.

Contemporary Medical Office Procedures. Doris D. Humphrey. 2nd ed. 1995. LC 95-6199. (Medical Assisting Ser.). 592p. (C). pap. text 55.95 (*0-8273-7420-8*) Delmar.

Contemporary Medical Physiology. Robert L. Vick. 1984. 1056p. (*0-201-08095-8*) Addison-Wesley.

Contemporary Metabolism, Vol. 2. Ed. by Norbert Freinkel. 1982. LC 79-643531. (Illus.). 564p. 95.00 (*0-306-40954-2*, Kluwer Plenum) Kluwer Academic.

***Contemporary Midwifery Practice.** Wickham. 2001. 29.95 (*0-7506-5427-9*) Buttrwrth-Heinemann.

Contemporary Models of Psychotherapy: A Comparative Analysis. Donald H. Ford & Hugh B. Urban. 2nd ed. 1998. LC 97-28994. 768p. 79.96 (*0-471-59638-8*) Wiley.

Contemporary Nephrology. Ed. by Saulo Klahr & Shaul G. Massry. Vol. 1. 1981. 736p. 125.00 (*0-306-40664-0*); Vol. 3. 1985. 792p. 125.00 (*0-306-41984-X*); Vol. 4. 1987. (Illus.). 774p. 125.00 (*0-306-42531-9*) Kluwer Academic (Kluwer Plenum).

Contemporary Nephrology, Vol. 5. S. Klahr & S. G. Massry. 1989. (Illus.). 596p. (C). text 125.00 (*0-306-43274-9*, Kluwer Plenum) Kluwer Academic.

Contemporary Nephrology Nursing. Ed. by Janet Parker & Gus Ostrum. 1998. (Illus.). 800p. 95.00 (*0-9653379-0-1*) Am Nephrology.

***Contemporary Neuropsychiatry.** Keoheo Miyoshi. 2001. LC 00-67934. (Illus.). xvi, 478p. 119.00 (*4-431-70300-4*) Spr-Verlag.

Contemporary Neuropsychology & the Legacy of Luria. E. Goldberg. 1990. 304p. (C). text 99.95 (*0-8058-0334-3*) L Erlbaum Assocs.

Contemporary Nursing: Issues, Trends & Management. Barbara Cherry & Susan Jacob. 1999. LC 98-40028. 587p. 29.95 (*0-323-00248-X*) Mosby Inc.

Contemporary Nursing: Issues, Trends & Management. Barbara Cherry et al. 1999. (Illus.). 587p. tchr. ed. (*0-323-00751-1*) Mosby Inc.

Contemporary Nursing Procedures. Carol A. Lindeman. 1999. pap. text (*0-7216-4208-X*) Saunders.

Contemporary Nutrition. Gordon M. Wardlaw. 1992. (*0-8016-6850-6*); 2nd annot. ed. 1994. tchr. ed. (*0-8151-9243-6*) Mosby Inc.

Contemporary Nutrition. Wardlaw. 5th ed. 2002. stu. ed. 17.74 net. (*0-07-231617-9*) McGraw.

Contemporary Nutrition: Issues - Insights. Wardlaw. 3rd ed. 1996. pap. 53.13 (*0-8151-9050-6*) Mosby Inc.

***Contemporary Nutrition: Issues & Insights with Foodworks.** Gordon M. Wardlaw. 2000. (C). 65.00 (*0-07-246815-7*) McGrw-H Hghr Educ.

Contemporary Nutrition Student Study Guide. Insel et al. 1991. 320p. pap. 15.95 (*0-8016-2340-5*) Mosby Inc.

Contemporary Nutrition Study Guide. Gordon M. Wardlaw. 3rd ed. 1996. (Illus.). 320p. (C). pap., stu. ed. 27.19 (*0-8151-9272-X*) McGrw-H Hghr Educ.

Contemporary Nutrition Support Practice: A Clinical Guide. Laura E. Matarese & Michele M. Gottschlich. Ed. by Maura Connor et al. 1998. LC 97-1437. (Illus.). 720p. (C). text 99.00 (*0-7216-5999-3*) Saunders.

Contemporary Nutrition Text. Inscl ct al. 1992. 44.95 incl. 3.5 hd (*0-8016-6873-5*); 44.95 incl. 5.25 hd (*0-8016-6874-3*) Mosby Inc.

***Contemporary Nutrition with NutriQuest 2.1.** Gordon M. Wardlaw. 4th ed. 2000. 65.00 (*0-07-246814-9*) McGrw-H Hghr Educ.

***Contemporary Occupational Therapy Practice Theorists.** Rosalie J. Miller. 1995. (*0-8342-2048-2*) PRO-ED.

Contemporary Oral & Maxillofacial Pathology. J. Philip Sapp et al. 1997. (Illus.). 448p. (*84-8174-291-0*) Mosby-Doyma Libros ESP. *Dist:* Mosby Inc.

Contemporary Oral & Maxillofacial Surgery. Larry J. Peterson. 3rd ed. 1997. LC 97-14848. (Illus.). 816p. (C). (gr. 13). text 69.00 (*0-8151-6699-0*, 25548) Mosby Inc.

Contemporary Oral Pathology. Philip Sapp & George Wysocki. 1996. (Illus.). 448p. (C). (gr. 13). text 61.00 (*0-8016-6918-9*, 06918) Mosby Inc.

Contemporary Orthodontics. William R. Proffit et al. 2nd ed. 1992. LC 92-22056. (Illus.). 688p. (C). (gr. 13). text 81.00 (*0-8016-6393-8*, 06393) Mosby Inc.

Contemporary Orthodontics. William R. Proffit & Henry W. Fields, Jr. 3rd ed. 1999. LC 99-24758. (Illus.). x, 742p. (C). text (*1-55664-553-8*) Mosby Inc.

Contemporary Orthodontics. William R. Proffit & Henry W. Fields, Jr. 3rd ed. 2000. (Illus.). 742p. (*84-8086-075-8*) Mosby-Doyma Libros ESP. *Dist:* Mosby Inc.

Contemporary Overview of Nitrate Therapy. Ed. by Jonathan Abrams. 1987. (Illus.). 32p. (Orig.). pap. (*0-943035-00-7*) CoMed Comm.

Contemporary Pediatric Nursing. Cathleen S. Opperman & Kathleen A. Cassandra. 1998. tchr. ed. (*0-8151-2899-1*); LC 97-42370. (Illus.). 576p. tchr. ed. (*0-8151-2897-5*, 30096); (Illus.). 224p. stu. ed. (*0-8151-2898-3*) Mosby Inc.

Contemporary Peridontics. Robert J. Genco et al. 1990. (Illus.). 752p. (C). (gr. 13). text 72.95 (*0-8016-1935-1*, 01935) Mosby Inc.

Contemporary Periodontal Instrumentation. Diane Schoen & Mary C. Dean. Ed. by Selma Ozmat. 1996. LC 95-36915. 304p. pap. text 42.00 (*0-7216-4551-8*) Saunders.

Contemporary Periodontics. Robert J. Genco & D. Walter Cohen. 2nd ed. 1999. (Illus.). 768p. (C). (gr. 13). text 72.95 (*0-8016-7978-8*, 07978) Mosby Inc.

Contemporary Perspectives on Psychotherapy with Lesbians & Gay Men. Ed. by Terry Stein & Carol J. Cohen. 1986. LC 86-692. (Critical Issues in Psychiatry Ser.). (Illus.). 286p. (C). 59.00 (*0-306-42161-5*, Plenum Trade) Perseus Pubng.

Contemporary Practical/Vocational Nursing. Corrine R. Kurzen. 4th ed. 2000. LC 00-44387. (Illus.). 448p. pap. text 26.95 (*0-7817-2593-3*) Lppncott W & W.

Contemporary Psychiatric-Mental Health Nursing. Ed. by Carol A. Glod. 1998. LC 97-46122. (Illus.). 705p. (C). text 54.95 (*0-8036-0293-6*) Davis Co.

Contemporary Psychoanalysis & Eastern Thought. John R. Suler. 1993. LC 92-30817. (SUNY Series, Alternatives in Psychology). 292p. (C). text 23.50 (*0-7914-1577-5*); pap. text 22.95 (*0-7914-1578-3*) State U NY Pr.

Contemporary Psychological Approaches to Depression: Theory, Research, & Treatment. R. E. Ingram. 1990. LC 90-43004. (Illus.). 208p. (C). 79.50 (*0-306-43690-6*, Plenum Trade) Perseus Pubng.

Contemporary Psychology & Effective Behavior. Morris. 7th ed. 1997. 208p. (C). pap., stu. ed. 30.00 (*0-673-38955-3*) Addson-Wesley Educ.

Contemporary Psychology & Effective Behavior, 7th Edition. Charles Morris & James C. Coleman. 7th ed. 1997. 546p. (C). pap. 69.80 (*0-673-46051-7*) Addson-Wesley Educ.

Contemporary Research on Renal Cell Carcinoma: Basic & Clinical Developments. Ed. by G. Staehler & S. Pomer. 1994. LC 93-23588. (Illus.). 170p. 103.00 (*0-387-57375-5*) Spr-Verlag.

Contemporary Rorschach Interpretation: A Casebook. Ed. by J. Reid Meloy et al. 1997. LC 96-49872. (Lea Series in Personality & Clinical Psychology Ser.). 450p. 55.00 (*0-8058-1920-7*) L Erlbaum Assocs.

Contemporary School Psychology. William G. Herron et al. 2nd ed. 1984. LC 83-15325. 405p. (gr. 1-12). pap. 19.50 (*0-910328-16-1*) Sulzburger & Graham Pub.

Contemporary Spiritual Classics: Albert Schweitzer. Compiled by Helen R. Neinast. 1989. LC 89-50644. 60p. pap. 3.00 (*0-8358-0605-7*) Upper Room Bks.

Contemporary Studies in Combat Psychiatry, 62. Ed. by Gregory Belenky. 1987. LC 86-33660. (Contributions in Military Studies Ser.: No. 62). 291p. 67.00 (*0-313-25513-X*, BYT/, Greenwood Pr) Greenwood.

Contemporary Themes in Psychiatry: A Tribute to Sir Martin Roth. Ed. by Kenneth Davison & Alan Kerr. 1989. 519p. pap. text (*0-902241-28-1*, 4128) Royal Coll Psych GBR. *Dist:* Parkwest Pubns.

Contemporary Theories & Systems in Psychology. Benjamin B. Wolman. 2nd ed. 1981. LC 80-21058. 652p. 85.00 (*0-306-40515-6*); pap. 39.50 (*0-306-40530-X*) Perseus Pubng (Plenum Trade).

Contemporary Theories in Psychoanalysis. Ed. by Robert J. Langs. 1996. 416p. (C). pap. text 35.95 (*0-89876-216-2*) Gardner Pr.

***Contemporary Therapy in Obstetrics & Gynecology.** Scott B. Ransom. 2001. LC 2001-31121. (*0-7216-9286-9*) Saunders.

Contemporary Topics in Developmental Psychology. Ed. by Nancy Weisenberg. 1987. LC 86-34026. (Personality Processes Ser.). 464p. 250.00 (*0-471-82913-7*) Wiley.

Contemporary Topics in Immunobiology Vol. 12: Immunobiology of Parasites & Parasitic Infections. Ed. by John J. Marchalonis. 1984. LC 79-179761. 518p. 95.00 (*0-306-41418-X*, Plenum Trade) Perseus Pubng.

Contemporary Topics in Immunobiology Vol. 15: Immune Complexes & Human Cancer, Vol. 15. Ed. by Fernando A. Salinas & Michael G. Hanna, Jr. 1985. LC 85-6315. 296p. 85.00 (*0-306-41955-6*, Plenum Trade) Perseus Pubng.

Contemporary Topics in Molecular Immunology, Vol. 8. Ed. by F. P. Inman & W. J. Mandy. 1981. LC 73-648513. 240p. 69.50 (*0-306-40661-6*, Plenum Trade) Perseus Pubng.

Contemporary Topics in Molecular Immunology, Vol. 9. Ed. by F. P. Inman & Thomas J. Kindt. 1983. LC 73-648513. 260p. 69.50 (*0-306-41304-3*, Plenum Trade) Perseus Pubng.

Contemporary Topics in Molecular Immunology Vol. 10: The Interleukins. Ed. by Steven Gillis & F. P. Inman. 1985. LC 73-648513. 312p. 85.00 (*0-306-41776-6*, Plenum Trade) Perseus Pubng.

Contemporary Treatment of Psychosis: Healing Relationships in the "Decade of the Brain" Ed. by Jon G. Allen & Dean T. Collins. 1996. LC 96-5658. 128p. pap. 25.00 (*1-56821-873-7*) Aronson.

Contemporary Treatments in Neurology. Neil Scolding. 2001. (Illus.). 446p. text 59.95 (*0-7506-3918-0*) Buttrwrth-Heinemann.

Content Analysis of Verbal Behavior: New Findings & Clinical Applications. Louis A. Gottschalk. 1995. 232p. text 49.95 (*0-8058-1558-9*) L Erlbaum Assocs.

Content & Process Specificity in the Effects of Prior Experiences. Ed. by Robert S. Wyer, Jr. & Thomas K. Srull. 1990. (Advances in Social Cognition Ser.: Vol. III). 208p. (C). 49.95 (*0-8058-0700-4*); pap. 27.50 (*0-8058-0714-4*) L Erlbaum Assocs.

Content Review for the NCLEX-PN. Sandra Smith. 6th ed. 1997. LC 97-139590. 509p. (C). pap. 29.95 (*0-8385-1516-9*) P-H.

Contents of Thought. Robert H. Grimm & Daniel D. Merrill. 1988. LC 88-4717. (Arizona Colloquim on Cognition Ser.). 211p. 45.50 (*0-8165-1064-4*) U of Ariz Pr.

Contested Issues of Ecosystem Management. Ed. by Piermaria Corona & Boris Zeide. 1999. LC 99-51660. (Journal of Sustainable Forestry Ser.: Vol. 9, Nos. 1/2). (Illus.). 180p. pap. text 24.95 (*1-56022-067-8*) Haworth Pr.

Context & Cognition. Ed. by Paul Light & George Butterworth. 1993. 192p. pap. 24.50 (*0-8058-1393-4*); text 39.95 (*0-8058-1392-6*) L Erlbaum Assocs.

Context & Development. Ed. by Robert Cohen & Alexander Siegel. 1991. 336p. (C). text 69.95 (*0-8058-0481-1*) L Erlbaum Assocs.

Context Color-Coded ICD-9-CM, 1997. Ed. by Context Software Staff. 5th ed. 1996. 650p. pap. text 44.95 (*1-57066-073-5*, 9727) Practice Mgmt Info.

Context Color-Coded ICD-9-CM 1998 annuals Context Software Staff. rev. ed. 1997. 890p. pap. text 44.95 (*1-57066-118-9*, 9827) Practice Mgmt Info.

Context Color-Coded ICD-9-CM, 1999 ADP Context Software Staff. rev. ed. 1998. 900p. pap. text 44.95 (*1-57066-092-1*, 9927) Practice Mgmt Info.

Context of Medicines in Developing Countries. Ed. by Sjaak Van der Geest & Susan R. Whyte. 1988. (C). lib. bdg. 173.50 (*1-55608-059-X*) Kluwer Academic.

Context of Self: A Phenomenological Inquiry Using Medicine As a Clue. Richard M. Zaner. 1981. LC 80-18500. (Series in Continental Thought : Vol. 1). (Illus.). xiv, 282p. text 24.95 (*0-8214-0443-1*) Ohio U Pr.

Contexts of Being: The Intersubjective Foundations of Psychological Life. Robert D. Stolorow & George E. Atwood. 1992. LC 92-21982. (Psychoanalytic Inquiry Ser.: Vol. 12). 160p. pap. text 29.95 (*0-88163-152-3*) Analytic Pr.

Contextual Family Therapy: Assessment & Intervention Procedures. Peter Goldenthal. 1993. LC 93-10551. (Practitioner's Resource Ser.). 90p. pap. 16.95 (*0-943158-79-6*, CFTBP, Prof Resc Pr) Pro Resource.

Contextualism & Understanding in Behavioral Science: Implications for Research & Theory. Ed. by Ralph L. Rosnow & Marianthi Georgoudi. 1986. 392p. 78.75 (*0-275-92121-2*, C2121, Praeger Pubs) Greenwood.

Continence: Promotion & Management by the Primary Health Care Team : Consensus Guidelines. Denise Button & Primary Health Care Team. 1998. LC 98-214881. (*1-86156-078-8*) Whurr Pub.

Continence with Biofeedback: New Treatment for Fecal Incontinence. Susan Trunnell. 1991. LC 91-75791. 173p. pap. 24.95 (*0-9630339-5-6*) Avantage.

Contingent Future Persons: On the Ethics of Deciding Who Will Live, or Not, in the Future. N. Fotion & Jan C. Heller. 1997. LC 97-18433. (Theology & Medicine Ser.). text 110.50 (*0-7923-4707-2*) Kluwer Academic.

Contingent Immaterialism: Meaning, Freedom, Time & Mind. Ben Mijuskovic. 1984. 214p. (Orig.). pap. (*90-6032-254-1*) B R Gruner NLD. *Dist:* Humanities.

Continued Management Concerns at the NIH: Hearing Before the Subcommittee on Oversight & Investigations of the Committee on Commerce, House of Representatives, One Hundred Fifth Congress, First Session, June 19, 1997. Contrib. by U. S. Congress, House Committee on Commerce, Subcommittee on Oversight and Investigations. 1997. LC 98-107112. (Illus.). (*0-16-055330-X*) USGPO.

Continuing Bonds: New Understandings of Grief. Ed. by Dennis Klass et al. 1996. LC 95-35022. (Death Education, Aging & Health Care Ser.). 260p. pap. 29.95 (*1-56032-339-6*) Hemisp Pub.

Continuing Care: For the Dying Patient, Family & Staff, 5. Ed. by Robert Debellis et al. 1985. LC 85-19165. (Foundation of Thanatology Ser.: Vol. 5). 190p. 62.50 (*0-275-91334-1*, C1334, Praeger Pubs) Greenwood.

Continuing Care: The Management of Chronic Disease. Ed. by John Hasler & Theo Schofield. 2nd ed. 1990. (Oxford General Practice Ser.: No. 19). (Illus.). 364p. pap. 42.50 (*0-19-261742-7*) OUP.

Continuing Care in a Community Hospital. Harold N. Willard et al. 1972. LC 75-186676. (Commonwealth Fund Publications). (Illus.). 208p. 29.00 (*0-674-16775-9*) HUP.

Continuing Care Retirement Communities: Political, Social & Financial Issues. Ian A. Morrison et al. 1986. LC 85-8669. (Journal of Housing for the Elderly: Vol. 3, No. 1-2). 188p. text 49.95 (*0-86656-384-9*) Haworth Pr.

Continuing Care Services No. 2: An Alternative to the Hospice for Preterminal & Terminal Patients, Vol. 8. 1980. 18.95 (*0-405-13098-8*) Ayer.

Continuing Challenge of Tuberculosis. 1995. lib. bdg. 250.75 (*0-8490-7569-6*) Gordon Pr.

Continuing Challenge of Tuberculosis. 1996. (Illus.). 148p. (Orig.). reprint ed. pap. text 30.00 (*0-7881-2991-0*) DIANE Pub.

Continuing Education in Management for Health Care Personnel. Donald K. White. 1975. LC 75-27158. 10.00 (*0-87914-028-3*, 567152) Hosp Res & Educ.

Continuing Education in Nursing: Strategies for Lifelong Learning. Patricia Dophlin & Barbara Hotzclaw. 1983. (C). pap. text 24.95 (*0-8359-1011-3*) P-H.

Continuing Education in Pharmacy. Ed. by Jack R. Arndt & Stephen J. Coons. 1987. LC 87-71365. (Illus.). 374p. (C). text 40.00 (*0-937526-13-4*) AACP Alexandria.

Continuing Medical Education: A Primer. Ed. by Adrienne B. Rosof & William C. Felch. 2nd ed. 1992. LC 91-24229. 256p. 68.00 (*0-275-94009-8*, C4009); pap. 18.95 (*0-275-94010-1*, B4010) Greenwood (Praeger Pubs).

Continuing Medical Education in the Community Hospital. James J. Bergin & Geraldine C. Holmes. 1979. LC 79-55326. (Illus.). 112p. text 22.00 (*0-935466-00-2*); pap. text 16.00 (*0-935466-01-0*) Pierson Pubs.

Continuing the Education of Health Workers: A Workshop Manual. F. Abbatt & A. Mejia. 1988. 185p. 35.00 (*92-4-154220-9*) World Health.

Continuing Trial of Treatment. Ed. by Stephen Frankel & Gilbert Lewis. 1988. (C). pap. text 61.00 (*0-7923-0078-5*); lib. bdg. 177.50 (*1-55608-076-X*) Kluwer Academic.

Continuities & Discontinuities in Development. Ed. by Robert N. Emde & Robert J. Harmon. 1984. LC 84-8225. (Topics in Developmental Psychobiology Ser.). 438p. 65.00 (*0-306-41563-1*, Plenum Trade) Perseus Pubng.

Continuity & Change in Psychoanalysis: Letters from Milan. Luciana Nissim-Momigliano. 1992. 192p. pap. text (*1-85575-009-0*) Karnac Bks GBR. *Dist:* Other Pr LLC.

Continuity & Crisis in the NHS. Ed. by Raymond Loveridge & Ken Starkey. 1992. 224p. (*0-335-15620-7*); pap. (*0-335-15599-5*) OpUniv Pr.

Continuity of Neural Functions from Prenatal to Postnatal Life. Ed. by Heinz F. Prechtl. 1991. LC 65-80476. (Clinics in Developmental Medicine Ser.: No. 94). (Illus.). 255p. (C). text (*0-521-41214-5*) Mc Keith Pr GBR. *Dist:* Cambridge U Pr.

Continuous Ambulatory Peritoneal Dialysis. Ed. by R. Gokal. 1987. (Illus.). 382p. text (*0-443-03634-9*) Church.

Continuous Ambulatory Peritoneal Dialysis: A Decade of Experience. Ed. by G. La Greca et al. 1991. (Contributions to Nephrology Ser.: Vol. 89). (Illus.). x, 288p. 49.75 (*3-8055-5307-2*) S Karger.

Continuous Ambulatory Peritoneal Dialysis: Host Defense, Nutrition & Ultrafiltration. Ed. by G. A. Coles et al. 1990. (Contributions to Nephrology Ser.: Vol. 85). (Illus.). viii, 172p. 29.75 (*3-8055-5215-7*) S Karger.

Continuous Ambulatory Peritoneal Dialysis (CAPD) Betty Bergerson & Christina M. Comty. 1983. 210p. ring bd. 30.00 (*1-56488-008-7*) Dialyrn.

Continuous Ambulatory Peritoneal Dialysis in the U. S. A. Ed. by A. S. Lindblad et al. 1989. (Developments in Nephrology Ser.). (C). text 207.50 (*0-7923-0179-X*) Kluwer Academic.

Continuous Arteriovenous Hemofiltration. Ed. by H. G. Sieberth & H. Mann. 1985. (Illus.). xii, 248p. 56.75 (*3-8055-4077-9*) S Karger.

Continuous Cell Lines: An International Workshop on Current Issues Held in Bethesda, MD, March 1991. Ed. by F. Brown et al. 1992. (Developments in Biological Standardization Ser.: Vol. 76). (Illus.). x, 354p. pap. 278.50 (*3-8055-5618-7*) S Karger.

Continuous Cell Lines As Substrates for Biologicals: Symposium Organized by IABS, Arlington, Va., May 1988. Ed. by Leonard Hayflick & W. Hennessen. 1989. (Developments in Biological Standardization Ser.: Vol. 70). (Illus.). x, 308p. pap. 61.00 (*3-8055-4940-7*) S Karger.

Continuous Challenge of Tuberculosis. 1994. lib. bdg. 250.00 (*0-8490-8548-9*) Gordon Pr.

Continuous Cultures of Cells Peter H. Calcott. 1981. 208p. 79.00 (*0-8493-5377-7*, QH585); 224p. 77.00 (*0-8493-5378-5*, QH585) Franklin (CRC Reprint).

Continuous Eligibility for Children under Medi-Cal: Cost Estimates for Six-Month & Twelve-Month Coverage Extension Options. unabr. ed. 1999. (Illus.). 140p. pap. (*1-929008-18-X*) CA HlthCare Fnd.

Continuous Extracorporeal Treatment in Multiple Organ Dysfunction Syndrome. Ed. by H. G. Sieberth et al. 1995. LC 95-23408. (Contributions to Nephrology Ser.: Vol. 116). (Illus.). x, 188p. 172.25 (*3-8055-6131-8*) S Karger.

Continuous Flow Analysis: Theory & Practice. William B. Furman. 1976. (Clinical & Biochemical Analysis Ser.: Vol. 3). (Illus.). 352p. text 185.00 (*0-8247-6320-3*) Dekker.

Continuous Hemofiltration. Ed. by H. G. Sieberth et al. 1991. (Contributions to Nephrology Ser.: Vol. 93). (Illus.). xii, 272p. 49.75 (*3-8055-5375-7*) S Karger.

Continuous Hemofiltration in the Intensive Care Unit. Ed. by Didier Journois. 1997. 248p. text 70.00 (*90-5702-121-8*, Harwood Acad Pubs) Gordon & Breach.

Continuous Improvement in the Healthcare Manufacturing Industry: A Practical Guide for Implementing an Improvement Program. Valerie Bland. 1999. LC 99-37163. (Illus.). xi, 165p. 149.00 (*1-57491-099-X*) IHS Health Grp.

Continuous Monitoring of Arterial Oxygen Partial Pressure: Journal: Biotelemetry & Patient Monitoring, Vol. 6, Nos. 1 & 2, 1979. Ed. by H. P. Kimmich. 1979. (Illus.). pap. 23.50 (*3-8055-0053-X*) S Karger.

Continuous Passive Motion: A Biological Concept for the Healing & Regeneration of Joint Tissues. Robert B. Salter. 1992. (Illus.). 400p. 125.00 (*0-683-07497-0*) Lppncott W & W.

Continuous Quality Improvement Fo Long-Term Care. Jennifer I. Cofer. 2nd ed. 1999. LC 00-701381. (Illus.). v, 169p. pap. text 87.00 (*1-57839-064-8*) Opus Communs.

Continuous Quality Improvement for Nutrition Care. Rita Jackson. 1992. (Illus.). 242p. (C). pap. text 37.00 (*0-9624150-2-2*) Amer Nutri-Tech.

Continuous Quality Improvement in EMS. American College of Emergency Physicians Staff. 1992. 80.00 (*0-07-000210-X*) McGraw.

Continuous Quality Improvement in Health Care: Theory, Implementation & Applications. Curtis P. McLaughlin & Arnold D. Kaluzny. 2nd ed. 1999. LC 99-20197. xxii, 659p. 62.00 (*0-8342-1655-8*) Aspen Pub.

Continuous Quality Improvement in Nursing. American Nurses Association Staff. Ed. & Intro. by Jacqueline Dienemann. 1992. LC 92-17870. 144p. (C). pap. 14.95 (*1-55810-075-X*, NP-80, Am Nurses Fnd) Am Nurses Pub.

Continuous Spikes & Waves During Slow Sleep. A. Beaumanoir. 1995. 272p. (*0-86196-488-8*) J Libbey Med GBR. *Dist:* Buttrwrth-Heinemann.

Continuous Transcutaneous Monitoring. R. Huch & G. Rooth. Ed. by A. Huch. 1987. LC 87-15358. (Advances in Experimental Medicine & Biology Ser.: Vol. 220). (Illus.). 342p. 79.50 (*0-306-42661-7*, Plenum Trade) Perseus Pubng.

Continuum of Care Treatment Planner. Chris E. Stout & Arthur E. Jongsma, Jr. 1997. LC 97-28834. 170p. pap. 44.95 (*0-471-19568-5*); pap. text 175.00 incl. disk (*0-471-19569-3*) Wiley.

Continuum of Long Term Care. Connie Evashwick. 2nd ed. 2001. LC 00-59046. (Delmar Series in Health Services Administration Ser.). (Illus.). 544p. (C). text 63.95 (*0-7668-1574-9*) Delmar.

Continuum of Long-Term Care: An Integrated Systems Approach. Ed. by Connie J. Evashwick. 1995. LC 94-48856. (Delmar Series in Health Services Administration Ser.). 445p. (C). mass mkt. 78.95 (*0-8273-6151-3*) Delmar.

Contours of Death & Disease in Early Modern England. Mary J. Dobson. 1997. (Studies in Population, Economy & Society in Past Time: No. 29). (Illus.). 668p. (C). text 100.00 (*0-521-40464-9*) Cambridge U Pr.

Contraception. Ed. by Donna Shoupe. 1993. LC 92-48671. (Clinical Perspectives in Obstetrics & Gynecology Ser.). 256p. (*3-540-97859-3*); (Illus.). 261p. 108.00 (*0-387-97859-3*) Spr-Verlag.

Contraception: A Guide on Birth Control Methods. Vern L. Bullough & Bonnie Bullough. 2nd ed. 1997. LC 97-23707. (Illus.). 216p. pap. text 22.00 (*1-57392-159-9*) Prometheus Bks.

Contraception: A User's Handbook. Anne Szarewski & John Guillebaud. 1994. LC 93-36749. (Illus.). 272p. (C). pap. 10.00 (*0-19-286164-6*) OUP.

Contraception: Science & Practice. Marchs Filshie & John Guillebaud. 1989. (Illus.). 376p. text (*0-7506-1186-3*) E A GBR. *Dist:* OUP.

Contraception: Your Questions Answered. John Guillebaud. 2nd ed. 1993. (Illus.). 372p. (Orig.). pap. text (*0-443-04070-2*) Church.

Contraception: Your Questions Answered. John Guillebaud. 3rd ed. 1999. 536p. (Orig.). (C). pap. text 34.95 (*0-443-06153-X*) Harcourt.

Contraception & Abortion from the Ancient World to the Renaissance. John M. Riddle. (Illus.). 1994. 256p. pap. 18.95 (*0-674-16876-3*); 1992. LC 91-33682. 272p. (C). 48.95 (*0-674-16875-5*) HUP.

Contraception & Fertility in the Southern Appalachians. Gilbert W. Beebe. 1972. LC 79-169373. (Family in America Ser.). (Illus.). 396p. reprint ed. 20.95 (*0-405-03849-6*) Ayer.

Contraception & Reproduction: Health Consequences for Women & Children in the Developing World. National Research Council Staff. 1989. 120p. pap. text 15.00 (*0-309-04094-9*) Natl Acad Pr.

Contraception Handbook. Everett. 1997. text (*0-7020-2001-X*) Bailliere Tindall.

Contraception Today: Pocketbook Edition. John Guillebaud. 4th ed. 2000. 104p. pap. (*1-85317-868-3*) Martin Dunitz GBR. *Dist:* Blackwell Sci.

Contraception Today: The Proceedings of the 4th Congress of the European Society of Contraception. G. Creatsas & European Society of Contraception Staff. Ed. by C. Coll Capdevila & L. Iglesias Cortit. 1998. LC 97-48549. (International Congress, Symposium, & Seminar Ser.: Vol. 14). (Illus.). 294p. lib. bdg. 85.95 (*1-85070-767-7*, B3252, Parthenon Pbng) CRC Pr.

Contraceptive Care: Meeting Individual Needs. Heather Montford. 1993. 256p. pap. 47.75 (*1-56593-213-7*, 0554) Singular Publishing.

Contraceptive Choice, Fertility, & Public Policy in Zimbabwe, 109. Duncan Thomas & John Maluccio. 1995. LC 94-30390. (Living Standards Measurement Study: No. 109). 56p. pap. 22.00 (*0-8213-3018-7*, 13018) World Bank.

Contraceptive Choices & Realities: Proceedings of the 5th Congress of the European Society of Contraception, 15. Ed. by R. H. W. Van Lunsen et al. 2000. LC 99-40630. (International Congress, Symposium, & Seminar Ser.: Vol. 15). (Illus.). 264p. lib. bdg. 148.95 (*1-85070-067-2*) CRC Pr.

Contraceptive Education: A Self-Instructional Course. Robert R. Wilson. 1974. 2.50 (*0-89055-121-9*) Carolina Pop Ctr.

Contraceptive Ethos. Stuart F. Spicker et al. 1987. 278p. (C). text 132.50 (*1-55608-035-2*) Kluwer Academic.

Contraceptive Method Mix: Guidelines for Policy & Service Delivery. 1994. LC 95-118070. (CHI, ENG & FRE.). viii, 143p. pap. text 32.00 (*92-4-154459-7*, 1150409) World Health.

Contraceptive Research & Development: Looking to the Future. Institute of Medicine Staff. Ed. by Polly F. Harrison & Allan Rosenfield. 1996. LC 96-26149. 536p. text 49.95 (*0-309-05442-7*) Natl Acad Pr.

Contraceptive Research & Development, 1984-1994: The Road from Mexico City to Cairo & Beyond. Ed. by P. F. Van Look & G. Perez-Palacios. 1995. (Illus.). 562p. text 95.00 (*0-19-563630-9*) OUP.

Contraceptive Research, Introduction & Use: Lessons from Norplant. Institute of Medicine Staff. 1998. LC 98-134174. 124p. (C). pap. text 26.00 (*0-309-05985-2*) Natl Acad Pr.

Contraceptive Revolution: An Era of Scientific & Social Development. Egon Diczfalusy. 1997. LC 96-34919. (Illus.). 256p. lib. bdg. 82.95 (*1-85070-748-0*, Parthenon Pbng) CRC Pr.

Contraceptive Steroids: Pharmacology & Safety. Ed. by A. T. Gregoire & Richard P. Blye. 1986. LC 86-20448. (Reproductive Biology Ser.). 410p. 95.00 (*0-306-42393-6*, Plenum Trade) Perseus Pubng.

Contraceptive Surgery for Men & Women. AVSC Staff & William M. Moss. 2nd ed. 1991. 182p. 12.95 (*0-929240-26-X*) EMIS.

Contraceptive Technology: Special Sections on Emergency Contraception & STI Treatment Guidelines. Robert A. Hatcher et al. 17th rev. ed. 1998. (Illus.). 880p. text 59.50 (*0-9664902-1-5*); pap. text 39.95 (*0-9664902-0-7*) Ardent Media.

Contraceptive Technology, 1988-1989: With a Special Section on AIDS & Family Planning. Robert A. Hatcher et al. rev. ed. 1988. (Illus.). 437p. pap. text 19.95 (*0-8290-1818-2*) Irvington.

Contraceptive Use & Controlled Fertility: Health Issues for Women & Children. National Research Council Staff. 1989. 172p. pap. text 18.00 (*0-309-04096-5*) Natl Acad Pr.

Contraceptive Use & Fertility in India: A Case Study of Gujarat. Pravin Visaria et al. 1995. LC 95-20193. 264p. 35.00 (*0-8039-9253-X*, 1709) Sage.

Contraceptive Use & the Quality, Price, & Availability of Family Planning in Nigeria. Bamikale J. Feyisetan & Martha Ainsworth. 1995. LC 94-3142. (Living Standards Measurement Study Working Papers: No. 108). 60p. pap. 22.00 (*0-8213-3017-9*, 13017) World Bank.

Contraceptives - Oral & Combinations: Index of New Information. Helen D. Dawson. Date not set. 160p. 57.50 (*0-7883-1928-0*); pap. 47.50 (*0-7883-1929-9*) ABBE Pubs Assn.

Contraceptives of the Future. R. V. Short & D. T. Baird. 1977. LC 77-371447. (Illus.). text 35.00 (*0-85403-087-5*) Scholium Intl.

Contraceptives-Postcoital & the Morning after Pill: Index of New Information. Helen D. Dawson. Date not set. 160p. 57.50 (*0-7883-1926-4*); pap. 47.50 (*0-7883-1927-2*) ABBE Pubs Assn.

Contract Pastoral Care & Education: The Trend of the Future? Ed. by Larry VandeCreek. 1999. LC 99-51929. (Journal of Health Care Chaplaincy Ser.: Vol. 9). 122p. (C). pap. text 19.95 (*0-7890-0826-2*); 39.95 (*0-7890-0793-2*) Haworth Pr (Haworth Pastrl).

Contractile Proteins in Muscle & Non-Muscle Cell Systems: Biochemistry, Physiology & Pathology. Ed. by Emanuele E. Alia et al. 1985. LC 85-12274. 752p. 150.00 (*0-275-91329-5*, C1329, Praeger Pubs) Greenwood.

Contracting a Cure: Patients & Healers in Early Modern Bologna. Gianna Pomata. 1998. LC 98-5982. 310p. 46.50 (*0-8018-5858-5*) Johns Hopkins.

Contracting & Negotiating Managed Care Agreements. 1996. 160p. pap. 45.00 (*0-89203-156-5*) Amer Acad Ortho Surg.

Contracting for Change: Contracts in Health, Social Care & Other Local Government Services. Kieron Walsh et al. 1997. LC 97-3699. (Illus.). 240p. (C). text 65.00 (*0-19-828945-6*) OUP.

Contracting for Health: Quasi-Markets & the National Health Service. Ed. by Robert Flynn & Gareth Williams. 1997. LC 97-4234. (Illus.). 190p. text 55.00 (*0-19-829022-5*) OUP.

Contracting for Managed Substance Abuse & mental Health Services: A Guide for Public Purchasers. Stephen Moss. 2000. 295p. reprint ed. pap. text 40.00 (*0-7567-0257-7*) DIANE Pub.

Contracting on a Capitated Basis: Managing Risk for Your Practice. American Psychological Association Staff et al. 1996. LC 96-23681. (Practitioner's Toolbox Ser.). 94p. pap. 29.95 (*1-55798-362-3*) Am Psychol.

Contracting with Organized Delivery Systems: Selecting, Evaluating & Negotiating Contracts. American Psychological Association Staff & Coopers and Lybrand Staff. 1995. LC 95-43415. (Practitioner's Toolbox Ser.). pap. 29.95 (*1-55798-348-8*) Am Psychol.

Contracts, Benefits, & Practice Management for the Veterinary Profession. James F. Wilson et al. 2000. xxvi, 422p. pap. text 89.95 (*0-9621007-3-0*) Priority Press.

Contraere Sexualempfindung see Perversions of the Sex Instinct

Contrast Agents in Liver Imaging, No. 25. Ed. by B. Hamm et al. 1995. LC 94-34131. (SERA Ser.: Vol. 25). 112p. (C). text 88.00 (*0-7923-3130-3*) Kluwer Academic.

Contrast Echocardiography. Jos R. Roelandt & Richard S. Meltzer. 1982. text 226.00 (*90-247-2531-3*) Kluwer Academic.

Contrast-Enhanced MRI of the Breast. S. H. Heywang-Koebrunner. 1991. (Illus.). 244p. 71.50 (*3-8055-5293-9*) S Karger.

Contrast-Enhanced MRI of the Breast. S. Heywang-Kobrunner & R. Beck. 2nd ed. 1996. (Medical Radiology Ser.). (Illus.). 200p. 125.00 (*3-540-58975-9*) Spr-Verlag.

Contrast Media. Ed. by Denis H. Carr. 1988. (Illus.). 227p. text (*0-443-03352-8*) Church.

Contrast Media in Magnetic Resonance Imaging. Val M. Runge. 1991. (Illus.). 176p. text 65.00 (*0-397-51270-8*) Lppncott W & W.

Contrast Media in Pediatric Radiology. Ed. by H. J. Kaufman. 1987. 118p. 52.25 (*3-8055-4440-5*) S Karger.

Contrast Media in Practice: Questions & Answers. Ed. by Peter Dawson & Wolfram Clauss. 2nd ed. 1999. LC 98-44436. (Illus.). 323p. pap. 80.00 (*3-540-64759-7*) Spr-Verlag.

Contrast Sensitivity, Vol. 5. Ed. by Robert Shapley & Dominic Man-Kit. 1993. (Illus.). 362p. 85.00 (*0-262-19339-6*, Bradford Bks) MIT Pr.

Contribution Al Estudio de los Aphyllophorales (Basidopmycotina) del Monteverde de las Islas Canarias: Tejera, Beltran. J. L. Rodrigues-Armas & E. B. Tejera. 1995. (Bibliotheca Mycologica: Vol. 160). (SPA., Illus.). ii, 456p. (*3-443-59062-4*) Gebruder Borntraeger DEU. *Dist:* Balogh.

Contribution of Long-Term Follow-up to the Prediction of Coronary Heart Disease. Ed. by Margaret Kornitzer & R. Goldberg. 1993. (Journal: Vol. 82, Nos. 2-3, 1993). (Illus.). 148p. pap. 45.25 (*3-8055-5790-6*) S Karger.

Contribution of Maternal Radionuclide Burdens to Prenatal Radiation Doses. 1997. lib. bdg. 250.95 (*0-8490-7714-1*) Gordon Pr.

Contribution of Nutrition to Human & Animal Health. Ed. by Elsie M. Widdowson & John C. Mathers. 1992. (Illus.). 423p. (C). text 100.00 (*0-521-42064-4*) Cambridge U Pr.

Contribution to Neuropsychological Assessment: A Clinical Manual. Arthur L. Benton et al. 2nd ed. 1994. LC 94-14767. (Illus.). 176p. pap. text 32.50 (*0-19-509179-5*) OUP.

Contributions of Harry Stack Sullivan. Ed. by Patrick Mullahy. 1995. LC 95-206848. (Master Work Ser.). 242p. pap. 45.00 (*1-56821-560-6*) Aronson.

Contributions of Physiology to the Understanding of Diabetes: Ten Essays in Memory of Albert E. Renold. G. R. Zahnd & C. B. Wollheim. 1997. LC 96-29827. (Illus.). 171p. 104.00 (*3-540-61385-4*) Spr-Verlag.

Contributions of Thought: The Collected Writings of William Garner Sutherland. William G. Sutherland. 1997. 400p. 35.00 (*0-915801-74-4*) Rudra Pr.

Contributions to a History of Developmental Psychology: International William T. Preyer Symposium. Ed. by Georg Eckardt et al. 1985. (New Babylon Studies in the Social Sciences: No. 44). x, 412p. pap. text (*3-11-009977-2*) Mouton.

Contributions to Autacoid Pharmacology: A Festschrift in Honour of Mauricio Rocha e Silva. Ed. by A. M. Rothschild. 1992. LC 92-10713. (Agents & Actions Supplements Ser.: Vol. 36). (Illus.). x, 286p. 90.00 (*0-8176-2617-4*) Birkhauser.

Contributions to Behavior - Genetic Analysis. Ed. by Gardner Lindzey & Delbert D. Thiessen. 1970. LC 73-92661. (Century Psychology Ser.). 34.50 (*0-89197-109-2*) Irvington.

Contributions to Developmental Neuropsychiatry. Paul Schilder. Ed. by Lauretta Bender. 1964. LC 64-23915. xi, 407p. 60.00 (*0-8236-1060-8*) Intl Univs Pr.

Contributions to Differential Psychology. Anne Anastasi. 1982. LC 82-9845. 258p. 49.95 (*0-275-90754-6*, C0754, Praeger Pubs) Greenwood.

Contributions to Group Theory. Ed. by Kenneth I. Appel et al. 1984. LC 84-18454. (Contemporary Mathematics Ser.: Vol. 33). 517p. pap. 61.00 (*0-8218-5035-0*, CONM/33) Am Math.

Contributions to Mathematical Psychology, Psychometrics, & Methodology. Ed. by Gerhard H. Fischer & Donald Laming. 1993. LC 93-31777. (Recent Research in Psychology Ser.). 421p. 106.00 (*0-387-94169-X*) Spr-Verlag.

Contributions to Medical Psychology Ed. by Stanley J. Rachman. 1984. 110.00 (*0-08-030855-4*, Pergamon Pr) Elsevier.

Contributions to Mental Pathology (1873). Isaac Ray. 1973. LC 73-9908. (History of Psychology Ser.). 576p. reprint ed. lib. bdg. 85.00 (*0-8201-1120-1*) Schol Facsimiles.

Contributions to Obstetrics & Gynecology. S. Shan Ratnam et al. 1991. (Illus.). Vol. 1. 258p. text (*0-443-04669-7*); Vol. 2. 232p. text (*0-443-04670-0*) Church.

Contributions to the Development of Human Deciduous Tooth Primordia. Ralf J. Radlanski. 1993. LC 92-48439.Tr. of Beitrage zur Gestaltentwicklung Menschlicher Zahnanlagen der Ersten Dentition. pap. text 58.00 (*0-86715-261-3*) Quint Pub Co.

Contributions to the Physical Anthropology of Central Asia & the Caucasus. M. G. Abdushelishvili et al. Ed. by Henry Field. Tr. by Barbara H. Heath. 1968. LC

79-158217. (Harvard University, Peabody Museum of Archaeology & Ethnology, Russian Translation Ser.: Vol. 3, No. 2). lib. bdg. 115.00 *(0-404-52645-4)* AMS Pr.

Contributions to the Physical Anthropology of the Soviet Union. Viktor V. Bunak et al. Tr. by William W. Howells. LC 60-1045. (Harvard University, Peabody Museum of Archaeology & Ethnology, Antiquities of the New World Ser.: Vol. 1, No. 2). reprint ed. lib. bdg. 47.50 *(0-404-52642-X)* AMS Pr.

Contributions to the Psychology of Addiction. Ed. by Gerard M. Schippers et al. 1991. 160p. *(90-265-1217-1)* Swets.

Contributions to the Racial Anthropology of the Near East. Carl C. Seltzer. 1940. (HU PMP Ser.). pap. 25.00 *(0-527-01237-8)* Periodicals Srv.

Contributions to the Theory of Natural Selection. Alfred R. Wallace. LC 72-1670. reprint ed. 55.00 *(0-404-08181-9)* AMS Pr.

Control: A History of Behavioral Psychology. John A. Mills. 1999. LC 98-19699. 256p. text 37.50 *(0-8147-5611-5)* NYU Pr.

Control & Automation in Anesthesia. Ed. by H. Schwilden & H. O. Stoeckel. 1995. LC 95-1211. *(0-387-58968-6)* Spr-Verlag.

Control & Automation in Anesthesia. H. O. Stoeckel & H. Schwilden. 1995. (Illus.). 272p. 107.00 *(3-540-58968-6)* Spr-Verlag.

Control & Diseases of Sodium Dependent Transport Proteins & Ion Channels, Vol. 1208. Y. Suketa et al. 2000. LC 2001-265637. (International Congress Ser.). (Illus.). 460p. 147.50 *(0-444-82986-5)* Elsevier.

Control & Management of Parturition. C. Sureau et al. 1987. (Colloque de L'INSERM Ser.). (ENG & FRE.). 288p. pap. 56.00 *(2-85598-311-8)* S M P F Inc.

Control & Removal of Radioactive Contamination in Laboratories. 1951. (Report Ser.: No. 8). pap. text 20.00 *(0-913392-00-6)* NCRP Pubns.

Control & Stimulation of Follicular Growth, Vol. 5. R. W. Shaw. 1993. (Advances in Reproductive Endocrinology Ser.). (Illus.). 175p. (C). lib. bdg. 74.95 *(1-85070-470-8,* Parthenon Pbng) CRC Pr.

Control Aspects of Biomedical Engineering. Ed. by M. Nalecz. 1987. (IFAC Ser.). (Illus.). 334p. 72.00 *(0-08-032553-X,* Pergamon Pr) Elsevier.

Control Aspects of Prosthetics & Orthotics: Proceedings of the IFAC Symposium, Columbus, Ohio, May, 1982. IFAC Symposium Staff & R. M. Campbell. 1983. (Illus.). 240p. *(0-08-029350-6)* Pergamon Repr GBR. *Dist:* Franklin.

Control de tu Estado de Animo: Manual de Tratamiento de Terapia Cognitiva Para Usuarios. Dennis Greenberger & Christine A. Padesky. Tr. by Jordi Cid. 1998. (Psicologia, Psiquiatria, Psicoterapia Ser.: Vol. 178). (SPA., Illus.). 254p. (C). pap. 21.00 *(1-57230-358-1)* Guilford Pubns.

Control High Blood Pressure Without Drugs: A Complete Hypertension Handbook. Robert Rowan & Constance Schrader. rev. ed. 2001. LC 2001-23068. (Illus.). 368p. pap. 14.00 *(0-684-87328-1,* Fireside) S&S Trade Pap.

Control Mechanisms in Cell - Type Conversion in Newt Lens Regeneration. T. Yamada. Ed. by A. Walsky. 1977. (Monographs in Developmental Biology: Vol. 13). (Illus.). 65.25 *(3-8055-2642-3)* S Karger.

Control Menopause Naturally see Controlling Hormones Naturally: My Journey for Solutions to PMS Menopause & Osteoporosis with...

Control of Air Pollution in the U. S. S. R. N. F. Izmerov. 1973. (Public Health Papers: No. 54). pap. text 9.00 *(92-4-130054-X,* 1110054) World Health.

Control of Arthropod Pests of Livestock: A Review of Technology. J. E. George. Ed. by S. E. Kunz & R. O. Drummond. 1988. LC 87-18187. (Pest Control Specialists & Agriculturalists Ser.). 272p. 146.00 *(0-8493-6860-X,* SF810, CRC Reprint) Franklin.

Control of Ascariasis: Report of a WHO Expert Committee, 1967. 1967. (Technical Report Ser.: No. 379). 47p. pap. text 5.00 *(92-4-120379-X,* 1100379) World Health.

Control of Breathing & Dyspnea: Proceedings of the International Symposium Held in Sendai, Japan, 27-28 October 1989. Ed. by T. Takishima & Neil S. Cherniack. 1991. (Advances in the Biosciences Ser.: No. 79). (Illus.). 402p. 190.25 *(0-08-040786-2,* Pergamon Pr) Elsevier.

Control of Breathing & Its Modeling Perspective. Ed. by Yoshiyuki Honda et al. 1992. LC 92-49245. (Illus.). 474p. (C). text 150.00 *(0-306-44300-7,* Kluwer Plenum) Kluwer Academic.

Control of Breathing During Development: Apnea of the Newborn & Sudden Infant Death Syndrome Colloquium, Nancy-Pont-a-Mousson, September 1994. Ed. by P. Vert et al. 1994. (Journal: Vol. 65, Nos. 3-4, 1994). (Illus.). 152p. pap. 103.50 *(3-8055-5975-5)* S Karger.

Control of Breathing During Sleep & Anesthesia. Ed. by W. A. Karczewski et al. 1988. LC 88-19689. (Illus.). 256p. 69.50 *(0-306-42993-4,* Plenum Trade) Perseus Pubng.

Control of Breathing in Health & Disease. Ed. by M. D. Altose & Y. Kawakami. 1999. LC 99-32707. (Lung Biology in Health & Disease Ser.). (Illus.). 800p. text 250.00 *(0-8247-9854-6)* Dekker.

Control of Breathing in Man. Ed. by B. J. Whipp. 1987. LC 87-19159. (Illus.). 134p. (C). text 44.95 *(0-8122-8095-4)* U of Pa Pr.

Control of Canine Genetic Diseases. George A. Padgett. 1998. LC 98-43170. 272p. pap. 27.95 *(0-87605-004-6,* Howell) Hungry Minds.

Control of Cardiac Rhythm: Basic Electrophysiology to Clinical Practice. E. M. Williams et al. 1997. LC 97-27241. (Illus.). 208p. text 105.00 *(0-397-58783-X)* Lppncott W & W.

Control of Cardiovascular Diseases in Developing Countries: Research, Development, & Institutional Strengthening. Institute of Medicine Staff. Ed. by Christopher P. Howson et al. 1998. LC 98-223563. 104p. pap. text 23.00 *(0-309-06137-7)* Natl Acad Pr.

Control of Cell Proliferation & Differentiation During Regeneration. Ed. by H. J. Anton. 1988. (Monographs in Developmental Biology: Vol. 21). (Illus.). x, 246p. 192.25 *(3-8055-4737-4)* S Karger.

Control of Chagas Disease: Report of a WHO Expert Committee. 1991. (Technical Reports: No. 811). (ENG, FRE & SPA.). vi, 95p. pap. text 14.00 *(92-4-120811-2,* 1100811) World Health.

Control of Cognitive Processes. Ed. by Stephen Monsell. 2000. LC 00-30732. (Attention & Performance Ser.: Vol. XVIII). (Illus.). xvi, 779p. (C). 90.00 *(0-262-13367-9,* Bradford Bks) MIT Pr.

Control of Communicable Diseases in Man. Ed. by Abram S. Benenson. 15th ed. 1990. 532p. 15.00 *(0-87553-170-9)* Am Pub Health.

Control of Communicable Diseases Manual. James E. Chin. 2000. (Illus.). pap. 30.00 *(0-87553-242-X)* Am Pub Health.

Control of Communicable Diseases Manual. Ed. by Abram S. Benenson. 16th rev. ed. 1995. 577p. 32.00 *(0-87553-228-4)*; 65.00 incl. cd-rom *(0-87553-225-X)*; pap. 22.00 *(0-87553-222-5)* Am Pub Health.

Control of Dual-Threat Agents: The Vaccines for Peace Programme. Ed. by Erhard Geissler & John P. Woodall. 1994. LC 94-235944. (SIPRI Chemical & Biological Warfare Studies: No. 15). 282p. pap. text 45.00 *(0-19-829172-8)* OUP.

Control of Enzyme Activity. Philip Cohen. 2nd ed. 1983. (Outline Studies in Biology). pap. 8.50 *(0-412-25560-X,* 6870) Chapman & Hall.

Control of Exposure of the Public to Ionizing Radiation in the Event of Accident or Attack. 1982. LC 82-81909. (Symposium Proceedings Ser.: No. 1). pap. text 30.00 *(0-913392-58-8)* NCRP Pubns.

Control of Foodborne Trematode Infections: Report of a WHO Study Group. 1995. LC 96-185716. (Technical Reports: No. 849). (CHI, FRE & SPA.). viii, 157p. pap. text 26.00 *(92-4-120849-X,* 1100849) World Health.

Control of Growth Factors & Prevention of Cancer. Ed. by Michael B. Sporn. 1992. (ESO Monographs). (Illus.). 74p. 72.95 *(0-387-55301-0)* Spr-Verlag.

Control of Head Movement. Ed. by Barry W. Peterson & Frances J. Richmond. 1988. (Illus.). 336p. text 55.00 *(0-19-504499-1)* OUP.

Control of Hereditary Diseases: Report of a WHO Scientific Group. 1996. (WHO Technical Reports: Vol. 865). 89p. pap. 14.40 *(92-4-120865-1,* 1100865) World Health.

Control of Hospital Infection. Ed. by E. J. L. Lowbury et al. 3rd ed. 1992. (Illus.). 400p. text *(0-412-28440-5)* E A GBR. *Dist:* OUP.

Control of Hospital Infection. Ed. by Graham A. J. Ayliffe et al. 4th ed. 2000. 416p. *(0-340-75911-9)* E A GBR. *Dist:* OUP.

Control of Human Movement. Mark L. Latash. 1993. LC 92-36991. (Illus.). 392p. text 54.00 *(0-87322-455-8,* BLAT0455) Human Kinetics.

Control of Immunogenesis by the Nervous System. Ed. by A. N. Gordienko. 1960. 192p. 3.5 hd 49.00 *(0-7065-0101-2)* Coronet Bks.

Control of Lymphatic Filariasis: A Manual for Health Personnel. WHO Staff. 1987. 89p. 15.00 *(92-4-154217-9)* World Health.

***Control of Pain & Anxiety in Dentistry.** J. P. Rood & P. Coulthard. 2001. (Illus.). 295p. pap. *(0-443-06200-5)* Church GBR. *Dist:* Saunders.

Control of Pain & Other Symptoms in Cancer Patients. Tor I. Tonnessen. Ed. by Jan V. Johannessen. Tr. by Allison Olsen from NOR. 1989. (Cancer Ser.). 66.95 *(0-89116-868-0)* Hemisp Pub.

Control of Particulate Matter Contamination in Healthcare Manufacturing, Vol. 1. Thomas A. Barber. 1998. LC 99-18307. (Illus.). xvii, 556p. 193.00 *(1-57491-072-8)* IHS Health Grp.

Control of Pesticides: A Survey of Existing Legislation. 1969. (International Digest of Health Legislation Offprints: Vol. 20, No. 4). 150p. pap. text 14.00 *(92-4-169204-9,* 1956902) World Health.

Control of Pre-Analytical Variation in Trace Element Determinations: Proposed Guideline (1994) Contrib. by Gillian Lockitch. 1994. 75.00 *(1-56238-262-4,* C38-P) NCCLS.

Control of Reproductive Functions in Domestic Animals. Wolfgang Jochle & Ross Lamond. 1981. (Current Topics in Veterinary Medicine & Animal Science Ser.: No. 7). (Illus.). text 153.00 *(90-247-2400-7)* Kluwer Academic.

Control of Schistosomiasis. 1985. (Technical Reports: No. 728). 113p. pap. text 10.00 *(92-4-120728-0,* 1100728) World Health.

Control of Schistosomiasis: Second Report of the WHO Expert Committee. 1993. (Technical Reports: No. 830). (CHI, ENG, FRE & SPA.). vii, 86p. pap. text 12.00 *(92-4-120830-9,* 1100830) World Health.

Control of the Cardiovascular & Respiratory Systems in Health & Disease: Proceedings of a Symposium Held at the University of California, Davis, April 8-9, 1994. Ed. by C. Tissa Kappagoda & Marc P. Kaufman. 1996. (Advances in Experimental Medicine & Biology Ser.: Vol. 381). (Illus.). 234p. 85.00 *(0-306-45121-2,* Kluwer Plenum) Kluwer Academic.

Control of the Hypothalamo-Pituitary-Adrenocortical Axis. Ed. by F. Clifford Rose. 1989. 468p. 65.00 *(0-8236-1070-5)* Intl Univs Pr.

Control of the Leishmaniases: Report of a WHO Expert Committee. 1990. (Technical Reports: No. 793). (ENG, FRE & SPA.). 158p. pap. text 18.00 *(92-4-120793-0,* 1100793) World Health.

Control of the Spread of Major Communicable Fish Diseases: Report of a Governmental Consultation on an International Convention for the Control of the Spread of Major Communicable Fish Diseases, Sc otland, 1974. 1974. (Fisheries Report Ser.: No. 149). 20p. pap. 8.00 Bernan Associates.

Control of the Spread of Major Communicable Fish Diseases: Report of the FAO-OIE Governmental Consultation on an International Convention for the Control of the Spread of Major Communicable Fish Diseases, OIE Headquarters, Paris, 1977. Incl. Control of the Spread of Major Communicable Fish Diseases: Report of a Governmental Consultation on an International Convention for the Control of the Spread of Major Communicable Fish Diseases, Sc otland, 1974. 20p. 1974. pap. 8.00 (Fisheries Report Ser.: No. 192). (ENG, FRE & SPA.). 48p. 1977. Set pap. 8.00 *(92-5-100275-4,* F839) Bernan Associates.

Control of the Thyroid Gland: Regulation of Its Normal Function & Growth. R. Ekholm et al. 1989. (Advances in Experimental Medicine & Biology Ser.: Vol. 261). (Illus.). 412p. 115.00 *(0-306-43380-X,* Plenum Trade) Perseus Pubng.

Control of Tuberculosis: A Survey of Existing Legislation. WHO Staff. 1963. (International Digest of Health Legislation Offprints: Vol. 14, No. 4). 46p. 3.00 *(92-4-169144-1)* World Health.

Control of Tumour Growth & Its Biological Bases. Ed. by W. Davis et al. 1984. (Developments in Oncology Ser.). text 256.50 *(0-89838-603-9)* Kluwer Academic.

Control of Uterine Contractility. Robert E. Garfield. 1993. 464p. 240.95 *(0-8493-6812-X,* QP262) CRC Pr.

Control of Virus Diseases. Ed. by N. J. Dimmock et al. 1990. (Society for General Microbiology Symposia Ser.: No. 45). 383p. (C). text 110.00 *(0-521-38562-8)* Cambridge U Pr.

Control of Virus Diseases. Ed. by Edouard Kurstak. 2nd exp. rev. ed. 1992. LC 92-49728. (Illus.). 456p. text 215.00 *(0-8247-8683-1)* Dekker.

Control of Vitamin A Deficiency & Xerophthalmia. 1982. (Technical Report Ser.: No. 672). 70p. pap. text 7.00 *(92-4-120672-1)* World Health.

Control over Intoxicant Use: Pharmacological, Psychological & Social Considerations: Special Issue of Journal of Drug Issues. Ed. by Norman E. Zinberg & Wayne Harding. 1982. LC 81-2333. 207p. 35.95 *(0-89885-064-9,* Kluwer Acad Hman Sci) Kluwer Academic.

Control Technology Assessment of Enzyme Formation Processes. 1995. lib. bdg. 251.95 *(0-8490-6682-4)* Gordon Pr.

Control Theory in the Practice of Reality Therapy: Case Studies. Ed. by Naomi Glasser. 1989. LC 89-45092. 336p. pap. 14.00 *(0-06-096400-6,* PL 6400) HarperCollins Pubs.

Control Therapy: An Integrated Approach to Psychotherapy, Health, & Healing. Deane H. Shapiro, Jr. & John Astin. 1998. LC 97-32851. (Personality Processes Ser.). 370p. 95.00 *(0-471-55278-X)* Wiley.

Control Your Child's Asthma: A Breakthrough Program for the Treatment & Management of Childhood Asthma. Harold J. Farber & Michael Boyette. 2001. LC 00-68253. (Illus.). xix, 256p. pap. 14.00 *(0-8050-6455-9,* Owl) H Holt & Co.

Control Your Depression. Peter M. Lewinsohn et al. 1978. 12.95 *(0-13-171702-2,* Spectrm) Hungry Minds.

***Control Your Diabetes for Life: Campaign Guide for Partners.** Frwd. by Charles M. Clark, Jr. 2001. (Illus.). 58p. (C). reprint ed. pap. text 20.00 *(0-7567-1034-0)* DIANE Pub.

Control Your Pain! 169 Painless Strategies for Taking Charge of Your Body. Robert H. Phillips. 1996. (Strategy Guidebooks Ser.). 52p. pap. 6.95 *(1-888614-00-5)* Balance Enter.

Controle el Dolor Antes de Que el Dolor le Controle a Usted. Margaret Caudill-Slosberg. Tr. by Isabel Custodio. 1997. (Psicologia, Psiquiatria, Psicoterapia Ser.: Vol. 175). (SPA., Illus.). 256p. pap. 19.95 *(1-57230-357-3)* Guilford Pubns.

Controlled Clinical Trial: An Analysis. Harris L. Coulter. 1991. LC 91-8016. 176p. (Orig.). pap. 12.00 *(0-916386-04-X)* Ctr Emp Med.

Controlled Clinical Trials in Neurological Disease. Ed. by Roger J. Porter & Bruce S. Schoenberg. 1990. 464p. text 234.00 *(0-7923-0613-9)* Kluwer Academic.

Controlled Drug Delivery Ed. by Stephen D. Bruck. 1983. LC 82-12921. 528p. 116.00 *(0-8493-5181-2,* RS201); 153.00 *(0-8493-5182-0,* RS201) Franklin (CRC Reprint).

Controlled Drug Delivery: Challenges & Strategies. Ed. by Kinam Park. 1997. LC 96-51016. (ACS Professional Reference Bk.). (Illus.). 720p. text 150.00 *(0-8412-3418-3)* Am Chemical.

Controlled Drug Delivery: Fundamentals & Applications. Joseph R. Robinson & H. L. Vincent Lee. 2nd ed. 1987. (Drugs & the Pharmaceutical Sciences Ser.: Vol. 29). (Illus.). 744p. text 299.00 *(0-8247-7588-0)* Dekker.

Controlled Eye Movements Versus Practice Exercises in Reading. Frederick L. Westover. LC 70-177648. (Columbia University, Teachers College. Contributions to Education Ser.: No. 917). reprint ed. 37.50 *(0-404-55917-4)* AMS Pr.

Controlled Killing of Exfoliated Colorectal Cancer Cells. Genc Basha. 1998. (Acta Biomedica Lovaniensia Ser.). (Illus.). 122p. pap. *(90-6186-887-4)* Leuven Univ BEL. *Dist:* Coronet Bks.

Controlled Release of Biological Active Agents. Richard E. Baker. 1987. LC 86-22422. 279p. 198.00 *(0-471-83724-5)* Wiley.

Controlled Release of Drugs: Polymers & Aggregate Systems. Ed. by Morton Rosoff. 1989. LC 88-19177. 315p. lib. bdg. 80.00 *(0-89573-321-8,* Wiley-VCH) Wiley.

Controlled-Release Technology: Pharmaceutical Applications. Ping I. Lee & William R. Good. 1987. LC 87-17447. (ACS Symposium Ser.: No. 348). (Illus.). 376p. 76.95 *(0-8412-1413-1)* Am Chemical.

Controlled Release Veterinary Drug Delivery: Biological & Pharmaceutical Considerations. Michael J. Rathbone & Robert Gurny. 2000. LC 00-42171. (Illus.). 392p. 179.00 *(0-444-82992-X)* Elsevier.

Controlling Cholesterol: Preventive Medicine Program. Kenneth H. Cooper. 1989. 416p. mass mkt. 6.99 *(0-553-27775-8)* Bantam.

Controlling Dangerous Pathogens: A Blueprint for U. S. - Russian Cooperation. Ed. by Christopher P. Howson. 1999. 78p. (C). pap. text 20.00 *(0-7881-7699-4)* DIANE Pub.

***Controlling Diabetes in Six Easy Steps.** Robinson. 2002. 256p. pap. *(0-312-28626-0)* St Martin.

Controlling Diabetes Naturally with Chinese Medicine: Diagnosis, Treatment & Prevention of Diabetes. Lynn M. Kuchinski. 1999. (Illus.). 173p. pap. 12.95 *(1-891845-06-3)* Blue Poppy Pr.

Controlling Diabetes the Easy Way. Joan R. Heilman & Stanley Mirsky. 3rd rev. ed. 1998. LC 97-23426. 256p. pap. 17.00 *(0-679-77803-9)* Random.

Controlling Drug Expenditure in Canada: The Ontario Experience. Paul K. Gorecki. 1992. (Illus.). 160p. (Orig.). pap. *(0-660-14437-9)* Can7 Govern Pub.

Controlling Health Professionals: The Future of Work & Organization in the National Health Service. Stephen Harrison & Christopher Pollitt. 1994. LC 93-2325. (State of Health Ser.). 160p. *(0-335-09644-1)*; pap. *(0-335-09643-3)* OpUniv Pr.

Controlling Herpes Naturally: A Holistic Approach to Prevention & Treatment. Michele Picozzi. 1998. LC 97-68478. (Illus.). 115p. pap. 12.95 *(0-9658600-0-0)* Southpaw Pr.

Controlling High Blood Pressure. Ed. by Frans H. Leenen et al. 1990. 176p. reprint ed. pap. 8.95 *(1-55958-087-9)* Prima Pub.

Controlling Hormones Naturally: My Journey for Solutions to PMS Menopause & Osteoporosis with... Melinda Bonk. Ed. by Lauri M. Aesoph & Laura K. Fraser. 1996. Orig. Title: Control Menopause Naturally. (Illus.). 240p. (Orig.). pap. 12.95 *(0-9650827-0-9)* MB Pubs.

Controlling Hospital Costs: The Role of Government Regulation. Paul L. Joskow. 1984. (Health & Public Policy Ser.). 224p. reprint ed. pap. 12.00 *(0-262-60012-9)* MIT Pr.

Controlling In-Plant Airborne Contaminants. John Constance. 1983. (Mechanical Engineering Ser.: Vol. 21). (Illus.). 368p. text 150.00 *(0-8247-1900-X)* Dekker.

Controlling Iodine Deficiency Disorders in Developing Countries, No. 5. David Phillips. 1989. (Practical Health Guide Ser.). (Illus.). 40p. (C). pap. *(0-85598-107-5)* Oxfam Pub GBR. *Dist:* Stylus Pub VA.

Controlling Medical Professionals: The Comparative Politics of Health Governance. Giorgio Freddi & James W. Bjorkman. 1988. (Modern Politics Ser.: Vol. 21). 250p. 69.95 *(0-8039-8198-8,* 6499) Sage.

Controlling Metallic Mercury Exposure in the Workplace: A Guide for Employers. Eileen P. Senn. 1997. (Illus.). 64p. (Orig.). pap. text 30.00 *(0-7881-3743-3)* DIANE Pub.

Controlling Movement: A Therapeutic Approach to Early Intervention. Margaret J. Baker et al. 1995. LC 91-115807. 352p. spiral bd. 110.00 *(0-8342-0192-5)* PRO-ED.

Controlling Occupational Exposure to Bloodborne Pathogens in Acute Care Facilities, Dentistry, Emergency Responders, & Long-Term Care Workers. 1995. 110p. (Orig.). (C). pap. text 40.00 *(0-7881-2324-6)* DIANE Pub.

***Controlling PMS: Natural Remedies for Better Living.** David Hazard. 2002. (Healthy Body, Healthy Soul Ser.). 112p. pap. 6.99 *(0-7369-0484-0)* Harvest Hse.

C
D

Controlling Public Health Nuisances: A Guide for Community Health Boards (in Minnesota) Warren Rodning. 1999. (Illus.). 84p. (C). reprint ed. pap. text 30.00 (*0-7881-8002-9*) DIANE Pub.

Controlling Reproduction. J. S. Hutchinson. 1993. (Illus.). 256p. (C). (gr. 13). pap. text 65.95 (*0-412-44310-4*) Chapman & Hall.

Controlling Reproduction: An American History. Ed. by Andrea Tone. 1996. LC 96-20020. (Worlds of Women Ser.: No. 2). 241p. 60.00 (*0-8420-2574-X*); pap. 19.95 (*0-8420-2575-8*) Scholarly Res Inc (SR Bks).

Controlling TB in Correctional Facilities. 1998. (Illus.). 82p. (C). reprint ed. pap. text 30.00 (*0-7881-4220-8*) DIANE Pub.

Controlling Technology: Genetic Engineering & the Law. Yvonne M. Cripps. 1980. LC 80-13754. 154p. 60.00 (*0-275-90465-2*, C0465, Praeger Pubs) Greenwood.

Controlling the Complement System for Novel Drug Development. Ed. by Helen Mazarakis. 1997. (Biomedical Library). pap. (*1-57936-025-4*) Drug & Market Dev.

Controlling the Smoking Epidemic: Report of the WHO Expert Committee on Smoking Control. 1979. (Technical Report Ser.: No. 636). 87p. pap. text 9.00 (*92-4-120636-5*, 1100636) World Health.

Controlling Unlawful Organizational Behavior: Social Structure & Corporate Misconduct. Diane Vaughan. LC 83-3489. (Studies in Crime & Justice). (Illus.). (C). 1993. xiv, 174p. 20.00 (*0-226-85171-0*); 1985. xiv, 188p. pap. text 10.95 (*0-226-85174-5*) U Ch Pr.

Controlling Waterborne Giardiasis. Ed. by Gary S. Logsdon. 1988. 118p. 5.00 (*0-87262-633-4*) Am Soc Civil Eng.

Controls: Brain & Nervous System. Sarah Angliss. 1999. (Human Machine Ser.). (Illus.). 32p. (J). lib. bdg. 16.95 (*1-929298-22-6*) Thameside Pr.

Controls from Within: Techniques for the Treatment of the Aggressive Child. Fritz Redl & David Wineman. 1965. LC 52-8161. pap. 17.95 (*0-02-926040-X*) Free Pr.

Controls of Eating. Carl Thompson. 1979. LC 79-17853. (Monographs in Pharmacology & Physiology: Vol. 4). 296p. text 48.95 (*0-88331-123-2*) R B Luce.

Controversial Issues in Health Care Policy. Jennie J. Kronenfeld. 1993. LC 92-35472. (Controversial Issues in Public Policy Ser.: Vol. 5). (Illus.). 200p. (C). pap. 31.95 (*0-8039-4878-6*, 4512) Sage.

Controversies about Inflammatory Diseases of the Pancreas. Ed. by C. Beglinger & U. Marbet. 1992. (Journal: Vol. 10, No. 6, 1992). (Illus.). iv, 56p. pap. 36.75 (*3-8055-5719-1*) S Karger.

Controversies & Innovations in Urological Surgery. Ed. by J. C. Gingell & P. H. Abrams. 1988. (Clinical Practice in Urology Ser.). (Illus.). 512p. 273.00 (*0-387-17491-5*) Spr-Verlag.

Controversies in Acute Pancreatitis: Symposium - Proceedings. Ed. by Louis F. Hollender. 1982. (Illus.). 344p. 79.95 (*0-387-11410-6*) Spr-Verlag.

Controversies in Alcoholism & Substance Abuse. Ed. by Barry Stimmel. 1986. LC 85-18233. (Advances in Alcohol & Substance Abuse Ser.: Vol. 5, No. 1 & 2). 236p. text 7.95 (*0-86656-539-6*) Haworth Pr.

Controversies in Cardiac Rehabilitation. Ed. by P. Mathes & M. J. Halhuber. 1982. (Illus.). 240p. 39.95 (*0-387-11234-0*) Spr-Verlag.

Controversies in Cardiovascular Anesthesia. Ed. by Philip Fyman & Alexander W. Gotta. 1988. (C). text 130.50 (*0-89838-985-2*) Kluwer Academic.

Controversies in Clinical Care. Ed. by V. Rosenoer & M. A. Rothschild. 1981. LC 80-21593. (Illus.). 312p. text 40.00 (*0-88331-125-9*) R B Luce.

Controversies in Clinical Thyroidology. Ed. by Joel I. Hamburger & J. M. Miller. 1981. (Illus.). 306p. 65.00 (*0-387-90569-3*) Spr-Verlag.

Controversies in Contemporary Psychoanalysis: Lectures from the Faculty of the New York Psychoanalytic Institute. Ed. by Manuel Furer et al. 1998. LC 96-30850. 204p. 32.50 (*0-8236-1065-9*, 01065) Intl Univs Pr.

Controversies in Diabetes & Pregnancy. Ed. by Lois Jovanovic. 1988. (Endocrinology & Metabolism Ser.: Vol. 2). (Illus.). 205p. 175.00 (*0-387-96622-6*) Spr-Verlag.

Controversies in Endourology. Arthur D. Smith. 1995. LC 94-25432. (Illus.). 496p. text 185.00 (*0-7216-5057-0*) Saunders.

Controversies in Managed Mental Health Care. Ed. by Arthur Lazarus. 1996. LC 95-47287. 480p. text 62.95 (*0-88048-115-3*, 8115) Am Psychiatric.

Controversies in Neuro-Oncology: 3rd International Symposium on Special Aspects of Radiotherapy, Berlin, April-May 1998. International Symposium on Special Aspects of Radiotherapy Staff. Ed. by T. Wiegel et al. 3rd ed. 1999. LC 99-28538. (Frontiers of Radiation Therapy & Oncology Ser.: Vol. 33). x, 380p. 212.25 (*3-8055-6834-7*) S Karger.

Controversies in Obesity, 5. Ed. by Barbara C. Hansen. 1983. LC 83-13678. (Endocrinology & Metabolism Ser.). 325p. 68.50 (*0-275-91393-7*, C1393, Praeger Pubs) Greenwood.

Controversies in Obstetric Anaesthesia, Vol. 2. Morgan. 2nd ed. 1993. 144p. pap. 32.50 (*0-340-55738-9*) Trafalgar.

Controversies in Oncology: Combination Therapy vs. Sequential Therapy for Breast Cancer. Gabriel N. Hortobagyi. 1997. (*1-57130-031-7*) Medicine Grp USA.

Controversies in Oral & Maxillofacial Surgery. Ed. by Philip Worthington & John R. Evans. 1993. (Illus.). 676p. text 157.00 (*0-7216-3099-5*) Saunders.

Controversies in Orthopaedic Sports Medicine. Kai-Ming Chang et al. 1997. LC 00-710405. (Illus.). 624p. 63.50 (*962-356-025-7*) Lppncott W & W.

Controversies in Pancreatic Islet Transplantation. Warnock. 2001. 450p. 200.00 (*0-471-97135-9*) Wiley.

Controversies in Psychoanalytic Method. Andre Haynal. 1990. (C). text 25.00 (*0-8147-3464-2*) NYU Pr.

Controversies in Psychology. Ed. by Andrew M. Colman. 1995. LC 95-18121. (Longman Essential Psychology Ser.). 128p. (C). pap. 35.20 (*0-582-27803-1*) Addison-Wesley.

Controversies in Reproductive Endocrinology & Fertility. Michael R. Soules. 1989. (Current Topics in Obstetrics & Gynecology Ser.). (Illus.). 352p. (C). (gr. 13). pap. 88.95 (*0-412-04631-8*) Chapman & Hall.

Controversies in Rheumatology. David A. Isenberg & Lori B. Tucker. 1997. 192p. (*1-85317-395-9*) Martin Dunitz GBR. *Dist:* Mosby Inc.

Controversies in Spine Surgery Vol. 2: Surgical Techniques & Medical Treatment. Ed. by Thomas A. Zdeblick & Edward C. Benzel. 2000. 330p. text 75.00 (*1-57626-143-3*) Quality Med Pub.

***Controversies in Surgery,** Vol. 4. Moshe Schein & Leslie Wise. 2001. LC 00-68783. (Illus.). 468p. 95.00 (*3-540-41103-8*) Spr-Verlag.

Controversies in the Management of Lymphomas. Ed. by John M. Bennett. 1983. (Cancer Treatment & Research Ser.). text 159.50 (*0-89838-586-5*) Kluwer Academic.

Controversies in the Practice of Medicine. Myrna Chandler Goldstein & Mark A. Goldstein. 2001. LC 00-61711. (Contemporary Controversies Ser.). (Illus.). 368p. 45.00 (*0-313-31131-5*, GR1131, Greenwood Pr) Greenwood.

Controversies in Therapeutics. Ed. by Peter Rubin. 1991. (Illus.). 78p. pap. text (*0-7279-0299-7*) BMJ Pub GBR. *Dist:* AIDC.

Controversies in Ultrasound. Ed. by John P. McGahan. 1986. (Clinics in Diagnostic Ultrasound Ser.: Vol. 20). (Illus.). 371p. pap. text (*0-443-08492-0*) Church.

***Controversies in Uro-Oncology: 5th International Symposium on Special Aspects of Radiotherapy, Berlin, May 2000.** Ed. by T. Wiegel et al. 2001. (Frontiers of Radiation Therapy & Oncology Ser.: Vol. 36). (Illus.). 161.75 (*3-8055-7217-4*) S Karger.

Controversies of Leukocyte-Poor Blood & Components. Leo J. McCarthy & Michael J. Baldwin. 1989. LC 89-17732. (Illus.). 104p. (C). text 7.00 (*0-915355-68-X*) Am Assn Blood.

Controversies of Surgical Sepsis. Stephen Karran. 1981. LC 80-81855. 352p. 110.00 (*0-275-91345-7*, C1345, Praeger Pubs) Greenwood.

Controversies on Countertransference. Ed. by Herbert S. Strean. 2001. LC 00-61063. 40.00 (*0-7657-0301-7*) Aronson.

Controversies on the Management of Urinary Stones. Ed. by L. Giuliani & P. Puppo. 1988. (Illus.). x, 254p. 163.50 (*3-8055-4760-9*) S Karger.

Controversy in Temporomandibular Disorders: A Clinicians' Guide to Critical Thinking. Allen J. Moses. 1997. (Illus.). vi, 172p. (Orig.). pap. text 70.00 (*0-9654416-0-1*) Futa Bk Pubs.

Convention on Human Rights & Biomedicine (Oviedo, 4.IV.1997) 1997. (Conventions & Agreements Ser.: No. 164). (ENG & FRE.). (*92-871-3223-2*) Council of Europe FRA. *Dist:* Manhattan Pub Co.

Conventional & Alternative Therapies for the Care of Chronic Conditions. Charlotte K. Eliopoulos. 1999. (Illus.). 347p. (C). (gr. 13). pap. text 32.95 (*0-8151-2793-6*, 31189) Mosby Inc.

Conventional Wisdom in Contemporary Refractive Care. Leonard Werner. 2001. 352p. pap. 49.99 (*0-7506-9912-4*) Buttrwrth-Heinemann.

Convergent Strabismus. L Evans. 1982. text 234.00 (*90-6193-806-6*) Kluwer Academic.

Converging Educational Perspectives (Perspectivas Educacionales Convergentes: An Anthology Based on the Pan American Conference on Graduate Nursing Education. Ed. by Nancy Jeffries. 1996. (ENG & SPA.). 315p. pap. 29.95 (*0-88737-689-4*, 19-6894, NLN Pr) Natl League Nurse.

Converging Themes in Psychotherapy: Trends in Psychodynamic Humanistic & Behavioral Practice. Ed. by Marvin R. Goldfried. 1982. 416p. 37.95 (*0-8261-3620-6*) Springer Pub.

Conversation Analysis of Therapeutics Discourse, 41. Jerry E. Gale. Ed. by Roy Freedle. 1991. LC 90-14423. (Advances in Discourse Processes Ser.: Vol. 41). 176p. 85.00 (*0-89391-705-2*, Ablex) Greenwood.

Conversation Analysis Profile for People with Aphasia (CAPPA) Anne Whitworth et al. 1997. 80p. spiral bd. 125.00 (*1-56593-910-7*, 1802) Singular Publishing.

Conversation Failure: Case Studies in Doctor-Patient Communication. Frederic W. Platt. 1992. LC 92-15049. 16.95 (*0-943685-16-8*) Essential Science.

Conversation, Language & Possibilities: A Postmodern Approach to Therapy. Harlene Anderson. 1997. LC 96-17802. 224p. 45.00 (*0-465-03805-0*) Basic.

Conversation Repair. Frederic W. Platt. 1995. LC 95-835. 24.95 (*0-316-71082-2*, Little Brwn Med Div) Lppncott W & W.

Conversational Management with Language-Impaired Children: Pragmatic Assessment & Intervention. Bonnie Brinton & Martin Fujiki. 1989. LC 89-17488. (Excellence in Practice Ser.). 240p. (C). 69.00 (*0-8342-0092-9*) PRO-ED.

Conversational Realities. John Shotter. 1993. (Inquiries in Social Construction Ser.). (Illus.). 208p. (C). 74.50 (*0-8039-8932-6*, 9561); pap. 25.95 (*0-8039-8933-4*, 9562) Sage.

Conversational Sign Language II: An Intermediate-Advanced Manual of American Sign Language. Willard J. Madsen. 1972. 236p. pap. text 13.95 (*0-913580-00-7*, Clerc Bks) Gallaudet Univ Pr.

Conversational Spanish for Health Professionals. Kelz. 3rd ed. 1998. (Medical Terminology Ser.). (SPA.). 384p. (C). pap. text 47.95 (*0-8273-6775-9*) Delmar.

Conversational Spanish for the Medical & Health Professions. Cynthia A. Teed et al. 1983. LC 82-15719. (ENG & SPA.). 255p. (C). pap. text 58.50 (*0-03-059287-9*) Harcourt Coll Pubs.

Conversations about Cancer. Michael Auerbach. 1998. 139p. pap. text 17.95 (*0-683-30432-1*) Lppncott W & W.

Conversations about Cancer: A Patient's Guide to Informed Decision Making. Michael Auerbach. 1996. LC 96-16212. 121p. pap. 24.95 (*0-683-30072-5*) Lppncott W & W.

Conversations about Illness: Family Preoccupations with Bulimia. Wayne A. Beach. 1996. LC 96-8103. (Everyday Communication Ser.). 160p. text 36.00 (*0-8058-1756-5*); pap. text 17.50 (*0-8058-1757-3*) L Erlbaum Assocs.

Conversations in Psychotherapy: Ways of Working with Individuals, Couples, & Families. R. V. Fitzgerald. 1992. LC 91-33335. 384p. 50.00 (*0-87668-561-0*) Aronson.

Conversations in the Cognitive Neurosciences. Ed. by Michael S. Gazzaniga. 1996. LC 96-28258. (Illus.). 201p. (C). pap. text 17.00 (*0-262-57117-X*, Bradford Bks) MIT Pr.

Conversations of Silence: A Memoir. S. Harold Nickerson. 1995. LC 94-45897. 226p. pap. 18.95 (*0-86534-231-8*) Sunstone Pr.

Conversations on Counselling: Between a Doctor & a Priest. Marcus Lefebure & Hans Schauder. 3rd ed. 1990. 288p. pap. (*0-567-29164-2*) T & T Clark GBR. *Dist:* Bks Intl VA.

Conversations on Therapy. David R. Grove & Jay Haley. 1993. LC 92-48451. 192p. (C). 22.95 (*0-393-70155-7*) Norton.

Conversations with an Alzheimer's Patient: An Interactional Sociolinguistic Study. Heidi E. Hamilton. 1994. 196p. (C). text 59.95 (*0-521-42101-2*) Cambridge U Pr.

Conversations with Anorexics: A Compassionate & Hopeful Journey Through the Therapeutic Process. Hilde Bruch. 1994. LC 94-70808. 238p. pap. 30.00 (*1-56821-261-5*) Aronson.

Conversations with Jean Piaget. Jean-Claude Bringuier. Tr. by Basia M. Gulati. 1989. (Illus.). xiv, 160p. pap. text 17.00 (*0-226-07505-2*, Midway Reprint) U Ch Pr.

Conversations with My Healers: My Journey to Wellness from Breast Cancer. Cynthia Ploski. 1996. 422p. pap. 18.95 (*1-57178-027-0*) Coun Oak Bks.

Conversations with Neil's Brain: Searching for the Narrator of Consciousness. William H. Calvin & George A. Ojemann. 1994. LC 93-23661. 343p. 23.08 (*0-201-63217-9*) Addison-Wesley.

Conversing with Uncertainty: Practicing Psychotherapy in a Hospital Setting. Rita W. McCleary. 1992. LC 92-17730. (Relational Perspectives Book Ser.: Vol. 1). 160p. text 29.95 (*0-88163-148-5*) Analytic Pr.

Conversion Coefficients for Use in Radiological Protection Against External Radiation. International Commission on Radiation Units and Measurements Staff. 1998. LC 98-12088. (ICRU Report Ser.: No. 57). 65.00 (*0-913394-56-4*) Intl Comm Rad Meas.

Converting & Merging Hospitals: Trustees Talk to Each Other. Harry Nelson & Ann F. Monroe. 1999. 28p. pap. (*1-887748-24-5*) Milbank Memorial.

Cookery Book: From the Lukas Clinic for Patients with Cancer or Pre-Cancerous Conditions. Society for Cancer Research Staff. Tr. by Anna R. Meuss from GER. 1988. 72p. (Orig.). pap. (*0-85440-716-2*) R Steiner Pr GBR. *Dist:* Anthroposophic.

***Cooking for Life: A Guide to Nutrition & Food Safety for the HIV-Positive Community.** Robert H. Lehmann. 2001. 244p. pap. 11.00 (*0-7881-9820-3*) DIANE Pub.

Cooking Healthy & Fast. Rachel Rudel. l.t. ed. 1994. 14.95 (*0-9642510-0-0*) Apple a Day.

Cooking Light, 1994. Oxmoor House Staff. 1993. LC 87-61020. 272p. 24.95 (*0-8487-1144-0*) Oxmoor Hse.

Cooking with Heart in Hand. Suzanne Ward et al. 1987. 256p. 13.95 (*0-9619445-0-1*) Heart in Hand Inc.

Cook's Healthy Handbook: Good Nutrition & Safety in Your Kitchen. Karen Eich Drummond et al. 1992. LC 92-21833. 320p. 32.95 (*0-471-55608-4*) Wiley.

Cooley's Anemia: 7th Symposium. Ed. by Alan R. Cohen. 1998. LC 98-17791. (Annals of the New York Academy of Sciences Ser.: No. 850). 527p. pap. 140.00 (*1-57331-122-7*) NY Acad Sci.

Cooley's Anemia Vol. 850: 7th Symposium, Vol. 850. Ed. by Alan R. Cohen. 1998. LC 98-17791. (Annals of the New York Academy of Sciences Ser.: No. 853). 527p. 140.00 (*1-57331-121-9*) NY Acad Sci.

Cooper-Clayton Method to Stop Smoking: New Hope for Heavy Smokers. Thomas M. Cooper & Richard R. Clayton. 1988. 160p. (Orig.). pap. 10.00 (*0-9621398-0-7*) SBC SBC.

Cooper Communications & Its Skills for Nursing & Health Care. Carol D. Cooper. 2000. (C). pap. text (*0-201-36059-4*) Addison-Wesley.

Cooperation Between the Sexes: Writings on Women & Men, Love & Marriage, & Sexuality. Alfred Adler. Ed. by Heinz Ludwig Ansbacher & Rowena R. Ansbacher. abr. ed. 1982. LC 82-7998. 192p. reprint ed. pap. 7.95 (*0-393-30019-6*) Norton.

Cooperation Between the Sexes: Writings on Women, Love, Marriage & Its Disorders. Alfred Adler. 1980. LC 76-23804. 480p. reprint ed. 25.00 (*0-87668-443-6*) Aronson.

Cooperation in Groups: Procedural Justice, Social Identity & Behavioral Engagement. Tom R. Tyler & Steven Blader. 2000. LC 00-32354. (Essays in Social Psychology Ser.). 208p. (*1-84169-006-6*) Psychol Pr GBR. *Dist:* Taylor & Francis.

Cooperative Healing: The Curative Properties of Human Radiations. L. E. Eeman. 1991. (Alternative Energy & Medicine Ser.). lib. bdg. 79.95 (*0-8490-4259-3*) Gordon Pr.

Cooperative Method of Natural Birth Control. Margaret Nofziger. 4th ed. 1992. LC 91-33429. (Illus.). 112p. pap. 8.95 (*0-913990-84-1*) Book Pub Co.

Cooperativity Theory in Biochemistry. T. L. Hill. 1985. (Molecular Biology, Biochemistry & Biophysics Ser.). (Illus.). 459p. 305.00 (*0-387-96103-8*) Spr-Verlag.

Cooper's Toxic Exposures Desk Reference. Andre R. Cooper, Sr. 1996. LC 96-35221. 2016p. pap. 199.00 (*1-56670-220-8*) Lewis Pubs.

Coordinated Care Options for Seniors: Congressional Hearing. Ed. by Bill Thomas. 2001. 102p. (C). reprint ed. pap. text 25.00 (*0-7567-0553-3*) DIANE Pub.

Coordinated Service Delivery Systems for the Elderly: New Approaches for Care & Referral in New York State. Ed. by Ruth Bennett et al. 1984. LC 83-13041. (Advanced Models & Practice in Aged Care Ser.: No. 2). 198p. text 39.95 (*0-86656-157-9*) Haworth Pr.

Coordinating Prenatal Care. Ian T. Hill & Janine M. Breyel. Ed. by Karen Glass. 1989. (Strategies for Improving State Perinatal Programs Ser.). 95p. (Orig.). pap. text 15.00 (*1-55877-058-5*) Natl Governor.

Coordination & Regulation of Movements. N. Bernstein. 1967. LC 66-25078. (*0-08-011940-9*) Pergamon Repr GBR. *Dist:* Franklin.

Coordinator of Community Mental Health Services. Jack Rudman. 1994. (Career Examination Ser.: C-1228). pap. 39.95 (*0-8373-1228-0*) Nat Learn.

Coordinator of Nursing Education. Jack Rudman. 1994. (Career Examination Ser.: C-1843). pap. 39.95 (*0-8373-1843-2*) Nat Learn.

Cope Program for Depression, Set. John H. Greist et al. 1999. (Illus.). 278p. pap. (*0-9702974-0-8*) Healthcare Sys.

COPE Starter Kit: COPE Program for Depression. John H. Greist et al. 1999. (Illus.). 33p. pap. (*0-9702974-1-6*) Healthcare Sys.

Cope's Early Diagnosis of the Acute Abdomen. William Silen. 20th ed. 2000. LC 99-40627. (Illus.). 336p. pap. text 29.95 (*0-19-513679-9*) OUP.

Coping: Attention Deficit Disorder: A Guide for Parents & Teachers. Mary E. Beugin. 1990. 173p. pap. 15.95 (*1-55059-013-8*) Temeron Bks.

Coping: The Psychology of What Works. C. R. Snyder. 1999. LC 98-30270. (Illus.). 368p. 29.95 (*0-19-511934-7*) OUP.

Coping & Health. Ed. by Seymour Levine & Holger Ursin. 1980. LC 79-28833. (NATO Conference Series III, Human Factors: Vol. 12). 372p. 85.00 (*0-306-40422-2*, Plenum Trade) Perseus Pubng.

Coping & Self-Concept in Adolescence. Ed. by H. A. Bosma & A. E. Jackson. 1990. (Illus.). 270p. 88.95 (*0-387-51897-5*, 3205) Spr-Verlag.

Coping, Behavior, & Adaption in Prison Inmates. E. Zamble & Frank Porporino. 1988. (Research in Criminology Ser.). (Illus.). 204p. 89.95 (*0-387-96613-7*) Spr-Verlag.

Coping in Medical School. Bernard Virshup. 1985. pap. 10.95 (*0-393-30253-9*) Norton.

Coping Skills Interventions for Children & Adolescents. Susan G. Forman. 1992. LC 92-25004. (Social & Behavioral Science - Education Ser.). 216p. 39.00 (*1-55542-493-7*) Jossey-Bass.

Coping Strategies for Burn Survivors & Their Families. Norman R. Bernstein et al. 1988. LC 87-7339. (Illus.). 159p. 55.00 (*0-275-92407-6*, C2407, Praeger Pubs) Greenwood.

Coping Successfully: A How-To Manual for Operational Improvement. Harry N. Dubin et al. 1981. 238p. (Orig.). text 27.50 (*0-8290-0262-6*); pap. text 15.95 (*0-8290-0270-7*) Irvington.

Coping Successfully: Cognitive Strategies for Older Caregivers. Susan S. Tebb. rev. ed. 1995. LC 95-3300. (Garland Studies on the Elderly in America). 153p. text 59.00 (*0-8153-1998-3*) Garland.

Coping with a Brain Tumor, Pt. I: From Diagnosis to Treatment. 1994. (*0-944093-30-2*) Am Brain Tumor.

Coping with a Brain Tumor, Pt. II: During & after Treatment. 1994. (*0-944093-31-0*) Am Brain Tumor.

Coping with a Hernia. David Delvin. 1998. LC 99-494989. (Fias Occasional Paper Ser.). 112p. pap. (*0-85969-783-5*) Sheldon Pr GBR. *Dist:* Intl Pubs Mktg.

Coping with a Myositis Disease. 2000. 154p. 13.95 (*0-9701671-0-5*, 2000-1) Kilpatrick Pubng.

Coping with AIDS: Psychological & Social Considerations in Helping People with HTLV-III Infection. 1991. lib. bdg. 78.75 (*0-8490-5141-X*) Gordon Pr.

Coping with Alzheimer's: A Caregiver's Emotional Survival Guide. Rose Oliver & Frances Bock. 1989. pap. 10.00 (*0-87980-424-6*) Wilshire.

Coping with Alzheimer's Disease & Other Dementing Illnesses. Mary N. Kindig & Molly Carnes. 1993. LC 93-2669. (Coping with Aging Ser.). (Illus.). 338p. (C). pap. text 18.95 (*1-56593-097-5*, 0401) Thomson Learn.

Coping with Anger. Gregory L. Little & Kenneth D. Robinson. 1997. 49p. pap. 10.00 (*0-940829-18-5*) Eagle Wing Bks.

Coping with Aphasia. Jon G. Lyon. 1997. LC 97-29700. (Coping with Aging Ser.). (Illus.). 422p. (Orig.). pap. 40.00 net. (*1-879105-75-6*, 0338) Thomson Learn.

Coping with Bowel & Bladder Problems. Barbara King & Judy Harke. 1994. LC 94-17284. (Coping with Aging Ser.). (Illus.). 254p. (C). pap. text 18.95 (*1-56593-068-1*, 0373) Thomson Learn.

Coping with Brain Injury: A Guide for Family & Friends. Ed. by Gordon M. Giles. 1996. LC 97-173815. (Illus.). 42p. (Orig.). pap. text 6.00 (*1-56900-036-0*, 1143) Am Occup Therapy.

Coping with Cancer: How to Fight & Treat Cancer with Vitamins, Minerals & Diet. John L. Sessions & Morton Walker. 1985. (Dr. Morton Walker Better Health Booklets Ser.). 56p. (Orig.). pap. 4.95 (*0-8159-5226-0*) Devin.

Coping with Cancer & Beyond: Cancer Treatment & Mental Health. Ed. by J. Ten Labije & H. Balner. 1991. (Publications of the Helen Dowling Institute for Biopsychosocial Medicine: Vol. 5). 194p. pap. (*90-265-1223-6*) Swets.

Coping with Cancer Stress. Ed. by Basil A. Stoll. 1986. lib. bdg. 105.00 (*0-89838-769-8*) Kluwer Academic.

Coping with Celiac, the Great Masquerader. Aileen M. Bennett. 1998. LC 98-93282. 160p. pap. 12.95 (*0-9665353-0-8*) A&G Pubg.

Coping with Cerebral Palsy: Answers to Questions Parents Often Ask. Jay Schleichkorn. 2nd ed. 1993. LC 92-27296. (For Interested Parents Ser.). 252p. (C). pap. text 26.00 (*0-89079-576-2*, 6576) PRO-ED.

Coping with Children in Stress. Ed. by Ved P. Varma. 1996. 176p. pap. (*1-85742-253-8*) Arena GBR. *Dist:* Ashgate Pub Co.

Coping with Chronic Fatigue Syndrome: Nine Things You Can Do. Fred Friedberg. 1995. LC 95-69480. 176p. pap. 13.95 (*1-57224-019-9*) New Harbinger.

***Coping with Chronic Heartburn.** Shimberg Elaine. 2002. 256p. mass mkt. (*0-312-98206-2*) St Martin.

Coping with Chronic Illness: Overcoming Powerlessness. Judith F. Miller. 3rd ed. 1999. LC 99-14320. (Illus.). xiv, 573p. (C). pap. text 39.95 (*0-8036-0298-7*) Davis Co.

Coping with Chronic Pain: A Guide to Patient Self-Management. Richard W. Hanson & Kenneth E. Gerber. LC 89-17204. 232p. 1993. pap. 24.00 (*0-89862-549-1*, 2549); 1989. 42.00 (*0-89862-396-0*) Guilford Pubns.

Coping with Chronic Stress. Ed. by Benjamin H. Gottlieb. 1997. LC 96-51879. (Series on Stress & Coping). 390p. (C). 52.50 (*0-306-45470-X*, Plenum Trade) Perseus Pubng.

Coping with Communication Challenges in Alzheimers Disease. Marie T. Rau. 1993. LC 92-41712. (Coping with Aging Ser.). (Illus.). 228p. (C). pap. 19.95 (*1-879105-76-4*, 0339) Thomson Learn.

Coping with Crisis: A Quick Reference. Scott Poland & Jami S. McCormick. 2000. LC 2001-272630. (Illus.). 132p. pap., tchr. ed. 15.00 (*1-57035-269-0*, 108PERT) Sopris.

Coping with Crisis: Understanding & Helping People in Need. Stephen Murgatroyd & Ray Woole. 1982. 180p. pap. (*0-335-09819-3*) OpUniv Pr.

Coping with Death & Dying: An Interdisciplinary Approach. Ed. by John T. Chirban. 1986. 108p. pap. text 18.00 (*0-8191-4985-3*) U Pr of Amer.

Coping with Diabetes. Pat Kelly. 1998. LC 97-49084. (Coping Ser.). 192p. (YA). (gr. 5 up). 17.95 (*0-8239-2549-8*, CODIAB) Rosen Group.

Coping with Difficult People in the Health Care Setting. William O. Umiker. 1994. LC 93-1079. (Practical Laboratory Management Ser.). (Illus.). 268p. pap. text 35.00 (*0-89189-361-X*) Am Soc Clinical.

Coping with Disruptive Behavior in Group Care. Eva M. Russo & Ann W. Shyne. 1980. LC 79-23739. 74p. (Orig.). (C). pap. 13.50 (*0-87868-137-X*, 1370) Child Welfare.

Coping with Drug Abuse: A Lifeline for Parents. Joe Baker. 1982. LC 82-12723. (Illus.). 60p. pap. 7.95 (*0-943690-00-5*) DARE.

Coping with Dual Disorders: Counseling Clients with Chemical Dependency & Mental Illness. Dennis C. Daley & Frances Campbell. 1989. 23p. pap. 4.25 (*0-89486-586-2*, 5218B) Hazelden.

Coping with Endometriosis. Lyle J. Breitkopf & Marion G. Bakoulis. 1988. LC 87-43148. (Illus.). 256p. stu. ed. 9.50 (*0-929655-63-X*) P-H.

Coping with Endometriosis. Jo Mears. 2000. pap. (*0-85969-748-7*) Sheldon Pr GBR. *Dist:* Intl Pubs Mktg.

Coping with Ethical Dilemmas in Psychotherapy. Martin Lakin. 1991. (Psychology Practitioner Guidebooks Ser.). 192p. text (*0-08-036451-9*); pap. text (*0-08-036450-0*) PPI GBR. *Dist:* Elsevier.

Coping with Food Intolerances: Surviving the Nineties. Dick Thom. 1995. LC 95-81909. 240p. pap. 14.95 (*0-9631918-0-2*) JELD Pub.

Coping with Head Injury: Information & Answers to Commonly Asked Questions. Christopher D. Strum et al. 1998. LC 98-28737. (Illus.). 314p. pap. 21.95 (*1-57626-096-8*, QMP) Quality Med Pub.

Coping with Headaches. Shirley Trickett. 2000. pap. (*0-85969-812-2*) Sheldon Pr GBR. *Dist:* Intl Pubs Mktg.

Coping with Hearing Loss: A Guide for Adults & Their Families. Susan V. Rezen & Carl Hausman. rev. ed. 1993. LC 92-36728. 224p. 17.95 (*0-942637-83-6*) Barricade Bks.

Coping with Hearing Loss & Hearing Aids. Debra A. Shimon. 1991. LC 91-26186. (Coping with Aging Ser.). (Illus.). 224p. (C). pap. 15.25 net. (*1-879105-45-4*, 0229) Thomson Learn.

Coping with Heart Surgery & Bypassing Depression: A Family's Guide to the Medical, Emotional, & Practical Issues. Carol Cohan et al. 1999. LC 97-21699. (Illus.). 280p. pap. 27.95 (*1-887841-07-5*, 60609, Psychosocial) Intl Univs Pr.

Coping with Hereditary Diseases. Marian B. Jacobs. 1999. LC 98-48064. (Coping Ser.). 192p. (YA). (gr. 7-12). lib. bdg. 18.95 (*0-8239-2823-3*, COHEDI) Rosen Group.

Coping with HIV Infection: Psychological & Existential Responses in Gay Men. Michael W. Ross & Lena Nilsson. 1999. LC 99-38194. (AIDS Prevention & Mental Health Ser.). 194p. 75.00 (*0-306-46220-6*, Kluwer Plenum) Kluwer Academic.

Coping with Illness. Helen Garvy. 1995. LC 95-67134. (Illus.). 240p. pap. 12.00 (*0-918828-18-X*) Shire Pr.

Coping with Impaired Mobility. Jane Mahoney & Reenie Euhardy. 1994. LC 93-40443. (Coping with Aging Ser.). 272p. pap. 18.95 (*1-879105-65-9*, 0329) Thomson Learn.

Coping with Life Crises: An Integrated Approach. R. H. Moos. 1986. LC 85-28149. (Stress & Coping Ser.). (Illus.). 444p. (C). 75.00 (*0-306-42133-X*, Plenum Trade) Perseus Pubng.

Coping with Life Crises: An Integrated Approach. Ed. by Rudolf H. Moos. 1986. LC 85-28149. (Stress & Coping Ser.). (Illus.). 444p. (C). pap. 45.00 (*0-306-42144-5*, Plenum Trade) Perseus Pubng.

Coping with Loss: A Guide for Caregivers. Shirley A. Locke. 1994. LC 94-7441. 238p. pap. 37.95 (*0-398-06244-7*); (C). text 54.95 (*0-398-05912-8*) C C Thomas.

Coping with Loss: Psychotherapeutic Use of Leave-Taking Rituals. Ed. by Onno Van der Hart. 1988. 300p. (C). 14.00 (*0-8290-2304-6*); text 32.95 (*0-8290-1596-5*) Irvington.

Coping with Loss of Independence. Michael J. Siebers et al. 1993. LC 92-42197. (Coping with Aging Ser.). (Illus.). 244p. (C). pap. 18.95 (*1-879105-60-8*, 0325) Thomson Learn.

Coping with Low Vision. Marshall E. Flax et al. 1993. LC 92-31826. (Coping with Aging Ser.). (Illus.). 214p. (Orig.). (C). pap. text 18.95 (*1-879105-71-3*, 0334) Thomson Learn.

Coping with Lyme Disease: A Practical Guide to Dealing with Diagnosis & Treatment. Denise Lang & Joseph Territo. 2nd ed. 1999. 283p. pap. text 15.00 (*0-7881-6073-7*) DIANE Pub.

Coping with Marital Transitions: A Family Systems Perspective. E. Mavis Hetherington et al. 1992. (Illus.). 250p. pap. text 19.50 (*0-226-33168-7*) U Ch Pr.

Coping with Mental Illness. Barbara Moe. 2000. LC 00-9904. (Coping Ser.). 138p. (J). (gr. 7-10). lib. bdg. 18.95 (*0-8239-3205-2*) Rosen Group.

Coping with Miscarriage: A Simple, Reassuring Guide to Emotional & Physical Healing. Mimi Luebbermann. 1996. 240p. per. 14.00 (*0-7615-0436-2*); 1994. LC 94-27377. 208p. 17.95 (*1-55958-503-X*) Prima Pub.

Coping with 'Morning' Sickness. Ee-Kheng Birks. 1993. 95p. pap. (*0-908569-76-9*) Univ Otago Pr NZL. *Dist:* Intl Spec Bk.

***Coping with Multiple Sclerosis.** Betty Burnett & Rob Gevertz. 2001. LC 00-12606. (Coping Ser.). (Illus.). 90p. (J). lib. bdg. 25.25 (*0-8239-3204-4*) Rosen Group.

Coping with Multisystem Complications. Sally A. Brozenec. 1998. LC 97-30022. 448p. pap. text 39.95 (*1-55664-484-1*) Mosby Inc.

Coping with Natural Disasters: The Role of Local Health Personnel & the Community. 1989. (ENG, FRE, RUS & SPA.). x, 97p. pap. text 18.00 (*92-4-154238-1*, 1150310) World Health.

Coping with Negative Life Events: Clinical & Social Psychological Perspectives. C. R. Snyder & C. E. Ford. 1987. LC 87-2483. (Stress & Coping Ser.). (Illus.). 436p. (C). 65.00 (*0-306-42432-0*, Plenum Trade) Perseus Pubng.

Coping with Prednisone: (*and Other Cortison-Related Medicines) It May Work Miracles, but How Do You Handle the Side Effects? Eugenia Zukerman. 1998. LC 97-6062. (Illus.). 208p. pap. 12.95 (*0-312-19570-2*, Tor Books) T Doherty Assocs.

Coping with Prednisone(*and Other Cortisone Related Medicines) It May Work Miracles, but How Do You Handle the Side Effects? Eugenia Zukerman & Julie Ingelfinger. 1997. LC 97-6062. 176p. 21.95 (*0-312-15502-6*) St Martin.

Coping with Psoriasis: A Patient's Guide to Treatment. David L. Cram. 2000. LC 00-8220. x, 132p. pap. 14.95 (*1-886039-47-X*) Addicus Bks.

Coping with Radiation Therapy: A Ray of Hope. Daniel Cukier & Virginia E. McCullough. 2nd ed. 1996. 240p. pap. 16.00 (*1-56565-436-6*, 04366W) Lowell Hse.

Coping with Rheumatism & Arthritis. Robert Youngson. 2000. pap. (*0-85969-785-1*) Sheldon Pr GBR. *Dist:* Intl Pubs Mktg.

Coping with Rheumatoid Arthritis: A Guide to Living with Arthritis for You & Your Family. Robert H. Phillips. 1988. LC 88-3450. 272p. pap. 9.95 (*0-89529-371-4*, Avery) Penguin Putnam.

Coping with Severe Mental Illness: Families Speak Out. Martha B. Mermier. 1993. LC 93-20490. (Studies in Health & Human Services: Vol. 23). 212p. text 89.95 (*0-7734-9285-2*) E Mellen.

Coping with Stomach Ulcers. Sheldon Press Staff. pap. (*0-85969-741-X*) Sheldon Pr GBR. *Dist:* Intl Pubs Mktg.

Coping with Stress: Insight from Eight Bible Leaders. Marilyn Kunz & Catherine Schell. rev. ed. 1997. (Neighborhood Bible Studies). 63p. pap. 5.99 (*1-880266-24-5*) Neighborhood Bible.

Coping with Stress at Work. Ed. by Judi Marshall & Cary L. Cooper. 1981. 236p. text (*0-566-02338-5*) Gower GBR. *Dist:* Ashgate Pub Co.

Coping with Stress in College. Mark Rowh. 1989. LC 89-51125. 306p. (C). pap. 9.95 (*0-87447-334-9*) College Bd.

Coping with Stress in the Health Professions: A Practical Guide. Philip Burnard. (Therapy in Practice Ser.: No. 21). 22.50 (*0-412-38910-X*) Chapman & Hall.

Coping with Surgery: A Guide to Self Help. Gary Boyd. 1990. 56p. (Orig.). pap. 6.95 (*0-910467-09-9*) Heritage Assocs.

Coping with Sustained Low Fertility in France & the Netherlands. N. Van Nimwegen et al. 1993. xii, 348p. pap. (*90-265-1343-7*) Swets.

Coping with the Biomedical Literature: A Primer for the Scientist & the Clinician. Ed. by Kenneth S. Warren. 1981. LC 81-5149. 233p. 72.95 (*0-275-91355-4*, C1355, Praeger Pubs) Greenwood.

Coping with the Final Tragedy: Dying & Grieving in Cross Cultural Perspective. Ed. by David Reese Counts & Dorothy Ayers Counts. 1991. (Perspectives on Death & Dying Ser.). 336p. text 48.95 (*0-89503-082-9*); 366p. pap. text 37.00 (*0-89503-081-0*) Baywood Pub.

Coping with Threatened Identities. Glynis M. Breakwell. 1987. 280p. 33.00 (*0-416-37120-5*, 9852) Routledge.

Coping with Thyroid Problems. Joan Gomez. 2000. pap. (*0-85969-687-1*) Sheldon Pr GBR. *Dist:* Intl Pubs Mktg.

Coping with Trauma: Theory, Prevention & Treatment. Rolf J. Kleber et al. 1998. viii, 320p. (*90-265-1227-9*) Swets.

Coping with Uncertainty: Behavioral & Developmental Perspectives. Ed. by David S. Palermo. 1989. (Penn State Series on Child & Adolescent Development). 224p. 45.00 (*0-8058-0157-X*) L Erlbaum Assocs.

Coping with Unhappy Children. Ed. by Ved P. Varma. 1993. LC 92-38453. (Education Ser.). 192p. pap. 31.95 (*0-304-32436-1*); text 80.00 (*0-304-32414-0*) Continuum.

Coping with Vision Loss: Maximizing What You Can See & Do. Bill Chapman. l.t. ed. 2001. LC 00-54688. (Illus.). 304p. 26.95 (*0-89793-317-6*); pap. 16.95 (*0-89793-316-8*) Hunter Hse.

Coping with War-Induced Stress: The Gulf War & the Israeli Response. Zahava Solomon. 1994. LC 94-43373. (Stress & Coping Ser.). (Illus.). 280p. (C). 42.50 (*0-306-44788-6*, Plenum Trade) Perseus Pubng.

Coping with Your Child's Chronic Illness. Singer Alesia Barrett. 1999. LC 96-36373. 95p. 9.95 (*1-885003-14-5*) R D Reed Pubs.

Copper & Lymphomas. M. Hrgovcic & C. Shullenberger. 1983. LC 83-14335. 264p. 149.00 (*0-8493-6331-4*, CRC Reprint) Franklin.

Copper & Zinc in Inflammation. Ed. by Kim D. Rainsford et al. 1989. (Inflammation & Drug Therapy Ser.). 160p. (C). text 106.00 (*0-7462-0079-X*) Kluwer Academic.

Copper & Zinc in Inflammatory & Degenerative Diseases. Ed. by K. D. Rainsford et al. 1998. LC 97-41393. 197p. 137.00 (*0-7923-4827-3*) Kluwer Academic.

Copper Bioavailabity & Metabolism. C Kies. 1989. (Advances in Experimental Medicine & Biology Ser.: Vol. 258). (Illus.). 314p. 85.00 (*0-306-43373-7*, Plenum Trade) Perseus Pubng.

Copper in Animals & Man. Howell. 1987. Vol. I. 136p. 83.00 (*0-8493-4685-1*); Vol. II. 152p. 91.00 (*0-8493-4686-X*) Franklin (CRC Reprint).

Copper Transport & Its Disorders: Molecular & Cellular Aspects. Ed. by A. Leone & J. F. B. Mercer. 1999. LC 98-46056. (Advances in Experimental Medicine & Biology Ser.: 448). (Illus.). 269p. (C). text 149.50 (*0-306-46045-9*, Kluwer Plenum) Kluwer Academic.

Coram's Children: The London Foundling Hospital in the Eighteenth Century. Ruth K. McClure. 1981. LC 80-21375. (Illus.). 322p. (C). 50.00 (*0-300-02465-7*) Yale U Pr.

Corazon Del Hombre (The Heart of Man) Erich Fromm. 1991. (SPA.). 182p. reprint ed. pap. 6.99 (*968-16-0334-6*) Fondo CA.

Cord Blood Characteristics: Role in Stem Cell Transplantation. Shara Cohen et al. 2000. (Illus.). 296p. (*1-85317-794-6*) Martin Dunitz GBR. *Dist:* Blackwell Sci.

Cordyceps: Tonic Food of Ancient China. Kenneth Jones. 1997. (Illus.). 52p. (Orig.). pap. 4.95 (*0-9625638-5-4*) Sylvan Pr WA.

Core Anatomy, Vol. 2. Christopher Dean. 1995. pap. text 21.00 (*0-7020-2041-9*) Saunders.

Core Anatomy: Head & Neck, Vol. 3. Dean. 1996. (C). pap. text 23.00 (*0-7020-2042-7*) Harcourt.

Core Anatomy for Students Vol. 1: The Limbs & Vertebral Column, Vol. 1. Christopher Dean & John Pegington. 1995. (Illus.). 208p. pap. text 21.00 (*0-7020-2040-0*) Saunders.

***Core Clinical Cases in Obstetrics & Gynecology: A Problem-Solving Approach.** Janesh Gupta et al. 2001. (Arnold Publication). (Illus.). 200p. (Orig.). pap. text (*0-340-76042-7*) E A GBR. *Dist:* OUP.

***Core Clinical Skills: How to Succeed in OSCEs in Medicine.** T. Dornan & Paul O'Neill. 2001. (Illus.). 340p. pap. (*0-443-06366-4*) Church GBR. *Dist:* Saunders.

Core Concepts in Health. Paul M. Insel & Walton T. Roth. 8th ed. 1999. LC 99-26823. xxvii, 692p. (C). pap. text 49.95 (*0-7674-1040-8*, 1040-8); 1997. LC 97-11273. xxviii, 688p. pap. text 49.95 (*1-55934-914-X*, 1914); 1999. LC 99-21055. xxi, 386p. pap. text (*0-7674-1204-4*, 1204-4) Mayfield Pub.

***Core Concepts in Health.** Ed. by Paul M. Insel et al. 9th ed. 2001. LC 2001-30399. (Illus.). xxiv, 420p. (*0-7674-2558-8*) Mayfield Pub.

Core Concepts in Health. Paul M. Insel et al. 9th ed. 2001. LC 00-66233. (Illus.). xxix, 698p. (*0-7674-2370-4*) Mayfield Pub.

Core Concepts in Health: Brief Edition. Paul M. Insel et al. 8th ed. 1997. LC 97-9311. xix, 442p. pap. text 37.95 (*1-55934-915-8*, 1915) Mayfield Pub.

Core Concepts in Health: Transparencies. Paul M. Insel & Walton T. Roth. 8th ed. 1998. trans. (*0-7674-0004-6*, 0004-6) Mayfield Pub.

Core Curriculum: Ultrasound. William E. Brant. 2001. LC 2001-37732. (Illus.). text 99.00 (*0-683-30733-9*) Lppncott W & W.

Core Curriculum for Critical Care Nursing. AACN Staff. Ed. by Thomas Eoyang. 5th ed. 1998. LC 97-36175. (Illus.). 752p. (C). pap. text 49.00 (*0-7216-5147-X*) Saunders.

Core Curriculum for Critical Care Nursing: Instructor's Manual. AACN Staff. 5th ed. (Illus.). 955p. tchr. ed. (*0-7216-8343-6*) Saunders.

Core Curriculum for Critical Care Nursing: Instructor's Resource Manual. Maurene A. Harvey. Ed. by Joann Grif Alspach. (Illus.). 2nd ed. 1991. 316p. pap. text, stu. ed. 28.00 (*0-7216-3500-8*); 4th ed. 1992. 345p. text, tchr. ed. 775.00 (*0-7216-3229-7*) Saunders.

Core Curriculum for Diabetes Education. M. Funnell et al. 3rd rev. ed. 1998. (Illus.). 1000p. pap. text 135.00 (*1-881876-04-7*) Am Assn Diabetes Ed.

Core Curriculum for Holistic Nursing. Barbara Montgomery Dossey. 1997. LC 96-36535. 800p. spiral bd. 50.00 (*0-8342-0870-9*, 20870) Aspen Pub.

Core Curriculum for Intravenous Nursing. Crudi & Patricia Larkin. 1984. 368p. text 26.00 (*0-397-54516-9*, Lippncott) Lppncott W & W.

Core Curriculum for Maternal-Newborn Nursing. Organization for Obstetric, Gynecologic and Neonatal. Ed. by Susan Mattson & Judy E. Smith. 1992. (Illus.). 816p. pap. text 63.00 (*0-7216-3122-3*) Saunders.

Core Curriculum for Neonatal Intensive Care Nursing. Organization for Obstetric, Gynecologic and Neonatal. Ed. by Patricia O. Beachy & Jane Deacon. 1992. (Illus.). 746p. pap. text 64.00 (*0-7216-3121-5*) Saunders.

Core Curriculum for Noenatal Intensive Care Nursing. Ed. by Patricia O'Neill. 2nd ed. 1998. LC 99-25873. (Illus.). xxi, 824p. (*0-7216-7489-5*) Saunders.

Core Curriculum for Oncology Nursing. Ed. by Jane C. Clark & Rose F. McGee. 2nd ed. 1992. (Illus.). 255p. pap. text, stu. ed. 31.95 (*0-7216-3487-7*) Saunders.

Core Curriculum for Oncology Nursing. Oncology Nursing Society Staff. Ed. by Joanne K. Itano & Karen N. Taoka. 3rd ed. 1998. LC 97-14399. (Illus.). 834p. pap. text 52.95 (*0-7216-7156-X*) Saunders.

***Core Curriculum for Orthopaedic Nursing.** Ed. by Delores C. Schoen. 4th rev. ed. 2001. 567p. text 79.00 (*1-892665-11-5*, P203-1) Natl Assn Ortho Nurse.

Core Curriculum for Pediatric Critical Care Nursing. American Association of Critical-Care Nurses Staff. Ed. by Margaret C. Slota. 1997. LC 97-9767. (Illus.). 830p. pap. text 45.00 (*0-7216-6114-9*) Saunders.

Core Curriculum for Perianesthesia Nursing Practice. American Society of PeriAnesthesia Nurses Staff. Ed. by Maura Connor. 4th ed. 1998. LC 98-28129. (Illus.). 600p. pap. text 47.00 (*0-7216-7896-3*) Saunders.

Core Curriculum for Perioperative Nursing. Billie Fernsebner. 1992. 168p. (Orig.). pap. 52.00 (*0-945970-02-1*) O R Manager.

Core Curriculum for Post Anesthesia Nursing Practice. Ed. by Kim Litwack. 3rd ed. 1994. LC 94-13579. (Illus.). 706p. (C). pap. text 49.00 (*0-7216-5051-1*) Saunders.

Core Curriculum for Professional Education in Pain. Task Force on Professional Education of the Intern. Ed. by Howard L. Fields. 2nd ed. 1995. LC 95-44088. 136p. pap. 16.00 (*0-931092-12-4*) Intl Assn Study Pain.

Core Curriculum for Surgical First Assisting. Ed. by Association of Surgical Technologists. 1993. 131p. (Orig.). (C). pap. text 65.00 (*0-926805-03-7*) Assn Surgical.

Core Curriculum for Surgical Technology. 4th ed. 1996. 179p. (C). pap. text 44.95 (*0-926805-14-2*) Assn Surgical.

Core Curriculum for the Nursing Care of Children & Their Families. Ed. by Marion E. Broome & Judy A. Rollins. 1998. LC 99-226706. 500p. text 69.00 (*0-9655310-3-1*) Jannetti Pubns.

Core Curriculum for the RN First Assistant. AORN Staff. Ed. by Jane C. Rothrock et al. rev. ed. 1994. (Illus.). 220p. pap. text 43.75 (*0-939583-86-0*) AORN.

Core Curriculum Gerontol Nursing. Ann Schmidt Luggen. 2nd ed. 2000. 475p. pap. text 55.95 (*0-323-01098-9*) Mosby Inc.

Core Curriculum in Professional Psychology. Ed. by Roger L. Peterson et al. 1991. 179p. pap. text 29.95 (*1-55798-143-4*) Am Psychol.

***Core Curriculum in Women's Health Nursing.** Association of Women's Health, Obstetric and Neonatal Nurses Staff. Ed. by Vicki Lucas & Eileen Breslin. 2001. (Illus.). 595p. pap. (*0-7216-7423-2*) Saunders.

Core Curriculum on Tuberculosis: What the Clinician Should Know. Ed. by Barry Leonard. 4th ed. 2000. (Illus.). 139p. (C). pap. text 30.00 (*0-7567-0116-3*) DIANE Pub.

Core Curriculum or Intravenous Nursing. Ann M. Corrigan et al. 2nd ed. 1999. LC 99-21557. (Illus.). 448p. text (*0-7817-2116-4*) Lppncott W & W.

Core Data for Epidemiological Studies of Nonmedical Drug Use. Hughes & J. Venulet. 1980. (WHO Offset Publication: No. 56). text (*92-4-170056-4*) World Health.

Core Management for HR Students & Practitioners. Peter W. Winfield et al. 2000. LC 99-86524. 552p. pap. text 47.95 (*0-7506-4549-0*) Buttrwrth-Heinemann.

Core Mathematics (Custom Publication) Leslie. 1991. pap. (*0-07-037220-9*) McGraw.

Core Pediatrics & Child Health. Diab Farhan Haddad et al. 2000. 410p. Price not set. (*0-443-05916-0*) Harcrt Hlth Sci Grp.

Core Readings in Psychiatry: An Annotated Guide to the Literature. Ed. by Michael H. Sacks et al. 2nd ed. 1995. 896p. text 89.95 (*0-88048-559-0*, 8559) Am Psychiatric.

Core Review for Critical Care Nursing. Joann Grif Alspach. 3rd ed. 1998. LC 98-9756. 206p. (C). pap. text 25.00 (*0-7216-5232-8*) Saunders.

Core Review for the NCLEX/CAT-RN. Margaret M. Dahlhauser. 2000. (Illus.). 441p. pap. 44.95 (*0-07-135339-9*) McGraw-Hill Prof.

Core Review in Emergency Nursing: A CEN Study Guide & Practice Examination. Pam Pourciau & Nancy G. Townsend. 2nd ed. 1989. 207p. (C). pap. text 19.95 (*0-9622174-4-1*) Nursing Knowledge.

***Core Review Study Disk for Critical Care Nursing.** Ed. by Joann Grif Alspach. 5th ed. 1999. pap. 56.00 incl. disk (*0-7216-8188-3*) Saunders.

Core Text of Acupuncture: A Contemporary Practice Manual for Professionals & Students. Kuei-Ming Wu. 2000. (Illus.). 240p. 49.95 (*1-58177-073-1*) Barrytown Ltd.

Core Textbook of Obstetrics & Gynecology. Kenneth L. Mattox. 1997. LC 96-49800. (Illus.). 624p. (C). (gr. 13). pap. text 36.95 (*0-8151-6035-6*, 24828) Mosby Inc.

Core Textbook of Pediatrics. Lawrence Taft. Date not set. (*0-393-71035-1*) Norton.

***Core Topics in General & Emergency Surgery: A Companion to Specialist Surgical Practice.** Simon Paterson-Brown. 2nd ed. 2001. (Illus.). 411p. pap. (*0-7020-2589-5*) W B Saunders GBR. *Dist:* Saunders.

Corectec's Comprehensive Set of Review Questions for Radiography. Gerald R. Cummings & Elizabeth Meixner. (C). 2nd ed. 1991. 300p. pap. text 18.50 (*1-880890-00-3*); 3rd ed. 1993. (Illus.). 284p. pap. text 22.00 (*1-880890-03-8*) Corectec.

***Corinne T. Netzer Carbohydrate Counter 2002.** Corinne T. Netzer. 7th rev. ed. 2001. 500p. mass mkt. 6.99 (*0-440-23682-7*) Dell.

Corinne T. Netzer Encyclopedia of Food Values. Corinne T. Netzer. 1992. 928p. 28.95 (*0-440-50367-1*) Dell.

***Corinne T. Netzer 2002 Calorie Counter.** Corinne T. Netzer. 2001. 288p. mass mkt. 6.99 (*0-440-23676-2*) Dell.

Corinne T. Netzer's Big Book of Miracle Cures. Corinne T. Netzer. 1999. LC 99-212487. 400p. mass mkt. 6.99 (*0-440-22609-0*) Dell.

***Cornea.** Douglas J. Coster. 2001. (Fundamentals in Clinical Ophthalmology Ser.). (Illus.). 200p. (*0-7279-1557-6*) BMJ Pub GBR. *Dist:* AIDC.

Cornea. Holland & Palay Krachmer. 1996. LC 96-223568. (Illus.). 2528p. (C). (gr. 13). text 399.00 (*0-8151-5249-3*, 24736) Mosby Inc.

Cornea. Ed. by Herbert E. Kaufman et al. 1988. (Illus.). 952p. text (*0-443-08374-6*) Church.

Cornea. Herbert E. Kaufman et al. 2nd rev. ed. 1997. LC 97-25706. (Illus.). 1168p. pap. text 285.00 (*0-7506-9928-0*) Buttrwrth-Heinemann.

Cornea: Its Examination in Contact Lens Practice. Nathan Efron. 2001. 206p. text 80.00 (*0-7506-4798-1*) Buttrwrth-Heinemann.

Cornea: Scientific Foundations & Clinical Practice. Ed. by Gilbert Smolin & Richard A. Thoft. 3rd ed. 1994. LC 93-4460. 784p. text 255.00 (*0-316-80270-0*) Lppncott W & W.

Cornea & Conjunctiva: Clinical Procedures. Chris J. Cakanac & Paul C. Ajamian. 1995. LC 95-17809. (Optometric Procedures Ser.). (Illus.). 118p. spiral bd. 44.99 (*0-7506-9582-X*) Buttrwrth-Heinemann.

Cornea & Refractive Surgery. Ed. by Daniel a. Long. 1998. (Illus.). ix, 307p. (*90-6299-140-8*) Kugler NLD. *Dist:* Lib Res.

Cornea Color Atlas. Palay & Palay Krachmer. 1995. (Illus.). 336p. (C). (gr. 13). text 174.00 (*0-8151-5147-0*, 24920) Mosby Inc.

Cornea in Normal Condition & in Groenouw's Macular Dystrophy. J. Francois & V. Victoria-Troncoso. 1980. (Illus.). x, 198p. text 141.50 (*90-6193-161-4*) Kluwer Academic.

Corneal Alterations with Contact Lens Wear. A. J. Rouwen. 1992. (Illus.). 168p. lib. bdg. (*90-6299-080-0*) Kugler NLD. *Dist:* Lib Res.

Corneal Angiogenesis: A Comprehensive Critical Review. G. K. Klintworth. 1990. (Illus.). 135p. 106.00 (*0-387-97440-7*) Spr-Verlag.

Corneal Disorders: Clinical Diagnosis & Management. Howard M. Leibowitz & George O. Waring. Ed. by Richard Lampert. 2nd ed. 1998. LC 97-44165. (Illus.). 1200p. (C). text 275.00 (*0-7216-5867-9*) Saunders.

Corneal Grafting: Principles & Practice. Thomas A. Casey et al. 2nd ed. 1984. (Illus.). 352p. text 180.00 (*0-7216-2448-0*) Saunders.

Corneal Healing Responses to Injuries & Refractive Surgeries. Ed. by T. Nishida. 1998. (Illus.). (*90-6299-157-2*) Kugler NLD. *Dist:* Lib Res.

Corneal Laser Surgery. James J. Saltz. 1995. (Illus.). 352p. (C). incl. Beta (*0-8151-8221-X*) Mosby Inc.

Corneal Physiology & Disposable Contact Lenses. Ed. by Hikaru Hamano & Herbert E. Kaufman. 1997. LC 97-4330. (Illus.). 184p. pap. text 105.00 (*0-7506-9927-2*) Buttrwrth-Heinemann.

Corneal Sensitivity: Measurement & Clinical Importance. J. Draeger. 1984. (Illus.). 155p. 61.95 (*0-387-81794-8*) Spr-Verlag.

Corneal Surgery: Theory, Technique & Tissue. Ed. by Frederick S. Brightbill. 2nd ed. 1992. LC 92-23630. (Illus.). 763p. (C). (gr. 13). text 225.00 (*0-8016-6487-X*, 06487) Mosby Inc.

Corneal Surgery: Theory, Technique & Tissue. Frederick S. Brightbill. 3rd ed. 1999. LC 99-19068. (Illus.). 848p. (C). (gr. 13). text 225.00 (*0-8151-1229-7*, 27235) Mosby Inc.

Corneal Topography: Measuring & Modifying the Cornea. Ed. by David J. Schanzlin & J. B. Robin. 1991. (Illus.). 185p. 181.00 (*0-387-97539-X*) Spr-Verlag.

Corneal Topography: The Clinical Atlas. Lucio Buratto. 1996.Tr. of Corneale Topografia. (Illus.). 476p. 135.00 (*1-55642-306-3*, 63063) SLACK Inc.

Corneal Topography: The State of the Art. James P. Gills et al. 1995. 352p. 135.00 (*1-55642-268-7*) SLACK Inc.

Corneale Topografia see Corneal Topography: The Clinical Atlas

Cornerstones of Leadership for Health Services Executives. Austin Ross. 1992. LC 91-35345. 220p. text 30.80 (*0-910701-58-X*, 0818) Health Admin Pr.

Corona & Related Viruses: Current Concepts in Molecular Biology & Pathogenesis: Proceedings of the Sixth International Symposium Held in Laval, Quebec, Canada, August 27-September 1, 1994. Vol. 380. Ed. by Pierre J. Talbot & Gary A. Levy. 1995. (Advances in Experimental Medicine & Biology Ser.: Vol. 380). (Illus.). 636p. (C). text 149.50 (*0-306-45117-4*, Kluwer Plenum) Kluwer Academic.

Coronary Angiography for the Interventionalist. George W. Vetrovec & Evelyne Goudreau. 1993. 140p. (gr. 13). 114.95 (*0-412-04461-7*) Chapman & Hall.

Coronary Angiography for the Interventionalist. George W. Vetrovec & Evelyne Goudreau. 1993. LC 92-48409. (*0-444-01667-8*) Elsevier.

Coronary Angioplasty. Susan D. Allen. Ed. by Colleen A. Holloran. 1992. (Illus.). 32p. pap. text 2.85 (*0-916999-12-2*) HERC Pubng.

Coronary Angioplasty. Ed. by David A. Clark. 2nd ed. 1991. 316p. 625.00 incl. VHS (*0-471-56109-6*, Wiley-Interscience); LC 90-13100. 162.00 (*0-471-56074-X*) Wiley.

Coronary Angioplasty: A Controlled Model for Ischemia. Ed. by Patrick W. Serruys & Greert T. Meester. 1986. (Developments in Cardiovascular Medicine Ser.). text 193.50 (*0-89838-819-8*) Kluwer Academic.

Coronary Arteriography. Herbert L. Abrams. 1982. 102.00 (*0-316-00469-3*, Little Brwn Med Div) Lppncott W & W.

Coronary Arteriography. King-Douglas. 2000. 99.00 (*0-07-134384-9*) McGraw.

Coronary Artery Anomalies: A Comprehensive Approach. Paolo Angelini. 1999. LC 99-10769. 208p. text 169.00 (*0-7817-1018-9*) Lppncott W & W.

Coronary Artery Bypass Surgery. Lawrence H. Patzelt & Nancy L. Berends. Ed. by Oliver D. Grin & Dorothy L. Bouwman. 1991. (Patient Education Ser.). (Illus.). 34p. (Orig.). pap. text 3.50 (*0-929689-41-0*) Ludann Co.

Coronary Artery Disease & Related Conditions Management: Clinical Pathways, Guidelines & Patient Education. Health & Administration Development Group Aspen Publishers Staff et al. Ed. by Jo Gulledge & Shawn Beard. 1995. LC 99-31850. (Chronic Disease Management Ser.). 289p. pap. 76.00 (*0-8342-1704-X*) Aspen Pub.

Coronary Artery Disease in Women: What All Physicians Need to Know. Pamela Charney. 1999. LC 98-28030. (Women's Health Ser.). (Illus.). 632p. pap. 43.00 (*0-943126-68-1*) Amer Coll Phys.

Coronary Artery Graft Disease: Mechanism & Prevention. Ed. by Thomas F. Luscher et al. 1994. LC 94-16135. (Illus.). 409p. 135.00 (*0-387-57438-7*) Spr-Verlag.

Coronary Artery Restenosis. Ed. by Ezra Deutsch & Robert Schwartz. 2000. (Contemporary Cardiology Ser.). 375p. 125.00 (*0-89603-740-1*) Humana.

Coronary Artery Stenosis. K. Gould. 1990. (Illus.). 323p. (C). (gr. 13). text 127.95 (*0-412-04501-X*) Chapman & Hall.

Coronary Artery Stenosis. K. Lance Gould. 2nd ed. 1999. LC 98-23776. (Illus.). 704p. 135.00 (*0-412-09141-0*, Chap & Hall NY) Chapman & Hall.

Coronary Artery Stenting. Ed. by Sheldon Goldberg & Igor F. Palacios. 2001. (Contemporary Cardiology Ser.). 450p. 125.00 (*0-89603-857-2*) Humana.

Coronary Artery Stenting. Ed. by Gary S. Roubin & S. Slyer. 1997. (Interventional Cardiology Ser.). 400p. 95.00 (*0-86542-283-4*) Blackwell Sci.

Coronary Balloon Angioplasty. Ed. by Ronald E. Vlietstra & David R. Holmes, Jr. 1993. LC 93-33051. (Series in Interventional Cardiology). (Illus.). 512p. 79.95 (*0-86542-295-8*) Blackwell Sci.

Coronary Blood Flow: Mechanics, Distribution, & Control. Joe A. Spaan. 1991. (Developments in Cardiovascular Medicine Ser.). 416p. text 264.50 (*0-7923-1210-4*) Kluwer Academic.

Coronary Bypass Surgery: A Guide for Patients. Timothy Denton & Jack M. Matloff. Ed. by Elliot Rapaport. 1996. (Cardiology Ser.). (Illus.). 32p. (Orig.). pap. 2.95 (*1-885274-33-5*) Health InfoNet Inc.

Coronary Bypass Surgery: The Late Results. Ed. by Karl E. Hammermeister. 1983. LC 82-13302. 452p. 89.95 (*0-275-91392-9*, C1392, Praeger Pubs) Greenwood.

Coronary Bypass Surgery in the Elderly: Ethical, Economical, & Quality of Life Aspects. Ed. by Paul J. Walter. 1995. LC 94-37708. (Developments in Cardiovascular Medicine Ser.). 280p. (C). text 144.00 (*0-7923-3188-5*) Kluwer Academic.

Coronary Care. William E. Boden & Robert J. Capone. 1984. (Blue Bk.). (Illus.). 224p. pap. text 38.00 (*0-7216-1072-2*) Saunders.

Coronary Care Manual: A Practical Guide to the Management of Acute Cardiac Problems & Their Subsequent Follow-Up. James Nolan & David P. Lipkin. 1993. LC 92-49665. (Pocket Medical Reference Ser.). (Illus.). 260p. pap. text 27.50 (*0-19-262314-1*); 134p. 25.95 (*0-19-262315-X*) OUP.

Coronary Care Medicine. Elliott M. Antman & John D. Rutherford. 1986. text 161.50 (*0-89838-788-4*) Kluwer Academic.

Coronary Care Nursing. Paul L. Huang et al. 2nd ed. 1989. 480p. pap. text 44.00 (*0-7216-2627-0*) Saunders.

Coronary Cinematography. Curtis E. Green. 1996. (*0-397-51300-3*) Lppncott W & W.

Coronary Circulation: From Basic Mechanisms to Clinical Implications. Ed. by Joe A. Spaan et al. 1987. (Developments in Cardiovascular Medicine Ser.). (C). lib. bdg. 129.50 (*0-89838-978-X*) Kluwer Academic.

Coronary Circulation & Myocardial Ischemia. Ed. by Michael R. Pinsky et al. 2000. LC 00-21646. (Update in Intensive Care & Emergency Medicine Ser.: Vol. 32). (Illus.). 192p. 109.00 (*3-540-62584-4*) Spr-Verlag.

Coronary Circulation in Physiological & Pathophysiological States. Ed. by M. Nakamura & Paul M. Vanhoutte. 1991. (Illus.). 178p. 69.00 (*0-387-70053-6*) Spr-Verlag.

Coronary Disease in Women. Ashton. 1998. text 69.95 (*0-443-07960-9*) Saunders.

Coronary Disease Management: Coronary Arteriography, Nitrates, & the Triple Pedicle Operation. William H. Sewell. 1969. LC 70-78062. (Illus.). 220p. 15.00 (*0-87527-072-7*) Green.

Coronary Excimer Laser Angioplasty: An Update. Ed. by K. R. Karsch & K. K. Haase. 1991. (Illus.). 160p. 55.00 (*0-387-91406-4*) Spr-Verlag.

Coronary Experience. John R. Singh. 2nd ed. 1980. LC 80-82823. (Illus.). 128p. (Orig.). text 9.95 (*0-9604672-0-3*) Mid Am Pr.

Coronary Heart Disease. Ed. by Gerald Sandler. (Practical Clinical Medicine Ser.). 1987. lib. bdg. 101.50 (*0-85200-692-6*); 1986. pap. text 59.00 (*0-85200-940-2*) Kluwer Academic.

Coronary Heart Disease: A Handbook for the Health Care Team. Grace M. Lindsay & Allan Gaw. 1996. LC 96-25835. text (*0-443-05460-6*) Church.

Coronary Heart Disease & Risk Factor Management: A Nursing Perspective. Nallini Jairath. Ed. by Robin Carter. 1999. LC 98-36804. (Illus.). 300p. (C). text 35.00 (*0-7216-6855-0*) Saunders.

Coronary Heart Disease in Women: Proceedings of an N. I. H. Workshop. Ed. by Nanette K. Wenger. 1987. (Illus.). x, 207p. (Orig.). 30.00 (*0-937716-26-X*) Haymkt-Doyma.

Coronary Heart Disease Prevention. Ed. by Frank G. Yanowitz. 1992. LC 92-22168. (Fundamental & Clinical Cardiology Ser.: Vol. 9). (Illus.). 488p. text 115.00 (*0-8247-8713-7*) Dekker.

Coronary Magnetic Resonance Angiography. Andre J. Duerinckx. 2000. LC 99-53567. (Illus.). xv, 342p. 198.00 (*0-387-94959-3*) Spr-Verlag.

Coronary Pressure. Nico H. Pijis & Bernard De Bruyne. 1997. LC 97-26047. (Developments in Cardiovascular Medicine Ser.: No. 195). 368p. text 167.00 (*0-7923-4672-6*) Kluwer Academic.

Coronary Prone Behavior. Ed. by T. M. Dembroski et al. 1978. LC 78-9947. (Illus.). 244p. 52.00 (*0-387-08876-8*) Spr-Verlag.

Coronary Restenosis. Ed. by Giora Z. Feuerstein. 1996. LC 96-43176. (Fundamental & Clinical Cardiology Ser.: Vol. 28). (Illus.). 504p. text 185.00 (*0-8247-9767-1*) Dekker.

Coronary Stenosis Morphology: Analysis & Implication. Ed. by Lloyd Klein. 1997. (Developments in Cardiovascular Medicine Ser.). 392p. (C). text 205.50 (*0-7923-9867-X*) Kluwer Academic.

Coronary Stenting: Current Perspectives. Michael Kutryk & Patrick W. Serruys. 1999. 318p. 59.95 (*1-85317-693-1*, M Dunitz) Scovill Paterson.

Coronary Stents. Ed. by U. Sigwart & G. I. Frank. 1992. LC 92-49671. (Illus.). 216p. 139.00 (*3-540-54541-7*); 179p. 181.00 (*0-387-54541-7*) Spr-Verlag.

Coronary Tone in Ischemic Heart Disease. Ed. by W. Kupper et al. 1984. (Developments in Cardiovascular Medicine Ser.). text 97.50 (*0-89838-646-2*) Kluwer Academic.

Coronaviridae. Ed. by Stuart G. Siddell. 1995. LC 95-32957. (Viruses Ser.). (Illus.). 446p. (C). text 105.00 (*0-306-44972-2*, Kluwer Plenum) Kluwer Academic.

Coronaviruses. Ed. by M. M. Lai & S. A. Stohlman. 1987. LC 87-22034. (Advances in Experimental Medicine & Biology Ser.: Vol. 218). (Illus.). 604p. 125.00 (*0-306-42672-2*, Plenum Trade) Perseus Pubng.

Coronaviruses: Molecular Biology & Virus-Host Interactions. H. Taude & J. F. Vautherot. 1994. LC 93-46630. (Advances in Experimental Medicine & Biology Ser.: Vol. 342). (Illus.). 490p. (C). text 145.00 (*0-306-44599-9*, Kluwer Plenum) Kluwer Academic.

Coronaviruses & Arteriviruses: Proceedings of the VIIth International Symposium Held in Segovia, Spain, May 10-15, 1997. Ed. by Luis Enjuanes et al. 1998. LC 98-8316. (Advances in Experimental Medicine & Biology Ser.: Vol. 440). (Illus.). 844p. (C). text 185.00 (*0-306-45910-8*, Kluwer Plenum) Kluwer Academic.

Coronaviruses & Their Diseases. Ed. by D. Cavanagh & T. D. Brown. 1990. (Advances in Experimental Medicine & Biology Ser.: Vol. 276). (Illus.). 670p. 149.50 (*0-306-43664-7*, Plenum Trade) Perseus Pubng.

Coroners' Reports, New York City, 1843-1849. Kenneth Scott. 1991. LC 90-63411. 320p. 26.95 (*1-877692-02-6*) NY Genealogical & Biographical.

Corporate Book Reserving for Postretirement Healthcare Benefits. Ed. by Dwight K. Bartlett. 1991. (Pension Research Council Publications). 128p. (C). text 30.95 (*0-256-09142-0*) U of Pa Pr.

Corporate Compliance: Self-Assessment & Planning. Greeley Company Staff & Horty, Springer and Mattern Staff. 1998. 60p. pap. text 32.00 (*1-57839-020-6*) Opus Communs.

Corporate Compliance in Home Health. Fay Rozovsky. 1998. LC 98-24887. 528p. pap. 61.00 (*0-8342-1173-4*, 11734) Aspen Pub.

Corporate Law for the Healthcare Provider: Organization, Operation, Merger & Bankruptcy. Ed. by Ann Huckstep et al. 1993. 251p. 55.00 (*0-918945-15-1*) Am Hlth Lawyers.

Corporate Practice of Medicine: Competition & Innovation in Health Care. James C. Robinson. 1999. LC 99-14072. (California/Milbank Series on Health & the Public Ser.: Vol. 1). xii, 261p. pap. 18.95 (*0-520-22076-5*) U CA Pr.

Corporate Practice of Medicine Prohibition in the Modern Era of Health Care. Francis J. Serbaroli. 1999. (Health Law & Business Ser.: Vol. No. 2800). pap. 95.00 (*1-55871-414-6*) BNA.

Corporate Therapy & Consulting, Vol. 5. Len Sperry. 1996. LC 96-24807. (Mental Health Practice under Managed Care Ser.: No. 5). 256p. pap. text 27.95 (*0-87630-820-5*) Brunner-Routledge.

Corporate Training for Medical Assisting. Boston Reed. 1998. 448p. (C). text 44.95 (*0-7668-0932-3*) Delmar.

Corporate Transformation of Health Care Pt. 1: Issues & Directions. Ed. by J. Warren Salmon. 1990. (Policy, Politics, Health & Medicine Ser.). 282p. pap. 33.75 (*0-89503-087-X*) Baywood Pub.

Corporate Transformation of Health Care Pt. 2: Perspectives & Implications. Ed. by J. Warren Salmon. 1993. (Policy, Politics, Health & Medicine Ser.). 269p. text 45.00 (*0-89503-103-5*) Baywood Pub.

C D

Corporate Venturing in Health Care. Price. 1989. (Orig.). pap. (*0-8273-4332-9*) Delmar.

Correct Food Combining for Easy Digestion: How to Get Rid of Indigestion, Gas, Bloating, Belching & Bad Breath. 1992. lib. bdg. 88.95 (*0-8490-8806-2*) Gordon Pr.

***CorrectCoder.** Yale Wasserman, D.M.D. Medical Publishers, Limited. 2001. per. 119.00 (*1-881072-63-0*) Y W DMD Med.

Correctional Psychiatry. Richard Rosner & R. B. Harmon. 1989. LC 88-657025. (Critical Issues in American Psychiatry & the Law Ser.: Vol. 6). (Illus.). 320p. (C). 80.00 (*0-306-43070-3*, Plenum Trade) Perseus Pubng.

Corrective & Protective Eyewear Markets: New Technologies Alter Marketing Strategies. Market Intelligence Staff. 1993. 297p. 1695.00 (*1-56753-481-3*) Frost & Sullivan.

Corrective & Reconstructive Rhinoplasty. H. J. Denecke & R. Meyer. Tr. by L. Oxtoby. 1967. (Plastic Surgery of Head & Neck Ser.: Vol. 1). (Illus.). 548p. 424.00 (*0-387-03757-8*) Spr-Verlag.

Corrective Osteotomies of the Lower Extremity after Trauma. Ed. by G. Hierholzer & K. H. Muller. Tr. by Terry C. Telger from GER. 1985. (Illus.). 407p. 158.00 (*0-387-15879-0*) Spr-Verlag.

Correlating Sensory Objective Measurements - STP 594. 1985. 133p. pap. 13.00 (*0-8031-0312-3*, STP594) ASTM.

Correlative Brain: Theory & Experiment in Neural Interaction. J. J. Eggermont. 1990. (Studies of Brain Function: Vol. 16). (Illus.). 307p. 195.00 (*0-387-52326-X*) Spr-Verlag.

Correlative Neuroanatomy. Stephen G. Waxman. 24th ed. 1999. (Lange Medical Bks.). (Illus.). 394p. pap. 34.95 (*0-8385-1583-5*) McGraw-Hill Prof.

Correlative Neuroradiology & Neuropathology: A Practical Guide to Interpretation. A. Wilkins & Clifton. 2000. 240p. pap. 129.00 (*0-412-54890-9*, Chap & Hall NY) Chapman & Hall.

Correlative Observations in Dementia. John S. Woodward. 1985. (Illus.). 110p. (Orig.). pap. text 14.00 (*0-9615638-0-X*) CA Med Pubns.

Correlative Urinalysis: The Body Knows Best. M. T. Morter, Jr. 1988. LC 87-51116. 200p. pap. 32.00 (*0-944994-02-4*); 150p. 32.00 (*0-944994-00-8*) BEST Research.

Correspondence of Sigmund Freud & Sandor Ferenczi: 1908-1914. Ed. by Andre Haynal et al. 1994. LC 93-17479. 622p. 48.00 (*0-674-17418-6*, Belknap) HUP.

Correspondence of Sigmund Freud & Sandor Ferenczi Vol. 2: 1914-1919. Ed. by Ernst Falzeder & Eva Brabant. Tr. by Peter T. Hoffer. 1996. LC 93-17479. (Illus.). 448p. 49.95 (*0-674-17419-4*) HUP.

Corridors of Deceit: The World of John Le Carre. Peter Wolfe. 1987. LC 87-70354. 282p. 32.95 (*0-87972-381-5*); pap. 16.95 (*0-87972-382-3*) Bowling Grn St Univ.

Corrosion & Degradation of Implant Materials: Second Symposium - STP 859. Ed. by Anna C. Fraker & Charles D. Griffin. 1985. LC 84-70337. (Illus.). 470p. text 62.00 (*0-8031-0427-8*, STP859) ASTM.

Corrositex: An in Vitro Test Method for Assessing Dermal Corrosivity Potential of Chemicals. Ed. by Robert Scala. 2000. (Illus.). 250p. pap. text 45.00 (*0-7567-0265-8*) DIANE Pub.

Corruption of Reality: A Unified Theory of Religion, Hypnosis & Psychopathology. John F. Schumaker. 1995. LC 94-41812. 289p. (C). 37.00 (*0-87975-935-6*) Prometheus Bks.

Corsini Encyclopedia of Psychology & Behavioral Science, Vol. 1. Ed. by W. Edward Craighead & Charles B. Nemeroff. 3rd ed. 2000. LC 99-58006. (Illus.). 496p. 175.00 (*0-471-24096-6*) Wiley.

Corsini Encyclopedia of Psychology & Behavioral Science W. Edward Craighead & Charles B. Nemeroff. 3rd ed. 2000. LC 99-58006. (Illus.). Vol. 2. 464p. 175.00 (*0-471-24097-4*); Vol. 3. 480p. 175.00 (*0-471-24098-2*); Vol. 4. 512p. 175.00 (*0-471-24099-0*) Wiley.

Cortex: Statistics & Geometry of Neuronal Connectivity. V. Braitenberg & A. Schuz. 2nd ed. 1998. (Studies Brain Function Ser.: Vol. 18). (Illus.). 262p. 99.00 (*3-540-63816-4*) Spr-Verlag.

Cortex Cerebri: Performance, Structural & Functional Organisation of the Cortex. O. Creutzfeldt. Tr. by Mary Creutzfeldt. 1995. LC 94-32583. (Illus.). 672p. text 129.50 (*0-19-852324-6*) OUP.

Cortical Circuits: Synaptic Organization & Cerebral Cortex - Structure, Function & Theory. Edward L. White. 1989. 264p. 71.00 (*0-8176-3402-9*) Birkhauser.

Cortical Functions. John D. Stirling. 1999. LC 99-31483. (Modular Psychology Ser.). (Illus.). 176p. pap. 12.99 (*0-415-19267-6*) Routledge.

Cortical Memory Functions. Charles M. Fair. 1992. (Illus.). x, 210p. 90.50 (*0-8176-3615-3*) Birkhauser.

Cortical Monkey & Healing. Majid Ali. 1995. 352p. pap. 14.99 (*1-879131-00-5*) Inst of Prev Med.

Cortical Neuron. Ed. by Michael J. Gutnick & Istvan Mody. 1995. LC 94-24546. (Illus.). 424p. text 79.50 (*0-19-508330-X*) OUP.

Cortical Plasticity: LTP & LTD. Ed. by Sam Fazeli & Graham L. Collingridge. 1998. LC 98-137866. (Molecular & Cellular Neurobiology Ser.). (Illus.). 266p. 78.50 (*1-872748-74-0*) OUP.

Cortico-Hippocampal Interplay & the Representation of Contexts in the Brain. R. Miller. 1991. (Studies of Brain Function: Vol. 17). (Illus.). 267p. 101.00 (*0-387-53109-2*) Spr-Verlag.

Corticonics: Neural Circuits of the Cerebral Cortex. M. Abeles. 1991. (Illus.). 294p. (C). text 80.00 (*0-521-37476-6*); pap. text 27.95 (*0-521-37617-3*) Cambridge U Pr.

Corticothalamic Projections & Sensorimotor Activities. T. Frigrjesi. 1972. 36.50 (*0-7204-7029-3*) Elsevier.

Cory Everson's Lifebalance: The Complete Mind/Body Program for a Leaner Body, Better Health & Self-Empowerment. Cory Everson. 1998. LC 98-26664. 256p. pap. 16.95 (*0-399-52444-4*, Perigee Bks) Berkley Pub.

Cosmeceuticals: Drugs vs. Cosmetics. Peter Elsner & Howard I. Maibach. 2000. LC 00-37682. (Illus.). xi, 369p. text 175.00 (*0-8247-0305-7*) Dekker.

Cosmetic & Pharmaceutical Applications of Polymers. Ed. by Charles G. Gebelein et al. 1991. (Illus.). 424p. (C). text 144.00 (*0-306-44088-1*, Kluwer Plenum) Kluwer Academic.

Cosmetic Blepharoplasty. Stephen L. Bosniak & Marian Zilkha. 2nd ed. 1998. LC 98-7633. (Illus.). 208p. text 179.00 (*0-397-58469-5*) Lppncott W & W.

Cosmetic Dentistry & the Latest Techniques. Hubert P. Sgambato. Ed. by Renee P. Heron. rev. ed. 1999. LC 88-92453. (Illus.). 200p. pap. 9.95 (*0-9621636-0-0*) H P Sgambato.

Cosmetic Dermatologic Surgery. Ed. by Leonard M. Dzubow. 1998. LC 97-51986. (Illus.). 320p. text 159.00 (*0-397-51740-8*) Lppncott W & W.

Cosmetic Dermatology. Robert Baran & Howard I. Maibach. 1994. (Illus.). 584p. (*0-683-00321-6*) Lppncott W & W.

Cosmetic Laser Surgery. Mitchel P. Goldman & Richard E. Fitzpatrick. 2000. LC 00-29216. (Illus.). xi, 239p. text (*0-8151-8674-6*, 31796) Mosby Inc.

Cosmetic Laser Surgery: A Practitioner's Guide. Tina S. Alster & David B. Apfelberg. 2nd ed. 1998. LC 98-3394. (Illus.). 393p. 252.00 (*0-471-25270-0*) Wiley.

Cosmetic Oculplastic Surgery: Eyelid, Forehead, & Facial Techniques. Allen M. Putterman. Ed. by Richard Lampert. 2nd ed. 1998. (Illus.). 400p. (C). text 145.00 (*0-7216-7076-8*) Saunders.

Cosmetic Oral & Maxillofacial. Bruce N. Epker. 1993. text (*0-397-51194-9*) Lppncott W & W.

Cosmetic Plastic Surgery. Betsy McCoy. Ed. by John M. Osborn. 1993. LC 92-62104. (Illus.). 176p. 24.95 (*0-9633816-0-1*) Paradise Sacramento.

Cosmetic Plastic Surgery: A Patient's Guide. Benjamin Gelfant. 1998. 160p. pap. (*0-9682626-0-0*) Flapartz CAN. *Dist:* Assoc Pubs Grp.

Cosmetic Safety: A Primer for Cosmetic Scientists. James H. Whittam. 1987. (Cosmetic Science & Technology Ser.: Vol. 5). (Illus.). 368p. text 210.00 (*0-8247-7538-4*) Dekker.

***Cosmetic Surgery: An Interdisciplinary Approach.** Ed. by Rhoda S. Narins. 2001. LC 2001-17436. (Basic & Clinical Dermatology Ser.: Vol. 20). (Illus.). xvi, 986p. text 250.00 (*0-8247-0302-2*) Dekker.

Cosmetic Surgery: The Consumer's Complete Easy Guide from Before to After. Cynthia E. Sutton & Wanda S. Lyon. 1992. LC 92-80816. (Illus.). 160p. (Orig.). pap. 16.95 (*0-9631071-0-0*) Swan Park.

Cosmetic Surgery of the Skin. William P. Coleman, 3rd & C. William Hanke. 2nd ed. 1997. LC 96-52513. (Illus.). 512p. (C). (gr. 13). text 169.00 (*0-8151-1460-5*, 29156) Mosby Inc.

Cosmetic Surgery Revolution in America: A Consumer's Survival Guide. Robert Scheer. 1992. (Illus.). 332p. pap. 14.95 (*0-945806-09-4*) Summit CA.

***Cosmetic Techniques: Index of New Information for Consumers, Reference & Research.** Ed. by Research and Development Division Staff & John C. Bartone. 2001. 180p. pap. 44.50 (*0-7883-2441-1*) ABBE Pubs Assn.

***Cosmetics: Index of New Information for Consumers, Reference & Research.** Ed. by Research and Development Division Staff & John C. Bartone. 2001. 180p. 47.50 (*0-7883-2414-4*); pap. 44.50 (*0-7883-2415-2*) ABBE Pubs Assn.

Cosmetics & Health: Index of Modern Information with Bibliography. Sandra O. Van Wertz. 1990. LC 88-47793. 150p. (Orig.). 47.50 (*1-55914-206-5*); pap. 44.50 (*1-55914-207-3*) ABBE Pubs Assn.

Cosmetics in Dermatology. Zoe K. Draelos. 1990. (Illus.). 214p. pap. text (*0-443-08644-3*) Church.

Cosmetics in Dermatology. Zoe D. Draelos. 2nd ed. 1995. LC 95-24705. 317p. text (*0-443-08965-5*) Church.

Cosmic Influences on Human Behaviour. Michel Gauquelin. 1985. 319p. pap. 12.50 (*0-943358-23-X*) Aurora Press.

Cosmo-Biological Birth Control. Shalila Sharamon & Bodo Baginski. 1989. 236p. (Orig.). pap. 14.95 (*0-941524-82-5*) Lotus Pr.

Cost Accounting for Health Care Organizations: Concepts & Applications. Steven A. Finkler & David M. Ward. 2nd ed. 1999. LC 98-31607. 800p. 180.00 (*0-8342-1012-6*, 10126) Aspen Pub.

Cost Analysis Module 8: Facilitator's Guide. Mary Millar. 1993. (Primary Health Care Management Advancement Programme Modules Ser.). 53p. pap. text (*1-882839-14-5*) Aga Khan Fnd.

Cost Analysis Module 8: User's Guide. Jack Reynolds. 1993. (Primary Health Care Management Advancement Programme Modules Ser.). 97p. pap. text (*1-882839-06-4*) Aga Khan Fnd.

Cost Analysis, Cost Recovery, Marketing & Fee-Based Services: A Guide for the Health Sciences Librarian. Ed. by M. Sandra Wood. 1985. LC 85-888. (Medical Reference Services Quarterly Ser.: Supp. Vol. 1). 268p. text 8.95 (*0-86656-353-9*) Haworth Pr.

Cost Analysis in Primary Health Care: A Training Manual for Programme Managers. Ed. by A. Creese & D. Parker. 1994. LC 95-202639. (ENG, FRE & SPA.). x, 147p. pap. text 25.00 (*92-4-154470-8*, 1150415) World Health.

Cost & Competition in American Medicine: Theory, Policy & Institutions. Les Seplaki. 1994. LC 94-22105. 498p. 81.00 (*0-8191-9639-8*); pap. 51.50 (*0-8191-9640-1*) U Pr of Amer.

Cost Benefit Analysis of Heroin Maintenance Treatment. Ed. by F. Gutzwiller & T. Steffen. 2nd ed. 2000. LC 99-24602. (Medical Prescription of Narcotics Ser.: Vol. 2). (Illus.). lx, 134p. 50.50 (*3-8055-6874-6*) S Karger.

Cost-Benefit Analysis of the Onchoceriasis Program (OCP) Aehyung Kim & Bruce Benton. 1995. LC 95-13778. (Technical Papers). 30p. pap. 22.00 (*0-8213-3235-X*, 13235) World Bank.

Cost Containment & New Priorities in Health Care: A Study of the European Community. Brian Abel-Smith. 1992. 160p. (*1-85628-319-4*) Avebry GBR. *Dist:* Ashgate Pub Co.

Cost Containment in the Clinical Laboratory. Evans et al. Ed. by Edith Helman. 1995. (Illus.). 264p. pap. 40.00 (*0-910224-16-1*) Berkeley Sci.

Cost Effective Diagnosis & Treatment of Coronary Artery Disease. Ed. by J. David Talky et al. 1997. LC 96-48407. (Topics in Clinical Cardiology Ser.). (Illus.). text (*0-89640-335-1*) Igaku-Shoin.

Cost Effective Diagnosis & Treatment of Coronary Artery Disease. J. David Talley et al. 1997. LC 96-48407. (Topics in Clinical Cardiology Ser.). (*4-260-14335-2*) Igaku-Shoin.

Cost-Effective Diagnostic Imaging: The Clinician's Guide. Zachary D. Grossman et al. 3rd ed. 1994. LC 95-102193. (Illus.). 480p. (C). (gr. 13). pap. text 47.95 (*0-8151-3440-1*, 24260) Mosby Inc.

Cost Effective Quality Control: Managing the Quality & Productivity of Analytical Processes. Ed. by Patricia L. Barry & James O. Westgard. 1986. (Illus.). 229p. reprint ed. 24.00 (*0-915274-35-3*, AACC Pr) Am Assn Clinical Chem.

Cost-Effective Surgical Management: Serving Two Masters. Ben E. Eiseman. 1987. (Illus.). 304p. text 77.00 (*0-7216-2102-3*) Saunders.

Cost-Effective Use of Once-Daily Ceftriaxone in the Treatment of Moderate to Severe Infections, Vol. 37, Supplement 3, 1991: Journal: Chemotherapy. Ed. by Vincent T. Andriole. 1991. (Illus.). iv, 28p. pap. 10.50 (*3-8055-5450-8*) S Karger.

Cost-Effectiveness in Health & Medicine. Ed. by Marthe R. Gold et al. 1996. LC 96-4753. (Illus.). 456p. (C). text 49.95 (*0-19-510824-8*) OUP.

Cost-Effectiveness in the Nonprofit Sector: Methods & Examples from Leading Organizations. Ed. by Gerald L. Schmaedick. 1993. LC 92-1746. 208p. 62.95 (*0-89930-627-6*, RES, Quorum Bks) Greenwood.

Cost Effectiveness of Psychotherapy: A Guide for Practitioners, Researchers, & Policymakers. Nancy E. Miller. 1999. LC 97-43075. (Illus.). 384p. text 55.00 (*0-19-511458-2*) OUP.

Cost-Effectiveness Study of Clinical Methods of Birth Control: With Special Reference to Puerto Rico. William J. Kelly. 1972. LC 72-79559. (Special Studies in International Economics & Development). 32.50 (*0-275-28637-1*) Irvington.

Cost Estimates for Expanded Substance Abuse Benefits for Medicaid-Eligible Pregnant Women. 1994. (Illus.). 210p. (Orig.). (C). pap. text 50.00 (*0-7881-1272-4*) DIANE Pub.

Cost Management in Long-Term Care Facilities. Mike Jacobs, Jr. 1986. 208p. (C). 49.50 (*0-929442-01-6*, 2208pp) Prof Prnting & Pub.

Cost of Cancer Treatment Study's Design & Methods. Dana P. Goldman et al. 2000. vii, 38p. pap. 8.00 (*0-8330-2848-0*, MR-1169) Rand Corp.

Cost of Tuberculosis Control in Minnesota: A Report to the Legislature. Ed. by Barry Leonard. 1999. 48p. (C). reprint ed. pap. text 20.00 (*0-7881-8195-5*) DIANE Pub.

Cost Outcome Methods for Mental Health. William A. Hargreaves et al. 1997. LC 97-80250. (Illus.). 242p. text 69.95 (*0-12-325155-9*) Morgan Kaufmann.

Cost Recovery in Public Health Services in Sub-Saharan Africa. Brian Nolan & Vincent Turbat. 1995. LC 95-14406. (EDI Technical Materials Ser.). 114p. pap. 22.00 (*0-8213-3240-6*, 13240) World Bank.

Cost Shifting in Health Care: Separating Evidence from Rhetoric. Michael A. Morrisey. 1994. LC 94-14605. 19.95 (*0-8447-3860-3*, AEI Pr) Am Enterprise.

Costing Human Resources. Wayne F. Cascio. 2nd ed. 1987. (SWC-Management). 288p. (C). mass mkt. 17.75 (*0-534-08034-0*) PWS Pubs.

Costing out Nursing: Pricing Our Product. Ed. by Franklin A. Shaffer. 1985. 272p. 18.95 (*0-88737-167-1*, 20-1982) Natl League Nurse.

Costs & Benefits in Health Care & Prevention: An International Approach to Priorities in Medicine. Ed. by U. Laaser et al. 1990. (Illus.). 180p. 34.95 (*0-387-52708-7*) Spr-Verlag.

Costs & Effectiveness of Prostate Cancer Screening in Elderly Men. 1998. (Illus.). 130p. reprint ed. pap. text 25.00 (*0-7881-3290-3*) DIANE Pub.

Costs of Excess Medical Claims for Automobile Personal Injuries. Allan Abrahamse et al. 1995. LC 95-221873. (Illus.). 28p. pap. text 6.00 (*0-8330-1649-0*, DB-139) Rand Corp.

Costs of Facility Development: A Comparative Analysis of Public & Private Sector Facility Development Processes & Costs. Jeffery A. Lackney et al. 1995. (Illus.). vi, 175p. (C). per. 20.00 (*0-938744-90-9*, R94-9) U of Wis Ctr Arch-Urban.

Costs of Illness & Benefits of Drug Treatment. Ed. by U. Abshagen & F. E. Munnich. 1990. (Clinical Pharmacology Ser.: Vol. 4). (Illus.). 112p. text (*3-88603-364-3*) W Zuckschwerdt DEU. *Dist:* Scholium Intl.

Costs of Medical Care: A Summary of Investigations on the Economic Aspects of the Prevention & Care of Illness, Vol. 27. Isidore S. Falk et al. 1972. LC 71-180568. (Medicine & Society in America Ser.). 652p. reprint ed. 37.95 (*0-405-03950-6*) Ayer.

Costs of Poor Health Habits. Willard G. Manning et al. 1991. (Illus.). 256p. (C). 42.00 (*0-674-17485-2*) HUP.

COTA Examination Review Guide. Caryn Johnson. 1997. LC 97-199931. (Illus.). 208p. (C). 28.95 (*0-8036-0278-2*) Davis Co.

COTA Examination Review Manual: A Practical Guide to Receiving Professional Certification. M. Teresa Mohler. 2nd ed. 1997. LC 97-8104. pap. 24.00 (*1-55642-346-2*) SLACK Inc.

Cotherapy with Individuals, Families & Groups. Ed. by Seymour Hoffman et al. 1995. LC 94-20885. 184p. pap. 35.00 (*1-56821-316-6*) Aronson.

Cotton Dust & Byssinosis. Shirley Inst. Staff. 1984. (C). (*0-7855-4571-9*) British Textile Tech GBR. *Dist:* St Mut.

Cotton Mather & American Science & Medicine: With Studies & Documents Concerning the Introduction of Inoculation or Variolation Ed. by I. Bernard Cohen. 1980. LC 79-7974. (Three Centuries of Science in America Ser.). (Illus.). lib. bdg. 82.95 (*0-405-12556-9*) Ayer.

Cotton Mather & American Science & Medicine: With Studies & Documents Concerning the Introduction of Inoculation or Variolation. I. Bernard Cohen. 1980. Vol. 1. 41.95 (*0-405-12520-8*); Vol. 2. 41.95 (*0-405-12521-6*) Ayer.

Cottone's Practical Infection Control in Dentistry. John A. Molinari & Geza Terezhalmy. 3rd ed. 2003. pap. text 39.95 (*0-683-30728-2*) Lppncott W & W.

Couch: Its Use & Meaning in Psychotherapy. Harold Stern. 1978. LC 77-15610. 215p. 32.95 (*0-87705-303-0*, Kluwer Acad Hman Sci) Kluwer Academic.

Cough & Other Respiratory Reflexes. J. Korpas & Z. Tomori. 1979. (Progress in Respiratory Research Ser.: Vol. 12). (Illus.). 142.75 (*3-8055-3007-2*) S Karger.

Coughs & Wheezes. Phyllis Speight. 1991. 105p. pap. (*0-85207-252-X*) C W Daniel GBR. *Dist:* Natl Bk Netwk.

Coughs & Wheezes: Their Treatment by Homoeopathy. Phyllis Speight. 80p. (Orig.). pap. 11.95 (*0-8464-4194-2*) Beekman Pubs.

Could It Be My Thyroid? Sheldon Rubenfeld. Ed. by Kathy Kobos. 1996. (Illus.). 193p. pap. 18.00 (*0-9660398-0-7*) S Rubenfeld.

Could It Be Stress? Reflections on Psychosomatic Illness. Cameron Macdonald. 1992. 192p. (C). pap. (*1-874640-10-6*) Argyll Pubng GBR. *Dist:* St Mut.

Could Your Kid Die "Laughing"? AIDS & Today's Adolescent. Carole Marsh. 1994. (Smart Sex Stuff Ser.). (Orig.). pap. 19.95 (*1-55609-225-3*); lib. bdg. 29.95 (*1-55609-262-8*) Gallopade Intl.

Council for International Organizations of Medical Sciences: Organization, Activities, Members. 1994. 90p. pap. text 10.00 (*92-9036-058-5*, 1840017) World Health.

Council of Judicial & Ethical Affairs: Reports on Managed Care. American Medical Association Staff. 1998. LC 00-500207. 100p. pap. text 32.95 (*0-89970-963-X*) AMA.

Council of Judicial & Ethical Affairs Reports on End-of-Life Care. Ed. by American Medical Association Staff. 1998. 100p. pap. 32.95 (*0-89970-962-1*) AMA.

Counseling: The Spiritual Dimension. Ed. by Mary T. Burke & Judith G. Miranti. 1995. LC 95-5667. (Illus.). 191p. pap. text 17.95 (*1-55620-145-1*, 72575) Am Coun Assn.

Counseling: Theory & Practice. Rickey L. George & Therese S. Cristiani. 4th ed. 1994. LC 94-11091. 320p. 90.00 (*0-205-15252-X*) Allyn.

Counseling - Guidance, Interventions, Skills, Management & Sex Infections: Index of New Information & Bibliography. Peter P. Richey. rev. ed. 1996. LC 96-3129. 157p. 57.50 (*0-7883-0972-2*); pap. 47.50 (*0-7883-0973-0*) ABBE Pubs Assn.

Counseling—Guidance, Intervention, Skills, Management & Sex Infections. Peter P. Richey. 1994. 150p. 57.50 (*0-7883-0146-2*); pap. 47.50 (*0-7883-0147-0*) ABBE Pubs Assn.

C D

*Counseling about Cancer: Strategies for Genetic Counselors.** Katherine Schneider. 2nd ed. 2001. 352p. pap. 39.95 (*0-471-37036-3*) Wiley.

Counseling Across Cultures. Ed. by Paul B. Pedersen et al. 4th ed. 1996. 484p. 81.95 (*0-8039-5748-3*, 4093); pap. 37.95 (*0-8039-5749-1*, 4094) Sage.

*Counseling Across Cultures.** Ed. by Paul Pedersen. 5th ed. 2002. LC 2001-5392. 84.95 (*0-7619-2085-4*); pap. 42.95 (*0-7619-2086-2*) Sage.

Counseling Adult Children of Alcoholics. Sandra Wilson. 1989. LC 89-37116. (Resources for Christian Counseling Ser.: Vol. 21). 312p. 22.99 (*0-8499-0581-8*) Nelson Ref & Elec Pub.

Counseling Adults in Transition: A Compassionate Approach. Ed. by Jane Goodman et al. 2nd ed. 1995. LC 95-7294. (Illus.). 320p. 42.95 (*0-8261-4231-1*) Springer Pub.

Counseling American Indians. Laurence Armand French. LC 96-39394. 216p. 2002. pap. 34.50 (*0-7618-0636-9*); 1997. 58.50 (*0-7618-0635-0*) U Pr of Amer.

Counseling American Minorities: A Cross-Cultural Perspective. Donald R. Atkinson et al. 4th ed. 1992. 400p. (C). text 31.50 net. (*0-697-10444-3*) Brown & Benchmark.

Counseling & AIDS. Gregg R. Albers. 1990. (Resources for Christian Counseling Ser.: Vol. 24). 224p. 22.99 (*0-8499-0695-4*) Nelson Ref & Elec Pub.

Counseling & Demonization: The Missing Link. Grayson H. Ensign & Edward Howe. 1989. 350p. pap. text 6.95 (*0-9613185-1-1*) Recovery Pubns.

Counseling & Development in a Multicultural Society. John A. Axelson. 2nd ed. 1993. LC 92-26095. 498p. 46.50 (*0-534-19902-X*) Brooks-Cole.

Counseling & Life-Style Development. R. Murray Thomas. 1990. 320p. (C). pap. 34.95 (*0-8039-3614-1*, 3512) Sage.

Counseling & Psychology for Health Professionals. Bayne. 1992. 250p. pap. 41.50 (*1-56593-117-3*, 0420) Singular Publishing.

Counseling & Psychotherapy. Les Parrott, III. 1996. LC 96-27915. 448p. (C). text 59.69 (*0-07-048581-X*) McGrw-H Hghr Educ.

Counseling & Psychotherapy. Dave Capuzzi et al. 2nd ed. 1998. LC 98-8649. 501p. (C). 76.00 (*0-13-569955-X*) P-H.

Counseling & Psychotherapy: A Multicultural Perspective. Mary B. Ivey et al. 4th ed. 1996. LC 96-15078. 448p. 77.00 (*0-205-19890-2*) Allyn.

Counseling & Psychotherapy: A Transpersonal Approach. Gay Hendricks & Barry K. Weinhold. 2nd ed. 1993. LC 91-77046. 233p. pap. 34.95 (*0-89108-224-7*, 9205) Love Pub Co.

Counseling & Psychotherapy: Classics on Theories & Issues Ed. by Ben N. Ard, Jr. 1993. LC 93-390. 274p. pap. text 39.95 (*0-7734-9932-6*); 248p. pap. text 39.95 (*0-7734-9934-2*) E Mellen.

Counseling & Psychotherapy: Excercises for Effective Counseling & Psychotherapy. Leslie Parrott, III. 1996. (C). pap., stu. ed. 29.06 (*0-07-048582-8*) McGrw-H Hghr Educ.

Counseling & Psychotherapy: Theories, Associated Research & Issues. Marty Sapp. 1996. LC 96-42213. 596p. pap. text 48.50 (*0-7618-0518-4*) U Pr of Amer.

Counseling & Psychotherapy of Work Dysfunctions. Rodney L. Lowman. 1993. LC 93-852. (Illus.). 333p. text 29.95 (*1-55798-204-X*); pap. text 24.95 (*1-55798-205-8*) Am Psychol.

Counseling & Psychotherapy with Children & Adolescents: Theory & Practice for School & Clinic Settings. Douglas T. Brown & H. Thompson Prout. 2nd ed. 1989. LC 89-62094. (Illus.). 434p. (C). text 49.50 (*0-88422-104-0*) Clinical Psych.

Counseling & Psychotherapy with Children & Adolescents: Theory & Practice for School & Clinic Settings. H. Thompson Prout & Douglas T. Brown. 3rd ed. 1998. LC 98-16412. 456p. 90.00 (*0-471-18236-2*) Wiley.

Counseling & Psychotherapy with College Students: A Guide to Treatment. Ed. by Joseph E. Talley & W. J. Rockwell. 1985. LC 85-16957. 208p. 60.00 (*0-275-90033-9*, C0033, Praeger Pubs) Greenwood.

Counseling & Psychotherapy with Persons with Mental Retardation & Borderline Intelligence. Ed. by Douglas C. Strohmer & H. Thompson Prout. 1994. LC 93-12016. 312p. lib. bdg. 34.95 (*0-88422-121-0*) Clinical Psych.

Counseling & Therapy for Children. Jim Gumaer. 1984. LC 83-48683. (Illus.). 384p. (C). 35.00 (*0-02-913350-5*) Free Pr.

Counseling & Therapy Skills. David G. Martin. 2nd ed. 1999. LC 00-709278. (Illus.). xiii, 313p. (C). pap. 23.95 (*1-57766-068-4*) Waveland Pr.

Counseling Chemically Dependent People with HIV Illness. Ed. by Michael Shernoff. 1992. (Journal of Chemical Dependency Treatment Ser.). 174p. LC 91-35376. pap. text 19.95 (*1-56023-016-9*, Harrington Park); LC 91-35375. lib. bdg. 49.95 (*1-56024-259-0*) Haworth Pr.

Counseling Children. Charles L. Thompson & Linda B. Rudolph. 2nd ed. 1988. LC 87-27670. 450p. (C). pap. 37.00 (*0-534-09000-1*) Brooks-Cole.

Counseling Children. Charles L. Thompson. 4th ed. 1995. LC 95-39260. (Counseling Ser.). 640p. mass mkt. 55.75 (*0-534-34002-4*) Brooks-Cole.

Counseling Children with Special Needs. Gill Brearley. 1997. LC 97-8094. 2995p. pap. 40.95 (*0-632-04151-X*) Blackwell Sci.

Counseling Clients with HIV Disease: Assessment, Intervention & Prevention. Mary Ann Hoffman. 1996. LC 95-37282. 324p. text 36.00 (*1-57230-063-9*, 0063) Guilford Pubns.

Counseling Depressed Women. Susan J. Dunlap. 1997. LC 97-14697. (Counseling & Pastoral Theology Ser.). pap. 16.00 (*0-664-25667-8*) Westminster John Knox.

Counseling Diverse Client Groups: An International Perspective on Human Social Functioning. Margaret R. Rodway. 1989. LC 89-9297. (Studies in Health & Human Services). 376p. lib. bdg. 99.95 (*0-88946-139-2*) E Mellen.

Counseling Elders & Their Families: Practical Techniques for Applied Gerontology. John J. Herr & John H. Weakland. 1979. LC 78-26365. (Adulthood & Aging Ser.: Vol. 2). 320p. 36.95 (*0-8261-2510-7*) Springer Pub.

Counseling Experience: Understanding & Living It. Michael E. Cavanagh. 1982. LC 81-17050. (Psychology-Counseling Ser.). 552p. (C). text 24.50 (*0-8185-0509-5*) Brooks-Cole.

Counseling Families: An Introduction to Marriage & Family Therapy. David L. Fenell & Barry K. Weinhold. 2nd rev. ed. 1997. 384p. (C). text 54.00 (*0-89108-245-X*, 9604) Love Pub Co.

Counseling for Psychosomatic Problems. Diana Sanders. 1996. LC 96-161016. (Counseling in Practice Ser.: Vol. 16). 160p. pap. 24.95 (*0-8039-7922-3*, 2936) Sage.

Counseling for Relapse Prevention. Terence T. Gorski & Merlene Miller. 1982. pap. 10.75 (*0-8309-0367-4*) Herald Pub Hse.

Counseling for Unplanned Pregnancy & Infertility. Everett L. Worthington. (Resources for Christian Counseling Ser.: Vol. 10). 284p. 22.99 (*0-8499-0588-5*) Nelson Ref & Elec Pub.

Counseling Gems: Thoughts for the Practitioner. J. Carnevale. 1989. LC 89-6588. vii, 176p. (Orig.). (C). pap. text 18.95 (*0-915202-88-3*) Accel Devel.

Counseling in Male Infertility. S. Lee. 1996. LC 95-43041. 224p. pap. 41.95 (*0-632-03906-X*) Blackwell Sci.

Counseling in Sports Medicine. Ed. by Richard Ray & Diane M. Wiese-Bjornstal. 1999. LC 98-40303. (Illus.). 376p. text 42.00 (*0-88011-527-0*, BRAY0527) Human Kinetics.

Counseling in the Asia-Pacific Region, 20. Ed. by Abdul H. Othman & Amir Awang. 1993. LC 92-45074. (Contributions in Psychology Ser.: No. 20). 168p. 67.00 (*0-313-28799-6*, GM8799, Greenwood Pr) Greenwood.

Counseling in the Rehabilitation Process: Community Services for Mental & Physical Disabilities. Gerald L. Gandy et al. 2nd ed. 1999. LC 99-19788. (Illus.). xxi, 336p. text 60.95 (*0-398-06969-7*) C C Thomas.

Counseling Individuals with Communication Disorders: Psychodynamic & Family Aspects. Walter J. Rollin. 2nd ed. 2000. LC 99-461973. 272p. text 49.99 (*0-7506-7178-5*) Buttrwrth-Heinemann.

Counseling Interactions with Traumatically Brain Injured Clients. Keith D. Cicerone. Ed. by Robert Fraser & David Clemmons. 1991. LC 91-73658. (Traumatic Brain Injury Rehabilitation Training Ser.). 46p. spiral bd. 36.95 (*1-878205-20-X*) St Lucie Pr.

Counseling Juvenile Offenders in Institutional Settings. Ed. by Sol Chaneles. 1983. (Journal of Offender Counseling, Services & Rehabilitation: Vol. 6, No. 3). 85p. pap. text 14.95 (*0-86656-170-6*) Haworth Pr.

Counseling Multiracial Families. Bea Wehrly et al. 1999. LC 99-6282. (Multicultural Aspects of Counseling Ser.). pap. 34.95 (*0-7619-1591-5*, 82662) Sage.

Counseling Older Adults. E. O'Leary. 1995. 224p. 45.00 (*1-56593-281-1*, 0605) Singular Publishing.

Counseling Older Persons: Careers, Retirement, Dying. Daniel Sinick. 1978. LC 77-21963. (New Vistas in Counseling Ser.: Vol. IV). 112p. 24.95 (*0-87705-312-X*, Kluwer Acad Hman Sci) Kluwer Academic.

Counseling Our Own: Lesbian-Gay Subculture Meets the Mental Health System. Charna Klein. 1986. (Illus.). 240p. (Orig.). (C). pap. 9.99 (*0-9617216-0-X*) Consult Serv NW.

Counseling Parents of Hearing-Impaired Children. David Luterman. 1979. text 15.00 (*0-316-53750-0*, Little Brwn Med Div) Lppncott W & W.

Counseling People with Communication Problems. Peggy Dalton. 1994. (Counseling in Action Ser.: Vol. 11). 192p. 57.95 (*0-8039-8894-X*, 9451); pap. 24.95 (*0-8039-8895-8*, 9452) Sage.

Counseling Persons with Communication Disorders & Their Families. David M. Luterman. 3rd ed. 1996. 196p. (C). pap. text 29.00 (*0-89079-680-7*, 7815) PRO-ED.

Counseling Persons with Physical Disabilities: Theoretical & Clinical Perspectives. Laura E. Marshak & Milton Seligman. 1993. LC 92-35809. 234p. (Orig.). (C). pap. text 29.00 (*0-89079-580-0*, 6594) PRO-ED.

*Counseling Problem Gamblers & Their Families: A Clinician's Guide.** Joseph W. Ciarrocchi. 2001. (Practical Resources for the Mental Health Professional Ser.). 224p. pap. 44.95 (*0-12-174653-4*) Acad Pr.

Counseling Psychology. Charles J. Gelso & Bruce R. Fretz. 1992. LC 91-13805. (William James Centennial Ser.). (Illus.). 480p. (C). text 89.00 (*0-03-027858-9*) Harcourt Coll Pubs.

Counseling Psychology. Charles A. Gelso & Bruce R. Fretz. 2nd ed. 2001. LC 00-105660. (Illus.). xx, 652p. (C). text 100.00 (*0-15-507156-4*) Harcourt Coll Pubs.

Counseling Skills for Health Professionals. Philip Burnard. 1989. (Therapy in Practice Ser.). 250p. pap. 15.95 (*0-412-32000-2*) Chapman & Hall.

Counseling Skills for Health Professionals. Philip Burnard. 3rd ed. 1999. LC 00-267407. (Illus.). ix, 256p. pap. (*0-7487-3976-9*) Nelson Thornes GBR. *Dist:* Intl Spec Bk.

Counseling Skills for Health Professionals. Philip Burnard. 2nd ed. 1994. 272p. 42.50 (*1-56593-312-5*, 0635) Singular Publishing.

Counseling Skills for Neurogenic Communication Disorders. Holland. 2001. pap. 40.00 net. (*0-7693-0117-7*) Singular Publishing.

Counseling Skills for Nurses. Verena Tschudin. 4th ed. 1995. pap. text 27.95 (*0-7020-1972-0*) Saunders.

Counseling Stutterers. Jane Fraser. 1982. (Publications on Stuttering: No. 18). 80p. pap. 2.00 (*0-933388-18-7*) Stuttering Fnd Am.

Counseling Supervision in Context. Michael Carroll & Elizabeth Holloway. 1998. LC 98-61426. (Counselling Supervision Ser.). (Illus.). ix, 206p. pap. 24.95 (*0-7619-5789-8*, 82342) Sage.

Counseling Techniques: An Outline & Overview. Frederick D. Harper & Gail C. Bruce. 1989. 225p. (C). pap. text 29.95 (*0-935392-04-1*) Douglass Pubs.

Counseling Techniques: Improving Relationships with Others, Ourselves, Our Families & Our Environment. Rosemary A. Thompson. 1996. LC 96-7064. 320p. 39.95 (*1-56032-397-3*) Taylor & Francis.

Counseling Techniques: Improving Relationships with Others, Ourselves, Our Families & Our Environment. Ed. by Rosemary A. Thompson. 1996. LC 96-7064. 320p. 79.95 (*1-56032-488-0*) Taylor & Francis.

Counseling Teenagers: The Complete Christian Guide to Understanding & Helping Adolescents. G. Keith Olson. 1984. 528p. (YA). (gr. 8-12). pap. 21.99 (*0-931529-67-0*) Group Pub.

Counseling the Alcoholic Group. Joseph F. Perez. 1986. 145p. text 22.95 (*0-89876-131-X*) Gardner Pr.

Counseling the Alcoholic Woman. Joseph F. Perez. 1993. 225p. (C). pap. text 24.95 (*1-55959-055-6*) Accel Devel.

Counseling the Bereaved: Conceptional Framework, Assessment & Counseling Strategies. Richard A. Dershimer. 1990. (Psychology Practitioner Guidebooks Ser.). 144p. text (*0-08-036816-6*); pap. text (*0-08-036815-8*) PPI GBR. *Dist:* Elsevier.

Counseling the Chemically Dependent: Theory & Practice. Rickey L. George & Therese S. Cristiani. 1990. LC 89-48178. 320p. (C). 93.00 (*0-13-181330-7*) P-H.

Counseling the Depressed. Archibald Hart. 1987. LC 86-28940. (Resources for Christian Counseling Ser.: Vol. 5). 275p. 22.99 (*0-8499-0582-6*) Nelson Ref & Elec Pub.

Counseling the Dying. Margaretta Bowers et al. 1990. LC 74-33146. (Downstate Psychoanalytic Institute Twenty-Fifth Anniversary Ser.). 192p. reprint ed. 20.00 (*0-87668-198-4*) Aronson.

Counseling the Female Alcoholic. Judith Goodman. 1999. 174p. pap. text 25.00 (*0-9663144-1-7*) Women & Addiction.

Counseling the Gifted: Developing the Whole Child. Cal Ross. 1990. pap. 6.00 (*0-89824-710-1*) Trillium Pr.

Counseling the Rainbow: Effectively Meeting the Needs of Gay & Lesbian Clients. Phil Travers. 2000. wbk. ed. 25.00 (*0-9701970-0-4*) My Life.

Counseling the Sick & Terminally Ill. Gregg R. Albers. (Resources for Christian Counseling Ser.: Vol. 20). 211p. 22.99 (*0-8499-0693-8*) Nelson Ref & Elec Pub.

Counseling the Terminally Ill: Sharing the Journey. George S. Lair. 1996. LC 96-12921. (Series in Death Education, Aging, & Health Care). 207p. (*1-56032-516-X*); 160p. pap. (*1-56032-517-8*) Tay Francis Ltd GBR. *Dist:* Taylor & Francis.

Counseling Today's Families. Herbert Goldenberg & Irene Goldenberg. 2nd ed. 1994. LC 93-29235. 330p. pap. 37.95 (*0-534-20526-7*); 3rd ed. 1997. LC 97-22977. 375p. pap. text 57.95 (*0-534-34655-3*) Brooks-Cole.

Counseling Troubled Older Adults: A Handbook for Pastors & Religious Caregivers. Harold George Koenig et al. 1997. LC 96-36718. 256p. 32.95 (*0-687-01731-9*) Abingdon.

Counseling with Choice Theory: The New Reality Therapy. William Glasser. 2001. 272p. pap. 13.00 (*0-06-095366-7*, Quil) HarperTrade.

Counseling with Native American Indians & Alaska Natives: Strategies for Helping Professionals. Roger D. Herring. 1999. LC 99-6396. (Multicultural Counseling Ser.). 89.95 (*0-7619-1386-6*, 82277) Sage.

Counseling with Parents of Handicapped Children: Guidelines for Improving Communication. Elizabeth J. Webster. 1977. 155p. text 31.00 (*0-8089-1036-1*, 794765, Grune & Strat) Harcrt Hlth Sci Grp.

Counseling Women: A Guide for Therapists. Helen V. Collier. 1982. (Illus.). 352p. 35.00 (*0-02-905840-6*) Free Pr.

Counseling Women over the Life Span. Judith A. Lewis et al. 1992. LC 91-77048. 307p. pap. 39.95 (*0-89108-222-0*, 9203) Love Pub Co.

Counselling: Approaches & Issues in Education. Helen Cowie & Andrea Pecherek. 1994. 176p. pap. (*1-85346-293-4*) David Fulton GBR. *Dist:* Taylor & Francis.

Counselling: Interdisciplinary Perspectives. Ed. by Brian Thorne & Wendy Dryden. 1993. LC 93-18531. x, 182p. pap. (*0-335-15678-9*) OpUniv Pr.

Counselling Adult Survivors of Child Sexual Abuse. Christiane Sanderson. 2nd ed. 1994. 288p. pap. 24.95 (*1-85302-252-7*) Taylor & Francis.

Counselling & Helping. Stephen Murgatroyd. 1986. (Psychology in Action Ser.). 170p. (C). pap. 19.95 (*0-901715-41-7*, 9910) Routledge.

Counselling & Therapy with Refugees & Victims of Trauma: Psychological Problems of Victims of War, Torture & Repression. Guus Van der Veer. 2nd ed. 1999. LC 97-45611. 206p. pap. 49.95 (*0-471-98227-X*) Wiley.

Counselling & Therapy with Refugees & Victims of Trauma: Psychological Problems of Victims of War, Torture, & Repression. Guus Van der Veer. 2nd ed. 1998. LC 97-45611. 206p. 100.00 (*0-471-98226-1*) Wiley.

Counselling Couples. Donald L. Bubenzer & John D. West. 1993. (Counselling in Action Ser.: Vol. 8). 160p. (C). 74.00 (*0-8039-8420-0*, 9157); pap. 25.95 (*0-8039-8421-9*, 9158) Sage.

Counselling Drug Users about HIV & AIDS. Geraldine Mulleady. 2nd ed. 1992. (Illus.). 224p. pap. 46.95 (*0-632-02939-0*) Blackwell Sci.

Counselling for Alcohol Problems. Richard Velleman. 1992. (Counselling in Practice Ser.). (Illus.). 160p. (C). 57.95 (*0-8039-8468-5*, 9227); pap. 24.95 (*0-8039-8469-3*, 9228) Sage.

Counselling for Anxiety Problems. Richard S. Hallam. 1992. (Illus.). 160p. (C). 57.95 (*0-8039-8460-X*, 9277); pap. 24.95 (*0-8039-8461-8*, 9278) Sage.

Counselling for Depression. Paul Gilbert. (Counselling in Practice Ser.). (Illus.). 1992. 160p. (C). 57.95 (*0-8039-8497-9*, 9171); 2nd ed. 2000. LC 00-269279. x, 228p. 74.00 (*0-7619-6576-9*, 85929) Sage.

Counselling for Fertility Problems. Jane Read. 1995. (Counselling in Practice Ser.). 240p. LC 95-67541. 57.95 (*0-8039-8949-0*, 1077); pap. 24.95 (*0-8039-8950-4*, 1078) Sage.

Counselling for Loss & Bereavement. Verena Tschudin. 1996. 190p. pap. text (*0-7020-2131-8*) W B Saunders GBR. *Dist:* Saunders.

Counselling for Sexual Abuse: A Therapist's Guide to Working with Adults, Children & Families. Kathy MacDonald et al. 1995. LC 96-141816. 336p. pap. text 49.95 (*0-19-558315-9*) OUP.

Counselling for Stress Problems. Windy Dryden & Stephen Palmer. 1994. (Counselling in Practice Ser.). 240p. LC 94-68660. 57.95 (*0-8039-8862-1*, 9483); pap. 25.95 (*0-8039-8863-X*, 9484) Sage.

Counselling for Toads: A Psychological Adventure. Robert De Board & Kenneth Grahame. 1998. LC 97-17524. (Illus.). 160p. (C). pap. 15.95 (*0-415-17429-5*) Routledge.

Counselling for Women. Janet Perry. 1993. LC 93-15402. (Counselling in Context Ser.). 128p. pap. (*0-335-19034-0*) OpUniv Pr.

Counselling Heroin & Other Drug Users. Paul Lockley. 1995. 315p. (C). pap. (*1-85343-304-7*) Free Assoc Bks GBR. *Dist:* Intl Spec Bk, NYU Pr.

Counselling in Health Care Settings. Robert Bor et al. 1998. LC 98-220788. 224p. 69.95 (*0-304-33985-7*); pap. 24.95 (*0-304-33986-5*) Continuum.

Counselling in HIV Infection & AIDS. J. Green & A. McCreaner. 2nd ed. 1996. 320p. pap. 39.95 (*0-632-03605-2*) Blackwell Sci.

Counselling in Independent Practice. Gabrielle Syme. 1994. LC 93-29252. (Counselling in Context Ser.). 128p. pap. (*0-335-19049-9*) OpUniv Pr.

Counselling in Medical Settings. Patricia East. 1995. LC 94-40669. (Counselling in Context Ser.). 160p. pap. (*0-335-19241-6*) OpUniv Pr.

Counselling in Obstetrics & Gynecology. Myra Hunter. 1994. (Communication & Counselling in Health Care Ser.). 160p. pap. text (*1-85433-119-1*) Brit Psychol Soc GBR. *Dist:* P H Brookes.

Counselling in the Voluntary Sector. Nicholas Tyndall. 1993. LC 93-18724. (Counselling in Context Ser.). (C). pap. (*0-335-19027-8*) OpUniv Pr.

Counselling Older People. Steve Scrutton. 1989. (C). (*0-340-42073-1*) Age Concern Eng GBR. *Dist:* St Mut.

Counselling Parents of Children with Chronic Illness or Disability. Hilton Davis. 1993. 144p. (Orig.). (C). text (*1-85433-091-8*) Brit Psychol Soc GBR. *Dist:* P H Brookes.

Counselling People with Cancer. Mary Burton & M. Watson. 1998. LC 97-34810. 214p. pap. 45.00 (*0-471-97813-2*) Wiley.

Counselling People with Disfigurement. Eileen Bradbury. 1996. LC 97-119022. (Communication & Counselling in Health Care Ser.). 138p. pap. text 28.00 (*1-85433-176-0*, 1760, BPS Bks) Stylus Pub VA.

Counselling Psychological Serv. D. Davies. 1997. LC 96-54224. (Counselling in Context Ser.). (*0-335-19165-7*); pap. (*0-335-19164-9*) OpUniv Pr.

Counselling Psychology: Integration of Theory, Research, & Supervised Practice. Petruska Clarkson. LC 97-9536. (Illus.). (C). 1998. xix, 337p. pap. 31.95 (*0-415-14523-6*); 1997. 360p. 89.95 (*0-415-14522-8*) Routledge.

Counselling Skills for Dietitians. Judy Gable. 1997. 208p. (Orig.). pap. 50.95 (*0-632-04261-3*) Blackwell Sci.

Counselling Skills for Doctors. Sam Smith & Kingsley Norton. 1999. LC 98-34015. x, 134p. (*0-335-20015-X*); (Illus.). 134p. pap. (*0-335-20014-1*) OpUniv Pr.

***Counselling Skills in Palliative Care.** John Davy & Susan Ellis. 160p. (Orig.). (C). (gr. 13). pap. 24.95 (*0-335-20312-4*) Routledge.

Counselling Skills Training: A Sourcebook of Activities for Trainers. Philip Burnard. 1993. 276p. (C). pap. text (*0-7494-0828-6*) Kogan Pg GBR. *Dist:* Nichols Pub.

***Counselling Survivors of Childhood Sexual Abuse.** Claire Burke Draucker. 2nd ed. 2000. LC 00-698192. (Counselling in Practice Ser.). 167p. 74.00 (*0-7619-6580-7*, 85933) Sage.

Counselling with Dreams & Nightmares. Delia Cushway & Robyn Sewell. 1992. (Counselling in Practice Ser.: Vol. 6). (Illus.). 160p. (C). 57.95 (*0-8039-8599-1*, 9115); pap. 24.95 (*0-8039-8600-9*, 9116) Sage.

Counselor & Client Notebooks: Large Size. Harvey Jackins. 1989. pap. 10.00 (*0-913937-39-8*) Rational Isl.

Counselor & Client Notebooks: Small Size. Harvey Jackins. 1989. pap. 10.00 (*0-913937-40-1*) Rational Isl.

Counselor & the Group: Integrating Theory, Training & Practice. James P. Trotzer. 2nd ed. 1989. LC 88-84112. 514p. (C). text 32.95 (*0-915202-87-5*) Accel Devel.

Counselor Intern's Handbook. Christopher Faiver et al. 1994. LC 94-18836. (Counseling Ser.). 165p. pap. 18.25 (*0-534-24870-5*) Brooks-Cole.

Counselor Preparation, 1993-95 Vol. 1: Programs & Personnel. Joseph W. Hollis & Richard A. Wantz. 8th ed. 1993. LC 80-644877. 566p. (C). pap. text 36.95 (*1-55959-045-9*) Accel Devel.

Counselor Preparation, 1993-95 Vol. II: Status, Trends, & Implications. Joseph W. Hollis & Richard A. Wantz. 8th ed. 1994. 250p. pap. text 27.95 (*1-55959-046-7*) Accel Devel.

Counselor Supervision: Principles, Process & Practice. Loretta Bradley. 3rd ed. 2000. LC 00-30469. (Accelerated Development Ser.). xxiv, 409p. 42.95 (*1-56032-873-8*) Taylor & Francis.

***Count on a Healthy Heart.** Annette Natow. 2002. 6.99 (*0-7434-2684-3*) PB.

Countdown to a Miracle: The Making of Me. Julie B. Carr. 1999. 296p. (YA). spiral bd. 12.95 (*0-9671428-0-6*) Motherly Way.

Counter-Dependency: The Flight from Intimacy. Barry K. Weinhold & Janae B. Weinhold. 1992. (Illus.). 251p. (Orig.). pap. 12.95 (*1-882056-00-0*) CICRCL Pr.

Countercurrent Chromatography: Theory & Practice. N. Bhushan Mandava. Ed. by Yoihciro Ito. 1988. (Chromatographic Science Ser.: Vol. 44). (Illus.). 752p. text 250.00 (*0-8247-7815-4*) Dekker.

Counterresistance. Gerald Schoenewolf. 1993. LC 93-3833. 320p. 50.00 (*1-56821-079-5*) Aronson.

Counterstrain Approaches in Osteopathic Manipulative Medicine. Harry Friedman et al. 2000. LC 00-131504. (Illus.). 98p. pap. 34.95 (*0-9701841-0-7*) S F I M M S Pr.

Countertransference. Ed. by Edmund Slakter. 1987. LC 87-21478. 257p. 50.00 (*0-87668-948-9*) Aronson.

Countertransference. Ed. by Herbert S. Strean. 1986. LC 86-22905. (Current Issues in Psychoanalytic Practice Ser.: Vol. 2, Nos. 3-4). 131p. text 29.95 (*0-86656-508-6*) Haworth Pr.

Countertransference. Benjamin Wolstein. 1995. LC 95-21055. (Master Work Ser.). 194p. pap. 35.00 (*1-56821-627-0*) Aronson.

Countertransference: The Therapist's Contribution to the Therapeutic Situation. Ed. by Lawrence J. Epstein & Arthur Feiner. 488p. reprint ed. 1993. LC 84-845014. pap. 60.00 (*1-56821-009-4*); 1990. LC 84-45014. 60.00 (*0-87668-662-5*) Aronson.

Countertransference: Theory, Technique, Teaching. Ed. by Athina Alexandris & Grigoris Vaslamatzid. 1993. 286p. pap. text (*1-85575-028-7*) Karnac Bks GBR. *Dist:* Other Pr LLC.

Countertransference & Older Clients. Bonnie Genevay. 1991. 192p. (C). pap. 31.95 (*0-8039-3851-9*, 3050) Sage.

Countertransference & Psychotherapeutic Technique: Teaching Seminars on Psychotherapy of the Borderline Adult. James F. Masterson. 1983. LC 83-3865. 320p. text 38.95 (*0-87630-334-3*) Brunner-Routledge.

Countertransference & Regression. L. Bryce Boyer. 1998. LC 97-51669. 288p. pap. 40.00 (*1-56821-706-4*) Aronson.

Countertransference & Related Subjects: Selected Papers. Harold F. Searles. 625p. 1999. pap. 39.95 (*0-8236-8021-5*, 21085); 1979. LC 77-92186. 82.50 (*0-8236-1085-3*) Intl Univs Pr.

Countertransference & the Treatment of Trauma. Constance J. Dalenberg. 2000. LC 00-24634. xii, 305p. text 39.95 (*1-55798-687-8*, 431-748A) Am Psychol.

Countertransference Enactment: How Institutions & Therapists Actualize Primitive Internal Worlds. Richard Shur. 1995. LC 93-11932. 272p. 50.00 (*1-56821-098-1*) Aronson.

Countertransference in Couples Therapy (Norton Professional Books) Ed. by Marion F. Solomon & Judith Siegel. 1997. LC 97-9583. 320p. 40.00 (*0-393-70244-8*) Norton.

Countertransference in Psychoanalytic Psychotherapy with Children & Adolescents. Ed. by John Tsiantis et al. 1996. LC 96-28231. (Efpp Clinical Monograph Ser.). 200p. 37.50 (*0-8236-1084-5*, BN01084) Intl Univs Pr.

Countertransference in Psychoanalytic Psychotherapy with Children & Adolescents. Ed. by John Tsiantis et al. 1996. 208p. pap. (*1-85575-111-9*) Karnac Bks GBR. *Dist:* Other Pr LLC.

Countertransference in Psychotherapy with Children & Adolescents. Ed. by Jerrold R. Brandell. 1992. LC 91-32229. 376p. 60.00 (*0-87668-481-9*) Aronson.

Countertransference in the Treatment of PTSD. Ed. by John P. Wilson & Jacob D. Lindy. 1994. LC 93-43029. 406p. 46.00 (*0-89862-369-3*, 2369) Guilford Pubns.

Countertransference Issues in Psychiatric Treatment. Glen O. Gabbard & Krin Gabbard. 1999. LC 99-10446. (Review of Psychiatry Ser.: Vol. 18). 12p. pap. text 27.50 (*0-88048-959-6*, 8959) Am Psychiatric.

Countertransference Triumphs & Catastrophes. Peter L. Giovacchini. LC 88-19471. 368p. 1993. pap. 60.00 (*0-87668-284-0*); 1988. 55.00 (*0-87668-879-2*) Aronson.

Counting for Something: Effective User Feedback in Mental Health Services. Ed. by Rob Leiper & Vida Field. 1993. 160p. (*1-85628-477-8*) Avebry GBR. *Dist:* Ashgate Pub Co.

Country Doctor's Book. Consumer Guide Editors. Ed. by B. Ted Boadway. 1997. 160p. mass mkt. 4.99 (*0-451-19423-3*, Sig) NAL.

Country Doctor's Book of Medical Wisdom & Cures. Michael J. Cummings. 1997. LC 97-150941. (Illus.). 160p. (*0-7853-2307-4*) Pubns Intl Ltd.

Country Folk Medicine. Elizabeth Janos. 1995. 160p. 6.98 (*0-88365-903-4*) Galahad Bks.

Country Medicines. Peter Rusholm. 1980. 15.00 (*0-85032-192-1*) St Mut.

Country Remedies: Traditional East Anglian Plant Remedies in the 20th Century. Gabrielle Hatfield. 1995. LC 95-182056. (Illus.). 160p. pap. 29.95 (*0-85115-563-4*, Boydell Pr) Boydell & Brewer.

Country Vet's Home Remedies for Cats. H. Ellen Whiteley. 1998. 192p. pap. 4.99 (*0-451-19526-4*, Sig) NAL.

Country Vet's Home Remedies for Dogs. William D. Fortney. 1998. 192p. pap. 4.99 (*0-451-19527-2*, Sig) NAL.

County Contracting for State Hospital Beds, Vol. 2. David Illig. 1995. 13p. pap. (*1-58703-037-3*) CA Res Bureau.

County Long-Term Care System Database, Camden County, New Jersey Model, 1992-1996. Text by Harmon T. Hicks. 1997. (Camden County Long Term Care Database Ser.). (Illus.). 100p. (*0-932965-35-0*) Old Cookbooks HT Hicks.

Couple & Family in Managed Care: Assessment, Evaluation & Treatment. Dennis A. Bagarozzi. 1996. LC 96-16041. (Mental Health Practice under Managed Care Ser.: No. 4). 176p. pap. text 21.95 (*0-87630-810-8*) Brunner-Routledge.

Couple & Family Therapy of Addiction. Jerome D. Levin. 1998. LC 97-29588. (Illus.). 368p. 60.00 (*1-56821-641-6*) Aronson.

Couple Therapy. Frank Bockus. 1993. LC 80-66920. 392p. pap. 50.00 (*1-56821-101-5*); 1980. LC 80-66923. 396p. 50.00 (*0-87668-412-6*) Aronson.

Couple Treatment. Judith C. Nelsen. 1998. LC 98-12033. 60.00 (*0-7657-0166-9*) Aronson.

Couple Who Fell in Hate: And Other Tales of Eclectic Psychotherapy. Gerald Schoenewolf. 1996. LC 95-32110. 288p. 45.00 (*1-56821-746-3*) Aronson.

Couples: A Medley of Models. Ed. by Barbara Jo Brothers. 1998. LC 98-8114. 157p. 29.95 (*0-7890-0531-X*) Haworth Pr.

Couples: Building Bridges. Ed. by Barbara J. Brothers. 1997. LC 96-12678. (Journal of Couples Therapy Ser.: Vol. 5, No. 4). 109p. (C). pap. 14.95 (*0-7890-0222-1*) Haworth Pr.

Couples & Change. Ed. by Barbara J. Brothers. 1996. LC 96-25514. 192p. 39.95 (*1-56024-828-9*) Haworth Pr.

Couples & Countertransference. Ed. by Barbara J. Brothers. 1995. LC 95-22643. 24.95 (*1-56024-746-0*) Haworth Pr.

Couples & the Tao of Congruence. Ed. by Barbara J. Brothers. 1997. LC 96-38931. (Journal of Couples Therapy Ser.: Vol. 6, Nos. 3-4). 168p. (C). pap. text 19.95 (*0-7890-0301-5*) Haworth Pr.

Couples Connecting: Prerequisites of Intimacy. Barbara Jo Brothers. 2000. LC 00-58133. 172p. (C). 29.95 (*0-7890-1165-4*) Haworth Pr.

Couples Connecting: Prerequisites of Intimacy. Ed. by Barbara Jo Brothers. 1999. LC 00-58133. 150p. (C). 49.95 (*0-7890-1164-6*) Haworth Pr.

Couples Group Psychotherapy: A Clinical Practice Model. Judith Coche & Erich Coche. 1990. LC 90-2216. 188p. text 29.95 (*0-87630-598-2*) Brunner-Routledge.

Couple's Guide to Fertility: The Complete Sympto-Thermal Method. R. J. Huneger & Rose Fuller. 1986. Orig. Title: Comprehensive Fertility Awareness & Natural Family Planning. 85p. reprint ed. pap. text 5.00 (*1-880220-00-8*) NW Family Srvs.

Couple's Guide to Fertility: Updated with the Newest Scientific Techniques That Can Help You Have a Baby. Gary S. Berger et al. rev. ed. 1994. LC 94-17765. 480p. pap. 16.95 (*0-385-47124-6*) Doubleday.

Couple's Hypnotic Dance: Creating Ericksonian Strategies in Marital Therapy. Carol J. Kershaw. 1991. LC 91-23466. 272p. text 36.95 (*0-87630-625-3*) Brunner-Routledge.

Couples Psychotherapy Treatment Planner. K. Daniel O'Leary et al. 1998. 272p. pap. 44.95 (*0-471-24711-1*); LC 98-15935. pap. text 175.00 incl. disk (*0-471-24710-3*) Wiley.

Couples, Sex, & Power: The Politics of Desire. Sally Foreman & Rudi Dallos. 1997. LC 97-12124. 160p. pap. (*0-335-19238-6*) OpUniv Pr.

Couples Therapy. Judith Siegel. 1995. LC 92-11152. 296p. reprint ed. pap. 40.00 (*1-56821-762-5*) Aronson.

Couples Therapy. Linda Berg-Cross. 2nd ed. 2001. LC 00-50552. pap. 49.95 (*0-7890-1454-8*); 456p. lib. bdg. 89.95 (*0-7890-1453-X*) Haworth Pr (Haworth Clinical).

Couples Therapy: A Nontraditional Approach. Daniel B. Wile. 1992. LC 93-103719. 248p. pap. 55.00 (*0-471-58989-6*) Wiley.

Couples Therapy: Feminist Perspectives. Ed. by Marcia Hill & Esther D. Rothblum. LC 96-39368. (Women & Therapy Monograph Ser.: Vol. 19, No. 3). 106p. (C). 1997. 29.95 (*0-7890-0017-2*); 1996. pap. text 14.95 (*1-56023-094-0*, Harrington Park) Haworth Pr.

Couples Therapy in Managed Care: Facing the Crisis. Ed. by Barbara Jo Brothers. 1999. LC 99-51401. (Journal of Couples Therapy Ser.: Vol. 8, Nos. 3/4). 130p. 39.95 (*0-7890-0788-6*) Haworth Pr.

Couples Therapy, Multiple Perspectives: In Search of Universal Threads. Intro. by Barbara J. Brothers. 1993. LC 92-32943. (Journal of Couples Therapy Ser.). (Illus.). 181p. lib. bdg. 39.95 (*1-56024-374-0*) Haworth Pr.

Couples, Trauma & Catastrophes. Ed. by Barbara Jo Brothers. 1998. LC 98-35597. 157p. 29.95 (*0-7890-0532-8*) Haworth Pr.

***Courage: One Woman's Dream & the Mighty Effort to Conquer Multiple Sclerosis.** Richard Trubo. 2001. LC 2001-37219. (Illus.). 320p. 27.50 (*1-56663-414-8*) I R Dee.

***Courage & Information for Life with Chronic Obstructive Pulmonary Disease: The Handbook for Patients, Families & Care Givers Managing COPD, Emphysema, Bronchitis.** Rick Carter et al. 2nd ed. 2001. pap. 29.95 (*1-882431-07-3*) New Technology.

***Courage to Care: A Caregiver's Companion Through the Stages of Alzheimer's.** Joanne Parrent. 2001. 320p. pap. 14.95 (*0-02-864202-3*) Mac USA.

Courage to Care: Responding to the Crisis of Children with AIDS. Ed. by Gary Anderson. 1990. pap. 15.95 (*0-87868-401-8*) Child Welfare.

Courage to Care: Responding to the Crisis of Children with AIDS. Ed. by Gary R. Anderson. 1990. 24.95 (*0-87868-384-4*, 3844) Child Welfare.

Courage to Fail: A Social View of Organ Transplants & Dialysis. Renee C. Fox & Judith P. Swazey. 2nd rev. ed. 2000. LC 2001-41589. (Illus.). 460p. pap. text 29.95 (*0-7658-0741-6*) Transaction Pubs.

Courage to Fail: A Social View of Organ Transplants & Dialysis. Renee C. Fox & Judith P. Swazey. rev. ed. 1979. LC 78-56332. (Illus.). xx, 438p. pap. text 6.95 (*0-226-25944-7*) U Ch Pr.

Courage to Grieve. Judy Tatelbaum. 1984. LC 84-47621. 192p. pap. 13.00 (*0-06-091185-9*, CN1185, Perennial) HarperTrade.

Courage to Heal - Third Edition - Revised & Expanded: A Guide for Women Survivors of Child Sexual Abuse. Ellen Bass & Laura Davis. 3rd rev. ed. 1994. LC 93-48353. 608p. pap. 22.50 (*0-06-095066-8*, Perennial) HarperTrade.

Course in Biology. Jeffrey J. Baker & Garland E. Allen. 3rd ed. 1979. LC 78-67451. (Life Sciences Ser.). text (*0-201-00308-2*) Addison-Wesley.

Course in Medical & Technical Terminology. Joseph R. Tebben. 2nd ed. 1997. (Illus.). 136p. (Orig.). (C). pap. text 21.33 (*0-8087-7851-X*) Pearson Custom.

Course of Instructions in the Biochemic Pathology of Disease: Includes Twelve Cell Salts of the Zodiac. George W. Carey. 1996. 31p. reprint ed. spiral bd. 11.50 (*0-7873-0145-0*) Hlth Research.

Course of Life Vol. 1: Infancy. Ed. by Stanley I. Greenspan & George H. Pollock. enl. rev. ed. 1989. LC 88-28465. 706p. 75.00 (*0-8236-1123-X*) Intl Univs Pr.

Course of Life Vol. 2: Early Childhood. Ed. by Stanley I. Greenspan & George H. Pollock. enl. rev. ed. 1990. (Course of Life Ser.: Vol. II). 429p. 70.00 (*0-8236-1124-8*, BN 01124) Intl Univs Pr.

Course of Life Vol. 3: Middle & Late Childhood. Ed. by Stanley I. Greenspan & George H. Pollock. enl. rev. ed. 1991. (Course of Life Ser.: Vol. III). 572p. 95.00 (*0-8236-1125-6*, BN 01125) Intl Univs Pr.

Course of Life Vol. 4: Adolescence. Ed. by Stanley I. Greenspan & George H. Pollock. enl. rev. ed. 1991. LC 88-28465. (Illus.). 530p. 77.50 (*0-8236-1126-4*) Intl Univs Pr.

Course of Life Vol. V: Early Adulthood, No. 5. Ed. by George H. Pollock & Stanley I. Greenspan. 1993. x, 420p. 62.50 (*0-8236-1127-2*) Intl Univs Pr.

Course of Life Vol. VI: Late Adulthood, No. 6. Ed. by George H. Pollock & Stanley I. Greenspan. 1993. 560p. 82.50 (*0-8236-1128-0*) Intl Univs Pr.

Course of Life Vol. VII: Completing the Journey. Ed. by George H. Pollock & Stanley I. Greenspan. 1998. LC 88-28465. (Course of Life Vol. VII Ser.: Vol. 7). 349p. 55.00 (*0-8236-1129-9*, BN 01129) Intl Univs Pr.

Coursebook on Language Disorders in Children. M. N. Hegde. 1995. 233p. (Orig.). (C). pap. text 49.95 (*1-56593-618-3*, 1286) Thomson Learn.

Coursebook on Scientific & Professional Writing for Speech-Language Pathology. M. N. Hegde. 2nd ed. 1998. LC 97-23984. (Singular Textbook Ser.). (Illus.). 436p. pap. text 53.95 (*1-56593-868-2*, 0574) Thomson Learn.

Court of Last Resort: Mental Illness & the Law. Carol A. Warren. LC 82-1839. (Illus.). (C). 1994. 27.50 (*0-226-87388-9*); 1984. 278p. pap. text 11.00 (*0-226-87389-7*) U Ch Pr.

Court-Ordered Insanity: Interpretive Practice & Involuntary Commitment. James A. Holstein. 1993. LC 92-35481. (Social Problems & Social Issues Ser.). 245p. pap. text 26.95 (*0-202-30449-3*); lib. bdg. 48.95 (*0-202-30448-5*) Aldine de Gruyter.

Court Reporters Guide to Medical Terminology. Nathaniel Weiss. 1996. 68p. pap. text 15.95 (*1-881859-18-5*) Natl Ct Report.

Courtroom Medicine: Abdominal Injuries, Vols. 10 & 10A. Jules R. Kalisch & Harold Williams. 1973. ring bd. 417.00 (*0-8205-1253-2*) Bender.

Courtroom Medicine: Death Marshall Houts & Irwin H. Haut. 1966. (Courtroom Medicine Ser.). ring bd. 781.00 (*0-8205-1236-2*) Bender.

Courtroom Medicine: The Low Back, Vols. 1, 1a & 1b. Leo Gelfand & Raoul D. Magana. 1962. (Courtroom Medicine Ser.). ring bd. 749.00 (*0-8205-1297-4*) Bender.

Courtroom Medicine, the Neck, Set, Vols. 2, 2a & 2b. Leon Wolfstone & Jack Leibman. 1965. (Courtroom Medicine Ser.). ring bd. 674.00 (*0-8205-1237-0*) Bender.

Couts Economiques de la Maladie pour les Menages au Milieu Rural du Burkina Faso. Ed. by Rainer Sauerborn et al. 1996. (Medizin in Entwicklungslandern Ser.: Bd. 41). (FRE.). xvi, 253p. 44.95 (*3-631-49651-6*) P Lang Pubng.

Covered Wagon Remedy Chest. (*0-937844-01-2*) Caverne Pub.

Covert Conditioning: A Review & Evaluation. Ed. by Hans J. Eysenck & Stanley J. Rachman. 1979. (Advances in Behaviour Research & Therapy Ser.: Vol. 2, No. 2). pap. 23.00 (*0-08-024271-5*, Pergamon Pr) Elsevier.

Cowan & Steel's Manual for the Identification of Medical Bacteria. Ed. by G. I. Barrow & R. K. Feltham. 3rd ed. 1993. (Illus.). 351p. (C). text 90.00 (*0-521-32611-7*) Cambridge U Pr.

Cows Can Be Purple. Sadie Dreikurs. 1986. pap. 9.95 (*0-918560-32-2*) Adler Sch Prof Psy.

Cox-Inhibitors: Pocketbook Edition. Bird. 2000. (*1-85317-795-4*) Martin Dunitz GBR. *Dist:* Blackwell Sci.

Coxsackieviruses: A General Update. M. Bendinelli & H. Friedman. 1988. LC 88-4234. (Infectious Agents & Pathogenesis Ser.). (Illus.). 450p. (C). text 120.00 (*0-306-42725-7*, Kluwer Plenum) Kluwer Academic.

Coyote Medicine: Lessons from Native American Healing. Lewis Mehl-Madrona. 304p. 1998. per. 13.00 (*0-684-83997-0*, Fireside); 1997. LC 96-32714. 24.00 (*0-684-80271-6*, Scribner Pap Fic) S&S Trade Pap.

CP Magnetic Resonance Imaging. Haacke. disk (*0-471-35344-2*) Wiley.

CP "Teach" Expert Coding Made Easy: 1995 Version. Patrice T. Morin-Spatz. 9th rev. ed. 1996. (Illus.). 368p. (C). text 48.00 (*0-923369-31-7*) MedBooks.

CP "Teach" Instructor's Manual. Patrice T. Morin-Spatz. 1996. (Illus.). 447p. (C). ring bd. 199.95 (*0-923369-33-3*) MedBooks.

CP "Teach" Student Workbook. Patrice T. Morin-Spatz. 9th rev. ed. 1996. (Illus.). 96p. (C). text 22.95 (*0-923369-32-5*) MedBooks.

CP "Teach" Workbook with Answers. Patrice T. Morin. 1996. (Illus.). 96p. pap. 29.95 (*0-923369-34-1*) MedBooks.

CPR. Ed. by National Safety Council Staff. 4th ed. 2000. LC 00-65548. (Illus.). 48p. (C). pap. text 15.95 (*0-7637-1331-7*, 1331-7) Jones & Bartlett.

CPR: 1992 Guidelines. National Safety Council Staff. 2nd ed. 1993. (Emergency Care Ser.). 120p. (C). pap. text, tchr. ed. 15.00 (*0-86720-811-2*) Jones & Bartlett.

Cpr: Resuscitation of the Arrested Heart. Ed. by Max H. Weil et al. 1998. LC 98-38027. (Illus.). 352p. (C). text 55.00 (*0-7216-4817-7*) Saunders.

CPR - Cardiopulmonary Resuscitation: Evaluating Performance & Potential. Mickey S. Eisenberg. Ed. by Lawrence Bergner. 1982. (Emergency Health Services Review Ser.: Vol. 1, No. 3). 70p. pap. text 19.95 (*0-917724-58-5*) Haworth Pr.

CPR for the Professional Rescuer. American Red Cross Staff. 1993. LC 92-41664. (Illus.). (*0-8016-0706-X*) Mosby Inc.

CPR Instructor's Manual. National Safety Council Staff. 2nd ed. 1997. (Emergency Care Ser.). (Illus.). 144p. pap. text, tchr. ed. 15.00 (*0-7637-0582-9*, 0582-9) Jones & Bartlett.

CPR Manual. National Safety Council Staff & Alton L. Thygerson. (First Aid Ser.). (C). 1992. pap. text 12.50

(0-86720-192-4); 1991. 10.00 (0-86720-233-5); 1991. (Illus.). VHS 195.00 (0-86720-159-2, 159-2) Jones & Bartlett.

CPR Manual: 1992 Guidelines. National Safety Council Staff. 1993. LC 92-40649. 128p. pap. text 13.75 (0-86720-784-1) Jones & Bartlett.

CPR Manual: SOS Version. National Safety Council Staff & SOS Staff. 1995. (Illus.). 31p. (C). pap. text 1.22 (0-7637-0037-1, 0037-1) Jones & Bartlett.

CPR Review Manual. National Safety Council Staff. (Emergency Care Ser.). (Illus.). 32p. (C). 1994. LC 93-46698. pap. text 3.75 (0-86720-849-X, 849-X); 2nd ed. 1998. pap. text 5.30 (0-7637-0894-1, 0894-1) Jones & Bartlett.

CPR Review Manual. Ed. by National Safety Council Staff. 3rd ed. 2002. LC 2001-50701. (Illus.). 32p. (C). pap. text 5.50 (0-7637-1466-6, 1466-6) Jones & Bartlett.

CPR Teaching Package. National Safety Council Staff. 2nd ed. 1997. (Emergency Care Ser.). 395.00 (0-7637-0560-8) Jones & Bartlett.

CPS Review Module: Behavioral Science in Business, No. 1. Betty L. Schroeder & Diane Routhier-Graf. 2nd ed. 1986. 200p. pap. text 19.95 (0-471-84353-9) P-H.

CPT: Beyond the Basics. Gail I. Smith. rev. ed. 2000. (Illus.). 144p. (C). pap. text 60.00 (1-58426-037-8, AC400800) Am Hlth Info.

***CPT & HCPCS Coding Made Easy: A Comprehensive Guide to CPT & HCPCS Coding for Health Care Professionals.** James B. Davis. Ed. by Kathryn Swanson. 5th ed. 2000. pap. text 39.95 (1-57066-183-9, ME127) Practice Mgmt Info.

CPT Coding & Regulatory Compliance for Laboratory. 1997. 129p. 99.00 (1-889115-15-0) Med Learn.

CPT Coding & Regulatory Compliance for Radiology. 1997. 130p. 99.00 (1-889115-16-9) Med Learn.

***CPT Coding Essentials 2001.** Ingenix, Inc. Staff. (Illus.). pap. 99.95 (1-56337-378-5) Ingenix Inc.

CPT Coding Handbook: With Answers, 1999 Edition. Rita A. Scichilone. 1999. 136p. pap. text 45.00 (1-55648-274-4) AHPI.

CPT Coding Handbook 1999: Without Answers. Rita A. Scichilone. 1999. 128p. pap. (1-55648-275-2) AHPI.

CPT Companion 2000: Frequently Asked Questins about CPT Coding. 2000. (Illus.). 49.95 (1-57947-031-9) AMA.

CPT Handbook for Psychiatrists. Chester W. Schmidt, Jr. 2nd ed. 1998. LC 98-17949. ix, 157p. spiral bd. 26.00 (0-88048-839-5, 8839) Am Psychiatric.

CPT 1999 Coder's Choice. Ed. by American Medical Association Staff. rev. ed. 1998. pap. text 54.95 (1-57066-095-6, 9901) Practice Mgmt Info.

CPT 1999 Codes on Disk. Ed. by American Medical Association Staff. rev. ed. 1998. pap. 149.95 incl. disk (1-57066-098-0, 9908) Practice Mgmt Info.

***CPT Plus! 2001: A Comprehensive Guide to Current Procedural Terminology.** annuals American Medical Association Staff. Ed. by Kathryn Swanson. 2001. 875p. pap. text 54.95 (1-57066-214-2, 21012) Practice Mgmt Info.

CPT, 2000. American Heart Association Staff. 1999. (C). ring bd. 60.00 (1-57947-019-X) Thomson Learn.

CPT 2000. Ed. by American Medical Association Staff. 1999. 54.95 (1-57066-157-X, 20002) Practice Mgmt Info.

CPT 2000: Spanish Edition. 1999. (SPA.). 640p. spiral bd. 51.95 (1-57947-030-0) AMA.

CPT 2000 Changes: An Insider's View. American Medical Association Staff. 2000. (Coding Ser.). (Illus.). 450p. pap. text 49.95 (1-57947-091-2) AMA.

CPT 2000 Coder's Choice. Ed. by American Medical Association Staff. 1999. (Illus.). pap. text 54.95 (1-57066-156-1, 20001) Practice Mgmt Info.

CPT 2000 Codes on Disk. Ed. by American Medical Association Staff. 1999. pap. text 149.95 incl. disk (1-57066-159-6, 20008) Practice Mgmt Info.

CPT 2000 Deluxe. Ed. by American Medical Association Staff. 1999. text 59.95 (1-57066-158-8, 20004) Practice Mgmt Info.

***CPT 2001: Coder's Choice.** annuals American Medical Association Staff. 520p. 2001. (Illus.). pap. text 59.95 (1-57066-189-8, 21001); 2000. spiral bd. 69.95 (1-57066-190-1, 21005); 2000. text 59.95 (1-57066-191-X, 21004) Practice Mgmt Info.

***CPT 2001: Timesaver Binder.** annuals American Medical Association Staff. 2000. 520p. ring bd. 64.95 (1-57066-193-6, 21003) Practice Mgmt Info.

CPT 2000 TimeSaver Binder. Ed. by American Medical Association Staff. 1999. ring bd. 59.95 (1-57066-160-X, 20003) Practice Mgmt Info.

***CPT 2002: Professional Edition.** 2001. 640p. pap. 74.95 (1-57947-221-4) AMA.

CPT/HCPCS for Physician Office Coding: 2000 Edition. Therese Jorwic. rev. ed. 2000. 144p. pap. text 60.00 (1-58426-035-1, AC401000) Am Hlth Info.

***CQ Researcher on Controversies in Medicine & Science.** CQ Editors. 2001. LC 00-65983. (Best of the CQ Researcher Ser.). (Illus.). 240p. 29.95 (1-56802-671-4, CQ Pr Lib Ref) CQ Pr.

CQI & the Renovation of an American Health Care System: A Culture under Construction. Mary J. Ryan & William P. Thompson. 1997. LC 97-3243. 216p. 27.00 (0-87389-417-0, H0960) ASQ Qual Pr.

CQI System for Healthcare: How the Williamsport Hospital Brings Quality to Life. Tim Mannello. 1995. LC 94-46508. 318p. 39.95 (0-527-76290-3) Product Pr.

Crack: Cocaine Squared. Christina Dye. rev. ed. 2000. pap. 0.50 (0-89230-214-3) Do It Now.

Crack & Other Addictions: Old Realities & New Challenges for Child Welfare. Child Welfare League of America Staff. 1990. 255p. pap. 14.95 (0-87868-409-3) Child Welfare.

Crack Babies: A National Epidemic. 1991. (Illus.). 37p. (Orig.). pap. text 15.00 (0-941375-37-4) DIANE Pub.

Crack Cocaine: A Challenge for Prevention. Ed. by Robert L. DuPont. 1994. (Illus.). 71p. (Orig.). (C). pap. text 25.00 (0-7881-0579-5) DIANE Pub.

Crack Cocaine: A Practical Treatment Approach for the Chemically Dependent. Barbara C. Wallace. 1991. LC 90-2683. 304p. text 43.95 (0-87630-604-0) Brunner-Routledge.

Crack, Cocaine, Methamphetamine & Ice: What Every One of Us Must Know about These Public Enemies. Leslie E. Moser. 1990. 336p. 19.95 (1-878938-00-2) Mlti-Media Prodns.

Crack, Powder Cocaine & Heroin: Drug Purchase & Use Patterns in Six U. S. Cities. K. Jack Riley. 1999. (Illus.). 39p. (C). pap. text 15.00 (0-7881-7627-7) DIANE Pub.

Crackdown on Cancer with Good Nutrition. Ruth Y. Long. 2nd rev. ed. 1991. 172p. reprint ed. pap. 10.00 (0-916243-15-X) Nutrit Educ.

Crackhouse: Notes from the End of the Line. Terence T. Williams. 1992. (Illus.). 192p. 17.95 (0-201-56759-8) Addison-Wesley.

Cracking the AP Psychology 2000-2001. Princeton Review Publishing Staff. 2000. (Princeton Review Ser.). 336p. pap. 17.00 (0-375-75480-6) PRP NY.

Cracking the Boards: USMLE Step 2. John Mariani. 2nd ed. 2000. 544p. pap. 29.95 (0-375-76164-0) PRP NY.

Cradle of Violence: Essays on Psychiatry, Psychoanalysis & Literature. Stephen Wilson. 1995. LC 95-14278. (Forensic Focus Ser.: No. 2). pap. 29.95 (1-85302-306-X) Taylor & Francis.

Craft of Psychotherapy: Twenty-Seven Studies. I. H. Paul. 1989. LC 89-17492. 320p. 55.00 (0-87668-826-1) Aronson.

Craft of Sociology: Epistemological Preliminaries. Pierre Bourdieu et al. 1991. xvi, 271p. (C). pap. 27.95 (3-11-011940-4); lib. bdg. 62.90 (3-11-013004-1) De Gruyter.

Craft of the Warrior. Robert L. Spencer. 1993. LC 93-8530. 211p. (Orig.). pap. 14.95 (1-883319-05-6) Frog Ltd CA.

Crafting Science: A Sociohistory of the Quest for the Genetics of Cancer. Joan H. Fujimura. 1996. LC 96-32222. (Illus.). 352p. 48.95 (0-674-17553-0) HUP.

Crafts in Therapy & Rehabilitation. Margaret Drake. 2nd ed. 1998. LC 98-42014. (Illus.). 272p. pap. 33.00 (1-55642-396-9, 33969) SLACK Inc.

Craig's Care of the Newly Born Infant. T. L. Turner et al. 8th ed. 1988. (Illus.). 600p. pap. text (0-443-03342-0) Church.

Crane-Style Chi Gong & Its Therapeutic Effects. Daoshing Ni. 1984. (Illus.). 68p. (Orig.). pap. 10.95 (0-937064-10-6) SevenStar Comm.

Cranial & Facial Adjusting Technique. abr. ed. 1988. 170p. spiral bd. 49.00 (0-917628-08-X) Coraco.

Cranial Computed Tomography in Infants & Children. Eric N. Faerber. 1991. (Clinics in Developmental Medicine Ser.: No. 93). (Illus.). 237p. (C). text (0-521-41213-7) Mc Keith Pr GBR. *Dist:* Cambridge U Pr.

Cranial Hemorrhage in the Full-Term Newborn Infant. Ed. by Paul Govaert. 1994. (Clinics in Developmental Medicine Ser.: No. 129). (Illus.). 223p. (C). text 69.95 (0-521-45149-3) Cambridge U Pr.

Cranial Manipulation Roots References. 1984. 113p. 18.00 (0-917628-03-9) Coraco.

Cranial Manipulation Theory & Practice: Osseous & Soft Tissue Approaches. L. Chaitow. 1999. text 99.00 (0-443-06439-3) Harcrt Hlth Sci Grp.

Cranial Manipulation Theory & Practice: Osseous & Soft Tissue Approaches. Leon Chaitow. 1999. LC 99-36445. (0-443-05803-2) Church.

Cranial Microsurgery: Approaches & Techniques. Laligam N. Sekhar et al. 1998. LC 97-25004. (Illus.). 704p. 299.00 (0-86577-698-9) Thieme Med Pubs.

Cranial MRI & CT. Ed. by S. Howard Lee et al. 4th ed. 1999. LC 97-28648. (Illus.). 875p. text 179.00 (0-07-037689-1) McGraw-Hill Prof.

Cranial Nerves. Andre LeBlanc. 2nd ed. 1996. (Illus.). 312p. 315.00 (3-540-58702-0) Spr-Verlag.

Cranial Nerves: Anatomy, Imaging, Vascularisation. Andre LeBlanc. Tr. by David Le Vay from FRE. 2nd enl. rev. ed. 1995. LC 95-8410. Orig. Title: Anatomy & Imaging of the Cranial Nerves. (Illus.). (0-387-58702-0) Spr-Verlag.

Cranial Nerves of the Coelacanth, Latimeria Chalumnae - Osteichtyes: Sarcoterygii: Actinistia-Comparisons with Other Cranista: Actinistia - Comparisons with Other Craniata. R. G. Northcutt & W. E. Bemis. 1993. (Journal: Vol. 42, Suppl. 1, 1993). (Illus.). x, 76p. 81.00 (3-8055-5802-3) S Karger.

Cranial Rhythmic Impulse Approaches in Osteopathic Manipulative Medicine. Harry Friedman et al. 2000. LC 00-133447. (SFIMMS Series in Neuromusculoskeletal Medicine). (Illus.). 253p. pap. 49.95 (0-9701841-2-3) S F I M M S Pr.

Cranial Sutures: Analysis, Morphology & Manipulative Strategies. Marc G. Pick. 1999. LC 98-74358. (Illus.). xxv, 469p. (C). 80.00 (0-939616-29-7) Eastland.

Cranicocerebral Trauma. Ed. by H. Krayenbuehl et al. 1981. (Progress in Neurological Surgery Ser.: Vol. 10). (Illus.). xiv, 402p. 259.25 (3-8055-0134-X) S Karger.

Cranio Cervical Syndrome. Howard Vernon. 2001. (Illus.). 280p. text 80.00 (0-7506-4495-8) Buttrwrth-Heinemann.

Craniofacial & Maxillofacial Surgery in Children & Young Adults. Jeffrey C. Posnick. Ed. by Allan Ross. 1999. LC 98-40586. (Illus.). 1195p. (C). text 395.00 (0-7216-7710-X) Saunders.

Craniofacial Anthropometry: Practical Measurement of the Head & Face for Clinical, Surgical & Research Use. John C. Kolar & Elizabeth M. Salter. 1996. LC 96-7346. (Illus.). 358p. text 76.95 (0-398-06616-7); pap. text 55.95 (0-398-06617-5) C C Thomas.

Craniofacial Deformities. D. J. David et al. 1989. (Illus.). 147p. 258.00 (0-387-96969-1, 2655) Spr-Verlag.

Craniofacial Growth During Adolescence. Ed. by Katherine A. Ribbens & D. S. Carlson. 1987. (Craniofacial Growth Ser.: Vol. 20). (Illus.). 226p. 49.00 (0-929921-16-X) UM CHGD.

Craniofacial Growth Series. Date not set. (0-929921-00-3) UM CHGD.

Craniofacial Growth Theory & Orthodontic Treatment. Donald H. Enlow et al. Ed. by David S. Carlson. 1990. (Craniofacial Growth Ser.: Vol. 23). (Illus.). 235p. 49.00 (0-929921-19-4) UM CHGD.

Craniofacial Identification in Forensic Medicine. Ed. by John G. Clement & David L. Ranson. 1998. LC 97-42826. (An Arnold Publication). (Illus.). 320p. text (0-340-60759-9) E A GBR. *Dist:* OUP.

Craniofacial Morphogenesis & Dysmorphogenesis. Ed. by K. L. Vig & A. R. Burdi. 1988. (Craniofacial Growth Ser.: Vol. 21). (Illus.). 221p. 39.00 (0-929921-17-8) UM CHGD.

Craniofacial Morphology of Pan Paniscus. D. L. Cramer. Ed. by F. S. Szalay. 1977. (Contributions to Primatology Ser.: Vol. 10). (Illus.). 41.75 (3-8055-2391-2) S Karger.

Craniofacial Morphology of the Sulawesi Macaques: Multivariate Analysis As a Tool in Systematics. Gene H. Albrecht. 1977. (Contributions to Primatology Ser.: Vol. 13). (Illus.). 64.50 (3-8055-2694-6) S Karger.

Craniofacial Prostheses: Anaplastology & Osseointegration. Per-Ingvar Branemark & Marcelo F. Oliveira. 1997. LC 96-50068. 136p. text 98.00 (0-86715-321-0) Quint Pub Co.

Craniofacial Surgery. Ernesto P. Caronni. 1985. 620p. 89.50 (0-316-12877-5, Little Brwn Med Div) Lppncott W & W.

Craniofacial Surgery. Kant Y. Lin et al. 2001. LC 00-66128. 395p. text (0-7216-8701-6) Saunders.

Craniofacial Surgery. Ed. by Daniel Marchac. 1987. (Illus.). 495p. 318.00 (0-387-16924-5) Spr-Verlag.

Craniofacial Trauma: An Interdisciplinary Approach. Ed. by Nicholas Jones. 1997. LC 97-7170. (Oxford Medical Publications). (Illus.). 224p. (C). text 98.50 (0-19-262856-9) OUP.

Craniofacial Trauma Imaging. Gentry. 1998. text (0-7216-5423-1) Saunders.

Craniology of the North Pacific Coast. Bruno Oetteking. LC 73-3533. (Jessup North Pacific Expedition Ser.: No. 11). reprint ed. 115.00 (0-404-58111-0) AMS Pr.

Craniomaxillofacial Fractures: Principles of Internal Fixation Using the AO-ASIF Techniques. Alex M. Greenberg. 1993. LC 92-2423. (Illus.). 211p. 165.00 (0-387-97902-6) Spr-Verlag.

Craniomaxillofacial Reconstructive & Corrective Bone Surgery: Principles of Internal Fixation Using AO-ASIF Techniques. Ed. by Alex M. Greenberg & J. Prein. 2000. LC 96-35162. (Illus.). 896p. 195.00 (0-387-94686-1) Spr-Verlag.

***Craniopharyngioma: Surgical Treatment.** Broggi. 1996. 160p. (C). 120.00 (3-540-75001-0) Spr-Verlag.

Craniopharyngioma: Surgical Treatment. Ed. by G. Broggi. 1995. (Illus.). 160p. pap. 102.00 (4-431-75001-0) Spr-Verlag.

Craniosacral Biodynamics: The Breath of Life, Biodynamics, & Fundamental Skills. Franklyn Sills. 2001. LC 00-67885. (Illus.). 500p. (C). pap. 25.00 (1-55643-354-9) North Atlantic.

Craniosacral Therapy. John E. Upledger & Jon Vredevoogd. 1983. LC 82-82505. (Illus.). 399p. 49.50 (0-939616-01-7) Eastland.

Craniosacral Therapy: Touchstone for Natural Healing. John E. Upledger. 2000. LC 00-45247. (Illus.). 150p. (C). pap. 14.95 (1-55643-368-9) North Atlantic.

Craniosacral Therapy Vol. II: Beyond the Dura. John E. Upledger. 1987. LC 82-82505. (Illus.). 260p. (C). text 45.00 (0-939616-05-X) Eastland.

Craniosacral Therapy in Practice: A Manual for Physical Therapists. 2002. 224p. pap. 49.95 (0-7506-4961-5) Buttrwrth-Heinemann.

Craniosynostosis. Ed. by Guido Galli. 1984. 280p. 158.00 (0-8493-5206-1, RJ482, CRC Reprint) Franklin.

Crash Course Gastroenterology. Emma Lam & Martin Lombard. 1999. text (0-7234-3153-1) Harcourt.

***Crash Course House Officer's Guide.** Danny Horton-Szar. 2001. (Illus.). 100p. pap. (0-7234-3197-3) Mosby Inc.

Crash Course in Motor Vehicle Injury Prevention: Participant Manual. Mary Jagin et al. Ed. by Laurie Flaherty & Susan MacLean. unabr. ed. 1996. (Illus.). 238p. (Orig.). pap. text 15.00 (0-935890-04-1) Emerg Nurses IL.

Crash Course in Motor Vehicle Injury Prevention & Campaign Safe & Sober Materials Set 1996. (Illus.). pap. 95.00 incl. sl. (0-935890-08-4) Emerg Nurses IL.

***Crash Course Surgery.** Helen Sweetland & James Cook. 2000. (Illus.). 288p. pap. 22.95 (0-7234-3154-X) Mosby Inc.

Crash Injuries - How & Why They Happen: A Primer For Anyone Who Cares About People in Cars. 1993. (0-9637057-0-9) Hyde Assocs.

Crashing the Boards. Benjamin Yeh. 2nd ed. 1999. LC 99-24903. (Illus.). 184p. pap. text 19.95 (0-7817-1977-1) Lppncott W & W.

Crassulacean Acid Metabolism, Vol. 114. Ed. by K. Winter & J. A. Smith. 1996. (Ecological Studies). (Illus.). 449p. 160.00 (0-387-58104-9) Spr-Verlag.

Crassulacean Acid Metabolism: Analysis of an Ecological Adaptation. M. Kluge & Irwin P. Ting. 1978. LC 78-12658. (Ecological Studies: Vol. 30). (Illus.). 210p. 71.95 (0-387-08979-9) Spr-Verlag.

Craving Brain. Ronald A. Ruden. 2nd ed. 2000. LC 2001-272141. (Illus.). 272p. pap. 13.00 (0-06-092899-9, Perennial) HarperTrade.

Craving for Ecstasy: How Our Passions Become Addictions & What We Can Do about Them. Harvey Milkman & Stanley Sunderwirth. 1998. LC 98-21171. 240p. reprint ed. pap. 16.00 (0-7879-4132-8) Jossey-Bass.

Crazy All the Time: Life, Lessons, & Insanity on the Psych Ward of Bellevue Hospital. Frederick L. Covan & Carol Kahn. 1994. LC 93-35900. 282p. 23.00 (0-671-79159-1) S&S Trade.

Crazy for You: The Making of Women's Madness. Jill Astbury. 1996. 240p. pap. 22.95 (0-19-553768-8) OUP.

Crazy Therapies: What are They? Do They Work? Margaret T. Singer. 1996. LC 96-16107. 263p. 23.00 (0-7879-0278-0) Jossey-Bass.

***Crazy Visitation: A Chronicle of Illness & Recovery.** Saundra Murray Nettles. 2001. LC 00-54493. xviii, 164p. 22.95 (0-8203-2299-7) U of Ga Pr.

CRC Desk Reference of Clinical Pharmacology. Manuchair S. Ebadi. 1997. LC 97-29883. (CRC Desk References Ser.). 528p. lib. bdg. 99.95 (0-8493-9683-2) CRC Pr.

CRC Handbook of Biochemistry & Molecular Biology: Cumulative Index. Ed. by Gerald D. Fasman. 3rd ed. 1977. 295p. 68.00 (0-8493-0511-X, CRC Reprint) Franklin.

CRC Handbook of Chromatography Vols. III-IV: Drugs. R. N. Gupta. 1988. 432p. 250.00 (0-8493-3094-7);Vol. 4. 392p. 250.00 (0-8493-3092-0, RS189);Vol. 5. 368p. 240.00 (0-8493-3093-9) CRC Pr.

CRC Handbook of Experimental Aspects of Oral Biochemistry. Ed. by Eugene P. Lazzari. 1983. 384p. 145.00 (0-8493-3162-5, QP146, CRC Reprint) Franklin.

CRC Handbook of Hospital Acquired Infections. Richard P. Wenzel. 1981. 656p. 357.00 (0-8493-0202-1, RA969, CRC Reprint) Franklin.

CRC Handbook of Human Immunology. Mary S. Leffell et al. 1997. LC 96-45395. 656p. 119.95 (0-8493-0134-3) CRC Pr.

CRC Handbook of Nutritive Value of Processed Food: Animal Foodstuffs, Vol. II. Ed. by Miloslav Rechcigl, Jr. 1982. 520p. 155.00 (0-8493-3953-7, TX551, CRC Reprint) Franklin.

CRC Handbook of Pharmacology of Aging see Handbook of Pharmacology of Aging

Create Your Own Perfumes Using Essential Oils. Christine Wildwood. 1995. 176p. pap. text (0-7499-1533-1) Piatkus Bks GBR. *Dist:* London Brdge.

Creatine. Richard A. Passwater. 1997. (Good Health Guides). 48p. pap. 3.95 (0-87983-868-X, 3868XK, Keats Pubng) McGraw-Hill Trade.

Creating a Healthier Community: The Story of Ashtabula County Medical Center. Michele K. Lehman. 1997. 144p. 20.00 (0-929690-32-X) Herit Pubs AZ.

Creating a Healthy Heart, I Did It Why Don't You. 1996. LC 97-185294. (Illus.). 180p. (Orig.). pap. 15.00 (0-9654590-0-4, 520) Hlthy Heart.

Creating a Memory of Causal Relationships: An Integration of Empirical & Explanation-Based Learning Methods. Michael J. Pazzani. 1990. 360p. 79.95 (0-8058-0629-6); stu. ed. 10.95 incl. disk (1-56321-037-1); stu. ed. 10.95 incl. disk (1-56321-038-X); stu. ed. 10.95 incl. disk (1-56321-039-8); 360p. pap. 34.50 (0-8058-0789-6) L Erlbaum Assocs.

Creating a Secure Workplace: Effective Policies & Practices in Health Care. Ed. by John R. Lion et al. 1996. LC 96-27340. (Illus.). 340p. (Orig.). pap. 69.95 (1-55648-167-5, 181150) AHPI.

Creating Abuse-Free Caregiving Environments for Children, the Disabled, & the Elderly: Preparing, Supervising & Managing Caregivers for the Emotional Impact of Their Responsibilities. Roger D. MacNamara. 1992. 270p. (C). text 51.95 (0-398-05761-3) C C Thomas.

Creating Alternatives to Depression in Our Schools: Assessment, Intervention & Prevention. S. Miezitis.

1992. LC 91-861. (Illus.). 457p. pap. text 37.00 (*0-88937-039-7*) Hogrefe & Huber Pubs.

Creating & Enhancing Patient & Family Resource Centers. 320p. ring bd. 50.00 (*0-9677733-3-4*) Inst Fmly Ctr.

Creating Beauty to Cure the Soul: Race & Psychology in the Shaping of Aesthetic Surgery. Sander L. Gilman. 1998. LC 98-23182. 179p. pap. 21.95 (*0-8223-2144-0*) Duke.

Creating Ceremonies: Innovative Ways to Meet Adoption Challenges. Cheryl A. Lieberman. 1999. LC 98-30945. 160p. pap. 23.95 (*1-891944-10-X*) Zeig Tucker Theisen.

Creating Change in Mental Health Organizations. George W. Fairweather et al. 1974. 200p. (*0-08-017833-2*) Pergamon Repr GBR. *Dist:* Franklin.

Creating Children's Advisory Councils. 164p. ring bd. 25.00 (*0-9677733-4-2*) Inst Fmly Ctr.

Creating Community: Integrating Elderly & Severely Mentally Ill Persons in Public Housing. Ed. by Dianne Cote. 2001. (Illus.). 164p. (C). reprint ed. pap. text 30.00 (*0-7567-0622-X*) DIANE Pub.

Creating Community-Responsive Physicians: Concepts & Models for Service-Learning in Medical Education. Ed. by Sarena D. Seifer et al. 2000. (Series on Service-Learning in the Disciplines). 292p. (C). pap. 28.50 (*1-56377-014-8*, SL09DS) Am Assn Higher Ed.

Creating Consumer Choice in Healthcare: Measuring & Communicating Health Plan Performance Information. Richard Curtis & Trisha Kurtz. 1998. LC 98-10363. 244p. 42.00 (*1-56793-080-8*) Health Admin Pr.

Creating Consumer Loyalty in Healthcare. R. Scott MacStravic. 1999. LC 99-26390. (Ache Management Ser.). 203p. pap. 40.00 (*1-56793-108-1*) Health Admin Pr.

Creating Excellence in Crisis Care: A Guide to Effective Training & Program Designs. Lee Ann Hoff & Kazimiera Adamowski. 1998. LC 98-18125. (Health Care Management Ser.). 256p. 38.00 (*0-7879-4071-2*) Jossey-Bass.

Creating Health Behavior Change: How to Develop Community-Wide Programs for Youth. Cheryl L. Perry. 1999. LC 99-6239. (Developmental Clinical Psychology & Psychiatry Ser.: Vol. 43). 140p. 74.95 (*0-7619-1226-6*, 82133) Sage.

Creating Hysteria: Women & Multiple Personality Disorder. Joan R. Acocella. 1999. LC 99-6358. 224p. 20.00 (*0-7879-4794-6*) Jossey-Bass.

Creating Mind: How the Brain Works. John E. Dowling. 1998. LC 98-9365. (Illus.). 224p. 24.95 (*0-393-02746-5*) Norton.

Creating Nursing's Future: Issues, Opportunities & Challenges. Eleanor J. Sullivan. 1999. LC 98-46292. (Illus.). 392p. pap. text 35.00 (*0-323-00239-0*) Mosby Inc.

Creating Sanctuary: Toward the Evolution of Sane Societies. 1997. LC 96-37298. 320p. (C). 80.00 (*0-415-91568-6*) Routledge.

Creating Sanctuary: Toward the Evolution of Sane Societies. Sandra Bloom. 1997. LC 96-37298. 320p. pap. 24.95 (*0-415-91858-8*) Routledge.

Creating Technology Strategies: How to Build Competitive Biomedical R&D. Alice M. Sapienza. 1997. LC 97-28682. (Illus.). 241p. 64.95 (*0-471-15370-2*, Wiley-Liss) Wiley.

Creating the Child: The Ethics, Law, & Practice of Assisted Procreation. Ed. by Donald Evans & Neil Pickering. 1996. LC 96-10812. lib. bdg. (*90-411-0207-8*);Set. lib. bdg. (*90-411-0209-4*) M Nijhoff NLD. *Dist:* Kluwer Academic.

Creating the Compliant Patient. Ed. by J. A. McNamara & C. A. Trotman. 1997. (Craniofacial Growth Ser.: Vol. 33). (Illus.). 206p. 59.00 (*0-929921-29-1*) UM CHGD.

Creating the Future: Innovative Programs & Structures in Academic Health Centers. Ed. by Clyde H. Evans & Elaine R. Rubin. 1999. LC 00-501118. 144p. 25.00 (*1-879694-15-8*) AAH Ctrs.

Creating the New American Hospital: A Time for Greatness. V. Clayton Sherman. 1993. LC 92-48943. (Health Management Ser.). 336p. 45.00 (*1-55542-514-3*) Jossey-Bass.

Creating Wholeness: A Self-Healing Workbook Using Dynamic Relaxation, Images, & Thoughts. Erik Peper & C. F. Holt. 1993. (Illus.). 232p. (C). spiral bd. 37.50 (*0-306-44172-1*, Plenum Trade) Perseus Pubng.

Creating Your Christian Engagement. John B. Ryan & Francis J. Lodato. 1994. LC 94-76020. 144p. (Orig.). pap. 6.95 (*0-89243-575-5*) Liguori Pubns.

Creation & Future Legacy of Stockpile Stewardship: Isotope Production, Applications & Consumption; Proceedings, Midyear Meeting of the Health Physics Society (32nd: 1999: Albuquerque, NM) Ed. by James M. Hylko & Randell L. Salyer. 1999. LC 98-89779. 308p. pap. text 35.95 (*0-944838-88-X*) Med Physics Pub.

Creation of a Medical Profession in Egypt, 1800-1922. Amira E. Sonbol. 1991. LC 91-7640. (Contemporary Issues in the Middle East Ser.). 256p. text 45.00 (*0-8156-2541-3*) Syracuse U Pr.

Creation of Dangerous Violent Criminals. Lonnie H. Athens. 1992. LC 91-43592. 120p. (C). text 23.95 (*0-252-01939-3*); pap. text 12.95 (*0-252-06262-0*) U of Ill Pr.

Creation of Dr. B: A Biography of Bruno Bettelheim. Richard Pollak. 1998. (Illus.). 480p. pap. 15.00 (*0-684-84640-3*, Touchstone) S&S Trade Pap.

Creation of Health: The Emotional, Psychological, & Spiritual Responses That Promote Health & Healing. C. Norman Shealy & Caroline Myss. 1998. LC 97-52687. (Illus.). 400p. pap. 15.00 (*0-609-80323-9*, Crown) Crown Pub Group.

Creation of Meaning in Clinical Social Work. Carolyn Saari. 1991. LC 91-24651. 216p. text 30.00 (*0-89862-772-9*, 2772) Guilford Pubns.

Creation of Violent Criminals. Lonnie H. Athens. 1989. 128p. 29.95 (*0-415-02837-X*) Routledge.

Creative Aging: Discovering the Unexpected Joys of Later Life Through Personality Type. Nancy Millner. 2000. LC 97-33177. 208p. (Orig.). pap. 16.95 (*0-89106-111-8*, 7780, Davies-Black Pub) Consulting Psychol.

Creative Caregiving. James R. Sherman. 1994. (Illus.). 80p. (Orig.). pap. 9.95 (*0-935538-17-8*) Pathway Bks.

Creative Childbirth: The Leclaire Method of Easy Birthing Through Hypnosis & Rational-Intuitive Thought. Michelle L. O'Neill. 1993. LC 92-81691. (Illus.). 105p. (Orig.). pap. 11.95 (*0-9633087-3-4*) Papyrus Pr.

Creative Collaboration in Psychotherapy: Making Room for Life. Roger A. Lewin. 1997. LC 97-5353. 208p. text 35.00 (*0-7657-0075-1*) Aronson.

Creative Computing in Health & Social Care. Fred E. Yates. 1996. LC 95-44665. 236p. pap. 79.95 (*0-471-95586-8*) Wiley.

Creative Cooking - The Low Fat Way: A Lifetime Approach to Delicious Healthy Living. Yvonne Jacob. Ed. by Jo Girard. 1989. (Illus.). 283p. (Orig.). pap. 19.95 (*0-9618415-3-2*) AZ Bariatric Phy.

Creative Counseling Techniques: An Illustrated Guide. Ed Jacobs. 1992. LC 92-32487. (Illus.). 158p. pap. 29.00 (*0-911907-06-8*, RO-2278) Psych Assess.

Creative Healing: How to Heal Yourself by Tapping Your Hidden Creativity. Mike Samuels & Mary R. Lane. 1998. LC 97-49821. 304p. pap. 18.00 (*0-06-251518-7*) Harper SF.

Creative Health & Health Enhancement: Individual Initiative & Responsibility for Self Health & Wellness. Stacey B. Day. 1982. LC 81-81300. (Monograph on Health Communications & Biopsychosocial Health). (Illus.). lib. bdg. 150.00 (*0-934314-07-1*, SBD/HES82SKI) Intl Found Biosocial Dev.

Creative Imagery. William Fezler. 1989. 288p. pap. 12.00 (*0-671-68238-5*, Fireside) S&S Trade Pap.

Creative Imagery for Nurse Healers: Nurse as Healer Series. Karilee H. Shames. 1995. LC 94-39827. (Nurse as Healer Ser.). 208p. pap. text 23.95 (*0-8273-6394-X*) Delmar.

Creative Intervention. Mary S. Hirschfeld. 1987. 14.95 (*0-9618024-0-5*) Counsel Voice.

Creative Journal: The Art of Finding Yourself. Lucia Capacchione. 1979. LC 78-51590. (Illus.). 180p. pap. 12.95 (*0-8040-0798-5*) Swallow.

Creative Living & Health Workbook: A New & Exciting System for Dealing with the Emotional & Physical Stress of Cancer. Rosemary Ross. 1989. 44p. pap. 8.95 (*0-9647382-1-X*); 1994. 36p. reprint ed. pap. 8.95 (*0-9647382-2-8*) R Ross.

Creative Long-Term Care Administration. Ed. by George K. Gordon & Ruth Stryker-Gordon. 3rd ed. 1994. LC 93-36918. (Illus.). 390p. (C). text 72.95 (*0-398-05898-9*) C C Thomas.

Creative Loving. Don Boone. 1994. 64p. (Orig.). pap. 9.95 (*1-56664-064-4*) WorldComm.

Creative Mastery in Hypnosis & Hypnoanalysis: A Festschrift for Erika Fromm. Ed. by Margot L. Fass & Daniel Brown. 1990. 352p. text 89.95 (*0-8058-0832-9*) L Erlbaum Assocs.

Creative Medical Teaching. Neal A. Whitman. 1990. 232p. text 30.00 (*0-940193-07-8*) Univ UT Sch Med.

Creative Menopause: Illuminating Women's Health & Spirituality. Farida Sharan. 2nd ed. 1995. LC 94-76389. (Illus.). 290p. (Orig.). reprint ed. pap. 17.95 (*1-57093-002-3*) Schl Nat Med.

Creative Myth & the Cosmic Hero: Text & Context in Ernest Becker's, The Denial of Death. Ronald V. Evans. 1992. LC 92-13192. (Reshaping of Psychoanalysis Ser.: Vol. 3). 145p. 35.95 (*0-8204-1845-5*) P Lang Pubng.

Creative Problem Solving for Health Care Professionals. Cecilia K. Golightly. 1981. LC 81-3631. 240p. 85.00 (*0-89443-371-7*) Aspen Pub.

Creative Problem Solving in Occupational Therapy. Ed. by Jeanne E. Lewin & Colleen A. Reed. 1998. LC 97-48862. (Illus.). 592p. pap. text 45.95 (*0-397-55233-5*) Lppncott W & W.

Creative Process: Reflections on the Invention of Art. Ed. & Intro. by Brewster Ghiselin. 1985. 259p. pap. 16.95 (*0-520-05453-9*) U CA Pr.

Creative Process in Gestalt Therapy. Joseph Zinker. 1978. LC 78-4820. (Giant Ser.). (Illus.). 282p. pap. 14.00 (*0-394-72567-0*, V-567) Knopf.

Creative Realities: The Search for Meanings. Maxine B. Junge. 1998. LC 98-5978. 378p. (C). 67.00 (*0-7618-1084-6*) U Pr of Amer.

Creative Scripts for Hypnotherapy. Marlene E. Hunter. 1994. LC 94-6138. 232p. pap. text 26.95 (*0-87630-742-X*) Brunner-Routledge.

Creative Side of Experimentation: Personal Perspectives from Leading Researchers in Motor Control, Motor Development, & Sport Psychology. Ed. by Conrad W. Snyder & Bruce Abernethy. 1992. LC 92-6234. (Illus.). 280p. text 22.00 (*0-87322-376-4*, BSNY0376) Human Kinetics.

Creative Social Work in Health Care: Challenges for the Profession. Ed. by Helen Rehr et al. 1998. LC 97-52579. 208p. 39.95 (*0-8261-1199-8*) Springer Pub.

Creative Teaching in Health. Donald A. Read & Walter H. Greene. 3rd ed. 1980. (Illus.). text 31.50 (*0-02-398700-6*, Macmillan Coll) P-H.

Creative Therapy Vol. I: 52 Exercises for Groups. Jane Dossick. 1988. LC 88-42577. (Illus.). 118p. pap. text 26.45 (*0-943158-50-8*, CTBP, Prof Resc Pr) Pro Resource.

Creative Therapy Vol. II: 52 More Exercises for Groups. Jane Dossick. 1990. LC 88-42577. (Illus.). 118p. pap. 26.45 (*0-943158-60-5*, CT2BP, Prof Resc Pr) Pro Resource.

Creative Therapy 2: Working with Parents. Kate Ollier & Angela Hobday. 2001. LC 2001-39201. (Practical Therapist Ser.). 192p. 21.95 (*1-886230-42-0*) Impact Pubs CA.

Creative Therapy II: Working with Parents. Kate Ollier & Angela Hobday. 2001. 128p. pap. (*0-86431-350-0*) Aust Council Educ Res AUS. *Dist:* Stylus Pub VA.

Creative Therapy with Children & Adolescents. Angela Hobday & Kate Ollier. 1999. LC 99-17409. (Practical Therapist Ser.). (Illus.). 192p. 21.95 (*1-886230-19-6*) Impact Pubs CA.

Creative Training: Sociodrama & Team-Building. Ron Wiener. 1997. LC 96-31276. 136p. pap. (*1-85302-422-8*) Jessica Kingsley GBR. *Dist:* Taylor & Francis.

Creative Use of Music in Group Therapy. Thomas A. Plach. 2nd ed. 1996. (Illus.). 84p. 33.95 (*0-398-06585-3*); pap. 21.95 (*0-398-06586-1*) C C Thomas.

Creative Visualization Workbook: Use the Power of Your Imagination to Create What You Want in Your Life. Shakti Gawain. 2nd rev. ed. 1995. 160p. pap., wbk. ed. 11.95 (*1-880032-75-9*) New Wrld Lib.

Creative Wellness: A Holistic Guide to Total Health. Michelle Lusson. 1987. 320p. (Orig.). mass mkt. 7.95 (*0-446-38225-6*) Warner Bks.

Creativity & Affect. Ed. by Melvin P. Shaw & Mark A. Runco. 1994. LC 94-1959. (Creativity Research Ser.). 298p. 77.00 (*0-89391-977-2*); pap. 39.50 (*1-56750-012-9*) Greenwood (Ablex).

Creativity & Culture: A Psychoanalytic Study of the Creative Process in the Arts, Sciences & Culture. Daniel Dervin. 1990. LC 88-46150. (Illus.). 408p. 55.00 (*0-8386-3366-8*) Fairleigh Dickinson.

Creativity & Disease: How Illness Affects Literature, Art & Music. Philip Sandblom. enl. rev. ed. 1997. LC 91-20217. (Illus.). 224p. pap. 21.95 (*0-7145-2941-9*) M Boyars Pubs.

Creativity & Madness: Psychological Studies of Art & Artists, Vol. I. Barry Panter et al. 1994. LC 94-94521. (Creativity & Madness Ser.: Vol. I). (Illus.). 320p. 24.95 (*0-9641185-1-3*) AIMED.

Creativity & Moral Vision in Psychology: Narratives on Identity & Commitment in a Postmodern Age. Lisa T. Hoshmand. 1998. LC 97-45464. (Psychology Ser.). pap. 36.95 (*0-7619-0378-X*, 2540) Sage.

Creativity & Moral Vision in Psychology: Narratives on Identity & Commitment in a Postmodern Age. Lisa Tsoi Hoshmand. 1998. LC 97-45464. (Psychology Ser.). 73.95 (*0-7619-0377-1*, 2539) Sage.

Creativity & Psychological Health. Frank Barron. 1990. 292p. (C). reprint ed. pap. text 16.95 (*0-930222-90-3*) Creat Educ Found.

Creativity & Psychotherapy: Proceedings of the International Congress of Psychopathology of Expression, 8th, Jerusalem, May 10-13, 1976. International Congress of Psychopathology of Expre. Ed. by Jakab Irene. 1978. (Journal: Vol. 21, Nos. 1-3). (Illus.). 64.50 (*3-8055-2766-7*) S Karger.

Creativity & the Art Therapist's Identity. Ed. by Roberta H. Shoemaker. 1976. (Conference Proceedings Ser.). 118p. (Orig.). pap. 7.00 (*1-882147-04-9*) Am Art Therapy.

Creativity Doesn't Die. Joan Parry & Marie Freudenberg. Ed. by Gwen Costa. 1990. LC 91-33875. pap. 13.95 (*0-87949-337-2*) Ashley Bks.

Creature Comfort: A Veterinarian's Journal. James D. Stowe. 1998. (Illus.). 282p. pap. text (*0-9682388-0-7*) Veredus.

Creature Totems: Nature Teacher Medicine. Twylah H. Nitsch. Ed. by Albert F. Rinebold. 1991. (Illus.). 130p. (Orig.). pap. 16.00 (*0-9626135-1-7*) Aware Tribe.

Credentialing & Privileges Manual. Margaret D. Bischel. 1997. (Illus.). 275p. ring bd. (*1-893826-03-1*) Apollo Managed.

Credentialing Desk Reference: 2000 Edition. Jack Zusman. 3rd ed. 1999. LC 00-698195. (Illus.). ix, 815p. pap. text 249.00 (*1-57839-066-4*) Opus Communs.

Credentialing Handbook. Christine S. Mobley & Sheryl K. Deutsch. 1999. LC 98-55685. 400p. 91.00 (*0-8342-0933-0*, 09330) Aspen Pub.

Credentialing in Counseling. Fred O. Bradley. 1991. 110p. pap. text 14.95 (*1-55620-087-0*, 72297) Am Coun Assn.

Credentialing Orientation Kit: Creating & Customizing Your Own Credentialing Handbook. Hugh Greeley. 1999. (Illus.). 56p. ring bd. 99.00 (*1-57839-063-X*) Opus Communs.

Credentialing Process - Physicians & Allied Health Professionals. Eric Joseph & Nancy Webster. 1998. pap. text 40.00 (*0-916499-53-7*) Care Educ Grp.

Credentials Review & Privileging: Questions & Answers for Ambulatory Care. Joint Commission on Accreditation of Healthcare Organizations. 1999. (Illus.). 154p. pap. 45.00 (*0-86688-602-8*, CR-100) Joint Comm Hlthcare.

Cresols. 1995. (Environmental Health Criteria Ser.: Vol. 168). 144p. (C). pap. 29.00 (*92-4-157168-3*, 1160168) World Health.

Crevicular Fluid. Geneve Cimasoni. 1974. (Monographs in Oral Science: Vol. 3). 121p. 48.75 (*3-8055-1699-1*) S Karger.

Crevicular Fluid Updated. Geneve Cimasoni. 1983. (Monographs in Oral Science: Vol. 12). (Illus.). viii, 152p. 101.00 (*3-8055-3705-0*) S Karger.

Crib Death: The Sudden Infant Death Syndrome. Warren G. Guntheroth. 3rd rev. ed. 1995. LC 95-7918. (Illus.). 456p. 72.00 (*0-87993-618-5*) Futura Pub.

Crime & Criminal Psychology: Index of New Information with Authors, Subjects, Research Categories & References. Clement K. Zaine. 1995. 160p. 57.50 (*0-7883-0742-8*); pap. 47.50 (*0-7883-0743-6*) ABBE Pubs Assn.

Crime & Its Repression. Gustav Aschaffenburg. Tr. by Adalbert Albrecht. 1968. LC 68-55767. (Criminology, Law Enforcement, & Social Problems Ser.: No. 11). reprint ed. 26.00 (*0-87585-011-1*) Patterson Smith.

Crime & the Mind, an Outline of Psychiatric Criminology. Walter Bromberg. 1982. LC 77-170192. 219p. reprint ed. lib. bdg. 86.50 (*0-8371-6249-1*, BRCM, Greenwood Pr) Greenwood.

Crime Investigations with Forensic Sciences: Index of New Information with Authors & Subjects. American Health Research Institute Staff. 1995. LC 95-16450. 57.50 (*0-7883-0432-1*) ABBE Pubs Assn.

Crime Society England 1750-1900. Clive Emsley. 1989. (Themes in British Social History Ser.). 287p. (C). pap. 40.00 (*0-582-49399-4*, 73603) Addison-Wesley.

Crime Victims Program Monitor. Jack Rudman. 1994. (Career Examination Ser.: C-3438). pap. 34.95 (*0-8373-3438-1*) Nat Learn.

Criminal Abortion. Horatio R. Storer & Franklin F. Heard. 1974. LC 73-20639. (Sex, Marriage & Society Ser.). 228p. reprint ed. 21.95 (*0-405-05820-9*) Ayer.

Criminal & Non-Criminal Homicide-Medical Guide-Book for Reference & Research. George A. Christos. 1997. 161p. 57.50 (*0-7883-1643-5*); pap. 47.50 (*0-7883-1644-3*) ABBE Pubs Assn.

Criminal Behavior: A Process Psychology Analysis. Nathaniel J. Pallone & James J. Hennessy. 1992. 436p. (C). text (*1-56000-044-9*) Transaction Pubs.

Criminal Court Consultation. Richard Rosner & R. B. Harmon. 1989. (Critical Issues in American Psychiatry & the Law Ser.: Vol. 5). (Illus.). 344p. (C). 80.00 (*0-306-43061-4*, Plenum Trade) Perseus Pubng.

Criminal Dangerousness & the Risk of Violence. Alfred B. Heilbrun, Jr. 1996. LC 96-19818. 234p. pap. text 33.00 (*0-7618-0409-9*); lib. bdg. 55.00 (*0-7618-0408-0*) U Pr of Amer.

Criminal Experiments on Human Beings in Auschwitz & War Research Laboratories: Twenty Women Prisoners' Accounts. Ed. by Lore Shelley. 1992. LC 91-40557. (Illus.). 420p. lib. bdg. 109.95 (*0-7734-9884-2*) E Mellen.

Criminal Justice in Action: The Core. Larry K. Gaines et al. 2000. LC 00-44918. (Illus.). xxiv, 392p. pap. 42.00 net. (*0-534-57456-4*) Wadsworth Pub.

Criminal Mentality. Gerald Locklin. 1976. pap. 2.50 (*0-88031-031-6*) Invisible-Red Hill.

Criminal Mind: A Study of Communication Between the Criminal Law & Psychiatry. Philip Roche. 1976. LC 76-28524. 299p. reprint ed. lib. bdg. 38.50 (*0-8371-9056-8*, ROCM, Greenwood Pr) Greenwood.

Criminal Personality Vol. I: A Profile for Change. Samuel Yochelson & Stanton E. Samenow. LC 75-13507. 552p. 1993. pap. 60.00 (*1-56821-105-8*); 1976. 75.00 (*0-87668-218-2*) Aronson.

Criminal Personality Vol. II: The Change Process. Samuel Yochelson & Stanton E. Samenow. 1994. LC 75-13507. 592p. reprint ed. pap. text 60.00 (*1-56821-349-2*) Aronson.

Criminal Personality Vol. III: The Drug User. Samuel Yochelson & Stanton E. Samenow. LC 75-13507. 1986. 372p. 60.00 (*0-87668-901-2*); 1994. 384p. reprint ed. pap. 45.00 (*1-56821-244-5*) Aronson.

Criminal Profiling: An Introduction to Behavioral Evidence Analysis. Brent E. Turvey. 1999. LC 98-89232. (Illus.). xxxiii, 462p. (C). 79.95 (*0-12-705040-X*) Acad Pr.

Criminal Psychology: A Manual for Judges, Practitioners & Student. Hans Gross. Tr. by Horace M. Kallen. 1968. LC 68-55772. (Criminology, Law Enforcement, & Social Problems Ser.: No. 13). reprint ed. 30.00 (*0-87585-013-8*) Patterson Smith.

Criminal Responsibility Evaluations: A Manual for Practice. David L. Shapiro. 1999. LC 98-54690. 180p. pap. 29.45 (*1-56887-046-9*, Prof Resc Pr) Pro Resource.

Criminally Insane: A Community Follow-Up of Mentally Ill Offenders. Terence P. Thornberry & Joseph E. Jacoby. 1979. LC 78-10703. (Studies in Crime & Justice). (Illus.). 312p. lib. bdg. 29.00 (*0-226-79818-6*) U Ch Pr.

Crises & Special Problems in Psychoanalysis & Psychotherapy. Leopold Bellak. 1994. LC 94-72438. (Master Work Ser.). 264p. pap. text 45.00 (*1-56821-351-4*) Aronson.

Crisis: Psychological First Aid for Recovery & Growth. Ann S. Kliman. 1986. LC 86-71118. 219p. reprint ed. 30.00 (*0-87668-929-2*) Aronson.

Crisis Admission Units & Emergency Psychiatric Services. J. Cooper. 1979. (Public Health in Europe Ser.: No. 11). 118p. 11.00 (*92-9020-130-4*, 1320011) World Health.

Crisis & Chaos: Life with the Combat Veteran. Colleen McCarty-Gould. 1998. LC 98-34038. 189p. pap. 18.95 (*1-56072-617-2*, Nova Kroshka Bks) Nova Sci Pubs.

Crisis at Adolescence: Object Relations Therapy with the Family. Ed. by Sally Box et al. 1994. LC 93-9010. (Library of Object Relations). 296p. 50.00 (*1-56821-094-9*) Aronson.

Crisis at the Front Line: The Effects of AIDS on Public Hospitals - A Twentieth Century Fund Paper. Dennis P. Andrulis. 1989. 93p. 18.95 (*0-87078-267-3*); pap. 8.95 (*0-87078-266-5*) Century Foundation.

Crisis Counseling. Howard W. Stone. enl. rev. ed. 1993. LC 92-39489. (Creative Pastoral Care & Counseling Ser.). 96p. (Orig.). pap. 15.00 (*0-8006-2760-1*, 1-2760, Fortress Pr) Augsburg Fortress.

Crisis Counseling Intervention & Prevention in the Schools. Ed. by Jonathan Sandoval. 1988. (Kratochwill-Yesseldyke School Psychology Ser.). 280p. text 34.50 (*0-89859-823-0*) L Erlbaum Assocs.

Crisis, Health & Medicine: A Social Critique. Vicente Navarro. 1986. 300p. (*0-422-60580-8*, 1006); pap. (*0-422-60170-5*, 9760) Tavistock GBR. *Dist:* Routldge.

Crisis in Black Sexual Politics. Nathan Hare & Julia Hare. 1989. 184p. pap. 15.00 (*0-9613086-2-1*) Black T T.

Crisis in Clinical AIDS Research. Mark Harrington. 1994. 33p. (Orig.). (C). pap. text 30.00 (*0-7881-1180-9*) DIANE Pub.

Crisis in Health Care, Vol. 63, No. 1. Ed. by Robert Emmet Long. 1991. pap. 25.00 (*0-8242-0811-0*) Wilson.

Crisis in Healthcare Financing: The Move Toward Universal Access. Market Intelligence Staff. 1992. 246p. (Orig.). 395.00 (*1-56753-045-1*) Frost & Sullivan.

Crisis in Modern Social Psychology: How to End It. Ian Parker. 1989. 176p. pap. 12.95 (*0-415-01494-8*, A3373) Routledge.

Crisis in the Public Sector—Challenge to the Public Health: American Public Health Association 1980 Meeting in Detroit, Michigan. Ed. by Oscar Gish. 1982. 48p. pap. 18.25 (*0-08-028948-7*, Pergamon Pr) Elsevier.

Crisis in the Workplace: Occupational Disease & Injury - (A Report to the Ford Foundation) Nicholas A. Ashford. 1976. LC 75-28424. 49.50 (*0-262-01045-3*) MIT Pr.

Crisis Intervention. Eric Lindemann. 1995. LC 94-47404. (Master Work Ser.). 302p. pap. 50.00 (*1-56821-468-5*) Aronson.

Crisis Intervention. Ed. by Lawrence Cohen et al. 2nd ed. 1982. (Community Psychology Ser.: Vol. IV). (Illus.). 222p. 38.95 (*0-89885-107-6*, Kluwer Acad Hman Sci) Kluwer Academic.

Crisis Intervention: A Handbook for Practice & Research. Karl A. Slaikeu. 2nd ed. 1990. LC 89-28374. 360p. (C). 99.00 (*0-205-12342-2*, H23427) Allyn.

Crisis Intervention: A Handbook of Immediate Person-to-Person Help. Kenneth France. 3rd ed. 1996. LC 95-47847. (Illus.). 310p. pap. 40.95 (*0-398-06580-2*); text 58.95 (*0-398-06579-9*) C C Thomas.

Crisis Intervention: A Manual for Education & Action. John P. Eddy et al. 1983. LC 83-6499. 134p. (C). pap. text 21.00 (*0-8191-3231-4*) U Pr of Amer.

Crisis Intervention: Theory & Methodology. Donna C. Aguilera. 8th ed. 1997. LC 97-20533. (Illus.). 360p. (C). (gr. 13). pap. text 33.00 (*0-8151-2604-2*, 31074) Mosby Inc.

Crisis Intervention & Counseling by Telephone. David Lester & Gene W. Brockopp. 1976. (Illus.). 336p. text 57.95 (*0-398-02641-6*) C C Thomas.

Crisis Intervention & Time-Limited Cognitive Treatment. Ed. by Albert R. Roberts. 1995. 320p. 74.95 (*0-8039-5629-0*, 4725); pap. 39.95 (*0-8039-5630-4*, 4726) Sage.

Crisis Intervention & Trauma Response: Theory & Practice. Barbara R. Wainrib & Ellin L. Bloch. 1998. LC 97-32184. (Illus.). 176p. 31.95 (*0-8261-1175-0*) Springer Pub.

Crisis Intervention in Criminal Justice/Social Service. Ed. by James E. Hendricks & Bryan Byers. 2nd ed. 1996. LC 95-50662. 430p. 77.95 (*0-398-06583-7*) C C Thomas.

Crisis Intervention in Practice: The Multidisciplinary Team & the Mental Health Social Worker. Richard Mitchell. 1993. (Studies of Care in the Community). 160p. (*1-85628-452-2*) Avebry GBR. *Dist:* Ashgate Pub Co.

Crisis Intervention in Residential Treatment: The Clinical Innovations of Fritz Redl. William C. Morse. 1991. LC 91-25834. (Residential Treatment for Children & Youth Ser.). (Illus.). 107p. lib. bdg. 29.95 (*1-56024-215-9*) Haworth Pr.

Crisis Intervention Strategies. Burl E. Gilliland & Richard K. James. 1988. LC 87-26133. 488p. (C). pap. 35.25 net. (*0-534-09054-0*) Brooks-Cole.

Crisis Intervention Strategies. Burl E. Gilliland & Richard James. 2nd ed. 1993. LC 92-10291. 611p. (C). text 35.75 (*0-534-19494-X*) Brooks-Cole.

Crisis Intervention Strategies. Burl E. Gilliland & Richard K. James. 3rd ed. 1996. LC 96-44872. (Counseling Ser.). 650p. (C). pap. 67.95 (*0-534-34568-9*) Brooks-Cole.

Crisis Intervention Strategies: For Chemical Abusers & Offenders. Gregory L. Little et al. 1998. 68p. (C). pap. 10.00 (*0-940829-20-7*) Eagle Wing Bks.

Crisis Intervention Strategies for School-Based Helpers. Ed. by Thomas N. Fairchild. 2nd ed. 1997. LC 97-8954. (Illus.). 496p. text 114.95 (*0-398-06768-6*); pap. text 96.95 (*0-398-06769-4*) C C Thomas.

Crisis Intervention Verbatim. Nira Kfir. 1989. 175p. 33.95 (*0-89116-837-0*) Hemisp Pub.

Crisis Management & Brief Treatment: Theory, Technique, & Applications. Ed. by Albert R. Roberts. 1996. LC 95-40746. 228p. (C). pap. text 42.95 (*0-8304-1429-0*) Thomson Learn.

Crisis Management in Anesthesiology. Ed. by David M. Gaba et al. 1993. LC 93-39076. (Illus.). 294p. pap. text (*0-443-08910-8*) Church.

Crisis OB. Judy Poole et al. 1994. text 99.00 (*0-8151-6835-7*) Mosby Inc.

Crisis Obstetrics: Emergency & Complicated Deliveries, Part 1. Judy Poole. 1994. 64p. (C). (gr. 13). pap. text 16.95 (*0-8151-6827-6*, 25470) Mosby Inc.

Crisis Obstetrics: Hemorrhage, Part 2. Judy Poole. 1994. 48p. (C). (gr. 13). pap. text 16.95 (*0-8151-6829-2*, 25472) Mosby Inc.

Crisis Obstetrics: Hypertension in Pregnancy, Part 3. Judy Poole. 1994. 40p. (C). (gr. 13). pap. text 16.95 (*0-8151-6832-2*, 25474) Mosby Inc.

Crisis of Competence: Transitional Stress & the Displaced Worker. Carl A. Maida et al. 1990. LC 89-15825. (Psychosocial Stress Ser.: No. 16). 224p. text 33.95 (*0-87630-559-1*) Brunner-Routledge.

Crisis of Meaning: How Gay Men Are Making Sense of AIDS. Steven S. Schwartzberg. 1996. LC 96-11004. 288p. 25.00 (*0-19-509627-4*) OUP.

Crisis of Public Health: Reflections for the Debate. 1993. (PAHO Scientific Publications: No. 540). (ENG & SPA.). vi, 246p. pap. text 56.00 (*92-75-11540-0*, 1610540) World Health.

Crisis Services & Hospital Crises: Mental Health at a Turning Point. Ed. by Dylan Tomlinson & K. Allen. 1999. LC 98-74638. ix, 180p. text 61.95 (*1-84014-389-4*) Ashgate Pub Co.

Criteria & Guidelines for Evaluation of Associate Degree Programs in Nursing. National League for Nursing Staff. rev. ed. 1991. 46p. pap. text 5.95 (*0-88737-535-9*, 23-2439) Natl League Nurse.

Criteria & Guidelines for Evaluation of Baccalaureate & Higher Degree Programs in Nursing. National League for Nursing Staff. 7th rev. ed. 1992. 74p. pap. text 6.95 (*0-88737-552-9*, 15-2474) Natl League Nurse.

Criteria & Guidelines for Evaluation of Diploma Programs in Nursing. National League for Nursing Staff. rev. ed. 1992. 50p. pap. text 5.95 (*0-88737-538-3*, 16-2444) Natl League Nurse.

Criteria & Guidelines for Evaluation of Practical Nursing Programs. National League for Nursing Staff. rev. ed. 1992. 64p. pap. text 5.95 (*0-88737-539-1*, 38-2445) Natl League Nurse.

Criteria & Guidelines for the Evaluation of Associate Degree Programs in Nursing, 1996. 1996. 34p. 7.95 (*0-88737-698-3*, 23-6983, NLN Pr) Natl League Nurse.

Criteria & Guidelines for the Evaluation of Baccalaureate & Higher Degree Programs in Nursing, 1996. 1996. 32p. 8.95 (*0-88737-701-7*, 15-7017, NLN Pr) Natl League Nurse.

Criteria & Guidelines for the Evaluation of Diploma Programs in Nursing, 1996. 1996. 24p. 7.95 (*0-88737-699-1*, 16-6991, NLN Pr) Natl League Nurse.

Criteria & Guidelines for the Evaluation of Practical Nursing Programs, 1996. 1996. 26p. 7.95 (*0-88737-700-9*, 38-7009, NLN Pr) Natl League Nurse.

Criteria & Methods for Quality Assurance & Medical X-Ray Diagnosis: British Journal of Radiology Supplement 18. 1985. pap. text (*0-905749-12-X*) Med Physics Pub.

Criteria (Dose Effect Relationships) for Organichlorine Pesticides: Report of a Working Group of Experts Prepared for the Commission of the European Communities. Ed. by M. Mercier. 1981. 400p. pap. (*0-08-023441-0*) Pergamon Repr GBR. *Dist:* Franklin.

Criteria for a Recommended Standard: Occupational Exposure to Respirable Coal Mine Dust. 1997. lib. bdg. 255.99 (*0-8490-8148-3*) Gordon Pr.

Criteria for Competence: Controversies in the Conceptualization & Assessment of Children's Abilities. Ed. by Michael Chandler & David Chapman. 1991. 296p. (C). text 59.95 (*0-8058-0606-7*) L Erlbaum Assocs.

Criteria for Drug Use Evaluation. Vol. 1. 1989. 137p. pap. 63.00 (*0-930530-95-0*); Vol. 2. 1990. 113p. pap. 63.00 (*0-930530-99-3*) Am Soc Hlth-Syst.

Criteria for Drug Use Evaluation, Vol. 3. ASHP Special Projects Division Staff. 1992. 176p. (Orig.). pap. 50.00 (*1-879907-19-4*) Am Soc Hlth-Syst.

Criteria for Evaluating an AIDS Curriculum. National Coalition of Advocates for Students Staff. rev. ed. 1992. 23p. reprint ed. pap. 4.00 (*1-880002-02-7*) Natl Coal Advocates.

Criteria for Short-Term Treatment of Acute Psychiatric Illness. American Academy of Child and Adolescent Psychiatry Staff & American Psychiatric Association Staff. 1998. LC 99-183946. 46p. pap. text 26.00 (*0-89042-412-8*, 2412) Am Psychiatric.

Criteria for the Life History, with Analyses of Six Notable Documents. John Dollard. 1977. (Select Bibliographies Reprint Ser.). reprint ed. 25.95 (*0-8369-6685-6*) Ayer.

Criterion-Referenced Articulation Profile. Larry J. Mattes. 1986. pap. text 45.00 (*0-930951-06-9*) Acad Comm.

Critical Analysis of Monoclonal Therapy in Transplantation. William J. Burlingham. 1991. 304p. lib. bdg. 139.00 (*0-8493-6821-9*, RC1235) CRC Pr.

Critical & High Acuity in Nursing Care. Audree Reynolds. 1994. (Outline Ser.). (Illus.). 300p. (C). per. 23.95 (*1-56930-028-3*) Delmar.

Critical & High Acuity Nursing Care. Audree Reynolds. 2nd rev. ed. 1999. (Outline Ser.). 250p. (C). per. 22.95 (*1-56930-094-1*) Delmar.

***Critical Appraisal for Psychiatrists.** Stephen Lawrie et al. 2001. (Illus.). 187p. (*0-443-07017-2*) Church GBR. *Dist:* Saunders.

Critical Appraisal of Epidemiological Studies & Clinical Trials. J. Mark Elwood. 2nd ed. 1998. (Illus.). 458p. pap. text 49.95 (*0-19-262744-9*) OUP.

Critical Appraisal of Fetal Surveillance. Ed. by Herman P. Van Geijn & Frans J. Copray. 1994. LC 94-10707. (International Congress Ser.: No. 1065). 720p. 229.00 (*0-444-89895-6*); pap. 130.00 (*0-444-82006-X*) Elsevier (Excerpta Medica).

Critical Calling: Reflections on Moral Dilemmas since Vatican II. Richard A. McCormick. 1989. LC 89-7622. 401p. (Orig.). pap. 29.95 (*0-87840-464-3*) Georgetown U Pr.

Critical Care. Stephen G. Jenkinson. 1990. (Contemporary Management in Internal Medicine Ser.: Vol. 1, No. 1). (Illus.). 219p. text (*0-443-08822-5*) Church.

Critical Care. Robert R. Kirby. 1997. LC 96-18844. (Atlas of Clinical Anesthesiology Ser.). text (*0-443-07906-4*) Church.

Critical Care. Robert J. Murtaugh. 2000. (Quick Look Veterinary Ser.). 23.95 (*1-889325-13-9*) Fence Crk Pubng.

Critical Care. Joseph M. Civetta et al. 3rd ed. 1996. 2,416p. text 225.00 (*0-397-51527-8*) Lppncott W & W.

Critical Care: Certification Practice Exams. Donald C. Ahrens. 4th rev. ed. 1997. LC 97-15239. 690p. (C). spiral bd. 52.95 (*0-8385-1474-X*, A-1474-4) McGraw-Hill Prof.

Critical Care: Standards, Audit & Ethics. Ed. by Jack Tinker et al. 1996. (Illus.). 424p. (*0-340-55424-X*) E A GBR. *Dist:* OUP.

Critical Care: State of the Art, Vol. 8. Ed. by Frank B. Cerra & William C. Shoemaker. 1987. (*0-936145-10-2*) SCCM Fullerton.

Critical Care Vol. 1: Atlas & Slides, Vol. 1. Ed. by R. D. Miller & R. R. Kirby. 1998. (*0-443-07972-2*) Church.

Critical Care & Emergency Drug Reference. Keen. 3rd ed. 1999. 624p. (C). (gr. 13). spiral bd. 26.95 (*0-8151-5055-5*) Mosby Inc.

Critical Care & Emergency Nursing. Sandra S. Huddleston & Sondra G. Ferguson. 3rd ed. 1997. LC 96-40890. (Springhouse Notes Ser.). 304p. pap. 26.95 (*0-87434-900-1*) Springhouse Corp.

Critical Care Assessment. Sharron E. Murray & Barbara S. White. 1999. LC 99-21517. xiii, 786p. pap. text (*0-7216-6585-3*) Saunders.

Critical Care Cardiology. Ed. by J. L. Anderson. 1988. (Progress in Critical Care Medicine Ser.: Vol. 3). (Illus.). vii, 260p. 113.25 (*3-8055-4734-X*) S Karger.

***Critical Care Cardiology in the Perioperative Period.** Ed. by J. L. Atlee, III & J. L. Vincent. 2001. (Topics in Anaesthesia & Critical Care Ser.). 120p. (C). pap. (*88-470-0133-1*) Spr-Verlag ITA. *Dist:* Spr-Verlag.

Critical Care Cases. Ed. by R. F. Armstrong & J. B. Salmon. 1997. (Illus.). 242p. pap. text 49.50 (*0-19-262583-7*) OUP.

Critical Care Core Review for Nurses. Nancy G. Townsend. 1988. (Illus.). 200p. (Orig.). (C). pap. text 19.50 (*0-9622174-0-9*); 3rd ed. pap. text 19.95 (*0-9622174-2-5*) Nursing Knowledge.

Critical Care Drugs: Handbook. Steven J. Zaloga et al. 2nd ed. 1996. LC 96-38859. (Illus.). 656p. (C). (gr. 13). pap. text 36.95 (*0-8151-9892-2*, 27875) Mosby Inc.

Critical Care Ethics: Treatment Decisions in American Hospitals. David F. Kelly. 1991. LC 90-62086. 224p. (Orig.). (C). pap. 12.95 (*1-55612-371-X*) Sheed & Ward WI.

Critical Care Examination Review. Joanne Noone & Laura G. Vonfrolio. 3rd ed. 1995. 415p. per. 24.95 (*0-9627246-9-6*) Power NY.

Critical Care Focus 3: Neurological Injury. Ed. by Helen F. Galley. 2000. (Illus.). 63p. pap. text (*0-7279-1596-7*) BMJ Pub GBR. *Dist:* AIDC.

Critical Care in Internal Medicine. Ed. by R. McCaffree. 1985. (Progress in Critical Care Medicine Ser.: Vol. 2). (Illus.). viii, 352p. 82.75 (*3-8055-3900-2*) S Karger.

Critical Care in Nursing. Welan. 2nd ed. 1998. pap. 250.00 (*0-323-00087-8*) Mosby Inc.

Critical Care Management - Case Studies: Tricks & Traps. Ed. by G. R. Park & M. R. Pinsky. 1997. (Illus.). 375p. pap. text (*0-7020-1909-7*) W B Saunders GBR. *Dist:* Saunders.

Critical Care Manual: Applied Physiology & Principles of Therapy, Vol. 1. Robert F. Wilson. 2nd ed. 1992. LC 92-9898. (Illus.). 781p. text 69.00 (*0-8036-9355-9*) Davis Co.

Critical Care Medicine. John J. Marini & Arthur P. Wheeler. 1989. 344p. (Orig.). pap. text 35.00 (*0-683-05554-2*) Lppncott W & W.

Critical Care Medicine: 2000 Edition. Matthew Brenner & Michael Safani. rev. ed. 1999. (Current Clinical Strategies Ser.). pap. 32.95 incl. cd-rom (*1-881528-78-2*) Current Clin Strat.

Critical Care Medicine: A Concise Review. Phillip Dellinger et al. 1995. 283p. pap. 65.00 (*0-916609-06-5*) Am Chest Phys.

Critical Care Medicine: Perioperative Management. Michael Murray. 1996. 600p. text 115.00 (*0-397-51637-1*) Lppncott W & W.

Critical Care Medicine: Perioperative Management. Michael J. Murray. 1996. LC 96-31453. 848p. text 149.00 (*0-397-51689-4*) Lppncott W & W.

Critical Care Medicine: Perioperative Management. Rosenthal. 1993. 39.00 (*0-316-75735-7*) Little.

Critical Care Medicine: Principles & Management. Roger C. Bone. 1994. (Illus.). 1800p. (C). (gr. 13). text 210.00 (*0-8016-7005-5*, 07005) Mosby Inc.

Critical Care Medicine: Principles of Diagnosis & Treatment. Joseph E. Parillo & R. Phillip Dellinger. 2nd ed. Date not set. 1695p. text (*0-323-01280-9*) Mosby Inc.

Critical Care Medicine: The Essentials. John J. Marini & Arthur P. Wheeler. 2nd ed. 1997. LC 96-46592. (Illus.). 640p. pap. 59.95 (*0-683-05555-0*) Lppncott W & W.

Critical Care Multidisciplinary Outcome Pathways. Kimberley A. Basham & Vickie A. Miracle. Ed. by Robin Carter. 1998. LC 98-5490. 512p. (C). pap. text 49.95 (*0-7216-7373-2*) Saunders.

Critical Care Nephrology. Ed. by Claudio Ronco & Rinaldo Bellomo. 1997. LC 97-17215. 1264p. 525.00 (*0-7923-4610-6*) Kluwer Academic.

Critical Care Neurology. Ed. by David Hugh Miller & Eric C. Raps. 1999. LC 98-54233. (Blue Books of Practical Neurology: Vol. 21). 440p. text 99.00 (*0-7506-9968-X*) Buttrwrth-Heinemann.

Critical Care Nurse. Jack Rudman. (Certified Nurse Examination Ser.: CN-18). pap. 27.95 (*0-8373-6118-4*) Nat Learn.

Critical Care Nursing. Linda Bucher & Sheila Melander. Ed. by Robin Carter. 1999. (Illus.). 285p. text, tchr. ed. (*0-7216-6918-2*) Saunders.

Critical Care Nursing. Linda Bucher & Sheila Melander. Ed. by Robin Carter et al. 1999. LC 98-7040. (Illus.). 1230p. (C). text (*0-7216-6917-4*) Saunders.

Critical Care Nursing. Sharon Decker. 2002. (C). pap. 18.75 net. (*0-7668-1386-X*) Delmar.

Critical Care Nursing. Sharon Decker. 2002. (C). pap. 49.50 net. (*0-7668-1384-3*) Thomson Learn.

Critical Care Nursing. Linda Valenti et al. 1997. LC 97-17480. (Lippincott's Review Ser.). 576p. pap. text 24.95 (*0-397-55455-9*) Lppncott W & W.

Critical Care Nursing. John M. Clochesy et al. 2nd ed. 1996. (Illus.). 1577p. text 103.00 (*0-7216-5674-9*) Saunders.

Critical Care Nursing. Moya Vazquez. 2nd ed. 1992. (Illus.). 528p. pap. text 33.00 (*0-7216-3212-2*) Saunders.

Critical Care Nursing: A History. Julie Fairman. 1998. (Illus.). 176p. (C). pap. text 15.95 (*0-8122-1536-2*) U of Pa Pr.

Critical Care Nursing: A History. Julie Fairman & Joan E. Lynaugh. 1998. LC 97-50184. (Studies in Health, Illness, & Caregiving). (Illus.). 175p. (C). text 27.50 (*0-8122-3258-5*) U of Pa Pr.

Critical Care Nursing: A Holistic Approach. Carolyn M. Hudak et al. 7th ed. 1997. LC 97-15951. 1,120p. text 63.95 (*0-7817-9195-2*) Lppncott W & W.

Critical Care Nursing: Assessment & Intervention. Sharon L. Roberts. 1995. LC 95-31492. 800p. (C). pap. text 49.95 (*0-8385-3604-2*, A3604-4, Apple Lange Med) McGraw.

Critical Care Nursing: Australian Perspectives. Ed. by Judith Romanini & John Daly. 1994. (Illus.). 1115p. text (*0-7295-1245-2*) Bailliere Tindall.

Critical Care Nursing: Clinical Companion. Sharon Decker et al. 2002. (C). pap. 20.25 net. (*0-7668-1387-8*) Thomson Learn.

Critical Care Nursing: Diagnosis & Management. Lynne A. Thelan et al. 3rd ed. 1998. tchr. ed. (*0-8151-4346-X*); 1997. LC 97-33345. (Illus.). 1296p. (C). (gr. 13). text 59.95 (*0-8151-3692-7*, 31034) Mosby Inc.

Critical Care Nursing Handbook. Joann Grif Alspach et al. Ed. by Joan M. Joyce. 1983. (Allied Health Professions Monograph). (Illus.). 269p. (C). 35.00 (*0-87527-318-1*) Green.

Critical Care Nursing of Infants & Children. Martha A. Curley et al. Ed. by Ilze Rader. 1996. LC 95-45034. (Illus.). 1126p. text 102.00 (*0-7216-3120-7*) Saunders.

Critical Care Nursing of the Elderly. Ed. by Terry T. Fulmer & Mary K. Walker. 1991. LC 91-4803. 376p. (C). text 43.95 (*0-8261-7050-1*) Springer Pub.

Critical Care Nursing of the Surgical Patient. S. Shekleton & Litwack. 1990. (Illus.). 680p. text 65.00 (*0-7216-3090-1*) Saunders.

Critical Care Nursing Review: Questions, Answers. Branum. 400p. pap. 23.95 (*0-8016-0789-2*) Mosby Inc.

Critical Care Obstetrics. Gary D. Hankins et al. Ed. by Stephen L. Clark & D. B. Cotton. 2nd ed. 1991. (Illus.). 752p. 99.95 (*0-86542-153-6*) Blackwell Sci.

Critical Care Obstetrics. Stephen L. Clark et al. 3rd ed. 1997. LC 97-5559. (Illus.). 720p. 120.95 (*0-86542-538-8*) Blackwell Sci.

Critical Care of the Burned Patient. Ed. by Lindsey T. Rylah. 1992. (Illus.). 222p. (C). text 64.95 (*0-521-39495-3*) Cambridge U Pr.

Critical Care of the Surgical Newborn. Ed. by Don K. Nakayama et al. 1997. LC 97-16497. (Illus.). 624p. 150.00 (*0-87993-653-3*) Futura Pub.

Critical Care of the Surgical Patient. Ed. by G. C. Hanson. 1997. (Illus.). 468p. text (*0-412-60350-0*) E A GBR. *Dist:* OUP.

Critical Care Oncology. Brenda K. Shelton & Stecker. 1998. (Nursing Ser.). 480p. (C). 49.95 (*0-86720-638-1*) Jones & Bartlett.

Critical Care Paramedic. Smith. 2000. pap. text (*0-7216-6807-0*) Saunders.

Critical Care Pearls, 2. Steven A. Sahn & John E. Heffner. 2nd ed. 1997. LC 97-23446. (Pearls Ser.). 479p. pap. 55.00 (*1-56053-224-6*) Hanley & Belfus.

Critical Care Pearls of Wisdom: Over 3000 Questions. Lenhardt. 1998. (Pearls of Wisdom Ser.). pap. 88.00 (*1-890369-16-0*) Boston Medical.

Critical Care Pediatrics: A Problem Oriented Approach. Sol S. Zimmerman & Joan H. Gildea. 1985. (Illus.). 500p. text 79.00 (*0-7216-1143-5*) Saunders.

Critical Care Physiology. Robert H. Bartlett. 1995. 304p. 72.95 (*0-316-08264-3*); LC 95-19794. text 69.95 (*0-316-08269-4*) Lppncott W & W.

Critical Care Plans: Guidelines for Advanced Medical-Surgical Care. Mary F. Moorhouse et al. 1987. LC 87-6740. 472p. 29.95 (*0-8036-6311-0*) Davis Co.

Critical Care Practice. John W. Hoyt et al. 1991. (Illus.). 592p. text 63.00 (*0-7216-4701-4*) Saunders.

Critical Care Procedures Performance Evaluation. American Association of Critical-Care Nurses Staff. 1994. LC 94-13892. (Illus.). 187p. text 74.00 (*0-7216-5441-X*) Saunders.

Critical Care Secrets: Questions You Will be Asked on Rounds, in the ICU, OR & ER & on Oral Exams. Polly E. Parsons & Jeanine P. Wiener-Kronish. 2nd ed. 1998. LC 98-21153. 550p. pap. 39.95 (*1-56053-274-2*) Hanley & Belfus.

Critical Care Skills: A Clinical Handbook. Barbara C. Mims et al. Ed. by Thomas Eoyang. 1996. LC 96-7418. (Illus.). 637p. pap. text 34.00 (*0-7216-4519-4*) Saunders.

Critical Care Toxicology. 2000. (Medical Reference Ser.). (Illus.). 1504p. text 175.00 (*0-8151-4387-7*, 31681) Mosby Inc.

Critical Care Toxicology. Robert Hoffman & Lewis R. Goldfrank. 1991. (Contemporary Management in Critical Care Ser.: Vol. 1, No. 3). (Illus.). 256p. text (*0-443-08830-6*) Church.

Critical Care Transport. University of Maryland Staff & Cindy Tait. 2001. (Illus.). 448p. (C). text 57.50 (*0-7637-1223-X*, 1223-X) Jones & Bartlett.

Critical Care Transport Field Guide. UMBC Cartographic Services Staff. 2001. (Illus.). 64p. (C). pap. text 18.95 (*0-7637-1580-8*, 1580-8) Jones & Bartlett.

Critical Caring: A Feminist Model for Pastoral Psychology. Valerie M. DeMarinis. 1993. LC 93-19485. 208p. text 23.00 (*0-664-22041-X*) Westminster John Knox.

Critical Challenges for Health Care Reform. Richard B. Saltman et al. 1998. LC 97-51880. (State of Health Ser.). 424p. (*0-335-19971-2*); pap. (*0-335-19970-4*) OpUniv Pr.

Critical Choices & Critical Care: Catholic Perspectives on Allocating Resources in Intensive Care Medicine. Ed. by Kevin W. Wildes. 1995. (Philosophy & Medicine Ser.: Vol. 51). 288p. (C). pap. text 50.50 (*0-7923-3701-8*) Kluwer Academic.

Critical Choices & Critical Care: Catholic Perspectives on Allocating Resources in Intensive Care Medicine. Ed. by Kevin W. Wildes. 1995. LC 95-1907. (Philosophy & Medicine Ser.: Vol. 51). 288p. (C). lib. bdg. (*0-7923-3382-9*) Kluwer Academic NLD. *Dist:* Kluwer Academic.

Critical Concepts in Fetal Monitoring. Awhonn. 2nd ed. 1997. VHS 24.95 (*0-683-40118-1*) Lppncott W & W.

Critical Concepts in Medical Practice Management: Working in a Managed Care Environment. Ed. by Robert Tallon. 1996. LC 95-43191. 370p. (Orig.). pap. text 44.95 (*0-07-600761-8*, ME103) Practice Mgmt Info.

Critical Decisions in Craniofacial Anomalies. Jeffrey L. Marsh. 2000. 400p. incl. cd-rom (*1-55009-072-0*) DEKR.

Critical Decisions in Headache Management. Rose M. Giammarco et al. 1998. LC 98-141278. (Illus.). 192p. incl. cd-rom (*1-55009-029-1*) DEKR.

Critical Decisions in Thrombosis & Hemostasis. Jeffrey S. Ginsberg et al. 1998. (Illus.). 356p. incl. cd-rom (*1-55009-043-7*) DEKR.

Critical Dictionary of Jungian Analysis. Andrew Samuels et al. 1986. 224p. pap. 16.95 (*0-7102-0915-0*, 09150); text 39.50 (*0-7102-0410-8*, 04108) Routledge (Routledge Thoemms).

Critical Dictionary of Jungian Anaylsis. Andrew Samuels. 1986. 171p. (C). pap. 27.95 (*0-415-05910-0*) Routledge.

Critical Dictionary of Psychology: Dictionnaire Critique De Psychiatrie. Barthold Berens de Haan. 1986. (FRE.). 304p. 39.95 (*0-8288-1788-X*, M2335) Fr & Eur.

Critical Evaluation of Alternatives to Acute Ocular Irritation Testing. Ed. by Alan M. Goldberg. 1987. (Alternative Methods in Toxicology Ser.: Vol. 4). 138p. 148.00 (*0-913113-09-3*) M Liebert.

Critical Evaluation of Cardiac Rehabilitation, Tel-Aviv, Nov.-Dec. 1975: Proceedings of the Meeting on Critical Evaluation of Cardiac Rehabilitation, Tel-Aviv, Nov.-Dec. 1975. Meeting on Critical Evaluation of Cardiac Rehabili. Ed. by J. J. Kellermann. 1977. (Bibliotheca Cardiologica Ser.: No. 36). (Illus.). 54.00 (*3-8055-2373-4*) S Karger.

Critical Evaluation of Cryptosporidium Research & Research Needs. Michelle M. Frey et al. 1998. LC 97-31911. (*0-89867-938-9*) Am Water Wks Assn.

Critical Evaluation of Research in Physical Therapy. Antoine Helewa et al. 1998. LC 99-51476. (Illus.). 319p. pap. 35.00 (*0-7216-7390-2*) Saunders.

Critical Evaluation of Strategies for a Successful Termination of Cardiopulmonary Bypass During Cardiac Surgery: Role of Pharmacologic Myocardial Protection; Appropriate Pharmacologic Support for the Postischemic Myocardium. Roland Demeyere. 1998. (Acta Biomedica Lovaniensia Ser.). (Illus.). 150p. pap. (*90-6186-892-0*) Leuven Univ BEL. *Dist:* Coronet Bks.

Critical Features of Piaget's Theory of the Development of Thought. Ed. by Frank B. Murray. 1972. LC 72-6359. 196p. pap. text 12.95 (*0-8422-0244-7*) Irvington.

Critical Gerontology: Perspectives from Political & Moral Economy. Ed. by Meredith Minkler & Carroll L. Estes. 1999. LC 97-37071. (Policy, Politics, Health & Medicine Ser.). 380p. pap. 39.00 (*0-89503-185-X*); text 59.00 (*0 89503 181 1*) Baywood Pub.

Critical Heart Disease in Infants & Children. Ed. by David G. Nichols et al. 1995. (Illus.). 1104p. (C). (gr. 13). text 185.00 (*0-8016-6929-4*, 06929) Mosby Inc.

Critical Incident Stress & Trauma in the Workplace. Gerald Lewis. 1994. 134p. (Orig.). pap. text 19.95 (*1-55959-054-8*) Accel Devel.

Critical Incident Stress Debriefing - Three-Fourths Inch. ASVP Staff. 1991. (gr. 13). 159.95 (*1-56200-401-8*) Mosby Inc.

Critical Incident Stress Debriefing-PAL. ASVP Staff. 1991. (gr. 13). 159.00 (*1-56200-402-6*) Mosby Inc.

Critical Incident Technique: A Bibliography. Ed. by Grace Fivars. 2nd ed. 1980. pap. 7.50 (*0-89785-662-7*) Am Inst Res.

Critical Incidents in Group Therapy. Jeremiah Donigian & Richard Malnati. 1986. LC 86-1011. (Psychology Ser.). 239p. (C). 27.75 (*0-534-06282-2*) Brooks-Cole.

Critical Incidents in Group Therapy. Jeremiah Donigian & Diana Hulse-Killacky. 2nd ed. 1998. (Counseling Ser.). 420p. pap. text 45.95 (*0-534-35727-X*) Brooks-Cole.

Critical Interventions in Psychotherapy. Haim Omer. 1994. LC 94-12384. 192p. 23.00 (*0-393-70182-4*) Norton.

Critical Issues, Developments, & Trends in Professional Psychology, Vol. 1. Ed. by Regis McNamara & Allan G. Barclay. 1982. LC 81-15863. 321p. 72.95 (*0-275-90860-7*, C08601, Praeger Pubs) Greenwood.

Critical Issues, Developments & Trends in Professional Psychology, Vol. 2. Ed. by J. Regis McNamara. 1984. LC 81-15863. 321p. 67.00 (*0-275-91227-2*, C12272, Praeger Pubs) Greenwood.

Critical Issues in American Nursing in the Twentieth Century: Perspectives & Case Studies. Ed. by Darwin H. Stapleton. 1994. 152p. (Orig.). (C). pap. 20.00 (*1-886511-02-0*) Fnd NY St Nurses.

Critical Issues in American Psychiatry & the Law, Vol. 2. Ed. by Richard Rosner. 1985. LC 81-9059. 324p. 80.00 (*0-306-41954-8*, Plenum Trade) Perseus Pubng.

Critical Issues in Clinical Practice. Jennifer Clegg. 1998. LC 98-61165. pap. 25.95 (*0-8039-7555-4*, 1274) Sage.

Critical Issues in Contemporary Health Care: Proceedings of the Eighth Bishops' Workshop. Ed. by Russell E. Smith. 1989. LC 89-22935. 354p. pap. 17.95 (*0-935372-27-X*) NCBC.

Critical Issues in Cytopathology. Ed. by Tilde S. Kline. 1996. LC 95-32576. (Illus.). 144p. pap. 39.50 (*0-89640-298-3*) Igaku-Shoin.

Critical Issues in Medical Technology. Ernest G. Cravalho. Ed. by Barbara J. McNeil. 1981. LC 81-7900. 447p. 28.00 (*0-86569-070-7*, Auburn Hse) Greenwood.

Critical Issues in Operating Room Management. Ed. by Mark A. Malangoni. 1997. LC 96-15605. cd-rom 299.00 (*0-397-51796-3*) Lppncott W & W.

Critical Issues in Personal Construct Psychotherapy. Ed. by L. M. Leitner & N. G. Dunnett. 1995. 330p. (C). pap. 19.95 (*0-89464-959-0*) Krieger.

Critical Issues in Psychology, Psychiatry & Physiology: A Memorial to W. Horsley Gantt. Ed. by F. J. McGuigan & Thomas A. Ban. 1987. (Monographs in Psychobiology: Vol. 2). xviii, 380p. text 108.00 (*2-88124-137-9*) Gordon & Breach.

***Critical Issues in Psychotherapy: Translating New Ideas into Practice.** Ed. by Brent D. Slife et al. 2001. LC 00-12405. xvii, 353p. 48.95 (*0-7619-2080-3*, 86087) Sage.

Critical Issues in Psychotherapy: Translating New Ideas into Practice. Brent D. Slife et al. 2001. LC 00-12405. xvii, 353p. pap. 39.95 (*0-7619-2081-1*, 86088) Sage.

Critical Issues in Qualitative Research Methods. Ed. by Janice M. Morse. 1993. (C). 81.95 (*0-8039-5042-X*, 4569); pap. 39.95 (*0-8039-5043-8*, 4570) Sage.

Critical Issues in Surgery: Proceedings of a Meeting Held in St. Thomas, U. S. Virgin Islands, November 9-11, 1992. Ed. by Aurel C. Cernaianu et al. 1995. LC 95-21518. 218p. 79.50 (*0-306-44918-8*, Kluwer Plenum) Kluwer Academic.

Critical Issues in the Treatment of Affective Disorders. Ed. by N. Brunello et al. 1995. LC 95-3161. (International Academy for Biomedical & Drug Research Ser.: Vol. 9). (Illus.). viii, 198p. 195.00 (*3-8055-6032-X*) S Karger.

Critical Issues in the Treatment of Schizophrenia. Ed. by G. Racagni et al. 1996. (International Academy for Biomedical & Drug Research Ser.: Vol. 10). (Illus.). vi, 206p. 198.25 (*3-8055-6199-7*) S Karger.

Critical Limb Ischemia Carotid Surgery. Ed. by S. Horsch & K. Ktenidis. 1999. (Illus.). 143p. (C). pap. (*3-7985-1075-X*) D Steinkopff DEU. *Dist:* Spr-Verlag.

Critical Literature Review of Clinical Effectiveness in Allied Health Practices. 1995. lib. bdg. 252.95 (*0-8490-6844-4*) Gordon Pr.

Critical Maneuvers in Urologic Surgery. George W. Yu. 1996. (Illus.). 1p. (C). (gr. 13). pap. text 160.00 incl. cd-rom, audio compact disk (*0-8151-2444-9*, 30818) Mosby Inc.

Critical Medical Anthropology. Merrill Singer & Hans Baer. 1995. (Critical Approaches in the Health Social Sciences Ser.). 416p. (C). 53.00 (*0-89503-124-8*) Baywood Pub.

Critical Moments in Qualitative Research. Joy Higgs et al. 2001. 232p. pap. 40.00 (*0-7506-5159-8*) Buttrwrth-Heinemann.

Critical Pathway Development Guide. Deborah K. Wall & Mitchell M. Proyect. 1997. LC 97-28928. (Illus.). 97p. pap. 40.00 (*0-944496-53-9*) Precept Pr.

Critical Pathway Implementation Guide. Deborah K. Wall & Mitchell M. Proyect. 1997. LC 97-23771. (Illus.). 128p. pap. 40.00 (*0-944496-54-7*) Precept Pr.

Critical Pathways: Current Bibliographies in Medicine: January 1988 Through December 1995. Ronald L. Gordner & Patricia Moritz. 1996. 57p. reprint ed. pap. text 25.00 (*0-7881-3343-8*) DIANE Pub.

Critical Pathways Implementation Guide. Eric Joseph. 1994. 145p. pap. text 40.00 (*0-916499-55-3*) Care Educ Grp.

Critical Pathways in Geriatric Care. Eric Joseph. 1994. 160p. (Orig.). pap. text (*0-916499-56-1*) Care Educ Grp.

Critical Pathways in Otolaryngology. Constantinides. 2001. (Illus.). 608p. pap. 89.00 (*0-86577-847-7*) Thieme Med Pubs.

Critical Pathways in Therapeutic Intervention: Upper Extremities. Saidoff & McDonnough. 1996. (Illus.). 368p. (C). (gr. 13). text 39.00 (*0-8151-4486-5*, 29952) Mosby Inc.

Critical Perspectives & Issues in Health Policy. Ed. by Ralph Straetz et al. 1980. (Orig.). pap. 15.00 (*0-918592-42-9*) Pol Studies.

Critical Psychological Issues: Judaic Perspectives. Reuven P. Bulka. 1992. 162p. (C). 51.50 (*0-8191-8476-4*); pap. 25.50 (*0-8191-8477-2*) U Pr of Amer.

Critical Psychology: Contributions to an Historical Science of the Subject. Ed. by Charles W. Tolman & Wolfgang Maiers. 1991. 280p. (C). text 54.95 (*0-521-39344-2*) Cambridge U Pr.

Critical Psychology: Interpretation of the Personal World. Edmund V. Sullivan. 1984. LC 83-20184. (PATH in Psychology Ser.). 212p. 60.00 (*0-306-41434-1*, Plenum Trade) Perseus Pubng.

Critical Psychophysical Passages in the Life of a Woman: A Psychodynamic Perspective. J. Offerman-Zuckerberg. 1988. LC 88-12615. (Illus.). 310p. (C). 54.50 (*0-306-42639-0*, Kluwer Plenum) Kluwer Academic.

Critical Reading for Primary Care. Ed. by Roger Jones & Ann-Louise Kinmonth. 1995. LC 94-28163. (Oxford General Practice Ser.: No. 28). (Illus.). 250p. pap. text 55.00 (*0-19-262381-8*) OUP.

Critical Reading for the Reflective Practitioner. Robert Clarke & Peter Croft. 1998. LC 99-182011. 336p. pap. text 38.50 (*0-7506-3939-3*) Buttrwrth-Heinemann.

Critical Review of Recent Literature on Toxicity of Cyanides to Fish. Peter Doudoroff. 1980. LC 80-68588. 71p. (Orig.). pap. 20.00 (*0-89364-039-5*, API 847-87000) Am Petroleum.

Critical Reviews in Tropical Medicine. Ed. by R. K. Chandra. LC 82-15129. Vol. 1. 1982. 412p. 95.00 (*0-306-40959-3*); Vol. 2. 1984. 290p. 85.00 (*0-306-41561-5*) Perseus Pubng (Plenum Trade).

Critical Social Welfare Issues: Tools for Social Work & Health Care Professionals. Ed. by Arthur J. Katz et al. 1997. LC 97-9241. 238p. 39.95 (*0-7890-0161-6*) Haworth Pr.

Critical Study of the American Nursing Home - the Final Solution. Ursula Adler. 1991. LC 91-8802. (Studies in Health & Human Services: Vol. 18). 242p. lib. bdg. 89.95 (*0-88946-383-2*) E Mellen.

Critical Success Factors in Biomedical Research & Pharmaceutical Innovation: The Joint Impact of Management Control & Contingencies on Performance & Effectiveness in Research Laboratories in Medical. . . S. W. Omta. 1995. LC 95-17479. 294p. text 129.00 (*0-7923-3563-5*) Kluwer Academic.

Critical Theories of Psychological Development. J. M. Broughton. 1987. LC 86-30383. (PATH in Psychology Ser.). (Illus.). 338p. (C). 62.50 (*0-306-42431-2*, Plenum Trade) Perseus Pubng.

Critical Thinking: An Interactive Tool for Learning Medical-Surgical Nursing. Eleanor V. Vanetzian. 2000. (Illus.). 633p. pap. text 29.95 (*0-8036-0616-8*) Davis Co.

Critical Thinking: Cases in Respiratory Care. Kathleen J. Wood. 1997. LC 97-10615. (Illus.). 151p. (C). pap. text 24.95 (*0-8036-0153-0*) Davis Co.

Critical Thinking: Developing Skills for Radiography. Kathryn S. Durand. 1999. LC 98-32464. (Illus.). xvii, 267p. pap. 29.99 (*0-8036-0343-6*) Davis Co.

Critical Thinking: Understanding & Evaluating Dental Research. Donald M. Brunette. 1996. LC 95-26777. (Illus.). 248p. pap. text 38.00 (*0-86715-301-6*) Quint Pub Co.

Critical Thinking Activities for Nursing. Marilyn Smith-Stoner. 1998. LC 98-3973. 192p. pap. text 22.95 (*0-7817-1619-5*) Lppncott W & W.

Critical Thinking Applied to Nursing. Mary A. Miller & Dorothy E. Babcock. 1996. tchr. ed. (*0-8151-6960-4*); 1995. LC 95-37174. (Illus.). 368p. (C). (gr. 13). pap. text 25.00 (*0-8151-6962-0*, 27243) Mosby Inc.

***Critical Thinking Approach to Skill Development & Competency Evaluation.** Donna Ignatavicius. 2001. (C). 300p. pap. text, tchr. ed. 19.95 (*0-9713433-1-4*); 320p. pap. text, stu. ed. 32.95 (*0-9713433-0-6*) Med Plastics Lab Inc.

Critical Thinking Assessment in Nursing Education Programs: An Aggregate Data Analysis. Noreen C. Facione & Peter A. Facione. 1997. LC 98-180614. (Illus.). x, 142p. (C). pap. text 49.50 (*1-891557-21-1*, 177) Calif Acad.

Critical Thinking Companion for Introductory Psychology. Jane S. Halonen. 1995. 144p. pap. text 9.95 (*1-57259-018-1*) Worth.

Critical Thinking in Clinical Practice: Improving the Accuracy of Judgments & Decisions about Clients. Eileen Gambrill. 1990. LC 89-24660. (Jossey-Bass Social & Behavioral Science Ser.). 432p. 46.00 (*1-55542-198-9*) Jossey-Bass.

***Critical Thinking in Medical-Surgical Settings: A Case Study Approach - Instructor's Resource Manual.** Maryl Winningham & Barbara Preusser. 2nd ed. 2001. (Illus.). pap. 250.00 (*0-323-01131-4*) Mosby Inc.

Critical Thinking in Nursing: A Practical Approach. Rosalinda A. Alfaro-Lefevre. 1995. (Illus.). pap., tchr. ed. (*0-7216-5902-0*); LC 94-25233. pap. text 22.00 (*0-7216-5897-0*) Saunders.

Critical Thinking in Nursing: A Practical Approach. Rosalinda A. Alfaro-Lefevre. Ed. by Thomas Eoyang. 2nd ed. 1999. LC 98-47454. (Illus.). 335p. (C). pap. text 24.95 (*0-7216-8277-4*) Saunders.

Critical Thinking in Nursing: An Interactive Approach. M. Gaie Rubenfeld & Barbara K. Scheffer. 2nd ed. 1999. LC 98-46410. 464p. pap. text 28.95 (*0-7817-1634-9*, Lippnctt) Lppncott W & W.

Critical Thinking in Nursing Case Studies Across the Curriculum. 2000. (*0-8053-8538-X*) Addison-Wesley.

Critical Thinking in Respiratory Care: A Problem Based Learning Approach. Shelley C. Mishoe & Melvin A. Welch, Jr. 2001. LC 00-65390. (Illus.). 528p. pap. 54.95 (*0-07-134474-8*) McGraw-Hill Prof.

Critical Thinking in the Medical Surgical Setting: A Case Study Approach. Maryl Winningham & Barbara Preusser. (Illus.). 456p. 1996. (*0-323-00723-6*); 1996. (*1-55664-560-0*); 1995. (C). (gr. 13). pap. text 24.95 (*0-8151-9419-6*, 27763) Mosby Inc.

Critical Thinking in the Medical-Surgical Setting: A Case Study Approach. Maryl Winningham & Barbara Preusser. 1996. tchr. ed. (*0-8151-9418-8*) Mosby Inc.

Critical Thinking in the Medical Surgical Setting: A Case Study Approach. Maryl Winningham. 2nd ed. 2000. (Illus.). 464p. pap. text 21.95 (*0-323-01154-3*) Saunders.

Critical Thinking Study Guide for Medical-Surgical Nursing Across the Health Care Continuum. Elaine Kennedy & Donna D. Ignatavicius. Ed. by Robin Carter et al. 3rd ed. 1999. 285p. stu. ed. (*0-7216-8257-X*) Saunders.

Critical Voices on Special Education: Problems & Progress Concerning the Mildly Handicapped. Ed. by Scott B. Sigmon. 1990. LC 89-38707. 265p. (C). text 22.50 (*0-7914-0319-X*); pap. text 21.95 (*0-7914-0320-3*) State U NY Pr.

Critically Ill Cardiac Patient: Multisystem Dysfunction & Management. Vladimir Kvetan. 1996. LC 96-19018. 432p. text 159.00 (*0-397-51465-4*) Lppncott W & W.

CritiControl: A Training Software. Ed. by NEC Corporation, Biological Simulators Inc. Staff et al. 1998. (ENG, FRE & GER.). 125.00 incl. cd-rom (*3-540-14682-2*) Spr-Verlag.

Critique of Psychoanalytic Reason: Hypnosis as a Scientific Problem from Lavoisier to Lacan. Leon Chertok & Isabelle Stengers. Tr. by Martha N. Evans from FRE. 1992. LC 91-22388. 356p. (C). 51.00 (*0-8047-1950-0*) Stanford U Pr.

Critique of Teachers' Ratings of High School Boys As an Indication of Later Neuropsychiatric Rejection for the Armed Services. Olive L. Ives. LC 71-176898. (Columbia University. Teachers College. Contributions to Education Ser.: No. 950). reprint ed. 37.50 (*0-404-55950-6*) AMS Pr.

Critique of the Foundations of Psychology: The Psychology of Psychoanalysis. Georges Politzer. Tr. by Maurice Apprey from FRE. 1994. LC 94-4139. 215p. (C). text 54.00 (*0-8207-0256-0*); pap. text 22.50 (*0-8207-0257-9*) Duquesne.

Critique, Resistance & Action: Working Papers in the Politics of Nursing. Ed. by David G. Allen et al. 1992. LC 92-48677. 224p. (C). pap. text 32.95 (*0-88737-563-4*) Natl League Nurse.

CRNA Guide to Ambulatory Anesthesia. John Aker & Chuck Biddle. 1997. (Illus.). 608p. 65.00 (*0-07-057127-9*) McGraw.

Crofton & Douglas's Respiratory Diseases. Anthony D. Seaton et al. 5th ed. 2000. LC 99-15579. (Illus.). 1698p. 299.00 (*0-86542-857-3*) Blackwell Sci.

Crohn's, Colitis, Hemorrhoids, & Me: A Patient's Story of Hope, Humor, & Living with Inflammatory Bowel Disease. Kathlene J. O'Leary. Ed. by Alan R. Danriquez. 1995. LC 95-78430. (Illus.). 128p. (Orig.). pap. 12.95 (*0-9647571-3-3*) Anderson Laguna.

Crohn's Disease. Ed. by Cosimo Prantera & Burton I. Korelitz. 1996. (Gastroenterology Ser.: Vol. 1). (Illus.). 624p. text 150.00 (*0-8247-9410-9*) Dekker.

Crohn's Disease: Treatment & Pathogenesis. 1987. 192p. 110.00 (*0-8493-6736-0*, RC862, CRC Reprint) Franklin.

Crohn's Disease & Ulcerative Colitis Fact Book. National Foundation for Ileitis and Colitis Staff. Ed. by Peter A. Banks et al. 1983. (Crohn's Disease Ulcerative Colitis Fact Book C Ser.: Vol. 1). (Illus.). 194p. pap. 18.95 (*0-684-17967-9*) Hungry Minds.

Cross - Cultural Contributions to Psychology. Ed. by L. H. Eckensberger et al. 1979. x, 442p. pap. (*90-265-0300-8*) Swets.

***Cross-Country Skiing: Olympic Handbook of Sports Medicine.** Heikki Rusko. 2001. (Handbooks of Sports Medicine & Science). (Illus.). 156p. pap. 29.95 (*0-632-05571-5*) Blackwell Sci.

Cross-Cultral Rehabilitation: An International Perspective. Ronnie Linda Leavitt. 1999. LC 99-233555. (Illus.). x, 413p. (C). pap. text (*0-7020-2245-4*) W B Saunders GBR. *Dist:* Saunders.

Cross-Cultural Anxiety, Vol. 3. Ed. by Charles D. Spielberger & Rogelio Diaz Guerrero. 1986. (Clinical & Community Psychology Ser.). (Illus.). 250p. (C). 63.95 (*0-89116-419-7*) Hemisp Pub.

Cross-Cultural Approach to Health Behavior. Ed. by L. Riddick Lynch. 1975. LC 73-84199. 364p. 38.50 (*0-8386-7439-9*); pap. 17.95 (*0-8386-1377-2*) Fairleigh Dickinson.

Cross-Cultural Caring: A Handbook for Health Professionals in Western Canada. Ed. by Nancy Waxler-Morrison et al. 1990. 284p. pap. 25.95 (*0-7748-0343-6*) U of Wash Pr.

Cross-Cultural Communication in the Health Sciences: Communicating with Migrant Patients. Anne Pauwels. 1996. LC 96-141837. 206p. (*0-7329-2953-9*); pap. (*0-7329-2954-7*) Macmill Educ AUS. *Dist:* Paul & Co Pubs.

Cross-Cultural Neuropsychological Assessment: Theory & Practice. Victor Nell. 1999. LC 99-32682. 250p. (*0-8058-3355-2*); 289p. pap. (*0-8058-3356-0*) L Erlbaum Assocs.

Cross-Cultural Nursing: Anthropological Approaches to Nursing. Ed. by J. M. Morse. 1989. vi, 144p. pap. text 35.00 (*2-88124-383-5*) Gordon & Breach.

Cross Cultural Nursing Care. Hoeman. 1995. (Professional Reference - Nursing Ser.). (C). pap. text 19.95 (*0-8273-6059-2*) Delmar.

***Cross-cultural Perspectives in Introductory Psychology.** William F. Price & Richley H. Crapo. 4th ed. 2001. 192p. pap. text 17.95 (*0-534-54654-4*) Wadsworth Pub.

Cross Cultural Perspectives in Medical Ethics: Readings. Robert M. Veatch. 2nd ed. 2000. LC 99-89318. (Illus.). 400p. (C). pap. text 38.95 (*0-7637-1332-5*, 1332-5) Jones & Bartlett.

Cross-Cultural Practice: Assessment, Treatment & Training. Sharon Gopaul-McNicol & Janet Brice-Baker. 1997. LC 97-8869. 192p. 95.00 (*0-471-14849-0*) Wiley.

Cross-Cultural Psychiatry: A Practical Guide. Dinesh Bhugra & Kamaldeep Bhui. 2000. 192p. (Orig.). pap. text (*0-7506-4353-6*) E A GBR. *Dist:* OUP.

Cross-Cultural Psychology. Eric Shiraev. 1996. (C). pap. 34.38 (*0-07-057802-8*) McGrw-H Hghr Educ.

Cross-Cultural Psychology: Research & Applications. John W. Berry et al. 1992. (Illus.). 475p. (C). pap. text 37.95 (*0-521-37761-7*) Cambridge U Pr.

Cross-Cultural Research in Human Development: A Life-Span Perspective. Ed. by Leonore L. Adler. 1989. LC 88-15536. (Illus.). 308p. 68.50 (*0-275-93048-3*, C3048, Praeger Pubs) Greenwood.

Cross-Cultural Study of Perception. Melville Jean Herskovits et al. rev. ed. 1969. LC 67-21404. spiral bd. 20.00 (*0-672-60811-1*) Irvington.

Cross-Cultural Training for Mental Health Professionals. Ed. by Harriet P. Lefley & Paul B. Pedersen. 1986. (Illus.). 360p. (C). 60.95 (*0-398-05257-3*) C C Thomas.

Cross Design Synthesis: A New Strategy for Medical Effectiveness Research. 1994. (Illus.). 121p. (Orig.). (C). pap. text 40.00 (*0-7881-0590-6*) DIANE Pub.

Cross-Examination of Medical Experts. Marshall Houts. 1982. (Art of Advocacy Ser.). 171.00 (*0-8205-1031-9*) Bender.

Cross Infection Control in General Dental Practice. Croser & Chipping. 1990. LC 93-31256. (Illus.). 118p. pap. text 34.00 (*0-86715-010-6*) Quint Pub Co.

Cross-Linguistic Evidence for Genetic Dysphasia. Ed. by Myrna Gopnik. 1998. (Folia Phoniatrica et Logopaedica Ser.: Vol. 51, No. 1 (1999)). (Illus.). 90p. pap. 34.00 (*3-8055-6820-7*) S Karger.

Cross Name Index to Medicinal Plants Anthony R. Torkelson. 1995. Set. 1200p. 1000.00 (*0-8493-2635-4*, 2635C2W); Vol. 1. 339p. 369.95 (*0-8493-2631-1*); Vol. 2. 396p. 369.95 (*0-8493-2632-X*); Vol. 3. 614p. 369.95 (*0-8493-2633-8*) CRC Pr.

Cross National Perspectives on Health Care Reform: Proceedings of the Second International Colloquium on Health Care & Health Care Reform. William R. Frey. 1995. LC 95-42472. 179p. 50.00 (*0-89941-986-0*, 308950) W S Hein.

Cross-over Experiments: Design, Analysis & Application. David A. Ratkowsky et al. 1992. (Statistics: Textbooks & Monographs Ser.: Vol. 135). (Illus.). 480p. text 175.00 (*0-8247-8892-3*) Dekker.

Cross-over Trials in Clinical Research: Statistics in Practice. Stephen Senn. 1993. 296p. 120.00 (*0-471-93493-3*) Wiley.

Cross Section of Nursing Research: Journal Articles for Discussion & Evaluation. Roberta J. Peteva. 2000. 194p. pap. text 24.95 (*1-884585-31-0*) Pyrczak Pub.

Cross-Sectional Abdominal Anatomy: CT, MRI, & Ultrasound. Kenneth Zirinsky & John A. Markisz. 1992. (Illus.). 1992p. pap. 35.00 (*0-89640-215-0*) Igaku-Shoin.

Cross-Sectional Anatomy for Computed Tomography. M. L. Farkas. 1988. (Illus.). 84p. 79.00 (*0-387-96714-1*) Spr-Verlag.

Cross-Sectional Anatomy of Acupoints. Eachou Chen. Tr. by Andrew Flower. 1995. LC 94-27579. text (*0-443-04974-2*) Church.

Cross Sectional Anatomy to Color & Study. Ray Poritsky. 1996. LC 96-2015. (Illus.). 160p. pap. 28.00 (*1-56053-169-X*) Hanley & Belfus.

Cross Sectional Atlas of Commonly Used Acupuncture Points of the Arm & Leg. Alex Holland. 1989. 200p. (Orig.). (C). pap. text 18.00 (*0-9622665-0-7*) A Holland.

Crossbreeding Beef Cattle: Series II. Ed. by Marvin Koger et al. 1973. LC 73-8847. 470p. 38.95 (*0-8130-0364-4*) U Press Fla.

Crossing Borders: Migration, Ethnicity & AIDS. Ed. by Mary Haour-Knipe & Richard Rector. 1996. LC 96-232435. (Social Aspects of AIDS Ser.). 224p. (*0-7484-0377-9*); pap. (*0-7484-0378-7*) Tay Francis Ltd GBR. *Dist:* Taylor & Francis.

Crossing Bridges: A Parent's Perspective on Coping after a Child Is Diagnosed with Autism/PDD. Viki Satkiewicz-Gayhardt et al. 1998. (Illus.). 64p. reprint ed. pap. 5.95 (*0-9650700-2-6*, PUP Bks) Potential Unltd.

Crossing Cultures in Mental Health. Ed. by Diane R. Koslow & Elizabeth P. Salett. 1989. 154p. (Orig.). pap. 9.95 (*0-933934-15-7*) NMCI Pubns.

Crossing the River: Creating a Conceptual Revolution in Community & Disability. David B. Schwartz. 1992. 238p. (C). pap. text 24.95 (*0-914797-82-4*) Brookline Bks.

Crossing the Road: A Guide to Teaching the Mentally Handicapped. P. D. Taylor & P. Robinson. 1984. 41p. 22.00 (*0-906054-12-5*) St Mut.

Crossing the Thin Line. Terence Williams. 1980. 20p. 2.00 (*0-89486-077-1*, 1213B) Hazelden.

Crossings: Preparing Ahead of Time, Vol I. Jayne Bremyer. 1985. 200p. pap. 4.95 (*0-931515-06-8*) Triumph Pr.

Crosslinguistic Study of Language Acquisition Ed. by Dan I. Slobin. 1986. (C). 976p. text 180.00 (*0-89859-367-0*); 400p. text 80.00 (*0-89859-799-4*) L Erlbaum Assocs.

Crossroads... A Journey of Commitment. Marianne E. Olson. 1999. (Illus.). 250p. pap. 14.95 (*0-9662512-1-0*) Planning Innovat.

Crossroads to Cure: The Homoeopath's Guide to Second Prescription. Nicola Henriques. 1998. pap. text 19.95 (*0-9663388-0-4*) Totality Pr.

Crowded Bed: An Effective Framework for Doing Couple Therapy. Toby Bobes. 1999. LC 98-22639. (Illus.). 208p. 27.00 (*0-393-70280-4*) Norton.

CRRT Abstracts Collection, 1995-1999. Ed. by R. L. Mehta. 1999. (Blood Purification, Abstracts 1995-1999 Ser.). cd-rom 50.50 (*3-8055-6856-8*) S Karger.

***CRRT Abstracts Collection 1995-2001.** Ed. by R. L. Mehta. 2001. (Abstracts 1995-2001 Ser.). cd-rom 50.50 (*3-8055-7226-3*) S Karger.

CRS Computer-Related Syndrome: The Prevention & Treatment of Computer-Related Injuries. Richard D. Smith. 1997. LC 97-6575. (Illus.). 146p. pap. 18.00 (*1-57392-145-9*) Prometheus Bks.

Crucial Controversies in Surgery, 1997: Perspectives on 15 Major Controversial Topics in General Surgery. Ed. by M. Schein & L. Wise. 1997. (Illus.). xxviii, 304p. text 98.00 (*3-8055-6615-8*) S Karger.

Crucial Controversies in Surgery, 1998: Perspectives on 15 Major Controversial Topics in General Surgery. Ed. by M. Schein & L. Wise. 1997. (Illus.). xxvi, 274p. text 98.00 (*3-8055-6616-6*) S Karger.

Crucial Ligaments. Ed. by John A. Feagin, Jr. 2nd ed. 1993. 720p. text (*0-443-08931-0*) Church.

Crucible of Experience: R. D. Laing & the Crisis of Psychotherapy. Daniel Burston. 2000. LC 99-57332. viii, 168p. 27.95 (*0-674-00217-2*) HUP.

Crude Black Molasses. Cyril Scott & John B. Lust. 1999. 92p. pap. 3.95 (*0-87904-010-6*) Lust.

Cruel Compassion: Psychiatric Control of Society's Unwanted. Thomas S. Szasz. 1998. LC 97-42659. 288p. pap. 19.95 (*0-8156-0510-2*) Syracuse U Pr.

Cruelest Death: The Enigma of Adolescent Suicide. David Lester. 1992. LC 92-34448. 160p. (Orig.). (C). pap. text 20.95 (*0-914783-64-5*) Charles.

Cruelty of Depression: On Melancholy. Jacques Hassoun. Tr. by David Jacobson. 2000. 105p. reprint ed. text 22.00 (*0-7881-6896-7*) DIANE Pub.

Cruelty, Violence & Murder: Understanding the Criminal Mind. Arthur Hyatt-Williams. 1998. LC 97-30757. (Illus.). 376p. 50.00 (*0-7657-0128-6*) Aronson.

Cruising Fundamentals. International Marine Publications Systems Staff. rev. ed. 1992. LC 93-248285. 136p. pap. 18.95 (*0-07-001519-8*, Ragged Mtn) McGraw-Hill Trade.

Crusade for Stroke Prevention. J. Crayton Pruitt. 1999. LC 99-6775. (Illus.). xx, 168p. (*1-879852-63-2*) Univ Tampa.

Crusader for Sex Education: Elisa Ottesen-Jensen, 1886-1973 in Scandinavia & on the International Scene. Doris H. Linder. 1996. LC 96-15161. 328p. (C). lib. bdg. 51.00 (*0-7618-0333-5*) U Pr of Amer.

Crush the Boards: The Ultimate USMLE Step 2 Review. Bruno Brochert & Adam Brochert. 1999. LC 99-42852. (Illus.). 224p. (C). pap. 28.00 (*1-56053-366-8*) Hanley & Belfus.

Cry for Help: The Professional Response. J. Kahn & E. Earle. 1982. LC 81-21110. (Pergamon International Library Science Technology Engineering & Social Studies). 130p. pap. text (*0-08-027437-4*) Pergamon Repr GBR. *Dist:* Franklin.

Cry of Mute Children: A Psychoanalytic Perspective of the Second Generation of the Holocaust. Ilany Kogan. 1995. (C). xiv, 178 p. pap. (*1-85343-322-5*); 170p. (*1-85343-321-7*) Free Assoc Bks GBR. *Dist:* Intl Spec Bk, NYU Pr.

Cry of the Eagle: Encounters with a Cree Healer. David E. Young et al. 1990. 260p. pap. text 20.95 (*0-8020-6820-0*) U of Toronto Pr.

Cry of the Invisible: Writings from the Homeless & Survivors of Psychiatric Hospitals. Ed. by Michael A. Susko. 1991. LC 90-82024. (Mental Health Ser.). (Illus.). 260p. 19.95 (*0-941401-05-7*); pap. 16.95 (*0-941401-04-9*) Conservatory.

Cry the Beloved Mind: A Voyage of Hope. Vernon M. Neppe. 2000. LC 98-67899. (Illus.). 367p. pap. 18.95 (*0-89716-823-2*) P B Pubng.

Cry Wolf: The Psychology of False Alarms. Shlomo Breznitz. 1984. 280p. text 49.95 (*0-89859-296-8*) L Erlbaum Assocs.

Crying As a Sign, a Symptom & a Signal: Clinical, Emotional & Developmental Aspects of Infant & Toddler Crying. Ed. by Ronald G. Barr et al. 2000. LC 00-421475. (Clinics in Developmental Medicine Ser.: No. 152). (Illus.). viii, 228p. (C). (*1-898683-21-2*) Mc Keith Pr GBR. *Dist:* Cambridge U Pr.

Crying Hands: Eugenics & Deaf People in Nazi Germany. Horst Biesold. 1999. LC 99-27291. (Illus.). xix, 230p. 39.95 (*1-56368-077-7*) Gallaudet Univ Pr.

Cryopreservation: Applications in Pharmaceuticals & Biotechnology. Ed. by Kenneth E. Avis & Carmen M. Wagner. 1998. LC 99-21101. (Drug Manufacturing Technology Ser.). 300p. 179.00 (*1-57491-090-6*) IHS Health Grp.

Cryopreservation & Low Temperature Biology in Blood Transfusion. Ed. by C. T. Sibinga et al. 1990. (C). text 91.50 (*0-7923-0908-1*) Kluwer Academic.

Cryopreservation of Plant Cells & Organs. Ed. by K. K. Kartha. 1985. 288p. lib. bdg. 203.00 (*0-8493-6102-8*, QK725) CRC Pr.

Cryosurgery of Maxillofacial Region: General Principles & Clinical Applications to Benign Lesions. Paul F. Bradley. 1986. LC 85-22421. 200p. 157.00 (*0-8493-5219-3*, CRC Reprint) Franklin.

Cryosurgery of Maxillofacial Region Vol. 2: Clinical Application Malignant Lesions & Comparison Lasers. Paul F. Bradley. 1986. LC 85-22421. 145.00 (*0-8493-5220-7*, CRC Reprint) Franklin.

Cryosurgery of the Maxillofacial Region, Set, Vols. I-II. Paul F. Bradley. 1986. 248.00 (*0-8493-5218-5*, RD523) CRC Pr.

Cryotherapy in Chest Medicine. J. P. Homasson & N. Bell. 1993. (Illus.). 126p. 121.00 (*0-387-59570-8*) Spr-Verlag.

Cryotherapy in Sport Injury Management. Kenneth L. Knight. 1995. LC 95-18201. (Illus.). 312p. pap. text 32.00 (*0-87322-771-9*, BKNI0771) Human Kinetics.

Cryptococcus Neoformans. Arturo Casadevall & John R. Perfect. 1998. LC 98-8693. (Illus.). 450p. 119.95 (*1-55581-107-8*) ASM Pr.

Cryptorchidism. Ed. by J. C. Job. 1979. (Pediatric & Adolescent Endocrinology Ser.: Vol. 6). pap. 86.25 (*3-8055-2998-8*) S Karger.

Cryptorchidism: Management & Implications. F. Hadziselimovic. 1982. (Illus.). 135p. 95.00 (*0-387-11881-0*) Spr-Verlag.

Cryptorchidism & Related Anomalies. Fray F. Marshall. Ed. by Jack S. Elder. 1982. LC 82-11302. 118p. 57.75 (*0-275-91374-0*, C1374, Praeger Pubs) Greenwood.

***Cryptorchildism, Environmental Impacts of Male Fertility: 4th International Symposium on Pediatric Andrology, Basel, November 2000.** Ed. by F. Hadziselimovic & B. Herzog. 2001. (Hormone Research Ser.: Vol. 55, No. 1). (Illus.). 56p. pap. 25.25 (*3-8055-7270-0*) S Karger.

Cryptosporidium & Cryptosporidiosis. Ronald Fayer. 1997. LC 96-24303. 272p. 129.95 (*0-8493-7695-5*) CRC Pr.

Crystallographically Determined Structures. Lennart Sjolin. 1996. (Medicine Ser.). pap. 89.95 (*0-412-10691-4*, VNR) Wiley.

CSF Analysis in Multiple Sclerosis. P. Livrea & E. Thompson. 1996. LC 96-26146. 152p. 96.00 (*3-540-75018-5*) Spr-Verlag.

CSR, RPR, RMR Written Knowledge Test Court Reporter Reference Workbook. Monette Benoit. 1995. (Court Reporter Reference Bks.: No. 2). pap. text, wbk. ed. 20.95 (*1-881149-01-3*) CRRB.

CT & MRI of the Abdomen & Pelvis: A Teaching File. Pablo R. Ros & Sylvester Lee. 1997. LC 97-1121. 360p. 99.00 (*0-683-18218-8*) Lppncott W & W.

CT & MRI of the Genitourinary Tract. Ed. by Stanford M. Goldman & Olga M. Gatewood. 1990. (Contemporary Issues in Computed Tomography Ser.: Vol. 13). (Illus.). 323p. text (*0-443-08657-5*) Church.

CT & Sonography of the Acute Abdomen. R. Brooke Jeffrey, Jr. & Philip W. Ralls. 2nd ed. 1995. (Illus.). 384p. text 175.00 (*0-7817-0287-9*) Lppncott W & W.

CT Densitometry in Osteoporosis: The Impact on Management of the Patient. L. E. Lampmann et al. 1984. (Series in Radiology). 124p. text 122.00 (*0-89838-633-0*) Kluwer Academic.

CT of Metastases. Francesco Ferrozzi et al. 1999. LC 99-32320. (Illus.). 225p. pap. 82.00 (*3-540-65097-0*) Spr-Verlag.

CT of the Abdomen. Y. Wang. 1986. LC 85-4243. 235.00 (*0-8493-6448-5*); 227.00 (*0-8493-6449-3*) Franklin (CRC Reprint).

CT of the Abdomen. Set. Ed. by Yen Wang. 1986. 178.00 (*0-8493-6447-7*, RC944) CRC Pr.

CT of the Immunocompromised Host. Ed. by Janet E. Kuhlman. 1990. (Contemporary Issues in Computed Tomography Ser.: Vol. 14). (Illus.). 194p. text (*0-443-08721-0*) Church.

CT Scan & MRI in Oncology. D. Buthiau & David Khayat. 1998. LC 97-45146. 435p. 165.00 (*3-540-62750-2*) Spr-Verlag.

CT Simulation for Radiotherapy. Shirish K. Jani. 1993. 172p. pap. text 38.95 (*0-944838-32-4*) Med Physics Pub.

CT Technique Guide. James J. Hickman, Jr. 1994. 75p. (*0-9642926-0-2*) J & L Prods.

CTG in Practice. Adam Balen & John Smith. 1992. (Illus.). 203p. (Orig.). pap. text (*0-443-04675-1*) Church.

Cuando el Medico Dice: Es Cancer. Mary B. Moster. 1987. (Serie Guia de Bolsillo - Pocket Guides Ser.).Tr. of When the Doctor Says "It's Cancer". (SPA.). 90p. pap. 2.79 (*0-8423-6515-X*, 498042) Editorial Unilit.

Cuando el SIDA Llega Al Hogar. Mignon M. Zylstra. 1997.Tr. of When AIDS Comes Home. (SPA.). 9.99 (*0-88113-469-4*, B001-4694) Caribe Betania.

Cuban Medicine. Roswell S. Danielson. 1978. LC 76-1768. 247p. text 44.95 (*0-87855-114-X*) Transaction Pubs.

Cube: Keep the Secret. Annie Gottlieb & Slobodan Pesic. 1995. LC 95-4174. 208p. pap. 14.00 (*0-06-251266-8*) Harper SF.

Cuentas Claras. Jorge Valdes. 2000. (SPA.). 320p. pap. 11.49 (*0-8297-2856-2*) Vida Pubs.

Cuerpo. Charles Colson. 1994.Tr. of Body. (SPA.). 464p. 11.99 (*0-88113-194-6*, B008-1946) Caribe Betania.

Cuerpos Sin Edad, Mentes Sin Tiempo. Deepak Chopra. 1997. LC 97-39028.Tr. of Ageless Bodies, Timeless Minds. (SPA.). 340p. pap. 15.00 (*0-609-80103-1*, RH9089, Three Riv Pr) Harmony Bks.

Culicine Mosquitoes of the Philippines. Mercedes Delfinado. 1966. (Memoir Ser.: No. 7). (Illus.). 252p. 50.00 (*1-56665-005-4*) Assoc Pubs FL.

Culpeper's Complete Herbal & English Physician. Nicholas Culpeper. enl. ed. 1987. (Illus.). reprint ed. 440p. pap. 12.50 (*0-916638-20-0*); 420p. text 35.00 (*0-916638-38-3*) Meyerbooks.

Culpeper's Herbal Remedies. Nicholas Culpeper. 1980. pap. 5.00 (*0-87980-025-9*) Wilshire.

Culpeper's Medicine. Graeme Tobyn. 1997. LC 97-3507. 256p. pap. 29.95 (*1-85230-943-1*) Element MA.

Cult Fictions: C. G. Jung & the Founding of Analytical Psychology. Sonu Shamdasani. 1998. LC 97-32830. 144p. pap. 20.95 (*0-415-18614-5*); (C). 63.95 (*0-415-18613-7*) Routledge.

Cult of Childhood. George Boas. 1966. LC 90-33312. (Dunquin Ser.: No. 18). 122p. reprint ed. pap. 13.50 (*0-88214-218-6*) Spring Pubns.

Cultivating Freud's Garden in France. Marion M. Oliner. 1988. LC 87-31908. 332p. 60.00 (*0-87668-995-0*) Aronson.

Cultivating Health: Cultural Perspectives on Health Promotion. Malcolm MacLachlan. 2000. LC 00-43549. (*0-471-49620-0*) Wiley.

Cultivating Health: Cultural Perspectives on Health Promotion. Malcolm Maclachlan. 2000. LC 00-43549. (Illus.). 250p. 80.00 (*0-471-97725-X*) Wiley.

Cultivating the Energy of Life. Liu Hua-Yang. Tr. by Eva Wong. 1998. LC 97-24079. 112p. pap. 11.95 (*1-57062-342-2*) Shambhala Pubns.

Cultivation of Marine Organisms & Its Importance for Marine Biology. Ed. by Otto Kinne & H. P. Bulnheim. 1973. (Helgolaender Wissenschaftliche Meeresuntersuchungen Ser.: Band 20). (Illus.). v, 721p. reprint ed. pap. (*3-87429-059-X*, 003077) Koeltz Sci Bks DEU. *Dist:* Lubrecht & Cramer.

Cults & Cons: The Exploitation of the Emotional Growth Consumer. Kenneth Cinnamon & Dave Farson. 1979. LC 79-1174. 128p. pap. text 27.95 (*0-88229-456-3*) Burnham Inc.

Cults & New Religious Movements: Task Force Report of the American Psychiatric Association. Ed. by Marc Galanter. 1989. LC 88-7817. 346p. text 19.95 (*0-89042-212-5*, 2212) Am Psychiatric.

Cults & Personality. Frank J. MacHovec. 1989. 210p. (C). text 49.95 (*0-398-05607-2*) C C Thomas.

Cultural & Demographic Aspects of Health Care in Sub-Saharan Africa. Ed. by Ezekiel Kalipeni & Philip Thiuri. 1996. 350p. (Orig.). pap. 35.00 (*1-879893-08-8*) IAAS Pubs.

Cultural & Sociological Aspects of Alcoholism & Substance Abuse. Ed. by Barry Stimmel. 1984. LC 84-12985. (Advances in Alcohol & Substance Abuse Ser.: Vol. 4, No.1). 84p. text 32.95 (*0-86656-367-9*) Haworth Pr.

Cultural Background of Personality. Ralph Linton. 1981. LC 80-29240. 157p. reprint ed. lib. bdg. 35.00 (*0-313-22783-7*, LICU, Greenwood Pr) Greenwood.

Cultural Clinical Psychology: Theory, Research, & Practice. Ed. by Shahe Kazarian & David R. Evans. 1998. LC 96-40844. (Illus.). 432p. pap. 39.95 (*0-19-510946-5*) OUP.

Cultural Cognition & Psychopathology. Ed. by John F. Schumaker & Tony Ward. 2000. LC 00-22888. (Illus.). 304p. 68.00 (*0-275-96604-6*, Praeger Pubs) Greenwood.

Cultural Competency in Health, Social & Human Services: Directions for the 21st Century. Pedro J. Lecca et al. 1998. LC 97-52279. (Illus.). 320p. pap. text 24.95 (*0-8153-2206-2*, SS1085) Garland.

Cultural Conceptions & Mental Illness: A Comparison of Germany & America. John M. Townsend. 1993. LC 77-22342. (Illus.). (C). lib. bdg. 14.00 (*0-226-81098-4*) U Ch Pr.

Cultural Context of Health, Illness & Medicine. Martha O. Loustaunau & Elisa J. Lobo. 1997. LC 97-16136. 232p. pap. 24.95 (*0-89789-548-7*, Bergin & Garvey) Greenwood.

Cultural Context of Health, Illness & Medicine. Martha O. Loustaunau & Elisa J. Sobo. 1997. LC 97-16136. 232p. 68.00 (*0-89789-487-1*, Bergin & Garvey) Greenwood.

Cultural Context of Infancy Vol. 2: Multicultural & Interdisciplinary Approaches to Parent-Infant Relations, 2. Ed. by Kevin Nugent et al. 1991. (Cultural Context of Infancy Ser.: Vol. 2). 384p. (C). 85.00 (*0-89391-627-7*, Ablex) Greenwood.

Cultural Diversity & Geriatric Care: Challenges to the Health Professions. Ed. by Darryl Wieland et al. 1995. LC 94-32666. (Gerontology & Geriatrics Education Ser.). (Illus.). 116p. 39.95 (*1-56024-710-X*) Haworth Pr.

Cultural Diversity in Health & Illness. Rachel E. Spector. 4th ed. 1996. LC 95-25684. xv, 407p. (C). pap. text 34.95 (*0-8385-1397-2*, A1397-7) Appleton & Lange.

Cultural, Ethnic, & Religious Reference Manual for Health Care Providers. Janice D. Andrews. 1995. 92p. ring bd. 59.95 (*0-9663552-1-0*) Jamarda NC.

Cultural Factors in Alcohol Research & Treatment of Drinking Problems. Ed. by D. W. Heath et al. 1981. (Journal of Studies on Alcohol: Suppl. No. 9). 15.00 (*0-911290-08-7*) Rutgers Ctr Alcohol.

Cultural Foods & Renal Diets: Section I: For the Clinical Dietitian; Section II: A Multilingual Guide for Renal Patients, Set. Chhaya Patel & Mary Denny. 1988. 565p. (C). pap. text 50.00 (*1-883146-53-4*) Coun Renal Nutrit.

Cultural Geography of Health Care. Wilbert M. Gesler. 1991. LC 90-44299. 256p. (C). pap. 19.95 (*0-8229-5490-7*) U of Pittsburgh Pr.

Cultural Images of Health: A Neglected Dimension. A. D'Houtaud. 1995. 177p. lib. bdg. 95.00 (*1-56072-228-2*) Nova Sci Pubs.

Cultural Issues in End-of-Life Decision Making. Kathryn Braun et al. 1999. LC 99-6734. (Health & Medical Ser.). 356p. 79.95 (*0-7619-1216-9*, 82035); pap. 37.95 (*0-7619-1217-7*, 82036) Sage.

Cultural Issues in the Treatment of Anxiety. Steven Friedman. 1997. LC 97-13509. 261p. text 35.00 (*1-57230-237-2*, 0237) Guilford Pubns.

Cultural Pluralism & Psychoanalysis: The Asian & North American Experience. Alan Roland. 1996. LC 96-30239. 228p. (C). pap. 23.95 (*0-415-91479-5*); 85.00 (*0-415-91478-7*) Routledge.

Cultural Psychiatry: Euro-International Perspectives. Ed. by A. T. Yilmaz et al. 2001. LC 00-66322. (Bibliotheca Psychiatrica Ser.: No. 169). (Illus.). vi, 188p. 77.50 (*3-8055-7048-1*) S Karger.

Cultural Psychology: An Once & Future Discipline. Michael Cole. 1998. 432p. pap. text 19.95 (*0-674-17956-0*) HUP.

Cultural Psychology: The Chicago Symposia on Human Development. Ed. by James W. Stigler et al. 1990. (Illus.). 637p. (C). pap. text 31.95 (*0-521-37804-4*) Cambridge U Pr.

Cultural Psychology & Qualitative Methodology: Theoretical & Empirical Considerations. Carl Ratner. 1997. LC 97-7783. (PATH in Psychology Ser.). (Illus.). 276p. (C). 45.00 (*0-306-45463-7*, Plenum Trade) Perseus Pubng.

Cultural Resistance: Challenging Beliefs about Men, Women, & Therapy. Ed. by Kathy Weingarten. 1995. 184p. 39.95 (*1-56024-748-7*); LC 95-24929. pap. 19.95 (*1-56023-081-9*, Harrington Park) Haworth Pr.

Cultural Theory & Psychoanalytic Tradition. David J. Fisher. 1991. 276p. (C). text 39.95 (*0-88738-387-4*) Transaction Pubs.

Culturally Affirmative Psychotherapy with Deaf Persons. Ed. by Neil S. Glickman & Michael A. Harvey. 1996. LC 95-49691. 300p. text 65.00 (*0-8058-1488-4*); pap. text 32.50 (*0-8058-1489-2*) L Erlbaum Assocs.

Culturally Competent Assessment for Family Violence. American Nurses Association Staff. 1998. LC 98-6511. pap. 18.95 (*1-55810-140-3*) Am Nurses Pub.

Culturally Competent Family Therapy: A General Model, 37. Shlomo Ariel. 1999. LC 99-11269. (Contributions in Psychology Ser.: Vol. 37). (Illus.). 272p. 68.00 (*0-313-31079-3*) Greenwood.

Culturally Diverse Children & Adolescents: Assessment, Diagnosis & Treatment. Ian A. Canino & Jeanne Spurlock. 1994. LC 93-50824. 196p. 27.95 (*0-89862-409-6*, C2409) Guilford Pubns.

Culturally Sensitive Caregiving & Childbearing Families. Leah Ramer. Ed. by Beverly S. Raff & Ellen Fiore. 1992. LC 92-13293. (Nursing Issues for the Twenty-First Century Ser.: No. 4, Module 1). pap. (*0-86525-054-5*) March of Dimes.

Culture: A Problem That Cannot Be Solved. Charles W. Nuckolls. 1998. LC 98-6856. 336p. pap. 22.95 (*0-299-15894-2*) U of Wis Pr.

Culture & AIDS. Ed. by Douglas A. Feldman. 1990. LC 90-30003. 224p. 62.50 (*0-275-93189-7*, C3189, Praeger Pubs) Greenwood.

Culture & Attachment: Perceptions of the Child in Context. Robin L. Harwood et al. 1997. LC 95-2023. (Culture & Human Development Ser.). 169p. pap. 21.00 (*1-57230-246-1*, 0246) Guilford Pubns.

Culture & Cognition: The Boundaries of Literary & Scientific Inquiry. Ronald Schleifer et al. 1992. LC 92-52770. 296p. (C). 45.00 (*0-8014-2632-4*); pap. 21.95 (*0-8014-9931-3*) Cornell U Pr.

Culture & Common Mental Disorders in Sub-Saharan Africa. Vikram Patel. 1998. (Volume in the Maudsley Monograph Ser.). 144p. (*0-86377-530-6*) Psychol Pr GBR. *Dist:* Taylor & Francis.

Culture & Depression: Studies in the Anthropology & Cross-Cultural Psychiatry of Affect & Disorder, Vol. 16. Ed. by Arthur Kleinman. 1985. LC 85-2535. (Culture & Depression Ser.: Vol. 16). 500p. pap. text 22.00 (*0-520-05883-6*) U CA Pr.

Culture & Family: Problems & Therapy. Wen-Shing Tseng & Jing Hsu. 1991. LC 90-21961. (Marriage & the Family Ser.). 274p. (C). text 49.95 (*1-56024-058-X*); pap. text 19.95 (*1-56024-059-8*) Haworth Pr.

Culture & Fertility: Anthropological Approaches to the Study of Reproduction. Ed. by Susan Greenhalgh. 1995. (Illus.). 320p. (C). text 69.95 (*0-521-47044-7*); pap. text 24.95 (*0-521-46999-6*) Cambridge U Pr.

Culture & Health: Psychological Perspectives on Problems & Practice. Malcolm MacLachlan. 1997. LC 97-8648. (Culture & Professional Practice Ser.). 332p. pap. 65.00 (*0-471-96626-6*) Wiley.

Culture & Human Fertility: A Study of the Relation of Cultural Conditions to Fertility in Non-Industrial & Transitional Societies. Frank Lorimer. 1970. LC 78-90549. 510p. reprint ed. lib. bdg. 85.00 (*0-8371-2152-3*, LOHF, Greenwood Pr) Greenwood.

Culture & Inference: A Trobriand Case Study. Edwin Hutchins. 1980. LC 80-13280. (Cognitive Science Ser.: No. 2). (Illus.). 153p. 31.00 (*0-674-17970-6*) HUP.

Culture & Interpersonal Morality. Joan Miller. Date not set. (New Directions in Social Psychology Ser.). 54.95 (*0-8133-1855-6*) Westview.

Culture & Mental Health: A Southern African View. Leslie Swartz. 1999. LC 00-501115. 336p. pap. text 39.95 (*0-19-570981-0*) OUP.

Culture & Nursing Care: A Pocket Guide. Pamela A. Minarik et al. 1996. pap. text 18.95 (*0-943671-15-9*) UCSF Schl Nursing.

Culture & Psychiatric Diagnosis: A DSM-IV Perspective. Ed. by Juan E. Mezzich et al. 1996. LC 95-26288. 432p. text 57.00 (*0-88048-553-1*, 8553) Am Psychiatric.

Culture & Psychology Reader. Ed. by Nancy R. Goldberger & Jody Veroff. 1995. 760p. (C). text 65.00 (*0-8147-3080-9*); LC 95-18843. pap. text 29.50 (*0-8147-3081-7*) NYU Pr.

Culture & Psychotherapy. Theodora M. Abel & Rhoda Metreaux. 1974. 24.95 (*0-8084-0368-0*); pap. 17.95 (*0-8084-0369-9*) NCUP.

Culture & Sexual Risk: Anthropological Perspectives on AIDS. Ed. by Han Ten Brummelhuis. 1995. LC 95-223554. 355p. text 65.00 (*2-88449-130-9*); pap. text 32.00 (*2-88449-131-7*) Gordon & Breach.

Culture & the Clinical Encounter: An Intercultural Sensitizer for the Health Professions. Rena C. Gropper. 1996. LC 95-52857. 184p. pap. text 19.95 (*1-877864-43-9*, 382) Intercult Pr.

Culture & the Development of Children's Action: A Theory of Human Development. Jaan Valsiner. 2nd ed. 1997. LC 96-46293. 364p. 55.00 (*0-471-13590-9*) Wiley.

Culture & Weight Consciousness. Mervat Nasser. 1997. LC 96-43021. 154p. (C). 63.95 (*0-415-16152-5*) Routledge.

Culture at Work in Aviation & Medicine: National, Organizational & Professional Influences. Robert L. Helmreich & Ashleigh C. Merritt. 1998. LC 98-2947. 250p. text (*0-291-39853-7*, TL553.H45) Ashgate Pub GBR. *Dist:* Ashgate Pub Co.

Culture-Bound Syndromes. Ed. by Ronald C. Simons & Charles C. Hughes. 1985. lib. bdg. 182.50 (*90-277-1858-X*) Kluwer Academic.

Culture Care Diversity & Universality: A Theory of Nursing. Ed. by Madeleine Leininger. 1991. LC 15-2402. (Illus.). 448p. (C). pap. text 32.95 (*0-88737-519-7*) Natl League Nurse.

Culture-Centered Counseling & Interviewing Skills: A Practical Guide. Allen E. Ivey & Paul B. Pedersen. 1993. LC 93-15372. 224p. 68.00 (*0-275-94668-1*, C4668); pap. 22.95 (*0-275-94669-X*, B4669) Greenwood (Praeger Pubs).

Culture-Centered Counseling Interventions: Striving for Accuracy. Paul B. Pedersen. 1997. LC 96-35663. 304p. (C). 81.95 (*0-7619-0249-X*, 2155); pap. 39.95 (*0-7619-0250-3*, 2156) Sage.

Culture Clash: The Making of Gay Sensibility. Michael Bronski. 1984. LC 84-50941. 254p. 30.00 (*0-89608-218-0*) South End Pr.

Culture, Curers & Contagion: Readings for Medical Social Science. Ed. by Norman Klein. 1979. LC 79-10888. (Anthropology Ser.). 256p. pap. text 14.95 (*0-88316-531-7*) Chandler & Sharp.

Culture, Curriculum & Community. Ed. by Virginia M. Fitzsimons & Mary L. Kelly. 1997. pap. 35.95 (*0-88737-743-2*, 14-7432, NLN Pr) Natl League Nurse.

Culture, Ecology & Politics In Gabon's Rainforest. James F. Barnes & Michael C. Reed. 1910. 360p. text 50.00 (*0-8133-3733-X*) Westview.

Culture, Ethnicity, & Mental Illness. Ed. by Albert C. Gaw. 1993. LC 92-10686. 640p. text 82.95 (*0-88048-359-8*, 8359) Am Psychiatric.

Culture, Experience & Pluralism: Essays on African Ideas of Illness & Healing. Ed. by A. Jacobson-Widding & David Westerlund. 1989. (Uppsala Studies in Cultural Anthropology: No. 13). 308p. (Orig.). pap. 48.50 (*91-554-2325-6*) Coronet Bks.

Culture, Health & Illness. C. Helman. 3rd ed. 1990. 344p. pap. (*0-7506-0478-6*) John Wright GBR. *Dist:* Buttrwrth-Heinemann.

Culture, Health & Illness. Cecil Helman. 4th ed. 2000. LC 99-89542. (Illus.). 336p. pap. (*0-7506-4786-8*) E A GBR. *Dist:* OUP.

Culture in Context. Weston La Barre. 1994. (C). text 40.00 (*1-885809-00-X*); pap. text 19.95 (*1-885809-01-8*) An LaBarre.

*__Culture in Psychology.__ Ed. by Corrine Squire. 2000. (Illus.). 240p. (Orig.). (C). (gr. 13). pap. 29.95 (*0-415-24354-8*) Routledge.

Culture Methodology for Legionella Species. Janet E. Stout. 1998. LC 98-96374. 13p. pap. 19.00 (*0-9649926-8-X*, 308) HC Info Res.

Culture of Addiction see Pathways: From the Culture of Addiction to the Culture of Recovery: A Travel Guide for Addiction Professionals

Culture of Adolescent Risk-Taking. Cynthia Lightfoot. 1997. LC 96-47250. (Culture & Human Development Ser.). 187p. pap. 21.00 (*1-57230-232-1*, 0232) Guilford Pubns.

Culture of Biomedicine. Ed. by D. Heyward Brock. 1984. LC 82-40438. (Studies in Science & Culture: Vol. 1). 200p. 32.50 (*0-87413-229-0*) U Delaware Pr.

Culture of Hematopoietic Cells. Ed. by R. Ian Freshney et al. 1994. LC 94-19025. (Culture of Specialized Cells Ser.). 296p. pap. 99.95 (*0-471-58830-X*, Wiley-Interscience) Wiley.

Culture of Honor: The Psychology of Violence in the South. Richard E. Nisbett & Dov Cohen. 1996. LC 96-166629. (New Directions in Social Psychology Ser.). 144p. (C). pap. text 18.00 (*0-8133-1993-5*) Westview.

Culture of Learning: Access, Retention, & Mobility of Minority Students in Nursing. Virginia M. Fitzsimmons & Mary L. Kelley. Date not set. LC 95-49578. 288p. pap. 25.95 (*0-88737-659-2*) Natl League Nurse.

Culture of Long Term Care: Nursing Home Ethnography. Ed. by J. Neil Henderson & Maria D. Vesperi. 1995. LC 94-42151. 264p. 72.50 (*0-89789-422-7*); pap. 22.95 (*0-89789-423-5*) Greenwood (Bergin & Garvey).

Culture of Pain. David B. Morris. 1991. LC 90-11305. (Illus.). 354p. text 45.00 (*0-520-07266-9*) U CA Pr.

Culture of Public Problems: Drinking-Driving & the Symbolic Order. Joseph R. Gusfield. LC 80-17007. 1992. lib. bdg. 22.00 (*0-226-31093-0*); 1984. 278p. pap. text 19.00 (*0-226-31094-9*) U Ch Pr.

Culture of Shame. Andrew P. Morrison. 1998. LC 98-16681. 240p. reprint ed. pap. 25.00 (*0-7657-0174-X*) Aronson.

Culture, Schooling, & Psychological Development, 4. Ed. by Liliana T. Landsmann & Sidney Strauss. 1991. (Human Development Ser.). 224p. (C). 77.00 (*0-89391-529-7*, Ablex) Greenwood.

Culture Shift: A Leader's Guide to Managing Change in Health Care. Ed. by Joan E. Lowery. 1997. LC 97-25187. 256p. 38.00 (*1-55648-208-6*) AHPI.

Culture Shock! A Traveller's Medical Guide. Paul Zakowich. 1995. (Culture Shock! Practical Guides). 240p. pap. text 12.95 (*1-55868-245-7*) Gr Arts Ctr Pub.

Culture, Society & Menstruation. Ed. by Virginia L. Olesen & Nancy F. Woods. 1986. LC 66-55252. 186p. 65.00 (*0-89116-557-6*) Hemisp Pub.

Culture's Consequences: International Differences in Work-Related Values. Geert Hofstede. LC 80-16327. (Cross-Cultural Research & Methodology Ser.: Vol. 5). (Illus.). 475p. 1984. pap. 44.95 (*0-8039-1306-0*, 5332); 1981. 96.95 (*0-8039-1444-X*, 7136) Sage.

Cultures of Change: Recovery & Relapse Prevention for Dually Diagnosed & Addicted Adolescents. Janice Gabe. 1993. 175p. (Orig.). pap. text 12.95 (*0-9639023-0-X*) Prof Resource.

Cultures of Healing: Correcting the Image of American Mental Health Care. Robert T. Fancher. 1997. 352p. pap. text 14.95 (*0-7167-3063-4*) W H Freeman.

Cumulated Index Medicus Vol. II: Nineteen Seventy. National Library of Medicine Staff. LC 74-8462. reprint ed. 1975. 48.95 (*0-405-18895-1*); Set. 1974. 360.00 (*0-405-06190-0*) Ayer.

Cumulated Index Medicus Vol. 9: Nineteen Sixty-Eight, Set. 1970. 8925p. 255.00 (*0-405-00975-5*) Ayer.

Cumulated Subject Index to Psychological Abstracts, 1927 to 1960. 1982. 940.00 (*0-8161-1352-1*, Macmillan Ref) Gale.

Cumulated Subject Index to Psychological Abstracts, 1961-1965, Supplement 1. 1980. suppl. ed. 390.00 (*0-8161-1295-9*, Macmillan Ref) Gale.

Cumulated Subject Index to Psychological Abstracts, 1966-1968, Supplement 2. 1980. suppl. ed. 515.00 (*0-8161-1289-4*, Macmillan Ref) Gale.

Cumulative Author Index to Psychological Index, 1894 to 1935, & Psychological Abstracts, 1927 to 1958 Compiled by Columbia University, New York Staff. 1970. 160.00 (*0-8161-0598-7*, Macmillan Ref) Gale.

Cumulative Index Vol. 45-57. Ed. by Pierre J. Vinken et al. 1990. 528p. 214.50 (*0-444-81277-6*, HCN/RCN 58/14) Elsevier.

Cumulative Index Medicus, Vol. 13 National Library of Medicine Staff. 1976. LC 74-8462. 455.00 (*0-405-06650-3*) Ayer.

Cumulative Index of the Journal of the American Psychoanalytic Association: 1953-1974, Vols. 1-22. American Psychoanalytic Association Staff. 1975. LC 75-37247. 102.00 (*0-8236-1111-6*); pap. 102.00 (*0-8236-1110-8*) Intl Univs Pr.

Cumulative Index to the Homeopathic Physician. Jay Yasgur. 1996. 330p. 75.00 (*1-886149-05-4*) Van Hoy Pubs.

Cumulative Record of Speech Skill Acquisition. Daniel Ling. 1977. LC 77-93949. pap. text 12.50 (*0-88200-115-9*, A1983) Alexander Graham.

Cumulative Subject Index, Vols. 61-74, 76-80. Ed. by Sidney P. Colowick & Anthan O. Kaplan. 1986. (Methods in Enzymology Ser.: Vol. 95). text 179.00 (*0-12-181995-7*) Acad Pr.

Cumulative Subject Index, Vols. 102-119, 121-134. Sidney P. Colowick & Nathan O. Kaplan. 1988. (Methods in Enzymology Ser.: Vol. 140). 288p. text 157.00 (*0-12-182040-8*) Acad Pr.

Cumulative Subject Index: Volumes 1-30. Ed. by Martha G. Dennis & Edward A. Dennis. 1975. (Methods in Enzymology Ser.: Vol. 33). text 199.00 (*0-12-181896-9*) Acad Pr.

Cumulative Subject Index: Volumes 228, 230-262. Ed. by John N. Abelson et al. 1996. (Methods in Enzymology Ser.: Vol. 265). (Illus.). 678p. text 95.00 (*0-12-182166-8*) Acad Pr.

Cumulative Subject Index: Volumes 31, 32, 34-60. Ed. by Sidney P. Colowick & Martha Dennis. 1982. (Methods in Enzymology Ser.: Vol. 75). text 188.00 (*0-12-181975-2*) Acad Pr.

Cumulative Trauma: Reducing the Risk. Dan MacLeod & H. Duane Saunders. Ed. by Richard A. Pollock. 1990. (Illus.). (Orig.). pap. text 2.75 (*0-9616461-7-9*) Saunders Grp.

Cumulative Trauma Disorder: A Legal Guide to CTD Prevention, Regulation & Liability. Ed. by CTDNews Staff. 1993. LC 93-25971. 125.00 (*0-9636246-2-8*) Andrews Pubns.

Cumulative Trauma Disorders. Arminius Cassvan et al. 1997. LC 97-2667. 264p. text 74.99 (*0-7506-9570-6*) Buttrwrth-Heinemann.

C D

Cumulative Trauma Disorders: A Manual for Musculoskeletal Diseases of the Upper Limbs. Ed. by Vern Putz-Anderson. 1988. 151p. 29.95 (*0-85066-405-5*) Taylor & Francis.

Cumulative Trauma Disorders: A Practical Guide to Prevention & Control. Wayne F. Peate & Karen A. Lunda. 1997. LC 96-37429. 238p. pap. text 75.00 (*0-86587-553-7*) Gov Insts.

Cumulative Trauma Disorders: Current Issues & Ergonomic. Kathy G. Parker. 1992. 160p. lib. bdg. 89.95 (*0-87371-322-2*, L322) Lewis Pubs.

Cumulative Trauma Disorders: Prevention, Evaluation & Treatment. Ed. by Michael Erdil & O. Bruce Dickerson. 1997. LC 96-34261. (Illus.). 736p. text 93.95 (*0-442-01074-5*, VNR) Wiley.

Cumulative Trauma Disorders: Prevention, Evaluation, & Treatment. Ed. by Michael Erdil & O. Bruce Dickerson. 1996. 719p. 120.00 (*0-471-28472-6*, VNR) Wiley.

Cumulative Trauma Disorders in the Workplace: Bibliography. 1996. 208p. (C). reprint ed. pap. text 35.00 (*0-7881-3379-9*) DIANE Pub.

Cumulative Trauma Disorders of the Hand & Wrist: An Ergonomics Guide. Thomas J. Armstrong & Ellen A. Lackey. 1994. (Ergonomics Guide Ser.). (Illus.). 24p. (Orig.). pap. text 8.00 (*0-932627-56-0*, 181-ER-94) Am Indus Hygiene.

Cunning Seeds. Cecil Sinnamon. 1990. 158p. (C). pap. (*0-908175-54-X*) Boolarong Pubns AUS. *Dist:* St Mut.

Cunningham's Manual of Practical Anatomy Vol. 1: Upper & Lower Limbs, Vol. 1. G. J. Romanes. 15th ed. 1986. (Illus.). 272p. (C). pap. text 27.50 (*0-19-263138-1*) OUP.

Cunningham's Manual of Practical Anatomy Vol. 2: Thorax & Abdomen, Vol. 2. G. J. Romanes. 15th ed. 1986. (Illus.). 304p. (C). pap. text 27.50 (*0-19-263139-X*) OUP.

Cunningham's Manual of Practical Anatomy Vol. 3: Head & Neck & Brain, Vol. 3. George J. Romanes. 15th ed. 1986. (Illus.). 352p. pap. text 27.50 (*0-19-263140-3*) OUP.

Cunningham's Textbook of Anatomy. G. J. Romanes. 12th ed. 1981. (Illus.). 1,090p. (C). text 79.50 (*0-19-263134-9*) OUP.

Cupid's Arrow: The Course of Love Through Time. Robert J. Sternberg. 1998. LC 97-52933. (Illus.). 226p. (C). text 44.95 (*0-521-47320-9*) Cambridge U Pr.

Curability of Insanity, a Series of Studies. Pliny Earle. 1972. LC 70-180573. (Medicine & Society in America Ser.). 236p. reprint ed. 19.95 (*0-405-03949-2*) Ayer.

Curable & Incurable Neurotics: Problems of "Neurotic" vs. "Malignant" Psychic Masochism. Edmund Bergler. 1993. LC 93-18828. 510p. reprint ed. 70.00 (*0-8236-1092-6*) Intl Univs Pr.

Curacion Espontanea. Andrew Weil. Tr. by Amelia Brito. 1995.Tr. of Spontaneous Healing. 412p. pap. 25.00 (*84-7953-115-0*) Hay House.

Curanderismo: Mexican American Folk Healing. Robert T. Trotter, 2nd & Juan A. Chavira. 2nd ed. 1997. LC 97-15784. 224p. pap. text 18.00 (*0-8203-1962-7*) U of Ga Pr.

Curative Eurythmy. Rudolf Steiner. 1990. 132p. reprint ed. pap. (*0-85440-398-1*, 871) R Steiner Pr GBR. *Dist:* Anthroposophic.

Curative Factors in Dynamic Psychotherapy. Samuel Slipp. 1993. LC 93-306763. 416p. pap. 50.00 (*1-56821-097-3*) Aronson.

Curative Measures: Body Cures for Mental Illness, 1900-1950s. Joel Braslow. 1997. LC 96-39469. (Medicine & Society Ser.: Vol. 8). 262p. text 45.00 (*0-520-20547-2*) U CA Pr.

Curativement Votre. Penny C. Royal. 1983. (Health Education Ser.). 128p. pap. 8.95 (*0-9609226-2-8*) Sound Nutri.

Curbside Consult: Infectious Diseases. Farrin A. Manian. 1997. LC 97-39640. (Illus.). 256p. (C). (gr. 13). pap. text 29.95 (*0-8151-2345-0*, 27220) Mosby Inc.

Cure: Faith. Dave Bowler & Bryan Dray. 1997. (Illus.). 198p. pap. (*0-330-34692-X*) Pan GBR. *Dist:* Trans-Atl Phila, Trafalgar.

Cure & Cult in Ancient Corinth: A Guide to the Asklepieion. Mabel L. Lang. 1977. (Illus.). 32p. pap. 3.00 (*0-87661-670-8*) Am Sch Athens.

Cure, Comfort & Safe Custody: Public Lunatic Asylums in Early 19th Century England. Leonard D. Smith. 1999. LC 98-26009. 99.95 (*0-7185-0094-6*) Bks Intl VA.

Cure Cottages of Saranac Lake: Architecture & History of a Pioneer Health Resort. Philip L. Gallos. 1985. LC 85-8697. (Illus.). 208p. reprint ed. 27.95 (*0-9615159-0-2*) Hist Saranac.

Cure Craft: Traditional Folk Remedies & Treatment from Antiquity to the Present Day. Keith Souter. 1995. 105p. pap. (*0-85207-282-1*) C W Daniel GBR. *Dist:* Natl Bk Netwk.

Cure for All Advanced Cancers. Hulda Regehr Clark. l.t. ed. 1999. LC 00-699599. (Illus.). vi, 610p. pap. 21.95 (*1-890035-16-5*) New Centry Pr.

Cure for All Cancers: With 100 Case Histories. Hulda Regehr Clark. 16th l.t. ed. 1993. (Illus.). 623p. pap. 19.95 (*1-890035-00-9*) New Centry Pr.

Cure for All Diseases: With Many Case Histories. Hulda Regehr Clark. 17th l.t. ed. 1995. (Illus.). 604p. pap. 21.95 (*1-890035-01-7*) New Centry Pr.

Cure for HIV & AIDS: With over 75 Case Histories. Hulda Regehr Clark. 7th l.t. ed. 1993. (Illus.). 543p. pap. 19.95 (*1-890035-02-5*) New Centry Pr.

Cure Is in the Kitchen. Sherry A. Rogers. 1991. 336p. pap. 14.95 (*0-9618821-3-1*) SandKey.

Cure of Childhood Leukemia: Into the Age of Miracles. John Laszlo. 1996. LC 94-47285. (Illus.). 300p. pap. 16.95 (*0-8135-2385-0*); (C). 29.95 (*0-8135-2186-6*) Rutgers U Pr.

Cure of High Blood Pressure by Respiratory Exercises. 1991. lib. bdg. 78.95 (*0-8490-4532-0*) Gordon Pr.

Cure of High Blood Pressure by Respiratory Exercises. Tirala. 1993. 71p. reprint ed. spiral bd. 11.00 (*0-7873-0882-X*) Hlth Research.

Cure of Imperfect Sight by Treatment Without Glasses. W. H. Bates. 1996. 313p. reprint ed. pap. 20.00 (*0-7873-0078-0*) Hlth Research.

Cure That Headache Naturally. Donald Bamer. 1989. 11p. pap. 2.95 (*0-913923-69-9*) Woodland UT.

Cure Your Allergies... And Life Your Life. Martin F. Healy. 2001. (Illus.). 144p. pap. (*0-85207-347-X*) C W Daniel GBR. *Dist:* Natl Bk Netwk.

Cure Your Own Allergies in Minutes. Jimmy Scott. 1989. pap. 12.95 (*0-945509-01-4*) Hlth Kinesiol Pubns.

Cured of Rheumatism Through Diet: A Natural & Sound Method for Patients to Cure Themselves of Rheumatic Pains Without Medicines. Jeanine Van Belle. 1994. 88p. pap. (*3-85068-392-3*) Ennsthaler AUT. *Dist:* Am Educ Systs.

Cures by Psychotherapy: What Effects Change? J. Martin Myers. 1984. LC 83-21195. 159p. 55.00 (*0-275-91445-3*, C1445, Praeger Pubs) Greenwood.

Cures for Chronic Disorders: Pathogenesis & Healing. Sharwar K. Kakar. 1993. LC 93-94982. (Illus.). 178p. (*0-9638976-0-8*) S K Kakar.

Cures out of Chaos: How Unexpected Discoveries Led to Breakthroughs in Medicine & Health. M. Lawrence Podolsky. 1998. 446p. text 65.00 (*90-5702-555-8*); pap. text 32.95 (*90-5702-556-6*) Gordon & Breach (Harwood Acad Pubs).

Curing Arthritis: More Ways to a Drug-Free Life. Margaret Hills. l.t. ed. 1992. 148p. (*1-85089-397-7*) ISIS Lrg Prnt GBR. *Dist:* Transaction Pubs.

Curing Arthritis: More Ways to a Drug-Free Life. Margaret Hills. 2000. pap. (*0-85969-628-6*) Sheldon Pr GBR. *Dist:* Intl Pubs Mktg.

Curing Arthritis Diet Book. Margaret Hills. 2000. pap. (*0-85969-604-9*) Sheldon Pr GBR. *Dist:* Intl Pubs Mktg.

Curing Arthritis Naturally with Chinese Medicine. Doug Frank. Ed. by Bob Flaws. 1997. LC 97-71728. (Illus.). 160p. pap. 12.95 (*0-936185-87-2*) Blue Poppy Pr.

Curing Cancer: Solving One of the Greatest Medical Mysteries of Our Time. Michael Waldholz. 1999. LC 97-24121. (Illus.). 320p. pap. 14.00 (*0-684-84802-3*) S&S Trade.

Curing Cancer: The Story of the Men & Women Unlocking the Secrets of Our Deadliest Illness. Michael Waldholz. 1997. LC 97-24121. 320p. 24.00 (*0-684-81125-1*) Simon & Schuster.

Curing Colic & Lactose Intolerance with Homeopathy. Jana Shiloh. 1988. 44p. (Orig.). reprint ed. pap. text 5.95 (*0-9619203-0-0*) Rocky Mtn Homeopathics.

Curing Depression Naturally with Chinese Medicine. Bob Flaws & Rosa Schnyer. 1999. LC 97-77990. (Illus.). 185p. pap. 12.95 (*0-936185-94-5*) Blue Poppy Pr.

Curing Everyday Ailments the Natural Way. Reader's Digest Editorial Staff. 2000. LC 99-21950. (Illus.). 384p. 35.00 (*0-7621-0240-3*) RD Assn.

Curing Fibromyalgia Naturally with Chinese Medicine. Bob Flaws. 2000. (Illus.). 182p. pap. 12.95 (*1-891845-09-8*) Blue Poppy Pr.

Curing Hay Fever Naturally with Chinese Medicine. Bob Flaws. 1997. LC 97-74484. (Illus.). 150p. pap. 12.95 (*0-936185-91-0*) Blue Poppy Pr.

Curing Health Care: New Strategies for Quality Improvement. Donald M. Berwick et al. 1990. LC 90-5229. (Health Management Ser.). 320p. 50.00 (*1-55542-294-2*) Jossey-Bass.

Curing IBS Naturally with Chinese Medicine. Jane Bean. 2000. LC 99-76040. (Illus.). v, 149p. pap. 12.95 (*1-891845-11-X*) Blue Poppy Pr.

***Curing Incurable Diseases Naturally: Cures Without Side Effects.** Dele Adebara. Ed. by Merille Weithers. unabr. ed. 2001. LC 00-91029. (Radiant Health Ser.: Vol. 2). 368p. pap. 19.95 (*0-942307-04-6*, Newbreed) Adebara & Honeycomb.

Curing Insomnia Naturally with Chinese Medicine. Bob Flaws. 1997. LC 97-71729. (Illus.). 160p. pap. 12.95 (*0-936185-86-4*) Blue Poppy Pr.

Curing PMS Naturally with Chinese Medicine. Bob Flaws. 1997. LC 97-71730. 176p. pap. 12.95 (*0-936185-85-6*) Blue Poppy Pr.

Curing the Incurable: How to Use Your Body's Natural Self-Healing Ability to Overcome MS & Other Diseases. Jacque C. Rigg. 1999. LC 98-73710. 301p. pap. 18.95 (*1-883697-17-4*) Hara Pub.

Curing the Incurables. John R. Christopher. 1991. pap. 2.00 (*1-879436-08-6*, 99108) Christopher Pubns.

Curing U. S. Health Care Ills. Bert Seidman. 1991. LC 91-62325. (Committee on New American Realities Ser.: No. 6). (Illus.). 104p. (Orig.). pap. 9.00 (*0-89068-108-2*, NAR6) Natl Planning.

Curiosity, Imagination & Play: On the Development of Spontaneous Cognitive & Motivational Processes. Ed. by Dietmar Gorlitz & Joachim F. Wohlwill. 1987. 416p. (C). text 89.95 (*0-89859-683-1*) L Erlbaum Assocs.

Curran's Atlas of Histopathology. Robert Curran. 4th ed. 2000. LC 99-88945. (Harvey Miller Publications). (Illus.). 288p. pap. text 45.00 (*0-19-263220-5*) OUP.

Current Advances in Ace Inhibition. Graham A. MacGregor. 3rd ed. 1993. text (*4-89370-071-5*) Church.

Current Advances in Ace Inhibition 2. Ed. by Graham A. MacGregor & Peter S. Sever. 2nd ed. 1991. (Illus.). 320p. text (*0-443-04600-X*) Church.

Current Advances in Basic & Clinical Microcirculatory Research. Ed. by G. Wolf-Heidegger. 1979. (Bibliotheca Anatomica Ser.: No. 18). (Illus.). 135.75 (*3-8055-3042-0*) S Karger.

Current Advances in Inpatient Psychiatric Care: A Handbook. Ed. by Douglas H. Ruben et al. 1993. LC 92-49214. 384p. lib. bdg. 87.50 (*0-313-28046-0*, RCP/, Greenwood Pr) Greenwood.

Current & Future Applications of Magnetic Resonance in Cardiovascular Disease. Ed. by Charles B. Higgins et al. 1998. LC 97-26138. (American Heart Association Monograph Ser.). (Illus.). 576p. 130.00 (*0-87993-681-9*) Futura Pub.

Current & Future Use of Registers in Health Information Systems. Eileen M. Brooke. 1974. (Offset Publications: No. 8). pap. text 14.00 (*92-4-170008-4*, 1120008) World Health.

Current & Potential Applications for Erythropoietin. Ed. by B. G. Durie. 1992. (Acta Haematologica Ser.: Vol. 87, Suppl. 1, 1992). (Illus.). vi, 34p. pap. 17.50 (*3-8055-5617-9*) S Karger.

Current Approaches in Drama Therapy. Ed. by Penny Lewis & David Read Johnson. 2000. LC 00-32612. (Illus.). xvi, 502p. pap. 59.95 (*0-398-07083-0*) C C Thomas.

Current Approaches to Bone Marrow Histopathology. Ed. by M. Corn & Stuart Roath. 1989. (Hematology Reviews & Communications Ser.: Vol. 3, Nos. 2-3). 114p. pap. text 255.00 (*3-7186-4974-8*) Gordon & Breach.

Current Approaches to Down's Syndrome. Ed. by David Lane & Brian Stratford. 1985. LC 85-8842. 447p. 80.00 (*0-275-90212-9*, C0212, Praeger Pubs) Greenwood.

Current Aspects & Concepts of Nursing, Coordinating, Bridging, & Rehabilitation in Organ Transplantation: Proceedings of the Fourth International Symposium on Nursing, Coordinating, Bridging, & Rehabilitation in Organ Transplantation Combined with the First International Meeting of Organ Recipients, Held in Bad Oeynhausen, Germany, 6-8 September 1994. Ed. by Michael M. Korner & Reiner Korfer. 1995. (International Congress Ser.: Vol. 1081). 302p. 163.00 (*0-444-82100-7*, Excerpta Medica) Elsevier.

Current Aspects of Blood Coagulation. Ed. by M. C. Shen et al. 1996. LC 93-23882. ix, 188p. text 59.00 (*4-431-70123-0*) Spr-Verlag.

Current Aspects of Blood Coagulation, Fibrinolysis, & Platelets. Ed. by Ming-Ching Shen et al. 1996. LC 93-23882. (Illus.). x, 190p. 59.00 (*0-387-70123-0*) Spr-Verlag.

Current Aspects of Pancreatic Diseases: Digestion, Supplement 1, 1987, Vol. 37. Ed. by H. G. Worning. 1987. (Illus.). iv, 68p. pap. 22.75 (*3-8055-4618-1*) S Karger.

Current Aspects of the Neurosciences, Vol. 3. Ed. by Neville N. Osborne. 1990. text 90.00 (*0-333-54833-7*) Intl Spec Bk.

Current Cancer Diagnosis & Treatment. I. Craig Henderson et al. 2001. 800p. (C). pap. text 45.00 (*0-8385-1461-8*, Apple Lange Med) McGraw.

Current Cancer Immunology. Ed. by V. Richards. 1980. (Progress in Experimental Tumor Research Ser.: Vol. 25). (Illus.). 126.25 (*3-8055-3033-1*) S Karger.

Current Cancer Research, 1989. 1990. 21.00 (*0-387-91366-1*) Spr-Verlag.

Current Cancer Research, 1994. 1996. 29.00 (*0-387-00989-2*) Spr-Verlag.

Current Cancer Research, 1997. Ed. by Deutsches Krebsforschungszentrum Staff. 1998. (Illus.). 280p. pap. 22.00 (*3-7985-1122-5*) Spr-Verlag.

Current Cancer Therapeutics. Kirkwood. 3rd ed. 1998. (C). pap. text (*0-443-06527-6*) Church.

Current Cardiovascular Drug Therapy. Franz H. Messerli. Ed. by Richard Zorab. 2nd ed. 1996. LC 95-1013. (Illus.). 1408p. text 115.00 (*0-7216-4814-2*) Saunders.

Current Cardiovascular Drugs. William H. Frishman. 1993. (Illus.). 304p. text 39.95 (*1-878132-11-3*) Current Med.

Current Cardiovascular Drugs. William H. Frishman. 2nd ed. 1994. (Illus.). 328p. text 39.95 (*1-878132-60-1*) Rapid Science.

Current Cardiovascular Drugs, Vol. 1. Ed. by William H. Fishman. 3rd ed. 2000. (Illus.). 352p. text (*1-57340-135-8*) Current Med.

Current Clinical Practice. Franz H. Messerli. 1987. (Illus.). 1000p. text 77.00 (*0-7216-1460-4*) Saunders.

Current Clinical Strategies CD-ROM Collection for PDAs & Desktops: 2002. Paul D. Chan. rev. ed. 2000. (Current Clinical Strategies Ser.). 1700p. pap. 49.95 incl. cd-rom (*1-881528-91-X*) Current Clin Strat.

Current Clinical Topics in Infectious Disease. Jack S. Remington & Morton N. Swartz. (Illus.). Vol. 17. 17th ed. 1997. (Current Clinical Topics in Infectious Diseases Ser.: Vol. 17). 336p. 79.95 (*0-86542-575-2*); Vol. 19. 1999. 87.95 (*0-632-04402-0*) Blackwell Sci.

Current Clinical Topics in Infectious Disease, Vol.16. Ed. by Jack S. Remington & Morton Swartz. 1996. (Illus.). 304p. 87.95 (*0-86542-477-2*) Blackwell Sci.

Current Clinical Topics in Infectious Diseases. Ed. by Jack S. Remington & Morton N. Swartz. (Illus.). 15. 1995. 300p. 79.95 (*0-86542-397-0*); Vol. 18. 18th ed. 1998. LC 80-643590. (Current Clinical Topics in Infectious Diseases Ser.: Vol. 18). 315p. 87.95 (*0-632-04398-9*) Blackwell Sci.

Current Clinical Topics in Infectious Diseases 12, Vol. 12. Ed. by Jack S. Remington & Morton N. Swartz. 1992. (Illus.). 352p. (C). 79.95 (*0-86542-207-9*) Blackwell Sci.

Current Clinical Topics in Infectious Diseases 13, Vol. 13. Jack S. Remington. 1993. (Illus.). 392p. 79.95 (*0-86542-278-8*) Blackwell Sci.

Current Clinical Topics in Infectious Diseases 14, Vol. 14. Ed. by Jack S. Remington & M. N. Swartz. 1994. (Illus.). 320p. 79.95 (*0-86542-359-8*) Blackwell Sci.

Current Clinical Topics in Infectious Diseases, Volume 20, Vol. 20. Jack S. Remington & Morton N. Swartz. 2000. (Illus.). 336p. 87.95 (*0-632-04427-6*) Blackwell Sci.

Current Clinical Topics in Orthopedics. Ed. by Michael S. Zeide & Sam W. Wiesel. 1987. (Illus.). 400p. text 50.00 (*0-07-072814-3*) McGraw.

Current Concept in the Therapy of Hypertension with Beta-Blockers. S. Chaithiraphan. 1980. (Journal: Vol. 66, Suppl. 1). (Illus.). vi, 62p. pap. 28.50 (*3-8055-0912-X*) S Karger.

Current Concepts in Childhood Spinal Muscular Atrophy. Ed. by L. Merlini et al. 1989. (Illus.). 227p. 120.00 (*0-387-82131-7*) Spr-Verlag.

Current Concepts in Clinical Cardiology. Ed. by J. H. Vogel. 1980. (Advances in Cardiology Ser.: Vol. 27). (Illus.). viii, 360p. 172.25 (*3-8055-0098-X*) S Karger.

Current Concepts in Contract Dermatitis. Ed. by Julian L. Verbov. 1987. (New Clinical Applications in Dermatology Ser.). (C). lib. bdg. 87.00 (*0-85200-687-X*) Kluwer Academic.

Current Concepts in Diagnosis & Management of Arrhythmias in Infants & Children. Ed. by Barbara J. Deal et al. 1998. LC 98-9638. (Illus.). 438p. 95.00 (*0-87993-687-8*) Futura Pub.

Current Concepts in Diagnosis & Treatment of Vitreoretinal Diseases. Ed. by G. Blankenship et al. 1981. (Developments in Ophthalmology Ser.: Vol. 2). (Illus.). xxviii, 408p. 256.75 (*3-8055-1672-X*) S Karger.

Current Concepts in Endovascular Surgery. Samuel S. Ahn et al. 1994. (Medical Intelligence Unit Ser.). 103p. 99.00 (*1-57059-000-1*, LN9000) Landes Bioscience.

Current Concepts in Parasitology. Ed. by Ronald C. Ko. 1989. (Illus.). 267p. (C). pap. (*962-209-236-5*) HK Univ Pr HKG. *Dist:* Intl Spec Bk, Coronet Bks.

Current Concepts in Parkinson's Disease Research. Ed. by J. S. Schneider & M. Gupta. 1993. LC 91-35314. (Illus.). 470p. text 89.00 (*0-920887-72-4*) Hogrefe & Huber Pubs.

Current Concepts in Pediatrics, Vol. 1, No. 1. Maureen O'Reilly. 1994. 4p. (Orig.). (*0-944036-97-X*) Medicine Grp USA.

Current Concepts in Positive Mental Health. Marie Jahoda. Ed. by Gerald N. Grob. 1980. LC 78-22567. (Historical Issues in Mental Health Ser.). reprint ed. lib. bdg. 18.95 (*0-405-11921-6*) Ayer.

Current Concepts in Primary & Revision Total Knee Arthroplasty. Ed. by John N. Insall et al. 1996. LC 95-47605. (Bristol-Myers Squibb/Zimmer Orthopaedic Symposium Ser.). 304p. text 115.00 (*0-397-51753-X*) Lppncott W & W.

Current Concepts in Radiology Management. Howard W. Schwartz. 1992. 144p. pap. 20.00 (*0-9634176-0-6*) Amer Hlthcare Radiol.

Current Concepts in Regional Anaesthesia. J. W. Van Kleef et al. 1984. (Developments in Critical Care, Medicine, & Anesthesiology Ser.). text 147.50 (*0-89838-644-6*) Kluwer Academic.

Current Concepts in Research of Gastrointestinal Motility: Selected Papers from an International Symposium in Aarhus, Denmark, July 1991 - Digestive Diseases Journal, Vol. 9, No. 6. Ed. by H. Gregersen et al. 1992. (Journal). (Illus.). iv, 130p. pap. 35.00 (*3-8055-5537-7*) S Karger.

Current Concepts in Spina Bifida & Hydrocephalus. Ed. by Carys M. Bannister & Brian Tew. 1992. (Clinics in Developmental Medicine Ser.: No. 122). 215p. (C). text 64.95 (*0-521-41279-X*) Cambridge U Pr.

Current Concepts in the Management of Pain in Cancer Patients. Ed. by Raymond J. Trudnowsky. 1982. 35.00 (*0-915340-10-0*) PJD Pubns.

Current Concepts in Virology: From Ivanofsky to the Present. Ed. by Brian W. Mahy & Dmitri K. Lvov. 1993. LC 93-3449. 350p. text 120.00 (*3-7186-0568-6*) Gordon & Breach.

Current Concepts of a New Animal Model: The Non Mouse. Ed. by N. Sakamoto et al. 1992. LC 92-14878. 176p. 168.00 (*0-444-89554-X*) Elsevier.

Current Concepts of CAPD Vol. 7, No. 2-3: Journal: Blood Purification, 1989. Ed. by R. A. Mactier & K. D. Nolph. 1989. (Illus.). 120p. pap. 74.00 (*3-8055-5009-X*) S Karger.

Current Concepts of Diagnosis & Treatment of Bone & Soft Tissue Tumors. Ed. by Hans K. Uhthoff. 1984. (Illus.). 430p. 117.00 (*0-387-12570-1*) Spr-Verlag.

Current Concepts of Somatization: Research & Clinical Perspectives. Ed. by Laurence J. Kirmayer & James M. Robbins. 1991. LC 90-14492. (PIP Ser.: No. 31). 230p. text 18.95 (*0-88048-198-6*, 8198) Am Psychiatric.

Current Concepts of Suicide. Ed. & Intro. by David Lester. 1990. LC 90-1600. 256p. (Orig.). pap. text 20.95 (*0-914783-45-9*) Charles.

Current Controversies & Issues in Personality. Lawrence A. Pervin. 2nd ed. 1984. LC 83-23246. 368p. (C). pap. 51.95 (*0-471-88086-8*) Wiley.

Current Controversies in Alcoholism. Ed. by Barry Stimmel. 1983. LC 83-207. (Advances in Alcohol & Substance Abuse Ser.: Vol. 2, No. 2). 82p. text 32.95 (*0-86656-225-7*) Haworth Pr.

Current Controversies in Orthodontics. Ed. by Birte Melsen. 1991. (Illus.). 314p. text 99.00 (*0-86715-174-9*) Quint Pub Co.

Current Controversies in Temporomandibular Disorders: Proceedings of the 10th Annual Squaw Valley Winter Seminar, Squaw Valley, California, January 23-27, 1991. Ed. by Charles McNeill. 1992. LC 92-49813. (Illus.). 190p. text 62.00 (*0-86715-252-4*) Quint Pub Co.

Current Controversies in Thoracic Surgery. Frederick C. Kittle. 1986. (Illus.). 285p. text 89.00 (*0-7216-5461-4*) Saunders.

Current Critical Care Diagnosis & Treatment. Frederick S. Bongard & Darryl Y. Sue. 2nd ed. 1999. (C). pap. text 45.00 (*0-8385-1454-5*) Appleton & Lange.

Current Critical Problems in Vascular Surgery. Ed. by Frank J. Veith. (Illus.). Vol. 2. 1990. 475p. 79.95 (*0-942219-19-8*); Vol. 3. 1992. 443p. 79.95 (*0-942219-24-4*); Vol. 4. 1992. 470p. 85.00 (*0-942219-39-2*); Vol. 5. 1993. 468p. 85.00 (*0-942219-54-6*); Vol. 6. 1994. 452p. 85.00 (*0-942219-42-2*) Quality Med Pub.

Current Dermatologic Therapy. Stuart Maddin. 2nd ed. 1991. text 72.00 (*0-7216-1053-6*) Saunders.

Current Developments in Animal Virology. S. Jameel. Ed. by Edward K. Wagner. 1996. (Illus.). 375p. lib. bdg. 97.00 (*1-886106-61-4*) Science Pubs.

Current Developments in Anthropological Genetics Vol. 2: Ecology & Population Structure. Ed. by Michael H. Crawford & James H. Mielke. 1982. LC 79-24900. (Illus.). 542p. 95.00 (*0-306-40842-2*, Plenum Trade) Perseus Pubng.

Current Developments in Health Psychology. Paul Bennett et al. 1990. 352p. text 95.00 (*3-7186-5064-9*, Harwood Acad Pubs) Gordon & Breach.

Current Developments in Psychopharmacology, Vol. VI. Ed. by Walter B. Essman & L. Valzelli. 1981. LC 75-642512. (Illus.). 339p. text 75.00 (*0-88331-128-3*) R B Luce.

Current Diabetology. F. Belfiore. 1985. (Frontiers in Diabetes Ser.: Vol. 6). viii, 284p. 154.00 (*3-8055-4029-9*) S Karger.

Current Diagnosis & Treatment. James O. Woolliscroft. 2nd ed. 1999. pap. (*1-57340-109-9*) Current Med.

Current Diagnosis & Treatment. James O. Woolliscroft. 2nd ed. 1998. 79.95 (*1-57340-114-5*) Mosby Inc.

Current Diagnosis & Treatment in Gastroenterology. J. Grendell et al. 1996. (Illus.). 746p. (C). pap. 54.95 (*0-8385-1448-0*, A1448-8, Apple Lange Med) McGraw.

Current Diagnosis & Treatment in Infectious Disease. Walter E. Wilson et al. 2001. (Lange Medical Bks.). (Illus.). 985p. pap. 69.95 (*0-8385-1494-4*) McGraw-Hill Prof.

Current Diagnosis & Treatment in Orthopedics. Harry B. Skinner. 2nd ed. 2000. (Lange Medical Bks.). (Illus.). 720p. pap. 54.95 (*0-8385-0363-2*) McGraw-Hill Prof.

Current Diagnosis & Treatment in Psychiatry. Michael H. Ebert et al. 2000. LC 00-268146. (Lange Medical Bks.). (Illus.). 640p. (C). pap. 54.95 (*0-8385-1462-6*) McGraw-Hill Prof.

Current Diagnosis & Treatment of Fractures. H. David Moehring & Adam Greenspan. 1999. LC 99-29747. x, 298p. (*1-57340-133-1*) Current Med.

Current Diagnosis in Neurology. Edward Feldman. 1994. (Illus.). 399p. (C). (gr. 13). text 88.00 (*0-8016-6963-4*, 06963) Mosby Inc.

Current Diagnosis 9. Rex B. Conn et al. Ed. by William Z. Borer & Ray Kersey. 9th ed. 1996. 1072p. text 120.00 (*0-7216-5843-1*) Saunders.

Current Dilemmas in Medical-Care Rationing: A Pragmatic Approach. Henry A. Shenkin. 1995. 118p. (C). lib. bdg. 35.00 (*0-7618-0238-X*) U Pr of Amer.

Current Directions in Insulin-Like Growth Factor Research. D. LeRoith & M. K. Raizada. 1994. LC 93-46649. (Advances in Experimental Medicine & Biology Ser.: Vol. 343). (Illus.). 430p. (C). text 130.00 (*0-306-44622-7*, Kluwer Plenum) Kluwer Academic.

Current Directions in Radiopharmaceutical Research & Development. Ed. by Stephen J. Mather. 1996. LC 96-38428. (Developments in Nuclear Medicine Ser.: Vol. 30). lib. bdg. 136.00 (*0-7923-4254-2*) Kluwer Academic.

Current Drug Handbook 1984-1986. H. Robert Patterson et al. 1984. text 42.00 (*0-7216-1223-7*) Saunders.

Current Emergency Diagnosis & Treatment. Charles E. Saunders & Mary T. Ho. 4th ed. 1995. (Illus.). 1015p. (C). pap. text 54.95 (*0-8385-1347-6*, A1347-2, Apple Lange Med) McGraw.

Current Emergency Diagnosis & Treatment. Saunders & Ho. 5th ed. 1999. (C). pap. text 45.00 (*0-8385-1450-2*) P-H.

Current Estimates from the National Health Interview Survey. 1994. lib. bdg. 255.00 (*0-8490-5820-1*) Gordon Pr.

Current Feminist Issues in Psychotherapy. Ed. by New England Association for Women in Psychology St. 1983. LC 82-15721. (Women & Therapy Ser.: Vol. 1, No. 3). 115p. text 29.95 (*0-86656-206-0*) Haworth Pr.

Current Gastroenterology, 19. 1999. 89.95 (*0-8151-8420-4*) Mosby Inc.

Current Genetic, Clinical & Morphological Problems. Ed. by W. Straub. 1981. (Developments in Ophthalmology Ser.: Vol. 3). (Illus.). vi, 218p. pap. 136.75 (*3-8055-2000-X*) S Karger.

Current Geriatric Therapy. Timothy R. Covington & J. Ingram Walker. 1984. (Illus.). 463p. text 99.00 (*0-7216-2743-9*) Saunders.

Current Hepatology, Vol. 19. 1999. 89.95 (*0-8151-8423-9*) Mosby Inc.

Current Indications for Growth Hormone Therapy. Ed. by Peter C. Hindmarsh. 1998. (Endocrine Development Ser.: Vol. 1). (Illus.). viii, 162p. 85.25 (*3-8055-6757-X*) S Karger.

Current Infectious Disease Drugs. Vincent T. Andriole. 1995. (Illus.). 324p. text 42.00 (*1-878132-71-7*) Current Med.

Current Investigations of the Microbiology of Yersiniae. T. Maruyama & M. Tsubokura. Ed. by T. Une et al. 1991. (Contributions to Microbiology & Immunology Ser.: Vol. 12). (Illus.). x, 316p. 274.00 (*3-8055-5370-6*) S Karger.

Current Issues in Alcohol-Drug Studies. Frwd. by Edith S. Gomberg. 1990. LC 89-24470. (Drugs & Society Ser.: Vol. 3, Nos. 3-4). (Illus.). 228p. text 49.95 (*0-86656-965-0*) Haworth Pr.

Current Issues in Cancer. G. M. Mead. 1992. (Illus.). 147p. pap. text (*0-7279-0775-1*) BMJ Pub GBR. *Dist:* AIDC.

Current Issues in Cardiology. Ed. by Jean R. McEwan. 1997. 245p. pap. text (*0-7279-1010-8*) BMJ Pub GBR. *Dist:* AIDC.

Current Issues in Clinical Lactation 2000. Kathleen Auerbach. 1999. (Illus.). 96p. (C). pap. text 34.95 (*0-7637-1024-5*, 1024-5) Jones & Bartlett.

***Current Issues in Clinical Lactation 2002.** Kathleen G. Auerbach. 2001. (Illus.). (C). text 36.95 (*0-7637-1822-X*, 1822-X, N L N Bart) Jones & Bartlett.

Current Issues in Clinical Psychology, Vol. 3. Ed. by E. Karas. 1987. LC 83-647976. 248p. 65.00 (*0-306-42603-X*, Plenum Trade) Perseus Pubng.

Current Issues in Cognitive Processes: The Tulane Flowerree Symposium. Chizuko Izawa. 1989. 440p. (C). pap. 49.95 (*0-8058-0669-5*) L Erlbaum Assocs.

Current Issues in Community Nursing Vol. 1: Primary Health Care in Practice. Ed. by J. Littlewood. 1995. (Illus.). 324p. pap. (*0-443-05185-2*) Church.

Current Issues in Developmental Psychology. Alex Fedde Kalverboer et al. 1999. LC 99-41412. 198p. 120.00 (*0-7923-5902-X*) Kluwer Academic.

Current Issues in Developmental Psychology: Biopsychological Perspectives. Ed. by A. F. Kalverboer et al. 1999. 198p. pap. 75.00 (*0-7923-5983-6*, Kluwer Acad) Kluwer Academic.

Current Issues in Infancy & Parenthood, Vol. 3. Ed. by Catherine A. Niven, RGN, BSc, PhD & Anne Walker. 1998. LC 98-16256. (Reproductive Psychology Ser.). 320p. pap. (*0-7506-2442-6*) E A GBR. *Dist:* OUP.

Current Issues in Lymphoma. Ed. by R. L. Katz & W. C. Pugh. 1994. (Journal: Vol. 4, No. 1). (Illus.). 58p. pap. 69.75 (*3-8055-6014-1*) S Karger.

Current Issues in Medical Device Quality Systems. Ed. by David Link & Ed McDonnell. 5th ed. 1996. LC 97-221321. pap. 225.00 (*1-57020-075-0*, GMP4-209) Assn Adv Med Instrn.

***Current Issues in Nurse Prescribing.** Ed. by Molly Courtenay. 2001. (Greenwich Medical Media Ser.). (Illus.). 160p. pap. (*1-84110-063-3*) Greenwich Med GBR. *Dist:* JAMCO Dist.

Current Issues in Nursing. Joanne C. McCloskey & Helen K. Grace. 5th ed. 1997. (Illus.). 736p. (C). (gr. 13). pap. text 39.00 (*0-8151-8594-4*, 28840) Mosby Inc.

Current Issues in Nursing. Joanne McCloskey Dochterman & Helen K. Grace. 6th ed. 2001. LC 00-48942. (Illus.). xxiii, 693p. 43.95 (*0-323-01276-0*) Mosby Inc.

Current Issues in Platelet Transfusion Therapy & Platelet Alloimmunity. Thomas S. Kickler & Jay H. Herman. 1999. LC 99-42924. 306p. pap. 119.00 (*1-56395-105-3*, AABB Pr) Am Assn Blood.

Current Issues in Platelet Transfusion Therapy & Platelet Alloimmunity. Ed. by Thomas S. Kickler & Jay H. Herman. 1999. (Illus.). 306p. (*3-8055-7060-0*) S Karger.

Current Issues in Rational-Emotive Therapy. Wendy Dryden. 1987. 220p. lib. bdg. (*0-7099-4557-4*) C Helm GBR. *Dist:* Routldge.

Current Issues in Women's Health. 1997. lib. bdg. 250.95 (*0-8490-6126-1*) Gordon Pr.

Current Issues in Women's Health: An FDA Consumer Special Report. (Illus.). 1994. 110p. pap. text 35.00 (*1-57979-015-1*); 1993. 63p. (C). pap. text 25.00 (*1-56806-936-7*); 2nd rev. ed. 1994. 111p. (YA). (gr. 12 up). pap. text 30.00 (*0-7881-0780-1*) DIANE Pub.

Current Knowledge in Reproductive Medicine, Vol. 1206. E. M. Coutinho & P. Spinola. 2000. LC 00-46242. (International Congress Ser.: No. 1206). (Illus.). 444p. 149.50 (*0-444-50419-2*) Elsevier.

Current Management in Child Neurology. Bernard L. Maria. 1999. LC 99-167190. 387 p. incl. cd-rom (*1-55009-070-4*) DEKR.

Current Management of Diabetes. Ralph Defronzo. 1997. LC 98-208447. (Illus.). 288p. (C). (gr. 13). text 59.95 (*0-8151-2757-X*, 22758) Mosby Inc.

Current Med Talk: A Dictionary of Medical Terms, Slang & Jargon. Joseph C. Segen. 2nd ed. 2002. 1300p. text 42.95 (*0-8385-1535-5*) McGraw-Hill Prof.

Current Medical Diagnosis & Treatment. Lawrence M. Tierney et al. 40th ed. 2000. LC 74-641062. (Current Medical Diagnosis & Treatment Ser.). (Illus.). 1794p. pap. 54.95 (*0-07-136466-8*) McGraw-Hill Prof.

***Current Medical Diagnosis & Treatment 2002 & Essentials of Diagnosis & Treatment.** Lawrence Tierney et al. 41st ed. 2001. (Illus.). pap. 75.00 (*0-07-139006-5*) McGraw-Hill Prof.

Current Medical Research in Eastern Africa. P. M. Tukei & A. R. Njogu. 1983. 292p. pap. 65.00 (*0-86346-040-2*, Tycooly Pub) Weidner & Sons.

Current Medical Terminology. Vera Pyle. Ed. by Sally C. Pitman. 6th rev. ed. 1996. LC 96-221591. pap. 37.00 (*0-934385-67-X*) Hlth Prof Inst.

Current Medical Terminology. Vera Pyle. 7th ed. 1999. LC 99-159074. pap. text (*0-934385-74-2*) Hlth Prof Inst.

Current Medicine. Lawson. 2nd ed. 1990. pap. text 41.00 (*0-443-04254-3*) Saunders.

Current Medicine 4: Royal College of Physicians of Edinburgh. Ed. by D. H. Lawson. 1994. (Illus.). 330p. pap. (*0-443-05040-6*) Church.

Current Medicine Three. Ed. by David A. Lawson. 3rd ed. 1991. (Illus.). 300p. (Orig.). pap. text (*0-443-04598-4*) Church.

Current Medtalk: Medical Terms, Slang & Jargon. Joseph Segen. 1996. LC 96-130050. 984p. (C). pap. text 44.95 (*0-8385-1464-2*, A1464-5, Apple Lange Med) McGraw.

Current Methodology in Experimental Hematology. Ed. by S. J. Baum. 1985. (Bibliotheca Haematologica Ser.: No. 48). (Illus.). vi, 418p. 215.75 (*3-8055-3722-0*) S Karger.

Current Methods in Muscle Physiology: Advantages, Problems, & Limitations. Ed. by Haruo Sugi. 1998. LC 97-41612. (Illus.). 384p. text 115.00 (*0-19-852397-1*) OUP.

Current Neurologic Drugs. Ed. by Lewis P. Rowland & Donald F. Klein. 1996. 360p. pap. text 53.00 (*1-878132-72-5*) Current Med.

Current Neurosurgery. Ed. by G. M. Teasdale & J. D. Miller. 1992. (Illus.). 351p. text (*0-443-04447-3*) Church.

Current Nutritional Therapy: A Clinical Reference. Ronald J. Grabowski. 1994. 360p. ring bd. 79.00 (*0-9640099-0-0*) Image Pr TX.

Current Obstetric & Gynecologic Diagnosis & Treatment. Alan H. DeCherney. 8th ed. 1996. (Current Obstetric & Gynecologic Diagnosis & Treatment Ser.). 1230p. (C). pap. text 54.95 (*0-8385-1447-2*, A1447-0, Apple Lange Med) McGraw.

Current Obstetric Medicine, 5. Richard V. Lee. 1999. 270p. text 69.95 (*0-8151-5553-0*) Mosby Inc.

Current Occular Therapy 4. Frederick T. Fraunfelder. 4th ed. 1994. (Illus.). 953p. text 98.00 (*0-7216-4913-0*) Saunders.

Current Ocular Therapy. Frederick T. Fraunfelder. 5th ed. Date not set. text (*0-7216-7781-9*) Saunders.

Current Oculomotor Research: Physiological & Psychological Aspects. Ed. by W. Becker et al. 1999. LC 98-31568. (Illus.). 492p. (C). text 135.00 (*0-306-46049-1*, Kluwer Plenum) Kluwer Academic.

Current Opinion in Cosmetic Dentistry. Gary Goldstein et al. 1993. (Illus.). 108p. (Orig.). pap. 59.95 (*1-870485-57-2*) Rapid Science.

Current Opinion in Dermatology. Mark V. Dahl. 3rd ed. 1996. (Illus.). 268p. text 110.00 (*1-85922-702-3*) Rapid Science.

Current Opinions in the Kyoto Cornea Club, Vol. II. Ed. by S. Kinoshita & Y. Ohashi. 1998. (Illus.). x, 107p. (*90-6299-150-5*) Kugler NLD. *Dist:* Lib Res.

Current Opinions in the Kyoto Cornea Club: Proceedings of the First Annual Meeting of the Kyoto Cornea Club; Kyoto, Japan, December 1-2, 1995. Kyoto Cornea Club Staff et al. 1997. LC 97-17663. (*90-6299-138-6*) Kugler NLD. *Dist:* Lib Res.

Current Oral & Maxillofacial Imaging. Thomas F. Razmus & Gail F. Williamson. 1996. text 37.00 (*0-7216-4005-2*) Saunders.

Current Orthopedic Diagnosis & Treatment. Ed. by James D. Heckman et al. 2000. LC 99-44555. (Illus.). 224p. text (*1-57340-141-2*) Current Med.

Current Paediatric Practice. Ed. by Peter G. Procopis & Geoff D. Kewley. 1991. (Illus.). 336p. pap. text (*0-7295-0397-6*) Bailliere Tindall.

Current Pediatric Drugs. Fredric D. Burg & Jeffrey A. Bourret. 1993. (Illus.). 224p. pap. text 31.00 (*0-7216-4574-7*) Saunders.

Current Perinatology. Ed. by Manohar L. Rathi. 1988. (Illus.). 283p. 125.00 (*0-387-96758-3*) Spr-Verlag.

Current Perinatology Two. Ed. by Manohar L. Rathi. 1990. (Illus.). 230p. 125.00 (*0-387-97214-5*) Spr-Verlag.

Current Perspectives in Hepatology: Festschrift for Hyman J. Zimmerman, M. D. L. B. Seeff & J. H. Lewis. 1989. (Illus.). 456p. (C). text 110.00 (*0-306-43063-0*, Kluwer Plenum) Kluwer Academic.

Current Perspectives in Human Physiology, 1998 Edition: Selected Readings. Ed. by Lauralee Sherwood. 3rd ed. 1997. LC 97-220295. (Biology Ser.). 224p. pap. text 19.95 (*0-314-20640-X*) West Pub.

Current Perspectives in Lithium Prophylaxis. Ed. by P. Berner et al. 1981. (Bibliotheca Psychiatrica Ser.: Vol. 161). (Illus.). viii, 248p. pap. 76.75 (*3-8055-1753-X*) S Karger.

Current Perspectives in Psychological, Legal & Ethical Issues Vol. 1: Children & Families. Ed. by Sandra A. Garcia & Robert Batey. 1991. 88.00 (*1-85302-084-2*) Taylor & Francis.

Current Perspectives in Psychological, Legal & Ethical Issues Vol. 1: Children & Families, Pt. A-Children & Families: Abuse & Endangerment. Ed. by Sandra A. Garcia & Robert Batey. 1991. 88.00 (*1-85302-083-4*) Taylor & Francis.

Current Perspectives in Psychological, Legal & Ethical Issues Vol. 1: Children & Families, Set. Ed. by Sandra A. Garcia & Robert Batey. 1991. 175.00 (*1-85302-082-6*) Taylor & Francis.

Current Perspectives in Toxicology. 1992. 93p. (C). (*0-85186-447-3*, RA1199) Royal Soc Chem GBR. *Dist:* Spr-Verlag.

Current Perspectives on Implantable Devices. Ed. by David F. Williams. Vol. 1. 1989. 317p. 128.50 (*0-89232-885-1*); Vol. 2. 1991. 291p. 128.50 (*1-55938-015-2*) Jai Pr.

Current Perspectives on Molecular & Cellular Oncology, Set, Vol. 1, Pts. A & B. Ed. by Demetrios Spandidos. 1992. 257.00 (*1-55938-355-0*) Jai Pr.

Current Perspectives on Molecular & Cellular Oncology Vol. 1, Pt. A: Mechanisms of Gene Regulation in Cancer, Vol. 1, Pt. A. Ed. by Demetrios Spandidos. 1992. 332p. 90.00 (*1-55938-486-7*) Jai Pr.

Current Perspectives on Molecular & Cellular Oncology Vol. 1, Pt. B: Cancer Genes & Their Clinical Implications, Vol. 1, Pt. B. Ed. by Demetrios Spandidos. 1992. 332p. 128.50 (*1-55938-487-5*) Jai Pr.

Current Perspectives on Nutrition & Health. Ed. by Kenneth K. Carroll. 1998. LC 00-700402. 312p. text (*0-7735-1698-0*); pap. text (*0-7735-1724-3*) McG-Queens Univ Pr CAN. *Dist:* CUP Services.

Current Perspectives on the Fetus as a Patient. Ed. by Frank A. Chervenak & Asim Kurjak. 1996. LC 96-17371. (Illus.). 666p. lib. bdg. 140.95 (*1-85070-742-1*, Parthenon Pbng) CRC Pr.

Current Pocket Reference: Pharmacoposia & Medical Notes, 1998. Larry T. Shepherd & Thomas J. Whalen. 1997. (Illus.). 120p. (C). text 8.75 (*0-9642193-4-4*) Specialty Cards.

Current Practice in Critical Illness. D. W. Ryan. 1996. (Illus.). 168p. 67.95 (*0-412-61790-0*) Chapman & Hall.

Current Practice in Critical Illness, Vol. 2. D. W. Ryan. 1997. (Illus.). 206p. (*0-412-61800-1*) E A GBR. *Dist:* OUP.

Current Practice in Critical Illness, Vol. 3. D.W. Ryan. 1999. (Illus.). 226p. text (*0-412-79300-8*) E A GBR. *Dist:* OUP.

Current Practice in Foot & Ankle Surgery, Vol. 2. Ed. by Glenn B. Pfeffer & Carol C. Frey. 1994. LC 92-49130. (Current Practice in Foot & Ankle Surgery Ser.: Vol. 2). (Illus.). 352p. text 55.00 (*0-07-049799-0*) McGraw-Hill Educ Grp.

Current Practice in Foot & Ankle Surgery, Vol. 1. Ed. by Glenn B. Pfeffer & Carol C. Frey. 1993. LC 92-49130. (Current Practice in Foot & Ankle Surgery Ser.). 304p. text 55.00 (*0-07-049732-X*) McGraw-Hill Med Pub.

Current Practice in Genitourinary Medicine. S. E. Barton. 1999. LC 99-213410. (Illus.). 296p. (*0-340-74084-1*) E A GBR. *Dist:* OUP.

Current Practice of Breast, Skin & Soft Tissue Surgery. Ed. by Barry A. Levine. 1994. LC 93-50590. pap. text (*0-443-08974-4*) Church.

Current Practice of Cardiothoracic Surgery. Barry A. Levine. 1994. LC 93-49075. pap. text (*0-443-08976-0*) Church.

Current Practice of Clinical Electroencephalography. David D. Daly & Timothy A. Pedley. 2nd ed. 1990. 848p. text 169.00 (*0-88167-635-7*) Lppncott W & W.

Current Practice of Clinical Electroencephalography. John S. Ebersole & Timothy A. Pedley. 3rd ed. 2002. text 149.00 (*0-7817-1694-2*) Lppncott W & W.

Current Practice of Dermatology. Jeffrey P. Callen. 1995. (Illus.). 200p. text 95.00 (*1-85922-801-1*) Current Med.

Current Practice of Dermatology. Jeffrey P. Callen. 1996. 188p. (C). pap. 125.00 (*0-8385-1505-3*, A-1505-5) McGraw-Hill Prof.

Current Practice of Fracture Treatment: New Concepts & Common Problems. Ed. by Ping-Chung Leung. 1994. (Illus.). 488p. 199.00 (*0-387-57367-4*) Spr-Verlag.

Current Practice of Gastrointestinal & Abdominal Surgery. Barry A. Levine. 1994. LC 93-50705. pap. text (*0-443-08975-2*) Church.

Current Practice of Medicine, Set. Ed. by Roger C. Bone. 1996. (Illus.). 2792p. text 195.00 (*0-443-07894-7*) Current Med.

Current Practice of Medicine: Dermatology. Jeffrey P. Callen. 1995. (Illus.). 200p. text 39.95 (*1-85922-688-4*) Current Med.

Current Practice of Medicine Vol. 2: Dermatology. Jeffrey P. Callen. 1995. (Illus.). 200p. text 39.95 (*0-443-07891-2*) Current Med.

Current Practice of Pediatric Surgery. Barry A. Levine. 1994. LC 93-49044. pap. text (*0-443-08978-7*) Church.

Current Practice of Surgery, Set. Ed. by Barry A. Levine et al. 1993. (Illus.). 2848p. text (*0-443-08767-9*) Church.

Current Practice of Surgery Essentials. Ed. by Barry A. Levine et al. 1994. LC 93-48804. pap. text (*0-443-08972-8*) Church.

Current Practice of Trauma Surgery. Barry A. Levine et al. 1994. LC 93-48362. pap. text (*0-443-08973-6*) Church.

Current Practice of Vascular Surgery. Ed. by Barry A. Levine. 1994. LC 93-50706. pap. text (*0-443-08977-9*) Church.

Current Problems & New Trends in Cystic Fibrosis. Ed. by M. Schoeni & R. Kraemer. 1981. (Monographs in Pediatrics: Vol. 14). (Illus.). xii, 216p. pap. 129.75 (*3-8055-3417-5*) S Karger.

Current Problems in Congenital Heart Disease. Ed. by W. Jay Eldredge et al. 1979. LC 78-15311. 220p. text 44.50 (*0-88331-129-1*) R B Luce.

Current Problems in Dermatology. Ed. by J. W. Mali. Vol. 3. 1970. 72.25 (*3-8055-0484-5*); Vol. 4. 1972. 83.50 (*3-8055-1248-1*); Vol. 5. 1973. 77.50 (*3-8055-1380-1*) S Karger.

Current Problems in Dermatology: Complete Set, Vol. 16 & 17. Ed. by Tobias Gedde-Dahl, Jr. & K. D. Wuepper. 1987. (Illus.). xvi, 472p. 361.75 (*3-8055-4407-3*) S Karger.

Current Problems in Leptospirosis Research: Report of a WHO Expert Group, 1967. 1967. (Technical Report Ser.: No. 380). 32p. pap. text 3.00 (*92-4-120380-3*, 1100380) World Health.

Current Problems of Cardiovascular Surgery: A Scientific Approach. Ed. by Z. G. Szabo. 1986. 196p. (C). (*963-05-4435-0*) Akade Kiado HUN. *Dist:* St Mut.

Current Progress in Perinatal Medicine: Proceedings of the World Congress of Perinatal Medicine, 1993, Rome & Florence, Italy. Ed. by Ermelando V. Cosmi & G. C. Di Renzo. 2nd ed. 1994. (Illus.). 902p. (C). lib. bdg. 104.95 (*1-85070-560-7*, Parthenon Pbng) CRC Pr.

Current Progress in the Understanding of Secondary Brain Damage from Trauma & Ischemia: Proceedings of the 6th International Symposium: Mechanisms of Secondary Brain Damage - Novel Developments, Mauls/Sterzing, Italy, February 1998. Ed. by A. Baethmann et al. 1999. LC 99-23445. (Acta Neurochirurgica Ser.: Vol. 73). (Illus.). 200p. 50.00 (*3-211-83313-7*) Spr-Verlag.

Current Protocals in Molecular Biology Vol. 3, Vol. 3. Roger Brent et al. Ed. by Frederick M. Ausubel. 1988. 1600p. 635.00 (*0-471-50338-X*) Wiley.

Current Protocols in Immunology. Ed. by John E. Coligan et al. 1991. LC 90-15726. 920p. pap. text 635.00 (*0-471-52276-7*) Wiley.

Current Protocols in Neuroscience Jacqueline N. Crawley. 1997. LC 97-14252. (Illus.). 700p. 395.00 (*0-471-16359-7*) Wiley.

Current Protocols in Pharmacology. Sam J. Enna. 1998. LC 97-43922. 700p. pap. 450.00 (*0-471-17197-2*) Wiley.

Current Psychiatric Diagnosis & Treatment. Lewis R. Baxter & Robert O. Friedel. 1998. LC 98-39106. 39.95 (*1-57340-121-8*) Current Med.

Current Psychiatric Therapies. Ed. by Jules H. Masserman. (Current Psychiatric Therapies Ser.). Vol. XV. 1975. LC 61-9411. 320p. text 91.00 (*0-8089-0881-2*, 792715); Vol. XVI. 1976. LC 61-9411. (Illus.). 368p. text 91.00 (*0-8089-0978-9*, 792716); Vol. XVIII. 1979. 320p. text 86.00 (*0-8089-1151-1*, 792718); Vol. 20. 1981. 432p. text 81.00 (*0-8089-1409-X*, 792720); Vol. 21. 1982. 352p. text 67.00 (*0-8089-1517-7*, 792721); Vol. 23. 1986. LC 79-2723. 320p. text 70.00 (*0-8089-1766-8*, 792723) Harcrt Hlth Sci Grp (Grune & Strat).

Current Psychiatric Therapy II, Vol. 2. David L. Dunner. Ed. by Judy Fletcher & Yolaine Lefebvre. 2nd ed. 1997. LC 96-16730. (Illus.). 624p. text 78.00 (*0-7216-5989-6*) Saunders.

Current Psychotherapeutic Drugs. Ed. by Donald F. Klein & Lewis P. Rowland. 1996. 192p. pap. text 39.95 (*0-87630-816-7*) Brunner-Routledge.

Current Psychotherapeutic Drugs. Ed. by Donald F. Klein & Lewis P. Rowland. 1995. 184p. pap. text 39.95 (*1-57340-079-3*) Current Med.

Current Radiation Oncology, Vol. 1. Ed. by Jeffrey S. Tobias & Patrick R. M. Thomas. 1994. (Illus.). 436p. (*0-340-56761-9*) E A GBR. *Dist:* OUP.

Current Radiation Oncology, Vol. 2. Jeffrey S. Tobias & Patrick R. M. Thomas. 1996. (Illus.). 496p. (*0-340-61387-4*) E A GBR. *Dist:* OUP.

Current Radiation Oncology, Vol. 3. Ed. by Jeffrey S. Tobias & Patrick R. Thomas. 1997. (Arnold Publication). (Illus.). 426p. (C). text 95.00 (*0-340-67739-2*) OUP.

Current Regulatory Issues in Medical Physics: Proceedings of an American College of Medical Physics Symposium, April 1992. Melissa Martin & James Smathers. 1992. 458p. pap. text 29.95 (*0-944838-29-4*) Med Physics Pub.

Current Research & Applications in Personality Theories. Larry A. Hjelle & Daniel J. Zeigler. 1992. (C). pap., stu. ed. 13.44 (*0-07-029084-9*) McGrw-H Hghr Educ.

Current Research & Clinical Management of Melanoma, Alk. paper. Ed. by Larry Nathanson. 1993. LC 93-9325. (Cancer Treatment & Research Ser.: Vol. 65). 400p. (C). text 291.50 (*0-7923-2152-9*) Kluwer Academic.

Current Research in Advanced Cockpit Display Concepts: A Special Issue of the International Journal of Aviation Psychology. Ed. by Lawrence Hettinger & Michael Haas. 2000. 89p. pap. 24.50 (*0-8058-9762-3*) L Erlbaum Assocs.

Current Research in Alzheimer Therapy. Ed. by Ezio Giacobini & Robert E. Becker. 1988. (Illus.). 366p. (C). text 94.95 (*0-8448-1555-1*) Taylor & Francis.

Current Research in Nephrology in Japan. Ed. by Y. Ueda. 1976. (Contributions to Nephrology Ser.: Vol. 4). 29.75 (*3-8055-2383-1*) S Karger.

Current Research in Neurosciences: Topical Problem in Psychiatry & Neurology. Ed. by E. Gruenthal et al. 1969. (Bibliotheca Psychiatrica Ser.: No. 143). pap. 61.75 (*3-8055-0331-8*) S Karger.

Current Research in Sports Sciences: An International Perspective. Ed. by Victor A. Rogozkin & Ron J. Maughan. 1996. (Illus.). 356p. (C). text 114.00 (*0-306-45319-3*, Kluwer Plenum) Kluwer Academic.

Current Respiratory Care. Kenneth F. MacDonnell & Maurice S. Segal. 1977. 489p. pap. text 15.95 (*0-316-54191-5*, Little Brwn Med Div) Lppncott W & W.

Current Review of Allergic Diseases. Michael A. Kaliner. 1998. (Illus.). 200p. 104.95 (*0-632-04383-0*) Blackwell Sci.

Current Review of Cerebrovascular Disease. Ed. by Marc Fisher & Julien Bogousslavsky. 1993. (Illus.). 196p. text 99.95 (*1-878132-14-8*) Current Med.

Current Review of Cerebrovascular Disease. Marc Fisher & Julien Bogousslausky. 2nd ed. 1995. (Illus.). 248p. text 105.00 (*1-878132-62-8*) Current Med.

Current Review of Complementary Medicine. Marc S. Micozzi. 1999. LC 99-12780. xiii, 167p. 49.95 (*1-57340-129-3*) Current Med.

Current Review of Diabetes. Simeon I. Taylor. 1999. LC 99-23880. 59.95 (*1-57340-132-3*) Current Med.

Current Review of Interventional Cardiology. Eric J. Topol & Patrick W. Serruys. 1993. (Illus.). 288p. text 149.95 (*1-878132-03-2*) Current Med.

Current Review of Interventional Cardiology: A Current Medicine Title. D. R. Holmes & P. W. Serrays. 2nd ed. 1997. 200p. text (*0-443-07951-X*) Church.

Current Review of Laparoscopy. David C. Brooks. 2nd ed. 1995. (Illus.). 248p. text 99.00 (*1-878132-61-X*) Rapid Science.

Current Review of Magnetic Resonance Imaging. Javier Beltran. 1995. (Illus.). 416p. text 99.95 (*1-878132-09-1*) Current Med.

Current Review of MRI. Javier Beltran. 1996. (Illus.). 400p. pap. 125.00 (*0-8385-1501-0*, A15014) McGraw-Hill Prof.

Current Review of Sports Medicine. Ed. by Robert J. Johnson & John Lombardo. 2nd ed. 1997. 200p. text 69.99 (*0-7506-9965-5*) Buttrwrth-Heinemann.

Current Role of Nitrates. Ed. by Chris Fellner. 1997. (Illus.). 20p. (Orig.). pap. (*1-57130-029-5*) Medicine Grp USA.

Current (Safety) Issues in the Screening of Donor Blood & the Preparation of Pure Blood Components. Ed. by S. Seidl et al. 1986. (Vox Sanguinis: Vol. 51, Suppl. 1, 1986). (Illus.). iv, 72p. pap. 28.75 (*3-8055-4346-8*) S Karger.

Current Science & Medicine: In Light of a Yeast Causal Hypothesis. Katherine E. Anderson. 1996. 30p. (Orig.). pap. 4.95 (*1-57876-903-5*) Triple U Enterprises.

Current Spleen Surgery. S. Uranus. 1995. (Illus.). 100p. text, lib. bdg. (*3-88603-431-3*) W Zuckschwerdt DEU. *Dist:* Scholium Intl.

Current Standards for the Evaluation of Pharmacological Care of BPH, Proceedings of a Symposium, Genoa, July 1992. Ed. by A. Jardin & F. Di Silverio. 1993. (Journal: Vol. 24, Suppl. 1, 1993). (Illus.). vi, 50p. pap. 24.50 (*3-8055-5827-9*) S Karger.

Current Status of Ankle Arthroplasty. Ed. by H. Kofoed. 1998. LC 98-26060. (Illus.). 168p. pap. 99.00 (*3-540-64653-1*) Spr-Verlag.

***Current Status of Carotid Bifurcation Angioplasty & Stenting.** Ed. by Frank J. Veith & M. Amor. 2001. LC 2001-17444. (Illus.). xiii, 291p. text 150.00 (*0-8247-0495-9*) Dekker.

Current Status of Centrally Acting Peptides: Proceedings of the Satellite Symposium of the International Congress of Pharmacology, Lucknow, India, July 8th, 1981, Vol. 38. International Congress of Pharmacology Staff. Ed. by B. N. Dhawan. 1982. LC 82-3825. (Illus.). 272p. 69.50 (*0-08-028008-0*, Pergamon Pr) Elsevier.

Current Status of Clinical Cardiology, 1990. Ed. by Desmond G. Julian. 1990. (C). text 118.50 (*0-7923-8936-0*) Kluwer Academic.

Current Status of Clinical Organ Transplantation. Ed. by George M. Abouna. 1984. LC 84-1553. (Developments in Surgery Ser.). text 206.50 (*0-89838-635-7*) Kluwer Academic.

Current Status of Diagnostic Cytology. Ed. by Peter Pfitzer & Ekkehard Grundmann. 1993. LC 93-11295. (Recent Results in Cancer Research Ser.: Vol. 133). 173p. 93.00 (*0-387-56618-X*); (Illus.). 175p. (*3-540-56618-X*) Spr-Verlag.

Current Status of Endometriosis: Research & Management: Proceedings of the 3rd World Congress of Endometriosis, Brussels, 1992. Ed. by I. Brosens & J. Donnez. 1993. LC 93-18078. (Illus.). ring bd. (*1-85070-454-6*, Parthenon Pbng) CRC Pr.

Current Status of Fetal Medicine & Its Future, 1989: Journal: Fetal Therapy, Vol. 4, Suppl. 1. Ed. by S. Mancuso. 1990. (Illus.). vi, 134p. pap. 42.75 (*3-8055-5284-X*) S Karger.

Current Status of Hemapheresis: Indications, Technology & Complications. Ed. by Robert G. Westphal & Duke O. Kasprisin. 1987. LC 87-14420. 124p. text 7.00 (*0-915355-45-0*) Am Assn Blood.

***Current Strategies & Advances in Headache Management.** Ed. by Seymour Diamond. 37p. pap. 25.00 (*0-8236-1103-5*, BN 01103) Intl Univs Pr.

Current Studies in Nephrology: Dialysis & Transplantation. Ed. by G. D'Amico & G. Colasanti. 1986. (Contributions to Nephrology Ser.: Vol. 48). (Illus.). vi, 206p. 29.75 (*3-8055-4141-4*) S Karger.

Current Studies in Otoneurology: Proceedings of the Barany Society Meeting, Toronto, Aug. 1971. Barany Society Meeting Staff. Ed. by H. O. Barber & J. M. Frederickson. 1973. (Advances in OtoRhinoLaryngology Ser.: Vol. 19). (Illus.). 134.00 (*3-8055-1448-4*) S Karger.

Current Surgical Diagnosis & Treatment. Lawrence W. Way. (Current Surgical Diagnosis & Treatment Ser.). (Illus.). (C). 10th ed. 1996. 1426p. pap. text 54.95 (*0-8385-1439-1*, A1439-7); 11th rev. ed. 2001. 1500p. pap. text 45.00 (*0-8385-1456-1*) McGraw (Apple Lange Med).

Current Surgical Practice, Vol. 6. M. Hobsley. 6th ed. 1993. 224p. pap. text (*0-340-55153-4*) E A GBR. *Dist:* Routldge.

Current Surgical Practice, Vol. 7. M. Hobsley. 1994. 208p. pap. 55.00 (*0-340-58913-2*) Trafalgar.

Current Surgical Therapy, Vol. 6. John L. Cameron. 6th ed. 1998. (Illus.). 1300p. (C). text 135.00 (*0-8151-2835-5*, 30964) Mosby Inc.

Current Techniques in Arthroscopy. J. Serge Parisien. 1994. (Illus.). 256p. text 149.95 (*1-878132-04-0*) Current Med.

Current Techniques in Arthroscopy. Illus. by Ann Saydlowski. 2nd ed. 1995. 240p. (C). text 125.00 (*1-878132-63-6*) Current Med.

Current Techniques in Arthroscopy. Parisien. 3rd ed. 1998. 99.00 (*0-86577-738-1*) Thieme Med Pubs.

Current Techniques in Equine Surgery & Lameness. Nathaniel A. White & James N. Moore. Ed. by Stephanie Donley. 2nd ed. 1998. LC 98-20446. (Illus.). 720p. (C). text 125.00 (*0-7216-4601-8*) Saunders.

Current Techniques in Interventional Radiology. Constantin Cope. 1993. (Illus.). 216p. text 99.95 (*1-878132-02-4*) Current Med.

Current Techniques in Interventional Radiology. Cope. 2nd ed. 1996. 200p. (C). pap. 125.00 (*0-8385-1503-7*) McGraw-Hill Prof.

Current Techniques in Interventional Radiology. Constantin Cope. 3rd ed. 1994. (Illus.). 208p. text 109.95 (*1-878132-59-8*) Current Med.

Current Techniques in Laparoscopy. David Brooks. 1993. (Illus.). 224p. text 149.95 (*1-878132-05-9*) Current Med.

Current Techniques in Modern Vascular Surgery. James S. T. Yao & William H. Pearce. 2000. (Illus.). 551p. text 185.00 (*0-07-136501-X*) McGraw-Hill Prof.

Current Techniques in Neurosurgery. Illus. by Lorie M. Manzardo. 1995. 240p. text 174.95 (*1-878132-01-6*) Current Med.

Current Techniques in Neurosurgery. Michael Salcman. 2nd ed. 1995. (Illus.). 248p. text 125.00 (*1-878132-58-X*) Rapid Science.

Current Techniques in Neurosurgery. Ed. by M. Salcman. 3rd ed. 1998. (Illus.). 253p. 165.00 (*0-387-98340-6*) Spr-Verlag.

Current Techniques in Ophthalmic Laser Surgery. Lawrence Singerman et al. 3rd ed. 1998. (Illus.). 200p. text 84.99 (*0-7506-7032-0*) Buttrwrth-Heinemann.

Current Techniques in Opthalmic Laser Surgery. William E. Benson et al. 2nd ed. 1995. (Illus.). 224p. text 139.95 (*1-878132-57-1*) Current Med.

Current Techniques in Small Animal Surgery. M. Joseph Bojrab et al. (Illus.). 3rd ed. 1989. LC 89-13005. 950p. text 105.00 (*0-8121-1193-1*); 4th ed. 1998. LC 97-22997. 1408p. 99.95 (*0-683-00890-0*) Lppncott W & W.

Current Techniques in Spinal Stabilization. Ed. by Richard G. Fessler & Regis W. Haid. 1996. (Illus.). 528p. text 125.00 (*0-07-020645-7*) McGraw-Hill Med Pub.

Current Themes in Psychiatry, Vol. 3. Ed. by Raghu N. Gaind & F. Fawzy. 1984. 400p. 35.00 (*0-88331-131-3*) R B Luce.

Current Themes in Psychiatry, Vol. 4. Ed. by Raghu N. Gaind et al. 1985. LC 84-643519. 283p. text 45.00 (*0-88331-132-1*) R B Luce.

Current Theories of Psychoanalysis. Ed. by Robert J. Langs. 1998. LC 98-13585. 356p. 55.00 (*0-8236-1094-2*, 01094) Intl Univs Pr.

Current Theories of Vascular Surgery. Ernst. 4th ed. 2000. text 179.00 (*0-323-00901-8*) Saunders.

Current Therapeutic Approaches to Panic & Other Anxiety Disorders. Giorgio Racagni et al. 1994. (International Academy for Biomedical & Drug Research Ser.: Vol. 8). (Illus.). vi, 206p. 195.75 (*3-8055-5989-5*) S Karger.

Current Therapy for Acute Coronary Ischemia. Ed. by Harold L. Lazar. 1993. LC 93-14925. (Illus.). 320p. 65.00 (*0-87993-555-3*) Futura Pub.

Current Therapy in Allergy, Immunology & Rheumatology. Laurence M. Lichtenstein & Anthony S. Fauci. 5th ed. 1996. (Illus.). 464p. (C). (gr. 13). text 92.95 (*0-8151-5396-1*, 25697) Mosby Inc.

Current Therapy in Cancer. Ed. by John F. Foley et al. 1994. (Illus.). 448p. text 79.00 (*0-7216-4578-X*) Saunders.

Current Therapy in Cancer. John F. Foley et al. Ed. by Marc Strauss. 2nd ed. 1999. LC 98-36144. (Illus.). 445p. text 124.50 (*0-7216-7548-4*) Saunders.

Current Therapy in Colon & Rectal Surgery. Victor W. Fazio & James M. Church. 2nd ed. 1999. (Illus.). 480p. (C). text (*1-55664-480-9*) Mosby Inc.

Current Therapy in Critical Care Medicine. Joseph E. Parrillo. 3rd ed. 1996. (Illus.). 448p. (C). (gr. 13). text 89.95 (*0-8151-7327-X*, 27780) Mosby Inc.

Current Therapy in Endocrinology & Metabolism, Vol. 6. C. Wayne Bardin. 6th ed. 1997. (Illus.). 704p. (C). (gr. 13). text 93.00 (*0-8151-2016-8*, 30566) Mosby Inc.

Current Therapy in Equine Medicine. N. Edward Robinson. Ed. by Lisette Bralow. 4th ed. 1997. (Illus.). 736p. text 95.00 (*0-7216-2633-5*) Saunders.

Current Therapy in Equine Medicine, Vol. 3. Ed. by N. Edward Robinson. 1991. (Illus.). 881p. text 126.00 (*0-7216-3475-3*) Saunders.

Current Therapy in Internal Medicine. Jerome P. Kassirer & Harry L. Greene. 4th ed. 1997. (Illus.). 1560p. (C). (gr. 13). text 110.00 (*0-8151-5480-1*, 28702) Mosby Inc.

Current Therapy in Large Animal Theriogenology: Large Animal Therapy. Robert S. Youngquist. Ed. by Stephanie Donley. 1997. LC 96-34064. 800p. text 126.00 (*0-7216-5396-0*) Saunders.

Current Therapy in Nephrology & Hypertension. Richard J. Glassock. 4th ed. 1998. (Illus.). 432p. (C). (gr. 13). text 89.00 (*0-8151-3733-8*, 24865) Mosby Inc.

Current Therapy in Neurologic Disease. Richard T. Johnson & Craig E. Griffin. 5th ed. 1996. (Illus.). 448p. (C). (gr. 13). text 89.95 (*0-8151-4873-9*, 29348) Mosby Inc.

***Current Therapy in Neurologic Disease.** Richard T. Johnson et al. 6th ed. (Illus.). 195p. text (*0-323-01472-0*) Saunders.

Current Therapy in Obstetrics & Gynecology. Ed. by Frederick P. Zuspan & Edward J. Quilligan. 4th ed. 1994. LC 94-3139. (Illus.). 480p. text 67.00 (*0-7216-5262-X*) Saunders.

Current Therapy in Obstetrics & Gynecology. Edward J. Quilligan & Frederick P. Zuspan. Ed. by William Schmitt et al. 5th ed. 1999. LC 99-16181. (Illus.). 525p. text (*0-7216-7579-4*) Saunders.

Current Therapy in Orthopaedics. McGinty & Jackson. 1991. (*1-55664-040-4*) Mosby Inc.

Current Therapy in Otolaryngology-Head & Neck Surgery, No. 6. George A. Gates. 6th ed. 1997. (Illus.). 560p. (C). (gr. 13). text 85.00 (*0-8151-3560-2*, 30085) Mosby Inc.

Current Therapy in Psychiatry: Physical Medicine & Rehabilitation. Ed. by Asa P. Ruskin. 1984. (Illus.). 608p. text 140.00 (*0-7216-7853-X*) Saunders.

Current Therapy in Sports Medicine. Joseph S. Torg. 3rd ed. 1994. 544p. (C). (gr. 13). text 99.95 (*1-55664-384-5*) Mosby Inc.

Current Therapy in Theriogenology Vol. 2: Diagnosis, Treatment & Prevention of Reproductive Diseases in Small & Large Animals. David A. Morrow. 2nd ed. 1986. LC 85-11937. (Illus.). 1143p. text 163.00 (*0-7216-6580-2*) Saunders.

Current Therapy in Vascular Surgery. Calvin B. Ernst & James C. Stanley. 3rd ed. 1995. (Illus.). 1040p. (C). (gr. 13). text 165.00 (*0-8151-3134-8*, 23653) Mosby Inc.

Current Therapy of Infectious Disease. David L. Schlossberg. 4th ed. 1996. (Illus.). 688p. (C). (gr. 13). text 99.95 (*0-8151-8220-1*, 27458) Mosby Inc.

Current Therapy of Infectious Diseases. David Schlossberg. 2nd ed. 2000. LC 00-57854. (Illus.). xl, 792p. 120.00 (*0-323-00907-7*) Mosby Inc.

Current Therapy of Trauma. Donald Trunkey. 4th ed. 1998. (Illus.). 408p. (C). (gr. 13). text 79.95 (*0-8151-6545-5*, 24038) Mosby Inc.

Current Therapy of Von Willebrand's Disease. Ed. by P. M. Mannucci. 1994. (Journal: Vol. 24, No. 5, 1994). (Illus.). 64p. pap. 46.25 (*3-8055-6078-8*) S Karger.

Current Thinking & Research in Brief Therapy Vol. 1: Solutions, Strategies, Narratives, Vol. 1. Ed. by William J. Matthews & John H. Edgette. 1997. 304p. 37.95 (*0-87630-819-1*) Brunner-Routledge.

Current Topics in Animal Learning: Brain, Emotion, & Cognition. Ed. by L. Dachowski. 1991. 456p. (C). text 89.95 (*0-8058-0441-2*) L Erlbaum Assocs.

Current Topics in Biomedical Research. Ed. by Reinhard Kurth & Walter K. Schwerdtfeger. 1992. LC 92-49916. (*3-540-54780-0*); (Illus.). 192p. 123.00 (*0-387-54780-0*) Spr-Verlag.

Current Topics in BRCA 1: A Breast Disease Book. Ed. by Edison T. Liu. 1998. (Breast Disease Ser.: Vols. 1 & 2). 140p. (YA). (gr. 12 up). pap. (*90-5199-394-3*) IOS Pr NLD. *Dist:* IOS Press.

Current Topics in Chinese Science: Section G: Medical Science, Vol. 2. 1984. 265p. pap. 73.00 (*0-677-06280-X*) Gordon & Breach.

Current Topics in Clinical Radiobiology of Tumors. Ed. by Hans-Peter Beck-Bornholdt. 1993. LC 93-22941. (Illus.). 152p. 134.00 (*0-387-56512-4*) Spr-Verlag.

Current Topics in Clinical Radiobiology of Tumors. Hans-Peter Beck-Bornholdt. 1993. LC 93-22941. (Illus.). 160p. (*3-540-56512-4*) Spr-Verlag.

Current Topics in Clinical Virology. Ed. by Peter Morgan-Capner. 1992. (Public Health Laboratory Service Publication). 314p. (C). pap. text 29.95 (*0-521-42710-X*) Cambridge U Pr.

Current Topics in Critical Care Medicine: Proceedings of the International Symposium, 3rd, Rio de Janeiro, November, 1974. International Symposium on Critical Care Staff. Ed. by William C. Shoemaker et al. 1976. (Current Topics in Critical Care Medicine Ser.: Vol. 1). (Illus.). 200p. 77.50 (*3-8055-2211-8*) S Karger.

Current Topics in Developmental Biology, Vol. 29. Ed. by Roger A. Pedersen. 1994. (Illus.). 369p. (C). text 94.00 (*0-12-153129-5*) Acad Pr.

Current Topics in Diabetes Research. Ed. by F. Belfiore et al. 1993. (Frontiers in Diabetes Ser.: Vol. 12). (Illus.). x, 286p. 259.25 (*3-8055-5779-5*) S Karger.

Current Topics in Intensive Care. Burchardi. 4th ed. 1997. pap. text (*0-7020-2161-X*) Bailliere Tindall.

Current Topics in Intensive Care, No. 1. Dobb. 1994. pap. text 55.00 (*0-7020-1677-2*) Saunders.

Current Topics in Intensive Care, No. 4. Ed. by R. P. Dellinger et al. 1997. 300p. pap. (*0-7020-2248-9*) W B Saunders GBR. *Dist:* Saunders.

Current Topics in Intensive Care, Vol. 2. Bion. 2nd ed. 1995. text 61.00 (*0-7020-1871-6*) Saunders.

Current Topics in Lung Cancer. Ed. by Paul A. Bunn, Jr. & U. Veronesi. 1991. (ESO Monographs). 82p. 56.95 (*0-387-54301-5*) Spr-Verlag.

Current Topics in Medical Mycology. Ed. by Michael R. McGinnis & M. Borgers. 1989. (Illus.). 424p. 232.00 (*0-387-96941-1*, 2540) Spr-Verlag.

Current Topics in Medical Mycology, Vol. 1. Ed. by Michael R. McGinnis. 1985. (Illus.). 359p. 132.00 (*0-387-96095-3*) Spr-Verlag.

Current Topics in Medical Mycology, Vol. 2. Michael R. McGinnis. 1987. (Illus.). 432p. 196.00 (*0-387-96543-2*) Spr-Verlag.

Current Topics in Medical Mycology, Vol. 4. Ed. by M. Borgers et al. 1991. (Illus.). 274p. 190.00 (*0-387-97504-7*) Spr-Verlag.

Current Topics in Medical Virology: Proceedings of the First Asia-Pacific Congress. Y. C. Chan & S. Doraisingham. 1989. 456p. text 130.00 (*9971-5-0806-0*) World Scientific Pub.

Current Topics in Membranes, Vol. 4. Ed. by W. James Nelson. 1996. text 85.00 (*0-12-153343-3*) Acad Pr.

Current Topics in Membranes Vol. 41: Cell Biology & Membrane Transport Processes. Ed. by Joseph F. Hoffman et al. 1994. (Illus.). 172p. text 94.00 (*0-12-153341-7*) Acad Pr.

Current Topics in Microbiology & Immunology. Ed. by A. Capron et al. 1994. (Molecular & Cellular Mechanisms Ser.: Vol. 189). (Illus.). 210p. 159.00 (*0-387-57259-7*) Spr-Verlag.

Current Topics in Microbiology & Immunology. Ed. by W. Arber et al. 1974. LC 15-12910. (Illus.). Vol. 66. 130p. 45.00 (*3-540-06831-7*); Vol. 67. iv, 162p. 55.00 (*3-540-06838-4*) Spr-Verlag.

Current Topics in Microbiology & Immunology, Vol. 75. W. Arber et al. 1976. LC 15-12910. (Illus.). 54.00 (*3-540-08013-9*) Spr-Verlag.

Current Topics in Microbiology & Immunology. Ed. by W. Arber et al. (Illus.). Vol. 76. 1977. LC 15-12910. 54.00 (*3-540-08238-7*); Vol. 90. 1980. 147p. 76.00 (*0-387-10181-0*); Vol. 91. 1981. 276p. 100.00 (*0-387-10722-3*) Spr-Verlag.

Current Topics in Microbiology & Immunology, Vol. 97. Ed. by W. Henle et al. 1981. (Illus.). 204p. 80.00 (*0-387-11118-2*) Spr-Verlag.

Current Topics in Microbiology & Immunology: Rotaviruses. Ed. by R. F. Ramig. 1994. (Illus.). 389p. 144.00 (*0-387-56761-5*) Spr-Verlag.

Current Topics in Microbiology & Immunology No. 187. C. E. Rupprecht et al. 1994. LC 15-12910. (Illus.). 361p. 160.00 (*0-387-57194-9*) Spr-Verlag.

Current Topics in Microbiology & Immunology V0l. 180: Pathogenesis of Shigellosis. Ed. by Michael B. Oldstone et al. 1992. (Illus.). 143p. 140.00 (*0-387-55058-5*) Spr-Verlag.

Current Topics in Microbiology & Immunology Vol. 157: Retroviruses, Strategies of Replication. Ed. by R. Swanstrom & P. K. Vogt. 1990. (Illus.). 259p. 66.00 (*0-387-51895-9*) Spr-Verlag.

Current Topics in Microbiology & Immunology Vol. 158: Viral Expression Vectors. Ed. by Michael B. Oldstone et al. 1992. (Illus.). 176p. 134.00 (*0-387-52431-2*) Spr-Verlag.

Current Topics in Microbiology & Immunology Vol. 163: Poxviruses. Ed. by Michael B. Oldstone et al. 1990. (Illus.). 256p. 99.00 (*0-387-52430-4*) Spr-Verlag.

Current Topics in Microbiology & Immunology Vol. 164: Human Diabetes: Genetics, Environmental & Autoimmune Etiology. Ed. by Michael B. Oldstone et al. 1990. (Illus.). 216p. 120.00 (*0-387-52652-8*) Spr-Verlag.

Current Topics in Microbiology & Immunology Vol. 165: Neuronal Growth Factors. Ed. by Michael B. Oldstone et al. 1991. (Illus.). 173p. 91.00 (*0-387-52654-4*) Spr-Verlag.

Current Topics in Microbiology & Immunology Vol. 166: Mechanisms in B-Cell Neoplasia 1990: Workshop at the National Cancer Institute, National Institutes of Health, Bethesda, MD, U.S.A., March 28-30, 1990. Ed. by Michael B. Oldstone et al. 1990. (Illus.). 380p. 129.00 (*0-387-52886-5*) Spr-Verlag.

Current Topics in Microbiology & Immunology Vol. 172: Transmissible Spongiform Encephalopathies, Scrapie, BSE & Related Human Disorders. Ed. by Michael B. Oldstone et al. 1991. (Illus.). 288p. 123.00 (*0-387-53883-6*) Spr-Verlag.

Current Topics in Microbiology & Immunology Vol. 174: Superantigens. Ed. by Michael B. Oldstone et al. 1991. (Illus.). 137p. 114.00 (*0-387-54205-1*) Spr-Verlag.

Current Topics in Microbiology & Immunology Vol. 175: ADP-Ribosylating Toxins. Ed. by Michael B. Oldstone et al. 1992. (Illus.). 148p. 126.00 (*0-387-54598-0*) Spr-Verlag.

Current Topics in Microbiology & Immunology Vol. 177: Hematopoietic Stem Cells: Animal Models & Human Transplantation. Ed. by Michael B. Oldstone et al. 1992. (Illus.). 251p. 129.00 (*0-387-54531-X*) Spr-Verlag.

Current Topics in Microbiology & Immunology Vol. 178: Membrane Defenses Against Attack by Complement & Perforins. Ed. by Michael B. Oldstone et al. 1992. (Illus.). 188p. 144.00 (*0-387-54653-7*) Spr-Verlag.

Current Topics in Microbiology & Immunology Vol. 183: Neutralization of Animal Viruses. Ed. by Michael B. Oldstone et al. 1993. (Illus.). 149p. 135.00 (*0-387-56030-0*) Spr-Verlag.

Current Topics in Microbiology & Immunology Vol. 193: Transacting Functions of Human Retroviruses. M. Potter & S. Olsnes. 1995. LC 15-12910. (Illus.). 249p. 145.00 (*0-387-57901-X*) Spr-Verlag.

Current Topics in Microbiology & Immunology Vol. 199: The Molecular Repertoire of Adenoviruses. M. Potter & S. Olsnes. 1995. (Illus.). Vol. I: Virion Structure & Infection. LC 15-12910. 336p. 145.00 (*3-540-58828-0*); Vol. II: Molecular Biology of Virus-Cell Interacti. 278p. 149.00 (*3-540-58829-9*) Spr-Verlag.

Current Topics in Microbiology & Immunology Vol. 204: Transposable Elements. Ed. by Hilary Koprowski et al. 1995. LC 15-12910. (Illus.). 234p. 153.00 (*3-540-59342-X*) Spr-Verlag.

Current Topics in Microbiology & Immunology Vol. 205: The CD4 Molecule. Ed. by D. R. Littman. 1995. (Illus.). 224p. 142.00 (*3-540-59344-6*) Spr-Verlag.

Current Topics in Microbiology & Immunology Vol. 206: Transgenic Models of Human Viral & Immunological Disease, No. 206. Ed. by Michael B. Oldstone et al. 1995. (Illus.). 350p. 164.00 (*3-540-59341-1*) Spr-Verlag.

Current Topics in Microbiology & Immunology Vol. 208: Transcriptional Control of Cell Growth: The E2F Gene Family, No. 208. Ed. by Hilary Koprowski et al. 1995. (Illus.). 144p. 153.00 (*3-540-60113-9*) Spr-Verlag.

Current Topics in Microbiology & Immunology Vol. 218: Adeno-Associated Virus (AAV) Vectors in Gene Therapy. Ed. by Kenneth I. Berns et al. 1996. (Illus.). 258p. 138.00 (*3-540-61076-6*) Spr-Verlag.

Current Topics in Microbiology & Immunology Vol. 219: Toxoplasma Gondii. Ed. by U. Gross et al. 1996. (Illus.). 274p. 138.00 (*3-540-61300-5*) Spr-Verlag.

Current Topics in Microbiology & Immunology, Vol. 161 Vol. 161: Picornaviruses. Michael B. Oldstone. 1990. (Illus.). 192p. 108.00 (*0-387-52429-0*) Spr-Verlag.

Current Topics in Mucosal Immunology 1993: Proceedings of the Tokyo International Symposium on Mucosal Immunology, Keidanren Kaikan. Ed. by Masharu Tsuchiya et al. 1994. LC 93-49045. (International Congress Ser.: No. 1047). 480p. 210.50 (*0-444-81586-4*, Excerpta Medica) Elsevier.

Current Topics in Neonatology, No. 2. Hansen. 2nd ed. 1997. 300p. pap. text (*0-7020-2104-0*) Bailliere Tindall.

*__Current Topics in Neonatology__, No. 4. Thomas N. Hansen & Neil McIntosh. 2000. 35.00 (*0-7020-2628-X*) Saunders.

*__Current Topics in Neonatology__, No. 3. Thomas N. Hansen & Neil McIntosh. 1999. (Illus.). 292p. pap. (*0-7020-2348-5*) W B Saunders GBR. *Dist:* Saunders.

Current Topics in Organizational Behavior Management. Ed. by Phillip K. Duncan. 1982. LC 82-11685. (Journal of Organizational Behavior Management: Vol. 3, No. 3). 111p. text 39.95 (*0-86656-198-6*) Haworth Pr.

Current Topics in Radiography. Paterson. 1995. pap. text 36.00 (*0-7020-1971-2*); 2nd ed. 1996. pap. text 41.00 (*0-7020-2202-0*) Saunders.

Current Topics in Rehabilitation Psychology. Charles Golden. 1984. 256p. text 41.95 (*0-8089-1641-6*, 791624, Grune & Strat) Harcrt Hlth Sci Grp.

Current Topics in Vector Research, Vol. 2. Ed. by Kerry F. Harris. 1984. 290p. 44.95 (*0-275-91433-X*, C14332, Praeger Pubs) Greenwood.

Current Topics in Vector Research, Vol. 4. Ed. by K. F. Harris. 1987. (Illus.). 213p. 161.00 (*0-387-96464-9*) Spr-Verlag.

Current Topics on Prostate Cancer Treatment. 1996. (Urologia Internationalis Ser.: Vol. 56, Suppl. 1, 1996). (Illus.). iv, 28p. pap., suppl. ed. 21.75 (*3-8055-6312-4*) S Karger.

Current Treatment in Dental Practice. Norman S. Levine. 1986. (Illus.). 533p. text 89.00 (*0-7216-1198-2*) Saunders.

Current Treatment of Ambulatory Asthma. Pref. by Guy A. Settipane. 1986. (Illus.). 250p. text 49.00 (*0-936587-01-6*) OceanSide Pubns.

Current Treatment of Anorexia Nervosa & Bulimia. Ed. by Pauline S. Powers & R. C. Fernandez. 1984. (Biobehavioral Medicine Ser.: Vol. 4). xvi, 348p. 85.25 (*3-8055-3879-0*) S Karger.

Current Treatments of Obsessive-Compulsive Disorder. Ed. by Michele T. Pato & Joseph Zohar. 1991. LC 90-14497. (Clinical Practice Ser.: No. 18). 198p. text 14.95 (*0-88048-351-2*, 8351) Am Psychiatric.

Current Trends in Audiology. Ed. by Herbert J. Oyer. 1996. (Journal: Vol. 48, No. 3, 1996). (Illus.). 58p. pap. 36.50 (*3-8055-6362-0*) S Karger.

Current Trends in Bone Grafting. Peter C. Leung. 1988. (Illus.). 108p. 85.95 (*0-387-50139-8*) Spr-Verlag.

Current Trends in Digestive Ultrasonography. Ed. by Lionello Gandolfi & Morimichi Fukuda. 1997. LC 97-15241. (Frontiers of Gastrointestinal Research Ser.: Vol. 24, 1997). (Illus.). x, 394p. 298.25 (*3-8055-6374-4*) S Karger.

Current Trends in Hand Surgery: Proceedings of the Sixth Congress of the International Federation of Societies for Surgery of the Hand, Held at Helsinki, 3-7 July 1995. Sixth Congress of the International Federation of Societies for Surgery of the Hand. Ed. by Martti Vastamaki. 1995. (International Congress Ser.: Vol. 1083). 680p. 298.25 (*0-444-81914-2*, Excerpta Medica) Elsevier.

Current Trends in Morphological Techniques. Ed. by John E. Johnson, Jr. 1981. 272p. 150.00 (*0-8493-5826-4*); 296p. 134.00 (*0-8493-5828-0*);I. 272p. 154.00 (*0-8493-5825-6*, QL927) Franklin (CRC Reprint).

Current Trends in Plant Virology: Proceedings of Group Discussions on Plant Virology, National Botanical Research Institute, Lucknow. Ed. by B. P. Singh & S. P. Raychaudhuri. 1982. xvi, 224p. (C). (*0-88065-220-9*) Today Tomorrow IND. *Dist:* Lubrecht & Cramer, Scholarly Pubns.

Current Trends in Platelet Transfusion: International COBE Meeting, Brussels, September 1994. Ed. by V. Kretschmer. 1996. (Infusionstherapie und Transfusionsmedizin Ser.: Vol. 23, Suppl. 1, 1996). (Illus.). 36p. pap. 28.75 (*3-8055-6307-8*) S Karger.

Current Trends in Surgery. Ed. by J. C. Pal. 1989. (C). Vol. I. (*0-89771-368-0*); Vol. II. (*0-89771-369-9*) Current Dist IND. *Dist:* St Mut.

Current Tumor Diagnosis: Applications Clinical Relevance, Research & Trends. Ed. by R. Klapdor. 1994. (7th Symposium on Tumor Markers Ser.). (Illus.). 907p. text (*3-88603-509-3*) W Zuckschwerdt DEU. *Dist:* Scholium Intl.

Current Update in Psychoimmunology. Ed. by G. Wieselmann. 1998. (Key Topics in Brain Research Ser.). (Illus.). 150p. pap. 64.00 (*3-211-83029-4*) Spr-Verlag.

Current Urologic Therapy Three. E. James Seidmon & Philop M. Hanno. 3rd ed. 1994. LC 94-6845. (Illus.). 608p. text 110.00 (*0-7216-5033-3*) Saunders.

Current Veterinary Practice: Small Animal Practice. Craig E. Griffin et al. 1992. (Illus.). 392p. (C). (gr. 13). text 115.00 (*0-8016-3384-2*, 03384) Mosby Inc.

Current Veterinary Therapy No. 3: Food Animal Practice. Jimmy L. Howard. 3rd ed. 1992. (Illus.). 1002p. (C). text 187.00 (*0-7216-3633-0*) Saunders.

Current Veterinary Therapy No. 4: Food Animal Practice. Jimmy L. Howard & Robert Smith. Ed. by Stephanie Donley. 4th ed. 1998. (Illus.). 704p. (C). text 135.00 (*0-7216-7654-5*) Saunders.

Current Veterinary Therapy Nine, Vol. 9. Robert W. Kirk. 1986. (Illus.). 1346p. text 115.00 (*0-7216-1500-7*) Saunders.

Current Veterinary Therapy Ten, Vol. 10. Robert W. Kirk. 1989. 1344p. text 115.00 (*0-7216-2858-3*) Saunders.

Currents in Alcoholism: Biochemical, Biological & Clinical Topics, Vol. I. Frank A. Seixas. 1977. 512p. text 83.00 (*0-8089-1007-8*, 793971, Grune & Strat) Harcrt Hlth Sci Grp.

Currents in Alcoholism: Psychological, Psychiatric, Sociological, Anthropological, & Epidemiological Studies. Ed. by Marc Galanter. Vol. II. 1977. 506p. text 83.00 (*0-8089-1008-6*, 793972); Vol. 4. 1978. 528p. text 83.00 (*0-8089-1101-5*, 793974) Harcrt Hlth Sci Grp (Grune & Strat).

Currents in Alcoholism: Recent Advances in Research & Treatment, Vol. 8. Ed. by Marc Galanter. 1981. LC 76-30552. 344p. text 83.00 (*0-8089-1458-8*, 793978, Grune & Strat) Harcrt Hlth Sci Grp.

Currents in American Medicine: A Developmental View of Medical Care & Education. Julius B. Richmond. 1969. LC 69-12733. (Commonwealth Fund Publications). 150p. 18.00 (*0-674-18015-1*) HUP.

Curriculum Building in Nursing: A Process. Em Oliva Bevis. 3rd ed. 1999. (Illus.). 200p. (C). pap. text 31.95 (*0-7637-0941-7*, 0941-7, N L N Bart) Jones & Bartlett.

Curriculum Building in Nursing: A Process. Em Oliva Bevis. 3rd ed. 1989. 304p. 30.95 (*0-88737-439-5*) Natl League Nurse.

Curriculum Development for Medical Education: A Six-Step Approach. David E. Kern et al. 1998. LC 97-51745. 176p. pap. text 25.95 (*0-8018-5844-5*) Johns Hopkins.

Curriculum for Primary Care Geriatrics. 1998. 174p. ring bd. (*1-891539-02-7*) U Chi Pritzker Schl.

Curriculum Guide for Public Safety & Emergency Response Workers: Prevention of Transmission of HIV & Hepatitis B Virus. 1995. lib. bdg. 250.95 (*0-8490-7527-0*) Gordon Pr.

Curriculum Guide for Public-Safety & Emergency-Response Workers: Prevention of Transmission of Human Immunodeficiency Virus & Hepatitis B Virus. 1994. (Illus.). 185p. (Orig.). (C). pap. text 50.00 (*0-7881-0322-9*) DIANE Pub.

Curriculum Guide to Managed Care. 1996. ring bd. 40.00 (*0-910329-88-5*, 0122017) Am Speech Lang Hearing.

Curriculum in Nursing Education. Ed. by Peta Allan & Moya Jolley. 1987. 208p. (C). (*0-7099-1462-8*) C Helm GBR. *Dist:* Routldge.

Curriculum Planning for ESN(S) Child, Vol. 1. N. B. Crawford. 1984. 80p. 40.00 (*0-906054-21-4*) St Mut.

Curriculum Planning in Nursing Education. (*0-340-51839-1*) E A GBR. *Dist:* Routldge.

Curriculum Revisited: An Update of Curriculum Design. Ed. by Elisabeth Pennington. 1986. 48p. 14.95 (*0-88737-338-0*, 15-2165) Natl League Nurse.

Curriculum Revolution: Community Building & Activism. 1991. 160p. 9.95 (*0-88737-517-0*) Natl League Nurse.

Curriculum Revolution: Mandate for Change. 1988. 256p. pap. 9.95 (*0-88737-404-2*, 15-224) Natl League Nurse.

Curriculum Revolution: Reconceptualizing Nursing Education. 1989. 152p. 9.95 (*0-88737-442-5*) Natl League Nurse.

Curriculums & Practical Aspects of Implementation: Preventive Health Services for Adolescents. John S. Wodarski & Lois A. Wodarski. 1992. 446p. (Orig.). (C). 79.00 (*0-8191-8574-4*); pap. 46.00 (*0-8191-8575-2*) U Pr of Amer.

Cursing Brain? The Histories of Tourette Syndrome. Howard I. Kushner. (Illus.). 320p. 2000. pap. 16.95 (*0-674-00386-1*); 1999. LC 98-38733. 29.95 (*0-674-18022-4*) HUP.

Curve: The Curve of Poor Medial Care for Blacks, Its Impact on Their Quality of Life & Future Solutions. Raymond Chukwu. 2000. pap. 12.95 (*1-878647-73-3*) APU Pub Grp.

Curve of Life: The Correspondence of Heinz Kohut, 1923-1981. Ed. by Geoffrey Cocks. 1994. LC 93-40922. 460p. 39.95 (*0-226-11170-9*) U Ch Pr.

*__Cushing's Syndrome a Patient Guide One Woman's Journey.__ Mary Walsh. Ed. by Mary Ellen Bissell. 2001. (Illus.). 12.95 (*0-9715707-0-1*) New Mill Pr.

Custody Dispute over Seven Human Embryos: The Testimony of Professor Jerome Lejeune, M. D., Ph. D. Intro. by John W. Brabner-Smith. 1990. 90p. (Orig.). (C). pap. 2.50 (*0-944561-19-5*) Chr Legal.

Custody of Children: A Behavioral Assessment Model. Richard A. Marafiote. 1985. LC 85-12217. (Illus.). 290p. (C). 78.00 (*0-306-41874-6*, Plenum Trade) Perseus Pubng.

Custom Ceramic Color: A Practical System. Ernst A. Hegenbarth. 1989.Tr. of Systematik der Individualien Keramischen Farbgestaltung. (Illus.). 109p. text 68.00 (*0-86715-216-8*) Quint Pub Co.

Custom-Made Child? Women-Centered Perspectives. Ed. by Helen B. Holmes et al. 1981. LC 80-83824. (Contemporary Issues in Biomedicine, Ethics & Society Ser.). 368p. 59.95 (*0-89603-024-5*) Humana.

Customer Oriented Laboratory. William O. Umiker. 2nd ed. 1996. LC 96-20371. (Practical Laboratory Management Ser.). 35.00 (*0-89189-405-5*) Am Soc Clinical.

Customer Service Revolution in Health Care. David Zimmerman et al. 1996. LC 95-43460. (Illus.). 224p. (C). text 42.50 (*0-7863-0893-1*, Irwn Prfssnl) McGraw-Hill Educ Grp.

Cutaneous Adnexal Tumors. Mark R. Wick et al. 1991. LC 91-17214. (Illus.). 238p. 135.00 (*0-89189-288-5*, 16-1-050-00) Am Soc Clinical.

Cutaneous Allergy. Ernest N. Charlesworth. 1996. LC 96-47622. (Illus.). 400p. 160.00 (*0-86542-370-9*) Blackwell Sci.

Cutaneous Antifungal Agents: Selected Compounds in Clinical Practice & Development. Ed. by Robert A. Fromtling & John W. Rippon. 1993. (Basic & Clinical Dermatology Ser.: Vol. 7). (Illus.). 488p. text 225.00 (*0-8247-9055-3*) Dekker.

Cutaneous Arteries of the Human Body. C. Manchot. 1983. (Illus.). 149p. 145.00 (*0-387-90792-0*) Spr-Verlag.

Cutaneous Clues to Systemic Diseases. H. L. Chan. 1986. (Illus.). 138p. (*9971-69-101-9*) Sngapore Univ Pr SGP. *Dist:* Coronet Bks.

Cutaneous Development, Aging & Repair. Ed. by G. Abatangelo & J. M. Davidson. 1989. (FIDIA Research Ser.: Vol. 18). 360p. 150.00 (*0-387-96995-0*, 2801) Spr-Verlag.

Cutaneous Drug Reactions: An Integral Synopsis of Today's Systemic Drugs. A. Krebs. 2nd rev. ed. 1992. (Illus.). viii, 570p. 431.50 (*3-8055-4939-3*) S Karger.

Cutaneous Fungal Infections. Boni E. Elewski. 2nd ed. 1998. LC 97-27801. (Illus.). xv, 371 p. 105.00 (*0-86542-527-2*) Blackwell Sci.

Cutaneous Fungal Infections. Ed. by Boni E. Elewski. 1992. LC 92-1430. (Topics in Clinical Dermatology Ser.). (Illus.). 272p. 75.00 (*0-89640-219-3*) Igaku-Shoin.

C D

Cutaneous Head & Neck Melanoma: Diagnosis & Treatment. Ed. by A. J. Balm & B. B. Kroon. 1994. (Journal: Vol. 3, No. 5, 1994). (Illus.). 58p. pap. 23.50 (*3-8055-6000-1*) S Karger.

Cutaneous Infestations & Insect Bites. Milton Orkin & Howard I. Maibach. 1985. LC 84-22977. (Dermatology Ser.: Vol. 4). (Illus.). 368p. text 175.00 (*0-8247-7273-3*) Dekker.

Cutaneous Infestations of Man & Animal. Ed. by Lawrence C. Parish et al. 1983. LC 82-18946. 392p. 83.50 (*0-275-91407-0*, C1407, Praeger Pubs) Greenwood.

Cutaneous Investigation in Health & Disease: Noninvasive Methods & Instrumentation. Ed. by Jean-Luc Leveque. 1988. (Basic & Clinical Dermatology Ser.: Vol. 1). (Illus.). 464p. text 210.00 (*0-8247-7967-3*) Dekker.

Cutaneous Laser Surgery. Ed. by Kenneth A. Arndt & Jeffrey S. Dover. 1997. LC 97-3099. (Illus.). 496p. text 145.00 (*0-316-05177-2*) Lppncott W & W.

Cutaneous Laser Surgery: Selective Photothermolysis, No. 2. Mitchel P. Goldman & Richard E. Fitzpatrick. 2nd ed. 1998. (Illus.). 554p. (C). (gr. 13). text 195.00 (*0-8151-3610-2*, 30072) Mosby Inc.

Cutaneous Lesions of the Lower Extremity. Gary L. Dockery. Ed. by Lisette Bralow. 1996. 304p. text 156.00 (*0-7216-5034-1*) Saunders.

Cutaneous Lymphoma. Ed. by W. A. Van Vloten. 1989. (Current Problems in Dermatology Ser.: Vol. 19). (Illus.). viii, 270p. 215.75 (*3-8055-5058-8*) S Karger.

Cutaneous Lymphomas, Pseudolymphomas & Related Disorders. G. Burg & O. Braun-Falco. 1983. (Illus.). 542p. 398.00 (*0-387-10467-4*) Spr-Verlag.

Cutaneous Manifestations of Rheumatic Diseases. Ed. by Richard D. Sontheimer & Thomas T. Provost. 1996. LC 95-3774. (Illus.). 528p. text 139.00 (*0-683-07852-6*) Lppncott W & W.

Cutaneous Medicine. Thomas T. Provost et al. 2000. 700p. incl. cd-rom (*1-55009-100-X*) DEKR.

Cutaneous Medicine & Surgery. Andreas Arndt. (Illus.). 400p. 1996. text 495.00 (*0-7216-6331-1*); 1995. text 425.00 (*0-7216-6333-8*) Saunders.

Cutaneous Medicine & Surgery: An Integrated Program in Dermatology, Set. Kenneth A. Arndt et al. 1996. (Illus.). text 635.00 incl. cd-rom (*0-7216-6332-X*) Saunders.

Cutaneous Medicine & Surgery: An Integrated Program in Dermatology, Set. June K. Robinson et al. 1995. LC 94-6429. (Illus.). 1600p. text 260.00 (*0-7216-4852-5*) Saunders.

Cutaneous Melanoma. Ed. by Charles M. Balch et al. 3rd ed. 1997. LC 97-29168. (Illus.). 650p. text 130.00 (*0-942219-85-6*) Quality Med Pub.

Cutaneous Melanoma of the Head & Neck. Robert P. Zitsch, III & Gregory J. Renner. 1996. LC 96-17692. (Self-Instructional Package Ser.). (Illus.). 81p. pap. text 25.00 (*1-56772-022-6*) AAO-HNS.

Cutaneous Neuroimmunomodulation: The Proopiomelanocortin System. Thomas A. Luger. 1999. LC 99-46380. (Annals of the New York Academy of Sciences Ser.: Vol. 885). (Illus.). xiv, 479p. pap. incl. 5.25 hd (*1-57331-201-0*) NY Acad Sci.

Cutaneous Neuroimmunomodulation: The Proopiomelanocortin System. Ed. by Thomas A. Luger et al. 1999. LC 99-46380. (Annals of the New York Academy of Sciences Ser.: Vol. 885). (Illus.). xiv, 479p. lib. bdg. 140.00 (*1-57331-200-2*) NY Acad Sci.

Cutaneous Oncology. Stanley J. Miller & Mary E. Maloney. 1997. LC 97-7305. 309.95 (*0-86542-517-5*) Blackwell Sci.

Cutaneous Pathology. Maize. 1998. LC 98-16468. (C). text 129.00 (*0-443-08717-2*) Saunders.

Cutaneous Surgery. Ronald G. Wheeland. 1993. (Illus.). 1104p. text 210.00 (*0-7216-3523-7*) Saunders.

Cutaneous Surgery: An Illustrated & Practical Approach. Ed. by Christopher Arpey et al. 1996. LC 96-34920. (Illus.). 325p. text 99.00 (*0-07-069619-5*) McGraw-Hill Educ Grp.

Cutaneous Surgical Anatomy of the Head & Neck. Eric A. Breisch & Hubert T. Greenway. 1991. (Practical Manuals in Dermatologic Surgery Ser.). (Illus.). 133p. pap. text (*0-443-08744-X*) Church.

Cutting: Understanding & Overcoming Self-Mutilation. Steven Levenkron. 1998. LC 98-10274. 256p. 25.00 (*0-393-02741-4*) Norton.

Cutting Costs in the Physician Practice. 2000. 128p. pap. 55.00 (*1-57947-161-7*) AMA.

Cutting Edge Medicine & Liaison Psychiatry: Psychiatric Problems of Organ Transplantation, Cancer, HIV/AIDS & Genetic Therapy: Proceedings of the 13th Tokyo Institute of Psychiatry International Symposium Held in Tokyo on 29-30 September 1998. Tokyo Institute of Psychiatry Staff et al. Ed. by Masaaki Matsushita & Isao Fukunishi. 1999. LC 99-23504. (International Congress Ser.). 256p. 127.00 (*0-444-50220-3*, Excerpta Medica) Elsevier.

Cutting-Edge Technologies for Preventing Restenosis. Ed. by CTB Emerging Technologies Group. 1995. 161p. (Orig.). pap. 877.00 (*1-887566-00-7*) CTB Intl.

Cutting More Ties That Bind: Letting Go of Fear, Anger, Guilt, & Jealousy So We Can Educate Our Children & Change Ourselves. Phyllis Krystal. 1993. LC 93-3964. (Illus.). 218p. (Orig.). pap. 12.95 (*0-87728-792-9*) Red Wheel ME.

Cutting the Ties That Bind: Growing up & Moving On. Phyllis Krystal. 1993. LC 93-3965. (Illus.). 192p. (Orig.). pap. 11.95 (*0-87728-791-0*) Red Wheel ME.

Cutting the Ties That Bind Workbook. Phyllis Krystal. 1995. LC 95-13493. (Illus.). 112p. (Orig.). pap. text 12.95 (*0-87728-841-0*) Red Wheel ME.

CVRMed-MRCAS 1997: First Joint Conference Computer Vision, Virtual Reality & Robotics in Medicine, Medical Robotics & Computer-Assisted Surgery, Grenoble, France, March 1997: Proceedings. Jocelyne Troccaz. 1997. LC 97-6604. (Lecture Notes in Computer Science: Vol. 120). 834p. pap. 106.00 (*3-540-62734-0*) Spr-Verlag.

CWLA Standards for Health Care Services for Children in Out-of-Home Care. Child Welfare League of America Staff. 1988. 58p. pap. 14.50 (*0-87868-378-X*, 3780) Child Welfare.

Cyanide & the Central Nervous System: Foreign Countries' Approaches to High-Level Waste Storage & Disposal. Gudrun Cassel. 1994. (Illus.). 101p. (Orig.). (C). pap. text 40.00 (*0-7881-1132-9*) DIANE Pub.

Cybermedicine: How Computing Empowers Doctors & Patients for Better Health Care. Warner V. Slack. 1998. (Illus.). 214p. text 24.00 (*0-7881-5705-1*) DIANE Pub.

Cybermedicine: How Computing Empowers Doctors & Patients for Better Health Care. Warner V. Slack. 1997. LC 97-3821. 214p. 25.00 (*0-7879-0343-4*) Jossey-Bass.

*__Cybermedicine: How Computing Empowers Doctors & Patients for Better Health Care.__ Warner V. Slack. 2nd rev. ed. 2001. LC 2001-2782. (Illus.). 224p. pap. 19.95 (*0-7879-5631-7*) Jossey-Bass.

Cybernetic Epistemology. Wyatt Woodsmall. 1998. (Advanced Neuro Linguistic Programming Applications Ser.). 60p. spiral bd. 35.00 (*1-892876-06-X*) Next Step Pr.

Cybernetic Systems of Limb Movements in Man, Animals & Robots. A. Morecki et al. 1985. LC 82-15717. 242p. 95.95 (*0-470-27374-7*) P-H.

Cybernetics of Prejudices in the Practice of Psychotherapy. Gianfranco Cecchin et al. 1994. 96p. pap. text (*1-85575-056-2*) Karnac Bks GBR. *Dist:* Other Pr LLC.

Cybersurgery: Advanced Technologies for Surgical Practice. Richard M. Satava & Jonathan M. Sackier. 1997. LC 97-17142. (Protocols in General Surgery Ser.). 224p. 105.00 (*0-471-15874-7*) Wiley.

Cyborgs & Citadels: Anthropological Interventions in Emerging Sciences & Technologies. Ed. by Gary L. Downey & Joseph Dumit. 1998. LC 97-20296. (Advanced Seminar Ser.). 328p. 55.00 (*0-933452-96-9*); pap. 24.95 (*0-933452-97-7*) Schol Am Res.

Cyclic Nucleotide Phosphodiesterases: Structure, Regulation, & Drug Action. Ed. by Joe Beavo & Miles D. Houslay. 1990. LC 90-11982. (Molecular Pharmacology Ser.). 358p. 295.00 (*0-471-92707-4*) Wiley.

Cyclic Nucleotides Part I: Biochemistry. Ed. by Jerry A. Nathanson & J. W. Kobabian. 1982. (Handbook of Experimental Pharmacology Ser.: Vol. 58, Pt. I). (Illus.). 736p. 344.00 (*0-387-10786-X*) Spr-Verlag.

Cyclic Nucleotides & Therapeutic Perspectives. G. Cehovic & G. A. Robison. 1979. (Advances in the Biosciences Ser.: 24). 256p. 50.00 (*0-08-023760-6*, Pergamon Pr) Elsevier.

Cyclodextrins in Pharmacy. Karl-Heinz Fromming. 1993. LC 92-46544. (Topics in Inclusion Science Ser.). 228p. (C). text 142.00 (*0-7923-2139-1*) Kluwer Academic.

Cyclooxygenase & Lipoxygenase Modulators in Lung Reactivity. Ed. by F. Berti et al. 1985. (Progress in Biochemical Pharmacology Ser.: Vol. 20). (Illus.). x, 146p. 115.75 (*3-8055-3974-6*) S Karger.

Cyclopedia of Formulas, Set. 1996. lib. bdg. 999.95 (*0-8490-5868-6*) Gordon Pr.

Cyclosporin: Mode of Action & Clinical Application. Ed. by Angus W. Thomson. 1989. (C). text 188.50 (*0-7462-0124-9*) Kluwer Academic.

Cyclosporin for Severe Psoriasis: The Italian Experience. Ed. by A. F. Finzi. 1993. (Journal: Vol. 187, Suppl. 1, 1993). (Illus.). iv, 44p. pap. 21.00 (*3-8055-5845-7*) S Karger.

Cyclostomata: An Annotated Bibliography. Ed. by L. J. Selley & F. W. Beamish. 1977. text 394.50 (*90-6193-562-8*) Kluwer Academic.

Cyhalothrin. 1990. (Environmental Health Criteria Ser.: No. 99). (ENG, FRE & SPA.). 106p. pap. text 23.00 (*92-4-154299-3*, 1160099) World Health.

Cystic Fibrosis. P. B. Davis. 1993. (Lung Biology in Health & Disease Ser.: Vol. 64). (Illus.). 576p. text 250.00 (*0-8247-8815-X*) Dekker.

Cystic Fibrosis. Michael E. Fritz et al. 1973. LC 73-13832. 198p. (C). text 24.50 (*0-8422-7133-3*) Irvington.

Cystic Fibrosis. Ed. by Margaret E. Hodson & D. Geddes. 1994. (Illus.). 456p. (*0-412-48440-4*) E A GBR. *Dist:* OUP.

*__Cystic Fibrosis.__ Judy Monroe. 2000. LC 00-12612. (Perspectives on Disease & Illness Ser.). (Illus.). (J). (gr. 5-12). lib. bdg. 23.93 (*0-7368-1026-9*, LifeMatters Bks) Capstone Pr.

Cystic Fibrosis. Ed. by Dennis J. Shale. 1996. 162p. pap. text (*0-7279-0826-X*) BMJ Pub GBR. *Dist:* AIDC.

Cystic Fibrosis. Ed. by J. O. Warner. 1992. (Illus.). 320p. text (*0-443-04716-2*) Church.

Cystic Fibrosis. M. E. Hodson. 2nd ed. 2000. LC 2001-268589. (Illus.). 480p. (*0-340-74208-9*) E A GBR. *Dist:* OUP.

Cystic Fibrosis: A Guide for Patient & Family. David M. Orenstein. 2nd ed. 1996. LC 96-27001. 480p. pap. text 29.95 (*0-397-51653-3*) Lppncott W & W.

*__Cystic Fibrosis: A State-of-the-Art Series.__ 2001. (Thematic Review Ser.: Vol. 67). (Illus.). iv, 72p. 30.50 (*3-8055-7224-7*) S Karger.

Cystic Fibrosis: Directory of Authors of New Medical & Scientific Reviews with Subject Index. Science and Life Consultants Association Staff. 1996. LC 96-12495. 57.50 (*0-7883-1042-9*); pap. 47.50 (*0-7883-1043-7*) ABBE Pubs Assn.

Cystic Fibrosis: Infection, Immunopathology & Host Response. Ed. by Richard B. Moss. 1990. 262p. 109.50 (*0-89603-192-6*) Humana.

Cystic Fibrosis: Medical Care. David M. Orenstein et al. 2000. LC 99-55489. (Illus.). 384p. pap. text 47.95 (*0-7817-1798-1*) Lppncott W & W.

Cystic Fibrosis: Nutritional & Intestinal Disorders. Ed. by Ross W. Shepherd & Geoffrey J. Cleghorn. 1989. 184p. 129.00 (*0-8493-6954-1*, RJ456) CRC Pr.

Cystic Fibrosis: The Facts. Ann Harris & Maurice Super. 3rd ed. 1995. LC 94-36967. (Facts Ser.). (Illus.). 138p. pap. 19.95 (*0-19-262543-8*) OUP.

Cystic Fibrosis in Adults. James R. Yankaskas & Michael R. Knowles. 1998. LC 98-29116. 528p. text 110.00 (*0-7817-1011-1*) Lppncott W & W.

*__Cystic Fibrosis in the 20th Century: People, Events & Progress.__ Ed. by Carl F. Doershuk. 2002. (Illus.). xvii, 403p. 35.95 (*0-9717064-0-9*) A M Pubng Ltd.

Cystic Fibrosis Methods & Protocols. Ed. by William R. Skach. 2002. (Methods in Molecular Medicine Ser.: Vol. 70). 688p. 145.00 (*0-89603-897-1*) Humana.

Cystic Fibrosis Pulmonary Infections: Lessons from Around the World. Ed. by A. Bauernfeind et al. 1996. (Respiratory Pharmacology & Pharmacotherapy Ser.). 333p. 190.00 (*0-8176-5027-X*) Birkhauser.

Cystic Fibrosis Pulmonary Infections: Lessons from Around the World. Ed. by M. I. Marks et al. 1996. (Respiratory Pharmacology & Pharmacotherapy Ser.). 333p. 190.00 (*3-7643-5027-X*) Birkhauser.

Cystic Kidney. Ed. by Kenneth D. Gardner, Jr. & Jay Bernstein. 1990. (Developments in Nephrology Ser.). (C). text 279.50 (*0-7923-0392-X*) Kluwer Academic.

Cytoarchitecture of the Human Brain Stem. J. Olszewsky & D. Baxter. 2nd ed. 1981. (Illus.). 200p. 242.75 (*3-8055-2210-X*) S Karger.

Cytochrome Oxidase in Neuronal Metabolism & Alzheimer's Disease: Proceedings of an International Symposium Held in New Orleans, Louisiana, October 28, 1997. Ed. by F. Gonzalez-Lima. 1998. LC 98-34611. 289p. 115.00 (*0-306-46024-6*, Kluwer Plenum) Kluwer Academic.

Cytochrome P-450. Ed. by Klaus Ruckpaul & Horst Rein. 1985. 398p. 88.00 (*0-85066-337-7*); pap. text 27.00 (*0-85066-970-7*) Taylor & Francis.

Cytochrome P-450 & Active Oxygen. I. A. Archakov & G. I. Bachmanova. 1990. 320p. (*0-85066-805-0*) Tay Francis Ltd GBR. *Dist:* Taylor & Francis.

Cytochrome P450. Ed. by Helmut Greim & John B. Schenkman. 1993. LC 92-21429. (Handbook of Experimental Pharmacology Ser.: Vol. 105). (Illus.). 739p. 447.00 (*0-387-55908-6*) Spr-Verlag.

Cytochromes C. G. W. Pettigrew & G. R. Moore. 1987. (Molecular Biology, Biochemistry & Biophysics Ser.). (Illus.). 282p. 186.00 (*0-387-17843-0*) Spr-Verlag.

Cytodiagnostic Urinalysis of Renal & Lower Urinary Tract Disorders. G. Berry Schumann et al. 1995. LC 93-24272. (Illus.). 216p. 139.00 (*0-89640-243-6*) Igaku-Shoin.

*__Cytogenetic & Molecular Analysis of Chromosomal Rearrangements Associated with Neuropsychiatric Disorders.__ Dmitry Tentler. 2001. (Comprehensive Summaries of Uppsala Dissertations from the Faculty of Medicine Ser.: No. 1091). (Illus.). 56p. pap. (*91-554-5149-7*) Acta Univ SWE. *Dist:* Coronet Bks.

Cytogenetic Aspects of Malignant Transformation. N. B. Atkin. Ed. by A Wolsky. 1976. (Experimental Biology & Medicine Ser.: Vol. 6). (Illus.). 200p. 64.50 (*3-8055-2330-0*) S Karger.

Cytogenetics of Vectors of Disease of Man: Report of a WHO Scientific Group, 1968. 1968. (Technical Report Ser.: No. 398). 41p. pap. text 5.00 (*92-4-120398-6*, 1100398) World Health.

Cytokeratins in Intracranial & Intraspinal Tissues. Michael Kasper. Ed. by F. Beck et al. 1992. LC 92-2224. (Advances in Anatomy, Embryology & Cell Biology Ser.: Vol. 126). (Illus.). 82p. 69.00 (*0-387-55161-1*); vi, 82p. pap. 69.00 (*3-540-55161-1*) Spr-Verlag.

Cytokine-Induced Tumour Immunogenicity: From Exogenous Molecules to Gene Therapy. Ed. by Guido Forni et al. 1994. (Illus.). 488p. (C). text 59.95 (*0-12-261520-4*) Acad Pr.

Cytokine Knockouts. Ed. by Scott K. Durum & Kathrin Muegge. 1997. LC 97-39690. (Contemporary Immunology Ser.). (Illus.). 512p. 150.00 (*0-89603-368-6*) Humana.

*__Cytokine-Regulated Eosinophil Migration in Inflammatory Disorders: Clinical & Experimental Studies.__ Maria Lampinen. 2000. (Comprehensive Summaries of Uppsala Disertations from the Faculty of Medicine: No. 971). (Illus.). 58p. (Orig.). pap. (*91-554-4849-6*) Uppsala Universitet SWE. *Dist:* Coronet Bks.

Cytokine Regulation of Humoral Immunity: Basic & Clinical Aspects. Ed. by Clifford M. Snapper. 1996. LC 95-23822. 456p. 245.00 (*0-471-95953-7*) Wiley.

Cytokine Therapeutics in Infectious Diseases. Steven Holland. 2001. text 159.00 (*0-7817-1625-X*) Lppncott W & W.

Cytokines. Ed. by Anthony Mire-Sluis et al. 1998. (Handbook of Immunopharmacology Ser.). (Illus.). 544p. (C). 99.95 (*0-12-498340-5*) Acad Pr.

Cytokines: Stress & Immunity. Nicholas P. Plotnikoff & Robert E. Faith. 1998. LC 98-34473. 384p. 104.95 (*0-8493-3150-1*) CRC Pr.

Cytokines & Adhesion Molecules in Lung Inflammation. Michel Chignard. 1996. LC 96-43703. (Annals of the New York Academy of Sciences Ser.). pap. 95.00 (*0-89766-980-0*); 297p. 95.00 (*0-89766-979-7*) NY Acad Sci.

Cytokines & Autoimmune Diseases. Ed. by Vijay K. Kuchroo et al. 2001. 416p. 145.00 (*0-89603-856-4*) Humana.

Cytokines & Autoimmunity. Fionula M. Brennan. 1996. LC 95-49399. (Medicine Ser.). pap. 89.95 (*0-412-10271-4*, VNR) Wiley.

Cytokines & Bone Metabolism. Maxine Gowen. 1991. 312p. lib. bdg. 210.00 (*0-8493-6268-7*, QP88) CRC Pr.

Cytokines & Growth Factors in Blood Transfusion: Proceedings of the Twenty-First International Symposium on Blood Transfusion, Groningen 1996, Organized by the Red Cross Blood Bank Noord-Nederland. Ed. by C. Smit Sibinga et al. 1997. LC 97-218096. (Developments in Hematology & Immunology Ser.: No. 32). 216p. text 92.50 (*0-7923-4787-0*) Kluwer Academic.

Cytokines & Inflammation. Edward S. Kimball. 1991. (Illus.). 368p. 195.00 (*0-8493-8806-6*, QR185) CRC Pr.

Cytokines & Pain. Ed. by L. R. Watkins & S. F. Maier. 1999. LC 98-42561. (Progress in Inflammation Research Ser.). 260p. 139.00 (*3-7643-5849-1*) Birkhauser.

Cytokines & Pain. Linda R. Watkins & Steven F. Maier. 1998. LC 98-42561. (PIR, Progress in Inflammation Research Ser.). 139.00 (*0-8176-5849-1*) Birkhauser.

Cytokines & the Abdominal Surgeon. Moshe Schein & Leslie Wise. 1998. LC 98-8811. 99.00 (*1-57059-536-4*) Landes Bioscience.

Cytokines & the Biotherapy of Infectious Diseases. Ed. by J. W. Van der Meer & B. J. Kullberg. 1995. LC 94-41689. (Biotherapy Ser.: Vol. 7, Issue 3-4). (C). text 92.50 (*0-7923-3267-9*) Kluwer Academic.

Cytokines & the CNS. Ed. by Richard M. Ransohoff & Etty N. Benveniste. 1996. LC 95-38135. 368p. 129.95 (*0-8493-2452-1*, 2452) CRC Pr.

Cytokines & the Heart: Molecular Mechanisms of Septic Cardiomyopathy. Ursula Muller-Werdan et al. 1996. LC 95-32356. (Medical Intelligence Unit Ser.). 231p. 99.00 (*1-57059-295-0*) Landes Bioscience.

Cytokines & the Heart: Molecular Mechanisms of Septic Cardiomyopathy. Ursula Muller-Werdan et al. 1996. (Medical Intelligence Unit Ser.). 260p. pap. 89.95 (*0-412-10111-4*, VNR) Wiley.

Cytokines & the Liver. Ed. by K. Decker. 1995. (Falk Symposium Ser.). 256p. (C). text 102.50 (*0-7923-8878-X*) Kluwer Academic.

Cytokines & Their Receptors Clinical Applications. Roberto Patarca. 1998. 99.95 (*0-8493-4020-9*) CRC Pr.

Cytokines in Animal Health & Disease. Ed. by Michael J. Myers & Michael P. Murtaugh. 1995. LC 95-13663. (Illus.). 480p. text 215.00 (*0-8247-9435-4*) Dekker.

Cytokines in Cancer Therapy. Ed. by L. Bergmann & Paris S. Mitrou. 1994. (Beitraege Zur Onkologie, Contributions to Oncology Ser.: Vol. 46). (Illus.). x, 392p. 121.75 (*3-8055-5809-0*) S Karger.

Cytokines in Health & Disease. Ed. by Daniel G. Remick & Jan S. Friedland. 2nd ed. 1997. LC 97-12544. (Illus.). 704p. text 225.00 (*0-8247-9823-6*) Dekker.

Cytokines in Hemopoiesis, Oncology, & AIDS II. Ed. by M. Freund et al. 1992. LC 92-29751. (Illus.). 784p. (*3-540-55242-1*); 238.00 (*0-387-55242-1*) Spr-Verlag.

Cytokines in Hemopoiesis, Oncology, & Immunology III. Ed. by Mathias Freund et al. 1994. LC 94-17634. 737p. 255.00 (*0-387-57753-X*) Spr-Verlag.

Cytokines in Human Multiple Myeloma. Bernard Klein et al. 1994. LC 94-37794. (Medical Intelligence Unit Ser.). 108p. 99.00 (*1-57059-042-7*, LN9042) Landes Bioscience.

Cytokines in Inflammatory Bowel Disease. Claudio Fiocchi. 1996. LC 95-33221. (Medical Intelligence Unit Ser.). 247p. 99.00 (*1-57059-124-5*) Landes Bioscience.

Cytokines in Inflammatory Bowel Disease. Claudio Fiocchi. 1996. (Medicine Ser.). pap. 89.95 (*0-412-10051-7*, VNR) Wiley.

Cytokines in Pulmonary Disease: Infection & Inflammation. Ed. by Steve Nelson & Thomas R. Martin. 2000. (Lung Biology in Health & Disease Ser.: Vol. 141). (Illus.). 624p. text 195.00 (*0-8247-1931-X*) Dekker.

Cytokines in Severe Sepsis & Septic Shock. Heinz Redl & Gunther Schlag. 1998. LC 98-37008. (PIR/Progress in Inflammation Research Ser.). xx, 369p. 179.00 (*0-8176-5877-7*); 179.00 (*3-7643-5877-7*) Birkhauser.

Cytokines in the Nervous System. Nancy J. Rothwell. 1996. LC 96-44039. (Neuroscience Intelligence Unit Ser.). 99.00 (*1-57059-392-2*, 0-412-13581-7) Landes Bioscience.

Cytokines in the Treatment of Hematopoietic Failure. Ed. by Arnold Ganser & Dieter Hoelzer. 1998. LC 98-39369. (Illus.). 416p. text 165.00 (*0-8247-0193-3*) Dekker.

Cytokines in Transfusion Medicine: A Primer. Ed. by Robertson D. Davenport & Edward L. Snyder. 1997. LC 97-35729. text 129.00 (*1-56395-080-4*) Am Assn Blood.

Cytokines in Transplantation. Anne Kelso. 1996. (Medicine Ser.). 192p. pap. 89.95 (*0-412-10361-3*) Chapman & Hall.

Cytokines in Transplantation. Anne Kelso & Andrew Clouston. 1995. (Medical Intelligence Unit Ser.). 194p. 99.00 (*1-57059-323-X*) Landes Bioscience.

Cytokines in Trauma & Hemorrhage. Harvey J. Sugerman & Eric J. DeMaria. 1997. (Medical Intelligence Unit Ser.). 174p. 99.00 (*1-57059-354-X*) Landes Bioscience.

Cytokines in Veterinary Medicine. Ed. by Virgil E. Schijns & Marian C. Horzinek. 1998. LC 98-141538. (Illus.). 352p. text 120.00 (*0-85199-209-9*) OUP.

Cytokines of the Lung. Ed. by Jason Kelley. 1992. LC 92-49726. (Lung Biology in Health & Disease Ser.: Vol. 61). (Illus.). 664p. text 235.00 (*0-8247-8703-X*) Dekker.

Cytokines Regulating the Allergic Response. Ed. by C. Muenster Sorg. 1989. (Cytokines Ser.: Vol. 2). (Illus.). 106p. 82.75 (*3-8055-5034-0*) S Karger.

Cytokines, Stress, Depression. Ed. by Robert Dantzer et al. 1999. LC 99-38077. (Illus.). 336p. (*0-306-46135-8*) Plenum.

Cytology. Edmund J. Messina. 1975. LC 74-79836. (Allied Health Ser.). pap. 7.65 (*0-672-61382-4*, Bobbs) Macmillan.

Cytology: Diagnostic Principles & Clinical Correlates. Edmund S. Cibas & Barbara S. Ducantman. 1995. (Illus.). 528p. text 115.00 (*0-7216-4069-9*) Saunders.

Cytology & Microscopic Anatomy. Horst-Dieter Dellmann & Jeanine A. Carithers. 1996. LC 95-14964. (National Veterinary Medical Series for Independent Study). (Illus.). 400p. 28.95 (*0-683-01467-6*) Lppncott W & W.

Cytology of the Central Nervous System. Dorothy L. Rosenthal. 1984. (Monographs in Clinical Cytology Ser.: Vol. 8). (Illus.). x, 206p. 85.25 (*3-8055-3808-1*) S Karger.

Cytology of Transudates & Exudates. E. Von Haam. 1977. (Monographs in Clinical Cytology Ser.: Vol. 5). 44.50 (*3-8055-2625-3*) S Karger.

Cytolytic Lymphocytes & Complement: Effectors of the Immune System. Eckhard R. Podack. 1988. Vol. I. 280p. 154.00 (*0-8493-6968-1*, QR185); Vol. II. 256p. 141.00 (*0-8493-6969-X*, 6969) Franklin (CRC Reprint).

Cytomegalovirus: A Hospitalization Diary. Herve Guibert. Tr. by Clara Orban & Elliot Weisenberg from FRE. 1996. LC 96-5410. 90p. lib. bdg. 33.00 (*0-7618-0305-X*) U Pr of Amer.

Cytomegalovirus: Biology & Infection. M. Ho. 2nd ed. 1991. LC 90-14345. (Illus.). 460p. (C). text 114.00 (*0-306-43654-X*, Kluwer Plenum) Kluwer Academic.

Cytomegalovirus & Immunity. J. D. Hamilton. 1982. (Monographs in Virology: Vol. 12). (Illus.). viii, 108p. 65.25 (*3-8055-3495-7*) S Karger.

Cytomegalovirus Infections of Man. U. Krech et al. 1971. (Illus.). 124p. 28.00 (*3-8055-1261-9*) S Karger.

Cytomegaloviruses. Ed. by Mark F. Stinski. 1997. (Journal: Vol. 39, No. 5-6, 1996). (Illus.). iv, 128p. pap. 75.00 (*3-8055-6500-3*) S Karger.

Cytomegloviruses. James B. Hanshaw. 1968. (Virology Monographs: Vol. 3). (Illus.). iv, 131p. 38.00 (*0-387-80891-4*) Spr-Verlag.

Cytopathology. Zuher M. Naib. 4th ed. 1995. LC 95-2408. 752p. text 115.00 (*0-316-59674-4*, Little Brwn Med Div) Lppncott W & W.

Cytopathology in Pediatrics. J. J. Buchino. 1991. (Monographs in Clinical Cytology Ser.: Vol. 13). (Illus.). x, 156p. 174.00 (*3-8055-5299-8*) S Karger.

Cytopathology of Malignant Effusions: Cytomorphologic Interpretation. Liang-Che & Tao. 1996. LC 95-35871. (ASCP Theory & Practice of Cytopathology Ser.: No. 5). (Illus.). 80.00 (*0-89189-395-4*) Am Soc Clinical.

Cytopathology of Pulmonary Disease. Dorothy L. Rosenthal. 1988. (Monographs in Clinical Cytology Ser.: Vol. 11). (Illus.). x, 238p. 116.75 (*3-8055-4740-4*) S Karger.

Cytopathology of Soft Tissue & Bone Tumors. S. I. Hajdu & Eva O. Hajdu. 1989. (Monographs in Clinical Cytology Ser.: Vol. 12). (Illus.). xvi, 348p. 208.75 (*3-8055-4814-1*) S Karger.

Cytopathology of the Breast. Shahla Masood. 1995. LC 95-39759. (Illus.). 116.00 (*0-89189-380-6*) Am Soc Clinical.

Cytopathology of the Central Nervous System. Sandra H. Bigner. 1994. 208p. 90.00 (*0-89189-362-8*) Am Soc Clinical.

Cytopathology of the Endometrium. Liang-Che Tao. 1993. LC 93-4916. (Illus.). 141p. 70.00 (*0-89189-363-6*) Am Soc Clinical.

Cytopathology of the Head & Neck. Lester J. Layfield et al. 1996. LC 96-36586. (ASCP Theory & Practice of Cytopathology Ser.). 115.00 (*0-89189-421-7*) Am Soc Clinical.

Cytopathology of the Lower Female Genital Tract: An Integrated Approach. Gerard J. Nuovo. 1994. LC 93-9608. (Illus.). 520p. 165.00 (*0-683-06595-5*) Lppncott W & W.

Cytopathology of the Uterine Cervix. Alexander Meisels. 1991. sl. 200.00 (*0-89189-341-5*) Am Soc Clinical.

Cytopathology of the Uterus. Alexander Meisels & Carol Morin. 2nd ed. 1996. LC 96-41995. (ASCP Theory & Practice of Cytopathology Ser.). 116.00 (*0-89189-383-0*) Am Soc Clinical.

Cytopathology of Tumours of the Nervous System. G. Andrioli & L. Rigobello. 1986. 100p. text (*1-57235-030-X*) Piccin Nuova.

Cytopathology Review Guide. E. Blair Holladay. 1998. (Illus.). 440p. pap. text 85.00 (*0-89189-398-9*) Am Soc Clinical.

Cytoplasmic Fate of Messenger RNA. Ed. by W. E. Muller & P. Jeanteur. 1996. LC 96-25885. (Progress in Molecular & Subcellular Biology Ser.). (Illus.). 280p. 157.00 (*3-540-61368-4*) Spr-Verlag.

Cytoskeletal & Extracellular Proteins. Ed. by U. Aebi & J. Engel. 1989. (Biophysics Ser.: Vol. 3). (Illus.). 366p. 172.00 (*0-387-50067-7*) Spr-Verlag.

Cytoskeletal Proteins in Tumor Diagnosis. Ed. by M. Osborn & K. Weber. 1989. (Current Communications in Molecular Biology Ser.). (Illus.). 244p. (C). pap. text 24.00 (*0-87969-325-8*) Cold Spring Harbor.

Cytoskeleton. M. Schliwa. 1986. (Cell Biology Monographs: Vol. 13). (Illus.). 340p. 124.95 (*0-387-81884-7*) Spr-Verlag.

Cytoskeleton Vol. 4: Altered Function in Pathological States. Ed. by J. E. Hesketh & Ian Pryme. Date not set. 128.50 (*1-55938-690-8*) Jai Pr.

Cytoskeleton in Normal & Pathologic Processes: Cell Biology. Ed. by Giulio Gabbiani. 1978. (Methods & Achievements in Experimental Pathology Ser.: Vol. 8). (Illus.). 85.25 (*3-8055-2917-1*) S Karger.

Cytoskeleton in Normal & Pathologic Processes: Cell Physiopathology. Ed. by Giulio Gabbiani. 1978. (Methods & Achievements in Experimental Pathology Ser.: Vol. 9). (Illus.). 129.75 (*3-8055-2919-8*) S Karger.

Cytosolic Calcium Measurements, Regulation & Biologic Significance in Epithelial Tissue. Ed. by Z. S. Agus & E. Kelepouris. 1988. (Journal: Vol. 14, No. 1, 1988). (Illus.). 96p. pap. 69.75 (*3-8055-4658-0*) S Karger.

Cytotest Two, 1992. 1993. 265.00 incl. sl. (*0-89189-345-8*) Am Soc Clinical.

Cytotoxic & Complement Mediated Reactions. Ed. by P. Dukor et al. 1980. (Par Pseudo-Allergic Reactions, Involvement of Drugs & Chemicals Ser.: Vol. 2). (Illus.). viii, 144p. 56.75 (*3-8055-0666-X*) S Karger.

Cytotoxic Anticancer Drugs - Models & Concepts for Drug Discovery & Development: Proceedings of the 22nd Annual Cancer Symposium, Detroit, Michigan, April 26-28, 1990. Ed. by Frederick A. Valeriote. 1992. (Developments in Oncology Ser.). 432p. (C). text 201.50 (*0-7923-1629-0*) Kluwer Academic.

Cytotoxic Cells: Basic Mechanisms & Medical Applications. Ed. by Michail V. Sitkovsky & Pierre A. Henkart. 1999. LC 99-34057. (Illus.). 496p. text 139.00 (*0-7817-1603-9*) Lppncott W & W.

Cytotoxic Drug Resistance Mechanisms. Robert Brown & Uta Boger-Brown. 1999. LC 98-43528. (Methods in Molecular Medicine Ser.: Vol. 28). (Illus.). 248p. 99.50 (*0-89603-603-0*) Humana.

Cytotoxic Drugs & the Granulopoietic System. Ed. by H. P. Lohrmann & W. Schreml. 1981. (Recent Results in Cancer Research Ser.: Vol. 81). (Illus.). 222p. 74.00 (*0-387-10962-5*) Spr-Verlag.

Cytotoxic Mediators of Inflammation & Host Defense. Ed. by M. L. Shin. 1988. (Progress in Allergy Ser.: Vol. 40). (Illus.). xii, 216p. 128.75 (*3-8055-4636-X*) S Karger.

Cytotoxic, Mutagenic & Carcinogenic Potential of Heavy Metals Related to Human Environment: Proceedings of the NATO Advanced Study Institute, Orzesieka, Poland, 15-26 June 1996. Ed. by Nick D. Hadjiliadis. 1997. LC 96-54478. (NATO Advanced Science Institutes Ser.). 652p. (C). text 298.00 (*0-7923-4432-4*) Kluwer Academic.

Cytotoxic T Cells in HIV & Other Retroviral Infections. Ed. by P. Racz et al. 1992. (Illus.). 178p. 167.00 (*3-8055-5469-9*) S Karger.

Cytotoxics Handbook. Ed. by Michael Allwood et al. 1997. (Illus.). 400p. (*0-917330-83-8*, T-276) Radcliff Med GBR. *Dist:* Am Pharm Assn.

Cytotoxics Handbook. M. C. Allwood & Patricia Wright. 3rd ed. 1997. LC 96-53119. (*1-85775-141-8*) Radcliffe Med Pr GBR. *Dist:* Balogh.

***Cytotoxics Handbook.** Ed. by Michael Allwood et al. 4th ed. 2001. 496p. (*1-85775-504-9*) Radcliffe Med Pr GBR. *Dist:* Balogh.

Czech-English, English-Czech Medical Dictionary. J. Paroubkova. 1991. (CZE & ENG.). 95.00 (*0-8288-7198-1*, F26310) Fr & Eur.

D

D & C: A Guide for Women. Courtland Robinson. Ed. by Edward E. Wallach. 1996. (Women's Health Ser.). (Illus.). 24p. (Orig.). pap. 2.95 (*1-885274-17-3*) Health InfoNet Inc.

D1: D2 Dopamine Receptors: Neuroscience & Psychopharmacology. Ed. by John L. Waddington. 1993. (Neuroscience Perspectives Ser.). (Illus.). 304p. text 78.00 (*0-12-729045-1*) Acad Pr.

D. O.'s: Osteopathic Medicine in America. Norman Gevitz. 1991. LC 82-47978. (Illus.). 200p. reprint ed. pap. text 19.95 (*0-8018-4321-9*) Johns Hopkins.

D-Phenothrin. 1990. (Environmental Health Criteria Ser.: No. 96). 64p. pap. text 16.00 (*92-4-154296-9*, 1160096) World Health.

D. W. Winnicott. Michael Jacobs. 1995. LC 95-71212. (Key Figures in Counselling & Psychotherapy Ser.). ix, 163p. pap. 25.95 (*0-8039-8596-7*, 9274) Sage.

***Dacie & Lewis's Practical Hematology.** S. M. Lewis et al. 9th ed. 2001. (Illus.). 595p. pap. (*0-443-06377-X*) Church GBR. *Dist:* Saunders.

Dactylology: Conversing with the Deaf & Dumb. A. Richardin. 1973. 59.95 (*0-87968-990-0*) Gordon Pr.

Dad Calls Me Jack: Boyhood in Midwest, 1920's Nostalgic. Eugene L. Vickery. 1986. (Illus.). 250p. (Orig.). pap. 11.95 (*0-937775-00-2*) Stonehaven Pubs.

Dahlin's Bone Tumors: General Aspects & Data on 11,087 Cases. K. Krishnan Unni. 5th ed. 1996. LC 95-38749. Orig. Title: Bone Tumors. 480p. text 179.00 (*0-397-51665-7*) Lppncott W & W.

Dailey's Notes on Blood. John F. Dailey. 2nd ed. 1998. (Illus.). 178p. (C). pap. text 18.00 (*0-7881-5232-7*) DIANE Pub.

Dailey's Notes on Blood: Self-Teaching Hematology, Immunology & Transfusion Therapy. John F. Dailey. Ed. by Jane E. Manley. 3rd ed. 1996. LC 93-214993. (Illus.). 173p. pap. text, stu. ed. 20.00 (*0-9631819-4-7*, DNB3) Med Cnslt Grp.

Dailey's Notes on Blood: Self-Teaching Hematology, Immunology, & Transfusion Therapy. John F. Dailey. 4th exp. ed. 2002. (Illus.). pap., stu. ed. 24.00 (*0-9631819-6-3*) Med Cnslt Grp.

Daily Activities after Your Total Knee Replacement. Janet V. Platt et al. 1992. (Illus.). 28p. (C). pap. text 6.00 (*0-910317-80-1*) Am Occup Therapy.

Daily Affirmations for Compulsive Eaters: Beyond Feast Or Famine. Susan Ward. 1990. LC 91-815335. 370p. (Orig.). pap. 7.95 (*1-55874-076-7*) Health Comm.

Daily Growth for Broader Experiences or Awareness, Achievements, Purposeful Relaxation & Comfort, Set-DG. Russell E. Mason. rev. ed. 1975. pap. 60.00 incl. audio (*0-89533-011-3*) F I Comm.

Daily Guide to a Better Marriage. Donald Moore. 1984. 32p. pap. 0.75 (*0-88144-021-3*) Christian Pub.

Daily Health in the Indian Ayurvedic System. Aja Thomas. 1984. 40p. (Orig.). pap. 4.00 (*0-9620108-0-4*) ATMA.

Daily Problem Solving Activities: Transitioning to Independence. Andrew K. Gruen & Lynn S. Gruen. 1994. LC 93-46014. 42.00 (*0-930599-94-2*) Thinking Pubns.

Daily Reflections: A Book of Reflections by AA Members for AA Members. Alcoholics Anonymous World Services, Inc., Staff. 1990. 382p. pap. 5.25 (*0-916856-37-2*) AAWS.

Daily Sensorimotor Training Activities. William T. Braly et al. 1968. tchr. ed. 8.95 (*0-914296-02-7*) Ed Activities.

Dairy Cattle Fertility & Sterility see Fertilidad y Esterilidad en Ganado Lechero

Dakin's Atlas of Melanoma Surgery. Richard W. Sagebiel & Keith Denkler. 1997. (Illus.). 400p. (*0-683-18101-7*) Lppncott W & W.

Dallas Doc: All the City & Country Critters in the Life of a Texas-style Vet. David Carlton. 1999. LC 99-49619. 178p. (Orig.). pap. 12.95 (*1-888843-53-5*) Bridgeline Pr.

***Damaged Bonds.** Michael Eigen. 2001. 200p. pap. (*1-85575-256-5*) Karnac Bks GBR. *Dist:* Other Pr LLC.

Damages: One Family's Legal Struggles in the World of Medicine. Barry Werth. 1999. 400p. reprint ed. pap. 13.00 (*0-425-16863-8*) Berkley Pub.

Damages: One Family's Legal Struggles in the World of Medicine. Barry Werth. 1998. LC 97-36949. 400p. 25.00 (*0-684-80769-6*) S&S Trade.

Damages for Personal Injuries & Death in Singapore & Malaysia. Michael F. Rutter. 1988. 1000p. 233.00 (*9971-70-060-3*, MICHIE) LEXIS Pub.

Dance - Movement Therapy Abstracts Vol. I: Doctoral Dissertations, Masters' Theses, & Special Projects. Ed. by Anne C. Fisher & Arlynne Stark. 1992. LC 92-72987. 300p. (Orig.). (C). pap. (*1-881766-01-2*) M Chace Mem Fund.

***Dance Against Time: The Brief, Brilliant Life of a Joffrey Dancer.** Diane Solway. 2001. (Illus.). 386p. reprint ed. 23.00 (*0-7881-9589-1*) DIANE Pub.

Dance & Other Expressive Art Therapies: When Words Are Not Enough. Ed. by Fran J. Levy. 1995. LC 95-16839. (Illus.). 273p. (C). 70.00 (*0-415-91228-8*); pap. 27.95 (*0-415-91229-6*) Routledge.

Dance & Stress: Resistance, Reduction & Euphoria. Judith L. Hanna. Ed. by James H. Humprey. 1988. LC 86-82028. (Stress in Modern Society Ser.: No. 13). 32.50 (*0-404-63264-5*) AMS Pr.

Dance Movement Therapy: Theory & Practice. Ed. by Helen Payne. 1992. LC 91-22938. 296p. (C). pap. 31.95 (*0-415-05660-8*, A5956) Routledge.

Dance Therapy Redefined: A Body Approach to Therapeutic Dance. Johanna Exiner & Denis Kelynak. 1994. LC 94-8556. (Illus.). 130p. (C). text 34.95 (*0-398-05913-6*) C C Thomas.

Dancing Among the Maenads Vol. 5: The Psychology of Comulsive Drug Use. Kevin Volkan. 1994. LC 93-23071. (Reshaping of Psychoanalysis Ser.: Vol. 5). XXII, 167p. (C). text 38.95 (*0-8204-2301-7*) P Lang Pubng.

Dancing Healers: A Doctor's Journey of Healing with Native Americans. Carl A. Hammerschlag. 61st ed. 1989. LC 87-45704. 176p. pap. 13.00 (*0-06-250395-2*, Perennial) HarperTrade.

Dancing in Fire. Wilbert Williams, Jr. 1999. LC 99-231716. 291p. (Orig.). reprint ed. pap. text 28.00 (*0-9627257-6-5*) Aye-Aye Arts.

Dancing in Limbo: Making Sense of Life after Cancer. Glenna Halvorson-Boyd & Lisa K. Hunter. 1995. LC 95-9135. (Health Psychology Ser.). 192p. 23.00 (*0-7879-0103-2*) Jossey-Bass.

Dancing Mania in the Middle Ages. Justus F. Hecker. 1977. 250.00 (*0-87968-992-7*) Gordon Pr.

Dancing Matrix: How Science Confronts Emerging Viruses. Robin M. Henig. 1994. LC 93-27553. (Illus.). 288p. pap. 13.00 (*0-679-73083-4*) Vin Bks.

Dancing on the Edge: A Story of Cancer, Courage, & the Resurrection of Life. Dorothy P. Doyle. 1996. LC 95-94707. 256p. pap. 14.95 (*0-9647763-5-9*) Hibiscus FL.

Dancing Prophets: Musical Experience in Tumbuka Healing. Steven M. Friedson. 1996. LC 95-44931. (Chicago Studies in Ethnomusicology). (C). 248p. pap. text 16.95 (*0-226-26502-1*); 239p. lib. bdg. 45.00 (*0-226-26501-3*) U Ch Pr.

Dancing the Last Mazurka: A Care Givers Journal. Gary T. Doyle. 1998. xii, 224p. mass mkt. 7.95 (*1-892589-11-7*) Madjec Jet.

Dancing the Wheel of Psychological Types. Mary E. Loomis. 1991. LC 90-25469. (Illus.). 214p. (Orig.). pap. 17.95 (*0-933029-49-7*) Chiron Pubns.

Dancing Through the Darkness: The Cognitive Treatment of Shame. Clarissa E. Steffen. Ed. by Richard J. Tippett. 1999. LC 99-93113. (Illus.). 125p. (Orig.). pap. 12.95 (*0-9670829-0-0*) Realizing Potential.

Dancing with the Family: A Symbolic-Experiential Approach. Carl A. Whitaker & William M. Bumberry. 1988. LC 87-36843. 256p. text 41.95 (*0-87630-496-X*) Brunner-Routledge.

Dancing with Tigers. Janet E. Lapp. 1994. LC 94-96110. 123p. pap. 10.95 (*1-885365-01-2*) Demeter Pr.

Danforth's Obstetrics & Gynecology. David N. Danforth & James R. Scott. 8th ed. 1999. LC 98 37809. (Illus.). 1,008p. text 139.00 (*0-7817-1206-8*) Lppncott W & W.

Danger & Defense: The Technique of Close Process Attention. Ed. by Marianne Goldberger. 1996. LC 95-17450. 408p. 65.00 (*1-56821-583-5*) Aronson.

Danger in the Comfort Zone: From Boardroom to Mailroom-How to Break the Entitlement Habit That's Killing American Business. Judith M. Bardwick. 1991. 200p. 21.95 (*0-8144-5059-8*, 040531) AMACOM.

Danger in the Land of Mavericks. Nelson A. Ossorio. 1995. (Orig.). pap. 11.95 (*1-56721-124-0*) Twenty-Fifth Cent Pr.

Dangerous Diagnostics: The Social Power of Biological Information. Dorothy Nelkin & Laurence Tancredi. 1994. LC 93-32571. 232p. pap. text 12.95 (*0-226-57129-7*) U Ch Pr.

Dangerous Families: Assessment & Treatment of Child Abuse. Peter Dale. 1987. 280p. (*0-422-60140-3*, 1129) Tavistock GBR. *Dist:* Routldge.

Dangerous Passage: The Social Control of Sexuality in Women's Adolescence. Constance A. Nathanson. 1991. LC 90-20580. (Health, Society, & Policy Ser.). 350p. 59.95 (*0-87722-824-8*) Temple U Pr.

Dangerous Sex Offenders: A Task Force Report of The American Psychiatric Association. American Psychiatric Association Staff. 1999. LC 98-50587. 224p. 29.95 (*0-89042-280-X*, 2280) Am Psychiatric.

Dangerous to Your Health: The Crisis of Medical Care in the United States. Vicente Navarro. 1993. (Cornerstone Bks.). 144p. pap. text 13.00 (*0-85345-865-0*) Monthly Rev.

Dangers of Immunization. Harold E. Buttram. 1987. 72p. (Orig.). pap. 4.00 (*0-916285-27-8*) Humanitarian.

Dangers of Socialized Medicine. Ed. by Jacob G. Hornberger & Richard M. Ebeling. 1994. 100p. (Orig.). pap. text 7.95 (*0-9640447-0-6*) Future of Freedom.

Daniel. Daymond R. Duck. 1998. LC 97-80894. (God's Word for the Biblically-Inept Ser.). (Illus.). 352p. pap. 16.95 (*0-914984-48-9*) Starburst.

Daniels & Worthingham's Muscle Testing: Techniques of Manual Examination. Helen J. Hislop & Jacqueline Montgomery. 6th ed. 1995. (Illus.). 400p. pap. text 41.95 (*0-7216-4305-1*) Saunders.

Danish/English-English/Danish Medical Dictionary. H. Baden. 1994. 913p. 140.00 (*0-7859-9559-5*) Fr & Eur.

Daredevils & Daydreams: New Perspectives on Attention Deficit/Hyperactivity Disorder. Barbara D. Ingersoll. 1997. LC 97-22397. 256p. pap. 11.95 (*0-385-48757-6*, Main St Bks) Doubleday.

Daring to Be Myself: A Case Study in Rational-Emotive Therapy. Windy Dryden & Joseph Yankura. 1992. 224p. pap. (*0-335-09341-8*) OpUniv Pr.

Daring to Care: Training Manual. Janet Lassman. 3rd ed. 1999. (Illus.). 506p. ring bd. 35.00 (*0-935890-27-0*) Emerg Nurses IL.

Dark Cures: Have Doctors Lost their Ethics? Paul DeParrie. 1998. LC 95-77223. 224p. pap. 11.99 (*1-56384-099-5*) Huntington Hse.

Dark Face of Science. John Vyvyan. 2nd ed. 1989. LC 86-33240. 208p. pap. 12.00 (*0-916288-22-6*) Micah Pubns.

Dark Night, Early Dawn: Steps to a Deep Ecology of Mind. Christopher M. Bache. 2000. LC 99-49013. 384p. (C). text 72.50 (*0-7914-4605-0*); (Illus.). pap. text 24.95 (*0-7914-4606-9*) State U NY Pr.

Dark Paradise: Opiate Addiction in America before 1940. David T. Courtwright. 1982. LC 81-6958. (Illus.). 280p. 39.50 (*0-674-19261-3*) HUP.

Dark Rapture: The Sex Life of the African Negro. Felix Bryk. Tr. by Arthur J. Norton. LC 72-9712. reprint ed. 39.50 (*0-404-57421-1*) AMS Pr.

***Dark Remedy: The Impact of Thalidomide & Its Revival As a Vital Medicine.** Trent D. Stephens & Rock Brynner. 2001. 240p. pap. text 16.00 (*0-7382-0590-7*) Perseus Bks Grp.

Dark Side of the Analytic Moon: A Memoir of Life in a Training Institute. Gerald Alper. 1997. LC 96-21099. 174p. 36.95 (*1-57309-017-4*); pap. 20.95 (*1-57309-016-6*) Intl Scholars.

Darstellung und Reaktionen Von Thiooxalsauren und Thiooxalsaurederivaten. Vol. 8. R. Mayer & W. Thiel. Ed. by Alexander Senning. 1988. (Sulfer Reports: Vol. 8, No. 1). (GER.). 58p. pap. text 90.00 (*3-7186-4807-5*) Gordon & Breach.

Dartmouth Atlas of Health Care. Dartmouth Medical School, Center for the Evaluative. 1996. LC 96-11510. 230p. (C). pap. 75.00 (*1-55648-163-2*, 70369); (Illus.). 350.00 (*1-55648-155-1*, 044100) AHPI.

Dartmouth Atlas of Health Care in the United States. 2nd ed. 1997. (*1-55648-186-1*) AHPI.

Dartmouth Atlas of Health Care 1998. Center for the Evaluative Clinical Sciences Staff. 1998. (Illus.). 328p. 350.00 (*1-55648-217-5*) OUP.

Darvon & Other Prescription Narcotics. Jim Parker. rev. ed. 1999. pap. 0.50 (*0-89230-147-3*) Do It Now.

Darwin: Competition & Cooperation. Ashley Montagu. 1973. LC 72-11332. 148p. reprint ed. lib. bdg. 35.00 (*0-8371-6657-8*, MODC, Greenwood Pr) Greenwood.

Darwinian Psychiatry. Michael McGuire & Alfonso Troisi. 1998. LC 98-2504. (Illus.). 360p. (C). text 45.00 (*0-19-511673-9*) OUP.

Darwiniana. Thomas Henry Huxley. LC 70-108122. reprint ed. 39.50 (*0-404-03468-3*) AMS Pr.

Darwinism. 4. J. R. Angell et al. 1977. LC 77-72191. (Contributions to the History of Psychology Ser.: Vol. IV, Pt. D, Comparative Psychology). 424p. lib. bdg. 83.50 (*0-313-26948-3*, U6948) Greenwood.

Darwinism: A Time for Funerals. Norman Macbeth. 1985. (Broadside Editions Ser.). 32p. (C). reprint ed. pap. 4.95 (*0-9609850-8-5*) Rob Briggs.

Darwinism: An Exposition of the Theory of Natural Selection, with Some of Its Applications. Alfred R. Wallace. LC 72-1666. reprint ed. 57.50 (*0-404-08182-7*) AMS Pr.

Darwinism & Determinism: The Role of Direction in Evolution. Anthony Ruffa. 1983. 25.95 (*0-8283-1732-1*) Branden Bks.

Darwin's Audubon: Science & the Liberal Imagination. Gerald Weissmann. 1998. LC 98-28473. (Illus.). 350p. (C). 28.95 (*0-306-45981-7*) Perseus Bks Grp.

***DASH Diet for Hypertension: Lower Your Blood Pressure in 14 Days - Without Drugs.** Thomas Moore et al. 2002. LC 2001-42946. 288p. 25.00 (*0-7432-0295-3*) Free Pr.

DAT - Dental Aptitude Test: Comprehensive Manual Self Study, No. 1. David M. Tarlow. 2nd rev. ed. 1999. (Illus.). 140p. (C). pap. text 19.95 (*1-57732-078-6*) Datar Pub.

DAT - Dental Aptitude Test: Comprehensive Review for Self Study. David M. Tarlow. 7th ed. 1996. (Illus.). (Orig.). pap., stu. ed. 19.95 (*1-57732-011-5*) Datar Pub.

DAT - Dental Aptitude Test No. 1: Practice Exam Annotated Answers. David M. Tarlow. 2nd rev. ed. 1999. 20p. (C). pap. text 6.95 (*1-57732-080-8*) Datar Pub.

DAT - Dental Aptitude Test No. 1: Practice Examination. David M. Tarlow. 2nd annot. rev. ed. 1999. 40p. (C). pap. text 18.95 (*1-57732-079-4*) Datar Pub.

DAT - Dental Aptitude Test No. 2: Practice Exam Annotated Answers. David M. Tarlow. 2nd rev. ed. 1999. 20p. (C). pap. text 6.95 (*1-57732-082-4*) Datar Pub.

DAT - Dental Aptitude Test No. 2: Practice Examination. David M. Tarlow. 2nd rev. ed. 1999. 40p. (C). pap. text 18.95 (*1-57732-081-6*) Datar Pub.

DAT - Dental Aptitude Test No. 3: Practice Exam Annotated Answers. David M. Tarlow. 2nd rev. ed. 1999. 20p. (C). pap. text 6.95 (*1-57732-084-0*) Datar Pub.

DAT - Dental Aptitude Test No. 3: Practice Examination. David M. Tarlow. 2nd rev. ed. 1999. 40p. (C). pap. text 18.95 (*1-57732-083-2*) Datar Pub.

DAT - Dental Aptitude Test No. 4: Practice Exam Annotated Answers. David M. Tarlow. 2nd rev. ed. 1999. 20p. (C). pap. text 6.95 (*1-57732-086-7*) Datar Pub.

DAT - Dental Aptitude Test No. 4: Practice Examination. David M. Tarlow. 2nd rev. ed. 1999. 40p. (C). pap. text 18.95 (*1-57732-085-9*) Datar Pub.

DAT - Dental Aptitude Test No. 5: Practice Exam Annotated Answers. David M. Tarlow. 2nd rev. ed. 1999. (C). pap. text 6.95 (*1-57732-088-3*) Datar Pub.

DAT - Dental Aptitude Test No. 5: Practice Examination. David M. Tarlow. 2nd rev. ed. 1999. 40p. (C). pap. text 18.95 (*1-57732-087-5*) Datar Pub.

DAT - Dental Aptitude Test - Core Content. David M. Tarlow. 2nd rev. ed. 1999. (Illus.). 400p. pap. 49.95 (*1-57774-006-8*) Educ Tsting Cnslts.

DAT (Dental Aptitude Test) Practice Examination. David M. Tarlow. 1992. (Practice Examination Ser.). 40p. No. 1. pap. 16.95 (*0-931572-16-9*); No. 2. pap. 16.95 (*0-931572-12-6*); No. 3. pap. 16.95 (*0-931572-13-4*); No. 4. pap. 16.95 (*0-931572-14-2*); No. 5. pap. 16.95 (*0-931572-15-0*) Datar Pub.

DAT Exam No. 1 Annotated Answers (Dental Aptitude Test) David M. Tarlow. 7th ed. 1996. (Orig.). pap. 5.95 (*1-57732-017-4*) Datar Pub.

DAT Exam No. 2 Annotated Answers (Dental Aptitude Test) David M. Tarlow. 7th ed. 1996. pap. 5.95 (*1-57732-018-2*) Datar Pub.

DAT Exam No. 3 Annotated Answers (Dental Aptitude Test) David M. Tarlow. 7th ed. 1996. (Orig.). pap. 5.95 (*1-57732-019-0*) Datar Pub.

DAT Exam No. 4 Annotated Answers (Dental Aptitude Test) David M. Tarlow. 7th ed. 1996. (Orig.). pap. 5.95 (*1-57732-020-4*) Datar Pub.

DAT Exam No. 5 Annotated Answers (Dental Aptitude Test) David M. Tarlow. 7th ed. 1996. (Orig.). pap. 5.95 (*1-57732-021-2*) Datar Pub.

DAT Exam No. 1 (Dental Aptitude Test) David M. Tarlow. 7th ed. 1996. (Orig.). pap. (*1-57732-012-3*); pap. (*1-57732-013-1*) Datar Pub.

DAT Exam No. 3 (Dental Aptitude Test) David M. Tarlow. 7th ed. 1996. (Illus.). (Orig.). pap. (*1-57732-014-X*) Datar Pub.

DAT Exam No. 5 (Dental Aptitude Test) David M. Tarlow. 7th ed. 1996. (C). pap. (*1-57732-016-6*) Datar Pub.

DAT Exam No. 4 (Dental Aptitude Test) David M. Tarlow. 7th ed. 1996. (Orig.). (C). pap. (*1-57732-015-8*) Datar Pub.

DAT Practice Examination: Annotated Master Answer Guide. David M. Tarlow. 1992. No. 1. 4.95 (*0-931572-37-1*); No. 3. 4.95 (*0-931572-39-8*); No. 4. 4.95 (*0-931572-40-1*); No. 5. 4.95 (*0-931572-41-X*) Datar Pub.

Data Acquisition & Measurement Techniques. Ed. by Angel Munez-Ruiz & Herman Vromans. 1998. LC 98-7662. (Illus.). 398p. 229.00 (*1-57491-068-X*) IHS Health Grp.

Data Analysis: A Basic Introduction. David Fruin. 1980. (*0-7855-0562-8*) Natl Inst Soc Work GBR. *Dist:* St Mut.

Data Analysis & Statistics for Nursing Research. Denise F. Polit. 1996. LC 95-83509. 512p. pap. 59.00 (*0-8385-6329-5*, A6329-5) P-H.

Data Analysis & Statistics for Nursing Research: Application Manual. Denise Polit. 1996. 196p. (C). pap. 30.40 (*0-8385-6334-1*, A6334-5) Appleton & Lange.

Data Base & Know Base. Ullman. 1991. (C). text (*0-7167-8185-9*) W H Freeman.

Data Cleaning Procedures for the 1993 Robert Wood Johnson Foundation Family Health Insurance Survey. Linda M. Andrews et al. 1997. LC 97-18144. pap. text 9.00 (*0-8330-2523-6*) Rand Corp.

Data in Medicine. Ed. by Robert S. Reneman & Jan Strackee. 1979. (Instrumentation & Techniques in Clinical Medicine Ser.: No. 1). text 162.50 (*90-247-2150-4*) Kluwer Academic.

Data in Modern Biology: Selected Papers from the 9th International CODATA Conference, Jerusalem, Israel, June 1984. Ed. by CODATA Staff. 1985. (Illus.). 63p. pap. 11.00 (*0-08-032483-5*, Pergamon Pr) Elsevier.

Data Interpretation for Paediatric Examinations. C. O'Callaghan & T. Stephenson. 1995. (Illus.). 188p. pap. (*0-443-05010-4*) Church.

Data Interpretation Questions & Case Histories Pt. 2: MRCP. Ed. by H. L. Beynon et al. 2nd ed. 1998. (Illus.). 232p. pap. (*0-443-05694-3*) Church.

Data Interpretation Questions in Paediatrics. Fiona Finlay et al. 1998. LC 98-21391. (Illus.). pap. 41.95 (*0-632-05044-6*) Blackwell Sci.

Data on the Abnormal Hemoglobins & Glucose-Six-Phosphate Dehydrogenase Deficiency in Human Populations. Frank B. Livingstone. 1973. (Technical Reports Ser.: No. 3). pap. 2.00 (*0-932206-12-3*) U Mich Mus Anthro.

Data Priorities for Population & Health in Developing Countries: Summary of a Workshop. National Research Council Staff. 1996. LC 97-104354. 40p. (C). pap. text 10.00 (*0-309-05626-8*) Natl Acad Pr.

Data Quality in Longitudinal Research. Ed. by David Magnusson & Lars R. Bergman. 1990. (Illus.). 297p. (C). text 80.00 (*0-521-38091-X*) Cambridge U Pr.

***Data Questions for the MRCPCH,** Pt. 2. James Robertson. rev. ed. 2001. (Illus.). 203p. pap. (*0-443-06474-1*) Church GBR. *Dist:* Saunders.

Data Structured Software Maintenance: The Warnier-Orr Approach. David A. Higgins. 1986. LC 86-72048. (Illus.). 212p. (Orig.). pap. 23.95 (*0-932633-03-X*) Dorset Hse Pub.

Databases for Cardiology. Ed. by Greert T. Meester & Francesco Pinciroli. 1991. (Developments in Cardiovascular Medicine Ser.). (C). text 306.50 (*0-7923-0886-7*) Kluwer Academic.

Databook of Anesthesia & Critical Care Medicine. P. A. Foster & J. Roelofse. 4th ed. 1987. 204p. 41.95 (*0-387-17794-9*) Spr-Verlag.

Databook on Nonfatal Injury: Incidence, Costs, & Consequences. Ted R. Miller et al. 1995. 200p. (C). lib. bdg. 51.00 (*0-87766-630-X*) Urban Inst.

Dates in Cardiology: A Chronological Record of Progress in Cardiology over the Last Millennium. H. Lee. 2000. (Landmarks in Medicine Ser.). (Illus.). 124p. 31.95 (*1-85070-499-6*); LC 99-54489. 130p. lib. bdg. 31.95 (*1-85070-498-8*) CRC Pr (Parthenon Pbng).

Dates in Gastroenterology: A Chronological Record of Progress in Gastroenterology over the Last Millennium. H. Lee. 2000. (Landmarks in Medicine Ser.). (Illus.). 100p. lib. bdg. 31.95 (*1-85070-502-X*, Parthenon Pbng) CRC Pr.

Dates in Medicine: A Chronological Record of Medical Progress over Three Millennia. A. Sebastian. 2000. LC 99-25481. (Illus.). 444p. 63.95 (*1-85070-095-8*, Parthenon Pbng) CRC Pr.

Dates in Neurology: A Chronological Record of Progress in Neurology over the Last Millennium. H. Lee. 2000. (Landmarks in Medicine Ser.). (Illus.). 164p. lib. bdg. 31.95 (*1-85070-529-1*, Parthenon Pbng) CRC Pr.

Dates in Obstetrics & Gynecology: A Chronological Record of Progress in Obstetrics & Gynecology over the Last Millennium. H. Lee. 2000. LC 99-57140. (Landmarks in Medicine Ser.). (Illus.). 130p. lib. bdg. 31.95 (*1-85070-516-X*, Parthenon Pbng) CRC Pr.

***Dates in Ophthalmology.** D. Albert. 2002. (Illus.). 130p. 49.95 (*1-84214-113-9*, Parthenon Pbng) CRC Pr.

Dates in Urology: A Chronological Record of Progress in Urology over the Last Millennium. H. Lee. 2000. LC 99-55487. (Landmarks in Medicine Ser.). (Illus.). 120p. lib. bdg. 31.95 (*1-85070-496-1*, Parthenon Pbng) CRC Pr.

Daughtering & Mothering: Female Subjectivity Reanalysed. Ed. by Janneke Van Mens-Verhulst et al. 1993. LC 93-14821. 454p. (C). pap. 27.95 (*0-415-08650-7*, B0899) Routledge.

Daughter's Seduction: Feminism & Psychoanalysis. Jane Gallop. LC 81-70709. 164p. 1984. pap. 16.95 (*0-8014-9235-1*); 1982. 35.00 (*0-8014-1493-8*) Cornell U Pr.

David Glendenning Cogan, M. D. The Howe Laboratory of Ophthalmology at Harvard Medical School, the Massachusetts Eye & Ear Infirmary, & the National Eye Institute. David G. Cogan. 1990. (Ophthalmology Oral History Ser.). (Illus.). xxvii, 284p. pap. 45.00 (*0-926886-05-3*) FAAO.

David Livingstone. J. H. Worchester. 1980. (Golden Oldies Ser.). 128p. (gr. 8 up). mass mkt. 5.99 (*0-8024-4782-1*, 378) Moody.

Davidson's Human Nutrition & Dietetics. Ed. by John Garrow & Philip James. 9th ed. 1993. (Illus.). pap. text (*0-443-04121-0*) Church.

Davidson's Principals & Practices of Medicine. Edwards. 17th ed. 1995. pap. text 52.00 (*0-443-04961-0*) Saunders.

Davidson's Principles & Practice of Medicine. Christopher R. Edwards. 16th ed. 1991. (Illus.). 1048p. pap. text (*0-443-04092-3*) Church.

Davies's Textbook of Adverse Drug Reactions. D. M. Davies. 5th ed. 1999. (Illus.). 992p. text (*0-412-82480-9*) E A GBR. *Dist:* OUP.

Davis Book of Medical Abbreviations. Sara L. Mitchell-Hatton. 1991. LC 91-9422. 1028p. pap. text 38.95 (*0-8036-6268-8*) Davis Co.

Davis' Drug Guide for Nurses. Judith Hopfer Deglin & April Hazard Vallerand. 7th ed. 2000. (Illus.). 1358p. 32.95 (*0-8036-0583-8*); pap. text 36.95 incl. disk (*0-8036-0582-X*) Davis Co.

Davis's Clinical Guide to Health Assessment. Ed. by Patricia G. Morton et al. 2nd ed. 1995. (Illus.). 340p. (C). pap. text 31.95 (*0-8036-0119-0*) Davis Co.

Davis's Drug Guide for Nurses Judith H. Deglin. 7th ed. 2000. 1358p. pap. 59.95 (*0-8036-0733-4*) Davis Co.

Davis's Electronic Drug Guide for Nurses: Includes Davis's Drug Guide for Nurses. Judith H. Deglin & April H. Vallerand. 1999. 1203p. (C). 49.95 incl. cd-rom (*0-8036-0495-5*) Davis Co.

Davis's Guide to IV Medications. April H. Vallerand & Judith H. Deglin. 3rd ed. 1995. LC 95-21035. (Illus.). 1101p. (C). pap. 29.95 (*0-8036-0092-5*) Davis Co.

Davis's Laboratory & Diagnostic Test Handbook. Marie S. Jaffe. 1997. LC 96-45650. 1494p. pap. 31.95 (*0-8036-0088-7*) Davis Co.

Davis's Manual of Critical Care Therapeutics. Kathleen M. Baldwin et al. 1995. LC 94-37605. (Illus.). 757p. (C). pap. text 33.95 (*0-8036-0574-9*) Davis Co.

Davis's Manual of Nursing Therapeutics for Diseases & Disorders. Ed. by Marilyn S. Sommers & Susan A. Johnson. 1996. LC 96-24491. (Illus.). 1132p. (C). pap. text 37.95 (*0-8036-0018-6*) Davis Co.

Davis's Manual of Psychosocial Nursing in General Patient Care. Linda M. Gorman et al. 1996. LC 95-48201. (Illus.). 617p. (C). pap. text 31.95 (*0-8036-0113-1*) Davis Co.

Davis's NCLEX-PN Review Book. Ed. by Patricia G. Beare et al. 2nd ed. 1998. LC 98-27802. (Illus.). 512p. pap. 31.95 (*0-8036-0403-3*) Davis Co.

Davis's NCLEX-RN Health Assessment Review Cards: Including Lab & Diagnostic Aspects. Patricia G. Beare. 1991. 320p. (C). 21.95 (*0-8036-0687-7*) Davis Co.

Davis's NCLEX-RN Nutrition Review Cards: The Passing Game. Patricia G. Beare. 1991. 176p. (C). pap. 17.95 (*0-8036-0673-7*) Davis Co.

Davis's NCLEX-RN Review. Patricia G. Beare. 3rd rev. ed. 2000. 676p. pap. text 34.95 (*0-8036-0577-3*) Davis Co.

Davis's Pharmacology Review for the NCLEX-RN. Joseph T. Catalano. 1999. LC 99-17377. (Illus.). 357p. pap. 27.95 (*0-8036-0404-1*, C3922) Davis Co.

Davis's Q & A for the NCLEX-RN. Patricia G. Beare & Patricia E. Thompson. 1998. LC 97-29247. (Illus.). 648p. (C). pap. text 31.95 (*0-8036-0282-0*) Davis Co.

Dawn of Modern Medicine. Albert H. Buck. LC 75-23687. reprint ed. 49.50 (*0-404-13240-5*) AMS Pr.

Dax's Case: Essays in Medical Ethics & Human Meaning. Lonnie D. Kleiver. 1989. 252p. 24.95 (*0-87074-277-9*) Phoenix Soc.

Dax's Case: Essays in Medical Ethics & Human Meaning. Lonnie D. Kliever. 1989. LC 88-42636. 252p. pap. 12.50 (*0-87074-278-7*) SMU Press.

Day at a Time: A Day at a Time. James Jennings. 1986. LC 93-46392. 384p. 8.95 (*1-56838-075-5*) Hazelden.

Day Brought Back My Night: Ageing & New Vision Loss. Stephen Ainlay. 1989. 176p. 29.95 (*0-415-00764-X*) Routledge.

Day by Day Diabetes: 1998 Calendar. Resa Levetan. 1997. 370p. pap. 9.95 (*1-883205-41-7*) Intl Med Pub.

Day Care Anaesthesia. Ed. by Ian Smith. 2001. (Fundamentals of Anaesthesia & Acute Medicine Ser.). (Illus.). 250p. pap. text (*0-7279-1422-7*) BMJ Pub GBR. *Dist:* AIDC.

Day Care Center Aide. Jack Rudman. 1994. (Career Examination Ser.: C-1235). pap. 23.95 (*0-8373-1235-3*) Nat Learn.

Day-Case Anaesthesia & Sedation: Anaesthesia & Sedation for Day-Case Procedures & Ambulatory Surgery. J. G. Whitwam. 1994. LC 93-34778. (Illus.). 440p. 99.95 (*0-632-03704-0*) Blackwell Sci.

Day Dreaming-Night Thinking: Roaming in Two Worlds. Colin P. Osborne, III. 1982. LC 81-84497. (Illus.). 80p. 7.50 (*0-9607332-2-1*) Ololon Pubns.

Day I Died: One Man's Successful Battle Back from the Dead. Jay Barbree. 1990. LC 90-53405. 296p. 19.95 (*0-88282-061-3*) New Horizon NJ.

Day Room: A Memoir of Madness & Mending. Kathleen Crowley. 1995. LC 94-46756. 178p. 19.95 (*0-9643348-0-1*) Kennedy Carlisle.

Day Surgery: A Handbook for Nurses. Elizabeth Sutherland. 1997. (Illus.). 220p. pap. text (*0-7020-1988-7*) W B Saunders GBR. *Dist:* Saunders.

Day Surgery: A Nursing Approach. Ed. by Debbie Hodge. 1998. 247p. (C). pap. text (*0-443-05343-X*) Church.

Day Surgery: Principles-Nursing. Heather Cahill. 1997. pap. text (*0-7020-2028-1*) Bailliere Tindall.

Day Treatment for Children with Emotional Disorders Vol. 1: Model in Action. S. G. Zimet & G. K. Farley. 1991. LC 91-2086. (Illus.). 296p. (C). 54.50 (*0-306-43743-0*, Plenum Trade) Perseus Pubng.

Day Treatment for Children with Emotional Disorders Vol. 2: Models Across the Country. S. G. Zimet & G. K. Farley. 1991. (Illus.). 248p. (C). 54.50 (*0-306-43744-9*, Plenum Trade) Perseus Pubng.

Days of Healing, Days of Joy: Daily Meditations for Adult Children. Earnie Larsen & Carole L. Hagarty. 1996. 400p. pap. 10.00 (*0-89486-455-6*, 5024A) Hazelden.

Daytop Village: A Therapeutic Community. Ed. by Louise S. Spindler et al. 1983. (Case Studies in Cultural Anthropology). (Illus.). 140p. (C). reprint ed. pap. 7.95 (*0-8290-0589-7*) Irvington.

DC 0-3 Casebook: A Guide to the Use of Zero to Three's Diagnostic Classification of Mental Health & Developmental Disorders of Infancy & Early Childhood in Assessment & Treatment Planning. Ed. by Alicia F. Lieberman et al. 1997. 350p. pap. 35.00 (*0-943657-38-5*) ZERO TO THREE.

DCR Budapest-Nashville in the Diagnosis & Classification of Functional Psychoses. Ed. by B. Pethoe. 1989. (Journal: Vol. 21, Nos. 4-5, 1988). (Illus.). 92p. pap. 65.25 (*3-8055-4970-9*) S Karger.

De Anima. Ed. by W. David Ross. 1956. (Oxford Classical Texts). 122p. text 24.95 (*0-19-814508-X*) OUP.

De Anima. Aristotle. Tr. & Intro. by Robert Drew Hicks. 1980. LC 75-13252. (History of Ideas in Ancient Greece Ser.). reprint ed. 47.95 (*0-405-07289-9*) Ayer.

De Anima With Passages from Book I, Bks. II-III. Aristotle. Tr. & Intro. by David W. Hamlyn. rev. ed. 1993. (Clarendon Aristotle Ser.). 212p. (C). pap. text 23.00 (*0-19-824085-6*) OUP.

De Animalibus Pt. 2, Bks. XI-XIV: Parts of Animals. Aristotle. Tr. by Michael Scot from ARA. 1998. (Aristoteles Semitico-Latinus Ser.: Vol. 10). 600p. 161.00 (*90-04-11070-4*) Brill Academic Pubs.

De Corporibus Marinis Lapidescentibus Quae Defossa Reperuntur Addita Dissertatione Fabii Columnae Glossopetris: On Petrified Marine Bodies Discovered Buried, to Which Is Appended a Dissertation by

Fabio Colonna on Tongue Stones. Agostino Scilla. Ed. by Stephen Jay Gould. 1980. LC 79-8349. (History of Paleontology Ser.). (LAT., Illus.). reprint ed. lib. bdg. 16.95 (*0-405-12742-1*) Ayer.

De Humani Corporis Fabrica Libri Septem see On the Fabric of the Human Body, Bk. 1, The Bones & Cartilages

De la Folie: Considerations Sur Cette Maladie. Etienne-Jean Georget. 1976. LC 75-16705. (Classics in Psychiatry Ser.). (FRE.). reprint ed. 44.95 (*0-405-07431-X*) Ayer.

De la Folie: Consideree Sous le Point de Vue Pathologique, Philosophique, Historique et Judiciai Re Louis-Florentin Calmeil. 1976. LC 75-16695. (Classics in Psychiatry Ser.). (FRE.). reprint ed. 87.95 (*0-405-07423-9*) Ayer.

De la Paralysie Consideree chez les Alienes. Louis-Florentin Calmeil. 1976. LC 75-16696. (Classics in Psychiatry Ser.). (FRE.). reprint ed. 39.95 (*0-405-07424-7*) Ayer.

De los Anteojos a la Cirugia Refractiva. Rogelio Herreman. (Ciencia para Todos Ser.). (SPA.). pap. 6.99 (*968-16-3151-X*) Fondo CA.

De Medicina Tr. by W. G. Spencer. (Loeb Classical Library: No. 292, 304, 336). 1. 1935. 504p. 18.95 (*0-674-99322-5*); 2. 1938. 360p. 18.95 (*0-674-99335-7*) HUP.

De Medicina, 3. Celsus. 1938. (Loeb Classical Library: No. 292, 304, 336). 656p. 18.95 (*0-674-99370-5*) HUP.

De Motu Cordis: Anatomical Studies on the Motion of the Heart & Blood. William Harvey. Tr. by Chauncey D. Leake. 5th ed. 1977. (Illus.). 186p. 39.95 (*0-398-00793-4*) C C Thomas.

De-NolR, Mucosal Protection & Peptic Ulcer Disease: Journal, Digestion, Supplement 2, 1987, Vol. 37. Ed. by Guido N. Tytgat. 1987. (Illus.). iv, 64p. 21.00 (*3-8055-4617-3*) S Karger.

De-Sensitization by Systematic Steps with Relaxation, Set-D. Russell E. Mason. 1975. pap. 35.00 incl. audio (*0-89533-005-9*) F I Comm.

Deaconess Heritage: One Hundred Years of Caring, Healing & Teaching. Ruth W. Rasche. 1994. 350p. pap. 9.95 (*0-9642849-0-1*) Deaconess Fnd.

Dead Reckoning: The Art of Forensic Detection. Jon J. Nordby. 1999. LC 99-40308. 304p. per. 49.95 (*0-8493-8122-3*) CRC Pr.

Dead Without a Fight: Diseases & Their Treatment in the Mexican War. Robert H. Dorian. 1998. 43p. pap. 7.95 (*0-9647895-3-1*) FLPB Pr.

Deadly Deception: The Proof That Sex & HIV Absolutely Do Not Cause AIDS. Robert E. Willner. 1994. 300p. 23.95 (*0-9642316-1-1*) Peltec Pubng.

Deadly Diet: Recovering from Anorexia & Bulimia. Terence J. Sandbek. 2nd rev. ed. 1993. LC 92-50707. 256p. pap. 14.95 (*1-879237-42-3*) New Harbinger.

Deadly Doctrine: Health, Illness & God-Talk. Wendell Watters. 1992. LC 92-29838. 198p. 35.00 (*0-87975-782-5*) Prometheus Bks.

Deadly Doses: A Writer's Guide to Poisons. Serita D. Stevens & Anne Klarner. 1990. LC 90-12227. (Howdunit Writing Ser.). 298p. pap. 16.99 (*0-89879-371-8*, 10177, Wrtrs Digest Bks) F & W Pubns Inc.

Deadly Drug Interactions: The People's Pharmacy Guide. Joe Graedon & Teresa Graedon. 1997. 447p. pap. 14.95 (*0-312-15510-7*, St Martin Griffin); 1995. LC 95-34800. (Illus.). 432p. 25.95 (*0-312-13243-3*); 1999. LC 99-204800. 510p. mass mkt. 6.99 (*0-312-96826-4*) St Martin.

Deadly Emotions: The Role of Anger, Hostility & Aggression in Health & Emotional Well-Being. Ernest H. Johnson. 1990. LC 90-35100. 240p. 67.00 (*0-275-93590-6*, C3590, Praeger Pubs) Greenwood.

Deadly Fashion: The Rise & Fall of Cigarette Smoking in North America. Roberta G. Ferrence. 1990. (Studies in Historical Demography). 300p. reprint ed. text 20.00 (*0-8240-4671-4*) Garland.

Deadly Feasts: The "Prion" Controversy & the Public's Health. Richard Rhodes. 1998. (Illus.). 272p. per. 13.00 (*0-684-84425-7*, Touchstone) S&S Trade Pap.

Deadly Feasts: Tracking the Secrets of a Terrifying New Plague. Richard Rhodes. 1997. LC 97-320. 259p. 24.00 (*0-684-82360-8*) S&S Trade.

Deadly Karate Blows - The Medical Implications. Brian Adams. rev. ed. 1986. LC 86-50088. 136p. (Orig.). reprint ed. pap. 10.95 (*0-86568-077-9*, 312) Unique Pubns.

Deadly Medicine: Why Tens of Thousands of Hearts Died in America's Worst Drug Disaster. Thomas J. Moore. 1995. LC 94-43501. 349p. 23.00 (*0-684-80417-4*) S&S Trade.

Deaf Adult Speaks Out. Leo M. Jacobs. 3rd rev. ed. 1989. LC 89-11787. 182p. pap. text 12.95 (*0-930323-61-0*) Gallaudet Univ Pr.

Deaf & Dumb. Edwin J. Mann. 1972. 59.95 (*0-8490-0002-5*) Gordon Pr.

Deaf-Blind Infants & Children: A Developmental Guide. John M. McInnes & Jacqueline A. Treffry. 1994. 480p. pap. text 17.95 (*0-8020-7787-0*) U of Toronto Pr.

Deaf Empowerment: Emergence, Struggle & Rhetoric. Katherine A. Jankowski. 1997. LC 97-11897. (Illus.). 206p. 34.95 (*1-56368-061-0*) Gallaudet Univ Pr.

Deaf Experience: An Anthology of Literature by & about the Deaf. Ed. by Trenton W. Batson & Eugene Bergman. 2nd ed. 1976. LC 76-27476. 384p. (C). (gr. 10-12). pap. 9.00 (*0-914562-03-7*) Merriam-Eddy.

Deaf Experience: Classics in Language & Education. Ed. by Harlan Lane. Tr. by Franklin Philip from FRE. 1984. (Illus.). 240p. 40.00 (*0-674-19460-8*) HUP.

Deaf Heritage: A Narrative History of Deaf America. Jack Gannon. 1981. (Illus.). 483p. (C). pap. 21.95 (*0-913072-38-9*) Natl Assn Deaf.

Deaf History Unveiled: Interpretations from the New Scholarship. Ed. by John V. Van Cleve. 1993. LC 93-12018. (Illus.). 316p. (C). text 39.95 (*1-56368-021-1*) Gallaudet Univ Pr.

Deaf Like Me. Thomas S. Spradley & James P. Spradley. 1985. LC 85-4468. 292p. reprint ed. pap. 12.95 (*0-930323-11-4*) Gallaudet Univ Pr.

Deaf Population of the United States. Jerome Schein & Marcus Delk. 1974. 4.95 (*0-913072-43-5*) Natl Assn Deaf.

Deaf Sport: The Impact of Sports Within the Deaf Community. David A. Stewart. 1991. LC 91-2056. 248p. (C). text 24.95 (*0-930323-74-2*) Gallaudet Univ Pr.

Deaf Way: Perspectives from the International Conference on Deaf Culture. Ed. by Bruce D. Snider et al. 1994. LC 94-17860. 944p. 95.00 (*1-56368-026-2*) Gallaudet Univ Pr.

Deafmutism. James K. Love. 1976. 250.00 (*0-87968-303-1*) Gordon Pr.

Deafmutism. Holger Mygind. 1976. 300.00 (*0-8490-0008-4*) Gordon Pr.

Deafmutism & the Education of Deafmutes by Lip-Reading & Articulation. Arthur Hartmann. 1976. 250.00 (*0-87968-090-3*) Gordon Pr.

Deafness: An Annotated Bibliography & Guide to Basic Materials. Ed. by Gail Kovalik et al. 1992. 244p. 30.00 (*0-8389-7578-X*) ASCLA.

Deafness & Mental Health. John C. Denmark. 1993. LC 94-181829. 160p. pap. 24.95 (*1-85302-212-8*) Taylor & Francis.

Deafness & Mental Health. Ed. by Laszlo K. Stein et al. 1981. 256p. text 42.00 (*0-8089-1347-6*, 794328, Grune & Strat) Harcrt Hlth Sci Grp.

Deafness & Vision Disorders: Anatomy & Physiology, Assessment Procedures, Ocular Anomalies & Educational Implications. Donald D. Johnson. 1999. LC 98-52323. (Illus.). xiii, 490p. 77.95 (*0-398-06945-X*) C C Thomas.

Deafness, Deprivation, & IQ. J. P. Braden. 1994. (Perspectives on Individual Differences Ser.). (Illus.). 242p. (C). 39.50 (*0-306-44686-3*, Plenum Trade) Perseus Pubng.

Deafness, Development & Literacy. Alec Webster. 1986. (Illus.). 180p. text 45.00 (*0-416-92050-0*, 9998); 288p. (C). pap. 24.95 (*0-416-92060-8*, 1010) Routledge.

***Dealing: Women in the Drug Economy.** Barbara A. Denton. 2001. 227p. pap. (*0-86840-627-9*) New South Wales Univ Pr AUS. *Dist:* U of Wash Pr.

Dealing Creatively with Death: A Manual of Death Education & Simple Burial. Ernest Morgan. 10th ed. 1984. LC 83-71373. (Simple Burial Ser.). 168p. (Orig.). pap. 9.00 (*0-914064-19-3*) Zinn Pub Grp.

Dealing Direct: A Strategy for Business-Provider Partnerships. E. Preston Gee & Allan Fine. 1997. LC 96-50461. (Illus.). 112p. (Orig.). pap. 32.50 (*1-55648-180-2*, 067104) AHPI.

Dealing, Feeling & Breathing Better with Asthma. P. D. Jordan. 1990. LC 89-82764. 96p. (Orig.). pap. text 11.95 (*0-929885-09-0*) Haypenny Pr.

Dealing with Anger. Sandy Livingstone & SL Discovery Consulting Services Staff. Ed. by Judith Johnson. 2nd rev. ed. 1997. (Illus.). 168p. pap. (*0-9681793-1-2*) SL Discovery Consult.

Dealing with Anger Problems: Rational-Emotive Therapeutic Interventions. Windy Dryden. Ed. by Harold H. Smith, Jr. 1990. LC 90-52986. (Practitioner's Resource Ser.). 60p. pap. 15.95 (*0-943158-59-1*, DAPBP, Prof Resc Pr) Pro Resource.

Dealing with Challenges in Psychotherapy & Counseling. Christiane Brems. 1999. LC 99-19539. (Counseling Ser.). 350p. pap. text 48.95 (*0-534-36471-3*) Brooks-Cole.

Dealing with Challenging Dialysis Patient Situations: A Resource Guide Designed Specifically for Nephrology Professionals. Mary Rau-Foster. 1999. xiv, 234p. 100.00 incl. disk (*1-930069-00-6*) F S C Pubng.

Dealing with Dementia: Optimizing Functional & Life-Quality Outcomes. Ed. by Anne M. Christner. 1997. 150p. (Orig.). pap. 69.00 (*1-884937-44-6*) Manisses Communs.

Dealing with Depression: Five Pastoral Interventions. Richard Dayringer. 1995. LC 94-33088. (Illus.). 182p. pap. 14.95 (*1-56024-967-6*, Harrington Park) Haworth Pr.

Dealing with Depression: Five Pastoral Interventions. Richard Dayringer & Byron Eicher. 1995. LC 94-33088. (Illus.). 175p. lib. bdg. 39.95 (*1-56024-933-1*) Haworth Pr.

Dealing with Depression in 12 Step Recovery. Jack O. 1990. LC 90-14047. (Fellow Travelers Ser.). 72p. (Orig.). pap. 4.95 (*0-934125-13-9*) Hazelden.

Dealing with Depression Naturally. Syd Baumel. 1995. LC 94-48656. 240p. (Orig.). pap. 19.95 (*0-87983-645-8*, Keats Pubng) McGraw-Hill Trade.

Dealing with Dilemma: A Manual for Genetic Counselors. P. T. Kelly. 1977. (Heidelberg Science Library). pap. 19.50 (*3-540-90237-6*) Spr-Verlag.

Dealing with Genes: The Language of Heredity. Paul Berg & Maxine Singer. 1992. (Illus.). 269p. (C). text 38.00 (*0-935702-69-5*) Univ Sci Bks.

Dealing with Medical Knowledge: Computers in Clinical Decision Making. Tibor Deutsch et al. 1994. LC 94-24011. (Illus.). 310p. (C). text 79.50 (*0-306-44849-1*, Kluwer Plenum) Kluwer Academic.

Dealing with Medical Malpractice: The British & Swedish Experience. Marilynn M. Rosenthal. 1988. LC 87-27245. xviii, 270p. (C). text 53.00 (*0-8223-0830-4*) Duke.

Dealing with the Problem of Low Self-Esteem: Common Characteristics & Treatment in Individual, Marital-Family & Group Psychotherapy. Robert P. Rugel. LC 94-33872. 228p. (C). 1995. (Illus.). pap. 37.95 (*0-398-05951-9*); 1994. text 50.95 (*0-398-05936-5*) C C Thomas.

Dealing with the Therapist's Vulnerability to Depression. Sheldon Heath. 1991. LC 90-15591. 192p. 40.00 (*0-87668-612-9*) Aronson.

Dear Dentist: Stop Being Your Own Worst Enemy. R. H. Schaper. 1994. LC 94-1885. (Illus.). 44.95 (*0-87814-418-8*) PennWell Corp.

Dear Diabetes Advisor. American Diabetes Association. 1997. LC 97-10397. (Illus.). 120p. pap. 11.95 (*0-945448-83-X*, 4813-01) Am Diabetes.

Dear Lucille: Breast Cancer: a Woman's Journal. Ilse E. Gilliland. 1994. pap. text (*1-886563-01-2*) Women in Process.

Dear Progeny. Michael F. Keleher. 1992. 720p. 40.00 (*0-9632949-0-3*) Value Quest Grp.

"Dear Teacher"! Eyes & Their Signals: A Handbook. Vera Ives. 1997. LC 97-36546. 31p. pap. 8.00 (*0-943599-96-2*) OEPF.

Death: 5 Sermons. Charles Haddon Spurgeon. 1978. pap. 4.00 (*1-56186-411-0*) Pilgrim Pubns.

Death: Medical, Spiritual & Social Care of the Dying. Ed. by H. M. Kuitert et al. 1997. 250p. (*90-5383-503-2*) VUB Univ Pr BEL. *Dist:* Paul & Co Pubs.

Death & Attitudes Towards Death. Stacey B. Day. 1984. LC 72-76821. Orig. Title: Proceedings A Symposium of the Bell Museum, Univ. of Minn. Med. School. 94p. (Orig.). reprint ed. 10.00 (*0-934314-76-4*) Intl Found Biosocial Dev.

Death & Dying: A Bibliography 1950-1974: Supplement, Vol. I: Suicide. G. Howard Poteet & Joseph C. Santora. 1978. LC 76-24093. xxii, 166p. 29.00 (*0-87875-108-4*) Whitston Pub.

Death & Dying: Values, Institutions, & Human Mortality. David W. Moller. 1996. (Illus.). 320p. (C). pap. text 23.95 (*0-19-504296-4*) OUP.

Death & Dying: Views from Many Cultures. Ed. by Richard A. Kalish. 1980. (Perspectives on Death & Dying Ser.: Vol. 1). 157p. (C). pap. 21.95 (*0-89503-012-8*) Baywood Pub.

Death & Dying, Life & Living. Charles A. Corr et al. 3rd ed. 1999. LC 99-30555. (Psychology Ser.). 688p. pap. text 66.95 (*0-534-36538-8*) Brooks-Cole.

Death & Dying Sourcebook: Basic Information for the Layperson about End-of-Life Care & Related Issues. Ed. by Annemarie Muth. 1999. LC 99-44810. (Health Reference Ser.). (Illus.). xiii, 641p. lib. bdg. 78.00 (*0-7808-0230-6*) Omnigraphics Inc.

Death & Ethnicity: A Psychocultural Study. Richard A. Kalish & David K. Reynolds. 1976. LC 81-65932. (Perspectives on Death & Dying Ser.: Vol. 4). 230p. (C). reprint ed. pap. text 29.95 (*0-89503-021-7*) Baywood Pub.

Death & Identity. Ed. by Robert Fulton & Robert Bendiksen. 3rd ed. 1994. LC 93-26364. 480p. (C). pap. text 24.95 (*0-914783-63-7*) Charles.

Death & Neurosis. Joachim E. Meyer. Tr. by Margarete Nunberg. 1975. LC 73-19951. 159p. (C). 35.00 (*0-8236-1130-2*) Intl Univs Pr.

Death & Post-Mortem Changes—Normal, Rare, Bizzare & Mysterious: Index of New Information. Willie S. Pelton. rev. ed. 1998. 157p. 57.50 (*0-7883-1462-9*); pap. 47.50 (*0-7883-1463-7*) ABBE Pubs Assn.

Death & Postmortem Changes-Normal, Rare, Bizarre & Mysterious: Index of New Information. Willis S. Pelton. 1994. 150p. 57.50 (*0-7883-0054-7*); pap. 47.50 (*0-7883-0055-5*) ABBE Pubs Assn.

Death & Trauma: The Traumatology of Grieving. Ed. by Charles R. Figley et al. 1997. LC 96-47172. (Series in Trauma & Loss). 250p. 69.95 (*1-56032-525-9*); pap. 26.95 (*1-56032-526-7*) Hemisp Pub.

Death Anxiety: The Loss of the Self. James B. McCarthy. 1980. text 27.95 (*0-89876-069-0*) Gardner Pr.

Death Anxiety Handbook. Ed. by Robert A. Neimeyer. 1994. (Series in Death Education, Aging, & Health Care). 312p. (*1-56032-282-9*) P Chapman GBR. *Dist:* Taylor & Francis.

Death Attitudes & the Older Adult. Adrian Tomer. 2000. LC 00-37859. (Series in Death, Dying & Bereavement). 264p. pap. 29.95 (*0-87630-989-9*) Brunner-Routledge.

Death Book: Terrors, Consolations, Contradictions & Paradoxes. Joseph A. Amato. 1985. 13.95 (*0-9614119-1-0*) Crossings Pr.

Death, Brain Death & Ethics. David Lamb. 1996. (Avebury Series in Philosophy). 144p. text (*1-85972-506-6*) Avebry GBR. *Dist:* Ashgate Pub Co.

Death by Deception: Unmasking Heart Failure. Dick Quinn et al. 1996. (Illus.). 225p. (Orig.). pap. 12.95 (*0-9653346-0-0*) R F Quinn.

Death by Denial: Studies of Suicide in Gay & Lesbian Teenagers. Ed. by Gary Remafedi. 1993. LC 95-120623. 205p. pap. 9.95 (*1-55583-260-1*) Alyson Pubns.

Death by Diet. Robert R. Barefoot. 1996. 144p. pap. 14.95 (*0-9633703-3-2*) Bokar Cnslts.

Death by Migration: Europe's Encounter with the Tropical World in the Nineteenth Century. Philip De Armond Curtin. 1989. (Illus.). 271p. (C). pap. text 19.95 (*0-521-38922-4*) Cambridge U Pr.

Death Deferred: How to Prolong Life & Postpone Death. H. Carrington. 1991. lib. bdg. 250.00 (*0-87700-945-7*) Revisionist Pr.

Death, Dying, & Euthanasia. Ed. by Dennis J. Horan & David Mall. 1980. LC 77-72189. 837p. pap. 21.95 (*0-313-27092-9*, P7092); lib. bdg. 95.00 (*0-313-27097-X*, U7097) Greenwood (Greenwood Pr).

Death, Dying & the Law. A. R. Forrest. Ed. by Vivienne Harpwood. 1996. (Medico-Legal Practitioner Ser.). 250p. pap. (*1-85941-015-4*) Cavendish Pubng GBR. *Dist:* Gaunt.

Death, Dying & the Law. Sheila A. McLean. 1996. LC 95-34897. (Medico-Legal Issues Ser.). (Illus.). 200p. text (*1-85521-657-4*) Dartmth Pub GBR. *Dist:* Ashgate Pub Co.

Death, Dying, Transcending. Ed. by Richard A. Kalish. 1980. (Perspectives on Death & Dying Ser.: Vol. 3). 160p. (C). pap. 21.95 (*0-89503-011-X*) Baywood Pub.

Death Education & Research: Critical Perspectives. Pref. by W. G. Warren. 1989. LC 88-37599. (Gerontology & Geriatrics Education Ser.: Vol. 9, Nos. 1 & 2). (Illus.). 212p. text 49.95 (*0-86656-814-X*) Haworth Pr.

Death Education for the Health Professional. Ed. by Jeanne Q. Benoliel. 1982. LC 81-20153. (Death Education, Aging & Health Care Ser.). (Illus.). 118p. text 60.95 (*0-89116-248-8*) Hemisp Pub.

Death in Abeyance: Illness & Therapies among the Tabwa of Zaire/Congo. Christopher Davis. 2000. LC 2001-326023. (International African Library: Vol. 23). (Illus.). x, 342p. pap. text (*0-7486-1305-6*) Edinburgh U Pr GBR. *Dist:* Col U Pr.

Death in the Family: Orphans of the HIV Epidemic. Ed. by Carol Levine. 1993. LC 93-21517. 10.00 (*1-881277-13-5*) United Hosp Fund.

Death in the School Community: A Handbook for Counselors, Teachers & Administrators. Martha Oates. 1993. LC 92-21966. 129p. (C). pap. text 31.95 (*1-55620-099-4*, 72040) Am Coun Assn.

Death Investigation: The Basics. Brad Randall. 1997. LC 97-2185. (Illus.). 150p. (Orig.). pap. 24.95 (*1-883620-24-4*) Galen AZ.

Death Investigation Evidence Manual. 1994. (Illus.). 132p. (Orig.). (C). pap. text 40.00 (*0-7881-0286-9*) DIANE Pub.

Death Log. James Romenesko. 1982. LC 82-90083. (Orig.). pap. 9.95 (*0-942724-00-3*) Police Beat Pr.

Death of an Adult Child: A Book for & about Bereaved Parents. Jeanne W. Blank. 1998. LC 97-9835. (Death, Value & Meaning Ser.). 324p. text 44.95 (*0-89503-178-7*) Baywood Pub.

Death of Medicine in Nazi Germany: Dermatology & Dermatopathology under the Swastika. Wolfgang Weyers. Ed. by A. Bernard Ackerman. 1998. (Illus.). 472p. pap. 18.95 (*1-56833-122-3*); 49.95 (*1-56833-121-5*) Madison Bks UPA.

Death of Psychoanalysis: Murder? Suicide? or Rumor Greatly Exaggerated. Robert M. Prince. 1998. LC 97-37074. xxv, 378p. pap. 50.00 (*0-7657-0147-2*) Aronson.

Death on Demand: Physician-Assisted Suicide in the United States a Legal Research Pathfinder. Cathleen DeSimone. 1996. LC 95-33290. (Legal Research Guides Ser.: Vol. 26). 57p. 42.00 (*0-89941-983-6*, 308910) W S Hein.

Death on Hemodialysis: Preventable or Inevitable? Ed. by E. A. Friedman. 1994. LC 93-42588. (Developments in Nephrology Ser.: Vol. 35). 224p. (C). text 127.50 (*0-7923-2652-0*) Kluwer Academic.

Death on Request U. S. A. Thomas S. Miles. 1999. 104p. pap. 11.00 (*0-8059-4573-3*) Dorrance.

Death Sentence of AIDS: A Comprehensive Source Book of Quotes by the World's Leading Physicians, Scientists & Researchers. Troy R. Mader. 1987. LC 87-72211. (Orig.). pap. 9.94 (*0-944402-00-3*) Cmmn Man Inst.

Death Stalks the Yakama: Epidemiological Transitions & Mortality on the Yakama Indian Reservation, 1888-1964. Clifford E. Trafzer. 1997. LC 96-52172. 220p. (Orig.). pap. 24.95 (*0-87013-463-9*) Mich St U Pr.

Death Talk: Conversations with Children & Families. G. Fredman. 1997. LC 98-150403. 176p. pap. (*1-85575-174-7*) Karnac Bks GBR. *Dist:* Other Pr LLC.

***Death Talk: The Case Against Euthanasia & Physician-Assisted Suicide.** Margaret A. Somerville. 2002. (Illus.). 464p. text (*0-7735-2201-8*); pap. text (*0-7735-2245-X*) McG-Queens Univ Pr.

Death Week: Exploring the Dying Process. Peter R. Prunkl & Rebecca L. Berry. 1988. (Death Education, Aging & Health Care Ser.). 240p. 89.95 (*0-89116-784-6*); pap. 33.95 (*0-89116-112-0*) Hemisp Pub.

Deathbed Observations by Physicians & Nurses. Karlis Osis. 4th ed. 1961. LC 61-18247. (Parapsychological Monographs: No. 3). pap. 7.00 (*0-912328-06-1*) Parapsych Foun.

Deaths in Custody: Caring for People at Risk. Alison Liebing. 1997. LC 97-175864. 226p. (*1-871177-85-5*); pap. (*1-871177-86-3*) Whiting & Birch GBR. *Dist:* Paul & Co Pubs.

Deaths of Man. Ed. by Edwin S. Shneidman. 1983. LC 83-12294. 256p. reprint ed. 40.00 (*0-87668-642-0*) Aronson.

Debates in Nephrology. Ed. by L. Minetti et al. 1982. (Contributions to Nephrology Ser.: Vol. 34). (Illus.). viii, 132p. pap. 29.75 (*3-8055-3535-X*) S Karger.

Decade of Lupus: Selections from Lupus News. Henrietta Aladjem. 1991. 288p. (Orig.). pap. text 12.00 (*0-9608660-9-4*) Lupus Found Am.

Decade of Progress. Ed. by Arnold Goldberg. 1994. (Progress in Self Psychology Ser.: Vol. 10). 296p. text 45.00 (*0-88163-179-5*) Analytic Pr.

Decade of the Plague: The Sociopsychological Ramifications of STDs. Marianne Wright. 1988. LC 88-2271. (Journal of Social Work & Human Sexuality: Vol. 6, No. 2). (Illus.). 162p. text 9.95 (*0-918393-53-1*, Harrington Park) Haworth Pr.

Decide for Yourself: A Book to Help You Make End of Life Decisions: Life Support, Living Will, Durable Power of Attorney for Health Care. Carolyn Brown et al. Ed. by Nancy R. Hull. 1993. LC 92-19858. (Illus.). 40p. pap. text 7.95 (*0-939838-34-6*) Pritchett & Hull.

Deciding for Others: The Ethics of Surrogate Decisionmaking. Allen Buchanan & Dan W. Brock. 1990. LC 89-33209. (Studies in Philosophy & Health Policy). 440p. (C). pap. text 29.95 (*0-521-31196-9*) Cambridge U Pr.

Deciding Who Lives: Fateful Choices in the Intensive-Care Nursery. Renee R. Anspach. LC 91-44245. 303p. 1997. pap. text 19.95 (*0-520-21213-4*); 1993. text 50.00 (*0-520-05268-4*) U CA Pr.

Deciphering Global Epidemics: Analytical Approaches to the Disease Records of World Cities, 1888-1912. Andrew Cliff et al. 1998. LC 97-27050. (Studies in Historical Geography: No. 26). (Illus.). 495p. (C). text 90.00 (*0-521-47266-0*); pap. text 31.95 (*0-521-47860-X*) Cambridge U Pr.

Deciphering Motivation in Psychotherapy. D. M. Allen. 1991. LC 91-2458. (Critical Issues in Psychiatry Ser.). (Illus.). 200p. (C). text 45.00 (*0-306-43790-2*, Kluwer Plenum) Kluwer Academic.

Deciphering the System: A Guide for Families of Young Children with Disabilities. Paula Beckman & Gayle B. Boyes. 1993. LC 93-7303. 208p. pap. text 14.95 (*0-914797-87-5*) Brookline Bks.

Decision Analysis in Medicine: Methods & Applications. Edward A. Patrick. 1979. 352p. 197.00 (*0-8493-5255-X*, R723, CRC Reprint) Franklin.

Decision Inventory Package. Hamid Noori & Frank Anatol. 1990. 58p. 167.00 incl. 5.25 hd (*0-444-98710-X*) Elsevier.

Decision Making & Age. A.T. Welford & James E. Birren. Ed. by Leon Stein. 1980. LC 79-8699. (Growing Old Ser.). (Illus.). reprint ed. lib. bdg. 19.95 (*0-405-12810-X*) Ayer.

Decision Making & Change in Human Affairs. Ed. by Helmut Jungermann & Gerard De Zeeuw. 1977. (Theory & Decision Library: No. 16). lib. bdg. 226.50 (*90-277-0855-X*) Kluwer Academic.

Decision Making & Judgement for Healthcare Professionals. Scott Bowman. 2001. (Illus.). 224p. pap. 32.50 (*0-7506-3841-9*) Buttrwrth-Heinemann.

Decision Making & Nursing Management. Ed. by Pruitt. 1989. (C). (*0-673-39855-2*) Addison-Wesley.

Decision Making & Problems Inc. Ed. by Andrew Grubb. 1994. LC 93-6187. 216p. 160.95 (*0-471-94236-7*) Wiley.

Decision Making for Women: Seeing Clearly, Planning Effectively, & Acting Decisively. Rita E. Watson. 1994. LC 94-29674. 216p. 23.95 (*1-56565-127-8*) Lowell Hse.

Decision Making in Anesthesiology. Ed. by Lois L. Bready. 3rd ed. 1999. LC 99-40692. (Illus.). 540p. (C). (gr. 13). text 65.95 (*0-8151-2455-4*, 31187) Mosby Inc.

Decision Making in Cardiothoracic Surgery. Laurens R. Pickard. 1989. 208p. text 120.00 (*0-7216-1168-0*) Saunders.

Decision Making in Community Health Nursing: A Workbook. Patricia Hamilton. 1985. (C). pap. text 15.95 (*0-316-34115-0*, Little Brwn Med Div) Lppncott W & W.

Decision Making in Critical Care. 2000. (Illus.). 368p. (C). (gr. 13). text 64.95 (*0-8151-4283-8*, 30565) Mosby Inc.

Decision Making in Dental Treatment Planning. Walter B. Hall et al. 2nd ed. 1998. (Illus.). 275p. (*84-8174-125-6*) Mosby-Doyma Libros ESP. *Dist:* Mosby Inc.

Decision Making in Dental Treatment Planning. Walter Hall et al. 2nd ed. 1998. LC 98-13366. (Illus.). 275p. text 65.00 (*0-8151-4194-7*, 25703) Mosby Inc.

Decision Making in Emergency Cardiology. William H. Montgomery & P. W. Atkins. 1991. 40.00 (*0-8016-3486-5*) Mosby Inc.

Decision-Making in Environmental Health: From Evidence to Action. C. Corvalban et al. 2000. LC 00-21614. (Illus.). xii, 278p. pap. 49.99 (*0-419-25950-3*, Spon) Routledge.

Decision Making in Gastroenterology, No. 2. Joel Seth Levine. 1992. 512p. (C). (gr. 13). text 79.95 (*1-55664-323-3*) Mosby Inc.

Decision Making in Gerontologic Nursing. Paula A. Loftis. 1993. 352p. (C). (gr. 13). pap. text 37.00 (*1-55664-186-9*) Mosby Inc.

Decision Making in Hematology. Brain. 1991. 89.00 (*1-55664-155-9*) Mosby Inc.

Decision Making in Long-Term Care: Factors in Planning. Ed. by Ruth E. Dunkle & May L. Wykle. 1988. 224p. 24.95 (*0-8261-5970-2*) Springer Pub.

Decision Making in Medicine. Harry L. Greene et al. 2nd ed. 1998. LC 98-28593. (Clinical Decision Making Ser.). text 69.95 (*0-323-00029-0*) Mosby Inc.

Decision Making in Medicine: An Algorithmic Approach. Harry L. Greene et al. 2nd ed. 1999. (Illus.). 637p. (*84-8174-103-5*) Mosby-Doyma Libros ESP. *Dist:* Mosby Inc.

Decision Making in Nursing. Rebecca A. Jones & Sharon E. Beck. 1995. LC 94-42417. (Nursing Education Ser.). 331p. (C). 62.95 (*0-8273-5684-6*) Delmar.

Decision Making in Oncology: Evidence-Based Management. Benjamin C. Djulbegovic. 1997. LC 97-3873. text (*0-443-08989-2*) Church.

Decision Making in Pediatric Neurologic Physical Therapy. Susan K. Campbell. Ed. by Andrew Allen. 1999. LC 98-38541. 335p. text (*0-443-07923-4*) Church.

Decision Making in Periodontology. Walter B. Hall. 3rd ed. 1997. LC 97-26209. (Illus.). 312p. (C). (gr. 13). text 56.95 (*0-8151-4193-9*, 25702) Mosby Inc.

Decision Making in Perioperative Nursing. Wells. 2nd ed. 44.00 (*1-55664-355-1*) Mosby Inc.

Decision Making in Psychiatry & the Law. Thomas G. Gutheil et al. 1991. 296p. 36.00 (*0-683-03801-X*) Lppncott W & W.

Decision-Making in Reconstructive Surgery: Upper Extremity. G. Germann et al. 1999. LC 99-36189. (Illus.). xvi, 240p. 199.00 (*3-540-64077-0*) Spr-Verlag.

Decision Making in the Post Anesthesia Care Unit. Cecil B. Drain. 1995. 288p. 29.95 (*0-8016-7875-7*) Mosby Inc.

Decision Making on the Outcomes in Sports Rehabilitation. Dinesh Kumbhare & John V. Basmajian. 2000. LC 99-48218. (Illus.). 350p. text Price not set. (*0-443-06546-2*) Saunders.

Decision-Related Research on the Organization of Service Delivery Systems in Metropolitan Areas: Public Health. Patrick O'Donoghue. 1979. LC 79-83820. (*0-89138-984-9*) ICPSR.

Decision-Related Research on the Organization of Service Delivery Systems in Metropolitan Areas: Solid Waste Management. E. Steven Savas. 1979. LC 79-83822. (*0-89138-982-2*) ICPSR.

Decision Support Systems in Critical Care. Ed. by M. Michael Shabot & Reed M. Gardner. 1993. LC 93-11902. (Computers & Medicine Ser.). (Illus.). 420p. 92.00 (*0-387-97799-6*) Spr-Verlag.

***Decisions for Health.** 1999. pap. 114.85 (*0-8172-8899-6*) Raintree Steck-V.

Decisions for Health Vivian Bernstein. 1997. (gr. 7-12). tchr. ed. 5.95 (*0-8114-7790-8*, JJ-7790-8); pap., tchr. ed. 5.95 (*0-8114-3302-1*, JJ-3302-1); tchr. ed., ring bd. 84.75 (*0-8114-7789-4*, JJ-7789-4) Raintree Steck-V.

Decisions for Health. Bruess & Richardson. 4th ed. 1995. pap. text, tchr. ed. 42.18 (*0-697-15226-X*); tchr. ed. 25.00 (*0-697-15225-1*); tchr. ed. 16.56 (*0-697-15228-6*) McGraw.

Decisions for Health Vivian Bernstein. 1997. (gr. 7-12). Bk. 1. pap., stu. ed. 11.28 (*0-8114-3300-5*, JJ-3300-5); Bk. 2. pap., stu. ed. 11.28 (*0-8114-3301-3*, JJ-3301-3) Raintree Steck-V.

Decisions for Your Life: Preventing Teenage Pregnancy. Girl Scouts of the U. S. A. Staff. 1989. (Contemporary Issues Ser.). 20p. pap. 1.75 (*0-88441-466-3*, 26-826) Girl Scouts USA.

Decisions Near the End of Life: Modules 1-7. Ed. by Mildred Z. Solomon et al. 1997. (Illus.). 206p. pap. 40.00 (*0-89292-292-3*, 5810) Educ Dev Ctr.

Decison Making for Incompetent Persons: The Law & Morality of Who Shall Decide. Shannon M. Jordan. 1985. 170p. (C). text 39.95 (*0-398-05150-X*) C C Thomas.

Decline & Fall of the Freudian Empire. Hans J. Eysenck. 1990. 224p. (C). lib. bdg. 24.00 (*1-878465-01-5*) Scott-Townsend Pubs.

Decline of the Global Village: How Specialization Is Changing the Mass Media. Ed. by James E. Grunig. 1976. LC 76-9295. (Illus.). 297p. pap. text 26.95 (*0-930390-29-6*) Gen Hall.

Decoding Darkness: The Search for the Genetic Causes of Alzheimer's Disease. Rudolph E. Tanzi et al. 2000. (Illus.). 320p. 26.00 (*0-7382-0195-2*) Perseus Pubng.

Decoding the Codes: A Comprehensive Guide to CPT, ICD, & HCPCS Coding Systems. Alex Toth. 1997. LC 97-38713. (HFMA Healthcare Financial Management Ser.). 320p. 75.00 (*0-7863-1246-7*, Irwn Prfssnl) McGraw-Hill Educ Grp.

Decoding the Past: The Psychohistorical Approach. Peter Loewenberg. 1996. 310p. (C). pap. text 24.95 (*1-56000-846-6*) Transaction Pubs.

Decommissioning & Restoration of Nuclear Facilities: 1999 Health Physics Society Summer School Proceedings. Ed. by Michael J. Slobodien. 1999. LC 99-62808. (Illus.). x, 660p. text 69.95 (*0-944838-18-9*) Med Physics Pub.

***Decommissioning Health Physics: A Handbook for MARSSIM Users.** E. W. Abelquist. 2001. (Illus.). 456p. 65.00 (*0-7503-0761-7*) Inst of Physics Pubng.

Decompressive Lumbar Laminectomy. Oliver D. Grin & Dorothy L. Bouwman. 1993. (Patient Education Ser.). (Illus.). 24p. (Orig.). pap. text 4.00 (*0-929689-60-7*) Ludann Co.

Deconstructing Developmental Psychology. Erica Burman. 1994. LC 93-5880. (Critical Psychology Ser.). 208p. (C). pap. 26.95 (*0-415-06438-4*) Routledge.

Deconstructing Psychopathology. Ian Parker et al. 1995. 176p. pap. 24.95 (*0-8039-7481-7*, 1878) Sage.

Deconstruction of Nursing. Ramprogus. 1995. 208p. 77.95 (*1-85972-101-X*) Ashgate Pub Co.

Deconstruction of Psychotherapy. Byram Karasu. 1996. LC 96-12693. 176p. 40.00 (*1-56821-821-4*) Aronson.

Decubitus Ulcer in Clinical Practice, Vol. XII. Ed. by Lawrence C. Parish et al. 1997. LC 96-31691. (Illus.). 241p. 118.00 (*3-540-61526-1*) Spr-Verlag.

Decubitus Ulcers of the Pelvic Region: Diagnostics & Surgical Therapy. N. Luscher. 1992. (Illus.). 152p. text 113.00 (*0-88937-049-4*) Hogrefe & Huber Pubs.

Deep Dyslexis. Ed. by Max Coltheart et al. 1988. (International Library of Philosophy, Psychology, & Scientific Method). 472p. (C). pap. text 27.50 (*0-7102-1235-6*, Routledge Thoemms) Routledge.

Deep Healing: The Essence of Mind/Body Medicine. Emmett E. Miller. 1997. LC 96-13953. 400p. pap. 12.95 (*1-56170-336-2*, 197) Hay House.

Deep Water Exercise for Health & Fitness. J. Glenn McWaters. 1988. LC 87-35861. (Illus.). 192p. (Orig.). 16.95 (*0-913581-07-0*); pap. 10.95 (*0-913581-08-9*) Publitec.

Deepening Shade: Psychological Aspects of Life-Threatening Illness. Barbara M. Sourkes. 1982. LC 81-16276. (Contemporary Community Health Ser.). 142p. pap. 12.95 (*0-8229-5337-4*) U of Pittsburgh Pr.

Deepening the Treatment. Jane S. Hall. 1998. LC 98-17723. 224p. 40.00 (*0-7657-0176-6*) Aronson.

Deeper Reaches of Love & Fear: The Birth of a New Psychology. David G. Mutchler. 1989. 250p. 18.95 (*0-922639-00-0*) Lakeshore Counsel.

Deer Life: A Deer Vet Tells His Story & Theirs. John Fletcher. 2000. (Illus.). 226p. (*0-575-07090-0*) VGO4.

Defeat Depression. Frank J. Bruno. 1997. LC 96-85333. (Life's Little Keys Ser.). 144p. pap. 10.95 (*0-02-861305-8*, Arc) Hungry Minds.

Defeating Depression: Lifting Yourself from Sadness into Joy. Dale R. Olen. 1992. (Illus.). 212p. (Orig.). pap. 5.95 (*1-56583-011-3*) JODA.

Defeating Depression: Run It Away! John Stewart. 1995. LC 94-61292. (Illus.). 120p. (Orig.). pap. 11.95 (*0-944482-10-4*) Except Bks NM.

Defective Delinquent & Insane. Henry A. Cotton. Ed. by Gerald N. Grob. 1980. LC 78-22557. (Historical Issues in Mental Health Ser.). (Illus.). reprint ed. lib. bdg. 19.95 (*0-405-11911-9*) Ayer.

Defendant: A Psychiatrist on Trial for Medical Malpractice. Sara C. Charles & Eugene Kennedy. 1985. 236p. 35.00 (*0-02-905910-0*) Free Pr.

Defenders of the Race: Jewish Doctors & Race Science in Fin-de-Siecle Europe. John M. Efron. 1994. LC 94-10413. (Illus.). 272p. 40.00 (*0-300-05440-8*) Yale U Pr.

Defending Against the Enemy: Coping with Parkinson's Disease. Eric Morgan. 1997. LC 95-72727. 128p. (Orig.). pap. 12.95 (*0-936609-36-2*) QED Ft Bragg.

Defending & Preventing Health Care Fraud Cases: An Attorney's Guide. Kevin J. Darken. 1999. LC 99-41031. 600p. 179.00 (*0-8342-1171-8*) Aspen Pub.

Defending Army. Ed. by Robert Somerville. 1994. LC 93-33512. (Journey Through the Mind & Body Ser.: Vol. 4). (Illus.). 144p. lib. bdg. 17.99 (*0-7835-1013-6*) Time-Life.

Defending the Breast Cancer Malpractice Case. Campbell F. Watts & David M. Elderkin. 1994. LC 94-34048. (Illus.). 530p. 95.00 (*0-13-349598-1*) Aspen Law.

Defense Against Alzheimer's Disease: A Rational Blueprint for Prevention. H. J. Roberts. 1995. LC 93-86995. (Illus.). 236p. 27.95 (*1-884243-00-2*) Sunshine Sentinel.

Defense & Resistance: Historical Perspectives & Current Concepts. Ed. by Harold P. Blum. 1985. LC 85-18028. 433p. 65.00 (*0-8236-1157-4*, 01157) Intl Univs Pr.

Defense Health Care: Effects of Mandated Cost Sharing on Uniformed Services Treatment Facilities Likely to Be Minor. 1996. (Illus.). 38p. (Orig.). (C). pap. text 25.00 (*0-7881-3617-8*) DIANE Pub.

Defense Health Care: Issues & Challenges Confronting Military Medicine. 1995. (Illus.). 66p. (Orig.). pap. text 35.00 (*0-7881-2047-6*) DIANE Pub.

Defense Health Care: Medical Costs & Other Issues May Affect Uniformed Services Treatment Facilities' Future. 1996. (Illus.). 37p. (Orig.). (C). pap. text 25.00 (*0-7881-3609-7*) DIANE Pub.

Defense Mechanisms in the Counseling Process. Arthur J. Clark. 1998. LC 97-45280. 255p. 73.95 (*0-7619-0660-6*, 80653); pap. 36.95 (*0-7619-0661-4*, 80654) Sage.

Defense of Mucosal Surfaces: Pathogenesis, Immunity & Vaccines. Ed. by Jean-Pierre Kraehenbuhl & Marian R. Neutra. 1998. (Current Topics in Microbiology & Immunology Ser.: Vol. 236). (Illus.). 306p. 149.00 (*3-540-64730-9*) Spr-Verlag.

Defense of the Ocular Surface. Feher Janos. 1994. (Pathophysiology of the Eye Ser.: No. 2). 169p. pap. (*963-05-6632-X*) Akade Kiado HUN. *Dist:* Intl Spec Bk, St Mut.

***Defense Vaccines: Force Protection or False Security? - Congressional Hearing.** Ed. by Dan Burton. 2001. (Illus.). 228p. reprint ed. pap. text 40.00 (*0-7567-1807-4*) DIANE Pub.

Defensive Medicine & Medical Malpractice. 1996. (Illus.). 182p. (C). reprint ed. pap. text 30.00 (*0-7881-3181-8*) DIANE Pub.

Defensive Medicine & Medical Malpractice. 1995. lib. bdg. 252.75 (*0-8490-7512-2*) Gordon Pr.

Defining Infants' Race & Ethnicity in a Study of Very Low Birthweight Infants. Donna O. Farley et al. 1993. LC 93-8807. pap. text 9.00 (*0-8330-1414-5*, MR-191-AHCPR) Rand Corp.

Defining Personhood: Toward the Ethics of Quality in Clinical Care. Sarah B. Merrill. 1998. LC 99-173197. (Value Inquiry Book Ser.). x, 222 p. (*90-420-0571-8*) Rodopi.

Defining the Legal Parent-Child Relationship in Alternative Reproductive Technology. 1991. 35p. 20.00 (*0-89707-667-2*, 513-0036) Amer Bar Assn.

Definite Medication. Eli G. Jones. 1996. 312p. reprint ed. spiral bd. 20.00 (*0-7873-0481-6*) Hlth Research.

Definition & Payment for Uncompensated Services & Special Problems of a Disproportionate Share. Uncompensated Services Task Force Staff & Richard L. Clarke. 1987. 17p. (Orig.). pap. 10.00 (*0-930228-54-5*) Hlthcare Fin Mgmt.

Definition of a Profession: The Authority of Metaphor in the History of Intelligence Testing, 1890-1930. JoAnne Brown. 1992. LC 92-1147. 216p. 52.50 (*0-691-08632-X*) Princeton U Pr.

Definition of Death: Contemporary Controversies. Stuart J. Younger et al. 1999. LC 98-20216. 368p. 56.00 (*0-8018-5985-9*) Johns Hopkins.

Definition of Quality & Approaches to Its Assessment. Avedis Donabedian. 1980. LC 80-15173. (Explorations in Quality Assessment & Monitoring Ser.: Vol. I). (Illus.). 178p. pap. text 30.00 (*0-914904-48-5*, 0824) Health Admin Pr.

Definition of Serious & Complex Medical Conditions. Institute of Medicine Staff. 1999. LC 00-500810. vi, 116p. pap. 29.50 (*0-309-06640-9*) Natl Acad Pr.

Definition of Suicide. Edwin S. Shneidman. 1995. LC 93-74372. (Master Work Ser.). 270p. pap. 40.00 (*1-56821-196-1*) Aronson.

Definitions & Diagnostic Criteria of Alcoholism. 1992. (Illus.). 65p. (Orig.). (C). pap. text 30.00 (*1-56806-130-7*) DIANE Pub.

Definitions of Quantities & Conventions Related to Blood pH & Gas Analysis (1994) National Committee for Clinical Laboratory Standards. 2nd ed. 1994. (Tentative Standard Ser.: Vol. 2). 75.00 (*1-56238-138-5*, C12-A) NCCLS.

Definitions of Time & Recovery in Paralytic Polio Convalescence. Fred Davis. 1993. (Reprint Series in Sociology). (C). reprint ed. pap. text 1.00 (*0-8290-2640-1*, S-366) Irvington.

Definitive Guide to Medical School Admission. Mark A. Goldstein & Myrna C. Goldstein. rev. ed. 1998. (Illus.). 192p. pap. 14.95 (*1-883280-09-5*) Font & Ctr Pr.

Definitive Work on the Origins of Human Lymphomas. Sergio DeCarvalho. 1985. LC 84-72903. 148p. 19.50 (*0-930376-40-4*) Chem-Orbital.

Deformable Models in Medical Image Analysis. Ajit Singh et al. 1998. LC 98-23491. 448p. 60.00 (*0-8186-8521-2*) IEEE Comp Soc.

Defy Aging: Develop the Mental & Emotional Vitality to Live Longer, Healthier & Happier Than You Ever Imagined. Michael P. Brickey. 2000. LC 00-91404. (Illus.). 416p. 24.95 (*0-9701555-0-6*) New Resour.

Defying the Gods: Inside the New Frontiers of Organ Transplants. Scott McCartney. 1994. LC 93-38976. 298p. 22.00 (*0-02-582820-7*) Macmillan.

Degenerative Dementias Other Than Alzheimer's Disease. Arthur W. Clark. 1998. LC 97-38212. 400p. pap. (*0-89089-713-1*) Carolina Acad Pr.

Degenerative Disease of the Cervical Spine. Ed. by Paul R. Cooper. 1994. (Neurosurgical Topics Ser.: Bk. 12). (Illus.). 175p. 95.00 (*1-879284-04-9*) Am Assn Neuro.

Degenerative Diseases of the Retina: Proceedings of the Sixth International Symposium Held in Jerusalem, Israel, November 4-9, 1994. Ed. by Robert E. Anderson et al. 1995. (Illus.). 428p. 120.00 (*0-306-45137-9*, Kluwer Plenum) Kluwer Academic.

Degenerative Retinal Diseases: Proceedings of the VIIth International Symposium Held in Sendai, Japan, October 5-9, 1996. Ed. by Matthew M. La Vail et al. 1997. LC 97-27725. 440p. 120.00 (*0-306-45701-6*, Kluwer Plenum) Kluwer Academic.

Degenerative Retinopathies: Advances in Clinical & Genetic Research. Peter Humphries et al. 1991. 560p. lib. bdg. 105.00 (*0-8493-0187-4*, RE661) CRC Pr.

Deglutition & Its Disorders: Anatomy, Physiology, Clinical Diagnosis, & Management. Ed. by Adrienne Perlman & Konrad Schulze-Delrieu. 1996. LC 96-17369. 546p. text 94.95 (*1-56593-621-3*, 1290) Thomson Learn.

DeGowin & DeGowin's Diagnostic Examination. Richard L. DeGowin. 6th ed. 1994. LC 93-38286. text 37.00 (*0-07-016338-3*) McGraw-Hill Med Pub.

Degradation of Dental Polymers. Jean-Francois Roulet. 1986. (Illus.). xiv, 228p. 172.25 (*3-8055-4320-4*) S Karger.

Dehydroepiandrosterone (DHEA) & Aging. Ed. by Francis L. Bellino et al. 1996. (Annals of the New York Academy of Sciences Ser.: Vol. 774). 350p. pap. 95.00 (*1-57331-005-0*) NY Acad Sci.

Dehydroepiandrostonerone (DHEA, Prasterone) Index of New Information for Research & Clinical Practice. Steven A. Gillikin. 1997. 133p. 57.50 (*0-7883-1374-6*); pap. 47.50 (*0-7883-1375-4*) ABBE Pubs Assn.

Deinstitutionalization: Program & Policy Development. Ed. by James M. Paul et al. 1977. (Special Education & Rehabilitation Monograph Ser.: No. 12). (C). 34.95 (*0-8156-0132-8*) Syracuse U Pr.

Deinstitutionalization & Community Adjustment of Mentally Retarded People. Ed. by Robert H. Bruininks et al. 1981. LC 80-70191. (Monographs of the American Association on Mental Retardation: No. 4). 412p. text 7.00 (*0-940898-10-1*) Am Assn Mental.

Deinstitutionalized Residential Care for the Mentally Disordered: The Soteria House Approach. Holly S. Wilson. 1982. 160p. text 26.00 (*0-8089-1427-8*, 794855, Grune & Strat) Harcrt Hlth Sci Grp.

Deinstitutionalizing Delinquent Youth. Michael Fabricant. 1980. LC 79-23023. 215p. pap. 11.95 (*0-87073-892-5*) Schenkman Bks Inc.

Deje de Fumar Brochure. 1994. (SPA.). 0.20 (*0-8151-3864-4*) Mosby Inc.

DeJong's the Neurologic Examination. Armin F. Haerer. 5th ed. 1992. (Illus.). 864p. text 115.00 (*0-397-51104-3*) Lppncott W & W.

De/La Pampa a los Estados Unidos see Challenging Dream of Heart Surgery: From the Pampas to Cleveland

Delaware Health Care in Perspective 2000. Ed. by Kathleen O'Leary Morgan & Scott E. Morgan. 2000. 21p. spiral bd. 19.00 (*0-7401-0207-9*) Morgan Quitno Corp.

Delaware Health Care Perspective, 1998. Ed. by Kathleen O'Leary Morgan & Scott E. Morgan. 1998. 20p. pap. 19.00 (*1-56692-807-9*) Morgan Quitno Corp.

Delay Law & New Class of Superelastic Shape Memory Materials & Implants in Medicine. Ed. by Victor E. Gunther. 2000. (Illus.). 448p. 49.99 (*0-9702353-0-5*) STT.

Delayed & Chronic Effects of Chemicals in the Workplace: Report on a WHO Meeting. 1982. (Euro Reports & Studies Ser.: No. 64). 48p. pap. text 4.00 (*92-890-1230-7*) World Health.

Delayed Diagnosis of Cancer. Phillip D. Minton & Dan J. Tennenhouse. 1995. iv, 109p. pap. 54.00 (*1-930548-01-X*) Tennenhouse Prof Pubns.

Delaying the Onset of Late-Life Dysfunction. Ed. by Robert N. Butler & Jacob A. Brody. 1995. LC 94-23931. (Illus.). 272p. 39.95 (*0-8261-8880-X*) Springer Pub.

Delicious & Easy Rice Flour Recipes: Gluten-Free: a Sequel to Gourmet Food on a Wheat-Free Diet. Marion N. Wood. 1981. 160p. spiral bd. 31.95 (*0-398-02441-3*) C C Thomas.

Delicious Herbal & Folk Remedies. Maria Kuman. 1997. (Illus.). pap. 20.00 (*1-893637-01-8*) Hlth & Hap.

Delicious Ways to Control Diabetes. 1999. (Illus.). 207p. 24.95 (*0-8487-1918-2*) Oxmoor Hse.

Delicious Ways to Control Diabetes Cookbook. 2001. (Illus.). 208p. 24.95 (*0-8487-2396-1*) Oxmoor Hse.

Delineation & Diagnosis of Craniofacial Syndromes: Effect on Case Management. 1994. 23p. pap. text 44.00 incl. VHS (*0-910329-78-8*, 0111848) Am Speech Lang Hearing.

Delinquency: The Problem & Its Prevention. D. H. Stott. 1982. LC 80-25928. 352p. (C). pap. 16.95 (*0-88331-133-X*) R B Luce.

Delinquency & Child Guidance: Selected Papers by August Aichhorn. August Aichhorn. Ed. by Otto Fleischmann et al. 1967. LC 64-8751. (Menninger Foundation Monograph Ser.: No. 1). 244p. 37.50 (*0-8236-1160-4*) Intl Univs Pr.

Delinquency & Drift. David Matza. 1990. 224p. pap. text 24.95 (*0-88738-804-3*) Transaction Pubs.

Delinquency & Psychopathology. Dorothy O. Lewis & David A. Balla. 1976. LC 76-44883. 240p. text 52.00 (*0-8089-0976-2*, 792525, Grune & Strat) Harcrt Hlth Sci Grp.

Delinquency, Crime, & Society. Ed. by James F. Short, Jr. 1978. LC 75-27895. (Illus.). 336p. pap. text 7.50 (*0-226-75469-3*, P772) U Ch Pr.

Delinquent Child & the Home. Sophonisba P. Breckinridge & Edith Abbott. 1974. LC 70-112525. (Rise of Urban America Ser.). reprint ed. 23.95 (*0-405-02438-X*) Ayer.

Delinquent Girls in Court: A Study of the Wayward Minor Court of New York. Paul W. Tappan. 1969. LC 69-14950. (Criminology, Law Enforcement, & Social Problems Ser.: No. 67). reprint ed. 24.00 (*0-87585-067-7*) Patterson Smith.

Delinquents & Criminals: Their Making & Unmaking. William Healy & Augusta F. Bronner. reprint ed. 20.00 (*0-404-03197-8*) AMS Pr.

Delinquents & Criminals, Their Making & Unmaking, Studies in Two American Cities. William Healy & Augusta F. Bronner. 1969. LC 69-14931. (Criminology, Law Enforcement, & Social Problems Ser.: No. 69). reprint ed. 10.00 (*0-87585-069-3*) Patterson Smith.

Delire et les Reves dans la Gradiva de W. Jenson. Sigmund Freud. 1991. (FRE.). pap. 11.95 (*0-7859-2825-1*) Fr & Eur.

Delirium: Acute Confusional States. Zbigniew J. Lipowski. 1990. 512p. text 79.00 (*0-19-506150-0*) OUP.

Delivering a Better Childbirth Experience: A Consumer's Guide to Nurse-Midwifery. Mary Gabay & Sidney M. Wolfe. 1995. 258p. (Orig.). (C). pap. 15.00 (*0-937188-01-8*) Pub Citizen.

Delivering Health Care Comprehensively. Richard Brotman et al. 1991. LC 91-1952. 192p. 60.00 (*0-275-93999-5*, C3999, Praeger Pubs) Greenwood.

Delivering Health Care in America: A Systems Approach. Leiyu Shi & Douglas A. Singh. 2nd ed. 2000. LC 00-40604. (Illus.). xv, 634p. pap. 57.00 (*0-8342-1764-3*, 17643) Aspen Pub.

Delivering Health Care to Homeless Persons: The Diagnosis & Management of Medical & Mental Health Conditions. Ed. by David Wood. 1992. LC 91-5074. 304p. 38.95 (*0-8261-7780-8*) Springer Pub.

Delivering Health Care to Refugees: Cross-Cultural Training to Enhance the Delivery of Quality Health Care to Culturally Diverse Persons. David Dunn, pseud. 1992. 32p. 5.00 (*0-940723-08-5*) SIIS.

Delivering High Technology Home Care: Issues for Decisionmakers. Ed. by Maxwell J. Mehlman & Stuart J. Youngner. 1991. LC 91-4741. 256p. 33.95 (*0-8261-7610-0*) Springer Pub.

Delivering Primary Health Care: Nurse Practitioners at Work. Michael Yedidia. 1981. LC 81-1946. 170p. (C). 45.00 (*0-86569-075-8*, Auburn Hse) Greenwood.

Delivering Quality Care to Nursing Home Residents: OBRA Regulations & Beyond. David A. Smith. 1995. (Geriatric Psychopathology Ser.). (Orig.). pap. text 49.95 (*1-884937-31-4*) Manisses Communs.

Delivering Quality in Midwifery. Rosemary Buckley. 1997. 153p. pap. text (*0-7020-2134-2*) Bailliere Tindall.

Delivery of Emergency Medical Services in Disasters: Assumptions & Realities. E. L. Quarantelli. 1985. LC 83-13028. 190p. (C). text 32.50 (*0-8290-0531-5*) Irvington.

Delivery of Psychological Services in the Schools: Concepts, Precesses & Issues. Ed. by Stephen N. Elliot & Joseph C. Witt. 1986. 448p. (C). text 89.95 (*0-89859-581-9*) L Erlbaum Assocs.

Delivery Strategies for Antisense Oligonucleotide Therapeutics. Ed. by Saghir Akhtar. 1995. 320p. 239.95 (*0-8493-4778-5*, 4778) CRC Pr.

Delivery Systems for Cancer Care. Susan L. Groenwald. 1991. (Illus.). (C). pap. text 22.50 (*0-86720-306-4*, 306-4) Jones & Bartlett.

Delivery Systems for Peptide Drugs. Ed. by S. S. Davis et al. 1987. LC 87-11036. (NATO ASI Series A, Life Sciences: Vol. 125). 380p. 110.00 (*0-306-42496-7*, Plenum Trade) Perseus Pubng.

Delmar Nursing Notes: Home Health Care, Safe. Booth. 1991. (Education Ser.). pap. 9.95 (*0-8273-4006-0*) Delmar.

Delmar Nursing Notes: Medical-Surgical Nursing. Booth. (Education Ser.). 1992. pap., tchr. ed. 8.00 (*0-8273-4011-7*); 1991. pap. 12.95 (*0-8273-4003-6*) Delmar.

Delmar Nursing Notes: NCLEX - RN Complete Prep. Booth. 1992. (Education Ser.). pap. 9.95 (*0-8273-4009-5*) Delmar.

Delmar Nursing Notes: Nursing Care Plans. Booth. 1991. (Education Ser.). pap. 9.95 (*0-8273-4004-4*) Delmar.

Delmar Nursing Notes: Nursing Ethics, Legal Aspects. Booth. 1991. (C). pap. text 9.95 (*0-8273-4008-7*) Delmar.

Delmar Nursing Notes: Pediatric/Geriatric. Booth. 1991. (Education Ser.). pap. 10.95 (*0-8273-4007-9*) Delmar.

Delmar Nursing Notes: Pharmacy & Medicine Administration. Booth. 1992. (Education Ser.). pap. 10.95 (*0-8273-4010-9*) Delmar.

Delmar Nursing Notes: Psychosocial/Cultural Nursing. Booth. 1991. (Education Ser.). pap. 10.95 (*0-8273-4005-2*) Delmar.

Delmar Nursing Notes: Women's Health. Booth. 1991. (Education Ser.). pap. 10.95 (*0-8273-4002-8*) Delmar.

Delmar's Administrative Medical Assisting. Lindh & Tamparo. 1997. 256p. (C). pap., wbk. ed. 17.95 (*0-8273-8529-3*) Delmar.

Delmar's Administrative Medical Assisting. Wilburta Q. Lindh et al. 1997. LC 97-21697. 416p. (C). pap. text 49.95 (*0-8273-8528-5*) Delmar.

Delmar's Administrative Medical Assisting. Pooler & Cerrato. 1997. 416p. text, wbk. ed. 18.95 (*0-8273-8526-9*) Delmar.

Delmar's Anatomy Coloring Book. Carr. 1998. (Allied Health Ser.). pap. 18.95 (*0-8273-5640-4*) Delmar.

Delmar's Clinical Handbook for the Health Care Professional. Michelle Heller & Connie Krebs. 1996. LC 96-20597. 256p. (C). pap. text 30.95 (*0-8273-7789-4*) Delmar.

Delmar's Clinical Lab Manual Series: Immunohematology. Sherly A. Whitlock. 1996. LC 96-28546. (Clinical Laboratory Manual Ser.). (Illus.). 160p. (C). pap. text, lab manual ed. 34.95 (*0-8273-6867-4*) Delmar.

Delmar's Clinical Lab Manual Series: Urinalysis. Sheryl Whitlock & John Flynn. 1996. LC 96-2564. (Clinical Laboratory Manual Ser.). (Illus.). 128p. (C). pap. text 34.95 (*0-8273-7196-9*) Delmar.

Delmar's Clinical Laboratory Manual Series: Hematology. Alan P. Russell. 1996. LC 96-18847. (Clinical Laboratory Manual Ser.). (Illus.). 272p. (C). pap. text 34.95 (*0-8273-6373-7*) Delmar.

Delmar's Clinical Medical Assisting. Wilburta Q. Lindh et al. 1997. LC 97-14957. 704p. (C). pap. text 52.95 (*0-8273-8525-0*) Delmar.

Delmar's Comprehensive Medical Assisting: Administrative & Clinical Competencies. Wilbuta Q. Lindh. 1997. LC 96-45520. (Medical Assisting Ser.). 1148p. (C). 65.95 (*0-8273-6764-3*) Delmar.

Delmar's Comprehensive Medical Terminology: A Competency Based Approach. Betty Davis Jones. 1998. LC 98-39257. (Illus.). 968p. pap. text 50.95 (*0-7668-0493-3*) Delmar.

Delmar's Concise Dictionary for Health-Related Professions. Hearl. 2000. (Dental Assisting Procedures Ser.). (C). pap. 16.00 net. (*0-7668-1122-0*) Delmar.

***Delmar's Dental Assisting.** 1999. 100p. pap. text 659.95 Delmar.

Delmar's Dental Assisting: A Comprehensive Approach. Donna J. Phinney & Judy Halstead. 1999. LC 98-55682. (Dental Assisting Procedures Ser.). 800p. (C). 61.95 (*0-8273-9073-4*) Delmar.

Delmar's Dental Assisting Exam Review. Thibodeaux. 1999. 288p. (C). pap. 23.50 net. (*0-8273-9071-8*) Thomson Learn.

***Delmar's Drug Reference for Health Care Professionals.** Sylvia Tindell Nobles. 2001. 992p. text 26.95 (*0-7668-2523-X*) Delmar.

Delmar's Fundamental & Advanced Nursing Skills. Gaylene Altman et al. 1999. LC 99-32852. 1440p. (C). pap. text 70.95 (*0-7668-0715-0*) Delmar.

Delmar's Fundamentals of Anatomy & Physiology. Rizzo. 2000. (Anatomy & Physiology). 496p. (C). pap. text 48.95 (*0-7668-0498-4*) Delmar.

***Delmar's Guide to Laboratory & Diagnostic Tests.** Rick Daniels. 2001. LC 2001-28082. (Illus.). xi, 1017p. (*0-7668-3112-4*) Delmar.

***Delmar's Guide to Laboratory & Diagnostic Tests.** Rick Daniels. 2001. 1200p. pap. 31.95 (*0-7668-1507-2*) Delmar.

Delmar's Medical Assisting Video Series: Instructor's Guide. 1994. 25p. 14.00 (*0-8273-6111-4*) Delmar.

Delmar's Medical Office Reference Manual. Doris D. Humphrey & Kathie Sigler. 3rd ed. 1997. 400p. pap., tchr. ed. (*0-8273-8171-9*) Delmar.

Delmar's Medical Office Reference Manual. Doris Humphrey et al. 3rd ed. 1996. LC 96-2941. (Illus.). 416p. (C). pap. text 36.95 (*0-8273-8169-7*) Delmar.

Delmar's Medical Transcription Handbook. Rachelle S. Blake. 2nd ed. 1997. LC 97-18408. 224p. (C). pap. text 35.95 (*0-8273-8325-8*) Thomson Learn.

Delmar's NCLEX-RN Review. Alice M. Stein. 4th ed. 1999. LC 99-12882. (NSNA Review Ser.). (Illus.). 1024p. pap. text 40.95 (*0-7668-1443-2*) Delmar.

Delmar's Nurses Drug Reference 96. Created by Delmar Staff. 1996. (Professional Reference - Nursing Ser.). 1440p. (C). pap. 26.95 (*0-8273-7540-9*) Delmar.

Delmar's Nursing Assistant Laser Disc. Barbara R. Hegner. 1994. (C). text 1746.50 (*0-8273-7039-3*) Delmar.

Delmar's Pharmacy Technician Exam Review. Patricia K. Anthony. 1999. LC 99-25102. (Allied Health Ser.). 192p. (C). pap. 20.00 (*0-7668-0743-6*) Delmar.

Delmar's Radiographic Positioning & Procedures Volume Vol. I: Workbook. Adams Greathouse. 1998. (Radiographic Technology Ser.). 300p. (C). wbk. ed., lab manual ed. 34.95 (*0-8273-6784-8*) Delmar.

Delmar's Radiographic Positioning And Procedures Volume 1: Basic Positioning & Procedures, Vol. 1. Greathouse. 1998. LC 97-43449. (Raciographic Technology Ser.). 725p. (C). 112.95 (*0-8273-6782-1*) Delmar.

Delmar's Radiographic Positioning & Procedures, Volume II: Advanced Imaging Procedures, Vol. II. Cowling. 1998. LC 97-43449. (Radiographic Technology Ser.). 425p. 75.95 (*0-8273-6317-6*) Delmar.

Delmar's Textbook of Basic Pediatric Nursing. Shapiro. abr. rev. ed. 1996. LC 96-21917. (LPN/LVN Nursing Ser.). 496p. pap. text 52.95 (*0-8273-7717-7*) Delmar.

Delmars Veterinary Guide: Small Animal Care. Delmar. 2000. (C). pap. 35.25 net. (*0-7668-1422-X*) Thomson Learn.

Delmar's Veterinary Technology Pocket Dictionary. Delmar Publishing Staff. 2000. LC 00-21729. xi, 268p. pap. 22.50 net. (*0-7668-1421-1*) Delmar.

Delta Sleep Inducing Peptide DSIP. 1984. (Journal: Vol. 23, No. 5). (Illus.). 76p. pap. 31.50 (*3-8055-4011-6*) S Karger.

Deltamethrin. 1990. (Environmental Health Criteria Ser.: No. 97). (ENG, FRE & SPA.). 133p. pap. text 26.00 (*92-4-154297-7*, 1160097) World Health.

Delusional Disorder: Paranoia & Related Illnesses. Alistair Munro. 1999. LC 98-17210. (Illus.). 276p. (C). text 80.00 (*0-521-58180-X*) Cambridge U Pr.

Delusional Misidentification Syndromes. G. N. Christodoulou. 1986. (Bibliotheca Psychiatrica Ser.: No. 164). (Illus.). x, 154p. 85.25 (*3-8055-4213-5*) S Karger.

Delusional Misidentification Syndromes. Ed. by Nils Retterstol et al. 1994. (Journal: Vol. 27, No. 3-5, 1994). (Illus.). 156p. pap. 126.25 (*3-8055-6082-6*) S Karger.

***Delusional Person Bodily Feelings in Psychosis.** Salomon Resnik. 2001. 260p. pap. (*1-85575-262-X*) Karnac Bks GBR. *Dist:* Other Pr LLC.

Delusions of Everyday Life. Leonard Shengold. 1995. LC 94-38368. 240p. 35.00 (*0-300-06268-0*) Yale U Pr.

Deluxe Family Medical Library. Set. Consumer Guide Editors. rev. ed. 1993. (Illus.). 29.95 (*1-56173-296-6*, 9006101) Pubns Intl Ltd.

***Deluxe Physician ICD-9-CM,** Vols. 1 & 2. Ingenix, Inc. Staff. (Illus.). pap. 71.95 (*1-56337-348-3*) Ingenix Inc.

Deluxe Physician ICD-9-CM, 1999-2000, Vols. 1-2. Medicode, Med-Index Division Staff. 1999. (C). pap. 56.00 (*1-56337-314-9*) Thomson Learn.

Demand for & Supply of Opiates for Medical & Scientific Needs: Special Report of the International Narcotics Control Board, 1989. 1989. 21p. 6.00 (*92-1-148079-5*, 89.XI.5) UN.

Demand for Health: A Theoretical & Empirical Investigation. Michael Grossman. 1972. (Occasional Papers: No. 119). 135p. pap. 35.10 (*0-87014-248-8*) Natl Bur Econ Res.

Demand for Health Care in Latin America: Lessons from the Dominican Republic & El Salvador. Ricardo A. Bitran & D. Keith McInnes. 1993. LC 93-18214. (EDI Seminar Ser.: No. 46). 66p. pap. 22.00 (*0-8213-2341-5*, 12341) World Bank.

Demand for Medical Care: Evidence from Urban Areas in Bolivia. Masako Ii. 1996. LC 96-927. (LSMS Working Papers: No. 123). 64p. pap. 22.00 (*0-8213-3565-0*, 13565) World Bank.

Demand for Military Health Care: Supporting Research for a Comprehensive Study of the Military Health-Care System. Susan D. Hosek et al. 1995. LC 95-11929. (Illus.). 159p. pap. text 13.00 (*0-8330-1637-7*, MR-407-1-OSD) Rand Corp.

Demand for Primary Health Services in the Third World. John S. Akin et al. 1985. LC 84-18153. (Illus.). 272p. 65.00 (*0-8476-7355-3*, R7355) Rowman.

Demanding Medical Excellence: Doctors & Accountability in the Information Age. Michael L. Millenson. 1997. LC 97-16677. 434p. 24.95 (*0-226-52587-2*) U Ch Pr.

Demanding Patients? Analysing the Use of Primary Care. Anne Rogers. 1998. (State of Health Ser.). 99.00 (*0-335-20091-5*) Taylor & Francis.

Demanding Patients? Analyzing the Use of Primary Care. Anne Rogers. 1998. LC 98-4299. (State of Health Ser.). x, 259p. pap. (*0-335-20090-7*) OpUniv Pr.

Dementia. Alistair Burns & Raymond Levy. 1994. LC 94-131499. (Illus.). 912p. 333.95 (*0-412-54740-6*, Chap & Hall NY) Chapman & Hall.

Dementia. Anthony J. Edwards. 1993. (Perspectives on Individual Differences Ser.). (Illus.). 316p. (C). 54.50 (*0-306-44286-8*, Plenum Trade) Perseus Pubng.

***Dementia.** Whalley & I. Emery Breitner. 2002. (Fast Facts Ser.). (Illus.). 64p. pap. (*1-899541-78-0*) Health Pr GBR. *Dist:* JAMCO Dist.

Dementia. Ed. by Peter J. Whitehouse. 1993. LC 92-49876. (Contemporary Neurology Ser.: No. 40). (Illus.). 514p. 90.00 (*0-8036-9271-4*) OUP.

Dementia. B. Mahendra. 2nd ed. 1987. text 119.00 (*0-7462-0044-7*) Kluwer Academic.

Dementia. Ed. by John O'Brien et al. 2nd ed. 2001. LC 2001-266306. (Illus.). 896p. 198.50 (*0-340-75916-X*) OUP.

Dementia: A Clinical Approach. Jeffrey L. Cummings & D. Frank Benson. 2nd ed. 1992. 560p. 99.00 (*0-7506-9065-8*) Buttrwrth-Heinemann.

Dementia: A Guide for Health Care Professionals. Simon B. Thompson. 1997. 176p. text (*1-85742-334-8*) Arena GBR. *Dist:* Ashgate Pub Co.

Dementia: Annotated Bibliography of the Dementia Associated Diseases & Diagnostic Tests. Jay B. Cohn. 1992. 437p. (Orig.). pap. text 40.00 (*0-935645-03-9*) AJFP.

Dementia: New Skills for Social Workers. Ed. by Alan Chapman & Mary Marshall. 1994. LC 93-38449. (Case Studies for Practice Ser.: No. 5). 160p. pap. 24.95 (*1-85302-142-3*) Taylor & Francis.

Dementia & Aging: Ethics, Values, & Policy Choices. Ed. by Robert H. Binstock et al. 1992. LC 92-6220. 208p. pap. text 20.95 (*0-8018-4545-9*) Johns Hopkins.

Dementia & Aging Adults with Intellectual Disabilities: A Handbook. Matthew P. Janicki & A. J. Dalton. 1998. LC 98-26774. (Illus.). xxix, 488p. 64.95 (*0-87630-915-5*); pap. 29.95 (*0-87630-916-3*) Brunner-Routledge.

Dementia & Communication. Ed. by Rosemary Lubinski. 1995. (Illus.). 320p. (C). pap. text 49.95 (*1-56593-084-3*, 1138) Singular Publishing.

Dementia & Homecare. Janet Askham & Catherine Thompson. 1989. (C). (*0-7855-6576-0*) Age Concern Eng GBR. *Dist:* St Mut.

Dementia & Normal Aging. Ed. by Felicia A. Huppert et al. 1994. (Illus.). 589p. (C). text 120.00 (*0-521-41393-1*) Cambridge U Pr.

Dementia Care: Keeping Intact & in Touch: A Search for Occupational Therapy Interventions. M. Catherine Conroy. 1996. LC 96-85505. 252p. text (*1-85972-036-6*) Avebury GBR. *Dist:* Ashgate Pub Co.

Dementia Care: Patient, Family, & Community. Ed. by Nancy L. Mace. 1991. LC 89-8106. 416p. reprint ed. pap. text 22.50 (*0-8018-4314-6*) Johns Hopkins.

Dementia Disorders: Advances & Prospects. Ed. by Cornelius L. Katona. 2nd ed. 1990. 232p. 92.50 (*0-412-32860-7*, A3988) Chapman & Hall.

Dementia in Close Up. Bere M. L. Miesen. 1999. LC 98-23238. 248p. (C). 78.95 (*0-415-12884-6*) Routledge.

Dementia in Close-up. Bere M. L. Miesen. 1999. LC 98-23238. 248p. (C). pap. 26.95 (*0-415-12885-4*) Routledge.

Dementia in Later Life: Research & Action. 1986. (Technical Reports: No. 730). 74p. pap. text 10.00 (*92-4-120730-2*, 1100730) World Health.

Dementia in Parkinsonism. Ed. by S. E. Daniel et al. 1998. (Illus.). 224p. 119.00 (*3-211-82960-1*) Spr-Verlag.

Dementia Praecox, or the Group of Schizophrenias. Eugen Bleuler. Tr. by Joseph Zinkin. 1966. (Monograph Series on Schizophrenia: No. 1). 548p. 72.50 (*0-8236-1180-9*) Intl Univs Pr.

Dementia Today. David Sutcliffe. 2000. 144p. pap. (*0-86242-283-3*) Age Concern Eng GBR. *Dist:* St Mut.

Dementia with Dignity. Barbara Sherman. rev. ed. 1991. (Illus.). 219p. pap. text 19.00 (*0-07-470184-3*) McGraw-Hill Med Pub.

Dementia with Lewy Bodies: Clinical, Pathological, & Treatment Issues. Ed. by Elaine Perry et al. 1996. LC 96-16710. (Illus.). 541p. (C). text 140.00 (*0-521-56188-4*) Cambridge U Pr.

Dementias. John H. Growdon & M. Rossor. 1998. LC 98-15850. (Blue Books of Practical Neurology). 472p. text 99.00 (*0-7506-9920-5*) Buttrwrth-Heinemann.

Dementias: Biological Bases & Clinical Approach to Treatment. Stefano Govoni et al. 1999. LC 98-54980. 325p. (C). pap. (*88-470-0048-3*) Spr-Verlag ITA. *Dist:* Spr-Verlag.

Dementias: Crossroads Between Neurology & Psychiatry: A Pathological Sequelae to Glutamate Neurotoxicity. Makram K. Girgis & Katherine Harris. 1992. (Illus.). 187p. pap. 27.50 (*0-87527-350-5*) Green.

Dementielle Hirnerkrankung im Alter. Ed. by W. Meier-Ruge. 1993. (Geriatrie fuer die Taegliche Praxis Ser.: Vol. 3). viii, 216p. pap. 28.00 (*3-8055-4509-6*) S Karger.

Dementing Brain Disease in Old Age. Ed. by W. Meier-Ruge. 1993. (Teaching & Training in Geriatric Medicine Ser.: Vol. 3). viii, 216p. pap. 31.50 (*3-8055-4478-2*) S Karger.

Democracy & DNA: The Social Progress of American Medicine. Gerald Weissman. 1996. LC 95-46250. 263p. 23.00 (*0-8090-9305-7*) Hill & Wang.

Democratic Participation & Health Care. Danny Pieters. 1994. 59p. pap. (*90-6215-410-7*) Maklu Uitgev BEL. *Dist:* Paul & Co Pubs.

Demographic & Programmatic Consequences of New Contraceptives. Ed. by S. Segal et al. 1989. LC 89-23083. (Reproductive Biology Ser.). (Illus.). 336p. (C). text 126.00 (*0-306-43384-2*, Kluwer Plenum) Kluwer Academic.

Demographic Changes Spur Contact Lens & Solutions Market: Frequent Replacement & Disposable Lenses Drive Mature Industry. 1992. 214p. 1495.00 (*1-56753-009-5*) Frost & Sullivan.

Demographic Modelling of the HIV-AIDS Epidemic. M. Artzrouni. 1992. 76p. pap. text 147.00 (*2-88124-567-6*) Gordon & Breach.

Demographic Trends in the European Region Health & Social Implications. A. Lopez & R. Cliquet. 1984. (WHO Regional Publications European Ser.: No. 17). 188p. pap. text 22.00 (*92-890-1108-4*) World Health.

Demography & Retirement in the 21st Century. Ed. by Anna M. Rappaport & Sylvester J. Schieber. 1993. LC 92-46552. 344p. 70.00 (*0-275-94248-1*, C4248, Praeger Pubs) Greenwood.

Demography & Vector-Borne Diseases. Ed. by Michael W. Service. 1989. 384p. lib. bdg. 252.95 (*0-8493-4961-3*, RA643) CRC Pr.

Demography of Health & Health Care. R. K. Thomas & Louis G. Pol. 1991. (Demographic Methods & Population Analysis Ser.). (Illus.). 376p. (C). 52.50 (*0-306-43981-6*, Plenum Trade) Perseus Pubng.

Demography of Health & Health Care. Louis G. Pol & Richard K. Thomas. 2nd ed. 2000. LC 00-22102. (Demographic Methods & Population Analysis Ser.). 382p. pap. 95.00 (*0-306-46336-9*, Kluwer Plenum) Kluwer Academic.

***Demography of Health & Health Care: Evolution & Innovation.** Louis G. Pol & Richard K. Thomas. 2nd ed. 2000. LC 00-22102. (Series on Demographic Methods & Population Analysis). 382p. 42.50 (*0-306-46337-7*, Kluwer Plenum) Kluwer Academic.

Demyelinating Diseases, No. 3. Ed. by Pierre J. Vinken et al. 1985. 660p. 364.00 (*0-444-90392-5*) Elsevier.

Dendritic Cells in Fundamental & Clinical Immunology: Proceedings of the 4th International Symposium Held in Venice, Italy, October 5-10, 1996, Vol. 3. Ed. by Paola Ricciardi-Castagnoli. 1997. LC 97-8041. (Advances in Experimental Medicine & Biology Ser.: Vol. 417). 610p. (C). text 149.50 (*0-306-45592-7*, Kluwer Plenum) Kluwer Academic.

Dendritic Cells in Fundamental & Clinical Immunology Vol. 1: Proceedings; International Symposium on Dendritic Cells in Fundamental & Clinical Immunology (2nd: 1992: Amsterdam, Netherlands), Vol. 1. E. W. Kamperdijk et al. 1993. LC 96-104186. (Advances in Experimental Medicine & Biology Ser.: Vol. 329). (Illus.). 668p. (C). text 145.00 (*0-306-44407-0*, Kluwer Plenum) Kluwer Academic.

Dendritic Cells in Fundamental & Clinical Immunology Vol. 2: Proceedings; International Symposium on Dendritic Cells in Fundamental & Clinical Immunology (3d: 1994: Annecy, France), Vol. 2. Ed. by Jacques Banchereau et al. 1995. (Advances in Experimental Medicine & Biology Ser.: Vol. 378). 592p. 145.00 (*0-306-45078-X*, Kluwer Plenum) Kluwer Academic.

Dengue & Dengue Hemorrhagic Fever in the Americas: Guidelines for Prevention & Control. 1994. (Scientific Publications: No. 548). 362p. text 20.00 (*92-75-11548-6*, 1610548) PAHO.

Dengue & Related Hemorrhagic Diseases. Susumu Hotta. 1969. LC 67-26013. (Illus.). 176p. 10.75 (*0-87527-043-3*) Green.

Dengue Fever & Dengue Hemorrhagic Fever. Ed. by D. J. Gubler & G. Kuno. 1998. LC 97-13184. (Illus.). 496p. text 135.00 (*0-85199-134-3*) OUP.

Dengue Haemorrhagic Fever: Diagnosis, Treatment & Control. 1986. 58p. pap. 13.00 (*92-4-154209-8*) World Health.

Dengue Haemorrhagic Fever: Diagnosis, Treatment, Prevention & Control. WHO Staff. 2nd ed. 1996. LC 98-163826. (*92-4-154500-3*) World Health.

Denial: A Clarification of Concepts & Research. E. L. Edelstein et al. 1989. (Illus.). 344p. (C). text 65.00 (*0-306-43058-4*, Kluwer Plenum) Kluwer Academic.

Denial of Death. Ernest Becker. 1985. LC 73-1860. pap. 14.95 (*0-02-902380-7*) Free Pr.

Denial of Stress. Ed. by Shlomo Breznitz. 1983. LC 82-13044. xiv, 316p. 50.00 (*0-8236-1185-X*) Intl Univs Pr.

Denn alles steht seit Ewigkeit geschrieben see Secret Medicine of the Pharoahs: Ancient Egyptian Medicine

Density Functional Theory of Molecules, Clusters & Solids. Ed. by D. E. Ellis. 1994. LC 94-30303. (Understanding Chemical Reactivity Ser.). 324p. (C). text 204.50 (*0-7923-3083-8*) Kluwer Academic.

Dental Acquisition Report, 1998. Irving Levin Associates, Inc. Staff. 1998. (Illus.). 125p. pap. 395.00 (*1-930625-03-0*) I Levin.

Dental Admission Test (DAT) Jack Rudman. (Admission Test Ser.: Vol. 12). 47.95 (*0-8373-5112-X*); 1994. pap. 27.95 (*0-8373-5012-3*) Nat Learn.

Dental Amalgam: A Scientific Review & Recommended Public Health Service Strategy for Research Education & Regulation. Ed. by James S. Benson. 1999. 183p. reprint ed. pap. text 30.00 (*0-7881-8056-8*) DIANE Pub.

Dental Anatomy. Gerald M. Cathey. 1972. (Dental Laboratory Technology Manuals Ser.). viii, 236p. pap. 34.95 (*0-8078-7905-3*) U of NC Pr.

Dental Anatomy: A Self-Instructional Program. Nancy S. Karst & Sarah K. Smith. 10th ed. 1997. LC 96-36841. (Illus.). 635p. (C). pap. 58.00 (*0-8385-1492-8*, A1492-6) P-H.

Dental Anatomy: Its Relevance to Dentistry. Ed. by Julian B. Woelfel. 4th ed. 1990. (Illus.). 438p. pap. 48.00 (*0-8121-1259-8*) Lppncott W & W.

Dental Anatomy: Its Relevance to Dentistry. Julian B. Woelfel & Rickne C. Scheid. 5th ed. 1997. LC 96-41063. (Illus.). 456p. pap. 44.95 (*0-683-30044-X*) Lppncott W & W.

***Dental Anatomy: Its Relevance to Dentistry.** Rickne C. Scheid & Julian B. Woelfel. 6th ed. 2001. LC 2001-38187. (Illus.). 468p. pap. text 47.00 (*0-7817-2797-9*) Lppncott W & W.

***Dental Anatomy & Occlusion.** Ed. by Khalid Choudhary. 2001. LC 2001-26175. (Pocket Brain Ser.). (Illus.). 92p. pap. 16.95 (*0-9651162-7-1*) Wysteria Ltd.

Dental Anatomy & Oral Histology. Arup K. Das. 1972. 260p. (*0-7855-2915-2*) Current Dist IND. *Dist:* St Mut.

Dental Anatomy & Oral Histology Review. A. K. Das. 1991. (C). (*0-89771-344-3*) Current Dist IND. *Dist:* St Mut.

Dental Aptitude Test (DAT) - Core Content. David M. Tarlow. 1996. (Medical Examinations Ser.). (Illus.). 560p. (Orig.). (C). pap. 49.95 (*1-57774-001-7*) Educ Tsting Cnslts.

Dental Aptitude Test Student Guide. David M. Tarlow & Marc L. Lichtenberg. 1993. LC 78-53093. (Illus.). pap. 12.95 (*0-931572-01-0*) Datar Pub.

Dental Asepsis: A Self-Instructional Guide, Bk. 5. Robert J. Whitacre et al. 3rd rev. ed. 1985. (Illus.). 128p. pap. 29.95 (*0-89939-051-X*) Stoma Pr.

Dental Assistant. Pauline C. Anderson. 1987. (Dental Assisting Procedures Ser.). 480p. (gr. 12). pap., tchr. ed. 10.00 (*0-8273-2753-6*) Delmar.

Dental Assistant. Jack Rudman. 1994. (Career Examination Ser.: C-205). pap. 29.95 (*0-8373-0205-6*) Nat Learn.

Dental Assistant. Pauline C. Anderson & Martha R. Burkard. 6th ed. 1994. 69p. pap., tchr. ed. 18.95 (*0-8273-5282-4*) Delmar.

Dental Assistant. Pauline C. Anderson et al. 6th ed. 1994. LC 93-40765. 784p. (C). pap. 56.95 (*0-8273-5281-6*) Delmar.

Dental Assistant. Ed. by Roger E. Barton et al. 6th ed. 1988. LC 87-31199. (Illus.). 655p. text 31.50 (*0-8121-1141-9*) Lppncott W & W.

Dental Assistant: Syllabus. E. A. Jacobson & Alma Jacobson. 1978. (gr. 10-12). pap. text 13.95 (*0-89420-046-1*, 198040); (J). 228.60 incl. audio (*0-89420-139-5*) Natl Book.

Dental Assistant Techniques. Betty Lorenzen. 1976. LC 74-18674. (Allied Health Ser.). (gr. 11-12). pap. (*0-672-61395-6*) Macmillan.

Dental Assisting. Jack Rudman. (Occupational Competency Examination Ser.: Vol. 15). 47.95 (*0-8373-5765-9*); 1994. pap. 27.95 (*0-8373-5715-2*) Nat Learn.

Dental Assisting Essentials. Pauline C. Anderson & Alice E. Pendleton. 7th ed. 2000. LC 00-50846. (Dental Assisting Procedures Ser.). (Illus.). 736p. (C). pap. text 67.95 (*0-7668-1113-1*) Delmar.

Dental Assisting Exam Preparation. Hazel O. Torres & Lois Mazzucchi-Ballard. 1993. LC 93-19477. 208p. pap. text 23.00 (*0-7216-3295-5*) Saunders.

Dental Assisting Test Preparation. Roberta Albano & Carol Giaquinto. 1995. LC 95-23664. (Brady/Prentice Hall Test Prep Ser.). 192p. pap. text 45.00 (*0-8359-4944-3*) P-H.

Dental Auxiliary Education Examination in Dental Materials. Jack Rudman. 1994. (College Level Examination Ser.: CLEP-47). pap. 27.95 (*0-8373-5347-5*) Nat Learn.

Dental Auxiliary Education Examination in Head, Neck & Oral Anatomy. Jack Rudman. 1994. (College Level Examination Ser.: CLEP-48). pap. 27.95 (*0-8373-5348-3*) Nat Learn.

Dental Auxiliary Education Examination in Oral Radiography. Jack Rudman. 1994. (College Level Examination Ser.: CLEP-49). pap. 27.95 (*0-8373-5349-1*) Nat Learn.

Dental Auxiliary Education Examination in Tooth Morphology & Function. Jack Rudman. 1994. (College Level Examination Ser.: CLEP-50). pap. 23.95 (*0-8373-5950-3*) Nat Learn.

Dental Auxillery Guide to Office Emergencies. Chernega. 1986. (C). pap. text 4.40 (*0-8273-2336-0*) Delmar.

Dental Back Office SOPs from Standard Operating Procedures for All Dentists. Marsha Freeman. 2000. 116p. ring bd. 60.00 incl. disk (*0-910167-67-2*, Dental Commun) Comm Unltd CA.

Dental Bibliography: A Reference Index to the Literature of Dental Science Wolf Weinberger. 1998. 262p. reprint ed. 65.00 (*1-57898-085-2*) Martino Pubng.

Dental Bookkeeping & Data Entry SOPs from Standard Operating Procedures for All Dentists. Marsha Freeman. 2000. 55p. ring bd. 60.00 (*0-910167-66-4*, Dental Commun) Comm Unltd CA.

Dental Care for Everyone: Problems & Proposals. James M. Dunning. 1976. (Illus.). 240p. 25.95 (*0-674-19790-9*) HUP.

Dental Care Today. Robert J. Kitson. 1993. (Illus.). 50p. (Orig.). pap. 7.95 (*0-9639767-0-2*) R J Kitson Pubng.

Dental Caries: A Treatable Infection. Walter J. Loesche. rev. ed. 1994. (Illus.). 550p. (C). pap. 39.95 (*0-9639689-0-4*) Automat Diag.

Dental Ceramics: Proceedings of the First International Symposium on Ceramics. Ed. by John W. McLean. 1983. (Illus.). 536p. text 160.00 (*0-86715-112-9*) Quint Pub Co.

Dental Charting: A Standard Approach. Jill Joroski-Graf. 1999. LC 99-30235. 320p. pap. text 28.95 (*0-7668-0625-1*) Delmar.

Dental Communication. David W. Chambers & Ronald G. Abrams. 1992. 295p. (C). pap. text 24.00 (*0-9632599-0-3*) Ohana Grp.

Dental Diagnostic Imaging: Diagnostic Features & Pathology. Ed. by Robert P. Langlais et al. 1997. LC 97-8630. (Illus.). 176p. text 55.95 (*0-398-06784-8*) C C Thomas.

Dental Drug Reference. Halstead Phinney. 1999. LC 99-30080. xxi, 487p. (C). pap. 26.50 net. (*0-7668-0115-2*) Delmar.

Dental Education at the Crossroads: Challenges & Change. Institute of Medicine Staff. Ed. by Marilyn J. Field. 1995. 360p. (Orig.). (C). text 49.95 (*0-309-05195-9*) Natl Acad Pr.

Dental Electronics & Equipment Markets: Dentists Look to Esthetics for New Revenues. Market Intelligence Staff. 1992. 314p. (Orig.). 1695.00 (*1-56753-031-1*) Frost & Sullivan.

Dental Enamel, Vol. 205. CIBA Foundation Staff & Hal. C. Slavkin. 1997. LC 96-42297. (CIBA Foundation Symposia Ser.). 284p. 128.00 (*0-471-96872-2*) Wiley.

Dental Ethics. Bruce Weinstein. 1993. (Illus.). 250p. pap. 29.95 (*0-8121-1444-2*) Lppncott W & W.

Dental Ethics at Chairside: Professional Principles & Practical Applications. David T. Ozar & David J. Sokol. 2nd ed. 1999. LC 99-37080. 288p. pap. text 38.00 (*0-87840-759-6*) Georgetown U Pr.

Dental First Aid for Families. Richard Diamond. 2000. LC 99-40278. (Idyll Arbor Personal Health Book Ser.). (Illus.). viii, 134p. pap. 10.00 (*1-882883-39-X*) Idyll Arbor.

Dental Front Office SOPs from Standard Operating Procedures for All Dentists. Marsha Freeman. 2000. 86p. ring bd. 60.00 (*0-910167-65-6*, Dental Commun) Comm Unltd CA.

Dental Handbook for Short-Term Mission Trips. Jack Shuler & Nardos Shuler. 2000. 30p. pap. 10.00 (*0-9666809-5-2*) Christ Med & Dental Assns.

Dental Health, Set. Helen Frost. 1998. (Illus.). (J). (ps-2). lib. bdg. 53.00 (*0-7368-0142-1*, Pebble Bks) Capstone Pr.

Dental Health Education: Lesson Planning & Implementation. Lori Gagliardi. 1998. LC 98-3597. 224p. pap. 29.33 (*0-8385-1574-6*) P-H.

Dental Health Education: Proceedings of the WHO Expert Committee, Geneva, 1969. WHO Staff. 1970. (Technical Reports: No. 449). pap. text 3.00 (*92-4-120449-4*, 1100449) World Health.

Dental Hygiene Aptitude Test (DHAT) Jack Rudman. (Admission Test Ser.: Vol. 32). 49.95 (*0-8373-5132-4*); 1994. pap. 29.95 (*0-8373-5032-8*) Nat Learn.

Dental Hygiene Care: Diagnosis & Care Planning. Laura Mueller-Joseph & Marie Petersen. 1995. LC 94-32214. (Health & Life Science Ser.). 272p. (C). 48.95 (*0-8273-5678-1*) Delmar.

Dental Hygiene Department SOPs from Standard Operating Procedures for All Dentists. Marsha Freeman. 2000. 59p. ring bd. 60.00 incl. disk (*0-910167-68-0*) Comm Unltd CA.

Dental Hygiene Infection Control. Stephen A. Eklund. 1998. pap. text (*0-7216-4623-9*) Saunders.

Dental Hygiene Theory & Practice. Darby. 2nd ed. 2001. text (*0-7216-9162-5*) Harcrt Hlth Sci Grp.

Dental Hygienist. Jack Rudman. 1994. (Career Examination Ser.: C-192). pap. 29.95 (*0-8373-0192-0*) Nat Learn.

Dental Hygienist's Guide to Nutritional Care. Judi R. Davis et al. Ed. by Selma Kaszczuk. 1998. LC 97-31211. (Illus.). 480p. pap. text 34.95 (*0-7216-5014-7*) Saunders.

Dental Implants: A Guide for the General Practitioner. Michael Norton. 1995. (Illus.). 148p. text 68.00 (*1-85097-037-8*) Quint Pub Co.

Dental Implants: Are They for Me? Thomas D. Taylor & William R. Laney. 2nd ed. 1993. LC 93-2019. (Illus.). 60p. pap. 26.00 (*0-86715-198-6*) Quint Pub Co.

Dental Implants: Fundamental & Advanced Laboratory Technology. Robert Winkelman & Kenneth Orh Orh. 1995. (Illus.). 209p. text (*0-7234-2040-8*) Martin Dunitz GBR. *Dist:* Mosby Inc.

Dental Implants: Principles & Practice. Charles A. Babbush. (Illus.). 1991. 320p. text 165.00 (*0-7216-2227-5*); 2nd ed. 2000. LC 00-52253. xvii, 532p. text 199.00 (*0-7216-7747-9*) Saunders.

Dental Informatics: Integrating Technology into the Dental Environment. Ed. by L. M. Abbey & J. Zimmerman. 1991. (Computers in Health Care Ser.). (Illus.). 348p. 92.00 (*0-387-97643-4*) Spr-Verlag.

Dental Kinesiology. George A. Eversaul. 1978. LC 78-66982. 57.50 (*0-9601978-1-8*) Health Res Las Vegas.

Dental Laboratory Procedures: Complete Dentures, 1. Ed. by Robert Morrow. 1985. 600p. (C). (gr. 13). text 99.95 (*0-8016-3519-5*, 03519) Mosby Inc.

Dental Laboratory Technology: Basic Sciences. 1993. lib. bdg. 299.95 (*0-8490-8905-0*) Gordon Pr.

Dental Laboratory Technology: Fixed & Special Prosthodontic & Orthodontic Appliances. 1993. lib. bdg. 333.75 (*0-8490-8906-9*) Gordon Pr.

Dental Laboratory Technology: Removable Prosthodontics. 1993. lib. bdg. 320.95 (*0-8490-8907-7*) Gordon Pr.

Dental Maintenance for Patients with Periodontal Disease. Thomas G. Wilson. 1989. (Illus.). 300p. text 68.00 (*0-86715-209-5*) Quint Pub Co.

Dental Malpractice: Legal & Medical Handbook. Norman L. Schafler. 3rd ed. 1998. pap. text, suppl. ed. 74.00 (*1-56706-984-3*) Aspen Pub.

Dental Management & Marketing SOPs from Standard Operating Procedures for All Dentists. Marsha Freeman. 2000. 143p. ring bd. 60.00 incl. disk (*0-910167-69-9*, Dental Commun) Comm Unltd CA.

Dental Management of Patients with HIV. Michael Glick. 1994. LC 94-30147. (Illus.). 320p. text 68.00 (*0-86715-288-5*) Quint Pub Co.

Dental Management of the Medically Compromised Patient. Donald A. Falace. Ed. by James W. Little. 5th ed. 1996. LC 96-24492. (Illus.). 688p. (C). (gr. 13). pap. text 44.00 (*0-8151-5634-0*, 25103) Mosby Inc.

Dental Materials. Prasanta K. Basu. 1985. (*0-7855-0814-7*) Current Dist IND. *Dist:* St Mut.

Dental Materials. Vanable. 2000. pap. text 42.61 (*0-8385-1576-2*, Medical Exam) Appleton & Lange.

Dental Materials: Biological Properties & Clinical Evaluation. Ed. by Ivar A. Mjor. 1985. 224p. 128.00 (*0-8493-6644-5*, RK652, CRC Reprint) Franklin.

Dental Materials: Properties & Manipulation. Robert G. Craig & William J. O'Brien. 6th ed. 1995. (Illus.). 304p. (C). (gr. 13). pap. text 35.00 (*0-8151-1919-4*, 25195) Mosby Inc.

Dental Materials: Properties & Manipulation. Robert G. Craig et al. 7th ed. 1999. (Illus.). tchr. ed. (*0-323-00521-7*); LC 99-31262. 352p. text 39.00 (*0-323-00512-8*) Mosby Inc.

Dental Materials: Properties & Selection. William J. O'Brien. 2nd ed. 1997. LC 96-48070. 434p. pap. text 58.00 (*0-86715-297-4*) Quint Pub Co.

Dental Materials & Technical Application. Karl F. Leinfelder et al. 3rd ed. 1980. (Dental Assisting Manuals Ser.: No. 6). ix, 145p. (C). pap. 24.95 (*0-8078-1380-X*) U of NC Pr.

Dental Mercury Detox. Sam Ziff et al. enl. rev. ed. 1997. 88p. pap. 5.95 (*0-941011-05-4*) Bio-Probe.

Dental Morphology: An Illustrated Guide. G. C. Van Beek. 2nd ed. 1983. (Illus.). 135p. pap. text (*0-7236-0666-8*) John Wright GBR. *Dist:* Buttrwrth-Heinemann.

Dental Morphology & Pathology of Prehistoric Guam. R. W. Leigh. 1929. (BMB Ser.). (Orig.). reprint ed. pap. 25.00 (*0-527-01668-3*) Periodicals Srv.

Dental Office Emergencies - A Quick Reference Guide: Medical Emergencies & Basic Cardiac Life Support (CPR) in Adults & Children. Ed. by Joseph Gargano et al. 1996. 72p. pap. 12.50 (*1-887272-10-0*) Amer Med Pub.

Dental Office Management. Sparks. 1996. (Dental Assisting Procedures Ser.). pap. 43.95 (*0-8273-6481-4*) Delmar.

Dental Office Procedures Manual. Ann Ehrlich. 3rd ed. 1993. (Illus.). 28.95 (*0-940012-34-0*) Colwell Syst.

Dental Pharmacology. Fred F. Cowan. 2nd ed. 1991. LC 90-13637. (Illus.). text 39.50 (*0-8121-1385-3*) Lppncott W & W.

Dental Practice & Research: Index of Modern Information. Ilonia M. Rekany. 1990. LC 88-47950. 150p. 47.50 (*1-55914-132-8*); pap. 44.50 (*1-55914-133-6*) ABBE Pubs Assn.

Dental Practice Management Encyclopedia. Carl M. Caplan. 1985. 280p. 10.00 (*0-87814-288-6*) PennWell Corp.

Dental Problems in Childhood. Ed. by David W. Kaplan. 1989. (Journal: Vol. 16, Nos. 3-4, 1989). (Illus.). 88p. pap. 48.00 (*3-8055-5112-6*) S Karger.

Dental Prosthetics. C. Barclay & A. D. Walmsley. 2nd ed. 1997. LC 97-18739. (Colour Guide Ser.). (*0-443-05813-X*) Harcrt Hlth Sci Grp.

Dental Public Health: Contemporary Practice for the Dental Hygienist. Christine Nathe. 2000. LC 00-55725. 316p. pap. 44.67 (*0-13-085157-4*) P-H.

Dental Pulp: Biologic Considerations in the Dental Procedures. I. B. Bender et al. 3rd ed. 1984. LC 65-7149. (Illus.). 358p. text 45.00 (*0-397-52107-3*, Lippncttt) Lppncott W & W.

Dental Radiographic Diagnosis. Kavas H. Thunthy. 2nd ed. 1996. LC 96-47747. 430p. 64.95 (*0-87814-706-3*) PennWell Corp.

Dental Radiography: An Introduction for Dental Hygienists & Assistants. Richard C. O'Brien. 4th ed. 1982. (Illus.). 296p. text 52.00 (*0-7216-6887-9*) Saunders.

Dental Radiography: Principles & Techniques. Joen I. Haring & Laura J. Lind. Ed. by Selma Ozmat. 1996. LC 95-30880. 496p. pap. text 41.95 (*0-7216-5596-3*) Saunders.

Dental Radiography, Lessons 1-14: Student Workbooks. Brown. 1985. (C). (gr. 13). spiral bd. 42.95 (*0-8016-2374-X*, 02374) Mosby Inc.

Dental Radiology. Pauline C. Anderson & Susan B. Clifford. 2nd rev. ed. LC 79-56352. (Dental Assisting Ser.). (Illus.). 152p. (C). (gr. 12). 1982. tchr. ed. 13.00 (*0-8273-1872-3*); 1981. mass mkt. 42.95 (*0-8273-1871-5*) Delmar.

Dental Radiology. Stephen R. Matteson et al. 4th rev. ed. 1988. LC 87-16258. (Dental Assisting Manuals Ser.). (Illus.). viii, 155p. (C). pap. 27.50 (*0-8078-4205-2*) U of NC Pr.

Dental Radiology: Understanding the X-ray Image. L. Brocklebank. 1997. (Illus.). 228p. (C). pap. text 65.00 (*0-19-262410-5*) OUP.

Dental Radiology Laboratory Manual. Sandra S. Olson. 1994. LC 94-8369. (Illus.). 256p. pap. text, lab manual ed. 28.00 (*0-7216-6455-5*) Saunders.

Dental Risk Prevention: Communicating & Record Keeping in Dental Practice. Jack A. Owens & Dan J. Tennenhouse. 1990. 171p. pap. 75.00 (*1-930548-02-8*) Tennenhouse Prof Pubns.

Dental Risk Prevention: For Dental Auxiliaries. Cara Miyasaki-Ching & Dan J. Tennenhouse. 1991. 143p. pap. 35.00 (*1-930548-03-6*) Tennenhouse Prof Pubns.

Dental Science in a New Age: A History of the National Institute of Dental Research. Ruth R. Harris. 1992. LC 90-15599. (History of Science & Technology Ser.). (Illus.). 496p. reprint ed. text 59.95 (*0-8138-1322-0*) Iowa U Pr.

Dental Self Help: New edition of Natural Dental Wellness. Soaring Bear. 2nd ed. 1983. 200p. pap. 19.95 (*0-9607518-1-5*) Dental-Info.

Dental Service & Oral Health: United States, 1989. 1992. LC 92-48918. (Vital & Health Statistics Ser. 10: Data from the National Health Interview Survey: No. 183). (*0-8406-0469-6*) Natl Ctr Health Stats.

Dental Services & Oral Health in the United States. 1997. lib. bdg. 250.95 (*0-8490-8119-X*) Gordon Pr.

Dental Services & Oral Health U. S. 1994. (Illus.). 95p. (Orig.). (C). pap. text 35.00 (*0-7881-1010-1*) DIANE Pub.

Dental Specialist, Set. 1992. lib. bdg. 1990.95 (*0-8490-8872-0*) Gordon Pr.

Dental Store Office Manual. Neil H. Shulkin. 1994. (Illus.). (Orig.). pap. 150.00 (*0-9640863-1-X*) Dental Store.

Dental Strategic Planning from Standard Operating Procedures for All Dentists. Marsha Freeman. 2000. 53p. ring bd. 20.00 (*0-910167-64-8*, Dental Commun) Comm Unltd CA.

Dental Team Management of Medical Emergency. Cassidy. 1999. text (*0-7216-5259-X*) Saunders.

Dental Terminology. Contrib. by Charline M. Dofka et al. 1999. LC 98-52154. (Illus.). 312p. pap. text 27.95 (*0-8273-9068-8*) Delmar.

Dentate Gyrus & Its Role in Seizures. Ed. by Charles E. Ribak et al. 1992. LC 92-18288. (Epilepsy Research Ser.: No. 7). 318p. 314.25 (*0-444-81447-7*) Elsevier.

Dentin & Dentinogenesis. Anders Linde. 1984. 168p. 96.00 (*0-8493-5201-0*, QM569);Vol. 1. LC 83-7714. 176p. 104.00 (*0-8493-5200-2*, QM569) Franklin (CRC Reprint).

Dentin/Pulp Complex: Proceedings of the International Conference on Dentin/Pulp Complex, 1995, & the International Meeting on Clinical Topics of Dentin/Pulp Complex. Ed. by Masaki Shimono et al. 1996. (Illus.). 377p. pap. text 90.00 (*4-87417-522-8*) Quint Pub Co.

Dentist. Jack Rudman. 1994. (Career Examination Ser.: C-193). pap. 49.95 (*0-8373-0193-9*) Nat Learn.

Dentistry. John Rowson & Adrian Slaney. Ed. by Walter Scott. 1996. LC 96-229460. (Medico-Legal Practitioner Ser.). 118p. (*1-85941-212-2*) Cavendish Pubng GBR. *Dist:* Gaunt.

Dentistry: An Illustrated History. Malvin E. Ring. 1985. (Illus.). 320p. 75.00 (*0-8109-1100-0*) Abrams.

Dentistry: An Illustrated History. Malvin E. Ring. 1985. (Illus.). 331p. (C). (gr. 13). text 49.95 (*0-8016-4146-2*, 04146) Mosby Inc.

Dentistry: An Illustrated History. Malvin E. Ring. 1986. (Illus.). 331p. (*84-8174-076-4*) Mosby-Doyma Libros ESP. *Dist:* Mosby Inc.

Dentistry: Creating a Profit Center. Coralee Eisner. 1999. LC 99-59462. (Blueprints for Your Bottom Line Ser.). (Illus.). xii, 119p. pap. (*1-58326-004-8*, AAHA Pr) Am Animal Hosp Assoc.

Dentistry, Dental Practice, & the Community. Ed. by Brian A. Burt & Stephen A. Eklund. 4th ed. 1992. (Illus.). 347p. pap. text 45.00 (*0-7216-3195-9*) Saunders.

Dentistry, Dental Practice & the Community. Brian A. Burt & Steven A. Ekland. Ed. by Judy Fletcher. 5th ed. 1999. LC 98-28551. (Illus.). 395p. (C). pap. text 36.95 (*0-7216-7309-0*) Saunders.

Dentistry for the Child & Adolescent. Ed. by Ralph E. McDonald & David R. Avery. 6th ed. 1993. LC 93-20508. (Illus.). 928p. (C). (gr. 13). text 70.00 (*0-8016-6705-4*, 06705) Mosby Inc.

Dentistry for the Child & Adolescent. Ralph E. McDonald & David R. Avery. 7th ed. 1999. (Illus.). 848p. (*84-8086-166-5*) Mosby-Doyma Libros ESP. *Dist:* Mosby Inc.

Dentistry in Industry: Index of New Information with Authors & Subjects. Science and Life Consultants Association Staff. 1992. 180p. 47.50 (*1-55914-710-5*); pap. 44.50 (*1-55914-711-3*) ABBE Pubs Assn.

Dentistry in Systemic Disease: Diagnostic & Therapeutic Approach to Patient Management. Ed. by Spencer W. Redding & Michael T. Montgomery. 1990. LC 89-64175. (Illus.). 348p. pap. text 21.95 (*0-945892-00-4*) JBK Pub.

Dentistry in the Twenty-First Century: A Global Perspective. Richard J. Simonsen. 1991. (Illus.). 262p. pap. text 22.00 (*0-86715-228-1*) Quint Pub Co.

Dentistry Journals & Serials: An Analytical Guide, 3. Aletha Kowitz. 1985. LC 85-17590. (Annotated Bibliographies of Serials: A Subject Approach Ser.: No. 3). 226p. lib. bdg. 62.50 (*0-313-24363-8*, KDJ/, Greenwood Pr) Greenwood.

Dentistry, Proplast & the Temporo-Mandibular Joint: Index & Reference Book of New Information. Erik F. Fenley. 1996. 150p. 57.50 (*0-7883-0916-1*); pap. 47.50 (*0-7883-0917-X*) ABBE Pubs Assn.

Dentistry Without Mercury. Sam Ziff & Michael F. Ziff. enl. rev. ed. 2000. 96p. 5.95 (*0-941011-04-6*) Bio-Probe.

Dentistry's Future: A Prescription for Success, Wealth & Joy. John A. Wilde. 1999. (Illus.). 464p. pap. 49.90 (*0-9648511-4-8*) Novel Pen.

Dentists' Handbook. Ellis J. Neiburger & S. Neiburger. 1993. LC 92-73278. (Illus.). 350p. (Orig.). pap. text 37.50 (*0-914555-01-4*) Andent Inc.

Dentist's Legal Advisor. William Otis Morris. 1994. LC 95-103734. 544p. (C). (gr. 13). text 51.95 (*0-8151-5867-X*, 25104) Mosby Inc.

Dentition & Dental Care, Vol. 3. Elderton. 1990. 515p. pap. text 78.50 (*0-433-00053-8*) Buttrwrth-Heinemann.

Dentition of Meroitic X-Group, & Christian Populations from Wadi Halfa, Sudan. David L. Greene. (Nubian Ser.: No. 1). reprint ed. 22.50 (*0-404-60685-7*) AMS Pr.

Dentofacial Deformities: Integrated Orthodontic, 1. John P. Stella & Fish. 2nd ed. 1995. (Illus.). 480p. (C). (gr. 13). text 149.00 (*0-8016-7729-7*, 07729) Mosby Inc.

Dentofacial Deformities: Integrated Orthodontic & Surgical Correction, 2. Bruce N. Epker & John P. Stella. 2nd ed. 1996. (Illus.). 656p. (C). (gr. 13). text 149.00 (*0-8151-3148-8*, 24201) Mosby Inc.

Dentofacial Deformities: Integrated Orthodontic & Surgical Correction, 4. Bruce E. Epker. 2nd ed. 1998. (Illus.). 682p. (C). (gr. 13). text 149.00 (*0-8151-2450-3*, 31048) Mosby Inc.

Dentofacial Deformities: Integrated Orthodontic Surgical Correction, 3. Bruce N. Epker & John P. Stella. 2nd ed. 1997. (Illus.). 656p. (C). (gr. 13). text 149.00 (*0-8151-3129-1*, 26227) Mosby Inc.

Dentofacial Growth & Growth Hormone Treatment in Short Children Born Small for Gestational Age. Ria Van Erum. 1998. (Acta Biomedica Lovaniensia Ser.: No. 159). (Illus.). 133p. pap. (*90-6186-844-0*) Leuven Univ BEL. *Dist:* Coronet Bks.

Dentofacial Orthopedics with Functional Appliances. T. M. Graber et al. 2nd ed. 1997. (Illus.). 544p. (*84-8174-331-3*) Mosby-Doyma Libros ESP. *Dist:* Mosby Inc.

Dentofacial Orthopedics with Functional Appliances. Thomas M. Graber & Thomas Rakosi. 2nd ed. 1997. LC 96-49801. (Illus.). 544p. (C). (gr. 13). text 94.95 (*0-8151-3558-0*, 26338) Mosby Inc.

Denver Metro Health Services Directory. 1996. 81p. pap. 40.00 (*1-57975-005-2*) Denver Metro Chamber.

Deoxyglucose Uptake & Oxygen Consumption: A Metabolic Approach to Cerebral Function. Ed. by M. Le Poncin-Lafitte & J. R. Rapin. 1981. (Journal: Vol. 20, No. 3). (Illus.). 170p. pap. 43.50 (*3-8055-3412-4*) S Karger.

***Department of Defense Anthrax Vaccine Immunization Program: Congressional Hearings.** Ed. by Steve Buyer. 2001. (Illus.). 362p. reprint ed. pap. text 45.00 (*0-7567-1030-8*) DIANE Pub.

Department of Health & Human Services' Proposed Budget for Fiscal Year 1998: Hearing Before the Subcommittee on Health & the Environment of the Committee on Commerce, House of Representatives, One Hundred Fifth Congress, First Session, February 12, 1997. U. S. Congress, House Committee on Commerce, Subcommittee on Health and the Environment. 1997. LC 97-174305. (Illus.). (*0-16-054326-6*) USGPO.

Department of Nursing Staff Education Manual. Massachusetts General Hospital Department of Nursi. Ed. by Cheryl B. Stetler et al. 1982. (C). pap. text 37.50 (*0-8359-4251-1*) P-H.

Department of Surgical Services Continuous Quality Improvement: Policy & Procedure Guideline Manual. Lea Johnson. 1992. 110.00 (*1-879575-24-8*) Acad Med Sys.

Department of Surgical Services Safety Management: Policy & Procedure Guideline Manual. Judith Smith. 1992. 90.00 (*1-879575-21-3*) Acad Med Sys.

Department of Surgical Services Standards - Nursing Care Plans: Policy & Procedure Guideline Manual. Judith Smith. 1992. 85.00 (*1-879575-20-5*) Acad Med Sys.

DePauw: A Pictorial History. Ed. by John J. Baughman. 1987. (Illus.). 234p. 30.00 (*0-936631-12-0*) DePauw Univ.

Dependency & Japanese Socialization: Psychoanalytic & Anthropological Investigations into "Amae" Frank A. Johnson. 1995. 452p. (C). pap. text 22.50 (*0-8147-4222-X*) NYU Pr.

Dependency or Interdependency in Old Age. Joep M. Munnichs et al. 1976. text 88.00 (*90-247-1895-3*) Kluwer Academic.

Dependent Elderly: Autonomy, Justice & Quality of Care. Ed. by Luke Gormally. 1992. 210p. (C). text 64.95 (*0-521-41531-4*) Cambridge U Pr.

Dependent Personality. Robert F. Bornstein. 1993. LC 92-49466. 241p. 35.00 (*0-89862-991-8*, 2991) Guilford Pubns.

Deployment: Hiding Behind Power Struggles As a Character Defense. Rena Moses-Hrushovski. 1994. LC 94-98. (Psychoanalytic Therapy Ser.). 344p. 60.00 (*1-56821-042-6*) Aronson.

Deportiva Fisioterapia y Entrenamiento Aletico. Daniel Arnheim. 2nd ed. 1994. (SPA.). 50.00 net. (*84-8086-073-1*) Mosby-Doyma Libros ESP. *Dist:* Mosby Inc.

Deposition, Retention & Dosimetry of Inhaled Radioactive Substances: Recommendations of the National Council on Radiation Protection & Measurements. National Council on Radiation Protection and Measure. 1997. LC 96-37944. (NCRP Reports: Vol. 125). (Orig.). pap. 40.00 (*0-929600-54-1*) NCRP Pubns.

Deprenyl: The Inside Story. Alastair Dow. 220p. (C). reprint ed. 19.95 (*0-9629285-0-X*) Easton CA.

Depressed Child: A Parent's Guide for Rescuing Kids. Douglas A. Riley. 2001. LC 00-62033. x, 208p. pap. 12.95 (*0-87833-187-5*) Taylor Pub.

Depressed Child & Adolescent: Developmental & Clinical Perspectives. Ed. by Ian M. Goodyer. 1995. (Cambridge Monographs on Child & Adolescent Psychiatry: 1). (Illus.). 378p. (C). text 90.00 (*0-521-43326-6*) Cambridge U Pr.

Depression. 1994. 21.95 (*0-387-57900-1*); 1993. 30.95 (*0-387-57133-7*) Spr-Verlag.

***Depression.** David S. Baldwin & Robert Hirschfeld. 2001. (Fast Facts Ser.). (Illus.). 64p. pap. (*1-899541-83-7*) Health Pr GBR. *Dist:* JAMCO Dist.

Depression. Guy BonGiovanni. 1983. 17p. (Orig.). (C). pap. 2.00 (*0-912981-04-0*) Hse BonGiovanni.

Depression. Constance L. Hammen. 1997. LC 98-106165. (Illus.). v, 218p. pap. (*0-86377-727-9*) Psychol Pr GBR. *Dist:* Taylor & Francis.

Depression. James B. Levenson. 2000. LC 99-57889. (Key Diseases Series). 340p. pap. text 35.00 (*0-943126-85-1*, 330300790) Amer Coll Phys.

Depression. B. Mahendra. 1987. text 176.50 (*0-85200-983-6*) Kluwer Academic.

Depression: A Cognitive Therapy Approach. Arthur Freeman. 1994. (Assessment & Treatment of Psychological Disorders Video Ser.). incl. VHS (*1-56784-400-6*) Newbridge Educ.

Depression: A Cognitive Therapy Approach - a Viewer's Manual. Arthur Freeman. 1994. (Assessment & Treatment of Psychological Disorders, a Video Ser.). incl. VHS (*1-56784-401-4*) Newbridge Educ.

Depression: A Guide for Patients. Michael Thase & A. John Rush. 1997. (Behavioral Health Ser.). 32p. pap. text 2.95 (*1-885274-38-6*) Health InfoNet Inc.

Depression: A Woman Doctor's Guide: Essential Facts & Up-to-the-Minute Information on Overcoming Depression. Jane S. Ferber & Suzanne LeVert. 2000. 256p. mass mkt. 6.99 (*1-57566-621-9*, Knsington) Kensgtn Pub Corp.

Depression: Causes & Cures. 1996. lib. bdg. 250.95 (*0-8490-5878-3*) Gordon Pr.

Depression: CE Booklet. Beth Harris. 1999. 34p. pap. text 39.95 (*0-7817-1898-8*) Lppncott W & W.

Depression: Comparative Studies of Normal, Neurotic & Psychotic Conditions. Edith Jacobson. 1971. LC 74-162056. 78p. 55.00 (*0-8236-1195-7*) Intl Univs Pr.

Depression: Neurobiological, Psychopathological & Therapeutic Advances. Adriaan Honig et al. 1997. LC 97-293. 672p. 235.00 (*0-471-96849-8*) Wiley.

Depression: Questions You Have...Answers You Need. Sandra Salmans. 1995. LC 94-39327. (Illus.). 192p. (Orig.). pap. 10.95 (*1-882606-14-0*) Peoples Med Soc.

Depression: The Dark Night of the Soul. Raymond E. Runde & Gregory Britton. 1990. 100p. pap. (*0-9628401-0-6*) Millers Pr.

Depression: The Evolution of Powerlessness. Paul Gilbert. 2nd ed. 1992. LC 92-1445. 576p. reprint ed. 47.95 (*0-89862-884-9*) Guilford Pubns.

Depression: The Way Out of Your Prison. Dorothy Rowe. 1984. (Illus.). 242p. pap. 10.95 (*0-7100-9586-4*, Routledge Thoemms); 2nd ed. 1996. LC 96-593. 272p. pap. 18.95 (*0-415-14482-5*) Routledge.

Depression - Theories & Treatments: Psychological, Biological, & Social Perspectives. Arthur Schwartz & Ruth M. Schwartz. 1993. LC 92-49525. (Illus.). 528p. (C). text 46.00 (*0-231-06818-2*) Col U Pr.

Depression & Aggression in Family Interaction. Gerald R. Patterson. 1990. 352p. (C). text 89.95 (*0-8058-0137-5*) L Erlbaum Assocs.

Depression & Antidepressants: A Guide. Dilek Sen et al. rev. ed. 1999. 48p. mass mkt. 4.95 (*1-890802-19-0*); 3rd rev. ed. 1997. vii, 47p. pap. 4.50 (*1-890802-08-5*) Madison Inst of Med.

Depression & Creativity. Andre Haynal. 1985. LC 84-27830. 290p. 45.00 (*0-8236-1201-5*, 01201) Intl Univs Pr.

Depression & Expressive Behavior. Jack D. Maser. 1987. 128p. (C). text 29.95 (*0-89859-999-7*) L Erlbaum Assocs.

Depression & Hope: New Insights for Pastoral Counseling. Howard W. Stone. 1998. LC 98-17840. 176p. pap. 17.00 (*0-8006-3139-0*, 1-3139, Fortress Pr) Augsburg Fortress.

Depression & Its Treatment. John H. Greist & James W. Jefferson. 2nd rev. ed. 1992. LC 92-9713. 157p. text 19.95 (*0-88048-527-2*, 8527) Am Psychiatric.

Depression & Its Treatment. John H. Greist & James W. Jefferson. 1985. 128p. mass mkt. 3.95 (*0-446-32718-2*) Warner Bks.

Depression & Mania: A Comprehensive Textbook. Ed. by Anastasios Georgotas & Robert Cancro. 1992. 728p. (C). pap. text 99.00 (*0-8385-1575-4*, A1575-8, Apple Lange Med) McGraw.

Depression & Mania: Friends Or Foes. Ty C. Colbert. 1995. LC 94-79289. (Illus.). 221p. (Orig.). pap. 13.95 (*0-9643635-5-0*) Kevco Pubg.

Depression & Natural Medicine. Rita Elkins. 2nd rev. ed. 1995. 228p. pap. text 11.95 (*1-885670-00-1*) Woodland UT.

Depression & Physical Illness. M. M. Robertson & Cornelius L. Katona. 1997. LC 96-37003. 576p. 189.95 (*0-471-96148-5*) Wiley.

Depression & Suicide in Children & Adolescents: Prevention, Intervention, & Postvention. Philip G. Patros. 1988. LC 88-14448. 360p. (C). 78.00 (*0-205-11670-1*, H16702) Allyn.

Depression & the Body. Alexander Lowen. 1993. pap. 14.95 (*0-14-019465-7*, Penguin Compass) Penguin Putnam.

Depression & the Social Environment: Research & Intervention with Neglected Populations. Ed. by Philippe Cappeliez & Robert J. Flynn. 1993. 448p. (*0-7735-0960-7*) McG-Queens Univ Pr CAN. *Dist:* CUP Services.

Depression As a Treatable Illness. 1994. lib. bdg. 250.00 (*0-8490-5702-7*) Gordon Pr.

Depression in Adults: The Latest Assessment & Treatment Strategies. Anton O. Tolman. 2001. LC 95-70155. (Condensed Reviews for Professionals Ser.). 96p. (C). pap. 14.95 (*1-887537-10-4*) Compact Clinicals.

Depression in Adults: The Latest Assessment & Treatment Strategies for Major Depressive Disorders. Anton O. Tolman. 2nd ed. 2001. (Condensed Reviews for

Professionals Ser.). 120p. (C). pap. 14.95 (*1-887537-16-3*) Compact Clinicals.

Depression in Children & Adolescents. Ed. by Kedar N. Dwivedi & Ved P. Varma. 1996. LC 97-110611. 168p. pap. 45.00 (*1-56593-835-6*) Singular Publishing.

Depression in Children & Adolescents. Ed. by Harold S. Koplewicz & Emily Klass. 1993. LC 92-28562. (Monographs in Clinical Pediatrics: Vol. 6). 238p. text 116.00 (*3-7186-5317-6*); pap. text 38.00 (*3-7186-5318-4*) Gordon & Breach.

Depression in Context. Neil Jacobson et al. 2001. LC 2001-18040. (Professional Book Ser.). xxx, 223p. 32.00 (*0-393-70350-9*) Norton.

Depression in Geriatric & Nursing Home Patients: A Treatment Manual. Michael Lichtenberg. 1998. LC 98-36843. (William Beaumont Hospital Speech & Language Pathology Ser.). pap. text 15.95 (*0-8143-2801-6*) Wayne St U Pr.

*__Depression in Late Life.__ Dan G. Blazer. 3rd ed. 2001. LC 2001-20649. (Illus.). viii, 485p. (*0-8261-1452-0*) Springer Pub.

Depression in Long Term & Residential Care: Advance in Research & Treatment. Robert L. Rubinstein & M. Powell Lawton. 1997. LC 97-16281. 272p. 47.95 (*0-8261-9550-4*) Springer Pub.

Depression in Marriage: A Model for Etiology & Treatment. Steven R. Beach et al. 1990. LC 90-2775. (Treatment Manuals for Practitioners Ser.). 242p. pap. 25.00 (*0-89862-216-6*, 2216) Guilford Pubns.

Depression in Old Age. Cornelius L. Katona. 1994. LC 93-46294. 160p. 137.95 (*0-471-94308-8*) Wiley.

Depression in Primary Care: Detection & Diagnosis. 1994. lib. bdg. 250.95 (*0-8490-5705-1*) Gordon Pr.

Depression in Primary Care: Detection, Diagnosis & Treatment of Major Depression, Set. 1994. lib. bdg. 625.95 (*0-8490-5703-5*) Gordon Pr.

Depression in Primary Care: Detection, Diagnosis, & Treatment Reference Guide for Clinicians. 1994. lib. bdg. 250.00 (*0-8490-5706-X*) Gordon Pr.

Depression in Primary Care: Treatment of Major Depression. 1994. lib. bdg. 260.75 (*0-8490-5704-3*) Gordon Pr.

Depression in Primary Care Vol. 1: Detection & Diagnosis. 1993. 176p. per. 8.00 (*0-16-042247-7*) USGPO.

Depression in Primary Care Vol. 2: Treatment of Major Depression. 1994. (Illus.). 175p. (C). pap. text 45.00 (*0-7881-0599-X*) DIANE Pub.

Depression in Primary Care Vol. 2: Treatment of Major Depression. 1993. 189p. per. 8.50 (*0-16-042249-3*) USGPO.

Depression in Schizophrenics. Ed. by R. Williams & J. T. Dalby. 1989. (Illus.). 272p. 75.00 (*0-306-43240-4*, Plenum Trade) Perseus Pubng.

Depression in the Elderly: A Multimedia Sourcebook, 36. John J. Miletich. 1997. LC 97-16238. (Bibliographies & Indexes in Gerontology Ser.: Vol. 36). 248p. lib. bdg. 72.95 (*0-313-30113-1*, Greenwood Pr) Greenwood.

Depression in the Elderly: Clinical Considerations & Therapeutic Approaches. Ed. by S. Kanowski. 1994. (Journal: Vol. 40, Suppl. 1, 1994). (Illus.). iv, 30p. pap. 15.75 (*3-8055-5964-X*) S Karger.

Depression in the Family. Ed. by Arthur Freeman et al. 1987. LC 86-22833. (Journal of Psychotherapy & the Family Ser.: Vol. 2, Nos. 3-4). 196p. text 49.95 (*0-86656-624-4*) Haworth Pr.

Depression in the Medically Ill: An Integrated Approach. Gary Rodin et al. 1991. LC 90-26064. 384p. text 48.95 (*0-87630-596-6*) Brunner-Routledge.

Depression in the Young: What We Can Do to Help Them. Trudy Carlson. 1998. LC 96-83676. 176p. (Orig.). pap. 9.95 (*0-9642443-5-7*) Benline Pr.

Depression in Young People. Ed. by Australian National Health and Medical Research Council Staff. 1997. 176p. pap. (*0-644-39771-3*) Aust Gov Pub AUS. *Dist:* Accents Pubns.

Depression Is a Treatable Illness: A Guide for Patients. 1994. lib. bdg. 256.95 (*0-8490-9056-3*) Gordon Pr.

Depression Prevention: Research Directions. Ed. by Ricardo F. Munoz. 1987. 301p. 76.95 (*0-89116-452-9*) Hemisp Pub.

Depression Runs in Families: The Social Context of Risks & Resilience in Children of Depressed Mothers. Constance L. Hammen. 1991. (Psychopathology Ser.). (Illus.). 275p. 87.95 (*0-387-97435-0*) Spr-Verlag.

Depression, Slide Kit. J. Thakore. 1998. 99.00 (*1-873413-81-5*, 8292) Merit Pub Intl.

Depression, the Mood Disease. Francis M. Mondimore. 1995. (Health Bks.). 256p. reprint ed. pap. 16.95 (*0-8018-5184-X*) Johns Hopkins.

Depression Workbook: A Guide for Living with Depression. Mary E. Copeland. 1992. LC 92-81725. (Illus.). 320p. pap. 19.95 (*1-879237-32-6*) New Harbinger.

Depressive Disorder in Childhood & Adolescence. Richard Harrington. 1995. 262p. pap. 70.00 (*0-471-96141-8*) Wiley.

Depressive Disorders. Mario Maj & N. Sartorius. 1999. LC 99-14217. (WPA Series in Evidence & Experience in Psychiatry: Vol. 1). 506p. 95.00 (*0-471-99905-9*) Wiley.

Depressive Disorders: Facts, Theories, & Treatment Methods. Ed. by Benjamin B. Wolman & George Stricker. 1990. (Personality Processes Ser.). 448p. 170.00 (*0-471-61819-5*) Wiley.

Depressive Illness. Ed. by Julien Mendlewicz et al. 1981. (Advances in Biological Psychiatry Ser.: Vol. 7). (Illus.). viii, 244p. pap. 64.50 (*3-8055-2482-X*) S Karger.

Depressive Illness: Prediction of Course & Outcome. Ed. by Tomas Helgason & R. J. Daly. 1988. (Illus.). 152p. 79.95 (*0-387-19090-2*) Spr-Verlag.

Depressive States & Their Treatment. Ed. by Vamik D. Volkan. 1985. LC 85-6216. 456p. 60.00 (*0-87668-743-5*) Aronson.

Depressive Stoerungen Erkennen und Behandeln: Leitfaden fuer Aerzte. S. Kasper et al. 1994. (Illus.). 64p. pap. 28.00 (*3-8055-5983-6*) S Karger.

Deprivation & Health in Scotland. Vera Carstairs. 1991. pap. text (*0-08-037979-6*) Aberdeen U Pr GBR. *Dist:* Macmillan.

Depth of Anesthesia. J. Gareth Jones. 1993. 39.00 (*0-316-47303-0*) Little.

Deputy Chief Medical Examiner. Jack Rudman. 1994. (Career Examination Ser.: C-2723). pap. 59.95 (*0-8373-2723-7*) Nat Learn.

Deputy Medical Examiner. Jack Rudman. 1994. (Career Examination Ser.: C-1245). pap. 44.95 (*0-8373-1245-0*) Nat Learn.

Derived Intervention Levels of Radionuclides in Food: Guidelines for Application after Widespread Radioactive Contamination. WHO Staff. 1988. 60p. 11.00 (*92-4-154233-0*) World Health.

Dermal Absorption & Toxicity Assessment. Roberts & Walters. 1998. (Illus.). 808p. text 250.00 (*0-8247-0154-2*) Dekker.

Dermal & Ocular Toxicology: Fundamentals & Methods. Ed. by David W. Hobson. 1991. 608p. lib. bdg. 159.00 (*0-8493-8811-2*, RL803) CRC Pr.

Dermal & Transdermal Drug Delivery. Robert Gurny & Teubner. 1993. 73.00 (*3-8047-1223-1*) CRC Pr.

Dermal Immune System. Brian J. Nickoloff. 1992. 352p. 189.00 (*0-8493-5941-4*, RL97) CRC Pr.

Dermatitis in Machinists: Causes & Solutions. E. O. Bennett. 1993. LC 92-75660. 240p. pap. 38.00 (*1-880319-09-8*) Biotech.

Dermatoglyphics: An International Bibliography (World Anthropology) Ed. by Jamshed Mavalwala. 1978. xvi, 306p. text (*90-279-7999-5*) Mouton.

Dermatoglyphics: Science in Transition. Chris C. Plato et al. 1991. (Birth Defects Original Article Ser.: No. 1903). 348p. 495.00 (*0-471-56104-5*, Wiley-Liss) Wiley.

Dermatologic Botany. Javier Avalos & Howard I. Maibach. 1999. LC 99-46442. (Dermatology: Clinical & Basic Science Ser.). 464p. 79.95 (*0-8493-7361-1*) CRC Pr.

Dermatologic Conditions. Eugene J. Barone et al. 1999. LC 99-26966. 432p. pap. text 39.95 (*0-683-30420-8*) Lppncott W & W.

Dermatologic Drug Therapy. Stephen E. Wolverton. 2001. LC 00-64105. (Illus.). xix, 954p. text 85.00 (*0-7216-7728-2*) Saunders.

Dermatologic Research Techniques. Ed. by Howard I. Maibach. 1995. LC 95-22841. (CRC Press Dermatology: Clinical & Basic Science Ser.). 288p. 119.95 (*0-8493-8373-0*, 8373) CRC Pr.

Dermatologic Surgery. Neal A. Swanson. 2001st ed. 2001. 84.95 (*0-8151-9040-9*, 29145) Mosby Inc.

Dermatologic Surgery: Textbook & Atlas. Perry Robins et al. Tr. by W. H. Burgdorf. 1996. (Illus.). 522p. 270.00 (*3-540-59453-1*) Spr-Verlag.

Dermatologic Surgery: Textbook & Atlas. Perry Robins et al. 1996. LC 96-3794. (Illus.). (*0-387-59453-1*) Spr-Verlag.

Dermatologic Surgical Suite: Design & Materials. Mary E. Maloney. 1990. (Practical Manuals in Dermatologic Surgery Ser.). (Illus.). 105p. pap. text (*0-443-08688-5*) Church.

Dermatological & Transdermal Formulations. Kenneth A. Walters. Date not set. (Drugs & the Pharmaceutical Sciences Ser.). (*0-8247-9889-9*) Dekker.

Dermatological Atlas of Black Skin. Coyle Connolly & Joseph Bikowski. 1998. (Illus.). 96p. 49.95 (*1-873413-61-0*, 8277) Merit Pub Intl.

Dermatological Differential Diagnosis & Pearls. H. Eliot Y. Ghatan. 1994. LC 94-9634. 330p. lib. bdg. 32.95 (*1-85070-524-0*, Parthenon Pbng) CRC Pr.

*__Dermatological Differential Diagnosis & Pearls.__ H. Eliot Y. Ghatan. 2nd ed. 2002. 340p. 35.95 (*1-84214-125-2*, Parthenon Pbng) CRC Pr.

Dermatological Formulations: Percutaneous Absorption. Brian W. Barry. 1983. (Drugs & the Pharmaceutical Sciences Ser.: Vol. 18). (Illus.). 496p. text 225.00 (*0-8247-1729-5*) Dekker.

Dermatological Phototherapy & Photodiagnostic Methods. Jean Krutmann. 2001. LC 00-63776. (Illus.). 485p. 90.00 (*3-540-67789-5*) Spr-Verlag.

Dermatological Signs of Internal Disease. Jeffrey P. Callen et al. 2nd ed. 1994. LC 94-30224. (Illus.). 436p. text 110.00 (*0-7216-5454-1*) Saunders.

Dermatological Surgery. Ed. by Julian L. Verbov. 1986. (New Clinical Applications in Dermatology Ser.). lib. bdg. 82.00 (*0-85200-934-8*) Kluwer Academic.

Dermatologie und Venerologie. Helmut Kerl et al. 1997. 374p. text 43.00 (*3-11-015123-5*) De Gruyter.

Dermatologie und Venerologie: Jahresversammlung der Schweizerischen Gesellschaft. 1976. (Journal: Vol. 153, No. 2). 21.75 (*3-8055-2632-6*) S Karger.

Dermatology. B. R. Allen. 1990. (Brainscan MCQs Ser.). 110p. 21.95 (*0-387-19607-2*) Spr-Verlag.

Dermatology. Ed. by Gene H. Nesbitt. 1987. (Contemporary Issues in Small Animal Practice Ser.: Vol. 8). (Illus.). 328p. text (*0-443-08447-5*) Church.

Dermatology. Milton Orkin et al. 1992. LC 92-105318. (Illus.). 696p. (C). pap. text 43.95 (*0-8385-1288-7*, A1288-8, Apple Lange Med) McGraw.

Dermatology. 2nd ed. 1984. (Medical Ser.). (Illus.). (C). pap. text 9.95 (*0-935920-19-6*, Ntl Pubs Blck) P-H.

Dermatology. J. D. Wilkinson & S. Shaw. 2nd ed. 1998. LC 97-42803. (Colour Guide Ser.). pap. text 16.95 (*0-443-05852-0*) Harcrt Hlth Sci Grp.

Dermatology. O. Braun-Falco et al. 2nd enl. rev. ed. 2000. (Illus.). 1600p. 235.00 (*3-540-59452-3*, B7292) Spr-Verlag.

Dermatology. Regents Staff. 3rd ed. 1993. LC 92-49125. (Regents - Prentice-Hall Medical Assistant Kit Ser.). 64p. pap. 16.40 (*0-13-105966-1*) P-H.

Dermatology, Set. Samuel L. Moschella & Harry J. Hurley. 3rd ed. 1992. (Illus.). 2767p. text 350.00 (*0-7216-3263-7*) Saunders.

Dermatology: Clinical Manual. Edward Bondi et al. 1992. (Illus.). 422p. (C). pap. 32.95 (*0-8385-1274-7*, A1274-8) McGraw-Hill Educ Grp.

Dermatology: Health Care Needs Assessment: The Epidemiologically Based Needs Assessment Reviews, Second Series. Andrew Stevens et al. 1997. LC 97-13350. (*1-85775-211-2*) Radcliffe Med Pr GBR. *Dist:* Balogh.

Dermatology & Dermatopathology: A Dynamic Interface. Paul Bozzo. 1998. LC 98-55499. 304p. text 129.00 (*0-397-58774-0*) Lppncott W & W.

Dermatology & Perinatal Infection. Arnold J. Rudolph. 1997. (Atlas of the Newborn Ser.: Vol. 4). (Illus.). incl. cd-rom (*1-55009-034-8*) DEKR.

Dermatology & Person-Threatening Illness: The Patient, the Family, the Staff. Ed. by Robert R. Walther et al. 1996. LC 96-16349. (Loss, Grief & Care Ser.: Vol. 7, Nos. 3/4). 227p. 49.95 (*1-56024-817-3*) Haworth Pr.

Dermatology & Syphilology of the Nineteenth Century. John T. Crissey & Lawrence C. Parish. 1981. LC 81-1954. 439p. 125.00 (*0-275-91343-0*, C1343, Praeger Pubs) Greenwood.

Dermatology at the Millennium: The Proceedings of the 19th World Congress of Dermatology. Ed. by D. Dyall-Smith & R. Marks. 1999. LC 99-10220. (Illus.). 812p. lib. bdg. 132.95 (*1-85070-005-2*) CRC Pr.

Dermatology Colour Guide. J. D. Wilkinson et al. 2nd ed. 1999. LC 98-54625. (C). pap. text (*0-443-05886-5*) Church.

Dermatology for Southern Africa. Heyl. 1990. pap. text 70.00 (*0-409-10191-5*) Buttrwrth-Heinemann.

*__Dermatology for The Boards & Wards.__ Carlos Ayala. 2001. LC 2001-25024. (Boards & Wards Ser.). (Illus.). viii, 61p. pap. 14.95 (*0-632-04572-8*) Blackwell Sci.

Dermatology (ICT) Gawkrodger. 2nd ed. 1997. (C). pap. text 29.00 (*0-443-05328-6*) Saunders.

Dermatology in General Medicine. Ed. by Thomas B. Fitzpatrick. 4th ed. 1. (*0-07-021207-4*); 2. (*0-07-021208-2*) McGraw.

Dermatology in General Medicine, Set. Ed. by Thomas B. Fitzpatrick et al. 4th ed. 1993. LC 92-48388. 3272p. text 350.00 (*0-07-909350-7*) McGraw-Hill Med Pub.

Dermatology in Pigmented Skin. Ed. by A. Moiin et al. 1998. (Illus.). 320p. (*0-443-05467-3*) Church.

Dermatology in Practice. Anthony Du Vivier. 1990. (Illus.). 220p. (gr. 13). text (*0-397-44698-5*, GM0094) Gower-Mosby.

*__Dermatology of the Lips.__ Crispian Scully et al. 2000. (Illus.). 178p. (*1-901865-74-6*) Isis Med GBR. *Dist:* Bks Intl VA.

Dermatology Office Manual. Richard L. Moss. 1995. (Office Manual Ser.). 221p. 149.50 (*1-890018-07-4*) Anadem Pubng.

Dermatology Pearls. Eleanor E. Sahn. 1999. LC 99-20512. (Pearls Ser.). 250p. pap. 65.00 (*1-56053-315-3*) Hanley & Belfus.

*__Dermatology Pocket Atlas.__ Anthony Du Vivier. 2001. (Illus.). 200p. pap. 33.95 (*0-632-05428-X*) Blackwell Sci.

Dermatology Progress & Perspectives: The Proceedings of the 18th World Congress of Dermatology. Ed. by W. H. Burgdorf et al. 1993. 1282p. lib. bdg. 162.95 (*1-85070-392-2*, Parthenon Pbng) CRC Pr.

*__Dermatology Self-Evaluation Program Vol. 2: Envelope & Scantron Sheet.__ American Academy of Dermatology Staff. 2001. pap. text (*0-7872-8372-X*) Kendall-Hunt.

Dermatology Self-Evaluation Program (DSEP) AAD Staff. 1997. 276p. pap. text 350.00 (*0-7872-2018-3*) Kendall-Hunt.

Dermatology Skills for Primary Care Vol. 1: Basic Skills. Daniel J. Trozak & Dan J. Tennenhouse. Ed. by Albert J. Finestone. 1998. (Illus.). x, 123p. 49.00 (*1-930548-04-4*) Tennenhouse Prof Pubns.

Dermatology Skills for Primary Care Vol. 2: Papular Lesions, Papulo-Squamous Lesions & Papulo-Vesicular Lesions. Daniel J. Trozak & Dan J. Tennenhouse. Ed. by Albert J. Finestone. 1998. (Illus.). x, 145p. 69.00 (*1-930548-05-2*) Tennenhouse Prof Pubns.

Dermatology Skills for Primary Care Vol. 3: Epidermal, Dermal & Epidermal/Dermal Lesions. Daniel J. Trozak & Dan J. Tennenhouse. Ed. by Albert J. Finestone. 1998. (Illus.). x, 119p. 69.00 (*1-930548-06-0*) Tennenhouse Prof Pubns.

Dermatology Skills for Primary Care Vol. 4: Epidermal & Dermal Lesions, Eczematous Lesions & Atrophies. Daniel J. Trozak & Dan J. Tennenhouse. Ed. by Albert J. Finestone. 1998. (Illus.). x, 129p. 69.00 (*1-930548-07-9*) Tennenhouse Prof Pubns.

Dermatology Skills for Primary Care Vol. 5: Pigmented, Pre-Malignant & Common Malignant Skin Lesions. Daniel J. Trozak & Dan J. Tennenhouse. Ed. by Albert J. Finestone. 1998. (Illus.). x, 163p. 69.00 (*1-930548-08-7*) Tennenhouse Prof Pubns.

Dermatology Skills for Primary Care Vol. 6: Vesiculo-Bullous & Papulo-Pustular Disorders. Daniel J. Trozak & Dan J. Tennenhouse. Ed. by Albert J. Finestone. 1998. (Illus.). x, 115p. 69.00 (*1-930548-09-5*) Tennenhouse Prof Pubns.

Dermatology Teaching File Vol. II: Gross & Microscopic Presentations. Ed. by Antoinette F. Hood & American Academy of Dermatology Staff. 2nd ed. 1995. (C). 232.00 (*0-8151-0082-5*) Mosby Inc.

Dermatology 2000: An Internet Resource Guide. Ed. by Dan Goldenson. 2000. 450p. pap. 24.95 (*0-9700525-0-2*) eMedguides.

Dermatopathology. George F. Murphy. 1995. LC 94-6843. (Illus.). 480p. text 135.00 (*0-7216-2418-9*) Saunders.

Dermatopathology of Systemic Diseases. Bruce R. Smoller & Thomas D. Horn. 2001. LC 00-44610. (Illus.). 416p. text 159.00 (*0-19-513038-3*) OUP.

Dermatopharmacology & Toxicology. Ed. by Howard I. Maibach & N. J. Lowe. 1984. (Models in Dermatology Ser.: No. 2). (Illus.). x, 370p. 217.50 (*3-8055-3947-9*) S Karger.

Dermatopharmacology of Topical Preparations: A Product Development-Oriented Approach. Ed. by B. Gabard et al. 1999. LC 99-23641. (Illus.). 370p. 105.00 (*3-540-64048-7*) Spr-Verlag.

Dermatophytes: Their Recognition & Identification. Ed. by Gerbert Rebell & David Taplin. rev. ed. 1974. LC 70-130448. (Illus.). vi, 124p. spiral bd. 22.95 (*0-87024-185-0*) U of Miami Pr.

Dermatosurgery. J. Petres & M. Hundeiker. 1978. 152p. 99.00 (*0-387-90296-1*) Spr-Verlag.

Dermatotoxicology. Ed. by Francis N. Marzulli & Howard I. Maibach. 4th ed. 1991. 800p. 136.00 (*1-56032-055-9*); 5th ed. 1996. 864p. 149.95 (*1-56032-356-6*) Hemisp Pub.

Dermatotoxicology Methods: The Laboratory Worker's Ready Reference. Ed. by Francis N. Marzulli & Howard I. Maibach. 1997. 400p. pap. 59.95 (*1-56032-672-7*) Hemisp Pub.

Dermotology of the Eye, Orbit & Adnexa. George E. White. 1994. pap. text 90.00 (*0-8385-1582-7*, A1582-4) Appleton & Lange.

Des Maladies Mentales: Considerees Sous les Rapports Medical Hygienique et Medico-Legal Etienne Esquirol. 1976. LC 75-16703. (Classics in Psychiatry Ser.). (FRE., Illus.). reprint ed. Set. 134.95 (*0-405-07464-6*); Vol. 1. 66.95 (*0-405-07465-4*); Vol. 2. 66.95 (*0-405-07466-2*) Ayer.

Descended & Cryptorchid Testis. Ed. by E. S. Hafez. 1980. (Clinics in Andrology Ser.: No. 3). (Illus.). 204p. text 176.50 (*90-247-2299-3*) Kluwer Academic.

Descent of Man & Selection in Relation to Sex. Charles Robert Darwin. 1981. LC 80-8679. (Illus.). 935p. reprint ed. pap. 29.95 (*0-691-02369-7*) Princeton U Pr.

Descent of the Testicles. Frier. 1993. 200p. text 125.00 (*0-340-55400-2*) Trafalgar.

Describing Learner Characteristics of Handicapped Children & Youth. Ed. by David A. Sabatino. 1978. 640p. text 55.00 (*0-8089-1127-9*, 793725, Grune & Strat) Harcrt Hlth Sci Grp.

Description of Advanced Clinical Practice (DACP) Cardiopulmonary. 1997. 30p. pap. 40.00 (*1-887759-77-8*, E-41) Am Phys Therapy Assn.

Description of Advanced Clinical Practice (DACP) Clinical Electrophysiologic. 1995. 20p. pap. 40.00 (*1-887759-78-6*, E-27) Am Phys Therapy Assn.

Description of Advanced Clinical Practice (DACP) Geriatric. 1998. 30p. pap. 40.00 (*1-887759-76-X*, E-45) Am Phys Therapy Assn.

Description of Advanced Clinical Practice (DACP) Neurologic. 1996. 80p. pap. 40.00 (*1-887759-75-1*, E-29) Am Phys Therapy Assn.

Description of Advanced Clinical Practice (DACP) Orthopaedic. 1994. 66p. pap. 40.00 (*1-887759-73-5*, E-46) Am Phys Therapy Assn.

Description of Advanced Clinical Practice (DACP) Pediatric. 1997. 30p. pap. 40.00 (*1-887759-74-3*, E-31) Am Phys Therapy Assn.

Description of Advanced Clinical Practice (DACP) Sports Physical Therapy. 1997. 26p. pap. 40.00 (*1-887759-72-7*, E-28) Am Phys Therapy Assn.

Description of the Retreat: An Institution Near York for Insane Persons of the Society of Friends Containing an Account of the Origin & Progress, the Modes of Treatment & a Statement of Cases. Samuel Tuke. 1996. LC 98-106997. pap. (*1-899209-04-2*) Process Pr GBR. *Dist:* Intl Spec Bk.

Descriptive Psychology. Franz Brentano. Ed. & Tr. by Benito Mueller. 1995. LC 94-44167. (International Library of Philosophy, Psychology, & Scientific Method).Tr. of Deskriptive Psychologie. 232p. (C). (gr. 13). 80.00 (*0-415-10811-X*, C0403) Routledge.

Desegregation of the Mentally Ill. J. Hoenig & Marian Hamilton. 1969. (International Library of Sociology & Social Reconstruction). 24.95 (*0-8464-0318-8*) Beekman Pubs.

Desert Camel. R. Yagil. 1985. (Comparative Animal Nutrition Ser.: Vol. 5). (Illus.). xii, 164p. 111.50 (*3-8055-4065-5*) S Karger.

Desert Wildlife. Edmund C. Jaeger. 1961. (Illus.). xii, 308p. pap. 15.95 (*0-8047-0124-5*) Stanford U Pr.

Design & Analysis. Geoffrey Keppel. 2nd ed. 1992. LC 92-1364. (Series of Books in Psychology). 626p. (C). pap. text 64.95 (*0-7167-2321-2*) W H Freeman.

Design & Analysis of Clinical Experiments. Joseph L. Fleiss. 1986. LC 99-10464. (Probability & Statistics Ser.). (Illus.). 448p. 125.00 (*0-471-82047-4*) Wiley.

Design & Analysis of Clinical Experiments. Joseph L. Fleiss. 1999. LC 99-10464. (Wiley Classics Library). (Illus.). 432p. pap. 69.95 (*0-471-34991-7*) Wiley.

Design & Analysis of Clinical Trials. Shein-Chung Chow & Jen-pei Liu. 1998. LC 97-28675. (Probability & Statistics Ser.). 672p. 150.00 (*0-471-13404-X*, Wiley-Interscience) Wiley.

Design & Analysis of Group-Randomized Trials. David M. Murray. 1998. (Monographs in Epidemiology & Biostatistics: No. 29). (Illus.). 480p. text 65.00 (*0-19-512036-1*) OUP.

Design & Analysis of Iron Supplementation Trials. Selwyn J. Baker & K. Ramachandran. Ed. by Edouard M. DeMaeyer & Samuel G. Kahn. 1984. (Illus.). 38p. (Orig.). pap. text 3.50 (*0-935368-44-2*) ILSI.

Design & Analysis of Research Studies. Bryan F. Manly. 1992. (Illus.). 369p. (C). pap. text 32.95 (*0-521-42580-8*) Cambridge U Pr.

Design & Analysis of Single Case Research. Ed. by Ronald D. Franklin et al. 1996. 392p. 99.95 (*0-8058-1618-6*) L Erlbaum Assocs.

Design & Estimation for the National Health Interview Survey, 1995-2004. Steven Botman & National Center for Health Statistics Staff. 2000. LC 00-37092. (Vital & Health Statistics Ser.). (Illus.). vi, 31p. (*0-8406-0562-5*) Natl Ctr Health Stats.

Design & Evaluation of Bioavailability & Bioequivalence Studies. Ramon Martinez-Pacheco & Angel Conchiero. Date not set. (Drugs & the Pharmaceutical Sciences Ser.). (*0-8247-9874-0*) Dekker.

***Design & Experimental Evaluation of Allergen-Derived Peptides for Specific Immunotherapy of Allergic Diseases.** Bo Wu. 2001. (Acta Biomedical Lovaniensia Ser.: No. 227). (Illus.). 145p. pap. (*90-5867-101-1*) Leuven Univ BEL. *Dist:* Coronet Bks.

Design & Operation of the National Hospital Discharge Survey. Charles F. Dennison et al. 2000. LC 00-64743. (Vital & Health Statistics Ser.). (Illus.). iv, 42p. (*0-8406-0565-X*) Natl Ctr Health Stats.

Design & Targeted Reactions of Oligonucleotide Derivative. Dmitri G. Knorre et al. 1993. LC 93-19678. 384p. 189.00 (*0-8493-4856-0*, QP628) CRC Pr.

Design & Use of Protocols: Proceedings of the Advances in Patient Care, Second Annual Conference, Feb. 15-22, 1975. Advances in Patient Care Conference Staff. Ed. by Marta Kallstrom & Stephen R. Yarnall. 1975. (Illus.). 294p. 18.00 (*0-917054-02-4*) Med Communications.

Design Concepts in Nutritional Epidemiology. Ed. by Barrie M. Margetts. 1991. (Illus.). 432p. text 69.95 (*0-19-261873-3*) OUP.

Design Concepts in Nutritional Epidemiology. 2nd ed. Ed. by Barrie Margetts & Michael Nelson. 2nd ed. 1997. LC 96-43448. (Illus.). 466p. pap. text 59.95 (*0-19-262739-2*) OUP.

Design Engineering of Biomaterials for Medical Devices. David Hill. 1998. LC 97-17449. (Biomaterials Science & Engineering Ser.). 480p. 285.00 (*0-471-96708-4*) Wiley.

Design for a Life: How Biology & Psychology Shape Human Behavior. Patrick Bateson & Paul Martin. 2001. 272p. pap. 14.00 (*0-684-86933-0*, Touchstone) S&S Trade Pap.

Design, Methods & Field Results of the 1996 Medical Expenditure Panel Survey Medical Provider Component. Steven R. Machlin. 2000. 12p. pap. (*1-58763-002-8*) Agency Healthcare.

Design of Analgesic Clinical Trials, Vol. 18. Mitchell B. Max et al. 1991. (Advances in Pain Research & Therapy Ser.: Vol. 18). 752p. text 159.00 (*0-88167-736-1*) Lppncott W & W.

Design of Cancer Chemotherapy. Ed. by E. Mihich & S. Eckhardt. 1980. (Antibiotics & Chemotherapy Ser.: Vol. 28). (Illus.). x, 194p. 77.50 (*3-8055-0411-X*) S Karger.

Design of Cardiac Pacemakers. Ed. by John G. Webster. 1995. LC 95-7390. 496p. 94.95 (*0-7803-1134-5*, PC5597) Inst Electrical.

Design of Clinical Engineering Quality Assurance & Risk Management Programs. 1989. 38p. pap. 55.00 (*0-910275-94-7*, MIR1-209) Assn Adv Med Instrn.

Design of Enzyme Inhibitors As Drugs, Vol. 2. Ed. by Merton Sandler & H. John Smith. 1994. (Illus.). 848p. text 150.00 (*0-19-262134-3*) OUP.

Design of Pulse Oximeters. John G. Webster. 1997. LC 97-37908. (Medical Science Ser.). (Illus.). 300p. 99.00 (*0-7503-0467-7*) Inst of Physics Pubng.

Design of Synthetic Inhibitors of Thrombin. G. Claeson et al. 1994. (Advances in Experimental Medicine & Biology Ser.: Vol. 340). (Illus.). 256p. (C). text 95.00 (*0-306-44593-X*, Kluwer Plenum) Kluwer Academic.

Design of the Electron Microscope Labora. Ed. by R. H. Alderson. 1975. (Practical Methods in Electron Microscopy Ser.: Vol. 4). 130p. pap. 35.50 (*0-7204-4260-5*, North Holland) Elsevier.

Design of the Electron Microscope Laboratory. Ed. by R. H. Alderson. 1975. (Practical Methods in Electron Microscopy Ser.: Vol. 4). pap. 21.00 (*0-444-10816-5*, North Holland) Elsevier.

Design Planning for Newborn Intensive Care: Resources for Family-Centered Practice. Jill H. Hall & Beverly H. Johnson. 1997. (Family-Centered Care Ser.). 100p. ring bd. 85.00 (*0-9642014-8-8*) Inst Fmly Ctr.

Designer Drugs. Lawrence Clayton. 1998. (Drug Abuse Prevention Library). 64p. (YA). (gr. 7 up). reprint ed. pap. 6.95 (*1-56838-209-X*) Hazelden.

Designer Vaccines: Principles for Successful Prophylaxis. H. P. Hughes & Manuel Campos. 1997. LC 97-34482. 224p. 129.95 (*0-8493-7676-9*) CRC Pr.

Designing a Capitation Payment Plan for Medicare End Stage Renal Disease Services. Donna O. Farley et al. 1994. LC 94-1869. pap. text 13.00 (*0-8330-1512-5*, MR-391-HCFA) Rand Corp.

Designing a Fair & Reasonable Basic Benefit Plan Using Clinical Guidelines. Ed. by David C. Hadorn & Deborah A. Lott. 1992. pap. (*0-9633681-0-9*) CA Public Emp Retire.

Designing a Laboratory. Ed. by Joseph H. Barker et al. 1989. 210p. 40.00 (*0-87553-150-4*) Am Pub Health.

Designing a Modern Microbiological/Biomedical Laboratory. Ed. by Jonathan Y. Richmond. 1997. LC 96-78611. 322p. (Orig.). pap. 65.00 (*0-87553-231-4*) Am Pub Health.

Designing & Conducting Behavioral Research. Clifford J. Drew & Michael L. Hardman. 1986. (General Psychology Ser.: No. 134). 311p. pap. (*0-08-033988-3*, Pergamon Pr) Elsevier.

Designing & Conducting Behavioral Research. Clifford J. Drew & Michael L. Hardman. 1985. (General Psychology Ser.: No. 134). (Illus.). 352p. text 70.00 (*0-08-031941-6*); pap. text 26.50 (*0-08-031940-8*) Elsevier (Pergamon Pr).

***Designing & Conducting Cost Effectiveness Analyses in Medicine & Health Care.** Peter Muennig. 2002. 368p. 65.00 (*0-7879-6013-6*) Wiley.

Designing & Conducting Health Surveys: A Comprehensive Guide. Lu Ann Aday. 2nd ed. 1996. LC 96-18108. 560p. 50.00 (*0-7879-0294-2*) Jossey-Bass.

Designing Babies: The Brave New World of Reproductive Technology. Roger Gosden. 2000. LC 99-17786. 260p. pap. text 14.95 (*0-7167-4168-7*) W H Freeman.

Designing Benefit Structures for Temporary Disability: A Guide for Policymakers & Designing Benefit Structures for Temporary Disability Richard B. Victor & Charles A. Fleischman. 1989. LC 89-24903. 50.00 (*0-935149-21-X*, WC-89-4) Workers Comp Res Inst.

Designing Clinical Evaluation Tools. Betty L. Battenfield. 1986. 43p. (Orig.). pap. 15.95 (*0-88737-290-2*, 23-2160) Natl League Nurse.

Designing Cost-Effective Employee Health Plans. Diana C. Walsh et al. 1982. (Studies in Productivity: Vol. 22). 63p. pap. 55.00 (*0-08-029503-7*) Work in Amer.

Designing for Aging: Patterns of Use. Sandra C. Howell. 1980. (Illus.). 329p. 40.00 (*0-262-08107-5*) MIT Pr.

Designing for Alzheimer's Disease: Strategies for Creating Better Care Environments. Elizabeth C. Brawley. 1997. LC 96-33457. (Healthcare & Senior Living Design Ser.). 340p. 85.00 (*0-471-13920-3*) Wiley.

Designing for the Disabled. Selwyn Goldsmith. 1977. (Illus.). (*0-900630-50-7*) Intl Spec Bk.

Designing Health Communication Campaigns: What Works? Thomas E. Backer et al. 1992. LC 92-6165. (Illus.). 200p. (C). pap. 32.95 (*0-8039-4332-6*, 3136) Sage.

Designing Program Evaluations. Linda T. Bilheimer. Ed. by Karen Glass. 1989. (Strategies for Improving State Perinatal Programs Ser.). 70p. (Orig.). pap. text 15.00 (*1-55877-060-7*) Natl Governor.

Designing Therapeutic Recreation Programs in the Community. Ed. by Marcia J. Carter et al. 1991. (Illus.). 354p. (Orig.). (C). pap. 25.00 (*0-88314-518-9*, A5189) AAHPERD.

Designing 21st Century Healthcare: Leadership in Hospitals & Healthcare Systems. John R. Griffith. 1998. LC 98-17721. 281p. 49.00 (*1-56793-087-5*) Health Admin Pr.

Designing Your Perfect Dental Practice: Foundations of Clinical Success. Jay M. Hislop. 1999. 292p. 69.00 (*0-910167-55-9*, Dental Commun) Comm Unltd CA.

Desire & the Femlae Therapist: Engendered Gazes in Psychotherapy & Art Therapy. Joy Schaverien. 1995. LC 94-48387. (Illus.). 240p. (C). (gr. 13). 89.95 (*0-415-08700-7*, C0036) Routledge.

Desk Reference for Asthma & Allergy. Hans-Uwe Simon. 2000. LC 99-58426. (Desk References Ser.). 400p. 79.95 (*0-8493-9684-0*) CRC Pr.

Desk Reference for Critical Care. Jonelle E. Wright & Brenda K. Shelton. 1993. (Nursing-Health Science Ser.). 1383p. (C). text 100.00 (*0-86720-325-0*) Jones & Bartlett.

Desk Reference for Hematology. N. K. Shinton. 1998. LC 98-12032. (CRC Desk References Ser.). 768p. 139.95 (*0-8493-9681-6*) CRC Pr.

Desk Reference for Neuroscience. I. Lockard. 2nd ed. 1991. (Illus.). 306p. 68.95 (*0-387-97715-5*) Spr-Verlag.

Desk Reference of Assessment Instruments in Speech & Language. Lonnie G. Harris. 1998. 393p. pap. text 62.00 (*0-12-784558-5*) Acad Pr.

Desk Reference to the Diagnostic Criteria from DSM-IV, No. IV. American Psychiatric Association Staff. 1994. LC 94-187643. (Dsm-IV Ser.). 358p. pap. 26.50 (*0-89042-064-5*, 2064) Am Psychiatric.

Desk Reference to the Diagnostic Criteria from DSM-IV-TR. American Psychiatric Association Staff. rev. ed. 2000. 496p. spiral bd. 26.50 (*0-89042-027-0*, 2027) Am Psychiatric.

Deskriptive Psychologie see Descriptive Psychology

Desktop Companion: To Physical Pathology. Roger Morrison. unabr. ed. 1998. text 75.00 (*0-9635368-2-6*) Hahnemann Clinic.

Desmopressin in Bleeding Disorders. G. Mariani & P. M. Mannucci. 1993. (NATO Advanced Science Institutes Ser.: Vol. 242). (Illus.). 372p. (C). text 125.00 (*0-306-44414-3*, Kluwer Plenum) Kluwer Academic.

Desorganisierte Mutterbindung Bei Einjahrigen Kindern: Die Motivationspsychologische Bedeutung der D-Klassifikation Im, Fremde-Situations-Test. Marina Zulauf-Logoz. 1997. (Psychoanalyse Im Dialog Ser.: Bd. 6). (GER.). 235p. 37.95 (*3-906759-49-0*) P Lang Pubng.

Desperate Disguises: Living in the Shadow of Psychiatric Illness. Jo Clancy. 1998. LC 97-21397. 197p. pap. 27.95 (*1-887841-09-1*, Psychosocial) Intl Univs Pr.

Desperate Remedy: The Search for a Cure for Parkinson's. Freed & Levay. 2001. text 24.95 (*0-7167-4177-6*) W H Freeman.

Desperately Seeking Solutions: Rationing Health Care. David J. Hunter. 1998. LC 97-28451. 176p. (C). pap. 57.60 (*0-582-28923-8*) Longman.

Despue's de un Ataque Cardi'aco: Qu'e Sigue? Julia A. Purcell et al. Ed. by Nancy R. Hull. Tr. by Olimpia De la Vega. 1994. LC 90-27143. (Illus.). 68p. pap. text 9.95 (*0-939838-30-3*) Pritchett & Hull.

Destinos: Spanish for Medical Professions. Ralph Kite. 1992. (C). pap., wbk. ed. 34.69 incl. audio (*0-07-911383-4*) McGrw-H Hghr Educ.

Destiny & Disease in Mental Disorders. C. M. Campbell. 1977. lib. bdg. 59.95 (*0-8490-1710-6*) Gordon Pr.

Destructive Behaviour in Developmental Disabilities: Diagnosis & Treatment. Ed. by Travis Thompson & David B. Gray. 1994. LC 93-43673. (Focus Editions Ser.: Vol. 170). 320p. (C). 86.95 (*0-8039-5582-0*, 4995); pap. 38.95 (*0-8039-5583-9*, 4996) Sage.

Destructive Narcissistic Pattern. Nina W. Brown. 1998. LC 97-27928. 200p. 57.75 (*0-275-96017-X*, Praeger Pubs) Greenwood.

Det Levende Spil see Garden in the Machine: The Emerging Science of Artificial Life

Detached Retinas. Thomas L. Vaultonburg. 1997. 70p. pap. 7.50 (*0-9670191-0-9*) Zom Log.

Detaching with Love. Carolyn W. Hazelden. 1984. 19p. (Orig.). pap. 2.00 (*0-89486-232-4*, 1253B) Hazelden.

Detachment: Seven Simple Steps. Judith M. Knowlton & Rebecca D. Chaitin. 1985. (Gifts of Growth Ser.). 56p. (Orig.). pap. 2.50 (*0-934391-00-9*) Quotidian.

Detailed Diagnoses & Procedures: National & Short Stay Hospital Surveys of Discharges, Set. 1992. lib. bdg. 550.95 (*0-8490-5330-7*) Gordon Pr.

Detailed Diagnoses & Procedures: National Hospital Discharge Survey. 1996. lib. bdg. 254.99 (*0-8490-6366-3*) Gordon Pr.

Detailed Diagnosis & Procedures: National Hospital Discharge Survey. 1994. lib. bdg. 251.95 (*0-8490-5821-X*) Gordon Pr.

Detecting Your Hidden Allergies. William G. Crook. 1988. (Illus.). 232p. (Orig.). pap. 11.95 (*0-933478-15-1*) Prof Bks Future Health.

Detection & Control of Ovulation. 1975. 208p. 110.00 (*0-7855-7175-2*) St Mut.

Detection & Measurement of Visual Impairment in Pre-Verbal Children. Ed. by Barrie Jay. 1986. (Documenta Ophthalmologica Proceedings Ser.). text 256.50 (*0-89838-789-2*) Kluwer Academic.

Detection & Prevention of Adverse Drug Reactions. Ed. by H. Bostrom & N. Ljungstedt. 1984. 294p. (Orig.). pap. text 48.50 (*91-22-00680-X*) Coronet Bks.

Detection & Quantitation of Rubella IgG Antibody: Evaluation & Performance Criteria for Multiple Component Test Products, Specimen Handling & Use of Test Products in the Clinical Laboratory; Approved Guideline (1997) 1997. 75.00 (*1-56238-335-3*, I/LA6-A) NCCLS.

Detection Methods for Cyanobacterial Toxins. Ed. by G. A. Codd et al. 1995. (Special Publications). 202p. (C). (*0-85186-961-0*, R6961) Royal Soc Chem GBR. *Dist:* Spr-Verlag.

Detection of Abnormal Hemoglobin Using Cellulose Acetate Electrophoresis. 2nd ed. 1994. (Approved Standard Ser.: Vol. 6). 75.00 (*1-56238-039-7*, H8-A2) NCCLS.

Detection of Dependence-Producing Drugs in Body Fluids: Proceedings of the WHO Expert Committee of Investigators, Geneva, 1974. WHO Staff. 1974. (Technical Reports: No. 556). pap. text 5.00 (*92-4-120556-3*, 1100556) World Health.

Detection of Malingering During Head Injury Litigation. Ed. by Cecil R. Reynolds. 1997. LC 97-34812. (Critical Issues in Neuropsychology Ser.). 304p. (C). 45.00 (*0-306-45655-9*, Plenum Trade) Perseus Pubng.

Detection of Mitochondrial Diseases. Ed. by Frank Norbert Gellerich & Stephan Zierz. 1997. LC 97-19828. (Developments in Molecular & Cellular Biochemistry Ser.: Vol. 21). 288p. text 275.00 (*0-7923-9925-0*) Kluwer Academic.

Detective Story: The Anatomy of the Cancer Problem. Solomon Tolmatsh. 2000. 128p. pap. 13.00 (*0-8059-4878-3*) Dorrance.

Detectors, Focal Plane Arrays & Imaging Devices II, Vol. 3553. Ed. by Pingzhi Liang et al. 1998. LC 98-226759. 48p. 89.00 (*0-8194-3014-5*) SPIE.

Determinants of Disability in Patients with Chronic Renal Failure. ECRI Health Technology Agency Staff. 2000. pap. (*1-58763-010-9*) Agency Healthcare.

Determinants of Expenditures for Physicians' Services in the United States. Victor R. Fuchs & Marcia J. Kramer. 1973. (Occasional Papers: No. 117). 72p. reprint ed. 20.00 (*0-87014-247-X*) Natl Bur Econ Res.

***Determinants of Health Care & Drug Utilisation: The Causes of Health Care Utilisation Study.** Ahmad Al-Windi. 2000. (Comprehensive Summaries of Uppsala Dissertations from the Faculty of Medicine Ser.: No. 965). (Illus.). 74p. (Orig.). pap. (*91-554-4836-4*) Uppsala Universitet SWE. *Dist:* Coronet Bks.

Determinants of Reproductive Change in Bangladesh: Success in a Challenging Environment. John Cleland et al. 1994. LC 94-16613. (Regional & Sectoral Studies). 200p. pap. 22.00 (*0-8213-2849-2*) World Bank.

Determinants of Substance Abuse: Biological, Psychological, & Environmental Factors. M. Galizio & S. A. Maisto. 1985. LC 85-3405. (Perspectives on Individual Differences Ser.). (Illus.). 454p. (C). 75.00 (*0-306-41873-8*, Plenum Trade) Perseus Pubng.

Determination of Absorbed Dose in a Patient Irradiated by Beams of X or Gamma Rays in Radiotherapy Procedures, No. 24. International Commission on Radiation Units and Measurements Staff. 1976. LC 76-22297. 40.00 (*0-913394-43-2*) Intl Comm Rad Meas.

Determination of Dose Equivalents from External Radiation Sources, Pt. II. 1988. LC 84-23053. (ICRU Report Ser.: No. 43). 50p. pap. text 50.00 (*0-913394-37-8*) Intl Comm Rad Meas.

Determination of Dose Equivalents Resulting from External Radiation Sources. International Commission on Radiation Units and Measurements Staff. 1985. LC 84-23053. (ICRU Report Ser.: No. 39). 10p. pap. text 30.00 (*0-913394-33-5*) Intl Comm Rad Meas.

Determination of Factor IX Coagulant Activity. 1986. (Proposed Guideline Ser.: Vol. 6). 75.00 (*1-56238-062-1*, H40-P) NCCLS.

Determination of Factor VIII Coagulant Activity. 1986. (Proposed Guideline Ser.: Vol. 6). 75.00 (*1-56238-060-5*, H34-P) NCCLS.

Determination of Food Carbohydrates. David A. Southgate. 1976. (Illus.). 57.75 (*0-85334-693-3*) Elsevier.

Determination of Nonregulated Status for Virus Resistance Squash, Vol. 69. 1996. (Illus.). 95p. (Orig.). (C). pap. text 40.00 (*0-7881-2554-0*) DIANE Pub.

Determination of Serum Iron & Total Iron-Binding Capacity: Proposed Standard (1990) Contrib. by Elkin Simson. 1990. 75.00 (*1-56238-047-8*, H17-P) NCCLS.

Determination of the Moments of Inertia of the Human Body & Its Limbs. W. Braune & O. Fischer. 1988. (Illus.). 84p. 68.95 (*0-387-18813-4*) Spr-Verlag.

Determination of the Position of a Momentary Impression. N. Trigant Burrow. Ed. by Stephen S. Colvin. 1909. (Of Psychol. Monos.: Vol. 11). 55.00 (*0-8115-1410-2*) Periodicals Srv.

Determination of von Willebrand Factor Antigen: Proposed Guideline, 1993) Contrib. by H. James Day. 1993. 75.00 (*1-56238-225-X*, H39-P) NCCLS.

Determined Dieter's Diary. Jan Rockin & Donna Rockin. 1985. (Illus.). 78p. (Orig.). pap. 3.25 (*0-9616081-0-2*) Rockin Enter.

Determined Survivors: Community Life among the Urban Elderly. Janice A. Smithers. 1985. 224p. (C). pap. text 16.00 (*0-8135-1080-5*) Rutgers U Pr.

Determining Ambulance Deployment in Santo Domingo, Dominican Republic. David J. Eaton et al. 1985. (Working Papers Ser.: No. 34). 39p. pap. 5.00 (*0-89940-514-2*) LBJ Sch Pub Aff.

Determining Risks to Health: Federal Policy & Practice. U. S. Department of Health & Human Services Staff. 1986. LC 85-26731. 200p. 50.00 (*0-86569-138-X*); pap. 19.95 (*0-86569-139-8*) Greenwood (Auburn Hse).

Determining the Future of Gerontological Nursing Education. Ed. by Christine Heine. 1992. 162p. (Orig.). (C). pap. text 15.95 (*0-88737-571-5*, 14-2508) Natl League Nurse.

Detox: Step One for the Alcoholic. Catherine Fellman. 1988. (American University Studies: Ser. XXIII, Vol. 1). X, 205p. (C). text 33.80 (*0-8204-0698-8*) P Lang Pubng.

***Detox Manual.** Suzannah Olivier. 2001. pap. 12.00 (*0-7432-1865-5*) S&S Trade.

***Detox Solution: The Missing Link to Radiant Health, Abundant Energy, Ideal Weight & Peace of Mind.** Patricia Fitzgerald. 2001. LC 2001-88962. (Illus.). 436p. pap. 19.95 (*0-9708299-0-6*) Illumination CA.

Detoxication & Drug Metabolism: Conjugation & Related Systems. Ed. by Sidney P. Colowick & William B. Jakoby. 1981. (Methods in Enzymology Ser.: Vol. 77). text 188.00 (*0-12-181977-9*) Acad Pr.

Detoxification: A Clinical Monograph. 1999. (Illus.). 42p. pap. 25.00 (*0-9624859-3-4*) HealthComm Intl.

Detoxification from Alcohol & Other Drugs: A Treatment Improvement Protocol. Ed. by Dorynne Czechowicz. 1999. 95p. (C). pap. text 20.00 (*0-7881-7597-1*) DIANE Pub.

Detoxification Treatment Manual. 1986. lib. bdg. 75.00 (*0-8490-3510-4*) Gordon Pr.

Detroit Receiving Hospital Emergency Medicine Handbook. William A. Berk. 3rd ed. 1995. 204p. pap. text 10.95 (*1-882663-01-2*) Plymouth VT.

Detroit Receiving Hospital Emergency Medicine Handbook. Ed. by William A. Berk. 4th rev. ed. 2000. 250p. pap. 14.95 (*1-882663-49-7*) Plymouth VT.

Deutsche Medizinische Inkunabeln. Karl Sudhoff. 1999. (GER.). 278p. reprint ed. 60.00 (*1-57898-134-4*) Martino Pubng.

***Deutsche und Oesterreichische Gesellschaft fur Hamatologie und Onkologie Band 23, Suppl. 7: Gemeinsame Jahrestagung, Graz, Oktober 2000.** Ed. by W. Linkesch. 2000. (GER.). x, 210p. 54.00 (*3-8055-7161-5*) S Karger.

Deutsches Archiv: Fur Geschichte der Medicin und Medicinische Geographie. Ed. by Heinrich Rohlfs & Gerhard Rohlfs. 1971. xxvii, 3896p. reprint ed. (*3-487-04127-8*) G Olms Pubs.

Developing a Chiropractic Practice. R. C. Schafer & D. C. FICC Staff. 1984. LC 83-73397. 75.00 (*0-9606618-5-9*) Am Chiro Assn.

Developing a Hospice Ethics Committee. National Hospice Organization. 1998. LC 99-163803. 78p. 11.85 (*0-931207-53-3*) Natl Hospice.

Developing a Hospital Emergency Preparedness Program. Gregg C. Beatty. rev. ed. 1990. (Management & Compliance Ser.: Vol. 2). (Illus.). 110p. reprint ed. ring bd. 110.00 (*0-87258-451-8*, 055201) Am Hospital.

Developing a Programme for Delayed Motor Development in Children. David Stewart. 1990. 69.95 (*1-85000-526-5*); pap. 34.95 (*1-85000-527-3*) Taylor & Francis (Falmer Pr).

Developing a Strategy for a Multiagency Response to Clandestine Drug Laboratories. 1994. (Illus.). 133p. (Orig.). (C). pap. text 40.00 (*0-7881-0581-7*) DIANE Pub.

Developing a Successful Physician - Hospital Organization. Jennings Ryan and Kolb, Inc. Staff. Ed. by Peter Straley. 1995. LC 95-10043. 204p. pap. 57.50 (*1-55648-136-5*, 164100) AHPI.

Developing Achievement Motivation in Adolescents: Education for Human Growth. Alfred S. Alschuler. 1973. LC 72-84336. 330p. 39.95 (*0-87778-037-4*) Educ Tech Pubns.

Developing Adaptive Work Behaviors. Ed. by William H. Burke. 1988. (Professional Series on Traumatic Brain Injury: Vol. 17). 52p. (Orig.). pap. 9.50 (*1-882855-24-8*) HDI Pubs.

Developing an Integrated Delivery System: Organizing a Seamless System of Care. American Psychological Association Staff & Coopers and Lybrand Staff. 1996. LC 96-4648. (APA Practitioner's Toolbox Ser.). pap. 29.95 (*1-55798-350-X*) Am Psychol.

Developing an Occupational Drug Abuse Program: Considerations & Approaches. 1986. lib. bdg. 79.95 (*0-8490-3512-0*) Gordon Pr.

Developing & Directing Counselor Education Laboratories. Ed. by Jane E. Myers. 1994. LC 94-3946. 216p. pap. text 33.95 (*1-55620-137-0*, 72583) Am Coun Assn.

Developing & Managing a Nursing Home Volunteer Program. Vicki Parsons. 1987. (C). 17.50 (*1-877735-32-9*, 2179pp) Prof Prnting & Pub.

Developing & Managing an Ambulatory Surgery Center. Jeanne M. Barkheimer et al. 2000. 109p. spiral bd. 41.00 (*1-56829-131-0*) M G M A.

***Developing & Sustaining a Patient & Family Advisory Council.** 148p. ring bd. 30.00 (*0-9677733-2-6*) Inst Fmly Ctr.

Developing Brain & Its Disorders: Proceedings of the 4th Annual Symposium on Development Disabilities, "Biological Aspects in the Pathogenesis of Developmental Disabilities," November 3-5, 1983, Tokyo. Ed. by Masataka Arima et al. 1985. (Illus.). viii, 314p. 139.25 (*3-8055-4010-8*) S Karger.

Developing Child. Bindler. 1999. pap. text 35.95 (*0-8385-1586-X*, Medical Exam) Appleton & Lange.

Developing Child. Owens. 2000. LC 2001-46581. (Psychology Ser.). pap. 52.00 net. (*0-534-36618-X*) Brooks-Cole.

Developing Child. Holly E. Brisbane. rev. ed. 1971. (Illus.). (gr. 9-12). text 20.64 (*0-02-663220-9*) Glencoe.

Developing Clinical Problem-Solving Skills: A Guide to More Effective Diagnosis & Treatment. Howard S. Barrows & Garfield C. Pickell. 1991. (Norton Medical Bks.). (Illus.). 264p. (C). pap. 19.95 (*0-393-71010-6*) Norton.

Developing Clinical Reasoning. Benamy. 1998. (Illus.). 132p. (C). text 47.00 (*0-12-784591-7*) Acad Pr.

Developing Cognitive & Creative Skills Through Art. Rawley A. Silver. 1978. 286p. text (*0-8391-1248-3*) Am Art Therapy.

Developing Cognitive-Behavioural Counselling. Michael J. Scott et al. 1995. (Developing Counselling Ser.). 144p. 57.95 (*0-8039-7893-6*, 9969) Sage.

Developing Cognitive Competence: New Approaches to Process Modeling. Ed. by Tony J. Simon & Graeme S. Halford. 1995. 400p. pap. 45.00 (*0-8058-1998-3*); text 89.95 (*0-8058-1289-X*) L Erlbaum Assocs.

Developing Collaborative Research in Primary Care. Ed. by Benjamin F. Crabtree et al. 1994. 340p. pap. 37.95 (*0-8039-5490-5*, 3658) Sage.

***Developing Community Nursing Practice.** Ed. by Sue Spencer et al. 2001. 192p. pap. (*0-335-20557-7*); LC 00-50178. text (*0-335-20558-5*) OpUniv Pr GBR. *Dist:* Taylor & Francis.

Developing Discipline: Selected Works of Margaret Newman. Margaret A. Newman. 1995. LC 94-23657. 320p. pap. 36.95 (*0-88737-638-X*) Natl League Nurse.

Developing Ericksonian Therapy: State of the Art. Jeffrey K. Zeig. Ed. by Stephen R. Lankton. 1988. LC 87-35533. 560p. text 57.95 (*0-87630-501-X*) Brunner-Routledge.

***Developing Family-Centered Vision, Mission & Philiosophy of Care Statements.** 56p. ring bd. 30.00 (*0-9677733-1-8*) Inst Fmly Ctr.

Developing Health Promotion Programs. David J. Anspaugh et al. 1999. LC 99-34740. 264p. (C). pap. 37.50 (*0-8151-4374-5*) McGrw-H Hghr Educ.

Developing Health Promotional Programs: HP 620. M. O'Donnell. 1989. 102p. (C). stu. ed. (*0-931657-14-8*) Learning Proc Ctr.

Developing Heart. 1997. LC 96-50463. 544p. text 135.00 (*0-397-58779-1*) Lppncott W & W.

Developing Heart. Ed. by Marianne J. Legato. 1984. text 141.00 (*0-89838-672-1*) Kluwer Academic.

Developing Heart: A History of Pediatric Cardiology. Ed. by Catherine A. Neill & Edward B. Clark. 1995. LC 95-3082. (Developments in Cardiovascular Medicine Ser.: Vol. 162). 176p. (C). text 70.50 (*0-7923-3375-6*) Kluwer Academic.

Developing Human: Clinical. Moore. 6th ed. 1998. (C). text 13.00 (*0-8089-2101-0*, Grune & Strat) Harcrt Hlth Sci Grp.

Developing Human: International Edition. Moore. 6th ed. 1998. (C). pap. text 33.00 (*0-8089-2064-2*, Grune & Strat) Harcrt Hlth Sci Grp.

Developing Individualized Activities for Language. Kay Campbell et al. 1995. 146p. pap. text 32.50 (*0-930951-98-0*) Acad Comm.

Developing Materials Management Job Descriptions. 1992. 150p. (Orig.). pap. 75.00 (*0-87258-630-8*, 142900) Am Hospital.

Developing Mental Health Services: A Foundation Training for Residential & Community Based Support Workers. Ed. by Liz Peretz & Chris Payne. 1994. (*0-902789-89-9*) Natl Inst Soc Work GBR. *Dist:* St Mut.

Developing Mind: Toward a Neurobiology of Interpersonal Experience. Daniel J. Siegel. 1999. LC 98-50993. 394p. 40.00 (*1-57230-453-7*, C0453) Guilford Pubns.

Developing Motivation. Ed. by William H. Burke. 2nd ed. 1996. (Professional Series on Traumatic Brain Injury: Vol. 11). 56p. (Orig.). pap. 9.50 (*1-882855-42-6*) HDI Pubs.

***Developing New Clinical Roles: A Guide for Health Professionals.** Debra Humphris & Abigail Masterson. 2001. (Illus.). 185p. pap. (*0-443-07071-7*) Church GBR. *Dist:* Saunders.

Developing New Contraceptives: Obstacles & Opportunities. Committee on Contraceptive Development, National R. 1990. 212p. text 24.95 (*0-309-04147-3*) Natl Acad Pr.

Developing Norm-Referenced Standardized Tests. Ed. by Lucy J. Miller. 1989. LC 88-36502. (Physical & Occupational Therapy in Pediatrics Ser.: Vol. 9, No. 1). (Illus.). 205p. text 49.95 (*0-86656-883-2*) Haworth Pr.

Developing Objectives for Healthy People 2010. Ed. by Barry Leonard. 1999. (Illus.). 180p. (C). pap. text 30.00 (*0-7881-7577-7*) DIANE Pub.

Developing Peer Leaders to Prevent the Spread of HIV: A Manual for Training College HIV Peer Health Educators. Jeffrey M. Gould. Ed. by Eric Engstrom & Kristen L. Glunz. 1995. 192p. (Orig.). pap. 35.00 (*1-882145-03-8*, 535) U WI Clearinghse.

Developing Performance Standards for Hospital Personnel. Lucia Berte. 1989. LC 89-17872. (Illus.). 92p. stu. ed. 25.00 (*0-89189-285-0*, 45-9-027-00) Am Soc Clinical.

Developing Person-Centered Counselling. Dave Mearns & Brian Thorne. 1994. 192p. 57.95 (*0-8039-8981-4*, 2885); pap. 24.95 (*0-8039-8982-2*, 2884) Sage.

Developing Person Through Childhood. Kathleen S. Berger & Ross A. Thompson. 1995. LC 94-62217. 624p. pap. text 56.95 (*1-57259-016-5*) Worth.

Developing Person Through Childhood & Adolescence. Kathleen S. Berger. 4th ed. 1995. 288p. pap. text, stu. ed. 17.95 (*1-57259-009-2*); LC 94-61333. 736p. text 69.95 (*1-57259-002-5*) Worth.

Developing Person Through the Lifespan. Berger. 5th ed. 2000. pap. text, stu. ed. 19.95 (*1-57259-944-8*) Worth.

Developing Positive Self-Images & Discipline in Black Children. Jawanza Kunjufu. 1984. LC 85-158270. (Illus.). 116p. pap. 8.95 (*0-913543-01-2*) African Am Imag.

Developing Professional Judgment in Health Care: Learning Through the Critical Appreciation of Practice. Della Fish et al. 1997. LC 97-30471. 256p. pap. text 40.00 (*0-7506-3123-6*) Buttrwrth-Heinemann.

Developing Programs to Control & Prevent Diabetes: An Analysis of the Problems. David C. Warner. 1982. LC 80-85242. (Policy Research Project Report Ser.: No. 43). 140p. pap. 5.00 (*0-89940-645-9*) LBJ Sch Pub Aff.

Developing Radiation Emergency Plans for Academic, Medical or Industrial Facilities. 1991. LC 91-23659. (Report Ser.: No. 111). 129p. pap. text 35.00 (*0-929600-20-7*) NCRP Pubns.

Developing Recreational Skills in Persons with Learning Disabilities. Lorraine Peniston. 1998. pap. 27.95 (*1-57167-134-X*) Sagamore Pub.

Developing Research in Nursing & Health: Quantitative & Qualitative Methods. Carol Noll Hoskins. 1998. LC 98-10333. (Teaching of Nursing Ser.). (Illus.). 144p. 35.95 (*0-8261-1185-8*) Springer Pub.

Developing Research in Primary Care. Ed. by Mike Saks et al. 2000. LC 00-364628. (Illus.). 168p. (*1-85775-397-6*) Radcliffe Med Pr GBR. *Dist:* Balogh.

Developing Responsive Human Services: New Perspectives about Residential Treatment Organizations. Jack Thaw & Anthony J. Cuvo. Ed. by Thomas R. Kratochwill & James E. Ysseldyke. 1986. (School Psychology Ser.). 336p. (C). 69.95 (*0-89859-612-2*) L Erlbaum Assocs.

Developing Role of Short-Lived Radionuclides in Nuclear Medical Practice: Proceedings. DOE Technical Information Center Staff. Ed. by Peter Paras & J. W. Thiessen. 1985. LC 84-26718. (Symposium Ser.). 571p. pap. 22.95 (*0-87079-518-X*, CONF-820523); fiche 9.00 (*0-87079-519-8*, CONF-820523) DOE.

Developing Safe, Effective & Reliable Medical Software. 1991. 46p. pap. 90.00 (*0-910275-56-4*, MDS-209) Assn Adv Med Instrn.

Developing Sanity in Human Affairs, 54. Ed. by Susan P. Kodish & Robert P. Holston. 1998. LC 97-37550. (Contributions to the Study of Mass Media & Communications Ser.: Vol. 54). 456p. 75.00 (*0-313-30613-3*, Greenwood Pr) Greenwood.

Developing School-Based Tobacco Use Prevention & Cessation Programs. Steve Sussman et al. 1994. 256p. 64.95 (*0-8039-4927-8*, 4723); pap. 34.95 (*0-8039-4928-6*, 4724) Sage.

Developing Self-Acceptance: A Brief, Educational & Small Group Approach. Windy Dryden. 1998. LC 97-38900. (Brief Therapy & Counselling Ser.). 240p. pap. 54.95 (*0-471-98099-4*) Wiley.

Developing Self Control. Ed. by William H. Burke. 2nd rev. ed. 1997. (HDI Professional Series on Traumatic Brain Injury: Vol. 14). (Illus.). 64p. pap. 9.50 (*1-882855-59-0*) HDI Pubs.

Developing Social Skills Ed. by William H. Burke. 2nd rev. ed. 1997. (HDI Professional Series on Traumatic Brain Injury). 64p. (Orig.). pap. 9.50 (*1-882855-57-4*) HDI Pubs.

Developing Sport Psychology Within Your Clinical Practice: A Practical Guide for Mental Health Professionals. Jack J. Lesyk. 1998. LC 97-45764. 240p. 42.00 (*0-7879-4046-1*) Jossey-Bass.

Developing Structure of Temperament & Personality from Infancy to Adulthood. Ed. by Charles F. Halverson et al. 1994. LC 93-50639. 464p. text 99.95 (*0-8058-1252-0*) L Erlbaum Assocs.

Developing Support Groups for Individuals with Early-Stage Alzheimer's Disease: Planning, Implementation & Evaluation. Robyn Yale. 1995. LC 95-6672. 256p. pap. text 28.50 (*1-878812-26-2*) Hlth Prof Pr.

Developing Technologies for Early Detection of Breast Cancer: A Public Workshop Summary. Laura Newman et al. 2000. 24p. pap. 12.00 (*0-309-07135-6*) Natl Acad Pr.

Developing the Information Infrastructure for Medicare Beneficiaries: Summary of a Workshop. Ed. by Valerie Tate Jopeck & Marion Ein Lewin. 1999. LC 00-687306. ix, 65p. 18.00 (*0-309-06388-4*) Natl Acad Pr.

Developing the TBI Rehab Plan. Ed. by William H. Burke. 1988. (Professional Series on Traumatic Brain Injury: Vol. 4). 48p. (Orig.). pap. 9.50 (*1-882855-11-6*) HDI Pubs.

Developing Transactional Analysis Counseling. Ian Stewart. 1996. (Developing Counselling Ser.). 224p. 57.95 (*0-8039-7901-0*, 2417); pap. 19.95 (*0-8039-7902-9*, 2418) Sage.

Developing Winning Strategies in Healthcare Industries: Dynamic Demographic & Regulatory Enivornments Demand Focus on Research & Corporate Structure. 1992. 218p. 1295.00 (*1-56753-024-9*) Frost & Sullivan.

Developing Your Career in Nursing. Ed. by Desmond Cormack. 1990. 250p. pap. 34.95 (*0-412-32130-0*, A4882) Chapman & Hall.

Developing Your Career in Nursing. Ed. by Robert Newell. 1996. LC 95-11758. pap. 25.95 (*0-304-33228-3*); text 90.00 (*0-304-33226-7*) Continuum.

Development - Evaluation - Drugs: From Laboratory Through Licensure to Market. Chi-Jen Lee. 1993. 240p. 131.95 (*0-8493-4447-6*, RM301) CRC Pr.

Development, Aging, & Disease: A New Rationale for an Intervention Strategy. Vladimir M. Vilman. Ed. & Tr. by John K. Young from RUS. 1994. LC 93-48915. 383p. text 116.00 (*3-7186-0552-X*) Gordon & Breach.

Development & Applications of a Decision Support System for Emergency Medical Services. David J. Eaton et al. 1988. (Working Papers Ser.: No. 46). 24p. pap. 5.00 (*0-89940-527-4*) LBJ Sch Pub Aff.

Development & Applications of Vaccines & Gene Therapy in AIDS. Ed. by G. Giraldo et al. 1996. LC 96-12691. (Antibiotics & Chemotherapy Ser.: Vol. 48). (Illus.). x, 246p. 234.00 (*3-8055-6256-X*) S Karger.

Development & Clinical Progress of DNA Vaccines: Paul-Ehrlich-Institut, Langen, October 1999. Ed. by F. Brown et al. 2000. (Developments in Biologicals Ser.). (Illus.). x, 214p. pap. 174.00 (*3-8055-7102-X*) S Karger.

Development & Clinical Uses of Haemophilus B Conjugate Vaccines, No. 11. Ed. by Ronald W. Ellis & Dan M. Granoff. 1994. LC 94-302. (Infectious Disease & Therapy Ser.: Vol. 11). (Illus.). 520p. text 225.00 (*0-8247-9186-X*) Dekker.

Development & Differentiation of the Nervous System: 21st Seiriken Conference, Okazaki, February 1996. Ed. by Kazuhiro Ikenaka et al. 1997. (Journal: Vol. 19, No. 1, 1997). (Illus.). 134p. pap. 48.75 (*3-8055-6444-9*) S Karger.

Development & Disabilities: Intellectual, Sensory, & Motor Impairments. Robert M. Hodapp. 1998. LC 97-49940. (Illus.). (C). 284p. text 54.95 (*0-521-48294-1*); 288p. pap. text 19.95 (*0-521-48338-7*) Cambridge U Pr.

Development & Dissemination of Model Systems for Hypertension Control in Organizational Settings. Andrea E. Foote & John C. Erfurt. 1974. 3.50 (*0-87736-322-6*) U of Mich Inst Labor.

Development & Diversity: New Applications in Art Therapy. Ed. by Doug Sandle. 1998. (Illus.). 200p. (*1-85343-401-9*); pap. (*1-85343-402-7*) Free Assoc Bks GBR. *Dist:* NYU Pr, Intl Spec Bk, Intl Spec Bk, NYU Pr.

Development & Environment: Proceedings. Conference on the Human Environment, Founex, Switz. Ed. by Maurice F. Strong. 1973. LC 72-75446. (Illus.). 225p. (Orig.). pap. text (*90-279-6990-6*) Mouton.

Development & Evaluation of Controlled Release Nasal Drug Delivery Systems of Apomorphine. Michael Ikechukwu Ugwoke. 1999. (Acta Biomedica Lovaniensia Ser.: Vol. 206). (Illus.). 206p. pap. (*90-6186-998-6*) Leuven Univ BEL. *Dist:* Coronet Bks.

Development & Integration of Behaviour: Essays in Honor of Robert Hinde. Ed. by Patrick Bateson. 1991. (Illus.). 516p. (C). text 95.00 (*0-521-40356-1*); pap. text 34.95 (*0-521-40709-5*) Cambridge U Pr.

Development & Learning: Conflict or Congruence? Lynn S. Liben. 1987. (Jean Piaget Symposia Ser.). 256p. 49.95 (*0-8058-0009-3*) L Erlbaum Assocs.

Development & Learning: Reconceptualizing the Intersection. Ed. by Deanna Kuhn. 1995. (Journal: Vol. 38, No. 6, 1995). (Illus.). 94p. pap. 46.25 (*3-8055-6257-8*) S Karger.

Development & Management of Ambulatory Care Programs: An Annotated Bibliography. 1995. 148p. (Orig.). (C). pap. text 40.00 (*0-7881-1825-0*) DIANE Pub.

Development & Management of Medical Groups. Gerald S. Benedict. 1996. 149p. (Orig.). pap. 44.95 (*1-56829-049-7*, 4856) M G M A.

Development & Meaning of Psychological Distance. Ed. by Rodney R. Cocking & K. Ann Renninger. 1993. 280p. text 59.95 (*0-8058-0747-0*) L Erlbaum Assocs.

Development & Organization of the Retina from Molecules to Function: Proceedings of a NATO ASI Held in Crete, Greece, June 18-28, 1997. Ed. by Leo M. Chalupa & Barbara L. Finlay. 1998. LC 98-21939. (NATO Advanced Science Institutes Ser.: Vol. 299). (Illus.). 356p. (C). text 125.00 (*0-306-45906-X*, Kluwer Plenum) Kluwer Academic.

Development & Plasticity of the Visual System. John R. Cronly-Dillon. 1991. 137.00 (*0-8493-7511-8*) CRC Pr.

Development & Policy Concerning Children with Special Needs. Ed. by Marion Perlmutter. 1983. (Minnesota Symposia on Child Psychology Ser.: Vol. 16). 272p. (C). text 59.95 (*0-89859-261-5*) L Erlbaum Assocs.

Development & Psychometric Characteristics of the Revised Illinois Test of Psycholinquistic Abilities. Samuel A. Kirk & John N. Paraskevopoulos. 1969. LC 69-19511. (Illus.). 243p. pap. text 15.00 (*0-252-00007-2*) U of Ill Pr.

Development & Recognition of the Transformed Cell. M. I. Greene & T. Hamaoka. 1987. LC 87-17175. (Illus.). 476p. (C). text 120.00 (*0-306-42636-6*, Kluwer Plenum) Kluwer Academic.

Development & Regeneration of Nervous System. Ed. by G. Calderini & Gino Toffano. 1982. (Journal: Vol. 5, No. 1). (Illus.). 116p. pap. 50.50 (*3-8055-3524-4*) S Karger.

Development & Regeneration of Skeletal Muscles. Ed. by B. Christ & R. Cihak. 1986. (Bibliotheca Anatomica Ser.: No. 29). (Illus.). viii, 224p. 155.75 (*3-8055-4227-5*) S Karger.

Development & Regeneration of the Nervous System. Ed. by S. Nona et al. 1992. (Eye & Brain: Biomedical & Clinical Aspects Ser.). (Illus.). 272p. (C). (gr. 13). pap. text 209.95 (*0-412-40280-7*, A9438) Chapman & Hall.

Development & Regenerative Potential of Cardiac Muscle. Ed. by John Oberpriller. 1991. xix, 463p. text 267.00 (*3-7186-0518-X*, Harwood Acad Pubs) Gordon & Breach.

Development & Repair of Cataract Induced by Ultraviolet Radiation. R. Michael. 2000. (Opthalmologica Ser.: Vol. 32, Suppl. 1 (2000)). (Illus.). vi, 120p. pap. 34.00 (*3-8055-7044-9*) S Karger.

Development & Structures of the Body Image Seymour Fisher. 1986. Set. text 125.00 (*0-89859-700-5*); Vol. 1. 344p. text 69.95 (*0-89859-684-X*); Vol. 2. 568p. text 99.95 (*0-89859-699-8*) L Erlbaum Assocs.

Development & Treatment of Childhood Aggression. Ed. by Debra Pepler & Kenneth H. Rubin. 1991. 488p. 95.00 (*0-8058-0370-X*) L Erlbaum Assocs.

Development During the Transition to Adolescence: The Minnesota Symposia on Child Psychology. Ed. by Megan R. Gunnar & W. Andrew Collins. 1988. (Minnesota Symposium on Child Psychology Ser.: Vol. 21). 232p. 49.95 (*0-8058-0194-4*) L Erlbaum Assocs.

Development, Genetics, & Psychology. Robert Plomin. 1986. 384p. (C). text 79.95 (*0-89859-630-0*) L Erlbaum Assocs.

Development in Adolescence. Ed. by W. Everaerd et al. 1983. text 141.50 (*0-89838-581-4*) Kluwer Academic.

Development in Adolescence. Harold E. Jones. 1943. (Century Psychology Ser.). (C). reprint ed. pap. text 11.95 (*0-89197-511-X*) Irvington.

Development in Adulthood. Lemme. 2nd ed. 1998. LC 98-17281. 544p. 78.00 (*0-205-27366-1*) Allyn.

Development in Context: Acting & Thinking in Specific Environments. Ed. by Robert H. Wozniak & Kurt Fischer. 1993. (Jean Piaget Symposia Ser.). 304p. text 69.95 (*0-8058-0769-1*) L Erlbaum Assocs.

Development in France. Baszan. 1985. (Social Science & Medicine Ser.). pap. 28.00 (*0-08-032655-2*, Pergamon Pr) Elsevier.

Development in Infancy: An Introduction. Marc H. Bornstein & Michael E. Lamb. 3rd ed. 1992. 704p. (C). text 75.63 (*0-07-006552-7*) McGrw-H Hghr Educ.

Development in Jeopardy: Clinical Responses to Infants & Families. Ed. by Emily Fenichel & Sally Provence. 1993. LC 93-2032. (Monograph Series of Zero to Three - National Center for Clinical Infant Programs). 340p. 50.00 (*0-8236-1227-9*) Intl Univs Pr.

Development, Methods, & Response Characteristics: National Mortality Followback Survey, 1986. 1992. LC 92-48960. (Vital & Health Statistics Ser.: Series 1, No. 29). (*0 8406 0471 8*) Natl Ctr Health Stats.

Development of a County-Based Public Health Data, Information & Resource Network: Framing the Concepts & Issues. Barry E. Gustin. 1997. LC 97-25873. 112p. pap. 40.00 (*1-889059-09-9*) Regent Pr.

Development of Aeromedical Evacuation in the USAF, 1909-1960. Robert Frank Futrell. 1960. (USAF Historical Studies: No. 23). Vol. 1. 446p. pap. text 56.95 (*0-89126-050-1*); Vol. 2. reprint ed. pap. text 50.95 (*0-89126-051-X*) MA-AH Pub.

Development of an Academic Surgeon: The Young Theodor Billroth (1829-1894) Karel B. Absolon. 1999. 115p. 49.50 (*1-57529-080-4*) Kabel Pubs.

Development of Aneurysms. Ed. by Richard R. Keen & Philip B. Dobrin. 2000. LC 99-36406. (Medical Intelligence Unit Ser.: Vol. 17). (Illus.). 235p. 99.00 (*1-58706-000-0*) Eurekah.

Development of Aneurysms. Richard R. Keen & Philip B. Dobrin. 1999. LC 99-36406. (Medical Intelligence Unit Ser.). 320p. 89.00 (*1-57059-648-4*) Landes Bioscience.

Development of Attachment & Affiliative Systems. Ed. by Robert N. Emde & Robert J. Harmon. 1982. LC 82-3818. (Topics in Developmental Psychobiology Ser.). 332p. 55.00 (*0-306-40849-X*, Plenum Trade) Perseus Pubng.

Development of Attention: Research & Theory. Ed. by J. T. Enns. 1990. (Advances in Psychology Ser.: No. 69). viv,570p. 201.50 (*0-444-88332-0*, North Holland) Elsevier.

Development of Behavioral States & the Expression of Emotions in Early Infancy: New Proposals for Investigation. Peter H. Wolff. 1987. LC 86-16066. (Illus.). viii, 296p. (C). 39.00 (*0-226-90520-9*) U Ch Pr.

Development of Biopharmaceutical Parenteral Dosage Forms. Ed. by John A. Bontempo. 1997. LC 97-15956. (Drugs & the Pharmaceutical Sciences Ser.: Vol. 85). (Illus.). 264p. text 150.00 (*0-8247-9981-X*) Dekker.

Development of Cancer Centres & Community Cancer Control Programmes: Report on a WHO Working Group. 1982. (Euro Reports & Studies Ser.: No. 70). 37p. pap. text 4.00 (*92-890-1236-6*) World Health.

Development of Children's Understanding of Space Relations Among Objects: The Coordination of Perspectives Task of Jean Piaget. Alfred J. Nigl. 1981. (European University Studies: Ser. 6, Vol. 62). 74p. 9.00 (*3-261-04872-7*) P Lang Pubng.

Development of Church Teaching on Prolonging Life. Kevin D. O'Rourke. 1988. 20p. pap. 3.00 (*0-87125-152-3*, 217) Cath Health.

Development of Cognition, Affect, & Social Relations Vol. 13: The Minnesota Symposium on Child Psychology. Ed. by W. Andrew Collins. 1980. LC 79-27560. (Illus.). 320p. text 49.95 (*0-89859-023-X*) L Erlbaum Assocs.

Development of Cognitive Anthropology. Roy D'Andrade. 1995. (Illus.). 286p. (C). text 59.95 (*0-521-45370-4*); pap. text 21.95 (*0-521-45976-1*) Cambridge U Pr.

Development of Coordination in Infancy. Ed. by Geert J. Savelsbergh. 1993. (Advances in Psychology Ser.: Vol. 97). 548p. 162.00 (*0-444-89328-8*, North Holland) Elsevier.

Development of Dialectical Operations: Journal: Human Development, Vol. 18, Nos. 1 & 2. Ed. by Klaus F. Riegel. 1976. (Illus.). vii, 241p. 33.25 (*3-8055-2225-8*) S Karger.

Development of Electronic Aids for the Visually Impaired. Ed. by P. L. Emiliani. 1986. (Documenta Ophthalmologica Proceedings Ser.). text 221.50 (*0-89838-805-8*) Kluwer Academic.

Development of Emotion Expression during the First Two Years of Life. Carol Z. Malatesta et al. 1989. (Child Development Monographs: No. 219 54: 1-2). 146p. pap. text 15.00 (*0-226-50285-6*) U Ch Pr.

Development of Emotion Regulation: Biological & Behavioral Considerations. Ed. by Nathan A. Fox. 1994. (Monographs of the Society for Research in Child Development: No. 240). 316p. pap. text 19.50 (*0-226-25940-4*) U Ch Pr.

Development of Emotion Regulation & Dysregulation. Ed. by Judy Garber & Kenneth A. Dodge. 1991. (Cambridge Studies in Social & Emotional Development). (Illus.). 352p. (C). text 69.95 (*0-521-36406-X*) Cambridge U Pr.

Development of Environmental Health Criteria for Urban Planning: Proceedings of the WHO Scientific Group, Geneva, 1971. WHO Staff. 1972. (Technical Reports: No. 511). pap. text 4.00 (*92-4-120511-3*, 1100511) World Health.

Development of Epstein-Barr Virus Vaccine. Ed. by Andrew J. Morgan. 1995. (Medical Intelligence Unit Ser.). 105p. text 99.00 (*1-57059-112-1*) Landes Bioscience.

Development of Eye-Hand Coordination Across the Life Span. Ed. by Chantal Bard et al. 1990. LC 89-22560. (Physical Activity, Growth & Motor Development Across the Lifespan Ser.). 396p. text 34.95 (*0-87249-628-7*) U of SC Pr.

Development of Fine Motor Coordination. Anne Henderson & Charlane Pehoski. 1994. (Illus.). 352p. (C). (gr. 13). text 45.00 (*0-8016-6917-0*, 06917) Mosby Inc.

Development of Forgetting & Reminiscence. Charles J. Brainerd et al. 1990. (Monographs for the Society for Research: Vol. 55, Nos. 3-4). 120p. pap. text 15.00 (*0-226-07095-6*) U Ch Pr.

Development of Gastrointestinal Functions in Mammals & Man. Otakar Koldovsky & W. Allan Walker. 1986. 250p. 40.00 (*0-03-061992-0*, Praeger Pubs) Greenwood.

Development of Gynaecological Surgery & Instruments. James Ricci. 1990. (Illus.). 594p. reprint ed. 165.00 (*0-930405-28-5*) Norman SF.

Development of Hand Skills in the Child. Ed. by Jane Case-Smith & Charlane Pehoski. 1992. (Illus.). 150p. (C). pap. text 37.00 (*0-910317-78-X*) Am Occup Therapy.

Development of Health Education in South-East Asia. J. Grossman. 1988. (SEARO Technical Publications Ser.: No. 10). 49p. pap. text 3.00 (*92-9022-149-6*) World Health.

Development of Health Psychology: An International Perspective. Ed. by M. A. Jansen. 1990. 92p. pap. text 71.00 (*3-7186-5021-5*, Harwood Acad Pubs) Gordon & Breach.

Development of Human Gene Therapy. Theodore Friedmann. 1998. LC 98-25205. (Monographs: Vol. 36). (Illus.). 744p. 134.00 (*0-87969-528-5*) Cold Spring Harbor.

Development of In Vitro & Ex Vivo Positron-Emitting Tracer Techniques & Their Application to Neurotrauma. Sven Sihver. 2000. (Comprehensive Summaries of Uppsala Dissertations from the Faculty of Medicine Ser.: Vol. 942). (Illus.). 52p. pap. (*91-554-4771-6*) Uppsala Universitet SWE. *Dist:* Coronet Bks.

Development of In Vitro Susceptibility Testing Criteria & Quality Control Parameters: Approved Guideline (1994), Vol. 10. Contrib. by William J. Novick, Jr. 1994. 95.00 (*1-56238-101-6*, M23-A) NCCLS.

Development of In Vitro Susceptibility Testing Criteria & Quality Control Parameters for Veterinary Antimicrobial Agents: Proposed Guideline (1996) 1996. 25.00 (*1-56238-310-8*, M37-P) NCCLS.

Development of Indicators for Monitoring Progress Towards Health for All by the Year 2000. 1981. text (*92-4-180004-6*) World Health.

Development of Infants Born at Risk. Deborah L. Holmes & Joseph F. Pasternak. 1984. 272p. (C). text 49.95 (*0-89859-283-6*) L Erlbaum Assocs.

Development of Infants of Drug Dependent Mothers. Anneloes Van Baar. 1991. xii, 132p. (*90-265-1189-2*) Swets.

Development of Infants with Disabilities & Their Families: Implications for Theory & Service Delivery. Jack P. Shonkoff et al. 1992. (Monographs of the Society for Research in Child Development: No. 232, Vol. 57, Nos. 6-7). 176p. (C). pap. text 15.00 (*0-226-75351-4*) U Ch Pr.

Development of Intelligence. Mike Anderson. 2000. (Studies in Developmental Psychology). 388p. pap. (*0-86377-845-3*) Psychol Pr GBR. *Dist:* Taylor & Francis.

Development of Intelligence in Children. Alfred Binet & Thomas Simon. 1975. LC 73-2962. (Classics in Psychology Ser.). reprint ed. 25.95 (*0-405-05135-2*) Ayer.

Development of Intersensory Perception: Comparative Perspectives. Ed. by David J. Lewkowicz & Robert Lickliter. 1994. 448p. text 99.95 (*0-8058-1217-2*) L Erlbaum Assocs.

Development of Iron Chelators for Clinical Use. Raymond J. Bergeron. 1993. 432p. 187.95 (*0-8493-8679-9*, RM666) CRC Pr.

Development of Language & Literacy in Young Children. Susanna Pflaum-Connor. 3rd ed. 1990. 256p. (C). pap. text 30.75 (*0-675-20447-X*, Merrill Coll) P-H.

Development of Long Term Retention. Ed. by M. L. Howe et al. 1992. (Illus.). 267p. 139.00 (*0-387-97734-1*) Spr-Verlag.

Development of Mathematical Skills. Chris Donlan. 2000. (Studies in Developmental Psychology). (Illus.). 352p. pap. (*0-86377-817-8*) Psychol Pr.

Development of Mature Walking. David Sutherland et al. 1991. (Clinics in Developmental Medicine Ser.: Nos. 104/105). (Illus.). 227p. (C). text (*0-521-41221-8*) Mc Keith Pr GBR. *Dist:* Cambridge U Pr.

Development of Medical Bibliography. Estelle Brodman. 1981. 226p. reprint ed. 8.25 (*0-912176-00-8*) Med Lib Assn.

Development of Medical Techniques & Treatments: From Leeches to Heart Surgery. Martin Duke. 1991. LC 90-4666. 270p. 37.50 (*0-8236-1232-5*) Intl Univs Pr.

Development of Medications for the Treatment of Opiate & Cocaine Addictions: Issues for the Government & Private Sector. National Institute on Drug Abuse, Institute of Med. Ed. by Carolyn E. Fulco et al. 1995. LC 95-118953. 272p. (Orig.). (C). pap. text 37.00 (*0-309-05244-0*) Natl Acad Pr.

Development of Metalinguistic Abilities in Children. David T. Hakes. 1980. (Language & Communication Ser.: Vol. 9). (Illus.). 119p. 34.95 (*0-387-10295-7*) Spr-Verlag.

***Development of Methods in CE, CE-MS & MS/MS: Applicatons in Pharmaceutical (sic), Biomedical & Forensic Sciences.** Emmy Javerfalk-Hoyes. 2001. (Comprehensive Summaries of Uppsala Dissertations from the Faculty of Pharmacy Ser.: No. 257). (Illus.). 38p. pap. (*91-554-5107-1*) Uppsala Universitet SWE. *Dist:* Coronet Bks.

Development of Modern Behavioural Psychology, Vol. 1. John McLeish. 1981. 228p. (Orig.). (C). pap. text 14.95 (*0-920490-20-4*) Temeron Bks.

Development of Motor Abilities During the First Three Years. Nancy Bayley. 1935. (SRCD M Ser.: Vol. 1, No. 1). pap. 25.00 (*0-527-01486-9*) Periodicals Srv.

Development of Newtonian Optics in England. Henry J. Steffens. 1977. (Illus.). 20.00 (*0-88202-048-X*, Sci Hist) Watson Pub Intl.

Development of Non-Myeloablative Transplants: Scientific Hypotheses. Marlies Van Hoef. 2000. 28p. pap. 24.95 (*0-9707183-0-6*) Transplant Creat.

Development of Novel Antimicrobial Agents: Emerging Strategies. Ed. by Karl Lohner. 2000. 296p. (*1-898486-23-9*) Horizon Sci GBR. *Dist:* Intl Spec Bk.

Development of Person-Context Relations. Ed. by Thomas A. Kindermann & Jaan Valsiner. 1995. 264p. text 49.95 (*0-8058-1568-6*) L Erlbaum Assocs.

Development of Plasma Derivatives for Clinical Use: Proceedings of the American Red Cross Symposium, Washington, October 1971 - Journal: Vox Sanguinis, Vol. 23, Nos. 1 & 2. American National Red Cross Staff. Ed. by G. A. Jamieson. 1972. (Illus.). pap. 46.75 (*3-8055-1483-2*) S Karger.

Development of Play. David Cohen. 2nd ed. 1993. LC 93-32142. (Concepts in Developmental Psychology Ser.). (C). 256p. pap. 27.95 (*0-415-09488-7*); 224p. text 69.95 (*0-415-09487-9*) Routledge.

Development of Prosocial Behavior. Ed. by Nancy Eisenberg. 1982. (Developmental Psychology Ser.). 416p. text 89.95 (*0-12-234980-6*) Acad Pr.

Development of Psychoanalysis. Sandor Ferenczi & Otto Rank. 1986. LC 86-7198. (Classics in Psychoanalysis Monographs: No. 4). 27.50 (*0-8236-1197-3*) Intl Univs Pr.

Development of Reasoning in Children with Normal & Defective Hearing, Vol. 24. Mildred C. Templin. 1975. LC 72-141551. (University of Minnesota Institute of Child Welfare Monographs: No. 24). 143p. reprint ed. lib. bdg. 48.00 (*0-8371-5898-2*, CWTR) Greenwood.

Development of Responsiveness to Steroid Hormones: Bat-Sheva Seminar on the Development of Responsiveness to Steroid Hormones Weizmann Institute of Science, Israel 18-26 Oct., 1978. Ed. by A. M. Kaye & Myra Kaye. 1980. LC 79-42938. (Advances in the Biosciences Ser.: Vol. 25). (Illus.). 483p. 69.50 (*0-08-024940-X*, Pergamon Pr) Elsevier.

Development of Social Cognition. Ed. by J. B. Pryor & J. D. Day. 1985. (Illus.). 268p. 86.95 (*0-387-96138-0*) Spr-Verlag.

Development of Social Skills by Blind & Visually Impaired Students: Exploratory Studies & Strategies. Ed. by Sharon Z. Sacks et al. 1992. LC 92-18638. 232p. pap. 39.95 (*0-89128-217-3*) Am Foun Blind.

Development of Spatial Cognition. Robert Cohen. 1985. 416p. 89.95 (*0-89859-543-6*) L Erlbaum Assocs.

Development of Specifications for Biotechnology Pharmaceutical Products: Symposium at Hyatt Regency, San Francisco, Calif., May 1996. Ed. by Fred Brown & James Fernandez. 1997. LC 98-100685. (Developments in Biological Standardization Ser.: Vol. 91, 1997). (Illus.). x, 122p. pap. 104.50 (*3-8055-6569-0*) S Karger.

Development of Speech. Paula Menyuk. 1972. LC 74-173981. (Studies in Communicative Disorders). pap. text 2.15 (*0-672-61276-3*, Bobbs) Macmillan.

Development of Speech Perception: The Transition from Speech Sounds to Spoken Words. Ed. by Judith Goodman & Howard C. Nusbaum. 1994. LC 93-11391. 360p. 60.00 (*0-262-07154-1*, Bradford Bks) MIT Pr.

Development of Standardized Clinical Evaluations in Mental Health. Ed. by Janice P. Burke et al. 1988. LC 88-656. (Occupational Therapy in Mental Health Ser.: Vol. 8, No. 1). (Illus.). 94p. text 39.95 (*0-86656-729-1*) Haworth Pr.

Development of the Central Nervous System in Vertebrates. S. C. Sharma & A. M. Goffinet. 1992. LC 92-49267. (NATO Advanced Science Institutes Ser.: Vol. 234). (Illus.). 284p. (C). text 105.00 (*0-306-44304-X*, Kluwer Plenum) Kluwer Academic.

Development of the Cerebral Cortex, No. 193. Colin Blakemore. 1996. LC 95-21512. (CIBA Foundation Symposia Ser.: Vol. 193). 246p. 128.00 (*0-471-95705-4*) Wiley.

Development of the Cranial Nerve Ganglia & Related Nuclei in the Rat. J. Altman & S. Bayer. 1982. (Advances in Anatomy, Embryology & Cell Biology Ser.: Vol. 74). (Illus.). 90p. 39.95 (*0-387-11337-1*) Spr-Verlag.

Development of the Craniofacial-Oral-Laryngeal Anatomy: A Review. Raymond D. Kent & Houri K. Vorperian. 1995. (Illus.). 96p. (Orig.). pap. 24.95 (*1-56593-425-3*, 1276) Thomson Learn.

Development of the Diencephalon of the Chinese Hamster: An Investigation of the Validity of the Criteria of Subdivision of the Brain. A. Keyser. 1973. (Journal: Vol. 83, Suppl.). (Illus.). pap. 31.50 (*3-8055-1593-6*) S Karger.

Development of the Digestive System in the North American Opossum, Didelphis Virginiana. W. J. Krause & J. H. Cutts. 1992. (Advances in Anatomy, Embryology & Cell Biology Ser.: Vol. 125). (Illus.). 151p. 96.00 (*0-387-55149-2*) Spr-Verlag.

Development of the Ego: Implications for Personality Theory, Psychopathology, & the Psychotherapeutic Process. Stanley Greenspan. 1989. LC 89-2237. 390p. 57.50 (*0-8236-1230-9*) Intl Univs Pr.

Development of the Eye: Experimental Studies. G. V. Lopashov & O. G. Stroeva. 1964. 182p. 3.5 hd 44.50 (*0-7065-0536-0*) Coronet Bks.

Development of the Gastrointestinal Tract. Ian R. Sanderson & W. Allan Walker. 1999. 400p. text incl. cd-rom (*1-55009-081-X*) DEKR.

Development of the Infant & Young Child: Normal & Abnormal. Ronald S. Illingworth. 9th ed. 1997. (Illus.). 364p. pap. text (*0-443-03840-6*) Church.

Development of the Mind: Psychoanalytic Papers on Clinical & Theoretical Problems. Jeanne Lampl-de Groot. 1965. LC 65-21749. 391p. 57.50 (*0-8236-1240-6*) Intl Univs Pr.

Development of the National Home & Hospice Care Survey. Barbara J. Haupt. 1994. LC 94-12450. (Vital & Health Statistics Ser.: Series 1, No. 33). 11.00 (*0-8406-0492-0*) Natl Ctr Health Stats.

Development of the Notion of Self: Understanding the Complexity of Human Interiority. William S. Schmidt. 1994. LC 93-20925. (Studies in the Psychology of Religion: Vol. 5). 416p. text 109.95 (*0-7734-9341-7*) E Mellen.

Development of the Rat Spinal Cord: Immuno- & Enzyme Histochemical Approaches. Martin Oudega et al. 1994. LC 93-44601. (Advances in Anatomy, Embryology & Cell Biology Ser.: Vol. 129). viii, 166p. pap. (*3-540-57173-6*); (Illus.). 166p. 108.00 (*0-387-57173-6*) Spr-Verlag.

Development of the Red Pulp in the Spleen. V. Grouls & B. Helpap. 1982. (Advances in Anatomy, Embryology & Cell Biology Ser.: Vol. 75). (Illus.). 71p. 34.95 (*0-387-11408-4*) Spr-Verlag.

Development of the Vascular System. Ed. by R. N. Feinberg et al. 1991. (Issues in Biomedicine Ser.: Vol. 14). (Illus.). viii, 192p. 191.50 (*3-8055-5285-8*) S Karger.

Development of the Vertebrate Retina. B. L. Finlay & D. R. Sengelaub. 1989. (Perspectives in Vision Research Ser.). (Illus.). 308p. (C). text 95.00 (*0-306-43060-6*, Kluwer Plenum) Kluwer Academic.

Development of the Vertebrate Skull. Gavin R. De Beer. LC 85-1081. (Illus.). reprint ed. 1998. xxiv, 760p. pap. text 27.00 (*0-226-13960-3*); 1995. xxiv, 730p. lib. bdg. 66.00 (*0-226-13958-1*) U Ch Pr.

Development of Therapeutic Skills. Mary Jo Bulbrook. 1980. text 14.95 (*0-316-11472-3*, Little Brwn Med Div) Lppncott W & W.

Development of Vegetable Oils in Human Nutrition. Ed. by R. Przbylski & B. McDonald. 1995. 144p. 70.00 (*0-935315-66-7*) Am Oil Chemists.

Development of X-Ray Analysis. Lawrence Bragg. Ed. by D. C. Phillips & H. Lipson. rev. unabr. ed. 1993. LC 92-39217. (Illus.). 270p. reprint ed. pap. text 8.95 (*0-486-67316-2*) Dover.

Development Psychology of Planning: Why, How, & When Do We Plan? Ed. by Sarah L. Friedman & Ellin K. Scholnick. 1997. LC 97-7420. 350p. 79.95 (*0-8058-1515-5*) L Erlbaum Assocs.

Development, Regeneration & Plasticity of the Autonomic Nervous System. Ed. by I. A. Hendry. 1992. (Autonomic Nervous System Ser.). xiv, 472p. text 184.00 (*3-7186-5138-6*, Harwood Acad Pubs) Gordon & Breach.

Development Through Health. Henry D. Molumphy. 1985. (Illus.). 16p. 1.00 (*0-918397-01-4*) Foster Parents.

Development Through Life: A Handbook for Clinicians. Ed. by Michael F. Rutter & Dale F. Hay. 1996. (Illus.). 640p. pap. 65.00 (*0-632-04192-7*) Blackwell Sci.

Development Through Life: A Handbook for Clinicians. Ed. by Michael Rutter & Dale F. Hay. 1994. (Illus.). 632p. (*0-632-03693-1*) Blckwell Science.

Development Through Life: A Psychosocial Approach. Barbara M. Newman. 5th ed. 1991. LC 90-25467. 708p. (C). text 49.95 (*0-534-15396-8*) Brooks-Cole.

Development Through Life: A Psychosocial Approach. Barbara M. Newman & Philip R. Newman. 6th ed. 1994. 763p. pap. 51.00 (*0-534-23334-1*) Brooks-Cole.

Development Through Life: Study Guide. Philip R. Newman. 6th ed. 1995. (Psychology Ser.). mass mkt., stu. ed. 17.75 (*0-534-23335-X*) Brooks-Cole.

Development Through the Lifespan. 1998. (C). (*0-205-28396-9*, Macmillan Coll) P-H.

Development Through the Lifespan. Laura E. Berk. 1997. LC 97-45631. 752p. 89.00 (*0-205-14684-8*) P-H.

Developmental Analysis of Cuba's Health Care System since 1959. Ed. by Theodore H. MacDonald. 1999. LC 99-22943. (Studies in Health & Human Services: Vol. 32). 13p. 99.95 (*0-7734-8049-8*) E Mellen.

*__Developmental Anatomy.__ Moore. 2000. (Illus.). (C). 20.80 (*0-8087-2622-6*) Pearson Custom.

Developmental & Acquired Dyslexia: Neuropsychological & Neurolinguistic Perspectives. Ed. by Che K. Leong. 1995. (Neuropsychology & Cognition Ser.). 300p. (C). text 148.50 (*0-7923-3166-4*) Kluwer Academic.

Developmental & Behavioral Characteristics of Preterm Infants. Lynn B. Hadley et al. 1999. LC 99-46984. vi, 32p. pap. 8.95 (*1-887571-06-X*) NICU Ink.

Developmental Approach to Problems of Acting Out. Ed. by Eveoleen N. Rexford. rev. ed. 1978. LC 77-17666. 223p. 35.00 (*0-8236-1221-X*) Intl Univs Pr.

Developmental Aspects of Health Compliance Behavior. Ed. by Suzanne B. Johnson et al. 1993. 368p. text 79.95 (*0-8058-1112-5*) L Erlbaum Assocs.

Developmental Aspects of Temporomandibular Joint Disorders. Ed. by J. A. McNamara et al. 1985. (Craniofacial Growth Ser.: Vol. 16). (Illus.). 298p. 59.00 (*0-929921-12-7*) UM CHGD.

Developmental Assessment & Intervention with Children & Adolescents. Ann Vernon. 1993. LC 93-13261. 168p. pap. text 33.95 (*1-55620-122-2*, 72560) Am Coun Assn.

Developmental Assessment in Clinical Child Psychology: A Handbook. J. H. Johnson & J. Goldman. 1990. (General Psychology Ser.). 304p. (*0-08-036446-2*) PPI GBR. *Dist:* Elsevier.

Developmental-Behavioral Disorders: Selected Topics. M. I. Gottlieb & J. E. Williams. (Critical Issues in Developmental & Behavioral Pediatrics Ser.). (Illus.). Vol. 1. 1988. 392p. text 85.00 (*0-306-42753-2*); Vol. 2. 1989. 310p. (C). text 85.00 (*0-306-43124-6*); Vol. 3. 1991. 390p. (C). text 102.00 (*0-306-43748-1*) Kluwer Academic (Kluwer Plenum).

Developmental Behavioral Neuroscience: The Minnesota Symposia on Child Psychology, Vol. 24. Ed. by Megan R. Gunnar & C. Nelson. 1992. (Minnesota Symposium on Child Psychology Ser.). 248p. (C). text 49.95 (*0-8058-0977-5*) L Erlbaum Assocs.

Developmental-Behavioral Pediatrics. Ed. by Melvin D. Levine et al. 2nd ed. 1992. (Illus.). 809p. text 155.00 (*0-7216-3189-4*) Saunders.

Developmental Biology Vol. 1: A Comprehensive Synthesis; Oogenesis. L. W. Browder. 1985. LC 85-3406. (Illus.). 644p. (C). text 120.00 (*0-306-41866-5*, Kluwer Plenum) Kluwer Academic.

Developmental Biology Vol. 1: Prenatal Growth. F. Falkner & J. M. Tanner. 2nd ed. 1986. LC 85-19397. (Human Growth Ser.). (Illus.). 518p. (C). text 120.00 (*0-306-41951-3*, Kluwer Plenum) Kluwer Academic.

Developmental Biology & Cancer. Ed. by Gisele M. Hodges & Charles Rowlatt. 1993. LC 93-9560. 560p. 225.00 (*0-8493-8869-4*, RC268) CRC Pr.

Developmental Biology Protocols, Vol. III. Ed. by Rocky S. Tuan & Cecilia W. Lo. 2000. (Methods in Molecular Biology Ser.: Vol. 137). (Illus.). 548p. spiral bd. 99.50 (*0-89603-576-X*) Humana.

Developmental Care of Premature. Young. 1996. pap. text 20.95 (*0-7020-2137-7*) Saunders.

Developmental Changes in Myocardial Inotropic Responsiveness. Michael Artman. 1994. (Medical Intelligence Unit Ser.). 118p. 99.00 (*1-57059-127-X*, LN9127) Landes Bioscience.

*__Developmental Co-Ordination, Disorder in Pre-School Children: Effects of Motor Skill Intervention, Parents' Descriptions, & Short-Term Follow-Up of Motor Status.__ Mia Pless. 2001. (Comprehensive Summaries of Uppsala Dissertations from the Faculty of Medicine Ser.: No. 1010). 43p. (*91-554-4963-8*) Uppsala Universitet SWE. *Dist:* Coronet Bks.

Developmental Cognitive Neuropsychology. Christine M. Temple. 1997. LC 97-202080. (Illus.). viii, 398p. (*0-86377-400-8*) Psychol Pr GBR. *Dist:* Taylor & Francis.

Developmental Cognitive Neuroscience: An Introduction. Mark H. Johnson. 1997. LC 96-16493. (Fundamentals of Cognitive Neuroscience Ser.: Vol. 1). 208p. pap. 29.95 (*0-631-20201-3*) Blackwell Pubs.

Developmental Concordance & Discordance During Puberty & Early Adolescence. D. M. Mort. 1953. (SRCD Ser.: Vol. 18, No. 1). 25.00 (*0-527-01557-1*) Periodicals Srv.

Developmental Conflicts & Diagnostic Evaluation in Adolescent Psychotherapy. Richard A. Gardner. 1999. LC 98-54479. 9376p. pap. 30.00 (*0-7657-0206-1*) Aronson.

Developmental Course of Marital Dysfunction. Ed. by Thomas N. Bradbury. 1998. LC 97-29630. (Cambridge Studies in Social & Emotional Development). (Illus.). 492p. (C). text 59.95 (*0-521-45190-6*) Cambridge U Pr.

Developmental Deviations & Personality: Theoretical Issues & Therapeutic Applications. D. R. Alexsandrowicz. 1989. xii, 126p. pap. text 62.00 (*2-88124-298-7*) Gordon & Breach.

Developmental Disabilities: A Handbook for Best Practices. Phillip J. McLaughlin & Paul Wehman. 1992. 328p. 38.00 (*1-56372-023-X*) PRO-ED.

Developmental Disabilities: A Handbook for Interdisciplinary Practice. Bruce Thyer & Nancy Kropf. 1995. 256p. pap. text 29.95 (*1-57129-003-6*) Brookline Bks.

Developmental Disabilities: A Handbook for Occupational Therapists. Ed. by Jerry A. Johnson & David A. Ethridge. 1990. LC 89-20012. (Occupational Therapy in Health Care Ser.: Vol. 6, Nos. 2 & 3). (Illus.). 249p. text 49.95 (*0-86656-959-6*) Haworth Pr.

Developmental Disabilities: A Neuropsychological Approach. David Freides. 1999. LC 00-25851. (Illus.). xiv, 586p. 84.95 (*1-55786-579-5*) Blackwell Pubs.

Developmental Disabilities: Psychosocial Aspects. George S. Baroff. 1991. LC 90-43702. (Illus.). 259p. (C). pap. text 29.00 (*0-89079-412-X*, 1590) PRO-ED.

Developmental Disabilities: Theory, Assessment & Intervention. Ed. by Michael Lewis & Lawrence Taft. 1982. 288p. text 35.00 (*0-88331-134-8*) R B Luce.

Developmental Disabilities in Infancy & Childhood Vol. II: The Spectrum of Developmental Disabilities. Arnold J. Capute & Pasquale J. Accardo. 2nd ed. 1996. LC 94-34249. 624p. text 110.00 (*1-55766-194-4*) P H Brookes.

Developmental Disabilities Program Aide. Jack Rudman. 1994. (Career Examination Ser.: C-864). pap. 23.95 (*0-8373-0864-X*) Nat Learn.

Developmental Disorders of Language. Betty B. Brown & Margaret Edwards. 1990. (Illus.). 234p. (Orig.). (C). pap. 39.95 (*1-879105-06-3*, A011) Thomson Learn.

Developmental Disorders of Language. Catherine Adams et al. 2nd ed. 1997. LC 97-2631. (Illus.). 256p. pap. 49.95 (*1-56593-863-1*, 1688) Singular Publishing.

Developmental Disorders of the Frontostriatal System: Neuropsychological, Neuropsychiatric & Evolutionary Perspectives. John L. Bradshaw. 2001. LC 00-40284. (Brain Damage, Behaviour & Cognition Ser.). (Illus.). xiii, 304p. (C). text (*1-84169-226-3*) Psychol Pr GBR. *Dist:* Taylor & Francis.

Developmental Dyslexia: Neural, Cognitive, & Genetic Mechanisms. Ed. by Christopher H. Chase et al. 1996. LC 96-10323. pap. 38.00 (*0-912752-39-4*) York Pr.

Developmental Dyslexia & Learning Disorders: Child Health & Development, Vol. 5. Ed. by D. J. Bakker et al. 1987. (Illus.). vi, 166p. 61.00 (*3-8055-4585-1*) S Karger.

Developmental Dysplasia of the Hip: Practical Guide to Screening. David Jones. 1998. LC 98-15742. (Illus.). 112p. pap. text 34.00 (*0-7506-2764-6*) Buttrwrth-Heinemann.

Developmental Dyspraxia & Adult-Onset Apraxia: A Lecture Prepared for Sensory Integration International. A. Jean Ayres. 1985. LC 88-151167. 85p. (Orig.). pap. 15.00 (*1-882068-00-9*) Sensory Integration.

Developmental Effects of Irradiation on the Brain of the Embryo & Fetus. Ed. by International Commission of Radiological Protectio. 1987. (International Commission on Radiological Protection Ser.: No. 49). (Illus.). 50p. pap. 32.00 (*0-08-035203-0*, Pergamon Pr) Elsevier.

Developmental Endocrinology: From Research to Clinical Practice. Ed. by Erica A. Eugster & Ora H. Pescovitz. 2001. LC 2001-51948. (Contemporary Endocrinology Ser.). 450p. 165.00 (*0-89603-860-2*) Humana.

Developmental Examination of Infants & Preschool Children. Dorothy F. Egan. 1991. (Clinics in Developmental Medicine Ser.: No. 112). (Illus.). 84p. (C). text (*0-521-41197-1*) Mc Keith Pr GBR. *Dist:* Cambridge U Pr.

Developmental Experiences: Treatment of Developmental Disorders in Children. David S. Levin. 1985. LC 84-24318. 352p. 60.00 (*0-87668-760-5*) Aronson.

Developmental Immunology. Edwin L. Cooper & Eric Nisbet-Brown. 1993. (Illus.). 496p. text 98.00 (*0-19-504353-7*) OUP.

Developmental Issues in the Clinical Treatment of Children. Ed. by Wendy K. Silverman & Thomas K. Ollendick. 1998. LC 98-20824. 510p. (C). 65.00 (*0-205-17001-3*) Allyn.

Developmental Motor Speech Disorders. Michael A. Crary. 1993. LC 93-3711. (Illus.). 298p. (Orig.). (C). pap. text 42.50 (*1-879105-92-6*, 0356) Thomson Learn.

Developmental Nephrology. Wallace W. McCrory. 1972. LC 72-75399. (Commonwealth Fund Publications). (Illus.). 230p. 37.50 (*0-674-20275-9*) HUP.

Developmental Neurobiology. M. Jacobson. 3rd ed. 1991. (Illus.). 786p. (C). text 105.00 (*0-306-43797-X*, Kluwer Plenum) Kluwer Academic.

Developmental Neurobiology of Breathing. Ed. by Gabriel G. Haddad & Jay P. Farber. 1991. (Lung Biology in Health & Disease Ser.: Vol. 53). (Illus.). 800p. text 255.00 (*0-8247-8459-6*) Dekker.

Developmental Neurobiology of the Autonomic Nervous System. Ed. by Phyllis M. Gootman. 1986. LC 86-3077. (Contemporary Neuroscience Ser.). (Illus.). 416p. 145.00 (*0-89603-080-6*) Humana.

Developmental Neurocognition - Speech & Face Processing in the First Year of Life: Proceedings of the NATO Advanced Research Workshop. Ed. by Benedict De Boysson-Bardies et al. 1993. LC 93-9598. (NATO Advanced Science Institutes Ser.: No. 69). 516p. (C). text 285.50 (*0-7923-2188-X*) Kluwer Academic.

Developmental Neuroimaging: Mapping the Development of Brain & Behavior. Ed. by G. Reid Lyon et al. 1996. LC 96-3067. (Illus.). 312p. text 139.95 (*0-12-686070-X*) Acad Pr.

Developmental Neuropathology. R. L. Friede. 1976. (Illus.). 550p. 71.00 (*0-387-81325-X*) Spr-Verlag.

Developmental Neuropathology. 2nd ed. 1996. (Illus.). 577p. 212.00 (*3-540-19280-8*) Spr-Verlag.

Developmental Neuropathology. R. L. Friede. 2nd ed. 1996. (Illus.). 625p. 198.50 (*0-387-19280-8*) Spr-Verlag.

Developmental Neuropathology in Etiology & Pathogenesis of Human Malformations: A Personal Contribution. Martin Lammens. 1997. (Acta Biomedica Lovaniensia Ser.: No. 154). (Illus.). 177p. pap. (*90-6186-825-4*) Almqvist & Wiksell SWE. *Dist:* Coronet Bks.

Developmental Neuropathology of Schizophrenia. Ed. by Sarnoff A. Mednick et al. 1992. (NATO Advanced Science Institutes Ser.: Vol. 217). (Illus.). 256p. (C). text 114.00 (*0-306-44081-4*, Kluwer Plenum) Kluwer Academic.

Developmental Neuropsychiatry: Assessment, Diagnosis & Treatment of Developmental Disorders, Vol. 2. James C. Harris. 1998. (Illus.). 624p. pap. text 47.50 (*0-19-513111-8*) OUP.

Developmental Neuropsychiatry: Fundamentals, Vol. 1. James C. Harris. 1995. LC 94-42699. (Illus.). 288p. text 49.95 (*0-19-506824-6*) OUP.

Developmental Neuropsychology. Otfried Spreen et al. 2nd ed. 1995. (Illus.). 688p. pap. text 45.00 (*0-19-506737-1*) OUP.

Developmental Neuropsychology: A Clinical Approach. Vicki Anderson et al. 2001. LC 00-42547. (Brain Damage, Behaviour & Cognition Ser.). (Illus.). 544p. (*0-86377-704-X*) Psychol Pr GBR. *Dist:* Taylor & Francis.

Developmental Neurotoxicity of Lead. Christopher Winder. 1984. text 164.00 (*0-85200-776-0*) Kluwer Academic.

Developmental Neurotoxicology. Gaylia J. Harry. 1994. 192p. 141.95 (*0-8493-4427-1*, RC347) CRC Pr.

Developmental Nutrition. Kretchmer. 1994. (*0-8493-8887-2*, CRC Reprint) Franklin.

Developmental Nutrition. Norman Kretchmer & Michael Zimmerman. 1996. 682p. 76.00 (*0-13-303744-4*) Allyn.

Developmental Optometry: The Optometric Appraisal of Vision Development & Visual Performance. G. N. Getman. Ed. by Sally M. Corngold. 2nd ed. 1992. LC 87-82198. (Introduction to Behavioral Optometry Ser.). (Illus.). 117p. reprint ed. pap. 18.00 (*0-943599-23-7*) OEPF.

Developmental Pathogenesis & Treatment of Borderline & Narcissistic Personalities. Donald B. Rinsley. 1989. LC 89-17506. 192p. 35.00 (*0-87668-828-8*) Aronson.

Developmental Patterning of the Vertebrate Limb. J. R. Hinchliffe et al. 1991. (NATO Advanced Science Institutes Ser.: Vol. 205). (Illus.). 462p. (C). text 145.00 (*0-306-43927-1*, Kluwer Plenum) Kluwer Academic.

Developmental Perspectives on Craniofacial Problems. Rebecca A. Eder. 1995. LC 93-31776. (Illus.). 303p. 137.00 (*0-387-94168-1*) Spr-Verlag.

Developmental Perspectives on Depression. Ed. by Dante Cicchetti & Sheree L. Toth. 1992. LC 92-18117. (Rochester Symposium on Developmental Psychopathology Ser.: Vol. 4). (Illus.). 418p. (C). 90.00 (*1-878822-16-0*) Univ Rochester Pr.

Developmental Perspectives on Trauma Vol. 8: Theory, Research & Intervention. Ed. by Dante Cicchetti & Sheree L. Toth. 1998. LC 97-24123. (Rochester Symposium on Developmental Psychopathology Ser.: Vol. 1056-6511). (Illus.). 632p. 120.00 (*1-878822-97-7*) Univ Rochester Pr.

Developmental Problems of Drug-Exposed Infants. Ed. by Louis M. Rossetti. 1992. (Illus.). 80p. (Orig.). (C). pap. text 24.95 (*1-56593-064-9*, 0370) Singular Publishing.

Developmental Processes Vol. I: Heinz Werner's Selected Writings Ed. by Sybil S. Barten & Margery B. Franklin. 1978. LC 77-92187. 562p. (Orig.). 50.00 (*0-8236-1250-3*) Intl Univs Pr.

Developmental Processes Vol. II: Heinz Werner's Selected Writings Ed. by Sybil S. Barten & Margery B. Franklin. 1978. LC 77-92187. 562p. (Orig.). 50.00 (*0-8236-1251-1*) Intl Univs Pr.

Developmental Processes in Normal & Diseased Muscle. Ed. by H. M. Eppenberger & J. Perriard. 1984. (Experimental Biology & Medicine Ser.: Vol. 9). (Illus.). x, 294p. 165.25 (*3-8055-3765-4*) S Karger.

Developmental Profiles: Birth to Six. K. Eilleen Allen. 1989. (Early Childhood Education Ser.). pap. 23.00 (*0-8273-3355-2*) Delmar.

Developmental Profiles: Pre-Birth Through Eight. K. Eileen Allen & Lynn R. Marotz. 2nd ed. 1994. LC 93-45861. (Illus.). 184p. (C). mass mkt. 35.95 (*0-8273-5814-8*) Delmar.

Developmental Profiles: Pre-Birth to Eight. K. Eileen Allen et al. 3rd ed. 1998. LC 98-26634. 192p. (C). pap. text 41.95 (*0-8273-8605-2*) Delmar.

Developmental Psychiatry. Ed. by Michael Rutter. 1987. LC 86-32058. 386p. pap. text 18.95 (*0-88048-271-0*, 8271) Am Psychiatric.

Developmental Psychoacoustics. Ed. by Lynne A. Werner & Edwin W. Rubel. 1992. LC 92-49922. 363p. text 19.95 (*1-55798-159-0*) Am Psychol.

Developmental Psychobiology & Behavioral Ecology. Ed. by Elliott M. Blass. 1988. LC 87-38501. (Handbook of Behavioral Neurobiology Ser.: Vol. 9). (Illus.). 476p. (C). text 115.00 (*0-306-42728-1*, Kluwer Plenum) Kluwer Academic.

Developmental Psychobiology & Clinical Neuropsychology. Ed. by R. W. Bell et al. 1984. (Interfaces in Psychology Ser.: No. 1). 133p. 24.95 (*0-89672-120-5*); pap. 14.95 (*0-89672-119-1*) Tex Tech Univ Pr.

Developmental Psychobiology, Developmental Neurobiology & Behavioral Ecology: Mechanisms & Early Principles. Ed. by Elliott M. Blass. 2001. LC 00-67113. (Handbook of Behavioral Neurobiology Ser.: Vol. 13). (Illus.). 638p. 140.00 (*0-306-46489-6*, Kluwer Plenum) Kluwer Academic.

Developmental Psychodiagnostic Assessment of Children & Adolescents. V. Krall. 1989. (Illus.). 270p. 35.00 (*0-89885-459-8*, Kluwer Acad Hman Sci) Kluwer Academic.

Developmental Psychologies of Jean Piaget & Psychoanalysis. Peter H. Wolff. 1960. (Psychological Issues Monographs: No. 5, Vol. 2, No. 1). 178p. (Orig.). 27.50 (*0-8236-1200-7*) Intl Univs Pr.

Developmental Psychology. Mark Bennett. 1999. LC 99-29808. (Illus.). xvi, 338p. 54.95 (*0-86377-577-2*) L Erlbaum Assocs.

Developmental Psychology. Cliffs Notes Staff. 2000. (Cliffs Quick Review Ser.). 240p. pap. 9.99 (*0-7645-8614-9*, Cliff) Hungry Minds.

Developmental Psychology. Florence L. Goodenough & Leona E. Tyler. 3rd ed. 1959. LC 59-6858. (Century Psychology Ser.). (Illus.). 30.50 (*0-89197-125-4*) Irvington.

Developmental Psychology: An Advanced Textbook. Ed. by Marc H. Bornstein & Michael E. Lamb. 3rd rev. ed. 1992. 856p. text 45.00 (*0-8058-1007-2*) L Erlbaum Assocs.

Developmental Psychology: An Advanced Textbook. Ed. by Marc H. Bornstein & Herbert Pierson. 4th ed. 1999. LC 98-44280. 664p. 49.95 (*0-8058-3072-3*) L Erlbaum Assocs.

Developmental Psychology: Childhood & Adolescence. David R. Shaffer. (C). 2nd ed. 1988. LC 88-10547. 680p. pap. 48.50 (*0-534-09444-9*); 3rd ed. 1993. LC 92-4061. 665p. pap., stu. ed. 16.50 (*0-534-16993-7*); 3rd ed. 1992. LC 92-4061. 665p. pap. 54.25 (*0-534-16992-9*) Brooks-Cole.

Developmental Psychology: Childhood & Adolescence. Shaffer. 5th ed. 1998. (Psychology Ser.). pap., stu. ed. 15.00 (*0-534-35889-6*); LC 98-23000. pap. 53.00 (*0-534-35592-7*) Brooks-Cole.

Developmental Psychology: Study Guide & Activities. David R. Shaffer. 4th ed. 1995. (Psychology Ser.). pap., stu. ed. 18.75 (*0-534-26439-5*) Brooks-Cole.

Developmental Psychology: Theory, Research, & Applications. David R. Shaffer. 1985. LC 84-12658. (Psychology Ser.). 700p. (C). pap. 34.00 (*0-534-02756-3*) Brooks-Cole.

Developmental Psychology of the Black Child. Amos N. Wilson. 1978. 216p. reprint ed. pap. text 12.95 (*0-933524-01-3*) Africana Res.

Developmental Psychology of Time. Ed. by William J. Friedman. 1982. (Developmental Psychology Ser.). text 99.95 (*0-12-268320-X*) Acad Pr.

Developmental Psychology Today. Elizabeth Hall et al. 6th ed. 1994. LC 93-9832. 640p. (C). 83.75 (*0-07-029338-4*) McGrw-H Hghr Educ.

Developmental Psychopathology. Ed. by H. Remschmidt & M. H. Schmidt. 1992. LC 90-4957. (Child & Youth Psychiatry: European Perspectives Ser.: Vol. 2). (Illus.). 200p. text 64.00 (*0-88937-051-6*) Hogrefe & Huber Pubs.

Developmental Psychopathology. Thomas M. Achenbach. 2nd ed. 1982. LC 82-2838. 770p. (C). 82.95 (*0-471-05536-0*) Wiley.

Developmental Psychopathology. Charles Wenar. 4th ed. 1999. LC 99-21568. (Illus.). 504p. text 82.81 (*0-07-069617-9*) McGrw-H Hghr Educ.

Developmental Psychopathology, Set. Ed. by Dante Cicchetti & Donald J. Cohen. Incl. Developmental Psychopathology: Theory & Methods. 787p. 250.00 (*0-471-53243-6*); Developmental Psychopathology Vol. 2: Risk, Disorder, & Adaptation. 928p. 250.00 (*0-471-53244-4*); (Illus.). LC 94-36391. (Personality Processes Ser.). 1695p. 1995. 500.00 (*0-471-53257-6*) Wiley.

Developmental Psychopathology: Epidemiology, Diagnostics & Treatment. Ed. by Cecilia A. Essau & Franz Petermann. 1997. 496p. text 60.00 (*90-5702-189-7*); pap. text 30.00 (*90-5702-190-0*) Gordon & Breach (Harwood Acad Pubs).

Developmental Psychopathology: From Infancy Through Adolescence. Charles Wenar. 3rd ed. 1994. LC 93-36673. (C). text 59.74 net. (*0-07-069286-6*) McGraw.

Developmental Psychopathology: Perspectives on Adjustment, Risk, & Disorder. Ed. by Suniya S. Luthar et al. 1997. (Illus.). 640p. (C). text 69.95 (*0-521-47142-7*); pap. text 28.95 (*0-521-47715-8*) Cambridge U Pr.

Developmental Psychopathology: Theory & Methods. Ed. by Dante Cicchetti & Donald J. Cohen. 1995. LC 94-36391. (Developmental Psychopathology Ser.: Vol. 1). (Illus.). 787p. 250.00 (*0-471-53243-6*) Wiley.

Developmental Psychopathology Vol. 2: Risk, Disorder, & Adaptation. Ed. by Dante Cicchetti & Donald J. Cohen. 1995. LC 94-36391. (Developmental Psychopathology Ser.: Vol. 2). (Illus.). 928p. 250.00 (*0-471-53244-4*) Wiley.

Developmental Psychopathology of Eating Disorders: Implications for Research, Prevention & Treatment. Ed. by Linda Smolak et al. 1996. 440p. pap. 45.00 (*0-8058-1747-6*); text 79.95 (*0-8058-1746-8*) L Erlbaum Assocs.

Developmental Psycohbiology & Developmental Neurobiology. E. M. Blass. 1986. LC 85-19276. (Handbook of Behavioral Neurobiology Ser.: Vol. 8). (Illus.). 348p. (C). text 95.00 (*0-306-42034-1*, Kluwer Plenum) Kluwer Academic.

Developmental Questionnaire for Infants Forty Weeks of Age: An Evaluation. Hilda Knobloch & Benjamin Pasamanick. 1972. (Society for Research in Child Development Monographs: Vol. 20, No. 2). reprint ed. pap. 25.00 (*0-527-01564-4*) Periodicals Srv.

Developmental Reading Disabilities: Language-Based Treatment Approach. Candace L. Goldsworthy. 2nd ed. 2002. pap. 40.00 net. (*0-7693-0100-2*) Singular Publishing.

Developmental Regulation in Adulthood: Age-Normative & Sociostructural Constraints As Adaptive Challenges. Jutta Heckhausen. 1998. LC 98-6509. (Illus.). 262p. (C). text 49.95 (*0-521-58144-3*) Cambridge U Pr.

Developmental Research Methods. Scott A. Miller. 2nd ed. 1997. LC 96-51752. 338p. 72.00 (*0-13-398892-9*) P-H.

Developmental Resource: A Behavioral Resource for Assessment & Programming Marilyn Cohen & Pamela Gross. 1978. 224p. text 36.00 (*0-8089-1122-8*, 790877); 256p. text 38.00 (*0-8089-1157-0*, 790878) Harcrt Hlth Sci Grp (Grune & Strat).

Developmental Scale of Cognition. Donald Ashurst et al. 1985. LC 84-73556. (Southern California Ordinal Scales of Development Ser.). 146p. stu. ed. 25.00 (*0-943292-17-4*) Foreworks.

Developmental Scale of Communication: Southern California Orginal Scales of Development. Donald Ashurst et al. 1985. LC 85-71210. 184p. stu. ed. 25.00 (*0-943292-18-2*) Foreworks.

Developmental Scale of Fine Motor Abilities. Donald Ashurst et al. 1985. LC 84-73557. (Southern California Ordinal Scales of Development Ser.). 92p. pap., stu. ed. 20.00 (*0-943292-21-2*) Foreworks.

Developmental Scale of Gross Motor Abilities. Donald Ashurst et al. 1985. LC 85-71209. (Southern California Ordinal Scales of Development Ser.). 70p. stu. ed. 20.00 (*0-943292-22-0*) Foreworks.

Developmental Scale of Practical Abilities. Donald Ashurst et al. 1985. LC 85-71211. (Southern California Ordinal Scales of Development Ser.). 62p. stu. ed. 20.00 (*0-943292-20-4*) Foreworks.

Developmental Scale of Social-Affective Behavior. Donald Ashurst et al. 1985. LC 84-73558. (Southern California Ordinal Scales of Development Ser.). 84p. stu. ed. 20.00 (*0-943292-19-0*) Foreworks.

Developmental Science. Ed. by Robert B. Cairns et al. 1996. (Cambridge Studies in Social & Emotional Development). (Illus.). 313p. (C). text 49.95 (*0-521-49585-7*) Cambridge U Pr.

Developmental Science & the Holistic Approach. Ed. by Lars R. Bergman et al. 1999. LC 99-55359. (Illus.). x, 484p. (*0-8058-3374-9*) L Erlbaum Assocs.

Developmental Screening & the Child with Special Needs. Cecil M. Drillien & Margaret B. Drummond. 1991. (Clinics in Developmental Medicine Ser.: No. 86). (Illus.). 284p. (C). text (*0-521-41206-4*) Mc Keith Pr GBR. *Dist:* Cambridge U Pr.

Developmental Screening in Early Childhood: A Guide. Samuel J. Meisels & Sally Atkins-Burnett. 1994. LC 94-68837. 60p. pap. text 5.00 (*0-912674-63-6*, NAEYC121) Natl Assn Child Ed.

Developmental Social Psychology: An Introduction. Kevin Durkin. 1995. (Illus.). 640p. (C). pap. 36.95 (*0-631-14829-9*) Blackwell Pubs.

Developmental Speech & Language Disorders. Dennis Cantwell & Lorian Baker. 1987. LC 86-26989. (Child Psychopathology Ser.). 214p. text 30.00 (*0-89862-400-2*) Guilford Pubns.

Developmental Stages in Human Embryos. Ronan O'Rahilly & Fabiola Muller. 1987. LC 87-70669. (Illus.). 320p. 52.00 (*0-87279-666-3*, 637) Carnegie Inst.

Developmental-Systemic Family Therapy with Adolescents. Ronald Jay Werner-Wilson. 2000. LC 00-38328. (Haworth Marriage & the Family Ser.). xiii, 240p. 69.95 (*0-7890-0118-7*); pap. text 24.95 (*0-7890-1205-7*) Haworth Pr (Haworth Clinical).

Developmental Technology of Gastrectomy & Vagotomy. Karel B. Absolon. rev. ed. 1995. (Illus.). 178p. pap. 34.50 (*0-930329-97-X*) Kabel Pubs.

Developmental Technology of Gastric Surgery. Karel B. Absolon. 1984. (Illus.). 152p. text 65.00 (*0-930329-01-5*); pap. text 42.50 (*0-930329-00-7*) Kabel Pubs.

Developmental Technology of Gastric Surgery. Karel B. Absolon. Ed. by Kabel Staff. 2nd rev. ed. 1986. (Illus.). 200p. 42.50 (*0-930329-08-2*) Kabel Pubs.

Developmental Theory & Clinical Process. Fred Pine. 1987. LC 84-20841. 272p. pap. 19.00 (*0-300-04002-4*, Y-661) Yale U Pr.

Developmental Therapy for Young Children with Autistic Characteristics. Ann W. Bachrach et al. 1978. LC 77-16370. (Illus.). 185p. pap. text 34.00 (*0-936104-61-9*, 1123) PRO-ED.

Developmental Therapy in the Classroom. Mary M. Wood et al. 2nd ed. 1986. LC 85-28277. 362p. pap. text 36.00 (*0-89079-104-X*, 1393) PRO-ED.

Developmental Time, Cultural Space: Studies in Psychogeography. Howard F. Stein. 1987. LC 87-5088. (Illus.). 256p. 26.95 (*0-8061-2070-3*) U of Okla Pr.

Developmental Toxicology: Mechanisms & Risk. Ed. by John M. McLachlan et al. 1987. (Banbury Reports: No. 26). (Illus.). 362p. (C). text 70.00 (*0-87969-226-X*) Cold Spring Harbor.

Developmental Toxicology: Risk Assessment & the Future. Ed. by Ronald D. Hood. 1990. 279p. 140.00 (*0-471-29079-3*, VNR) Wiley.

Developmental View of the Psychoanalytic Process: Follow up Studies & Their Consequences. Nathan Schlessinger & Fred Robbins. 1983. LC 83-225. (Emotions & Behavior Monographs: No. 1). xiii, 228p. (C). 37.50 (*0-8236-1257-0*) Intl Univs Pr.

Developments & Controversies in Gastrointestinal Motility: Journal. Ed. by Sami R. Achem et al. 1997. (Journal: Vol. 15, Suppl. 1, 1997). (Illus.). iv, 138p. pap. 41.75 (*3-8055-6521-6*) S Karger.

Developments & Ethical Considerations in Toxicology. Ed. by Michael I. Weitzner. 1993. (Special Publications). 212p. (C). (*0-85186-435-X*, R6435) Royal Soc Chem GBR. *Dist:* Spr-Verlag.

Developments & Research on Aging. Ed. by Erdman B. Palmore. 1993. LC 92-25737. 456p. lib. bdg. 92.50 (*0-313-27785-0*, PDV, Greenwood Pr) Greenwood.

Developments in Analytical Methods in Pharmaceutical, Biomedical, & Forensic Sciences. Ed. by G. Piemonte et al. 1988. LC 87-7180. 340p. 85.00 (*0-306-42695-1*, Plenum Trade) Perseus Pubng.

Developments in Antibiotic Treatment of Respiratory Infections: New Perspectives in Clinical Microbiology, No. 4. Ed. by Ralph Van Furth. 1981. 240p. text 126.50 (*90-247-2493-7*) Kluwer Academic.

Developments in Cancer Chemotherapy. Ed. by Robert I. Glazer. Vol. I. 1984. 296p. 170.00 (*0-8493-5778-0*, RC271); Vol. II. 1988. 224p. 122.00 (*0-8493-5770-5*, RC271) Franklin (CRC Reprint).

Developments in Clinical & Experimental Neuropsychology. Ed. by J. R. Crawford & D. M. Parker. 1989. (Illus.). 346p. 85.00 (*0-306-43244-7*, Plenum Trade) Perseus Pubng.

Developments in Cognitive Psychotherapy. Windy Dryden & Peter Trower. 1988. 288p. (C). 69.95 (*0-8039-8134-1*, 7079) Sage.

Developments in Dementia & Functional Disorders in the Elderly. Ed. by Raymond Levy & Robert Howard. 1995. LC 94-47442. 232p. (*1-871816-27-0*) Wrightson Biomed GBR. *Dist:* Taylor & Francis.

Developments in Drugs Used in Anesthesia. Ed. by J. Spierdijk et al. 1982. text 121.50 (*90-6021-492-7*) Kluwer Academic.

Developments in Environmental Control & Public Health. Ed. by A. Porteous. (Illus.). 311p. Vol. 1. 1979. 83.00 (*0-85334-834-0*); Vol. 2. 1981. 83.00 (*0-85334-941-X*) Elsevier.

Developments in Family Therapy: Theories & Applications Since 1948. Ed. by Sue Walrond-Skinner. 1981. 248p. (Orig.). pap. 18.95 (*0-7100-0812-0*, Routledge Thoemms) Routledge.

Developments in Fertility Control: Proceedings of the WHO Scientific Group, Geneva, 1968. WHO Staff. 1969. (Technical Reports: No. 424). pap. text 5.00 (*92-4-120424-9*, 1100424) World Health.

Developments in Geriatric Psychiatry, Vol. 76. Ed. by Lon S. Schneider. 1998. pap. 28.00 (*0-7879-9878-8*) Jossey-Bass.

Developments in Infant Observation: The Tavistock Model. Susan Reid & Tavistock Clinic Staff. 1997. LC 96-43621. 248p. (C). 84.95 (*0-415-14940-1*); pap. 29.95 (*0-415-14941-X*) Routledge.

Developments in Ophthalmology Vol. 6: Diagnostic Techniques & Clinical Questions. Ed. by W. Straub. 1982. (Illus.). viii, 140p. 100.00 (*3-8055-3431-0*) S Karger.

Developments in Pediatric Psychosocial Oncology. B. F. Last & A. M. Van Veldhuizen. 1992. 184p. pap. (*90-265-1131-0*) Swets.

Developments in Psychotherapy: Historical Perspectives. Windy Dryden. 1996. 256p. 74.50 (*0-8039-7911-8*, 2959); pap. 27.95 (*0-8039-7912-6*, 2958) Sage.

Developments in Radioimmunoassay & Related Procedures. International Atomic Energy Agency Staff. 1992. 601p. pap. (*92-0-000392-3*, STI/PUB/879) IAEA AUT. *Dist:* Bernan Associates.

Developments in the Field of Drug Abuse: Proceedings. National Association for the Prevention of Addiction. Ed. by Edward C. Senay. 1975. 1130p. text 79.95 (*0-87073-388-5*) Transaction Pubs.

Developments In the Management of Chemotherapy-Induced Nausea & Vomiting: A Workshop Held At Lake Tahoe Nevada, April 11, 1987. David Basedow. 1987. (Illus.). 24p. (Orig.). (*0-944036-00-7*) Medicine Grp USA.

Developments in the Science & Practice of Toxicology: Proceedings of the Third International Congress of Toxicology, San Diego, CA, August 28 - September 3, 1983. Ed. by A. Wallace Hayes et al. 1984. (Developments in Toxicology & Environmental Science Ser.: Vol. 11). 614p. 202.75 (*0-444-80547-8*) Elsevier.

Developments of Cancer Chemotherapy. Ed. by K. Lapis. 1980. (Journal: Vol. 37, Suppl. 1). (Illus.). iv, 120p. pap. 28.75 (*3-8055-1588-X*) S Karger.

Deviance: Rulemakers & Rulebreakers. Nancy A. Heitzeg. 1995. 500p. (C). pap. text 60.95 (*0-314-04471-X*) Wadsworth Pub.

Deviance & Moral Boundaries: Witchcraft, the Occult, Science Fiction, Deviant Sciences & Scientists. Nachman Ben-Yehuda. 1985. LC 85-1167. x, 260p. 25.00 (*0-226-04335-5*) U Ch Pr.

Deviance & Psychopathology: The Sociology & Psychology of Outsiders. Robert Endleman. 1989. LC 88-13949. 308p. (C). lib. bdg. 37.50 (*0-89464-344-4*) Krieger.

Deviant Behavior. Erich Goode. 6th ed. 2000. LC 00-46524. (Illus.). 480p. 62.00 (*0-13-082578-6*) P-H.

Deviant Behavior: Patterns, Sources, & Control. S. Palmer & J. A. Humphrey. 1990. LC 88-23264. (Illus.). 312p. (C). 54.50 (*0-306-43285-4*, Plenum Trade) Perseus Pubng.

Deviant Behavior: Readings in the Sociology of Norm Violations. Ed. by Clifton D. Bryant. 1989. 250p. 59.95 (*0-89116-696-3*); pap. 45.95 (*0-89116-779-X*) Hemisp Pub.

Devices & Desires: A History of Contraceptives in America. Andrea Tone. 2001. LC 00-50547. (Illus.). xvii, 366p. 30.00 (*0-8090-3817-X*) Hill & Wang.

Devices & Desires: Gender, Technology & American Nursing. Margarete Sandelowski. 2000. LC 00-32588. (Studies in Social Medicine). (Illus.). 362p. 45.00 (*0-8078-2579-4*) U of NC Pr.

Devil's Claw Root: And Other Natural Remedies for Arthritis. Rachel Carston. 3rd rev. ed. 1994. LC 94-910296. (Kaufmann Foods Ser.). (Illus.). 110p. pap. 10.95 (*0-920470-36-X*) Alive Bks.

Devils, Drugs & Doctors: A Wellcome History of Medicine. Brian Bracegirdle. 1991. pap. text 9.95 (*0-642-09877-8*) Seven Hills Bk.

Devil's Flu: The World's Deadliest Influenza Epidemic & the Scientific Hunt for the Virus That Caused It. Pete Davies. 2000. LC 00-36963. 306p. pap. 14.00 (*0-8050-6622-5*, Owl) H Holt & Co.

Dewhurst's Textbook of Obstetrics & Gynaecology for Postgraduates. C. R. Whitfield. 5th ed. 1995. 800p. 195.00 (*0-632-02547-6*) Blackwell Sci.

Dewhurst's Textbook of Obstetrics & Gynaecology for Postgraduates. Keith Edmonds & John Dewhurst. 6th ed. 1999. LC 98-42393. ix, 622p. 198.95 (*0-86542-651-1*) Blackwell Sci.

Dhanwantari: A Complete Guide to the Ayurvedic Life. Harish Johari. 1998. LC 98-7312. (Illus.). 240p. pap. 14.95 (*0-89281-618-X*, Heal Arts VT) Inner Tradit.

DHEA: A Comprehensive Review. Ed. by J. H. H. Thijssen & H. Nieuwenhuyse. 1999. LC 99-10458. (Illus.). 176p. lib. bdg. 69.95 (*1-85070-061-3*) CRC Pr.

DHEA: The Ultimate Rejuvenating Hormone. Hasnain Walji. 1996. LC 96-43991. 144p. (Orig.). pap. 9.95 (*0-934252-70-X*) Hohm Pr.

DHEA: The Youth & Health Hormone. C. Norman Shealy. Ed. by Phyllis Herman. 1996. (Good Health Guides). 48p. pap. 3.95 (*0-87983-695-4*, 36954K, Keats Pubng) McGraw-Hill Trade.

DHEA: Unlocking the Secrets to the Fountain of Youth. Beth M. Ley & Richard N. Ash. 1997. (Orig.). rev. ed. LC 95-96059. 208p. pap. 14.95 (*0-9642703-3-1*); 2nd rev. ed. LC 97-22004. (GER, JPN & SPA.). 256p. pap. 14.95 (*0-9642703-8-2*) B L Pubns.

DHEA & Sex Steroids: Intracrinology in Target Tissues. Fernand Labrie et al. 1996. 319p. text 75.00 (*1-898099-10-3*) Blackwell Sci.

DHEA Discovery: Wonder Hormone of the 90'S. Beverly Greenberg. 1997. 105p. pap. text 12.95 (*0-9654601-0-X*) Majesty Pr.

Di Fiore's Atlas of Histology with Functional Correlations. Victor P. Eroschenko. 9th ed. 2000. LC 00-20713. (Illus.). xv, 363p. pap. text 45.00 (*0-7817-2676-X*); 384p. spiral bd. 45.00 (*0-683-30749-5*) Lppncott W & W.

Dia-Logo Therapy: Psychonarration & the Pardes. Mordechai Rotenberg. 1991. LC 90-44250. 192p. 59.95 (*0-275-92943-4*, C2943, Praeger Pubs) Greenwood.

Diabetes. James W. Anderson. 1987. 224p. mass mkt. 5.99 (*0-446-34399-4*) Warner Bks.

Diabetes. Maria Barnwell. 1994. (Outline Ser.). 300p. (Orig.). (C). per. 23.95 (*1-56930-031-3*) Delmar.

Diabetes. Dorling Kindersley Publishing Staff. Ed. by David R. Goldmann. 2000. LC 99-76861. (ACP Home Medical Guides Ser.). (Illus.). 96p. pap. 6.95 (*0-7894-5200-6*, D K Ink) DK Pub Inc.

Diabetes. Draznin. 1999. (C). text (*0-7216-8219-7*) Saunders.

Diabetes. Andrew J. Krentz. 1996. LC 96-6471. (Colour Guide Ser.). (Illus.). pap. text 16.95 (*0-443-05080-5*) Harcrt Hlth Sci Grp.

Diabetes. Leslie. 1989. text 99.00 (*0-443-04069-9*) Saunders.

Diabetes. Mary D. Litchford & Laura Yordy. 1995. (C). pap. 6.00 (*1-880989-53-0*) Case Sftware.

Diabetes. Massachusetts General Hospital Staff et al. 1997. LC 96-24842. (Illus.). 320p. pap. 14.00 (*0-8129-2320-0*) Random.

Diabetes. Polaino. 1997. (SPA.). pap. text (*84-270-1422-8*) Planeta Edit.

Diabetes. Sue Vander Hook. 2000. LC 98-43883. (Understanding Illness Ser.). lib. bdg. 16.95 (*1-58340-023-0*) Smart Apple.

Diabetes. Douglas Wetherill et al. 2000. LC 00-699789. (What You Should Know Ser.). (Illus.). viii, 136p. pap. 6.99 (*1-55870-552-X*, Betrwy Bks) F & W Pubns Inc.

***Diabetes.** Douglas L. Wetherill & Dean J. Kereiakes. 2nd ed. 2001. (What You Should Know Ser.). (Illus.). 136p. pap. 8.99 (*0-632-04531-0*) Blackwell Sci.

Diabetes, sets. Ed. by Stanley G. Korenman & C. Ronald Kahn. 1999. LC 98-35631. (Atlas of Clinical Endocrinology Ser.: Vol. 2). (Illus.). 212p. 125.00 (*0-632-04399-7*) Blackwell Sci.

Diabetes: A Guide to Living Well. Ernest Lowe & Gary Arsham. 3rd ed. 1997. LC 99-159057. 384p. (Orig.). pap. 14.95 (*1-56561-112-8*) Wiley.

Diabetes: Beating the Odds: The Doctor's Guide to Reducing Your Risk. Elliot J. Rayfield & Cheryl Solimini. 2000. LC 92-14725. (Illus.). 198p. pap. 13.00 (*0-201-57784-4*) Perseus Bks Grp.

Diabetes: Caring for Your Emotions As Well As Your Health. Jerry Edelwich & Archie Brodsky. 1986. LC 86-10868. 256p. 17.95 (*0-201-10609-4*) Addison-Wesley.

Diabetes: Clinical Management. Ed. by Robert Tattersall & Edwin Gale. 1990. (Illus.). 382p. text (*0-443-02273-9*) Church.

Diabetes: Clinical Science in Practice. Ed. by R. D. Leslie & David C. Robbins. 1995. (Illus.). 508p. (C). text 110.00 (*0-521-45029-2*) Cambridge U Pr.

Diabetes: Current & Future Trends in Therapeutics & Diagnostics. Stanley A. Shapiro & Marvin Silverberg. Ed. by Susan C. DiClemente. 1998. (Illus.). 415p. 4950.00 (*1-57936-123-4*, 1984) International Business.

Diabetes: Don't Fear It. Beat It!: My Story, My Message, My Mission. Martin M. Mandel. l.t. ed. 1997. (Illus.). 175p. (Orig.). pap. 19.95 (*0-9657143-0-6*) Neuro Diabetic.

***Diabetes: How to Combine the Best of Traditional & Alternative Therapies.** Milton Hammerly. 2001. 352p. pap. 7.95 (*1-58062-481-2*) Adams Media.

Diabetes: Instructor's Guide. Mary D. Litchford & Laura Yordy. 1991. (C). tchr. ed. 139.00 incl. 5.25 hd (*1-880989-10-7*); tchr. ed. 139.00 incl. 3.5 hd (*1-880989-11-5*); tchr. ed. 139.00 incl. 3.5 hd (*1-880989-09-3*); tchr. ed. 139.00 incl. 5.25 hd (*1-880989-08-5*) Case Sftware.

Diabetes: Its Etiology & Control with Ayurvedic Herbs. Muhammed Majeed. 1998. pap. text (*0-9647856-3-3*) Nutrisci Pubs.

Diabetes: Practical & Easy-to-Follow Advice. Catherine Steven. 1998. LC 97-48332. (Your Child Ser.). 122p. pap. 9.95 (*1-86204-208-X*) Element MA.

Diabetes: Questions You Have, Answers You Need. Paula Brisco. rev. ed. 1997. LC 96-49561. 192p. pap. 12.95 (*1-882606-53-1*) Peoples Med Soc.

Diabetes: Recipes for Health. Azmina Govindji & Jill Myers. 2001. pap. (*0-00-710318-2*) Thorsons GBR. *Dist:* Natl Bk Netwk.

***Diabetes: The Complete Guide.** Rowan Hillson. 2002. 256p. pap. (*0-09-182701-9*) Random GBR. *Dist:* Trafalgar.

Diabetes: The Facts That Let You Regain Control of Your Life. Charles Kilo et al. 1987. LC 87-6136. 208p. pap. 16.95 (*0-471-85801-3*) Wiley.

Diabetes: Vital Health Information for African Americans. Lester Henry, Jr. & Kirk A. Johnson. 1999. (Black Health Library Guides). 192p. mass mkt. 5.99 (*1-57566-452-6*) Kensgtn Pub Corp.

Diabetes Vol. II: A Guide for Patients. Mayer Davidson. 1996. (Endocrinology Ser.). pap. text 2.95 (*1-885274-32-7*) Health InfoNet Inc.

Diabetes - Type I: A Guide for Patients. Mayer Davidson. 1996. (Endocrinology Ser.). (Illus.). 32p. (Orig.). pap. 2.95 (*1-885274-64-5*) Health InfoNet Inc.

Diabetes: A Guide to Living Well: A Program of Individualized Self-Care. Ernest Lowe. 3rd ed. 1997. 384p. pap. 14.95 (*0-471-34677-2*) Wiley.

Diabetes A to Z: What You Need to Know about Diabetes - Simply Put Treatment & Self Care. American Diabetes Association. 4th ed. 1999. LC 99-46249. (Illus.). 202p. pap. 14.95 (*1-58040-035-3*, 00353Q) Am Diabetes.

Diabetes A to Z: What You Need to Know about Diabetes-Simply Put. American Diabetes Association. 3rd ed. 1998. LC 97-30806. 202p. pap. 11.95 (*0-945448-96-1*, 4801-01) Am Diabetes.

Diabetes & Artherosclerosis: Molecular Basis & Clinical Aspects. Ed. by Boris Draznin & Robert H. Eckel. 1993. (Illus.). 385p. (gr. 13). text 101.95 (*0-412-04431-5*) Chapman & Hall.

Diabetes & Atherosclerosis. Ed. by Robert W. Stout. 1992. (Developments in Cardiovascular Medicine Ser.). (C). text 229.00 (*0-7923-1310-0*) Kluwer Academic.

Diabetes & Atherosclerosis: Molecular Basis & Clinical Aspects. Ed. by Boris Draznin & Robert H. Eckel. 1993. LC 92-48854. (*0-444-01665-1*) Elsevier.

Diabetes & Brief Illness. Marion J. Franz & Judy O. Joynes. 1987. pap. 2.00 (*0-937721-04-2*) Wiley.

Diabetes & Cardiovascular Disease. Ed. by Michael T. Johnstone & Aristidis Veves. 2001. LC 00-539800. (Contemporary Cardiology Ser.). 472p. 125.00 (*0-89603-755-X*) Humana.

Diabetes & Cardiovascular Disease: A Practical Primer. Thomas D. Giles et al. 2000. (Illus.). pap. text (*0-9704788-0-1*) Inst of Pro Edu.

Diabetes & Doing Your Best. Nick Walters. 1990. (Illus.). 112p. (Orig.). 7.95 (*0-911071-01-6*) Olde Maryland.

Diabetes & Endocrinology in Clinical Practice. Turnbridg. 1991. 340p. pap. 39.95 (*0-340-54561-5*) Trafalgar.

Diabetes & Exercise: Guidelines for Safe & Enjoyable Activity. Marion J. Franz. Ed. by Michael P. Moore. 1988. (Illus.). 20p. 2.50 (*0-937721-05-0*) Wiley.

Diabetes & Hemostasis. J. Van de Loo. 1987. (Journal: Vol. 17, No. 1). (Illus.). vi, 90p. pap. 75.00 (*3-8055-4448-0*) S Karger.

Diabetes & Hypoglycemia: How You Can Benefit from Diet, Vitamins, Minerals, Herbs, Exercise & Other Natural Methods. Michael T. Murray. 1994. LC 93-36307. (Getting Well Naturally Ser.). 176p. pap. 12.95 (*1-55958-426-2*) Prima Pub.

Diabetes & Its Management. Peter J. Watkins et al. 5th ed. 1996. LC 95-31623. (Illus.). 320p. pap. 54.95 (*0-86542-863-8*) Blackwell Sci.

Diabetes & Lipids: Pocketbook Edition. Reckless. 2nd ed. 2000. (*1-85317-614-1*) Martin Dunitz GBR. *Dist:* Blackwell Sci.

Diabetes & Pregnancy: An International Approach to Diagnosis & Management. Ed. by Anne Dornhorst & David R. Hadden. 1996. LC 96-13798. (Practical Diabetes Ser.). 424p. 125.00 (*0-471-96204-X*) Wiley.

Diabetes & Pregnancy: Teratology, Toxicity & Treatment. Ed. by Lois Jovanovic et al. 1986. LC 85-31705. 451p. 105.00 (*0-275-92092-5*, C2092, Praeger Pubs) Greenwood.

Diabetes & Pregnancy: What to Expect. American Diabetes Association. 3rd rev. ed. 1996. LC 96-142307. (Illus.). 72p. pap. 9.95 (*0-945448-05-8*, 4903-01) Am Diabetes.

Diabetes & Primary Eye Care. A. Ariffin et al. 1992. (Modern Optometry Ser.). (Illus.). 224p. 70.00 (*0-632-03142-5*) Blackwell Sci.

Diabetes & Protein Glycation: Clinical & Pathophysiologic Relevance. Margo P. Cohen. 1996. (Illus.). x, 275p. (Orig.). pap. 35.00 (*0-9654654-0-3*) J C Press.

Diabetes & Protein Glycosylation. M. P. Cohen. 1986. (Illus.). 170p. 61.00 (*0-387-96297-2*) Spr-Verlag.

Diabetes & the Adolescent. George A. Werther & John M. Court. 1998. 89.95 (*0-9587142-1-5*) Blackwell Sci.

Diabetes & the Heart. Ed. by Kenneth G. Taylor. 1992. LC 92-18892. (Oxford Medical Publications). pap. 25.00 (*0-19-263026-1*) OUP.

Diabetes & the Kidney. Ed. by A. Heidland. 1989. (Contributions to Nephrology Ser.: Vol. 73). (Illus.). 232p. 29.75 (*3-8055-4968-7*) S Karger.

Diabetes Annual. Ed. by S. M. Marshall et al. 1998. (Diabetes Annual Ser.: Vol. 11). 280p. 172.00 (*0-444-82895-8*) Elsevier.

Diabetes Annual. Ed. by S. M. Marshall & R. A. Rizza. 1996. (Diabetes Annual Ser.: Vol. 10). 404p. 232.00 (*0-444-82426-X*) Elsevier.

Diabetes Annual. Ed. by S. M. Marshall et al. 7th ed. 1993. 384p. 221.00 (*0-444-89694-5*); 9. 1995. 368p. 231.50 (*0-444-82055-8*) Elsevier.

Diabetes Annual, Vol. 8. Ed. by S. M. Marshall & P. H. Home. 1994. 502p. text 243.25 (*0-444-81788-3*) Elsevier.

Diabetes Annual 12. Ed. by S. M. Marshall et al. 1999. (Diabetes Annual Ser.). (Illus.). 422p. 182.50 (*0-444-82896-6*) Elsevier.

Diabetes As a Disease of Civilization: The Impact of Culture Change on Indigenous Peoples. Ed. by Jennie R. Joe & Robert S. Young. 1993. LC 93-10649. (New Babylon Studies in the Social Sciences: No. 50). (Illus.). vi, 527p. (C). lib. bdg. (*3-11-013474-8*) Mouton.

Diabetes at the Beginning of the New Millennium. Alberto Signori & Umberto DiMario. 2000. LC 00-48589. (Illus.). 392p. 125.00 (*0-471-49299-X*) Wiley.

Diabetes Carbohydrate & Calorie Counter. Annette B. Natow & Jo-Ann Heslin. Ed. by Sally Peters. 1991. 265p. mass mkt. 6.99 (*0-671-69565-7*) PB.

Diabetes Care for Babies, Toddlers, & Preschoolers: A Reassuring Guide. Jean Betschart. 1998. 96p. pap. 14.95 (*0-471-34676-4*) Wiley.

Diabetes Care Markets: Revenue & Cost-Savings Forecasts. 1998. (Illus.). 198p. spiral bd. 695.00 (*1-889713-20-1*, DCM-201) Feedback Rsch.

Diabetes Caring for Patients in the Community. Ed. by Joan R. Mcdowell & Derek Gordon. 1996. LC 96-25833. 273p. text (*0-443-05295-6*) Church.

Diabetes Complicating Pregnancy: The Joslin Clinic Method. Ed. by Florence M. Brown & John W. Hare. 2nd ed. 1995. LC 95-8383. 232p. 120.00 (*0-471-11031-0*) Wiley.

Diabetes Control & the Kosher Diet. Ada P. Kahn. 1985. LC 84-51535. 180p. pap. 9.95 (*0-930121-00-7*) Wordscope Inc.

Diabetes Cure: A Medical Approach That Can Slow, Stop, Even Cure Type 2 Diabetes. Vern Cherewatenko & Paul Perry. 1999. LC 98-43193. 288p. 25.00 (*0-06-019210-0*, Cliff Street) HarperTrade.

Diabetes Dictionary. 1994. (Illus.). 64p. (Orig.). (C). pap. text 20.00 (*0-7881-1023-3*) DIANE Pub.

Diabetes: Do Your Level Best: Start Controlling Your Blood Sugar Today. 1997. 60p. pap. text 35.00 (*1-57979-157-3*) DIANE Pub.

Diabetes Doesn't Have to Be a Death Sentence see Life to the Fullest: Stories of People Coping with Diabetes

***Diabetes Educagtion & Management in Home Care: A Handbook for Nurses.** Linda C. Pearce. Ed. by Kate Kuha & Marcia Barnette. 2000. LC 00-143222. (Illus.). 141p. (C). pap. (*1-930304-10-2*) Home Care Univ.

Diabetes Education Course. Competence Assurance Systems Staff. 1986. (Illus.). pap. text 75.00 (*0-89147-064-6*) CAS.

Diabetes Education Goals. Ed. by American Diabetes Association Staff. 1995. LC 95-10032. (Practical Approaches in Diabetes Care Ser.). pap. 24.95 (*0-945448-49-X*, 5502-01) Am Diabetes.

Diabetes Eye Care Sourcebook. Donald S. Fong & Robin D. Ross. 1998. LC 98-9903. 320p. 30.00 (*1-56565-875-2*, 08752W) Lowell Hse.

Diabetes Eye Care Sourcebook. Donald S. Fong & Robin D. Ross. 1999. (Illus.). 320p. pap. 16.95 (*0-7373-0133-3*, 01333W) NTC Contemp Pub Co.

Diabetes Fact Book. Theodore G. Duncan. 1983. 160p. pap. 6.95 (*0-684-18033-2*); 1982. 144p. 11.95 (*0-684-17449-9*) Gale (Macmillan Ref).

***Diabetes Food & Nutrition Bible: A Complete Guide to Planning, Shopping, Cooking & Eating.** Hope S. Warshaw & Robyn Webb. 2001. LC 00-22343. (Illus.). 320p. pap. 18.95 (*1-58040-037-X*) Am Diabetes.

Diabetes from the Inside Out: A Resource Manual. Char Gast. l.t. ed. 1992. (Illus.). 215p. 21.25 (*0-9632453-0-9*); 29p. 2.00 (*0-9632453-1-7*) Diabetes Educ.

Diabetes Guide. K. Johansen & S. Dagogo-Jack. 1992. (Illus.). 121p. 25.00 (*0-387-54429-1*) Spr-Verlag.

***Diabetes in Adolescent Girls: Endocrine Influences on Metabolic Control with Special Regard to the GH-IGF-I Axis.** Maria Halldin Stenlid. 2001. (Comprehensive Summaries of Uppsala Dissertations from the Faculty of Medicine Ser.: No.). (Illus.). 99p. (*91-554-5014-8*) Uppsala Universitet SWE. *Dist:* Coronet Bks.

Diabetes in America. Ronald E. Aubert et al. 2nd ed. 1996. (Illus.). 782p. (C). pap. text 75.00 (*0-7881-2662-8*) DIANE Pub.

Diabetes in Childhood & Adolescence. Ed. by David W. Kaplan. 1986. (Journal: Vol. 12, No. 4, 1983-85). (Illus.). iv, 72p. pap. 41.75 (*3-8055-4400-6*) S Karger.

Diabetes in Children: A Guide for the Family. Ed. by Mayer Davidson. 1996. (Pediatric Ser.). (Illus.). 32p. (Orig.). pap. text 2.95 (*1-885274-31-9*) Health InfoNet Inc.

Diabetes in Color/No More Black & White. 2nd rev. ed. 1999. 56p. pap. (*0-9671168-1-3*) F Thibodeau.

Diabetes in Elderly People. Ed. by Colin M. Kesson & Paul V. Knight. 1990. 200p. pap. 22.95 (*0-412-32870-4*, A4450) Chapman & Hall.

Diabetes in Europe. Williams. 224p. (*0-86196-130-7*) J Libbey Med GBR. *Dist:* Bks Intl VA.

***Diabetes in Focus.** Patel. 1999. (*0-85369-401-X*) Pharmaceutical Pr GBR. *Dist:* Rittenhouse.

Diabetes in Hispanic Americans: Current Research & Education Programs. 1994. (Illus.). 107p. (Orig.). (C). pap. text 30.00 (*0-7881-1084-5*) DIANE Pub.

Diabetes in Juveniles: Proceedings of the 2nd Beilinson, Symposium on the Various Faces in Juveniles, Jerusalem, Israel. International Beilinson Symposium Staff. Ed. by Zvi Laron. 2nd ed. 1977. (Illus.). 64.50 (*3-8055-2698-9*) S Karger.

Diabetes in Native Americans: The Eastern Tribes. 1996. (Illus.). 126p. (Orig.). pap. text 35.00 (*0-7881-2784-5*) DIANE Pub.

Diabetes in Pregnancy. Jo M. Kendrick et al. 2nd ed. 1998. LC 97-42386. pap. 10.00 (*0-86525-079-0*) March of Dimes.

Diabetes in the Family. Dorothy Born. 1982. LC 81-18024. (Illus.). pap. 9.95 (*0-13-208463-5*) P-H.

Diabetes in the U. S. A Strategy for Prevention. 1993. 61p. (Orig.). (C). pap. text 35.00 (*0-7881-0112-9*) DIANE Pub.

Diabetes Insipidus in Man. Ed. by P. Czernichow & A. D. Robinson. 1985. (Frontiers of Hormone Research Ser.: Vol. 13). (Illus.). x, 326p. 143.50 (*3-8055-3921-5*) S Karger.

Diabetes Is Not a Piece of Cake: Prescribed for Family, Friends & Co-workers of Folks with Diabetes. Janet Meirelles. 1994. LC 94-75824. (Illus.). pap. 15.95 (*1-884929-75-3*) Lincoln Pubng.

Diabetes Management: Clinical Pathways, Guidelines & Patient Education. Health & Administration Development Group Aspen Publishers Staff. Ed. by Jo Gulledge & Shawn Beard. 1995. LC 99-31853. (Chronic Disease Management Ser.). 306p. pap. 79.00 (*0-8342-1703-1*) Aspen Pub.

Diabetes Management: Step by Step. Michael Dracquer et al. 1997. LC 98-18760. (Illus.). 64p. pap. 38.95 (*0-632-04848-4*) Blackwell Sci.

Diabetes Management in the 1980s: The Role of Home Blood Glucose Monitoring & New Insulin Delivery Systems. Charles M. Peterson. 1982. LC 82-80561. 328p. 84.00 (*0-275-91377-5*, C1377, Praeger Pubs) Greenwood.

***Diabetes Matters in Primary Care.** Ruth Chambers et al. 2001. 184p. pap. (*1-85775-424-7*) Radcliffe Med Pr GBR. *Dist:* Balogh.

Diabetes Meal Planning Made Easy. Hope S. Warshaw. 1996. 192p. pap. 14.95 (*0-945448-61-9*, 4706-01) Am Diabetes.

Diabetes Medical Nutrition Therapy: A Professional Guide to Management & Nutrition Education Resources. Harold J. Holler & Joyce Green Pastors. 1997. 290p. pap. 24.95 (*0-88091-146-8*) Am Dietetic Assn.

Diabetes Mellitus. 1985. (Technical Reports: No. 727). 113p. pap. text 9.00 (*92-4-120727-2*, 1100727); 1965. (Technical Report Ser.: No. 310). 44p. pap. text 3.00 (*92-4-120310-2*) World Health.

Diabetes Mellitus. Ed. by K. Oberdisse. 1977. (Handbuch der Inneren Medicine Ser.: Vol. 7/2). 392.00 (*0-387-07741-3*) Spr-Verlag.

***Diabetes Mellitus.** Campbell & Lebovitz. 2nd ed. 2001. (Fast Facts Ser.). (Illus.). 96p. pap. (*1-899541-88-8*) Health Pr GBR. *Dist:* JAMCO Dist.

Diabetes Mellitus, Vol. 5. Ed. by Harold Rifkin & Philip Raskin. 1980. (Illus.). 391p. text 22.95 (*0-87619-747-0*) P-H.

Diabetes Mellitus: A Fundamental & Clinical Text. Derek LeRoith et al. 2nd ed. 2000. 1,088p. text 259.00 (*0-7817-2058-3*) Lppncott W & W.

Diabetes Mellitus: A Source Guide. 1991. lib. bdg. 250.00 (*0-8490-4893-1*) Gordon Pr.

Diabetes Mellitus: Diagnosis & Treatment. Mayer B. Davidson. Ed. by Richard Zorab. 4th ed. 1998. LC 97-50320. (Illus.). 544p. pap. text 65.00 (*0-7216-6403-2*) Saunders.

Diabetes Mellitus: Etiopathogenesis & Metabolic Aspects. Ed. by F. Belfiore et al. 1984. (Frontiers in Diabetes Ser.: Vol. 4). (Illus.). x, 282p. 184.50 (*3-8055-3771-9*) S Karger.

Diabetes Mellitus: Management & Complications. Ed. by Jerrold M. Olefsky & Robert S. Sherwin. 1985. (Contemporary Issues in Endocrinology & Metabolism Ser.: Vol. 1). (Illus.). 399p. text (*0-443-08379-7*) Church.

Diabetes Mellitus: Pathophysiology & Therapy. Ed. by W. Creutzfeldt & Pierre J. Lefebvre. 1989. (Illus.). 400p. 117.00 (*0-387-50506-7*) Spr-Verlag.

Diabetes Mellitus & Pathology of the Heart: Diabetes & Diseased Arteries. Sokolov E. Ivanovich. 1999. LC 99-70042. (Illus.). 352p. 29.95 (*0-9667937-5-7*) Medical Trading Ctr.

Diabetes Mellitus in Pregnancy: Principles & Practice. Ed. by E. Albert Reece & Donald R. Coustan. 1988. (Illus.). 652p. text (*0-443-08470-X*); 2nd ed. 1995. LC 95-12415. text (*0-443-08979-5*) Church.

Diabetes Mellitus in the Elderly. Ed. by James W. Cooper. 1999. LC 99-12436. (Illus.). 84p. 39.95 (*0-7890-0682-0*, Pharmctl Prods) Haworth Pr.

Diabetes 1994: Proceedings of the 15th International Diabetes Federation Congress, Kobe, 6-11, November 1994. Ed. by Shigeaki Baba & Toshio Kaneko. 1995. LC 95-14961. (International Congress Ser.: 1100). 1302p. 383.00 (*0-444-81725-5*) Elsevier.

Diabetes Nursing Care: Overview & Management. Sandra Winter. 4th rev. ed. 1999. LC 00-701548. (Clinical Nursing Ser.). (Illus.). 240p. pap. (*1-57801-033-0*) Western Schls.

Diabetes, Obesity & Hyperlipidemias: The Plurimetabolic Syndrom; Proceedings of the European Symposium on Metabolism, Padova, 24-26 May, 1993. Ed. by G. Crepaldi et al. 1993. LC 93-38467. (International Congress Ser.: No. 1039). 310p. 206.50 (*0-444-81639-9*, Excerpta Medica) Elsevier.

Diabetes 101: A Pure & Simple Guide for People Who Use Insulin. Betty P. Brackenridge. 3rd ed. 1998. LC 99-158831. (Illus.). 224p. pap. 12.95 (*1-56561-156-X*) Wiley.

Diabetes 101: A Pure & Simple Guide for People Who Use Insulin. Betty Page Brackenridge & Richard O. Dolinar. 3rd ed. 1998. 224p. pap. 12.95 (*0-471-34675-6*) Wiley.

Diabetes Patient Education Manual. Simon B. Weavers et al. 1999. LC 99-23529. (Illus.). ring bd. 189.00 (*0-8342-1275-7*) Aspen Pub.

Diabetes Patient Education Manual: Aspen Reference Group. 169.00 (*0-8342-1611-6*) Aspen Pub.

Diabetes Prediction, Prevention, & Genetic Counseling. Ed. by Jerry P. Palmer. 1996. LC 95-38949. (Practical Diabetes Ser.). 462p. 132.50 (*0-471-95525-6*) Wiley.

Diabetes Prevention & Care in the Villages of Alaska. Cynthia Schraer et al. 1993. (Illus.). 228p. (Orig.). (C). pap. text 45.00 (*1-56806-489-6*) DIANE Pub.

Diabetes Product Markets: Product Penetration Increases with Patient Awareness. Market Intelligence Staff. 1992. 300p. 1995.00 (*1-56753-404-X*) Frost & Sullivan.

Diabetes-Related Programs for Black Americans: A Resource Guide. 1994. (Illus.). 107p. (Orig.). (C). pap. text 35.00 (*0-7881-1027-6*) DIANE Pub.

Diabetes Research: A Guide for Postgraduates. Bernard Tuch et al. 2000. 156p. 35.00 (*90-5702-461-6*, Harwood Acad Pubs) Gordon & Breach.

Diabetes Revised. Jerry Edelwich. 2nd rev. ed. 1998. pap. (*0-201-36089-6*) Addison-Wesley.

Diabetes Self-Care Method: The Breakthrough Program of Self-Management That Will Help You Lead a Better, Freer, More Normal Life. Charles M. Peterson & Lois Jovanovic-Peterson. rev. ed. 1990. (Illus.). 144p. reprint ed. pap. 12.95 (*0-929923-29-4*) Lowell Hse.

Diabetes Self-Care Method: The Breakthrough Program of Self-Management That Will Help You Lead a Better, Freer, More Normal Life. Charles M. Peterson & Lois Jovanovic-Peterson. 2nd rev. ed. 1998. LC 98-231434. (Illus.). 176p. pap. 16.00 (*0-7373-0017-5*, 00175W) NTC Contemp Pub Co.

***Diabetes Sourcebook.** Diana W. Guthrie & Richard A. Guthrie. 5th ed. 2002. 352p. pap. 16.95 (*0-7373-0642-4*, Contemporary) McGraw-Hill Trade.

Diabetes Sourcebook: Basic Consumer Health Information about Diabetes & Related Disorders. Ed. by Karen Bellenir. 2nd rev. ed. 1998. LC 98-45983. (Health Reference Ser.). (Illus.). xiii, 688p. lib. bdg. 78.00 (*0-7808-0224-1*) Omnigraphics Inc.

Diabetes Sourcebook: Basic Information about Insulin-Dependent & Non-Insulin Dependent Diabetes Mellitus. Ed. by Peter D. Dresser & Karen Bellenir. 1994. LC 94-39437. (Health Reference Ser.: Vol. 3). 825p. lib. bdg. 78.00 (*1-55888-751-2*) Omnigraphics Inc.

Diabetes Sourcebook: Today's Methods & Ways to Give Yourself the Best Care. Diana W. Guthrie & Richard A. Guthrie. 3rd ed. 2000. 286p. reprint ed. pap. text 16.00 (*0-7881-6916-5*) DIANE Pub.

Diabetes Sourcebook: Today's Methods & Ways to Give Yourself the Best Care. Diana W. Guthrie & Richard A. Guthrie. 4th rev. ed. 1999. LC 99-20148. (Illus.). 311p. pap. 15.95 (*0-7373-0084-1*, 008411W) NTC Contemp Pub Co.

Diabetes Travel Guide. Davida F. Kruger. 2001. LC 00-50219. vii, 172p. pap. 15.95 (*1-58040-041-8*) Am Diabetes.

Diabetes 2E PB: Caring for Your Emotions as Well as Your Health, 2. Jerry Edelwich & Archie Brodsky. 2nd rev. ed. 2000. LC 98-87224. 336p. pap. text 15.00 (*0-7382-0021-2*) Perseus Bks Grp.

***Diabetes Type 2: The Complete Food Management Program.** Sherri Shafer. 2001. LC 2001-51346. 368p. pap. 18.95 (*0-7615-3252-8*, Prima Health) Prima Pub.

Diabetes Type II & What to Do. Virginia Valentine et al. LC 92-37694. 1993. 180p. 21.95 (*1-56565-034-4*, Anodyne); 2nd ed. 1998. 204p. pap. 16.00 (*1-56565-865-5*, 08655W) Lowell Hse.

Diabetes Type 2 & What to Do. Virginia Valentine & Barbara Toohey. 3rd ed. 2000. LC 00-64243. xxi, 250p. pap. 16.95 (*0-7373-0493-6*) Lowell Hse.

Diabetes und Graviditaet. Ed. by A. Reist et al. 1975. (Fortschritte der Geburtshilfe & Gynaekologie Ser.: Vol. 54). (GER., Illus.). pap. 16.75 (*3-8055-2144-8*) S Karger.

Diabetes, Visual Impairment, & Group Support: A Guidebook. Judith Caditz. 1989. LC 89-90678. (Illus.). 77p. pap. text 12.95 (*0-9622368-1-0*) Ctr Partially.

Diabetes, Visual Impairment & Group Support: A Guidebook. Judith Caditz. l.t. ed. 1989. LC 89-90678. (Illus.). 114p. pap. text 12.95 (*0-9622368-0-2*) Ctr Partially.

Diabetes Without Fear. Joseph I. Goodman & W. Watts Biggers. 1979. pap. 4.99 (*0-380-43562-4*, Avon Bks) Morrow Avon.

Diabetes Youth Curriculum: A Toolbox for Educators: Resource & Activities Guide - "The Toolbox", Bk. 2. Patricia M. Moynihan. Ed. by Patricia B. Raab. 1988. LC 88-7112. (Illus.). 260p. ring bd. 55.00 (*0-937721-50-6*) Wiley.

Diabetes Youth Curriculum Bk. 1: A Toolbox for Educators: The Curriculum. Patricia M. Moynihan et al. 1988. LC 88-7111. (Illus.). 136p. (Orig.). pap. text 95.00 (*0-937721-49-2*) Wiley.

***Diabetic Adolescents & Their Families: Stress, Coping, & Adaptation.** Inge Seiffge-Krenke. 2001. LC 00-68949. 368p. text 64.95 (*0-521-79200-2*) Cambridge U Pr.

Diabetic Always: Insulin No More - or Any Other Darn Pills. Julian Goldstein. 1994. 111p. (Orig.). pap. 11.95 (*1-884295-03-7*) Ananta Prnting.

Diabetic Angiopathy. Tooke. 1999. (Illus.). 464p. pap. 129.95 (*0-412-73440-0*, Chap & Hall NY) Chapman & Hall.

Diabetic Angiopathy. J. E. Tooke. 1999. LC 99-24158. (Illus.). 320p. (*0-340-74102-3*) E A GBR. *Dist:* OUP.

Diabetic Angiopathy in Children. Ed. by B. Weber. 1981. (Pediatric & Adolescent Endocrinology Ser.: Vol. 9). (Illus.). xvi, 380p. 172.25 (*3-8055-1574-X*) S Karger.

Diabetic Athlete. Sheri Colberg. 2000. LC 00-31907. (Illus.). 272p. pap. 17.95 (*0-7360-3271-1*) Human Kinetics.

Diabetic Complications. Ed. by Kenneth Shaw. 1996. LC 96-10648. (Practical Diabetes Ser.). 244p. 120.00 (*0-471-96678-9*) Wiley.

Diabetic Cookbook. 1994. (Illus.). 96p. 7.98 (*0-7853-0177-1*, 2022700) Pubns Intl Ltd.

Diabetic Diet Exchange Lists. Margaret B. Salmon. 1980. (Illus.). pap. 3.50 (*0-918662-02-8*) Techkits.

Diabetic Diet Exchange Lists for Low Sodium Diets. Margaret B. Salmon. 1980. (Illus.). pap. 2.50 (*0-918662-06-0*) Techkits.

Diabetic Diet Exchange Lists in Spanish see Dieta Diabetica Para Buena Salud: (Diabetic Diet Exchange Lists)

Diabetic Doctor Looks at Diabetes: His & Yours. Peter A. Lodewick. 1997. pap. text 14.95 (*1-890203-00-9*) DiaBetes Care Ctr.

Diabetic Doctor Looks at Diabetes: His & Yours. Peter A. Lodewick. 1998. LC 98-4119. 336p. pap. 16.00 (*1-56565-940-6*, 09406W) Lowell Hse.

Diabetic Doctor Looks at Diabetes: His & Yours. Peter A. Lodewick. 1984. (Illus.). 204p. pap. 7.95 (*0-910117-00-4*) RMI.

Diabetic Eye Disease: Identification & Co-Management. Alicja Rudnicka & Jennifer Birch. 2000. LC 99-44005. (Illus.). 147p. text 55.00 (*0-7506-3781-1*) Buttrwrth-Heinemann.

Diabetic Foot. John E. McDermott. 1995. 70p. pap. 38.00 (*0-89203-119-0*) Amer Acad Ortho Surg.

Diabetic Foot: An Illustrated Guide to Management. William Jeffcoat & MacFarlane. 1995. (Illus.). 192p. (*0-412-54410-5*) E A GBR. *Dist:* OUP.

***Diabetic Foot: Medical & Surgical Management.** Ed. by Aristidis Veves et al. 2001. 512p. 125.00 (*0-89603-925-0*) Humana.

Diabetic Low-Fat & No-Fat Meals in Minutes: More Than 250 Delicious, Easy & Healthy Recipes. M. J. Smith. 1998. 368p. pap. 19.95 (*1-56561-158-6*) Wiley.

Diabetic Macro- & Microangiopathy. Julian Mincu. 1975. LC 73-82434. (C). 150.00 (*3-11-004533-8*) De Gruyter.

Diabetic Man. Peter A. Lodewick et al. 3rd rev. ed. 1999. LC 99-21681. 368p. pap. 17.95 (*0-7373-0085-X*, 0085XW) NTC Contemp Pub Co.

Diabetic Man: A Guide to Health & Success in All Areas of Your Life. Peter A. Lodewick et al. 1992. 336p. pap. 15.00 (*0-929923-78-2*) Lowell Hse.

Diabetic Microangiopathy. Ed. by H. Abe & M. Hoshi. 1983. (Frontiers in Diabetes Ser.: Vol. 3). (Illus.). xii, 500p. 240.00 (*3-8055-3787-5*) S Karger.

Diabetic Nephropathy: Strategy for Therapy. Ed. by Eli A. Friedman & Charles M. Peterson. 1985. text 146.50 (*0-89838-735-3*) Kluwer Academic.

Diabetic Nepropathy. Hasslacher. 2001. (Practical Diabetes Ser.). 336p. 85.00 (*0-471-48992-1*) Wiley.

Diabetic Neuropathy. Peter J. Dyck et al. 1987. (Illus.). 336p. (C). text 110.00 (*0-7216-2125-2*) Saunders.

Diabetic Neuropathy. Peter J. Dyck & P. K. Thomas. Ed. by Allan Ross. 2nd ed. 1998. LC 97-39762. (Illus.). xiv, 560p. (C). text 125.00 (*0-7216-6182-3*) Saunders.

Diabetic Neuropathy - New Concepts & Insights: Proceedings of the 3rd International Symposium on Diabetic Neuropathy, Kanagawa, 3-5 November 1994. International Diabetes Federation Congress Staff. Ed. by N. Hotta. 1995. LC 95-17702. (International Congress Ser.: No. 1084). 472p. 217.50 (*0-444-82098-1*) Elsevier.

Diabetic Patients Handbook: The Easy Guide to Managing Your Diabetes. 1999. 120p. pap. 14.95 (*0-9675498-0-9*) Worldwide Educ.

Diabetic Pregnancy. J. M. Brudenell et al. 1989. (Current Reviews in Obstetrics & Gynaecology Ser.). (Illus.). 147p. pap. text (*0-443-02792-7*) Church.

Diabetic Renal-Retinal Syndrome Vol. 5: 21st Century Management Now. Eli A. Friedman & Francis A. L'Esperance. 1998. LC 98-15927. 284p. (*0-7923-5049-9*) Kluwer Academic.

Diabetic Retinopathy. Riaskoff. 1976. pap. (*90-6193-554-7*) Kluwer Academic NLD. *Dist:* Kluwer Academic.

Diabetic Retinopathy. O. Paul van Bijsterveld. 2000. (Illus.). 264p. (*1-85317-625-7*) Martin Dunitz GBR. *Dist:* Blackwell Sci.

Diabetic Retinopathy: A Guide For Primary Care Teams. William Alexander. Ed. by Blackwell Science Incorporated Staff. 1998. (Illus.). 10p. pap. 35.95 (*0-632-05171-X*) Blackwell Sci.

Diabetic Woman: All Your Questions Answered. Lois Jovanovic-Peterson et al. 2nd rev. ed. 1996. LC 95-49952. 288p. (Orig.). 14.95 (*0-87477-829-8*, Tarcher Putnam) Putnam Pub Group.

Diabetic's Book: All Your Questions Answerable. June Biermann & Barbara Toohey. 4th rev. ed. 1998. LC 98-4630. 272p. 13.95 (*0-87477-924-3*) Putnam Pub Group.

Diabetic's Book: All Your Questions Answered. June Bierman & Barbara Toohey. 3rd rev. ed. 1994. 256p. 12.95 (*0-87477-773-9*, Tarcher Putnam) Putnam Pub Group.

Diabetic's Jet Ejectors: Diabetic Gun for Personal Insulin Injection. C. Chicka & Anthony C. Chimpa. 1989. LC 88-92324. (Illus.). 78p. (Orig.). pap. 9.95 (*0-922958-03-3*) H W Parker.

Diabetic's Total Health Book. June Biermann & Barbara Toohey. 3rd rev. ed. 1992. 272p. 13.95 (*0-87477-689-9*, Tarcher Putnam) Putnam Pub Group.

Diagnose in der Inneren Medizin. J. Brod & A. J. Knell. 2nd ed. 1985. (GER., Illus.). xiv, 362p. pap. 24.50 (*3-8055-4148-1*) S Karger.

Diagnosing & Treating Arrhythmias Made Easy. Glenn N. Levine. 1998. LC 98-3821. 85p. 10.00 (*1-57626-106-9*) Quality Med Pub.

Diagnosing & Treating Co-Dependence: A Guide for Professionals Who Work with Chemical Dependents, Their Spouses & Children. Timmen L. Cermak. 1986. LC 86-16119. (Professional Ser.). 112p. (Orig.). pap. 14.00 (*0-935908-32-3*, 3272, HazeldenJohnson Inst) Hazelden.

***Diagnosing Cancer in Primary Care.** Nicholas Summerton. 1999. 184p. pap. (*1-85775-307-0*) Radcliffe Med Pr GBR. *Dist:* Balogh.

Diagnosing Early Glaucoma with Nerve Fiber Layer Examination. Harry A. Quigley. 1996. LC 95-644. (Illus.). 192p. pap. text 58.95 (*0-89640-295-9*) Igaku-Shoin.

Diagnosing Learning Disorders: A Neuropsychological Framework. Bruce F. Pennington. 1991. LC 91-9558. 224p. 31.00 (*0-89862-563-7*, 2563) Guilford Pubns.

Diagnosing Male Infertility: New Possibilities & Limits. Ed. by Giovanni M. Colpi & D. Pozza. 1992. (Progress in Reproductive Biology & Medicine Ser.: Vol. 15). (Illus.). x, 250p. 214.00 (*3-8055-5443-5*) S Karger.

Diagnosis: A Brief Introduction. Reuben D. Glass. 1996. (Illus.). 134p. pap. text 24.00 (*0-19-553963-X*) OUP.

Diagnosis: Cataract. Robert T. Lacy. 1982. LC 82-73668. (Illus.). (Orig.). pap. 7.95 (*0-9611782-0-5*) Britton Inc.

***Diagnosis: Heart Disease.** John Farquhar. 2002. 176p. pap. 12.95 (*0-393-32235-1*) Norton.

Diagnosis: Philosophical & Medical Perspectives. Nathaniel Laor & Joseph Agassi. 1990. 280p. (C). lib. bdg. (*0-7923-0845-X*) Kluwer Academic NLD. *Dist:* Kluwer Academic.

Diagnosis: The Moral Authority of Medicine. Abby L. Wilkerson. 1998. LC 98-8217. 208p. 45.00 (*0-8014-3448-3*); pap. 16.95 (*0-8014-8459-6*) Cornell U Pr.

Diagnosis - Cancer: Your Guide Through the First Few Months. Wendy S. Harpham. rev. ed. 1997. LC 97-9291. 192p. 23.00 (*0-393-04620-6*); (Illus.). pap. 13.00 (*0-393-31691-2*) Norton.

Diagnosis & Assessment in Autism. E. Schopler & G. B. Mesibov. 1988. LC 88-19675. (Current Issues in Autism Ser.). (Illus.). 348p. (C). text 59.00 (*0-306-42889-X*, Kluwer Plenum) Kluwer Academic.

Diagnosis & Bone & Joint Disorders. Donald Resnick. 4th ed. Date not set. (Illus.). 5495p. text (*0-7216-8921-3*) Saunders.

Diagnosis & Classification in Psychiatry: A Critical Appraisal of DSM-III. Gary L. Tischler. 1987. (Illus.). 560p. text 105.00 (*0-521-32366-5*) Cambridge U Pr.

Diagnosis & Clinical Measurement in Psychiatry. Ed. by J. K. Wing et al. 1999. (Illus.). 166p. (C). text 57.95 (*0-521-43477-7*) Cambridge U Pr.

Diagnosis & Comprehensive Management of Myofascial Pain. Ed. by Edward S. Rachlin. 1993. LC 93-36499. (Illus.). 552p. (C). (gr. 13). text 85.00 (*0-8016-6817-4*, 06817) Mosby Inc.

Diagnosis & Differential Diagnosis of Breast Calcifications. Marton Lanyi. 252p. 1988. 140.00 (*3-540-16949-0*); 1987. (Illus.). 165.00 (*0-387-16949-0*) Spr-Verlag.

Diagnosis & Evaluation in Speech Pathology. William O. Haynes & Rebekah H. Pindzola. 5th ed. 1997. LC 97-19808. 451p. 78.00 (*0-205-27212-6*) Allyn.

Diagnosis & Exercise Management of Musculoskeletal. Shirley Sahrmann. 1999. (Illus.). 350p. (gr. 13). text 42.00 (*0-8016-7205-8*, 07205) Mosby Inc.

Diagnosis & Injection Techniques in Orthopaedic Medicine. Thomas A. Dorman & Thomas Ravin. 1991. (Illus.). 328p. 60.00 (*0-683-02630-5*) Lppncott W & W.

Diagnosis & Management in Vision Care. John F. Amos. 1987. (Illus.). 729p. pap. text 74.99 (*0-7506-9669-9*) Buttrwrth-Heinemann.

Diagnosis & Management of Acoustic Neuroma. Peter S. Roland & Bradley F. Marple. 1998. LC 98-14985. (Self-Instructional Package Ser.). (Illus.). 108p. pap. text 25.00 (*1-56772-060-9*, 5506320) AAO-HNS.

Diagnosis & Management of Asthma. Mani S. Kavuru & Herbert P. Wiedemann. 2nd rev. ed. 1998. 224p. per. 21.95 (*1-884735-26-6*) Prof Comms.

Diagnosis & Management of Bone Infections. Ed. by Luis E. Jauregui. 1995. LC 94-43569. (Infectious Disease & Therapy Ser.: No. 16). (Illus.). 480p. text 185.00 (*0-8247-8868-0*) Dekker.

Diagnosis & Management of Breast Cancer. Marc E. Lippman et al. 1988. (Illus.). 480p. text 98.00 (*0-7216-1958-4*) Saunders.

Diagnosis & Management of Breast Disease. Ed. by Richard E. Blackwell & James C. Grotting. 1996. LC 96-5096. 664p. 54.95 (*0-86542-405-5*) Blackwell Sci.

Diagnosis & Management of Cutaneous Malignant Melanoma. Daniel F. Roses et al. 1983. (Major Problems in Clinical Surgery Ser.: Vol. 27). (Illus.). 336p. text 142.00 (*0-7216-7706-1*) Saunders.

Diagnosis & Management of Deep Neck Infections. Daniel D. Rabuzzi et al. 3rd ed. 1993. (Self-Instructional Package Ser.). (Illus.). 61p. pap. text 25.00 (*1-56772-006-4*) AAO-HNS.

Diagnosis & Management of Disorders of the Spinal Cord. Robert R. Young & Robert M. Woolsey. 1995. LC 94-30370. (Illus.). 464p. text 93.00 (*0-7216-5447-9*) Saunders.

Diagnosis & Management of Endocrine-Related Tumors. Richard J. Santen & Andrea Manni. 1984. LC 84-1557. (Cancer Treatment & Research Ser.). 400p. text 187.00 (*0-89838-636-5*) Kluwer Academic.

***Diagnosis & Management of Hypertension.** G. Mancia. 2001. (Illus.). 655p. pap. (*0-443-06195-5*) Church GBR. *Dist:* Saunders.

Diagnosis & Management of Immunologic Deficiencies in Infectious Diseases. Louis Saravolatz et al. 12p. (Orig.). pap. text (*1-878294-05-9*) Health Dimensions.

Diagnosis & Management of Inhalant Allergy. Elaine R. Radford & Gary D. Becker. 3rd ed. 1993. (Self-Instructional Package Ser.). (Illus.). 93p. (Orig.). pap. text 25.00 (*1-56772-004-8*) AAO-HNS.

Diagnosis & Management of Liver Disease. Ed. by Ralph E. Kirsch et al. 1995. LC 94-69670. (Illus.). 352p. (Orig.). pap. 93.95 (*0-412-57570-1*, Chap & Hall NY) Chapman & Hall.

Diagnosis & Management of Male Sexual Dysfunction. Ed. by John J. Mulcahy. 1997. LC 96-22329. (Topics in Clinical Urology Ser.). (Illus.). 240p. 79.50 (*0-89640-322-X*) Igaku-Shoin.

Diagnosis & Management of Malignant Solid Tumors in Infants & Children. Daniel M. Green. 1985. (Developments in Oncology Ser.). text 186.00 (*0-89838-750-7*) Kluwer Academic.

Diagnosis & Management of Melanoma in Clinical Practice. Ed. by N. Kirkham et al. 1992. (Illus.). 190p. 122.00 (*0-387-19717-6*) Spr-Verlag.

Diagnosis & Management of Ocular Motility Disorders. Alec M. Ansons & Helen Davis. 3rd rev. ed. 2001. LC 00-23115. (Illus.). 568p. 168.95 (*0-632-04798-4*) Blackwell Sci.

Diagnosis & Management of Oculoplastic & Orbital Disorders: Proceedings of the 43rd Annual Symposium, New Orleans, LA, February 18-20, 1994. Ed. by Thomas C. Naugle, Jr. et al. 1995. LC 95-46564. (*90-6299-132-7*) Kugler NLD. *Dist:* Lib Res.

Diagnosis & Management of Orbital Tumors. Jerry A. Shields. 1989. text 210.00 (*0-7216-2791-9*) Saunders.

Diagnosis & Management of Paediatric Respiratory Disease. Robert Dinwiddie. 1990. (Illus.). 299p. text (*0-443-02744-7*); 2nd ed. 1997. text (*0-443-05084-8*) Church.

Diagnosis & Management of Pain in Patients with Cancer. Ronald M. Kanner. 1988. (Pain & Headache Ser.: Vol. 10). (Illus.). viii, 104p. 60.00 (*3-8055-4690-4*) S Karger.

Diagnosis & Management of Peptic Ulcer Disease. Gary Gitnick. 2nd rev. ed. 1997. 203p. per. 21.95 (*1-884735-30-4*) Prof Comms.

Diagnosis & Management of Peripheral Nerve Disorders. Jerry R. Mendell et al. 2000. LC 99-48702. (Contemporary Neurology Ser.: Vol. 59). (Illus.). 720p. text 165.00 (*0-19-513301-3*) OUP.

Diagnosis & Management of Renal Disease & Hypertension. Ed. by Anil K. Mandal & J. Charles Jennette. 2nd ed. 1994. LC 93-73562. (Illus.). 548p. (C). 98.50 (*0-89089-557-0*) Carolina Acad Pr.

Diagnosis & Management of Seizures in Children. George L. Holmes. 1987. (Major Problems in Clinical Pediatrics Ser.). (Illus.). 320p. pap. text 62.00 (*0-7216-1188-5*) Saunders.

***Diagnosis & Management of Special Populations.** Dominick M. Maino. 2001. (Illus.). 328p. reprint ed. pap. text (*0-943599-37-7*) OEPF.

Diagnosis & Masked Depression. Stanley Lesse. 1996. LC 84-45119. 392p. pap. 60.00 (*1-56821-871-0*) Aronson.

Diagnosis & Misdiagnosis of Back Pain. Julie Zimmerman. 1991. LC 90-85649. (Illus.). 160p. (Orig.). pap. 9.95 (*1-879418-02-9*) Biddle Pub.

Diagnosis & Nonsurgical Management of Osteoarthritis. Kenneth D. Brandt. 2nd ed. 2000. 328p. per. 24.95 (*1-884735-57-6*) Prof Comms.

Diagnosis & Procedure Combinations in Hospital Inpatient Data. Sarah Q. Duffy et al. 1996. 128p. (Orig.). (C). pap. text 35.00 (*0-7881-3716-6*) DIANE Pub.

Diagnosis & Psychopharmacology of Childhood & Adolescent Disorders. Ed. by Jerry M. Weiner. 2nd ed. 1995. LC 95-24343. 519p. 120.00 (*0-471-04262-5*) Wiley.

Diagnosis & Rehabilitation of Pediatric Head Injuries. Mahalick. 1998. 36.75 net. (*1-56593-175-0*) Thomson Learn.

Diagnosis & Risk Prediction of Dental Caries. Per Axelsson. 2000. LC 99-55485. (Series on Preventive Dentistry). (Illus.). viii, 307p. text 118.00 (*0-86715-362-8*) Quint Pub Co.

Diagnosis & Severity of Drug Abuse & Drug Dependence. Blaine. 1996. lib. bdg. 252.75 (*0-8490-6893-2*) Gordon Pr.

Diagnosis & Severity of Drug Abuse & Drug Dependence. Ed. by Jack D. Blaine et al. 1997. (Illus.). 84p. (C). reprint ed. pap. text 25.00 (*0-7881-4602-5*) DIANE Pub.

Diagnosis & Staging of Neoplasms of the Digestive Tract. Morton Meyers. 1997. LC 97-26538. 608p. text 225.00 (*0-397-51757-2*) Lppncott W & W.

Diagnosis & Surgical Treatment of Mediastinal Tumors & Pseudotumors. I. Besznyak et al. 1984. (Illus.). 336p. 112.25 (*3-8055-3582-1*) S Karger.

Diagnosis & Therapy of Acute Leukemia in Adults. J. M. Rowe. 1995. 144p. text 50.00 (*3-7186-5559-4*, Harwood Acad Pubs) Gordon & Breach.

Diagnosis & Therapy of Coronary Artery Disease. Ed. by Peter F. Cohn. 1985. text 186.00 (*0-89838-693-4*) Kluwer Academic.

Diagnosis & Therapy of Spinal Tumors. Ed. by P. R. Algra et al. 1997. LC 97-18905. (Medical Radiology Ser.). (Illus.). 244p. 180.00 (*3-540-58861-2*) Spr-Verlag.

Diagnosis & Treatment for Aortic & Peripheral Arterial Aneurysms. Keith D. Calligaro et al. Ed. by Richard Lambert. 1998. LC 98-5823. (Illus.). 336p. (C). text 98.00 (*0-7216-7675-8*) Saunders.

Diagnosis & Treatment of Acute Radiation Injury: Proceedings. International Atomic Energy Agency Staff & World Health Organization Staff. 1961. (ENG, FRE & RUS., Illus.). 425p. pap. text 24.00 (*92-4-156024-X*, 1150032) World Health.

Diagnosis & Treatment of Anxiety Disorders: A Physician's Handbook. Ed. by Thomas J. McGlynn & Harry L. Metcalf. 2nd ed. 1991. 144p. spiral bd. 18.50 (*0-88048-523-X*, 8523) Am Psychiatric.

Diagnosis & Treatment of Autism. C. Gillberg. 1989. LC 89-71050. (Illus.). 460p. (C). text 120.00 (*0-306-43481-4*, Kluwer Plenum) Kluwer Academic.

Diagnosis & Treatment of Chronic Depression. James H. Kocsis & Daniel N. Klein. 1995. LC 95-2539. 178p. 30.00 (*0-89862-849-0*, C2849) Guilford Pubns.

Diagnosis & Treatment of Chronic Pain. Nelson H. Hendler et al. 2nd ed. 1989. 29.95 (*0-88416-615-5*) Mosby Inc.

Diagnosis & Treatment of Depression in Late Life: Results of the NIH Consensus Development Conference. Ed. by Lon S. Schneider et al. 1994. LC 93-4216. 535p. text 22.95 (*0-88048-556-6*, 8556) Am Psychiatric.

Diagnosis & Treatment of Dermatology, Set. Ed. by Barry W. Hancock. 2nd ed. 1996. 198p. pap. text (*1-85775-093-4*, RA645) Radcliffe Med Pr GBR. *Dist:* Balogh.

Diagnosis & Treatment of Diseases in Ayurveda, Pt. 3. Dash Kashyap. 1984. (C). (*0-8364-2483-2*) Concept IND. *Dist:* S Asia.

Diagnosis & Treatment of Diseases in Ayurveda, Pt. 4. Vaidya B. Dash & Lalitesh Kashyap. 1987. (*81-7022-024-6*) Concept IND. *Dist:* S Asia.

Diagnosis & Treatment of Diseases in Ayurveda, Pt. V. Bhagwan Dass. 1991. (*81-7022-348-2*) Concept IND. *Dist:* S Asia.

Diagnosis & Treatment of Diseases in Ayurveda, Vols. 1-3. Bhagwan Dass. 1988. (C). (*0-7855-2281-6*) Scientific GBR. *Dist:* St Mut.

Diagnosis & Treatment of Drug & Alcohol Abuse. Ed. by Sidney Cohen & James F. Callahan. 1986. LC 85-24833. 305p. text 69.95 (*0-86656-479-9*) Haworth Pr.

Diagnosis & Treatment of Early Melanoma. 1995. lib. bdg. 250.99 (*0-8490-6727-8*) Gordon Pr.

Diagnosis & Treatment of Functional Infertility. Bruno Lunenfeld et al. 3rd ed. 1993. (Illus.). 216p. pap. 85.00 (*3-89412-129-7*) Blackwell Sci.

Diagnosis & Treatment of Global Aphasia. Michael Collins. 1991. (Illus.). 194p. (Orig.). (C). reprint ed. pap. text 45.00 (*1-879105-23-3*, A013) Singular Publishing.

Diagnosis & Treatment of Hearing Impairment in Children. Dennis G. Pappas. 2nd ed. 1998. LC 98-5580. (Singular Audiology Text Ser.). (Illus.). 288p. pap. text 68.95 (*1-56593-865-8*, 1690) Thomson Learn.

Diagnosis & Treatment of Lead Poisoning. Ed. by J. Julian Chisolm, Jr. et al. 1976. 213p. text 42.50 (*0-8422-7262-3*) Irvington.

Diagnosis & Treatment of Lung Cancer. Frank C. Detterbeck et al. 2001. LC 00-30059. (Illus.). xiv, 480p. text 165.00 (*0-7216-9192-7*) Saunders.

Diagnosis & Treatment of Mental Illness: An Introduction. Jonathan P. Beard et al. 1989. LC 88-5507. (Illus.). 216p. 34.95 (*0-8143-1920-3*); pap. 18.95 (*0-8143-1921-1*) Wayne St U Pr.

Diagnosis & Treatment of Minimal Brain Dysfunction in Children: A Clinical Approach. Ed. by Ruth Ochroch. 1981. LC 80-15858. 303p. 45.95 (*0-87705-503-3*, Kluwer Acad Hman Sci) Kluwer Academic.

Diagnosis & Treatment of Multiple Personality Disorder. Frank W. Putnam. 1989. LC 88-11217. (Foundations of Modern Psychiatry Ser.). 351p. 42.00 (*0-89862-177-1*) Guilford Pubns.

C D

Diagnosis & Treatment of Odontogenic Infections: A Self-Instructional Guide, Bk. 9. Thomas H. Hohl et al. Ed. by James R. Hooley & Robert J. Whitacre. 1983. (Illus.). 288p. pap. 44.50 (*0-89939-090-0*) Stoma Pr.

Diagnosis & Treatment of Old Age Dementias. Ed. by T. A. Ban & H. Peter Lehmann. 1989. (Modern Problems of Pharmacopsychiatry Ser.: Vol. 23). (Illus.). viii, 112p. 62.75 (*3-8055-4844-3*) S Karger.

Diagnosis & Treatment of Parkinson's Disease - State of the Art. Ed. by Horst Przuntek & Thomas Mueller. 1999. LC 99-19306. (Journals of Neural Transmission: Suppl. 56). (Illus.). 150p. 119.00 (*3-211-83276-9*); pap. 91.00 (*3-211-83275-0*) Spr-Verlag.

Diagnosis & Treatment of Pituitary Insufficiency. S. W. J. Lambert. 1998. 79.95 (*1-901978-00-1*) Blackwell Sci.

Diagnosis & Treatment of Prevalent Diseases of North American Indian Populations. Melvin Lee et al. 1974. (American Indian Health Ser.: Vol. 1). 302p. text 30.50 (*0-8422-7215-1*) Irvington.

Diagnosis & Treatment of Prevalent Diseases of North American Indian Populations. Max J. Miller et al. 1974. (American Indian Health Ser.: Vol. 2). 250p. text 27.50 (*0-8422-7216-X*) Irvington.

C
D

Diagnosis & Treatment of Radiation Injuries. International Atomic Energy Agency Staff. 1998. (Safety Report Ser.). (Illus.). 59p. pap. (*92-0-100498-2*, STI/PUB/1040) IAEA AUT. *Dist:* Bernan Associates.

Diagnosis & Treatment of Shock: Diagnosis & Treatment. Max H. Weil et al. 2nd ed. 1994. LC 92-48454. (Illus.). 468p. (*0-683-08897-1*) Lppncott W & W.

Diagnosis & Treatment of Skin Infections. Marwali Harahap. 1997. LC 97-7108. (Illus.). 488p. 180.00 (*0-632-04757-7*) Blackwell Sci.

Diagnosis & Treatment of Symptoms of the Respiratory Tract. Ed. by Richard S. Irwin et al. 1997. LC 97-10812. (Illus.). 656p. 125.00 (*0-87993-657-6*) Futura Pub.

Diagnosis & Treatment of Temporomandibular Joint & Myofascial Pain Dysfunctions. Errol Lader. Tr. by Calvin Hogue. 1983. LC 83-50819. (Illus.). 150p. pap. text 75.00 (*0-9610782-4-3*) Vadare.

Diagnosis & Treatment of the Lower Extremities: Nonoperative Orthopaedic Medicine & Manual Therapy. Dos Winkel et al. 1997. LC 96-36871. 688p. 94.00 (*0-8342-0902-0*) Aspen Pub.

Diagnosis & Treatment of the Spine: Nonoperative Orthopaedic Medicine & Manual Therapy. Dos Winkel et al. 1998. LC 95-31860. 992p. 135.00 (*0-8342-0731-1*, 20731) PRO-ED.

Diagnosis & Treatment of the Unborn Child. Maria I. New et al. 1999. (Illus.). 186p. 100.00 (*1-928649-00-9*) Idelson Gnocchi Pub.

Diagnosis & Treatment of the Upper Extremities: Nonoperative Orthopaedic Medicine & Manual Therapy. Dos Winkel et al. 1991. LC 96-46879. 592p. 85.00 (*0-8342-0901-2*) PRO-ED.

Diagnosis & Treatment of the Young Male Victim of Sexual Abuse. William Breer. 1992. (Illus.). 236p. (C). text 50.95 (*0-398-05816-4*) C C Thomas.

Diagnosis & Treatment of Turbinate Dysfunction. Richard L. Goode & Edmund Pribitkin, 2nd. 2nd ed. 1995. LC 95-37147. (Self-Instructional Package Ser.). (Illus.). 73p. (Orig.). pap. text 25.00 (*1-56772-019-6*) AAO-HNS.

Diagnosis & Treatment of Voice Disorders. Sergey K. Korovin & Gould. Ed. by John S. Rubin & Robert T. Sataloff. 1995. LC 95-3243. (Illus.). 536p. 185.00 (*0-89640-276-2*) Igaku-Shoin.

Diagnosis & Treatment Planning in Counseling. Linda Seligman. 1986. LC 85-19728. (Illus.). 353p. (C). pap. 23.95 (*0-89885-262-5*, Kluwer Acad Hman Sci) Kluwer Academic.

Diagnosis & Treatment Product for Immune Diseases, No. C-141. Business Communications Co., Inc. Staff. 1991. 162p. 2750.00 (*0-89336-832-6*) BCC.

Diagnosis, Assessment & Management. Ed. by Andrew N. Nicolaides & Abdul-Majeed Salmasi. 1991. (Developments in Cardiovascular Medicine Ser.). (C). text 249.00 (*0-7923-1188-4*) Kluwer Academic.

Diagnosis Cancer: A Prescription for Creating Your Own Life-Saving Miracle. Robert Rykovich. 2000. LC 98-87122. xxi, 160p. pap. 17.95 (*1-58501-006-5*) CeShore Pubg.

Diagnosis Color - Pediatrics. Taylor. 1997. text (*0-7234-2494-2*) Wolfe Publishing GBR. *Dist:* Mosby Inc.

Diagnosis Color - Sexually Transmitted Diseases, '97. Wisdom. 2nd ed. 1997. text (*0-7234-2496-9*) Wolfe Publishing GBR. *Dist:* Mosby Inc.

***Diagnosis, Conceptualization, & Treatment Planning for Adults: A Step-By-Step Guide.** Ed. by Michel Hersen & Linda Krug Porzelius. 2001. LC 2001-40312. (Illus.). x, 339p. (*0-8058-3491-5*); pap. (*0-8058-3492-3*) L Erlbaum Assocs.

Diagnosis, Dimensions, & the DSM IV Special Issues Journal of Abnormal Psychology: The Science of Classification, Vol. 100, No. 3. Ed. by David H. Barlow. 1991. 150p. text 20.00 (*1-55798-135-3*) Am Psychol.

Diagnosis Documentation & Coding: The Key to Reimbursement & Capitation. Dennis M. Adams. 1997. LC 96-48064. 144p. (C). 40.00 (*0-7863-1000-6*, Irwn Prfssnl) McGraw-Hill Educ Grp.

Diagnosis, Fitting & Care of the Keratoconus Patient. Karla Zadnik et al. 1999. LC 98-50994. (Contact Lens Update Ser.). 96p. pap. text 34.99 (*0-7506-9676-1*) Buttrwrth-Heinemann.

Diagnosis for Disaster: The Devastating Truth about False Memory Syndrome & Its Impact on Accusers & Families. Claudette Wassil-Grimm. 1996. 320p. pap. 13.95 (*0-87951-638-0*) Overlook Pr.

Diagnosis from the Spine. B. H. Jones. 1996. 255p. spiral bd. 18.50 (*0-7873-0478-6*) Hlth Research.

Diagnosis Heart Disease: Answers to Your Questions About Recovery & Lasting Health. John Farquhar & Gene A. Spiller. 2001. LC 00-62210. (Illus.). xii, 164p. 25.95 (*0-393-05012-2*) Norton.

Diagnosis in a Multicultural Context: A Casebook for Mental Health Professionals. Freddy A. Paniagua. 2000. LC 00-9855. xvii, 252p. 64.95 (*0-7619-1788-8*, 83427) Sage.

Diagnosis in Andrology. Ed. by J. Bain & E. S. Hafez. 1980. (Clinics in Andrology Ser.: No. 4). (Illus.). 255p. text 195.50 (*90-247-2365-5*) Kluwer Academic.

Diagnosis in Color: Medical Mycology. Gillian Midgley et al. 1997. 155p. text (*0-7234-2450-0*) Wolfe Publishing GBR. *Dist:* Mosby Inc.

Diagnosis in Color: Ob/Gyn. Symonds. 1997. (*0-7234-2987-1*) Wolfe Publishing GBR. *Dist:* Mosby Inc.

Diagnosis in Color: Physical Signs in General Medicine. Michael Zatouroff. 2nd ed. 1996. 448p. pap. (*0-7234-2587-6*) Mosby Inc.

Diagnosis in Color: Physical Signs in General Medicine. Michael Zatouroff. 2nd ed. 1996. 448p. (*84-8174-283-X*) Mosby-Doyma Libros ESP. *Dist:* Mosby Inc.

Diagnosis in Color: Skin Signs in Clinical Medicine. John A. Savin et al. 1997. (Illus.). 256p. 32.00 (*0-7234-2240-0*) Mosby Inc.

Diagnosis in Colour Cardiology. Adam D. Timmis & Stephen Brecker. 1997. 328p. (*0-7234-2551-5*) Martin Dunitz GBR. *Dist:* Mosby Inc.

Diagnosis in Colour Physical. Michael Zatouroff. 2nd ed. 1996. text 70.00 (*0-7234-2326-1*) Mosby Inc.

Diagnosis in Pediatric Hematology. Smith. 1996. text 157.00 (*0-443-05106-2*) Saunders.

Diagnosis in Speech-Language Pathology. Ed. by Bruce J. Tomblin et al. 1994. LC 93-23600. 472p. 49.95 (*1-56593-147-5*, 0506) Thomson Learn.

Diagnosis Is Cancer: A Psychological & Legal Resource Handbook for Cancer Patients, Their Families & Helping Professionals. Edward J. Larschan & Richard J. Larschan. 1986. LC 86-207718. 144p. pap. 9.95 (*0-915950-77-4*) Bull Pub.

Diagnosis of Acute Abdominal Pain, No. 2E. F. T. DeDombal. 1990. (Illus.). 274p. text (*0-443-03487-7*) Church.

Diagnosis of Alcohol Abuse. Ed. by Ronald R. Watson. 1989. 288p. 127.00 (*0-8493-6381-0*, RC565) CRC Pr.

Diagnosis of Bone & Joint Disorders, Set. Donald Resnick. 3rd ed. 1994. LC 93-48321. (Illus.). text 725.00 (*0-7216-5066-X*) Saunders.

Diagnosis of Cholecystoses. J. H. Ruijs. 1977. pap. text 94.00 (*90-247-1932-1*) Kluwer Academic.

Diagnosis of Deep Vein Thrombosis & Pulmonary Embolism. Ed. by G. Agnelli & H. R. Bueller. 1994. (Journal: Vol. 25, No. 1-2, 1995). (Illus.). 88p. pap. 96.75 (*3-8055-6116-4*) S Karger.

Diagnosis of Defective Colour Vision. Jennifer Birch. 2nd ed. 2001. LC 00-66722. (Illus.). 160p. pap. text 55.00 (*0-7506-4174-6*) Buttrwrth-Heinemann.

Diagnosis of Defective Colour Vision. Jennifer Birch. 1993. LC 92-48986. (Oxford Medical Publications). (Illus.). 204p. (*0-19-261870-9*) OUP.

Diagnosis of Depression. J. P. Feighner & W. F. Boyer. 1991. LC 91-24508. (Perspectives in Psychiatry Ser.). 214p. 215.00 (*0-471-92891-7*, Wiley-Interscience) Wiley.

Diagnosis of Disease by Observation of the Eye: Includes Answers to Diagnosis Questions, Pt. II, Vol. I. Peter J. Thiel. 1997. 100p. reprint ed. spiral bd. 10.00 (*0-7873-0862-5*) Hlth Research.

Diagnosis of Diseases of the Breast. Lawrence W. Bassett et al. Ed. by Lisette Bralow. 1996. LC 95-51372. 448p. text 152.00 (*0-7216-3796-5*) Saunders.

Diagnosis of Diseases of the Chest. Robert G. Fraser et al. 3rd ed. Vol. 1. 1988. (Illus.). 728p. text 120.00 (*0-7216-3870-8*); Vol. 2. 1989. 900p. text 120.00 (*0-7216-3871-6*) Saunders.

Diagnosis of Diseases of the Chest, Vol. 4. Robert G. Fraser & J. A. Pare. 3rd ed. 1990. LC 76-20932. (Illus.). text 120.00 (*0-7216-3873-2*) Saunders.

Diagnosis of Endometrial Biopsies & Curetting: A Practical Approach. Michael T. Mazur & Robert J. Kurman. LC 94-10428. 1997. (Illus.). 260p. 92.00 (*0-387-94230-0*); 1994. 158.00 (*3-540-94230-0*) Spr-Verlag.

Diagnosis of Genitourinary Disease. Martin I. Resnick & Robert A. Older. 2nd ed. 1997. (Illus.). 688p. text 149.00 (*0-86577-573-7*) Thieme Med Pubs.

Diagnosis of Heart Disease. N. O. Fowler. 1991. (Illus.). 429p. 110.00 (*0-387-97428-8*) Spr-Verlag.

Diagnosis of Herbicide Damage to Crops. D. J. Eagle & D. J. Caverly. 1981. (Illus.). 65.00 (*0-8206-0294-9*) Chem Pub.

Diagnosis of Human Peroxisomal Disorders: A Handbook. Ed. by F. Roels. 1997. 232p. (C). pap. text 98.00 (*0-7923-3855-3*) Kluwer Academic.

Diagnosis of Human Viruses by Polymerase Chain Reaction Technology. Ed. by Yechiel Becker & G. Darai. 1992. LC 92-49412. (Frontiers of Virology Ser.: Vol. 1). (Illus.). 426p. 154.00 (*0-387-55461-0*) Spr-Verlag.

Diagnosis of Metabolic Bone Disease. Paul Grech et al. 1986. (Illus.). 384p. text 115.00 (*0-7216-2151-1*) Saunders.

Diagnosis of Mycotoxicoses. Ed. by J. L. Richard & J. R. Thurston. 1986. (Current Topics in Veterinary Medicine & Animal Science Ser.). lib. bdg. 270.50 (*0-89838-751-5*) Kluwer Academic.

Diagnosis of Non-Palpable Breast Lesions: Ultrasonographical Controlled Fine Needle Aspiration. Jacqueline Mouriquand et al. 1993. LC 93-13055. (Illus.). x, 72p. 75.00 (*3-8055-5747-7*) S Karger.

Diagnosis of Onychomycosis & Other Nail Disorders: A Pictorial Atlas. C. Ralph Danial, 3rd. 1995. LC 95-46880. (Illus.). 89p. 46.00 (*0-387-94625-X*) Spr-Verlag.

Diagnosis of Persistent Viral Infections. Joachim Kuehn. 1997. (Journal: Vol. 39, No. 3, 1996). (Illus.). 88p. pap. 60.00 (*3-8055-6458-9*) S Karger.

Diagnosis of Salivary Gland Disorders. Ed. by K. Graamans & H. P. Van Den Akker. 1991. (C). text 126.50 (*0-7923-1384-4*) Kluwer Academic.

Diagnosis of the Orthodontic Patient. F. McDonald & A. J. Ireland. 1998. (Illus.). 278p. pap. text 49.50 (*0-19-262889-5*) OUP.

Diagnosis of the Temporomandibular Joint. Richard W. Katzberg & Per-Lennart Westesson. 1993. (Illus.). 416p. text 155.00 (*0-7216-2368-9*) Saunders.

Diagnosis Related Groups. Ed. by Peter Allen. 1984. 200p. pap. 995.00 (*0-931634-38-5*) FIND-SVP.

Diagnosis Related Groups in Europe: Uses & Perspectives. M. Casas & M. Wiley. 1993. LC 93-33225. 225p. 69.95 (*0-387-57168-X*) Spr-Verlag.

Diagnosis Unknown: Our Journey to an Unconventional Cure. Randy Smith. 1997. LC 97-212641. 256p. (Orig.). pap. 12.95 (*1-57174-065-1*) Hampton Roads Pub Co.

Diagnostic Advances: Molecular Medicine in the Diagnosis & Prognosis of Genito-Urinary Malignancies. Ed. by Kenneth J. Pienta. 1996. LC 96-30169. (Cancer Treatment & Research Ser.). 280p. (C). text 260.00 (*0-7923-4164-3*) Kluwer Academic.

Diagnostic Analysis of the Casebooks of Ticehurst House Asylum, 1845-1890. Trevor H. Turner. 1993. (Psychological Medicine Monograph Supplements Ser.: No. 21). (Illus.). 76p. (C). pap. text 23.95 (*0-521-42986-2*) Cambridge U Pr.

Diagnostic & Interventional Catherization in Cogenital Heart Disease. James E. Lock et al. 1987. 208p. (C). text 139.00 (*0-89838-831-7*) Kluwer Academic.

Diagnostic & Interventional Catheterization in Congenital Heart Disease. James E. Lock et al. 2nd ed. 2000. LC 99-27712. x, 377p. (*0-7923-8597-7*) Kluwer Academic.

Diagnostic & Interventional Radiology: A Clinical Manual. Gaylord et al. 1989. 336p. pap. text 41.00 (*0-7216-2333-6*) Saunders.

Diagnostic & Interventional Radiology in Surgical Practice. Ed. by Peter Armstrong & M. L. Wastie. 1997. LC 96-86529. (Companion Series to Bailey & Love's Short Practice of Surgery). (Illus.). 592p. (*0-412-61960-1*) E A GBR. *Dist:* OUP.

Diagnostic & Laboratory Cards. Linda Skidmore-Roth. 3rd rev. ed. 1998. (C). 27.95 (*1-56930-065-8*) Delmar.

Diagnostic & Laboratory Testing in Psychiatry. Ed. by Mark S. Gold & A. L. Pottash. 1986. LC 85-24465. (Critical Issues in Psychiatry Ser.). (Illus.). 300p. (C). text 78.00 (*0-306-42054-6*, Kluwer Plenum) Kluwer Academic.

Diagnostic & Management Guidelines for Mental Disorders in Primary Care: ICD-10 Chapter V Primary Care Version. World Health Organization, Geneva, Switzerland Sta. 1996. LC 96-931353. (Illus.). 104p. spiral bd. 24.50 (*0-88937-148-2*) Hogrefe & Huber Pubs.

Diagnostic & Operative Arthroscopy. James R. Andrews & Laura A. Timmerman. Ed. by Richard Lampert. 1997. (Illus.). 496p. text 190.00 (*0-7216-5690-0*) Saunders.

Diagnostic & Operative Arthroscopy of the Temporomandibular Joint. Joseph P. McCain. 1996. (Illus.). 321p. (C). (gr. 13). text 149.00 (*0-8016-6074-2*, 06074) Mosby Inc.

Diagnostic & Operative Fetoscopy. R. A. Quintero. 2001. (Illus.). 200p. lib. bdg. 129.95 (*1-85070-714-6*, Parthenon Pbng) CRC Pr.

Diagnostic & Operative Hysteroscopy: A Text Atlas. Michael S. Baggish & Jacques Barbot. 2nd ed. 1998. LC 99-190767. (Illus.). 432p. (C). (gr. 13). text 169.00 (*0-8151-0457-X*, 26931) Mosby Inc.

Diagnostic & Statistical Manual of Mental Disorders: Primary Care Version (DSM-IV-PC) American Psychiatric Association Staff. 4th ed. 1995. 208p. pap. text 29.50 (*0-89042-407-1*, 2407); LC 95-30607. spiral bd. 42.95 (*0-89042-406-3*, 2406) Am Psychiatric.

Diagnostic & Statistical Manual of Mental Disorders: Primary Care Version-International Version (DSM-IV-PC, International Version) American Psychiatric Association Staff. 4th ed. 1996. LC 95-49850. 252p. pap. text 29.50 (*0-89042-408-X*, 2408) Am Psychiatric.

Diagnostic & Statistical Manual of Mental Disorders, DSM-IV-TR: Text Revision. American Psychiatric Association Staff. 4th rev. ed. 2000. LC 00-24852. xxxvii, 943p. 64.95 (*0-89042-024-6*, 2024) Am Psychiatric.

Diagnostic & Surgical Arthroscopy in the Horse. C. Wayne McIlwraith. 2nd ed. 1990. LC 89-2463. (Illus.). 227p. text 98.50 (*0-8121-1186-9*) Lppncott W & W.

Diagnostic & Therapeutic Advances in Hematologic Malignancies. Martin S. Tallman & Leo I. Gordon. 1998. LC 98-26890. (Cancer Treatment & Research Ser.). 377p. (*0-7923-8206-4*) Kluwer Academic.

Diagnostic & Therapeutic Advances in Pediatric Oncology. Ed. by David O. Walterhouse & Susan L. Cohn. 1998. LC 97-25313. (Cancer Treatment & Research Ser.). 400p. 349.00 (*0-7923-9978-1*) Kluwer Academic.

Diagnostic & Therapeutic Antibodies. Ed. by Andrew J. T. George & Catherine E. Urch. 2000. LC 99-36821. (Methods in Molecular Medicine Ser.: Vol. 40). (Illus.). 492p. 99.50 (*0-89603-798-3*) Humana.

Diagnostic & Therapeutic Assessments in Alzheimer's Disease. Ed. by C. G. Gottfries et al. 1991. 248p. (*1-871816-12-2*) Wrightson Biomed GBR. *Dist:* Taylor & Francis.

Diagnostic & Therapeutic Cardiac Catheterization. Carl J. Pepine et al. 3rd ed. 1998. LC 97-21511. (Illus.). 1,329p. 129.00 (*0-683-30125-X*) Lppncott W & W.

Diagnostic & Therapeutic Cardiovascular Interventions II. Ed. by George S. Abela. 1992. 66.00 (*0-8194-0788-7*, 1642) SPIE.

Diagnostic & Therapeutic ERCP: Technical Aspects & Atlas. Neuhaus Von Bernard & Bernard Hogemann. Tr. by Konrad H. Soergel & Michael J. Schmalz. 1992. (Illus.). 328p. 170.00 (*0-683-06433-9*) Lppncott W & W.

Diagnostic & Therapeutic Musculoskeletal Procedures. Jacqueline Hodge. 1997. LC 96-45275. (On Call In...Ser.). 342p. (*1-57059-417-1*) Landes Bioscience.

Diagnostic & Therapeutic Problems in Connective Tissue Diseases. R. A. Asherson et al. 1988. (C). text 126.00 (*0-7462-0051-X*) Kluwer Academic.

Diagnostic & Therapeutic Radiology. Gibbs. 1999. pap. text 49.95 (*0-8385-1605-X*, Medical Exam) Appleton & Lange.

***Diagnostic & Treatment Centres: ACD, Central Middlesex Hospital - An Evaluation.** 2001. 92p. pap. (*0-11-322463-X*) Statnry Office GBR. *Dist:* Balogh.

Diagnostic Angiography: Monographs in Clinical Radiology. Saadoon Kadir. 1986. (Illus.). 734p. text 155.00 (*0-7216-1055-2*) Saunders.

Diagnostic Approach to Organizational Behavior. Judith R. Gordon. 3rd ed. 1991. 800p. text 51.00 (*0-205-12090-3*, H20902) Allyn.

Diagnostic Assays for Colon Cancer. Abulkalam Shamsuddin. 1991. (Illus.). 168p. 87.00 (*0-8493-6540-6*, RC280, CRC Reprint) Franklin.

Diagnostic Atlas of Ear, Nose & Throat Diseases. Lee. 2001. 400p. pap. 59.00 (*0-86577-851-5*) Thieme Med Pubs.

Diagnostic Atlas of the Heart. Ed. by Joseph S. Alpert & J. Willis Hurst. 1993. LC 92-48357. (*1-56375-016-3*) Gower-Mosby.

Diagnostic Atlas of the Heart. Ed. by J. Willis Hurst et al. 1994. sl. 936.00 (*0-7817-0059-0*); 576p. text 199.00 (*0-7817-0058-2*) Lppncott W & W.

Diagnostic Bacteriology: A Study Guide. Margaret Bartelt. 1999. LC 99-32887. (Illus.). 516p. (C). pap. text, stu. ed. 31.95 (*0-8036-0301-0*) Davis Co.

Diagnostic Bacteriology Protocols. Ed. by Jenny Howard & David M. Whitcombe. 1995. LC 95-15032. (Methods in Molecular Biology Ser.: Vol. 46). (Illus.). 293p. 99.50 (*0-89603-297-3*) Humana.

Diagnostic Breast Imaging: Mammography, Sonography, Magnetic Resonance Imaging, & Interventional Procedures. Sylvia H. Heywang-Kobrunner et al. 1997. (GER., Illus.). 448p. 99.00 (*0-86577-636-9*) Thieme Med Pubs.

Diagnostic Breast Pathology: A Text & Colour Atlas. A. Ahmed. 1992. (Illus.). 151p. (C). (*0-443-03185-1*) Church.

Diagnostic Bronchoscopy: A Teaching Manual. Peter Stradling. 6th ed. 1991. (Illus.). 184p. text (*0-443-04293-4*) Church.

Diagnostic Challenges: 150 Cases to Test Your Clinical Skills. Marshall Goldberg. 1998. LC 98-4112. 398p. pap. 39.95 (*0-683-30694-4*) Lppncott W & W.

Diagnostic Clinical Neuropsychology. Erin D. Bigler. rev. ed. 1988. (Illus.). 288p. text 47.50 (*0-292-71537-4*) U of Tex Pr.

Diagnostic Clinical Neuropsychology. Erin D. Bigler & Pamelia F. Clement. 3rd ed. 1997. LC 95-50220. (Illus.). 438p. 75.00 (*0-292-70841-6*) U of Tex Pr.

***Diagnostic Coding Essentials 2001.** Ingenix, Inc. Staff. (Illus.). pap. 99.95 (*1-56337-379-3*) Ingenix Inc.

Diagnostic Criteria for Functional Psychoses. P. Berner et al. 2nd ed. 1992. 284p. (C). text 80.00 (*0-521-42315-5*) Cambridge U Pr.

Diagnostic Cytology of the Dog & Cat. Rick L. Cowell et al. 2nd ed. 1998. LC 98-14959. (Illus.). 352p. (C). (gr. 13). text 89.95 (*0-8151-0362-X*, 31755) Mosby Inc.

Diagnostic Cytology of the Urinary Tract. N. D. Holmqvist. Ed. by G. L. Wied. 1977. (Monographs in Clinical Cytology Ser.: Vol. 6). (Illus.). 41.00 (*3-8055-2685-7*) S Karger.

Diagnostic Cytology of the Urinary Tract: With Histopathologic & Clinical Correlations. Leopold G. Koss. 1995. 416p. text 169.00 (*0-397-51475-1*) Lppncott W & W.

Diagnostic Cytopathology. Ed. by Winifred Gray. 1995. LC 95-11346. 975p. text (*0-443-04557-7*) Church.

Diagnostic Cytopathology. McKee. 1996. text (*0-7234-2449-7*) Wolfe Publishing GBR. *Dist:* Mosby Inc.

Diagnostic Cytopathology. Paul Richman. 1994. 400.00 (*1-56815-031-8*) Mosby Inc.

Diagnostic Cytopathology of Breast. Clive Wells & Hani Zakhour. 1999. 257p. 160.00 (*0-443-05204-2*) Saunders.

Diagnostic Decisions in Neurology. Klaus Poeck. 1985. LC 85-18801. 168p. 39.00 (*0-387-15779-4*) Spr-Verlag.

Diagnostic Dermatopathology. Richard A. Jacoby & William Halmi. 1992. pap. text 90.00 (*0-07-032243-0*) McGraw.

Diagnostic Dilemma: Exploring Risk Management Solutions. RiskCare Staff & Ed Bartlett. 1999. 99p. pap. 150.00 (*1-893929-10-8*) RiskCare.

Diagnostic Dysmorphology: An Approach to the Patient with Multiple Congenital Anomalies. J. M. Aase. 1990. (Illus.). 308p. (C). text 59.50 (*0-306-43444-X*, Kluwer Plenum) Kluwer Academic.

Diagnostic Electrocardiographic Devices. 1991. 39p. pap. 90.00 (*0-910275-68-8*, EC11-113) Assn Adv Med Instrn.

Diagnostic Electron Microscopy: A Text-Atlas. Richard G. Dickersin. 1988. LC 87-30997. (Illus.). 640p. 110.00 (*0-89640-137-5*) Igaku-Shoin.

Diagnostic Electron Microscopy: A Text-Atlas. Richard G. Dickersin. 2nd ed. 2000. LC 99-32439. (Illus.). 704p. 275.00 (*0-387-98388-0*) Spr-Verlag.

Diagnostic Electron Microscopy in Practical Dermatology. J. Daroczy & I. Racz. 1987. 213p. (C). (*963-05-4152-1*) Akade Kiado HUN. *Dist:* Intl Spec Bk, St Mut.

Diagnostic Electronics & Imaging Equipment Markets: A Detailed Database on a 13 Billion Dollar Market. Market Intelligence Staff. 1992. 370p. 995.00 (*1-56753-086-9*) Frost & Sullivan.

Diagnostic Endocrinology. Ed. by W. Tabb Moore & Richard C. Eastman. 2nd ed. 1996. LC 95-35681. (Illus.). 512p. (C). (gr. 13). text 95.00 (*0-8151-5957-9*, 24090) Mosby Inc.

Diagnostic Errors in Primary Care: 84 Case Illustrations. David S. Rubsamen. 1999. xii, 218p. 29.00 (*0-933994-21-4*) Comstock Bon.

Diagnostic Evaluation of the Knee. M. Strobel & H. W. Stedtfeld. 1990. (Illus.). 356p. 185.00 (*0-387-50710-8*) Spr-Verlag.

Diagnostic Function Tests in Chemical Pathology. P. T. Lascelles & D. Donaldson. 1990. 224p. lib. bdg. 82.00 (*0-7462-0108-7*); (C). pap. text 73.50 (*0-7462-0107-9*) Kluwer Academic.

Diagnostic Gene Detection & Quantification Technologies for Infectious Agents & Human Genetic Diseases. Ed. by Shelley A. Minden. 1997. (IBC Library Ser.). (Illus.). (Orig.). pap. (*1-57936-038-6*, 948) Drug & Market Dev.

Diagnostic Guide to Clinical Gastroenterology. Ed. by D. Kumar & J. Christensen. 1996. (Illus.). 468p. (*0-443-05130-5*) Church.

Diagnostic Hematology. Rodak. 1995. 380.00 (*0-7216-4736-7*) Harcourt.

Diagnostic Hematology. Bernadette F. Rodak. 1995. LC 94-11097. (Illus.). 608p. text 62.95 (*0-7216-4727-8*) Saunders.

Diagnostic Hematology: A Pattern Approach. Doyen T. Nguyen & Lawrence W. Diamond. 2001. LC 99-25098. (Arnold Publication). (Illus.). 480p. incl. cd-rom (*0-7506-4247-5*) OUP.

Diagnostic Hematopathology. Braylan. 1997. 145.00 (*0-397-51516-2*, B2827) Lppncott W & W.

Diagnostic Histopathology of the Bone Marrow. James A. Strauchen. 1996. (Illus.). 368p. text 129.50 (*0-19-509756-4*) OUP.

Diagnostic Histopathology of the Breast. David L. Page & Thomas J. Anderson. 1988. (Illus.). 362p. text (*0-443-02240-2*) Church.

Diagnostic Histopathology of the Breast - 2. D. L. Page & T. J. Anderson. 1998. (Illus.). 400p. text (*0-443-04758-8*) Church.

Diagnostic Histopathology of the Lymph Node. James A. Strauchen. 1998. (Illus.). 432p. text 139.50 (*0-19-511860-X*) OUP.

Diagnostic Histopathology of Tumors Ed. by Christopher D. Fletcher. 1995. LC 94-24321. text (*0-443-04295-0*) Church.

Diagnostic Imaging. P. Armstrong & M. L. Wastie. 3rd ed. 1992. (Illus.). 456p. 75.00 (*0-632-03093-3*) Blackwell Sci.

Diagnostic Imaging. Peter Armstrong & Marin L. Wastie. 4th ed. 1998. LC 97-23281. (Illus.). 460p. 78.95 (*0-86542-696-1*) Blackwell Sci.

Diagnostic Imaging: An Algorithmic Approach. Ronald L. Eisenberg. 2nd ed. 1987. LC 65-9491. text 95.00 (*0-397-58300-1*, Lippnctt) Lppncott W & W.

Diagnostic Imaging: MCQs. Richard E. Wright et al. 1992. 224p. pap. text (*0-7020-1597-0*) W B Saunders GBR. *Dist:* Saunders.

Diagnostic Imaging Asia, No. 2. William H. Straub. 1989. 10.95 (*0-316-81889-5*, Little Brwn Med Div) Lppncott W & W.

Diagnostic Imaging-Endoscopy. Brosens. 1997. text (*0-7020-2105-9*) Bailliere Tindall.

Diagnostic Imaging for Reproductive Failure. Lisa B. Schwartz et al. 1998. LC 97-12274. (Illus.). 252p. lib. bdg. 96.95 (*1-85070-561-5*, Parthenon Pbng) CRC Pr.

Diagnostic Imaging in Clinical Cardiology. Joao A. Lima. 1998. (Illus.). 360p. (*1-85317-309-6*) Martin Dunitz GBR. *Dist:* Mosby Inc.

Diagnostic Imaging in Gynecology. Olive. 1998. text (*0-7216-5890-3*) Saunders.

Diagnostic Imaging in Medicine. Richard Reba et al. 1983. text 282.00 (*90-247-2798-7*) Kluwer Academic.

Diagnostic Imaging in Ophthalmology. Ed. by C. Gonzalez et al. 1985. (Illus.). 576p. 385.00 (*0-387-96140-2*) Spr-Verlag.

Diagnostic Imaging Methods in Hepatology. Ed. by H. Lutz & L. Demling. 1984. text 225.00 (*0-85200-807-4*) Kluwer Academic.

Diagnostic Imaging of Child Abuse. Paul K. Kleinman. 2nd ed. 1998. LC 98-13525. (Illus.). 464p. (C). (gr. 13). text 95.00 (*0-8151-5139-X*, 26818) Mosby Inc.

Diagnostic Imaging of the Acute Abdomen. D. Beyer & U. Modder. 1988. (Illus.). 453p. 169.00 (*0-387-17520-2*) Spr-Verlag.

Diagnostic Imaging of the Dog & Cat: Self Assessment Picture Tests in Veterinary Medicne. Christopher R. Lamb. 1994. (Illus.). 144p. (C). (gr. 13). pap. text 32.95 (*0-8151-5323-6*, 22956) Mosby Inc.

Diagnostic Imaging of the Head & Neck. Anton N. Hasso. 2002. text 169.00 (*0-397-51537-5*) Lppncott W & W.

Diagnostic Imaging of the Jaws. Robert P. Langlais et al. 1994. (Illus.). 715p. (C). pap. text 62.95 (*0-683-04849-X*) Lppncott W & W.

Diagnostic Imaging of the Liver, Biliary Tract, & Pancreas. S. Sakuma et al. 1987. (Illus.). 340p. 91.00 (*0-387-16667-X*) Spr-Verlag.

Diagnostic Imaging of the Lung. Ed. by Charles E. Putman. 1990. (Lung Biology in Health & Disease Ser.: Vol. 46). (Illus.). 752p. text 275.00 (*0-8247-8318-2*) Dekker.

Diagnostic Imaging of the Premature Infant. Ed. by Rodrigo Dominguez. 1991. (Illus.). 288p. text (*0-443-08740-7*) Church.

Diagnostic Imaging Review. Gordon K. Gamsu & Maitray Patel. Ed. by Lisette Bralow. 1998. LC 97-41325. 544p. (C). pap. text 89.00 (*0-7216-3801-5*) Saunders.

Diagnostic Immunocytochemistry & Electron Microscopy. Hossein Yazdi & Irving Dardick. 1992. LC 91-20908. (Guides to Clinical Aspiration Biopsy Ser.). (Illus.). 344p. text 97.00 (*0-89640-214-2*) Igaku-Shoin.

Diagnostic Immunohistochemistry of the Skin: An Illustrated Text. I. Kanitkas. 1999. LC 97-69683. (Illus.). 328p. text (*0-412-72390-5*) E A GBR. *Dist:* OUP.

Diagnostic Immunopathology. Ed. by Robert B. Colvin et al. 2nd ed. 1994. LC 93-41659. 848p. text 279.00 (*0-7817-0020-5*) Lppncott W & W.

Diagnostic Immunopathology: Laboratory Practice & Clinical Application. Heddy Zola et al. 1996. (Illus.). 325p. (C). pap. text 29.95 (*0-521-43331-2*) Cambridge U Pr.

Diagnostic Interviewing. Samuel M. Turner. Ed. by M. Hersen. 2nd ed. 1994. (Illus.). 416p. (C). 49.50 (*0-306-44755-X*, Plenum Trade) Perseus Pubng.

Diagnostic Laryngology: Adults & Children. Benjamin. 2nd ed. 1989. (Illus.). 192p. text 152.00 (*0-7216-2838-9*) Saunders.

Diagnostic Liver Pathology. Christopher S. Foster. 1994. (C). text 300.00 incl. disk (*1-56815-010-5*) Mosby Inc.

Diagnostic Manual for Parasitic Infections. Gunnel Huldt. 2000. 89.95 (*0-8493-9234-9*) CRC Pr.

Diagnostic Medical Parasitology. Lynne S. Garcia. 4th ed. 2001. LC 00-56919. 718p. 124.95 (*1-55581-200-7*) ASM Pr.

Diagnostic Medical Sonography: Echocardiography. Mark Allen et al. 2nd ed. 1998. LC 98-10883. 672p. text 110.00 (*0-397-55262-9*) Lppncott W & W.

Diagnostic Medical Ultrasound Examination Review. B. Peters & G. P. Kocheril. 2nd ed. 1988. (Allied Health Ser.). 300p. pap. 37.00 (*0-444-01334-2*) Elsevier.

Diagnostic Methods & Syndrome Identification. Ed. by Chen Ping & Xu Hongwen. Date not set. LC 96-78111. (Advanced Traditional Chinese Medicine Ser.: Vol. 3). 450p. 77.00 (*90-5199-297-1*, 297-1) IOS Press.

Diagnostic Methods in Clinical Thyroidology. Ed. by Joel I. Hamburger. 1989. (Illus.). 261p. 127.00 (*0-387-96923-3*) Spr-Verlag.

Diagnostic Methods in Clinical Virology. Norman R. Grist & Urquhart. 3rd ed. 1979. (Illus.). 240p. (C). (gr. 13). 27.00 (*0-632-00152-6*, B-2007-4) Mosby Inc.

Diagnostic Microbiology. Connie Mahon. 1995. pap. text, lab manual ed. 22.00 (*0-7216-4029-X*) Saunders.

Diagnostic Microbiology & Cytology of the Eye. Kathleen A. Byrne et al. 1995. LC 94-28598. 199p. spiral bd. 74.99 (*0-7506-9607-9*) Buttrwrth-Heinemann.

Diagnostic Molecular Biology. Theodore E. Mifflin et al. 1993. text 47.50 (*0-07-041933-7*) McGraw.

Diagnostic Molecular Microbiology: Principles & Applications. Ed. by David H. Persing et al. 1993. LC 92-38523. (Illus.). 700p. spiral bd. 79.95 (*1-55581-056-X*) ASM Pr.

Diagnostic Monitoring of Skill & Knowledge Acquisition. Ed. by N. Frederickson et al. 1990. 528p. (C). text 125.00 (*0-89859-992-X*) L Erlbaum Assocs.

Diagnostic Neuropathology. Julio H. Garcia. Ed. by Herbert Budka. 1997. LC 96-48279. (Illus.). 824p. (C). (gr. 13). text 169.00 (*0-8151-5562-X*, 29740) Mosby Inc.

Diagnostic Neuropathology. Harry V. Vinters. 1998. LC 98-15854. (Diagnostic Pathology Ser.). (Illus.). 688p. text 225.00 (*0-8247-9888-0*) Dekker.

Diagnostic Neuropathology. Julio Garcia. Vol. 2. 1990. 75.00 (*0-938607-16-2*); Vol. 3. Date not set. (*0-938607-32-4*) Field & Wood Inc Medical.

Diagnostic Neuroradiology: A Text/Atlas. Anne G. Osborn. 1993. (Illus.). 960p. (C). text 260.00 (*0-8016-7486-7*, 04008) Mosby Inc.

Diagnostic Nuclear Medicine. Ed. by C. Schiepers et al. 2000. LC 99-33012. (Medical Radiology Ser.). (Illus.). 304p. 175.00 (*3-540-63467-3*) Spr-Verlag.

Diagnostic Nuclear Medicine Alexander Gottschalk et al. 2nd ed. 1988. (Illus.). 1288p. 260.00 (*0-683-03670-X*) Lppncott W & W.

Diagnostic Obstetrical Ultrasound. John P. McGahan & Manuel Porto. 1994. (Illus.). 544p. text 115.00 (*0-397-51320-8*) Lppncott W & W.

Diagnostic Parasitology for Veterinary Technicians. Charles M. Hendrix. 1999. (C). text 20.56 (*84-8174-392-5*) Harcourt.

Diagnostic Parasitology for Veterinary Technicians. Charles M. Hendrix. 2nd ed. 1998. LC 97-34819. (Illus.). 352p. (C). (gr. 13). pap. text 32.95 (*0-8151-8544-8*, 28921) Mosby Inc.

Diagnostic Pathology of Infectious Diseases. Gail Woods. 1993. (Illus.). 656p. text 105.00 (*0-8121-1604-6*) Lppncott W & W.

Diagnostic Pathology of Infectious Diseases, Vol. 1/2. Daniel Connor et al. 1997. LC 96-31452. 1707p. (C). text 320.00 (*0-8385-1601-7*, A1601-2) McGraw-Hill Prof.

Diagnostic Pathology of Liver & Biliary Tract. Boris H. Ruebner. 2nd ed. 1991. 164.00 (*1-56032-060-5*) Hemisp Pub.

Diagnostic Pathology of the Intestinal Mucosa. W. O. Dobbins. 1989. (Illus.). x, 217p. 189.00 (*0-387-97059-2*, 3051) Spr-Verlag.

Diagnostic Patterns in Nuclear Medicine. Edward B. Silberstein et al. 1998. LC 98-7932. 250p. 63.00 (*0-932004-69-5*) Soc Nuclear Med.

Diagnostic Pediatric Imaging. C. M. Hall & S. Lingam. 1986. (Illus.). 416p. 79.95 (*0-387-16202-X*) Spr-Verlag.

Diagnostic Picture Tests in Clinical Infectious Diseases. Nick J. Beeching & Fred J. Nye. 1996. 124p. pap. 18.00 (*0-7234-2451-9*, 70082) Mosby Inc.

Diagnostic Picture Tests in Dermatology. G. M. Levene & S. K. Goolamali. 1986. (Illus.). 128p. (C). text 19.00 (*0-8151-5407-0*, 09893) Mosby Inc.

Diagnostic Picture Tests in ENT. Bull. 1990. (C). (gr. 13). 16.00 (*0-8151-1310-2*, 22500) Mosby Inc.

Diagnostic Picture Tests in Gastroenterology. Sarner. 1991. (*0-8151-7516-7*) Mosby Inc.

Diagnostic Picture Tests in Hematology. Alastair J. Bellingham. 1994. 128p. (C). (gr. 13). pap. text 20.95 (*0-8151-5224-8*, 23041) Mosby Inc.

Diagnostic Picture Tests in Hematology. Alastair J. Bellingham & Henry Hambly. 1994. LC 94-23606. (Illus.). 118p. text 15.00 (*0-7234-1936-1*) Mosby Inc.

Diagnostic Picture Tests in Hypertension. Graham A. MacGregor. 1996. (*0-7234-2477-2*) Martin Dunitz GBR. *Dist:* Mosby Inc.

Diagnostic Picture Tests in Infectious Diseases. Ronald T. Emond & H. A. K. Rowl. 1987. (Illus.). 128p. (YA). 19.95 (*0-8151-3111-9*, 09504) Mosby Inc.

Diagnostic Picture Tests in Pediatric Dentistry. Rock. 1988. LC 87-29472. 19.95 (*0-8151-7381-4*) Mosby Inc.

Diagnostic Picture Tests in Pediatric Dentistry. N. P. Rock. 1988. (C). (gr. 13). (*0-7234-0984-6*) Wolfe Publishing GBR. *Dist:* Mosby Inc.

Diagnostic Picture Tests in Renal Disease. Graeme R. Catto et al. 1994. (Illus.). 128p. pap. 21.00 (*0-7234-1973-6*) Mosby Inc.

Diagnostic Picture Tests in Sexually Transmitted Diseases. Patrick K. Taylor. 1994. (Illus.). 128p. pap. 22.00 (*0-7234-1965-5*) Mosby Inc.

Diagnostic Problems in Clinical Ophthalmology. Ed. by Curtis Margo et al. 1993. LC 92-49132. (Illus.). 896p. text 102.00 (*0-7216-3659-4*) Saunders.

Diagnostic Problems in Dermatology. Neil H. Cox & Clifford M. Lawrence. 2nd ed. 1998. 42.95 (*0-7234-2790-9*) Mosby Inc.

Diagnostic Procedures for Bacterial Infections. Ed. by Berttina B. Wentworth. 7th ed. 1988. LC 87-19306. 886p. 80.00 (*0-87553-149-0*) Am Pub Health.

Diagnostic Procedures for Mycotic & Parasitic Infections. Ed. by Berttina B. Wentworth. 7th ed. 1988. 650p. 75.00 (*0-87553-156-3*) Am Pub Health.

Diagnostic Procedures for Viral, Rickettsial & Chlamydial Infections. Ed. by Nathalie J. Schmidt & Richard W. Emmons. 6th ed. 1989. 1244p. 85.00 (*0-87553-155-5*) Am Pub Health.

Diagnostic Procedures for Viral, Rickettsial & Chlamydial Infections. Ed. by Edwin H. Lennette et al. 7th ed. 1995. LC 96-147851. 633p. (C). pap., lab manual ed. 96.00 (*0-87553-220-9*) Am Pub Health.

Diagnostic Procedures in Pancreatic Disease. Ed. by P. Malfertheiner et al. 1997. LC 97-5281. (Illus.). 444p. 69.00 (*3-540-61821-X*) Spr-Verlag.

Diagnostic Procedures in Veterinary Bacteriology & Mycology. Ed. by Gary R. Carter & John R. Cole, Jr. 5th ed. 1990. 620p. text 45.00 (*0-12-161775-0*) Acad Pr.

Diagnostic Psychological Testing. David Rapaport et al. rev. ed. 1968. LC 68-16993. 562p. 75.95 (*0-8236-1260-0*) Intl Univs Pr.

Diagnostic Pulmonary Pathology. Ed. by Phillip Cagle. 2000. (Illus.). 792p. text 215.00 (*0-8247-0168-2*) Dekker.

Diagnostic Radiography: A Concise Practical Manual. Glenda J. Bryan. 4th ed. 1987. LC 87-8072. (Illus.). 500p. pap. text (*0-443-02992-X*) Church.

Diagnostic Radiology & Ultrasonography of the Dog & Cat. J. Kevin Kealy et al. 3rd ed. 2000. LC 99-42000. (Illus.). xiii, 436p. text 99.00 (*0-7216-5090-2*) Saunders.

Diagnostic Radiology in Emergency Medicine. Peter Rosen et al. (C). (gr. 13). 1994. (SPA.). 674p. text 110.00 (*84-8086-047-2*); 1991. (Illus.). 704p. text 145.00 (*0-8016-6267-2*, 06267) Mosby Inc.

Diagnostic Radiology of the Brain: CT, DSA, NMR. Ruth G. Ramsey. 2nd ed. 1984. (Advanced Exercises in Diagnostic Radiology Ser.: Vol. 9). (Illus.). 320p. pap. text 65.00 (*0-7216-1177-X*) Saunders.

Diagnostic Radiology of the Dog & Cat. J. Kevin Kealy. 2nd ed. 1987. (Illus.). 528p. text 85.00 (*0-7216-1853-7*) Saunders.

Diagnostic Radiology of the Horse Pt. 2: Diseases of the Hind Limb, Vol. 2. Dik & Gunsser. 1989. (Illus.). 148p. text 165.00 (*0-7216-2959-8*) Saunders.

Diagnostic Radiology of the Horse Pt. 3: Diseases of the Head, Neck & Throat, Vol. 3. Dik & Gunsser. 1990. (Illus.). 172p. text 176.00 (*0-7216-3448-6*) Saunders.

Diagnostic Reasoning: Case Analysis in Primary Care Practice. Jean M. Nagelkerk. 2001. LC 00-45809. (Illus.). 415p. pap. 39.95 (*0-7216-8692-3*) Saunders.

***Diagnostic Reasoning: Case Analysis in Primary Care Practice - Case Study Answers for Instructor's Manual.** Jean M. Nagelkerk. 2001. pap. 75.00 (*0-7216-9255-9*) Saunders.

Diagnostic Renal Pathology. Solez. 1997. (*0-443-08980-9*, S2132) Church.

Diagnostic Sonography: Principles & Clinical Applications. Arthur C. Fleischer & Donna M. Kepple. 2nd ed. 1995. (Illus.). 608p. text 184.00 (*0-7216-3764-7*) Saunders.

Diagnostic Strategies for Common Medical Problems. Rober J. Panzer. 2nd ed. 1999. LC 98-34279. 674p. pap. 45.00 (*0-943126-74-6*) Amer Coll Phys.

Diagnostic Strategies for Internal Medicine. Charles J. Grodzin et al. 1995. LC 95-32579. (Illus.). 816p. (C). (gr. 13). pap. text 56.95 (*0-8151-0642-4*, 24689) Mosby Inc.

Diagnostic Summary Form. Boder. 1982. text 14.00 (*0-8089-1449-9*, 790639, Grune & Strat) Harcrt Hlth Sci Grp.

Diagnostic Surgical Pathology. Stephen S. Sternberg. 3rd ed. 1999. LC 98-49375. 2,784p. text 349.00 (*0-397-58792-9*) Lppncott W & W.

Diagnostic Surgical Pathology of the Head & Neck. Ed. by Douglas R. Gnepp. 1999. LC 99-22687. (Illus.). xi, 888p. text 360.75 (*0-7216-6856-9*) Saunders.

Diagnostic Techniques in Equine Medicine. Ed. by F. G. Taylor & M. Hillyer. 1996. (Illus.). 350p. text (*0-7020-1663-2*) W B Saunders GBR. *Dist:* Saunders.

Diagnostic Techniques in Pulmonary Disease, Part 2. Marvin A. Sackner. 1981. (Lung Biology in Health & Disease Ser.: Vol. 16). (Illus.). 424p. text 175.00 (*0-8247-1182-3*) Dekker.

Diagnostic Techniques in Urology. O'Reilly et al. 1990. (Illus.). 640p. text 240.00 (*0-7216-3116-9*) Saunders.

Diagnostic Test Cards. Springhouse Publishing Company Staff. 1996. 392p. pap. 27.95 (*0-87434-844-7*) Springhouse Corp.

Diagnostic Testing & Nursing Implications: A Case Study Approach. Kathleen D. Pagana & Timothy J. Pagana. 5th ed. 1998. LC 98-34086. (Illus.). 640p. text 36.95 (*0-323-00289-7*) Mosby Inc.

Diagnostic Testing in Emergency Medicine. Allan B. Wolfson & Paul M. Paris. Ed. by Sandra Valkhoff & Judy Fletcher. 1996. LC 95-33470. (Illus.). 560p. pap. text 42.00 (*0-7216-4539-9*) Saunders.

Diagnostic Testing in Neurology. Randolph W. Evans. 1999. LC 99-25745. (Illus.). 525p. text (*0-7216-7603-0*) Saunders.

Diagnostic Testing of Deaf Children. A. Van Uden. 1983. viii, 216p. (*90-265-0436-5*) Swets.

Diagnostic Tests & Nursing Implications. V. F. Valasek. 1983. 704p. 1.00 (*0-07-066805-1*) McGraw.

Diagnostic Tests in Endocrinology & Diabetes. Ed. by Pierre-Marc G. Bouloux & Lesley H. Rees. 1993. LC 93-20474. (Diagnostic Tests Ser.). 328p. pap. (*0-412-35200-1*) E A GBR. *Dist:* OUP.

Diagnostic Tests in Nephrology. J. Bradley. 1999. (Illus.). 332p. pap. (*0-340-74085-X*) E A GBR. *Dist:* OUP.

***Diagnostic Tests Made Incredibly Easy!** Contrib. by Springhouse Corporation Staff. 2001. LC 2001-49609. 404p. pap. 34.95 (*1-58255-137-5*) Springhouse Corp.

Diagnostic Transmission Electron Microscopy of Tumors: With Clinicopathological, Immunohistochemical, & Cytogenic Correlations. Robert A. Erlandson. 1993. LC 93-1632. 880p. text 239.00 (*0-7817-0042-6*) Lppncott W & W.

Diagnostic Ultrasonics. McDicken. 4th ed. 1998. text 105.00 (*0-443-05465-7*) Saunders.

Diagnostic Ultrasonics: Principles & Use of Instruments. W. N. McDicken. 3rd ed. 1990. (Illus.). 367p. text (*0-443-04132-6*) Church.

Diagnostic Ultrasonography (Second Series) Test & Syllabus. Thomas L. Lawson et al. 1994. LC 94-16701. (Professional Self-Evaluation Program Ser.: Vol. 38). (Illus.). 940p. 220.00 (*1-55903-038-0*) Am Coll Radiology.

Diagnostic Ultrasound. Stewart C. Bushong. 1999. LC 99-10455. (Essentials of Medical Imaging Ser.). (Illus.). 150p. pap. 19.95 (*0-07-012017-X*) McGraw-Hill Prof.

Diagnostic Ultrasound. Rumack et al. 2nd ed. 1997. LC 97-41915. (Illus.). 1952p. (C). (gr. 13). text 250.00 (*0-8151-8683-5*, 28974) Mosby Inc.

Diagnostic Ultrasound: A Logical Approach. John P. McGahan. 1,312p. 320.00 incl. cd-rom (*0-7817-1565-2*) Lppncott W & W.

Diagnostic Ultrasound: A Logical Approach. Ed. by John P. McGahan & Barry B. Goldberg. 1997. LC 97-2677. (Illus.). 1,312p. text 235.00 (*0-397-51614-2*) Lppncott W & W.

Diagnostic Ultrasound: A Logical Approach. John P. McGahan & Barry B. Goldberg. 1997. 1200p. (*0-397-58473-3*) Lppncott W & W.

***Diagnostic Ultrasound: Physics & Equipment.** Hoskins et al. 2002. (Illus.). 256p. pap. (*1-84110-042-0*) Greenwich Med GBR. *Dist:* JAMCO Dist.

***Diagnostic Ultrasound: Principles & Instruments.** Frederick W. Kremkau. 6th ed. 2002. LC 2001-34481. (*0-7216-9330-X*) Saunders.

Diagnostic Ultrasound: Principles, Instruments & Exercises. Frederick W. Kremkau. Ed. by Andrew Allen. 5th ed. 1998. LC 97-36858. (Illus.). 640p. text 49.95 (*0-7216-7143-8*) Saunders.

Diagnostic Ultrasound Applied to Ob-Gyn. Rudy E. Sabbagha. 3rd ed. 1993. 752p. text 139.00 (*0-397-51241-4*) Lppncott W & W.

Diagnostic Ultrasound Applied to Obstetrics & Gynecology. Rudy E. Sabbagha et al. 2nd ed. 1987. LC 65-8634. (Illus.). 608p. text 95.00 (*0-397-50699-6*, Lippnctt) Lppncott W & W.

Diagnostic Ultrasound in Gastroenterology: Instrumentation, Clinical Problems & Atlas. L. Bolondi et al. 1984. 544p. text (*1-57235-054-7*) Piccin Nuova.

Diagnostic Ultrasound of the Lower Abdomen. A. Tranta et al. 1985. 198p. text (*1-57235-024-5*) Piccin Nuova.

Diagnostic Ultrasound Test & Syllabus, Vol. 23. Michael L. Manco-Johnson et al. 1988. (Professional Self-Evaluation & Continuing Education Program Ser.). (Illus.). 700p. 165.00 (*1-55903-023-2*) Am Coll Radiology.

Diagnostic Ultrastructural Pathology. Date not set. text (*0-8493-9498-8*) CRC Pr.

Diagnostic Ultrastructural Pathology: A Self-Evaluation & Self-Teaching Manual. Feroze N. Ghadially. 2nd ed. 1997. LC 00-265420. 176p. pap. (*0-7506-9894-2*) E A GBR. *Dist:* OUP.

Diagnostic Ultrastructural Pathology I: Text Atlas Case Studies, Vol. 1. Ann M. Dvorak. 1992. 512p. 156.95 (*0-8493-4404-2*, RB643) CRC Pr.

Diagnostic Ultrastructural Pathology II: A Text-Atlas of Case Studies Emphasizing Respiratory & Nervous Systems, Vol. 2. Ed. by Ann M. Dvorak & Rita A. Monahan-Earley. 1995. LC 94-47018. (Diagnostic Ultrastructural Pathology II Ser.: Vol. 2). 416p. 344.95 (*0-8493-4490-5*, 4490) CRC Pr.

Diagnostic Ultrastructural Pathology III: A Text-Atlas of Case Studies Emphasizing Endocrine & Hematopoietic Systems, Vol. 3. Ann M. Dvorak & Rita A. Monahan-Earley. 1995. LC 94-47673. 464p. 314.95 (*0-8493-9474-0*, 9474) CRC Pr.

Diagnostic Vascular Ultrasound. Ed. by Doris Neuerburg-Heusler et al. 1992. 376p. (*0-340-55399-5*) E A GBR. *Dist:* OUP.

Diagnostic Virology Protocols. John R. Stephenson & Alan Warnes. 1998. LC 98-21040. (Methods in Molecular Medicine Ser.: Vol. 12). (Illus.). 384p. 119.50 (*0-89603-479-8*); spiral bd. 99.50 (*0-89603-401-1*) Humana.

Diagnostical Hysteroscopy: A Practical Guide. Thomas Roemer & Wolfgang Straube. 1996. vi, 102p. (Orig.). (C). pap. text 60.00 (*3-11-015056-5*) De Gruyter.

Diagnostico de Enfermeria. Mija Kim. 2nd ed. 1990. (SPA.). pap. text 29.95 (*0-07-104011-0*) McGraw.

Diagnostico En Enfermeria. Kim. 5th ed. 1994. (C). text (*84-8086-089-8*) Mosby-Doyma Libros.

Diagnostics: An A to Z Nursing Guide to Laboratory Tests & Diagnostic Procedures. Springhouse Publishing Company Staff. 2000. LC 00-61884. (Illus.). x, 981p. 44.95 (*1-58255-075-1*) Springhouse Corp.

Diagnostics According to F. X. Mayr: Criteria of Good, Marginal & Ill Health. Erich Rauch. Tr. by David M. Fogg from GER. 1993. (Illus.). 129p. (Orig.). pap. text (*2-8043-4004-X*) Edits Haug Intl BEL. *Dist:* Medicina Bio.

Diagnostics & Vaccines for Parasitic Diseases. Ed. by M. Tiru & W. Hennessen. 1986. (Developments in Biological Standardization Ser.: Vol. 62). viii, 162p. pap. 61.00 (*3-8055-4266-6*) S Karger.

Diagnostics of Adrenal Cortex Diseases: Integrated Approach Luigi Troncone. 1986. 188.00 (*0-8493-6359-4*, RC659) CRC Pr.

Diagnostics of Adrenal Cortex Diseases Vol. 2: Integrated Approach. Luigi Troncone. 1986. LC 85-25522. 288p. 162.00 (*0-8493-6361-6*, CRC Reprint) Franklin.

Diagnostik des Hodentumors und Seiner Metastasen. Ed. by L. Weissbach & Roswitha Bussar-Maatz. 1987. (Beitraege Zur Onkologie, Contributions to Oncology Ser.: Vol. 28). (GER., Illus.). x, 194p. 58.50 (*3-8055-4614-9*) S Karger.

Diagnostik und Therapie der Erektilen Dysfunktion mit Vasoaktiven Substanzen. Ed. by U. Wetterauer & C. G. Stief. 1990. (GER., Illus.). viii, 156p. (C). lib. bdg. 75.40 (*3-11-012183-2*) De Gruyter.

Diagnostik und Therapie des Prostatakarzinoms. Ed. by H. Goettinger. 1979. (Beitraege zur Urologie Ser.: Vol. 1). (GER.). pap. 28.75 (*3-8055-0294-X*) S Karger.

Dialectics: Humanistic Rationale for Behavior & Development. Ed. by Joseph F. Rychlak. 1976. (Contributions to Human Development Ser.: Vol. 2). 150p. 42.75 (*3-8055-2288-6*) S Karger.

Dialectics of Schizophrenia. Philip Thomas. 1998. 270p. (*1-85343-362-4*); pap. (*1-85343-361-6*) Free Assoc Bks GBR. *Dist:* Intl Spec Bk, NYU Pr.

Dialogical Self: Meaning As Movement. Hubert J. Hermans et al. 1993. LC 93-16702. (Illus.). 195p. text 69.95 (*0-12-342320-1*) Acad Pr.

Dialogue & the Interpretation of Illness: Conversations in a Cameroon Village. Robert Pool. 1994. LC 93-4290. (Explorations in Anthropology Ser.). 296p. (*0-85496-873-3*); pap. (*1-85973-016-7*) Berg Pubs GBR. *Dist:* NYU Pr.

Dialogue Concerning Contemporary Psychodynamic Therapy. Richard D. Chessick. 1997. LC 95-32111. 200p. pap. 30.00 (*1-56821-371-9*) Aronson.

Dialogue in Children. T. Slama-Cazacu. 1977. (*90-279-7754-2*) Mouton.

Dialogue of Hope: Talking Our Way Through Cancer. Charles Downes & Peggy Downes. 1993. LC 93-84083. (Illus.). 136p. pap. 10.00 (*0-931104-37-8*) SunInk Pubn.

Dialogue of Touch: Developmental Play Therapy. Viola A. Brody. 1997. LC 97-9432. (Master Work Ser.). 400p. (C). pap. 45.00 (*0-7657-0088-3*) Aronson.

Dialogue of Touch: Developmental Play Therapy. Viola A. Brody. 1993. 373p. (C). pap. text 20.00 (*0-9646232-0-X*) V A Brody.

Dialogue with B. F. Skinner. Richard I. Evans. 1981. LC 81-15377. 140p. 45.00 (*0-275-90612-4*, C0612, Praeger Pubs) Greenwood.

Dialogue with Erich Fromm. Richard I. Evans. 1981. LC 81-15376. 136p. 45.00 (*0-275-90614-0*, C0614, Praeger Pubs) Greenwood.

Dialogue with Erik Erikson. Richard I. Evans. 1995. LC 95-14657. (Master Work Ser.). 184p. pap. 35.00 (*1-56821-561-4*) Aronson.

Dialogue with Jean Piaget. Richard I. Evans. 1981. LC 81-15374. 189p. 55.00 (*0-275-90619-1*, C0619, Praeger Pubs) Greenwood.

Dialogue with R. D. Laing. Richard I. Evans. 1981. LC 81-15372. 170p. 60.00 (*0-275-90617-5*, C0617, Praeger Pubs) Greenwood.

Dialogues: The Dying & the Living. Austin H. Kutscher & Lillian G. Kutscher. 1979. 20.95 (*0-405-12511-9*) Ayer.

Dialogues in Neurological Surgery. Ed. by Mark N. Hadley & Daniel L. Barrow. 1995. (Illus.). 280p. pap. 65.00 (*0-942219-76-7*) Quality Med Pub.

Dialogues in Perception. Bela Julesz. 1994. LC 94-8883. 298p. 55.00 (*0-262-10052-5*, Bradford Bks) MIT Pr.

Dialogues on the Psychology of Language & Thought: Conversations with Noam Chomsky, Charles Osgood, Jean Piaget, Ulric Neisser, & Marcel Kinsbourne. Ed. by Robert W. Rieber. 1983. LC 82-42850. (Cognition & Language Ser.). 174p. 42.50 (*0-306-41185-7*, Plenum Trade) Perseus Pubng.

***Dialysing for Life: The Development of the Artificial Kidney.** Ed. by Jacob Van Noordwijk. 2001. LC 00-52048. (Illus.). xii, 114p. pap. 16.00 (*0-7923-6840-1*) Kluwer Academic.

Dialysing for Life: The Development of the Artificial Kidney. Jacob Van Noordwijk. 2001. LC 00-52048. (Illus.). xii, 114p. pap. 52.00 (*0-7923-6762-6*) Kluwer Academic.

Dialysis Acess: Current Practice. J. A. Akoh. 1999. 300p. (*1-86094-169-9*) Imperial College.

Dialysis Amyloid. Ed. by Charles Van Ypersele & Tilman B. Drueke. 1996. (Oxford Clinical Nephrology Ser.). (Illus.). 290p. (C). text 99.00 (*0-19-262494-6*) OUP.

Dialysis & Transplantation. William F. Owens et al. 1999. LC 98-53548. (Illus.). xiv, 682p. text (*0-7216-7687-1*) Saunders.

Dialysis as Treatment of End-Stage Renal Disease/Transplantation as Treatment of End-Stage Renal Disease Ed. by Robert W. Schrier et al. 1999. LC 98-29127. (Atlas of Diseases of the Kidney Ser.: Vol. 5). (Illus.). 131.95 (*0-632-04391-1*) Blackwell Sci.

***Dialysis, Dialyzers & Sorbents: Where Are We Going?** Ed. by C. Ronco & J. F. Winchester. 2001. LC 2001-29613. (Contributions to Nephrology Ser.: Vol. 133). (Illus.). viii, 199p. 198.25 (*3-8055-7225-5*) S Karger.

Dialysis Prescription Vol. 16, No. 1: American Journal of Nephrology, 1996. Ed. by G. Schulman. 1995. (Journal: Vol. 16, No. 1, 1996). (Illus.). 90p. pap. 32.25 (*3-8055-6250-0*) S Karger.

Dialysis-Related Amyloidosis. Ed. by K. Maeda & T. Shinzato. 1995. (Contributions to Nephrology Ser.: Vol. 112). (Illus.). viii, 176p. 172.25 (*3-8055-6046-X*) S Karger.

Dialysis Therapy. Ed. by Allen R. Nissenson & Richard N. Fine. 2nd ed. 1993. LC 92-49507. (Illus.). 417p. 55.00 (*1-56053-058-8*) Hanley & Belfus.

Dialysis Therapy in the 1990s. Ed. by H. Tanaka. 1991. (Contributions to Nephrology Ser.: Vol. 82). (Illus.). 116p. 29.75 (*3-8055-5188-6*) S Karger.

Dialysis, Transplantation, Nephrology: Proceedings European Dialysis & Transplant Assoc. Volume 13. Ed. by Brian Robinson. 1977. (Illus.). 65.00 (*0-8464-0328-5*) Beekman Pubs.

Dialysis, Transplantation, Nephrology: Proceedings, European Dialysis & Transplant Association. Brian Robinson. 1978. (Illus.). 65.00 (*0-8464-0329-3*) Beekman Pubs.

Dialysis, Transplantation, Nephrology: Proceedings, European Dialysis & Transplant Association, Vol. 15. Ed. by Brian Robinson. 1979. (Illus.). 662p. 65.00 (*0-8464-1087-7*) Beekman Pubs.

Dialysis, Transplantation, Nephrology: Proceedings, European Dialysis & Transplant Association, Vol. 16. Ed. by J. H. Robinson et al. 1979. (Illus.). 785p. 65.00 (*0-8464-1067-2*) Beekman Pubs.

Dialysis, Transplantation, Nephrology: Proceedings of the European Dialysis & Transplant Association, Tel Aviv, 1974, Vol. 11. European Dialysis and Transplant Association Staff. Ed. by John Moorhead. 1975. (Illus.). 600p. 65.00 (*0-8464-0326-9*) Beekman Pubs.

Diamond & Dalessio's the Practicing Physician's Approach to Headache. Merle L. Diamond & Glen D. Solomon. Ed. by Ray Kersey. 6th ed. 1999. LC 98-7039. (Illus.). 270p. text 45.00 (*0-7216-6999-9*) Saunders.

***Diamond-Blackfan Anemia: Mapping & Identification of the Disease Gene.** Peter Gustavsson. 2000. (Comprehensive Summaries of Uppsala Dissertations from the Faculty of Medicine Ser.: No. 974). (Illus.). 47p. pap. (*91-554-4861-5*) Uppsala Universitet SWE. *Dist:* Coronet Bks.

Diapering & Infant Skin Care: Journal, Pediatrician, Supplement 1, 1987, Vol. 14. Ed. by A. L. Norins. 1987. (Illus.). iv, 52p. pap. 19.25 (*3-8055-4615-7*) S Karger.

Diarrhea. Michael Gracey. 1991. 344p. lib. bdg. 139.00 (*0-8493-8819-8*, RC862) CRC Pr.

Diarrhea & Malnutrition: Interactions, Mechanisms, & Interventions. Ed. by Lincoln C. Chen & Nevin S. Scrimshaw. 1983. LC 82-18894. 334p. 85.00 (*0-306-41046-X*, Plenum Trade) Perseus Pubng.

Diarrheal Diseases. Ed. by Michael Field. 1992. 538p. (C). pap. text 125.00 (*0-8385-1684-X*, A1684-8, Apple Lange Med) McGraw.

Diarrhoea & PHC. Ed. by Ivan Wolffers. 1992. (Orig.). pap. text (*90-5383-042-1*) VU Univ Pr NLD. *Dist:* Paul & Co Pubs.

Diary of a Drug Fiend. Aleister Crowley. 1970. LC 79-142495. 384p. pap. 12.50 (*0-87728-146-7*) Red Wheel ME.

Diary of a Drug Fiend. Aleister Crowley. 1989. 384p. reprint ed. lib. bdg. 26.95 (*0-89966-593-4*) Buccaneer Bks.

Diary of a Midwife: The Power of Positive Childbearing. Juliana Van Olphen-Fehr. 1998. LC 98-3358. 240p. pap. 23.95 (*0-89789-588-6*, Bergin & Garvey) Greenwood.

Diary of a Southern Queen: An HIV Plus Vision Quest. J. Michael Clark. 1990. LC 90-44705. 108p. (Orig.). pap. 8.00 (*0-930383-17-6*) Monument Pr.

Diary of Courage: Coping with Life-Threatening Illness. Mary W. Priest. 1990. 176p. (Orig.). pap. 9.95 (*0-89407-099-1*) Strawberry Hill.

Diary of Sigmund Freud, 1929-1939: A Record of the Final Decade. Sigmund Freud. 1992. (Illus.). 256p. 65.00 (*0-684-19329-9*) Scribner.

Diastematomyelia. F. B. Maroun. 1976. LC 75-17393. (Illus.). 144p. 12.50 (*0-87527-143-X*) Green.

Diastereoselective Reactions of Sulfoximines, Vol. 12. S. G. Pyne. 1992. (Sulfur Reports). 93p. pap. text 85.00 (*3-7186-5315-X*, Harwood Acad Pubs) Gordon & Breach.

Diastolic Relaxation of the Heart: The Biology of Diastole in Health & Disease. Ed. by William Grossman & Beverly H. Lorell. 2nd ed. 1994. LC 93-35878. 368p. (C). text 176.50 (*0-7923-2611-3*) Kluwer Academic.

Dibenzanthracenes & Environmental Carcinogenesis. Walter Karcher. 1992. (Monographs on Cancer Research). 281p. (C). text 130.00 (*0-521-30382-6*) Cambridge U Pr.

Diccionari Enciclopedic de Medicina. Enc Catalana Staff. 1990. (CAT.). 1730p. 195.00 (*0-7859-6297-2*, 8477390932) Fr & Eur.

Diccionario Atlas de Anatomia Humana. Nicola Piscitelli. 2nd ed. 1980. (SPA., Illus.). 256p. pap. 29.95 (*0-7859-5106-7*) Fr & Eur.

***Diccionario Breve de Medicina de Blakiston.** Ed. by J. A. Inestrillas. (SPA.). 1380p. pap. (*968-435-062-7*, PMM627) Ediciones Cientificas MEX. *Dist:* Continental Bk.

Diccionario de Bacteriologia Humana. Giuseppe Nicoletti. 1989. (SPA.). 320p. pap. (*0-7859-6034-1*, 8440435959) Fr & Eur.

Diccionario de Biologia Animal. Carlos A. Aguayo & Virgilio Biaggi. 1982. LC 76-41882. (SPA.). 581p. 15.00 (*0-8477-2318-6*) U of PR Pr.

Diccionario de Enfermeria. John M. Last. 15th ed. 1984. (SPA.). 400p. pap. 19.95 (*0-7859-5929-7*, 8434523728) Fr & Eur.

Diccionario de Epidemiologia. John M. Last. 1989. (SPA.). 216p. 49.95 (*0-7859-3356-5*, 8434523728) Fr & Eur.

Diccionario de Especialidades en Analises Clinicos. Emilio R. Ster. 2nd ed. 1990. (SPA.). 520p. pap. 95.00 (*0-7859-6419-3*, 8487368026) Fr & Eur.

Diccionario de Especialidades Farmaceuticas. Ed. by Medical Economics Staff. 46th rev. ed. 2000. LC 95-49012. (SPA., Illus.). 1900p. 89.00 (*1-56363-359-0*) Med Econ.

Diccionario de Especialidades Farmaceuticas, 2001, Vol. 47. Medical Economics Staff & PLM Staff. 47th rev. ed. 2001. (SPA.). 1,850p. 89.00 (*1-56363-382-5*) Med Econ.

***Diccionario de Especialidades Farmaceuticas 2002.** Medical Economics Staff & PLM Staff. 48th ed. 2002. (SPA.). 2300p. (*968-460-237-5*) PLM.

Diccionario de Especialidades Odontolgicas. Emilio S. Rosenstein. 1989. (SPA.). 360p. 85.00 (*0-7859-3446-4*) Fr & Eur.

Diccionario de Farmacologia. W. C. Bowman. 1989. (SPA.). 250p. pap. 125.00 (*0-7859-6394-4*, 8486193206) Fr & Eur.

Diccionario de Immunologia. Francisco L. Corbian. 1991. (SPA.). 256p. pap. 25.95 (*0-7859-6502-5*) Fr & Eur.

Diccionario de Immunologia. W. J. Herbert & P. C. Wilkinson. 1974. (SPA.). 256p. 45.00 (*0-7859-0648-7*, S50055) Fr & Eur.

Diccionario de la Diabetes. Ed. by Barry Leonard. 1998. (SPA., Illus.). 65p. (C). pap. text 20.00 (*0-7881-7136-4*) DIANE Pub.

Diccionario de la Psicologia. Norberth Sillamy. 4th ed. 1974. (SPA.). 344p. 14.95 (*0-8288-5982-5*, S12360) Fr & Eur.

Diccionario de la Tecnicas de Grupo. Anne A. Schutzsenberger. 1974. (SPA.). 260p. pap. 19.95 (*0-8288-5983-3*, S50365) Fr & Eur.

Diccionario de Medicina. Ed. by E. Dabout. (SPA.). 24.95 (*0-7859-0587-1*, S-37586) Fr & Eur.

Diccionario de Medicina. Andre Duranteau. 1987. (SPA.). 396p. 39.95 (*0-7859-5809-6*) Fr & Eur.

Diccionario de Medicina de Urgencia: Dictionary of Emergency Medicine. Cedel Staff. 2nd ed. 1977. (SPA.). 208p. 9.95 (*0-8288-5318-5*, S13672) Fr & Eur.

Diccionario de Medicina Gran Vox. Vox Staff. 1990. (SPA.). 382p. 150.00 (*0-7859-6170-4*, 8471533448) Fr & Eur.

Diccionario de Medicina Mosby. 1995. (SPA.). 1448p. 275.00 (*0-7859-9781-4*) Fr & Eur.

Diccionario de Medicos Puertorriquenos Que Se Man Distinguico Fuera de la Medicina. Soto Arana. (SPA.). 22.50 (*0-8288-8094-8*, S5070) Fr & Eur.

Diccionario de Medicos Puertorriquenos Que Se Man Distinguico Fuera de la Medicina. Arana Soto. (SPA.). 17.50 (*0-8288-9020-X*, S5070) Fr & Eur.

Diccionario de Optometria. Michel Millodot. 1990. (SPA.). 304p. (*0-7859-6039-2*, 8440464142) Fr & Eur.

Diccionario de Psicoanalisis Clasico. Friedrich W. Doucet. 1974. (SPA.). 232p. pap. 24.95 (*0-8288-5985-X*, S50069) Fr & Eur.

Diccionario de Psicologia Evolutiva y da le Educacion. Rom Harre. 1990. (SPA.). 320p. 65.00 (*0-7859-6229-8*, 8475096077) Fr & Eur.

Diccionario de Psicologia Sexual. Georges Bastin. 2nd ed. 1978. (SPA.). 412p. pap. 39.95 (*0-7859-5086-9*, S13099) Fr & Eur.

Diccionario de Psicopedagogia y Psiqiatria del Nino: French - Spanish. Robert Lafon. 5th ed. 1993. (FRE & SPA.). 1056p. lib. bdg. (*0-7859-3677-7*, 8428107556) Fr & Eur.

Diccionario de Psiquiatria. Raymond Battegay. 1989. (SPA.). 680p. 150.00 (*0-7859-5827-4*, 8425415802) Fr & Eur.

Diccionario de Psiquiatria. James A. Brussel & George L. Cantzlaar. (SPA.). 306p. pap. 49.50 (*0-7859-0781-5*, S50209) Fr & Eur.

Diccionario de Psiquiatria, Vol. 1. Antoine Porot. 3rd ed. 1977. (SPA.). 650p. 59.95 (*0-7859-5924-6*, 8433566695) Fr & Eur.

Diccionario de Psiquiatria: Dictionary of Psychiatry, Set. Antoine Porot. 3rd ed. 1977. (SPA.). 650p. 125.00 (*0-8288-5320-7*, S50071) Fr & Eur.

Diccionario de Terminos y Frases Medicas: English-Spanish/Espagnol-Ingles. 1996. (ENG & SPA.). 400p. (*84-283-2273-2*) Paraninfo ESP. *Dist:* IBD Ltd, Distribks Inc.

C D

Diccionario de Terminos y Frases Medicas Ingles-Espano/Espanol-Ingles. 1996. (ENG & SPA.). 49.95 (*0-7859-9479-3*) Fr & Eur.

Diccionario de Traumatologia Jims. Jims Staff. 1991. (SPA.). 288p. pap. 59.95 (*0-7859-6111-9*, 88470923463) Fr & Eur.

Diccionario de Vitaminas. Leonard Mervyn. 1985. (CAT & SPA.). 240p. pap. 24.95 (*0-7859-4920-8*) Fr & Eur.

Diccionario del Psicoanalisis. Jean Laplanche & Jean-Bertrand Pontalis. Ed. by Fernando Cervantes Gimeno. 3rd deluxe ed. 1977. (SPA.). 558p. 65.50 (*0-7859-0894-3*, S-31445) Fr & Eur.

Diccionario Enciclopedico de la Vida Sexual, Set. Jesus Noguer More. 1974. (SPA.). 792p. 250.00 (*0-8288-5987-6*, S50029) Fr & Eur.

Diccionario Enciclopedico de Medicina "Jims" L. Braier. 4th ed. 1980. (ENG, FRE, GER, ITA & LAT.). 125.00 (*0-8288-0580-6*, S33099) Fr & Eur.

Diccionario Enciclopedico Ilustrado de Medicina. Emalsa Staff. 26th ed. 1987. (SPA.). 1760p. 225.00 (*0-7859-6242-5*, 8476054122); Set. 1985. (SPA.). 595.00 (*0-7859-6241-7*, 8476052235); Vol. 1. 1985. (SPA.). 650p. 225.00 (*0-7859-6238-7*, 8476052200); Vol. 2. 1985. 650p. 225.00 (*0-7859-6239-5*, 8476052219); Vol. 3. 1985. (SPA.). 650p. 225.00 (*0-7859-6240-9*, 8476052227) Fr & Eur.

Diccionario Familiar de Medicina Natural: Colloquial Dictionary of Natural Medicine. Emmerick-Armand Maury & Chantal De Rudder. 1981. (SPA.). 441p. 19.95 (*0-8288-1867-3*, S37815) Fr & Eur.

Diccionario Humano. Reta M. Iribarren. 2nd ed. 1975. (SPA.). 552p. pap. 19.95 (*0-8288-5823-3*, S50088) Fr & Eur.

Diccionario Medico. F. Beer-Poitevin. 1979.Tr. of Medical Dictionary. (SPA.). 352p. 95.00 (*0-8288-4776-2*, S3751) Fr & Eur.

Diccionario Medico. Salvat Staff. 1990. (SPA.). 738p. pap. 45.00 (*0-7859-5930-0*, 8434524775) Fr & Eur.

Diccionario Medico. Luigi Segatore & Gianangelo Poli. 7th ed. 1982. (SPA.). 1200p. 95.00 (*0-7859-5104-0*) Fr & Eur.

Diccionario Medico: De Bosillo. Prologue by Jose M. Mascaro Y Porcar. 2nd deluxe ed. 1974. (SPA.). 632p. 39.95 (*0-8288-5997-3*, S13673) Fr & Eur.

Diccionario Medico de Bolsillo. Salvat Staff. 1989. (SPA.). 640p. pap. 36.95 (*0-7859-5928-9*, 8434517892) Fr & Eur.

Diccionario Medico Dorland (Bolsillo) Newman W. Dorland. 1988. (SPA.). 900p. pap. 45.00 (*0-7859-6243-3*, 8476152825) Fr & Eur.

Diccionario Medico Illustrado. Newman W. Dorland. 27th ed. 1991. (SPA., Illus.). text 55.00 (*0-07-104004-8*) McGraw.

Diccionario Medico Labor para la Familia. H. Mommsen. (SPA.). 1979. (*0-8288-4775-4*, S50063); 6th ed. 1982. 880p. 150.00 (*0-7859-5093-1*) Fr & Eur.

Diccionario Medico Teide. Teide Staff. 1988. (SPA.). 660p. 39.95 (*0-7859-5893-2*, 8430780165) Fr & Eur.

Diccionario Monografico de Medicina y Salud. Ed. by Vox Staff. deluxe ed. 1979.Tr. of Monographic Dictionary of Medicine & Health. (SPA.). 24.95 (*0-8288-4778-9*, S36145) Fr & Eur.

Diccionario Mosby de Medicina y Ciencias de la Salud (Mosby's Pocket Dictionary of Medicine, Nursing & Allied Health) 1996. (SPA.). text (*84-8086-140-1*) Mosby-Doyma Libros ESP. *Dist:* Mosby Inc.

Diccionario Practico de Psicopatologia. Yves Poinso. 1976. (SPA.). 324p. 29.95 (*0-8288-5618-4*, S50194); pap. 29.95 (*0-8288-5619-2*, S50186) Fr & Eur.

Diccionario Pschyrembel de Ginecologia y Obstetricia. 1988. (SPA., Illus.). xii, 295p. lib. bdg. 52.35 (*3-11-011876-9*) De Gruyter.

Diccionario Tecnologico de Salud Publica Veterinaria. Moreno L. Saez. 1990. (SPA.). 166p. pap. 21.95 (*0-7859-6219-0*, 8473600975) Fr & Eur.

Diccionario Terminologico de Ciencias Medicas. Cientificas y Tecnic Staff. 1991. (SPA.). 1424p. 150.00 (*0-7859-6042-2*, 8445800701) Fr & Eur.

Diccionario Terminologico de Ciencias Medicas. Salvat Staff. 13th ed. 1978.Tr. of Terminological Dictionary of the Medical Sciences. (SPA.). 1088p. 250.00 (*0-7859-5048-6*) Fr & Eur.

Diccionario Visual Altea del Cuerpo Humano. Equipo Dorling Staff. 1992. (SPA.). 64p. pap. 45.00 (*0-7859-5997-1*, 8437245184) Fr & Eur.

Dictations: On Haunted Writing. Avital Ronell. 1993. LC 93-8475. 205p. pap. 15.00 (*0-8032-8945-6*, Bison Books) U of Nebr Pr.

Dictionaire de Pratique Gerontologique. Yves Kagan. 1996. (FRE.). 840p. 150.00 (*0-7859-9257-X*) Fr & Eur.

Dictionaire des Termes Odontostomatologiques. Louis Verchere. 3rd ed. 1992. (FRE.). 200p. 65.00 (*0-8288-9475-2*, M15415) Fr & Eur.

Dictionaire Francais-Anglais, Anglais-Francais de Medecine Physique de Reedaptaticn Ponctionelles. Herman L. Kamenetz & Georgette Kamenetz. 1972. (ENG & FRE.). 192p. 39.95 (*0-8288-6366-0*, M-6325) Fr & Eur.

Dictionar de Mecanica. Artexim. 1980. (FRE & RUM.). (*0-8288-2161-5*, M15837) Fr & Eur.

Dictionaries of Psychology Ed. by Ian Stuart-Hamilton. 1995. 800p. (*1-85302-342-6*) Jessica Kingsley GBR. *Dist:* Taylor & Francis.

Dictionary Catalog of the Applied Life Studies Library, First Supplement, Set. 1982. (C). 315.00 (*0-8161-0390-9*, Macmillan Ref) Gale.

Dictionary Catalog of the London School of Hygren & Tropical Medicine. 1994. 175.00 (*0-7838-2224-3*, Macmillan Ref) Gale.

Dictionary Catalogue of the London School of Hygiene & Tropical Medicine, Set. University of London Staff. 1970. 705.00 (*0-8161-0703-3*, Macmillan Ref) Gale.

Dictionary Clinical Medicine. Stephan Dressler. 1990. (ENG & GER.). 841p. 115.00 (*0-89573-993-3*, Wiley-VCH) Wiley.

Dictionary Clinical Medicine English, German. S. Dressler. 1990. (ENG & GER.). 400p. lib. bdg. 195.00 (*0-8288-3408-3*, 3527154639) Fr & Eur.

Dictionary for Brain Tumor Patients. 1993. (*0-944093-27-2*) Am Brain Tumor.

Dictionary for Clinical Trials. Simon Day. 1999. LC 99-11151. (Illus.). 228p. 124.95 (*0-471-98611-9*); pap. 34.95 (*0-471-98596-1*) Wiley.

Dictionary for Lupus Patients. Ed. by Linda K. Rohner. 1993. 60p. pap. text 9.95 (*0-9638245-0-3*) Mtn Gem Pubng.

Dictionary for Nurses. J. Delamare. 1996. Orig. Title: Dictionnaire de l'Infirmiere. 512p. pap. (*2-224-02293-X*) Maloine FRA. *Dist:* IBD Ltd.

Dictionary for Physicians. F. Lejeune & Werner E. Bunjes. 2nd ed. 1968. (ENG & GER.). 459p. 175.00 (*0-7859-0829-3*, M-7106) Fr & Eur.

Dictionary for the Mental Health Professional: Psychiatrists, Psychologists. Dorothy H. Mills. 1993. 250p. 24.95 (*0-8288-1871-1*, S50021) Fr & Eur.

Dictionary for Veterinary Science & Biosciences. Roy Mack. 1987. (ENG & GER.). 324p. pap. 85.00 (*0-8288-2385-5*, M4375) Fr & Eur.

Dictionary-Handbook of Nuclear Medicine & Clinical Imaging. Ed. by Mario P. Iturralde. 1990. 576p. 157.95 (*0-8493-3233-8*, RC78) CRC Pr.

Dictionary Medicale: French/German/French. H. Unseld. 1993. (FRE & GER.). 707p. 125.00 (*0-320-00588-7*) Fr & Eur.

Dictionary Medicaments Conseil Grand Public. Thera. 10th ed. 1998. (FRE.). 125.00 (*0-320-00225-X*) Fr & Eur.

Dictionary of Abbreviations, Acronyms, Synonyms & Symbols Used in Medicine. Samuel A. Tsur. 1999. LC 99-30739. 646p. 166.00 (*0-444-82904-0*) Elsevier.

Dictionary of Abbreviations in Medical Science. Rolf Heister. 1989. (ENG & GER.). 287p. lib. bdg. 85.00 (*0-8288-3587-X*, F122440) Fr & Eur.

Dictionary of Abbreviations in Medical Sciences. Rolf Heister. 1989. 287p. 52.95 (*0-387-50487-7*) Spr-Verlag.

***Dictionary of Acronyms & Synonyms in Medicine.** David Allison & Nicola Strickland. 2001. 220p. pap. (*1-901865-47-9*) Isis Med.

Dictionary of Acupuncture Terms, Concepts & Points. Ralph Alan Dale. 1993. LC 93-90608. (Illus.). 431p. pap. 69.00 (*1-877589-11-X*) Dialectic Pubng.

Dictionary of Adult Emergency Medicine see Dictionnaire des Urgences Medicales de l'Adulte

Dictionary of AIDS-Related Terminology. Jeffrey T. Huber. 1993. 172p. 45.00 (*1-55570-117-5*) Neal-Schuman.

Dictionary of Alcohol Use & Abuse: Slang, Terms & Terminology. Compiled by Ernest L. Abel. 1985. LC 84-22521. 189p. lib. bdg. 75.00 (*0-313-24631-9*, ABA/, Greenwood Pr) Greenwood.

Dictionary of Alternative Medicine. Joseph Segen. 1997. LC 98-112697. 407p. (C). pap. 54.95 (*0-8385-1620-3*, A-1620-2) McGraw-Hill Prof.

Dictionary of Alternative Medicine. Segen. 2nd ed. 2000. pap. text 31.95 (*0-8385-1621-1*, Medical Exam) Appleton & Lange.

Dictionary of American Medical Biography Ed. by Joseph Carvalho et al. 1984. LC 82-21110. Set. 1028p. lib. bdg. 195.00 (*0-313-21378-X*, KDA/); Vol. 1. 600p. lib. bdg. 100.00 (*0-313-24333-6*, KDA/01); Vol. 2. 600p. lib. bdg. 100.00 (*0-313-24334-4*, KDA/02) Greenwood.

Dictionary of American Nursing Biography. Ed. by Martin Kaufman et al. 1988. LC 87-25454. 472p. lib. bdg. 75.00 (*0-313-24520-7*, KAU/, Greenwood Pr) Greenwood.

Dictionary of Animal Health Terminology. Ed. by Roy Mack. 1992. LC 92-9212. (ENG, FRE, GER, LAT & SPA.). 434p. 143.50 (*0-444-88085-2*) Elsevier.

Dictionary of Animal Health Terminology in English, French, Spanish, German & Latin. Office International des Epizooties Staff. Ed. by Roy Mack. 1992. (ENG, FRE, GER, LAT & SPA.). 426p. 250.00 (*0-8288-9215-6*) Fr & Eur.

Dictionary of Antibiotics & Related Substances. Ed. by B. W. Bycroft. 1997. 964p. ring bd. 1024.95 (*0-412-25450-6*) Chapman & Hall.

Dictionary of Bach Flower Remedies. T. H. Jones. 1976. 105p. pap. (*0-85207-145-0*) C W Daniel GBR. *Dist:* Natl Bk Netwk.

Dictionary of Behavior Therapy Techniques. Ed. by Alan S. Bellack & Michel Hersen. 1985. (General Psychology Ser.: No. 132). 304p. 60.00 (*0-08-030168-1*); pap. 26.50 (*0-08-030167-3*) Elsevier (Pergamon Pr).

***Dictionary of Behavioral Assessment Techniques.** Ed. by Michel Hersen & Alan S. Bellack. 2002. (Foundations of Psychology). 590p. reprint ed. pap. text Price not set. (*0-9712427-2-0*) E Werner Pubns.

Dictionary of Behavioral Assessment Techniques. Ed. by Michel Hersen & Alan S. Bellack. 1988. (General Psychology Ser.: No. 147). 588p. 110.00 (*0-08-031975-0*, Pergamon Pr) Elsevier.

Dictionary of Biological Psychology. James W. Kalat. 1994. (Psychology Ser.). mass mkt. 6.00 (*0-534-26010-1*) Brooks-Cole.

Dictionary of Biology. Guenther Haensch & Gisela Haberkamp de Anton. 2nd enl. rev. ed. 1981. (ENG, FRE, GER & SPA.). 692p. 190.00 (*0-444-41968-3*) Elsevier.

***Dictionary of Biomedical Science.** Peter J. Gosling. 2001. 512p. (C). (gr. 13). pap. 25.95 (*0-415-23723-8*); text 90.00 (*0-415-24138-3*) Routledge.

Dictionary of Cat Symptoms. Glanze. 1992. 21.95 (*0-13-208695-6*) P-H.

Dictionary of Chemistry, Vol. 1. Richard R. Ernst. 1961. (ENG & GER.). 95.00 (*0-8288-6818-2*, M7037) Fr & Eur.

Dictionary of Child Psychiatry & Psychology: Diccionario de Psicologia y Psiquiatria Infantil. Alberto L. Merani. 1983. (SPA.). 176p. 28.50 (*0-8288-2221-2*, S39839) Fr & Eur.

Dictionary of Clinical Medicine. Stephan Dressler. 1991. (ENG & GER.). 878p. lib. bdg. 115.00 (*0-89573-992-5*, Wiley-VCH) Wiley.

Dictionary of Clinical Pharmacology for Doctors & Pharmacists: Woerterbuch der Klinischen Pharmakologie Fuer Mediziner und Pharmazeuten. R. K. Liedtke. 1980. (ENG & GER.). 245p. 49.95 (*0-8288-1838-X*, M15389) Fr & Eur.

Dictionary of Clinical Tests. Olivera Potparic & J. Gibson. 1993. (Illus.). 262p. lib. bdg. 52.95 (*1-85070-416-3*, Parthenon Pbng) CRC Pr.

Dictionary of Cognitive Psychology. Ed. by Ian Stuart-Hamilton. 1995. 250p. 49.95 (*1-85302-202-0*) Taylor & Francis.

Dictionary of Concepts in General Psychology, Vol. 7. John A. Popplestone & Marion W. McPherson. 1988. LC 88-3120. (Reference Sources for the Social Sciences & Humanities Ser.: No. 7). 391p. lib. bdg. 90.00 (*0-313-23190-7*, PGP/, Greenwood Pr) Greenwood.

Dictionary of Concepts in NMR. S. W. Homans. 2nd rev. ed. 1993. (Oxford Paperback Reference Ser.). (Illus.). 380p. pap. text 39.95 (*0-19-854765-X*) OUP.

Dictionary of Congenital Malformations & Disorders. Olivera Potparic & John Gibson. 1995. (Illus.). 192p. (C). lib. bdg. 60.95 (*1-85070-577-1*, Parthenon Pbng) CRC Pr.

Dictionary of Counseling. Colin Feltham. 1993. 228p. pap. 62.25 (*1-56593-261-7*, 0544) Singular Publishing.

Dictionary of Dental Pharmacology see Dictionnaire de Pharmacologie Dentaire

Dictionary of Dermatologic Terms. Robert L. Carter. 4th ed. 1992. 408p. 24.95 (*0-683-14691-2*) Lppncott W & W.

Dictionary of Developmental Disabilities Terminology. Pasquale J. Accardo & Barbara Y. Whitman. 1996. LC 95-47373. (Illus.). 368p. 55.95 (*1-55766-245-2*); text 35.95 (*1-55766-112-X*) P H Brookes.

Dictionary of Disaster Medicine & International Relief, English-German/German-English. Sisvan Gunn. 1996. (ENG & GER.). 304p. 95.00 (*0-7859-9526-9*) Fr & Eur.

Dictionary of Dog Symptoms. Glanze. 1992. 21.95 (*0-13-208703-0*) P-H.

Dictionary of Dog Symptoms. Glanze. 1992. pap. 12.95 (*0-13-208711-1*, Fireside) S&S Trade Pap.

Dictionary of Dream Interpretation. Gerald Schoenewolf. 1997. LC 96-31855. 320p. 50.00 (*0-7657-0041-7*) Aronson.

Dictionary of Drug Abuse Terms & Terminology. Ernest L. Abel. 1984. LC 83-22867. 137p. lib. bdg. 49.95 (*0-313-24095-7*, ADD/, Greenwood Pr) Greenwood.

Dictionary of Drugs. Satish Anand & Raj Kumar. 1990. (*81-7041-240-4*) Anmol IND. *Dist:* S Asia.

Dictionary of Drugs: Chemical Data, Set. 1990. 1550p. (gr. 13). ring bd. (*0-412-27300-4*, Chap & Hall CRC) CRC Pr.

Dictionary of Eldercare Terminology. Walter Feldesman & United Seniors Health Cooperative Staff. 1997. LC 97-490. 49.95 (*0-944847-19-6*) United Sr Hlth Co-op.

Dictionary of Emergency Homeopathy: Dictionnaire Homeopathique d'Urgentce. Louis Pommier. 13th ed. 1985. (ENG & FRE.). 765p. 75.00 (*0-7859-4836-8*, M6461) Fr & Eur.

Dictionary of Endocrinology & Related Biomedical Sciences. Constance R. Martin. 1995. (Illus.). 792p. text 85.00 (*0-19-506033-4*) OUP.

Dictionary of Epilepsy: Part I - Definitions. H. Gastaut. 1973. pap. text 20.00 (*92-4-154027-3*, 1150033) World Health.

Dictionary of Eponymic Names of Diseases & Syndromes. E. P. Mezhenina. 1982. 182p. 19.95 (*0-8288-1858-4*, M15443) Fr & Eur.

Dictionary of Evidence-Based Medicine. Alain Li Wan Po. 1998. LC 99-170133. 176p. pap. (*1-85775-305-4*) Radcliffe Med Pr GBR. *Dist:* Balogh.

Dictionary of Eye Terminology. Barbara Cassin & Sheila A. Solomon. Ed. by Melvin L. Rubin. 3rd rev. ed. 1997. (Illus.). 288p. spiral bd. 24.95 (*0-937404-44-6*) Triad Pub FL.

Dictionary of Family Therapy. Jacques Miermont. Ed. by Hugh Jenkins. Tr. by Chris Turner from FRE. 1995. (Illus.). 600p. (C). text 111.95 (*0-631-17048-0*) Blackwell Pubs.

Dictionary of Food Ingredients. Robert S. Igoe & Yiu H. Hui. 3rd ed. 1995. LC 95-4648. 216p. (C). (gr. 13). 45.00 (*0-412-07281-5*) Kluwer Academic.

Dictionary of Gene Technology. Gunter Kahl. 1994. 551p. 149.95 (*3-527-30005-8*, Wiley-VCH) Wiley.

Dictionary of Gene Technology Terms. Yong-He Zhang & M. Zhang. 2001. LC 00-62431. (Illus.). 504p. pap. 69.95 (*1-85070-015-X*, Parthenon Pbng) CRC Pr.

Dictionary of General Psychology: Basic Terminology & Key Concepts. Charles A. Heidenreich. rev. ed. 1970. (C). pap. text 7.95 (*0-8403-0171-5*) Heidenreich.

Dictionary of Gerontology. Diana K. Harris. 1988. LC 87-25142. 216p. lib. bdg. 55.00 (*0-313-25287-4*, HGE/, Greenwood Pr) Greenwood.

Dictionary of Gerontology & Geriatrics: In English, with Definitions, & Japanese (Transliterated & in Japanese Characters) S. Sri Kantha. 300p. (*0-444-82666-1*) Elsevier.

Dictionary of Gynecology: Dictionnaire de Gynecologie. Henri Rozenbaum. 1981. (ENG & FRE.). 312p. 85.00 (*0-8288-1826-6*) Fr & Eur.

Dictionary of Health Physics & Nuclear Sciences Terms. Rex J. Borders. Ed. by K. Paul Steinmeyer. 1991. 440p. 95.00 (*0-9630191-0-4*) RSA Pubns.

Dictionary of Helminthology & Plant Nematology. Ed. by G. I. Pozniak. 1979. (ENG & RUS.). 108p. 35.00 (*0-8288-4786-X*) Fr & Eur.

Dictionary of Homeopathic Medical Terminology see Yasgur's Homeopathic Dictionary & Holistic Health Reference

Dictionary of Human Oncology: A Concise Guide to Tumors. Olivera Potparic & J. Gibson. 1994. LC 93-35740. 173p. lib. bdg. 60.95 (*1-85070-472-4*, Parthenon Pbng) CRC Pr.

Dictionary of Hypnotism. Anita Evangelista. 1991. LC 90-36941. 288p. lib. bdg. 65.00 (*0-313-25967-4*, EVH/, Greenwood Pr) Greenwood.

Dictionary of Immunology. Ed. by W. John Herbert et al. 4th ed. 1995. (Illus.). 192p. text 42.00 (*0-12-752025-2*) Acad Pr.

Dictionary of Infections & Infectious Diseases. Olivera Potparic & J. Gibson. 1995. 156p. (C). lib. bdg. 38.95 (*1-85070-607-7*, Parthenon Pbng) CRC Pr.

Dictionary of International Medical Abbreviations. Maurice A. Touati. 1994. 474p. 60.00 (*0-7859-8755-X*) Fr & Eur.

Dictionary of International Medical Abbreviations. Maurice A. Touati. 1994. 474p. (*2-85608-058-8*) La Maison Du Dict FRA. *Dist:* IBD Ltd.

Dictionary of Key Words in Psychology. Frank J. Bruno. 1988. 274p. pap. 14.95 (*0-7102-1394-8*, A3116, Routledge Thoemms) Routledge.

Dictionary of Kleinian Thought. R. D. Hinshelwood. 1991. LC 90-28363. 520p. 50.00 (*0-87668-556-4*) Aronson.

Dictionary of Managed Behavioral Health Care: "A" Is for "Access" Jodi Aronson. 1997. LC 97-17437. 50p. pap. 9.95 (*0-87630-846-9*) Brunner-Routledge.

Dictionary of Medical Acronyms & Abbreviations. Stanley Jablonski. 3rd ed. 1997. LC 97-80820. pap. 19.95 (*1-56053-264-5*) Hanley & Belfus.

Dictionary of Medical & Surgical Syndromes. J. Gibson & Olivera Potparic. 1991. (Illus.). 202p. (C). lib. bdg. 52.95 (*1-85070-338-8*, Parthenon Pbng) CRC Pr.

Dictionary of Medical Archaeology. K. Krishna Murthy. 1996. (C). (*81-85067-93-7*) Sundeep Prak IND. *Dist:* S Asia.

Dictionary of Medical Derivations: The Real Meaning of Medical Terms. William Casselman et al. 1998. LC 97-26856. (Illus.). 436p. 46.95 (*1-85070-771-5*, Parthenon Pbng) CRC Pr.

Dictionary of Medical Engineering. Roald Albert. 1998. (ENG, FRE, GER & RUS.). 550p. 160.00 (*3-86117-051-5*) Routledge.

***Dictionary of Medical Eponyms.** Robert D. Edwards et al. 2001. (Illus.). 400p. ring bd. 37.95 (*1-85070-333-7*, Parthenon Pbng) CRC Pr.

Dictionary of Medical Eponyms. B. G. Firkin & J. A. Whitworth. 2nd ed. 1996. (Illus.). 452p. (C). 64.95 (*1-85070-477-5*, Parthenon Pbng) CRC Pr.

Dictionary of Medical Equipment. Malcolm Brown et al. 1997. (Illus.). 312p. (C). (gr. 13). pap. 128.95 (*0-412-28290-9*) Chapman & Hall.

Dictionary of Medical Imaging: French-English, English-French. Dorothy Nakos. 1995. (ENG & FRE.). 108p. 49.95 (*0-7859-9752-0*) Fr & Eur.

Dictionary of Medical Laboratory Diagnostics, English, French, German: English, French, German. Ursula Spranger. 1993. (ENG, FRE & GER.). 439p. 295.00 (*0-7859-8826-2*) Fr & Eur.

Dictionary of Medical Management Terms & Initialisms. Ed. by Wesley Curry. 1998. LC 97-78155. 178p. pap. 48.00 (*0-924674-62-8*) Am Coll Phys Execs.

Dictionary of Medical Objects. 1983. 1344p. 360.00 (*0-387-12138-2*) Spr-Verlag.

Dictionary of Medical Siglas: Dictionnaire des Sigles Medicaux. J. P. Poinsotte. 1982. (ENG & FRE.). 146p. pap. text 24.95 (*0-8288-4420-8*, M9772) Fr & Eur.

Dictionary of Medical Sociology. William C. Cockerham & Ferris J. Ritchey. 1997. LC 96-36575. 200p. lib. bdg. 75.00 (0-313-29269-8, Greenwood Pr) Greenwood.

Dictionary of Medical Syndromes. Sabina I. Magalini & Sergio C. Magalini. 4th ed. 1996. LC 96-41119. 976p. text 125.00 (0-397-58418-0) Lppncott W & W.

Dictionary of Medical Terms. (C). pap. (1-85986-010-9) OUP.

Dictionary of Medical Terms, English-Spanish, Spanish-English. 7th ed. 1991. (ENG & SPA.). 872p. 150.00 (0-7859-4904-6) Fr & Eur.

Dictionary of Medical Terms in Galen. Richard J. Durling. 1993. LC 92-39986. (Studies in Ancient Medicine: No. 5). (ENG & GRE.). xiii, 344p. 148.00 (90-04-09754-6) Brill Academic Pubs.

Dictionary of Medications see Dictionnaire des Medicaments

Dictionary of Medicine. Klaus P. Eschenbach. 1983. (ENG & GER.). 606p. 49.95 (0-8288-0568-7, M6454) Fr & Eur.

Dictionary of Medicine. Ed. by Peter Hodgson Collin. 2nd rev. ed. 1998. 450p. 55.00 (1-57958-074-2) Fitzroy Dearborn.

Dictionary of Medicine. Peter Collin Publishing Staff. 3rd ed. 2000. 460p. pap. (1-901659-45-3) P Collin.

Dictionary of Medicine: French-English/English-French. Svetolik P. Djordjevic. 2001. LC 00-63753. (ENG & FRE.). xi, 1149p. 179.50 (1-887563-53-9) Schreiber Pub.

Dictionary of Medicine: Russian - French. G. Bejenar. (FRE & RUS.). lib. bdg. 75.00 (0-8288-2615-3, F12776) Fr & Eur.

Dictionary of Medicine, German & English. Jurgen Nohring. 1987. (ENG & GER.). 848p. 195.00 (0-8288-0572-5, M1735) Fr & Eur.

Dictionary of Mental Health. Richard B. Fisher. 1983. (Illus.). 268p. pap. 12.00 (0-586-08339-1) Academy Chi Pubs.

Dictionary of Modern Herbalism: A Comprehensive Guide to Practical Herbal Therapy. Simon Y. Mills. 1997. 224p. reprint ed. 7.98 (1-56731-223-3, MJF Bks) Fine Comms.

Dictionary of Modern Herbalism: The Complete Guide to Herbs & Herbal Therapy. Simon Y. Mills. 1985. 208p. pap. 12.95 (0-89281-238-9, Heal Arts VT) Inner Tradit.

Dictionary of Modern Medicine: A Sourcebook of Current Medical Expressions, Jargon & Technical Terms. J. C. Segen. 1992. (Illus.). 800p. (C). lib. bdg. 82.95 (1-85070-321-3, Parthenon Pbng) CRC Pr.

Dictionary of Natural Foods. William L. Esser. 1983. LC 83-72140. (Illus.). pap. 9.95 (0-914532-30-8) Amer Natural Hygiene.

Dictionary of Natural Healing. Deborah R. Mitchell. 1998. LC 98-195262. (Dictionary of Natural Healing Ser.: Vol. 1). 272p. pap. 5.99 (0-312-96516-8, Tor Books) T Doherty Assocs.

Dictionary of Natural Products: Terms in the Field of Pharmacognosy Relating to Natural, Medicinal, & Pharmaceutical Materials & the Plants, Animals & Minerals from Which They Are Derived. George M. Hocking. 1997. LC 97-321. 1024p. 139.50 (0-937548-31-6) Plexus Pub.

Dictionary of Nursing. Churchill Livingstone. 17th ed. 1996. pap. text (0-443-05534-3) Church.

Dictionary of Nursing Theory & Research. Bethel A. Powers & Thomas R. Knapp. 2nd ed. 1995. 224p. 81.95 (0-8039-5625-8, 4951); pap. 39.95 (0-8039-5626-6, 4952) Sage.

Dictionary of Nutrition & Dietetics. Karen E. Drummond. 1996. (Culinary Arts Ser.). 391p. 60.00 (0-471-29370-9, VNR) Wiley.

Dictionary of Nutrition & Food Technology. Arnold E. Bender. 6th ed. 1990. 336p. text 82.95 (0-408-03753-9) Buttrwrth-Heinemann.

Dictionary of Obstetrics & Gynecology. 1988. (Illus.). xxi, 277p. (C). lib. bdg. 52.35 (3-11-011875-0) De Gruyter.

Dictionary of Odontological Materials & Products: Dictionnaire des Materiels, Materiaux et Produits Odontologiques. 1986. (FRE.). 876p. 150.00 (0-8288-1785-5) Fr & Eur.

Dictionary of Ophthalmic Optics. Arthur H. Keeney et al. Ed. by Robert E. Hagman, Jr. 1994. LC 94-38287. (Illus.). 345p. pap. text 44.99 (0-7506-9592-7) Buttrwrth-Heinemann.

Dictionary of Pediatric Dermatology: Dictionnaire de Dermatologie Pediatrique. J. L. Bonafe. 1985. (ENG & FRE.). 175.00 (0-8288-1790-1, M15583) Fr & Eur.

Dictionary of Pharmaceutical Medicine. Gerhard Nahler. 1994. LC 94-11648. 177p. 34.95 (0-387-82557-6) Spr-Verlag.

Dictionary of Pharmaceutical Medicine: English-German, German-English. Gerhard Nahler. 1994. (ENG & GER.). 177p. 69.95 (0-7859-9985-X) Fr & Eur.

Dictionary of Pharmacological Agents: Properties & Synonyms. Ian Morton & Judith Hall. 1999. LC 99-42527. (0-7514-0499-3) Kluwer Academic.

Dictionary of Pharmacology & Allied Topics. Ed. by D. R. Laurence. 2nd ed. 1998. LC 98-33476. 386p. 161.50 (0-444-82591-6); 373p. pap. 39.50 (0-444-50050-2) Elsevier (Excerpta Medica).

Dictionary of Philosophy & Psychology: 1901-1902 Edition Ed. by James M. Baldwin. 2nd ed. 1998. (Illus.). 1576p. 295.00 (1-85506-596-7) Thoemmes Pr.

Dictionary of Plant Toxins: Phytotoxins, Vol. 1. Ed. by Jeffrey B. Harborne et al. 1996. LC 96-11164. 540p. 565.00 (0-471-95107-2) Wiley.

Dictionary of Practical Materia Medica 1980. 2585p. (C). text 224.95 (0-8464-1004-4) Beekman Pubs.

Dictionary of Practical Materia Medica. John Henrik Clarke. 1980. 175.00 (0-85032-139-5) St Mut.

Dictionary of Practical Materia Medica. John H. Clark. 3rd ed. 1991. 1635p. 225.00 (0-8464-4505-0) Beekman Pubs.

Dictionary of Principal Medications: Dictionnaire des Medicaments Principaux. Lagier Lechat. 1982. (FRE & SPA.). 528p. 110.00 (0-8288-1815-0, M15386) Fr & Eur.

Dictionary of Procurement Terms. 1992. 108p. pap. (0-644-12783-X) AGPS Pr AUS. *Dist:* Intl Spec Bk.

Dictionary of Prosthetic Rehabilitation. Ed. by David Trainor et al. 1998. (Illus.). 288p. (Orig.). pap. 35.00 (1-886236-18-6) ABI Prof Pubns.

Dictionary of Protopharmacology: Therapeutic Practices 1700-1850. J. Worth Estes. 1990. (Illus.). 220p. 39.95 (0-88135-068-0, Sci Hist) Watson Pub Intl.

Dictionary of Psychiatry & Medical Psychology: Woerterbuch der Psychiatrie und Medizinischen Psychologie. Uwe H. Peters. 4th ed. 1990. (ENG, FRE & GER.). 676p. 69.95 (0-8288-0586-5, M 6972) Fr & Eur.

Dictionary of Psychoanalysis: Diccionario de Psicoanalisis. Pierre Fedida. 3rd ed. 1988. (ENG & SPA.). 176p. pap. (0-7859-4967-4) Fr & Eur.

Dictionary of Psychological Medicine Daniel H. Tuke. 1976. LC 75-16737. (Classics in Psychiatry Ser.). reprint ed. Set. 121.95 (0-405-07457-3); Vol. 1. 60.95 (0-405-07458-1); Vol. 2. 60.95 (0-405-07459-X) Ayer.

Dictionary of Psychological Testing, Assessment & Treatment. Ian Stuart-Hamilton. 1996. 300p. pap. text (1-85302-147-4) Jessica Kingsley GBR. *Dist:* Taylor & Francis.

Dictionary of Psychology. V. V. Davydov. 1983. (RUS.). 448p. 29.95 (0-8288-2210-7, M15381) Fr & Eur.

Dictionary of Psychology. W. D. Frohlich & J. Drever. 1983. (ENG & GER.). 443p. 49.95 (0-8288-2206-9, M4649) Fr & Eur.

Dictionary of Psychology. J. P. Chaplin. 2nd rev. ed. 1985. 528p. mass mkt. 7.99 (0-440-31925-0, LE) Dell.

Dictionary of Psychology: Diccionario de Psicologia. Friedrich Dorsch. 6th ed. 1991. (ENG & SPA.). 1040p. 125.00 (0-7859-4966-6) Fr & Eur.

Dictionary of Psychology & Psychiatry, Set. R. Haas. 1988. (ENG & GER.). 906p. 188.00 (0-88937-037-0) Hogrefe & Huber Pubs.

Dictionary of Psychology & Psychiatry: English-German, Vol. 1. Ed. by Roland Haas. 1980. LC 81-463989. (ENG & GER.). 466p. (C). text 88.00 (0-88937-000-1) Hogrefe & Huber Pubs.

Dictionary of Psychology & Psychiatry: German-English, Vol. 2. Ed. by Roland Haas. 1988. LC 81-463989. (ENG & GER.). 440p. (C). text 116.00 (0-88937-013-3) Hogrefe & Huber Pubs.

Dictionary of Psychology in 3 Languages see Dictionnaire de Psychologie en Trois Langues

Dictionary of Psychology with Thesaurus. William Verplanck. (0-89197-729-5) Irvington.

Dictionary of Public Health Promotion & Education: Terms & Concepts. Naomi N. Modeste. 1996. LC 95-35417. 194p. 64.95 (0-7619-0002-0, 1533); pap. 31.95 (0-7619-0003-9, 1534) Sage.

Dictionary of Radiation Protection, Radiobiology & Nuclear Medicine. Ralf Sube. 1986. (ENG, FRE, GER & RUS.). 475p. 195.00 (0-8288-0588-1, F 96000) Fr & Eur.

Dictionary of Radiologic Terminology. Alphons Jacob & Herbert L. Jackson. 1982. 118p. (C). 17.50 (0-87527-216-9) Green.

Dictionary of Radiological Engineering. Gustav F. Neuder & Heinz M. Ullrich. 1979. (ENG, FRE & GER.). (C). pap. text 53.10 (3-11-007807-4) De Gruyter.

Dictionary of Rational Emotive Behavior Therapy. Dryden. 1994. 174p. pap. 39.95 (1-56593-508-X, 1174) Singular Publishing.

Dictionary of Rational Emotive Behaviour Therapy. Windy Dryden & Michael Neenan. 22.95 (1-897635-71-0, B152) Inst Rational-Emotive.

Dictionary of Rehabilitation. M. G. Eisenberg. 1995. LC 94-48400. (Illus.). 392p. 43.95 (0-8261-8890-7) Springer Pub.

Dictionary of Sports Injuries & Disorders. Olivera Potparic & J. Gibson. 1996. 156p. 38.95 (1-85070-686-7, Parthenon Pbng) CRC Pr.

Dictionary of Steroids: Chemical Data Structure, Set. Ed. by D. N. Kirk et al. 1991. 1824p. (gr. 13). ring bd. 1044.95 (0-412-27060-9, A5565, Chap & Hall CRC) CRC Pr.

Dictionary of Street Alcohol & Drug Terms. Peter Johnson et al. 4th ed. 1993. 200p. (Orig.). (C). pap. 30.00 (0-941375-48-X) DIANE Pub.

Dictionary of Substances & Their Effects: Index. Richardson. 1996. 320p. (C). (0-85404-814-6) Royal Soc Chem GBR. *Dist:* Spr-Verlag.

Dictionary of Symbols & Imagery. 1984. 530p. 127.50 (0-7204-8021-3) Elsevier.

Dictionary of Symptoms. Joan Gomez. rev. ed. 1992. LC 82-42525. (Illus.). 383p. pap. 8.95 (0-8128-6230-9, Scrbrough Hse) Madison Bks UPA.

Dictionary of Syndromes & Inherited Disorders. Ed. by Patricia Gilbert. 3rd ed. 2000. 373p. lib. bdg. 45.00 (1-57958-226-5) Fitzroy Dearborn.

Dictionary of Technical Medical Terms: Diccionario de los Terminos Tecnicos de Medicina. M. Garnier & Valery Delamare. 20th ed. 1981. (ENG & SPA.). 1114p. 39.95 (0-8288-1866-5, S60551) Fr & Eur.

Dictionary of Technical Medical Terms: Dictionnaire des Termes Techniques de Medecine. Valery Delamare & M. Garnier. 21st ed. 1984. (ENG & FRE.). 880p. 95.00 (0-8288-1806-1) Fr & Eur.

Dictionary of the Bach Flower Remedies. T. W. Jones. 18th ed. 48p. pap. 7.95 (0-8464-4192-6) Beekman Pubs.

Dictionary of the Biochemistry of Food & Nutrition. Jean Adrian et al. 1981.Tr. of Dictionnaire de Biochimie Alimentaire et de Nutriition. (ENG & FRE.). 320p. 125.00 (0-8288-4440-2, M9626) Fr & Eur.

Dictionary of the History of Medicine. Anton Sebastian. 1999. LC 98-32249. (Illus.). 788p. 99.95 (1-85070-021-4) CRC Pr.

Dictionary of the Pharmach Vol. 1: Woerterbuch der Pharmazie: Biologie, Chemie, Technologie. H. Auterhoff. 1981. (ENG & GER.). 532p. 95.00 (0-8288-1835-5, M15388) Fr & Eur.

Dictionary of the Rheumatic Diseases: Health Status Measurement, Vol. III. American College of Rheumatology, Glossary Committ. 1988. 80p. (C). pap. text (0-911059-03-2) Cntct Assocs Intl.

Dictionary of Theoretical Concepts in Biology. Keith E. Roe & Richard G. Frederick. 1981. LC 80-19889. 380p. 50.00 (0-8108-1353-X) Scarecrow.

Dictionary of Toxicology. Ed. by Robert A. Lewis. 1996. LC 96-35759. 1127p. 79.95 (1-56670-223-2, L1223) Lewis Pubs.

Dictionary of Toxicology. Ernest Hodgson et al. 2nd ed. 1998. 608p. 130.00 (1-56159-216-1) Nature Pubg Grp.

Dictionary of Ultrasound. Ed. by S. Schering. 1996. (Illus.). 168p. 49.95 (0-632-04171-4) Blackwell Sci.

Dictionary of Veterinary & Zoological Terms: Dictionnaire des Termes Veterinaires et Zootech-Niques. Martial Villemin. 3rd ed. 1984. 470p. 95.00 (0-8288-2384-7, M4674) Fr & Eur.

Dictionary of Veterinary Epidemiology. Ed. by Bernard Toma et al. 1999. LC 99-24920. (Illus.). 300p. pap. 59.95 (0-8138-2639-X) Iowa U Pr.

Dictionary of Veterinary Medicine & Biosciences, German-English, English-German, 4 Language Index. Roy Mack. 2nd ed. 1996. (ENG, FRE, GER & LAT.). 824p. 195.00 (0-7859-9807-1) Fr & Eur.

Dictionary of Veterinary Medicine, English, French, German, Russian. Gotthard Ilchmann. 1993. (ENG, FRE, GER & RUS.). 414p. 295.00 (0-7859-9987-6) Fr & Eur.

Dictionary of Veterinary Medicine German-English - English-German. R. Mack. 2nd ed. 1997. (ENG & GER.). 823p. (3-8263-3055-2) Blckwell Wissenschafts DEU. *Dist:* IBD Ltd.

Dictionary of Veterinary Medicine in English, French, German & Russian. Gotthard Ilchmann. 1993. (ENG, FRE, GER & RUS.). 414p. 175.00 (0-7859-9347-9) Fr & Eur.

Dictionary of Visual Science. David Cline et al. 3rd ed. 1980. LC 78-14640. 736p. 40.00 (0-8019-6778-3); 4th ed. 1989. LC 88-20235. (Illus.). 848p. text 55.00 (0-8019-7862-9) NP-Chilton.

Dictionnaire Abrege des Termes de Medecine. Jacques Delamare. 1990. (FRE.). (0-7859-7822-4, 2-224-01940-8) Fr & Eur.

Dictionnaire Anglais-Francais des Sciences Medicales & Paramedicales see Medical & Paramedical Dictionary English-French

Dictionnaire Atlas d'Anatomie, Set. Pierre Kamina. 1984. (FRE.). lib. bdg. 395.00 (0-8288-2620-X, 2224009321) Fr & Eur.

Dictionnaire Bilingue de l'Edition: French-English, English-French. Philippe Schuwer. 1993. (ENG & FRE.). 447p. pap. 95.00 (0-7859-4837-6, M6508) Fr & Eur.

Dictionnaire Chinois-Francais des Termes Medicaux Usuels. L'Hygiene Populaire Staff. 1990. (CHI & FRE.). (0-7859-8702-9, 7117006668) Fr & Eur.

Dictionnaire Clinique des Therapies Familiales Systemiques. Jean-Claude Benoit et al. 1988. (FRE.). (0-7859-7935-2, 2-7101-0694-9) Fr & Eur.

Dictionnaire Conseil des Medicaments Vendus Sans Ordonnance. Jean-Paul Giroud & Charles Hagege. 1987. (FRE.). (0-7859-7877-1, 2-268-00440-6) Fr & Eur.

Dictionnaire de Biochimie Alimentaire et de Nutruition see Dictionary of the Biochemistry of Food & Nutrition

Dictionnaire de Cardiologie. Masson Staff. 1986. (FRE.). 352p. 135.00 (0-7859-7827-5, 2225802521) Fr & Eur.

Dictionnaire de Cardiologie. Paul E. Valere. 1986. (FRE.). 352p. 95.00 (0-8288-1829-0, F28480) Fr & Eur.

Dictionnaire de Dermatologie. Francois Daniel. 1990. (FRE.). 760p. lib. bdg. 225.00 (0-8288-2593-9) Fr & Eur.

Dictionnaire de Genetique. Philippe L'Heritier. 1979. (FRE.). 272p. pap. 69.95 (0-7859-7824-0, 2225526575) Fr & Eur.

Dictionnaire de Graphologie et des Termes Psychologiques Correspondants. Augusto Vels. 1993. (FRE.). 659p. pap. 95.00 (0-7859-7987-5, 2733904221) Fr & Eur.

Dictionnaire de Gynecologie et D'Obstetrique: Termes Usuels S'Hier et D'Aujourd'Hui. Alain Mavel. 1990. (FRE.). 592p. pap. (0-7859-0499-9, 2718404957) Fr & Eur.

Dictionnaire de la Medecine Larousse. Larousse Staff. 1990. (FRE.). pap. 16.95 (0-7859-7850-X, 2253037842) Fr & Eur.

Dictionnaire de la Nouvelle Dietetique. Albert-Francois Creff. 1984. (FRE.). 607p. 69.95 (0-7859-8631-6, 222104276x) Fr & Eur.

Dictionnaire de l'Homeopathie. J. Boulet. 1998. (FRE.). 69.95 (0-320-00227-6) Fr & Eur.

Dictionnaire de l'Infirmiere see Dictionary for Nurses

Dictionnaire de Matiere Medicale Homeopathique. Andre O. Julian. 1981. (FRE.). 496p. 150.00 (0-8288-1811-8) Fr & Eur.

Dictionnaire de Medecine du Sport. Philippe Most. 1987. (FRE.). 274p. pap. 95.00 (0-7859-7828-3, 2225810176) Fr & Eur.

Dictionnaire de Medecine Flammarion. Serge Kernbaum. 5th ed. 1994. (FRE.). 1024p. 95.00 (0-8288-2613-7, M6123) Fr & Eur.

Dictionnaire de Medicaments Conseil, Grand Public. 9th ed. 1997. (FRE.). 492p. pap. (2-85270-631-8) SEMP FRA. *Dist:* IBD Ltd.

Dictionnaire de Medicaments de Conseil Grand Public. 1997. (FRE.). 88.00 (0-7859-9723-7) Fr & Eur.

Dictionnaire de Medecine Chinoise Traditionelle. Jean-Francois Borsarello. 1984. (FRE.). 248p. 225.00 (0-7859-7826-7, 2225800855) Fr & Eur.

Dictionnaire de Pathologies Professionelles et Medecine du Travail. Frejaville Hachet. 1988. (FRE.). 1004p. 195.00 (0-7859-7819-4, 2224017243) Fr & Eur.

Dictionnaire de Pharmacologie Dentaire. Roger Viellefosse. 1970.Tr. of Dictionary of Dental Pharmacology. (FRE.). 228p. 49.95 (0-8288-6516-7, M-6550) Fr & Eur.

Dictionnaire de Psychanalyse. Elisabeth Roudinesco. 1997. (FRE.). 1200p. 125.00 (0-7859-9473-4) Fr & Eur.

Dictionnaire de Psychologie. Roland Doron. 1991. (FRE.). 776p. pap. 175.00 (0-7859-7744-9, 2130435513) Fr & Eur.

Dictionnaire de Psychologie en Trois Langues Hubert C. Duijker & Maria Van Sijswijk. 1977.Tr. of Dictionary of Psychology in 3 Languages. (ENG, FRE & GER.). 416p. ring bd. 165.00 (0-7859-0938-9, M-4661) Fr & Eur.

Dictionnaire de Psychologie en Trois Langues, Vol. 2. Hubert C. Duijker. 1977.Tr. of Dictionary of Psychology in 3 Languages. (ENG & GER.). 356p. ring bd. 165.00 (0-7859-4782-5, M4660) Fr & Eur.

Dictionnaire d'Epidemiologie. Jammal. 1988. (FRE.). 171p. pap. 65.00 (0-7859-7820-8, 2224018029) Fr & Eur.

Dictionnaire d'Epidemiologie. Annette Leclerc et al. 1990. (FRE.). 143p. (0-7859-0506-5, 2876710382) Fr & Eur.

Dictionnaire des Articles Medico-Chirurgicaux, Articles de Pansements. ETIM Staff. 1988. (FRE.). 1200p. 295.00 (0-7859-8231-0, 2905201045) Fr & Eur.

Dictionnaire des Difficultes du Francais Medical. S. Querin. 1998. (FRE.). 69.95 (0-320-00212-8) Fr & Eur.

Dictionnaire des Eponymes Medicaux: French-English. Henri Van Hoof. 1993. (ENG & FRE.). 405p. pap. 105.00 (0-7859-8187-X, 2877230716) Fr & Eur.

Dictionnaire Des Examens Biologiques et Investigations Paracliniques. Herve Durand. 3rd ed. 1991. (FRE.). 488p. pap. 110.00 (0-7859-7917-4, 2704006687) Fr & Eur.

Dictionnaire des Malades: Choix des Examens Complementaires. Herve Durand. 1989. (FRE.). 316p. pap. 79.95 (0-7859-7916-6, 2704005982) Fr & Eur.

Dictionnaire des Medicaments. Vittorio Fattorusso. 1992. (FRE.). 1000p. 79.95 (0-7859-7832-1, 2225826935) Fr & Eur.

Dictionnaire des Medicaments. Maurice Neuman. 1971.Tr. of Dictionary of Medications. (FRE.). 432p. pap. 35.00 (0-8288-6446-2, M-6424) Fr & Eur.

Dictionnaire des Medicaments. Jean Thuillier. 1990. (FRE.). 940p. pap. 55.00 (0-7859-7809-7, 2221067916) Fr & Eur.

Dictionnaire des Medicaments Conseil. Jean-Marie Hardre. 5th ed. 1992. (FRE.). 513p. pap. 85.00 (0-7859-8074-1, 2852704366) Fr & Eur.

Dictionnaire des Medicaments Veterinaires et des Parapharmacies Animales. Etienne Meisonnier. 6th ed. 1992. (FRE.). 1328p. pap. 110.00 (0-7859-8659-6, 286326091x) Fr & Eur.

Dictionnaire des Pierres Utilisees en Lithotheraphies. R. Boschiere. 1998. (FRE.). 24.95 (0-320-00263-2) Fr & Eur.

Dictionnaire des Signes et des Symptomes en Homeopathie et des Remedes Correspondent. Yves Le Penven. 1986. (FRE.). 412p. 95.00 (0-7859-7818-6, 2224011733) Fr & Eur.

Dictionnaire des Substances Chimiques Reglementees. Afnor Staff. 1987. (FRE.). 812p. pap. 395.00 (0-7859-7738-4, 2124201115) Fr & Eur.

Dictionnaire des Termes d'Anatomie, d'Embryologie et d'Histologie. Ernst Lovasy. 1954. (FRE.). 624p. 65.00 (0-8288-6871-9, M-6380) Fr & Eur.

Dictionnaire des Termes de Medecine. Marcel Garnier. (FRE.). 23rd ed. 1992. 1068p. 105.00 (*0-7859-7823-2*, 2224021259); 24th ed. 1995. 1080p. 125.00 (*0-7859-9927-2*) Fr & Eur.

Dictionnaire des Termes Medicaux Francais - Neerlandais & Neerlandais - Francais. R. Vanden Driessche. 1989. (DUT & FRE.). 1884p. 395.00 (*0-8288-9474-4*, 2870170408) Fr & Eur.

Dictionnaire des Termes Veterinaires et Animlaiers: French-English, English-French. Roy Mack. 1991. (ENG & FRE.). 576p. 195.00 (*0-7859-8134-9*, 2863260863) Fr & Eur.

Dictionnaire des Terms Odonto-Stomatologiques. L. Verchore. 3rd ed. 1992. (FRE.). 196p. pap. (*2-225-82677-3*) Masson FRA. *Dist:* IBD Ltd.

Dictionnaire des Urgences Medicales de l'Adulte. Arnaud Cenac et al. 2nd ed. 1989.Tr. of Dictionary of Adult Emergency Medicine. (FRE.). 416p. ring bd. 85.00 (*0-7859-4621-7*, F126640) Fr & Eur.

Dictionnaire d'Homeopathie Pediatrique a l'Usage des Familles et des Medecins de Famille. Herman Leduc. 1990. (FRE.). 494p. pap. 79.95 (*0-7859-7910-7*, 2700211057) Fr & Eur.

Dictionnaire d'ORL (Oto-Rhino-Laryngologie) d'Orthophonie et de Chirurgie Maxillo-Faciale: French with English Translations. Yves Guerrier. 1993. (ENG & FRE.). 351p. pap. 225.00 (*0-7859-7957-3*, 2718406399) Fr & Eur.

Dictionnaire d'Oto-Rhino-Laryngologie Augustin Larrauri. 1971. (ENG, FRE, GER, ITA & SPA.). 95.00 (*0-8288-6442-X*, M-6338) Fr & Eur.

Dictionnaire du Diabetique. Philippe Renou. 1991. (FRE.). 320p. 79.95 (*0-8288-9478-7*) Fr & Eur.

Dictionnaire Encyclopedie Pediatric en Medecine du Sport. P. Pilardeau. 1998. (FRE.). 110.00 (*0-320-00392-2*) Fr & Eur.

Dictionnaire Encyclopedique Medical. Maurice Rapin. 1986. (FRE.). 395.00 (*0-7859-8636-7*, 225710482x) Fr & Eur.

Dictionnaire Etim-Freisz 1990. ETIM Staff. 7th ed. 1990. (FRE.). (*0-7859-8232-9*, 2-905201-06-1) Fr & Eur.

Dictionnaire Europeen des Medicaments et Leurs Equivalents. Christian Gariot. 2nd ed. 1991. (FRE.). 1699p. 295.00 (*0-8288-9522-8*) Fr & Eur.

Dictionnaire Familial des Medecines Naturelles. Emmerick-Armand Maury & Chantal De Rudder. 1982. (FRE.). 105.00 (*0-8288-9523-6*, M6832) Fr & Eur.

Dictionnaire Familial d'Homeopathie. Emmerick-Armand Maury. 1991. (*0-7859-7896-8*, 2-501-01546-0) Fr & Eur.

Dictionnaire Familial D'Homeopathie. Emmerick-Armand Maury. 1982. (FRE.). (*0-7859-7938-7*, 2-7113-0026-9) Fr & Eur.

Dictionnaire Francais-Anglais et Anglais-Francais des Termes Medicaux et Biologiques. Pierre Lepine. 2nd ed. 1974. (ENG & FRE.). 896p. 175.00 (*0-8288-6027-0*, M4665) Fr & Eur.

Dictionnaire Francais de Medicine et de Biologie, Vol. 3. A. Mauila et al. 1972. (FRE.). 1200p. 195.00 (*0-7859-0746-7*, M-6394) Fr & Eur.

Dictionnaire Francais de Medicine et de Biologie, Vol. 4. H. Lambert et al. 1975. (FRE.). 580p. 1195.00 (*0-8288-5856-X*, M15420) Fr & Eur.

Dictionnaire Francais de Medicine et de Biologie: Annexes, Vol. 4. H. Lambert et al. 1975. (FRE.). 580p. 325.00 (*0-7859-4432-X*, 2225287767) Fr & Eur.

Dictionnaire Homeopathique. Louis Pommier. 1986. (FRE.). 19.95 (*0-7859-7851-8*, 2-253-03815-6) Fr & Eur.

Dictionnaire Illustre de Rhumathologie. A. K. Bhalla & P. L. Williams. 1990. (FRE.). 352p. 150.00 (*0-8288-9535-X*) Fr & Eur.

Dictionnaire Inespere de Fifty-Five Termes Visites par Jacques Lacan. Oreste Saint-Drome. 1994. (FRE.). (*0-7859-7630-2*, 2020213508) Fr & Eur.

Dictionnaire International des Abreviations Medicales. Maurice A. Touati. 1994. (FRE.). (*0-7859-8106-3*, 2-85608-058-8) Fr & Eur.

Dictionnaire Maloine de l'Infirmiere et Aide-Memoire des Pri. B. F. Cape & P. Dobson. 1979. (FRE.). 49.95 (*0-7859-7816-X*, 2224005210) Fr & Eur.

Dictionnaire Medecine Flammarion. J. Hamburger. 6th ed. 1998. (FRE.). 95.00 (*0-320-00352-3*) Fr & Eur.

Dictionnaire Medical. 1998. (FRE.). 89.95 (*0-320-00184-9*) Fr & Eur.

Dictionnaire Medical. Georges Bellicha & Pierre Bellicha. 1987. (FRE.). 480p. pap. 79.95 (*0-7859-7701-5*, 2040163506) Fr & Eur.

Dictionnaire Medical. Ludmila Manuila. 5th ed. 1991. (FRE.). 504p. pap. 39.95 (*0-7859-7833-X*, 2225827958) Fr & Eur.

Dictionnaire Medical. Alexandre Manuila. 6th ed. 1994. (FRE.). 544p. 49.95 (*0-7859-9279-0*) Fr & Eur.

Dictionnaire Medical: Allemand - Francais, Francais - Allemand. Dieter W. Unseld. 1992. (FRE & GER.). 550p. lib. bdg. 150.00 (*0-7859-3644-0*, 2856080502) Fr & Eur.

Dictionnaire Medical Chinois-Francois. 1993. (CHI & FRE.). 1599p. 140.00 (*0-7859-5675-1*, 7117011556) Fr & Eur.

Dictionnaire Medical de l'Infirmiere. J. Quevauvilliers & Leon Perlemuter. 4th rev. ed. 1992. (FRE.). 1344p. 130.00 (*0-7859-4749-3*, M1900) Fr & Eur.

Dictionnaire Medical de Poche. Ludmila Manuila et al. 1994. (FRE.). (*0-7859-7862-3*, 2-253-08521-9) Fr & Eur.

Dictionnaire Medical du Chirugien-Dentiste. Patrick Girard. Date not set. 250.00 (*0-7859-9582-X*) Fr & Eur.

Dictionnaire Medical Illustre De Semiologie Patronymique. Maloine Staff. 1979. (FRE.). 49.95 (*0-8288-4798-3*, M6149) Fr & Eur.

Dictionnaire Pratique de Droit Medicale. J. Pouletti. 1982. (FRE.). 424p. 110.00 (*0-8288-4421-6*, M9773) Fr & Eur.

Dictionnaire Pratique de l'Acupuncture et de l'Acupressure. Pierre Crepon. 1980.Tr. of Practical Dictionary of Acupuncture & Accupressure. (FRE.). 192p. 39.95 (*0-8288-1797-9*, M8979); (*0-7859-7968-9*, 2-7256-1308-6) Fr & Eur.

Dictionnaire Pratique de l'Alimentation. Andre Levy & Jacqueline Duffour. 1987. (FRE.). 69.95 (*0-7859-7914-X*, 2-7021-1649-3) Fr & Eur.

Dictionnaire Pratique de Pharmacologie: Clinique. Yvan Touitou & Leon Perlemuter. 1976. (FRE.). 1204p. 250.00 (*0-8288-5655-9*, M6536) Fr & Eur.

Dictionnaire Pratique de Therapeutique Canine et Feline. Robert Moraillon et al. 3rd rev. ed. 1992. (FRE.). 195.00 (*0-7859-7831-3*, 2-225-82579-3) Fr & Eur.

Dictionnaire Pratique de Therapeutique Canine et Feline. Robert Moraillon & Yves Legeay. 4th ed. 1997. (FRE.). 544p. 195.00 (*0-320-00431-7*) Fr & Eur.

Dictionnaire Pratique de Therapeutique Pediatrique. Robert Steinschneider. 1980.Tr. of Practical Dictionary of Pediatric Therapeutics. (FRE.). 824p. 125.00 (*0-8288-1828-2*, F58400) Fr & Eur.

Dictionnaire Pratique des Medicaments. Larousse Staff. 1989. (FRE.). (*0-7859-8609-X*, 203510128X) Fr & Eur.

Dictionnaire Raisonne des Termes d'Entreprises du Medicaments. A. Beresniak. 1998. (FRE.). 95.00 (*0-320-00267-5*) Fr & Eur.

Dictionnaire Termes de Medecine. Garnier & Delamare. 1998. (FRE.). 25p. 95.00 (*0-320-00367-1*) Fr & Eur.

Dictionnaire Usuel de Psychologie. N. Sillamy. 1991. (FRE.). 784p. 130.00 (*0-7859-4747-7*, M15538) Fr & Eur.

Dictionnaire Vidal. Jean-Paul Vidal. 68th ed. 1994.Tr. of French Physician Desk's Reference. (FRE.). 2296p. 295.00 (*0-8288-9541-4*) Fr & Eur.

Dictionnaire Vidal: 1995 Edition. 71st ed. 1995.Tr. of French Physician's Desk Reference. (FRE.). 295.00 (*0-7859-9877-2*) Fr & Eur.

Dictionnaire Vidal, 1996 Edition. 72nd ed. 1996.Tr. of French Physician's Desk Reference. (FRE.). 350.00 (*0-7859-9806-3*) Fr & Eur.

Dictionnaire Vidal 1999. annuals Ed. by Vidal Staff. 1998.Tr. of French Physician's Desk Reference. (FRE.). 350.00 (*0-320-03695-2*) Fr & Eur.

Dictionnaire Vidal (French Physicians Desk Refrence) 1998. Date not set. (FRE.). 350.00 (*0-7859-9594-3*) Fr & Eur.

Dictionnaire Vidal 1997: French Physician's Desk Reference. 73rd ed. 1997. (FRE.). 350.00 (*0-7859-9551-X*) Fr & Eur.

Dictionnaire Vidal 2000. annuals Ed. by French and European Staff. 1999.Tr. of French Physician's Desk Reference. (FRE.). 350.00 (*0-320-03689-8*) Fr & Eur.

Dictionnaires des Maladies. Jean P. Barbier & Francois C. Hugues. 1973. (FRE.). 528p. 59.95 (*0-7859-0725-4*, M6022) Fr & Eur.

Did Trojans Use Trojans? A Trip Inside the Corner Drugstore. Vince Staten. 2000. 208p. pap. 12.00 (*0-684-85433-3*, Fireside) S&S Trade Pap.

Did Your Eyes Deceive You? Expert Psychological Testimony on the Unreliability of Eyewitness Identification. F. Woocher. 1978. (Monographs: No. CR-41). 4.00 (*1-55524-042-9*) Ctr Respon Psych.

Diderot's Holism: Philosophical Anti-Reductionism & Its Medical Background. Timo Kaitaro. Ed. by Georg Gimpl & Juha Manninen. 1997. (European Studies in the History of Science & Ideas: Vol. 4). 283p. pap. 54.95 (*0-8204-2948-1*) P Lang Pubng.

Diet - In Life, Food, Old Age & Research: Index of New Information with Authors & Subjects. Melba J. Milligan. rev. ed. 1996. LC 96-7238. 179p. 57.50 (*0-7883-1034-8*); pap. 47.50 (*0-7883-1035-6*) ABBE Pubs Assn.

Diet - Investigations, Research & Results: Index of New Information with Authors & Subjects. Melba J. Milligan. 1993. 180p. 47.50 (*1-55914-844-6*); pap. 44.50 (*1-55914-845-4*) ABBE Pubs Assn.

Diet & Arthritis: A Comprehensive Guide to Controlling Arthritis Through Diet. Gail Darlington & Linda Gamlin. 1998. 448p. pap. (*0-09-178577-4*) Vermilion GBR. *Dist:* Trafalgar.

Diet & Breast Cancer. American Institute for Cancer Research Staff. 1994. (Advances in Experimental Medicine & Biology Ser.: Vol. 364). (Illus.). 200p. (C). text 79.50 (*0-306-44895-5*, Kluwer Plenum) Kluwer Academic.

Diet & Cancer. Udo Renzenbrink. pap. (*0-85440-766-9*, 415) R Steiner Pr GBR. *Dist:* Anthroposophic.

Diet & Cancer: Markers, Prevention & Treatment. M. M. Jacobs. 1994. (Advances in Experimental Medicine & Biology Ser.: Vol. 354). (Illus.). 274p. (C). text 89.50 (*0-306-44723-1*, Kluwer Plenum) Kluwer Academic.

Diet & Cancer: Molecular Mechanisms of Interactions. Ed. by American Institute for Cancer Research Staff. 1995. LC 95-17694. (Advances in Experimental Medicine & Biology Ser.: Vol. 375). 236p. 89.50 (*0-306-45067-4*, Kluwer Plenum) Kluwer Academic.

Diet & Health in Europe - the Evidence. Ed. by G. B. Brubacher. 1991. (Journal: Vol. 35, Suppl. 1, 1991). (Illus.). iv, 120p. pap. 38.50 (*3-8055-5400-1*) S Karger.

Diet & Health of Isolated Populations. G. R. Wadsworth. 1984. 232p. 130.00 (*0-8493-6101-X*, RC623, CRC Reprint) Franklin.

Diet & Heart Disease. British Nutrition Foundation Staff. Ed. by Margaret Ashwell. 2nd ed. 1996. LC 96-86099. 96p. (*0-412-79130-7*) Kluwer Academic.

Diet & Nutrition Activities. Patricia R. Toner. 1993. LC 93-4965. (Just for the Health of It!: Unit 2). (Illus.). 160p. (YA). (gr. 7-12). pap., tchr. ed. 19.95 (*0-87628-265-6*) Ctr Appl Res.

Diet & Nutrition Sourcebook: Basic Consumer Health Information about Dietary Guidelines... Ed. by Karen Bellenir. 2nd ed. 1999. LC 99-17687. (Health Reference Ser.). (Illus.). xiii, 650p. lib. bdg. 78.00 (*0-7808-0228-4*) Omnigraphics Inc.

Diet & Nutrition Sourcebook: Basic Information about Nutrition, Including the Dietary Guidelines for Americans, the Food Guide Pyramid & More. Ed. by Dan R. Harris. 1996. LC 96-9512. (Health Reference Ser.: Vol. 15). 662p. lib. bdg. 78.00 (*0-7808-0084-2*) Omnigraphics Inc.

Diet & Obesity. Ed. by G. A. Bray et al. 1989. (Illus.). xiv, 248p. 139.25 (*3-8055-4980-6*) S Karger.

Diet & Physical Efficiency: Influence of Frequency of Meals Upon Physical Efficiency & Industrial Productivity. Howard W. Haggard & Leon A. Greenberg. Ed. by Leon Stein. 1977. LC 77-70500. (Illus.). lib. bdg. 23.95 (*0-405-10171-6*) Ayer.

Diet & the Aetiology of Cancer. Ed. by A. B. Miller. 1989. (ESO Monographs). (Illus.). 73p. 73.95 (*0-387-50681-0*) Spr-Verlag.

Diet-Behavior Relationships: Focus on Depression. Larry Christensen. 1996. LC 96-4665. 209p. (Orig.). pap. text 29.95 (*1-55798-325-9*, 431-7580) Am Psychol.

Diet, Demography & Disease: Changing Perspectives on Anemia. Ed. by Patricia Stuart-Macadam & Susan Kent. 202nd ed. 1992. LC 92-11086. (Evolutionary Foundations of Human Behavior Ser.). 294p. lib. bdg. 63.95 (*0-202-01189-5*) Aldine de Gruyter.

Diet Diary: The Culinary Companion for a New You! Andrew Ludy. 1984. (Illus.). 193p. (Orig.). pap. 4.95 (*0-943912-01-6*) Landing Pr.

Diet for a Strong Heart. Michio Kushi. 1986. LC 86-24864. (Illus.). 566p. pap. 14.95 (*0-312-00120-7*) St Martin.

Diet, Hormones & Cancer: Methodological Issues for Prospective Studies. E. Riboli & R. Saracci. 1988. (IARC Scientific Publications Ser.: No. 4). 159p. text 30.00 (*92-832-1415-3*) World Health.

Diet, Lifestyle, & Mortality in China: A Study of the Characteristics of 65 Chinese Counties. Junshi Chen et al. Ed. by T. Colin Campbell et al. 1990. LC 89-38882. (Illus.). 920p. 195.00 (*0-8014-2453-4*) Cornell U Pr.

Diet, Lipoproteins & Coronary Heart Disease: A Biochemical Perspective. E. H. Mangiapane & A. M. Salter. 1999. 180p. pap. (*1-897676-81-6*) Nottingham Univ Pr GBR. *Dist:* St Mut.

Diet Manual. Newark Beth Israel Medical Center, Dietary Departm. 1980. LC 80-82889. 92p. (Orig.). pap. 10.00 (*0-937714-00-3*) Newark Beth.

Diet Manual: A Compilation of Food Allowances Prescribed in Normal & Abnormal States of Health for the Use of Physicians, Paramedical Personnel & Trainees. 1991. lib. bdg. 79.95 (*0-8490-5053-7*) Gordon Pr.

Diet, Nutrition, & Cancer. National Research Council Staff. 1982. 496p. pap. text 29.95 (*0-309-03280-6*) Natl Acad Pr.

Diet, Nutrition & Cancer: A Critical Evaluation. Ed. by Bandaru S. Reddy & Leonard A. Cohen. 1986. LC 85-15172. 184p. 109.00 (*0-8493-6332-2*, RC268, CRC Reprint); 208p. 112.00 (*0-8493-6333-0*) Franklin.

Diet, Nutrition & Cancer: Proceedings of the 16th International Symposium of the Princess Takamatsu Cancer Research Fund, Japan, 1985. Ed. by Y. Hayaishi et al. 1986. 344p. lib. bdg. (*90-6764-085-9*) VSP NLD. *Dist:* Coronet Bks.

Diet, Nutrition & Chronic Disease: Lessons from Contrasting Worlds. Prakash S. Shetty & Klim McPherson. 1997. LC 96-50379. 318p. 130.00 (*0-471-97133-2*) Wiley.

Diet, Nutrition & Dental Research. Ed. by M. E. Curzon & J. M. Ten Cate. 1990. (Journal: Vol. 24, Suppl. 1, 1990). (Illus.). iv, 80p. pap. 36.75 (*3-8055-5305-6*) S Karger.

Diet, Nutrition & Health. K. K. Carroll. 1990. 368p. (C). text (*0-7735-0733-7*); pap. text (*0-7735-0741-8*) McG-Queens Univ Pr CAN. *Dist:* CUP Services.

Diet, Nutrition & Immunity. L. Kabbash. 1994. 282p. 154.95 (*0-8493-6744-1*) CRC Pr.

Diet, Nutrition, & the Prevention of Chronic Diseases: Report of a WHO Study Group. 1990. (Technical Reports: No. 797). (FRE, RUS & SPA.). 203p. pap. text 26.00 (*92-4-120797-3*, 1100797) World Health.

Diet Reference Manual. Massachusetts General Hospital Department of Nursing Staff. Ed. by Ruth D. Palombo & Mary Carey. 1984. 240p. spiral bd. 17.50 (*0-316-54947-9*) Lppncott W & W.

Diet Selection: An Interdisciplinary Approach to Foraging Behaviour. Ed. by R. N. Hughes. 1993. LC 92-27323. pap. 73.95 (*0-632-03559-5*) Blackwell Sci.

Diet Therapy. Sue R. Williams. 1994. LC 94-21373. (*0-8016-9128-1*) Mosby Inc.

Diet Therapy. Sue Rodwell Williams. 1994. LC 94-21373. (Illus.). 304p. (C). (gr. 13). pap. text 46.00 (*0-8151-9128-6*, 24880) Mosby Inc.

***Diet Therapy for the Dietary Manager.** Dietary Managers Assn. Drummond Staff. abr. ed. 2001. pap. text (*0-7872-8124-7*) Kendall-Hunt.

Diet Therapy in Traditional Chinese Medicine. Ed. by Liu Chi-Lin. 1995. LC 94-44954. ix, 252p. pap. text (*0-443-04967-X*) Church.

Dieta Diabetica Para Buena Salud: (Diabetic Diet Exchange Lists) Margaret B. Salmon. 1979.Tr. of Diabetic Diet Exchange Lists in Spanish. (ENG & SPA., Illus.). pap. 2.50 (*0-918662-05-2*) Techkits.

Dietary Excesses & Health Disease Implications. John J. Anderson. 1984. (Illus.). pap. 18.95 (*0-938938-13-4*) Health Sci Comm.

Dietary Factors & Birth Defects. Ed. by Raghubir P. Sharma. 1993. LC 93-12186. 380p. (Orig.). pap. text 28.50 (*0-934394-08-3*) AAASPD.

Dietary Fat & Cancer: Genetic & Molecular Interactions. Ed. by American Institute for Cancer Research Staff. 1997. LC 97-4389. (Advances in Experimental Medicine & Biology Ser.: Vol. 422). (Illus.). 268p. (C). text 107.00 (*0-306-45683-4*, Kluwer Plenum) Kluwer Academic.

Dietary Fats & Health. Ed. by Edward G. Perkins & Willard Visek. 1983. 978p. 40.00 (*0-935315-07-1*) Am Oil Chemists.

Dietary Fats & Thrombosis: Proceedings of the Inserm Symposium at Lyon, 1973. Inserm-International Symposium Staff. Ed. by S. Renaud & A. Nordoy. 1974. (Journal: Vol. 2, Nos. 1-4). (Illus.). 200p. 73.25 (*3-8055-1712-2*) S Karger.

Dietary Fats, Lipids, Hormones & Tumorigenesis: New Horizons in Basic Research. Ed. by David Heber & David Kritchevsky. 1996. LC 96-22307. (Illus.). 182p. 90.00 (*0-306-45317-7*, Kluwer Plenum) Kluwer Academic.

Dietary Fats, Prostanoids & Arterial Thrombosis. G. Hornstra. 1982. text 155.50 (*90-247-2667-0*) Kluwer Academic.

Dietary Fiber: Basic & Clinical Aspects. Ed. by George V. Vahouny & David Kritchevsky. 1986. LC 85-19159. 586p. 125.00 (*0-306-42028-7*, Plenum Trade) Perseus Pubng.

Dietary Fiber: Chemistry, Physiology & Health Effects. D. Kritchevsky et al. 1990. LC 90-6710. (Illus.). 512p. (C). text 135.00 (*0-306-43310-9*, Kluwer Plenum) Kluwer Academic.

Dietary Fiber Analysis & Applications. Sungsoo Cho et al. 1997. 202p. pap. 79.00 (*0-935584-62-5*) AOAC Intl.

Dietary Fiber, Calories & Cancer: Index of Modern Authors & Subjects with Guide for Rapid Research. Joseph M. Bahr. 1992. LC 92-36369. 47.50 (*1-55914-958-2*); pap. 44.50 (*1-55914-959-0*) ABBE Pubs Assn.

Dietary Fiber in Health & Disease. Ed. by George V. Vahouny & David Kritchevsky. 1982. LC 82-7549. (GWUMC Department of Biochemistry & Molecular Biology Annual Spring Symposium Ser.). 344p. 85.00 (*0-306-40926-7*, Plenum Trade) Perseus Pubng.

Dietary Fiber in Health & Disease: Proceedings of the Fifth Washington Symposium Held in Washington, D. C., March 26-29, 1996. Ed. by David Kritchevsky & Charles Bonfield. 1997. LC 97-36252. (Advances in Experimental Medicine & Biology Ser.: Vol. 427). 340p. (C). text 95.00 (*0-306-45703-2*, Kluwer Plenum) Kluwer Academic.

Dietary Fiber Research. Z. Madar & S. H. Odes. 1990. (Progress in Biochemical Pharmacology Ser.: Vol. 24). (Illus.). viii, 148p. 116.75 (*3-8055-5043-X*) S Karger.

Dietary Fibre: Nutritional Function in Health & Disease. Ed. by M. I. Gurr & N. G. Asp. 1994. LC 95-232368. (Illus.). 23p. pap. 12.50 (*0-944398-24-3*) ILSI.

Dietary Fibre - A Component of Food: Nutritional Function in Health & Disease. Ed. by T. F. Scheizer et al. 1992. (ILSI Human Nutrition Reviews Ser.). (Illus.). 354p. 206.00 (*0-387-19718-4*) Spr-Verlag.

Dietary Imbalances, Metabolism & Disease: The Southeast Asian Perspective. John Candlish. 1990. 164p. (Orig.). pap. (*9971-69-145-0*) Singapore Univ Pr SGP. *Dist:* Coronet Bks.

Dietary Influences on Cancer: Traditional & Modern. Ed. by R. Schoental. 1982. 272p. 154.00 (*0-8493-5647-4*, RC262, CRC Reprint) Franklin.

Dietary Iron & Iron Overload (Hemosiderosis) Illness: Index of New Information. Lawrence C. Hallahan. 1998. 57.50 (*0-7883-1834-9*); pap. 47.50 (*0-7883-1835-7*) ABBE Pubs Assn.

Dietary Management of Young Children with Acute Diarrhoea: A Practical Manual for District Programme Managers. D. B. Jelliffe & E. F. Jelliffe. 2nd ed. 1991. (ENG, FRE & SPA.). 29p. pap. text 8.00 (*92-4-154428-7*, 1152316) World Health.

Dietary Minerals & Cardiovascular Disease. Ed. by B. M. Altura & Bella T. Altura. 1983. (Journal: Vol. 1, No. 3-6). (Illus.). vi, 188p. pap. 113.25 (*3-8055-3682-8*) S Karger.

Dietary Minerals & Dangerous Influences: Index of Modern Authors & Subjects with Guide for Rapid Research. Judy P. Payter. rev. ed. 149p. 1996. LC 96-3124. 57.50 (*0-7883-1120-4*); 1996. LC 96-3124. pap. 47.50 (*0-7883-1121-2*); 1995. LC 90-56319. 57.50 (*0-7883-0244-2*); 1995. LC 90-56319. pap. 47.50 (*0-7883-0245-0*) ABBE Pubs Assn.

Dietary Phytochemicals in Cancer Prevention & Treatment: Proceedings of the American Institute for Cancer Research's Sixth Annual Research Conference Held in Washington, D. C., August 31-September 1, 1995. Ed. by American Institute for Cancer Research Staff. 1996. LC 96-24704. (Advances in Experimental Medicine & Biology Ser.: Vol. 401). (Illus.). 324p. (C). text 114.00 (*0-306-45365-7*, Kluwer Plenum) Kluwer Academic.

Dietary Policies & Procedures. Karen Walton. 1991. 109p. (C). 29.50 (*1-877735-09-4*, 2111PP) Prof Prnting & Pub.

Dietary Proteins, Cholesterol Metabolism & Atherosclerosis. Ed. by M. Sugano & Anton C. Beynen. 1990. (Monographs on Atherosclerosis: Vol. 16). (Illus.). viii, 164p. 151.50 (*3-8055-5193-2*) S Karger.

Dietary Reference Intakes: A Risk Assessment Model for Establishing Upper Intake Levels. Institute of Medicine Staff. 1999. LC 99-212474. 82p. pap. 18.00 (*0-309-06348-5*) Natl Acad Pr.

***Dietary Reference Intakes: Applications in Dietary Assessment.** Contrib. by Institute of Medicine Staff. 2001. LC 00-69187. (Illus.). xvii, 287p. 54.95 (*0-309-07311-1*) Natl Acad Pr.

Dietary Reference Intakes: Definition & Plan for Review of Dietary Antioxidants & Related Compounds. Institute of Medicine Staff. 1998. LC 99-172157. 24p. pap. text 10.00 (*0-309-06187-3*) Natl Acad Pr.

Dietary Reference Intakes: Thiamin, Riboflavin, Niacin, Vitamin B6, Folate, Vitamin B12, Pantothenic Acid, Biotin & Choline. Institute of Medicine Staff & Food and Nutrition Board Staff. 2000. LC 00-28380. 592p. (C). 64.95 (*0-309-06411-2*) Natl Acad Pr.

Dietary Reference Intakes for Calcium, Phosphorous, Magnesium, Vitamin D & Fluoride. Institute of Medicine Staff & Joyce L. Vedral. 1999. LC 97-33777. (Dietary Reference Intakes Ser.). 448p. 54.95 (*0-309-06350-7*); pap. 34.95 (*0-309-06403-1*) Natl Acad Pr.

Dietary Reference Intakes for Thiamin, Riboflavin, Niacin, Vitamin B6, Folate, Vitamin B12, Pantothenic Acid, Biotin & Choline. Institute of Medicine Staff & Food and Nutrition Board Staff. 2000. LC 00-28380. (Dietary Reference Intakes Ser.). 592p. (C). pap. 44.95 (*0-309-06554-2*) Natl Acad Pr.

Dietary Research & Guidance in Health & Disease. Ed. by Geoffrey H. Bourne. 1986. (World Review of Nutrition & Dietetics Ser.: Vol. 48). (Illus.). viii, 270p. 202.75 (*3-8055-4341-7*) S Karger.

Dietary Restriction: Implications for the Design & Interpretation of Toxicity & Carcinogenicity Studies. Ed. by R. Hart et al. 1995. LC 95-77852. (Illus.). 385p. pap. 60.00 (*0-944398-34-0*) ILSI.

***Dietary Supplements: Index of New Information & Guide-Book for Consumers, Reference & Research.** Ed. by Research and Development Division Staff & John C. Bartone. 2001. 180p. 47.50 (*0-7883-2576-0*); pap. 44.50 (*0-7883-2577-9*) ABBE Pubs Assn.

Dietary Supplements: Uncertainties in Analyses Underlying FDA's Proposed Rule on Ephedrine Alkaloids. William Scanlon & Nye Stevens. 2000. 79p. pap. text 20.00 (*0-7881-8798-8*) DIANE Pub.

Dietary Tannins: Consequences & Remedies. D. K. Salunkhe et al. 1989. 208p. 195.00 (*0-8493-6811-1*, RA1242) CRC Pr.

Dieter's Dictionary & Problem Solver: An A to Z Guide to Nutrition, Health & Fitness. Victoria Zak & Peter Vash. 1998. (Illus.). 394p. text 20.00 (*0-7881-5539-3*) DIANE Pub.

Dieter's Directory: A Comprehensive Guide to Diets. Dean Kimmel. 1993. LC 89-82277. 93p. (Orig.). pap. 12.95 (*0-9621446-1-4*) Corbin Hse.

Dietetic Service Operation Handbook: Practical Applications in Geriatric Care. Karen S. Kolasa. 1994. LC 92-49635. 69.95 (*1-56022-027-9*) Haworth Jrnl Co-Edits.

Diethylhexyl Phthalate. 1992. (Environmental Health Criteria Ser.: No. 131). (ENG, FRE & SPA.). 141p. pap. text 29.00 (*92-4-157131-4*, 1160131) World Health.

Dieting for an Emperor: A Translation of Books 1 & 4 of Oribasius' Medical Compilations with an Introduction & Commentary. Mark D. Grant. 1997. LC 97-29918. (Studies in Ancient Medicine: No. 15). (ENG & GRE., Illus.). 328p. 117.50 (*90-04-10790-8*) Brill Academic Pubs.

Dietitian. Jack Rudman. 1994. (Career Examination Ser.: C-196). pap. 27.95 (*0-8373-0196-3*) Nat Learn.

Dietitian's Handbook of Enteral & Parenteral Nutrition. Annalynn Skipper. 2nd rev. ed. 1998. LC 97-40065. 465p. 72.00 (*0-8342-0920-9*, 20920) Aspen Pub.

Dietitian's Patient Education Resource Manual. ACPE Staff. 2nd ed. 2000. LC 2001-22413. (ENG & SPA., Illus.). 528p. 199.00 (*0-8342-1925-5*) Aspen Pub.

Dietitian's Reference for Renal Nutrition. Helen N. Sanders et al. 2nd ed. 1990. (Illus.). 150p. (C). pap. 35.00 (*1-880864-00-2*) F S H.

Diets Don't Work: Now You Can Become "Naturally Thin" Step-by-Step When All Else Fails. Bob Schwartz. 3rd ed. 1995. LC 96-83096. pap. 12.95 (*0-942540-16-6*) Breakthru Pub.

Diets for Reducing Obesity Including Diet Therapy Research: Index of New Information for Reference & Practice. Pat L. Widmer. 1997. (Illus.). 150p. 57.50 (*0-7883-1236-7*); pap. 47.50 (*0-7883-1237-5*) ABBE Pubs Assn.

Diets Still Don't Work: How to Lose Weight Step-by-Step Even after You've Failed at Dieting. Bob Schwartz. 1990. 202p. pap. 9.95 (*0-942540-04-2*) Breakthru Pub.

Diets to Help Arthritis. MacFarlane. 1981. pap. (*0-7225-2871-X*) Thorsons GBR. *Dist:* Natl Bk Netwk.

Dietwalk: The Doctor's Fast & Easy 3 Day Superdiet & Fitness Plan. Fred A. Stutman. 1983. LC 83-61033. (Illus.). 200p. pap. 8.95 (*0-934232-02-4*) Med Manor Bks.

Difenacoum. 1995. (Health & Safety Guides Ser.: No. 95). 25p. (C). pap. 4.50 (*92-4-151095-1*, 1860095) Am Soc Clinical.

Difference & Pathology: Stereotypes of Sexuality, Race, & Madness. Sander L. Gilman. 1985. LC 85-7809. (Illus.). 304p. (C). pap. 18.95 (*0-8014-9332-3*) Cornell U Pr.

Difference & Subjectivity. Francis Jacques. Tr. by Andrew Rothwell from FRE. 1991. 384p. (C). 50.00 (*0-300-04830-0*) Yale U Pr.

Difference Equations with Public Health Applications. Lemuel A. Moybe & Asha Seth Kapadia. 2000. LC 00-40473. (Biostatistics Ser.). (Illus.). xiii, 392p. text 165.00 (*0-8247-0447-9*) Dekker.

Differences in Common: Straight Talk on Mental Retardation, Down Syndrome, & Life. Marilyn Trainer. 1991. LC 90-50503. 231p. (Orig.). pap. 14.95 (*0-933149-40-9*) Woodbine House.

Differences in Medicine: Unraveling Practices, Techniques & Bodies. Ed. by Marc Berg & Annemarie Mol. 1998. LC 97-37836. (Body, Commodity, Text Ser.). (Illus.). 272p. pap. 17.95 (*0-8223-2174-2*) Duke.

Differences in Medicine: Unraveling Practices, Techniques & Bodies. Marc Berg & Annemarie Mol. 1998. LC 97-37836. (Body, Commodity, Text Ser.). (*0-8223-2162-9*) Duke.

Differences in Nursing Care: Area A. Jack Rudman. (Regents External Degree Ser.: Vol. 21). 43.95 (*0-8373-5671-7*); 1994. (ACT Proficiency Examination Program Ser.: Vol. PEP-43). pap. 23.95 (*0-8373-5543-5*); 1994. pap. 23.95 (*0-8373-5621-0*) Nat Learn.

Differences in Nursing Care: Area B. Jack Rudman. (Regents External Degree Ser.: Vol. 22). 43.95 (*0-8373-5672-5*); 1994. pap. 23.95 (*0-8373-5622-9*); 1994. (ACT Proficiency Examination Program Ser.: Vol. PEP-44). pap. 23.95 (*0-8373-5544-3*) Nat Learn.

Differences in Nursing Care: Area C. Jack Rudman. (Regents External Degree Ser.: Vol. 23). 43.95 (*0-8373-5673-3*); 1994. (ACT Proficiency Examination Program Ser.: Vol. PEP-45). pap. 23.95 (*0-8373-5545-1*); 1994. pap. 23.95 (*0-8373-5623-7*) Nat Learn.

Differences in Nursing Care, Area A. Jack Rudman. (ACT Proficiency Examination Program Ser.: Vol. 43). 43.95 (*0-8373-5593-1*) Nat Learn.

Differences in Nursing Care, Area B. Jack Rudman. (ACT Proficiency Examination Program Ser.: Vol. 44). 43.95 (*0-8373-5594-X*) Nat Learn.

Differences in Nursing Care, Area C. Jack Rudman. (ACT Proficiency Examination Program Ser.: Vol. 45). 43.95 (*0-8373-5595-8*) Nat Learn.

Different Drum: Community Making & Peace. Scott Peck. 1988. 336p. pap. 12.00 (*0-671-66833-1*, Touchstone) S&S Trade Pap.

Different Existence: Principles of Phenomenological Psychopathology. Jan H. Van den Berg. 1972. LC 72-182104. 152p. pap. text 16.50 (*0-8207-0244-7*) Duquesne.

Different Kind of Diplomacy: A Source Book for International Health Volunteers. Ed. by Jack C. Fisher & Debra Armstrong. 1987. (Illus.). 200p. (Orig.). (C). pap. 10.95 (*0-9618734-0-X*) PSRF Pub.

Different Kind of Health: Finding Well-Being Despite Illness. Blair Justice. 1998. LC 97-42433. 310p. lib. bdg. 22.00 (*0-9605376-4-3*) Peak Pr.

Differential Approaches in Microsurgery of the Brain. Wolfgang Seeger. 1985. (Illus.). 428p. 214.00 (*0-387-81857-X*) Spr-Verlag.

Differential Diagnose der Medizinisch-Klinischen Symptome: Differential Diagnosis of Symptoms in Clinical Medicine, Set. H. Vogl. 2nd ed. 1981. (GER.). 1120p. 95.00 (*0-8288-1842-8*) Fr & Eur.

Differential Diagnoses in Neuroradiology. Ed. by J. Randy Jinkins. 1998. (Illus.). 400p. text 98.00 (*0-07-032942-7*) McGraw-Hill Med Pub.

Differential Diagnosis. Jeremiah A. Barondess & Charles C. Carpenter. 1994. (Illus.). 993p. 75.00 (*0-8121-1446-9*) Lppncott W & W.

Differential Diagnosis & Management for the Chiropractor: Protocols & Algorithms. Thomas A. Souza. 2nd ed. 2000. LC 00-58282. (Illus.). 959p. 89.00 (*0-8342-1728-7*, 17287) Aspen Pub.

Differential Diagnosis & Treatment in Social Work. Ed. by Francis J. Turner. 3rd rev. ed. 1983. LC 82-48390. (Illus.). 897p. (C). 37.95 (*0-02-932990-6*) Free Pr.

Differential Diagnosis & Treatment in Social Work. Ed. by Francis J. Turner. 4th ed. 1995. LC 95-16212. 1440p. 45.00 (*0-02-874007-6*) Free Pr.

Differential Diagnosis & Treatment of Movement Disorders. Tolosa & Koller. 1998. 224p. pap. text 140.00 (*0-7506-7050-9*) Buttrwrth-Heinemann.

Differential Diagnosis for Primary Practice. Jennifer R. Jamison. 1999. LC 98-20743. (*0-443-06264-1*) Church.

Differential Diagnosis for the Orthopedic Physical Therapist. James D. Meadows. 1999. LC 98-49161. (Illus.). 350p. pap. 44.95 (*0-07-041235-9*) McGraw-Hill Prof.

Differential Diagnosis in Abdominal Ultrasound. R. A. Bisset & A. N. Khan. 1990. (Illus.). 374p. pap. text (*0-7020-1483-4*) W B Saunders GBR. *Dist:* Saunders.

Differential Diagnosis in Chest X-Rays. F. Burgener & M. Kormano. 1996. (Illus.). 192p. 73.00 (*0-86577-677-6*) Thieme Med Pubs.

Differential Diagnosis in Computed Tomography. Francis A. Burgener & Martti Kormano. 1995. (Illus.). 440p. text 169.00 (*0-86577-547-8*) Thieme Med Pubs.

Differential Diagnosis in Conventional Gastrointestinal Radiology. F. Burgener & Kormano. 1996. (Illus.). 240p. 79.00 (*0-86577-676-8*) Thieme Med Pubs.

Differential Diagnosis in Conventional Radiology. Francis A. Burgener & Martti Kormano. 2nd rev. ed. 1991. text 169.00 (*0-86577-346-7*) Thieme Med Pubs.

Differential Diagnosis in Dermatology. Richard Ashton & Barbara Leppard. 2nd ed. 1993. pap. (*1-870905-42-3*) Radcliffe Med Pr GBR. *Dist:* Balogh.

Differential Diagnosis in Dermatology. Richard Ashton & Barbara Leppard. 2nd ed. 1993. 115.00 (*1-870905-47-4*, Radcliffe Med Pr) Scovill Paterson.

Differential Diagnosis in Dermatopathology. A. Bernard Ackerman et al. (Illus.). No. I. 2nd ed. 1992. LC 91-8881. text 125.00 (*0-8121-1383-7*); Vol. 3. 1992. LC 92-23655. 202p. 125.00 (*0-8121-1580-5*); Vol. 4. 1994. 228p. text 125.00 (*0-8121-1676-3*) Lppncott W & W.

Differential Diagnosis in Head & Neck Imaging. Thomas J. Vogl. 1998. LC 98-36571. 139.00 (*3-13-115411-X*); (Illus.). 400p. 139.00 (*0-86577-811-6*) Thieme Med Pubs.

Differential Diagnosis in Magnetic Resonance Imaging. Francis A. Burgener & Martti Kormano. 2002. (Illus.). 448p. 149.00 (*0-86577-720-9*) Thieme Med Pubs.

Differential Diagnosis in Neuro-Oncology. Jerzy Hildebrand & Michael Brada. 2001. LC 00-50161. (Illus.). 310p. text (*0-19-263213-2*) OUP.

Differential Diagnosis in Neurology & Neurosurgery: A Clinician's Pocket Guide. Sotirios A. Tsementzis. 2000. LC 99-23138. (Illus.). 336p. pap. 35.00 (*0-86577-830-2*) Thieme Med Pubs.

Differential Diagnosis in Obstetric & Gynecologic Ultrasound. R. A. Bisset et al. 1996. (Illus.). 350p. text (*0-7020-2171-7*) W B Saunders GBR. *Dist:* Saunders.

Differential Diagnosis in Ophthalmology. Vernon. 1999. 192p. pap. 39.95 (*0-8385-1707-2*) McGraw-Hill Prof.

Differential Diagnosis in Otorhinolaryngology: Symptoms, Syndromes, & Interdisciplinary Issues. Hans H. Naumann. 1993. LC 93-26903.Tr. of Differentialdiagnostik in der Hals-Nasen Ohren-Heilkunde. 99.00 (*0-86577-507-9*) Thieme Med Pubs.

Differential Diagnosis in Pathology: Bone & Joint Disorders. Edward F. McCarthy. 1996. LC 95-48167. (Illus.). 184p. 98.50 (*0-89640-313-0*) Igaku-Shoin.

Differential Diagnosis in Pathology: Breast Disorders. Ayten Someren & G. Whitaker Sewell. 1997. LC 96-3027. (Differential Diagnosis in Pathology Ser.). (Illus.). 200p. 130.00 (*0-89640-314-9*) Igaku-Shoin.

Differential Diagnosis in Pathology: Liver Disorders. Swan N. Thung & Michael A. Gerber. 1995. LC 95-3691. 192p. 79.50 (*0-89640-268-1*) Igaku-Shoin.

Differential Diagnosis in Pathology: Pulmonary Disorders. Anthony A. Gal & Michael N. Koss. 1997. LC 96-40066. (Differential Diagnosis in Pathology Ser.). (*4-260-14329-8*) Igaku-Shoin.

Differential Diagnosis in Pediatric Radiology. K. D. Ebel & H. Blickmann. 1998. LC 98-23692. (Illus.). 840p. 199.00 (*0-86577-713-6*) Thieme Med Pubs.

Differential Diagnosis in Pediatric Radiology. M. Gruenebaum. 1986. xx, 140p. pap. 42.75 (*3-8055-4249-6*) S Karger.

Differential Diagnosis in Pediatrics. H. Ewerbeck. 1980. 471p. 85.00 (*0-387-90474-3*) Spr-Verlag.

Differential Diagnosis in Physical Therapy: Musculoskeletal & Systemic Conditions. Catherine C. Goodman & Teresa E. Snyder. 2nd ed. 1994. LC 93-49789. (Illus.). 512p. pap. text 48.00 (*0-7216-5267-0*) Saunders.

Differential Diagnosis in Primary Care. R. Douglas Collins. 2nd ed. 1987. LC 65-9814. (Illus.). 538p. text 55.00 (*0-397-50816-6*, Lippnctt) Lppncott W & W.

Differential Diagnosis in Primary Eye Care. Debra Bezan et al. 1998. 496p. text 89.99 (*0-7506-9462-9*) Buttrwrth-Heinemann.

***Differential Diagnosis in Surgical Pathology.** Meryl Haber et al. (Illus.). 730p. text (*0-7216-9053-X*) Saunders.

Differential Diagnosis of Acute Pain: By Body Region. Stanley L. Wiener. 1993. (Illus.). 845p. text 74.95 (*0-07-070177-6*) McGraw-Hill Prof.

Differential Diagnosis of Arrhythmias. Dale Davis. Ed. by Lisa Biello. 2nd ed. 1997. (Illus.). 288p. pap. text 31.50 (*0-7216-4477-5*) Saunders.

Differential Diagnosis of Bone Tumors. Adam Greenspan & Remagen. 1997. LC 97-37501. (Illus.). 448p. text 250.00 (*0-397-51710-6*) Lppncott W & W.

Differential Diagnosis of Chronic Pain by Body Region. Stanley L. Weiner. 1999. (Illus.). 816p. text 75.00 (*0-07-070183-0*) McGraw-Hill Med Pub.

Differential Diagnosis of Common Complaints. Robert H. Seller. Ed. by Ray Kersey. (Illus.). 3rd ed. 1996. LC 95-24440. 416p. pap. text 34.00 (*0-7216-5808-3*); 4th ed. 1999. LC 99-27918. xii, 442p. pap. text (*0-7216-8017-8*) Saunders.

Differential Diagnosis of Diseases of the Chest Robert G. Fraser et al. 3rd ed. (Illus.). 1990. 3460p. text 480.00 (*0-7216-3879-1*); Vol. 3. 1989. 819p. text 120.00 (*0-7216-3872-4*) Saunders.

Differential Diagnosis of Diseases of the Oral Mucosa. Wolfgang Bengel et al. 1988. (Illus.). 361p. text 78.00 (*0-86715-204-4*) Quint Pub Co.

Differential Diagnosis of Eye Disease. H. Pau. Tr. by Frederick C. Blodi from GRE. 2nd enl. rev. ed. 1988. (Illus.). 560p. 159.00 (*0-86577-264-9*) Thieme Med Pubs.

Differential Diagnosis of Lymphoid Disorders. Tsieh Sun & Myron Susin. 1996. LC 95-19893. (Illus.). 248p. 98.50 (*0-89640-289-4*) Igaku-Shoin.

Differential Diagnosis of Neuromusculoskeletal Disorders. Lawrence H. Wyatt. 1994. LC 94-1815. 300p. pap. 56.00 (*0-8342-0550-5*) Aspen Pub.

Differential Diagnosis of Oral & Maxillofacial Lesions. Norman K. Wood & Paul W. Goaz. 5th ed. 1996. LC 96-7855. (Illus.). 672p. (C). (gr. 13). text 78.00 (*0-8151-9432-3*, 26259) Mosby Inc.

Differential Diagnosis of Oral & Maxillofacial Lesions. Norman K. Wood & Paul W. Goaz. 5th ed. 1997. (Illus.). 672p. (*84-8174-293-7*) Mosby-Doyma Libros ESP. *Dist:* Mosby Inc.

Differential Diagnosis of Vertigo: Equilibrium in Patients & Research. Claus-Frenz Claussen. 1980. (Proceedings of the 8th Scientific Meeting of the NES, Turku-Finland, 1979 Ser.). 617p. 92.30 (*3-11-008298-5*) De Gruyter.

Differential Diagnosis Pediatric Radiology. Leonard E. Swischuk & Susan D. John. 2nd ed. 1994. (Illus.). 480p. text 125.00 (*0-683-08046-6*) Lppncott W & W.

Differential Diagnosis Small Mammals. Radrobe & Meredith. 2001. 256p. pap. text 63.00 (*0-7506-4250-5*) Buttrwrth-Heinemann.

Differential Diagnosis Soft Tissue Tumors. Andrew Rosenberg. 1998. (Illus.). 128p. (*0-89640-323-8*) Igaku-Shoin.

Differential Forecasts of Achievement & Their Use in Educational Counseling. Ralph R. Wolf. 1972. (Psychology Monographs General & Applied: Vol. 51). reprint ed. pap. 55.00 (*0-8115-1450-1*) Periodicals Srv.

Differential Psychopharmacology on Anxiolytics & Sedatives. Ed. by J. R. Boissier et al. 1979. (Modern Problems of Pharmacopsychiatry Ser.: Vol. 14). (Illus.). 47.00 (*3-8055-2777-2*) S Karger.

Differential Therapy of Depression: Possibilities & Limitations. Ed. by H. Hippius & N. Matussek. 1986. (Advances in Pharmacotherapy Ser.: Vol. 2). (Illus.). x, 238p. 161.75 (*3-8055-4049-3*) S Karger.

Differential Treatment of Drug & Alcohol Abusers. Ed. by Carl S. Davis & Marlin R. Schmidt. 1977. LC 76-54203. 19.95 (*0-88280-048-5*) ETC Pubns.

Differentialdiagnosen der Pilzvergiftungen, mit Bestimmungsschluesselein fuer Mediciner und Mykologen. R. Flammer. 1980. LC 88-5921. (GER., Illus.). 92p. text 17.50 (*3-437-10636-8*) Lubrecht & Cramer.

Differentialdiagnostik in der Hals-Nasen Ohren-Heilkunde see Differential Diagnosis in Otorhinolaryngology: Symptoms, Syndromes, & Interdisciplinary Issues

Differentialdiagnostisches Kompendium: Symptome - Befunde - Krankheiten - Laborwerte - EKG-Befunde - Roentgenbefunde. Jan Horny. 1994. (Illus.). x, 172p. pap. 28.00 (*3-8055-6075-3*) S Karger.

Differentiated Lymphocyte Functions. Ed. by Alain L. De Weck. 1981. (Progress in Allergy Ser.: Vol. 28). (Illus.). x, 286p. 126.25 (*3-8055-1834-X*) S Karger.

Differentiating Normal & Abnormal Personality. Ed. by Stephen Strack & Maurice Lorr. 1994. LC 94-28761. (Illus.). 464p. (C). 58.95 (*0-8261-8550-9*) Springer Pub.

Differentiating Nursing Practice: Into the Twenty-First Century. Pamela H. Mitchell et al. 1991. 452p. (Orig.). (C). pap. 25.00 (*1-55810-065-2*, G-182, Am Acad Nursing) Am Nurses Pub.

Differentiation of Human Oral Stratified Epithelia. H. E. Schroeder. 1981. (Illus.). xii, 308p. 138.50 (*3-8055-1462-X*) S Karger.

Differentiation of Iris Markings: With Illustrated Atlas & Indications of Treatment for Advanced Students of Iris Diagnosis, No. 2. 1986. (Illus.). text (*3-87306-013-2*) Inst Fund Rsch DEU. *Dist:* Medicina Bio.

Differix Internal Medicine. Martin Von Planta. 1996. 224p. (gr. 13). pap. 28.95 (*0-412-63510-0*) Chapman & Hall.

Difficult Art: A Critical Discourse on Psychotherapy. Aldo Carotenuto. Tr. by Joan Tambureno from ITA. 1992. LC 92-7870. 312p. (Orig.). pap. 5.95 (*0-933029-64-0*) Chiron Pubns.

Difficult Cardiology. Graham Jackson. 3rd ed. 1998. 432p. (*1-85317-406-8*) Martin Dunitz GBR. *Dist:* Mosby Inc.

Difficult Cardiology: Practical Management & Decision Making. Ed. by George G. Jackson. 1990. (Illus.). 360p. 110.00 (*0-387-91387-4*) Spr-Verlag.

Difficult Connection: The Therapeutic Relationship in Sex Offender Treatment. Geral T. Blanchard. Ed. by Euan Bear. 1998. 76p. (Orig.). (C). pap. text 12.00 (*1-884444-15-6*) Safer Soc.

Difficult Diabetes. Geoff Gill et al. 2000. LC 00-56419. (Illus.). xi, 308p. 146.95 (*0-632-05324-0*) Blackwell Sci.

Difficult Diagnosis in Surgical Pathology. Noel Weidner. 1995. LC 95-19481. (Illus.). 864p. text 165.00 (*0-7216-6464-4*) Saunders.

Difficult Medical Management. Robert B. Taylor. 1990. (Illus.). 768p. text 105.00 (*0-7216-8768-7*) Saunders.

Difficult Moments in Child Psychotherapy. S. Gabel et al. 1988. LC 88-25188. (Illus.). 230p. (C). 45.00 (*0-306-42971-3*, Kluwer Plenum) Kluwer Academic.

Difficult Patient. Joe Duxbury. 2000. 192p. pap. text 35.00 (*0-7506-3838-9*) Buttrwrth-Heinemann.

Difficult Patient. Eric Sohr. 1996. (Illus.). 120p. (Orig.). pap. text 11.95 (*0-940780-27-5*) MedMaster.

Difficult Patient: Managing/Understanding Dental Anxiety. Arthur A. Weiner. 2nd rev. ed. 1994. LC 94-66750. 77p. pap. 23.00 (*0-9641828-0-7*) Reniew Pubng.

Difficult Patient: Psychotherapeutic Strategies: A Special Issue of Journal of Contemporary Psychotherapy. Ed. by Sherman O. Schacter. 1988. 92p. pap. 16.95 (*0-89885-429-6*, Kluwer Acad Hman Sci) Kluwer Academic.

***Difficult-to-Treat Psychiatry Patient.** Ed. by Mantosh J. Dewan & Ronald Pies. 2001. LC 00-69519. 448p. pap. 53.95 (*0-88048-949-9*, 8949) Am Psychiatric.

Difficult Vaginal Hysterectomy: A Surgical Atlas. Mitchell S. Hoffman & William N. Spellacy. 1994. LC 94-5703. (Illus.). 133p. 94.00 (*0-387-94273-4*) Spr-Verlag.

Difficulties in the Analytic Encounter. J. Klauber. 1991. 267p. pap. (*0-946960-52-6*) Karnac Bks GBR. *Dist:* Other Pr LLC.

Difficulties in the Analytic Encounter. John Klauber. 1981. LC 80-69670. (Classical Psychoanalysis & Its Applications Ser.). 272p. 40.00 (*0-87668-430-4*) Aronson.

Difficulties in Tracheal Intubation. L. P. Latto. 2nd ed. 1996. (Illus.). 395p. (C). text 82.95 (*0-7020-2116-4*) Harcourt.

Diffraction Methods for Biological Macromolecules, Pt. A. Ed. by Sidney P. Colowick & Nathan O. Kaplan. 1985. (Methods in Enzymology Ser.: Vol. 114). text 188.00 (*0-12-182014-9*) Acad Pr.

Diffuse Lung Disorders: A Comprehensive Clinical-Radiological Overview. Ed. by Miriam Sperber. 1998. LC 97-53117. (Illus.). 528p. 199.00 (*3-540-76202-7*) Spr-Verlag.

Diffusion & Membrane Technology. Sidney B. Tuwiner. 1962. LC 62-20783. (ACS Monograph: No. 156). 39.95 (*0-8412-0284-2*) Am Chemical.

Diffusion Chamber Culture: Hemopoiesis, Cloning of Tumors, Cytogenetic & Carinogenic Assays. Eugene P. Cronkite & A. L. Carstens. 1980. (Illus.). 277p. 67.95 (*0-387-10064-4*) Spr-Verlag.

Diffusion-Controlled Stress Relaxation of Swollen Rubber-Like Networks. D. E. Knibbe. 1968. 60p. pap. text 112.00 (*0-677-61185-4*) Gordon & Breach.

Diffusion of Influenza: Patterns & Paradigms. Gerald F. Pyle. 1986. LC 86-1780. (Illus.). 240p. (C). 64.00 (*0-8476-7429-0*, R7429) Rowman.

Diffusion of Medical Innovations: An Applied Network Analysis. M. L. Fennell & R. B. Warnecke. 1988. LC 88-2475. (Environment, Development, & Public Policy Ser.). (Illus.). 300p. (C). text 63.00 (*0-306-42752-4*) Plenum.

Diffusion Processes Ed. by J. N. Sherwood et al. 1971. 444p. 198.00 (*0-677-14830-5*) Gordon & Breach.

Diffusion Processes & Related Topics in Biology. Luigi M. Ricciardi. 1977. LC 77-7464. (Lecture Notes in Biomathematics: Vol. 14). (Illus.). 200p. 32.00 (*0-387-08146-1*) Spr-Verlag.

Diflubenzuron. 1995. (Health & Safety Guides Ser.: No. 99). 28p. (C). pap. text 4.50 (*92-4-151099-4*, 1860099) Am Soc Clinical.

Dig Up Bones. Nikos M. Linardakis. 1998. (Digging Up the Bones Ser.). (Illus.). 128p. pap. 19.95 (*0-07-038214-X*) McGraw-Hill Prof.

Digestibility & Amino Acid Availability in Cereals & Oilseeds. Ed. by John W. Finley & Daniel T. Hopkins. 1985. LC 85-72941. 304p. 99.00 (*0-913250-40-6*) Am Assn Cereal Chem.

Digestion & Dyspepsia, 1874. R. T. Trall. 1996. (Illus.). 160p. reprint ed. pap. 14.00 (*1-56459-809-8*) Kessinger Pub.

Digestion & the Structure & Function of the Gut. D. F. Magee & A. F. Dalley. 1986. (Continuing Education Ser.: Vol. 8). (Illus.). viii, 360p. 128.75 (*3-8055-4204-6*) S Karger.

Digestive Disease Pathology. Shaw Watanabe. Vol. 2. 1989. 65.00 (*0-938607-25-1*); Vol. 3. Date not set. (*0-938607-38-3*) Field & Wood Inc Medical.

Digestive Diseases. Albert Mendeloff & James P. Dunn. 1971. LC 71-158432. (Vital & Health Statistics Monographs). (Illus.). 190p. 31.00 (*0-674-20580-4*) HUP.

Digestive Diseases & Disorders Sourcebook: Basic Consumer Health Information about Diseases & Disorders That Impact the Upper & Lower Digestive Systems. Ed. by Karen Bellenir. 1999. LC 99-45761. (Health Reference Ser.). (Illus.). 300p. lib. bdg. 48.00 (*0-7808-0327-2*) Omnigraphics Inc.

Digestive Diseases of the U. S. Epidemiology & Impact. Ed. by James E. Everhart. 1995. (Illus.). 799p. (Orig.). (C). pap. text 75.00 (*0-7881-2604-0*) DIANE Pub.

Digestive Enzymes. Earl R. Mindell & Jeffrey S. Bland. 1983. (Good Health Guides). 31p. pap. 3.95 (*0-87983-331-9*, 33319K, Keats Pubng) McGraw-Hill Trade.

Digestive Health: And Your Optimal Wellness. Jonathan Silver. 1999. (Living Longer, Living Stronger Ser.). (Illus.). 12.00 (*1-892870-08-8*) Best Years Inc.

Digestive System. Thomas Braem. 1994. (Organs of the Human Anatomy: Vol. 2). 80p. (C). spiral bd. 15.95 (*1-878576-27-5*) Flash Anatomy Inc.

***Digestive System.** Margaret Smith & Dion Morton. 2001. (Illus.). 155p. (*0-443-06245-5*) Church GBR. *Dist:* Saunders.

Digestive System. Thomas C. Jones et al. 2nd ed. LC 96-27162. (Monographs in Pathology of Laboratory Animals). (Illus.). 1997. 488p. 289.00 (*3-540-61373-0*); 1996. 450p. 320.00 (*0-944398-75-8*) Spr-Verlag.

Digestive System Vol. 3, Pt. III: Liver, Biliary Tract & Pancreas, Vol. 3, Pt. 3. Illus. by Frank H. Netter. 1957. LC 53-2151. 38.00 (*0-914168-05-3*) Icon Lrning Systs.

Digestive System Physiology. 2nd ed. 256p. pap. (*0-340-56020-7*) E A GBR. *Dist:* Routldge.

Digestive Tract Surgery: A Text & Atlas. Ed. by Richard H. Bell, Jr. et al. 1995. LC 95-981. 1,688p. text 250.00 (*0-397-51344-5*) Lppncott W & W.

Digestive Tract Tumors. Ed. by Kiyoshi Inokuchi et al. 1986. LC 86-42515. (Gann Monographs on Cancer Research: No. 31). (Illus.). 288p. (C). text 126.00 (*0-306-42297-2*) Plenum.

Digger's Guide to Medicinal Plants. Allen Lockard & Alice Q. Swanson. 1998. LC 98-84753. (Illus.). 96p. pap. 9.95 (*0-9663398-1-9*) Ameri Botan.

Digging up the Bones Wilson et al. Ed. by Nikos. 1995. (Illus.). 600p. (C). pap. 96.00 (*1-884084-13-3*) Michaelis Med.

Digging up the Bones: Pharmacology. Nikos M. Linardakis. 2nd ed. 1996. LC 96-157441. pap. 17.95 (*1-884084-23-0*) Michaelis Med.

Digging up the Bones... Pharmacology, Microbiology, Pathology & Biochemistry Nikos M. Linardakis. 1994. 400p. (Orig.). (C). pap. text 16.00 (*1-884084-00-1*); pap. text 16.00 (*1-884084-01-X*); pap. text 16.00 (*1-884084-02-8*); pap. text (*1-884084-04-4*);Set. pap. text 64.00 (*1-884084-10-9*) Michaelis Med.

Digging up the Bones... Vol. 5: Behavioral Science. Nikos M. Linardakis. 1995. (Illus.). 80p. (C). pap. text 16.00 (*1-884084-11-7*) Michaelis Med.

Digital Analysis of Bitemark Evidence. C. Michael Bowers & Raymond Johansen. 2000. (Illus.). vi, 110p. pap. 29.95 (*0-9677866-0-6*) Forensic Imaging Inst.

Digital Biosignal Processing. R. Weitkunat. 1991. (Techniques in the Behavioral & Neural Sciences Ser.: Vol. 5). 602p. pap. 84.00 (*0-444-89144-7*) Elsevier.

Digital Biosignal Processing. Ed. by R. Weitkunat. 1991. (Techniques in the Behavioral & Neural Sciences Ser.: No. 5). 602p. 290.00 (*0-444-81140-0*) Elsevier.

Digital Cardiac Imaging. Ed. by Andrew J. Buda & Edward J. Delp. 1985. text 208.00 (*0-89838-697-7*) Kluwer Academic.

Digital Doctors. Marshall Ruffin. 1999. LC 98-89673. 220p. pap. 45.00 (*0-924674-63-6*) Am Coll Phys Execs.

Digital EEG in Clinical Practice. Peter K. Wong. 1995. LC 95-32100. 320p. text 105.00 (*0-397-51635-5*) Lppncott W & W.

Digital Hearing Aid Handbook. Chasin. 2000. pap. 49.95 (*1-56593-978-6*, C3969) Thomson Learn.

Digital Imaging in Health Care. 1987. 174p. 48.00 (*92-1-116380-3*, E.86.II.E.29) UN.

Digital Mammography: Proceedings of the 2nd International Workshop on Digital Mammography, York, England, 10-12 July 1994. Ed. by Alastair G. Gale. 1994. LC 94-32879. (International Congress Ser.: Vol. 1069). 434p. 227.25 (*0-444-81916-9*) Elsevier.

Digital Mammography '96: Proceedings of the 3rd International Workshop on Digital Mammography, Chicago, 9-12 June 1996. Kunmio Doi. 1996. LC 96-44173. (International Congress Ser.: Vol. 1119). 494p. 223.50 (*0-444-82431-6*) Elsevier.

Digital Signal Processing Hearing Aids. Kuk. 2000. pap. 34.95 (*1-56593-974-3*, K2334) Thomson Learn.

Digital Subtraction Angiography. Arina Van Breda & Barry T. Katzen. 1986. 240p. 52.00 (*0-316-10774-3*, Little Brwn Med Div) Lppncott W & W.

Digital Techniques in Echocardiography. Ed. by Jos R. Roelandt. 1987. (Developments in Cardiovascular Medicine Ser.). text 184.00 (*0-89838-861-9*) Kluwer Academic.

Dignostic Imaging Eye Orbit. Weber. 1999. pap. text 110.00 (*0-8385-1610-6*) P-H.

Dihlmann: Gelenksilhoette. 1995. 204.00 (*0-387-57523-5*) Spr-Verlag.

Dihydropyridines: Progress in Pharmacology & Therapy. Ed. by W. E. Busse et al. 1993. LC 93-21268. (Illus.). 130p. 51.95 (*0-387-57308-9*) Spr-Verlag.

Dilemma of Ritual Abuse: Cautions & Guides for Therapists. Ed. by George A. Fraser. 1997. LC 96-30140. (Clinical Practice Ser.). (Illus.). 268p. text 39.50 (*0-88048-478-0*, 8478) Am Psychiatric.

***Dilemma of the Sexual Offender.** George B. Palermo & Mary Ann Farkas. 2001. LC 2001-27393. (American Series in Behavioral Science & Law). 252p. text 49.95 (*0-398-07199-3*); pap. text 33.95 (*0-398-07200-0*) C C Thomas.

Dilemmas & Difficulties in the Management of Psychiatric Patients. Ed. by Keith E. Hawton & Philip Cowen. 1990. (Illus.). 272p. 75.00 (*0-19-261883-0*); 270p. pap. 38.95 (*0-19-261944-6*) OUP.

Dilemmas in Community Mental Health Practice: Choice or Control. Rachel Perkins & Julie Repper. 1998. LC 98-169278. 160p. pap. (*1-85775-181-7*) Radcliffe Med Pr GBR. *Dist:* Balogh.

Dilemmas in General Practice: Hot Topics for the MRCGP & Beyond. Edward Warren. 1997. 240p. pap. text 37.50 (*0-7506-3233-X*) Buttrwrth-Heinemann.

Dilemmas in Health Care. Ed. by Basiro Davey & Jennie Popay. rev. ed. 1993. LC 92-44760. (Health & Disease Ser.: Bk. 7). pap. (*0-335-19119-3*) OpUniv Pr.

Dilemmas of Brief Psychotherapy. James P. Gustafson. 1995. LC 95-24190. (Illus.). 252p. (C). 42.50 (*0-306-44975-7*, Plenum Trade) Perseus Pubng.

Dimension of Nursing Management. S. W. Booyens. 2nd ed. 1998. 719p. pap. (*0-7021-4211-5*) Juta & Co ZAF. *Dist:* Intl Spec Bk.

Dimensional Adjectives. Ed. by Manfred Bierwisch & E. K. Lang. 1989. (Language & Communication Ser.: Vol. 26). (Illus.). 523p. 128.00 (*0-387-50633-0*, 3157) Spr-Verlag.

Dimensional Analysis for Meds. Anna M. Curren & Laurie D. Munday. 1998. LC 98-177565. (Illus.). (C). pap. text 36.95 (*0-918082-08-0*) WI Pubns Inc.

***Dimensional Analysis for Meds.** Anna M. Curren. 2nd ed. 2001. LC 2001-47128. (*0-7668-5938-X*) Delmar.

Dimensions Characteristics & Roles in Client Care. Barbara L. Mandleco. 1998. (C). pap. text (*0-8053-7190-7*) Addison-Wesley.

***Dimensions in Empathic Therapy.** Ed. by Peter Roger Breggin et al. 2001. LC 2001-40010. pap. (*0-8261-1513-6*) Springer Pub.

Dimensions in Professional Development. Caroline Reynolds. 4th ed. 1993. LC 92-18247. (C). mass mkt. 43.95 (*0-538-61416-1*) S-W Thomson.

Dimensions in Wholistic Healing: New Frontiers in the Treatment of the Whole Person. Ed. by Herbert A. Otto & James W. Knight. 1979. LC 78-27071. 568p. text 46.95 (*0-88229-513-6*) Burnham Inc.

Dimensions of Community Mental Health Care. Ed. by M. P. Weller & M. Muijen. 1994. (Illus.). 348p. pap. text (*0-7020-1612-8*) W B Saunders GBR. *Dist:* Saunders.

Dimensions of Food. Vickie A. Vaclavik et al. 4th ed. 1998. LC 97-27378. 279p. pap. 40.00 (*0-412-14731-9*) Chapman & Hall.

Dimensions of HIV Prevention: Needle Exchange. Ed. by Jeff Stryker & Mark D. Smith. 1993. (Illus.). 182p. (Orig.). pap. text 5.00 (*0-944525-14-8*) H J Kaiser.

Dimensions of Hospital Industry Student Workbook. Drummond. 1993. pap. 22.95 (*0-442-01473-2*, VNR) Wiley.

Dimensions of Human Sexuality, Test Item File/QIF. Curtis O. Byer & Shainberg. 4th ed. 1994. 13.43 (*0-697-12604-8*) McGraw.

Dimensions of Human Sexuality. Curtis O. Byer & Shainberg. 4th ed. 1993. stu. ed. 12.25 net. (*0-697-24423-7*, WCB McGr Hill) McGrw-H Hghr Educ.

Dimensions of Learning Disability. Gates. 1996. pap. text 41.00 (*0-7020-1916-X*) Saunders.

Dimensions of New Contraceptives, Norplant & Women: A Publication from the Kaiser Forums Sponsored by the Henry J. Kaiser Family Foundation. Ed. by Sarah E. Samuels & Mark D. Smith. 1992. 123p. (Orig.). pap. text 5.00 (*0-944525-11-3*) H J Kaiser.

Dimensions of Nursing Management. S. W. Booyens. 1993. pap. (*0-7021-2988-7*) Juta & Co ZAF. *Dist:* Intl Spec Bk, Gaunt.

Dimensions of Personality. Hans J. Eysenck. 1998. LC 97-13292. 320p. pap. text 29.95 (*1-56000-985-3*) Transaction Pubs.

Dimensions of Personality. Procidano. 1999. (C). text 53.50 (*0-15-500127-2*) Harcourt Coll Pubs.

Dimensions of Professional Nursing. Lucie Y. Kelly. 6th ed. 1991. (Illus.). 760p. text (*0-08-040303-4*) PPI GBR. *Dist:* McGraw.

Dimensions of Professional Nursing. Lucie Young Kelly & Lucille A. Joel. 8th ed. 1999. LC 98-50589. (Illus.). 750p. pap. 39.00 (*0-07-034440-X*) McGraw-Hill Prof.

Dimensions of Psychoanalysis. Ed. by Joseph Sandler. 1990. 281p. 40.00 (*0-8236-1293-7*) Intl Univs Pr.

Dimensions of Psychotherapy: An Experimental & Clinical Approach. Donald R. Stieper & Daniel N. Wiener. 1965. LC 65-22494. 42.50 (*0-89197-622-1*) Irvington.

Dimensions of Radionics. David V. Tansley. 1977. 224p. (C). pap. 22.95 (*0-8464-1005-2*) Beekman Pubs.

Dimensions of Radionics. David V. Tansley. 1980. (*0-85032-156-5*) C W Daniel GBR. *Dist:* Natl Bk Netwk.

Dimensions of Radionics: Techniques of Instrumented Distant Healing. David V. Tansley & Malcolm Rae. 2nd ed. 1992. (Illus.). 222p. reprint ed. pap. 17.95 (*0-914732-29-3*) Bro Life Inc.

Dimensions of Self Experience, Vol. 5. Ed. by Arnold Goldberg. 1989. (Progress in Self Psychology Ser.). 320p. text 45.00 (*0-88163-086-1*) Analytic Pr.

Dimensions of Social Life: Essays in Honor of David G. Mandelbaum. Ed. by Paul Hockings. 1987. (New Babylon Studies in the Social Sciences: No. 48). (Illus.). xiv, 712p. (C). lib. bdg. (*0-89925-292-3*) Mouton.

Dimensions of State Mental Health Policy. Ed. by Christopher G. Hudson & Arthur J. Cox. 1990. LC 90-7595. 320p. 72.50 (*0-275-93252-4*, C3252, Praeger Pubs) Greenwood.

Dimensions of the Cancer Problem. Fikri M. Meleka. 1983. xii, 144p. pap. 42.75 (*3-8055-3622-4*) S Karger.

Dimethyl Sulfate. 1985. (Environmental Health Criteria Ser.: No. 48). 55p. pap. text 13.00 (*92-4-154188-1*, 1160048) World Health.

***Dimethyl Sulfoxide (DMSO) Index of New Information for Therapy, Clinical Uses, Research & Reference.** Ed. by Research and Development Division Staff & John C. Bartone. 2001. 180p. 47.50 (*0-7883-2402-0*); pap. 44.50 (*0-7883-2403-9*) ABBE Pubs Assn.

Dimethylformamide. 1991. (Environmental Health Criteria Ser.: No. 114). (ENG, FRE & SPA.). 124p. pap. text 24.00 (*92-4-157114-4*, 1160114) World Health.

Diminished Mind: One Family's Extraordinary Battle with Alzheimer's. Jean Tyler. 1990. 16.95 (*0-8306-3465-7*) McGraw-Hill Educ Grp.

Dimorphic Fungi in Biology & Medicine. H. Vanden Bossche et al. 1993. (Illus.). 440p. (C). text 125.00 (*0-306-44493-3*, Kluwer Plenum) Kluwer Academic.

Dimorphism in Human Pathogenic & Apathogenic Yeasts. Ed. by J. F. Ernst & A. Schmidt. 2000. (Contributions to Microbiology Ser.: Vol. 5). (Illus.). x, 246p. 172.25 (*3-8055-6986-6*) S Karger.

Dinh Duong Tri Lieu: Nutrition Therapy. Thu T. Nguyen. 1993. LC 92-62316. (Illus.). 928p. 59.00 (*0-9635459-0-6*) N X Phuong.

Dinosaur Brains: Dealing with All Those Impossible People at Work. Albert J. Bernstein & Sydney C. Rozen. 1989. LC 88-22336. 272p. 29.95 (*0-471-61808-X*) Wiley.

Dioxin Perspectives: A Pilot Study on the International Information Exchange on Dioxins & Related Compounds. Ed. by E. W. Bretthauer et al. 1991. (NATO Challenges of Modern Society Ser.: Vol. 16). (Illus.). 800p. (C). text 258.00 (*0-306-43916-6*, Kluwer Plenum) Kluwer Academic.

Dioxins & Agent Orange: Index of New Information with Clinical & Research Results. Jerome W. Shawn. 1995. LC 95-15410. 57.50 (*0-7883-0502-6*); pap. 47.50 (*0-7883-0503-4*) ABBE Pubs Assn.

Dioxins & Health. Ed. by Arnold J. Schecter. 1994. (Illus.). 732p. (C). text 135.00 (*0-306-44785-1*, Kluwer Plenum) Kluwer Academic.

Dioxins & the Immune System: Mechanisms & Consequences of Interference. Ed. by C. Esser & E. Gleichmann. 1994. (Journal: Vol. 11, No. 2-3, 1994). (Illus.). 114p. pap. 83.50 (*3-8055-6060-5*) S Karger.

Dipeptides As New Substrates in Nutrition Therapy Peptide als neue Substrate in der Ernaehrungstherapie. Ed. by S. A. Adibi et al. 1987. (Beitraege zur Infusionstherapie und Klinische Ernaehrung Ser.: Vol. 17). (Illus.). viii, 196p. 55.00 (*3-8055-4613-0*) S Karger.

Diplegic Child: Evaluation & Management. Ed. by Michael D. Sussman. 1992. 496p. 85.00 (*0-89203-068-2*) Amer Acad Ortho Surg.

Dipyrone: Recent Investigations on Its Mode of Action, Pharmacokinetics, & Clinical Use. Ed. by Kay Brune. 1992. LC 92-49454. 56p. 32.00 (*0-8176-2804-5*) Spr-Verlag.

Dipyrone: Recent Investigations on Its Mode of Action, Pharmacokinetics, & Clinical Use, Berlin, October 24, 1991. Ed. by Kay Brune. 1992. LC 92-49454. vii, 45p. (*3-7643-2804-5*) Birkhauser CHE. *Dist:* Princeton Arch.

Dire Mastery: Discipleship from Freud to Lacan. Francois Roustang. Tr. by Ned Lukacher from FRE. 1986. LC 86-20572. 162p. pap. text 7.50 (*0-88048-259-1*, 8259) Am Psychiatric.

Direct & Allosteric Control of Glutamate Receptors. Ed. by Michael G. Palfreyman et al. 1994. LC 94-7075. (Series on Pharmacology & Toxicology). 192p. lib. bdg. 149.00 (*0-8493-8307-2*, 8307) CRC Pr.

Direct & Indirect Costs of Diabetes in the United States in 1992. American Diabetes Association. 1993. 32p. pap. 19.95 (*0-945448-32-5*, 5701-01) Am Diabetes.

Direct Contracting Manual. 1994. 250.00 (*0-937925-94-2*, DCM) Capitol Publns.

Directed Drug Delivery: A Multidisciplinary Approach. Ed. by Ronald T. Borchardt et al. 1985. LC 85-2291. (Experimental Biology & Medicine Ser.: Vol. 7). (Illus.). 384p. 145.00 (*0-89603-089-X*) Humana.

Directing Health Messages Toward African Americans: Attitudes Toward Health Care & the Mass Media. Judith L. Sylvester. Ed. by John G. Bruhn. 1997. LC 97-42742. (Health Care Policy in the United States Ser.). (Illus.). 304p. text 72.00 (*0-8153-3051-0*) Garland.

Directing the Clinical Lab. D. Hardwick. 1990. 44.95 (*0-938607-27-8*) Field & Wood Inc Medical.

C
D

Direction: The Essential Dimension. Charles W. Williams. 1960. 15.00 (*0-8315-0003-4*) Speller.

Direction for the Health of Magistrates & Students. Gulielmus Gratarolus. Tr. by Thomas Newton. 1972. LC 72-38192. (English Experience Ser.: No. 462). 172p. reprint ed. 30.00 (*90-221-0462-1*) Walter J Johnson.

Directional Hearing. Ed. by William A. Yost & G. Gourevitch. 1987. (Illus.). 305p. 98.00 (*0-387-96493-2*) Spr-Verlag.

Directions 1996: Directory of Health & Human Care Services in San Diego County. Resource Center, United Way of San Diego County Staff. 1995. 700p. 38.00 (*0-9629793-4-1*) United Way SD.

Directions for New Anti-Asthma Drugs. S. O'Donnell & C. G. Persson. 1988. (Agents & Actions Supplements Ser.: No. 23). 246p. 107.00 (*0-8176-1957-7*) Birkhauser.

Directions 1997: Directory of Health & Human Care Services in San Diego County. Resource Center, United Way of San Diego County Staff. unabr. ed. 1996. 676p. 38.00 (*0-9629793-5-X*) United Way SD.

Directive Group Therapy: Innovative Mental Health Treatment. Kathy Kaplan. 1988. LC 88-42754. 165p. (C). pap. 27.00 (*1-55642-050-1*) SLACK Inc.

Director of Drug Treatment Services. Jack Rudman. 1994. (Career Examination Ser.: C-2821). pap. 39.95 (*0-8373-2821-7*) Nat Learn.

Director of Environmental Health Services. Jack Rudman. 1994. (Career Examination Ser.: C-3136). pap. 39.95 (*0-8373-3136-6*) Nat Learn.

Director of Nursing Care. Jack Rudman. 1994. (Career Examination Ser.: C-2859). pap. 39.95 (*0-8373-2859-4*) Nat Learn.

Director of Patient Services. Jack Rudman. 1994. (Career Examination Ser.: C-2724). pap. 39.95 (*0-8373-2724-5*) Nat Learn.

Directors of Development: Influences on the Development of Children's Thinking. Ed. by Lynn Okagaki & Robert J. Sternberg. 1991. 304p. pap. 34.50 (*0-8058-0628-8*); text 59.95 (*0-8058-0627-X*) L Erlbaum Assocs.

Directory of Agents Being Tested for Carcinogenicity, No. 17. 1996. 247p. pap. 45.00 (*92-832-1317-3*, 1780017) World Health.

Directory of Agents Being Tested for Carcinogenicity, No. 16. Compiled by M. J. Ghess et al. 1994. x, 293p. pap. text 45.00 (*92-832-1316-5*, 1740016) World Health.

Directory of Authors of New Medical & Scientific Reviews of Contraception with Subject Index. Science and Life Consultants Association Staff. rev. ed. 1998. 145p. 57.50 (*0-7883-2080-7*); pap. 47.50 (*0-7883-2081-5*) ABBE Pubs Assn.

Directory of Biomedical & Life Science Online Databases. Cuadra Staff & Elsevier Science Publishing Staff. 1987. 29.95 (*0-444-01196-X*) Elsevier.

Directory of Biomedical Research in France see Annuaire de la Recherche Biomedicale

Directory of Certified Clinical Specialists in Physical Therapy. 1999. 160p. pap. 21.00 (*1-887759-22-0*, CERT-1) Am Phys Therapy Assn.

Directory of Certified Surgical Technologists & Certified First Assistants, 1995. LCC-ST Staff. Ed. by Nadine A. Davis. 1995. pap. text (*0-9622332-5-0*) Liaison Coun.

Directory of Community Blood Centers, 1997. American Association of Blood Banks Staff. 1997. 118p. pap. (*3-8055-6784-7*) S Karger.

Directory of Community Substance Abuse Programs in Virginia. 1993. 56p. (Orig.). (C). pap. text 25.00 (*0-7881-0045-9*) DIANE Pub.

Directory of Complementary & Alternative Medicine. Ed. by Hugh P. Greeley & Anne M. Banas. 1999. (Illus.). 530p. pap. text 149.00 (*1-57839-065-6*) Opus Communs.

Directory of Credentials in Counseling & Psychotherapy. Daniel R. Martin & J. Richard Cookerly. 1989. (Reference Bks.). 270p. 40.00 (*0-8161-9062-3*, Hall Reference) Macmillan.

Directory of Drugs in Clinical Trials. CenterWatch Editorial Staff. 2000. 656p. pap. 399.00 (*0-9673029-3-5*) CenterWatch.

***Directory of Drugs in Clinical Trials.** Ed. by Kristen Eschmann. 2nd rev. ed. 2001. 599.99 (*1-930624-18-2*) CenterWatch.

Directory of Educational Software for Nursing: Addendum. Christine Bolwell. 1995. 229p. (C). 39.95 (*1-888418-00-1*) FITNE.

***Directory of Ethnic Minority Professionals in Psychology.** American Psychological Association Staff. 4th ed. 2001. LC 2001-22592. xv, 315p. pap. 24.95 (*1-55798-824-2*, 407-873) Am Psychol.

Directory of Facial Prosthetic Resources: A Guide to the Literature, Products & Suppliers for the Facial Prosthetic Community. Ed. by Robert E. McKinstry. 1998. pap. 55.00 incl. disk (*1-886236-13-5*) ABI Prof Pubns.

Directory of Federal Aid for Health & Allied Fields. 1982. 47.50 (*0-916270-35-1*) Ready Ref Pr.

Directory of Federal Aid for the Handicapped. 1982. 47.50 (*0-916270-30-0*) Ready Ref Pr.

Directory of Graduate Programs in Clinical Child & Pediatric Psychology. Kenneth J. Tarnowski & Susan J. Simonian. 1997. 98p. pap. (*0-8058-2958-X*) L Erlbaum Assocs.

Directory of Grants for Medical Study & Research in the U. S. A. Ed. by Susan Offerman. 10th rev. ed. 2000. 165p. pap. 52.00 (*1-930459-01-7*) Overseas.

Directory of Health Care Professionals. 1996. (*1-57372-021-6*); 1995. (*1-880678-67-5*) Solucient.

Directory of Health Care Professionals, 1997. HCIA Staff. 1996. pap. 299.00 (*1-57372-051-8*, H2308) Solucient.

Directory of Healthcare Group Purchasing Organizations, 2001. Medical Economics Staff. rev. ed. 2000. (Directory of Healthcare Group Purchasing Organizations Ser.). (Illus.). 500p. 325.00 (*1-56363-391-4*, PDR) Med Econ.

Directory of Healthcare Professionals, 1998. 1997. pap. 299.00 (*1-57372-092-5*) Solucient.

Directory of Historians of Islamic Medicine & Allied Sciences. Sami K. Hamarneh. 1997. 358p. (C). text 25.00 (*0-934905-87-8*, Library of Islam) Kazi Pubns.

Directory of Holistic Medicine & Alternate Health Care Services in the U. S. Ed. by Shirley Linde & Donald J. Carrow. 1986. LC 85-13193. 264p. pap. 6.95 (*0-932090-18-4*) Mosby Inc.

Directory of Holistic Practitioners for the Greater Boston Area. Ed. by David I. Weiss et al. 1987. LC 87-90042. 106p. (Orig.). pap. 6.00 (*0-9618049-0-4*) D I Weiss.

Directory of Hospital Personnel, 1987. Ed. by William J. Feinberg. 1986. 1100p. (Orig.). pap. text 259.00 (*0-938184-18-0*) Whole World.

Directory of Hospital Personnel, 2001. Medical Economics Staff. rev. ed. 2000. (Directory of Hospital Personnel Ser.). (Illus.). 2,400p. 325.00 (*1-56363-390-6*, PDR) Med Econ.

Directory of Information Resources for the Handicapped. 47.50 (*0-916270-28-9*) Ready Ref Pr.

Directory of International & National Medical Societies. G. Zeitak. 1982. 350p. pap. 115.00 (*0-08-027991-0*, Pergamon Pr) Elsevier.

Directory of International Grants & Fellowships in the Health Sciences. (Orig.). 1996. 118p. pap. text 40.00 (*1-57979-250-2*); 1994. 100p. (C). pap. text 30.00 (*0-7881-0343-1*) DIANE Pub.

***Directory of International Grants & Fellowships in the Health Sciences.** Pref. by Gerald T. Keusch. 2001. 110p. reprint ed. pap. text 25.00 (*0-7567-1766-3*) DIANE Pub.

Directory of International Grants & Fellowships in the Health Sciences (1996) Ed. by Philip E. Schambra. 1998. 118p. (C). pap. text 25.00 (*0-7881-7298-0*) DIANE Pub.

Directory of Internet Sources for Health Professionals. Griffin. 1998. LC 98-30169. 500p. (C). 32.95 (*0-7668-0485-2*) Delmar.

Directory of Internship & Post-Doctoral Fellowships in Clinical Child/Pediatric Psychology. Susan J. Simonian & Kenneth J. Tarnowski. 1997. 194p. pap. (*0-8058-2957-1*) L Erlbaum Assocs.

Directory of Licensed Mental Health Care Providers, 1995-1996: Middle Tennessee Edition. Council of Community Services Staff. 1996. 120p. spiral bd. 8.00 (*1-888334-00-2*) Coun Commun Serv.

Directory of Living Aids for the Handicapped. 1984. 47.50 (*0-916270-41-6*) Ready Ref Pr.

Directory of Medical Internet Site Addresses: With Emphasis on Authority, Responsibility, & Sponsorship. Michael D. Gainey & Milton C. Heuston. 3rd rev. ed. 1999. Orig. Title: The Doctor's Directory of Medical Internet Addresses. 114p. pap. text 29.95 (*0-9675465-0-8*) Heuston Consult.

Directory of Medical Management Software. Gary Knox. 1997. 149p. pap. 39.95 (*1-887212-11-6*) AQC Resource.

Directory of Medical Rehabilitation Facilities, 1997. 1997. pap. 195.00 (*1-57372-050-X*) Solucient.

Directory of Medical Specialists from Kerala India. A. Enas Enas. 1986. 140p. (Orig.). pap. 25.00 (*0-9616232-0-9*) EA Enas.

Directory of Minority Health Data Resources of the Public Health Service. 1995. lib. bdg. 253.99 (*0-8490-7570-X*) Gordon Pr.

Directory of Minority Nursing Faculty, 1996. 4th ed. 1996. 375p. 150.00 (*0-923950-13-3*) Tucker IL.

Directory of Newsletters Related to Health, Medicine, Nutrition, & Sports. Ed. by Greg Landry & Nancy Landry. 1988. 48p. (Orig.). (*0-929363-00-0*) G Landry.

Directory of Nursing Homes, 1997. 1997. pap. 249.00 (*1-57372-052-6*) Solucient.

Directory of Nursing Homes, 1998. 1997. pap. 249.00 (*1-57372-100-X*) Solucient.

Directory of Nursing Preceptorships in the United States. Linda K. Fetters & W. R. Hudson. 2nd ed. 1988. 485p. pap. (*0-929599-00-4*) FimCo Bks.

Directory of Nursing Preceptorships in the United States. Linda K. Fetters & Hudson Fetters. 3rd ed. 1990. 600p. pap. 50.00 (*0-929599-01-2*) FimCo Bks.

Directory of On-Going Research in Cancer Epidemiology, 1983. G. Wagner. Ed. by Calum S. Muir. 1986. (IARC Scientific Publications Ser.: No. 50). 740p. pap. 32.00 (*0-19-723050-4*) OUP.

Directory of On-Going Research in Cancer Epidemiology, 1984. Ed. by Calum S. Muir & G. Wagner. 1985. (IARC Scientific Publications Ser.: No. 62). 748p. pap. 26.50 (*0-19-723062-8*) OUP.

Directory of Online Healthcare Databases. Karen Peterkin & Donald V. Black. 5th rev. ed. 1990. 80p. spiral bd. 35.00 (*0-931712-10-6*) Alpine Guild.

Directory of Perioperative Nursing Courses, 1996. rev. ed. 1995. 86p. (C). pap. text 12.50 (*0-939583-91-7*) AORN.

Directory of Physician Groups & Networks. Contrib. by Russell Perkins. 1999. 220p. 345.00 (*1-880874-50-4*) Dorland Hlthcare.

Directory of Physicians in the U. S. 36th ed. 1998. 695.00 (*0-89970-913-3*) AMA.

Directory of Physicians in the United States 37th ed. 2000. 7000p. 695.00 (*1-57947-067-X*) AMA.

Directory of Programs & Services for Older People with Impaired Vision. 1996. (Aging & Vision Ser.). 29.95 (*0-9603444-1-1*, P960) Lighthouse NYC.

Directory of Psychiatry Residency Training Programs. American Psychiatric Association, Department of Education Staff. 7th ed. 1997. 752p. pap. text 31.00 (*0-89042-708-9*, 2708) Am Psychiatric.

Directory of Psychological Tests in the Sport & Exercise Sciences. Ed. by Andrew C. Ostrow. 2nd ed. 1996. LC 96-86376. 570p. (C). text 46.00 (*1-885693-06-0*) Fit Info Tech.

Directory of Resources for Aging, Gerontology & Retirement. Ed. by Michael R. Gabriel. 2nd ed. 1986. 250p. lib. bdg. 75.00 (*0-933474-41-5*) Media Mktg Group.

Directory of the APA, 1993. Ed. by John A. Lazo. 1993. 1952p. 70.00 (*1-55798-210-4*) Am Psychol.

Directory of the European Medical Device & Biomaterials Industry. O'Donnell. 1995. LC 96-114298. pap. (*1-85617-276-7*) Elsvr Adv Tech GBR. *Dist:* Elsevier.

Directory of the Medical Library Association, 1989-1990. Medical Library Association Staff. 1989. 151p. pap. 43.75 (*0-912176-27-X*) Med Lib Assn.

Directory of the Medical Library Association, 1990-1991. Medical Library Association Staff. 1990. 168p. pap. 43.75 (*0-912176-31-8*) Med Lib Assn.

Directory of the Medical Library Association, 1991-1992. Medical Library Association Staff. 1991. 175p. pap. 95.00 (*0-912176-32-6*) Med Lib Assn.

Directory of the Medical Library Association, 1993-1994. Medical Library Association Staff. 1993. 200p. pap. 150.00 (*0-912176-35-0*) Med Lib Assn.

Directory of the Medical Library Association 1994-1995. Medical Library Staff. 1996. 224p. pap. 150.00 (*0-912176-36-9*) Med Lib Assn.

Directory of Unpublished Experimental Mental Measures, Vol. 6. Bert A. Goldman & David F. Mitchell. 1995. 387p. pap. 29.95 (*1-55798-289-9*) Am Psychol.

Directory of Unpublished Experimental Mental Measures, Vols. 4-5. Ed. by Bert A. Goldman et al. 1996. 534p. pap. text 29.95 (*1-55798-351-8*) Am Psychol.

Directory of Unpublished Experimental Mental Measures Vol. 1: Through 1970, Vol. 1. Ed. by Bert A. Goldman & John Saunders. 1974. LC 73-17342. 223p. (C). 49.95 (*0-87705-130-5*, Kluwer Acad Hman Sci) Kluwer Academic.

Directory of Unpublished Experimental Mental Measures, 1973: 1973-1974, Vol. 3. Ed. by Bert A. Goldman & John C. Busch. 1982. LC 73-17342. 448p. 49.95 (*0-89885-095-9*, Kluwer Acad Hman Sci) Kluwer Academic.

Directory of Vendors for Group Practice. 1993. text 75.00 (*1-56829-038-1*, Irwn Prfssnl) McGraw-Hill Educ Grp.

Directory of Vendors for Group Practice. Timothy Carse & Jeffrey Slater. 1993. text 75.00 (*0-07-413111-7*, Irwn McGrw-H) McGrw-H Hghr Educ.

Directory of Workers' Compensation Managed Care Organizations, 1997. Ed. by Ashli Towler. 3rd ed. 1996. 350p. pap. 179.00 (*1-56925-058-8*, WCD3) Capitol Publns.

Dirofilariasis. Ed. by Peter L. Boreham & Richard B. Atwell. 1988. (Parasitologists & Veterinarians Ser.). 272p. 148.00 (*0-8493-6488-4*, SF992, CRC Reprint) Franklin.

Dirt & Disease: Polio Before FDR. Naomi Rogers. 1992. LC 91-32642. (Health & Medicine in American Society Ser.). (Illus.). 276p. (C). text 45.00 (*0-8135-1785-0*); pap. text 17.95 (*0-8135-1786-9*) Rutgers U Pr.

Dirty Details: The Days & Nights of a Well Spouse. Marion Deutsche Cohen. 1996. LC 95-42473. (Illus.). 165p. (C). lib. bdg. 49.95 (*1-56639-425-2*); pap. 18.95 (*1-56639-426-0*) Temple U Pr.

Dirty Words: Psychoanalytic Insights. Ariel C. Arango. 1989. LC 89-6745. 240p. 40.00 (*0-87668-855-5*) Aronson.

Disabilities Sourcebook: Basic Consumer Health Information about Physical & Psychiatric Disabilities. Ed. by Dawn D. Matthew. 2000. LC 99-56930. (Health Reference Ser.). (Illus.). xii, 616p. lib. bdg. 78.00 (*0-7808-0389-2*) Omnigraphics Inc.

Disability: Situation, Strategies & Policies. 1987. 59p. pap. 7.00 (*92-1-130116-5*, E.86.IV.9) UN.

Disability & Chronic Fatigue Syndrome: Clinical, Legal & Patient Perspectives. Ed. by Nancy G. Klimas & Roberto Patarca-Montero. 1998. LC 97-42720. (Journal of Chronic Fatigue Syndrome Ser.: Vol. 3). 116p. pap. 14.95 (*0-7890-0501-8*, Hawrth Medical) Haworth Pr.

Disability & Chronic Fatigue Syndrome: Clinical, Legal & Patient Perspectives. Ed. by Nancy Klimas & Roberto Patarca-Montero. 1998. LC 97-42720. (Journal of Chronic Fatigue Syndrome Ser.). 116p. 29.95 (*0-7890-0393-7*, Hawrth Medical) Haworth Pr.

Disability & Dependency. Len Barton. 1989. 69.95 (*1-85000-616-4*); pap. 34.95 (*1-85000-617-2*) Taylor & Francis.

Disability & Society: Emerging Issues & Insights. Len Barton. 1996. LC 95-46007. (Longman Sociology Ser.). 304p. (C). pap. 57.60 (*0-582-29166-6*) Longman.

Disability & Sport. Karen P. DePauw & Susan J. Gavron. 1995. LC 94-25215. (Illus.). 312p. text 40.00 (*0-87322-848-0*, BDEP0848) Human Kinetics.

Disability & the City: International Perspectives. Rob Imrie. 1996. (Urban & Regional Development Ser.). 192p. pap. (*1-85396-273-2*, 84276) P Chapman GBR. *Dist:* Sage.

Disability & Work: Incentives, Rights, & Opportunities. Weaver. 1991. 150p. (C). 19.75 (*0-8447-3738-0*) Am Enterprise.

Disability Business: Political Economy of Rehabilitation in America. Gary L. Albrecht. 1992. (Library of Social Research: Vol. 190). 320p. (C). pap. 37.95 (*0-8039-3631-1*, 7714) Sage.

Disability Determination: The Administrative Process & the Role of Medical Personnel, 13. Frank S. Bloch. 1992. LC 91-33483. (Studies in Social Welfare Policies & Programs: No. 13). 248p. 58.00 (*0-313-27638-2*, BNP/, Greenwood Pr) Greenwood.

Disability Evaluation. Ed. by Stephen L. Demeter et al. 1996. LC 95-25683. (Illus.). 656p. (C). (gr. 13). text 79.95 (*0-8151-2400-7*, 23962) Mosby Inc.

Disability Evaluation: Practical Guide for Physicians. Michel Lacerte. 1995. 180p. lib. bdg. 49.95 (*1-57444-037-3*, SL0373) St Lucie Pr.

Disability Evaluation Guide for People with Interstitial Cystitis: Writing Medical Reports to the Social Security Administration. Douglas M. Smith. Ed. by Barbara W. Smith. 1997. (Illus.). 58p. pap. 12.95 (*1-878140-08-6*) Phys Dis Servs.

Disability Evaluation of the Musculoskeletal System. Charles H. Epps, Jr. 1993. text (*0-397-50922-7*) Lppncott W & W.

Disability Fact Finder: Nursing Management of Individuals with Disabilities. Audrey Schmerzler & Jane Walsh. 1998. LC 98-22077. 240p. spiral bd. 34.95 (*0-7817-1702-7*) Lppncott W & W.

***Disability Management & Physical Rehabilitation.** David Clifton, Jr. 2001. (Illus.). 415p. (*0-7216-8474-2*) Saunders.

***Disability, Society & the Individual.** Smart. 1999. tchr. ed. (*0-8342-1923-9*) PRO-ED.

Disability, Society & the Individual. Julie F. Smart. 1999. LC 00-58285. xv, 357p. pap. 49.00 (*0-8342-1601-9*, 16019) PRO-ED.

Disability, Stigma, & Recovery: The Patient As Anthropologist. Jimmie R. Rankin. 1997. (Literature of a Patient Response Ser.). 75p. pap. 14.95 (*1-883938-13-9*) Dry Bones Pr.

Disabled Children: Challenging Social Exclusion. Laura Middleton. 1999. LC 99-34782. (Working Together for Children, Young People & Their Families Ser.). pap. 50.95 (*0-632-05055-1*) Blackwell Sci.

Disabled Children & Developing Countries. Ed. by Pam Zinkin & Helen McConachie. 1995. (Clinics in Developmental Medicine Ser.: No. 136). 59.95 (*0-521-68304-1*) Cambridge U Pr.

Disabled in the Soviet Union: Past & Present, Theory & Practice. Ed. by William O. McCagg & Lewis H. Siegelbaum. 1989. LC 89-40206. (Russian & East European Studies). 310p. text 49.95 (*0-8229-3622-4*) U of Pittsburgh Pr.

Disabled Learner. Ed. by Paul Satz & J. L. Ross. 1973. (Modern Approaches to the Diagnosis & Instruction of Multi-Handicapped Children Ser.: Vol. 8). xvi, 298p. 38.75 (*90-237-4107-2*) Taylor & Francis.

Disabled Parents: Dispelling the Myths. Michele Wates. 1997. LC 97-28927. (National Childbirth Trust Guide Ser.). 176p. pap. (*1-85775-257-0*) Radcliffe Med Pr GBR. *Dist:* Balogh.

Disabled Persons: Their Education & Rehabilitation. Oscar M. Sullivan & Kenneth O. Snortum. Ed. by William R. Phillips & Janet Rosenberg. 1980. LC 79-6925. (Physically Handicapped in Society Ser.). reprint ed. lib. bdg. 61.95 (*0-405-13132-1*) Ayer.

Disabled Soldier. Douglas C. McMurtrie. Ed. by William R. Phillips & Janet Rosenberg. 1980. LC 79-6921. (Physically Handicapped in Society Ser.). (Illus.). reprint ed. lib. bdg. 25.95 (*0-405-13140-2*) Ayer.

Disabled Village Children: A Guide for Health Workers, Rehabilitation Workers & Families. David B. Werner. 1987. LC 86-81738. (Illus.). 672p. (Orig.). pap. 22.00 (*0-942364-06-6*) Hesperian Found.

Disabled We Stand. Allan T. Sutherland. 1988. LC 83-49408. 159p. pap. 10.00 (*0-253-21255-3*) Brookline Bks.

Disappearance of Introspection. William Lyons. 1988. 211p. pap. 15.95 (*0-262-62062-6*); 1986. 224p. 25.00 (*0-262-12115-8*) MIT Pr (Bradford Bks).

***Disappearing & Reviving: Sandor Ferenczi in the History of Psychoanalysis.** Andre Haynal. 2001. 168p. pap. (*1-85575-254-9*) Karnac Bks GBR. *Dist:* Other Pr LLC.

Disarming the Past: How an Intimate Relationship Can Heal Old Wounds. Jerry M. Lewis & John T. Gossett. 1999. LC 98-33362. x, 221p. 35.95 (*1-891944-06-1*) Zeig Tucker Theisen.

Disaster: A Psychological Essay. Martha Wolfenstein. Ed. by Robert J. Kastenbaum. 1977. LC 76-19595. (Death & Dying Ser.). reprint ed. lib. bdg. 25.95 (*0-405-09589-9*) Ayer.

Disaster & Disaster Stress. A. J. P. Taylor. Ed. by James H. Humphrey. 1989. LC 86-82025. (Studies in Modern Society: No. 10). 32.50 (*0-404-63262-9*) AMS Pr.

Disaster & Mass Trauma: Global Perspectives on Post Disaster Mental Health Management. Anie S. Kalayjian. Ed. by Joseph Jaeger. 1995. LC 95-61475. 294p. (C). pap. 29.95 (*1-880254-32-8*) Vista.

Disaster Beliefs & Emergency Planning. Charles E. Faupel et al. 1985. 259p. text 29.50 (*0-8290-1361-X*) Irvington.

Disaster Medicine. David E. Hogan & Jonathan L. Burstein. 2002. text 79.95 (*0-7817-2625-5*) Lppncott W & W.

Disaster Medicine: Proceedings of the International Conference, Cape Town, August 1979. Ed. by A. G. Macmahon & M. Jooste. 1980. 248p. (C). text (*0-86961-122-4*) A A Balkema NLD. *Dist:* Ashgate Pub Co.

Disaster Medicine & International Relief: Multilingual Dictionary. S. W. Gunn. 1993. (ARA, ENG, FRE & SPA.). 190p. (C). pap. text 81.00 (*0-7923-2256-8*) Kluwer Academic.

Disaster Mitigation Guidelines for Hospitals & Other Health Care Facilities in the Caribbean. 1993. (Illus.). 78p. (Orig.). (C). pap. text 30.00 (*1-56806-973-1*) DIANE Pub.

Disaster Recovery Planning Manual: Assessing Risks & Developing a Comprehensive Plan for the Healthcare Organization. Geoffrey H. Wold & Robert F. Shriver. 1994. 200p. text 125.00 (*1-55738-602-1*, Irwn Prfssnl) McGraw-Hill Educ Grp.

Disaster Response & Recovery: A Handbook for Mental Health Professionals. Diane Meyers. 1996. (Illus.). 144p. (C). reprint ed. pap. text 40.00 (*0-7881-3126-5*) DIANE Pub.

Disasters: Hospital Planning. P. E. Savage. 1979. (*0-08-024914-0*) Pergamon Repr GBR. *Dist:* Franklin.

Disasters: Mental Health Interventions. John D. Weaver. 1995. LC 95-3891. (Crisis Management Ser.). 220p. pap. 27.45 (*1-56887-011-6*, DMHBP, Prof Resc Pr) Pro Resource.

Discharge Planning: A Practitioner's Guide to Policies, Procedures & Protocols, Guideline Manual. Jacqueline J. Birmingham. 1992. 90.00 (*1-879575-25-6*) Acad Med Sys.

Discharge Planning for Home Health Care: A Multidisciplinary Approach. Barbara Stover Gingerich & Deborah A. Ondeck. 1994. 258p. ring bd. 132.00 (*0-8342-0572-6*, 20572) Aspen Pub.

Discharge Planning for the Elderly: A Guide for Nurses. Kimberly Dash et al. 1996. LC 95-25626. (Illus.). 280p. 35.95 (*0-8261-9230-0*) Springer Pub.

Discharge Planning Handbook. Judith W. Rorden. 1990. (Illus.). 384p. pap. text 39.00 (*0-7216-2845-1*) Saunders.

Discipline of Medicine: Proceedings of the Symposium, May 25 & 26, 1993. A. Querido et al. 1994. LC 94-27792. 206p. pap. (*0-444-85772-9*) Royal Netherlands Acad NLD. *Dist:* Elsevier.

Disciplines of Delight: The Psychoanalysis of Popular Culture. Barry Richards. 1994. LC 95-137211. 200p. (C). pap. (*1-85343-325-X*) Free Assoc Bks GBR. *Dist:* Intl Spec Bk.

Disciplining Reproduction: Modernity, American Life Sciences, & "The Problem of Sex" Adele Clarke. 1998. LC 97-1114. (Illus.). 438p. text 50.00 (*0-520-20720-3*) U CA Pr.

Disclosure Processes in Children & Adolescents. Ed. by Ken J. Rotenberg. 1995. LC 95-23746. (Cambridge Studies in Social & Emotional Development). (Illus.). 247p. (C). text 44.95 (*0-521-47098-6*) Cambridge U Pr.

Discontinuation of Hospice Care: Ethical Issues. National Hospice Organization, Ethics Committee. 1993. 15p. 15.75 (*0-931207-22-3*) Natl Hospice.

Discontinuous Conduction in the Heart. Ed. by Peter M. Spooner et al. 1997. LC 97-23561. (American Heart Association Monograph Ser.). (Illus.). 592p. 95.00 (*0-87993-669-X*) Futura Pub.

Discourse Ability & Brain Damage. Ed. by Yves Joanette & H. Brownell. 1989. (Neuropsychology Ser.). (Illus.). 258p. 115.00 (*0-387-97044-4*, 2992) Spr-Verlag.

Discourse Analysis & Applications: Studies in Adult Clinical Populations. Ed. by Ronald L. Bloom et al. 1994. 264p. text 55.00 (*0-8058-1365-9*) L Erlbaum Assocs.

Discourse & Institutional Authority: Medicine, Education & Law. Ed. by Sue Fisher et al. 1986. LC 85-22888. (Advances in Discourse Processes Ser.: Vol. 19). 272p. (C). pap. 42.50 (*0-89391-367-7*);19. 85.00 (*0-89391-282-4*) Greenwood (Ablex).

Discourse in the Social Sciences: Strategies for Translating Models of Mental Illness, 40. Jonathan D. Moreno & Barry Glassner. 1981. LC 81-7092. (Contributions in Sociology Ser.: No. 40). (Illus.). 160p. 59.95 (*0-313-23159-1*, GLM/) Greenwood.

Discourse of Medicine. Elliot G. Mishler. Ed. by Cynthia Wallat & Judith Green. 1985. LC 84-16832. (Language & Learning for Human Service Professions Ser.: Vol. 3). 224p. 77.00 (*0-89391-276-X*); pap. 39.50 (*0-89391-277-8*) Greenwood (Ablex).

Discourse of the Causes, Natures & Cure of Phrensie, Madness or Distraction from a Treatise of Dreams & Visions. Thomas Tryon. 1973. LC 92-22977. (Augustan Reprints Ser.: No. 160). reprint ed. 14.50 (*0-404-70160-4*, RC340) AMS Pr.

Discourse on the Plague. Richard Mead. 9th enl. rev. ed. LC 75-23742. reprint ed. 45.00 (*0-404-13297-9*) AMS Pr.

Discourse upon the Duties of a Physician. Samuel Bard. 1996. LC 96-9412. 32p. reprint ed. 9.95 (*1-55709-446-2*) Applewood.

Discourse upon the Institution of Medical Schools in America. John Morgan. 1975. LC 74-26276. (History, Philosophy, & Sociology of Science Ser.). reprint ed. 17.95 (*0-405-06604-X*) Ayer.

Discourses of Counselling: HIV Counselling As Social Interaction. David Silverman. 1996. 224p. 74.50 (*0-8039-7661-5*, 1621); pap. 25.95 (*0-8039-7662-3*, 16222) Sage.

Discover a New World of Healing: Answers for Successful Living in These Times. Robin Llast. 1992. (Illus.). 234p. (Orig.). pap. text 12.95 (*0-929240-52-9*) EMIS.

Discover Ayurveda: A First-Step Handbook to Better Health. Angela Hope-Murray. 1997. LC 97-61010. (First-Step Handbook to Better Health Ser.). 128p. (Orig.). pap. 8.95 (*1-56975-081-5*) Ulysses Pr.

Discover Magazine & Introduction to Psychology. Peterson. 1997. (C). pap. 74.00 (*0-673-52189-3*) Addson-Wesley Educ.

Discover Osteopathy: A First-Step Handbook to Better Health. Peta Sneddon & Paolo Cosechi. 1997. LC 97-60158. Orig. Title: Healing with Osteopathy. (Illus.). 132p. pap. 8.95 (*1-56975-115-3*) Ulysses Pr.

***Discover the Beta Glucan Secret: For Immune Enhancement, Cancer Prevention & Treatment, Cholesterol Reduction, Glucose Regulation & Much More!** Beth M. Ley. 2nd ed. 2001. LC 00-13128. (Health Learning Handbook Ser.). 32p. pap. 3.95 (*1-890766-18-6*) B L Pubns.

Discoverers for Medicine. William H. Woglom. 1977. LC 78-156733. (Essay Index Reprint Ser.). reprint ed. 19.95 (*0-8369-2432-0*) Ayer.

Discoveries in Head Trauma. Ed. by Lynn M. Savage. 1996. (Biomedical Library). 111p. pap. 595.00 (*1-57936-003-3*) Drug & Market Dev.

Discoveries in the Human Brain: Neuroscience Prehistory, Brain Structure & Function. Louise H. Marshall & Horace W. Magoun. 1997. LC 97-42118. (Illus.). 336p. 79.50 (*0-89603-435-6*) Humana.

***Discovering Health Issues & Strategies.** Thomps & Levinthal. 2001. 404p. 48.00 (*0-536-63208-1*) Pearson Custom.

Discovering Homeopathy: Your Introduction to the Science & Art of Homeopathic Medicine. Dana Ullman. 2nd rev. ed. 1991. LC 87-28149. Orig. Title: Homeopathy: Medicine for the 21st Century. 277p. pap. 14.95 (*1-55643-108-2*) North Atlantic.

Discovering Lifetime Fitness: Concepts of Exercise & Weight Control. George B. Dintiman et al. Ed. by Marshall. 2nd ed. 1988. 312p. (C). mass mkt. 37.25 (*0-314-48120-6*) West Pub.

Discovering Neurons: The Experimental Basis of Neuroscience. Ed. by Carol A. Paul et al. 1997. LC 97-24523. (Illus.). 456p. (C). pap. text 40.00 (*0-87969-455-6*); text 100.00 (*0-87969-454-8*) Cold Spring Harbor.

Discovering New Medicines: Careers in Pharmaceutical Research & Development. Ed. by Peter D. Stonier. 1995. LC 94-16151. 406p. pap. 65.00 (*0-471-94194-8*) Wiley.

Discovering Nutrition. Helen Kowtaluk. 1985. (Illus.). (gr. 6-8). stu. ed. 2.99 (*0-02-667900-0*); pap., tchr. ed. 20.84 (*0-02-667910-8*); 2nd ed. text 37.96 (*0-02-667810-1*); 2nd ed. stu. ed. 7.27 (*0-02-667890-X*) Glencoe.

Discovering Psychology. Hockenbury. 2nd ed. 2000. text, stu. ed. 44.00 (*0-7167-5161-5*) Worth.

Discovering the Brain. Sandra Ackerman. 1991. 194p. 22.95 (*0-309-04529-0*) Natl Acad Pr.

Discovering the History of Psychiatry. Ed. by Mark S. Micale & Roy Porter. 1994. LC 93-12244. 480p. text 49.50 (*0-19-507739-3*) OUP.

Discovering the Self Through Drama & Movement: The Sesame Approach. Ed. by Jenny Pearson. 1996. 350p. text (*1-85302-384-1*) Jessica Kingsley GBR. *Dist:* Taylor & Francis.

Discovering the Soul: The Amazing Findings of a Psychiatrist & His Patients. Robert G. Jarmon. 1997. LC 96-38945. 215p. (Orig.). pap. 14.95 (*0-87604-370-8*, 486) ARE Pr.

Discovering Your Subpersonalities: Our Inner World & the People in It. John Rowan. 1993. LC 93-14812. (Illus.). 192p. (C). pap. 24.95 (*0-415-07366-9*, A7634) Routledge.

Discovery & Explanation in Biology & Medicine. Kenneth F. Schaffner. 1993. LC 93-21826. (Science & Its Conceptual Foundations Ser.). (Illus.). 652p. (C). pap. text 27.95 (*0-226-73592-3*); lib. bdg. 55.00 (*0-226-73591-5*) U Ch Pr.

Discovery of Insulin. Michael Bliss. 1996. 304p. pap. (*0-7710-1560-7*) McCland & Stewart.

Discovery of Insulin. Michael Bliss. 1984. LC 82-50911. (Illus.). 304p. (C). pap. text 18.00 (*0-226-05898-0*) U Ch Pr.

Discovery of Insulin. Michael Bliss. 3rd ed. 2000. LC 00-363200. (Illus.). 478p. pap. 21.95 (*0-8020-8344-7*) U of Toronto Pr.

Discovery of Magnetic Health. George J. Washnis & Richard Z. Hricak. 1993. 356p. pap. text 21.95 (*0-9639560-1-9*) Nova Pubng.

"Discovery" of Sudden Infant Death Syndrome: Lessons in the Practice of Political Medicine. Abraham B. Bergman. 1988. LC 87-34542. 257p. pap. 12.50 (*0-295-96601-7*) U of Wash Pr.

Discovery of Sudden Infant Death Syndrome: Lessons in the Practice of Political Medicine. Abraham B. Bergman. 1986. LC 85-30778. (Illus.). 254p. 78.75 (*0-275-92059-3*, C2059, Praeger Pubs) Greenwood.

Discovery of Talent: The Walter Van Dyke Bingham Lectures on the Development of Exceptional Abilities & Capacities. Ed. by Dael L. Wolfle. 1969. LC 69-18046. 338p. 46.50 (*0-674-21235-5*) HUP.

Discovery of the Unconscious: The History & Evolution of Dynamic Psychiatry. Henri F. Ellenberger. 1981. LC 79-94287. (Illus.). 932p. 65.00 (*0-465-01673-1*) Basic.

Discrete Mathematical Problems with Medical Applications: DIMACS Workshop Discrete Mathematical Problems with Medical Applications, December 8-10, 1999, DIMACS Center. DIMACS Workshop Discrete Mathematical Problems with Medical Applications Staff et al. 2000. LC 00-45118. (DIMACS Series in Discrete Mathematics & Theoretical Computer Science: Vol. 55). (Illus.). ix, 219p. text 69.00 (*0-8218-2096-6*) Am Math.

Discriminative Properties of Reinforcement Schedules: Quantitative Analyses of Behavior, Vol. 1. Ed. by Michael L. Commons & J. A. Nevin. 1985. 480p. 99.95 (*0-89859-831-1*) L Erlbaum Assocs.

Discursive Mind. Rom Harre & Grant Gillett. 1994. LC 93-43672. 200p. (C). 49.95 (*0-8039-5501-4*, 3669); pap. 23.95 (*0-8039-5502-2*, 3670) Sage.

Discursive Psychology. Derek Edwards & Jonathan Potter. 1992. (Inquiries in Social Construction Ser.: Vol. 8). (Illus.). 208p. (C). 74.50 (*0-8039-8442-1*, 9433); pap. 25.95 (*0-8039-8443-X*, 9434) Sage.

Discursive Psychology in Practice. Rom Harre & Peter Stearns. 1995. LC 95-70196. (Rethinking Psychology Ser.). 240p. 74.50 (*0-8039-7736-0*, 1393); pap. 26.50 (*0-8039-7737-9*, 1394) Sage.

Discussing Death: A Guide to Death Education. Gretchen Mills et al. 1976. LC 75-17885. pap. 14.95 (*0-88280-027-2*); (gr. 3-12). 14.95 (*0-88280-026-4*) ETC Pubns.

Discussions on Ego Identity. Ed. by Jane Kroger. 1993. 280p. text 59.95 (*0-8058-1329-2*) L Erlbaum Assocs.

Disease: Identification, Prevention & Control. Barbara P. Hamann. 2nd ed. 2000. LC 00-37253. (Illus.). xi, 451p. (C). pap. text 63.75 (*0-8151-2847-9*) McGrw-H Hghr Educ.

Disease: In Search of Remedy. Peter M. Marcuse. 1996. LC 95-19707. 168p. 26.95 (*0-252-02215-7*) U of Ill Pr.

Disease & Class: Tuberculosis & the Shaping of Modern North American Society. Georgina D. Feldberg. 1995. (Health & Medicine in American Society Ser.). (Illus.). 320p. (C). LC 96-31547. text 52.00 (*0-8135-2217-X*); pap. text 18.95 (*0-8135-2218-8*) Rutgers U Pr.

Disease & Demography in the Americas. Ed. by John W. Verano & Douglas H. Ubelaker. 1994. LC 91-32713. (Illus.). 352p. (C). reprint ed. pap. text 34.95 (*1-56098-401-5*) Smithsonian.

Disease & Distinctiveness in the American South. Ed. by Todd L. Savitt & James H. Young. 1988. LC 87-30238. (Illus.). 232p. pap. 17.95 (*0-87049-685-9*) U of Tenn Pr.

Disease & Empire: Military Medicine in the Conquest of Africa. Philip De Armond Curtin. 1998. LC 98-22027. (Illus.). 272p. (C). text 54.95 (*0-521-59169-4*); pap. text 19.95 (*0-521-59835-4*) Cambridge U Pr.

Disease & History. Frederick F. Cartwright & Michael Biddiss. 2nd expurg. rev. ed. 2000. (Illus.). 220p. 29.95 (*0-7509-2315-6*) Sutton Publng.

Disease & Its Control: The Shaping of Modern Thought. Robert P. Hudson. 1987. LC 87-9340. 276p. pap. 18.95 (*0-275-92779-2*, B2779, Praeger Pubs); 12. 1983. LC 82-21135. (Contributions in Medical History Ser.: No. 12). 259p. 59.95 (*0-313-23806-5*, HHD/, Greenwood Pr) Greenwood.

Disease & Its Impact on Modern European History. Vincent J. Knapp. 1989. LC 88-13946. (Studies in Health & Human Services: Vol. 10). 392p. lib. bdg. 99.95 (*0-88946-135-X*) E Mellen.

Disease & Medical Care in the Mountain West: Essays on Region, History, & Practice. Ed. by Martha Hildreth & Bruce Moran. 1998. LC 97-26959. (Wilbur S. Shepperson Series in History & Humanities). (Illus.). 208p. text 39.95 (*0-87417-304-3*) U of Nev Pr.

Disease & Representation: Images of Illness from Madness to AIDS. Sander L. Gilman. 1988. (Illus.). 49.95 (*0-8014-2119-5*); 347p. pap. 19.95 (*0-8014-9476-1*) Cornell U Pr.

Disease & Social Diversity: The European Impact on the Health of Non-Europeans. Stephen J. Kunitz. 1996. (Illus.). 224p. (C). pap. text 29.95 (*0-19-510869-8*) OUP.

Disease & Society in Provincial Massachusetts: Collected Accounts 1736-1939. Ernest Caulfield. 1979. (Medicine & Society in America Ser.). 25.95 (*0-405-03948-4*, 15700) Ayer.

Disease & the Soul Vol. 2: Archetypal Perspectives on Pathology. Benjamin Sells. 2000. 181p. pap. 18.50 (*0-88214-377-8*) Spring Pubns.

Disease Concept of Alcoholism. E. M. Jellinek. 1960. pap. 19.95 (*0-8084-0419-9*) NCUP.

Disease Concept of Alcoholism. E. M. Jellinek. 1960. LC 60-9206. pap. 12.95 (*0-910724-12-1*) Rutgers Ctr Alcohol.

Disease Connection: Are Mental "Illness," Alcoholism, & Drug Addiction Really Diseases? Erwin A. Gaede. 1996. LC 94-90810. 98p. (Orig.). pap. 9.00 (*1-56002-544-1*, Univ Edtns) Aegina Pr.

Disease Control Priorities in Developing Countries. Ed. by Dean T. Jamison et al. 1993. LC 92-48723. 1. (*0-19-520885-4*); 2. (*0-19-520886-2*) OUP.

Disease Control Priorities in Developing Countries: A Summary. Ed. by Dean T. Jamison et al. 1993. LC 93-29945. 40p. pap. 22.00 (*0-8213-2480-2*, 12480) World Bank.

Disease Data Book. J. Fry et al. 1986. text 124.00 (*0-85200-922-4*) Kluwer Academic.

Disease Dynamics: Systems & Control: Foundations & Applications. Ed. by Alexander Asachenkov et al. 1993. LC 93-40316. (Illus.). xv, 316p. 105.00 (*0-8176-3692-7*) Birkhauser.

Disease, Ecology & Health: Readings in Medical Geography. Ed. by Rais Akhtar. 1990. (*81-7033-095-5*) Rawat Pubns IND. *Dist:* S Asia.

Disease Fighters since 1950. Ray Spangenburg & Diane Moser. 1996. LC 96-5571. (Global Profiles Ser.). (Illus.). 160p. (gr. 5-12). 19.95 (*0-8160-3319-6*) Facts on File.

Disease (Fourth Series) Test & Syllabus. Donald Resnick et al. 1989. (Professional Self-Evaluation & Continuing Education Program Ser.: Vol. 25). (Illus.). 900p. (C). 165.00 (*1-55903-025-9*) Am Coll Radiology.

Disease-Free at 60 Plus: Hundreds of Life-Preserving Tips & Techniques to Defy Heart Trouble, Cancer, & Stroke. Doug Dollemore et al. 1997. LC 96-46765. 416p. 27.95 (*0-87596-342-0*) Rodale Pr Inc.

Disease Handbook for Child Care Providers. Ed. by Geraldine Sylvester. 1999. (Illus.). 108p. reprint ed. pap. text 25.00 (*0-7881-8165-3*) DIANE Pub.

Disease in Milk, the Remedy Pasteurization: The Life Work of Nathan Straus. Lina G. Straus. Ed. by Barbara G. Rosenkrantz. 1977. LC 76-40650. (Public Health in America Ser.). (Illus.). reprint ed. lib. bdg. 34.95 (*0-405-09833-2*) Ayer.

Disease in Populations in Transition: Anthropological & Epidemiological Perspectives. Alan C. Swedlund et al. 1990. LC 89-18513. 400p. 70.00 (*0-89789-175-9*, H175, Bergin & Garvey) Greenwood.

Disease in the Civil War: Natural Biological Warfare in 1861-1865. Paul E. Steiner. 1968. 260p. 45.95 (*0-398-01852-9*) C C Thomas.

Disease in the Popular American Press: The Case of Diphtheria, Typhoid Fever, & Syphilis, 1870-1920, 24. Terra Ziporyn. 1988. LC 88-5585. (Contributions in Medical Studies Ser.: No. 24). 208p. 62.50 (*0-313-26035-4*, ZDE/, Greenwood Pr) Greenwood.

Disease Management. Roy C. Lilley. 1998. LC 97-41339. 172p. 84.95 (*0-471-97503-6*) Wiley.

Disease Management: Directions for 2000. pap. text (*0-86471-067-4*) Adis Intl NZL. *Dist:* Lppncott W & W.

Disease Management Handbook. 64p. pap. text (*0-86471-056-9*) Adis Intl NZL. *Dist:* Lppncott W & W.

Disease Mechanisms in Small Animal Surgery. M. Joseph Bojrab et al. 2nd ed. 1992. (Illus.). 1271p. text 125.00 (*0-8121-1491-4*) Lppncott W & W.

Disease, Medicine & Empire. Ed. by Roy M. MacLeod & Milton Lewis. 1989. 302p. (C). lib. bdg. 79.95 (*0-415-00685-6*) Routledge.

Disease, Medicine & Society in England, 1550-1860. Roy Porter. 2nd ed. 1995. (New Studies in Economic & Social History: Vol. 3). (C). 84p. text 39.95 (*0-521-55262-1*); 92p. pap. text 11.95 (*0-521-55791-7*) Cambridge U Pr.

Disease, Metabolism & Reproduction in the Toxic Response to Drugs & Other Chemicals: Proceedings of the European Society of Toxicology Meeting Held in Rome, March 28-30, 1983. P. L. Chambers et al. 1984. (Archives of Toxicology Ser.: Suppl. 7). (Illus.). 400p. 111.00 (*0-387-12452-7*) Spr-Verlag.

Disease Mongers: How Doctors, Drug Companies & Insurers Are Making You Feel Sick. Lynn Payer. 1994. LC 92-12513. 292p. pap. 12.95 (*0-471-00737-4*) Wiley.

Disease, Mortality & Population in Transition. Alex Mercer. 1991. 69.00 (*0-7185-1344-4*) St Martin.

Disease of Aging. Hans J. Kugler & Earl R. Mindell. 1984. (Good Health Guides). 32p. (Orig.). pap. 3.95 (*0-87983-366-1*, 33661K, Keats Pubng) McGraw-Hill Trade.

Disease of Alcoholism. David L. Ohlms. Ed. & Intro. by GWC, Inc. Staff. rev. ed. 1997. (Illus.). 30p. 2.50 (*1-56168-025-7*, B101) GWC Inc.

Disease of Cultivable Freshwater Fishes & Their Control. N. M. Chakrabarthi. 1994. 180p. pap. (*0-7855-0405-2*) Intl Bks & Periodicals IND. *Dist:* St Mut.

Disease of Inebriety from Alcohol, Opium & Other Narcotic Drugs: Its Etiology, Pathology Treatment & Medico-Legal Relations. American Association for the Study and Cure of Inebriety. Ed. by Gerald N. Grob. 1981. LC 80-1210. (Addiction in America Ser.). reprint ed. lib. bdg. 40.95 (*0-405-13566-1*) Ayer.

Disease of One's Own: Psychotherapy, Addiction, & the Emergence of Co-Dependency. John S. Rice. 1996. 253p. pap. text 24.95 (*0-7658-0454-9*) Transaction Pubs.

Disease of Society: Cultural & Institutional Responses to AIDS. Ed. by Dorothy Nelkin et al. 1991. 295p. (C). text 54.95 (*0-521-40411-8*); pap. text 19.95 (*0-521-40743-5*) Cambridge U Pr.

Disease, Pain, & Suicidal Behavior. Elsebeth Stenager & Egon Stenager. 1997. LC 97-15308. (Illus.). 128p. 39.95 (*0-7890-0111-X*); pap. 14.95 (*0-7890-0295-7*) Haworth Pr (Hawrth Medical).

C
D

Disease Patterns. Ed. by G. Jasmin & M. Cantin. 1975. (Methods & Achievements in Experimental Pathology Ser.: Vol. 7). 112.25 (*3-8055-2155-3*) S Karger.

Disease Prevention: Health Facts. Lucas Stang & Kathleen R. Miner. 1994. LC 93-43465. 12.95 (*1-56071-182-5*, H302) ETR Assocs.

Disease Prevention & Health Promotion: A Handbook for Physicians. Ed. by John H. Holbrook. 1985. LC 85-25983. 266p. 72.95 (*0-275-91303-1*, C1303, Praeger Pubs) Greenwood.

Disease Prevention & Treatment: Scientific Protocols That Integrate Mainstream & Alternative Medicine. Life Extension Staff and Medical Advisary Board Staff et al. 3rd rev. ed. 2000. 946p. pap. 34.95 (*0-9658777-4-4*) Life Ext Media.

Disease Prevention Research. 1995. lib. bdg. 255.95 (*0-8490-7577-7*) Gordon Pr.

Disease Prevention Research: A Bibliography. 1996. lib. bdg. 255.95 (*0-8490-5979-8*) Gordon Pr.

Disease Prevention Through Immunization: The Beginning of Health Care Reform. 1993. (Illus.). 30p. (Orig.). (C). pap. text 25.00 (*0-7881-0034-3*) DIANE Pub.

Disease Prevention Through Vector Control: Guidelines for Relief Organizations. Madeline C. Thomson. 1995. (Practical Health Guide Ser.: No. 10). 96p. (C). pap. (*0-85598-306-X*) Oxfam Pub GBR. *Dist:* Stylus Pub VA.

Disease Staging Clinical Criteria. Ed. by Joseph S. Gonnella et al. 4th ed. 1994. 994p. (*0-9641308-0-7*) MEDSTAT Systs.

Disease State Management Vol. I: Clinical Guidelines for the Primary Physician. Margaret D. Bischel. 1997. (Illus.). 163p. ring bd. 195.00 (*1-893826-05-8*) Apollo Managed.

Disease State Management, Clinical Behavioral Vol. II: Health Guidelines. Margaret D. Bischel. 1997. 195p. ring bd. 195.00 (*1-893826-06-6*) Apollo Managed.

Disease Susceptibility: Medical Subject Analysis with Reference Bibliography. Shirley L. Mettler. rev. ed. 1992. 150p. LC 85-48180. 47.50 (*1-55914-896-9*); LC 92-31212. pap. 44.50 (*1-55914-897-7*) ABBE Pubs Assn.

Disease, the Individual & Society. Gerald Gordon et al. 1968. pap. 25.95 (*0-8084-0107-6*) NCUP.

Disease Transmission by Insects: Its Discovery & 90 Years of Effort to Prevent It. James R. Busvine. 1993. LC 92-48241. pap. (*3-540-55457-2*); (Illus.). 361p. 86.00 (*0-387-55457-2*) Spr-Verlag.

Diseases. Grolier Educational Staff. 1996. LC 96-27606. (Illus.). 1024p. (gr. 7-12). lib. bdg. 295.00 (*0-7172-7617-1*) Grolier Educ.

Diseases. SPC Staff. 1997. LC 97-24667. (Healthcare Professional Guides: Vol. 3). 384p. spiral bd. 26.95 (*0-87434-913-3*) Springhouse Corp.

Diseases: Finding the Cure. Robert Mulcahy. 1996. LC 95-42739. (Innovators Ser.). (Illus.). 144p. (YA). (gr. 5-12). lib. bdg. 21.95 (*1-881508-28-5*) Oliver Pr MN.

Diseases Affecting the Eye & the Kidney. Ed. by Lucian S. Regenbogen & H. E. Eliahou. 1993. (Illus.). xviii, 458p. 389.75 (*3-8055-5660-8*) S Karger.

Diseases & Disorders: A Nursing Therapeutics Manual. Marilyn Sawyer Sommers. 2nd ed. 2002. LC 2001-47710. (Illus.). 1056p. per. 39.95 (*0-8036-0811-X*) Davis Co.

Diseases & Disorders Bk. II: The World's Best Anatomical Charts Collection. Anatomical Chart Company Staff. 2000. (Illus.). 35p. pap. 15.95 (*1-889241-08-3*, DIS-35) Anatomical Chart.

Diseases & Disorders of the Domestic Fowl & Turkey. C. J. Randall. 2nd ed. 1996. 92.95 (*0-7234-1628-1*) Iowa U Pr.

Diseases in Antiquity: A Survey of the Diseases, Injuries & Surgery of Early Populations. Don R. Brothwell & A. T. Sandison. 1967. (Illus.). 792p. 131.95 (*0-398-00233-9*) C C Thomas.

Diseases in the Ancient Greek World. Mirko D. Grmek. Tr. by Mireille Muellner & Leonard Muellner. 1991. LC 88-45412. 472p. reprint ed. pap. text 25.95 (*0-8018-4225-5*) Johns Hopkins.

Diseases in Wax: The History of the Medical Moulage. Thomas Schnalke. Tr. by Kathy Spatschek from GER. 1995. LC 95-3773. (Illus.). 226p. text 180.00 (*0-86715-306-7*) Quint Pub Co.

Diseases of Amphibians & Reptiles. Ed. by Gerald L. Hoff et al. 1984. LC 84-8385. 794p. 145.00 (*0-306-41711-1*, Plenum Trade) Perseus Pubng.

Diseases of Bones & Joints. P. Byers et al. 1994. LC 93-74499. (Illus.). 576p. 200.95 (*0-412-48010-7*) Chapman & Hall.

Diseases of Cage & Aviary Birds. Ed. by Walter J. Rosskopf, Jr. & Richard Woerpel. 3rd ed. 1996. LC 96-2665. (Illus.). 1100p. 75.00 (*0-683-07382-6*) Lppncott W & W.

Diseases of Cattle in the Tropics. Miodrag Ristic. 1981. pap. text 126.50 (*90-247-2495-3*); lib. bdg. 230.00 (*90-247-2399-X*) Kluwer Academic.

Diseases of Children in the Subtropics & Tropics. 4th ed. 1104p. (*0-340-50633-4*) E A GBR. *Dist:* Routldge.

Diseases of Dairy Cattle. William C. Rebhun. 1995. LC 94-44191. (Illus.). 544p. 59.00 (*0-683-07193-9*) Lppncott W & W.

Diseases of Domestic Guinea Pigs. V. C. G. Richardson. 2nd ed. 2000. LC 99-86938. (Library of Veterinary Practice). (Illus.). 162p. pap. text (*0-632-05209-0*) Blckwell Science GBR. *Dist:* Iowa U Pr.

Diseases of Famous Composers. F. H. Franken. unabr. ed. Date not set.Tr. of Frankheiten Grosser Komponisten. 79.50 (*1-57529-010-3*) Kabel Pubs.

Diseases of Fish. Lionel E. Mawdesley-Thomas et al. 1974. 277p. (C). text 27.50 (*0-8422-7178-3*) Irvington.

Diseases of Hematopoietic System: Proceedings of the 45th Annual Anatomic Pathology Slide Seminar of ASCP. Ed. by Philip H. Lieberman & Robert A. Good. 1981. LC 81-4946. (Anatomic Pathology Slide Seminar Ser.). (Illus.). 121p. pap. text 35.00 (*0-89189-085-8*, 50-1-046-00) Am Soc Clinical.

Diseases of Infection: An Illustrated Textbook. Norman R. Grist et al. 2nd ed. 1993. LC 92-16185. (Illus.). 472p. text 78.50 (*0-19-262308-7*) OUP.

Diseases of Livestock. Tom G. Hungerford. 9th ed. 1991. 1942p. text 175.00 (*0-07-031280-X*) McGraw-Hill Med Pub.

Diseases of Memory, 1. Theodule A. Ribot. Tr. by W. H. Smith & M. M. Snell. 1977. LC 77-72191. (Contributions to the History of Psychology Ser.: Vol. 1, Pt. C, Medical Psychology). 134p. reprint ed. lib. bdg. 75.00 (*0-313-26940-8*, U6940, Greenwood Pr) Greenwood.

Diseases of Oral Mucosa & the Mouth. Bork. 1996. text 99.00 (*0-7216-4039-7*) Saunders.

Diseases of Poultry. B. W. Calnek. 10th ed. 1997. LC 97-2161. (Illus.). 1146p. 139.95 (*0-8138-0427-2*) Iowa U Pr.

Diseases of Pregnancy & Childbirth. Ed. by Philip K. Wilson. 1996. LC 96-794. (Childbirth Ser.: Vol. 5). (Illus.). 496p. reprint ed. text 94.00 (*0-8153-2234-8*) Garland.

Diseases of Sheep. W. B. Martin & I. D. Aitken. 3rd ed. 2000. LC 99-36665. (Illus.). 528p. text (*0-632-05139-6*) Blckwell Science GBR. *Dist:* Iowa U Pr.

Diseases of Small Domestic Rodents. V. C. Richardson. 1997. LC 97-6214. (Library of Veterinary Practice). (Illus.). 224p. 39.95 (*0-632-04132-3*) Blackwell Sci.

Diseases of Swine. Ed. by Barbara Straw et al. 8th ed. 1999. LC 98-48548. (Illus.). 1230p. text 154.95 (*0-8138-0338-1*) Iowa U Pr.

Diseases of Swine. Barbara E. Straw. 8th ed. 1999. LC 99-25432. (*0-632-05256-2*) Blackwell Sci.

Diseases of the Abdomen & Pelvis: Diagnostic Imaging & Interventional Techniques. R. Scully. Ed. by G. K. von Schultess. 1999. LC 99-24354. 286p. pap. 82.00 (*88-470-0058-0*) Spr-Verlag.

Diseases of the Aorta. Joseph Lindsay. 1993. (Illus.). 370p. 75.00 (*0-8121-1694-1*) Lppncott W & W.

Diseases of the Arterial Wall. Ed. by J. P. Camilleri et al. 1989. (Illus.). 693p. 477.00 (*0-387-17492-3*) Spr-Verlag.

Diseases of the Breast Test & Syllabus, Vol. 24. Stephen A. Feig et al. 1988. (Professional Self-Evaluation & Continuing Education Program Ser.). (Illus.). 650p. 165.00 (*1-55903-024-0*) Am Coll Radiology.

Diseases of the Cat. G. Wilkinson & P. Scott. 1966. LC 66-18239. (*0-08-011723-6*) Pergamon Repr GBR. *Dist:* Franklin.

Diseases of the Cat & Their Management. Wilkinson. 1987. 69.00 (*0-86793-032-2*) CRC Pr.

Diseases of the Colon & Rectum. Him-che Yeung. 1993. 100p. pap. text 10.00 (*0-9639715-0-6*) Inst Chinese Med.

Diseases of the Digestive System: International Nomenclature of Diseases. 1990. (International Nomenclature of Diseases Ser.: Vol. 4). xvi, 269p. pap. text 18.00 (*92-4-154409-0*, 1820004) World Health.

Diseases of the Digestive Sytem. 1990. (International Nomenclature of Diseases Ser.: No. 4). pap. text 20.00 (*92-9036-041-0*) World Health.

Diseases of the Ear. Ed. by Harold Ludman & Tony Wright. 6th ed. 1998. LC 97-26916. (An Arnold Publication). (Illus.). 608p. (*0-340-56441-5*) E A GBR. *Dist:* OUP.

Diseases of the Ear: A Pocket Atlas. M. F. Hawke & A. W. McCombe. 1995. (Illus.). 112p. 39.95 (*1-896251-02-1*) Manticore Pubs.

Diseases of the External Ear. William Lawson et al. 3rd ed. 1995. (Illus.). 352p. text 99.00 (*0-7216-5667-6*) Saunders.

Diseases of the External Eye & Adnexa: A Text & Atlas. H. Bruce Ostler. 1993. (Illus.). 864p. 250.00 (*0-683-06651-X*) Lppncott W & W.

Diseases of the Eye & Ear Consequent on Inherited Syphilis: A Clinical Memoir. Jonathan Hutchinson. 1979. LC 78-27655. 272p. reprint ed. lib. bdg. 32.50 (*0-88275-838-1*) Krieger.

Diseases of the Eye & Skin: A Color Atlas. H. Bruce Ostler et al. 1996. (Illus.). 352p. text 150.00 (*0-683-06653-6*) Lppncott W & W.

Diseases of the Female Genital System: International Nomenclature of Diseases. 1992. xii, 126p. pap. text 23.00 (*92-4-154423-6*, 1820008) World Health.

Diseases of the Fetus & Newborn: Pathology, Imaging, Genetics & Management. Ed. by G. B. Reed et al. 2nd ed. 1994. 1728p. (*0-412-39160-0*) E A GBR. *Dist:* OUP.

Diseases of the Gastroesophageal Mucosa: The Acid-Related Disorders. Ed. by James W. Freston. 2001. (Clinical Gastroenterology Ser.). 208p. 99.50 (*0-89603-965-X*) Humana.

Diseases of the Gastrointestinal Tract: Proceedings of the Fifty Fifth Annual Anatomic Pathology Slide Seminar of the ASCP. Ed. by Roger C. Haggitt et al. 1991. LC 91-4560. 126p. 35.00 (*0-89189-336-9*, 50-1-056-00) Am Soc Clinical.

Diseases of the Gastrointestinal Tract & Liver. David J. Shearman & Niall D. Finlayson. 2nd ed. 1989. (Illus.). 1350p. text (*0-443-03110-X*) Church.

Diseases of the Gastrointestinal Tract & Liver. Ed. by David J. C. Shearman et al. 3rd ed. 1997. text (*0-443-05147-X*, S1021) Church.

Diseases of the Goat. John G. Matthews. 2nd rev. ed. 1999. LC 99-34208. (Illus.). 364p. pap. (*0-632-05167-1*) Blckwell Science GBR. *Dist:* Iowa U Pr.

Diseases of the Gut & Pancreas. Ed. by J. J. Misiewicz & R. E. Pounder. 2nd ed. 1994. (Illus.). 1176p. 225.00 (*0-632-02783-5*) Blackwell Sci.

Diseases of the Hair & Scalp. Rodney Dawber. 3rd ed. 1997. LC 96-45303. (Illus.). 640p. 246.95 (*0-86542-866-2*) Blackwell Sci.

Diseases of the Hair & the Scalp. Ludmila Bartosova et al. 1984. (Current Problems in Dermatology Ser.: Vol. 12). (Illus.). x, 252p. 71.50 (*3-8055-3783-2*) S Karger.

Diseases of the Head & Neck, Nose & Throat. Ed. by Andrew S. Jones et al. 1998. LC 97-27629. (An Arnold Publication). 984p. (*0-340-64610-1*) E A GBR. *Dist:* OUP.

Diseases of the Heart. Julian. 2nd ed. 1996. text 131.00 (*0-7020-1756-6*) Saunders.

Diseases of the Hip, Knee, & Ankle Joints. Hugh O. Thomas. deluxe ed. 1991. (Illus.). 283p. lthr. 375.00 (*0-930405-52-8*); reprint ed. 125.00 (*0-930405-31-5*) Norman SF.

Diseases of the Human Body. Carol D. Tamparo & Marcia A. Lewis. 3rd ed. 2000. LC 99-54159. (Illus.). 423p. (Orig.). pap. text 32.95 (*0-8036-0564-1*) Davis Co.

Diseases of the Human Carotid Body. D. Heath & P. Smith. 1991. (Illus.). 205p. 211.00 (*0-387-19687-0*) Spr-Verlag.

Diseases of the Kidney Ed. by Robert W. Schrier & Carl W. Gottschalk. 6th ed. 1996. LC 96-1831. Set. 3,276p. text 439.00 (*0-316-77456-1*); Vol. 1. 133.31 (*0-316-77447-2*, Little Brwn Med Div); Vol. 2. 133.31 (*0-316-77448-0*, Little Brwn Med Div); Vol. 3. 133.31 (*0-316-77446-4*, Little Brwn Med Div) Lppncott W & W.

Diseases of the Kidney, the Lower Urinary Tract, & the Male Genital System: International Nomenclature of Diseases. 1992. xiii, 180p. pap. text 20.00 (*92-4-154441-4*, 1820007) World Health.

Diseases of the Lips: An Illustrated Guide. Robert Jackson. 2000. (Illus.). 126p. 42.95 incl. audio compact disk (*1-896918-00-X*) Manticore Pubs.

Diseases of the Liver. Ed. by B. R. Bacon & A. M. Di Bisceglie. 1998. LC 98-52043. (Illus.). 512p. text (*0-443-05712-5*) Church.

Diseases of the Liver. Ed. by Leon Schiff & Eugene R. Schiff. 6th ed. 1987. LC 65-9111. (Illus.). 1536p. text 150.00 (*0-397-50747-X*, Lippncott) Lppncott W & W.

Diseases of the Liver, In Two Volumes. Eugene R. Schiff. 8th ed. 1998. LC 98-11708. (Illus.). xxi, 1641p. text 279.00 (*0-397-58769-4*) Lppncott W & W.

Diseases of the Liver & Bile Ducts: Diagnosis & Treatment. George Y. Wu & Jonathan Israel. 1998. LC 98-23699. (Current Clinical Practice Ser.). (Illus.). 456p. 125.00 (*0-89603-431-3*) Humana.

Diseases of the Liver & Bile Ducts: Proceedings of the Fifty Fourth Annual Anatomic Pathology Slide Seminar of the ASCP. Ed. by Jurgen Ludwig & Kamal G. Ishak. 1989. LC 89-17874. 133p. 35.00 (*0-89189-294-X*, D50-1-055-00) Am Soc Clinical.

***Diseases of the Liver & Biliary System.** Sheila Sherlock. 2001. LC 2001-52704. (Illus.). 736p. 170.00 (*0-632-05582-0*) Blackwell Sci.

Diseases of the Liver & Biliary System. Sheila Sherlock & James Dooley. 10th ed. 1996. LC 96-23961. (Illus.). 704p. 208.95 (*0-86542-906-5*) Blackwell Sci.

Diseases of the Liver & Biliary System in Children. Deirdre A. Kelly. 1999. LC 98-52864. (Illus.). 400p. 198.95 (*0-632-04802-6*) Blackwell Sci.

Diseases of the Liver & Biliary Tract with Standardization of Nomenclature Diagnostic Criteria & Diagnostic Methodology: Proceedings of the International Association for the Study of the Liver Quadrennial Meeting, 5th, Acapulco, October 1974. International Association for the Study of Pain. Ed. by Carroll M. Leevy. 1976. (Illus.). 250p. 52.25 (*3-8055-2276-2*) S Karger.

Diseases of the Liver & Billiary Tract: Standardization of Nomenclature, Diagnostic Criteria Diagnostic Methodology. Ed. by Carroll M. Leevy et al. 1979. 49.95 (*0-7194-0006-6*) Coronet Bks.

Diseases of the Liver & the Bile Ducts: New Aspects & Clinical Implications : Proceedings of the Falk Symposium 107 Held in Prague, Czech Republic, September 12-13, 1998. Ed. by J. Spicak. 1999. LC 99-229855. (Falk Symposium Ser.: Vol. 107). xiii, 246p. (*0-7923-8751-1*) Kluwer Academic.

Diseases of the Lower Respiratory Tract International Nomenclature of Diseases, 3. 1979. (International Nomenclature of Diseases Ser.: No. 3). pap. text 25.00 (*92-9036-001-1*) World Health.

Diseases of the Lymphatic System: Diagnosis & Therapy. Ed. by D. W. Molander. 1983. (Illus.). 500p. 224.00 (*0-387-90850-1*) Spr-Verlag.

Diseases of the Motor System. Pierre J. Vinken et al. 1991. (Handbooks of Clinical Neurology: Vol. 59(15)). 530p. 248.50 (*0-444-81278-4*) Elsevier.

Diseases of the Nails & Their Management. Ed. by Robert Baran & R. P. R. Dawber. 2nd ed. 1994. LC 93-41599. (Illus.). 528p. 195.00 (*0-632-03754-7*) Blackwell Sci.

Diseases of the Nerves Ed. by Pierre J. Vinken & George W. Bruyn. Pt. 1. 1996. 95.00 (*0-444-10017-2*); Pt. 2. 1971. 216.50 (*0-444-10018-0*) Elsevier.

***Diseases of the Nervous System.** Ed. by Arthur K. Asbury et al. 3rd ed. 2002. LC 2001-43713. 1500p. text 375.00 (*0-521-79351-3*) Cambridge U Pr.

Diseases of the Nervous System, Pt. I. Pierre J. Vinken & George W. Bruyn. 1991. Elsevier.

Diseases of the Nervous System: Clinical Neurobiology Ed. by Arthur K. Asbury et al. 2nd ed. 1991. (Illus.). 1780p. text 335.00 (*0-7216-3208-4*) Saunders.

Diseases of the Nervous System in Childhood. Jean Aicardi. 2nd rev. ed. 1998. LC 98-172809. (Clinics in Developmental Medicine Ser.). (Illus.). 1100p. (C). text (*1-898683-16-6*) Mc Keith Pr GBR. *Dist:* Cambridge U Pr.

Diseases of the Nose, Throat & Ear. Bernard H. Coleman. 14th ed. 1992. (Illus.). 304p. (Orig.). pap. text (*0-443-04563-1*) Church.

Diseases of the Nose, Throat, Ear, Head & Neck. John Jacob Ballenger. 14th ed. 1991. LC 90-6143. (Illus.). 1376p. text 199.50 (*0-8121-1345-4*) Lppncott W & W.

Diseases of the Oral Mucosa: A Color Atlas. Manfred Strassburg & Gerdt Knolle. Tr. by Hannelore T. Loevy from GER. 2nd ed. 1993. LC 93-31256. (Illus.). 800p. text 210.00 (*0-86715-210-9*, B2109) Quint Pub Co.

Diseases of the Patellofemoral Joint. John Fulkerson. 2nd ed. 1990. 320p. 69.00 (*0-683-03382-4*) Lppncott W & W.

Diseases of the Retina: New Approaches in the Diagnosis & Therapy of Macular & Retinal Diseases, Leipzig, November 1996. Ed. by Peter Wiedemann & Leon Kohen. 1997. (Opthalmologica Ser.: Vol. 29, No. 5, 1997). (Illus.). 124p. pap. 50.50 (*3-8055-6577-1*) S Karger.

Diseases of the Retina & Uvea. Ed. by S. Mishima. 1982. (Journal: Vol. 185, No. 3). (Illus.). 72p. pap. 41.75 (*3-8055-3563-5*) S Karger.

Diseases of the Retina & Vitreous. Richard F. Spaide. Ed. by Richard Lampert. 1999. LC 98-4296. (Illus.). 365p. text (*0-7216-8005-4*) Saunders.

Diseases of the Salivary Glands Including Dry Mouth & Sj Ogren's Syndrome: Diagnosis & Treatment. Isaac Van der Waal & Leo M. Sreebny. 1996. LC 96-22209. (Illus.). 144p. 82.95 (*3-540-61380-3*) Spr-Verlag.

Diseases of the Sinuses: A Comprehensive Textbook of Diagnosis & Treatment. Ed. by M. Eric Gershwin & Gary Incaudo. 1996. LC 95-39511. (Illus.). 608p. 170.00 (*0-89603-317-1*) Humana.

Diseases of the Sinuses: Diagnosis & Endoscopic Management. David W. Kennedy & James Zinreich. 2000. 600p. incl. cd-rom (*1-55009-045-3*) DEKR.

Diseases of the Skeletal Muscle. Contrib. by Robert Wortmann. 2000. LC 99-31927. 400p. text 99.00 (*0-7817-1614-4*) Lppncott W & W.

***Diseases of the Skin: A Color Atlas & Text.** Gary M. White & Neil H. Cox. 2000. (Illus.). 528p. text 199.00 (*0-7234-3155-8*) Mosby Inc.

Diseases of the Small Intestine in Childhood. John W. Smith. 1975. (Illus.). 259p. pap. 29.00 (*0-8464-1089-3*) Beekman Pubs.

Diseases of the Throat & Lungs & Principles of Hygeiotherapy. R. T. Trall & S. W. Dodds. 1994. 126p. reprint ed. spiral bd. 12.00 (*0-7873-1193-6*) Hlth Research.

Diseases of the Thyroid. Ed. by Lewis E. Braverman. 1997. LC 97-11636. (Contemporary Endocrinology Ser.: Vol. 2). (Illus.). 408p. 145.00 (*0-89603-414-3*) Humana.

Diseases of the Thyroid. D. C. Evered. 1976. 182p. pap. 29.00 (*0-8464-1462-7*) Beekman Pubs.

Diseases of the Thyroid: Pathophysiology & Management. M. H. Wheeler & J. H. Lazarus. 1994. (Illus.). 448p. (gr. 13). (*0-412-43030-4*) E A GBR. *Dist:* OUP.

Diseases of the Veins. Norman L. Browse. 704p. text (*0-7131-4523-4*) E A GBR. *Dist:* Routldge.

Diseases of the Veins: Pathology, Diagnosis, & Treatment. Norman L. Browse et al. 1988. (Illus.). 704p. text 149.50 (*0-683-13006-4*) Lppncott W & W.

Diseases of the Wistar Rat. Mary J. Tucker. 1997. LC 97-179499. 288p. (*0-7484-0521-6*) Tay Francis Ltd GBR. *Dist:* Taylor & Francis.

Diseases of Wild Waterfowl. Gary A. Wobeser. 2nd ed. 1997. LC 97-1133. (Illus.). 336p. 79.50 (*0-306-45590-0*, Kluwer Plenum) Kluwer Academic.

Diseases of Women & Easy Childbirth. J. H. Tilden. 1996. 195p. reprint ed. spiral bd. 15.00 (*0-7873-0878-1*) Hlth Research.

Diseases of Women & Easy Childbirth, 1912. J. H. Tilden. 1996. 196p. reprint ed. pap. 14.95 (*1-56459-876-4*) Kessinger Pub.

Disenfranchised Grief. Kenneth J. Doka. 1989. 347p. 46.95 (*0-669-17081-X*) Lxngtn Bks.

Disenfranchised Grief: Recognizing & Treating Hidden Sorrow. Kenneth J. Doka. 1998. LC 98-14145. pap. (*0-7879-4376-2*) Jossey-Bass.

Disillusionment. Ed. by Charles Boer et al. 1995. (Spring Journal: Vol. 58). 176p. (Orig.). pap. 17.50 (1-882670-06-X) Spring Jrnl.

Disinfectants: Do They Work? 1994. (Illus.). 68p. (Orig.). (C). pap. text 25.00 (0-7881-0630-9) DIANE Pub.

Disinfecting Plumbing Systems of Legionella: Solving Problems Without Overspending. Matthew R. Freije. 1998. LC 98-92504. 25p. pap. 19.00 (0-9649926-2-0, 303) HC Info Res.

Disinfection & Sterilization: Index of Modern Authors & Subjects with Guide for Rapid Research. Luther S. Zachery. rev. ed. 1994. 57.50 (0-7883-0190-X); pap. 47.50 (0-7883-0191-8) ABBE Pubs Assn.

Disinfection, Sterilization & Preservation. Seymour S. Block. 5th ed. 2000. LC 00-41221. (Illus.). xxii, 1481p. text 225.00 (0-683-30740-1) Lppncott W & W.

Disjointed Life. Corbett Woodall. 1980. pap. 10.95 (0-434-87796-4) Trafalgar.

Disney Encyclopedia of Baby & Child Care Judith Palfrey et al. Ed. by Genell Subak-Sharpe. 1999. LC 99-217326. (Illus.). 672p. (J). pap. 19.95 (0-7868-8297-2) Hyperion.

Disordered Body: Epidemic Disease & Cultural Transformation. Suzanne E. Hatty & James Hatty. 1999. LC 99-17302. (SUNY Series in Medical Anthropology). 299p. (C). text 58.50 (0-7914-4365-5); pap. text 19.95 (0-7914-4366-3) State U NY Pr.

Disordered Couple. Ed. by Jon Carlson & Len Sperry. 1997. LC 97-24085. xxiii, 342p. 45.95 (0-87630-815-9) Brunner-Routledge.

Disordered Defecation. Ed. by H. G. Gooszen et al. 1987. (Developments in Surgery Ser.). (C). text 184.00 (0-89838-891-0) Kluwer Academic.

***Disordered Mind & Brain.** Peter F. Liddle. 2001. 320p. (1-901242-65-X) Royal Coll Psych GBR. *Dist:* Balogh.

Disordered Mother or Disordered Diagnosis? Munchausen by Proxy Syndrome. David B. Allison & Mark S. Roberts. 1998. LC 98-34172. 336p. 49.95 (0-88163-290-2) Analytic Pr.

Disordered Thinking & Schizophrenic Psychopathology. Martin Harrow & Donald M. Quinlan. 1985. LC 78-13649. (C). text 44.95 (0-89876-099-2) Gardner Pr.

Disorderly Eaters: Texts in Self-Empowerment. Ed. by Lilian R. Furst & Peter W. Graham. 1992. (Illus.). 288p. pap. 23.95 (0-271-00871-7) Pa St U Pr.

Disorders & Dysfunctions of the Self. Ed. by Dante Cicchetti & Sheree L. Toth. 1994. LC 93-24573. (Rochester Symposium on Developmental Psychopathology Ser.: Vol. 5). 460p. (C). 100.00 (1-878822-31-4) Univ Rochester Pr.

Disorders, Diagnosis & Therapy, Vol. 2. Norman Kretchmer et al. 1987. x, 364p. text 195.00 (3-7186-0345-4) Gordon & Breach.

Disorders of Affect Regulation: Alexithymia in Medical & Psychiatric Illness. Graeme J. Taylor et al. 1999. (Illus.). 382p. pap. text 44.95 (0-521-77850-6) Cambridge U Pr.

Disorders of Articulation: Aspects of Dysarthria & Verbal Dyspraxia. M. Edwards. 1984. (Disorders of Human Communication Ser.: Vol. 7). (Illus.). 134p. 59.95 (0-387-81787-5) Spr-Verlag.

Disorders of Eating Behaviour: A Psychoneuroendocrine Approach - Proceedings of the International Symposium, September 1985, Pavia, Italy. Ed. by E. Ferrari & F. G. Brambilla. 1986. (Advances in the Biosciences Ser.: No. 60). (Illus.). 426p. 100.50 (0-08-032024-4, Pergamon Pr) Elsevier.

Disorders of Feeding & Swallowing in Infants & Children. Ed. by David N. Tuchman & Rhonda S. Walter. 1993. LC 93-19636. (Illus.). 280p. (Orig.). (C). pap. text 75.00 (1-56593-092-4, 0396) Thomson Learn.

Disorders of Fluid & Electrolyte Balance: Diagnosis & Treatment. Jules B. Puschett. 1985. (Illus.). 259p. (Orig.). pap. text (0-443-08318-5) Church.

Disorders of Growth & Development Ed. by David W. Kaplan. 1988. (Journal: Vol. 14, Nos. 3 & 4, 1987). (Illus.). iv, 84p. pap. 43.50 (3-8055-4801-X); 96p. pap. 49.75 (3-8055-4799-4) S Karger.

Disorders of Hemoglobin: Genetics, Pathophysiology & Clinical Management. Ed. by Martin H. Steinberg et al. 2000. (Illus.). 1282p. (C). text 275.00 (0-521-63266-8) Cambridge U Pr.

Disorders of Hemostasis. Oscar D. Ratnoff & Charles D. Forbes. Ed. by Richard Zorab. 3rd ed. 1996. LC 95-2349. (Illus.). 576p. text 154.00 (0-7216-5273-5) Saunders.

Disorders of Hemostasis & Thrombosis: A Clinical Guide. William E. Hathaway & Scott H. Goodnight, Jr. 1993. (Illus.). 592p. pap. 48.00 (0-07-027015-5) McGraw-Hill Educ Grp.

Disorders of Higher Nervous Activity. Ed. by Pierre J. Vinken & George W. Bruyn. 1969. 161.75 (0-444-10300-7) Elsevier.

Disorders of Learning in Childhood. Archie A. Silver & Rose A. Hagin. 1990. LC 89-28492. (Child & Adolescent Mental Health Ser.). 704p. 275.00 (0-471-50828-4) Wiley.

Disorders of Lipid Metabolism. G. V. Marinetti. 1990. LC 89-72205. (Illus.). 240p. (C). text 69.50 (0-306-43431-8, Kluwer Plenum) Kluwer Academic.

Disorders of Mental Status: Dementia, Encephalopathy, Coma, Syncope. Karl E. Misulis. 1998. LC 97-50382. 303p. pap. text 39.99 (0-7506-9988-4) Buttrwrth-Heinemann.

Disorders of Movement: Clinical, Pharmacological & Physiological Aspects. Ed. by Niall Quinn & Peter Jenner. 1989. 567p. text 178.00 (0-12-569685-X) Acad Pr.

Disorders of Narcissism: Diagnostic, Clinical, & Empirical Implications. Ed. by Elsa Ronningstam. 1997. LC 97-902. 304p. text 44.50 (0-88048-701-1, 8701) Am Psychiatric.

Disorders of Narcissism: Diagnostic, Clinical & Empirical Implications. Elsa Ronningstam. 2000. LC 99-59531. pap. 35.00 (0-7657-0259-2) Aronson.

Disorders of Personality: DSM-IVTM & Beyond. Theodore Millon et al. 2nd ed. 1995. LC 95-9045. (Interscience Monograph Ser.). 832p. 140.00 (0-471-01186-X) Wiley.

Disorders of Smell & Taste - The Most Common Complaints. Hawkes. 2001. LC 2001-58613. (Most Common Complaints Ser.). 208p. pap. 24.99 (0-7506-7287-0) Buttrwrth-Heinemann.

Disorders of Speech Perception & Symbolic Behavior. Ed. by Pierre J. Vinken & George W. Bruyn. 1969. 188.75 (0-444-10301-5) Elsevier.

Disorders of Syntactic Comprehension. David N. Caplan & Nancy Hildebrandt. 1988. (Issues in the Biology of Language & Cognition Ser.). 288p. 49.95 (0-262-03132-9, Bradford Bks) MIT Pr.

Disorders of Taste & Smell. Charles P. Kimmelman. 2nd rev. ed. 1996. LC 96-28185. (Self-Instructional Package Ser.). (Illus.). 62p. pap. text 25.00 (1-56772-024-2) AAO-HNS.

Disorders of the Anterior Segment. Epstein. 2000. text (0-7216-5761-3) Saunders.

Disorders of the Autonomic Nervous System. David Robertson. 1995. xvi, 434p. text 132.00 (3-7186-5146-7, Harwood Acad Pubs) Gordon & Breach.

Disorders of the Brain & Mind. Ed. by Maria A. Ron & Anthony S. David. 1999. (Illus.). 388p. pap. text 44.95 (0-521-77851-4) Cambridge U Pr.

Disorders of the Cardiovascular System. 368p. pap. (0-340-53593-8) E A GBR. *Dist:* Routldge.

Disorders of the Cervical Spine. Martin B. Camins & Patrick F. O'Leary. 1992. (Illus.). 656p. 155.00 (0-683-01401-3) Lppncott W & W.

Disorders of the Cervical Spine: Diagnosis & Medical Management. John H. Bland. 2nd ed. 1994. LC 93-33171. text 105.00 (0-7216-5015-5) Saunders.

Disorders of the Endocrine System. Robert D. Utiger. 1991. (0-8151-8941-9) Mosby Inc.

Disorders of the Foot & Ankle: Medical & Surgical Management, Set. Melvin H. Jahss. 2nd ed. 1990. (Illus.). 3392p. text 525.00 (0-7216-1327-6) Saunders.

***Disorders of the Hair & Scalp.** Farrell et al. 2000. (Fast Facts Ser.). (Illus.). 88p. pap. (1-899541-03-9) Health Pr GBR. *Dist:* JAMCO Dist.

Disorders of the Heel, Rearfoot & Ankle. Rock G. Positano. Ed. by Marc Strauss. 1999. LC 98-54193. (Illus.). 555p. (C). text (0-443-07838-6) Church.

Disorders of the Horse & What to Do about Them. Elsie V. Hanauer. 1974. pap. 5.00 (0-87980-281-2) Wilshire.

Disorders of the Lymph Nodes & Related Organs: Based on the Proceedings of the 58th Annual Anatomic Pathology Slide Seminar of the American Society of Clinical Pathologists. Nancy L. Harris et al. 1994. LC 94-25191. 35.00 (0-89189-365-2) Am Soc Clinical.

Disorders of the Pancreas: Controversies in Diagnosis & Management. Ed. by Gerard P. Burns & Simmy Bank. 1991. (Illus.). 450p. (0-08-040317-4) PPI GBR. *Dist:* McGraw.

Disorders of the Pancreas: Current Issues in Diagnosis & Management. Ed. by Gerard P. Burns & Simmy Bank. 1992. (Illus.). 506p. text 82.00 (0-07-105402-2) McGraw-Hill Med Pub.

Disorders of the Patellofemoral Joint. John P. Fulkerson. 3rd ed. 1996. LC 96-18023. (0-683-03396-4) Lppncott W & W.

Disorders of the Patellofemoral Joint. John P. Fulkerson et al. 3rd ed. 1997. LC 96-18023. (Illus.). 384p. text 120.00 (0-683-03392-1) Lppncott W & W.

Disorders of the Pelvic Floor. Philip Caushaj et al. 1996. (Illus.). 350p. text 89.00 (1-57626-008-9) Quality Med Pub.

Disorders of the Self: New Therapeutic Horizons - The Masterson Approach. Ed. by James F. Masterson & Ralph Klein. 1995. 448p. 51.95 (0-87630-786-1) Brunner-Routledge.

Disorders of the Shoulder: Diagnosis & Management. Joseph P. Iannotti. 1999. LC 98-37040. 1,168p. text 229.00 (0-7817-1320-X) Lppncott W & W.

Disorders of the Shoulder: Diagnosis & Management. Joseph P. Iannotti & Gerald R. Williams, Jr. 1999. 1,168p. 359.00 (0-7817-1996-8) Lppncott W & W.

Disorders of the Spine: A Coding System for Diagnoses. Ed. by North American Spine Society Staff & David F. Fardon. 1991. LC 91-71142. 132p. (Orig.). text 30.00 (1-56053-014-6) Hanley & Belfus.

Disorders of the Spleen. Alfred Cuschieri. 1994. (Illus.). 256p. 135.00 (0-632-03314-2) Blackwell Sci.

Disorders of the Spleen, Vol. 20. Barbara C. Wolf & Richard S. Neiman. 1989. text 99.00 (0-7216-2503-7) Saunders.

Disorders of the Spleen: Pathophysiology & Management. Schwartz et al. 1989. (Hematology Ser.: Vol. 10). (Illus.). 488p. text 210.00 (0-8247-7933-9) Dekker.

Disorders of the Vestibular System. M. Halmagyi. Ed. by Robert W. Baloh. 1996. LC 95-12313. (Illus.). 712p. (C). text 135.00 (0-19-509006-3) OUP.

Disorders of Thrombosis. Russell Hull & Graham F. Pineo. Ed. by Richard Zorab. 1995. LC 95-4086. (Illus.). 448p. text 145.00 (0-7216-5278-6) Saunders.

Disorders of Tubular Transport: Physiologic & Clinical Correlations. Ed. by J. A. Arruda & N. A. Kurtzman. 1981. (Journal: Vol. 5, Nos. 2-4). (Illus.). 144p. pap. 91.50 (3-8055-2515-X) S Karger.

Disorders of Voice. Margaret Greene. 1972. LC 77-183113. (Studies in Communicative Disorders). (C). pap. (0-672-61279-8, Bobbs) Macmillan.

Disorders of Voluntary Muscle. Ed. by J. A. Walton. 5th ed. 1988. (Illus.). 1166p. text (0-443-03882-1) Church.

Disorders of Voluntary Muscle. Ed. by John Walton et al. 6th ed. 1994. LC 94-3177. text (0-443-04624-7) Church.

Disorders of Water, Electrolytes & Acid Base/Acute Renal Failure Ed. by Robert W. Schrier et al. 1998. LC 98-29127. (Atlas of Diseases of the Kidney Ser.: Vol. 1). (Illus.). 131.95 (0-632-04385-7) Blackwell Sci.

Disorders with Defective Hearing. Ed. by V. Colletti & S. D. Stephens. 1985. (Advances in Audiology Ser.: Vol. 3). (Illus.). viii, 216p. 142.75 (3-8055-3965-7) S Karger.

Dispatches from the Freud Wars: Psychoanalysis & Its Passions. John Forrester. 1997. LC 96-38678. 320p. 27.95 (0-674-53960-5) HUP.

Dispelling the Myths about Addiction: Strategies to Increase Understanding & Strengthen Research. Institute of Medicine Staff. 1997. LC 97-69691. 218p. pap. 39.95 (0-309-06401-5) Natl Acad Pr.

Dispensaries, Their Management & Development: A Book for Administrators, Public Health Workers. Michael M. Davis, Jr. & Andrew R. Warner. Ed. by Barbara G. Rosenkrantz. 1977. LC 76-25658. (Public Health in America Ser.). (Illus.). reprint ed. lib. bdg. 36.95 (0-405-09813-8) Ayer.

Dispensary: With a Short Account of the Proceedings of the College of Physicians, London, in Relation to the Sick Poor (1697) & Claremont (1715) Samuel Garth. 1975. LC 74-23391. 160p. reprint ed. lib. bdg. 50.00 (0-8201-1145-7) Schol Facsimiles.

Dispensing of Medication. Robert F. King. 9th ed. 1984. LC 84-61218. 28.95 (0-912734-08-6) Mack Pub.

Dispensing Optician Manual: An Introduction to Vision Care for the New Ophthalmic Technician. A. J. Zelada. 1987. (Illus.). 146p. (C). 43.95 (0-398-05359-6) C C Thomas.

Dispersion of Ventricular Repolarization: State of the Art. Ed. by S. Bertil Olsson et al. 2000. LC 00-37552. (Illus.). 300p. 125.00 (0-87993-458-1) Futura Pub.

Disposable ECG Electrodes. 2nd ed. 1991. 9p. pap. 62.00 (0-910275-61-0, EC12-209) Assn Adv Med Instrn.

Disposable Medical Product Markets: PPE Demand Creates Specialty Products. Market Intelligence Staff. 1992. 299p. 1495.00 (1-56753-417-1) Frost & Sullivan.

Disposable Medical Product Markets, Vol. Two: Respiratory Disease & Infection Control Dominiate Trends for Growth. Market Intelligence Staff. 1993. 297p. 1495.00 (1-56753-474-0) Frost & Sullivan.

Disposition of Toxic Drugs & Chemicals in Man. Randall C. Baselt. 1999. (Illus.). 900p. text 119.00 (0-9626523-3-4) Chem Toxicol Inst.

Disposition of Toxic Drugs & Chemicals in Man. Randall C. Baselt & Robert H. Cravey. 4th ed. 1994. (Illus.). 1000p. text 99.50 (0-9626523-1-8) Chem Toxicol Inst.

Disputed Issues in Renal Failure Therapy. Ed. by M. J. Lysaght et al. 1985. (Contributions to Nephrology Ser.: Vol. 44). (Illus.). xii, 294p. 29.75 (3-8055-3938-X) S Karger.

Disquectomia Cervical Anterior. Oliver D. Grin & Dorothy L. Bouwman. Ed. by Laura C. Kienbaum. Tr. by Hector BeltrandelRio & Marisa BeltrandelRio from ENG. 1993. (Patient Education Ser.). (SPA., Illus.). 18p. (Orig.). pap. text 3.50 (0-929689-58-5) Ludann Co.

Disruptive Behavior Disorders in Childhood. Ed. by Donald K. Routh. 1994. (Illus.). 256p. (C). 45.00 (0-306-44695-2, Plenum Trade) Perseus Pubng.

Disruptive Behavior Disorders in Children: Treatment-Focused Assessment. Michael J. Breen & Thomas S. Altepeter. 1990. LC 90-3817. 288p. 35.00 (0-89862-439-8, 2439) Guilford Pubns.

Disruptive Behavior Disorders in Children & Adolescents. Ed. by Robert L. Hendren et al. 1999. LC 99-10438. (Review of Psychiatry Ser.: Vol. 18). 214p. 27.50 (0-88048-960-X) Am Psychiatric.

Dissection & Tissue Culture Manual of the Nervous System. Ed. by Abraham Shahar et al. 1989. LC 89-8234. 398p. pap. 160.00 (0-471-56237-8) Wiley.

Dissection Guide & Atlas to the Fetal Pig. David G. Smith & Michael P. Schenk. 1997. (Illus.). 114p. pap. text 19.95 (0-89582-363-2) Morton Pub.

Dissection Manual: Companion to Rohen - Yokochi Color Atlas of Anatomy. Jack L. Wilson. 3rd ed. 1993. LC 92-49400. (Illus.). 288p. 39.50 (0-89640-230-4) Igaku-Shoin.

Dissector for Gross Anatomy. Larsen. 1999. pap. text (0-7216-4647-6) Saunders.

Dissector for Netter's Atlas of Human Anatomy Vols. I-II: Dissections - Discussions. Frank H. Netter. 1997. (0-914168-20-7) Icon Lrning Systs.

Disseminated Intravascular Coagulation. Ed. by T. Abe & M. Yamamaka. 1983. (Bibliotheca Haematologica Ser.: No. 49). (Illus.). xiv, 356p. 171.50 (3-8055-3726-3) S Karger.

Disseminated Intravascular Coagulation & Related Syndromes. Ed. by Roger L. Bick. 1983. 144p. 88.00 (0-8493-6636-4, RC647, CRC Reprint) Franklin.

Dissemination of Health Information: A Case Study in Adult Learning. Jacob J. Feldman. 1966. LC 66-14570. (Monographs in Social Research: No. 11). 15.00 (0-202-27001-7) Natl Opinion Res.

Dissenting Doctors in Medicine. 1991. lib. bdg. 77.75 (0-8490-4667-X) Gordon Pr.

Dissertatio de Effervescentia et Fermentatione see Dissertations on the Mechanics of Effervescence & Fermentation & on the Mechanics of the Movement of the Muscles by John Bernoulli

Dissertation on Speech. J. C. Amman. Tr. by C. Baker. 1966. 5.00 (0-934454-29-9) Lubrecht & Cramer.

Dissertation on the Disorder of Death: That State of the Frame Under the Signs of Death Called Suspended Animation. Walter Whiter. Ed. by Robert J. Kastenbaum. 1977. LC 76-19598. (Death & Dying Ser.). reprint ed. lib. bdg. 42.95 (0-405-09592-9) Ayer.

Dissertation on the Functions of the Nervous System. Georg Prochaska. Tr. by T. Laycock. LC 78-72819. (Brainedness, Handedness, & Mental Abilities Ser.). reprint ed. 34.50 (0-404-60888-4) AMS Pr.

Dissertation upon Genius. William Sharpe. 1973. LC 72-13112. (History of Psychology Ser.). 168p. reprint ed. lib. bdg. 50.00 (0-8201-1110-4) Schol Facsimiles.

Dissertations on the Mechanics of Effervescence & Fermentation & on the Mechanics of the Movement of the Muscles by John Bernoulli. Ed. by Paul G. Maquet et al. Tr. by Paul G. Maquet from LAT. 1997. LC 97-8258. (Transactions Ser.: Vol. 87, Pt. 3).Tr. of Dissertatio de Effervescentia et Fermentatione. 160p. pap. 18.00 (0-87169-873-0, T873-map) Am Philos.

Dissociation. Herbert Spiegel. 1998. 29.95 (0-465-01676-6) Basic.

Dissociation: Clinical & Theoretical Perspectives. Ed. by Steven Jay Lynn & Judith W. Rhue. 1994. LC 94-12041. 477p. 60.00 (0-89862-186-0, 2186) Guilford Pubns.

Dissociation: Culture, Mind & Body. Ed. by David Spiegel. 1994. LC 93-47478. 227p. text 34.50 (0-88048-557-4, 8557) Am Psychiatric.

Dissociation in Children & Adolescents: A Developmental Perspective. Frank W. Putnam. 1997. LC 97-20444. 423p. 44.00 (1-57230-219-4, 0219) Guilford Pubns.

Dissociation of a Personality: A Biographical Study in Abnormal Psychology. Morton Prince. 1969. LC 69-10148. 575p. reprint ed. lib. bdg. 35.00 (0-8371-1988-X, PRAP, Greenwood Pr) Greenwood.

Dissociation of Trauma: Theory, Phenomenology & Technique. Ira Brenner. 2000. LC 00-46124. xiv, 256p. 40.00 (0-8236-1289-9) Intl Univs Pr.

Dissociative Child: Diagnosis, Treatment & Management. Ed. by Joyanna L. Silberg. 2nd rev. ed. 1998. LC 98-30902. 400p. text 45.00 (1-886968-06-3, SIDC) Sidran Pr.

Dissociative Disorders: A Clinical Review. Ed. by David Spiegel. 1993. LC 92-82037. x, 134p. (Orig.). (C). pap. 13.95 (0-9629164-1-2) Sidran Pr.

Dissociative Identity Disorder: Diagnosis, Clinical Features & Treatment of Multiple Personality. Colin A. Ross. 2nd ed. 1996. LC 96-23334. 464p. 95.00 (0-471-13265-9) Wiley.

Distancing: A Guide to Avoidance & Avoidant Personality Disorder. Martin D. Kantor. 1993. LC 93-294. 200p. 67.00 (0-275-94408-5, C4408, Praeger Pubs) Greenwood.

***Distant Metastases from Head & Neck Cancer: A Multi-Institutional View.** Ed. by A. Ferlito. 2001. (Special Issue Ser.: Vol. 63). (Illus.). 80p. pap. 34.00 (3-8055-7276-X) S Karger.

***Distant Wanderers: The Search for Planets Beyond the Solar System.** Bruce G. Dorminey & Robert Kirby. 2001. LC 2001-47132. (Illus.). 225p. 29.95 (0-387-95074-5, Copernicus) Spr-Verlag.

Distinctive Approach to Psychological Research: The Influence of Stanley Schachter. Ed. by Neil Grunberg et al. 1987. 248p. text 49.95 (0-89859-910-5) L Erlbaum Assocs.

Distinctive Characteristics of Re-Evaluation Counseling. Harvey Jackins. 1973. pap. 2.00 (0-911214-26-7) Rational Isl.

Distinctive Characteristics of Re-Evaluation Counseling: Chinese Translation. Sun Jian-Min. 1987. pap. 1.00 (0-913937-31-2) Rational Isl.

Distinguishing Psychological from Organic Disorders: Screening for Psychological Masquerade. Robert L. Taylor. 2000. 256p. pap. (1-85343-521-X) Free Assoc Bks GBR. *Dist:* Intl Spec Bk.

Distinguishing Psychological from Organic Disorders: Screening for Psychological Masquerade. Robert L. Taylor. 1990. LC 90-9477. 256p. 35.95 (0-8261-6950-3) Springer Pub.

Distraction of the Craniofacial Skeleton. Ed. by Joseph G. McCarthy. 1998. LC 97-13230. (Illus.). 459p. 163.00 (0-387-94912-7) Spr-Verlag.

Distractive Joint Manipulation. Thomas F. Bergmann et al. 1997. LC 96-40215. (Illus.). 304p. (C). (gr. 13). text 82.00 (0-8151-0900-8, 28148) Mosby Inc.

Distributed Cognitions: Psychological & Educational Considerations. Ed. by Gavriel Salomon. 1993. LC 92-41220. (Learning in Doing). (Illus.). 297p. (C). text 59.95 (*0-521-41406-7*) Cambridge U Pr.

Distribution & Functions of Mental Imagery. George H. Betts. LC 76-176560. (Columbia University. Teachers College. Contributions to Education Ser.: No. 26). reprint ed. 37.50 (*0-404-55026-6*) AMS Pr.

Distribution of Cataracts in the Population & Influencing Factors. Ed. by K. Sasaki & Otto Hockwin. 1991. (Developments in Ophthalmology Ser.: Vol. 21). (Illus.). viii, 182p. 161.00 (*3-8055-5335-8*) S Karger.

***Distribution of Organs for Transportation: Expectations & Practices.** Richard P. Kusserow. 2001. (Illus.). 105p. (C). pap. text 20.00 (*0-7567-1636-5*) DIANE Pub.

Distribution of Subcutaneous Fat in Childhood & Adolescence. E. L. Reynolds. 1950. (SRCD Ser.: Vol. 15, No. 2). 25.00 (*0-527-01551-2*) Periodicals Srv.

District Administrator, Public Health. Jack Rudman. 1994. (Career Examination Ser.: C-3006). pap. 44.95 (*0-8373-3006-8*) Nat Learn.

District Hospitals: Guidelines for Development. 1992. (WHO Regional Publications, Western Pacific Ser.: No. 4). xi, 189p. pap. text 61.00 (*92-9061-103-0*, 1510004) World Health.

Disturbance of Homeostasis. N. Das. 1988. (C). (*0-7855-4651-0*) Current Dist IND. *Dist:* St Mut.

Disturbance of Homeostasis. Ed. by N. Das. 1987. (C). (*0-89771-342-7*) Current Dist IND. *Dist:* St Mut.

Disturbances of Lower & Higher Visual Capacities Caused by Occipital Damage: With Special Reference to the Psychopathological, Pedagogical, Industrial, & Social Implications. W. Poppelreuter. Tr. by J. Zihl. 1991. (History of Neuroscience Ser.: No. 2).Tr. of Psychischen Schadigungen Durch Kopfschuss in Kriege, 1914-16. (Illus.). 392p. 47.50 (*0-19-852190-1*) OUP.

Disturbances of Nervous Function. Ed. by Pierre J. Vinken & George W. Bruyn. 1969. 272.50 (*0-444-10298-1*) Elsevier.

Disturbances of Water & Electrolyte Metabolism. Ed. by J. Bahlmann & J. Brod. 1980. (Contributions to Nephrology Ser.: Vol. 21). (Illus.). pap. 29.75 (*3-8055-0215-X*) S Karger.

Disturbed Children: Assessment Through Team Process. Menninger Clinic Children's Division Staff. 1995. LC 95-21246. (Master Work Ser.). 318p. pap. 50.00 (*1-56821-649-1*) Aronson.

Disturbed Violent Offender. Hans Toch & Kenneth Adams. rev. ed. 1994. LC 94-27951. 252p. pap. text 19.95 (*1-55798-260-0*, 431-6470) Am Psychol.

Disulfiram & Its Metabolite, Dithiocarb: Pharmacology & Status in the Treatment of Alcoholism, Human Immunodeficiency Virus Infections & Heavy Metal Intoxication. P. K. Gessner & T. Gessner. 1992. 176p. (C). (gr. 13). text 309.95 (*0-412-36010-1*, A4752) Chapman & Hall.

Ditch Medicine: Advanced Field Procedures for Emergencies. Hugh L. Coffee. 1993. (Illus.). 224p. pap. 25.00 (*0-87364-717-3*) Paladin Pr.

DIU: Guide Pratique a l'Intention des Programmes de Planification Familiale. Ed. by Noel McIntosh et al. rev. ed. 1992. (FRE., Illus.). 160p. pap. text 15.00 (*0-929817-03-6*) JHPIEGO.

DIU: Pautas para Su Uso en los Programas de Planificacion Familiar. Ed. by Noel McIntosh et al. 2nd ed. 1996. (SPA., Illus.). pap. text 15.00 (*0-929817-36-2*) JHPIEGO.

Diuretic Agents: Clinical Physiology & Pharmacology. Ed. by Donald W. Seldin & Gerhard H. Giebisch. 1997. LC 97-25926. (Illus.). 666p. text 79.95 (*0-12-635690-4*) Morgan Kaufmann.

Diuretica. Ed. by H. Herken. 1969. (Handbook of Experimental Pharmacology Ser.: Vol. 24). (Illus.). xix, 764p. 232.00 (*0-387-04520-1*) Spr-Verlag.

Diuretics. O. S. Better et al. Ed. by R. F. Gregor et al. 1995. LC 95-3116. (Handbook of Experimental Pharmacology Ser.: Vol. 117). (*0-387-58965-1*) Spr-Verlag.

Diuretics. Ed. by R. F. Greger et al. 1996. (Handbook of Experimental Pharmacology Ser.: Vol. 117). (Illus.). 496p. 396.00 (*3-540-58965-1*) Spr-Verlag.

Diuretics: Physiology, Pharmacology & Clinical Use. John H. Dirks & Roger A. Sutton. 1986. (Illus.). 396p. text 104.00 (*0-7216-1243-1*) Saunders.

Diurnal Distribution in Cardiovascular Disease: Prognosis & Therapy. Ed. by John E. Deanfield & Philippe Sellier. 1994. (Journal: Vol. 85, Suppl. 2, 1994). (Illus.). iv, 32p. pap. 10.50 (*3-8055-6092-3*) S Karger.

Divalproex & Manic Depression: A Guide. James W. Jefferson & John H. Greist. 31p. 2000. pap. 5.95 (*1-890802-24-7*); 1999. mass mkt. 4.95 (*1-890802-20-4*) Madison Inst of Med.

***Dive: First Responder.** Richard A. Clinchy, III. 2nd ed. 2002. (Illus.). (C). pap. text 36.25 (*0-7637-1792-4*, 1792-4) Jones & Bartlett.

Diver Health Occupation Computer Test Bank. Louise M. Simmers. 3rd ed. 1993. (Health Occupations Ser.). pap. 61.50 (*0-8273-5904-7*) Delmar.

Diverse Families, Competent Families: Innovations in Research & Preventive Intervention Practice. Ed. by Janet F. Gillespie & Judy Primavera. 2000. LC 00-40928. (Illus.). 224p. 49.95 (*0-7890-0797-5*); pap. 24.95 (*0-7890-0830-0*) Haworth Pr.

Diverse Techniques of Analysis by 27 Eminent Clinicians. Ed. by Benjamin B. Wolman. 1995. LC 94-49232. (Master Work Ser.). 610p. pap. 60.00 (*1-56821-493-6*) Aronson.

Diversification & Conversion Strategies for Rural Hospitals. Scott Mason et al. 1989. 52p. (Orig.). pap. 35.00 (*0-87258-524-7*, 184207) Am Hospital.

Diversification in Toxicology - Man & Environment: Proceedings of the 1997 EUROTEX Meeting Held in Arhus, Denmark, June 25-28, 1997. Ed. by J. P. Seiler et al. 1997. LC 97-44576. (Archives of Toxicology Ser.: Supplementa 20). (Illus.). 482p. 139.00 (*3-540-63660-9*) Spr-Verlag.

Diversified Health Occupations. Louise M. Simmers. (Orig.). 2nd ed. 1988. LC 82-73084. (Illus.). 560p. pap., tchr. ed. 15.25 (*0-8273-3045-6*); 2nd ed. 1988. pap., wbk. ed. 20.50 (*0-8273-3046-4*); 2nd ed. 1988. LC 92-14881. (Illus.). 560p. pap. 32.95 (*0-8273-3044-8*); 3rd ed. 1993. LC 92-14881. 623p. pap. 38.95 (*0-8273-4971-8*); 3rd ed. 1993. 76p. tchr. ed. 23.50 (*0-8273-4972-6*); 3rd ed. 1993. LC 92-14881. 559p. pap., stu. ed. 21.50 (*0-8273-4973-4*) Delmar.

Diversified Health Occupations. Simmers. 4th ed. 1997. (Health Occupations Ser.). tchr. ed. 16.95 (*0-8273-7826-2*) Delmar.

Diversified Health Occupations. Louise Simmers. 4th ed. 1997. (Health Occupations Ser.). 140.95 (*0-8273-7824-6*) Delmar.

Diversified Health Occupations. Louise M. Simmers. 4th ed. (Health Occupations Ser.). (Orig.). 1997. 608p. wbk. ed. 23.95 (*0-8273-7827-0*); 1997. 49.95 (*0-8273-7825-4*); 1996. LC 96-13882. 768p. mass mkt. 62.95 (*0-8273-7823-8*) Delmar.

Diversified Health Occupations Essentials. Louise M. Simmers. (Health Occupations Ser.). 1997. 66.95 (*0-8273-7822-X*); 1997. 272p. wbk. ed. 18.95 (*0-8273-7820-3*); 1997. 13.40 (*0-8273-7818-1*); 1997. 134.95 (*0-8273-7819-X*); 1997. 15.00 (*0-8273-7821-1*); 1996. LC 96-14034. 768p. text 43.95 (*0-8273-7817-3*) Delmar.

Diversified Health Occupations Teacher's Resource Kit. Louise M. Simmers. 3rd ed. 1993. pap. 131.95 (*0-8273-4974-2*) Delmar.

Diversity & Complexity in Feminist Therapy: Women in Therapy, Vol. 9, Nos. 1-3. Ed. by Laura S. Brown & Maria P. Root. 1994. LC 90-31160. 355p. text 49.95 (*0-86656-997-9*) Haworth Pr.

Diversity & Direction in Psychoanalytic Technique. Fred Pine. 1997. LC 97-37013. 224p. 30.00 (*0-300-07344-5*) Yale U Pr.

Diversity & Unity in Cross-Cultural Psychology. Ed. by R. Rath et al. 1982. vi, 374p. pap. (*90-265-0431-4*) Swets.

Diversity in Auditory Mechanics. 1997. 432p. lib. bdg. 60.00 (*981-02-2712-4*) World Scientific Pub.

Diversity in College Settings: New Directions for College Mental Health. Yvonne M. Jenkins. 1998. LC 98-5920. 256p. (C). 80.00 (*0-415-91305-5*); pap. 24.95 (*0-415-91306-3*) Routledge.

Diversity in Psychotherapy: The Politics of Race, Ethnicity & Gender. Jean L. Chin et al. 1993. LC 93-18240. 224p. 67.00 (*0-275-94180-9*, C4180, Praeger Pubs) Greenwood.

Diversity Leadership. Janice Dreachslin & Portia L. Hunt. 1996. LC 96-16820. (Management Ser.). 256p. 42.00 (*1-56793-046-8*) Health Admin Pr.

Diversity of Bacterial Respiratory Systems Christopher J. Knowles. 1980. 256p. 113.95 (*0-8493-5400-5*, QR89) CRC Pr.

Diversity of Bacterial Respiratory Systems Christopher J. Knowles. 1980. 272p. 156.00 (*0-8493-5399-8*, QR89, CRC Reprint) Franklin.

Diversity of Mammalian Cerebral Cortex: 11th Annual Karger Workshop, Miami Beach, October 1999. Ed. by T. M. Preuss. 2000. (Brain, Behavior & Evolution Ser.: Vol. 55, No. 6). (Illus.). vi, 70p. pap. 25.25 (*3-8055-7145-3*) S Karger.

Diverticulitis. Arthur White. 1998. (New Self Help Ser.). (Illus.). 112p. pap. (*0-7225-1549-9*) Thorsons GBR. *Dist:* Natl Bk Netwk.

Divided Children. Lynn Jay & Steve Jay. 1982. LC 81-71019. 128p. (Orig.). pap. 5.25 (*0-87516-474-9*) DeVorss.

Divided Legacy. Set. Harris L. Coulter. 1973. 200.00 (*0-916386-00-7*) Ctr Emp Med.

Divided Legacy: A History of the Schism in Medical Thought. The Patterns Emerge: Hippocrates to Paracelsus Harris L. Coulter. 1994. LC 73-75718. 537p. 50.00 (*0-916386-01-5*) Ctr Emp Med.

Divided Legacy: The Conflict Between Homoeopathy & the American Medical Association. Harris L. Coulter. LC 73-75718. (Science & Ethics in American Medicine 1800-1910 Ser.: Vol. III). 552p. (Orig.). reprint ed. 1982. 50.00 (*0-938190-57-1*); 2nd ed. 1973. pap. 20.00 (*0-913028-96-7*) North Atlantic.

Divided Legacy Vol. II: A History of the Schism in Medical Thought. The Origins of Modern Western Medicine: J.B. Van Helmont to Claude Bernard Harris L. Coulter. 1973. LC 73-75718. 50.00 (*0-916386-02-3*) Ctr Emp Med.

Divided Legacy Vol. 2: The Origins of Modern Medicine: J. B. Van Helmont to Claude Bernard. Harris L. Coulter. 1988. 785p. 50.00 (*1-55643-035-3*) North Atlantic.

Divided Legacy: A History of the Schism in Medical Thought Vol. 4: The Bacteriological Age, Twentieth Century Medicine. Harris L. Coulter. 1994. LC 73-75718. 776p. 50.00 (*1-55643-170-8*) North Atlantic.

Divided Self: An Existential Study in Sanity & Madness. R. D. Laing. 1999. LC 99-220349. 78.95 (*0-415-19818-6*) Routledge.

Divided Staffs, Divided Selves: A Case Approach to Mental Health Ethics. Ed. by Stanley J. Reiser et al. 1987. LC 86-28416. (Illus.). 164p. pap. text 19.95 (*0-521-31890-4*) Cambridge U Pr.

Dividing of Soul & Spirit. Bill Freeman. 1984. (Illus.). 32p. pap. 1.00 (*0-914271-03-2*) Mnstry Pubns.

Divination, Magic & Healing: The Book of Jewish Folklore. Ronald H. Isaacs. 1998. LC 97-48. 208p. 25.00 (*0-7657-9951-0*) Aronson.

Divine Farmer's Materia Medica: A Translation of the Shen Nong Ben Cao Jing. Ed. by Bob Flaws. Tr. by Yang Shou-Zhong from CHI. 1998. LC 97-77991. Orig. Title: Shen Nong Ben Cao Jing. 205p. pap. text 21.95 (*0-936185-96-1*) Blue Poppy Pr.

Divine Origin of the Craft of the Herbalist. E.A. Wallis Budge. 2001. (Library of Arcana). text (*0-7103-0730-6*) Kegan Paul Intl GBR. *Dist:* Col U Pr.

Divine Origin of the Craft of the Herbalist. E.A. Wallis Budge. unabr. ed. 1996. LC 95-49175. (Illus.). 112p. reprint ed. pap. text 4.95 (*0-486-29169-3*) Dover.

Divine Prescription/Science of Health & Healing. Gunther Paulien. 1995. LC 94-61325. 560p. otabind 19.95 (*1-57258-017-8*) TEACH Servs.

Divinely Responding Classic: A Translation of the Shen Ying Jing from the Zhen Jin Da Cheng. Yang Ji-zhou. Ed. by Bob Flaws. Tr. by Yang Ji-zhou et al. 1994. LC 93-74979. (Great Masters Ser.). 165p. (Orig.). pap. 18.95 (*0-936185-55-4*) Blue Poppy Pr.

Diving & Subaquatic Medicine. Carl Edmonds et al. 3rd ed. 1994. (Illus.). 580p. pap. (*0-7506-2131-1*) E A GBR. *Dist:* OUP.

***Diving & Subaquatic Medicine.** Carl Edmonds et al. 4th ed. 2001. (Arnold Publication). (Illus.). 672p. text 98.50 (*0-340-80630-3*) OUP.

Diving Medicine. Alfred A. Bove. 3rd ed. 1997. LC 96-16714. text 69.00 (*0-7216-6056-8*) Saunders.

Diving Medicine for Scuba Divers. Carl Edmonds et al. rev. ed. 1997. (Illus.). 316p. pap. 32.00 (*0-9590306-6-2*) Aqua Quest.

Divorce & New Beginnings: A Complete Guide to Recovery, Solo Parenting, Co-Parenting & Stepfamilies. Genevieve Clapp. 2nd ed. 2000. LC 00-25516. (Illus.). 400p. pap. 19.95 (*0-471-32648-8*) Wiley.

Divorce Group Counseling Program. M. S. Prokop. rev. ed. 1996. wbk. ed. 209.95 incl. audio (*0-933879-34-2*) Alegra Hse Pubs.

Divorce Mediation: A Practical Guide for Therapists & Counselors. John M. Haynes. 1981. LC 80-25065. 208p. 29.95 (*0-8261-2590-5*) Springer Pub.

Divorce Shock: Perspectives on Counseling & Therapy. Ed. by Adrian R. Tiemann et al. 1992. LC 92-5969. 224p. (Orig.). (C). pap. text 21.95 (*0-914783-61-0*) Charles.

Divulging of Useful Truths in Physick: The Medical Agenda of Robert Boyle. Barbara B. Kaplan. 1993. LC 92-48468. 232p. (C). 42.00 (*0-8018-4601-3*) Johns Hopkins.

XIXes Journees Nationales de Neonatologie, 1999. 1999. (Progres en Neonatologie Ser.: Vol. 19). (Illus.). xiii, 342p. 197.50 (*3-8055-6913-0*) S Karger.

Dizionario Medico: Inglese-Italiano/Italiano-Inglese. Mario Lucchesi. 1987. (ENG & ITA.). 1460p. 160.00 (*0-913298-52-2*) S F Vanni.

Dizionario Medico Poliglotta. E. Veillon & Albert Nobel. deluxe ed. (ENG, FRE, GER, ITA & SPA.). 295.00 (*0-7859-0803-X*, M-9636) Fr & Eur.

Dizionario Medico Ragionato Inglese-Italiano: Regionato English-Italian Medical Dictionary. M. Lucchesi. 1978. (ENG & ITA.). 1489p. 150.00 (*0-8288-5206-5*, M9353) Fr & Eur.

Dizziness. B. Todd Troost. 2001. (Most Common Complaints Ser.). (Illus.). 200p. pap. 25.00 (*0-7506-7133-5*) Buttrwrth-Heinemann.

Dizziness & Balance Disorders: An Interdisciplinary Approach to Diagnosis, Therapy Treatment & Rehabilitation. Ed. by I. Kaufman Arenberg. 1993. LC 93-38841. (Illus.). lib. bdg. (*90-6299-100-9*) Kugler NLD. *Dist:* Lib Res.

Dizziness, Hearing Loss, & Tinnitus. Robert W. Baloh. 1997. LC 97-42657. (Illus.). 240p. (C). 49.50 (*0-8036-0330-4*) OUP.

DK Healthcare: HRT. Miriam Stoppard. 1999. LC 98-28521. (Healthcare Ser.). (Illus.). 96p. pap. 7.95 (*0-7894-3756-2*) DK Pub Inc.

DMT - The Spirit Molecule: A Doctor's Revolutionary Research into the Biology of Near-Death & Mystical Experiences. Rick Strassman. 2000. LC 00-50498. (Illus.). xviii, 358p. pap. 16.95 (*0-89281-927-8*, Heal Arts VT) Inner Tradit.

DNA Adducts: Identification & Biological Significance. Ed. by K. Hemminki et al. 1994. LC 95-113575. (IARC Scientific Publications Ser.: No. 125). (Illus.). 488p. pap. text 95.00 (*92-832-2125-7*) OUP.

DNA Alterations in Cancer: Genetic & Epigenetic Changes. Ed. by Melanie Ehrlich. 2000. LC 99-56013. (Illus.). 525p. 116.00 (*1-881299-19-8*) Eaton Pub Co.

DNA & Chromosomes. 1994. (Symposia on Quantitative Biology Ser.: Vol. LVIII). (Illus.). 950p. (C). pap. text 50.00 (*0-87969-066-6*) Cold Spring Harbor.

DNA & the I Ching: The Tao of Life. Johnson F. Yan. 1991. LC 91-193504. 160p. (Orig.). pap. 14.95 (*1-55643-097-3*) North Atlantic.

DNA Arrays: Methods & Protocols. Ed. by Jang B. Rampal. 2001. LC 00-40791. (Methods in Molecular Biology Ser.: Vol. 170). (Illus.). xi, 264p. 89.50 (*0-89603-822-X*) Humana.

DNA Damage & Repair Vol. II: DNA Repair in Higher Eukaryotes. Jac A. Nickoloff & Merl F. Hoekstra. 1998. LC 97-28562. (Contemporary Cancer Research Ser.). (Illus.). 656p. 145.00 (*0-89603-500-X*) Humana.

DNA Damage & Repair Vol. III: Advances from Phage to Humans. Ed. by Merl F. Hoekstra & Jac A. Nickoloff. 2001. (Contemporary Cancer Research Ser.: Vol. 3). (Illus.). 432p. 135.00 (*0-89603-803-3*) Humana.

DNA Double Helix & the Chemistry of Cancer. Ramaswamy H. Sarma & M. H. Sarma. 1988. (Illus.). 272p. reprint ed. lib. bdg. 40.00 (*0-940030-26-8*) Adenine Pr.

DNA Fingerprinting Methods in Infectious Diseases. Ed. by David R. Soll. 2001. (Infectious Disease Ser.). 350p. 99.50 (*0-89603-752-5*) Humana.

DNA Healing Techniques. Robert V. Gerard et al. Ed. by Tony Stubbs. 3rd ed. 1998. LC 99-195856. (Illus.). 112p. pap. 9.95 (*1-880666-77-4*) Oughten Hse.

DNA Methylation & Cancer. Ed. by P. A. Jones & P. K. Vogt. 2000. (Current Topics in Microbiology & Immunology Ser.: Vol. 249). (Illus.). 224p. 129.00 (*3-540-66608-7*) Spr-Verlag.

DNA Methylation & Cellular Differentiation. J. H. Taylor. 1984. (Cell Biology Monographs: Vol. 11). (Illus.). 150p. 79.95 (*0-387-81761-1*) Spr-Verlag.

DNA Ploidy & Cell Cycle Analysis in Pathology, Vol. 1. Jeffrey S. Ross. 1996. LC 95-38361. (Illus.). 176p. pap. 55.00 (*0-89640-301-7*) Igaku-Shoin.

DNA Polymorphisms As Disease Markers. Ed. by David J. Galton & G. Assmann. 1991. (NATO Advanced Science Institutes Ser.: Vol. 214). (Illus.). 168p. (C). text 102.00 (*0-306-44039-3*, Kluwer Plenum) Kluwer Academic.

DNA Probes for Infectious Diseases. Ed. by Fred C. Tenover. 1988. 320p. 229.00 (*0-8493-6176-1*, QR69) CRC Pr.

DNA-Protein Interactions: Principles & Protocols. Ed. by Tom Moss. 2nd ed. 2001. LC 00-54100. (Methods in Molecular Biology Ser.: Vol. 148). (Illus.). xvii, 638p. 89.50 (*0-89603-671-5*) Humana.

DNA Provirus: Howard Temin's Scientific Legacy. Geoffrey M. Cooper et al. 1995. LC 95-12355. 99.95 (*1-55581-098-5*) ASM Pr.

DNA Repair Mechanism. 1996. (Illus.). 384p. 112.00 (*3-540-59208-3*) Spr-Verlag.

DNA Replication & the Cell Cycle: Colloquium der Gesellschaft fur Biologische Chemie 9-11 April 1992 in Mosbach - Baden. Ed. by E. Fanning et al. 1993. LC 92-26845. (Illus.). 256p. 175.00 (*0-387-54729-0*) Spr-Verlag.

DNA Sequencing Protocols. Ed. by Colin A. Graham & Alison J. M. Hill. 2nd ed. 2001. LC 00-33483. (Methods in Molecular Biology Ser.: Vol. 167). (Illus.). x, 244p. 99.50 (*0-89603-716-9*) Humana.

DNA Simplified II: The Illustrated Hitchhiker's Guide to DNA. Daniel H. Farkas. 1999. (Illus.). 128p. pap. 20.00 (*1-890883-13-1*, 202865) Am Assn Clinical Chem.

DNA Technology & Forensic Science. Ed. by John Ballantyne et al. 1989. (Banbury Reports: No. 32). (Illus.). 430p. lib. bdg. 95.00 (*0-87969-232-4*) Cold Spring Harbor.

DNA Tumor Viruses: Control of Gene Expression & Replication. Ed. by Michael Botchan et al. 1986. LC 86-50649. (Cancer Cells Ser.). 620p. (Orig.). pap. 75.00 (*0-87969-192-1*) Cold Spring Harbor.

DNA Tumor Viruses: Oncogenic Mechanisms. Ed. by Giuseppe Barbanti-Brodano et al. 1996. (Infectious Agents & Pathogenesis Ser.). (Illus.). 452p. (C). text 115.00 (*0-306-45151-4*, Kluwer Plenum) Kluwer Academic.

DNA Vaccines: Methods & Protocols. Ed. by Douglas B. Lowrie & Robert Whalen. 2000. LC 98-55325. (Methods in Molecular Medicine Ser.: Vol. 29). (Illus.). 550p. 119.50 (*0-89603-580-8*) Humana.

***Do Financial Incentives Make a Difference? A Comparative Study of the Effect of Performance-Based Reimbursement in Swedish Health Care.** Ewa Forsberg. 2001. (Comprehensive Summaries of Uppsala Dissertations from the Faculty of Medicine Ser.: No. 1077). 54p. pap. (*91-554-5123-3*) Acta Univ SWE. *Dist:* Coronet Bks.

Do HMO's Cut Costs' & Lives? Emerita T. Gueson. 1997. LC 96-90337. 300p. 32.99 (*0-9653861-0-4*) Theresevision.

Do It Yourself Babymaking. Courtney Hafela. 1997. 200p. 14.95 (*0-9660181-3-3*) Two Blond Gdes.

Do-It-Yourself Health: 1,001 Tips You Can Use to Feel Better & Stay Well. Time-Life Books Editors. 1999. LC 97-10716. (Illus.). 400p. pap. 14.95 (*0-7835-4939-3*) Time-Life.

Do It Yourself Psychotherapy Book. Martin Shepard. 17.95 (*0-88411-978-5*); pap. 12.95 (*0-88411-979-3*) Amereon Ltd.

Do It Yourself Psychotherapy Book. Martin Shepard. 1986. 194p. pap. 6.95 (*0-932966-23-3*) Permanent Pr.

Do No Harm: The Libby Zion Case; How Doctors Killed Her & Then Blamed the Victim. Warren Hinckle & John J. Simon. 1995. (Illus.). 224p. 22.95 (*1-882206-12-6*) Argonaut Pr.

Do No Harm: The Scientific, Ethical, Legal & Spiritual Revelation of Somatidian Orthobiology & 714X. Gaston Naessens et al. 1995. LC 95-24978. (*0-09-647030-5*) Writers & Res.

Do Tell Someone! Inner Turmoils Surrounding Sexual Abuse Victims. Yvonnia M. Houston. Ed. by Kathy Robinson. 1991. LC 90-84068. 165p. 16.95 (*0-9628235-0-3*); lib. bdg. 16.95 (*0-9628235-1-1*) Shane CA.

Do They Grow Out of It? Long-Term Outcomes of Childhood Disorders. Ed. by Lily T. Hechtman. 1996. LC 95-46924. 303p. text 42.00 (*0-88048-703-8*, 8703) Am Psychiatric.

Do We Care? Renewing Canada's Commitment to Health. Directions for Canadian Health Care Conference Staff et al. 1999. LC 2001-431168. (Illus.). 166p. (*0-7735-1878-9*) McG-Queens Univ Pr.

Do We Still Need Doctors? John D. Lantos. 1997. 24.95 (*0-415-91853-7*); LC 97-11424. 214p. 29.95 (*0-415-91852-9*) Routledge.

Do We Still Need Doctors? Physician's Personal Account of Practicing Medicine Today. John D. Lantos. 1999. LC 99-25174. (Reflective Bioethics Ser.). 214p. pap. 17.95 (*0-415-92495-2*) Routledge.

Do You Have Any Questions? Vol. 1: A Woman Doctor Answers the 100 Most Asked Questions in Pregnancy. Mary J. Bovo. Ed. by Christine O'Brien. unabr. ed. 1997. (Illus.). 108p. (Orig.). pap. 6.95 (*1-889972-73-8*) Newpt Media.

Do You Really Need Eyeglasses? Marilyn B. Rosanes-Berrett. enl. ed. 1990. (Illus.). 140p. 20.95 (*0-88268-107-9*); pap. 10.95 (*0-88268-104-4*) Station Hill Pr.

Do Your Level Best: Start Controlling Your Blood Sugar Today. Ed. by Barry Leonard. 2000. (Illus.). 60p. pap. text 20.00 (*0-7567-0126-0*) DIANE Pub.

Dobzhansky's Genetics of Natural Populations: I-XLIII. Theodosius Dobzhansky. Ed. by Richard C. Lewontin et al. 1981. LC 81-2073. 1024p. text 112.00 (*0-231-05132-8*) Col U Pr.

Doc. Howard W. Roberts. 1987. LC 86-90702. (Illus.). 176p. 11.95 (*0-9617971-0-X*) Circuit Writer.

Doc: Then & Now With a Montana Physician. R. E. Losee. 1996. mass mkt. 5.99 (*0-8041-1415-3*) Ivy Books.

Doc: Then & Now with a Montana Physician. R. E. Losee. 1994. LC 94-28555. (Illus.). 232p. 22.95 (*1-55821-323-6*, Lyons) Globe Pequot.

Doc Graham: Sandhills Doctor. Duane Hutchinson. 2nd ed. 1995. LC 95-32718. (Illus.). 160p. (gr. 6-12). pap. 8.95 (*0-934988-26-9*) Foun Bks.

Doc Susie: The True Story of a Country Physician in the Colorado Rockies. Virginia Cornell. 1991. (Illus.). 240p. 23.95 (*0-9627896-4-X*); pap. 14.95 (*0-9627896-5-8*) Manifest Pubns.

Doctor-Activist: Physicians Fighting for Social Change. Ed. by Ellen L. Bassuk. 1996. (Illus.). 276p. (C). 27.95 (*0-306-45176-X*, Kluwer Plenum) Kluwer Academic.

Dr. Amarnick's Mind over Matter Pain Relief Program. Claude Amarnick. 1995. LC 95-81679. 204p. 24.95 (*1-880539-37-3*); pap. 9.95 (*1-880539-36-5*) Garrett FL.

Dr. Ambedkar Life & Mission. Dhananjay V. Keer. 1990. reprint ed. (*0-86132-145-6*) Popular Prakashan IND. *Dist:* S Asia.

Doctor & Christian Marriage. H. P. Dunn. 1992. LC 92-15244. pap. 9.95 (*0-8189-0642-1*) Alba.

Doctor & Patient. Silas W. Mitchell. 1972. LC 71-180584. (Medicine & Society in America Ser.). 182p. reprint ed. 19.95 (*0-405-03961-1*) Ayer.

Doctor & the Law: A Practical Guide for the Canadian Physician. Emson. 2nd ed. 1989. 256p. 68.00 (*0-409-88875-3*, UK, MICHIE) LEXIS Pub.

Doctor & the Soul: From Psychotherapy to Logotherapy. Viktor E. Frankl. 3rd ed. 1986. LC 85-40681. 336p. pap. 13.00 (*0-394-74317-2*) Vin Bks.

Doctor & the Word. Reginald Cherry. 1998. pap. 12.99 (*0-88419-513-9*) Creation House.

Dr. Anderson's High-Fiber Fitness Plan. James W. Anderson & Nancy J. Gustafson. 1994. LC 93-45451. 264p. 19.95 (*0-8131-1867-0*) U Pr of KY.

Dr. Anne's Cancer Journal. Robert L. Owen. 1990. LC 90-81824. 414p. pap. 14.00 (*1-882657-06-3*) Health Digest.

Doctor Assisted Suicide: And the Euthanasia Movement. Ed. by Gary E. McCuen. 2nd rev. ed. 1999. (Ideas in Conflict Ser.). (Illus.). 178p. (YA). (gr. 8-12). text 15.95 (*0-86596-178-6*) G E M.

Doctor at Calvary: The Passion of Our Lord Jesus Christ As Described by a Surgeon. Pierre Barbet. Tr. by Earl of Wicklow from FRE. 1993. (Illus.). 192p. reprint ed. text 15.75 (*0-912141-04-2*) Roman Cath Bks.

Doctor at Nagasaki: My First Assignment Was Mercy Killing. Masao Sciotsuki. Tr. by Simul International Inc. Staff from JPN. 1987. 191p. pap. (*4-333-01250-3*) Kosei Pub Co JPN. *Dist:* Tuttle Pubng.

Doctor at War: The Story of Colonel Martin Herford - The Most Decorated Doctor of World War Two. Matthew Hall. 1995. 256p. 24.95 (*1-897817-54-1*) Seven Hills Bk.

Dr. Atkins' Diet Revolution: The High Calorie Way to Stay Thin Forever. Robert C. Atkins. 1981. 336p. mass mkt. 7.50 (*0-553-27157-1*) Bantam.

Dr. Atkins' Health Revolution: How Complementary Medicine Can Extend Your Life. Robert C. Atkins. 1990. LC 88-12827. 448p. mass mkt. 6.99 (*0-553-28360-X*) Bantam.

***Dr. Atkins' New Diet Revolution.** Robert C. Atkins. rev. ed. 2002. 464p. mass mkt. 7.99 (*0-06-001203-X*) Morrow Avon.

Dr. Atkins' Vita-Nutrient Solution: Nature's Answer to Drugs. Robert C. Atkins. 1998. LC 97-42790. 448p. 24.00 (*0-684-81849-3*) S&S Trade.

Doctor Bernard de Gordon: Professor & Practitioner. Luke E. Demaitre. 1980. (Studies & Texts Ser.: Vol. 51). xii, 236p. (C). pap. text (*0-88844-051-0*) Pontif Inst.

Dr. Bernstein's Diabetes Solution: A Complete Guide to Achieving Normal Blood Sugars. Richard K. Bernstein & Timothy J. Aubert. 1997. LC 96-37900. (Illus.). 416p. 25.95 (*0-316-09344-0*) Little.

Dr. Bob & the Good Oldtimers. 1989. (SPA.). 5.20 (*0-916856-22-4*) AAWS.

Dr. Bob & the Good Oldtimers: A Biography, with Recollections of Early A.A. in the Midwest. 1980. LC 80-65962. (Illus.). 373p. 3.45 (*0-916856-07-0*) AAWS.

Doctor Book Home Remedy Children. Prevention Magazine Editors. 1994. mass mkt. 8.99 (*0-553-85057-1*) Bantam.

Dr. Braly's Food Allergy & Nutrition Revolution. James Braly. 1992. LC 92-27994. 544p. pap. 17.95 (*0-87983-590-7*, 35907K, Keats Pubng) McGraw-Hill Trade.

Dr. Breath: The Story of Breathing Coordination. Carl Stough & Reece Stough. 1981. LC 81-82800. 255p. reprint ed. 22.00 (*0-940830-00-0*) Stough Inst.

Dr. Bruce Miller's "The Nutrition Guarantee" Bruce Miller. 1998. LC 97-45347. (Illus.). 480p. pap. 17.99 (*1-56530-283-4*) Summit TX.

Doctor Business: How to Boost Practice Growth & Strengthen Long-Term Relationships. Hal Alpiar. Ed. by Gregg Rogers. 1994. LC 94-3563. (Illus.). 232p. 39.95 (*1-57066-003-4*, ME056) Practice Mgmt Info.

Dr. Carl Robinson's Basic Baby Care: A Guide for New Parents for the First Year. Carl D. Robinson. 1998. LC 97-75474. (Illus.). 160p. pap. 10.95 (*1-57224-105-5*) New Harbinger.

Dr. Chan's Cancer Healing Vol. 10: Cancer Prevention & Self-Healing. Y. C. Chan. Ed. & Photos by R. S. Yu. 1997. LC 97-75491. (Illus.). 39.00 (*0-9658744-2-7*) ACOM.

Dr. Chi's Method of Fingernail & Tongue Diagnosis Vol. I. Tsu-Tsair Chi. Ed. by Chi's Enterprise Staff. unabr. ed. 1997. (Illus.). 201p. pap. 39.95 (*0-9657847-9-7*) Chis Enterprise.

Dr. Christopher Talks on Rejuvenation Through Elimination. John R. Christopher. 1994. pap. 2.00 (*1-879436-06-X*, 99106) Christopher Pubns.

Dr. Christopher's Three-Day Cleansing Program. John R. Christopher. 1994. 32p. pap. 2.00 (*1-879436-04-3*, 99104) Christopher Pubns.

Dr. Dave. Clark S. Sturges. 1993. 87p. pap. 15.00 (*0-915685-08-6*) Devil Mountain Bks.

Dr. Deal's Delicious Detox Diet & Wellness Lifestyle. Grady A. Deal. 1991. 240p. pap. 15.00 (*0-9631405-3-1*) Liv Wellness.

Dr. Dean Ornish's Program for Reversing Heart Disease Without Drugs or Surgery. Dean Ornish. 1992. LC 91-91878. (Illus.). 672p. pap. 15.00 (*0-345-37353-7*) Ballantine Pub Grp.

Dr. Dean Ornish's Program for Reversing Heart Disease: The Only System Scientifically Proven to Reverse Heart Disease Without Drugs or Surgery. Dean Ornish. 2002. 736p. mass mkt. 7.99 (*0-8041-1947-3*); 704p. pap. 18.00 (*0-345-43808-6*) Ballantine Pub Grp (Ballantine).

Dr. Dean Ornish's Program for Reversing Heart Disease: The Only System Scientifically Proven to Reverse Heart Disease Without Drugs or Surgery. Dean Ornish. 1996. LC 95-94897. 638p. mass mkt. 6.99 (*0-8041-1038-7*) Ivy Books.

Dr. Deely, You Do Great Things: The Medicine of Laughter. Nicholas Deely. 1995. 100p. pap. text 12.95 (*0-9648669-0-0*) Denali Desgns.

Doctor Dilemma: Public Policy & the Changing Role of Physicians under Ontario Medicare. Samuel E. Shortt. 1998. 152p. (*0-7735-1793-6*); 148p. pap. (*0-7735-1794-4*) McG-Queens Univ Pr.

Doctor Discusses Care of the Back. Paul Neimark & Gerald Berkowitz. 1990. pap. 6.00 (*0-910304-04-1*) Budlong.

Doctor Discusses Learning to Live with Heart Trouble. Arthur J. Snider & I. J. Adatto. 1991. (Illus.). pap. 6.00 (*0-910304-15-7*) Budlong.

Doctor Discusses Menopause & Estrogens. M. Edward Davis & Dona Z. Meilach. 1994. (Illus.). pap. 6.00 (*0-910304-26-2*) Budlong.

Doctor Dock: Teaching & Learning Medicine at the Turn of the Century. Horace W. Davenport. 1987. (Illus.). 250p. text 45.00 (*0-8135-1190-9*) Rutgers U Pr.

Dr. D's Handbook for Men over 40: A Guide to Health, Fitness, Living & Loving in the Prime of Life. Peter Dorsen. 1998. LC 98-230244. 260p. 23.95 (*1-56561-130-6*) Wiley.

Dr. Earl Mindell's What You Should Know about Natural Health for Women. Earl L. Mindell. 1996. LC 96-19146. (Dr. Earl Mindell Ser.). 96p. (Orig.). mass mkt. 4.95 (*0-87983-754-3*, Keats Pubng) McGraw-Hill Trade.

Dr. Edward Taub's Seven Steps to Self-Healing Pack. Edward Taub. 1998. LC 96-7819. (Illus.). 168p. 24.95 (*0-7894-1082-6*) DK Pub Inc.

Dr. Folkman's War: Angiogenesis & the Struggle to Defeat Cancer. Robert Cooke. 2001. LC 00-34165. (Illus.). 384p. 25.95 (*0-375-50244-0*) Random.

Doctor for the People: Two Thousand Years of General Practice in Britain. John Cule. 1980. (Illus.). text 88.00 (*0-906141-29-X*) Kluwer Academic.

Doctor from Bugtussle. Wendell W. Wilson. 1995. (Orig.). pap. 14.95 (*0-9647202-1-3*);Vol. 1. 329p. 25.00 (*0-9647202-2-1*) Hillbilly Bks.

Dr. Generic Will See You Now: 33 Ways You Can Survive Managed Care. Oscar London. 1996. LC 95-26085. 160p. (Orig.). pap. 11.95 (*0-89815-816-8*) Ten Speed Pr.

Dr. George: An Account of the Life of a Country Doctor. George T. Mitchell. 1993. LC 93-16589. (Illus.). 400p. pap. 21.95 (*0-8093-1916-0*) S Ill U Pr.

Dr. Gollup's Survival Guide for New Parents. Howard J. Gollup. 3rd ed. 1995. LC 94-72909. (Illus.). 160p. (Orig.). pap. 11.95 (*0-9643482-0-9*) Iguana Med Bks.

Dr. Heinerman's Encyclopedia of Nature's Vitamins & Minerals. John Heinerman. 1997. LC 97-25868. 416p. (C). text 27.95 (*0-13-258500-6*) P-H.

***Doctor, His Patient & the Illness.** Michael Balint. 2001. (Books-on-Demand Ser.). 315p. reprint ed. pap. text 37.95 (*0-8236-8028-2*, 21380) Intl Univs Pr.

Doctor, His Patient & the Illness. Michael Balint. 2nd ed. 1963. 395p. 62.50 (*0-8236-1380-1*) Intl Univs Pr.

Dr. Humor's Health Book: Old Cures - New Jokes. J. Edward Thornberg. 1986. (Illus.). 56p. (Orig.). pap. 3.00 (*0-929082-07-9*) Natl Hall Humor.

***Dr. Ian Smith's Guide to Medical Websites.** Ian K. Smith. 2001. LC 2001-46000. 272p. pap. 15.00 (*0-8129-9181-8*) Random Trade.

Doctor in Colonial America. annuals Zachary B. Friendenberg. 1998. 256p. pap. 17.95 (*1-887750-93-2*) Rutledge Bks.

Doctor in Gray - Hunter Holmes McGuire. John W. Schildt. 1987. (Illus.). 137p. text 13.50 (*0-936772-05-0*) Antietam.

Doctor in History. Howard W. Haggard. 1977. LC 79-99342. (Essay Index Reprint Ser.). 32.95 (*0-8369-1654-9*) Ayer.

Doctor in Medicine & Other Papers on Professional Subjects. Stephen Smith. 1972. LC 74-180590. (Medicine & Society in America Ser.). 318p. reprint ed. 25.95 (*0-405-03972-7*) Ayer.

Doctor-in-My-Pocket. Russell Dollinger. 1995. (SPA.). 264p. spiral bd. 11.95 (*0-945585-05-5*) Booksmythe.

Doctor in the House: Your Best Guide to Effective Medical Self-Care. John C. Harbert. 1994. LC 93-33242. (Illus.). 520p. 39.50 (*0-89603-219-1*) Humana.

Doctor in the XIVth Army. Charles Evans. 1998. (Illus.). 224p. (*0-85052-597-7*) Leo Cooper GBR. *Dist:* Trans-Atl Phila, Combined Pub.

Dr. Jensen's Guide to Diet & Detoxification. Bernard Jensen. 2nd ed. 2000. LC 00-43450. (Dr. Bernard Jensen Library). (Illus.). ix, 114p. pap. 12.95 (*0-658-00275-9*) NTC Contemp Pub Co.

Dr. Jensen's Nature Has a Remedy. Bernard Jensen. 2nd ed. 2000. LC 00-69022. (Dr. Bernard Jensen Library). 256p. pap. 16.95 (*0-658-00272-4*) NTC Contemp Pub Co.

Doctor Jessie, the Odyssey of a Woman Physician. Jessie L. Brodie. 1991. (Illus.). 395p. (Orig.). (C). 22.50 (*0-945490-03-8*); pap. 12.50 (*0-945490-04-6*) Carolina Pacific.

Doctor Jim's Odyssey. James W. Pleasant. 1994. LC 94-60592. 138p. pap. 8.00 (*0-912400-14-5*) Western Res Pr.

Doctor Johann Weyer: Ein Rheinischer Arzt der Erste Bekampfer Des Hexenwahns Beitrag Zur Geschicte der Aufklarung und der Heilkunde. Carl Binz. 2nd rev. ed. 1976. LC 75-16683. (Classics in Psychiatry Ser.). (GER.). reprint ed. 19.95 (*0-405-07415-8*) Ayer.

Dr. John Willard's Catalyst Altered Water. Beth M. Ley. 1992. 64p. (Orig.). pap. 3.95 (*91-49-59100-2*) B L Pubns.

Dr. Johnston's Essays on the Physiological & Psychological Characteristics of the Homeopathic Materia Media - Nux Vomica. Linda Johnston. 1998. 200p. pap. 20.00 (*1-877691-26-7*) C Kent Agency.

Doctor Judas: A Portrayal of the Opium Habit. William R. Cobbe. Ed. by Gerald N. Grob. 1981. LC 80-1218. (Addiction in America Ser.). reprint ed. lib. bdg. 33.95 (*0-405-13574-2*) Ayer.

Dr. K. M. Nadkarni's Indian Materia Medica. Ed. by K. M. Nadkarni. 1988. (C). (*0-8364-2337-2*) Popular Prakashan IND. *Dist:* S Asia.

Dr. Kellon's Guide to First Aid for Horses. Eleanor M. Kellon. 1989. (Illus.). 254p. spiral bd. 29.95 (*0-914327-29-1*) Breakthrgh NY.

Dr. Kidd's Guide to Herbal Cat Care. Randy Kidd. 2000. LC 00-61873. (Doctor Kidds Guides Ser.). (Illus.). iv, 203p. pap. 14.95 (*1-58017-188-5*, 67188) Storey Bks.

Dr. Kinsey & the Institute for Sex Research. Wardell B. Pomeroy. 1982. LC 82-4924. 496p. 18.00 (*0-300-02916-0*) Yale U Pr.

Doctor Looks at Life: From a Christian Perspective - An Examination of the Forces That Threaten Human Dignity. Frank Pedreira. 1999. LC 98-87119. 192p. pap. 14.95 (*1-56315-164-2*) SterlingHse.

Dr. Miles: The Life of Dr. Franklin L. Miles (1845-1929) Martha M. Pickrell. 1998. LC 97-77133. 120p. pap. 12.00 (*1-57860-023-5*) Guild Pr Emmis Pubng.

Doctor Minor-a Sketch of the Life of Dr. Thomas T. Minor, 1844-1889. T. M. Pelly. (Shorey Historical Ser.). 142p. reprint ed. pap. 10.00 (*0-8466-0204-0*, S204) Shoreys Bkstore.

Dr. Mom. Marianne E. Neifert et al. 1987. 544p. pap. 7.99 (*0-451-16311-7*, Sig) NAL.

Dr. Mom: Success Stories of an Herbalist Student. Sandra K. Ellis & David Christopher. 2nd rev. ed. 1996. 89p. pap. 7.95 (*1-879436-14-0*, 99509) Christopher Pubns.

Dr. Montessori's Own Handbook. Maria Montessori. 1988. LC 65-14827. (Illus.). 192p. (C). pap. 12.00 (*0-8052-0921-2*) Schocken.

***Dr. Murray's Total Body Tune-Up.** Michaltel T. Murray. 2001. 432p. reprint ed. pap. 15.95 (*0-553-37952-6*, Spectra) Bantam.

Doctor, My Bill Is Too High. Charles L. Pelton. 1978. (Illus.). 18.00 (*0-931470-01-3*); pap. 14.95 (*0-931470-00-5*) Fam Health Media.

Doctor of Their Own: The History of Adolescent Medicine. Heather M. Prescott. 1998. LC 97-52222. 272p. 36.50 (*0-674-21461-7*) HUP.

***Doctor Olds of Twillingate: Portrait of an American Surgeon in Newfoundland.** Gary Saunders. 1995. 368p. pap. (*1-55081-092-8*) Breakwater Bks.

Doctor-Patient Handbook. Bernard Jensen. 1978. pap. 12.99 (*0-932615-10-4*) B Jensen.

Doctor-Patient Interaction. Ed. by Walburga von Raffler-Engel. 1989. LC 89-17883. (Pragmatics & Beyond New Ser.: Vol. No. 4). xxxvii, 294p. 98.00 (*1-55619-079-4*); pap. 31.95 (*1-55619-080-8*) J Benjamins Pubng Co.

Doctor-Patient Relationship in Pharmacotherapy: Improving Treatment Effectiveness. Allan Tasman et al. 2000. LC 00-37114. 182p. 30.00 (*1-57230-596-7*, 8R0596) Guilford Pubns.

***Dr. Patrick Walsh's Guide to Surviving Prostate Cancer.** Patrick C. Walsh & Janet Farrar Worthington. 2002. 480p. pap. (*0-446-67914-3*) Warner.

Dr. Patrick Walsh's Guide to Surviving Prostate Cancer: Give Yourself a Second Opinion. Patrick C. Walsh & Janet Farrar Worthington. 2001. LC 2001-26260. (Illus.). 480p. 25.95 (*0-446-52640-1*) Warner Bks.

Dr. Pitcairn's Complete Guide to Natural Health for Dogs & Cats. Richard H. Pitcairn & Susan H. Pitcairn. rev. ed. 1995. LC 94-44229. (Illus.). 383p. pap. 17.95 (*0-87596-243-2*) Rodale Pr Inc.

Doctor, Please Close the Door: A Book on Living Wills, Powers of Attorney, Terminal Care & the Right to Die with Dignity! Kenneth A. Bartholomew. 1994. LC 93-39045. 96p. pap. 9.95 (*0-942963-45-8*) Distinctive Pub.

Doctor Rabelais. Dominic B. Lewis. 1969. LC 69-10117. 274p. reprint ed. lib. bdg. 72.50 (*0-8371-0145-X*, LEDR, Greenwood Pr) Greenwood.

Dr. Rechtschaffen's Diet for Lifetime Weight Control & Better Health. Joseph S. Rechtschaffen & Robert Carola. rev. ed. 1995. LC 94-42187. 224p. pap. 10.00 (*1-56836-077-0*) Kodansha.

Dr. Richard Marrs' Fertility Book: America's Leading Fertility Expert Tells You Everything You Need to Know about Getting Pregnant. Richard P. Marrs et al. 1998. (Illus.). 528p. pap. 15.95 (*0-440-50803-7*, Delta Trade) Dell.

Dr. Rinse Formula: How to Prevent Hardening of the Arteries. Morton Walker. 1984. (Dr. Morton Walker Good Health Guides Ser.). (Illus.). 56p. (Orig.). pap. 3.95 (*0-8159-6721-7*) Devin.

Dr. Rosenfeld's Guide to Alternative Medicine: What Works, What Doesn't - And What's Right for You. Isadore Rosenfeld. 1999. 342p. reprint ed. text 26.00 (*0-7881-6290-X*) DIANE Pub.

Dr. Rosenfeld's Guide to Alternative Medicine: What Works, What Doesn't - And What's Right for You. Isadore Rosenfeld. 1997. LC 97-90458. 384p. pap. 13.95 (*0-449-00074-5*) Fawcett.

Dr. Salov's Secrets for Good Vision & Good Health: Alternatively, Naturally & Organically. Leslie H. Salov. 1998. (Illus.). 120p. pap. 74.95 (*0-9666126-0-4*) J Patterson.

Dr. Scott's Knee Book: Symptoms, Diagnosis, Treatment Knee Problems Ligaments Tendinitis. W. Norman Scott & Carol Colman. 1996. LC 95-45405. (Illus.). 208p. per. 12.00 (*0-684-81104-9*) S&S Trade Pap.

Doctor Speaks on Sexual Expression in Marriage. Donald W. Hastings. 2nd ed. 1971. 190p. 18.50 (*0-316-35017-6*, Little Brwn Med Div) Lppncott W & W.

Dr. Spock's Baby & Child Care. Benjamin M. Spock. 1989. pap. 12.95 (*0-671-69054-X*) PB.

Dr. Spock's Baby & Child Care. Benjamin M. Spock & Michael B. Rothenberg. Ed. by Gina Centrello. 6th rev. ed. 1992. LC 91-5105. mass mkt. 18.00 (*0-671-75967-1*); 864p. per. 7.99 (*0-671-76060-2*) PB.

Dr. Spock's Baby & Child Care. Benjamin Spock & Steven J. Parker. 7th rev. ed. 1998. (Illus.). 939p. per. 18.00 (*0-671-53763-6*, Pocket Books) PB.

Dr. Spock's Baby & Child Care Fiftyith Anniversary Spanish Edition. Benjamin Spock. 6th anniv. ed. 1997. (SPA., Illus.). 896p. mass mkt. 7.99 (*0-671-56881-7*, Pocket Books) PB.

Dr. Susan Love's Breast Book. Susan M. Love. 1991. pap. 16.00 (*0-201-57097-1*) Addison-Wesley.

Dr. Susan Love's Breast Book. Susan M. Love & Karen Lindsey. 1990. 18.95 (*0-201-09665-X*) Addison-Wesley.

Dr. Susan Love's Breast Book. Susan M. Love. 2nd ed. 1995. pap. 17.00 (*0-201-31599-8*) Addison-Wesley.

Dr. Susan Love's Breast Book. Susan M. Love & Karen Lindsey. 3rd rev. ed. 2000. (Illus.). 720p. pap. text 20.00 (*0-7382-0235-5*) Perseus Bks Grp.

Dr. Susan Love's Hormone Book: Making Informed Choices about Menopause. Susan M. Love & Karen Lindsey. 1998. LC 96-35120. (Illus.). 375p. pap. 15.00 (*0-8129-6392-X*, Crown) Crown Pub Group.

Doctor the Jokes on You. Charles L. Cleek. 1997. (Illus.). 44p. pap. (*0-9660543-2-6*) GIFTGO.

Doctor, the Patient & the Group: Balint Revisited. Enid Balint et al. 1993. LC 92-49166. 176p. pap. (*0-415-08053-3*) Routledge.

Doctor-to-Doctor: Avoiding Financial Suicide. Gary D. Steinman. 1998. LC 98-71744. 124p. per. 12.95 (*0-9665105-0-X*) Baffin Bks.

Doctor Veterinarian Board Review, Bk. II. Sam H. Basilious. 1991. (Illus.). 504p. (Orig.). (C). pap. 75.00 (*0-9630843-1-3*) Infoconnect.

Doctor Veterinarian Quick Review, Bk. I. Sam H. Basilious. 1991. (Illus.). 232p. (Orig.). (C). pap. 42.50 (*0-9630843-0-5*) Infoconnect.

Doctor, What Should I Eat? Nutrition Prescriptions for Ailments in Which Diet Can Really Make a Difference. Isadore Rosenfeld. 1996. LC 95-41965. 560p. pap. (*0-446-67261-0*) Warner.

Doctor What Should I Eat? Nutrition Prescriptions for Ailments in Which Diet Can Really Make a Difference. Isadore Rosenfeld. 2000. 528p. reprint ed. mass mkt. (*0-446-60922-6*) Warner.

Dr. Whitaker's Guide to Natural Healing: America's Leading "Wellness Doctor" Shares His Secrets for Lifelong Health. Julian M. Whitaker. LC 93-50780. (Illus.). 432p. 1996. pap. 18.95 (*0-7615-0669-1*); 1994. 24.95 (*1-55958-495-5*) Prima Pub (Prima Health).

Doctor Who Cures Cancer. William K. Eidem. 1997. LC 97-13695. (Illus.). 400p. 26.95 (*1-890410-01-2*) Sullivan & Foster.

Dr. Willis in Japan, 1862-1877: A British Medical Pioneer. Hugh Cortazzi. 1985. LC 85-1334. (Illus.). 273p. (C). text (*0-485-11264-7*) Athlone Pr GBR. *Dist:* Transaction Pubs, Humanities.

Doctor with Big Shoes: Missionary Experiences in China & Africa. Henry S. Nelson. 1995. LC 95-70539. (Illus.). 288p. (Orig.). pap. 17.95 (*1-881576-45-0*) Providence Hse.

Doctora: The Journal of an American Doctor Practicing Medicine on the Amazon River. Linnea Smith. 1998. LC 98-40076. (SPA.). 240p. pap. 14.95 (*1-57025-140-1*) Pfeifer-Hamilton.

Doctorate in Mental Health: An Experiment in Mental Health Professional Education. Ed. by Robert S. Wallerstein. 1991. 298p. (C). pap. text 40.00 (*0-8191-8317-2*); lib. bdg. 67.00 (*0-8191-8316-4*) U Pr of Amer.

Doctoring: The Nature of Primary Care Medicine. Eric J. Cassell. 1997. 224p. (C). 27.50 (*0-19-511323-3*) OUP.

Doctors. Mary K. Dornhoffer. 2000. LC 00-8617. (Community Workers Ser.). (Illus.). 32p. (J). (gr. k-3). lib. bdg. 19.93 (*0-7565-0008-7*) Compass Point.

Doctors: The Biography of Medicine. Sherwin B. Nuland. 2nd ed. 1995. pap. 16.00 (*0-679-76009-1*) Vin Bks.

Doctors Advice on Alternative Medicine. Marc S. Micozzi. 2000. 600p. pap. text 29.95 (*0-9670772-9-X*) Integratv Med Commn.

Doctors Afield & Afar. William V. McDermott. 2000. LC 99-50053. (Illus.). 175p. (*0-87233-126-1*) Bauhan.

Doctor's Always In: A Guide to 1100+ Best Health & Medical Information Sites on the Internet. Jay S. Schneider & Theodore I. Lidsky. 1999. 400p. pap. 24.95 (*0-9664949-0-3*) Neuroinfo.

Doctors & Diseases in the Roman Empire. Ralph Jackson. 1988. LC 88-40206. (Illus.). 224p. 37.95 (*0-8061-2167-X*) U of Okla Pr.

Doctors & Hospitals: Legal Duties. Meagher et al. 1991. 448p. text 81.00 (*0-409-89767-1*, MICHIE) LEXIS Pub.

Doctors & Management in the National Health Service. Gordon Marnoch. 1996. LC 96-19931. (Health Services Management Ser.). 208p. (*0-335-19345-5*); pap. (*0-335-19344-7*) OpUniv Pr.

***Doctors & Patients: Doomed to Destruction.** Yulian Rafes. Ed. by Steven Sedlis et al. 2001. LC 2001-52851. (*1-56700-177-7*) Begell Hse.

Doctors & Rules. Joseph M. Jacob. 1988. (Sociology of Professional Values Ser.). 250p. (C). lib. bdg. 65.00 (*0-415-00688-0*) Routledge.

Doctors & Rules. Joseph M. Jacob. 2nd ed. 1998. LC 98-27095. 300p. pap. text 24.95 (*0-7658-0477-8*) Transaction Pubs.

Doctors & the Law: Defendants & Expert Witnesses. Hiller B. Zobel & Stephen N. Rous. 1993. LC 92-16344. 224p. 22.95 (*0-393-03450-X*) Norton.

Doctors & the Law: Medical Jurisprudence in Nineteenth-Century America. James C. Mohr. 1996. LC 95-48061. (Illus.). 330p. (C). pap. text 18.95 (*0-8018-5398-2*) Johns Hopkins.

Doctors & the State: The Politics of Health Care in France & the United States. David Wilsford. 1991. LC 90-13995. 375p. text 54.95 (*0-8223-1082-1*); pap. text 59.95 (*0-8223-1092-9*) Duke.

Doctors & the State: The Struggle for Professional Control in Zimbabwe. Dorothy Mutizwa-Manigza. 1999. LC 99-72335. (Making of Modern Africa Ser.). 274p. (*1-84014-914-0*) Ashgate Pub GBR. *Dist:* Ashgate Pub Co.

Doctors & Their Feelings: A Pharmacology of Medical Caring. Benjamin Maoz et al. 1992. LC 91-29032. 168p. 60.00 (*0-275-93990-1*, C3990, Praeger Pubs) Greenwood.

Doctors & Their Patients: A Social History. Edward Shorter. 1991. 330p. (C). pap. text 24.95 (*0-88738-871-X*) Transaction Pubs.

Doctors & Their Practice Patterns: Index of New Information. Niccola D. Dejo. 1998. 57.50 (*0-7883-1818-7*); pap. 47.50 (*0-7883-1819-5*) ABBE Pubs Assn.

Doctors at War. Ed. by Morris Fishbein. 1977. LC 72-4477. (Essay Index Reprint Ser.). reprint ed. 46.95 (*0-8369-2943-8*) Ayer.

Doctors Book, Home. Prevention Magazine Editors. 1995. mass mkt. 8.99 (*0-553-85152-7*) Bantam.

***Doctors Book of Food Remedies.** Selene Yeager & Editors of Prevention Health Books Staff. 2002. (SPA., Illus.). 768p. 29.95 (*1-57954-348-0*) Rodale Pr Inc.

Doctors Book of Herbal Home Remedies. Prevention Magazine Health Book Staff. 2001. 608p. pap. 16.95 (*1-57954-463-0*) Rodale Pr Inc.

Doctors' Book of Home Remedies. Sid Kirchheimer. 1995. (Doctors' Book of Home Remedies Ser.: Vol. II). 720p. mass mkt. 6.99 (*0-553-56984-8*) Bantam.

Doctors' Book of Home Remedies. Prevention Magazine Editors. 1991. 752p. mass mkt. 6.99 (*0-553-29156-4*) Bantam.

Doctor's Book of Home Remedies. Prevention Magazine Editors. 1995. mass mkt. 8.99 (*0-553-85158-6*) Bantam.

Doctor's Book of Home Remedies. Ed. by Prevention Magazine Health Book Staff. 1990. LC 89-38656. 688p. 27.95 (*0-87857-873-0*, 05-627-0) Rodale Pr Inc.

Doctors' Book of Home Remedies: Thousands of Tips & Techniques Anyone Can Use to Heal Everyday Health Problems. Prevention Magazine Health Book Staff. 1993. LC 94-48050. (SPA.). 739p. 26.95 (*0-87596-182-7*) Rodale Pr Inc.

Doctor's Book of Home Remedies for Airborne Allergies. Ed. by Prevention Magazine Health Book Staff. 2000. LC 00-25360. ix, 134p. pap. 12.95 (*1-57954-211-5*) Rodale Pr Inc.

Doctor's Book of Home Remedies for Children. Prevention Magazine Editors. 1995. 528p. mass mkt. 6.99 (*0-553-56985-6*) Bantam.

Doctors' Book of Home Remedies for Children. Prevention Magazine Health Book Staff. 1995. LC 94-45592. (SPA., Illus.). 450p. 26.95 (*0-87596-266-1*) Rodale Pr Inc.

Doctors Book of Home Remedies for Children: From Allergies & Animal Bites to Toothache & TV Addiction, Hundreds of Doctor-Proven Techniques & Tips to Care for Your Kid. Denise Foley. 1999. LC 93-5854. 464p. pap. 16.95 (*1-57954-063-5*) Rodale Pr Inc.

Doctors Book of Home Remedies for Colds & Flu: Incredible Tips to Get You On Your Feet Fast-From the Leading Experts. Ed. by Mary S. Kittel. 2000. LC 99-55328. 144p. pap. 12.95 (*1-57954-210-7*) Rodale Pr Inc.

Doctors Book of Home Remedies for Depression: Tips to Brighten Your Mood Through Herbs, Diet & Lifestyle. Prevention Magazine Health Book Staff. 2001. LC 00-10496. (Doctors' Book of Home Remedies Ser.). (Illus.). 144p. pap. 9.99 (*1-57954-232-8*) Rodale Pr Inc.

Doctor's Book of Home Remedies for Dogs & Cats. Hoffman. 1996. 139.75 (*0-87596-382-X*) St Martin.

Doctor's Book of Home Remedies for Dogs & Cats. Prevention Magazine Health Book Staff. 1998. LC 95-46481. (Illus.). 448p. pap. 16.95 (*1-57954-010-4*) Rodale Pr Inc.

Doctor's Book of Home Remedies for Managing Menopause: Over 100 Tips from Leading Experts to Reduce the Stress. Ed. by Prevention Magazine Editors. 2001. LC 00-9751. (Doctors' Book of Home Remedies Ser.). pap. 9.99 (*1-57954-234-4*) Rodale Pr Inc.

Doctor's Book of Home Remedies for Men. Mens Health Books Staff. 1999. 89.85 (*1-57954-108-9*) Rodale Pr Inc.

Doctors' Book of Home Remedies for Men. Ed. by Prevention Magazine Editors. 2000. 944p. mass mkt. 7.50 (*0-553-58234-8*) Bantam.

Doctor's Book of Home Remedies for Men: From Heart Disease & Headaches to Flabby Abs & Road Rage, over 2,000 Simple Solutions. Jack Croft. 2000. (Illus.). 688p. pap. 17.95 (*1-57954-261-1*) Rodale Pr Inc.

Doctor's Book of Home Remedies for Men: From Heart Disease & Headaches to Flabby Abs & Road Rage, over 2,000 Simple Solutions. Ed. by Jack Croft. 1999. LC 98-46311. (Doctors' Book of Home Remedies Ser.). (Illus.). 672p. 29.95 (*0-87596-529-6*) Rodale Pr Inc.

Doctor's Book of Home Remedies for Preventing Disease. Ed. by Hugh O'Neill. 1998. LC 98-44629. xviii, 637p. 29.95 (*0-87596-415-X*) Rodale Pr Inc.

Doctors' Book of Home Remedies for Preventing Disease. Prevention Magazine Health Book Staff. 2000. 864p. mass mkt. 6.99 (*0-553-58233-X*) Bantam.

Doctors Book of Home Remedies for Seniors: An A-to-Z Guide to Staying Physically Active, Mentally Sharp & Disease-Free. Ed. by Doug Dollemore & Prevention Health Books for Seniors Staff. 2000. LC 99-11451. pap. 17.95 (*1-57954-012-0*) Rodale Pr Inc.

Doctor's Book of Home Remedies for Seniors: An A-to-Z Guide to Staying Physically Active, Mentally Sharp & Disease Free. Doug Dollemore & Prevention Magazine Editors. 1999. LC 99-11451. (Illus.). 29.95 (*1-57954-011-2*) Rodale Pr Inc.

Doctor's Book of Home Remedies for Sharper Memory. Prevention Magazine Health Book Staff. 2000. LC 00-36602. ix, 118p. pap. 12.95 (*1-57954-233-6*) Rodale Pr Inc.

Doctor's Book of Home Remedies for Stronger Bones: Tips to Stop Osteoporosis & Reverse the Loss that Affects Every Woman over 30. Ed. by Mary S. Kittel. 2000. LC 99-56548. 144p. pap. 12.95 (*1-57954-209-3*) Rodale Pr Inc.

Doctor's Book of Home Remedies for Women. Ed. by Prevention Magazine Editors. 1998. 720p. reprint ed. mass mkt. 7.50 (*0-553-57693-3*) Bantam.

Doctor's Book of Home Remedies for Women. 3rd ed. 1996. 83.85 (*0-87596-438-9*) Rodale Pr Inc.

Doctors Book of Home Remedies for Women: Women Doctors Reveal over 2,000 Self-Help Tips on the Health Problems That Concern Women the Most. Sharon Faelten & Prevention Magazine Editors. 1996. LC 96-22163. 688p. 27.95 (*0-87596-343-9*) Rodale Pr Inc.

Doctor's Book of Home Remedies II. Sid Kirchheimer. 2nd ed. 1996. (SPA.). 29.95 (*0-87596-335-8*) Rodale Pr Inc.

Doctor's Book of Symptoms & Treatments: Your Guide to Aches, Pains & Other Physical Problems: Illnesses, Medical Tests & Surgeries. Gary J. Martin & Northwestern University Staff. 1997. LC 98-183700. 400 p. (*0-7853-2594-8*) Pubns Intl Ltd.

Doctors, Bureaucrats & Public Health in France, 1888-1902. Martha Hildreth. 1987. (Modern European History Ser.). 368p. text 15.00 (*0-8240-8037-8*) Garland.

Doctor's Case: The Life & Survival of a Physician Turned Patient. Kurland. 2002. text 24.95 (*0-7167-4290-X*) W H Freeman.

Doctors' Case Against the Pill. Barbara Seaman. 25th anniv. ed. 1995. LC 95-12085. 272p. 24.95 (*0-89793-182-3*); pap. 14.95 (*0-89793-181-5*) Hunter Hse.

Doctor's Cholesterol & Low Salt Diet Guide. Sylvan R. Lewis. 1980. (Illus.). 128p. (Orig.). pap. 2.00 (*0-936320-02-8*) Compact Books.

Doctor's Communication Handbook. Peter Tate. 1995. pap. (*1-85775-011-X*); 2nd ed. 1997. LC 97-17082. (*1-85775-256-2*) Radcliffe Med Pr GBR. *Dist:* Balogh.

***Doctor's Communication Handbook.** Peter Tate. 3rd ed. 2001. 184p. pap. (*1-85775-550-2*) Radcliffe Med Pr GBR. *Dist:* Balogh.

Doctors' Competence in Clinics & Hospitals: Index of New Information. 1998. 57.50 (*0-7883-1822-5*); pap. 47.50 (*0-7883-1823-3*) ABBE Pubs Assn.

Doctor's Complete Guide to Vitamins & Minerals. Mary Dan Eades. 2000. LC 00-710462. xiv, 559p. mass mkt. 6.99 (*0-440-23645-2*) Dell.

Doctors Cry, Too: Essays from the Heart of a Physician. Frank H. Boehm. 2001. LC 00-54020. xxv, 160p. 17.95 (*1-56170-816-X*) Hay House.

Doctor's Cure. Michael Loes et al. 1998. LC 98-4273. 224p. pap. 12.95 (*0-87983-929-5*, 39295K, Keats Pubng) McGraw-Hill Trade.

Doctors' Dilemma: In Vitro Fertilization. Veritas Publications Staff. 1989. pap. (*1-85390-051-6*) Veritas Pubns IRL. *Dist:* St Mut.

Doctor's Dilemma: Stress & the Role of the Carer. John W. Holland. 1995. 250p. (C). pap. (*1-85343-306-3*) Free Assoc Bks GBR. *Dist:* Intl Spec Bk, NYU Pr.

Doctor's Dilemmas. Louis S. Lasagne. 1977. LC 70-105025. (Essay Index Reprint Ser.). 25.95 (*0-8369-1669-7*) Ayer.

Doctors' Dilemmas: Medical Ethics & Contemporary Science. John Dawson & Melanie Phillips. 1985. 224p. (Orig.). pap. 12.95 (*0-416-01121-7*, 9342) Routledge.

Doctor's Directory of Medical Internet Addresses see Directory of Medical Internet Site Addresses: With Emphasis on Authority, Responsibility, & Sponsorship

Doctors, Dollars & Death: Bad Medicine in America. Oliver S. Owen. 1994. 115p. (Orig.). (C). pap. text 17.50 (*0-87527-508-7*) Green.

Doctor's Guide to Chronic Fatigue Syndrome: Understanding, Treating & Living with CFIDS. David S. Bell. 1993. LC 93-37533. (Illus.). 256p. 21.00 (*0-201-62616-0*) Addison-Wesley.

Doctor's Guide to Chronic Fatigue Syndrome: Understanding, Treating & Living with CFIDS. David S. Bell. 2000. 304p. pap. 15.00 (*0-201-40797-3*) Perseus Bks Grp.

Doctor's Guide to Diabetes & Your Child: New Therapies for Type 1 & Type 2. Allan E. Sosin et al. 2000. 240p. pap. 14.00 (*1-57566-576-X*, Knsington) Kensgtn Pub Corp.

***Doctor's Guide to Herbs & Supplements.** Robert S. DiPaola & Timothy Gower. 2001. LC 2001-24842. (Illus.). 224p. pap. 15.00 (*0-8050-6665-9*, Owl) H Holt & Co.

Doctor's Guide to Over-the-Counter Drugs. Ed. & Compiled by Brenda Adderly. 1998. LC 98-208738. (Illus.). 885p. (Orig.). mass mkt. (*0-446-60525-5*) Warner.

Doctor's Guide to Partnership Accounts. E. J. Parker. 1984. 76p. (*0-7212-0698-0*) Regency Pr GBR. *Dist:* St Mut.

Doctor's Guide to Therapeutic Touch: Enhancing the Body's Energy to Promote Healing. Susan Wager. 1996. LC 96-7240. 144p. pap. 12.00 (*0-399-52250-6*) Berkley Pub.

Doctors in Blue: The Medical History of the Union Army in the Civil War. George Worthington Adams. 1996. LC 96-22219. (Illus.). 253p. pap. 17.95 (*0-8071-2105-3*) La State U Pr.

Doctors in Canada: The Changing World of Medical Practice. Bernard R. Blishen. 1991. 224p. text 50.00 (*0-8020-5926-0*); pap. text 19.95 (*0-8020-6866-9*) U of Toronto Pr.

Doctors in Elizabethan Drama. Percival M. Yearsley. LC 75-23772. reprint ed. 34.50 (*0-404-13398-3*) AMS Pr.

Doctors in Gray: The Confederate Medical Service. H. H. Cunningham. 1990. (Illus.). 20.50 (*0-8446-0566-2*) Peter Smith.

***Doctor's Internet Handbook.** Kiley Robert. 2000. 76p. pap. (*1-85315-370-2*) Royal Soc of Medicine Pr Ltd GBR. *Dist:* Balogh.

***Doctor's Life: Unique Stories.** William T. Close. 2nd ed. 2001. (Illus.). 210p. pap. 15.95 (*0-9703371-0-8*) Meadowlark Springs.

Doctor's Little Book of Answers: 600 Medical Facts Everyone Should Know. Celia Brown. 1996. LC 95-39609. 176p. pap. 9.95 (*0-7615-0325-0*) Prima Pub.

Doctor's Little Book of Wisdom. William W. Forgey. 1995. LC 95-8833. 160p. pap. 5.95 (*1-57034-016-1*) Globe Pequot.

Doctor's Little Instruction Book. Robert A. Norman. 2000. 65 p. pap. 9.95 (*1-891576-00-3*) North Shore Pr.

Doctors' Marriages: A Look at the Problems & Their Solutions. M. F. Meyers. 2nd ed. 1994. (Illus.). 284p. (C). text 39.00 (*0-306-44618-9*, Kluwer Plenum) Kluwer Academic.

Doctors, Nurses & Medical Practitioners: A Bio-Bibliographical Sourcebook. Ed. by Lois N. Magner. 1997. LC 97-2232. 384p. lib. bdg. 87.50 (*0-313-29452-6*, Greenwood Pr) Greenwood.

Doctors of Modernity: Darwin, Marx, & Freud. R. F. Baum. 1986. 200p. (Orig.). pap. 8.95 (*0-89385-215-5*) Sugden.

Doctors on Horseback: Pioneers of American Medicine. James T. Flexner. 2nd ed. 1993. LC 92-19615. (Illus.). xiv, 370p. (C). reprint ed. pap. 22.50 (*0-8232-1379-X*) Fordham.

Doctors on the Edge: General Practitioners, Health & Learning, in the Inner-City. Linden West. 2000. 340p. (*1-85343-523-6*); pap. (*1-85343-522-8*) Free Assoc Bks GBR. *Dist:* Intl Spec Bk.

Doctors Only: The Evolving Image of the American Physician, 25. Richard Malmsheimer. 1988. LC 88-5685. (Contributions in Medical Studies Ser.: No. 25). 185p. 57.95 (*0-313-23465-5*, MAD/, Greenwood Pr) Greenwood.

Doctors Orders: Go Fishing. 2000. 224p. pap. (*0-9704254-0-6*) First Pubs Grp.

Doctors, Patients & Society: Power & Authority in Medical Care. Ed. by Martin S. Staum & Donald E. Larsen. 1982. 285p. (C). pap. (*0-88920-111-0*) W Laurier U Pr.

Doctors, Patients & the Law. Date not set. pap. 47.95 (*0-8464-4168-3*) Beekman Pubs.

Doctors, Patients & the Law. Ed. by C. Dyer. 1992. (Illus.). 240p. pap. 39.95 (*0-632-03442-4*) Blackwell Sci.

Doctor's Proven New Home Cure for Arthritis. Giraud W. Campell. 1989. 224p. (C). pap. text 10.95 (*0-13-216375-6*) P-H.

***Doctor's Story.** 2001. (Illus.). 320p. (*1-878326-10-4*) East Hall Pr.

Doctor's Tale: The Work of Hospital Doctors in England & Wales. HMSO Staff. 1995. 92p. pap. (*0-11-886149-2*, HM61492) Statnry Office GBR. *Dist:* Bernan Associates.

Doctors Talking with Patients - Patients Talking with Doctors: Improving Communication in Medical Visits. Debra L. Roter & Judith A. Hall. LC 92-17633. 224p. 1992. 55.00 (*0-86569-048-0*, T048); 2nd ed. 1993. pap. 21.95 (*0-86569-234-3*) Greenwood (Auburn Hse).

Doctor's 30-Day Cholesterol Blitz. Leslie C. Norins & Rainey Norins. 1996. LC 96-213590. 350p. 12.95 (*1-888266-00-7*) Adv Hlth Inst.

Doctors under Fire. Emerita T. Gueson. Ed. by Laurie McBrinn & Frank A. Gerolamo. 2nd ed. 1998. 115p. reprint ed. pap. 15.95 (*0-9653861-4-7*) Theresevision.

Doctor's Vitamin & Mineral Encyclopedia. Sheldon S. Hendler. 1991. 496p. per. 15.00 (*0-671-74092-X*) S&S Trade.

Doctor's Walking Diet: How to Lose Weight Without Dieting. Fred A. Stutman. 1982. LC 81-90742. 128p. pap. 7.95 (*0-934232-01-6*) Med Manor Bks.

Doctor's Wealth Protection Guide. David B. Mandell et al. 1999. (Illus.). 315p. pap. 35.00 (*1-890415-11-1*) Guardian Pub.

Doctors Who Followed Christ: 32 Biographies of Historic Physicians & Their Christian Faith. Dan Graves. 1999. LC 99-57356. 256p. pap. 12.99 (*0-8254-2734-7*) Kregel.

Doctors Who Kill. Max Haines. 1999. mass mkt. 6.99 (*0-451-18393-2*, Sig) NAL.

Doctors Who Rape: Malpractice & Misogyny. Pauline Trumpi. 1997. LC 97-5625. 342p. reprint ed. 34.95 (*0-87047-108-2*) Schenkman Bks Inc.

Doctors with Buggies, Snowshoes & Planes. Louise Shadduck. 1993. LC 95-105713. (Illus.). 500p. pap. 19.95 (*0-9634839-1-9*) Tamarack Bks.

Doctors' Wives: The Truth about Marriage to a Doctor. Cynthia S. Smith. 1994. pap. 5.50 (*1-56171-150-0*) SPI.

Doctrine of Signatures: A Defense of Theory in Medicine. Scott Buchanan. 2nd ed. 1990. 248p. text 34.95 (*0-252-01782-X*); LC 90-11127. pap. text 16.95 (*0-252-06150-0*) U of Ill Pr.

Documentary History of Biochemistry, 1770-1940. Mikulas Teich & Dorothy M. Needham. 1992. LC 91-36678. (Illus.). 756p. 85.00 (*0-8386-3487-7*) Fairleigh Dickinson.

Documentation: The Language of Nursing. Erma L. Coty et al. 2000. 256p. (C). spiral bd. 31.95 (*0-8385-1723-4*) P-H.

Documentation & Coding Strategies for the Long-Term Care PPS. Ed. by Jennifer I. Cofer. 1999. (Illus.). 112p. pap. text 79.00 (*1-57839-004-4*) Opus Communs.

Documentation & Information Management in Home Care & Hospice Programs. Susan C. Miller. 1996. (Illus.). 348p. pap. text 50.00 (*1-58426-011-4*, AB101697) Am Hlth Info.

***Documentation & Reimbursement for Home Care & Hospice Programs.** Prinny Rose Abraham. 2001. (AHIMA's Documentation Ser.). 496p. pap. text 72.00 (*1-58426-043-2*) Am Hlth Info.

Documentation & Reimbursement for Physician Offices. LaVonne Wieland & Lynn Kuehn. rev. ed. 1999. Orig. Title: Physician Office Health Records. (Illus.). 128p. (C). pap. text 50.00 (*1-58426-023-8*, AB303499) Am Hlth Info.

Documentation Field Guide. Ron Milewski & Rick Lang. 1999. LC 98-38471. (Illus.). 72p. (C). pap. text 18.95 (*0-7637-0879-8*, 0879-8) Jones & Bartlett.

Documentation for Physical Therapist Assistants. Marianne Lukan. (Illus.). 2001. LC 2001-28198. 208p. pap. 25.95 (*0-8036-0837-3*); 1996. LC 96-20735. 204p. (C). pap. text 23.95 (*0-8036-0187-5*) Davis Co.

Documentation for the Survey of Pesticide Use During the Gulf War: The Survey Instrument. Dalia M. Spektor et al. 2000. LC 00-62578. (Illus.). iii, 204p. pap. 25.00 (*0-8330-2900-2*) Rand Corp.

Documentation Manual for Speech Language Pathology. Gloria B. Nelson. 2001. 240p. ring bd. 115.00 (*0-8342-0991-8*, 20991) Aspen Pub.

Documentation Manual for Writing SOAP Notes in Occupational Therapy. Sherry Borcherding. 2000. (Illus.). 256p. pap. text 24.00 (*1-55642-441-8*) SLACK Inc.

Documentation of Joint Motion: International Standard Neutral-Zero-Measuring, SFTR Recording & Application of the Plurimeter. John J. Gerhardt. 1988. (Illus.). 60p. (C). pap. text (*0-9621736-0-6*) Isomed.

Documentation of Joint Motion: International Standard Neutral Zero Measuring, SFTR Recording & Application of the Plurimeter. John J. Gerhardt. 2nd rev. ed. 1989. (Illus.). 61p. (Orig.). reprint ed. spiral bd. (*0-9621736-1-4*) Isomed.

Documentation of the Threshold Limit Values & Biological Exposure Indices. 6th ed. 1999. (Illus.). (C). pap. text 550.00 (*0-936712-96-1*) Am Conf Govt Indus Hygienist.

Documentation Requirements for the Acute Care Patient Record. Barbara A. Glondys. rev. ed. 1999. (Illus.). 382p. pap. text 62.00 (*1-58426-030-0*, AB100799) Am Hlth Info.

Documentation Requirements in Non-Acute Care Facilities & Organizations. B. J. Manger. 2001. LC 00-56681. (Illus.). 220p. pap. 37.95 (*1-84214-001-9*) CRC Pr.

Documentation Skills for Quality Patient Care. R. Fay Yocum. Ed. by Esther Silverman. 1993. LC 93-79567. 184p. (Orig.). (C). pap. 18.95 (*0-9637649-7-7*) Awareness Prods.

Documentation Skills for Quality Patient Care. Fay Yocum. 2nd rev. ed. 1999. 300p. pap. (*0-9637649-6-9*) Awareness Prods.

Documentation Skills for Quality Patient Care: Narrative Notes Supplement. Fay Yocum. 1994. 16p. (C). pap. text, suppl. ed. 5.99 (*0-9637649-8-5*) Awareness Prods.

Documenting Hospital Meetings. Eric Joseph & Nancy Webster. 1998. 108p. (Orig.). pap. text 40.00 (*0-916499-60-X*) Care Educ Grp.

Documenting Psychotherapy: Essentials for Mental Health Practitioners. Mary E. Moline et al. 1997. LC 97-4884. 176p. 67.95 (*0-8039-4691-0*, 3365); pap. 32.95 (*0-8039-4692-9*, 3366) Sage.

Documenting Sensorimotor Progress: A Pediatric Therapist's Guide. Georgia A. Degangi. 1998. 157p. pap. text 42.00 (*0-12-784554-2*) Acad Pr.

***DOD's Mandatory Anthrax Vaccine Immunization Program for Military Personnel: Congressional Hearing.** Ed. by Christopher Shays. 2001. 200p. (C). reprint ed. pap. text 40.00 (*0-7567-1086-3*) DIANE Pub.

Does AIDS Hurt? Educating Your Children about AIDS. Marcia Quackenbush & Sylvia Villarreal. 2nd ed. 1992. LC 92-25691. 17.95 (*1-56071-084-5*) ETR Assocs.

Does Anyone Hear Our Cries for Help? Strategies for Successful Living in Difficult Situations. Bertie Ryan Synowiec. rev. ed. 1995. (Successful Living Ser.). 120p. pap. 9.95 (*1-885335-03-2*) Positive Support.

Does God Help? Developmental & Clinical Aspects of Religious Belief. Ed. by Akhtar Salman & Henri Parens. 2001. LC 00-67595. pap. 40.00 (*0-7657-0319-X*) Aronson.

Does It Run in the Family? A Consumer's Guide to DNA Testing for Genetic Disorders. Doris T. Zallen. 1997. LC 96-49677. 200p. 24.95 (*0-8135-2446-6*) Rutgers U Pr.

Does My Child Have a Speech Problem? Katherine I. Martin. 1997. LC 96-35302. 224p. pap. 16.95 (*1-55652-315-7*) Chicago Review.

Does My Child Need a Therapist? Colleen Alexander-Roberts & Mark T. Snyder. 1997. LC 96-29588. 224p. (Orig.). pap. 12.95 (*0-87833-942-6*) Taylor Pub.

Does Psychiatry Need a Public Philosophy? Ed. by Don S. Browning & Ian S. Evison. 1991. 131p. (Orig.). text 36.95 (*0-8304-1244-1*) Burnham Inc.

Does Stress Cause Psychiatric Illness? Ed. by Carolyn M. Mazure. 1994. (Progress in Psychiatry Ser.: Vol. 46). 315p. text 39.50 (*0-88048-482-9*, 8482) Am Psychiatric.

Does Your Child Have Epilepsy? James E. Jan et al. 2nd ed. 1991. LC 90-27089. (For Interested Parents Ser.). (Illus.). 201p. pap. text 24.00 (*0-89079-456-1*, 1948) PRO-ED.

Does Your Doctor Charge Too Much? The Consumers Guide to Physicians Fees. James Davis. 1997. LC 97-5172. 275p. (Orig.). pap. 12.95 (*1-885987-02-1*, ME071, Health Info Pr) Practice Mgmt Info.

Dog Anatomy. Robert F. Way. 1974. LC 74-75114. (Illus.). pap. 5.95 (*0-88376-054-1*) Dreenan Pr.

Dog & Cat. Stanley H. Done. 1996. (Color Atlas of Veterinary Anatomy Ser.: Vol. 3). (Illus.). 464p. (*0-7234-2441-1*) Wolfe Publishing GBR. *Dist:* Mosby Inc.

Dog & Cat Nutrition: A Handbook for Students, Veterinarians, Breeders & Owners. Andrew T. Edney. 1982. (Illus.). 124p. text 35.00 (*0-08-028891-X*); pap. text 16.25 (*0-08-028890-1*) Elsevier (Pergamon Pr).

Dog First Aid. Sid Gustafson. 1998. 128p. pap. 6.95 (*1-56044-658-7*) Falcon Pub Inc.

Dog Language: An Encyclopedia of Canine Behavior. Roger Abrantes. Tr. by Sarah Whitehead from DAN. 1997.Tr. of Hundesprog. (Illus.). 295p. pap. 19.95 (*0-9660484-0-7*) Wakan Tanka.

Dog Owner's Encyclopedia of Veterinary Medicine. A. Hart. 1970. 19.95 (*0-87666-287-4*, H-934) TFH Pubns.

Dog Owner's Healthcare Guide. Lowell J. Ackerman. 1996. (Illus.). 432p. 39.95 (*0-7938-0183-4*, TS214) TFH Pubns.

Dog Owner's Home Veterinary Handbook. Delbert G. Carlson & James M. Giffin. 2nd rev. ed. 1992. (Illus.). 448p. pap. 25.00 (*0-87605-537-4*, Howell) Hungry Minds.

Dog Owner's Home Veterinary Handbook. James M. Giffin. 3rd ed. 1999. LC 99-62755. (Illus.). 560p. pap. 29.95 (*0-87605-201-4*, Howell) Hungry Minds.

Dogs: Homoeopathic Remedies. George MacLeod. 1990. 156p. pap. 20.95 (*0-8464-1334-5*) Beekman Pubs.

Dogs: Homoeopathic Remedies. George MacLeod. 1989. 128p. pap. (*0-85207-218-X*) C W Daniel GBR. *Dist:* Natl Bk Netwk.

Dog's Drugstore: A Dog Owner's Guide to Nonprescription Drugs & Their Safe Use in Veterinary Home Care. Richard W. Redding & M. L. Papurt. 2000. LC 00-27487. (Illus.). xvi, 234p. 23.95 (*0-312-20888-X*) St Martin.

Dohrmann Kaspar Pischel, M. D. American Links with Germanic Ophthalmology, Retinal Detachment Surgery, San Francisco. Dohrmann K. Pischel. 1988. (Ophthalmology Oral History Ser.). (Illus.). xxii, 142p. (Orig.). (C). pap. 35.00 (*0-926866-00-1*) FAAO.

Doing Better & Feeling Worse. Ed. by John H. Knowles. 1977. 287p. pap. 10.95 (*0-393-06423-9*) Norton.

Doing Child & Adolescent Psychotherapy... The Ways & Whys. Richard Bromfield. 1999. LC 99-12391. (Illus.). ix, 297p. 40.00 (*0-7657-0220-7*) Aronson.

Doing Contextual Therapy: An Intergrated Model for Working with Individuals, Couples & Families. Peter Goldenthal. 1996. LC 95-42742. 180p. 29.00 (*0-393-70208-1*) Norton.

Doing Counselling Research. John McLeod. 1994. 224p. 74.50 (*0-8039-7803-0*, 7883); pap. 25.95 (*0-8039-7804-9*, 7884) Sage.

Doing Family Therapy: Craft & Creativity in Clinical Practice. Robert Taibbi. 1996. LC 96-29005. (Guilford Family Therapy Ser.). 226p. pap. 22.00 (*1-57230-181-3*, 0181) Guilford Pubns.

Doing Good: The Life of Toronoto's General Hospital. J. T. H. Connor. 2000. LC 2001-339464. (Illus.). xi, 342p. text 60.00 (*0-8020-4774-2*) U of Toronto Pr.

Doing Legal Research: A Guide for Social Scientists & Mental Health Professionals. Roberta A. Morris et al. 1997. LC 96-35664. (Applied Social Research Methods Ser.: Vol. 43). 139p. 69.95 (*0-8039-3428-9*, 6717); pap. 26.95 (*0-8039-3429-7*, 6753) Sage.

Doing More Good Than Harm: The Evaluation of Health Care Interventions. Ed. by Kenneth S. Warren & Frederick Mosteller. 1994. LC 94-2873. (Annals Ser.: Vol. 703). 341p. pap. 90.00 (*0-89766-834-0*) NY Acad Sci.

Doing More with Less: Using Long-Term Skills in Short-Term Treatment. Barbara Dane. 2001. LC 00-56938. 60.00 (*0-7657-0296-7*) Aronson.

Doing Psychological Research. Joseph Horvat & Stephen Davis. 1997. LC 97-29377. 192p. pap. text 29.00 (*0-13-243692-2*) P-H.

Doing Psychology Experiments. David W. Martin. 2nd ed. 1984. LC 84-14987. 246p. (C). mass mkt. 19.50 (*0-534-03807-7*); 3rd ed. 1991. (C). pap. 24.75 (*0-534-14490-X*); 4th ed. 1995. LC 94-47424. 304p. mass mkt. 28.50 (*0-534-33840-2*) Brooks-Cole.

Doing Psychotherapy. Michael F. Basch. 1980. LC 79-3084. 188p. pap. 44.00 (*0-465-01684-7*) Basic.

Doing Psychotherapy Effectively. Mona S. Weissmann & Daniel A. Giacomo. 1997. LC 97-25027. 176p. 21.00 (*0-226-89167-4*) U Ch Pr.

Doing Right: A Practical Guide to Ethics for Physicians & Medical Trainees. Ed. by Philip Hebert. 1996. 220p. pap. text 32.50 (*0-19-541104-8*) OUP.

Doing Right: Everyday Medical Ethics. Solomon Papper. 1983. 148p. 30.95 (*0-316-69044-9*, Little Brwn Med Div) Lppncott W & W.

Doing Social Psychology: Laboratory & Field Exercises. Ed. by Glynis M. Breakwell et al. 1988. (Illus.). 328p. text 64.95 (*0-521-34015-2*); pap. text 22.95 (*0-521-33563-9*) Cambridge U Pr.

Doing the Dissertation: The Nuts & Bolts of Psychological Research. Brian T. Yates. 1982. (Illus.). 232p. pap. 32.95 (*0-398-04650-6*) C C Thomas.

Doing What Counts for Patient Safety: Federal Actions to Reduce Medical Errors. 2000. (Report of the Quality Interagency Coordination Task Force Ser.). pap. (*1-58763-000-1*) Agency Healthcare.

Doing What Works in Brief Therapy: A Strategic Solution Focused Approach. Ellen K. Quick. 1996. LC 95-25308. (Illus.). 244p. pap. text 44.95 (*0-12-569660-4*) Acad Pr.

Dolan's Critical Care Nursing: Clinical Management Through the Nursing Process. Susan D. Ruppert et al. 2nd ed. 1996. (Illus.). 1123p. text 61.95 (*0-8036-0025-9*) Davis Co.

Domestic Accidents. E. Maurice Backett. 1965. (Public Health Papers: No. 26). (ENG, FRE, RUS & SPA.). 137p. pap. text 6.00 (*92-4-130026-4*, 1110026) World Health.

Domestic 007 - Eliminating Hidden Killers in Your Home: Ridding Your Home of Harmful Chemicals & Cancer-Causing Agents. Maryla W. Records. Ed. by Cynthia Lane. 1997. LC 96-38137. (Illus.). 102p. (Orig.). pap. 18.95 (*0-9655793-0-1*) Earth-Wise.

Domestic Violence: A Nursing Concern - 1 Hour. G. Rumay Alexander. Ed. by M. Rosanna Rodriguez. Tr. by Kathy Johnson. 2nd rev. ed. 1998. (Illus.). 22p. pap. 12.95 (*1-57801-022-5*) Western Schls.

Domestic Violence: A Nursing Concern - 3 Hour. G. Rumay Alexander & M. Rosanna Rodriguez. Tr. by Kathy Johnson. 1998. (Illus.). 46p. pap. 19.95 (*1-57801-021-7*) Western Schls.

Domestic Violence & Child Abuse Sourcebook: Basic Information about Spousal/Partner... Ed. by Helene Henderson. 2000. LC 00-58436. (Health Reference Ser.). (Illus.). xx, 1064p. 78.00 (*0-7808-0235-7*) Omnigraphics Inc.

Domestic Violence & Health Care: What Every Professional Needs to Know. Sherri L. Schornstein. 1997. LC 96-35629. 208p. pap. 32.95 (*0-8039-5959-1*, 1506) Sage.

Domesticated Drug. Ed. by George L. Maddox. 1970. 29.95 (*0-8084-0108-4*); pap. 24.95 (*0-8084-0109-2*) NCUP.

Domestication of the Savage Mind. Ed. by Jack Goody. 1977. (Themes in the Social Sciences Ser.). (Illus.). 192p. pap. text 19.95 (*0-521-29242-5*) Cambridge U Pr.

Dominance & Reproduction in Baboons (Papio Cynocephalus) A Quantitative Analysis. G. Hausfater. Ed. by H. Kuhn et al. 1975. (Contributions to Primatology Ser.: Vol. 7). (Illus.). viii, 149p. pap. 63.50 (*3-8055-2139-1*) S Karger.

Dominance Factor: How Knowing Your Dominant Eye, Ear, Brain, Hand & Foot Can Improve Your Learning. Carla Hannaford. 1997. LC 97-498. (Illus.). 176p. (Orig.). pap. 14.95 (*0-915556-31-6*) Great Ocean.

Dominant Issues in Medical Sociology. Compiled by Howard D. Schwartz. 3rd ed. 1994. LC 93-5516. 576p. (C). text 54.06 (*0-07-055732-2*) McGrw-H Hghr Educ.

Domjan & Burkhard's the Principles of Learning & Behavior. Michael P. Domjan & Barbara Burkhard. 2nd ed. 1985. LC 85-5276. (Psychology). 365p. (C). mass mkt. 46.00 (*0-534-05208-8*) Brooks-Cole.

Donde No Hay Doctor see Where There Is No Doctor: A Village Health Care Handbook

Donde No Hay Doctor: Una Guia Para los Campesinos Que Viven Lejos De los Centros Medicos. Jane Maxwell et al. Ed. by Elizabeth De Avila. 1995. LC 95-39889. (SPA., Illus.). 518p. pap. 17.00 (*0-942364-01-5*) Hesperian Found.

Donkeys: Their Care & Management. M. R. De Wesselow. 1969. pap. 20.00 (*0-87556-076-8*) Saifer.

Donor-Acceptor Approach to Molecular Interactions. Viktor Gutmann. 1978. LC 77-25012. 296p. 85.00 (*0-306-31064-3*, Plenum Trade) Perseus Pubng.

Donor-Acceptor Bond. E. N. Guryanova et al. 1975. 366p. 3.5 hd 76.00 (*0-7065-1515-3*) Coronet Bks.

Donor Insemination. Ed. by Christopher L. Barratt & Ian Cooke. 1993. (Illus.). 241p. (C). text 69.95 (*0-521-40433-9*) Cambridge U Pr.

Donor Recruitment: Strategies for Success. Ed. by Leslie Botos & Carolyn Mihalko. 1996. LC 96-21201. (Illus.). 233p. (Orig.). spiral bd. 69.00 (*1-56395-059-6*, PC97-PR9606) Am Assn Blood.

Donor Recruitment/Public Relations Manual, Vol. 2. Ed. by Carolyn Mihalko. 1992. (Illus.). pap. text 25.00 (*1-56395-017-0*) Am Assn Blood.

Don't Accept Me as I Am: Helping Retarded People to Excel. Reuven Feuerstein et al. LC 88-17618. (Illus.). 342p. (C). 24.95 (*0-306-42964-0*) Da Capo.

Don't Be Afraid of EKGs. Jeffrey Stephen Halsell. 2001. (Illus.). 175p. pap. 24.95 (*0-8036-0754-7*) Davis Co.

Don't Be Mistreated! Marci Cunningham. Ed. by P. Rodriguez. 1987. (Natural Health Ser.). 100p. (Orig.). pap. text 5.95 (*0-938833-03-0*) Backwoods Bks.

Don't Butter Me Up: The Handbook for a Low Fat Eating Plan that Will Melt Your Fat Away Forever! Rebecca Harvin. 1993. (Illus.). 175p. pap. 14.95 (*0-9641477-0-X*) Rebecca Entpses.

Don't Count Me Out: A Different Perception of Fear. Joann Czyz. 1995. 272p. 16.95 (*0-9645587-0-X*); pap. 12.95 (*0-9645587-1-8*) LAF Pub.

Don't Forget to Smile or How to Stay Sane & Fit over Ninety. Ruth Stout. Date not set. (*0-912846-21-6*) Bookstore Pr.

Don't Lose Your Patients! Responding to Clients Who Want to Quit Treatment. Herbert S. Strean. 1998. LC 98-17725. 256p. 40.00 (*0-7657-0171-5*) Aronson.

Don't Panic: The Psychology of Emergency Egress & Ingress. Jerome Chertkoff & Russell H. Kushigian. 1999. LC 98-47812. 160p. 55.00 (*0-275-96268-7*, Praeger Pubs) Greenwood.

Don't Panic Revised Edition: Taking Control of Anxiety Attacks. R. Reid Wilson. rev. ed. 1996. LC 96-181518. 400p. pap. 15.00 (*0-06-095160-5*) HarperCollins Pubs.

Don't Read This Book. Neal Starkman. 1992. LC 92-30922. pap. text 10.00 (*0-935529-54-3*) Comprehen Health Educ.

Don't Think about Monkeys: Extraordinary Stories by People with Tourette Syndrome. Ed. by Adam W. Seligman & John S. Hilkevich. 1992. LC 92-15489. 200p. (Orig.). pap. 12.95 (*1-878267-33-7*) Hope Pr CA.

Don't Water the Stick: The Path of the Psyche. Bernard Willemsen. 2nd ed. 1998. LC 98-900240. 156p. pap. (*0-9680351-1-6*) Quasar.

Doody's Health Science Book Review Annual, 1993. Ed. by Daniel J. Doody. 1994. 654p. 295.00 (*1-885234-00-7*) Doody Pubng.

Doody's Health Sciences Book Review Annual, 1994-1995. Daniel J. Doody. 1995. (Doody's Health Sciences Book Review Annual Ser.). 1000p. 150.00 (*1-885234-02-3*) Doody Pubng.

Doody's Rating Service: A Buyer's Guide to the 250 Best Health Sciences Books, 1993. Intro. by Daniel J. Doody. 1994. 200p. 49.95 (*1-885234-01-5*) Doody Pubng.

Doody's Rating Service: A Buyer's Guide to the 250 Best Health Sciences Books, 1994-1995. Doody. 1995. (Doody's Rating Service Ser.). 200p. pap. 45.00 (*1-885234-03-1*) Doody Pubng.

Doody's Rating Service: A Buyer's Guide to the 250 Best Health Sciences Books 1997. Intro. by Daniel J. Doody. 1997. (Illus.). 250p. pap. 50.00 (*1-885234-07-4*) Doody Pubng.

Dopamine & Mental Depression: Proceedings of the Biannual Capo Boi Conference on Neuroscience, June 1989, Villasimius, Italy. Ed. by Gian L. Gessa & G. Serra. 1990. (Advances in the Biosciences Ser.: Vol. 77). (Illus.). 216p. 153.00 (*0-08-040762-5*, Pergamon Pr) Elsevier.

Dopamine Receptor Agonists. Ed. by Stanely T. Crooke & George H. Poste. 1984. LC 84-8290. (New Horizons in Therapeutics Ser.). 414p. 95.00 (*0-306-41654-9*, Plenum Trade) Perseus Pubng.

Dopamine Receptors & Transporters, Pharmacology, Structure & Function: Pharmacology, Structure & Function. Hyman B. Niznik. 1994. LC 93-42705. (Illus.). 704p. text 250.00 (*0-8247-9158-4*) Dekker.

Dopaminergic System. 1985. (Basic & Clinical Aspects of Neuroscience Ser.). (Illus.). 39p. 26.95 (*0-387-13700-9*) Spr-Verlag.

Dopaminergic System: Evolution from Biology to Clinical Aspects. Liana Bolis et al. 2000. LC 00-53466. 224p. text 110.00 (*0-7817-3266-2*) Lppncott W & W.

Doped up, Knocked up, & ... Locked Up? The Criminal Prosecution of Women Who Use Drugs During Pregnancy. Valerie Green. 1993. LC 92-35296. (Children of Poverty Ser.). 128p. text 20.00 (*0-8153-1125-7*) Garland.

Doping: Proceedings, International Seminar Organ. University Ghent Brussels, May 1964. A. Schaepdryv & M. Hebbelinck. 1965. LC 65-12294. (*0-08-011046-0*) Pergamon Repr GBR. *Dist:* Franklin.

Doppler Color Flow Imaging. Joseph A. Kisslo et al. 1987. (Illus.). 184p. text (*0-443-08563-3*) Church.

Doppler Color Imaging, Vol. 27. Ed. by Christopher R. Merritt. 1992. (Clinics in Diagnostic Ultrasound Ser.: Vol. 27). (Illus.). 282p. text (*0-443-08763-6*) Church.

***Doppler Tissue Imaging Echocardiography.** M. A. Garcia-Fernandez et al. 1998. (Illus.). 176p. (*84-486-0187-4*) McGraw-Hill Interamer ESP. *Dist:* McGraw.

Doppler Ultrasound: Physics, Instrumental, & Clinical Applications. D. H. Evans. 2nd ed. 2000. LC 99-33585. (Illus.). 456p. 240.00 (*0-471-97001-8*) Wiley.

Doppler Ultrasound in Gynecology. Ed. by Asim Kurjak & A. C. Fleischer. 1997. LC 97-41399. (Progress in Obstetric & Gynecological Sonography Ser.). (Illus.). 176p. (C). lib. bdg. 85.95 (*1-85070-623-9*, Parthenon Pbng) CRC Pr.

Doppler Ultrasound in Obstetrics. Ed. by K. Marsal & B. J. Trudinger. 2001. (Progress in Obstetric & Gynecological Sonography Ser.). (Illus.). 150p. 78.00 (*1-85070-644-1*, Parthenon Pbng) CRC Pr.

Doppler Ultrasound in Obstetrics & Gynecology. Dev Maulik. 1996. LC 96-11916. (Illus.). 639p. 185.00 (*0-387-94240-8*) Spr-Verlag.

Doppler Ultrasound in Perinatal Medicine. Ed. by J. Malcolm Pearce. 1992. (Illus.). 358p. text 98.00 (*0-19-262019-3*) OUP.

Dora: An Analysis of a Case of Hysteria. Sigmund Freud. 1963. pap. 5.95 (*0-02-076250-X*) Hungry Minds.

Dorland's Cardiology Speller. Newman W. Dorland. 1992. 287p. pap. text 26.00 (*0-7216-3748-5*) Saunders.

Dorland's Cardiology Word Book for Medical Transcriptionists. Newman W. Dorland. 2000. 605p. 32.00 (*0-7216-9151-X*) Saunders.

Dorland's Dentistry Speller. Newman W. Dorland. 1993. LC 92-13389. 192p. pap. text 19.00 (*0-7216-4572-0*) Saunders.

Dorland's Dermatology Speller. Newman W. Dorland. Date not set. pap. text (*0-7216-4932-7*) Saunders.

Dorlands Gastroenterology Speller. Newman W. Dorland. 1993. LC 92-13353. 192p. pap. text 26.00 (*0-7216-4568-2*) Saunders.

Dorland's Hematology - Oncology Speller. Newman W. Dorland. 1993. LC 92-13352. 255p. pap. text 22.95 (*0-7216-3750-7*) Saunders.

Dorland's Illustrated Medical Dictionary. Newman W. Dorland. 29th ed. 2000. LC 00-6383. (Dorland's Illustrated Medical Dictionary Ser.). (Illus.). 2175p. (C). 49.95 (*0-7216-6254-4*) Harcrt Hlth Sci Grp.

Dorland's Medical Abbreviations. Newman W. Dorland. 1992. LC 92-11623. 309p. pap. text 27.00 (*0-7216-3751-5*) Saunders.

Dorland's Medical Speller. Newman W. Dorland. 1991. 1493p. pap. text 34.50 (*0-7216-3599-7*) Saunders.

Dorland's Neurology Speller. Newman W. Dorland. 1999. pap. text 20.00 (*0-7216-4933-5*) Saunders.

Dorland's Neurology Word Book for Medical Transcriptionists. Contrib. by Saunders, W.B., Publishing Staff. 2000. 220p. 32.00 (*0-7216-9078-5*) Saunders.

Dorland's Ob/Gyn Speller. Newman W. Dorland. 1999. pap. text 20.00 (*0-7216-4934-3*) Saunders.

Dorland's Orthopedic Speller. Newman W. Dorland. 1993. LC 92-13380. 320p. pap. text 26.00 (*0-7216-3752-3*) Saunders.

Dorland's Pathology Speller. Newman W. Dorland. 1999. pap. text 20.00 (*0-7216-4935-1*) Saunders.

Dorland's Pocket Medical Dictionary. Newman W. Dorland. 26th ed. 2001. 912p. pap. text 29.95 (*0-7216-8281-2*) Harcrt Hlth Sci Grp.

Dorland's Pocket Medical Dictionary. Newman W. Dorland. 25th ed. 1995. 816p. pap. text 24.00 (*0-7216-5738-9*) Saunders.

Dorland's Podiatry Speller. Newman W. Dorland. 1999. pap. text 20.00 (*0-7216-4936-X*) Saunders.

Dorland's Psychiatry/Psychology Speller. Newman W. Dorland. 1992. 272p. pap. text 23.00 (*0-7216-3749-3*) Saunders.

Dorland's Radiology/Diagnostic Imaging Speller. Newman W. Dorland. 1999. pap. text 20.00 (*0-7216-4937-8*) Saunders.

Dorland's Rheumatology Speller. Newman W. Dorland. 1999. pap. text 20.00 (*0-7216-4938-6*) Saunders.

Dorland's Spanish-English Illustrated Medical Dictionary. 1992. (ENG & SPA.). 265.00 (*0-7859-9739-3*) Fr & Eur.

Dorland's Spanish English Illustrated Medical Dictionary. Newman W. Dorland. 27th ed. 1992. (ENG & SPA., Illus.). 250.00 (*0-7859-7485-7*, 8476158920) Fr & Eur.

Dorothea Dix: New England Reformer, Vol. 127. Thomas J. Brown. 1998. LC 97-44207. (Harvard Historical Studies: Vol. 127). 432p. 35.00 (*0-674-21488-9*) HUP.

Dorothea Orem: Self-Care Deficit Theory of Nursing. Donna L. Hartweg. 1991. (Notes on Nursing Theories Ser.: Vol. 4). (Illus.). 70p. (C). pap. 14.95 (*0-8039-4299-0*, 3042) Sage.

D.O.'s: Osteopathic Medicine in the Mountains. Penny Ellis & Alayne R. Steiger. 1986. (Illus.). (Orig.). 12.00 (*0-9617546-0-5*); pap. 7.00 (*0-9617546-1-3*) WV Soc Osteo Med.

Do's & Dont's for Family Members: How to Pull Your Life Together When You're Suffering. Terence Williams. 1982. 24p. pap. 3.75 (*0-89486-221-9*, 1235B) Hazelden.

Dosage & Solutions Calculations: The Dimensional Analysis Way. Alice J. Smith. 1989. (Illus.). 400p. (C). (gr. 13). pap. text 24.95 (*0-8016-5146-8*, 05146) Mosby Inc.

Dosage Calculation Apple Software. Luzerne. 3rd ed. 1990. (Education Ser.). pap. 125.00 (*0-8273-2788-9*) Delmar.

Dosage Calculations. June L. Olsen & Eugenia B. Murray. 1991. LC 91-4828. (Nursetest Ser.). (Illus.). 304p. pap. 21.95 (*0-87434-301-1*) Springhouse Corp.

Dosage Calculations. Gloria D. Pickar. 2nd ed. 1987. LC 82-71146. (Illus.). 128p. (C). reprint ed. disk 160.00 (*0-8273-2778-1*); 4th ed. 1993. 153p. tchr. ed. 14.00 (*0-8273-5741-9*); 4th ed. 1993. LC 92-23154. pap. 27.20 (*0-8273-4982-3*); 5th ed. 1996. 176p. tchr. ed. 14.95 (*0-8273-6781-3*) Delmar.

Dosage Calculations: A Ratio- Proportion Approach. Pickar. 1998. LC 98-3830. 400p. (C). pap. text 43.95 (*0-7668-0630-8*) Delmar.

Dosage Calculations: A Simplified Approach. Billie E. Wilson & Margret T. Shannon. 3rd ed. 1996. LC 96-20502. 190p. (C). pap. 34.20 (*0-8385-9297-X*, A-9297-1) P-H.

Dosage Calculations, 6E. Gloria D. Pickar. 6th ed. 1999. LC 98-32460. (Nursing Education Ser.). 496p. (C). pap. text 47.95 (*0-7668-0504-2*) Delmar.

Dosage Calculations for Veterinary Programs. Boufford. 2000. (C). pap. text 29.95 net. (*0-7668-0756-8*) Delmar.

Dosage Calculations IBM Software. Luzerne. 3rd ed. 1990. (Education Ser.). 125.00 (*0-8273-2785-4*) Delmar.

Dosage Calculations in SI Units. Maureen J. Osis. 3rd ed. 1995. (Illus.). 192p. (C). (gr. 13). spiral bd. 17.00 (*0-8151-6549-8*, 23838) Mosby Inc.

Dosage Calculations in SI Units, No. 2. Karlis Osis. 1990. (Illus.). 192p. spiral bd. 15.95 (*0-8016-3753-8*) Mosby Inc.

Dosage Calculations Made Incredibly Easy. Springhouse Publishing Company Staff. 1997. LC 97-26128. (Made Incredibly Easy Ser.). (Illus.). 304p. pap. 34.95 (*0-87434-904-4*) Springhouse Corp.

Dosage Calculations Manual. Catherine M. Todd & Belle Erickson. 3rd ed. 1996. LC 96-32692. (Illus.). 304p. pap. 27.95 (*0-87434-845-5*) Springhouse Corp.

***Dosage Calculations Using Dimensional Analysis.** Joyce Chappelear & Donna Thomas. 2000. 36.00 (*0-323-00980-8*) Mosby Inc.

Dosages & Solutions: A Programmed Approach to Meds & Math. Emily F. Cornett & Dorothy M. Blume. 5th ed. 1991. LC 91-9455. (Illus.). 273p. (C). pap. 21.95 (*0-8036-1981-2*) Davis Co.

Dose & Risk in Diagnostic Radiology How Big? How Little? Edward W. Webster. 1992. LC 92-49772. (Taylor Lectures: No. 16). 40p. (Orig.). pap. text 25.00 (*0-929600-26-6*) NCRP Pubns.

Dose & Timing: The Pillars of Successful Chemotherapy. Giovanni Rosti & European School of Oncology Staff. 1998. LC 98-17786. (Oncology Scientific Updates Ser.). 140p. 90.00 (*0-444-82968-7*) Elsevier.

Dose & Volume Specification for Reporting Interstitial Therapy. International Commission on Radiation Units and Measurements Staff. 1997. LC 97-40863. (ICRU Report Ser.: Vol. 58). 35.00 (*0-913394-57-2*) Intl Comm Rad Meas.

Dose Limits for Individuals Who Receive Exposure from Radionuclide Therapy Patients. Pref. by Charles B. Meinhold. 1995. LC 95-3556. (NCRP Commentaries Ser.: No. 11). 21p. (Orig.). pap. text 20.00 (*0-929600-42-8*) NCRP Pubns.

Dose Makes the Poison: A Plain-Language Guide to Toxicology. M. Alice Ottoboni. 2nd ed. 1997. 256p. pap. 44.95 (*0-471-28837-3*, VNR) Wiley.

Dose of Sanity: Mind, Medicine & Misdiagnosis. Sydney Walker, III. 1997. LC 95-46671. 272p. pap. 16.95 (*0-471-19262-7*) Wiley.

Dose-Response Relationship of Drugs. Ed. by J. Kuhlmann & W. Wingender. 1990. (Clinical Pharmacology Ser.: Vol. 3). (Illus.). 225p. text (*3-88603-366-X*) W Zuckschwerdt DEU. *Dist:* Scholium Intl.

Double: A Psychoanalytic Study. Otto Rank. 1989. 112p. reprint ed. pap. text (*0-946439-58-3*) Karnac Bks GBR. *Dist:* Other Pr LLC.

Double Axe: Cancer & the Mind. Abq Milo. 1996. (Illus.). 14p. (Orig.). pap., wbk. ed. 2.00 (*0-9653664-0-5*) Balanced Way.

Double Bind: Women Affected by Alcohol & Other Drugs. Ed. by Dorothy Broom. 1995. 235p. pap. (*1-86373-724-3*) Allen & Unwin Pty AUS. *Dist:* Paul & Co Pubs.

Double Contrast Barium Enema: The Genoa Approach. Giorgio Cittadini. 1997. LC 97-40608. 150p. 75.00 (*88-470-0003-3*) Spr-Verlag.

Double Contrast Gastrointestinal Radiology. Ed. by Igor Laufer & Marc S. Levine. 2nd ed. 1992. (Illus.). 713p. text 179.00 (*0-7216-5649-8*) Saunders.

Double Contrast Gastrointestinal Radiology. Igor Laufer et al. 3rd ed. 2000. LC 99-29019. (Illus.). 605p. text (*0-7216-8211-1*) Saunders.

Double Contrast Imaging of the Small Intestine. G. Salerno & V. Alessi. 1988. 184p. text (*1-57235-036-9*) Piccin Nuova.

Double Contrast Radiology of the Aesophagus. G. Rossetti et al. 1985. 154p. text (*1-57235-035-0*) Piccin Nuova.

Double Helix: A Norton Critical Edition. James Dewey Watson. Ed. by Gunther S. Stent. 1980. (Critical Editions Ser.). (Illus.). 298p. (C). pap. text 8.00 (*0-393-95075-1*) Norton.

Double Helix: A Personal Account of the Discovery of the Structure of DNA. James Dewey Watson. 1969. (Illus.). 143p. mass mkt. 6.99 (*0-451-62787-3*, Ment) NAL.

Double Jeopardy: Chronic Mental Illness & Substance Use Disorders. Ed. by Anthony F. Lehman & Lisa B. Dixon. 1995. LC 00-500876. (Chronic Mental Illness Ser.: Vol. 3). 304p. text 43.00 (*3-7186-0599-6*, Harwood Acad Pubs) Gordon & Breach.

Double Vision: An East-West Collaboration for Coping with Cancer. Alexandra D. Todd & John A. Todd. 1998. 190p. reprint ed. text 20.00 (*0-7881-5187-8*) DIANE Pub.

Doubt & Certainty in Science: A Biologist's Reflections on the Brain. John Z. Young. 1982. LC 81-20226. (Illus.). 168p. reprint ed. lib. bdg. 60.00 (*0-313-23364-0*, YODC, Greenwood Pr) Greenwood.

Doubting Disease: Help for Scrupulosity & Religious Compulsions. Joseph W. Ciarrocchi. 1995. LC 94-25222. (Integration Bks.). 208p. (Orig.). pap. 14.95 (*0-8091-3553-1*) Paulist Pr.

Douglas-Stromme's Operative Obstetrics. Frederick P. Zuspan & Edward J. Quilligan. 5th ed. 1992. 751p. (C). pap. text 159.00 (*0-8385-7404-1*, A7404-5, Apple Lange Med) McGraw.

Down & Dirty Guide to Adult ADD. Michael Gordon & F. Daniel McClure. 1996. 208p. pap. 16.95 (*0-9627701-9-1*) GSI Pubns.

Down Below. Leonora Carrington. 1982. (Illus.). 56p. pap. 14.00 (*0-941194-17-5*) Black Swan Pr.

Down from Troy: A Doctor Comes of Age. Richard Selzer. 1993. LC 93-11302. pap. 10.95 (*0-316-78065-0*, Little Brwn Med Div) Lppncott W & W.

Down Home Gynecology. Marvin Jaffee & Mary S. Jaffee. 1989. LC 88-71122. (Illus.). 160p. (Orig.). pap. 9.00 (*0-916383-63-6*) Aegina Pr.

Down Syndrome. Ann Garcia. 1995. pap. 9.95 (*0-9630158-0-X*) Baker-Hill.

Down Syndrome. Salvatore Tocci. 2000. LC 99-31019. (Venture Ser.). (Illus.). 144p. (YA). (gr. 8-12). lib. bdg. 18.95 (*0-531-11589-5*) F Watts.

Down Syndrome: A Promising Future, Together. Terry J. Hassold & David Patterson. LC 98-3117. (Illus.). 1999. 312p. pap. 19.95 (*0-471-29687-2*); Vol. 1. 1998. 293p. 69.95 (*0-471-29686-4*) Wiley.

Down Syndrome: Birth to Adulthood (Giving Families an Edge) John E. Rynders & J. Margaret Horrobin. 1996. LC 94-76444. 356p. pap. 39.95 (*0-89108-236-0*, 9502) Love Pub Co.

Down Syndrome: Living & Learning in the Community. Ed. by Lynn Nadel & Donna M. Rosenthal. 1995. LC 94-37595. 312p. 87.50 (*0-471-02192-X*); pap. 24.95 (*0-471-02201-2*) Wiley.

Down Syndrome: Moving Through Life. Ed. by Yvonne Burns. 1993. 235p. pap. 44.75 (*1-56593-140-8*, 0452) Singular Publishing.

Down Syndrome: Successful Parenting of Children with Down Syndrome. John F. Unruh. 1994. LC 94-193820. (Illus.). 112p. pap. 13.95 (*0-9615332-4-2*) Fern Ridge Pr.

Down Syndrome: The Facts. Mark Selikowitz. 2nd ed. 1997. (Facts Ser.). (Illus.). 204p. pap. 19.95 (*0-19-262662-0*) OUP.

Down Syndrome & Alzheimer Disease. Ed. by Lynn Nadel & Charles J. Epstein. 1992. LC 92-18114. (Progress in Clinical & Biological Research Ser.: Vol. 379). 334p. 225.00 (*0-471-58841-5*) Wiley.

Down Syndrome Behind the Dykes: Research in the Netherlands. E. A. de Graaf & A. Vermeer. Ed. by H. A. Heymans et al. 1999. LC 99-194698. 208p. pap. (*90-5383-610-1*) VU Univ Pr NLD. *Dist:* Paul & Co Pubs.

Down-to-Earth Approach to Being a Nurse Educator. Victoria Schoolcraft. 1993. LC 93-34776. (Teaching of Nursing Ser.: Vol. 16). (Illus.). 224p. (C). text 31.95 (*0-8261-8130-9*) Springer Pub.

Down with Gloom: COPE Program for Depression. John H. Greist et al. 1999. (Illus.). 16p. pap. (*0-9702974-5-9*) Healthcare Sys.

Downey & Darlings Physiology. Ed. by Erwin G. Gonzalez. 2001. LC 00-63084. 976p. text 99.00 (*0-7506-7179-3*) Buttrwrth-Heinemann.

Down's Syndrome: Children Growing Up: a Longitudinal Perspective. Janet Carr. 1995. LC 94-46986. (Illus.). 216p. (C). pap. text 37.95 (*0-521-46933-3*) Cambridge U Pr.

Down's Syndrome: Psychological, Psychobiological, & Socio-Educational Perspectives. Ed. by Jean A. Rondal et al. 1996. (Illus.). 264p. (Orig.). (C). pap. text 45.00 (*1-56593-740-6*, 1444) Thomson Learn.

Dozen Dangers to Your Baby's Brain & How to Reduce Those Dangers. 1987. 12p. (*1-55672-025-4*) US HHS.

Draft Compliance Program Guidance for Individual & Small Group Physician Practices. 10th ed. 2000. 150p. pap. text 45.00 (*1-58383-112-6*, PHYCOMPO) Robert D Keene.

Dragon Within the Gates: The Once & Future AIDS Epidemic. Stephen C. Joseph. 1993. LC 93-21941. 272p. pap. 9.95 (*0-7867-0033-5*) Carroll & Graf.

Dragons Touch: Weaknesses of the Human Anatomy. Hei Long. 1983. (Illus.). 184p. pap. 14.00 (*0-87364-271-6*) Paladin Pr.

Drainage in Homeopathy. Emmerick-Armand Maury. 1982. 105p. pap. (*0-85032-069-0*) C W Daniel GBR. *Dist:* Natl Bk Netwk.

Drainage in Homoeopathy. Emmerick-Armand Maury. 1980. (C). pap. 8.95 (*0-8464-1007-9*) Beekman Pubs.

Drama & Healing: The Roots of Drama Therapy. Roger Grainger. 1995. pap. (*1-85302-337-X*) Jessica Kingsley GBR. *Dist:* Taylor & Francis.

Drama & Intelligence: A Cognitive Theory. Richard Courtney. 1990. 208p. (C). text (*0-7735-0766-3*) McG-Queens Univ Pr CAN. *Dist:* CUP Services.

Drama As Therapy: Theatre As Living. Philip Jones. 1996. 352p. (C). pap. 29.95 (*0-415-09970-6*, C0324) Routledge.

Drama for All: Developing Drama in the Curriculum with Pupils with Special Educational Needs. Melanie Peter. 1994. 96p. pap. (*1-85346-315-9*) David Fulton GBR. *Dist:* Taylor & Francis.

Drama Therapy Activities for Parents & Children: An Exercise Handbook. Pam B. Dunne. 2nd ed. 1992. 53p. pap. 18.00 (*1-888657-05-7*) Drama Thrpy Inst.

Drama Within: Psychodrama & Experiential Therapy. Tian Dayton. 1994. LC 94-16374. 275p. (Orig.). pap. 14.95 (*1-55874-296-4*, 2964) Health Comm.

Dramatherapy. Ed. by Sue Jennings. 3rd ed. 1997. LC 95-26386. (C). 376p. pap. 29.95 (*0-415-13141-3*);No. 3. 368p. 84.95 (*0-415-13140-5*) Routledge.

Dramatherapy: Theory & Practice 2. Ed. by Sue Jennings. 2nd ed. 1992. 224p. (C). (gr. 13). pap. 29.95 (*0-415-05214-9*, A6532) Routledge.

Dramatherapy with Children & Adolescents. Ed. by Sue Jennings. 1995. LC 94-18586. (Illus.). 240p. (C). pap. 29.95 (*0-415-11041-6*, B4544) Routledge.

Dramatherapy with People with Learning Disabilities. Anna Chesner. 1994. 200p. pap. 29.50 (*1-85302-208-X*) Taylor & Francis.

Dramatic Approaches to Brief Therapy. Alida Gersie. 1995. 320p. text 29.95 (*1-85302-271-3*) Taylor & Francis.

Dramatic Play in Childhood: Rehearsal for Life. Virginia G. Koste. 1995. LC 95-5132. (Illus.). 144p. pap. 17.50 (*0-435-08669-3*, 08669) Heinemann.

Draw-a-Person Catalogue for Interpretative Analysis. William H. Urban. 1963. 72p. pap. 39.50 (*0-87424-044-1*, W-44) Western Psych.

Draw a Story: Screening for Depression & Age or Gender Differences. Rawley A. Silver. 2nd rev. ed. 1993. LC 93-72384. (Illus.). 112p. (C). pap. text 25.00 (*0-9621429-4-8*) Ablin Pr.

Drawing Blood: Technology & Disease Idenity in Twentieth-Century America. Keith Wailoo. 1999. (Henry E. Sigerist Series in the History of Medicine). 304p. pap. text 18.95 (*0-8018-6181-0*) Johns Hopkins.

Drawing on Difference: Art Therapy with People Who Have Learning Difficulties. Mair Rees. 1998. LC 97-38891. (Illus.). (C). 280p. 89.95 (*0-415-15479-0*); 264p. pap. 27.95 (*0-415-15480-4*) Routledge.

Drawing the Line: Life, Death & Ethical Choices in an American Hospital. Samuel Gorovitz. 1991. 224p. (C). text 30.00 (*0-19-504428-2*) OUP.

Drawing the Line: Life, Death & Ethical Choices in an American Hospital. Samuel Gorovitz. 1993. LC 93-26163. 195p. pap. 16.95 (*1-56639-149-0*) Temple U Pr.

Drawing the Soul: Models & Schemas in Psychoanalysis. Ed. by Bernard Burgoyne. 2000. 260p. pap. (*1-900877-02-3*) Rebus Pr Ltd GBR. *Dist:* Intl Spec Bk.

Drawings from a Dying Child: Insights into Death from a Jungian Perspective. Judi Bertoia. 1993. LC 92-15267. (Illus.). 176p. (C). text 49.95 (*0-415-07218-2*, A7169) Routledge.

***DRCOG - MCQs & OSCEs: How to Pass First Time.** Una Coales. 2001. 263p. pap. (*1-85315-506-3*) Royal Soc of Medicine Pr Ltd GBR. *Dist:* Balogh.

Dread Disease: Cancer & Modern American Culture. James T. Patterson. 1987. (Illus.). 416p. pap. 20.50 (*0-674-21626-1*); LC 87-160. 42.50 (*0-674-21625-3*) HUP.

Dream ... the Journey: Lorain Community Hospital. Margaret Finnerty. Ed. by Amy Phillips & Rodney Nelson. 1993. 96p. (C). (*0-929690-20-6*) Herit Pubs AZ.

Dream Analysis: Notes of the Seminar Given in 1928-1930, Vol. 1. Carl Gustav Jung. Ed. by William McGuire. 1984. LC 82-42787. (Dream Analysis Ser.: No. XCIX-1). (Illus.). 780p. 95.00 (*0-691-09896-4*) Princeton U Pr.

Dream Analysis in Psychotherapy. Lillie Weiss. 1992. (Practitioner Guidebook Ser.). (C). pap. text 36.50 (*0-205-14499-3*, H4499, Longwood Div) Allyn.

Dream Analysis in Psychotherapy. Lillie Weiss. 1986. LC 85-26040. (Psychology Practitioner Guidebooks). 144p. text 28.00 (*0-08-033162-9*, J115); pap. text 14.95 (*0-08-033161-0*) Elsevier (Pergamon Pr).

Dream & an Honor: The Life & Times of Dr. Alan J. Snider. Alan J. Snider. Ed. by Jayne A. Branch. 1996. 84p. (*0-9649148-0-8*) Sun Coast Hosp.

Dream & Existence. Michel Foucault & Ludwig Binswanger. Ed. by Keith Hoeller. 1992. LC 92-41852. (Studies in Existential Psychology & Psychiatry).Tr. of Reve et l'existence; Traum und Existenz. 112p. (Orig.). (C). pap. 12.50 (*0-391-03783-8*) Brill Academic Pubs.

Dream Fulfillment. Maria C. Gear et al. 1988. LC 88-408. 230p. 50.00 (*0-87668-912-8*) Aronson.

Dream Images: A Call to Mental Arms. Ed. by Jayne Gackenbach & A. Sheikh. 1991. (Imagery & Human Development Ser.). 320p. text 45.95 (0-89503-074-8); pap. text 35.00 (0-89503-056-X) Baywood Pub.

Dream in Clinical Practice. Ed. by Joseph M. Natterson. 1980. LC 80-65142. 498p. 40.00 (0-87668-402-9) Aronson.

***Dream in Psychoanalysis.** Leon L. Altman. rev. ed. 2001. (Books-on-Demand Ser.). 280p. reprint ed. pap. text 29.95 (0-8236-8030-4, 21431) Intl Univs Pr.

Dream in Psychoanalysis. Leon L. Altman. rev. ed. 1975. LC 75-13572. 280p. 42.50 (0-8236-1431-X) Intl Univs Pr.

Dream Interpretation. Thomas French & Erica Fromm. 1985. LC 86-30131. (Classics in Psychoanalysis Monographs: No. 5). 235p. 35.00 (0-8236-1435-2, BN#01435) Intl Univs Pr.

Dream Interpretation for Beginners. Michele Simmons & Chris McLaughlin. 1995. (Headway Lifeguides Ser.). 144p. pap. (0-340-60150-7) Hodder & Stought Ltd GBR. *Dist:* Lubrecht & Cramer, Trafalgar.

Dream-Life: A Re-Examination of the Psycho-Analytical Theory & Technique. Donald Meltzer. 1983. 185p. pap. (0-902965-17-4) Clunie Pr GBR. *Dist:* Other Pr LLC.

Dream, Mirror of Conscience: A History of Dream Interpretation from 2000 B.C. & a New Theory of Dream Synthesis. Werner Wolff. 1972. LC 70-152618. (Illus.). 348p. reprint ed. lib. bdg. 65.00 (0-8371-6053-7, WODR, Greenwood Pr) Greenwood.

Dream of the Moving Statue. Kenneth Gross. 1993. LC 92-52755. (Illus.). 272p. 39.95 (0-8014-2702-9) Cornell U Pr.

Dream Portrait: A Study of Nineteen Sequential Dreams As Indicators of Pretermination. Alma Bond et al. 1992. LC 91-35421. 200p. (C). 30.00 (0-8236-1438-7) Intl Univs Pr.

Dream Reader: Psychoanalytic Articles on Dreams. Ed. by Toni M. Alston et al. 1993. LC 93-17645. xviii, 772p. 115.00 (0-8236-1452-2) Intl Univs Pr.

Dream Spoilers: A Quadriplegic's Nightmare. Elizabeth R. Means. 1996. LC 97-123443. (Orig.). pap. 12.95 (0-9652561-0-3) Pelican Pr CA.

Dream Studies & Telepathy. Montague Ullman & Stanley Krippner. 1970. LC 71-113639. (Parapsychological Monographs: No. 12). pap. 7.00 (0-912328-16-9) Parapsych Foun.

Dream Symbolism. Manly P. Hall. 1979. pap. 7.95 (0-89314-392-8) Philos Res.

Dream Telepathy: Experiments in Nocturnal ESP. Montague Ullman et al. 2nd ed. 1989. LC 88-39093. (Illus.). 280p. lib. bdg. 45.00 (0-89950-349-7) McFarland & Co.

Dream Theatres of the Soul: Empowering the Feminine Through Jungian Dreamwork. Jean B. Raffa. 1994. LC 93-36669. 224p. pap. 15.95 (1-880913-10-0) Innisfree Pr.

Dream Work: Techniques for Discovering the Creative Power of Dreams. Jeremy Taylor. 1997. LC 82-62411. 280p. reprint ed. pap. 17.95 (0-8091-2525-0) Paulist Pr.

Dream Work in Psychotherapy & Self-Change. Alvin R. Mahrer. 1990. 372p. 34.95 (0-393-70089-5) Norton.

Dreaming: A Cognitive Psychological Analysis. David Foulkes. 1985. 232p. (C). text 45.00 (0-89859-553-3) L Erlbaum Assocs.

Dreaming: Anthropological & Psychological Interpretations. Ed. by Barbara Tedlock. 1992. (Advanced Seminar Ser.). (Illus.). 320p. reprint ed. pap. 24.95 (0-933452-81-0) Schol Am Res.

Dreaming the End of the World: Apocalypse as a Rite of Passage. Michael O. Hill. 1994. LC 94-22586. 200p. pap. 18.00 (0-88214-364-6) Spring Pubns.

Dreaming Way. Patricia Reis et al. 2000. LC 00-64454. (Illus.). 448p. pap. 29.95 (1-888602-11-2) Chiron Pubns.

Dreams. Carl Gustav Jung. Tr. by R. F. C. Hull. 1974. LC 72-11949. (Bollingen Ser.: No. 20). (Illus.). 354p. pap. 17.95 (0-691-01792-1) Princeton U Pr.

Dreams: A Key to Self-Knowledge. Zygmunt a. Piotrowski & Albert M. Biele. 1986. 200p. text 39.95 (0-89859-691-2) L Erlbaum Assocs.

Dreams Across the Lifespan. Raymond E. Rainville. 1988. 234p. (C). pap. text 22.95 (0-89641-177-X) American Pr.

Dreams & Emotional Adaptation: A Clinical Notebook for Psychotherapists. Robert J. Langs. 1998. LC 98-38986. 206p. 32.95 (1-891944-05-3) Zeig Tucker Theisen.

Dreams & Memories. Joan T. Sherman. 1994. (Illus.). 64p. pap. 19.95 (0-9642424-0-0) Hearts Desire.

Dreams & Nightmares: A Book of Gestalt Therapy Sessions. Jack Downing. 2nd ed. 1996. 192p. reprint ed. pap. 20.00 (0-939266-27-X) Gestalt Journal.

Dreams & Professional Personhood: The Contexts of Dream Telling & Dream Interpretation among American Psychotherapists. Mary T. Dombeck. 1991. LC 90-9780. (SUNY Series in Dream Studies). 271p. (C). pap. text 22.95 (0-7914-0589-3) State U NY Pr.

Dreams & the Growth of Personality: Expanding Awareness in Psychotherapy. Ernest L. Rossi. 1972. 232p. (C). (0-08-016787-X) Pergamon Repr GBR. *Dist:* Franklin.

Dreams As a Tool in Psychodynamic Psychotherapy: Traveling the Royal Road to the Unconscious. Vincenzo Conigliaro. 1997. LC 96-29393. 426p. 62.50 (0-8236-1439-5) Intl Univs Pr.

Dreams of a Woman: An Analyst's Inner Journey. Sheila Moon. 1983. LC 83-10826. (Illus.). 207p. 27.50 (0-938434-17-9); pap. 13.95 (0-938434-14-4) Sigo Pr.

Dreisbach's Handbook of Poisoning: Prevention, Diagnosis & Treatment. B. True. Ed. by R. H. Dreisbach. 13th ed. 2001. LC 2001-36722. (Illus.). 638p. per. 49.95 (1-85070-038-9, Parthenon Pbng) CRC Pr.

***DRG Guidebook 2001.** Ingenix, Inc. Staff. spiral bd. 89.95 (1-56329-703-5) Ingenix Inc.

***DRG Companion 2001: Formerly DRG Optimizer.** Ingenix, Inc. Staff. spiral bd. 139.95 (1-56329-732-9) Ingenix Inc.

***DRG Compliance Auditor 2001.** Ingenix, Inc. Staff. spiral bd. 69.95 (1-56329-702-7) Ingenix Inc.

DRG Handbook, 1998. 1998. pap. 399.00 (1-57372-090-9) Solucient.

Dried BCG Vaccine. Y. Obayashi. 1955. (Monographs: No. 28). (ENG & FRE.). 220p. pap. text 18.00 (92-4-140028-5, 1140028) World Health.

Drink Moderately & Live Longer: Understanding the Good of Alcohol. Morris E. Chafetz & Marion C. Chafetz. 1995. LC 95-94. pap. 9.95 (0-8128-8560-0) Madison Bks UPA.

Drink Water for Live: Your Journey to Better Health. Deanna DeLong. 1998. (Illus.). 36p. pap. 25.00 (1-892972-00-X) Creative Market.

Drinkers, Drinking & Alcohol-Related Mortality & Hospitalizations: A Statistical Compendium. M. M. Hyman et al. 1980. 12.50 (0-911290-05-2) Rutgers Ctr Alcohol.

Drinking among Teen-Agers. George L. Maddox & Bevode C. McCall. 1964. pap. 15.95 (0-8084-0413-X) NCUP.

Drinking among Teen-Agers. George L. Maddox & Bevode C. McCall. 1964. LC 64-63392. (Monographs: No. 4). 14.95 (0-911290-31-1) Rutgers Ctr Alcohol.

Drinking & Damage: Theoretical Advances & Implications for Prevention. B. G. Frankel & P. C. Whitehead. 1981. LC 80-620052. (Monographs: No. 14). 8.00 (0-911290-09-5) Rutgers Ctr Alcohol.

Drinking & Intoxication: Selected Readings in Social Attitudes & Controls. Ed. by Raymond G. McCarthy. 1963. LC 59-5289. pap. 13.95 (0-911290-28-1) Rutgers Ctr Alcohol.

Drinking, Community & Civilization: The Account of a New Jersey Interview Study. H. Fallding & C. Miles. 1974. LC 73-620137. (Monographs: No. 9). 4.00 (0-911290-41-9) Rutgers Ctr Alcohol.

Drinking, Driving, & You: A Guide to Making Choices & Understanding Consequences. 1995. 32p. pap. 5.50 (1-56246-032-3, 3134, HazeldenJohnson Inst) Hazelden.

Drinking Habits Among Alcoholics. Salme Ahlstrom-Laakso. 1975. (Finnish Foundation for Alcohol Studies: Vol. 21). 8.00 (951-9191-18-6) Rutgers Ctr Alcohol.

Drinking Habits Among Northern Youth: A Cross-National Study in the Scandinavian Capitals. Kettil Bruun & Ragnar Hauge. 1963. (Finnish Foundation for Alcohol Studies: Vol. 12). 4.00 (951-9192-04-2) Rutgers Ctr Alcohol.

Drinking Water & Cardiovascular Disease, Vol. 1. Ed. by Edward J. Calabrese et al. 1980. LC 80-81669. 327p. 47.00 (0-930376-16-1) Chem-Orbital.

Drinking Water & Health. National Research Council Staff. Vol. 5. 1983. 157p. pap. text 18.95 (0-309-03381-0); Vol. 6. 1986. 457p. pap. text 39.95 (0-309-03687-9) Natl Acad Pr.

Drinking Water & Health: Selected Issues in Risk Assessment, Vol. 9. National Research Council Staff. 1989. 284p. pap. text 29.95 (0-309-03897-9) Natl Acad Pr.

Drinking Water & Health, Vol. 7: Disinfectants & Disinfectant By-Products. National Research Council Staff. 1987. 212p. pap. text 19.95 (0-309-03741-7) Natl Acad Pr.

Drinking Water & Health, Vol. 8: Pharmacokinetics in Risk Assessment. National Research Council Staff. 1987. 512p. pap. text 43.50 (0-309-03775-1) Natl Acad Pr.

Drinking Water Health Advisory: Pesticides. U. S. Environmental Protection Agency Staff. 1989. (Illus.). 900p. lib. bdg. 125.00 (0-87371-235-8, L235) Lewis Pubs.

Drinking Water Health Advisory: Volatile Organic Compounds. U. S. Environmental Protection Agency Staff. 1990. 272p. 79.95 (0-87371-436-9, L436) Lewis Pubs.

Drinking Water Microbiology. Ed. by G. A. McFeters. 1990. (Contemporary Bioscience Ser.). (Illus.). 502p. 115.00 (0-387-97162-9, 3531) Spr-Verlag.

Dripps-Eckenhoff-Vandam Introduction to Anesthesia. David E. Longnecker & Frank L. Murphy. Ed. by Lesley Day. 9th ed. 1996. LC 96-70362. 480p. text 49.95 (0-7216-6279-X) Saunders.

Drive, Ego, Object, & Self: A Synthesis for Clinical Work. Fred Pine. 1990. LC 89-43168. 288p. 45.00 (0-465-01722-3) Basic.

Driven to Distraction: Recognizing & Coping with Attention Deficit Disorder from Childhood through Adulthood. Edward M. Hallowell. 1995. LC 94-40712. 336p. pap. 14.00 (0-684-80128-0, Touchstone) S&S Trade Pap.

C D

Drives, Affects, Behavior Ed. by Rudolph M. Loewenstein. 1960. LC 53-11056. Vol. 1. 399p. 60.00 (0-8236-1480-8); Vol. 2. 502p. 75.00 (0-8236-1500-6) Intl Univs Pr.

Driving Force: The Natural Magic of Magnets. James D. Livingston. 1997. (Illus.). 336p. pap. 14.95 (0-674-21645-8) HUP.

Drogen & Alkohol Series Vol. 3: Folgestudien und Therapieabbruch. Ed. by D. Ladewig. 1984. (GER., Illus.). vi, 174p. pap. 50.50 (3-8055-3874-X) S Karger.

Drogengefaehrdung als Zeiterscheinung. Ed. by K. Heymann. 1973. (Psychologische Praxis Ser.: No. 47). 64p. pap. 15.75 (3-8055-1556-1) S Karger.

Drogenkunde. Heinz A. Hoppe. 8th ed. (C). 1. 1975. 250.00 (3-11-003849-8); Vol. 2. 1977. 100.00 (3-11-006660-2) De Gruyter.

Drogenpraevention: Der Strafrechtliche Beitrag. H. U. Stoos. 1978. (Sozialmedizinische und Paedagogische Jugendkunde Ser.: Vol. 15). (GER., Illus.). 21.00 (3-8055-2874-4) S Karger.

Droit a la Sante: Au-Dela de la Grossesse et de la Reproduction. Jennifer Kitts & Janet Hatcher Roberts. 1996. LC 96-980323.Tr. of Health Gap. (FRE., Illus.). x, 257p. pap. (0-88936-796-5) IDRC-CRDI CAN. *Dist:* Stylus Pub VA.

Droit & Genie Genetique. Ed. by S. Soumastre et al. 1994. 190p. 44.00 (2-906077-47-X) Elsevier.

Drug Absorption Enhancement: Concepts, Possibilities, Limitations, & Trends. Ed. by A. G. De Boer. 1994. LC 93-38330. (Drug Targeting & Delivery Ser.: Vol. 3). 430p. text 146.00 (3-7186-5492-X) Gordon & Breach.

Drug Abuse. 1990. (PAHO Scientific Publications: No. 522). (ENG & SPA.). xi, 198p. pap. text 50.00 (92-75-11522-2, 1610522) World Health.

Drug Abuse: A Family's Guide to Detection, Treatment & Education. A. James Giannini. 1999. LC 98-42762. (Illus.). 300p. pap. 12.95 (1-885987-11-0, Health Info Pr) Practice Mgmt Info.

Drug Abuse: Foundation for a Psychosocial Approach. George J. Hubba. Ed. by Seymour Eiseman & John Wingard. 1984. 268p. (C). pap. text 33.95 (0-89503-039-X) Baywood Pub.

Drug Abuse: Its Natural History & the Effectiveness of Current Treatments. Marvin R. Burt. 1979. LC 77-13464. 362p. text 44.95 (0-87073-995-6) Transaction Pubs.

Drug Abuse: Why It Happens & How to Prevent It. Russel R. Allinson. 1984. LC 84-7369. 130p. (Orig.). pap. 9.95 (0-9612990-1-0) Valley Publishing.

Drug Abuse & Alcoholism: Current Critical Issues. Ed. by Sidney Cohen. 1981. LC 79-25648. 62p. pap. text 9.95 (0-917724-10-0) Haworth Pr.

Drug Abuse & Drug Counseling. Thomas Weisman. 1974. LC 73-17748. reprint ed. 20.00 (0-87668-125-9) Aronson.

Drug Abuse & Social Policy in America: The War That Must Be Won Barry Stimmel. 1996. LC 95-52541. 228p. pap., tchr. ed. 19.95 (0-7890-0128-4) Haworth Pr.

Drug Abuse & Society: The Indian Scenario. Saroj Prashant. 1993. (Illus.). xii, 219p. 17.95 (1-881338-34-7) Nataraj Bks.

Drug Abuse & the American Adolescent. 1986. lib. bdg. 79.95 (0-8490-3520-1) Gordon Pr.

Drug Abuse & the Elderly: An Annotated Bibliography. Douglas H. Ruben. 1984. LC 83-20463. 269p. 35.00 (0-8108-1677-6) Scarecrow.

Drug Abuse & the Law Sourcebook, Set. Gerald F. Uelmen & Victor G. Haddox. 1983. LC 81-21711. (Criminal Law Ser.). ring bd. 240.00 (0-87632-370-0) West Group.

Drug Abuse Bibliography for 1970. Compiled by Jean C. Advena. 1971. LC 79-116588. 202p. 10.00 (0-87875-016-9) Whitston Pub.

Drug Abuse Bibliography for 1971. Compiled by Jean C. Advena. 1972. LC 79-116588. 451p. 15.00 (0-87875-025-8) Whitston Pub.

Drug Abuse Bibliography for 1974. Compiled by Charles W. Triche, III & Diane Samson Triche. 1976. LC 79-116588. 456p. 18.00 (0-87875-077-0) Whitston Pub.

Drug Abuse Bibliography for 1976. Compiled by Charles W. Triche, III & Diane Samson Triche. 1979. LC 79-116588. (Annual Bibliography Ser.: No. 7). 386p. 22.50 (0-87875-127-0) Whitston Pub.

Drug Abuse Bibliography for 1977. Whitston Publishing Company Inc. Staff. 1980. LC 79-116588. 734p. 42.50 (0-87875-176-9) Whitston Pub.

Drug Abuse Bibliography for 1978-1979. 1983. 1863p. Pt. I. 50.00 (0-87875-269-2); Pt. II. 50.00 (0-87875-270-6) Whitston Pub.

Drug Abuse Bibliography for 1983, Vol. 14. Compiled by Polly T. Goode. 1986. LC 79-116588. xxiii, 478p. 45.00 (0-87875-321-4) Whitston Pub.

Drug Abuse Bibliography for 1984. Compiled by Polly T. Goode. 1987. LC 79-116588. 763p. 63.50 (0-87875-322-2) Whitston Pub.

Drug Abuse Bibliography for 1986. Compiled by Bonnie L. Clements. 1989. LC 79-116588. 1240p. 120.00 (0-87875-372-9) Whitston Pub.

Drug Abuse Bibliography for 1991. Compiled by Bonnie L. Clements. 1993. LC 79-116588. 601p. 65.00 (0-87875-445-8) Whitston Pub.

Drug Abuse Bibliography for 1987. Compiled by Bonnie L. Clements. 1991. LC 79-116588. 695p. 75.00 (0-87875-406-7) Whitston Pub.

Drug Abuse Bibliography for 1988. Compiled by Bonnie L. Clements. 1991. LC 79-116588. 791p. 85.00 (0-87875-412-1) Whitston Pub.

Drug Abuse Bibliography for 1980, No. 10. Compiled by Elizabeth Goode. 1984. LC 79-116588. xxxii, 689p. 48.50 (0-87875-285-4) Whitston Pub.

Drug Abuse Bibliography for 1989. Compiled by Bonnie L. Clements. 1992. xxxiv, 593p. 65.00 (0-87875-434-2) Whitston Pub.

Drug Abuse Bibliography for 1972. Compiled by Jean C. Advena. 1974. LC 79-116588. 514p. 18.00 (0-87875-046-0) Whitston Pub.

Drug Abuse Bibliography for 1973. Compiled by Jean C. Advena. 1975. LC 79-116588. xlii, 410p. 18.00 (0-87875-057-6) Whitston Pub.

Drug Abuse Bibliography for 1978-1979, Set. Compiled by Elizabeth Goode. 1983. 1546p. 100.00 (0-87875-222-6) Whitston Pub.

Drug Abuse Counselor. Jack Rudman. 1994. (Career Examination Ser.: C-2725). pap. 29.95 (0-8373-2725-3) Nat Learn.

Drug Abuse Education Group Leader. Jack Rudman. 1994. (Career Examination Ser.: C-1259). pap. 29.95 (0-8373-1259-0) Nat Learn.

Drug Abuse Educator. Jack Rudman. 1994. (Career Examination Ser.: C-1597). pap. 29.95 (0-8373-1597-2) Nat Learn.

Drug Abuse from the Family Perspective. 1986. lib. bdg. 79.95 (0-8490-3511-2) Gordon Pr.

Drug Abuse Group Worker. Jack Rudman. 1994. (Career Examination Ser.: C-1260). pap. 27.95 (0-8373-1260-4) Nat Learn.

Drug Abuse Handbook. Steven B. Karch. 1997. LC 97-45100. 1152p. 110.00 (0-8493-2637-0) CRC Pr.

Drug Abuse in Sports: An Annotated Bibliography. Betty Weiner. 1985. (CompuBibs Ser.: No. 10). 34p. pap. 10.00 (0-914791-09-5, 997) Vantage Info.

Drug Abuse Is a Major Problem. Ted Kowalski. 1994. (C). pap. text (0-8013-1333-3) Longman.

Drug Abuse, Mental Health & Delinquency. 1986. lib. bdg. 79.95 (0-8490-3499-X) Gordon Pr.

Drug Abuse Prevention & Community Readiness: Training Facilitator's Manual. Joseph Wheeler & Elaine Cardenas. 1998. (Illus.). 325p. (C). pap. text 45.00 (0-7881-7370-7) DIANE Pub.

Drug Abuse Rehabilitation Counselor. Jack Rudman. 1994. (Career Examination Ser.: C-2929). pap. 29.95 (0-8373-2929-9) Nat Learn.

Drug Abuse Secretarial Aide. Jack Rudman. 1994. (Career Examination Ser.: C-1261). pap. 23.95 (0-8373-1261-2) Nat Learn.

Drug Abuse Sourcebook: Basic Consumer Health Information about Illicit Substances of Abuse & the Diversion of Prescription Medications. Ed. by Karen Bellenir. 2nd ed. 2000. LC 00-55071. (Health Reference Ser.). (Illus.). xii, 629p. lib. bdg. 78.00 (0-7808-0242-X) Omnigraphics Inc.

Drug Abuse Technician. Jack Rudman. 1994. (Career Examination Ser.: C-1405). pap. 27.95 (0-8373-1405-4) Nat Learn.

Drug Abuse Technician Trainee. Jack Rudman. 1994. (Career Examination Ser.: C-1406). pap. 23.95 (0-8373-1406-2) Nat Learn.

Drug Abuse Treatment. Ed. by Ronald R. Watson. 1992. LC 92-1691. (Drug & Alcohol Abuse Reviews Ser.: No. 4). (Illus.). 224p. 89.50 (0-89603-233-7) Humana.

Drug Abuse Treatment: The Implementation of Innovative Approaches, 45. Ed. by Frank M. Tims et al. 1994. LC 94-11221. (Contributions in Criminology & Penology Ser.: No. 45). 280p. 72.50 (0-313-28906-9, Greenwood Pr) Greenwood.

Drug Abuse Treatment Client Characteristics. 1994. (Illus.). 105p. (Orig.). (C). pap. text 30.00 (0-7881-0433-0) DIANE Pub.

Drug Abuse Treatment Evaluation: Strategies, Progress, & Prospects. 1986. lib. bdg. 250.00 (0-8490-3504-X) Gordon Pr.

Drug Abuse Treatment in Prisons & Jails. 1995. lib. bdg. 253.95 (0-8490-6812-6) Gordon Pr.

Drug Abuse Treatment System: Prospects for Reform. John G. Haaga & Elizabeth A. McGlynn. 1993. LC 93-1445. pap. text 13.00 (0-8330-1377-7, MR-226-DPRC) Rand Corp.

Drug Abusers in Prisons: Managing Their Health Problems: Report on a WHO Meeting. 1990. (WHO Regional Publications: No. 27). 52p. pap. text 10.00 (92-890-1118-1, 1310027) World Health.

Drug Action in the Central Nervous System. Paul M. Carvey. 1997. LC 97-14183. (Illus.). 432p. text 57.50 (0-19-509333-X); pap. text 32.50 (0-19-509334-8) OUP.

Drug Addict As a Patient. Marie Nyswander. 1956. LC 55-12227. 192p. text 56.00 (0-8089-0351-9, 793150, Grune & Strat) Harcrt Hlth Sci Grp.

***Drug Addict Trivia Game: Drug Prevention Game.** Ed. by Thomas J. Rundquist. 2001. (Illus.). 47p. pap. text 29.96 (1-884239-55-2) Nova Media.

Drug Addiction: The Problem, Treatment Services Development & Management. Richard E. Isralowitz & Darwin Telias. 1998. LC 98-14908. 176p. 60.00 (0-275-96128-1, Praeger Pubs) Greenwood.

Drug Addiction & AIDS. Ed. by N. Loimer et al. 1991. (Illus.). 431p. 82.95 (0-387-82298-4) Spr-Verlag.

C
D

Drug Addiction & Related Clinical Problems. Ed. by Alessandro Tagliamonte & Icro Maremmani. 1995. LC 95-5162. (Illus.). 250p. 77.95 (*3-211-82674-2*) Spr-Verlag.

Drug Addiction Research & the Health of Women. Ed. by Cora L. Wetherington & Adele B. Roman. 1999. (Illus.). 581p. pap. text 50.00 (*0-7881-8053-3*) DIANE Pub.

Drug Addiction Research & the Health of Women: Executive Summary. Ed. by Cora L. Wetherington & Adele B. Roman. 1999. 142p. pap. text 25.00 (*0-7881-8054-1*) DIANE Pub.

Drug Addiction Treatment Research: German & American Perspectives. Ed. by Gerhard Buhringer & Jerome J. Platt. 1992. 550p. (C). lib. bdg. 94.50 (*0-89464-628-1*) Krieger.

Drug Addicts: Are They Out of Control? John C. Brady, II. Ed. by Nancy McFall. 1991. LC 90-71961. 240p. (Orig.). (C). 14.95 (*0-936029-24-2*); pap. text 10.95 (*0-936029-25-0*) Western Bk Journ.

Drug Allergy & Protocols for Management of Drug Allergies. Roy Patterson et al. 2nd ed. 1995. LC 94-69157. 43p. (C). pap. 38.50 (*0-936587-06-7*) OceanSide Pubns.

Drug Analysis: Keynote & Plenary Papers from the First International Symposium, June 1983, Brussels, Belgium. Ed. by A. F. Fell. 1984. 200p. pap. 22.00 (*0-08-031441-4*, Pergamon Pr) Elsevier.

Drug & Alcohol Abuse: A Clinical Guide to Diagnosis & Treatment. Marc A. Schuckit. 4th ed. 1995. LC 94-48434. (Critical Issues in Psychiatry Ser.). (Illus.). 390p. (C). text 41.00 (*0-306-44864-5*, Kluwer Plenum) Kluwer Academic.

Drug & Alcohol Abuse in Children & Adolescence. Ed. by David W. Kaplan. 1987. (Journal: Vol. 14, No. 1-2, 1987). (Illus.). 92p. pap. 48.00 (*3-8055-4631-9*) S Karger.

Drug & Alcohol Abuse in the Workplace: A Guide to the Issues. J. Michael Walsh & Stephen C. Yohay. 1987. LC 87-60167. (Monograph Ser.). (Orig.). pap. 25.00 (*0-916559-08-4*) EPF.

Drug & Alcohol Abuse Prevention. Ed. by Ronald R. Watson. 1991. LC 90-28904. (Drug & Alcohol Abuse Reviews Ser.: No. 1). 418p. 104.50 (*0-89603-179-9*) Humana.

Drug & Alcohol Community Coordinator. Jack Rudman. 1994. (Career Examination Ser.: C-2776). pap. 34.95 (*0-8373-2776-8*) Nat Learn.

Drug & Alcohol Counselor. Jack Rudman. 1994. (Career Examination Ser.: C-2741). pap. 29.95 (*0-8373-2741-5*) Nat Learn.

Drug & Alcohol Program Coordinator. Jack Rudman. 1994. (Career Examination Ser.: C-2775). pap. 34.95 (*0-8373-2775-X*) Nat Learn.

Drug & Alcohol Rehabilitation Programs Industry. 2000. 20p. 59.00 (*1-891084-41-0*) Mktdata Ent.

Drug & Enzyme Targeting, Pt. A. Ed. by Sidney P. Colowick & Nathan O. Kaplan. 1985. (Methods in Enzymology Ser.: Vol. 112). text 188.00 (*0-12-182012-2*) Acad Pr.

Drug & Hormonal Resistance in Breast Cancer: Cellular & Molecular Mechanics. Robert B. Dickson. Ed. by M. E. Lippman. 1995. 448p. (C). 95.00 (*0-13-224858-1*) P-H.

Drug & Hormone Resistance in Neoplasia: Basic Concepts, Vol. I. Ed. by Nicholas Bruchovsky & James H. Goldine. 1983. LC 96-2084. (Illus.). 208p. 118.00 (*0-8493-6516-3*, RC271, CRC Reprint) Franklin.

Drug & Natural Medicine Advisor: The Complete Guide to Alternative & Conventional Medications. Time-Life Books Editors. 1999. LC 97-3309. (Illus.). 896p. (Orig.). pap. 19.95 (*0-7835-4938-5*) Time-Life.

Drug Bioscreening: Drug Evaluation Techniques in Pharmacology. Emmanuel Thompson. 1990. LC 89-70662. 384p. 40.00 (*0-89573-730-2*, Wiley-VCH) Wiley.

Drug Biotechnology Regulation: Scientific Basis & Practices. Yuan-Yuan H. Chiu & John L. Gueriguian. 1991. (Bioprocess Technology Ser.: Vol. 13). (Illus.). 568p. text 199.00 (*0-8247-8420-0*) Dekker.

Drug Calculations: Process & Problems for Clinical Practice. Meta Brown & Joyce L. Mulholland. 5th ed. 1995. LC 95-39518. (Illus.). 336p. (C). (gr. 13). pap. text 29.00 (*0-8151-0508-8*, 24413) Mosby Inc.

Drug Calculations for Nurses. 256p. pap. (*0-340-60479-4*) E A GBR. *Dist:* Routldge.

Drug Card Workbook. Perspective Press. 2000. 160p. (Orig.). (C). pap., wbk. ed. 20.95 (*0-89582-540-6*) Morton Pub.

Drug Cards for Pharmaceutical Reference. Saunders. 2000. pap. text 31.95 (*0-7216-8567-6*) Saunders.

Drug Charts in Basic Pharmacology. Jonathan D. Baum et al. 2000. 310p. pap. text 18.95 (*0-942447-37-9*) Med Surveill.

Drug Classification Cards. Springhouse Publishing Company Staff. 2nd ed. 1995. 160p. 26.95 (*0-87434-783-1*) Springhouse Corp.

Drug Comparison Handbook. Robert Reilly. 3rd rev. ed. 1998. LC 98-232107. 550p. (C). per. 41.95 (*1-56930-075-5*) Delmar.

Drug Consultant & Interaction Guide. Mark C. Rathgerber. 1992. (C). (gr. 13). 15.95 (*1-878060-04-X*) GW Medical.

Drug Control & System Improvement: Formula Grant Application, Hawaii. 1993. (Illus.). 125p. (Orig.). (C). pap. text 30.00 (*1-56806-499-3*) DIANE Pub.

Drug Control Policy: Essays in Historical & Comparative Perspective. Ed. by William O. Walker, III. 1992. LC 91-45160. (Issues in Policy History Ser.: Vol. 1). 184p. pap. 20.95 (*0-271-00843-1*) Pa St U Pr.

Drug Data Handbook. 244p. pap. text (*0-86471-038-0*) Adis Intl NZL. *Dist:* Lppncott W & W.

Drug Delivery Devices: Fundamentals & Applications. Ed. by Praveen Tyle. 1988. (Drugs & the Pharmaceutical Sciences Ser.: Vol. 32). (Illus.). 640p. text 255.00 (*0-8247-7836-7*) Dekker.

Drug Delivery in Cancer Treatment II. Ed. by L. Domellof. 1989. (ESO Monographs). (Illus.). 107p. 108.00 (*0-387-51055-9*) Spr-Verlag.

Drug Delivery in Cancer Treatment III: Home Care Symptom Control, Economy, Brain Tumours. Ed. by L. Domellof & U. Veronesi. 1990. (ESO Monographs). (Illus.). 125p. 118.00 (*0-387-52951-9*) Spr-Verlag.

Drug Delivery Systems. Vasant V. Ranade & Mannfred A. Hollinger. 1995. LC 95-17154. (CRC Pharmacology & Toxicology: Basic & Clinical Aspects Ser.). 384p. 139.95 (*0-8493-8542-3*, 8542) CRC Pr.

***Drug Delivery Systems: Technologies, Trends & Market Opportunities.** Pamela Bassett. Ed. by Susan C. DiClemente. 3rd rev. ed. 1998. (Illus.). 1542p. spiral bd. (*1-57936-118-8*, 997, D&MD Reports) International Business.

Drug Delivery Systems in Cancer Therapy. Ed. by Dennis M. Brown. 2001. (Cancer Drug Discovery & Development Ser.). 400p. 140.00 (*0-89603-888-2*) Humana.

***Drug Delivery to the Lung.** Ed. by Hans Bisgaard et al. 2001. (Lung Biology in Health & Disease Ser.). 511p. 175.00 (*0-8247-0541-6*) Dekker.

Drug Dependence: A Methodology for Evaluating Treatment & Rehabilitation. A. Arif et al. 1987. (Offset Publications: No. 98). 67p. pap. text 12.00 (*92-4-170098-X*, 1120098) World Health.

Drug Dependence & Alcohol-Related Problems: A Manual for Community Health Workers with Guidelines for Trainers. 1986. 38p. pap. text 9.00 (*92-4-154212-8*, 1150254) World Health.

Drug Dependence & Emotional Behavior: Neurophysiological & Neurochemical Approaches. A. V. Valdman. Tr. by L. R. Sandler from RUS. 1986. LC 86-8127. (Illus.). 510p. (C). text 162.00 (*0-306-10984-0*, Kluwer Plenum) Kluwer Academic.

Drug Depletion & Nutrient Replacement Therapy. Derrick DeSilva. 2000. 450p. pap. 29.95 (*1-930256-01-9*) Integratv Med Commn.

Drug Development. Ed. by Charles E. Hamner, Jr. 1982. 264p. 151.00 (*0-8493-6310-1*, RS122, CRC Reprint) Franklin.

Drug Development. Ed. by Charles E. Hamner. 2nd ed. 1990. 320p. 225.00 (*0-8493-6319-5*, RS192) CRC Pr.

Drug Development Assay Approaches: Including Molecular Imprinting & Biomarkers. Ed. by E. Reid & H. M. Hill. 1998. (Special Publications). 300p. (C). (*0-85404-748-4*) Royal Soc Chem GBR. *Dist:* Spr-Verlag.

Drug Development for Life Cycle Management in Women. Vanaja V. Ragavan & Judith Jones. 1998. LC 97-42810. 496p. 185.00 (*0-471-96850-1*) Wiley.

Drug Development Process: Increasing Efficiency & Cost-Effectiveness. Peter G. Welling et al. 1996. LC 96-24681. (Drugs And The Pharmaceutical Sciences ;: Vol. 76). (Illus.). 472p. text 175.00 (*0-8247-9727-2*) Dekker.

Drug, Device & Diagnostic Manufacturing: The Ultimate Resource Handbook. Carol DeSain. 2nd ed. 1992. 429p. 149.00 (*0-935184-38-4*) IHS Health Grp.

Drug, Diet & Disease, Vol. 1. Ed. by C. Ionnides & D. V. P. Lewis. 1995. LC 94-30694. (Biochemistry & Biotechnology Ser.). 304p. text 105.00 (*0-13-027400-3*) P-H.

Drug Dilemma. Sidney Cohen. 2nd ed. 1975. (Health, Physical Education & Recreation Ser.). 144p. 17.95 (*0-07-011587-7*); pap. text (*0-07-011588-5*) McGraw.

Drug Discovery: A Casebook & Analysis. Robert A. Maxwell & Shohreh B. Eckhardt. 1990. LC 90-4915. 463p. 129.50 (*0-89603-180-2*) Humana.

Drug Discovery & Development of Anti-Cancer Agents. Ed. by Michael Williams & Jeffrey B. Malick. 1987. LC 87-3343. (Illus.). 467p. 145.00 (*0-89603-108-X*) Humana.

Drug Discovery & Evaluation: Pharmacological Assays. H. Gerhard Vogel & Wolfgang H. Vogel. 1997. LC 96-27977. 757p. 199.00 (*3-540-60291-7*) Spr-Verlag.

Drug Discovery Approaches for Developing Cosmeceuticals - Advanced Skin Care & Cosmetic Products. 1997. (Biomedical Library). pap. (*1-57936-032-7*) Drug & Market Dev.

Drug Discovery from Nature. Ed. by S. Grabley & R. Thiericke. 2000. (Springer Desktop Editions in Chemistry Ser.). 348p. pap. 42.95 (*3-540-66947-7*) Spr-Verlag.

Drug Discovery from Nature. Ed. by Susanne Grabley & Ralf Thiericke. 1998. LC 98-42182. (Illus.). 366p. 129.00 (*3-540-64844-5*) Spr-Verlag.

Drug Discovery Technologies. Colin R. Clark & Walter H. Moos. 1990. 283p. 113.00 (*0-470-21604-2*) P-H.

***Drug Discovery Technologies & Strategies: Genomics, Protemics & the Need for Speed.** James W. Hawkins et al. Ed. by Lynn M. Savage. 2001. (Illus.). 53p. spiral bd. 595.00 (*1-57936-158-7*, 9013) International Business.

Drug Discovery Technology: Interdisciplinary Approaches to Accelerate Drug Development. Wendy Hori. 1997. (Biomedical Library). pap. 895.00 (*1-57936-023-8*) Drug & Market Dev.

Drug Disposition & Metabolism. Ed. by G. R. Wilkinson & M. D. Rawlins. 1985. text 225.00 (*0-85200-902-X*) Kluwer Academic.

Drug Dissolution & Bioavailability (Seminar Notes - Oct. 1993) 1994. 520p. ring bd. 144.95 (*1-56676-125-5*) CRC Pr.

Drug Dosage Calculations for the Emergency Care Provider. Alan A. Mikolaj. 1996. LC 96-16998. 156p. pap. text 49.00 (*0-8359-4994-X*) P-H.

Drug Dosage in Renal Insufficiency. Gunter Seyffart. 1991. 680p. (C). text 355.50 (*0-7923-0964-2*) Kluwer Academic.

Drug Dosages & Solutions. Geraldine A. Medici. 2nd ed. 1988. 384p. (C). pap. 36.40 (*0-8385-1775-7*, A1775-4) Appleton & Lange.

Drug Dosages & Solutions: A Workbook. Mary A. Norville. 3rd ed. 1994. LC 93-41308. (Illus.). 320p. (C). pap. 38.00 (*0-8385-1613-0*, A1613-7) P-H.

***Drug-Drug Interactions.** Rodrigues. 2001. (Drug & the Pharmaceutical Sciences Ser.). (*0-8247-0283-2*) Dekker.

Drug Dynamics for Analytical, Clinical & Biological Chemists. Benjamin J. Gudzinowicz. 1984. (Drugs & the Pharmaceutical Sciences Ser.: Vol. 26). (Illus.). 192p. text 135.00 (*0-8247-7239-3*) Dekker.

Drug Education. Daniel A. Girdano & Dorothy E. Dusek. 4th ed. 1987. 350p. (C). pap. text 32.18 net. (*0-07-554988-3*) McGraw.

Drug Education: Content & Methods. Daniel A. Girdano & Dorothy Dusek-Girgano. 3rd ed. 1980. (Illus.). 352p. (C). pap. text 12.00 (*0-394-34876-1*) Random.

Drug Education in Schools. Christine Eiser & R. J. Eiser. 1988. (Recent Research in Psychology Ser.). (Illus.). 156p. 69.95 (*0-387-96792-3*) Spr-Verlag.

Drug Education in Schools: The Need for New Impetus - Report by Advisory Council. HMSO Staff. 1993. 94p. pap. (*0-11-341081-6*, HM10816) Statnry Office GBR. *Dist:* Bernan Associates.

Drug Effects on Laboratory Test Results. Ed. by G. Siest. 1980. (Developments in Clinical Biochemistry Ser.: No. 2). (Illus.). 338p. text 148.50 (*90-247-2419-8*) Kluwer Academic.

Drug Effects on Psychomotor Performance. Randall C. Baselt. 2000. LC 00-133235. 475p. text 107.00 (*0-9626523-4-2*) Biomedical Pubns.

Drug Epidemiology & Post-Marketing Surveillance. B. L. Strom & G. P. Velo. 1992. (NATO Advanced Science Institutes Ser.: Vol. 224). (Illus.). 170p. (C). text 85.00 (*0-306-44099-7*, Kluwer Plenum) Kluwer Academic.

Drug Eruption Reference Manual. Jerome Z. Litt & Walter A. Pawlak, Jr. 1993. 470p. (*0-9634973-2-4*); 1993. 470p. (*0-9634973-3-2*); 1992. 400p. ring bd. 100.00 (*0-9634973-1-6*); 1992. 400p. ring bd. 100.00 (*0-9634973-0-8*); 4th ed. 1995. 670p. per. (*0-9634973-4-0*) Wal-Zac Ent.

***Drug Eruption Reference Manual.** Jerome Z. Litt. 6th ed. 2002. (Illus.). 500p. 148.95 (*1-84214-178-3*, Parthenon Pbng) CRC Pr.

Drug Eruption Reference Manual, 1997. Jerome Z. Litt. 6th ed. 1997. (Illus.). 536p. 163.95 (*1-85070-907-6*, Parthenon Pbng) CRC Pr.

***Drug Eruption Reference Manual on Disk.** J. Z. Litt. 2001. 74.95 (*1-84214-097-3*, Parthenon Pbng) CRC Pr.

Drug Eruption Reference Manual, 2000. Jerome Z. Litt. 5th ed. 2000. LC 99-58758. (Illus.). 712p. lib. bdg. 163.95 (*1-85070-788-X*, Parthenon Pbng) CRC Pr.

Drug Etiology of Agranulocytosis & Aplastic Anemia. David W. Kaufman et al. 1991. (Monographs in Epidemiology & Biostatistics: No. 18). (Illus.). 432p. text 89.00 (*0-19-505983-2*) OUP.

Drug Evaluation in Angina Pectoris. Ed. by Diegoi ARdissino et al. 1994. LC 94-12345. (Developments in Cardiovascular Medicine Ser.: Vol. 158). 288p. (C). text 133.50 (*0-7923-2897-3*) Kluwer Academic.

Drug Evaluations. American Medical Association, Department of Drugs Staff. 6th ed. 1986. 1770p. text 68.00 (*0-03-012647-9*) Saunders.

Drug-Exposed Infants: A Generation at Risk. 1994. (Illus.). 48p. (Orig.). (C). pap. text 15.00 (*0-7881-0270-2*) DIANE Pub.

Drug Facts & Comparisons. Facts and Comparisons Staff. 4080p. 279.00 (*0-932686-00-1*) Facts & Comparisons.

Drug Facts & Comparisons 1997. Steven K. Hebel. Date not set. 3400p. text 450.00 (*0-932686-04-4*); text 450.00 (*0-932686-06-0*) Lppncott W & W.

***Drug Facts & Comparisons 2002 Pocket Ver.** Ed. by Facts and Comparisons Staff. 6th ed. 2001. (Drug Facts & Comparisons). 1150p. per. 59.95 (*1-57439-115-1*) Facts & Comparisons.

Drug Formularies & Pharmaceutical Industry: Thriving in the Managed Care Era. Timothy F. Donohue & Curtis R. Sprouse. 1995. 179p. (Orig.). pap. 175.00 (*1-882615-23-9*) Parexel Intl.

Drug Free Parent Booklet. Joyce McKay et al. 1989. (Drug Free Ser.). pap. text 14.95 (*0-88671-296-3*, 5110) Am Guidance.

Drug Free Teachers Guide. Joyce L. McKay et al. 1989. (Drug Free Ser.). 29.95 (*0-88671-295-5*, 5101) Am Guidance.

Drug-Free Therapeutic Community: An Evaluation. Robert Brook & Paul Whitehead. 1980. LC 79-20477. 158p. 32.95 (*0-87705-383-9*, Kluwer Acad Hman Sci) Kluwer Academic.

Drug Guide for Critical Care & Emergency Nursing. April H. Vallerand & Judith H. Deglin. 1990. 500p. pap. 27.95 (*0-8036-8845-8*) Davis Co.

Drug Guide for Paramedics. Richard A. Cherry & Bryan Bledsoe. 2001. LC 00-58011. 288p. spiral bd. 15.00 (*0-13-028798-9*) P-H.

Drug Guide 2000. Medicode, Med-Index Division Staff. 1999. (C). 89.95 (*1-56337-307-6*) Thomson Learn.

***Drug Guide 2001.** Ingenix, Inc. Staff. pap. 99.95 (*1-56337-327-0*) Ingenix Inc.

Drug Guidebook 2000. St. Anthony's Publishing Staff. 1999. (C). pap. 64.00 (*1-56329-657-8*) Thomson Learn.

Drug Guidelines for Emergency Medical Intervention. Ed. by Gary A. Holt & Agatha Underhill. 1991. LC 90-63765. 152p. pap. 19.95 (*0-944496-16-4*) Precept Pr.

Drug Handbook: A Nursing Process Approach. Rosalinda A. Alfaro-Lefevre et al. 1991. 734p. (C). pap. 48.00 (*0-201-09278-6*) Addison-Wesley.

Drug Identification Bible. Tim Marnell. 1997. 700p. (Orig.). pap. 34.95 (*0-9635626-2-2*) Amera-Chem.

Drug Induced Dysfunction in Psychiatry. Matcheri S. Keshavan et al. 1991. 73.95 (*0-89116-961-X*) Hemisp Pub.

Drug-Induced Headache. Ed. by H. C. Diener & M. Wilkinson. 1988. (Advances in Applied Neurological Sciences Ser.: Vol. 5). (Illus.). 173p. 71.95 (*0-387-18762-6*) Spr-Verlag.

Drug-Induced Hepatic Injury. Ed. by B. H. Stricker & P. Spoelstra. 1985. (Drug Induced Disorders Ser.: Vol. 1). 314p. 165.00 (*0-444-90342-9*) Elsevier.

Drug-Induced Hepatic Injury. B. H. Stricker. 2nd rev. ed. 1992. LC 92-49765. (Drug Induced Disorders Ser.: Vol. 5). 550p. 207.00 (*0-444-81303-9*) Elsevier.

Drug-Induced Hepatotoxicity. George Feuer. Ed. by R. G. Cameron et al. 1996. (Handbook of Experimental Pharmacology Ser.: Vol. 121). (Illus.). 681p. 398.00 (*3-540-60201-1*) Spr-Verlag.

Drug-Induced Infertility & Sexual Dysfunction. Robert Forman et al. 1996. (Illus.). 165p. (C). text 54.95 (*0-521-46563-X*) Cambridge U Pr.

Drug-Induced Injury to the Digestive System. Ed. by M. Guslandi & P. C. Braga. 1993. LC 93-43578. (Illus.). 226p. 140.00 (*0-387-56656-2*) Spr-Verlag.

Drug Induced Liver Disease. Geoffrey C. Farrell et al. 1994. text (*0-443-04368-X*) Church.

Drug Induced Ocular Side Effects. Frederick T. Fraunfelder. 5th ed. 2000. LC 00-41391. 704p. 64.99 incl. cd-rom (*0-7506-7274-9*) Buttrwrth-Heinemann.

Drug-Induced Ocular Side Effects & Drug Interactions. F. T. Fraunfelder. 3rd ed. 1988. LC 88-13647. 675p. text 59.50 (*0-8121-1191-5*) Lppncott W & W.

Drug Induced Ocular Side Effects & Ocular Toxicology. Ed. by Otto Hockwin. 1987. (Concepts in Toxicology Ser.: Vol. 4). (Illus.). xii, 424p. 259.25 (*3-8055-4371-9*) S Karger.

Drug Industries: Index of New Information with Authors, Subjects & References. Science and Life Consultants Association Staff. 1997. 155p. 57.50 (*0-7883-1482-3*); pap. 47.50 (*0-7883-1483-1*) ABBE Pubs Assn.

Drug Information. Patrick M. Malone & Mosdell. 2nd ed. 2000. LC 00-55919. 716p. pap. 39.95 (*0-8385-1577-0*) McGraw-Hill Prof.

Drug Information: A Guide to Current Resources. Bonnie Snow. 2nd ed. LC 99-31655. (Illus.). xv, 752p. 1999. pap. 50.00 (*0-8108-3321-2*); 1998. text 75.00 (*0-8108-3320-4*) Scarecrow.

Drug Information for the Health Professions. Ed. by I. Welt. Vol. 1. 1969. xiv, 466p. text 348.00 (*0-677-13460-6*); Vol. 2. 1970. xii, 390p. text 348.00 (*0-677-14090-8*) Gordon & Breach.

Drug Information Handbook for the Criminal Justice Professional. Marcelline Burns et al. 1998. 925p. pap. 29.75 (*0-916589-60-9*) Lexi-Comp.

Drug Infusions in Anesthesiology. Ed. by Robert J. Fragen. 2nd ed. 1995. 304p. text 99.00 (*0-7817-0265-8*) Lppncott W & W.

Drug Injecting & HIV Infection: Global Dimensions & Local Responses. Ed. by Andrew Ball et al. 1998. LC 98-203733. (Social Aspects of AIDS Ser.). 294p. (*1-85728-824-6*) UCL Pr Ltd GBR. *Dist:* Taylor & Francis.

Drug Interaction Alert. D. I. Quinn & R. O. Day. 44p. pap. text (*0-86471-040-2*) Adis Intl NZL. *Dist:* Lppncott W & W.

Drug Interaction & Lethality Analysis. Ed. by Marshall N. Brunden et al. 1988. LC 87-30917. 192p. 100.00 (*0-8493-5743-8*, RM302, CRC Reprint) Franklin.

Drug Interaction Facts: Bundled Version. Facts and Comparisons Staff. Ed. by David S. Tatro. 1392p. cd-rom 160.00 (*1-57439-015-5*) Facts & Comparisons.

***Drug Interaction Facts 2002.** Ed. by Facts and Comparisons Staff. 2001. 1430p. per. 79.95 (*1-57439-111-9*) Facts & Comparisons.

Drug Interaction Studies During Drug Development. J. Kuhlmann. 1994. (Clinical Pharmacology Ser.: Vol. 11). (Illus.). 73p. text (3-88603-519-0) W Zuckschwerdt DEU. *Dist:* Scholium Intl.

Drug Interactions: Protecting Yourself from Dangerous Drug, Medication & Food Combinations. Melanie Apel Gordon. 1999. LC 98-44974. (Drug Abuse Prevention Library). (Illus.). 64p. (YA). (gr. 7-12). lib. bdg. 17.95 (0-8239-2825-X, DRINTE) Rosen Group.

Drug Interactions: The Effects of Alcohol & Meprobamate Applied Singly & Jointly in Human Subjects. Ed. by J. A. Carpenter. 1975. (Journal of Studies on Alcohol: Suppl. No. 7). 10.00 (0-911290-02-8) Rutgers Ctr Alcohol.

Drug Interactions & Updates. Philip D. Hansten & John R. Horn. 7th ed. 1991. xi, 500p. text 75.00 (0-8121-1381-0) Lppncott W & W.

Drug Interactions in Infectious Diseases. Ed. by Stephen C. Piscitelli & Keith A. Rodvold. 2000. LC 00-35037. (Infectious Disease Ser.). (Illus.). xii, 363p. 99.50 (0-89603-750-9) Humana.

Drug Interactions in Psychiatry. Domenic A. Ciraulo. 2nd ed. 1995. (Illus.). 352p. pap. 42.95 (0-683-01944-9) Lppncott W & W.

Drug Interactions Monographs, 1996: (Applied Therapeutics) Hansten. 1996. 70.00 (0-915486-29-6) Applied Therapeutics.

Drug Interference & Drug Management in Clinical Chemistry: Proceedings of the 3rd International Colloquium on Prospective Biology, Pont-a-Mousson, Oct. 1975. International Colloquium on Prospective Biology Staff. Ed. by D. S. Young & G. Siest. 1976. 250p. 85.25 (3-8055-2360-2) S Karger.

Drug Labeling in Developing Countries. 1993. (Illus.). 193p. (C). pap. text 50.00 (0-7881-0109-9) DIANE Pub.

Drug Legalization. Scott Barbour. 2000. LC 99-48084. (Current Controversies Ser.). 192p. pap. 13.96 (0-7377-0335-0, Greenhaven Pr) Gale.

Drug Library Teacher's Guide. rev. ed. 1999. LC 95-14144. (Illus.). 25p. (YA). (gr. 6-12). tchr. ed., ring bd. 7.15 (0-89490-963-0) Enslow Pubs.

Drug Lords... America's Pharmaceutical Cartel. Tonda R. Bian. 1998. LC 96-92687. (Illus.). 192p. (Orig.). per. 12.95 (0-9654568-0-3) No Barriers.

Drug Master Files: Global Harmonization of Quality Standards. H. Moller & Oeser. 1992. 66.00 (3-8047-1207-X) CRC Pr.

Drug Measurement & Drug Effect in Laboratory Health Science: Proceedings of the 4th International Colloquium on Prospective Biology, Pont-a-Mousson, October 1978. International Colloquium on Prospective Biology Staff. Ed. by G. Siest & D. S. Young. 1979. (Illus.). 115.75 (3-8055-3045-5) S Karger.

Drug Mechanisms. Ed. by M. E. Caplis et al. 1985. (Journal: Vol. 3, No. 2-3). (Illus.). 96p. pap. 73.25 (3-8055-4051-5) S Karger.

Drug Metabolism: Molecular Approaches & Pharmacological Implications: Proceedings of the 9th European Workshop on Drug Metabolism Held at Pont-a-Mousson, France June 11-15 1984. Ed. by G. Siest. 1985. (Illus.). 242p. 52.50 (0-08-031995-5, Pergamon Pr) Elsevier.

Drug Metabolism - Towards the Next Millennium. Ed. by N. Gooderhan et al. 1998. LC 97-75198. (Biomedical & Health Research Ser.: Vol. 25). 213p. 86.00 (90-5199-378-1) IOS Press.

Drug Metabolism Concepts. Ed. by Donald M. Jerina. 1977. LC 77-2279. (ACS Symposium Ser.: No. 44). 27.95 (0-8412-0370-9) Am Chemical.

***Drug Misuse.** Keene. 1996. pap. 35.95 (0-412-64280-8) Chapman & Hall.

Drug Monitoring & Pharmacokinetic Data. Hugo C. Pribor et al. 1980. LC 79-90657. 190p. 29.50 (0-930376-10-2) Chem-Orbital.

Drug-Nutrient Interactions. T. K. Basu. 1988. 180p. lib. bdg. 55.00 (0-7099-3203-0) Routledge.

Drug Permeation Enhancement: Theory & Applications. Ed. by Dean S. Hsieh. 1993. (Drugs & the Pharmaceutical Sciences Ser.: Vol. 62). (Illus.). 448p. text 199.00 (0-8247-9015-4) Dekker.

Drug Plants of India. V. S. Agarwal. 1984. (C). (0-7855-2276-X) Scientific GBR. *Dist:* St Mut.

Drug Policy & Human Nature: Psychological Perspectives on the Prevention, Management, & Treatment of Illicit Drug Abuse. Ed. by Warren K. Bickel & Richard J. DeGrandpre. 1996. LC 96-28284. (Illus.). 322p. 49.50 (0-306-45241-3, Kluwer Plenum) Kluwer Academic.

Drug Prescribing in Renal Failure: Dosing Guidelines for Adults. George R. Aronoff et al. 4th ed. 1999. LC 98-44099. 176p. (C). pap. text 28.00 (0-943126-76-2) Amer Coll Phys.

Drug Prevention - Just Say Now. Peter Stoker. 1992. 176p. pap. (1-85346-235-7) David Fulton GBR. *Dist:* Taylor & Francis.

Drug Prevention Curricula: A Guide to Selection & Implementation. 1995. 65p. (C). pap. text 25.00 (0-7881-2371-8) DIANE Pub.

Drug Prevention Curricula: A Guide to Selection & Implementation. 1991. lib. bdg. 75.00 (0-8490-5048-0) Gordon Pr.

Drug Problems in the Sociocultural Context a Basis for Policies & Programme Planning. G. Edwards & A Arif. 1980. (Public Health Papers: No. 73). 258p. pap. text 18.00 (92-4-130073-6, 1110073) World Health.

Drug Product Liability Marden G. Dixon & Frank C. Woodside. 1974. ring bd. 728.00 (0-8205-1257-5) Bender.

Drug Products for Clinical Trials: An International Guide to Formulation-Production-Quality Control. Ed. by Rhodes & Monkhouse. 1997. LC 97-31539. (Drugs & the Pharmaceutical Sciences Ser.: Vol. 87). (Illus.). 408p. text 185.00 (0-8247-9852-X) Dekker.

Drug Profile on Anabolic Steroids. rev. ed. 2000. 5.95 (0-89230-239-9) Do It Now.

Drug Profile on Cocaine. rev. ed. 2000. pap. 5.95 (0-89230-172-4) Do It Now.

Drug Profile on Drugs & Sexuality. rev. ed. 2000. 5.95 (0-89230-240-2) Do It Now.

Drug Profile on Heroin. rev. ed. 2000. pap. 5.95 (0-89230-176-7) Do It Now.

Drug Profile on Inhalants. rev. ed. 2000. pap. 5.95 (0-89230-174-0) Do It Now.

Drug Profile on Minor Tranquilizers. rev. ed. 2000. 5.95 (0-89230-238-0) Do It Now.

Drug-Protein Binding: Esteve Foundation Symposium I. Ed. by Marcus S. Reidenberg & Sergio Erill. 1985. LC 85-12479. (Clinical Pharmacology & Therapeutics Ser.: Vol. 6). 380p. 49.95 (0-275-90010-X, C0010, Praeger Pubs) Greenwood.

Drug Reactions & the Liver. Ed. by M. Davis et al. 1981. 300p. (C). pap. 69.00 (0-8464-1220-9) Beekman Pubs.

Drug Receptor Interactions in Antimicrobial Chemotherapy: Proceedings. Symposium, Vienna, Sept. 4-6, 1974. Ed. by J. Drews & F. E. Hahn. 1975. (Topics in Infectious Diseases Ser.: Vol. 1). (Illus.). 340p. 29.95 (0-387-81311-X) Spr-Verlag.

Drug Receptor Subtypes & Ingestive Behavior. Ed. by Steven J. Cooper & Peter G. Clifton. 1996. (Illus.). 416p. text 95.00 (0-12-187620-9) Acad Pr.

Drug Regimen Compliance. Jean-Michel Metry & Urs A. Meyer. 1999. LC 98-28130. (Illus.). 212p. (C). 155.00 (0-471-97122-7) Wiley.

Drug Regimen Review: A Process Guide for Pharmacists, 1992. Ed. by Gary Ermn. 2nd ed. 1992. 372p. ring bd. 83.00 (0-934322-11-2) Am Soc Consult Phar.

Drug Regulatory Affairs: Administrative Enforcement Regulations by the Food & Drug Administration. 2000. (Professional Ser.: Vol. 1). 300p. pap. text (1-893091-50-3, 2000(AE)300/091-50-3) F R Parker.

Drug Regulatory Affairs: Good Clinical Practices (GCP) Regulations of the Food & Drug Administration. 2000. 300p. pap. text (1-893091-03-1) F R Parker.

Drug Regulatory Affairs: Good Laboratory Practices (GLP) Regulations of the Food & Drug Administration. 2000. (Professional Ser.: Vol. 5). 300p. pap. text (1-893091-54-6, 2000(GL)300/091-54-6) F R Parker.

Drug Regulatory Affairs: Life Threatening Illness Drugs Regulations of the Food & Drug Administration. 2000. (Professional Ser.: Vol. 7). 300p. pap. text (1-893091-56-2, 2000(LT)300/091-57-2) F R Parker.

Drug Regulatory Affairs: Orphan Drug Regulations of the Office of Orphan Drugs Public Health Service. 2000. (Professional Ser.: Vol. 6). 300p. pap. text (1-893091-58-9, 2000(OD)300/091-57-9) F R Parker.

Drug-Related Problems in Geriatric Nursing Home Patients. James W. Cooper. 1991. (Pharmaceutical Sciences Ser.). 101p. text 39.95 (1-56024-085-7); pap. text 19.95 (1-56024-086-5) Haworth Pr.

Drug Research on Human Subjects: A Source Guide. 1991. lib. bdg. 76.00 (0-8490-4842-7) Gordon Pr.

Drug Residues in Food-Producing Animals. Ed. by Myron A. Mehlman & Jerry Brunton. 1980. LC 79-91220. 150p. pap. 22.00 (0-930376-11-0) Chem-Orbital.

Drug Residues in Foods: Pharmacology, Food Safety & Analysis. Nikolaos A. Botsoglou & Dimitrious J. Fletouris. 2000. LC 00-49718. (Food Science & Technology Ser.: Vol. 102). (Illus.). xv, 1194p. text 225.00 (0-8247-8959-8) Dekker.

Drug Resistance. Ed. by William N. Hait. 1996. LC 96-7538. (Cancer Treatment & Research Ser.: Vol. 87). 418p. (C). text 419.50 (0-7923-4022-1) Kluwer Academic.

Drug Resistance in Cancer: Mechanisms & Models. J. H. Goldie & A. J. Coldman. 1998. LC 97-41916. (Illus.). 256p. (C). text 85.00 (0-521-48273-9) Cambridge U Pr.

Drug Resistance in Cancer Therapy. Ed. by Robert F. Ozols. 1989. (C). text 168.50 (0-7923-0244-3) Kluwer Academic.

Drug Resistance in Leukemia & Lymphoma Ed. by R. Pieters et al. 2nd ed. 1997. (Advances in Blood Disorders Ser.). 504p. text 150.00 (3-7186-5934-4, Harwood Acad Pubs) Gordon & Breach.

Drug Resistance in Leukemia & Lymphoma 3. Ed. by G. J. Kaspers et al. 1999. LC 98-43929. (Advances in Experimental Medicine & Biology Ser.: Vol. 457). (Illus.). 638p. 165.00 (0-306-46055-6, Kluwer Plenum) Kluwer Academic.

Drug Resistance in Mammalian Cells Ed. by Radhey S. Gupta. 1989. Vol. I. LC 89-466. 304p. 159.00 (0-8493-6921-5, RC271); Vol. II. 320p. 173.00 (0-8493-6922-3, RC271) Franklin (CRC Reprint).

Drug Resistance in Oncology. Samuel D. Bernal. 1997. LC 97-22375. (Basic & Clinical Oncology Ser.: Vol. 13). (Illus.). 416p. text 185.00 (0-8247-9295-5) Dekker.

Drug Resistance in the Treatment of Cancer. Ed. by Herbert M. Pinedo & Giuseppe Giaccone. 1998. (Cancer Ser.). (Illus.). 339p. (C). text 105.00 (0-521-47321-7) Cambridge U Pr.

Drug Resistance on Leukemia & Lymphoma: The Clinical Value of Laboratory Studies. Ed. by G. J. Kaspers et al. 1993. LC 93-20039. 436p. text 201.00 (3-7186-5387-7) Gordon & Breach.

***Drug-Resistant Tuberculosis: From Molecules to Macro-Economics.** Ed. by P. D. O. Davies. 2001. LC 2001-52647. (Annals of the New York Academy of Sciences Ser.: Vol. 953). (1-57331-388-2); pap. (1-57331-389-0) NY Acad Sci.

Drug Safety Assessment in Clinical Trials. Gene Soquero Gilbert. 1993. (Statistics: Textbooks & Monographs: Vol. 138). (Illus.). 456p. text 195.00 (0-8247-8893-1) Dekker.

Drug Safety in Pregnancy. F. I. Caird & P. J. Scott. 1990. (Drug Induced Disorders Ser.: No. C1). xxii,520p. 311.50 (0-444-90362-3, Excerpta Medica) Elsevier.

Drug Screen Manual: The Tests, the Technology, the Risks, the Reality. John Mrozek. 1998. LC 98-234088. 64p. pap. 18.00 (0-87364-982-6) Paladin Pr.

Drug Side Effects, Drug-Drug Interactions, Drug Resistance, & Patient Compliance in the Management of Hypertension. Ed. by Michael J. Horan & Lot B. Page. 1988. LC 73-2002. (Hypertension Ser.: No. 5). 106p. 12.00 (0-87493-654-3) Am Heart.

Drug Stability: Principles & Practices. Jens T. Carstensen. 2nd exp. rev. ed. 1995. LC 95-12770. (Drugs & the Pharmaceutical Sciences Ser.: Vol. 68). (Illus.). 616p. text 185.00 (0-8247-9635-7) Dekker.

***Drug Stability: Principles & Practices.** Ed. by Christopher T. Rhodes et al. 3rd ed. 2000. LC 00-31584. (Drugs & the Pharmaceutical Sciences Ser.: Vol. 107). (Illus.). 688p. text 185.00 (0-8247-0376-6) Dekker.

Drug Studies in the Elderly: Methodological Concerns. N. R. Cutler & P. K. Narang. 1986. LC 86-18738. (Illus.). 464p. (C). text 120.00 (0-306-42311-1, Kluwer Plenum) Kluwer Academic.

Drug Surveillance: International Cooperation Past, Present, & Future: Proceedings of the XXVIIth CIOMS Conference. Ed. by Z. Bankowski & J. F. Dunne. 1994. LC 95-155443. viii, 198p. pap. text 25.00 (92-9036-059-3, 1830027) World Health.

Drug Susceptibility in the Chemotherapy of Mycobacterial Infections. Leonid Heifets. 1991. 224p. 149.00 (0-8493-6716-6, QR201) CRC Pr.

Drug Synergism & Dose-Effect Data Analysis. Ronald J. Tallarida. 2000. LC 00-31433. 264p. (C). 59.95 (1-58488-045-7, Chap & Hall CRC) CRC Pr.

Drug-Taking Behavior among School-Aged Youth: The Alaska Experience & Comparisons with Lower-48 States. Intro. by Bernard Segal. 1990. LC 89-29119. (Drugs & Society Ser.: Vol. 4, Nos. 1-2). (Illus.). 168p. text 39.95 (0-86656-966-9) Haworth Pr.

***Drug Targeting: Organ-Specific Strategies.** Grietje Molema & Dirk Meijer. 2001. 300p. 130.00 (3-527-29989-0) Wiley.

Drug Targeting: Strategies, Principles & Applications. Ed. by G. E. Francis & Christina Delgado. 2000. (Methods in Molecular Medicine Ser.: Vol. 25). (Illus.). 320p. 99.50 (0-89603-531-X) Humana.

***Drug Targeting Technology.** Ed. by Hans Schreier. 2001. LC 2001-42174. (Drugs & the Pharmaceutical Sciences Ser.). (Illus.). x, 294p. 150.00 (0-8247-0580-7) Dekker.

Drug Testing. John J. Fay. 1990. 432p. 54.95 (0-409-90239-X) Buttrwrth-Heinemann.

Drug Testing: A Workplace Guide to Designing Practical Policies & Winning Arbitrations. 1990. LC 90-15136. 95.00 (1-55871-186-4, BSP 176) BNA PLUS.

Drug Testing: Issues & Options. Ed. by Robert H. Coombs & Louis J. West. 1991. 272p. text 47.95 (0-19-505414-8) OUP.

Drug Testing: What Every Mariner Should Know about Chemical Tests for Drugs & Alcohol. Alan E. Spears. 1996. (Sea Code Ser.). 96p. (Orig.). pap. text 12.95 (0-939837-04-8) Paradise Cay Pubns.

Drug Testing in Hair. Ed. by Pascal Kintz. 1996. LC 95-47255. 304p. 94.95 (0-8493-8112-6) CRC Pr.

Drug Testing in Sports. Ed. by David L. Black. 1995. 238p. (Orig.). pap. 60.00 (0-912474-20-3) Preston Pubns.

Drug Testing in the Workplace: A Resource Manual & Benchmarking Report on Nationwide Practices & Trends. Executive KnowledgeWorks Staff. 1987. (Illus.). 300p. ring bd. 550.00 (0-943353-02-5) Exec Knowledge.

Drug Testing Legal Manual Kevin B. Zeese. 1988. LC 87-37516. (Criminal Law Ser.). ring bd. 210.00 (0-87632-586-X) West Group.

Drug Testing Methods Assessment & Evaluation. Tom Mieczkowski. 1999. LC 98-51465. (Methods in Analytical Toxicology Ser.). 392p. 69.95 (0-8493-7884-2) CRC Pr.

Drug Testing Programs by Public Employers: Suggested Guidelines. 1988. 12p. pap. 3.95 (0-89707-380-0, 533-0035-01) Amer Bar Assn.

***Drug Therapy & Breastfeeding.** Thomas Hale. 2002. LC 2001-56117. (Illus.). 100p. lib. bdg. 44.95 (1-84214-110-4, Parthenon Pbng) CRC Pr.

Drug Therapy & the Elderly: A Complete Guide for Healthcare Professionals to Optimizing Drug Therapy for Elderly Clients. Alvin K. Swonger & Patricia M. Burbank. 1995. LC 94-29758. (Illus.). 344p. (C). pap. text 47.95 (0-86720-716-7, 716-7) Jones & Bartlett.

Drug Therapy Decision Making Guide. Marc S. Levine et al. 1995. (Illus.). 574p. pap. text 49.95 (0-7216-4215-2) Saunders.

Drug Therapy for Asthma: Research & Clinical Practice. Murphy. Ed. by John Jenne. 1987. (Lung Biology in Health & Disease Ser.: Vol. 31). (Illus.). 1152p. text 295.00 (0-8247-7633-X) Dekker.

Drug Therapy for Behavior Disorders: An Introduction. Kenneth D. Gadow et al. 1991. (Psychology Practitioner Guidebooks Ser.). 192p. text (0-08-034950-1); pap. text (0-08-034949-8) PPI GBR. *Dist:* Elsevier.

Drug Therapy for Headache. Ed. by Michael Gallagher. 1990. (Infectious Disease & Therapy Ser.: Vol. 6). (Illus.). 296p. text 145.00 (0-8247-8179-1) Dekker.

Drug Therapy in Dialysis Patients. Ed. by K. Schaefer & Eberhard Ritz. 1986. (Journal: Vol. 3, Nos. 1-3, 1985). (Illus.). 97.50p. pap. 89.75 (3-8055-4288-7) S Karger.

Drug Therapy in Emergency Medicine. Ed. by Joseph P. Ornato & Edgar R. Gonzalez. 1990. (Illus.). 607p. text (0-443-08599-4) Church.

Drug Therapy in Old Age. Charles F. George. 1998. LC 97-21352. 686p. 285.00 (0-471-94149-2) Wiley.

Drug Therapy in Pregnancy. Jerome Yankowitz & Jennifer R. Niebyl. 3rd ed. 2001. LC 00-52016. 336p. text 49.95 (0-683-30708-8) Lppncott W & W.

Drug Therapy in Reproductive Endocrinology. Jean Ginsburg. 1996. (Illus.). 400p. (0-340-61385-8) E A GBR. *Dist:* OUP.

Drug Therapy in Rheumatology Nursing Sarah Ryan. 1999. 298p. pap. text (1-86156-114-8) Whurr Pub.

Drug Therapy of the Rheumatic Diseases see Treatment of the Rheumatic Diseases: Companion to the Textbook of Rheumatology

Drug Toxicity & Metabolism in Pediatrics. Ed. by Sam Kacew. 1989. 320p. lib. bdg. 190.00 (0-8493-4564-2, RJ560) CRC Pr.

Drug Toxicity in Embryonic Development I: Advances in Understanding Mechanisms of Birth Defects. Robert J. Kavlock & George P. Daston. 1996. LC 96-24471. (Illus.). Vol. I. 624p. 445.00 (3-540-61259-9); Vol. II. 485p. 398.50 (3-540-61261-0) Spr-Verlag.

Drug Toxicodynamics. D. E. Johnson. Date not set. (Drugs & the Pharmaceutical Sciences Ser.). (0-8247-9873-2) Dekker.

Drug Toxicokinetics. Ed. by Peter G. Welling & Felix A. De La Iglesia. 1993. LC 93-16817. (Drug & Chemical Toxicology Ser.: Vol. 9). (Illus.). 432p. text 199.00 (0-8247-9019-7) Dekker.

Drug Transport Across the Blood-Brain Barrier: In Vitro & In Vivo Techniques. Ed. by A. G. De Boer & Win Sutanto. 1997. 236p. text (90-5702-032-7) GBSP NLD. *Dist:* Gordon & Breach.

Drug Treatment Considerations in the Elderly. 112p. pap. text (0-86471-055-0) Adis Intl NZL. *Dist:* Lppncott W & W.

Drug Treatment in Dementia. Roy Jones. 2000. LC 99-88086. (Illus.). 128p. pap. 41.95 (0-632-05492-1) Blackwell Sci.

Drug Treatment in Intestinal Helminthiasis. A. Davis. 1973. pap. text 16.00 (92-4-156036-3, 1150035) World Health.

Drug Treatment in Obstetrics: A Handbook of Prescribing. D. F. Hawkins et al. 2nd ed. 1991. (Illus.). 320p. (Orig.). (C). (gr. 13). pap. 66.95 (0-412-34900-0) Chapman & Hall.

Drug Treatment in Psychiatry. Trevor Silverstone & Paul Turner. (Social & Psychological Aspects of Medical Practice Ser.). 4th rev. ed. 1988. 304p. 29.95 (0-415-00264-8); 5th ed. 1995. LC 94-9633. 288p. (C). pap. 31.95 (0-415-10610-9, B4113); 5th ed. 1994. LC 94-9633. 288p. (C). 89.95 (0-415-10609-5, B4108) Routledge.

Drug Treatment of Hyperlipidemia. Ed. by Basil M. Rifkind. 1991. (Fundamental & Clinical Cardiology Ser.: Vol. 1). (Illus.). 280p. text 125.00 (0-8247-8512-6) Dekker.

Drug Treatment of Migraine & Other Headaches. Ed. by H. C. Diener. 2000. LC 00-23281. (Monographs in Clinical Neuroscience: Vol. 17). (Illus.). x, 371p. 191.50 (3-8055-6971-8) S Karger.

Drug Treatment of Sexual Dysfunction. Ed. by T. A. Ban & F. A. Freyhan. 1980. (Modern Problems of Pharmacopsychiatry Ser.: Vol. 15). (Illus.). vi, 194p. 85.25 (3-8055-2906-6) S Karger.

***Drug Treatment Practice in Diabetes Mellitus During 1975-1994: Population-Based Pharmaco-Epidemiological Studies.** Jan Stalhammar. 2000. (Comprehensive Summaries of Uppsala Dissertations from the Faculty of Medicine: No. 976). (Illus.). 61p. (Orig.). pap. (91-554-4869-0) Uppsala Universitet SWE. *Dist:* Coronet Bks.

Drug Use & Abuse. Stephen A. Maisto. 2nd ed. 1994. (C). pap. text, tchr. ed. 49.75 (0-15-502524-4) Harcourt Coll Pubs.

Drug Use & Abuse. Gerard Joseph Connors et al. 3rd ed. 1998. LC 98-85987. (Illus.). xv, 480p. (C). pap. 72.50 (0-15-508356-2) Harcourt Coll Pubs.

C
D

Drug Use & Abuse: Instructor's Manual & Test Bank. Maisto. 3rd ed. 1998. (C). pap. text, tchr. ed. 30.00 (*0-15-507148-3*) Harcourt Coll Pubs.

Drug Use & Psychological Theory. Ed. by Stanley W. Sadava. 1987. LC 87-14929. (Drugs & Society Ser.: Vol. 1, No. 4). 126p. text 3.95 (*0-86656-678-3*) Haworth Pr.

Drug Use in America: Problem in Perspective & Report of National Commission on Marijuana & Drug Abuse. Shafer. 1975. text 30.00 (*0-8422-7239-9*) Irvington.

Drug Use in America: Social, Cultural & Political Perspectives. Peter Venturelli. 1994. (Health Science Ser.). (Illus.). 352p. (C). pap. text 41.95 (*0-86720-752-3*, 752-3) Jones & Bartlett.

Drug Use in Assisted Suicide & Euthanasia. Ed. by Margaret Pabst Battin & Arthur G. Lipman. 1996. LC 95-49632. (Journal of Pharmaceutical Care in Pain & Symptom Control Ser.: Vol. 3, Nos. 3/4 & Vol. 4, Nos. 1/2). 360p. pap. 29.95 (*1-56024-843-2*); 59.95 (*1-56024-814-9*) Haworth Pr (Pharmctl Prods).

Drug Use in Pregnancy: Mother & Child. Ed. by Ira J. Chasnoff. 1986. text 124.00 (*0-85200-949-6*) Kluwer Academic.

Drug Use Measurement: Strengths, Limitations, & Recommendations for Improvement. 1994. (Illus.). 85p. (Orig.). (C). pap. text 25.00 (*0-7881-0370-9*) DIANE Pub.

Drug Use Prevention: Health Facts. Lucas Stang & Kathleen R. Miner. 1994. LC 93-43599. 12.95 (*1-56071-185-X*, H305) ETR Assocs.

Drug User: Documents 1840-1960. Ed. by John Strausbaugh & Donald Blaise. 1991. 242p. (Orig.). pap. 10.95 (*0-922233-05-5*) Blast Bks.

Drug User: Personality Issues, Factors, & Theories. Ed. by Stanley Einstein. 1983. LC 82-18905. (Illus.). 214p. 90.00 (*0-306-40913-5*, Plenum Trade) Perseus Pubng.

Drug Users & the Criminal Justice System. 1986. lib. bdg. 79.95 (*0-8490-3514-7*) Gordon Pr.

Drug Utilization Studies: Methods & Uses. Ed. by M. N. Dukes. 1993. (WHO Regional Publications: No. 45). viii, 218p. pap. text 36.00 (*92-890-1308-7*, 1310045) World Health.

Drugless Treatment for Deafness & Partial Deafness: Osteopathic, Somapathic, Naturopathic, Chiropractic & Mechano-Therapic. C. H. Murray & M. S. Murray. 1991. (Alternative Medicine Ser.). lib. bdg. 69.95 (*0-8490-4263-1*) Gordon Pr.

Drugs. Ed. by James F. Fixx. 1971. LC 78-169196. (Great Contemporary Issues Ser.). (Illus.). 757p. 35.00 (*0-405-01290-X*) Ayer.

Drugs. Payne. 1991. 13.75 (*0-697-40328-9*, WCB McGr Hill) McGrw-H Hghr Educ.

Drugs. Ray. 7th ed. 1996. tchr. ed. 28.12 (*0-8151-7301-6*) Mosby Inc.

Drugs: Photochemistry & Photostability. Ed. by A. Albini & E. Fasani. 1998. 354p. 120.00 (*0-85404-743-3*) Spr-Verlag.

Drugs: The Effects on Patterns of Consciousness. John-Roger. 1976. LC 76-16594. pap. 5.00 (*0-914829-09-2*) Mandeville LA.

Drugs Across the Spectrum. Raymond Goldberg. Ed. by Baxter Staff. 1994. LC 93-29267. 400p. (C). pap. text 37.00 (*0-314-02790-4*) West Pub.

Drugs Affecting Kidney Function & Metabolism. Ed. by K. D. Edwards. 1972. (Progress in Biochemical Pharmacology Ser.: Vol. 7). 165.25 (*3-8055-1386-0*) S Karger.

Drugs Affecting Lipid Metabolism. Ed. by A. L. Catapano et al. 1993. LC 93-5111. (Medical Science Symposia Ser.: Vol. 2). 544p. (C). lib. bdg. 200.00 (*0-7923-2232-0*) Kluwer Academic.

Drugs Affecting Lipid Metabolism. Ed. by Antonio M. Gotto et al. 1996. LC 96-30284. (Medical Science Symposia Ser.: Vol. 10). 700p. text 307.50 (*0-7923-4167-8*) Kluwer Academic.

Drugs Affecting the Renin-Angiotensin-Aldosterone System Use of Angiotensin Inhibitors: Proceedings. Ed. by K. D. Edwards & G. S. Stokes. 1977. (Progress in Biochemical Pharmacology Ser.: Vol. 12). 123.50 (*3-8055-2410-2*) S Karger.

Drugs Affecting the Respiratory System. Ed. by Davis L. Temple, Jr. 1980. LC 79-24958. (ACS Symposium Ser.: No. 118). 43.95 (*0-8412-0536-1*) Am Chemical.

Drugs Against Men. Henry S. Williams. Ed. by Gerald N. Grob. 1981. LC 80-1253. (Addiction in America Ser.). reprint ed. lib. bdg. 19.95 (*0-405-13623-4*) Ayer.

Drugs, Alcohol & Pregnancy. Christina Dye. rev. ed. 2000. pap. 3.50 (*0-89230-190-2*) Do It Now.

Drugs, Alcohol, & Tobacco: Totally Awesome Teaching Strategies. Randy M. Page et al. Ed. by Mary Baker & Ann Turpie. 2nd rev. ed. 1994. LC 94-76120. (Illus.). 594p. pap. text 55.00 (*0-9630009-5-0*) Everyday Learn.

Drugs, Alcohol, Pregnancy & Parenting. Ed. by Ira J. Chasnoff. 1988. (C). text 95.50 (*0-7462-0095-1*) Kluwer Academic.

Drugs & AIDS. Danielle Hain. rev. ed. 1999. pap. 0.50 (*0-89230-220-8*) Do It Now.

Drugs & Alcohol: Simple Facts about Alcohol/Drug Combinations. Jennifer James. rev. ed. 2000. pap. 0.50 (*0-89230-193-7*) Do It Now.

Drugs & Anesthesia: Pharmacology for Anesthesiologists. Margaret Wood & Alastair J. Wood. 3rd ed. 1996. 85.00 (*0-683-09254-5*) Lppncott W & W.

Drugs & Behavior. Baumeister. 1919. (Psychology Ser.). mass mkt. 53.95 (*0-534-34484-4*) Wadsworth Pub.

Drugs & Behavior. Fred Leavitt. 3rd ed. 1995. 424p. 86.95 (*0-8039-4783-6*, 4527); LC 94-35078. (Illus.). pap. 47.95 (*0-8039-4784-4*, 4527) Sage.

Drugs & Cosmetics Act, 1940 Together with Drugs & Cosmetics Rules, 1945, Drugs (Price Control) Order, 1987. Vijay Malik. 1993. (C). (*81-7012-514-6*) Eastern Book IND. *Dist:* St Mut.

Drugs & Diagnostic Tests. Sailly. 1986. (Social Science & Medicine Ser.). pap. 25.25 (*0-08-034047-4*, Pergamon Pr) Elsevier.

Drugs & Disabilities: Handle with Care. Karen Green McGowan. 2nd ed. 2000. (Illus.). 564p. pap. 49.95 (*1-928752-17-9*) Mc Gowan Pubns.

Drugs & Driving: A Survey of the Relationship of Adverse Drug Reactions, & Drug-Alcohol Interaction to Driving Safety. G. Milner. Ed. by G. S. Avery. 1971. (Monographs on Drugs: Vol. 1). (Illus.). xi, 124p. 26.25 (*3-8055-1242-2*) S Karger.

Drugs & Drug Eruptions in Health & Disease: Index of New Information. Sara L. Hasche. Date not set. 160p. 57.50 (*0-7883-1876-4*); pap. 47.50 (*0-7883-1877-2*) ABBE Pubs Assn.

Drugs & Handwriting. Patricia Wellingham-Jones. 1991. (Illus.). 92p. (C). pap. 16.00 (*0-939221-08-X*) PWJ Pubg.

Drugs & Hormones in Brain Development. Ed. by M. Schlumpf & Walter Lichtensteiger. 1983. (Monographs in Neural Sciences: Vol. 9). (Illus.). viii, 244p. 143.50 (*3-8055-3514-7*) S Karger.

Drugs & Human Behavior. Palfai & Jankiewic. 2nd ed. 1996. tchr. ed. 19.68 (*0-697-12714-1*) McGraw.

Drugs & Human Behavior. Tibor Palfai & Henry Jankiewicz. 2nd ed. 1996. LC 96-83185. 560p. (C). pap. 60.63 (*0-697-12713-3*) McGrw-H Hghr Educ.

Drugs & Human Behavior. David M. Grilly. 3rd ed. 1997. LC 97-29265. 388p. pap. text 63.67 (*0-205-26501-4*) P-H.

Drugs & Human Lactation: A Comprehensive Guide to the Content & Consequences of Drugs, Micronutrients, Radiopharmaceuticals, & Environmental & Occupational Chemicals in Human Milk. 2nd ed. 1996. LC 96-38943. 722p. 259.00 (*0-444-81981-9*) Elsevier.

Drugs & Information Control: The Role of Men & Manipulation in the Control of Drug Trafficking. 23. Jerald W. Cloyd. 1982. LC 81-6675. (Contributions in Legal Studies Ser.: No. 23). 195p. 55.00 (*0-313-22178-2*, CDS/, Greenwood Pr) Greenwood.

Drugs & Life. Harry H. Avis. 3rd ed. 1995. tchr. ed. 14.68 (*0-697-22291-8*, WCB McGr Hill) McGrw-H Hghr Educ.

Drugs & Narcotics in History. Ed. by Roy Porter & Mikulas Teich. 1997. (Illus.). 239p. pap. text 24.95 (*0-521-58597-X*) Cambridge U Pr.

Drugs & Nutrients: The Interactive Effects. Daphne A. Roe & T. Colin Campbell. 1984. (Drugs & the Pharmaceutical Sciences Ser.: Vol. 21). (Illus.). 624p. text 255.00 (*0-8247-7054-4*) Dekker.

Drugs & Nutrients to Improve Your Brain Power, Increase Productivity & Job Performance. 1992. lib. bdg. 88.95 (*0-8490-5529-6*) Gordon Pr.

Drugs & Pain. Joann Rodgers. 1987. (Encyclopedia of Psychoactive Drugs Ser.: No. 2). (Illus.). 128p. (YA). (gr. 7 up). lib. bdg. 19.95 (*1-55546-212-X*) Chelsea Hse.

Drugs & Pharmacology for Nurses. S. J. Hopkins. 11th ed. 1992. (Illus.). 612p. pap. text (*0-443-04389-2*); 12th rev. ed. 1995. LC 95-7245. pap. text (*0-443-05249-2*) Church.

Drugs & Pregnancy. Larry C. Gilstrap & B. Little. 1992. (Illus.). 447p. (C). (gr. 13). pap. 104.95 (*0-412-04561-3*) Chapman & Hall.

Drugs & Pregnancy. Ed. by Larry C. Gilstrap & Bertis B. Little. 1992. LC 92-14733. (*0-444-01655-4*) Elsevier.

Drugs & Pregnancy. Larry C. Gilstrap et al. 2nd ed. 1999. LC 97-7948. 552p. (*0-412-12201-4*) E A GBR. *Dist:* OUP.

Drugs & Pregnancy: It's Not Worth the Risk. Paddy S. Cook. rev. ed. 1991. LC 86-70944. 36p. pap. 3.00 (*0-942348-17-6*) Am Council Drug Ed.

Drugs & Protocols Common to Prehospital & Emergency Care. P. Howard Cummings. 1993. (Nursing-Health Science Ser.). (Illus.). 459p. (C). pap. text 35.95 (*0-86720-214-9*, 214-9) Jones & Bartlett.

Drugs & Renal Disease. Ed. by William M. Bennett. 2nd ed. 1986. (Monographs in Clinical Pharmacology: Vol. 2). (Illus.). 205p. text (*0-443-08403-3*) Church.

Drugs & Sex: A Bibliography. Compiled by Ernest L. Abel. 1983. LC 83-5656. 129p. lib. bdg. 59.00 (*0-313-23941-X*, ADS/, Greenwood Pr) Greenwood.

Drugs & Society. Glen Hanson & Peter Venturelli. 4th ed. 1995. LC 94-46298. (Health Science Ser.). (Illus.). 528p. pap. text 49.95 (*0-86720-830-9*, 830-9) Jones & Bartlett.

Drugs & Society: A Biological Perspective. Patricia Witters-Jones & Weldon L. Witters. 1983. LC 82-21738. (Illus.). 400p. (C). pap. text 25.00 (*0-86720-367-6*, 367-6) Jones & Bartlett.

Drugs & Society: Contemporary Social Issues. Ed. by Louis Miller & Stanley Einstein. 1976. 317p. text 34.95 (*0-87855-273-1*) Transaction Pubs.

Drugs & Solutions: A Programmed Introduction. Claire B. Keane & Sybil M. Fletcher. 4th ed. 1980. (Illus.). 166p. pap. text 28.00 (*0-7216-5343-X*) Saunders.

Drugs & the Brain. Edward Edelson. 1987. (Encyclopedia of Psychoactive Drugs Ser.: No. 2). (Illus.). 128p. (YA). (gr. 7 up). lib. bdg. 19.95 (*1-55546-209-X*) Chelsea Hse.

Drugs & the Brain. Solomon H. Snyder. 1996. (Illus.). 228p. (C). pap. text 19.95 (*0-7167-6017-7*) W H Freeman.

Drugs & the Brain: A Scientific American Book. Solomon H. Snyder. 1986. 228p. text 32.95 (*0-7167-5015-5*) W H Freeman.

Drugs & the Delivery of Oxygen to Tissues. 1989. 296p. 203.00 (*0-8493-6656-9*, RC700) CRC Pr.

Drugs & the Elderly: Clinical, Social, & Policy Perspectives. Helene L. Lipton & Philip R. Lee. 1988. LC 87-33574. 280p. 51.00 (*0-8047-1295-6*) Stanford U Pr.

Drugs & the Eye. Janet Vale & Barry Cox. 3rd ed. 1999. 132p. pap. text 32.50 (*0-7506-1041-7*) Buttrwrth-Heinemann.

Drugs & the Higher Consciousness: A New Model for Solving the Drug Problem. 1991. lib. bdg. 78.95 (*0-8490-4653-X*) Gordon Pr.

Drugs & the Human Body. Liska. 5th ed. 1997. pap. text, tchr. ed. (*0-13-598152-2*) P-H.

Drugs & the Human Body: With Implications for Society. Ken Liska. 4th ed. 1993. (Illus.). 464p. (C). pap. text 45.33 (*0-02-371091-8*, Macmillan Coll) P-H.

Drugs & the Kidney. Graeme R. Catto. 1990. 176p. text 107.00 (*0-7923-8918-2*) Kluwer Academic.

Drugs & the Kidney. Ed. by K. D. Edwards. 1974. (Progress in Biochemical Pharmacology Ser.: Vol. 9). 300p. 95.75 (*3-8055-1693-2*) S Karger.

Drugs & the Liver: High Risk Patients & Transplantation. Ed. by D. Galmarini et al. 1993. LC 93-1383. (Medical Science Symposia Ser.: Vol. 4). 204p. (C). text 112.00 (*0-7923-2307-6*) Kluwer Academic.

Drugs & the Older Population. Peter Crome. 2000. LC 00-61417. (Illus.). xxi, 704p. (*1-86094-099-4*) Imperial College GBR. *Dist:* World Scientific Pub.

Drugs & the Peptic Ulcer. C. J. Pfeiffer. 1982. Vol. 1. 224p. 127.00 (*0-8493-6211-3*, RC821); Vol. 2. 280p. 156.00 (*0-8493-6212-1*) Franklin (CRC Reprint).

Drugs & the Performance Horse. Thomas Tobin. 1981. (Illus.). 488p. 74.95 (*0-398-04446-5*) C C Thomas.

Drugs & Their Effects on Neurodiagnostics. American Journal of END Technology Staff. rev. ed. 1997. LC 99-188506. (Illus.). 171p. spiral bd. 25.00 (*1-57797-010-1*) ASET.

Drugs & Their Usage. William D. Grimley et al. 1998. 264p. pap. text 15.00 (*1-886532-08-7*) Christian Vet.

Drugs & Women. Paul N. August. 1987. (Encyclopedia of Psychoactive Drugs Ser.: No. 2). (Illus.). 128p. (YA). (gr. 7 up). lib. bdg. 19.95 (*1-55546-227-8*) Chelsea Hse.

Drugs & You: Adverse Drug Experience Reporting - What You Should Know! 2000. 300p. pap. (*1-893091-60-0*, 2000(AD)300/091-60-0) F R Parker.

Drugs & Your Brain. Beatrice Grabish. 1998. (Drug Abuse Prevention Library). 64p. (YA). (gr. 7 up). reprint ed. pap. 6.95 (*1-56838-214-6*) Hazelden.

Drugs As Tools in Neurotransmitter Research. Ed. by Alan A. Boulton et al. 1989. LC 88-32044. (Neuromethods Ser.: Vol. 12). (Illus.). 532p. 145.00 (*0-89603-122-5*) Humana.

Drugs, Athletes & Physical Performance. J. A. Thomas. 1988. LC 88-22381. (Illus.). 254p. (C). text 57.50 (*0-306-42888-1*, Kluwer Plenum) Kluwer Academic.

Drugs Available Abroad: A Guide to Therapeutic Drugs Available & Approved for Use Outside the U. S. 1990. 120.00 (*0-8103-7177-4*) Gale.

Drugs, Behavior, & Modern Society. Charles F. Levinthal. 2nd ed. 1998. LC 98-15221. 390p. pap. text 65.00 (*0-205-27703-9*) Allyn.

***Drugs, Behavior & Modern Society: Exam Copy with Web Edition CD-ROM.** Charles F. Levinthal. 2nd ed. 1999. (*0-205-31346-9*, 1346L-5) Allyn.

***Drugs, Behavior & Modern Society: Instructor's Manual & Test Bank.** Charles F. Levinthal. 2nd ed. 1999. tchr. ed. (*0-205-28648-8*, T8648-2) Allyn.

Drugs Between Research & Regulations. Ed. by C. Steichele et al. 1986. 300p. 55.00 (*0-387-91265-7*) Spr-Verlag.

Drugs, Biogenic Amines & Body Temperature: Proceedings of the Pharmacology of Thermoregulation Symposium, 3rd, Banff, Alberta, Sept. 1976. Pharmacology of Thermoregulation Symposium Staff et al. Ed. by K. E. Cooper. 1977. (Illus.). 101.00 (*3-8055-2395-5*) S Karger.

Drugs, Crime, & the Justice System. 1993. (Illus.). 310p. (Orig.). (C). pap. text 40.00 (*1-56806-417-9*) DIANE Pub.

Drugs, Daydreaming, & Personality: A Study of College Youth. Bernard Segal et al. 1980. LC 80-10094. 254p. 49.95 (*0-89859-042-6*) L Erlbaum Assocs.

Drugs, Disease & the Periodontium. Robin A. Seymour & Peter A. Heasman. 1992. (Illus.). 228p. 98.00 (*0-19-261992-6*) OUP.

Drugs, Diseases & Anesthesia. Ronald Stern. 1996. LC 96-27496. 522p. pap. text 45.00 (*0-397-58736-8*) Lppncott W & W.

Drugs, Doctors, Demons & Disease. Perry A. Sperber. 1973. LC 70-111808. 294p. 15.50 (*0-87527-127-8*) Green.

Drugs for Children. 1988. text 30.00 (*92-890-1048-7*) World Health.

Drugs for Control of Epilepsy: Actions on Neuronal Networks Involved in Seizure Disorders. Carl L. Faingold. 1991. 560p. 139.00 (*0-8493-5059-X*, RC374) CRC Pr.

Drugs for Infants & Children: Report on the 10th European Symposium on Clinical Pharmacological Evaluation in Drug Control. 1982. (Euro Reports & Studies Ser.: No. 66). 34p. pap. text 4.00 (*92-890-1232-3*) World Health.

Drugs for Mental Illness see Medicine & Mental Illness

Drugs for the Elderly. 1985. 147p. pap. text 25.00 (*92-890-1020-7*, 1340019) World Health.

Drugs for the Elderly. Ed. by L. Offerhaus. 1997. LC 98-177897. (WHO Regional Publications, European Ser.: No. 71). 155p. pap. 28.80 (*92-890-1335-4*, 1310071) Am Soc Clinical.

Drugs for the Gut. Walt. 1997. (Illus.). 350p. pap. text 35.00 (*0-7020-1802-3*) Saunders.

Drugs for the Heart. Lionel H. Opie. 4th rev. ed. 1997. pap. text 35.00 (*0-7216-7525-5*) Saunders.

Drugs for the Treatment of Parkinson's Disease. Ed. by D. B. Calne. 1989. (Handbook of Experimental Pharmacology Ser.: Vol. 88). (Illus.). 599p. 415.00 (*0-387-50041-3*, 2034) Spr-Verlag.

Drugs from Plants. Trevor I. Williams. 1980. lib. bdg. 49.95 (*0-8490-3162-1*) Gordon Pr.

Drugs from the Sea. Ed. by N. Fusetani. 2000. LC 00-30966. (Illus.). vi, 158p. 121.00 (*3-8055-7098-8*) S Karger.

Drugs in America. Ansley Hamid. 1995. LC 98-25990. 327p. pap. 48.00 (*0-8342-1060-6*, 10606) Aspen Pub.

***Drugs in America: A Historical Reader.** Ed. by David F. Musto. 2002. 432p. pap. 22.00 (*0-8147-5663-8*) NYU Pr.

Drugs in America: A Social History, 1800-1980. H. Wayne Morgan. 1982. LC 81-14531. (Illus.). 248p. pap. 17.95 (*0-8156-2282-1*) Syracuse U Pr.

Drugs in Anesthesia: Mechanisms of Action. Stanley A. Feldman. Ed. by Cyril F. Scurr. 1988. 464p. (*0-683-13022-6*) E A GBR. *Dist:* Williams & Wilkins.

Drugs in Anesthesia & Intensive Care. Martin Sasada & Sue Smith. 2nd ed. 1997. LC 97-193987. 414p. pap. 39.50 (*0-19-262872-0*) OUP.

Drugs in Combination with Other Therapies. Ed. by Milton Greenblatt. 1975. LC 75-25846. (Seminars in Psychiatry Ser.). 224p. text 56.00 (*0-8089-0908-8*, 791727, Grune & Strat) Harcrt Hlth Sci Grp.

Drugs in Competitive Athletics. John Savory & Shipe. 1991. 49.00 (*0-632-03181-6*) CRC Pr.

Drugs in Inflammation. Ed. by W. B. Van den Berg & Michael J. Parnham. 1991. (Agents & Actions Supplements Ser.: Vol. 32). 264p. 161.50 (*0-8176-2504-6*) Birkhauser.

Drugs in Litigation: Damage Awards Involving Prescription & Nonprescription Drugs, 1994 Edition. 1994. 936p. pap. 70.00 (*1-55834-173-0*, MICHIE) LEXIS Pub.

Drugs in Litigation: Damage Awards Involving Prescription & Nonprescription Drugs, 1995. Michie Company Editorial Staff. 1995. 936p. pap. 62.00 (*1-55834-226-5*, 71208-12, MICHIE) LEXIS Pub.

Drugs in Modern Society. Carroll. 4th ed. 1996. tchr. ed. 15.31 (*0-697-22298-5*, WCB McGr Hill) McGrw-H Hghr Educ.

Drugs in Nursing Practice. C. R. Henney. 4th ed. 1993. (Illus.). 384p. (Orig.). pap. text (*0-443-04378-7*) Church.

Drugs in Nursing Practice. Henney. 5th ed. 1995. pap. text 27.00 (*0-443-05235-2*) Saunders.

Drugs in Perspective. Richard Fields. 4th ed. 2000. LC 00-58728. (Illus.). xxi, 346p. pap. 28.25 net. (*0-697-29426-9*) McGraw.

Drugs in Perspective. Richard Fields. (C). 2nd ed. 1994. 400p. pap. 46.88 (*0-697-15236-7*); 3rd ed. 1997. LC 96-80077. 416p. text 32.00 net. (*0-697-29425-0*, WCB McGr Hill) McGrw-H Hghr Educ.

***Drugs in Perspective with PowerWeb: Drugs.** Richard Fields. 4th ed. 2000. pap. 53.75 (*0-07-246697-9*) McGrw-H Hghr Educ.

Drugs in Pregnancy & Lactation: A Reference Guide to Fetal & Neonatal Risk. Gerald G. Briggs et al. 5th ed. 1998. LC 97-42686. 1,200p. 99.00 (*0-683-30262-0*) Lppncott W & W.

Drugs in Psychiatric Practice. Peter Tyrer et al. 1997. LC 97-25188. (Illus.). 320p. text 85.00 (*0-7506-2251-2*) Buttrwrth-Heinemann.

Drugs in the Management of Heart Disease. Ed. by A. Breckenridge. 1984. text 127.50 (*0-85200-724-8*) Kluwer Academic.

Drugs in the Workplace: Research & Evaluation Data. 1993. (Illus.). 246p. (Orig.). (C). pap. text 45.00 (*1-56806-892-1*) DIANE Pub.

Drugs in the Workplace: Research & Valuation Data. 1990. lib. bdg. 250.00 (*0-8490-4002-7*) Gordon Pr.

Drugs in Western Pacific Societies. Ed. by Lamont Lindstrom. 1987. (ASAO Monographs: No. 11). (Illus.). 314p. (Orig.). (C). 32.00 (*0-8191-6123-3*) U Pr of Amer.

Drugs of Abuse. 1991. lib. bdg. 250.00 (*0-8490-4944-X*) Gordon Pr.

Drugs of Abuse: Chemistry, Pharmacology, Immunology, & AIDS. 1993. lib. bdg. 256.95 (*0-8490-8917-4*) Gordon Pr.

Drugs of Abuse & Addiction: Neurobehavioral Toxicology. Raymond J. Niesink. 1998. LC 98-39869. (Pharmacology & Toxicology Ser.). (Illus.). 368p. 99.95 (*0-8493-7803-6*) CRC Pr.

Drugs of Abuse & Immune Function. Ed. by Ronald R. Watson. 1990. 248p. 129.00 (*0-8493-6747-6*, RC582) CRC Pr.

Drugs of Abuse & Neurobiology. Ronald R. Watson. 1992. 368p. lib. bdg. 119.00 (*0-8493-7934-2*, RC347) CRC Pr.

Drugs of Abuse Digest: A Prevention Guide for the Family, School & Workplace. Allan R. Pringle et al. rev. ed. 1998. (Illus.). 112p. pap. 12.95 (*0-935847-11-1*) Inst Subs Abuse Res.

Drugs of Abuse, Immunity & AIDS. Ed. by Herman Friedman et al. 1993. (Advances in Experimental Medicine & Biology Ser.: Vol. 335). (Illus.). 300p. (C). text 89.50 (*0-306-44566-2*, Kluwer Plenum) Kluwer Academic.

Drugs of Abuse, Immunity & Immunodeficiency. Ed. by H. Friedman. 1991. (Advances in Experimental Medicine & Biology Ser.). (Illus.). 330p. (C). text 132.00 (*0-306-43890-9*, Plenum Trade) Perseus Pubng.

Drugs of Abuse, Immunity, & Infections. Ed. by Herman Friedman et al. 1995. 208p. 199.95 (*0-8493-7637-8*, 7637) CRC Pr.

Drugs of Abuse, Immunomodulation & AIDS: Proceedings of the Fifth Annual Symposium Held in Nashville, Tennessee, June 12-14, 1997. Ed. by Herman Friedman et al. 1998. LC 98-18199. (Advances in Experimental Medicine & Biology Ser.: Vol. 437). (Illus.). 332p. 95.00 (*0-306-45838-1*, Kluwer Plenum) Kluwer Academic.

Drugs of Abuse (1996) Ed. by Carol Gibson. 1996. (Illus.). 54p. (Orig.). pap. text 40.00 (*0-7881-2849-3*) DIANE Pub.

Drugs of Natural Origin: Economic & Policy Aspects of Discovery, Development, & Marketing. Anthony Artuso. 1997. LC 97-19503. (Illus.). 201p. (C). 39.95 (*0-7890-0123-3*); pap. 24.95 (*0-7890-0414-3*) Haworth Pr (Pharmctl Prods).

Drugs of Pediatric Emergencies. American Academy of Pediatrics Staff. 1998. 54p. pap. 12.95 (*1-58110-014-0*) Am Acad Pediat.

Drugs of the Future. William A. Check. 1987. (Encyclopedia of Psychoactive Drugs Ser.: No. 2). (Illus.). 128p. (YA). (gr. 7 up). lib. bdg. 19.95 (*1-55546-208-1*) Chelsea Hse.

Drugs Policy in Developing Countries. Najmi Kanji et al. 1992. (C). (*1-85649-059-9*); (*1-85649-060-2*) Zed Books GBR. *Dist:* St Martin.

Drugs, Society & Behavior, 2000-2001. Hugh Wilson. 15th ed. 2000. (Annual Editions Ser.). 240p. (C). pap. 17.50 (*0-07-236538-2*) McGrw-H Hghr Educ.

Drugs, Society, & Human Behavior. Oakley S. Ray & Charles Ksir. 8th ed. 1998. LC 98-7758. 39.14 net. (*0-07-059307-8*) McGraw.

Drugs, Systemic Diseases, & the Kidney. Ed. by Alberto Amerio et al. 1989. (Illus.). 418p. 105.00 (*0-306-43219-6*, Plenum Trade) Perseus Pubng.

Drugs That Enslave: The Opium, Morphine, Chloral & Hashish Habits. Harry H. Kane. Ed. by Gerald N. Grob. 1981. LC 80-1236. (Addiction in America Ser.). reprint ed. lib. bdg. 23.95 (*0-405-13595-5*) Ayer.

Drugs, the Brain & Behavior. Hand. 1999. (C). pap. text 48.50 (*0-15-505769-3*) Harcourt Coll Pubs.

Drugs, the Brain, & Behavior: The Pharmacology of Abuse & Dependence. John Brick & Carlton K. Erickson. 1998. LC 97-39232. pap. 19.95 (*0-7890-0275-2*); xv, 186 p. 49.95 (*0-7890-0274-4*) Haworth Pr (Hawrth Medical).

Drugs, Therapy & Professional Power: Problems & Pills. Ernest Keen. 1998. LC 97-41933. 248p. 67.00 (*0-275-96200-8*, Praeger Pubs) Greenwood.

Drugs under Patent, 1997. FOI Services. 1997. 250p. pap. 89.00 (*1-880626-16-0*, Y149520) FOI Services.

Drugs, What They Are- How They Look- What They Do. Frank Gannon. 1971. LC 70-148361. 20.00 (*0-89388-005-1*) Okpaku Communications.

Drugspeak: The Analysis of Drug Discourse. John Booth Davies. 1997. 220p. pap. text 20.00 (*90-5702-192-7*, Harwood Acad Pubs) Gordon & Breach.

Drum & Stethoscope: Integrating Ethnomedicine & Biomedicine in Bolivia. Joseph W. Bastien. 1992. LC 92-53602. (Illus.). 320p. 34.95 (*0-87480-386-1*) U of Utah Pr.

***Drumbeat for Mother Earth: Persistent Organic Pollutants Threatening Indigenous Peoples.** 2000. pap., tchr. ed. 250.00 incl. VHS (*1-56029-817-0*) Bullfrog Films.

Drunken Synapse: Studies of Alcohol-Related Disorders. Yuan Liu & W. A. Hunt. 1999. LC 99-23706. (C). text (*0-306-46111-0*, Kluwer Plenum) Kluwer Academic.

Dry All Night: The Picture Book Technique That Stops Bedwetting. Alison Mack. 1990. LC 88-32524. (Illus.). 175p. pap. 16.95 (*0-316-54225-3*) Little.

Dry Bones Breathe: Gay Men Creating Post-AIDS Identities & Cultures. Eric Rofes. 1998. LC 98-9555. 352p. (C). 49.95 (*0-7890-0470-4*); pap. 24.95 (*1-56023-934-4*) Haworth Pr (Harrington Park).

Dry Drunk Syndrome. R. J. Solberg. rev. ed. 1983. 20p. (Orig.). pap. 2.00 (*0-89486-172-7*, 1251B) Hazelden.

Dry Eye: A Comprehensive Guide. Ed. by M. A. Lemp & R. Marquardt. 1992. (Illus.). 249p. 155.00 (*0-387-53308-7*) Spr-Verlag.

Dryden Interviews: Dialogues on the Psychotherapeutic Process. Dryden. 1992. 152p. pap. 48.00 (*1-56593-526-8*, 0315) Singular Publishing.

Dryden on Counseling, Vol. 3. Dryden. 1991. 180p. pap. 47.75 (*1-56593-529-2*, 0309) Singular Publishing.

Dryden on Counseling Vol. 1: Seminal Papers. Dryden. 1991. 164p. pap. 47.75 (*1-56593-527-6*, 0307) Singular Publishing.

Dryden on Counseling Vol. 2: A Dialogue. Dryden. 1991. 84p. pap. 40.00 (*1-56593-528-4*, 0308) Singular Publishing.

DSM-IV Case Studies: A Clinical Guide to Differential Diagnosis. Allen J. Frances & Ruth Ross. 1996. LC 95-38067. (Dsm-IV Ser.). 400p. 47.00 (*0-88048-416-0*, 8416); pap. text 33.00 (*0-88048-434-9*, 8434) Am Psychiatric.

DSM-IV Crosswalk: Guidelines for Coding Mental Health Information. Andrea Albaum-Feinstein. 1999. 132p. pap. text 60.00 (*1-58426-000-9*, AC200298) Am Hlth Info.

DSM-IV Diagnosis in the Schools. Alvin E. House. 1998. LC 98-19601. (Guilford School Practitioner Ser.). 230p. 30.00 (*1-57230-346-8*, 0346) Guilford Pubns.

DSM-IV Guidebook. Allen J. Frances et al. 1995. LC 95-38067. 442p. pap. text, stu. ed. 44.50 (*0-88048-430-6*, 8430) Am Psychiatric.

DSM-IV Handbook for Differential Diagnosis. Michael B. First et al. 1995. LC 95-4141. 200p. pap. text 28.50 (*0-88048-431-4*, 8431) Am Psychiatric.

DSM-IV KSO Coding Update, 1996: (1996 Edition - Includes ICD-9-CM Codes Effective October 1, 1996) American Psychiatric Association Staff et al. 1996. LC 96-38257. 72p. 10.00 (*0-89042-409-8*, 2409) Am Psychiatric.

DSM-IV Made Easy: The Clinician's Guide to Diagnosis. James Morrison. 1995. LC 94-34302. (Illus.). 594p. 55.00 (*0-89862-568-8*, 2568) Guilford Pubns.

DSM-IV Personality Disorders. Ed. by W. John Livesley. 1995. LC 94-25319. (Diagnosis & Treatment of Mental Disorders Ser.). 516p. text 60.00 (*0-89862-257-3*, 2257) Guilford Pubns.

DSM-IV Sourcebook, Vol. 1. American Psychiatric Association Staff. 1994. (Dsm-IV Sourcebook Ser.: Vol. 1). 768p. pap. text 78.00 (*0-89042-070-X*, 2070) Am Psychiatric.

DSM-four Sourcebook, Vol. 1. Thomas A. Widiger. Ed. by Ruth Ross & Michael B. First. 1994. LC 93-48304. (Dsm-IV Sourcebook Ser.: Vol. 1). 768p. text 129.00 (*0-89042-065-3*, 2065) Am Psychiatric.

DSM-IV Sourcebook. American Psychiatric Association Staff. (Dsm-IV Sourcebook Ser.: Vol. 2). Vol. 2. 2nd ed. 1995. LC 93-48304. 1184p. text 129.00 (*0-89042-069-6*, 2069); Vol. 2. 2nd ed. 1995. 1184p. pap. text 78.00 (*0-89042-071-8*, 2071); Vol. 3. 3rd ed. 1997. LC 93-48304. 912p. text 129.00 (*0-89042-073-4*, 2073); Vol. 3. 3rd ed. 1997. 912p. pap. text 78.00 (*0-89042-074-2*, 2074) Am Psychiatric.

DSM-IV-TR Diagnostic & Statistical Manual of Mental Disorders: Text Revision. American Psychiatric Association Staff. 4th rev. ed. 2000. LC 00-24852. 1082p. pap. 49.95 (*0-89042-025-4*, 2025) Am Psychiatric.

DSM-III-R Casebook of Treatment Selection. Samuel Perry et al. 2nd ed. 1990. LC 90-1317. 416p. text 49.95 (*0-87630-572-9*) Brunner-Routledge.

DSM-IV Casebook: A Learning Companion to the Diagnostic & Statistical Manual of Mental Disorders. Robert L. Spitzer et al. 4th ed. 1994. LC 94-10598. (Dsm-IV Ser.). 576p. text 54.95 (*0-88048-674-0*, 8674); pap. text 38.50 (*0-88048-675-9*, 8675) Am Psychiatric.

DSM-IV Casebook of Treatment Selection. John F. Clarkin et al. 3rd ed. 1997. text (*0-87630-746-2*) Brunner-Routledge.

DSM-IV Clinical Vignettes. 210.00 (*0-87630-783-7*) Brunner-Routledge.

***DSM-IV-TR Case Studies: A Clinical Guide to Differential Diagnosis.** Ed. by Allen J. Frances & Ruth Ross. 2002. 408p. pap. 39.95 (*1-58562-055-6*, 62055) Am Psychiatric.

DSM-IV Training Guide. William H. Reid & Michael G. Wise. 1995. 384p. LC 95-9947. pap. text 26.95 (*0-87630-763-2*, 7632); 50.00 (*0-87630-768-3*) Brunner-Routledge.

DSM-IV Training Guide for Diagnosis of Childhood Disorders. Judith L. Rapoport & Deborah R. Ismond. 1996. 384p. text 49.95 (*0-87630-770-5*); 2nd ed. pap. text 26.95 (*0-87630-766-7*) Brunner-Routledge.

DSM-IV Training Program Complete, Set. Reid. 1995. text 425.00 incl. VHS, sl. (*0-87630-771-3*); text 425.00 incl. trans., VHS (*0-87630-772-1*) Brunner-Routledge.

DTV Medical Dictionary: DTV Woerterbuch der Medizin, Set. Herbert Schaldach & Maxim Zetkin. 7th rev. ed. 1985. (GER.). 1597p. 75.00 (*0-8288-1844-4*, M7342) Fr & Eur.

DTV Woerterbuch zur Psychologie. Werner Von Frohlich. (GER.). 39.95 (*0-7859-8353-8*, 3423032855) Fr & Eur.

Dual Brain: Hemispheric Specialization in Humans. Ed. by D. Frank Benson & Eran Zaidel. 1985. LC 85-24955. 430p. 55.00 (*0-89862-643-9*) Guilford Pubns.

Dual Brain, Religion & the Unconscious. Sim C. Liddon. 1989. LC 89-3765. 265p. 37.00 (*0-87975-523-7*) Prometheus Bks.

Dual Diagnosis: Challenges of Serving Mentally Ill Substance Abusers. Marjorie Beggs. 1998. 48p. pap. 8.95 (*0-936434-99-6*, Study Ctr Pr) SF Study Ctr.

Dual Diagnosis: Counseling the Mentally Ill Substance Abuser. Katie Evans & J. Michael Sullivan. 1990. LC 90-3036. 191p. pap. 19.95 (*0-89862-450-9*) Guilford Pubns.

Dual Diagnosis: Counseling the Mentally Ill Substance Abuser. Katie Evans et al. 1990. LC 90-3036. 191p. text 49.95 (*0-89862-436-3*) Guilford Pubns.

Dual Diagnosis: Evaluation, Treatment, Training & Program Development. Ed. by J. Solomon et al. 1994. 346p. (C). text 49.50 (*0-306-44543-3*, Kluwer Plenum) Kluwer Academic.

***Dual Diagnosis: Substance Misuse & Psychiatric Disorders.** Hussein Rassool. 2001. 224p. pap. 44.95 (*0-632-05621-5*) Blackwell Sci.

Dual Diagnosis & Treatment: Substance Abuse & Comorbid Medical & Psychiatric Disorders. Ed. by Henry R. Kranzler & Bruce J. Rounsaville. 1997. LC 97-42395. (Medical Psychiatry Ser.). (Illus.). 608p. text 150.00 (*0-8247-9895-3*) Dekker.

Dual Diagnosis in Substance Abuse. Ed. by Mark Gold & Andrew E. Slaby. 1991. (Illus.). 352p. text 135.00 (*0-8247-8457-X*) Dekker.

Dual Diagnosis of Major Mental Illness & Substance Disorder, Vol. 50. Ed. by Kenneth Minkoff & Robert Drake. 1991. LC 87-646993. (New Directions for Mental Health Services Ser.: No. MHS 50). 120p. pap. 28.00 (*1-55542-794-4*) Jossey-Bass.

Dual Diagnosis Recovery Sourcebook: A Physical, Mental & Spiritual Approach to Addiction with an Emotional Disorder. Dennis C. Ortman. 2001. LC 00-65538. 304p. pap. 18.95 (*0-7373-0319-0*, 03190W) McGraw-Hill Prof.

Dual Disorders: Counseling Clients with Chemical Dependency & Mental Illness. Dennis C. Daley et al. 2nd ed. 1990. LC 92-48321. 141p. pap. 18.95 (*0-89486-449-1*, 5023A) Hazelden.

Dual Disorders: Essentials for Assessment & Treatment. David F. O'Connell. 1997. LC 97-10777. 250p. (C). pap. 19.95 (*0-7890-0249-3*); pap. 19.95 (*0-7890-0401-1*) Haworth Pr.

Dual Disorders Recovery Book. Hazelden Publishing Staff. 1993. LC 92-34149. 242p. pap. 10.00 (*0-89486-849-7*, 1500) Hazelden.

Dual Process Model of Impression Formation, Vol. 1. Ed. by Robert S. Wyer, Jr. & Thomas K. Srull, Jr. 1988. (Advances in Social Cognition Ser.). 208p. 39.95 (*0-89859-888-5*); pap. 22.50 (*0-89859-673-4*) L Erlbaum Assocs.

Duality & Unity of the Brain: Unified Functioning & Specialization of the Hemispheres. Ed. by David Ottoson. 1987. LC 87-42720. (Wenner-Gren International Symposia Ser.: Vol. 47). 516p. 125.00 (*0-306-42720-6*, Plenum Trade) Perseus Pubng.

Duality of the Mind. A. L. Wigan. ltd. ed. 1985. LC 85-50042. 368p. 48.00 (*0-934710-12-0*) Rachelle Simon.

Dually Diagnosed: A Therapist's Guide to Helping the Substance Abusing, Psychologically Disturbed Patient. Dennis C. Ortman. 1997. LC 96-29280. 40.00 (*1-56821-770-6*) Aronson.

Duane's Clinical Ophthalmology Loose Leaf Reference Services Staff. Ed. by William S. Tasman et al. (Illus.). ring bd. 495.00 (*0-06-148007-X*) Lppncott W & W.

Dubois' Lupus Erythematosus. Daniel Wallace & Bevra H. Hahn. 4th ed. 1992. (Illus.). 1000p. text 129.00 (*0-8121-1558-9*) Lppncott W & W.

Dubois' Lupus Erythematosus. Ed. by Daniel J. Wallace et al. 5th ed. 1997. LC 96-8020. 1,008p. text 179.00 (*0-683-08665-0*) Lppncott W & W.

Duchenne Muscular Dystrophy. Alan E. Emery. 2nd ed. 1993. LC 92-49084. (Oxford Monographs on Medical Genetics: No. 24). (Illus.). 408p. (C). text 110.00 (*0-19-262370-2*) OUP.

Duden Grosse Woerterbuch Deutsch Vol. 5: O-So. Drosdowksi. 1980. (GER.). 527p. 95.00 (*0-7859-7553-5*, 3411013605) Fr & Eur.

Due Consideration: Controversy in the Age of Medical Miracles. Arthur Caplan. 1997. LC 97-29022. 296p. pap. 16.95 (*0-471-18344-X*) Wiley.

Duke-Elder's Practice of Refraction. Contrib. by David Abrams. 10th ed. 1993. LC 92-49141. 301p. text (*0-443-03856-2*) Church.

Duke Longitudinal Studies of Normal Aging 1955-1980: Overview of History, Design & Findings. Ewald W. Busse & George L. Maddox. 1985. 192p. 26.95 (*0-8261-4150-1*) Springer Pub.

Duke Radiology Boards Review. James Provenzale. 1997. LC 97-34795. 608p. pap. text 99.00 (*0-397-51613-4*) Lppncott W & W.

Dukes' Physiology of Domestic Animals. Ed. by Melvin J. Swenson & William O. Reece. 11th ed. 1993. LC 92-56781. (Comstock Bk.). (Illus.). 992p. 75.00 (*0-8014-2804-1*) Cornell U Pr.

Duncan's Dictionary for Nurses. Helen Duncan. 2nd ed. 1989. 816p. 73.95 (*0-8261-6201-0*); pap. 36.95 (*0-8261-6200-2*) Springer Pub.

Duodenal Ulcer. Ed. by Henry Weiner. 1971. (Advances in Psychosomatic Medicine Ser.: Vol. 6). 65.00 (*3-8055-1159-0*) S Karger.

Duplex & Phlebology. Michael Schadeck. 1999. (Illus.). 143p. 60.00 (*1-928649-01-7*) Idelson Gnocchi Pub.

Duplex Doppler Ultrasound. Ed. by Kenneth J. Taylor & D. Eugene Strandness, Jr. 1989. (Clinics in Diagnostic Ultrasound Ser.: Vol. 26). (Illus.). 182p. text (*0-443-08646-X*) Church.

Duplex Scanning in Vascular Disorders. D. Eugene Strandness, Jr. 2nd ed. 1993. LC 93-12955. 352p. text 125.00 (*0-7817-0014-0*) Lppncott W & W.

Duplex Sonography. E. G. Grant & E. M. White. 1991. (Illus.). 265p. 170.00 (*0-387-96564-5*) Spr-Verlag.

DuPont Guerry III, M. D. Ophthalmologist, Richmond, Virginia & the Medical College of Virginia. DuPont Guerry, 3rd. 1993. (Ophthalmology Oral History Ser.). (Illus.). xxiv, 240p. pap. 35.00 (*1-56055-067-8*) FAAO.

Dupuytren's Disease: Pathobiochemistry & Clinical Management. Ed. by A. Berger. 1994. LC 93-34322. (Illus.). 319p. 129.00 (*0-387-57239-2*) Spr-Verlag.

Durability of Macromolecular Materials. Ed. by Ronald K. Eby. 1979. LC 78-31777. (ACS Symposium Ser.: No. 95). 54.95 (*0-8412-0485-3*) Am Chemical.

***Durability of Vascular & Endovascular Surgery: Management & Progression of Vascular Disease.** Ed. by R. M. Greenhalgh. 1999. (Illus.). 524p. text (*0-7020-2540-2*) W B Saunders GBR. *Dist:* Saunders.

Dust Between My Toes: An Amish Boy's Journey. Wayne M. Weaver. 1997. LC 96-39479. (Illus.). 256p. 21.95 (*1-888683-37-6*) Wooster Bk.

Dutch Annual of Psychoanalysis, 1993. Han Groen-Prakken & A. Ladan. 1993. 304p. (*90-265-1368-2*) Swets.

Dutch-English, English-Dutch Medical Dictionary. Mostert. 3rd ed. 1990. (DUT & ENG.). 206p. 75.00 (*0-7859-7519-5*, 9031310786) Fr & Eur.

Dutch/English-English-Dutch Medical Dictionary. P. L. Kerkhof. Date not set. (DUT & ENG.). 150.00 (*0-7859-9591-9*) Fr & Eur.

Dutcher's Hematologic Morphology. Dutcher. 1994. text 500.00 (*1-56815-023-7*) Mosby Inc.

Duties to Others. Ed. by Courtney S. Campbell & B. Andrew Lustig. 1994. LC 93-40310. (Theology & Medicine Ser.: Vol. 4). 332p. (C). lib. bdg. (*0-7923-2638-5*) Kluwer Academic NLD. *Dist:* Kluwer Academic.

Dwell in Possibility: Selected Writings of Pierre Turquet. Ed. by W. Gordon Lawrence & Robert Gosling. 2000. pap. (*1-899209-05-0*) Process Pr GBR. *Dist:* Intl Spec Bk.

Dworkin-Culatta Oral Mechanism Examination. James P. Dworkin & Richard Culatta. 1980. (Illus.). 76p. (Orig.). (C). 13.00 (*0-938820-00-1*) Edgewood KY.

Dyadic Transaction: An Investigation into the Nature of the Psychotherapeutic Process. Samuel Eisenstein et al. 1994. LC 93-23866. 180p. (C). text 34.95 (*1-56000-136-4*) Transaction Pubs.

Dying: A Psychoanalytic Study with Special Reference to Individual Creativity & Defensive Organization. Tor-Bjorn Haggland. 1978. LC 77-92179. 259p. 40.00 (*0-8236-1510-3*) Intl Univs Pr.

Dying & Death in Law & Medicine: A Forensic Primer for Health & Legal Professionals. Arthur S. Berger. 1992. LC 92-18875. 240p. 67.00 (*0-275-93928-6*, C3928, Praeger Pubs) Greenwood.

Dying & Disabled Children: Dealing with Loss & Grief. Ed. by Harold M. Dick et al. 1989. LC 88-15364. (Loss, Grief & Care Ser.: Vol. 2, Nos. 3 & 4). (Illus.). 153p. text 39.95 (*0-86656-759-3*) Haworth Pr.

Dying, Death & Bereavement. Inge B. Corless,R.N. et al. 1994. (Nursing-Health Science Ser.). 432p. (C). pap. text 41.25 (*0-86720-631-4*) Jones & Bartlett.

Dying, Death & Loss in Long-Term Care. Marylou Hughes. 1993. 190p. (Orig.). (C). 22.50 (*1-877735-42-6*, 2226PP) Prof Prnting & Pub.

Dying for a Drink: A Pastor & a Physician Talk about Alcoholism. Alexander DeJong & Martin Doot. 1999. LC 98-49965. 76p. pap. 8.00 (*0-8028-4622-X*) Eerdmans.

Dying for Care. Harry Van Bommel. 1992. 180p. (Orig.). pap. (*1-55021-073-4*) NC Ltd CAN. *Dist:* U of Toronto Pr.

Dying from Dioxin: A Citizen's Guide to Reclaiming Our Health & Rebuilding Democracy. Lois M. Gibbs & Citizens Clearinghouse for Hazardous Waste Staff. 1995. LC 95-23589. 360p. 40.00 (*0-89608-526-0*); pap. 20.00 (*0-89608-525-2*) South End Pr.

Dying in Care. Wayne Minnick. 2002. 184p. pap. 13.95 (*0-88739-413-2*) Creative Arts.

Dying of Enoch Wallace: Life, Death & the Changing Brain. Ira B. Black. 2000. LC 2001-265187. (Illus.). 260p. text 24.95 (*0-07-136208-8*) McGraw-Hill Prof.

Dying 101: A Short Course on Living for the Terminally ill. G. Cason-Reiser et al. 1996. LC 96-92022. 224p. 19.95 (*0-9649938-0-5*) Push the Envelope.

Dying Patient. Howard E. Freeman. Ed. by Orville G. Brim, Jr. et al. 1970. LC 77-104181. 45.00 (*0-87154-155-6*) Russell Sage.

Dying Patient. Orville G. Brim, Jr. et al. 1981. LC 80-20141. 390p. (C). reprint ed. pap. text 24.95 (*0-87855-684-2*) Transaction Pubs.

Dying to Be Thin: Understanding & Defeating Anorexia Nervosa & Bulimia. Ira M. Sacker & Marc A. Zimmer. 1987. 288p. reprint ed. pap. 14.95 (*0-446-38417-8*) Warner Bks.

Dying to Care? Work, Stress & Burnout in HIV/AIDS Careers. David Miller. 2000. LC 99-42155. (*1-85728-820-3*) UCL Pr Ltd GBR. *Dist:* Taylor & Francis.

Dying to Care? Work, Stress & Burnout in HIV/AIDS Carers. David Miller. 2000. LC 99-42155. (Social Aspects of AIDS Ser.). (*1-85728-821-1*) UCL Pr Ltd GBR. *Dist:* Taylor & Francis.

Dying to Know: Public Release of Information about Quality of Health Care. Martin V. Marshall et al. 2001. LC 00-59110. (Nuffield Trust Ser.: No. 12). (Illus.). 137p. pap. 25.00 (*0-8330-2891-X*) Rand Corp.

Dying to Please: Anorexia Nervosa & Its Cure. Avis Rumney. 1983. LC 83-9443. 128p. (Orig.). (gr. 10-12). per. 25.00 (*0-89950-083-8*) McFarland & Co.

Dying to Quit: Why We Smoke & How We Stop. Janet Brigham. 1998. LC 98-17906. 308p. 29.95 (*0-309-06409-0*) Natl Acad Pr.

Dying to Smoke: One Family's Struggle with America's Deadliest Drug. Wendy Kirchner. Ed. by Writers Edge, Inc. Staff. 1997. LC 97-91041. (Illus.). 172p. pap. 9.95 (*0-9659188-0-7*) Starr Publ.

Dying Too Soon: How Cost-Effectiveness Analysis Can Save Lives. Tammy O. Tengs. 1996. 26p. pap. 10.00 (*1-56808-072-7*, 204) Natl Ctr Pol.

Dying Well: A Guide to Enabling a Good Death. Julia Neuberger. 1999. 186p. pap. (*1-898507-26-0*) Books For Midwives Pr GBR. *Dist:* Buttrwrth-Heinemann, Balogh.

Dying with AIDS-Living with AIDS. Leslie. 1993. (Illus.). 76p. pap. (*0-919754-46-5*, Muses Co) J G Shillingford Pub.

Dynamic Aspects of Cell Surface Organization. Ed. by Garth, L. Nicolson & George H. Poste. 1980. (Cell Surface Reviews Ser.: Vol. 3). 368.25 (*0-7204-0623-4*) Elsevier.

Dynamic Aspects of Conformation Changes in Biological Macromolecules: Proceedings of the Societe de Chimie Physique, 23rd. Societe de Chemie Physique Staff. Ed. by C. Sadron. 1973. LC 72-97962. 400p. text 239.50 (*90-277-0334-5*) Kluwer Academic.

Dynamic Aspects of Dental Pulp: Molecular Biology, Pharmacology & Pathophysiology. Ed. by R. Inoki et al. 1990. 250p. pap. 224.95 (*0-412-35860-3*, A4930) Chapman & Hall.

Dynamic Assessment in Couple Therapy. William J. Hiebert et al. 1993. LC 93-11168. 132p. pap. 18.95 (*0-669-24863-0*) Free Pr.

Dynamic Assessment of Young Children. David Tzuriel. 2001. LC 00-67110. (Series on Human Exceptionality). (Illus.). xvi, 241p. 59.50 (*0-306-46510-8*, Kluwer Plenum) Kluwer Academic.

Dynamic Biological Networks: The Stomatogastric Nervous System. Ed. by Ronald M. Harris-Warrick et al. 1992. (Bradford-Computational Neuroscience Ser.). (Illus.). 248p. 65.00 (*0-262-08214-4*, Bradford Bks) MIT Pr.

Dynamic Cardiomyoplasty: The Mechanisms & Optimization of Programming. Carlos M. Li et al. 1997. LC 97-29969. (Current Clinical Practices in Dynamic Cardiomyoplasty Ser.: Vol. 1). (Illus.). 67p. pap. 15.00 (*0-87993-686-X*) Futura Pub.

Dynamic Clinical Studies with Radioisotopes: Proceedings. Ed. by Ralph M. Kniseley et al. 1964. (AEC Symposium Ser.). 634p. pap. 6.25 (*0-87079-181-8*, TID-7678); fiche 6.50 (*0-87079-182-6*, TID-7678) DOE.

Dynamic Concepts in Psychology. Mitterer. 1993. (C). pap. text, tchr. ed. 35.00 (*0-15-500935-4*) Harcourt Coll Pubs.

Dynamic EMG Evaluation: Interpreting Postural Dysfunction Barbara J. Headley. 1990. (Illus.). 87p. (Orig.). pap. 14.00 (*0-929538-06-4*) Innovat Systems.

Dynamic Knowledge Interaction. Toyoaki Nishida. 2000. LC 00-23087. (International Series on Computational Intelligence Ser.). 296p. 89.95 (*0-8493-0113-0*) CRC Pr.

Dynamic Living Workbook. Aileen Ludington & Hans Diehl. rev. ed. 1995. LC 95-7074. Orig. Title: Lifestyle Capsules. 112p. pap. 5.99 (*0-8280-0942-2*) Review & Herald.

Dynamic Measures of Low Back Performance. William S. Marras et al. 1993. 20p. (C). pap. 8.00 (*0-932627-52-8*, 174-ER-93) Am Indus Hygiene.

Dynamic Modeling in the Health Sciences. James L. Hargrove. 1998. LC 97-39337. (Modeling Dynamic Systems Ser.). (Illus.). 321p. 62.95 (*0-387-94996-8*) Spr-Verlag.

Dynamic Monoclonal & Polyclonal Antibody Business. 1992. 138p. 2650.00 (*0-89336-914-4*, C-088R) BCC.

Dynamic Muscular Relaxation. Harry D. Lawson. 1991. LC 86-17410. (Illus.). 150.00 (*0-87949-270-8*) Ashley Bks.

Dynamic Nurse-Patient Relationship. Ida O. Pelletier. 1990. 128p. 12.50 (*0-88737-489-1*) Natl League Nurse.

Dynamic Psychiatry: Explorations in Psychotherapy, Psychoanalysis, & Psychosomatic Medicine. Pietro Castelnuovo-Tedesco. 1991. LC 90-4927. (Emotions & Behavior Monographs: No. 10). 474p. 70.00 (*0-8236-1515-4*) Intl Univs Pr.

Dynamic Psychiatry & the Sense of Justice. Warren H. Gorman. 1974. LC 70-96982. (Illus.). 320p. 22.50 (*0-87527-106-5*) Green.

Dynamic Psychology. Robert S. Woodworth. 1980. LC 73-2998. (Classics in Psychology Ser.). reprint ed. 21.95 (*0-405-05172-7*) Ayer.

Dynamic Psychotherapy: An Introductory Approach. Marc H. Hollender & Charles V. Ford. 1990. LC 90-77. 229p. text 34.50 (*0-88048-319-9*, 8319) Am Psychiatric.

Dynamic Psychotherapy Explained. Patricia Hughes. 1999. LC 99-206272. 176p. pap. (*1-85775-336-4*) Radcliffe Med Pr GBR. *Dist:* Balogh.

Dynamic Psychotherapy with the Borderline Patient. William N. Goldstein. 1996. LC 96-4641. 312p. 50.00 (*1-56821-817-6*) Aronson.

Dynamic Radiology of the Abdomen. 1995. 155.00 (*0-387-94613-6*) Spr-Verlag.

Dynamic Radiology of the Abdomen: Normal & Pathologic Anatomy. M. A. Meyers. 4th ed. 1993. (Illus.). 680p. (*3-540-94022-7*) Spr-Verlag.

Dynamic State of Muscle Fibers: Proceedings of the Int'l Symposium Oct. 1-6, 1989, Konstanz, Fed. Rep. of Germany. Ed. by Dirk Pette. 1990. (Illus.). xxiv, 729p. (C). lib. bdg. 288.50 (*3-11-012168-9*) De Gruyter.

Dynamic Strength. Harry Wong. 1980. LC 80-53545. (Illus.). 144p. pap. 6.95 (*0-86568-013-2*, 209) Unique Pubns.

Dynamic Surface Tensiometry in Medicine. Valery N. Kazakov. 2000. LC 00-22813. (Studies in Interface Science). (Illus.). 388p. 204.00 (*0-444-50411-7*) Elsevier.

Dynamic Therapies for Psychiatric Disorders: Axis I. Ed. by Jacques P. Barber et al. 1995. LC 94-42944. 460p. 55.00 (*0-465-01742-8*) Basic.

Dynamic Therapy in Brief Hospitalization. John M. Oldham & L. Mark Russakoff. 1987. LC 87-12629. 235p. 40.00 (*0-87668-965-9*) Aronson.

Dynamic Therapy of the Older Patient. Wayne A. Myers. 1984. LC 83-25772. (Dynamic Thrpy Older Patient CL. Ser.). 270p. 45.00 (*0-87668-623-4*) Aronson.

Dynamical Disease: Mathematical Analysis of Human Illness. J. Milton. 1995. LC 95-18267. 224p. pap. 53.95 (*1-56396-370-1*, AIP Pr) Spr-Verlag.

Dynamically Oriented Art Therapy: Its Principles & Practice. Margaret Naumburg. 1987. (Illus.). 168p. (C). reprint ed. 36.95 (*0-9613309-1-0*) Magnolia St Pub.

Dynamics & Evolution of Transposable Elements. Pierre Capy & Thierry Langin. 1997. 200p. 89.95 (*0-412-12091-7*) Landes Bioscience.

Dynamics & Indeterminism in Developmental & Social Processes. Ed. by Alan Fogel et al. 1996. LC 96-34678. 280p. 69.95 (*0-8058-1805-7*); pap. text 32.50 (*0-8058-1806-5*) L Erlbaum Assocs.

Dynamics & Treatment of Alcoholism: Essential Papers. Ronna H. Weiss. Ed. by Jerome D. Levin. 1994. LC 93-8825. 464p. 60.00 (*1-56821-072-8*) Aronson.

Dynamics in Psychology. Wolfgang Kohler. 1973. pap. 2.95 (*0-87140-277-7*); 1940. (C). 6.00 (*0-87140-902-X*) Liveright.

Dynamics of Acute Bacterial Diseases Epidemiological Models & Their Application in Public Health. B. Cvjetanovic & B. Grab. 1978. (Bulletin Supplement Ser.: No. 56). 143p. text 12.00 (*92-4-068561-8*) World Health.

Dynamics of Aggression: Biological & Social Processes in Dyads & Groups. Michael Potegal & John Knutson. 1994. 352p. text 75.00 (*0-8058-0729-2*) L Erlbaum Assocs.

Dynamics of Art as Therapy with Adolescents. Bruce L. Moon. LC 98-37400. (Illus.). 1999. 260p. text 55.95 (*0-398-06923-9*); 1998. xxii, 237p. pap. text 41.95 (*0-398-06924-7*) C C Thomas.

Dynamics of Art Psychotherapy. Harriet Wadeson. 1994. LC 94-236038. 336p. pap. 65.00 (*0-471-11464-2*) Wiley.

Dynamics of Cell & Tissue Motion. Ed. by W. Alt et al. 1997. LC 97-39810. (Mathematics & Biosciences in Interaction Ser.). xvi, 336p. 69.50 (*3-7643-5781-9*) Birkhauser.

Dynamics of Cell Ultrastructure. Judy M. Strum. 1996. (Imagedisc Library Ser.). text 500.00 (*0-8151-8535-9*) Mosby Inc.

Dynamics of Clinical Dietetics. Marion Mason et al. 1989. LC 81-16160. 354p. text 32.95 (*0-8273-4298-5*) Delmar.

Dynamics of Clinical Rehabilitative Exercise: Dynamics of Clinical Rehabilitative Exercise. Stephen M. Ordet & Leonard S. Grand. 1991. (Illus.). 304p. 55.00 (*0-683-06654-4*) Lppncott W & W.

Dynamics of Creation. Anthony Storr. 1985. LC 85-47639. 264p. reprint ed. pap. 8.95 (*0-689-70700-2*, 334) Atheneum Yung Read.

Dynamics of Crisis Intervention: Loss as the Common Denominator. Juliann Whetsell Mitchell. 1999. LC 98-34004. 299p. 62.95 (*0-398-06915-8*); 312p. pap. 49.95 (*0-398-06916-6*) C C Thomas.

Dynamics of Development & the Therapeutic Process. Richard Lasky. 1993. LC 92-17808. 488p. 60.00 (*0-87668-565-3*) Aronson.

Dynamics of Dispensing, Vol. III. William A. Borover. 1983. (Illus.). per. 48.00 (*0-9606398-3-7*) Gracie Ent.

Dynamics of Drug Abuse. Diana Fishbein & Susan Pease. 1995. LC 95-24215. 480p. pap. text 67.00 (*0-205-13967-1*) Allyn.

Dynamics of Group Psychotherapy. S. R. Slavson & Mortimer Schiffer. 1979. LC 78-68010. 830p. 40.00 (*0-87668-372-3*) Aronson.

Dynamics of Hemostasis & Thrombosis. Ed. by Marcus B. Simpson, Jr. & Daniel B. Brubaker. 1995. LC 95-40739. (Illus.). 183p. (C). 55.00 (*1-56395-043-X*) Am Assn Blood.

Dynamics of Homosexuality. Major J. Baisden, Jr. 1975. LC 75-31. 199p. 6.95 (*0-912984-02-3*) Allied Res Soc.

Dynamics of Human Adjustment. Percival M. Symonds. 1970. LC 72-94620. 666p. reprint ed. lib. bdg. 95.00 (*0-8371-3148-0*, SYHA, Greenwood Pr) Greenwood.

Dynamics of Human Biologic Tissues. Dean P. Currier & Roger M. Nelson. 1992. (Contemporary Perspectives in Rehabilitation Ser.: Vol. 8). (Illus.). 276p. (C). text 35.00 (*0-8036-2298-8*) Davis Co.

Dynamics of Human Communication: A Laboratory Approach. Gail E. Myers & Michele T. Myers. 6th ed. 1991. 480p. (C). text 52.50 (*0-07-044231-2*) McGrw-H Hghr Educ.

Dynamics of Human Reproduction: Biology, Biometry, Demography. James W. Wood. 1994. LC 93-36613. (Evolutionary Foundations of Human Behavior Ser.). (Illus.). 669p. pap. text 44.95 (*0-202-01180-1*); lib. bdg. 79.95 (*0-202-01179-8*) Aldine de Gruyter.

Dynamics of Personality. Lewis R. Wolberg & John P. Kildahl. 1970. LC 75-91600. 336p. text 59.00 (*0-8089-0539-2*, 794876, Grune & Strat) Harcrt Hlth Sci Grp.

Dynamics of Sensory & Cognitive Processing by the Brain. Ed. by E Baser. 1988. (Brain Dynamics Ser.). (Illus.). 406p. 121.00 (*0-387-16994-6*) Spr-Verlag.

Dynamics of Stress: Physiological, Psychological, & Social Perspectives. M. H. Appley & R. A. Trumbull. 1986. LC 86-25175. (Illus.). 360p. (C). 65.00 (*0-306-42252-2*, Plenum Trade) Perseus Pubng.

Dynamics of the Singing Voice. Meribeth Bunch. 196p. 3rd ed. 1995. LC 94-35638. pap. 39.00 (*0-387-82623-8*); 4th ed. 1997. LC 97-5468. (Illus.). 49.00 (*3-211-82985-7*) Spr-Verlag.

Dynamics of Therapy in a Controlled Relationship. Jessie Taft. 1990. 20.50 (*0-8446-3045-4*) Peter Smith.

Dynamik, Koronardurchblutung und Sauerstoffverbrauch des Normalen und Kranken Herzens: Experimentell-Pharmakologische Untersuchungen und Herzkatheterstudien am Patienten. B. E. Strauer. 1995. (Illus.). 124p. pap. 34.00 (*3-8055-2152-9*) S Karger.

Dysfunction & Heart Failure. William Gaasch & Martin M. Lewinter. 1993. LC 93-9991. (Illus.). 498p. text 89.50 (*0-8121-1509-0*) Lppncott W & W.

Dysfunctional by Design: The Rebirth of Cultural Survivors: Self-Help for African-American Substance Abusers. William Green. 1995. 136p. (Orig.). pap. 12.00 (*1-886094-10-1*) Chicago Spectrum.

Dysfunctional Uterine Bleeding. Ed. by R. W. Shaw. 1990. (Advances in Reproductive Endocrinology Ser.: Vol. 2). (Illus.). 164p. (C). lib. bdg. 74.95 (*1-85070-296-9*, Parthenon Pbng) CRC Pr.

Dyslexia. Pete Sanders & Steve Myers. 1999. LC 98-44971. (What Do You Know About... Ser.). (Illus.). 32p. (J). (gr. 1-3). 22.90 (*0-7613-0915-2*, Copper Beech Bks) Millbrook Pr.

***Dyslexia.** Thomson. 1997. pap. 28.95 (*0-412-59690-3*) Chapman & Hall.

Dyslexia: A Cognitive Developmental Perspective. Margaret Snowling. 2nd ed. 2000. LC 00-29241. (Illus.). xiv, 253p. 62.95 (*0-631-22144-1*); pap. 26.95 (*0-631-20574-8*) Blackwell Pubs.

Dyslexia: A Global Issue. Ed. by Rattihalli N. Malatesha & Harry A. Whitaker. 1983. (NATO Advanced Science Institutes Ser.). text 306.00 (*90-247-2909-2*) Kluwer Academic.

***Dyslexia: A Multidisciplinary Approach.** Ed. by P. Thomson. 1996. (Illus.). (Orig.). pap. (*0-7487-5793-7*) Nelson Thornes GBR. *Dist:* Intl Spec Bk.

Dyslexia: A Neuroscientific Approach. Frank H. Duffy & Norman Geschwind. 1985. 223p. 57.00 (*0-316-19454-9*, Little Brwn Med Div) Lppncott W & W.

Dyslexia: A Practitioner's Handbook. Gavin Reid. 2nd ed. 1998. LC 97-17407. 264p. pap. 65.00 (*0-471-97391-2*) Wiley.

Dyslexia: An Annotated Bibliography, 5. Ed. by Martha M. Evans. 1982. LC 81-20319. (Contemporary Problems of Childhood Ser.: No. 5.). (Illus.). 644p. lib. bdg. 85.00 (*0-313-21344-5*, EVD/, Greenwood Pr) Greenwood.

Dyslexia: An Introductory Guide. James Doyle. 1995. (Illus.). 218p. pap. 39.95 (*1-56593-604-3*, 1254) Thomson Learn.

Dyslexia: Biology, Cognition & Intervention. Ed. by Charles Hulme & Margaret Snowling. 1997. LC 97-176156. (Illus.). 302p. pap. 39.95 (*1-56593-892-5*, 1744) Thomson Learn.

Dyslexia: Interdisciplinary Approaches to Reading Disabilities. Herman Goldberg et al. 1982. 217p. text 28.00 (*0-8089-1484-7*, 791628, Grune & Strat) Harcrt Hlth Sci Grp.

Dyslexia: Neuropsychological Theory, Research, & Clinical Differentiation. Morris Cohen & George W. Hynd. 1989. (C). pap. text 81.95 (*0-205-10117-8*) Allyn.

Dyslexia: Neuropsychological Theory, Research, & Clinical Differentiation. Morris Cohen & George W. Hynd. 1983. (Illus.). 304p. (C). text 38.00 (*0-8089-1584-3*, 792110, Grune & Strat) Harcrt Hlth Sci Grp.

Dyslexia: Practical & Easy-to-Follow Advice. Robin Temple. 1999. LC 98-36694. (Your Child Ser.). 128p. pap. 9.95 (*1-86204-314-0*) Element MA.

Dyslexia & Development: Neurobiological Aspects of Extra-Ordinary Brains. Ed. by Albert M. Galaburda. 1993. LC 92-49952. (Illus.). 368p. 57.50 (*0-674-21940-6*) HUP.

Dyslexia & Hyperlexia. P. G. Aaron. 1989. (C). lib. bdg. 128.00 (*1-55608-079-4*) Kluwer Academic.

Dyslexia & Hyperlexia: Diagnosis & Management of Developmental Reading Disabilities. P. G. Aaron. 1994. (Neuropsychology & Cognition Ser.). 319p. (C). pap. text 73.00 (*0-7923-3155-9*) Kluwer Academic.

Dyslexia & Reading Disabilities. Helmer Muckelbust et al. 1972. 224p. text 29.50 (*0-8422-7005-1*) Irvington.

***Dyslexia & Vision.** Bruce J. W. Evans. 2001. 150p. (Orig.). (C). pap. (*1-86156-242-X*) Whurr Pub GBR. *Dist:* Taylor & Francis.

Dyslexia at College. Timothy R. Miles. 1987. 160p. 12.95 (*0-416-39670-4*) Routledge.

Dyslexia in Practice: A Guide for Teachers. Janet Townend & Martin Turner. 2000. LC 99-43454. (Illus.). xx, 349p. 65.00 (*0-306-46251-6*) Plenum.

Dyslexia Matters: A Celebratory Contributed Volume to Honour Professor T.R. Miles. Ed. by Gerald Hales. 1994. (Education). (Illus.). 236p. (Orig.). (C). pap. 29.99 (*1-56593-367-2*, 0740) Thomson Learn.

Dyslexia Reconsidered: A Cognitive-Developmental Perspective. Margaret Snowling. 1987. 250p. (Orig.). pap. text 28.95 (*0-631-14433-1*) Blackwell Pubs.

Dyslexia, Speech & Language: A Practitioner's Handbook. Ed. by Margaret Snowling & Joy Stackhouse. 1996. (Illus.). 272p. (Orig.). pap. 59.95 (*1-56593-306-0*, 1248) Singular Publishing.

Dyslipoproteinaemias & Diabetes. Ed. by R. W. James & D. Pometta. 1985. (Monographs on Atherosclerosis: Vol. 13). (Illus.). viii, 180p. 129.75 (*3-8055-4139-2*) S Karger.

Dyspepsia. Richard V. Heatley & Peter Moncur. 2000. LC 99-44002. (Illus.). 288p. 152.95 (*0-632-05458-1*) Blackwell Sci.

Dyspepsia. David A. Johnson et al. 2000. LC 00-44765. (Key Diseases Ser.). 200p. pap. text 35.00 (*0-943126-97-5*, 330300100) Amer Coll Phys.

***Dyspepsia.** Lancaster et al. 2000. (Fast Facts Ser.). (Illus.). 78p. pap. (*1-899541-92-6*) Health Pr GBR. *Dist:* JAMCO Dist.

Dysphagia: A Continuum of Care. Barbara Sonies. 1997. LC 96-42145. 300p. 58.00 (*0-8342-0785-0*) PRO-ED.

Dysphagia: Competencies, Controversies, & Costs. Adrienne L. Pearlman. 1997. 38.00 incl. audio (*1-58041-007-3*, 0112076) Am Speech Lang Hearing.

Dysphagia: Diagnosis & Management. Michael E. Groher. 3rd ed. 1997. LC 96-47477. 388p. text 59.99 (*0-7506-9730-X*) Buttrwrth-Heinemann.

Dysphagia: Update on Assessment & Treatment of Swallowing Disorders. Ed. by J. Logemann. 1999. (Folia Phoniatrica et Logopaedica Ser.: Vol. 51, Nos. 4-5 (1999)). (Illus.). 102p. pap. 34.00 (*3-8055-6944-0*) S Karger.

Dysphagia & the Child with Developmental Disabilities: Medical Clinical & Family Intervention. Susan R. Rosenthal & Justine J. Sheppard. 1994. (Illus.). 432p. (Orig.). (C). pap. text 95.95 (*1-56593-089-4*, 0394) Thomson Learn.

Dysphagia Assessment & Treatment Planning: A Team Approach. Rebecca Leonard & Katherine Kendall. 1997. LC 97-23885. (Dysphagia Ser.). (Illus.). 328p. (Orig.). pap. 65.00 (*1-56593-749-X*, 1458) Thomson Learn.

Dysphagia Care: Team Approach. Nadine O'Sullivan. 1990. (Team Approach with Acute & Long Term Patients). (Illus.). 112p. (Orig.). (C). pap. 29.95 (*0-9633234-0-7*) Cottage Sq Pr.

Dysphagia Care Team Approach with Acute & Long Term Patients. Nadine O'Sullivan. Ed. by Arthur C. Turner. 2nd ed. 1995. (Illus.). 212p. (C). pap. 20.97 (*0-9633234-1-5*) Cottage Sq Pr.

Dysphagia Challenge, Techniques for the Individual. Pam Womack. Ed. by Jody Vogelzang & Nancy Bishop. 3rd rev. ed. 1999. 72p. pap. 12.00 (*0-9671338-0-7*) Challenge Bks.

Dysphagia in the Elderly. Musson. 2002. pap. 48.50 net. (*1-56593-858-5*) Thomson Learn.

Dysplasia & Cancer in Colitis: Proceedings of the Symposium Held June 1-4, 1989, Baltimore, MD. Ed. by Robert H. Riddell. 1991. 296p. 155.00 (*0-444-01570-1*) P-H.

Dyspnea. HPNA Staff. 1999. 40p. pap. text 15.00 (*0-7872-6010-X*) Kendall-Hunt.

Dyspnea. Donald A. Mahler. 1997. LC 97-42473. (Lung Biology in Health & Disease Ser.). (Illus.). 432p. text 195.00 (*0-8247-9814-7*) Dekker.

Dysrhythmia Recognition & Management. Karen Fenstermacher. Ed. by Robin Carter. 3rd ed. 1998. LC 98-5491. (Illus.). 224p. (C). pap. text 25.00 (*0-7216-7923-4*) Saunders.

Dysthymia & the Spectrum of Chronic Depressions. Hagop S. Akiskal. Ed. by Giovanni B. Cassano. 1997. LC 97-11003. 228p. text 35.00 (*1-57230-089-2*, 0089) Guilford Pubns.

Dystonia: The Disease That Distorts. Eugene Smith. 1997. LC 96-68617. pap. text 15.00 (*0-89716-621-3*) P B Pubng.

Dystonia 3, Vol. 78. Stanley Fahn & C. David Marsden. 1998. 400p. text 169.00 (*0-7817-1538-5*) Lppncott W & W.

Dystrophin: Gene, Protein & Cell Biology. Ed. by Susan C. Brown & Jack A. Lucy. 1997. LC 96-37800. (Illus.). 356p. (C). text 100.00 (*0-521-55033-5*) Cambridge U Pr.

E

E. C. Rosenow (1875-1966) & Associates—A Reference Manual: Medical Guide of the Future. S. H. Shakman. rev. ed. 1998. LC 98-96131. 200p. pap. text 49.95 (*1-892506-08-4*) Inst of Science.

E Dickersons Secrets of Pro Power P. Eric Dickerson & Richard G. Walsh. rev. ed. 1999. (Illus.). 224p. reprint ed. pap. 9.95 (*1-56743-018-X*, Amistad) HarperTrade.

***E-Drugs: Who Regulates Internet Pharmacies?: Congressional Hearing.** Ed. by James M. Jeffords. 2001. (Illus.). 165p. (C). pap. text 35.00 (*0-7567-1230-0*) DIANE Pub.

E-Healthcare: Harness the Power of Internet e-Commerce & e-Care. Douglas E. Goldstein. 2000. LC 99-58554. 491p. pap. 95.00 (*0-8342-1365-6*) Aspen Pub.

E-M Coding Made Easy! Ed. by Kathryn M. Swanson. 3rd ed. 1998. 242p. ring bd. 44.95 (*1-57066-085-9*, ME085) Practice Mgmt Info.

***e-Pharmacy: A Guide to the Internet CareZone.** Mark R. Jacobs. 2001. LC 2001-53742. 200p. pap. 35.00 (*1-58212-029-3*) Am Pharm Assn.

e-Pharmacy: A Guide to the Internet CareZone. Mark R. Jacobs. 2001. LC 00-48090. (Illus.). xx, 165p. pap. text 35.00 net. (*1-58212-014-5*) Am Pharm Assn.

***E-Therapy.** Robert Hsiung. 250p. pap. 25.00 (*0-393-70370-3*) Norton.

E-Z Abegeez: Arterial Blood Gases. Gregory L. Culver. 1998. LC 98-90061. pap. 10.95 (*0-533-12697-5*) Vantage.

EAP Digest Annual 1981-1982. 1983. 147p. (Orig.). pap. text 21.00 (*0-9610026-1-1*) Perf Resource Pr.

Ear, Vol. 2. J. A. Jahrsdoerfer. Ed. by Hans H. Naumann. 2nd ed. 1996. (Illus.). 500p. text 189.00 (*0-86577-660-1*) Thieme Med Pubs.

Ear: A Comprehensive Textbook of Otology & Neurotology. Rinaldo F. Canalis & Paul R. Lambert. 2000. LC 99-16731. (Illus.). xxv, 900p. text 199.00 (*0-7817-1558-X*) Lppncott W & W.

Ear Book: A Parent's Guide to Common Ear Disorders of Children. David R. Marty. 1987. (Illus.). 132p. pap. 16.95 (*0-943023-12-2*); lib. bdg. 23.95 (*0-943023-11-4*) Lang E N T Pub.

Ear Identification. Alfred V. Iannarelli. rev. ed. 1989. (Forensic Identification Ser.). (Illus.). 220p. (C). reprint ed. 62.50 (*0-9623178-0-2*) Paramont Pub.

Ear Infections in Your Child. Kenneth Grundfast & Cynthia J. Carney. 1989. 296p. pap. 12.95 (*0-446-38931-5*) Warner Bks.

Ear, Nose & Throat. R. Youngs & Nicholas D. Stafford. 1988. (Colour Aids Ser.). (Illus.). 112p. pap. text (*0-443-03198-3*) Church.

Ear, Nose, & Throat, & Head & Neck Surgery: An Illustrated Colour Text. R. S. Dhillon & C. A. East. 2nd ed. 1999. LC 99-11695. (*0-443-05955-1*) Church.

Ear, Nose & Throat Diseases. K. P. Gibbin & P. J. Bradley. 1989. (MCQs Brain Scan Ser.). 156p. 28.95 (*0-387-19559-9*, 2927) Spr-Verlag.

Ear, Nose, & Throat Diseases: A Pocket Reference. Walter Becker et al. 2nd ed. 1994. 32.00 (*0-86577-536-2*) Thieme Med Pubs.

Ear, Nose & Throat Disorders. Barbara A. Sigler. 1993. LC 93-23154. (Mosby's Clinical Nursing Ser.). (Illus.). 320p. (C). (gr. 13). text 37.00 (*0-8016-8011-5*, 08011) Mosby Inc.

Ear, Nose & Throat Disorders Sourcebook: Basic Information about Disorders of the Ears, Nose, Sinus Cavities, Pharynx & Larynx. Ed. by Linda M. Ross. 1997. LC 98-29719. (Health Reference Ser.). 576p. lib. bdg. 78.00 (*0-7808-0206-3*) Omnigraphics Inc.

***Ear, Nose & Throat Emergencies: Diagnosis & Management.** Farrell & Lavy. 2001. pap. text 45.00 (*0-7506-3832-X*) Buttrwrth-Heinemann.

Ear, Nose & Throat, Head & Neck Surgery. R. S. Dhillon & C. A. East. 1994. (Illus.). 128p. pap. text (*0-443-04299-3*) Church.

Ear, Nose & Throat Surgery. John R. Cherry, III. Ed. by Walter Scott. 1997. LC 97-167502. (Medico-Legal Practitioner Ser.). 582p. (*1-85941-210-6*) Cavendish Pubng GBR. *Dist:* Gaunt.

Ear to the Chest: The Evolution of the Stethoscope. M. D. Blaufox. 2001. LC 2001-36721. (Illus.). 120p. lib. bdg. 74.95 (*1-85070-278-0*, Parthenon Pbng) CRC Pr.

Earache in Children: A Guide for Parents. Bluestone & Stool. 1995. (Pediatrics Ser.). (Illus.). 24p. pap. 2.95 (*1-885274-10-6*) Health InfoNet Inc.

***Earl Mindell's Food as Medicine: What You Can Eat to Help Prevent Everything from Colds to Heart Disease to Cancer.** Earl Mindell. 2002. 400p. mass mkt. 7.99 (*0-7432-2662-3*) PB.

Earl Mindell's New & Revised Vitamin Bible. Earl L. Mindell. 1989. 384p. mass mkt. 5.95 (*0-446-35643-3*) Warner Bks.

Earl Mindell's Safe Eating. Earl L. Mindell. 1988. 288p. mass mkt. 5.99 (*0-446-34670-5*) Warner Bks.

***Earl Mindell's Secret Remedies.** Earl Mindell. 2002. 304p. mass mkt. 7.99 (*0-7432-2660-7*, Fireside) S&S Trade Pap.

Earl Mindell's Shaping up with Vitamins. Earl L. Mindell. 1988. 320p. mass mkt. 5.99 (*0-446-30952-4*) Warner Bks.

Earliest Childhood Memories: Theory & Application to Clinical Practice, Vol. 1. Arnold R. Bruhn. 1990. LC 90-7079. 192p. 45.00 (*0-275-92699-0*, C2699, Praeger Pubs) Greenwood.

Earliest Printed Literature on Syphilis: Being Ten Tractates from the Years 1495-1498. Karl Sudhoff. LC 75-23762. reprint ed. 60.00 (*0-404-13368-1*) AMS Pr.

Early Adolescence: Perspectives on Research, Policy, & Intervention. Ed. by Richard M. Lerner. 1993. (Penn State Series on Child & Adolescent Development). 528p. text 99.95 (*0-8058-1164-8*) L Erlbaum Assocs.

Early Adolescence & the Search for Self. Douglas Schave & Barbara Schave. 1989. LC 88-27514. 161p. 52.95 (*0-275-92765-2*, C2765, Praeger Pubs) Greenwood.

Early Adolescence to Early Adulthood: The Best of ALCD, Vol. 5. Ed. by William M. Cruickshank & Joanne M. Kliebhan. 1984. LC 83-17968. (Best of ACLD Ser.). (Illus.). 208p. pap. text 19.95 (*0-8156-2301-1*) Syracuse U Pr.

Early American Home Remedies. 1968. (Americana Bks.). (Illus.). 3.00 (*0-911410-20-1*) Applied Arts.

Early American Medical Imprints: A Guide to Works Printed in the United States, 1668-1880. Robert B. Austin. 1999. 240p. reprint ed. 50.00 (*1-57898-139-5*) Martino Pubng.

Early American Medical Imprints 1668-1820. Robert B. Austin. 1987. 240p. reprint ed. pap. text 15.00 (*0-915497-01-8*) Printers Devil.

Early American Medical Imprints, 1668-1820: A Guide to Works Printed in the U. S. Robert B. Austin. 1981. LC 81-12077. 240p. 175.00 (*0-89235-078-4*, PSM) Gale.

Early American Medical Imprints, 1668-1820: Subject, Name & Format Index to the Microfilm Collection. Compiled by Bertha Almagro. 1981. 23p. (C). pap. text 55.00 (*0-89235-027-X*, PSM) Gale.

Early Aphasia Therapy: For the Clinic & Home. Emily Pietz Porter. 2000. (Illus.). 250p. spiral bd. 49.00 (*1-883315-53-0*) Imaginart Intl.

Early Black American Leaders in Nursing: Architects for Integration & Equality. Althea T. Davis. 1999. LC 98-52865. (National League for Nursing Ser.). (Illus.). 256p. (C). pap. text 34.95 (*0-7637-1009-1*, 1009-1, N L N Bart) Jones & Bartlett.

Early Breast Cancer: Its History & Results of Treatment. C. M. Mansfield. Ed. by A. Wolsky. 1976. (Experimental Biology & Medicine Ser.: Vol. 5). (Illus.). 120p. 42.75 (*3-8055-2300-9*) S Karger.

Early Child Care in Britain, Vol. 5. M. Pringle & Sandhya Naidoo. 1975. LC 74-80075. (International Monographs on Early Child Care). (Illus.). xii, 175p. text 104.00 (*0-677-05200-6*) Gordon & Breach.

Early Child Care in France. M. David & I. Lezine. 1975. (International Monographs on Early Child Care). xvi, 148p. text 129.00 (*0-677-05210-3*) Gordon & Breach.

Early Child Care in Sweden, Vol. 2. Ragnar Berfenstam & Inger William-Olsson. 1973. (International Monographs on Early Child Care). xii, 156p. text 117.00 (*0-677-04890-4*) Gordon & Breach.

Early Child Development: Investing in Our Children's Future. Ed. by M. E. Young. 1997. LC 97-6217. (International Congress Ser.: Vol. 1137). 352p. 162.50 (*0-444-82605-X*) Elsevier.

Early Childhood Autism. I. A. Van Berckelaer-Onnes. 1983. (Modern Approaches to the Diagnosis & Instruction of Multi-Handicapped Children Ser.: Vol. 17). x, 166p. (*90-265-0451-9*) Swets.

Early Childhood Caries: A Team Approach to Prevention & Treatment. Peter Milgrom & Philip Weinstein. 1998. (Illus.). 200p. pap. text 39.95 (*1-880291-02-9*) Cont Dental Educ.

Early Childhood Development: Prebirth Through Age Eight. Franz Anselmo. 2nd ed. 1994. LC 94-13382. 576p. (C). pap. 73.00 (*0-02-303607-9*, Macmillan Coll) P-H.

Early Childhood Development & Care - An Australian Perspective: A Special Issue of the Journal Early Child Development & Care. Ed. by W. Schiller. 1989. 186p. pap. text 238.00 (*0-677-26040-7*) Gordon & Breach.

Early Childhood Disturbances, the Infantile Neurosis, & the Adult Disturbances. Humberto Nagera. 1966. LC 66-17526. (Psychoanalytic Study of the Child Monographs: No. 2). 96p. 27.50 (*0-8236-1520-0*) Intl Univs Pr.

Early Childhood Parenting Skills. Richard R. Abidin. 1996. (Illus.). pap., wbk. ed. 15.00 (*0-911907-25-4*) Psych Assess.

Early Childhood Parenting Skills for the Mental Health Professional. Richard R. Abidin. 1996. (Illus.). pap. 34.00 (*0-911907-24-6*) Psych Assess.

Early Chinese Medical Literature: The Mawangdui Medical Manuscripts. Tr. by Donald Harper from CHI. 1997. LC 96-47823. (Sir Henry Wellcome Asian Ser.). 549p. 161.50 (*0-7103-0582-6*) Col U Pr.

Early Clinical Diagnosis. Gerald Sandler & J. Fry. 1986. text 206.50 (*0-85200-921-6*) Kluwer Academic.

Early Colorectal Cancer: Detection of Depressed Types Colorectal Carcinomas. Shin'ei Kudo. 1997. LC 96-30135. (Illus.). 174p. 139.00 (*0-89640-330-0*) Igaku-Shoin.

Early Conceptions & Tests of Intelligence. Joseph Peterson. 1970. LC 70-98868. 320p. reprint ed. lib. bdg. 69.95 (*0-8371-2836-6*, PETI, Greenwood Pr) Greenwood.

Early CT Diagnosis of Hemispheric Brain Infarction, Vol. VII. R. Von Kummer et al. 1996. LC 95-24344. (Illus.). 101p. pap. 69.95 (*3-540-60056-6*) Spr-Verlag.

Early Detection & Localization of Lung Tumors in High Risk Groups. Ed. by P. R. Band. 1982. (Recent Results in Cancer Research Ser.: Vol. 82). (Illus.). 190p. 76.00 (*0-387-11249-9*) Spr-Verlag.

Early Detection & Management of Cerebral Palsy. Ed. by H. Galjaard et al. 1987. (Topics in the Neurosciences Ser.). (C). text 151.50 (*0-89838-890-2*) Kluwer Academic.

Early Detection & Treatment of Liver Cancer. Ed. by Kunio Okuda et al. 1991. (Gann Monographs on Cancer Research: No. 38). 240p. (*0-7484-0036-2*) Tay Francis Ltd GBR. *Dist:* Taylor & Francis.

Early Detection of Cancer: A Report. WHO Staff. 1969. (Technical Reports: No. 422). 35p. pap. text 5.00 (*92-4-120422-2*, 1100422) World Health.

Early Detection of Dental Caries: Proceedings of the 1st Annual Indiana Conference. Ed. by George K. Stookey. 1996. LC 96-79094. (Illus.). 348p. text (*0-9655149-0-0*) IN Univ Schl Dentstry.

Early Detection of Psychiatric Disorders in Children. H. Van Engeland. 1990. 88p. pap. (*90-265-0949-9*) Swets.

Early Development & Education of the Child. Willi Hoffer. 1980. LC 76-5230. (Early Development Education Child C Ser.). 240p. 45.00 (*0-87668-154-2*) Aronson.

Early Development of Xenopus Laevis: An Atlas of the Histology. Ed. by P. Hausen & M. Riebesell. 1991. (Illus.). 142p. 189.00 (*0-387-53740-6*) Spr-Verlag.

Early Developmental Stages of Substance Abuse. Ed. by H. U. Wittchen & C. B. Nelson. 1998. (European Addiction Research Ser.: Vol. 4, Nos. 1-2, 1998). (Illus.). 84p. pap. 60.00 (*3-8055-6674-3*) S Karger.

Early Diagnosis & Interventional Therapy in Cerebral Palsy: An Interdisciplinary Approach. Alfred L. Scherzer. 3rd ed. 2000. LC 00-50086. (Pediatric Habilitation Ser.: Vol. 11). (Illus.). xi, 355p. text 55.00 (*0-8247-6006-9*) Dekker.

Early Diagnosis & Prevention of Genetic Diseases. L. N. Went et al. 1975. text 85.50 (*90-6021-237-1*) Kluwer Academic.

Early Diagnosis & Therapy in Cerebral Palsy: A Primer on Infant Developmental Problems. Alfred L. Scherzer & Tscharnuter. 2nd rev. ed. 1990. (Pediatric Habilitation Ser.: Vol. 6). (Illus.). 376p. text 55.00 (*0-8247-8109-0*) Dekker.

Early Diagnosis of Alzheimer's Disease. Ed. by Leonard F. M. Scinto & Kirk R. Daffner. 2000. LC 99-25252. (Current Clinical Neurology Ser.). (Illus.). xiii, 359p. 99.50 (*0-89603-452-6*) Humana.

Early Diagnosis of Cancer in General Practice. K. Holtedahl. 1990. (Illus.). 122p. 27.95 (*0-387-51252-7*, 3495) Spr-Verlag.

Early Diagnosis of Coronary Heart Disease: Proceedings of the Paavo Nurmi Symposium, 2nd, Porvoo, September 1971. Paavo Nurmi Symposium Staff. Ed. by P. I. Halonen & A. Louhija. 1972. (Advances in Cardiology Ser.: Vol. 8). 68.00 (*3-8055-1352-6*) S Karger.

Early Diagnosis of Hearing Loss. Ed. by Sanford E. Gerber & George T. Mencher. 1978. 384p. text 42.00 (*0-8089-1153-8*, 791547, Grune & Strat) Harcrt Hlth Sci Grp.

Early Drug Courts: Case Studies in Judicial Innovation. W. Clinton Terry, III. 1999. LC 98-25361. (Drugs, Health, & Social Policy Ser.). xi, 191p. 59.95 (*0-7619-0723-8*, 81457) Sage.

Early Embryonic Somatic Movements in Birds & Mammals Other Than Man. George E. Coghill. 1940. (SRCD M Ser.: Vol. 5, No. 2). pap. 25.00 (*0-527-01514-8*) Periodicals Srv.

Early Focus: Working with Young Blind & Visually Impaired Children & Their Families. Ed. by Rona L. Pogrund et al. 1992. LC 92-17874. 160p. pap. 32.95 (*0-89128-215-7*) Am Foun Blind.

Early Freud & Late Freud: Reading Anew Studies on Hysteria & Moses & Monotheism. Ilse Grubrich-Simitis. 29th ed. 1997. LC 97-12958. (New Library of Psychoanalysis). (Illus.). 136p. (C). 73.95 (*0-415-14843-X*) Routledge.

Early Freud & Late Freud: Reading Anew Studies on Hysteria of Moses & Monotheism. Ilse Grubrich-Simitis. 29th ed. 1997. LC 97-12958. (New Library of Psychoanalysis: Vol. 29). (Illus.). 152p. (C). pap. 24.95 (*0-415-14844-8*) Routledge.

Early Heart Attack Care. National Safety Council Staff. 1998. (Emergency Care Ser.). pap. 1.25 (*0-7637-0421-0*) Jones & Bartlett.

Early Hominid Activities at Olduvai. Richard B. Potts. 1988. (Evolutionary Foundations of Human Behavior Ser.). (Illus.). 407p. (C). lib. bdg. 59.95 (*0-202-01176-3*) Aldine de Gruyter.

Early Identification of Children at Risk: An International Perspective. Ed. by William K. Frankenburg et al. 1985. LC 85-12340. (Topics in Developmental Psychobiology Ser.). (Illus.). 414p. (C). 108.00 (*0-306-41946-7*, Plenum Trade) Perseus Pubng.

Early Influences Shaping the Individual. Ed. by Spyros Doxiadis. 1989. (NATO ASI Series A, Life Sciences: Vol. 160). (Illus.). 348p. 89.50 (*0-306-43140-8*, Plenum Trade) Perseus Pubng.

Early Interaction Between Animal Viruses & Cells. K. Lonberg-Holm & L. Philipson. Ed. by Joseph L. Melnick. 1974. (Monographs in Virology: Vol. 9). (Illus.). 160p. 77.50 (*3-8055-1764-5*) S Karger.

Early Intervention. Patricia M. Blasco. 2000. LC 99-49319. 348p. (C). 64.00 (*0-205-19443-5*) Allyn.

Early Intervention, Evaluation, & Assessment Ed. by Joy D. Osofsky & Hiram E. Fitzgerald. 1999. LC 99-11893. (World Association for Infant Mental Health Ser.: Vol. 2). (Illus.). 575p. 220.00 (*0-471-18944-8*) Wiley.

Early Intervention for Children & Their Families: Preventing Infant Deaths & Diseases. 1992. (Illus.). 110p. (Orig.). (C). pap. text 35.00 (*1-56806-018-1*) DIANE Pub.

Early Intervention for Special Populations of Infants & Toddlers. Ed. by Louis M. Rossetti & Jack E. Kile. 1997. LC 96-49788. 318p. 39.95 (*1-56593-798-8*, 1560) Thomson Learn.

Early Intervention I: Working with Infants & Toddlers. Ed. by Katharine G. Butler. 1993. LC 93-36266. 240p. pap. 44.00 (*0-8342-0584-X*) PRO-ED.

Early Intervention in Transition: Current Perspectives on Programs for Handicapped Children. Ed. by Kofi Marfo. 1991. LC 91-15312. 368p. 77.00 (*0-275-93470-5*, C3470, Praeger Pubs) Greenwood.

Early Intervention Programs for Infants. Robert Hess et al. Ed. by Howard A. Moss. 1982. LC 82-15608. (Prevention in Human Services Ser.: Vol. 1, No. 4). 122p. text 39.95 (*0-917724-54-2*) Haworth Pr.

Early Intervention Series: Materials for Training Personnel Serving Families of Deaf & Hard of Hearing Infants & Young Children, Set. Ed. by Valerie Schuyler. 1993. 300p. (C). ring bd. 570.00 incl. VHS (*0-9618297-3-7*) Hearing & Speech.

Early Intervention Services for Infants & Toddlers with Disabilities. 1991. 34p. 10.00 (*1-55516-693-8*, 6631) Natl Conf State Legis.

Early Intervention with High-Risk Children: Freeing Prisoners of Circumstance. Ed. by Arthur B. Zelman. 1996. LC 96-16403. 376p. 50.00 (*0-7657-0008-5*) Aronson.

Early Interventions in Acute Myocardial Infarction. Ed. by Elliott Rapaport. 1989. (Developments in Cardiovascular Medicine Ser.). (C). text 181.00 (*0-7923-0175-7*) Kluwer Academic.

Early Language. Peter DeVilliers & Jill DeVilliers. 1979. LC 78-9862. (Developing Child Ser.). (Illus.). 160p. pap. text 14.50 (*0-674-22141-9*) HUP.

Early Language Development: Implications for Clinical & Educational Practice. John Harris. 1991. (Illus.). 352p. (C). pap. 31.95 (*0-415-01417-4*, A4628) Routledge.

Early Man. Ed. by George G. MacCurdy. 1977. LC 77-86770. (Essay Index Reprint Ser.). 32.95 (*0-8369-1184-9*) Ayer.

Early Management of Hearing Loss. Ed. by George T. Mencher & Sanford E. Gerber. 1980. (Illus.). 468p. text 36.50 (*0-8089-1346-8*, 792879, Grune & Strat) Harcrt Hlth Sci Grp.

Early Markers in Parkinson's & Alzheimer's Diseases. Ed. by P. Dostert et al. 1991. (New Vistas in Drug Research Ser.: Vol. 1). (Illus.). 310p. 111.00 (*0-387-82223-2*) Spr-Verlag.

Early Medical History of Pinellas Peninsula. Frederick Eberson. 1978. LC 78-50560. (Illus.). 192p. 15.00 (*0-912760-67-2*) Valkyrie Pub Hse.

Early Medieval Medicine: With Special Reference to France & Charters. Loren C. MacKinney. 1979. 25.95 (*0-405-10613-0*) Ayer.

Early Phase Drug Evaluation in Man. John Ogrady. 1990. 115.00 (*0-8493-7708-0*, RM301) CRC Pr.

Early Phases of Personality Development: A Non-Normative Study of Infant Behavior. Sybelle K. Escalona & Mary Leitch. 1952. (SRCD M Ser.: Vol. 17, No. 1). pap. 25.00 (*0-527-01554-7*) Periodicals Srv.

Early Physicians of the West. Frederick Eberson. 1979. LC 79-63659. 144p. 10.00 (*0-912760-92-3*) Valkyrie Pub Hse.

Early Pregnancy, Vol. 10. Ed. by Jean-Michel Foidart et al. 1997. LC 97-28673. (Trophoblast Research Ser.). (*1-58046-017-8*) Univ Rochester Pr.

Early Pregnancy Failure. Ed. by H. J. Huisjes & T. Lind. 1990. (Illus.). 288p. text (*0-443-03775-2*) Church.

Early Pregnancy Loss. Ed. by R. W. Beard & Frank Sharp. 1988. (Illus.). 442p. 101.00 (*0-387-19530-0*) Spr-Verlag.

Early Psychological Development & Experience. J. McVicker Hunt. 1978. (Heinz Werner Lectures: No. 10). pap. 7.50 (*0-914206-06-0*) Clark U Pr.

Early Recognition & Intervention in Nutritional Dependent Diseases. Frueherkennung und Behandlung Ernaehrungsbedingter Krankheiten. Ed. by J. C. Somogyi & D. Hoetzel. 1992. (Bibliotheca Nutritio et Dieta Ser.: No. 50). (Illus.). xiv, 98p. 128.75 (*3-8055-5628-4*) S Karger.

Early Recognition of Child Abuse & Neglect: A Quick Reference Guide. Ed. by Gabriel J. Otterman & Diana M. Elliot. 1996. (Illus.). 34p. (Orig.). spiral bd. 9.95 (*1-887272-06-2*) Amer Med Pub.

Early Recognition of Domestic Violence: A Quick Reference Guide. Ed. by Jennifer L. Robertson & Linda R. Chambliss. 1997. LC 98-109797. (Abuse: No. 3). (Illus.). 40p. (Orig.). pap. 9.95 (*1-887272-09-7*) Amer Med Pub.

E
F
G

Early Recognition of Elder Abuse. Ed. by Andrew D. Weinberg & Jeanne Y. Wei. 1995. LC 95-201870. (Abuse). 36p. (Orig.). spiral bd. 9.95 (*1-887272-05-4*) Amer Med Pub.

Early Recollections & Life of Dr. James Still. James Still. 1977. LC 72-164394. (Black Heritage Library Collection). reprint ed. 29.95 (*0-8369-8853-1*) Ayer.

Early Recollections & Life of Dr. James Still. James Still. 1970. LC 72-107522. 274p. reprint ed. lib. bdg. 35.00 (*0-8371-3769-1*, SER&) Greenwood.

Early Signs of Nutritional Deficiencies. Ed. by J. C. Somogyi. 1976. (Bibliotheca Nutritio et Dieta Ser.: No. 23). (Illus.). 150p. 85.25 (*3-8055-2314-9*) S Karger.

Early Social Cognition: Understanding Others in the First Months of Life. Ed. by Philippe Rochat. 1999. LC 98-24653. 352p. 79.95 (*0-8058-2829-X*) L Erlbaum Assocs.

Early Stage Alzheimer's Care: A Guide for Community-Based Programs. Diane Weddington. 1994. LC 94-30812. 176p. 29.95 (*0-8261-8640-8*) Springer Pub.

***Early Stages of Schizophrenia.** Ed. by Robert B. Zipursky & S. Charles Schulz. 2001. LC 2001-34343. 320p. (*0-88048-840-9*, 8840) Am Psychiatric.

Early Supplementary Feeding & Cognition: Effect over Two Decades. Ernesto Pollitt et al. 1993. (Monographs of the Society for Research on Child Development). 128p. pap. text 15.00 (*0-226-67453-3*) U Ch Pr.

Early Vascular Complications in Children with Diabetes Mellitus. Ed. by B. Weber. 1988. (Pediatric & Adolescent Endocrinology Ser.: Vol. 17). xiv, 284p. 186.25 (*3-8055-4485-5*) S Karger.

Early Vision & Beyond. Ed. by Thomas V. Papathomas et al. 1995. LC 94-3117. 284p. 70.00 (*0-262-16146-X*, Bradford Bks) MIT Pr.

Early Warning: Cases & Ethical Guidance for Presymptomatic Testing in Genetic Diseases, Medical Ethics. David H. Smith et al. 1998. LC 98-3978. (Medical Ethics Ser.). (Illus.). 240p. 29.95 (*0-253-33401-2*) Ind U Pr.

Earth, Air, Fire & Water. Camille Hayward. 1993. 49p. (Orig.). pap. 6.00 (*0-944920-05-5*) Bellowing Ark Pr.

Earth Honoring: The New Male Sexuality. Robert Lawlor. 1989. 256p. 16.95 (*0-89281-254-0*, Destiny Bks) Inner Tradit.

Earth Medicine: Revealing Hidden Teachings of the Native American Medicine Wheel. Kenneth Meadows. 1996. 333p. pap. 16.95 (*1-85230-668-8*) Element MA.

Earth Medicine Earth Foods. Weiner. 1982. 18.95 (*0-02-625610-X*) Macmillan.

Earthly Bodies & Heavenly Hair: Natural & Healthy Personal Care for Every Body. Dina Falconi. 1998. LC 97-69510. (Illus.). 242p. pap. 17.95 (*1-886101-04-3*) Ceres Pr.

Earthmagic: Using New England Medicinal Herbs. Corinne Martin. Ed. by Ed Francis & Sylvia Dovner. 1990. (Illus.). 250p. (Orig.). pap. 12.95 (*0-9623199-1-0*) Dirigo Bks.

Easeful Death? Perspectives on Death, Dying & Euthanasia. Ed. by John Morgan. 1996. LC 97-106308. 218p. pap. (*1-86287-222-8*) Federation Pr AUS. *Dist:* Gaunt.

Easily Missed Fractures & Corner Signs in Radiology. Hans O. Riddervold. 1991. (Illus.). 416p. 150.00 (*0-87993-502-2*) Futura Pub.

Easing Anxiety & Stress Naturally. Susan M. Lark. Ed. by Phyllis Herman. 1996. (Good Health Guides). 48p. pap. 3.95 (*0-87983-728-4*, 37284K, Keats Pubng) McGraw-Hill Trade.

Easing Labor Pain: The Complete Guide to a More Comfortable & Rewarding Birth. Adrienne B. Lieberman. Ed. by Dan Rosenberg. rev. ed. 1992. LC 92-382. (Illus.). 288p. 19.95 (*1-55832-044-X*); pap. 14.95 (*1-55832-043-1*) Harvard Common Pr.

Easing the Ache: Gay Men Recovering from Compulsive Behaviors. Guy Kettelhack. 1998. LC 97-52185. 204p. reprint ed. pap. 14.95 (*1-56838-235-9*) Hazelden.

Easing the Transition from Hospital to Home: Postpartum Discharge Planning & Homecare Services. Kathleen Simpson. Ed. by Lynn G. Wellman et al. 1996. LC 95-51198. pap. (*0-86525-068-5*) March of Dimes.

East African Doctors: A History of the Modern Profession. John Iliffe. 1998. LC 97-51551. (African Studies: No. 95). (Illus.). 350p. (C). text 69.95 (*0-521-63272-2*) Cambridge U Pr.

East & West: Acupunture, an Alternative to Suffering. M. J. Cunningham & I. Yen Yang. 1994. LC 93-93901. (Illus.). 80p. pap. 8.00 (*1-56002-340-6*, Univ Edtns) Aegina Pr.

East Asian Medicine in Urban Japan: Varieties of Medical Experience. Margaret M. Lock. 1979. (Comparative Studies of Health Systems & Medical Care: Vol. 3). (Illus.). pap. text 22.50 (*0-520-05231-5*) U CA Pr.

East-West Healing: Integrating Chinese & Western Medicines for Optimal Healing. Mary Loo & Jack Maguire. 2001. LC 00-68601. (Illus.). 336p. 24.95 (*0-471-35603-4*) Wiley.

East-West Life Expectancy Gap in Europe - Environmental & Non-Environmental Determinants: Proceedings of the NATO Advanced Research Workshop, Surrey, U. K., March 20-22, 1995. Shona Kelly et al. Ed. by Clyde Hertzman. 1996. LC 96-31912. (NATO Advanced Science Institutes Ser.). 256p. (C). text 161.50 (*0-7923-4207-0*) Kluwer Academic.

Easy ACLS Preparatory Manual. James Paturas & Andrew D. Weinberg. 1995. (Emergency Care Ser.). (Illus.). 240p. (C). pap. text 33.75 (*0-86720-819-8*, 819-8) Jones & Bartlett.

Easy Coder Internal Medicine. Contrib. by Paul K. Tanaka. 1997. LC 99-205902. (*1-56781-130-2*) Unicor Medical.

Easy Coder 2000. Paul K. Tanaka. rev. ed. 1999. 657p. 59.00 (*1-56781-208-2*) Unicor Medical.

Easy Coder 2000 - Cardiology. Paul K. Tanaka. rev. ed. 1999. 260p. 59.00 (*1-56781-432-8*) Unicor Medical.

Easy Coder 2000 - Chiropractic. Paul K. Tanaka. rev. ed. 1999. 239p. 59.00 (*1-56781-552-9*) Unicor Medical.

Easy Coder 2000 - Dermatology. Paul K. Tanaka. rev. ed. 1999. 274p. 59.00 (*1-56781-083-7*) Unicor Medical.

Easy Coder 2000 - ENT. Paul K. Tanaka. rev. ed. 1999. 232p. 59.00 (*1-56781-006-3*) Unicor Medical.

Easy Coder 2000 - Family Practice. Paul K. Tanaka. rev. ed. 1999. 59.00 (*1-56781-109-4*) Unicor Medical.

Easy Coder 2000 - Internal Medicine. Paul K. Tanaka. rev. ed. 1999. 516p. 59.00 (*1-56781-133-7*) Unicor Medical.

Easy Coder 2000 - OB Gyn. Paul K. Tanaka. rev. ed. 1999. 316p. 59.00 (*1-56781-159-0*) Unicor Medical.

Easy Coder 2000 - Ophthalmology. Paul K. Tanaka. rev. ed. 1999. 208p. 59.00 (*1-56781-059-4*) Unicor Medical.

Easy Coder 2000 - Optometry. Paul K. Tanaka. rev. ed. 1999. 208p. 59.00 (*1-56781-529-4*) Unicor Medical.

Easy Coder 2000 - Urology. Paul K. Tanaka. rev. ed. 1999. 232p. 59.00 (*1-56781-455-7*) Unicor Medical.

Easy Coder 2000 Including Volume 3. Paul K. Tanaka. rev. ed. 1999. 976p. 59.00 (*1-56781-479-4*) Unicor Medical.

Easy Does It: A Book of Daily 12 Step Meditations. Intro. by Bill Pittman. 400p. (Orig.). pap. 8.95 (*0-934125-12-0*) Hazelden.

Easy Gourmet Menus to Lower Your Fat Thermostat. Howard Gifford. 1991. 264p. pap. 13.95 (*0-912547-08-1*) Vitality Hse Int Inc.

Easy Guide to Ayurveda. Roy E. Davis. 1996. pap. 4.95 (*0-87707-249-3*) CSA Pr.

Easy OMT. W. H. Howard, III. 1993. 320p. (C). text 69.50 (*0-9636688-0-3*) Specialty Pub.

Easy-to-Chew & Easy-on-Salt. Rosalie N. Norris & Janet C. Powell. 1982. LC 81-65460. 176p. 10.95 (*0-8453-4718-7*, Cornwall Bks) Assoc Univ Prs.

Eat Away Illness: How to Age-Proof Your Body with Antioxidant Foods. Carlson Wade. 2nd enl. rev. ed. 1992. LC 92-18098. 352p. (C). text 24.95 (*0-13-224809-3*) P-H.

Eat Better, Feel Better: A Visual Directory of Foods & the Nutrients They Contain, Plus a Unique Section on Combating Common Ailments. Mary Deirdre Donovan. 1998. LC 97-32143. (Illus.). 176p. 29.95 (*1-882606-68-X*); pap. 18.95 (*1-882606-28-0*) Peoples Med Soc.

Eat, Drink & Be Healthy: The Harvard Medical School Guide to Healthy Eating. Ed. by Walter C. Willett et al. 2001. LC 2001-20565. (Illus.). 304p. 25.00 (*0-684-86337-5*) S&S Trade.

***Eat, Drink & Be Healthy: The Harvard Medical School Guide to Healthy Eating.** Walter C. Willett. 2002. (Illus.). pap. 13.00 (*0-7432-2322-5*, Fireside) S&S Trade Pap.

Eat, Drink & Sleep Smoke-Free. Ed. by Catherine Mooney. 1995. (Illus.). 258p. (Orig.). pap. (*1-899583-00-9*) JARR UK GBR. *Dist:* Seven Hills Bk.

Eat Fat, Be Healthy: Understanding the Heart-Stopper Gene & When a Low-Fat Diet Can Kill You. Matthew J. Bayan. 2000. LC 99-45721. (Illus.). 224p. 23.00 (*0-684-86527-0*) Scribner.

Eat Fat, Be Healthy: When a Low-Fat Diet Can Kill You. Matthew J. Bayan. 2001. 224p. pap. 12.00 (*0-684-86528-9*, Fireside) S&S Trade Pap.

Eat for Life: The Food & Nutrition Board's Guide to Reducing Your Risk of Chronic Disease. Institute of Medicine Staff & National Academy of Sciences Staff. Ed. by Catherine E. Woteki & Paul R. Thomas. 1992. LC 91-37837. 192p. 18.95 (*0-309-04049-3*) Natl Acad Pr.

Eat Right, Be Bright. Arthur Winter & Ruth Winter. 1989. mass mkt. 4.95 (*0-312-91553-5*) St Martin.

Eat Right for Your Type: The Individualized Diet Solution to Staying Healthy, Living Longer & Achieving Your Ideal Weight. Peter J. D'Adamo & Catherine Whitney. 1997. LC 96-35510. (Illus.). 392p. 24.95 (*0-399-14255-X*, G P Putnam) Penguin Putnam.

Eat to Compete: The Guide to Sports Nutrition. Marilyn S. Peterson. 2nd ed. 1996. (Illus.). 384p. (C). (gr. 13). pap. text 33.95 (*0-8151-6786-5*, 26811) Mosby Inc.

Eat to Live Long & Well: Master the Essential Fats. Edward Siguel. 1999. (Illus.). 600p. pap. 34.95 (*0-9642534-1-0*) Nutrek Pr.

Eat to Win: The Sports Nutrition Bible. Robert Haas. 1985. 384p. pap. 5.99 (*0-451-15509-2*, Sig) NAL.

Eat Well for a Healthy Menopause: The Low-Fat, High-Nutrition Guide. Elaine Magee. 1997. 288p. pap. 5.99 (*0-471-19360-7*) Wiley.

Eat Well for a Healthy Menopause: The Low-Fat, High-Nutrition Guide. Elaine Moquette-Magee. 1996. LC 95-41711. 288p. pap. 15.95 (*0-471-12250-5*) Wiley.

Eat Well for Fifty Dollars a Week. Rhonda Barfield. 1993. (Illus.). 144p. (Orig.). pap. 9.95 (*0-9635782-0-0*) Lilac Pub.

Eat Well, Live Longer: A Manual for a Healthy Heart. Marita Westberg. (*0-7043-3219-1*) Quartet GBR. *Dist:* Charles River Bks.

Eat Well, Stay Well: 500 Delicious Recipes Made with Healing Foods. Reader's Digest Editorial Staff. 1998. LC 98-28078. (Illus.). 450p. 29.95 (*0-7621-0124-5*) RD Assn.

Eat Your Colors: Maximize Your Health by Eating the Right Foods for Your Body Type. Marcia Zimmerman. 2001. LC 2001-16917. (Illus.). 304p. pap. 14.00 (*0-8050-6728-0*, Owl) H Holt & Co.

Eat Your Way to Health. Anne Smith. 1.50 (*0-9601262-1-X*) FairMail Serv.

Eaters' Easy Guide to Natural Diet & Nutrition: Sources of Energy-Producing Foods. 1992. lib. bdg. 250.00 (*0-8490-8805-4*) Gordon Pr.

***Eating & Drinking in Labour.** Penny Champion & Carol McCormick. 2001. LC 2001-43862. 128p. pap. 24.99 (*0-7506-5315-9*) Buttrwrth-Heinemann.

Eating & Growth Disorders in Infants & Prepubertal Children. Joseph L. Woolston. 1991. (Developmental Clinical Psychology & Psychiatry Ser.: Vol. 24). 152p. (C). 74.95 (*0-8039-3683-4*, 7561);No. 24. pap. 34.95 (*0-8039-3684-2*, 7562) Sage.

Eating Defensively: Food Safety Advice for People with AIDS. 1991. (AIDS Ser.). lib. bdg. 250.00 (*0-8490-5148-7*) Gordon Pr.

Eating Disorder among Athletes: Theory, Issues & Research. Ed. by David R. Black. 1991. 92p. pap. 17.00 (*0-88314-497-2*) AAHPERD.

Eating Disorder Sourcebook. Carolyn Costin. 2nd ed. 1997. 304p. reprint ed. pap. 15.00 (*1-56565-853-1*, Anodyne) Lowell Hse.

Eating Disorder Sourcebook: A Comprehensive Guide to the Causes, Treatments & Prevention. Carolyn Costin. 2nd ed. 1999. LC 99-37565. xxiv, 328p. pap. 16.95 (*0-7373-0102-3*, 01023W) NTC Contemp Pub Co.

Eating Disorder Sourcebook: Everything You Need to Know about Anorexia, Bulimia, & Other Eating Disorders. Carolyn Costin. 1996. 304p. 17.00 (*1-56565-463-3*) Lowell Hse.

Eating Disorders. W. Stewart Agras. 1987. 144p. (C). pap. text 53.95 (*0-205-14263-X*, H4263, Longwood Div) Allyn.

Eating Disorders. Ed. by A. James Giannini & Andrew E. Slaby. 1993. LC 93-20481. (Illus.). 286p. 140.00 (*0-387-94002-2*) Spr-Verlag.

Eating Disorders. L. George Hsu. 1990. LC 89-17179. (Child Psychopathology Ser.). 248p. 35.00 (*0-89862-401-0*, 2401) Guilford Pubns.

Eating Disorders: A Guide for Health Professionals. Thompson. 1993. 326p. pap. 47.75 (*1-56593-182-3*, 0497) Singular Publishing.

Eating Disorders: A Guide to Medical Care & Complications. Philip S. Mehler. 2000. LC 99-27939. 304p. pap. text 19.95 (*0-8018-6277-9*) Johns Hopkins.

Eating Disorders: A Reference Sourcebook. Raymond Lemberg & Leigh Cohn. 2nd rev. ed. 1998. LC 98-48506. (Illus.). 272p. pap. 49.95 (*1-57356-156-8*, Oryx) Greenwood.

Eating Disorders: Feminist, Historical, Cultural, Psychological Aspects: A Bibliography. Ed. by Joan Nordquist. 1989. (Contemporary Social Issues: A Bibliographic Ser.: No. 15). 60p. (C). pap. 20.00 (*0-937855-29-4*) Ref Rsch Serv.

Eating Disorders: Management of Obesity, Bulimia & Anorexia Nervosa. W. Stewart Agras. 1987. (Psychology Practitioner Guidebooks). 146p. 28.00 (*0-08-033646-9*); pap. 14.95 (*0-08-033645-0*) Elsevier (Pergamon Pr).

Eating Disorders: New Directions in Treatment & Recovery. Barbara P. Kinoy. 1994. LC 93-50149. 50.00 (*0-231-09694-1*); 166p. pap. 19.50 (*0-231-09695-X*) Col U Pr.

Eating Disorders: New Directions in Treatment & Recovery. Ed. by Barbara P. Kinoy. 2nd ed. 2000. LC 00-55497. xxii, 195p. text 49.50 (*0-231-11852-X*); pap. text 19.50 (*0-231-11853-8*) Col U Pr.

Eating Disorders: Obesity, Anorexia Nervosa, & the Person Within. Hilde Bruch. 1979. LC 72-89189. 400p. pap. 28.00 (*0-465-01782-7*) Basic.

***Eating Disorders: Prevalence, Incidence & Prospective Risk Factors for Eating Disorders among Young Adult Women in the General Population.** Ata Ghaderi. 2001. (Comprehensive Summaries of Uppsala Dissertations from the Faculty of Social Sciences Ser.: No. 99). 79p. pap. (*91-554-4924-7*) Uppsala Universitet SWE. *Dist:* Coronet Bks.

Eating Disorders & Marriage: The Couple in Focus. D. Blake Woodside et al. Ed. by Paul E. Garfinkel & David M. Garner. 1993. (Eating Disorders Monographs: No. 8). (Illus.). 224p. text 31.95 (*0-87630-705-5*) Brunner-Routledge.

Eating Disorders in Adolescence: Anorexia & Bulimia Nervosa, Vol. 3. Ed. by Hans-Christoph Steinhausen. 1995. LC 95-547. (International Studies on Childhood & Adolescence). xviii, 374p. (C). lib. bdg. 74.95 (*3-11-014347-X*) De Gruyter.

Eating Disorders Throughout the Life Span. Ed. by Howard L. Field & Barbara B. Domangue. 1987. LC 87-16955. 176p. 55.00 (*0-275-92212-X*, C2212, Praeger Pubs) Greenwood.

Eating Do's & Don'ts for Nutritional Management of Carpal Tunnal Syndrome. Mary Lawler. 2000. XII,68p. pap. 7.00 (*0-9702211-0-X*) MTL Pubns.

Eating Expectantly: A Practical & Tasty Approach to Prenatal Nutrition. Bridget Swinney & Tracy Anderson. rev. ed. 2000. LC 00-28403. (Illus.). xii, 398p. pap. (*0-88166-371-9*) Meadowbrook.

Eating Expectantly: The Practical & Tasty Guide to Prenatal Nutriton. Bridget Swinney & Tracey Anderson. 10th ed. 1996. LC 96-21804. 320p. (*0-88166-257-7*) Meadowbrook.

Eating for A's: A Delicious Twelve-Week Nutrition Plan to Improve Your Child's Academic & Athletic Performance. Barbara F. Meyer et al. Ed. by Sally Peters. 1991. 288p. (Orig.). pap. 9.00 (*0-671-72814-8*) PB.

Eating for IBS: 175 Delicious, Nutritious, Low-Fat, Low-Residue Recipes to Stabilize the Touchiest Tummy. Heather Van Vorous. 2000. LC 00-56219. (Illus.). xxi, 279p. pap. 16.95 (*1-56924-600-9*) Marlowe & Co.

Eating for Two: The Complete Guide to Nutrition During Pregnancy. Mary A. Hess & Anne E. Hunt. 1992. LC 91-47161. 256p. pap. 13.95 (*0-02-065441-3*) Hungry Minds.

Eating Hints: Recipes & Tips For Better Nutrition During Cancer Treatment. 1986. lib. bdg. 75.00 (*0-8490-3788-3*) Gordon Pr.

Eating Hints: Recipes & Tips for Better Nutrition During Cancer Treatment. Ed. by Yale-New Haven Medical Center Staff. 1992. (Illus.). 86p. (Orig.). (C). pap. text 20.00 (*0-941375-30-7*) DIANE Pub.

Eating Hints for Cancer Patients. rev. ed. 1995. (Illus.). 94p. (Orig.). pap. text 20.00 (*0-7881-2597-4*) DIANE Pub.

Eating Illness Workbook. Joan Ebbitt. 1987. pap. 8.95 (*1-56838-067-4*) Hazelden.

Eating Out Nutrition Guide. Natow. 1998. 384p. mass mkt. 6.99 (*0-671-89471-4*) PB.

Eating Positive: A Nutrition Guide & Recipe Book for People with HIV/AIDS. Jeffrey T. Huber & Kris Riddlesperger. 1997. LC 97-28285. 110p. 29.95 (*0-7890-0103-9*); pap. text 14.95 (*1-56023-893-3*) Haworth Pr (Harrington Park).

Eating Right. 1987. (Fitness, Health & Nutrition Ser.). (Illus.). 144p. 17.27 (*0-8094-6163-3*); lib. bdg. 23.27 (*0-8094-6164-1*) Time-Life.

Eating, Sleeping, & Sex: Perspectives in Behavioral Medicine. Ed. by Albert J. Stunkard & Andrew Baum. 1989. 272p. 49.95 (*0-8058-0280-0*) L Erlbaum Assocs.

Eating to Lower Your Blood Cholesterol. 1991. lib. bdg. 59.95 (*0-8490-5020-0*); 1990. lib. bdg. 75.00 (*0-8490-3997-5*) Gordon Pr.

Eating with Your Heart in Mind. 1995. (Illus.). 36p. pap. text 30.00 (*1-57979-020-8*) DIANE Pub.

Eating Your Way to Health: Dietotherapy in Traditional Chinese Medicine. 1996. 181p. pap. (*7-119-01885-X*) Beijing Foreign Lang CHN. *Dist:* China Bks.

Ebers Papyrus: Oldest Medical Book in the World. Cyril Bryan. (African Studies). reprint ed. 25.00 (*0-938818-27-9*) ECA Assoc.

Ebola. William T. Close. 1995. LC 95-205102. 404p. mass mkt. 5.99 (*0-8041-1432-3*) Ivy Books.

EC Study-Lessons Learnt from Emergencies after Accidents in Ireland Involving Dangerous Substances: EUR 15565. D. R. Maxwell. 1994. 98p. pap. (*92-826-7516-5*) Comm Europ Commun BEL. *Dist:* Bernan Associates.

ECAT Essay Procedures: A Manual of Laboratory Techniques. Ed. by J. Jespersen et al. 1992. 240p. (C). lib. bdg. 133.00 (*0-7923-8987-5*) Kluwer Academic.

Ecce Homo: An Annotated Bibliographic History of Physical Anthropology, 2. Compiled by Frank Spencer. 1986. LC 86-19417. (Bibliographies & Indexes in Anthropology Ser.: No. 2). 518p. lib. bdg. 100.00 (*0-313-24056-6*, SPE/, Greenwood Pr) Greenwood.

Eccentric & Bizarre Behaviors. Louis R. Franzini & John M. Grossberg. 1995. LC 94-36298. 256p. pap. 19.95 (*0-471-54520-1*) Wiley.

Eccentric Muscle Training in Sports & Orthopaedics. Mark Albert. 2nd ed. 1995. LC 95-7871. text (*0-443-08987-6*) Church.

ECG Assessment & Interpretation. Bradford C. Lipman & Toni Cascio. 1994. (Illus.). 295p. pap. 26.95 (*0-8036-5646-7*) Davis Co.

ECG-Challenger: Electrocardiography Case Studies, Quiz & Atlas. 1999. 175.00 incl. cd-rom (*1-889244-09-0*); 175.00 incl. cd-rom (*1-889244-11-2*) Chllnger.

ECG Criteria & ACLS Handbook. O'Keefe et al. 1998. (Illus.). 202p. (C). pap. text 12.95 (*1-890114-03-0*) Physicians Pr.

ECG Diagnosis: A Self-Assessment Workbook. Edward K. Chung & Brad Spellberg. 2000. (Illus.). 200p. pap., wbk. ed. 32.95 (*0-86542-587-6*) Blackwell Sci.

ECG Diagnosis Simplified. Edward K. Chung. Ed. by Steven Gross. 1995. (Illus.). 300p. (C). pap. text 34.95 (*1-887174-00-1*) DevCom.

ECG for the Small Animal Practitioner. Larry P. Tilley & Naomi L. Burtnick. rev. ed. 1999. (Made Easy Ser.). (Illus.). 104p. spiral bd. 31.00 (*1-893441-00-8*) Teton New.

ECG in Anesthesia & Critical Care. Daniel M. Thys & Joel A. Kaplan. 1987. (Illus.). 264p. pap. text (*0-443-08426-2*) Church GBR. *Dist:* Saunders.

ECG in Emergency Decision Making. Conover & Hein J. Wellens. 1991. 272p. pap. text 36.95 (*0-7216-3214-9*) Saunders.

ECG in Practice. John R. Hampton. 3rd ed. 1997. LC 96-29704. im. lthr. (*0-443-05679-X*); pap. text (*0-443-05680-3*) Church.

ECG Interpretation. Randall. 2000. (Quicklook Medicine Ser.). 19.95 (*1-889325-79-1*) Fence Crk Pubng.

ECG Interpretation. Springhouse Publishing Company Staff. 1991. LC 90-38614. (Clinical Skillbuilders Ser.). (Illus.). 183p. spiral bd. 28.95 (*0-87434-309-7*) Springhouse Corp.

ECG Interpretation for Emergency Medicine: A Self Assessment Guide. Francis Morris. 1997. LC 97-25514. 160p. pap. (*0-7506-3019-1*) E A GBR. *Dist:* OUP.

ECG Interpretation Made Incredibly Easy. Ed. by Patricia Schull. 1997. LC 97-2965. (Made Incredibly Easy Ser.). (Illus.). 292p. (Orig.). pap. 34.95 (*0-87434-887-0*) Springhouse Corp.

ECG Made Easy. John R. Hampton. 5th ed. 1997. (*0-443-05695-1*); LC 97-5637. pap. text (*0-443-05681-1*) Church.

ECG Manual for the Veterinary Technician. N. Joel Edwards. 1993. LC 92-25705. (Illus.). 224p. spiral bd. 27.95 (*0-7216-3083-9*) Saunders.

ECG-SAP I: Electrocardiography Self-Assessment Program. Ed. by Jay W. Mason. 1995. LC 95-75848. (Illus.). 102p. pap. 95.00 (*1-882764-12-9*, ECGPR) Am Coll Cardiology.

ECG-SAP II: Electrocardiography Self-Assessment Program II. Ed. by Jay W. Mason. 1997. LC 97-94681. (Illus.). 97p. pap. 120.00 (*1-882764-19-6*) Am Coll Cardiology.

ECG Workbook: A Review & Discussion of ECG Findings & Abnormalities. Glenn N. Levine & Philip J. Podrid. 1995. LC 95-128715. (Illus.). 544p. 74.00 (*0-87993-597-9*) Futura Pub.

ECG Workout: Exercises in Arrhythmia Interpretation. Jane Huff. 3rd ed. 1996. LC 96-29037. 352p. pap. text 28.95 (*0-397-55371-4*) Lppncott W & W.

***ECG Workout: Exercises in Arrhythmia Interpretation.** Jane Huff. 4th ed. 2001. LC 2001-50393. 368p. pap. text 28.95 (*0-7817-3192-5*) Lppncott W & W.

ECGs by Example. Jenkins. 1998. (C). pap. text 24.95 (*0-443-05697-8*) Saunders.

***ECG's Made East.** Barbara Achlert. 2nd ed. 2001. (Illus.). 110p. (*0-323-00473-3*) Mosby Inc.

ECG's Made Easy. Barbara Aehlert. (Illus.). tchr. ed. (*0-8151-1380-3*); LC 95-176348. suppl. ed. (*0-8151-0092-2*); 1995. 272p. (C). (gr. 13). pap. text, tchr. ed. 28.00 (*0-8151-0093-0*, 26655) Mosby Inc.

***ECG's Made Easy.** Barbara Aehlert. 2nd ed. 2001. (Illus.). 110p. (*0-323-01433-X*) Mosby Inc.

***ECG's Made Easy: Including Pocket Guide.** Barbara Aehlert. 2nd ed. 2001. (Illus.). 335p. (*0-323-01432-1*) Mosby Inc.

ECGs Made Easy: With Pocket Reference. Barbara Aehlert. 1995. (Illus.). 400p. spiral bd. 31.00 (*0-8151-0094-9*, 26654) Mosby Inc.

Echidnas. M. Griffiths. 1968. LC 68-21385. (Illus.). (*0-08-012650-2*) Pergamon Repr GBR. *Dist:* Franklin.

Echinacea. Rita Elkins. 1996. (Woodland Health Ser.). 32p. pap. text 3.95 (*1-885670-13-3*) Woodland UT.

Echo Manual. Jae Oh & James Seward. 2nd ed. 1998. LC 98-19451. 288p. text 145.00 (*0-7817-1205-X*) Lppncott W & W.

Echo-Morphologic Correlates: The Adult Heart. S. Brecker & R. H. Anderson. 2000. (Series on Echocardiographic Diagnosis of Congenital Heart Disease). (Illus.). 28p. pap. (*1-86094-240-7*) Imperial College GBR. *Dist:* World Scientific Pub.

Echo-Morphologic Correlates: The Normal Heart. Robert H. Anderson. 1998. 32p. (*1-86094-110-9*) Imperial College GBR. *Dist:* World Scientific Pub.

Echo-Planar Imaging: Theory, Technique & Application. F. Schmitt et al. 1998. LC 98-10705. (Illus.). 676p. 189.00 (*3-540-63194-1*) Spr-Verlag.

***Echocardiogram Made Easy.** S. Kaddoura. 2001. (Illus.). 140p. pap. (*0-443-06188-2*) Church GBR. *Dist:* Saunders.

Echocardiographer's Pocket Reference. Terry Reynolds. 180p. 34.95 (*0-9635767-0-4*); 2nd ed. (Illus.). 450p. (*0-9635767-9-8*) AZ Heart Inst.

Echocardiographic Anatomy. Ivan D'Cruz. 1996. 563p. (C). pap. text 125.00 (*0-8385-2037-5*, A2037-8, Apple Lange Med) McGraw.

Echocardiographic Diagnosis of Cardiac Malformations. Roberta G. Williams. 1986. 86.00 (*0-316-94132-8*, Little Brwn Med Div) Lppncott W & W.

Echocardiographic Diagnosis of Congenital Heart Disease: An Embryologic & Anatomic Approach. Lilliam V. Valdes-Cruz & Raul O. Cayre. 1998. LC 98-26987. 592p. text 205.00 (*0-7817-1433-8*) Lppncott W & W.

Echocardiography. Harvey Feigenbaum. 5th ed. 1994. LC 92-48436. (Illus.). 707p. 125.00 (*0-8121-1692-5*) Lppncott W & W.

Echocardiography: A Practical Guide for Reporting. Helen Rimmington & John Chambers. 1998. LC 97-35746. (Illus.). 96p. 29.95 (*1-85070-011-7*, Parthenon Pbng) CRC Pr.

Echocardiography: An International Review. Ed. by John Chambers & M. J. Monaghan. 1994. (Illus.). 226p. (C). 98.00 (*0-19-262091-6*) OUP.

Echocardiography & Cardiovascular Function: Tools for the Next Decade. Julio E. Erez et al. 1997. LC 97-4338. (Developments in Cardiovascular Medicine Ser.). 288p. text 104.50 (*0-7923-9884-X*) Kluwer Academic.

Echocardiography for the Neonatologist. Ed. by Jonathan Skinner et al. 2000. (Illus.). 243p. pap. (*0-443-05480-0*) Church GBR. *Dist:* Saunders.

Echocardiography in Cardiac Interventions. Ed. by I. Cikes. 1989. (Developments in Cardiovascular Medicine Ser.). (C). text 420.50 (*0-7923-0088-2*) Kluwer Academic.

***Echocardiography in Clinical Practice.** J. Chambers. 2001. LC 2001-50050. (Illus.). 98p. 64.95 (*1-84214-108-2*, Parthenon Pbng) CRC Pr.

Echocardiography in Congenital Heart Disease Made Simple. S. Y. Ho et al. 1999. (Cardiopulmonary Medicine Ser.). (Illus.). 150p. 48.00 (*1-86094-124-9*) World Scientific Pub.

Echocardiography in Coronary Artery Disease. Ed. by Richard S. Meltzer et al. 1988. (Developments in Cardiovascular Medicine Ser.). (C). text 179.50 (*0-89838-979-8*) Kluwer Academic.

Echocardiography in Ischemic Heart Disease. M. Herregods. 1994. 154p. (Orig.). pap. (*90-6186-628-6*) Leuven Univ BEL. *Dist:* Coronet Bks.

Echocardiography in Pediatric Heart Disease. Serwer & A. Rebecca Snider. 2nd ed. 1997. LC 96-37370. (Illus.). 608p. (C). (gr. 13). text 175.00 (*0-8151-7851-4*, 24092) Mosby Inc.

Echocardiography in Primary Care. John Chambers. 1996. (Illus.). 78p. lib. bdg. 49.95 (*1-85070-909-2*, Parthenon Pbng) CRC Pr.

Echocardiography of Congenital Heart Disease. Lilliam Valdes-Cruz et al. 1997. 700p. text (*0-7817-0278-X*) Lppncott W & W.

Echocardiography Review. Barton A. Bean & Kathleen A. Oss. 1989. LC 89-18089. pap. 55.00 (*0-941022-16-1*) Davies Pubng.

Echocardiology. N. Bom. 1977. text 155.50 (*90 247 2009 5*) Kluwer Academic.

Echocardiology. Ed. by Charles T. Lancee. 1979. (Developments in Cardiovascular Medicine Ser.: No. 1). text 220.00 (*90-247-2209-8*) Kluwer Academic.

Echocardiology: Developments in Cardiovascular Medicine, No. 13. Ed. by H. Rijsterborgh. 1981. 504p. text 211.50 (*90-247-2491-0*) Kluwer Academic.

Echoenhancers & Transcranial Color Duplex Sonography. Ulrich Bogdahn et al. 1998. LC 98-30068. 195.00 (*0-632-05227-9*) Blackwell Sci.

Echoes of the Call Identity & "...Ideology" "...Among" American Missionaries in Ecuador. Jeffrey Swanson. 1995. LC 94-9012. (Illus.). 224p. text 60.00 (*0-19-506823-8*) OUP.

Echography in Ophthalmology. J. Poujol. 1986. (gr. 13). 34.00 (*0-89352-228-7*, MA228) Mosby Inc.

Echolalia: An Adult's Story of Tourette Syndrome. Adam W. Seligman. 1991. LC 91-13102. 165p. (Orig.). pap. 11.95 (*1-878267-31-0*) Hope Pr CA.

Echo's Subtle Body: Contributions to an Archetypal Psychology. Patricia Berry. 1982. LC 82-19506. 200p. pap. 17.00 (*0-88214-313-1*) Spring Pubns.

Eclectic Dispensatory of Botanical Therapeutics, Vol. 2. Ed. by Kathryn Rosson. 1996. 600p. text 125.00 (*1-888483-08-3*) Eclectic Med.

Eclectic Materia Medica, Pharmacology, & Therapeutics. Harvey W. Felter. 1992. 743p. reprint ed. 95.00 (*1-888483-03-2*) Eclectic Med.

Eclectic Psychotherapy: A Systematic Approach. Larry E. Beutler. 1983. (General Psychology Ser.: No. 118). 270p. 47.50 (*0-08-028842-1*, Pergamon Pr) Elsevier.

Eclipses: Behind the Borderline Personality Disorder. Melissa F. Thornton. 1997. LC 97-74498. (Illus.). 160p. pap. 13.00 (*0-9659392-2-7*) Monte Sano.

ECMO: Extracorporeal Cardiopulmonary Support in Critical Care. Ed. by Joseph B. Zwischenberger & Robert Bartlett. 1996. (Illus.). xv, 717p. pap. text 60.00 (*0-9656756-0-2*); 2nd rev. ed. pap. text 60.00 (*0-9656756-1-0*) Extracorporeal Life Support.

Ecobehavioral Analysis & Developmental Disabilities. Ed. by S. R. Schroeder. 1990. (Disorders of Human Learning, Behavior, & Communication Ser.). (Illus.). 256p. 126.00 (*0-387-97146-7*) Spr-Verlag.

Ecobehavioral Family Interventions in Development Disabilities. John R. Lutzker & Randy Campbell. 1994. LC 94-3954. (Special Education Ser.). 126p. 20.75 (*0-534-24396-7*) Brooks-Cole.

Ecobichon. Donald J. Ecobichon. 1992. (Basic Toxicity Testing Ser.). lib. bdg. 69.95 (*0-8493-4299-6*, CRC Reprint) Franklin.

ECOG, OAE & Intraoperative Monitoring: Proceedings of the First International Conference, Wurzburg, Germany, September 20-24, 1992. Ed. by D. Hohmann. 1993. LC 93-26892. (*90-6299-097-5*) Kugler NLD. *Dist:* Lib Res.

Ecogenetics: Genetic Predisposition to the Toxic Effects of Chemicals. Ed. by Philippe Grandjean et al. 1991. (Illus.). 250p. (gr. 13). pap. 155.95 (*0-412-39290-9*, A5564) Chapman & Hall.

EcoHerbalist's Fieldbook: Wildcrafting in the Mountain West. Gregory L. Tilford. 2nd ed. 1994. LC 93-80091. (Illus.). 295p. pap. 20.95 (*0-9638638-7-8*) Mtn Weed Pub.

Ecological & Biological Effects of Air Pollution. G. M. Woodwell et al. 1973. 39.50 (*0-8422-7138-4*) Irvington.

Ecological & Sociological Studies of Gelada Baboons. Ed. by M. Kawai. 1978. (Contributions to Primatology Ser.: Vol. 16). (Illus.). 128.75 (*3-8055-2873-6*) S Karger.

Ecological Approach to Visual Perception. James J. Gibson. 1979. 336p. pap. 45.00 (*0-89859-959-8*) L Erlbaum Assocs.

Ecological Implications of Body Size. Robert H. Peters. 1986. 345p. pap. text 31.95 (*0-521-28886-X*) Cambridge U Pr.

Ecological Inference. Laura I. Langbein & Allan J. Lichtman. 1978. LC 77-93283. (Quantitative Applications in the Social Sciences Ser.: Vol. 10). 70p. pap. 14.95 (*0-8039-0941-1*, 407010) Sage.

Ecological Perception Research, Visual Communication, & Aesthetics. Ed. by K. Landwehr. 1990. (Recent Research in Psychology Ser.). 143p. 38.95 (*0-387-52200-X*) Spr-Verlag.

Ecological Perspective in Family-Centered Therapy. Ed. by Margaret R. Rodway & Barry Trute. 1993. LC 93-29860. (Studies in Health & Human Services: Vol. 19). 364p. text 99.95 (*0-7734-9362-X*) E Mellen.

Ecological Perspectives on Carcinogens & Cancer Control: Proceedings of the International Conference, September, 1976. International Conference, Cremona Staff. Ed. by C. C. Stock et al. 1978. (Progress in Biochemical Pharmacology Ser.: Vol. 14). (Illus.). 83.50 (*3-8055-2684-9*) S Karger.

Ecological Psychology: Concepts & Methods for Studying the Environment of Human Behavior. Roger G. Barker. 1968. LC 68-21287. vi, 242p. 51.00 (*0-8047-0658-1*) Stanford U Pr.

Ecological Relationships & Evolution of the Rickettsiae, Vol. I. Nyven J. Marchette. 1982. 176p. 104.00 (*0-8493-6125-7*, QR353, CRC Reprint) Franklin.

Ecological Relationships & Evolution of the Rickettsiae, Vol. II. Ed. by Nyven J. Marchette. 1982. 192p. 165.00 (*0-8493-6126-5*, QR353, CRC Reprint) Franklin.

Ecological Statistical Studies on Environmental Pollution & Chronic Disease in Metropolitan Areas of the U. S. Richard J. Hickey et al. 1970. (Discussion Papers: No. 35). pap. 10.00 (*1-55869-029-8*) Regional Sci Res Inst.

Ecological Studies on Insect Parasitism: An Original Anthology. Ed. by Frank N. Egerton, 3rd. 1978. LC 77-73820. (History of Ecology Ser.). lib. bdg. 26.95 (*0-405-10389-1*) Ayer.

Ecological Validity of Neuropsychological Testing. Ed. by Robert J. Sbordone & Charles Long. 1996. LC 94-73034. 530p. lib. bdg. 99.95 (*1-57444-024-1*) St Lucie Pr.

Ecology: A Textbook. Hermann Remmert. 1980. (Illus.). 289p. 53.95 (*0-387-10059-8*) Spr-Verlag.

Ecology & Control of Vectors in Public Health: Proceedings of the WHO Expert Committee on Insecticides, 21st, Geneva, 1974. WHO Staff. 1975. (Technical Reports: No. 561). pap. text 6.00 (*92-4-120561-X*, 1100561) World Health.

Ecology & Environmental Management of Lyme Disease. Ed. by Howard S. Ginsberg. 1993. LC 92-24221. (Illus.). 224p. (C). text 40.00 (*0-8135-1928-4*) Rutgers U Pr.

Ecology & Mental Health. Ed. by C. Muller. 1975. (Journal: Vol. 7, Nos. 4 & 5). 100p. 48.75 (*3-8055-2212-6*) S Karger.

Ecology of Aggression. A. P. Goldstein. 1994. LC 94-26532. (Social-Clinical Psychology Ser.). (Illus.). 208p. (C). 39.50 (*0-306-44741-X*, Plenum Trade) Perseus Pubng.

Ecology of Disaster: An Application of a Conceptual Model. Charles E. Faupel. 1985. 245p. text 29.50 (*0-8290-1350-4*); pap. text 19.95 (*0-8290-1532-9*) Irvington.

Ecology of Fish & Wildlife. Lawrence D. Burton. 1995. LC 94-44242. (Agriculture Ser.). (Illus.). 432p. (J). text 55.95 (*0-8273-6065-7*) Delmar.

Ecology of Graduate Medical Education: Improving the Quality of Residency Programs. Ed. by Alexander J. Walt et al. 1993. 154p. lib. bdg. 44.95 (*0-934277-18-4*) Am Bd Med Spec.

Ecology of Health: Issues & Alternatives. Jennifer Chesworth. 1996. LC 95-32538. (Illus.). 288p. 81.95 (*0-8039-7302-0*, 1213); xiv, 337p. pap. 39.95 (*0-8039-7303-9*, 1214) Sage.

Ecology of Human Development: Experiments by Nature & Design. Urie Bronfenbrenner. LC 78-27232. 368p. 1981. pap. 20.50 (*0-674-22457-4*); 1979. 39.95 (*0-674-22456-6*) HUP.

Ecology of Infectious Diseases in Natural Populations. Ed. by Bryan Grenfell & Andrew Dobson. 1995. (Publications of the Newton Institute: No. 7). 533p. (C). text 80.00 (*0-521-46502-8*) Cambridge U Pr.

Ecology of Marine Parasites. Klaus Rohde. 1982. LC 81-12934. (Australian Ecology Ser.). (Illus.). 245p. (C). pap. 24.95 (*0-7022-1670-4*) Intl Spec Bk.

Ecology of Mycobacteria. Jindrich Kazda. 2000. 80p. pap. (*0-7923-6197-0*) Kluwer Academic NLD. *Dist:* Kluwer Academic.

Ecology of Pathogenic Bacteria. B. A. Van der Zeijst et al. LC 97-196434. 304p. pap. (*0-444-85802-4*) Royal Netherlands Acad NLD. *Dist:* Elsevier.

Ecology of Stress. Ed. by Stevan E. Hobfoll. 1988. (Series in Health Psychology & Behavioral Medicine). 350p. 79.95 (*0-89116-637-8*); pap. 47.95 (*0-89116-845-1*) Hemisp Pub.

Ecology of the Body: Styles of Behavior in Human Life. Joseph Lyons. 1987. LC 87-9080. 339p. (C). text 49.95 (*0-8223-0710-3*) Duke.

Econometrics of Health Care. G. Duru. 1991. (C). lib. bdg. 191.50 (*0-7923-0766-6*) Kluwer Academic.

Economic & Medicinal Plant Research, Vol. 6. Ed. by H. Wagner & Norman R. Farnsworth. 1994. (Economic & Medicinal Plant Research Ser.: Vol. 6). (Illus.). 329p. text 94.00 (*0-12-730067-8*) Acad Pr.

Economic Approach to Human Behavior. Gary Stanley Becker. 1978. LC 75-43240. 320p. reprint ed. pap. text 17.00 (*0-226-04112-3*, P803) U Ch Pr.

Economic Aspects of AIDS & HIV-Infection. Ed. by D. Schwefel et al. 1990. (Health Systems Research Ser.). (Illus.). 364p. 99.00 (*0-387-52135-6*) Spr-Verlag.

Economic Aspects of Diabetes: Selected Annotations. 1993. 82p. (Orig.). (C). pap. text 35.00 (*0-7881-0111-0*) DIANE Pub.

Economic Aspects of Health. Victor R. Fuchs. 1982. LC 81-15938. (Conference Report / National Bureau of Economic Research Ser.). 344p. (C). lib. bdg. 42.00 (*0-226-26785-7*) U Ch Pr.

Economic Aspects of the Liquor Problem. John Koren. Ed. by Gerald N. Grob. 1981. LC 80-1261. (Addiction in America Ser.). reprint ed. lib. bdg. 32.95 (*0-405-13599-8*) Ayer.

Economic Botany of the Himalayan Regions. E. T. Atkinson. 1988. (C). (*0-7855-2279-4*) Scientific GBR. *Dist:* St Mut.

Economic Change, Social Welfare, & Health in Europe. Ed. by L. S. Levin et al. 1995. (WHO Regional Publications: No. 54). xii, 131p. pap. text 26.10 (*92-890-1318-4*, 1310054) World Health.

Economic Consequences of Traumatic Spinal Cord Injury. Ed. by Monroe Berkowitz et al. 1992. 212p. pap. 89.95 (*0-939957-44-2*) Demos Medical.

Economic Effects of Health Reform. C. Eugene Steuerle. 1994. (Special Studies in Health Reform). 28p. (Orig.). pap. 9.95 (*0-8447-7019-1*, AEI Pr) Am Enterprise.

Economic Evaluation & Health Promotion. Ceri Phillips. 1997. LC 96-80385. 144p. text (*1-85972-487-6*) Avebry GBR. *Dist:* Ashgate Pub Co.

Economic Evaluation in Healthcare. 196p. pap. text (*0-86471-062-3*) Adis Intl NZL. *Dist:* Lppncott W & W.

Economic Evaluation of Epilepsy Management. Ed. by Pachlatko & R. G. Beran. 1996. 112p. (*0-86196-556-6*) J Libbey Med GBR. *Dist:* Buttrwrth-Heinemann.

Economic Evaluation of Mental Health Care. Martin Knapp. 1995. 264p. pap. (*1-85742-211-2*) Arena GBR. *Dist:* Ashgate Pub Co.

Economic Evaluation of Mental Health Care. Ed. by Martin Knapp. 1995. 264p. (*1-85742-207-4*) Arena GBR. *Dist:* Ashgate Pub Co.

Economic Evolution of American Health Care: From Marcus Welby to Managed Care. David Dranove. 2000. LC 00-39975. 211p. 27.95 (*0-691-00693-8*) Princeton U Pr.

Economic Impact of Worksite Health Promotion. Association for Worksite Health Promotion Staff. Ed. by Joseph P. Opatz. 1993. LC 93-19102. (Illus.). 272p. text 34.00 (*0-87322-436-1*, BOPA0436) Human Kinetics.

Economic Implications of Rising Health Care Costs. 1992. (Illus.). 63p. (Orig.). (C). pap. text 30.00 (*1-56806-140-4*) DIANE Pub.

Economic Issues Related to the Health Care Industry. Ed. by S. Y. Wu & M. A. Zaidi. 1980. (Journal: Vol. 5, Nos. 5-6). (Illus.). pap. 33.25 (*3-8055-0473-X*) S Karger.

Economic Plants of India. V. S. Agarwal. 1988. (C). (*0-7855-2275-1*) Scientific GBR. *Dist:* St Mut.

Economic Report on Veterinarians & Veterinary Practices. Center for Info. Management Staff. 3rd ed. 1996. (Illus.). 229p. (Orig.). pap. 96.00 (*1-882691-10-5*) Am Veterinary Med Assn.

Economic Scarcity & Healthcare Quality: Tradeoffs in Delineations & Dilemmas. Les Seplaki. 1997. LC 96-44639. (Illus.). 272p. (*1-85521-841-0*) Dartmth Pub GBR. *Dist:* Ashgate Pub Co.

Economics. Dale B. Truett. 1987. stu. ed. 12.95 (*0-8016-2393-6*) Mosby Inc.

Economics & Episodic Disease: The Benefits of Preventing a Giardiasis Outbreak. Winston Harrington et al. 1991. LC 91-2129. 228p. (C). 24.00 (*0-915707-59-4*) Resources Future.

Economics & Mental Health. Ed. by Richard G. Frank & Willard G. Manning, Jr. 1992. LC 92-11603. (Illus.). 368p. pap. text 20.95 (*0-8018-4546-7*) Johns Hopkins.

Economics & Nursing: Critical Professional Issues. Cyril F. Chang et al. 2000. LC 00-31474. (Illus.). 507p. (C). text 49.95 (*0-8036-0465-3*) Davis Co.

Economics for Health Sector Analysis: Concepts & Cases. Mead Over. 1992. (EDI Seminar Ser.). 224p. pap. 22.00 (*0-8213-1335-5*, 11335) World Bank.

E
F
G

Economics, Medicine & Health Care. Gavin H. Mooney. 2nd ed. 1992. 170p. (C). 80.50 (*0-389-20991-0*) Rowman.

Economics of Health Ed. by A. J. Culyer. 1991. (International Library of Critical Writings in Economics: Vol. 12). 840p. text 335.00 (*1-85278-176-9*) E Elgar.

Economics of Health: An Introduction. John G. Cullis & Peter A. West. 1992. (Modern Revivals in Economics Ser.). 336p. (*0-7512-0026-3*) Gregg Revivals GBR. *Dist:* Ashgate Pub Co.

Economics of Health & Health Care. Sherman Folland et al. 2nd ed. 1996. LC 96-23953. 688p. 86.00 (*0-13-565987-6*) P-H.

Economics of Health & Medical Care. Philip Jacobs. 4th ed. 1996. 432p. 65.00 (*0-8342-0803-2*) Aspen Pub.

Economics of Health & Medical Care. Jacobs & Rappoport. 5th ed. 2001. 464p. 68.00 (*0-8342-1937-9*) Aspen Pub.

Economics of Health & Nutrition: Some Aspects of Growth & Welfare. K. Rani Gopal. 1987. (C). (*81-85076-18-9*) Chugh Pubns IND. *Dist:* S Asia.

Economics of Health Care. Ed. by Jacques van der Gaag et al. 1982. LC 82-3699. 420p. 88.00 (*0-275-90918-2*, C0918, Praeger Pubs) Greenwood.

Economics of Health Care: A Reference Handbook. Michael D. Rosko & Robert W. Broyles. 1988. LC 87-36101. 448p. lib. bdg. 110.00 (*0-313-25416-8*, REH/, Greenwood Pr) Greenwood.

Economics of Health in Developing Countries. Ed. by Kenneth Lee & Anne Mills. 1983. (Illus.). 256p. 39.95 (*0-19-261385-5*) OUP.

Economics of Health Reconsidered. Thomas Rice. 1998. 251p. pap. text 40.00 (*1-56793-077-8*, EHRS-1019) Health Admin Pr.

Economics of Medicare Reform. Andrew J. Rettenmaier & Thomas R. Saving. 2000. LC 00-43722. (Illus.). ix, 183p. (C). pap. text 17.00 (*0-88099-211-5*); 34.00 (*0-88099-212-3*) W E Upjohn.

***Economics of Mental Health Care: Industry, Government & Community Issues.** Ruth F. G. Williams. 2001. 294p. (*0-7546-1714-9*) Ashgate Pub GBR. *Dist:* Ashgate Pub Co.

Economics of Mental Health Services, Vol. 8. Ed. by Richard M. Scheffler et al. 1988. (Advances in Health Economics & Health Services Research Ser.). 305p. 73.25 (*0-89232-735-9*) Jai Pr.

Economics of Mental Illness. Rashi Fein. Ed. by Gerald N. Grob. 1980. LC 78-22559. (Historical Issues in Mental Health Ser.). (Illus.). reprint ed. lib. bdg. 18.95 (*0-405-11913-5*) Ayer.

Ecophysiological Adaptation Strategies of Intertidal Marine Macroalgae: Ein Neues Artenkonzept. Rachel Einav. 1993. (Dissertationes Botanicae Ser.: Band 208). (GER., Illus.). 75p. pap. (*3-443-64120-2*) Gebruder Borntraeger DEU. *Dist:* Balogh.

Ecosystem Health: Principles & Practice. David J. Rapport et al. 1998. LC 97-27825. (Illus.). 304p. pap. 52.95 (*0-632-04368-7*) Blackwell Sci.

Ecosystem Homeostasis. P. Trojan. 1984. pap. text 107.50 (*90-6193-622-5*) Kluwer Academic.

Ecosystems. Gordon Dickinson & Kevin J. Murphy. 1997. LC 97-18303. (Introduction to Environment Ser.). (Illus.). 208p. (C). 70.00 (*0-415-14512-0*) Routledge.

Ecstasy: Dance, Trance, & Transformation. Nicholas Saunders. 1996. 279p. pap. text 19.95 (*0-932551-20-3*) Quick Am Pub.

Ecstasy: The Clinical Pharmacological & Neurotoxicological Effects of the Drug MDMA. Ed. by Stephen J. Peroutka. 1989. (Topics in Neurosciences Ser.). (C). text 160.50 (*0-7923-0305-9*) Kluwer Academic.

Ecstasy: The Complete Guide - A Comprehensive Look at the Risks & Benefits of MDMA. Ed. by Julie Holland. 2001. LC 2001-2945. (Illus.). 464p. pap. 19.95 (*0-89281-857-3*, Park St Pr) Inner Tradit.

Ecstasy & Agony: Living with Mood Swings. David Grounds & June Armstrong. 1995. 174p. (Orig.). pap. (*0-85091-520-1*) Lothian Pub AUS. *Dist:* Seven Hills Bk.

Ecstatic Antibodies: Resisting the AIDS Mythology. Ed. by Sunil Gupta & Tessa Boffin. 1990. (Illus.). 198p. text 44.95 (*1-85489-005-0*); pap. text 17.95 (*1-85489-014-X*) Routledge.

Ecstatic Imagination: Psychedelic Experiences & the Psychoanalysis of Self-Actualization. Dan Merkur. 1998. LC 97-20414. (C). 226p. text 59.50 (*0-7914-3605-5*); 218p. pap. text 20.95 (*0-7914-3606-3*) State U NY Pr.

Ectopic Pregnancy: Diagnosis & Management. Isabel Stabile. 1996. (Illus.). 170p. (C). pap. text 19.95 (*0-521-49612-8*) Cambridge U Pr.

Ectopic Pregnancy: Pathophysiology & Clinical Management. C. M. Fredericks et al. 1989. 231p. 94.95 (*0-89116-807-9*) Hemisp Pub.

***Ecuador Gender Review: Issues & Recommendations.** Maria Correia & Bernice van Bronkhorst. 2000. LC 00-49533. (World Bank Country Study Ser.). xv, 81p. (*0-8213-4778-0*) Wrld Bank.

Eczema. Patsy Westcott. 2000. (Illus.). 128p. pap. 16.95 (*1-56649-183-5*) Welcome Rain.

Eczema: Practical & Easy-to-Follow Advice. Maggie Jones. 1998. LC 97-48333. (Your Child Ser.). 128p. pap. 9.95 (*1-86204-209-8*) Element MA.

Eczema in Childhood: The Facts. David J. Atherton. 1994. LC 94-7384. (Facts Ser.). (Illus.). 274p. pap. 19.95 (*0-19-262398-2*) OUP.

Eczema in Children: A Guide for Parents. David & Bernard Cohen. Ed. by Frank A. Oski. 1999. (Pediatrics Ser.). (Illus.). 24p. pap. 2.95 (*1-885274-09-2*) Health InfoNet Inc.

Edgar Cayce Handbook for Health Through Drugless Therapy. Harold J. Reilly. 1988. 348p. pap. 14.95 (*0-87604-215-9*, 2073) ARE Pr.

Edgar Cayce Home Medicine Guide. Pref. by Gladys D. Turner. rev. ed. 1982. (Medicines for the New Age Ser.). 136p. pap. 10.95 (*0-87604-139-X*, 315) ARE Pr.

Edgar Cayce on Healing. Mary E. Carter & William A. McGarey. 1988. 208p. mass mkt. 3.95 (*0-446-35250-0*) Warner Bks.

Edgar Cayce Primer. Herbert B. Puryear. 1982. 272p. (Orig.). mass mkt. 6.99 (*0-553-25278-X*) Bantam.

Edgar Cayce Products: Twenty Years of Research. Ed. by Carol Baraff. 1979. 79p. 2.50 (*1-882545-02-8*) Herit Pubns.

Edgar Cayce Remedies. William A. McGarey. 1983. 288p. mass mkt. 6.99 (*0-553-27427-9*) Bantam.

Edgar Cayce Way of Overcoming Multiple Sclerosis - Vibratory Medicine. Dudley Delany. 4th l.t. rev. ed. 1998. LC 97-93411. (Illus.). 120p. pap. 10.95 (*0-9657903-3-9*, A04) Meridian VA.

Edgar Cayce's ESP: Who He Was, What He Said & How It Came True. Kevin J. Todeschi. 2001. LC 00-26646. xv, 153p. pap. 12.95 (*0-87604-469-0*) ARE Pr.

Edgar Cayce's Guide to Colon Care: The First Step to Vibrant Health. Sandra Duggan. 1995. (Illus.). 225p. (Orig.). pap. 19.95 (*0-917483-32-4*) InnerVision.

Edgar Cayce's Holistic Health Program. Daniel Redwood. 1996. (Good Health Guides). 48p. pap. 3.95 (*0-87983-661-X*, 3661XK, Keats Pubng) McGraw-Hill Trade.

Edgar Cayce's on Rejuvenation of the Body. John Van Auken. 1997. LC 96-3217. (A.R.E. Membership Ser.). 91p. pap. 9.95 (*0-87604-359-7*, 463) ARE Pr.

Edge of Experience: Borderline & Psychosomatic Patients in Clinical Practice. Ed. by Grigoris Vaslamatzis & Andreas Rabavilas. 2000. 120p. pap. (*1-85575-238-7*) Karnac Bks GBR. *Dist:* Other Pr LLC.

EDI: A Guide for Integrating Electronic Data Interchange in Today's Healthcare Facility. James J. Moynihan & Marcia L. McLure. 1995. 216p. (C). text 45.00 (*1-55738-624-2*, Irwn Prfssnl) McGraw-Hill Educ Grp.

EDI: A Guide for the Healthcare Professional. James J. Moynihan. 1993. LC 93-16554. (Illus.). 98p. per. 24.95 (*1-882198-17-4*) Hlthcare Fin Mgmt.

Edible & Medical Plants of Northwest Montana. Crystal L. Cox. 1999. 114p. pap. 12.00 (*1-892930-01-3*) Nakaii Pubg.

***Edible & Medicinal Wild Plants of Minnesota & Wisconsin.** Matthew Alfs. 2001. (Illus.). 474p. pap. 45.00 (*0-9612964-3-7*) Old Theology Bk Hse.

Edible Oilseeds: Growth, Area Responses & Prospects. K. N. Ninan. 1989. (C). (*81-204-0397-5*) Oxford IBH IND. *Dist:* S Asia.

Edinburgh & Dore Lectures on Mental Science. Thomas Troward. 1989. 206p. reprint ed. pap. 14.95 (*0-87516-614-8*) DeVorss.

Educated Guesses: Making Policy About Medical Screening Tests. Louise B. Russell. 1994. LC 93-8768. pap. text 12.95 (*0-520-08366-0*) U CA Pr.

Educating Able Learners: Programs & Promising Practices. June Cox et al. 1985. LC 85-7405. (Illus.). 261p. pap. 13.95 (*0-292-70387-2*) U of Tex Pr.

Educating All Handicapped Children. Ed. by Robert Heinich. 1979. LC 78-12749. 384p. 39.95 (*0-87778-131-1*) Educ Tech Pubns.

Educating Beginning Practitioners: Challenges for Health Professional Education. Joy Higgs & Helen Edwards. 1999. LC 99-11381. 320p. pap. text 65.00 (*0-7506-3773-0*) Buttrwrth-Heinemann.

Educating Children with Severe Maladaptive Behaviors. William Stainback & Susan B. Stainback. 1980. 307p. text 40.00 (*0-8089-1269-0*, 794298, Grune & Strat) Harcrt Hlth Sci Grp.

Educating Disturbed Adolescents: Theory & Practice. Payton Towns. 1981. (Current Issues in Behavioral Psychology Ser.). 225p. text 35.00 (*0-8089-1312-3*, 794642, Grune & Strat) Harcrt Hlth Sci Grp.

Educating Doctors: Crisis in Medical Education, Research, & Practice. Stewart G. Wolf. 1997. LC 96-29359. 217p. text 32.95 (*1-56000-301-4*) Transaction Pubs.

Educating for Health & Prevention: A History of the Department of Community & Preventive Medicine of the (Woman's) Medical College of Pennsylvania. Bonnie E. Blustein. 1993. LC 93-5822. (Illus.). 160p. (C). 15.00 (*0-88135-148-2*); pap. text 9.95 (*0-88135-185-7*) Watson Pub Intl (Sci Hist).

Educating for Professionalism: Creating a Culture of Humanism in Medical Education. Ed. by Delese Wear & Janet Bickel. 2000. LC 00-44344. (Illus.). xvii, 215p. text 42.95 (*0-87745-741-7*) U of Iowa Pr.

Educating Gifted Children at Hunter College Elementary School. Gertrude H. Hildreth et al. 1970. LC 72-98228. (Illus.). 272p. reprint ed. lib. bdg. 68.50 (*0-8371-3941-4*, HIEG, Greenwood Pr) Greenwood.

Educating Medical Teachers. George E. Miller. 1980. (Commonwealth Fund Publications). (Illus.). 243p. 26.95 (*0-674-23775-7*) HUP.

Educating Professional Psychologists: History & Guiding Conception. Donald R. Peterson. 1997. LC 97-14077. 281p. pap. 29.95 (*1-55798-420-4*, 431-7880) Am Psychol.

Educating RNs for the Baccalaureate: Programs & Issues. Ed. by Barbara K. Redman et al. 1990. LC 90-9533. (Teaching of Nursing Ser.: Vol. 12). 248p. 39.95 (*0-8261-7210-5*) Springer Pub.

Educating the Creative Arts Therapist: A Profile of the Profession. Shaun McNiff. 1986. 296p. (C). text 49.95 (*0-398-05172-0*) C C Thomas.

Educating the Dentist of the Future: The Pennsylvania Experiment. D. Walter Cohen et al. 1985. LC 84-19602. 224p. text 36.50 (*0-8122-7947-6*) U of Pa Pr.

Educating the Emotions: Bruno Bettelheim & Psychoanalytic Development. N. M. Szajnberg. 1991. (Illus.). 248p. (C). 47.50 (*0-306-43942-5*, Plenum Trade) Perseus Pubng.

Educating the Future GP: The Course Organizer's Handbook. Patrick McEvoy. 2nd ed. 1998. LC 98-27318. (*1-85775-281-3*) Radcliffe Med Pr GBR. *Dist:* Balogh.

Educating Young Children Prenatally Exposed to Drugs & at Risk. 1993. 90p. pap. text 30.00 (*1-57979-141-7*) DIANE Pub.

Educating Young Children Prenatally Exposed to Drugs & at Risk: Report & Resource Compendium. Shirley A. Jackson. 1995. (Illus.). 80p. (Orig.). (C). pap. text 20.00 (*0-7881-2350-5*) DIANE Pub.

Education & Career Opportunities in Alternative Medicine: All You Need to Find Your Calling in the Healing Professions. Rosemary Jones. 1998. LC 97-52165. 360p. pap. 18.95 (*0-7615-1244-6*, Prima Health) Prima Pub.

Education & Epilepsy: Proceedings of an International Workshop on Education & Epilepsy. A. P. Aldenkamp & G. Stores. 1988. x, 146p. (*90-265-0885-9*) Swets.

Education & Health. Ed. by P. J. Kelly & J. L. Lewis. 1987. LC 86-25525. (Science & Technology Education & Future Human Needs Ser.: Vol. 5). (Illus.). 314p. (*0-08-033946-8*) Pergamon Repr GBR. *Dist:* Franklin.

Education & Occupations of Cripples: Juveniles & Adults. Ed. by William R. Phillips & Janet Rosenberg. 1980. LC 79-6924. (Physically Handicapped in Society Ser.). reprint ed. lib. bdg. 19.95 (*0-405-13131-3*) Ayer.

Education & Physical Growth. J. M. Tanner. 2nd ed. 1979. LC 78-8809. 144p. 27.50 (*0-8236-1531-6*) Intl Univs Pr.

Education & Training for Family Planning in Health Services: Proceedings of the WHO Scientific Group, Geneva, 1971. WHO Staff. 1972. (Technical Reports: No. 508). pap. text 5.00 (*92-4-120508-3*, 1100508) World Health.

Education & Training in Occupational Health, Safety & Ergonomics. 1981. (Technical Report Ser.: No. 663). 48p. pap. text 3.00 (*92-4-120663-2*) World Health.

Education & Training of Engineers for Environmental Health. J. Cassel et al. 1970. 152p. pap. text 20.00 (*92-4-156004-5*, 1150038) World Health.

Education & Training of Health Sciences Librarians. 1995. (Illus.). 50p. (Orig.). (C). pap. text 20.00 (*0-7881-2442-0*) DIANE Pub.

Education & Training of Nurse Teachers & Managers with Special Regard to Primary Health Care: Report of a WHO Expert Committee, 1984. WHO Staff. 1984. (Technical Report Ser.: No. 708). 54p. 7.00 (*92-4-120708-6*) World Health.

Education & Training of Senior Managers in the National Health Service. 1977. pap. 30.00 (*0-8464-0355-2*) Beekman Pubs.

Education & Training Policies in Occupational Safety & Health & Ergonomics: International Symposium. 1982. (Occupational Safety & Health Ser.: No. 47). (ENG & FRE.). viii, 389p. (Orig.). pap. 31.50 (*92-2-003002-0*) Intl Labour Office.

Education & Treatment in Human Sexuality, the Training of Health Professions: Proceedings of the WHO Expert Committee, Geneva, 1971. WHO Staff. 1975. (Technical Reports). pap. text 6.00 (*92-4-120572-5*, 1100572) World Health.

Education Begins Before Birth. Omraam M. Aivanhov. 1982. (Izvor Collection: Vol. 203). (Illus.). 168p. pap. 6.95 (*0-911857-02-8*) Prosveta USA.

Education for Health: A Manual on Health Education in Primary Health Care. 1988. (CHI, ENG, FRE & SPA.). viii, 261p. pap. text 34.00 (*92-4-154225-X*, 1150297) World Health.

Education for Health Manpower in the Middle East. Ed. by R. E. Nassif & J. D. Thaddeus. 1967. pap. 12.95 (*0-8156-6006-5*) Am U Beirut.

Education for More Synergistic Practice of Medicine & Public Health. Ed. by Mary Hager. 1999. 287p. (*0-9614362-1-2*) J Macy Foun.

Education for Positive Mental Health: A Review of Existing Research & Recommendations for Future Studies. James A. Davis. 1965. LC 64-15607. (Monographs in Social Research: No. 5). 15.00 (*0-202-09009-4*) Natl Opinion Res.

Education for the Health Professions: Policies for the 1980s. Peter F. Regan & Hans G. Schultze. 1983. 93p. (Orig.). pap. text 23.50 (*91-22-00627-3*) Coronet Bks.

Education Groups for Men Who Batter: The Duluth Model. Ellen Pence & Michael Paymar. 1993. LC 92-35954. 212p. 28.95 (*0-8261-7990-8*) Springer Pub.

Education in Ayurveda: A Re-Constructional Analysis. Bernd Pflug. 1992. (Illus.). xiii, 213p. (C). (*81-212-0399-6*) Gyan Publishing Hse IND. *Dist:* Nataraj Bks.

Education in Community Psychology: Models for Graduate & Undergraduate Programs. Ed. by Clifford R. O'Donnell & Joseph R. Ferrari. 1997. LC 97-759. 107p. 39.95 (*0-7890-0315-5*) Haworth Pr.

***Education in Heart.** Mills. 2001. 253p. (*0-7279-1620-3*) BMJ Pub.

Education of Audiologists & Speech-Language Pathologists. Ed. by Judith A. Rassi & Margaret D. McElroy. 1992. LC 92-16758. 496p. text 49.50 (*0-912752-30-0*) York Pr.

Education of Engineers in Environmental Health: Report of a WHO Expert Committee, 1967. 1967. (Technical Report Ser.: No. 367). 26p. pap. text 3.00 (*92-4-120376-5*, 1100376) World Health.

Education of Medical Students: Ten Stories of Curriculum Change. Frwd. by Jordan J. Cohen & Daniel M. Fox. 2000. 248p. pap. (*1-887748-40-7*) Milbank Memorial.

Education of the Handicapped: Laws, Legislative Histories & Administrative Documents, Set. Ed. by Bernard D. Reams. 1982. LC 82-81360. (Federal Legislative Histories of the Law of Disabled Persons Ser.: Part 2). lib. bdg. 2850.00 (*0-89941-157-6*, 302020) W S Hein.

Education of the Medical Student in Thanatology. Bernard Schoenberg. 1981. 20.95 (*0-405-13824-5*) Ayer.

Education of the Self: A Trainer's Manual. Gerald Weinstein et al. 1982. LC 76-9529. (Mandala Series in Education). 155p. pap. 12.95 (*0-8290-0976-0*) Irvington.

Educational Alternatives for Students with Learning Disabilities. Ed. by S. A. Vogel. 1994. (Illus.). 228p. 59.95 (*0-387-97668-X*) Spr-Verlag.

Educational & Emotional Adjustments of Stuttering Children. Elizabeth V. McDowell. LC 74-177022. (Columbia University. Teachers College. Contributions to Education Ser.: No. 314). reprint ed. 37.50 (*0-404-55314-1*) AMS Pr.

Educational Audiology for the Hard-of-Hearing Child. Ed. by Frederick G. Berg et al. 1985. LC 79-549. 256p. text 35.50 (*0-8089-1771-4*, 790549, Grune & Strat) Harcrt Hlth Sci Grp.

Educational Audiology for the Limited-Hearing Infant & Preschooler: An Auditory-Verbal Program. Doreen Pollack et al. 3rd ed. 1997. LC 96-49202. (Illus.). 410p. pap. text 69.95 (*0-398-06751-1*) C C Thomas.

Educational Audiology Handbook. Cheryl D. Johnson et al. 2000. 554p. pap. 129.95 incl. cd-rom (*0-7693-0120-7*); 1997. LC 97-11045. xi, 532p. 16.95 incl. disk (*1-56593-891-7*, 1742) Singular Publishing.

Educational Audiology Handbook. Cheryl D. Johnson et al. 1997. LC 97-11045. (Singular Audiology Text Ser.). (Illus.). 544p. pap. text 101.95 (*1-56593-823-2*, 1598) Thomson Learn.

Educational Audiology Handbook. Cheryl DeConde Johnson et al. 2000. pap. text 52.95 (*0-7693-0119-3*) Singular Publishing.

Educational Challenge: Meeting the Needs of Students with Brain Injury. Dana S. DeBoskey. 1995. (Illus.). 120p. (Orig.). pap. 14.50 (*1-882855-37-X*) HDI Pubs.

Educational Commission for Foreign Medical Graduates English Test (ECFMG-ET) Jack Rudman. (Admission Test Ser.: Vol. 43). 49.95 (*0-8373-5143-X*); 1994. pap. 29.95 (*0-8373-5043-3*) Nat Learn.

Educational Commission for Foreign Medical Graduates Examination (ECFMG) Jack Rudman. (Admission Test Ser.: Vol. 24). 89.95 (*0-8373-5124-3*) Nat Learn.

Educational Commission for Foreign Veterinary Graduates Examination (ECFVG) Pt. I: Anatomy, Physiology, Pathology. Jack Rudman. (Admission Test Ser.: Vol. 49A). 59.95 (*0-8373-6982-7*); 1994. pap. 39.95 (*0-8373-6957-6*) Nat Learn.

Educational Commission for Foreign Veterinary Graduates Examination (ECFVG) Pt. II: Pharmacology, Therapeutics, Parasitology, Hygiene. Jack Rudman. (Admission Test Ser.: Vol. 49B). 59.95 (*0-8373-6983-5*); 1994. pap. 39.95 (*0-8373-6958-4*) Nat Learn.

Educational Commission for Foreign Veterinary Graduates Examination (ECFVG) Pt. III: Physical Diagnosis, Medicine, Surgery. Jack Rudman. (Admission Test Ser.: Vol. 49C). 59.95 (*0-8373-6984-3*); 1994. pap. 39.95 (*0-8373-6959-2*) Nat Learn.

Educational Design & Cognitive Science. Ed. by Robert Glaser. 2000. (Advances in Instructional Psychology Ser.: Vol. 5). 392p. 89.95 (*0-8058-2549-5*) L Erlbaum Assocs.

Educational Handbook for Health Personnel. J. J. Guilbert. 6th rev. ed. 1987. (WHO Offset Publications: No. 35). (ENG, FRE & SPA.). 390p. pap. text 50.00 (*92-4-170635-X*, 1120035) World Health.

Educational Health & Safety Manual. Paul M. Stewart. 1993. LC 93-11371. 416p. 89.95 (*1-56670-044-2*, L1044) Lewis Pubs.

Educational Imperatives for Oral Health Personnel: Change or Decay?: Report of a WHO Expert Committee. 1990. (Technical Reports: No. 794). (ENG, FRE & SPA.). 43p. pap. text 6.00 (*92-4-120794-9*, 1100794) World Health.

Educational Outcomes: Assessment of Quality - A Compendium of Measurement Instruments-Baccalaureate Programs. 1988. 72p. pap. 7.50 (*0-88737-430-1*, 18-2254); 104p. pap. 7.50 (*0-88737-433-6*, 18-2267); 56p. pap. 7.50 (*0-88737-434-4*, 18-2268) Natl League Nurse.

Educational Outcomes: Assessment of Quality - A Directory of Student Outcome Measurements. 1987. 51p. 7.50 (*0-88737-392-5*) Natl League Nurse.

Educational Outcomes: Assessment of Quality - A Measurement Instrument Prototype. 1988. 44p. pap. 7.50 (*0-88737-431-X*, 18-2255) Natl League Nurse.

Educational Outcomes of Associate Degree Nursing Programs. NLN Council of Associate Degree Programs Staff. 1990. 10p. 5.95 (*0-88737-495-6*, 23-2348) Natl League Nurse.

Educational Process in Nursing Staff Development. Joann Grif Alspach. 1994. LC 94-20732. (*0-8016-0060-X*) Mosby Inc.

Educational Process in Nursing Staff Development: Applications to Critical. Joann Grif Alspach. 2nd ed. 1994. (Illus.). 340p. (C). (gr. 13). text 51.95 (*0-8016-7422-0*, 00060) Mosby Inc.

Educational Program Development for Employees in Health Care Agencies. June Dyche. 1982. 384p. (Orig.). pap. text 23.50 (*0-9609732-0-6*) Tri-Oak.

Educational Psychology. Jack Rudman. 1994. (Dantes Subject Standardized Tests Ser.: Vol. DANTES-13). pap. 27.95 (*0-8373-6613-5*); (ACT Proficiency Examination Program Ser.: Vol. PEP-28). pap. 23.95 (*0-8373-5528-1*) Nat Learn.

Educational Psychology Kelvin Seifert. 1990. (C). pap., tchr. ed. 3.16 (*0-395-48869-9*); pap., tchr. ed., suppl. ed. 3.96 (*0-395-48867-2*) HM.

Educational Psychology. Edward Lee Thorndike. 456p. 100.00 (*1-85506-701-3*) Thoemmes Pr.

Educational Psychology Kelvin Seifert. 2nd ed. 1990. (C). pap. 67.16 (*0-395-43235-9*); pap., stu. ed. 20.36 (*0-395-48868-0*) HM Soft Schl Col Div.

Educational Psychology Gage. 5th ed. 1991. (C). pap. text 62.36 (*0-395-62837-7*); pap. text, stu. ed. 21.56 (*0-395-58896-0*) HM.

Educational Psychology: A Developmental Approach. Richard C. Sprinthall & Norman A. Sprinthall. 4th ed. 1987. 680p. (C). pap. text 31.95 (*0-394-36297-7*) Random.

Educational Psychology: A Developmental Approach. Norman A. Sprinthall et al. 6th ed. 1994. (C). pap. text, stu. ed. 13.75 (*0-07-060555-6*) McGraw.

Educational Psychology: A Practitioner-Researcher Model of Teaching. Contrib. by Richard D. Parsons & Stephanie Lewis Hinson. 2000. LC 00-24140. (Illus.). xxi, 537p. (*0-534-55701-5*) Wadsworth Pub.

***Educational Psychology: Grade Aid Workbook.** Sternberg. 2001. 240p. suppl. ed. 20.00 (*0-205-35420-3*) Allyn.

Educational Psychology: Mastering Principles & Applications. Janice T. Gibson & Louis A. Chadler. 1988. pap. text 44.00 (*0-205-11360-5*, H13600) Allyn.

Educational Psychology: Theory & Practice. Robert E. Slavin. 6th ed. 1999. LC 99-20561. 596p. (C). pap. text 78.00 (*0-205-29270-4*, Longwood Div) Allyn.

Educational Psychology: Windows on Classrooms. Paul D. Eggen & Donald Kauchak. 5th ed. 2000. LC 00-26983. (Illus.). 728p. pap. 78.00 (*0-13-017176-X*) P-H.

Educational Psychology: Windows on Teaching. Thomas K. Crowl et al. 1996. 36p. (C). per. 38.75 (*0-697-38003-3*) Brown & Benchmark.

Educational Psychology 1995/96. Cauley et al. 10th annot. ed. 1996. tchr. ed. 13.12 (*0-697-31556-8*, WCB McGr Hill) McGrw-H Hghr Educ.

Educational Psychology 2000-2001. Kathleen Cauley et al. 15th ed. 2000. (Annual Editions Ser.). 240p. (C). pap. 17.50 (*0-07-236547-1*) McGrw-H Hghr Educ.

Educational Rhythmics in Practice: Starting & Running a Programme with the Mentally Handicapped. S. Moule et al. 1984. 24p. 60.00 (*0-906054-14-1*) St Mut.

Educational Services in Health Sciences Libraries. Ed. by Francesca Allegri & Alison Bunting. 1995. (Current Practice in Health Science Librarianship Ser.: Vol. 2). 196p. (C). 35.00 (*0-8108-3004-3*) Scarecrow.

Educational Significance of Left-Handedness. Ralph Haefner. LC 73-178804. (Columbia University. Teachers College. Contributions to Education Ser.: No. 360). reprint ed. 37.50 (*0-404-55360-5*) AMS Pr.

Educational Slide Graphics for the Vascular Laboratory. Claudia B. Rumwell. 1988. 20p. ring bd. 115.00 (*0-941022-13-7*) Davies Pubng.

Educationally Retarded Child: Comprehensive Assessment & Planning for Slow Learners & Educable Mentally Retarded Pupils. Nadine M. Lambert et al. 1974. LC 74-5099. (Illus.). 256p. text 45.00 (*0-8089-0836-7*, 792430, Grune & Strat) Harcrt Hlth Sci Grp.

Educator's Guide to AIDS: Law, Medicine & Policy. Barbara Harty-Golder & D. Parker Young. Ed. by Donald D. Gehring. 1994. LC 89-25250. (Higher Education Administration Ser.). 142p. (Orig.). pap. 17.95 (*0-912557-12-5*) Coll Admin Pubns.

Educator's Guide to AIDS & Other STD's. Stephen R. Sroka. 1989. (Illus.). 100p. tchr. ed. 30.00 (*0-9622034-0-8*) Hlth Educ Consults.

Educators Guide to Difficult Parents. Jerry Wilde. 2000. LC 99-55100. (*1-56072-763-2*, Nova Kroshka Bks) Nova Sci Pubs.

Educator's Guide to Preventing Child Sexual Abuse. Ed. by Mary Nelson & Kay Clark. 1986. 250p. pap. text 19.95 (*0-941816-17-6*) ETR Assocs.

Educators' Guide to Teaching Successful Problem-Solving & Test-Taking for Beginning Nursing Students. Patricia A. Hoefler. Ed. by Amelia R. Hummel. 1995. (Illus.). 80p. pap. text 29.95 (*1-56533-019-6*, IBK10) M E D S Inc.

EEG Activation & Artifacts. American Journal of END Technology Staff. 2nd ed. 1996. (Illus.). 241p. per. 28.00 (*1-57797-006-3*) ASET.

EEG in Clinical Practice. John R. Hughes. 2nd ed. 1994. (Illus.). 242p. text 59.99 (*0-7506-9511-0*) Buttrwrth-Heinemann.

EEG Montages & Polarity. American Journal of EEG Technology Staff & American END Society Committee. 1996. (Illus.). iv, 174p. per. 25.00 (*1-57797-002-0*) ASET.

EEG of Mental Activities. Ed. by D. Giannitrapani & Luigi Murri. 1988. (Illus.). viii, 204p. 155.75 (*3-8055-4812-5*) S Karger.

EEG Technician. Jack Rudman. 1994. (Career Examination Ser.: C-1263). pap. 39.95 (*0-8373-1263-9*) Nat Learn.

EEG Technician Curriculum: EEG 110, 111, 112, 114, 120. K. Ballinger et al. 1994. 515p. (C). ring bd. (*0-933195-76-1*) CA College Health Sci.

Effect of Added Thiamine on Learning. Ruth F. Harrell. LC 70-176841. (Columbia University. Teachers College. Contributions to Education Ser.: No. 877). reprint ed. 37.50 (*0-404-55877-1*) AMS Pr.

Effect of Aging in Oral Mucosa & Skin. Ed. by Christopher A. Squier. 1994. LC 94-5993. 192p. lib. bdg. 179.00 (*0-8493-9403-1*, 9403) CRC Pr.

Effect of Cancer on Quality of Life. David Osoba. 1991. 368p. lib. bdg. 139.00 (*0-8493-6977-0*, SB324) CRC Pr.

Effect of Carbohydrates on Lipid Metabolism. Ed. by I. MacDonald. 1973. (Progress in Biochemical Pharmacology Ser.: Vol. 8). (Illus.). 125.25 (*3-8055-1600-2*) S Karger.

Effect of Delay of Intervening Events on Reinforcement Value: Quantitative Analyses of Behavior, Vol. 5. Ed. by Michael L. Commons et al. 1986. (Roitblat-Bever-Olton: Comparative Cognition & Neuroscience Ser.). 344p. text 69.95 (*0-89859-800-1*) L Erlbaum Assocs.

Effect of Diet on Tumor Development in Animals. V. Mohr & J. P. Lewkowski. 1988. LC 88-10680. 144p. 100.00 (*0-89573-453-2*, Wiley-VCH) Wiley.

Effect of Exercise on Several Systems of Aging Mice. Ed. by D. Gershon. 1987. (Journal: Vol. 33, No. 1, 1987). (Illus.). 56p. pap. 48.00 (*3-8055-4584-3*) S Karger.

Effect of Female Sex Hormones on Fetal Development & Infant Health. 1981. (Technical Report Ser.: No. 657). 76p. pap. text 5.00 (*92-4-120657-8*) World Health.

Effect of Immunological & Non-Immunological Factors on Corneal Graft Survival. H. J. Volker-Dieben. 1984. (Monographs in Ophthalmology). text 160.50 (*90-6193-808-2*) Kluwer Academic.

Effect of Intensity of Light, State Adaptation of the Eye. Louise L. Sloan. 1972. (Psychology Monographs General & Applied: Vol. 38). reprint ed. 55.00 (*0-8115-1437-4*) Periodicals Srv.

Effect of Manual Guidance upon Maze Learning. Katherine E. Ludgate. 1972. (Psychology Monographs General & Applied: Vol. 33). reprint ed. 55.00 (*0-8115-1432-3*) Periodicals Srv.

Effect of Radiation on Human Heredity. 1957. (ENG & FRE., Illus.). 168p. pap. text 14.00 (*92-4-156023-1*, 1150040) World Health.

Effect of Radiation on Human Heredity: Investigations of Areas of High Natural Radiation. 1959. (Technical Report Ser.: No. 166). 47p. pap. text 3.00 (*92-4-120166-5*) World Health.

Effect of Stress on Dreams. Louis Breger et al. 1971. LC 74-160287. (Psychological Issues Monographs: No. 27, Vol. 7, No. 3). 214p. pap. 32.50 (*0-8236-1535-9*) Intl Univs Pr.

Effect of Tamoxifen on the Uterus in Postmenopausal Breast Cancer Patients. Patrick Neven. 1998. (Acta Biomedica Lovaniensia Ser.). (Illus.). 160p. pap. (*90-6186-895-5*) Leuven Univ BEL. *Dist:* Coronet Bks.

Effect of Welding on Health III (EWH III-83) 1983. (Illus.). 50p. pap. 48.00 (*0-87171-226-1*) Am Welding.

Effecting Change in Psychotherapy. Stephen A. Appelbaum. 1995. LC 81-65786. (Master Work Ser.). 256p. pap. 45.00 (*1-56821-600-9*) Aronson.

Effective AIDS Education on Campus, Vol. 57. Ed. by Richard P. Keeling. 1992. LC 85-644751. (New Directions for Student Services Ser.: No. SS 57). 112p. pap., stu. ed. 27.00 (*1-55542-761-8*) Jossey-Bass.

Effective Approaches to Patients' Behavior. Gladys B. Lipkin & Roberta G. Cohen. 4th ed. 1992. LC 91-4806. 312p. (C). pap. text 33.95 (*0-8261-1496-2*) Springer Pub.

Effective Approaches to Patients Behavior: A Guide Book for Health Care Professionals, Patients & Their Caregivers. Gladys B. Lipkin & Roberta G. Cohen. 5th ed. 1998. LC 97-52092. 360p. 56.95 (*0-8261-1497-0*) Springer Pub.

Effective Approaches to Patient's Behavior: A Guide Book for Health Care Professionals, Patients, & Their Caregivers. Gladys B. Lipkin & Roberta G. Cohen. 5th ed. 1998. LC 97-52092. xi, 379p. pap. 34.95 (*0-8261-1498-9*) Springer Pub.

Effective Brief Therapy: A Clinician's Guide. Michel Hersen. 2000. LC 00-103148. (Practical Resources for the Mental Health Professional Ser.). (Illus.). xv, 458p. pap. 49.95 (*0-12-343530-7*) Acad Pr.

Effective Business Psychology. Andrew J. DuBrin. 2nd ed. 1984. (C). text 40.33 (*0-8359-1570-0*) P-H.

Effective Choices for Diagnostic Imaging in Clinical Practice: Report of a WHO Scientific Group. 1990. (Technical Reports: No. 795). (CHI, ENG, FRE & RUS.). 131p. pap. text 14.40 (*92-4-129685-2*, 1100795) World Health.

Effective Choices for Diagnostic Imaging in Clinical Practice: Report of a WHO Scientific Group, 1988. WHO Staff. 1990. (Technical Report Ser.: No. 795). 131p. 16.00 (*92-4-120795-7*) World Health.

Effective Clinical Neurologist. Joshua Hollander & Louis Caplan. 2nd ed. 2001. 328p. pap. text 49.99 (*0-7506-7226-9*) Buttrwrth-Heinemann.

Effective Clinical Practice. Andrew Miles & Myriam Lygon. 1996. 224p. (Orig.). pap. 47.95 (*0-632-03908-6*) Blackwell Sci.

Effective Closing Argument. Peter C. Lagarias. 1991. 817p. suppl. ed. 100.00 (*0-87473-434-7*, 64195-10, MICHIE) LEXIS Pub.

Effective Communication in Practice. J. Pye & W. Jago. 1998. (Illus.). 240p. pap. (*0-443-05993-4*) Church.

Effective Communication Skills for Health Professionals: A Manual for Writers. Philip Burnard. 1992. LC 92-20116. (Therapy in Practice Ser.: Vol. 32). 232p. pap. 46.50 (*1-56593-014-2*, 0257) Singular Publishing.

***Effective Communications for Health Professionals.** Diane Herschfelt & Sharon Brill. (Illus.). 2001. pap., tchr. ed. (*0-7216-8457-2*); 2000. 255p. pap. (*0-7216-8456-4*) Saunders.

Effective Communications for Nutrition in Primary Health Care. (United Nations University Publications Ser.). 208p. 20.00 (*92-808-0634-3*, E.88.III.A.3) UN.

Effective Community Mental Health Services. Peter Huxley. 1990. 243p. text (*1-85628-040-3*) Avebry GBR. *Dist:* Ashgate Pub Co.

Effective Counseling Approaches for Chemical Abusers & Offenders. Gregory L. Little et al. 1997. 104p. (C). pap. 12.00 (*0-940829-19-3*) Eagle Wing Bks.

Effective Counseling Strategies for Dietary Management. Patricia A. Hodges & Connie E. Vickery. 1988. LC 88-7487. 213p. (C). 87.00 (*0-8342-0031-7*) Aspen Pub.

Effective Dental Assisting. Shirley P. Schwarzrock & James R. Jensen. 6th ed. 1982. 848p. (C). text 79.50 net. (*0-697-05664-3*) Brown & Benchmark.

Effective Dental Assisting. Shirley P. Schwarzrock & James R. Jensen. 7th ed. 1990. 640p. (C). text 120.00 (*0-697-11315-9*) McGrw-H Hghr Educ.

Effective Dental Assisting. Shirley P. Schwarzrock & Lorraine Schwarzrock. 7th ed. 1990. 640p. (C). spiral bd., wbk. ed. 50.63 (*0-697-11317-5*) McGrw-H Hghr Educ.

Effective Documentation for Physical Therapists. Darlene L. Stewart & Susan H. Abeln. 1993. (Illus.). 312p. (C). (gr. 13). text 52.00 (*0-8016-6359-8*, 06359) Mosby Inc.

Effective Electrotherapy Application, a Physical Therapist's Manual. Nancy Avena. 1999. 163p. (C). pap. 24.95 (*0-9670978-0-0*) Avena Pubg.

Effective Group Practice in Midwifery. Ed. by Lesley Page. 1994. LC 94-26761. (Illus.). 224p. pap. 34.95 (*0-632-03825-X*) Blackwell Sci.

Effective Gynecological Day Surgery. D. Healy. 1999. LC 98-71424. (Illus.). 168p. text (*0-412-79010-6*) E A GBR. *Dist:* OUP.

***Effective Health Care Manager.** Charles R. McConnell. 5th ed. 2002. LC 2001-53631. 52.00 (*0-8342-2083-0*) Aspen Pub.

Effective Heat & Power Strategies for Healthcare Premises. 1994. 74p. pap. (*0-11-321735-8*, HM17358) Statnry Office GBR. *Dist:* Bernan Associates.

Effective Hemodiafiltration: New Methods. Ed. by K. Maeda & T. Shinzato. 1994. (Contributions to Nephrology Ser.: Vol. 108). (Illus.). viii, 136p. 49.75 (*3-8055-5886-4*) S Karger.

Effective Hemostasis in Cardiac Surgery: A Society of Cardiovascular Anesthesiologists Monograph. Norig Ellison & David R. Jobes. 1988. text 75.00 (*0-7216-2757-9*) Saunders.

Effective Interaction with Patients. Ann Faulkner. 2nd ed. 1998. LC 97-25788. pap. text (*0-443-05876-8*) Church.

Effective Intervention with the Language Impaired Child. Martha L. Cole & Jack T. Cole. 2nd ed. 1988. LC 88-19003. 301p. (C). 71.00 (*0-87189-798-9*) PRO-ED.

Effective Language in Health & Social Work. R. Pugh. 1996. LC 95-71376. (Illus.). 184p. (Orig.). pap. 54.25 (*1-56593-324-9*, 0654) Singular Publishing.

Effective Leadership & Management in Nursing. Eleanor J. Sullivan. 4th ed. 1996. 192p. (C). pap. text 33.00 (*0-8053-7231-8*) Addison-Wesley.

Effective Leadership & Management in Nursing. Eleanor J. Sullivan et al. 5th ed. 2000. LC 00-51490. (Illus.). 384p. pap. 38.95 (*0-8053-2833-5*) P-H.

Effective Management in Nursing. Eleanor J. Sullivan & Phillip J. Decker. 1985. 500p. (C). pap. text (*0-201-06208-9*, Health Sci) Addison-Wesley.

Effective Management in Nursing. Eleanor Sullivan. 4th ed. 1996. 467p. (C). pap. text 52.00 (*0-8053-7871-5*) Addison-Wesley.

Effective Management in Therapeutic Recreation Service. Gerald S. O'Morrow & Marcia J. Carter. 1997. LC 96-61938. 412p. text 39.95 (*0-910251-87-8*, ETR91) Venture Pub PA.

***Effective Management of Musculoskeletal Injury: A Clinical Ergonomics Approach to Prevention, Treatment, & Rehabilitation.** Andrew Wilson. 2001. LC 2001-28165. (*0-443-06353-2*) Church.

Effective Management of Occupational & Environmental Health & Safety Programs: A Practical Guide. Royce Moser. 2nd ed. 1999. LC 99-21243. 80.00 (*1-883595-25-8*) OEM Health.

Effective Management of Private Health Care. Byrne. 1990. pap. text (*0-582-04283-6*) Addison-Wesley GBR. *Dist:* Trans-Atl Phila.

Effective Management of Volunteer Programs. Marlene Wilson. 1996. LC 75-39384. (Illus.). (Orig.). (C). pap. text 14.95 (*0-9603362-0-6*) Volunteer Mgmt.

Effective Medical Testifying: A Courtroom Handbook for Physicians. Kenneth K. Nakano et al. 1997. LC 97-34806. 227p. pap. text 39.99 (*0-7506-9986-8*) Buttrwrth-Heinemann.

Effective Medical Treatment of Heroin Addiction. 1998. lib. bdg. 250.75 (*0-8490-9087-3*) Gordon Pr.

Effective Menu Planning for the Elderly Nutrition Program. Gerontological Nutritionists Staff et al. 1991. LC 91-26184. spiral bd. 12.95 (*0-88091-090-9*, 0165) Am Dietetic Assn.

Effective Nurse: Leader & Manager. Laura M. Douglass. 5th ed. 1995. LC 95-19342. (Illus.). 448p. (C). (gr. 13). pap. text 36.00 (*0-8151-2779-0*, 25188) Mosby Inc.

Effective Nursing Leadership: A Practical Guide. Virginia Baillie & Louise Trygstad. Ed. by Tatiana I. Cordoni. 1988. 348p. (C). 70.00 (*0-8342-0036-8*, 20036) Aspen Pub.

Effective Outpatient Treatment for Adolescents: Principles, Practices & a Program Model for Working with Adolescents. David Gust & Ted Smith. 1994. LC 94-216665. pap. 21.95 (*1-55691-106-8*, 068) Learning Pubns.

Effective Pain Management. Rita Tamerius. 5th ed. 1994. LC 94-60262. 234p. (C). pap. 49.95 (*1-878025-62-7*) Western Schls.

Effective Patient Education: A Guide to Increased Compliance. Donna R. Falvo. 2nd ed. 1994. 340p. 79.00 (*0-8342-0382-0*, 20382) Aspen Pub.

Effective Presentations for Healthcare Professionals. Lisa Hadfield-Law. 1999. 128p. pap. text 32.50 (*0-7506-3843-5*) Buttrwrth-Heinemann.

Effective Psychotherapist. Annellen M. Simpkins. Ed. by Alex Simpkins. text (*0-8290-1370-9*) Irvington.

Effective Psychotherapist: Conclusions from Practice & Research. David Brenner. 1982. (General Psychology Ser.: No. 105). 160p. text 35.00 (*0-08-028056-0*); pap. text 16.95 (*0-08-028055-2*) Elsevier (Pergamon Pr).

Effective Psychotherapy: The Silent Dialogue. Robert J. Decker. 1988. 177p. 78.95 (*0-89116-679-3*) Hemisp Pub.

Effective Psychotherapy for Low-Income & Minority Patients. F. X. Acosta et al. 1982. LC 82-9053. (Illus.). 182p. (C). pap. 35.00 (*0-306-40879-1*, Plenum Trade) Perseus Pubng.

Effective Psychotherapy for Patient & Therapist. Jules Meisler. 1991. LC 91-2881. 208p. 62.50 (*0-275-93985-5*, C3985, Praeger Pubs) Greenwood.

Effective Psychotherapy with Borderline Patients: Case Studies. Robert J. Waldinger & John G. Gunderson. 1989. 232p. text 12.95 (*0-88048-272-9*, 8272) Am Psychiatric.

Effective Risk Communication: The Role & Responsibility of Government & Nongovernment Organizations. Vincent T. Covello et al. 1989. (Contemporary Issues in Risk Analysis Ser.: Vol. 4). (Illus.). 366p. (C). 110.00 (*0-306-43075-4*, Plenum Trade) Perseus Pubng.

Effective Supervision: A Task-Oriented Model for the Mental Health Professions. D. Eugene Mead. 1990. LC 90-2257. 200p. text 27.95 (*0-87630-600-8*) Brunner-Routledge.

Effective Technology: Integration for Disabled Children: The Family Perspective. M. Margalit. 1990. (Illus.). 226p. 59.95 (*0-387-97256-0*) Spr-Verlag.

Effective Therapy: Choosing the Right Therapy That Works for You. Michael J. Hurd. 1997. LC 97-3285. 352p. pap. text 16.95 (*0-935016-23-6*) Liv Resources.

Effective Treatments for PTSD: Practice Guidelines from the International Society for Traumatic Stress Studies. Ed. by Edna B. Foa et al. 2000. LC 00-26468. 388p. 44.00 (*1-57230-584-3*, 8R0584) Guilford Pubns.

Effective Upper & Lower Extremity Prostheses: A Special Issue of the Journal Automedica. Ed. by C. A. Phillips. 1989. 276p. pap. text 875.00 (*0-677-25830-5*) Gordon & Breach.

Effective Use of Group Therapy in Managed Care. Ed. by K. Roy MacKenzie. 1994. (Clinical Practice Ser.: No. 29). 31.00 (*0-88048-492-6*, 8492) Am Psychiatric.

Effective Use of Health Care Information: A Review of Recent Research. Peter Merrylees. 1997. LC 97-228546. (British Library Research Ser.). 262 p. (*1-85739-230-2*) Bowker.

Effectiveness & Costs of Osteoporosis Screening & Hormone Replacement Therapy, Set. 1997. lib. bdg. 608.95 (*0-8490-6372-8*) Gordon Pr.

*__Effectiveness & Efficiency: Random Reflections on Health Services.__ Admiral Lord Cochrane. 1999. 120p. pap. (1-85315-394-X) Royal Soc of Medicine Pr Ltd GBR. Dist: Balogh.

Effectiveness of CQI in Healthcare: Stories from a Global Perspective. Ed. by Vahe Kazandjian. 1997. LC 97-20201. 288p. 45.00 (0-87389-415-4, H0958) ASQ Qual Pr.

Effectiveness of Drug Abuse Treatment: Dutch & American Perspectives. Ed. by Jerome J. Platt et al. 1990. 344p. 55.00 (0-89464-266-9) Krieger.

Effectiveness of Drug Abuse Treatment: Implications for Controlling HIV Infections. 1991. lib. bdg. 75.00 (0-8490-4337-9) Gordon Pr.

Effectiveness of Innovative Approaches in the Treatment of Drug Abuse, 49. Ed. by Frank M. Tims, Jr. et al. 1997. LC 96-18222. (Contributions in Criminology & Penology Ser.: Vol. 49). 280p. 72.50 (0-313-30065-8, Greenwood Pr) Greenwood.

Effectiveness of Methadone Maintenance Treatment: Patients, Programs, Services & Outcome. J. C. Ball & A. Ross. 1991. (Illus.). 283p. 92.00 (0-387-97423-7) Spr-Verlag.

Effects - Immune Cells & Inflammation on Smooth Muscle & Enteric Ner. Ed. by Snape. 1990. 312p. 170.00 (0-8493-0174-2, RC802) CRC Pr.

Effects of A-Bomb Radiation on the Human Body. Ed. by Itsuzo Shigematsu et al. Tr. by Brian Harrison. 1995. (Illus.). 432p. text 55.00 (3-7186-5418-0, Harwood Acad Pubs) Gordon & Breach.

Effects of a Severely Mentally Retarded Child on Family Integration. B. Farber. 1959. (SRCD M Ser.: Vol. 24, No. 2). pap. 25.00 (0-527-01578-4) Periodicals Srv.

*__Effects of Acute Metabolic Interventions on Hemodynamics, Endothelial Function & Forearm Glucose Uptake.__ Andreas Furgmann. 2001. (Comprehensive Summaries of Uppsala Dissertations from the Faculty of Medicine Ser.: No. 1040). (Illus.). 60p. (91-554-5032-6) Uppsala Universitet SWE. Dist: Coronet Bks.

Effects of Aging & Environment on Vision. Ed. by D. A. Armstrong et al. 1991. (Illus.). 232p. (C). text 114.00 (0-306-43920-4, Kluwer Plenum) Kluwer Academic.

Effects of Aging on Regulation of Cerebral Blood Flow & Metabolism. Ed. by C. Fieschi et al. 1984. (Monographs in Neural Sciences: Vol. 11). (Illus.). xiv, 258p. 142.75 (3-8055-3805-7) S Karger.

Effects of Aging on Regulation of Cerebral Blood Flow & Metabolism: Abstracts. Ed. by C. Fieschi & C. W. Loeb. 1983. (Journal: Vol. 22, Suppl. 2). (Illus.). x, 64p. pap. 45.25 (3-8055-3732-8) S Karger.

Effects of Anaesthetics upon Cerebral Circulation & Metabolism. J. B. Madsen & G. E. Cold. 1991. (Illus.). 160p. 77.95 (0-387-82198-8) Spr-Verlag.

*__Effects of Anti-Psychotics on GABA Neurons in the Basal Ganglia of the Rat.__ Jiang Yu. 2000. (Comprehensive Summaries of Uppsala Dissertations from the Faculty of Medicine Ser.: No. 912). (Illus.). 46p. pap. (91-554-4673-6) Uppsala Universitet SWE. Dist: Coronet Bks.

Effects of Autism on the Family. E. Schopler & G. B. Mesibov. 1984. (Current Issues in Autism Ser.). (Illus.). 384p. (C). 59.00 (0-306-41533-X, Plenum Trade) Perseus Pubng.

Effects of Bisulphite & the Stability of Adrenaline. Goran Nilsson. 1986. (Dissertations from the Faculty of Science & Technology Ser.: No. 2). (Illus.). vii, 98p. pap. text (91-554-1888-0) Uppsala Universitet SWE. Dist: Coronet Bks.

Effects of Changing the Staffing in Military Treatment Facilities. Jacob A. Klerman et al. 1998. LC 96-20307. (Illus.). 81p. pap. 13.00 (0-8330-2380-2, MR-631-OSD) Rand Corp.

Effects of Child Abuse & Neglect: Issues & Research. Ed. by Raymond H. Starr, Jr. & David A. Wolfe. 1991. LC 91-20247. 304p. pap. 45.00 (0-89862-759-1, 2759) Guilford Pubns.

Effects of Clinical Nursing Specialization: A Controlled Organizational Experiment. Basil S. Georgopoulos & Luther Christman. 1991. LC 90-13639. (Studies in Health & Human Services: Vol. 14). 613p. lib. bdg. 129.95 (0-88946-271-2) E Mellen.

Effects of Drugs on Clinical Laboratory Tests Donald S. Young. 5th rev. ed. 2000. 2200p. pap. 199.00 (1-890883-24-7, 209) Am Assn Clinical Chem.

Effects of Drugs on Communication Disorders. Deanie Vogel & John E. Carter. 1994. (Clinical Competence Ser.). (Illus.). 180p. (C). pap. 45.00 (1-56593-072-X, 0377) Thomson Learn.

Effects of Drugs on Communication Disorders. Deannie Vogel et al. 2nd ed. 1999. LC 99-10766. (Clinical Competence Ser.). (Illus.). 350p. pap. 45.00 (1-56593-996-4, 1974) Thomson Learn.

Effects of Drugs on Human Functioning. Ed. by S. Streufert & F. M. Gengo. 1993. (Progress in Basic & Clinical Pharmacology Ser.: Vol. 9). (Illus.). xii, 184p. 215.00 (3-8055-5632-2) S Karger.

Effects of Drugs on the Fetus & Nursing Infant: A Handbook for Health Care Professionals. J. M. Friedman & Janine E. Polifka. 1996. LC 95-46371. 672p. (Orig.). (C). pap. text 55.00 (0-8018-5345-1) Johns Hopkins.

Effects of Early Parent Death. John Birtchnell et al. 1973. (Attitudes Toward Death Ser.: Vol. 1). 177p. (C). text 37.00 (0-8422-7145-7) Irvington.

Effects of Extracellular Adenosine & ATP on Cardiomyocytes. Amir Pelleg & Luiz Belardinelli. 1999. LC 97-46653. (Molecular Ser.). (Illus.). 221p. 99.00 (1-57059-524-0) Landes Bioscience.

Effects of Fatty Acids & Lipids in Health & Disease. Ed. by Claudio Galli et al. 1994. LC 94-27985. (World Review of Nutrition & Dietetics Ser.: Vol. 76). (Illus.). xii, 152p. 156.75 (3-8055-6040-0) S Karger.

Effects of Ginkgo Biloba Extract (EGb 761) on the Central Nervous System: Proceedings of the International Symposium, Montreux, Switzerland, 20 April 1991. Y. Christen et al. (Advances in Ginkgo Biloba Extract Research Ser.). 184p. pap. 66.00 (2-906077-28-3) Elsevier.

Effects of Health Programs on Child Mortality in Sub-Saharan Africa. National Research Council Staff. Ed. by Douglas C. Ewbank & James N. Gribble. 1993. (Population Dynamics of Sub-Saharan Africa Ser.). 208p. (Orig.). (C). pap. text 33.00 (0-309-04941-5) Natl Acad Pr.

Effects of Heating on Foodstuffs. Ed. by R. J. Priestly. 1979. (Illus.). 410p. 106.25 (0-85334-797-2) Elsevier.

Effects of High Altitude on Human Birth: Observations on Mothers, Placentas, & the Newborn in Two Peruvian Populations. Jean McClung. 1969. LC 72-91629. 168p. 17.95 (0-674-24065-0) HUP.

Effects of Ionizing Radiation: Atomic Bomb Survivors & Their Children (1945-1995) Ed. by Leif E. Peterson & Seymour Abrahamson. 1997. LC 97-52238. 379p. 79.95 (0-309-06402-3, Joseph Henry Pr) Natl Acad Pr.

Effects of Litigation on Health Care Costs. Ed. by Mary A. Baily & Warren I. Cikins. 1985. LC 85-70875. (Dialogues on Public Policy Ser.). 85p. pap. text 10.95 (0-8157-0757-6) Brookings.

Effects of Low-Power Light on Biological Systems III. Ed. by Giovanni F. Bottiroli et al. 1997. LC 98-164535. (Europto Ser.: Vol. 3198). 132p. 69.00 (0-8194-2630-X) SPIE.

Effects of Maternal Alcohol & Drug Abuse on the Newborn. Ed. by Barry Stimmel. 1982. LC 82-9393. (Advances in Alcohol & Substance Abuse Ser.: Vol. 1, Nos. 3 & 4). 157p. text 49.95 (0-917724-92-5) Haworth Pr.

Effects of Mineral Dusts on Cells. Ed. by B. T. Mossman & R. O. Begin. 1989. (NATO ASI Ser.: Vol. 30). (Illus.). 470p. 172.00 (0-387-50422-2, 3117) Spr-Verlag.

Effects of Music: A Series of Essays: International Library of Psychology, Philosophy, & Scientific Method. Ed. by Max Schoen. 1977. LC 68-20330. (Essay Index Reprint Ser.). 25.95 (0-8369-0854-6) Ayer.

Effects of Neurologic & Psychiatric Drugs on the Fetus & Nursing Infant: A Handbook for Health Care Professionals. J. M. Friedman & Janine E. Polifka. 1998. LC 97-49682. 653p. pap. text 57.00 (0-8018-5962-X) Johns Hopkins.

Effects of Nicotine on Biological Systems. Ed. by F. Adlkofer & K. Thurau. 1991. (Advances in Pharmacological Sciences Ser.). 664p. 172.00 (0-8176-2519-4) Birkhauser.

Effects of Organochlorines on Bone Tissue Morphology, Composition & Strength. Monica Linden. 2000. (Comprehensive Summaries of Uppsala Dissertations from the Faculty of Science & Technology Ser.: No. 528). (Illus.). 63p. pap. (91-554-4701-5) Uppsala Universitet SWE. Dist: Coronet Bks.

Effects of Polyelectrolyte Conformation, Charge Density & Ion Specificity in Polyelectrolyte & Polyelectrolyte-Drug Interaction. Andreas M. Hugerth. 2000. (Comprehensive Summaries of Uppsala Dissertations from the Faculty of Pharmacy Ser.: No. 227). (Illus.). 37p. pap. (91-554-4724-4) Uppsala Universitet SWE. Dist: Coronet Bks.

Effects of Preanalytical Variables on Clinical Laboratory Tests. Donald S. Young. 2nd rev. ed. 1997. 1285p. pap. 147.00 (0-915274-88-4, 202679, AACC Pr) Am Assn Clinical Chem.

Effects of Psychological Therapy. G. Terence Wilson. 2nd enl. ed. 1980. (FEBS Ser.: Vol. 24). 400p. (0-08-024675-3) Pergamon Repr GBR. Dist: Franklin.

Effects of Psychotherapy, Vol. II. Michael J. Lambert. 1982. (Psychotherapy Research Review Ser.). 288p. 42.95 (0-89885-099-1, Kluwer Acad Hman Sci) Kluwer Academic.

Effects of Psychotherapy with Children & Adolescents. John R. Weisz & Bahr Weiss. 1993. (Developmental Clinical Psychology & Psychiatry Ser.: Vol. 27). (Illus.). 120p. (C). 74.95 (0-8039-4388-1, 4869); pap. 34.95 (0-8039-4389-X, 4870) Sage.

*__Effects of Public Financing on Public Health Infrastructure: Congressional Hearing.__ Ed. by Sam Brownback. 2001. 75p. pap. text 20.00 (0-7567-1712-4) DIANE Pub.

Effects of Substance Abuse Treatment on AIDS Risk Behavior. Ed. by Edward Gottheil. 2000. 165p. pap. 19.95 (0-7890-0774-6, Hawrth Medical) Haworth Pr.

Effects of Substance Abuse Treatment on AIDS Risk Behavior. Ed. by Edward L. Gottheil. 1998. LC 98-51374. 126p. 49.95 (0-7890-0696-0, Hawrth Medical) Haworth Pr.

Effects of the Use of Methylphenidate in the Treatment of Attention Deficit Hyperactivity Disorder Diagnosed Children. 1994. (Illus.). 83p. (Orig.). (C). pap. text 25.00 (0-7881-0228-1) DIANE Pub.

Effects of Undernutrition on Children's Behavior. David E. Barrett & Deborah A. Frank. 1987. (Food & Nutrition in History & Anthropology Ser.: Vol. 6). xxvi, 348p. text 157.00 (2-88124-190-5) Gordon & Breach.

Effects of Welding on Health (EWH-79) 1979. (Illus.). 121p. pap. 48.00 (0-87171-180-X) Am Welding.

Effects of Welding on Health II (EWH II-81) 1981. (Illus.). 45p. pap. 48.00 (0-87171-212-1) Am Welding.

Effects of Welding on Health IV (EWH IV-83) 1983. (Illus.). 37p. pap. 48.00 (0-87171-230-X) Am Welding.

Effects of Welding on Health VI (EWH VI-89) 1989. (Illus.). 64p. pap. 48.00 (0-87171-298-9) Am Welding.

Effects of Welding on Health VII (EWH VII-90) 1990. (Illus.). 57p. 48.00 (0-87171-344-6) Am Welding.

Effects on the Baby of Maternal Analgesia & Anaesthesia. Ed. by Felicity Reynolds. 1993. (Illus.). 292p. text (0-7020-1574-1) W B Saunders GBR. Dist: Saunders.

Efferent Auditory System: Structure & Function. Tony L. Sahley et al. 1997. LC 97-1170. (Illus.). 240p. (Orig.). pap. 65.00 (1-56593-857-7, 1676) Thomson Learn.

Efficacy & Cost-Effectiveness of Psychotherapy. David Spiegel. 1999. LC 98-26812. (Clinical Practice Ser.: Vol. 45). 12p. 29.50 (0-88048-769-0) Am Psychiatric.

*__Efficacy & Radiation Safety in Interventional Radiology: A Focus for Health Education.__ World Health Organisation Staff. 2001. 90p. pap. 39.00 (92-4-154529-1) World Health.

Efficacy of Caries Preventive Strategies. Ed. by M. E. Curzon & J. M. Ten Cate. 1993. (Journal: Vol. 27, Suppl. 1, 1993). (Illus.). iv, 96p. pap. 26.25 (3-8055-5816-3) S Karger.

Efficacy of Myocardial Infarction Therapy: An Evaluation of Clinical Trials Evidence. Ira S. Nash & Valentin Fuster. 1999. LC 99-10224. (Illus.). 520p. text 195.00 (0-8247-1932-8) Dekker.

Efficiency & Economy in Animal Physiology. Ed. by Robert W. Blake. 1992. 199p. (C). text 59.95 (0-521-40066-X) Cambridge U Pr.

Efficiency & Performance in Health Sciences: Medical Analysis Index with Reference Bibliography. American Health Research Institute Staff. rev. ed. 1994. LC 94-34918. 131p. 57.50 (0-7883-0360-0); pap. 47.50 (0-7883-0361-9) ABBE Pubs Assn.

Efficiency Improving Innovations in Social Care of the Elderly. Ewan Ferlie et al. 1989. text (0-566-07049-9) Avebry GBR. Dist: Ashgate Pub Co.

Efficiency of Voice Production. Schutte. 1991. 208p. pap. 34.95 (1-56593-057-6, 0362) Singular Publishing.

Efficiency, Science Management, & Hospital Standardization: An Anthology of Sources. Ed. by Edward T. Morman. 1989. (Medical Care in the United States Ser.). 288p. reprint ed. text 25.00 (0-8240-8338-5) Garland.

Egan's Fundamentals of Respiratory Care. Sheldon et al. 5th ed. 1990. (Illus.). 1056p. (C). (gr. 13). pap. text, stu. ed. 14.95 (0-8016-5059-3) Mosby Inc.

Egan's Fundamentals of Respiratory Care. Craig L. Scanlan et al. 7th ed. 1998. LC 98-4101. (Illus.). 1128p. (C). (gr. 12). text 69.95 (0-8151-2798-7, 31173) Mosby Inc.

Egan's Fundamentals of Respiratory Care. Stephen F. Wehrman. 7th ed. 1998. (Illus.). 248p. stu. ed. (0-8151-2891-6) Mosby Inc.

EGF Receptor in Tumor Growth & Progession. R. B. Lichtner & R. N. Harkins. 1996. LC 96-41508. (Ernst Schering Research Foundation Ser.: Vol. 19). (Illus.). 288p. 65.00 (3-540-61720-5) Spr-Verlag.

Ego & Analysis of Defense. Paul Gray. 1994. LC 93-49005. 288p. 50.00 (1-56821-192-9) Aronson.

Ego & Archetype: Individuation & the Religious Function of the Psyche. Edward F. Edinger. 1992. LC 90-53380. (C. G. Jung Foundation Bks.). 336p. reprint ed. pap. 20.00 (0-87773-576-X) Shambhala Pubns.

Ego & His Own. Max Stirner. 1984. lib. bdg. 250.00 (0-87700-639-3) Revisionist Pr.

Ego & Reality in Psychoanalytic Theory: A Proposal Regarding the Independent Ego Energies. Robert W. White. LC 63-19631. 209p. 1963. (Psychological Issues Monographs: Vol. 11, No. 3). 32.50 (0-8236-1540-5); 1986. (Psychological Issues Ser.: Vol. 3). reprint ed. pap. text 32.50 (0-8236-1560-X, 01560) Intl Univs Pr.

Ego & Self in Weekly Psychotherapy. Gene Bocknek. 1991. LC 90-4923. 360p. 55.00 (0-8236-1545-6) Intl Univs Pr.

Ego & the Dynamic Ground: A Transpersonal Theory of Human Development. Michael Washburn. 2nd rev. ed. 1995. LC 94-1379. 272p. (C). pap. text 20.95 (0-7914-2256-9) State U NY Pr.

Ego & the Mechanisms of Defense. Anna Freud. rev. ed. 1967. LC 66-30463. (Writings of Anna Freud: Vol. 2). 191p. 35.00 (0-8236-6871-1); pap. 27.95 (0-8236-8035-5, 26871) Intl Univs Pr.

Ego & the Self. Percival M. Symonds. 1968. LC 68-23331. (Century Psychology Ser.). 229p. reprint ed. lib. bdg. 72.50 (0-8371-0243-X, SYES, Greenwood Pr) Greenwood.

Ego at the Center of Clinical Technique. Fred Busch. 1995. LC 94-46740. (Critical Issues in Psychoanalysis Ser.). 280p. 50.00 (1-56821-471-5) Aronson.

Ego Boundaries. Bernard Landis. 1970. LC 70-138248. (Psychological Issues Monographs: No. 24, Vol. 6, No. 4). 177p. 27.50 (0-8236-1570-7) Intl Univs Pr.

Ego Defenses: Theory & Measurement. Ed. by Hope R. Conte & Robert Plutchik. 1994. LC 94-7484. (Einstein Psychiatry Publication Ser.: No. 10). (Illus.). 340p. (0-471-05233-7) Interscience GBR. Dist: Wiley.

Ego Development & Psychopathology. David Ausubel. 1996. LC 96-6118. 313p. text 49.95 (1-56000-266-2) Transaction Pubs.

Ego Development & the Personality Disorders. David P. Ausubel. 1953. LC 52-2222. 576p. text 70.00 (0-8089-0023-4, 790270, Grune & Strat) Harcrt Hlth Sci Grp.

Ego Function Assessment (EFA) A Manual. Leopold Bellak. 1989. LC 88-26291. (Orig.). (C). pap. 10.50 (0-918863-02-3) CPS Inc.

Ego, Hunger & Aggression: A Revision of Freud's Theory & Method. Frederick Perls. 1992. 286p. reprint ed. pap. 25.00 (0-939266-18-0) Gestalt Journal.

Ego Identity: A Handbook for Psychosocial Research. James E. Marcia et al. 1993. (Illus.). 400p. (3-540-94033-2); LC 93-2919. 391p. 119.00 (0-387-94033-2) Spr-Verlag.

Ego Mechanisms of Defense: A Guide for Clinicians & Researchers. George E. Vaillant. 1992. LC 91-33137. 306p. text 42.00 (0-88048-404-7, 8404) Am Psychiatric.

Ego Psychology: Theory & Practice. Gertrude Blanck & Rubin Blanck. 2nd ed. 1994. LC 93-15638. 322p. 43.50 (0-231-08292-4) Col U Pr.

Ego Psychology & the Problem of Adaptation. Heinz Hartmann. Tr. by David Rapaport. 1964. LC 58-13783. (Journal of the American Psychoanalytic Association Monograph Ser.: No. 1). 121p. 27.50 (0-8236-1600-2) Intl Univs Pr.

Ego Psychology Two: Developmental Psychology. Gertrude Blanck & Rubin Blanck. 1979. LC 78-10956. (Illus.). 274p. text 44.00 (0-231-04470-4) Col U Pr.

Egoscue Method of Health Through Motion: A Revolutionary Program That Let's You Rediscover the Body's Power to Rejuvenate Itself. Pete Egoscue. 1993. LC 92-52558. (Illus.). 224p. reprint ed. pap. 13.00 (0-06-092430-6, Perennial) HarperTrade.

Ehrlichiosis: A Vector-Borne Disease of Animals & Humans. Ed. by Jim C. Williams & Ibulaimu Kakoma. 1990. 184p. text 124.00 (0-7923-0691-0) Kluwer Academic.

Eicosanoids & Other Bioactive Lipids in Cancer & Radiation Injury. Ed. by Kenneth V. Honn et al. 1991. (C). text 204.50 (0-7923-1303-8) Kluwer Academic.

Eicosanoids & Other Bioactive Lipids in Cancer, Inflammation, & Radiation Injury: Proceedings of the 2nd International Conference, September 17-21, 1991, Berlin, FRG. Ed. by Santosh Nigam et al. 1992. LC 92-23659. (Developments in Oncology Ser.: Vol. 71). 848p. (C). text 272.50 (0-7923-1870-6) Kluwer Academic.

Eicosanoids & Other Bioactive Lipids in Cancer, Inflammation, & Radiation Injury: Proceedings of the Fourth International Conference Held in Hong Kong, October 4-7, 1995, Vol. 3. Ed. by Kenneth V. Honn et al. 1997. LC 97-4119. (Advances in Experimental Medicine & Biology Ser.: Vol. 407). (Illus.). 616p. 149.50 (0-306-45487-4, Kluwer Plenum) Kluwer Academic.

Eicosanoids & Other Bioactive Lipids in Cancer, Inflammation, & Radiation Injury 2 Pts. A-B: Proceedings of the Third International Conference Held in Washington, D. C., October 13-16, 1993, Vol. 2A & B. Ed. by Kenneth V. Honn et al. 1998. LC 96-36444. (Advances in Experimental Medicine & Biology Ser.: Vol. 400). (Illus.). 1098p. 270.00 (0-306-45360-6, Kluwer Plenum) Kluwer Academic.

Eicosanoids & Other Bioactive Lipids in Cancer, Inflammation & Radiation Injury 4. Lawrence J. Marnett & S. K. Nigam. 1999. LC 99-40840. (Advances in Experimental Medicine & Biology Ser.). (0-306-46138-2, Kluwer Plenum) Kluwer Academic.

Eicosanoids & the Gastrointestinal Tract. Ed. by K. Hillier. 1988. (C). text 147.00 (0-85200-957-7) Kluwer Academic.

Eicosanoids & the Skin. Ed. by Thomas Ruzicka. 1990. 224p. lib. bdg. 229.00 (0-8493-6032-3, RL96) CRC Pr.

Eicosanoids, Apolipoproteins, Lipoprotein Particles, & Atherosclerosis. Ed. by C. L. Malmendier & P. Alaupovic. 1988. LC 88-28929. (Advances in Experimental Medicine & Biology Ser.: Vol. 243). (Illus.). 372p. 89.50 (0-306-43037-1, Plenum Trade) Perseus Pubng.

Eicosanoids, Aspirin, & Asthma. Andrzej Szczeklik et al. 1998. LC 98-5319. (Lung Biology in Health & Disease Ser.). (Illus.). 648p. text 195.00 (0-8247-0146-1) Dekker.

Eicosanoids in Inflammatory Conditions of the Lung, Skin & Joints. Ed. by Martin K. Church & C. Robinson. 1988. (C). text 147.00 (0-85200-958-5) Kluwer Academic.

Eicosanoids in the Cardiovascular & Renal Systems. Ed. by P. V. Halushka & D. E. Mais. 1988. (C). text 164.50 (0-85200-959-3) Kluwer Academic.

Eide und Bekenntnisse in der Medizin. J. Kleeberg. 1979. (Illus.). pap. 20.00 (3-8055-3041-2) S Karger.

Eidetic Imagery & Typological Methods of Investigation. Erich Jaensch. Ed. by Oscar Oeser. 1970. LC 78-98232. 136p. reprint ed. lib. bdg. 55.00 (*0-8371-3963-5*, JAEI, Greenwood Pr) Greenwood.

Eidetic Parents Test: Desk Volume. Akhter Ahsen. 1989. LC 89-62539. 96p. stu. ed. 19.95 (*0-913412-01-5*) Brandon Hse.

Eidetic Parents Test & Analysis. Akhter Ahsen. 1972. 256p. 35.00 (*0-913412-02-3*) Brandon Hse.

***800 Individual Statement Questions for the MRCPsych.** M. Mathews. 2001. 200p. pap. (*1-85315-505-5*) Royal Soc of Medicine Pr Ltd GBR. *Dist:* Balogh.

Eight Hundred Year Old Book of Indian Medicine & Formulas. E. Sharpe. 1986. 136p. reprint ed. (*0-8364-1767-4*) Manohar IND. *Dist:* S Asia.

Eight Language Dictionary of Medical Technology. Ed. by Ronald Albert & Harry Hahnewald. 1979. LC 78-40828. (*0-08-023763-0*) Pergamon Repr GBR. *Dist:* Franklin.

Eight Simple Qigong Exercises for Health: The Eight Pieces of Brocade. Jwing-Ming Yang. 2nd rev. ed. 1997. LC 97-60896. (Qigong Health & Healing Ser.). (Illus.). 112p. pap. 14.95 (*1-886969-52-3*, B010R/523) YMAA Pubn.

Eight Ways to Take an Active Role in Your Health: Steps You Can Take to Keep Yourself Healthy. Bill Little. 2000. LC 95-2546. 224p. pap. 9.99 (*0-87788-382-3*, H Shaw Pubs) Waterbrook Pr.

8 Weeks to a Healthy Dog. Shawn Messonnier. 1998. (Pet Care Naturally Ser.). 64p. pap. 4.95 (*0-87983-969-4*, Keats Pubng) McGraw-Hill Trade.

Eight Weeks to Optimum Health. Andrew Weil. 1998. LC 97-97069. 276p. pap. 13.95 (*0-449-00026-5*) Fawcett.

Eight Weeks to Optimum Health: A Proven Program for Taking Full Advantage of Your Body's Natural Healing Power. Andrew Weil. 1997. LC 96-51918. (Illus.). 288p. 23.00 (*0-679-44715-6*) Knopf.

Eighteen Seventy-Nine & All That: Essays in the Theory & History of Psychology. Mary Henle. 1986. LC 85-22432. pap. text 20.50 (*0-231-06171-4*) Col U Pr.

Eighth Annual Report on Carcinogens: 1998 Summary. Ed. by Barry Leonard. 1999. (Illus.). 252p. (C). pap. text 50.00 (*0-7881-8396-6*) DIANE Pub.

Eighth HGH Symposium: Mannheim, April 1997. Ed. by J. Girard & J. S. Christiansen. 1997. (Hormone Research Ser.: Vol. 48, Suppl. 5, 1997). (Illus.). iv, 122p. pap. 55.00 (*3-8055-6606-9*) S Karger.

Eighth International Symposium on Cerebral Hemodynamics, Muenster, September 1994: Abstracts. Ed. by E. B. Ringelstein. 1994. (Journal: Vol. 4, Suppl. 3, 1994). xxii, 26p. pap. 21.00 (*3-8055-6065-6*) S Karger.

Eighth International Symposium on Endocrinology & Development, Telfs, Austria, October 1991. Ed. by A. Attanasio. 1992. (Hormone Research Ser.: Vol. 38, Suppl. 2, 1992). (Illus.). iv, 88p. pap. 40.00 (*3-8055-5740-X*) S Karger.

Eighth International Symposium on Gastrointestinal Hormones, Timmendorfer Strand, Baltic Sea, September 1990, Abstracts. Ed. by W. Creutzfedt & F. Stoeckmann. 1990. (Journal: Vol. 46, Suppl. 1, 1990). (Illus.). ii, 138p. pap. 42.75 (*3-8055-5291-2*) S Karger.

Eighth Symposium by the 6 Winners of the Grants from Sandoz Foundation for Gerontological Research, Makuhari, June 1996. Ed. by Hajime Orimo. 1997. (Journal: Vol. 43, Suppl. 1, 1997). (Illus.). iv, 54p. pap. 21.75 (*3-8055-6489-9*) S Karger.

81st Annual Meeting of the Endocrine Society Program & Abstract Book 1999. 1300p. (C). pap. text 90.00 (*1-879225-35-2*) Endocrine Soc.

Eighty Puerto Rican Families in New York City: Health & Disease Studied in Context. Beatrice B. Berle. 1975. LC 74-14221. (Puerto Rican Experience Ser.). (Illus.). 356p. reprint ed. 29.95 (*0-405-06211-7*) Ayer.

80629 a Mengele Experiment. Gene Church. 2nd rev. ed. 1996. LC 96-6247. 296p. pap. 12.95 (*0-9644293-2-2*) Route Sixty-Six.

Einfuehrung in die Praktische Biochemie. Ed. by H. Aebi et al. 3rd ed. 1982. xii, 462p. pap. 65.25 (*3-8055-3448-5*) S Karger.

Einfuehrung in die Ultraschalldiagnostik: Kurzgefasstes Lehrbuch & Atlas. Ed. by W. G. Zoller et al. 2nd rev. ed. 1994. (Illus.). x, 266p. 86.25 (*3-8055-5974-7*) S Karger.

Einfuhrung in die Psychopharmakologie see Psychopharmacology: An Introduction

Ejercicios de Rehabilitacion el Hogar: Mano. Illus. by Dan Winter. 1992. (SPA.). 16p. (Orig.). (C). pap. 4.20 (*0-910317-84-4*) Am Occup Therapy.

Ejercicios de Rehabilitacion para el Hogar: Hombro, Antebrazo, Codo, Muneca. Illus. by Dan Winter. 1992. (SPA.). 16p. (Orig.). (C). pap. 4.20 (*0-910317-83-6*) Am Occup Therapy.

EKG & Heart Murmurs. Peter Warinner. 1998. LC 98-31026. (Pocket Brain Ser.: No. 1). (Illus.). 60p. pap. 12.95 (*0-9651162-3-9*) Wysteria Ltd.

***E.K.G. in a Heartbeat.** Karen Ellis. 2001. 96p. spiral bd. 16.00 (*0-13-061440-8*) P-H.

***EKG Plain & Simple: From Rhythm Strips to 12-Leads.** Karen Ellis. 2001. 576p. pap. 46.67 (*0-13-019745-9*) P-H.

EKG Pocket Survival Guide. Thomas M. Masterson et al. 1993. (Illus.). 54p. (Orig.). (C). pap. text 7.50 (*0-9634063-8-8*) Intl Med Pub.

EKG Technician. Marshall. 1990. LC 89-70794. 272p. pap. 59.00 (*0-89303-702-8*) P-H.

EKG Technician. Jack Rudman. 1994. (Career Examination Ser.: C-1264). pap. 39.95 (*0-8373-1264-7*) Nat Learn.

EKG Video-Workbook. Springhouse Publishing Company Staff. 1992. (Illus.). 144p. pap. text 39.95 incl. VHS (*0-87434-370-4*) Springhouse Corp.

Elastin & Elastases, Vol. I. Ed. by Robert Ladislas & William Hornebeck. 1989. 328p. 229.00 (*0-8493-6428-0*, QP552) CRC Pr.

Elastin & Elastases, Vol. 2. Ed. by Ladislas Robert & William Hornebeck. 1989. 280p. 225.00 (*0-8493-6429-9*, QP552) CRC Pr.

Elbow. Ed. by Bernard F. Morrey. 1993. LC 93-4630. (Master Techniques in Orthopaedic Surgery Ser.). (Illus.). 368p. text 195.00 (*0-7817-0036-1*) Lppncott W & W.

Elbow: Endoprosthetic Replacement & Non-Endoprosthetic Procedures. Ed. by W. Ruther. 1995. (Illus.). 240p. 175.00 (*3-540-59245-8*) Spr-Verlag.

Elbow: Traumatic Lesions. Ed. by L. Celli. Tr. by A. Warr from ITA. 1991. (Illus.). 194p. 182.00 (*0-387-82244-5*) Spr-Verlag.

Elbow & Its Disorders. Bernard F. Morrey. 2nd ed. 1993. (Illus.). 944p. text 199.00 (*0-7216-6794-5*) Saunders.

Elbow & Its Disorders. Bernard F. Morrey. 3rd ed. 2000. LC 99-33416. (Illus.). 925p. text (*0-7216-7752-5*) Saunders.

Elbow in Sport: Injury, Treatment, & Rehabilitation. Todd S. Ellenbecker & Angelo Mattalino. 1996. LC 96-31956. (Illus.). 216p. text 35.00 (*0-87322-897-9*, BELL0897) Human Kinetics.

Elder Abuse: A Decade of Shame & Inaction. 1995. (Illus.). 88p. (C). pap. text 20.00 (*0-7881-2355-6*) DIANE Pub.

Elder Abuse: Concepts, Theories & Interventions. Gerald A. Bennett & Paul Kingston. 1993. LC 93-32199. (Therapy in Practice Ser.). 47.75 (*1-56593-038-X*, 0432) Singular Publishing.

Elder Abuse: Conflict in the Family. Ed. by Karl A. Pillemer & Rosalie S. Wolf. 1986. LC 86-14014. 381p. 37.95 (*0-86569-133-9*); pap. 22.95 (*0-86569-134-7*) Greenwood (Auburn Hse).

Elder Care Handbook: Resources & Guidance for Persons Helping Older Family Members. Ronald L. Burdon. 1995. 92p. pap. 11.95 (*0-9647559-1-2*) Am Wellness.

Elder Care in Occupational Therapy. Sandra C. Lewis. 1989. LC 87-43265. 502p. pap. 36.00 (*1-55642-037-4*) SLACK Inc.

Elder Care Today & Tomorrow: Hearing Before the Special Committee on Aging, United States Senate, One Hundred Fifth Congress, Second Session, Washington, D.C, April 27, 1998. U. S. Government Staff. 1998. LC 98-211758. iii, 140 p. (*0-16-057246-0*) USGPO.

***Elder Law.** Margaret C. Jasper. 2nd ed. 2001. (Oceana's Legal Almanac Ser.). 174p. 25.50 (*0-379-11354-6*) Oceana.

Elder Mistreatment: Deciding Who Is at Risk, 21. Tanya F. Johnson. 1991. LC 90-43380. (Contributions to the Study of Aging Ser.: No. 21). 216p. 60.00 (*0-313-26409-0*, JRK/, Greenwood Pr) Greenwood.

Elder Suicide: Research, Theory, & Treatment. John L. McIntosh et al. 1994. LC 94-4604. (Illus.). 260p. pap. text 19.95 (*1-55798-242-2*) Am Psychol.

Elder Suicide: Research, Theory & Treatment. John L. McIntosh et al. 1994. (Illus.). 260p. text 24.95 (*1-55798-240-6*) Am Psychol.

Eldercare: A Practical Guide to Clinical Geriatrics. Ed. by Mary O'Hara-Devereaux et al. 1981. (Illus.). 368p. text 54.00 (*0-8089-1285-2*, 793190, Grune & Strat) Harcrt Hlth Sci Grp.

Eldercare: Coping with Late-Life Crisis. James A. Kenny & Stephen Spicer. 1989. LC 88-63504. (Golden Age Bks.). 152p. (Orig.). pap. 21.00 (*0-87975-517-2*) Prometheus Bks.

Eldercare in New York: The Consumer's Guide for Long-Term Health Care. Friends and Relatives of Institutionalized Aged Staff. 7th rev. ed. 1998. 384p. pap. 30.00 (*0-9652790-1-4*) Frnds & Relatives.

Elderly Americans: Health, Housing, & Nutrition Gaps Between the Poor & Nonpoor. 1993. (Illus.). 63p. (Orig.). (C). pap. text 30.00 (*1-56806-898-0*) DIANE Pub.

Elderly Care: A World Perspective. Ken Tout. 1993. 350p. pap. 54.25 (*1-56593-141-6*, 0453) Singular Publishing.

Elderly Care Medicine. Gurcharan S. Rai & Stephen Webster. 2000. (Medico-Legal Practitioner Ser.). 223p. (*1-85941-529-6*) Cavendish Pubng GBR. *Dist:* Gaunt.

Elderly Care Source Book: Comprehensive Guide to Long Term Care Facilities in Connecticut. Ann H. Maier. 1996. 532p. (Orig.). pap. 85.00 (*0-9626513-1-1*) Maier Pubns.

Elderly in Eleven Countries. E. Heikkinen & Waters. 1983. (Public Health in Europe Ser.: No. 21). 231p. pap. text 20.00 (*92-890-1157-2*) World Health.

Elderly in 2005: Health & Care: Updated Scenarios on Health & Aging, 1990-2005. Scenario Committee on Aging Staff & National Institute of Public Health and the Environment. 1994. LC 94-9741.Tr. of Ouderen in Het Jaar 2005. pap. text 94.00 (*0-7923-2783-7*) Kluwer Academic.

***Elderly Medicine: Specialist Guide.** Ed. by Gurcharan S. Rai & Graham Mulley. 2001. 420p. pap. (*90-5823-234-4*, Harwood Acad Pubs) Gordon & Breach.

Elderly Patient. W. B. Wright. 1986. 236p. 29.95 (*0-387-16856-7*) Spr-Verlag.

Elderly Patient in General Practice. Ed. by W. Meier-Ruge. 1988. (Teaching & Training in Geriatric Medicine Ser.: Vol. 1). viii, 256p. pap. 31.50 (*3-8055-4476-6*) S Karger.

Elderly People, Their Medicines, & Their Doctors. Ann Cartwright & Christopher Smith. 1988. 240p. text 79.50 (*0-415-00684-8*) Routledge.

Elderly Uncooperative Patient. Ed. by T. L. Brink. 1987. LC 86-26997. (Clinical Gerontologist Ser.: Vol. 6, No. 2). 194p. text 39.95 (*0-86656-604-X*) Haworth Pr.

Elderly with Chronic Mental Illness. Ed. by Enid Light & Barry D. Lebowitz. 1991. 384p. 49.95 (*0-8261-7280-6*) Springer Pub.

Elders at Risk: Abstracts of the Psychological & Behavioral Literature on Elder Abuse, Victimization, & Suicide, 1967-1993. Ed. by John F. Santos & Verna R. Walker. 1993. LC 93-40554. (Bibliographies in Psychology Ser.: No. 13). 103p. pap. 19.95 (*1-55798-231-7*) Am Psychol.

Elecrocardigraphy: The Monitoring & Diagnostic Leads. Richard Wiederhold. 2nd ed. 1999. LC 98-26495. (Illus.). 415p. (C). pap. text (*0-7216-7337-6*) Saunders.

Elective Incisions & Scar Revision. Albert F. Borges. 1973. 55.00 (*0-316-10269-5*, Little Brwn Med Div) Lppncott W & W.

Elective Mutism: A Handbook for Educators, Counsellors, & Health Care Professionals. Norman H. Hadley. 1994. LC 93-27859. (Neuropsychology & Cognition Ser.: Vol. 5). 260p. (C). lib. bdg. 169.50 (*0-7923-2418-8*) Kluwer Academic.

Electric & Electromagnetic Stimulation of Bone Growth. T. J. Van Rens. 1985. (Reconstruction Surgery & Traumatology Ser.: Vol. 19). (Illus.). vi, 154p. 121.00 (*3-8055-3939-8*) S Karger.

Electric & Magnetic Fields: An EPA Perspective on Research Needs & Priorities for Improving Health Risk Assessment. 1994. 65p. (Orig.). (C). pap. text 40.00 (*0-7881-0382-2*) DIANE Pub.

Electric & Magnetic Fields: Invisible Risks? Leonard A. Sagan. 1996. 250p. pap. text 19.95 (*2-88449-217-8*) Gordon & Breach.

Electric Injuries Including Lightning: Index of New Information with Authors & Subjects. John C. Bartone. 1996. LC 96-12481. 57.50 (*0-7883-0778-9*); pap. 47.50 (*0-7883-0779-7*) ABBE Pubs Assn.

Electric Injuries Including Lightning: Index of New Information with Authors & Subjects. J. C. Bartone, II. rev. ed. 1994. pap. 47.50 (*0-7883-0161-6*) ABBE Pubs Assn.

Electric Injuries Including Lightning: Index of New Information with Authors & Subjects. John C. Bartone, II. rev. ed. 1994. 57.50 (*0-7883-0160-8*) ABBE Pubs Assn.

Electrical Activity of the Archicortex. G. Buzsaki & C. H. Vanderwolf. 1985. 414p. (C). (*963-05-4159-9*) Akade Kiado HUN. *Dist:* St Mut.

Electrical Bioimpedance Methods: Applications to Medicine & Biotechnology. Pere J. Riu. 1999. LC 99-22308. (Annals of the New York Academy of Sciences Ser.: Vol. 873). (Illus.). xi, 545p. pap. (*1-57331-191-X*) NY Acad Sci.

Electrical Defibrillation. W. A. Tacker & Leslie A. Geddes. 1980. 208p. 129.00 (*0-8493-5359-9*, RC684, CRC Reprint) Franklin.

Electrical Injury: A Multidisciplinary Approach to Therapy, Prevention, & Rehabilitation. Ed. by Raphael C. Lee et al. 1994. LC 94-9282. (Annals Ser.: Vol. 720). 299p. 95.00 (*0-89766-864-2*); pap. 95.00 (*0-89766-865-0*) NY Acad Sci.

Electrical Nerve Stimulation: Theory, Experiments & Applications. F. Rattay. 1991. (Illus.). 264p. 84.95 (*0-387-82247-X*) Spr-Verlag.

Electrical Safety & Hazards in Hospitals. William J. Curran et al. 1974. 205p. (C). text 19.50 (*0-8422-7135-X*) Irvington.

Electrical Sensitivity Handbook: How Electromagnetic Fields (EMFS) Are Making People Sick. Lucinda Grant. 1995. LC 95-60142. 100p. (Orig.). pap. 23.00 (*0-9635407-2-6*) Weldon Pub.

Electrical Stimulation Vol. 1: Enhancement of Muscle Function. 1993. 245p. pap. 34.00 (*0-912452-84-6*, P-89) Am Phys Therapy Assn.

Electrical Stimulation Vol. 2: Management of Pain. 1993. 252p. pap. 34.00 (*0-912452-85-4*, P-90) Am Phys Therapy Assn.

Electrical Stimulation Vol. 3: Effects on Circulation & Wound Healing. 1993. 164p. pap. 30.00 (*0-912452-86-2*, P-91) Am Phys Therapy Assn.

Electrical Stimulation Vol. 4: Iontophoresis, Management of Paralysis, & Use for Other Medical Disorders. 1993. 154p. pap. 25.00 (*0-912452-87-0*, P-92) Am Phys Therapy Assn.

Electrical Stimulation & Auditory Management of Cochlear Implants. Shallop. 1998. 27.00 net. (*1-56593-218-8*) Singular Publishing.

Electrical Systems for Health Care Facilities. Hugh O. Nash, Jr. 1992. (Management & Compliance Ser.: Vol. 7). (Illus.). 144p. ring bd. 110.00 (*0-87258-608-1*, 055206) Am Hospital.

Electrical Therapy of Cardiac Arrhythmias. Franklin B. Saksena & Goldshlager. 1989. (Illus.). 760p. text 142.00 (*0-7216-2451-0*) Saunders.

Electrical Trauma: The Pathophysiology, Manifestations, & Clinical Management. Ed. by R. C. Lee et al. 1992. (Illus.). 456p. (C). text 110.00 (*0-521-38345-5*) Cambridge U Pr.

Electrically Assisted Transdermal & Topical Drug Delivery Metabolism & Molecular Physiology of Saccharomyces. Ajay K. Banga. 1998. LC 98-214657. (Series in Pharmaceutical Sciences). 95.00 (*0-7484-0687-5*) Taylor & Francis.

Electricity & Magnetism in Biology & Medicine. Ferdinando Bersani. 1999. LC 98-47483. 996p. (C). text (*0-306-46041-6*, Kluwer Plenum) Kluwer Academic.

Electricity & Magnetism in Biology & Medicine. Ed. by Martin Blank. 1993. (Illus.). 50.00 (*0-911302-67-0*) San Francisco Pr.

Electrified Potentials in Biological Membrane Transport. Erich Heinz. 1981. (Molecular Biology, Biochemistry & Biophysics Ser.: Vol. 33). (Illus.). 85p. 53.00 (*0-387-10928-5*) Spr-Verlag.

Electro-Acupuncture: Its Clinical Applications in Therapy. Pedro Chan. 1974. (Illus.). 15.00 (*0-914322-06-0*); pap. 8.50 (*0-914322-05-2*) Chans Corp.

Electro-Oculography-Its Clinical Importance: Proceedings. Ed. by R. Taeumer. 1976. (Bibliotheca Ophthalmologica Ser.: No. 85). 130p. 55.75 (*3-8055-2301-7*) S Karger.

***Electroactive Polymer (EAP) Actuators as Artificial Muscles.** Yoseph Bar-Cohen. 2001. LC 00-69854. (Monographs: Vol. 98). (Illus.). xiv, 671p. (*0-8194-4054-X*) SPIE.

***Electroacupuncture.** Mayor. 2001. (Illus.). 347p. (*0-443-06369-9*) Church GBR. *Dist:* Saunders.

Electroacupuncture Primer. F. Werner & Reinhold Voll. Tr. by Hartwig Schuldt from GER. 1979. (Illus.). 164p. pap. text (*3-88136-073-5*) ML-Verlag DEU. *Dist:* Medicina Bio.

Electrocardiagrams: A Systematic Method of Reading Them. Michael L. Armstrong. 5th ed. (Illus.). 328p. pap. 38.00 (*0-07-470248-3*) McGraw-Hill Educ Grp.

Electrocardiografia Clinica. C. Castellano. 1996. (C). text 34.00 (*84-8174-133-7*) Mosby Inc.

Electrocardiogram in Acute Myocardial Infarction. Ed. by Ian P. Clements. 1998. LC 97-50183. (Illus.). 272p. 65.00 (*0 87993 693 2*) Futura Pub.

Electrocardiograph Technician. Jack Rudman. 1994. (Career Examination Ser.: C-1269). pap. 39.95 (*0-8373-1269-8*) Nat Learn.

Electrocardiographic Body Surface Mapping. Ed. by Raymond Van Dam & A. T. Van Oosterom. 1986. (Developments in Cardiovascular Medicine Ser.). text 193.50 (*0-89838-834-1*) Kluwer Academic.

Electrocardiographic Data Acquisition & Applications for Cardiac Dysrhythmia Monitoring. 1983. 27p. pap. 30.00 (*0-910275-19-X*, TU1-209) Assn Adv Med Instrn.

Electrocardiographic Diagnosis of Tachycardias. Ed. by Clifford J. Garratt et al. 1994. LC 94-38170. (Clinical Approaches to Tachyarrhythmias Ser.: Vol. 2). (Illus.). 64p. 16.00 (*0-87993-598-7*) Futura Pub.

Electrocardiographic Interpretation: A Self-Study Approach to Clinical Electrocardiography. Emanuel Stein. 1991. (Illus.). 701p. 155.00 incl. audio (*0-8121-1380-2*); text, stu. ed. 39.95 incl. audio (*0-8121-1378-0*) Lppncott W & W.

Electrocardiography: A Programmed Text. S. G. Owen. rev. ed. 1973. 180p. pap. 18.00 (*0-316-67724-8*, Little Brwn Med Div) Lppncott W & W.

Electrocardiography: Biophysical Measurements. Charles A. Rawlings. 1991. 129p. (C). 28.00 (*0-9627449-1-3*) SpaceLabs.

Electrocardiography: The Monitoring Lead. Richard Wiederhold. 1989. (Illus.). 336p. pap., tchr. ed. (*0-7216-3004-9*); pap. text, tchr. ed. 38.95 (*0-7216-2979-2*) Saunders.

Electrocardiography & Cardiac Drug Therapy. Ed. by V. Hombach et al. 1989. (Developments in Cardiovascular Medicine Ser.). 366p. (C). text 223.00 (*0-89838-395-1*) Kluwer Academic.

Electrocardiography in Clinical Practice. L. S. Ramaiah & Chou. Ed. by Richard Zorab. 4th ed. 1996. (Illus.). 736p. text 104.00 (*0-7216-5647-1*) Saunders.

Electrocardiography of Clinical Arrhythmias. Charles Fisch & Suzanne B. Knoebel. 2000. LC 99-54158. (Illus.). 432p. 49.00 (*0-87993-446-8*) Futura Pub.

Electrocardiography of Rate-Modulated Pacemaker Rhythms. Paul A. Levine et al. 1990. (Illus.). 90p. (Orig.). (C). pap. 40.00 (*0-9626364-0-1*); pap. 40.00 (*0-9626364-1-X*) Siemens Pacesetter.

Electrocardiography of Tachycardias. Niraj Varma & Vassillos P. Vassilikos. 1993. LC 92-49019. 416p. (gr. 13). pap. 429.95 (*0-412-48000-X*) Chapman & Hall.

Electrocardiography Pocket Book. D. J. Rowlands. 1993. 160p. (C). pap. text 22.00 (*0-7923-8805-4*) Kluwer Academic.

Electrocardiology: Eighteenth International Congress. J. Jagielski & M. Gornicki. 1992. 400p. text 121.00 (*981-02-0947-9*) World Scientific Pub.

Electrocardiology No. II: Physiological, Pathophysiology & Diagnostical Research Proceedings, 2nd International Congress, Varna, Oct., 1975.

International Congress on Electrocardiology Staff. Ed. by H. Abel & Z. Pavlov. 1977. (Advances in Cardiology Ser.: Vol. 19). 121.75 (*3-8055-2377-7*) S Karger.

Electrocardiology No. III: Proceedings of the International Congress on Electrocardiology & Vectorcardiography, 17th, Brussels, June, 1976. International Congress of Electrocardiology and Vect. Ed. by F. Kornreich. 1977. (Advances in Cardiology Ser.: Vol. 21). (Illus.). 117.50 (*3-8055-2650-4*) S Karger.

Electrocardiology No. VI. Ed. by H. Abel. 1981. (Advances in Cardiology Ser.: Vol. 28). (Illus.). xii, 248p. 136.75 (*3-8055-1185-X*) S Karger.

Electrocardiology 1993. P. W. MacFarlane & P. Rautarharju. 1994. LC 95-108388. 364p. text 86.00 (*981-02-1793-5*) World Scientific Pub.

Electrocardiology 92. P. W. MacFarlane & F. De Padva. 1993. 400p. text 121.00 (*981-02-1387-5*) World Scientific Pub.

Electrocardiology, 1996: From the Cell to the Body Surface. 1997. 500p. text 61.00 (*981-02-3109-1*) World Scientific Pub.

Electrochemical Data. Brian E. Conway. 1971. LC 69-10078. (Illus.). 374p. reprint ed. lib. bdg. 75.00 (*0-8371-1630-9*, COED, Greenwood Pr) Greenwood.

Electroconvulsive Therapy. Richard Ambrams. 3rd ed. 1997. LC 96-36870. (Illus.). 392p. text 59.50 (*0-19-510944-9*) OUP.

Electroconvulsive Therapy: A Programmed Text. John L. Beyer et al. 2nd ed. 1998. LC 97-3184. 211p. 36.00 (*0-88048-813-1*, 8813) Am Psychiatric.

Electrocorticography: Current Trends & Future Perspectives. L. Felipe Quesney et al. 1998. LC 98-21791. (Electroencephalography & Clinical Neurophysiology Ser.). 170p. 139.50 (*0-444-82509-6*) Elsevier.

Electrodermal Activity. W. Boucsein. 1992. (Behavioral Psychophysiology Ser.). (Illus.). 456p. (C). text 89.50 (*0-306-44214-0*, Kluwer Plenum) Kluwer Academic.

Electrodiagnosis in Clinical Neurology. Michael J. Aminoff. 3rd ed. 1992. (Illus.). 822p. text (*0-443-08795-4*) Church.

Electrodiagnosis in Clinical Neurology. Michael J. Aminoff. Ed. by Allan Ross. 4th ed. 1999. LC 98-52731. (Illus.). 700p. text (*0-443-07549-2*) Church.

Electrodiagnosis in Clinical Neurology. Michael J. Aminoff. 4th ed. 1999. text (*0-443-06507-1*) Harcourt.

Electrodiagnosis, Toxic Agents & Vision. Ed. by J. Francois & A. De Rouck. 1978. text 171.00 (*90-6193-155-X*) Kluwer Academic.

Electrodiagnostic Medicine. Daniel Dumitru. 1995. (Illus.). 1233p. 153.00 (*1-56053-071-5*) Hanley & Belfus.

Electroencephalograms of Normal Children. C. E. Henry. 1944. (SRCD M Ser.: Vol. 9, No. 3). pap. 25.00 (*0-527-01532-6*) Periodicals Srv.

Electroencephalography: Basic Principles, Clinical Applications, & Related Fields. Ed. by Ernst Niedermeyer & Fernando L. Da Silva. 3rd rev. ed. 1993. LC 93-3005. (Illus.). 1,189p. text 189.00 (*0-683-06511-4*) Lppncott W & W.

Electroencephalography: Basic Principles, Clinical Applications & Related Fields. Ernst Niedermeyer & F. H. Lopes da Silva. 4th ed. 1998. LC 97-48637. 1,226p. text 235.00 (*0-683-30284-1*) Lppncott W & W.

Electrogastrography: Methodology, Validation & Applications. Robert M. Stern & Kenneth L. Koch. 1985. LC 84-22312. 240p. 67.00 (*0-275-91326-0*, C1326, Praeger Pubs) Greenwood.

Electrogenesis of BioPotentials in the Cardiovascular System. Nicholas Sperelakis. 1995. LC 95-2188. (Developments in Cardiovascular Medicine Ser.: Vol. 164). 392p. (C). text 127.00 (*0-7923-3398-5*) Kluwer Academic.

Electrographic Imaging in Medicine & Biology. Ion Dumitrescu & Julian N. Kenyon. (Illus.). 316p. pap. 38.95 (*0-8464-4189-6*) Beekman Pubs.

Electrolysis, Thermolysis & the Blend: The Principles & Practice of Permanent Hair Removal. Arthur R. Hinkel & Richard W. Lind. 1968. LC 68-19191. (Illus.). 34.00 (*0-9600284-1-2*) Arroway.

Electrolyte & Acid-Base Companion: A Visual Guide to the Anatomy of the Stick Figure. Sarah Faubel & Joel Topf. Date not set. (Illus.). 550p. (Orig.). pap. 21.95 (*0-9640124-2-1*) Alert & Oriented.

Electrolyte Data Collection: Conductivities, Transference Numbers & Limiting Ionic Conductivities of Solutions of Aproptic, Protophobic Solvents. J. Barthel et al. Ed. by Gerhard Kreysa. 1995. (Dechema Chemistry Data Ser.: Vol. 12, Pt, 1C). 546p. lib. bdg. (*3-926959-69-X*) Dechema DEU. *Dist:* Scholium Intl.

Electrolyte Metabolism in Severe Infantile Malnutrition. J. Garrow & R. Smith. 1956. (*0-08-012623-5*) Pergamon Repr GBR. *Dist:* Franklin.

Electrolytes & Acute Renal Failure. Ed. by G. Eknoyan. 1991. (Journal: Vol. 17, No. 2). (Illus.). 76p. pap. 59.25 (*3-8055-5505-9*) S Karger.

Electrolytes, Body Fluids & Acid Base Balance. Eccles. 1994. 144p. pap. text 19.95 (*0-340-56754-6*) Trafalgar.

Electromagnetic Compatability in Medical Equipment: A Guide for Designers & Installers. William D. Kimmel & Darryl Gerke. 1995. LC 95-25000. 256p. 89.95 (*0-7803-1160-4*, PC5633) Inst Electrical.

Electromagnetic Compatibility in Medical Equipment: A Guide for Designers & Installers. William D. Kimmel & Daryl D. Gerke. 1995. LC 95-25000. (Illus.). 288p. 169.00 (*0-935184-80-5*) IHS Health Grp.

Electromagnetic Fields & Cancer: A Report to the People. 1992. 31p. (Orig.). (C). pap. text 20.00 (*1-56806-090-4*) DIANE Pub.

Electromagnetic Fields & Circadian Rhythmicity. Ed. by Russell J. Reiter et al. 1993. (Circadian Factors in Human Health & Performance Ser.). vii, 210p. 66.00 (*0-8176-3552-1*) Birkhauser.

Electromagnetic Non-Destructive Evaluation (II) Ed. by R. Albanese. 1997. LC 97-75199. (Studies in Applied Electromagnetics & Mechanics: Vol. 14). 450p. 113.00 (*90-5199-375-7*) IOS Press.

***Electromagnetic Radiation & the Human Body: Effects, Diagnostics & Therapeutic Technologies.** Nikolaos Uzunoglu & Konstantina S. Nikita. 2001. (Electrical Engineering & Applied Signal Processing Ser.). 350p. 99.95 (*0-8493-0960-3*, 0960) CRC Pr.

Electromagnetics in Medicine & Biology. Ed. by C. T. Brighton & S. R. Pollack. 1991. (Illus.). 37.50 (*0-911302-65-4*) San Francisco Pr.

Electromyographer's Handbook. Thomas T. Thompson. 1982. pap. text 19.00 (*0-316-84185-4*, Little Brwn Med Div) Lppncott W & W.

Electromyography. No. 5. Ed. by H. P. Ludin. 1995. LC 93-36498. (Handbooks of Electroencephalography & Clinical Neurophysiology: Vol. 5). 732p. 265.00 (*0-444-81256-3*) Elsevier.

Electromyography & Neuromuscular Disorders: Clinical-Electrophysiologic Correlations. Barbara E. Shapiro. 1997. LC 97-22494. 581p. text 140.00 (*0-7506-9724-5*) Buttrwrth-Heinemann.

Electromyography for Experimentalists. Gerald E. Loeb & Carl Gans. 1986. LC 85-28934. (Illus.). xx, 394p. pap. text 28.00 (*0-226-49015-7*) U Ch Pr.

Electromyography in Clinical Practice: Clinical & Electrodiagnostic Aspects of Neuromuscular Disease. Michael J. Aminoff. 3rd ed. 1997. LC 97-25846. text (*0-443-07681-2*) Church.

Electromyography of Jaw Reflexes in Man. Ed. by D. Van Steenberghe & A. De Laat. 1989. 466p. (Orig.). pap. (*90-6186-325-2*) Leuven Univ BEL. *Dist:* Coronet Bks.

Electron Microscopic Cytochemistry in Biomedicine. Kazuo Ogawa. 1992. 816p. lib. bdg. 297.00 (*0-8493-6012-9*, RB46) CRC Pr.

Electron Microscopic Immunocytochemistry. Ed. by Julia M. Polak & John V. Priestley. 1992. (Modern Methods in Pathology Ser.). (Illus.). 282p. spiral bd. 64.50 (*0-19-963248-0*) OUP.

Electron Microscopy & Alzheimer's Disease. Ed. by J. Metuzals. 1986. (Illus.). 20.00 (*0-911302-57-3*) San Francisco Pr.

Electron Microscopy at Molecular Dimensions. Ed. by W. Daumeister. 1980. (Proceedings in Life Sciences Ser.). (Illus.). 353p. 86.95 (*0-387-10131-4*) Spr-Verlag.

Electron Microscopy for the Fine Needle Aspiration of Tumors: A Primer: Vademecum. Ed. by G. Quinonez. 1997. LC 97-34984. (Systems Publications). (Illus.). vi, 192p. 98.00 (*3-8055-6604-2*) S Karger.

Electron Microscopy in Dermatology—Basic & Clinical Research: Proceedings for the Joint Meeting for the Society for Cutaneous Ultrastructure Research & the Japanese Society for Ultrastructural Cutaneous Biology, Nara, Japan, 25-27 October 1993. Ed. by Yasumasa Ishibashi et al. 1994. LC 94-2264. (International Congress Ser.: Vol. 1045). 484p. 236.50 (*0-444-81589-9*) Elsevier.

Electron Microscopy in Forensic, Occupational & Environmental Health Sciences. Ed. by Samarendra Basu & James R. Millette. 1986. LC 86-25290. 294p. 75.00 (*0-306-42466-5*, Plenum Trade) Perseus Pubng.

Electron Microscopy in Medicine & Biology. Ed. by P. D. Gupta et al. 2000. LC 99-56992. (Illus.). 200p. 75.00 (*1-57808-085-1*) Science Pubs.

Electron Microscopy in Viral Diagnosis. Erskine L. Palmer & Mary L. Martin. 1988. 194p. 199.00 (*0-8493-4747-5*, QR387) CRC Pr.

Electron Microscopy Methods & Protocols. M. A. Nasser. Hajibagheri. 1999. LC 98-37685. (Methods in Molecular Biology Ser.: Vol. 117). 296p. 99.50 (*0-89603-640-5*) Humana.

Electron Microscopy of the Lung. Schraufnagel. 1990. (Lung Biology in Health & Disease Ser.: Vol. 48). (Illus.). 608p. text 275.00 (*0-8247-8319-0*) Dekker.

Electron Paramagnetic Resonance of Exchange Coupled Systems. A. Bencimi & Dante Gatteschi. 1990. (Illus.). 287p. 127.00 (*0-387-50944-5*, 2772) Spr-Verlag.

Electroneurophysiology & Psychopathology. Ed. by Dargut Kemali et al. 1981. (Advances in Biological Psychiatry Ser.: Vol. 6). (Illus.). viii, 200p. pap. 48.00 (*3-8055-2420-X*) S Karger.

Electronic Atlas of Dermatology. Saunders. 1996. 285.00 (*0-7216-6224-2*) Saunders.

***Electronic British National Formulary.** Mehta. 2001. (*0-85369-495-8*); No. 39. 2000. (British National Fomulary Ser.: Vol. 39). cd-rom (*0-85369-463-X*); No. 40. 2000. cd-rom (*0-85369-466-4*) Pharmaceutical Pr GBR. *Dist:* Rittenhouse.

Electronic Classroom Manager to Accompany Community Health Nursing: Caring in Action. Hitchcock. 1999. 176p. tchr. ed. 75.00 (*0-7668-0217-5*) Delmar.

Electronic Companion to Complete Nutrition. Paul Insel. Ed. by Walter Escobar. 1998. (Electronic Companion Ser.). (Illus.). 300p. pap. text (*1-58032-005-8*) Cogito Lrning.

Electronic Data Interchange: The Physicians' Guide. American Medical Association Staff. pap. 29.95 (*0-89970-764-5*, OP205996WE) AMA.

Electronic Database of Cancer Incidence in Five Continents: CI5VII, Vol. VII. Ed. by J. Ferlay et al. 1998. (IARC Scientific Publications Ser.). (Illus.). 63p. pap. text 130.00 (*92-832-1449-8*) OUP.

Electronic Health Records: Changing the Vision. Gretchen Murphy et al. Ed. by Maureen Pfeiffer. 721st ed. 1999. LC 98-37968. (Illus.). xxiv, 627p. text 75.00 (*0-7216-7386-4*) Saunders.

Electronic House Calls: 21st Century Options. 1995. 27p. (Orig.). (C). pap. text 30.00 (*0-7881-2558-3*) DIANE Pub.

Electronic Image Bank-General Psychology. Brown Widdison. 2nd ed. 1995. (*0-697-29647-4*, WCB McGr Hill) McGrw-H Hghr Educ.

***Electronic Image Collection to Accompany Women's Health During the Childbearing Years.** Peggy S. Matteson. 2001. (*0-323-00920-4*) Mosby Inc.

Electronic Imaging in Medicine: Proceedings of an International Conference Held in San Antonio, Texas, March 27-April 1, 1983. Ed. by Gary D. Fullerton et al. 1984. (American Association of Physicists in Medicine Symposium Ser.: No. 11). 500p. 70.00 (*0-88318-454-0*) Am Inst Physics.

Electronic Mail & Office Automation in the Health Occupations: Index of New Information. Elliot D. Kass. 1994. 150p. 57.50 (*0-7883-0074-1*); pap. 47.50 (*0-7883-0075-X*) ABBE Pubs Assn.

Electronic Mail & Office Automation in the Health Professions: Index of New Information. Elliot D. Kass. 1996. LC 96-3125. 57.50 (*0-7883-0760-6*); pap. 47.50 (*0-7883-0761-4*) ABBE Pubs Assn.

Electronic Medical Record Infrastructures: An Overview of Critical Standards & Classifications. Christopher G. Chute. 1997. 320p. 49.00 (*0-387-94864-3*) Spr-Verlag.

Electronic Monitoring of the Fetal Heart. Jacqui Williams. 1996. LC 96-142811. 112p. pap. text 29.90 (*1-898507-11-2*) Buttrwrth-Heinemann.

Electronic Spatial Sensing for the Blind: Contributions from Perception, Rehabilitation, & Computer Vision. Ed. by David H. Warren & Edward R. Strelow. 1985. text 274.00 (*90-247-3238-7*) Kluwer Academic.

Electronically Controlled Drug Delivery. Bret Berner & Steven M. Dinh. 1998. LC 98-15824. (Illus.). 272p. lib. bdg. 129.95 (*0-8493-7681-5*) CRC Pr.

Electropharmacology. Ed. by George M. Eckert et al. 1990. 432p. lib. bdg. 259.00 (*0-8493-5409-9*, RM301) CRC Pr.

Electrophy of the Heart. David Ward. 1993. 99.50 (*0-7131-4507-2*) Routledge.

Electrophysiologic Basis of ECG & Cardiac Arrhythmias. Borys Surawicz. 1995. (Illus.). 560p. 92.00 (*0-683-08015-6*); 1994. LC 94-7820. (*0-8121-1591-0*) Lppncott W & W.

Electrophysiologic Correlates of Psychopathology. Ed. by L. Goldstein & Dargut Kemali. 1988. 49.95 (*0-915340-16-X*) PJD Pubns.

Electrophysiologic Evaluation in Otolaryngology. Ed. by B. R. Alford et al. 1997. LC 97-985. (Advances in OtoRhinoLaryngology Ser.: Vol. 53, 1997). (Illus.). viii, 212p. 169.00 (*3-8055-6427-9*) S Karger.

Electrophysiologic Testing. Richard N. Fogoros. (Practical Cardiac Diagnosis Ser.). (Illus.). 2nd ed. 1995. 256p. pap. 42.95 (*0-86542-392-X*); 3rd ed. 1999. LC 98-53197. pap. 48.95 (*0-632-04325-3*) Blackwell Sci.

Electrophysiological Correlates of Psychopathology(Advances in Biological Psychiatry), Vol. 9. 1982. (Illus.). x, 90p. pap. 42.75 (*3-8055-3525-2*) S Karger.

Electrophysiological Disorders. Camm. 2001. text (*0-443-06570-5*) Harcrt Hlth Sci Grp.

Electrophysiological Kinesiology: Proceedings of ISEK Conference, Florence, Italy 28-6 - 2-7. Ed. by Antonio Pedotti. 1992. LC 92-53264. (Studies in Health Technology & Informatics: Vol. 5). 412p. (YA). (gr. 12 up). 130.00 (*90-5199-095-2*) IOS Press.

Electrophysiology & Layout of the Auditory Nervous System. J. Donald Harris. 1974. LC 73-18092. (Studies in Communicative Disorders). (C). pap. text (*0-672-61286-0*, Bobbs) Macmillan.

Electrophysiology & Pharmacology of the Heart: A Clinical Guide. Dangman & Dennis S. Miura. 1991. (Illus.). 784p. text 250.00 (*0-8247-8449-9*) Dekker.

Electrophysiology in Neurotoxins. Lowndes. 1987. Vol. I. 128p. 81.00 (*0-8493-4694-0*); Vol. II. 152p. 90.00 (*0-8493-4695-9*) Franklin (CRC Reprint).

Electrophysiology of Gland Cells. O. H. Peterson. 1981. LC 80-40303. (Physiological Society Monographs: No. 36). text 157.00 (*0-12-552150-2*) Acad Pr.

Electrophysiology of Intellectual Functions. D. Giannitrapani. 1984. (Illus.). xvi, 248p. 142.75 (*3-8055-3878-2*) S Karger.

Electrophysiology of Mind: Event-Related Brain Potentials & Cognition. Ed. by Michael D. Rugg & Michael G. Coles. 1996. (Oxford Psychology Ser.: No. 25). (Illus.). 238p. pap. text 34.95 (*0-19-852416-1*) OUP.

Electrophysiology of Neuroendocrine Cells. Ed. by Hans Scherubl & Jurgen Hescheler. 1995. LC 95-4036. 384p. 169.95 (*0-8493-2477-7*, 2477) CRC Pr.

Electrophysiology of Single Cardiac Cells. Ed. by D. Nobel & T. Powell. 1987. 252p. text 116.00 (*0-12-520040-4*) Acad Pr.

Electrophysiology of the Neuron: An Interactive Tutorial: Macintosh Version. John Huguenard & David A. McCormick. 1994. (Illus.). 80p. (C). 24.95 incl. disk (*0-19-509167-1*) OUP.

Electrophysiology of the Neuron: An Interactive Tutorial: MS-DOS Version; A Companion to Neurobiology by Gordon Shepherd. John Huguenard & David A. McCormick. 1994. LC 93-39004. (Illus.). 80p. (C). 24.95 incl. disk (*0-19-509111-6*) OUP.

Electropotentials in the Clinical Assessment of Breast Neoplasia. Ed. by J. M. Dixon. 1995. LC 95-39600. (ESO Monographs). (Illus.). 80p. 78.95 (*3-540-60348-4*) Spr-Verlag.

Electroshock: Its Brain Disabling Effects. Peter R. Breggin. 1979. 256p. 32.95 (*0-8261-2710-X*) Springer Pub.

Electroshock: Restoring the Mind. Max Fink. 1999. LC 98-45789. 176p. 22.00 (*0-19-511956-8*) OUP.

Electroshock Treatment over Four Decades: The Case Against. Robert F. Morgan et al. Ed. by Robert F. Morgan. 1999. LC 00-500416. 99p. pap. 25.00 (*1-885679-02-5*) Morgan Fnd Pubs.

Electrosurgery of the Skin. Sheldon V. Pollack. 1990. (Practical Manuals in Dermatologic Surgery Ser.). (Illus.). 93p. pap. text (*0-443-08683-4*) Church.

Electrosurgical Devices. AAMI Staff. 2nd ed. 1993. (Illus.). 34p. pap. text 90.00 (*1-57020-019-X*, HF18-209) Assn Adv Med Instrn.

Electrotherapeutic Terminology in Physical Therapy. rev. ed. 2000. (Illus.). 48p. pap. 34.00 (*1-887759-88-3*) Am Phys Therapy Assn.

Electrotherapy. Fish. 1995. (C). pap. text (*0-7216-6713-9*) Saunders.

Electrotherapy Clinical Procedures. Theresa Nalty. 2000. LC 00-55030. (Illus.). 312p. pap. 44.95 (*0-07-134317-2*) McGraw-Hill Prof.

Electrotherapy in Rehabilitation. Ed. by Meryl R. Gersh. (Illus.). 1991. LC 91-28188. (Contemporary Perspectives in Rehabilitation Ser.: Vol. 7). 413p. 39.95 (*0-8036-4025-0*); 2nd ed. 2000. 450p. (C). 38.00 (*0-8036-0252-9*) Davis Co.

Electrotherapy of the Heart: Technical Aspects in Cardiac Pacing. Max Shaldach. 1992. LC 92-2219. (Illus.). 272p. 59.00 (*3-540-55333-9*) Spr-Verlag.

Elektronik Foster Overvakning see Fetal Heart Rate Monitoring: A Practical Guide

Element Guide to Anorexia/Bulimia. Julia Buckroyd. 1996. LC 95-47431. (Element Guide Ser.). 144p. pap. 9.95 (*1-85230-776-5*) Element MA.

Element Guide to Anxiety, Panic Attacks & Phobias: Your Questions Answered. Elaine Sheehan. 1996. LC 95-40160. (Element Guide Ser.). 144p. pap. 9.95 (*1-85230-773-0*) Element MA.

Element Guide to Childhood Trauma: Your Questions Answered. Ursula Markham. 1998. LC 97-38012. (Element Guide Ser.). 128p. pap. 9.95 (*1-86204-181-4*) Element MA.

Element Guide to Depression: Your Questions Answered. Sue Breton. 1996. LC 95-42156. (Element Guide Ser.). 144p. pap. 9.95 (*1-85230-775-7*) Element MA.

Elemental Industrial Hygiene Home Study Course. D. Jeff Burton. 1992. 360p. (*0-9623160-0-8*) IVE Inc.

Elementary Dictionary of Medicine: Dictionnaire Elementaire de Medicine. Andre Duranteau. 1981. (FRE.). 576p. 59.95 (*0-8288-1803-7*, M15411) Fr & Eur.

Elementary Economic Evaluation in Health Care. Ed. by Tom Jefferson et al. 2000. 132p. pap. (*0-7279-1478-2*) BMJ Pub GBR. *Dist:* AIDC.

Elementary Principles of Behavior. Richard W. Malott et al. 3rd ed. 1996. LC 96-21581. pap. text 61.00 (*0-13-533571-X*) P-H.

Elementary Radiesthesia & the Use of the Pendulum. F. A. Archdale. 1996. 32p. spiral bd. 10.00 (*0-7873-0039-X*) Hlth Research.

Elementary School Health Inst. Pollock. 3rd ed. 1994. tchr. ed. 31.87 (*0-8151-6746-6*) Mosby Inc.

Elementary Statistical Methods in Psychology & Education. Paul J. Blommers & Robert A. Forsyth. 2nd ed. 1983. LC 83-6978. (Illus.). 584p. (C). reprint ed. pap. text 30.50 (*0-8191-2684-5*) U Pr of Amer.

Elementary Statistical Methods in Psychology & Education: Study Manual. Paul J. Blommers & Robert A. Forsyth. 2nd ed. 1984. (Illus.). 268p. reprint ed. pap. text 24.00 (*0-8191-4122-4*) U Pr of Amer.

Elementary Statistics. Janet T. Spence et al. 5th rev. ed. 1991. LC 91-34514. 400p. (C). 110.00 (*0-13-253261-1*) P-H.

Elementary Statistics for Psychology Students. Charles F. Hinderliter. 1996. 462p. (C). pap. 72.50 (*0-07-029017-2*) McGrw-H Hghr Educ.

Elementary Textbook of Ayurveda: Medicine with a Six Thousand Year Old Tradition. Frank J. Ninivaggi. unabr. ed. 2001. LC 00-51725. (Illus.). xvii, 286p. pap. text 28.75 (*1-887841-33-4*, 61624, Psychosocial) Intl Univs Pr.

Elementary Textbook of Psychoanalysis. Charles Brenner. rev. ed. 1974. 272p. reprint ed. pap. 13.00 (*0-385-09884-7*) Doubleday.

EFG

Elementary Textbook of Psychoanalysis. Charles Brenner. enl. rev. ed. 1973. LC 72-86658. x, 280p. 45.00 (*0-8236-1621-5*) Intl Univs Pr.

Elementary Treatise on Human Physiology. 4. Francois Magendie. Tr. by John Revere from FRE. 1978. LC 77-72191. (Contributions to the History of Psychology Ser.: Vol. IV, Pt. E, Physiological Psychology). 280p. reprint ed. lib. bdg. 75.00 (*0-313-26952-1*, U6952, Greenwood Pr) Greenwood.

Elemente der Psychophysik. Set. Gustav T. Fechner. 589p. 210.00 (*1-85506-657-2*) Thoemmes Pr.

Elements Vol. II: Symptoms of Disease. Ingrid Naiman. 7th ed. 1997. (Astrology of Healing Ser.). (Illus.). 183p. reprint ed. pap. 35.00 (*1-882834-02-X*) Seventh Ray.

Elements & Dimensions of an Ericksonian Approach. Ed. by Stephen R. Lankton. 1985. LC 85-17454. (Ericksonian Monographs: No. 1). 152p. text 28.95 (*0-87630-411-0*) Brunner-Routledge.

Elements of Acoustic Phonetics. Peter Ladefoged. 2nd ed. 1995. LC 95-9057. 224p. lib. bdg. 39.95 (*0-226-46763-5*); pap. text 15.00 (*0-226-46764-3*) U Ch Pr.

Elements of Anatomy & Physiology. Stanley Jacob & Clarice Ashworth. 2nd ed. 1989. (Illus.). 336p. pap., tchr. ed. (*0-7216-5077-5*) Saunders.

Elements of Anatomy & Physiology. Stanley W. Jacob & Clarice A. Francone. 2nd ed. 1989. 352p. pap. text 29.00 (*0-7216-5089-9*) Saunders.

Elements of Applied Psychology. Ed. by Peter Spurgeon et al. 1994. LC 93-19277. x, 386p. text 71.00 (*3-7186-5120-3*) Gordon & Breach.

Elements of Clinical Research in Psychiatry. James E. Mitchell et al. 2000. LC 99-48422. 224p. 34.50 (*0-88048-802-6*, 8802) Am Psychiatric.

Elements of Counseling. Scott T. Meier. 1988. LC 88-18754. 85p. (C). pap. 9.00 (*0-534-09900-9*) Brooks-Cole.

Elements of Crime: Psycho-Social Interpretation. Boris Brasol. 2nd ed. 1969. LC 69-16226. (Criminology, Law Enforcement, & Social Problems Ser.: No. 93). reprint ed. 28.00 (*0-87585-093-6*) Patterson Smith.

Elements of Crisis Intervention. James L. Greenstone & Sharon C. Leviton. 1996. LC 92-36153. 112p. pap. 18.00 (*0-534-19908-9*) Brooks-Cole.

Elements of Danger: Protect Yourself Against the Hazards of Modern Dentistry. Morton Walker & Victor Zeines. 1999. LC 99-71623. (Illus.). 384p. pap. 14.95 (*1-57174-146-1*) Hampton Roads Pub Co.

Elements of Dental Materials: For Dental Hygienists & Dental Assistants. Ralph W. Phillips & B. Keith Moore. 5th ed. 1993. LC 93-12562. (Illus.). 352p. pap. text 36.95 (*0-7216-4298-5*) Saunders.

Elements of Digital Radiology. H. K. Huang. 1987. 416p. text 59.95 (*0-13-264136-4*, Busn) P-H.

Elements of Dreamwork. Strephon Kaplan-Williams. 1997. (Elements of Ser.). (Illus.). 144p. pap. 9.95 (*1-86204-030-3*) Element MA.

Elements of Fracture Fixation. A. J. Thakur. 1997. LC 97-9090. text (*0-443-05547-5*) Church.

Elements of Human Cancer. Geoffrey M. Cooper. (Biology Ser.). (Illus.). (C). 1992. 368p. text 48.95 (*0-86720-191-6*, 191-6); 2nd ed. 2001. 416p. text 53.95 (*0-7637-0619-1*, 0619-1) Jones & Bartlett.

Elements of Medical Genetics. Alan E. Emery & Robert F. Mueller. 8th ed. 1992. (Illus.). 349p. pap. text (*0-443-04524-0*) Church.

Elements of Medical Jurisprudence, 1823 Theodoric R. Beck. fac. ed. 1997. LC 96-35845. 125.00 (*1-886363-24-2*) Lawbk Exchange.

Elements of Medical Statistics. F. Bisset Hawkins. 1989. (Resources in Medical History Ser.). (*81-205-0091-1*) Oxford IBH IND. *Dist:* S Asia.

Elements of Medical Statistics. F. Bisset Hawkins. 1989. 20.00 (*0-88135-094-X*, N Watson) Watson Pub Intl.

Elements of Medical Terminology. April Applegate. 1994. 46.50 net. incl. audio (*0-8273-6552-7*) Delmar.

Elements of Medical Terminology. April Applegate & Valerie Overton. 1994. 218p. tchr. ed. 20.00 (*0-8273-6674-4*) Delmar.

Elements of Medical Terminology. April Applegate et al. 1994. LC 93-32985. 388p. (C). pap. 44.95 (*0-8273-6406-7*) Delmar.

Elements of Molecular Neurobiology. C. U. Smith. 2nd ed. 1996. LC 95-32004. 534p. pap. 64.95 (*0-471-96079-9*) Wiley.

Elements of Nursing. Nancy Roper. 3rd ed. 1990. (Illus.). 376p. pap. text (*0-443-03950-X*) Church.

Elements of Pathology. Gurel. 1998. pap. text (*0-7216-6024-X*) Saunders.

Elements of Pediatric Physiotherapy. Ed. by Pamela M. Eckersley. 1993. (Illus.). 416p. (Orig.). pap. text (*0-443-03894-5*) Church.

Elements of Pharmaceutical Pricing. E. M. Kolassa. 1997. LC 97-10137. 118p. 39.95 (*0-7890-0333-3*); pap. 19.95 (*0-7890-0334-1*) Haworth Pr (Pharmctl Prods).

Elements of Pharmacology. Gurel. 1998. pap. text (*0-7216-6025-8*) Saunders.

Elements of Pharmacology: A Primer on Drug Action. P. J. Bentley. 1981. LC 80-26624. (Illus.). 168p. pap. text 19.95 (*0-521-28074-5*) Cambridge U Pr.

Elements of Physiological Psychology. Pandey. 1995. pap. text, stu. ed. (*0-07-055570-2*) McGraw.

Elements of Physiological Psychology. Allen M. Schneider & Barry Tanskis. 1994. LC 94-21354. (C). text, stu. ed. 65.00 (*0-07-911488-1*) McGrw-H Hghr Educ.

Elements of Physiological Psychology. Barry Tarshis & Allen M. Schneider. 1994. (C). text 44.74 net. (*0-07-055569-9*) McGraw.

Elements of Psychological Medicine. Daniel Noble. LC 78-72815. (Brainedness, Handedness, & Mental Abilities Ser.). reprint ed. 45.00 (*0-404-60885-X*) AMS Pr.

Elements of Psychology. George C. Robertson. Ed. by C. A. Davids. LC 78-72820. (Brainedness, Handedness, & Mental Abilities Ser.). reprint ed. 39.50 (*0-404-60889-2*) AMS Pr.

Elements of Psychology. David Krech & Richard Crutchfield. 4th ed. 1982. LC 81-19302. (C). text 24.00 (*0-394-32417-X*); stu. ed. 9.00 (*0-394-32916-3*) Knopf (KnopfC).

Elements of Psychopathology: The Mechanisms of Defense. Robert White & Robert M. Gilliland. 1975. (Illus.). 208p. text 32.95 (*0-8089-0913-4*, 794825, Grune & Strat) Harcrt Hlth Sci Grp.

Elements of Psychophysical Theory. Jean-Claude Falmagne. 1985. (Illus.). 480p. text 75.00 (*0-19-503493-7*) OUP.

Elements of Quality in Pharmaceutical Care. Charles P. Coe. 1992. 350p. (Orig.). pap. (*1-879907-18-6*) Am Soc Hlth-Syst.

Elements of Radiobiology. Joseph Selman. 1983. (Illus.). 324p. (C). 42.95 (*0-398-04753-7*) C C Thomas.

Elements of Research in Physical Therapy. Dean Currier. 3rd ed. 1990. (Illus.). 352p. 35.00 (*0-683-02248-2*) Lppncott W & W.

Elements of Stuttering. Courtney Stromsta. 1986. LC 86-90366. (Illus.). 256p. (Orig.). (C). pap. 19.50 (*0-9620355-4-8*) Atsmorts Pub.

Elements of the Helping Process: A Guide for Clinicians. Raymond Fox. 1993. 216p. pap. 19.95 (*1-56024-157-8*) Haworth Pr.

Elements of Toxicology. K. Pandey & J. P. Shukla. 1991. (C). (*81-85484-26-0*) Classical Pubng IND. *Dist:* S Asia.

Elephant Medicine & More: Musings of a Medical Educator. Herbert L. Fred. 1989. LC 88-39602. (Illus.). 202p. (C). 2.00 (*0-86554-078-0*, MUP/H277) Mercer Univ Pr.

Elevated Dining: Cuisine Art of Healing with Vegetables, Vitamins Minerals & Gems. Robert Rison. Ed. by Chris Allen. 1993. (Illus.). 88p. (Orig.). pap. 16.95 (*0-9625706-3-X*) ECLAT Bks.

11-14 Week Scan: The Diagnosis of Fetal Abnormalities. Ed. by K. H. Nicolaides et al. 1999. LC 99-52488. (Diploma in Fetal Medicine Ser.). (Illus.). 204p. 69.95 (*1-85070-743-X*, Parthenon Pbng) CRC Pr.

11th National ACCP Pulmonary Board Review. Prakash. Ed. by American College of Chest Physicians Staff. 1996. 580p. pap. text 65.00 (*0-916609-09-X*) Am Chest Phys.

Eli Lilly: A Life, 1885-1977. James H. Madison. 1989. (Illus.). xiii, 342p. 24.95 (*0-87195-047-2*) Ind Hist Soc.

Elimination Pneumoconiosis among Coal Mine Workers: Report of the Secretary of Labor's Advisory Committee. David H. Wegman. 1997. 160p. (Orig.). (C). pap. text 40.00 (*0-7881-4519-3*) DIANE Pub.

Elisa: Enzyme-Linked Immunosorbent Assay in Veterinary Research & Diagnosis. R. C. Wardley & J. R. Crowther. 1982. text 176.50 (*90-247-2769-3*) Kluwer Academic.

Elizabeth Blackwell, M. D., 1821-1910: A Biography. Nancy A. Sahli. 1981. 60.95 (*0-405-14106-8*) Ayer.

Ellenberg & Rifkin's Diabetes Mellitus: Theory & Practice. Daniel Porte & Robert S. Sherwin. 5th ed. 1998. LC 96-17517. 1423p. (C). text 225.00 (*0-8385-2041-3*) McGraw-Hill Prof.

Ellenhorn's Medical Toxicology: A Synopsis with Review Questions. Seth Schonwald. 2001. LC 00-52018. 912p. pap. text 89.95 (*0-7817-2613-1*) Lppncott W & W.

Else Frenkel-Brunswik: Selected Papers. Else Frenkel-Brunswick. Ed. by Nanette Heiman & Joan Grant. 1974. LC 73-8079. (Psychological Issues Monographs: No. 31, Vol. 8, No. 3). 333p. (C). 50.00 (*0-8236-1645-2*) Intl Univs Pr.

Elsevier's Dictionary of Cancer. M. P. Mayar. 1999. 500p. (*0-444-82950-4*) Elsevier.

Elsevier's Dictionary of Cosmetic Science. H. E. Philippsborn. 2000. LC 00-37197. (ENG, FRE, GER & POR., Illus.). 644p. 170.00 (*0-444-50171-1*, Pergamon Pr) Elsevier.

Elsevier's Dictionary of Pharmaceutical & Technique Vol. 2: Materia Medica. A. Sliosberg. 1980. (ENG, FRE, GER, ITA & LAT.). 552p. 350.00 (*0-8288-9316-0*) Fr & Eur.

Elsevier's Dictionary of Pharmaceutical Science & Techniques Vol. 1: Pharmaceutical Technology. A. Sliosberg. 1980. (ENG, FRE, GER, ITA & SPA.). 686p. reprint ed. 350.00 (*0-8288-9315-2*) Fr & Eur.

Elsevier's Dictionary of Public Health. Nick J. Deblock. 1976. (DUT, ENG, FRE, GER & ITA.). 196p. 175.00 (*0-8288-9309-8*, M7948) Fr & Eur.

Elsevier's Encyclopaedic Dictionary of Medicine Pt. D: Therapeutic Substances. A. F. Dorian. 1990. (ENG, FRE, GER, ITA & SPA.). 504p. 173.00 (*0-444-42826-7*) Elsevier.

Elsevier's Encyclopaedic Dictionary of Medicine Vol. 1: General Medicine, Defined in English. A. F. Dorian. 1989. (ENG, FRE, GER, ITA & SPA.). 1176p. reprint ed. 495.00 (*0-8288-9310-1*, M1710) Fr & Eur.

Elsevier's Encyclopaedic Dictionary of Medicine Vol. 2: Anatomy, Defined in English. A. F. Dorian. 1988. (ENG, FRE, GER, ITA & SPA.). 602p. 350.00 (*0-8288-9311-X*, M1715) Fr & Eur.

Elsevier's Encyclopaedic Dictionary of Medicine Vol. 3: Biology, Genetics & Biochemistry, Defined in English. A. F. Dorian. 1989. (ENG, FRE, GER, ITA & SPA.). 708p. 375.00 (*0-8288-9312-8*) Fr & Eur.

Elsevier's Encyclopaedic Dictionary of Medicine Vol. 4: Therapeutic Substances, Defined in English. A. F. Dorian. 1990. (ENG, FRE, GER, ITA & SPA.). 492p. 295.00 (*0-8288-9313-6*, M1730) Fr & Eur.

Elsevier's Encyclopedia Dictionary of Medicine: In English (With Definitions), French, German, Italian, & Spanish; Part A: General Medicine. A. F. Dorian. 1987. 1188p. 288.00 (*0-444-42823-2*) Elsevier.

Elsevier's Encyclopedia Dictionary of Medicine Part B: Anatomy - in English (with definitions), French, German, Italian, & Spanish. A. F. Dorian. 1988. 616p. 212.50 (*0-444-42824-0*) Elsevier.

Elsevier's Encyclopedic Dictionary of Medicine: In English (with Definitions), French, German, Italian, & Spanish. Part C: Biology, Genetics & Biochemistry. A. F. Dorian. 1989. 720p. 217.50 (*0-444-87293-0*) Elsevier.

Elsevier's Medical Dictionary. A. Sliosberg. 1991. (ENG, FRE, GER, ITA & SPA.). 1452p. reprint ed. 450.00 (*0-8288-9314-4*, M7956) Fr & Eur.

Elsevier's Medical Dictionary in Five Languages. A. Sliosberg. 2nd rev. ed. 1982. LC 72-97436. (ENG, FRE, GER, ITA & SPA.). 1464p. 292.50 (*0-444-41103-8*) Elsevier.

Elsevier's Medical Terminology for the Practicing Nurse. Sally F. Vanderwerf. 1998. LC 96-39427. 468p. 149.50 (*0-444-82470-7*) Elsevier.

Elusive Quest: Accountability in Hospitals. Carolyn L. Wiener. 2000. LC 99-59684. (Social Problems & Social Issues Ser.). xvi, 256p. pap. text 25.95 (*0-202-30631-3*); lib. bdg. 52.95 (*0-202-30630-5*) Aldine de Gruyter.

***E/M Fast Finder 2001.** Ingenix, Inc. Staff. pap. 29.95 (*1-56337-357-2*) Ingenix Inc.

Embarazo: Relajacion y Acondicio-Namiento Sicologico. Editorial America, S. A. Staff. Ed. by Maria E. Del Real. 1990. (SPA., Illus.). 232p. (Orig.). pap. (*0-944499-66-X*) Editorial Amer.

Embarazo, la Infancia y la Ninez: Pregnancy, Infant & Childcare. Marvin Pietruszka. 1992. 426p. pap. 7.95 (*0-934249-03-2*) Quail Valley.

Embarrassing Medical Problems: Everything You Always Wanted to Know but Were Afraid to Ask Your Doctor. Margaret Stearn. 2001. (Illus.). 208p. pap. 14.95 (*1-57826-067-1*, Red Brick) Hatherleigh.

EMBASE List of Journals Indexed. Date not set. 276p. pap. text 50.00 (*0-444-82423-5*) Elsevier.

Embedded Self: A Psychoanalytic Guide to Family Therapy. Mary-Joan Gerson. 1996. LC 95-37630. 288p. text 45.00 (*0-88163-158-2*) Analytic Pr.

Embodied Progress: A Cultural Account of Assisted Conception. Sarah Franklin. 1997. LC 96-7491. 264p. (C). 90.00 (*0-415-06766-9*); pap. 26.95 (*0-415-06767-7*) Routledge.

Embodied Selves: An Anthology of Psychological Texts 1830-1890. Ed. by Jenny B. Taylor & Sally Shuttleworth. 1998. LC 97-19676. (Illus.). 450p. text 85.00 (*0-19-871041-0*); pap. text 19.95 (*0-19-871042-9*) OUP.

***Embodied Theories.** Ernesto Spinelli & Sue A. Marshall. 2001. 192p. pap. 24.95 (*0-8264-5208-6*) Continuum.

Embodient, Morality, & Medicine. Ed. by Lisa S. Cahill & Margaret A. Farley. 1995. LC 94-46674. (Theology & Medicine Ser.: Vol. 6). 236p. (C). lib. bdg. (*0-7923-3342-X*) Kluwer Academic NLD. *Dist:* Kluwer Academic.

Embodiment & Experience: The Existential Ground of Culture & Self. Ed. by Thomas J. Csordas. 1995. LC 93-45993. (Cambridge Studies in Medical Anthropology: Vol. 2). (Illus.). 306p. (C). pap. text 22.95 (*0-521-45890-0*) Cambridge U Pr.

Embodying Bioethics: Recent Feminist Advances. Ed. by Anne Donchin & Laura M. Purdy. 1999. LC 98-28146. (New Feminist Perspectives Ser.). 288p. text 76.00 (*0-8476-8924-7*) Rowman.

Embolotherapy. Douglas M. Coldwell. 1997. LC 96-29621. (Radiologic Interventions Ser.). (Illus.). 256p. (*0-89640-328-9*) Igaku-Shoin.

Embolotherapy. Douglas M. Coldwell. 1997. LC 96-29621. (Radiologic Interventions Ser.). 185p. 59.00 (*0-683-30268-X*) Lppncott W & W.

Embrace of Spirit: A Woman's View of Mind - Body Healing. Marcy A. Witkin-Lupo. 1998. LC 00-500799. 196p. pap. 13.95 (*0-9656811-3-0*) Four Seasons.

Embrace the Dawn: One Woman's Story of Triumph over Epilepsy. Andrea L. Davidson. 1989. LC 88-92687. (Illus.). 144p. (Orig.). pap. 10.95 (*0-9621761-1-7*) Sylvan Creek Pr.

Embracing the Wolf: A Lupus Victim & Her Family Learn to Live with Chronic Disease. Joanna B. Permut. Ed. by Alexa M. Selph. 1989. LC 88-91193. 192p. 14.95 (*0-87797-166-8*) Cherokee.

Embryo: Normal & Abnormal Development & Growth. Ed. by M. G. Chapman et al. 1991. (Illus.). 263p. 124.00 (*0-387-19630-7*) Spr-Verlag.

Embryo as a Patient. A. Kurjak & F. A. Chervenak. 2001. LC 2001-35177. (Illus.). 262p. 119.95 (*1-84214-020-5*, Parthenon Pbng) CRC Pr.

Embryo Experimentation: Ethical, Legal & Social Issues. Ed. by Peter Albert David Singer et al. (Illus.). 279p. (C). 1992. pap. text 19.95 (*0-521-43588-9*); 1990. text 54.95 (*0-521-38359-5*) Cambridge U Pr.

Embryo Research-Development, Uses, Storage, Ethics & Legal Decisions: Index of New Information. Oliver O. Bodey. 1997. (Illus.). 150p. 57.50 (*0-7883-1392-4*); pap. 47.50 (*0-7883-1393-2*) ABBE Pubs Assn.

Embryogenesis of the Human Skull: An Anatomic & Radiographic Atlas. Robert Shapiro & Franklin Robinson. 1980. LC 78-5714. (Commonwealth Fund Publications). (Illus.). 101p. 56.00 (*0-674-24790-6*) HUP.

Embryology. R. E. Coalson. Ed. by J. Tomasek. 2nd ed. 1992. (Oklahoma Notes). (Illus.). 128p. 12.95 (*0-387-97776-7*) Spr-Verlag.

Embryology. Ronald W. Dudek & James D. Fix. 2nd ed. 1998. LC 98-22361. (Board Review Ser.). (Illus.). 250p. pap. text 27.95 (*0-683-30272-8*) Lppncott W & W.

Embryology: Review for New National Boards. Raymond F. Gasser et al. 1997. (Illus.). 221p. pap. 25.00 (*0-8036-0724-5*) Davis Co.

Embryology & Anomalies of the Facial Nerve & Their Surgical Implications. Robert T. Sataloff. 1991. (Illus.). 172p. (Orig.). (C). text 65.00 (*1-56593-491-1*, 1134) Singular Publishing.

Embryology & Anomalies of the Facial Nerve & Their Surgical Implications. Robert T. Sataloff. 1996. 176p. (Orig.). 104.00 (*0-88167-728-0*) Lppncott W & W.

Embryology & Teratology of the Heart & the Great Arteries. Ed. by L. H. Van Mierop & A. Opperheimer-Dekker. Tr. by C. Bruins. 1978. (Boerhaave Ser.: No. 13). text 126.50 (*90-6021-424-2*) Kluwer Academic.

Embryology for Surgeons. John E. Skandalakis & Stephen W. Gray. 2nd ed. 1994. (Illus.). 960p. 195.00 (*0-683-07756-2*) Lppncott W & W.

Embryology of Behavior. Arnold L. Gesell. 1991. (Classics in Developmental Medicine Ser.: No. 3). (Illus.). 274p. (C). text (*0-521-41328-1*) Mc Keith Pr GBR. *Dist:* Cambridge U Pr.

Embryology of the Eye & Its Adnexae. Y. R. Barisbak. 1992. (Developments in Ophthalmology Ser.: Vol. 24). (Illus.). viii, 142p. 143.50 (*3-8055-5511-3*) S Karger.

***Embryology of the Eye & Its Adnexae.** Y. Robert Barishak. 2nd rev. ed. 2001. LC 2001-18983. (Illus.). 132p. 85.00 (*3-8055-7179-8*) S Karger.

Embryology of the Human Locomotor System. Hans K. Uhthoff. 1990. (Illus.). 166p. 190.00 (*0-387-52028-7*) Spr-Verlag.

Embryonic Human Brain: An Atlas of Developmental Stages. Ronan O'Rahilly & Fabiola Muller. 1994. LC 93-33438. (Illus.). 352p. 240.00 (*0-471-58845-8*, Wiley-Interscience) Wiley.

Embryonic Human Brain: An Atlas of Developmental Stages. Ronan O'Rahilly et al. 2nd ed. 1999. LC 98-42193. (Illus.). 464p. 199.95 (*0-471-25450-9*) Wiley.

Embryonic Medicine & Therapy. Ed. by Eric Jauniaux et al. 1997. LC 97-33445. (Illus.). 546p. (C). text 145.00 (*0-19-262729-5*) OUP.

Embryonic Mortality in Domestic Species. Ed. by Rodney D. Geisert & Michael T. Zavy. 1994. LC 93-47293. 236p. lib. bdg. 189.00 (*0-8493-7634-3*) CRC Pr.

Embryonic Mortality in Farm Animals. Ed. by J. M. Sreenan & M. G. Diskin. 1985. (Current Topics in Veterinary Medicine & Animal Science Ser.). text 176.50 (*0-89838-772-8*) Kluwer Academic.

Embryonic Motility & Sensitivity. William Preyer. 1937. (SRCD Ser.: Vol. 2, No. 6). 25.00 (*0-527-01499-0*) Periodicals Srv.

Embryonic Stem Cells. Nos. 3-4. Ed. by A. M. Wobus & K. R. Boheler. 1999. (Cells Tissues Organs Ser.: Vol. 165). (Illus.). iv, 132p. pap. 39.25 (*3-8055-6975-0*) S Karger.

Embryos: Color Atlas of Development. Ed. by Jonathan B.L. Bard. 1993. (Illus.). 224p. text 89.00 (*0-7234-1740-7*) CRC Pr.

Embryos, Ethics, & Woman's Rights: Exploring the New Reproductive Technologies. Elaine H. Baruch. Ed. by Amadeo F. D'Adamo et al. 1988. LC 87-38148. (Women & Health Ser.: Vol. 13, Nos. 1-2). 259p. pap. 19.95 (*0-918393-45-0*, Harrington Park) Haworth Pr.

Embryos, Ethics, & Women's Rights Exploring the New Reproductive Technologies. Ed. by Elaine Hoffman Baruch et al. 1988. LC 87-38147. (Women & Health Ser.: Vol. 13, Nos. 1-2). (Illus.). 259p. text 49.95 (*0-86656-707-0*) Haworth Pr.

Embryos, Genes & Birth Defects. Peter Thorogood. 1997. LC 96-46036. 370p. 225.00 (*0-471-97196-0*) Wiley.

Embryos, Genes & Birth Defects. Ed. by Peter V. Thorogood. 1997. LC 96-46036. 370p. pap. 115.00 (*0-471-95565-5*) Wiley.

EMDR: The Breakthrough Therapy for Overcoming Anxiety, Stress, & Trauma. Francine Shapiro & Margot S. Forrest. 1998. 304p. pap. 16.00 (*0-465-04301-1*) Basic.

Emergence: Labeled Autistic. Temple Grandin & Margaret M. Scariano. 1996. LC 96-10511. 192p. pap. (*0-446-67182-7*) Warner.

E F G

Emergence & Adaptation: Studies in Speech Communication & Language Development. Ed. by R. D. Diehl et al. 2000. (Phonetica Ser.: Vol. 57). (Illus.). 244p. pap. 48.75 (3-8055-7147-X) S Karger.

Emergence of a Discipline: Rochester Symposium on Developmental Psychopathology, Vol. 1. Ed. by Dante Cicchetti. 1990. 320p. 89.95 (0-8058-0553-2) L Erlbaum Assocs.

Emergence of Bacterial Genetics. Thomas D. Brock. 1990. (Illus.). 346p. 55.00 (0-87969-350-9) Cold Spring Harbor.

Emergence of Personality. Ed. by Joel Aronoff et al. 1987. 272p. 35.95 (0-8261-6120-0) Springer Pub.

Emergence of Roman Catholic Medical Ethics in North America: An Historical-Methodological-Bibliographical Study. David F. Kelly. 1979. LC 79-66372. (Texts & Studies in Religion: Vol. 3). 520p. lib. bdg. 119.95 (0-88946-877-X) E Mellen.

Emergence of Women into the 21st Century. Patricia L. Munhall & Virginia M. Fitzsimons. 1995. (Women's Issues Ser.). 300p. pap. 31.95 (0-88737-662-2) Natl League Nurse.

*__Emergencias de la Nunez.__ Marin Child Care Council. 2001. (SPA., Illus.). 44p. pap. 14.95 (0-923521-27-5) Bull Pub.

Emergencies in Mental Health Practice: Evaluation & Management. Ed. by Phillip M. Kleespies. 450p. 2000. pap. 24.95 (1-57230-551-7, C0551); 1997. LC 97-33643. 50.00 (1-57230-255-0, C0255) Guilford Pubns.

Emergencies in Obstetrics & Gynaecology. K. L. Stevens. 1995. LC 93-49710. (Handbooks in Emergency Medicine Ser.: Vol. 8). (Illus.). 276p. text 62.00 (0-19-262470-9); pap. text 31.50 (0-19-262051-7) OUP.

Emergencies of the Head & Neck. David W. Eisele & Shelly McQuone. 1999. (Illus.). 400p. (C). text (1-55664-470-1) Mosby Inc.

Emergency! The Active Horseman's Book of Emergency Care. Karen E. Hayes. 1995. LC 95-20091. (Illus.). 213p. 32.95 (0-939481-42-1) Half Halt Pr.

Emergency Abdominal Surgery. R. C. Williamson & M. J. Cooper. 1990. (Clinical Surgery International Ser.: Vol. 17). (Illus.). 288p. text (0-443-03907-0) Church.

Emergency Abdominal Surgery: In Infancy, Childhood & Adult Life. Peter F. Jones. 3rd ed. 1999. LC 98-71425. (Illus.). 384p. text (0-412-81950-3) E A GBR. Dist: OUP.

Emergency Anaesthesia. pap. text (0-7131-4505-6) E A GBR. Dist: Routldge.

Emergency Anaesthesia. Ed. by Anthony P. Adams et al. 2nd ed. 1998. LC 97-21355. (An Arnold Publication). (Illus.). 456p. pap. (0-340-69219-7) E A GBR. Dist: OUP.

Emergency Anesthesia. Anthony P. Adams et al. 1987. (Illus.). 361p. text 54.00 (0-03-013297-5) Saunders.

Emergency Asthma. Barry E. Brenner. 1999. LC 98-56653. (Clinical Allergy & Immunology Ser.: No. 13). (Illus.). 600p. text 175.00 (0-8247-1945-X) Dekker.

Emergency Bulletin: A Guide to Drug Treatment Programs in New York City. 1995. (Orig.). pap. 10.00 (0-9650675-0-5) Drugs Dont Wrk.

Emergency Cardiac Care. Robert S. Huszar. 2nd ed. 1982. LC 81-65693. (Illus.). 448p. pap. 35.00 (0-87619-863-9) P-H.

Emergency Cardiac Maneuvers: A Rescuer's Handbook. Carl E. Bartecchi. 2nd ed. 1990. pap. 7.95 (0-929240-15-4) EMIS.

Emergency Care. Harvey D. Grant et al. 3rd ed. 1982. (Illus.). 512p. tchr. ed. 14.95 (0-89303-429-0); stu. ed. 8.95 (0-89303-186-0); pap. text 18.95 (0-89303-116-X) P-H.

Emergency Care. Limmer. Ed. by Michael F. O'Keefe. 8th ed. 1997. LC 97-14615. 912p. pap. text 59.00 (0-8359-5089-1); (Illus.). text 54.00 (0-8359-5073-5) P-H.

Emergency Care: Instructor's Resource Manual. Grant Staff & Murray. 8th ed. 1997. pap., tchr. ed. 54.00 (0-8359-5144-8) P-H.

Emergency Care: Principles & Practice for the EMT-Paramedic. Alan B. Gazzaniga et al. 2nd ed. 1982. (Illus.). text 37.00 (0-8359-1675-8) P-H.

Emergency Care: Self-Assessment. Tim Hodgetts. 1997. 241p. pap. text (0-7020-2345-0) Bailliere Tindall.

Emergency Care: Textbook for Paramedics. Ed. by Ian Greaves et al. 1997. text 63.00 (0-7020-1975-5) Saunders.

Emergency Care: The Core Curriculum. Richard V. Aghababian. 1998. LC 97-44162. 1,536p. pap. text 139.00 (0-316-00753-6) Lppncott W & W.

Emergency Care & Transport Section 1: Instructor's Resource Kit. American Academy of Orthopaedic Surgeons Staff. 6th ed. 1995. (Emergency Care Ser.). (Illus.). spiral bd. 15.00 (0-89203-135-2, 135-2) Jones & Bartlett.

Emergency Care & Transport Section 2: Instructor's Resource Kit. American Academy of Orthopaedic Surgeons Staff. 6th ed. 1995. (Emergency Care Ser.). (Illus.). spiral bd. 15.00 (0-89203-136-0, 136-0) Jones & Bartlett.

Emergency Care & Transport Section 3: Instructor's Resource Kit. American Academy of Orthopaedic Surgeons Staff. 6th ed. 1995. (Emergency Care Ser.). (Illus.). spiral bd. 15.00 (0-89203-137-9, 137-9) Jones & Bartlett.

Emergency Care & Transport Section 4: Instructor's Resource Kit. American Academy of Orthopaedic Surgeons Staff. 6th ed. 1995. (Emergency Care Ser.). (Illus.). spiral bd. 15.00 (0-89203-138-7, 138-7) Jones & Bartlett.

Emergency Care & Transport Section 8: Instructor's Resource Kit. American Academy of Orthopaedic Surgeons Staff. 6th ed. 1995. (Emergency Care Ser.). (Illus.). spiral bd. 15.00 (0-89203-142-5, 142-5) Jones & Bartlett.

Emergency Care & Transport Basic: Instructor's Resource Kit. American Academy of Orthopaedic Surgeons Staff. 6th ed. 1995. (Emergency Ser.). (Illus.). spiral bd. 15.00 (0-89203-134-4, 134-4) Jones & Bartlett.

*__Emergency Care & Transport of the Sick & Injured.__ American Academy of Orthopaedic Surgeons Staff. 6th ed. 1998. (Illus.). 328p. (C). pap. text, stu. ed. 29.95 (0-7637-0748-1, 0748-1) Jones & Bartlett.

Emergency Care & Transport of the Sick & Injured. American Academy of Orthopaedic Surgeons Staff. Ed. by Lynn Crosby & David Lewallen. 6th ed. 1995. (Emergency Care Ser.). (Illus.). 766p. pap. text 56.95 (0-89203-105-0, 105-0) Jones & Bartlett.

Emergency Care & Transportation of the Sick & Injured. AAOS Staff. Ed. by James D. Heckman. 5th rev. ed. 1993. (Illus.). 589p. text 59.95 (0-89203-127-1, 127-1) Jones & Bartlett.

Emergency Care & Transportation of the Sick & Injured. Ed. by James D. Heckman. 5th rev. ed. 1993. LC 91-75604. (Illus.). 889p. pap. text 56.95 (0-89203-049-6, 049-6) Jones & Bartlett.

Emergency Care & Transportation of the Sick & Injured. American Academy of Orthopaedic Surgeons Staff. Ed. by Lynn Crosby & David Lewallen. 6th ed. 1995. (Emergency Care Ser.). (Illus.). 766p. text 59.95 (0-89203-106-9, 106-9) Jones & Bartlett.

Emergency Care & Transportation of the Sick & Injured. American Academy of Orthopaedic Surgeons Staff. (Emergency Care Ser.). (Illus.). (C). 6th rev. ed. 1997. 784p. text 56.95 (0-89203-165-4, 165-4); 6th rev. ed. 1997. pap. text 56.95 (0-89203-164-6, 164-6); 7th ed. 1999. LC 98-20963. 992p. text 59.95 (0-7637-1044-X, 1044-X) Jones & Bartlett.

Emergency Care & Transportation of the Sick & Injured. Lenworth M. Jacobs et al. 7th ed. 1999. LC 98-20963. (Illus.). 992p. (C). pap. text 56.95 (0-7637-0796-1, 0796-1) Jones & Bartlett.

Emergency Care & Transportation of the Sick & Injured: CyberClass Edition. American Academy of Orthopaedic Surgeons Staff. 7th ed. 1999. (Illus.). (C). pap. text 73.95 (0-7637-1104-7) Jones & Bartlett.

Emergency Care & Transportation of the Sick & Injured: Instructor Question Bank. American Academy of Orthopaedic Surgeons Staff. 6th rev. ed. 1997. (Emergency Care Ser.). (Illus.). pap. text 39.95 (0-89203-180-8, 180-8) Jones & Bartlett.

*__Emergency Care & Transportation of the Sick & Injured: Student Review Manual.__ AAOS Staff. 8th ed. 2001. pap. 33.95 (0-7637-1945-5, 1945-5) Jones & Bartlett.

*__Emergency Care & Transportation of the Sick & Injured: Student Workbook.__ AAOS Staff. 8th ed. 2001. pap., stu. ed., wbk. ed. 33.95 (0-7637-1943-9, 1943-9) Jones & Bartlett.

*__Emergency Care & Transportation of the Sick & Injured: Thirtieth Anniversary Edition.__ AAOS Staff et al. 8th ed. 2001. LC 2001-52032. (Illus.). (C). pap. text, stu. ed. 54.95 (0-7637-1666-9, 1666-9) Jones & Bartlett.

Emergency Care & Transportation of the Sick & Injured Instructor Workbook. American Academy of Orthopaedic Surgeons Staff. 5th ed. 1994. (Emergency Care Ser.). (Illus.). 290p. pap. text, tchr. ed. 49.95 (0-89203-054-2, 054-2) Jones & Bartlett.

Emergency Care for Cats & Dogs: First Aid for Your Pets. Craton R. Burkholder. LC 87-3726. (Illus.). 1995. 172p. pap. 15.95 (0-935576-18-5); 1987. 176p. 23.95 (0-935576-19-3) Kesend Pub Ltd.

Emergency Care for Hazardous Materials Exposure, Vol. 2. Alvin C. Bronstein & Phillip L. Currance. 2nd ed. 1994. LC 94-7953. (Emergency Care for Hazardous Materials Exposure Ser.: Vol. 2). (Illus.). 656p. (C). (gr. 13). pap. text 25.95 (0-8016-7813-7, 07813) Mosby Inc.

Emergency Care in the Streets. Nancy L. Caroline. 3rd ed. 1987. 25.50 (0-316-12879-1, Little Brwn Med Div); 5th ed. 1995. LC 94-30822. (Illus.). 1,104p. pap. text 54.95 (0-316-12891-0) Lppncott W & W.

Emergency Care of Children. Sharon W. Thompson. 1990. 400p. 51.25 (0-86720-417-6) Jones & Bartlett.

Emergency Care of the Elder Person: Nurse's Edition. Jeanne M. Lewis et al. Ed. by Jeanne M. Lewis. 1996. (Illus.). 351p. text, tchr. ed. 40.00 (0-935890-10-6) Emerg Nurses IL.

Emergency Care of the Elder Person (Nurse's Edition) Ed. by Jeanne M. Lewis. unabr. ed. Date not set. (Regional Conference Ser.). (Illus.). ring bd. 475.00 (0-935890-22-X) Emerg Nurses IL.

Emergency Care of the Woman. Mark D. Pearlman & Judith E. Tintinalli. 1997. LC 97-36815. (Illus.). 792p. text 79.95 (0-07-049127-5) McGraw-Hill Prof.

*__Emergency Care Technician.__ Emergency Nurses Association Staff. 2001. LC 2001-50795. (Illus.). (C). pap. text 53.95 (0-7637-1913-7, 1913-7) Jones & Bartlett.

Emergency Childborth: A Manual for the Non-Medically Trained. Gregory J. White. Ed. by Gordon Carson et al. 1998. LC 93-86848. (Illus.). 72p. reprint ed. spiral bd. 15.95 (0-934426-87-2) NAPSAC Reprods.

Emergency Childcare: A Pediatrician's Guide. Peter R. Greenspan & Suzanne LeVert. 1997. LC 96-96168. (Orig.). pap. 5.99 (0-380-77635-9, Avon Bks) Morrow Avon.

Emergency Contraception: The Nation's Best Kept Secret. Robert A. Hatcher et al. 1995. (Illus.). 235p. (Orig.). pap. 12.95 (0-9638875-3-X) Bridging The Gap.

Emergency CT Scans of the Head: A Practical Atlas. A. Adam Cwinn & Steven Grahovac. 1998. LC 97-42384. (Illus.). 224p. text 69.95 (0-8151-2621-2, 31882) Mosby Inc.

Emergency Dental Care: Diagnosis & Management of Urgent Dental Problems. Ed. by Donald A. Falace. 1994. LC 93-42675. (Illus.). 395p. 55.00 (0-683-03007-8) Lppncott W & W.

Emergency Department Clinical Information Systems: A Guide Selection & Implementation. Ed. by Marsha Zimmerman et al. unabr. ed. 1996. 74p. (Orig.). pap. 45.00 (0-935890-06-8, P29) Emerg Nurses IL.

Emergency Department Management: Principles & Application. Salluzzo. Ed. by Thom A. Mayer. 1996. (Illus.). 912p. (C). (gr. 13). text 120.00 (0-8151-7751-8, 25532) Mosby Inc.

Emergency Department Patient Classification Systems Manual. Ed. by Christopher L. Laurent. 2nd ed. 1995. ring bd. 48.00 (0-935890-54-8) Emerg Nurses IL.

Emergency Department Technician. Marianne McBrien. 1995. LC 94-71971. (Clinical Allied Healthcare Ser.). (Illus.). 540p. (C). spiral bd. 44.95 (0-89262-432-9) Career Pub.

Emergency Department Technician: Instructor's Guide. Marianne McBrien. Ed. by Kay Cox. 1997. (Clinical Allied Healthcare Ser.). (Illus.). 422p. (C). (gr. 12). tchr. ed., ring bd. 99.95 (0-89262-440-X) Career Pub.

Emergency Departments: Unevenly Affected by Growth & Change in Patient Use. 1993. (Illus.). 72p. (Orig.). (C). pap. text 25.00 (1-56806-316-4) DIANE Pub.

Emergency Diagnostic Tests for Cardiac Ischemia. Robert J. Zalenski et al. 1997. LC 96-52002. 192p. pap. 19.95 (0-632-04304-0) Blackwell Sci.

Emergency Drug Therapy. Barsan et al. 1990. (Illus.). 672p. text 105.00 (0-7216-2584-3) Saunders.

Emergency Dysrhythmias & Electrocardiograph Injury Patterns. Brown. 2nd ed. 2001. 500p. (C). pap. 36.95 (0-7668-1988-4) Delmar.

Emergency Encounters. James M. Mannon. 1992. (Illus.). (C). pap. text 29.95 (0-86720-189-4, 189-4) Jones & Bartlett.

Emergency First Aid Care. Frank J. Poliafico. 1996. pap., stu. ed. 32.60 (0-89303-183-6) P-H.

Emergency First Aid for Your Cat. Tamara S. Shearer. Ed. by Stanford Apseloff. 1995. LC 95-71696. (Illus.). 326p. (Orig.). pap. 14.95 (0-9647934-1-5) OH Distinct Pub.

Emergency First Aid for Your Child. Consumer Guide Editors. 1993. (Illus.). 128p. spiral bd. 9.98 (0-88176-815-4, 3203000) Pubns Intl Ltd.

Emergency First Aid for Your Dog. Tamara S. Shearer. Ed. by Stanford Apseloff. 1996. LC 96-67366. (Illus.). 314p. (Orig.). pap. 14.95 (0-9647934-2-3) OH Distinct Pub.

Emergency First Aid Guide. National Safety Council Staff. 1996. (Illus.). 32p. (C). pap. text 200.00 (0-86720-543-1, 543-1) Jones & Bartlett.

Emergency First Care. Frank J. Poliafico. 1995. 160p. pap. text 24.40 (0-89303-181-X) P-H.

Emergency Guide for Dental Auxiliaries. Janet B. Chernega. 1986. LC 86-24303. 198p. (C). pap. 29.95 (0-8273-2335-2); 2nd ed. 1994. LC 93-41955. 179p. (C). pap. 46.95 (0-8273-4109-1); 3rd ed. 2001. 224p. text 48.95 (0-7668-1887-X) Delmar.

Emergency Health Management after Natural Disaster. 1981. (Scientific Publications: No. 407). 74p. pap. text 8.00 (92-75-11407-2) PAHO.

Emergency Imaging. Ed. by R. Brooke Jeffery, Jr. 1999. LC 98-31217. 224p. pap. text 55.00 (0-7817-1592-X) Lppncott W & W.

Emergency Imaging of the Acutely Ill or Injured Child. Leonard E. Swischuk. 4th ed. 2000. LC 00-20040. 624p. text 159.00 (0-683-30710-X) Lppncott W & W.

Emergency Incident Rehabilitation. Edward T. Dickinson & Michael A. Wieder. 1999. LC 99-39052. (Illus.). 129p. pap. text 32.00 (0-8359-5375-0) Globe Fearon.

Emergency Interventional Radiology. M. Pinson Neal. 1989. 115.00 (0-316-59927-1, Little Brwn Med Div) Lppncott W & W.

Emergency Management of Cardiovascular Disease. Richard V. Aghababian. 1994. LC 94-22739. 275p. text (0-7506-9633-8) E A GBR. Dist: OUP.

Emergency Management of Pediatric Trauma. Thom Mayer. 1985. (Illus.). 531p. text 135.00 (0-7216-6189-0) Saunders.

Emergency Management of the Injured Hand. G. R. Wilson et al. 1997. LC 96-35095. (Oxford Handbooks in Emergency Medicine Ser.: No. 17). (Illus.). 166p. text 89.50 (0-19-262824-0); pap. text 42.50 (0-19-262823-2) OUP.

Emergency Medical Care: A Manual for the Paramedic in the Field 1992. lib. bdg. 300.00 (0-8490-8863-1); Set. 1990. lib. bdg. 600.00 (0-8490-4010-8) Gordon Pr.

Emergency Medical Care: Basic Sc. Beebe & Funk. 2001. (C). pap., wbk. ed. 19.50 net. (0-7668-1493-9) Thomson Learn.

Emergency Medical Care for Disaster. 1991. lib. bdg. 79.95 (0-8490-5112-6); 1986. lib. bdg. 79.95 (0-8490-3604-6) Gordon Pr.

Emergency Medical Consent: Medical Consent for a Minor. LawPak Staff. 1994. (Illus.). 72p. (Orig.). pap. 7.95 (1-879421-03-8) LawPak.

Emergency Medical Dispatch Guide: Manager's Guide. 2nd ed. 1997. (Illus.). 69p. spiral bd. 60.00 (1-57927-033-6) APCO Inst.

Emergency Medical Dispatch Implementation Guide. 4th ed. 1997. (Illus.). 24p. spiral bd. (1-57927-032-8) APCO Inst.

Emergency Medical Dispatch Legal Issues. 1998. (Training in a Box Ser.). 48p. ring bd. 49.00 (1-57927-040-9) APCO Inst.

Emergency Medical Dispatch Program, Basic EMD Course: Instructor Manual. 4th ed. 1997. (Illus.). 243p. tchr. ed., ring bd. 60.00 (1-57927-031-X) APCO Inst.

Emergency Medical Dispatch Program, Basic EMD Course: Student Manual. 4th ed. 1997. (Illus.). 243p. stu. ed., spiral bd. 60.00 (1-57927-030-1) APCO Inst.

Emergency Medical Dispatch Respiratory Emergencies. 1998. (Training in a Box Ser.). 48p. ring bd. 49.00 (1-57927-039-5) APCO Inst.

Emergency Medical Dispatch Roles & Responsibilites. 1998. (Training in a Box Ser.). 48p. ring bd. 49.00 (1-57927-041-7) APCO Inst.

Emergency Medical Procedures for the Outdoors. Patient Care Publications Staff. 3rd ed. 1987. LC 87-18508. (Illus.). 120p. reprint ed. pap. 7.95 (0-89732-051-4) Menasha Ridge.

Emergency Medical Response to Hazardous Materials Incidents. Armando S. Bevelacqua & Richard H. Stilp. 1996. LC 96-34053. (Career Education Ser.). 522p. pap. text 63.95 (0-8273-7829-7) Delmar.

Emergency Medical Services: Behavioral & Planning Perspectives. John H. Noble et al. 1973. LC 73-9940. 595p. 59.95 (0-87705-117-8, Kluwer Acad Hman Sci) Kluwer Academic.

Emergency Medical Services Dispatcher 1992. lib. bdg. 375.00 (0-8490-8865-8) Gordon Pr.

Emergency Medical Services First Responder Training Course 1992. lib. bdg. 350.00 (0-8490-8867-4) Gordon Pr.

Emergency Medical Services for Children. Institute of Medicine Staff. Ed. by Jane S. Durch & Kathleen N. Lohr. 1993. LC 93-8084. 416p. text 49.95 (0-309-04888-5) Natl Acad Pr.

Emergency Medical Services for Children. Kelly Perez. 1998. LC 98-213930. 60p. 20.00 (1-55516-604-0, 6663) Natl Conf State Legis.

Emergency Medical Services for Children: The Role of the Primary Care Provider. American Academy of Pediatrics Staff. 1992. 266p. pap. 44.95 (0-910761-37-X) Am Acad Pediat.

Emergency Medical Services in Travis County, Texas: An Assessment of Cost, Demand, & Performance. David J. Eaton et al. 1996. (Special Project Reports: Vol. SP-EMS). 135p. pap. 18.00 (0-89940-902-4) LBJ Sch Pub Aff.

Emergency Medical Services Instructor Training Program 1992. lib. bdg. 375.00 (0-8490-8862-3) Gordon Pr.

Emergency Medical Technician: Ambulance 1992. lib. bdg. 400.00 (0-8490-8869-0) Gordon Pr.

Emergency Medical Technician: Intermediate 1992. lib. bdg. 355.00 (0-8490-8868-2) Gordon Pr.

Emergency Medical Technician: Paramedic 1992. lib. bdg. 375.00 (0-8490-8866-6) Gordon Pr.

Emergency Medical Technician & Paramedic Training: Perspectives on Status & Trends. Barbara R. Bennett. Ed. by Lenworth M. Jacobs. 1983. (Emergency Health Services Review Ser.: Vol. 2, No. 1). 66p. pap. text 19.95 (0-917724-51-8) Haworth Pr.

Emergency Medical Technician B VT 02 Med/Legal/ Ethics. Debbie G. Stoy. 1995. pap. text 75.00 (0-8151-7962-6) Mosby Inc.

Emergency Medical Technician Instructor's Manual. Nancy L. Caroline. 2nd ed. 1987. tchr. ed. 18.50 (0-316-12881-3, Little Brwn Med Div) Lppncott W & W.

Emergency Medical Technicians - Paramedic Examination (EMT) Jack Rudman. (Admission Test Ser.: Vol. 70). 69.95 (0-8373-5170-7) Nat Learn.

Emergency Medical Technicians-Paramedic Examination (EMT) Jack Rudman. 1994. (Admission Test Ser.: ATS-70). pap. 49.95 (0-8373-5070-0) Nat Learn.

Emergency Medical Therapeutics. Gideon Bosker. 2nd ed. 1995. (C). 36.95 (0-8151-0992-X, 28453) Mosby Inc.

Emergency Medical Therapy. Bosker. 2nd ed. 1999. pap. text 39.95 (1-55664-485-X) Mosby Inc.

Emergency Medical Therapy. Mickey S. Eisenberg et al. 4th ed. 1995. LC 94-39975. (Illus.). 800p. pap. text 49.95 (0-7216-5162-3) Saunders.

Emergency Medical Treatment. Nancy L. Caroline. 3rd ed. 1991. 644p. pap. text 39.00 (0-316-12886-4) Lppncott W & W.

E F G

Emergency Medical Treatment: A Text for EMT-As & EMT-Intermediates. Nancy L. Caroline. 2nd ed. 1987. 24.00 (*0-316-12878-3*); tchr. ed. 7.95 (*0-316-12880-5*); stu. ed. 15.50 (*0-316-12882-1*) Lppncott W & W (Little Brwn Med Div).

Emergency Medical Treatment: Adults. Stephen Vogel et al. 1991. pap. 7.95 (*0-916363-05-8*) Beechwood Hlthbks.

Emergency Medical Treatment: Infants. Stephen Vogel & David H. Manhoff. 1989. (Illus.). 28p. pap. text 7.95 (*0-916363-01-5*) Beechwood Hlthbks.

Emergency Medical Treatment: Infants, Children & Adults: A Handbook on What to Do in an Emergency to Keep Someone Alive Until Help Arrives. Stephen Vogel & David H. Manhoff. enl. rev. ed. 1990. (Illus.). 78p. pap. 12.95 (*0-916363-10-4*) Beechwood Hlthbks.

Emergency Medical Treatment: Intermediate. Bruce R. Shade & Mikel A. Rothenberg. 1997. LC 96-41315. (Illus.). 576p. (C). (gr. 13). text 39.95 (*0-8151-8003-9*, 26333) Mosby Inc.

Emergency Medical Treatment: Intermediate. Bruce R. Shade et al. 1997. (C). pap., tchr. ed. (*0-8151-8022-5*); pap. text, wbk. ed. (*0-8151-8004-7*) Mosby Inc.

Emergency Medicine. Birnbaumer. 2000. pap. text (*0-7216-6452-0*) Saunders.

Emergency Medicine. Linas Dzuikas. 1999. 304p. text 50.00 (*0-07-452910-2*) McGraw-Hill Med Pub.

Emergency Medicine. John M. Howell. Ed. by Judy Fletcher. 1997. LC 96-43967. (Illus.). 1856p. text 195.00 (*0-7216-5825-3*) Saunders.

Emergency Medicine. Scott H. Plantz & Jonathan N. Adler. 1997. LC 97-21471. (National Medical Series for Independent Study). 800p. pap. text 32.00 (*0-683-18107-6*) Lppncott W & W.

Emergency Medicine. Yeh. 1999. text (*0-7216-4113-X*) Saunders.

Emergency Medicine. A. 2nd ed. 1992. 87.50 (*0-316-55186-4*, Little Brwn Med Div) Lppncott W & W.

Emergency Medicine. Lidia Pousada et al. 2nd ed. 1996. (House Officer Ser.). (Illus.). 423p. pap. text 29.95 (*0-683-06963-2*) Lppncott W & W.

Emergency Medicine, Vol. 2. A. 1992. 87.50 (*0-316-55187-2*, Little Brwn Med Div) Lppncott W & W.

Emergency Medicine: A Comprehensive Study Guide. Judith E. Tintinalli et al. 5th ed. 1999. LC 99-10685. (Illus.). 2127p. text 149.00 (*0-07-065351-8*) McGraw-Hill Prof.

Emergency Medicine: An Approach to Clinical Problem Solving. Hamilton et al. 1990. (Illus.). 1184p. text 134.00 (*0-7216-4487-2*) Saunders.

Emergency Medicine: Concepts & Clinical Practice. Peter Rosen. 1999. (Illus.). 1661p. (C). text 365.00 incl. cd-rom (*0-323-00461-X*) Mosby Inc.

Emergency Medicine: Concepts & Clinical Practice. Roger M. Barkin & Peter Rosen. 4th ed. 1997. LC 97-33346. (Illus.). 3312p. (C). (gr. 13). text 255.00 (*0-8151-3774-5*, 29223) Mosby Inc.

Emergency Medicine: Pretest Self-Assessment & Review. Ed. by Jesse A. Cole & Scott H. Plantz. 1990. LC 89-12937. (Pretest Specialty Level Ser.). (Illus.). 211p. pap. 45.00 (*0-07-050323-0*) McGraw-Hill Prof.

Emergency Medicine: Review & Self Assessment. John M. Howell et al. Ed. by Judy Fletcher. 1999. LC 98-19199. 365p. pap. 35.00 (*0-7216-5821-0*) Saunders.

Emergency Medicine: Self Assessment & Review. Harold A. Thomas, Jr. et al. 4th ed. 1999. LC 98-52912. (Illus.). 300p. (C). text (*0-323-00538-1*) Mosby Inc.

Emergency Medicine: Steps 2 & 3. Southland Staff. 3rd rev. ed. 1998. 201p. (C). pap., wbk. ed. 30.00 (*1-888628-19-7*) Southlnd Tutor.

Emergency Medicine: The Principles of Practice. Ed. by Gordian W. Fulde. 3rd ed. 1998. (Illus.). 479p. (C). pap. text 58.00 (*0-8036-0481-5*) Davis Co.

Emergency Medicine Asia. Jon L. Jenkins. 1986. 8.95 (*0-316-46054-0*, Little Brwn Med Div) Lppncott W & W.

Emergency Medicine Asia. Jenkins. 3rd ed. 1995. 34.95 (*0-316-46003-6*, Little Brwn Med Div) Lppncott W & W.

Emergency Medicine Asia, No. 2. Jon L. Jenkins. 1990. 10.95 (*0-316-46057-5*, Little Brwn Med Div) Lppncott W & W.

Emergency Medicine Clinical Manual. Scott H. Plantz & Jonathan N. Adler. 1997. LC 98-42719. (National Medical Series for Independent Study). 320p. pap. text 16.95 (*0-683-30349-X*) Lppncott W & W.

Emergency Medicine Companion Handbook. David M. Cline et al. 5th ed. 1999. (Illus.). 1055p. pap. 39.95 (*0-07-012039-0*) McGraw-Hill Prof.

Emergency Medicine in Small Animal Practice. 1997. LC 97-178479. (Illus.). 365p. pap. text 68.00 (*1-884254-32-2*) Vet Lrn Syst.

Emergency Medicine ISE. Jon L. Jenkins. 1986. 14.95 (*0-316-46053-2*); No. 2. 1990. 15.95 (*0-316-46056-7*) Lppncott W & W (Little Brwn Med Div).

Emergency Medicine Pearls. Adam J. Singer et al. 2nd ed. 2000. (Illus.). 304p. pap. 21.95 (*0-8036-0755-5*); 2001. 288p. pap. 21.95 (*0-8036-0775-X*) Davis Co.

Emergency Medicine Pearls of Wisdom. Scott H. Plantz. 4th ed. 1997. pap. text 84.00 (*1-890369-00-4*) Boston Medical.

Emergency Medicine Pearls of Wisdom Oral Board Review. Gossman et al. 1998. pap. text 84.00 (*1-890369-01-2*) Boston Medical.

Emergency Medicine Pretest. Kristi L. Koenig. 2nd ed. 2000. LC 99-59151. (Illus.). 256p. pap. 49.95 (*0-07-135144-2*) McGraw-Hill Prof.

Emergency Medicine Question Pearls of Wisdom. Kreplick. 1998. (Pearls of Wisdom Ser.). pap. 42.00 (*1-890369-03-9*) Boston Medical.

Emergency Medicine Residencies. Ed. by Rebecca A. Anwar. 1981. (Emergency Health Services Review Ser.: Vol. 1, No. 1). 129p. pap. text 19.95 (*0-917724-57-7*) Haworth Pr.

Emergency Medicine Risk Management: A Comprehensive Review. American College of Emergency Physicians Staff. 1991. 132.00 (*0-07-000214-2*) McGraw.

Emergency Medicine Secrets. Vincent J. Markovchick & Peter T. Pons. 2nd rev. ed. 1998. LC 98-43419. (Secrets Ser.). (Illus.). 475p. pap. 39.95 (*1-56053-253-X*) Hanley & Belfus.

Emergency Mental Health Services in the Community. Ed. by Michael Phelan et al. 1995. (Studies in Social & Community Psychiatry). (Illus.). 375p. (C). text 90.00 (*0-521-45251-1*) Cambridge U Pr.

Emergency Neurology: Principles & Practice. Ed. by Sid M. Shah & Kevin M. Kelly. 1999. LC 98-19188. (Illus.). 634p. (C). text 160.00 (*0-521-49688-8*) Cambridge U Pr.

Emergency Nurse Pediatric Course Pocket Review. R. Warren Crow, Jr. et al. Ed. by Steven Tressa-Weber. 2000. 300p. spiral bd. (*0-935890-73-4*) Emerg Nurses IL.

Emergency Nursing: A Physiologic & Clinical Perspective. Ed. by Stephanie Kitt. 2nd ed. 1994. LC 94-23208. (Illus.). 766p. text 68.00 (*0-7216-5204-2*) Saunders.

Emergency Nursing: An Essential Guide for Patient Care. Judy Selfridge-Thomas. Ed. by Barbara N. Cullen. 1996. LC 96-23285. (Illus.). 223p. pap. text 23.00 (*0-7216-4703-0*) Saunders.

Emergency Nursing: Principles & Practice. Lorene Newberry & Susan B. Sheehy. 4th ed. 1997. LC 97-17575. (Illus.). 848p. (C). (gr. 13). text 59.95 (*0-8151-7678-3*, 24508) Mosby Inc.

Emergency Nursing: With Certification Preparation & Review. Nedell Lanros. 4th ed. 1997. LC 97-456. (Illus.). 692p. (Orig.). (C). pap. text 54.95 (*0-8385-0437-X*, A0437-2, Apple Lange Med) McGraw.

Emergency Nursing Pediatric Course Instructor Course Manual. Ed. by Nancy Eckle et al. 2nd ed. 1999. spiral bd. (*0-935890-58-0*) Emerg Nurses IL.

Emergency Nursing Pediatric Course Instructor Supplemental Manual. Ed. by Nancy Eckle et al. 2nd ed. 1999. spiral bd. (*0-935890-57-2*) Emerg Nurses IL.

Emergency Nursing Pediatric Course Provider Manual. Ed. by Nancy Eckle et al. 2nd ed. pap. (*0-935890-56-4*) Emerg Nurses IL.

Emergency Nursing Procedure. Jean A. Proehl. Ed. by Terri Wood. 2nd ed. 1999. LC 98-36264. (Illus.). 540p. text 65.00 (*0-7216-7589-1*) Saunders.

Emergency Nursing Standards of Care & Quality Improvement. Judy Selfridge-Thomas & Shelia Sanning Shea. 1994. LC 93-48330. (Illus.). 125p. pap. text 41.00 (*0-7216-5453-3*) Saunders.

Emergency Ophthalmology. Hung Cheng et al. 1997. 344p. pap. (*0-7279-0861-8*) BMJ Pub GBR. *Dist:* AIDC.

Emergency Orthopaedics & Trauma. Andrew Unwin & Kirsten Jones. 1995. LC 96-113925. 288p. pap. (*0-7506-2034-X*) E A GBR. *Dist:* OUP.

Emergency Orthopedics: The Extremities. Robert R. Simon & Steven J. Koenigsknecht. 4th ed. 2000. LC 00-20715. (Illus.). 620p. (C). text 99.00 (*0-8385-2210-6*) McGraw-Hill Prof.

Emergency Orthopedics: The Spine. Robert Galli et al. 1992. (Illus.). 294p. (C). pap. text 95.00 (*0-8385-2203-3*, A2203-6, Apple Lange Med) McGraw.

Emergency Pediatric Management. Lozon. 1999. pap. text (*0-7216-7651-0*) Saunders.

Emergency Pediatric Radiology. Ed. by L. W. Brady et al. 1999. LC 98-40967. (Medical Radiology Ser.). (Illus.). 464p. 249.00 (*3-540-63882-2*) Spr-Verlag.

***Emergency Pediatric Radiology.** Ed. by H. M. L. Carty et al. 2002. (Medical Radiology Ser.). 450p. 89.95 (*3-540-42292-7*) Spr-Verlag.

Emergency Pediatrics: A Guide to Ambulatory Care. Roger M. Barkin & Peter Rosen. 5th ed. 1998. LC 98-26889. pap. text 169.00 (*0-323-00326-5*) Mosby Inc.

Emergency Pediatrics: A Guide to Ambulatory Care. Roger M. Barkin & Peter Rosen. 5th ed. 1999. (Illus.). 960p. pap. (*84-8086-138-X*) Mosby-Doyma Libros ESP. *Dist:* Mosby Inc.

Emergency Pharmacology. David E. Gangeness & Roger D. White. Ed. by Gideon Bosker. 1984. LC 83-21404. 320p. pap. text 27.95 (*0-89303-430-4*) P-H.

Emergency Planning. 1983. (Advanced Health Physics Training Ser.). (Illus.). 220p. ring bd. 95.00 (*0-87683-208-7*) GP Courseware.

Emergency Plastic Surgery. Greco. 1991. 69.95 (*0-316-32562-7*, Little Brwn Med Div) Lppncott W & W.

Emergency Procedures. Michael S. Jastremski & Marc Dumas. 1992. (Illus.). 400p. pap. text 55.00 (*0-7216-5127-5*) Saunders.

Emergency Procedures & Techniques. Robert R. Simon & Barry E. Brenner. 3rd ed. 1994. LC 93-20416. (Illus.). 488p. 69.95 (*0-683-07738-4*) Lppncott W & W.

Emergency Psychiatry. Juan E. Mezzich & Ben A. Zimmer. 1990. LC 88-13599. 475p. 67.50 (*0-8236-1647-9*) Intl Univs Pr.

Emergency Psychiatry: Concepts, Methods, & Practices. Ed. by Ellen L. Bassuk & Ann W. Birk. 1984. LC 84-11709. (Critical Issues in Psychiatry Ser.). 468p. 69.50 (*0-306-41655-7*, Plenum Trade) Perseus Pubng.

Emergency Psychiatry & Mental Health Policy: An International Point of View. Michel De Clercq et al. 1998. LC 98-34614. pap. 62.00 (*0-444-50016-2*, Excerpta Medica) Elsevier.

Emergency Psychiatry for the House Officer. William R. Dubin & R. Stolberg. 1981. (Illus.). 166p. (Orig.). pap. text 19.50 (*0-88331-139-9*) R B Luce.

Emergency Radio Dispatching: 911 Dispatchers Guide Procedures, Safety, Technology. Sue Pivetta. 150p. pap. text 10.95 (*1-882960-07-6*) Prof Pride.

Emergency Radiology. Helen C. Redman et al. 1992. (Illus.). 554p. text 120.00 (*0-7216-7491-7*) Saunders.

Emergency Radiology. Earl Reisdorff et al. Ed. by David T. Schwartz. 1999. LC 98-36343. (Illus.). 672p. text 149.00 (*0-07-050827-5*) McGraw-Hill Prof.

Emergency Radiology. James T. Rhea & Eric Vansonnenberg. 1988. 256p. 72.95 (*0-316-74200-7*, Little Brwn Med Div) Lppncott W & W.

Emergency Radiology in Childhood: Syllabus. European Society for Pediatric Radiology Staff et al. 1998. LC 98-23326. (*88-470-0029-7*) Springer Pub.

Emergency Radiology of the Pelvis & Lower Extremities, Vol. 17. E. Paul Nance et al. 1983. (Advanced Exercises in Diagnostic Radiology Ser.). (Illus.). 176p. pap. text 53.00 (*0-7216-6653-1*) Saunders.

Emergency Radiology (Second Series) Test & Syllabus. Kent R. Donovan et al. 1997. LC 97-33316. (Professional Self-Evaluation Program Ser.). (*1-55903-041-0*) Am Coll Radiology.

Emergency Respiratory Care. Gina M. Buldra. 2002. (C). pap. 16.00 net. (*0-7668-1985-X*) Delmar.

Emergency Response. American Red Cross Staff. (gr. 13). rev. ed. 1997. (C). pap. text 5.00 (*0-8151-2635-2*, 31634); 2nd ed. 1996. LC 96-41118. pap. text 32.00 (*0-8151-1260-2*) Mosby Inc.

Emergency Response Instructor's Notebook. American Red Cross Staff. 1993. 85.00 (*0-8016-9015-3*) Mosby Inc.

Emergency Response Planning. Paul A. Erickson. 1999. LC 98-85211. 32p. (C). text 79.95 (*0-12-241540-X*) Harcourt.

Emergency Response to Crisis. Jeffrey Mitchell & H. L. Resnik. 1981. (Illus.). 256p. (C). text 24.95 (*0-87619-856-6*) P-H.

Emergency Room. Caroline B. Cooney. 1994. (Point Ser.). 10.55 (*0-606-06361-7*) Turtleback.

Emergency Room: Doctors Tell Their Stories. Ed. by Dan Sachs. 1996. LC 96-8254. 272p. (gr. 8). 22.95 (*0-316-76592-9*) Little.

Emergency Room Care. Charles Eckert. 4th ed. 1981. 27.50 (*0-316-20878-7*, Little Brwn Med Div) Lppncott W & W.

Emergency Services Reimbursement. 1997. 292p. 149.00 (*1-889115-18-5*) Med Learn.

Emergency Squad Volunteers: Professionalism in Unpaid Work. Gloria M. Nemerowicz & Joann Gora. 1985. LC 85-12310. 176p. 55.00 (*0-275-90206-4*, C0206, Praeger Pubs) Greenwood.

Emergency Survival Guide: You Can Survive Anything. Michael Borofka. 1994. LC 94-60498. (Illus.). 135p. (Orig.). pap. 11.95 (*0-9640856-0-7*) M Borofka.

Emergency Transport of the Perinatal Patient. Mhairi G. MacDonald. 1989. 55.00 (*0-316-54198-2*, Little Brwn Med Div) Lppncott W & W.

Emergency Treatment of Acute Respiratory Disease. Llewellyn W. Stringer. 3rd ed. 1981. LC 81-12238. (Illus.). 192p. pap. text 11.95 (*0-87619-862-0*) P-H.

***Emergency Triage.** Manchester Triage Group Staff. 2nd ed. 2002. 170p. pap. (*0-7279-1542-8*) BMJ Pub GBR. *Dist:* AIDC.

Emergency Triage - Manchester Triage Group. Ed. by Kevin Mackway-Jones. 1996. 156p. pap. text (*0-7279-1126-0*, 340300460) BMJ Pub GBR. *Dist:* AIDC.

Emergency Vascular Practice. Anthony D. Chant & Aires A. D'Sa. LC 97-152687. (Illus.). 294p. (*0-340-56170-X*) E A GBR. *Dist:* OUP, Routldge.

Emergency War Surgery. 1984. lib. bdg. 300.00 (*0-87700-539-7*) Revisionist Pr.

Emergency War Surgery. Ed. by Thomas E. Bowen & Ronald F. Bellamy. rev. ed. 1994. (Illus.). 446p. (C). text 60.00 (*0-7881-0291-5*) DIANE Pub.

Emergent & Urgent Neurology. William J. Weiner. 2nd ed. 1998. LC 98-42015. 592p. text 110.00 (*0-397-51857-9*) Lppncott W & W.

Emergent Care in Transplant Patients. George Perdrizet & Alan J. Smally. 2001. (Vademecum Ser.). spiral bd. 45.00 (*1-57059-581-X*) Landes Bioscience.

Emergent Evolution. Conwy L. Morgan. 2nd ed. LC 77-27209. (Gifford Lectures: 1922). reprint ed. 42.50 (*0-404-60468-4*) AMS Pr.

Emergent Field Medicine. Vanrooyen et al. 2001. (Illus.). 900p. pap. 80.00 (*0-07-135142-6*) McGraw-Hill Prof.

Emergent Literacy: Writing & Reading. Ed. by William Teale et al. 1986. LC 86-1037. (Writing Research Ser.: Vo. 6). 248p. (C). 77.00 (*0-89391-301-4*, Ablex) Greenwood.

Emergent Management of Trauma. Scaletta. 2nd ed. 2000. LC 2001-268096. (Illus.). 619p. pap. 44.95 (*0-07-134568-X*) McGraw-Hill Prof.

Emergicare Cards. Springhouse Publishing Company Staff. 2nd ed. 1995. 26.95 (*0-87434-814-5*) Springhouse Corp.

***Emerging Bacterial Pathogens.** Ed. by I. Muhldorfer & K. P. Schafer. 2001. LC 2001-46238. (Contributions to Microbiology Ser.: Vol. 8). (Illus.). xiv, 214p. 195.75 (*3-8055-7218-2*) S Karger.

Emerging Dimensions of Sexology: Selected Papers from the 6th World Congress, 2. Ed. by R. Taylor Segraves et al. 1984. LC 83-26890. (Sexual Medicine Ser.: Vol. 2). 355p. 78.75 (*0-275-91451-8*, C1451, Praeger Pubs) Greenwood.

Emerging Electromagnetic Medicine. Ed. by M. E. O'Connor et al. 1990. (Illus.). 307p. 97.00 (*0-387-97224-2*) Spr-Verlag.

Emerging Field of Sociobibliography: The Collected Essays of Ilse Bry, 19. Ed. by Lois Afflerbach & Marga Franck. 1977. LC 76-28644. (Contributions in Librarianship & Information Science Ser.: No. 19). 251p. 72.50 (*0-8371-9289-7*, BRB/, Greenwood Pr) Greenwood.

Emerging Infections. Ed. by Richard M. Krause et al. 1998. LC 97-45688. (Biomedical Update Ser.). (Illus.). 440p. text 84.95 (*0-12-425930-8*) Morgan Kaufmann.

Emerging Infections, Vol. 1. W. Michael Scheld et al. 1997. (Emerging Infections Ser.). (Illus.). 300p. pap. 79.95 (*1-55581-121-3*) ASM Pr.

Emerging Infections. Ed. by W. Michael Scheld et al. (Illus.). Vol. 2. 1998. 330p. pap. 79.95 (*1-55581-141-8*); Vol. 4. 2000. 300p. pap. 79.95 (*1-55581-197-3*) ASM Pr.

***Emerging Infections**, Vol. 5. Ed. by W. Michael Scheld et al. 2001. 250p. pap. 79.95 (*1-55581-216-3*) ASM Pr.

Emerging Infections: Microbial Threats to Health in the United States. Ed. by Joshua Lederberg et al. 1992. LC 92-26480. 312p. (C). pap. text 34.95 (*0-309-04741-2*) Natl Acad Pr.

Emerging Infectious Disease Test Markets. Ed. by CTB Diagnostics Intelligence Staff. 1995. 170p. (Orig.). pap., spiral bd. 867.00 (*1-887566-01-5*, REI-01) CTB Intl.

Emerging Issues & Methods in Personality Assessment. John A. Schinka & Roger L. Greene. 1997. LC 97-27324. (*0-8058-2676-9*) L Erlbaum Assocs.

Emerging Issues in Family Support. Valerie J. Bradley et al. 1992. (AAMD Monographs). 160p. (Orig.). (C). pap. text 22.95 (*0-940898-29-2*) Am Assn Mental.

Emerging Issues in Forensic Psychology: From Clinic to the Courthouse, Vol. 69. E. Benedek. 1996. pap. 28.00 (*0-7879-9901-6*) Jossey-Bass.

Emerging Issues in Mental Health & Aging. Ed. by Margaret Gatz. 1995. LC 95-23748. 379p. pap. 14.95 (*1-55798-317-8*) Am Psychol.

Emerging Legal Issues in Blood Banking & Transfusion Medicine. Ed. by Karen S. Lipton & Edward Wolf. 1998. LC 98-3649. 202p. pap. text (*1-56395-079-0*) Am Assn Blood.

Emerging Markets for Drugs & Vaccines for AIDS-Related Infections, No. C-170. 1993. (Illus.). 157p. 2650.00 (*1-56965-002-0*) BCC.

Emerging Minds: The Process of Change in Children's Thinking. Robert S. Siegler. 1996. LC 95-42099. (Illus.). 288p. text 40.00 (*0-19-507787-3*) OUP.

Emerging Opportunities in Peripheral Neuropathy Vol. I, 1999: ENS Satellite Symposium, Nice, June 1998. Ed. by Vera Bril & Gerard Said. 1999. (European Neurology Ser.: Vol. 41). (Illus.). iv, 44p. pap. 25.25 (*3-8055-6843-6*) S Karger.

Emerging Perspectives on Assessment of Exceptional Children. Ed. by Randy E. Bennett & Charles A. Maher. 1986. LC 86-3128. (Special Services in the Schools Ser.: Vol. 2, Nos. 2 & 3). 193p. text 39.95 (*0-86656-410-1*) Haworth Pr.

Emerging Policies for Biomedical Research. William N. Kelley et al. 1993. (Health Policy Annual Ser.: Vol. III). (Illus.). 250p. (Orig.). pap. 20.00 (*1-879694-06-9*) AAH Ctrs.

Emerging Problems in Human Nutrition. Ed. by J. C. Somogyi et al. 1987. (Bibliotheca Nutritio et Dieta Ser.: No. 40). (Illus.). viii, 140p. 115.00 (*3-8055-4497-9*) S Karger.

Emerging Profession: Philadelphia Doctors, 1860-1900. Leo O'Hara. 1989. (Medical Care in the United States Ser.: Vol. 10). 270p. text 25.00 (*0-8240-8339-3*) Garland.

Emerging Self: A Developmental, Self, & Object Relations Approach to the Treatment of the Closet Narcissistic Disorder of the Self. James F. Masterson. 1993. LC 93-1604. 340p. text 39.95 (*0-87630-721-7*) Brunner-Routledge.

Emerging Strategies in Neuroprotection. Ed. by H. Lal & Paul J. Marangos. 1992. (Advances in Neuroprotection Ser.). (Illus.). xviii, 359p. 120.00 (*0-8176-3544-0*) Birkhauser.

Emerging Systems in Long Term Care Vol. 4: Advances in Long Term Care. Ed. by Paul R. Katz et al. 1999. 200p. 43.95 (*0-8261-6833-7*) Springer Pub.

Emerging Targets in Antibacterial & Antifungal Chemotherapy. Ed. by Joyce Sutcliffe & Nafsika H. Georgopapadakou. 1991. 544p. (C). (gr. 13). pap. text 125.95 (*0-412-02711-9*, A4646, Chap & Hall NY) Chapman & Hall.

Emerging Theories of Human Communication. Ed. by Branislav Kovacic. 1997. LC 96-43768. (SUNY Series in Human Communication Processes). 220p. (C). text 57.50 (*0-7914-3451-6*); pap. text 19.95 (*0-7914-3452-4*) State U NY Pr.

Emerging Treatments in Neurology: Centenary Issues, 1897-1997. Ed. by Julien Bogousslavsky. 1997. (European Neurology Ser.: Vol. 38, No. 3, 1997). 120p. pap. 60.00 (*3-8055-6612-3*) S Karger.

Emerging Trends for EAPS in the 21st Century. Nan Van den Bergh. 2000. LC 00-46153. (Employee Assistance Quarterly Ser.: vol. 16, Nos. 1/2). 145p. (C). pap. text 24.95 (*0-7890-1020-8*) Haworth Pr.

Emerging Trends in Physician's Office Diagnostic Testing. Ed. by Peter Allen. 1985. 150p. pap. text 1475.00 (*0-931634-61-X*) FIND-SVP.

Emerging Viruses: AIDS & Ebola - Nature, Accident or Intentional? Leonard G. Horowitz. 1996. LC 95-61123. (Illus.). 544p. 29.95 (*0-923550-12-7*) Tetrahedron Pub.

Emery & Rimoin's Principles & Practice of Medical Genetics Ed. by D. L. Rimoin et al. 3rd ed. 1996. LC 96-216363. (Illus.). 2756p. (*0-443-04851-7*) Church.

Emery's Elements of Medical Genetics. Robert F. Mueller & Ian D. Young. 10th ed. 1998. LC 97-35527. (*0-443-05951-9*) Church.

Emery's Elements of Medical Genetics. Robert F. Mueller et al. 10th ed. 1998. LC 97-35527. (C). pap. text (*0-443-05902-0*) Church.

Emery's Elements of Medical Genetics. Robert F. Mueller et al. 11th ed. 2000. LC 00-46275. (*0-443-07125-X*) Harcrt Hlth Sci Grp.

Emesis in Anti-Cancer Treatment: Mechanisms & Treatment. Ed. by P. L. Andrews & G. J. Sanger. 1993. LC 92-49072. (Illus.). 272p. (gr. 13). 161.95 (*0-412-37250-9*) Chapman & Hall.

Emf & Light Therapies. John J. Williams. unabr. ed. 1999. (Illus.). 15p. pap. 15.00 (*0-934274-89-4*) Consumertronics.

EMF Science Review Symposium Breakout Group Reports for Clinical & in Vivo Laboratory Findings. Ed. by Judy Fleming et al. 1998. (Illus.). 180p. (C). pap. text 30.00 (*0-7881-7499-1*) DIANE Pub.

EMF Science Review Symposium Breakout Group Reports for Epidemiological Research Findings. Ed. by Mary S. Wolfe. 1998. (Illus.). 125p. pap. text 25.00 (*0-7881-7368-5*) DIANE Pub.

EMG Manual. Joe F. Jabre & Earl R. Hackett. 1983. (Illus.). 140p. 32.95 (*0-398-04837-1*) C C Thomas.

EMIC (Emergency Maternity & Infant Care) A Study of Administrative Experience. Nathan Sinai & Odin W. Anderson. 1974. LC 74-1704. (Children & Youth Ser.: Vol. 23). 234p. reprint ed. 26.95 (*0-405-05981-7*) Ayer.

Eminent Doctors, Set. George T. Bettany. 1977. LC 76-39663. (Essay Index Reprint Ser.). 46.95 (*0-8369-2747-8*) Ayer.

Emmanuel Movement: The Origins of Group Treatment & the Assault on Lay Psychotherapy. Sanford Gifford. 1997. (Francis Countway Library of Medicine). (Illus.). 180p. 19.95 (*0-674-25111-3*) HUP.

Emmett's Clinical Urography David M. Witten et al. 4th ed. 1977. LC 76-19614. (Illus.). 1. text 155.00 (*0-7216-9472-1*); 2. text 155.00 (*0-7216-9473-X*); 3. text 155.00 (*0-7216-9474-8*); Set. 2279p. 410.00 (*0-7216-9471-3*) Saunders.

Emociones, la Saludy y la Mujer de Hoy. Abel Delgado. 2000. LC 99-52074. (Guides to Improve Your Health Ser.). (SPA.). 192p. pap. 12.95 (*1-57954-203-4*) Rodale Pr Inc.

Emory University Comprehensive Board Review in Internal Medicine. Sidney F. Stein & Juha P. Kokko. 1999. LC 00-266411. (Illus.). 960p. pap. 99.00 (*0-07-061500-4*) McGraw-Hill Educ Grp.

Emotion: A Comprehensive Phenomenology of Theories & Their Meanings for Therapies. James Hillman. 1992. LC 91-39163. 318p. reprint ed. pap. 24.00 (*0-8101-1020-2*) Northwestern U Pr.

Emotion & Adaptation. Richard S. Lazarus. 1994. (Illus.). 576p. reprint ed. pap. text 35.00 (*0-19-509266-X*) OUP.

Emotion & Social Judgments: An Introductory Review. Ed. by Joseph P. Forgas. 1998. (Social Psychology Ser.: No. 23). (Illus.). 310p. pap. 26.95 (*0-08-040235-6*) Routledge.

Emotion & Spirit. Neville Symington. 1998. 216p. pap. (*1-85575-203-4*) Karnac Bks GBR. *Dist:* Other Pr LLC.

Emotion at Work. Rob B. Briner. 1999. 128p. pap. text 39.95 (*0-86377-991-3*) L Erlbaum Assocs.

Emotion, Cognition, & Representation: Rochester Symposium on Developmental Psychopathology VI. Ed. by Dante Cicchetti & Sheree L. Toth. 1995. LC 94-46745. (Rochester Symposium on Developmental Psychopathology Ser.: Vol. 6). (Illus.). 360p. (C). 90.00 (*1-878822-49-7*) Univ Rochester Pr.

Emotion, Cognition, Health & Development in Children & Adolescents. Ed. by Elizabeth J. Susman et al. 1992. (Penn State Series on Child & Adolescent Development). 192p. text 39.95 (*0-8058-0548-6*) L Erlbaum Assocs.

Emotion in Psychotherapy. Leslie S. Greenberg & Jeremy D. Safran. 1990. LC 86-22892. (Guilford Clinical Psychology & Psychotherapy Ser.). 338p. pap. 35.00 (*0-89862-522-X*, 2522) Guilford Pubns.

Emotion in the Human Face: Guidelines for Research & an Integration of Findings. Paul Ekman & W. Friesen. 1972. LC 71-140578. (Pergamon General Psychology Ser.). (*0-08-016643-1*) Pergamon Repr GBR. *Dist:* Franklin.

Emotion, Inhibition, & Health. Ed. by Harald C. Traue & James W. Pennebaker. 1993. LC 92-48708. (Illus.). 280p. text 49.00 (*0-88937-060-5*) Hogrefe & Huber Pubs.

Emotion, Psychotherapy & Change. Ed. by Jeremy D. Safran & Leslie S. Greenberg. 1991. LC 90-14130. 372p. 45.00 (*0-89862-556-4*, 2556) Guilford Pubns.

Emotional Abuse. Marti T. Loring. 1994. LC 94-10293. 160p. 29.95 (*0-02-919343-5*) Jossey-Bass.

Emotional Abuse: The Trauma & the Treatment. Marti T. Loring. 1998. LC 98-20964. (Psychology Ser.). 160p. reprint ed. pap. 23.00 (*0-7879-4377-0*) Jossey-Bass.

Emotional Abuse of the Child. Dorothy L. Renn. 1988. LC 87-92179. 16.95 (*0-87212-216-6*) Libra.

Emotional Aftermath of the Persian Gulf War: Veterans, Families, Communities, & Nations. Ed. by Robert J. Ursano & Ann E. Norwood. 1996. 608p. text 74.95 (*0-88048-652-X*, 8652) Am Psychiatric.

Emotional & Behavioral Disorders: Theory & Practice. Margaret C. Coleman. 3rd ed. 1995. LC 95-5505. 416p. 83.00 (*0-205-16632-6*) Allyn.

Emotional & Behavioural Difficulties: Theory to Practice. Paul Cooper et al. 1994. LC 93-25943. 176p. (C). text 59.95 (*0-415-07198-4*) Routledge.

Emotional & Psychological Abuse of Children. Kieran O'Hagan. 1992. LC 92-23834. 160p. (C). 88.00 (*0-335-09889-4*); pap. 32.50 (*0-335-09884-3*) U of Toronto Pr.

Emotional & Psychological Responses to Anesthesia & Surgery. Ed. by Frank Guerra & J. Antonio Aldrete. 1980. 288p. text 47.00 (*0-8089-1195-3*, 791747, Grune & Strat) Harcrt Hlth Sci Grp.

Emotional & Sensory Processing Problems: Assessment & Treatment Approaches for Young Children & Their Families. S. Poisson & G. DeGangi. 1991. 139p. pap. text 20.00 (*1-880341-00-X*) R S Lourie Ctr.

Emotional Armoring: An Introduction to Psychiatric Orgone Therapy. Morton Herskowitz. 1998. 347p. pap. text 26.95 (*3-8258-3555-3*) Transaction Pubs.

Emotional Aspects of Heart Disease. Harold Geist. 1977. LC 76-16319. 12.95 (*0-87212-062-7*) Libra.

Emotional Aspects of Pituitary Disease. Ed. by M. A. Weitzner et al. 1998. (Psychotherapy & Psychosomatics Ser.: Vol. 67, No. 3). (Illus.). 78p. pap. 41.75 (*3-8055-6664-6*) S Karger.

Emotional Brain. Joseph LeDoux. 1998. 384p. per. 14.00 (*0-684-83659-9*) S&S Trade.

Emotional Brain: Physiology, Neuroanatomy, Psychology, & Emotion. P. V. Simonov. 1986. LC 86-15098. (Emotions, Personality, & Psychotherapy Ser.). (Illus.). 274p. (C). 85.00 (*0-306-42363-4*, Plenum Trade) Perseus Pubng.

Emotional Care of the Facially Burned & Disfigured. Norman R. Bernstein. 1976. pap. 16.50 (*0-316-09193-6*, Little Brwn Med Div) Lppncott W & W.

Emotional Computer. Jose A. Jauregui. Tr. by Eduardo Jauregui & Pablo Jauregui. 1995. LC 94-44904. 256p. pap. 22.95 (*0-631-19844-X*) Blackwell Pubs.

Emotional Contagion. Elaine Hatfield et al. 1993. (Studies in Emotion & Social Interaction). 250p. text 49.95 (*0-521-44498-5*); pap. text 18.95 (*0-521-44948-0*) Cambridge U Pr.

Emotional Development. Thompson. 2001. 33.50 net. (*0-07-231686-1*) McGraw.

Emotional Development, Theory & Applications: A Neo-Piagetian Perspective. Henry Dupont. 1994. LC 93-43067. 152p. 60.00 (*0-275-94839-0*, Praeger Pubs) Greenwood.

Emotional Disorders in Physically Ill Patients. Robert Roessler & Norman Decker. 1986. LC 85-15120. (Illus.). 269p. 35.95 (*0-89885-254-4*, Kluwer Acad Hman Sci) Kluwer Academic.

Emotional Disturbance in Adopted Adolescents: Origins & Development. Ruth G. McRoy et al. 1988. LC 87-1053. 226p. 67.00 (*0-275-92913-2*, C2913, Praeger Pubs) Greenwood.

Emotional Disturbances & Juvenile Delinquency. Guy E. Swanson. Ed. by Harriet Zuckerman & Robert K. Merton. 1980. LC 79-9033. (Dissertations on Sociology Ser.). lib. bdg. 23.95 (*0-405-13000-7*) Ayer.

Emotional Eating: What You Need to Know Before Starting Your Next Diet. Edward Abramson. 1998. LC 97-45845. 208p. pap. 19.00 (*0-7879-4047-X*) Jossey-Bass.

Emotional Experience of Learning & Teaching. Isca Salzberger-Wittenberg et al. 1999. LC 00-269299. (Routledge Education Books). xii, 155p. pap. (*1-85575-230-1*) Karnac Bks GBR. *Dist:* Other Pr LLC.

Emotional Expression. Gary Collier. 1985. 264p. text 49.95 (*0-89859-505-3*) L Erlbaum Assocs.

Emotional Expression in Infancy: A Biobehavioral Study. Robert N. Emde et al. 1976. LC 76-4609. (Psychological Issues Monographs: No. 37). 210p. 32.50 (*0-8236-1651-7*); pap. 27.50 (*0-8236-1650-9*) Intl Univs Pr.

Emotional Expression in Psychotherapy. Robert Pierce et al. 1983. LC 83-5604. 356p. 29.95 (*0-89876-015-1*) Gardner Pr.

Emotional Fatigue: Causes & Cures. 1996. lib. bdg. 251.75 (*0-8490-5903-8*) Gordon Pr.

Emotional First Aid. Sean Haldane. 1989. pap. 6.95 (*0-8290-3177-4*) Irvington.

Emotional First Aid. Sean Haldane. 1985. 151p. 12.95 (*0-88282-004-4*) New Horizon NJ.

Emotional First Aid: A Crisis Handbook. Sean Haldane. 1996. 152p. pap. text 11.95 (*1-886449-33-3*) Barrytown Ltd.

Emotional First Aid: A Crisis Handbook. Sean Haldane. 1988. LC 88-20061. 151p. pap. 9.95 (*0-88268-071-4*) Station Hill Pr.

Emotional Fitness: Discovering Our Natural Healing Power. Janice Berger & Harry Hall. 2000. 256p. pap. 22.95 (*0-13-018182-X*) P-H.

Emotional Flooding: An Official Publication of the National Institute for the Psychotherapies. Ed. by Paul T. Olsen. 1976. LC 74-12620. (New Directions in Psychotherapy Ser.: Vol. I). 270p. 35.95 (*0-87705-239-5*, Kluwer Acad Hman Sci) Kluwer Academic.

Emotional Growth: Psychoanalytic Studies of the Gifted & a Great Variety of Other Individuals, Vol. I. Phyllis Greenacre. 1975. LC 75-129768. ix, 396p. 65.00 (*0-8236-1655-X*) Intl Univs Pr.

Emotional Healing with Homeopathy: A Self-Help Manual. Peter Chappell. 1994. LC 94-15322. pap. 13.95 (*1-85230-487-1*) Element MA.

Emotional Intimacy: Overlooked Requirement for Survival. Alan M. Dahms. 1972. LC 72-78443. (Illus.). 154p. (C). 8.95 (*0-87108-184-9*) Publishers Consult.

Emotional Motor System. Ed. by G. Holstege et al. 1996. LC 96-17075. (Progress in Brain Research Ser.: Vol. 107). 642p. 225.00 (*0-444-81962-2*) Elsevier.

Emotional Needs of Young Children & Their Families: Using Psychoanalytic Ideas in the Community. Ed. by Marion Bower & Judith Trowell. 1996. LC 95-16139. 320p. (C). pap. 27.95 (*0-415-11613-9*) Routledge.

Emotional Options: How to Use the Option Method. Mandy Evans. 1990. 56p. (Orig.). pap. 5.95 (*1-878639-03-X*) Yes You Can Pr.

Emotional Problems in Children & Young People. Linda Winkley. Ed. by Cedric Cullingford. 1996. LC 97-127198. (Children, Teachers & Learning Ser.). 208p. 80.00 (*0-304-32571-6*); pap. 33.95 (*0-304-32569-4*) Continuum.

Emotional Problems in Later Life: Intervention Strategies for Professional Caregivers. Dan Blazer. 2nd ed. 1997. LC 97-39495. 280p. 39.95 (*0-8261-7561-9*) Springer Pub.

Emotional Release for Children. Mark Pearson & Patricia Nolan. 1996. LC 96-147023. 212p. pap. (*0-86431-162-1*) Aust Council Educ Res AUS. *Dist:* Stylus Pub VA.

Emotional Rescue: The Theory & Practice of a Feminist Father. Isaac D. Balbus. 1997. LC 97-28024. (Thinking Gender Ser.). 256p. (C). 85.00 (*0-415-91917-7*); pap. 22.95 (*0-415-91918-5*) Routledge.

Emotional Risk Factors: The New Science of Health & Illness. Dorthy E. Dusek & Daniel A. Girdano. rev. ed. 1995. LC 92-80753. 174p. pap. 12.95 (*0-9633305-2-7*) Paradox CO.

Emotional Tie: Psychoanalysis, Mimesis, & Affect. Mikkel Borch-Jacobsen. 1993. LC 92-20356. 216p. pap. 17.95 (*0-8047-2037-1*) Stanford U Pr.

Emotional Understanding: Studies in Psychoanalytic Epistemology. Donna M. Orange. 1995. LC 95-32107. 226p. 35.00 (*1-57230-010-8*, 0010) Guilford Pubns.

Emotional Vertigo: Between Anxiety & Pleasure. Danielle Quinodoz. Tr. by Arnold Pomerans from FRE. 1997. LC 97-12260. 216p. (C). (New Library of Psychoanalysis). 85.00 (*0-415-14835-9*); (New Library of Psychoanalysis: Vol. 28). pap. 31.95 (*0-415-14836-7*) Routledge.

Emotionally Abused & Neglected Child: Identification, Assessment & Intervention. Dorota Iwaniec. 1995. LC 95-9879. (Child Care & Protection Ser.). 222p. pap. 70.00 (*0-471-95579-5*) Wiley.

Emotionally Normal Heart Attack. Richard D. Tenney. 1998. LC 97-41667. 128p. pap. 14.95 (*1-56072-500-1*, Nova Kroshka Bks) Nova Sci Pubs.

Emotions. Ed. by Y. Oomura. 1986. (Illus.). xiv, 446p. 233.25 (*3-8055-4405-7*) S Karger.

Emotions. Purdy. 1994. (C). pap. text 38.36 (*0-395-66539-6*) HM.

Emotions. Ed. by Robert Somerville. 1994. (Journey Through the Mind & Body Ser.). (Illus.). 144p. lib. bdg. 17.99 (*0-7835-1061-6*) Time-Life.

Emotions. Ed. by Robert Somerville. 1999. LC 94-8885. (Illus.). 144p. (*0-7835-1060-8*) Time-Life Bks GBR. *Dist:* AOL Time Warner.

Emotions: Current Issues & Future Directions. Ed. by Tracy J. Mayne & George A. Bonanno. 1920. LC 00-61689. (Emotions & Social Behavior Ser.). (Illus.). 421p. text 48.00 (*1-57230-622-X*, C0622) Guilford Pubns.

Emotions: Essays on Emotion Theory. Ed. by Stephanie Van Goozen et al. 1994. 320p. pap. 36.00 (*0-8058-1208-3*); text 69.95 (*0-8058-1207-5*) L Erlbaum Assocs.

Emotions: Outline of a Theory. Jean-Paul Sartre. Tr. by Bernard Frechtman from FRE. 96p. pap. 7.95 (*0-8065-0904-X*, Citadel Pr) Kensgtn Pub Corp.

Emotions & Behaviour: A Systems Approach. Ed. by K. V. Sudakov et al. 1989. (Systems Research in Physiology Ser.: Vol. 2). 496p. text 376.00 (*2-88124-711-3*) Gordon & Breach.

Emotions & Bodily Changes: A Survey of Literature on Psychosomatic Interrelationships, 1910-1953. Helen F. Dunbar. 4th ed. 1976. LC 75-16699. (Classics in Psychiatry Ser.). reprint ed. 99.95 (*0-405-07426-3*) Ayer.

Emotions & Bodily Responses: A Psychophysiological Approach. William W. Grings & Michael E. Dawson. 1978. (Behavioral Biology & International Ser.). text 55.00 (*0-12-303750-6*) Acad Pr.

Emotions & Psychopathology. Ed. by Manfred Clynes & Jaak Panksepp. 1988. LC 88-12508. (Illus.). 340p. 89.50 (*0-306-42916-0*, Plenum Trade) Perseus Pubng.

Emotions & the Dual Brain. Ed. by G. Gainotti & C. Caltagirone. 1989. (Experimental Brain Research Ser.: Vol. 18). (Illus.). 264p. 86.95 (*0-387-18873-8*) Spr-Verlag.

Emotions & the Enneagram: Working Through Your Shadow Life Script. Margaret F. Keyes. rev. ed. 1992. LC 91-75329. Orig. Title: Out of the Shadows, Emotions & the Enneagram. (Illus.). 178p. pap. 14.95 (*1-882042-09-3*) Molysdatur Pubns.

Emotions & the Will, 5. Alexander Bain. 1977. LC 77-72191. (Contributions to the History of Psychology Ser.: No. 5, Pt. A, Orientations). 638p. reprint ed. lib. bdg. 95.00 (*0-313-26929-7*, U6929, Greenwood Pr) Greenwood.

Emotions Anonymous. rev. ed. 1995. LC 95-60130. 240p. 15.00 (*0-9607356-3-1*) Emotions Anony Intl.

Emotions in Health & Illness: Applications to Clinical Practice. Ed. by Craig Van Dyke & Zegans Temoshok. 1984. (Mind & Medicine Ser.). text 49.00 (*0-8089-1659-9*, 794688, Grune & Strat) Harcrt Hlth Sci Grp.

Emotions in Health & Illness: Theoretical & Research Foundations. Ed. by Lydia Temoshok. 1983. 288p. text 49.00 (*0-8089-1581-9*, 794562, Grune & Strat) Harcrt Hlth Sci Grp.

Emotions in Ideal Human Development. Ed. by Leonard Cirillo et al. 1989. 184p. 39.95 (*0-8058-0473-0*) L Erlbaum Assocs.

Emotions in Personality & Psychopathology. Ed. by Carroll E. Izard. 1979. LC 78-10958. (Illus.). 618p. 85.00 (*0-306-40093-6*, Plenum Trade) Perseus Pubng.

Emotions in Social Life: Critical Themes & Contemporary Issues. Gillian Bendelow & Simon J. Williams. 1997. LC 97-11499. 368p. (C). 95.00 (*0-415-13798-5*); pap. 31.95 (*0-415-13799-3*) Routledge.

Emotions in the Practice of Psychotherapy: Clinical Implications of Affect Theories. Robert Plutchik. 2000. LC 00-41612. (Illus.). xiii, 229p. 39.95 (*1-55798-694-0*, 431-757A) Am Psychol.

Emotions of a Physician. Mariella Fischer-Williams. 1993. LC 92-75099. 223p. (Orig.). (C). pap. 14.95 (*0-936400-02-1*) Gearhart-Edwards.

Emotions, the Social Bond & Human Reality: Part-Whole Analysis. Thomas J. Scheff. 1997. LC 96-51847. (Studies in Emotion & Social Interaction). (Illus.). 260p. (C). text 59.95 (*0-521-58491-4*); pap. text 21.95 (*0-521-58545-7*) Cambridge U Pr.

Empathic Accuracy. William Ickes. 1997. LC 96-32416. 352p. text 48.00 (*1-57230-161-9*, 0161) Guilford Pubns.

Empathic Attunement: The "Technique" of Psychoanalytic Self Psychology. Crayton E. Rowe & David S. MacIsaac. 1989. LC 88-8069. 328p. 50.00 (*0-87668-857-1*) Aronson.

Empathic Attunement: The "Technique" of Psychoanalytic Self Psychology. Crayton E. Rowe, Jr. & David S. MacIsaac. 1996. LC 88-8069. 336p. pap. 40.00 (*0-87668-551-3*) Aronson.

Empathic Brief Psychotherapy. Barbara B. Seruya. 1997. LC 97-638. 168p. 35.00 (*0-7657-0067-0*) Aronson.

***Empathic Healer.** Michael J. Bennett. 2001. LC 00-111402. (Practical Resources for the Mental Health Professional Ser.). 200p. 44.95 (*0-12-088662-6*) Acad Pr.

Empathic Practitioner: Empathy, Gender, & Medicine. Ed. by Ellen S. More & Maureen A. Milligan. 1994. LC 94-10061. 265p. (C). text 45.00 (*0-8135-2118-1*); pap. text 20.00 (*0-8135-2119-X*) Rutgers U Pr.

Empathic Reader: A Study of the Narcissistic Character & the Drama of the Self. J. Brooks Bouson. 1989. LC 89-4695. 216p. (C). lib. bdg. 30.00 (*0-87023-678-4*) U of Mass Pr.

Empathy: Development, Training & Consequences. Arnold P. Goldstein & Gerald Y. Michaels. 1985. 304p. (C). text 59.95 (*0-89859-538-X*) L Erlbaum Assocs.

Empathy & the Practice of Medicine. Howard Spiro. 1996. pap. text 17.00 (*0-300-06670-8*) Yale U Pr.

Empathy in the Helping Relationship. Ed. by Ruth MacKay et al. 1989. LC 89-11408. 208p. 29.95 (*0-8261-6140-5*) Springer Pub.

Empathy Reconsidered: New Directions in Psychotherapy. Ed. by Arthur C. Bohart & Leslie S. Greenberg. 1997. LC 97-3398. 477p. text 49.95 (*1-55798-410-7*, 431-7860) Am Psychol.

Empirical Approaches to Psychosocial Aspects of Disability. Ed. by Myron G. Eisenberg & Roy Glueckauf. 1991. 288p. text 32.95 (*0-8261-7600-3*) Springer Pub.

Empirical Approaches to Synergetics in Psychology: Self-Organization & Clinical Psychology. Ed. by W. Tschacher et al. 1992. LC 92-19036. (Synergetics Ser.: Vol. 58). (Illus.). 472p. 95.00 (0-387-55502-1) Spr-Verlag.

Empirical Perspectives on the Psychoanalytic Unconscious. Ed. by Robert F. Bornstein & Joseph M. Masling. 1997. LC 97-37667. 291p. 49.95 (1-55798-463-8, 431-6970) Am Psychol.

Empirical Studies of Professional Practice, Vol. 1. Alan Carr. 2000. LC 99-54657. (Studies in Health & Human Services: Vol. 36). (Illus.). xii, 246p. 89.95 (0-7734-7831-0) E Mellen.

Empirical Studies of the Therapeutic Hour. Ed. by Robert F. Bornstein & Joseph M. Masling. 1998. LC 98-36423. (Empirical Studies of Psychoanalytic Theories; Vol. 8). 321p. 49.95 (1-55798-526-X, 431-607A) Am Psychol.

Empirically Based Assessment of Child & Adolescent Psychopathology: Practical Applications. Thomas M. Achenbach & Stephanie H. McConaughy. 2nd ed. 1996. LC 96-10137. (Developmental Clinical Psychology & Psychiatry Ser.: Vol. 13). 256p. pap. 39.95 (0-8039-7248-2, 1174) Sage.

***Empirically Supported Cognitive Therapies: Current Status & Future Directions (Tentative)** Ed. by William J. Lyddon & John V. Jones, Jr. 2001. LC 2001-20070. (Illus.). xiii, 258p. (0-8261-2299-X) Springer Pub.

Empirically Supported Therapies: Best Practice in Professional Psychology. Keith S. Dobson & Kenneth D. Craig. 1998. LC 98-19759. (Banff International Behavioral Science Ser.). 317p. 86.95 (0-7619-1075-1, 81637); pap. 36.95 (0-7619-1076-X, 81638) Sage.

Employee Benefits: A Guide for Health Care Professionals. Aspen Health Law and Compliance Center Staff. 1998. LC 98-9617. (Aspen Health Law Center Current Issues Ser.). 160p. pap. 48.00 (0-8342-1158-0, 11580) Aspen Pub.

Employee Guide to Carpal Tunnel Syndrome in Industry. Tel-A-Train, Inc. Staff. 1990. stu. ed. 3.50 (1-56355-153-5) Tel-A-Train.

Employee Guide to Respirator Safety. Tel-A-Train, Inc. Staff. 1988. stu. ed. 3.50 (1-56355-162-4) Tel-A-Train.

Employee Guide to the Care & Use of APR's. Tel-A-Train, Inc. Staff. 1988. stu. ed. 3.50 (1-56355-165-9) Tel-A-Train.

Employee Testing Vol. II: Resource Guide. 1990. 95.00 (1-55871-174-0) BNA PLUS.

Employer-Based Health Insurance: High Costs, Wide Variation Threaten System. 1993. (Illus.). 60p. (Orig.). (C). pap. text 35.00 (1-56806-905-7) DIANE Pub.

Employer-Based Health Plans: Issues, Trends, & Challenges Posed by ERISA. 1996. (Illus.). 64p. (Orig.). pap. text 30.00 (0-7881-3141-9) DIANE Pub.

Employer Checkup: How to Choose & Manage Employee Health Benefits. Brenda B. Thompson. 1999. LC 99-87091. 88p. 47.00 (0-925773-51-4) M Lee Smith.

Employer Health Plan Accountability: Do Plan Participants Have Adequate Protections?: Congressional Hearing. Ed. by John A. Boehner. 2000. 139p. (C). pap. text 35.00 (0-7567-0521-5) DIANE Pub.

Employer-Provided Health Benefits: Coverage, Provisions & Policy Issues. Employee Benefit Research Institute Staff & Deborah J. Chollet. 1984. LC 84-3977. (Orig.). pap. 24.95 (0-86643-033-4) Empl Benefit Res Inst.

Employer-Sponsored Health Insurance: State & National Estimates. National Center for Health Statistics Staff. 1997. LC 97-32968. (0-8406-0539-0, PHS 98-1017) Natl Ctr Health Stats.

Employer's Back Injury Prevention Handbook. Bruce A. Lepore & Chris N. Lepore. 1984. (Illus.). 164p. (C). pap. 24.95 (0-9613365-0-1) Bridgeview.

Employer's Guide to Hiring Relief & Part-Time Veterinarians. Carin A. Smith. rev. ed. 1999. 100p. ring bd., wbk. ed. 79.00 (1-885780-11-7) Smith Vet Srvs.

Employment & Distributional Effects of Mandated Benefits. June E. O'Neill & Dave M. O'Neill. 1994. (Studies in Health Reform). 35p. (Orig.). pap. 9.95 (0-8447-7021-3, AEI Pr) Am Enterprise.

Employment in Community Psychology: The Diversity of Opportunity. Clifford R. O'Donnell & Joseph R. Ferrari. 2000. LC 00-28115. 140p. pap. 24.95 (0-7890-1036-4) Haworth Pr.

Employment Issues & Multiple Sclerosis. Phillip D. Rumrill, Jr. 1996. LC 96-22536. (Illus.). 180p. (Orig.). pap. 29.95 (1-888799-03-X) Demos Medical.

Employment Law in the NHS. Viv Du-Feu & Owen Warnock. 1995. (Medico-Legal Practitioner Ser.). 173p. pap. (1-85941-016-2) Cavendish Pubng GBR. *Dist:* Gaunt.

Employment Relationship: A Psychological Perspective. Peter Herriot. 2001. LC 00-59234. (1-84169-239-5) Psychol Pr GBR. *Dist:* Taylor & Francis.

Empowered Laboratory Team: A Survival Kit for Supervisors, Team Leaders, & Team Professionals. William O. Umiker. 1996. (Practical Laboratory Management Ser.). 35.00 (0-89189-384-9) Am Soc Clinical.

Empowering Children to Cope with Difficulty & Build Muscles for Mental Health. Eric L. Dlugokinski & Sandra F. Allen. 1996. LC 96-35133. 160p. pap. 22.95 (1-56032-497-X) Accel Devel.

Empowering Families, Helping Adolescents: Family-Centered Treatment of Adolescents with Alcohol, Drug Abuse, & Mental Health Problems. Ed. by Wendy Snyder & Theodora Ooms. 1998. (Illus.). 204p. (C). pap. text 35.00 (0-7881-2624-5) DIANE Pub.

Empowering Survivors of Abuse: Health Care, Battered Women & Their Children. Jacquelyn Campbell. 1998. LC 98-25308. (Series on Violence Against Women). 74.95 (0-7619-1121-9, 81631); pap. 32.95 (0-7619-1122-7, 81632) Sage.

Empowerment in Community Care. Ed. by R. Jack. 1995. 320p. pap. 39.95 (1-56593-421-0, 1087) Singular Publishing.

Empowerment Through Health Education: Organization, Administration, & the Practice of Comprehensive Health Education in Developing Countries & Multicultural Settings. Martin A. Ayim. 2nd ed. 1998. 385p. pap. text 35.00 (0-9659474-0-8) Vita Pr.

Emptied Soul: On the Nature of the Psychopath. Adolf Guggenbuhl-Craig. 2000. (Classics in Archetypal Psychology Ser.: Vol. 1). 156p. pap. 15.00 (0-88214-371-9) Spring Pubns.

Empty Arms: Coping with Miscarriage, Stillbirth & Infant Death. Sherokee Ilse. 1990. 88p. pap. 9.95 (0-9609456-6-0) Wntergrn.

Empty Arms: Emotional Support for Those Who Have Suffered Miscarriage or Stillbirth. Pamela W. Vredevelt. 1994. 171p. pap. 9.99 (0-88070-810-7, Multnomah Bks) Multnomah Pubs.

Empty Arms - Coping with Miscarriage, Stillbirth & Infant Loss see Brazos Vacios: Como Vivir con el Aborto la Muerte Prenatala y la Muerte Infantil

Empty Beds: History of Vermont State Hospital. Marsha R. Kincheloe & Herbert G. Hunt, Jr. 1989. LC 89-91284. (Illus.). 254p. (Orig.). (C). text 13.00 (0-9622832-0-7); pap. text 10.00 (0-9622832-1-5) M Kincheloe.

Empty Cradle: Infertility in America from Colonial Times to the Present. Margaret Marsh. 1999. (Henry E. Sigerist Series in the History of Medicine). (Illus.). 344p. pap. text 19.95 (0-8018-6176-4) Johns Hopkins.

Empty Fortress: Infantile Autism & the Birth of the Self. Bruno Bettelheim. 1972. LC 67-10886. (Illus.). 496p. reprint ed. pap. 16.95 (0-02-903140-0) Free Pr.

Empty Laugh Book. Intro. by Sally C. Pitman. 1981. (Orig.). pap. text 15.00 (0-935229-07-8) Am Assoc Med.

Empty Your Bucket: Practical Steps to Overcome Allergy & Allergic Asthma. Stephen Astor. 1993. LC 92-80164. (Illus.). 312p. (Orig.). pap. 14.95 (0-915001-10-1) Two As Pub.

Emptying Beds: The Work of an Emergency Psychiatric Unit. Lorna A. Rhodes. (Comparative Studies of Health Systems & Medical Care: Vol. 27). (Illus.). 199p. 1995. pap. text 17.95 (0-520-20351-8); 1991. LC 90-11161. text 40.00 (0-520-07054-2) U CA Pr.

EMS: Emergency Medical Services, Agenda for the Future, Implementation Guide. 1999. 118p. per. 14.00 (0-16-050038-9) USGPO.

***EMS & the Law.** AAOS Staff. 2001. pap. 24.95 (0-7637-2068-2, 2068-2) Jones & Bartlett.

EMS & the Law. Scott Henderson. 2002. (C). pap. 37.33 (0-8359-4913-3) P-H.

EMS Drug Manual: A Field Guide for Emergency Care Personnel. Peter A. Dillman. (Orig.). 1987. LC 87-91752. 150p. pap. text 9.50 (0-9619221-0-9); 1990. pap. text 9.50 (0-9619221-1-7) Dillman Pub.

***EMS Field Guide: ALS Version.** Paul LeSage et al. 13th rev. ed. 2001. (Illus.). 114p. spiral bd. 16.50 (1-890495-10-7) InforMed OR.

***EMS Field Guide: BLS - Intermediate Version.** Jon Tardiff et al. 3rd rev. ed. 2001. (Illus.). 98p. spiral bd. 16.50 (1-890495-11-5) InforMed OR.

EMS Field Protocal Manual. Jonathan D. Apfelbaum. 1999. (Illus.). 300p. spiral bd. 23.95 (1-56930-091-7) Delmar.

EMS Incident Management System: Operations for Mass Casualty & High Impact Incidents. Hank T. Christen & Paul M. Maniscalco. 1998. LC 97-53270. 240p. (C). 54.00 (0-89303-972-1, Prentice Hall) P-H.

EMS Medical Directors' Handbook. National Association of EMS Physicians Executive Staff. 2nd ed. 1994. (Illus.). 512p. (gr. 13). pap. text 46.95 (0-8016-6580-9, 06580) Mosby Inc.

***EMS Medication Field Guide: Pocket Field Guide.** Peter A. Dillman. 2nd rev. ed. 2001. (Illus.). 210p. (C). pap. text 24.95 (0-7637-1795-9, 1795-9) Jones & Bartlett.

EMS Medication Pocket Field Guide. Peter A. Dillman. 2nd ed. 2000. (Illus.). 210p. (C). pap. text 21.95 (0-7637-1225-6, 1225-6) Jones & Bartlett.

EMS Pocket Drug Manual. Peter A. Dillman. 1991. 171p. pap. 16.25 (0-86720-171-1) Jones & Bartlett.

EMS Report Writing: A Pocket Reference. Todd Stanford. 1991. LC 91-3470. 112p. pap. text 26.00 (0-89303-823-7, 740803) P-H.

EMS Response to Hazardous Materials Incidents. L. Scott Ulin & D. R. Stutz. 1993. (Illus.). 450p. pap. text 32.95 (0-913019-06-2) BRADCOMM.

EMS Skill Sheets. Randy Miller et al. Ed. by Steve Mercer. 1994. 176p. (C). ring bd. 59.95 (1-884225-01-2) Communs Skills.

EMS Street Strategies: Effective Patient Interaction. Stephen M. Soreff & Robert T. Cadigan. 1992. (Illus.). 218p. (C). pap. 18.95 (0-8036-7979-3) Thomson Learn.

EMS Stress: An Emergency Responder's Handbook for Living Well. Ray Shelton & Jack Kelly. 1994. LC 94-78604. (Illus.). 256p. (Orig.). pap. 16.95 (0-8151-7512-4, 24613) Jems Comm.

EMT. American College of Emergency Physicians Staff. 1999. LC 00-698643. (Illus.). xxv, 640p. (gr. 13). text 38.95 (0-8151-0100-7, 24559) Mosby Inc.

EMT: Prehospital Care. Mark C. Henry & Edward R. Stapleton. Ed. by Selma Kaszczuk. 2nd ed. 1997. LC 96-30207. (Illus.). 768p. pap. text 41.00 (0-7216-6101-7) Saunders.

EMT - Basic Student Review Manual. American Academy of Orthopaedic Surgeons Staff. 3rd ed. 1999. (Illus.). 328p. (C). pap. text, stu. ed. 29.95 (0-7637-1026-1, 1026-1) Jones & Bartlett.

EMT & Paramedic Quick Reference. Norman E. McSwain et al. 1994. (Illus.). 336p. (C). pap. text (1-884225-02-0) Communs Skills.

EMT-B National Standards Review Self Test. C. D. Miller & Brent Q. Hafen. 2nd ed. 1997. LC 97-37172. 464p. pap. text 42.00 (0-8359-5155-3) P-H.

EMT-B Vitals & History Vt04. Debbie G. Stoy. 1995. 75.00 (0-8151-7964-2) Mosby Inc.

EMT B Vt05 Lifting/moving. Debbie G. Stoy. 1995. 75.00 (0-8151-7965-0) Mosby Inc.

EMT B VT03 Human Body. Debbie G. Stoy. 1995. 75.00 (0-8151-7963-4) Mosby Inc.

EMT-Basic Field Care: A Case-Based Approach. American Academy of Orthopaedic Surgeons Staff. 1998. (Illus.). 66p. (C). pap. text 21.95 (0-7637-0880-1, 0880-1) Jones & Bartlett.

EMT-Basic Field Care: A Case-Based Approach. American College of Emergency Physicians Staff. 1999. pap. text, wbk. ed. 16.95 (0-8151-0102-3) Mosby Inc.

EMT-Basic Field Care: A Case-Based Approach. American College of Emergency Physicians Staff. 2000. pap. text (0-323-01152-7) Saunders.

EMT-Basic Field Care: A Case-Based Approach. Jon Krohmer & American College of Emergency Physicians Staff. 1999. tchr. ed. (0-8151-0101-5) Mosby Inc.

EMT Basic National Standards Review Self Test. C. D. Miller. 1992. 256p. pap. 39.80 (0-89303-875-X) Appleton & Lange.

EMT-Basic National Standards Review Self Test. Charly D. Miller & David White. 2nd ed. 1994. LC 94-12398. 256p. (C). pap. 27.00 (0-89303-002-3) P-H.

EMT Basic Pearls of Wisdom: Over 1500 Questions. Haskell & Kruse. 1999. (Pearls of Wisdom Ser.). pap. 22.00 (1-58409-003-0) Boston Medical.

EMT-Basic Student Workbook. American Academy of Orthopaedic Surgeons Staff. 7th ed. 1999. (Illus.). 448p. (C). pap. text, stu. ed. 33.95 (0-7637-0804-6, 0804-6) Jones & Bartlett.

EMT-D Prehospital Defibrillation. Kenneth Stults. 1986. (Illus.). 192p. pap. text 49.00 (0-89303-433-9) P-H.

EMT Handbook of Emergency Care. D. J. Arneson & Maureen L. Bruce. 1986. LC 65-8592. (Illus.). 320p. text 19.00 (0-397-54595-9, Lippnctt) Lppncott W & W.

EMT-Intermediate Self Assessment Examination Review Manual. Joseph J. Mistovich. 2001. LC 00-51644. (Health Review Ser.). 256p. (C). pap. 22.67 (0-8359-5019-0) Globe Fearon.

EMT Introduction. Debbie G. Stoy. 1995. pap. 75.00 (0-8151-7961-8) Mosby Inc.

EMT Manual. Michael K. Copass et al. 3rd ed. 1998. LC 97-47600. (Illus.). 432p. (C). pap. text 29.00 (0-7216-6965-4) Saunders.

EMT Paramedic National Standards. Charly D. Miller. 3rd ed. 1996. LC 96-38269. 411p. pap. text 42.00 (0-8359-5102-2) P-H.

EMT-Paramedic National Standards Review Self Test. Charly D. Miller & David White. LC 92-49915. (0-89303-955-1) Brady Pub.

EMT-Paramedic Pretest Self Assessment & Review. Richard E. Westfal et al. 2000. LC 00-28748. (Illus.). 336p. pap. 29.95 (0-07-134156-0) McGraw-Hill Prof.

EMT Prehospital Care. Ed. by Mark C. Henry & Edward R. Stapleton. (Illus.). 1992. pap. text, tchr. ed. 55.00 (0-7216-4619-0); 1992. 886p. pap. text 39.00 (0-7216-1301-2); 2nd ed. 1997. 810p. pap., tchr. ed. 49.95 (0-7216-7412-7) Saunders.

EMT Prepares: One Hundred Role-Playing Scenarios. Susan Rubinsky et al. 1993. 311p. (C). ring bd. 59.95 (1-884225-00-4) Communs Skills.

EMT Recertification Practice Exams. LC 94-77026. 208p. pap. 24.95 (0-938329-75-8) Info Guides.

EMT Review Manual. Brent Q. Hafen & Keith J. Karren. 2nd ed. 1994. LC 93-21373. (Illus.). 384p. pap. 28.33 (0-89303-200-X) P-H.

EMT Review Manual. Donald J. Ptacnik. 5th ed. 2000. pap. text (0-7216-5081-3) Saunders.

EMT Review Manual: Self-Assessment Practice Tests for Basic Life Support Skills. Donald J. Ptacnik. 4th ed. 1993. 326p. pap. text 26.00 (0-7216-5043-0) Saunders.

EMT Teaching: A Common-Sense Approach. Richard A. Cherry. 1997. LC 97-32499. 160p. pap. 67.00 (0-89303-007-4) P-H.

EMTALA Answer Book. Mark M. Moy. 3rd ed. 2000. LC 00-33183. xxviii, 328p. pap. 73.00 (0-8342-1877-1, 18771) Aspen Pub.

EMTB. American Academy of Orthopaedic Surgeons Staff. (Illus.). (C). 6th rev. ed. 1998. 784p. pap. text 56.95 (0-7637-0803-8, 0803-8); 7th ed. 1998. pap. text 10.00 (0-7637-0906-9); 7th ltd. ed. 1999. 992p. text, tchr. ed. 77.50 (0-7637-1070-9, 1070-9) Jones & Bartlett.

***EMTB.** AAOS Staff. 7th ed. Date not set. (C). Section 1. (Illus.). pap. text 15.00 (0-7637-1027-X, 1027-X); Section 3. (Illus.). pap. text 15.00 (0-7637-1029-6, 1029-6); Section 4. (Illus.). pap. text 15.00 (0-7637-1030-X, 1030-X); Section 5. pap. text 15.00 (0-7637-1031-8, 1031-8); Section 6. (Illus.). pap. text 15.00 (0-7637-1032-6, 1032-6); Section 7. (Illus.). pap. text 15.00 (0-7637-1033-4, 1033-4); Section 8. (Illus.). pap. text 15.00 (0-7637-1034-2, 1034-2) Jones & Bartlett.

EMTB: Student Workbook. American Academy of Orthopaedic Surgeons Staff. 6th ed. 1997. (Emergency Care Ser.). (Illus.). pap. text, stu. ed. 33.95 (0-89203-166-2, 166-2) Jones & Bartlett.

EMTB Supplements Folder. American Academy of Orthopaedic Surgeons Staff. 7th ed. 1999. (Illus.). (C). pap. text, suppl. ed. (0-7637-1143-8) Jones & Bartlett.

En la Frontera de la Vida: Los Virus. Armando Aranda Anzaldo. (Ciencia para Todos Ser.). (SPA.). pap. 6.99 (968-16-4811-0) Fondo CA.

Enabling & Empowering Families: Principles & Guidelines for Practice. Carl J. Dunst et al. 1989. (Illus.). 220p. pap. 24.95 (0-914797-59-X) Brookline Bks.

Enabling Change-When Your Child Returns from Treatment. Jane Nakken. 1985. 24p. pap. 2.00 (0-89486-264-2, 1271B) Hazelden.

Enamel Microabrasion. Theodore P. Croll. 1991. LC 91-112. (Illus.). 102p. text 65.00 (0-86715-243-5) Quint Pub Co.

Encapsulation & Controlled Release. Ed. by David R. Karsa & R. A. Stephenson. 1993. (Special Publications). 186p. (0-85186-615-8, R6615) Royal Soc Chem GBR. *Dist:* Spr-Verlag.

Enchanted Self: A Positive Therapy. Barbara Becker Holstein. 1997. LC 99-458455. 144p. 55.00 (90-5702-502-7); 224p. pap. text 18.00 (90-5702-503-5) Gordon & Breach (Harwood Acad Pubs).

Enchantment & Intervention in Family Therapy: Training in Ericksonian Approaches. Stephen R. Lankton & Carol H. Lankton. 1986. LC 86-4240. 336p. text 39.95 (0-87630-428-5) Brunner-Routledge.

Enciclopedia de Antibioticos. John S. Glasby. 1978. (SPA.). 700p. pap. 53.95 (0-8288-5210-3, S50564) Fr & Eur.

Enciclopedia de Frutas, Vegetales y Hierbas. John Heinerman. 2000. (SPA., Illus.). 519p. pap. 14.00 (0-7352-0194-3) PH Pr.

Enciclopedia de Jugos Curativos. John Heinerman. 2000. (SPA.). 350p. pap. 14.00 (0-7352-0190-0) PH Pr.

Enciclopedia de la Medicina y la Salud, Set. Servagrup Staff. 11th ed. 1990. (SPA.). 1250.00 (0-8288-8228-2, 8486017068) Fr & Eur.

Enciclopedia de la Psicologia, Set. Denis Huisman. 1977. (SPA.). 3212p. 595.00 (0-8288-5408-4, S50546) Fr & Eur.

Enciclopedia de la Salud. Castells A. Roca et al. 6th ed. 1974. (SPA.). 1043p. 70.00 (0-7859-0868-4, S-13678) Fr & Eur.

Enciclopedia de la Salud y la Belleza: Encyclopedia of Health & Beauty. Simona Morini. 1977. (SPA.). 448p. pap. 19.95 (0-8288-5409-2, S50037) Fr & Eur.

Enciclopedia de la Sexualidad. Fernando Montes. 1975.Tr. of Span.. 944p. 44.95 (0-8288-5865-9, S32223) Fr & Eur.

Enciclopedia de la Vida Sexual y Conyugal. Kurt et al. 1975. (SPA.). 504p. pap. 17.25 (0-7859-0889-7, S-13880) Fr & Eur.

Enciclopedia de las Hierbas y de las Plantas Medicinales: Encyclopedia of Medicinal Herbs & Plants. Tina Cecchini. 4th ed. 1990. (SPA.). 536p. (0-7859-5053-2) Fr & Eur.

Enciclopedia de Remedios Caseros Naturales. Myra Cameron. 2000. (SPA.). 525p. pap. 14.00 (0-7352-0211-7) PH Pr.

Enciclopedia Familiar de la Medicina y la Salud. Servagrup Staff. 11th ed. 1990. (SPA.). 1250.00 (0-8288-7573-1, 8486017157) Fr & Eur.

Enciclopedia Heinerman de Frutas, Vegetales, y Herbas. John Heinerman. 1998. LC 98-13114. (SPA.). 560p. (C). text 24.95 (0-13-863754-7) P-H.

Enciclopedia Medica 1989. (ITA.). 1265p. 250.00 (0-913298-81-6) S F Vanni.

Enciclopedia Medica Familiar, Set. Nauta Staff. 5th ed. 1979. (SPA.). 448p. pap. 75.00 (0-8288-4742-8, S50532) Fr & Eur.

Enciclopedia Medica para la Familia Moderna. Frank Beer-Poitevin. 1985. (SPA.). 368p. Vol. 1. pap. 125.00 (0-7859-5030-3); Vol. 2. pap. 125.00 (0-7859-6397-9, 8486452023); Vol. 3. pap. 125.00 (0-7859-6398-7, 8486452031) Fr & Eur.

Enciclopedia Pediatrica, Set. Helmut Opitz & F Schmid. 1974. (SPA.). 13429p. 1495.00 (0-8288-6036-X, S50558) Fr & Eur.

Enciclopedia Pediatrica Vol. 1, Pt. 1: Historia De. Helmut Opitz & F Schmid. 1973. 960p. 275.00 (0-7859-6113-5, 8471121352) Fr & Eur.

Enciclopedia Pediatrica Vol. 1, Pt. 2: Fisio-Patologia del Recien. Helmut Opitz & F Schmid. 1974. 570p. 275.00 (0-7859-6115-1, 8471121433) Fr & Eur.

Enciclopedia Pediatrica Vol. 2, Pt. 2: Terapeutica Pediatrica. Helmut Opitz & F Schmid. 1971. 806p. 275.00 (0-7859-6117-8, 8471121875) Fr & Eur.

Enciclopedia Pediatrica Vol. 3: Immunologia. Pediatria Social. Helmut Opitz & F Schmid. 1969. 1366p. 295.00 (*0-7859-6118-6*, 8471121883) Fr & Eur.

Enciclopedia Pediatrica Vol. 4: Metabolismo, Nutricion, Digestion. Helmut Opitz & F Schmid. 1967. 1376p. 295.00 (*0-7859-6119-4*, 8471121891) Fr & Eur.

Enciclopedia Pediatrica Vol. 5: Enfermedades Infecciosas. Helmut Opitz & F Schmid. 1967. 1398p. 295.00 (*0-7859-6120-8*, 8471121905) Fr & Eur.

Enciclopedia Pediatrica Vol. 6: Enfermedades de los Tejidos De. Helmut Opitz & F Schmid. 1970. 1353p. 295.00 (*0-7859-6121-6*, 8471121913) Fr & Eur.

Enciclopedia Pediatrica Vol. 7: Enfermedades del Aparato Respirato. Helmut Opitz & F Schmid. 1968. 1450p. 295.00 (*0-7859-6122-4*, 8471121921) Fr & Eur.

Enciclopedia Pediatrica Vol. 8, Pt. 1: Neurologia, Psicologia. Helmut Opitz & F Schmid. 1971. 1136p. 275.00 (*0-7859-6481-9*) Fr & Eur.

Enciclopedia Pediatrica Vol. 8, Pt. 2: Tumores en la Infancia. Helmut Opitz & F Schmid. 1974. 840p. 275.00 (*0-7859-6114-3*, 8471121417) Fr & Eur.

Enciclopedia Pediatrica Vol. 9: Ojos, Nariz, Dientes, Piel. Helmut Opitz & F Schmid. 1972. 997p. 295.00 (*0-7859-6112-7*, 8471121174) Fr & Eur.

Enciclopedia Vida Sexual, Set. Gilbert Tordjman. 1978. (SPA.). 1048p. 295.00 (*0-8288-5231-6*, S50565) Fr & Eur.

Encounter: Group Sensitivity Training Experience. Carl Goldberg. 1971. LC 70-133292. 25.00 (*0-87668-035-X*) Aronson.

Encounter with Children. Suzanne D. Dixon & Martin T. Stein. 3rd ed. 1999. LC 99-44552. 666p. pap. text 49.95 (*0-323-00253-6*) Mosby Inc.

Encountering Freud: The Politics & Histories of Psychoanalysis. Paul Roazen. 1990. 405p. text 44.95 (*0-88738-295-9*) Transaction Pubs.

Encounters with Aging: Mythologies of Menopause in Japan & North America. Margaret M. Lock. 1995. LC 93-21379. 439p. pap. text 22.50 (*0-520-20162-0*) U CA Pr.

Encounters with Biomedicine: Case Studies in Medical Anthropology. Ed. by Hans A. Baer. 1987. (Health, Society, & Culture Ser.: Vol. 1). xxvi, 350p. text 158.00 (*2-88124-195-6*) Gordon & Breach.

Encounters with Children: A Practical Guide to Pediatric Behavior & Development. Suzanne D. Dixon & Martin T. Stein. 2nd ed. 1991. (Illus.). 480p. (C). (gr. 13). pap. text 59.95 (*0-8016-1432-5*, 01432) Mosby Inc.

Encounters with Parapsychology. Ed. by R. A. McConnell. 1982. LC 81-90032. (Illus.). ix, 235p. pap. 12.00 (*0-9610232-1-X*) McConnell.

Encounters with Qi: Exploring Chinese Medicine. David Eisenberg & Thomas L. Wright. rev. ed. 1995. LC 95-234224. (Illus.). 256p. pap. 12.95 (*0-393-31213-5*, Norton Paperbks) Norton.

Encounters with the Soul: Active Imagination as Developed by C. G. Jung. Barbara Hannah. 1981. LC 81-5316. 254p. 35.00 (*0-938434-04-7*); pap. 18.95 (*0-938434-02-0*) Sigo Pr.

Encouragement Packet. Elizabeth A. Einstein & Linda Albert. 1986. (Strengthening Stepfamilies Ser.). pap. 17.95 (*0-88671-219-X*, 6473) Am Guidance.

Encouraging the Use of Nurse-Midwives: A Report for Policymakers. Mary Gabay & Sidney M. Wolfe. 1995. 72p. (Orig.). (C). pap. 15.00 (*0-937188-02-6*) Pub Citizen.

Encyclopaedia of Indian Medicine Vol. 1: Historical Perspectives. S. K. Rao. 1985. (C). (*0-8364-2322-4*) Popular Prakashan IND. *Dist:* S Asia.

Encyclopaedia of Indian Medicine Vol. 2: Basic Concepts. S. K. Rao. 1987. (C). (*0-8364-2323-2*) Popular Prakashan IND. *Dist:* S Asia.

Encyclopaedia of Indian Medicine Vol. 3: Clinical Examination & Diagnostic Methods. S. K. Rao. 1987. (C). (*0-8364-2324-0*) Popular Prakashan IND. *Dist:* S Asia.

Encyclopaedia of Medical Ignorance: The Mind & Body in Health & Disease. Ed. by R. Duncan & Miranda Weston-Smith. 1984. LC 83-4785. (Illus.). 240p. (*0-08-024515-3*, 37) Pergamon Repr GBR. *Dist:* Franklin.

Encyclopedia Chiropractica. Paul Smallie. 1990. 172p. (Orig.). (C). spiral bd. (*0-9614296-7-4*) Wrld-Wide Bks.

Encyclopedia Medica del Hogar. American Medical Association Staff. 1991. text 60.00 (*0-07-104016-1*) McGraw.

Encyclopedia Mosby de Medicina y Enfermeria, Set. C. V. Mosby. 1990. (SPA.). 495.00 (*0-8288-8235-5*, 8477642184) Fr & Eur.

Encyclopedia of Aging. Ed. by George L. Maddox. 2nd ed. 1995. LC 95-24029. (Illus.). 1256p. 159.00 (*0-8261-4841-7*) Springer Pub.

Encyclopedia of Aging George L. Maddox. 3rd ed. 2001. LC 00-49663. (Illus.). 1408p. (*0-8261-4842-5*) Springer Pub.

Encyclopedia of Aging & the Elderly. F. Hampton Roy & Charles Russell. 1992. (Illus.). 320p. lib. bdg. 50.00 (*0-8160-1869-3*) Facts on File.

Encyclopedia of AIDS: A Social, Political, Cultural & Scientific Record of the HIV Epidemic. Ed. by Raymond A. Smith. 1998. LC 98-200474. (Illus.). 650p. 125.00 (*1-57958-007-6*) Fitzroy Dearborn.

Encyclopedia of Allergies. Myron A. Lipkowitz & Tova Navarra. 2nd rev. ed. 2001. LC 00-49490. (Library of Health & Living). 352p. 66.00 (*0-8160-4404-X*, Checkmark) Facts on File.

Encyclopedia of Alternative Medicine: A Complete Family Guide to Complementary Therapies. Jennifer Jacobs. 1996. LC 96-18786. (Illus.). 320p. pap. text 24.95 (*1-885203-36-5*) Jrny Editions.

Encyclopedia of Anesthesia Practice. Steven M. Yentis et al. Ed. by Thomas B. Feeley. 1996. LC 95-47196. 435p. pap. text 89.99 (*0-7506-9699-0*) Buttrwrth-Heinemann.

Encyclopedia of Associations Vol. 2: Association Periodicals Science, Medicine & Technology Publications. Robert C. Thomas & Denise M. Allard. 1987. 650p. 85.00 (*0-8103-2062-2*) Gale.

Encyclopedia of Bioethics. Warren T. Reich. 2nd ed. 1995. Vol. 1. 100.00 (*0-02-897353-4*); Vol. 2. 100.00 (*0-02-897354-2*); Vol. 3. 100.00 (*0-02-897356-9*); Vol. 5. 100.00 (*0-02-897352-6*) Macmillan.

Encyclopedia of Biopharmaceutical Statistics. Contrib. by Shein-Chung Chow et al. 2000. LC 99-54245. (Illus.). 552p. text 165.00 (*0-8247-6001-8*) Dekker.

Encyclopedia of Biostatistics, Set. Ed. by Peter Armitage & Ted Colton. 1998. LC 98-10160. 4898p. 3775.00 (*0-471-97576-1*) Wiley.

Encyclopedia of Birth Control. Vern L. Bullough. 2001. LC 2001-1345. 0349p. lib. bdg. 85.00 (*1-57607-181-2*) ABC-CLIO.

Encyclopedia of Blindness & Vision Impairment. Jill Sardegna & T. Otis Paul. 1991. LC 90-3374. (Facts on File Ser.). 340p. (C). 50.00 (*0-8160-2153-8*) Facts on File.

Encyclopedia of Bodybuilding! The Ultimate A-Z Book on Muscle Building. Gerard Thorne & Phil Embleton. 1997. LC 95-920923. (Illus.). 640p. pap. (*1-55210-001-4*) MuscleMag Intl CAN. *Dist:* BookWorld.

Encyclopedia of Bodywork: From Acupressure to Zone Therapy. Elaine Stillerman. 1997. (Illus.). 336p. pap. 19.95 (*0-8160-3646-2*) Facts on File.

Encyclopedia of Cancer Joseph R. Bertino. 1996. LC 96-3046. text 184.00 (*0-12-093231-8*); text 183.00 (*0-12-093232-6*); text 183.00 (*0-12-093233-4*) Acad Pr.

Encyclopedia of Cancer Ed. by Joseph R. Bertino. 1996. LC 96-3046. (Illus.). 2133p. text 578.00 (*0-12-093230-X*) Acad Pr.

Encyclopedia of Childbearing: Critical Perspectives. Barbara Katz Rothman. 1992. LC 92-14975. (Illus.). 472p. 74.50 (*0-89774-648-1*, Oryx) Greenwood.

Encyclopedia of Clinical Trial. Ed. by Carol K. Redmond & Theodore Colton. 2001. LC 2001-17865. (Reference Series in Biostatistics). (Illus.). 522p. 245.00 (*0-471-82211-6*) Wiley.

Encyclopedia of Complementary Health Practice. Ed. by Carolyn C. Clark et al. 1999. LC 99-25832. (Illus.). 664p. text 119.00 (*0-8261-1237-4*) Springer Pub.

Encyclopedia of Controlled Drug Delivery, Set. Edith Mathiowitz. 1999. LC 99-24907. 1057p. 695.00 (*0-471-14828-8*) Wiley.

Encyclopedia of Criminology & Deviant Behavior Clifton D. Bryant. 2000. LC 00-58558. (Illus.). 3000p. 495.00 (*1-56032-772-3*) Taylor & Francis.

Encyclopedia of Deafness & Hearing Disorders. Carol Turkington & Allen E. Sussman. 1992. (Illus.). 288p. lib. bdg. 45.00 (*0-8160-2267-4*) Facts on File.

Encyclopedia of Depression. Roberta Roesch. 2nd ed. 1991. 270p. (C). 45.00 (*0-8160-1936-3*) Facts on File.

Encyclopedia of Drugs & Alcohol. Jerome Jaffe. 1995. Vol. 1. 100.00 (*0-02-897196-5*); Vol. 2. 100.00 (*0-02-897197-3*); Vol. 3. 100.00 (*0-02-897198-1*); Vol. 4. 100.00 (*0-02-897199-X*) Macmillan (Hall Reference).

Encyclopedia of Elder Care: The Comprehensive Resource on Geriatric & Social Care. Mathy D. Mezey. 2001. LC 00-61890. xl, 824p. (*0-8261-1368-0*) Springer Pub.

Encyclopedia of Emulsion Technology, Vol. 2. Paul Becher. 1985. (Illus.). 536p. text 235.00 (*0-8247-1877-1*) Dekker.

Encyclopedia of Energy Healing: A Complete Guide to Using the Major Forms of Healing for Body, Mind & Spirit. Andy Baggott. 2000. (Illus.). 192p. pap. 17.95 (*0-8069-9328-6*, OCC011000) Sterling.

Encyclopedia of Epidemics. Jo Hays. 2003. lib. bdg. 150.00 (*1-57607-257-6*) ABC-CLIO.

Encyclopedia of Epidemiology. Mitchell H. Gail & Jacques Benichou. 2000. LC 00-42285. (Reference Series in Biostatistics). (Illus.). 1000p. 395.00 (*0-471-86641-5*) Wiley.

Encyclopedia of Evolving Techniques in Dynamic Psychotherapy: The Movement to Multiple Models. Irving Solomon. 1992. LC 92-11362. 424p. 60.00 (*0-87668-511-4*) Aronson.

Encyclopedia of Fears & Anxieties. James Wynbrandt & Mark D. Ludman. 2nd ed. 1999. LC 99-56020. (Facts on File Ser.). (Illus.). viii, 568p. lib. bdg. 65.00 (*0-8160-3989-5*) Facts on File.

Encyclopedia of Fertility & Infertility. Carol Turkington & Michael M. Alper. 2001. LC 00-67749. (Library of Health & Living). (Illus.). 71.50 (*0-8160-4154-7*) Facts on File.

Encyclopedia of Food Microbiology, Set. Ed. by Richard Robinson et al. 2000. LC 98-87954. (Illus.). 2467p. 925.00 (*0-12-227070-3*) Acad Pr.

Encyclopedia of Food Science, Food Technology, & Nutrition Ed. by Robert MacRae et al. 1993. LC 92-15557. (Illus.). 1. text 314.00 (*0-12-226851-2*); 2. text 314.00 (*0-12-226852-0*); 3. text 314.00 (*0-12-226853-9*); 4. text 314.00 (*0-12-226854-7*); 5. text 314.00 (*0-12-226855-5*); 6. text 314.00 (*0-12-226856-3*); 7. text 314.00 (*0-12-226857-1*); 8. text 314.00 (*0-12-226858-X*) Acad Pr.

Encyclopedia of Food Science, Food Technology & Nutrition, Set. Ed. by Robert MacRae et al. 1993. LC 92-15557. (Illus.). 5500p. text 2414.00 (*0-12-226850-4*) Acad Pr.

Encyclopedia of Genetics Ed. by Sydney Brenner & Jeffrey K. Miller. 2001. 2800p. 845.00 (*0-12-227080-0*) Acad Pr.

Encyclopedia of Gerontology. Ed. by James E. Birren. 1996. LC 95-47195. (Illus.). Vol. 1. text 175.00 (*0-12-226861-X*); Vol. 2. text 175.00 (*0-12-226862-8*) Acad Pr.

Encyclopedia of Gerontology: Age, Aging & the Aged Ed. by James E. Birren. 1996. LC 95-47195. (Illus.). 1474p. text 350.00 (*0-12-226860-1*) Acad Pr.

Encyclopedia of Healing Therapies. Anne Woodham & David Peters. 1997. LC 97-16171. (Illus.). 336p. pap. 39.95 (*0-7894-1984-X*) DK Pub Inc.

Encyclopedia of Herbal Medicine. Andrew Chevallier. 2000. (Illus.). 336p. 40.00 (*0-7894-6783-6*) DK Pub Inc.

Encyclopedia of Home Remedies. John Tish. Ed. by Frieda Nelson. 1997. 437p. 24.95 (*1-884350-59-3*) Alpha Pubng.

Encyclopedia of Human Behavior Ed. by Vangipuram S. Ramachandran. 1994. LC 93-34371. (Illus.). 2765p. text 685.00 (*0-12-226920-9*);1. text 165.00 (*0-12-226921-7*) Acad Pr.

Encyclopedia of Human Emotions, Set. Ed. by David Levinson et al. 1999. LC 99-31198. (Illus.). 768p. 240.00 (*0-02-864766-1*, Macmillan Ref) Gale.

Encyclopedia of Human Emotions, Vol. 2. David Levinson & James J. Ponzetti, Jr. 1999. LC 99-31198. (Illus.). 130.00 (*0-02-864767-X*); 195.00 (*0-02-864768-8*) S&S Trade.

Encyclopedia of Human Nutrition Michelle Sadler. 1998. LC 97-16267. (Illus.). xlix, 1973p. (C). text 310.00 (*0-12-226695-1*); text 310.00 (*0-12-226696-X*) Acad Pr.

Encyclopedia of Human Nutrition Michelle Sadler. 1998. LC 97-16267. (Illus.). xlix, 1973p. (C). text 305.00 (*0-12-226697-8*) Harcourt.

Encyclopedia of Immunology. Peter J. Delves & Ivan M. Roitt. 2nd ed. 1998. (C). LC 96-39910. text 250.00 (*0-12-226766-4*); LC 96-39910. text 250.00 (*0-12-226767-2*); text 250.00 (*0-12-226768-0*) Acad Pr.

Encyclopedia of Immunology Ed. by Peter J. Delves & Ivan M. Roitt. 2nd ed. 1998. LC 96-39910. (Illus.). 2516p. (C). text 972.00 (*0-12-226765-6*) Morgan Kaufmann.

Encyclopedia of Immunology, Vol. 4. Delves. 2nd ed. 1998. text 250.00 (*0-12-226769-9*) Harcourt.

Encyclopedia of Infectious Diseases. Carol Turkington & Bonnie Ashby. 1998. LC 97-50440. (Facts on File Ser.). 400p. 50.00 (*0-8160-3512-1*) Facts on File.

Encyclopedia of Medical Devices & Instrumentation, Vol. 4. John G. Webster. 1988. 3022p. 1140.00 (*0-471-82936-6*) Wiley.

Encyclopedia of Medical Organizations & Agencies. 11th ed. 2001. (Encyclopedia of Medical Organizations & Agencies Ser.). 1600p. 285.00 net. (*0-7876-3414-X*) Gale.

Encyclopedia of Medical Tests. Micheal B. Brodin. 1997. LC 98-189593. 592p. per. 6.99 (*0-671-53537-4*) S&S Trade.

Encyclopedia of Medicinal Plants: A Practical Reference Guide to More Than 550 Herbs, Oils, & Medicinal Plants. Andrew Chevallier. 1996. LC 96-15192. (Illus.). 336p. 39.95 (*0-7894-1067-2*) DK Pub Inc.

Encyclopedia of Memory & Memory Disorders. Richard Noll & Carol Turkington. 1994. LC 94-1590. (Facts on File Ser.). 280p. 45.00 (*0-8160-2610-6*) Facts on File.

Encyclopedia of Mental Health. Ed. by Howard S. Friedman. 1998. LC 98-84208. (C). text 180.00 (*0-12-226678-1*); text 185.00 (*0-12-226676-5*) Acad Pr.

Encyclopedia of Mental Health Ed. by Howard S. Friedman. 1998. LC 98-84208. (Illus.). 2398p. (C). text 600.00 (*0-12-226675-7*) Morgan Kaufmann.

Encyclopedia of Mental Health. Ada P. Kahn & Jan Fawcett. 1993. LC 92-35148. (Facts on File Ser.). 480p. 50.00 (*0-8160-2694-7*) Facts on File.

***Encyclopedia of Mental Health.** Ada P. Kahn & Jan Fawcett. 2nd ed. 2001. LC 00-69511. (*0-8160-4062-1*) Facts on File.

Encyclopedia of Mind Enhancing Foods, Drugs & Nutritional Substances. David W. Group. 2000. LC 00-58678. (Illus.). 221p. lib. bdg. 45.00 (*0-7864-0853-7*) McFarland & Co.

Encyclopedia Of Molecular Biology Vol. 5: Plasmids - Synthetic Peptide & Nonpeptide Combinatorial Libraries, Vol. 5. Ed. by Robert A. Meyers. 1997. (Illus.). 517p. 460.00 (*3-527-28475-3*, Wiley-VCH) Wiley.

Encyclopedia of Molecular Biology & Molecular Medicine Vol. 4: Mass Spectrometry High Speed DNA Fragment Sizing - Plasma Lipoprotein, Vol. 4. Ed. by Robert A. Meyers. 1996. (Illus.). 509p. 460.00 (*3-527-28474-5*, Wiley-VCH) Wiley.

Encyclopedia of Molecular Biology & Molecular Medicine Vol. 6, Vol. 6. Ed. by Robert A. Meyers. 1997. (Illus.). 512p. 460.00 (*3-527-28476-1*, Wiley-VCH) Wiley.

Encyclopedia of Molecular Medicine. Creighton. 2001. Vol. 1. text (*0-471-37497-0*); Vol. 2. text (*0-471-37498-9*); Vol. 3. text (*0-471-37496-2*) Wiley.

Encyclopedia of Native American Healing. William S. Lyon. 1996. LC 96-26860. 360p. lib. bdg. 70.00 (*0-87436-852-9*) ABC-CLIO.

Encyclopedia of Native American Healing. William S. Lyon. 1998. LC 96-26860. (Illus.). 416p. pap. 18.95 (*0-393-31735-8*) Norton.

Encyclopedia of Natural Healing: The Authoritative Reference to Alternative Health & Healing. Siegfrid Cursche. 1997. (Illus.). 1472p. 59.95 (*0-920470-75-0*) Alive Bks.

Encyclopedia of Natural Health & Healing for Children: The Complete Guide to Safe & Effective Home Treatments. Marcea Weber. 1994. LC 93-23572. (Illus.). 288p. pap. 16.95 (*1-55958-435-1*, Prima Health) Prima Pub.

Encyclopedia of Natural Medicine. Michael Murray & Joseph E. Pizzorno. 2nd rev. ed. 1997. LC 97-50569. 960p. pap. 24.95 (*0-7615-1157-1*, Prima Health) Prima Pub.

Encyclopedia of Natural Remedies. Louise Tenney. 1995. 410p. pap. 17.95 (*0-913923-98-2*) Woodland UT.

Encyclopedia of Nursing Care Quality, Set, Vols. 1-3. Patricia Schroeder. 1995. 758p. 190.00 (*0-8342-0219-0*, 20219) Aspen Pub.

Encyclopedia of Nursing Care Quality Vol. 2: Approaches to Nursing Standards, Vol. 2. Patricia Schroeder. 1991. 224p. 77.00 (*0-8342-0214-X*, 20214) Aspen Pub.

Encyclopedia of Nursing Care Quality Vol. 3: Monitoring & Evaluation in Nursing, Vol. 3. Patricia Schroeder. 1991. 296p. 77.00 (*0-8342-0217-4*, 20217) Aspen Pub.

Encyclopedia of Nursing Research. Ed. by Joyce J. Fitzpatrick. 1998. LC 98-15853. (Illus.). 750p. 100.00 (*0-8261-1170-X*) Springer Pub.

Encyclopedia of Nutrition & Good Health. Robert A. Ronzio. 1997. 486p. LC 96-17858. 49.50 (*0-8160-2665-3*); reprint ed. pap. text 19.95 (*0-8160-3755-8*) Facts on File.

Encyclopedia of Nutritional Supplements: The Essential Guide for Improving Your Health Naturally. Michael Murray. 1996. LC 96-3804. (Illus.). 576p. pap. 22.95 (*0-7615-0410-9*, Prima Health) Prima Pub.

Encyclopedia of Obesity & Eating Disorders. Dana K. Cassell & Felix E. Larocca. 1994. LC 92-18289. (Facts on File Ser.). 272p. lib. bdg. 45.00 (*0-8160-1985-1*) Facts on File.

Encyclopedia of Pharmaceutical Technology. James Swarbrick & James C. Boylan. (Illus.). Vol. 1. 1988. text 195.00 (*0-8247-2800-9*); Vol. 2. 1989. 512p. text 195.00 (*0-8247-2801-7*); Vol. 3. 1990. 512p. text 195.00 (*0-8247-2802-5*); Vol. 4. 1991. 344p. text 195.00 (*0-8247-2803-3*); Vol. 5. 1991. 500p. text 195.00 (*0-8247-2804-1*); Vol. 6. 1992. 504p. text 195.00 (*0-8247-2805-X*); Vol. 7. 1992. 506p. text 195.00 (*0-8247-2806-8*); Vol. 9. 1993. 488p. text 195.00 (*0-8247-2808-4*) Dekker.

Encyclopedia of Pharmaceutical Technology. Ed. by James Swarbrick & James C. Boylan. (Illus.). Vol. 10. 1994. 560p. text 195.00 (*0-8247-2809-2*); Vol. 14. 1996. 472p. text 195.00 (*0-8247-2813-0*) Dekker.

Encyclopedia of Pharmaceutical Technology, Vol. 16. Ed. by Swarbrick & Boylan. 1997. (Illus.). 504p. text 195.00 (*0-8247-2815-7*) Dekker.

Encyclopedia of Pharmaceutical Technology, Vol. 19, Suppl. 2. Ed. by James Swarbrick & James C. Boylan. 1999. LC 88-25664. (Illus.). 500p. text 195.00 (*0-8247-2818-1*) Dekker.

Encyclopedia of Pharmaceutical Technology: Hydrolysis of Drugs to Lipids in Pharmaceutical Dosage Forms, Vol. 8. Ed. by James Swarbrick & James C. Boylan. 1993. (Illus.). 520p. text 195.00 (*0-8247-2807-6*) Dekker.

Encyclopedia of Pharmaceutical Technology: Index for Volumes 1-16, Vol. 17. Ed. by James Swarbrick & James C. Boylan. 1997. (Illus.). 500p. text 195.00 (*0-8247-2816-5*) Dekker.

Encyclopedia of Pharmaceutical Technology: Nuclear Medicine & Pharmacy to Permeation Enhancement Through Skin, Vol. 11. Ed. by James Swarbrick & James C. Boylan. 1994. (Illus.). 544p. text 195.00 (*0-8247-2810-6*) Dekker.

Encyclopedia of Pharmaceutical Technology: Pharmaceutical Packaging to Prescribing of Drugs, Vol. 12. Ed. by James Swarbrick & James C. Boylan. 1995. (Illus.). 512p. text 195.00 (*0-8247-2811-4*) Dekker.

Encyclopedia of Pharmaceutical Technology: Supplement 1, Vol. 18. Ed. by James Swarbrick & James C. Boylan. 1998. (Illus.). 500p. text, suppl. ed. 195.00 (*0-8247-2817-3*) Dekker.

Encyclopedia of Pharmaceutical Technology: Thermal Analysis of Drugs & Drug Products to Unit Processes in Pharmacy: Fundamentals, Vol. 15. Ed. by James Swarbrick & James C. Boylan. 1996. (Illus.). 448p. text 195.00 (*0-8247-2814-9*) Dekker.

Encyclopedia of Phobias, Fears & Anxieties. Ronald M. Doctor & Ada P. Kahn. 1989. 500p. 50.00 (*0-8160-1798-0*) Facts on File.

Encyclopedia of Physical Education, Fitness & Sports. Thomas K. Cureton. 49.95 (*0-88314-293-7*) Natl Assn Sport.

Encyclopedia of Practice & Financial Management. Ed. by Lawrence Farber et al. 3rd ed. 1997. (Illus.). 1125p. text 69.95 (*1-878487-89-2*, ME060) Practice Mgmt Info.

Encyclopedia of Psychiatry, Psychology & Psychoanalysis. Benjamin B. Wolman. 1996. LC 95-41116. 688p. 160.00 (*0-8050-2234-1*) H Holt & Co.

Encyclopedia of Psychoactive Drugs: Series 2 Ed. by Jack H. Mendelson & Nancy K. Mello. 1989. (Illus.). 3328p. (YA). (gr. 7 up). lib. bdg. 359.10 (*1-55546-202-2*) Chelsea Hse.

Encyclopedia of Psychoative Substances. Richard Rudgley. 2000. (Illus.). 320p. pap. 15.95 (*0-312-26317-1*) St Martin.

Encyclopedia of Psychological Disorders Carol C. Nadelson. 1998. (Encyclopedia of Psychological Disorders Ser.). 160.65 (*0-7910-4902-7*) Chelsea Hse.

Encyclopedia of Psychological Medicine: Enciclopedia de Psicologia Medica. Stephen Krauss. 1981. (SPA.). 580p. 65.00 (*0-8288-2217-4*, S21333) Fr & Eur.

Encyclopedia of Psychology Ed. by Alan E. Kazdin. 2000. LC 99-55239. (Illus.). 4160p. 750.00 (*1-55798-187-6*) OUP.

Encyclopedia of Psychology Ed. by Raymond J. Corsini. 2nd ed. 1994. (C). Vol. 1. 576p. 225.00 (*0-471-55823-0*); Vol. 2. 544p. 225.00 (*0-471-55822-2*); Vol. 3. 608p. 225.00 (*0-471-55824-9*); Vol. 4. 680p. 225.00 (*0-471-55821-4*) Wiley.

Encyclopedia of Radiographic Positioning. Ed. by Steven B. Dowd & Bettye G. Wilson. 1995. (Illus.). 1249p. tchr. ed. (*0-7216-4288-8*) Saunders.

Encyclopedia of Radiographic Positioning, Set. Steven B. Dowd & Bettye G. Wilson. 1995. LC 94-13891. (Illus.). 2016p. text 145.00 (*0-7216-4202-0*) Saunders.

Encyclopedia of Reproduction. Ed. by Ernst Knobil & Jimmy D. Neill. 1998. LC 98-84463. (C). Vol. 1. text 125.00 (*0-12-227021-5*); Vol. 2. text 125.00 (*0-12-227022-3*); Vol. 3. text 125.00 (*0-12-227023-1*); Vol. 4. text 125.00 (*0-12-227024-X*) Acad Pr.

Encyclopedia of Reptiles & Amphibians. John F. Breen. 1974. (Illus.). 576p. text 39.95 (*0-87666-220-3*, H-935) TFH Pubns.

Encyclopedia of Schizophrenia & Psychotic Disorders. Richard Noll. 1992. 368p. lib. bdg. 50.00 (*0-8160-2240-2*) Facts on File.

Encyclopedia of Sleep & Sleep Disorders. Michael Thorpy & Jan Yager. 1990. 304p. 50.00 (*0-8160-1870-7*) Facts on File.

Encyclopedia of Sports Science & Medicine. John Zumerchik. 1997. LC 96-47502. (Encyclopedia of Sports Science & Medicine Ser.: Vol. 1). Vol. 1. 115.00 (*0-02-864665-7*); Vol. 2. 115.00 (*0-02-864666-5*) Gale (Macmillan Ref).

Encyclopedia of Stress Ed. by George Fink. 2000. LC 99-62774. (Illus.). 2400p. 550.00 (*0-12-226735-4*) Acad Pr.

Encyclopedia of the Alkaloids, Vol. 4. John S. Glasby. 1983. LC 75-17753. 398p. 125.00 (*0-306-41217-9*, Plenum Trade) Perseus Pubng.

Encyclopedia of the History of Science, Technology, & Medicine in Non-Western Cultures. Ed. by Helaine Selin. 1997. LC 96-36625. 1150p. (C). lib. bdg. 420.00 (*0-7923-4066-3*) Kluwer Academic.

Encyclopedia of Therapeutic Exercises see Miracle Exercises That Can Save Your Life!

Encyclopedia of Tibetan Medicine. 1994. LC 94-900815. (C). (*81-7030-396-6*) Sri Satguru Pubns IND. *Dist:* S Asia.

Encyclopedia of Tibetan Medicine: Being the Tibetan Text of Rgyud Bzi & Sanskrit Restoration of Amtrta Htrdaya Arsteagnga Guhyopadebsa Tantra & Expository Translation in English / Bhagavan D. Dash. 1994. LC 94-900815. (Indian Medical Science Ser.). (ENG & TIB.). 58.00 (*81-7030-397-4*) S Asia.

Encyclopedia of Toxicology, Set. Ed. by Philip Wexler. 3rd ed. 1998. LC 98-84114. (Illus.). 1500p. (C). text 499.95 (*0-12-227220-X*) Acad Pr.

Encyclopedia of U. S. Biomedical Policy. Ed. by Robert H. Blank & Janna Merrick. 1996. LC 95-33969. 384p. lib. bdg. 95.00 (*0-313-28641-8*, Greenwood Pr) Greenwood.

Encyclopedia of Understanding Alcohol & Other Drugs Robert O'Brien & Morris Chafetz. 1998. LC 98-22491. (Facts on File Ser.). (Illus.). 505p. 195.00 (*0-8160-3970-4*) Facts on File.

Encyclopedia of Virology Allan Granoff. Ed. by Robert G. Webster. 2nd ed. 1999. LC 00-267938. (Illus.). lxxxii, 1997p. 925.00 (*0-12-227030-4*) Acad Pr.

Encyclopedia of Vitamins, Minerals, & Supplements. Tova Navarra & Myron A. Lipowitz. LC 95-12645. 304p. 1997. pap. 17.95 (*0-8160-3241-6*); 1995. 35.00 (*0-8160-3183-5*) Facts on File.

Encyclopedia of Women's Health Issues. Kathlyn Gay. 2001. LC 2001-37342. (Illus.). 320p. 69.95 (*1-57356-303-X*, Oryx) Greenwood.

Encyclopedia on Radiographic Positioning, Vol. 1. Dowd. 1995. (Illus.). 625p. (C). text 90.00 (*0-7216-5745-1*) Harcourt.

Encyclopedia on Radiographic Positioning, Vol. 2. Dowd. 1995. (Illus.). 624p. (C). 85.00 (*0-7216-5746-X*) Harcrt Hlth Sci Grp.

Encyclopedic Dictionary of AIDS-Related Terminology: Make Sense Out of Confusing HIV/AIDS Terminology! Ed. by Jeffrey T. Huber et al. 2000. LC 00-38919. v, 246p. (C). pap. 24.95 (*0-7890-1207-3*, Haworth Info Pr) Haworth Pr.

Encyclopedic Dictionary of AIDS-Related Terminology: Make Sense Out of Confusing HIV/AIDS Terminology! Ed. by Jeffrey T. Huber & Mary L. Gillaspy. 2000. LC 00-38919. v, 246p. (C). 59.95 (*0-7890-0714-2*, Haworth Info Pr) Haworth Pr.

Encyclopedic Dictionary of Genetics: With German Equivalents & German, English Index. R. J. King. 1990. (ENG & GER.). 809p. lib. bdg. 350.00 (*0-8288-3588-8*, F115270) Fr & Eur.

Encyclopedic Dictionary of Medical Terms, Set. B. V. Petrovskij. 1982. 125.00 (*0-8288-1859-2*, M15410) Fr & Eur.

Encyclopedic Dictionary of Roman Law. Adolf Berger. 2001. LC 00-67774. (*1-58477-142-9*) Lawbk Exchange.

Encyclopedic Dictionary of Sports Medicine. David F. Tver & Howard F. Hunt. 1986. (Advanced Industrial Technology Ser.). 340p. 35.00 (*0-412-01361-4*, 9949, Chap & Hall NY) Chapman & Hall.

Encyclopedic Handbook of Alcoholism. Ed. by E. Mansell Pattison & Edward Kaufman. 1982. LC 81-24196. 1256p. 120.00 (*0-89876-017-8*) Gardner Pr.

Encyclopedic Handbook of Biomaterials & Bioengineering. Ed. by Donald L. Wise et al. 1995. LC 95-21232. (Illus.). text 995.00 (*0-8247-9593-8*);Set. 3744p. text 995.00 (*0-8247-9649-7*);Vol. 1. text 995.00 (*0-8247-9595-4*) Dekker.

Encyclopedic Handbook of Biomaterials & Bioengineering: Part A: Materials, Vol. 2. Ed. by Donald L. Wise & Debra J. Trantolo. 1995. (Illus.). 1912p. text 995.00 (*0-8247-9594-6*) Dekker.

Encyclopedic Handbook of Biomaterials & Bioengineering: Part B: Applications, Vol. 2. Ed. by Donald L. Wise & Debra J. Trantolo. 1995. (Illus.). 1832p. text 995.00 (*0-8247-9596-2*) Dekker.

Encyclopedic Handbook of Private Practice. Ed. by Eric Margenau. 1990. LC 87-19624. 1050p. text 120.00 (*0-89876-151-4*) Gardner Pr.

Encyclopedic Reference of Cancer Research. Ed. by Manfred Schwab. 2001. LC 2001-49122. (Illus.). 1500p. 195.00 incl. cd-rom (*3-540-66527-7*) Spr-Verlag.

Encyclopedic Reference of Vascular Biology & Pathology. Andreas Bikfalvi. 2000. 466p. 195.00 incl. cd-rom (*3-540-65289-2*) Spr-Verlag.

Encyclopedie de la Vie Sexuelle, 3: De la Physiologie a la Psychologie, 14-16 Ans. Jean Cohen et al. 1973. (FRE.). 160p. 22.95 (*0-8288-6281-8*, M-6074) Fr & Eur.

Encyclopedie de la Vie Sexuelle, 4: De la Physiologie a la Psychologie, 17-18 Ans. Jean Cohen et al. 1973. (FRE.). 48p. 26.50 (*0-7859-0737-8*, M-6075) Fr & Eur.

Encyclopedie de la Vie Sexuelle, 5: De la Physiologie a la Psychologie, Adultes. Jean Cohen et al. 1973. (FRE.). 48p. 32.95 (*0-8288-6283-4*, M-6076) Fr & Eur.

Encyclopedie Medecines Douces (Natural Medicine) Auzou. 1998. (FRE.). 228p. 69.95 (*0-320-00669-7*) Fr & Eur.

Encyclopedie Medicale de la Famille, Set. Lidis Staff. 1976. (FRE.). 1200p. 650.00 (*0-8288-5688-5*, M6221) Fr & Eur.

Encyclopedie Veterinaire, Set. K. Wamberg. 1974. (ENG & FRE.). 2900p. pap. 695.00 (*0-8288-6042-4*, M6566) Fr & Eur.

End of Cancer. John Lubecki. 2nd ed. (Illus.). 198p. reprint ed. (*1-884030-00-9*) Better Hlth Bks.

End of Life: Guidelines for Health Professionals Concerning Death Certificates, Autopsies & Organ & Tissue Donations. New York Academy of Medicine Staff. Ed. by Charles Hirsch & Jacqueline Messite. rev. ed. 1994. (Illus.). pap. text 10.00 (*0-924143-03-7*) NY Acad Med.

End-of-Life Care & Hospital Legal Counsel: Current Involvements & Future Trends. Connie Zuckerman. 1999. LC 99-202739. vi, 33p. pap. (*1-887748-22-9*) Milbank Memorial.

End-of-Life Decisions: A Psychosocial Perspective. Ed. by Maurice Steinberg & Stuart J. Younger. 1998. LC 97-52636. 330p. text 44.50 (*0-88048-756-9*, 8756) Am Psychiatric.

End-of-Life Decisions: Facing the Challenges of Medical & Ethical Choices. Ed. by Anne M. Christner. 1995. 56p. (Orig.). pap. 29.95 (*1-884937-36-5*) Manisses Communs.

End of Medicine: How I Learned to Quit Worrying & Love My Disease. Kaare Bursell. 2000. 212p. pap. 15.00 (*0-9700262-7-7*, 1) K Bursell.

End of Obesity. Samuel N. Grief & Sophie Ares-Grief. Ed. by Joyce Griffith. 1998. (Illus.). 220p. pap. 14.95 (*0-9660563-0-2*) G&G Pub.

End of the Empty Organism: Neurobiology & the Sciences of Human Action. Elliott White. 1992. LC 92-3571. (Human Evolution, Behavior, & Intelligence Ser.). 168p. 60.00 (*0-275-94368-2*, C4368, Praeger Pubs) Greenwood.

End-Stage Renal Disease: Choosing a Treatment That's Right for You. 1994. (Illus.). 37p. (Orig.). (C). pap. text 15.00 (*0-7881-1235-X*) DIANE Pub.

End Stage Renal Disease: Choosing the Right Treatment. 1997. lib. bdg. 250.95 (*0-8490-8145-9*) Gordon Pr.

End User Searching in the Health Sciences. Ed. by M. Sandra Wood et al. 1986. LC 86-9886. (Medical Reference Services Quarterly Ser.: Supp. Vol. 2). 290p. 49.95 (*0-86656-465-9*) Haworth Pr.

End Your Back & Neck Pain. Tennant & Hall. rev. ed. 1996. (Illus.). 160p. mass mkt. 6.99 (*0-7704-2712-X*) Bantam.

End Your Carpal Tunnel Pain Without Surgery: A Daily Program to Prevent & Treat Carpal Tunnel. Kate Montgomery. 1998. LC 98-9366. (Illus.). 192p. pap. 14.95 (*1-55853-591-8*) Rutledge Hill Pr.

Endangered Lives: Public Health in Victorian Britain. Anthony S. Wohl. 1983. (Illus.). 416p. 35.00 (*0-674-25241-1*) HUP.

Endangered Medical Record: Ensuring Its Integrity in the Age of Informatics. Vergil N. Slee et al. 2000. LC 99-20388. 640p. pap. 49.95 (*0-9615255-2-5*) Tringa Pr.

Endangered Sex: Neglect of Female Children in Rural North India. Barbara Miller. 1981. LC 81-3226. (Illus.). 192p. 32.50 (*0-8014-1371-0*) Cornell U Pr.

Ended Beginnings: Healing Childbearing Losses. Claudia Panuthos & Catherine Romeo. 1984. LC 84-12284. (Illus.). 236p. 29.95 (*0-89789-053-1*, Bergin & Garvey) Greenwood.

Endemic Areas of Tropical Infections. D. Stuerchler. 2nd rev. ed. 1988. LC 88-8977. 450p. (C). text 34.00 (*0-920887-35-X*) Hogrefe & Huber Pubs.

Endemic Cretinism. Basil S. Hetzel & Peter O. Pharoah. 1971. 133p. 42.00 (*0-7855-0625-X*) St Mut.

Endemic Diseases & Risk Factors. 1988. (Illus.). 36p. 34.95 (*0-387-18847-9*) Spr-Verlag.

Endemic Goitre & Thyroid Function in Central Africa. F. Delange. Ed. by Frank Falkner et al. 1974. (Monographs in Pediatrics: Vol. 2). (Illus.). xvi, 160p. 64.50 (*3-8055-1687-8*) S Karger.

Ending the Cycle of Abuse: The Stories of Women Abused As Children & the Group Therapy Techniques That Helped Them Heal. Philip G. Ney & Anna Peters. 1995. LC 94-28150. 272p. 23.95 (*0-87630-752-7*) Brunner-Routledge.

Ending the HIV Epidemic: Community Strategies in Disease Prevention & Health Promotion. Ed. by Steven Petrow et al. 1990. LC 90-6384. 140p. pap. 24.95 (*1-56071-030-6*) ETR Assocs.

Endings & Beginnings: Law, Medicine & Society in Assisted Life & Death. Larry I. Palmer. 2000. LC 99-54876. 160p. 45.00 (*0-275-96681-X*, Praeger Pubs) Greenwood.

Endless Energy. L. Kenton. 1993. (*0-09-177753-4*) Random GBR. *Dist:* Trafalgar.

Endless Journey: A Head-Trauma Victim's Remarkable Rehabilitation. Janet A. Stumbo. unabr. ed. 1998. LC 98-3439. xiii, 209p. pap. 22.95 (*0-943599-26-1*) OEPF.

Endo Nasal, Aural & Allied Techniques: Ear, Eye, Nose & Throat. Thomas T. Lake. 1996. 109p. reprint ed. spiral bd. 11.00 (*0-7873-0521-9*) Hlth Research.

Endocardial Endothelium: Functional Morphology. Luc J. Andries. 1994. LC 93-45589. (Medical Intelligence Unit Ser.). 121p. 99.00 (*1-57059-072-9*, LN9072) Landes Bioscience.

Endocardial Lead Extraction. Peter H. Belott. 1998. LC 98-4104. (Illus.). 160p. pap., tchr. ed. 115.00 incl. VHS (*0-87993-671-1*) Futura Pub.

Endocavitary MRI of the Pelvis. Ed. by Nandita M. deSouza. 2000. 184p. 60.00 (*90-5823-100-3*, Harwood Acad Pubs) Gordon & Breach.

Endocrine Advances in Neonatology. Christine Vanhole. 1998. (Acta Biomedica Lovaniensia Ser.). (Illus.). 165p. pap. (*90-6186-890-4*) Leuven Univ BEL. *Dist:* Coronet Bks.

Endocrine & Hormonal Toxicology. Philip W. Harvey et al. 1999. LC 98-30335. (Illus.). 596p. 250.00 (*0-471-97086-7*) Wiley.

Endocrine & Metabolic Effects of Lithium. John H. Lazarus. 1986. LC 85-28308. (Illus.). 220p. (C). text 90.00 (*0-306-42057-0*, Kluwer Plenum) Kluwer Academic.

Endocrine & Metabolic Emergencies. Ed. by Allan B. Wolfson. 1990. (Contemporary Issues in Emergency Medicine Ser.). (Illus.). 221p. text (*0-443-08626-5*) Church.

Endocrine & Metabolic Testing Manual. Ed. by Robert F. Dons. 2nd ed. 1994. LC 94-10461. 192p. spiral bd. 83.95 (*0-8493-7657-2*) CRC Pr.

Endocrine & Metabolic Testing Manual. Robert F. Dons. 3rd ed. 1997. LC 97-27641. 304p. spiral bd. 84.95 (*0-8493-7606-8*) CRC Pr.

Endocrine & Metabolism. Engelking. 2000. (Quick Look Veterinary Ser.). 23.95 (*1-889325-14-7*) Fence Crk Pubng.

Endocrine & Metabolism Diseases & Disorders Sourcebook: Basic Information for the Layperson about Pancreatic & Insulin-Related Disorders. Ed. by Linda M. Ross. 1998. LC 98-6657. (Health Reference Ser.: Vol. 36). (Illus.). xii, 574p. lib. bdg. 78.00 (*0-7808-0207-1*) Omnigraphics Inc.

Endocrine & Neuroendocrine Mechanisms of Aging. Richard C. Adelman & George S. Roth. 1982. 232p. 99.95 (*0-8493-5811-6*, QP187) CRC Pr.

Endocrine & Nutritional Control of Basic Biological Functions. Ed. by Hendrik Lehnert et al. 1993. LC 91-35313. (Neuronal Control of Bodily Function Ser.: Vol. 7). (Illus.). 580p. text 138.00 (*0-88937-076-1*) Hogrefe & Huber Pubs.

Endocrine & Organ Specific Autoimmunity. George S. Eisenbarth. 1998. LC 98-40838. (Medical Intelligence Unit Ser.: Vol. 13). 271p. 99.00 (*1-57059-538-0*) Landes Bioscience.

Endocrine Aspects of Disease Processes: (Conference Selye) G. Jasmin et al. 1968. LC 68-14063. (Illus.). 468p. 22.75 (*0-87527-020-4*) Green.

Endocrine Autoimmunity & Associated Conditions. Anthony P. Weetman. 1998. LC 98-15828. (Immunology & Medicine Ser.). 292p. 157.00 (*0-7923-5042-1*) Kluwer Academic.

Endocrine Causes of Seasonal & Lactational Anestrus in Farm Animals. Ed. by Franz Ellendorf & F. Elsaesser. 1985. (Current Topics in Veterinary Medicine & Animal Science Ser.). text 154.00 (*0-89838-738-8*) Kluwer Academic.

Endocrine Cell Culture. Ed. by Stephen Bidey. 1998. LC 98-14244. (Handbooks in Practical Animal Cell Biology). (Illus.). 166p. (C). text 74.95 (*0-521-59399-9*) Cambridge U Pr.

Endocrine Diagnosis: Clinical & Laboratory Approach. William F. Streck & Dean H. Lockwood. 1983. 330p. 48.00 (*0-316-81960-3*, Little Brwn Med Div) Lppncott W & W.

Endocrine Disorders: A Guide to Diagnosis. Richard A. Donald. 1984. (Basic & Clinical Endocrinology Ser.: Vol. 4). (Illus.). 760p. text 250.00 (*0-8247-1913-1*) Dekker.

Endocrine Disorders in Thalassemia: Physiological Therapeutic Aspects. M. Maggiolini et al. LC 94-23058. 1996. (Illus.). 208p. 99.00 (*3-540-58390-4*); 1994. 86.00 (*0-387-58390-4*) Spr-Verlag.

Endocrine Disrupters: Advances in Measuring & Analyzing Their Effects. Ed. by Paul Guttry. 1997. (Biomedical Library). pap. (*1-57936-026-2*) Drug & Market Dev.

Endocrine Disruption. Ana Soto. 1997. 191p. pap. text 105.00 (*90-5699-523-5*) Gordon & Breach.

Endocrine Disruptors: Effects of Male & Female Reproductive Systems. Rajesh K. Naz. 1999. LC 98-36723. (Illus.). 384p. 129.95 (*0-8493-3164-1*) CRC Pr.

Endocrine Disturbance. Ed. by Helen F. Galley et al. 2001. (Critical Care Focus Ser.: Vol. 4). (Illus.). 80p. pap. text (*0-7279-1582-7*) BMJ Pub GBR. *Dist:* AIDC.

Endocrine Function & Aging. Ed. by H. J. Armbrecht et al. 1989. (Illus.). 236p. 81.95 (*0-387-97007-X*) Spr-Verlag.

Endocrine Functions & Aging: International Henri-Pierre Klotz Days of Clinical Endocrinology, 37th International Symposium, Paris, May 1994. Ed. by M. Vallotton. 1995. (Journal: Vol. 43, No. 1-3, 1995). (Illus.). 112p. pap. 141.00 (*3-8055-6124-5*) S Karger.

Endocrine Imaging. Martin P. Sandler. 1992. (Illus.). 461p. (C). pap. text 149.00 (*0-8385-2206-8*, A2206-9, Apple Lange Med) McGraw.

Endocrine Management of Benign Gynecologic Disease. Alvin Goldfarb. 1997. LC 97-42608. (Illus.). 224p. (*0-412-12671-0*) E A GBR. *Dist:* OUP.

Endocrine Management of Cancer. Ed. by Basil A. Stoll. 1988. (Limited Volume Ser.: Vols. 1 & 2). (Illus.). xvi, 424p. Complete Set. 218.50 (*3-8055-4687-4*); Vol. 1: Biological Bases. 116.75 (*3-8055-4685-8*); Vol. 2: Contemporary Therapy. 126.25 (*3-8055-4686-6*) S Karger.

Endocrine Management of Infertility. T. J. Wilkin. 1988. xii, 102p. kivar 106.00 (*3-7186-4827-X*) Gordon & Breach.

Endocrine Methods. Ed. by John A. Thomas. 1996. (Illus.). 458p. text 85.00 (*0-12-688460-9*) Acad Pr.

Endocrine Neoplasms. Andrew Arnold. 1997. LC 96-49030. (Cancer Treatment & Research Ser.). 786p. text 412.50 (*0-7923-4354-9*) Kluwer Academic.

Endocrine Oncology. Ed. by Stephen P. Ethier. 2000. LC 00-40912. (Contemporary Endocrinology Ser.). (Illus.). 408p. 145.00 (*0-89603-621-9*) Humana.

***Endocrine Pathology.** Virginia A. Livolsi & Sylvia Asa. (Illus.). 635p. text (*0-443-06595-0*) Saunders.

Endocrine Pathology. Ricardo V. Lloyd. 1990. (Illus.). 275p. 114.00 (*0-387-97166-1*) Spr-Verlag.

Endocrine Pathology of the Gut & Pancreas. Yogeshwar Dayal. 1991. (Illus.). 328p. lib. bdg. 202.00 (*0-8493-5993-7*, RC280) CRC Pr.

Endocrine Pathology Update. Cecilia M. Fenoglio-Preiser. 1990. 85.00 (*0-938607-18-9*) Field & Wood Inc Medical.

Endocrine Pathophysiology. C. Niewoehner. 1997. (Pathophysiology Ser.). pap. 30.95 (*1-889325-02-3*) Blackwell Sci.

Endocrine Pathophysiology: A Problem-Oriented Approach. Ronald A. Arky & William M. Kettyle. 1998. LC 98-18408. (Illus.). 352p. pap. text 32.95 (*0-397-51376-3*) Lppncott W & W.

Endocrine Physiology. Susan P. Porterfield. 1996. (Illus.). 272p. (C). (gr. 13). pap. text 31.00 (*0-8151-8492-1*, 28438) Mosby Inc.

Endocrine Regulation of Early Embryonic Development & Implantation: Tokyo Conference of Reproductive Physiology II, Tokyo, August 1994. Ed. by A. Miyake & H. Suginami. 1995. (Journal: Vol. 44, Suppl. 2, 1995). (Illus.). iv, 50p. pap. 26.25 (*3-8055-6169-5*) S Karger.

Endocrine Regulation of Human Gestation: Proceedings of the WHO Scientific Group, Geneva, 1970. WHO Staff. 1971. (Technical Reports: No. 471). pap. text 5.00 (*92-4-120471-0*, 1100471) World Health.

Endocrine Rhythms: Roles of the Sleep-Wake Cycle, the Circadian Clock & the Environment: Diagnostic & Therapeutic Implications 40th International Henri-Pierre Klotz Symposium on Clinical

Endocrinology, Paris, May 1997. Ed. by Georges Copinschi & Eve Van Cauter. 1998. (Hormone Research Ser.: Vol. 49, Nos. 3-4). (Illus.). 98p. pap. 85.25 (*3-8055-6666-2*) S Karger.

Endocrine Role of the Pineal Gland. Sue A. Binkley. 1988. (Illus.). 288p. (C). pap. text 48.00 (*0-13-277146-2*) P-H.

Endocrine Secrets: Questions You Will Be Asked on Rounds, in the Clinic, on Oral Exams. Ed. by Michael T. McDermott. 2nd ed. 1998. LC 97-81435. (Secrets Ser.). (Illus.). 350p. pap. 39.95 (*1-56053-268-8*) Hanley & Belfus.

Endocrine Society Clinical Endocrinology Update: 1995 Syllabus. Ed. by Ed W. Dillmann. 1995. (Illus.). 382p. (C). pap. text 55.00 (*1-879225-20-4*) Endocrine Soc.

Endocrine Society Forty-Sixth Annual Postgraduate Assembly Syllabus, 1994. Ed. by Lawrence A. Leiter. 1994. (Illus.). 350p. (C). pap. text 35.00 (*1-879225-15-8*) Endocrine Soc.

Endocrine Society Forty-Third Postgraduate Assembly Syllabus, 1991: Annual Postgraduate Assembly Syllabus, 43rd. Faculty of Endocrine Society. Ed. by Paul I. Jagger. 1991. (Illus.). 512p. (C). pap. text 10.00 (*1-879225-03-4*) Endocrine Soc.

Endocrine Society Introduction to Molecular & Cellular Research, 1995. Ed. by Marvin C. Gershengorn & Henry M. Kronenberg. 1995. (Illus.). 180p. (C). pap. text 45.00 (*1-879225-16-6*) Endocrine Soc.

Endocrine Society Introduction to Molecular & Cellular Research, 1996. Ed. by Henry M. Kronenberg. 1996. (Illus.). 180p. (Orig.). (C). pap. text 60.00 (*1-879225-21-2*) Endocrine Soc.

***Endocrine Surgery.** Ed. by John R. Farndon. 2001. 405p. (*0-7020-2594-1*) W B Saunders GBR. *Dist:* Saunders.

Endocrine Surgery. Richard Prinz. 1999. (Vademecum Ser.). spiral bd. 45.00 (*1-57059-574-7*) Landes Bioscience.

Endocrine Surgery of the Head & Neck. Phillip Pellitteri. 2001. 400p. pap. 150.00 (*0-7693-0091-X*) Singular Publishing.

Endocrine System. Thomas Braem. 1994. (Organs of the Human Anatomy: Vol. 8). 88p. (C). spiral bd. 15.95 (*1-878576-34-8*) Flash Anatomy Inc.

Endocrine System. Goodman. 2000. (Integrated Medical Sciences Ser.). 25.95 (*1-889325-32-5*) Fence Crk Pubng.

Endocrine System. Ed. by Ulrich Mohr. 1994. (Illus.). 88p. pap. text 30.00 (*92-832-0126-4*) OUP.

Endocrine System. Ed. by T. C. Jones et al. 2nd ed. 1996. LC 95-31393. (Illus.). xvi, 400p. 320.00 (*0-944398-64-2*, 398642) ILSI.

Endocrine System. Ed. by W. S. Symmers & P. D. Lewis. 3rd ed. 1996. (Systemic Pathology Ser.: No. 12). (Illus.). 314p. text (*0-443-03116-9*) Church.

Endocrine System, Vol. 4. Ed. by Bruce S. McEwen. 2000. LC 98-12003. (Handbook of Physiology Ser.). (Illus.). 574p. text 150.00 (*0-19-511252-0*) OUP.

Endocrine System Course. Competence Assurance Systems Staff. 1981. (Illus.). pap. text 45.00 (*0-89147-063-8*) CAS.

Endocrine Therapy & Growth Regulation of Breast Cancer. Ed. by U. Eppenberger & A. Goldhirsch. 1989. (Recent Results in Cancer Research Ser.: Vol. 113). (Illus.). 92p. 76.00 (*0-387-50456-7*) Spr-Verlag.

Endocrine Therapy of Breast Cancer. Ed. by U. Eppenberger. 1986. (Beitraege Zur Onkologie, Contributions to Oncology Ser.: Vol. 23). (Illus.). viii, 96p. 43.50 (*3-8055-4324-7*) S Karger.

Endocrine Therapy of Breast Cancer VI. Ed. by A. Howell. 1994. LC 93-48231. (Monographs of the European School of Oncology). (Illus.). 99p. 76.95 (*0-387-57690-8*) Spr-Verlag.

Endocrine Toxicology. Ed. by Christopher K. Atterwill & J. D. Flack. 1992. (Illus.). 489p. (C). text 110.00 (*0-521-40225-5*) Cambridge U Pr.

Endocrine Toxicology. Sokol. 1994. (*0-8493-8894-5*, CRC Reprint) Franklin.

Endocrine Toxicology. J. A. Thomas & Howard D. Colby. 2nd ed. 1996. LC 95-39059. (Target Organ Toxicology Ser.). 352p. 150.00 (*1-56032-613-1*) Taylor & Francis.

Endocrine Tumors. Orio H. Clark et al. 2000. (ACS Atlas of Clinical Oncology Ser.). 300p. incl. cd-rom (*1-55009-134-4*) DEKR.

Endocrine Tumors. Naguib A. Samaan. Ed. by Ernest L. Mazzaferri. 1993. LC 92-49583. (Illus.). 896p. 275.00 (*0-86542-267-2*) Blackwell Sci.

Endocrine Tumors of the Pancreas. Ed. by M. Mignon & Randall T. Jensen. 1994. LC 94-27027. (Frontiers of Gastrointestinal Research Ser.: Vol. 23). (Illus.). xii, 482p. 323.50 (*3-8055-5953-4*) S Karger.

Endocrines & Aging. O. H. Robertson et al. 1972. 232p. text 49.50 (*0-8422-7029-9*) Irvington.

Endocrinological Aspects of Alcoholism. Ed. by F. S. Messiha & G. S. Tyner. 1981. (Progress in Biochemical Pharmacology Ser.: Vol. 18). (Illus.). xii, 232p. 135.00 (*3-8055-2689-X*) S Karger.

Endocrinology. Mac E. Hadley. 1984. (Illus.). 592p. (C). text 45.00 (*0-13-277137-3*) P-H.

Endocrinology. Andrew Levy & Stafford L. Lightman. 1997. LC 97-7853. (Oxford Core Texts). (Illus.). 398p. pap. text 37.50 (*0-19-262766-X*) OUP.

Endocrinology. Ed. by S. M. McCann. 1988. (People & Ideas Ser.). (Illus.). 484p. text 75.00 (*0-19-520718-1*) OUP.

Endocrinology. Peter H. Wise. 1986. LC 85-21306. (Colour Aids Ser.). (Illus.). 108p. (Orig.). pap. text (*0-443-03374-9*) Church.

Endocrinology. Peter H. Wise. 1994. LC 94-5219. (Colour Guide Ser.). (Orig.). pap. text 16.95 (*0-443-04979-3*) Harcrt Hlth Sci Grp.

Endocrinology. 2nd ed. 1984. (Medical Ser.). (Illus.). (C). 12.95 (*0-935920-20-X*, Ntl Pubs Blck) P-H.

Endocrinology. Warner M. Burch. 3rd ed. 1994. (House Officer Ser.). (Illus.). 200p. pap. text 29.95 (*0-683-01131-6*) Lppncott W & W.

Endocrinology. P. H. Regents. 3rd ed. 1993. 64p. pap. 16.91 (*0-13-035502-X*) P-H.

Endocrinology Leslie J. Degroot & Larry Jameson. 4th ed. 2000. 2925p. text 495.00 (*0-7216-7840-8*) Saunders.

Endocrinology. Ed. by Leslie J. DeGroot et al. 3rd ed. 1994. LC 93-8208. 1. (*0-7216-4263-2*); 2. (*0-7216-4264-0*); 3. (*0-7216-4265-9*); Set. text 475.00 (*0-7216-4262-4*) Saunders.

Endocrinology: A Nursing Approach. Norma C. Muthe. 1981. pap. 13.00 (*0-316-59160-2*, Little Brwn Med Div) Lppncott W & W.

***Endocrinology: An Integrated Approach.** S. S. Nussey & S. A. Whitehead. 2001. 376p. pap. (*1-85996-252-1*) Bios Sci GBR. *Dist:* Spr-Verlag.

Endocrinology: Basic & Clinical Principles. Ed. by P. Michael Conn & Shlomo Melmed. 1997. LC 96-43898. (Illus.). 460p. 135.00 (*0-89603-349-X*) Humana.

Endocrinology: Key Questions Answered. John Laycock & Peter Wise. 1997. LC 98-107373. (Illus.). 332p. pap. text 35.00 (*0-19-262846-1*) OUP.

Endocrinology Section 7: Cellular Mechanisms, Vol. I. Ed. by P. Michael Conn & H. Maurice Goodman. 1998. LC 98-12003. (Handbook of Physiology Ser.). (Illus.). 616p. text 165.00 (*0-19-510935-X*) OUP.

Endocrinology & Metabolism. Aldo Pinchera et al. 2001. (Clinical Medicine Ser.). (Illus.). 700p. pap. 79.95 (*0-07-709520-0*) McGraw-Hill Prof.

Endocrinology & Metabolism in the Elderly. Ed. by J. E. Morley & Stanley G. Korenman. 1992. (Current Issues in Endocrinology & Metabolism Ser.). (Illus.). 592p. 150.00 (*0-86542-148-X*) Blackwell Sci.

Endocrinology & Reproduction. Mary Thompson & Rachakonda Nagabhushanam. Ed. by Milton Fingerman et al. 1997. (Recent Advances in Marine Biotechnology Ser.). 536p. 125.00 (*1-886106-53-3*) Science Pubs.

Endocrinology for Primary Care. Ernest L. Mazzaferri. 1999. text 49.00 (*0-7216-6044-4*) Saunders.

Endocrinology of Aging. Ed. by John E. Morley & Lucretia Van den Berg. 2000. LC 99-31970. (Contemporary Endocrinology Ser.: Vol. 20). 280p. 99.50 (*0-89603-756-8*) Humana.

Endocrinology of Aging. Ed. by W. A. Scherbaum & W. G. Rossmanith. 1995. x, 176p. (Orig.). (C). pap. text 113.85 (*3-11-014591-X*) De Gruyter.

Endocrinology of Breast Cancer. Andrea Manni. 1999. LC 98-33989. (Contemporary Endocrinology Ser.: Vol. 11). (Illus.). 408p. 145.00 (*0-89603-591-3*) Humana.

Endocrinology of Cancer David P. Rose. Vol. 1. 1979. 160p. 91.00 (*0-8493-5337-8*, RC271); Vol. 2. 1979. 160p. 98.00 (*0-8493-5338-6*); Vol. 3. 1982. 208p. 119.00 (*0-8493-5339-4*, RC271) Franklin (CRC Reprint).

Endocrinology of Cardiovascular Function. Ellis R. Levin. 1998. LC 98-12410. (Endocrine Updates Ser.). 189.95 (*0-7923-8217-X*) Kluwer Academic.

Endocrinology of Critical Disease. Ed. by K. Patrick Ober. 1997. LC 97-198438. (Contemporary Endocrinology Ser.: Vol. 4). (Illus.). 336p. 140.00 (*0-89603-422-4*) Humana.

Endocrinology of Embryo-Endometrium Interactions. Ed. by Stanley R. Glasser et al. 1994. (Illus.). 428p. (C). text 125.00 (*0-306-44809-2*, Kluwer Plenum) Kluwer Academic.

***Endocrinology of Paturition: Basic Science & Clinical Application.** Ed. by R. Smith. 2001. (Frontiers of Hormone Research Ser.: Vol. 27). (Illus.). xiv, 316p. 260.00 (*3-8055-7195-X*) S Karger.

Endocrinology of Pregnancy. Fuller W. Bazer. 1998. LC 98-3059. (Contemporary Endocrinology Ser.: Vol. 9). (Illus.). 592p. 175.00 (*0-89603-462-3*) Humana.

Endocrinology of Puberty: Journal: Hormone Research, Vol. 36, Nos. 3 & 4, 1991. Ed. by J. Girard. 1992. (Illus.). 76p. pap. 85.25 (*3-8055-5597-0*) S Karger.

Endocrinology of Reproduction & Fertility: Practical Diagnosis & Treatment. Daniel Spratt & Nanette Santoro. 1999. (Contemporary Endocrinology Ser.). 500p. 125.00 (*0-89603-554-9*) Humana.

Endocrinology of the Lung: Development & Surfactant Synthesis. Ed. by Carole R. Mendelson. 2000. LC 99-52787. (Contemporary Endocrinology Ser.). (Illus.). 360p. 139.50 (*0-89603-676-6*) Humana.

Endocrinology of the Vasculature. Ed. by J. R. Sowers. 1996. LC 96-172071. (Contemporary Endocrinology Ser.: Vol. 1). (Illus.). 408p. 170.00 (*0-89603-363-5*) Humana.

Endocrinology of Thermal Injury: Pathophysiologic Mechanisms & Clinical Interpretation. Rajko Dolecek et al. Ed. by George Vaughan. 1990. LC 89-12668. (Illus.). 469p. text 85.00 (*0-8121-1127-3*) Lppncott W & W.

Endocrinology 2000: An Internet Resource Guide. Ed. by Dan Goldenson. 2000. pap. 24.95 (*0-9700525-1-0*) eMedguides.

Endocytobiology: Endosymbiosis & Cell Research. Ed. by H. Schenk et al. 1980. 1060p. (C). text 146.15 (*3-11-008299-3*) De Gruyter.

Endocytobiology II: Intracelluar Space Oligogenetic Ecosystem. 1983. LC 83-20973. (Illus.). xxv, 1071p. 226.95 (*3-11-008660-3*) De Gruyter.

Endocytosis. Ed. by Ira H. Pastan & Mark C. Willingham. 1985. LC 85-3436. 344p. 89.50 (*0-306-41853-3*, Plenum Trade) Perseus Pubng.

Endocytosis: From Cell Biology to Health, Disease & Therapy. Ed. by Pierre J. Courtoy et al. 1992. LC 92-2176. (NATO ASI Ser.: Vol. 62). (Illus.). 529p. 341.00 (*0-387-53146-7*) Spr-Verlag.

Endocytosis & Exocytosis in Host Defence. Ed. by L. Edebo et al. 1981. (Monographs in Allergy: Vol. 17). (Illus.). viii, 272p. pap. 142.75 (*3-8055-1865-X*) S Karger.

Endodontic Surgery. C. R. Stockdale. 1993. (Illus.). 122p. text 56.00 (*1-85097-020-3*) Quint Pub Co.

Endodontic Therapy, Vol. 5. Franklin S. Weine. 5th ed. 1995. (Illus.). 880p. (C). (gr. 13). text 85.00 (*0-8016-7963-X*, 07963) Mosby Inc.

Endodontics. Ed. by John I. Ingle & Jerry F. Taintor. 4th ed. 1994. (Illus.). 960p. text 90.00 (*0-683-04310-2*) Lppncott W & W.

Endodontics. John I. Ingle & Leif K. Bakland. 5th ed. 2002. 700p. text 74.95 (*0-683-30696-0*) Lppncott W & W.

Endodontics in Clinical Practice. F. J. Harty. 3rd ed. 1990. (Dental Practitioners' Handbook Ser.: Vol. 24). (Illus.). 366p. pap. 80.00 (*0-7236-1955-7*) Buttrwrth-Heinemann.

Endodontics in Clinical Practice. Ed. by F. J. Harty et al. 4th ed. 1997. LC 96-30102. (Dental Practitioners' Handbook Ser.: Vol. 24). 296p. pap. text 70.00 (*0-7236-1020-7*) Buttrwrth-Heinemann.

***Endodontology.** Bergenholtz. 2002. text (*87-16-12185-6*) Black Mksgaard DNK. *Dist:* Iowa U Pr.

Endogene Opiate in der Gynaekologischen Endokrinologie. Ed. by Eduard Gitsch. 1987. (Journal: Vol. 27, Suppl. 1, 1987). (Illus.). iv, 56p. pap. 20.00 (*3-8055-4625-4*) S Karger.

Endogenous Mediators of Gastrointestinal Damage. Ed. by John L. Wallace. 1989. 232p. 190.00 (*0-8493-4574-X*, RC5453) CRC Pr.

Endogenous Peptides & Centrally Acting Drugs. Ed. by A. Levy et al. 1980. (Progress in Biochemical Pharmacology Ser.: Vol. 16). (Illus.). xvi, 160p. 71.50 (*3-8055-0831-X*) S Karger.

Endogenous Regulatory Peptides: Chemistry, Biology & Medical Significance. J. Menyhart. 1989. (Illus.). 923p. (C). (*963-05-5592-1*) Akade Kiado HUN. *Dist:* Intl Spec Bk, St Mut.

Endogenous Sleep Substances & Sleep Regulation. Ed. by Shojiro Inoue & A. A. Borbely. 1985. (Taniguchi Symposia on Brain Sciences Ser.: No. 8). 276p. lib. bdg. (*90-6764-058-1*) VSP NLD. *Dist:* Coronet Bks.

Endoluminal Ultrasound. Barry B. Goldberg & Ji-Bin Liu. 1998. 368p. (*1-85317-236-7*) Martin Dunitz GBR. *Dist:* Mosby Inc.

Endoluminal Vascular Prostheses. Ed. by Timothy A. Chuter et al. 2nd ed. 2001. (Illus.). (*0-87993-642-8*) Futura Pub.

Endolymphatic Duct & Sac: Journal: Oto-Rhino-Laryngology, Vol. 54, No. 4, 1992. Ed. by M. Anniko. 1992. (Illus.). 60p. pap. 58.50 (*3-8055-5640-3*) S Karger.

Endometrial Ablation. Ed. by B. Victor Lewis & Adam L. Magos. 1993. LC 92-21014. 232p. text (*0-443-04587-9*) Church.

Endometrial Cancer. Ed. by Earl A. Surwit & David S. Alberts. 1989. (Cancer Treatment & Research Ser.). (C). text 142.50 (*0-7923-0286-9*) Kluwer Academic.

Endometrial Cancers. Ed. by M. Bolla. 1986. (Illus.). x, 270p. 128.75 (*3-8055-4211-9*) S Karger.

Endometriosi: Italian. P. L. Venturini. 2001. 156p. (*1-84214-068-X*, Parthenon Pbng) CRC Pr.

Endometriosis. Julia Older. 1985. (Illus.). 240p. pap. 10.95 (*0-684-18505-9*) Hungry Minds.

Endometriosis: A Natural Approach. Jo Mears. 1997. (Illus.). 184p. (Orig.). pap. 9.95 (*1-56975-088-2*) Ulysses Pr.

Endometriosis: Contemporary Concepts of Clinical Management. Robert S. Schenken. 1988. LC 65-10317. (Illus.). 320p. text 59.50 (*0-397-50866-2*, Lippncott) Lppncott W & W.

Endometriosis: Current Understanding & Management. Ed. by Robert W. Shaw. 1995. LC 94-36488. 304p. 99.95 (*0-86542-821-2*) Blackwell Sci.

Endometriosis: The Enigmatic Disease. Stephen Corson. 1992. 257p. pap. 12.95 (*0-929240-42-1*) EMIS.

Endometriosis & Infertility & Traditional Chinese Medicine: A Laywoman's Guide. Bob Flaws. 1989. (Illus.). 115p. (Orig.). pap. 10.95 (*0-936185-14-7*) Blue Poppy Pr.

Endometriosis Sourcebook. Endometriosis Association Staff & Mary Lou Ballweg. 1995. LC 95-24526. (Illus.). 496p. pap. 16.95 (*0-8092-3263-4*, 326340, Contemporary) McGraw-Hill Trade.

Endometriosis Survival Guide: Your Guide to the Latest Treatment Options & the Best Coping Strategies. Margot J. Fromer. 1998. LC 98-66707. (Illus.). 199p. pap. 13.95 (*1-57224-152-7*) New Harbinger.

Endometriosis Today: Proceedings of the Vth World Congress, Yokohama, Japan, 21-24 October, 1996 Ed. by Hiroshi Minaguchi. 1997. LC 97-15483. (International Congress, Symposium, & Seminar Ser.). (Illus.). 496p. lib. bdg. 145.95 (*1-85070-901-7*, Parthenon Pbng) CRC Pr.

Endometrium: A Clinico-Pathologic Approach. Debra S. Heller. 1994. LC 93-39684. (Illus.). 240p. 79.50 (*0-89640-244-4*) Igaku-Shoin.

Endometrium & Endometriosis. Michael P. Diamond & Kevin G. Osteen. 1997. LC 97-12678. (Illus.). 704p. 145.00 (*0-86542-502-7*) Blackwell Sci.

Endometrium as a Target for Contraception. H. M. Beier et al. 1996. LC 96-29098. (Ernst Schering Research Foundation Ser.). (*0-387-61257-2*); (Illus.). 229p. 79.50 (*3-540-61257-2*) Spr-Verlag.

Endomyocardial Biopsy Techniques & Applications. Ed. by John J. Fenoglio, Jr. 1982. 176p. 103.00 (*0-8493-5630-X*, RC683, CRC Reprint) Franklin.

Endomyocardial Fibrosis. Ed. by M. S. Vallathan et al. 1993. (Illus.). 318p. text 41.95 (*0-19-563237-0*) OUP.

Endoprosthetics: Commemorative Volume for Dr. Otto Frey-Zund. Ed. by E. W. Morscher. 1995. LC 95-30520. (Illus.). 400p. 160.00 (*3-540-58499-4*) Spr-Verlag.

Endoscope & Peripheral Equipment Markets. Market Intelligence Staff. 1994. 310p. 1995.00 (*0-7889-0044-7*) Frost & Sullivan.

Endoscopes & Peripheral Equipment Markets: Technology Pays off - Less Invasive Procedures Benefit Physicians & Patients. Market Intelligence Staff. 1992. 319p. 1895.00 (*1-56753-175-X*) Frost & Sullivan.

Endoscopic Accessory Markets: A Fresh Look: New Instruments for New Procedures. Market Intelligence Staff. 1993. 268p. 1895.00 (*1-56753-449-X*) Frost & Sullivan.

Endoscopic Anatomy for Neurosurgery. Alex Perneczky et al. 1993. (Illus.). 350p. text 399.00 (*0-86577-490-0*) Thieme Med Pubs.

Endoscopic Anatomy of the Middle Ear. Manfred Tschabitscher & Clemens Klug. 2000. (Illus.). 140p. 149.00 (*3-211-82973-3*) Spr-Verlag.

Endoscopic Anatomy of the Paranasal Sinuses. Peter S. Hechl et al. 1997. LC 97-12722. (Illus.). 200p. 210.00 (*3-211-82922-9*) Spr-Verlag.

Endoscopic & Laparoscopic Ultrasonography for Surgeons: Colon, Rectum & Anus. Jeffrey W. Milsom et al. 1997. LC 96-52546. (*4-260-14338-7*) Igaku-Shoin.

Endoscopic Approach to Bilio-Pancreatic Disease. L. Familiari. 1988. 196p. text (*1-57235-023-7*) Piccin Nuova.

Endoscopic Approaches to Cancer Diagnosis & Treatment. Ed. by Yanao Oguro & Kunio Takagi. 1990. (Gann Monographs on Cancer Research: No. 37). 172p. (*0-7484-0016-8*) Tay Francis Ltd GBR. *Dist:* Taylor & Francis.

Endoscopic Control of Gastrointestinal Hemorrhage. Ed. by John P. Papp. 1981. 200p. 119.00 (*0-8493-6295-4*, RC802, CRC Reprint) Franklin.

Endoscopic Diagnosis in Gastroenterology: Fourth Extended & Illustrated Edition of Terminology, Definitions, & Diagnostic Criteria in Digestive Endoscopy. Zdenek Maratka. 4th exp. ed. 1999. (Illus.). 260p. text 40.00 (*0-926592-20-3*) Normed Verlag.

***Endoscopic Diagnosis of the Female Lower Urinary Tract.** Geoffrey W. Cundiff & Alfred E. Bent. 1999. (Illus.). 157p. (*0-7020-2352-3*) W B Saunders GBR. *Dist:* Saunders.

Endoscopic Evaluation & Treatment of Swallowing Disorders. Susan E. Langmore. 2000. LC 00-56811. (Illus.). 224p. 89.00 (*0-86577-838-8*) Thieme Med Pubs.

Endoscopic Facial Plastic Surgery. Gregory S. Keller. 1997. LC 96-45493. (Illus.). 176p. (C). (gr. 13). text 99.95 (*0-8151-5192-6*, 26549) Mosby Inc.

Endoscopic Feto-Placental Surgery: From Animal Experiments to Early Human Applications. Jan A. Deprest. 1999. (Acta Biomedica Lovaniensia Ser.: Vol. 198). (Illus.). 164p. pap. (*90-6186-963-3*) Leuven Univ BEL. *Dist:* Coronet Bks.

Endoscopic Gastric Surgery. Ed. by E. Hanisch et al. 1999. (Illus.). 144p. 85.00 (*3-540-65333-3*) Spr-Verlag.

Endoscopic Interpretation. Loren Laine. 2nd ed. 1998. LC 97-16692. 800p. text 185.00 (*0-7817-0290-9*) Lppncott W & W.

Endoscopic Laser Surgery Handbook. Ed. by Stanley M. Shapshay. 1987. (Science & Practice of Surgery Ser.: Vol. 10). (Illus.). 520p. text 175.00 (*0-8247-7711-5*) Dekker.

Endoscopic Laser Surgery of the Trachea & Esophagus. W. Steiner. 2000. (Illus.). 145p. 105.00 (*0-86577-904-X*) Thieme Med Pubs.

Endoscopic Management of Gynecologic Disease. Ed. by G. David Adamson & Daniel C. Martin. 1995. LC 94-48584. (Illus.). 464p. text 169.00 (*0-7817-0281-X*) Lppncott W & W.

Endoscopic Paranasal Sinus Surgery. Dale H. Rice & Steven D. Schaefer. 2nd ed. 1992. LC 92-17094. (Illus.). 272p. text 149.00 (*0-88167-946-1*) Lppncott W & W.

Endoscopic Plastic Surgery. John Bostwick, III et al. 1994. LC 94-40344. (Illus.). 584p. 325.00 (*0-942219-65-1*) Quality Med Pub.

Endoscopic Plastic Surgery. John Bostwick, 3rd et al. 2nd ed. 2000. (Illus.). 350p. 275.00 (*1-57626-005-4*) Quality Med Pub.

Endoscopic Sclerotherapy of Esophageal Varices, 1. Ed. by Michael V. Sivak, Jr. 1984. LC 84-4864. (Gastroenterology Ser.: Vol. 1). 157p. 57.75 (*0-275-91453-4*, C1453, Praeger Pubs) Greenwood.

Endoscopic Sinus Surgery. Howard L. Levine & Mark May. 1993. LC 92-49512. (Rhinology & Sinusology Ser.). (Illus.). 256p. 149.00 (*0-86577-474-9*) Thieme Med Pubs.

Endoscopic Sinus Surgery. Terence M. Davidson. 2nd rev. ed. 1998. LC 98-36304. (Self-Instructional Package Ser.). (Illus.). 164p. pap. text 25.00 (*1-56772-068-4*, 5506515) AAO-HNS.

Endoscopic Sinus Surgery: A Practical Approach. S. K. Kaluskar. 1997. LC 96-17383. (Illus.). 128p. 140.00 (*3-540-19989-6*) Spr-Verlag.

Endoscopic Sinus Surgery: New Horizons. Nikhil J. Bhatt. 1997. LC 97-20818. (Illus.). 196p. (Orig.). 159.95 (*1-56593-897-6*, 1766) Thomson Learn.

***Endoscopic Spine Surgery: Thoracoscopic, Laparoscopic, Retroperitoneoscopic.** Angela Olinger & Ulrich Hildebrandt. 2001. (Illus.). 130p. (*3-540-66487-4*) Spr-Verlag.

Endoscopic Staining in Early Diagnosis of Esophageal Cancer. Ed. by Mitsuo Endo & Hiroko Ide. 1991. text (*4-7622-4668-9*) Busn Ctr Acad JPN. *Dist:* Intl Spec Bk.

Endoscopic Surgery. Peter Ball. 1997. LC 96-44663. (Perioperative Nursing Ser.). (Illus.). 224p. (C). (gr. 13). text 54.95 (*0-8151-0600-9*, 27473) Mosby Inc.

Endoscopic Surgery. Ed. by Frederick L. Greene & Jeffrey L. Ponsky. 1994. LC 93-4600. text 163.00 (*0-7216-4504-6*) Saunders.

Endoscopic Surgery for Gynecologists. Ed. by Chris Sutton & Michael P. Diamond. 2nd ed. 1998. (Illus.). 670p. (C). text (*0-7020-2250-0*) W B Saunders GBR. *Dist:* Saunders.

***Endoscopic Surgery for Gynecologists.** Ed. by Chris Sutton & Michael P. Diamond. 2nd ed. 1998. (Illus.). 724p. text (*0-7020-2489-9*) W B Saunders GBR. *Dist:* Saunders.

Endoscopic Surgery in Children. Ed. by N. M. A. Bax et al. 1999. LC 99-10448. (Illus.). 509p. 129.00 (*3-540-64073-8*) Spr-Verlag.

Endoscopic Surgery of the Paranasal Sinuses & Anterior Skull Base. E. M. Wigand. 1990. (Illus.). 160p. text 119.00 (*0-86577-369-6*) Thieme Med Pubs.

Endoscopic Techniques in Plastic & Aesthetic Surgery. Ed. by Oscar M. Ramirez & Rollin K. Daniel. 1995. LC 95-16149. (Illus.). 352p. 327.00 (*0-387-94466-4*) Spr-Verlag.

Endoscopic Ultrasonography. Frank Gress & Ishan Bhattacharya. 2000. LC 00-56421. (Illus.). 200p. 104.95 (*0-86542-565-5*) Blackwell Sci.

Endoscopic Ultrasonography in Gastroenterology. Keiichi Kawai. 1988. LC 88-8429. (Illus.). 170p. 98.00 (*0-89640-151-0*) Igaku-Shoin.

Endoscopy. Ed. by Gunther O. Schlag & W. Wayand. 1995. LC 94-37089. (Fibrin Sealing in Surgical & Nonsurgical Fields Ser.: Vol. 8). xiv, 117p. (*3-540-58282-7*) Spr-Verlag.

Endoscopy & Biopsy in Gastroenterology. P. Fruehmorgen & M. Claasen. 1980. (Illus.). 198p. 57.95 (*0-387-09645-0*) Spr-Verlag.

Endoscopy in Neuro-Otology. Jacques Magnan & M. Sanna. 1999. LC 98-32395. (Illus.). 119p. 129.00 (*0-86577-828-0*) Thieme Med Pubs.

Endoscopy of Paranasal Sinuses. 1983. 118.00 (*0-387-92115-X*) Spr-Verlag.

Endoscopy of the Central & Peripheral Nervous System. Wesley King et al. 1997. LC 97-33644. (Illus.). 344p. 179.00 (*0-86577-690-3*) Thieme Med Pubs.

Endoscopy of the Colon, Rectum & Anus. Jame M. Church. 1995. (Illus.). 448p. 129.50 (*0-89640-264-9*) Igaku-Shoin.

Endoscopy Pancreatic Disease: Diagnosis & Therapy. Alberto Tittobello & Pier Alberto Testoni. 1998. text 130.00 (*0-7234-2481-0*) Mosby Inc.

Endosonography. Ed. by Bruno D. Fornage. 1990. (C). text 248.50 (*0-7923-0047-5*) Kluwer Academic.

Endosonography in Obstetrics & Gynecology. G. Bernaschek et al. 1990. (Illus.). 187p. 181.00 (*0-387-50328-5*) Spr-Verlag.

Endosseous Implants: Scientific & Clinical Aspects. Ed. by Georg Watzek. 1996. LC 95-38989. (Illus.). 407p. text 210.00 (*0-86715-302-4*) Quint Pub Co.

Endosseous Implants for Maxillofacial Reconstruction. Michael S. Block & John N. Kent. 1995. LC 94-21278. (Illus.). 624p. text 195.00 (*0-7216-3958-5*) Saunders.

Endothelial Cell: A Pluripotent Control Cell of the Vessel Wall. Ed. by D. G. Thilo-Koerner & R. I. Freshney. 1983. (Illus.). viii, 208p. 101.00 (*3-8055-3708-5*) S Karger.

Endothelial Cell Biology in Health & Disease. N. Simionescu & M. Simionescu. 1988. LC 88-15935. (Illus.). 478p. (C). 130.00 (*0-306-42751-6*, Kluwer Plenum) Kluwer Academic.

Endothelial Cell Dysfunctions. N. Simionescu & M. Simionescu. 1991. (Illus.). 592p. (C). text 125.00 (*0-306-43863-1*, Kluwer Plenum) Kluwer Academic.

Endothelial Cell Function in Diabetic Microangiopathy: Problems in Methodology & Clinical Aspects. Ed. by F. Belfiore et al. 1990. (Frontiers in Diabetes Ser.: Vol. 9). (Illus.). 212p. pap. 168.75 (*3-8055-5052-9*) S Karger.

Endothelial Cell Vesicles. Ed. by F. Hammersen & K. Messmer. 1985. (Mikrozirkulation in Forschung und Klinik Ser.: Vol. 9). (Illus.). x, 174p. pap. 68.75 (*3-8055-4070-1*) S Karger.

Endothelial Function in Hypertension. David J. Webb & P. Vallance. 1997. LC 97-17213. (Illus.). 154p. 95.00 (*3-540-62943-2*) Spr-Verlag.

Endothelial Mechanisms of Vasomotor Control: With Special Reference to the Coronary Circulation. Ed. by H. Drexler et al. 1991. 352p. 63.00 (*0-387-91392-0*) Spr-Verlag.

Endothelial Regulation of Vascular Tone. Ed. by Una S. Ryan & Gabor M. Rubanyi. 1991. (Illus.). 416p. text 199.00 (*0-8247-8578-9*) Dekker.

Endothelial Vasoactive Substances & Cardiovascular Disease. T. F. Luescher. 1988. (Illus.). xiv, 134p. 125.75 (*3-8055-4675-0*) S Karger.

Endothelialization of Vascular Grafts. Ed. by P. P. Zilla et al. 1987. (Illus.). vi, 258p. 172.25 (*3-8055-4557-6*) S Karger.

Endothelin. Gabor M. Rubanyi. 1992. (Clinical Physiology Ser.). (Illus.). 306p. text 70.00 (*0-19-506641-3*) OUP.

Endothelin Receptors & Signaling Mechanisms. David M. Pollock & Robert F. Highsmith. 1998. LC 98-10421. (Molecular Biology Intelligence Unit Ser.). 189p. (*1-57059-487-2*) Landes Bioscience.

Endothelin Receptors From the Gene to the Human: From the Gene to the Brain. Ed. by Robert R. Ruffolo, Jr. 1995. LC 94-40203. (Pharmacology & Toxicology: Basic & Clinical Aspects Ser.). 304p. ring bd. 224.95 (*0-8493-5938-4*, 5938) CRC Pr.

Endothelins. W. G. Nayler. 1990. (Illus.). 208p. 95.00 (*0-387-52856-3*) Spr-Verlag.

Endothelins in Biology & Medicine. Ed. by John P. Huggins & John T. Pelton. 1996. LC 96-27766. 400p. 199.95 (*0-8493-6975-4*) CRC Pr.

Endothelium & Anesthetics. Roland Hofbauer. 2000. (Illus.). 120p. (*3-902104-02-3*) VICER Pubg AUT. *Dist:* VICER Pub.

Endothelium-Derived Contracting Factors. Ed. by G. M. Rubanyi & P. M. Vanhoutte. 1990. (Illus.). x, 238p. 177.50 (*3-8055-5092-8*) S Karger.

Endothelium-Derived Factors & Vascular Functions: Proceedings of the Fourth International Symposium on Endothelium-Derived Factors, Tokyo, 7-9 December 1993. Ed. by Tomoh Masaki. 1994. LC 94-16819. (International Congress Ser.: No. 1051). 270p. 191.50 (*0-444-81669-0*, Excerpta Medica) Elsevier.

Endothelium-Derived Relaxing Factors. Ed. by G. M. Rubanyi & P. M. Vanhoutte. 1990. (Illus.). x, 336p. 245.25 (*3-8055-5091-X*) S Karger.

Endothelium in Cardiovascular Disease: Pathophysiology, Clinical Presentation, & Pharmacology. Ed. by Thomas F. Luscher. 1995. (Illus.). 197p. 139.00 (*3-540-59352-7*) Spr-Verlag.

Endothelium in Clinical Practice. Ed. by Gabor M. Rubanyi & Victor J. Dzau. 1997. LC 96-49906. (Fundamental & Clinical Cardiology Ser.: Vol. 29). (Illus.). 576p. text 210.00 (*0-8247-9809-0*) Dekker.

Endothelium, Nitrix Oxide, & Atherosclerosis: From Basic Mechanisms to Clinical Implications. Ed. by Julio A. Panza & Richard O. Cannon. 1999. LC 99-15251. (Illus.). 320p. 75.00 (*0-87993-436-0*) Futura Pub.

Endotoxin. Ed. by H. Friedman et al. 1990. (Illus.). 734p. 145.00 (*0-306-43241-2*, Plenum Trade) Perseus Pubng.

Endotoxin & Sepsis: Molecular Mechanisms of Pathogenesis, Host Resistance & Therapy. Ed. by Jack Levin et al. 1998. LC 97-50215. 398p. 170.00 (*0-471-19432-8*, Wiley-Liss) Wiley.

Endotoxin & the Lungs. Kenneth L. Brigham. 1994. (Lung Biology in Health & Disease Ser.: Vol. 77). (Illus.). 575p. text 225.00 (*0-8247-9222-X*) Dekker.

Endotoxin in Health & Disease. Ed. by Helmut Brade. 1999. LC 99-29165. (Illus.). 968p. text 225.00 (*0-8247-1944-1*) Dekker.

Endotracheal Tubes. Springhouse Publishing Company Staff. 1992. (Procedures Video Ser.). 36.95 incl. VHS (*0-87434-374-7*) Springhouse Corp.

Endourology. Ed. by U. Jonas et al. 1988. (Illus.). 170p. 94.95 (*0-387-18415-5*) Spr-Verlag.

Endovascular Grafting: Advanced Treatment for Vascular Disease. Ed. by Michael L. Marin & Larry H. Hollier. 2000. LC 00-26470. (Endovascular Intervention Ser.: Vol. 1). (Illus.). xvi, 192p. 85.00 (*0-87993-457-3*) Futura Pub.

Endovascular Grafting Techniques. Juan C. Parodi et al. 1998. (Illus.). 300p. (*0-683-06769-9*) Lppncott W & W.

Endovascular Grafting Techniques. Juan Carlos Parodi et al. 1998. LC 98-28509. 300p. text 129.00 (*0-683-30209-4*) Lppncott W & W.

Endovascular Intervention: Basic Concepts & Techniques. Ed. by Frank J. Criado. 1999. LC 99-29255. (Illus.). 208p. 79.00 (*0-87993-415-8*) Futura Pub.

***Endovascular Intervention: New Tools & Techniques for the 21st Century.** Ed. by Frank J. Criado. 2001. LC 2001-54466. (Endovascular Intervention Ser.: Vol. 3). (Illus.). (*0-87993-495-6*) Futura Pub.

Endovascular Skills: Guidewires, Catheters, Arteriography, Balloon Angioplasty & Stents. Peter Schneider. 2001. (Illus.). 248p. text 85.00 (*1-57626-140-9*) Quality Med Pub.

Endovascular Skills: Guidewires, Catheters, Arteriography, Balloon Angioplasty, Stents. Peter A. Schneider. 1997. LC 97-26332. 223p. 85.00 (*1-57626-079-8*) Quality Med Pub.

Endovascular Surgery. Rosenwasse. 1999. text (*0-7216-7313-9*) Saunders.

Endovascular Surgery. Samuel S. Ahn & Wesley S. Moore. 2nd ed. 1992. (Illus.). 612p. text 175.00 (*0-7216-4370-1*) Saunders.

Endovascular Surgery for Aortic Aneurysms. Ed. by Brian Hopkinson et al. 1997. (Illus.). 260p. text (*0-7020-2148-2*) W B Saunders GBR. *Dist:* Saunders.

***Endovascular Therapy for Atherosclerotic Renal Artery Stenosis: Present & Future.** Ed. by Michael R. Jaff. 2001. LC 2001-40233. (Endovascular Intervention Ser.: Vol. 2). (Illus.). 160p. 75.00 (*0-87993-470-0*) Futura Pub.

Endovascular Treatment of Cerebral Lesions. Pierre L. Lasjaunias & Alejandro Berenstein. 1992. (Surgical Neuroangiography Ser.: Vol. 4). (Illus.). 344p. 198.00 (*3-540-17500-8*) Spr-Verlag.

Endovascular Treatment of Craniofacial Lesions. Pierre L. Lasjaunias & Alejandro Berenstein. 1996. (Surgical Neuroangiography Ser.: Vol. 2). (Illus.). 434p. 220.00 (*3-540-16535-5*) Spr-Verlag.

Endovascular Treatment of Intracranial Aneurysms. J. V. Byrne & G. Guglielmi. 1997. LC 97-28768. (Illus.). 248p. 130.00 (*3-540-62764-2*) Spr-Verlag.

Endrin. 1992. (Environmental Health Criteria Ser.: No. 130). (ENG, FRE & SPA.). 241p. pap. text 45.00 (*92-4-157130-6*, 1160130) World Health.

Ends & Means: The National Conference on Continuing Education in Nursing, 1970. Ed. by Ruth W. McHenry. 1971. LC 70-157408. (Notes & Essays Ser.: No. 69). pap. 2.50 (*0-87060-041-9*, NES 69) Syracuse U Cont Ed.

Ends of Human Life: Medical Ethics in a Liberal Polity. Ezekiel J. Emanuel. 1991. 320p. (C). 42.50 (*0-674-25325-6*) HUP.

Ends of Time: Life & Work in a Nursing Home. Joel S. Savishinsky. 1991. LC 91-10660. 304p. 72.50 (*0-89789-226-7*, H226); pap. 24.00 (*0-89789-229-1*) Greenwood (Bergin & Garvey).

Endurance in Sports. Ed. by Roy J. Shepard & Per Olaf Astrand. 2nd ed. 2000. LC 99-38456. (Encyclopedia of Sports Medicine Ser.: Vol 2). (Illus.). 1008p. 131.95 (*0-632-05348-8*) Blackwell Sci.

Enduring Grief: True Stories of Personal Loss. Ed. by Florence Selder et al. 1996. LC 95-38130. 272p. pap. 25.95 (*0-914783-69-6*) Charles.

Enduring Issues in American Nursing. Ellen D. Baer. 2000. LC 00-63528. (Illus.). x, 377p. (*0-8261-1373-7*) Springer Pub.

Enediyne Antibiotics as Antitumor Agents. Ed. by Donald B. Borders & Terrence W. Doyle. 1994. LC 94-37776. (Illus.). 478p. text 185.00 (*0-8247-8938-5*) Dekker.

Enemies Within & Without. Arthur O'Neill. 1994. LC 95-165992. pap. (*1-86324-413-1*) LaTrobe Univ AUS. *Dist:* Intl Spec Bk.

Enemy Is Us: How to Defeat Drug Abuse & End the "War on Drugs" Robert H. Dowd. LC 96-94697. 193p. 1996. 17.95 (*0-9653999-7-4*); 1997. reprint ed. pap. 8.95 (*0-9653999-8-2*) Hefty Pr.

Enemy Within: The High Cost of Living Near Nuclear Reactors. Jay Gould. 1996. LC 96-789. 224p. (Orig.). pap. 14.95 (*1-56858-066-5*) FWEW.

"Energestische" Medizin: Gibt es Nur Physikalische Wirkprinzipien? Ed. by Brigitte Ausfeld-Hafter et al. 1998. (Komplementare Medizin Im Interdisziplinaren Diskurs Ser.: Vol. 1). (Illus.). 225p. pap. 32.95 (*3-906759-84-9*) P Lang Pubng.

Energetic Approaches to Emotional Healing. Dorothea Hover-Kramer & Karilee H. Shames. 1996. LC 96-35567. (Illus.). 240p. pap. text 23.95 (*0-8273-8417-3*) Delmar.

Energetics of Personality: Defining a Self. John G. Geier & Dorothy E. Downey. 1989. LC 88-83729. (Aristos Ser.: Vol. 1). 577p. 29.95 (*0-927634-03-1*); pap. 24.95 (*0-927634-01-5*) Aristos Pub Hse.

Energetics of Western Herbs: Treatment Strategies Integrating Western & Oriental Herbal Medicine. Peter Holmes. 3rd rev. ed. 1997. (Illus.). 442p. Vol. 1. pap. 50.00 (*1-890029-06-8*); Vol. 2. pap. 50.00 (*1-890029-07-6*) Snow Lotus.

Energies of Consciousness: Exploration in Acupuncture, Auras & Kirlian Photography. Ed. by Stanley Krippner & Daniel Rubin. 1975. (Social Change Ser.). xvi, 250p. text 168.00 (*0-677-05190-5*) Gordon & Breach.

***Energizing Fibromyalgia.** R. Paul St. Armand & Claudia Craig Marek. 2002. 320p. pap. (*0-446-67730-2*) Warner Bks.

Energy: Nutrition of Women. Ed. by Geoffrey H. Bourne. 1987. (World Review of Nutrition & Dietetics Ser.: Vol. 52). (Illus.). x, 266p. 211.50 (*3-8055-4664-5*) S Karger.

Energy & Protein Requirements: Report of a Joint FAO-WHO-UNU Expert Consultation. 1985. (Technical Reports: No. 724). 206p. pap. text 17.00 (*92-4-120724-8*, 1100724) World Health.

Energy & Protein Requirements: Report of the FAO-WHO Ad Hoc Expert Committee, Rome, 1971. FAO-WHO Ad Hoc Expert Committee. 1973. (Technical Reports: No. 522). pap. text 8.00 (*92-4-120522-9*, 1100522) World Health.

Energy Conservation in Health Care Facilities. Daniel Hunt. 1983. (Illus.). 300p. text 43.00 (*0-915586-66-5*) Fairmont Pr.

Energy Conservation in Transport: New Engines & Flywheels. H. Ehringer et al. 1983. text 94.00 (*90-277-1579-3*) Kluwer Academic.

Energy Diagnostic & Treatment Methods. Fred P. Gallo. 2000. LC 99-49653. (Professional Book Ser.). (Illus.). 240p. 35.00 (*0-393-70312-6*) Norton.

Energy Medicine. Laurence E. Badgley. 1985. (Illus.). 173p. 40.00 (*0-941523-02-0*) Human Energy Pr.

Energy Medicine: The Scientific Basis. James L. Oschman. 2000. 272p. pap. (*0-443-06261-7*) Church.

Energy Metabolism in Brain Function & Neuroprotection Vol. 20, Nos. 4-5: Symposium, Waterville Valley, N.H., July 1997. Ed. by Mary C. McKenna & John Edmond. 1998. (Developmental Neuroscience Ser.: Vol. 20, Nos. 4-5). (Illus.). 230p. pap. 49.00 (*3-8055-6691-3*) S Karger.

Energy Metabolism in Farm Animals: Effects of Housing, Stress & Disease. Ed. by M. W. A. Verstegen & A. M. Henken. 1987. (Current Topics in Veterinary Medicine & Animal Science Ser.). (C). text 278.50 (*0-89838-974-7*) Kluwer Academic.

Energy Metabolism, Nutrition & Growth in Premature Infants. Ed. by G. Duc. 1988. (Journal: Vol. 52, Supplement 1). vi, 148p. pap. 46.25 (*3-8055-4731-5*) S Karger.

Energy Metabolism of Farm Animals. Ed. by K. J. McCracken et al. 1998. (CAB International Publication). (Illus.). 480p. (C). text 100.00 (*0-85199-276-5*) OUP.

Energy Now: Simple Ways to Gain Vitality, Overcome Tension, & Achieve Harmony & Balance by Unlocking the Energy Secrets of East & West. Emma Mitchell. 1998. LC 98-6835. (Illus.). 160p. 17.95 (*0-02-862675-3*, Macmillan Ref) Gale.

Energy Nutrition in Ruminants. E. R. Orskov & M. Ryle. 1990. pap. 191.95 (*1-85166-439-4*) Elsevier.

Energy Psychology: Explorations at the Interface of Energy, Cognition, Behavior, & Health. Fred P. Gallo. 1998. LC 98-15822. (Innovations in Psychology Ser.). 288p. 39.95 (*1-57444-184-1*) CRC Pr.

***Energy Psychology in Psychotherapy.** Ed. by Fred P. Gallo. 2002. 544p. 65.00 (*0 393 70346 0*) Norton.

***Energy-Related Metabolites During & after Myocardial Ischemia & Retroperfusion of the Coronary Sinus: An Experimental Study in the Pig with the Microdialysis Technique & Extracorporeal Circulation.** Vitas Zemgulis. 2001. (Comprehensive Summaries of Uppsala Dissertations from the Faculty of Medicine Ser.: No. 1070). (Illus.). 73p. pap. (*91-554-5108-X*) Uppsala Universitet SWE. *Dist:* Coronet Bks.

Energy Tapping: How to Rapidly Eliminate Anxiety, Depression, Cravings & More Using Energy Psychology. Fred P. Gallo & Harry Vincenzi. 2000. (Illus.). 214p. pap. 14.95 (*1-57224-195-0*) New Harbinger.

Enfermedad de Alzheimer see Alzheimer's Disease: A Primer for Caregivers

Enfermedad Llamada Sida: Guia para el Instructor. Betty M. Hubbard. 1991. (Illus.). 58p. (gr. 5-7). pap. 10.00 (*0-88314-502-2*, A5022) AAHPERD.

Enfermedades Ano-Rectales: Dia. Lopez-Rios. 1998. (SPA.). (C). text 95.82 (*84-8174-327-5*) Harcourt.

Enfermeria Atencion Maxilofaci. Jaffe. 1998. (C). text 29.31 (*84-8174-317-8*) Mosby Inc.

Enfermeria en la Consulta Externa Hospitalaria. T. Soy Andrade. 1991. (SPA.). 407p. pap. (*84-7978-003-7*) Ediciones Diaz ESP. *Dist:* IBD Ltd.

Enfermeria Gerontologica. Burke. 2nd ed. 1998. (C). text (*84-8174-308-9*) Mosby-Doyma Libros ESP. *Dist:* Mosby Inc.

Enfermeria Oncologica. Otto. 3rd ed. 1999. (C). text 80.28 (*84-8174-427-1*) Mosby Inc.

Eng Manual. Gans. 2003. pap. 60.95 (*1-56593-954-9*, G2441) Thomson Learn.

***Engaged Youth: Supportive Frameworks for Commitment,** Vol. 93. Mimi Michaelson et al. 2001. (J-B CAD Single Issue Child & Adolescent Development Ser.: Vol. 1). 112p. pap. 28.00 (*0-7879-5777-1*) Wiley.

Engaging the Immediate: Kierkegaard's Indirect Communication & Psychotherapy. Katherine M. Ramsland. 1989. LC 87-46432. 136p. 29.50 (*0-8387-5152-0*) Bucknell U Pr.

Engendering Psychology: Bringing Women into Focus. Florence Denmark et al. 1999. LC 99-19908. 527p. pap. text 57.00 (*0-205-14685-6*) Allyn.

Engineering a Hospital Turnaround: Proven Strategies for Reinvigorating Financial & Operating Performance. Ed. by Richard A. Baehr. 1993. LC 93-9622. (Illus.). 228p. pap. 45.00 (*1-55648-102-0*, 001120) AHPI.

Engineering Approach to Occupational Safety & Health in Business & Industry: An Instructional Aid. Richard L. Shell & Rodney J. Simmons. 1990. 230p. ring bd. 27.00 (*0-89806-109-1*, EAOSHT) Eng Mgmt Pr.

Engineering Aspects of Vector Control Operations: First Report of the WHO Expert Committee on Vector

Biology & Control. 1977. (Technical Report Ser.: No. 603). 40p. pap. text 6.00 (*92-4-120603-9*, 1100603) World Health.

Engineering Disability: Public Policy & Compensatory Technology. Sandra J. Tanenbaum. 1986. LC 85-19684. (Health, Society, & Policy Ser.). 184p. 32.95 (*0-87722-403-X*) Temple U Pr.

Engineering Field Reference Manual. AIHA Engineering Committee. 1984. 132p. 42.50 (*0-932627-08-0*) Am Indus Hygiene.

Engineering Medical Waste-to-Energy Systems. Frank B. Cross & Howard E. Hesketh. 1995. 160p. 39.95 (*1-56676-219-7*) CRC Pr.

Engineering Physiology: Physiologic Bases of Human Factors-Ergonomics. K. H. Kroemer et al. 1986. (Advances in Human Factors-Ergonomics Ser.: No. 4). 248p. 111.00 (*0-444-42693-0*) Elsevier.

***Engineering Psychology & Cognitive Ergonomics.** Ed. by Don Harris. 2001. (Engineering Psychology & Cognitive Ergonomics Ser.: Vol. 6). 382p. text (*0-7546-1338-0*) Ashgate Pub GBR. *Dist:* Ashgate Pub Co.

***Engineering Psychology & Cognitive Ergonomics,** Vol. 5. Don Harris. 2001. 482p. text (*0-7546-1337-2*) Ashgate Pub GBR. *Dist:* Ashgate Pub Co.

Engineering Theory in Orthopaedics: An Introduction. M. Green et al. 1988. 120p. 36.95 (*0-470-21261-6*) P-H.

Engines of Empowerment: Using Information Technology to Create Healthy Communities & Challenge Public Policy. Nancy Milio. 1996. LC 95-43993. 304p. pap. 22.00 (*1-56793-038-7*, 0973) Health Admin Pr.

***English - Russian & Russian - English Medical Dictionary.** A. Yu. Bolotina & E. O. Yakusheva. 3rd ed. 2001. (ENG & RUS.). 541p. (*5-88721-207-1*) Russo RUS. *Dist:* Coronet Bks.

English - Russian Dictionary of Aerospace, Medicine, Psychology & Ergonomics. A. A. Gurjian et al. 1997. (ENG & RUS.). 443p. 49.95 (*0-8285-5469-2*) Firebird NY.

***English - Russian Dictionary of Psychology.** Ed. by E. V. Nikoshkova. 2nd ed. 2001. (ENG & RUS.). 351p. (*5-88721-200-4*) Russo RUS. *Dist:* Coronet Bks.

English & German Dictionary of Medicine. Jurgen Nohring. 2nd ed. 1986. (ENG & GER.). 708p. 195.00 (*0-8288-0571-7*, M 14674) Fr & Eur.

English & Spanish Dictionary for the Dental Professional. Dorothy H. Mills. 1988. (ENG & SPA.). 255p. 24.95 (*0-8288-1870-3*, S50376) Fr & Eur.

English & Spanish Medical Words & Phrases. Springhouse Publishing Company Staff. 2nd ed. 1999. LC 98-34572. (ENG & SPA., Illus.). 224p. pap. 27.95 (*0-87434-961-3*) Springhouse Corp.

English-Arabic Medical Pocket Dictionary. K. A. Shihabi. 1983. (ARA & ENG.). 343p. pap. 19.95 (*0-8288-0557-1*, F 20041) Fr & Eur.

English-Chinese & Chinese-English Dictionary of Traditional Chinese Medicine. Wen-Hwa Zhang. (CHI & ENG.). pap. (*7-5357-1656-3*) China Intl Bk CHN. *Dist:* Distribks Inc.

English-Chinese Medical Dictionary. Commercial Press Staff. 1980. 1665p. 150.00 (*0-8288-0558-X*, M9264); 1977. (CHI & ENG.). 292p. pap. 39.95 (*0-8288-5428-9*, M9253) Fr & Eur.

English for Medicine: English fuer Mediziner. R. Sprigade. 4th ed. 1987. (ENG & GER.). 29.95 (*0-8288-0562-8*, M12194) Fr & Eur.

English-French Dictionary of Medical & Paramedical Sciences. W. J. Gladstone. 4th ed. 1996. (ENG & FRE.). 1280p. 250.00 (*0-7859-9458-0*) Fr & Eur.

English-French Dictionary of the Medical Sciences: Dictionnaire Anglais-Francais des Sciences Medicales. William J. Gladstone. 3rd ed. 1990. (ENG & FRE.). 1110p. 225.00 (*0-8288-0565-2*, M6277) Fr & Eur.

English-French Lexicon of Childhood Problems: Lexique Anglais-Francais de l'Enfant en Difficulte. M. Nadeau & D. Levesque. 1982. (ENG & FRE.). 454p. pap. 35.00 (*0-8288-0938-0*, M8670) Fr & Eur.

English-German Dictionary of Medicine. G. Hofig & P. Schulze. 1992. (ENG & GER.). 255p. 49.00 (*0-8288-7382-8*, 3861170361) Fr & Eur.

English-German Medical & Pharmaceutical Dictionary. Werner E. Bunjes. 696p. 195.00 (*0-8288-1832-0*, M7106) Fr & Eur.

English-German Medical Dictionaries. Peter Hodgson Collin. 1992. (ENG & GER.). 620p. 62.50 (*0-8288-7563-4*, 3125179904) Fr & Eur.

English-German/German-English Dictionary of Drug Epidemiology. Annekatrin Bertelsmann. 1993. (ENG & GER.). 182p. 125.00 (*0-7859-9963-9*) Fr & Eur.

English-Greek Dictionary of Biology & Medical Terms. Patargias. (ENG & GRE.). 413p. pap. 95.00 (*0-7859-9051-8*) Fr & Eur.

English-Hungarian - Hungarian-English Medical Dictionary. 1989. (ENG & HUN.). 37.50 (*0-87557-116-6*) Saphrograph.

English-Hungarian Medical Dictionary. P. Veghelyi. 1981. 820p. 39.95 (*0-8288-1881-9*) Fr & Eur.

English-Hungarian Medical Dictionary. P. Veghelyi & M. Kuntner. 2nd ed. 1988. 942p. 39.95 (*0-8288-4404-6*, M96350) Fr & Eur.

English-Hungarian Medical Dictionary. Ed. by P. Veghelyi & T. Csink. 5th ed. 1991. 820p. (*963-205-260-9*) Akade Kiado HUN. *Dist:* IBD Ltd.

English-Italian Dictionary of Medical Phraseology. V. Marino. 1985. 526p. 184.00 (*88-299-0279-9*) IBD Ltd.

English-Italian Phraseological Medical Dictionaries. V. Marino. 1985. (ENG & ITA.). 526p. 115.00 (*0-7859-7516-0*, 8828902795) Fr & Eur.

English-Japanese-English Medical Dictionary. Seo. 1985. (FRE & JPN.). 231p. 125.00 (*0-8288-1848-7*, F18130) Fr & Eur.

English Malady. George Cheyne. 1976. LC 76-49853. (History of Psychology Ser.). 304p. reprint ed. 50.00 (*0-8201-1281-X*) Schol Facsimiles.

English Medicine in the Anglo-Saxon Times. Joseph F. Payne. LC 75-23749. (Illus.). reprint ed. 30.00 (*0-404-13355-X*) AMS Pr.

English Medieval Hospital. Elizabeth Prescott. 1992. (Illus.). 288p. 45.00 (*1-85264-054-5*) Trafalgar.

English Midwives: Their History & Prospects. James H. Aveling. LC 75-23678. reprint ed. 42.50 (*0-404-13231-6*) AMS Pr.

English-Polish Medical Dictionary. Przemyslaw Slomski. 1987. (ENG & POL.). 1266p. 95.00 (*0-8288-0575-X*, M3503) Fr & Eur.

English-Polish Medical Dictionary. Przemyslaw Stomski. 1991. 1266p. (C). (*0-89771-895-X*) Collets GBR. *Dist:* St Mut.

English-Polish Medical Dictionary. Przemyslaw Slomski. 2nd ed. 1991. (ENG & POL.). 1264p. 150.00 (*0-7859-9336-3*) Fr & Eur.

English-Russian & Russian-English Medical Dictionary. A. I. Bolotina & E. O. Yakusheva. 1998. 544p. (C). 37.50 (*0-8285-5486-2*) Firebird NY.

English Russian Dictionary of Immunology & Immunogenetics. S. V. Suchkov. 1990. (ENG & RUS.). 95.00 (*0-8288-3972-7*, F39624) Fr & Eur.

English-Russian Dictionary of Immunology & Immunogenetics. Ed. by S. V. Suchkov. 1990. 436p. (C). (*0-89771-896-8*) Collets GBR. *Dist:* St Mut.

English-Russian Dictionary of Medical & Biological Abbreviations A-Z. G. N. Akzhigitov. 1992. 426p. (C). 32.95 (*0-8285-5162-6*) Firebird NY.

English-Russian Dictionary of Psychology. E. V. Nikoshkova. 1998. 352p. (C). 28.95 (*0-8285-5495-1*) Firebird NY.

English-Russian Medical Dictionary. G. N. Akzhigitov. 1992. 604p. (C). 29.95 (*0-8285-4998-2*) Firebird NY.

English-Russian Medical Dictionary. Azhighitov. 1993. (ENG & RUS.). 604p. reprint ed. 24.95 (*0-8288-7580-4*, F33450) Fr & Eur.

English-Somali Phrase Book of Common & Medical Terms. Wayne F. Peate. Ed. by Phyllis W. Heald. 2nd ed. 1993. 101p. pap. text 17.95 (*1-883023-07-6*) Comp Occup.

English-Spanish Dictionary for Doctors & Medical Students: Diccionario Ingles-Espanol para Medicos y Estudiantes de Medicina. Anselmo Garrido. 3rd ed. 1987. 780p. 95.00 (*0-7859-5035-4*) Fr & Eur.

English-Spanish Dictionary of Medical Abbreviations. J. A. Garrido. 1983. 221p. 39.95 (*0-8288-1862-2*, F65783) Fr & Eur.

English-Spanish Dictionary of Medical Terms. Erich Ruiz Torres. 8th ed. 1995. (ENG & SPA.). 652p. 125.00 (*0-7859-9751-2*) Fr & Eur.

English-Spanish Glossary for Health Aids: Glosario Espanol-Ingles Para los Auxiliares De Salud. Ed. by Barry Leonard. 7th rev. ed. 2000. (Illus.). 89p. (C). pap. text 20.00 (*0-7567-0242-9*) DIANE Pub.

English-Spanish, Spanish-English Medical Vocabulary: Vocabulario Ingles-Espanol, Espanol-Ingles de Medicina. Francisco Ruiz Torres. 1979. (ENG & SPA.). 300p. pap. 24.95 (*0-8288-4845-9*, S50091) Fr & Eur.

English-Spanish/Spanish-English Medical Dictionary. Ed. by Glenn T. Rogers. 2nd ed. 1997. LC 96-50377. (ENG & SPA.). 230p. pap. 19.95 (*0-07-053680-5*) McGraw-Hill Prof.

English-Swedish - Swedish-English Dictionary of Medicine. Peter Hodgson Collin. 1992. 684p. 25.94 (*0-7859-8714-2*) Fr & Eur.

English-Swedish Dictionary of Medicine: With Swedish-English Glossary. Peter Hodgson Collin. 1993. (ENG & SWE.). 697p. 68.00 (*0-7859-8772-X*) Fr & Eur.

English-Swedish Dictionary of Medicine: With Swedish-English Glossary. Peter Hodgson Collin & M. B. Myrman. 1993. (ENG & SWE.). 697p. (*0-948549-23-8*) P Collin.

English-Turkish Medical Dictionary. P. Tuglaci. 1990. (ENG & TUR.). 923p. (*975-09-0192-4*) ABC Kitabevi TUR. *Dist:* IBD Ltd.

English-Turkish Medical Dictionary. P. Tuglaci. 1990. (ENG & TUR.). 923p. 65.00 (*0-7859-7532-2*) Fr & Eur.

English/German Dictionary of Medicine & Veterinary Medicine. Fritz-Jurgen Nohring. 3rd ed. 1996. (ENG & GER.). 750p. 295.00 (*0-7859-9345-2*) Fr & Eur.

English/German Medical Dictionary. Peter Reuter. 1994. (ENG & GER.). 295.00 (*0-7859-9984-1*) Fr & Eur.

Enhance Your Life Experience. Joseph B. Strauss. 1996. (Illus.). 200p. (Orig.). pap. 8.00 (*1-890419-00-1*) Fnd Chiropractic Educ.

Enhancing Autonomy in Long-Term Care: Concepts & Strategies. Ed. by Lucia Gamroth et al. 1995. LC 94-35281. (Illus.). 264p. 41.95 (*0-8261-8680-7*) Springer Pub.

Enhancing Children's Communication: Research Foundations for Intervention. Ed. by Ann P. Kaiser & David B. Gray. 1992. (Communication & Language Intervention Ser.: Vol. 2). 448p. (C). text 43.00 (*1-55766-076-X*) P H Brookes.

Enhancing Children's Wellness. Roger P. Weissberg et al. 1997. LC 97-4750. (Issues in Children's & Families' Lives Ser.). pap. 37.95 (*0-7619-1092-1*, 81596) Sage.

Enhancing Decision Making in the National Health Service: The Role of Decision Support Systems. Steve Cropper & Paul Forte. 1997. LC 96-51488. (Health Services Management Ser.). (*0-335-19635-7*) OpUniv Pr.

Enhancing Fertility Naturally: Holistic Therapies for a Successful Pregnancy. Nicky Wesson. 1999. LC 99-13567. (Illus.). 192p. pap. 14.95 (*0-89281-832-8*, Heal Arts VT) Inner Tradit.

Enhancing Health Service Management: The Role of Decision Support Systems. S. Cropper. 1997. LC 96-51488. (Health Services Management Ser.). pap. (*0-335-19634-9*) OpUniv Pr.

Enhancing Human Traits: Ethical & Social Implications. Ed. by Erik Parens et al. 1998. LC 98-16197. (Hastings Center Studies in Ethics). 288p. 49.95 (*0-87840-703-0*) Georgetown U Pr.

Enhancing Primary Care of Elderly People. F. Ellen Netting & Frank G. Williams. 1998. LC 98-21725. (Garland Reference Library of Social Science: Vol. 1142). 272p. 57.00 (*0-8153-2531-2*); pap. text 24.95 (*0-8153-2532-0*) Garland.

Enhancing Primary Care Systems Through Federally Qualified Health Centers. L. Carl Volpe & Janine M. Breyel. Ed. by Karen Glass. 1991. 85p. (Orig.). pap. text 15.00 (*1-55877-129-8*) Natl Governor.

Enhancing Psychodynamic Therapy with Cognitive-Behavioral Techniques. Ed. by Terry B. Northcut & Nina R. Heller. 1998. LC 98-21443. 376p. 50.00 (*0-7657-0181-2*) Aronson.

Enhancing Self-Concept in Early Childhood: Theory & Practice. Shirley C. Samuels. 1977. LC 76-58348. 312p. 43.95 (*0-87705-316-2*, Kluwer Acad Hman Sci) Kluwer Academic.

Enhancing Teaching & Learning. 1998. (Resource Guide Ser.). 99p. pap. 17.00 (*1-887759-25-5*, P-85) Am Phys Therapy Assn.

Enhancing the Abilities of Persons with Alzheimer's & Related Dementias: A Nursing Perspective. Pam Dawson et al. 1993. LC 93-12113. 184p. 32.95 (*0-8261-7790-5*) Springer Pub.

Enhancing the Accountability of Alternative Medicine. Frwd. by Samuel L. Milbank & Daniel M. Fox. 1998. (Illus.). 44p. pap. (*1-887748-18-0*) Milbank Memorial.

Enhancing the Lives of Adults with Disabilities: An Orientation Manual. Dale DiLeo. 2nd rev. ed. 1993. LC 93-61405. 104p. pap. 20.00 (*1-883302-02-1*) Trning Res.

Enhancing the Quality of Prenatal Services. Ian T. Hill & Trude Bennett. Ed. by Karen Glass. 1990. (Strategies for Improving State Perinatal Programs Ser.). 70p. (Orig.). pap. text 15.00 (*1-55877-059-3*) Natl Governor.

Enhancing the Self-Esteem of the Nursing Home Resident. Marylou Hughes. 1987. 110p. (C). 17.50 (*1-877735-16-7*, 2129PP) Prof Prnting & Pub.

Enhancing Your Knowledge of HCA. Robert Haacker & Patricia Berry. 1998. 89.00 incl. audio (*0-929442-48-2*, 2502PP) Prof Prnting & Pub.

Enigma of Anna O. The Remarkable Story of Visionary, Writer, Feminist & Social Worker Bertha Pappenheim. Melinda G. Guttmann. 2001. LC 00-44507. (Illus.). 413p. 27.95 (*1-55921-285-3*) Moyer Bell.

Enigma of Health: The Art of Healing in a Scientific Age. Hans Georg Gadamer. Tr. by Jason Geiger & Nick Walker. 1996. LC 95-74982. 220p. (Orig.). pap. 14.95 (*0-8047-2692-2*) Stanford U Pr.

Enigma of Slow Viruses: Facts & Artefacts. P. P. Liberski. 1993. LC 92-48419. (Archives of Virology Ser.: No. 6). (*3-211-82427-8*); (Illus.). 272p. 197.00 (*0-387-82427-8*) Spr-Verlag.

Enigma of Suicide. George H. Colt. 1992. LC 90-19859. 576p. pap. 25.75 (*0-671-76071-8*, Touchstone) S&S Trade Pap.

Enigma of the Oceanic Feeling: Revisioning the Psychoanalytic Theory of Mysticism. William B. Parsons. 1999. LC 97-18199. 264p. text 45.00 (*0-19-511508-2*) OUP.

Enigma of Woman: Women in Freud's Writings. Sarah Kofman. Tr. by Catherine Porter from FRE. 1985. LC 85-47702. 240p. (C). pap. 18.95 (*0-8014-9898-8*) Cornell U Pr.

Enjoying Good Health. Gloria Rose. 1987. 320p. (Orig.). 12.50 (*0-944785-00-X*) Herm Barr Pub.

Enjoying Life with Chronic Obstructive Pulmonary Disease. Thomas L. Petty & Louise M. Nett. (*1-886128-04-9*) Laennec Pub.

Enjoying Sex. Miriam Stoppard. 1998. LC 97-48493. (DK Healthcare Ser.). (Illus.). 96p. pap. 7.95 (*0-7894-3093-2*) DK Pub Inc.

Enkephalins & Endorphins: Stress & the Immune System. N. P. Plotnikoff et al. 1986. LC 85-23234. (Illus.). 458p. (C). text 120.00 (*0-306-42226-3*, Kluwer Plenum) Kluwer Academic.

Enlightened Eating: Understanding & Changing Your Relationship with Food. Rebecca Ruggles Radcliffe. 1996. 172p. 18.95 (*0-9636607-0-5*) EASE.

Enneagram Intelligences: Understanding Personality for Effective Teaching & Learning. Janet Levine. 1999. LC 98-20129. 320p. 65.00 (*0-89789-561-4*); pap. 24.95 (*0-89789-562-2*) Greenwood (Bergin & Garvey).

Enneagram Personality Portraits: Enhancing Professional Relationships. Patrick J. Aspell & Dee D. Aspell. 1997. LC 96-45887. (Enneagram Personality Portraits Ser.). 150p. 34.00 (*0-7879-0883-5*, Pffr & Co) Jossey-Bass.

Enneagram Psychology Series: Emotions & the Enneagram; The Enneagram Relationship Workbook; The Enneagram & Psychodrama (Video) Margaret F. Keyes. 1995. (Illus.). 358p. (C). pap. 60.00 incl. VHS (*1-882042-13-1*) Molysdatur Pubns.

Enneatypes in Psychotherapy. Claudio Naranjo. 1995. LC 94-77115. 160p. (Orig.). pap. 14.95 (*0-934252-47-5*) Hohm Pr.

Enough Already! The Overtreatment of Early Breast Cancer. George Goldberg. 1996. LC 96-67117. xii, 240p. (Orig.). pap. 13.50 (*0-9651435-3-8*) Paracelsus Pr.

Enough Is Enough: How & When to Stop Taking Psychiatric Drugs. Peter Breggin. 1998. (*0-201-32810-0*) Addison-Wesley.

ENPC Pocket Review. Pamela Baker et al. 1994. (Illus.). spiral bd. 22.00 (*0-935890-37-8*) Emerg Nurses IL.

Enrichment Triad Model: A Guide for Developing Defensible Programs for the Gifted & Talented. Joseph S. Renzulli. 1977. (Illus.). 88p. (gr. k-12). pap. 9.95 (*0-936386-01-0*, 685) Creative Learning.

***Ensuring Access to Affordable Health Care: Congressional Hearing.** Ed. by James M. Jeffords. 2001. 71p. (C). pap. text 25.00 (*0-7567-0916-4*) DIANE Pub.

Ensuring Image Quality Student Workbook. Phillips. 1987. 96p. (C). (gr. 13). pap. text, wbk. ed. 17.95 (*0-8016-3906-9*, 03906) Mosby Inc.

Ensuring Quality Cancer Care. National Cancer Policy Board Staff et al. Ed. by Maria E. Hewitt & Joseph V. Simone. 1999. LC 99-6488. 256p. pap. 34.95 (*0-309-06480-5*, Joseph Henry Pr) Natl Acad Pr.

Ent: Colour Guide. Nicholas D. Stafford & Robin Youngs. 1994. LC 93-20831. (*0-443-04954-8*) Church.

Ent: Colour Guide. Nicholas D. Stafford & Robin Youngs. 2nd ed. 2000. LC 99-29017. (Colour Guide Ser.). 122p. (*0-443-06146-7*) Saunders.

Ent: Colour Guide. Picture Tests. G. W. McGarry & G. G. Browning. 1999. LC 99-36938. (Colour Guide Ser.). (Illus.). 134p. text (*0-443-06235-8*) Saunders.

ENT & Oral Surgery of the Dog & Cat: Veterinary Practitioner Handbook. J. G. Lane. 1982. 296p. pap. text 25.50 (*0-7236-0659-5*) Buttrwrth-Heinemann.

ENT for Primary Care Providers. Gayle Ellen Woodson. 2000. LC 00-38811. (Illus.). 289p. text (*0-7216-7431-3*) Saunders.

ENT Practice for the GP's Surgery. Andrew J. Coley & Nicholas J. Kay. 1992. (Illus.). 98p. (Orig.). pap. text (*0-443-04813-4*) Church.

ENT Secrets. Ed. by Bruce W. Jafek & Anne K. Stark. 1996. LC 96-19319. (Secrets Ser.). (Illus.). 475p. pap. 39.95 (*1-56053-159-2*) Hanley & Belfus.

Enter the Physician: The Transformation of Domestic Medicine, 1760-1860. Lamar R. Murphy. 1991. LC 90-10887. (History of American Science & Technology Ser.). 336p. text 39.95 (*0-8173-0514-9*) U of Ala Pr.

Enteral Feeding in Long Term Care. Keith N. Apelgren & Richard E. Dean. 1990. LC 90-60436. 125p. pap. 22.95 (*0-944496-13-X*) Precept Pr.

Enteral Feedings in the Nursing Home. Donna Du Bois. 1988. (Illus.). 111p. (Orig.). (C). 13.50 (*1-877735-20-5*, 2135PP) Prof Prnting & Pub.

Enteral Nutrition. Stacey J. Bell et al. 1993. text 54.95 (*0-442-01342-6*) Chapman & Hall.

Enteral Nutrition. Ed. by George L. Blackburn et al. 1995. LC 93-47999. (Series in Clinical Nutrition). (Illus.). 350p. 73.00 (*0-412-98471-7*) Aspen Pub.

Enteral Nutrition: Handbook for Dietitians & Health Professionals. University of Iowa Hospitals and Clinics, Dietary Department Staff. 1990. LC 90-4452. (Illus.). 96p. pap. text 19.95 (*0-8138-0006-4*) Iowa U Pr.

Enteric Fevers: Causing Organisims & Host's Reactions. A. Olitzki. Ed. by A. Grumbach. 1971. (Bibliotheca Microbiologica Ser.: Vol. 10). pap. 126.25 (*3-8055-1237-6*) S Karger.

Enteric Infection: Intestinal Helminths, Vol. 2. Ed. by M. J. Farthing et al. 1995. LC 95-185471. (Illus.). 336p. (*0-412-39140-6*) E A GBR. *Dist:* OUP.

Enteric Infections. 1964. (Technical Report Ser.: No. 288). 35p. pap. text 5.00 (*92-4-120288-2*) World Health.

Enteric Infections & Immunity. Ed. by L. J. Paradise et al. 1996. LC 96-2981. (Infectious Agents & Pathogenesis Ser.). (Illus.). 256p. (C). text 95.00 (*0-306-45242-1*, Kluwer Plenum) Kluwer Academic.

Enteric Infections in Man & Animals. Ed. by Irene B. Hillary & W. Hennessen. 1983. (Developments in Biological Standardization Ser.: Vol. 53). (Illus.). xii, 356p. pap. 61.00 (*3-8055-3714-X*) S Karger.

Enteric Physiology of the Transplanted Intestine. Micael G. Sarr & Nadey S. Hakim. 1994. LC 94-1206. (Medical Intelligence Unit Ser.). 99.00 (*1-57059-010-9*) Landes Bioscience.

Enteric Viruses in Water. Ed. by Joseph L. Melnick. 1984. (Monographs in Virology: Vol. 15). (Illus.). x, 238p. 142.75 (*3-8055-3803-0*) S Karger.

Entering the Child's Mind: The Clinical Interview in Psychological Research & Practice. Herbert P.

Ginsburg. 1997. LC 97-5635. (Illus.). 293p. (C). text 59.95 (*0-521-49685-3*); pap. text 22.95 (*0-521-49803-1*) Cambridge U Pr.

Entering the World: The De-Medicalization of Childbirth. Michel Odent. Tr. by Christine Hauch et al from FRE. 1989. LC 83-6079. (Open Forum Ser.). (Illus.). 154p. reprint ed. pap. 8.95 (*0-7145-2801-3*) M Boyars Pubs.

Entero-Insular Axis. Ed. by W. Creutzfeldt. 1980. (Frontiers of Hormone Research Ser.: Vol. 7). (Illus.). x, 310p. 100.00 (*3-8055-0795-X*) S Karger.

Enterobacteria. J. Michael Janda & Sharon L. Abbott. 1998. LC 97-42726. (Illus.). 400p. text 129.00 (*0-397-51723-8*) Lppncott W & W.

Enterobacterial Vaccines: Proceedings of the International Symposium, 27th, Bern, 1969. International Symposium on Enterobacterial Vaccine. Ed. by R. H. Regamey et al. 1971. (Immunobiological Standardization Symposia Ser.: Vol. 15). 26.25 (*3-8055-1143-4*) S Karger.

Entity Possession: Freeing the Energy Body of Negative Influence: A Medical Doctor's Extraordinary Work with the Root Causes of Obsessive Behavior. Samual Sagan. 1997. LC 97-16061. (Illus.). 192p. pap. 14.95 (*0-89281-612-0*) Inner Tradit.

Entomopathogenic Nematodes in Biological Control. Ed. by Randy Gaugler & Harry K. Kaya. 1990. 72.95 (*0-8493-4541-3*, SB933) CRC Pr.

Entrapment in Escalating Conflicts. J. Brockner & J. Z. Rubin. 1985. (Social Psychology Ser.). (Illus.). 335p. 107.00 (*0-387-96089-9*) Spr-Verlag.

Entrapment Neuropathies. David M. Dawson et al. 1983. 307p. 49.50 (*0-316-17742-3*, Little Brwn Med Div) Lppncott W & W.

Entrapment Neuropathies. David M. Dawson. 2nd ed. 1990. 94.95 (*0-316-17743-1*, Little Brwn Med Div) Lppncott W & W.

Entrapment Neuropathies. David M. Dawson et al. 3rd ed. 1998. LC 98-25819. 496p. text 125.00 (*0-316-17733-4*) Lppncott W & W.

Entre Mujeres: Su Recuperacion Fisica y Emocional Despues de la Mastectomia. Rosalind Benedet. Tr. by Casa Hispana Staff. 1999. (SPA., Illus.). 92p. pap. 12.00 (*0-9637917-2-9*) Benedet Pbng.

Entrepreneuring: A Nurse's Guide to Starting a Business. Gerry Vogel & Nancy Doleysh. 2nd ed. 1994. 367p. pap. 31.95 (*0-88737-611-8*, 14-2635, NLN Pr) Natl League Nurse.

Entry Level Exam Review for Respiratory Care. Wojciechowski. 2nd ed. 2000. (Respiratory Care Ser.). 368p. (C). pap. text 58.95 (*0-7668-0779-7*) Delmar.

Entry Level Exam Review for Respiratory Care: Guidelines for Success. William V. Wojciechowski. 1995. LC 94-28909. (Health & Life Science Ser.). 288p. (C). mass mkt. 48.95 (*0-8273-6686-8*) Delmar.

Entry-Level Respiratory Care Review: Study Guide & Workbook. Gary Persing. Ed. by Lisa Biello. 2nd ed. 1995. (Illus.). 272p. pap. text, stu. ed., wbk. ed. 40.95 (*0-7216-6426-1*) Saunders.

Entry Strategies in School Consultation. Edward S. Marks. 1995. LC 94-27760. (Guilford School Practitioner Ser.). 287p. 37.00 (*0-89862-368-5*, 2368) Guilford Pubns.

Entwicklung der Paediatrischen Haematologie und Onkologie. Ed. by H. P. Wagner. 1980. (Paediatrische Fortbildungskurse fuer die Praxis Ser.: Vol. 50). (GER., Illus.). pap. 28.75 (*3-8055-0229-X*) S Karger.

Entwicklungstendenzen in Ernaehrung und Diaetetik - Future Trends in Nutrition & Dietetics: Proceedings of the Symposium, Zuerich, March 1973. Symposium, Zuerich Staff. Ed. by P. Kopp. 1975. (Bibliotheca Nutritio et Dieta Ser.: No. 21). (ENG & GER.). 200p. pap. 84.50 (*3-8055-1737-8*) S Karger.

Entwined Lives: Twins & What They Tell Us about Human Behavior. Nancy L. Segal. 2000. LC 99-59376. 416p. pap. 16.00 (*0-452-28057-5*, Plume) Dutton Plume.

Entzuendung und Rheologie der Leukozyten. Ed. by K. Messmer & F. Hammersen. 1985. (GER., Illus.). x, 136p. pap. 61.75 (*3-8055-4071-X*) S Karger.

Enucleation, Evisceration & Exenteration of the Eye. Michael E. Migliori. 1999. LC 98-50637. 256p. text 105.00 (*0-7506-9495-5*) Buttrwrth-Heinemann.

Enumeration of Chinese Materia Medica. Hu Shiu-Ying. 2nd rev. ed. Date not set. LC 00-268831. (CHI & ENG., Illus.). 288p. (C). (*962-201-803-3*) Chinese Univ HKG. *Dist:* U of Mich Pr.

Enuresis Research Today: 1st International Enuresis Symposium, Kyoto, September 1997 - Proceedings. Ed. by Hiroki Watanabe. 1998. (European Urology Ser.: Vol. 33, Suppl. 3, 1998). (Illus.). iv, 62p. pap. 28.75 (*3-8055-6687-5*) S Karger.

Environment & Aging Theory: A Focus on Housing, 26. Ed. by Rick J. Scheidt & Paul G. Windley. 1998. LC 97-37968. (Contributions to the Study of Aging Ser.: Vol. 26). 208p. 62.95 (*0-313-28389-3*, Greenwood Pr) Greenwood.

Environment & Behavior Studies: Emergence of Intellectual Traditions. I. Altman & K. Christensen. 1990. LC 90-7098. (Human Behavior & Environment Ser.: Vol. 11). (Illus.). 392p. (C). 80.00 (*0-306-43468-7*, Plenum Trade) Perseus Pubng.

Environment & Health: The European Charter & Commentary. 1990. (WHO Regional Publications, European Ser.: No. 35). (ENG, FRE, GER & RUS.). x, 154p. pap. text 26.00 (*92-890-1126-2*, 1310035) World Health.

Environment & Health in Europe. Theakeston. 1995. (Illus.). 592p. 129.00 (*0-419-20560-8*, Spon) Routledge.

Environment & Psychopathology. Ed. by A. M. Ghadirian & H. E. Lehmann. 1993. LC 92-49539. 208p. 35.95 (*0-8261-7460-4*) Springer Pub.

Environment, Drugs & Thermoregulation: International Symposium on the Pharmacology of Thermoregulation, 5th, Saint-Paul-de-Vence, November 1982. P. Lomax & E. Schoenbaum. 1983. (Illus.). xvi, 224p. 68.75 (*3-8055-3654-2*) S Karger.

Environment, Health & Population Displacement: Development & Change in Mozambique's Diarrhoeal Disease Ecology. Andrew E. Collins. 1998. LC 97-77896. (Making of Modern Africa Ser.). (Illus.). 315p. text (*1-84014-329-0*) Ashgate Pub GBR. *Dist:* Ashgate Pub Co.

Environment Medical Emergency. Carolyn Steedman. 1994. (Illus.). 220p. pap. text 31.50 (*0-19-262392-3*) OUP.

Environment of the Teeth. Ed. by D. B. Ferguson. 1982. (Frontiers of Oral Physiology Ser.: Vol. 3). (Illus.). x, 174p. 85.25 (*3-8055-2577-X*) S Karger.

Environmental & Community Health: Health Facts. Nora J. Krantzler & Kathleen R. Miner. 1994. LC 93-44548. 12.95 (*1-56071-189-2*, H309) ETR Assocs.

Environmental & Health Monitoring in Occupational Health: Proceedings of the WHO Expert Committee, Geneva, 1973. WHO Staff. 1973. (Technical Reports: No. 535). pap. text 5.00 (*92-4-120535-0*, 1100535) World Health.

Environmental & Occupational Cancer: Scientific Update. Ed. by Myron A. Mehlman. 1990. LC 89-6864. 348p. 65.00 (*0-911131-17-5*) Specialist Journals.

Environmental & Occupational Health in Central & Eastern Europe: Recent Developments One Day Seminar: Institute of Pathology & Experimental Cancer Research, Semmelweiss University, Budapest, June, 1996. Ed. by John A. Hoskins & Szende Bela. 1997. (Indoor & Build Environment Ser.: Vol. 6, No. 4, 1997). (Illus.). 60p. pap. 29.75 (*3-8055-6619-0*) S Karger.

Environmental & Occupational Medicine. William N. Rom. 3rd ed. 1998. LC 97-42366. 1,920p. text 225.00 (*0-316-75578-8*) Lppncott W & W.

Environmental Aspects of Cancer: The Role of Macro & Micro Components of Foods. Ernest L. Wynder et al. 1983. 294p. 81.00 (*0-917678-17-6*) Food & Nut Pr.

Environmental Asthma. Robert K. Bush. 2000. LC 00-60191. (Lung Biology in Health & Disease Ser.: Vol. 153). (Illus.). xvi, 370p. text 165.00 (*0-8247-0301-4*) Dekker.

Environmental Cancer: A Political Disease? S Robert Lichter & Stanley Rothman. 1998. LC 98-25559. (Illus.). 208p. 40.00 (*0-300-07306-2*) Yale U Pr.

Environmental Carcinogens: Methods of Analysis & Exposure Measurement, Vol. 12: Indoor Air. Ed. by B. Seifert et al. 1994. (IARC Scientific Publications Ser.: No. 109). (Illus.). 398p. text 90.00 (*92-832-2109-5*) OUP.

Environmental Change & Human Health - Symposium No. 175. Ed. by Alexander J. Zehnder. 1993. (CIBA Foundation Symposia Ser.: No. 175). 282p. 128.00 (*0-471-93842-4*) Wiley.

Environmental Change & Resulting Impact on Health. 1964. (Technical Report Ser.: No. 292). 23p. pap. text 3.00 (*92-4-120292-0*) World Health.

Environmental Chemical Exposures & Immune System Integrity. Ed. by E. Burger et al. 1987. LC 87-618327. (Advances in Modern Environmental Toxicology Ser.: Vol. 13). (Illus.). 259p. 65.00 (*0-911131-14-0*) Specialist Journals.

Environmental Chemistry. Peter O'Neill. 1985. (Illus.). 176p. (C). text 60.00 (*0-04-551085-7*); pap. text 19.95 (*0-04-551086-5*) Routledge.

Environmental Concept Development in Children. Pravakar Rout. 1988. (C). (*81-7024-206-1*) Ashish Pub Hse IND. *Dist:* S Asia.

Environmental Contexts of AIDS. Marie A. Muir. 1991. LC 90-7705. 232p. 67.00 (*0-275-93618-X*, C3618, Praeger Pubs) Greenwood.

Environmental Emergencies. Nelson. 1985. pap. text 37.00 (*0-7216-1163-X*) Saunders.

Environmental Emergencies. Charles E. Stewart. 1989. (Illus.). 424p. 49.00 (*0-683-07932-8*) Lppncott W & W.

Environmental Endocrine Disruptors. Ed. by Louis J. Guillette, Jr. 1998. LC 99-35847. (Illus.). x, 355p. 89.95 (*1-56032-571-2*) Hemisp Pub.

Environmental Endocrine Disruptors: A Handbook of Property Data. Lawrence H. Keith. 1997. LC 97-17406. 1232p. 195.00 (*0-471-19126-4*) Wiley.

Environmental Epidemiology. Ed. & Intro. by Frederick C. Kopfler. 1986. (Illus.). 304p. lib. bdg. 79.95 (*0-87371-073-8*, L073) Lewis Pubs.

Environmental Epidemiology. Paul E. Leaverton. Ed. by Louis Masse et al. 1982. LC 82-5335. 176p. 57.95 (*0-275-91369-4*, C1369, Praeger Pubs) Greenwood.

Environmental Epidemiology: Effects of Environmental Chemicals on Human Health. Ed. by William M. Draper. 1994. LC 94-28456. (Advances in Chemistry Ser.: No. 241). (Illus.). 272p. 90.00 (*0-8412-2517-6*); pap. 60.00 (*0-8412-2933-3*) Am Chemical.

Environmental Epidemiology: Epidemiological Investigation of Community Environmental Health Problems. Ed. by John R. Goldsmith. 1986. 280p. 182.00 (*0-8493-5468-4*, RA964) CRC Pr.

Environmental Epidemiology Vol. 1: Public Health & Hazardous Wastes. National Research Council Staff. 1992. LC 91-28051. (Environmental Epidemiology Ser.). 296p. text 29.95 (*0-309-04496-0*) Natl Acad Pr.

Environmental Epidemiology Vol. 2: Use of the Gray Literature & Other Data in Environmental Epidemology. Committee on Environmental Epidemiolgy, National R. 1997. 200p. 39.95 (*0-309-05737-X*) Natl Acad Pr.

Environmental Epidemiology for the Busy Clinician. Stanley H. Schuman. 1997. 240p. pap. text 50.00 (*90-5702-510-8*) Gordon & Breach.

Environmental Exposure from Chemicals. Ed. by W. Brock Neely & Gary E. Blau. 1985. 256p. 146.00 (*0-8493-6165-6*, TD196, CRC Reprint) Franklin.

Environmental Exposure from Chemicals, Vol. 2. W. Brock Neely & Gary E. Blau. 1989. LC 84-7765. 192p. 96.00 (*0-8493-6166-4*, TD196) Franklin.

Environmental Goitrogenesis. Ed. by Eduardo Gaitan. 1989. 256p. lib. bdg. 189.00 (*0-8493-6728-X*, RC656) CRC Pr.

Environmental Hazards: Toxic Wastes & Hazardous Materials. E. Willard Miller & Rudy M. Miller. 1991. LC 91-14545. (Contemporary World Issues Ser.). 268p. lib. bdg. 39.50 (*0-87436-596-1*) ABC-CLIO.

Environmental Hazards & Human Health. Richard B. Philp. 1995. LC 94-38920. 320p. lib. bdg. 85.00 (*1-56670-133-3*, L1133) Lewis Pubs.

Environmental Health. Dade W. Moeller. (Illus.). 1992. 332p. (C). 49.95 (*0-674-25858-4*); 1997. LC 96-43287. 512p. 56.00 (*0-674-25859-2*) HUP.

Environmental Health. Monroe T. Morgan. 2nd ed. 1996. (Health Sciences Ser.). (Illus.). 317p. (C). pap. text 44.95 (*0-89582-373-X*) Wadsworth Pub.

Environmental Health: Impact of Pollutants, Vol. 1. Ed. by J. Rose. 1990. (Environmental Topics Ser.). ix, 456p. text 165.00 (*2-88124-738-5*) Gordon & Breach.

Environmental Health: New Directions. Jacqueline Shields. 1990. LC 90-63344. 282p. (C). 45.00 (*0-911131-88-4*) Specialist Journals.

Environmental Health & Risk Assessment, 1990-1994. Susan Maret. 1995. LC 95-39621. (CPL Bibliographies Ser.: No. 325). 114p. 10.00 (*0-86602-325-9*, Sage Prdcls Pr) Sage.

Environmental, Health, & Safety Auditing Handbook. Lee Harrison. 2nd ed. 1995. LC 94-39110. 647p. text 74.50 (*0-07-026904-1*) McGraw-Hill Prof.

Environmental Health Decision Making: The Policies of Disease Prevention. Jens Steensberg. 1989. 327p. (Orig.). pap. 69.00 (*91-22-01260-5*) Coronet Bks.

Environmental Health Engineering in the Tropics: An Introductory Text. Sandy Cairncross & Richard G. Reachem. 2nd ed. 1993. LC 92-41230. 320p. pap. 85.00 (*0-471-93885-8*) Wiley.

Environmental Health for All: Risk Assessment & Risk Communication for National Environmental Health Action Plans. David J. Briggs et al. 1998. LC 98-40849. (NATO Science Ser.). (*0-7923-5453-2*) Kluwer Academic.

Environmental Health Hazards: Recognition & Avoidance. Donald E. Waite. 1994. LC 94-182912. 610p. 21.95 (*0-9640831-0-8*) Environ Health.

Environmental Health in Urban Development: Report of a WHO Expert Committee. 1991. (Technical Reports: No. 807). (ENG, FRE & SPA.). 65p. pap. text 11.00 (*92-4-120807-4*, 1100807) World Health.

Environmental Health Law. Wright. 1997. 352p. (Orig.). pap. text 42.95 (*0-412-48510-9*, Chap & Hall NY) Chapman & Hall.

Environmental Health Law in Scotland. Francis McManus. 1989. 262p. text (*0-566-07036-7*) Avebry GBR. *Dist:* Ashgate Pub Co.

Environmental Health Management after Natural Disasters. 1982. (Technical Publications: Vol. 430). 67p. 8.00 (*92-75-11430-7*) PAHO.

Environmental Health Procedures. Bassett. 3rd ed. 1992. (Architecture Ser.). text 69.50 (*0-412-39490-1*) Chapman & Hall.

Environmental Health Procedures. W. H. Bassett. 3rd ed. 1991. LC 91-45976. 464p. pap. 59.95 (*0-442-31530-9*); 4th ed. 1995. LC 95-67915. 512p. text 72.00 (*0-412-56190-5*, Chap & Hall NY) Chapman & Hall.

***Environmental Health Risk.** Ed. by C.A. Brebbia & D. Fayzieva. 2001. 328p. (*1-85312-875-9*) WIT Pr GBR. *Dist:* Computational Mech MA.

Environmental Health Risks & Public Policy: Decision Making in Free Societies. David V. Bates. 1994. LC 94-2410. (Jessie & John Danz Lectures). xii, 117p. 30.00 (*0-295-97336-6*); (Illus.). 117p. pap. 12.95 (*0-295-97337-4*) U of Wash Pr.

Environmental Health Sciences. Mancy. Date not set. 69.95 (*0-87371-028-2*) Lewis Pubs.

Environmental Health Sciences Chemistry. Gershon J. Shugar. 1992. (Illus.). 422p. 69.95 (*0-925760-58-7*) SciTech Pubs.

Environmental Health Services: A Survey of Administrative & Legal Provisions. R. Dean. 1983. (Public Health in Europe Ser.). 220p. pap. text 19.00 (*92-890-1155-6*) World Health.

Environmental Health Technician. Jack Rudman. 1994. (Career Examination Ser.: C-2652). pap. 29.95 (*0-8373-2652-4*) Nat Learn.

***Environmental Hormones: The Scientific Basis of Endocrine Disruption.** Ed. by John A. McLachian et al. 2001. LC 2001-51397. (Annals of the New York Academy of Sciences Ser.: Vol. 948). 200p. 120.00 (*1-57331-348-3*) NY Acad Sci.

Environmental Hygiene. Ed. by N. H. Seemayer & W. Hadnagy. 1988. (Illus.). 214p. 65.00 (*0-387-19354-5*) Spr-Verlag.

Environmental Hygiene III. Ed. by N. H. Seemayer & W. Hadnagy. 1992. LC 92-21699. (Illus.). 275p. 119.00 (*0-387-54844-0*) Spr-Verlag.

Environmental Impact on the Airways: From Injury to Repair, No. 93. Ed. by Jacques Chretien & Daniel Dusser. 1996. LC 96-13129. (Lung Biology in Health & Disease Ser.: Vol. 93). (Illus.). 600p. text 215.00 (*0-8247-9485-0*) Dekker.

Environmental Impacts on Human Health: The Agenda for Long-Term Research & Development. Ed. by Sidney Draggan et al. 1987. 264p. 62.95 (*0-275-92338-X*, C2338, Praeger Pubs) Greenwood.

Environmental Justice: Research, Education, & Health Policy Needs. Institute of Medicine Staff. 1998. LC 99-199872. 210p. (C). text 34.95 (*0-309-06407-4*) Natl Acad Pr.

Environmental Land & Marine Pollution & Their Control. Ed. by G. R. Chatwal et al. 1989. (*81-7041-208-0*) Anmol IND. *Dist:* S Asia.

Environmental Management for Vector Control. 1980. (Technical Report Ser.: No. 649). 75p. pap. text 5.00 (*92-4-120649-7*) World Health.

Environmental Management in Healthcare Facilities 1998. Kathryn D. Wagner. Ed. by Lisa Biello. 1998. LC 97-704. (Illus.). 512p. (C). text 175.00 (*0-7216-6444-X*) Saunders.

Environmental Medical Emergencies. David J. Steedman. 1994. (Handbooks in Emergency Medicine Ser.: No. 10). (Illus.). 220p. text 59.95 (*0-19-262393-1*) OUP.

Environmental Medicine: Integrating a Missing Element into Medical Education. Institute of Medicine Staff. Ed. by Andrew M. Pope & David P. Rall. 1995. LC 94-74838. 992p. (Orig.). (C). text 49.00 (*0-309-05140-1*) Natl Acad Pr.

Environmental Medicine: Principles & Practice. Brooks. 1995. (Illus.). 864p. (C). (gr. 13). text 96.00 (*0-8016-6469-1*, 06469) Mosby Inc.

Environmental Metal Pollutants, Reactive Oxygen Intermediaries & Genotoxicity: Molecular Approaches to Determine Mechanisms of Toxicity. Maria E. Ariza et al. 1999. LC 98-55187. (*0-7923-8448-2*) Kluwer Academic.

Environmental Neurotoxicology. National Research Council Staff. 1992. 168p. pap. text 24.95 (*0-309-04531-2*) Natl Acad Pr.

Environmental Physiology of Animals. P. J. Willmer et al. 2000. LC 99-23146. (Illus.). x, 644p. pap. 71.95 (*0-632-03517-X*) Blackwell Sci.

Environmental Physiology of Fishes. Ed. by M. A. Ali. 1981. LC 80-22156. (NATO ASI Series A, Life Sciences: Vol. 35). 734p. 135.00 (*0-306-40574-1*, Plenum Trade) Perseus Pubng.

Environmental Pollution & Health Hazards in India. R. Kumar. 1987. (C). (*81-7024-095-6*) Ashish Pub Hse IND. *Dist:* S Asia.

Environmental Problems & Human Behavior. Gerald T. Gardner & Paul C. Stern. 1995. LC 95-36564. 300p. pap. text 65.00 (*0-205-15605-3*, H5606-4) Allyn.

Environmental Psychology. Paul A. Bell. 5th ed. 2001. LC 00-105961. (Illus.). xvii, 634p. (C). text 94.50 (*0-15-508064-4*) Harcourt Coll Pubs.

Environmental Psychology: An Psycho-Social Introduction. Mirilia Bonnes & Gianfranco Secchiaroli. 1995. 240p. (C). pap. 26.50 (*0-8039-7906-1*, 9954) Sage.

Environmental Psychology: Behaviour & Experience in Context. Tony Cassidy. 1997. LC 97-202071. (Illus.). vi, 282p. (*0-86377-480-6*) Psychol Pr GBR. *Dist:* Taylor & Francis.

Environmental Psychology: Directions & Perspectives. Ed. by Nickolaus R. Feimer & Scott Geller. 1983. LC 83-2174. 356p. 65.00 (*0-275-90975-1*, C0975, Praeger Pubs) Greenwood.

Environmental Radiation Measurements. 1976. LC 76-51565. (Report Ser.: No. 50). 251p. pap. text 50.00 (*0-913392-32-4*) NCRP Pubns.

Environmental Radiation Surveillance Laboratory: A Guide to Design, Layout, Staff & Equipment Requirements. P. R. Kamath. 1970. pap. text 5.00 (*92-4-154012-5*, 1150039) World Health.

Environmental Respiratory Diseases. Ed. by Edward M. Cordasco et al. 1994. (Industrial Health & Safety Ser.). 619p. 225.00 (*0-471-29072-6*, VNR) Wiley.

Environmental Sampling for Hazardous Wastes. Ed. by Glenn E. Schweitzer & John A. Santolucito. 1984. LC 84-20480. (ACS Symposium Ser.: No. 267). 144p. lib. bdg. 38.95 (*0-8412-0884-0*) Am Chemical.

Environmental Specimen Banking & Monitoring As Related to Banking. Ed. by Robert A. Lewis et al. 1983. 370p. text 211.50 (*0-89838-621-7*) Kluwer Academic.

Environmental Tobacco Smoke. Ed. by H. Kasuga. 1993. LC 93-21945. 133p. 59.00 (*0-387-94122-3*) Spr-Verlag.

Environmental Tobacco Smoke & Mortality: A Detailed Review of Epidemiological Evidence Relating Environmental Tobacco Smoke to the Risk of Cancer, Heart Disease & Other Causes of Death in Adults Who Have Never Smoked. P. N. Lee. 1992. (Illus.). xx, 224p. 155.00 (*3-8055-5529-6*) S Karger.

Environmental Tobacco Smoke in the Workplace. 1995. lib. bdg. 252.75 (*0-8490-7528-9*) Gordon Pr.

Environmental Toxicants. Lippmann. 2nd ed. 1998. (Environmental Health Ser.). pap. 114.95 (*0-442-02670-6*, VNR) Wiley.

Environmental Toxicants: Human Exposures & Their Health Effects. Ed. by Morton Lippmann. 1991. 699p. text 120.95 (*0-442-00549-0*, VNR) Wiley.

Environmental Toxicology. Wayne G. Landis. 1994. 352p. 75.00 (*0-87371-515-2*, L515) Lewis Pubs.

Environmental Toxicology & Chemistry. Donald G. Crosby. 1998. LC 97-22438. (Topics in Environmental Chemistry Ser.). (Illus.). 352p. (C). text 62.95 (*0-19-511713-1*) OUP.

Environmental Toxicology & Pharmacology of Human Development. Sam Kacew & George H. Lambert. 1997. LC 96-43034. 336p. 99.00 (*1-56032-448-1*) Taylor & Francis.

Environmental Toxins: Psychological, Behavioral, & Sociocultural Aspects, 1973-1989. Ed. by Cheryl B. Travis et al. 1989. 144p. pap. 25.00 (*1-55798-063-2*) Am Psychol.

Environmental UV Photobiology. A. R. Young et al. 1993. LC 93-6129. (Illus.). 502p. (C). 125.00 (*0-306-44443-7*, Plenum Trade) Perseus Pubng.

Environmental Variables in Animal Experimentation: Proceedings of the American Association fo Laboratory Animal Science, New Jersey, 1970. American Association of Laboratory Animal Science Staff. Ed. by Hulda Magalhaes. 1974. LC 72-3526. (Illus.). 146p. 15.00 (*0-8387-1231-2*) Bucknell U Pr.

Environmental Vision: Interactions of the Eye, Vision & the Environment. Donald G. Pitts & Robert N. Kleinstein. 1993. (Illus.). 422p. text 99.00 (*0-7506-9051-8*) Buttrwrth-Heinemann.

Environmentally Induced Disorders Sourcebook: Basic Information about Diseases & Syndromes Linked to Indoor & Outdoor Environments. Ed. by Allan R. Cook. 1997. LC 97-14614. (Health Reference Ser.: Vol. 28). (Illus.). 632p. 78.00 (*0-7808-0083-4*) Omnigraphics Inc.

Environmentally Induced Illnesses: Ethics, Risk Assessment & Human Rights. Thomas A. Kerns. 2001. LC 00-66235. 304p. per. 39.95 (*0-7864-0827-8*) McFarland & Co.

Environments for People with Dementia: Annotated Bibliography. Mylinda Barisas et al. 1995. viii, 96p. (C). per. 15.00 (*0-938744-82-8*, R93-2) U of Wis Ctr Arch-Urban.

***Enzinger & Weiss' Soft Tissue Tumors.** Sharon W. Weiss & John R. Goldblum. 4th ed. 2001. (Illus.). 1344p. (*0-323-01200-0*) Mosby Inc.

Enzootic Bovine Leukosis & Bovine Leukemia Virus. Ed. by A. Burny & M. Mammerickx. 1986. (Developments in Veterinary Virology Ser.). text 161.50 (*0-89838-846-5*) Kluwer Academic.

Enzymatic Peptide Synthesis. W. Kullmann. 1987. LC 86-29898. 91.00 (*0-8493-6841-3*, CRC Reprint) Franklin.

Enzymdiagnostik bei Herz-Leber-und Pankreaserkrankungen. L. Adolph & Rita Lorenz. 1978. (GER.). 15.75 (*3-8055-2872-8*) S Karger.

Enzyme Activation in Blood-Perfused Artificial Organs. Ed. by H. Schmid-Schonbein et al. 1984. (Developments in Hematology & Immunology Ser.). text 179.50 (*0-89838-704-3*) Kluwer Academic.

Enzyme Activities of Human Tissue. 1970. (Enzymologia Biologica et Clinica Ser.: Vol. 11, Nos. 1-2). reprint ed. pap. 46.25 (*3-8055-0824-7*) S Karger.

Enzyme Cure. Lita Lee et al. 1998. LC 98-38395. (Illus.). 304p. pap. 18.95 (*1-887299-22-X*) AlternMed Bks.

Enzyme Diagnosis in Diseases of the Heart, Liver & Pancreas. A. L. Adolph & Rita Lorenz. 1982. (Illus.). 124p. pap. 24.50 (*3-8055-3079-X*) S Karger.

Enzyme Engineering XIV. Ed. by Allen I. Laskin et al. 1998. LC 98-41795. (Annals of the New York Academy of Sciences Ser.: Vol. 864). 665p. (*1-57331-149-9*); pap. (*1-57331-150-2*) NY Acad Sci.

Enzyme Handbook, Vol. 8. D. Stephan et al. 1994. 1008p. 220.00 (*0-387-57837-4*) Spr-Verlag.

Enzyme Handbook: Class 1.5-1.1.2 - Oxidoreductases, Vol. 7. Ed. by M. Salzmann et al. 1993. 833p. 220.00 (*0-387-57246-5*) Spr-Verlag.

Enzyme Handbook Vol. 11: Class 2.1-2.3 Transferases, Vol. 11. Ed. by D. Stephan & D. W. Schomburg. 1996. 700p. 213.00 (*3-540-60295-X*) Spr-Verlag.

Enzyme-Immunoassay. Edward T. Maggio. 1980. 304p. 173.00 (*0-8493-5617-2*, QP519, CRC Reprint) Franklin.

Enzyme Immunoassays: From Concept to Product Development. S. S. Deshpande. 1996. 464p. (C). (gr. 13). 120.00 (*0-412-05601-1*) Kluwer Academic.

Enzyme Induction in Aging & Protein Synthesis. Richard C. Adelman et al. 1974. LC 74-6131. 172p. text 39.00 (*0-8422-7222-4*) Irvington.

Enzyme Kinetics: Behavior & Analysis of Rapid Equilibrium & Steady State Enzyme Systems. Irwin H. Segel. 1975. LC 74-26546. 992p. 198.00 (*0-471-77425-1*) Wiley.

Enzyme Kinetics & Mechanism, Pt. C. Ed. by Sidney P. Colowick & Nathan O. Kaplan. 1982. (Methods in Enzymology Ser.: Vol. 87). 752p. text 188.00 (*0-12-181987-6*) Acad Pr.

Enzyme Kinetics & Mechanism, Pt. A. Ed. by Daniel L. Purich. 1979. LC 54-9110. (Methods in Enzymology Ser.: Vol. 63). 547p. text 121.00 (*0-12-181963-9*) Acad Pr.

Enzyme Kinetics & Mechanisms, Part E. Sidney P. Colowick. 1999. LC 79-18746. (Methods in Enzymology Ser.: Vol. 308). 404p. 99.95 (*0-12-182209-5*) Acad Pr.

Enzyme Patterns in Fetal, Adult & Neo-Plastic Rat Tissues. W. E. Knox. 2nd ed. 1976. 42.75 (*3-8055-2357-2*) S Karger.

Enzyme-Prodrug Strategies for Cancer Therapy. Ed. by R. G. Melton & R. J. Knox. 1999. LC 98-37682. (Illus.). 255p. (C). text 125.00 (*0-306-45895-0*, Kluwer Plenum) Kluwer Academic.

Enzyme Purification & Related Techniques. Ed. by William B. Jakoby. 1971. (Methods in Enzymology Ser.: Vol. 22). text 209.00 (*0-12-181885-3*) Acad Pr.

Enzyme Regulation & Metabolic Diseases. F. Belfiore. 1981. (Illus.). xxiv, 880p. 216.75 (*3-8055-0005-X*) S Karger.

Enzyme Structure. Ed. by C. H. Hirs et al. 1967. (Methods in Enzymology Ser.: Vol. 11). text 209.00 (*0-12-181860-8*) Acad Pr.

Enzyme Structure. Ed. by C. H. Hirs & Serge N. Timasheff. (Methods in Enzymology Ser.: Vol. 26). Pt. C. 1972. text 199.00 (*0-12-181889-6*); Pt. D. 1973. text 209.00 (*0-12-181890-X*); Pt. B. 1972. text 199.00 (*0-12-181888-8*) Acad Pr.

Enzyme Structure, Pt. H. Ed. by C. H. W. Hirs & Serge N. Timasheff. 1979. (Methods in Enzymology Ser.: Vol. 61). 577p. text 121.00 (*0-12-181961-2*) Acad Pr.

Enzyme Structure. Ed. by Sidney P. Colowick & Nathan O. Kaplan. (Methods in Enzymology Ser.: Vol. 91). Vol. 91, Pt. I. 1983. text 188.00 (*0-12-181991-4*); Vol. 117, Pt. J. 1985. text 188.00 (*0-12-182017-3*) Acad Pr.

Enzyme Structure, Vol. 130, Pt. K. Ed. by Sidney P. Colowick et al. 1986. (Methods in Enzymology Ser.: Vol. 130). text 167.00 (*0-12-182030-0*) Acad Pr.

Enzyme Tests in Diagnosis. Ed. by Donald W. Moss & Sydney B. Rosalki. 1996. (Illus.). 304p. pap. (*0-340-55245-X*) E A GBR. *Dist:* OUP.

Enzyme Therapy Basics: Powerful Remedies for Women. Friedrich W. Dittmar & Jutta Wellmann. 2000. LC 99-37531. (Illus.). 160p. pap. 14.95 (*0-8069-2031-9*) Sterling.

Enzymes: Principles, New Technologies & Applications. Subramanian. 1993. 240.00 (*0-8493-0154-8*) CRC Pr.

***Enzymes Vol. 22: Co- & Posttranslational Proteolysis of Proteins.** Ed. by R. E. Dalbey. 3rd ed. 2001. LC 00-107123. 509p. 125.00 (*0-12-122723-5*) Acad Pr.

Enzymes - Tools & Targets. Ed. by Ellen Schmidt et al. 1988. (Advances in Clinical Enzymology Ser.: Vol. 6). viii, 272p. 240.00 (*3-8055-4688-2*) S Karger.

Enzymes & Isoenzymes in Pathogenesis & Diagnosis. Ed. by D. M. Goldberg et al. 1987. (Advances in Clinical Enzymology Ser.: Vol. 5). (Illus.). viii, 162p. 147.00 (*3-8055-4344-1*) S Karger.

Enzymes in Anesthesiology. Ed. by F. F. Foldes. 1978. (Illus.). 60.00 (*3-540-90241-4*) Spr-Verlag.

Enzymes in Carbohydrate Synthesis. Ed. by Mark D. Bednarski & Ethan S. Simon. 1991. LC 91-18662. (ACS Symposium Ser.: No. 466). (Illus.). 131p. text 45.00 (*0-8412-2097-2*) Am Chemical.

Enzymes in Food & Beverage Processing. Ed. by Robert L. Ory & Allen J. St. Angelo. 1977. LC 77-6645. (ACS Symposium Ser.: No. 47). 38.95 (*0-8412-0375-X*) Am Chemical.

Enzymes in Health & Disease: Proceedings of the Inaugural Scientific Meeting of the International Society for Clinical Enzymology, London, September 1977. Inaugural Scientific Meeting of the International Society for Clinical Enzymology Staff. Ed. by J. H. Wilkinson. 1978. (Illus.). 85.25 (*3-8055-2853-1*) S Karger.

Enzymes in Industry & Medicine. Gordon F. Bickerstaff. 1987. LC 87-169847. pap. text (*0-7131-2935-2*) E A.

Enzymes of Lipid Metabolism II. Ed. by Louis Freysz et al. 1986. LC 86-22702. (NATO ASI Series A, Life Sciences: Vol. 116). 870p. 155.00 (*0-306-42404-5*, Plenum Trade) Perseus Pubng.

Methods of Enzymatic Analysis, Enzymes 1: Oxidoreductases & Transferases, Vol. 3, Enzymes 1: Oxidoreductases, Transferases. Ed. by Hans U. Bergmeyer. 3rd ed. 1983. LC 84-105641. 606p. 305.00 (*3-527-26043-9*, Wiley-VCH) Wiley.

Enzymology. D. L. Purich. Vol. 73. 1999. 283p. 150.00 (*0-471-24644-1*); Vol. 74. 2000. 392p. 140.00 (*0-471-34921-6*) Wiley.

Enzymology & Medicine. D. W. Moss & P. J. Butterworth. 1974. (Illus.). pap. text 60.00 (*0-272-00094-9*) St Mut.

Enzymology & Molecular Biology of Carbonyl Metabolism, Vol. 4. H. Weiner et al. 1993. LC 92-48366. (Advances in Experimental Medicine & Biology Ser.: Vol. 328). (Illus.). 654p. (C). text 155.00 (*0-306-44357-0*, Kluwer Plenum) Kluwer Academic.

Enzymology & Molecular Biology of Carbonyl Metabolism 3. Ed. by Henry Weiner et al. 1991. (Advances in Experimental Medicine & Biology Ser.: Vol. 284). (Illus.). 370p. (C). text 138.00 (*0-306-43812-7*, Kluwer Plenum) Kluwer Academic.

Enzymology & Molecular Biology of Carbonyl Metabolism 5: Proceedings of the Seventh International Workshop Held in Palmerston North, New Zealand, July 3-7, 1994. Ed. by Henry Weiner et al. 1995. LC 95-7575. (Advances in Experimental Medicine & Biology Ser.: Vol. 372). 454p. 130.00 (*0-306-44989-7*, Kluwer Plenum) Kluwer Academic.

Enzymology of Plasminogen Activation. Ed. by R. Machovich & W. G. Owen. 1988. (Journal: Vol. 40, No. 2-3, 1988). (Illus.). 116p. pap. 75.00 (*3-8055-4854-0*) S Karger.

Enzymology of the Liver. Ed. by L. Van de Reis. 1976. (Frontiers of Gastrointestinal Research Ser.: Vol. 2). (Illus.). xii, 292p. 133.25 (*3-8055-2220-7*) S Karger.

Eosinofils in Allergy & Inflammation. Ed. by Gerald J. Gleich & A. Barry Kay. 1993. (Clinical Allergy & Immunology Ser.: Vol. 2). (Illus.). 528p. text 230.00 (*0-8247-9121-5*) Dekker.

Eosinophils: A Comprehensive Review & Guide to the Scientific & Medical Literature. Christopher J. Spry. 1989. (Illus.). 502p. text 89.00 (*0-19-261408-8*) OUP.

Eosinophils: Biological & Clinical Aspects. Ed. by Sohei Makino & Takeshi Fukuda. 1992. 464p. 256.00 (*0-8493-6822-7*, RB145, CRC Reprint) Franklin.

Eosinophils in Allergy. Ed. by S. Makino & Takeru H. Ishikawa. 1995. (Journal: Vol. 108, Suppl. 1, 1995). (Illus.). 56p. pap. 26.25 (*3-8055-6216-0*) S Karger.

Eosinophils in Allergy & Related Dieases: Workshop, Tokyo, June 1997: Proceedings, Vol.117. Ed. by Takeshi Fukuda et al. 1998. (International Archives of Allergy & Immunology Ser.: Vol. 117, Suppl. 1 (1998)). (Illus.). vi, 82p. pap. 37.50 (*3-8055-6792-8*) S Karger.

Eosinophils in Allergy & Related Diseases: Proceedings of a Workshop, Tokyo, June 1995. Ed. by Sohei Makino et al. 1996. (Journal: Vol. 111, Supplement 1, 1996). (Illus.). iv, 70p. pap. 32.25 (*3-8055-6397-3*) S Karger.

Eosinophils in Allergy & Related Diseases: Proceedings of a Workshop, Tokyo, June 1996. Ed. by Sohei Makino et al. 1997. (International Archives of Allergy & Immunology Ser.: Vol. 114, Suppl. 1). (Illus.). iv, 90p. pap. 41.00 (*3-8055-6580-1*) S Karger.

Eosinophils in Allergy & Related Diseases: Proceedings of a Workshop, Tokyo, June 1999. Ed. by T. Ishikawa et al. 2000. (International Archives of Allergy & Immunology Ser.: Vol. 122). (Illus.). iv, 68p. pap. 25.25 (*3-8055-7103-8*) S Karger.

Eosinophils in Allergy & Related Dieases: Workshop, Tokyo, June 1998: Proceedings. Ed. by S. Makino et al. 1999. (International Archives of Allergy & Immunology Ser.: Vol. 120, Suppl. 1). (Illus.). iv, 106p. pap. 34.00 (*3-8055-6992-0*) S Karger.

***Eosinophils in Allergy & Related Diseases: Workshop, Tokyo, June 2000 - Proceedings.** Ed. by S. Makino et al. 2001. (International Archives of Allergy & Immunology Ser.: Vol. 125). (Illus.). iv, 72p. pap., suppl. ed. 25.25 (*3-8055-7241-7*) S Karger.

Eosinophils in Allergy Research. Ed. by Takeru H. Ishikawa & S. Makino. 1994. (Journal: Vol. 104, Suppl. 1, 1994). (Illus.). iv, 66p. pap. 30.50 (*3-8055-5978-X*) S Karger.

Eosinophils in Asthma. Ed. by John Morley & I. Colditz. 1989. (Perspectives in Asthma Ser.: No. 4). 300p. text 83.00 (*0-12-506452-7*) Acad Pr.

Ephedrine - Medical Biology & Adverse Effects on Health: Index of New Information. Science and Life Consultants Staff. 1997. 160p. 57.50 (*0-7883-1762-8*); pap. 47.50 (*0-7883-1763-6*) ABBE Pubs Assn.

EPIC Study - German Part: European Prospective Investigation into Cancer & Nutrition. Ed. by H. Boeing. 1999. (Annals of Nutrition & Metabolism Ser.: Vol. 43, No. 4). (Illus.). 76p. pap. 25.25 (*3-8055-7016-3*) S Karger.

Epidemic. Brian Ward. 2000. LC 00-27948. (Eyewitness Books Ser.). (Illus.). 64p. (gr. 4-7). (J). 15.95 (*0-7894-6296-6*, D K Ink); pap. 19.99 (*0-7894-6989-8*) DK Pub Inc.

Epidemic. Contrib. by Brian R. Ward. 2000. LC 00-27948. (*0-7894-6297-4*) DK Pub Inc.

Epidemic! The World of Infectious Disease. Ed. by Rob DeSalle. 1999. LC 99-14127. (American Museum of Natural History Ser.). (Illus.). 256p. pap. text 19.95 (*1-56584-546-3*) New Press NY.

Epidemic Models: Their Structure & Relation to Data. Ed. by Denis Mollison. 1995. (Publications of the Newton Institute: No. 5). (Illus.). 442p. (C). text 100.00 (*0-521-47536-8*) Cambridge U Pr.

Epidemic of Acquired Immune Deficiency Syndrome (AIDS) & Kaposi's Sarcoma. Ed. by G. Giraldo & Elke Beth. 1984. (Antibiotics & Chemotherapy Ser.: Vol. 32). (Illus.). viii, 164p. 112.25 (*3-8055-3876-6*) S Karger.

Epidemic of Health Care Worker Injury: An Epidemiology. William Charney & Guy Fragala. 1998. LC 98-36748. 248p. 74.95 (*0-8493-3382-2*) CRC Pr.

Epidemic Versus Sporadic MRSA: Relative Importance in an Endemic Situation & Relationship to Nasal Adherence. Annette Schuermans. 1998. (Acta Biomedica Lovaniensia Ser.). (Illus.). 121p. pap. (*90-6186-878-5*) Leuven Univ BEL. *Dist:* Coronet Bks.

***Epidemic/Epizootic West Nile Virus in the United States: Revised Guidelines for Surveillance, Prevention & Control.** Ed. by Duane J. Gubler. 2001. 104p. (C). pap. text 25.00 (*0-7567-1444-3*) DIANE Pub.

Epidemics: Opposing Viewpoints. Ed. by William Dudley. 1998. LC 98-28458. (Opposing Viewpoints Ser.). (Illus.). 188p. (YA). (gr. 9-12). pap. 16.20 (*1-56510-940-6*); lib. bdg. 26.20 (*1-56510-941-4*) Gale (Greenhaven Pr).

Epidemics & Crowd Diseases: Introduction to the Study of Epidemiology. Major Greenwood. Ed. by Barbara G. Rosenkrantz. 1977. LC 76-40628. (Public Health in America Ser.). (Illus.). reprint ed. lib. bdg. 36.95 (*0-405-09821-9*) Ayer.

Epidemics & Disease Outbreaks: Index of New Information for Reference & Research. Joseph D. Pratt. 1997. (Illus.). 150p. 57.50 (*0-7883-1060-7*); pap. 47.50 (*0-7883-1061-5*) ABBE Pubs Assn.

Epidemics & Ideas: Essays on the Historical Perception of Pestilence. Ed. by Terence Ranger & Paul A. Slack. 1996. (Past & Present Publications). 357p. (C). pap. text 24.95 (*0-521-55831-X*) Cambridge U Pr.

Epidemics in the Modern World. Joann P. Krieg. 1992. LC 92-14090. (Twayne's Literature & Society Ser.). 200p. pap. 13.95 (*0-8057-8859-X*); text 26.95 (*0-8057-8852-2*) Macmillan.

Epidemics Resulting from Wars. Friedrich Prinzing. Ed. by Harold Westergaard. 1977. lib. bdg. 59.95 (*0-8490-1781-5*) Gordon Pr.

Epidemien und das Corpus Hippocraticum: Voruntersuchung zu einer Geschichte der koischen Aerzteschule. Karl Deichgraeber. 1971. (GER.). 187p. (C). reprint ed. 84.60 (*3-11-003635-5*) De Gruyter.

Epidemiologic Field Methods in Psychiatry: The Nimh Epidemiologic Catchment Area Program. Ed. by William W. Eaton & Larry G. Kessler. 1985. text 83.00 (*0-12-228250-7*) Acad Pr.

Epidemiologic Methods for Detection of Teratogens. Ed. by Marcus A. Klingberg & Josephine A. Weatherall. 1979. (Contributions to Epidemiology & Biostatistics Ser.: Vol. 1). pap. 72.25 (*3-8055-2889-2*) S Karger.

Epidemiologic Methods for Health Policy. Robert A. Spasoff. 1999. LC 98-50116. (Illus.). 240p. text 39.95 (*0-19-511499-X*) OUP.

Epidemiologic Research: Principles & Quantitative Methods. David G. Kleinbaum et al. 1982. (Industrial Health & Safety Ser.). 560p. 130.00 (*0-471-28985-X*); (Illus.). 544p. text 77.95 (*0-534-97950-5*) Wiley (VNR).

Epidemiologic Studies in Psychosomatic Medicine. Ed. by F. Reichsman. 1977. (Advances in Psychosomatic Medicine Ser.: Vol. 9). (Illus.). 49.75 (*3-8055-2654-7*) S Karger.

Epidemiologic Study of the Elderly. Ed. by Robert B. Wallace & Robert F. Woolson. 1992. (Illus.). 400p. text 68.00 (*0-19-506120-9*) OUP.

Epidemiologic Surveillance after Natural Disasters. 1999. (Technical Publications: Vol. 420). 106p. 8.00 (*92-75-11420-X*) PAHO.

Epidemiological & Statistical Aspects of the AIDS Epidemic. Ed. by David R. Cox et al. 1989. (Philosophical Transactions of the Royal Society, Series B: Vol. 325). (Illus.). 144p. reprint ed. pap. text 53.00 (*0-85403-390-4*) Scholium Intl.

Epidemiological Aspects of Cutaneous Malignant Melanoma. Ed. by Richard P. Gallagher & J. Mark Elwood. 1994. LC 94-3133. (Developments in Oncology Ser.: Vol. 73). 344p. (C). text 176.50 (*0-7923-2740-3*) Kluwer Academic.

Epidemiological Concepts in Clinical Pharmacology. Ed. by H. Kewitz et al. 1987. (Illus.). 148p. 53.50 (*0-387-16291-7*) Spr-Verlag.

Epidemiological Imagination: A Reader. Ed. by John R. Ashton. 1994. LC 94-858. (*0-335-19101-0*); pap. (*0-335-19100-2*) OpUniv Pr.

Epidemiological Methods in the Study of Chronic Diseases: Eleventh Report of the WHO Expert Committee on Health Statistics. Ed. by WHO Staff. 1967. (Technical Report Ser.: No. 365). 31p. pap. text 3.00 (*92-4-120365-X*, 1100365) World Health.

Epidemiological Practices in Research on Small Effects. Ed. by Hans Hoffmeister et al. 1998. LC 98-9322. (Illus.). 132p. 85.00 (*3-540-63345-6*) Spr-Verlag.

Epidemiological Research Methods. Don Mcneil. 1996. LC 96-190443. 316p. 149.95 (*0-471-96195-7*); pap. 69.95 (*0-471-96196-5*) Wiley.

***Epidemiological Studies.** Alan J. Silman & Gary J. Macfarlane. 2002. 220p. text 80.00 (*0-521-81097-3*); pap. text 28.95 (*0-521-00939-1*) Cambridge U Pr.

Epidemiological Studies: A Practical Guide. Alan J. Silman. 1996. (Illus.). 189p. (C). text 74.95 (*0-521-43371-1*); pap. text 27.95 (*0-521-43979-5*) Cambridge U Pr.

Epidemiological Studies on Social & Medical Conditions of the Elderly: Report on a Survey. A. Svanborg & G. Bergstrom. 1982. (Euro Reports & Studies Ser.: No. 62). 38p. pap. text 4.00 (*92-890-1228-5*) World Health.

Epidemiological Study of Demographic Factors Associated with Infant Mortality in Bridgeport, Connecticut, 1981-1984. Gail M. Andrenyak. 1990. (Studies in Historical Demography). 150p. reprint ed. text 10.00 (*0-8240-4959-4*) Garland.

Epidemiologisches Untersuchungsprogramm Bille-Siedlung. Ed. by Behorde Arbeit. 1997. (Illus.). 714p. pap. 95.95 (*3-631-30040-9*) P Lang Pubng.

Epidemiology. David Christie et al. 1987. 116p. (C). pap. *(0-86840-186-2)* New South Wales Univ Pr AUS. *Dist:* Intl Spec Bk.

Epidemiology. Leon Gordis. Ed. by Larry McGrew. 1996. LC 95-16680. (Illus.). 288p. pap. text 26.50 *(0-7216-5137-2)* Saunders.

Epidemiology. Staffan E. Norell. 1995. (Illus.). 328p. text, wbk. ed. 49.95 *(0-19-507490-4)* OUP.

Epidemiology. Leon Gordis. 2nd ed. 2000. LC 00-38809. (Illus.). xii, 308p. pap. text 29.95 *(0-7216-8338-X)* Saunders.

Epidemiology: Beyond The Basics. Moyses Szklo & F. Javier Nieto. 1999. text 55.00 *(0-8342-1909-3)* Aspen Pub.

Epidemiology: Beyond the Basics. Moyses Szklo & F. Javier Nieto. 1999. LC 99-29768. 495p. pap. 58.00 *(0-8342-0618-8)* Aspen Pub.

Epidemiology: Principles & Practice. Brian MacMahon & Dimitrios Trichopoulos. 2nd ed. 1996. LC 96-5095. 288p. text 49.95 *(0-316-54222-9,* Little Brwn Med Div) Lppncott W & W.

Epidemiology: Progress in Public Health. Ed. by Gabriel Scally. 1997. 302p. pap. *(0-443-05938-1)* Royal Soc of Medicine Pr Ltd GBR. *Dist:* Balogh.

Epidemiology: Study Design & Data Analysis. Mark Woodward. 1999. LC 99-13286. 516p. 79.95 *(0-8493-0398-2,* Chap & Hall CRC) CRC Pr.

Epidemiology & Biology of Multiple Myeloma. Ed. by G. I. Obrams & M. Potter. 1991. (Illus.). 192p. 48.95 *(0-387-54061-X)* Spr-Verlag.

Epidemiology & Control of African Trypanosomiasis. 1986. (Technical Reports: No. 739). 124p. pap. text 16.00 *(92-4-120739-6,* 1100739) World Health.

Epidemiology & Control of Nematodiasis in Cattle: Current Topics in Veterinary Medicine & Animal Science, No. 9. Ed. by P. Nansen et al. 1981. 616p. text 249.00 *(90-247-2502-X)* Kluwer Academic.

Epidemiology & Control of Schistosomiasis: Report of a WHO Expert Committee. Ed. by WHO Staff. 1980. (Technical Report Ser.: No. 643). 63p. pap. text 4.00 *(92-4-120643-8,* 1100643) World Health.

Epidemiology & Control of Schistosomiasis: Report of a WHO Expert Committee, 1967. Ed. by WHO Staff. 1967. (Technical Report Ser.: No. 372). 35p. pap. text 5.00 *(92-4-120372-2,* 1100372) World Health.

Epidemiology & Etiology of Insulin-Dependent Diabetes in the Young. Ed. by Claire Levy-Marschal & P. Czernichow. 1992. (Pediatric & Adolescent Endocrinology Ser.: Vol. 21). (Illus.). xii, 242p. 208.75 *(3-8055-5521-0)* S Karger.

Epidemiology & Health Policy. Sol Levine & Abraham M. Lilienfeld. 1987. (Contemporary Issues in Health, Medicine & Social Policy Ser.). 290p. text *(0-422-78000-6)* Tavistock GBR. *Dist:* Routldge.

Epidemiology & Mental Illness. Richard J. Plunkett & John E. Gordon. Ed. by Gerald N. Grob. 1980. LC 78-22581. (Historical Issues in Mental Health Ser.). reprint ed. lib. bdg. 18.95 *(0-405-11933-X)* Ayer.

Epidemiology & Non-Drug Treatment of Head Pain. Ed. by A. P. Friedman & M. E. Granger. 1978. (Pain & Headache Ser.: Vol. 5). (Illus.). 54.00 *(3-8055-2803-5)* S Karger.

Epidemiology & Prevention of Cardiovascular Diseases: A Global Public Health Challenge. Darwin R. Labarthe. 1998. LC 97-45221. 704p. 78.00 *(0-8342-0659-5,* 06595) Aspen Pub.

Epidemiology & Prevention of Cardiovascular Diseases in Elderly People: Report of a WHO Study Group. Ed. by WHO Staff. 1995. LC 96-137208. (Technical Reports: No. 853). (FRE & SPA.). v, 67p. (C). pap. text 14.00 *(92-4-120853-8,* 1100853) World Health.

Epidemiology & Public Health. Norman Vetter & Ian Matthews. 1998. LC 99-36781. (C). pap. text *(0-443-05704-4)* Saunders.

Epidemiology & Screening of Diabetes. Mario Morsiani. 1989. LC 88-7249. 320p. 163.00 *(0-8493-4971-0,* RC660, CRC Reprint) Franklin.

Epidemiology & the Delivery of Health Care Services: Methods & Applications. Ed. by Denise M. Oleske. 1995. LC 95-9426. (Illus.). 252p. (C). text 54.00 *(0-306-44968-4,* Kluwer Plenum) Kluwer Academic.

Epidemiology, Biostatistics & Preventive Medicine. James F. Jekel et al. Ed. by Bill Schmitt. 1996. LC 95-42002. (STARS Ser.). (Illus.). 352p. pap. text 31.95 *(0-7216-5258-1)* Saunders.

Epidemiology, Biostatistics & Preventive Medicine. David L. Katz. Ed. by William Schmitt. rev. ed. 1996. LC 96-29335. (Illus.). 256p. pap. text 20.95 *(0-7216-4084-2)* Saunders.

Epidemiology, Causes & Prevention of Skin Diseases. J. J. Grob et al. 1997. LC 96-39073. (Illus.). 384p. 208.95 *(0-632-04256-7)* Blackwell Sci.

Epidemiology for Public Health Practice. Robert H. Friis & Thomas A. Sellers. 2nd ed. 1999. LC 99-11560. 506p. pap. 52.00 *(0-8342-1178-5)* Aspen Pub.

Epidemiology for the Health Sciences: A Primer on Epidemiologic Concepts & Their Uses. Donald F. Austin & S. Benson Werner. 1982. (Illus.). 88p. pap. 18.95 *(0-398-02949-0)* C C Thomas.

Epidemiology for the Uninitiated. D. Coggin. Ed. by Geoffrey Rose & D. J. Barker. 3rd ed. 1993. (Illus.). 80p. pap. text *(0-7279-0770-0)* BMJ Pub GBR. *Dist:* AIDC.

Epidemiology for the Uninitiated. D. Coggan et al. 4th ed. 1997. 80p. pap. text *(0-7279-1102-3)* BMJ Pub GBR. *Dist:* AIDC.

Epidemiology, Health, & Society: Selected Papers. Mervyn W. Susser. 1987. (Illus.). 320p. text 45.00 *(0-19-505020-7)* OUP.

Epidemiology in Anaesthesia. J. N. Lunn. 1988. 184p. *(0-683-13056-0)* E A GBR. *Dist:* Williams & Wilkins.

Epidemiology in Health Care. Barbara G. Valanis. 3rd ed. 1998. LC 98-15835. 464p. (C). pap. 50.00 *(0-8385-2227-0,* A-2227-5) P-H.

Epidemiology in Health Services Management. G. E.Alan Dever. 1984. 350p. (C). 80.00 *(0-89443-850-6)* Aspen Pub.

Epidemiology in Health Services Management. Dever. 2nd ed. 2001. 350p. text 68.00 *(0-8342-1873-9)* Aspen Pub.

Epidemiology in Medical Practice. D. J. Barker et al. 5th ed. 1997. LC 97-29782. 170p. pap. text *(0-443-05620-X)* Church.

Epidemiology in Medicine, Set. Charles Hennekens & Julie Buring. 1987. 400p. pap. text 47.95 *(0-316-35636-0)* Lppncott W & W.

Epidemiology in Military & Veteran Populations: Proceedings of the Second Biennial Conference. Institute of Medicine Staff. Ed. by William F. Page. 1991. 112p. text 19.00 *(0-309-04548-7)* Natl Acad Pr.

Epidemiology in Nursing Practice. Gail Harkness. 1994. LC 95-120319. (Illus.). 320p. (C). (gr. 13). pap. text 36.00 *(0-8016-2052-X,* 02052) Mosby Inc.

Epidemiology in Occupational Health. 1995. lib. bdg. 255.99 *(0-8490-7500-9)* Gordon Pr.

Epidemiology in Primary Health Care. F. Shattock et al. 1990. 332p. (C). *(81-85017-41-7)* Interprint IND. *Dist:* St Mut.

Epidemiology Kept Simple: An Introduction to Classic & Modern Epidemiology. B. Burt Gerstman. 1998. LC 97-42365. 320p. pap. 49.95 *(0-471-24029-X,* Wiley-Liss) Wiley.

Epidemiology of Air Pollution: Report on a Symposium. P. Lawther et al. 1962. (Public Health Papers: No. 15). 31p. pap. text 1.00 *(92-4-130015-9,* 1110015) World Health.

Epidemiology of Allergic Diseases. Ed. by M. L. Burr. 1993. (Monographs in Allergy: Vol. 31). (Illus.). viii, 216p. 239.25 *(3-8055-5601-2)* S Karger.

Epidemiology of Allergic Diseases. Ed. by H. D. Schlumberger. 1987. (Monographs in Allergy: Vol. 21). (Illus.). viii, 288p. 156.75 *(3-8055-4543-6)* S Karger.

Epidemiology of Alzheimer's Disease: From Gene to Prevention. Ed. by Richard Mayeux & Yves Christen. 1999. LC 98-54192. (Research & Perspectives in Alzheimer's Disease Ser.). (Illus.). 144p. 95.00 *(3-540-65413-5)* Spr-Verlag.

Epidemiology of Alzheimer's Disease & Related Disorders. Anthony F. Jorm. 1990. 234p. 55.95 *(0-442-31315-2);* 250p. pap. 73.50 *(0-412-31520-3,* A4449) Chapman & Hall.

Epidemiology of Arterial Blood Pressure. Ed. by Hugo Kesteloot & J. V. Joossens. 1980. (Developments in Cardiovascular Medicine Ser.: No. 8). (Illus.). 525p. text 249.00 *(90-247-2386-8)* Kluwer Academic.

Epidemiology of Blindness & Eye Disease. Ed. by H. G. Krumpaszky & V. Klauss. 1996. (Journal: Vol. 210, No. 1, 1996). (Illus.). 84p. pap. 69.75 *(3-8055-6315-9)* S Karger.

Epidemiology of Cancer. Ed. by Geoffrey J. Bourke. 1983. LC 84-70185. 374p. text 29.95 *(0-914783-03-3)* Charles.

Epidemiology of Cancer of the Digestive Tract. P. Correa & W. Haenszel. 1982. text 171.00 *(90-247-2601-8)* Kluwer Academic.

Epidemiology of Cancer of the Lung. 1960. (Technical Report Ser.: No. 192). 13p. pap. text 3.00 *(92-4-120192-4)* World Health.

Epidemiology of Childhood Disorders. Ivan B. Pless. 1994. (Illus.). 552p. text 79.50 *(0-19-507516-1)* OUP.

Epidemiology of Childhood Hyperactivity. Eric A. Taylor et al. 1991. (Maudsley Monographs: No. 33). 158p. 59.95 *(0-19-262172-6)* OUP.

Epidemiology of Drug Addiction: Three Studies, 1924 to 1926, An Original Anthology. Ed. by Gerald N. Grob. 1981. LC 80-1205. (Addiction in America Ser.). (Illus.). lib. bdg. 23.95 *(0-405-13559-9)* Ayer.

Epidemiology of Eye Disease. Ed. by Gordon J. Johnson et al. 1999. LC 97-75070. (Illus.). 464p. pap. text *(0-412-84500-8)* E A GBR. *Dist:* OUP.

Epidemiology of Human Reproduction. T. Kallen. 1988. (Illus.). 224p. lib. bdg. 195.00 *(0-8493-6452-3,* RA1224) CRC Pr.

Epidemiology of Infertility: Proceedings of the WHO Scientific Group, Geneva, 1975. WHO Staff. 1975. (Technical Reports: No. 582). pap. text 6.00 *(92-4-120582-2)* World Health.

Epidemiology of Leprosy in Relation to Control: Report of a WHO Study Group, 1985. WHO Staff. 1985. (Technical Report Ser.: No. 716). 60p. 7.00 *(92-4-120716-7)* World Health.

Epidemiology of Lung Cancer. Jonathan M. Samet. 1994. LC 93-46314. (Lung Biology in Health & Disease Ser.: Vol. 74). (Illus.). 568p. text 215.00 *(0-8247-8853-2)* Dekker.

Epidemiology of Mental Disorders. 1960. (Technical Report Ser.: No. 185). 29p. pap. text 3.00 *(92-4-120185-1)* World Health.

Epidemiology of Mental Disorders & Psychosocial Problems: Dementia. A. S. Henderson. 1994. (CHI, ENG & FRE.). x, 62p. pap. text 17.00 *(92-4-156164-5,* 1152407) World Health.

Epidemiology of Mental Disorders & Psychosocial Problems: Personality Disorders. G. De Girolamo et al. Ed. by World Health Organization Staff. 1993. (CHI & FRE.). xi, 66p. pap. text 17.00 *(92-4-156160-2,* 1151407) World Health.

Epidemiology of Mental Disorders & Psychosocial Problems: Schizophrenia. R. Warner & G. De Girolamo. 1995. LC 96-227635. (FRE.). 139p. (C). pap. 28.80 *(92-4-156171-8,* 1153407) World Health.

Epidemiology of Musculoskeletal Disorders. Jennifer L. Kelsey. 1982. (Monographs in Epidemiology & Biostatistics). (Illus.). 275p. (C). text 39.95 *(0-19-503117-2)* OUP.

Epidemiology of Natural Disasters. J. Seaman et al. 1984. (Contributions to Epidemiology & Biostatistics Ser.: Vol. 5). (Illus.). viii, 180p. 128.75 *(3-8055-3779-4)* S Karger.

Epidemiology of Neurologic & Sense Organ Disorders. Leonard T. Kurland et al. 1973. LC 72-90644. (Vital & Health Statistics Monographs). (Illus.). 470p. 44.50 *(0-674-25875-4)* HUP.

Epidemiology of Neurological Diorders. Ed. by C. N. Martyn & R. A. Hughes. 1998. (Illus.). 248p. *(0-7279-1149-X)* BMJ Pub GBR. *Dist:* AIDC.

Epidemiology of Neurological Disorders. Lawrence W. Svenson. 1999. 85.00 *(0-8493-2669-9)* CRC Pr.

Epidemiology of Occupational Health. Sven Hernberg. 1991. 256p. lib. bdg. 95.00 *(0-87371-636-1,* L636) Lewis Pubs.

Epidemiology of Occupational Health. Ed. by M. Karvonen & M. I. Mikheev. 1986. (WHO Regional Publications, European Ser.: No. 20). 392p. pap. text 48.00 *(92-890-1111-4,* 1310020) World Health.

Epidemiology of Oral Health. Walter J. Pelton et al. 1969. LC 77-88811. (Vital & Health Statistics Monographs, Am). (Illus.). 189p. 27.50 *(0-674-25885-1)* HUP.

Epidemiology of Peripheral Vascular Disease. Ed. by F. G. Fowkes. 1991. (Illus.). 366p. 164.00 *(0-387-19696-X)* Spr-Verlag.

Epidemiology of Prostate Disease. Ed. by Michael Garraway. 1995. (Illus.). 293p. 114.00 *(0-387-57708-4);* LC 95-6469. *(3-540-57708-4)* Spr-Verlag.

Epidemiology of Quality. Vahe A. Kazandjian & Elizabeth Sternberg. 1995. 330p. 72.00 *(0-8342-0533-5,* 20533) Aspen Pub.

Epidemiology of Road Traffic Accidents. 1976. (WHO Regional Publications, European Ser.: No. 2). 38p. pap. text 6.00 *(92-9020-102-9,* 1310002) World Health.

Epidemiology of the Cerebral Palsies. Ed. by Fiona Stanley & Eva Alberman. 1991. (Clinics in Developmental Medicine Ser.: No. 87). (Illus.). 188p. (C). text *(0-521-41207-2)* Mc Keith Pr GBR. *Dist:* Cambridge U Pr.

Epidemiology of the Rheumatic Diseases. Alan J. Silman & Marc C. Hochberg. 1994. LC 93-33168. (Oxford Medical Publications). (Illus.). 514p. text 79.50 *(0-19-262356-7)* OUP.

Epidemiology of Work Related Diseases. Ed. by J. C. McDonald. 1995. 500p. text *(0-7279-0856-1)* BMJ Pub GBR. *Dist:* AIDC.

Epidemology of Pychogenic Disorders. H. Schepank. 1987. (Illus.). 176p. 42.95 *(0-387-18027-3)* Spr-Verlag.

Epidermal Growth Factors & Cytokines. Ed. by Thomas A. Luger & Thomas Schwarz. 1993. LC 93-27742. (Basic & Clinical Dermatology Ser.: Vol. 10). (Illus.). 504p. text 225.00 *(0-8247-9102-9)* Dekker.

Epidermal Keratinocyte Differentiation & Fibrillogenesis. Ed. by M. Prunieras. 1981. (Frontiers of Matrix Biology Ser.: Vol. 9). (Illus.). viii, 192p. 104.50 *(3-8055-0893-X)* S Karger.

Epidermolysis Bullosa: Basic & Clinical Aspects. Ed. by A. N. Lin & D. M. Carter. 1992. (Illus.). 302p. 170.00 *(0-387-97796-1)* Spr-Verlag.

Epidermolysis Bullosa: Clinical, Epidemiologic & Laboratory Advances, & the Findings of the National Epidermolysis Bullosa Registry. National Epidermolysis Bullosa Registry U.S. Staff. Ed. by Jo-David Fine et al. 1999. LC 98-41894. (Illus.). 510p. 110.00 *(0-8018-6024-5)* Johns Hopkins.

Epididymis & Fertility: Biology & Pathology. Ed. by C. G. Bollack & A. Clavert. 1981. (Progress in Reproductive Biology & Medicine Ser.: Vol. 8). (Illus.). x, 174p. 103.50 *(3-8055-2157-X)* S Karger.

Epididymis as a Chloride-Secreting Organ. Anskar Y. Leung. 1995. 173p. (Orig.). (C). pap. *(962-201-673-1)* Chinese Univ HKG. *Dist:* Coronet Bks.

Epidurals for Childbirth. Anne May. 1994. LC 94-8975. (Oxford Medical Publications). (Illus.). 216p. text 59.95 *(0-19-262439-3);* pap. text 29.50 *(0-19-262438-5)* OUP.

Epigenesis of Mind: Essays on Biology & Cognition. Ed. by Susan Carey & Rochel Gelman. 1991. LC 90-49812. (Jean Piaget Symposia Ser.). 360p. text 69.95 *(0-8058-0438-2)* L Erlbaum Assocs.

Epigenetic Mechanisms of Gene Regulation. Ed. by Vincenzo E. Russo et al. 1996. LC 96-85974. (Monographs: Vol. 32). (Illus.). 672p. (C). text 129.00 *(0-87969-490-4)* Cold Spring Harbor.

Epilepsie-Francais, Vol. 8. Larousse Staff. 1976. 160.00 *(0-7859-5585-2,* 2030009083) Fr & Eur.

Epilepsies. Ed. by Pierre J. Vinken & George W. Bruyn. 1974. 293.50 *(0-444-10457-7)* Elsevier.

Epilepsies. Pierre J. Vinken et al. 1974. (Handbooks of Clinical Neurology: Vol. 15). 860p. 381.00 *(0-7204-7215-6)* Elsevier.

Epilepsies: Etiologies & Prevention. Ed. by Prakash Kotagal & Hans O. Luders. 1998. LC 98-85529. (Illus.). 587p. (C). 159.95 *(0-12-422150-5)* Acad Pr.

Epilepsies Pt. 1, Pt. 1. Ed. by P.J. Vinken et al. 1999. LC 00-21830. (Handbooks of Clinical Neurology). (Illus.). 452p. 187.00 *(0-444-82810-9,* Excerpta Medica) Elsevier.

Epilepsies 2. Roger J. Porter et al. 1997. LC 96-50470. (Blue Bks. of Practical Neurology: Vol. 18). 384p. text 95.00 *(0-7506-9824-1)* Buttrwrth-Heinemann.

Epilepsy. J. Majkowski. 1981. (Monographs in Neural Sciences: Vol. 5). (Illus.). xvi, 304p. pap. 81.75 *(3-8055-0635-X)* S Karger.

Epilepsy. Cal Orey & Joan Hustace Walker. 1999. LC 98-39298. (Essential Guide to Natural Pet Care Ser.: Vol. 4). (Illus.). 64p. pap. 6.95 *(1-889540-34-X)* Bowtie Press.

Epilepsy. J. Sander & Yvonne Hart. 1997. (Questions & Answers Ser.). (Illus.). 188p. pap. 17.95 *(1-873413-80-7)* Merit Pub Intl.

Epilepsy. Sue Vander Hook. 2000. LC 99-39170. (Understanding Illness Ser.). (J). lib. bdg. 16.95 *(1-58340-025-7)* Smart Apple.

Epilepsy. Adrienne Richard & Joel Reiter. rev. ed. 1995. LC 95-3651. 288p. pap. 14.95 *(0-8027-7465-2)* Walker & Co.

***Epilepsy.** Brodie & Schachter. 2nd ed. 2001. (Fast Facts Ser.). (Illus.). 82p. pap. *(1-899541-69-1)* Health Pr GBR. *Dist:* JAMCO Dist.

Epilepsy. Ed. by A. Hopkins et al. 2nd ed. 1995. (Illus.). 696p. *(0-412-54330-3)* E A GBR. *Dist:* OUP.

Epilepsy: 199 Answers (A Doctor Responds to His Patients' Questions) Andrew N. Wilner. 1996. (Illus.). 128p. (Orig.). pap. 19.95 *(1-888799-09-9)* Demos Medical.

Epilepsy: A Behavior Medicine Approach to Assessment & Treatment in Children: A Handbook for Professionals Working with Epilepsy. JoAnne C. Dahl. 1993. LC 92-49951. (Illus.). 187p. pap. 38.00 *(0-88937-106-7)* Hogrefe & Huber Pubs.

Epilepsy: A Comprehensive Textbook. Jerome Engel, Jr. 1997. LC 96-31052. 3,092p. text 475.00 *(0-397-51639-8)* Lppncott W & W.

Epilepsy: A Comprehensive Textbook. Jerome Engel, Jr. et al. 1997. 3,092p. 550.00 *(0-7817-2099-0)* Lppncott W & W.

Epilepsy: A Handbook. Buchanan. 1995. pap. text 25.00 *(0-7020-2014-1)* Saunders.

Epilepsy: A Personal Approach. Nancy C. Schumacher. 1985. LC 85-1965. 200p. 18.95 *(0-87073-469-5);* pap. 11.95 *(0-87073-494-6)* Schenkman Bks Inc.

Epilepsy: A Source Guide. 1991. lib. bdg. 66.95 *(0-8490-4832-X)* Gordon Pr.

Epilepsy: Diagnosis & Management. Ed. by Thomas R. Browne & Robert G. Feldman. 1983. 376p. 75.00 *(0-316-11114-7,* Little Brwn Med Div) Lppncott W & W.

Epilepsy: Facts about Fits. Roy G. Beran. 1999. 116p. pap. 42.00 *(0-8036-0401-7)* Davis Co.

Epilepsy: Frequency, Causes & Consequences. Alan Hauser & Dale Hesdorffer. 1990. 392p. text 94.95 *(0-939957-32-9)* Demos Medical.

Epilepsy: Models, Mechanisms & Concepts. Ed. by Philip A. Schwartzkroin. 1993. (Illus.). 558p. (C). text 120.00 *(0-521-39298-5)* Cambridge U Pr.

Epilepsy: Patient & Family Guide. Orrin Devinsky. 2nd ed. 2001. LC 2001-37243. (Illus.). 448p. per. 24.95 *(0-8036-0498-X)* Davis Co.

Epilepsy: Practical & Easy-to-Follow Advice. Fiona Marshall. 1999. LC 98-36449. (Your Child Ser.). 128p. pap. 9.95 *(1-86204-315-9)* Element MA.

Epilepsy: Problem Solving in Clinical Practice. Ed. by Dieter A. Schmidt & Steven C. Schachter. 1999. 489p. *(1-85317-504-8)* Martin Dunitz GBR. *Dist:* Blackwell Sci.

***Epilepsy: Questions & Answers.** J. W. Sanders & Yvonne Hart. 2nd ed. 2001. (Illus.). 158p. pap. 29.95 *(1-873413-87-4)* Merit Pub Intl.

Epilepsy: Recent View on Its Theory, Diagnosis & Therapy of Epilepsy. Ernest Niedermeyer. 1970. (Modern Problems of Pharmacopsychiatry Ser.: Vol. 4). 90.50 *(3-8055-0529-9)* S Karger.

Epilepsy: The Facts. Anthony Hopkins & Richard E. Appleton. 2nd ed. 1996. (Facts Ser.). (Illus.). 168p. pap. 19.95 *(0-19-262548-9)* OUP.

Epilepsy: Your Guide to Complementary Therapies, Alternative Techniques & Conventional Treatments. Fiona Marshall. 1998. LC 98-4675. (Natural Way Ser.). 128p. pap. 5.95 *(1-86204-194-6)* Element MA.

Epilepsy A to Z: A Glossary of Epilepsy Terminology. Peter W. Kaplan et al. 1995. LC 95-4234. 340p. pap. 34.95 *(0-939957-75-2)* Demos Medical.

Epilepsy & Developmental Disabilities. Devinsky. 2001. 496p. 125.00 *(0-7506-7273-0)* Buttrwrth-Heinemann.

Epilepsy & Law. Ed. by Roy G. Beran & A. Carmi. 1998. 266p. pap. 40.00 *(965-7077-01-X,* 324080) W S Hein.

Epilepsy & Other Neurological Disorder in Coeliac Disease. Gobbi. 1997. 392p. text 114.00 *(0-86196-537-X)* Buttrwrth-Heinemann.

E F G

Epilepsy & Pregnancy: Maternal & Fetal Aspects. Ed. by Torbjorn Tomson et al. 1997. LC 97-9933. 288p. (*1-871816-36-X*) Wrightson Biomed GBR. *Dist:* Taylor & Francis.

Epilepsy & Sudden Death. Schraeder & Marie Lathers. 1990. (Neurological Disease & Therapy Ser.: Vol. 7). (Illus.). 552p. text 225.00 (*0-8247-8308-5*) Dekker.

Epilepsy & the Corpus Callosum. Ed. by Alexander G. Reeves. 1985. LC 85-3465. 520p. 135.00 (*0-306-41848-7*, Plenum Trade) Perseus Pubng.

Epilepsy & the Corpus Callosum 2: Proceedings of the Second International Conference Held in Hanover, New Hampshire, August 14-18, 1991. Ed. by Alexander G. Reeves & David W. Roberts. 1995. (Advances in Behavioral Biology Ser.: Vol. 45). (Illus.). 322p. 110.00 (*0-306-45134-4*, Kluwer Plenum) Kluwer Academic.

Epilepsy & the Family. Richard Lechtenberg. (Illus.). 240p. 1986. pap. text 16.00 (*0-674-25889-4*); 1984. 29.00 (*0-674-25888-6*) HUP.

Epilepsy & the Oral Manifestations of Phenytoin Therapy. Thomas M. Hassell. 1981. (Monographs in Oral Science: Vol. 9). (Illus.). xiv, 206p. pap. 129.75 (*3-8055-1008-X*) S Karger.

Epilepsy Diet Treatment: An Introduction to the Ketogenic Diet see Ketogenic Diet: A Treatment for Epilepsy

Epilepsy Handbook: The Practical Management of Seizures. Robert J. Gumnit. 2nd ed. 1994. LC 94-18362. 208p. pap. text 39.95 (*0-7817-0176-7*) Lppncott W & W.

Epilepsy in Children. Ed. by S. Wallace. 1995. (Illus.). 672p. (*0-412-56860-8*) E A GBR. *Dist:* OUP.

Epilepsy in Children. Jean Aicardi. 2nd ed. 1993. (International Review of Child Neurology Ser.). 576p. text 129.00 (*0-7817-0111-2*) Lppncott W & W.

Epilepsy in Children & Adolescents. Ed. by Albert P. Aldenkamp et al. 1995. LC 95-90097. 336p. 189.95 (*0-8493-7659-9*, 7659) CRC Pr.

Epilepsy in Clinical Practice: A Case Studies Approach. Andrew N. Wilner. 2000. LC 00-54407. 296p. pap. text 34.95 (*1-888799-34-X*) Demos Medical.

Epilepsy in Primary Care: A Team Approach to Effective Management. Simon J. Ellis & Linda Baddeley. 2002. 240p. pap. 39.99 (*0-7506-4954-2*) Buttrwrth-Heinemann.

Epilepsy Parent & Family Networks Resource Manual. Epilepsy Foundation of America Staff. 1992. 202p. pap. 19.95 (*0-916570-10-X*) Epilepsy Foundation of America.

Epilepsy, Pregnancy & the Child. Sibylle Ried & Gertrud Beck-Managetta. 1996. 96p. (Orig.). pap. text 19.95 (*0-632-04164-1*) Blackwell Sci.

Epilepsy State of the Art, 1993. H. Lechner. Ed. by G. Scollo-Lavizzari. 1994. (Journal: Vol. 34, Suppl. 1, 1994). (Illus.). iv, 90p. pap. 41.00 (*3-8055-6038-9*) S Karger.

Epilepsy Surgery. Hans Otto Loders & Youssef G. Comair. 2nd ed. 2000. 1,088p. text 235.00 (*0-7817-1442-7*) Lppncott W & W.

Epilepsy Surgery: Case Rounds. Kost Elisevich & Brien Smith. 2002. text 120.00 (*0-7817-1727-2*) Lppncott W & W.

Epileptic & Crippled Child & Adult. Charity Organisation Society Staff. Ed. by William R. Phillips & Janet Rosenberg. 1980. LC 79-6899. (Physically Handicapped in Society Ser.). reprint ed. lib. bdg. 19.95 (*0-405-13109-7*) Ayer.

Epileptic Focus. H. G. Wieser et al. 1987. (Current Problems in Epilepsy Ser.: Vol. 3). 240p. (*0-86196-062-9*) J Libbey Med GBR. *Dist:* Bks Intl VA.

Epileptic Seizures. Hans Luders & Soheyl Noachtar. 1999. LC 98-53144. (Illus.). xix, 796p. text 85.00 (*0-443-08959-0*) Saunders.

Epileptic Seizures & Syndromes. Wolf. 1994. 688p. (*0-86196-430-6*) J Libbey Med GBR. *Dist:* Buttrwrth-Heinemann.

Epileptic Sydromes in Infancy. Roger. 1992. 432p. (*0-86196-320-2*) J Libbey Med GBR. *Dist:* Buttrwrth-Heinemann.

Epileptic Syndromes in Infancy, Childhood & Adolescence. Ed. by J. Roger et al. 1985. (Current Problems in Epilepsy Ser.: Vol. 2). (*0-86196-045-9*) J Libbey Med GBR. *Dist:* Bks Intl VA.

Epileptic Syndromes in Infancy, Childhood & Adolescence. J. Roger. 3rd ed. 2001. 99p. (*0-86196-611-2*) John Libby GBR. *Dist:* Buttrwrth-Heinemann.

Epileptogenic & Excitotoxic Mechanisms. Avanzini. 1993. 168p. (*0-86196-386-5*) J Libbey Med GBR. *Dist:* Buttrwrth-Heinemann.

***Epilspsy.** Robert J. DeLorenzo. (Fast Facts Ser.). (*1-899541-27-6*) Health Pr GBR. *Dist:* JAMCO Dist.

Episiotomy: Challenging Obstetric Interventions. Ian D. Graham. 1997. LC 96-43827. (Illus.). 192p. pap. 40.95 (*0-632-04145-5*) Blackwell Sci.

Episiotomy & the Second Stage of Labor. Ed. by Sheila Kitzinger & Penny Simkin. 2nd ed. 1986. LC 84-61122. (Illus.). 133p. pap. 7.95 (*0-937604-07-0*, Pennypr) Intl Childbirth.

Epistemology & Psychology of Functions. Jean Piaget et al. Tr. by Javier Castellanos & Vivian Anderson. 1977. (Synthese Library: No. 83). 219p. lib. bdg. 112.00 (*90-277-0804-5*) Kluwer Academic.

***Epitaph & an Elegy for a Prostate Pt. 1: Incontinence, Impotence & Artifical Urinary Sphincter.** Gene Washington. 2001. 283p. 25.00 (*0-7388-6926-0*); pap. 16.00 (*0-7388-6927-9*) Xlibris Corp.

Epitaph for Merlin & Perhaps for Medicine. Sylvan L. Weinberg. 1984. LC 83-62808. 94p. pap. 9.95 (*0-914783-01-7*) Charles.

Epitaphs for the Living: Words & Images in the Time of AIDS. Billy Howard. 1989. LC 88-43252. (Illus.). 160p. 35.00 (*0-87074-289-2*) SMU Press.

Epithelial Hyperplastic Lesions of the Larynx. V. Kambic. 1995. 284p. 198.50 (*0-444-82273-9*) Elsevier.

Epithelial-Mesenchymal Interactions in Cancer. Ed. by I. D. Goldberg & E. M. Rosen. (EXS Ser.: No. 74). 1996. 298p. 89.50 (*3-7643-5117-9*); 1995. 89.50 (*0-8176-5117-9*) Birkhauser.

Epithelial-Mesenchymal Interactions in Development. Roger H. Sawyer. Ed. by John F. Fallon. 1983. LC 82-13160. 252p. 68.00 (*0-275-91074-1*, C1074, Praeger Pubs) Greenwood.

Epithelial-Mesenchymal Transitions, Pt. 1. Ed. by M. Ferguson & Don Newgreen. 1996. (Journal: Vol. 154, No. 1, 1995). (Illus.). 98p. pap. 91.50 (*3-8055-6303-5*) S Karger.

Epithelial Secretion of Water & Electrolytes. Ed. by J. A. Young & P. Y. Wong. 1990. (Illus.). 379p. 190.00 (*0-387-51627-1*) Spr-Verlag.

Epithelial Transport & Barrier Function: Pathomechanisms in Gastrointestinal Disorders. Jhorg-Dieter Schulzke. 2000. LC 00-51126. (Annals of the New York Academy of Sciences Ser.: Vol. 915). (Illus.). xii, 375p. pap. (*1-57331-260-6*) NY Acad Sci.

Epithelial Tumors of the Thymus: Pathology, Biology & Treatment. Ed. by Alexander Marx & Hans K. Muller-Hermelink. 1997. LC 97-1867. 411p. (C). text 120.00 (*0-306-45591-9*, Kluwer Plenum) Kluwer Academic.

Epitome of Practical Surgery for Field & Hospital. Edward Warren. 1989. LC 88-60669. (American Civil War Surgery Ser.: No. 6). 401p. reprint ed. 60.00 (*0-930405-09-9*) Norman SF.

Eponymic Dictionary of Psychiatric Terminology. V. M. Bleikher. 1980. 238p. 14.95 (*0-8288-1857-6*, M15372) Fr & Eur.

Eponyms in Orthopaedics & Rheumatology. Moll. 1995. (Illus.). (C). (gr. 13). 22.00 (*0-412-27200-8*) Chapman & Hall.

Eponyms in Psychology: A Dictionary & Biographical Sourcebook. Leonard Zusne. 1987. LC 87-255. 360p. lib. bdg. 95.00 (*0-313-25750-7*, ZPS/, Greenwood Pr) Greenwood.

Eponyms of Behavioral Optometry. Homer H. Hendrickson. Ed. by Sally M. Corngold. 1992. (Illus.). 150p. (C). lib. bdg. 18.00 (*0-943599-24-5*) OEPF.

EPSAP II: Electrophysiology Self-Assessment Program. Ed. by Gerald V. Naccarelli et al. 2000. LC 99-67738. 595p. pap. 645.00 (*1-58397-007-X*) Am Coll Cardiology.

Epstein-Barr Virus & Human Cancer. T. Osato et al. 1998. LC 98-164993. (Gann Monographs on Cancer Research). viii, 190 p. (*4-7622-1874-X*) Jap Sci Soc Pr.

Epstein-Barr Virus & Human Cancer. Ed. by Toyoro Osato et al. 1998. (Gann Monographs on Cancer Research: No. 45, 1998). (Illus.). viii, 190p. 243.50 (*3-8055-6663-8*) S Karger.

Epstein-Barr Virus & Human Disease. Ed. by D. V. Ablashi et al. 1987. LC 87-16869. (Experimental Biology & Medicine Ser.: Vol. 15). 530p. 145.00 (*0-89603-130-6*) Humana.

Epstein-Barr Virus & Human Disease - 1988. Ed. by D. V. Ablashi et al. (Experimental Biology & Medicine Ser.: Vol. 24). 1991. LC 91-20857. (Illus.). 496p. 155.00 (*0-89603-221-3*); 1989. LC 89-15445. 549p. 155.00 (*0-89603-165-9*) Humana.

Epstein-Barr Virus & Malignancy. Ed. by Richard F. Ambinder & Sally L. Glaser. 1999. 500p. 125.00 (*0-89603-701-0*) Humana.

Epstein-Barr Virus Products. Ed. by Joanna B. Wilson & Gerhard H. W. May. 2001. LC 2001-16991. (Methods in Molecular Biology Ser.: Vol. 174). (Illus.). 438p. 135.00 (*0-89603-690-1*) Humana.

Equal Partnering: A Feminine Perspective. Ed. by Barbara J. Brothers. 1992. LC 92-13454. (Journal of Couples Therapy Ser.). (Illus.). 109p. pap. 9.95 (*1-56023-017-7*, Harrington Park); text 24.95 (*1-56024-260-4*) Haworth Pr.

Equal Partners - Good Friends: Empowering Couples Through Therapy. Claire Rabin. 1996. LC 95-42247. (Illus.). 296p. (C). 85.00 (*0-415-11614-7*); pap. 25.99 (*0-415-11615-5*) Routledge.

Equal Treatment for People with Mental Retardation: Having & Raising Children. Martha A. Field & Valerie A. Sanchez. 2000. LC 99-35786. (Illus.). 448p. 49.95 (*0-674-80086-9*) HUP.

Equilibration in the Natural & Restored Dentition. Hyman Smukler. 1991. (Illus.). 136p. text 48.00 (*0-86715-224-9*) Quint Pub Co.

Equilibration, Mind & Brain: Toward an Integrated Psychology. E. J. Parkins. 1990. LC 90-32179. 216p. 60.95 (*0-275-93609-0*, C3609, Praeger Pubs) Greenwood.

Equine Acupressure, a Working Manual. Nancy A. Zidonis et al. Ed. by Ella Bittel. 1998. (Illus.). 152p. spiral bd. 29.95 (*0-9645982-2-1*) Tallgrass Pubs.

Equine Acute Abdomen. Ed. by Nathaniel A. White. 1990. LC 89-12795. (Illus.). 434p. 89.50 (*0-8121-1175-3*) Lppncott W & W.

Equine Anesthesia: Monitoring & Emergency Therapy. Muir & John A. E. Hubbell. 1991. (Illus.). 528p. (C). (gr. 13). text 74.95 (*0-8016-3576-4*, 03576) Mosby Inc.

Equine Behavioural Problems. Marsden. 2000. text 79.00 (*0-7020-1891-0*) Saunders.

Equine Body Language. Victoria Vidal. Date not set. 100p. pap. 8.95 (*1-885351-81-X*) Cheval Intl.

Equine Breeding Management & Artificial Insemination. Juan C. Samper. Ed. by Stephanie Donley. 1999. LC 98-34632. (Illus.). 300p. (C). text 55.00 (*0-7216-7012-1*) Saunders.

***Equine Cardiology.** Chris Brown. 2001. (Illus.). 415p. (*0-7216-9209-5*) Saunders.

Equine Cardiology. Mark Patteson. 1995. LC 95-661. (Illus.). 224p. pap. (*0-632-03299-5*) Blckwell Science.

Equine Clinical Nutrition. Lon D. Lewis. 1995. (Illus.). 650p. 79.95 (*0-683-04962-3*) Lppncott W & W.

Equine Color Genetics. D. Phillip Sponenberg. 1996. LC 96-33961. (Illus.). 192p. text 44.95 (*0-8138-2905-4*) Iowa U Pr.

Equine Dermatology. Fadok. 1999. text (*0-7216-2571-1*) Saunders.

Equine Dermatology Handbook. Pascoe. 1998. (Illus.). 255p. (C). text 45.00 (*0-7020-1968-2*) Saunders.

Equine Diagnostic Ultrasonography. Norman W. Rantanen & Angus O. McKinnon. 1997. LC 97-33085. (Illus.). 696p. 129.00 (*0-683-07123-8*) Lppncott W & W.

Equine Diagnostic Ultrasound. Virginia B. Reef. Ed. by Stephanie Donley. 1998. LC 97-48247. (Illus.). 400p. (C). text 125.00 (*0-7216-5023-6*) Saunders.

Equine Diseases. H. J. Wintzer. 1986. (Illus.). 450p. 180.00 (*0-387-91225-8*) Spr-Verlag.

Equine Drugs & Vaccines. Eleanor M. Kellon. 1994. (Illus.). 350p. spiral bd. 56.00 (*0-914327-55-0*) Breakthrgh NY.

Equine Endoscopy. Josie L. Traub-Dargatz & Christopher Brown. 2nd ed. 1996. LC 96-27784. (Illus.). 264p. (C). (gr. 13). text 125.00 (*0-8151-8858-7*, 25286) Mosby Inc.

Equine Foot. C. MacGregor. 2000. (Illus.). 510p. text (*0-7020-1766-3*) W B Saunders GBR. *Dist:* Saunders.

Equine Fracture Repair. Alan J. Nixon. 1995. LC 94-32748. (Illus.). 352p. text 104.00 (*0-7216-6754-6*) Saunders.

Equine Infectious Diseases No. 5: Proceedings of the Fifth International Conference. Ed. by David G. Powell. 1989. LC 88-27670. 312p. text 70.00 (*0-8131-1676-7*) U Pr of KY.

Equine Infectious Diseases II: Proceedings of the International Conference, 2nd, Paris, 1969. International Conference on Equine Infectious Dise. Ed. by J. T. Bryans & H. Gerber. 1970. 65.25 (*3-8055-0825-5*) S Karger.

Equine Injury & Therapy. Mary W. Bromiley. 2nd ed. 1993. LC 93-26995. (Illus.). 192p. pap. 34.95 (*0-632-03608-7*) Blackwell Sci.

Equine Internal Medicine. Reed. 1997. LC 95-48272. text 135.00 (*0-7216-3524-5*) Saunders.

Equine Lameness. Christine King & Richard A. Mansmann. Ed. by Don M. Wagoner. 1997. LC 00-710223. (Illus.). 900p. 85.00 (*0-935842-12-8*) Equine Res.

Equine Lameness. Schneider. 1997. pap. text (*0-7216-5036-8*) Saunders.

Equine Manual. Higgins. 1995. text 99.00 (*0-7020-1572-5*) Saunders.

Equine Massage Therapy: A Practical Guide. Jean-Pierre Hourdebaigt. 1997. LC 95-13806. (Illus.). 240p. pap. 27.95 (*0-87605-998-1*, Howell) Hungry Minds.

Equine Medical Disorders. A. M. Johnston. 2nd ed. 1994. LC 93-46065. (Library of Veterinary Practice). (Illus.). 224p. pap. (*0-632-03841-1*) Blckwell Science.

Equine Medicine: Surgery & Repair. Mair et al. 1997. (Illus.). 507p. text 89.00 (*0-7020-1725-6*) Saunders.

Equine Medicine & Management, Vol. 1. Cody W. Faerber. 2nd ed. 2000. 195p. reprint ed. ring bd. 74.95 (*0-9701159-0-3*) Animal Hlth.

Equine Medicine & Surgery. Edgar D. Mayhew et al. 5th ed. 1998. LC 98-24941. (Illus.). 2076p. (gr. 13). text 239.00 (*0-8151-1743-4*, 28580) Mosby Inc.

Equine Medicine Secrets. Catherine J. Savage. 1998. LC 98-40692. (Secrets Ser.). (Illus.). 350p. pap. 39.95 (*1-56053-263-7*) Hanley & Belfus.

Equine Musculoskeletal Ultrasound. Smith. 1998. text 70.00 (*0-7020-1894-5*) Saunders.

Equine Nutrition. Derek Cuddeford. 1997. (Illus.). 160p. (*1-85223-852-6*) Crowood Pr GBR. *Dist:* Trafalgar.

Equine Nutrition & Feeding. D. L. Frape. 1989. (Illus.). 390p. text (*0-582-45014-4*) Church.

Equine Nutrition & Feeding. David Frape. 2nd ed. LC 97-34539. (Illus.). 1999. 564p. pap. (*0-632-05303-8*); 1997. 400p. (*0-632-04105-6*) Blckwell Science GBR. *Dist:* Iowa U Pr.

Equine Perinatology. Vaala. Date not set. (C). text (*0-7216-8109-3*) Saunders.

Equine Physiology. Beth Maloney. 1999. (*0-85131-735-9*) J A Allen GBR. *Dist:* St Mut.

Equine Practice. William E. Boden. 1991. pap. text 48.00 (*0-7020-1521-0*) Saunders.

Equine Practice 3. William E. Boden. 3rd ed. 1997. 233p. pap. text 55.00 (*0-7020-2332-9*) Saunders.

Equine Radiography. Joe P. Morgan et al. 1991. (Venture Series in Veterinary Medicine). (Illus.). 384p. (C). text 92.95 (*0-8138-0257-1*) Iowa U Pr.

Equine Reproduction. Angus McKinnon & James Voss. 1992. LC 91-29283. (Illus.). 1,137p. text 110.00 (*0-8121-1427-2*) Lppncott W & W.

Equine Reproductive Physiology: Breeding & Stud Management. Mina D. Morel. 1993. (Illus.). 450p. text (*0-85236-255-2*) Farming Pr GBR. *Dist:* Diamond Farm Bk.

Equine Respiratory Disorders. Ed. by Jill Beech. 1991. LC 90-5885. (Illus.). 458p. 89.50 (*0-8121-1325-X*) Lppncott W & W.

Equine Science. Rick Parker. 1997. LC 96-35298. 660p. 61.95 (*0-8273-7136-5*); (C). pap. text, tchr. ed., lab manual ed. 13.95 (*0-8273-8098-4*); (C). pap. text, lab manual ed. 18.95 (*0-8273-8097-6*) Delmar.

Equine Science, Health & Performance: The Essentials. Sarah Pilliner & Zoe Davies. 1996. LC 96-11750. 240p. pap. 46.95 (*0-632-03913-2*) Blackwell Sci.

Equine Sports Medicine. Ed. by William E. Jones et al. 1989. LC 87-21289. (Illus.). 329p. 80.00 (*0-8121-1100-1*) Lppncott W & W.

Equine Surgery. Jorg A. Auer. 2nd ed. 1992. text 240.00 (*0-7216-2860-5*) Saunders.

Equine Surgery. Jorg A. Auer & John A. Stick. Ed. by Stephanie Donley. 2nd ed. 1999. LC 98-43180. (Illus.). 955p. text 155.00 (*0-7216-7733-9*) Saunders.

Equine Surgery & Medicine, Vol. 1. Ed. by John Hickman. 1985. (Animal Care, Health & Welfare Ser.). text 176.00 (*0-12-347221-0*) Acad Pr.

Equine Surgery & Medicine, Vol. 2. John Hickman. 1987. (Animal Care, Health & Welfare Ser.). text 176.00 (*0-12-347222-9*) Acad Pr.

Equine Training Log & Health Care Diary. Michael Scott. 1997. pap. 19.95 (*0-9662677-2-9*) Massage-Muscle.

***Equine Veterinary Nursing Manual.** Ed. by Karen Coumbe. 2001. LC 2001-25149. (*0-632-05727-0*) Blackwell Sci.

Equine Wound Management. Ted S. Stashak. 1991. LC 90-13484. (Illus.). 278p. 75.00 (*0-8121-1185-0*) Lppncott W & W.

Equipment for Diagnostic Radiography. E. Forster. 1985. pap. text 73.50 (*0-85200-437-0*); lib. bdg. 122.50 (*0-85200-928-3*) Kluwer Academic.

Equipment for Older or Disabled People & the Law. Michael Mandelstam. 1996. LC 97-135389. 200p. pap. (*1-85302-352-3*) Jessica Kingsley GBR. *Dist:* Taylor & Francis.

Equipment for Vector Control. 3rd ed. 1990. (Illus.). x, 310p. pap. text 51.00 (*92-4-154403-1*, 1153041) World Health.

Equipment Theory for Respiratory Care. Gary C. White. 1992. text 48.95 (*0-8273-3860-0*); 2nd ed. 1996. 192p. 18.00 (*0-8273-7697-9*); 2nd ed. 1996. 176p. (C). pap., wbk. ed. 16.95 (*0-8273-7547-6*); 2nd ed. 1995. 688p. (C). pap. 48.00 (*0-8273-6482-2*); 3rd ed. 1999. 224p. tchr. ed. 20.95 (*0-7668-0461-5*); 3rd ed. 1998. LC 98-28026. 720p. (C). 78.95 (*0-7668-0460-7*) Delmar.

Equivalence of Medical Qualifications & the Practice of Medicine: A Survey of Existing Legislation. WHO Staff. 1967. (International Digest of Health Legislation Offprints: Vol. 18, No. 3). 47p. 5.00 (*92-4-169183-2*) World Health.

ER Intern Pocket Survival Guide. Todd C. Rothenhaus & Thomas M. Masterson. 1992. 78p. (Orig.). (C). pap. text 7.50 (*0-9634063-2-9*) Intl Med Pub.

Eradication of Infectious Diseases. P. Yekutiel. 1980. (Contributions to Epidemiology & Biostatistics Ser.: Vol. 2). (Illus.). pap. 56.75 (*3-8055-3068-4*) S Karger.

Eradication of Infectious Diseases: Report of the Dahlem Workshop on the Eradication of Infectious Diseases, Berlin, March 16-22, 1997. Walter Dowdle & David Hopkins. 1998. LC 97-41829. (Dahlem Workshop Reports). 238p. 159.95 (*0-471-98089-7*) Wiley.

Eradication of Smallpox from India. R. Basu & Z. Jezek. 1979. (WHO Regional Publications, South-East Asia Ser.: No. 5). 346p. text 30.00 (*92-9022-105-4*) World Health.

Erasing Scars: Herpes & Healing. James D. Okun & Evangilita Goodmere. Ed. by Ed Roberts et al. 1997. LC 96-92867. (Illus.). 180p. (YA). pap. 15.95 (*0-9649093-0-8*) Jane Pubns.

ERCP & It's Applications. Ed. by Ira M. Jacobson. 1997. LC 97-23060. (Illus.). 288p. text 139.00 (*0-397-51664-9*) Lppncott W & W.

Erectile Disorders: Assessment & Treatment. Ed. by Raymond C. Rosen & Sandra R. Leiblum. 1992. LC 91-38062. 378p. text 45.00 (*0-89862-792-3*) Guilford Pubns.

***Erectile Dysfunction.** Evans & Kell. 2000. (Patient Pictures Ser.). (Illus.). 33p. pap. (*1-899541-11-X*) Health Pr GBR. *Dist:* JAMCO Dist.

Erectile Dysfunction. Ed. by U. Jonas et al. 1991. (Illus.). 336p. 206.00 (*0-387-52748-6*) Spr-Verlag.

***Erectile Dysfunction.** Kirby et al. 3rd ed. 2002. (Fast Facts Ser.). (Illus.). 64p. pap. (*1-903734-05-3*) Health Pr GBR. *Dist:* JAMCO Dist.

Erectile Dysfunction: Integrating Couple Therapy, Sex Therapy & Medical Treatment. Gerald R. Weeks & Nancy Gambescia. 2000. LC 99-58041. (Professional Bks. for Psychotherapists). 208p. 30.00 (*0-393-70330-4*) Norton.

Erektionsstoerungen: Organbefund & Psychodynamik. Ed. by W. Weidner et al. 1988. (Beitraege zur Urologie Ser.: Vol. 5). (Illus.). x, 234p. 95.00 (*3-8055-4789-7*) S Karger.

Erg, Ver & Psychophysics. Theodore Lawwill. 1977. (Documenta Ophthalmologica Proceedings Ser.: Vol. 13). text 191.50 (*90-6193-153-3*) Kluwer Academic.

ErgAerobics: Why Does Working at My Computer Hurt So Much? Perry Bonomo & Daniel Seldler. 1998. LC 99-163013. (Illus.). 128p. pap. 14.95 (*0-9664090-0-0*) Erg Aerobics.

Ergometrie bei Herzkranken. Elektrokardiogramm, Herzschlagfrequenz und Blutdruck bei Belastungsuntersuchungen. F. L. Schmidt. 1977. (GER.). 71.50 (*3-8055-2409-9*) S Karger.

Ergonomic Interventions to Prevent Musculoskeletal Injuries in Industry. American Conference of Governmental Industrial Hygenists Staff. 1987. (Illus.). 216p. lib. bdg. 84.95 (*0-87371-103-3*, L103) Lewis Pubs.

Ergonomics & Cumulative Trauma Disorders: A Handbook for Occupational Therapists. Denise K. Claiborne et al. 1999. LC 98-50553. 10p. (Orig.). pap. 39.95 (*0-7693-0024-3*, 2026) Thomson Learn.

Ergonomics & Musculoskeletal Disorders: Research on Manual Materials Handling, 1983-1996. Ed. by Waldemar Karwowski et al. 1997. LC 97-31460. 312p. (C). pap. text 50.00 (*0-945289-09-X*) Human Factors.

Ergonomics for Therapists. Ed. by Karen Jacobs & Carl M. Bettencourt. 1994. LC 94-35496. (Illus.). 256p. 45.00 (*0-7506-9530-7*) Buttrwrth-Heinemann.

Ergonomics for Therapists. King. 1995. (Nursing Education Ser.). text 39.95 (*0-8273-6058-4*) Delmar.

Ergonomics in Back Pain: A Guide to Prevention & Rehabilitation. Tarek M. Khalil et al. 1993. 223p. 130.00 (*0-471-28544-7*); 240p. text 70.95 (*0-442-01375-2*) Wiley (VNR).

Ergonomics in Clinical Practice: Prevention & Rehabilitation. Berg et al. 1998. LC 97-34808. 369p. text 54.99 (*0-7506-9714-8*) Buttrwrth-Heinemann.

Ergonomics of Manual Wheelchair Propulsion: State of the Art. Ed. by L. H. Van der Woude et al. 1992. LC 92-75337. 365p. (YA). (gr. 12 up). pap. 110.00 (*90-5199-118-5*) IOS Press.

Eric Berne. Ian Stewart. 1992. (Key Figures in Counselling & Psychotherapy Ser.). (Illus.). 160p. (C). 57.95 (*0-8039-8466-9*, 9683); pap. 25.95 (*0-8039-8467-7*, 9684) Sage.

Erich Fromm: His Life & Ideas: An Illustrated Biography. Rainer Funk. 2000. LC 00-21987. (Illus.). 175p. 29.95 (*0-8264-1224-6*) Continuum.

Erich Fromm & Critical Criminology: Beyond the Punitive Society. Kevin Anderson & Richard Quinney. 2000. LC 99-6327. x, 176p. 34.95 (*0-252-02514-8*) U of Ill Pr.

Erich Fromm Reader. Erich Fromm. 1994. LC 93-47511. 152p. (C). text 45.00 (*0-391-03856-7*); pap. 15.00 (*0-391-03851-6*) Brill Academic Pubs.

Erich Lindemann: A Biographical Sketch. Elizabeth B. Lindemann. 1987. LC 87-80018. (Illus.). (Orig.). pap. 14.40 (*0-9618299-0-7*) E B Lindemann.

Ericksonian Approaches: A Comprehensive Manual. Rubin Battind & Thomas L. South. 1999. 300p. (*1-899836-31-4*) Crown Hse GBR. *Dist:* LPC Group.

Ericksonian Hypnotherapeutic Group Inductions. Ed. by Hildegard Klippstein. 1991. LC 90-2531. 384p. text 41.95 (*0-87630-588-5*) Brunner-Routledge.

Ericksonian Methods: The Essence of the Story. Ed. by Jeffrey K. Zeig. 1994. LC 93-46938. 540p. text 69.95 (*0-87630-738-1*) Brunner-Routledge.

Ericksonian Monographs No. 10: Difficult Contexts for Therapy. Ed. by Stephen R. Lankton & Jeffrey K. Zeig. 1994. LC 94-5346. (Ericksonian Monographs: No. 10). 160p. text 28.95 (*0-87630-749-7*) Brunner-Routledge.

Erik Erikson: An Introduction. Richard Stevens. 1983. 160p. pap. (*0-335-10114-3*) OpUniv Pr.

Erik H. Erikson: The Growth of His Work. Robert Coles. 1987. (Quality Paperbacks Ser.). 462p. pap. 12.95 (*0-306-80291-0*) Da Capo.

Erik H. Erikson: The Power & Limits of a Vision. Paul Roazen. 1997. LC 97-19207. (Master Work Ser.). 258p. pap. text 40.00 (*0-7657-0094-8*) Aronson.

Erinnerungen, Gedanken und Meinungen see Memories, Thoughts & Convictions

Erin's Daughters in America: Irish Immigrant Women in the Nineteenth Century. Hasia R. Diner. 1983. LC 83-183. (Studies in Historical & Political Science: No. 2). 208p. pap. text 18.95 (*0-8018-2872-4*) Johns Hopkins.

Erisa: A Quarter Century of Providing Workers Health Insurance: Congressional Hearingpt. Ed. by John A. Boehner. 2000. (Illus.). 155p. pap. text 35.00 (*0-7567-0102-3*) DIANE Pub.

Ernaehrung und Alkoholismus. Ed. by J. C. Somogyi. 1976. (Bibliotheca Nutritio et Dieta Ser.: Vol. 24). (GER., Illus.). 75.00 (*3-8055-2376-9*) S Karger.

Ernaehrung und Gesundheit. L. Arab et al. 1981. (Beitraege zur Infusionstherapie und Klinische Ernaehrung Ser.: Band 7). (GER., Illus.). xii, 204p. pap. 28.75 (*3-8055-2384-X*) S Karger.

Ernaehrung und Stoffwechsel: Die Adipositas im Kindesalter. Ed. by E. Bern Rossi. 1975. (Paediatrische Fortbildungskurse fuer die Praxis Ser.: Band 42). (GER., Illus.). 113p. 30.50 (*3-8055-2158-8*) S Karger.

Ernaehrung und Tumorerkrankungen. Ed. by Peter Schauder. 1991. (GER., Illus.). xii, 702p. 105.25 (*3-8055-5383-8*) S Karger.

Erogeneity & Libido. Robert Fliess. 1970. LC 57-9327. (Psychoanalytic Ser.: Vol. 1). 325p. pap. 24.95 (*0-8236-8039-8*, 217000) Intl Univs Pr.

Eros & Civilization: A Philosophical Inquiry into Freud. Herbert Marcuse. 1974. LC 66-3219. 320p. reprint ed. pap. 17.00 (*0-8070-1555-5*) Beacon Pr.

Eros & Evil: The Sexual Psychopathology of Witchcraft. R. E. Masters. LC 79-8114. reprint ed. 36.50 (*0-404-18427-8*) AMS Pr.

Eros & Modernization: Sylvester Graham, Health Reform, & the Origins of Victorian Sexuality in America. Jayme A. Sokolow. 1983. LC 82-71644. 216p. 32.50 (*0-8386-3147-9*) Fairleigh Dickinson.

Eros Plays: Parts & Pieces from a Left-Handed Psychology. Jerry C. Godard. 1990. 148p. (C). pap. text 24.50 (*0-8191-7965-5*); lib. bdg. 45.50 (*0-8191-7964-7*) U Pr of Amer.

Erosion of Autonomy in Long-Term Care. Charles W. Lidz et al. 1992. LC 92-6085. 216p. text 39.95 (*0-19-507394-0*) OUP.

Erosion of Childhood. Valerie Suransky Polakow. LC 81-16227. 256p. 1997. pap. text 9.95 (*0-226-78007-4*); 1982. lib. bdg. 15.00 (*0-226-78006-6*) U Ch Pr.

Erotic Preference, Gender Identity, & Aggression in Men: New Research Studies. Ed. by Ron Langevin. 1984. 376p. text 79.95 (*0-89859-445-6*) L Erlbaum Assocs.

Errors & Pitfalls in Diagnostic Cytology. Leopold G. Koss & James Linder. 1997. (International Academy of Pathology Monographs Ser.: Vol. 39). (Illus.). 270p. (*0-683-18327-3*) Lppncott W & W.

Errors in Abdominal Radiology. Manuel Viamonte, Jr. 1992. (Illus.). 91p. 75.95 (*0-387-54080-6*) Spr-Verlag.

Errors in Chest Radiography. Manuel Viamonte, Jr. 1991. (Illus.). 135p. 81.95 (*0-387-52906-3*) Spr-Verlag.

Errors in Uroradiology. Manuel Viamonte, Jr. 1992. LC 92-10890. (Illus.). 127p. 82.95 (*0-387-54504-2*) Spr-Verlag.

Erste Zionistenkongress von 1897: In Basel Habe Ich den Judenstaat Gegrundet 100 Jahre Erster Zionistenkongress, Basel, August 1897. Ed. by Heiko Haumann et al. 1997. (GER., Illus.). xii, 404p. pap. 59.25 (*3-8055-6491-0*) S Karger.

ER/Trauma CheckMate. Angela G. Clarkson & Anne M. Larson. 3rd rev. ed. 2000. (Critical Care CheckMate Ser.). 170p. vinyl bd. (*0-9700484-6-7*) NNCC.

***Erythrocyte Engineering for Drug Delivery & Targeting.** Mauro Magnani. 2002. LC 2001-6817. (Biotechnology Intelligence Unit Ser.: Vol. 6). 115p. 119.00 (*1-58706-061-2*); pap. 69.00 (*1-58706-117-1*) Eurekah.

Erythrocyte Protoporphyrin Testing: Approved Guideline (1996) Contrib. by Patricia H. Field & Noel V. Stanton. 1996. 75.00 (*1-56238-306-X*, C42-A) NCCLS.

Erythrocytes As Drug Carriers in Medicine: Proceedings of the Sixth Meeting of the International Society for the Use of Resealed Erythrocytes Held in Irsee, Germany, July 25-28, 1996. Ed. by Ulrich Sprandel & James L. Way. 1997. LC 97-16221. 158p. (C). text 75.00 (*0-306-45599-4*, Kluwer Plenum) Kluwer Academic.

Erythropoetin in Clinical Applications. Mark B. Garnick. 1990. (Illus.). 360p. text 125.00 (*0-8247-8377-8*) Dekker.

Erythropoietin. Ed. by Wolfgang Jelkmann & A. J. Gross. 1989. (Illus.). 180p. 95.00 (*0-387-50955-0*) Spr-Verlag.

Erythropoietin: From Molecular Structure to Clinical Application. Ed. by C. A. Baldamus & K. M. Koch. 1989. (Contributions to Nephrology Ser.: Vol. 76). (Illus.). x, 350p. 29.75 (*3-8055-5035-9*) S Karger.

Erythropoietin in Renal & Non-Renal Anemias. Ed. by H. J. Gurland et al. 1991. (Contributions to Nephrology Ser.: Vol. 88). (Illus.). x, 362p. 49.75 (*3-8055-5272-6*) S Karger.

Erythropoietin in the Nineties. Ed. by R. M. Schaefer et al. 1991. (Contributions to Nephrology Ser.: Vol. 87). (Illus.). viii, 114p. 29.75 (*3-8055-5267-X*) S Karger.

Es Werde Licht: Praktischer Leitfaden fur Dinshahs 12-Farben Chromotherapie. Darius Dinshah. 1989.Tr. of Let There Be Light. (GER., Illus.). 191p. 15.00 (*0-933917-03-1*) Dinshah Hlth Soc.

Escape from Anxiety & Stress. Tom McLellan et al. 1988. LC 85-31378. (Encyclopedia of Psychoactive Drugs Ser.: No. 1). (Illus.). 124p. (YA). (gr. 7-11). lib. bdg. 19.95 (*0-87754-772-6*) Chelsea Hse.

Escape from Depression. David Goliath. (Illus.). 1986. 13.95 (*0-936407-00-X*); 2nd abr. rev. ed. 1999. LC 86-855. 240p. pap. 11.95 (*0-936407-02-6*) Ordinary Man.

Escape from Freedom. Erich Fromm. 1976. 336p. mass mkt. 5.99 (*0-380-01167-0*, Avon Bks) Morrow Avon.

Escape the Drug Scene. LaDean Griffin. pap. 3.95 (*0-89036-141-X*) Liahona Pub Trust.

Escapism. Yi-Fu Tuan. 1998. LC 98-5366. (Illus.). 264p. 47.00 (*0-8018-5926-3*) Johns Hopkins.

Escherichia Coli: Mechanisms of Virulence. Ed. by Max Sussman. 1997. (Illus.). 655p. (C). text 130.00 (*0-521-45361-5*) Cambridge U Pr.

Escherichia Coli in Domestic Animals & Humans. Ed. by C. L. Gyles. 1994. (Illus.). 688p. text 160.00 (*0-85198-921-7*) OUP.

Escherichia Coli 0157: Bibliography. January 1993-December 1993. Ellen K. Miller. 1995. 64p. (Orig.). (C). pap. text 35.00 (*0-7881-2179-0*) DIANE Pub.

Escherichia Coli 0157:H7: Other Shiga Toxin-Producing E. Coli Strains. James B. Kaper & Alison D. O'Brien. 1998. LC 98-2732. (Illus.). 500p. 99.95 (*1-55581-129-9*) ASM Pr.

E6 & E7 Oncoproteins of Human Papillomaviruses. Massimo Tommasino. 1997. (Molecular Biology Intelligence Unit Ser.). 181p. pap. 89.95 (*0-412-13361-X*) Chapman & Hall.

E6 & E7 Oncoproteins of Human Papillomaviruses. Massimo Tommasino. 1997. LC 97-19205. (Molecular Biology Intelligence Unit Ser.). 181p. 99.00 (*1-57059-456-2*) Landes Bioscience.

ESO Ecstasy Program: Better, Safer Sexual Intimacy & Extended Orgasmic Response. Alan P. Brauer et al. 1991. LC 82-50863. (Illus.). 228p. pap. 12.99 (*0-446-39178-6*) Warner Bks.

Esogetics: The Sense & Nonsense of Sickness & Pain. Peter Mandel. Tr. by S. Kristen & J. Allanach from GER. 1993. (Illus.). 182p. (Orig.). pap. text 25.00 (*3-925806-71-7*) Medicina Bio.

Esophageal & Gastric Emptying. Ed. by Andre Dubois & Donald Castell. 1984. LC 84-1895. 168p. 101.00 (*0-8493-6367-5*, OP150, CRC Reprint) Franklin.

Esophageal & Thoracic Surgery Atlas. Pearsons. 1995. (C). text 475.00 (*0-443-08984-1*) Saunders.

Esophageal Carcinoma: State of the Art. Ed. by J. Lange & J. Rhudiger Siewert. 2000. LC 99-56373. (Recent Results in Cancer Research Ser.: Vol. 155). (Illus.). 200p. 106.00 (*3-540-65323-6*) Spr-Verlag.

Esophageal Manometry in Clinical Investigation. R. D. Henderson. 1983. LC 82-24673. 258p. 72.95 (*0-275-91395-3*, C1395, Praeger Pubs) Greenwood.

Esophageal Mucosa: 300 Questions—300 Answers. Ed. by R. Giuli et al. 1994. LC 94-38852. (International Congress Ser.: No. 1052). 1268p. 333.00 (*0-444-81753-0*) Elsevier.

Esophageal Mucosal Defence Vol. 56, Suppl. 1: Recent Advances. Ed. by C. Scarpignato et al. 1995. (Journal: Vol. 56, Suppl. 1, 1995). (Illus.). iv, 62p. pap. 28.75 (*3-8055-6210-1*) S Karger.

Esophageal Surgery. F.Griffith Pearson et al. 1995. LC 94-24093. text (*0-443-08832-2*) Church.

Esophageal Surgery. Pearson. 2nd ed. Date not set. (C). text (*0-443-07605-7*) Church.

Esophagus. Ed. by Leo Van der Reis. 1978. (Frontiers of Gastrointestinal Research Ser.: Vol. 3). (Illus.). 85.25 (*3-8055-2700-4*) S Karger.

Esophagus: Medical & Surgical Management. Lucius Hill et al. 1988. (Illus.). 400p. text 135.00 (*0-7216-2348-4*) Saunders.

Esophagus - Stomach - GI Bleeding. Charles E. Brady, III. 1991. (Contemporary Management in Internal Medicine Ser.: Vol. 1, No. 3). (Illus.). 218p. text (*0-443-08824-1*) Church.

Esophagus & Pharynx. Ed. by Roy C. Orlando. 1997. LC 96-18669. (Gastroenterology & Hepatology Ser.: Vol. 5). (Illus.). 233p. text (*0-443-07855-6*) Church GBR. *Dist:* Saunders.

Esophagus, Stomach & Duodedum. Ed. by K. Kremer et al. 1989. (Illus.). 380p. text 189.00 (*0-86577-291-6*) Thieme Med Pubs.

Esoteric Anthropology: The Mysteries of Man. Thomas L. Nichols. 1972. LC 75-180585. (Medicine & Society in America Ser.). (Illus.). 350p. reprint ed. 24.95 (*0-405-03962-X*) Ayer.

ESP Experiments with LSD Twenty-Five & Psilocybin. Roberto Cavanna & Emilio Servadio. 1964. LC 64-24271. (Parapsychological Monographs: No. 5). pap. 5.00 (*0-912328-08-8*) Parapsych Foun.

ESP in Relation to Rorschach Test Evaluation. Gertrude R. Schmeidler. 1960. LC 60-2760. (Parapsychological Monographs: No. 2). pap. 6.00 (*0-912328-04-5*) Parapsych Foun.

ESPE-Symposium, Copenhagen, June 1988: Cryptorchidism, Pt. II. Ed. by R. Sharpe et al. 1989. (Journal: Vol. 30, Nos. 4-5, 1988). 88p. pap. 75.75 (*3-8055-5004-9*) S Karger.

ESPE-Symposium, Copenhagen, June 1988: Growth & Development in Children Treated for Cancer, Pt. I. Ed. by S. Shalet et al. 1989. (Journal: Vol. 30, Nos. 2-3, 1988). 84p. pap. 75.75 (*3-8055-5003-0*) S Karger.

Esprit du Remede Homeopathique see Spirit of Homeopathic Medicines: Essential Insights to 300 Remedies

Essai de Psychologie. Charles Bonnet. 1978. (FRE.). xlii, 390p. reprint ed. 95.00 (*3-487-06526-6*) G Olms Pubs.

Essais de Psychoanalyse. Sigmund Freud. 1989. (FRE.). pap. 14.95 (*0-7859-3040-X*, 2228882054) Fr & Eur.

Essay, Medical, Philosophical, & Chemical on Drunkenness & Its Effects on the Human Body, 1804. Thomas Trotter. Ed. by Roy Porter. 1989. (Tavistock Classic Reprints in the History of Psychiatry Ser.). 272p. 42.50 (*0-415-00636-8*) Routledge.

Essay of Health & Long Life. George Cheyne. Ed. by Robert J. Kastenbaum. 1979. LC 78-22191. (Aging & Old Age Ser.). reprint ed. lib. bdg. 25.95 (*0-405-11808-2*) Ayer.

Essay on Fevers. John Huxham. Ed. by Saul Jarcho. 1988. LC 86-11912. 15.95 (*0-88135-083-4*) Watson Pub Intl.

Essay on Stress. Morris Halle & Jean-Roger Vergnaud. 1990. 287p. reprint ed. pap. 22.00 (*0-262-58105-1*) MIT Pr.

Essay on the Disorders of Old Age, & on the Means for Prolonging Human Life. Anthony Carlisle. Ed. by Robert J. Kastenbaum. 1979. LC 78-22183. (Aging & Old Age Ser.). reprint ed. lib. bdg. 16.95 (*0-405-11802-3*) Ayer.

Essay on the Nature & Conduct of the Passions & Affections, 1742. Francis Hutcheson. 3rd ed. 1969. LC 76-81361. (History of Psychology Ser.). 378p. reprint ed. 50.00 (*0-8201-1058-2*) Schol Facsimiles.

Essays in General Psychology: Seven Danish Contributions. Ed. by Niels Engelsted et al. 1989. 146p. (C). pap. (*87-7288-277-8*) Aarhus Univ Pr DNK. *Dist:* David Brown.

Essays in Honor of Robert E. Moyers. Ed. by W. Stuart Hunter & David S. Carlson. 1992. (Craniofacial Growth Ser.: Vol. 24). (Illus.). 260p. 59.00 (*0-929921-20-8*) UM CHGD.

Essays in Medical Anthropology. Ed. by Roger Pearson. 1981. (Mankind Quarterly Monographs: No. 2). (Orig.). (C). pap. 12.00 (*0-941694-01-1*) Inst Study Man.

Essays in Medical Sociology Elizabeth Blackwell. 1974. LC 73-180555. (Medicine & Society in America Ser.). 580p. reprint ed. 36.95 (*0-405-03935-2*) Ayer.

Essays in Medical Sociology: Journeys into the Field. Renee C. Fox. 1988. 548p. text 49.95 (*0-88738-148-0*); pap. text 24.95 (*0-88738-682-2*) Transaction Pubs.

Essays in Psychology. William James. Ed. by Frederick Burkhardt et al. 1984. LC 83-8452. (Works of William James: Eleventh Title: Vol. 13). (Illus.). 512p. 56.00 (*0-674-26714-1*) HUP.

Essays in Schizophrenia. Bernard H. Shulman. 2nd ed. 1983. LC 82-72136. 191p. pap. 14.95 (*0-918560-29-2*) Adler Sch Prof Psy.

Essays in the Economics of Health & Medical Care. Ed. by Victor R. Fuchs. 1972. (Human Resources & Social Institutions Ser.: No. 1). 261p. text 68.40 (*0-87014-236-4*) Natl Bur Econ Res.

Essays in Theoretical Psychology. Fred Vollmer. 1990. 160p. (*82-560-0647-1*) Solum Verlag NOR. *Dist:* Intl Spec Bk.

Essays in Therapeutic Jurisprudence. David B. Wexler & Bruce J. Winick. 1991. LC 91-74075. 336p. 34.95 (*0-89089-459-0*) Carolina Acad Pr.

Essays Inspired by Theodore Jacobs's "The Use of the Self" Ed. by Bornstein. 1997. (Psychoanalytic Inquiry Ser.: Vol. 17, No. 1). pap. 20.00 (*0 88163 936 2*) Analytic Pr.

Essays, Medical, Philosophical & Chemical on Drunkenness. Thomas Trotter. Ed. by Gerald N. Grob. 1981. LC 80-1251. (Addiction in America Ser.). reprint ed. lib. bdg. 22.95 (*0-405-13620-X*) Ayer.

Essays of a Biologist. Julian S. Huxley. 1977. LC 72-111838. (Essay Index Reprint Ser.). 23.95 (*0-8369-1613-1*) Ayer.

Essays on AIDS: Introduction to the Influence of a Virus on Politics. James H. Boykin. 1994. LC 93-91068. 90p. (Orig.). lib. bdg. 6.94 (*1-880833-01-8*) Boykin.

Essays on Analytical Music Therapy. Mary Priestley. 1994. 358p. (C). pap. text 30.00 (*0-9624080-2-6*) Barcelona Pubs.

Essays on Anthropology & International Health. Mark Nichter. 1989. (C). pap. text 61.00 (*0-7923-0158-7*); lib. bdg. 196.50 (*0-7923-0005-X*) Kluwer Academic.

Essays on DNA in Clinical Medicine. Ed. by T. J. Wilkin. 1987. x, 96p. text 74.00 (*3-7186-0360-8*); 96p. pap. text 41.00 (*3-7186-0361-6*) Gordon & Breach.

Essays on Economic Psychology. Ed. by Hermann Brandstatter & Werner Guths. 1994. LC 94-31029. (Illus.). 291p. 120.00 (*0-387-58283-5*); 140.00 (*3-540-58283-5*) Spr-Verlag.

Essays on Ego Psychology: Selected Problems in Psychoanalytic Theory. Heinz Hartmann. 1965. LC 64-14655. 508p. 75.00 (*0-8236-1740-8*) Intl Univs Pr.

Essays on Maimonides. Ed. by Salo W. Baron. LC 79-160004. reprint ed. 32.50 (*0-404-00658-2*) AMS Pr.

Essays on Medical Education. Stephen Abrahamson. 1996. LC 96-17730. 162p. lib. bdg. 36.50 (*0-7618-0366-1*) U Pr of Amer.

Essays on Mind. Donald O. Hebb. 1980. LC 79-24993. (Illus.). 176p. text 29.95 (*0-89859-017-5*) L Erlbaum Assocs.

Essays on Nursing Leadership. Claire M. Fagin. 2000. LC 00-30055. xviii, 212p. (*0-8261-1357-5*) Spr-Verlag.

Essays on Otherness. Jean Laplanche & John Fletcher. LC 98-11837. (Warwick Studies in European Philosophy). (C). 1999. vii, 279p. pap. 26.95 (*0-415-13108-1*); 1998. 272p. 90.00 (*0-415-13107-3*) Routledge.

Essays on Spiritual Psychology. Carolyn Blackmer. Ed. & Intro. by Stephen Larsen. 1991. LC 87-60495. (Illus.). 68p. pap. 10.95 (*0-87785-135-2*) Swedenborg.

Essays on State Medicine. Henry W. Rumsey. Ed. by Barbara G. Rosenkrantz. 1977. LC 76-40641. (Public Health in America Ser.). reprint ed. lib. bdg. 35.95 (*0-405-09829-4*) Ayer.

Essays on the Anatomy & Physiology of Lymphoid Tissues. Ed. by Z. Trnka & R. N. Cahill. 1979. (Monographs in Allergy: Vol. 16). (Illus.). pap. 126.25 (*3-8055-3059-5*) S Karger.

Essays on the Changes of the Human Body at Its Different Ages. Thomas Jameson. Ed. by Robert J. Kastenbaum. 1979. LC 78-22203. (Aging & Old Age Ser.). reprint ed. lib. bdg. 32.95 (*0-405-11818-X*) Ayer.

E
F
G

Essays on the History of Medicine Presented to Karl Sudhoff on the Occasion of His Seventieth Birthday, Vol. 26. Ed. by C. Singer & Henry E. Sigerist. 1977. LC 68-8459. (Essay Index Reprint Ser.). 30.95 (0-8369-0431-1) Ayer.

Essays on the Rise & Decline of Bedside Medicine. Mark D. Altschule. 1988. (Illus.). 458p. text 32.50 (0-8121-1226-1) Lppncott W & W.

Essays on Women, Medicine & Health. Ann Oakley. 1993. LC 93-246217. 256p. (0-7486-0441-3); pap. (0-7486-0450-2) Edinburgh U Pr GBR. *Dist:* Col U Pr.

Essays Plans for Anaesthesia Exams. Maher Michel et al. 1993. (Illus.). 192p. (Orig.). pap. text (0-443-04395-7) Church.

Essays Stimulated by Joseph Lichtenberg's Psychoanalysis & Motivation Vol. 15, No. 4, 1995: A Special Issue of Psychoanalytic Inquiry. Shane. 1995. pap. 19.95 (0-88163-993-1) L Erlbaum Assocs.

Essays That Will Get You into Medical School. Dan Kaufman. 1998. LC 98-28189. 240p. pap. 10.95 (0-7641-0611-2) Barron.

Essence of a Single-Session Success. Ed. by Stephen R. Lankton & Kristina K. Erickson. 1993. LC 93-11832. (Ericksonian Monographs: No. 9). 184p. text 28.95 (0-87630-727-6) Brunner-Routledge.

Essence of Abnormal Psychology. David S. Holmes. 1998. LC 97-37758. pap. (0-13-748633-2) P-H.

Essence of Anesthesia Practice. Michael F. Roizen & Lee A. Fleisher. Ed. by Lew Reines. 1996. LC 96-24185. (Illus.). 620p. pap. text 55.00 (0-7216-5972-1) Saunders.

Essence of Bach Flowers: Traditional & Transpersonal Use & Practice. Rachelle Hasnas. 1999. LC 98-53511. pap. 16.95 (0-89594-969-5) Crossing Pr.

Essence of Chinese Medical. Yip F. Li. 1995. 218p. pap. text 20.00 (0-9649931-9-8) Yip Fun Li.

Essence of Cognitive Psychology. Helen Gavin. 1998. LC 97-44936. tchr. ed. (0-13-796459-5) P-H.

Essence of Liu Feng-Wu's Gynecology. Liu Feng-Wu. Ed. & Tr. by Bob Flaws from CHI. Tr. by Shuai Xue-Zhong from CHI. 1998. LC 97-77996. xi, 335p. pap. text 24.95 (0-936185-88-0) Blue Poppy Pr.

Essence of Nectar, Vol. 1. Karen Moawad & Hummingbird Associates Staff. 1995. pap. (0-9647903-0-0) Hummingbrd Assocs.

Essence of Organic Chemistry. Jane M. Cram & Donald J. Cram. 1978. LC 77-73957. (Chemistry Ser.). text (0-201-01031-3) Addison-Wesley.

Essence of Phenomenology & Its Meaning for the Scientific Study of Religion. Thomas Ryba. 1991. (Toronto Studies in Religion). (Illus.). XVII, 269p. (C). text 47.95 (0-8204-0742-9) P Lang Pubng.

Essential AIDS Fact Book. Paul H. Douglas & Laura Pinsky. 1989. pap. 3.95 (0-671-67853-1) PB.

Essential AIDS Fact Book: Newly Revised & Updated. Laura Pinsky & Paul H. Douglas. rev. ed. 1996. LC 95-50007. 144p. pap. 7.00 (0-671-55287-2) S&S Trade.

Essential AIDS Fact Book: What You Need to Know to Protect Yourself, Your Family, All Your Loved Ones. Paul H. Douglas & Laura Pinsky. 1987. pap. 3.95 (0-671-64772-5) PB.

Essential Albert Ellis: Seminal Writings on Psychotherapy. Ed. by Windy Dryden. 1990. LC 89-26338. 336p. 38.95 (0-8261-6940-6) Springer Pub.

Essential Allergy. Niels Mygind et al. 2nd rev. ed. 1996. LC 95-14201. (Essentials Ser.). 496p. 78.95 (0-632-03645-1) Blackwell Sci.

Essential Allies: Families As Advisors Elizabeth S. Jeppson & Josie Thomas. 1995. 76p. (Orig.). (C). pap. text 15.00 (0-9642014-1-0) Inst Fmly Ctr.

Essential Anaesthesia for Medical Students. Mark Heining et al. 1996. (Arnold Publication). (Illus.). 160p. pap. 24.95 (0-340-61386-6) OUP.

Essential Anatomy. Lumley. 4th ed. 1987. pap. text 39.00 (0-443-03573-3) Saunders.

Essential Anatomy & Some Clinical Applications. J. S. Lumley et al. 5th ed. 1995. LC 94-18967. text (0-443-04808-8) Church.

Essential Anatomy Dissector: Following Grant's Method. John T. Hansen. 1998. LC 98-3759. 190p. spiral bd. 27.95 (0-683-30575-1) Lppncott W & W.

***Essential Anatomy Dissector: Following Grant's Method.** John T. Hansen. 2nd ed. 2001. LC 2001-50349. spiral bd. 32.95 (0-7817-3283-2) Lppncott W & W.

Essential Anatomy for Anesthesia. Sue M. Black. 1998. (0-443-05054-6) Church.

Essential Arnold Lazarus. Dryden. 1991. 246p. pap. 48.00 (1-56593-573-X, 0305) Singular Publishing.

Essential Aspects of Atopic Dermatitis. G. Rajka. 1989. (Illus.). 261p. 133.00 (0-387-51165-2) Spr-Verlag.

Essential Atlas of Gastroenterology & Hepatology for Primary Care. Ed. by Mark Feldman. 1998. LC 97-35820. 125.00 (0-632-04394-6) Blackwell Sci.

Essential Atlas of Gastroenterology & Hepatology for Primary Care. Ed. by Mark Feldman. 1998. (Illus.). 250p. pap. 115.00 (1-57340-026-2) Current Med.

Essential Atlas of Infectious Diseases for Primary Care. Gerald L. Mandell & Thomas P. Bleck. 1997. LC 96-45957. text (0-443-07961-7) Church.

Essential Cardiac Technology. Laurence Pillar. 1996. 260p. text 55.00 (3-7186-5896-8); pap. text 30.00 (3-7186-5897-6) Gordon & Breach (Harwood Acad Pubs).

Essential Cardiology. Clive Rosendorff. 2000. LC 99-89412. (Illus.). xv, 895p. (C). pap. text 79.50 (0-7216-8144-1) Saunders.

Essential Cardiology. Adam D. Timmis et al. 3rd ed. 1997. LC 97-14105. (Essentials Ser.). (Illus.). 378p. pap. 57.95 (0-632-04843-3) Blackwell Sci.

***Essential Chemistry for Safe Aromatherapy.** David Lowe & Sue Clarke. 2001. (Illus.). 205p. pap. (0-443-06485-7) Church GBR. *Dist:* Saunders.

Essential Child Psychiatry. Peter Hoare. 1993. LC 93-19374. pap. text (0-443-04464-3) Church.

Essential Clinical Anatomy. Keith L. Moore & Anne M.R. Agur. 1995. LC 94-36235. (Illus.). 656p. pap. 45.00 (0-683-06128-3); 3rd ed. 1992. 930p. 83.00 (0-683-06136-4) Lppncott W & W.

Essential Clinical Immunology. Helen M. Chapel et al. 4th ed. 1999. LC 98-40975. (Illus.). 351p. pap. 52.95 (0-632-04972-3) Blackwell Sci.

Essential Clinical Pathology. Dinah V. Parums. 1996. LC 41-50522. (Essentials Ser.). 707p. pap. 74.95 (0-632-03088-7) Blackwell Sci.

Essential Clinical Physiology. Ed. by Moore-Gillon & Forgacs. 2000. (Illus.). 352p. (Orig.). (C). (gr. 13). pap. 36.95 (0-412-48910-4, Chap & Hall NY) Chapman & Hall.

Essential Coloproctology for Nurses. Theresa Porrett & Norma Daniel. 1999. LC 99-494978. 438p. (1-86156-085-0) Whurr Pub.

Essential Community Medicine: Including Relevant Social Services. R. J. Donaldson & L. J. Donaldson. 1983. 600p. text 37.50 (0-85200-373-0) Kluwer Academic.

Essential Concepts for Healthy Living. Sandra Alters & Wendy Schiff. 1998. LC 97-52730. pap. text 49.95 (0-534-35732-6) Brooks-Cole.

***Essential Concepts for Healthy Living.** Alters & Schiff. 2nd ed. 2001. (Illus.). (C). 15.00 (0-7637-1926-9, 1926-9) Jones & Bartlett.

Essential Concepts for Healthy Living with InfoTrac. Sandra M. Alters-Gottfried. 1998. (Health Sciences Ser.). 30.00 incl. cd-rom (0-534-36376-8) Brooks-Cole.

Essential Diagnostic Microbiology. Elmer W. Koneman et al. 1994. LC 93-35744. (Illus.). 544p. text 45.95 (0-397-51215-5) Lppncott W & W.

Essential Drugs for Primary Health Care: A Manual for Health Workers in South-East Asia. 1988. (SEARO Regional Health Papers: No. 16). 109p. pap. text 10.00 (92-9022-185-2) World Health.

Essential Elements in Early Intervention: Visual Impairment & Multiple Disabilities. Ed. by Deborah Chen. 1998. LC 99-41221. (Illus.). xx, 503p. pap. 34.95 (0-89128-305-6) Am Foun Blind.

Essential Elements of Obstetric Care at First Referral Level. 1991. (CHI, ENG & FRE.). vii, 72p. pap. text 14.00 (92-4-154424-4, 1150364) World Health.

Essential Emergency Care. Georgia O'Keeffe. 1995. pap., tchr. ed., suppl. ed. 44.00 (0-8359-4975-3) P-H.

Essential Endocrinology. John F. Laycock & Peter H. Wise. 3rd ed. 1996. (Illus.). 418p. pap. text 37.95 (0-19-262471-7) OUP.

Essential Endocrinology: A Primer for Nonspecialists. C. R. Kannan. 1986. LC 86-4925. (Illus.). 548p. 114.00 (0-306-42172-0, Kluwer Plenum) Kluwer Academic.

Essential Endodontology: Prevention & Treatment of Apical Periodontitis. Dag Rstavik & Thomas R. Pittford. 1998. LC 98-25953. (0-632-04089-0) Blackwell Sci.

Essential ENT Practice: A Clinical Text. Rogan Corbridge. 1998. LC 98-3603. (Illus.). 192p. pap. text (0-340-67704-X) E A GBR. *Dist:* OUP.

Essential Exercises for Breast Cancer Survivors: How to Live Stronger & Feel Better. Amy Halverstadt & Andrea Leonard. 2000. LC 00-40719. (Illus.). xii, 209p. 29.95 (1-55832-178-0) Harvard Common Pr.

Essential Facts-Health Care Practice Management: A Legal & Business Guide for Practitioners. Daniel N. Steven. 1995. 500p. 135.00 (0-7913-2527-X) Warren Gorham & Lamont.

***Essential Fats for Athletes.** Michael Colgan. (Progressive Health Ser.). 24p. 3.99 (1-896817-08-4) Apple Pubg Co.

Essential Fatty Acids in Health & Disease. Edward N. Siguel. 1994. LC 94-67872. (Illus.). 400p. pap. 28.95 (0-9642534-0-2) Nutrek Pr.

Essential Flower Essence Handbook: Remedies for Inner Well-Being. Lila Devi. 2nd ed. 1997. LC 97-41535. 368p. reprint ed. pap. 13.95 (1-56170-511-X, 874) Hay House.

Essential Fromm: Life Between Having & Being. Erich Fromm. Ed. by Rainer Funk. 1995. 137p. pap. 19.95 (0-09-474450-5) Trans-Atl Phila.

Essential General Surgical Oncology. Ed. by I. Taylor et al. 1996. (Illus.). 460p. text (0-443-05045-7) Church.

Essential Guide to Chronic Illness: The Active Patient's Handbook. James W. Long. 2000. 625p. pap. text 20.00 (0-7881-6903-3) DIANE Pub.

Essential Guide to Cosmetic Laser Surgery. Tina S. Alster & Lydia Preston. 1997. (Illus.). 200p. (Orig.). pap. 16.00 (1-887110-09-7) Allian Pubng.

***Essential Guide to Geriatric Medicine.** Ranjit N. Ratnaike. 2001. (Illus.). 1152p. 95.00 (0-07-470801-5, Apple Lange Med) McGraw.

Essential Guide to Group Practice in Mental Health: Clinical, Legal & Financial Fundamentals. Simon H. Budman & Brett N. Steenbarger. 1997. LC 97-20098. (Clinician's Toolbox Ser.). 318p. text 50.00 (1-57230-254-2, C0254) Guilford Pubns.

Essential Guide to Mental Health. Gorman. 1998. LC 96-2878. 416p. pap. 16.95 (0-312-18715-7) St Martin.

Essential Guide to Nutrition & the Foods We Eat. Jean A. Thompson Pennington. 1999. LC 98-41937. (Harper Resource Book Ser.). (Illus.). 240p. pap. 15.95 (0-06-273346-X, Perennial) HarperTrade.

Essential Guide to Prescription Drugs, 1999. James J. Rybacki. 1999. (Illus.). 1120p. pap. 20.00 (0-06-273635-3) HarperCollins Pubs.

Essential Guide to Prescription Drugs 2000: Everything You Need to Know for Safe Drug Use. James Long. 2000. LC 87-657561. (Essential Guide to Prescription Drugs Ser.). (Illus.). 1216p. pap. 20.00 (0-06-273683-3) HarperCollins Pubs.

Essential Guide to Prescription Drugs 1998: Everything You Need to Know for Safe Drug Use. James J. Rybacki & James W. Long. 1997. 1152p. 50.00 (0-06-271606-9, Harper Ref) HarperCollins Pubs.

Essential Guide to Prescription Drugs 2001: Everything You Need to Know for Safe Drug Use. James J. Rybacki. 2001. LC 87-657561. (Essential Guide to Prescription Drugs Ser.). (Illus.). 1273p. pap. 20.00 (0-06-095816-2) HarperCollins Pubs.

***Essential Guide to Prescription Drugs 2002.** James J. Rybacki. 2002. 1360p. pap. 19.95 (0-06-001165-3) HarperCollins Pubs.

***Essential Guide to Prescription Drugs 2002: Everything You Need to Know for Safe Drug Use.** James J. Rybacki. 2002. 1360p. 54.95 (0-06-001164-5) HarperCollins Pubs.

Essential Guide to Prescription Drugs 2000: Everything You Need to Know for Safe Drug Use, Vol. 1. James J. Rybacki. 2000. LC 87-657561. (Essential Guide Ser.). (Illus.). 1216p. 50.00 (0-06-271613-1, HarpRes) HarpInfo.

Essential Guide to Psychiatric Drugs. Jack M. Gorman. 1997. (Illus.). 397p. reprint ed. pap. text 20.00 (0-7881-5005-7) DIANE Pub.

Essential Guide to Psychiatric Drugs. Jack M. Gorman. rev. ed. 1995. LC 95-161715. 416p. mass mkt. 6.99 (0-312-95458-1) St Martin.

Essential Guide to Psychiatric Drugs. Jack M. Gorman & J. Bowen. 3rd rev. ed. 1997. LC 97-17659. 398p. pap. 16.95 (0-312-16824-1) St Martin.

Essential Guide to Vitamins & Minerals: Second Edition, Revised & Updated. Elizabeth Somer & Health Media of America Staff. 2nd rev. ed. 1996. (Illus.). 464p. (Orig.). pap. 18.00 (0-06-273345-1, Harper Ref) HarperCollins Pubs.

Essential Haematology. A. Victor Hoffbrand et al. 4th ed. 2001. LC 00-23594. (At a Glance Ser.). (Illus.). 448p. pap. 44.95 (0-632-05153-1) Blackwell Sci.

***Essential Health Psychology.** Mark Forshaw. 2002. (Arnold Publication). (Illus.). 224p. text (0-340-75971-2) OUP.

Essential Histology. David H. Cormack. 1993. LC 92-13416. 448p. spiral bd. 41.95 (0-397-51062-4) Lppncott W & W.

Essential Histology Review. Frank J. Wilson et al. 1996. LC 96-1559. 293p. 21.95 (0-86542-487-X) Blackwell Sci.

Essential HIV Treatment Fact Book. Laura Pinsky et al. Ed. by Gina Centrello. 1992. LC 92-1716. 464p. per. 14.00 (0-671-72528-9) PB.

Essential Humility of Marriage: Honoring the Third Identity in Couple Therapy. Terry D. Hargrave. 2000. LC 00-25245. x, 223p. 36.95 (1-891944-36-3) Zeig Tucker Theisen.

Essential Hypertension, No. 2. Ed. by K. Aoki. 1990. (Illus.). 416p. 176.00 (0-387-70044-7) Spr-Verlag.

Essential Hypertension: A Strategy for Individualized Treatment. Timothy N. Caris. 1990. LC 89-64149. 130p. (Orig.). pap. 11.95 (0-945892-01-2) JBK Pub.

Essential Illustrated Neurosurgery. A. Fortuna et al. 2001. (Illus.). 250p. 99.00 (88-470-0126-9) Spr-Verlag.

Essential Immunology Review. Peter J. Delves & Ivan M. Roitt. 1995. LC 95-202673. 256p. pap. 19.95 (0-86542-458-6) Blackwell Sci.

Essential Jung. Carl Gustav Jung. Ed. by Anthony Storr. 1983. LC 82-61441. 448p. pap. 16.95 (0-691-02455-3) Princeton U Pr.

Essential Life Choices, Concepts & Strategies. Eleanor Whitney. 1989. (Health Sciences Ser.). stu. ed. 14.75 (0-314-52519-X) Brooks-Cole.

Essential Medical Genetics. J. Michael Connor & M. A. Ferguson-Smith. 5th ed. 1997. LC 96-45181. (Essentials Ser.). (Illus.). 288p. pap. 49.95 (0-86542-666-X) Blackwell Sci.

Essential Medical Ophthalmology: A Problem Oriented Approach. John Ferris. 2001. 304p. pap. text 79.95 (0-7506-4937-2) Buttrwrth-Heinemann.

Essential Medical Physiology. Ed. & Contrib. by Leonard R. Johnson. 2nd ed. 1997. LC 97-13703. (Illus.). 880p. text 65.00 (0-397-58401-6) Lppncott W & W.

Essential Medical Procedures. Ed. by Peter J. Toghill. (Illus.). 160p. pap. (0-340-63187-2) E A GBR. *Dist:* OUP, Routldge.

Essential Medical Term: Instructor's Manual. Christine Stanfield & Pogorzala. 2nd ed. 1996. (Health Science Ser.). (Illus.). 204p. (C). pap. text, tchr. ed. 20.95 (0-7637-0190-4, 0190-4) Jones & Bartlett.

Essential Medical Terminology. Peggy S. Stanfield. 1991. tchr. ed. 95.00 (0-86720-341-2) Jones & Bartlett.

Essential Medical Terminology. Peggy S. Stanfield & Yiu H. Hui. 2nd ed. 1996. LC 95-37952. (Health Science Ser.). (Illus.). 352p. (C). pap. text 47.95 (0-86720-743-4, 743-4) Jones & Bartlett.

***Essential Medication Guidebook to Healthy Aging: An Easy-to-Use Reference to Medications Taken for Common Conditions.** Les Paul & Becky Nagle. Ed. by Merck-Medco Editors. 2002. 880p. pap. 18.95 (0-345-45137-6, Ballantine) Ballantine Pub Grp.

Essential Medicine. John V. Jones & C. R. Tomson. 2nd ed. 1998. LC 97-29680. (C). pap. text (0-443-05811-3) Church.

Essential Microbiology for Dentistry. Lakshman P. Samaranayake. 1996. LC 95-40805. 357p. pap. text (0-443-04989-0) Church.

***Essential Microbiology for Dentistry.** Lakshman P. Samaranayake. 2001. (Illus.). 351p. pap. (0-443-06461-X) Church GBR. *Dist:* Saunders.

Essential Midwifery. Henders. 1997. 454p. mass mkt. (0-7234-2439-X) Wolfe Publishing GBR. *Dist:* Mosby Inc.

Essential Moreno: Writings on Psychodrama, Group Method, & Spontaneity. Ed. by Jonathan Fox. 1987. 264p. (C). pap. 37.95 (0-8261-5821-8) Springer Pub.

Essential Neurology. Ian M. Wilkinson. (Essentials Ser.). (Illus.). 2nd ed. 1993. LC 93-16238. 272p. pap. 39.95 (0-632-03516-1); 3rd ed. 1999. LC 98-36148. pap. 41.95 (0-86542-854-9) Blackwell Sci.

Essential Neurosurgery. Andrew H. Kaye. 1991. (Illus.). 407p. pap. text (0-443-04350-7); 2nd ed. 1997. LC 96-26151. text (0-443-05347-2) Church.

Essential Nursing. Barbara Kozier et al. Ed. by Debra Hunter. 1989. 954p. (C). pap. text 9.95 (0-201-17869-9) Addison-Wesley.

Essential Nursing Assistant in Long Term Care. Badasch. 2nd ed. 1994. 280p. pap. text 41.95 (0-8273-5633-1) Delmar.

Essential Nutrients in Carcinogenesis. Ed. by Lionel A. Poirier et al. 1986. LC 86-25356. (Advances in Experimental Medicine & Biology Ser.: Vol. 206). 572p. 125.00 (0-306-42471-1, Plenum Trade) Perseus Pubng.

Essential Nutrition. John A. Allocca. 2nd rev. ed. 1997. (Illus.). 223p. pap. text 19.95 (0-9659987-0-3) Allocca Biotech.

***Essential Nutrition for Anti-Aging & Anti-Cancer.** John A. Allocca. rev. ed. 2001. (Illus.). 250p. 19.95 (0-9659987-5-4) Allocca Biotech.

Essential Obstetrics & Gynaecology. E. M. Symonds & Ian M. Symonds. 3rd ed. 1997. LC 97-10852. pap. text (0-443-05453-3) Church.

Essential of Human Anatomy, Vol. 1: Thorax & Abdomen. Ed. by A. K. Datta. 1986. (C). (0-7855-6117-X) Current Dist IND. *Dist:* St Mut.

Essential of Human Anatomy, Vol. 2: Head, Neck & Brain. A. K. Datta. 1989. (C). (0-7855-6116-1) Current Dist IND. *Dist:* St Mut.

Essential of Medical Microbiology B. Banerjee. 2nd ed. 1988. (C). (0-7855-6118-8) Current Dist IND. *Dist:* St Mut.

Essentials of MMPI-2 Assessment. David S. Nichols. 2001. LC 00-47991. (Essentials of Psychological Assessment Ser.). 384p. pap. 34.95 (0-471-34533-4) Wiley.

Essentials of MMPI-2 & MMPI-A Interpretation. James Neal Butcher & Carolyn L. Williams. 1992. 384p. (C). 44.95 (0-8166-2100-4) U of Minn Pr.

Essential of Neonatal Medicine. Malcolm I. Levene & David Tudehope. 2nd ed. 1993. LC 92-49090. (Essentials Ser.). 448p. pap. 49.95 (0-632-03558-7) Blackwell Sci.

***Essential Oil Safety: A Guide for Health Care Professionals.** Robert Tisserand & Tony Balacs. 2nd ed. 2001. (Illus.). 305p. (0-443-06241-2) Church GBR. *Dist:* Saunders.

Essential Oncology of the Lymphocyte. I. J. Forbes & A. S. Leong. 1987. (Illus.). 376p. 87.00 (0-387-17493-1) Spr-Verlag.

Essential Orthopaedics & Trauma. David J. Dandy. 1989. (Illus.). 456p. pap. text (0-443-04003-6) Church.

Essential Other: A Developmental Psychology of Self. Robert M. Galatzer-Levy & Bertram J. Cohler. 1993. LC 92-56171. 416p. 57.00 (0-465-02066-6) Basic.

Essential Otolaryngology. K. J. Lee. 6th ed. 1994. LC 94-34211. (Illus.). 1209p. (C). pap. text 75.00 (0-8385-2214-9, A2214-3) Appleton & Lange.

Essential Otolaryngology. K. J. Lee. 7th ed. 1998. LC 98-29768. 1232p. pap. text 79.95 (0-8385-2270-X, Apple Lange Med) McGraw.

Essential over 35 Pregnancy Guide: Everything You Need to Know about Becoming a Mother Later in Life. Ellen R. Lavin & Samuel H. Wood. 1998. LC 97-37542. pap. 11.00 (0-380-78819-5, Avon Bks) Morrow Avon.

Essential Paediatrics. Ed. by David Hull & Derek I. Johnston. 1999. LC 99-27755. xii, 382p. (0-443-05958-6) Church.

Essential Papers on Addiction. Daniel L. Yalisove. 1997. LC 97-10332. (Essential Papers in Psychoanalysis). text 75.00 (0-8147-9672-9); 550p. pap. text 27.50 (0-8147-9677-X) NYU Pr.

Essential Papers on Borderline Disorders. Ed. by Michael H. Stone. 1986. (Essential Papers in Psychoanalysis). 580p. (C). pap. text 27.50 (0-8147-7850-X) NYU Pr.

Essential Papers on Countertransference. Ed. by Benjamin Wolstein. 1988. (Essential Papers in Psychoanalysis). 400p. (C). text 75.00 (*0-8147-9220-0*); pap. text 27.50 (*0-8147-9221-9*) NYU Pr.

Essential Papers on Depression. Ed. by James C. Coyne. 1986. LC 85-21498. (Essential Papers in Psychoanalysis). 496p. (C). pap. text 27.50 (*0-8147-1399-8*) NYU Pr.

Essential Papers on Dreams. Ed. by Melvin R. Lansky. 1992. (Essential Papers in Psychology). 488p. (C). text 75.00 (*0-8147-5061-3*); pap. text 27.50 (*0-8147-5062-1*) NYU Pr.

Essential Papers on Literature & Psychoanalysis. Ed. by Emanuel Berman. 1993. (Essential Papers in Psychoanalysis). 550p. (C). text 75.00 (*0-8147-1184-7*); pap. text 27.50 (*0-8147-1185-5*) NYU Pr.

Essential Papers on Masochism. Ed. by Margaret Ann Fitzpatrick Hanly. 1995. (Essential Papers in Psychoanalysis). 550p. (C). text 75.00 (*0-8147-3495-2*); pap. text 27.50 (*0-8147-3496-0*) NYU Pr.

Essential Papers on Object Loss. Ed. by Rita V. Frankiel. 1994. LC 93-37084. (Essential Papers in Psychoanalysis). (C). text 75.00 (*0-8147-2607-0*); 547p. pap. text 27.50 (*0-8147-2621-6*) NYU Pr.

Essential Papers on Object Relations. Ed. by Peter Buckley. 1986. (Essential Papers in Psychoanalysis). 512p. (C). pap. text 27.50 (*0-8147-1080-8*) NYU Pr.

Essential Papers on Post Traumatic Stress Disorder. Ed. by Mardi J. Horowitz. 1999. LC 98-34012. (Essential Papers in Psychoanalysis). 550p. pap. text 27.50 (*0-8147-3559-2*) NYU Pr.

Essential Papers on Psychosis. Ed. by Peter Buckley. 1988. (Essential Papers in Psychoanalysis). 384p. (C). text 75.00 (*0-8147-1096-4*); pap. text 27.50 (*0-8147-1097-2*) NYU Pr.

Essential Papers on Short-Term Dynamic Therapy. Ed. by James E. Groves. 1996. (Essential Papers in Psychoanalysis). 450p. (C). text 75.00 (*0-8147-3076-0*); LC 95-37145. pap. text 27.50 (*0-8147-3083-3*) NYU Pr.

Essential Papers on Suicide. John T. Maltsberger. 1996. LC 96-21405. (Essential Papers in Psychoanalysis). 648p. (C). pap. text 27.50 (*0-8147-5550-X*) NYU Pr.

Essential Papers on the Psychology of Aging. Ed. by M. Powell Lawton & Timothy A. Salthouse. 1998. LC 98-12220. (Essential Papers in Psychoanalysis). 803p. pap. text 29.50 (*0-8147-5126-1*) NYU Pr.

Essential Papers on Transference. Ed. by Aaron H. Esman. 1990. (Essential Papers in Psychoanalysis). 528p. (C). text 75.00 (*0-8147-2176-1*); pap. text 27.50 (*0-8147-2177-X*) NYU Pr.

Essential Papers on Transference Analysis. Ed. by Gregory P. Bauer. 1993. LC 93-8962. 240p. pap. 45.00 (*0-87668-529-7*) Aronson.

Essential Pathology. Emanuel Rubin & John L. Farber. 3rd ed. 2000. LC 00-42037. (Illus.). 800p. pap. text 59.95 (*0-7817-2395-7*) Lppncott W & W.

Essential Pathology for Dental Students. William Lawler et al. 1987. 160p. pap. text (*0-443-02910-5*) Church.

Essential Pediatric Dermatology, Vol. 1. J. A. Keipert. 1990. 280p. text 184.00 (*3-7186-0505-8*) Gordon & Breach.

Essential Pediatric MCQs. Derek I. Johnston & David M. Hull. 2nd ed. 1989. 160p. pap. text (*0-443-03446-X*) Church.

Essential Pediatric MCQS. Johnston. 3rd ed. 1995. pap. text 21.95 (*0-443-05245-X*) Saunders.

Essential Pediatric Nursing. James & Sandra R. Mott. Ed. by Debra Hunter. 1988. 1315p. (C). pap. text 9.95 (*0-201-14197-3*) Addison-Wesley.

Essential Pediatric Radiology. Steve Chapman. 1999. (Illus.). 360p. text (*0-7020-2150-4*) W B Saunders GBR. *Dist:* Saunders.

Essential Pediatric Surgery. Spencer W. Beasley et al. 1996. (Arnold Publication). (Illus.). 200p. 89.50 (*0-340-56017-7*) OUP.

Essential Pediatrics. O. P. Ghai. 1990. 456p. (C). (*81-85017-50-6*) Interprint IND. *Dist:* St Mut.

Essential Pediatrics. Ed. by David M. Hull & Derek I. Johnston. 3rd ed. 1993. (Illus.). 304p. pap. text (*0-443-04782-0*) Church.

Essential Pediatrics. David Hull & Derek I. Johnston. 4th ed. 1999. LC 99-27755. xii, 382p. (*0-443-05959-4*) Church.

Essential Physics of Medical Imaging. Jerrold T. Bushberg et al. 1993. LC 93-34268. 742p. 89.95 (*0-683-01140-5*); 575p. 55.00 (*0-683-01040-9*) Lppncott W & W.

Essential Practice in Patient-Centered Care. Ed. by K. W. Fulford et al. 1995. LC 95-35999. 240p. pap. 49.95 (*0-632-03903-5*) Blackwell Sci.

Essential Procedures for Clinical Microbiology. Henry D. Isenberg. 1998. LC 97-25189. (Illus.). 854p. pap. 99.95 (*1-55581-125-6*) ASM Pr.

Essential Psychiatry. Nicholas D. Rose. 2nd ed. 1994. LC 93-34958. (Essentials Ser.). 336p. pap. 46.95 (*0-632-03737-7*) Blackwell Sci.

Essential Psychoanalysis: A Contemporary Introduction. Robert M. Galatzer-Levy & Bertram J. Cohler. Date not set. 224p. 25.00 (*0-465-06491-4*) Basic.

Essential Psychology. R. B. Burns. 2nd ed. 1991. 416p. pap. text 59.00 (*0-7923-8957-3*) Kluwer Academic.

Essential Psychology for Nurses & Other Health Professionals. Graham Russell. 1999. LC 98-36107. xiv, 203p. 80.00 (*0-415-18888-1*); xiv, 203 p. pap. 26.95 (*0-415-18889-X*) Routledge.

Essential Psychopathology & Its Treatment. Jerrold S. Maxmen & Nicholas G. Ward. 2nd ed. 1995. LC 94-38839. (Illus.). 400p. (C). 45.00 (*0-393-70173-5*) Norton.

Essential Psychopharmacology: Neuroscientific Basis & Practical Applications. Stephen M. Stahl. (Illus.). (C). 2000. LC 99-89281. 660p. text 175.00 (*0-521-64154-3*); 1996. 391p. text 125.00 (*0-521-56011-X*); 1996. LC 00-265510. 391p. pap. text 59.95 (*0-521-42620-0*); 2nd ed. 2000. 576p. 300.00 incl. cd-rom (*0-521-79560-5*); 2nd ed. 2000. LC 99-89281. 660p. pap. text 64.95 (*0-521-64615-4*) Cambridge U Pr.

Essential Psychopharmacology of Depression & Bipolar Disorder. Stephen M. Stahl. 2000. (Illus.). 198p. (C). pap. text 29.95 (*0-521-78645-2*) Cambridge U Pr.

Essential Psychosocial Inservices for Nursing Home Personnel. Marylou Hughes. 1992. 385p. (C). 65.00 (*1-877735-37-X*, 2193PP) Prof Prnting & Pub.

Essential Psychotherapies: Theory & Practice. Ed. by Alan S. Gurman & Stanley B. Messer. LC 95-297. 534p. 1997. pap. 36.00 (*1-57230-223-2*, 0223); 1995. 55.00 (*1-57230-018-3*, 0018) Guilford Pubns.

Essential Radiology: Clinical Presentation, Pathophysiology, Imaging. Richard B. Gunderman. 1997. LC 97-31577. (Illus.). 576p. pap. text 49.00 (*0-86577-684-9*) Thieme Med Pubs.

Essential Readings in Case Management. Catherine M. Mullahy. 2nd ed. 1998. LC 98-14420. 307p. pap. 34.00 (*0-8342-1139-4*, 11394) Aspen Pub.

Essential Readings in Holistic Nursing. Cathie E. Guzzetta. 1998. LC 98-12132. 384p. pap. 32.00 (*0-8342-1132-7*, 11327) Aspen Pub.

Essential Readings in Nursing Managed Care. Susan Odegaard Turner. 1999. LC 98-50336. 368p. pap. 33.00 (*0-8342-1326-5*, 13265) Aspen Pub.

Essential Readings in Rehabilitation Outcomes Measurement: Application, Methodology, & Technology. Edward A. Dobrzykowski, Jr. 1997. LC 98-20405. 304p. pap. 55.00 (*0-8342-1194-7*) PRO-ED.

Essential Reiki: A Complete Guide to an Ancient Healing Art. Diane Stein. 1995. (Illus.). 158p. pap. 18.95 (*0-89594-736-6*) Crossing Pr.

Essential Reproduction. Martin H. Johnson & Barry J. Everitt. 5th rev. ed. 2000. LC 99-20350. (Illus.). xvi, 285p. pap. 52.95 (*0-632-04287-7*) Blackwell Sci.

Essential Skills, Bk. 1. Pauk. pap. Price not set. (*0-89061-220-X*) NTC Contemp Pub Co.

Essential Skills & Strategies in the Helping Process. Robert E. Doyle. 1992. LC 91-24852. 336p. (C). text 53.95 (*0-534-17328-4*) Brooks-Cole.

Essential Skills in Clinical Medicine. Charles L. Bardes. 1995. LC 95-19189. (Illus.). 397p. (C). pap. text 28.95 (*0-8036-0014-3*) Davis Co.

Essential Skills in Family Therapy: From the First Interview to Termination. JoEllen Patterson et al. 1998. LC 97-41754. (Guilford Family Therapy Ser.). 250p. pap. 32.00 (*1-57230-307-7*, 0307) Guilford Pubns.

Essential Skin Pathology. Phillip H. McKee. 1999. LC 98-47945. 59.95 (*0-7234-3067-5*) Mosby Inc.

Essential Social Psychology. Donald C. Pennington et al. 2nd ed. 1999. LC 00-697984. (Illus.). xiv, 443p. pap. text 24.95 (*0-340-54846-0*) OUP.

Essential Spanish for Pharmacists. Glenn R. Kisch. 1999. 56p. pap. text 12.00 (*1-58212-003-X*) Am Pharm Assn.

Essential Subtleties on the Silver Sea: The Yin-Hai Jing-Wei: A Chinese Classic on Apthalmology. Tr. by Paul U. Unschuld & Jurgen Kovacs. 1994. LC 97-138. (Comparative Studies of Health Systems & Medical Care: Vol. 38). (Illus.). 525p. 70.00 (*0-520-08058-0*) U CA Pr.

Essential Surgery. H. George Burkitt et al. 1990. (Illus.). 771p. pap. text (*0-443-03593-8*) Church.

***Essential Surgery: Problems, Diagnosis & Management.** George Burkitt & Clive R. G. Quick. 3rd ed. 2001. LC 2001-28718. (Illus.). 655p. (*0-443-06375-3*) Church GBR. *Dist:* Saunders.

Essential Surgical Immunology. Pierce A. Grace et al. 1996. 192p. pap. text 60.00 (*0-7506-0875-7*) Buttrwrth-Heinemann.

Essential Surgical Practice. Alfred Cuschieri et al. Ed. by A. R. Moossa. 3rd ed. 1995. LC 94-24687. (Illus.). 1656p. text 165.00 (*0-7506-1850-7*) Buttrwrth-Heinemann.

Essential Surgical Practice. Alfred Cuschieri. 4th ed. 2000. 1700p. 210.00 (*0-7506-3729-3*) Buttrwrth-Heinemann.

Essential Surgical Practice: Basic Surgical Training. Alfred Cuschieri. 4th ed. 2000. 600p. (*0-7506-4780-9*) E A GBR. *Dist:* OUP.

Essential Urology. Nigel Bullock et al. 2nd ed. 1993. LC 93-20138. (Illus.). 384p. pap. text (*0-443-04807-X*) Church.

Essential Vascular Surgery. Ed. by Alun H. Davies et al. 1999. 418p. text 38.00 (*0-7020-2326-4*) Saunders.

Essential/Nursing Assistant Long Term Care CTB. Badasch. 2nd ed. 1994. (Home Care Aide Ser.). 41.95 (*0-8273-6393-1*) Delmar.

Essentials: Walsh & Hoyt's Clinical Neuro-Opthalmology. Neil R. Miller & Nancy J. Newman. 5th ed. 1998. LC 98-21736. 730p. pap. 75.00 (*0-683-30682-0*) Lppncott W & W.

Essentials Emergency Care. Daniel Limmer et al. Ed. by Edward T. Dickinson. 2nd ed. 1998. LC 98-24803. (Illus.). xv, 528p. pap. text 38.00 (*0-8359-5181-2*) P-H.

Essentials for Directors of Social Work Programs in Health Care. Alice M. Scesny. 1991. LC 90-14462. 78p. (Orig.). pap. 37.00 (*0-87258-559-X*, 187104) Am Hospital.

Essentials for Health & Wellness. Gordon Edlin et al. 1997. LC 96-48503. (Health Science Ser.). (Illus.). 384p. (C). pap. text 40.00 (*0-7637-0318-4*, 0318-4) Jones & Bartlett.

Essentials for Nurse Assistant. Grubbs. 1998. LC 98-27544. 576p. pap. text 46.67 (*0-8359-4973-7*) P-H.

Essentials for Nursing Assistants. Sheila A. Sorrentino. 1997. (Illus.). 400p. (gr. 13). pap. text 23.95 (*0-8151-1566-0*, 30002) Mosby Inc.

Essentials for Nursing Assisted Long-Term Care. Badasch. 1990. (Home Care Aide Ser.). pap., tchr. ed. 8.00 (*0-8273-3990-9*) Delmar.

Essentials for Nursing Assisted Long-Term Care. Shirely A. Badasch. 1990. (Home Care Aide Ser.). pap. 27.95 (*0-8273-3989-5*) Delmar.

Essentials for Ophthalmic Lens Work. Clifford W. Brooks. 2001. 400p. 70.00 (*0-7506-7213-7*); 1983. (Illus.). 267p. text 69.99 (*0-7506-9248-0*) Buttrwrth-Heinemann.

Essentials for Post Graduate Surgery. Louis Fligelstone & Alun Huw Davies. 2000. 350p. pap. text 39.95 (*0-443-06025-8*) Saunders.

Essentials for the Activity Professional in Long Term Care. Susan E. Lanza. 1996. LC 96-19631. (Home Care Aide Ser.). (Illus.). 320p. pap. text 72.95 (*0-8273-7387-2*) Delmar.

Essentials for the Nursing Assistant in Long Term Care. Shirley A. Badasch & Doreen S. Chesebro. 1994. 512p. pap. 40.40 net. (*0-8273-8786-5*); 1994. 334p. (C). stu. ed., wbk. ed. 18.00 (*0-8273-5632-3*); 2nd ed. 512p. (C). pap. 41.95 (*0-8273-5631-5*) Delmar.

***Essentials in Autopsy: Practice I.** Ed. by G. N. Rutty. 2001. LC 2001-34160. (Illus.). x, 254p. 129.00 (*1-85233-349-9*) Spr-Verlag.

Essentials in Emergency Nursing Pamela Baker et al. Date not set. (Illus.). 145p. pap. text 250.00 (*0-935890-26-2*) Emerg Nurses IL.

Essentials in Hemodial. Jungers. 1978. pap. text (*90-247-2103-2*) M Nijhoff NLD. *Dist:* Kluwer Academic.

Essentials in Pressure Monitoring: Blood & Other Body Fluids. Jozef Cywinski. 1980. (Tardieu Ser.: No. 3). (Illus.). 120p. pap. text 59.00 (*90-247-2385-X*) Kluwer Academic.

Essentials of Abdomen & Thorax. Asim Kumar Datta & B. C. Roy. 1983. (*0-7855-7514-6*) Current Dist IND. *Dist:* St Mut.

Essentials of Abnormal Psychology. 1999. (*0-13-022050-7*) P-H.

Essentials of Abnormal Psychology. Robert E. Emery. 1999. LC 99-41291. (Illus.). 531p. pap. 62.67 (*0-13-083330-4*) P-H.

Essentials of Abnormal Psychology: Practice Test & Review Manual. Emery. 2000. 216p. pap. 22.00 (*0-13-022064-7*) P-H.

Essentials of Abnormal Psychology: Test Item File. 2000. 450p. (*0-13-022059-0*) P-H.

Essentials of Accident & Emergency Care. John Lourie et al. 1987. (Illus.). 132p. pap. (*0-443-03903-8*) Church.

Essentials of Advanced Cardiac Life Support: Program Review & Exam Preparation. Tony Brainard. 1997. LC 96-48081. 320p. (C). pap. 31.80 (*0-8385-0259-8*, A0259-0) P-H.

Essentials of Aggression Management in Health Care. Steven S. Wilder & Chris Sorensen. 2000. LC 00-46523. (Illus.). 152p. pap. 38.40 (*0-13-013130-X*) P-H.

Essentials of Anaesthetic Equipment. B. Al-Shaikh & S. Stacey. 1995. (Illus.). 147p. pap. (*0-443-05069-4*) Church.

***Essentials of Anatomic Pathology: A Practical Guide with Emphasis on Diffential Diagnosis & Diagnostic Criteria.** Ed. by Liang Cheng & David G. Bostwick. 2002. 880p. pap. 99.50 (*1-58829-118-9*) Humana.

Essentials of Anatomy & Physiology. Dale P. Layman. 1998. (Allied Health Ser.). pap. 37.95 (*0-8273-6116-5*) Delmar.

Essentials of Anatomy & Physiology. Bartholomew & Martini. 2nd ed. 1999. 464p. text, stu. ed. 26.67 (*0-13-082193-4*) PH School.

Essentials of Anatomy & Physiology. Rodney Seeley & Trent D. Stephens. 2nd ed. 1996. (C). (*0-8151-8187-6*) Mosby Inc.

Essentials of Anatomy & Physiology. Valerie C. Scanlon & Tina Sanders. 3rd ed. 1998. LC 98-25201. (Illus.). 589p. pap. 36.95 (*0-8036-0407-6*) Davis Co.

Essentials of Anesthesiology. David C. Chung & Arthur M. Lam. Ed. by Lesley Day. 3rd ed. 1996. 400p. pap. text 32.00 (*0-7216-6675-2*) Saunders.

Essentials of Antimicrobial Pharmacology: A Guide to Fundamentals for Practice. Ed. by Paul H. Axelsen. 2001. 152p. pap. 24.50 (*0-89603-842-4*) Humana.

Essentials of Art Therapy Training & Practice. Bruce L. Moon. 1992. (Illus.). 188p. (C). text 41.95 (*0-398-05794-X*) C C Thomas.

Essentials of Aspiration Biopsy Cytology. Gia-Khanh Nguyen. 1991. LC 90-5005. (Illus.). 200p. pap. 39.50 (*0-89640-188-X*) Igaku-Shoin.

Essentials of Audiology. Stanley A. Gelfand. 1996. LC 96-43591. (Illus.). 512p. (C). text 42.00 (*0-86577-621-0*) Thieme Med Pubs.

Essentials of Behavioral Research: Methods & Data Analysis. Robert Rosenthal & Ralph L. Rosnow. 2nd ed. 1991. (Psychology Ser.). 736p. (C). text 96.25 (*0-07-053929-4*) McGrw-H Hghr Educ.

Essentials of Biostatics. Robert C. Elston & William D. Johnson. 2nd ed. 1993. LC 93-31126. (Illus.). 328p. (C). pap. text 33.95 (*0-8036-3123-5*) Davis Co.

Essentials of Body Computed Tomography. R. Kristina Gedgaudas-McClees. 1989. 256p. text 83.00 (*0-7216-8890-X*) Saunders.

Essentials of Canine & Feline Electrocardiography: Interpretation & Treatment. Larry P. Tilley. 3rd ed. 1992. LC 91-35007. (Illus.). 470p. text 99.00 (*0-8121-1443-4*) Lppncott W & W.

Essentials of Cardiology. A. D. Timmis & A. W. Nathan. 2nd ed. 1992. LC 92-22044. (Essentials Ser.). (Illus.). 368p. pap. 49.95 (*0-632-03367-3*) Blackwell Sci.

Essentials of Cardiopulmonary Physical Therapy. Ed. by Ellen Hillegass & H. Steven Sadowsky. (Illus.). 1993. LC 92-49848. 608p. text 69.00 (*0-7216-3609-8*); 2nd ed. 2001. LC 00-56293. xvii, 868p. text 64.95 (*0-7216-7288-4*) Saunders.

Essentials of Cardiovascular Medicine. Mark Freed & Cindy Grines. unabr. ed. 1994. 628p. (C). pap. text 29.92 (*0-9633886-2-2*) Physicians Pr.

Essentials of CAS Assessment. Jack A. Naglieri. 1999. LC 98-40739. (Essentials of Psychological Assessment Ser.). (Illus.). 224p. pap. 34.95 (*0-471-29015-7*, J223-Y3H) Wiley.

Essentials of Castaneda's Interventional Radiology. Hector Ferral et al. 1998. LC 00-32742. 448p. text 69.95 (*0-683-30094-6*) Lppncott W & W.

Essentials of Cell Biology. Brown et al. 250p. (*1-55664-228-8*) Mosby Inc.

***Essentials of Chemical Dependence.** Gary Lawson. 3rd ed. 1996. tchr. ed. (*0-8342-1933-6*) PRO-ED.

***Essentials of Chemical Dependency.** Gary Lawson. 2nd ed. 2000. tchr. ed. (*0-8342-0828-8*) PRO-ED.

Essentials of Chemical Dependency Counseling. Gary W. Lawson et al. 3rd ed. 2000. LC 00-33161. (Illus.). xii, 504p. pap. 49.00 (*0-8342-1824-0*, 18240) PRO-ED.

Essentials of Child Psychiatry. Helen Margaret Connell. 2nd ed. 1985. (Illus.). 354p. (C). (gr. 13). 23.95 (*0-86793-144-2*, B-1017-6) Mosby Inc.

Essentials of Chinese Diagnostics. Manfred Porkert. 1983. (Illus.). 292p. reprint ed. pap. 16.00 (*0-912379-00-6*) Ctr Traditional Acupuncture.

Essentials of Clinical Anatomy. Ralph Ger & Peter H. Abrahams. 1986. (Illus.). 350p. (Orig.). pap. (*0-443-03963-1*) Church.

Essentials of Clinical Anatomy. Ed. by Ralph Ger et al. 2nd ed. 1996. (Illus.). 558p. (Orig.). 43.95 (*1-85070-635-2*, Parthenon Pbng) CRC Pr.

Essentials of Clinical Dental Assisting. Cara M. Miyasaki-Ching & Joseph E. Chasteen. 5th ed. 1996. (Illus.). 480p. (C). (gr. 13). pap. text 46.00 (*0-8151-6211-1*, 25549) Mosby Inc.

Essentials of Clinical Epilepsy. Alan H. Guberman & Joseph Bruni. 2nd ed. 1999. LC 98-50640. 224p. pap. text 49.99 (*0-7506-7109-2*) Buttrwrth-Heinemann.

Essentials of Clinical Examination: A Question & Answer Guide for Students. Donald G. McLarty. 1991. 158p. pap. text (*0-7020-1512-1*) W B Saunders GBR. *Dist:* Saunders.

Essentials of Clinical Geriatrics. Robert L. Kane et al. 3rd ed. 1994. pap. text 30.00 (*0-07-112989-8*) McGraw.

Essentials of Clinical Geriatrics. Robert L. Kane et al. 3rd ed. 1993. LC 93-20533. (Illus.). 608p. text 32.00 (*0-07-033473-0*) McGraw-Hill Med Pub.

Essentials of Clinical Geriatrics. Robert L. Kane et al. 4th ed. 1999. LC 98-55689. (Illus.). 621p. pap. 39.95 (*0-07-034458-2*) McGraw-Hill Prof.

Essentials of Clinical Immunology. Helen M. Chapel & Mansel Haeney. 3rd ed. 1993. (Essentials Ser.). (Illus.). 352p. pap. 49.95 (*0-632-03366-5*) Blackwell Sci.

Essentials of Clinical MRI. Ed. by Theo H. Falke. 1987. (Radiology Ser.). (C). text 176.50 (*0-89838-353-6*) Kluwer Academic.

Essentials of Clinical Neurology. Weisberg. 3rd ed. 1996. (Illus.). 800p. (C). (gr. 13). text 38.00 (*0-8151-9129-4*, 24830) Mosby Inc.

Essentials of Clinical Neurophysiology. Karl E. Misulis. 2nd ed. 1997. LC 96-50458. 378p. pap. text 49.99 (*0-7506-9887-X*) Buttrwrth-Heinemann.

Essentials of Clinical Pharmacology in Nursing. Ed. by Bradley R. Williams & Charold L. Baer. 2nd ed. 1993. LC 93-11294. 208p. tchr. ed., suppl. ed. (*0-87434-525-1*) Springhouse Corp.

Essentials of Clinical Pharmacology in Nursing. Bradley R. Williams & Charold L. Baer. 3rd ed. 1998. LC 97-34614. (Illus.). 896p. pap. 49.95 (*0-87434-931-1*) Springhouse Corp.

Essentials of Clinical Pharmacology in Nursing: Instructor's Manual & Test Bank. Bradley R. Williams & Charold L. Baer. 3rd ed. 1998. 224p. pap. text, tchr. ed. 44.95 (*0-87434-939-7*) Springhouse Corp.

Essentials of Clinical Psychiatry: Based on The American Psychiatric Press Textbook of Psychiatry. Ed. by Robert E. Hales & Stuart C. Yudofsky. 3rd ed. 1999. LC 98-31874. 1092p. text 75.00 (*0-88048-848-4*, 8848) Am Psychiatric.

E
F
G

Essentials of Clinical Psychopharmacology. Ed. by Charles B. Nemeroff & Alan F. Schatzberg. 2001. LC 00-55834. 752p. pap. 75.00 (1-58562-017-3, 62017) Am Psychiatric.

Essentials of Complementary & Alternative Medicine. Wayne B. Jonas & Jeffrey S. Levin. 1998. LC 98-22365. (Illus.). 604p. pap. text 59.95 (0-683-30674-X) Lppncott W & W.

Essentials of Computers for Nurses. Virginia K. Saba & Kathleen Ann McCormick. 3rd ed. 2000. LC 00-20237. (Illus.). 555p. pap. 49.95 (0-07-134900-6) McGraw-Hill Prof.

Essentials of Consultation-Liaison Psychiatry: Based on the American Psychiatric Press Textbook of Consultation-liaison Psychiatry. Ed. by James R. Rundell & Michael G. Wise. 1999. LC 98-54234. 688p. pap. 60.00 (0-88048-801-8) Am Psychiatric.

Essentials of Cranio-Sacral Osteopathy. Ronald R. McCatty. unabr. ed. 1988. (Illus.). 336p. pap. (0-906798-90-6) Ashgrove Pr GBR. *Dist:* Words Distrib.

Essentials of Critical Care Pharmacology. Bart Chernow. 2nd ed. 1994. (Illus.). 640p. 65.00 (0-683-01529-X) Lppncott W & W.

Essentials of Dental Assisting. Ann Ehrlich. 1992. (C). pap. text 42.95 (0-7216-3262-9) Harcourt.

Essentials of Dental Assisting. Ann Ehrlich et al. 2nd ed. 1996. (Illus.). 654p. pap., tchr. ed. (0-7216-6397-4) Saunders.

Essentials of Dental Assisting. Ann Ehrlich et al. Ed. by Selma Kaszczuk. 2nd ed. 1996. LC 96-20544. (Illus.). 576p. pap. text 41.95 (0-7216-6396-6) Saunders.

Essentials of Dental Radiography & Radiology. Eric Whaites. (Dental Ser.). (Illus.). (Orig.). 1993. 346p. pap. text (0-443-04212-8); 2nd ed. 1996. 416p. pap. (0-443-05349-9) Church.

Essentials of Dental Radiology for Dental Assistants & Hygienists. Orlen N. Johnson et al. 6th ed. 1998. LC 98-6878. 496p. (C). pap. 53.00 (0-8385-2222-X) P-H.

Essentials of Dermatology. J. L. Burton. 3rd ed. 1990. (Illus.). 308p. pap. (0-443-04082-6) Church.

Essentials of Diagnostic Imaging. Gary M. Guebert et al. 1994. LC 93-44003. (Illus.). 272p. (C). (gr. 13). text 71.00 (0-8016-7455-7, 01995) Mosby Inc.

Essentials of Diagnostic Microbiology. Rodgers. 1998. (Medical Lab Technician Ser.). (C). wbk. ed. 24.95 (0-8273-7390-2); 49.95 (0-8273-7391-0) Delmar.

Essentials of Diagnostic Microbiology. Vantage. Ed. by Lisa Anne Shimeld. 1998. LC 98-17226. (Medical Lab Technician Ser.). 750p. (C). pap. text 75.95 (0-8273-7388-0) Delmar.

Essentials of Diagnostic Microbiology - IML. Shimeld. 1998. (Medical Lab Technician Ser.). 112p. text, tchr. ed. 19.95 (0-8273-7389-9) Delmar.

Essentials of Drug Therapy. Johnson. 1991. (Illus.). 448p. pap. text 41.00 (0-7216-3020-0) Saunders.

Essentials of Educational Psychology. Ladislav Duric. 1990. (Educational Sciences Ser.). 160p. pap. 23.00 (1-85302-054-0) Taylor & Francis.

Essentials of Electrodiagnostic Medicine. William W. Campbell. 1998. LC 98-14102. 338p. text 89.00 (0-683-30239-6) Lppncott W & W.

Essentials of Emergency Care: A Refresher for the Practicing EMT-B. Michael F. O'Keefe et al. Ed. by Edward T. Dickinson. 1995. LC 95-19433. 496p. pap. text 46.67 (0-8359-4963-X) P-H.

Essentials of Emergency Medicine. Douglas Rund et al. 2nd ed. 1996. LC 96-17608. (Illus.). 912p. (C). (gr. 13). pap. text 59.95 (0-8151-7146-3, 24599) Mosby Inc.

Essentials of Endocrinology. C. Brook & N. Marshall. 3rd ed. 1996. (Essentials Ser.). (Illus.). 256p. pap. (0-632-03622-2) Blckwell Science.

Essentials of Epidemiology in Public Health. Ann Aschengram & Seage. 2000. 275p. 45.00 (0-8342-0626-9) Aspen Pub.

Essentials of Exercise Physiology. William D. McArdle et al. 2nd ed. 2000. LC 99-48195. 679p. pap. text 55.95 (0-683-30507-7) Lppncott W & W.

Essentials of Experimental Surgery. J. S. P. Lumley. 1997. 262p. text 199.00 (0-407-01395-4) Buttrwrth-Heinemann.

Essentials of Experimental Surgery: Gastroenterology. Ed. by S. Lindkaer Jensen et al. 1996. 784p. text 220.00 (3-7186-5496-2, Harwood Acad Pubs) Gordon & Breach.

Essentials of Facial Growth. Donald H. Enlow & Mark G. Hans. Ed. by Larry McGrew. 1996. LC 96-16720. 400p. pap. text 47.00 (0-7216-6106-8) Saunders.

Essentials of Family Medicine. Ed. by Philip D. Sloane et al. 2nd ed. 1993. LC 92-48801. (Illus.). 432p. pap. 34.00 (0-683-07759-7) Lppncott W & W.

Essentials of Family Medicine. Philip D. Sloane et al. 3rd ed. 1998. LC 97-42734. 732p. 42.95 (0-683-30147-0) Lppncott W & W.

Essentials of Family Practice. Robert E. Rakel. Ed. by Ray Kersey. 2nd ed. 1998. LC 97-34009. (Illus.). 576p. (C). pap. text 49.95 (0-7216-5868-7) Saunders.

Essentials of Family Therapy: A Therapist's Guide to Eight Approaches. William M. Walsh & James A. McGraw. 1996. LC 95-75401. 154p. pap. 24.95 (0-89108-239-5, 9504) Love Pub Co.

Essentials of First Aid & CPR. National Safety Council Staff. 2nd ed. 1997. (Emergency Care Ser.). (Illus.). 160p. (C). pap. text 22.50 (0-7637-0434-2, 0434-2) Jones & Bartlett.

Essentials of Florida Mental Health Law. S. Behnke et al. 2000. LC 99-54664. (Professional Book Ser.). (Illus.). 240p. 35.00 (0-393-70309-6) Norton.

Essentials of Food Microbiology. John Garbutt. 1997. LC 97-186975. (Arnold Publication). (Illus.). 256p. (Orig.). pap. 34.50 (0-340-67701-5) OUP.

Essentials of Functional Sinus Surgery. Heinz Stammberger & Michael Hawke. 2nd ed. 1993. LC 93-4631. 300p. (gr. 13). text 123.00 (1-55664-386-1) Mosby Inc.

Essentials of General, Organic & Biological Chemistry. D. H. Wolfe. 1986. 656p. (C). pap. text, stu. ed. 28.12 (0-07-071417-7) McGraw.

Essentials of General Surgery. Peter F. Lawrence. 3rd ed. 1999. 664p. LC 99-37812. pap. text 42.95 (0-683-30133-0); 75.00 (0-7817-2817-7) Lppncott W & W.

Essentials of Geriatric Medicine. Alex Ming. 1997. (Illus.). 440p. (962-356-015-X) Lppncott W & W.

Essentials of Geriatric Psychiatry: A Guide for Health Professionals. Ed. by Lawrence W. Lazarus et al. 1988. 272p. 38.95 (0-8261-5990-7) Springer Pub.

Essentials of Gerontological Nursing: Adaptation to the Aging Process. Ed. by Angela S. Staab & Linda C. Hodges. 2nd ed. 1995. LC 93-783. 576p. pap. text 29.95 (0-397-54973-3) Lppncott W & W.

Essentials of Glycobiology. Ed. by Ajit Varki et al. 1999. LC 99-17198. (Illus.). 668p. lib. bdg. 175.00 (0-87969-559-5) Cold Spring Harbor.

Essentials of Gynaecological Care. Lawton. 1999. 392p. pap. (0-412-79290-7) E A GBR. *Dist:* OUP.

Essentials of Head & Neck Oncology. Ed. by L. G. Close et al. 1998. LC 97-42730. (Illus.). 400p. pap. 59.00 (0-86577-740-3) Thieme Med Pubs.

Essentials of Head, Neck & Brain. Asim Kumar Datta & B. C. Roy. 1983. (0-7855-0788-4) Current Dist IND. *Dist:* St Mut.

Essentials of Health & Wellness. Gordon Edlin & Kelli M. Brown. 1997. (Health Science Ser.). 256p. pap. 10.00 incl. cd-rom (0-7637-0513-6) Jones & Bartlett.

Essentials of Health & Wellness: Test Bank. Gordon Edlin & Kelli M. Brown. 1997. (Health Science Ser.). (Illus.). 176p. pap. text 10.00 (0-7637-0498-9, 0498-9) Jones & Bartlett.

Essentials of Health Care in Old Age. Gerald J. Bennet & Shah B. Ebrahim. 2nd ed. 1995. 256p. pap. (0-340-61372-6) E A GBR. *Dist:* OUP.

Essentials of Health Care Management. Arnold D. Kaluzny & Stephen M. Shortell. 1996. LC 95-52993. (Health Services Administration Ser.). 464p. (C). 73.95 (0-8273-7145-4) Delmar.

Essentials of Health Care Marketing. Eric N. Berkowitz. 1995. LC 95-40372. 432p. pap. 60.00 (0-8342-0687-0) Aspen Pub.

Essentials of Health Services. Stephen J. Williams. (Delmar Series in Health Services Administration Ser.). 1994. LC 94-25469. 175p. mass mkt. 47.95 (0-8273-6969-7); 2nd ed. 2000. 288p. pap. text 47.95 (0-7668-1885-3) Delmar.

Essentials of HIV-AIDS. Research and Education Association Staff. 1995. LC 94-68527. 100p. pap. text 5.95 (0-87891-984-8) Res & Educ.

Essentials of Homeopathic Therapeutics. W. A. Dewey. 1993. 286p. spiral bd. 18.00 (0-7873-0285-6) Hlth Research.

Essentials of Homoeopathic Prescribing. H. Fergie Woods. 1980. 35.00 (0-85032-134-4) St Mut.

Essentials of Hospital Care. P. A. Howarth et al. 1997. 304p. pap. (1-85996-006-5) Bios Sci GBR. *Dist:* Coronet Bks.

Essentials of Hospital Risk Management. Ed. by Barbara J. Youngberg. 1989. (Health Care Administration Ser.). 268p. (C). 91.00 (0-8342-0098-8) Aspen Pub.

Essentials of Human Anatomy. Russell T. Woodburne & William E. Burkel. 9th ed. 1994. LC 92-49098. (Illus.). 736p. text 52.95 (0-19-507727-X) OUP.

Essentials of Human Anatomy & Physiology. John W. Hole, Jr. 5th ed. 1994. (C). text, stu. ed. 54.50 net. (0-697-25533-6); 160p. text, stu. ed. 16.00 net. (0-697-24396-6); 608p. per. 45.00 (0-697-22925-4); 344p. text, stu. ed. 33.50 net. (0-697-16047-5); 192p. text, stu. ed. 25.62 (0-697-16046-7) McGrw-H Hghr Educ (WCB McGr Hill).

Essentials of Human Anatomy & Physiology. John W. Hole, Jr. & Nancy Ann Sickles Corbett. 6th ed. 1997. 192p. (C). pap., stu. ed. 33.13 (0-697-32920-8, WCB McGr Hill) McGrw-H Hghr Educ.

Essentials of Human Anatomy & Physiology. John W. Hole, Jr. et al. 6th ed. 1997. 640p. (C). text 68.12 (0-697-28251-1); LC 96-78736. per. 65.00 (0-697-28252-X) McGrw-H Hghr Educ (WCB McGr Hill).

Essentials of Human Anatomy & Physiology: School Version. Elaine Marieb. 5th ed. 1997. 560p. text 49.00 (0-8053-4195-1) Addison-Wesley.

Essentials of Human Anatomy, Vol. I: Thorax-Abdomen. A. K. Datta. 1991. (C). (0-89771-347-8) Current Dist IND. *Dist:* St Mut.

Essentials of Human Anatomy, Vol. II: Head, Neck & Brain. Ed. by A. K. Datta. 1990. (C). (0-89771-348-6) Current Dist IND. *Dist:* St Mut.

Essentials of Human Diseases & Conditions. Margaret S. Frazier et al. 1996. (Illus.). pap., tchr. ed. (0-7216-5308-1) Saunders.

Essentials of Human Diseases & Conditions. Margaret S. Frazier et al. Ed. by Margaret Biblis. 1996. LC 95-19484. (Illus.). 544p. pap. text 27.00 (0-7216-5279-4) Saunders.

***Essentials of Human Diseases & Conditions.** Margaret Schell Frazier et al. 2nd ed. 2000. LC 99-57048. (Illus.). 544p. pap. 35.95 (0-7216-8475-0) Saunders.

Essentials of Human Embryology. A. K. Datta. 1991. (C). (0-89771-346-X) Current Dist IND. *Dist:* St Mut.

Essentials of Human Embryology. William J. Larsen. 1998. LC 97-17953. (Illus.). 406p. pap. text (0-443-07514-X) Church GBR. *Dist:* Saunders.

Essentials of Human Embryology. D. Datta. 2nd ed. 1990. (C). (0-7855-4654-5) Current Dist IND. *Dist:* St Mut.

Essentials of Human Nutrition. Ed. by Jim Mann & A. Stewart Trusell. 1998. (Illus.). 658p. pap. text 59.95 (0-19-262756-2) OUP.

Essentials of Human Parasitology. Heelan & Ingersoll. 2001. (C). pap., wbk. ed., lab manual ed. 14.50 net. (0-7668-1285-5) Delmar.

Essentials of Human Parasitology. Judith S. Heelan & Frances W. Ingersoll. 2001. (C). text 47.95 (0-7668-1284-7) Thomson Learn.

Essentials of Human Sexuality. Bryan Strong. 2nd ed. Date not set. pap. text, tchr. ed. (0-8299-0525-1); 1980. mass mkt. 42.00 (0-8299-0418-2) West Pub.

Essentials of Hypnosis. Michael D. Yapko. 4th ed. 1994. LC 94-30541. (Basic Principles Into Practice Ser.: No. 4). 192p. pap. 19.95 (0-87630-761-6) Brunner-Routledge.

Essentials of Immediate Medical Care. C. J. Eaton. 2nd ed. 1998. (Illus.). 700p. pap. (0-443-05345-6) Church.

Essentials of Immunohematology. John C. Flynn, Jr. Ed. by Selma Kaszczuk. 1997. LC 97-36859. (Illus.). 450p. text 35.00 (0-7216-6812-7) Saunders.

Essentials of Immunology & Serology. Stanley. (Medical Lab Technician Ser.). (C). 2002. 448p. text 47.95 (0-7668-1064-X); 2001. pap., wbk. ed. 16.00 (0-7668-1065-8) Delmar.

Essentials of Industrial & Organizational Psychology. William C. Howell & Robert L. Dipboye. 3rd ed. 1986. 414p. (C). pap. 43.95 (0-534-10588-2) Brooks-Cole.

Essentials of Internal Medicine in Clinical Podiatry. Bennett G. Zier. 1990. (Illus.). 576p. text 110.00 (0-7216-1400-0) Saunders.

Essentials of Laparoscopy. Ed. by Nathaniel J. Soper et al. 1993. LC 93-27517. (Illus.). 285p. text 40.00 (0-942219-53-8) Quality Med Pub.

Essentials of Learning Electrocardiography: A Complete Course for the Non-Cardiologist. Jules Constant. 4th ed. 1997. LC 97-5800. (Illus.). 232p. lib. bdg. 38.95 (1-85070-921-1, Parthenon Pbng) CRC Pr.

Essentials of Long-Term Care Administration. Seth B. Goldsmith. 1994. 384p. 67.00 (0-8342-0567-X, 20567) Aspen Pub.

Essentials of Low Vision Practice. Richard L. Brilliant. 1998. LC 98-4114. 480p. text 99.00 (0-7506-9307-X) Buttrwrth-Heinemann.

Essentials of Managed Health Care. Peter R. Kongstvedt. 4th ed. 2000. LC 00-33199. 912p. pap. 72.00 (0-8342-1862-3, 18623) Aspen Pub.

Essentials of Managed Health Care: Includes Study Guide. Peter R. Kongstvedt. 4th ed. 2000. 67.00 (0-8342-1985-9) Aspen Pub.

Essentials of Maternal & Neonatal Nursing. Aileen MacLaren & Carole A. Kenner. 1992. 208p. pap., tchr. ed. (0-87434-472-7) Springhouse Corp.

***Essentials of Maternal & Pediatric Nursing.** Lois White. 2001. LC 2001-55520. (0-7668-6300-X) Delmar.

Essentials of Maternal-Fetal Medicine. Ed. by G. Ashmead. 1997. LC 96-35128. (Illus.). 410p. (0-412-08681-6) E A GBR. *Dist:* OUP.

Essentials of Maternal-Newborn Nursing. Patricia A. Ladewig et al. Ed. by Debra Hunter. 2nd ed. 1990. 889p. (C). text 56.95 (0-201-13238-9) Addison-Wesley.

Essentials of McTimoney Chiropractic: The Gentle Art of Whole Body Alignment. Andrews & Courtney. 1999. pap. (0-7225-3747-6) Thorsons GBR. *Dist:* Natl Bk Netwk.

Essentials of Mechanical Ventilation. Ed. by Dean Hess & Robert Kacmarek. 1996. (Illus.). 269p. text 49.95 (0-07-028436-9) McGraw-Hill Prof.

Essentials of Medical Assisting. Fremgen. 1997. LC 97-41972. (C). 49.27 (0-8359-5122-7) P-H.

Essentials of Medical Assisting: Administrative & Clinical Competition. 1998. 576p. text, tchr. ed. 26.00 (0-8359-5275-4) Globe Fearon.

Essentials of Medical Electricity. E. Reginald Morton. 1991. lib. bdg. 88.95 (0-8490-5014-6) Gordon Pr.

Essentials of Medical Imaging: Anatomy & Physiology. Evelyn F. Burns. Ed. by Stewart C. Bushong. 1998. LC 98-24889. (Essentials of Medical Imaging Ser.). (Illus.). 130p. pap. 19.95 (0-07-009231-1) McGraw-Hill Educ Grp.

Essentials of Medical Microbiology. Wesley A. Volk et al. 5th ed. 1995. LC 95-16385. 736p. pap. text 45.00 (0-397-51308-9) Lppncott W & W.

Essentials of Medical Statistics. Betty Kirkwood. 2nd ed. 1997. 288p. pap. text 36.95 (0-86542-871-9) Blackwell Sci.

Essentials of Medical-Surgical Nursing. Ed. by Susan C. DeWit. 4th ed. 1998. (Illus.). 1085p. stu. ed. (0-7216-6922-0); pap., tchr. ed. 19.95 (0-7216-6921-2) Saunders.

Essentials of Medical-Surgical Nursing. Susan C. DeWit. Ed. by Ilze Rader. 4th ed. 1998. LC 97-36860. (Illus.). 1088p. text 47.50 (0-7216-6920-4) Saunders.

***Essentials of Medical-Surgical Nursing: ExaMaster.** Susan C. DeWit. 1998. (Illus.). (0-7216-7973-0) Saunders.

***Essentials of Medical Surgical Nursing: Test Manual.** Susan C. DeWit. 4th ed. 1998. (Illus.). (0-7216-7974-9) Saunders.

Essentials of Medical Syndromes. S. K. Gupta. 1986. (81-204-0078-X) Oxford IBH IND. *Dist:* S Asia.

Essentials of Medical Terminology. Davies. 1997. LC 97-42612. 300p. (C). pap. text 36.95 (0-314-12811-5) West Pub.

***Essentials of Medical Terminology.** Juanita J. Davies. 1998. 300p. pap. text 51.95 incl. audio (0-8273-9431-4); 2nd ed. 2001. LC 2001-37125. 416p. pap. text 34.95 (0-7668-3110-8) Delmar.

Essentials of Medical Transcription: Modular Approach. Ed DeStafano. 2000. LC 00-57377. 350p. pap. text 45.00 (0-7216-8694-X) Saunders.

Essentials of Medical Ultrasound: A Practical Introduction to the Principles, Techniques & Biomedical Applications. Ed. by Michael H. Repacholi & Deirdre A. Benwell. 1982. LC 80-85522. (Medical Methods Ser.). (Illus.). 330p. 140.00 (0-89603-028-8) Humana.

Essentials of Medicinal Chemistry. Andrejus Korolkovas. 2nd ed. 1988. LC 87-33992. 1216p. 298.00 (0-471-88356-5) Wiley.

Essentials of Medicine & Surgery for Dental Students. A. C. Kennedy et al. 5th ed. 1989. (Dental Ser.). (Illus.). 216p. pap. text (0-443-04087-7) Church.

Essentials of Medicine in Ancient China & Japan: Yasuyori Tamba's Ishimpo. Set. Emil C. Hsia et al. 1986. (Illus.). 224.50 (90-04-07808-8) Brill Academic Pubs.

Essentials of Mental Health Care: Planning & Interventions. Barbara B. Bauer & Signe S. Hill. 1986. (Illus.). 203p. pap. text 25.00 (0-7216-1367-5) Saunders.

Essentials of Mental Health Nursing. J. Sue Cook & Karen L. Fontaine. Ed. by Mark McCormick. 2nd ed. 1991. (Illus.). 768p. (C). text 45.25 net. (0-201-12597-8) Addison-Wesley.

Essentials of Mental Health Nursing. Karen L. Fontaine & J. Sue Fletcher. 3rd ed. 1994. LC 94-32934. text 41.95 (0-201-31370-7) Addison-Wesley.

Essentials of Microscopic Hematology. Takeo Nomura & Shimpei Furusawa. 1991. (Illus.). 120p. pap. 43.50 (0-89640-205-3) Igaku-Shoin.

Essentials of Modern Hospital Safety. William Charney & Joseph Schirmer. (Illus.). 1990. 384p. 95.00 (0-87371-198-X, RA969); Vol. 2. 2nd ed. 1993. 368p. 104.95 (0-87371-584-5, L584) Lewis Pubs.

Essentials of Modern Hospital Safety, Vol. 3. Ed. by William Charney. 1994. 512p. lib. bdg. 85.00 (1-56670-083-3, L1083) Lewis Pubs.

Essentials of Mucosal Immunology. Ed. by Martin Kagnoff & Hiroshi Kiyono. 1996. LC 96-14720. (Illus.). 611p. pap. text 59.95 (0-12-394330-2) Acad Pr.

Essentials of Musculoskeletal Care. American Academy of Pediatrics Staff & American Academy of Orthopaedic Surgeons Staff. Ed. by Robert K. Snider. 1997. LC 98-117881. (Illus.). 725p. 100.00 (0-89203-162-X) Amer Acad Ortho Surg.

Essentials of Neonatal Medicine. Malcolm I. Levene et al. 3rd ed. 2000. LC 99-38947. (Illus.). 352p. pap. 49.95 (0-632-05163-9) Blackwell Sci.

Essentials of Neural Science. Kandel. 1997. text 95.00 (0-8385-2262-9, Apple Lange Med) McGraw.

Essentials of Neural Science: A Behavior Study Guide/Problem Book. Ronald Calabrese et al. 1997. (Illus.). 364p. (C). pap. text, stu. ed. 34.95 (0-8385-2221-1, A2221-8, Apple Lange Med) McGraw.

Essentials of Neural Science & Behavior. Eric R. Kandel et al. 1996. LC 94-42332. 540p. (C). pap. text 74.95 (0-8385-2245-9, A2245-7, Apple Lange Med) McGraw.

Essentials of Neurochemistry. Gaynor C. Wild & Edward C. Benzel. 1994. LC 93-47356. (Illus.). 240p. (C). text 78.95 (0-86720-862-7, 862-7) Jones & Bartlett.

Essentials of Neuroimaging. Kirkwood. 2nd ed. 1995. LC 95-20537. text (0-443-08946-9, K5279) Church.

Essentials of Neurology. Lord Walton. 6th ed. 1990. (Illus.). 340p. pap. text (0-443-03986-0) Church.

Essentials of Neuropsychological Assessment. Ed. by Lawrence C. Hartlage et al. 1987. 248p. (C). 34.95 (0-8261-4470-5) Springer Pub.

Essentials of New York Mental Health Law. S. Behnke et al. 1999. (Professional Book Ser.). 35.00 (0-393-70308-8) Norton.

Essentials of Nonverbal Communication. Mark L. Knapp. 1980. LC 79-17769. 264p. (Orig.). (C). pap. text 34.50 (0-03-049861-9) Harcourt Coll Pubs.

Essentials of Nuclear Medicine. M. V. Merrick. 2nd ed. 1997. LC 97-34666. (Illus.). 350p. pap. 89.00 (3-540-76205-1) Spr-Verlag.

Essentials of Nuclear Medicine Imaging. Fred A. Mettler et al. Ed. by Lisette Bralow. 4th ed. 1997. LC 97-14400. (Illus.). 512p. text 69.00 (0-7216-5121-6) Saunders.

Essentials of Nuclear Medicine Physics. Rachel A. Powsner & Edward R. Powsner. 1998. LC 98-21578. (Illus.). 256p. pap. 47.95 (0-632-04314-8) Blackwell Sci.

Essentials of Nurse Anesthesia. Ed. by Laura W. McIntosh. 1996. LC 96-23810. (Illus.). 550p. pap. 49.00 (*0-07-076537-5*) McGraw-Hill Prof.

Essentials of Nursing Care. Susan C. DeWit. 2001. pap. text, stu. ed. 23.75 (*0-7216-6929-8*); LC 00-24804. (Illus.). xxvi, 942p. text 53.25 (*0-7216-6923-9*) Saunders.

Essentials of Nursing Leadership & Management. Ruth M. Tappen et al. 1997. LC 97-39633. 256p. pap. 26.95 (*0-8036-0244-8*); 2nd ed. 2001. LC 2001-17399. (Illus.). xiii, 278p. pap. 31.95 (*0-8036-0817-9*) Davis Co.

Essentials of Nursing Management: Concepts & Context of Practice. Barbara J. S. Barnum & Catherine O. Mallard. 1988. Orig. Title: First Line Patient Care Management. 326p. (C). reprint ed. 61.00 (*0-8342-0018-X*, 20018) Aspen Pub.

Essentials of Nursing Research. Lucille E. Notter & Jacqueline R. Hott. 5th rev. ed. 1994. LC 93-38407. (Illus.). 224p. pap. text 27.95 (*0-8261-1598-5*) Springer Pub.

Essentials of Nursing Research: Methods, Appraisal, & Utilization. Denise F. Polit & Bernadette P. Hungler. 5th ed. 2000. LC 00-44369. (Illus.). 544p. text 40.00 (*0-7817-2557-7*) Lppncott W & W.

Essentials of Nutrition. C. Schmidt. 1987. 313p. pap. 11.95 (*0-938250-22-1*) Bio-Dynamic Farm.

Essentials of Nutrition & Diet Therapy. Yiu H. Hui. 1985. LC 84-25753. (Nursing-Health Science Ser.). (Illus.). 500p. (C). pap. text, tchr. ed. 10.00 (*0-534-04381-X*, 381-X) Jones & Bartlett.

Essentials of Nutrition & Diet Therapy. Yiu H. Hui. 1985. LC 84-25753. (Nursing-Health Science Ser.). (Illus.). 240p. (C). pap. text 39.95 (*0-534-04380-1*, 380-1) Jones & Bartlett.

Essentials of Nutrition & Diet Therapy. Williams. 6th ed. 1997. (C). (gr. 13). text, stu. ed. 48.95 (*0-8151-9489-7*, 30465) Mosby Inc.

Essentials of Nutrition & Diet Therapy: Edition/Nutritrac Package, Set. Sue R. Williams. 7th ed. 1998. (Illus.). 657p. (C). text incl. cd-rom (*0-323-00398-2*) Mosby Inc.

Essentials of Nutrition & Diet Therapy: Nutritrac Package. Sue R. Williams. 7th ed. 1998. (Illus.). (C). stu. ed. (*0-323-00639-6*) Mosby Inc.

Essentials of Nutrition & Diet Therapy: Nutritrac Package: Includes Test Bank. Sue R. Williams. 7th ed. 1998. (Illus.). (C). tchr. ed. (*0-323-00634-5*) Mosby Inc.

Essentials of Nutrition & Diet Therapy: Study Guide. Williams. 5th ed. 1990. 312p. pap. text 14.95 (*0-8016-5262-6*) Mosby Inc.

Essentials of Nutrition & Diet Therapy: Study Guide. S. R. Williams. 6th ed. 1994. 320p. (C). (gr. 13). pap. text 19.95 (*0-8016-7996-6*, 07996) Mosby Inc.

Essentials of Obstetrics & Gynecology. Neville F. Hacker & J. George Moore. Ed. by William Schmitt. 3rd ed. 1998. LC 97-15482. (Illus.). 752p. pap. text 35.00 (*0-7216-7473-9*) Saunders.

Essentials of Oral Histology & Embryology. James K. Avery & Pauline F. Steele. 2nd ed. 1999. LC 99-25601. (Illus.). 256p. (C). text (*0-323-00460-1*) Mosby Inc.

Essentials of Oral Histology & Embryology. Leslie P. Gartner. 2nd ed. 1986. (Illus.). 124p. (C). pap. text 17.50 (*0-910841-04-7*) Jen Hse Pub Co.

Essentials of Oral Histology & Embryology: A Clinical Approacch. James K. Avery. 1991. 224p. (C). (gr. 13). pap. text 38.95 (*1-55664-188-5*) Mosby Inc.

Essentials of Oral Pathology & Oral Medicine. R. A. Cawson & E. W. Odell. 6th ed. 1998. LC 97-28646. pap. text (*0-443-05348-0*) Church.

Essentials of Oral Physiology. Robert M. Bradley. 1994. 208p. (C). pap. text 39.00 (*1-55664-088-9*) Mosby Inc.

Essentials of Orthopaedic Surgery. Sam W. Wiesel & John N. Delahay. Ed. by Richard Lampert. 2nd ed. 1997. LC 96-41700. (Illus.). 368p. pap. text 36.95 (*0-7216-6671-X*) Saunders.

Essentials of Otolaryngology. Frank E. Lucente & Steven M. Sobol. Ed. by Har-Ed Gady. 4th ed. 1999. LC 99-21310. 512p. pap. text 39.95 (*0-7817-1463-X*) Lppncott W & W.

***Essentials of Outcome Assessment.** Benjamin Ogles et al. 2002. (Essentials of Mental Health Practice Ser.). 304p. pap. (*0-471-41998-2*) Wiley.

Essentials of Outdoor First-Aid: Student Manual. Robert J. Koester. 1996. 90p. (Orig.). pap. text, wbk. ed. 10.00 (*1-879471-24-8*) DBS Prodns.

Essentials of Oxygenation. Thomas Ahrens & Kim Rutherford. 1992. (Nursing-Health Science Ser.). (Illus.). 194p. (C). text 59.95 (*0-86720-332-3*, 332-3) Jones & Bartlett.

Essentials of Pain Medicine & Regional Anesthesia. Honorio Benzon et al. Ed. by Allan Ross. 1999. LC 98-24849. 495p. (C). pap. text (*0-443-06509-8*) Church.

Essentials of Parasitology. Marvin C. Meyer et al. 5th ed. 1991. 320p. (C). text 42.50 net. (*0-697-12310-3*, WCB McGr Hill) McGrw-H Hghr Educ.

Essentials of Pathology. Ed. by Malcolm J. Mitchinson et al. 1995. LC 95-14348. 352p. pap. 48.95 (*0-632-02944-7*) Blackwell Sci.

Essentials of Pathology for Dentistry. R. F. McMahon & P. Sloan. 1998. (Illus.). 224p. pap. (*0-443-05706-0*) Church.

Essentials of Pathophysiology. Ed. by Christian E. Kaufman, Jr. & Patrick A. McKee. 1996. LC 95-26499. 816p. pap. text 39.95 (*0-316-48405-9*) Lppncott W & W.

Essentials of Pathophysiology: Concepts & Applications for Health Care Professionals. Thomas J. Nowak & A. Gordon Handford. 1994. 688p. (C). text 63.50 net. (*0-697-13314-1*, WCB McGr Hill) McGrw-H Hghr Educ.

Essentials of Pathophysiology: Concepts & Applications for Health Care Professionals. Nowak. 3rd ed. 2002. 68.74 net. (*0-07-027255-7*) McGraw.

Essentials of Pathophysiology: Concepts & Applications of Healing. Nowak & Handford. 1994. trans. 10.93 (*0-697-26625-7*) McGrw-H Hghr Educ.

***Essentials of Pathophysiology of Pharmacy: An Integrated Approach.** Martin M. Zdanowicz. 2002. 59.95 (*1-58716-036-6*) CRC Pr.

Essentials of Pediatric Intensive Care. Daniel L. Levin & Frances C. Morris. 2nd ed. 1997. LC 96-53381. text (*0-443-05932-2*) Church.

Essentials of Pediatric Intensive Care. Daniel L. Levin & Frances C. Morriss. 2nd ed. 1997. LC 96-53381. text (*0-443-05931-4*) Church.

Essentials of Pediatric Intensive Care, Set. Daniel L. Levin & Frances C. Morriss. Ed. by Judy Fletcher. 2nd ed. 1999. LC 96-53381. (Illus.). 1890p. pap. text (*0-443-05930-6*) Church.

Essentials of Pediatric Intensive Care, Set. Ed. by Daniel L. Levin & Frances C. Morriss. 2nd ed. 1996. (Illus.). 1600p. pap. 89.00 (*0-942219-84-8*) Quality Med Pub.

Essentials of Pediatric Intensive Care - A Pocket Companion. Ed. by D. L. Levin & F. C. Morris. 2nd ed. 1998. pap. (*0-443-07613-8*) Church.

Essentials of Pediatric Nursing. Lucille L. Whaley & Donna L. Wong. 3rd ed. 1988. (Illus.). 482p. trans. 100.00 (*0-8016-2863-6*) Mosby Inc.

Essentials of Pediatric Nursing. Donna L. Wong. 5th ed. 1999. (Illus.). 1278p. 63.00 incl. cd-rom (*0-323-01058-X*) Mosby Inc.

Essentials of Pediatric Oncology Nursing: A Core Curriculum. Ed. by Marilyn Hockenberry-Eaton. 1998. LC 98-73093. (Illus.). pap. text 84.00 (*0-9666193-0-7*) Assn Pediatric.

Essentials of Pediatric Radiology. Edward Burton & Alan Brody. 1999. LC 98-34484. 109.00 (*3-13-115681-3*) Thieme Med Pubs.

Essentials of Pediatric Radiology. Edward M. Burton. 1999. LC 98-34484. (Illus.). 528p. 109.00 (*0-86577-802-7*) Thieme Med Pubs.

Essentials of Pediatrics. Frank A. Oski. 1996. LC 96-38508. 788p. pap. text 39.95 (*0-397-51514-6*) Lppncott W & W.

Essentials of Periodontics. Phillip M. Hoag & Elizabeth A. Pawlak. 4th ed. 1989. (Illus.). 272p. (C). (gr. 13). pap. text 39.95 (*0-8016-2228-X*, 02228) Mosby Inc.

Essentials of Perioperative Nursing: A Self-Learning Guide. Cynthia Spry. 2nd ed. 1996. LC 96-18621. 300p. 75.00 (*0-8342-0581-5*, 20581) Aspen Pub.

Essentials of Peritoneal Dialysis. Ramesh Khanna et al. 1993. LC 92-17615. lib. bdg. 57.00 (*0-7923-1813-7*) Kluwer Academic.

Essentials of Person-Environment-Correspondence Counseling. Lloyd H. Lofquist & Rene V. Dawis. 1991. (Illus.). 192p. pap. 16.95 (*0-8166-2066-0*); text 42.95 (*0-8166-1889-5*) U of Minn Pr.

Essentials of Pharmacology. Cedric M. Smith & Alan M. Reynard. 1995. LC 94-11096. (Illus.). 694p. pap. text 39.00 (*0-7216-5531-9*) Saunders.

Essentials of Pharmacology. Ruth Woodrow. 2nd ed. 1992. pap. 32.95 (*0-8273-4599-2*) Delmar.

Essentials of Pharmacology for Health Occupations. Ruth Woodrow. 3rd ed. 1996. (Medical Assisting Ser.). 96p. tchr. ed. 17.95 (*0-8273-7023-7*); LC 96-18216. (Illus.). 544p. (C). pap. text 51.95 (*0-8273-7022-9*) Delmar.

***Essentials of Pharmacology for Health Occupations.** Ruth Woodrow. 4th ed. 2001. LC 2001-47100. 576p. text 51.95 (*0-7668-3890-0*) Delmar.

Essentials of Pharmacy Management. Dennis H. Tootelian & Ralph M. Gaedeke. 1993. LC 92-44282. (Illus.). 432p. (gr. 13). text 54.00 (*0-8016-6513-2*, 06513) Mosby Inc.

Essentials of Pharmocology - Health Occupations Instructors Guide. Ruth Woodrow. 2nd ed. 1992. pap. 16.00 (*0-8273-4601-8*) Delmar.

***Essentials of Physical Medicine & Rehabilitation.** Walter P. Frontera & Julie K. Silver. 2001. LC 2001-51752. (Illus.). 800p. 95.00 (*1-56053-443-5*) Hanley & Belfus.

Essentials of Pig Anatomy & Horowitz-Kramer Atlas of the Musculoskeletal Anatomy of the Pig. Wolfgang O. Sack. 1982. LC 81-71150. (Illus.). x, 192p. text 21.00 (*0-9601152-2-6*) Veterinary Textbks.

Essentials of Plastic Surgery. William M. Cocke, Jr. et al. 1979. 15.00 (*0-316-14921-7*, Little Brwn Med Div) Lppncott W & W.

Essentials of Postgraduate Psychiatry. Ed. by Peter Hill et al. 2nd ed. 1986. 832p. text 99.95 (*0-8089-1697-1*, 791984, Grune & Strat) Harcrt Hlth Sci Grp.

Essentials of Postgraduate Psychiatry. Ed. by Robin Murray et al. 3rd ed. 1997. (Illus.). 869p. text 130.00 (*0-521-44396-2*); LC 96-44256. 864p. (C). pap. text 59.95 (*0-521-57801-9*) Cambridge U Pr.

Essentials of Prenatal Diagnosis. Ed. by Joe L. Simpson & Sherman Elias. 1993. (Illus.). 431p. text (*0-443-08780-6*) Church.

***Essentials of Psychiatric/Mental Health Nursing.** Mary C. Townsend. 2nd ed. 2001. LC 2001-54778. 692p. per. 39.95 (*0-8036-0920-5*) Davis Co.

Essentials of Psychiatric Nursing. Taylor. 14th ed. 1993. text 52.00 (*0-8151-8920-6*) Mosby Inc.

Essentials of Psychiatric Nursing. Cecelia M. Taylor. 14th ed. 1994. stu. ed. (*0-8151-8918-4*) Mosby Inc.

Essentials of Psychiatric Nursing. Cecelia Monet Taylor. 14th ed. 1993. (Illus.). 560p. (C). (gr. 13). text 46.00 (*0-8016-7814-5*, 07814) Mosby Inc.

Essentials of Psychiatric Nursing: Includes Testbank. Cecelia M. Taylor. 14th ed. 1994. tchr. ed. (*0-8151-8839-0*) Mosby Inc.

Essentials of Psychiatric/Mental Health Nursing. Mary C. Townsend. 1999. LC 98-42616. 827p. (C). pap. text 33.95 (*0-8036-0413-0*) Davis Co.

Essentials of Psychiatry. Ed. by Eric R. Marcus & Janis L. Cutler. 1998. LC 97-42379. xiv, 351p. (C). pap. text 32.00 (*0-7216-6721-X*) Saunders.

Essentials of Psychiatry. Puri. 1995. pap. text 21.00 (*0-7020-1877-5*) Saunders.

Essentials of Psychoanalysis. Herbert S. Strean. 1994. LC 94-2891. (Basic Principles into Practice Ser.: Vol. 2). 176p. pap. text 22.95 (*0-87630-737-3*) Brunner-Routledge.

Essentials of Psychological Testing. Lee J. Cronbach. 5th ed. 1997. 726p. (C). lib. bdg. 123.00 (*0-06-041418-9*) Addson-Wesley Educ.

Essentials of Psychology. Carol Tavris & Carole Wade. 1998. LC 98-8510. 626p. (C). pap. text 59.00 (*0-321-01285-2*) Addson-Wesley Educ.

Essentials of Psychology. Robert A. Baron & Michael J. Kalsher. 2nd ed. 1998. LC 97-47474. 580p. pap. text 57.00 (*0-205-28146-X*) Allyn.

Essentials of Psychology. Dennis L. Coon. 5th ed. Date not set. pap. text, stu. ed. 15.75 (*0-314-83332-3*); 5th ed. 1991. (C). mass mkt. (*0-314-89884-0*); 6th ed. Date not set. pap. text, stu. ed. 17.25 (*0-314-03686-5*); 7th ed. 1996. LC 96-35206. pap. 44.50 net. (*0-314-20479-2*) West Pub.

Essentials of Psychology: Exploration & Application. Dennis L. Coon. Ed. by Clyde Perlee. 6th ed. 1993. LC 93-32251. 600p. (C). mass mkt. 39.25 (*0-314-02768-8*) West Pub.

Essentials of Psychology: Exploration & Application. Dennis L. Coon. 7th ed. 1996. LC 96-35206. 682p. pap. 45.50 (*0-314-20629-9*) West Pub.

Essentials of Psychology: Exploration & Application. Dennis Coon. 8th ed. 1999. LC 99-24490. (Psychology Ser.). (Illus.). 665p. pap. text 54.95 (*0-534-36291-5*) Brooks-Cole.

Essentials of Psychology (Case) with InfoTrac. Dennis L. Coon. 7th ed. 1998. (Psychology Ser.). pap. 46.50 (*0-534-36331-8*) Brooks-Cole.

Essentials of Psychology Exploration & Application. Dennis L. Coon. 6th ed. 1994. (Psychology Ser.). 33.75 (*0-314-04189-3*) Brooks-Cole.

Essentials of Psychology I. Research and Education Association Staff. 1996. LC 94-65261. 96p. pap. text 6.95 (*0-87891-930-9*) Res & Educ.

Essentials of Psychology with InfoTrac. Dennis L. Coon. 7th ed. 1998. (Psychology Ser.). pap. 31.00 (*0-534-36332-6*) Brooks-Cole.

Essentials of Psychotherapy. Rex Haigh et al. 1999. LC 99-20515. (Arnold Publication). (Illus.). 424p. pap. 60.00 (*0-7506-2655-0*) OUP.

Essentials of Pulmonary Medicine. Herbert P. Wiedemann. Date not set. (Illus.). 512p. pap. text 50.00 (*0-07-070104-0*) McGraw-Hill Med Pub.

Essentials of Radiologic Imaging. John H. Juhl. 7th ed. 1998. LC 97-50110. 1,408p. text 159.00 (*0-397-58421-0*) Lppncott W & W.

Essentials of Radiology. Fred A. Mettler, Jr. Ed. by Lisette Bralow. 1995. LC 95-17721. (Illus.). 384p. pap. text 39.95 (*0-7216-6744-9*) Saunders.

Essentials of Radiology Physics. Charles A. Kelsey. 1985. (Illus.). 474p. pap. 47.50 (*0-87527-354-8*) Green.

Essentials of Renal Physiology. Alluru S. Reddi. 1999. LC 98-74967. (Illus.). 350p. pap. text (*0-9669823-0-4*) College Book.

Essentials of Respiratory Care. Robert M. Kacmarek. 3rd ed. 1990. 712p. (C). (gr. 13). text 57.95 (*0-8151-4956-5*, 20119) Mosby Inc.

Essentials of Rheumatology. H. L. Currey. 2nd ed. 1988. (Illus.). 200p. pap. text (*0-443-03913-5*) Church.

Essentials of Safe Dentistry for the Medical Compromised Patient. McCarthy. 1989. 272p. text 46.00 (*0-7216-6233-1*) Saunders.

Essentials of Skeletal Radiology Terry R. Yochum & Lindsay J. Rowe. (Illus.). In Two Volumes. 2nd ed. 1996. LC 95-33501. 1,800p. text 225.00 (*0-683-09330-4*, RC930); Set. 1986. 1136p. 189.00 (*0-683-09329-0*) Lppncott W & W.

Essentials of Spinal Microsurgery. John A. McCulloch & Paul H. Young. 3rd ed. 1998. LC 99-22923. (Illus.). xv, 431p. pap. text 39.95 (*0-7817-1607-1*) Lppncott W & W.

Essentials of Sports Medicine. G. McLatchie et al. 2nd ed. 1993. (Illus.). 272p. (Orig.). pap. text (*0-443-04541-0*) Church.

Essentials of Stochastic Processes. Rick Durrett. Ed. by G. Casella et al. 1999. LC 99-14733. (Texts in Statistics). (Illus.). 304p. 77.95 (*0-387-98836-X*) Spr-Verlag.

Essentials of Surgery. Becker. 2000. (C). pap. text (*0-7216-8186-7*) Saunders.

Essentials of Surgery: Scientific Principles & Practice. Lillemoe et al. Ed. by Lazar J. Greenfield. 1997. LC 97-2444. (Illus.). 864p. spiral bd. 52.95 (*0-397-51532-4*) Lppncott W & W.

Essentials of Surgical Critical Care: Clinical Cases & Practical Solutions (Case Book) Ed. by Jerome H. Abrams & Frank B. Cerra. 1992. LC 92-48762. (Illus.). 184p. pap. 25.00 (*0-942219-32-5*) Quality Med Pub.

Essentials of the Orthopaedic Examination. Hammer. 1995. (Illus.). 128p. pap. text (*0-340-61382-3*) E A GBR. *Dist:* OUP.

Essentials of Total Fitness: Exercise, Nutrition, & Wellness - Examination Copy. Scott K. Powers & Stephen L. Dodd. 1996. 272p. (C). pap. (*0-205-26447-6*, T6447-1) Allyn.

Essentials of Toxicology. Ted A. Loomis & A. Wallace Hayes. 4th ed. 1996. LC 78-9005. (Illus.). 282p. text 35.00 (*0-12-455625-6*) Acad Pr.

Essentials of Traditional Chinese Pediatrics. Compiled by Cao Jiming et al. 1990. 260p. pap. 9.95 (*0-8351-2368-5*) China Bks.

***Essentials of Traumatic Injuries to the Teeth: A Step-by-Step Treatment Guide.** Jens O. Andreasen & Frances M. Andreasen. 2nd ed. 2000. (Illus.). 200p. 89.00 (*0-323-01353-8*) Mosby Inc.

Essentials of Tropical Infections: Principles, Pathogens & Practice for the Clinician. Richard L. Guerrant et al. 2000. LC 00-65824. (Illus.). xxiv, 664p. (C). text 79.00 (*0-443-07909-9*) Saunders.

Essentials of Ultrasonography. William Zwiebel. 1997. LC 96-18778. text 89.00 (*0-7216-6947-6*) Saunders.

Essentials of Ultrasonography: A Practical Guide. D. Pickuth. 1995. (Illus.). 150p. 87.95 (*3-540-58973-2*) Spr-Verlag.

Essentials of Ultrasound. Michael R. Williamson. Ed. by Sandra Valkoff. 1995. (Illus.). 320p. text 49.95 (*0-7216-6642-6*) Saunders.

Essentials of Ultrasound Physics. James A. Zagzebski. 1996. LC 96-199893. (Illus.). 240p. (C). (gr. 13). pap. text 43.00 (*0-8151-9852-3*, 25468) Mosby Inc.

Essentials of Understanding Psychology. Robert S. Feldman. 2nd abr. ed. 1994. LC 93-37332. (C). pap. text 27.25 net. (*0-07-021236-8*) McGraw.

***Essentials of Understanding Psychology.** 4th ed. 1999. (C). stu. ed. 51.25 (*0-07-240254-7*) McGrw-H Hghr Educ.

Essentials of Veterinary Anesthesia & Analgesia. Ed. by John C. Thurmon. 1999. LC 99-14445. 320p. pap. text 42.95 (*0-683-30107-1*) Lppncott W & W.

Essentials of Veterinary Bacteriology & Mycology. G. R. Carter. 4th ed. 1990. LC 90-42674. (Illus.). 280p. 46.00 (*0-8121-1369-1*) Lppncott W & W.

Essentials of Veterinary Hematology. Nemi C. Jain. 1993. (Illus.). 417p. text 59.95 (*0-8121-1437-X*) Lppncott W & W.

Essentials of Veterinary Microbiology. G. R. Carter et al. 5th ed. 1995. LC 94-29049. (Illus.). 394p. 49.95 (*0-683-01473-0*) Lppncott W & W.

Essentials of Veterinary Ophthalmology. Kirk N. Gelatt. 2000. LC 00-25601. (Illus.). xii, 595p. pap. text 75.00 (*0-683-30077-6*) Lppncott W & W.

Essentials of Writing Biomedical Research. Mimi Zeiger. 2nd ed. 1999. LC 99-20851. (Illus.). 440p. pap. 45.00 (*0-07-134544-2*) McGraw-Hill Prof.

Essentials Researcher's Handbook. Tarling. 1997. pap. text (*0-7020-2115-6*) Bailliere Tindall.

Essiac: A Native Herbal Cancer Remedy. Cynthia B. Olsen et al. 2nd ed. 1998. LC 98-35978. (Illus.). pap. 12.50 (*1-890941-00-X*) Kali Pr.

Essiac Essentials. Sheila Snow & Mali Klein. 2000. pap. 12.00 (*1-57566-563-8*, Knsington) Kensgtn Pub Corp.

Essiac Handbook. James Percival. 1994. (Illus.). 24p. pap. 5.00 (*0-9651484-9-1*) Rideout Pub.

Essiac Report: Canada's Remarkable Unknown Cancer Remedy. Richard Thomas. (Illus.). 256p. (Orig.). 29.95 (*0-9639818-3-8*); text 29.95 (*0-9639818-2-X*); pap. text 19.95 (*0-9639818-0-3*); lib. bdg. 29.95 (*0-9639818-1-1*) Alternat Treatment.

Establishing a Forensic Psychiatric Practice: A Practical Guide. Steven H. Berger. 1997. LC 97-10232. 160p. 29.00 (*0-393-70252-9*) Norton.

Establishing & Implementing Universal Newborn Hearing Screening Programs. Brandt Culpepper. 2000. 250p. pap. 49.95 (*1-56593-895-X*, 1750) Thomson Learn.

Establishing Dysphagia Programs: A Speech-Language Pathologist's Guide. Rehab Choice Incorporated Staff. 1993. (Illus.). 96p. (Orig.). (C). pap. text 43.95 (*0-937857-38-6*, 1521) Speech Bin.

Establishing Health Priorities in the Developing World. Julia A. Walsh. 1988. 151p. (C). pap. text 27.00 (*0-944903-02-9*) Adams Pub Group.

Establishing Preventive Services. Ed. by Roger P. Weissberg et al. 1997. LC 97-4687. (Issues in Children's & Families' Lives Ser.: Vol. 9). pap. 37.95 (*0-7619-1090-5*, 81594) Sage.

Estate Planning for Those Receiving or about to Receive Medicaid Benefits. Thomas E. Webb, Jr. 1990. (Estate Planning for the Elderly Ser.). (C). 75.00 (*0-943843-02-2*) Bristol Hunter.

Esthetic Approach to Metal Ceramic Restorations for the Mandibular Anterior Region. Klaus Muterthies. 1990. (Illus.). 94p. text 58.00 (*1-85097-016-5*) Quint Pub Co.

E F G

Esthetic Composite Bonding: Techniques & Materials. Ronald E. Jordan. 2nd ed. 1992. LC 92-49805. (Illus.). 371p. (C). (gr. 13). text 155.00 (*0-8016-6980-4*, 06980) Mosby Inc.

Esthetic Denistry & Ceramic Restoration. Bernard Touati. 1998. (Illus.). 424p. 199.95 (*1-85317-159-X*) Thieme Med Pubs.

Esthetic Dentistry: A Clinical Approach to Techniques & Materials. B. Dale & K. W. Aschheim. 1992. (Illus.). 510p. text 135.00 (*0-8121-1467-1*) Lppncott W & W.

Esthetic Dentistry: A Clinical Approach to Techniques & Materials. Kenneth W. Aschheim & Barry G. Dale. 2nd ed. 2000. LC 00-48046. (Illus.). xii, 606p. text 180.00 (*0-323-00162-9*) Mosby Inc.

Esthetic in Orthodontics & Orthognathic Surgery: Contemporary Planning & Treatment. David M. Sarver. 1997. LC 97-21247. (Illus.). 304p. (C). (gr. 13). text 132.00 (*0-8151-7997-9*, 26665) Mosby Inc.

Esthetic Maxillofacial Surgery. Bruce N. Epker. 1993. (Illus.). 700p. text 225.00 (*0-8121-1759-X*) Lppncott W & W.

Esthetic Restorations: Improved Dentist-Laboratory Communication. Paul J. Muia. 1993. LC 92-48524. (Illus.). 280p. text 110.00 (*0-86715-226-5*) Quint Pub Co.

Esthetics & Prosthetics: An Interdisciplinary Consideration of the State of the Art. Ed. by Jens Fischer. 1999. LC 98-31213. (Illus.). x, 207p. text 89.00 (*0-86715-324-5*) Quint Pub Co.

Esthetics & the Treatment of Facial Form. Ed. by James A. McNamara. 1993. (Craniofacial Growth Ser.: Vol. 28). (Illus.). 216p. 55.00 (*0-929921-24-0*) UM CHGD.

Esthetics in Comprehensive Denistry. McGuire. 1997. text (*0-7216-6011-8*) Saunders.

Esthetics in Dentistry Vol. I: Principles, Communications, Treatment Methods. Ronald E. Goldstein. 2nd ed. 1998. LC 98-215744. 470p. incl. cd-rom (*1-55009-047-X*) DEKR.

Esthetics of Anterior Fixed Prosthodontics. Gerard Chiche & Alain Pinault. 1994. LC 93-25776. (Illus.). 204p. text 98.00 (*0-86715-258-3*) Quint Pub Co.

Esthetique du Mouvement see Aesthetics of Movement

Estimated Useful Lives of Depreciable Hospital Assets. American Hospital Association Staff. 1983. LC 83-8767. (*0-87258-409-7*) Am Hospital.

Estimated Useful Lives of Depreciable Hospital Assets: 1993 Edition. rev. ed. 1993. 36p. pap. 25.00 (*1-55648-101-2*, 061170) AHPI.

Estimating Eye Care Provider Supply & Workforce Requirements. Paul P. Lee et al. 1995. LC 95-18056. 164p. pap. 9.00 (*0-8330-1652-0*, MR-516-AAO) Rand Corp.

Estimating Human Exposure to Air Pollutants: GEMS: Global Environmental Monitoring System. WHO Staff. 1982. (WHO Offset Publications: No. 69). 59p. 8.00 (*92-4-170069-6*) World Health.

Estimation de la Mortalite de Juene Enfant (0-5 and) Pour Guider les Actions de Sante dans les Pays en Developpement. P. Cantrelle et al. 1987. (Colloque de L'INSERM Ser.: No. 145). 570p. lib. bdg. 42.00 (*2-85598-306-1*) S M P F Inc.

Estimation of Blood Velocities Using Ultrasound: A Signal Processing Approach. Jorgen A. Jensen. 1996. (Illus.). 336p. (C). text 90.00 (*0-521-46484-6*) Cambridge U Pr.

Estimation of the Time since Death in the Early Postmortem Period. Claus Henssge et al. 1995. 272p. (*0-340-57319-8*) E A GBR. *Dist:* OUP.

Estrogen. Lila Nachtigall & Joan R. Heilman. 2nd ed. 1995. LC 95-6222. 208p. pap. 12.00 (*0-06-092602-3*, Perennial) HarperTrade.

Estrogen: Answers to All Your Questions about Hormone Replacement Therapy & Natural Alternatives. Mark Stolar. 1997. LC 97-93168. pap. 5.99 (*0-380-79076-9*, Avon Bks) Morrow Avon.

Estrogen: How & Why It Can Save Your Life. Adam Romoff & Ina Yalof. 1999. LC 98-31174. 144p. 16.00 (*1-58238-012-0*, Golden Adult) St Martin.

Estrogen: Is It Right for You?: A Thorough, Factual Guide to Help You Decide. Paula Dranov. 1993. (Illus.). 160p. pap. 11.75 (*0-671-78130-8*, Fireside) S&S Trade Pap.

Estrogen: The Natural Way. Nina Shandler. 1998. LC 96-39670. (Illus.). 336p. pap. 14.95 (*0-375-75141-6*) Villard Books.

Estrogen: Yes or No? Morris Notelovitz. 1993. 173p. mass mkt. 4.50 (*0-312-95105-1*) St Martin.

Estrogen & Breast Cancer. W. R. Miller. 1996. (Medical Intelligence Unit Ser.). 207p. 99.00 (*1-57059-047-8*) Landes Bioscience.

Estrogen & Breast Cancer. W. R. Miller. 1996. (Medical Intelligence Unit Ser.). 207p. pap. 89.95 (*0-412-10371-0*, VNR) Wiley.

Estrogen & Breast Cancer: A Warning to Women. Carol A. Rinzler. 2nd rev. ed. 1996. LC 96-33977. (Illus.). 240p. pap. 14.95 (*0-89793-198-X*) Hunter Hse.

Estrogen Answer Book: 150 Most-Asked Questions about Hormone Replacement Therapy. Ruth S. Jacobowitz. 1999. LC 98-25178. 272p. pap. 12.00 (*0-316-45808-2*, Back Bay) Little.

Estrogen-Antiestrogen Action & Breast Cancer Therapy. Ed. by V. Craig Jordan. 1986. LC 92-25829. (Illus.). 512p. text 50.00 (*0-299-10480-X*) U of Wis Pr.

Estrogen Decision: A Self-Help Program. Susan M. Lark. 1994. (Women's Health Ser.). 316p. pap. 14.95 (*0-917010-56-6*) Celestial Arts.

Estrogen Deficiency & Deprivation: Index of New Information with Authors & Subjects. Virginia L. Jensen. 1992. 180p. 47.50 (*1-55914-706-7*); pap. 44.50 (*1-55914-707-5*) ABBE Pubs Assn.

Estrogen-Dependent Tumors: Conference on the Treatment of Hormone-Dependent Tumors, Tokyo, January 1998. Ed. by Hiroyuki Mori. 1998. (Oncology Ser.: Vol. 55, Suppl. 1). (Illus.). iv, 60p. pap. 24.50 (*3-8055-6768-5*) S Karger.

Estrogen Receptor As Target for Rational Drug Design. Erwin Von Angerer. 1995. LC 95-21355. (Molecular Biology Intelligence Unit Ser.). 159p. 99.00 (*1-57059-288-8*) Landes Bioscience.

Estrogen Replacement Education Course. Competence Assurance Systems Staff. 1984. (Illus.). pap. text 65.00 (*0-89147-108-1*) CAS.

Estrogens: Directory of Authors of New Medical & Scientific Reviews with Subject Index. Science and Life Consultants Association Staff. 1995. 160p. 57.50 (*0-7883-0582-4*); pap. 47.50 (*0-7883-0583-2*) ABBE Pubs Assn.

Estrogens & Anti-Estrogens: Basic & Clinical Aspects. Ed. by David W. Dempster et al. 1997. (Illus.). 320p. text 120.00 (*0-397-51719-X*) Lppncott W & W.

Estrogens & Brain Function: Neural Analysis of a Hormone-Controlled Mammalian Reproductive Behavior. D. W. Pfaff. 1980. (Illus.). 281p. 97.00 (*0-387-90487-5*) Spr-Verlag.

Estrogens & Progestogens in Clinical Practice. Ed. by I. S. Fraser et al. 1998. (Illus.). 800p. text (*0-443-04706-5*) Church.

Estrogens, Estrogen Receptor & Breast Cancer. Ed. by Fritz F. Parl. 2000. LC 99-64854. (Biomedical & Health Research Ser.: Vol. 36). (Illus.). viii, 263p. 115.00 (*0-9673355-4-X*) IOS Press.

Estrogens in the Post-Menopause: Proceedings of the Workers Conference, Geneva October 1974. Estrogens in the Post-Menopause Workshop Staff. Ed. by Pieter A. Van Keep & C. Lauritzen. 1975. (Frontiers of Hormone Research Ser.: Vol. 3). x, 234p. 66.25 (*3-8055-2187-1*) S Karger.

Estrogens, Progestins & Their Antagonists. Edward J. Pavlik. Date not set. LC 96-3059. (*3-7643-3947-0*); 1996. LC 96-3059. 256p. 95.00 (*0-8176-3947-0*); 1996. LC 96-30592. 600p. 170.00 (*0-8176-3948-9*) Birkhauser.

Estrogens, Progestins & Their Antagonists. Ed. by Edward J. Pavlik. 1996. LC 96-3059. 344p. 95.00 (*0-8176-3854-7*) Birkhauser.

Esvitaf Vitamin Status in Three Groups of French Adults: Control, Obese Subjects, Alcohol Drinkers. A. Lemoine et al. 1986. (Journal: Vol. 30, Suppl. 1, 1986). (ENG & FRE., Illus.). 96p. pap. 25.25 (*3-8055-4244-5*) S Karger.

Eternal Wisdom & Health with Light on the Scriptures. William Estep. 1998. 786p. reprint ed. pap. 45.00 (*0-7661-0415-X*) Kessinger Pub.

Eternally Wounded Woman: Women, Exercise, & Doctors in the Late Nineteenth Century. Patricia A. Vertinsky. 1994. LC 93-37145. 288p. (C). pap. text 16.95 (*0-252-06372-4*) U of Ill Pr.

Eternally Young: A Guide to Aging Well. Shawn A. McGivney & Joseph H. McGivney. 1989. LC 89-85373. (Illus.). (Orig.). pap. text 9.95 (*0-9623941-0-6*) Ageless Pub.

Eterohepatic Circulation of Bile Acids & Sterol Metabolism. Ed. by G. Paumgartner et al. 1985. (Falk Symposium Ser.: No. 42). text 225.00 (*0-85200-905-4*) Kluwer Academic.

Ethel Browning's Toxicity & Metabolism of Industrial Solvents: Hydrocarbons, Vol. 1. Ed. by R. Snyder. 2nd ed. 1987. 416p. 292.00 (*0-444-90434-4*); 269.00 (*0-444-90391-7*) Elsevier.

Ethical & Legal Dilemmas in Occupational Therapy. Diana M. Bailey. Ed. by Sharan L. Schwartzberg. 1994. LC 94-33914. 184p. 22.95 (*0-8036-0567-6*) Davis Co.

Ethical & Legal Issues for Imaging Professionals. Simon Towsley-Cook. 1998. LC 98-23571. (Illus.). 336p. (C). pap. text 26.00 (*0-8151-2966-1*, 31847) Mosby Inc.

Ethical & Legal Issues in Home Health & Long-Term Care: Challenges & Solutions. Dennis A. Robbins & Mangum. 1996. LC 96-5377. 254p. 69.00 (*0-8342-0783-4*) Aspen Pub.

Ethical & Moral Dimensions of Care. Ed. by Madeleine M. Leininger. 1986. LC 90-38404. (Human Care & Health Ser.). 116p. (C). pap. text 22.95 (*0-8143-2332-4*) Wayne St U Pr.

Ethical & Religious Directions for Catholic Health Care Services. U. S. Catholic Conference Staff. 1995. 16p. pap. 1.95 (*1-57455-034-9*) US States Conference.

Ethical Approaches in Epidemiologic Research, Vol. VII. Ed. by Laurence R. Tancredi. 1986. (Psychosocial Epidemiology Ser.). 208p. (C). pap. text 18.00 (*0-8135-1157-7*) Rutgers U Pr.

Ethical Aspects of Health Care for the Elderly: An Annotated Bibliography, 17. Marshall B. Kapp. 1992. LC 92-17776. (Bibliographies & Indexes in Gerontology Ser.: No. 17). 200p. lib. bdg. 57.75 (*0-313-27490-8*, KEG, Greenwood Pr) Greenwood.

Ethical Challenges in Managed Care: A Casebook. Ed. by Karen G. Gervais et al. 1999. LC 98-44645. 384p. text 60.00 (*0-87840-718-9*); 372p. pap. text 29.95 (*0-87840-719-7*) Georgetown U Pr.

Ethical Choices: Case Studies for Medical Practice. Lois Snyder. 1996. LC 96-5405. 121p. 22.00 (*0-943126-43-6*) Amer Coll Phys.

Ethical Confrontation in Counseling. John C. Hoffman. LC 78-11799. 1996. lib. bdg. 13.00 (*0-226-34785-0*); 1993. pap. text 4.95 (*0-226-34786-9*) U Ch Pr.

Ethical Considerations in the Business Aspects of Health Care. Woodstock Theological Center Seminar in Business E. 1995. LC 95-5133. 56p. pap. 5.95 (*0-87840-587-9*) Georgetown U Pr.

Ethical Considerations of Healthcare Delivery: HSM 510 Course Study Guide. Jacquelyn Hall. rev. ed. 1993. 380p. (C). (*0-933195-23-0*) CA College Health Sci.

Ethical Decision-Making: A Guide for Therapists. Julius Sim. 1997. LC 97-25705. 216p. pap. text 40.00 (*0-7506-2173-7*) Buttrwrth-Heinemann.

Ethical Decision Making for Perinatal Nurses. Karen Duderstadt & Kathleen Lagana. Ed. by Lynn G. Wellman. 1995. (*0-86525-065-0*) March of Dimes.

Ethical Decision Making in Nursing. Haddad. 1998. (C). pap. text 29.95 (*0-7216-7422-4*) Saunders.

Ethical Decision Making in Nursing, Vol. 2. Gladys L. Husted & James H. Husted. 2nd ed. 1994. (Illus.). 352p. (C). (gr. 13). pap. text 32.00 (*0-8016-7774-2*, 07774) Mosby Inc.

Ethical Decision Making in Therapy: Feminist Perspectives. Elizabeth S. Rave & Carolyn C. Larsen. 1995. LC 95-18762. 284p. 35.00 (*0-89862-089-9*, 2089) Guilford Pubns.

Ethical Dilemmas: A Values Guide for Medical Students. George A. Kanoti. 2000. LC 00-8059. (Surviving Medical School Ser.). (Illus.). xii, 107p. pap. 36.95 (*0-7619-1799-3*, 83414) Sage.

Ethical Dilemmas: Crises in Faith & Modern Medicine. Ed. by John T. Chirban. 1994. LC 93-34746. 172p. (Orig.). (C). 58.00 (*0-8191-9337-2*) U Pr of Amer.

Ethical Dilemmas: Crises in Faith & Modern Medicine. Ed. by John T. Chirban. 2002. LC 93-34746. 172p. pap. 35.00 (*0-8191-9338-0*) U Pr of Amer.

Ethical Dilemmas & Nursing Practice. Anne J. Davis et al. 4th ed. 1996. LC 96-41638. 252p. (C). pap. 47.00 (*0-8385-2283-1*, A-2283-8) P-H.

Ethical Dilemmas in Assisted Reproduction. Ed. by F. Shenfield & Claude Sureau. 1997. LC 97-19650. (Studies in Profertility: Vol. 7). (Illus.). 104p. lib. bdg. 71.95 (*1-85070-916-5*, S3625, Parthenon Pbng) CRC Pr.

Ethical Dilemmas in Contemporary Nursing Practice. Ed. by Gladys B. White. 1992. 154p. (Orig.). (C). pap. text 37.50 (*1-55810-074-1*, NP-81) Am Nurses Pub.

Ethical Dilemmas in Modern Medicine: A Physician's Viewpoint. Erich H. Loewy. 1986. LC 86-23460. (Studies in Health & Human Services: Vol. 8). 352p. lib. bdg. 99.95 (*0-88946-133-3*) E Mellen.

Ethical Dimensions in the Health Professions. Ruth B. Purtilo. 2nd ed. 1993. LC 92-49438. (Illus.). 288p. pap. text 30.00 (*0-7216-3550-4*) Saunders.

Ethical Dimensions in the Health Professions. Ruth Purtilo. Ed. by Andrew Allen. 3rd ed. 1998. LC 98-44276. (Illus.). 300p. (C). pap. text 30.00 (*0-7216-7799-1*) Saunders.

Ethical Dimensions of Geriatric Care. Stuart F. Spicker et al. 1987. 332p. (C). text 151.50 (*1-55608-027-1*) Kluwer Academic.

Ethical Dimensions of Pharmaceutical Care. Ed. by Amy M. Haddad & Robert A. Buerki. LC 96-17373. (Journal of Pharmacy Teaching Ser.: Vol. 5, Nos. 1/2). 183p. (C). 1997. pap. 14.95 (*0-7890-0204-3*); 1996. 39.95 (*1-56024-835-1*) Haworth Pr (Pharmctl Prods).

Ethical Emotivism. S. A. Satris. 1986. 214p. (C). text 118.00 (*90-247-3413-4*) Kluwer Academic.

Ethical Guidelines in the Conduct, Dissemination & Implementation of Nursing Research. Mary Silva. 1995. 60p. pap. text 21.95 (*1-55810-109-8*, D-95) Am Nurses Pub.

Ethical Implications of Behaviour Modification—with Special Reference to Mental Handicap. John Hattersley et al. 1984. 51p. 50.00 (*0-906054-07-9*) St Mut.

Ethical Implications of Primary Prevention. Ed. by Robert Hess et al. 1991. (Prevention in Human Services Ser.). 132p. text 39.95 (*1-56024-019-9*) Haworth Pr.

Ethical Issues & Decision in Feeding. Julie O. Maillet. 1989. 30p. stu. ed. 10.25 (*0-88091-051-8*, 1219) Am Dietetic Assn.

Ethical Issues in Advanced Nursing. Martha A. Bartter. 2001. 160p. pap. 29.95 (*0-7506-4955-0*) Buttrwrth-Heinemann.

Ethical Issues in Behavioral Research. Allan J. Kimmel. 1996. LC 95-37163. 320p. (C). 60.95 (*1-55786-394-6*); pap. 28.95 (*1-55786-395-4*) Blackwell Pubs.

Ethical Issues in Biomedical Publication. Anne Hudson Jones & Faith McLellan. 2000. LC 99-44900. 384p. pap. text 23.95 (*0-8018-6315-5*) Johns Hopkins.

Ethical Issues in Cancer Patient Care. Ed. by Peter Angelos. 2000. LC 99-49245. (Cancer Treatment & Research Ser.). (Illus.). x, 152p. (*0-7923-7726-5*) Kluwer Academic.

Ethical Issues in Developmental Disabilities. Ed. by Linda J. Hayes et al. 1994. (Illus.). 208p. (C). text 41.95 (*1-878978-16-0*) Context Pr.

Ethical Issues in Drug Testing, Approval & Pricing: The Clot-Dissolving Drugs. Baruch A. Brody. 1995. LC 94-4479. (Illus.). 280p. text 39.50 (*0-19-508831-X*) OUP.

Ethical Issues in Family Therapy. Ed. by Sue Walrond-Skinner & David H. Watson. 1987. LC 87-4562. 224p. (C). lib. bdg. 49.95 (*0-7102-1196-1*, Routledge Thoemms) Routledge.

Ethical Issues in HIV Vaccine Trials in Developing Nations. Thomas A. Kerns. 1997. LC 96-25611. 249p. text 45.00 (*0-312-16397-5*) St Martin.

Ethical Issues in Managed Health Care Organizations. Seminar in Business Ethics Staff. 1999. LC 98-51558. ix, 42p. (*0-87840-728-6*) Georgetown U Pr.

***Ethical Issues in Maternal-Fetal Medicine.** Ed. by Donna Dickenson. 2001. LC 2001-25633. 352p. text 80.00 (*0-521-66266-4*); pap. text 28.95 (*0-521-66474-8*) Cambridge U Pr.

Ethical Issues in Medicine Sourcebook: Basic Information about Controversial Treatment Issues. Ed. by Helene Henderson. 2002. (Health Reference Ser.). (Illus.). 600p. lib. bdg. 78.00 (*0-7808-0237-3*) Omnigraphics Inc.

Ethical Issues in Mental Health. Ed. by Philip J. Barker & Steve Baldwin. 1991. 200p. (C). pap. text 29.95 (*0-412-32950-6*, A5586) Chapman & Hall.

Ethical Issues in Mental Health Research with Children & Adolescents. Ed. by Kimberly Hoagwood et al. 1996. LC 97-100451. 250p. pap. text 32.50 (*0-8058-1953-3*); text 59.95 (*0-8058-1952-5*) L Erlbaum Assocs.

Ethical Issues in Modern Medicine. John Arras & Bonnie Steinbock. 5th ed. 1998. LC 98-16724. 784p. pap. text 51.95 (*0-7674-0016-X*) Mayfield Pub.

Ethical Issues in Neurology. James L. Bernat. 1994. LC 94-19096. 364p. text 63.00 (*0-7506-9501-3*); 2nd ed. 2001. 520p. 74.99 (*0-7506-7312-5*) Buttrwrth-Heinemann.

Ethical Issues in Nursing. Ed. by Geoffrey Hunt. 1994. LC 93-34921. (Professional Ethics Ser.). 240p. (C). pap. 26.95 (*0-415-08145-9*, B3908) Routledge.

***Ethical Issues in Palliative Care: Reflections & Considerations.** Ed. by Patricia Webb. 2000. 144p. pap. (*1-898507-27-9*) Books For Midwives Pr GBR. *Dist:* Balogh.

Ethical Issues in Pharmacy. Bruce D. Weinstein. 1996. LC 95-83225. 344p. (Orig.). (C). pap. 29.95 (*0-915486-25-3*) Applied Therapeutics.

Ethical Issues in Preventive Medicine. Ed. by Spyros Doxiadis. 1985. 120p. lib. bdg. (*90-247-3232-8*) M Nijhoff NLD. *Dist:* Kluwer Academic.

Ethical Issues in Research. Ed. by Darwin Cheney. 1993. 258p. 39.00 (*1-55572-016-1*) Univ Pub Group.

Ethical Issues in the Use of Animals in Research: A Special Issue of Ethics & Behavior, Vol. 7, No. 2. Ed. by Kenneth D. Pimple et al. 1997. 100p. pap. 20.00 (*0-8058-9860-3*) L Erlbaum Assocs.

Ethical Issues of HIV Infection in the Health Care & Social Settings (Recommendation), No. R(89)14. Council of Europe Staff. 1990. (*92-871-1780-2*) Council of Europe FRA. *Dist:* Manhattan Pub Co.

Ethical Issues of Molecular Genetics in Psychiatry. Ed. by R. J. Sam et al. 1991. (Illus.). 176p. 79.00 (*0-387-53675-2*) Spr-Verlag.

***Ethical Patient Care: A Casebook for Geriatric Health Care Teams.** Ed. by Mathy Doval Mezey. 2001. LC 2001-335. (*0-8018-6769-X*); 392p. pap. text 24.95 (*0-8018-6770-3*) Johns Hopkins.

Ethical Policy in Mental Health Care: The Goals of Psychiatric Intervention. Lawrence P. Tancredi & Andrew E. Slaby. 1977. LC 77-1996. 20.00 (*0-88202-102-8*) Watson Pub Intl.

Ethical Practice in Clinical Medicine. William J. Ellos. 1991. 224p. (C). (gr. 13). pap. 25.99 (*0-415-05070-7*, A5082) Routledge.

Ethical Practice in Psychiatry & the Law. Richard Rosner & R. Weinstock. 1990. LC 88-657025. (Critical Issues in American Psychiatry & the Law Ser.: Vol. 7). (Illus.). 366p. (C). 95.00 (*0-306-43476-8*, Plenum Trade) Perseus Pubng.

Ethical Practice of Psychology in Organizations. Ed. by Rodney L. Lowman. 1998. LC 97-47450. 299p. pap. 24.95 (*1-55798-486-7*, 431-2070) Am Psychol.

Ethical Practices in Pharmacy: A Guidebook for Pharmacy Technicians. Robert A. Buerki & Louis D. Vottero. 1997. 55p. pap. text 9.50 (*0-931292-28-X*) Am Inst Hist Pharm.

Ethical Principle in Catholic Health Care. Edward James Furton & Veronica McLoud Dort. 1999. LC 99-51420. (Short Essays in Catholic Medical Ethics Ser.). (*0-935372-42-3*) NCBC.

Ethical Principles in the Conduct of Research with Human Participants. Committee for the Protection of Human Participants. 1982. 80p. pap. 12.95 (*0-912704-82-9*) Am Psychol.

Ethical Problem in Clinical Practice. Holm. 1998. (Illus.). 224p. text (*0-7190-5050-2*) Manchester Univ Pr GBR. *Dist:* St Martin.

Ethical Problem in Clinical Practice: The Ethical Reasoning. Soren Holm. 1998. LC 97-13570. (*0-7190-5049-9*) Manchester Univ Pr GBR. *Dist:* St Martin.

Ethical Problems in Dialysis & Transplantation. Carl M. Kjellstrand. 1992. (Developments in Nephrology Ser.). 264p. (C). lib. bdg. (*0-7923-1625-8*) Kluwer Academic NLD. *Dist:* Kluwer Academic.

E
F
G

Ethical Problems in Pediatrics. 1990. (Journal: Vol. 17, No. 2, 1990). 72p. pap. 41.00 (*3-8055-5175-4*) S Karger.

Ethical Questions in Brain & Behavior. Ed. by D. W. Pfaff. 1983. (Illus.). 158p. 82.95 (*0-387-90870-6*) Spr-Verlag.

Ethical Questions in Dentistry. James Rule & Robert Veacht. 1993. LC 92-48228. 282p. pap. text 28.00 (*0-86715-203-6*) Quint Pub Co.

Ethical Responsibility in Pharmacy Practice. Robert A. Buerki & Louis D. Vottero. 1994. 194p. (Orig.). (C). pap. text 15.00 (*0-931292-25-5*) Am Inst Hist Pharm.

Ethical Use of Touch in Psychotherapy. Mic Hunter & Jim Struve. 1997. LC 97-4799. 232p. 74.95 (*0-7619-0360-7*, 2609); pap. 32.95 (*0-7619-0361-5*, 2610) Sage.

Ethical Way: Challenges & Solutions for Managed Behavioral Healthcare. H. Steven Moffic. 1997. LC 96-53565. (Jossey-Bass Managed Behavioral Healthcare Library). 234p. 44.00 (*0-7879-0841-X*) Jossey-Bass.

Ethico-Embryonic Theories of Abortion & Development in Africa. Ngolela W. Kabongo. 1982. (Illus.). 200p. (Orig.). pap. 7.95 (*0-943324-01-7*) Omenana.

Ethics. Perrin. 2000. (Nursing Concepts Ser.). 22.95 (*1-889325-52-X*) Fence Crk Pubng.

Ethics: The Heart of Health Care. David Seedhouse. 2nd ed. 1998. LC 97-46064. 250p. pap. 36.95 (*0-471-97592-3*) Wiley.

Ethics & Basic Law for Medical Imaging Professionals. Bettye G. Wilson. 1997. LC 96-53384. (Illus.). 184p. (C). pap. text 21.95 (*0-8036-0152-2*) Davis Co.

Ethics & Community in the Health Care Profession. Michael Parker. 1999. LC 98-35439. (Professional Ethics Ser.). 80.00 (*0-415-15027-2*); 208p. pap. 26.95 (*0-415-15028-0*) Routledge.

Ethics & Critical Care Medicine. Ed. by John C. Moskop & Loretta M. Kopelman. 1985. (Philosophy & Medicine Ser.: No. 19). 256p. text 107.00 (*90-277-1820-2*) Kluwer Academic.

***Ethics & Economics of Assisted Reproduction: The Cost of Longing.** Maura A. Ryan. 2001. LC 2001-23258. (Moral Traditions & Moral Arguments Ser.). 192p. 44.95 (*0-87840-871-1*) Georgetown U Pr.

Ethics & Economics of Health Care. George M. Hall. 1992. (Illus.). 144p. (Orig.). pap. text 19.50 (*0-87527-495-1*) Green.

Ethics & Epidemiology. Ed. by Steven S. Coughlin & Thomas L. Beauchamp. 1996. 320p. (C). text 52.50 (*0-19-510242-8*) OUP.

Ethics & Epidemiology: International Guidelines. Ed. by Z. Bankowski et al. 1991. (Proceedings of the XXVth CIOMS Conference Ser.). (ENG & FRE.). viii, 191p. pap. text 25.00 (*92-9036-048-8*, 1830025) World Health.

Ethics & Human Genetics. D. C. Wertz & J. C. Flechter. 1989. (Illus.). 536p. 152.00 (*0-387-19224-7*) Spr-Verlag.

Ethics & Human Genetics: (Proceedings of the 2nd Symposium on Bioethics, Strasbourg, 30 November-2 December, 1993) 1994. (Bioethics Ser.). (*92-871-2541-4*) Council of Europe FRA. *Dist:* Manhattan Pub Co.

Ethics & Issues in Contemporary Nursing. Burkhardt-Nathaniel et al. 1998. LC 97-38418. 416p. (C). pap. text 49.95 (*0-8273-7702-9*) Delmar.

Ethics & Jurisprudence. Ann Ehrlich. 1983. 7.95 (*0-940012-07-3*) Colwell Syst.

Ethics & Law in Health Care & Research, Vol. 5, Vol. 5. Ed. by Peter Byrne. 1990. LC 90-13504. 204p. 189.95 (*0-471-92806-2*) Wiley.

Ethics & Law in Mental Health Administration. Walter E. Barton & Gail M. Barton. 1984. LC 84-4610. xxi, 378p. 55.00 (*0-8236-1765-3*) Intl Univs Pr.

Ethics & Law in the Study of AIDS. Ed. by H. Fuenzalida-Puelma et al. 1992. (PAHO Scientific Publications: No. 530). (ENG & SPA.). x, 273p. pap. text 52.00 (*92-75-11530-3*, 1610530) World Health.

***Ethics & Medical Decision-Making.** Ed. by Michael D. A. Freeman. 2001. LC 00-69961. (International Library of Medicine, Ethics, & Law). 550p. (*0-7546-2112-X*) Ashgate Pub GBR. *Dist:* Ashgate Pub Co.

Ethics & Mental Retardation. Loretta M. Kopelman & John C. Moskop. 1984. 274p. text 152.50 (*90-277-1630-7*) Kluwer Academic.

Ethics & Midwifery: Issues in Contemporary Practice. Lucy Frith. 1996. LC 96-25888. 288p. pap. text 47.50 (*0-7506-3056-6*) Buttrwrth-Heinemann.

Ethics & Perinatology: Issues & Perspectives. Ed. by Amnon Goldworth et al. 1995. (Illus.). 506p. text 58.50 (*0-19-262379-6*) OUP.

Ethics & Psychiatry: Toward Professional Definition. Allen R. Dyer. 1988. LC 87-1337. 176p. text 12.95 (*0-88048-225-7*, 8225) Am Psychiatric.

Ethics & Regulation of Clinical Research. Robert J. Levine. 2nd ed. 1988. LC 87-28955. pap. 26.00 (*0-300-04288-4*) Yale U Pr.

Ethics & Research on Human Subjects: International Guidelines. Ed. by Z. Bankowski & R. J. Levine. 1993. (Proceedings of the XXVth CIOMS Conference Ser.). ix, 291p. pap. text 25.00 (*92-9036-054-2*, 1830026) World Health.

Ethics & the Discovery of the Unconscious. John H. Riker. 1997. LC 96-41498. (Series in Transpersonal & Humanistic Psychology). 254p. (C). text 50.50 (*0-7914-3425-7*); pap. text 17.95 (*0-7914-3426-5*) State U NY Pr.

Ethics & the Elderly. Mark R. Wicclair. 1993. LC 92-49054. 272p. (C). text 38.50 (*0-19-505315-X*) OUP.

Ethics & the Law in Intensive Care. Nicholas A. Pace & Sheila McLean. 1996. (Illus.). 208p. (C). text 69.50 (*0-19-262520-9*) OUP.

Ethics & Uncertainty: The Economics of John M. Keynes & Frank H. Knight. William B. Greer. 2000. LC 00-34833. 160p. 75.00 (*1-84064-445-1*) E Elgar.

Ethics & Values for Care Workers. G. V. Tadd. 1998. LC 97-41491. 148p. pap. 36.95 (*0-632-04814-X*) Blackwell Sci.

Ethics & Values in Health Care Management. Souzy Dracopoulou. 1999. LC 98-16654. 224p. (C). 70.00 (*0-415-14644-5*); pap. 26.95 (*0-415-14645-3*) Routledge.

Ethics & Values in Long Term Health Care. Ed. by Patricia J. Vilani. 1994. LC 94-35455. 121p. 39.95 (*1-56024-698-7*) Haworth Pr.

Ethics & Values in Psychotherapy. Alan C. Tjeltveit. 1998. LC 98-8506. 85.00 (*0-415-15663-7*); 352p. pap. 29.95 (*0-415-15664-5*) Routledge.

Ethics Casebook for Hospitals: Practical Approaches to Everyday Cases. Mark G. Kuczewski & Rosa L. Pinkus. 1999. LC 98-44652. 219p. pap. 23.95 (*0-87840-723-5*) Georgetown U Pr.

Ethics, Computing, & Medicine: Informatics & the Transformation of Health Care. Ed. by Kenneth W. Goodman. 1997. LC 97-10265. 192p. (C). pap. text 29.95 (*0-521-46905-8*) Cambridge U Pr.

Ethics Consultation: A Practical Guide. John La Puma & David Schieder Mayer. 1994. LC 93-28098. (Illus.). 248p. (C). pap. text 47.95 (*0-86720-797-3*, 797-3) Jones & Bartlett.

Ethics for Addiction Professionals. LeClair Bissell & James Royce. 1987. LC 94-32433. 60p. (Orig.). pap. 10.00 (*0-89486-454-8*) Hazelden.

Ethics for Doctors, Nurses, & Patients. H. P. Dunn. 1994. LC 93-44150. 158p. pap. 8.95 (*0-8189-0688-X*) Alba.

Ethics for Everyone: A Practical Guide to Interdisciplinary Biomedical Ethics Education. Linda C. Grafius. 1995. LC 95-3469. 223p. pap. 61.95 (*1-55648-134-9*) AHPI.

Ethics for Health Care. Catherine Anne Berglund. 1999. LC 99-206857. (Illus.). 240p. pap. text 39.95 (*0-19-554172-3*) OUP.

Ethics for Health Information Managers. Toth. 1997. (Allied Health Ser.). tchr. ed. 12.00 (*0-8273-7182-9*) Delmar.

Ethics for Marriage, Family & Child Counselors: A Commentary on the California Association of Marriage & Family Therapists. Federico C. Grosso. 2nd ed. 1997. LC 97-94449. 180p. pap. text 25.00 (*0-9654534-2-1*) F C Grosso.

Ethics for Psychologists: A Commentary on the APA Ethics Code. Bruce E. Bennett et al. 1994. LC 94-36224. 254p. (Orig.). pap. text 24.95 (*1-55798-259-7*, 431-2050) Am Psychol.

Ethics in Action: A Workbook for Nurses. Kevin D. Kendrick. 1999. (Illus.). 160p. (Orig.). pap. 38.25 (*1-56593-760-0*, 1478) Singular Publishing.

Ethics in an Epidemic: AIDS, Morality & Culture. Timothy F. Murphy. 1994. LC 94-8248. text 45.00 (*0-520-08636-8*) U CA Pr.

Ethics in Applied Developmental Psychology: Emerging Issues in an Emerging Field, 4. Warren W. Tryon & Irving E. Sigel. 1990. (Advances in Applied Developmental Psychology Ser.: Vol. 4). 335p. (C). 77.00 (*0-89391-598-X*, Ablex) Greenwood.

Ethics in Clinical Practice. Judith C. Ahronheim et al. 2nd ed. 1999. LC 99-42872. 464p. 62.00 (*0-8342-1075-4*, 10754) Aspen Pub.

Ethics in Counseling & Psychotherapy: Perspectives on Issues & Decision Making. William VanHoose & Louis V. Paradise. 1979. LC 79-15429. 160p. (gr. 1-12). pap. 11.00 (*0-910328-25-0*) Sulzburger & Graham Pub.

Ethics in Counseling & Psychotherapy: Standards, Research, & Emerging Issues. Elizabeth R. Welfel. 1997. LC 97-41217. (Counseling Ser.). 512p. pap. text 45.95 (*0-534-34302-3*) Brooks-Cole.

Ethics in Emergency Medicine. Kenneth V. Iserson et al. 2nd ed. 1995. LC 95-12227. 450p. pap. 39.95 (*1-883620-14-7*) Galen AZ.

Ethics in Epidemiology & Clinical Research: Annotated Readings. Ed. by Steven S. Coughlin. 1995. LC 95-7873. 272p. (C). pap. text 35.00 (*0-917227-08-5*) Epidemiology.

Ethics in Forensic Science & Medicine: Guidelines for the Forensic Expect & the Attorney. Ed. by Melvin A. Shiffman. 2000. LC 99-47828. 326p. 62.95 (*0-398-07024-5*); pap. text 47.95 (*0-398-07025-3*) C C Thomas.

***Ethics in General Practice: A Practical Handbook for Personal Development.** Ann Orme-Smith & John Spicer. 2001. 280p. pap. (*1-85775-328-3*) Radcliffe Med Pr GBR. *Dist:* Balogh.

Ethics in Health Education. Ed. by Spyros Doxiadis. 1990. 230p. 415.00 (*0-471-92606-X*) Wiley.

Ethics in Health Services Management. Kurt Darr. 3rd ed. 1997. LC 96-26874. pap. text 35.95 (*1-878812-36-X*) Hlth Prof Pr.

Ethics in HIV-Related Psychotherapy: Clinical Decision Making in Complex Cases. Ed. by John R. Anderson & Robert L. Barret. 2000. LC 00-59350. 376p. 39.95 (*1-55798-722-X*, 431-2320) Am Psychol.

Ethics in Long-Term Care. Robert Haacker. 1998. 32.50 (*0-929442-29-6*, 2207PP) Prof Prnting & Pub.

Ethics in Medical Research: A Handbook of Good Practice. Trevor Smith. 1999. LC 98-36842. 422p. (C). pap. text 47.95 (*0-521-62619-6*) Cambridge U Pr.

Ethics in Medicine. Milton D. Heifetz. 1996. LC 96-17892. 264p. pap. text 24.00 (*1-57392-073-8*) Prometheus Bks.

Ethics in Mental Health Practice. Ed. by David K. Kentsmith et al. 1986. LC 79-2276. 336p. text 40.95 (*0-8089-1738-2*, 792276, Grune & Strat) Harcrt Hlth Sci Grp.

***Ethics in Midwifery.** Shirley Jones. 2nd ed. 2001. 185p. pap. 29.95 (*0-7234-3172-8*) Mosby Inc.

Ethics in Neurobiological Research with Human Subjects. Ed. by Adil E. Shamoo. 1996. LC 99-458422. 280p. text 79.00 (*2-88449-161-9*) Gordon & Breach.

Ethics in Nursing. Davis. 1986. (International Journal of Nursing Studies: Vol. 22). pap. 27.50 (*0-08-033969-7*, Pergamon Pr) Elsevier.

Ethics in Nursing. Martin Benjamin & Joy Curtis. 3rd ed. 1992. 264p. pap. text 26.50 (*0-19-506748-7*) OUP.

Ethics in Nursing: An Annotated Bibliography. Terry Pence. 2nd ed. 1986. 255p. pap. 12.95 (*0-88737-192-2*, 20-1936) Natl League Nurse.

Ethics in Nursing: An Anthology. Ed. by Terry Pence & Janice Cantrall. 1990. 344p. pap. 34.95 (*0-88737-461-1*) Natl League Nurse.

Ethics in Nursing: The Caring Relationship. Verena Tschudin. 2nd rev. ed. 1992. 192p. pap. text 47.50 (*0-7506-0346-1*) Buttrwrth-Heinemann.

Ethics in Nursing Practice. Graham Rumbold. 3rd ed. 1999. LC 98-31648. xi, 275p. pap. text 24.00 (*0-7020-2312-4*) Saunders.

Ethics in Obstetrics & Gynecology. Laurence B. McCullough & Frank A. Chervenak. 1994. LC 93-6426. (Illus.). 296p. (C). text 41.50 (*0-19-506005-9*) OUP.

Ethics in Physical Therapy Pt. 2: The Patient & Society. 1998. 220p. pap. 40.00 (*1-887759-66-2*) Am Phys Therapy Assn.

Ethics in Psychiatric Research: A Resource Manual on Human Subjects Research. Ed. by Harold A. Pincus et al. 1999. LC 98-17948. 334p. 79.00 (*0-89042-281-8*, 2281) Am Psychiatric.

Ethics in Psychology: Professional Standards & Cases. Ed. by Patricia C. Keith-Spiegel & Gerald P. Koocher. 1995. 522p. text 36.00 (*0-8058-2128-7*) L Erlbaum Assocs.

Ethics in Psychology: Professional Standards & Cases. Patricia C. Keith-Spiegel & Gerald P. Koocher. 1985. 544p. (C). text (*0-07-554879-8*) McGraw.

Ethics in Psychology: Professional Standards & Cases, Vol. 3. Gerald P. Koocher & Patricia Keith-Spiegel. 2nd ed. 1998. LC 97-28322. (Oxford Textbooks in Clinical Psychology Ser.). (Illus.). 528p. text 49.95 (*0-19-509201-5*) OUP.

Ethics in Reproductive & Perinatal Medicine: A New Framework. Carson Strong. 1997. LC 96-18957. 256p. 40.00 (*0-300-06832-8*) Yale U Pr.

Ethics in Reproductive Medicine. Ed. by David R. Bromham et al. 1992. (Illus.). 232p. 89.95 (*0-387-19698-6*) Spr-Verlag.

Ethics in the Hospital Setting. Ed. by Bruce D. Weinstein. 1986. 118p. pap. 12.50 (*0-937058-23-8*) West Va U Pr.

Ethics Intelligence & Discipline. Alan C. Walter. Ed. by Beverly Miles. 1991. 32p. (Orig.). pap. text 12.97 (*1-57569-030-6*) Wisdom Pubng.

Ethics, Law & Medical Practice. Kerry Breen et al. 1997. LC 97-179968. 386p. pap. (*1-86448-407-1*) Allen & Unwin Pty AUS. *Dist:* Paul & Co Pubs.

Ethics, Law & Nursing. Nina Fletcher & Janet Holt. Ed. by Margaret Brazier. 1995. LC 94-27746. text (*0-7190-4049-3*) Manchester Univ Pr GBR. *Dist:* St Martin.

Ethics, Law & Nursing. Nina Fletcher & Janet Holt. Ed. by Margaret Brazier. 1995. LC 94-27746. 243p. pap. (*0-7190-4050-7*) Manchester Univ Pr GBR. *Dist:* St Martin.

Ethics, Legal Medicine & Forensic Pathology. Vernon D. Plueckhahn. 1983. (Illus.). 287p. 44.95 (*0-522-84252-6*) Intl Spec Bk.

Ethics, Legal Medicine & Forensic Pathology. Vernon D. Plueckhahn & Stephen M. Cordner. 1991. 440p. (*0-522-84445-6*) Melbourne Univ Pr AUS. *Dist:* Paul & Co Pubs.

Ethics, Legalities, Professional Practice Issues in Marriage & Family Therapy. Joyce H. Vesper & Gregory W. Brock. 1990. 200p. (C). 81.00 (*0-205-12831-9*, H28319) Allyn.

Ethics of Animal & Human Experimentation. De Deyn. 388p. (*0-86196-429-2*) J Libbey Med GBR. *Dist:* Bks Intl VA.

Ethics of Biomedical Research: An International Perspective. Baruch A. Brody. 1998. 400p. text 49.95 (*0-19-509007-1*) OUP.

Ethics of Care & the Ethics of Cure. Ed. by Jean Watson & Marilyn A. Ray. 1988. 64p. pap. 8.95 (*0-88737-418-2*, 15-2237) Natl League Nurse.

Ethics of Diagnosis. Ed. by Jose L. Peset. 1992. LC 91-35370. (Philosophy & Medicine Ser.). 320p. (C). lib. bdg. (*0-7923-1544-8*) Kluwer Academic NLD. *Dist:* Kluwer Academic.

Ethics of Electronic Patient Records: A Foundational Inquiry. Eike-Henner W. Kluge. 2001. LC 00-49779. (International Healthcare Ethics Ser.: Vol. 6). (Illus.). vi, 182p. (*0-8204-5259-9*) P Lang Pubng.

Ethics of Health Care. Edge. 2nd ed. 1998. LC 98-27212. (Allied Health Ser.). 240p. (C). text 49.95 (*0-7668-0518-2*) Delmar.

Ethics of Health Care: A Guide for Clinical Practice. Raymond S. Edge & John R. Groves. 1994. 222p. (C). mass mkt. 42.95 (*0-8273-5454-1*) Delmar.

Ethics of Health Care: A Textbook. Benedict Ashley & Kevin D. O'Rourke. 2nd ed. 1994. LC 93-36677. 288p. (C). pap. 24.95 (*0-87840-548-8*) Georgetown U Pr.

Ethics of Health Care: Dilemmas of Technology & Techniques in Health Care & Psychotherapy. Ed. by Henry L. Lennard & Suzanne H. Lennard. 1979. LC 79-57022. 174p. (Orig.). pap. 16.00 (*0-935824-01-4*) Gondolier.

Ethics of Health Care - IML. Edge. 2nd ed. 1998. 96p. tchr. ed. 21.95 (*0-7668-0519-0*) Delmar.

Ethics of Health Care Facilitators Guide: A Guide for Clinical Practice. Raymond S. Edge & John R. Groves. 1994. 87p. tchr. ed. 18.00 (*0-8273-5456-8*) Delmar.

Ethics of Human Cloning. Leon R. Kass. 1998. LC 98-18223. 121p. 16.95 (*0-8447-4050-0*) Am Enterprise.

Ethics of Managed Care: A Pragmatic Approach. Mary Anderlik. 2001. LC 00-54015. (Medical Ethics Ser.). x, 293p. 39.95 (*0-253-33848-4*) Ind U Pr.

Ethics of Medical Choice. Ed. by Jon Elster. 1995. 168p. pap. 15.00 (*1-85567-211-1*); text 39.00 (*1-85567-249-9*) St Martin.

***Ethics of Medical Research on Humans.** Claire Foster. 2001. 176p. text 74.95 (*0-521-64196-9*); pap. text 24.95 (*0-521-64573-5*) Cambridge U Pr.

Ethics of New Reproductive Technologies: The Glover Report to the European Commission. Jonathan Glover et al. 1989. 160p. 28.00 (*0-87580-147-1*) N Ill U Pr.

Ethics of Opium. Ellen N. LaMotte. Ed. by Gerald N. Grob. 1981. LC 80-1260. (Addiction in America Ser.). reprint ed. lib. bdg. 22.95 (*0-405-13601-3*) Ayer.

Ethics of Organ Transplantation. Wayne N. Shelton. 2001. LC 00-66277. (Advances in Bioethics Ser.: Vol. 7). (Illus.). 406p. 98.00 (*0-7623-0764-1*) Jai Pr.

Ethics of Psychiatry: Insanity, Rational Autonomy, & Mental Health Care. Ed. by Rem B. Edwards. 2nd rev. ed. 1997. LC 96-36439. 553p. pap. 29.00 (*1-57392-113-0*) Prometheus Bks.

Ethics of Psychoanalysis. Thomas Szasz. 1988. 250p. reprint ed. pap. 16.95 (*0-8156-0229-4*) Syracuse U Pr.

Ethics of Reproductive Technology. Ed. by Kenneth D. Alpern. 1992. 376p. (C). pap. text 27.95 (*0-19-507435-1*) OUP.

Ethics of Research Involving Human Subjects: Facing the 21st Century. Ed. by Harold Y. Vanderpool. 1996. 544p. 59.00 (*1-55572-036-6*) Univ Pub Group.

Ethics of Terminal Care: Orchestrating the End of Life. Erich H. Loewy & Roberta Springer Loewy. 2000. LC 00-41588. xv, 181p. 55.00 (*0-306-46435-7*) Kluwer Academic.

Ethics of the Ordinary in Healthcare: A Reflection for the Powerful. John A. Worthley. 1997. LC 97-3040. 50.00 (*1-56793-056-5*) Health Admin Pr.

Ethics of Withdrawal of Life-Support Systems: Case Studies in Decision Making in Intensive Care. Douglas N. Walton. 1987. LC 87-2459. 272p. pap. 19.95 (*0-275-92710-5*, B2710, Praeger Pubs) Greenwood.

Ethics of Withdrawal of Life-Support Systems: Case Studies on Decision Making in Intensive Care, 23. Douglas N. Walton. 1983. LC 82-15662. (Contributions in Philosophy Ser.: No. 23). 257p. 64.00 (*0-313-23752-2*, WLS/, Greenwood Pr) Greenwood.

Ethics, Trade-Offs & Medical Radiation. Eugene L. Saenger. 1982. (Taylor Lectures: No. 6). 20.00 (*0-913392-59-6*) NCRP Pubns.

Ethik, Technik, Konzepte. Ed. by U. Laffer & M. Duerig. 1988. (Basler Beitraege zur Chirurgie Ser.: Vol. 1). (Illus.). x, 138p. pap. 50.50 (*3-8055-4926-1*) S Karger.

Ethnic Americans for the Health Professional. Norma J. Downes. 2nd ed. 1997. LC 97-178620. 256p. (C). per. 44.95 (*0-7872-3653-5*, 41365301) Kendall-Hunt.

Ethnic Diseases Sourcebook: Basic Consumer Health Information for Ethnic & Racial Minority Groups in the United States. Joyce Brennfleck Shannon. 2001. LC 00-52853. (Health Reference Ser.). (Illus.). xiii, 664p. lib. bdg. (*0-7808-0336-1*) Omnigraphics Inc.

Ethnic Elderly & Long-Term Care. Ed. by Charles M. Barresi & Donald E. Stull. 1992. LC 92-6066. 312p. 39.95 (*0-8261-7370-5*) Springer Pub.

Ethnic Health Collections in the United States, 13. Tyson Gibbs. 1996. LC 95-50402. (Bibliographies & Indexes in Medical Studies: Vol. 13). 160p. lib. bdg. 57.95 (*0-313-29740-1*, Greenwood Pr) Greenwood.

Ethnic Health Handbook: A Factfile for Health Care Professionals. Ed. by Ghada Karmi. 1995. LC 95-38399. 132p. pap. 36.95 (*0-632-04042-4*) Blackwell Sci.

Ethnic Issues in Adolescent Mental Health. Arlene R. Stiffman. 1990. LC 90-8735. (Illus.). 360p. (C). pap. 34.95 (*0-8039-3985-X*, 3328) Sage.

Ethnic Minorities: Social Psychological Perspectives. Ed. by Jan P. Van Oudenhoven. 1989. 288p. (*90-265-0988-X*) Swets.

Ethnic Minority Elderly: Task Force Report of the American Psychiatric Association. American Psychiatric Association Task Force Staff. 1993. LC 93-27940. 192p. text 11.95 (*0-89042-247-8*, 2247) Am Psychiatric.

E F G

Ethnic Minority Perspectives on Clinical Training & Services in Psychology. Ed. by Hector F. Myers et al. 1991. 194p. pap. 14.95 (*1-55798-120-5*) Am Psychol.

Ethnic Psychiatry. C. B. Wilkinson. 1986. LC 86-8181. (Critical Issues in Psychiatry Ser.). (Illus.). 214p. (C). 45.00 (*0-306-42306-5*, Plenum Trade) Perseus Pubng.

Ethnic Rhinoplasty. Steven M. Hoefflin. 1997. LC 97-7621. (Illus.). 198p. 181.00 (*0-387-94691-8*) Spr-Verlag.

Ethnic Skin: Medical Surgical. Bernett L. Johnson et al. 1998. LC 97-45884. (Illus.). 304p. (C). (gr. 13). text 95.00 (*0-8151-5687-1*, 29160) Mosby Inc.

Ethnic Validity, Ecology, & Psychotherapy: A Psychosocial Competence Model. F. B. Tyler et al. 1991. (Applied Clinical Psychology Ser.). (Illus.). 360p. (C). 57.50 (*0-306-43870-4*, Plenum Trade) Perseus Pubng.

Ethnicity & Aging: Mental Health Issues. Ed. by Shirley A. Lockery & Susan A. Schoenrock. 1990. LC 90-71303. 73p. (C). pap. text 8.00 (*1-879167-00-X*) SDSU Coll Hlth Hum Servs.

Ethnicity & Family Therapy. Ed. by Monica McGoldrick et al. (Guilford Family Therapy Ser.). 1982. LC 81-20198. 600p. text 43.95 (*0-89862-040-6*); 2nd ed. 1996. LC 96-7923. 717p. text 62.00 (*0-89862-959-4*, 2959) Guilford Pubns.

Ethnicity & Gerontological Social Work. Ed. by Rose Dobrof. 1987. LC 86-29464. (Journal of Gerontological Social Work Ser.: Vol. 9, No. 4). 143p. text 39.95 (*0-86656-646-5*) Haworth Pr.

Ethnicity & Health. Ed. by Winston A. Van Horne. 1988. LC 88-51124. (Ethnicity & Public Policy Ser.: Vol. 7). xiii, 212p. (Orig.). (C). text 25.00 (*0-942672-12-7*) UWI IRE.

Ethnicity & Medical Care. Alan Harwood. 1981. LC 80-19339. (Commonwealth Fund Publications). (Illus.). 537p. (C). 42.50 (*0-674-26865-2*) HUP.

Ethnicity & Organizational Diversity: A Study of Social Cognition & Psychological Climate Perception. Wendy V. Chung. 1996. LC 96-41350. 168p. lib. bdg. 42.00 (*0-7618-0528-1*) U Pr of Amer.

Ethnicity & the Dementias. Gwen Yeo & Dolores Gallagher-Thompson. 1996. 250p. pap. text 24.95 (*1-56032-437-6*) Hemisp Pub.

Ethnicity & the Dementias. Gwen Yeo & Dolores Gallagher-Thompson. 1996. 261p. text 69.95 (*1-56032-436-8*) Taylor & Francis.

Ethnicity, Disability, & Chronic Illness. Contrib. by W. I. U. Ahmad. 2000. LC 99-41465. (*0-335-19983-6*) OpUniv Pr GBR. *Dist:* Taylor & Francis.

Ethnicity Immigration & Psychopathology. Ed. by Ihsan Al-Issa & Michel Tousignant. 1997. LC 97-14149. (Series on Stress & Coping). 316p. (C). 49.50 (*0-306-45479-3*, Plenum Trade) Perseus Pubng.

Ethnobotany & Medicinal Plants: Bibliography: January 1990-June 1991. Susan A. McCarthy. 1993. 107p. (C). reprint ed. pap. text 30.00 (*1-56806-929-4*) DIANE Pub.

Ethnobotany & Medicinal Plants Bibliography: July 1991-July 1992. Susan McCarthy. 1993. 134p. (Orig.). (C). pap. text 30.00 (*1-56806-620-1*) DIANE Pub.

Ethnobotany & the Search for New Drugs. Derek J. Chadwick et al. 1994. LC 94-28300. (CIBA Foundation Symposia Ser.: 185). (Illus.). 290p. 128.00 (*0-471-95024-6*) Wiley.

Ethnocultural Aspects of Posttraumatic Stress Disorders: Issues, Research, & Clinical Applications. Ed. by Anthony J. Marsella et al. 1996. LC 95-40252. (Illus.). 576p. 49.95 (*1-55798-319-4*) Am Psychol.

Ethnoepidemiology on Cancer, Vol. 44. Ed. by Kazuo Tajima & Tashiro Sonoda. 1996. LC 95-34200. (Gann Monographs on Cancer Research). 89.95 (*0-8493-7779-X*) CRC Pr.

Ethnography: Theory & Applications in Health Research. Marlene De Laine. 1997. (Illus.). 369p. (C). pap. text 58.00 (*0-8036-0393-2*) Davis Co.

Ethnography of Fertility & Birth. Ed. by Carol P. MacCormack. 2nd rev. ed. 1994. (Illus.). 283p. (C). pap. text 15.50 (*0-88133-817-6*) Waveland Pr.

Ethnomedical Systems in Africa: Patterns of Traditional Medicine in Rural & Urban Kenya. Charles M. Good. 1987. LC 86-26998. 354p. text 42.00 (*0-89862-779-6*) Guilford Pubns.

Ethnomedicine. M. Nichter. 1990. i, 172p. text 93.00 (*2-88124-470-X*) Gordon & Breach.

Ethnopharmacologie (Ethnopharmacology) Sources, Methodes, Objectifs (Sources, Methods, Objectives) J. Fleurentin et al. 1991. (ENG & FRE.). 494p. pap. (*2-7099-1038-1*) LInstitut Francais FRA. *Dist:* Balogh.

Ethnopsychiatry: The Cultural Construction of Professional & Folk Psychiatries. Ed. by Atwood D. Gaines. 1992. LC 91-5076. (SUNY Series in Medical Anthropology). 506p. (C). text 25.50 (*0-7914-1021-8*) State U NY Pr.

Ethnoveterinary Medicine: An Annotated Bibliography. Evelyn Mathias-Mundy & Constance M. McCorkle. 1989. (Bibliographies in Technology & Social Change Ser.: No. 6). 209p. (C). pap. 18.00 (*0-945271-16-6*) ISU-CIKARD.

Ethnoveterinary Research & Development. Constance M. McCorkle et al. 1996. (Studies in Indigenous Knowledge & Development). 450p. pap. (*1-85339-326-6*) Intermed Tech GBR. *Dist:* Stylus Pub VA.

Ethological Psychiatry: Psychopathology in the Context of Evolutionary Biology. Ed. by M. T. McGuire & L. A. Fairbanks. 1964. (Seminars in Psychiatry Ser.). (Illus.). 230p. text 49.00 (*0-8089-0988-6*, 792840, Grune & Strat) Harcrt Hlth Sci Grp.

Ethology: The Mechanisms & Evolution of Behavior. James L. Gould. 1982. (Illus.). 61p. (C). text 40.00 (*0-393-01488-6*) Norton.

Ethology & Psychopharmacology. Ed. by S. J. Cooper & C. A. Hendrie. 1995. LC 94-15718. 370p. 294.95 (*0-471-95213-3*) Wiley.

Ethology of Farm Animals: A Comprehensive Study of Behavioural Features of the Common Farm Animals. Ed. by A. F. Fraser. 1985. (World Animal Science Ser.: Vol. A5). 500p. 314.00 (*0-444-42359-1*) Elsevier.

Ethology-the Biological Study of Animal Behavior. Remy Chauvin. Tr. by Joyce Diamanti from FRE. 1977. LC 76-46818. 245p. (Orig.). 37.50 (*0-8236-1770-X*) Intl Univs Pr.

Ethopharmacology of Agonistic Behaviour in Animals & Humans. Ed. by B. Olivier et al. 1987. (Topics in the Neurosciences Ser.). (C). text 176.50 (*0-89838-972-0*) Kluwer Academic.

Ethylbenzene. 1996. (Environmental Health Criteria Ser.: No. 186). 101p. (Orig.). pap. text 27.00 (*92-4-157186-1*, 1160186) World Health.

Ethylene Oxide. 1985. (Environmental Health Criteria Ser.: No. 55). 79p. pap. text 15.00 (*92-4-154195-4*, 1160055) World Health.

Ethylene Oxide Sterilization Residuals. 1995. 30p. pap. 62.00 (*1-57020-048-3*, 10993-7-209) Assn Adv Med Instrn.

Etica Medica. Elena Lugo. 1984. 173p. (C). pap. text 24.95 (*1-881375-13-7*) Libreria Univ.

Etica y Psicoanalisis. E. Fromm. (Breviarios Ser.). (SPA.). pap. 8.99 (*968-16-0325-7*) Fondo CA.

ETIM Dental Dictionary. ETIM Staff. 1989. (FRE.). 920p. 150.00 (*0-8288-7291-0*, 2905201053) Fr & Eur.

Etiology & Morphogenesis of Congenital Heart Disease: Twenty Years of Progress in Genetics & Developmental Biology. Ed. by Edward B. Clark et al. 2000. LC 00-28826. (Illus.). xxv, 389p. 150.00 (*0-87993-447-6*) Futura Pub.

Etiology & Pathogenesis of Down Syndrome. Ed. by Charles J. Epstein et al. 1995. LC 95-21511. (Progress in Clinical & Biological Research Ser.: Vol. 393). 280p. 215.00 (*0-471-12317-X*) Wiley.

Etiology & Pathogenesis of Viral Infections, Vol. 3. V. M. Zhdanov & Dmitri K. Lvov. 1989. (Virology Reviews Ser.: Sec. E: Soviet Medical Reviews, Vol. 3, Pt. 1). viii, 148p. pap. text 182.00 (*3-7186-4911-X*) Gordon & Breach.

Etiology & Prevention of Communication Disorders. Sanford E. Gerber. 2nd ed. 1998. LC 98-12128. 328p. pap. text 77.95 (*1-56593-947-6*, 1902) Thomson Learn.

Etiology, Concept & Prophylaxis of Childbed Fever. Ignaz Semmelweis. Tr. by K. Codell Carter. 1983. LC 83-47758. (Wisconsin Publications in the History of Science & Medicine: No. 2). (GER.). 288p. (Orig.). pap. 12.95 (*0-299-09364-6*) U of Wis Pr.

Etiology of Breast & Gynecological Cancers, Vol. 396. Ed. by C. Marcelo Aldaz et al. 1997. LC 96-40180. 296p. 247.00 (*0-471-16901-3*) Wiley.

Etiology of Bulimia Nervosa: The Individual & Family Context. Ed. by Janis H. Crowther et al. 1992. 252p. 57.95 (*1-56032-206-3*) Hemisp Pub.

Etiology of Cancer in Man. Ed. by Arthur S. Levine. 1989. (Cancer Growth & Progression Ser.). (C). text 207.50 (*0-89838-995-X*) Kluwer Academic.

Etiology of Dementia of Alzheimer's Type. Ed. by A. S. Henderson & J. H. Henderson. 1988. LC 88-20473. 268p. 290.00 (*0-471-92075-4*) Wiley.

Etiology of Drug Abuse: Implications for Prevention. 1986. lib. bdg. 250.00 (*0-8490-3495-7*) Gordon Pr.

Etiology of Hodgkin's Disease: Proceedings of a NATO ARW Held in Loch Lomond, Scotland, May 2-5, 1994. Ed. by Ruth F. Jarrett. 1996. (NATO ASI Ser.: Vol. 280). (Illus.). 238p. 95.00 (*0-306-45205-7*) Plenum.

Etiology of Inherited Disorders. C. B. Kerr et al. 1974. LC 73-11118. 196p. (C). text 22.00 (*0-8422-7151-1*) Irvington.

Etiology of Parkinson's Disease, No. 40. Ed. by Ellenberg et al. 1995. (Neurological Disease & Therapy Ser.: Vol. 40). (Illus.). 600p. text 225.00 (*0-8247-8823-0*) Dekker.

Etiology of Vision Disorders: A Neuroscience Model. Joseph N. Trachtman. Ed. by Sally M. Corngold & Monika Goodwin. 1991. (Illus.). 140p. (C). lib. bdg. 18.00 (*0-943599-22-9*) OEPF.

Etiology, Pathology & Treatment of Hepatocellular Carcinoma in North America. Ed. by Edward Tabor et al. 1991. (Advances in Applied Biotechnology Ser.: Vol. 13). (Illus.). 384p. (*0-943255-17-1*) Portfolio Pr Corp.

Etiopathogenetic Hypotheses of Schizophrenia. Ed. by C. L. Cazzulio. 1987. 208p. (C). text 124.00 (*0-85200-843-0*) Kluwer Academic.

Etoile du Nord: An Account of Owen Harding Wangensteen (1898-1981), Surgeon-Teacher-Scholar. Leonard F. Peltier & J. Bradley Aust. 1994. LC 94-78654. (Illus.). 165p. (Orig.). pap. text 20.00 (*1-880696-07-X*) Am Coll Surgeons.

Etudes et Essais sur le Droit International Humanitaire et sur les Principes de la Croix-Rouge en l'Honneur de Jean Pictet: Studies & Essays on International Humanitarian Law & Red Cross Principles in Honor of Jean Pictet. International Committee of the Red Cross et al. 1985. LC 84-22631. pap. text 42.50 (*90-247-3199-2*) Kluwer Academic.

EU Electro-Medical Equipment. Intro. by Melinda C. Bailey. 1996. 81p. 64.95 (*1-57172-060-X*) Intl Qual.

EU Human Medicinal Products Directive. Intro. by Melinda C. Bailey. 1996. 162p. 94.95 (*1-57172-064-2*) Intl Qual.

EU Human Medicinal Products Testing Directive. Intro. by Melinda C. Bailey. 1996. 150p. 99.95 (*1-57172-065-0*) Intl Qual.

EU Medical Device Compendium. Intro. by Melinda C. Bailey. 1996. 897p. 595.00 (*1-57172-067-7*) Intl Qual.

EU Medicinal Product Compendium. Intro. by Melinda C. Bailey. 1996. 950p. 695.00 (*1-57172-069-3*) Intl Qual.

EU Medicinal Product Labeling Directive. Intro. by Melinda C. Bailey. Date not set. 95p. 79.95 (*1-57172-070-7*) Intl Qual.

EU Veterinary Medicinal Products Directive. Intro. by Melinda C. Bailey. 1995. 119p. 99.95 (*1-57172-042-1*) Intl Qual.

EUCAMBIS: Immunology & Aging in Europe. Ed. by G. Pawelec. 1999. LC 99-68067. (Biomedical & Health Research Ser.: Vol. 29). (Illus.). v, 137p. 73.00 (*90-5199-434-6*) IOS Press.

Eudralex - The Rules Governing Medicinal Products in the European Union Vol. 6: Notice to Applicants: Veterinary Medical Products European Communities Commission, Directorate-General for Industry, Pharmaceuticals and Cosmetics. 1999. 340p. pap. (*0-11-985351-5*) Statnry Office GBR. *Dist:* Balogh.

Eudralex - The Rules Governing Medicinal Products in the European Union Vol. 7: Guidelines: Veterinary Medicinal Products European Communities Commission, Directorate-General for Industry, Pharmaceuticals and Cosmetics. 1999. pap. (*0-11-985366-3*) Statnry Office GBR. *Dist:* Balogh.

Eugene N. Marais & the Problem of the Animal Psyche. Carole E. Baumann. 1985. 10.00 (*0-7855-1875-4*) St Mut.

Eugenical Sterilization. American Neurological Association Staff. Ed. by Gerald N. Grob. 1980. LC 78-22556. (Historical Issues in Mental Health Ser.). (Illus.). reprint ed. lib. bdg. 19.95 (*0-405-11910-0*) Ayer.

Eugenics: Index to Modern Information with Bibliography. Ruth G. Parrish. 1997. 193p. 57.50 (*0-7883-1639-7*) ABBE Pubs Assn.

Eugenics in Michigan Without Due Process: Coercised Sterilization in the 1960's & 1970's in Michigan Hospitals. Thomas J. Rundquist. unabr. ed. 1996. (Illus.). 60p. (Orig.). 29.95 (*1-884239-09-9*) Nova Media.

Eukaryotic DNA Replication. Ed. by Thomas Kelly & Bruce Stillman. 1988. LC 88-2558. (Cancer Cells Ser.: Vol. 6). (Illus.). 423p. pap. text 85.00 (*0-87969-308-8*) Cold Spring Harbor.

Eukaryotic Gene Regulation Gerald M. Kolodny. 1981. Vol. 1. 192p. 102.95 (*0-8493-5225-8*, QH450); Vol. 2. 240p. 99.50 (*0-8493-5226-6*) CRC Pr.

Eukaryotism & Symbiosis: Intertaxonic Combination vs. Symbiotic Adaptation. Ed. by H. E. Schenk et al. 1997. LC 97-40171. (Illus.). 530p. 138.00 (*3-540-63375-8*) Spr-Verlag.

Euro-Barometer 38.0: European Court of Justice, Passive Smoking, & Consumer Issues, September-October 1992. Karlheinz Reif & Anna Melich. 2nd ed. 1995. LC 92-70498. 976p. pap. (*0-89138-864-8*) ICPSR.

Euro-Barometer Twenty-Nine: Environmental Problems & Cancer, March-April 1988. Karlheinz Reif & Anna Melich. 1990. LC 90-85881. 472p. (*0-89138-869-9*) ICPSR.

Euro-Barometer 27: The Common Agricultural Policy & Cancer, March-May 1987. Ronald Inglehart et al. 1989. LC 89-811139. (Euro-Barometers Ser.). 378p. (*0-89138-874-5*) ICPSR.

Euro-Qual Program: Toward a Quality System for European Orthodontic Professionals. Ter G. Heege. 1997. LC 97-70590. (Biomedical & Health Research Ser.: Vol. 14). 248p. pap. 79.00 (*90-5199-330-7*) IOS Press.

Eurocare 2: Survival of Cancer Patients in Europe in the Late Eighties. Ed. by F. Berrino et al. 2000. (IARC Scientific Publications Ser.: 151). 572p. pap. text 69.00 (*92-832-2151-6*) OUP.

Eurodoc. 1997. text 109.00 (*3-540-14624-5*) Spr-Verlag.

EUROMAT 99: Materials for Medical Engineering. Ed. by H. Stallforth. 2000. 266p. 99.95 (*3-527-30123-2*) Wiley.

Europaisches Medizinisches Woerterbuch: German-English-Spanish-French-Italian. Schattauer Staff. 1991. (ENG, FRE & GER.). 1022p. 195.00 (*0-7859-7036-3*) Fr & Eur.

Europe Adrift. John Newhouse. 2000. 339p. reprint ed. text 27.00 (*0-7881-6996-3*) DIANE Pub.

European Agreement on the Exchange of Therapeutic Substances of Human Origin (1983) & Additional Protocol (1990) Council of Europe Staff. 1990. (Conventions & Agreements Ser.: Nos. 26 & 109). (ENG & FRE.). (*92-871-1799-3*) Council of Europe FRA. *Dist:* Manhattan Pub Co.

European Agreement on the Exchange of Tissue-Typing Reagents. Council of Europe Staff. 1987. (Conventions & Agreements Ser.: No. 84). (ENG & FRE.). (*92-871-0130-2*) Council of Europe FRA. *Dist:* Manhattan Pub Co.

European Agreement on the Instruction & Education of Nurses. Council of Europe Staff. 1978. (Conventions & Agreements Ser.: No. 59). (ENG & FRE.). (*92-871-0106-X*) Council of Europe FRA. *Dist:* Manhattan Pub Co.

European Anatomical Congress: Sixth Congress Abstracts. Ed. by W. Lierse. 1981. (Journal: Vol. 3, No. 1-2). 176p. pap. 137.50 (*3-8055-3463-9*) S Karger.

European Anatomical Congress / Congres Europeen Anatomique / Europaischer Anatomen-Kongress: 4th Congress, Basel, August/September 1977: Abstracts. European Anatomical Congress, Staff. 1977. (Acta Anatomica Ser.: Vol. 99, No. 3). 79.25 (*3-8055-2776-4*) S Karger.

European Anatomical Congress, Eighth, Antwerp, September 1987. Ed. by D. W. Scheuermann et al. 1987. (Journal: Vol. 130, No. 1, 1987). (Illus.). 108p. pap. 80.00 (*3-8055-4663-7*) S Karger.

European Anesthetic Product Markets. Market Intelligence Staff. 1994. 3800.00 (*0-7889-0120-6*) Frost & Sullivan.

European Anti-Epilepsy Product Markets. 1995. LC 98-168689. 205p. spiral bd. 3950.00 (*0-7889-0364-0*, 3079-49) Frost & Sullivan.

European Anti-Infective Markets: Companies Forced to Rethink Strategies. 1996. 243p. spiral bd. 3900.00 (*0-7889-0573-2*, 3327-44) Frost & Sullivan.

European Anti-Parkinson's Pharmaceutical Markets. Ed. by Frost and Sullivan Staff. 1995. 367p. spiral bd. 3900.00 (*0-7889-0394-2*, 3162-45) Frost & Sullivan.

European Anticoagulant & Thrombolytic Markets. Frost and Sullivan Staff. 1996. 382p. spiral bd. 3950.00 (*0-7889-0582-1*, 3331-45) Frost & Sullivan.

European Antiviral Drug & Vaccine Markets. Market Intelligence Staff. 1994. 400p. 3800.00 (*0-7889-0016-1*) Frost & Sullivan.

European Arthritis Markets. Market Intelligence Staff. 1994. LC 97-213401. 230p. 3800.00 (*0-7889-0153-2*) Frost & Sullivan.

European Association of Urology: 12th Congress, Paris, September 1996 - Abstracts. Ed. by Laurent Boccon-Gibod et al. 1996. (Journal: Vol. 30, Suppl. 2, 1996). (Illus.). 310p. pap. 135.00 (*3-8055-6387-6*) S Karger.

European Association of Urology: 13th Congress, Barcelona, March 1998: Abstracts. 1998. (European Urology Ser.: Vol. 33, Suppl. 1). xiv, 192p. pap. 89.75 (*3-8055-6646-8*) S Karger.

***European Association of Urology: XVIth Congress, Geneva, April 2001 - Abstracts.** Ed. by Scientific Committee of the EAU Congress Members. 2001. (European Urology Ser.: Vol. 39, Suppl. 5). xviii, 216p. pap. 48.75 (*3-8055-7215-8*) S Karger.

European Association of Urology: XVth Congress, Brussels, April 2000: Abstracts. Ed. by Members of the Scientific Committee of the XVth EAU Congress. 2000. (European Urology Ser.: Vol. 37, Suppl. 2). (Illus.). xvi, 176p. pap. 45.25 (*3-8055-7068-6*) S Karger.

European Association of Urology (EAU) 9th Congress, Amsterdam , June Abstracts. Ed. by Adolphe Steg et al. 1990. (Journal: Vol. 18, Supplement 1, 1990). (Illus.). viii, 480p. pap. 168.75 (*3-8055-5237-8*) S Karger.

European Association of Urology (EAU) XIVth Congress, Stockholm, April 1999: Abstracts, Vol. 1 & 2. Ed. by Members of the Scientific Committee of the XIVth EAU Congress. 1999. (European Urology Ser.: Vol. 35, Suppl. 2). xiv, 192p. pap. 45.25 (*3-8055-6850-9*) S Karger.

European Biotechnology Pharmaceutical Markets: The Lucrative Business of Genetic Engineering. Market Intelligence Staff. 1993. 450p. (Orig.). 3500.00 (*1-56753-623-9*) Frost & Sullivan.

European Clinical Diagnostics Industry Manufacturers & Suppliers: Detailed Profiles of 148 Industry Leaders. Market Intelligence Staff. 1993. (Orig.). 1500.00 (*1-56259-621-7*) Frost & Sullivan.

European Co-Operation Concerning Epidemiological Studies in the Field of Mental Health. Council of Europe Staff. 1993. (*92-871-2100-1*) Council of Europe FRA. *Dist:* Manhattan Pub Co.

European Community Atlas of Avoidable Death. Ed. by Walter W. Holland. 2nd ed. 1993. (CEC Health Services Research Ser.: No. 9, Vol. 2). (Illus.). 196p. 110.00 (*0-19-262206-4*) OUP.

European Community Medical Device Directives: Certification, Quality Assurance & Liability. James W. Kolka et al. 1992. 224p. pap. 75.00 (*1-883337-25-9*) CEEM Inc.

European Conference on Microcirculation: 20th Conference, Paris, August/September 1998: Abstracts. Ed. by P. H. Carpentier. 1998. (Journal of Vascular Research: Vol. 35, Suppl. 2 (1998)). 114p. pap. 29.75 (*3-8055-6747-2*) S Karger.

European Conference on Microcirculation: 21st Conference, Stockholm, June 2000: Abstracts. 2000. (Journal of Vascular Research: Vol. 37). iv, 88p. pap. 34.00 (*3-8055-7122-4*) S Karger.

European Conference on Microcirculation, 6th, Aalborg, 1970. Conference on Microcirculation, 6th, Aalborg, 1970. Ed. by J. Ditzel & D. H. Lewis. 1971. (Illus.). 204.50 (*3-8055-1234-1*) S Karger.

European Congress of the International Hepato-Pancreato-Billiary Association (IHPBA) Congress, Budapest, May 1999: Abstracts. Ed. by P. K. Kupcsulik et al. 1999. (Digestive Surgery Ser.: Vol. 16). 138p. pap. 39.25 (*3-8055-6887-8*) S Karger.

European Congress on Ballistocardiography & Cardiovascular Dynamics, 8th, Ljubliana, 1971. European Congress on Ballistocardiography and Cardiovascular Dynamics Staff. Ed. by G. Juznic. (Bibliotheca Cardiologica Ser.: No. 30). Pt. 1. 1973. 73.25 (*3-8055-1374-7*); Pt. 2. 1974. 100.00 (*3-8055-1375-5*) S Karger.

European Cytogenetics Conference: 1st Conference, Athens, June 1997: Abstracts. Ed. by Vladislva Baranov et al. 1997. (Cytogenetics & Cell Genetics Ser.: Vol. 77, No. 1-2, 1997). 168p. pap. 64.50 (*3-8055-6549-6*) S Karger.

European Dental Surgery Furniture & Equipment Markets. Frost and Sullivan Staff. 1996. LC 98-168755. 421p. spiral bd. 3900.00 (*0-7889-0426-4*, 3070-54) Frost & Sullivan.

European Diagnostic Products: Competitive Benchmarking. Ed. by Frost and Sullivan Staff. 1997. 570p. spiral bd. 1950.00 (*0-7889-0733-6*, 3402-53) Frost & Sullivan.

European Dietary Supplement Markets. Market Intelligence Staff. 1995. 266p. spiral bd. 3800.00 (*0-7889-0188-5*, 3005-88) Frost & Sullivan.

European Drug Delivery System Markets. Market Intelligence Staff. 1994. 400p. 3800.00 (*0-7889-0005-6*) Frost & Sullivan.

European Drug Directory. Charles Garlot. 2nd ed. 1992. (ENG & FRE.). 2034p. 335.00 (*0-7859-9280-4*) Fr & Eur.

European Drug Index. N. F. Muller & R. P. Dessing. 2nd ed. 1992. 1380p. 315.00 (*0-444-89733-X*) Elsevier.

European Fluid & Drug Delivery Systems Market: Extensive Forecasts Document Country Differences & Usage Trends. Market Intelligence Staff. 1992. 344p. 1895.00 (*1-56753-078-8*) Frost & Sullivan.

European Generic Drugs Market. Market Intelligence Staff. 1993. 207p. 3900.00 (*1-56753-509-7*) Frost & Sullivan.

European Handbook of Dermatological Treatments. Ed. by A. D. Katsambast & T. M. Lotti. 1999. LC 98-42394. (Illus.). 872p. 119.00 (*3-540-64045-2*) Spr-Verlag.

European Health Care Reform: Analysis of Current Strategies. R. Saltman & J. Figueras. 1997. (WHO Regional Publications, European Ser.: No. 72). 322p. text 50.00 (*92-890-1336-2*) World Health.

European Hospital Furniture Markets: Introduction of Day Surgery & Development of Computer Technologies Revive Industry. Frost and Sullivan Staff. 1995. LC 98-168646. 448p. 3900.00 (*0-7889-0292-X*, 3080-54) Frost & Sullivan.

European Hospital Infection Control Equipment & Supply Market: Governmental Responses to AIDS Stimulate Product Demand. Market Intelligence Staff. 1992. 350p. 1895.00 (*1-56753-080-X*) Frost & Sullivan.

European Immunotherapeutics Markets. Market Intelligence Staff. 1994. 334p. 3800.00 (*0-7889-0017-X*) Frost & Sullivan.

European Implantable & Interventional Cardiovascular Device Markets. Frost & Sullivan. 1997. 227p. spiral bd. 3900.00 (*0-7889-0630-5*, 3404-541) Frost & Sullivan.

European In Vitro Cancer Diagnostic Markets. 1996. 281p. spiral bd. 3900.00 (*0-7889-0561-9*, 3326-53) Frost & Sullivan.

European Intra-Ocular Lens Markets. Market Intelligence Staff. 1994. 104p. 1750.00 (*0-7889-0004-8*) Frost & Sullivan.

European Market for Alzheimer's Drugs. Ed. by Frost and Sullivan Staff. 1995. 439p. spiral bd. 3800.00 (*0-7889-0369-1*, 3163-45) Frost & Sullivan.

European Market for Livestock & Poultry Vaccines. Ed. by Frost and Sullivan Staff. 1997. 365p. spiral bd. 3950.00 (*0-7889-0676-3*, 3338-42) Frost & Sullivan.

European Market for X-Ray Diagnostic Images. Market Intelligence Staff. 1993. 3900.00 (*1-56753-501-1*) Frost & Sullivan.

European Markets for Medical Diagnostic Ultrasound Equipment. Ed. by Frost and Sullivan Staff. 1997. 333p. spiral bd. 3950.00 (*0-7889-0690-9*, 3413-50) Frost & Sullivan.

European Medical Device Directive: Self-Certification of Class I Devices. John S. Adcock. 1997. 120p. wbk. ed. 295.00 (*1-56993-001-5*) HISTECH.

European Medical Device Manufacturers: Competitive Benchmarking. Ed. by Frost and Sullivan Staff. 1997. 687p. spiral bd. 1995.00 (*0-7889-0695-X*, 3406-54) Frost & Sullivan.

European Medical Diagnostic Ultrasound Equipment Markets. Market Intelligence Staff. 1995. 430p. 3800.00 (*0-7889-0189-3*, 1968-50) Frost & Sullivan.

European Medical Dictionary: English, French, German, Italian, Spanish. 1991. (ENG, FRE, GER, ITA & SPA.). 1022p. 195.00 (*0-7859-9989-2*) Fr & Eur.

European Medical Imaging Contrast Media Markets. Frost and Sullivan Staff. 1996. 271p. spiral bd. 3950.00 (*0-7889-0471-X*, 3261-50) Frost & Sullivan.

European Medicines Research: Perspectives in Pharmacotoxicology & Pharmcovigilance. Ed. by G. N. Fracchia. 1994. LC 94-7542. (Biomedical & Health Research Ser.: Vol. 7). 421p. 99.00 (*90-5199-154-1*) IOS Press.

European Meeting on Complement in Human Disease, Innsbruck, March 1997: Proceedings & Abstracts. Ed. by Reinhard Wuerzner & Manfred P. Dierich. 1997. (Journal: Vol. 14, No. 1, 1997). (Illus.). 112p. pap. 41.75 (*3-8055-6492-9*) S Karger.

European Minimally Invasive Surgical Equipment Markets. Market Intelligence Staff. 1994. 324p. 3800.00 (*1-56753-974-2*) Frost & Sullivan.

European Mobility Aid & Associated Paramedical Product Markets. Market Intelligence Staff. 1994. 385p. 3800.00 (*1-56753-971-8*) Frost & Sullivan.

European Non Isotopic Immunoassay Product Markets. Market Intelligence Staff. 1994. 374p. (Orig.). 3800.00 (*1-56753-891-6*) Frost & Sullivan.

European Nuclear Medical Imaging Equipment Markets. Frost & Sullivan. 1996. 189p. spiral bd. 3900.00 (*0-7889-0626-7*, 3335-50) Frost & Sullivan.

European Nutrition Conference: 2nd Conference, Munich, September 1976: Abstracts. European Nutrition Conference Staff. Ed. by N. Zoellner et al. 1976. (Journal: Vol. 20, No. 3). 32.25 (*3-8055-2441-2*) S Karger.

European Ophthalmic Diagnostic Markets. Market Intelligence Staff. 1994. 94p. 1750.00 (*0-7889-0003-X*) Frost & Sullivan.

European Ophthalmic Laser Markets. Market Intelligence Staff. 1994. 113p. 1750.00 (*0-7889-0002-1*) Frost & Sullivan.

European Orthopaedic Soft Goods & Braces Markets. Frost and Sullivan Staff. 1995. 420p. spiral bd. 3950.00 (*0-7889-0404-3*, 3269-58) Frost & Sullivan.

European Orthopaedic Soft Goods & Cast Room Markets. Market Intelligence Staff. 1994. (Orig.). 3800.00 (*0-7889-0125-7*) Frost & Sullivan.

European Ostomy & Urine Incontinence Product Markets. Ed. by Frost and Sullivan Staff. 1997. 354p. spiral bd. 3950.00 (*0-7889-0708-5*, 3329-51) Frost & Sullivan.

European OTC Sensory Organ Treatment Markets. Frost and Sullivan Staff. 1995. LC 98-168737. 330p. spiral bd. 3800.00 (*0-7889-0313-6*, 1964-45) Frost & Sullivan.

European over the Counter Cough & Cold Medicine Markets. Market Intelligence Staff. 1994. 392p. 3800.00 (*0-7889-0141-9*) Frost & Sullivan.

European Pancreatic Club: EPC 14th Meeting, Essen, Sept.-Oct. 1982, Abstracts. Ed. by H. Goebell. 1982. (Journal: Vol. 25, No. 1). 80p. pap. 50.50 (*3-8055-3633-X*) S Karger.

European Pancreatic Club, 23rd Meeting, Lund, September 1991 Abstracts: Journal: Digestion, Vol. 49, No. 1. Ed. by I. Ihse & A. Andren-Sandberg. 1991. 64p. pap. 38.50 (*3-8055-5492-3*) S Karger.

European Pancreatic Club EPC, 15th Meeting, Verona, Sept.-Oct. 1983: Abstracts, Vol. 28, No. 1. Ed. by L. A. Scuro. 1983. (Journal). 76p. pap. 50.50 (*3-8055-3792-1*) S Karger.

European Pancreatic Club, (EPC), 16th Meeting, Cascais, Sept. 1984. Ed. by O. Bordalo. 1984. (Journal: Vol. 30, No. 2). (Illus.). 66p. pap. 50.50 (*3-8055-3956-8*) S Karger.

European Pancreatic Club (EPC) 17th Meeting, Manchester, September 1985: Abstracts. Ed. by Lynn M. Case. 1985. (Illus.). 76p. pap. 50.50 (*3-8055-4203-8*) S Karger.

European Pancreatic Club EPC, 18th Meeting, Nijmegen, September 1986: Abstracts. Ed. by J. J. De Pont. 1986. (Journal: Vol. 35, No. 1). 68p. pap. 50.50 (*3-8055-4456-1*) S Karger.

European Pancreatic Club EPC, 20th Meeting, Budapest, August 1988, Abstracts. Ed. by M. Papp. 1988. (Journal: Vol. 40, No. 2, 1988). 68p. pap. 50.50 (*3-8055-4902-4*) S Karger.

European Pancreatic Club EPC, 21st Meeting, Glasgow, September 1989. Ed. by C. W. Imrie. 1989. 64p. pap. 36.75 (*3-8055-5087-1*) S Karger.

European Pancreatic Club EPC, 26th Meeting, Bologna, September 1994: Abstracts, No. 55. Ed. by L. Gullo. 1994. (Journal: No. 5). 78p. pap. 84.50 (*3-8055-6056-7*) S Karger.

European Pancreatic Club, EPC, 27th Meeting, Barcelona, June-July 1995, Abstracts. Ed. by L. Fernandez-Cruz. 1995. (Journal: Vol. 56, No. 4, 1995). (Illus.). 70p. pap. 89.75 (*3-8055-6200-4*) S Karger.

European Pancreatic Club EPC, Abstracts 24th Meeting, Ulm, October 1992: Journal: Digestion, Vol. 52, No. 2, 1992. Ed. by H. G. Beger & M. W. Buechler. 1992. 76p. pap. 36.75 (*3-8055-5693-4*) S Karger.

European Pancreatic Club EPC, Nineteenth Meeting, Marseille, September 1987 Abstracts: Journal: Digestion, Vol. 38, No. 1. Ed. by H. Sarles. 1987. 68p. pap. 49.75 (*3-8055-4662-9*) S Karger.

European Pancreatic Club, EPC Twenty-Fifth Meeting, Paris, October 1993: Abstracts. Ed. by C. Roze & P. Bernades. 1993. (Journal: Vol. 54, No. 5, 1993). (Illus.). 62p. pap. 85.25 (*3-8055-5876-7*) S Karger.

European Pancreatic Club EPC, Twenty-Second Meeting, Basel, October 1990: Abstracts. Ed. by C. Beglinger. 1990. (Journal: Vol. 46, No. 3, 1990). 72p. pap. 38.50 (*3-8055-5315-3*) S Karger.

European Pancreatic Club Meeting (EPC) 29th Meeting, London, July 1997: Abstracts & Papers of the Young Researcher's Corner. Ed. by Giovanni Mann et al. 1997. (Digestion Ser.: Vol. 58, Suppl. 2, 1997). (Illus.). iv, 98p. pap. 44.50 (*3-8055-6552-6*) S Karger.

European Pharmaceutical Technical & Regulatory Compendium. John Sharp. 1994. 275p. 99.00 (*0-935184-57-0*) IHS Health Grp.

European Pharmacopoeia. European Pharmacopoeia Commission Staff. 2001. (*0-11-986421-5*) Statnry Office GBR. *Dist:* Balogh.

European Pharmacopoeia: Including 1998 Supplement. 1997. Vol. 97F. 3rd ed. (*92-871-2990-8*); Vol. 1998A. (*92-871-3311-5*) Council of Europe FRA. *Dist:* Manhattan Pub Co.

***European Pharmacopoeia: Supplement 4.1.** 2001. pap. (*0-11-986435-5*) Statnry Office GBR. *Dist:* Balogh.

European Pharmacopoeia Binder, Pts. 5-8. 1983. (*0-85369-001-4*) Pharmaceutical Pr GBR. *Dist:* Rittenhouse.

European Protocol on Dosimetry in Mammography, Vol. 16263. European Commission Staff. 1996. 84p. pap. (*92-827-7289-6*, CG-NA-16263-ENC) Comm Europ Commun BEL. *Dist:* Bernan Associates.

European Radiopharmaceutical Markets. 1995. 428p. spiral bd. 3800.00 (*0-7889-0370-5*, 3167-53) Frost & Sullivan.

European Rapid Microbiology Product Marekts. Frost & Sullivan. 1996. 453p. spiral bd. 3950.00 (*0-7889-0602-X*, 3337-55) Frost & Sullivan.

European Refraction Correction Markets. Market Intelligence Staff. 1994. 103p. 1750.00 (*0-7889-0001-3*) Frost & Sullivan.

European Rehabilitation Support Product Markets. Market Intelligence Staff. 1995. 374p. spiral bd. 3800.00 (*0-7889-0181-8*, 1977-58) Frost & Sullivan.

European Renal & Hemodialysis Equipment & Supplies Market. Frost and Sullivan Staff. 1996. 441p. spiral bd. 3950.00 (*0-7889-0462-0*, 3267-57) Frost & Sullivan.

European Resuscitation Council Guidelines for Resuscitation. Leo Bossaert & European Resuscitation Council Staff. 1998. LC 98-22179. 228p. 62.00 (*0-444-82957-1*) Elsevier.

European Review of Social Psychology. Wolfgang Stroebe. 2000. 336p. pap. (*0-471-89968-2*) Wiley.

European Review of Social Psychology, Vol. 8. Ed. by Wolfgang Stroebe & Miles Hewstone. 1998. 318p. 250.00 (*0-471-97949-X*) Wiley.

European RX to OTC Switching Markets. Market Intelligence Staff. 1994. 154p. 3800.00 (*0-7889-0102-8*) Frost & Sullivan.

Europcan Septic & Scpticacmia Markcts. Ed. by Frost and Sullivan Staff. 1997. 258p. spiral bd. 3950.00 (*0-7889-0675-5*, 3403-44) Frost & Sullivan.

European Septicaemia & Septic Shock Therapy Markets: Increasing Numbers of Patients Paralleled by Decreasing Treatment Costs. Market Intelligence Staff. 1993. 285p. 3800.00 (*1-56753-558-5*) Frost & Sullivan.

European Society for Developmental Pharmacology: Diablerets Proceedings, 1st Congress, 1988. Ed. by J. P. Guignard. 1990. (Journal: Vol. 13, Nos. 2-4, 1989). 150p. pap. 100.00 (*3-8055-5116-9*) S Karger.

European Society for Developmental Pharmacology, 3rd Congress, Borgholm-Sweden, May 1992. Ed. by J. P. Guignard. 1993. (Journal: Vol. 18, No. 3-4, 1992). (Illus.). iv, 116p. pap. 90.50 (*3-8055-5780-9*) S Karger.

European Society for Developmental Pharmacology, Proceedings of the 2nd Congress, Como, May 1990. Ed. by J. P. Guignard. 1991. (Journal: Vol. 15, No. 2-3, 1990). (Illus.). 116p. pap. 79.25 (*3-8055-5317-X*) S Karger.

European Society for Pediatric Endocrinlogy (EPSE) 37th Annual Meeting, Florence, September 1998:Abstracts, No. 50. Ed. by Giorgio Givannelli. 1998. (Hormone Research Ser.: No. 3). (Illus.). vi, 162p. pap. 73.25 (*3-8055-6776-6*) S Karger.

European Society for Pediatric Endocrinology, 29th Annual Meeting (ESPE), Abstracts, Vienna, September 1990: Journal: Hormone Research, Vol. 33, Suppl. 3, 1990. Ed. by H. Frisch. 1990. (Illus.). vi, 68p. pap. 32.25 (*3-8055-5288-2*) S Karger.

European Society for Pediatric Endocrinology (ESPE) 35th Annual Meeting, Montpellier, September 1996: Abstracts. Ed. by C. Sultan. 1996. (Hormone Research Ser.: Vol. 46). (Illus.). vi, 142p. pap. 64.50 (*3-8055-6375-2*) S Karger.

European Society for Pediatric Endocrinology (ESPE) 38th Annual Meeting, Warsaw, August 1999: Abstracts. Ed. by T. E. Romer. 1999. (Hormone Research Ser.: Vol. 51, Suppl. 2). (Illus.). viii, 154p. pap. 45.25 (*3-8055-6959-9*) S Karger.

European Society for Pediatric Endocrinology (ESPE) 39th Annual Meeting, Brussels, September 2000: Abstracts. J. P. Bourguignon & R. Rooman. Ed. by M. Maes. 2000. (Hormone Research Ser.: Vol. 53). (Illus.). viii, 192p. pap. 45.25 (*3-8055-7121-6*) S Karger.

European Society for Pediatric Endocrinology (ESPE) Proceedings from the 31st Annual Meeting, Zaragoza, Spain, September 1992. Ed. by A. Ferrandez Longas & J. Girard. 1993. (Journal: Vol. 38, No. 5-6, 1992). (Illus.). 96p. pap. 89.75 (*3-8055-5815-5*) S Karger.

European Society for Pediatric Endocrinology (ESPE) 30th Annual Meeting, Berlin, August 1991 - Abstracts: Journal: Hormone Research, Vol. 35, Suppl. 2, 1991. Ed. by V. Hesse. 1991. vi, 68p. pap. 29.75 (*3-8055-5462-1*) S Karger.

European Society for Pediatric Endocrinology (ESPE), 34th Annual Meeting, Edinburgh, June 1995 Abstracts. Ed. by A. Aynsley-Green & Christopher J. Kelnar. 1995. (Journal: Vol. 44, Suppl. 1, 1995). viii, 110p. pap. 52.25 (*3-8055-6174-1*) S Karger.

European Society for Pediatric Endocrinology (ESPE) & Lawson Wilkins Pediatric Endocrinology Society (LWPES) Abstracts: Third Joint Meeting, Jerusalem, October - November 1989. Ed. by Z. Laron. 1989. (Journal: Vol. 31, Suppl. 1). viii, 84p. 40.00 (*3-8055-5117-7*) S Karger.

European Society for Pediatric Endocrinology (ESPE) & the Lawson Wilkins Pediatric Endocrine Society (LWPES) 5th Joint Meeting, Stockholm, June 1997: Abstracts. Ed. by Martin Ritzen. 1997. (Hormone Research Ser.: Vol. 48, Suppl. 2, 1997). xiv, 212p. pap. 98.25 (*3-8055-6546-1*) S Karger.

European Society for Surgical Research: Abstracts, 10th, Paris, 1975. European Society for Surgical Research Staff. Ed. by J. P. Cachera. 1976. (Journal: Vol. 8, Suppl. 2). 39.25 (*3-8055-2397-1*) S Karger.

European Society for Surgical Research: Abstracts, 12th Congress, Warsaw 1977 - Journal: European Surgical Research, Vol. 9, Suppl. 1. European Society for Surgical Research Staff. Ed. by Waldemar L. Olszewski. 1977. 32.25 (*3-8055-2746-2*) S Karger.

European Society for Surgical Research: Abstracts, 13th, Helsinki, May 1978 - Journal: European Surgical Research, Vol. 10. European Society for Surgical Research Staff. Ed. by M. Lempinen et al. 1978. pap. 34.00 (*3-8055-2922-8*) S Karger.

European Society for Surgical Research: Abstracts, 22nd Congress, Aarhus, Denmark, May 1987. Ed. by J. C. Djurhuus et al. 1988. (Journal: Vol. 19, Suppl. 1, 1987). 128p. pap. 41.75 (*3-8055-4624-6*) S Karger.

European Society for Surgical Research - Abstracts, 24th Congress, Brussels, May 1989: Journal: European Surgical Research, Vol. 21, Supplement 2, 1989. Ed. by B. Hemptinne et al. 1989. x, 104p. pap. 35.00 (*3-8055-5057-X*) S Karger.

European Society for Surgical Research, 18th Congress, Athens 1983: Abstracts. Ed. by G. Androulakis & C. Pissiotis. 1983. (Journal: Vol. 15, Suppl. 1). (Illus.). iv, 120p. pap. 39.25 (*3-8055-3781-6*) S Karger.

European Society for Surgical Research, 19th Congress, Zurich 1984: Abstracts. Ed. by G. K. Uhlschmid. 1984. (Journal: Vol. 16). 124p. pap. 39.25 (*3-8055-3901-0*) S Karger.

European Society for Surgical Research, 20th Congress, Rotterdam 1985: Abstracts. Ed. by H. J. Jeekel. 1985. (Journal: Vol. 17; Suppl. 1). xii, 118p. pap. 39.25 (*3-8055-4078-7*) S Karger.

European Society for Surgical Research, 21st Congress, Nancy 1986 Abstracts. Ed. by R. Benichoux & M. Merle. 1986. (Journal: Vol. 18, Suppl. 1, 1986). (Illus.). xii, 112p. pap. 38.50 (*3-8055-4383-2*) S Karger.

European Society for Surgical Research, 25th Congress, Berlin GDR, May 1990 Abstracts. Ed. by D. Attig et al. 1990. (Illus.). x, 110p. pap. 52.25 (*3-8055-5221-1*) S Karger.

European Society for Surgical Research, Congress, Bologna, 23rd, May 1988: Abstracts. Ed. by G. Ussia. 1988. (Journal: Vol. 20, Suppl. 1). xviii, 196p. (Orig.). pap. 46.25 (*3-8055-4826-5*) S Karger.

European Society for Surgical Research (ESSR) 34th Congress of the European Society for Surgical Research, Bern, April 1999: Abstracts. Ed. by M. W. Buchler & H. U. Baer. 1999. (European Surgical Research Ser.: Vol. 31, Suppl. 1 (1999)). xxxii, 244p. pap. 47.00 (*3-8055-6892-4*) S Karger.

European Society for Surgical Research (ESSR) 35th Congress, Malmo, June 2000: Abstracts. Ed. by C. Vagianos et al. 2000. (European Surgical Research Ser.: Vol. 32). xvi, 118p. pap. 39.25 (*3-8055-7093-7*) S Karger.

European Society for Surgical Research (ESSR) Abstracts from 33rd Congress, Padua, Italy April 22 - 25, 1998. Ed. by Paolo Rigotti et al. 1998. (European Surgical Research Ser.: Vol. 30, Suppl. 1). xii, 134p. pap. 44.50 (*3-8055-6699-9*) S Karger.

European Society for Surgical Research (ESSR), 28th Congress, Turku - Finland, May 1993 Abstracts. Ed. by H. Aro & J. Niinikoski. 1993. (Journal: Vol. 25, Suppl. 1, 1993). (Illus.). xii, 124p. pap. 41.75 (*3-8055-5794-9*) S Karger.

European Society for Surgical Research (ESSR) 30th Congress, Amsterdam, May 1995: Abstracts. Ed. by T. M. van Gulik et al. 1995. (Journal: Vol. 27, Suppl. 1, 1995). (Illus.). xii, 130p. pap. 43.50 (*3-8055-6202-0*) S Karger.

European Society for Surgical Research (ESSR) Abstracts, 27th Congress, May 1992, Zaragoza, Spain: Journal: European Surgical Research, Vol. 24, Suppl. 2, 1992. Ed. by J. R. Morandeira et al. 1992. (Illus.). xii, 124p. pap. 41.75 (*3-8055-5615-2*) S Karger.

European Society for Surgical Research Festchrift, 20 Years. Ed. by W. Brendel & K. Messmer. 1986. (Journal: Vol. 18, No. 3-4, 1986). (Illus.). 144p. pap. 108.00 (*3-8055-4384-0*) S Karger.

European Society for Surgical Research Twenty-Sixth Congress, Salzburg, Austria, May 1991: Abstracts. Ed. by H. W. Waclawiczek et al. 1991. xiv, 150p. pap. 50.50 (*3-8055-5421-4*) S Karger.

European Society of Human Genetics: Abstracts. Ed. by G. J. Van Ommen. 1996. (Journal: Vol. 4, Suppl. 1, 1996). (Illus.). iv, 188p. pap., suppl. ed. 31.50 (*3-8055-6317-5*) S Karger.

European Society of Neurosonology & Cerebral Hemodynamics: 4th Meeting, Venice, April 1999: Abstracts. Ed. by E. M. Zanette et al. 1999. (Cerebrovascular Diseases Ser.: Vol. 9, Suppl. 2 (1999)). (Illus.). iv, 60p. pap. 25.25 (*3-8055-6869-X*) S Karger.

European Society of Neurosonology & Cerebral Hemodynamics: 5th Meeting, Graz, Austria, May 2000: Abstracts. Ed. by K. Niederkorn et al. 2000. (Cerebrovascular Diseases Ser.: Vol. 10, Suppl. 1, 2000). x, 48p. pap. 25.25 (*3-8055-7109-7*) S Karger.

European Society Surgical Research, 16th Congress, Garmisch-Partenkirchen, April 1981. Ed. by K. Messmer et al. 1981. (Journal: Vol. 13, Suppl. 1). (Illus.). viii, 104p. pap. 35.75 (*3-8055-2644-X*) S Karger.

European Society Surgical Research, 17th Congress, Stresa, May 1982: Abstracts. Ed. by R. Dionigi et al. 1982. (Journal: Vol. 14, No. 2). (Illus.). 120p. pap. 39.25 (*3-8055-3558-9*) S Karger.

European Special & Dietetic Food Markets. Ed. by Frost and Sullivan Staff. 1997. 324p. spiral bd. 3950.00 (*0-7889-0730-1*, 3369-88) Frost & Sullivan.

European Stroke Conference: Abstracts from 7th Conference, Edinburgh, U. K. May 27 - 30, 1998. Ed. by Michael Hennerici. 1998. (Cerebrovascular Diseases Ser.: Vol. 8, Suppl. 4). xii, 110p. pap. 46.25 (*3-8055-6712-X*) S Karger.

European Stroke Conference: Abstracts of the 8th Conference, Venice, April, 1999. Ed. by M. G. Hennerici. 1999. (Cerebrovascular Diseases Ser.: Vol. 9, Suppl. 1 (1999)). (Illus.). 130p. pap. 39.25 (*3-8055-6871-1*) S Karger.

European Stroke Conference: Abstracts of the 9th European Stroke Conference, Vienna, Austria, May 2000. Ed. by M. G. Hennerici. 2000. (Cerebrovascular Diseases Ser.: Vol. 10, Suppl. 2). xii, 116p. pap. 39.25 (*3-8055-7096-1*) S Karger.

European Stroke Conference - 6th Conference, Amsterdam, May 1997: Abstracts. Ed. by M. G. Hennerici. 1997. (Cerebrovascular Diseases Ser.: Vol. 7, Suppl. 4, 1997). (Illus.). x, 94p. pap. 41.00 (*3-8055-6538-0*) S Karger.

European Studies on the Incidence of Dementing Diseases: A Report of the EURODEM Research Group - Neuroepidemiology Journal, 1992, Vol. 11, Suppl. 1. Ed. by L. J. Launer et al. 1992. (Illus.). vi, 122p. pap. 39.25 (*3-8055-5593-8*) S Karger.

European Surgical Disposable Product Markets: Challenges & Opportunities in Eight Regions & Seven Products Sectors. Frost and Sullivan Staff. 1995. LC 98-168609. 522p. spiral bd. 3800.00 (*0-7889-0291-1*, 1966-51) Frost & Sullivan.

European Synthetic Lubricant Markets. Market Intelligence Staff. 1994. 184p. 3800.00 (*0-7889-0154-0*) Frost & Sullivan.

European Technical Conference on the Control of Infectious Diseases Through Vaccination Programmes. 1960. (Technical Report Ser.: No. 198). 21p. pap. text 3.00 (*92-4-120198-3*) World Health.

European Uninterruptible Power Supply & Power Conditioning Markets. Market Intelligence Staff. 1993. 250p. (Orig.). 3900.00 (*1-56753-885-1*) Frost & Sullivan.

European Union: Active Implantable Medical Device. Intro. by Melinda C. Bailey. 1996. 75p. 64.95 (*1-57172-058-8*) Intl Qual.

European Union: EMEA Authorization Directive. Intro. by Melinda C. Bailey. 1996. 153p. 94.95 (*1-57172-068-5*) Intl Qual.

European Union: Good Laboratory Practices. Intro. by Melinda C. Bailey. 1996. 84p. 69.95 (*1-57172-061-8*) Intl Qual.

European Union: In-Vitro Diagnostic Directive. Intro. by Melinda C. Bailey. 1996. 118p. 99.95 (*1-57172-066-9*) Intl Qual.

European Union Biomedical & Health Research: The EU Biomed 1 Program. A. Baert. 1995. LC 94-7731. (Biomedical & Health Research Ser.: Vol. 9). 1000p. 130.00 (*90-5199-173-8*) IOS Press.

Eurythmy: Essays & Anecdotes in Art, Education & Therapy. Ed. by Eva Lauterbach. 1981. LC 80-22938. (Illus.). 256p. (Orig.). pap. 15.95 (*0-935690-01-8*) Schaumburg Pubns.

Eustachian Tube & Middle Ear Diseases. Iwao Honjo. 1989. (Illus.). 182p. 166.00 (*0-387-70033-1*) Spr-Verlag.

Eustachian Tube & Middle Ear Diseases, Clinical Aspects. Ed. by Jacob Sade. 1991. LC 91-20840. (Illus.). 417p. lib. bdg. (*90-6299-079-7*) Kugler NLD. *Dist:* Lib Res.

***Euthanasia.** Lisa Yount. 2001. LC 2001-33778. (Contemporary Issues Companion Ser.). 174p. 31.20 (*0-7377-0829-8*); pap. 19.95 (*0-7377-0828-X*) Gale (Greenhaven Pr).

Euthanasia: Killing or Caring? Rita L. Marker. 1992. (Orig.). (C). pap. 2.00 (*0-919225-36-5*) Life Cycle Bks.

Euthanasia: Moral & Pastoral Perspectives. Richard M. Gula. 1995. LC 94-34075. 96p. pap. 5.95 (*0-8091-3539-6*) Paulist Pr.

Euthanasia: Opposing Viewpoints. Ed. by Carol Wekesser. rev. ed. 1995. (Opposing Viewpoints Ser.). (Illus.). 214p. lib. bdg. 26.20 (*1-56510-244-4*, 2444, Greenhaven Pr) Gale.

Euthanasia: Or, Medical Treatment in Aid of an Easy Death. William Munk. Ed. by Robert J. Kastenbaum. 1979. LC 76-19584. (Death & Dying Ser.). reprint ed. lib. bdg. 21.95 (*0-405-09580-5*) Ayer.

Euthanasia: The Good of the Patient, the Good of Society. Ed. by Robert I. Misbin. 1992. 245p. 35.00 (*1-55572-017-X*) Univ Pub Group.

Euthanasia: The Moral Issues. Ed. by Robert M. Baird & Stuart E. Rosenbaum. 1989. LC 89-24042. (Contemporary Issues Ser.). 216p. (Orig.). (C). pap. 19.00 (*0-87975-555-5*) Prometheus Bks.

***Euthanasia - Death, Dying & the Medical Duty.** G. R. Dunstan & P. J. Lachmann. 1996. (British Medical Bulletin Ser.: Vol. 52, No. 2). 171p. pap. (*1-85315-278-1*) Royal Soc of Medicine Pr Ltd GBR. *Dist:* Balogh.

Euthanasia & Assisted Suicide: Psychosocial Issues. Samuel I. Greenberg. 1997. LC 97-16298. (American Behavioral Science & Law Ser.). 188p. text 56.95 (*0-398-06785-6*) C C Thomas.

Euthanasia & Other Medical Decisions Concerning the End of Life. P. J. Van der Maas et al. 1992. (Health Policy Monographs: Vol. 2). 262p. 159.00 (*0-444-89278-8*) Elsevier.

Euthanasia & Physician-Assisted Suicide, Killing or Caring. Contrib. by Michael Manning. 1998. LC 98-17655. 96p. pap. 8.95 (*0-8091-3804-2*, 3804-2) Paulist Pr.

Euthanasia & the Newborn: Conflicts Regarding Saving Lives. Ed. by Richard C. McMillan et al. 1987. (Philosophy & Medicine Ser.: No. 24). 340p. lib. bdg. 117.50 (*90-277-2299-4*) Kluwer Academic.

Euthanasia & the Newborn: Conflicts Regarding Saving Lives. Richard C. McMillan et al. 1987. LC 86-33835. (Philosophy & Medicine Ser.: Vol. 24). 343p. (C). pap. text 64.50 (*1-55608-039-5*) Kluwer Academic.

Euthanasia, Clinical Practice & the Law. Ed. by Luke Gormally. 256p. pap. text (*0-906561-08-6*) Linacre Centre GBR. *Dist:* St Augustines Pr.

Euthanasia Controversy, 1812-1974: A Bibliography with Select Annotations. Charles W. Triche, III & Diane Samson Triche. annot. ed. 1975. LC 75-8379. ix, 242p. 40.00 (*0-87875-071-1*) Whitston Pub.

Euthanasia Is Not the Answer: A Hospice Physician's View. David Cundiff. 1992. LC 92-17245. 190p. 29.95 (*0-89603-237-X*) Humana.

Euthanasia, Right or Wrong? (Or Tell-Tale Signs of Murders) Isaac I. Omoike. 1995. LC 94-90564. 169p. (Orig.). (C). pap. text 19.95 (*0-9632236-3-1*) I Omoike Bks.

Euthenics: The Science of Controllable Environment: A Plea for Better Conditions As a First Step Toward Higher Human Efficiency. Ellen H. Richards. Ed. by Barbara G. Rosenkrantz. 1977. LC 76-40639. (Public Health in America Ser.). (Illus.). reprint ed. lib. bdg. 19.95 (*0-405-09827-8*) Ayer.

Evacuated Tubes for Blood Specimen Collection. National Committee for Clinical Laboratory Standards. 3rd ed. 1991. (Approved Standard Ser.). 75.00 (*1-56238-107-5*, H1-A3) NCCLS.

Evacuation of the Sick & the Wounded. 1990. lib. bdg. 79.95 (*0-87700-897-3*) Revisionist Pr.

Evaluating AIDS Prevention Programs. National Research Council Staff. Ed. by Susan L. Coyle et al. exp. ed. 1991. 392p. (Orig.). (C). pap. 39.95 (*0-309-04281-X*) Natl Acad Pr.

Evaluating Alternative Cancer Therapies: A Guide to the Science & Politics of an Emerging Medical Field. David J. Hess. 1999. LC 98-7541. 288p. (C). text 35.00 (*0-8135-2594-2*) Rutgers U Pr.

Evaluating & Improving Written Expression: A Practical Guide for Teachers. Beverly Salas et al. 3rd ed. 1997. LC 97-1537. 250p. spiral bd. 39.00 (*0-89079-715-3*, 8438) PRO-ED.

Evaluating & Negotiating Compensation Arrangements: Understanding the Process & Ensuring You. American Medical Association Staff. 1998. LC 00-265882. (Career Development Ser.). 69p. pap. text 39.95 (*0-89970-894-3*) AMA.

Evaluating & Testing in Nursing Eduction. Marilyn H. Oermann & Kathleen B. Gaberson. 1998. LC 97-42741. (Teaching of Nursing Ser.). (Illus.). 336p. 43.95 (*0-8261-9950-X*) Springer Pub.

Evaluating & Treating Adult Children of Alcoholics: A Guide for Professionals, Vol. I: Evaluation. Timmen L. Cermak. 1990. 225p. text 24.95 (*0-935908-64-1*, 3269, HazeldenJohnson Inst) Hazelden.

Evaluating & Treating Adult Children of Alcoholics: A Guide for Professionals, Vol. II: Treatment. Timmen L. Cermak. 1991. 316p. text 24.95 (*0-935908-66-8*, 3270, HazeldenJohnson Inst) Hazelden.

Evaluating Care Management for Older People. Ed. by Judith Phillips & Bridget Penhale. 1995. LC 95-32046. 250p. pap. (*1-85302-317-5*) Jessica Kingsley GBR. *Dist:* Taylor & Francis.

Evaluating Children for the Courts Using Psychological Tests. Stanley Kissel & Nelson W. Freeling. 1990. 102p. (C). text 32.95 (*0-398-05647-1*) C C Thomas.

Evaluating Competencies: Forensic Assessments & Instruments. Thomas Grisso. 1986. LC 85-28190. (Perspectives in Law & Psychology Ser.: Vol. 7). (Illus.). 414p. (C). 57.50 (*0-306-42126-7*, Plenum Trade) Perseus Pubng.

Evaluating Costs & Outcomes: Demonstrating the Value of Rehabilitation Services. Diane E. Watson. 1999. LC 00-500747. (Illus.). xi, 179p. pap. (*1-56900-138-3*) Am Occup Therapy.

Evaluating Couples: A Handbook for Practitioners. Mark A. Karpel. 1994. LC 94-32970. 368p. 40.00 (*0-393-70180-8*) Norton.

Evaluating Critical Care: Using Health Services Research to Improve Quality. Ed. by William J. Sibbald et al. 2000. LC 00-57414. (Update in Intensive Care & Emergency Medicine Ser.: Vol. 35). (Illus.). 400p. 149.00 (*3-540-67776-3*) Spr-Verlag.

Evaluating Family Mental Health: History, Epidemiology & Treatment Issues. J. J. Schwab et al. 1994. (Critical Issues in Psychiatry Ser.). (Illus.). 452p. (C). text 69.50 (*0-306-44436-4*, Kluwer Plenum) Kluwer Academic.

Evaluating Health Care Information Systems: Methods & Applications. Ed. by James G. Anderson et al. 1993. LC 93-27074. (Illus.). 320p. (C). pap. 42.95 (*0-8039-4936-7*, 4202) Sage.

Evaluating Health Interventions: An Introduction to Evaluation of Health Treatments, Services, Policies & Organizational Interventions. John Ovretveit. 1997. LC 97-8733. (*0-335-19965-8*); 336p. pap. (*0-335-19964-X*) OpUniv Pr.

Evaluating Health Maintenance Organizations: A Guide for Employee Benefits Managers. Perry Moore. 1991. LC 91-4719. 208p. 62.95 (*0-89930-557-1*, MHG/, Quorum Bks) Greenwood.

Evaluating Health Projects: Lessons from the Literature. Susan Strout et al. 1997. LC 97-1485. (Discussion Paper Ser.: No. 356). 132p. pap. 22.00 (*0-8213-3881-1*, 13881) World Bank.

Evaluating Health Risks: An Economic Approach. Per-Olov Johansson. 1995. (Illus.). 200p. (C). text 59.95 (*0-521-47285-7*); pap. text 19.95 (*0-521-47878-2*) Cambridge U Pr.

Evaluating Health Services' Effectiveness: A Guide for Health Professionals, Service Managers & Policy Makers. Ed. by A. S. St. Leger et al. 1991. 224p. pap. (*0-335-09356-6*) OpUniv Pr.

Evaluating HIV Prevention Interventions. Joanne E. Mantell et al. 1997. LC 96-53003. (Volume in AIDS Prevention & Mental Health Ser.). (Illus.). 310p. (C). text 45.00 (*0-306-45476-9*, Kluwer Plenum) Kluwer Academic.

Evaluating HIV/AIDS Treatment Programs: Innovative Methods & Findings. Ed. by George J. Huba et al. 2000. LC 00-47218. (Drugs & Socity Monograph: Vol. 16, Nos. 1-2). (Illus.). 284p. 49.95 (*0-7890-1190-5*) Haworth Pr.

Evaluating in Practice. Ian Shaw. 1996. 224p. (*1-85742-232-5*) Arena GBR. *Dist:* Ashgate Pub Co.

Evaluating Managed Mental Health Services: The Fort Bragg Experiment. Leonard Bickman et al. 1995. (Illus.). 219p. 42.50 (*0-306-45044-5*, Plenum Trade) Perseus Pubng.

Evaluating Medical School Courses: A User-Centered Handbook. Neal A. Whitman & Thomas W. Cockayne. 2nd ed. 1984. 35p. (C). reprint ed. pap. text 10.00 (*0-940193-02-7*) Univ UT Sch Med.

Evaluating Medical Tests: Objective & Quantitative Guidelines. Helena C. Kraemer. 1992. (Illus.). 288p. (C). 67.95 (*0-8039-4611-2*, 3653); pap. 34.95 (*0-8039-4612-0*, 3654) Sage.

Evaluating Mental Health Practice: Methods & Applications. Ed. by Derek Milne. 1987. 288p. lib. bdg. (*0-7099-4626-0*) C Helm GBR. *Dist:* Routldge.

Evaluating Mental Health Services: How Do Programs for Children "Work" in the Real World? Carol T. Nixon & Denine A. Northrup. 1997. LC 96-35681. (Children's Mental Health Services Annual Ser.: Vol. 3). 312p. 66.95 (*0-7619-0795-5*, 80815); pap. 31.95 (*0-7619-0796-3*, 80816) Sage.

Evaluating Noncognitive Skills & Clinical Performance. 1982. 24.95 (*0-934277-00-1*) Am Bd Med Spec.

Evaluating Nursing Interventions: A Theory-Driven Approach. Souraya Sidani & Carrie J. Braden. 1997. LC 97-21227. 210p. 66.95 (*0-7619-0315-1*, 2337); pap. 32.95 (*0-7619-0316-X*, 2338) Sage.

Evaluating Palliative Care: Establishing the Evidence Base. Margaret Robbins. 1998. (Illus.). 192p. pap. text 32.50 (*0-19-262621-3*) OUP.

Evaluating Preventive Care: Report on a Workshop. Louise B. Russell. 1987. LC 87-9304. 107p. text 26.95 (*0-8157-7626-8*); pap. text 9.95 (*0-8157-7625-X*) Brookings.

Evaluating Primary Health Care in South-East Asia. 1984. (SEARO Technical Publications Ser.). 217p. pap. text 7.00 (*92-9022-143-7*) World Health.

Evaluating Psychological Information: Sharpening Your Critical Thinking Skills. Bell. 3rd ed. 1998. 64p. pap. text 12.00 (*0-205-28635-6*) Allyn.

Evaluating Radiographs. Quinn B. Carroll. 1993. LC 93-8350. (Illus.). 374p. (C). 46.95 (*0-398-05878-4*) C C Thomas.

Evaluating Research in Communicative Disorders. Nicholas Schiavetti & Dale Metz. 3rd rev. ed. 1996. LC 96-23757. (Illus.). 446p. (C). 73.00 (*0-205-19396-X*) Allyn.

Evaluating, Selecting & Using Assistive Technology. Jan J. Galvin & Marcia J. Scherer. 1995. LC 96-15711. 304p. pap. 70.00 (*0-8342-0664-1*, 20664) PRO-ED.

Evaluating Sleep in Infants & Children. Stephen H. Sheldon. 1995. 288p. text 89.00 (*0-397-51628-2*) Lppncott W & W.

Evaluating Stress Vol. 2: A Book of Resources. Ed. by Carlos P. Zalaquett & Richard J. Wood. 1998. (Illus.). 378p. 69.50 (*0-8108-3522-3*) Scarecrow.

Evaluating the Cost-Effectiveness of Counselling in Health Care. Nancy Rowland & Keith Tolley. 1995. LC 94-47491. 256p. (C). pap. 29.95 (*0-415-07661-7*, C0326); (gr. 13). 90.00 (*0-415-07660-9*, C0325) Routledge.

Evaluating the Health Care System: Effectiveness, Efficiency, & Equity. Lu Ann Aday. 2nd ed. 1998. LC 98-12225. 334p. 45.00 (*1-56793-079-4*) Health Admin Pr.

Evaluating the National Health Service Reforms. Ray Robinson & Julia Le Grand. 1994. (Reshaping the Public Sector Ser.: Vol. 8). 275p. (C). 34.95 (*1-56000-194-1*); pap. 24.95 (*1-56000-796-6*) Transaction Pubs.

Evaluating the NHS. D. Powell. 1997. LC 96-39950. (State of Health Ser.). pap. (*0-335-19530-X*) OpUniv Pr.

Evaluating the Quality of Health Care: What Research Offers Decision Makers. Lee Greenfield et al. 1996. LC 97-140825. 32p. (Orig.). pap. (*1-887748-04-0*) Milbank Memorial.

Evaluating the Reliability of Biokinetic & Dosimetric Models & Parameters Used to Assess Individual Doses for Risk Assessment Purposes. National Council on Radiation Protection and Measure. 1998. LC 98-4408. (NCRP Commentaries Ser.: Vol. 15). 119p. pap. 30.00 (*0-929600-58-4*) NCRP Pubns.

Evaluation: Obtaining & Interpreting Data. Ed. by Jim Hinojosa & Paula Kramer. 1998. LC 98-145738. 299p. pap. text 36.00 (*1-56900-090-5*, 1174) Am Occup Therapy.

Evaluation & Accountability in Clinical Training. B. A. Edelstein & E. Berler. 1987. (Illus.). 400p. (C). 85.00 (*0-306-42510-6*, Plenum Trade) Perseus Pubng.

Evaluation & Care of Severely Disturbed Children & Their Families. Leon Hoffman. 1982. text 22.50 (*0-88331-141-0*) R B Luce.

Evaluation & Control of Meat Quality in Pigs. P. V. Tarrant et al. 1987. (Current Topics in Veterinary Medicine & Animal Science Ser.). text 306.50 (*0-89838-854-6*) Kluwer Academic.

Evaluation & Decision Making for Health Services. James E. Veney & Arnold D. Kaluzny. 3rd ed. 1998. LC 98-18954. 436p. 60.00 (*1-56793-088-3*) Health Admin Pr.

Evaluation & Diagnostic Test in Neuromuscular Disorders. Bertorini. 2001. 400p. 80.00 (*0-7506-7290-0*) Buttrwrth-Heinemann.

***Evaluation & Habilitation of the Hearing-Impaired Child.** Darius Kohan & Laurie Hanin. 2001. LC 00-52576. (Illus.). 102p. pap. 30.00 (*1-56772-031-5*, 5506370) AAO-HNS.

Evaluation & Installation of Surgical Laser Systems. Ed. by David B. Apfelberg. 1986. (Illus.). 324p. 133.00 (*0-387-96385-5*) Spr-Verlag.

Evaluation & Management of Early HIV Infection: Clinical Practice Guideline. 1994. (Illus.). 196p. (Orig.). (C). pap. text 50.00 (*0-7881-1088-8*) DIANE Pub.

Evaluation & Management of Gait Disorders. Ed. by Barney S. Spivack. 1994. LC 94-24238. (Neurological Disease & Therapy Ser.: Vol. 35). (Illus.). 368p. text 180.00 (*0-8247-9586-5*) Dekker.

Evaluation & Management of the Thyroid Nodule: A Practical Approach. Scott R. Schoem et al. 1998. LC 98-6429. (Self-Instructional Package Ser.). (Illus.). 112p. pap. text 25.00 (*1-56772-064-1*) AAO-HNS.

Evaluation & Management Percentages & Policies. 10th ed. 2000. 150p. pap. text 79.00 (*1-58383-113-4*, EMPAPO) Robert D Keene.

Evaluation & Performance Criteria for Multiple Component Test Products Intended for the Detection & Quantitation of Rubella IgG Antibody: Tentative Guideline (1992) Contrib. by Laurence P. Skendzel. 1992. 75.00 (*1-56238-158-X*, I/LA6-T) NCCLS.

Evaluation & Rehabilitation of the Shoulder: An Integration of the Guide to Physical Therapist Practice. Brian J. Tovin & Bruce H. Greenfield. 2001. LC 00-65752. (Contemporary Perspectives in Rehabilitation Ser.). (Illus.). 464p. (C). 45.00 (*0-8036-0262-6*) Davis Co.

Evaluation & Testing of Drugs for Mutagenicity, Principles & Problems: Proceedings of the WHO Scientific Group, Geneva, 1971. WHO Staff. 1971. (Technical Reports: No. 482). pap. text 3.00 (*92-4-120482-6*, 1100482) World Health.

Evaluation & Treatment of Adolescents & Children. Ed. & Frwd. by Diane Gibson. 1987. LC 87-25109. (Occupational Therapy in Mental Health Ser.: Vol. 7, No. 2). 114p. text 3.95 (*0-86656-658-9*) Haworth Pr.

Evaluation & Treatment of Chronic Pain. Ed. by Gerald M. Aronoff. (Illus.). 2nd rev. ed. 1992. 608p. 99.00 (*0-683-00261-9*); 3rd ed. 1998. LC 98-22557. 730p. text 149.00 (*0-683-30149-7*) Lppncott W & W.

Evaluation & Treatment of Eating Disorders. Ed. by Diane Gibson. 1986. LC 85-24856. (Occupational Therapy in Mental Health Ser.: Vol. 6, No. 1). 150p. 39.95 (*0-86656-541-8*) Haworth Pr.

E F G

Evaluation & Treatment of Mild Traumatic Brain Injury. Ed. by Nils R. Varney & Richard J. Roberts. 1999. LC 98-33439. 552p. 99.95 (*0-8058-2393-X*); pap. 49.95 (*0-8058-2394-8*) L Erlbaum Assocs.

Evaluation & Treatment of Myopathies. Robert C. Griggs et al. 1995. LC 94-10338. (Contemporary Neurology Ser.: No. 44). (Illus.). 464p. 135.00 (*0-8036-4410-8*) OUP.

Evaluation & Treatment of Postpartum Emotional Disorders. Ann L. Dunnewold. 1997. LC 96-47166. (Practitioner's Resource Ser.). 112p. pap. 17.95 (*1-56887-024-8*, ETPEBP, Prof Resc Pr) Pro Resource.

Evaluation & Treatment of Swallowing Disorders. Jerilyn A. Logemann. (Illus.). 1983. LC 90-52769. 249p. (C). text 38.00 (*0-89079-274-7*, 1729); 2nd rev. ed. 1998. LC 97-20659. 510p. text 42.00 (*0-89079-728-5*, 8483) PRO-ED.

Evaluation & Treatment of the Aging Face. Ed. by Melvin L. Elson. 1995. LC 94-14223. (Illus.). 341p. 155.00 (*0-387-94237-8*) Spr-Verlag.

Evaluation & Treatment of the Infertile Male. Ed. by Grace M. Centola & Kenneth Ginsburg. 1996. (Illus.). 336p. (C). text 90.00 (*0-521-45059-4*) Cambridge U Pr.

Evaluation & Treatment of the Psychogeriatric Patient. Intro. by Diane Gibson. 1991. (Occupational Therapy in Mental Health Ser.). 113p. text 39.95 (*1-56024-052-0*) Haworth Pr.

Evaluation & Treatment of Urinary Incontinence. Ed. by Jerry G. Blaivas. 1996. (Topics in Clinical Urology Ser.). (Illus.). 208p. 69.00 (*0-89640-306-8*) Igaku-Shoin.

Evaluation, Diagnosis & Treatment of Occlusal Problems. Ed. by Peter E. Dawson. 2nd ed. 1988. (Illus.). 632p. (C). (gr. 13). text 145.00 (*0-8016-2788-5*, 02788) Mosby Inc.

Evaluation Fundamentals: Guiding Health Programs, Research, & Policies. Arlene Fink. 1993. (Illus.). 256p. (C). 71.95 (*0-8039-4838-7*, 4335); pap. 37.95 (*0-8039-4839-5*, 4336) Sage.

Evaluation in Education, Vol. 4, No. 3. Ed. by B. H. Choppin. 1981. LC 77-81507. (Illus.). 93p. pap. 25.00 (*0-08-027134-0*, Pergamon Pr) Elsevier.

Evaluation in Education, Vol. 8. Ed. by Herbert J. Walberg & T. Neville Postlethwaite. 1985. (International Review Ser.). (Illus.). 288p. (*0-08-032732-X*) PPL GBR. *Dist:* Elsevier.

Evaluation in Health Promotion. Ed. by David Scott & Ros Weston. 1998. 224p. pap. (*0-7487-3313-2*) Nelson Thornes GBR. *Dist:* Intl Spec Bk, Trans-Atl Phila.

Evaluation in Occupational Health Practice. Ewa Menckel & Peter Westerholm. 1999. LC 99-29660. (Arnold Publication). 256p. 72.00 (*0-7506-4303-X*) OUP.

Evaluation in the Health Services. 1972. 75p. 90.00 (*0-7855-7184-1*) St Mut.

Evaluation Methods & Analytical Performance Characteristics of Immunological Assays for Human Immunoglobulin E (IGE) Antibodies of Defined Allergen Specificities: Approved Guideline (1997) 1997. 65.00 (*1-56238-343-4*, I/LA20-A) NCCLS.

Evaluation Methods in Laboratory Medicine. Ed. by Rainer Haeckel. 1992. LC 92-49050. 315p. pap. 215.00 (*3-527-30002-3*, Wiley-VCH) Wiley.

Evaluation Methods in Medical Informatics. Charles P. Friedman & Jeremy Wyatt. 1996. LC 96-1841. (Computers & Medicine Ser.). (Illus.). 330p. 69.00 (*0-387-94228-9*) Spr-Verlag.

Evaluation of a Cancer Information Telephone Facility: Can-Dial. Gregg S. Wilkinson et al. 1984. LC 84-26399. 144p. 60.00 (*0-275-91348-1*, C1348, Praeger Pubs) Greenwood.

Evaluation of a Medicaid-Eligibility Expansion in Florida: Developing the Database. Ellen R. Harrison et al. 1996. LC 96-47872. 22p. (Orig.). pap. 15.00 (*0-8330-2462-0*, MR-702-HCFA/MOD) Rand Corp.

Evaluation of a Preventative Program in Young Children with Rampant Caries Treated under General Anaesthesia. Sotiria Gizani. 1998. (Acta Biomedica Lovaniensia Ser.). (Illus.). 150p. pap. (*90-6186-898-X*) Leuven Univ BEL. *Dist:* Coronet Bks.

***Evaluation of Alginate Microcapsules for Use in Transplantation of Islets of Langerhans.** Aileen King. 2001. (Comprehensive Summaries of Uppsala Dissertations from the Faculty of Medicine Ser.: No. 1072). (Illus.). 43p. pap. (*91-554-5113-6*) Acta Univ SWE. *Dist:* Coronet Bks.

Evaluation of Beta Blocker & Calcium Antagonist Drugs. Joel Morganroth & E. Neil Moore. 1982. text 176.50 (*90-247-2642-5*) Kluwer Academic.

Evaluation of Beta-Blockers, Calcium Antagonists, Nitrates & Alternative Therapies for Stable Angina. Kathryn M. McDonald et al. 2000. (Evidence Report/Technology Assessment Ser.: No. 10). 128p. pap. (*1-58763-006-0*) Agency Healthcare.

Evaluation of Cancer Screening. Ed. by Jocelyn Chamberlain & Sue Moss. 1995. LC 95-23890. (Focus on Cancer Ser.). 204p. 46.00 (*3-540-19957-8*) Spr-Verlag.

Evaluation of Cardiac Contractility. Ed. by Ruthard Jacob. 1990. 155p. pap. (*0-89574-307-8*) Gustav Fischer DEU. *Dist:* Lubrecht & Cramer, Balogh.

Evaluation of Cardiac Function by Echocardiography. Ed. by W. Bleifeld et al. 1980. (Illus.). 198p. 53.00 (*0-387-10045-8*) Spr-Verlag.

Evaluation of Certain Food Additives. (Technical Report Ser.: No. 669). 1981. 48p. pap. text 3.00 (*92-4-120669-1*); 1980. 45p. pap. text 3.00 (*92-4-120648-9*); 1980. 38p. pap. text 3.00 (*92-4-120653-5*) World Health.

Evaluation of Certain Food Additives: Twenty-First Report of the Joint FAO/WHO Expert Committee on Food Additives. 1978. (Technical Report Ser.: No. 617). 41p. pap. text 5.00 (*92-4-120617-9*, 1100617) World Health.

Evaluation of Certain Food Additives & Contaminants. 1982. (Technical Report Ser.: No. 683). 51p. pap. text 5.00 (*92-4-120683-7*) World Health.

Evaluation of Certain Food Additives & Contaminants: 44th Report of the Joint FAO-WHO Expert Committee on Food Additives. 1995. (Technical Report Ser.: Vol. 859). (FRE & SPA.). 54p. (C). pap. 11.00 (*92-4-120859-7*, 1100859) World Health.

Evaluation of Certain Food Additives & Contaminants: Forty-First Report of the Joint FAO-WHO Expert Committee on Food Additives. 1993. (Technical Reports: No. 837). (ENG, FRE & SPA.). viii, 53p. pap. text 10.00 (*92-4-120837-6*, 1100837) World Health.

Evaluation of Certain Food Additives & Contaminants: Report of the Joint FAO-WHO Expert Committee on Food Additives, 29th. 1986. (Technical Reports: No. 733). 60p. pap. text 9.00 (*92-4-120733-7*, 1100733) World Health.

Evaluation of Certain Food Additives & Contaminants: Thirty-Seventh Report of the Joint FAO-WHO Expert Committee on Food Additives. 1991. (Technical Reports: No. 806). (ENG, FRE & SPA.). 49p. pap. text 10.00 (*92-4-120806-6*, 1100806) World Health.

Evaluation of Certain Food Additives & Contaminants: Twenty-Second Report of the Joint FAO/WHO Expert Committee on Food Additives. 1978. (Technical Report Ser.: No. 631). 39p. pap. text 5.00 (*92-4-120631-4*, 1100631) World Health.

Evaluation of Certain Veterinary Drug Residues in Food: 43rd Report of the Joint FAO-WHO Expert Committee on Food Additives. 1995. (Technical Reports: Vol. 855). (FRE & SPA.). 59p. (C). pap. 12.00 (*92-4-120855-4*, 1100855) World Health.

Evaluation of Certain Veterinary Drug Residues in Food: 45th Report of a WHO Scientific Group, Report 34. 1996. (WHO Technical Reports: Vol. 864). 66p. (Orig.). pap. 10.80 (*92-4-120864-3*, 1100864) World Health.

Evaluation of Certain Veterinary Drug Residues in Food: Fortieth Report of the Joint FAO-WHO Expert Committee on Food Additives. 1993. (Technical Reports: No. 832). (ENG, FRE & SPA.). vi, 62p. pap. text 10.00 (*92-4-120832-5*, 1100832) World Health.

Evaluation of Certain Veterinary Drug Residues in Food: Forty-Second Report of the Joint FAO-WHO Expert Committee on Food Additives. 1995. (Technical Reports: No. 851). (FRE & SPA.). viii, 42p. (C). pap. text 10.00 (*92-4-120851-1*, 1100851) World Health.

Evaluation of Certain Veterinary Drug Residues in Food: Thirty-Eighth Report of the Joint FAO-WHO Expert Committee on Food Additives. 1991. (Technical Reports: No. 815). vi, 64p. pap. text 9.00 (*92-4-120815-5*, 1100815) World Health.

Evaluation of Certain Veterinary Drug Residues in Food: Thirty-Fourth Report of the Joint FAO/WHO Expert Committee on Food Additives. WHO Staff. 1989. (Technical Report Ser.: No. 788). 68p. 9.00 (*92-4-120788-4*) World Health.

Evaluation of Certain Veterinary Drug Residues in Food: Thirty-Second Report of the Joint FAO-WHO Expert Committee on Food Additives, 1988. 1988. (Technical Report Ser.: No. 763). 40p. pap. text 6.00 (*92-4-120763-9*, 1100763) World Health.

Evaluation of Certain Veterinary Drug Residues in Food: Thirty-Sixth Report of the Joint FAO-WHO Expert Committee on Food Additives. 1990. (Technical Reports: No. 799). (CHI, ENG, FRE & SPA.). 68p. pap. text 9.00 (*92-4-120799-X*, 1100799) World Health.

Evaluation of Clinical Nursing. J. M. Mellish. 1987. 72p. pap. text 25.00 (*0-409-10256-3*) Buttrwrth-Heinemann.

Evaluation of Clinical Systems for Invasive Blood Pressure Monitoring. 1992. 58p. pap. 90.00 (*0-910275-07-6*, TIR9-209) Assn Adv Med Instrn.

Evaluation of Community Health Centres. M. I. Roemer. 1972. (Public Health Papers: No. 48). pap. text 5.00 (*92-4-130048-5*, 1110048) World Health.

Evaluation of Continuing Education in the Health Professions. Stephen Abrahamson. 1985. lib. bdg. 80.50 (*0-89838-168-1*) Kluwer Academic.

Evaluation of Dependence Liability & Dependence Potential of Drugs: Proceedings of the WHO Scientific Group, Geneva, 1974. WHO Staff. 1975. (Technical Reports: No. 577). pap. text 7.00 (*92-4-120577-6*, 1100577) World Health.

Evaluation of Dependence-Producing Drugs. 1964. (Technical Report Ser.: No. 287). 25p. pap. text 3.00 (*92-4-120287-4*) World Health.

Evaluation of Drug Treatment Programs. Ed. by Barry Stimmel. 1983. LC 82-21194. (Advances in Alcohol & Substance Abuse Ser.: Vol. 2, No 1). 123p. text 39.95 (*0-86656-194-3*) Haworth Pr.

Evaluation of Educational Programmes in Nursing. M. Allen. 1977. 67p. 12.00 (*92-4-156054-1*) World Health.

Evaluation of Exposure to Airborne Particles in the Work Environment. WHO Staff. 1984. (WHO Offset Publications: No. 80). 75p. 9.00 (*92-4-170080-7*) World Health.

Evaluation of Family Planning in Health Services: Proceedings of the WHO Expert Committee, Geneva, 1974. WHO Staff. 1975. (Technical Reports: No. 569). pap. text 7.00 (*92-4-120569-5*, 1100569) World Health.

Evaluation of Federal Funding Policies & Programs & Their Relationship to the Chiropractic Profession. Ruth S. Hanft et al. 1991. 140p. pap. (*0-9631715-0-X*) Fnd Chiro Educ Res.

Evaluation of Food Additives - Some Enzymes, Modified Starches & Certain Other Substances: Toxicological Evaluations & Specifications & a Review of the Technological Efficacy of Some Antioxidants: Report of the FAO-WHO Expert Committee on Food Additives, 15th, Rome, 1971. FAO-WHO Expert Committee on Food Additives. 1972. (Technical Reports: No. 488). pap. text 4.00 (*92-4-120488-5*, 1100488) World Health.

Evaluation of Food Additives - Specifications for the Identity & Purity of Food Additives & Their Toxicological Evaluation: Some Extraction Solvents & Certain Other Substances & a Review of the Technological Efficacy of Some Antimicrobial Agent: Report of the FAO-WHO Expert Committee on Food Additives, 14th, Geneva, 1970. FAO-WHO Expert Committee on Food Additives. 1971. (Technical Reports: No. 462). pap. text 5.00 (*92-4-120462-1*, 1100462) World Health.

Evaluation of Forensic DNA Evidence. National Research Council Staff. rev. ed. 1996. LC 96-25364. 270p. text 37.95 (*0-309-05395-1*) Natl Acad Pr.

Evaluation of "Freestyle": See the Field: A Television Series to Reduce Sex-Role Stereotypes. Jerome Johnston et al. 1980. 308p. (Orig.). pap. 16.00 (*0-87944-256-5*) Inst Soc Res.

Evaluation of Growth Hormone Secretion. Ed. by Z. Laron & O. Butenandt. 1983. (Pediatric & Adolescent Endocrinology Ser.: Vol. 12). (Illus.). viii, 200p. 132.25 (*3-8055-3623-2*) S Karger.

Evaluation of Health Promotion, Health Education, & Disease Prevention Programs. Richard Windsor et al. 2nd ed. 1994. LC 93-32540. xxi, 451p. text 56.95 (*1-55934-243-9*, 1243) Mayfield Pub.

Evaluation of Industrial Disability. Packard Thurber. Ed. by California Medical Association Staff & Industrial Accident Commission. 2nd ed. 1960. (Illus.). 64p. pap. text 15.00 (*0-19-501143-0*) OUP.

Evaluation of Joint Motion: Methods of Measurement & Recording. Dortha Esch & Marvin Lepley. 1974. LC 73-93576. (Illus.). 50p. pap. 12.95 (*0-8166-0714-1*) U of Minn Pr.

Evaluation of Local HIV Service Delivery: Issues, Approaches & Strategies under Title I, the Ryan White Care Act. Kay Eilbert & Rebecca Hines. 1997. (Illus.). 52p. (C). reprint ed. pap. text 30.00 (*0-7881-4044-2*) DIANE Pub.

Evaluation of Mercury, Lead, Cadmium & Food Additives Amaranth, Diethylpyrocarbonate, & Octyl Gallate. FAO-WHO Joint Expert Committee on Food Additives. 1972. (WHO Food Additives Ser.: No. 4). 84p. pap. text 6.00 (*92-4-166004-X*, 1270004) World Health.

Evaluation of Methods for the Treatment of Mental Disorders: Report of a WHO Scientific Group. 1991. (Technical Reports: No. 812). (ENG, FRE, RUS & SPA.). v, 79p. pap. text 10.00 (*92-4-120812-0*, 1100812) World Health.

Evaluation of Myocardial Perfusion in Man. Ed. by C. Vigorito & F. Rengo. 1989. (Bibliotheca Cardiologica Ser.: No. 44). (Illus.). vi, 202p. 152.25 (*3-8055-4882-6*) S Karger.

Evaluation of National Health Interview Survey Diagnostic Reporting. Ed. by W. Sherman Edwards et al. 1993. LC 93-29687. (Vital & Health Statistics Ser.: Series 2, No. 120). (*0-8406-0486-6*) Natl Ctr Health Stats.

Evaluation of New Antiarrhythmic Drugs. Ed. by Joel Morganroth. 1981. 340p. text 126.50 (*90-247-2474-0*) Kluwer Academic.

Evaluation of Nutrition Education in Africa: Community Research in Uganda, 1971-1972. Jan Hoorweg & Ian Dowell. 1979. pap. text (*90-279-7617-1*) Mouton.

Evaluation of Orthopedic & Athletic Injuries. Chad Starkey & Jeff Ryan. 1995. LC 95-24692. (Illus.). 564p. (C). 53.95 (*0-8036-0048-8*) Davis Co.

Evaluation of Outcomes in Brain Injury Rehabilitation. Simon Fleminger. 1999. 384p. 69.95 (*0-86377-648-5*) L Erlbaum Assocs.

Evaluation of People Reporting Occupational Hearing Loss. Medical Aspects of Noise, 1994 Subcommittee. 1998. LC 97-43725. (Monograph Ser.). (Illus.). 62p. pap. text 15.00 (*1-56772-059-5*, S206275) AAO-HNS.

Evaluation of Performance. B. Hannover. 1988. (Recent Research in Psychology Ser.). (Illus.). 164p. 76.95 (*0-387-96768-0*) Spr-Verlag.

Evaluation of Radiation Emergencies & Accidents: Selected Criteria & Data. Edward J. Vallario. 1974. (Technical Reports: No. 152). (Illus.). 136p. (Orig.). pap. (*92-0-125074-6*, IDC152) IAEA AUT. *Dist:* Bernan Associates.

Evaluation of Recent Changes in the Financing of Health Services: Report of a WHO Study Group. 1993. (Technical Reports: No. 829). (ENG, FRE & SPA.). v, 74p. pap. text 10.00 (*92-4-120829-5*, 1100829) World Health.

Evaluation of Renal Function & Disease with Radionuclides. Ed. by M. Donald Blaufox. 2nd rev. ed. 1989. (Illus.). xviii, 418p. 241.00 (*3-8055-4933-4*) S Karger.

Evaluation of Sexual Disorders: Psychological & Medical Aspects. Helen S. Kaplan et al. 1983. LC 83-2749. 304p. text 52.95 (*0-87630-329-7*) Brunner-Routledge.

Evaluation of Ten Randomly Chosen Animal Models of Human Disease. Stephen R. Kaufman et al. 1990. (Perspectives on Animal Research Ser.: Vol. 1, Supplement). 131p. 15.00 (*0-9623858-2-4*); pap. 10.00 (*0-9623858-3-2*) Med Res Modern.

Evaluation of the Injured: How Not to Make the Situation Worse. Arthur J. Varley, Jr. 1991. LC 91-61191. (Illus.). 80p. (Orig.). (*0-9629739-0-4*) SPORT Found.

Evaluation of the Linearity of Quantitative Analytical Methods. 1986. (Proposed Guideline Ser.: Vol. 6). 85.00 (*1-56238-019-2*, EP6-P) NCCLS.

Evaluation of the Psychiatric Patient: A Primer. S. L. Halleck. 1991. (Critical Issues in Psychiatry Ser.). (Illus.). 224p. (C). text 42.50 (*0-306-43749-X*, Kluwer Plenum) Kluwer Academic.

Evaluation of the Sexually Abused Child: A Medical Textbook & Photographic Atlas. Ed. by Astrid Heger et al. 2nd ed. 2000. LC 99-13480. (Illus.). 262p. text 69.50 incl. cd-rom (*0-19-513126-6*) OUP.

Evaluation of the Strategy for Health for All by the Year 2000: Seventh Report on the World Health Situation. 1986. Vol. 4: South-East Asia Region. 106p. pap. 15.00 (*92-4-160274-0*); Vol. 7: Western Pacific Region. 163p. pap. 24.00 (*92-4-160277-5*) World Health.

Evaluation of the Teratogenic Potential of Chemicals in the Rat. H. Fritz Basel & K. Giese Basel. 1990. (Journal: Vol. 40, Suppl. 1, 1990). (Illus.). iv, 28p. pap. 11.50 (*3-8055-5177-0*) S Karger.

Evaluation of Therapeutic Recreation Through Quality Assurance. Bob Riley. 1987. LC 87-50299. 103p. text 16.95 (*0-910251-18-5*) Venture Pub PA.

Evaluation of Two-Week Doctor Visit Reporting in the National Health Interview Survey. 1996. LC 96-16763. (Vital & Health Statistics Ser.: Series 2, No. 123). (*0-8406-0515-3*) Natl Ctr Health Stats.

Evaluation, Stabilization & Transport of the Critically Ill Child. Byron Yl Aoki. 1992. (Illus.). 512p. (C). (gr. 13). pap. text 42.95 (*0-8151-0114-7*, 22560) Mosby Inc.

Evaluation Treatment & Prevention of Musculoskeletal Disorders Set, 2 vols., Set. H. Duane Saunders et al. 3rd rev. ed. 1995. LC 84-91301. (Illus.). 811p. (C). text 99.95 (*1-879190-09-5*) Saunders Grp.

Evaluation, Treatment & Prevention of Musculoskeletal Disorders Vol. I: Spine. H. Duane Saunders et al. 3rd rev. ed. 1995. LC 84-91301. (Illus.). 396p. (C). text 59.95 (*1-879190-06-0*) Saunders Grp.

Evaluation, Treatment & Prevention of Musculoskeletal Disorders Vol. 2: Extremeties. John P. Tomberlin & H. Duane Saunders. 3rd rev. ed. 1995. LC 84-91301. (Illus.). 415p. (C). text 59.95 (*1-879190-07-9*) Saunders Grp.

Evaluations of Adolescent Personality by Adolescents. Caroline M. Tryon. 1939. (SRCD M Ser.: Vol. 4, No. 4). pap. 25.00 (*0-527-01511-3*) Periodicals Srv.

Evaluations of Drug Interactions. Ed. by Frederic J. Zucchero et al. rev. ed. 1990. (EDI Ser.). 1700p. (C). reprint ed. 185.00 (*0-9626616-0-0*) First Data.

Evaluations of Some Pesticide Residues in Food 1975. WHO Staff. 1976. (WHO Pesticide Residues Ser.: No. 5). 409p. 32.00 (*92-4-166505-X*) World Health.

Evaluative Process in Psychiatric Occupational Therapy. Barbara J. Hemphill. 1991. LC 81-86210. 424p. reprint ed. pap. 35.00 (*1-55642-204-0*) SLACK Inc.

Even in America. Zalman Plotkin. 1998. (Illus.). 120p. pap. 10.00 (*0-8059-4299-8*) Dorrance.

Even Paranoids Have Enemies: New Perspectives on Paranoia & Persecution. Joseph H. Berke. 1998. LC 97-26882. 248p. (C). 80.00 (*0-415-15557-6*); pap. 25.99 (*0-415-15558-4*) Routledge.

Even the Rat Was White: A Historical View of Psychology. Robert V. Guthrie. 2nd ed. 1997. LC 97-12003. 282p. (C). pap. text 41.00 (*0-205-14993-6*) Allyn.

Event Cognition: An Ecological Perspective. Ed. by Vickie McCabe & Gerald J. Balzano. 1986. (Ecological Psychology Ser.). 304p. (C). text 59.95 (*0-89859-811-7*) L Erlbaum Assocs.

Event Knowledge: Structure & Function in Development. Ed. by Katherine Nelson. 1986. 288p. (C). text 59.95 (*0-89859-657-2*) L Erlbaum Assocs.

Event-Related Brain Potentials: Basic Issues & Applications. Ed. by John W. Rohrbaugh et al. 1990. (Illus.). 402p. text 95.00 (*0-19-504891-1*) OUP.

Event Theory: A Piaget-Freud Integration. Irene Fast et al. 1985. 192p. (C). text 39.95 (*0-89859-618-1*) L Erlbaum Assocs.

Ever Get Depressed. Katie Ton. 1977. (Uplook Ser.). pap. 0.99 (*0-8163-0280-4*) Pacific Pr Pub Assn.

***Ever 2001: European Association for Vision & Eye Research, Joint European Research Meeting in Ophthalmology & Vision, Alicante, October 2001: Abstracts.** Ed. by L. Missotten. 2001. (Illus.). 204p. pap. 48.75 (*3-8055-7330-8*) S Karger.

Ever Yours, Florence Nightingale: Selected Letters. Florence Nightingale. Ed. by Martha Vicinus & Bea Nergaard. 1990. (Illus.). 480p. text 36.50 (*0-674-27020-7*) HUP.

Every Birth Is Different: The Truth about Pregnancy & Birth. Pat Thomas. 1998. 256p. pap. (*0-7472-7737-0*) Headline Bk Pub GBR. *Dist:* Trafalgar.

Every Child a Wanted Child: Clarence James Gamble & His Work in the Birth Control Movement. Doone Williams & Greer Williams. Ed. by Emily P. Flint. 1978. (Historical Publications: No. 4). (Illus.). 464p. 25.00 (*0-674-27025-8*) HUP.

Every-Day Courage Therapy. Linus Mundy. 1995. LC 95-75102. (Elf-Help Bks.). 80p. pap. 4.95 (*0-87029-274-9*) Abbey.

Every Day Gets a Little Closer: A Twice-Told Therapy. Irvin D. Yalom & Ginny Elkin. 1990. LC 74-78308. 256p. pap. 16.00 (*0-465-02118-2*) Basic.

Every Man His Own Doctor: Popular Medicine in Early America. James N. Green et al. 1998. (Illus.). 64p. pap. 10.00 (*0-914076-93-0*) Lib Co Phila.

Every Nurses Guide to Physical Assessment: A Primary Care Focus. Ed. by Peggy Raish & Billie J. Klaus. 1989. LC 86-34007. (Red Bks.). 500p. pap. text 33.95 (*0-8273-4213-6*) Delmar.

Every Person's Guide to Antioxidants. John R. Smythies. 1998. LC 98-6810. 180p. 35.00 (*0-8135-2574-8*); pap. 16.00 (*0-8135-2575-6*) Rutgers U Pr.

Every Pregnant Woman's Guide to Preventing Premature Birth. Barbara Luke. 1996. pap. (*0-8129-2830-X*, Crown) Crown Pub Group.

Every Woman Has a Right to Know the Dangers of Legal Abortion. Ann Saltenberger. 3rd ed. 1983. 237p. (Orig.). 12.95 (*0-937930-06-7*); pap. 6.95 (*0-937930-04-0*) Sun Life.

***Every Woman's Guide to Health & Fitness.** Lisa Callahan. 2002. pap. 19.95 (*1-58574-009-8*, Lyons) Globe Pequot.

Every Woman's Herbal. John R. Christopher & Cathy Gileadi. 1994. LC 90-20536. (Illus.). 225p. per. 14.95 (*1-879436-10-8*, 99110) Christopher Pubns.

Every Woman's Inheritance. 1997. pap. 15.00 (*0-9655679-9-0*) BodyGuide.

Everybody: The Healthy Eating Handbook. Derek Llewellyn-Jones. 1993. LC 92-19159. 5.99 (*0-19-286155-7*) OUP.

Everybody's Different: Understanding & Changing Our Reactions to Disabilities. Nancy B. Miller & Catherine C. Sammons. 1999. LC 98-51018. 384p. pap. 21.95 (*1-55766-359-9*, 3599) P H Brookes.

Everybody's Guide to Homeopathic Medicines: Safe & Effective Remedies for You & Your Family. Stephen Cummings & Dana Ullman. 3rd rev. ed. 1997. LC 96-31021. 304p. (Orig.). 16.95 (*0-87477-843-3*, Tarcher Putnam) Putnam Pub Group.

Everyday Aids & Appliances. Ed. by Graham Mulley. 1989. (Illus.). 111p. pap. text (*0-7279-0241-5*) BMJ Pub GBR. *Dist:* AIDC.

Everyday Biological Stress Mechanisms: International Symposium on Scientifically Based Biological Assessment of Long-Term Stress in Daily Life, Wenner-Gren Foundations, Stockholm, April 2000. Ed. by Torres Theorell. 2001. LC 2001-29139. (Advances in Psychosomatic Medicine Ser.: Vol. 22). (Illus.). vi, 156p. 98.25 (*3-8055-7191-7*) S Karger.

Everyday Cognition: Its Development in Social Context. Ed. by Barbara Rogoff & Jean Lave. 1984. (Illus.). 320p. 44.00 (*0-674-27030-4*) HUP.

Everyday Drugs & Pregnancy: Alcohol, Tobacco & Caffeine. Christina Dye. rev. ed. 2000. pap. 0.50 (*0-89230-192-9*) Do It Now.

Everyday Ethics: Resolving Dilemmas in Nursing Home Life. Ed. by Rosalie A. Kane & Arthur L. Caplan. 1989. 352p. 44.95 (*0-8261-6640-7*) Springer Pub.

Everyday Health-Related Behavior in Adolescence. Donna Spruijt-Metz. 1999. LC 00-501101. (Studies in Adolescent Development). (Illus.). xvii, 221p. 49.95 (*0-86377-518-7*) L Erlbaum Assocs.

Everyday Initiations: How to Survive Crises Using Rituals. Rudiger Dahlke. 1999. LC 98-16528. 384p. pap. 16.95 (*1-885394-23-3*) Bluestar Communs.

Everyday Miracles: Homeopathy in Action. Linda Johnston. 1991. (Illus.). 274p. pap. 17.95 (*1-877691-00-3*) C Kent Agency.

Everyday Mysteries: Existential Dimensions of Psychotherapy. Emmy Van Deurzen-Smith. 1997. LC 96-16314. (Illus.). 320p. (C). 89.95 (*0-415-08704-X*); pap. 29.95 (*0-415-08705-8*) Routledge.

Everyday Pediatrics for Parents. Elmer R. Grossman. 1996. 472p. text 21.95 (*0-89087-813-7*) Celestial Arts.

Everyday Problems in Dermatology: The Cosmetic Connection: 2nd International Meeting on Cosmetic Dermatology, Rome, Italy, May 19-22, 1987. Ed. by F. J. Ebling. 1991. (Cosmetic Dermatology Ser.: No. 2). (Illus.). 425p. text (*0-87936-018-6*) Intl Ediemme ITA. *Dist:* Scholium Intl.

Everyone Here Spoke Sign Language: Hereditary Deafness on Martha's Vineyard. Nora E. Groce. 1985. LC 85-5451. 192p. reprint ed. pap. 16.00 (*0-674-27041-X*) HUP.

Everyone's Children: A Pediatrician's Story of an Inner-City Practice. Claire McCarthy. 1998. LC 97-28289. 224p. 23.00 (*0-684-81876-0*) Scribner.

Everyone's Guide to Cancer Therapy: How Cancer Is Diagnosed, Treated, & Managed Day to Day. Malin Dollinger et al. 3rd rev. ed. 1998. LC 97-34123. (Illus.). 848p. 29.95 (*0-8362-3617-3*); pap. 21.95 (*0-8362-3709-9*) Andrews McMeel.

Everything Alternative Medicine Book: The Latest Research & Proven Techniques to Get You Feeling Better. Nancy Faass. Date not set. (Everything Ser.). (Illus.). 304p. pap. 12.95 (*1-58062-435-9*) Adams Media.

Everything Get Ready for Baby Book: From Buying the Right Gear to Learning the Best Lullabies. Katina Jones. 1998. LC 97-45898. (Everything Ser.). (Illus.). 290p. pap. 12.95 (*1-55850-844-9*) Adams Media.

***Everything in Its Place: My Trials & Triumphs with Obsessive Compulsive Disorder.** Marc Summers & Eric Hollander. 2002. 213p. reprint ed. 22.00 (*0-7567-5395-3*) DIANE Pub.

***Everything Smart Nutrition Mini Book: What's Healthy, What's Not... The Best Foods for You & Your Family.** Barbara Ravage. 2001. (Everything Mini Book Ser.). (Illus.). 192p. pap. 4.95 (*1-58062-606-8*) Adams Media.

Everything Women of Color Should Know About Cosmetic Surgery. R. Jan Adams. 2000. LC 00-40241. (Illus.). xiii, 210p. 24.95 (*0-312-25310-9*) St Martin.

Everything You Need to Know about AIDS. Barbara Taylor. Ed. by Ruth C. Rosen. rev. ed. 1998. LC 00-266279. (Need to Know Library). (Illus.). 64p. (YA). (gr. 7-12). lib. bdg. 17.95 (*0-8239-2833-0*, NTAIDS) Rosen Group.

Everything You Need to Know about Babies. Linda McDonald. 1978. LC 77-21017. (Illus.). pap. 12.95 (*0-916198-04-9*) Oaklawn Pr.

Everything You Need to Know About Chemical Dependence: Vernon Johnson's Complete Guide for Families. Vernon Johnson. 1990. 496p. pap. 22.95 (*0-935908-53-6*, P011, HazeldenJohnson Inst) Hazelden.

***Everything You Need to Know about Chemotherapy.** Magdalena Alagna. 2001. LC 00-11392. (Need to Know Library). (Illus.). 64p. (YA). (gr. 6 up). lib. bdg. 23.95 (*0-8239-3394-6*) Rosen Group.

Everything You Need to Know about Diseases. Springhouse Publishing Company Staff. Ed. by Matthew Cahill, Advertising Staff. 1995. LC 95-6697. (Illus.). 928p. 26.95 (*0-87434-822-6*) Springhouse Corp.

Everything You Need to Know about Drugs. Springhouse Publishing Company Staff. 1996. LC 96-16575. 912p. pap. 27.95 (*0-87434-864-1*) Springhouse Corp.

Everything You Need to Know about Going to the Gynecologist. Shifra N. Diamond. 1999. (Need to Know Library). (Illus.). 64p. (YA). (gr. 7-12). lib. bdg. 17.95 (*0-8239-2839-X*, NTGOGY) Rosen Group.

Everything You Need to Know about Lyme Disease & Other Tick-Borne Disorders. Karen Vanderhoof-Forschner. 1997. LC 97-10073. (Illus.). 256p. pap. 15.95 (*0-471-16061-X*) Wiley.

Everything You Need to Know about Measles & Rubella. Trisha Hawkins. 2000. LC 00-9721. (Need to Know Library). (Illus.). 64p. (J). (gr. 4-8). lib. bdg. 17.95 (*0-8239-3322-9*) Rosen Group.

Everything You Need to Know about Medical Tests. SPC Staff. 1996. LC 95-10232. 768p. pap. 27.95 (*0-87434-933-8*) Springhouse Corp.

Everything You Need to Know about Medical Treatments. Springhouse Publishing Company Staff. Ed. by Matthew Cahill, Advertising Staff. 1995. LC 95-10231. 640p. 26.95 (*0-87434-821-8*); LC 95-10232. 768p. 26.95 (*0-87434-823-4*) Springhouse Corp.

Everything You Need to Know about Old Age Psychiatry. Robert Howard. 1999. LC 99-14082. 85.00 (*1-871816-38-6*) Taylor & Francis.

Everything You Need to Know about Prozac. Angelo T. Scotti et al. 1991. 160p. mass mkt. 5.50 (*0-553-29192-0*) Bantam.

Everything You Need to Know to Understand & Live with Depression. Charles D. Mellon. 1996. (Illus.). 112p. pap. 11.85 (*0-9653362-2-0*) Genetics Heritage.

Everything You've Always Wanted to Know about Energy But Were Too Weak to Ask. Naura Hayden. rev. ed. 1984. 182p. 12.95 (*0-942104-03-X*) Bibli O Phile Pub Co.

Everywoman's Book. Paavo O. Airola. 1984. (Illus.). 640p. 17.95 (*0-932090-00-1*); pap. 14.95 (*0-932090-10-9*) Health Plus.

Eve's Herbs: A History of Contraception & Abortion in the West. John M. Riddle. 1997. LC 96-40383. (Illus.). 384p. 43.50 (*0-674-27024-X*) HUP.

***Eve's Rib: What You Must Know about the New Women's Medicine & How It Can Save Your Life.** Marianne J. Legato. 2002. 288p. 23.00 (*0-609-60830-4*) Harmony Bks.

Evidence-Based & Cost-Effective Medicine for the Uninitiated. Tony Lockett. 1997. LC 97-49. 104p. pap. (*1-85775-235-X*) Radcliffe Med Pr GBR. *Dist:* Balogh.

Evidence-Based Asthma Management. J. Mark FitzGerald et al. 1999. (Evidence-Based Ser.). 360p. incl. cd-rom (*1-55009-114-X*) DEKR.

Evidence-Based Cardiology. Peter J. Sharis & Christopher P. Cannon. 1999. LC 99-38949. 384p. pap. text 39.95 (*0-7817-1613-6*) Lppncott W & W.

Evidence Based Cardiology. Ed. by Salim Yusuf et al. 1998. 1200p. text (*0-7279-1171-6*) BMJ Pub GBR. *Dist:* AIDC.

***Evidence-Based Clinical Pearls in Internal Medicine.** Todd B. Ellerin & Luis A. Diaz. 2001. LC 2001-16486. 176p. pap. text 24.95 (*0-7817-3280-8*) Lppncott W & W.

Evidence-Based Counselling & Psychological Therapies: Research & Applications. Nancy Rowland & Stephen Goss. 2000. LC 00-21257. xvi, 216p. pap. (*0-415-20507-7*) Routledge.

Evidence-Based Decision Making for Community Health Programs. Catherine A. Jackson et al. 1998. LC 97-46934. xv, 85p. pap. 15.00 (*0-8330-2573-2*, MR-933) Rand Corp.

Evidence Based Dementia. Nawab Qizilbash et al. 2001. (Illus.). 448p. 129.95 (*0-632-05296-1*) Blackwell Sci.

Evidence-Based Diabetes Management. Hertzel C. Gerstein & R. Brian Haynes. 2000. (Evidence-Based Ser.). 360p. incl. cd-rom (*1-55009-124-7*) DEKR.

Evidence-Based Diagnosis: A Handbook of Clinical Prediction Rules. M. Ebell. 2000. LC 00-26571. (Illus.). 408p. pap. 49.95 incl. cd-rom (*0-387-95025-7*) Spr-Verlag.

Evidence-Based Family Medicine. Walter W. Rosser & M. Sharon Shafir. 1997. (Evidence-Based Ser.). 180p. incl. cd-rom (*1-55009-053-4*) DEKR.

Evidence-Based Gastroenterology. E. Jan Irvine & Richard H. Hunt. 2000. (Evidence-Based Ser.). 400p. incl. cd-rom (*1-55009-105-0*) DEKR.

Evidence Based Gastroenterology & Hepatology. Ed. by John McDonald et al. 1999. (Illus.). 608p. text (*0-7279-1182-1*) BMJ Pub GBR. *Dist:* AIDC.

***Evidence Based Healthcare.** J. A. Muir Gray. 2nd ed. 2001. (Illus.). 295p. pap. (*0-443-06288-9*) Church GBR. *Dist:* Saunders.

***Evidence Based Hypertension.** Ed. by Cynthia D. Mulrow. 2001. (Illus.). 256p. pap. (*0-7279-1438-3*) BMJ Pub GBR. *Dist:* AIDC.

***Evidence-Based Infertility Treatment.** S. Daya. 2002. 350p. 86.95 (*1-84214-116-3*, Parthenon Pbng) CRC Pr.

Evidence Based Medicine. Sackett. 1996. pap. text 26.95 (*0-443-05686-2*) Saunders.

Evidence-Based Medicine: A Framework for Clinical Practices. Daniel J. Friedland. 1998. (Illus.). 263p. (C). pap. 34.95 (*0-8385-2476-1*, A-2476-8, Apple Lange Med) McGraw.

Evidence-Based Medicine: A Framework for Clinical Practices. 2nd ed. Date not set. (C). text 26.95 (*0-8385-2306-4*) P-H.

***Evidence Based Medicine Toolkit.** Heneghan & Badenoch. 2002. 72p. pap. (*0-7279-1601-7*) BMJ Pub.

Evidence Based Medicine Workbook: Critical Appraisal for Clinical Problem Solving. Robert A. Dixon et al. 1997. LC 96-24355. (Arnold Publication). 224p. pap. 35.00 (*0-7506-2590-2*) OUP.

Evidence Based on General Practice. Ridsdale. 1995. pap. text 29.95 (*0-7020-1611-X*) Saunders.

Evidence-Based Otitis Media. Richard M. Rosenfeld & Charles D. Bluestone. 1999. (Evidence-Based Ser.). 420p. text incl. cd-rom (*1-55009-083-6*) DEKR.

***Evidence Based Paediatric Oncology.** Pinkerton et al. 2002. 300p. pap. (*0-7279-1440-5*) BMJ Pub GBR. *Dist:* AIDC.

Evidence-Based Palliative Care. Huda Abu-Saad & Annemie Courtens. 2001. LC 00-52913. (Illus.). 184p. pap. 47.95 (*0-632-05818-8*) Blackwell Sci.

***Evidence-Based Patient Choice: Inevitable or Impossible?** Ed. by Adrian Edwards & Glyn Elwyn. 2001. 330p. (Orig.). pap. 45.00 (*0-19-263194-2*) OUP.

Evidence-Based Pediatrics. William Feldman. 1999. (Evidence-Based Ser.). 450p. incl. cd-rom (*1-55009-087-9*) DEKR.

Evidence-Based Perioperative & Critical Care Vol. 1: Gynecology: Guidelines for Clinical Decision-Making. Steven A. Vasilev. 2000. LC 99-28929. (Illus.). 697p. 167.00 (*0-471-24788-X*) Wiley.

Evidence Based Practice: A Primer. Mary Law. 2001. (Illus.). 250p. pap. text 30.00 (*1-55642-453-1*) SLACK Inc.

Evidence-Based Practice: A Primer for Health Care Professionals. Martin Dawes. 2000. LC 99-29502. x, 254p. (*0-443-06126-2*) Saunders.

***Evidence Based Practice in Primary Care.** Chris Silagy & Andrew Haines. 2nd ed. 2001. (Illus.). 206p. pap. text (*0-7279-1568-1*) BMJ Pub GBR. *Dist:* AIDC.

***Evidence-Based Primary Care Handbook.** Mark Gabbay. 1999. 328p. pap. (*1-85315-415-6*) Royal Soc of Medicine Pr Ltd GBR. *Dist:* Balogh.

Evidence Based Resource in Anaesthesia & Analgesia. Ed. by Martin Tramer. 2001. 240p. pap. text (*0-7279-1437-5*) BMJ Pub GBR. *Dist:* AIDC.

Evidence-Based Surgery. Toby Gordon & John L. Cameron. 1999. (Evidence-Based Ser.). 450p. incl. cd-rom (*1-55009-116-6*) DEKR.

Evidence Based Symptom Control in Palliative Care: Systemic Reviews & Validated Clinical Practice Guidelines for 15 Common Problems in Patients with Life Limiting Disease. Ed. by Arthur G. Lipman et al. 2000. LC 00-32388. (Journal of Pharmaceutical Care in Pain & Symptom Control Ser.: No. 7). (Illus.). xvii, 247p. 59.95 (*0-7890-1013-5*); (C). pap. 29.95 (*0-7890-1014-3*) Haworth Pr.

Evidence-Guided Prescribing of the Pill. Ed. by Philip C. Hannaford & Anne M. Webb. 1996. (Illus.). 364p. lib. bdg. 71.95 (*1-85070-747-2*, Parthenon Pbng) CRC Pr.

***Evidence in Mental Health Care.** Ed. by Stefan Priebe & Mike Slade. 2002. LC 2001-52545. (*0-415-23692-4*) Brunner-Routledge.

Evidence or Person: Testing the Eyewitness. R. Buckhout & K. W. Ellison. 1977. (Monographs: No. CR-23). 4.00 (*1-55524-024-0*) Ctr Respon Psych.

Evil We Do: The Psychoanalysis of Destructive People. Carl Goldberg. 2000. LC 00-42166. 259p. 25.00 (*1-57392-839-9*) Prometheus Bks.

Evocative Images: The Thematic Apperception Test & the Art of Projection. Ed. by Lon Gieser & Morris I. Stein. 1999. LC 99-25182. 231p. 39.95 (*1-55798-579-0*, 431-727A) Am Psychol.

Evocativeness: The Therapist's Second Voice. Stephen A. Appelbaum. 2000. LC 00-28853. viii, 325p. 45.00 (*0-7657-0246-0*) Aronson.

Evoked & Event-Related Potentials in Hearing Research & Clinical Application. Ed. by Valeria Csepe & Risto Naatanen. 1997. (Audiology & Neuro-Otology Ser.: Vol. 2, No. 5, 1997). (Illus.). 138p. pap. 36.50 (*3-8055-6605-0*) S Karger.

Evoked Potential Audiometry: Fundamentals & Applications. William M. Aldrich et al. 1998. LC 98-23831. 260p. 78.00 (*0-13-299603-0*) P-H.

Evoked Potential Manual. Ed. by E. J. Colon et al. 1983. text 199.50 (*0-89838-614-4*) Kluwer Academic.

Evoked Potential Manual: A Practical Guide to Clinical Applications. Ed. by E. J. Colon & S. L. Visser. 2nd rev. ed. 1990. (C). text 257.50 (*0-7923-0791-7*) Kluwer Academic.

Evoked Potentials. Ed. by B. L. Grundy & R. M. Villani. 1989. (Illus.). 200p. 62.95 (*0-387-82059-0*) Spr-Verlag.

Evoked Potentials in Clinical Medicine. Keith H. Chiappa. 3rd ed. 1997. LC 96-47700. 720p. text 115.00 (*0-397-51659-2*) Lppncott W & W.

Evolution. Colin Patterson. 2nd ed. 1999. LC 98-41312. (Comstock Book Ser.). 176p. 39.95 (*0-8014-3642-7*); (Illus.). pap. 18.95 (*0-8014-8594-0*) Cornell U Pr.

Evolution & Application of Clinical Theory: Perspective from Four Psychologies. Judith M. Mishne. 1993. LC 92-39586. (Illus.). 444p. 40.00 (*0-02-921635-4*) Free Pr.

Evolution & Dissolution of the Nervous System. John H. Jackson. 119p. 55.00 (*1-85506-669-6*) Thoemmes Pr.

Evolution & Eradication of Infectious Diseases. Aidan Cockburn. 1983. LC 83-10883. 255p. reprint ed. lib. bdg. 48.50 (*0-313-24118-X*, COEV, Greenwood Pr) Greenwood.

Evolution & Human Behavior. John Cartwright. 2000. LC 99-87600. (Illus.). xxiv, 376p. (C). 60.00 (*0-262-03281-3*, Bradford Bks) MIT Pr.

Evolution & Memory. Caleb Gattegno. 1976. pap. 10.00 (*0-87825-072-7*) Ed Solutions.

Evolution & Modification of Behavior. Konrad Lorenz. 1997. LC 65-24436. vi, 128p. reprint ed. pap. text 12.00 (*0-226-49334-2*, Midway Reprint) U Ch Pr.

Evolution & the Genetics of Populations: Genetic & Biometric Foundations, Vol. 1. Sewall Wright. 1968. LC 67-25533. x, 470p. lib. bdg. 46.00 (*0-226-91049-0*) U Ch Pr.

Evolution & the Genetics of Populations: Theory of Gene Frequencies, Vol. 2. Sewall Wright. 1969. LC 67-25533. (Evolution & the Genetics of Populations Ser.: Vol. 2). vii, 520p. lib. bdg. 50.50 (*0-226-91050-4*) U Ch Pr.

Evolution & the Genetics of Populations: Variability Within & among Natural Populations, Vol. 4. Sewall Wright. 1978. LC 67-25533. (Evolution & the Genetics of Populations Ser.: Vol. 4). (Illus.). x, 590p. lib. bdg. 43.00 (*0-226-91052-0*) U Ch Pr.

***Evolution & the Origin of Life: Index of New Information & Guide-Book for Consumers, Reference & Research.** Hans Hermann Schmidt. 2002. 180p. pap. 47.50 (*0-7883-2477-2*) ABBE Pubs Assn.

Evolution & Trends in Peritoneal Dialysis. Ed. by L. L. Scarpioni & S. Ballocchi. 1990. (Contributions to Nephrology Ser.: Vol. 84). (Illus.). x, 110p. 29.75 (*3-8055-5206-8*) S Karger.

Evolution & Variation of Multigene Families. T. Ohta. 1980. (Lecture Notes in Biomathematics: Vol. 37). 131p. 34.95 (*0-387-09998-0*) Spr-Verlag.

Evolution Emerging: A Survey of Changing Patterns from Primeval Life to Man William K. Gregory. 1974. LC 73-17822. (Natural Sciences in America Ser.). (Illus.). 1808p. reprint ed. Set. 134.95 (*0-405-05738-5*); Vol. 1. 66.95 (*0-405-05739-3*); Vol. 2. 66.95 (*0-405-05740-7*) Ayer.

Evolution, Genetics & Eugenics. Ed. by Horatio H. Newman. 1970. LC 69-14010. (Illus.). 620p. reprint ed. lib. bdg. 89.50 (*0-8371-1880-8*, NEEV, Greenwood Pr) Greenwood.

Evolution in Health & Diseaase. Ed. by Stephen Stearns. 1999. LC 98-21522. (Illus.). 344p. pap. text 45.00 (*0-19-850445-4*) OUP.

Evolution in Urodynamics Multidisciplinary Treatment of GU Tumors: Urologia Internationalis Journal, Vol. 47, Suppl. 1. Ed. by U. Jonas. 1991. (Urologia Internationalis Ser.). (Illus.). iv, 152p. pap. 68.00 (*3-8055-5318-8*) S Karger.

Evolution Mitochondrialer Gene: Strukturanalyse Von Gruppe I Intronen Im Chondriom des Ascomyceten Podospora Anserina. Thomas Karsch. 1988. (Bibliotheca Mycologica: Vol. 124). (GER., Illus.). x, 112p. *(3-443-59025-X)* Gebruder Borntraeger DEU. *Dist:* Balogh.

Evolution of British General Practice, 1850-1948. Anne Digby. 1999. LC 98-51327. (Illus.). 390p. text 80.00 *(0-19-820513-9)* OUP.

Evolution of Cancer. Shinichi Okuyama & Hitoshi Mishina. 1990. text *(0-86008-460-4)* U of Tokyo JPN. *Dist:* Col U Pr.

Evolution of Canine Social Behavior. Roger Abrantes. 1997. (Illus.). 80p. pap. 11.95 *(0-9660484-1-5)* Wakan Tanka.

Evolution of Cardiac Surgery. Harris B. Shumacker, Jr. 1992. LC 91-35312. (Illus.). 496p. 59.95 *(0-253-35221-5)* Ind U Pr.

Evolution of Consciousness. Euan MacPhail. 1998. (Illus.). 272p. pap. text 29.95 *(0-19-850324-5)* OUP.

Evolution of Epidemiologic Ideas. Ed. by Sander Greenland. 1987. LC 87-3320. 190p. (Orig.). pap. text 21.00 *(0-917227-02-6)* Epidemiology.

Evolution of Fish Species Flocks. Ed. by Anthony A. Echelle & Irv Kornfield. 1994. LC 84-51502. 257p. (C). 30.00 *(0-89101-058-0)*; pap. 14.95 *(0-89101-057-2)* U Maine Pr.

Evolution of Genetic Systems: Brookhaven Symposium in Biology, No. 23. Harold Smith. 1972. LC 74-181433. viii, 580p. text 382.00 *(0-677-12230-6)* Gordon & Breach.

Evolution of Human Sexuality. Donald Symons. 1981. (Illus.). 368p. pap. text 26.95 *(0-19-502907-0)* OUP.

Evolution of Immune Reactions. Peter Sima & Vaclav Vetvicka. 1990. (Illus.). 280p. lib. bdg. 225.00 *(0-8493-6593-7*, QR182) CRC Pr.

Evolution of Love. Ada Lampert. 1997. LC 97-11073. (Human Evolution, Behavior, & Intelligence Ser.). 144p. 55.00 *(0-275-95907-4*, Praeger Pubs) Greenwood.

Evolution of Man: Essays. Grafton E. Smith. 2nd ed. LC 77-86438. reprint ed. 34.50 *(0-404-16677-6)* AMS Pr.

Evolution of Meningococcal Disease, Set. Ed. by Neylan A. Vedros. 1987. 187.00 *(0-8493-4643-6*, RC124, CRC Reprint) Franklin.

Evolution of Meningococcal Disease, Vol. 1. Neylan A. Vedros. 1987. LC 87-18406. 152p. reprint ed. 92.00 *(0-8493-4644-4*, CRC Reprint) Franklin.

Evolution of Meningococcal Disease, Vol. 2. N. Vedros. 1987. LC 87-18406. 160p. reprint ed. 95.00 *(0-8493-4645-2*, CRC Reprint) Franklin.

Evolution of Microsurgery. Ed. by Ph. Sourdille. 1991. (Developments in Ophthalmology Ser.: Vol. 22). (Illus.). x, 168p. 148.00 *(3-8055-5333-1)* S Karger.

Evolution of Modern Medicine: A Series of Lectures Delivered at Yale University on the Silliman Foundation in April, 1913. William Osler. 1980. LC 77-140610. (Medicine & Society in America Ser.). (Illus.). 264p. reprint ed. 22.00 *(0-405-02805-9)* Ayer.

Evolution of Operant Learning & Memory. W. F. Angermeier. 1984. (Illus.). xii, 204p. text 165.25 *(3-8055-3736-0)* S Karger.

Evolution of Preventive Medicine. Arthur Newsholme. LC 75-23748. reprint ed. 37.50 *(0-404-13354-1)* AMS Pr.

Evolution of Psychoanalytic Technique. Ed. by Martin S. Bergmann & Frank R. Hartman. 1990. 520p. text 76.00 *(0-231-07420-4)* Col U Pr.

Evolution of Psychological Theory: A Critical History of Concepts & Presuppositions. Richard Lowry. 2nd ed. 1982. 256p. pap. text 28.95 *(0-202-25135-7)*; lib. bdg. 51.95 *(0-202-25134-9)* Aldine de Gruyter.

Evolution of Psychology: Fifty Years of the American Psychologist. Ed. by Joseph M. Notterman. LC 97-37081. 783p. 1998. pap. 34.95 *(1-55798-484-0)*; 1997. 39.95 *(1-55798-473-5)* Am Psychol.

Evolution of Psychotherapy. Ed. by Jeffrey K. Zeig. 1987. LC 86-23263. 650p. text 67.95 *(0-87630-440-4)* Brunner-Routledge.

Evolution of Psychotherapy: The Second Conference. Jeffrey K. Zeig. 1992. 352p. text 67.95 *(0-87630-677-6)* Brunner-Routledge.

Evolution of Psychotherapy: The Third Conference. Ed. by Jeffrey K. Zeig. 1996. 384p. 68.95 *(0-87630-813-2)* Brunner-Routledge.

***Evolution of Psychotherapy: The Third Conference.** Ed. by Jeffrey K. Zeig. 2001. (Illus.). 358p. reprint ed. 35.00 *(0-7881-9880-7)* DIANE Pub.

Evolution of Respiratory Processes: A Comparative Approach. Lenfant Wood & C. L. Lenfant. 1979. LC 79-4051. (Lung Biology in Health & Disease Ser.: Vol. 13). (Illus.). 392p. text 175.00 *(0-8247-6793-4)* Dekker.

Evolution of Self Psychology. Ed. by Arnold Goldberg. 1991. (Progress in Self Psychology Ser.: Vol. 7). 264p. text 45.00 *(0-88163-130-2)* Analytic Pr.

Evolution of Sickness & Healing. Horacio Fabrega, Jr. 1997. LC 96-29318. (Illus.). 379p. text 48.00 *(0-520-20609-6)* U CA Pr.

Evolution of Sleep. Ida G. Karmanova. 1982. (Illus.). xii, 164p. 83.50 *(3-8055-3530-9)* S Karger.

Evolution of Social Systems. J. P. Scott. 1989. (Monographs in Psychology: Vol. 3). xii, 356p. text 198.00 *(2-88124-317-7)*; pap. text 117.00 *(2-88124-358-4)* Gordon & Breach.

Evolution of the Aging Self: The Sociatal Impact on the Aging Process. K. Warner Schaie & Jon Hendricks. 2000. LC 00-27398. xiv, 348p. *(0-8261-1363-X)* Springer Pub.

Evolution of the Brain: Creation of the Self. John C. Eccles. 1991. 304p. (C). pap. 29.95 *(0-415-03224-5*, A5341) Routledge.

Evolution of the First Nervous Systems. Ed. by P. A. Anderson. 1990. LC 90-34441. (NATO Advanced Science Institutes Ser.: Vol. 188). (Illus.). 446p. (C). text 156.00 *(0-306-43529-2*, Kluwer Plenum) Kluwer Academic.

Evolution of the Human Pelvis in Relation to the Mechanics of the Erect Posture. Edward Reynolds. 1931. (HU PMP Ser.: Vol. 11, No. 5). pap. 25.00 *(0-527-01222-X)* Periodicals Srv.

Evolution of the Immune System. Charlemagne. 1992. 95.00 *(0-8493-8885-6*, CRC Reprint) Franklin.

Evolution of the Psyche. Ed. by D. H. Rosen & M. C. Luebbert. 1999. LC 98-24561. (Human Evolution, Behavior, & Intelligence Ser.). 248p. 62.50 *(0-275-96312-8*, Praeger Pubs) Greenwood.

Evolution of Vertebrate Endocrine Systems. A. Epple. Ed. by Peter K. Pang. 1980. (Graduate Studies: No. 21). 404p. (Orig.). 35.00 *(0-89672-077-2)*; pap. 25.00 *(0-89672-076-4)* Tex Tech Univ Pr.

Evolution Theory, Set. August Weismann. Tr. by J. Arthur Thomson & Margaret R. Thomson from GER. LC 72-1665. (Illus.). 864p. reprint ed. 135.00 *(0-404-08188-6)* AMS Pr.

***Evolutionary Algorithms in Molecular Design.** Ed. by David E. Clark. 2000. (Methods & Principles in Medicinal Chemistry Ser.). 288p. 145.00 *(3-527-30155-0)* Wiley.

Evolutionary Aspects of Nutrition & Health: Diet, Exercise, Genetics & Chronic Disease. Ed. by A. P. Simopoulos. 1999. LC 99-20310. (World Review of Nutrition & Dietetics Ser.: Vol. 84 (1999)). (Illus.). 146p. 172.25 *(3-8055-6827-4)* S Karger.

Evolutionary Biology of Hearing. Ed. by Arthur N. Popper et al. 1991. (Illus.). 859p. 165.00 *(0-387-97588-8)* Spr-Verlag.

Evolutionary Dynamics of Genetic Diversity: Proceedings of a Symposium Held in Manchester, England, March 29-30, 1983. Ed. by G. S. Mani. 1984. (Lecture Notes in Biomathematics: Vol. 53). 312p. 44.95 *(0-387-12903-0)* Spr-Verlag.

Evolutionary History of the Primates. Frederick S. Szalay & Eric Delson. 1980. LC 78-20051. text 79.95 *(0-12-680150-9)* Acad Pr.

Evolutionary Mechanisms in Sex Determination. Stephen S. Wachtel. 1989. LC 88-5011. 320p. 187.00 *(0-8493-4830-7*, QH600, CRC Reprint) Franklin.

Evolutionary Medicine. Euclid O. Smith. Ed. by Wenda R. Trevathan & James J. McKenna. 1999. LC 98-17323. (Illus.). 496p. pap. text 40.00 *(0-19-510356-4)* OUP.

Evolutionary Medicine. Ed. by Wenda R. Trevathan et al. 1999. LC 98-17323. (Illus.). 496p. text 75.00 *(0-19-510355-6)* OUP.

Evolutionary Origins of Developmental Psychology, Set. Ed. by Robert H. Wozniak. 1995. 3070p. (C). 782.00 *(0-415-13115-4)* Routledge.

Evolutionary Origins of Developmental Psychology: Annualk General & Linguistic Psychology 1920-1952, Set. Ed. by C.K. Ogden. 2nd ed. 1995. LC 96-163002. 6500p. (C). 2599.00 *(0-415-12779-3)* Routledge.

***Evolutionary Perspectives on Human Reproductive Behavior.** Ed. by Dori LeCroy & Peter Moller. 2001. 230p. pap. 26.00 *(0-8018-6696-0)* NY Acad Sci.

Evolutionary Psychiatry: A New Beginning. Anthony Stevens & John Price. (Illus.). 1996. LC 96-11334. 288p. (C). 89.95 *(0-415-13839-6)*; 1996. LC 96-11334. 288p. (C). pap. 29.99 *(0-415-13840-X)*; 2nd ed. 2000. LC 99-86488. xiv, 310p. pap. *(0-415-21979-5)* Routledge.

Evolutionary Psychiatry: A New Beginning. Contrib. by Anthony Stevens & John Price. 2nd ed. 2000. LC 99-86488. (Illus.). xiv, 310p. *(0-415-21978-7)* Routledge.

Evolutionary Theory: The Unfinished Synthesis. Robert G. Reid. 1985. 416p. (C). 49.95 *(0-8014-1831-3)* Cornell U Pr.

Evolutionary Visions of the Future. Ed. by Bela H. Banathy. 1985. (Illus.). 96p. pap. *(0-08-032563-7)* PPL GBR. *Dist:* Elsevier.

Evolving Concepts in Gastrointestinal Motility. Ed. by Malcolm C. Champion & William C. Orr. 1996. LC 96-13281. 110.95 *(0-86542-944-8)* Blackwell Sci.

Evolving Female: Women in Psychosocial Context. Carol L. Heckerman. 1980. LC 79-4240. 368p. pap. 24.95 *(0-87705-411-8*, Kluwer Acad Hman Sci) Kluwer Academic.

Evolving Health Care Delivery System: Necessary Changes to Providers of Care, Consumers & Patients. Ed. by Jennie J. Kronenfeld. 1997. (Research in the Sociology of Health Care Ser.: Vol. 14). 78.50 *(0-7623-0244-5)* Jai Pr.

Evolving HIM Careers: Seven Roles for the Future. 1999. (Illus.). 120p. pap. text 20.00 *(1-58426-033-5*, AB102299) Am Hlth Info.

Evolving Possibilities: Selected Works of Bill O'Hanlon. William Hudson O'Hanlon et al. 1999. LC 99-28379. 210p. pap. text 29.95 *(0-87630-980-5)* Brunner-Routledge.

Evolving Self: Problem & Process in Human Development. Robert Kegan. 1983. (Illus.). 336p. pap. 19.50 *(0-674-27231-5)* HUP.

Evolving the Mind: On the Nature of Matter & the Origin of Consciousness. A. G. Cairns-Smith. 1998. (Illus.). 337p. (C). reprint ed. pap. text 16.95 *(0-521-63755-4)* Cambridge U Pr.

Evolving Therapist: Ten Years of the Family Therapy Networker. Ed. by Richard Simon et al. 1992. LC 91-43237. 592p. pap. 26.95 *(0-89862-268-9)* Guilford Pubns.

Exacta Medica: Reference Tables & Data for the Medical & Nursing Professions. Ian R. Entwistle. 2nd ed. 1998. LC 97-34192. (C). pap. text *(0-443-05894-6)* Church.

Exacta Paediatrica: Reference Tables & Data for Medical & Nursing Professions. Ian R. Entwistle. 2nd ed. 1998. LC 97-34008. 61p. pap. text *(0-443-05895-4)* Church.

Exacta Paediatrica: Reference Tables & Data for the Medical & Nursing Professions. Ed. by Ian R. Entwistle. 1991. (Illus.). 40p. (Orig.). pap. text *(0-443-04627-1)* Church.

Exam Master for Medical-Surgical Nursing Across the Health Care Continuum. Donna D. Ignatavicius et al. Ed. by Robin Carter. 3rd ed. 1999. 1935p. *(0-7216-6984-0)* Saunders.

Exam Review & Study Guide for Perinatal-Pediatric Respiratory Care. Robert Harwood. 1998. (Illus.). 350p. (C). pap. text 34.95 *(0-8036-0347-9)* Davis Co.

Exam Study Guide for Vet Techs. Blais. 1998. pap. text *(0-7216-4971-8)* Harcourt.

Examaster for Linton, Matteson, & Maebius: Introductory Nursing Care of Adults. Nancy K. Maebius & Adrianne D. Linton. Date not set. (Illus.). 100p. *(0-7216-8075-5)* Saunders.

ExaMaster for LPN/LVN Maternity & Pediatrics. Rosner et al. Ed. by Terri Wood. 1999. cd-rom *(0-7216-8270-7)* Saunders.

EXAMaster for Mental Health Nursing: The Nurse-Patient Journey. Verna B. Carson & Elizabeth N. Arnold. Ed. by Thomas Eoyang. 1997. pap. text *(0-7216-6838-0)* Saunders.

Examaster Nuclear Medicine Image. Owens. 1998. *(0-7216-6153-X)* Saunders.

Examaster to Accompany Principles of Imaging Science & Protection. Michael A. Thompson et al. 1995. (Illus.). 544p. text 275.00 *(0-7216-5941-1)* Saunders.

Examaster to Accompany Sorensen & Luckmann's Basic Nursing: A Psychophysiologic Approach. Verolyn B. Bolander. 3rd ed. 1994. text *(0-7216-5253-0)* Saunders.

EXAMaster to Accompany the Medical Assistant: Administrative & Clinical. Kinn & Woods. Ed. by Adrianne Williams. 8th ed. 1999. *(0-7216-7300-7)* Saunders.

Examaster to Physical Examination & Health Assessment. Janice Donaldson Hausauer. 3rd ed. 2000. *(0-7216-8432-7)* Saunders.

Examination & Diagnosis of Muskuloskeletal Disorders: History - Physical Examination - Imaging Techniques - Arthroscopy. W. M. Castro & J. Jerosch. 2000. (Illus.). 400p. 119.00 *(0-86577-741-1)* Thieme Med Pubs.

Examination in Physical Therapy Practice: Screening for Medical Disease. Ed. by William G. Boissonnault. 2nd ed. 1995. text *(0-443-08956-6)* Church.

Examination Medicine: A Guide to Physician Training. Nicholas J. Talley & Simon O'Connor. 3rd ed. 1996. (Illus.). 285p. pap. 60.00 *(0-8036-0274-X)* Davis Co.

Examination Notes in Psychiatry. Glynn Harrison & J. M. Bird. Ed. by Peter F. Buckley. 3rd ed. 1995. 413p. pap. *(0-7506-1427-7)* E A GBR. *Dist:* OUP.

Examination Notes in Psychiatry: Basic Sciences. Gin S. Malhi & Alexander Mitchell. 1999. LC 99-37335. (Illus.). 280p. pap. *(0-7506-4088-X)* E A GBR. *Dist:* OUP.

Examination Obstetics & Gynecology. Judith Goh & Michael Flynn. 1996. 246p. pap. 47.00 *(0-8036-0373-8)* Davis Co.

Examination of Knee Ligament, Vol. 1. 1986. 385.00 *(0-387-92587-2)*; 410.00 *(0-387-92588-0)*; 451.00 *(0-387-92592-9)* Spr-Verlag.

Examination of the Back: An Introduction. John K. Paterson & Loic Burn. 1986. text 73.50 *(0-85200-930-5)* Kluwer Academic.

Examination of the Child with Minor Neurological Dysfunction. Bert C. Touwen. 2nd ed. 1991. (Clinics in Developmental Medicine Ser.: Vol. 71). (Illus.). 141p. (C). text *(0-521-41200-5)* Mc Keith Pr GBR. *Dist:* Cambridge U Pr.

Examination of the Cranial & Peripheral Nerves. Orrin Devinsky & Edward Feldmann. 1987. (Illus.). 118p. text *(0-443-08562-5)* Church.

Examination Paediatrics. Wayne Harris et al. 1992. 370p. pap. *(0-86433-064-2)* Taylor & Francis.

Examination Preparation: A Complete Guide for the Physical Therapist. Scott Giles & Ronda Sanders. Ed. by Therese Giles. rev. ed. 1998. 174p. per., wbk. ed. 33.95 *(1-890989-08-8)* Mainely Phys.

***Examining Asylum Seekers: A Health Professional's Guide to Medical & Psychological Evaluation of Torture.** Physicians For Human Rights Staff. 2001. 200p. 10.00 *(1-879707-36-5)* Phy Human Rights.

Examining Holistic Medicine. Ed. by Douglas Stalker & Clark N. Glymour. LC 85-63039. (Illus.). 406p. (C). reprint ed. 1989. pap. 25.00 *(0-87975-553-9)*; 1985. 42.00 *(0-87975-303-X)* Prometheus Bks.

Examining Patients: An Introduction to Clinical Medicine. Peter J. Toghill. 2nd ed. 1995. (Illus.). 352p. pap. *(0-340-58966-3)* E A GBR. *Dist:* OUP.

Examples Illustrating the Use of Frank Leads. A. H. Lemmerz. 1972. (Illus.). 48p. pap. 10.50 *(3-8055-1294-5)* S Karger.

Exceeding the Boundaries: Understanding Exceptional Lives. Judy W. Wood & Andrea M. Lazzari. 1997. LC 96-76432. 608p. (C). text 94.95 *(0-15-501743-8)* Wadsworth Pub.

Excel in Health Care. Alan C. Gillies & Phil Baugh. 1994. (Illus.). 240p. (Orig.). pap. text 75.95 *(0-412-59760-8*, Chap & Hall NY) Chapman & Hall.

Excellence & Expertise in Nursing. Bronwyn Paterson. 1995. (C). pap. *(0-7300-1266-2*, NPR300) Deakin Univ AUS. *Dist:* St Mut.

Excellence in Health Care Management. Alison Morton-Cooper et al. 1996. LC 96-21528. 256p. (Orig.). pap. 41.95 *(0-632-04032-7)* Blackwell Sci.

Excelling: The Nutritional Way to Good Health. Cecilia Maguire. 1985. (Excelling Ser.). 109p. (gr. 7-12). 10.97 *(0-8239-0635-3)* Rosen Group.

Exceptional Brain: Neuropsychology of Talent & Special Abilities. Ed. by Loraine Obler & Deborah Fein. 1988. LC 86-27136. 522p. 60.00 *(0-89862-701-X)* Guilford Pubns.

Exceptional Child. Kaplan Staff. Date not set. pap. text, tchr. ed. *(0-314-06304-8)*; 1996. stu. ed. 13.00 *(0-314-06305-6)* West Pub.

Exceptional Child: A Guidebook for Churches & Community Agencies. Ed. by James L. Paul. 1983. LC 82-16914. 176p. text 45.00 *(0-8156-2287-2)*; pap. text 19.95 *(0-8156-2288-0)* Syracuse U Pr.

Exceptional Child in the Family-Helping Parents of Exceptional Children. Alan O. Ross. 1964. LC 64-13170. 230p. text 42.00 *(0-8089-0389-6*, 793660, Grune & Strat) Harcrt Hlth Sci Grp.

Exceptional Children: A Developmental View. Marvin D. Wyne & Peter D. O'Connor. 1979. (C). pap. text 45.16 *(0-669-06297-9)* HM Trade Div.

Exceptional Language Development in Down Syndrome: Implications for the Cognition-Language Relationship. Jean A. Rondal. 1995. (Cambridge Monographs & Texts in Applied Psycholinguistics). (Illus.). 367p. (C). text 90.00 *(0-521-36167-2)*; pap. text 32.95 *(0-521-36966-5)* Cambridge U Pr.

Exceptional People: A Guide for Understanding. Schwartz. 1991. (C). text 36.25 net. *(0-07-055962-7)* McGraw.

Excercise Physiology. Robergs. 2nd ed. 1999. pap. text 55.62 net. *(0-07-235392-9)* McGraw.

Exercise Physiology CPS 1615. Joseph Libonati. 1998. text 14.19 *(1-56870-304-X)* RonJon Pub.

***Excerpts from a Family Medical Dictionary.** Rebecca Brown. 2001. 103p. pap. 45.00 *(1-58249-007-4)* Grey Spider.

Excerpts from Classics in Allergy (& Immunology) Ed. by Sheldon Cohen & Max Samter. 1992. 224p. 69.50 *(0-88372-006-X)* OceanSide Pubns.

Excess Catecholamine Syndrome: From Cause to Therapy, Symposium-Stuttgart, Germany, June 29, 1995. Heinz Rupp & International Society for Molecular Nutrition and Th. 1996. LC 96-39362. lib. bdg. *(0-7923-4328-X)* Kluwer Academic.

Excess Face Height Malocclusion: Etiology, Diagnosis & Treatment. Sten Linder-Aronson & Donald G. Woodside. 2000. LC 00-27818. (Illus.). xiv, 106p. *(0-86715-389-X)* Quint Pub Co.

Excessive Venery, Masturbation & Continence. Joseph W. Howe. 1974. LC 73-20629. (Sex, Marriage & Society Ser.). 298p. reprint ed. 25.95 *(0-405-05805-5)* Ayer.

Exchange Lists for Meal Planning. American Diabetes Association & American Dietetic Association Staff. rev. ed. 1995. (Illus.). 32p. pap. *(0-945448-09-0*, 5601) Am Diabetes.

Exchange Lists for Weight Management. American Diabetes Association & American Dietetic Association Staff. 1995. (Illus.). 31p. pap. *(0-945448-17-1*, 5603) Am Diabetes.

Exchanging Voices: A Collaborative Approach to Family Therapy. Lynn Hoffman. 1993. (Systemic Thinking & Practice Ser.). 240p. pap. text *(1-85575-052-X)* Karnac Bks GBR. *Dist:* Brunner-Routledge.

Excimer: Fundamentals & Clinical Use. Harold A. Stein et al. 2nd ed. 1997. LC 97-10945. (Illus.). 260p. pap. text 49.00 *(1-55642-338-1*, 63381) SLACK Inc.

Excimer Laser for Corneal Disease. Peter Hersh & Michael D. Wagoner. 1998. LC 97-16429. (Illus.). 200p. pap. 85.00 *(0-86577-686-5)* Thieme Med Pubs.

Excimer Laser Phototherapeutic Keratectomy. Dimitri T. Azar et al. 1997. LC 96-40065. *(4-260-14332-8)* Igaku-Shoin.

Excimer Laser Therapy Phototherapeutic Keratectomy. Ed. by Dimitri T. Azar et al. 1997. (Illus.). 225p. *(0-89640-332-7)* Igaku-Shoin.

Excimer Lasers in Ophthalmology. McGhee. 1997. LC 97-166783. 453p. text 99.00 incl. audio *(0-7506-9785-7*, M3574) Buttrwrth-Heinemann.

E
F
G

Excipient Toxicity & Safety. Myra L. Weiner & Lois A. Kotkoskie. 1999. LC 99-51474. (Drugs & the Pharmaceutical Sciences Ser.). (Illus.). 392p. text 165.00 (*0-8247-8210-0*) Dekker.

Excipients & Delivery Systems for Pharmaceutical Formulations. Ed. by David R. Karsa & Ronald A. Stephenson. 1995. (Special Publications). 200p. (*0-85404-715-8*, R4715) Royal Soc Chem GBR. *Dist:* Spr-Verlag.

Excision & Reconstruction in Head & Neck Surgery. Ed. by David S. Soutar & Rammohan M. Tiwari. 1994. LC 93-20833. text (*0-443-04526-7*) Church.

Excitation - Contraction Coupling & Cardiac Contractile Force. Donald M. Bers. 1991. (Developments in Cardiovascular Medicine Ser.). 258p. (C). lib. bdg. 118.50 (*0-7923-1186-8*) Kluwer Academic.

Excitation-Contraction Coupling & Cardiac Contractile Force. Donald M. Bers. 1993. (Developments in Cardiovascular Medicine Ser.). 288p. (C). pap. text 61.00 (*0-7923-2479-X*) Kluwer Academic.

Excitation-Contraction Coupling in Skeletal, Cardiac & Smooth Muscle. G. B. Frank et al. 1992. (Advances in Experimental Medicine & Biology Ser.: Vol. 311). (Illus.). 480p. (C). text 135.00 (*0-306-44194-2*, Kluwer Plenum) Kluwer Academic.

Excitation-Contraction Coupling in the Heart. Andrew C. Zygmunt. 1994. 118p. 89.95 (*1-57059-040-0*, LN9040) CRC Pr.

Excitatory Amino Acids: Clinical Results with Antagonists. Ed. by Paul Herrling. 1997. (Illus.). 224p. text 99.95 (*0-12-546820-2*) Morgan Kaufmann.

Excitatory Amino Acids: From Genes to Therapy. P. H. Seeburg et al. 1998. LC 97-51340. (Schering, Ernst, Research Foundation Workshop Ser.). (Illus.). 240p. 79.95 (*3-540-63387-1*) Spr-Verlag.

Excitatory Amino Acids: Their Role in Neuroendocrine Function. Ed. by Darrell W. Brann & Virendra B. Mahesh. 1995. LC 95-36659. 336p. 224.95 (*0-8493-7662-9*, 7662) CRC Pr.

Excitatory Amino Acids & Brain Ischemia: Pharmacological & Clinical Aspects, Proceedings of the Biannual Capo Boi Conference on Neuroscience, June 1989, Villasimius, Italy. Giovanni Biggio et al. 1990. (Advances in the Biosciences Ser.: No. 78). 156p. 100.00 (*0-08-040783-8*, Pergamon Pr) Elsevier.

Excitatory Amino Acids & Epilepsy. Ed. by Robert Schwarcz & Yehezkel Ben-Ari. 1986. LC 86-22614. (Advances in Experimental Medicine & Biology Ser.: Vol. 203). 748p. 135.00 (*0-306-42402-9*, Plenum Trade) Perseus Pubng.

Excitatory Amino Acids & Neuronal Plasticity. Ed. by Yehezkel Ben-Ari. 1990. LC 90-7177. (Advances in Experimental Medicine & Biology Ser.: Vol. 268). (Illus.). 540p. (C). text 174.00 (*0-306-43534-9*, Kluwer Plenum) Kluwer Academic.

Excitatory & Inhibitory States of the Brain. B. N. Klosovskii & E. N. Kosmarskaya. 1963. 464p. 3.5 hd 105.00 (*0-7065-0270-1*) Coronet Bks.

Excited States in Organic Chemistry & Biochemistry. Ed. by Bernard Pullman & Nathan Goldblum. 1977. (Jerusalem Symposia on Quantum Chemistry & Biochemistry Ser.: No. 10). text 171.00 (*90-277-0853-3*) Kluwer Academic.

Excitotoxins: The Taste That Kills. Russell L. Blaylock. 1996. LC 96-52323. (Illus.). pap. 17.95 (*0-929173-25-2*) Health Press.

Excruciating History of Dentistry: Toothsome Tales & Oral Oddities from Babylon to Braces. James Wynbrandt. 1998. LC 98-9794. 288p. 23.95 (*0-312-18576-6*) St Martin.

Excrutiating History of Dentistry. James Wynbrandt. 2000. (Illus.). 2556p. pap. 14.95 (*0-312-26319-8*) St Martin.

Executive Control & the Frontal Lobe: Current Issues. Ed. by Werner X. Schneider et al. 2000. LC 00-57361. (Illus.). vi, 138p. 69.00 (*3-540-67676-7*) Spr-Verlag.

Executive Guide to Case Management Strategies. Marjorie A. Satinsky. 1995. 149p. pap. 56.00 (*1-55648-128-4*, 027102) AHPI.

Executive Skills for Medical Faculty. Neal A. Whitman et al. 1989. 117p. (Orig.). pap. text 20.00 (*0-940193-06-X*) Univ UT Sch Med.

Executive's & Professional Employment Contracts. Art Cowan. 1990. 120p. pap. 39.50 (*1-55943-072-9*, MICHIE) LEXIS Pub.

Executive's Guide to Health & Fitness. Kenneth H. Franklin. 1985. (Illus.). 14.95 (*0-910187-04-5*) Economics Pr.

Executives in Crisis: Recognizing & Managing the Alcoholic, Drug-Addicted, or Mentally Ill Executive. Jeffrey L. Speller. 1989. LC 89-45571. (Management-Human Resource Ser.). 164p. 40.00 (*1-55542-175-X*) Jossey-Bass.

***Exemplary Practices in Employment Services for People with Psychiatric Disabilities.** Elaine Viccora et al. 2001. 72p. (C). reprint ed. pap. text 20.00 (*0-7567-0623-8*) DIANE Pub.

Exemplary Social Intervention Programs for Members & Their Families. Ed. by David Guttman & Marvin B. Sussman. 1995. LC 94-30137. (Marriage & the Family Ser.: Vol. 21, Nos. 1/2). (Illus.). 179p. (C). 39.95 (*1-56024-707-X*) Haworth Pr.

Exercise: Benefits, Limits & Adaptations. Ed. by Donald Macleod et al. 1987. 416p. pap. text 27.50 (*0-419-14140-5*, Spon) Routledge.

Exercise: Pulmonary Physiology & Pathophysiology. Wasserman & Brian J. Whipp. 1991. (Lung Biology in Health & Disease Ser.: Vol. 52). (Illus.). 584p. text 230.00 (*0-8247-8230-5*) Dekker.

Exercise - Immunology. Bente K. Pedersen. 1997. (Medical Intelligence Unit Ser.). 250p. pap. 89.95 (*0-412-13501-9*) Chapman & Hall.

Exercise Activities for the Elderly. Kay Flatten et al. 1988. (Adulthood & Aging Ser.). 224p. pap. 31.95 (*0-8261-5910-9*) Springer Pub.

Exercise & Arthritis: A Guide to Pain-Free Movement. Margaret Hills. 1997. LC 97-17033. (Illus.). 128p. pap. text 10.95 (*1-882606-33-7*) Peoples Med Soc.

Exercise & Circulation in Health & Disease. Ed. by Bengt Saltin et al. 1999. LC 99-24144. 360p. 62.00 (*0-88011-632-3*) Human Kinetics.

Exercise & Disease. Ronald R. Watson. 1992. 240p. 141.95 (*0-8493-7912-1*, RM725) CRC Pr.

Exercise & Disease Management. Brian C. Leutholtz. 1999. LC 99-26886. (CRC Series in Exercise Physiology Ser.). 240p. 149.95 (*0-8493-8713-2*) CRC Pr.

Exercise & Heart Failure. Ed. by Gary J. Balady & Ileana L. Pina. 1997. LC 97-6841. (American Heart Association Monograph Ser.). (Illus.). 368p. 75.00 (*0-87993-667-3*) Futura Pub.

Exercise & Mental Health. William P. Morgan & Stephen E. Goldston. 1987. (Series in Health Psychology & Behavioral Medicine). 196p. 56.95 (*0-89116-564-9*) Hemisp Pub.

Exercise & Nutrition in Preventative Cardiology. David A. Leaf. 1991. 296p. (C). text 27.00 net. (*0-697-14839-4*) Brown & Benchmark.

Exercise & Oxygen Toxicity. Ed. by Chandan K. Sen et al. 1994. LC 94-40584. 536p. 256.25 (*0-444-81765-4*) Elsevier.

Exercise & Sport in Diabetes. William A. Burr & Dinesh K. Nagi. 1999. LC 99-32280. (Diabetes in Practice Ser.). (Illus.). 208p. 95.00 (*0-471-98496-5*) Wiley.

Exercise & Sport Sciences Reviews (ESSR), Vol. 25. Holloszy. 1997. (Illus.). 500p. (Orig.). 60.00 (*0-683-18333-8*) Lppncott W & W.

Exercise & Sport Sciences Reviews (ESSR), Vol. 26. annuals American College of Sports Medicine Staff. Ed. by Douglas R. Seals. 2001. LC 98-23508. 425p. 60.00 (*0-683-18346-X*) Lppncott W & W.

Exercise & Sports Science Reviews 1991, Vol. 19. John D. Holloszy. 1991. (Illus.). 545p. 49.00 (*0-683-00048-9*) Lppncott W & W.

Exercise & Sports Sciences Review, Vol. 17. Ed. by Kent B. Pandolf. 1989. (American College of Sports Medicine Ser.). (Illus.). 584p. pap. 46.95 (*0-683-00046-2*) Lppncott W & W.

Exercise & Sports Sciences Review, Vol. 18. Kent B. Pandolf. 1990. (Illus.). 480p. 46.95 (*0-683-00047-0*) Lppncott W & W.

Exercise & the Heart: Clinical Concepts. Victor F. Froelicher. 3rd ed. 1993. (Illus.). 408p. (C). (gr. 13). text 74.95 (*0-8016-6819-0*, 06819) Mosby Inc.

Exercise & the Heart in Health & Disease. Ed. by Roy J. Shephard & H. S. Miller. 2nd exp. rev. ed. 1998. (Fundamental & Clinical Cardiology Ser.). (Illus.). 656p. text 195.00 (*0-8247-0227-1*, 0227-1) Dekker.

Exercise, Calories, Fat & Cancer. M. M. Jacobs. 1992. LC 92-49867. (Advances in Experimental Medicine & Biology Ser.: Vol. 322). (Illus.). 318p. (C). text 95.00 (*0-306-44256-6*, Kluwer Plenum) Kluwer Academic.

Exercise Designed for the Aging. Francis D. Meyer. 1985. (Exercise & Care of Aging Body Ser.). (Illus.). 181p. pap. text 5.95 (*0-9615720-0-0*) FDM Distributor.

Exercise Echocardiography: A Book & Videotape. Ed. by Linda J. Crouse & Paul H. Kramer. 1991. (Illus.). 112p. 95.00 incl. VHS (*0-87993-520-0*) Futura Pub.

Exercise Education: A Personal Approach to Weight Control & Wellness. Myrna M. Schild. 1990. (Illus.). 112p. (Orig.). pap. 9.95 (*0-9624958-2-4*) Auto Review Pub.

Exercise Exchange Program: The Unique System That Allows You to Design Your Own Diet & Workout Every Day for a Lifetime of Good Health. James M. Rippe. 1993. LC 91-26196. (Illus.). 384p. pap. 18.25 (*0-671-79453-1*, Fireside) S&S Trade Pap.

Exercise for a Healthy Pregnancy & Birth. Linda Barr & Catherine P. Monserrat. rev. ed. 1992. (Illus.). 17p. reprint ed. pap. 2.95 (*0-945886-09-8*) New Futures.

Exercise for the Prevention & Treatment of Illness. Ed. by Linn Goldberg & Dianne L. Elliot. 1994. LC 93-46467. (Contemporary Exercise & Sports Medicine Ser.). (Illus.). 344p. (C). pap. 79.00 (*0-8036-4163-X*) Davis Co.

Exercise Handouts for Rehabilitation. Carole B. Lewis & Therese McNerney. 2000. (Aspen Series on Physical Therapy). spiral bd. 99.00 (*0-8342-0372-3*, 20372) PRO-ED.

Exercise in Diagnosis & Treatment of Coronary Heart Disease. Ed. by J. J. Kellermann. 1977. (Cardiology Ser.: Vol. 62, No. 3 (1977)). (Illus.). 26.25 (*3-8055-2805-1*) S Karger.

Exercise in Health & Disease. Pollock. 3rd ed. 1999. text 55.00 (*0-7216-7321-X*) Saunders.

Exercise in Health & Disease: Evaluation & Prescription for Prevention & Rehabilitation. Bruce Pollock & D. W. Wilmore. 2nd ed. 1990. (Illus.). 736p. text 60.00 (*0-7216-2948-2*) Saunders.

Exercise in Modern Medicine: Testing & Prescription in Health & Disease. Barry A. Franklin et al. 1988. (Illus.). 328p. 49.00 (*0-683-03350-6*) Lppncott W & W.

Exercise in Pregnancy. Raul Artal-Mittelmark et al. 2nd ed. 1990. (Illus.). 352p. 69.00 (*0-683-00258-9*) Lppncott W & W.

Exercise in Rehabilitation Medicine. Ed. by Walter R. Frontera et al. 1999. LC 98-53986. (Illus.). xii, 484p. text 84.00 (*0-88011-839-3*, BFRO0839) Human Kinetics.

Exercise in the Clinical Management of Diabetes. Barbara Campaigne & Richard M. Lampman. 1994. LC 93-43321. (Illus.). 224p. text 37.00 (*0-87322-634-8*, BCAM0634) Human Kinetics.

Exercise Induced Asthma. E. R. McFadden. 1999. LC 98-56648. (Lung Biology in Health & Disease Ser.). (Illus.). 410p. text 175.00 (*0-8247-9904-6*) Dekker.

Exercise Manual for Head & Neck Patients. 1981. 5.00 (*0-940876-05-1*) City Hope.

Exercise Manual for Mastectomy Patients, Auxillary Node Disection Patients. 1981. 5.00 (*0-940876-04-3*) City Hope.

Exercise, Nutrition & the Older Woman: Wellness for Women over Fifty. Maria Fiatarone-Singh. 2000. LC 00-20810. (Illus.). 624p. 89.95 (*0-8493-0258-7*) CRC Pr.

Exercise on Prescription: Cardiovascular Activity for Health. John Buckley et al. 1998. LC 98-28353. 248p. pap. text 32.50 (*0-7506-3288-7*) Buttrwrth-Heinemann.

Exercise Packet for CPT Coding. 1997. 500p. (C). pap. text 120.00 (*1-889115-26-6*) Med Learn.

Exercise Physiology. Scott K. Powers & Edward T. Howley. 3rd ed. 1996. LC 96-83127. 624p. (C). text 49.50 net. (*0-697-25798-3*) Brown & Benchmark.

Exercise Physiology. Victor L. Katch et al. 4th ed. 1996. 437p. pap., stu. ed. 17.95 (*0-683-18103-3*) Lppncott W & W.

Exercise Physiology: Energy, Nutrition & Human Performance. William D. McArdle et al. 3rd ed. 1990. 853p. text 57.95 (*0-8121-1351-9*); 4th ed. 1996. (Illus.). 850p. 62.95 (*0-683-05731-6*) Lppncott W & W.

Exercise Physiology: For Health, Fitness & Performance. Sharon A. Plowman & Denise L. Smith. 1997. (C). tchr. ed. (*0-205-19862-7*, H9862-7) Allyn.

Exercise Physiology: For Health, Fitness & Performance - Examination Copy. Sharon A. Plowman & Denise L. Smith. 1996. 592p. (C). (*0-205-26443-3*, T6443-0) Allyn.

Exercise Physiology Text & Study Guide Set. William D. McArdle et al. 1997. 69.95 (*0-683-30051-2*) Lppncott W & W.

Exercise Prescription & the Back. 2000. LC 00-55029. 254p. (C). text 54.95 (*0-8385-2325-0*) McGraw-Hill Prof.

Exercise Prescription for the High-Risk Cardiac Patient. Ray W. Squires. 1998. LC 97-42640. (Illus.). 216p. text 36.00 (*0-87322-980-0*, BSQU0980) Human Kinetics.

Exercise Psychology: The Influence of Physical Exercise on Psychological Processes. Ed. by Peter Seraganian. 1992. LC 92-5498. (Health Psychology & Behavioral Medicine Ser.). 432p. 200.00 (*0-471-52701-7*) Wiley.

Exercise Testing & Exercise Prescription for Special Cases: Theoretical Basis & Clinical Application. Ed. by James S. Skinner. 2nd ed. 1993. LC 92-10383. (Illus.). 395p. 49.00 (*0-8121-1440-X*) Lppncott W & W.

Exercise Testing & Prescription: A Health-Related Approach. David C. Nieman. 4th ed. 1998. LC 98-10359. xii, 708p. pap. text 55.95 (*0-7674-0474-2*) Mayfield Pub.

Exercise Testing & Training in the Elderly Cardiac Patient. Mark A. Williams. 1993. LC 93-34283. (Current Issues in Cardiac Rehabilitation Ser.: Vol. 1). 136p. pap. text 23.00 (*0-87322-621-6*, BWIL0621) Human Kinetics.

Exercise Tests in Relation to Cardiovascular Function: Report of a WHO Meeting, 1968. 1968. (Technical Report Ser.: No. 388). 30p. pap. text 4.00 (*92-4-120388-9*, 1100388) World Health.

Exercise Throughout the Life Cycle: A Comprehensive Handbook. Richard R. Suminski. 1999. (Exercise Physiology Ser.). 59.95 (*0-8493-8711-6*) CRC Pr.

Exercise, Training & the Immune Response. Roy J. Shephard. 1997. LC 96-72242. 460p. pap. 75.00 (*1-884125-65-4*) Cooper Pubng.

***Exercises for Chemotherapy Patients: Getting Well Faster Through Exercise.** Harry Raftopolous. 2002. 160p. 14.95 (*1-57826-093-0*) Hatherleigh.

Exercises for the Elderly. Robert H. Jamieson. l.t. ed. 1982. LC 85-9781. (Illus.). 158p. pap. 6.95 (*0-8008-2564-0*) Taplinger.

Exercises in Diagnostic Imaging. Sarah Burnett & Asif Saifuddin. 1997. 150p. text (*90-5702-017-3*); pap. text (*90-5702-018-1*) GBSP NLD. *Dist:* Gordon & Breach.

Exercises in Diagnostic Radiology: Chest, Abdomen, Bone & Clinical Skills: A Problem-Based Text. Judith K. Amorosa et al. 3rd ed. 1992. (Illus.). 380p. pap. text 38.95 (*0-7216-3129-0*) Saunders.

Exercises in Fetal Monitoring. Barry S. Schifrin. 1990. (Illus.). 192p. (C). (gr. 13). spiral bd. 40.00 (*0-8151-7565-5*, 20330) Mosby Inc.

Exercises in Health Information: Management of Strategic Resources. Mervat Abdelhak. 1996. 784p. pap. text, wbk. ed. 23.00 (*0-7216-5133-X*) Saunders.

Exercises in Oral Radiographic Interpretation. Robert P. Langlais & Myron J. Kasle. 3rd ed. 1992. (Illus.). 281p. pap. text 47.00 (*0-7216-4468-6*) Saunders.

Exercises in Positioning. Kathy McQuillen-Martensen. 1996. LC 95-17703. 438p. pap. text 39.95 (*0-7216-4981-5*) Saunders.

Exercises in Radiological Diagnosis of the Cervico-Occipital Joint. A. Wackenheim. Tr. by M. T. Wackenheim from FRE. 1985. LC 85-14691. (Exercises in Radiological Diagnosis Ser.). (Illus.). 192p. 35.95 (*0-387-15327-6*) Spr-Verlag.

Exercises in Sonography. Reva Arnez Curry. 1995. 492p. (C). pap. text 42.00 (*0-7216-4962-9*) Harcrt Hlth Sci Grp.

Exercising Through Your Pregnancy. James T. Clapp, III. 1998. LC 98-12426. (Illus.). 256p. pap. 16.95 (*0-87322-941-X*, BCLA0941) Human Kinetics.

Exercising Your Way to Better Mental Health. Larry M. Leith. 1998. LC 97-61333. (Illus.). 120p. 14.95 (*1-885693-09-5*) Fit Info Tech.

Exercising Your Wellpower for Optimal Physical Health. Raymond Cole & Steve Bhaerman. 1984. (Illus.). 233p. (Orig.). pap. 9.95 (*0-917073-00-2*) Wellpower.

Exhausting Our Options. Leonie J. Archer. 1992. 132p. 29.95 (*0-948061-72-3*, P7483) PennWell Corp.

Existence. Ed. by Rollo May et al. 1994. LC 94-71311. (Master Work Ser.). 456p. pap. 40.00 (*1-56821-271-2*) Aronson.

Existential - Dialectical Marital Therapy: Breaking the Secret Code of Marriage. Israel W. Charny. 1992. LC 91-43195. (Frontiers in Couples & Family Therapy Ser.: No. 5). 352p. text 39.95 (*0-87630-636-9*) Brunner-Routledge.

Existential Art Therapy: The Canvas Mirror. Bruce L. Moon. 2nd ed. 1995. LC 95-3655. (Illus.). 230p. (C). text 55.95 (*0-398-05999-3*); pap. text 37.95 (*0-398-06514-4*) C C Thomas.

Existential Counseling in Practice. Emmy Van Deurzen-Smith. 1987. 256p. (C). 74.50 (*0-8039-8126-0*, 7016); pap. 24.95 (*0-8039-8127-9*, 7017) Sage.

Existential Foundations of Medicine & Psychology. Medard Boss. 1995. LC 84-2822. 340p. pap. text 60.00 (*1-56821-420-0*) Aronson.

Existential Hypnotherapy. Mark E. King & Charles M. Citrenbaum. 1993. LC 93-25048. (Clinical & Experimental Hypnosis Ser.). 175p. 30.00 (*0-89862-344-8*, 2344) Guilford Pubns.

Existential-Phenomenological Perspectives in Psychology: Exploring the Breadth of Human Experience. R. S. Valle & S. Halling. 1989. LC 88-39126. (Illus.). 376p. (C). 70.00 (*0-306-42979-9*); pap. 37.50 (*0-306-43044-4*) Perseus Pubng (Plenum Trade).

Existential Psychology. Ed. by Rollo May. 2nd ed. 1969. 128p. (C). pap. 20.31 (*0-07-553578-5*) McGrw-H Hghr Educ.

Existential Psychology. Rollo May. 1990. pap. 9.95 (*0-394-30743-7*) Random.

Existential Psychotherapy. Irvin D. Yalom. 1980. LC 80-50553. 524p. pap. 52.00 (*0-465-02147-6*) Basic.

Existential Psychotherapy & the Interpretations of Dreams. Clark Moustakas. 1995. LC 93-40807. 232p. reprint ed. pap. 40.00 (*1-56821-771-4*) Aronson.

Existential Self in Society. Ed. by Joseph A. Kotarba & Andrea Fontana. LC 84-166. (Illus.). (C). 1992. 272p. lib. bdg. 25.00 (*0-226-45140-2*); 1987. 242p. pap. text 13.50 (*0-226-45141-0*) U Ch Pr.

Existential Time-limited Thera. Freddie Strasser & Alison Strasser. 1997. LC 97-222179. 222p. pap. 60.00 (*0-471-97571-0*) Wiley.

Existentialist Approach to Psychotherapy with Adults & Children. Hanna Colm. 1966. (Illus.). 240p. text 45.00 (*0-8089-0102-8*, 790882, Grune & Strat) Harcrt Hlth Sci Grp.

Exocrine Pancreatic Cancer. Ed. by H. Baumel & B. Deixonne. 1986. (Illus.). 214p. 146.00 (*0-387-16530-4*) Spr-Verlag.

Exogenous & Endogenous Influences on Metabolic & Neural Control Vol. 2: Abstracts: Proceedings of the Third Congress of the European Society for Comparative Physiology & Biochemistry, August 31-September 3, 1981, Noorwijkerhout, Netherlands. Ed. by A. D. Addink & N. Spronk. 1982. (Illus.). 260p. (*0-08-028845-6*) Pergamon Repr GBR. *Dist:* Franklin.

Exogenous Dermatology: Advances in Skin-Related Allergology, Bioengineering, Pharmacology, & Toxicology. Ed. by A. J. Bircher et al. 1995. LC 95-13572. (Current Problems in Dermatology Ser.: Vol. 22). (Illus.). xviii, 242p. 224.50 (*3-8055-6062-1*) S Karger.

Exogenous Dermatoses: Environmental Dermatitis. Torkil Menne. 1990. 472p. 135.95 (*0-8493-5969-4*, RC593) CRC Pr.

Exotic Deviance: Medicalizing Cultural Idioms. Robert E. Bartholomew. 2000. LC 00-51878. xviii, 280p. 59.95 (*0-87081-597-0*); 288p. pap. 29.95 (*0-87081-598-9*) Univ Pr Colo.

Exotic Medicine Library. Ed. by Branson W. Ritchie et al. 1994. (Illus.). 2400p. (C). text 225.00 incl. cd-rom (*0-9636996-2-8*) Zoological Educ.

Exotic Pet Guide Update 2. Shawn P. Messonnier. 2000. 39.95 (*0-323-00042-8*) Mosby Inc.

Exotic Pleasures Fascicle III: Curious Scientific & Medical Observations. Engelbert Kaempfer. Tr. by Robert W. Carrubba from LAT. 1995. LC 94-29042. (Library of Renaissance Humanism). (Illus.). 280p. (C). 50.00 (*0-8093-1976-4*) S Ill U Pr.

Exotic Viral Infections. Ed. by James Porterfield. 1996. (Illus.). 416p. (C). 209.95 (*0-412-63030-3*, Chap & Hall NY) Chapman & Hall.

Expanded Family Life Cycle: Individual, Family, & Social Perspectives. Elizabeth A. Carter et al. 3rd ed. 1998. LC 98-15208. 541p. (C). 81.00 (*0-205-20009-5*) Allyn.

Expanded Programme on Immunization in South-East Asia. 1986. (SEARO Regional Health Papers: No. 12). 377p. pap. text 20.00 (*92-9022-181-X*, 1580012) World Health.

Expanding Access to Investigational Therapies for HIV Infection & AIDS. Institute of Medicine Staff. 1991. 84p. (C). pap. text 19.00 (*0-309-04490-1*) Natl Acad Pr.

Expanding Face of AIDS: Implications for Social Work Practice. Ed. by Vincent J. Lynch et al. 1993. LC 92-42902. 288p. 55.00 (*0-86569-205-X*, T205, Auburn Hse) Greenwood.

Expanding Health Coverage for Children: Matching Federal Policies & State Strategies. Frwd. by Sandy Praeger. 1998. LC 98-124749. (Illus.). 48p. pap. (*1-887748-19-9*) Milbank Memorial.

Expanding Horizons in Medical Social Work. Ed. by Dora Goldstine. 1993. LC 54-11423. lib. bdg. 17.50 (*0-226-30164-8*) U Ch Pr.

Expanding Indications for the New Macrolides, Azalides & Streptogramins. Ed. by Stephen H. Zinner et al. 1997. LC 97-12233. (Illus.). 720p. text 225.00 (*0-8247-0056-2*) Dekker.

Expanding Nursing Knowledge: Understanding & Reseaching Your Own Practice. Gary Rolfe. 1998. LC 97-36320. (Illus.). 224p. pap. text 35.00 (*0-7506-3013-2*) Buttrwrth-Heinemann.

Expanding Role of Folates & Fluoropyrimidines in Cancer Chemotherapy. Ed. by Y. Rustum & J. J. McGuire. 1989. LC 88-38105. (Illus.). 346p. 79.50 (*0-306-43100-9*, Plenum Trade) Perseus Pubng.

Expanding Role of Medical Physics in Diagnostic Imaging: (1997 AAPM Summer School) Ed. by G. Donald Frey & Perry Sprawls. 1997. (AAPM Monograph Ser.: No. 23). 592p. text (*1-888340-09-6*) AAPM.

Expanding the Employer-Provided Health Insurance System: Effects on Workers & Their Employers. Sheila R. Zedlewski. 1991. LC 91-6616. (Urban Institute Report: No. 91-3). (Illus.). 106p. (C). pap. text 19.50 (*0-87766-509-5*); lib. bdg. 46.00 (*0-87766-508-7*) Urban Inst.

Expanding the Medicaid Program in Texas: Funding Issues & Alternatives. Anne Dunkelberg. 1988. (Special Project Reports: Vol. SP-EMP). 237p. reprint ed. pap. 10.00 (*0-89940-861-3*) LBJ Sch Pub Aff.

Expanding the Role of Medical Physics in Nuclear Medicine. Ed. by G. D. Frey et al. 1991. (American Association Physicists in Medicine Monographs: No. 18). 376p. 75.00 (*0-88318-915-1*) Am Inst Physics.

Expanding the Role of the Nurse: The Scope of Professional Practice. Ed. by Geoffrey Hunt & Paul Wainright. 1994. LC 93-46835. 240p. pap. 41.95 (*0-632-03604-4*) Blackwell Sci.

Expansion of the Use of Immunization in Developing Countries: Proceedings of the WHO Seminar, 1st, Kumasi, Ghana, 1974. WHO Staff. 1975. (Offset Publications: No. 16). pap. text 12.00 (*92-4-170016-5*, 1120016) World Health.

Expansions of Feminist Family Theory Through Diversity. Ed. by Rhea V. Almeida. 1994. LC 94-175. (Journals of Feminist Family Therapy). (Illus.). 134p. (C). lib. bdg. 39.95 (*1-56024-667-7*) Haworth Pr.

Expectancy: A Guide for Pregnant Women. Ellen Farhang & Kenneth Farhang. 1986. LC 86-70733. (Illus.). 208p. 12.95 (*0-9617497-0-9*); pap. 8.95 (*0-9617497-1-7*) Alamitos Hlth Pubns.

***Expectant Mothers & Substance Abuse Intervention & Treatment Challenges for State Government: Congressional Hearing.** Ed. by Mark E. Souder. 2001. reprint ed. pap. text 35.00 (*0-7567-1818-X*) DIANE Pub.

Expectant Parent's Guide to Preventing a Cesarean Section. Carl Jones. 1991. LC 90-1299. 176p. pap. 15.75 (*0-89789-223-2*); (Illus.). 55.00 (*0-89789-222-4*, H222) Greenwood (Bergin & Garvey).

Expected Miracles: Surgeons at Work. Joan Cassell. 1991. 259p. 59.95 (*0-87722-804-3*); pap. 22.95 (*0-87722-838-8*) Temple U Pr.

Expecting the Best: The Journey Toward a Healthy Pregnancy. Kathy King. 1992. 92p. pap. text (*1-884153-07-0*) Prk Nicollet.

Expecting Trouble: The Myth of Prenatal Care in America. Thomas H. Strong, Jr. 2000. LC 00-8927. ix, 243p. 24.95 (*0-8147-9767-9*) NYU Pr.

Expedition Medicine. Ed. by Bent Juel-Jensen. 1993. (C). (*0-907649-61-0*) Expedit Advisory Ctr GBR. *Dist:* St Mut.

Experience of Alzheimer's Disease: Life Through a Tangled Veil. Steven Sabat. 2001. LC 2001-18140. (Illus.). 368p. pap. 26.95 (*0-631-21666-9*) Blackwell Pubs.

Experience of Anxiety: A Casebook. James O. Palmer. Ed. by Michael J. Goldstein. 2nd ed. 1975. 312p. (C). pap. text 22.95 (*0-19-501921-0*) OUP.

Experience of Circumcision in Immigrant Somali Women. Carol D. Christiansen. 1997. 19.95 (*0-88737-727-0*, 14-7270, NLN Pr) Natl League Nurse.

Experience of Hypnosis. Ernest R. Hilgard. 1968. LC 68-25372. 353p. pap. 8.95 (*0-15-629552-0*, Harvest Bks) Harcourt.

Experience of Place. Tony Hiss. 1991. LC 91-50006. (Illus.). 256p. pap. 13.00 (*0-679-73594-1*) Vin Bks.

Experience of Psychiatric Hospital Closure: An Anthropological Study. Christine M. Perring. 1993. (Studies of Care in the Community). 231p. (*1-85628-422-0*) Avebry GBR. *Dist:* Ashgate Pub Co.

Experience of Psychopathology: Investigating Mental Disorders in Their Natural Settings. Ed. by Marten W. De Vries. 1992. 447p. (C). text 100.00 (*0-521-40339-1*) Cambridge U Pr.

Experience of Recovery. Ed. by LeRoy Spaniol & Martin Koehler. 1994. 89p. pap. text 10.00 (*1-878512-04-8*) Boston Univ Ctr Psy Rehab.

Experiences in Management & Organizational Behavior. Donald D. Bowen et al. 4th ed. 1996. LC 96-29422. 432p. pap. 44.95 (*0-471-30826-9*) Wiley.

Experiences in Personality: Research, Assessment & Change. Matthew R. Merrens & Gary G. Brannigan. 1997. LC 97-15015. 240p. pap. 29.95 (*0-471-13937-8*) Wiley.

Experiences of Counselling in Action. Dave Mearns & Windy Dryden. 1989. (Counselling in Action Ser.). 160p. (C). pap. 24.95 (*0-8039-8193-7*, 7142) Sage.

Experiences of Counselling in Action. Ed. by Dave Mearns & Windy Dryden. 1989. (Counselling in Action Ser.). 160p. (C). 52.50 (*0-8039-8192-9*) Sage.

Experiences of Schizophrenia: An Integration of the Personal, Scientific & Therapeutic. Michael Robbins. 1993. LC 92-48311. 511p. 65.00 (*0-89862-997-7*, 2997) Guilford Pubns.

Experiences with Primary Health Care in Zambia. Ed. by J. M. Kasonde & J. D. Martin. 1994. LC 96-142219. (Public Health in Action Ser.: No. 2). (ENG & FRE.). vii, 118p. pap. text 26.00 (*92-4-156169-6*, 1390002) World Health.

Experiencing: A Humanistic Theory of Psychology & Psychiatry. Alvin R. Mahrer. 1989. 1204p. pap. 47.00 (*0-7766-0245-4*) Paul & Co Pubs.

Experiencing & Explaining Disease. Basiro Davey. 1985. 148p. pap. (*0-335-15055-1*) OpUniv Pr GBR. *Dist:* Raincoast Bk.

Experiencing & Explaining Disease. Ed. by Basiro Davey & Clive Seale. 1996. LC 95-44211. (Health & Disease Ser.: Bk. 8). 224p. pap. (*0-335-19208-4*) OpUniv Pr.

***Experiencing & Explaining Disease.** Ed. by Basiro Davey & Clive Seale. 2001. (Health & Disease Ser.). 224p. pap. (*0-335-20837-1*) OpUniv Pr GBR. *Dist:* Taylor & Francis.

Experiencing Cancer: Quality of Life in Treatment. Kristen C. Schou & Jenny Hewison. 1998. LC 98-18404. viii, 197p. (*0-335-19892-9*); 192p. pap. (*0-335-19891-0*) OpUniv Pr.

Experiencing HIV: Personal, Family & Work Relationships. Barry D. Adam & Alan Sears. 1996. LC 96-19248. 182p. 52.00 (*0-231-10120-1*); 224p. pap. 17.50 (*0-231-10121-X*) Col U Pr.

Experiencing Hypnosis: Therapeutic Approaches to Altered States. Milton H. Erickson & Ernest L. Rossi. 1981. LC 80-26957. 300p. 49.50 (*0-8290-0246-4*) Irvington.

Experiencing Social Psychology: Readings & Projects. Ayala M. Pines & Christina Maslach. 3rd ed. 1993. LC 92-11918. (Series in Social Psychology). 352p. (C). pap. 38.75 (*0-07-040773-8*) McGraw-H Hghr Educ.

Experiencing Youth: First-Person Accounts. George W. Goethals & Dennis Klos. 2nd ed. 1987. 480p. (C). reprint ed. pap. text 43.00 (*0-8191-5688-4*) U Pr of Amer.

Experiential Psychotherapy: A Symphony of Selves. Richard E. Felder & Avrum G. Weiss. 1991. 196p. (C). pap. text 32.00 (*0-8191-8194-3*) U Pr of Amer.

Experiential Psychotherapy: Basic Practices. Alvin R. Mahrer. 1989. 572p. pap. 33.00 (*0-7766-0244-6*) Paul & Co Pubs.

Experiential Psychotherapy Within Families. Walter Kempler. 2nd ed. 1991. 274p. reprint ed. pap. 25.00 (*0-9600808-2-1*) Kempler Inst.

Experiment & Interpretation: A Pathologist Reflects on Thirty Years of Cancer Research. Myer H. Salaman. 1995. LC 94-22351. 264p. (C). text (*0-485-11470-4*) Athlone Pr GBR. *Dist:* Transaction Pubs, Humanities.

Experiment Perilous: Physicians & Patients Facing the Unknown. Renee C. Fox. 1997. LC 97-9857. 290p. pap. text 24.95 (*1-56000-949-7*) Transaction Pubs.

Experimental & Applied Physiology. Richard G. Pflanzer. 5th ed. 1994. 384p. (C). text 38.00 net. (*0-697-13786-4*, WCB McGr Hill) McGrw-H Hghr Educ.

Experimental & Clinical Amblyopia. Ed. by E. Auerbach. 1977. (Documenta Ophthalmologica Proceedings Ser.: Vol. 11). pap. text 107.50 (*90-6193-151-7*) Kluwer Academic.

Experimental & Clinical Aspects of Proteinuria. Ed. by M. Weise. 1981. (Contributions to Nephrology Ser.: Vol. 24). (Illus.). x, 166p. pap. 29.75 (*3-8055-1655-X*) S Karger.

Experimental & Clinical Evaluation of the Tuberculostatics, Capeomycin, Isoxyl, Myambutol, Rifampicin: Proceedings of the International Colloquium, Borstel, 1968. International Colloquium Borstel Staff. Ed. by E. Freerksen. 1970. (Antibiotics & Chemotherapy Ser.: Vol. 16). (Illus.). 151.50 (*3-8055-0481-0*) S Karger.

Experimental & Clinical Hepatology. Ed. by Christoph E. Broelsch-Houssin & O. Zelder. 1986. text 178.50 (*0-85200-929-1*) Kluwer Academic.

Experimental & Clinical Neurotoxicology. Ed. by Peter S. Spencer & Herbert H. Schaumberg. 2nd ed. 2000. LC 98-18540. (Illus.). 1352p. text 195.00 (*0-19-508477-2*) OUP.

Experimental & Clinical Photoimmunology, Vol. 2. R. Daynes & G. R. Krueger. 1983. LC 82-14695. 208p. 120.00 (*0-8493-5371-8*, CRC Reprint) Franklin.

Experimental & Clinical Photoimmunology, Vol. III. Ed. by R. Daynes & Gerald Krueger. 1985. 256p. 132.00 (*0-8493-5372-6*, QR182, CRC Reprint) Franklin.

Experimental & Clinical Progress in Cancer Chemotherapy. Ed. by Franco M. Muggia. 1985. (Cancer Treatment & Research Ser.). text 146.50 (*0-89838-679-9*) Kluwer Academic.

***Experimental & Clinical Studies on the Antiemetic Effects of Propofol.** Bengt Hammas. 2001. (Comprehensive Summaries of Uppsala Dissertations from the Faculty of Medicine Ser.: No. 1028). 39p. (*91-554-5001-6*) Uppsala Universitet SWE. *Dist:* Coronet Bks.

Experimental & Genetic Rat Models of Chronic Renal Failure. Ed. by N. Gretz & M. Strauch. 1993. (Illus.). x, 344p. 215.75 (*3-8055-5499-0*) S Karger.

Experimental & Surgical Technique in the Rat. H. B. Waynforth & P. A. Flecknell. 2nd ed. 1992. (Illus.). 400p. 90.00 (*0-12-738851-6*) Acad Pr.

Experimental & Theoretical Studies of Consciousness - Symposium No. 174. Ed. by Thomas Nagel. 1993. (CIBA Foundation Symposia Ser.: No. 174). 326p. 150.00 (*0-471-93866-1*) Wiley.

Experimental Animal in Biomedical Research, Vol. 1. Bernard Rollin. 1990. 464p. 294.95 (*0-8493-4981-8*, HV4915) CRC Pr.

Experimental Animal in Biomedical Research, Vol. 2. Bernard E. Rollin. 1995. LC 90-1698. (Experimental Animal in Biomedical Research Ser.: Vol. II). 560p. 239.95 (*0-8493-4982-6*) CRC Pr.

Experimental Aspects of Normal & Diabetic Pregnancy. Ed. by E. Herrera & J. Girard. 1987. (Journal: Vol. 51, No. 2,). (Illus.). 68p. pap. 40.00 (*3-8055-4560-6*) S Karger.

Experimental Basis for Absorbed-Dose Calculations in Medical Use of Radionuclides. 1985. LC 85-7292. (Report Ser.: No. 83). 109p. pap. text 35.00 (*0-913392-76-6*) NCRP Pubns.

Experimental Cardiopulmonary Cerebral Resuscitation. Ala Nozari. 2000. (Comprehensive Summaries of Uppsala Dissertations from the Faculty of Medicine Ser.: No. 931). (Illus.). 59p. pap. (*91-554-4726-0*) Uppsala Universitet SWE. *Dist:* Coronet Bks.

Experimental Colon Carcinogenesis. Ed. by Herman Autrup & Gary M. Williams. 1983. 320p. 180.00 (*0-8493-5543-5*, RC280, CRC Reprint) Franklin.

Experimental Comparison of Statistical & Case History Methods of Attitude Research. Samuel A. Stouffer. Ed. by Harriet Zuckerman & Robert K. Merton. 1980. LC 79-9031. (Dissertations on Sociology Ser.). lib. bdg. 25.95 (*0-405-12997-1*) Ayer.

Experimental Design: Procedures for Behavioral Sciences. Roger E. Kirk. 3rd ed. 1994. LC 94-20548. (Psychology Ser.). 928p. 137.95 (*0-534-25092-0*) Brooks-Cole.

Experimental Design & Analysis in Animal Sciences. T. R. Morris. 1999. LC 99-22857. 224p. pap. text 40.00 (*0-85199-349-4*) OUP.

Experimental Dimension of Psychology. Alan Richardson. 1987. LC 83-23335. 244p. pap. text (*0-7022-1937-1*) Univ Queensland Pr AUS. *Dist:* Intl Spec Bk.

Experimental Endodontics. Ed. by Larz S. Spangberg. 1989. 224p. 169.00 (*0-8493-4737-8*, RK351) CRC Pr.

Experimental Endolymphatic Hydrops. P. R. Ruding. 1988. (Illus.). 89p. pap. (*90-5103-011-8*) SPB Acad Pub NLD. *Dist:* Balogh.

Experimental Foundations of Behavioral Medicine: Conditioning Approaches. Robert Ader et al. 1988. (Perspectives in Behavioral Medicine Ser.). 240p. 59.95 (*0-8058-0139-1*) L Erlbaum Assocs.

Experimental Foundations of Modern Immunology. William P. Clark. 4th ed. 1991. LC 90-13085. 506p. text 83.95 (*0-471-51707-0*) Wiley.

Experimental Hematology Today. Ed. by S. J. Baum & G. D. Ledney. 1977. (Illus.). 251p. 142.00 (*0-387-90208-2*) Spr-Verlag.

Experimental Hematology Today 1978. Ed. by S. J. Baum & G. D. Ledney. 1978. LC 78-8054. (Illus.). 256p. 142.00 (*0-387-90323-2*) Spr-Verlag.

Experimental Hematology Today, 1979. Ed. by S. J. Baum & G. D. Ledney. 1979. (Illus.). 267p. 211.00 (*0-387-90380-1*) Spr-Verlag.

Experimental Hematology Today, 1980. Ed. by S. J. Baum et al. 1981. (Illus.). xiv, 342p. 142.25 (*3-8055-1705-X*) S Karger.

Experimental Hematology Today, 1981. Ed. by S. J. Baum et al. 1981. (Illus.). xiv, 250p. 142.25 (*3-8055-2255-X*) S Karger.

Experimental Hematology Today, 1982. Ed. by S. J. Baum et al. 1982. (Illus.). xx, 270p. 172.25 (*3-8055-3486-8*) S Karger.

Experimental Hematology Today, 1988. Ed. by S. J. Baum et al. 1989. (Illus.). 182p. 126.00 (*0-387-96932-2*) Spr-Verlag.

Experimental Hematology Today, 1989. Ed. by N. C. Gorin & L. Douay. 1990. (Illus.). 115p. 126.00 (*0-387-97246-3*) Spr-Verlag.

Experimental Hypertension & Therapeutic Progress: Vasodilation & Beyond. B. Garthoff. 1995. (Illus.). 110p. 99.00 (*3-540-58545-1*); (*0-387-58545-1*) Spr-Verlag.

Experimental Introductory Chemistry in 2 Pts. Robert G. Lowman et al. 1981. (Illus.). 274p. pap. text 14.95 (*0-89641-096-X*) American Pr.

Experimental Learning in Action. Philip Burnard. 1991. 190p. (*1-85628-261-9*) Avebry GBR. *Dist:* Ashgate Pub Co.

Experimental Leukemia & Mammary Cancer: Induction, Prevention, Cure. Charles B. Huggins. 1979. LC 78-25790. (Illus.). 238p. 27.00 (*0-226-35860-7*) U Ch Pr.

Experimental Liver Transplantation. Naoshi Kamada. 1988. LC 87-24281. 192p. 97.00 (*0-8493-6832-4*, QR188, CRC Reprint) Franklin.

Experimental Malignant Hyperthermia. Ed. by C. H. Williams. 1987. (Illus.). 166p. 98.00 (*0-387-96554-8*) Spr-Verlag.

Experimental Medicine. Claude Bernard. 2nd ed. 1999. LC 99-25208. 226p. pap. text 29.95 (*0-7658-0615-0*) Transaction Pubs.

Experimental Methods in Psychology. Gustav Levine & Stanley Parkinson. 1994. 496p. text 39.95 (*0-8058-1438-8*) L Erlbaum Assocs.

Experimental Microbiology for the Health Sciences. Samuel J. Deal et al. 4th ed. 1976. spiral bd. 24.00 (*0-8087-0436-2*) Pearson Custom.

Experimental Models in Antimicrobial Chemotherapy, Vol. 1. Oto Zak & Merle A. Sande. 1986. text 146.00 (*0-12-775401-6*) Acad Pr.

Experimental Models of Diabetes. John H. McNeill. 1999. LC 99-190807. (Illus.). 424p. 149.95 (*0-8493-1667-7*) CRC Pr.

Experimental Pedagogy & the Psychology of the Child. Edouard Claparede. Tr. by Mary Louch & Henry Holman from FRE. 1975. LC 74-21404. (Classics in Child Development Ser.). 344p. reprint ed. 31.95 (*0-405-06457-8*) Ayer.

Experimental Psychology. Donald H. McBurney. (C). 1983. 289p. mass mkt. 26.75 (*0-534-01319-8*); 2nd ed. 1989. 410p. mass mkt. 53.50 (*0-534-12084-9*) Brooks-Cole.

Experimental Psychology. Anne Myers. 2nd ed. 1986. LC 86-10728. (Psychology Ser.). 386p. (C). mass mkt. 48.50 (*0-534-06618-6*) Brooks-Cole.

Experimental Psychology. Anne Myers & Christine Hansen. 4th ed. 1996. LC 96-5045. (Psychology Ser.). 567p. (C). spiral bd. 94.95 (*0-534-33979-4*) Brooks-Cole.

Experimental Psychology. Barry Kantowitz. 5th ed. Date not set. pap. text, tchr. ed. (*0-314-03296-7*) West Pub.

Experimental Psychology. Barry H. Kantowitz. 5th ed. Date not set. pap. text, stu. ed. 21.75 (*0-314-03648-2*) West Pub.

Experimental Psychology: A Computerized Laboratory Course. Ian W. Bushnell & Jim T. Mullin. 1988. 272p. pap. text, stu. ed. 24.50 (*0-86377-058-4*) L Erlbaum Assocs.

Experimental Psychology: Contemporary Methods & Applications. Irwin P. Levin et al. 1994. 432p. (C). text 80.31 (*0-697-12794-X*, WCB McGr Hill) McGrw-H Hghr Educ.

Experimental Psychology: Rationale, Procedures & Issues. Siu L. Chow. 1987. 325p. (C). pap. text 23.95 (*0-920490-68-9*) Temeron Bks.

Experimental Psychology: Research, Design & Analysis. Douglas W. Matheson. 3rd ed. 1978. LC 77-25185. 390p. (C). text 43.25 (*0-03-089891-9*) Harcourt Coll Pubs.

Experimental Psychology: Understanding Psychological Research. Barry H. Kantowitz et al. Ed. by Schiller. 5th ed. 1993. LC 93-21503. 500p. (C). text 60.25 (*0-314-02730-0*) West Pub.

Experimental Psychology: Understanding Psychological Research. Barry H. Kantowitz et al. 6th ed. 1996. LC 96-3082. 650p. mass mkt. 79.95 (*0-314-09973-5*) West Pub.

Experimental Psychology & Pedagogy. Rudolf Schulze. 392p. 100.00 (*1-85506-699-8*) Thoemmes Pr.

Experimental Psychology, Cognition & Human Aging. Donald H. Kausler. 2nd ed. 1991. (Illus.). 800p. 218.00 (*0-387-97327-3*) Spr-Verlag.

Experimental Psychopharmacology. O'Hanlon. 2000. 500p. 185.00 (*0-471-49045-8*) Wiley.

Experimental Research. Olf. 1994. pap. text 50.00 (*0-443-05270-0*) Saunders.

***Experimental Research on Radiofrequency Tissue Ablation as an Alternative in Cancer Therapy.** Yi Miao. 2000. (Acta Biomedical Lovaniensia Ser.: No. 224). (Illus.). 132p. pap. (*90-5867-096-1*) Leuven Univ BEL. *Dist:* Coronet Bks.

Experimental Research on Trichloroethylene Carcinogenesis. Ed. by Cesare Maltoni et al. 1986. LC 86-61069. (Archives of Research on Industrial Carcinogenesis Ser.: Vol. 5). (Illus.). 393p. 220.00 (*0-911131-40-X*) Specialist Journals.

E F G

Experimental Skin Grafts & Transplantation Immunity. D. L. Ballantyne & John M. Converse. 1979. (Illus.). 196p. 127.00 (*0-387-90425-5*) Spr-Verlag.

Experimental Slips & Human Error: Exploring the Architecture of Volition. B. J. Baars. 1992. (Cognition & Language). (Illus.). 366p. (C). 65.00 (*0-306-43866-6*, Plenum Trade) Perseus Pubng.

Experimental Sociology of Architecture: A Guide to Theory, Research & Literature. Guy C. Ankerl. 1981. (New Babylon Studies in the Social Sciences: No. 36). 550p. (*90-279-3219-0*); pap. (*90-279-3440-1*) Mouton.

Experimental Studies of the Differential Effect in Life Setting. P. Sailaja & K. R. Rao. 1973. LC 72-84013. (Parapsychological Monographs: No. 13). pap. 5.00 (*0-912328-20-7*) Parapsych Foun.

Experimental Study in Measuring & Modifying Assertive Behavior in Young Children. Gertrude Chittenden. 1942. (SRCD M Ser.: Vol. 7, No. 1). pap. 25.00 (*0-527-01522-9*) Periodicals Srv.

Experimental Study of Psychopathic Delinquent Women. Edith R. Spaulding. 1969. LC 69-14947. (Criminology, Law Enforcement, & Social Problems Ser.: No. 60). (Illus.). reprint ed. 30.00 (*0-87585-060-X*) Patterson Smith.

Experimental Study of the Eidetic Type. Heinrich Kluver. 1975. LC 74-21418. (Classics in Child Development Ser.). (Illus.). 166p. reprint ed. 19.95 (*0-405-06468-3*) Ayer.

Experimental Techniques in Fracture. Ed. by Jonathan S. Epstein. 1993. 514p. 125.00 (*1-56081-641-4*, Wiley-VCH) Wiley.

Experimental Techniques in Human Neuropsychology. Ed. by H. Julia Hannay. 1988. (Illus.). 608p. pap. text 35.00 (*0-19-505471-7*) OUP.

Experimental Telepathy. Rene Warcollier. Tr. by Josephine B. Gridley & Maud K. Murphy from FRE. 1975. LC 75-7411. (Perspectives in Psychical Research Ser.). (Illus.). reprint ed. 25.95 (*0-405-06997-9*) Ayer.

Experimental Therapeutics in Addiction Medicine. Ed. by Stephen Magura & Andrew Rosenblum. 1995. LC 94-43278. (Journal of Addictive Diseases Ser.). (Illus.). 256p. lib. bdg. 49.95 (*1-56024-699-5*) Haworth Pr.

Experimental Therapies for Eating Disorders. Ed. by Lynne M. Hornyak & Ellen K. Baker. 1989. LC 88-24518. 339p. 42.00 (*0-89862-740-0*) Guilford Pubns.

Experimental Toxicology: The Basic Issues. Ed. by Diana Anderson & D. M. Conning. 2nd ed. 1993. 580p. (C). (*0-85186-451-1*, R6451) Royal Soc Chem GBR. *Dist:* Spr-Verlag.

Experimental Transplantation Models in Small Animals. Ed. by Marjorie K. Green & Thomas E. Mandel. 1995. LC 93-48557. 494p. text 143.00 (*3-7186-5523-3*) Gordon & Breach.

Experimental Tumors in Monkeys. Dzhemali Beniashvili. 1994. 176p. lib. bdg. 139.00 (*0-8493-5383-1*) CRC Pr.

Experimentally Induced Chronic Intoxication & Withdrawal in Alcoholics. Ed. by Jack H. Mendelson. 1964. (Journal of Studies on Alcohol: Suppl. No. 2). 5.00 (*0-911290-00-1*) Rutgers Ctr Alcohol.

Experimentation with Human Beings: The Authority of the Investigator, Subject, Professions, & State in the Human Experimentation Process. Jay Katz. 1972. LC 70-188394. 1160p. 85.00 (*0-87154-438-5*) Russell Sage.

Experimenting in the Hearing & Speech Sciences, 1978. Barry Voroba. 1978. LC 78-63106. (Illus.). 204p. (C). 21.95 (*0-9601970-2-8*); pap. 14.95 (*0-9601970-1-X*); ring bd. 29.95 (*0-9601970-0-1*) Starkey Labs.

Experimenting with the Mind: Readings in Cognitive Psychology. Ed. by Lloyd Komatsu. 1994. LC 93-23715. (Psychology Ser.). 607p. pap. 22.50 (*0-534-21600-5*) Brooks-Cole.

Experiments & Demonstrations in Exercise Physiology. Wayne E. Sinning. 1975. LC 74-4591. (Illus.). 162p. (C). pap. text 16.00 (*0-7216-8313-4*) SCP.

Experiments & Demonstrations in Physical Therapy: An Inquiry Approach to Learning. DiCarlo. 1998. LC 98-41442. 144p. (C). pap. text 28.40 (*0-13-095686-4*, Macmillan Coll) P-H.

Experiments & Observations on the Gastric Juice & Physiology of Digestion: With a Biographical Essay, "William Beaumont: A Pioneer American Physiologist" William Beaumont & William Osler. unabr. ed. 1996. LC 96-23124. (Illus.). 320p. reprint ed. pap. text 10.95 (*0-486-69213-2*) Dover.

Experiments in Biochemistry. Jane M. Magill & John B. Moore, Jr. 1978. (Illus.). 100p. spiral bd. 10.95 (*0-89641-007-2*) American Pr.

Experiments in Environmental Chemistry. P. D. Vowles & D. W. Connell. 1980. LC 80-40270. (Pergamon Series on Environmental Science: Vol. 4). (Illus.). 108p. (*0-08-024010-0*) Pergamon Repr GBR. *Dist:* Franklin.

Experiments in Hearing. George Von Bekesy. 1989. LC 89-45810. 760p. pap. 26.00 (*0-88318-630-6*) Acoustical Soc Am.

Experiments in Metabolism. Jane M. Magill & John B. Moore, Jr. 1979. (Illus.). 100p. spiral bd. 10.95 (*0-89641-013-7*) American Pr.

Experiments in Psychology: A Microcomputer Laboratory. William S. Bainbridge. 1986. 80p. (C). pap. text 16.50 (*0-534-04043-8*) Brooks-Cole.

Experiments in Social Interaction. Ed. by Michael Argyle. 1993. (Benchmark Ser.). 336p. (*1-85521-371-0*) Dartmth Pub GBR. *Dist:* Ashgate Pub Co.

Experiments on Embryos. Ed. by Anthony Dyson & John Harris. 1989. 224p. 49.95 (*0-415-00749-6*, A3624) Routledge.

Experiments with Drugs: Studies Relation Personality Learning Theory & Drug Action. Hans J. Eysenck. 1963. LC 61-11548. (*0-08-013823-3*) Pergamon Repr GBR. *Dist:* Franklin.

Expert Committee on Addiction-Producing Drugs. 1961. (Technical Report Ser.: No. 211). 16p. pap. text 3.00 (*92-4-120211-4*) World Health.

Expert Committee on Biological Standardization. 1963. (Technical Report Ser.: No. 259). 60p. pap. text 3.00 (*92-4-120259-9*) World Health.

Expert Committee on Health Education of the Public. 1954. (Technical Report Ser.: No. 89). 41p. pap. text 5.00 (*92-4-120089-8*) World Health.

Expert Committee on Malaria. 1957. (Technical Report Ser.: No. 123). 84p. pap. text 5.00 (*92-4-120123-1*) World Health.

Expert Committee on Medical Assessment of Nutritional Status. 1963. (Technical Report Ser.: No. 258). 67p. pap. text 5.00 (*92-4-120258-0*) World Health.

Expert Committee on Rabies. (Technical Report Ser.: No. 201). 1960. 28p. pap. text 3.00 (*92-4-120201-7*); 1954. 69p. pap. text 3.00 (*92-4-120082-0*) World Health.

Expert Committee on Training of Health Personnel in Health Education of the Public. 1958. (Technical Report Ser.: No. 156). 40p. pap. text 6.00 (*92-4-120156-8*) World Health.

Expert Consultations in Gynecological Cancers. Ed. by Maurie Markman & Jerome L. Belinson. 1996. LC 96-43175. (Basic & Clinical Oncology Ser.: Vol. 11). (Illus.). 528p. text 95.00 (*0-8247-9768-X*) Dekker.

Expert Critiquing Systems. P. L. Miller. 1986. (Illus.). 175p. 46.00 (*0-387-96291-3*) Spr-Verlag.

Expert Guide to Allergy & Immunology. Ed. by Raymond G. Slavin & Robert E. Reisman. 1999. LC 98-28031. (Expert Guide Ser.). (Illus.). 236p. pap. 35.00 (*0-943126-73-8*) Amer Coll Phys.

Expert Guide to Infectious Disease. James Tan. 2001. LC 00-69964. (ACP Expert Guide Ser.). (Illus.). pap. text 55.00 (*0-943126-98-3*) Amer Coll Phys.

Expert Guide to Oncology. Jacob D. Bitran. 1999. LC 99-44526. (Illus.). 232p. pap. text 35.00 (*0-943126-88-6*) Amer Coll Phys.

Expert Guide to Otolaryngology. Ed. by Karen Calhoun. 2001. LC 2001-22524. (ACP Expert Guides Ser.). (Illus.). xii, 707p. pap. text 45.00 (*0-943126-99-1*, 330301100) Amer Coll Phys.

Expert Medical Witness. Rosalind Winfield. 1989. 150p. pap. (*1-86287-012-8*) Federation Pr AUS. *Dist:* Gaunt.

Expert Pain Management. Springhouse Publishing Company Staff. 1996. LC 96-3089. (Illus.). 416p. (Orig.). pap. 29.95 (*0-87434-777-7*) Springhouse Corp.

Expert Rapid Response. Mosby-Year Book Staff. 1998. LC 98-20962. 140.00 (*0-323-00377-X*) Mosby Inc.

Expert Systems & Decision Support in Medicine. Ed. by O. Rienhoff & B. Schneider. 1988. (Lecture Notes in Medical Informatics: Vol. 36). 591p. 103.00 (*0-387-50317-X*) Spr-Verlag.

Expert 10-Minute Physical Examinations. 1997. LC 97-16571. (Illus.). 320p. (C). (gr. 13). spiral bd. 36.95 (*0-8151-2039-7*, 32016) Mosby Inc.

Expert Third Molar Extractions. Soichiro Asanami & Yasunori Kasazaki. 1990. (Illus.). 109p. text 42.00 (*4-87417-308-X*) Quint Pub Co.

Expertise at Work: A Special Issue of the European Journal of Work & Organizational Psychology. Sabine Sonnentag. 1999. 128p. pap. text 39.95 (*0-86377-972-7*) Taylor & Francis.

Expertise in Nursing Practice: Caring, Clinical, Judgment & Ethics. Patricia Benner et al. 1995. LC 95-31425. (Illus.). 432p. 46.95 (*0-8261-8700-5*) Springer Pub.

Expertise in Physical Therapy Practice. Gail M. Jensen et al. 1999. LC 99-22320. 294p. text 44.99 (*0-7506-9040-2*) Buttrwrth-Heinemann.

Experts Speak, 1996 Vol. 1: The Role of Nutrition in Medicine. Kirkham R. Hamilton. Ed. by Kris Simpson et al. 1996. (Orig.). pap. text 35.00 (*0-9628840-9-X*) ITServices.

Expiscations in Cross-Cultural Psychology. Ed. by J. B. Deregowski et al. 1983. viii, 456p. pap. (*90-265-0450-0*) Swets.

Explaining Cardiac Surgery: Patient Assessment & Care. Ed. by Russell Millner & Tom Treasure. 1995. 250p. (Orig.). pap. text (*0-7279-0853-7*) BMJ Pub GBR. *Dist:* AIDC.

Explaining Emotions. Ed. by Amelie O. Rorty. 1980. LC 78-62859. (Topics in Philosophy; 5 Ser.: Vol. V). 543p. pap. text 22.50 (*0-520-03921-1*) U CA Pr.

***Explaining Endometriosis.** Lorraine Henderson & Ros Wood. 2001. 192p. pap. (*1-86508-133-7*) Allen & Unwin Pty AUS. *Dist:* IPG Chicago.

Explaining Epidemics: And Other Studies in the History of Medicine. Charles E. Rosenberg. 1992. 367p. (C). text 54.95 (*0-521-39340-X*); pap. text 24.95 (*0-521-39569-0*) Cambridge U Pr.

Explaining One's Self to Others: Reason-Giving in a Social Context. Ed. by Margaret L. McLaughlin et al. 1992. (Communication Ser.). 320p. text 59.95 (*0-8058-0799-3*) L Erlbaum Assocs.

Explanation & Cognition. Ed. by Frank C. Keil & Robert A. Wilson. 2000. LC 99-87946. (Illus.). x, 396p. 40.00 (*0-262-11249-3*, Bradford Bks) MIT Pr.

Explanation & Experiment in Social Psychological Science. J. D. Greenwood. 1988. 264p. 79.95 (*0-387-96799-0*) Spr-Verlag.

Explanation, Causation & Psychological Theories. 1989. xxviii, 300p. pap. (*90-265-0979-0*) Swets.

Explanation of the Fashion & Use of Instruments of Chirurgery. Ambroise Pare. Tr. by H. Crooke. 1969. LC 75-26045. (English Experience Ser.: No. 141). 64p. reprint ed. 35.00 (*90-221-0141-X*) Walter J Johnson.

Explanation Patterns: Understanding Mechanical & Creatively. Roger C. Schank. 1986. 256p. text 49.95 (*0-89859-768-4*) L Erlbaum Assocs.

Explanations, Accounts & Illusions: A Critical Analysis. John McClure. 1991. (European Monographs in Social Psychology). 196p. (C). text 54.95 (*0-521-38532-6*) Cambridge U Pr.

Explanations in Search of Facts, a Critique of "A Study of Physicians' Fees" Keith B. Leffler. 1978. (LEC Occasional Paper). pap. text 2.50 (*0-916770-08-7*) Law & Econ U Miami.

Exploding Self: The Creative & Destructive Nucleus of the Personality. Joseph Redfearn. 1992. LC 91-38084. 312p. pap. 16.95 (*0-933029-60-8*) Chiron Pubns.

Exploitation of a Desire: Women's Experiences with In-Vitro Fertilisation. Renate Klein. 1989. (C). (*0-7300-0287-X*) Deakin Univ AUS. *Dist:* St Mut.

***Exploracion Clinica Ortopedica (Clinical Orthopaedic Examination)** Ronald McRae. 4th ed. 1997. (SPA., Illus.). 308p. pap. (*84-8174-347-X*) Mosby-Doyma Libros ESP. *Dist:* Saunders.

Exploracion Pediatrica. Joyce K. Engel. 2nd ed. 1994. (Illus.). 384p. (C). text (*84-8086-085-5*) Mosby-Doyma Libros ESP. *Dist:* Mosby Inc.

Explorations in Cognitive Neuropsychology. Alan J. Parkin. 1996. (Illus.). 288p. (C). pap. 31.95 (*0-631-19473-8*) Blackwell Pubs.

Explorations in Cognitive Neuropsychology. Alan J. Parkin. 1999. 296p. 59.95 (*0-86377-633-7*); pap. 29.95 (*0-86377-634-5*) L Erlbaum Assocs.

Explorations in Criminal Psychopathology: Clinical Syndromes with Forensic Implications. Louis B. Schlesinger. 1996. LC 96-33869. (Illus.). 366p. text 81.95 (*0-398-06622-1*); pap. text 54.95 (*0-398-06623-X*) C C Thomas.

Explorations in Cross-Cultural Psychology. Douglass R. Price-Williams. 1975. LC 74-28740. (Publications in Anthropology & Related Fields). 144p. 7.50 (*0-88316-515-5*) Chandler & Sharp.

Explorations in Developmental Biology. Chandler Fulton & Attila Klein. 1976. (Illus.). 720p. 59.50 (*0-674-27852-6*) HUP.

Explorations in Family Nursing. Dorothy A. Whyte. 1997. LC 96-35163. (C). 224p. pap. 26.95 (*0-415-13350-5*); (Illus.). 248p. 80.00 (*0-415-13349-1*) Routledge.

Explorations in Marital & Family Therapy: Selected Papers of James L. Framo. James L. Framo. 1982. 320p. 46.95 (*0-8261-3400-9*) Springer Pub.

Explorations in Nonverbal & Vocal Behavior. George Mahl. 1987. 440p. 89.95 (*0-89859-757-9*) L Erlbaum Assocs.

Explorations in Psychoanalysis. Ralph R. Greenson. 1978. LC 77-90230. 578p. 85.00 (*0-8236-1810-2*) Intl Univs Pr.

Explorations in Psychoneuroimmunology. Ruth Lloyd et al. 1987. 176p. text 34.50 (*0-8089-1854-0*, 792578, Grune & Strat) Harcrt Hlth Sci Grp.

Explorations in Temperament: International Perspectives on Theory & Measurement. J. Strelau & A. Angleitner. 1991. (Perspectives on Individual Differences Ser.). (Illus.). 358p. (C). 80.00 (*0-306-43782-1*, Plenum Trade) Perseus Pubng.

Explorations in the History of Psychology in America. Ed. by Josef M. Brozek. 1984. LC 81-72024. (Illus.). 336p. 45.00 (*0-8387-5039-7*) Bucknell U Pr.

Explorations in Women's Health: A Workbook. Nora Howley & Maureen Edwards. 1998. (Illus.). 160p. (C). pap. text, wbk. ed. 28.95 (*0-7637-0868-2*, 0868-2) Jones & Bartlett.

Explorations into the Self. M. Fordham. 1985. 249p. (*1-85575-078-3*) Karnac Bks GBR. *Dist:* Other Pr LLC.

Explorations on Martha Rogers' Science of Unitary Human Beings. Violet M. Malinski. 1987. LC 86-14138. 240p. (C). pap. text 48.00 (*0-8385-2493-1*, A2493-3) Appleton & Lange.

Exploratory Case Study of the Operating Room. 1994. (Illus.). 76p. (Orig.). (C). pap. text 30.00 (*0-7881-1271-6*) DIANE Pub.

Exploring Abnormal Psychology. John M. Neale et al. 1995. LC 95-20152. 608p. 86.95 (*0-471-59673-6*) Wiley.

Exploring Adolescent Happiness: Commitment, Purpose & Fulfillment. Zipora Magen. 1998. LC 98-8973. 248p. 73.95 (*0-7619-0730-0*, 80983); pap. 36.95 (*0-7619-0731-9*, 80984) Sage.

***Exploring Animal Behavior: Readings from American Scientist.** Ed. by Paul W. Sherman & John Alcock. 3rd ed. 2001. LC 2001-20701. pap. 21.95 (*0-87893-814-1*) Sinauer Assocs.

Exploring Applied Psychology: Origins & Critical Analyses. Ed. by Thomas K. Fagan & Gary R. VandenBos. 1993. 208p. pap. text 14.95 (*1-55798-206-6*) Am Psychol.

Exploring Biology. Pamela S. Camp et al. 2nd ed. 1984. (C). pap. text, stu. ed. 61.50 (*0-03-063373-7*) SCP.

Exploring Brain Functional Anatomy with Positron Tomography - Symposium No. 163. CIBA Foundation Staff. Ed. by R. Porter. 1992. LC 91-40214. (CIBA Foundation Symposia Ser.: No. 163). 298p. 128.00 (*0-471-92970-0*, Wiley-Interscience) Wiley.

Exploring Brain Functions: Models in Neuroscience. T. A. Poggio & D. A. Glaser. 1993. LC 00-92. (Life Sciences Research Reports: No. 52). 358p. 305.00 (*0-471-93602-2*) Wiley.

Exploring Careers in Dentistry. Jessica A. Rickert. rev. ed. 1988. (Careers in Depth Ser.). 154p. (gr. 7-12). lib. bdg. 16.95 (*0-8239-0801-1*) Rosen Group.

Exploring Cognition: Damaged Brains & Neural Networks. Ed. by Gillian Cohen et al. 2000. 432p. (*1-84169-217-4*) Psychol Pr GBR. *Dist:* Taylor & Francis.

Exploring Collaborative Research in Primary Care. Ed. by Benjamin F. Crabtree et al. 1994. 340p. 76.95 (*0-8039-5489-1*, 3657) Sage.

Exploring Developmental Theories: Toward a Structural Model to Account for Behavioral Development. Frances D. Horowitz. 1987. 224p. text 45.00 (*0-89859-937-7*); pap. text 24.50 (*0-89859-938-5*) L Erlbaum Assocs.

Exploring Health: A Problem-Based Inquiry. Fred Garman. 1999. 190p. (C). pap. 15.63 (*0-07-236500-5*) McGrw-H Primis Cstm.

Exploring Health Careers. Maureen McCutcheon. 1993. (C). pap. text, tchr. ed. 10.00 (*0-8273-6117-3*); 1993. LC 92-14924. 317p. (C). mass mkt. 43.95 (*0-8273-4897-5*); rev. ed. 1993. 133p. text, tchr. ed. 12.75 (*0-8273-4898-3*); 2nd ed. 1998. 96p. pap. text, tchr. ed. 14.00 (*0-8273-8534-X*); 2nd ed. 1998. LC 97-26075. (Illus.). 352p. (J). 44.95 (*0-8273-8533-1*) Delmar.

Exploring Individual & Organizational Boundaries. W. Gordon Lawrence. 1999. 278p. reprint ed. pap. (*1-85575-232-8*) Karnac Bks GBR. *Dist:* Other Pr LLC.

Exploring Jupiter: The Astrological Key to Progress, Prosperity & Potential. Stephen Arroyo. Ed. by Barbara McEnerney. 1995. (Illus.). 316p. (Orig.). pap. 14.95 (*0-916360-58-X*) CRCS Pubns CA.

Exploring Medical Anthropology. Donald Joralemon. 1998. LC 98-23502. 158p. pap. 30.00 (*0-205-27006-9*) Allyn.

Exploring Medical Language. Myrna LaFleur Brooks & Winnifred K. Starr. 3rd ed. 1994. tchr. ed. (*0-8151-4600-0*); text (*0-323-00110-6*) Mosby Inc.

Exploring Medical Language. Myrna LaFleur Brooks. 4th ed. 1998. (Illus.). 704p. 38.00 (*0-323-00040-1*) Mosby Inc.

***Exploring Medical Language.** Myrna LaFleur Brooks. 4th ed. 1998. (Illus.). 675p. 43.00 incl. audio (*0-323-00070-3*) Mosby Inc.

Exploring Medical Language: A Student-Directed Approach. Myrna LaFleur Brooks. 5th ed. 2001. text (*0-323-01218-3*) Mosby Inc.

***Exploring Medical Language: Computerized Testbank.** Myrna LaFleur Brooks. 4th ed. 1998. (*0-323-00076-2*) Mosby Inc.

***Exploring Medical Language: Text/Audiotape/Dictionary Package.** Myrna LaFleur Brooks. 4th ed. 1998. (Illus.). 65.00 incl. audio (*0-323-00072-X*) Mosby Inc.

Exploring Medical Language: Text/Dictionary. Myrna LaFleur Brooks. 4th ed. 1998. (Illus.). text (*0-323-00071-1*) Mosby Inc.

Exploring New Vistas in Health Care. Ed. by John M. Virgo. 1985. LC 85-80123. 400p. (Orig.). (C). pap. 25.00 (*0-914943-01-4*) IHEMI.

Exploring Our Environmental Connections. Ed. by Eleanor Schuster & Carolyn Brown. 1994. 345p. pap. 38.95 (*0-88737-628-2*) Natl League Nurse.

Exploring Physiology. Goodall. 1994. LC 94-234020. pap. text 19.00 (*0-443-04817-7*) Saunders.

Exploring Psychology. Myers. 2nd ed. 1992. 548p. (gr. 11-12). pap. text, stu. ed. 14.95 (*0-87901-605-1*); text 49.95 (*0-87901-578-0*) Worth.

Exploring Psychology. David Myers. 3rd ed. 1995. LC 95-61216. 544p. pap. text 49.95 (*1-57259-069-6*) Worth.

Exploring Psychology. Richard O. Straub. 3rd ed. 1995. 480p. pap. text, stu. ed. 16.95 (*1-57259-051-3*) Worth.

Exploring Psychology: Instructor's Resources. Martin Bolt. 3rd ed. 1996. tchr. ed., ring bd. (*1-57259-053-X*) Worth.

Exploring Rural Medicine: Current Issues & Concepts. Ed. by Barbara Yawn et al. 1993. (Illus.). 416p. (C). 76.95 (*0-8039-4851-4*, 4937); pap. 36.95 (*0-8039-4852-2*, 4938) Sage.

Exploring Sacred Landscapes: Religious & Spiritual Experiences in Psychotherapy. Ed. by Mary Lou Randour et al. 1993. LC 92-49511. 216p. (C). text 49.50 (*0-231-07000-4*) Col U Pr.

Exploring Social Behavior: Investigations in Social Psychology. James A. Schellenberg. 1995. LC 92-22210. 240p. pap. text 38.00 (*0-205-13861-6*) Allyn.

Exploring Sport & Exercise Psychology. Ed. by Judy L. Van Raalte & Britton W. Brewer. 1996. LC 96-11811. (Illus.). 487p. (C). pap. text 29.95 (*1-55798-355-0*) Am Psychol.

Exploring the Biomedical Revolution: A Look at the Work of Front-Line Scientists & How They Are Changing Medicine. Howard Hughes Medical Institute Staff. 2000. LC 2001-39476. (Illus.). 432p. pap. 19.95 (*0-8018-6398-8*) Johns Hopkins.

Exploring the Biomedical Revolution: A Look at the Work of Frontline Scientists & How They Are Changing Medicine. Howard Hughes Medical Institute Staff. 2000. 432p. 45.00 (*0-8018-6587-5*) Johns Hopkins.

Exploring the Function of the Intact Kidney, Vol.6. Ed. by Robert J. Unwin. 1998. (Reprint of Experimental Nephrology Ser.). (Illus.). 94p. pap. 29.75 (*3-8055-6765-0*) S Karger.

Exploring the History of Medicine. John H. Tiner. 1999. LC 99-70076. (Exploring Ser.). (Illus.). 160p. (YA). (gr. 5-9). pap. 13.99 (*0-89051-248-5*) Master Bks.

Exploring the Jungle: A Teacher's Guide to Preparing for Health Careers. Sherry Makely & Lana Christian. 1996. (Illus.). 38p. pap. 12.95 (*0-9652954-2-7*) Pine Ridge Publns.

Exploring the Skills of Mental Health Nurses. Harry Gijbels & Philip Burnard. 1995. 128p. (*1-85628-662-2*) Avebry GBR. *Dist:* Ashgate Pub Co.

Exploring the Spectrum of Autism & Pervasive Developmental Disorders: Intervention Strategies. Carolyn Murray-Slutsky & Betty A. Paris. 2000. LC 00-8445. 469p. pap. 49.00 (*0-12-784469-4*) Acad Pr.

Exploring the Speech-Language Connection. Rhea Paul. 1998. LC 97-29523. (Communication & Language Intervention Ser.: Vol. 8). 344p. 42.00 (*1-55766-325-4*) P H Brookes.

Exploring Theories of Sickness & Misfortune among the Hasandowa: Narratives As Points of Entry into Beja Cultural Knowledge. Frode Jacobsen. 1997. LC 97-37375. (Illus.). 280p. (*0-7103-0591-5*) Kegan Paul Intl GBR. *Dist:* Col U Pr.

Explosions, Bombs, Blasts, Property Damage & Injury Types: Index of New Information & Bibliography. Lloyd H. Granner. 1996. 150p. pap. 47.50 (*0-7883-0987-0*) ABBE Pubs Assn.

Explosive Growth in Fluid & Drug Delivery Markets: New Product Introductions Generate Rapid Growth. 1992. 272p. 1895.00 (*1-56753-004-4*) Frost & Sullivan.

Exportable U Conn Generalist Faculty Development in Geriatrics. Gail Sullivan. 1998. 100p. ring bd. 100.00 (*1-891509-02-0*) Univ CT Hlth.

***Exposure & Human Health Reassessment of 2, 3, 7, 8 - Tetrachlorodibenzo - p - Dioxin (TCDD) & Related Compunds Pt. 1, Vol. 2: Sources of Dioxin - Like Compounds in the United States.** Ed. by Barry Leonard. 2001. (Illus.). 600p. pap. text 75.00 (*0-7567-1649-7*) DIANE Pub.

Exposure Assessment for Epidemiology & Hazard Control. American Conference of Governmental Industrial Hygenists Staff. 1990. 336p. lib. bdg. 95.00 (*0-87371-197-1*, L197) Lewis Pubs.

Exposure of the American People to Iodine-131 from Nevada Nuclear-Bomb Tests: Review of the National Cancer Institute Report & Public Health Implications of Exposure. National Research Council Staff & Institute of Medicine Staff. 1999. LC 98-83277. (Illus.). xv, 272p. (C). pap. 35.00 (*0-309-06175-X*) Natl Acad Pr.

Exposure of the Pregnant Patient to Diagnostic Radiations: A Guide to Medical Management. Louis K. Wagner et al. 2nd rev. ed. 1997. LC 96-50271. (Illus.). 259p. text 69.95 (*0-944838-72-3*) Med Physics Pub.

Exposure of the U. S. Population from Diagnostic Medical Radiation. 1989. LC 88-25316. (Report Ser.: No. 100). 105p. (Orig.). pap. text 40.00 (*0-929600-01-0*) NCRP Pubns.

Exposures from the Uranium Series with Emphasis on Radon & Its Daughters. Intro. by Warren K. Sinclair. 1984. LC 84-3420. (Report Ser.: No. 77). 134p. pap. text 40.00 (*0-913392-67-7*) NCRP Pubns.

Expressed Emotion in Families: Its Significance for Mental Illness. Julian Leff & Christine Vaughn. 1985. LC 84-549. 241p. 34.50 (*0-89862-058-9*) Guilford Pubns.

Expression of Attitude. R. J. Eisner. 1987. (Recent Research in Psychology Ser.). (Illus.). 86p. 63.95 (*0-387-96562-9*) Spr-Verlag.

Expression of Developmentally Regulated Genes in the Nervous System. Ed. by A. T. Campagnoni. 1990. (Journal: Vol. 12, No. 4-5, 1990). (Illus.). 128p. pap. 81.00 (*3-8055-5313-7*) S Karger.

Expression of Human Apolipoprotein E4 in the Central Nervous System of Transgenic Mice: Towards a Model for Alzheimer's Disease. Ina Tesseur. 2000. (Illus.). 122p. (*90-5867-008-2*) Leuven Univ BEL. *Dist:* Coronet Bks.

Expression of Knowledge: Neurobehavioral Transformation into Action. Ed. by Robert L. Isaacson & Norman E. Spear. 1982. LC 82-13253. 442p. 75.00 (*0-306-40927-5*, Plenum Trade) Perseus Pubng.

Expression of Recombinant Genes in Eukaryotic Systems. Sidney P. Colowick. 1999. (Methods in Enzymology Ser.: Vol. 306). 394p. 99.95 (*0-12-182207-9*) Acad Pr.

Expression of the Alpha-2-Macroglobulin Receptor System & the Amyloid Precursor Protein Family in Embryos & in Adult Brain of Wild Type & Transgenic Mice. Kristin Lorent. 1997. (Acta Biomedica Lovaniensia Ser.: Vol. 148). (Illus.). 151p. pap. (*90-6186-810-6*) Leuven Univ BEL. *Dist:* Coronet Bks.

Expression of the Emotions in Man. Ed. by Peter H. Knapp. 1963. LC 63-22481. 351p. 52.50 (*0-8236-1820-X*) Intl Univs Pr.

Expression of the Emotions in Man & Animals. Charles Robert Darwin. 1965. LC 65-17286. (Illus.). 386p. pap. text 17.00 (*0-226-13656-6*, P526) U Ch Pr.

***Expressions of Mercury-Selenium Interaction in Vitro.** Peter Frisk. 2001. (Comprehensive Summaries of Uppsala Dissertations from the Faculty of Medicine Ser.: No. 988). (Illus.). 62p. pap. (*91-554-4913-1*) Uppsala Universitet SWE. *Dist:* Coronet Bks.

Expressive & Functional Therapies in the Treatment of Multiple Personality Disorder. Ed. by Estelle S. Kluft. 1993. (Illus.). 332p. (C). text 71.95 (*0-398-05826-1*) C C Thomas.

Expressive & Receptive Fingerspelling for Hearing Adults. La Vera M. Guillory. 1982. pap. 3.00 (*0-87511-055-X*) Claitors.

Expressive Arts Therapies in Schools: A Supervision & Program Development Guide. Karen Frostig. 1998. LC 98-13491. (Illus.). 108p. spiral bd. 21.95 (*0-398-06868-2*) C C Thomas.

Expressive Processes in Group Counseling: Theory & Practice. Nina W. Brown. 1996. LC 95-45417. 168p. 58.00 (*0-275-95509-5*, Praeger Pubs) Greenwood.

Expressive Therapy with Elders & the Disabled: Touching the Heart of Life. Ed. by Jules C. Weiss. 1984. LC 84-571. (Activities, Adaptation & Aging Ser.: Vol. 5, Nos. 1-2). (Illus.). 213p. text 49.95 (*0-86656-266-4*) Haworth Pr.

Expressiveness of the Body & the Divergence of Greek & Chinese Medicine. Shigehisa Kuriyama. 1999. LC 98-37210. (Illus.). 256p. 27.50 (*0-942299-88-4*) Zone Bks.

Exquisite Specificity: The Monoclonal Antibody Revolution. Alberto Cambrosio & Peter Keating. 1995. LC 95-16982. (Illus.). 272p. text 59.95 (*0-19-509741-6*) OUP.

Exstrophy-Epispadias Complex: Research Concepts & Clinical Applications. John P. Gearhart & Ranjiv Mathews. 1999. LC 99-16120. (C). text (*0-306-46128-5*, Kluwer Plenum) Kluwer Academic.

Extemporaneous Ophthalmic Preparations. Pharmacists in Ophthalmic Practice, Inc. Staff. Ed. by Richard G. Closson & Lois A. Reynolds. 1993. LC 93-72671. (Illus.). 347p. (Orig.). pap. 37.50 (*0-915486-18-0*) Applied Therapeutics.

Extend Your Lifespan: How You Can Live a Long & Healthy Life. Gary A. Holt et al. Date not set. (Illus.). 646p. 34.50 (*0-931541-52-9*) Mancorp Pub.

Extended Care Center: Role Play Peacegames. David W. Felder. 1996. 44p. pap. text 8.95 (*0-910959-67-6*) Wellington Pr.

Extended (Experiential) Awareness, Purposeful Relaxation, Differential (Multiple) Bodily Feeling States & Communication, Set-EA. Russell E. Mason. 1975. (Train-Ascendance Ser.). pap. 55.00 incl. audio (*0-89533-013-X*, GT-LE) F I Comm.

***Extended Matching Questions for the MRCS.** Auplish & Hossain-Ibrahim. 2001. (Greenwich Medical Media Ser.). 140p. pap. (*1-84110-062-5*) Greenwich Med GBR. *Dist:* JAMCO Dist.

Extending Access to Health Care Through Public-Private Partnerships: The Prosalud Experience. Carlos J. Cuellar et al. 2000. LC 99-52798. (Stubbs Monograph Ser.: No. 2). (Illus.). xiv, 130p. pap. 15.00 (*0-913723-63-0*) Mgmt Sci Health.

Extending Family Practice Medical Services to 24 Hours in Rural Areas: Studies of a Demonstration Model. John B. Dekock. 1975. (Illus.). pap. 7.95 (*0-916552-05-5*) Acoma Bks.

Extending Horizons: Psychoanalytic Psychotherapy with Children, Adolescents & Families. Ed. by Rolene Szur & Sheila Miller. 1992. 496p. pap. text (*0-946439-88-5*, RC) Karnac Bks GBR. *Dist:* Other Pr LLC.

Extending Life, Enhancing Life: A National Research Agenda on Aging. Institute of Medicine Staff. 1991. 164p. text 22.95 (*0-309-04399-9*) Natl Acad Pr.

Extending Medicare Reimbursement in Clinical Trials. Ed. by Institute of Medicine Staff. 2000. LC 00-269522. ix, 76p. pap. 18.00 (*0-309-06888-6*) Natl Acad Pr.

Extending Primary Care: Polyclinics, Resource Centres, Hospital-at-Home. Ed. by Pat Gordon & Janet Hadley. 1996. (*1-85775-029-2*) Radcliffe Med Pr GBR. *Dist:* Balogh.

Extending Psychological Frontiers: Selected Works of Leon Festinger. Ed. by Stanley Schachter & Michael S. Gazzaniga. 1990. LC 89-24204. 640p. 45.00 (*0-87154-275-7*) Russell Sage.

Extending SAS Survival Analysis Techniques for Medical Research. Alan Cantor. 1999. LC 98-149814. 208p. (C). pap. 34.95 (*1-55544-954-9*, BR55504) SAS Publ.

Extensile Exposure. Henry. 3rd ed. 1995. text 85.00 (*0-443-05191-7*) Saunders.

External & Internal Reporting by Hospitals: Accounting Reports & Financial Statements. L. Vann Seawell. 1984. (Illus.). 390p. (Orig.). per. 45.00 (*0-930228-21-9*) Hlthcare Fin Mgmt.

External Eye Disease: A Colour Atlas. Mark T. Watts et al. 1992. (Illus.). 105p. text (*0-443-04446-5*) Church.

External Fixation: Joint Deformities & Bone Fractures. M. V. Volkov & O. V. Oganesyan. Tr. by Micheal Burov from RUS. 1987. LC 85-19699. (Illus.). 300p. (C). 60.00 (*0-8236-1795-5*) Intl Univs Pr.

External Fixation in the Hand & Upper Extremity. Ed. by William H. Seitz, Jr. Date not set. (Illus.). 272p. text 85.00 (*0-07-056292-X*) McGraw-Hill Med Pub.

External Manifestations of Systemic Infections. Ed. by Robert Fekety & Gerald L. Mandell. 1996. LC 96-15291. (Atlas of Infectious Diseases Ser.: Vol. 8). (Illus.). 237p. text (*0-443-07760-6*) Church GBR. *Dist:* Saunders.

External Neuroanatomy of Old World Monkeys (Cercopithecoidea) Dean Folk. Ed. by F. S. Szalay. 1978. (Contributions to Primatology Ser.: Vol. 15). (Illus.). 51.50 (*3-8055-2834-5*) S Karger.

Externalization of Consciousness & the Psychopathology of Everyday Life, 17. Stephen T. Deberry. 1990. LC 90-36638. (Contributions in Psychology Ser.: No. 17). 232p. 65.00 (*0-313-27280-8*, DEG, Greenwood Pr) Greenwood.

Extinctive Prescription. M. Loubser. 1996. LC 97-162762. 239p. (*0-7021-3717-0*) Juta & Co ZAF. *Dist:* Gaunt.

Extra & Intracellular Calcium & Phosphate Regulation. Felix Bronner. 1992. 176p. lib. bdg. 99.50 (*0-8493-0188-2*, QP535) CRC Pr.

Extra-Intracranial Bypass Operation for Prevention & Treatment of Stroke. G. Kletter. 1979. (Illus.). 75.95 (*0-387-81522-8*) Spr-Verlag.

Extra-Oral Radiography. Abramovitc. 1994. (C). text (*0-7216-2941-5*) Saunders.

Extra-Sensory Perception. J. B. Rhine. 1997. pap. 15.95 (*0-8283-1464-0*) Branden Bks.

Extra Treatises Based on Investigation & Inquiry: A Translation of Zhu Dan-Xi's Ge Zhi Yu Lun. Zhu Dan-xi. Ed. by Bob Flaws. Tr. by Yang Shou-zhong & Duan Wu-jin from CHI. 1994. LC 93-74980. (Great Masters Ser.). (Illus.). 135p. (Orig.). pap. 16.95 (*0-936185-53-8*) Blue Poppy Pr.

Extracellular Matrix: Chemistry, Biology & Pathobiology with Emphasis on the Liver. Ed. by Mark A. Zern & Lola M. Reid. 1993. LC 92-48485. (Illus.). 624p. text 250.00 (*0-8247-8830-3*) Dekker.

***Extracellular Matrix as a Regulator of Cell Behavior: Biological Effects of Hyaluronan Biosynthesis & Catabolism.** Mehdi Rahmanian. 2001. (Comprehensive Summaries of Uppsala Dissertations from the Faculty of Medicine Ser.: Vol. 1047). (Illus.). 58p. (*91-554-5050-4*) Uppsala Universitet SWE. *Dist:* Coronet Bks.

Extracellular Matrix in Neural Development & Regeneration: Journal: Developmental Neuroscience, Vol. 11, No. 4-5, 1989. Ed. by S. Carbonetto. 1989. (Illus.). 156p. pap. 94.00 (*3-8055-5056-1*) S Karger.

Extracellular Matrix in the Kidney. T. Hayashi. Ed. by H. Koide. 1994. (Contributions to Nephrology Ser.: Vol. 107). (Illus.). x, 226p. 49.75 (*3-8055-5833-3*) S Karger.

Extracellular Matrix Protocols. Ed. by Charles Streuli & Michael Grant. 2000. LC 00-26153. (Methods in Molecular Biology Ser.: Vol. 139). (Illus.). xiv, 370p. 89.50 (*0-89603-624-3*) Humana.

Extracellular Microbial Polysaccharides. Ed. by Paul A. Sandford & Allen Laskin. 1977. LC 77-6368. (ACS Symposium Ser.: No. 45). 32.95 (*0-8412-0372-5*) Am Chemical.

Extracerebral Collections. Ed. by Robert L. McLaurin. 1986. (Advances in Neurotraumatology Ser.: Vol. 1). (Illus.). 255p. 97.00 (*0-387-81876-6*) Spr-Verlag.

Extrachromosomal Inheritance in Bacteria. Ed. by A. Cohen et al. 1980. (Contributions to Microbiology & Immunology Ser.: Vol. 6). pap. 92.25 (*3-8055-2943-0*) S Karger.

Extracoronary Atherosclerosis. Ed. by A. Ventura et al. 1986. (Monographs on Atherosclerosis: Vol. 14). (Illus.). x, 238p. 135.00 (*3-8055-4162-7*) S Karger.

Extracorporeal Life Support. Ed. by Robert M. Arensman & J. Cornish. 1992. (Illus.). 416p. 125.00 (*0-86542-197-8*) Blackwell Sci.

Extracorporeal Reconstruction of Blood in Clinical Practice, Vol. 6. L. V. Borzova. 1993. (Soviet Medical Reviews Series, Section C: Hematology Reviews: Vol. 6, Pt. 1). 114p. pap. text 161.00 (*3-7186-5395-8*) Gordon & Breach.

Extracorporeal Renal Surgery & Autotransplantation. Dagfinn Albrechtsen. Ed. by Inge B. Brekke & Audum Flatmark. 1997. LC 97-17144. (Illus.). 149p. 128.00 (*3-540-62761-8*) Spr-Verlag.

Extracorporeal Shock Wave Lithotripsy. Ed. by Christian Chaussy. 2nd enl. rev. ed. 1986. (Illus.). viii, 156p. 71.50 (*3-8055-4360-3*) S Karger.

Extracorporeal Shock Waves in Orthopaedics. Ed. by W. Siebert & M. Buch. Tr. by John Chinnery from ENG. 1997. LC 97-28728. (ENG & GER., Illus.). 256p. pap. text 63.00 (*3-540-63092-9*) Spr-Verlag.

Extract from the United States Army X-Ray Manual. U. S. Army Medical Department Staff. 1988. 210p. reprint ed. 45.00 (*0-916973-05-0*) Burnell Co.

Extraction of Natural Products with Near-Critical Solvents. Ed. by M. B. King & T. R. Bott. 1993. 256p. pap. (*0-7514-0069-6*, A6877) B Acad & Prof GBR. *Dist:* Routldge.

Extrageniculostriate Mechanisms Underlying Visually-Guided Orientation Behavior. Masao Norita et al. 1996. LC 96-41410. (Progress in Brain Research Ser.). 462p. 198.50 (*0-444-82347-6*) Elsevier.

Extragenital Effects of Oral Contraceptives. Ed. by Max Elstein. 1997. (Illus.). 68p. lib. bdg. 38.95 (*1-85070-939-4*, Parthenon Pbng) CRC Pr.

Extrahepatic Manifestations in Liver Diseases: Proceedings of the 69th Falk Symposium Held at Basel, Switzerland, October 15-17, 1992. Ed. by R. D. Schmid et al. 1993. LC 93-15126. (Falk Symposium Ser.). 416p. (C). text 174.50 (*0-7923-8821-6*) Kluwer Academic.

Extramural Grant Program 1996 Chicago, June 1996: Abstracts. Ed. by Debra Adenau. 1997. (Journal: Vol. 15, Suppl. 1, 1997). (Illus.). xii, 130p. pap. 42.75 (*3-8055-6510-0*) S Karger.

Extramural Grant Program Meeting: Abstracts. Ed. by L. W. Henderson. 1993. (Journal: Vol. 11, No. 1, 1993). (Illus.). 84p. pap. 44.50 (*3-8055-5788-4*) S Karger.

Extramural Grant Program Meeting, Chicago, Ill., June 1994 Abstracts. Ed. by Mary K. Zentz. 1994. (Journal: Vol. 11, No. 5, 1993). (Illus.). 82p. pap. 44.50 (*3-8055-5951-8*) S Karger.

Extramural Grant Program Meeting, Chicago, Illinois, June 1994, Abstracts Vol. 13, No. 1-2: Abstracts. Ed. by Debra Adenau. 1995. (Journal: Vol. 13, No. 1 - 2, 1994). (Illus.). 106p. pap. 48.00 (*3-8055-6117-2*) S Karger.

Extramural Grant Program, 1997: Chicago, June 1997 - Abstracts. Ed. by Debra L. Adenau. 1998. (Blood Purification Ser.: Vol. 16, Suppl. 1, 1998). (Illus.). vi, 122p. pap. 39.25 (*3-8055-6676-X*) S Karger.

Extranodal Lymphomas. Peter G. Isaacson. 1994. text (*0-443-04039-7*) Church.

Extraordinary Disorders of Human Behavior. Ed. by Claude T. Friedmann & Robert A. Faguet. 1982. LC 82-12286. (Critical Issues in Psychiatry Ser.). 340p. 69.50 (*0-306-40875-9*, Plenum Trade) Perseus Pubng.

Extraordinary Healing: Transforming Your Consciousness, Your Energy System & Your Life. Marilyn Gordon. 2000. (Illus.). 284p. pap. 18.95 (*0-9627762-1-1*) WiseWord Pub.

Extraordinary Measures. Archer. 1998. (C). text 50.00 (*0-15-501357-2*) Harcourt Coll Pubs.

Extraordinary Minds. Howard Gardner. 1998. LC 96-45069. (MasterMinds Ser.). 192p. pap. 14.00 (*0-465-02125-5*) Basic.

Extraordinary Play with Ordinary Things: Recycling Everyday Materials to Build Motor Skills. Barbara Sher. 1998. 165p. pap. text 45.00 (*0-12-784564-X*) Acad Pr.

Extraordinary Silence: The Emergence of a Deeply Disturbed Child. David C. Cipolloni. 1993. LC 93-15184. 160p. 49.95 (*0-89789-357-3*, H357, Bergin & Garvey) Greenwood.

Extraordinary Vessels. Kiiko Matsumoto & Stephen Birch. Ed. by Robert L. Felt. 1993. 220p. (Orig.). pap. text 22.00 (*0-912111-35-6*) Paradigm Publns.

Extraperitoneal Laparoscopic Surgery. Christopher G. Eden. 1997. LC 96-50088. (Illus.). 176p. 165.00 (*0-86542-623-6*) Blackwell Sci.

Extrapolations: Demonstrations of Ericksonian Therapy. Ed. by Stephen R. Lankton & Jeffrey K. Zeig. 1989. LC 89-37590. (Ericksonian Monographs: No. 6). 136p. text 28.95 (*0-87630-567-2*) Brunner-Routledge.

Extrapyramidal Disorders. Ed. by Pierre J. Vinken et al. 1987. (Revised Ser.: Vol. 5). 708p. 323.00 (*0-444-90420-4*) Elsevier.

Extrapyramidal Sensory, Convulsive & Behavioral Disorders. Ed. by E. A. Spiegel & H. T. Wycis. 1971. (Advances in Stereoencephalotomy Ser.: Vol. 5). 82.75 (*3-8055-1148-5*) S Karger.

Extraretinal Photoreception in Circadian Rhythms & Related Phenoma: Proceedings of a Symposium, Vancouver. Ed. by Michael Menaker. 1976. pap. 26.00 (*0-08-020965-3*, Pergamon Pr) Elsevier.

Extrasensory Ecology: Parapsychology & Anthropology. Ed. by Joseph K. Long. 1977. LC 77-6367. 437p. 37.00 (*0-8108-1036-0*) Scarecrow.

Extrasensory Perception. Ed. by Fabian Gudas. 1975. LC 75-7385. (Perspectives in Psychical Research Ser.). reprint ed. 19.95 (*0-405-07033-0*) Ayer.

Extreme Aged in America: A Portrait of an Expanding Population, 3. Ira Rosenwaike & Barbara Logue. 1985. LC 85-8014. (Contributions to the Study of Aging Ser.: No. 3). (Illus.). 253p. 55.00 (*0-313-24857-5*, REA/, Greenwood Pr) Greenwood.

Extreme Fear, Shyness & Social Phobia: Origins, Biological Mechanisms & Clinical Outcomes. Ed. by Louis A. Schmidt & Jay Schulkin. 1999. LC 98-51459. (Series in Affective Science). (Illus.). 344p. text 45.00 (*0-19-511887-1*) OUP.

Extreme Stress & Communities: Impact & Intervention. Marten W. De Vries. Ed. by Stevan E. Hobfoll. 1995. LC 95-14392. (Proceedings of the NATO Advanced Research Workshop on 'Stress & Communities' Ser.: Vol. 80). 560p. (C). lib. bdg. 276.00 (*0-7923-3468-X*) Kluwer Academic.

Extremely Hazardous Substances: Superfund Chemical Profiles USEPA Staff. 1989. LC 88-28279. 1800p. 157.00 (*0-8155-1166-3*) Noyes.

Extremities: Basic Evaluation & Mobilization Techniques. Freddy M. Kaltenborn. Ed. by Eileen Volowitz & Dennis Morgan. 5th ed. 1999. (Illus.). 270p. (C). pap. text 39.95 (*82-7054-043-9*, 608) Orthopedic Phys.

Extremities: Muscles & Motor Points. John H. Warfel. 6th ed. 1993. (Illus.). 140p. pap. text 19.95 (*0-8121-1582-1*) Lppncott W & W.

Eye, Vols. 14 & 14A. Loring F. Chapman & Edward A. Dunlap. 1981. (Courtroom Medicine Ser.). ring bd. 465.00 (0-8205-1214-1) Bender.

Eye: Basic Sciences in Practice. Forrester. 1995. text 82.95 (0-7020-1790-6) Saunders.

Eye & Brain: The Psychology of Seeing. Richard L. Gregory. (Illus.). 1990. 260p. pap. 14.95 (0-691-02456-1); 5th ed. 1997. LC 99-175857. 288p. pap. 19.95 (0-691-04837-1) Princeton U Pr.

Eye & Ear. Ed. by Thomas C. Jones et al. 1991. (Monographs in Pathology of Laboratory Animals). (Illus.). 170p. 259.00 (0-387-54044-X) Spr-Verlag.

Eye & Ocular Adnexae. Robert H. Sagerman & David H. Abramson. 1982. (Illus.). 242p. pap. 135.00 (0-08-027467-6, H230, Pergamon Pr) Elsevier.

Eye & Skin Disease. Ed. by Mark J. Mannis et al. 1995. LC 95-14343. (Illus.). 736p. text 179.00 (0-7817-0269-0) Lppncott W & W.

Eye & Visual Optical Instruments. George Smith & David A. Atchison. 1997. (Illus.). 830p. (C). pap. text 59.95 (0-521-47820-0) Cambridge U Pr.

Eye Book: A Complete Guide to Eye Disorders & Health. Gary H. Cassel et al. (Johns Hopkins Press Health Bks.). (Illus.). 1998. LC 97-35348. 384p. 44.95 (0-8018-5835-6); 1998. LC 97-35348. 384p. pap. 18.95 (0-8018-5847-X); 2001. LC 00-55275. 528p. pap. 19.95 (0-8018-6520-4) Johns Hopkins.

Eye Book: A Specialist's Guide to Your Eyes & Their Care. Ben Esterman. 1977. LC 77-11660. (Illus.). (C). 10.95 (0-915556-04-9) Great Ocean.

Eye Book: Eyes & Eye Problems Explained. Ian Grierson. 2000. (Illus.). 224p. pap. (0-85323-755-7) Liverpool Univ Pr GBR. *Dist:* Intl Spec Bk.

Eye Care for Children: Guidelines. George L. Spaeth. 1985. LC 85-12258. 111p. 52.50 (0-275-91300-7, C1300, Praeger Pubs) Greenwood.

Eye Care for Infants & Young Children. Bruce D. Moore. 1997. LC 97-2666. 474p. pap. text 69.99 (0-7506-9646-X) Buttrwrth-Heinemann.

Eye Care in Developing Nations. Larry Schwab. 3rd ed. 1999. LC 99-19269. (1-56055-043-0) Am Acad Ophthal.

Eye Disease in Clinical Practice: A Concise Colour Atlas. Peter Shah et al. 2000. (Illus.). 160p. 49.95 incl. cd-rom (1-900887-03-7, Manticore Europe) Manticore Pubs.

Eye Diseases in Hot Climates. John Sandford-Smith. 3rd ed. 1997. LC 97-5631. (Illus.). 352p. pap. text 90.00 (0-7506-2544-9) Buttrwrth-Heinemann.

Eye, Ear, Nose & Throat Disorders. Hirsch. 1992. 29.95 (0-8016-1917-3) Mosby Inc.

Eye Emergencies: Diagnosis & Management. Lennox Webb. 1995. LC 94-38580. (Illus.). 196p. pap. text 40.00 (0-7506-2015-3) Buttrwrth-Heinemann.

Eye Guidance in Reading, Driving & Scene Perception. Geoffrey Underwood. 1998. LC 98-7314. 300p. 121.00 (0-08-043361-8) Elsevier.

Eye in Clinical Medical. Joseph B. Michelson & Mitchell H. Friedlaender. 1996. 54.95 (0-7234-2147-1) Mosby Inc.

Eye in Clinical Practice. Peggy Frith. 2nd ed. 2001. LC 00-60808. (Illus.). pap. 79.00 (0-632-05895-1) Blackwell Sci.

Eye in Contact Lens Wear. John Larke. 2nd rev. ed. 1997. LC 96-38860. 224p. text 95.00 (0-7506-1518-4) Buttrwrth-Heinemann.

Eye in General Practice. C. R. Jackson & R. D. Finlay. 9th ed. 1991. 178p. pap. (0-443-04381-7) Church.

Eye in General Practice. R. D. Finlay et al. 10th ed. 1997. LC 97-25704. 216p. pap. text 57.50 (0-7506-3691-2) Buttrwrth-Heinemann.

Eye in Pediatric Disease. Morin. 1991. (Illus.). 400p. 60.00 (0-8016-3553-5) Mosby Inc.

***Eye in Primary Care: A Symptom-Based Approach.** Hunter Maclean. 2001. (Illus.). 176p. pap. 32.50 (0-7506-5288-8) Buttrwrth-Heinemann.

Eye Injuries: An Illustrated Guide. Elizabeth Eagling & Michael J. Roper-Hall. 1986. LC 65-73281. (Gower Bk.). (Illus.). 190p. 89.00 (0-397-58301-X, GM0114) Lppncott W & W.

Eye Know How. Scott Fraser et al. 2001. 240p. pap. text (0-7279-1413-8) BMJ Pub GBR. *Dist:* AIDC.

Eye Movement Basics for the Clinician. Kenneth J. Ciuffreda & Barry Tannen. 1994. (Illus.). 280p. (C). (gr. 13). text 45.00 (0-8016-6843-3, 06843) Mosby Inc.

Eye Movement Desensitization & Reprocessing: Basic Principles, Protocols & Procedures. Francine Shapiro. 1995. LC 94-41750. 398p. text 46.00 (0-89862-960-8, C2960) Guilford Pubns.

Eye Movement Disorders. Ed. by E. A. Sanders & R. J. De Keizer. 1987. (Monographs in Ophthalmology). (C). text 221.50 (0-89838-874-0) Kluwer Academic.

Eye Movement Research: Mechanisms, Processes & Applications. Ed. by John M. Findlay et al. 1995. LC 94-42061. (Studies in Visual Information Processing: No. 6). 582p. 133.00 (0-444-81473-6) Elsevier.

Eye Movements & Their Role in Visual & Cognitive Processes. Ed. by E. Kowler. 1990. (Reviews of Oculomotor Research Ser.: No. 4). 496p. 282.00 (0-444-81254-7) Elsevier.

Eye Movements & Visual Cognition: Scene Perception & Reading. Ed. by Keith Rayner & H. A. Whitaker. 1992. (Neuropsychology Ser.). (Illus.). 486p. 151.00 (0-387-97711-2) Spr-Verlag.

Eye Movements in Reading. Gunnar Lennerstrand & J. Ygge. 1994. LC 94-19379. (Wenner-Gren International Ser.: Vol. 64). 390p. 173.50 (0-08-042509-7, Pergamon Pr) Elsevier.

Eye Movements, Surprise Reactions & Cognitive Development. K. M. Wilton & F. J. Boersma. 1973. (Modern Approaches to the Diagnosis & Instruction of Multi-Handicapped Children Ser.: Vol. 13). 78p. 20.00 (90-237-4117-X) Taylor & Francis.

Eye of the Centaur: A Visionary Guide into Past Lives. Barbara H. Clow. 2nd ed. 1990. LC 89-6929. (Mind Chronicles Trilogy Ser.). (Illus.). 244p. pap. 12.95 (0-939680-60-2) Bear & Co.

Eye Opener. 380p. 10.00 (0-89486-023-2, 1020A) Hazelden.

Eye Pathology: An Atlas & Basic Text. Ralph C. Eagle. Ed. by Richard Lampert. 1999. LC 99-11310. (Illus.). 595p. text 125.00 (0-7216-7809-2) Saunders.

Eye Surgery: An Introduction to Operative Technique. Georg Eisner. 2nd ed. 1990. 318p. 179.00 (3-540-17407-9) Spr-Verlag.

Eye Surgery: An Introduction to Operative Technique. Terry C. Telger. 2nd rev. ed. 1990. (Illus.). 318p. 159.00 (0-387-17407-9) Spr-Verlag.

Eyecare Business Marketing & Strategy. Gary Moss. 2001. LC 00-49806. (Illus.). 336p. pap. text 44.99 (0-7506-7238-2) Buttrwrth-Heinemann.

Eyelid Myoclinia with Absences. Duncan. 1996. 130p. text 31.00 (0-86196-550-7) Buttrwrth-Heinemann.

Eyelid Surgery. Rathbun. 1990. 200.00 (0-316-73437-3, Little Brwn Med Div) Lppncott W & W.

Eyelid Surgery: Principles & Techniques. Clinton D. McCord, Jr. et al. 1995. LC 95-12660. (Illus.). 400p. text 159.00 (0-7817-0293-3) Lppncott W & W.

Eyes & the Mind: Psychophysiological Approach to Psychiatric Disorders Through Visual & Ocular Functions. Ed. by T. Kojima & E. Matsushima. 2000. LC 00-700387. (Illus.). xii, 215p. 213.25 (3-8055-7075-9) S Karger.

Eyes Have It. Ed. by Jim Jenks. 1986. (Illus.). 44p. pap. 3.95 (0-913923-45-1) Woodland UT.

Eyes Have It: A Self-Help Manual for Better Vision. Earlyne Chaney. 1987. LC 86-23438. (Illus.). 176p. reprint ed. pap. 9.95 (0-87728-621-3) Red Wheel ME.

Eyewear: Gli Occhiali. Franca Acerenza. 1997. LC 96-50007. (Bella Cosa Ser.). 144p. pap. 12.95 (0-8118-1870-5) Chronicle Bks.

Eyewitness Memory. Ed. by Charles P. Thompson et al. 1997. LC 97-8625. 300p. (0-8058-2794-3) L Erlbaum Assocs.

Eyewitness Testimony. Elizabeth F. Loftus. 1996. LC 95-51176. 272p. pap. text 18.50 (0-674-28777-0) HUP.

EZ ECG's. American Safety Video Publishers, Inc. Staff. 1994. (Illus.). 96p. (0-8151-0033-7) Mosby Inc.

F

F. A. Davis's Review for the Radiography Examination. Jennifer S. Thomas. 1999. LC 99-43605. (Illus.). 286p. pap. text 35.95 (0-8036-0460-2) Davis Co.

F. D. A. User Fees: Current Measures Not Sufficient for Evaluating Effect on Public Health. 1995. (Illus.). 43p. (Orig.). (C). pap. text 20.00 (0-7881-2085-9) DIANE Pub.

F. I. G. O. Manual of Human Reproduction, Vols. 1-3. Ed. by A Rosenfield & Mahmoud F. Fathalla. 1989. (Illus.). text 90.00 (1-85070-190-3, Parthenon Pbng) CRC Pr.

FAA Medical Certification: Guidelines for Pilots. Richard B. Reinhart. 3rd ed. 1997. LC 97-18886. 264p. pap. 24.95 (0-8138-2769-8) Iowa U Pr.

FAA Medical Certification: The New Rules. Richard O. Reinhart. 2nd ed. 1996. LC 91-31005. (Illus.). 272p. pap. text 24.95 (0-07-052251-0) McGraw.

Faber Book of Madness. Ed. by Roy Porter. 1993. 480p. pap. 18.00 (0-571-14388-1) Faber & Faber.

Faber Guide to Long Term Care Nursing Procedures. Linda Faber-Czingula. 2nd rev. ed. 1993. 225p. ring bd. 75.00 (1-890118-02-8, QualityCare Pub) Convalescnt Cnslts.

Fabrication, Testing, Reliability & Applications of Semiconductor Lasers III, Vol. 3285. Ed. by Mahmoud Fallahi et al. 1998. 240p. 69.00 (0-8194-2724-1) SPIE.

Face & Mind. Ed. by Andrew W. Young. 1998. (Oxford Cognitive Science Ser.: No. 2). (Illus.). 416p. pap. text 26.00 (0-19-852420-X) OUP.

Face-Lift (Rhytidoplasty) Index of New Information with Authors, Subjects & References. Christopher L. Clemons. 1997. 150p. 57.50 (0-7883-1366-5); pap. 47.50 (0-7883-1367-3) ABBE Pubs Assn.

Face Lifting by Exercise. Senta M. Runge. 9th rev. ed. 1992. LC 56-6321. (Illus.). 25.00 (0-9601042-1-6) Allegro Pub.

Face, Nose & Facial Skull, Vol. 1. Ed. by Hans H. Naumann et al. 2nd ed. 1995. LC 95-11552. 299.00 (0-86577-586-9) Thieme Med Pubs.

Face to Face: A Guide to AIDS Counseling. James W. Dilley et al. 1995. LC 89-20217. 350p. text 16.95 (0-89087-583-9) Celestial Arts.

Face to Face: Men & Women Talk Freely about Their Plastic Surgery. James Nolan. 1998. LC 96-79213. (Illus.). 120p. pap. 14.95 (1-885221-44-4) BookPartners.

Face to Face: The Small Group Experience & Interpersonal Growth. Gerard Egan. 1973. LC 72-90673. 162p. (C). 31.95 (0-8185-0075-1) Brooks-Cole.

Face to Face with Distress: The Professional Use of Self in Psychosocial Care. Elizabeth Barnes. 1997. LC 97-25272. 4p. pap. text 34.00 (0-7506-3617-3) Buttrwrth-Heinemann.

Face Value: Coping with Facial Disfigurement. Linda R. Shafritz. 1994. 81p. pap. 10.00 (0-9646774-0-7) Face Value.

Facelift Naturally: The At-Home or Anywhere, Painless, Natural Facelift for Men & Women That Really Works! Julia M. Busch. rev. ed. 1993. LC 93-90243. (Illus.). 128p. per. 14.95 (0-9632907-9-7) Anti Aging Pr.

Facercise: The Dynamic Muscle-Toning Program for Renewed Vitality & a More Youthful Appearance. Carole Maggio & Kyle Roderick. 1995. LC 94-43974. (Illus.). 85p. pap. 12.95 (0-399-51960-2, Perigee Bks) Berkley Pub.

Faces in a Cloud: Intersubjectivity in Personality Theory. Ed. by George E. Atwood et al. 1994. LC 93-14932. 224p. 45.00 (1-56821-050-7) Aronson.

Faces in a Cloud: Subjectivity in Personality Theory. Robert D. Stolorow & George E. Atwood. 1979. LC 78-24754. 218p. 40.00 (0-87668-305-7) Aronson.

Faces of Medicine. Wim Steen & P. J. Thung. 1988. 244p. lib. bdg. (90-247-3673-0) Kluwer Academic NLD. *Dist:* Kluwer Academic.

Faces of Women & Aging. Ed. by Ellen Cole & Esther D. Rothblum. 1993. LC 93-6593. (Women & Therapy Ser.: Vol. 14, Nos. 1-2). (Illus.). 225p. pap. 19.95 (1-56023-042-8, Harrington Park); lib. bdg. 49.95 (1-56024-435-6) Haworth Pr.

Facets of Emotion. Klaus R. Scherer. 1988. 280p. 49.95 (0-8058-0141-3); pap. 29.95 (0-8058-0142-1) L Erlbaum Assocs.

Facial Clefts & Craniosynostosis: Principles & Management. Timothy A. Turvey et al. 1995. LC 95-7122. (Illus.). 928p. text 205.00 (0-7216-3783-3) Saunders.

Facial Contouring. Ed. by Edward O. Terino & Robert S. Flowers. 1999. LC 99-48220. (Illus.). 400p. (C). (gr. 13). text 199.00 (0-8151-8731-9, 24501) Mosby Inc.

Facial Danger Zones: Avoiding Nerve Injury in Facial Plastic Surgery. Brooke R. Seckel. 1993. LC 93-39123. (Illus.). 52p. text 85.00 (0-942219-59-7) Quality Med Pub.

Facial Expressions - Anatomy & Analysis: Index of Modern Authors & Subjects with Guide for Rapid Research. Judy J. Hallcrest. 1991. LC 90-56323. 150p. 47.50 (1-55914-432-7); pap. 44.50 (1-55914-433-5) ABBE Pubs Assn.

Facial Expressions & Smiling: Index of New Information. Mary B. Schneply. 1996. 150p. pap. 47.50 (0-7883-0957-9) ABBE Pubs Assn.

Facial Growth & Facial Orthopedics. Frans P. Van der Linden. 1986. LC 85-16964. (Continuing Dental Education Ser.). (Illus.). 245p. (Orig.). pap. text 58.00 (1-85097-004-1, 1595) Quint Pub Co.

Facial Harmony: Standards for Orthognathic Surgery & Orthodontics. Rijnko Brons. 1998. LC 98-10901. (Illus.). 166p. text 78.00 (0-86715-331-8) Quint Pub Co.

Facial Nerve. Ed. by D. Castro. 1990. LC 89-24517. (Illus.). 579p. lib. bdg. (90-6299-058-4) Kugler NLD. *Dist:* Lib Res.

Facial Nerve. Mark May & Barry M. Schaitkin. 2nd ed. 1999. LC 99-34435. (Illus.). 912p. 199.00 (0-86577-821-3) Thieme Med Pubs.

Facial Nerve - an Update on Clinical & Basic Neuroscience Research: Proceedings of the VIIth International Symposium on the Facial Nerve Cologne, June 9-13, 1992. Ed. by E. Stennert. 1994. (Illus.). 464p. 274.00 (0-387-57686-X) Spr-Verlag.

***Facial Plastic & Reconstructive Surgery.** Ed. by Ira D. Papel. 2nd ed. 2002. LC 2001-54041. (3-13-124811-4) Thieme Med Pubs.

Facial Plastic & Reconstructive Surgery. Ira D. Papel et al. 2nd ed. 2001. LC 2001-54041. (Illus.). 608p. 149.00 (0-86577-918-X) Thieme Med Pubs.

Facial, Plastic & Reconstructive Surgery: Surgery of the Face & Neck. Sykes. 1998. LC 98-9868. 704p. text 269.00 (0-397-51289-9, T0454) Lppncott W & W.

Facial Plastic Surgery. Willett. 1997. LC 97-3531. 350p. (C). text 169.00 (0-8385-2524-5, A-2524-5) McGraw-Hill Prof.

Facial Reconstruction by Prosthetic Means. Edward Watts. 1989. (C). (0-89771-748-1) Assn Brit Dispen Opticians GBR. *Dist:* St Mut.

Facial Rejuvenation. Paul Carniol. 2000. LC 99-59535. (Illus.). 464p. 199.00 (0-471-31846-9) Wiley.

Facial Skin Resurfacing. Thomas J. Baker et al. 1997. LC 97-28725. 230.00 (0-942219-77-5); (Illus.). 250p. 275.00 incl. VHS (1-57626-085-2, QMP) Quality Med Pub.

Facilitated Communication Training. Rosemary Crossley. 1994. LC 93-44306. (Special Education Ser.). 235p. (C). pap. 15.95 (0-8077-3327-X) Tchrs Coll.

Facilitating Change in Mental Health. Bill Lemmer & Martin Smits. 1990. 236p. pap. 25.50 (0-412-33010-5, A4458) Chapman & Hall.

Facilitating Client Change in Rational Emotive Behavior Therapy. Dryden. 1995. 163p. pap. 35.00 (1-56593-512-8, 1182) Singular Publishing.

Facilitating Cognitive Development: International Perspectives, Programs & Practices. Ed. by Milton Schwebel & Charles A. Maher. 1996. LC 86-14850. (Special Services in the Schools Ser.: Vol. 3, Nos. 1 & 2). 209p. text 49.95 (0-86656-415-2) Haworth Pr.

Facilitating Emotional Change: The Moment-by-Moment Process. Leslie S. Greenberg et al. LC 93-7562. 346p. 1996. pap. 24.00 (1-57230-201-1, 0201); 1995. 39.95 (0-89862-994-2, 2994) Guilford Pubns.

Facilitating Environment. M. Gerard Fromm & Bruce L. Smith. 1997. 660p. 80.00 (0-8236-1825-0, BN#01825) Intl Univs Pr.

Facilitating Hearing And Listening In Young Children. Carol A. Flexer. 2nd rev. ed. 1999. LC 98-42099. (Illus.). 310p. pap. text 57.95 (1-56593-989-1, 1958) Thomson Learn.

Facilitating Partnership: A Winnicottian Approach for Social Workers & Other Helping Professionals. Jeffrey S. Applegate & Jennifer M. Bonovitz. 1995. LC 94-49143. 296p. 55.00 (1-56821-494-4) Aronson.

Facilitating Post-Traumatic Growth: A Clinician's Guide. Lawrence G. Calhoun & Richard G. Tedeschi. 1999. LC 99-18525. (Personality & Clinical Psychology Ser.). 176p. 24.95 (0-8058-2412-X) L Erlbaum Assocs.

Facilitating Psychotherapy. Sidney Levin. Ed. by Lois Levin. 1987. 221p. text 32.95 (0-8290-2137-X) Irvington.

Facilitating Self Care Practices in the Elderly. Barbara J. Horn. 1990. LC 90-4244. (Home Health Care Services Quarterly Ser.: Vol. 11, Nos. 1 & 2). 185p. text 39.95 (1-56024-013-X) Haworth Pr.

Facilitating Social-Emotional Development in Multiply Handicapped Children. Ed. by Eugene T. McDonald & Diane L. Gallagher. 1985. 285p. (Orig.). (C). pap. text (0-9613558-0-8) Home Merciful SFCC.

Facilitating Treatment Adherence: A Practitioner's Guidebook. D. Meichenbaum & D. C. Turk. 1987. LC 87-15397. (Illus.). 310p. (C). 44.50 (0-306-42638-2, Plenum Trade) Perseus Pubng.

Facilitating Wellness: Inside the Miracle of Hypnosis. Julie Griffin. Ed. by Roger F. Meads. 1997. LC 96-60030. (Illus.). 224p. (Orig.). pap. 11.95 (1-57691-001-6) TWT Pubng.

Facilitation Techniques Based on NDT Principles. Lois Bly & Allison Whiteside. 1997. LC 98-121487. (Illus.). (0-7616-4400-8, Thrpy Skill Bldrs) Commun Skill.

Facilitation Techniques in Therapeutic Recreation. John Dattilo. 2000. LC 99-69164. (Illus.). xiv, 498p. text 35.95 (1-892132-13-3, FAC115) Venture Pub PA.

Facilitative Management in Rehabilitation Counseling. J. Bozarth & S. Rubin. 1972. pap. 10.40 (0-87563-053-7) Stipes.

Facing & Avoiding Urological Complications of Prostate Cancer: Proceedings of a Satellite Symposium, Held at the XIIth Congress of the European Association of Urology, Paris, September 1996. Ed. by Claude C. Schulman. 1997. (European Urology Ser.: Vol. 31, Suppl. 3, 1997). (Illus.). iv, 30p. pap. 21.75 (3-8055-6488-0) S Karger.

Facing & Fighting Fatigue: A Practical Approach. Benjamin H. Natelson. 1998. LC 97-30094. 208p. 40.00 (0-300-06848-4); 203p. pap. 16.95 (0-300-07401-8) Yale U Pr.

Facing Death. Ed. by Howard M. Spiro et al. 1998. LC 96-2487. (Illus.). 240p. 35.00 (0-300-06349-0) Yale U Pr.

Facing Death: Conversations with a Cancer Patient. Gill L. McLean. 1993. LC 93-21524. (Illus.). 224p. (Orig.). pap. text (0-443-04667-0) Church.

Facing Depression. Lawson. 1997. pap. (0-340-69066-6) Hodder & Stought Ltd GBR. *Dist:* Lubrecht & Cramer, Trafalgar.

Facing Forward: A Guide for Cancer Survivors. 1994. (Illus.). 45p. (Orig.). (C). pap. text 15.00 (0-7881-0332-6) DIANE Pub.

Facing Forward: A Guide for Cancer Survivors - Coping with the Physical, Psychological & Financial Effects Including Insurance Coverage & Employment Concerns. 1991. lib. bdg. 75.95 (0-8490-5150-9) Gordon Pr.

Facing It: AIDS Diaries & the Death of the Author. Ross Chambers. (Illus.). 160p. 2001. (C). pap. text 16.95 (0-472-08748-7, 08748); 1998. LC 98-9005. text 32.50 (0-472-10958-8, 10958) U of Mich Pr.

Facing it Out. Robin Anderson & Anna Darlington. 1999. LC 98-35023. (Tavistock Clinic Ser.). 90.00 (0-415-92262-3); 256p. pap. 25.95 (0-415-92263-1) Routledge.

Facing Shame: Families in Recovery. Merle A. Fossum & Marilyn J. Mason. 1989. (Professional Bks.). (Illus.). pap. 13.00 (0-393-30581-3) Norton.

Facing the Challenge of Liability in Psychotherapy Practice: Practicing Defensively (A1) Lawrence E. Hedges. 2000. LC 00-30638. (Illus.). xx, 391p. 112.50 (0-7657-0290-8) Aronson.

Facing the Fire: Experiencing Expressing Anger Appropriately. John Lee & Bill Stott. 1993. LC 92-46216. 256p. pap. 14.95 (0-553-37240-8) Bantam.

Facing the Pancreatic Dilemma: Update of Medical & Surgical Pancreatology. Ed. by P. Pederzoli et al. 1994. LC 94-35004. (Illus.). 504p. 186.00 (0-387-58284-3) Spr-Verlag.

Facing the Wolf: Inside the Process of Deep Feeling Therapy. Theresa S. Alexander. 2000. 176p. reprint ed. 21.00 (*0-7881-9305-8*) DIANE Pub.

Facing up to AIDS. John Mordaunt. 1990. LC 89-85265. 141p. (Orig.). 16.95 (*0-86278-182-5*); pap. 9.95 (*0-86278-191-4*) Dufour.

Fact & Fable in Psychology. Joseph Jastrow. 1977. (Select Bibliographies Reprint Ser.). reprint ed. 25.95 (*0-8369-6694-5*) Ayer.

Facticity: A Door to Mental Health & Beyond. Ragini E. Michaels. 1991. (Illus.). 256p. (Orig.). pap. 16.95 (*0-9628686-0-4*) Facticity Tr.

Factor Eight - von Willebrand Factor: Biochemical, Methodological, & Functional Aspects, Vol. 1. Ed. by M. J. Seghatchian & G. F. Savidge. 1989. 360p. 216.00 (*0-8493-6828-6*, RC642) CRC Pr.

Factor Seven, a Written Symposium. Ed. by H. C. Hemker. 1983. (Journal: Vol. 13, No. 3). (Illus.). viii, 64p. pap. 48.75 (*3-8055-3757-3*) S Karger.

Factor VIII - Von Willebrand Factor, Vol. 2. M. J. Seghatchian. 1989. 376p. 219.00 (*0-8493-6829-4*) CRC Pr.

Factoring Utilization Review: A Step-by-Step Approach to Behavioral Health Treatment Authorizations. Walter Shepperd. 1998. v, 109p. pap. 30.00 (*0-9660256-2-8*) W Shepperd.

Factors Affecting Contraceptive Use in Sub-Saharan Africa. National Research Council Staff. 1993. (Population Dynamics of Sub-Saharan Africa Ser.). 272p. (Orig.). (C). pap. text 35.00 (*0-309-04944-X*) Natl Acad Pr.

Factors Affecting Demand for Primary Health Care Services by Residents in Nursing Homes & Residential Care Homes. Charles Crosby et al. 2001. LC 00-48055. (Studies in Health & Human Services: Vol. 39). (Illus.). xvii, 117p. 79.95 (*0-7734-7627-X*) E Mellen.

Factors Affecting Human Fertility in Nonindustrial Societies: A Cross-Cultural Study. Moni Nag. 1968. LC 68-22204. (Yale University Publications in Anthropology Reprints Ser.: No. 66). 227p. pap. 20.00 (*0-87536-514-0*) HRAFP.

Factors Determining Human Behavior. Ed. by Robert K. Merton. 1974. LC 73-14153. (Perspectives in Social Inquiry Ser.). 186p. reprint ed. 13.95 (*0-405-05500-5*) Ayer.

Factors in the Sex Life of Twenty-Two Hundred Women. Katharine B. Davis. 1977. LC 70-169379. (Family in America Ser.). 456p. reprint ed. 33.95 (*0-405-03856-9*) Ayer.

Factors Influencing Fertility in the Post-Partum Cow. H. Karg & E. Schallenberger. 1982. text 249.00 (*90-247-2715-4*) Kluwer Academic.

Factors Influencing the Economical Application of Food Irradiation. International Atomic Energy Agency Staff. 1973. (Panel Proceedings Ser.). (Illus.). 137p. pap. (*92-0-111373-0*, ISP331) IAEA AUT. *Dist:* Bernan Associates.

Factors Regulating the Immune Response: Proceedings of the WHO Scientific Group, Geneva, 1969. WHO Staff. 1970. (Technical Reports: No. 448). 88p. pap. text 7.00 (*92-4-120448-6*, 1100448) World Health.

Facts about AIDS & Other Sexually Transmitted Diseases: Sexual Decisions of Responsible Adults. Jerry L. Bogner. 1987. LC 87-13208. 108p. 14.95 (*0-943323-00-2*); pap. 6.95 (*0-943323-01-0*) Bogners Limited.

Facts about Alternative Medicine: Twenty of the Most Common Alternative Treatments. Ed. by Time-Life Books Editors. 1999. LC 98-2854. (Time-Life Medical Guides). (Illus.). 144p. (gr. 11). pap. 6.95 (*0-7370-1106-8*, Time Life) Henninger Prod.

Facts about Birth Control. Judie Brown. 1997. (Illus.). 74p. pap. 5.00 (*1-890712-13-2*, LG02) Amer Life League.

Facts about Hearing & Hearing Aids. 1984. lib. bdg. 79.95 (*0-87700-534-6*) Revisionist Pr.

Facts & Fairy Tales about Female Labour, Family & Fertility: A Seven-Country Comparison, 1850-1990. Hettie A. Pott-Buter. 1993. 370p. (C). text (*90-5356-045-9*) Amsterdam U Pr NLD. *Dist:* U of Mich Pr.

Facts & Figures of Cancer in the European Community. D. M. Parkin & A. Kricker. 1993. 51p. pap. text 9.00 (*92-832-1437-4*, 1760004) World Health.

Facts & Figures of Medical Sciences. L. G. Gupta. 1990. 214p. (C). (*81-85017-46-8*) Interprint IND. *Dist:* St Mut.

Facts & Ideas from Anywhere. William C. Roberts. 2000. 192p. 39.00 (*0-87993-463-8*) Futura Pub.

Facts & Research in Gerontology, 1992: Epidemiology, Vol. 3. Ed. by Bruno J. Vellas & J. L. Albarede. 1992. 279p. 43.95 (*0-8261-8170-8*) Springer Pub.

Facts & Research in Gerontology, 1993: Nutrition. Ed. by Bruno J. Vellas. 1993. 336p. 44.95 (*0-8261-8172-4*) Springer Pub.

Facts of Hormone Replacement Therapy. D. W. Sturdee. 2002. (Illus.). 150p. lib. bdg. 39.95 (*1-85070-807-X*, Parthenon Pbng) CRC Pr.

Facts of Life: The Creation of Sexual Knowledge in Britain, 1650-1950. Lesley Hall & Roy Porter. 1995. LC 94-21091. (Illus.). 415p. 50.00 (*0-300-06221-4*) Yale U Pr.

Facts on File Encyclopedia of Black Women in America: Science, Health & Medicine, Vol. 12. Ed. by Darlene Clark Hine. 1997. (Facts on File Ser.). (Illus.). 208p. 29.95 (*0-8160-3428-1*) Facts on File.

Faculty Guide for Discovering Psychology Telecourse. David G. Myers. 3rd ed. 1996. tchr. ed. (*1-57259-191-9*) Worth.

Faculty Practice Plans: Models for a New Health Care Age. Ed. by James E. Casanova. 1997. LC 97-71052. 150p. pap. 48.00 (*0-924674-54-7*) Am Coll Phys Execs.

Fading Away: The Experience of Transition in Families with Terminal Illness. Betty Davies et al. 1995. (Death, Value & Meaning Ser.). 150p. pap. 30.95 (*0-89503-127-2*) Baywood Pub.

Fading Memories: An Adolescent's Guide to Alzheimer's Disease. 1997. (Illus.). 54p. pap. 5.00 (*1-930181-06-X*) A H A F.

***Faecal Incontinence: Aspects of Diagnosis & Treatment.** Asbjorn Osterberg. 2000. (Comprehensive Summaries of Uppsala Dissertations from the Faculty of Medicine Ser.: No. 899). (Illus.). 83p. pap. (*91-554-4628-0*) Uppsala Universitet SWE. *Dist:* Coronet Bks.

Faecal Incontinence & Related Problems in the Older Adult. Barrett. 1993. 323p. 55.00 (*0-340-54361-2*) Trafalgar.

Failed Back Syndrome: Etiology & Therapy. H. A. Wilkinson. 2nd ed. 1991. (Illus.). 254p. 115.00 (*0-387-97617-5*) Spr-Verlag.

Failure Free Activities for the Alzheimer's Patient: A Guidebook for Caregivers. Carmel Sheridan. 1987. LC 87-70051. 187p. (Orig.). pap. 10.95 (*0-943873-05-3*) Elder Bks.

Failure in the Restored Dentition: Management & Treatment. Michael D. Wise. 1995. (Illus.). 766p. text 240.00 (*1-85097-033-5*, B8811) Quint Pub Co.

Failure of Apoptosis & Cancer Metastasis. Gennadi V. Glinsky. 1998. LC 98-11142. (Medical Intelligence Unit Ser.). 180p. (*1-57059-478-3*) Landes Bioscience.

Failure of Private Hospital Regulation. Lauren Dame & Sidney M. Wolfe. 1996. 52p. (Orig.). pap. 15.00 (*0-937188-47-6*) Pub Citizen.

***Failure of Psychiatry: A Marxist Critique.** Robinson. 2001. 82p. pap. 19.95 (*0-8464-5266-9*) Beekman Pubs.

Failures in Family Therapy. Ed. by Sandra B. Coleman. 1985. LC 84-19325. (Family Therapy Ser.). 401p. text 47.50 (*0-89862-048-1*) Guilford Pubns.

***Failures in Psychoanalytic Treatment.** Ed. by Joseph Reppen & Martin Schulman. unabr. ed. 2001. 365p. pap. text 39.95 (*0-8236-1835-8*, 21835) Intl Univs Pr.

***Fainting Phenomenon: Understanding Why People Faint & What Can Be Done about It.** Blair P. Grubb & Mary Carole McMann. 2001. LC 2001-33211. (Illus.). v, 138p. (*0-87993-491-3*) Futura Pub.

Fair Price for Health Services: Opinion to the Ministre de la Sante et des Services Sociaux. Quebec Government Staff. 1996. LC 96-181721. 48p. (*2-550-25732-4*) Gvt Quebec.

Fair Sex, Savage Dreams: Race, Psychoanalysis, Sexual Difference. Jean Walton. 2001. LC 00-64691. (Illus.). 248p. 18.95 (*0-8223-2611-6*); 54.95 (*0-8223-2603-5*) Duke.

Fairbairn, Then & Now. Ed. by Neil J. Skolnick & David E. Scharff. 1998. LC 97-47789. (Relational Perspectives Bks.: Vol. 10). 320p. 45.00 (*0-88163-262-7*) Analytic Pr.

Fairy Tale at Forty: Curing My Incurable Disease, a True Story. Mary A. Celente. 1995. 283p. (Orig.). pap. 25.00 (*0-9648167-1-7*) Trends Res Inst.

Fairy Tales in Psychotherapy: The Creative Use of Old & New Tales. Erich Franzke. 1989. LC 88-22059. 150p. (C). pap. 29.50 (*0-920887-42-2*) Hogrefe & Huber Pubs.

Faith & Medicine. William Mast. 1995. 78p. (Orig.). pap. text (*0-9648937-0-3*) W Mast.

Faith & the Professions. Thomas L. Shaffer. 1987. LC 87-863. 337p. (C). text 19.50 (*0-88706-561-9*) State U NY Pr.

Faith Factor: Proof of the Healing Power of Prayer. Dale Matthews & Connie Clark. 1999. LC 97-52337. 320p. pap. 13.95 (*0-14-027575-4*) Penguin Putnam.

***Faith, Healing & Miracles.** Frederick Flach. 2001. 300p. reprint ed. pap. 15.95 (*1-57826-100-7*) Hatherleigh.

Faith Healing & Speaking in Tongues. H. L. Heijkoop. 40p. pap. 2.95 (*0-88172-083-6*) Believers Bkshelf.

Faith in Action: Medical Missionaries in Central America. Mike Billington & Cari DeSantis. 1997. LC 97-91255. (Illus.). 104p. pap. 25.00 (*0-9660486-0-1*) White Rose Bks.

Faith, Medical Alchemy & Natural Philosophy: Johann Moriaen, Reformed Intelligencer, & Hartlib Circle. John T. Young. 1999. LC 98-73999. (History of Medicine in Context Ser.). 18p. text (*1-84014-282-0*) Ashgate Pub GBR. *Dist:* Ashgate Pub Co.

Faith of Biology & the Biology of Faith: Order, Meaning & Free Will in Modern Medical Science. Robert Pollack. 2000. LC 00-55594. (Series in Science & Religion). xvi, 125p. (*0-231-11507-5*) Col U Pr.

Faith of Biology & the Biology of Faith: Order, Meaning, & Free Will in Modern Medical Science. Robert Pollack. 2000. LC 00-55594. (Columbia Series in Science & Religion). xvi, 125p. 19.95 (*0-231-11506-7*) Col U Pr.

Faith, Spirituality & Medicine: Toward the Making of the Healing Practitioner. Dana E. King. 2000. LC 00-38329. pap. (*0-7890-1206-5*); (Illus.). xvii, 126p. (C). 49.95 (*0-7890-0724-X*); (Illus.). xvii, 126p. (C). pap. 15.95 (*0-7890-1115-8*) Haworth Pr (Haworth Pastrl).

Faith That Heals (How to Develop) Fenwicke L. Holmes. 1991. 100p. pap. 10.00 (*0-89540-124-X*, SB-124) Sun Pub.

Faithful Choices: An Adult Program in Clinical Ethics & Religious Values. Wayne B. Arnason. 1998. LC 98-140095. (*1-55896-362-6*) Unitarian Univ.

Fallacy of Medicine. Hattie M. Baker. 1996. 9p. reprint ed. spiral bd. 8.00 (*0-7873-0064-0*) Hlth Research.

Fallen Angel: The Status Insularity of the Female Alcoholic. Florence V. Ridlon. 1988. LC 86-47992. 184p. 30.00 (*0-8387-5115-6*) Bucknell U Pr.

Falling Apart & Other Fallacies: Stories of Survival & Recovery. Pat H. Fulbright. 1993. LC 93-14913. 192p. pap. 16.00 (*1-880837-27-7*) Smyth & Helwys.

Falling in Old Age: Prevention & Management. Rein Tideiksaar. 2nd ed. 1996. LC 96-3017. (Springer Series on Adulthood & Aging). (Illus.). 408p. 48.95 (*0-8261-5291-0*) Springer Pub.

Falling Sickness: A History of Epilepsy from the Greeks to the Beginnings of Modern Neurology. Owsei Temkin. 2nd ed. 1994. (Softshell Bks.). (Illus.). 488p. (C). reprint ed. pap. text 26.50 (*0-8018-4849-0*) Johns Hopkins.

Falling Through the Cracks: AIDS & the Urban Poor. Victor Ayala. 1996. LC 95-70518. 125p. (Orig.). pap. 17.95 (*0-9644437-0-8*) Social Change Pr.

Falling Through the Safety Net: Insurance Status & Access to Health Care. Joel S. Weissman & Arnold M. Epstein. 1994. 208p. (C). pap. text 18.95 (*0-8018-4917-9*) Johns Hopkins.

Fallopian Tube. 1994. LC 93-34147. 139.00 (*3-540-19763-X*) Spr-Verlag.

Fallopian Tube: Clinical & Surgical Aspects. Ed. by J. Gedes Grudzinskas et al. 1994. LC 93-34147. (Illus.). 320p. 119.00 (*0-387-19763-X*) Spr-Verlag.

Falls, Balance & Gait Disorders in the Elderly. Bruno J. Vellas et al. 1992. 206p. pap. 49.00 (*2-906077-26-7*) Elsevier.

Falls-Immobility & Restraints, Package. Ann L. Hendrich. 1996. 32p. (*0-8151-4253-6*) Mosby Inc.

Falls-Immobility & Restraints Resources Manual. Ann L. Hendrich. 1996. 384p. (*0-8151-4256-0*) Mosby Inc.

Falls in Epileptic & Non Epileptic Seizures During Childhood. A. Beaumanoir. 1997. 232p. (*0-86196-540-X*) J Libbey Med GBR. *Dist:* Buttrwrth-Heinemann.

Falls in Older Persons: Prevention & Management. Rein Tideiksaar. 2nd ed. 1998. LC 98-5138. (Illus.). 176p. pap. 23.50 (*1-878812-44-0*) Hlth Prof Pr.

Falls in Older Persons: Prevention & Management in Hospitals & Nursing Homes. Rein Tideiksaar. 1993. 135p. pap. text 39.95 (*0-9637866-0-1*) Tactilitics.

Falls in the Elderly. Joanna H. Downton. 1993. 168p. pap. (*0-340-54848-7*) E A GBR. *Dist:* OUP.

False Hopes: Overcoming the Obstacles to a Sustainable, Affordable Medicine. David Callahan. 1999. LC 98-52987. 330p. pap. 17.00 (*0-8135-2674-4*) Rutgers U Pr.

False Hopes: Why America's Quest for Perfect Health Is a Recipe for Failure. Daniel Callahan. 1998. LC 97-40541. 336p. 24.00 (*0-684-81109-X*, Scribner Pap Fic) S&S Trade Pap.

False-Memory Creation in Children & Adults: Theory, Research & Implications. David F. Bjorklund. 1999. LC 99-55909. (Illus.). x, 254p. (C). 59.95 (*0-8058-3169-X*) L Erlbaum Assocs.

Familia Saludable. Abel Delgado. 2000. LC 00-37263. (SPA., Illus.). 192p. pap. 12.95 (*1-57954-205-0*) Rodale Pr Inc.

Familial Adenomatous Polyposis & other Polyposis Syndromes. James P. Thomson. Ed. by Robin K. Phillips et al. 1994. 260p. (*0-340-56755-4*) E A GBR. *Dist:* OUP.

Familial & Hereditary Tumors. M. Ponz De Leon. 1994. LC 94-13711. (Recent Results in Cancer Research Ser.: Vol. 136). (Illus.). 347p. 137.00 (*0-387-57633-9*) Spr-Verlag.

Familial Brain Tumours. Cornelis C. Tijssen et al. 1982. text 176.50 (*90-247-2691-3*) Kluwer Academic.

Familial Cancer. Ed. by H. Mueller & W. Weber. 1985. (Illus.). xx, 292p. 161.00 (*3-8055-4245-3*) S Karger.

Familial Cancer & Prevention: Molecular Epidemiology: A New Strategy Toward Cancer Control. Ed. by Joji Utsunomiya et al. 1999. LC 98-20473. (UICC Ser.). (Illus.). 559p. 220.95 (*0-471-24937-8*, Wiley-Liss) Wiley.

Familial Cancer Control. Ed. by W. Weber & U. Veronesi. 1992. LC 92-2420. (Monographs of the European School of Oncology). (Illus.). 126p. 84.95 (*0-387-55570-6*) Spr-Verlag.

Familial Cancer Management. Ed. by Walter Weber et al. 1996. 256p. 209.95 (*0-8493-4782-3*, 4782) CRC Pr.

Families & Communities Responding to AIDS. Ed. by Peter Aggleton et al. 1999. LC 00-266838. (Social Aspects of AIDS Ser.). (Illus.). x, 226p. (*1-85728-999-4*); pap. (*1-85728-965-X*) UCL Pr Ltd GBR. *Dist:* Taylor & Francis.

Families & Family Therapy. Salvador Minuchin. 1974. LC 73-89710. 268p. 34.50 (*0-674-29236-7*) HUP.

Families & Forgiveness: Healing Wounds in the Intergenerational Family. Terry D. Hargrave. 1994. LC 93-43736. (Illus.). 256p. text 39.95 (*0-87630-735-7*) Brunner-Routledge.

Families & Groups. Robin Hall. 1992. LC 92-28828. (Skills for Caring Ser.). 48p. pap. text (*0-443-04528-3*) Church.

Families & Health. William J. Doherty & Thomas L. Campbell. 1988. (Family Studies Ser.: Vol. 10). 160p. (C). 76.95 (*0-8039-2992-7*, 6783); pap. 31.95 (*0-8039-2993-5*, 6784) Sage.

Families & Health Care. Ed. by Barbara A. Elliott & Sharon J. Price. 1993. (Vision 2010 Ser.: Vol. 1, No. 1). (Illus.). 44p. (Orig.). (C). pap. text 19.95 (*0-916174-39-5*) Natl Coun Family.

Families & Health Care: Psychosocial Practice. Kathleen Ell & Helen Northen. 1990. LC 89-18560. (Modern Applications of Social Work Ser.). 332p. pap. text 28.95 (*0-202-36060-1*); lib. bdg. 51.95 (*0-202-36059-8*) Aldine de Gruyter.

Families & Larger Systems: A Family Therapist's Guide Through the Labyrinth. Evan Imber-Black. LC 87-31343. (Family Therapy Ser.). 228p. 1992. pap. 22.00 (*0-89862-109-7*, 2109); 1988. 39.95 (*0-89862-100-3*) Guilford Pubns.

Families & Mental Health Treatment: A Compendium of Articles from Psychiatric Services & Hospital & Community Psychiatry. Intro. by Lisa B. Dixon. 1998. LC 99-192267. 72 p. (*0-89042-413-6*) Amer Psych Assn.

Families & Mental Illness: New Directions in Professional Practice. Diane T. Marsh. 1992. LC 91-33605. 288p. 70.00 (*0-275-94018-7*, C4018, Praeger Pubs) Greenwood.

Families & Mental Retardation: New Directions in Professional Practice. Diane T. Marsh. 1992. LC 91-38306. 272p. 68.00 (*0-275-94014-4*, C4014, Praeger Pubs) Greenwood.

Families & the Gravely Ill: Roles, Rules & Rights, 23. Richard Sherlock & C. Mary Dingus. 1988. LC 87-32264. (Contributions in Medical Studies Ser.: No. 23). 201p. 60.00 (*0-313-25615-2*, SKF/, Greenwood Pr) Greenwood.

Families & the Interpretation of Dreams: Awakening the Intimate Web. Edward B. Bynum. 1993. LC 92-17827. (Illus.). 252p. lib. bdg. 7.95 (*1-56024-336-8*) Haworth Pr.

Families & Their Children with Down's Syndrome. Elizabeth Byrne et al. 1988. 160p. text 47.50 (*0-415-00607-4*) Routledge.

Families as Allies in Treatment of the Mentally Ill: New Directions for Mental Health Professionals. Ed. by Harriet P. Lefley & Dale L. Johnson. 1990. LC 89-17778. 284p. text 14.95 (*0-88048-298-2*, 8298) Am Psychiatric.

Families Coping with Schizophrenia: A Practitioner's Guide to Family Groups. Jacqueline M. Atkinson & Denise A. Coia. 1995. LC 94-33593. 294p. pap. 75.00 (*0-471-94181-6*) Wiley.

Families Facing Death: A Guide for Healthcare Profesionals & Volunteers. Elliott J. Rosen. rev. ed. 1998. LC 97-42590. 272p. pap. 28.00 (*0-7879-4050-X*) Jossey-Bass.

Families, Health & Illness. Carol B. Danielson & Brenda Hamel-Bissec. 1992. (Illus.). 427p. (C). (gr. 13). pap. text 35.00 (*0-8016-0360-9*, 00360) Mosby Inc.

Families Helping Families: Living with Schizophrenia. Families of the Mentally Ill Collective. 1987. 192p. mass mkt. 6.95 (*0-380-70354-8*, Avon Bks) Morrow Avon.

Families, Illness & Disability: An Integrative Treatment Model. John S. Rolland. 1994. LC 94-206. 304p. 47.00 (*0-465-02915-9*) Basic.

Families in Perpetual Crises. Richard Kagan & Shirley Schlosberg. 1989. LC 88-37919. 208p. 22.95 (*0-393-70066-6*) Norton.

Families Living with Drugs & HIV: Intervention & Treatment Strategies. Ed. by Richard P. Barth et al. 1993. LC 92-1693. 384p. pap. 26.00 (*0-89862-150-X*) Guilford Pubns.

Families of Handicapped Children: Needs & Supports Across the Life-Span. Ed. by Rebecca R. Fewell & Patricia F. Vadasy. 1986. LC 85-12167. 475p. (Orig.). pap. text 35.00 (*0-936104-84-8*, 1365) PRO-ED.

Families of Schizophrenic Patients: Cognitive Behavioral Intervention. Christine Barrowclough & Nicholas Tarrier. 1992. LC 92-32395. 276p. pap. 51.00 (*1-56593-021-5*, 0264) Thomson Learn.

Families of the Mentally Ill: Coping & Adaptation. Ed. by Agnes B. Hatfield & Harriet P. Lefley. 1987. LC 86-22878. 340p. pap. 24.00 (*0-89862-918-7*, 2918) Guilford Pubns.

Families, Physicians, & Children with Special Health Needs: Collaborative Medical Education Models. Rosalyn B. Darling & Margo I. Peter. 1994. LC 93-40559. 224p. 67.00 (*0-86569-226-2*, Auburn Hse) Greenwood.

Families, Services & Confusion in Old Age. Enid Levin et al. 1989. 338p. text (*0-566-05714-X*) Avebry GBR. *Dist:* Ashgate Pub Co.

Families That Abuse: Diagnosis & Therapy. Stefano Cirillo & Paola DiBlasio. Tr. by Joachim Neugroschel. 1992. 192p. 22.95 (*0-393-70122-0*) Norton.

Family: A Focal Point in Health Education. Ed. by Iago Galdston. 1969. LC 58-14314. (Illus.). 216p. (Orig.). (C). reprint ed. pap. 24.95 (*0-8236-8049-5*) Intl Univs Pr.

Family: Family, Youth, Aging & Death & Dying. 2000. (Enduring Issues Ser.). ring bd. 100.00 (*0-89777-224-5*) SIRS Pubng.

Family: Proceedings. Congress of Psychosomatic Obstetrics and Gynecology. Ed. by H. Hirsh et al. 1975. 600p. 153.25 (*3-8055-2206-1*) S Karger.

Family Addiction: An Analytical Guide. Douglas H. Ruben. 1993. LC 92-27787. (Reference Books on Family Issues: Vol. 21). 384p. text 66.00 (*0-8153-0031-X*) Garland.

Family Affair: Helping Families Cope with Mental Illness. Group for the Advancement of Psychiatry Staff. 1986. LC 86-18866. (GAP Reports: No. 119). 102p. text 28.95 (*0-87630-444-7*); pap. text 15.95 (*0-87630-443-9*) Brunner-Routledge.

Family & Child Mental Health: Selected Readings. Ed. by John Touliatos & Byron W. Lindholm. 1973. 32.50 (*0-8422-5096-4*) Irvington.

Family & Friends Guide to Diabetes: Everything You Need to Know. Eve Gehling. 2000. LC 99-39650. (Illus.). 282p. (C). pap. 15.95 (*0-471-34801-5*) Wiley.

Family & HIV. Robert Bor. 1994. LC 95-145079. (Sexual Politics Ser.). 208p. pap. (*0-304-32985-1*) Cassell GBR. *Dist:* LPC InBook.

Family & HIV Today. Robert Bor & Jonathan Elford. 1998. 300p. 75.00 (*0-304-70405-9*); 304th ed. pap. 24.95 (*0-304-70188-2*) Continuum.

Family & Human Adaptation. Theodore Lidz. 1963. LC 63-20457. 126p. 27.50 (*0-8236-1880-3*); pap. 24.95 (*0-8236-8051-7*, 21880) Intl Univs Pr.

Family & Human Development Across Cultures: A View from the Other Side. Cigdem Kagitcibasi. 1996. 248p. pap. 27.50 (*0-8058-2077-9*); text 59.95 (*0-8058-2076-0*) L Erlbaum Assocs.

Family & Population Control. Rueben Hill et al. pap. 21.95 (*0-8084-0130-0*) NCUP.

Family & Schizophrenia. John G. Howells & Wahuih Guirguis. 1985. LC 84-9087. 346p. 50.00 (*0-8236-1850-1*, 01850) Intl Univs Pr.

Family & Support Systems Across the Life Span. S. K. Steinmetz. 1988. (Illus.). 292p. (C). 66.00 (*0-306-42792-3*, Plenum Trade) Perseus Pubng.

Family & the Depression: A Study of One Hundred Chicago Families. Ruth S. Cavan & Katherine H. Ranck. 1977. LC 79-102229. (Select Bibliographies Reprint Ser.). 26.95 (*0-8369-5114-X*) Ayer.

Family & the School: A Joint Systems Approach to Problems with Children. Ed. by Emilia Dowling & Elsie Osborne. 2nd ed. 1994. LC 93-44329. 224p. (C). text 49.95 (*0-415-10127-1*, B3918) Routledge.

Family Approach to Psychiatric Disorders. Richard A. Perlmutter. 1996. LC 96-5703. 416p. text 52.95 (*0-88048-714-3*, 8714) Am Psychiatric.

Family Art Psychotherapy: A Clinical Guide & Casebook. Helen B. Landgarten. 1987. LC 86-28380. (Illus.). 320p. text 38.95 (*0-87630-456-0*) Brunner-Routledge.

Family Assessment: A Guide to Methods & Measures. Harold D. Grotevant & Cindy I. Carlson. 1989. LC 88-12041. 500p. 58.00 (*0-89862-733-8*, 2733) Guilford Pubns.

Family Assessment: Effective Uses of Personality Tests with Couples & Families. A. Rodney Nurse. 1999. LC 98-37415. (Couples & Family Dynamics & Treatment Ser.). (Illus.). 324p. (Orig.). 95.00 (*0-471-15397-4*) Wiley.

Family Assessment: Rationale, Methods, & Future Directions. T. Jacob & D. L. Tennenbaum. 1988. LC 88-2319. (Applied Clinical Psychology Ser.). (Illus.). 220p. (C). 49.50 (*0-306-42755-9*, Plenum Trade) Perseus Pubng.

Family-Based Palliative Care. Ed. by Jane M. Kirschling. 1990. LC 90-39008. (Hospice Journal). 123p. text 39.95 (*1-56024-039-3*) Haworth Pr.

Family-Based Services: A Solution-Focused Approach. Insoo K. Berg. 1994. LC 93-46043. 192p. (C). 27.00 (*0-393-70162-X*) Norton.

Family Based Treatment in Communicative Disorders: A Systemic Approach. James R. Andrews & Mary A. Andrews. 1990. (C). text 25.00 (*0-9626939-0-1*) Janelle Pubns.

Family Birthplace: Planning & Designing Today's Obstetric Facilities. Judith A. Smith. 1995. LC 95-36647. 118p. pap. 50.00 (*1-55648-147-0*, 043184) AHPI.

Family Building Through Egg & Sperm Donation: Medical, Legal & Ethical Issues. Machelle M. Seibel & Susan L. Crockin. 1996. LC 95-31221. (Medical Ser.). (Illus.). 320p. (C). text 76.95 (*0-86720-483-4*, 483-4) Jones & Bartlett.

Family Care Homes for the Mentally Ill. 1993. (Illus.). 40p. (Orig.). (C). pap. text 30.00 (*1-56806-721-6*) DIANE Pub.

Family Care of Mental Patients: A Review of Systems of Family Care in America & Europe. Horatio M. Pollock. 1976. LC 75-17236. (Social Problems & Social Policy Ser.). (Illus.). reprint ed. 21.95 (*0-405-07505-7*) Ayer.

Family Care of Schizophrenia: A Problem-Solving Approach to the Treatment of the Mentally Ill. Ian R. Falloon et al. 1984. LC 82-108352. (Guilford Family Therapy Ser.). 451p. text 50.00 (*0-89862-049-X*) Guilford Pubns.

Family Care of Schizophrenia: A Problem-Solving Approach to the Treatment of the Mentally Illness. Ian R. Falloon et al. 1987. LC 82-108352. (Family Therapy Ser.). 451p. pap. 30.00 (*0-89862-923-3*, 2923) Guilford Pubns.

Family Caregiver's Guide: Planning & Decision-Making for the Elderly. James A. Wilkinson. 1998. LC 98-20198. 160p. pap. 16.95 (*1-57749-077-0*) Fairview Press.

Family Caregiver's Guide: The Home Health Care Efficiency System that Really Works. Joan E. Foyder. 1987. LC 86-82135. (Illus.). 85p. (Orig.). pap. text 14.95 (*0-9617392-0-7*) Futuro Ohio.

Family Caregiving: Agenda for the Future. Ed. by Marjorie H. Cantor. 1994. (Critical Debates in an Aging Society Ser.). 149p. (Orig.). (C). pap. 19.95 (*0-9640387-0-6*) Am Soc Aging.

Family Caregiving Across the Lifespan. Ed. by Eva Kahana et al. 1994. LC 93-43663. (Family Caregiver Applications Ser.: Vol. 44). 380p. (C). 78.95 (*0-8039-4430-6*, 3505); pap. 38.95 (*0-8039-4431-4*, 3506) Sage.

Family Caregiving in Mental Illness, No. 7. Harriet P. Lefley. 1996. (Family Caregiver Applications Ser.: Vol. 7). pap. 38.95 (*0-8039-5721-1*, 4072) Sage.

Family-Centered Early Intervention for Commmunication Disorders: Prevention & Treatment. Gail D. Kilburg. 1997. (Excellence in Practice Ser.). 309p. 60.00 (*0-8342-0294-8*) PRO-ED.

Family Centered Maternity & Newborn Care: A Basic Text. Celeste R. Phillips. 4th ed. 1995. (Illus.). 464p. (C). (gr. 13). pap. text 34.95 (*0-8151-6794-6*, 25335) Mosby Inc.

Family-Centered Maternity-Newborn Care. Phillips. 4th ed. 1996. (Illus.). 96p. (C). (gr. 13). tchr. ed., spiral bd. (*0-8151-6793-8*, 25334) Mosby Inc.

Family-Centered Nursing Care of Children. Ed. by Cecily L. Betz et al. 2nd ed. 1994. (Illus.). 2346p. tchr. ed. (*0-7216-4573-9*) Saunders.

Family-Centered Nursing Care of Children. Cecily L. Betz et al. 2nd ed. 1994. LC 93-2268. (Illus.). 2272p. reprint ed. text 68.00 (*0-7216-4489-9*) Saunders.

Family-Centered Services in Residential Treatment: New Approaches for Group Care. John Y. Powell. 2000. LC 00-38856. (Illus.). xvii, 146p. pap. 17.95 (*0-7890-1022-4*) Haworth Pr.

Family-Centered Services in Residential Treatment: New Approaches for Group Care. Ed. by John Y. Powell. 2000. LC 00-38856. (Illus.). xvii, 146p. 39.95 (*0-7890-1021-6*) Haworth Pr.

Family Context of Adolescent Drug Use. Ed. by Robert H. Coombs. LC 88-10965. (Journal of Chemical Dependency Treatment Ser.: Vol. 1, No. 2). (Illus.). 273p. (Orig.). 1989. text 49.95 (*0-86656-799-2*); 1988. pap. text 24.95 (*0-86656-828-X*) Haworth Pr.

Family Cookbook, Vol. 1. American Dietetic Association Staff & American Diabetes Association. rev. ed. 1987. LC 87-42674. 392p. 23.00 (*0-13-024901-7*, 0840) Am Dietetic Assn.

Family Counseling: Strategies & Issues. Ed. by Jon Carlson & Judith A. Lewis. 1991. pap. 32.00 (*0-89108-219-0*, 9102) Love Pub Co.

Family Counseling Casebook. John C. Gunzburg. 1991. (Illus.). 272p. text 42.00 (*0-07-452817-3*) McGraw-Hill Med Pub.

Family Crucible: The Intense Experience of Family Therapy. Augustus Y. Napier & Carl A. Whitaker. 1988. LC 74-1872. 320p. pap. 14.00 (*0-06-091489-0*, PL-1489, Perennial) HarperTrade.

Family Diagnosis. John G. Howells & A. Winnifred Brown. 1986. LC 85-18175. 350p. 50.00 (*0-8236-1870-6*, 01870) Intl Univs Pr.

Family Doctor: Good Advice for Better Health. E. R. Fox. 1993. 440p. (Orig.). pap. 12.95 (*0-9639027-3-3*) Gatewood Pr.

Family Doctors & Economic Incentives. Nick Bosanquet & Brenda Leese. 1989. 150p. text (*1-85521-009-6*) Dartmth Pub GBR. *Dist:* Ashgate Pub Co.

Family Doctors Guide to Understanding & Preventing Cancer Vol. 1: Environmental Risks & Solutions. Sita R. Kaura. 1992. (Illus.). 279p. 24.95 (*0-9650621-1-2*) Manisha Pr.

Family Dynamics for Physicians: Guidelines to Assessment & Treatment. Russell J. Sawa. 1985. LC 85-21374. (Studies in Health & Human Services: Vol. 4). 346p. lib. bdg. 99.95 (*0-88946-129-5*) E Mellen.

Family Dynamics in Individual Psychotherapy: A Guide to Clinical Strategies. Ellen F. Wachtel & Paul L. Wachtel. LC 85-27242. 258p. 1985. 49.95 (*0-89862-663-3*); 1991. reprint ed. pap. 23.00 (*0-89862-462-2*, 2462) Guilford Pubns.

Family Education in Mental Illness. Agnes B. Hatfield. 1990. LC 89-71487. 211p. 49.95 (*0-89862-427-4*) Guilford Pubns.

Family Emergency Plan, Vol. I. Barry G. Crockett & Lynette B. Crockett. 1990. LC 89-91819. (Illus.). 80p. pap. 11.95 (*0-915131-89-7*) Crockett Pub Co.

Family Encyclopedia of Natural Healing. John Heinerman & Lendon Smith. 2000. 302p. 19.95 (*1-55517-492-2*, Bonneville Bks) CFI Dist.

Family Evaluation: An Approach Based on Bowen Theory. Michael E. Kerr & Murray Bowen. 1988. (Professional Bks.). (Illus.). 400p. 35.00 (*0-393-70056-9*) Norton.

Family Face of Schizophrenia: True Stories of Mental Illness with Practical Counsel from America's Leading Experts. Patricia Backlar. 1995. LC 94-30061. 14.95 (*0-87477-790-9*, Tarcher Putnam) Putnam Pub Group.

Family Focused Behavioral Pediatrics. William L. Coleman. 2001. LC 00-67526. (Core Handbooks in Pediatrics Ser.). (Illus.). xi, 322p. pap. text 29.95 (*0-7817-2857-6*) Lppncott W & W.

Family Focused Care. Jean R. Miller & Ellen Janosik. 1979. (Illus.). text 32.95 (*0-07-042060-2*) McGraw.

Family Games. Mara S. Palazzoli et al. Tr. by Veronica Kleiber. 1989. 285p. 27.95 (*0-393-70070-4*) Norton.

Family Games: General Models of Psychotic Processes in the Family. M. S. Palazzoli et al. 1988. 302p. pap. (*0-946439-53-2*) Karnac Bks GBR. *Dist:* Other Pr LLC.

Family Genetic Sourcebook. Benjamin A. Pierce. 1990. LC 89-24884. 340p. pap. 14.95 (*0-471-61709-1*) Wiley.

Family Guide to Homeopathy: Symptoms & Natural Solutions. Andrew Lockie. 1993. LC 93-15113. (Illus.). 464p. 16.00 (*0-671-76771-2*, Fireside) S&S Trade Pap.

Family Guide to Reflexology. Ann Gillanders. 1998. LC 97-73864. (Illus.). 144p. pap. 12.95 (*0-316-31484-6*, Back Bay) Little.

***Family Guide to Stroke, Treatment, Recovery & Prevention.** Louis R. Caplan et al. 2001. (Illus.). reprint ed. 23.00 (*0-7567-5175-6*) DIANE Pub.

Family Guide to Surviving Stroke & Communication Disorders. Dennis C. Tanner. 1998. LC 98-26258. 273p. (C). pap. text 25.00 (*0-205-28538-4*) Allyn.

Family Handbook of Medical Tests. Carole Horn & Carol Eron. 1985. 256p. 9.95 (*0-399-51140-7*) Berkley Pub.

Family Healing: Strategies for Hope & Understanding. Minuchin. 1998. pap. 15.00 (*0-684-85573-9*) S&S Trade.

Family Healing: Tales of Hope & Renewal from Family Therapy. Salvador Minuchin & Michael P. Nichols. 1998. 287p. (C). text 23.00 (*0-7881-5599-7*) DIANE Pub.

Family Healing: Tales of Hope & Renewal from Family Therapy. Salvador Minuchin & Michael P. Nichols. 1994. 304p. pap. 12.00 (*0-671-88099-3*, Touchstone) S&S Trade Pap.

Family Health: A Holistic Approach to Social Work Practice. Ed. by John T. Pardeck & Francis K. O. Yuen. 1999. LC 98-47756. 208p. 58.00 (*0-86569-268-8*, Auburn Hse) Greenwood.

Family Health: From Data to Policy. Ed. by Gerry E. Hendershot & Felicia B. LeClere. 1993. LC 93-86892. 126p. (Orig.). (C). pap. 16.95 (*0-916174-37-9*) Natl Coun Family.

Family Health & Emergency Guide: First Aid & Home Treatments for Over 50 Everyday Injuries & Illnesses, Including, Allergies, Burns, Flu, Insect. Ed. by Time-Life Books Editors. 1999. LC 98-13141. (Time-Life Medical Guides). (Illus.). 144p. (gr. 11). pap. 6.95 (*0-7370-1104-1*, Time Life) Henninger Prod.

Family Health & Medical Guide. Ira J. Chasoff & Jeffrey W. Ellis. 1998. 608p. pap. 7.99 (*0-451-19433-0*) NAL.

Family Health Care. Russell J. Sawa. 1992. (Illus.). 320p. (C). 64.95 (*0-8039-4748-8*, 4747); pap. 32.95 (*0-8039-4749-6*, 4748) Sage.

Family Health Care Debra P. Hymovich & Martha U. Barnard. 1979. (Illus.). 1. pap. text 26.95 (*0-07-031675-9*); 2. pap. text 26.95 (*0-07-031676-7*) McGraw.

Family Health for Dummies. Charles B. Inlander et al. 1998. LC 98-89041. (For Dummies Ser.). 408p. pap. 19.99 (*0-7645-5121-3*) Hungry Minds.

Family Health Guide to Homeopathy. Barry Rose. 1995. LC 93-3586. (Illus.). 310p. text 34.95 (*0-89087-695-9*) Celestial Arts.

Family Health Psychology. Ed. by T. John Akamatsu et al. 1992. LC 92-6333. (Series in Applied Psychology: Social Issues & Questions). 240p. 69.95 (*1-56032-247-0*) Taylor & Francis.

Family Healthcare Nursing: Theory, Practice & Research. Shirley H. Hansen. 2nd rev. ed. 2000. LC 00-31483. (Illus.). 496p. pap. text 37.95 (*0-8036-0598-6*) Davis Co.

Family Herbal: A Guide to Natural Health Care for Yourself & Your Children from Europe's Leading Herbalists. Barbara Theiss & Peter Theiss. rev. ed. 1993. LC 93-13856. (Illus.). 288p. pap. 19.95 (*0-89281-484-5*, Heal Arts VT) Inner Tradit.

Family Heritage. Valerie S. Peacock. 2nd ed. 1982. 94p. reprint ed. 9.95 (*0-939909-00-6*) Scribe Write.

Family Home Care: Critical Issues for Services & Policies. Ed. by Robert Perlman. 1983. LC 83-81. (Home Health Care Services Quarterly Ser.: Vol. 3, Nos. 3 & 4). 294p. text 49.95 (*0-86656-220-6*) Haworth Pr.

Family Homeopath: Safe, Natural & Effective Health Care for You & Your Children. Robin Hayfield. 1995. LC 95-8366. (Illus.). 144p. pap. 16.95 (*0-89281-532-9*, Heal Arts VT) Inner Tradit.

Family Homeopathy. Paul Callinan. Ed. by Don R. Bensen. 1995. LC 95-25132. 344p. 24.95 (*0-87983-687-3*, 36873K, Keats Pubng) McGraw-Hill Trade.

Family in Clinical Psychiatry. Sidney Bloch et al. 1994. LC 93-45494. (Medical Publications). (Illus.). 312p. 79.50 (*0-19-262311-7*); pap. text 36.50 (*0-19-262310-9*) OUP.

Family in Family Medicine: Graduate Curriculum & Teaching Strategies. Ed. by Society for Teachers of Family Medicine, Task Forc. 1981. 109p. 5.00 (*0-942295-03-X*) Soc Tchrs Fam Med.

Family in Family Medicine: Graduate Curriculum & Teaching Strategies. Compiled & Des. by STFM Task Force on the Family in Family Medicine S. 2nd ed. 1989. 269p. 15.00 (*0-942295-20-X*, 30) Soc Tchrs Fam Med.

Family in Medical Practice. Ed. by M. A. Crouch & L. Roberts. 1986. (Illus.). 256p. 37.00 (*0-387-96372-3*) Spr-Verlag.

Family in Mourning: A Guide for Health Professionals. Charles E. Hollingsworth & Robert O. Pasnau. 1977. (Seminars in Psychology Ser.). 240p. text 56.00 (*0-8089-1020-5*, 792055, Grune & Strat) Harcrt Hlth Sci Grp.

Family Interaction & Psychopathology: Theories, Methods, & Findings. T. Jacob. 1987. LC 87-2570. (Applied Clinical Psychology Ser.). (Illus.). 684p. (C). 100.00 (*0-306-42357-X*, Plenum Trade) Perseus Pubng.

***Family Interventions in Mental Illness: International Perspectives.** Ed. by Harriet P. Lefley & Dale L. Johnson. 2001. LC 2001-32931. 264p. 69.00 (*0-275-96954-1*, Praeger Pubs) Greenwood.

Family Interventions Throughout Chronic Illness & Disability. Ed. by Paul W. Power et al. 1988. (Series on Rehabilitation: No. 7). 336p. 43.95 (*0-8261-5580-4*) Springer Pub.

Family Is the Patient: Using Family Interviews in Children's Medical Care. Bayard W. Allmond et al. 1998. LC 98-33474. 384p. pap. 29.95 (*0-683-30288-4*) Lppncott W & W.

Family Issues in Pediatric Psychology. Ed. by Michael Roberts & Jan L. Wallander. 1992. 288p. pap. text 32.50 (*0-8058-0854-X*) L Erlbaum Assocs.

Family Kaleidoscope. Salvador Minuchin. 1984. 248p. 22.00 (*0-674-29230-8*) HUP.

Family Life: Process & Practice. Robert J. Janosik & Elta Green. 1991. 62.50 (*0-86720-318-8*) Jones & Bartlett.

Family Life of Psychotherapists: Clinical Implications. Ed. by Florence W. Kaslow. 1987. LC 87-25107. (Journal of Psychotherapy & the Family Ser.: Vol. 3, No. 2). 160p. (C). text 49.95 (*0-86656-683-X*) Haworth Pr.

Family Massage Manual. Zhaoguang Chen. Tr. by Yong Zhao from CHI. 1992. (Illus.). 149p. (Orig.). pap. 6.95 (*0-8351-2571-8*) China Bks.

Family Medical Advisor: The Complete Guide to Alternative & Conventional Treatments. Parenting Magazine Editors. 2001. LC 00-45575. pap. (*0-7835-0909-X*) Time-Life.

Family Medical & Health Guide. Consumer Guide Editors. 1993. (Illus.). 384p. pap. 9.98 (*1-56173-451-9*, 4005500) Pubns Intl Ltd.

Family Medical & Prescription Drug Guide. Consumer Guide Editors. 1993. (Illus.). 864p. 39.95 (*0-7853-0084-8*, 3211400) Pubns Intl Ltd.

Family Medical Dictionary. Justus J. Schifferes. 1983. mass mkt. 6.99 (*0-671-74191-8*) PB.

Family Medical Dictionary: Diccionario Medico Familiar. Reader's Digest Editorial Staff. 1981. (SPA.). 756p. 95.00 (*0-8288-1878-9*, S34982) Fr & Eur.

Family Medical Emergency Library. Manoff. 1996. (C). (gr. 13). pap. 12.04 (*0-8151-2503-8*, 31238) Mosby Inc.

Family Medical Group: A MediSoft for Windows Simulation. 1999. tchr. ed. 20.00 incl. disk (*0-02-804873-3*) Glencoe.

Family Medical Group: A MediSoft for Windows Simulation. Deborah Jones et al. 1999. LC 98-47126. (*0-02-804872-5*) Glencoe.

Family Medical Guide: The Illustrated Medical & Health Advisor. Consumer Guide Editors et al. 1993. (Illus.). 576p. 9.98 (*0-7853-0184-4*, 3212000) Pubns Intl Ltd.

Family Medical History. Hugh W. Johnston et al. Ed. by Kris Jordan. 1994. 130p. 14.95 (*1-883681-99-5*) Lrning Thrgh Ent.

Family Medical Record: An Interactive Guide to Getting the Best Care. Maria Hester et al. 2000. LC 99-45539. (Illus.). 224p. pap. 14.95 (*0-471-34792-2*) Wiley.

Family Medicine. David R. Rudy & Kurt Kurowski. 1997. LC 96-37442. (House Officer Ser.). 936p. pap. 29.95 (*0-683-18243-9*) Lppncott W & W.

Family Medicine. Jeffrey G. Hirsch. Ed. by Rita R. Claudet. 2nd ed. 1996. LC 96-1058. (Oklahoma Notes). 290p. pap. 24.95 (*0-387-94638-1*) Spr-Verlag.

Family Medicine: 2000 Edition. Paul D. Chan. rev. ed. 1999. (Current Clinical Strategies Ser.). pap. 46.95 incl. cd-rom (*1-881528-80-4*) Current Clin Strat.

Family Medicine: A New Approach to Health Care. Ed. by Betty E. Cogswell & Marvin B. Sussman. 1982. LC 81-6980. (Marriage & the Family Ser.: Vol. 4, Nos. 1-2). 187p. text 39.95 (*0-917724-25-9*) Haworth Pr.

Family Medicine: Principles & Practice. Robert B. Taylor. 5th ed. 1997. LC 96-29794. (Illus.). 1128p. 145.00 (*0-387-94958-5*) Spr-Verlag.

Family Medicine: The Maturing of a Discipline. Ed. by William J. Doherty et al. 1987. LC 86-29501. (Marriage & the Family Ser.: Vol. 10, Nos. 3-4). 236p. text 49.95 (*0-86656-625-2*) Haworth Pr.

Family Medicine, Year 2000 Edition: Current Clinical Strategies. Paul D. Chan. rev. ed. 1999. (Current

Clinical Strategies Ser.). 300p. pap. 26.95 (*1-881528-79-0*) Current Clin Strat.

Family Meeting Handbook: Achieving Family Harmony Happily. Robert Slagle. 1985. LC 84-82425. (Illus.). 170p. pap. 7.95 (*0-9614218-0-0*) Family Relat.

Family Mental Health Encyclopedia. Frank J. Bruno. 1989. LC 88-33968. 422p. 32.50 (*0-471-63573-1*) Wiley.

Family Myths: Psychotherapy Implications. Stephen A. Anderson & Dennis A. Bagarozzi. 1989. LC 88-30091. (Journal of Psychotherapy & the Family Ser.: Vol. 4, Nos. 3-4). (Illus.). 213p. text 49.95 (*0-86656-775-5*) Haworth Pr.

Family Nurse: Companion of the Frugal Housewife. Lydia Maria Child. 1997. LC 97-84. 288p. reprint ed. 12.95 (*1-55709-461-6*) Applewood.

Family Nurse Practitioner. Jack Rudman. 1994. (Certified Nurse Examination Ser.: CN-2). pap. 27.95 (*0-8373-6102-8*) Nat Learn.

Family Nurse Practitioner Certification Examination: Adult Health. Margaret A. Fitzgerald. 2nd ed. 2000. (Illus.). 508p. pap. text, stu. ed. 39.95 (*0-8036-0593-5*) Davis Co.

Family Nurse Practitioner Certification Prep Exams. Amelie Hollier et al. 2nd rev. ed. 1998. 293p. (C). pap. text 39.95 (*1-892418-02-9*) APEA.

Family Nurse Practitioner Certification Review. Kidd Robinson et al. 1998. LC 98-23492. (Illus.). 768p. (C). (gr. 13). pap. text 54.95 (*0-8151-5581-6*, 31784) Mosby Inc.

Family Nurse Practitioner Certification Review. JoAnn Zerwekh & Jo C. Claborn. Ed. by Robin Carter. 1998. LC 98-34772. 300p. (C). pap. text 39.95 (*0-7216-7743-6*) Saunders.

Family Nurse Practitioner Certification Review & Clinical Reference Guide. Ed. by Virginia Millonig. 2001. 1300p. 69.95 (*1-878028-28-6*) Hlth Lead Assoc.

Family Nurse Practitioner Certification Review Book: Comprehensive Outline & Study Guide. Amelie Hollier et al. 2nd rev. ed. 1999. (C). 51.95 (*1-892418-05-3*) APEA.

Family Nurse Practitioner Certification Review Books: A Comprehensive Study Guide. Abr. by Amelie Hollier et al. 1998. 800p. pap. text 121.95 (*1-892418-01-0*) APEA.

Family Nurse Practitioner Certification Review Guide Set, Set. Ed. by Virginia Millenig et al. 2nd ed. 1998. pap. text 130.00 (*1-878028-24-3*) Hlth Lead Assoc.

Family Nurse Practitioner Certification Study Question Book Set, Set. Sally K. Miller. 1999. LC 99-22759. 900p. pap. text 70.00 (*1-878028-26-X*) Hlth Lead Assoc.

Family Nurse Practitioner Pearls of Wisdom: Over 3000 Questions. Michael Krieger et al. Date not set. (Pearls of Wisdom Ser.). pap. 32.00 (*1-890369-04-7*) Boston Medical.

***Family Nurse Practitioner Preview & Resource Manual (FNP)** Nurse Practitioner Alternatives in Education, Inc. Staff. 2001. 2001p. (C). pap. text (*1-55810-171-3*) Am Nurses Pub.

Family Nurse Practitioner Review Course. Michael Gibbs & Anne Nichols. 2000. 250p. 199.95 incl. cd-rom (*0-9679170-0-X*) NPeducationcom.

Family Nursing. C. Luise Riehl. 1974. (Illus.). 384p. (C). text 23.20 (*0-02-663760-X*) Glencoe.

Family Nursing: Research Theory & Practice. Marilyn M. Friedman. 4th ed. 1997. LC 97-2151. 672p. (C). pap. 52.00 (*0-8385-2525-3*, A-2525-2) P-H.

Family Nursing: The Case of Cystic Fibrosis. Dorothy Whyte. 1994. 229p. (*1-85628-524-3*) Avebry GBR. *Dist:* Ashgate Pub Co.

Family Nursing Practice. Beth Vaughan-Cole et al. 1997. LC 97-18481. (Illus.). 352p. (C). pap. text 35.00 (*0-7216-6492-X*) Saunders.

Family-of-Origin Therapy: An Intergenerational Approach. James L. Framo. 1992. LC 91-29310. 272p. text 41.95 (*0-87630-590-7*) Brunner-Routledge.

Family of Origin Therapy & Diversity. 1997. LC 96-47173. 62.95 (*1-56032-463-5*) Hemisp Pub.

Family of Origin Therapy & Diversity. Searight. 1997. LC 96-47173. pap. 31.95 (*1-56032-464-3*) Hemisp Pub.

Family of the Retarded Child. John N. Carver & Nellie E. Carver. 1972. LC 72-85384. (Segregated Settings & the Problems of Change Ser.: No. 2). 156p. 14.95 (*0-8156-8079-1*) Syracuse U Pr.

Family Organization & Crisis: Maintenance of Integration in Families with a Severely Mentally Retarded Child. B. Farber. 1960. (SRCD M Ser.: Vol. 25, No. 1). pap. 25.00 (*0-527-01583-0*) Periodicals Srv.

Family-Oriented Primary Care. S. McDaniel et al. 1997. (Illus.). 387p. 69.00 (*0-387-97056-8*) Spr-Verlag.

Family Partnership in Hospital Care: The Cooperative Care Concept. Ed. by Anthony J. Grieco et al. 1994. LC 94-10518. 304p. 37.95 (*0-8261-8490-1*) Springer Pub.

Family Placements. British Institute of Mental Handicap Staff. 1985. 36p. 25.00 (*0-906054-52-4*) St Mut.

Family Placements for Mentally Handicapped Children. John Hattersley et al. 1985. 66p. 29.00 (*0-906054-22-2*) St Mut.

Family Planning. Ed. by Mahmoud F. Fathalla et al. 1989. (F. I. G. O. Manual of Human Reproduction Ser.: Vol. 2). (Illus.). 237p. text 35.00 (*1-85070-193-8*, Parthenon Pbng) CRC Pr.

Family Planning & Population: A Compendium of International Statistics. Ed. by John A. Ross et al. 1993. LC 93-93706. 202p. pap. 25.00 (*0-87834-078-5*) Population Coun.

Family Planning & Reproductive Health Services in Ghana: An Annotated Bibliography, 18. Ed. by Yaw Oheneba-Sakyi. 1994. LC 94-10358. (African Special Bibliographic Ser.: No. 18). 176p. lib. bdg. 59.95 (*0-313-28900-X*, Greenwood Pr) Greenwood.

Family Planning & Reproductive Rights: A Feminist Report. Ed. by Elizabeth Hayes et al. 1997. LC 97-28038. (C). pap. (*1-85649-452-7*) Zed Books GBR. *Dist:* St Martin.

Family Planning & the Law. Kenneth M. Norrie. 1991. 220p. text (*1-85521-035-5*) Dartmth Pub GBR. *Dist:* Ashgate Pub Co.

Family Planning at Your Fingertips: Adapted from the Pages of Contraceptive Technology. Robert A. Hatcher et al. Ed. by Deborah Kowal. 1993. LC 93-7618. (Illus.). 420p. (C). pap. text 19.95 (*0-8290-3168-5*); lib. bdg. 29.95 (*0-8290-3172-3*) Irvington.

Family Planning Counseling: A Curriculum Prototype, Participant's Handbook. AVSC International Staff. 1995. LC 94-48622. 79p. (Orig.). pap., stu. ed. 8.00 (*1-885063-09-1*) EngenderHlth.

Family Planning Counseling: A Curriculum Prototype, Trainer's Package. AVSC International Staff. 1995. LC 94-48622. ring bd. 75.00 (*1-885063-10-5*) EngenderHlth.

Family Planning Counseling & Voluntary Sterilization: A Guide for Managers. Georgeanne S. Neamatalla & Pamela B. Harper. rev. ed. 1994. 55p. pap. text 8.00 (*1-885063-05-9*) EngenderHlth.

Family Planning in Haryana: Analysis of a State Program in India. Nancy C. Henley & Sagar C. Jain. 1977. LC 77-11989. pap. 5.00 (*0-89055-125-1*) Carolina Pop Ctr.

Family Planning in Health Services: A Report. WHO Staff. 1971. (Technical Reports: No. 476). 65p. pap. text 7.00 (*92-4-120476-1*, 1100476) World Health.

Family Planning in India. K. G. Jolly. 1986. 287p. (*0-8364-1930-8*) Hindustan IND. *Dist:* S Asia.

Family Planning in the Education of Nurses & Midwives. L. M. Turnbull & H. Pizurki. 1973. (Public Health Papers: No. 53). pap. text 5.00 (*92-4-130053-1*, 1110053) World Health.

Family Planning Legislation. B. Swartz. 1983. (Euro Reports & Studies Ser.: No. 85). 86p. pap. text 8.00 (*92-890-1251-X*) World Health.

Family Planning Library Manual. Gloria A. Roberts. 5th enl. rev. ed. 1994. LC 93-84534. (Illus.). 148p. (Orig.). pap. text 15.00 (*0-934586-72-1*) Plan Parent.

Family Planning Manager's Handbook: Basic Skills & Tools for Managing Family Planning Programs. Ed. by James A. Wolff et al. 1991. LC 91-7252. (Library of Management for Development, Management). (Illus.). 374p. spiral bd. 24.95 (*0-931816-72-6*) Kumarian Pr.

Family Planning Manager's Handbook: Basic Skills & Tools for Managing Family Planning Programs. Ed. by James A. Wolff et al. (Illus.). (Orig.). 1997. (ARA.). pap. 25.00 (*0-913723-41-X*); 1995. 374p. pap. 25.00 (*0-913723-33-9*) Mgmt Sci Health.

Family Planning on a Crowded Planet. Yates Wilson. 1983. LC 82-24160. 96p. reprint ed. lib. bdg. 59.75 (*0-313-22680-6*, YAFP, Greenwood Pr) Greenwood.

Family Planning Programme in India. Shanta K. Chandra. 1987. (*81-7099-023-8*) Mittal Pubs Dist IND. *Dist:* S Asia.

Family Planning Sourcebook: Basic Information about Planning for Pregnancy & Contraception. Ed. by Amy Marcaccio. 2001. LC 00-53029. (Health Reference Ser.). (Illus.). xv, 520p. lib. bdg. 78.00 (*0-7808-0379-5*) Omnigraphics Inc.

Family Play Therapy. Ed. by Charles E. Schaefer & Lois J. Carey. 1994. LC 93-47160. (Child Therapy Ser.). 336p. 45.00 (*1-56821-150-3*) Aronson.

Family Practice: Brief Systems Methods for Social Work. Cynthia Franklin & Catheleen Jordan. 1998. LC 98-16953. 416p. pap. text 50.95 (*0-534-16182-0*) Brooks-Cole.

Family Practice & Preventive Medicine: Health Promotion in Primary Care. Ed. by Joseph W. Hess et al. 1983. LC 82-15718. 448p. (C). 55.95 (*0-89885-131-9*, Kluwer Acad Hman Sci) Kluwer Academic.

Family Practice Board Certification Review. D. Kanjilal. 1999. (Illus.). 1000p. LC 99-22060. text 149.00 (*1-58141-040-9*); LC 99-22060. text 299.00 incl. cd-rom (*1-58141-044-1*); cd-rom 199.00 (*1-58141-042-5*) Rivercross Pub.

Family Practice Board Review. Robert L. Bratton. 1998. LC 97-48636. 300p. 69.95 (*0-683-30504-2*) Lppncott W & W.

Family Practice Desk Reference. Ed. by Charles E. Driscoll et al. 3rd ed. 1995. LC 95-19477. (Illus.). 784p. (C). (gr. 13). text 54.95 (*0-8151-2201-2*, 24423) Mosby Inc.

Family Practice in the Nineteen Eighties: A Second Decade of Essays. G. Gayle Stephens. 1990. 201p. 18.95 (*0-942295-18-8*, 36) Soc Tchrs Fam Med.

Family Practice Office Manual. Edward T. Bope & William A. Verhoff. 1994. (Office Manual Ser.). 246p. 115.00 (*1-890018-05-8*) Anadem Pubng.

Family Practice Pearls of Wisdom: Over 3000 Questions. Schwer et al. 1998. (Pearls of Wisdom Ser.). pap. 88.00 (*1-890369-02-0*) Boston Medical.

Family Practice Review: A Problem Oriented Approach. Richard W. Swanson. 3rd ed. 1996. 736p. (C). (gr. 13). text 64.95 (*0-8151-8624-X*, 25692) Mosby Inc.

Family Practice Sourcebook. Contrib. by Mosby Staff. 2000. 510p. pap. 59.00 (*1-55664-469-8*) Mosby Inc.

Family Practice, Specialty Board Review. Ernest Yuh-Ting Yen. 6th ed. 1998. LC 98-3615. 250p. (C). pap. 54.95 (*0-8385-8739-9*) McGraw-Hill Prof.

Family Practice Two Thousand. Berg. 2000. (Illus.). 550p. text 66.95 (*0-8151-6858-6*, 31731) Mosby Inc.

Family Practice Two Thousand & One. Berg. 2001. 66.95 (*0-8151-2035-4*, 31732) Mosby Inc.

Family Practitioner's Survival Guide to the Business of Medicine. Robert W. Katz. 1997. LC 98-4003. pap. 75.00 (*0-8342-1152-1*) Aspen Pub.

Family Practitioners Survival Guide to the Business of Medicine. Katz. 1998. No. 2. (*0-8342-1135-1*); No. 3. (*0-8342-1136-X*) Aspen Pub.

Family Problem Solving. William J. Reid. 1985. 360p. text 46.00 (*0-231-06056-4*) Col U Pr.

Family Processes & Schizophrenia. Ed. by Elliot G. Mishler & Nancy E. Waxler. 1983. LC 84-45085. 336p. 50.00 (*0-87668-711-7*) Aronson.

Family Psychiatry in the Kibbutz: Collected Papers of Mordecai Kaffman, with Esther Elizur Talmon, & Avigail Sivan-Sher. Ed. by Mordecai Kaffman. 1985. (Special Issue of International Journal of Family Therapy: Vol. 6, No. 4). 132p. pap. 16.95 (*0-89885-252-8*, Kluwer Acad Hman Sci) Kluwer Academic.

Family Psychology Two: Theory, Therapy, Enrichment & Training. Luciano L'Abate. 1988. 300p. (Orig.). (C). 30.50 (*0-8191-6680-4*) U Pr of Amer.

Family Psychopathology: The Relational Roots of Dysfunctional Behavior. Luciano L'Abate. 1998. LC 98-13462. 528p. text 60.00 (*1-57230-369-7*, C0369) Guilford Pubns.

Family Reconstruction: Long Day's Journey into Light. William F. Nerin. 1986. (Professional Bks.). (Illus.). 222p. 22.95 (*0-393-70017-8*) Norton.

Family Recovery Workbook: For Families Affected by Chemical Dependency, Set. Dennis C. Daley. 1987. 32p. (Orig.). 3.50 (*0-943519-03-9*, B1903) Sulzburger & Graham Pub.

Family Resources: The Hidden Partner in Family Therapy. Ed. by Mark A. Karpel. 1986. LC 86-14922. (Guilford Family Therapy Ser.). 479p. 55.00 (*0-89862-069-4*) Guilford Pubns.

Family Rights: Advances in Medico-Legal Ethics. Alexander M. Smith & Elaine Sutherland. 1991. 192p. (*0-7486-0204-6*) Edinburgh U Pr GBR. *Dist:* Col U Pr.

Family Rights: Family Law & Medical Advances. Alexander M. Smith & Elaine Sutherland. 1992. 144p. pap. (*0-7486-0239-9*) Edinburgh U Pr GBR. *Dist:* Col U Pr.

Family Sexual Abuse: Frontline Research & Evaluation. Michael Q. Patton. 1991. (Illus.). 248p. 64.95 (*0-8039-3960-4*, 3071) Sage.

Family Sexual Abuse: Frontline Research & Evaluation. Michael Quinn Patton. 1991. (Illus.). 248p. pap. 32.95 (*0-8039-3961-2*, 3072) Sage.

Family Stress, Coping & Social Support. Hamilton I. McCubbin et al. 1982. (Illus.). 294p. (C). text 50.95 (*0-398-04692-1*) C C Thomas.

Family Stress Management. Pauline Boss. 1988. (Family Studies Ser.: Vol. 8). 150p. (C). 76.95 (*0-8039-2380-5*); 2nd ed. pap. 31.95 (*0-8039-2381-3*, 5648) Sage.

Family Support Programs & Rehabilitation: A Cognitive-Behavioral Approach to Traumatic Brain Injury. Hamish P. Godfrey & Louise M. Smith. 1995. LC 95-19332. (Critical Issues in Neuropsychology Ser.). 236p. (C). text 36.50 (*0-306-44932-3*, Kluwer Plenum) Kluwer Academic.

Family Systems Approach to Individual Psychotherapy. David M. Allen. 1995. LC 94-70369. 392p. pap. 60.00 (*1-56821-246-1*) Aronson.

Family Systems, Family Therapy: Applications for Clinical Practice. Ed. by Joan D. Atwood. 2001. LC 00-59673. (Journal of Prevention & Intervention in the Community Monograph: Vol. 21, No. 1). 188p. 39.95 (*0-7890-0798-3*); 165p. (C). pap. text 19.95 (*0-7890-0831-9*) Haworth Pr.

Family Systems in Medicine. Ed. by Christian N. Ramsey, Jr. 1989. LC 88-24477. (Guilford Family Therapy Ser.). (Illus.). 615p. 79.95 (*0-89862-103-8*) Guilford Pubns.

Family Systems Therapy: An Integration. Stephen J. Schultz. LC 83-15516. 512p. 40.00 (*0-87668-645-5*) Aronson.

Family Systems Therapy: Developments in the Milan-Systemic Therapies. Elsa Jones. 1993. LC 92-30568. (Family Psychology Ser.). 280p. pap. 125.00 (*0-471-93825-4*) Wiley.

***Family Therapy.** Lynn Hoffman. 2001. LC 2001-44331. 320p. 35.00 (*0-393-70380-0*) Norton.

Family Therapy. John E. Bell. 1995. LC 74-22276. 436p. reprint ed. pap. 60.00 (*1-56821-506-1*) Aronson.

Family Therapy. Irene Goldenberg & Herbert Goldenberg. 2nd ed. 1985. (C). pap., wbk. ed. 13.25 (*0-534-04687-8*) Brooks-Cole.

Family Therapy: A Bibliography, 4. Ed. by Alice W. Lubin et al. 1988. LC 88-18682. 470p. lib. bdg. 95.00 (*0-313-26172-5*, LFT/, Greenwood Pr) Greenwood.

Family Therapy: A Social Work Approach. George Thorman. 1997. LC 97-16699. (Illus.). 150p. text 46.95 (*0-398-06787-2*); pap. text 31.95 (*0-398-06788-0*) C C Thomas.

Family Therapy: A Systemic Behavioral Approach. Ed. by Joan Atwood. 1999. (Social Welfare Ser.). 356p. (C). pap. text 48.95 (*0-8304-1300-6*) Thomson Learn.

Family Therapy: A Triadic-Based Approach. Gerald H. Zuk. rev. ed. 1981. LC 80-24708. 351p. pap. 24.95 (*0-87705-955-1*); text 45.95 (*0-87705-430-4*) Kluwer Academic (Kluwer Acad Hman Sci).

Family Therapy: An Interactional Approach. Maurizio Andolfi. 1979. LC 78-27741. 186p. 37.50 (*0-306-40200-9*, Plenum Trade) Perseus Pubng.

Family Therapy: An Overview. Irene Goldenberg & Herbert Goldenberg. (Psychology Ser.). (C). 2nd ed. 1985. LC 84-21387. 365p. pap. 34.00 (*0-534-04686-X*); 3rd ed. 1991. LC 89-78294. 432p. text 36.75 (*0-534-13746-6*) Brooks-Cole.

Family Therapy: An Overview. Irene Goldenberg et al. 5th ed. 1999. LC 99-20853. (Counseling Ser.). (Illus.). 500p. spiral bd. 72.95 (*0-534-35757-1*) Wadsworth Pub.

Family Therapy: Combining Psychodynamic & Family Systems Approaches. Ed. by John W. Pearce & Leonard Friedman. 1980. 185p. text 24.00 (*0-8089-1245-3*, 793271, Grune & Strat) Harcrt Hlth Sci Grp.

Family Therapy: Concepts & Methods. Michael P. Nichols & Richard C. Schwartz. 5th ed. 2000. LC 99-86266. (Illus.). 570p. 78.00 (*0-205-31737-5*) Allyn.

Family Therapy: Ensuring Treatment Efficacy. Jon Carlson et al. 1996. LC 96-32435. (Counseling Ser.). 256p. (C). spiral bd. 70.95 (*0-534-16698-9*) Brooks-Cole.

Family Therapy: Full Length Case Studies. Peggy Papp. 1977. LC 77-16641. pap. text 24.95 (*0-89876-019-4*) Gardner Pr.

Family Therapy: Fundamentals of Theory & Practice. William A. Griffin. 1993. LC 93-4316. (Basic Principles into Practice Ser.: Vol. 1). 204p. pap. text 26.95 (*0-87630-719-5*) Brunner-Routledge.

Family Therapy: History, Theory, & Practice. Samuel T. Gladding. 2nd ed. 1997. LC 96-39579. 507p. 72.00 (*0-13-836396-X*) P-H.

Family Therapy: The Major Contributions. Ed. by Robert J. Green & James L. Framo. 1982. LC 81-14325. 620p. 82.50 (*0-8236-1885-4*) Intl Univs Pr.

Family Therapy: The Treatment of Natural Systems. Sue Walrond-Skinner. 1976. (Library of Social Work). pap. 13.95 (*0-7100-8705-5*, Routledge Thoemms) Routledge.

Family Therapy: Theory & Practice. Joseph H. Brown & Dana N. Christensen. 1986. LC 85-24271. (Psychology-Counseling Ser.). 312p. (C). pap. 38.00 (*0-534-05580-X*) Brooks-Cole.

Family Therapy: Theory & Practice. Ed. by Philip J. Guerin, Jr. 1976. LC 76-8409. text 37.50 (*0-89876-020-8*) Gardner Pr.

Family Therapy: Theory & Practice. Joseph H. Brown & Dana N. Christensen. 2nd ed. 1998. LC 98-22364. (Counseling Ser.). (Illus.). 360p. spiral bd. 58.95 (*0-534-34651-0*) Brooks-Cole.

Family Therapy & Evaluation Through Art. Hanna Y. Kwiatkowska. 1978. (Illus.). 304p. text 55.95 (*0-398-03729-9*) C C Thomas.

Family Therapy & Family Medicine: Toward the Primary Care of Families. William J. Doherty & Macaran A. Baird. 1983. LC 82-3135. (Family Therapy Ser.). 302p. text 45.00 (*0-89862-041-4*, 2041) Guilford Pubns.

Family Therapy & Major Psychopathology. Melvin R. Lansky. 1981. (Seminars in Psychiatry Ser.). (Illus.). 431p. text 47.00 (*0-8089-1360-3*, 792441, Grune & Strat) Harcrt Hlth Sci Grp.

Family Therapy & Mental Health: Innovations in Theory & Practice. Ed. by Malcolm M. MacFarlane. 2001. LC 00-66457. (Haworth Marriage & the Family Ser.). 395p. (C). 69.95 (*0-7890-0880-7*, Haworth Clinical) Haworth Pr.

Family Therapy & Research: An Annotated Bibliography. Ira Glick et al. 2nd ed. 1981. 308p. text 59.00 (*0-8089-1431-6*, 791588, Grune & Strat) Harcrt Hlth Sci Grp.

Family Therapy & Sibling Position. Walter Toman. 1992. LC 87-33664. 256p. reprint ed. 45.00 (*0-87668-966-7*) Aronson.

Family Therapy & Systemic Practice: Readings on Child Protection, Clinical Techniques & Empirical Foundations. Alan Carr. 1997. 328p. (C). 68.50 (*0-7618-0912-0*); pap. 40.50 (*0-7618-0913-9*) U Pr of Amer.

Family Therapy Basics. Mark Worden. 1996. LC 93-29240. 167p. pap. 21.50 net. (*0-534-23076-8*) Brooks-Cole.

Family Therapy Basics. Worden. 2nd ed. 1998. LC 98-17047. (Counseling Ser.). 220p. pap. text 32.95 (*0-534-35769-5*) Brooks-Cole.

Family Therapy for Suicidal People. Joseph Richman. 1985. 224p. 33.95 (*0-8261-5010-1*) Springer Pub.

Family Therapy in Clinical Practice. Murray Bowen. LC 84-45863. 584p. 1978. 65.00 (*0-87668-761-3*); 1994. reprint ed. pap. 65.00 (*1-56821-011-6*) Aronson.

Family Therapy in Schizophrenia. Ed. by William R. McFarlane. 1983. LC 82-11742. (Guilford Family Therapy Ser.). 355p. 45.00 (*0-89862-042-2*) Guilford Pubns.

E F G

Family Therapy Moment with Ijoy. Lucille W. Ijoy. 1997. (Illus.). 200p. pap. (*1-891251-03-1*) Motivat Inst Phila.

Family Therapy of Drug Abuse & Addiction. M. Duncan Stanton & Thomas C. Todd. 1982. LC 81-6602. (Guilford Family Therapy Ser.). 474p. 55.00 (*0-89862-037-6*, 2037) Guilford Pubns.

Family Therapy of Drug & Alcohol Abuse. Edward Kaufman & Pauline Kaufmann. 2nd ed. 1998. 276p. (C). pap. text 87.00 (*0-205-13430-0*) Allyn.

Family Therapy of Neurobehavioral Disorders. Judith Johnson & McCown, William and Associates Staff. 1997. LC 96-25535. 332p. (C). pap. text 24.95 (*0-7890-0192-6*) Haworth Pr.

Family Therapy of Neurobehavioral Disorders: Integrating Neuropsychology & Family Therapy. Judith Johnson et al. 1997. LC 96-25535. 332p. (C). lib. bdg. 49.95 (*0-7890-0077-6*) Haworth Pr.

Family Therapy Sourcebook. Fred P. Piercy et al. 2nd ed. 1996. LC 96-34673. 475p. 44.95 (*1-57230-150-3*, 0150); pap. 29.00 (*1-57230-151-1*, 0151) Guilford Pubns.

Family Therapy Supervision: Recent Developments in Practice. Ed. by Rosemary Whiffen & John Byng-Hall. 1982. 268p. text 44.00 (*0-8089-1462-6*, 794815, Grune & Strat) Harcrt Hlth Sci Grp.

Family Therapy Techniques. Salvador Minuchin & H. Charles Fishman. 1990. LC 80-25392. (Illus.). 303p. 35.95 (*0-674-29410-6*) HUP.

Family Therapy with Couples: The Family-of-Origin Approach. David S. Freeman. 1992. LC 91-33209. 416p. 60.00 (*0-87668-471-1*) Aronson.

Family Therapy with Ethnic Minorities. Ho Man Keung. 1987. LC 86-29717. (Sourcebooks for the Human Services: Vol. 5). 320p. (C). pap. 39.95 (*0-8039-2678-2*, 5968) Sage.

Family Transitions: Continuity & Change over the Life Cycle. Ed. by Celia J. Falicov. 1991. LC 87-28119. (Guilford Family Therapy Ser.). 476p. reprint ed. pap. 27.00 (*0-89862-484-3*, 2484) Guilford Pubns.

Family Violence: A Clinical & Legal Guide. Ed. by Sandra J. Kaplan. 1996. LC 95-628. 368p. text 48.50 (*0-89042-010-6*, 2010) Am Psychiatric.

Family Violence: Responding to Signs of Abuse in Your Patients. Faith S. Schaefer. Ed. by Milton E. Burglass. 1995. (Illus.). 78p. (Orig.). pap. text 21.00 (*1-879772-05-1*) Health Studies.

Family Wellness Guide: From Mother Earth with Love. Tara Fellner. 1998. LC 97-48325. (Illus.). 256p. pap. 18.95 (*1-885203-62-4*) Jrny Editions.

Family with a Handicapped Child: Understanding & Treatment. Milton Seligman. 1983. 317p. (C). pap. text 32.95 (*0-8089-1561-4*, 793988, Grune & Strat) Harcrt Hlth Sci Grp.

Family's Guide to Selecting, Financing & Asserting Rights in a Nursing Home. Teresa Meuer & Betsy Abramson. 1986. 31p. 15.00 (*0-932622-09-7*) Ctr Public Rep.

Famine, Disease & the Social Order in Early Modern Society. Ed. by John Walter & Roger S. Schofield. 1991. (Studies in Population, Economy & Society in Past Time). (Illus.). 349p. (C). pap. text 31.95 (*0-521-40613-7*) Cambridge U Pr.

Famotidine: A Further Development in the Modern Treatment of Peptic Ulcer Disease. Ed. by A. Bettarello. 1985. (Journal: Vol. 32, Suppl. 1, 1985). (Illus.). 72p. pap. 19.25 (*3-8055-4254-2*) S Karger.

Famous & Very Important Persons: Medical, Psychological & Psychiatric Bibliography 1960-1984. Johan Schioldann-Nielsen. 1986. 186p. (Orig.). pap. text (*87-7492-577-6*) Odense Univ.

Fanconi Anemia, Clinical, Cytogenetic & Experimental Aspects. Ed. by T. M. Schroeder-Kurth et al. 1989. (Illus.). 264p. 93.00 (*0-387-50401-X*) Spr-Verlag.

Fan's Guide to Baseball Fever: The Official Medical Reference. Thomas Singer & Stuart A. Copans. 1992. (Illus.). 139p. (Orig.). pap. 10.95 (*1-55935-083-0*) Elijim Pubns.

Fantastic Antone Succeeds! Experiences in Educating Children with Fetal Alcohol Syndrome. Judith S. Kleinfeld & Siobhan Wescott. 1993. LC 93-8839. (Illus.). xii, 368p. 30.00 (*0-912006-71-4*); pap. 20.00 (*0-912006-65-X*) U of Alaska Pr.

Fantastic Fit for Everybody. Gale G. Hazen. 1998. LC 97-33932. (Rodale Sewing Book Ser.). (Illus.). 256p. 29.95 (*0-87596-792-2*) Rodale Pr Inc.

Fantasy Bond: The Structure of Psychological Defenses. Robert W. Firestone & Joyce Catlett. 1985. 406p. 38.95 (*0-89885-234-X*); pap. 22.95 (*0-89885-330-3*) Kluwer Academic (Kluwer Acad Hman Sci).

Fantasy, Myth, & Reality: Essays in Honor of Jacob A. Arlow. Ed. by Harold P. Blum et al. 1988. LC 88-12766. 520p. 75.00 (*0-8236-1887-0*, BN 01887) Intl Univs Pr.

FAO-WHO Expert Committee on Brucellosis. 1986. (Technical Reports: No. 740). 133p. pap. text 18.00 (*92-4-120740-X*, 1100740) World Health.

FAQs All about Sports Nutrition. Daniel Gastelu. 1999. 96p. mass mkt. 2.99 (*0-89529-990-9*, Avery) Putnam Pub Group.

Far Side of Madness. John W. Perry. 1974. LC 89-21572. (Jungian Classics Ser.: No. 12). 180p. reprint ed. pap. 17.00 (*0-88214-511-8*) Spring Pubns.

Farm Animal Well-Being: Stress Physiology, Animal Behavior & Environmental Design. Solon A. Ewing et al. 1998. LC 98-9445. 357p. (C). 98.00 (*0-13-660200-2*) P-H.

Farmacia Natural. James A. Duke. 2000. LC 98-6318. (SPA., Illus.). 640p. pap. 17.95 (*1-57954-262-X*) Rodale Pr Inc.

Farmworkers in California. Alicia Bugarin & Elias Lopez. 1998. 79p. pap. (*1-58703-085-3*, CRB-98-007) CA Res Bureau.

Farquharson's Textbook of Operative Surgery. Ed. by R. F. Rintoul. 8th ed. 1995. LC 94-43499. 714p. text (*0-443-04712-X*) Church.

Farrier & His Craft. Leslie Prince. 1990. 280p. (*0-85131-353-1*) J A Allen GBR. *Dist:* Trafalgar, St Mut.

Farther Reaches of Human Nature. Abraham H. Maslow. 1993. LC 93-23973. 432p. pap. 14.95 (*0-14-019470-3*, Penguin Compass) Penguin Putnam.

Fashion for Disabled People. Nellie Thornton. 1990. (Illus.). 128p. 22.95 (*0-7134-6129-2*) Trafalgar.

Fashions in Eyeglasses. Richard Corson. 1980. (Illus.). reprint ed. (*0-7206-3282-X*) P Owen Ltd GBR. *Dist:* Dufour.

Fast Magnetic Resonance Body Imaging. Hiroto Hatabu & H. Imhof. 2000. LC 00-34127. (Illus.). 132p. 351.50 (*0-444-50516-4*) Elsevier.

Fast Neutrons & High-LET Particles in Cancer Therapy: Clinical Status. Ed. by R. Engenhart et al. 1998. LC 98-10677. (Recent Results in Cancer Research Ser.: Vol. 150). (Illus.). 230p. 119.00 (*3-540-57632-0*) Spr-Verlag.

Fast Oscillations in Cortical Circuits. Roger D. Traub et al. 1999. LC 98-34707. (Computational Neuroscience Ser.). (Illus.). 308p. 55.00 (*0-262-20118-6*, Bradford Bks) MIT Pr.

Fast Reactions. Ed. by Kenneth Kustin. 1970. (Methods in Enzymology Ser.: Vol. 16). text 209.00 (*0-12-181873-X*) Acad Pr.

FastCare for a Healthy Heart: The Easy Health & Wellness Guide. FastMark Editorial Staff & American Academy of Family Physicians Staff. 1997. (FastCare, the Easy Health & Wellness Guides Ser.). (Illus.). 16p. 4.95 (*1-887562-14-1*, Accordia Pr) FastMark.

FastCare for Allergies & Asthma: The Easy Health & Wellness Guide. FastMark Editorial Staff & American Academy of Allergies, Asthma and Immunology Staff. 1997. (FastCare, the Easy Health & Wellness Guides Ser.). 16p. 4.95 (*1-887562-18-4*) FastMark.

FastCare for Diabetes: The Easy Health & Wellness Guides. FastMark Editorial Staff & American Diabetes Association. 1997. (FastCare, the Easy Health & Wellness Guides Ser.). 16p. 4.95 (*1-887562-22-2*, Accordia Pr) FastMark.

FastCare for Fitness: The Easy Health & Wellness Guide. FastMark Editorial Staff & American Academy of Family Physicians Staff. 1997. (FastCare, the Easy Health & Wellness Guides Ser.). (Illus.). 16p. 4.95 (*1-887562-16-8*, Accordia Pr) FastMark.

FastCare for Seniors. 1996. (Illus.). 16p. (Orig.). pap. 4.95 (*1-887562-10-9*) FastMark.

Faster, Better Healing: How to Combine the World's Most Powerful Cures to Remedy Common Ailments As Quickly As Possible. Arden Moore et al. 1999. LC 98-31951. (Prevention's New Approaches to Health Ser.). (*1-57954-059-7*) Rodale Pr Inc.

Fasting Girls: The Emergence of Anorexia Nervosa As a Modern Disease. Joan Jacobs Brumberg. 1988. LC 87-25092. (Illus.). 376p. 40.00 (*0-674-29501-3*) HUP.

Fasting Girls: The History of Anorexia Nervosa. Joan Jacobs Brumberg. 2000. LC 00-28210. (*0-375-72453-2*); (Illus.). xvii, 374p. pap. 14.00 (*0-375-72448-6*) Vin Bks.

Fat - A Fate Worse Than Death? Women, Weight & Appearance. Ruth R. Thone. 1997. LC 97-4041. 212p. 39.95 (*0-7890-0178-0*); pap. 17.95 (*1-56023-908-5*) Haworth Pr.

Fat Attack Plan. Annette B. Natow & JoAnn Heslin. Ed. by Claire Zion. 1991. 400p. reprint ed. mass mkt. 6.99 (*0-671-73426-1*) PB.

Fat Chance Diet Book. Junius Quail. 1983. LC 82-62878. 64p. pap. 3.95 (*0-9610764-0-2*) Quail Prods.

Fat Fat Fat: A Threefold Look at Fat Control. Jack D. Osman. 1985. LC 84-81813. (Illus.). 134p. (Orig.). pap. 7.95 (*0-918275-00-8*) Fat Control.

Fat Free, Flavor Full: Dr. Gabe Mirkin's Guide to Losing Weight & Gaining Life. Gabe Mirkin. 1995. LC 94-37919. (Fat Free, Flavor Full Ser.: Vol. 1). 336p. (gr. 8). 21.95 (*0-316-57440-6*) Little.

Fat Is a Family Affair see Obesidad Es un Problema Familiar

Fat Is a Family Affair. Judi Hollis. 1996. 106p. pap. 11.00 (*0-89486-263-4*, 1091A) Hazelden.

Fat Management: The Thermogenic Factor. Daniel B. Mowrey. 1995. (Illus.). 359p. (Orig.). pap. text 16.95 (*0-936261-07-2*) Victory Pubns.

Fat Oppression & Psychotherapy: A Feminist Perspective. Ed. by Esther D. Rothblum & Laura S. Brown. 1990. LC 89-19860. (Women & Therapy Ser.: Vol. 8, No. 3). 103p. text 39.95 (*0-86656-954-5*) Haworth Pr.

Fat Production & Consumption: Technologies & Nutritional Implications. Ed. by Corrado L. Galli & E. Fedeli. 1987. LC 87-14124. (NATO ASI Series A, Life Sciences: Vol. 131). (Illus.). 346p. 89.50 (*0-306-42591-2*, Plenum Trade) Perseus Pubng.

Fat Reduction: Trim Fat from Your Life. Consumer Guide Editors. 1993. (Illus.). 160p. spiral bd. 9.98 (*0-7853-0187-9*, 3211800) Pubns Intl Ltd.

Fat-Storing Cells & Liver Fibrosis: Proceedings of the 71st Falk Symposium Held in Florence, Italy, July 1-3, 1993. Falk Symposium 71 Staff. Ed. by C. Surrenti et al. 1994. LC 93-40475. 400p. (C). text 174.50 (*0-7923-8842-9*) Kluwer Academic.

Fat to Fit Without Dieting. Jeanne Rhodes. 1990. LC 90-35875. (Illus.). 288p. pap. 14.95 (*0-8092-4158-7*, 415870, Contemporary) McGraw-Hill Trade.

Fat to Muscle Diet. Victoria Zak et al. 1988. 100p. pap. 6.99 (*0-425-11060-5*) Berkley Pub.

Fatal Asthma. Albert L. Sheffer. 1998. LC 98-11381. (Lung Biology in Health & Disease Ser.). (Illus.). 640p. text 215.00 (*0-8247-0155-0*) Dekker.

Fatal Attractions: Protein Aggregates in Neurodegenerative Disorders. Ed. by V. M. Y. Lee et al. 2000. LC 00-28458. (Research & Perspectives in Alzheimer's Disease Ser.). (Illus.). 172p. 95.00 (*3-540-67172-2*) Spr-Verlag.

Fatal Genes. Robert C. Nienkemper. 1999. 351p. pap. 7.50 (*1-892614-15-4*, BWP-FG) Briarwood VA.

Fatal Injuries to Workers in the United States, 1980-1989: A Decade of Surveillance: National & State Profiles. E. Lynn Jenkins & Suzanne M. Kisner. 1996. (Illus.). 340p. (C). reprint ed. pap. text 50.00 (*0-7881-3561-9*) DIANE Pub.

Fatal Workplace Injuries in 1992: A Collection of Data & Analysis. 1994. (Illus.). 92p. (Orig.). (C). pap. text 35.00 (*0-7881-1200-7*) DIANE Pub.

Fatbook. Howard Lamb. 1982. 133p. ring bd. 39.95 (*0-9609150-0-1*) H Lamb.

Fate of the Male Germ Cell: Proceedings of a Symposium Held in Hamburg, Germany, December 5-7, 1996. Ed. by Richard Ivell & Adolf-Friedrich Holstein. 1997. LC 97-27283. (Advances in Experimental Medicine & Biology Ser.: Vol. 424). 348p. (C). text 95.00 (*0-306-45696-6*, Kluwer Plenum) Kluwer Academic.

Father-Daughter Incest. Judith L. Herman. (Illus.). 272p. 1982. LC 81-2534. pap. text 16.00 (*0-674-29506-4*); 1981. 20.00 (*0-674-29505-6*) HUP.

Father-Infant Relationship: Observational Studies in the Family Settings. Ed. by Frank A. Pedersen. 1980. LC 79-20514. (Praeger Special Studies). 185p. 35.95 (*0-275-90535-7*, C0535, Praeger Pubs) Greenwood.

Father Knows Best: The Use & Abuse of Power in Freud's Case of Dora. Robin T. Lakoff & James C. Coyne. 1992. (Athene Ser.). 160p. (C). text 36.00 (*0-8077-6267-9*); pap. text 16.95 (*0-8077-6266-0*) Tchrs Coll.

Fathering Behaviors: The Dynamics of the Man-Child Bond. Wade C. Mackey. 1985. LC 85-6599. (Perspectives in Developmental Psychology Ser.). (Illus.). 220p. (C). 59.00 (*0-306-41868-1*, Plenum Trade) Perseus Pubng.

Fathering the ADHD Child: A Book for Fathers, Mothers & Professionals. Edward H. Jacobs. 1997. LC 97-2061. 312p. 40.00 (*0-7657-0068-9*) Aronson.

Fatherloss: How Sons of All Ages Come to Terms with the Death of Their Dads. Neil Chethik. 2001. LC 00-44965. xii, 304p. 24.95 (*0-7868-6532-6*) Hyperion.

Fathers & Adolescents: Developmental & Clinical Perspectives. Shmuel Shulman & Inge Seiffge-Krenke. 1997. LC 96-16341. (Adolescence & Society Ser.). 264p. (C). 78.95 (*0-415-11791-7*); pap. 26.95 (*0-415-11792-5*) Routledge.

Fathers & Developmental Psychopathology. Vicky Phares. 1995. LC 95-20363. (Personality Processes Ser.). 405p. 110.00 (*0-471-59940-9*) Wiley.

Fathers As Primary Caregivers, 17. Brenda Geiger. 1996. LC 95-41688. (Contributions in Family Studies Ser.: Vol. 17). 168p. 58.00 (*0-313-29919-6*, Greenwood Pr) Greenwood.

Father's Story: The Story of a Son's Battle with AIDS. Edmund Hansen. 1996. LC 95-95363. 128p. pap. 9.95 (*0-7880-0663-0*, Fairway Pr) CSS OH.

Fathers Who Fail: Shame & Psychopathology in the Family System. Melvin R. Lansky. 1992. LC 92-18664. 264p. 45.00 (*0-88163-105-1*) Analytic Pr.

Fatherson: A Self Psychology of the Archetypal Masculine. Alfred Collins. 1994. LC 93-26635. 168p. (Orig.). pap. 4.95 (*0-933029-75-6*) Chiron Pubns.

Fatigue. Lauren B. Krupp. 2001. (Most Common Complaints Ser.). (Illus.). 200p. pap. 25.00 (*0-7506-7038-X*) Buttrwrth-Heinemann.

Fatigue: Causes, Treatment & Prevention. Phylis A. Austin et al. 1989. 61p. pap. 4.95 (*1-878726-22-6*) Fam Hlth Pubns.

Fatigue: Causes, Treatment & Prevention. Phylis A. Austin et al. 1989. (Illus.). 62p. pap. 4.95 (*0-942658-10-8*) NLB.

Fatigue: Neural & Muscular Mechanisms. Ed. by Simon C. Gandevia et al. 1995. LC 95-43970. (Advances in Experimental Medicine & Biology Ser.: Vol. 384). (Illus.). 556p. (C). text 135.00 (*0-306-45139-5*, QP321, Kluwer Plenum) Kluwer Academic.

Fatigue: Sleep Management. Robert J. Koester. 1997. LC 47-67951. (Illus.). 58p. lib. bdg. 14.95 (*1-879471-29-9*); pap. text, stu. ed., wbk. ed. 9.95 (*1-879471-18-3*) DBS Prodns.

Fatigue: Sleep Management Instructor's Manual. Robert J. Koester. 1997. (Illus.). (Orig.). 180p. pap. text 110.00 (*1-879471-17-5*); trans. 200.00 (*1-879471-19-1*) DBS Prodns.

***Fatigue & Cancer/Fatigue und Krebs: 2. Internationales Symposium, Koln, Februar 2001: Abstracts.** Ed. by H. Flechtner & J. H. Ruffer. 2001. (Onkologie Ser.: Vol. 24, Suppl. 2). vi, 18p. pap. 27.00 (*3-8055-7231-X*) S Karger.

Fatigue in Cancer: A Multidimensional Approach. Ed. by Maryl Winningham & Margaret B. Burke. 1999. LC 98-43133. (Illus.). 464p. (C). text 68.95 (*0-7637-0630-2*, 0630-2) Jones & Bartlett.

***Fatigue in Cancer: A Workbook for Regaining Energy & Strength.** Nancy Howe. 2001. (Illus.). (C). pap. text, wbk. ed. 31.95 (*0-7637-1803-3*, 1803-3, N L N Bart) Jones & Bartlett.

Fatigue in Patients with Cancer: Analysis & Assessment. Agnes Glaus. Ed. by P. Schlag & H. J. Senn. 1998. LC 97-38312. (Recent Results in Cancer Research Ser.: Vol. 145). (Illus.). 183p. 109.00 (*3-540-63556-4*) Spr-Verlag.

Fats of Life. Caroline M. Pond. 1998. LC 97-46515. (Illus.). 343p. (C). text 59.95 (*0-521-58321-7*); pap. text 21.95 (*0-521-63577-2*) Cambridge U Pr.

***Fatty Acid Composition in Skeletal Muscle: Influence of Physical Activity & Dietary Fat Quality.** Agneta Andersson. 2001. (Comprehensive Summaries of Uppsala Dissertations from the Faculty of Medicine Ser.: No. 1059). (Illus.). 78p. pap. (*91-554-5078-4*) Acta Univ SWE. *Dist:* Coronet Bks.

Fatty Acids: Physiological & Behavioral Functions. Ed. by David I. Mostofsky et al. 2001. LC 00-67293. (Nutrition & Health Ser.). (Illus.). 435p. 165.00 (*0-89603-942-0*) Humana.

Fatty Acids in Foods & Their Health Implications. Ed. by Ching Kuang Chow. 1992. (Food Science & Technology Ser.: Vol. 53). (Illus.). 896p. text 275.00 (*0-8247-8622-X*) Dekker.

Faulkner's Search for a South. Walter Taylor. 1982. LC 81-16127. 256p. text 27.50 (*0-252-00943-6*) U of Ill Pr.

Faulk's Basic Forensic Psychiatry. J. H. Stonehouse & Malcolm Faulk. 3rd ed. 1999. LC 99-34502. pap. 69.95 (*0-632-05019-5*) Blackwell Sci.

Favorite Counseling & Therapy Techniques: 51 Therapists Share Their Most Creative Strategies. Howard Rosenthal. 1997. LC 97-27881. 202p. pap. 22.95 (*1-56032-667-0*) Accel Devel.

Faxing Safeguards: Guidelines for Transmitting Patient Health Information. Mary D. Brandt. 1997. 34p. pap. text 32.00 (*1-58426-005-X*, AB101097) Am Hlth Info.

***Faye Brown's ICD-9-CM Coding Handbook: With Answers.** Faye Brown. 2001. 416p. pap. 66.00 (*1-55648-291-4*) AHPI.

***Faye Brown's ICD-9-CM Coding Handbook: Without Answers.** Faye Brown. 2001. 408p. pap. 56.00 (*1-55648-292-2*) AHPI.

***Fc Receptors & Feedback Enhancement of Antibody Responses.** Sara Wernersson. 2000. (Comprehensive Summaries of Uppsala Dissertations from the Faculty of Medicine Ser.: No. 907). (Illus.). 59p. pap. (*91-554-4654-X*) Uppsala Universitet SWE. *Dist:* Coronet Bks.

Fc Receptors & Feedback Regulation by Antibodies. Mikael Karlsson. 1999. (Comprehensive Summaries of Uppsala Dissertations from the Faculty of Medicine Ser.: 901). (Illus.). 64p. (Orig.). pap. (*91-554-4633-7*) Uppsala Universitet SWE. *Dist:* Coronet Bks.

FC Receptors & the Action of Antibodies. Ed. by Henry Metzger. 1990. (Illus.). 368p. 99.95 (*1-55581-016-0*) ASM Pr.

FC Receptors Symposium: Journal: Immunologic Research, Vol. 11, Nos. 3-4, 1992. Ed. by R. G. Lynch. 1992. (Illus.). iv, 144p. pap. 35.00 (*3-8055-5695-0*) S Karger.

FDA & Worldwide Quality System Requirements Guidebook for Medical Devices. Compiled by Kimberly A. Trautman. 1996. LC 96-43156. 210p. 45.00 (*0-87389-377-8*, H0965) ASQ Qual Pr.

FDA Drug Approval: Review Time Has Decreased in Recent Years. 1996. (Illus.). 44p. (Orig.). (C). pap. text 20.00 (*0-7881-2767-5*) DIANE Pub.

***FDA Inside & Out.** Suzanne Parisian. 2001. LC 2001-116097. xix, 647p. text 289.00 (*0-9707109-1-7*) Fast Horse.

FDA Inspections: A Guide for Medical Device & Diagnostic Manufacturers. John S. Adcock. 1997. LC 97-50. 178p. 149.00 (*1-57491-046-9*) IHS Health Grp.

FDA Investigations Operations Manual. Department of Health and Human Services, Food and Drug Administration Staff. 1994. 541p. pap. text 85.00 (*0-86587-416-6*) Gov Insts.

FDA Oversight: Blood Safety & the Implications of Pool Sizes in the Manufacture of Plasma Derivatives: Hearing Before the Subcommittee on Human Resources of the Committee on Government Reform & Oversight, House of Representatives, One Hundred Fifth Congress, First Session, July 31, 1997. Contrib. by U. S. Congress, House Committee on Government Reform and Oversight, Subcommittee on Human Resources. 1998. LC 98-142574. (Illus.). (*0-16-056103-5*) USGPO.

FDA Regulation of Medical Devices. Bradley M. Thompson. 1995. (Illus.). 497p. 249.00 (*0-935184-79-1*) IHS Health Grp.

FDA Warning Letters 1996 Vol. 2: Medical Devices, Medical Equipment & Diagnostic Products. Ed. by Michael H. Anisfeld & Francisco Torres. 1997. (Illus.). ring bd. 194.00 (*1-57491-057-4*) IHS Health Grp.

FDI Lexicon of English Dental Terms. L. J. Baume. 1985. (ENG, FRE, GER & SPA.). 400p. 75.00 (*0-8288-7607-X*) Fr & Eur.

Fear & Defence. Ed. by P. F. Brain & Antonio L. Zichichi. 1990. (Ettore Majorana International Life Sciences Ser.: Vol. 8). x, 420p. text 162.00 (*3-7186-5015-0*) Gordon & Breach.

Fear, Avoidance & Phobias: A Fundamental Analysis. Ed. by M. Ray Denny. 1991. 456p. pap. 49.95 (*0-8058-0317-3*); text 89.95 (*0-8058-0316-5*) L Erlbaum Assocs.

Fear, Love & Worship. C. FitzSimons Allison. 1983. 4.95 (*0-8164-2020-3*, SP17) Harper SF.

Fear of Being Fat. C. Philip Wilson. LC 82-11338. 384p. reprint ed. pap. (*1-56821-012-4*) Aronson.

***Fear of Intimacy.** Robert W. Firestone & Joyce Catlett. 2001. 358p. pap. 24.95 (*1-55798-720-3*) Am Psychol.

Fear of Life. Alexander Lowen. 1981. 274p. pap. 6.95 (*0-02-077330-7*) Macmillan.

Fear of the Feminine & Other Essays on Feminine Psychology: Five Essays. Erich Neumann. Tr. by Boris Matthews et al from GER. 1994. LC 93-32444. (Essays of Erich Neumann Ser.: Vol. 4). 524p. pap. 19.95 (*0-691-03473-7*) Princeton U Pr.

Fearful Symmetry: The Development & Treatment of Sadomasochism. Jack Novick et al. 1995. LC 95-31774. (Critical Issues in Psychoanalysis Ser.: Vol. 3). 432p. 45.00 (*1-56821-652-1*) Aronson.

Fearfully & Wonderfully Made. Paul Brand & Philip Yancey. 1980. (Illus.). 224p. 12.95 (*0-310-35450-1*, 10241) Zondervan.

Fearless Living. Judith L. Marquart. 192p. (Orig.). pap. 9.95 (*0-935236-48-1*) Genl Med Pub.

Fears of Childhood: A Guide to Recognizing & Reducing Fearful States in Children. Edward P. Sarafino. 1986. 212p. pap. 19.95 (*0-89885-296-X*, Kluwer Acad Hman Sci) Kluwer Academic.

Fears, Phobias & Panic: A Self-Help Guide to Agoraphobia. Maureen Sheehan. 1988. 104p. (Orig.). pap. 23.95 (*0-8464-1490-2*) Beekman Pubs.

Fears, Phobias & Rituals: Panic, Anxiety & Their Disorders. Isaac M. Marks. 1987. (Illus.). 704p. text 55.00 (*0-19-503927-0*) OUP.

Fears Related to Death & Suicide. Marvin J. Feldman et al. 1974. LC 73-12803. (Thanatology Ser.). 221p. (C). text 37.00 (*0-8422-7149-X*) Irvington.

Feasibility of Health Maintenance Organizations in Texas. Lynn Anderson. 1975. (Policy Research Project Report Ser.: No. 11). 110p. pap. 3.00 (*0-89940-607-6*) LBJ Sch Pub Aff.

Feasibility of New Epidemiologic Studies of Low Level Arsenic. Allan H. Smith. 1998. LC 98-25667. (*0-89867-961-3*) Am Water Wks Assn.

Feather in My Wig: Ovarian Cancer: Cured Twelve Years & Going Strong. Barbara R. Van Billiard. 1998. LC 98-46047. 169p. pap. 12.50 (*0-914339-69-9*) P E Randall Pub.

Featherless Chickens, Laughing Women & Serious Stories. Jeannie B. Thomas. 1997. LC 96-51753. 45.00 (*0-8139-1723-9*) U Pr of Va.

Febrile Neutropenia. Jean Klastersky. 1997. LC 96-21660. (Illus.). 130p. 34.00 (*3-540-61230-0*) Spr-Verlag.

February Man: Evolving Consciousness & Identity in Hypnotherapy. Milton H. Erickson & Ernest L. Rossi. 1989. LC 88-38964. 288p. text 37.95 (*0-87630-545-1*) Brunner-Routledge.

Fed up & Hungry: Women, Oppression & Food. Ed. by Marilyn Lawrence. pap. (*0-7043-4008-9*) Womens Press GBR. *Dist:* Trafalgar.

Federal Anti-Kickback Law. W. Bradley Tully. 1996. (Health Law & Business Ser.: No. 1500). 125.00 (*1-55871-334-4*) BNA.

***Federal Desk Reference.** Ingenix, Inc. Staff. pap. 99.95 (*1-56337-377-7*) Ingenix Inc.

Federal Food Safety Inspection System: Dangerous to Your Health? 1992. (Illus.). 70p. (Orig.). (C). pap. text 25.00 (*1-56806-029-7*) DIANE Pub.

Federal Health Dollar: 1969-1976. Michael S. Koleda et al. 1976. LC 76-48764. 72p. 6.95 (*0-89068-002-7*) Natl Planning.

Federal Information Sources in Health & Medicine: A Selected Annotated Bibliography, 1. Ed. by Natalie Schatz. 1988. LC 88-226. (Bibliographies & Indexes in Medical Studies: No. 1). 323p. lib. bdg. 89.50 (*0-313-25530-X*, CFD/) Greenwood.

Federal Laws of the Mentally Handicapped: Laws, Legislative Histories, & Administrative Documents,, Set. Ed. by Bernard D. Reams. 1981. LC 81-83898. (Legislative Histories of the Law of Disabled persons Ser.: Part 1). 2200.00 (*0-89941-106-1*, 302010) W S Hein.

Federal Medical Malpractice Insurance at Community & Migrant Health Centers: Estimated Savings, Insurance Costs & Claims Experience. 1994. (Illus.). 60p. (Orig.). (C). pap. text 25.00 (*0-7881-0379-2*) DIANE Pub.

Federal Personnel: Issues on the Need for the Public Health Service's Commissioned Corps. 1996. (Illus.). 45p. (Orig.). (C). pap. text 25.00 (*0-7881-3610-0*) DIANE Pub.

Federal Priorities in Funding Alcohol & Drug Abuse Programs. Ed. by Barry Stimmel. 1983. LC 83-6111. (Advances in Alcohol & Substance Abuse Ser.: Vol. 2, No. 3). 79p. text 39.95 (*0-86656-195-1*) Haworth Pr.

Federal Regulation of Methadone Treatment. Ed. by Adam Yarmolinsky & Richard A. Rettig. 1995. LC 94-74890. 252p. (Orig.). (C). pap. text 33.00 (*0-309-05240-8*) Natl Acad Pr.

Federal Self-Referral Law. W. Bradley Tully & David P. Henninger. 1997. (Health Law & Business Ser.: No. 2400). 125.00 (*1-55871-355-7*) BNA.

Federalism & Health Policy: The Development of Health Systems in Canada & Australia. Gwendolyn Gray. 1991. 320p. text 50.00 (*0-8020-5904-X*); pap. text 19.95 (*0-8020-6862-6*) U of Toronto Pr.

Fee Scale for Physician Services: Medicare's New Approach. Paul L. Grimaldi. 1992. 50p. 10.00 (*0-930228-76-6*) Hlthcare Fin Mgmt.

Feeble-Mindedness. Henry H. Goddard. 1977. LC 76-39391. (Select Bibliographies Reprint Ser.). reprint ed. 48.95 (*0-8369-9907-X*) Ayer.

Feeble-Mindedness: Its Causes & Consequences. Henry H. Goddard. 1973. LC 73-2401. (Mental Illness & Social Policy; the American Experience Ser.). reprint ed. 47.95 (*0-405-05207-3*) Ayer.

Feed, Need, Greed. Food and Nutrition Group Staff. Ed. by Sue Tafler & Connie Phillips. 1980. (Illus.). 108p. (Orig.). pap. 5.00 (*0-9607314-0-7*) Sci People.

Feed Your Kids Well: How to Help Your Child Lose Weight & Get Healthy. Fred Pescatore. 1998. LC 98-13103. (Illus.). 304p. 22.95 (*0-471-24855-X*) Wiley.

Feedback Mechanisms in Blood Coagulation & Their Inhibition by Heparins: Journal: Haemostasis, Vol. 21, No. 4, 1991. Ed. by H. C. Hemker. 1991. 88p. pap. 43.50 (*3-8055-5525-3*) S Karger.

Feeding & Swallowing Disorders in Infants. Wolf. 1998. (C). pap. text 69.50 (*0-12-784567-4*) Acad Pr.

Feeding Frenzy: Organizational Deviance in the Texas Psychiatric Hospital Industry. Henry Vandenburgh. 1999. LC 98-54356. 128p. 46.00 (*0-7618-1337-3*); pap. 25.50 (*0-7618-1338-1*) U Pr of Amer.

Feeding Problems & Eating Disorders in Children & Adolescents, Vol. 5. Peter J. Cooper. 1992. (Monographs in Clinical Pediatrics). xiii, 205p. text 132.00 (*3-7186-5158-0*, Harwood Acad Pubs) Gordon & Breach.

***Feeding Problems in Children: A Practical Guide.** Ed. by Angela Southall & Anthony Schwartz. 2000. 296p. pap. (*1-85775-208-2*) Radcliffe Med Pr GBR. *Dist:* Balogh.

Feeding System of the Pigeon (Columba Livia L) G. A. Zweers. 1982. (Advances in Anatomy, Embryology & Cell Biology Ser.: Vol. 73). (Illus.). 108p. 38.00 (*0-387-11332-0*) Spr-Verlag.

Feeding the Body, Nourishing the Soul: Essentials of Eating for Physical, Emotional & Spiritual Well-Being. Deborah Kesten. 1997. LC 97-24324. 224p. (Orig.). pap. 14.95 (*1-57324-068-0*) Conari Press.

Feeding the Disabled Child. Peter B. Sullivan & Lewis Rosenbloom. 1996. (Clinics in Developmental Medicine Ser.: No. 140). (Illus.). 256p. (C). (*1-898683-08-5*) Mc Keith Pr GBR. *Dist:* Cambridge U Pr.

Feeding the Hungry Heart: The Experience of Compulsive Eating. Geneen Roth. 1993. LC 93-13035. 242p. reprint ed. pap. 12.95 (*0-452-27083-9*, Plume) Dutton Plume.

Feeding to Win II. Equine Research, Inc. Research Staff. Ed. by Don M. Wagoner. 1992. (Illus.). 544p. (C). text 65.00 (*0-935842-00-4*) Equine Res.

Feeding Your Child: Infant to Toddler. Lewis Barnesa. Ed. by Frank A. Oski. 1995. (Pediatrics Ser.). (Illus.). 32p. pap. 2.95 (*1-885274-13-0*) Health InfoNet Inc.

Feeds & Nutrition. M. E. Ensminger et al. 1990. LC 89-83516. (Illus.). 1552p. 89.45 (*0-941218-08-2*) Ensminger.

Feel Full Diet. Steven R. Peikin. 1987. LC 86-47927. 288p. 17.95 (*0-689-11789-2*) Atheneum Yung Read.

***Feel Good: Understand Your Emotions.** Kathy Feeney. 2001. LC 00-12536. (Your Health Ser.). 24p. (J). (-3). lib. bdg. 18.60 (*0-7368-0972-4*, Bridgestone Bks) Capstone Pr.

Feel Good Book. 1992. mass mkt. 0.99 (*0-440-60203-3*) Dell.

Feel-Good Food: A Guide to Intuitive Eating. Susie Miller & Karen Knowler. 2000. (Illus.). pap. (*0-7043-4546-3*) Womens Press GBR. *Dist:* Trafalgar.

Feeling & Emotion: A History of Theories. Harry N. Gardiner. 1970. LC 74-98223. 445p. reprint ed. lib. bdg. 38.50 (*0-8371-3683-0*, GAFE, Greenwood Pr) Greenwood.

Feeling & Healing Your Emotions: A Christian Psychiatrist Shows How to Grow in Wholeness. Conrad W. Baars. 1979. 275p. pap. 8.99 (*0-88270-510-5*) Bridge-Logos.

Feeling As a Way of Knowing: A Practical Guide for Working with Emotional Experience. Sibylle Artz. 1999. (Illus.). 108p. pap. (*1-895579-34-1*) Trifolium Inc CAN. *Dist:* ACCESS Pubs Network.

Feeling Dizzy: Understanding & Treating Dizziness, Vertigo & Other Balance Disorders. Brian W. Blakley. 1997. LC 95-6609. 244p. pap. 14.95 (*0-02-861680-4*) Hungry Minds.

Feeling Dizzy: Understanding & Treating Vertigo, Dizziness, & Other Balance Disorders. Brian W. Blakeley & Mary E. Siegel. 1995. LC 95-6609. (Illus.). 256p. 21.95 (*0-02-860009-6*) Macmillan.

Feeling Fit. Aileen Ludington. 1997. LC 97-29250. 238p. pap. 12.99 (*0-8280-1284-9*) Review & Herald.

Feeling Good: An Alternative Approach to Health Care. Darice A. Angwin. Date not set. 100p. (Orig.). pap. text 9.95 (*0-9648088-0-3*) Sunset Intl.

Feeling Good: The New Mood Therapy. David D. Burns. 1999. LC 91-92428. 736p. pap. 15.00 (*0-380-73176-2*, Avon Bks) Morrow Avon.

Feeling Good Again: The Most Powerful Medicine Is What You Can Do for Yourself. Larry Feldman. 1993. 128p. pap. 9.95 (*1-883855-00-4*) St Georges Pr.

Feeling Great! Wellness Program for Older Adults. Jules C. Weiss. 1988. LC 88-23326. (Activities, Adaptation & Aging Ser.: Vol. 12, Nos. 3 & 4). (Illus.). 218p. text 39.95 (*0-86656-821-2*); pap. text 19.95 (*0-86656-854-9*) Haworth Pr.

Feeling Right When Things Go Wrong. Bill Borcherdt. 1998. LC 98-35775. 272p. pap. 22.45 (*1-56887-036-1*, FRBP, Prof Resc Pr) Pro Resource.

Feeling the Sound. K. S. Roskam. 1992. (Illus.). pap. 15.00 (*0-911302-69-7*) San Francisco Pr.

Feelings - The Three R's: Receiving, Reflecting, Responding. Judith Tindall & Shirley Salmon. 1993. LC 92-75958. viii, 200p. ring bd. 39.95 (*1-55959-044-0*) Accel Devel.

Feelings & Emotions: Proceedings of the International Symposium, 2nd, Mooseheart, Ill, 1948. International Symposium on Feelings and Emotions Staff. 1977. (Essay Index Reprint Ser.). reprint ed. 29.95 (*0-8369-2599-8*) Ayer.

Feelings & Emotions: The Wittenberg Symposium. Ed. by Martin L. Reymert. 1974. LC 73-2986. (Classics in Psychology Ser.). reprint ed. 28.95 (*0-405-05158-1*) Ayer.

Feet First: A Guide to Foot Reflexology. Laura Norman & Thomas Cowan. 1988. (Illus.). 336p. pap. 16.00 (*0-671-63412-7*, Fireside) S&S Trade Pap.

Feldman Understanding Psychology & the Interactive E-Source. 5th ed. 1999. (C). pap., stu. ed. 72.19 (*0-07-239999-6*) McGrw-H Hghr Educ.

Feline Behavior: A Guide for Veterinarians. Bonnie V. Beaver. 2nd ed. 1992. (Illus.). 272p. pap. text 34.00 (*0-7216-3992-5*) Saunders.

Feline Husbandry: Disease & Management in the Multiple-Cat Environment. Niels C. Pedersen et al. 1991. LC 90-81326. (Illus.). 453p. text 43.95 (*0-939674-29-7*) Am Vet Pubns.

Feline Immunology & Immunodeficiency. Ed. by B. J. Willett & O. Jarrett. 1995. (Illus.). 370p. text 125.00 (*0-19-854777-3*) OUP.

Feline Leukemia. Ed. by Richard G. Olsen. 1981. LC 80-24314. 184p. 107.00 (*0-8493-6070-6*, SF986, CRC Reprint) Franklin.

Feline Medicine. Wolf. 1996. (C). text (*0-7216-5844-X*) Saunders.

Feline Medicine & Therapeutics. Ed. by E. A. Chandler et al. (Illus.). 718p. pap. 69.95 (*0-632-04133-1*) Blackwell Sci.

Feline Medicine & Therapeutics. E. A. Chandler et al. 2nd ed. 1994. (Illus.). 720p. 96.95 (*0-632-03361-4*) Blackwell Sci.

Feline Patient: Essentials of Diagnosis & Treatment. Gary D. Norsworthy. 1998. LC 97-13122. 559p. 52.00 (*0-683-06556-4*) Lppncott W & W.

Feline Practice. William E. Boden. 1991. pap. text 39.00 (*0-7020-1523-7*) Saunders.

Feline Practice No. 2. Edward Boden. 2nd ed. 1996. (Illus.). 218p. pap. text 49.00 (*0-7020-2081-8*) Saunders.

***Felix Semon, 1849-1921: A Victorian Laryngologist.** Donald Harrison. 2000. (History of Medicine Ser.). (Illus.). 243p. (*1-85315-413-X*) Royal Soc of Medicine Pr Ltd GBR. *Dist:* Balogh.

Fellowship Short Answer Papers. F. Smiddy. 1995. 336p. pap. 38.95 (*0-632-03815-2*) Blackwell Sci.

Felt Meanings of the World: A Metaphysics of Feeling. Quentin Smith. 1986. LC 85-9532. 352p. 25.95 (*0-911198-76-8*) Purdue U Pr.

Female Adolescence. Katherine Dalsimer. 1987. LC 85-26389. 160p. pap. 17.00 (*0-300-04031-8*) Yale U Pr.

Female Alcoholic. Judith Goodman. 1998. LC 98-60139. 205p. pap. text 25.00 (*0-9663144-0-9*) Women & Addiction.

Female Athlete. Ed. by J. Borms et al. 1982. (Medicine & Sport Science Ser.: Vol. 15). (Illus.). xiv, 218p. 108.00 (*3-8055-2739-X*) S Karger.

Female Authority: Empowering Women Through Psychotherapy. Polly Young-Eisendrath & Florence L. Wiedemann. 1990. LC 86-27145. 242p. reprint ed. pap. 22.00 (*0-89862-460-6*, 2460) Guilford Pubns.

Female Body. Prevention Magazine Editors. 1996. (Illus.). 432p. pap., tchr. ed. 27.95 (*0-87596-290-4*) Rodale Pr Inc.

Female Body: An Owner's Manual: a Head-to-Toe Guide to Good Health & Good Looks - at Any Age. Ed. by Prevention Magazine Health Book Staff. 1996. LC 96-13237. (Illus.). 432p. pap. 19.95 (*0-87596-400-1*) Rodale Pr Inc.

Female Breast & Its Disorders: Essentials of Diagnosis & Management. George W. Mitchell. 1990. (Illus.). 384p. 75.00 (*0-683-06100-3*) Lppncott W & W.

Female Disorders. Valerie Edge. 1993. (Illus.). 320p. (C). (gr. 13). text 36.00 (*0-8016-8013-1*, 08013) Mosby Inc.

Female Disorders & Symptoms. Eli Pieters. 1984. 2.95 (*0-8062-1671-9*) Eli Mail.

Female Experience: Three Generations of British Women Psychoanalysts on Work with Women. Ed. by Joan Raphael-Leff & Rosine J. Perelberg. 1997. LC 96-40328. 328p. (C). 89.95 (*0-415-15769-2*); pap. 31.95 (*0-415-15770-6*) Routledge.

***Female Fertility & the Body-Fat Connection.** Rose E. Frisch. 2001. LC 2001-53859. (Women in Culture & Society Ser.). 176p. 18.00 (*0-226-26545-5*) U Ch Pr.

Female Genital System. Ed. by Ulrich Mohr. 1997. (Illus.). 94p. pap. text 29.50 (*92-832-0129-9*) OUP.

Female Heart: The Truth about Women & Coronary Artery Disease. Marianne J. Legato. 1991. pap. 19.95 (*0-13-321811-2*) P-H.

Female Heart: The Truth about Women & Coronary Artery Disease. Marianne J. Legato & Carol Colman. 1992. (Illus.). 272p. pap. 21.00 (*0-671-76110-2*) S&S Trade.

Female Heart: The Truth about Women & Heart Disease. Marianne J. Legato. 2000. 272p. pap. 13.00 (*0-688-18065-5*, Quil) HarperTrade.

Female Infertility. Ed. by P. J. Keller. 1978. (Contributions to Gynecology & Obstetrics Ser.: Vol. 4). (Illus.). 60.00 (*3-8055-2791-8*) S Karger.

Female Pelvic Floor: Disorders of Function & Support. Ed. by Linda T. Brubaker et al. 1996. LC 96-2454. (Illus.). 309p. (C). text 89.00 (*0-8036-0075-5*) Davis Co.

Female Pelvic Floor Disorders: Investigation & Management. Ed. by J. Thomas Benson. 1992. LC 91-31999. (Illus.). 750p. (C). 109.00 (*0-393-71013-0*) Norton.

Female Pelvic Organs. 1997. LC 96-49628. (Guides to Clinical Aspiration Biopsy Ser.). (*4-260-14319-0*) Igaku-Shoin.

Female Pelvic Organs. Ed. by Suzanne M. Selvaggi. 1997. LC 96-49628. (Guides to Clinical Aspiration Biopsy Ser.). (Illus.). 153p. (*0-89640-319-X*) Igaku-Shoin.

Female Psychology: A Partially Annotated Bibliography. Carole Dilling & Barbara L. Claster. 1985. 326p. pap. text 25.00 (*0-9616028-0-5*) NYCCWMH.

Female Psychology: An Annotated Psychoanalytic Bibliography. Eleanor Schuker & Nadine Levinson. 1991. LC 91-4562. 704p. text 69.95 (*0-88163-087-X*) Analytic Pr.

Female Reproductive Aging, Vol. 9. Ed. by E. R. Te Velde et al. 2000. LC 00-25520. (Studies in Profertility: Vol. 9). (Illus.). 316p. lib. bdg. 88.95 (*1-85070-676-X*, Parthenon Pbng) CRC Pr.

Female Reproductive Health. N. Manassiev & M. Whitehead. 2002. (Illus.). 300p. lib. bdg. 79.95 (*1-85070-491-0*, Parthenon Pbng) CRC Pr.

Female Sexuality. Marie Bonaparte. 1971. 225p. (Orig.). pap. 24.95 (*0-8236-8050-9*, 021900) Intl Univs Pr.

Female Sexuality: Contemporary Engagements. Adrienne Applegarth. Ed. by Donna Bassin. 1998. LC 97-34280. (Illus.). xx, 507p. 60.00 (*0-7657-0081-6*) Aronson.

Female Sterilization: A Guide to Provision of Services. 1992. (ENG, FRE & SPA.). x, 197p. pap. text 41.00 (*92-4-154434-1*, 1150383) World Health.

Female Sterilization: Guidelines for the Development of Services. 1980. (Offset Publications: No. 26). pap. text 4.00 (*92-4-170026-2*, 1120026) World Health.

Female Stress Incontinence. Ed. by U. Ulmsten. 1983. (Contributions to Gynecology & Obstetrics Ser.: Vol. 10). (Illus.). viii, 72p. pap. 48.00 (*3-8055-3665-8*) S Karger.

Female Stress Syndrome Survival Guide. Georgia Witkin. 3rd ed. 2000. LC 00-30492. 336p. 24.95 (*1-55704-415-5*) Newmarket.

Female Subjects in Black & White: Race, Psychoanalysis, Feminism. Ed. by Elizabeth Abel et al. 1997. LC 96-23683. (Illus.). 425p. text 55.00 (*0-520-20629-0*); pap. text 22.50 (*0-520-20630-4*) U CA Pr.

Female Urinary Incontinence. Attila Tanko. 1994. 156p. (*963-05-6530-7*) Akade Kiado HUN. *Dist:* Intl Spec Bk.

Female Urinary Incontinence, 2. N. O. Sjoberg. 2000. LC 99-55263. (Swedish Consensus of Obstetrics & Gynecology Ser.: Vol. 2). (Illus.). 208p. lib. bdg. 82.95 (*1-85070-493-7*, Parthenon Pbng) CRC Pr.

Female Urology. Shlomo Raz. Ed. by Sandra Valkoff. 2nd ed. 1996. LC 95-17714. 656p. text 180.00 (*0-7216-6723-6*) Saunders.

Females & Autonomy: A Life-Span Perspective. Margot B. Nadien & Florence Denmark. 1998. LC 98-12181. 176p. pap. text 48.00 (*0-205-19856-2*) Allyn.

Feminine Personality & Conflict. Judith M. Bardwick et al. 1981. LC 80-24191. (Contemporary Psychology Ser.). 102p. reprint ed. lib. bdg. 35.00 (*0-313-22504-4*, BAFP, Greenwood Pr) Greenwood.

Feminine Psychology. Karen Horney. 1993. 272p. pap. 10.95 (*0-393-31080-9*) Norton.

Feminine Sensuality. Alcira Miriam Alizade. 1999. LC 00-687290. (Illus.). xiv, 184p. pap. (*1-85575-097-X*) Karnac Bks GBR. *Dist:* Other Pr LLC.

Femininities, Masculinities, Sexualities: Freud & Beyond. Nancy Julia Chodorow. 1994. LC 93-39481. (Blazer Lectures: Vol. 1990). 144p. 25.00 (*0-8131-1872-7*) U Pr of KY.

Femininity. Susan Brownmiller. 1985. pap. 11.00 (*0-449-90142-4*, Columbine) Fawcett.

Femininity & Domination: Studies in the Phenomenology of Oppression. Sandra L. Bartky. 1990. (Thinking Gender Ser.). 176p. (C). (gr. 13). pap. 19.95 (*0-415-90186-3*, A3598) Routledge.

E F G

Femininity & Shame: Women, Men & Giving Voice to the Feminine. Barbara L. Eurich-Rascoe et al. 1997. LC 96-52829. 184p. pap. 31.00 (0-7618-0678-4) U Pr of Amer.

Femininity & Shame: Women, Men & Giving Voice to the Feminine. Barbara L. Eurich-Rascoe et al. 2001. LC 96-52829. 184p. 55.00 (0-7618-0677-6) U Pr of Amer.

Femininity Played Straight: Gender, Sexuality, Subjectivity. Biddy Martin. 1997. LC 96-892. 288p. (C). 80.00 (0-415-91680-1); pap. 20.95 (0-415-91681-X) Routledge.

Feminism & Bioethics: Beyond Reproduction. Ed. by Susan M. Wolf. 1996. 416p. pap. 29.95 (0-19-509556-1) OUP.

Feminism & Its Discontents: A Century of Struggle with Psychoanalysis. Mari Jo Buhle. 1999. LC 97-32397. 432p. 37.00 (0-674-29868-3) HUP.

Feminism & Nursing: An Historical Perspective on Power, Status, & Political Activism. Joan I. Roberts. 1995. LC 94-33756. 400p. pap. 28.95 (0-275-95120-0, Praeger Pubs) Greenwood.

Feminism & Nursing: An Historical Perspective on Power, Status & Political Activism. Joan I. Roberts & Thetis M. Group. 1995. LC 94-33756. 400p. 82.50 (0-275-94916-8, Praeger Pubs) Greenwood.

Feminism & Psychoanalysis. Ed. by Richard Feldstein & Judith Roof. 1989. LC 88-43235. 392p. 49.95 (0-8014-2298-1) Cornell U Pr.

Feminism & Psychoanalysis: A Critical Dictionary. Ed. by Elizabeth Wright. 1992. (Blackwell Reference Ser.). 288p. (C). pap. 29.95 (0-631-18347-7) Blackwell Pubs.

Feminism & Sexuality. Ed. by Stevi Jackson et al. 1996. LC 95-13809. (Gender & Culture Reader Ser.). 320p. 58.00 (0-231-10708-0) Col U Pr.

Feminism in Nursing. Gray. 1998. (Professional Reference - Nursing Ser.). pap. 20.95 (0-8273-6966-2) Delmar.

Feminism Within the Science & Health Professions: Overcoming Resistance. Sue V. Rosser. 1988. (Athene Ser.). 168p. text 36.50 (0-08-035558-7); pap. text 16.95 (0-08-035557-9) Elsevier (Pergamon Pr).

Feminist Approaches to Art Therapy. Ed. by Susan Hogan. 1997. LC 96-52368. (Illus.). 296p. (C). pap. 29.95 (0-415-14840-5) Routledge.

Feminist Approaches for Men in Family Therapy. Ed. by Michele Bograd. 1991. (Journal of Feminist Family Therapy Ser.: Vol. 2 Nos. 3 & 4). 279p. text 49.95 (1-56024-128-4); pap. text 19.95 (1-56023-000-2, Harrington Park) Haworth Pr.

Feminist Approaches to Art Therapy. Ed. by Susan Hogan. 1997. LC 96-52368. (Illus.). 296p. (C). 89.95 (0-415-14839-1) Routledge.

Feminist Ethics in Psychotherapy. Ed. by Hannah Lerman & Natalie Porter. 1990. LC 90-9625. 288p. 39.95 (0-8261-6290-8) Springer Pub.

Feminist Groupwork. Sandra Butler. 1991. (Gender & Psychology Ser.: Vol. 3). 208p. (C). pap. 24.95 (0-8039-8210-0, 7223) Sage.

Feminist Perspectives in Medical Ethics. Ed. by Helen B. Holmes & Laura M. Purdy. 1992. LC 91-17749. (Illus.). 340p. text 42.00 (0-253-32848-9); pap. text 15.95 (0-253-20695-2, MB-695) Ind U Pr.

Feminist Perspectives on Eating Disorders. Patricia Fallon et al. 1993. LC 93-23951. 465p. 45.00 (0-89862-180-1) Guilford Pubns.

Feminist Perspectives on Family Care: Policies for Gender Justice. Nancy R. Hooyman & Judith Gonyea. 1995. (Family Caregiver Applications Ser.: Vol. 6). 416p. (C). pap. 38.95 (0-8039-5143-4, 4422) Sage.

Feminist Psychotherapies: Integration of Therapeutic & Feminist Systems. Ed. by Mary A. Dutton-Douglas et al. 1989. LC 88-16705. (Developments in Clinical Psychology Ser.: Vol. 9). 320p. (C). 73.25 (0-89391-387-1, Ablex) Greenwood.

Feminist Social Psychologies: International Perspectives. Sue Wilkinson. 1996. LC 96-8815. 192p. (0-335-19355-2); pap. (0-335-19354-4) OpUniv Pr.

Feminist Theories & Feminist Psychotherapies: Origins, Themes & Variations. Carolyn Z. Enns. 1997. LC 97-1571. 346p. 49.95 (1-56024-980-3); pap. 24.95 (1-56023-873-9) Haworth Pr.

Feminist Therapy As a Political Act. Ed. by Marcia Hill. 1998. LC 98-12812. 129p. 29.95 (0-7890-0517-4, Harrington Park) Haworth Pr.

Feminizing Hormonal Therapy for the Transgendered. Sheila Kirk. 1996. 96p. pap. 14.95 (1-887796-01-0) Together Lifeworks.

Feminizing the Fetish: Psychoanalysis & Narrative Obsession in Turn-of-the-Century France. Emily Apter. Ed. by William Pietz. 1991. LC 91-55067. (Illus.). 296p. 49.95 (0-8014-2653-7); pap. 19.95 (0-8014-9952-6) Cornell U Pr.

Feminizing Venereal Disease: The Body of the Prostitute in Nineteenth-Century Medical Discourse. Mary Spongberg. 1997. LC 96-21227. 240p. (C). text 50.00 (0-8147-8060-1) NYU Pr.

Fenbufen. Ed. by W. M. O'Brien. 1982. (Journal: Vol. 25, Suppl. 1). (Illus.). iv, 96p. pap. 45.25 (3-8055-3542-2) S Karger.

Fenceless Field: Essays on Psychoanalysis & Analytical Psychology. Michael S. Fordham. Ed. by Roger Hobdell. 1998. 296p. (C). pap. 29.95 (0-415-18615-3) Routledge.

***Feng Shui & Health: Using Feng Shui to Disarm Illness, Accelerate Recovery, & Create Optimal Healing.** Nancy SantoPietro. 2002. LC 2001-34067. (Illus.). 448p. pap. 15.95 (0-609-80661-0, Three Riv Pr) Harmony Bks.

Fenitrothion. 1992. (Environmental Health Criteria Ser.: No. 133). (ENG, FRE & SPA.). 184p. pap. text 36.00 (92-4-157133-0, 1160133) World Health.

Fenvalerate. 1990. (Environmental Health Criteria Ser.: No. 95). 121p. pap. text 24.00 (92-4-154295-0, 1160095) World Health.

Feral Cats: Notes for Veterinary Surgeons. Ed. by Universities Federation for Animal Welfare Staff. 1981. 16.00 (0-7855-1104-0) St Mut.

Feral Children & Clever Animals: Reflections on Human Nature. Douglas K. Candland. 1993. LC 93-59. (Illus.). 432p. (C). text 35.00 (0-19-507468-8) OUP.

Ferenczi's Turn in Psychoanalysis. Ed. by Peter L. Rudnytsky et al. 1996. LC 96-10022. 450p. (C). text 50.00 (0-8147-7475-X) NYU Pr.

Ferenczi's Turn in Psychoanalysis. Peter L. Rudnytsky et al. 2000. LC 96-10022. 450p. pap. text 20.00 (0-8147-7545-4) NYU Pr.

Ferret Husbandry Medicine & Surgery. John Henry Lewington. 2000. LC 00-44424. (Illus.). 289p. pap. text 75.00 (0-7506-4251-3) Buttrwrth-Heinemann.

Ferrets, Rabbits & Rodents: Clinical Medicine & Surgery. Elizabeth V. Hillyer & Katherine Quesenberry. Ed. by Sandra Valkoff. 1996. LC 95-37114. (Illus.). 384p. pap. text 42.00 (0-7216-4023-0) Saunders.

Ferri's Clinical Advisor: Instant Diagnosis & Treatment. Fred F. Ferri. 2000. 89.95 incl. cd-rom (0-323-00972-7) Mosby Inc.

Ferri's Clinical Advisor Package. Fred F. Ferri. 1999. (Illus.). 89.95 (0-323-00529-2) Mosby Inc.

***Ferri's Clinical Advisor 2001: Instant Diagnosis & Treatment.** Fred F. Ferri. 2001. (Illus.). 1375p. text 120.00 incl. cd-rom (0-323-00974-3) Mosby Inc.

Ferri's Clinical Advisor 2001: Instant Diagnosis & Treatment. Fred F. Ferri. 3rd ed. 2001. (Illus.). 1375p. text 54.95 (0-323-00973-5) Mosby Inc.

Ferri's Patient. Ferri. 1998. LC 98-36345. (Illus.). 848p. pap. text, tchr. ed. 49.95 (0-8151-8397-6, 31697) Mosby Inc.

Fertile Ground. Ben Mezrich. 2001. 288p. mass mkt. 6.99 (0-06-109798-5) HarperCollins Pubs.

Fertilidad y Esterilidad en Ganado Lechero. Tr. by Abelardo Martinez. 1996.Tr. of Dairy Cattle Fertility & Sterility. (SPA., Illus.). 79p. (Orig.). pap. text 12.00 (0-932147-29-1, Hoards Dairyman) Hoard & Sons Co.

Fertility Analysis Through Extension of Stable Population Concepts & Stochastic Model of Human Reproduction, Vol. 2. J. R. Rele. 1976. LC 76-5439. (Population Monograph: No. 11). reprint ed. lib. bdg. 55.00 (0-8371-8826-1, REFA, Greenwood Pr) Greenwood.

Fertility & Chromosome Pairing: Recent Studies in Plants & Animals. Ed. by Christopher B. Gillies. 1989. 176p. lib. bdg. 256.00 (0-8493-6039-0, QH485) CRC Pr.

Fertility & Conception: An Essential Guide for Childless Couples. John J. Stangel. 1980. pap. 7.95 (0-452-22732-1, Z5316, Plume) Dutton Plume.

Fertility & Conception: The Essential Guide to Maximizing Your Fertility & Conceiving a Healthy Baby. Karen Trewinnard. 1999. LC 98-48577. 192p. 22.50 (1-58238-016-3, Whitman Coin) St Martin.

Fertility & Differential Fertility. Babu R. Kesarwani. 1989. (81-7169-001-7) Commonwealth IND. Dist: S Asia.

Fertility & Family Planning in Greater Bombay. J. R. Rele & Tara Kanitkar. 1980. 217p. (0-940500-87-6) Popular Prakashan IND. Dist: Asia Bk Corp.

Fertility & Family Planning in Rural Areas. A. K. Sharma. 1987. (0-8364-2243-0) Mittal Pubs Dist IND. Dist: S Asia.

Fertility & Obstetrics in Cattle. David E. Noakes. 2nd ed. 1997. LC 96-43821. (Library of Veterinary Practice). (Illus.). 176p. pap. (0-632-04083-1) Blckwell Science GBR. Dist: Iowa U Pr.

Fertility & Reproductive Medicine. Ed. by Roger D. Kempers & A. F. Haney. 1998. 864p. 250.00 (0-444-50068-5) Elsevier.

Fertility & Resources. Ed. by John Landers & Vernon Reynolds. 1990. (Society for the Study of Human Biology Symposium Ser.: No. 31). 207p. (C). text 64.95 (0-521-39526-7) Cambridge U Pr.

Fertility & Sterility: A Current Overview. Ed. by B. Hedon et al. 1995. LC 95-23865. (International Congress, Symposium, & Seminar Ser.: Vol. 12). (Illus.). 498p. lib. bdg. 104.95 (1-85070-694-8, HO955, Parthenon Pbng) CRC Pr.

Fertility & Sterility: Progress in Research & Practice. Ed. by O. Rodriquez Armas et al. 1994. LC 93-46623. (International Congress, Symposium, & Seminar Ser.: Vol. 5). 599p. 137.95 (1-85070-501-1, Parthenon Pbng) CRC Pr.

Fertility Awareness & Natural Family Planning Resource Directory, 1991. Ed. by Suzannah C. Doyle. 2nd rev. ed. 1991. 200p. reprint ed. pap. 40.00 (0-9628284-1-6) FA Services.

Fertility Awareness Handbook: The Natural Guide to Avoiding or Achieving Pregnancy. Barbara Kass-Annese & Hal Danzer. 5th rev. ed. 1992. LC 91-44714. (Illus.). 160p. pap. 11.95 (0-89793-096-7) Hunter Hse.

Fertility Awareness Self-Instruction Course. Suzannah C. Doyle. 1989. (Illus.). 185p. (Orig.). stu. ed. 45.00 (0-9628284-2-4) FA Services.

Fertility, Biology & Behavior: An Analysis of the Proximate Determinants (Monograph) Ed. by John Bongaarts & Robert G. Potter. 1983. (Studies in Population). 216p. text 70.00 (0-12-114380-5) Acad Pr.

Fertility Control. Stephen L. Corson et al. 1984. 400p. 49.95 (0-316-15748-1, Little Brwn Med Div) Lppncott W & W.

Fertility Control. Ed. by Stephen L. Corson & R. J. Derman. 2nd ed. 1995. (Illus.). 526p. lib. bdg. 27.95 (0-9697978-0-X, Parthenon Pbng) CRC Pr.

Fertility Control: New Techniques, New Policy Issues, 32. Robert H. Blank. 1991. LC 91-13115. (Contributions in Medical Studies Ser.: No. 32). 176p. 58.00 (0-313-27640-4, BKF, Greenwood Pr) Greenwood.

Fertility Control: Update & Trends. Ed. by Thomas Rabe & Benno Runnebaum. 1998. LC 98-33842. (Illus.). 268p. 99.00 (3-540-64763-5) Spr-Verlag.

Fertility Control in India. M. E. Khan & C. V. Prasad. 1980. (0-8364-0628-1) Manohar IND. Dist: S Asia.

Fertility Controlled: The British Argument for Family Limitation. Charles E. Rosenberg & Carroll-Smith Rosenberg. 1974. LC 73-20644. (Sex, Marriage & Society Ser.). 137p. reprint ed. 18.95 (0-405-05799-7) Ayer.

Fertility Counselling. Sue Mack. 1996. pap. text 28.00 (0-7020-1977-1) Saunders.

Fertility, Cycles & Nutrition: Can What You Eat Affect Your Menstrual Cycles & Your Fertility? Marilyn M. Shannon. 3rd ed. 2001. LC 91-76812. 202p. per. 12.95 (0-926412-09-4) Couple to Couple.

Fertility Decline in Developing Countries, 1960-1997: An Annotated Bibliography, 3. Renbee Stapleton. 1999. LC 98-51612. (Bibliographies & Indexes in Geography Ser.: Vol. 3). 160p. lib. bdg. 65.00 (0-313-30242-1) Greenwood.

Fertility Decline in the Less Developed Countries. Ed. by Nick Eberstadt. 1981. LC 80-23528. 370p. 78.75 (0-275-90606-X, C0606, Praeger Pubs) Greenwood.

Fertility, Family Planning, & Women's Health: New Data from the 1995 National Survey of Family Growth. J. Abma et al. 1998. (Illus.). 114p. (C). pap. text 30.00 (0-7881-7193-3) DIANE Pub.

Fertility, Family Planning & Women's Health: New Data from the 1995 National Survey of Family Growth. Joyce C. Abma & National Center for Health Statistics Staff. 1997. LC 97-3229. (Vital & Health Statistics Ser.: Series 23, No. 19). (0-8406-0526-9) Natl Ctr Health Stats.

Fertility Guide. John C. Jarrett, 2nd & Deidra T. Rausch. 1998. (Illus.). 200p. pap. 14.95 (0-929173-29-5) Health Press.

Fertility Management: Contraception in Practice. C. J. Roux. 1995. pap. (0-7021-3254-3) Juta & Co ZAF. Dist: Intl Spec Bk.

Fertility of American Women. 1994. (Illus.). 84p. (Orig.). (C). pap. text 30.00 (0-7881-0506-X) DIANE Pub.

Fertility of American Women. 1994. (Orig.). lib. bdg. 250.00 (0-8490-5735-3) Gordon Pr.

Fertility Patient Ho. Peggy Robin. 1993. LC 92-41043. 448p. pap. 15.00 (0-688-11732-5, Quil) HarperTrade.

Fertility Plan: A Holistic Program to Conceiving a Healthy Baby. Helen Caton et al. 2000. LC 99-53242. (Illus.). 144p. per. 15.00 (0-684-86944-6) S&S Trade.

***Fertility Problems: A Simple Guide.** Ruth Chambers. 1999. 128p. pap. (1-85775-302-X) Radcliffe Med Pr GBR. Dist: Balogh.

Fertility Regulation & the Public Health: Selected Papers of Christopher Tietze. Ed. by S. L. Tietze & R. Lincoln. 1987. (Illus.). 351p. 99.00 (0-387-96450-9) Spr-Verlag.

Fertility Revolution: A Supply-Demand Analysis. Richard A. Easterlin & Eileen M. Crimmins. 1985. LC 85-1163. xx, 230p. 29.95 (0-226-18029-8) U Ch Pr.

Fertility Sourcebook: Everything You Need to Know. M Sara Rosenthal. 1996. 272p. pap. 16.00 (1-56565-455-2) Lowell Hse.

Fertility Transition & Women's Life Course in Mexico. 61p. pap. 10.00 (92-1-151263-8, E.94.XIII.5) UN.

Fertilization & Embryonic Development In Vitro. Ed. by Luigi Mastroianni, Jr. et al. 1981. LC 81-13829. 382p. 85.00 (0-306-40783-3, Plenum Trade) Perseus Pubng.

Fertilization in Mammals. Ed. by Barry D. Bavister et al. 1990. (Serono Symposia, U. S. A. Ser.). (Illus.). 492p. (C). text 80.00 (1-878601-03-2) Serono Symposia USA.

***Fertiltiy Handbook: A Guide to Getting Pregnant.** C. Maud Doherty & Melanie Morrissey Clark. 2001. LC 2001-6010. 160p. pap. 14.95 (1-886039-55-0) Addicus Bks.

Festschrift for B. F. Skinner. Ed. by Peter B. Dews. 1977. LC 76-133193. (Century Psychology Ser.). (Orig.). (C). reprint ed. 42.00 (0-89197-497-0) Irvington.

Festschrift for Jacques Chretien: Journal: Respiration, Vol. 57, No. 3, 1990. Ed. by G. J. Huchon. 1990. (Illus.). 100p. pap. 54.00 (3-8055-5340-4) S Karger.

Festschrift for Joel D. Kopple on the Occasion of His 60th Birthday. Ed. by Garabed Eknoyan. 1998. (Mineral & Electrolyte Metabolism Ser.: Vol. 24, No. 4). (Illus.). 100p. pap. 52.25 (3-8055-6653-0) S Karger.

Festschrift fuer W. E. Schreiner: Abschieds-Symposium, Universitaets-Frauenklinik Zuerich, September, 1988. Ed. by R. A. Steiner. 1989. (Journal: Vol. 29, Suppl. 1, 1989). (Illus.). iv, 96p. pap. 30.50 (3-8055-5106-1) S Karger.

Festschrift Zum 75. Geburtstag Von Prof. Dr. Med. Karl-Heinz Vosteen. Ed. by W. Arnold. 2000. (Oto-Rhino-Laryngologia Nova Ser.: Vol. 9, No. 3-4). (GER.). 34p. pap. 34.00 (3-8055-7047-3) S Karger.

Fetal Adrenal Hyperplasia: Its Relationship to Late Toxemia. William B. Patterson. 1973. LC 73-90025. (Illus.). 81p. 6.00 (0-9606968-0-6) W B Patterson.

Fetal Alcohol Abuse Syndrome. Ernest L. Abel. 1998. LC 98-26505. (Illus.). 242p. (C). text 42.50 (0-306-45666-4, Kluwer Plenum) Kluwer Academic.

Fetal Alcohol Exposure & Effects: A Comprehensive Bibliography. Compiled by Ernest L. Abel. 1985. LC 85-9864. 309p. lib. bdg. 82.50 (0-313-24632-7, AFC/, Greenwood Pr) Greenwood.

Fetal Alcohol Syndrome. Hazelden Publishing Staff. 1996. pap. 4.75 (0-89486-951-5) Hazelden.

Fetal Alcohol Syndrome. Amy Nevitt. rev. ed. 1998. LC 95-10884. (Drug Abuse Prevention Library). (Illus.). 64p. (YA). (gr. 7-12). lib. bdg. 17.95 (0-8239-2829-2, DRFEAL) Rosen Group.

Fetal Alcohol Syndrome: An Annotated & Comprehensive Bibliography Ernest L. Abel. 144p. I. 1981. 83.00 (0-8493-6192-3, RG629); II. 1982. 117.00 (0-8493-6193-1); III. 1982. 117.00 (0-8493-6194-X) Franklin (CRC Reprint).

Fetal Alcohol Syndrome: An Annotated Bibliography. Ernest L. Abel. 1985. LC 85-25594. 170p. 65.00 (0-275-92028-3, C2028, Praeger Pubs) Greenwood.

Fetal Alcohol Syndrome: Diagnosis, Epidemiology, Prevention & Treatment. Institute of Medicine Staff. Ed. by Kathleen Stratton et al. 1996. LC 95-49289. 232p. text 39.95 (0-309-05292-0) Natl Acad Pr.

Fetal Alcohol Syndrome: From Mechanism to Prevention. Ed. by Ernest L. Abel. 1996. LC 96-19080. 352p. 139.95 (0-8493-7685-8) CRC Pr.

Fetal Alcohol Syndrome & Fetal Alcohol Effects. Ernest L. Abel. 1984. LC 83-26898. (Illus.). 256p. (C). 49.00 (0-306-41427-9, Plenum Trade) Perseus Pubng.

Fetal Alcohol Syndrome Information Packet: Early Childhood Research Project. Ed. by Enoch Gordis. 2000. 61p. (C). pap. text 20.00 (0-7881-8906-9) DIANE Pub.

Fetal Alcohol Syndrome the Man-Made Disease for Babies & Children: Index of New Information. American Health Research Institute Staff. 1998. 160p. 57.50 (0-7883-1900-0); pap. 47.50 (0-7883-1901-9) ABBE Pubs Assn.

***Fetal & Early Childhood Environment: Long-Term Health Implications.** M. Marmot & M. Wadsworth. 1997. (British Medical Bulletin Ser.: Vol. 53, No. 1). 224p. pap. (1-85315-318-4) Royal Soc of Medicine Pr Ltd GBR. Dist: Balogh.

Fetal & Infant Origins of Adult Disease. Ed. by D. J. Barker. 1992. (Illus.). 343p. text (0-7279-0743-3) BMJ Pub GBR. Dist: AIDC.

Fetal & Neonatal Haematology. Ian M. Hann. 1991. text 110.00 (0-7020-1406-0) Saunders.

Fetal & Neonatal Neurology & Neurosurgery. Ed. by Malcolm I. Levene et al. 1988. (Illus.). 640p. text (0-443-03713-2); 2nd ed. 1995. LC 94-24322. text (0-443-04910-6) Church.

***Fetal & Neonatal Neurology & Neurosurgery.** Malcolm Levene et al. 3rd ed. 2001. (Illus.). 751p. (0-443-06379-6) Church GBR. Dist: Saunders.

Fetal & Neonatal Pathology. A. J. Barson. 1982. 72.95 (0-275-91359-7, C1359, Praeger Pubs) Greenwood.

Fetal & Neonatal Pathology. Jean W. Keeling. 2nd ed. 1993. (Illus.). 699p. 185.00 (3-540-19711-7) Spr-Verlag.

Fetal & Neonatal Pathology. Ed. by Jean W. Keeling. 2nd ed. 1993. LC 92-2323. (Illus.). 699p. 209.00 (0-387-19711-7) Spr-Verlag.

Fetal & Neonatal Physiology. Richard A. Polin & William W. Fox. 2nd ed. 1997. LC 96-31628. (0-7216-6017-7); (0-7216-6018-5) Saunders.

Fetal & Neonatal Physiology, Set. Richard A. Polin & William W. Fox. Ed. by Judy Fletcher. 2nd ed. 1997. LC 96-31628. (Illus.). 2496p. text 415.00 (0-7216-6016-9) Saunders.

Fetal & Perinatal Neurology. Ed. by Y. Fukuyama et al. 1992. (Illus.). viii, 388p. 252.25 (3-8055-5398-6) S Karger.

Fetal Anomalies: Ultrasound Diagnosis & Postnatal Management. Ed. by Max Maizels et al. 2001. LC 00-43433. 286p. 159.95 (0-471-38052-0) Wiley.

Fetal Behaviour: Developmental & Perinatal Aspects. Ed. by Jan G. Nijhuis. 1992. LC 92-12913. (Illus.). 306p. text 79.95 (0-19-262089-4) OUP.

Fetal Bovine Serum: Approved Guideline (1995) 1995. 95.00 (1-56238-276-4, M25-A) NCCLS.

Fetal Cardiac Function. Ed. by D. Arduini et al. 1994. (Illus.). 140p. (C). lib. bdg. 85.95 (1-85070-467-8, Parthenon Pbng) CRC Pr.

***Fetal Cells & Fetal DNA in Maternal Blood: New Developments for a New Millenium 11th Fetal Cell Workshop, Basel, April 2000: Proceedings.** S. Hahn & W. Holzgreve. 2001. (Illus.). viii, 160p. 85.25 (3-8055-7222-0) S Karger.

Fetal Cells in Maternal Blood: Prospects for Noninvasive Prenatal Diagnosis. Ed. by Joe L. Simpson & Sherman

E F G

Elias. 1994. (Annals of the New York Academy of Sciences Ser.: Vol. 731). pap. 80.00 (*0-89766-889-8*) NY Acad Sci.

Fetal Development: A Psychobiological Perspective. Ed. by Jean-Pierre Lecanuet et al. 1995. LC 94-44324. 524p. text 99.95 (*0-8058-1485-X*) L Erlbaum Assocs.

Fetal Development: Directory of Authors of New Medical & Scientific Reviews with Subject Index. Science and Life Consultants Association Staff. 1995. 160p. 57.50 (*0-7883-0574-3*); pap. 47.50 (*0-7883-0575-1*) ABBE Pubs Assn.

Fetal Disorders: A Multidisciplinary Approach. Boris M. Petrikovsky. 1998. LC 98-6113. (Illus.). 320p. 120.00 (*0-471-19152-3*) Wiley.

Fetal Echocardiography. Julia A. Drose. Ed. by Andrew Allen. 1998. LC 97-18557. (Illus.). 352p. text 65.00 (*0-7216-6284-6*) Saunders.

Fetal Echocardiography. Darla B. Hess. 1998. LC 98-3614. 450p. text 139.00 (*0-8385-2577-6*) McGraw-Hill Prof.

Fetal Echocardiography: Principles & Applications. C. S. Kleinman. 2002. (*0-87993-262-7*) Futura Pub.

Fetal Electrocardiography. E. Malcolm Symonds et al. 1999. (Series in Cardiopulmonary Medicine Ser.). 200p. pap. text (*1-86094-171-0*) Imperial College GBR. *Dist:* World Scientific Pub.

Fetal Endocrinology. Ed. by T. Zondek et al. 1978. (Contributions to Gynecology & Obstetrics Ser.: Vol. 5). (Illus.). pap. 68.75 (*3-8055-2926-0*) S Karger.

Fetal Growth. Ed. by Frank Sharp et al. 1989. (Illus.). 428p. 143.00 (*0-387-19562-9*) Spr-Verlag.

Fetal Growth & Development. Ed. by Alan D. Bocking & Richard Harding. 2001. (Illus.). 294p. (C). text 80.00 (*0-521-64237-X*); pap. text 28.95 (*0-521-64543-3*) Cambridge U Pr.

Fetal Growth & the Placenta: From Implantation to Delivery. Ed. by Henning Schneider et al. 1993. LC 93-784. (Trophoblast Research Ser.: No. 7). (Illus.). 313p. (C). 110.00 (*1-878822-26-8*) Univ Rochester Pr.

Fetal Growth Retardation: Diagnosis & Treatment. Ed. by Asim Kurjak & John M. Beazley. 1989. 240p. lib. bdg. 127.00 (*0-8493-4765-3*, RG629) CRC Pr.

Fetal Heart Rate As a Behavioral Indicator. Lester W. Sontag. 1938. (SRCD M Ser.: Vol. 3, No. 4). pap. 25.00 (*0-527-01504-0*) Periodicals Srv.

Fetal Heart Rate Monitoring. Ed. by W. Kunzel. 1985. (Illus.). 244p. 126.00 (*0-387-15313-6*) Spr-Verlag.

Fetal Heart Rate Monitoring. Roger K. Freeman et al. 2nd ed. 1991. (Illus.). 240p. 79.00 (*0-683-03381-6*) Lppncott W & W.

Fetal Heart Rate Monitoring: A Practical Guide. Ingemar Ingemarsson et al. 1993. LC 92-48525.Tr. of Elektronik Foster Overvakning. (ENG & SWE., Illus.). 340p. text 68.00 (*0-19-262269-2*) OUP.

Fetal Hypoxia. Ed. by Ph. Arbeille et al. 1999. LC 99-32279. (Progress in Obstetric & Gynecological Sonography Ser.). (Illus.). 146p. 85.95 (*1-85070-012-5*, Parthenon Pbng) CRC Pr.

Fetal Islet Transplantation: Implications for Diabetes. Ed. by Charles M. Peterson et al. 1988. (Illus.). 205p. 178.00 (*0-387-96587-4*) Spr-Verlag.

Fetal Islet Transplantation: Proceedings of the Second International Sansum Symposium on Human Fetal Islet Transplantation Held in Santa Barbara, California, October 27-30, 1994. International Sansum Symposium on Human Fetal Isle. Ed. by Charles M. Peterson et al. 1995. LC 95-13980. (Illus.). 202p. (C). text 85.00 (*0-306-45066-6*, Kluwer Plenum) Kluwer Academic.

Fetal Medicine: Prenatal Diagnosis & Management. Ed. by Andre Boue. Tr. by Michel Vekemans & Lola Cartier. 1995. LC 93-39528. (Oxford Monographs on Medical Genetics). (Illus.). 304p. (C). text 98.50 (*0-19-261904-7*) OUP.

Fetal Medicine: Principles & Practice. Frank A. Manning. 1995. LC 94-44480. 596p. (C). pap. text 495.00 (*0-8385-2572-5*, A2572-4, Apple Lange Med) McGraw.

Fetal Medicine: The Clinical Care of the Fetus as a Patient. Ed. by Frank A. Chervenak & A. Kurjak. 1999. LC 99-26995. (Illus.). 402p. lib. bdg. 93.95 (*1-85070-072-9*) CRC Pr.

Fetal Monitoring in Practice. D. M. Gibo & Sabaratnam Arulkumaran. 2nd ed. 1997. LC 97-31071. 240p. pap. text 40.00 (*0-7506-3432-4*) Buttrwrth-Heinemann.

Fetal Monitoring Interpretation. Micki Cabaniss. 1993. LC 65-9897. (Illus.). 592p. text 99.00 (*0-397-50824-7*, Lippnctt) Lppncott W & W.

Fetal Monitoring Interpretation. Micki L. Cabaniss. 2nd ed. 1998. text (*0-397-51860-9*) Lppncott W & W.

Fetal, Neonatal & Infant Cardiac Disease. James H. Moller & William A. Neal. 1992. (Illus.). 1061p. (C). pap. text 225.00 (*0-8385-2575-X*, A2575-7, Apple Lange Med) McGraw.

Fetal, Neonatal & Infant Monitoring Markets. Market Intelligence Staff. 1994. 364p. (Orig.). 2195.00 (*0-7889-0074-9*) Frost & Sullivan.

Fetal Pathology. Jean W. Keeling. 1994. text (*0-443-04426-0*) Church.

Fetal Patient: Multi Approach to Management. Bianchi et al. 2000. (Illus.). 1081p. (C). text 145.00 (*0-8385-2570-9*) McGraw-Hill Prof.

Fetal Positions: Individualism, Science, Visuality. Karen Newman. 1996. LC 95-41182. (Writing Science Ser.). xi, 157p. 46.00 (*0-8047-2647-7*); 157p. pap. 18.95 (*0-8047-2648-5*) Stanford U Pr.

Fetal Research & Applications: A Conference Summary. Institute of Medicine, Fetal Research and Applications Staff. 1994. LC 94-67254. 116p. (Orig.). (C). pap. text 24.00 (*0-309-05176-2*) Natl Acad Pr.

Fetal Sonographic Biometry: A Guide to Normal & Abnormal Measurements. D. Bettelheim et al. 1997. LC 96-33682. (Illus.). 346p. lib. bdg. 107.95 (*1-85070-725-1*, Parthenon Pbng) CRC Pr.

Fetal Sonography. Terry J. DuBose. 1995. LC 95-5452. (Illus.). 416p. text 75.00 (*0-7216-5432-0*) Saunders.

Fetal Therapy: Invasive & Transplacental. Ed. by Nicholas M. Fisk & Kenneth J. Moise. 1997. LC 96-13127. 385p. (C). text 130.00 (*0-521-46133-2*) Cambridge U Pr.

Fetal Therapy: State of the Art. Mark I. Evans & Lawrence D. Platt. 2001. LC 99-36191. (Illus.). 138p. 94.95 (*1-85070-064-8*, Parthenon Pbng) CRC Pr.

Fetal Well Being: Physiological Basis & Methods - Clinical Assessment. Ed. by Miriam Katz. 1990. 200p. lib. bdg. 95.00 (*0-8493-6052-8*, RG) CRC Pr.

Fetus. Harris J. Finberg et al. 1997. (Illus.). 115p. pap. 64.00 (*1-930047-00-2*, TF) Am Inst Ultrasound.

Fetus & Neonate: Physiology & Clinical Applications. Ed. by Mark A. Hanson et al. 1993. (Illus.). 454p. (C). text 110.00 (*0-521-41187-4*) Cambridge U Pr.

Fetus & Neonate: Physiology & Clinical Applications. Ed. by Mark A. Hanson et al. 1993. (Illus.). 454p. (C). pap. text 39.95 (*0-521-42327-9*) Cambridge U Pr.

Fetus & Neonate: Physiology & Clinical Applications, Vol. 2. Ed. by Mark A. Hanson et al. 1995. LC 93-31377. (Illus.). 414p. (C). text 100.00 (*0-521-41765-1*) Cambridge U Pr.

Fetus as a Patient: Advances in Diagnosis & Therapy. Ed. by Asim Kurjak & Frank A. Chervenak. 1994. LC 94-7115. 562p. lib. bdg. 107.95 (*1-85070-558-5*, Parthenon Pbng) CRC Pr.

Fetus As a Patient: Ninth International Congress, Fuji-Yoshida, November-December 1993 Abstracts. 1993. (Journal: Vol. 8, Suppl. 2, 1993). (Illus.). xiv, 100p. pap. 30.50 (*3-8055-5890-2*) S Karger.

Fetus As Medical Patient: Moral Dilemmas in Prenatal Diagnosis from a Catholic Perspective. Alfred Cioffi. 1995. LC 94-24378. 334p. (C). 49.50 (*0-8191-9780-7*) U Pr of Amer.

Fetus into Man: Physical Growth from Conception to Maturity. James M. Tanner. enl. rev. ed. 1990. (Illus.). 288p. 39.50 (*0-674-30702-X*); pap. 19.95 (*0-674-30692-9*) HUP.

FEU Class '61 Yearbook: Medical Alumni. J. B. Nolasco. Ed. by Philip S. Chua. 1994. LC 94-94310. (Illus.). 153p. 65.00 (*0-9641472-4-6*) P S Chua.

FEU United Class Nineteen Sixty-One: Thirty-Third Anniversary Yearbook. Philip S. Chua & J. B. Nolasco. 1994. LC 94-94310. 152p. pap. (*0-9641472-2-X*); pap. text (*0-9641472-3-8*); (*0-9641472-5-4*); (*0-9641472-6-2*); (*0-9641472-7-0*); (*0-9641472-8-9*) P S Chua.

Fever & Antipyresis: The Role of the Nervous System. Keith E. Cooper. 1995. (Illus.). 198p. (C). text 59.95 (*0-521-41924-7*) Cambridge U Pr.

Fever Coast Log. Chaplin. 1991. 18.95 (*0-13-194234-4*) P-H.

Fever in Pediatric Practice. Sahib El-Radhi & James Carroll. 1994. LC 93-39209. 272p. 50.00 (*0-632-03513-7*) Blackwell Sci.

Fevered Lives: Tuberculosis in American Culture since 1870. Katherine Ott. 1996. LC 96-26830. (Illus.). 256p. 27.95 (*0-674-29910-8*) HUP.

Feverfew: Natural Headache Relief. Deanne Tenney. 1998. (Woodland Health Ser.). 23p. pap. 3.95 (*1-58054-012-0*) Woodland UT.

FHA Hospital Mortgage Insurance Program: Health Care Trends & Portfolio Concentration Could Affect Program Stability. 1996. (Illus.). 53p. (Orig.). (C). pap. text 25.00 (*0-7881-3485-X*) DIANE Pub.

FHP: The Evolution of a Managed Care Health Maintenance Organization, 1955-1992. Robert Gumbiner. 1995. LC 95-79744. 448p. pap. (*0-9645847-0-0*) R Gumbiner.

Fiber Optic Medical & Fluorescent Sensors & Applications. Ed. by D. R. Hansmann et al. 1992. 56.00 (*0-8194-0794-1*, 1648) SPIE.

Fiber-Reinforced Composites in Clinical Dentistry. Martin A. Freilich. 2000. LC 99-46512. 106p. text 68.00 (*0-86715-373-3*) Quint Pub Co.

Fiber Toxicology. Ed. by David B. Warheit. 1993. (Illus.). 526p. text 99.00 (*0-12-735430-1*) Acad Pr.

Fiberoptic Airway Endoscopy in Anesthesia & Critical Care see Fiberoptic Endoscopy & the Difficult Airway

Fiberoptic Endoscopy & the Difficult Airway. Ed. by Andranik Ovassapian. 2nd rev. ed. 1996. LC 96-4639. Orig. Title: Fiberoptic Airway Endoscopy in Anesthesia & Critical Care. 304p. text 169.00 (*0-7817-0272-0*) Lppncott W & W.

Fiberoptic Rhinolaryngoscopy. John C. Selner et al. 2nd ed. 1989. (Illus.). stu. ed. 120.00 (*0-9622943-0-6*) ARI CO.

***Fibreoptic Intubation.** Hawkins. 2001. (Greenwich Medical Media Ser.). (Illus.). 82p. pap. incl. cd-rom (*1-84110-060-9*) Greenwich Med GBR. *Dist:* JAMCO Dist.

Fibrin Sealant in Operative Medicine. Ed. by Gunther O. Schlag & H. Redl. (Illus.). Vol. 6. 1986. 210p. 52.95 (*0-387-17280-7*); Vol. 7. 1987. 236p. 48.95 (*0-387-17281-5*) Spr-Verlag.

Fibrin Sealing in Surgical & Nonsurgical Fields. Ed. by Gunther O. Schlag. 1995. (Cardiovascular Surgery Ser.: Vol. 61). (Illus.). 215p. 64.95 (*3-540-58381-5*) Spr-Verlag.

Fibrin Sealing in Surgical & Nonsurgical Fields, 4. Gunther O. Schlag & P. Bosch. 1994. (Advances in Pharmacological Sciences Ser.). (Illus.). 201p. 74.95 (*0-387-58009-3*) Spr-Verlag.

Fibrin Sealing in Surgical & Nonsurgical Fields Vol. 1. Ed. by Gunther O. Schlag & H. Redl. 1994. LC 94-5663. (Illus.). 149p. 86.95 (*0-387-57511-1*) Spr-Verlag.

Fibrin Sealing in Surgical & Nonsurgical Fields Vol. 2: General & Abdominal Surgery, Pediatric Surgery. Ed. by H. W. Waclawiczek et al. 1999. (Illus.). 224p. 112.00 (*0-387-57742-4*) Spr-Verlag.

Fibrinogen, Vol.2: Structure-Functional Aspects - Metabolism. Ed. by Haverkate et al. 1983. (Proceedings Workshop on Fibrinogen Ser.). (Illus.). 343p. 111.55 (*3-11-008986-6*) De Gruyter.

Fibrinogen, Thrombosis, Coagulation & Fibrinolysis. Ed. by C. Y. Liu & Shu Chien. 1990. LC 90-14299. (Advances in Experimental Medicine & Biology Ser.: Vol. 281). (Illus.). 460p. (C). text 162.00 (*0-306-43726-0*, Kluwer Plenum) Kluwer Academic.

Fibrinolysis. Daniel L. Kline & K. N. Reddy. 1980. 256p. 145.00 (*0-8493-5425-0*, QP93, CRC Reprint) Franklin.

Fibrinolysis in Disease: The Malignant Process, Interventions in Thrombogenic Mechanisms, & Novel Treatment Modalities. Pia Glas-Greenwalt. 1995. 280p. 224.95 (*0-8493-6080-3*, 6080) CRC Pr.

Fibrinolysis, Thrombosis, & Hemostasis. Sol Sherry. 1992. 59.50 (*0-8121-1502-3*) Lppncott W & W.

Fibroid Tumors & Endometriosis: A Self-Help Program. Susan M. Lark. 1993. (Women's Health Ser.). 264p. pap. 12.95 (*0-917010-54-X*) Celestial Arts.

Fibroid Tumors & Endometriosis: Self Help Book. Susan M. Lark. 3rd rev. ed. 1995. LC 95-17689. 272p. text 16.95 (*0-89087-773-4*) Celestial Arts.

Fibroids: A Guide for Women. Andrew Friedman. Ed. by Edward E. Wallach. 1996. (Women's Health Ser.). (Illus.). 32p. pap. 2.95 (*1-885274-24-6*) Health InfoNet Inc.

Fibroids: The Complete Guide to Taking Charge of Your Physical, Emotional & Sexual Well-Being. Joanna Skilling. 2000. (Illus.). 288p. pap. 15.95 (*1-56261-494-0*) Marlowe & Co.

Fibromyalgia: A Handbook for Self Care & Treatment. Janet A. Hulme. 1995. 112p. 14.95 (*0-9644848-0-3*) Phoenix Pubng Co.

***Fibromyalgia: A Journey Towards Healing.** Chanchal Cabrera. 2002. LC 2001-55965. 304p. pap. 16.95 (*0-658-00305-4*, Contemporary) McGraw-Hill Trade.

Fibromyalgia: My Journey to Wellness. Claire Musickant. 1999. LC 99-64037. (Illus.). iii, 220p. pap. 17.95 (*0-89716-931-X*) P B Pubng.

Fibromyalgia: Relief from Chronic Muscle Pain. Illus. by Paul Davidson. 1999. 107p. 69.95 incl. audio (*0-9653493-2-2*) HlthRd Prods.

Fibromyalgia: Simple Relief Through Movement. Stacie Bigelow. 2000. LC 00-699095. 144p. pap. 14.95 (*0-471-34802-3*) Wiley.

Fibromyalgia - A Comprehensive Approach: What You Can Do about Chronic Pain & Fatigue. Miryam E. Williamson. 1996. LC 96-3251. (Illus.). 224p. pap. 14.95 (*0-8027-7484-9*) Walker & Co.

Fibromyalgia - Managing the Pain: Understanding the Syndrome & Managing Its Pain. Mark J. Pellegrino. 2nd ed. 1997. LC 97-205620. (Illus.). 102p. (Orig.). pap. 12.45 (*1-890018-10-4*) Anadem Pubng.

Fibromyalgia a Handbook for Self Care & Treatment: Five Types, Five Tests, Five Treatments. Janet A. Hueme. 3rd rev. ed. 2001. (Illus.). 220p. pap. 14.95 (*1-928812-01-5*) Phoenix Pubg.

Fibromyalgia Advocate: Getting the Support You Need to Cope with Fibromyalgia & Myofascial Pain Syndrome. Devin J. Starlanyl. 1998. LC 98-66701. (Illus.). 381p. pap. 18.95 (*1-57224-121-7*) New Harbinger.

Fibromyalgia & Chronic Myofascial Pain Syndrome: A Survival Manual. Devin J. Starlanyl & Mary E. Copeland. 1996. LC 95-72229. (Illus.). 432p. pap. 19.95 (*1-57224-046-6*) New Harbinger.

Fibromyalgia & Chronic Myofascial Pain Syndrome: A Survival Manual. Devin J. Starlanyl & Mary Ellen Copeland. 2nd ed. 2001. (Illus.). 432p. pap. 19.95 (*1-57224-238-8*) New Harbinger.

Fibromyalgia & Muscle Pain: What Causes It, How It Feels & What to Do about It. Leon Chaitow. 1996. 220p. pap. 11.95 (*0-7225-3098-6*) Harper SF.

Fibromyalgia Chef. Mark J. Pellegrino. 1997. (Illus.). 203p. pap. 15.50 (*1-890018-16-3*) Anadem Pubng.

Fibromyalgia, Chronic Fatigue Syndrome, & Repetitive Strain Injury: Current Concepts in Diagnosis, Management, Disability, & Health Economics. Ed. by Andrew Chalmers et al. 1995. LC 95-30842. (Journal of Musculoskeletal Pain: Vol. 3, No. 2). 49.95 (*1-56024-744-4*, Hawrth Medical) Haworth Pr.

Fibromyalgia Cookbook: A Daily Guide to Becoming Healthy Again. Mary Moeller. Ed. by Karl Moeller. 1998. (Illus.). 163p. reprint ed. pap. 14.95 (*0-9660190-8-3*) Fibromyalgia Solns.

Fibromyalgia Help Book: Practical Guide to Living Better with Fibromyalgia. Jenny Fransen & I. John Russell. 1996. LC 97-136216. (Illus.). 239p. pap. 18.95 (*0-9615221-4-3*) Smith Hse Pr.

Fibromyalgia Relief Book: 213 Ideas for Improving Your Quality of Life. Miryam E. Williamson. 1998. LC 98-15697. 224p. pap. 14.95 (*0-8027-7553-5*) Walker & Co.

Fibromyalgia Supporter: Everything Your Loved One Needs to Know. Mark J. Pellegrino. 1997. (Illus.). 90p. pap. 15.50 (*1-890018-11-2*) Anadem Pubng.

Fibromyalgia Survivor: Specific Steps for Coping with Fibromyalgia. Mark J. Pellegrino. 1995. LC 97-205623. (Illus.). 119p. (Orig.). pap. 19.50 (*0-9646891-2-X*) Anadem Pubng.

Fibromyalgia Syndrome. Stogner. 1998. (Illus.). 117p. (C). pap. text 55.00 (*0-12-784580-1*) Acad Pr.

Fibromyalgia Syndrome: Current Research & Future Directions in Epidemiology, Pathogenesis & Treatment. Ed. & Intro. by Stanley R. Pillemer. 1994. LC 94-35454. (Illus.). 200p. lib. bdg. 39.95 (*1-56024-714-2*, Hawrth Medical) Haworth Pr.

Fibromyalgia Syndrome - Getting Healthy. Jeanne Melvin. 1996. (Illus.). 60p. (Orig.). pap. text 6.00 (*1-56900-041-7*, 1144) Am Occup Therapy.

***Fibromyalgia Syndrome in Women - A Stress Disorder? Neurobiological & Hormonal Aspects.** Ulla Maria Anderberg. 1999. (Comprehensive Summaries of Uppsala Dissertations from the Faculty of Medicine Ser.: No. 815). (Illus.). 77p. pap. (*91-554-4366-4*) Uppsala Universitet SWE. *Dist:* Coronet Bks.

Fibronolysis & Urokinase. Ed. by Tilsner Volkmar & H. Lenau. 1981. LC 80-41295. (Serono Symposia Ser.: No. 31). text 199.00 (*0-12-691150-9*) Acad Pr.

Fibrositis & Myofibrositis. 1996. lib. bdg. 250.96 (*0-8490-5882-1*) Gordon Pr.

Field, Camp, Hospital & Prison in the Civil War: 1863-1865. Charles A. Humphreys. 1977. LC 75-146860. (Select Bibliographies Reprint Ser.). reprint ed. 32.95 (*0-8369-5627-3*) Ayer.

Field Crop Diseases. Robert Nyvall. 3rd ed. 1999. LC 99-18995. (Illus.). 1054p. text 129.95 (*0-8138-2079-0*) Iowa U Pr.

Field Dependence in Psychological Theory Research & Application: Two Symposia in Memory of Herman A. Witkin. Ed. by Mario Bertini et al. 1985. 152p. (C). text 39.95 (*0-89859-668-8*) L Erlbaum Assocs.

Field Dependence-Independence: Bio-Psycho-Social Factors Across the Life Span. Ed. by J. Demick & Seymour Wapner. 1991. 448p. (C). text 89.95 (*0-8058-0950-3*) L Erlbaum Assocs.

Field Epidemiology. Ed. by Michael B. Gregg et al. 1996. (Illus.). 288p. text 47.50 (*0-19-507207-3*) OUP.

Field, Form & Fate: Patterns in Mind, Psyche & Nature. Michael Conforti. 1999. LC 99-16065. (Seminar Ser.: Vol. 18). 256p. pap. 19.00 (*0-88214-118-X*) Spring Pubns.

Field Guide for Human Skeletal Identification. Kenneth A. Bennett. 2nd ed. 1993. LC 93-14458. (Illus.). 124p. (C). spiral bd. 38.95 (*0-398-05884-9*) C C Thomas.

Field Guide for International Health Project Planners & Managers, 001. Gregory P. Loos. 1993. 80p. pap. (*1-85756-159-7*) Janus Pubng GBR. *Dist:* Paul & Co Pubs.

Field Guide to Clinical Dermatology. David H. Frankel. 1999. LC 99-22603. 240p. pap. text 29.95 (*0-7817-1730-2*) Lppncott W & W.

Field Guide to Germs. Wayne Biddle. 1996. LC 96-13621. (Illus.). 224p. pap. 13.95 (*0-385-48426-7*) Doubleday.

Field Guide to Medicinal & Useful Plants of the Upper Amazon. James L. Castner et al. 1998. LC 97-77509. (Illus.). 160p. pap. 35.00 (*0-9625150-7-8*) Feline Pr.

Field Guide to Medicinal Plants. Roger T. Peterson et al. 1990. (Peterson Field Guides Ser.). (Illus.). 384p. pap. 18.00 (*0-395-92066-3*) HM.

Field Guide to Medicinal Wild Plants. Bradford Angier. 1992. 320p. (C). (*81-7002-033-6*) Himalayan Bks IND. *Dist:* St Mut.

Field Guide to Medicinal Wild Plants. Bradford Angier. 1978. LC 78-19112. (Illus.). 320p. pap. 18.95 (*0-8117-2076-4*) Stackpole.

Field Guide to the Chest X-Ray. Wallace T. Miller & Wallace T. Miller, Jr. 1999. LC 99-17626. 186p. pap. text 29.95 (*0-7817-2028-1*) Lppncott W & W.

Field Guide to the Difficult Patient Interview. Frederic W. Platt & Geoffrey H. Gordon. 1999. LC 99-19265. 196p. pap. text 29.95 (*0-7817-2044-3*) Lppncott W & W.

Field Guide Wilderness Medicine. Paul S. Auerbach et al. 1998. LC 98-29514. (Illus.). 576p. (C). (gr. 13). pap. text 34.95 (*0-8151-0926-1*, 28913) Mosby Inc.

Field Manual in Athletic Training. Marcia K. Anderson & Malissa Martin. 1998. LC 98-15945. (Illus.). 409p. 29.95 (*0-683-30235-3*) Lppncott W & W.

***Field Manual of Horse Health: Basic Veterinary Care for Working Equids.** Ed. by David Hadrill. 2001. 208p. pap. (*1-85339-486-6*) Intermed Tech GBR. *Dist:* Stylus Pub VA.

Field of Play: A Guide for the Theory & Practice of Music Therapy. Carolyn B. Kenny. 1989. xvi, 160p. (Orig.). pap. text 16.00 (*0-917930-50-9*); lib. bdg. 36.00 (*0-917930-97-5*) Ridgeview.

Field's Medico-Legal Guide: For Doctors & Lawyers. George W. Field. 1983. 291p. reprint ed. 42.00 (*0-8377-0543-6*, Rothman) W S Hein.

Fields of Group Psychotherapy. Ed. by S. R. Slavson. 1956. LC 64-15375. 338p. 50.00 (*0-8236-1940-0*); pap. 24.95 (*0-8236-8053-3*, 21940) Intl Univs Pr.

Fields of Poison: California Farmworkers & Pesticides. Margaret Reeves et al. Tr. by Victor Reyes. 1999. (ENG & SPA., Illus.). 103p. (C). pap. text 20.00 (*0-7881-8418-0*) DIANE Pub.

Fieldwork Anthology: A Classic Research & Practice Collection. Ed. by Christine R. Privott. 1998. LC 98-139903. 468p. pap. text 40.00 (*1-56900-092-1*, 1176) Am Occup Therapy.

Fieser & Fieser's Reagents for Organic Synthesis, Vol. 9. Fieser and Fieser's Staff. 1981. (Fieser's Reagents for Organic Synthesis Ser.: Vol. 9). 608p. 115.00 (*0-471-05631-6*) Wiley.

***15 Minute Auditor for Physician Practices 2001.** Ingenix, Inc. Staff. pap. 89.95 (*1-56337-356-4*) Ingenix Inc.

Fifteen-Minute Hour: Applied Psychotherapy for the Primary Care Physician. Marian R. Stuart & Joseph A. Lieberman, III. 2nd ed. 1993. LC 92-48985. 224p. 72.50 (*0-275-94498-0*, C4498); pap. 20.95 (*0-275-94499-9*, B4499) Greenwood (Praeger Pubs).

Fifth Conference on Superoxide & Superoxide Dismutase. Ed. by G. Czapski. 1991. (Free Radical Research Communications Ser.). 460p. pap. text 1050.00 (*3-7186-5125-4*, Harwood Acad Pubs) Gordon & Breach.

Fifth International Symposium on Inflammatory Bowel Diseases. Ed. by D. Rachmilewitz. 1998. (Falk Symposium Ser.). 256p. 146.00 (*0-7923-8743-0*) Kluwer Academic.

Fifth Psychoactive Drug Usage Guide. Intro. by William S. Appleton. 1991. 105p. (C). pap. text 19.95 (*0-933171-00-5*) Phys Postgrad.

Fifth Report of the Joint National Committee on Detection, Evaluation & Treatment of High Blood Pressure. 1995. (Illus.). 51p. (Orig.). (C). pap. text 30.00 (*0-7881-1824-2*) DIANE Pub.

Fifth Symposium by the Nine Winners of the Grants from Sandoz Foundation for Gerontological Research: Annual Meeting of the Japan Gerontological Society, Sapporo, Japan, September 1993, No. 40. Ed. by H. Orimo. 1994. (Journal: Supplement 2, 1994). (Illus.). iv, 72p. pap. 33.25 (*3-8055-6044-3*) S Karger.

50 Cases in Health Care Law. Paul Lombardo. 1999. (*0-89089-843-X*) Carolina Acad Pr.

Fifty-Five Ways to Beat Colds & Flu. Charles B. Inlander & Cynthia K. Moran. 1994. LC 94-32102. 96p. 14.95 (*0-8027-1304-1*); pap. 7.95 (*0-8027-7447-4*) Walker & Co.

Fifty Simple Things You Can Do to Save Your Life. UCLA School of Public Health Staff. 1992. 132p. pap. 5.95 (*1-879682-11-7*) Bathroom Reader.

Fifty-Sixth Evac Hospital: Letters of a WWII Army Doctor. Lawrence D. Collins. 1995. LC 94-45516. (War & the Southwest Ser.: No. 4). (Illus.). 304p. 29.95 (*0-929398-83-1*) UNTX Pr.

52 Simple Steps to Natural Health: A Week-by-Week Guide to More Healthful Living. Natural Health Magazine Editors & Mark Mayell. Ed. by Claire Zion. 1995. 464p. per. 14.00 (*0-671-88061-6*) PB.

52 Ways to Live a Long & Healthy Life. Laura Lewis. Ed. by Ann Moyer & Mike Towle. 1993. LC 99-197756. 300p. pap. 8.95 (*1-56530-066-1*) Summit TX.

Fifty Ways to Avoid Malpractice: A Guidebook for Mental Health Professionals. Robert H. Woody. 1988. LC 88-42814. 158p. pap. 23.45 (*0-943158-54-0*, FWBP, Prof Resc Pr) Pro Resource.

50 Ways to Cope with Diabetes. Ed. by Nal-Dutton Staff. 1996. pap. 4.99 (*0-451-18585-4*, Sig) NAL.

50 Ways to Ease Back Pain. 9.98 (*0-7853-0679-X*) Pubns Intl Ltd.

Fifty Ways to Keep Your Child Safe: Physically, Emotionally, Medically, Environmentally. Susan K. Golant. 1992. 204p. pap. 10.95 (*1-56565-019-0*) Lowell Hse.

50 Ways to Manage Type 2 Diabetes. M Sara Rosenthal. 2001. LC 00-66002. 192p. pap. 12.95 (*0-7373-0540-1*) McGraw-Hill Prof.

50 Ways to Prevent Colon Cancer. M Sara Rosenthal. 2000. LC 00-35216. (Illus.). xv, 111p. pap. 14.95 (*0-7373-0459-6*, 04596W) Lowell Hse.

50 Ways to Relieve Heartburn, Reflux & Ulcers. M Sara Rosenthal. 2001. LC 00-66001. 192p. pap. 14.95 (*0-7373-0472-3*, Contemporary) McGraw-Hill Prof.

Fifty Years a Country Doctor. Hull Cook. 1998. LC 97-50636. 203p. pap. 12.00 (*0-8032-6389-9*) U of Nebr Pr.

Fifty Years of LSD: Current Status & Perspectives of Hallucinogens. Ed. by A. Pletscher & D. Ladewig. 1994. LC 94-8290. (Illus.). 238p. 82.95 (*1-85070-569-0*, Parthenon Pbng) CRC Pr.

Fifty Years of Personality Psychology. K. H. Craik et al. 1993. (Perspectives on Individual Differences Ser.). (Illus.). 324p. (C). 59.50 (*0-306-44291-4*, Plenum Trade) Perseus Pubng.

Fight Against Fears: An Intimate Account of a Woman's Psychoanalysis. Lucy Freedman. 1994. 332p. pap. 12.95 (*0-8038-9358-2*) Hastings Hse.

Fight Alzheimer's Naturally. Cathy Picoulin. 1999. LC 97-41569. 192p. pap. 14.00 (*0-7615-1261-6*) Prima Pub.

Fight Back & Win: How to Get HMOs & Health Insurance to Pay Up. William M. Shernoff. 1998. LC 99-167186. 156p. 9.95 (*0-88723-172-1*) Boardroom.

Fight the Good Fight. Philip Bedsworth & Joyce Bedsworth. 1991. LC 91-20148. 128p. (Orig.). pap. 7.99 (*0-8361-3568-7*) Herald Press.

Fighters of Fate. Jay A. Myers. 1977. LC 79-84329. (Essay Index Reprint Ser.). 23.95 (*0-8369-1099-0*) Ayer.

Fighting Back Against HIV: Self-Help for the Newly Diagnosed. Peter Tatchell. 1997. (AIDS Awareness Ser.). 224p. (*0-304-33278-X*) Cassell GBR. *Dist:* LPC InBook.

Fighting Cancer: A Survival Guide. Jonathan Chamberlain. 1998. 342p. pap. (*0-7472-7728-1*) Headline Bk Pub GBR. *Dist:* Trafalgar.

Fighting Chance: Journeys Through Childhood Cancer. Harry Connolly et al. 1998. LC 97-14834. (Illus.). 144p. 27.95 (*0-9656342-5-6*) Woodholme Hse.

Fighting Disease: Hundreds of Strategies for Preventing, Treating, & Curing Common Illnesses & Conditions. Ed. by Prevention Magazine Health Book Staff. 1996. LC 94-24202. (Family Home Remedies Collection). 136p. 6.95 (*0-87596-263-7*) Rodale Pr Inc.

Fighting Drug Abuse with Acupuncture: The Treatment That Works. Ellinor R. Mitchell. 1995. LC 95-69800. (Illus.). 224p. (Orig.). pap. 17.95 (*1-881896-12-9*) Pacific View Pr.

Fighting for America's Minds: Unraveling the Mysteries of Alzheimer's Disease. 1995. 122p. pap. 2.00 (*1-930181-08-6*) A H A F.

Fighting for Darla: Challenges for Family Care & Professional Responsibility: the Case Study of a Pregnant Adolescent with Autism. Ellen Brantlinger. 1994. 176p. (C). pap. 18.95 (*0-8077-3356-3*); text 37.00 (*0-8077-3357-1*) Tchrs Coll.

Fighting for Life. S. Josephine Baker. 1974. LC 74-1664. (Children & Youth Ser.). (Illus.). 280p. reprint ed. 28.95 (*0-405-05945-0*) Ayer.

Fighting for Life: American Military Medicine in World War II. Albert E. Cowdrey. LC 94-8280. 392p. 1998. per. 18.75 (*0-684-86379-0*); 1994. 29.95 (*0-02-906835-5*) Free Pr.

Fighting for Life: An Introduction to the Intensive Care Unit. Kieron Saunders. 1996. LC 96-4811. (Illus.). 122p. pap. 21.95 (*0-19-262572-1*) OUP.

Fighting for Your Life: How to Survive a Life-Threatening Illness. Jerome Wolfe. Ed. by William Hamilton. 2001. LC 99-68349. xviii, 373p. pap. 14.95 (*0-9676296-0-8*, FFYL2000) W Hamilton.

Fighting Infection: Conquests of the Twentieth Century. Harry F. Dowling. 1977. LC 77-8307. (Commonwealth Fund Publications). 336p. 41.00 (*0-674-30075-0*) HUP.

Fighting Prostate Problems. Aaron Katz. 2001. pap. (*0-312-28001-7*) St Martin.

Fighting Sudden Cardiac Death: A Worldwide Challenge. Ed. by Etienne Aliot et al. 2000. LC 00-37655. (Illus.). xxii, 724p. 125.00 (*0-87993-460-3*) Futura Pub.

Fighting the Silent Killer: How Men & Women Can Prevent & Cope with Heart Disease Today. Peter Cohn & Joan Cohn. 1993. LC 93-31115. (Illus.). 240p. pap. 24.00 (*1-56881-021-0*) AK Peters.

Fighting with Food: Overcoming Bulimia Nervosa. G. F. Huon & L. B. Brown. 1989. 125p. pap. (*0-86840-051-3*) New South Wales Univ Pr AUS. *Dist:* Intl Spec Bk.

Figments of Reality: The Evolution of the Curious Mind. Ian Stewart & Jack Cohen. 1997. LC 96-49357. (Illus.). 339p. (C). text 39.95 (*0-521-57155-3*) Cambridge U Pr.

Figural Synthesis. Ed. by Peter C. Dodwell & Terrence M. Caelli. 1984. 318p. (C). 49.95 (*0-89859-382-4*) L Erlbaum Assocs.

Figurative Language & Thought. Albert N. Katz et al. 1998. LC 98-19101. (Counterpoints Ser.). (Illus.). 208p. text 55.00 (*0-19-510962-7*); pap. text 24.95 (*0-19-510963-5*) OUP.

Fijian Medicinal Plants. R. C. Cambie & J. Ash. 1994. LC 94-117116. 356p. (*0-643-05404-9*) CSIRO AUS. *Dist:* Accents Pubns.

Filariasis. CIBA Foundation Staff. 1987. LC 86-28154. (CIBA Foundation Symposia Ser.: No. 127). 316p. 128.00 (*0-471-91093-7*) Wiley.

Filgrastim in Clinical Practice. Ed. by George Morstyn. 2nd ed. 1998. LC 98-3974. (Illus.). 680p. text 215.00 (*0-8247-0057-0*) Dekker.

Filicide: The Murder, Humiliation, Mutilation, & Abandonment of Children by Parents. Arnaldo Rascovsky. Tr. by Susan H. Rogers. 1995. LC 94-46705.Tr. of Filicidio. 304p. pap. 45.00 (*1-56821-456-1*) Aronson.

Filicidio see Filicide: The Murder, Humiliation, Mutilation, & Abandonment of Children by Parents

Filing Your Medicare - Medigap Claims & Get Quicker Payments: A Handbook. 1991. lib. bdg. 75.00 (*0-8490-4245-3*) Gordon Pr.

Filmless Radiology. Ed. by Eliot L. Siegel & Robert M. Kolodner. 1998. LC 98-3823. (Health Informatics Ser.). (Illus.). 452p. 65.00 (*0-387-98515-8*) Spr-Verlag.

Filth-Diseases & Their Prevention. John Simon. Ed. by Barbara G. Rosenkrantz. 1977. LC 76-40644. (Public Health in America Ser.). reprint ed. lib. bdg. 19.95 (*0-405-09830-8*) Ayer.

Filth-Inhabiting Flies of Guam. George E. Bohart & J. Linsley Gressitt. 1951. (BMB Ser.: No. 204). (Illus.). 25.00 (*0-527-02312-4*) Periodicals Srv.

Filtration in the Biopharmaceutical Industry. Theodore H. Meltzer & Maik W. Jornitz. 2nd ed. 1998. LC 97-43494. (Illus.). 952p. text 250.00 (*0-8247-9896-1*) Dekker.

Filtration in the Pharmaceutical Industry. Theodore H. Meltzer. 1986. (Advances in Parenteral Science Ser.: Vol. 3). (Illus.). 1120p. text 295.00 (*0-8247-7519-8*) Dekker.

Fimbriae: Aspects of Adhesion Genetics, Biogenesis & Vaccines. Ed. by Per Klemm. 1994. 292p. 229.00 (*0-8493-4894-3*, QR78) CRC Pr.

Fimetariales of Ohio (Probably III of the Ascomycetes of Ohio) Robert Stratton. 1921. (Bulletin Ser.: No. 12). pap. text 3.00 (*0-86727-011-X*) Ohio Bio Survey.

Final Accounting: Philosophical & Empirical Issues in Freudian Psychology. Edward Erwin. 1995. LC 95-8338. (Illus.). 350p. 50.00 (*0-262-05050-1*, Bradford Bks) MIT Pr.

***Final Acts of Love: Families, Friends & Assisted Dying.** Stephen Jamison. 2002. 279p. reprint ed. pap. 14.00 (*0-7567-5394-5*) DIANE Pub.

Final Analysis: The Making & Unmaking of a Psychoanalyst. Jeffrey M. Masson. 1990. 18.22 (*0-201-52368-X*) Addison-Wesley.

Final Analysis: The Making & Unmaking of a Psychoanalyst. Jeffrey M. Masson. 1998. 224p. pap. 14.00 (*0-671-02572-4*, PB Trade Paper) PB.

Final Contributions to the Problems & Methods of Psycho-Analysis. S. Ferenczi. 1994. 447p. (*1-85575-087-2*) Karnac Bks GBR. *Dist:* Other Pr LLC.

Final Exit: The Practicalities of Self-Deliverance & Assisted Suicide for the Dying. Derek Humphry. 1998. 192p. reprint ed. text 17.00 (*0-7881-5607-1*) DIANE Pub.

Final Exit: The Practicalities of Self-Deliverance & Assisted Suicide for the Dying. Derek Humphry. 2nd rev. ed. 1997. LC 96-32756. 240p. pap. 13.95 (*0-440-50785-5*, Dell Trade Pbks) Dell.

Final FRCA: Multiple Choice Questions. Michael D. Brunner et al. 2000. 320p. pap. text 32.00 (*0-7506-4214-9*) Buttrwrth-Heinemann.

Final Freedom: Pioneering Sexual Addiction Recovery. Douglas Weiss. 1998. LC 97-91762. 180p. pap. 22.95 (*1-881292-37-1*) Discov CO.

Final Lectures. Karen Horney. 1991. pap. 6.95 (*0-393-30755-7*) Norton.

Final Legacies. William D. Hartt. 1998. LC 98-38436. lib. bdg. 27.00 (*1-56072-482-X*, Nova Kroshka Bks) Nova Sci Pubs.

Final MB: A Guide to Success in Clinical Medicine. H. R. Dalton & N. J. Reynolds. 2nd ed. 1997. LC 96-25827. pap. text (*0-443-05332-4*) Church.

Final MB: A Guide to Success in Clinical Medicine. H. R. Dalton. 3rd ed. 2001. LC 00-46274. (*0-443-07006-7*) Harcrt Hlth Sci Grp.

Final Remedy. Daniel Steven. 384p. mass mkt. (*0-06-101041-3*, Harp PBks) HarperCollins Pubs.

Final Report: American Psychological Association Task Force on the Mental Health Response to the Oklahoma City Bombing. John R. Tassey. 1998. (Illus.). 108p. (C). pap. text 35.00 (*0-7881-4830-3*) DIANE Pub.

Final Report of the Michigan Commission on Death & Dying. Howard Brody et al. 1997. 205p. reprint ed. pap. text 35.00 (*0-7881-4681-5*) DIANE Pub.

Final Report of the Pooling Project on CHD. (AHA Monograph Ser.: No. 60). pap. 4.80 (*0-87493-095-2*, 73-046A) Am Heart.

Final Report of the Task Force on Quality in Australian Health Care. Ed. by Australian Health Ministers' Advisory Council Staff. 1996. (Illus.). pap. (*0-644-39703-9*) Aust Gov Pub AUS. *Dist:* Accents Pubns.

Finally There's Help for Yeast Infections. Cheryl M. Ufkin. 1996. 1.95 (*1-889868-03-5*) Shiloh Press.

Finals in Surgery: A Guide to Success in Clinical Examinations in Surgery. Alastair M. Thompson & Kenneth G. Park. 1997. LC 96-52896. text (*0-443-05768-0*) Church.

***Finals in Surgery: A Guide to Success in Clinical Surgery.** Alastair M. Thompson & Kenneth G. A. Park. 2nd ed. 2001. (Illus.). 243p. pap. (*0-443-07005-9*) Church GBR. *Dist:* Saunders.

Finance Principles for the Health Information Manager. Rose Dunn. 1999. (Illus.). 254p. pap. text 62.00 (*1-58426-006-8*, AB120899) Am Hlth Info.

Financial Aid Guide, 1994-1995. Shirley A. Wells. 1994. 107p. (C). pap. text 10.00 (*1-56900-010-7*) Am Occup Therapy.

Financial Analysis & Decision Making for Healthcare Organizations. Louis C. Gapenski. 1996. LC 96-45343. 408p. 65.00 (*0-7863-1033-2*, Irwn Prfssnl) McGraw-Hill Educ Grp.

Financial Condition of New York City Voluntary Hospitals: The First Year of NYPHRM. Susan Nesbitt & Melvin I. Krasner. 1985. (Papers: No. 2). 24p. 5.00 (*0-934459-10-X*) United Hosp Fund.

Financial Management, 1990, Level 2. 1990. 124p. ring bd. 63.00 (*1-879907-10-0*, P315) Am Soc Hlth-Syst.

Financial Management for Health Care Administrators. Ronald J. Hy. 1989. LC 89-3448. 177p. 57.50 (*0-89930-373-0*, HFM/, Quorum Bks) Greenwood.

Financial Management for Medical Groups: A Resource for New & Experienced Managers. Ernest J. Pavlock. 2nd rev. ed. 2000. 714p. 82.00 (*1-56829-021-7*) M G M A.

Financial Management for Nurse Managers & Executives. Steven A. Finkler & Christine T. Kovner. 1993. (Illus.). 616p. tchr. ed. (*0-7216-3631-4*); text 55.00 (*0-7216-3285-8*) Saunders.

Financial Management for Pharmacists: A Decision-Making Approach. Norman V. Carroll. 1991. LC 90-5886. 236p. pap. text 34.00 (*0-8121-1341-1*); 2nd ed. 1997. LC 97-8492. 273p. pap. 39.00 (*0-683-30119-5*) Lppncott W & W.

Financial Management in a Managed Care Environment. Claudia Campbell et al. 1998. LC 98-3061. 400p. (C). pap. text 66.95 (*0-8273-8133-6*) Delmar.

Financial Management in a Managed Care Environment - IML. Campbell et al. 1998. 94p. tchr. ed. 16.00 (*0-8273-8134-4*) Delmar.

Financial Management in Health Care Organizations. Robert A. McLean. 1997. LC 96-23085. (Health Services Administration Ser.). 400p. 73.95 (*0-8273-5595-5*) Delmar.

Financial Management in Health Services. Mary Courtney. 1997. 453p. pap. 82.00 (*0-8036-0338-X*) Davis Co.

Financial Management in the NHS: A Manager's Handbook. Howard J. Mellett et al. 1993. LC 93-34382. 64.95 (*0-412-47320-8*, Chap & Hall NY) Chapman & Hall.

Financial Management of Hospitals. V. M. Levy. 3rd ed. 1985. xxii, 510p. pap. (*0-455-20296-6*); 4th ed. 1992. 486p. pap. (*0-455-21060-8*) LawBk Co AUS. *Dist:* Gaunt.

Financial Management of Hospitals & Healthcare Organizations. Michael Nowicki. 1998. LC 98-36556. 300p. 52.00 (*1-56793-092-1*) Health Admin Pr.

Financial Management of the Medical Practice: The Physician's Handbook for Successful Budgeting, Forecasting & Cost Accounting. Lauretta Mink & Max Reiboldt. Ed. by Kay Stanley. 1996. (Practice Success Ser.). 54.00 (*0-89970-758-0*, OP701195AFR) AMA.

Financial Manager's Guide to Managed Care & Integrated Delivery Systems: Strategies for Contracting & Reimbursement. Paul R. DeMuro. 94th ed. 1995. LC 95-223117. 200p. (C). text 45.00 (*1-55738-623-4*, Irwn Prfssnl) McGraw-Hill Educ Grp.

Financial Planning for Health for All by the Year 2000. 1984. (SEARO Technical Publications Ser.: No. 5). 236p. pap. text 7.00 (*92-9022-144-5*) World Health.

Financial Planning for Long Term Care: A Guide for Lawyers, Caregivers, & Consumers. Ira S. Schneider & Ezra Huber. 1989. (Insight Bk.). 192p. 28.95 (*0-89885-417-2*, Kluwer Acad Hman Sci) Kluwer Academic.

Financial Trends & Insights into Managed Care. John Esposito. 1999. 360p. spiral bd. 203.50 (*1-882364-41-4*, Amer Busn Pub) Hlth Res Pub.

Financial Valuation of Your Practice. Linda G. Ginsberg. 1991. (Illus.). 384p. (C). text 49.95 (*1-878487-31-0*, ME028) Practice Mgmt Info.

Financially Competitive Healthcare Organization: The Executive's Guide to Strategic Financial... Kaufman. 1993. (C). text 60.00 (*1-55738-606-4*, Irwn Prfssnl) McGraw-Hill Educ Grp.

Financing & Organization of Universal Healthcare. Herbert Dorken. 1994. (Report to the National Academies of Practice Healthcare Utilization & Costs Ser.: Vol. 3). pap. text (*0-9637577-1-7*) Fnd Behav Hlth.

Financing Health Care. Catriona Waddington & Hilary Goodman. 1992. 80p. (C). pap. text (*0-7855-6995-2*) Oxfam Pubns GBR. *Dist:* St Mut.

Financing Health Care: Issues & Options for China. World Bank Staff. 1997. LC 97-207679. (Illus.). 92p. pap. 22.00 (*0-8213-4048-4*, C14048) World Bank.

Financing Health Care in Sub-Saharan Africa, 164. Ronald J. Vogel. 1993. LC 93-7713. (Contributions in Afro-American & African Studies Ser.: No. 164). 248p. 72.50 (*0-313-28993-X*, GM8993, Greenwood Pr) Greenwood.

Financing Health Services in Developing Countries: An Agenda for Reform. 1987. (Policy Study Ser.). 99p. pap. 22.00 (*0-8213-0900-5*, 10900) World Bank.

Financing Health Services Through User Fees & Insurance: Case Studies from Sub-Saharan Africa. R. Paul Shaw & Martha Ainsworth. 1996. LC 95-23626. (World Bank Discussion Papers: Vol. 294). 254p. pap. 22.00 (*0-8213-3396-8*, 13396) World Bank.

Financing Healthcare in the Nineteen Nineties. John Appleby. 1992. (State of Health Ser.). 160p. pap. (*0-335-09776-6*) OpUniv Pr.

Financing Rural Health Care. Ed. by LaVonne A. Straub & Norman L. Walzer. 1988. LC 87-29271. 2524p. 70.00 (*0-275-92900-0*, C2900, Praeger Pubs) Greenwood.

Financing Services for Homeless People with Mental Illnesses: Annotated Bibliography. annot. ed. 1995. 30p. (Orig.). (C). pap. text 20.00 (*0-7881-2583-4*) DIANE Pub.

Financing Your Practice: Using Business Planning & Financial Management to Your Advantage. American Psychological Association Staff. 1996. (Practitioner's Toolbox Ser.). 29.95 (*1-55798-361-5*) Am Psychol.

Finasteride, MSD: Innovation in the Management of Benign Prostatic Hyperplasia. Ed. by J. E. Altwein & L. J. Denis. 1993. (Journal: Vol. 25, Suppl. 1, 1994). (Illus.). iv, 36p. pap. 17.50 (*3-8055-5914-3*) S Karger.

FIND, Inc. Living Skills Inventories for Individuals with Deaf-Blindness. FIND, Inc. Staff. 1990. 85p. 30.00 (*0-9626896-0-2*) DeafBlind Srvcs.

Finding a Lump in Your Breast: Where to Go...What to Do. Judy C. Kneece. 1996. (Illus.). 156p. pap. 14.95 (*1-886665-04-4*) EduCare Pub.

Finding Comfort in the Zone: Encouragement & Deliverance for Women Dealing with Breast Cancer. Sheila A. Stover. Ed. by Cynthia Thompkins. 1997. (Illus.). 63p. pap. 12.00 (*0-9659846-0-5*) SAS Inc.

Finding Consciousness in the Brain: A Neurocognitive Approach. Ed. by Peter G. Grossenbacher. 2000. LC 98-51348. (Advances in Cognitive Research Ser.: Vol. 8). (Illus.). xiv, 326p. pap. 38.95 (*1-55619-188-X*) J Benjamins Pubng Co.

Finding Flow: The Psychology of Engagement with Everyday Life. Mihaly Csikszentmihalyi. 1998. LC 97-2008. (MasterMinds Ser.). 192p. pap. text 14.00 (*0-465-02411-4*) Basic.

Finding Love: Counselling for Couples in Crisis. Gabriel Kiely. 1989. 144p. pap. (*1-85371-026-1*) Poolbeg Pr IRL. *Dist:* Dufour.

Finding Meaning in Life: Logotherapy. William S. Sahakian. Ed. by Reuven P. Bulka et al. 1995. LC 95-11818. (Master Work Ser.). 396p. pap. 50.00 (*1-56821-558-4*) Aronson.

Finding Nursing in the Library: A Student Manual of Information Retrieval & Utilization Skills. Dennis C. Tucker & Joyce N. Giger. 1991. LC 90-50484. (Illus.). 78p. (C). pap. text 16.00 (*1-55605-172-7*) Wyndham Hall.

Finding Out about Asperger Syndrome, High-Functioning Autism & PDD. Gunilla Gerland. 1999. LC 99-40289. (*1-85302-840-1*) Jessica Kingsley.

Finding Resources for Healthy Heart Programs at Work. Ed. by Barry Leonard. 1998. (Illus.). 92p. pap. text 20.00 (*0-7881-7290-5*) DIANE Pub.

Finding Solutions to Social Problems: Behavioral Strategies for Changes. Ed. by Mark A. Mattaini & Bruce A. Thyer. 1996. LC 96-9216. (Illus.). 427p. text 39.95 (*1-55798-367-4*); pap. text 19.95 (*1-55798-390-9*) Am Psychol.

Finding Strength in Weakness: Help & Hope for Families Battling Chronic Fatigue Syndrome. Lynn Vanderzalm. 1995. 288p. pap. 10.99 (*0-310-20004-0*) Zondervan.

Finding the Evidence: A Gateway to the Literature in Child & Adolescent Mental Health. Ed. by Angela Scott et al. 2nd ed. 2001. 203p. pap. (*1-901242-68-4*) Royal Coll Psych GBR. *Dist:* Balogh.

Finding the Healer Within: Taking Control of Your Health. Beth Moran & Kkakthy Schultz. 1996. 234p. pap. 19.95 (*0-88737-681-9*) Natl League Nurse.

Finding the Right Treatment: Modern & Alternative Medicine: A Comprehensive Guide to Getting the Best of Both Worlds. annuals Jacqueline Krohn & Frances Taylor. 1999. LC 98-28774. (Illus.). xvi, 494p. (J). (ps-3). pap. 24.95 (*0-88179-166-0*) Hartley & Marks.

Finding the Source of Medical Information: A Thesaurus-Index to the Reference Collection. Ed. by Barbara S. Shearer & Geneva L. Bush. 1985. LC 84-22474. 225p. lib. bdg. 75.00 (*0-313-24094-9*, SBF/, Greenwood Pr) Greenwood.

Finding the Way Home: A Compassionate Approach to Illness. Gayle Heiss. 1997. LC 96-24392. 328p. 24.95 (*0-936609-35-4*) QED Ft Bragg.

Finding the Words Vol. I: Participant Manual - From the "A Path to Responsibility" Treatment Program. G. Richard Kishur. 1994. 166p. pap. text, stu. ed. 19.95 (*1-885473-01-X*) Wood N Barnes.

Finding True Magic: Transpersonal Hypnotherapy/NLP: A Radical Synthesis of Eastern & Western Perspectives & Techniques. Jack Elias. 1997. (Illus.). 296p. (Orig.). pap. 24.95 (*0-9655210-0-1*) Five Wisdoms Pubns.

Finding Ways: Recovering from Rheumatoid Arthritis Through Alternative Medicine. Barbara J. Nies. 1997. LC 96-92944. 272p. (Orig.). pap. 19.95 (*0-9653648-6-0*) Synchrony Pub.

Finding Words for Your Feelings. Lois F. Timmins. 1985. 14p. (Orig.). (C). pap. 4.00 (*0-931814-06-5*) Comn Studies.

Finding Your Balance see Healing Hip, Joint, & Knee Pain: A Mind-Body Guide to Recovery from Surgery & Injuries

Findings & Current Opinion in Cognitive Neuroscience. Ed. by Larry R. Squire & Stephen M. Kosslyn. 1998. LC 97-28491. (Illus.). 388p. pap. 39.95 (*0-262-69204-X*) MIT Pr.

Findings from Two Decades of Family Planning Research. John A. Ross & Elizabeth Frankenberg. 1993. LC 93-86577. 108p. pap. 12.00 (*0-87834-080-7*) Population Coun.

Fine Afferent Nerve Fibers & Pain. Ed. by R. F. Schmidt et al. 1987. LC 87-15625. 499p. 200.00 (*0-89573-668-3*, Wiley-VCH) Wiley.

Fine Art of Prescribing Glasses Without Making a Spectacle of Yourself. Benjamin Milder & Melvin L. Rubin. 2nd ed. 1991. (Illus.). 544p. text 78.00 (*0-937404-02-0*) Triad Pub FL.

Fine Art of Therapy. Ed. by Linda Gantt. 1980. (Conference Proceedings Ser.). 125p. (Orig.). pap. 7.00 (*1-882147-12-X*) Am Art Therapy.

Fine Black Lines: Reflections on Facing Cancer, Fear, & Loneliness. Lois T. Hjelmstad. 1993. LC 93-78394. (Illus.). 165p. (Orig.). pap. 14.95 (*0-9637139-5-7*) Mulberry Hill.

Fine Needle Aspiration Biopsy. Frable. 2nd ed. 1998. text (*0-7216-4888-6*) Harcourt.

Fine-Needle Aspiration Biopsy (FNAB) Techniques: Approved Guideline, 1996. Contrib. by Kenneth D. McClatchey. 1996. 75.00 (*1-56238-305-1*, GP20-A) NCCLS.

Fine Needle Aspiration Biopsy of the Head & Neck. Celeste N. Powers & William J. Frable. 1996. (Illus.). 253p. (*0-7506-9503-X*) E A GBR. *Dist:* OUP.

Fine Needle Aspiration Biopsy of the Liver. Martha B. Pitman & Wanda M. Szyfelbein. 1994. LC 94-15909. (Illus.). 144p. (*0-7506-9463-7*) E A GBR. *Dist:* OUP.

Fine Needle Aspiration Biopsy of the Pancreas. Barbara A. Centeno & Martha Bishop Pitman. 1998. LC 97-52016. 200p. (*0-7506-9725-3*) E A GBR. *Dist:* OUP.

Fine-Needle Aspiration Cytodiagnosis: A Color Atlas. Carlo Ravetto & P. Boccato. 1984. 210p. text (*1-57235-031-8*) Piccin Nuova.

Fine-Needle Aspiration Cytodiagnosis: A Color Atlas. Carlo Ravetto & Paolo Boccato. 1984. (Illus.). 212p. text 160.00 (*0-407-01054-8*) Buttrwrth-Heinemann.

Fine Needle Aspiration Cytology of Superficial Organs & Body Sites. Jan F. Silverman & Kim R. Geisinger. Ed. by Marc Strauss. 1999. LC 99-71799. (Illus.). 320p. text (*0-443-07963-3*) Church.

Fine Needle Aspiration Cytology of the Thorax & Abdomen. J. F. Silverman & K. R. Geisinger. 1996. (Illus.). 304p. (*0-443-07763-0*) Church.

Fine Needle Aspiration Cytopathology. Ed. by Jennifer A. Young. 1993. LC 92-48545. 368p. 199.00 (*0-632-02393-7*) Blackwell Sci.

Fine Needle Aspiration of Palpable Masses. Michael W. Stanley & Torsten Lowhagen. 1993. (Illus.). 156p. text (*0-7506-9455-6*) E A GBR. *Dist:* OUP.

Fine Structure of the Developing Epithelial Attachment of Human Teeth. H. E. Schroeder & M. A. Listgarten. 2nd rev. ed. 1977. (Monographs in Developmental Biology: Vol. 2). (Illus.). 50.50 (*3-8055-2647-4*) S Karger.

Fine Structure of the Nervous System: The Neurons & Their Supporting Cells. Alan A. Peters et al. 3rd ed. 1990. (Illus.). 528p. text 69.50 (*0-19-506571-9*) OUP.

Fine Tuning: An Auditory-Visual Training Program: Primary - Intermediate Level. Ray H. Barsch. Ed. by Betty Lou Kratoville. 1995. (Illus.). 176p. (Orig.). stu. ed. 15.00 (*1-57128-000-6*, 000-6) Acad Therapy.

Fine Tuning Bk. 1: An Auditory-Visual Training Program: Intermediate - Advanced Level. Ray H. Barsch. Ed. by Betty Lou Kratoville. 1995. 224p. stu. ed. 15.00 (*1-57128-001-4*, 001-4) Acad Therapy.

Finger Bone & Joint Injuries. Ed. by Peter Bruser & Alain Gilbert. 1999. 383p. (*1-85317-690-7*) Martin Dunitz.

Fingers & Thumbs: Toys & Activities for Children with Hand-Function Problems. Roma Lear. 1999. LC 00-500856. 134p. pap. text 25.00 (*0-7506-2524-4*) Buttrwrth-Heinemann.

Fire & the Rose: Human Core Needs & Personal Transformation. Robert G. Turner, Jr. Date not set. LC 95-38489. (Illus.). vi, 240p. pap. text (*0-936015-78-0*) Pocahontas Pr.

Fire in the Valley: The Traditional Chinese Medical Diagnosis & Treatment of Vaginal Diseases. Bob Flaws. 1991. LC 91-72618. 171p. (Orig.). (C). pap. text 18.95 (*0-936185-25-2*) Blue Poppy Pr.

Fire Inside: Distinguishing Heartburn & Related Symptoms. M. Michael Wolfe & Thomas J. Nesi. 1996. LC 95-10737. 224p. 23.00 (*0-393-03863-7*) Norton.

Fire Service Emergency Care. Edward T. Dickinson. 1998. LC 98-25811. 896p. pap. text 59.00 (*0-8359-5133-2*); (Illus.). 871p. 48.00 (*0-8359-5279-7*) P-H.

Fire Service First Responder. IFSTA Committee. Ed. by Gene P. Carlson & Lynne C. Murnane. 1987. LC 86-83301. (Illus.). 340p. (Orig.). pap. text 25.00 (*0-87939-070-0*) IFSTA.

Fire Warning & Safety Systems. William E. Koffel & David M. Birk. 1992. (Management & Compliance Ser.: Vol. 4). (Illus.). 202p. ring bd. 110.00 (*0-87258-511-5*, 055203) Am Hospital.

Firearms: A Handbook for Health Professionals. David C. Stolinsky & Timothy W. Wheeler. 1999. 28p. pap. 7.00 (*0-930783-02-6*, Dr for Respons Gun) Claremont Inst.

Firearms & Gunshot Wounds: Index of Modern Information. John C. Bartone, II. 1990. LC 88-47970. 150p. 47.50 (*1-55914-198-0*); pap. 44.50 (*1-55914-199-9*) ABBE Pubs Assn.

Firefighter & Paramedic Burnout. Gerald L. Fishkin. 1990. pap. 14.95 (*0-15-631060-0*) Harcourt.

Firepower in the Lab: Automation in the Fight Against Infectious Diseases & Bioterrorism. C. Kumar Patel. 2000. LC 2001-24533. (Illus.). ix, 299p. 69.95 (*0-309-06849-5*, Joseph Henry Pr) Natl Acad Pr.

Firesetting Children: Risk Assessment & Treatment. George A. Sakheim & Elizabeth Osborn. 1994. (Orig.). pap. 14.95 (*0-87868-579-0*) Child Welfare.

Firewalk: The Psychology of Physical Immunity. Jonathan Sternfield. 1992. LC 90-81448. (Illus.). 240p. pap. 12.95 (*0-936399-04-X*) Berkshire Hse.

Firewater Myths: North American Indian Drinking & Alcohol Addiction. Joy H. Leland. 1976. LC 75-620113. (Monographs: No. 11). 6.00 (*0-911290-43-5*) Rutgers Ctr Alcohol.

First 50 Years: The American Board of Physical Medicine & Rehabilitation. Ed. by Gordon M. Martin & Joachim L. Opitz. 1997. LC 97-71225. (Illus.). 75p. text 100.00 (*0-9657664-0-3*) ABPMR.

First a Dream: The History of Boston's Jewish Hospitals, 1896-1928. Arthur J. Linenthal. 1990. LC 90-82277. (Illus.). xxii, 727p. 33.00 (*0-9626606-0-4*) A J Linenthal.

First Aid. Bureau of Mines Staff. 1997. pap. 6.25 (*1-883205-20-4*) Intl Med Pub.

First Aid. National Safety Council Staff. (Emergency Care Ser.). (C). 1993. 178p. tchr. ed. 395.00 (*0-86720-780-9*); 1993. 176p. pap., tchr. ed. 15.00 (*0-86720-781-7*); 1993. (Illus.). 176p. pap. text 19.95 (*0-86720-755-8*, 755-8); 2nd ed. 1997. LC 97-20507. (Illus.). 144p. pap. text 22.95 (*0-7637-0418-0*, 0418-0) Jones & Bartlett.

First Aid. Ed. by National Safety Council Staff. 4th ed. 2000. LC 00-65547. (Illus.). 136p. (C). pap. text 22.95 (*0-7637-1321-X*, 1321-X) Jones & Bartlett.

First Aid: A Pocket Guide. Christopher Van Tilburg. 4th ed. 2001. (Illus.). 44p. pap. 3.50 (*0-89886-719-3*) Mountaineers.

First Aid: Emergency Care for Dogs & Cats. Roger W. Gfeller & Michael W. Thomas. 1994. 108p. pap. 19.95 (*0-9644637-0-9*) Pet Care Bks.

First Aid: Index of Modern Information. Janette K. Ruppert. rev. ed. 1991. LC 91-7266. 150p. 47.50 (*1-55914-352-5*); pap. 44.50 (*1-55914-353-3*) ABBE Pubs Assn.

First Aid: Instructor's Resource Manual. National Safety Council Staff. 2nd ed. 1997. (Illus.). 128p. pap. text 15.00 (*0-7637-0715-5*, 0715-5) Jones & Bartlett.

First Aid: Responding to Emergencies. American Red Cross Staff. 2nd ed. 1996. (gr. 13). 45.00 (*0-8151-0956-3*); pap. text 4.50 (*0-8151-0957-1*) Mosby Inc.

First Aid: Responding to Emergencies Instructor's. American Red Cross Staff. 1991. 250.00 (*0-8016-9029-3*); 416p. 6.25 (*0-8016-9023-4*); (gr. 13). disk 250.00 (*0-8016-9030-7*) Mosby Inc.

First Aid: Student Syllabus. Eva M. Bushman. 1979. (YA). (gr. 9-12). text 84.95 incl. audio (*0-89420-207-3*, 380000); pap. text 8.95 (*0-89420-075-5*, 380020) Natl Book.

First Aid Level 1: SOS Version. National Safety Council Staff & SOS Staff. 1995. (Illus.). 96p. (C). pap. text 3.65 (*0-7637-0039-8*, 0039-8) Jones & Bartlett.

First Aid - CPR Infants & Children: Instructor's Manual. National Safety Council Staff. 2nd ed. 1994. (Emergency Care Ser.). (Illus.). 128p. (C). pap. text 15.00 (*0-86720-838-4*, 838-4) Jones & Bartlett.

First Aid Afloat. Robert Haworth. 1993. 96p. (C). text (*0-906754-88-7*) Fernhurst Bks GBR. *Dist:* Motorbooks Intl, St Mut.

First Aid & Beyond: A Handbook of Homeopathic First Aid for Active Adults & Families. Suzette Hanzarotta. Ed. by Gail Burgess. 1998. (Illus.). 100p. pap. 12.95 (*0-9661285-0-8*) Natural Med.

First Aid & CPR. National Safety Council Staff. 1998. (Illus.). 104p. (C). pap. text, tchr. ed. 15.00 (*0-7637-0947-6*, 0947-6); 1991. (Illus.). 288p. (C). pap. text, tchr. ed. 10.00 (*0-86720-195-9*, 195-9); 2nd ed. 1993. LC 92-42883. (Illus.). tchr. ed. 795.00 (*0-86720-802-3*, 802-3); 2nd ed. 1993. LC 92-42883. pap., tchr. ed. 10.00 (*0-86720-791-4*) Jones & Bartlett.

First Aid & CPR. National Safety Council Staff. 4th ed. 2001. (Illus.). (C). 15.00 (*0-7637-1925-0*, 1925-0) Jones & Bartlett.

First Aid & CPR. Alton L. Thygerson & National Safety Council Staff. 4th ed. (Illus.). 2001. LC 00-65535. 152p. pap. 5.25 (*0-7637-1335-X*); 2000. LC 00-49739. 488p. (C). pap. text 40.00 (*0-7637-1319-8*, 1319-8) Jones & Bartlett.

First Aid & CPR. National Safety Council Staff. 1990. 96p. Level 1. pap. 7.50 (*0-86720-154-1*); Level 1. pap., tchr. ed. 11.00 (*0-86720-157-6*); Set. tchr. ed. 650.00 (*0-86720-161-4*) Jones & Bartlett.

First Aid & CPR: Academic Version. National Safety Council Staff. 1991. 288p. tchr. ed. 795.00 (*0-86720-194-0*); 1991. 288p. pap. 30.00 (*0-86720-193-2*); 2nd ed. 1993. LC 92-42883. pap. text 33.75 (*0-86720-785-X*) Jones & Bartlett.

First Aid & CPR: Advanced. National Safety Council Staff. 3rd ed. 1997. LC 96-21029. (Illus.). 496p. pap. text 40.00 (*0-7637-0183-1*, 0183-1) Jones & Bartlett.

First Aid & CPR: Basic. Alton L. Thygerson & National Safety Council Staff. 2000. LC 00-49738. (Illus.). vi, 58p. pap. text 12.95 (*0-7637-1684-7*, 1684-7) Jones & Bartlett.

First Aid & CPR: Infants & Children. National Safety Council Staff. 2nd ed. 1994. 208p. pap. 31.95 (*0-86720-835-X*); 3rd ed. 1998. LC 97-41585. (Illus.). 224p. (C). pap. text 29.95 (*0-7637-0633-7*, 0633-7) Jones & Bartlett.

First Aid & CPR: Instructor's Teaching Package. National Safety Council Staff. 3rd ed. 1997. tchr. ed., ring bd. 794.95 (*0-7637-0197-1*) Jones & Bartlett.

First Aid & CPR: Level 2. National Safety Council Staff. 2nd ed. 1994. 192p. pap. 12.00 (*0-86720-825-2*) Jones & Bartlett.

First Aid & CPR: Level 3. National Safety Council Staff. 2nd ed. 1994. LC 93-23167. 288p. pap. 21.00 (*0-86720-824-4*) Jones & Bartlett.

First Aid & CPR: Test Bank. National Safety Council Staff. 2nd ed. 1994. LC 92-42883. pap., tchr. ed. 50.00 (*0-86720-801-5*) Jones & Bartlett.

First Aid & CPR: Web Enhanced. National Safety Council Staff. 3rd ed. 1998. (Illus.). 468p. (C). pap. text 40.00 (*0-7637-0833-X*, 0833-X) Jones & Bartlett.

First Aid & CPR Advanced. National Safety Council Staff. 1997. (Emergency Care Ser.). 488p. pap. 33.75 (*0-7637-0530-6*) Jones & Bartlett.

First Aid & CPR Essentials. Ed. by National Safety Council Staff. 4th ed. 2000. LC 00-65536. (Illus.). 151p. (C). pap. text 22.50 (*0-7637-1324-4*, 1324-4) Jones & Bartlett.

First Aid & CPR for Infants & Children. National Safety Council Staff. (First Aid Ser.). (C). 1992. 200p. pap., tchr. ed. 15.00 (*0-86720-759-0*); 1992. (Illus.). 224p. sl. 194.95 (*0-86720-761-2*, 761-2); 1992. 224p. pap. text 22.50 (*0-86720-249-1*); First Aid. 1991. 224p. VHS 325.00 (*0-86720-273-4*) Jones & Bartlett.

First Aid & CPR for Infants & Children: Instructor's Teaching Package. National Safety Council Staff. 2nd ed. 1993. (First Aid Ser.). (Illus.). 224p. (C). tchr. ed., ring bd. 450.00 (*0-86720-800-7*, 800-7) Jones & Bartlett.

First Aid & CPR Standard. National Safety Council Staff. 3rd ed. 1997. LC 96-47633. (Emergency Care Ser.). 160p. pap. 11.25 (*0-7637-0329-X*) Jones & Bartlett.

First Aid & CPR Standard: SOS Version. National Safety Council Staff. 1997. (Emergency Care Ser.). 160p. pap. 18.75 (*0-7637-0555-1*) Jones & Bartlett.

First Aid & Emergencies: Index of Modern Authors & Subjects in Current Research. Janette K. Ruppert. 1991. 160p. 47.50 (*1-55914-466-1*); pap. 44.50 (*1-55914-467-X*) ABBE Pubs Assn.

First Aid & Emergency Care Workbook. Alton L. Thygerson. (Illus.). 352p. (C). 1988. tchr. ed., ring bd. 295.00 (*0-86720-097-9*, 097-9); 1987. pap. text, tchr. ed. 10.00 (*0-86720-085-5*, 085-5) Jones & Bartlett.

First Aid & Safety for Day Care Providers. James L. Paturas & Michael J. Werdmann. Ed. by Steven E. Reinberg. 1994. (Illus.). 100p. (C). pap. text 15.00 (*1-884225-03-9*) Communs Skills.

First Aid & Safety for Day Care Provider's Instructor's Guide. Steven E. Reinberg. 1994. (Illus.). 50p. (C). ring bd. 110.00 incl. sl., fiche (*1-884225-04-7*) Communs Skills.

First Aid Book. rev. ed. 1993. (Illus.). 237p. (C). pap. text 35.00 (*0-7881-0064-5*) DIANE Pub.

First Aid Children: Quick Parent Guide. National Safety Council Staff. 1996. (Emergency Care Ser.). 32p. (C). pap. text 10.00 (*0-86720-546-6*) Jones & Bartlett.

First Aid Companion. Robert Haworth. 2000. (Illus.). 24p. spiral bd. (*1-898660-60-3*, 128414AE) Fernhurst Bks GBR. *Dist:* Motorbooks Intl.

First Aid Companion for Dogs & Cats. Amy Shojai. 2001. LC 00-11856. (Illus.). viii, 439p. pap. 19.95 (*1-57954-365-0*) Rodale Pr Inc.

First Aid CPR: Academic. National Safety Council Staff. 3rd ed. 1996. (Emergency Care Ser.). (Illus.). 152p. pap. text, tchr. ed. 15.00 (*0-7637-0200-5*, 0200-5) Jones & Bartlett.

First Aid CPR: Test Bank. National Safety Council Staff. 3rd ed. 1996. (Emergency Care Ser.). (Illus.). 272p. pap. text 50.00 (*0-7637-0199-8*, 0199-8) Jones & Bartlett.

First Aid CPR Infant Child. National Safety Council Staff. 2nd ed. 1996. (Illus.). 196p. (C). pap. text 22.50 (*0-86720-833-3*) Jones & Bartlett.

First Aid CPR Standard. National Safety Council Staff. 1997. (Emergency Care Ser.). 136p. pap., tchr. ed. 15.00 (*0-7637-0520-9*) Jones & Bartlett.

First Aid CPR Transition Kit. National Safety Council Staff. 1997. (Emergency Care Ser.). 295.00 (*0-7637-0553-5*) Jones & Bartlett.

First Aid Essentials. Alton L. Thygerson. 1989. (Illus.). 224p. (C). pap. text 15.00 (*0-86720-116-9*, 116-9) Jones & Bartlett.

First Aid Fast. American Red Cross Staff. 1996. pap. text 5.00 (*0-8151-0908-3*); 1994. (Illus.). 84p. (gr. 13). pap. text 5.00 (*0-8151-0258-5*) Mosby Inc.

First Aid for Colleges & Universities. Brent Q. Hafen. 7th ed. 1999. 10p. (C). pap. text (*0-205-31460-0*) Allyn.

First Aid for Colleges & Universities. Brent Q. Hafen et al. 7th ed. 1998. LC 98-31203. 518p. pap. text 53.00 (*0-205-29123-6*) P-H.

First Aid for Disaster Stress Trauma Victims: A Guide & Self-Help Manual for the Lay Person Treating Disaster Stress Trauma Victims. Ralph W. Ritchie. 1995. LC 95-92032. (Emergency Procedures Ser.). 81p. (Orig.). ring bd. 11.95 (*0-939656-18-3*) Ritchie Unltd.

First Aid for Dogs. Bruce Fogle. 1997. LC 96-3400. 208p. pap. 9.95 (*0-14-025541-9*) Penguin Putnam.

First Aid for Horses. Charles H. Denning, Jr. 1981. pap. 7.00 (*0-87980-189-1*) Wilshire.

First Aid for Horses. Jacqueline Duke. cd-rom 39.95 (*1-58150-028-9*) Blood-Horse.

First Aid for Soldiers: An Army Field Manual. Department of the Army Staff. 1982. lib. bdg. 250.00 (*0-87700-402-1*) Revisionist Pr.

First Aid for the Emergency Medicine Clerkship. Latha Stead et al. 2001. (First Aid for the Clinical Clerkship Ser.). (Illus.). 300p. pap. 29.95 (*0-07-136426-9*) McGraw-Hill Prof.

E F G

First Aid for the Match. Vikas Bhushan et al. 1996. 162p. (C). pap. 29.95 (0-8385-2596-2) McGraw-Hill Educ Grp.

***First Aid for the Medicine Clerkship.** Latha Stead et al. 2001. (Illus.). 300p. pap. 29.95 (0-07-136421-8) McGraw-Hill Prof.

First Aid for the NCLEX-PN Success. Donald L. Anderson. 1998. LC 97-77501. 272p. (C). pap. 29.95 (0-8385-2601-2, A-2601-1) P-H.

First Aid for the NCLEX-RN Computerized Adaptive Testing. Donald L. Anderson. 2nd ed. 1996. LC 96-21847. 342p. (C). pap. 29.95 (0-8385-2600-4, A2600-3) P-H.

First Aid for the Neurology Clinical Clerkship. Latha Stead. 2000. (Clinical Clerkship Ser.). 200p. pap. 24.95 (0-07-136419-6) McGraw-Hill Educ Grp.

First Aid for the Office & Workplace. Shirley M. Baldwin. 1991. (Illus.). 192p. pap. 15.00 (0-87527-483-8) Green.

First Aid for the Psychiatry Clinical Clerkship. Latha Stead. 2000. LC 2001-56202. (Clinical Clerkship Ser.). 200p. pap. 24.95 (0-07-136420-X) McGraw-Hill Educ Grp.

First Aid for the USMLE II. Angelka Go & Curet. 1995. (C). pap. text 23.95 (0-8385-2591-1, A2591-4) Appleton & Lange.

First Aid for the USMLE Step 1 2001. Vikas Bhushan et al. 11th ed. 2000. (Clinical Clerkship Ser.). (Illus.). 481p. pap. 34.95 (0-07-136454-4) McGraw-Hill Prof.

***First Aid for the USMLE Step 2.** Tao Le et al. 3rd ed. 2001. 430p. pap. 29.95 (0-07-137770-0) McGraw-Hill Prof.

First Aid for the USMLE Step 2: A Student to Student Guide. Vikas Bhushan et al. 2nd ed. 1999. (Illus.). 3200p. pap. 29.95 (0-8385-2604-7) McGraw-Hill Educ Grp.

***First Aid for the USMLE Step 2: A Student to Student Guide.** Tao Le et al. 3rd ed. 2001. (Illus.). 430p. pap. 29.95 (0-07-137673-9, Apple Lange Med) McGraw.

First Aid for the Wards. Vikas Bhushan et al. 1997. 302p. (C). pap. 29.95 (0-8385-2595-4, A-2595-5) McGraw-Hill Prof.

First Aid Guide. National Safety Council Staff. (Illus.). 2nd ed. 1993. 64p. (C). pap. text 200.00 (0-86720-803-1, 803-1); Certification Cards. 1991. 1p. pap. 10.00 (0-86720-234-3) Jones & Bartlett.

First Aid Handbook. National Safety Council Staff. 1994. (Illus.). 208p. (C). text 14.95 (0-86720-943-7, 943-7) Jones & Bartlett.

First Aid Handbook. National Safety Council Staff & Alton L. Thygerson. 1995. LC 94-21032. (Illus.). 208p. (C). pap. text 10.95 (0-86720-846-5, 846-5) Jones & Bartlett.

First Aid in Counselling. Ed. by C. L. Mitton. 1977. 224p. pap. (0-567-22304-3) T & T Clark GBR. *Dist:* Bks Intl VA.

First Aid in the Workplace. Grant B. Goold. 1994. pap., tchr. ed. 32.60 (0-89303-907-1) P-H.

1st Aid in the Workplace. Goold & Dubhoff. 2nd ed. 1997. pap., tchr. ed. 32.60 (0-8359-5119-7) P-H.

First Aid in the Workplace. Grant B. Goold. 2nd ed. 1997. LC 97-12174. 144p. pap. text 24.40 (0-8359-5109-X) P-H.

First-Aid Kit for Mothers: Fill Your Pockets Full of Miracles. Nancy Swan Drew. 2000. LC 99-56534. (Illus.). xxii, 234p. text 18.95 (0-89087-861-7) Celestial Arts.

First Aid Manual: A Comprehensive Guide to Treating Emergency Victims of All Ages in Any Situation. American College of Emergency Physicians Staff. 2001. LC 00-53103. (Illus.). 288p. pap. 14.95 (0-7894-7205-8) DK Pub Inc.

First Aid Manual: General First Aid for Dogs. Siegfried Zahn. 1984. (Illus.). 106p. (Orig.). pap. 7.00 (0-912183-02-0) Univelt Inc.

First Aid Manual for Chemical Accidents. Marc J. Lefevre. 2nd ed. 1989. 272p. pap. 60.95 (0-442-20490-6); pap. 84.95 (0-471-28855-1) Wiley (VNR).

First Aid Pamphlet. Mountaineers Staff. 1996. 36p. 1.10 (0-89886-070-9) Mountaineers.

First Aid Pocket Guide. National Safety Council Staff. Date not set. 132p. pap. 47.70 (0-86720-538-5) Jones & Bartlett.

First Aid Procedures & Lifesaving Techniques & Outback Skills & Survival Techniques. Ron Dawson et al. 1995. 56p. spiral bd. (0-9647141-0-8) Ron L Dawson.

First Aid Quick. National Safety Council Staff. 1996. (Emergency Care Ser.). 32p. (C). pap. text 10.00 (0-86720-545-8) Jones & Bartlett.

First Aid to the Battlefront: Life & Letters to Sir Vincent Kennett-Barrington (1844-1903) Ed. by Peter Norris. 1992. (Illus.). 224p. (0-7509-0016-4) Sutton Pub Ltd GBR. *Dist:* Intl Pubs Mktg.

First Aid When Help Is Delayed. American Red Cross Staff. 1996. LC 96-7932. (0-8151-1576-8) Mosby Inc.

First Aid with Herbs. John Heinerman. Ed. by Richard A. Passwater & Earl R. Mindell. 1983. (Good Health Guides). 32p. pap. 3.95 (0-87983-304-1, 33041K, Keats Pubng) McGraw-Hill Trade.

First Aid Yourself: Essential Breast Cancer Websites. Betsy Dance. 2000. (Essential Websites Ser.). 128p. pap. 15.95 (0-9639531-8-4) Hope Springs.

First AIDS: Frank Facts for Kids. Carole Marsh. 1994. (Smart Sex Stuff Ser.). (Orig.). pap. 19.95 (1-55609-205-9); lib. bdg. 29.95 (1-55609-153-2) Gallopade Intl.

First Amendment Book: A Guide for Abortion Providers & Their Attorneys. NAF Legal Clearinghouse Staff. rev. ed. 1992. pap. text 15.00 (0-9601326-9-4) Natl Abort Fed.

First American Medical Association Reports on Public Hygiene in American Cities: An Original Anthology. Ed. by Barbara G. Rosenkrantz. 1977. LC 76-40663. (Public Health in America Ser.). reprint ed. lib. bdg. 21.95 (0-405-09872-3) Ayer.

First & Foremost in Community Health Centres: The Community Health Centre at Sault Ste. Marie & the CHC Alternatives. Jonathan Lomas. 1985. 215p. 30.00 (0-8020-5635-0); pap. 13.95 (0-8020-6532-5) U of Toronto Pr.

First Annual Conference on Improving Clinical Data Bases for Health Policy Development: A Meeting of Health Data Professionals. Ed. by Philip Graitcer. 1996. LC 96-79256. (Illus.). 130p. (Orig.). pap. (0-9655476-0-4) Multinatl Busn Serv.

***First Class Man in Every Particular: Dr. Sami I. Haddad (1890-1957)** Farid S. Haddad. 2001. (1-886465-05-3) Shad Board.

First Compendium of Social Network Research Focusing on Children & Young Adults: Social Networks of Children, Adolescents & College Students. Ed. by Suzanne Salzinger et al. 1988. 344p. (C). text 69.95 (0-89859-979-2) L Erlbaum Assocs.

First-Contact Mental Health Care. 1984. (Euro Reports & Studies Ser.: No. 92). 74p. pap. text 8.00 (92-890-1258-7) World Health.

First Contributions to Psycho-Analysis. S. Ferenczi. 1994. 337p. (1-85575-085-6) Karnac Bks GBR. *Dist:* Other Pr LLC.

First Course in Applied Behavior Analysis. Chance. 1997. LC 97-25987. (Psychology Ser.). 485p. pap. text 66.95 (0-534-33936-0) Brooks-Cole.

First Do No Harm: A Practical Guide to Medication Safety & JCAHO Compliance. Ed. by David Beardsley. 1998. LC 99-212067. (Illus.). 150p. pap. text 87.00 (1-57839-035-4) Opus Communs.

First, Do No Harm: Wrestling with the New Medicine's Life & Death Dilemmas. Bruce Hilton. 1991. LC 90-42190. 144p. pap. text 12.00 (0-687-13050-6) Abingdon.

First Drawings: Genesis of Visual Thinking. Sylvia Fein. 1993. (Illus.). 149p. 40.00 (0-917388-03-8); 139p. (YA). pap. text 26.00 (0-917388-04-6) Exelrod Pr.

First Due Company Officer Drill Guide. J. Steven Kidd & John Czajkowski. 1997. LC 97-212128. (Illus.). 544p. text 49.00 (0-8151-4551-9, 30220) Mosby Inc.

First Episode on Psychosis. Kathy J. Aitchison et al. 1999. 138p. pap. (1-85317-435-1) Martin Dunitz.

First Essene: Edmond Bordeaux Szekely's Last Seminar. Edmond B. Szekely. 1981. (Illus.). 240p. pap. 9.50 (0-89564-018-X) IBS Intl.

First Examination of the Newborn: A Practical Guide. Helen Baston & Heather Durward. 2000. (Illus.). 208p. 85.00 (0-415-19184-X); pap. 25.99 (0-415-19185-8) Routledge.

First Fifty Years, 1944- 1994, Society of Obstetricians & Gynaecologists of Canada. Harry Oxorn. 1994. 362p. lib. bdg. 63.95 (1-85070-562-3, Parthenon Pbng) CRC Pr.

***First Five Minutes: An Injury Prevention & Pediatric Emergency Care Handbook.** Grant Goold & Paul Marmen. 2002. 180p. pap. 26.67 (0-13-014573-4) P-H.

First Foods. rev. ed. 1980. 8p. (SPA.). (0-910869-03-0); pap. 2.00 (0-910869-02-2) Soc Nutrition Ed.

First Forty Years: The University of Alabama School of Medicine. Max Heldman. 1988. (Illus.). 86p. 35.00 (0-9621672-0-7) UASM.

First Freudians. Ed. by Hendrik M. Ruitenbeek. rev. ed. 1973. LC 73-77278. 288p. 50.00 (0-87668-694-3) Aronson.

First Group Psychotherapy Book. Edward L. Pinney, Jr. 1995. LC 95-17203. (Master Work Ser.). 224p. pap. 40.00 (1-56821-617-3) Aronson.

First Horseman. John Case. 1999. LC 99-90174. 384p. mass mkt. 6.99 (0-345-43579-6) Ballantine Pub Grp.

First International Moxifloxacin Symposium - Berlin 1999. Ed. by Lionel A. Mandell. 1999. LC 99-45431. (Illus.). 160p. 59.00 (3-540-66476-9) Spr-Verlag.

First International Symposium on Current Issues of Drug Abuse Testing. Jordi Segura & Rafael De La Torre. 1991. (Illus.). 216p. lib. bdg. 110.00 (0-8493-4283-X, HV5823) CRC Pr.

First International Symposium on the On-X Prosthetic Heart Valve Abstract Book. Ed. by Silent Partners, Inc. Staff. 1999. 32p. pap. (1-878353-49-7) Silent Partners.

First Interview: A Guide for Clinicians. James Morrison. 1993. LC 92-48703. 317p. text 35.00 (0-89862-992-6) Guilford Pubns.

First Interview: Revised for DSM-IV. Ed. by James Morrison et al. rev. ed. 1994. LC 94-32119. 317p. 40.00 (0-89862-569-6, 2569) Guilford Pubns.

First Japan Conference on Endometriosis: Pathogenesis & Progression of Endometriosis: Proceedings of the First Japan Conference on Endometriosis Held at the Hakone Prince Hotel, Kanagawa, Japan, on May 9, 1998. Ed. by H. Hoshiai et al. 1999. (Gynecologic & Obstetric Investigation Ser.: Vol. 47, Supplement 1, 1999). (Illus.). iv, 48p. suppl. ed. 25.25 (3-8055-6858-4) S Karger.

First Line Patient Care Management see Essentials of Nursing Management: Concepts & Context of Practice

First Look. Amelia Davis. 2000. LC 00-8763. (Illus.). 87p. 34.95 (0-252-02602-0); pap. 16.95 (0-252-06925-0) U of Ill Pr.

First Lox Workshop Symposium - Rationale & Study Design: Proceedings of the First Lox Workshop on Long Term Portable Oxygen Treatment in Severe Disabled COPD, Germany, Berlin, November 1990. Ed. by W. Mitlehner et al. 1992. (Journal: Vol. 59, Suppl. 2, 1992). (Illus.). vi, 46p. pap. 22.75 (3-8055-5645-4) S Karger.

First Nine Months of Life. Geraldine Lux Flanagan. 1992. 149p. reprint ed. pap. 4.95 (0-919225-26-8) Life Cycle Bks.

First Nine Months of Life. Geraldine Lux Flanagan. 2nd ed. 1982. (Illus.). 96p. pap. 11.00 (0-671-45975-9) S&S Trade.

First Opinion: Wholistic Health Care for the 21st Century. Barbara Condron. 1998. 320p. (Orig.). pap. 15.00 (0-944386-18-0) SOM Pub.

First Person Plural: My Life As a Multiple. Cameron West. 1999. 350p. mass mkt. 7.50 (0-7868-8978-0); LC 98-25740. 304p. (J). 23.95 (0-7868-6390-0) Hyperion.

First Relationship: Infant & Mother. Daniel N. Stern. Ed. by Jerome S. Bruner et al. 1977. (Developing Child Ser.). (Illus.). 160p. pap. text 12.95 (0-674-30432-2) HUP.

First Research Seminar of the ISME Commission on Music Therapy & Music in Special Education. Ed. by Rosalie R. Pratt & Helmut Moog. 1989. (Illus.). 165p. per. 11.95 (0-918812-60-7, ST 192) MMB Music.

First Responder. AAOS/NSC Staff. 1995. (Illus.). 376p. pap. text 46.95 (0-86720-530-X, 530-X) Jones & Bartlett.

First Responder. American Academy of Orthopaedic Surgeons Staff & National Safety Council Staff. 2nd ed. 1997. LC 96-48546. (Emergency Care Ser.). (Illus.). 544p. (C). pap. text 47.95 (0-86720-541-5, 541-5) Jones & Bartlett.

First Responder. J. David Bergeron & Gloria J. Bizjak. 4th ed. 1995. LC 95-11230. 544p. pap. 40.00 (0-8359-4964-8) P-H.

First Responder. Bergeron & Bizjak. 5th ed. 1998. pap., tchr. ed. 36.80 (0-8359-5273-8) P-H.

First Responder. Brent Q. Hafen & Karren. 5th ed. 1997. pap., wbk. ed. 25.67 (0-8359-5143-X); pap., tchr. ed. 36.80 (0-8359-5142-1) P-H.

***First Responder.** Bergeron & Bizjak. 6th ed. 2001. 224p. stu. ed., suppl. ed. 32.00 (0-13-032487-6) P-H.

First Responder: A Skills Approach. Keith J. Karren et al. 4th ed. 1994. LC 94-19139. 544p. pap. text 50.67 (0-89303-038-4) P-H.

First Responder: A Skills Approach. Brent Q. Hafen. 5th ed. 1997. LC 97-24631. 560p. pap. text 50.67 (0-8359-5106-5) P-H.

First Responder: Instructor's Manual. American Academy of Orthopaedic Surgeons Staff & National Safety Council Staff. 2nd ed. 1997. (Emergency Care Ser.). (Illus.). 192p. (C). pap. text, tchr. ed. 39.95 (0-7637-0464-4, 0464-4) Jones & Bartlett.

First Responder: Student Workbook. American Academy of Orthopaedic Surgeons Staff & National Safety Council Staff. 2nd ed. 1997. (Emergency Care Ser.). (Illus.). 168p. (C). pap. text, stu. ed., wbk. ed. 33.95 (0-7637-0477-6, 0477-6) Jones & Bartlett.

First Responder: Teaching Package. American Academy of Orthopaedic Surgeons Staff & National Safety Council Staff. 2nd ed. 1997. (Emergency Care Ser.). (Illus.). 3p. (C). tchr. ed. 495.00 (0-7637-0478-4, 0478-4) Jones & Bartlett.

First Responder: Test Bank. American Academy of Orthopaedic Surgeons Staff & National Safety Council Staff. 2nd ed. 1997. (Emergency Care Ser.). (Illus.). 168p. (C). pap. text 50.00 (0-7637-0465-2, 0465-2) Jones & Bartlett.

First Responder Coursebook. 2002. (Medical Examination Review Bks.). 500p. (C). pap. 42.61 (0-8385-6372-4, Medical Exam) Appleton & Lange.

First Responder in Action: A Practical Approach. Candace Brown-Nixon & Robert Nixon. 1985. (Illus.). 517p. pap. text 35.00 (0-8359-2055-0) P-H.

1st Responder Skills Approach. Keith J. Karren & Hafen. 4th ed. 1995. tchr. ed. 33.70 (0-89303-039-2) Mosby Inc.

First Responder Training Series Instructor's Manual. Walt A. Stoy. 1997. (Illus.). 408p. tchr. ed. (0-8151-8280-5) Mosby Inc.

First Sandoz Symposium on the Treatment of Parkinson's Disease, Tokyo, October 1992. Ed. by Y. Mizuno. 1993. (Journal: Vol. 33, Suppl. 1, 1993). (Illus.). vi, 70p. pap. 33.25 (3-8055-5829-5) S Karger.

First Session in Brief Therapy. Ed. by Simon H. Budman et al. 1992. LC 92-1533. 370p. 42.00 (0-89862-138-0) Guilford Pubns.

***First Session with Children & Adolescents.** Alvin E. House. 2002. LC 2001-55659. 270p. 32.00 (1-57230-750-1) Guilford Pubns.

First Step: Guidelines on Care & Recovery Following Colostomy Surgery. Kay Marshall. 2nd ed. 1990. (Illus.). pap. text (0-916999-06-8) HERC Pubng.

First Steps in Aromatherapy. 1996. pap. 11.95 (0-8464-4478-X) Beekman Pubs.

First Steps in Psychotherapy. Ed. by W. Brautigam et al. 1985. 164p. 54.95 (0-387-15042-0) Spr-Verlag.

First Steps in the Art of Intervention: A Guidebook for Trainees in the Helping Professions. David G. Martin & Allan D. Moore. 1995. LC 94-33769. 500p. text 60.95 (0-534-22272-2) Brooks-Cole.

***First Steps into the Clinical Practice of Psychotherapy.** Maxa Ott. 2001. LC 2001-22556. 50.00 (0-7657-0320-3) Aronson.

First Steps Towards an International Harmonization of Veterinary Biologicals: 1993 & Free Circulation of Vaccines Within the E.E.C. Ed. by F. Brown & P. Vannier. 1992. (Developments in Biological Standardization Ser.: Vol. 79). (Illus.). x, 238p. pap. 182.75 (3-8055-5650-0) S Karger.

First Symposium by the Six Winners of the Grants from Sandoz Foundation for Gerontological Research: Annual Meeting of the Japan Gerontological Society, Nagoya, Japan, November 1989 - Journal: Gerontology, Vol. 36, Suppl. 1, 1990. Ed. by H. Orimo. 1990. (Illus.). vi, 50p. pap. 24.50 (3-8055-5240-8) S Karger.

First Ten Years of the World Health Organization. 1958. (Illus.). viii, 538p. text 15.00 (92-4-156014-2, 1150180) World Health.

First Things: Reading the Maternal Imaginary. Mary Jacobus. 1995. LC 95-17589. 256p. (C). pap. 28.95 (0-415-90384-X) Routledge.

First 30 Years of the ESPR: The History of Pediatric Radiology in Europe. Ed. by Herbert J. Kaufmann et al. 1995. LC 93-13095. 37.95 (0-387-56541-8) Spr-Verlag.

First Three Years of Childhood. Bernard Perez. Ed. by Alice M. Christie. 1975. LC 74-21425. (Classics in Child Development Ser.). 330p. reprint ed. 31.95 (0-405-06474-8) Ayer.

First Trimester Fetal Diagnosis. Ed. by M. Fraccaro et al. 1985. LC 85-17362. (Illus.). 355p. 158.00 (0-387-15785-9) Spr-Verlag.

First Words: Selected Addresses from NLN 1894-1933. Ed. by Nettie Birnbach & Sandra B. Lewenson. 1991. 408p. 28.95 (0-88737-526-X) Natl League Nurse.

***First Year - I. B. S. - Irritable Bowel Syndrome: An Essential Guide for the Newly Diagnosed.** Heather Van Vorous. 2002. LC 2001-41044. (First Year Ser.). 272p. pap. 14.95 (1-56924-547-9) Marlowe & Co.

First-Year Baby Care. Paula Kelly. 1989. LC 83-8361. (Illus.). 144p. pap. 7.00 (0-88166-125-2) Meadowbrook.

First Year Baby Care. Ed. by Paul Kelly. rev. ed. 1989. 136p. pap. 7.00 (0-671-69206-2) Meadowbrook.

First Year of Life. H. B. Valman. 1989. (Illus.). 99p. pap. (0-7279-0224-5) BMJ Pub GBR. *Dist:* AIDC.

First Year of Life. Charlotte M. Buhler. Tr. by Pearl Greenberg & Rowena Ripin. 1975. LC 74-21402. (Classics in Child Development Ser.). 296p. reprint ed. 26.95 (0-405-06455-1) Ayer.

First Year of Life. H. B. Valman. 4th ed. 1995. pap. text (0-7279-0897-9) BMJ Pub GBR. *Dist:* AIDC.

First Year of Life: A Psychoanalytic Study of Normal & Deviant Development of Object Relations. Rene A. Spitz & W. Godfrey Cobliner. 1966. LC 68-18382. 394p. 60.00 (0-8236-1960-5) Intl Univs Pr.

First Year of Nursing: Real World Stories from America's Nurses. Ed. by Barbara Finkelstein. 1996. 160p. 19.95 (0-8027-1296-7); LC 96-12903. pap. 10.95 (0-8027-7428-8) Walker & Co.

First Year Physics for Radiographers. G. A. Hay & D. J. Hughes. 3rd ed. 1983. (Illus.). 343p. text (0-7020-0969-5) Bailliere Tindall.

Fiscal Survival of Community Mental Health in the 80's: Sharing Demonstrated Methods to Increase Revenues & Decrease Expenses: A Special Issue of Community Mental Health Journal, Vol. 21, No. 4. Ed. by James E. Sorenson. 1986. 98p. pap. 16.95 (0-89885-298-6, Kluwer Acad Hman Sci) Kluwer Academic.

Fish & Shellfish Farming in Coastal Waters. P. H. Milne. 1978. 70.00 (0-7855-6919-7) St Mut.

Fish Disease: Diagnosis & Treatment. Edward J. Noga. 2000. LC 99-58466. (Illus.). ix, 367p. 99.95 (0-8138-2558-X) Iowa U Pr.

Fish Diseases, Set. Wilhelm Schaperclaus. 5th enl. rev. ed. 1992. (Illus.). 1432p. (C). text (90-6191-950-9) A A Balkema NLD. *Dist:* Ashgate Pub Co.

Fish Diseases & Disorders Vol. 1: Protozoan & Matazoan Infection, Vol. 1. Ed. by P. T. Woo. 20th ed. 1995. LC 98-27553. 816p. text 185.00 (0-85198-823-7) OUP.

Fish Diseases & Water Chemistry. John Gratzek et al. 1993. (Aquariology Ser.). (Illus.). 150p. 19.95 (1-56465-108-8, 16858) Tetra Pr.

Fish, Fiber, & Fitness: Magic Keys to a Healthy, Vigorous, Happy Life. Edwin L. Morris. Ed. by Aubrey R. McKinney. 1989. (Adventures in Science Ser.). (Illus.). 160p. 24.95 (0-914587-05-6) Helix Pr.

Fish, Fish Oil & Human Health. Ed. by J. C. Frolich & C. Von Schacky. 1991. (Clinical Pharmacology Ser.: Vol. 5). (Illus.). 160p. text (3-88603-426-7) W Zuckschwerdt DEU. *Dist:* Scholium Intl.

Fish Medicine. Michael K. Stoskopf. 1992. LC 91-41386. (Illus.). 902p. text 125.00 (0-7216-2629-7) Saunders.

Fish Nutrition in Aquaculture. Sena S. De Silva & Trevor A. Anderson. 1994. LC 94-72448. (Chapman & Hall Aquaculture Ser.). 319p. (C). (gr. 13). pap. text 119.95 (0-412-55030-X) Chapman & Hall.

Fish Oil & Vascular Disease. Ed. by R. De Caterina & E. B. Schmidt. 1992. LC 92-49797. (Topics in Cardiovascular Diseases Ser.). (3-540-19792-3); (Illus.). 136p. 65.00 (0-387-19792-3) Spr-Verlag.

Fish Oils in Health, Disease & Health: Index of New Information with Authors, Subjects, & Bibliography. Johann D. Westervelt. 1995. LC 95-16707. 57.50 (0-7883-0666-9); pap. 47.50 (0-7883-0667-7) ABBE Pubs Assn.

Fish Oils Update. Richard A. Passwater. 1987. (Good Health Guides). 31p. pap. 3.95 (0-87983-432-3, 34323K, Keats Pubng) McGraw-Hill Trade.

Fish Pathology. R. J. Roberts. 2000. 472p. text (0-7020-2563-1) W B Saunders GBR. *Dist:* Saunders.

Fish Physiology. Ed. by W. S. Hoar & D. J. Randall. Vol. 2. 1969. text 104.00 (0-12-350402-3); Vol. 7. 1979. text 104.00 (0-12-350407-4) Acad Pr.

Fish Respiration. Ed. by Steve F. Perry et al. 1998. (Fish Physiology Ser.: Vol. 17). (Illus.). 356p. (C). 89.95 (0-12-350441-4) Acad Pr.

Fish Vaccination. Ed. by A. E. Ellis. 1988. 300p. text 62.00 (0-12-237485-1) Acad Pr.

Fish Vaccinology: Symposium Organized & Sponsored by the International Association of Biological Standardization, National Centre for Veterinary Contract Research & Commercial Services, Ltd., & National Veterinary Institute, Soria Moria Hotel, Oslo, June 1996. Ed. by R. Gudding et al. 1997. (Developments in Biological Standardization Ser.: Vol. 90, 1997). (Illus.). xiv, 490p. pap. 378.25 (3-8055-6482-1) S Karger.

Fish Viruses & Fish Viral Diseases. Ken Wolf. 1988. LC 87-47968. (Comstock Bk.). (Illus.). 480p. 80.00 (0-8014-1259-5) Cornell U Pr.

Fishbein's Illustrated Medical & Health Encyclopedia Ed. by Morris Fishbein & Justin Fishbein. 1983. LC 77-79746. (Home Library Edition). (Illus.). 39.95 (0-87475-245-0) Websters Unified.

Fisher King & the Handless Maiden: Understanding the Wounded Feeling Function in Masculine & Feminine Psychology. Robert A. Johnson. 1995. LC 92-53213. 128p. pap. 12.00 (0-06-250648-X) Harper SF.

Fisher's Contact Dermatitis. Robert L. Rietschel & Joseph F. Fowler, Jr. 5th ed. 2000. LC 00-45339. ix, 862p. text 125.00 (0-7817-2252-7) Lppncott W & W.

Fishman's Pulmonary Diseases & Disorders. Alfred P. Fishman & Jack A. Elias. 3rd ed. 1997. LC 96-26303. (0-07-021181-7) McGraw.

Fishman's Pulmonary Diseases & Disorders. Ed. by Alfred P. Fishman et al. 3rd ed. 1997. LC 96-26303. (Illus.). Vol. 1. text (0-07-021179-5); Vol. 2. text (0-07-021180-9) McGraw-Hill Med Pub.

Fishman's Pulmonary Diseases & Disorders, Set. Ed. by Alfred P. Fishman et al. 3rd ed. 1997. LC 96-26303. (Illus.). 3088p. text 415.00 (0-07-911167-X) McGraw-Hill Prof.

Fisica en la Medicina. Pina Barba & Maria Cristina. (Ciencia para Todos Ser.). (SPA.). 6.99 (968-16-2652-4) Fondo CA.

Fison's Retinal Detachment Surgery. Ed. by Arthur M. Lim. 1978. (Illus.). 68.00 (3-8055-2862-0) S Karger.

Fit & Pregnant: The Pregnant Woman's Guide to Exercise. Joan M. Butler. 1996. LC 95-32263. (Illus.). 180p. pap. 16.00 (0-937921-55-6) Acorn Pub.

Fit & Well: Core Concepts & Labs in Fitness & Wellness. Thomas D. Fahey et al. 3rd ed. 1998. LC 98-21016. 448p. (C). pap. text 30.95 (0-7674-0535-8) Mayfield Pub.

Fit & Well: Core Concepts & Labs in Physical Fitness & Wellness. Thomas D. Fahey et al. 4th ed. 2000. LC 00-23785. (Illus.). (0-7674-1679-1) Mayfield Pub.

Fit Back. 1988. (Fitness, Health & Nutrition Ser.). (Illus.). 144p. 17.27 (0-8094-6114-5); lib. bdg. 23.27 (0-8094-6115-3) Time-Life.

Fit-Famous. Ron Barnes. 1994. (Orig.). pap. 14.95 (0-9641773-1-5) Colo Cowboy.

Fit, Firm & Fifty: A Fitness Guide for Men-Women over 50. Jay Lehr & Ken Swanson. 1990. 328p. lib. bdg. 24.95 (0-87371-399-0, L399) Lewis Pubs.

Fit for Life. Harvey Diamond & Marilyn Diamond. 1987. LC 84-40457. 352p. mass mkt. 7.99 (0-446-30015-2) Warner Bks.

Fit or Fat Target Diet. Covert Bailey. 1989. LC 84-532. 144p. pap. 11.00 (0-395-51082-1) HM.

Fit Testing of Respirator Facepieces. John P. Hale. 1990. 50p. (Orig.). pap. text 35.00 (0-9626831-0-8) Respirator Support.

Fitness: Health Facts. Nora J. Krantzler & Kathleen R. Miner. 1994. LC 93-46061. 12.95 (1-56071-180-9, H300) ETR Assocs.

***Fitness after 50: It's Never Too Late to Start!** Walter H. Ettinger, Jr. et al. 2001. (Illus.). 308p. reprint ed. 25.00 (0-7881-9706-1) DIANE Pub.

Fitness & Health. Alton L. Thygerson. 1989. 352p. (Orig.). pap. 28.75 (0-86720-119-3) Jones & Bartlett.

Fitness & Wellness. Seiger et al. 1996. 54.74 net. (0-697-39579-0, WCB McGr Hill) McGrw-H Hghr Educ.

Fitness & Wellness Concepts. Corbin & Lindsey. 2nd ed. 1997. text 18.00 (0-697-29574-5) McGraw.

Fitness & Wellness for Life. William E. Prentice. 6th ed. 1998. LC 98-3936. 30.25 (0-07-109260-9) McGraw.

Fitness for Life. Philip E. Allsen. 7th ed. 2000. pap. text 18.00 (0-697-29672-5) McGraw.

Fitness for Sport. Rex Hazeldine. 1991. (Skills of the Game Ser.). (Illus.). 128p. pap. (1-85223-085-1) Crowood Pr GBR. *Dist:* Trafalgar.

Fitness for the Busy Executive in Only Ten Minutes a Day: A Lifetime Program to Stay in Shape for Your Best Top Level Performance. Oh. Date not set. (Life Management Ser.). pap. 20.00 (0-89896-243-9) Larksdale.

Fitness Made Easy. George McGlynn. 1990. 304p. text (0-697-11015-X) Brown & Benchmark.

Fitness of a Nation. Roy J. Shephard. 1986. (Medicine & Sport Science Ser.: Vol. 22). (Illus.). x, 186p. 153.25 (3-8055-4319-0) S Karger.

Fitness Tracker. Espiritu. 1992. 66.50 net. (0-697-15282-0) McGraw.

Fitness Unfolding: How to Begin & Maintain a Quality, Healthy Lifestyle. Tips, Guidelines, & Resources. Sydney Meredith. 1991. 233p. (Orig.). pap. 13.95 (0-911107-01-0) Markbks.

Fitness Wellness. Ballahue. 3rd ed. 1995. 36.74 net. (0-697-23731-1, WCB McGr Hill) McGrw-H Hghr Educ.

Fitness Without Exercise. Bryant A. Stamford. 1991. mass mkt. 12.95 (0-446-39222-7) Warner Bks.

Fits & Faints. J. B. Stephenson. 1991. (Clinics in Developmental Medicine Ser.: No. 109). (Illus.). 202p. (C). text (0-521-41196-3) Mc Keith Pr GBR. *Dist:* Cambridge U Pr.

Fits & Starts: A Genealogy of Hysteria in Modern France. Martha N. Evans. 1991. LC 91-55063. 272p. 37.50 (0-8014-2643-X) Cornell U Pr.

Fits, Faints & Falls in Old Age. M. S. Kataria. 1985. (Modern Geriatric Medicine Ser.). text 119.00 (0-85200-802-3) Kluwer Academic.

Fitting Guide for Rigid & Soft Contact Lenses. Harold A. Stein & Bernard J. Slatt. 3rd ed. 1989. (Illus.). 648p. (C). (gr. 13). text 85.00 (0-8016-5182-4, 05182) Mosby Inc.

Fitzpatrick's Dermatology in General Medicine Ed. by Irwin M. Freedberg et al. 5th ed. 1999. LC 98-37070. (Illus.). 3002p. text 350.00 (0-07-912938-2) McGraw-Hill Med Pub.

Fitzpatrick's Dermatology in General Medicine. Irwin M. Freedberg & Thomas Fitzpatrick. 5th ed. 1998. LC 98-37070. (0-07-021942-7); (0-07-021943-5) McGraw.

Five Centuries of Veterinary Medicine: A Short-Title Catalog of the Washington State University Veterinary History Collection. Compiled by J. Fred Smithcors & Ann Smithcors. 1997. LC 96-35493. (Illus.). 160p. pap. text 19.95 (0-87422-141-2) Wash St U Pr.

Five Centuries of Veterinary Medicine: A Short-Title Catalog of the Washington State University Veterinary History Collection. Washington State University Staff. 1997. LC 96-35493. (Illus.). 160p. text 36.00 (0-87422-142-0) Wash St U Pr.

5-Day Miracle Diet. Adele Puhn. 1998. mass mkt. 6.99 (0-345-91314-0) Ballantine Pub Grp.

5 Steps to Selecting the Best Alternative Medicine: A Guide to Complementary & Integrative Healthcare. Mary Morton & Michael Morton. 1996. LC 96-36134. 352p. pap. 16.95 (1-880032-94-5) New Wrld Lib.

Five Elements & Ten Stems: Nan-Ching Theory, Diagnosis, & Practice. Kiiko Matsumoto & Stephen Birch. Ed. by Robert L. Felt. 1993. (Illus.). 236p. reprint ed. pap. text 18.95 (0-912111-25-9) Paradigm Publns.

Five-Factor Model of Personality: Theoretical Perspectives. Ed. by Jerry S. Wiggins. 1996. LC 96-4859. 216p. text 35.00 (1-57230-068-X, 0068) Guilford Pubns.

Five-HT Antagonists As Psychoactive Drugs. Ed. by R. H. Rech & G. A. Gudelsky. 1988. LC 88-61898. (Illus.). 308p. 50.00 (0-916182-06-1) NPP Bks.

5-HTP: The Natural Way to Overcome Depression, Obesity & Insomnia. Michael T. Murray. 1999. 304p. reprint ed. pap. 12.95 (0-553-37946-1) Bantam.

5-HTP: The Seratonin Connection; the Exciting New Approach to Overcoming Depression, Reducing Anxiety, & Controlling Your Appetite. Othniel Seiden. 1998. LC 98-23313. 224p. pap. 14.95 (0-7615-1661-1, Prima Health) Prima Pub.

500 Formulas for Aromatherapy: Mixing Essential Oils for Every Use. Carol Schiller & David Schiller. 1994. LC 93-39895. (Illus.). 128p. pap. 12.95 (0-8069-0584-0) Sterling.

***501 Delicious Heart Healthy Recipes.** 2001. (Illus.). 496p. 19.95 (0-8487-2499-2) Oxmoor Hse.

Five Hundred Tips for Coping with Chronic Illness. Pamela D. Jacobs. rev. ed. 1994. LC 94-18785. 260p. pap. 11.95 (1-885003-04-8) R D Reed Pubs.

Five-Hydroxytryptamine in Psychiatry: A Spectrum of Ideas. M. Sandler et al. 1991. (Illus.). 368p. 85.00 (0-19-262011-8) OUP.

Five-Hydroxytryptamine-Three Receptor Antagonists. Francis D. King. 1993. 384p. 249.00 (0-8493-5463-3) CRC Pr.

Five Kids & a Monkey Investigate a Vicious Virus Vol. 1: Complete with Unit Study & Poster! Nina Riccio. 1997. (Five Kids & a Monkey Ser.). (Illus.). 32p. (J). (gr. 2-6). pap. 12.95 (0-9653955-7-X) Creative Attic.

Five Lectures on Psycho-Analysis. Sigmund Freud. Ed. by James Strachey. 1990. 73p. reprint ed. pap. 8.95 (0-393-00847-9) Norton.

Five Lessons on the Psychoanalytic Theory of Jacques Lacan. Juan-David Nasio. Tr. by David Pettigrew & Francois Raffoul from FRE. 1998. LC 97-35886. (Series in Psychoanalysis & Culture). 192p. (C). text 21.50 (0-7914-3831-7); (Illus.). pap. text 20.95 (0-7914-3832-5) State U NY Pr.

Five-Lipoxygenase Products in Asthma. Ed. by Jeffrey M. Drazen & Sven-Erik Dahl. 1998. LC 98-26626. (Lung Biology in Health & Disease Ser.). (Illus.). 496p. text 165.00 (0-8247-0167-4) Dekker.

5 Minute Clinical Consult for Dental Professionals. Ed. by James R. Hupp. 1996. LC 95-41086. 640p. 53.95 (0-683-04279-3) Lppncott W & W.

5-Minute Clinical Consult. H. Winter Griffith & M. Dambro. 1997. cd-rom 59.95 (0-683-30157-8, OP916897) Lppncott W & W.

Five-Minute Clinical Consult, 1994. Ed. by H. Winter Griffith & Mark R. Dambro. 1993. LC 92-48691. 1224p. text 52.95 (0-8121-1753-0) Lppncott W & W.

Five Minute Clinical Consult, 1995. Mark R. Dambro. Ed. by Jo Griffith. 1994. 1252p. 52.95 (0-683-03741-2) Lppncott W & W.

5 Minute Consult in Medical Toxicology. Richard C. Dart. 1998. 752p. text 79.95 (0-683-30202-7) Lppncott W & W.

5 Minute Emergency Medicine Consult. Peter Rosen et al. 1998. LC 99-22602. (Illus.). 1,290p. text 79.95 (0-683-30177-2) Lppncott W & W.

Five Minute Health Advisor. Mark R. Dambro & Bruce Goldfarb. 1998. LC 97-24984. 527p. pap. 19.95 (0-683-30435-6) Lppncott W & W.

5 Minute Massage: Quick & Simple Exercises to Reduce Tension & Stress. Robert Robert Staff. 1995. LC 95-12946. Orig. Title: Stressbusters Five Minute Massage. (Illus.). 96p. pap. 12.95 (0-8069-4200-2) Sterling.

5 Minute Ocular Consult: A Color Atlas. Daniel Gold & Richard A. Lewis. 1998. (Illus.). 750p. (0-683-03600-9) Lppncott W & W.

Five Minute Orthopaedic Consult. Paul D. Sponseller. 1998. LC 98-3652. (Illus.). 400p. text 79.95 (0-683-30088-1) Lppncott W & W.

5-Minute Patient Advisor. Mark R. Dambro & Bruce Goldfarb. 2000. LC 00-49326. xlviii, 1344p. pap. text 49.95 (0-7817-3067-8) Lppncott W & W.

5 Minute Pediatric Consult. M. William Schwartz et al. 2nd ed. 2000. LC 99-34055. (Illus.). 1,072p. text 64.95 (0-683-30744-4) Lppncott W & W.

5 Minute Pediatric Consultant. Schwartz. 2nd ed. 2000. 1,072p. 129.95 incl. cd-rom (0-683-30295-7) Lppncott W & W.

5-Minute Pediatric Patient Advisor. M. William Schwartz & Bruce Goldfarb. 2000. LC 00-58630. xv, 167p. pap. text 39.95 (0-7817-2987-4) Lppncott W & W.

5-Minute Urology Consult. Leonard G. Gomella. 2000. 832p. text 89.95 (0-7817-2284-5) Lppncott W & W.

***5-Minute Veterinary Consult: Canine & Feline PDA.** Larry P. Tilley & Francis W. K. Smith, Jr. 2001. 85.00 (0-7817-3459-2); 85.00 (0-7817-3460-6) Lppncott W & W.

5 Minute Veterinary Consult: Equine. Christopher Brown & Joseph Bertone. 2001. LC 2001-50328. 1,184p. text 89.00 (0-683-30605-7) Lppncott W & W.

5 Minute Veterinary Consultant. Larry P. Tilley. 2nd ed. 2000. LC 99-98181. (Illus.). 1,488p. text 85.00 (0-683-30461-5) Lppncott W & W.

Five Patients. Michael Crichton. 1989. 272p. mass mkt. 6.99 (0-345-35464-8) Ballantine Pub Grp.

Five Senses. rev. ed. 1992. 3.00 (0-939418-44-4) Ferguson-Florissant.

Five Stages of Getting Well. Judy E. Allen. 1993. 221p. (Orig.). pap. 14.95 (0-9627954-0-2) LifeTime OR.

Five Stages of Managed Care: Strategies for Providers, HMOs, & Suppliers. Russell C. Coile, Jr. 1997. LC 96-44119. (Orig.). pap. 48.00 (1-56793-050-6) Health Admin Pr.

Five Standards for Safe Childbearing. David Stewart et al. 4th ed. 1998. 536p. (Orig.). reprint ed. pap. text 19.95 (0-934426-72-4) NAPSAC Reprods.

Five States That Could Not Wait: Lessons for Health Reform from Hawaii, Oregon, Minnesota... Daniel M. Fox. 1995. pap. 24.95 (1-55786-607-4) Blackwell Pubs.

5 Steps to a PMS Free Life: Proven to Stop the Monthly Rollercoaster, Conquer Stress & Awaken Energy. George J. Kallins & Gloria Keeling. 2000. (Illus.). 150p. pap. 15.95 (0-9678988-0-3) Village Healer.

Five Years of Laparoscopic Cholecystectomy: A Reappraisal. Ed. by M. W. Buechler et al. 1996. (Progress in Surgery Ser.: Vol. 22, 1996). (Illus.). viii, 216p. 159.25 (3-8055-6271-3) S Karger.

Five Years Without Food: The Food Allergy Survival Guide How to Overcome Your Food Allergies & Recover Good Health. Nicolette M. Dumke. 1998. LC 97-93899. 320p. (Orig.). pap. 19.95 (1-887624-04-X) Adapt Bks.

Fixation, Dehydration & Embedding of Biological Specimens. A. M. Glauert. (Practical Methods in Electron Microscopy Ser.: Vol. 3, No. 1). 1984. 208p. pap. 32.00 (0-7204-4257-5); 1975. pap. 21.50 (0-444-10666-9) Elsevier.

Fixation Factor, in Alcohol Addition: An Hypothesis Derived from a Comparative Study of Irish-Jewish Social Norms. Robert F. Bales. Ed. by Harriet Zuckerman & Robert K. Merton. 1980. LC 79-8971. (Dissertations on Sociology Ser.). lib. bdg. 44.95 (0-405-12948-3) Ayer.

Fixed Orthodontic Appliances: Principles & Practice. J. K. Williams et al. 1995. LC 95-5741. (Illus.). 176p. 100.00 (0-7236-1001-0) Buttrwrth-Heinemann.

"Fixed Period" Controversy: Prelude to Modern Ageism, an Original Anthology. Ed. by Gerald J. Gruman & Robert J. Kastenbaum. 1979. LC 78-22186. (Aging & Old Age Ser.). lib. bdg. 19.95 (0-405-11804-X) Ayer.

Fixed Restorative Techniques. Henry V. Murray & Troy B. Sluder. Ed. by Roger E. Barton. enl. rev. ed. 1989. LC 88-39479. (Dental Laboratory Technology Manuals Ser.). (Illus.). viii, 364p. reprint ed. pap. 59.95 (0-8078-4250-8) U of NC Pr.

Fixing Health Budgets: Experience from Europe & North America. Ed. by Howard Glennerster et al. 1997. LC 95-52087. 254p. 125.00 (0-471-96497-2) Wiley.

Flap Reconstruction Surgery. Khouri. 1999. text (0-7216-5191-7) Harcourt.

Flaps: Decision Making in Clinical Practice. Franklin L. Elliott. 1996. LC 96-23107. (Illus.). 294p. 195.00 (0-387-94738-8) Spr-Verlag.

Flaps in Head & Neck Reconstruction. Ian T. Jackson. 1985. (Illus.). 464p. (C). (gr. 13). text 150.00 (0-8016-2380-4, 02380) Mosby Inc.

Flaps in Limb Reconstruction. Alain C. Masquelet & Alain Gilbert. 1995. (Illus.). 256p. text 159.00 (0-397-51420-4) Lppncott W & W.

Flash Facts for the USMLE 2 & 3. Kaiser. 1997. 200p. (C). pap. 29.95 (0-8385-2606-3, A-2606-0) McGraw-Hill Prof.

Flavins & Flavoproteins: Proceedings of the Eighth International Symposium, Brighton, England, July 9-13, 1984. Ed. by R. C. Bray et al. 1985. (Illus.). xxxiv, 923p. (Orig.). 257.70 (3-11-009879-2) De Gruyter.

Fleeting Memories: Cognition of Brief Visual Stimuli. Ed. by Veronika Coltheart. 1999. LC 98-36547. (Cognitive Psychology: A Bradford Book Ser.). (Illus.). 300p. 35.00 (0-262-03261-9, Bradford Bks) MIT Pr.

Flesh & Blood. 1980. LC 80-65769. (Illus.). (Orig.). pap. 17.50 (0-936618-01-9) Genotype.

Flesh of My Flesh: The Ethics of Cloning Humans: A Reader. Stephen Jay Gould et al. Ed. by Gregory F. Pence. 1998. LC 98-11287. 160p. pap. 12.95 (0-8476-8982-4) Rowman.

Flesh of My Flesh: The Ethics of Cloning Humans: A Reader. Ed. by Gregory E. Pence. 1998. LC 98-11287. 160p. 54.50 (0-8476-8981-6) Rowman.

Flexible Bodies: The Role of Immunity in American Culture from the Days of Polio to the Age of AIDS. Emily Martin. 1995. LC 93-39065. (Illus.). 336p. (C). pap. text 13.00 (0-8070-4627-2) Beacon Pr.

Flexible Endoscopy of the Urinary Tract. Ralph V. Clayman. 2001. (Illus.). 350p. pap. text 90.00 (0-942219-98-8) Quality Med Pub.

Flexible Sigmoidoscopy. Ed. by Ronald Katon et al. 1985. 192p. text 74.00 (0-8089-1701-3, 792251, Grune & Strat) Harcrt Hlth Sci Grp.

Flexible Sigmoidoscopy. Douglas K. Rex & Blair S. Lewis. 1995. LC 95-22330. 200p. pap. 46.95 (0-86542-369-5) Blackwell Sci.

Flexible Sigmoidoscopy Indications & Techniques. Wu. 1991. (0-8151-9071-9) Mosby Inc.

Flexible Work Arrangements: Managing the Work-Family Boundary. Raymond H. Gottlieb et al. 1998. LC 97-34185. (Work, Well-Being, & Stress Ser.). (Illus.). 204p. pap. 80.00 (0-471-96228-7) Wiley.

Flexner: Seventy-Five Years Later: A Current Commentary on Medical Education. Ed. by Charles Vevier. 1987. 124p. 38.00 (0-8191-6140-3) U Pr of Amer.

Flexor Tendon Injuries. Lawrence H. Schneider. 1985. (Illus.). 183p. 80.00 (0-316-77401-4, Little Brwn Med Div) Lppncott W & W.

Flight for Life: A Matter of Life & Death. Opal Cavitt. Ed. by Marie Hassell. 1990. (Illus.). 157p. 29.95 (1-878394-12-6) Sanuk.

Flight Nursing: Principles & Practice. Renee S. Holleran & National Flight Nurses Association Staff. 2nd ed. 1996. LC 96-230087. (Illus.). 752p. (C). (gr. 13). text 66.95 (0-8151-7471-3, 28278) Mosby Inc.

Flight Nursing Core Curriculum. Pamela J. Adams et al. Ed. by Debra T. Krupa. unabr. ed. 1997. 845p. pap. text 45.00 (0-935890-12-2) Emerg Nurses IL.

Flint's Emergency Treatment & Management. Harvey D. Cain. 7th ed. 1985. (Illus.). 842p. text 65.00 (0-7216-2313-1) Saunders.

Flip & See ECG. Elizabeth C. Cohn & Mary Gilroy-Doohan. 1995. (Illus.). 120p. pap. text 21.95 (0-7216-5834-2) Saunders.

Flock: The Autobiography of a Multiple Personality. Joan F. Casey & Lynn Wilson. 1992. 320p. pap. 12.95 (0-449-90732-5, Columbine) Fawcett.

Flooding & Implosive Therapy: Direct Therapeutic Exposure in Clinical Practice. Ed. by Patrick A. Boudewyns & Robert H. Shipley. 1983. LC 83-2380. 248p. 49.50 (0-306-41155-5, Plenum Trade) Perseus Pubng.

E
F
G

Floor Plan Book: Veterinary Hospital & Boarding Kennel Planning & Design, Vol. 2. E. John Knapp. 1996. (Illus.). 301p. pap. 89.95 (*0-935078-59-2*) Veterinary Hlthcare.

Floppy Infant. Ed. by Victor Dubowitz. 2nd ed. 1993. (Clinics in Developmental Medicine Ser.: Vol. 76). 158p. (C). text (*0-521-41203-X*) Mc Keith Pr GBR. *Dist:* Cambridge U Pr.

Flora Medica: Botanical Account of More Important Plants Used in Medicine. L. Lindley. 1988. (C). (*0-7855-2295-6*) Scientific GBR. *Dist:* St Mut.

Flora Mycologica Argentina: Hongos II (Fungi II) J. Raithelhuber. 1988. (SPA., Illus.). 287p. pap. 35.00 (*3-9801550-2-1*) Lubrecht & Cramer.

Florence Nightingale. Basil Miller. 1987. LC 87-71602. (Women of Faith Ser.). 128p. reprint ed. mass mkt. 4.99 (*0-87123-985-X*) Bethany Hse.

Florence Nightingale: An Environmental Adaptation Theory. Louise C. Selanders. 1993. (Notes on Nursing Theories Ser.: Vol. 9). (Illus.). 38p. (C). pap. 14.95 (*0-8039-4860-3*, 4736) Sage.

***Florence Nightingale: An Introduction to Her Life & Family.** Ed. by Lynn McDonald. 2001. (Collected Works of Florence Nightingale: Vol. 1). 512p. text 75.00 (*0-88920-387-3*) Wilfrid Laurier.

Florence Nightingale: Saint, Reformer, or Rebel? Raymond G. Hebert. 1981. LC 80-28473. 246p. pap. 13.50 (*0-89874-127-0*) Krieger.

Florence Nightingale & Her Era: A Collection of New Scholarship. Vern Bullough et al. 1990. LC 89-25949. 400p. text 20.00 (*0-8240-6998-6*, SS629) Garland.

Florence Nightingale & the Nursing Legacy: Building the Foundation of Modern Nursing & Midwifery. Monica Baly. 2nd ed. 1998. LC 98-70738. (Illus.). 256p. 19.95 (*1-891696-01-7*) BainBridgeBooks.

Florence Nightingale Jones in Tender Loving Comedy. Thelma Canarecci & Laura Canarecci. 1986. LC 86-50693. (Illus.). 100p. pap. 9.95 (*0-9617081-0-7*) Power NY.

Florida Health Care in Perspective 1999. Ed. by Kathleen O'Leary Morgan & Scott E. Morgan. 1999. 21p. spiral bd. 19.00 (*0-7401-0058-0*) Morgan Quitno Corp.

Florida Health Care in Perspective 2000. Ed. by Kathleen O'Leary Morgan & Scott E. Morgan. 2000. 21p. spiral bd. 19.00 (*0-7401-0208-7*) Morgan Quitno Corp.

Florida Health Care Reference, 1994-95. Richard F. Polangin & Ernest Feigenbaum. Ed. by Creston Nelson-Morrill. 1994. LC 95-122389. 320p. pap. 12.95 (*1-879919-88-5*) HealthTrac.

Florida Healthcare & Legal Guide. Joseph M. Taraska. 1995. 500p. lib. bdg. 125.00 (*1-57444-036-5*, SL0365) St Lucie Pr.

Florida Project Development Manual: A Guide to Planning, Design & Construction of Healthcare Facilities in the State of Florida. Kenneth N. Dickerman et al. 1994. (Illus.). 216p. pap. 39.95 (*1-881556-03-4*) Hlth Facility.

Flouride the Aging Factor: How to Avoid the Devastating Effects of Flouride. John Yiamouyiannis. 3rd ed. 1993. (Illus.). 300p. pap. 14.95 (*0-913571-03-2*) Health Act Pr.

Flourishing Yin: Gender in China's Medical History, 960-1665. Charlotte Furth. 1998. LC 97-38116. (Illus.). 343p. pap. 18.95 (*0-520-20829-3*); text 48.00 (*0-520-20828-5*) U CA Pr.

Flow Cytogenetics. Ed. by Joe W. Gray. 1990. (Analytical Cytology Ser.). 312p. text 94.00 (*0-12-296110-2*) Acad Pr.

Flow Cytometry & Cell Sorting. Ed. by A Radbruch. 1996. (Illus.). 223p. 79.95 (*0-387-55594-3*) Spr-Verlag.

Flow Cytometry & Clinical Diagnosis. David F. Keren et al. 1994. 665p. 35.00 (*0-89189-346-6*) Am Soc Clinical.

Flow Cytometry in Hematology. Ed. by Ole D. Laerum & R. Bjerknes. 1992. (Analytical Cytology Ser.). (Illus.). 272p. text 115.00 (*0-12-432940-3*) Acad Pr.

Flow Dependent Regulation of Vascular Function. Ed. by John A. Bevan et al. 1995. (Clinical Physiology Ser.). (Illus.). 384p. text 89.50 (*0-19-507842-X*) OUP.

Flow Diagrams in Advanced Cancer & Other Disease. C. Regnard & J. M. Hockley. 1996. 120p. pap. (*0-340-61389-0*) E A GBR. *Dist:* OUP.

Flow Injection Analysis of Pharmaceuticals: Automation in the Laboratory. J. Martinez Calatayud. 1996. LC 97-116588. 250p. (*0-7484-0445-7*) Tay Francis Ltd GBR. *Dist:* Taylor & Francis.

Flower Dolls: Essays in Child Psychotherapy. Francoise Dolto & John Howe. 1998. 224p. (Orig.). pap. 22.95 (*0-7145-3026-3*) M Boyars Pubs.

Flower Essence Repertory. Patricia A. Kaminski & Richard A. Katz. rev. ed. 1994. LC 91-90677. (Illus.). 416p. pap. 19.95 (*0-9631306-1-7*) Flower Essence.

Flower Essences. Carol Rudd. 1998. LC 98-6434. (Illustrated Guides Ser.). (Illus.). 144p. pap. 19.95 (*1-86204-167-9*) Element MA.

Flower Remedies: Natural Healing with Flower Essences. Christine Wildwood. 1996. (Health Essentials Ser.). (Illus.). 128p. pap. 9.95 (*1-85230-336-0*) Element MA.

Flower Remedy Book: A Comprehensive Guide to over 700 Remedies. Jeffrey Shapiro. 1999. LC 98-39493. xii, 282p. pap. text 19.95 (*1-55643-296-8*) North Atlantic.

Flowering of a Waratah: A History of Australian Neurology & of the Australian Association... Mervyn J. Eadie. 2000. LC 2001-320801. (Illus.). 264p. (*0-86196-606-6*) John Libby GBR. *Dist:* Buttrwrth-Heinemann.

Flowers & Silver MCAT. James Flowers. 4th ed. 1998. LC 95-4454. (Princeton Review Ser.). (Illus.). 1072p. pap. 50.00 (*0-375-75003-7*) Random.

Flowers Can Heal Vol. 1: Essences Vibrational Therapy. Gilda Lee. 1997. (Illus.). (Orig.). pap. 11.00 (*0-9695954-0-9*) In The Pink.

Flowers of Ecstasy & Immortality: The Folklore, Medicinal & Psychopharmacology of Sacred Lotus & Water Lily Plants of Both Egypt & India. David Spess. 2000. (Ethnopharmacology Ser.). (Illus.). 300p. 49.95 (*0-935548-10-6*) Codex Pr.

Flu: The Story of the Great Influenza Pandemic of 1918 & the Search for the Virus That Caused It. Gina Kolata. l.t. ed. 2000. LC 00-25171. (G. K. Hall Nonfiction Ser.). 455p. 28.95 (*0-7838-9019-2*, Macmillan Ref) Gale.

Fluff My Pillow, Bend My Straw: The Evolution & Undoing of a Nurse. Joan Brady. Ed. by Mary L. Diecker. 1992. LC 92-61477. (Illus.). 195p. pap. 14.95 (*1-880254-02-6*) Vista.

Fluid & Drug Delivery System Markets: Patients on the Move: Patches, Ambulatory Packs & Implants. Market Intelligence Staff. 1993. 305p. 2295.00 (*1-56753-502-X*) Frost & Sullivan.

Fluid & Electrolyte Abnormalities in Exocrine Glands in Cystic Fibrosis. Ed. by P. M. Quinton et al. 1982. (Illus.). 15.00 (*0-911302-45-X*) San Francisco Pr.

Fluid & Electrolyte Balance. Norma Milligan Metheny. 4th ed. 2000. LC 99-42877. (Illus.). 456p. pap. text 29.95 (*0-7817-2072-9*) Lppncott W & W.

Fluid & Electrolytes. 1994. (Illus.). 96p. pap. text, wbk. ed. 9.95 (*0-87434-724-6*) Springhouse Corp.

Fluid & Electrolytes. Priscilla LeMone. 2nd ed. 1999. 55p. (C). pap. 9.95 (*0-8053-8128-7*) Benjamin-Cummings.

Fluid & Solute Transport in the Airspaces of the Lungs. Ed. by Richard M. Effros & H. K. Chang. 1993. (Lung Biology in Health & Disease Ser.: Vol. 70). (Illus.). 568p. text 245.00 (*0-8247-8849-4*) Dekker.

Fluid Balance & Volume Resuscitation for Beginners: A Practical Guide. Ed. by G. R. Park & P. G. Roe. 2000. (Illus.). 150p. pap. text (*1-900151-54-5*) Greenwich Med GBR. *Dist:* OUP, JAMCO Dist.

Fluid Dynamics As a Localizing Factor for Atherosclerosis. Ed. by C. Diehm et al. 1983. (Illus.). 230p. 45.00 (*0-387-12393-8*) Spr-Verlag.

Fluid, Electrolyte, & Acid-Base Balance: A Case Study Approach, No. 1. Mima M. Horne et al. 1990. (Illus.). 464p. (C). (gr. 13). pap. text 27.95 (*0-8016-5479-3*, 05479) Mosby Inc.

Fluid, Electrolyte & Acid-Base Disorders. Allen I. Arieff & Ralph A. DeFronzo. 2nd ed. 1995. LC 95-19811. 946p. text (*0-443-08774-1*) Church.

Fluid Electrolyte & Acid-Base Regulation: Physiology & Pathophysiology. Jack L. Keyes. 1990. LC 84-21925. (Life Science Ser.). 288p. (C). pap. text 40.00 (*0-86720-389-7*) Jones & Bartlett.

Fluid Exchanges: Artists & Critics in the Age of AIDS. James Miller. 1992. LC 92-195657. 700p. pap. 22.95 (*0-8020-6824-3*); 810p. text 50.00 (*0-8020-5892-2*) U of Toronto Pr.

Fluid Physiology & Pathology in Traditional Chinese Medicine. Steven Clavey. 1995. LC 94-39411. text (*0-443-04362-0*) Church.

Fluid Therapy, Electrolytes, & Acid-Base Balance in Veterinary Practice. Sam B. Basilious. 1993. (Veterinary Medicine Ser.). (Illus.). 350p. (Orig.). (C). text 99.99 (*0-9630843-9-9*); text 399.99 incl. disk (*0-9630843-8-0*); text, stu. ed. 49.99 (*0-9630843-6-4*) Infoconnect.

Fluid Therapy in Small Animal Practice. Stephen P. DiBartola. (Illus.). (C). 1992. 736p. text 89.00 (*0-7216-3182-7*); 2nd ed. 1999. LC 99-46857. xii, 611p. text 89.00 (*0-7216-7739-8*) Saunders.

Fluids & Electrolytes. Sheryl A. Innerarity & June L. Stark. 3rd ed. 1997. LC 96-40891. (Springhouse Notes Ser.). 192p. pap. 26.95 (*0-87434-902-8*) Springhouse Corp.

Fluids & Electrolytes. Juha P. Kokko & Richard L. Tannen. Ed. by Ray Kersey. 3rd ed. 1996. LC 95-17723. 800p. text 180.00 (*0-7216-5318-9*) Saunders.

Fluids & Electrolytes: A Practical Approach. Carla A. Lee et al. 4th ed. 1996. (Illus.). 360p. pap. 28.95 (*0-8036-5531-2*) Davis Co.

Fluids & Electrolytes in the Surgical Patient. Carlos Pestana. 5th ed. 1999. LC 99-40625. 192p. pap. text 49.95 (*0-7817-2425-2*) Lppncott W & W.

Fluids & Electrolytes Made Incredibly Easy. Ed. by Patricia Shaw. 1997. LC 96-47450. (Made Incredibly Easy Ser.). (Illus.). 328p. (Orig.). pap. 34.95 (*0-87434-886-2*) Springhouse Corp.

Fluids & Electrolytes with Clinical Applications: A Programmed Approach. Joyce L. Kee & Betty J. Paulanka. 5th ed. 1994. LC 93-46613. 645p. (C). pap. 42.95 (*0-8273-5134-8*) Delmar.

Fluids & Electrolytes with Clinical Applications: A Programmed Approach. Joyce Kee & Betty Paulanka. 6th abr. rev. ed. 1999. LC 98-37022. 672p. spiral bd. 43.95 (*0-7668-0332-5*) Delmar.

***Fluids, Electrolytes & Acid-Base Balance: Review & Rationales.** Mary A. Hogan & Daryle Wane. 2001. 288p. pap. 24.95 (*0-13-030454-9*) P-H.

Fluorescein & ICG Angiography: Textbook & Atlas. Gisbert Richard. Tr. by Frederick C. Blodi. 2nd ed. 1998. LC 97-34734. (Illus.). 412p. 169.00 (*0-86577-712-8*) Thieme Med Pubs.

Fluorescein & Indocyanine Green Angiography: Technique & Interpretation. Joseph W. Berkow. 2nd ed. 1997. LC 97-19753. (Ophthalmology Monographs). (*1-56055-044-9*) Am Acad Ophthal.

Fluorescein Angiography: Technique, Interpretation, & Application. Max Nanjiani. 1992. (Illus.). 144p. 79.50 (*0-19-261932-2*) OUP.

Fluorescein Angiography-Angiographie Fluoresceinique: Proceedings of the International Symposium, Albi, 1969. International Symposium on Fluorescein Angiography. Ed. by P. Amalric. 1972. (Illus.). 600p. 152.25 (*3-8055-1264-3*) S Karger.

Fluorescein Angiography in the Anterior Eye Segment. S. N. Fyodorov. 1991. 172.00 (*0-8493-7129-5*, RE78) CRC Pr.

Fluorescein Angiography. Harney. 1994. text (*0-7234-2044-0*) Wolfe Publishing GBR. *Dist:* Mosby Inc.

Fluorescence & Phosphorescence Spectroscopy: Physicochemical Principles & Practice. Stephen G. Schulman. 1977. (*0-08-020499-6*) Pergamon Repr GBR. *Dist:* Franklin.

Fluoridation: The Great Dilemma. George L. Waldbott et al. 1978. (Illus.). 14.95 (*0-87291-097-0*) Coronado Pr.

Fluoride in Preventive Dentistry. James R. Mellberg & Louis W. Ripa. 1983. (Illus.). 1288p. text 84.00 (*0-86715-102-1*) Quint Pub Co.

Fluorides & Dental Fluorosis. H. M. Myers. 1978. (Monographs in Oral Science: Vol. 7). (Illus.). 34.00 (*3-8055-1412-3*) S Karger.

Fluorides & Human Health. P. Adler et al. 1970. (Monographs: No. 59). 364p. pap. text 42.00 (*92-4-140059-5*, 1140059) World Health.

Fluorides & Oral Health: Report of a WHO Expert Committee on Oral Health Status & Fluoride Use. 1994. LC 95-130398. (WHO Technical Reports: No. 846). (CHI, ENG, FRE & SPA.). v, 37p. pap. text 8.00 (*92-4-120846-5*, 1100846) World Health.

Fluorinated Carbohydrates: Chemical & Biochemical Aspects. Ed. by N. F. Taylor. 1988. LC 88-19332. (ACS Symposium Ser.: No. 374). (Illus.). x, 214p. 49.95 (*0-8412-1492-1*) Am Chemical.

Fluorine-Containing Amino Acids: Synthesis & Properties. Ed. by V. P. Kukhar & V. A. Soloshonok. 1995. LC 94-13954. 422p. 355.00 (*0-471-95203-6*) Wiley.

Fluorine Coupling Constants. James W. Emsley & L. Phillips. 1977. LC 66-17931. (Progress in Nuclear Magnetic Resonance Spectroscopy Ser.: Vol. 10: 3-4). (*0-08-019464-8*) Pergamon Repr GBR. *Dist:* Franklin.

Fluorometric Analysis in Biomedical Chemistry: Trends & Techniques Including HPLC Applications. Norio Ichinose et al. 1991. LC 90-12271. (Chemical Analysis Monographs: Vol. 109). 225p. 170.00 (*0-471-52258-9*) Wiley.

Fluoroscopy Manual for Pain Management. Tina McKay Best. 2000. (Illus.). 178p. pap. text 80.00 (*0-9678176-0-9*) Pain Mgmt.

Fluoxetine (Prozac, Fluoxetine HCl) Index of New Information with Authors & Subjects. American Health Research Institute Staff. 1992. LC 92-54234. 150p. 47.50 (*1-55914-616-8*); pap. 44.50 (*1-55914-617-6*) ABBE Pubs Assn.

Flux Control in Biological Systems: From Enzymes to Populations & Ecosystems. Ed. by Ernst-Detlef Schulze. 1994. (Physiological Ecology Ser.). (Illus.). 494p. text 136.00 (*0-12-633070-0*) Acad Pr.

Flying Honeybee: Aspects of Energetics. Ed. by Werner Nachtigall. 1989. (BIONA Report Ser.: No. 6). (ENG & GER.). 148p. pap. text 41.00 (*0-89574-289-6*) Gustav Fischer DEU. *Dist:* Lubrecht & Cramer, Balogh.

Flynn's Hand Surgery. Jesse B. Jupiter. 4th ed. 1990. (Illus.). 1037p. 150.00 (*0-683-04490-7*) Lppncott W & W.

FMGEMS Examination Review: Clinical Sciences, Vol. 2. B. A. Allen et al. 3rd ed. 1986. 226p. pap. 27.00 (*0-444-01042-4*) Elsevier.

FMLA Guide: Practical Solutions to Administration & Management. Alexander Consulting Group. 1995. LC 95-33566. (Illus.). 583p. (C). text 50.00 (*0-7863-0535-5*, Irwn Prfssnl) McGraw-Hill Educ Grp.

Foal in the Womb. A. W. Marrable. 1990. (Illus.). 142p. pap. (*0-85131-345-0*) J A Allen GBR. *Dist:* St Mut.

Focal Group Psychotherapy: For Mental Health Professionals. Ed. by Matthew McKay & Kim Paleg. 1994. LC 92-54160. 544p. text 59.95 (*1-879237-18-0*) New Harbinger.

Focal Peripheral Neuropathies. John D. Stewart. 3rd ed. 2000. LC 99-33661. (Illus.). 592p. text 110.00 (*0-7817-1717-5*) Lppncott W & W.

Focus Charting: Documentation for Patient Centered Care. Susan Lampe. 7th rev. ed. 1997. 431p. pap. (*1-886624-06-2*, B250) Creative Nursing.

Focus on Anesthetics for Patients. S. Samra. 2001. (Focus on Ser.). 100p. pap. text 19.95 (*1-873413-27-0*) Merit Pub Intl.

Focus on Angiotensin-Converting Enzyme Inhibition. Ed. by J. Rosenthal. 1990. (Journal: Vol. 8, Suppl. 1, 1990). (Illus.). iv, 52p. pap. 17.50 (*3-8055-5258-0*) S Karger.

Focus on Beta-Adrenergic Blockade: Journal: Clinical Physiology & Biochemistry, Supplement 2, 1990, Vol. 8. Ed. by J. Rosenthal. 1991. (Illus.). iv, 56p. pap. 18.50 (*3-8055-5329-3*) S Karger.

Focus on Eating Disorders. M. Sean O'Halloran. 1993. LC 93-37136. (Teenage Perspectives Ser.). 297p. lib. bdg. 39.50 (*0-87436-692-5*) ABC-CLIO.

Focus on Electrocardiograph. Gareth Mallon. 2001. (Focus on Ser.). (Illus.). 100p. pap. text 23.95 (*1-873413-04-1*) Merit Pub Intl.

***Focus on Glaucoma: A Community Guide & 2001 Resource Directory.** Ed. by Barry Leonard. 2001. (Illus.). 60p. (C). pap. 25.00 (*0-7567-0938-5*) DIANE Pub.

Focus on Group Psychotherapy: Clinical Essays. Saul Scheidlinger. 1982. LC 82-53. 264p. 40.00 (*0-8236-1990-7*) Intl Univs Pr.

Focus on Health. ABC Staff et al. 1993. 160p. (C). pap. text 29.33 (*0-13-007121-8*) P-H.

Focus on Health. Dale B. Hahn & Wayne A. Payne. 3rd ed. 1997. 14.06 (*0-8151-3385-5*) Mosby Inc.

Focus on Health: Issues & Events of 1978 from the New York Times Information Bank. Ed. by Arthur Levin & Mitchell Rapoport. 1980. LC 78-31464. (News in Print Ser.). lib. bdg. 30.95 (*0-405-12874-6*) Ayer.

Focus on Health: Issues & Events of 1979. Ed. by Helen Zelon. 1981. LC 80-1719. (News in Print Ser.). (Illus.). lib. bdg. 30.95 (*0-405-12879-7*) Ayer.

***Focus on Health with Healthquest 3.0 & Learning to Go.** Dale B. Hahn & Wayne A. Payne. 5th ed. 2001. pap. 47.50 incl. audio compact disk (*0-07-253066-9*) McGrw-H Hghr Educ.

***Focus on Health with Healthquest 2.0.** 5th ed. 2001. 35.75 incl. cd-rom (*0-07-246694-4*) McGraw.

Focus on Pathophysiology. Barbara L. Bullock & Reet Henze. 1999. LC 99-16400. 1,264p. pap. text 56.95 (*0-7817-1736-1*) Lppncott W & W.

Focus on Physical Impairments. Nicholas Karolides, Jr. 1990. LC 90-47032. (Teenage Perspectives Ser.). 332p. lib. bdg. 39.50 (*0-87436-428-0*) ABC-CLIO.

Focus on Practical - Vocational Nursing. 1997. (Nursing DataSource, 1997 Ser.: Vol. III). 80p. 35.00 (*0-88737-753-X*, 19-753X, NLN Pr) Natl League Nurse.

Focus on Psychodrama: The Therapeutic Aspects of Psychodrama. Peter F. Kellerman. 1992. 160p. pap. text 27.00 (*1-85302-127-X*) Taylor & Francis.

Focus on Psychopharmacologic Interventions in Late Life. Ed. by Ira Katz et al. 1999. (Annual Review of Gerontology & Geriatrics Ser.: Vol. 19). (Illus.). 288p. text 54.00 (*0-8261-6502-8*) Springer Pub.

Focus on Pulmonary Pharmacology & Toxicology, Vol. I. Ed. by Mannfred A. Hollinger. 1988. 176p. 94.00 (*0-8493-4191-4*, RC, CRC Reprint) Franklin.

Focus on Pulmonary Pharmacology & Toxicology, Vol. 2. Mannfred A. Hollinger. 1990. (Illus.). 208p. 131.00 (*0-8493-4192-2*, CRC Reprint) Franklin.

Focus on the Family Complete Book of Baby & Child Care. Paul C. Reisser & Focus on the Family Staff. 1997. LC 97-23617. 928p. 29.99 (*0-8423-0889-X*) Tyndale Hse.

Focus on the Future: The Next Ten Years. Ed. by Linda Gantt & Audrey Evans. 1979. (Conference Proceedings Ser.). 151p. (Orig.). pap. 6.00 (*1-882147-10-3*) Am Art Therapy.

Focus on Vision. Robert A. Weale. 1983. (Illus.). 208p. pap. 20.50 (*0-674-30701-1*) HUP.

Focused Expressive Psychotherapy: Freeing the Overcontrolled Patient. Roger J. Daldrup et al. 1988. LC 88-21183. 233p. 33.00 (*0-89862-729-X*, 2729) Guilford Pubns.

Focused Psychotherapy: A Casebook of Brief, Intermittent Psychotherapy Throughout the Lifecycle. Nick Cummings & Mike Sayama. 1995. LC 95-19865. 272p. text 32.95 (*0-87630-789-6*) Brunner-Routledge.

Focusing Hypothesis: The Theory of Left Hemisphere Lateralised Language Re-examined. Alison Wray. 1992. LC 92-36730. (Studies in Speech Pathology & Clinical Linguistics: Vol. No. 3). xiv, 207p. 65.00 (*1-55619-389-0*) J Benjamins Pubng Co.

Focusing on Modern Microscopy: An Introduction from General Principles to Bioimaging. Alberto Diaspro. 2000. 352p. 79.95 (*0-7803-3414-0*, PC5687-QOE) Inst Electrical.

Focusing-Oriented Psychotherapy: A Manual of the Experiential Method. Eugene T. Gendlin. LC 96-4755. (Practicing Professional Ser.). 317p. 1998. pap. 22.00 (*1-57230-376-X*, C0376); 1996. 39.95 (*0-89862-479-7*, C2479) Guilford Pubns.

***Folate & Human Development.** Ed. by Edward J. Massaro & John M. Rogers. 2002. LC 2001-51863. 375p. 119.00 (*0-89603-936-6*) Humana.

Folate in Health & Disease, No. 1. Ed. by Lynn B. Bailey. 1994. LC 94-35431. (Clinical Nutrition in Health & Disease Ser.: Vol. 1). (Illus.). 488p. text 195.00 (*0-8247-9280-7*) Dekker.

Folates & Cobalamines. Ed. by B. A. Cooper & J. Zittoun. 1989. (Illus.). 264p. 126.00 (*0-387-50653-5*) Spr-Verlag.

Foldable Intraocular Lenses: Evolution, Clinicopathologic Correlations & Complications. David J. Apple et al. 2000. LC 00-29134. (Illus.). 288p. 95.00 (*1-55642-435-3*) SLACK Inc.

Folic Acid & the Amazing B Vitamins. Glenn S. Rothfeld. 2000. LC 00-699757. vi, 186p. pap. 6.99 (*0-425-17369-0*) Berkley Pub.

Folic Acid (Pteroylglutamic Acid) - In Health, Deficiency & Therapy: Index of New Information with Authors, Subjects & References. Spencer D. Bradshaw. 1996.

150p. pap. 47.50 (*0-7883-1323-1*); 1998. 149p. 57.50 (*0-7883-2068-8*); 1998. 149p. pap. 47.50 (*0-7883-2069-6*) ABBE Pubs Assn.

Folie a Deux: An Experience of One-to-One Therapy. Rosie Alexander. 1995. (C). pap. (*1-85343-317-9*); 190p. (*1-85343-316-0*) Free Assoc Bks GBR. *Dist:* Intl Spec Bk, NYU Pr.

Folk Cures. Sue Turber. 1979. 48p. bds. 28.00 (*0-88014-014-3*) Mosaic Pr OH.

Folk Healer: The Mexican-American Tradition of Curanderismo. Eliseo Torres et al. Ed. by Carolyn Banks & Clark Magruder. 1984. (Illus.). 64p. (Orig.). pap. 4.95 (*0-9612008-1-2*) Nieves Pr.

Folk Medicine. D. C. Jarvis. 1985. 192p. mass mkt. 5.99 (*0-449-20880-X*, Crest) Fawcett.

Folk Medicine. D. C. Jarvis. 1996. 192p. 7.98 (*0-88365-940-9*) Galahad Bks.

Folk-Medicine: A Chapter in the History of Culture. William G. Black. 1972. (Folk-Lore Society, London Monographs: Vol. 12). reprint ed. pap. 30.00 (*0-8115-0504-9*) Periodicals Srv.

Folk Medicine: The Art & the Science. Ed. by Richard P. Steiner. 1985. LC 85-22904. (Illus.). viii, 215p. text 40.00 (*0-8412-0939-1*); pap. text 29.95 (*0-8412-0946-4*) Am Chemical.

Folk Medicine from Around the World. John Heinerman. 1997. 320p. (C). 27.95 (*0-13-397761-7*, Macmillan Coll) P-H.

Folk Medicine in Modern Egypt: Being the Relevant Parts of the Tibb al-Rukka, or Old Wives' Medicine, of 'Abd al-Rahman Isma'il. Abd al-Rahman Isma'il. LC 77-87651. (Anthropology Ser.). (Illus.). reprint ed. 32.50 (*0-404-16407-2*) AMS Pr.

Folk Medicine of the Delaware & Related Algonkian Indians. Gladys Tantaquidgeon. 1972. LC 73-620801. (Pennsylvania Historical & Museum Commission Anthropological Ser.: No. 3). (Illus.). 145p. pap. 9.95 (*0-911124-70-5*) Pa Hist & Mus.

Folk Medicine Plants: Used in Pennsylvania Dutch Country. Paul R. Wieand. 1992. 52p. reprint ed. pap. 6.50 (*0-9617210-5-7*) Remembrance.

Folk Remedies: Healing Wisdom from Days Gone By. Paul Bergner & David Hufford. 1999. LC 99-208427. (Consumer Guide Ser.). (Illus.). 384p. pap. 7.99 (*0-451-19903-0*) NAL.

Folk Remedies for Common Ailments. Anne McIntyre. 1994. (Illus.). 96p. (Orig.). pap. 12.95 (*1-55013-611-9*) Firefly Bks Limited.

Folk Remedies from Around the World: An International Collection of Time-Honored, All Natural Treatment for Common Illness. John Heinerman. 2000. (Illus.). 320p. pap. 15.00 (*0-7352-0170-6*) PH Pr.

Folk Remedies That Work: Revised Edition of Live & Be Well. Joan Wilen & Lydia Wilen. 1996. LC 96-5224. 352p. pap. 13.00 (*0-06-095164-8*) HarperCollins Pubs.

Folk Wisdom & Mother Wit: John Lee - An African American Herbal Healer. 161. Arvilla Payne-Jackson & John Lee. 1993. LC 92-46396. (Contributions in Afro-American & African Studies Ser.: No. 161). 192p. 60.00 (*0-313-28868-2*, GM8868, Greenwood Pr) Greenwood.

Follicle Stimulating Hormone: Regulation of Secretion & Molecular Mechanisms of Action. Ed. by M. Hunzicker-Dunn & N. L. Schwartz. 1992. (Serono Symposia Ser.). (Illus.). 420p. 141.00 (*0-387-97630-2*) Spr-Verlag.

Follicular Dendritic Cells in Normal & Pathological Conditions. Ernst Heinen. 1996. LC 95-20664. (Molecular Biology Intelligence Unit Ser.). 201p. 89.95 (*1-57059-309-4*) Landes Bioscience.

Follicular Growth & Ovulation Rate in Farm Animals. Ed. by J. F. Roche & D. O'Callaghan. 1987. (Current Topics in Veterinary Medicine & Animal Science Ser.). text 176.50 (*0-89838-855-4*) Kluwer Academic.

Follies & Fallacies in Medicine. Petr Skrabanek & James McCormick. 1990. LC 90-8827. 147p. (C). 34.00 (*0-87975-630-6*) Prometheus Bks.

Follow-Up Management of the High-Risk Infant. H. William Taeusch & Michael W. Yogman. 1987. 368p. 47.95 (*0-316-83106-9*, Little Brwn Med Div) Lppncott W & W.

Follow-Up of Cancer: A Handbook for Physicians. Ed. by David S. Fischer et al. 4th ed. 1995. LC 95-31124. 208p. pap. text 37.95 (*0-397-51533-2*) Lppncott W & W.

Food: Its Influence As a Factor in Disease & Health (1914) J. H. Tilden. 1996. 561p. reprint ed. pap. 31.00 (*1-56459-897-7*) Kessinger Pub.

Food—Good, Bad, Cancer Potential & the Delaney Clause: Index of New Information & Medical Research Bible. American Health Research Institute Staff. 1994. 180p. 57.50 (*0-7883-0142-X*); pap. 47.50 (*0-7883-0143-8*) ABBE Pubs Assn.

Food Acceptance & Nutrition. Ed. by J. Solms et al. 1988. (Food Science & Technology Ser.). 490p. text 104.00 (*0-12-654430-1*) Acad Pr.

Food Addiction: The Body Knows. Kay Sheppard. 1993. 190p. pap. 9.95 (*1-55874-276-X*) Health Comm.

Food Additive Toxicology. Ed. by Joseph A. Maga & Anthony T. Tu. 1994. (Illus.). 552p. text 215.00 (*0-8247-9245-9*) Dekker.

Food Additives: A Source Guide. 1991. lib. bdg. 77.96 (*0-8490-4833-8*) Gordon Pr.

Food Additives - Reports of Adverse, Hostile, Aggressive & Harmful Reactions, Including Psychologic Distress: Index of New Information with Authors, Subjects & Bibliography. Josepha M. Karnola. 1993. 180p. 47.50 (*1-55914-834-9*); pap. 44.50 (*1-55914-835-7*) ABBE Pubs Assn.

Food Additives & Hyperactive Children. C. Keith Conners. 1980. LC 80-66. 182p. 35.00 (*0-306-40400-1*, Plenum Trade) Perseus Pubng.

Food Additives, Student Syllabus. Ronald B. Froehlich. 1978. (gr. 9-12). pap. text 6.95 (*0-89420-076-3*, 168008) Natl Book.

Food Additives Toxicology, Regulation & Properties. 1996. 32p. lib. bdg. 349.00 (*0-8493-8580-6*) CRC Pr.

Food, Agriculture & Education. Ed. by A. N. Rao. 1987. LC 86-25243. (Science & Technology Education & Future Human Needs Ser.: Vol. 6). (Illus.). 254p. (*0-08-033948-4*) Pergamon Repr GBR. *Dist:* Franklin.

Food Alert! The Ultimate Sourcebook for Food Safety. Morton Satin. 1999. LC 98-33431. (Sourcebks.). (Illus.). xiii, 306p. 27.95 (*0-8160-3935-6*); pap. 14.95 (*0-8160-3936-4*) Facts on File.

Food Allergies. American Dietetic Association Staff. 1998. 112p. pap. 8.95 (*0-471-34714-0*) Wiley.

Food Allergies. Merri L. Dobler. 1991. pap. 5.50 (*0-88091-096-8*, 0882) Am Dietetic Assn.

Food Allergies & Adverse Reactions. Judy E. Perkin. 1990. LC 90-684. 294p. 83.00 (*0-8342-0170-4*) Aspen Pub.

Food Allergies Made Simple. Illus. by Phylis A. Austin et al. 1985. pap. 4.95 (*0-942658-08-6*) NLB.

Food Allergies Made Simple: The Complete Manual for Diagnosis, Treatment, & Prevention of Food Allergies. Phylis A. Austin et al. 1985. 85p. reprint ed. pap. 4.95 (*1-878726-05-6*) Fam Hlth Pubns.

Food Allergy. Richard J. Trevino. Ed. by Jacquelynne P. Corey. 1997. LC 96-49624. (American Academy of Otolaryngic Allergy Monograph Ser.). (Illus.). 120p. pap. text 32.00 (*0-86577-618-0*) Thieme Med Pubs.

Food Allergy. Dean D. Metcalfe et al. 2nd ed. 1996. LC 96-43618. (Illus.). 600p. text 99.95 (*0-86542-432-2*) Blackwell Sci.

Food Allergy: A Practical Approach to Diagnosis & Management. Chiaramonte. Ed. by Arlene Schneider et al. 1988. (Clinical Pediatrics Ser.: Vol. 5). (Illus.). 504p. text 185.00 (*0-8247-7652-6*) Dekker.

Food Allergy: A Primer for People. S. Allan Bock. 1983. LC 83-72531. 72p. pap. 5.00 (*0-9612332-0-6*) AJ Pub Co.

***Food Allergy & Intolerance.** Jonathan Brostoff. 2nd ed. 2001. (Illus.). 1115p. (*0-7020-2038-9*) W B Saunders GBR. *Dist:* Saunders.

Food Allergy & Other Adverse Reactions to Food. M. H. Lessof. 1994. (Illus.). 22p. pap. text 12.50 (*0-944398-19-7*) ILSI.

Food Allergy Book: The Complete Guide to Understanding & Relieving Your Food Allergies. William E. Walsh. 2000. LC 00-24608. 304p. pap. 16.95 (*0-471-38268-X*) Wiley.

Food Allergy Book: The Foods That Cause You Pain & Discomfort & How to Eliminate Them from Your Diet. William E. Walsh. 3rd ed. 1995. LC 94-96717. Orig. Title: Treating Food Allergy, My Way!. 203p. pap. 12.95 (*0-9631544-7-8*) ACA Pubns.

Food Allergy Cure: A New Solution to Food Cravings, Obesity, Depression, Headaches, Arthritis & Fatigue. Ellen W. Cutler. 2001. LC 00-58084. (Illus.). 352p. 24.00 (*0-609-60639-5*) Harmony Bks.

Food Allergy News Cookbook. Anne Munoz-Furlong. rev. ed. 1996. LC 92-97152. 156p. text 20.00 (*1-882541-00-6*) Food Allergy.

Food & Animal Borne Diseases Sourcebook: Basic Information about Diseases That Can Be Spread to Humans Through the Ingestion of Contaminated Food or Water or by Contact with Infected Animals. Ed. by Karen Bellenir & Peter D. Dresser. 1995. LC 95-21240. (Health Reference Ser.: Vol. 7). 535p. 78.00 (*0-7808-0033-8*) Omnigraphics Inc.

Food & Cancer Prevention: Chemical & Biological Aspects. Ed. by K. W. Waldron et al. 1993. (Special Publications). 476p. (C). (*0-85186-455-4*) Royal Soc Chem GBR. *Dist:* Spr-Verlag.

Food & Culture in America: A Nutrition Handbook. Pamela G. Kittler & Kathryn P. Sucher. 2nd ed. 1997. LC 97-4468. 400p. 53.95 (*0-314-20487-3*) Wadsworth Pub.

***Food & Diet Additives: Index of New Information Including Adverse Tissue & Organ Reactions.** Ed. by Research and Development Division Staff & John C. Bartone. 2001. (Illus.). 180p. 47.50 (*0-7883-2570-1*); pap. 44.50 (*0-7883-2571-X*) ABBE Pubs Assn.

Food & Diet: Reports of Harmful & Unfavorable Effects Including Illness & Cancer: Index of New Information with Authors & Subjects. M. L. Dillard. rev. ed. 1994. LC 94-31245. 57.50 (*0-7883-0184-5*); pap. 47.50 (*0-7883-0185-3*) ABBE Pubs Assn.

Food & Diet: Reports of Harmful & Unfavorable Effects Including Illness & Cancer: Index of New Information with Authors & Subjects. Miladie L. Dillard. rev. ed. 1994. LC 94-31245. 171p. 57.50 (*0-7883-0232-9*); pap. 47.50 (*0-7883-0233-7*) ABBE Pubs Assn.

Food & Drug Administration Management Concerns: Hearing Before the Subcommittee on Oversight & Investigations of the Committee on Commerce, House of Representatives, 105th Congress, Second Session, April 1, 1998. 1998. LC 98-167892. iii, 71p. (*0-16-056498-0*) USGPO.

Food & Drug Administration's Quality Systems Regulations for Medical Devices: Effective Date, June 1, 1997. U. S. Food and Drug Administration Staff. 1997. LC 96-45447. (Handi-Regs Ser.: No. 9603). pap. 3.95 (*0-940701-78-2*) Keystone Pr.

Food & Drug Interactions: A Professional's Guide to Protect You & Your Family. Ed. by Gary A. Holt. rev. ed. 1997. LC 97-37129. 414p. pap. 22.95 (*0-944496-59-8*) Precept Pr.

Food & Food Additive Intolerance in Childhood. T. J. David. 2nd ed. 2002. (Illus.). 384p. (Orig.). pap. text 54.95 (*0-86542-663-5*) Blackwell Sci.

Food & Free Radicals: Proceedings of the First Symposium Held in Yamagata, Japan, June 16, 1994. Ed. by Midori Hiramatsu. 1997. LC 97-7267. (Illus.). 180p. (C). text 79.50 (*0-306-45493-9*, Kluwer Plenum) Kluwer Academic.

Food & Health: Science & Technology. Ed. by Gordon G. Birch & K. J. Parker. 1976. (Illus.). xii, 532p. 144.00 (*0-85334-875-8*) Elsevier.

Food & Health Data: Their Use in Nutrition Policy-Making. Ed. by W. Backer & E. Helsing. 1991. (WHO Regional Publications: No. 34). (ENG, FRE & GER.). xii, 171p. pap. text 26.00 (*92-890-1125-4*, 1310034) World Health.

Food & Immunology. Ed. by Leif Hambraeus et al. 1977. 204p. lib. bdg. 47.00 (*91-22-00092-5*) Coronet Bks.

Food & Its Dangerous Ingredients for Health & Safety in America: Index of New Information with Authors & Subjects. Mary R. Bartone. 1995. LC 95-15405. 57.50 (*0-7883-0756-8*); pap. 47.50 (*0-7883-0757-6*) ABBE Pubs Assn.

Food & Nutrition: Customs & Culture. Paul Fieldhouse. 1985. LC 85-21276. 256p. pap. (*0-7099-1079-7*) C Helm GBR. *Dist:* Routldge.

Food & Nutrition in the Middle East, 1970-1986: An Annotated Bibliography, 3. Compiled by Gail G. Harrison et al. 1988. LC 87-34023. (Bibliographies & Indexes in Science & Technology Ser.: No. 3). 266p. lib. bdg. 78.75 (*0-313-26188-1*, HFN/, Greenwood Pr) Greenwood.

Food & Nutrition Strategies in National Development: Report of the FAO-WHO Expert Committee on Nutrition, 9th, Rome, 1977. FAO-WHO Expert Committee on Nutrition. 1976. (Technical Reports: No. 584). pap. text 7.00 (*92-4-120584-9*, 1100584) World Health.

Food & Our Bones: The Natural Way to Prevent Osteroporosis. Annemarie Colbin. 1998. LC 97-53118. 320p. pap. 13.95 (*0-452-27806-6*, Plume) Dutton Plume.

Food & the Gut Reaction: Intestinal Health Through Diet. Elaine Gottschall. 1987. (Illus.). 146p. pap. (*0-9692768-0-X*) Kirkton Pr.

Food, Body & the Self. Deborah Lupton. 1996. (C). pap. 25.95 (*0-8039-7648-8*, 1604) Sage.

Food Borne Carcinogens: Heterocyclic Amines. Minako Nago & Takashi Sugimura. 2000. LC 99-56525. (Current Toxicology Ser.). (Illus.). 390p. 145.00 (*0-471-98399-3*) Wiley.

Food-Borne Disease - Methods of Sampling & Examination in Surveillance Programmes: Proceedings of the WHO Scientific Group, Geneva, 1973. WHO Staff. 1974. (Technical Reports: No. 543). pap. text 5.00 (*92-4-120543-1*, 1100543) World Health.

Food-Borne Infections & Intoxication. Ed. by Hans Riemann & Frank L. Bryan. 2nd ed. 1979. LC 79-14935. (Food Science & Technology Ser.). text 146.00 (*0-12-588360-9*) Acad Pr.

Food, Brain Chemistry & Behavior. Jeffrey Fortuna. 1997. 238p. (C). pap. text 46.00 (*0-536-00277-0*) Pearson Custom.

Food-Calorie Intake & Effects on Diet, Energy & Metabolism: Index of New Information with Authors & Subjects. Andrew R. Morton. rev. ed. 1997. LC 94-34922. 163p. 57.50 (*0-7883-0444-5*) ABBE Pubs Assn.

Food Chemicals Codex. Institute of Medicine, Committee on Food Chemicals. 4th rev. ed. 1998. 882p. ring bd. 195.00 (*0-309-05394-3*) Natl Acad Pr.

Food Code: 1999 Recommendations of the United States Public Health Service, Food & Drug Administration. U. S. Department of Health & Human Services Staff et al. 1999. (Illus.). 525p. spiral bd. 40.00 (*0-934213-68-2*, PB99-115925) Natl Tech Info.

Food Combining Made Easy. 1998. pap. 4.95 (*0-9606948-0-3*) Willow Pub.

Food Commodities-Catering, Processing, Storing. Bernard Davis. 1978. pap. 19.95 (*0-434-90297-7*) Trafalgar.

Food Contamination from Environmental Sources. Ed. by Jerome O. Nriagu & Milagros S. Simmons. 1990. LC 89-5671. (Environmental Science & Technology Ser.). 785p. 350.00 (*0-471-50891-8*) Wiley.

Food Cures: The Chinese System. 1992. (Alternative Medicine Ser.). lib. bdg. 79.99 (*0-8490-5398-6*) Gordon Pr.

Food Demand Analysis: Problems, Issues & Empirical Evidence. Ed. by Robert Raunikar & Chung-Liang Huang. 1987. LC 86-30534. 302p. (C). text 39.95 (*0-8138-1841-9*) Iowa U Pr.

Food, Drug & Insecticide Administration: Its History, Activities & Organization. Gustavus A. Weber. LC 72-3066. (Brookings Institution. Institute for Government Research. Service Monographs of the U. S. Government: No. 50). reprint ed. 37.50 (*0-404-57150-6*) AMS Pr.

Food, Eating & Obesity: The Psychological Basis of Appetite & Weight Control. P. Rogers & D. J. Mela. 1995. LC 97-68946. (Illus.). 240p. 109.00 (*0-412-71920-7*) Aspen Pub.

Food, Ecology & Culture Vol. 1: Readings in the Anthropology of Dietary Practices. Ed. by J. K. R. Robson. 1980. x, 144p. text 168.00 (*0-677-16090-9*) Gordon & Breach.

Food Energy in Tropical Ecosystems. Ed. by Dorothy J. Cattle & Karl H. Schwerin. 1985. (Food & Nutrition in History & Anthropology Ser.: Vol. 4). xxvi, 290p. text 134.00 (*2-88124-036-4*) Gordon & Breach.

Food Enzymes: Structures & Mechanism. Dominic W. S. Wong. 1995. LC 94-42926. 390p. (C). 109.00 (*0-412-05691-7*) Aspen Pub.

Food Enzymes for Health & Longevity. Edward Howell. 2nd ed. 1994. LC 94-75625. (Illus.). 222p. (Orig.). pap. 10.95 (*0-941524-28-0*) Lotus Pr.

Food Factors for Cancer Prevention. H. Ohigashi. 1997. LC 97-16526. (Illus.). 700p. 263.00 (*4-431-70196-6*) Spr-Verlag.

Food for Life. Richard Bohannon et al. 1998. LC 98-15348. 336p. pap. 16.95 (*0-8092-2845-9*, 284590, Contemporary) McGraw-Hill Trade.

Food for Life. Ed. by Ralph W. Gerard. 1965. LC 52-14880. pap. text 3.25 (*0-226-28790-4*, P527) U Ch Pr.

Food for Life: The Macrobiotic Approach to Discovering Personal Balance. Seymour A. Koblin. 1990. (Illus.). 110p. (Orig.). pap. 15.95 (*0-9625000-1-1*) Soulstar Creations.

Food for Recovery: The Next Step. Joseph D. Beasley & Susan Knightly. 1994. LC 93-25244. 14.00 (*0-517-58694-0*, Crown) Crown Pub Group.

Food for Solitude: Menus & Meditations to Heal Body, Mind & Soul. Francine Schiff. 1992. pap. 16.95 (*1-85230-181-3*) Element MA.

***Food Fortification in Canada: Experience & Issues in Controlling Micronutrient Malnutrition.** Mahshid Lotfi. 2001. (Micronutrient Initiative Ser.). 80p. pap. (*1-894217-16-0*) IDRC-CRDI CAN. *Dist:* Stylus Pub VA.

Food Habits & Customs: Index of Authors & Subjects with Guide for Rapid Research. Glenn J. Kuffner. 1994. LC 94-35174. 57.50 (*0-7883-0490-9*); pap. 47.50 (*0-7883-0491-7*) ABBE Pubs Assn.

Food Hydrocolloids, Vol. III. Ed. by Martin Glicksman. 1986. 304p. 189.95 (*0-8493-6043-9*, TP453) CRC Pr.

Food Hypersensitivity & Adverse RXNs: A Practical Guide for Diagnosis & Management. M. Frieri & B. Kettelhutt. 1999. LC 99-29662. (Clinical Allergy & Immunology Ser.). (Illus.). 520p. text 195.00 (*0-8247-9903-8*) Dekker.

Food Inspector. Jack Rudman. 1994. (Career Examination Ser.: C-2543). pap. 29.95 (*0-8373-2543-9*) Nat Learn.

Food Intake & Energy Expenditure. Ed. by Margriet S. Westerterp-Plantenga et al. 1994. LC 93-46315. 416p. 83.95 (*0-8493-9228-4*) CRC Pr.

Food Irradiation. International Atomic Energy Agency Staff. 1966. (Proceedings Ser.). (ENG, FRE, RUS & SPA., Illus.). 957p. pap. (*92-0-010166-6*, ISP127) IAEA AUT. *Dist:* Bernan Associates.

Food Irradiation Now. Ganmaster. 1982. 22.00 (*90-247-2763-4*) Kluwer Academic.

Food Mania & Over-Eating: Index of Modern Authors & Subjects with Guide for Rapid Research. Melba J. Milligan. 1991. LC 90-56314. 160p. 47.50 (*1-55914-416-5*); pap. 44.50 (*1-55914-417-3*) ABBE Pubs Assn.

Food Microbiology Protocols. Ed. by John F. T. Spencer & Alicia L. Ragout de Spencer. 2000. LC 00-21718. (Methods in Biotechnology Ser.: Vol. 14). (Illus.). xiv, 495p. 99.50 (*0-89603-867-X*) Humana.

***Food-Mood-Body Connection.** Gary Null. 2001. 496p. pap. 19.95 (*1-58322-257-X*) Seven Stories.

Food, Nutrition & Diet. Marie V. Krause & Kathleen Mahan. 9th ed. 1996. pap. text, stu. ed. 18.95 (*0-7216-6816-X*) Saunders.

Food, Nutrition & Health. Ed. by Miloslav Rechcigl. 1973. (World Review of Nutrition & Dietetics Ser.: Vol. 16). (Illus.). 350p. 156.75 (*3-8055-1398-4*) S Karger.

Food, Nutrition & the Young Child. Jeanette Endres & Robert E. Rockwell. 4th ed. 1993. LC 93-25602. (Illus.). 416p. (C). pap. 55.00 (*0-02-333721-4*, Macmillan Coll) P-H.

Food Phytochemicals for Cancer Prevention Vol. 1: Fruits & Vegetables. Mou-Tuan Huang et al. 1994. LC 93-33775. (ACS Symposium Ser.: Vol. 546). 439p. 115.00 (*0-8412-2768-3*) Am Chemical.

Food Phytochemicals for Cancer Prevention Vol. 2: Teas, Spices & Herbs. Ed. by Chi-Tang Ho et al. 1994. LC 93-33774. (ACS Symposium Ser.: Vol. 547). 382p. 105.00 (*0-8412-2769-1*) Am Chemical.

Food Poisoning. John P. Monahan. 1984. LC 83-63604. 125p. pap. 11.95 (*0-916093-00-X*) Med-Info Bks.

Food Poisoning & Food Hygiene. Betty C. Hobbs & R. J. Gilbert. 4th ed. 1978. 344p. 33.00 (*0-917678-06-0*) Food & Nut Pr.

Food Poisoning Prevention in Australia. Highfield Publications Staff. 1989. (C). (*0-89771-807-0*) Highfield Pubns GBR. *Dist:* St Mut.

Food Power: A Doctor's Guide to Common Sense Nutrition. E. Earle Arnow. 1972. LC 75-185419. (Illus.). 305p. text 32.95 (*0-911012-37-0*) Burnham Inc.

Food Preservation by Irradiation 1978. (Illus.). 595p. pap. (*92-0-010278-6*, ISP470-1) IAEA AUT. *Dist:* Bernan Associates.

Food Process Engineering Vol. 1: Food Processing Systems. Ed. by P. Linko et al. 1980. (Illus.). xii, 981p. 255.75 (*0-85334-896-0*) Elsevier.

Food Process Engineering Vol. 2: Enzyme Engineering in Food Processing. Ed. by P. Linko et al. 1980. (Illus.). vii, 328p. 93.75 (*0-85334-897-9*) Elsevier.

Food Proteins. Ed. by John E. Kinsella & William G. Soucie. 1990. 440p. 85.00 (*0-935315-26-8*) Am Oil Chemists.

Food Safety. Julie Miller Jones. 1992. (Illus.). 453p. 99.00 (*0-9624407-3-6*) Eagan Pr.

***Food Safety: Actions Needed by USDA & FDA to Ensure That Companies Promptly Cary Out Recalls.** Rosellen McCarthy & Jay L. Scott. Ed. by Lawrence J. Dyckman. 2001. 51p. (C). pap. 25.00 (*0-7567-0903-2*) DIANE Pub.

Food Safety: Oversight of the Centers for Disease Control Monitoring of Foodborne Pathogens: Congressional Hearing. Ed. by Christopher Shays. 1999. 174p. reprint ed. pap. text 25.00 (*0-7881-8294-3*) DIANE Pub.

Food Safety: Oversight of the Centers for Disease Control Monitoring of Foodborne Pathogens: Hearing Before the Subcommittee on Human Resources & Intergovernmental Relations of the Committee on Government Reform & Oversight, House of Representatives, One Hundred Fourth Congress, Second Session, May 23, 1996. Contrib. by U. S. Congress, House Committee on Government Reform & Oversight, Subcommittee on Human Resources and Intergovernmental Relations. 1997. LC 98-132518. (Illus.). (*0-16-055673-2*) USGPO.

Food Safety & Sanitation. Barbara Border. 1979. (Careers in Home Economics Ser.). (Illus.). text 17.80 (*0-07-006511-X*) McGraw.

Food Safety for Professionals: A Reference. Mildred M. Cody & Mary Keith. 1991. LC 91-29325. stu. ed., spiral bd. 17.00 (*0-88091-091-7*, 0181) Am Dietetic Assn.

Food Science & Human Nutrition. Ed. by George Charalambous. 1992. LC 92-9175. (Developments in Food Science Ser.: Vol. 29). 822p. 372.50 (*0-444-88834-9*) Elsevier.

Food Science & Nutritional Health: An Introduction. Theodore P. Labuza & John Erdman. 1984. (Illus.). 558p. pap. text, tchr. ed. (*0-314-78015-7*) West Pub.

Food Science, Nutrition & Health. 6th ed. 400p. pap. (*0-340-60483-2*) E A GBR. *Dist:* Routldge.

Food Sensitivity Diet. Doug A. Kaufmann & Racquel Skolnik. 1984. 224p. 15.95 (*0-88191-003-1*) Freundlich.

Food Service Manual for Health Care Institutions, 1994. Brenda A. Byers et al. 94th rev. ed. 1994. LC 94-7495. 556p. pap. 48.00 (*1-55648-114-4*, 046172) AHPI.

Food Smart: A Man's Plan to Fuel up for Peak Performance. Jeff Bredenberg et al. 1996. (Men's Health Life Improvement Guides: Vol. 1). (Illus.). 176p. pap. 14.95 (*0-87596-280-7*) Rodale Pr Inc.

Food Sweeteners - Aspartame & Its Adverse Reactions, Strange Symptoms, Illness Behavior & Controversy: Index of New Information with Authors & Subjects. Miladie L. Dillard. rev. ed. 1994. 157p. 57.50 (*0-7883-0446-1*); pap. 47.50 (*0-7883-0447-X*) ABBE Pubs Assn.

Food Technology in the Year Two Thousand. Ed. by S. E. Lindroth & S. S. Rynaenen. 1990. (Bibliotheca Nutritio et Dieta Ser.: No. 47). (Illus.). xiv, 22p. 115.00 (*3-8055-5243-2*) S Karger.

Food Values of Poi, Taro & Limu. C. D. Miller. 1969. (BMB Ser.: No. 37). reprint ed. pap. 25.00 (*0-527-02140-7*) Periodicals Srv.

Foodborne Bacterial Pathogens. Doyle. 1989. (Food Science & Technology Ser.: Vol. 31). (Illus.). 816p. text 250.00 (*0-8247-7866-9*) Dekker.

Foodborne Disease Handbook Ed. by Y. H. Hui. 2nd ed. 2000. LC 00-60172. (Illus.). 704p. text 195.00 (*0-8247-0337-5*); 536p. text 195.00 (*0-8247-0338-3*); 840p. text 195.00 (*0-8247-0343-X*) Dekker.

***Foodborne Disease Handbook** Ed. by Y. H. Hui et al. 2nd exp. ed. (Illus.). 2760p. text 680.00 (*0-8247-0597-1*) Dekker.

Foodborne Disease Handbook Y. H. Hui. 2nd exp. rev. ed. 2000. LC 00-60172. (Illus.). 680p. text 195.00 (*0-8247-0344-8*) Dekker.

Foodborne Disease Handbook: Diseases Caused by Viruses, Parasites & Fungi, Vol. 1. Ed. by Y. H. Hui et al. 1994. (Diseases Caused by Bacterial Ser.). (Illus.). 632p. text 215.00 (*0-8247-9063-4*) Dekker.

Foodborne Disease Handbook: Diseases Caused by Viruses, Parasites & Fungi, Vol. 2. Ed. by Y. H. Hui et al. 1994. (Illus.). 702p. text 215.00 (*0-8247-9165-7*) Dekker.

Foodborne Disease Handbook Vol. 3: Diseases Caused by Hazardous Substances. Ed. by Y. H. Hui et al. 1994. LC 94-10139. (Illus.). 688p. text 215.00 (*0-8247-9166-5*) Dekker.

Foodborne Diseases. Ed. by Dean O. Cliver. 1990. 395p. text 63.00 (*0-12-176558-X*) Acad Pr.

Foodborne Illness. 160p. (*0-340-55570-X*) E A GBR. *Dist:* Routldge.

Foodborne Microorganisms & Their Toxins (IFT) Merle D. Pierson & Norman J. Stern. 1986. LC 99-49286. (IFT Basic Symposium Ser.: Vol. 1). (Illus.). 488p. text 125.00 (*0-8247-7607-0*) Dekker.

Foodborne Pathogens. Ed. by Ronald G. Labbe & Santos Garcia. 2001. LC 2001-26958. (Illus.). 400p. 99.95 (*0-471-35034-6*) Wiley.

Foodborne Pathogens. Alan V. Varnam. 1991. (Illus.). 557p. (gr. 13). text 120.95 (*0-8151-8976-1*, 21899) Mosby Inc.

Foodborne Pathogens: Hazards, Risk Analysis & Control. Ed. by Clive Blackburn & Peter McClure. 2001. 288p. (*1-85573-454-0*) Woodhead Pubng GBR. *Dist:* Am Educ Systs.

Foods & Moods. Richard Crews. 1993. 88p. (Orig.). pap. 8.95 (*0-945864-47-7*) Columbia Pacific U Pr.

Foods & Nutrition: Syllabus. Mary A. Plummer. 1976. (gr. 10-12). pap. text 7.95 (*0-89420-001-1*, 167070) Natl Book.

Foods & Nutrition: Syllabus. Mary A. Plummer. 1976. (J). pap. 58.10 incl. audio (*0-89420-147-6*, 167040) Natl Book.

Foods & Nutrition Encyclopedia M. E. Ensminger et al. 1983. (Illus.). 2432p. 99.00 (*0-941218-05-8*) Pegus Pr.

Foods & Nutrition Encyclopedia, Set. Audrey H. Ensminger et al. 2nd ed. 1993. LC 93-36692. 2432p. 382.00 (*0-8493-8980-1*, TX849) CRC Pr.

Foods & Nutrition Encyclopedia, Vol. 2. M. E. Ensminger et al. 2nd ed. 1993. LC 93-36692. 1216p. 246.95 (*0-8493-8982-8*) CRC Pr.

Foods, Fads & Foolishness. W. F. Wines. rev. ed. 1982. (Illus.). 165p. reprint ed. pap. 5.95 (*0-911579-00-1*) Fleur-Di-Lee.

Foods, Nutrition & Dental Health Vol. 1: Cariogenicity of Foods, Beverages, Confections & Chewing Gum: The Role of Sugar & Other Foods in Dental Caries & What Can Industry Do? Ed. by John J. Hefferren & Henry M. Koehler. 1981. 425p. 56.00 (*0-930376-21-8*) Chem-Orbital.

Foods, Nutrition & Immunity: Effects of Dairy & Fermented Milk Products. Ed. by M. Paubert-Braquet et al. 1992. (Dynamic Nutrition Research Ser.: Vol. 1). (Illus.). viii, 126p. 106.25 (*3-8055-5605-5*) S Karger.

Foods, Nutrition & Sports Performance: An International Scientific Concensus, Held 4-6 February, 1991. Ed. by Clyde Williams & John T. Devlin. 1992. LC 92-13358. (Illus.). 194p. (C). pap. 41.95 (*0-419-17890-2*, Spon) Routledge.

Foot. B. Regnauld. Tr. by Reginald A. Elson from FRE. 1986. (Illus.). 633p. 430.00 (*0-387-13222-8*) Spr-Verlag.

Foot, Set. Ed. by Basil Helal & Derek Wilson. 1988. (Illus.). 1376p. text (*0-443-02981-4*) Church.

Foot: A New Approach to Structure & Function. G. D. Stainsby. 2000. (Illus.). 256p. (*0-7506-2950-9*) E A GBR. *Dist:* OUP.

***Foot: An Illustrated Guide to Clinical Assessment.** Colin Thomson. 2001. (Illus.). 211p. pap. (*0-443-06495-4*) Church GBR. *Dist:* Saunders.

Foot: Examination & Diagnosis. Ian J. Alexander. 2nd ed. 1997. LC 96-40478. pap. text (*0-443-07656-1*) Church.

Foot & Ankle. Ed. by Kenneth A. Johnson. LC 93-20598. (Master Techniques in Orthopaedic Surgery Ser.). (Illus.). 1994. sl. 625.00 (*0-7817-0209-7*); 1993. 544p. text 199.00 (*0-7817-0030-2*) Lppncott W & W.

Foot & Ankle: A Sectional Imaging Atlas. David P. Mayer et al. 1993. LC 93-9264. (Illus.). 228p. text 120.00 (*0-7216-3199-1*) Saunders.

Foot & Ankle: Clinical Application. A. L. Logan. 1994. 194p. pap. 68.00 (*0-8342-0605-6*) Aspen Pub.

Foot & Ankle Disorders Mark Myerson. 1999. LC 99-11880. (Illus.). xv, 1511p. text 299.00 (*0-7216-7155-1*) Harcourt.

Foot & Ankle in Sport. Donald E. Baxter. 1994. (Illus.). 400p. (C). (gr. 13). text 155.00 (*0-8016-6890-5*, 06890) Mosby Inc.

Foot & Ankle Pain. Henry L. Feffer et al. 1988. (Illus.). 711p. 85.00 (*0-87473-410-X*, 62005-10, MICHIE) LEXIS Pub.

Foot & Ankle Pain. Rene Cailliet. 3rd ed. 1996. LC 96-46127. (Pain Ser.). (Illus.). 287p. (C). pap. text 24.95 (*0-8036-0216-2*) Davis Co.

Foot & Ankle Radiology. Christman. 1999. text 115.00 (*0-443-08782-2*) Saunders.

Foot & Ankle Secrets. Lawrence B. Harkless & Kim Felder-Johnson. 1997. LC 97-19922. (Secrets Ser.). (Illus.). 250p. pap. 39.95 (*1-56053-211-4*) Hanley & Belfus.

Foot & Ankle Trauma. Ed. by Barry L. Scurran. 2nd ed. 1995. LC 95-38028. 888p. text (*0-443-08937-X*) Church.

Foot & Ankle Trauma & Reconstruction. Mark Myerson. 1997. (Illus.). 480p. text 99.00 (*0-07-044328-9*) McGraw.

Foot Book. John S. Gould. 1988. (Illus.). 346p. 69.50 (*0-683-03727-7*) Lppncott W & W.

Foot Book: Relief for Overused, Abused & Ailing Feet. Glenn Copeland. 1992. LC 91-43125. 208p. pap. 14.95 (*0-471-55840-0*) Wiley.

Foot Care Book. William P. Fiegel. 1982. (Runner's World Ser.). pap. 9.95 (*0-02-499510-X*, Macmillan Coll) P-H.

Foot Care Revolution: How to Walk Away from a Foot Operation on Your Own Two Feet. Dennis F. Augustine. 2nd ed. 1993. (Illus.). 213p. reprint ed. pap. 15.00 (*0-9636736-1-0*) Gldn Gate Pub.

Foot Function: A Programmed Text. Michael O. Seibel. 1988. (Illus.). 264p. 45.00 (*0-683-07651-5*) Lppncott W & W.

Foot in Both Worlds. Arthur Guirdham. 224p. (Orig.). pap. 26.95 (*0-8464-4182-9*) Beekman Pubs.

Foot in Diabetes. G. James Sammarco. 1991. LC 90-13338. (Illus.). 235p. text 53.50 (*0-8121-1358-6*) Lppncott W & W.

Foot in the Door. John J. Pelizza. 1985. (Stress Management & Personal Growth Ser.). (Illus.). 152p. (Orig.). pap. 10.95 (*0-9614872-0-8*) Pelizza & Assocs.

Foot Injuries: Index of New Information. James A. Triferro. 1999. 191p. 57.50 (*0-7883-1916-7*); pap. text 47.50 (*0-7883-1917-5*) ABBE Pubs Assn.

Foot Orthoses & Other Forms of Conservative Foot Care. Thomas C. Michaud. 1993. LC 92-48944. (*0-06-830597-4*); (Illus.). 270p. 80.00 (*0-683-05974-2*) Lppncott W & W.

Foot Orthotics in Therapy & Sport. Skip Hunter et al. 1995. LC 95-2243. (Illus.). 152p. pap. text 42.00 (*0-87322-829-4*, BHUN0829) Human Kinetics.

Foot Reflexology: A Visual Guide for Self-Treatment. Jurgen Jora. 1991. 79p. pap. 16.95 (*0-312-05864-0*) St Martin.

Football (Soccer) Association Guide to the Treatment & Rehabilitation of Injuries in Sports. William J. Armour. 1984. (Illus.). 224p. 29.95 (*0-434-02751-0*) Trafalgar.

Footprints: A History of St. Paul Red Cross. June W. Dahl. 1981. (Illus.). 233p. 10.00 (*0-9605584-0-3*) Red Cross St Paul.

Footrot & Foot Abscess of Ruminants. Ed. by J. R. Egerton et al. 1989. 272p. 127.00 (*0-8493-5861-2*, SF906) CRC Pr.

For a Blissful Baby: Healthy & Happy Pregnancy with Maharishi Vedic Medicine. Kumuda Reddy et al. 2001. (Illus.). 250p. pap. 16.95 (*1-929297-01-7*) Samhita Prodns.

For & Against Psychoanalysis. Stephen Frosh. 1997. LC 97-9748. 288p. (C). 80.00 (*0-415-13138-3*); pap. 20.99 (*0-415-13139-1*) Routledge.

For Dentists Only: How to Protect Your Practice, Property & Savings from Lawsuits & Other Creditor Risks. David B. Mandell. 1997. LC 99-210164. (Illus.). 305p. ring bd. (*1-890415-06-5*) Guardian Pub.

For Doctors Only: How to Protect Your Practice, Property & Savings from Lawsuits & Other Creditor Threats. David B. Mandell. 1996. LC 97-90452. (Illus.). 297p. (Orig.). pap. (*1-890415-00-6*) Guardian Pub.

For Formulation Chemists Only, Vol. 2. Ed. by Esam M. Morsy. (F2CO Ser.). 1992. 148p. pap. text 95.00 (*0-937425-03-6*); 1991. (Illus.). 144p. pap. 95.00 (*0-937425-14-1*) C I T A Intl.

For Health's Sake: A Critical Analysis of Medical Care in the United States. Howard R. Grossman. 1977. LC 77-23828. 221p. 21.95 (*0-87015-222-X*) Pacific Bks.

For Love or Money: The Fee in Feminist Therapy. Ed. by Marcia Hill & Ellyn Kaschak. 1999. LC 99-51402. (Women & Therapy Monograph Ser.: Vol. 22, No. 3). 113p. 39.95 (*0-7890-0955-2*); pap. 15.95 (*0-7890-0956-0*) Haworth Pr.

For Non-Smokers Only! Antonio R. Saqueton. 1981. LC 81-69803. (Illus.). 258p. 24.95 (*0-941616-05-3*) ARS Pub.

For Our Kids' Sake: How to Protect Your Child Against Pesticides in Food. Ann W. Garland & Natural Resources Defense Council Staff. 1990. LC 89-12376. (Guides). pap. 6.95 (*0-87156-613-3*) Sierra.

For-Profit Healthcare Revolution: The Growing Impact of Investor-Owned Health Systems in America. E. Preston Gee & Sandy Lutz. 1995. LC 95-23203. 208p. (C). text 32.50 (*1-55738-650-1*, Irwn Prfssnl) McGraw-Hill Educ Grp.

For Radiation Imaging. Mosby Staff. 1998. text 1150.00 (*0-8151-6948-5*) Mosby Inc.

For the Bereaved: The Road to Recovery. Ed. by Austin H. Kutscher et al. 1990. LC 89-22190. 282p. pap. 18.95 (*0-914783-32-7*) Charles.

For the Love of Teddi: The Story Behind Camp Good Days & Special Times The 2001 Edition. Lou Buttino. 2001. LC 00-65570. (Illus.). 208p. 24.95 (*0-275-97341-7*, C7341, Praeger Trade) Greenwood.

For the Patient's Good: The Restoration of Beneficence in Health Care. Edmund D. Pellegrino & David C. Thomasma. 1988. 256p. text 41.50 (*0-19-504319-7*) OUP.

For the Record: Protecting Electronic Health Information. Committee on Maintaining Privacy and Secruity in Hea. 1997. LC 97-65240. 288p. 29.95 (*0-309-05697-7*, Joseph Henry Pr) Natl Acad Pr.

For the Record: Risk Management Issues in Medical Records & Documentation. RiskCare Staff. 1997. 97p. pap. text 135.00 (*1-893929-01-9*) RiskCare.

For the World to Hear: Biography of Dr. Howard P. House. Sydney Hyman. 1990. LC 89-15615. (Illus.). 432p. 20.00 (*0-932727-34-4*) Hope Pub Hse.

For Those We Love: A Spiritual Perspective on AIDS. Ed. by Joanne Lucid. 2nd enl. ed. 1990. (Illus.). 96p. (Orig.). pap. 7.50 (*1-879035-01-4*) AIDS Ministry.

For Those Who Live: Helping Children Cope with the Death of a Brother or Sister. Kathy La Tour. 1983. 145p. 9.95 (*0-9612870-0-4*) K LaTour.

For Whose Protection? Reproductive Hazards & Exclusionary Policies in the United States & Britain. Sally J. Kenney. 1993. 408p. (C). pap. text 22.95 (*0-472-08176-4*, 08176) U of Mich Pr.

For Women Only: Chinese Herbal Formulas. Hong-yen Hsu. 1993. pap. 4.95 (*0-941942-06-6*) Orient Heal Arts.

***For Women Only! Your Guide to Health Empowerment.** Gary Null & Barbara Seaman. 2001. LC 2001-41073. 1600p. pap. 29.95 (*1-58322-278-2*) Seven Stories.

For Women Only! Your Guide to Health Empowerment. Gary Null & Barbara Seaman. 2000. LC 99-39822. (Illus.). xxiv, 1571p. 49.95 (*1-58322-015-1*) Seven Stories.

For Your Back. H. Duane Saunders. Ed. by Robin Saunders. 1983. (Illus.). (Orig.). pap. text 4.00 (*0-9616461-1-X*) Saunders Grp.

For Your Neck. Ed. by Robin Saunders & Beth Solheim. 2nd ed. 1986. (Illus.). (Orig.). pap. text 4.00 (*0-9616461-3-6*) Saunders Grp.

Foraging Vol. 6: Qualitative Analysis of Behavior. Ed. by Michael L. Commons & A. Kacelnick Shettleworth. 1987. (Comparative Cognition & Neuroscience Ser.). 312p. text 69.95 (*0-89859-550-9*) L Erlbaum Assocs.

Forbidden Medicine: Is Effective Non-Toxic Cancer Treatment Being Suppressed? Ellen Hodgson Brown. 1998. LC 98-203415. x, 329p. (*1-879854-28-7*) Christian Servs Pub.

***Force Program: The Proven Way to Fight Cancer Through Physical Activity & Exercise.** Jeffrey Berman et al. 2001. LC 2001-35328. (Illus.). 208p. 24.00 (*0-345-44088-9*, Ballantine) Ballantine Pub Grp.

Forced into Treatment: The Role of Coercion in Clinical Practice. Committee on Government Policy, Group for the Adva. 1993. LC 93-26825. (Reports). xii, 133p. 23.00 (*0-87318-205-7*) Grp Adv Psych.

Forced Movements, Tropisms & Animal Conduct. Jacques Loeb. 1990. (Illus.). 17.75 (*0-8446-4776-4*) Peter Smith.

Forced Normalization & Alternative Psychoses of Epilepsy. Michael R. Trimble & Bettina Schmitz. 1998. LC 98-7538. 235p. (*1-871816-37-8*) Wrightson Biomed GBR. *Dist:* Taylor & Francis.

Forecasting in Cardiology. E. Stoupel. 1976. 144p. text 36.50 (*0-7065-1550-1*) Coronet Bks.

Forecasting the Cost of Chemical Dependency Treatment under Managed Care: The Washington State Study. Chris Hansen. 1997. (Illus.). 84p. (C). reprint ed. pap. text 25.00 (*0-7881-4600-9*) DIANE Pub.

Forecasting the Health of Elderly Populations. Ed. by Kenneth G. Manton et al. 1993. LC 92-48819. (Series in Statistics in the Health Sciences). (Illus.). 371p. 105.00 (*0-387-97953-0*) Spr-Verlag.

Forefoot Reconstruction. L. S. Barouk. 1999. (Illus.). 150p. (C). incl. audio compact disk (*2-287-59656-9*) Spl France Editions FRA. *Dist:* Spr-Verlag.

Forefront of Pediatric Pathology. Ronald Jaffe et al. 1990. 155.00 (*1-56032-010-9*) Hemisp Pub.

Foreign Body Prevention, Detection & Control: A Practical Approach. Peter J. Wallin & Peter Haycock. 1998. LC 98-70585. 359p. (*0-7514-0416-0*) B Acad & Prof GBR. *Dist:* Aspen Pub.

Foreign Compound Metabolism in Mammals, Vol. 6. Royal Society of Chemistry Staff. 1989. 185.00 (*0-85186-058-3*) CRC Pr.

Foreign Medical Graduates Examination in Medical Science (FMGEMS) Rudman. (Admission Test Ser.: ATS-74). pap. 69.95 (*0-8373-5074-3*) Nat Learn.

Foreign Medical Graduates Examination in Medical Science (FMGEMS) Pt. I: Basic Medical Sciences. Jack Rudman. (Admission Test Ser.: Vol. 74A). 69.95 (*0-8373-6990-8*); 1994. pap. 49.95 (*0-8373-6965-7*) Nat Learn.

Foreign Medical Graduates Examination in Medical Science (FMGEMS) Pt. II: Clinical Sciences. Jack Rudman. (Admission Test Ser.: Vol. 74B). 69.95 (*0-8373-6991-6*);Pt. 2. 1994. pap. 49.95 (*0-8373-6966-5*) Nat Learn.

Foreign Medical Graduates in the United States. Harold Margulies & Lucille S. Bloch. 1990. LC 69-18040. (Commonwealth Fund Publications). (Illus.). 186p. 27.50 (*0-674-30875-1*) HUP.

Foreign Pharmacy Graduates Equivalency Examination (FPGEE) Jack Rudman. (Admission Test Ser.: Vol. 82). 69.95 (*0-8373-5182-0*); 1994. pap. 49.95 (*0-8373-5082-4*) Nat Learn.

Foreign Substances & Nutrition. R. Tarjan. Ed. by J. C. Somogyi. 1980. (Bibliotheca Nutritio et Dieta Ser.: No. 29). (Illus.). viii, 132p. pap. 72.25 (*3-8055-0621-X*) S Karger.

Foremost Physician, the Farseeing Physician. E. Ted Chandler & Robert L. Bloomfield. 1983. LC 83-82069. 14.00 (*0-9612242-0-7*) Harbinger Med Pr NC.

Forensic Analysis of the Skull: Craniofacial Analysis, Reconstruction, & Identification. M. Yasar Iscan & Richard P. Helmer. 1993. LC 93-6838. 276p. 135.00 (*0-471-56078-2*) Wiley.

EFG

Forensic & Clinical Applications of Solid Phase Extraction. Michael J. Telepchak et al. 1999. (Forensic Science & Medicine Ser.). (Illus.). 400p. 99.50 (*0-89603-648-0*) Humana.

Forensic Applications of the MMPI-2, No. 2. Yossef S. Ben-Porath et al. 1995. LC 95-12873. (Applied Psychology Ser.: Vol. 2). 248p. (C). 53.95 (*0-8039-7013-7*, 7574) Sage.

Forensic Aspects in Pediatric Pathology. Ed. by J. E. Dimmick & D. B. Singer. 1995. LC 72-88828. (Perspectives in Pediatric Pathology Ser.: Vol. 19). (Illus.). vi, 178p. 189.75 (*3-8055-6194-6*) S Karger.

Forensic Aspects of Sleep. Colin Sharpiro & Alexander M. Smith. 1997. LC 96-48755. 216p. 130.00 (*0-471-96998-2*) Wiley.

Forensic Assessment with the Millon Inventories. Joseph T. McCann & Frank J. Dyer. 1996. LC 96-7349. (Illus.). 241p. text 38.00 (*1-57230-055-8*, 0055) Guilford Pubns.

Forensic Dentistry. Ed. by Paul G. Stimson & Curtis A. Mertz. 1997. LC 98-150823. 320p. 94.95 (*0-8493-8103-7*) CRC Pr.

Forensic Diatomology & Drowning. Michael S. Pollanen. 1997. LC 98-142915. 170p. 154.50 (*0-444-82844-3*) Elsevier.

Forensic DNA Technology. Mark A. Farley & James J. Harrington. 1990. 272p. 124.95 (*0-87371-265-X*, L265) Lewis Pubs.

Forensic Documentation Sourcebook: A Comprehensive Collection of Forms & Records for Forensic Mental Health Practice. Theodore H. Blau. 1998. LC 98-16154. (Illus.). 224p. pap. text 95.00 incl. disk (*0-471-25459-2*) Wiley.

Forensic Engineering Reconstruction of Accidents. John F. Brown & Kenneth S. Obenski. 1990. (Illus.). 270p. pap. 38.95 (*0-398-06605-1*) C C Thomas.

Forensic Epidemiology. Sana Loue. 1998. LC 98-3783. (Medical Humanities Ser.). (Illus.). 254p. 39.95 (*0-8093-2222-6*) S Ill U Pr.

Forensic Evaluation of Juveniles. Thomas Grisso. 1998. LC 98-14684. 286p. 39.95 (*1-56887-037-X*, FEJBP, Prof Resc Pr) Pro Resource.

Forensic Evaluation of Traumatic Brain Injury: A Handbook for Clinicians & Attorneys. Gregory J. Murrey et al. 2000. LC 00-21760. (Illus.). 168p. 99.95 (*0-8493-2035-6*) CRC Pr.

Forensic Evidence Analysis & Crime Scene Investigation, Vol. 2941. Ed. by John Hicks et al. 1997. LC 96-69891. 154p. 46.00 (*0-8194-2343-2*) SPIE.

Forensic Histopathology. W. Janssen. Tr. by S. Forster from GER. 1986. (Illus.). 360p. 215.00 (*0-387-12466-7*) Spr-Verlag.

Forensic Laboratories: Handbook for Facility Planning, Design, Construction & Moving. Ed. by Alim A. Fatah & Kathleen M. Higgins. 1999. (Illus.). 250p. (C). pap. text 35.00 (*0-7881-7624-2*) DIANE Pub.

Forensic Mass Spectrometry. Ed. by Jehuda Yinon. 1987. 240p. 217.00 (*0-8493-5366-1*, HV8073) CRC Pr.

Forensic Medical Investigator. Jack Rudman. 1994. (Career Examination Ser.: C-2936). pap. 39.95 (*0-8373-2936-1*) Nat Learn.

Forensic Medicine. I. Gordon et al. 3rd ed. 1987. (Illus.). 464p. text (*0-443-03440-0*) Church.

Forensic Medicine. Keith Simpson & Bernard Knight. 9th ed. 1988. 360p. pap. (*0-683-13077-3*) E A GBR. *Dist:* Williams & Wilkins.

Forensic Medicine: An Illustrated Reference. J. K. Mason. 1993. LC 92-48550. (Illus.). 213p. (gr. 13). pap. 381.95 (*0-412-43300-1*) Chapman & Hall.

***Forensic Medicine: Clinical & Pathological Aspects.** Payne-James & Busittil. 2002. (Illus.). 600p. (*1-84110-026-9*) Greenwich Med GBR. *Dist:* JAMCO Dist.

Forensic Medicine - A Handbook for Professionals. Alan A. Watson. 1989. text (*0-566-05513-9*) Dartmth Pub GBR. *Dist:* Ashgate Pub Co.

Forensic Medicine & the Law: An Introduction. David Ranson. 1997. LC 97-158187. 200p. pap. (*0-522-84469-3*) Melbourne Univ Pr AUS. *Dist:* Paul & Co Pubs.

Forensic Medicine for Lawyers. J. K. Mason. 3rd ed. 1995. 490p. pap. (*0-406-04999-8*, MFML3, MICHIE) LEXIS Pub.

Forensic Medicine for Lawyers. J. K. Mason. 1978. 453p. 35.00 (*0-7236-0455-X*) W S Hein.

Forensic Medicine Sourcebook: Basic Consumer Information for the Layperson about Forensic Medicine. Ed. by Annemarie Muth. 1999. LC 99-26967. (Health Reference Ser.). xiii, 574p. 78.00 (*0-7808-0232-2*) Omnigraphics Inc.

***Forensic Mental Health - Issues in Practice.** Colin Dale et al. 2001. (Illus.). 315p. (*0-7020-2441-4*) W B Saunders GBR. *Dist:* Saunders.

***Forensic Mental Health Assessment: A Casebook.** Kirk Heilbrun et al. 2002. 672p. text 55.00 (*0-19-514568-2*) OUP.

Forensic Mental Health Assistant. Jack Rudman. 1994. (Career Examination Ser.: C-3058). pap. 29.95 (*0-8373-3058-0*) Nat Learn.

Forensic Mental Health Care. Ed. by Dave Mercer. 2000. 315p. 28.00 (*0-443-06140-8*) Harcrt Hlth Sci Grp.

Forensic Neuropsychology. Ed. by Charles J. Golden & Mary A. Strider. 1986. LC 86-21176. (Nebraska Neuropsychology Symposia Ser.: Vol. 1). 200p. 54.50 (*0-306-42394-4*, Plenum Trade) Perseus Pubng.

Forensic Neuropsychology: Conceptual Foundations & Clinical Practice. Jose A. Valciukas. 1995. LC 94-20581. (Illus.). 330p. lib. bdg. 49.95 (*1-56024-402-X*) Haworth Pr.

Forensic Neuropsychology: Fundamentals & Practice. Ed. by Jerry J. Sweet. 1999. LC 99-22363. (Studies on Neuropsychology, Development & Cognition: No. 2). 500p. (*90-265-1544-8*) Swets.

Forensic Neuropsychology: Legal & Scientific Bases. Ed. by Hans O. Doerr & Albert S. Carlin. 1991. LC 91-16389. 242p. 35.00 (*0-89862-770-2*, 2770) Guilford Pubns.

Forensic Nursing & Mental Disorder: Clinical Practice. Lorraine Conlon. Ed. by Norman McClelland. 2001. LC 00-54371. (Illus.). 160p. pap. text 45.00 (*0-7506-4309-9*) Buttrwrth-Heinemann.

Forensic Nursing & Multidisciplinary Care of the Mentally Disordered Offender. Ed. by David Robinson & Alyson Kettles. 1999. LC 99-42863. (Forensic Focus Ser.: Vol. 14). (Illus.). 320p. (*1-85302-753-7*) Jessica Kingsley GBR. *Dist:* Taylor & Francis.

Forensic Odontology. Mark L. Bernstein & James A. Cottone. 1999. 79.95 (*0-8493-9525-9*) CRC Pr.

Forensic Osteological Analysis: A Book of Case Studies. Ed. by Scott I. Fairgrieve. 1999. LC 99-10981. (Illus.). xxiii, 340p. text 72.95 (*0-398-06963-8*) C C Thomas.

Forensic Osteology: Advances in the Identification of Human Remains. Ed. by Kathleen J. Reichs. 2nd ed. 1998. LC 97-24812. (Illus.). 584p. text 98.95 (*0-398-06804-6*) C C Thomas.

Forensic Pathology. (*0-340-55391-X*) E A GBR. *Dist:* Routldge.

Forensic Pathology. Dominic J. Di Maio. 1992. (Practical Aspects of Criminal & Forensic Investigation Ser.). 528p. 94.95 (*0-8493-9503-8*) CRC Pr.

Forensic Pathology. Vincent J. Di Maio & Suzanna E. Dana. 1998. LC 98-4300. 176p. spiral bd. 45.00 (*1-57059-495-3*) Landes Bioscience.

Forensic Pathology. D. J. Dimaio. 1992. (Practical Aspects of Criminal & Forensic Investigation Ser.). 65.00 (*0-444-01506-X*, RA1063) CRC Pr.

Forensic Pathology. David J. Williams. 1998. LC 96-45555. (Colour Guide Ser.). pap. text 16.95 (*0-443-05388-X*) Harcrt Hlth Sci Grp.

Forensic Pathology. Bernard Knight. 2nd ed. 1996. (Arnold Publication). (Illus.). 648p. (C). 189.50 (*0-340-58897-7*) OUP.

Forensic Pathology in Criminal Cases. Michael A. Graham & Randy Hanzlick. 1997. LC 98-100223. 401p. 100.00 (*1-55834-685-6*) LEXIS Pub.

Forensic Pharmacology: Medicines, Mayhem & Malpractice. R. E. Ferner. 1996. (Illus.). 264p. (C). text 59.95 (*0-19-854826-5*) OUP.

***Forensic Pharmacology of Drugs of Abuse.** Olaf Drummer. 2001. (Arnold Publication). 416p. (*0-340-76257-8*) E A GBR. *Dist:* OUP.

Forensic Psychiatry. A. Carmi. Ed. by Amihay Levy & David Nachshon. 1999. (Psychiatry, Law & Ethics Ser.: Bk. 1). 377p. pap. 55.00 (*965-7077-05-2*, 324090) W S Hein.

Forensic Psychiatry. John Gunn & Pamela Taylor. 1993. (Illus.). 784p. 205.00 (*0-7506-0349-6*) Buttrwrth-Heinemann.

Forensic Psychiatry. John Gunn & Taylor. 2nd ed. 2000. 1100p. (*0-7506-4183-5*) E A GBR. *Dist:* OUP.

Forensic Psychiatry: A Practical Guide for Lawyers & Psychiatrists. Robert L. Sadoff. 2nd ed. 1988. 262p. text 61.95 (*0-398-05421-5*) C C Thomas.

Forensic Psychiatry: Study Guide Questions & Answers. Fritz Thenor. 1997. LC 98-101206. xv, 276 p. (*0-9660427-0-0*) Prometheus Pubg.

Forensic Psychiatry, Race & Culture. Suman Fernando et al. 1998. LC 97-42754. 304p. (C). 89.95 (*0-415-15321-2*); pap. 29.95 (*0-415-15322-0*) Routledge.

Forensic Psychology. Lionel Haward. 1981. 280p. 40.95 (*0-7134-2475-3*) Trafalgar.

Forensic Psychology: Practitioner's Guide. Gisli H. Gudjonsson & Lionel Haward. 1998. LC 97-42955. (C). 240p. pap. 29.95 (*0-415-13291-6*); 256p. (gr. 13). 89.95 (*0-415-13290-8*) Routledge.

Forensic Psychology for the Journeyman Clinician. Ed. by R. M. Costello & S. L. Schneider. 1991. 350p. (C). pap. text (*0-9630867-0-7*) TX Psych Found.

Forensic Psychotherapy: Crime, Psychodynamics & the Offender Patient. Christopher Cordess. 1995. 1100p. 299.00 (*1-85302-240-3*) Taylor & Francis.

Forensic Radiology. B. G. Brogdon. 1998. LC 97-43645. 496p. 99.95 (*0-8493-8105-3*) CRC Pr.

Forensic Science: An Introduction to Criminalistics. Peter R. DeForest et al. 1983. (Criminology Ser.). (Illus.). 512p. (C). text 82.19 (*0-07-016267-0*) McGrw-H Hghr Educ.

Forensic Science Handbook, Vol. 2. Richard Saferstein. 1987. 492p. 190.00 (*0-13-326877-2*); 1982. (Illus.). 768p. (C). 190.00 (*0-13-326850-0*) P-H.

Forensic Sciences in Clinical Medicine: A Case Study Approach. William R. Anderson. 1998. (Illus.). 272p. text 189.00 (*0-397-58777-5*) Lppncott W & W.

Forensic Scientist I (Toxicology) Jack Rudman. 1994. (Career Examination Ser.: C-2937). pap. 34.95 (*0-8373-2937-X*) Nat Learn.

Forensic Scientist II (Toxicology) Jack Rudman. 1994. (Career Examination Ser.: C-2938). pap. 34.95 (*0-8373-2938-8*) Nat Learn.

Forensic Taphonomy: The Postmortem Fate of Human Remains. Ed. by William D. Haglund & Marcella H. Sorg. 1996. LC 96-33308. 672p. 99.95 (*0-8493-9434-1*) CRC Pr.

Forensics. Kemtec Staff. 1997. (Illus.). 120p. text 99.95 (*1-58100-003-0*) Beckley Cardy.

Forest Pharmacy: Medicinal Plants in American Forests. Steven Foster. 1995. (Forest History Society Issues Ser.). (Illus.). vi, 58p. (Orig.). pap. 6.95 (*0-89030-051-8*) Forest Hist Soc.

Forever Healthy: Introduction to Maharishi Ayur-Veda Health Care. Kumuda Reddy et al. 1997. LC 98-142454. (Illus.). 198p. pap. 14.95 (*1-57582-021-8*) Samhita Enterprises.

Forever Young: Twenty Years Younger in 20 Weeks. Stuart M. Berger. 1990. 272p. mass mkt. 4.95 (*0-380-70696-2*, Avon Bks) Morrow Avon.

Forfar & Arneil's Textbook of Pediatrics. Ed. by A. G. Campbell & N. McIntosh. 5th ed. 1997. (Illus.). 2000p. (*0-443-05393-6*) Church.

Forget Perfect. Lisa Earle McCleod & JoAnn Swan Neely. 2001. LC 00-68473. 288p. pap. 13.95 (*0-399-52715-X*, Perigee Bks) Berkley Pub.

***Forgetting: Alzheimer's, Portrait of an Epidemic.** David Shenk. 2001. LC 2001-28012. 304p. 24.95 (*0-385-49837-3*) Doubleday.

Forgetting Whose We Are: Alzheimer's Disease & the Love of God. David Keck. 1996. LC 96-15344. 256p. (Orig.). pap. text 24.00 (*0-687-02088-3*) Abingdon.

Forging a Women's Health Research Agenda: Policy Issues for the 1990s. Ed. by Jeri A. Sechzer et al. 1995. LC 94-42248. (Annals Ser.: Vol. 736). text (*0-89766-893-6*); pap. text 60.00 (*0-89766-894-4*) NY Acad Sci.

***Forging Links for Health Research: Perspectives from the Council on Health Research for Development.** Nancy Johnson et al. 2000. xii, 293p. pap. (*0-88936-935-6*) IDRC-CRDI CAN. *Dist:* Stylus Pub VA.

Forging Partnerships to Eliminate Tuberculosis. Ed. by Barry Leonard. 2000. (Illus.). 67p. (C). reprint ed. pap. text 20.00 (*0-7567-0093-0*) DIANE Pub.

Forgive & Remember: Managing Medical Failure. Charles L. Bosk. 1981. LC 78-16596. 248p. pap. text 11.00 (*0-226-06680-0*) U Ch Pr.

Forgotten Ages, Forgotten Problems: Adolescents' Health. Phyllis L. Ellickson et al. 1993. LC 93-8687. pap. text 13.00 (*0-8330-1409-9*, MR-141-RC) Rand Corp.

Forgotten Children of the AIDS Epidemic. Ed. by Shelley Geballe et al. 1995. LC 94-34758. 283p. 35.00 (*0-300-06270-2*); pap. 14.95 (*0-300-06271-0*) Yale U Pr.

Forgotten Man: A Combat Doctor's Tour of Duty in Hell. Carl Bancoff. 1992. pap. 4.95 (*1-56171-095-4*) SPI.

Forgotten Man: Understanding the Male Psyche. Reuben Fine. 1987. LC 87-61. (Current Issues in Psychoanalytic Practice Ser.: Vol. 3, Nos. 2-4). 423p. text 79.95 (*0-86656-383-0*) Haworth Pr.

Forgotten People: Positive Approaches to Dementia Care. Jonathan Parker & Bridget Penhale. 1998. LC 97-49445. 150p. text (*1-85742-414-X*) Ashgate Pub GBR. *Dist:* Ashgate Pub Co.

Forgotten Traditions in Ancient Chinese Medicine. Hsu Ta-chun. Ed. by Robert L. Felt. Tr. by Paul U. Unschuld from CHI. 1998. 416p. (C). pap. text 63.00 (*0-912111-24-0*) Paradigm Publns.

Forgotten Traditions of Ancient Chinese Medicine: A Chinese View from the 18th Century. Paul Unschuld. 1998. 403p. pap. text 29.95 (*0-912111-56-9*, Paradgm Pubns) Redwing Bk Co.

Form & Function: A Contribution to the History of Animal Morphology. E. S. Russell. 1992. LC 82-8575. (Phoenix Fiction Ser.). xlii, 384p. (C). pap. text 12.00 (*0-226-73173-1*) U Ch Pr.

Form & Function in the Brain & Spinal Cord: Perspectives of a Neurologist. Stephen G. Waxman. 2000. (Issues in Clinical & Cognitive Neuropsychology Ser.). (Illus.). 582p. 45.00 (*0-262-23210-3*, Bradford Bks) MIT Pr.

Form & Pattern in Human Evolution. Charles E. Oxnard. 1998. 228p. lib. bdg. 20.50 (*0-226-64251-8*) U Ch Pr.

Form, Sound, Colour & Healing. Theo Gimbel. 2nd ed. (Illus.). 192p. pap. 29.95 (*0-8464-4181-0*) Beekman Pubs.

Formal Methods in Developmental Psychology. J. Bisanz et al. 1987. LC 96-35385. (Cognitive Development Ser.). (Illus.). 412p. 172.00 (*0-387-96441-X*) Spr-Verlag.

Formaldehyde. 1989. (Environmental Health Criteria Ser.: No. 89). 219p. pap. text 36.00 (*92-4-154289-6*, 1160089) World Health.

Formaldehyde Sensitivity & Toxicity. Susan E. Feinman. 1988. 240p. 209.00 (*0-8493-4789-0*, RC598) CRC Pr.

Formation & Regeneration of Nerve Connections. Ed. by Sansar C. Sharma & James W. Fawcett. 1992. LC 92-49631. xii, 260p. 120.50 (*0-8176-3563-7*) Birkhauser.

Formation & Transformation of the Perceptual World. Ivo Kohler. 1964. LC 64-18328. (Psychological Issues Monographs: No. 12, Vol. 3, No. 4). 173p. pap. 27.50 (*0-8236-2000-X*) Intl Univs Pr.

Formation of the American Medical Profession: The Role of Institutions, 1780-1860. Joseph F. Kett. 1980. LC 80-14326. 217p. reprint ed. lib. bdg. 72.50 (*0-313-22428-5*, KEFO, Greenwood Pr) Greenwood.

Forming a Moral Community, a Resource for Healthcare Ethics Committees: Forming a Moral Community, a Methodology for Case Review. John D. Golenski. 1992. 161p. (C). 30.00 (*1-882674-00-6*) Bioethics Cnslt.

Forming Winning Strategies: An Integrated Theory of Habitual Domains. P. L. Yu. 1990. (Illus.). 392p. 53.95 (*0-387-52689-7*) Spr-Verlag.

Forms for Behavior Analysis with Children. Joseph R. Cautela et al. 1983. LC 82-62572. 208p. spiral bd. 39.95 (*0-87822-267-7*, 2677) Res Press.

Forms of Brief Therapy. Ed. by Simon H. Budman. rev. ed. 1983. LC 81-2779. 482p. pap. 30.00 (*0-89862-900-4*, 2900) Guilford Pubns.

Forms of Feeling: The Heart of Psychotherapy. Robert F. Hobson. 1988. 300p. pap. text (*0-422-78880-5*) Tavistock GBR. *Dist:* Routldge.

Formshaping Movements in Neurogenesis. Ed. by Carl-Olof Jacobson & Ted Ebendal. 1979. (Illus.). 259p. text 77.00 (*91-22-00272-3*) Coronet Bks.

Formulary Monograph Service. Facts and Comparisons Staff. ring bd. 510.00 (*0-932686-57-5*) Facts & Comparisons.

Formulary of Tibetan Medicine. Vaidya B. Dash. 1988. (C). (*81-85132-04-6*) Classics India Pubns IND. *Dist:* S Asia.

Formulas for Healthful Living. Francis Brinker. Ed. by Kathryn Rosson. (Illus.). 1996. LC 95-83568. 240p. pap. 12.95 (*1-888483-00-8*); Vol. 2. 2nd rev. ed. 1998. LC 97-78424. 244p. pap. 12.95 (*1-888483-01-6*) Eclectic Med.

Formulating Strategies for Health for All by the Year 2000: Guiding Principles & Essential Issues. 1979. text (*92-4-180002-X*) World Health.

Formulation & Delivery of Proteins & Peptides. Ed. by Jeffrey L. Cleland & Robert Langer. 1994. LC 94-3789. (ACS Symposium Ser.: No. 567). (Illus.). 340p. 100.00 (*0-8412-2959-7*) Am Chemical.

Formulation As a Basis for Planning Psychotherapy Treatment. Mardi J. Horowitz. 1997. LC 96-35388. 168p. text 29.50 (*0-88048-749-6*, 8749) Am Psychiatric.

Formulation, Characterization & Stability of Protein Drugs: Case Histories. Ed. by Rodney Pearlman & Y. John Wang. 1996. LC 96-38784. (Pharmaceutical Biotechnology Ser.: Vol. 9). (Illus.). 460p. (C). text 114.00 (*0-306-45332-0*, Kluwer Plenum) Kluwer Academic.

Formulation of AIDS Policies: Legal Considerations for Schools. Matthew Welker & Sarah Pell. 1992. (Monograph). 134p. text 20.00 (*1-56534-049-3*) Ed Law Assn.

Formulation of Veterinary Dosage Forms. Gregory E. Hardee & J Desmond Baggot. 2nd ed. 1998. LC 97-44120. (Drugs & the Pharmaceutical Sciences Ser.). (Illus.). 536p. text 195.00 (*0-8247-9878-3*) Dekker.

***Formulations, Release & Skin Penetration of Topical Anesthetics.** Katayoun Welin-Berger. 2001. (Comprehensive Summaries of Uppsala Dissertations from the Faculty of Pharmacy Ser.: No. 258). (Illus.). 53p. pap. (*91-554-5115-2*) Uppsala Universitet SWE. *Dist:* Coronet Bks.

Forrest General Medical Center. Connerly Lott. 2nd ed. 1997. 208p. text, tchr. ed. 18.00 (*0-8273-8181-6*) Delmar.

Forrest General Medical Center: Advanced Medical Terminology & Transcription Course. Donna Conerly & Wanda Lott. 1986. (C). pap. 32.95 (*0-538-11310-3*, K31); 299.95 (*0-538-11316-2*) S-W Thomson.

Forrest General Medical Center: Advanced Medical Terminology & Transcription Course. Conerly Lott. 2nd ed. 1997. 240p. (C). pap. text 55.95 (*0-8273-8179-4*) Delmar.

***Forrest's Principles & Practice of Surgery.** O. J. Garden et al. 4th ed. 2001. LC 2001-28717. (Illus.). 685p. pap. (*0-443-06493-8*) Church GBR. *Dist:* Saunders.

Forsaken Garden: Four Conversations on the Deep Meaning of Environmental Illness. Nancy Ryley. 1998. LC 98-15996. (Illus.). 256p. pap. 16.00 (*0-8356-0771-2*, Quest) Theos Pub Hse.

***Forschungsfreiheit und Forschungskontrolle in der Medizin - Zur Geplanten Revision der Deklaration von Helsinki.** Ed. by Erwin Deutsch & Jochen Taupitz. 2000. (Veroffentlichungen des Instituts fur Deutsches, Europalsches und Internationales Medizinrecht, Gesundheitsrecht und Bioethik der Universitaten Heidelberg und Mannheim Ser.: Bd. 2).Tr. of Freedom & Control of Biomedical Research - The Planned Revision of the Declaration of Helsinki. (GER.). xii, 466p. pap. 99.00 (*3-540-67253-2*) Spr-Verlag.

Forsyth Experiment: An Alternative System for Dental Care. Ralph Lobene & Alix Kerr. 1979. (Illus.). 162p. (C). 25.95 (*0-674-31035-7*) HUP.

Fortbildungstagung und Jahrestagung der Oesterreichischen Gesellschaft Fuer Gynaekologie und Geburtshilfe, Gmunden, Juni 1992. Ed. by E. Reinold. 1992. (Gynaekologische Rundschau Journal: Vol. 32, Suppl. 1). (Illus.). iv, 160p. pap. 48.75 (*3-8055-5725-6*) S Karger.

Fortieth Anniversary of the Iowa Child Welfare Research Station, 1917-1957. Iowa Child Welfare Research Station, State Univers. 1959. (SRCD M Ser.: Vol. 24, No. 5). pap. 25.00 (*0-527-01581-4*) Periodicals Srv.

Fortress NHS: A Philosophical Review of the National Health Service. David Seedhouse. 1994. LC 93-30021. 188p. pap. 80.00 (*0-471-93909-9*) Wiley.

Fortschritte der Chemie Organischer Naturstoffe, Vol. 44. Laszlo Zechmeister. 1983. (Illus.). 326p. 145.00 (*0-387-81754-9*) Spr-Verlag.

Fortschritte der Chemie Organischer Naturstoffe: Band 33. Ed. by W. Herz et al. 1976. (Illus.). 211.95 (*0-387-81357-8*) Spr-Verlag.

Forty-Five in the Family: The Story of a Home for Children. Eva E. Burmeister. 1970. LC 76-100147. 247p. reprint ed. lib. bdg. 72.50 (*0-8371-3259-2*, BUFA, Greenwood Pr) Greenwood.

Forty-Seven Hundred: The Story of the Mount Sinai Hospital School of Nursing. Janie B. Nowak. 1981. LC 81-5202. (Illus.). 160p. 15.00 (*0-914016-79-2*) Phoenix Pub.

Forty Something Forever: A Consumer's Guide to Chelation Therapy & Other Heart-Savers. Arline Brecher & Harold Brecher. 1992. (Illus.). 377p. pap. 6.95 (*0-927839-46-6*) HlthSavers Pr.

Forty Studies That Changed Psychology: Explorations into History of Psychological Research. Roger R. Hock. 2nd ed. 1995. LC 94-36763. 336p. pap. text 24.20 (*0-13-339896-X*) P-H.

Forty Studies That Changed Psychology: Explorations into the History of Psychological Research. Roger R. Hock. 3rd ed. 1998. LC 98-11270. 336p. (C). (gr. 1 up). pap. text 27.00 (*0-13-922725-3*) P-H.

43 Practical Medicare Compliance Strategies for Physician Group Practices. Ed. by AIS Editorial Staff. 1999. 43p. spiral bd. 47.00 (*0-929156-62-5*) Atlantic Info Services Inc.

Forty Years - & Counting: A Nurse's Story. Harold M. Updike. 1994. 12.95 (*0-533-10791-1*) Vantage.

Forty Years in Phrenology: Embracing Recollections of History, Anecdote & Experience. Nelson Sizer. LC 74-29301. reprint ed. 29.50 (*0-404-13425-4*) AMS Pr.

Forum 1982 Fuer Experimentelle und Klinische Urologie. Ed. by H. W. Bauer et al. 1983. (Beitraege zur Urologie Ser.: Band 3). (Illus.). x, 324p. pap. 87.00 (*3-8055-3718-2*) S Karger.

Forum of Modern Obstetrical Practice: Journal: Gynecologic Investigations, Vol. 1, Suppl. Ed. by W. L. Herrmann & W. L. Heinrichs. 1971. pap. 12.25 (*3-8055-1144-2*) S Karger.

Fosfestrol, Honvanr, St 52r, Honvolr, A Review of New Pharmacokinetic & Clinical Data. Ed. by Gerald P. Murphy & H. Oelschlager. 1988. (Urologia Internationalis Ser.: Vol. 42, Suppl., 1988). iv, 60p. 21.00 (*3-8055-4903-2*) S Karger.

Fosfomycin Trometamol Single Dose: Significance & Management of Lower UTI's - Journal: Chemotherapy, Vol. 36, Suppl. 1, 1990. Ed. by H. C. Neu. 1990. (Illus.). iv, 56p. pap. 18.50 (*3-8055-5325-0*) S Karger.

Foster Family Care for Persons with Mental Retardation. Sharon Borthwick-Duffy et al. 1992. (AAMD Monographs). 200p. (Orig.). (C). pap. 22.95 (*0-940898-27-6*) Am Assn Mental.

Fostering Emotional Well-Being in the Classroom. Randy M. Page & Tana S. Page. 1993. LC 92-31112. (Health Science Ser.). (Illus.). 304p. (C). pap. text 44.95 (*0-86720-753-1*, 753-1) Jones & Bartlett.

Fostering Friendship: Pair Therapy for Treatment & Prevention. Ed. by Robert L. Selman et al. 1997. LC 97-8970. (Modern Applications of Social Work Ser.). 337p. pap. text 26.95 (*0-202-36096-2*) Aldine de Gruyter.

Fostering Healing & Growth: A Psychoanalytic Social Work Approach. Joyce Edward & Jean Sanville. 1996. LC 95-30910. 512p. 50.00 (*1-56821-723-4*) Aronson.

Fostering Learning in Small Groups: A Practical Guide. Jane Westberg & Hilliard Jason. 1996. LC 96-1996. (Series on Medical Education). (Illus.). 310p. 41.95 (*0-8261-9330-7*) Springer Pub.

Foucault, Health & Medicine. Alan R. Petersen & Robin Bunton. 1997. LC 96-43375. 288p. (C). 85.00 (*0-415-15177-5*); pap. 29.95 (*0-415-15178-3*) Routledge.

Foulkeways: The Treasure & the Dream. Blanche P. Zimmerman. 1992. LC 92-71095. (Illus.). 176p. 14.95 (*0-923687-17-3*) Celo Valley Bks.

Found: A Place for Me: The Development, Diagnosis & Treatment of Manic-Depressive Structure. Sandra G. Landsman. 1985. (Illus.). xvi, 149p. (Orig.). pap. text 14.95 (*0-935571-01-9*) Treehouse.

Foundation Health & Social Care. Liam Clarke & Peter Waltham. 1995. 320p. (Orig.). pap. (*0-7487-2082-0*) Nelson Thornes GBR. *Dist:* Trans-Atl Phila.

Foundation of Allied Health Sciences. Frederick C. Ross et al. 4th ed. 1996. 88p. (C). stu. ed., spiral bd. 15.94 (*0-697-25153-5*) McGrw-H Hghr Educ.

Foundation of Allied Health Sciences: An Introduction to Chemistry & Cell Biology. Frederick C. Ross. 4th ed. 1996. LC 95-79337. 240p. (C). pap. 45.63 (*0-697-25151-9*) McGrw-H Hghr Educ.

Foundation of Neurobiology. Delcomyn Staff. 1997. 64.95 incl. cd-rom (*0-7167-3295-5*) W H Freeman.

Foundation of Physiological Psychology. Neil R. Carlson. 1988. 620p. (C). text 50.00 (*0-205-11261-7*, H12610) Allyn.

Foundation of the Allied Health Sciences. Frederick C. Ross et al. 4th ed. 1996. (C). spiral bd., lab manual ed. 36.25 (*0-697-25154-3*) McGrw-H Hghr Educ.

Foundational Analysis: Presuppositions in Experimental Psychology. Pertti Saariluoma. 1997. LC 97-205318. (Progress in Psychology Ser.). 216p. (C). 73.95 (*0-415-14585-6*) Routledge.

Foundational Guide to Art Therapy. Ilse E. Gilliland. 1985. 64p. (C). pap. text (*1-886563-00-4*) Women in Process.

Foundational Issues in Natural Language Processing. Ed. by Peter Sells et al. 1991. (Bradford - System Development Benchmark Ser.). (Illus.). 240p. 35.00 (*0-262-19303-5*, Bradford Bks) MIT Pr.

Foundations: Adult Health Nursing. Barbara L. Christensen & Elaine O. Kockrow. 3rd ed. 1998. (Illus.). 828p. (C). text (*0-323-00316-8*) Mosby Inc.

Foundations & Clinical Applications of Nutrition: A Nursing Approach. Michele Grodner et al. (Illus.). tchr. ed. (*0-8151-3582-3*); 1996. pap. text, stu. ed. (*0-8151-3563-7*) Mosby Inc.

Foundations & Clinical Applications of Nutrition: A Nursing Approach. Michelle Grodner et al. 2nd ed. 1999. (Illus.). (C). tchr. ed. (*0-323-00718-X*); LC 00-269915. xix, 868p. text (*0-323-00390-7*) Mosby Inc.

***Foundations & Clinical Applications of Nutrition: A Nursing Approach - Computerized Test Bank (Win/Mac)** Michele Grodner et al. 2000. (Illus.). pap. 500.00 incl. audio compact disk (*0-323-00715-5*) Mosby Inc.

Foundations for a Psychology of Education. Ed. by Alan M. Lesgold & Robert Glaser. 1988. 328p. 69.95 (*0-8058-0296-7*) L Erlbaum Assocs.

Foundations for Care Giving. American Red Cross Staff. 1993. 24.95 (*0-8016-8105-7*) Mosby Inc.

Foundations for Caregiving Instructor's Manual. American Red Cross Staff. 1993. 544p. (*0-8151-0013-2*) Mosby Inc.

Foundations for Caregiving Skills Book. American Red Cross Staff. 1993. 288p. pap. text 12.50 (*0-8016-6514-0*) Mosby Inc.

Foundations for Conceptual Research in Psychoanalysis. Anna Ursula Dreher. 2000. LC 00-59731. (Monograph Series of the Psychoanalysis Unit of University College London & the Anna Freud Centre: No. 5). xi, 208p. 32.50 (*0-8236-1994-X*) Intl Univs Pr.

Foundations for Gathering & Interpreting Behavioral Data. Robert T. Maleske. 1994. LC 94-15947. (Illus.). 464p. mass mkt. 56.25 (*0-534-23742-8*) Brooks-Cole.

Foundations for Osteopathic Medicine. Ed. by Robert C. Ward et al. 1997. LC 96-16610. (Illus.). 1,200p. text 120.00 (*0-683-08792-4*) Lppncott W & W.

Foundations Maternal-Newborn. Gorrie. 2nd ed. 1998. (C). pap. text, stu. ed. (*0-7216-8656-7*) EHS.

Foundations of Aphasia Rehabilitation. Michel Paradis. 1993. LC 93-1040. 464p. 142.00 (*0-08-041940-2*, Pergamon Pr) Elsevier.

Foundations of Aversion Therapy. Norman H. Hadley. 1985. LC 84-18001. 145p. text 20.00 (*0-88331-145-3*) R B Luce.

Foundations of Behavioral Neuroscience. Shavit & Hasson. 2001. 22.00 (*0-7167-5201-8*) Worth.

Foundations of Behavioral Research. Frederick N. Kerlinger. 3rd ed. 1986. LC 85-8693. 768p. (C). text 100.50 (*0-03-041761-9*) Harcourt Coll Pubs.

Foundations of Binocular Vision: A Clinical Perspective. Ralph P. Garzia. 2000. LC 99-88757. (Illus.). 368p. (C). text 64.95 (*0-8385-2670-5*) McGraw-Hill Prof.

Foundations of Bioenergetics. Harold J. Morowitz. 1978. 55.00 (*0-12-507250-3*) Ox Bow.

Foundations of Bioethics. H. Tristram Engelhardt. 2nd ed. 1996. 464p. text 42.50 (*0-19-505736-8*) OUP.

Foundations of Biological Psychology. 2000. 224p. (*0-13-010913-4*) P-H.

Foundations of Biology. Felix Mainx. 1993. (Foundations of the Unity of Science Ser.: Vol. 1, No. 9). pap. text 2.25 (*0-226-57584-5*) U Ch Pr.

Foundations of Cardiac Pacing: An Illustrated Practical Guide to Rate Variable Pacing, Nos. 1 & 2. Ed. by Richard Sutton et al. 1999. (Bakken Research Center Ser.: Vol. 1, Pt. 2). (Illus.). 12p. 98.00 (*0-87993-381-X*) Futura Pub.

Foundations of Cardiac Pacing Vol. 1, Pt. 1: An Illustrated Practical Guide to Basic Pacing. Richard Sutton & Ivan M. Bourgeois. 1991. (Bakken Research Center Ser.). (Illus.). 352p. 65.00 (*0-87993-337-2*) Futura Pub.

Foundations of Cellular Neurophysiology. Daniel Johnston & Samuel Maio-sin Wu. 1994. LC 93-49890. (Illus.). 710p. 71.50 (*0-262-10053-3*, Bradford Bks) MIT Pr.

Foundations of Chinese Medicine: A Comprehensive Text for Acupuncturists & Herbalists. Giovanni Maciocia. 1989. LC 88-20339. (Illus.). 528p. (*0-443-03980-1*) Church.

Foundations of Chiropractic: Subluxation. Meridel I. Gatterman. 1995. LC 95-9902. (Illus.). 464p. (gr. 13). text 71.00 (*0-8151-3543-2*, 23878) Mosby Inc.

Foundations of Clinical & Counseling Psychology. Judith Todd. 3rd ed. 1998. pap. text 65.50 (*0-321-02512-1*) Addson-Wesley Educ.

Foundations of Clinical & Counseling Psychology. Judith Todd & Arthur C. Bohart. 3rd ed. 1998. LC 98-4648. 589p. (C). text 93.00 (*0-321-01395-6*) Allyn.

Foundations of Clinical Neuropsychology. Charles J. Golden & Peter J. Vicente. 1983. LC 83-16097. (Illus.). 520p. (C). text 120.00 (*0-306-41286-1*, Kluwer Plenum) Kluwer Academic.

Foundations of Clinical Psychiatry. Ed. by Sidney Bloch & Bruce Singh. 1994. LC 94-165714. 488p. (C). pap. (*0-522-84531-2*) Melbourne Univ Pr AUS. *Dist:* Paul & Co Pubs.

Foundations of Clinical Psychology. Ed. by Salvatore Cullari. 1998. LC 97-38141. 448p. (C). 94.00 (*0-205-26202-3*) Allyn.

Foundations of Clinical Psychology: Instructor's Manual & Test Bank. Salvatore Cullari. 1997. 160p. (C). text, tchr. ed. (*0-205-28008-0*, T8008-9) Allyn.

Foundations of Clinical Research. Carol A. Saunders et al. 1998. (Illus.). 88p. pap. 100.00 (*0-9663593-0-5*) Ctr for Clin Res.

Foundations of Clinical Research: Applications to Practice. Leslie G. Portney & Mary P. Watkins. 1998. (Illus.). 752p. (C). pap. text 55.47 (*0-8385-1065-5*, A1065-0) Appleton & Lange.

Foundations of Clinical Research: Applications to Practice. Leslie G. Portney & Mary P. Watkins. 2nd ed. 1999. LC 99-55198. (Illus.). 742p. (C). 63.00 (*0-8385-2695-0*) P-H.

Foundations of Cognitive Science. Ed. by Michael I. Posner. 1989. LC 89-32116. 896p. 105.00 (*0-262-16112-5*) MIT Pr.

Foundations of Cognitive Therapy: Theoretical Methods & Practical Applications. Ed. by Nicolas Hoffmann. Tr. by Elizabeth Lachman from GER. 1984. LC 84-4853. 250p. (C). 54.50 (*0-306-40681-0*, Plenum Trade) Perseus Pubng.

Foundations of Conditioning & Learning. Ed. by Gregory A. Kimble. 1967. LC 67-10442. (Century Psychology Ser.). (Illus.). 49.50 (*0-89197-172-6*) Irvington.

Foundations of Dance - Movement Therapy: The Life & Work of Marian Chace. Ed. by Susan Sandel et al. rev. ed. 1993. (Illus.). 472p. pap. 20.00 (*1-881766-02-0*) M Chace Mem Fund.

Foundations of Electronic Fetal Monitoring. Awhonn. 1998. cd-rom 695.00 (*0-683-40245-5*) Lppncott W & W.

Foundations of Epidemiology. David E. Lilienfield & Paul D. Stolley. 3rd ed. 1994. (Illus.). 384p. text 55.00 (*0-19-505035-5*); pap. text 34.50 (*0-19-505036-3*) OUP.

Foundations of Ethology. Konrad Lorenz. 1981. (Illus.). 380p. 107.00 (*0-387-81623-2*) Spr-Verlag.

Foundations of Gerontology. Jack Rudman. 1994. (ACT Proficiency Examination Program Ser.: PEP-54). pap. 23.95 (*0-8373-5904-X*) Nat Learn.

Foundations of Gestalt Theory. Christian Von Ehrenfels et al. Ed. by Barry Smith. 1988. (Resources Library Ser.). 495p. 119.00 (*3-88405-060-5*) Philosophia Pr.

Foundations of Health. Charles A. Bucher et al. 1967. LC 67-10700. (Illus.). 19.95 (*0-8290-2398-4*) Irvington.

Foundations of Inorganic, Organic & Biological Chemistry: A Medical Perspective. Robert L. Caret et al. 1994. 94p. (C). text, stu. ed. 15.50 net. (*0-697-26037-2*, WCB McGr Hill) McGrw-H Hghr Educ.

Foundations of Integrated Care: Facing the Challenges of Change. Marjorie A. Satinsky. 1998. LC 97-17763. 292p. 48.00 (*1-55648-207-8*) AHPI.

Foundations of Intellectual Assessment: The WAIS-III & Other Tests in Clinical Practice. Robert J. Gregory. 1998. LC 98-21398. 251p. (C). 63.00 (*0-205-19833-3*) Allyn.

Foundations of Laboratory Safety. S. R. Rayburn. 1989. (Contemporary Bioscience Ser.). (Illus.). 418p. 95.00 (*0-387-97125-4*) Spr-Verlag.

Foundations of Maternal-Newborn Nursing. Trula Myers Gorrie et al. 2nd ed. 1998. LC 97-18556. (Illus.). 992p. (C). text 57.95 (*0-7216-8652-4*) Saunders.

Foundations of Maternal Newborn Nursing: Instructor's Manual & Test Questions, Instructor's Manual & Test Questions. Trula M. Gorrie et al. 1994. (Illus.). tchr. ed. (*0-7216-4034-6*) Saunders.

Foundations of Medical Imaging. Z. H. Cho et al. 1993. LC 92-26906. 600p. 135.00 (*0-471-54573-2*) Wiley.

***Foundations of Mental Health Care: Instructor's Resource Manual.** Michelle Morrison-Valfre. 2nd ed. 2001. (Illus.). pap. (*0-323-01344-9*) Mosby Inc.

Foundations of Mental Health Counseling. William J. Weikel & Artis J. Palmo. 2nd ed. 1996. LC 96-21358. (Illus.). 446p. text 93.95 (*0-398-06669-8*); pap. text 71.95 (*0-398-06670-1*) C C Thomas.

Foundations of Mental Health Nursing. Morrison & Michelle. 1997. LC 96-42058. (Illus.). 592p. (C). (gr. 13). pap. text 29.95 (*0-8151-6964-7*, 27246) Mosby Inc.

Foundations of Neuropsychology: An Historical Reader. Ed. by R. W. Rieber. 1987. LC 78-72822. 32.50 (*0-404-60891-4*) AMS Pr.

Foundations of Neuroscience. Marcus Jacobson. (Illus.). 400p. (C). 1995. LC 95-5742. text 44.50 (*0-306-45165-4*); 1993. LC 93-5742. text 85.00 (*0-306-44540-9*) Kluwer Academic (Kluwer Plenum).

Foundations of Noninvasive Cardiovascular Diagnostic Processes. Ed. by Dhanjoo N. Ghista. 1980. (Advances in Cardiovascular Physics Ser.: Vol. 4). (Illus.). 85.25 (*3-8055-2923-6*) S Karger.

Foundations of Normal & Therapeutic Nutrition. T. Randall Lankford & Paula M. Jacobs-Steward. 1989. pap. text 34.95 (*0-8273-4282-9*) Delmar.

Foundations of Normal Nutrition. T. Randall Lankford. 2nd ed. 1994. (Nursing Education Ser.). tchr. ed. 18.95 (*0-8273-6543-8*) Delmar.

Foundations of Nursing. Patrick J. Leahy. 1998. (C). pap. text, stu. ed. 19.95 (*0-7216-5251-4*) Harcourt.

Foundations of Nursing. Christensen. 3rd ed. 1998. (Illus.). 828p. pap. text 35.00 (*0-323-00160-2*) Mosby Inc.

Foundations of Nursing. Goodner. 3rd ed. 1998. pap. text, stu. ed. (*0-323-00155-6*) Mosby Inc.

Foundations of Nursing: Caring for the Whole Person. White. 2000. pap. text, stu. ed. 16.00 net. (*0-7668-0827-0*) Delmar.

Foundations of Nursing: Caring for the Whole Person. Ed. by Lois White. 2000. LC 99-59937. 1856p. text 73.95 (*0-7668-0826-2*) Delmar.

Foundations of Nursing Knowledge. Rodgers. 2002. pap. text (*0-7216-8010-0*) Saunders.

Foundations of Nursing Practice: A Nursing Process Approach. Julia M. Leahy & Patricia E. Kizilay. Ed. by Thomas Eoyang. 1998. LC 97-9768. (Illus.). 1216p. text 57.95 (*0-7216-3881-3*) Saunders.

***Foundations of Nursing Practice: A Nursing Process Approach, ExaMaster.** Julia M. Leahy & Patricia E. Kizilay. 1998. (*0-7216-7830-0*) Saunders.

Foundations of Nursing Research. Rose M. Nieswiadomy. 3rd ed. 1997. 190p. (C). pap., tchr. ed. 26.67 (*0-8385-2697-7*, A-2697-9) Appleton & Lange.

Foundations of Nursing Research. Rose M. Nieswiadomy. 3rd ed. 1997. LC 97-37912. 470p. (C). pap. 45.00 (*0-8385-2696-9*, A-2696-1) P-H.

***Foundations of Nursing Research.** Rose M. Nieswiadomy. 4th ed. 2001. 400p. pap. 39.93 (*0-13-033991-1*, Prentice Hall) P-H.

Foundations of Nursing Theory: Contributions of 12 Key Theorists. Chris M. McQuiston & Adele A. Webb. 1995. 650p. 91.95 (*0-8039-7136-2*, 2681); pap. 46.95 (*0-8039-7137-0*, 2680) Sage.

Foundations of Nutritional Medicine: A Sourcebook of Clinical Research. Melvyn R. Werbach. 1997. LC 96-90623. 330p. text 49.95 (*0-9618550-6-1*) Third Line Pr.

Foundations of Object Relations Family Therapy. Ed. by Jill S. Scharff. 1991. LC 89-19472. 512p. 75.00 (*0-87668-946-2*) Aronson.

Foundations of PE & Sports. Wuest. 12th ed. 1995. tchr. ed. (*0-8151-9466-8*) Mosby Inc.

Foundations of Perceptual Theory. Ed. by Sergio C. Masin. 1993. LC 93-11012. (Advances in Psychology Ser.: Vol. 99). 434p. 153.00 (*0-444-89496-9*, North Holland) Elsevier.

Foundations of Personality: Combining Elements, Crosses & Houses with Jungian Psychological Concepts. Karen Hamaker-Zondag. 1994. LC 94-17757. (Illus.). 336p. (Orig.). pap. 14.95 (*0-87728-808-9*) Red Wheel ME.

Foundations of Personality: Proceedings of the NATO Advanced Research Workshop on Basic Issues in Personality. Ed. by Joop Hettema. 1993. LC 93-9801. (NATO Advanced Science Institutes Ser.). 296p. (C). lib. bdg. 188.00 (*0-7923-2231-2*) Kluwer Academic.

Foundations of Physical Education, Exercise & Sport Sciences. William C. Adams. 1990. LC 90-37084. (Illus.). 296p. text 36.95 (*0-8121-1359-4*) Lppncott W & W.

Foundations of Physical Rehabilitation. Doreen Bauer. 1989. (Illus.). 238p. pap. text (*0-443-03716-7*) Church.

Foundations of Physiological Psychology: Neuroscience Animation 2.0. 2nd ed. 2000. (*0-205-33052-5*) Allyn.

Foundations of Psychiatric Mental Health Nursing. Ed. by Elizabeth M. Varcarolis. 2nd ed. 1994. (Illus.). tchr. ed. (*0-7216-3769-8*) Saunders.

Foundations of Psychiatric Mental Health Nursing. Elizabeth M. Varcarolis. Ed. by Ilze Rader. 3rd ed. 1997. LC 97-7150. (Illus.). 960p. text 51.95 (*0-7216-8643-5*) Saunders.

***Foundations of Psychiatric Mental Health Nursing: ExaMaster.** Elizabeth M. Varcarolis. 3rd ed. 1998. (*0-7216-8646-X*) Saunders.

Foundations of Psychiatry. Davis et al. 1990. (Illus.). 336p. text 52.00 (*0-7216-1341-1*) Saunders.

Foundations of Psychoanalysis: A Philosophical Critique. Adolf Grunbaum. 1984. LC 83-9264. (Pittsburgh Series in Philosophy & History of Science Ser.: No. 2). 256p. pap. text 18.95 (*0-520-05017-7*) U CA Pr.

Foundations of Psychodrama: History, Theory & Practice. Adam Blatner & Allee Blatner. 3rd ed. 1988. 224p. pap. 33.95 (*0-8261-6040-9*); 4th ed. 2000. LC 99-59299. (Illus.). xxi, 285p. pap. 42.95 (*0-8261-6041-7*) Springer Pub.

Foundations of Psychological Research: A Basic Question. Ken Rosenberg & Helen Daly. 1993. LC 92-70921. (Illus.). 420p. (C). pap. text 74.50 (*0-03-055558-2*) Harcourt Coll Pubs.

Foundations of Psychology. Jared S. Moore. 1977. text 19.95 (*0-8369-8189-8*, 8327) Ayer.

Foundations of Psychology. Nicky Hayes. 3rd ed. 2000. (*1-86152-589-3*) ITBP GBR. *Dist:* Thomson Learn.

Foundations of Psychology: An Introductory Text. Nicky Hayes. 1994. LC 93-24314. 1136p. (C). text 62.95 (*0-415-01560-X*) Routledge.

Foundations of Psychology: Some Personal Views. David Rogers. 1984. LC 84-13374. 256p. 67.00 (*0-275-91253-1*, C1253, Praeger Pubs) Greenwood.

Foundations of Psychopathology. John C. Nemiah. 1966. 352p. pap. text 24.50 (*0-19-501137-6*) OUP.

Foundations of Psychotherapy: Theory & Practice. Ed. by Bruce Bongar & Larry E. Beutler. 1995. LC 94-12593. (Textbooks in Clinical Psychology Ser.). (Illus.). 520p. (C). text 57.95 (*0-19-508215-X*) OUP.

Foundations of Rehabilitation Teaching: With Persons Who Are Blind or Visually Impaired. Paul E. Ponchillia & Susan V. Ponchillia. 1996. LC 94-32260. (Illus.). 432p. text 59.95 (*0-89128-939-9*) Am Foun Blind.

Foundations of Respiratory Care. Ed. by David J. Pierson & Robert M. Kacmarek. 1992. LC 92-17459. (Illus.). 1045p. (C). text (*0-443-08509-9*) Church.

Foundations of Respiratory Care. Wyka. 2001. LC 2001-42530. 1216p. (C). text 69.95 (*0-7668-0893-9*) Delmar.

Foundations of Sensory Science. Ed. by W. W. Dawson & Jay M. Enoch. 1984. (Illus.). 577p. 244.00 (*0-387-12967-7*) Spr-Verlag.

Foundations of the Neuron Doctrine. Gordon M. Shepherd. 1991. (History of Neuroscience Ser.: No. 6). (Illus.). 352p. text 39.95 (*0-19-506491-7*) OUP.

Foundations of the Vocational Rehabilitation Process. Stanford E. Rubin & Richard T. Roessler. 4th ed. 1995. LC 94-6130. 460p. (C). pap. text 37.00 (*0-89079-601-7*, 6786) PRO-ED.

Foundations of Voice & Speech Rehabilitation Following Laryngeal Cancer. Philip C. Doyle. 1994. LC 94-7648. (Illus.). 309p. (Orig.). (C). pap. text 55.00 (*1-56593-109-2*, 0412) Thomson Learn.

Foundations of Your Private Practice Vol. 2: The Complete Book of Clinical Forms for an Effective Private Practice. Michael I. Gold et al. 1994. LC 93-12015. (Foundations of Your Private Practice Ser.: Vol. 2). 192p. 74.95 (*0-89793-125-4*) Hunter Hse.

Foundations of Your Private Practice Vol. 3: Clinical Forms. Michael I. Gold. 1994. 80p. ring bd. 50.00 (*0-89793-126-2*) Hunter Hse.

Founders of Child Neurology. Ed. by Stephen Ashwal. 1990. (Illus.). 952p. 125.00 (*0-930405-26-9*) Norman SF.

Founders of Humanistic Psychology. Roy J. DeCarvalho. 1991. LC 91-444. 232p. 67.00 (*0-275-94008-X*, C4008, Praeger Pubs) Greenwood.

Founders of Modern Medicine. Mechnikov et al. Tr. by D. Berger. 1977. LC 78-142669. (Essay Index Reprint Ser.). 25.95 (*0-8369-2111-9*) Ayer.

Founders of Neurology: One Hundred Forty-Six Biographical Sketches by Eighty-Nine Authors. Webb Haymaker et al. 2nd ed. 1970. (Illus.). 640p. 100.95 (*0-398-00809-4*) C C Thomas.

Founders of Nutrition Science: Biographical Articles from the Journal of Nutrition. Ed. by William J. Darby & Thomas H. Jukes. 1992. (Illus.). 1200p. 95.00 (*0-943029-02-3*) Am Soc Nutr Sci.

Fountain of Health: An A-Z of Traditional Chinese Medicine. Charles Windridge. Ed. by Wu Xiaochun. 1995. (Illus.). 658p. pap. (*1-85158-635-0*) Mainstream Pubng GBR. *Dist:* Trafalgar.

Fountain of Youth: Secrets of Health, Rejuvenation & Long Life. Jonathon D. Miller. 2000. pap. 6.98 (*0-935815-05-8*) Lifecircle.

Fountain of Youth: Slowing the Aging Process. Stephen Redmond. 1995. (Illus.). 308p. (Orig.). pap. 14.95 (*0-9643754-0-0*) Ridgeback Pr.

Four Approaches to Counselling & Psychotherapy. Windy Dryden. 1999. LC 98-37422. vi, 210p. 85.00 (*0-415-13992-9*) Routledge.

Four Archetypes. Carl Gustav Jung. Ed. by G. Adler. Tr. by R. F. C. Hull. 1971. (Bollingen Ser.: Vol. 20). 182p. pap. 12.95 (*0-691-01766-2*) Princeton U Pr.

Four Centuries of Clinical Chemistry. Rosenfeld. 1999. 580p. text (*90-5699-645-2*) GBSP NLD. *Dist:* Gordon & Breach.

Four False Pillars of Biopsychiatry. Ty C. Colbert. 1997. (Illus.). 50p. (Orig.). pap. 9.95 (*0-9643635-6-9*) Kevco Pubg.

Four Fundamental Concepts of Psychoanalysis. Jacques Lacan. 1998. (Seminar of Jacques Lacan Ser.: Bk. XI). 304p. pap. 18.95 (*0-393-31775-7*) Norton.

Four-Handed Dentistry: A Handbook of Clinical Application & Ergonomic Concepts. Betty Ladley Finkbeiner. 2000. LC 00-57110. 56p. pap. 20.00 (*0-13-030413-1*) P-H.

***400 MCQs in Paediatrics for the MRCPCH**, Pt. 1. Nagi G. Barakat & Guy's and St. Thomas Hospital Staff. 2001. 200p. pap. (*1-85315-491-1*) Royal Soc of Medicine Pr Ltd GBR. *Dist:* Balogh.

400+ Times Improved PET Efficiency for Lower-Dose Radiation, Lower-Cost Cancer Screening: A Method & Appartus for Cancer Screening Requiring Only the Radiation Equivalent to that Received During Two Intercontinental Flights. 2000. 230p. per. Price not set. (*0-9702897-0-7*) Three D Comp.

Four Hundred Self-Assessment Picture Tests in Clinical Medicine. Wolfe. 1984. (C). (gr. 13). 32.00 (*0-8151-9403-X*, 09956) Mosby Inc.

4-in-1 Master Coder: General Surgery. Robert M. Jensen. rev. ed. 1996. LC 96-76004. 400p. (Orig.). pap. text 39.95 (*0-07-600799-5*, 9646) Practice Mgmt Info.

4-in-1 Master Coder: Orthopedic Surgery. Robert M. Jensen. rev. ed. 1996. LC 96-76002. 425p. (Orig.). pap. text 39.95 (*0-07-600801-0*, 9647) Practice Mgmt Info.

4-in-1 Master Coder: Otolaryngology. Robert M. Jensen. rev. ed. 1996. LC 96-76003. 260p. (Orig.). pap. text 39.95 (*0-07-600800-2*, 9648) Practice Mgmt Info.

4 in 1 Master Coder: Plastic & Reconstructive Surgery. Robert M. Jensen. 1996. LC 96-10896. (*0-07-666802-9*) McGraw.

4-in-1 Master Coder: Plastic & Reconstructive Surgery. Robert M. Jensen. rev. ed. 1996. 350p. (Orig.). pap. text 39.95 (*0-07-600802-9*, 9649) Practice Mgmt Info.

Four Levels of Healing: A Guide to Balancing the Spiritual, Mental, Emotional & Physical Aspects of Life. Shakti Gawain. 1997. LC 97-67259. 112p. 16.00 (*1-882591-30-5*) New Wrld Lib.

Four Minute Neurologic Exam. Stephen Goldberg. 1999. (Illus.). 58p. pap. text 12.95 (*0-940780-05-4*) MedMaster.

Four Paws Five Directions: A Guide to Chinese Medicine for Cats & Dogs. Cheryl Schwartz. 1996. LC 96-15931. (Illus.). 412p. text 25.95 (*0-89087-790-4*) Celestial Arts.

Four Roads to Ruin: Your Health in the Twenty-First Century. Karl Loren. 1995. (Illus.). 400p. (Orig.). 19.95 (*1-882537-06-8*) Bigelow Charter.

Four Score & Five: Recollections & Reflections. Anna Hudesman. 1981. LC 79-92326. 200p. 7.95 (*0-88437-021-6*) Psych Dimensions.

Four Strong Winds: Understanding the Growing Challenges to Health Care. Michael B. Decter. 2000. LC 2001-270965. (Illus.). xii, 307p. (*0-7737-3224-1*) Stoddart Publ CAN. *Dist:* General Distrib Services.

Four Treatises. Ed. by George S. Rosen. Tr. by C. Lillian Temkin et al. 1996. LC 96-30930. 256p. reprint ed. pap. text 17.95 (*0-8018-5523-3*) Johns Hopkins.

Fourier & Wavelet Analysis with Applications to Signal Processing & Medicine. James S. Walker. Date not set. 79.95 (*0-8493-9043-5*, 9043) CRC Pr.

Fourteen Day Stress Cure: A New Approach for Dealing with Stress That Can Change Your Life Forever. Mort Orman & Frank Reuter. 1991. 350p. pap. 13.95 (*0-942540-06-9*) Breakthru Pub.

Fourteen Ounces of Prevention: A Casebook for Practitioners. Ed. by Richard H. Price et al. 1988. LC 88-14471. 191p. pap. 29.95 (*1-55798-036-5*) Am Psychol.

XIV Akademische Tagung Deutschsprechender Hochschullehrer in der Gynaekologie & Geburtshilfe. Ed. by R. Winter & E. Reinold. 1996. (Journal: Vol. 35, Suppl. 1, 1995). (Illus.). xii, 164p. pap., suppl. ed. 78.25 (*3-8055-6306-X*) S Karger.

Fourteenth International Complement Workshop, Cambridge, U. K., September 1991 Abstracts: Complement & Inflammation Journal, Vol. 8, Nos. 3-4. Ed. by P. J. Lachmann et al. 1991. (Journal). 136p. pap. 81.75 (*3-8055-5472-9*) S Karger.

XIVth International Congress "The Fetus As a Patient" XIIth International Congress "Fetal Cardiology" Amsterdam, May 1998 - Abstracts. Ed. by H. P. Van Geijn et al. 1998. (Fetal Diagnosis & Therapy Ser.: Vol. 13, Suppl. 1). 176p. pap. 76.50 (*3-8055-6678-6*) S Karger.

***4th Decennial Conference on Nosocomial & Health Care Associated Infections.** Ed. by Joseph E. McDade. 2001. (Illus.). 197p. (C). pap. text 35.00 (*0-7567-1228-9*) DIANE Pub.

Fourth Estate. Robert E. McDaniel. 1992. (Orig.). pap. 9.95 (*0-9623475-6-6*) Zanni Pubs.

Fourth Generation of Managed Behavioral Health Pt. I: What Does It Look Like? Barbara B. Seltzer. Ed. by Anne M. Christner. 1995. 180p. (Orig.). pap. 99.00 (*1-884937-34-9*) Manisses Communs.

Fourth Generation of Managed Care Pt. II: What Does It Look Like? Barbara B. Seltzer. Ed. by Anne M. Christner. 1997. (Orig.). pap. 99.00 (*1-884937-35-7*) Manisses Communs.

Fourth International Symposium on Bovine Leukosis. Ed. by O. C. Straub. 1982. text 239.50 (*90-247-2604-2*) Kluwer Academic.

Fourth International Symposium on Resistance Arteries, Warren, Vermont, January 1994: Abstracts. Ed. by M. J. Mulvany. 1993. (Journal: Vol. 31, Suppl. 1, 1994). ii, 60p. pap. 26.25 (*3-8055-5919-4*) S Karger.

Fourth International Visual Field Symposium, 1980. Ed. by Erik L. Greve & Guy Verriest. 1981. (Documenta Ophthalmologica Proceedings Ser.: Vol. 26). 416p. text 239.50 (*90-6193-165-7*) Kluwer Academic.

Fourth National Health Policy Forum Healthy Children 2000: Obstacles & Opportunities April 24-25, 1992. 1993. 155p. pap. 12.00 (*1-883848-00-8*) Nat Acad Practice.

Fourth Symposium by the Five Winners of the Grants from Sandoz Foundation for Gerontological Research, Annual Meeting of the Japan Gerontological Society, Kanazawa, Japan, November 1992. Ed. by H. Orimo. 1993. (Journal: Vol. 39, Suppl. 1, 1993). (Illus.). vi, 38p. pap. 14.00 (*3-8055-5823-6*) S Karger.

Fourth WHO Scientific Group on Trachoma Research. 1966. (Technical Report Ser.: No. 330). 24p. pap. text 3.00 (*92-4-120330-7*) World Health.

Fractal Physiology & Chaos in Medicine. Bruce J. West. 1990. 288p. (C). text 74.00 (*981-02-0127-3*); pap. text 40.00 (*981-02-0128-1*) World Scientific Pub.

Fractals & Chaos Simplified for the Life Sciences. Larry S. Liebovitch. 1998. LC 97-20874. 288p. (C). pap. 37.95 (*0-19-512024-8*) OUP.

Fractals in Biology & Medicine. Ed. by F. F. Nonnenmacher et al. 1994. LC 93-44016. 397p. 73.50 (*0-8176-2989-0*) Birkhauser.

Fractals in Biology & Medicine, Vol. II. Ed. by G. A. Losa et al. 1998. (Illus.). 350p. text 75.00 (*3-7643-5715-0*) Birkhauser.

Fractals of Brain, Fractals of Mind: In Search of a Symmetry Bond. Ed. by Earl MacCormac & Maxim I. Stamenov. 1996. LC 96-17605. (Advances in Consciousness Research Ser.: Vol. 7). x, 359p. pap. 38.95 (*1-55619-187-1*) J Benjamins Pubng Co.

Fractional Oxyhemoglobin, Oxygen Content & Saturation & Related Quantities in Blood: Terminology, Measurement & Reporting; Tentative Guideline (1992) Contrib. by Sharon Ehrmeyer. 1992. 75.00 (*1-56238-160-1*, C25-T) NCCLS.

Fractionation in Radiotherapy. Howard Thames & J. H. Hendry. 1987. 200p. 119.00 (*0-85066-374-1*) Taylor & Francis.

Fracture Management for Primary Care. M. Patricia Eiff et al. Ed. by Richard Lampert. 1998. LC 97-22940. (Illus.). 293p. pap. text 55.00 (*0-7216-6394-X*) Saunders.

Fracture Non-Unions. Ed. by Berton R. Moed & Tracy Watson. 1999. (Illus.). 256p. (*0-7506-2231-8*) E A GBR. *Dist:* OUP.

Fracture to the Acetabulum. E. Letournel & R. Judet. 1981. (Illus.). 428p. 175.00 (*0-387-09875-5*) Spr-Verlag.

Fractured Marketplace for Standardized Testing. Walter M. Haney et al. 1993. LC 93-21880. (Evaluation in Education & Human Services Ser.). lib. bdg. 82.00 (*0-7923-9338-4*) Kluwer Academic.

Fractured Minds: A Case-Study Approach to Clinical Neuropsychology. Jenni A. Ogden. 1996. (Illus.). 304p. pap. text 32.50 (*0-19-508814-X*) OUP.

Fractured Scaphoid. Timothy Herbert. 1990. (Illus.). 202p. text 79.95 (*0-942219-06-6*) Quality Med Pub.

Fractures: Diagnosis & Treatment. Ed. by H. David Moehring & Adam Greenspan. 2000. (Hazelden Chronic Illness Ser.). 298p. text 199.00 (*0-07-135902-8*) McGraw-Hill Prof.

Fractures: Directory of Authors of New Medical & Scientific Reviews with Subject Index. Science and Life Consultants Association Staff. 1995. 160p. 57.50 (*0-7883-0576-X*); pap. 47.50 (*0-7883-0577-8*) ABBE Pubs Assn.

Fractures & Dislocations. P. J. Gregg et al. 1996. (Illus.). 1024p. 357.95 (*0-632-02303-1*) Blackwell Sci.

Fractures & Dislocations: A Manual of Orthopaedic Trauma. Ari Ben-Yishay et al. 1994. (Illus.). 212p. (Orig.). pap. 45.00 (*0-9642813-0-9*) Hosp For Joint Diseases.

Fractures & Dislocations - Closed Management. John F. Connolly. 1995. (Illus.). 1264p. text 150.00 (*0-7216-2601-7*) Saunders.

Fractures & Dislocations of the Hand. Jesse Jupiter & Neil Ford-Jones. 1999. text (*0-7234-2645-7*) Martin Dunitz GBR. *Dist:* Mosby Inc.

Fractures & Orthopaedics. David F. Paton. 2nd ed. 1992. LC 92-12316. (Student Notes Ser.). (Illus.). 248p. pap. text (*0-443-04707-3*) Church.

Fractures in Children. Ed. by G. Chapchal. 1979. (Reconstruction Surgery & Traumatology Ser.: Vol. 17). (Illus.). x, 182p. 68.75 (*3-8055-3013-7*) S Karger.

Fractures in Children. Walter P. Blount. 1977. LC 76-11. 294p. reprint ed. 33.50 (*0-88275-392-4*) Krieger.

Fractures of the Acetabulum. E. Letournel & R. Judet. Ed. & Tr. by Reginald A. Elson. 2nd enl. rev. ed. 1997. LC 92-48836. (Illus.). 756p. 250.00 (*0-387-52189-5*) Spr-Verlag.

Fractures of the Distal Radius. Ed. by Harris Gellman. 1998. LC 98-21744. (Monograph Ser.). (Illus.). 104p. pap. 38.00 (*0-89203-204-9*) Amer Acad Ortho Surg.

Fractures of the Distal Radius. Jesse B. Jupiter & Diego L. Fernandez. 1995. LC 94-45533. (Illus.). 351p. 145.00 (*0-387-94239-4*) Spr-Verlag.

Fractures of the Facial Skeleton. Andrew E. Brown & Peter Banks. 2001. 196p. pap. text 55.00 (*0-7236-1034-7*) Buttrwrth-Heinemann.

***Fractures of the Facial Skeleton.** Maisel. 2001. (Illus.). 19-p. (*1-901865-12-6*) Isis Med GBR. *Dist:* Bks Intl VA.

Fractures of the Foot & Ankle. Gumann. Date not set. text (*0-7216-7655-3*) Saunders.

Fractures of the Limbs: The Relationship Between Mechanism & Treatment. Robert Soeur. Tr. by Thomas J. Fairbank from FRE. 1982. (Illus.). 848p. 161.95 (*0-398-04659-X*) C C Thomas.

Fractures of the Wrist & Hand. Terry S. Axelrod. 1997. 112p. 69.00 (*3-540-61811-2*) Spr-Verlag.

Fractures with Soft Tissue Injuries. Ed. by H. Tscherne & L. Gotzen. Tr. by T. C. Telger from GER. 1984. (Illus.). 164p. 85.00 (*0-387-13082-9*) Spr-Verlag.

Fragen an Meister Arion (Franz Bardon) see Franz Bardon: Questions & Answers

Fragile Alliance: An Orientation to the Psychiatric Treatment of the Adolescent. John E. Meeks & William Bernet. 4th ed. 1996. LC 90-4107. 616p. 59.50 (*1-57524-005-X*) Krieger.

Fragile Community: Living Together with AIDS. Mara B. Adelman & Lawrence R. Frey. 1996. LC 96-28452. (Everyday Communication Ser.). 136p. (C). pap. text 16.50 (*0-8058-1844-8*) L Erlbaum Assocs.

***Fragile Lives: Death, Dying & Care.** Beverly McNamara. 2001. 192p. pap. (*0-335-20899-1*) OpUniv Pr GBR. *Dist:* Taylor & Francis.

Fragile Revolution: Consumers & Psychiatric Survivors Confront the Power of the Mental Health System. Barbara Everett. 2000. 251p. pap. (*0-88920-342-3*) W Laurier U Pr CAN. *Dist:* Wilfrid Laurier.

Fragile Self: The Structure of Narcissistic Disturbance. Phil Mollon. 1993. 220p. pap. 48.00 (*1-56593-245-5*, 0316) Singular Publishing.

Fragile Species. Lewis Thomas. 1993. 208p. pap. 10.00 (*0-02-054555-X*) Macmillan.

Fragile X Child. Ed. by Betty B. Schopmeyer & Fonda Lowe. 1992. LC 92-17229. (Illus.). 232p. (Orig.). (C). pap. text 45.00 (*1-879105-83-7*, 0346) Thomson Learn.

Fragile X Syndrome: Diagnosis, Treatment & Research. Ed. by Randi J. Hagerman & Amy Cronister. 2nd ed. 1996. LC 95-25991. (Illus.). 384p. (C). pap. text 37.50 (*0-8018-5388-5*) Johns Hopkins.

Fragile X, 2000 Vol. 8: Current Research & Treatment. Randi Hagerman. 2000. (Belle Curve Informational Ser.). 3.50 (*1-893601-32-3*, BC15-8) Belle Curve.

Fragmentation & Consensus: Communitarianism & Casuist Bioethics. Mark G. Kuczewski. 1999. LC 97-6087. 192p. reprint ed. 55.00 (*0-87840-648-4*) Georgetown U Pr.

Fragments of an Analysis With Freud. Joseph Wortis. 1984. LC 83-24328. 232p. 50.00 (*0-87668-656-0*) Aronson.

Fragments of Genius: Investigations of the Strange Feats of Mentally Retarded Idiots Savants. Michael J. Howe. 1989. (Cognitive Psychology Ser.). 200p. 29.95 (*0-415-00781-X*) Routledge.

Fragmin. Ed. by E. W. Salzman & S. Sherry. 1986. (Journal: Vol. 16, Suppl. 2, 1986). (Illus.). iv, 72p. pap. 24.50 (*3-8055-4347-6*) S Karger.

Fragrant Mind: Aromatherapy for Personality, Mind, Mood & Emotion. Valerie Ann Worwood. 1996. LC 96-6316. 448p. pap. 19.95 (*1-880032-91-0*) New Wrld Lib.

Frail Elderly: Problems, Needs & Community Responses. Carole Cox. 1993. LC 92-38000. 224p. 59.95 (*0-86569-031-6*, T031); pap. 21.95 (*0-86569-228-9*, R228) Greenwood (Auburn Hse).

Frames of Mind: The Theory of Multiple Intelligences. Howard Gardner. 2nd anniv. ed. 1993. LC 92-53248. 480p. reprint ed. pap. 20.00 (*0-465-02510-2*) Basic.

Frames of Reference for Pediatric Occupational Therapy. Paula M. Kramer & Jim Hinojosa. 1993. (Illus.). 576p. 48.00 (*0-683-04779-5*) Lppncott W & W.

Frames of Reference for the Assessment of Learning Disabilities: New Views on Measurement Issues. Ed. by Reid Lyon. 1994. LC 93-30854. 672p. text 55.00 (*1-55766-138-3*) P H Brookes.

Framework for a Comprehensive Health & Safety Program in the Hospital Environment. 1995. lib. bdg. 250.99 (*0-8490-7563-7*); 1994. lib. bdg. 250.00 (*0-8490-8549-7*) Gordon Pr.

Framework for the Imaginary: Clinical Explorations in Primitive States of Being. Judith L. Mitrani. 1996. LC 95-35054. 328p. 45.00 (*1-56821-479-0*) Aronson.

Framework of Systemic Organization: A Conceptual Approach to Families & Nursing. Marie-Luise Friedemann. 1995. LC 95-21327. 336p. 64.95 (*0-8039-4913-8*, 4341); pap. 32.95 (*0-8039-4914-6*, 4342) Sage.

Frameworks for Sport Psychologists: Enhancing Sport Performance. Karen Lee Hill. 2000. LC 00-38894. (Illus.). xviii, 205p. pap. 28.00 (*0-7360-0014-3*) Human Kinetics.

Framing Disease: Studies in Cultural History. Ed. by Charles E. Rosenberg & Janet Golden. 1992. LC 91-19164. (Health & Medicine in American Society Ser.). 450p. (C). text 48.00 (*0-8135-1756-7*); pap. text 17.00 (*0-8135-1757-5*) Rutgers U Pr.

Frances Tustin. Sheila Spensley. 1995. LC 94-15681. (Makers of Modern Psychotherapy Ser.). 176p. (C). pap. 26.95 (*0-415-09263-9*, B4157) Routledge.

Frank M. Engle Lectures, 1978-1997. Ed. by Roger C. Bird. 1998. LC 98-73516. 1000p. (C). text 35.00 (*1-57996-008-1*) Amer College.

Frankheiten Grosser Komponisten see Diseases of Famous Composers

Franklin Institute Illinois' First Medical School. Rodney B. Nelson, III. 1991. (Illus.). v, 94p. (Orig.). pap. 9.95 (*0-9625624-2-4*) Grant Hse Pr.

Frantz Fanon & the Psychology of Oppression. H. A. Bulhan. 1985. LC 85-19101. (PATH in Psychology Ser.). (Illus.). 314p. (C). text 71.00 (*0-306-41950-5*, Kluwer Plenum) Kluwer Academic.

Franz Bardon: Questions & Answers. Dieter Ruggeberg. Tr. by Gerhard Hanswille from GER. 1998. Orig. Title: Fragen an Meister Arion (Franz Bardon). 100p. per. 14.95 (*1-885928-11-4*) Merkur Pubng.

Franzoezich fur Mediziner: Medizinisches Woerterbuch. Christian Bamberg. 1992. (FRE & GER.). 398p. 75.00 (*0-7859-7113-0*, 38243118IX) Fr & Eur.

Fraser & Pare's Diagnosis & Diseases of the Chest Richard S. Fraser et al. Ed. by Lisette Bralow. 4th ed. 1999. LC 98-36145. (Illus.). xlii, 3190p. text (*0-7216-6194-7*) Saunders.

E F G

Fraser & Pare's Diagnosis of Diseases of the Chest, Set. Contrib. by Richard S. Fraser. 4th ed. 1999. LC 98-36145. (Illus.). xlii, 3190p. (*0-7216-6195-5*) Saunders.

Fraud: The Hidden Cost of Health Care. Ed. by Amanda Sheedy. 1996. LC 97-177004. 286p. pap. text 30.00 (*1-879143-32-1*) Health Ins Assn Am.

Fraud: The Hidden Cost of Health Care Study Manual. 1996. 54p. pap., stu. ed. 10.00 (*1-879143-33-X*) Health Ins Assn Am.

Fraud & Abuse in Healthcare. Larry Manson. Date not set. 175.00 (*1-57018-124-1*) BNA Books.

Fraud & Misconduct in Medical Research. Ed. by Stephen Lock & Frank Wells. 1993. 202p. text (*0-7279-0757-3*); 2nd ed. 1996. text (*0-7279-0996-7*) BMJ Pub GBR. *Dist:* AIDC.

Fraud & Root Canals: Medicine's Greatest Fraud; Dentistry, Deception, Quackery. S. Hale Shakman. 1998. LC 98-96132. 130p. pap. text 19.95 (*1-892506-01-7*) Inst of Science.

Fraud Auditing & Forensic Accounting: New Tools & Technique. G. Jack Bologna et al. 2nd ed. 1995. LC 95-5510. 272p. 110.00 (*0-471-10646-1*) Wiley.

Fraud, Malpractice, Pretense & Deception in the Medical Arts & Sciences: Index of Authors, Subjects & Investigations. Roy R. Zimmerman. 1991. LC 90-56241. 220p. 47.50 (*1-55914-268-5*); pap. 44.50 (*1-55914-269-3*) ABBE Pubs Assn.

Fraud, Waste, Abuse & Safe Harbors: A Guide for the Healthcare Professional. Jonathan P. Tomes. 1993. LC 91-35487. 102p. (Orig.). per. 24.95 (*1-882198-01-8*) Hlthcare Fin Mgmt.

FRCA: Passing the Primary Examination. Hugh Williams et al. 1996. LC 97-121845. 160p. pap. text 40.00 (*0-7506-3108-2*, RD81) Buttrwrth-Heinemann.

Frcr Part 1, Pt. I. P. J. Butler et al. 1991. (Brainscan MCQs Ser.). 192p. 31.95 (*0-387-19620-X*) Spr-Verlag.

Free Association: Method & Process. Anton O. Kris. 1996. (Gestalt Institute of Cleveland Book Ser.). 144p. text 24.95 (*0-88163-253-8*) Analytic Pr.

Free Associations: Memories of a Psychoanalyst. Ernest Jones. 1990. 271p. pap. text 24.95 (*0-88738-833-7*) Transaction Pubs.

Free Circulation of Physicians within the European Community. Leon Hurwitz. 1990. (Illus.). 148p. text (*0-566-07064-2*) Avebry GBR. *Dist:* Ashgate Pub Co.

Free Fall to-? Ed. by Francis Pigott. 1989. (C). text (*0-902662-01-5*) R K Pubns GBR. *Dist:* St Mut.

Free for All? Lessons from the Rand Health Insurance Experiment. Joseph P. Newhouse & Insurance Experiment Group Staff. 1994. LC 93-1356. (Illus.). 592p. (C). 60.00 (*0-674-31846-3*) HUP.

Free from Addictions see Libre de Addiciones

Free Hand: Enfranchising the Education of Deaf Children. Ed. by Margaret Walworth et al. 1992. 204p. pap. 16.95 (*0-932666-40-X*) T J Pubs.

Free Health Care. Matthew Lesko. 1995. 603p. pap. 19.95 (*1-878346-34-2*) Info USA.

Free Living Amebas: Natural History, Preventions, Diagnosis, Pathology, & Treatment of Disease. Ed. by A. Julio Martinez. 1985. 168p. 99.00 (*0-8493-6631-3*, QR201, CRC Reprint) Franklin.

Free Money for Nursing Education: A Guide to Scholarships & Loans Available to Nursing Students. Reginald Williams. 1997. LC 97-182500. 64p. (Orig.). pap. 19.95 (*1-57502-498-5*, PO1485) Morris Pubng.

Free of the Shadows: Recovering from Sexual Violence. Caren Adams & Jennifer Fay. 1990. 224p. pap. 12.95 (*0-934986-70-3*) New Harbinger.

Free Radical Damage & Its Control. Ed. by Catherine A. Rice-Evans & Roy H. Burdon. 1994. LC 93-40154. 408p. 178.50 (*0-444-89716-X*) Elsevier.

Free-Radical Mechanisms of Ischemic & Reperfusion Injuries of Various Organs. M. V. Bilenko. 2000. LC 00-25271. (Illus.). 347p. lib. bdg. 79.00 (*1-56072-800-0*) Nova Sci Pubs.

Free Radical Mechanisms of Tissue Injury. Mary Trinen Moslen. 1992. 240p. 149.00 (*0-8493-5161-8*, RB170) CRC Pr.

Free Radical Reactions in Medicine. Janos Feher et al. 1987. (Illus.). 199p. 114.00 (*0-387-17855-4*) Spr-Verlag.

Free Radical Toxicology. Kendall B. Wallace. 1997. LC 96-37786. (Target Organ Toxicology Ser.). 352p. 125.00 (*1-56032-632-8*) Hemisp Pub.

Free Radicals: From Basic Science to Medicine. Ed. by Guiseppe Poli et al. 1993. LC 93-16440. (Molecular & Cell Biology Updates Ser.). x, 528p. 152.50 (*0-8176-2763-4*) Birkhauser.

Free Radicals & Iron: Chemistry, Biology & Medicine. Martyn Symons & John Gutteridge. 1998. LC 98-18401. (Illus.). 258p. text 115.00 (*0-19-855892-9*) OUP.

Free Radicals & the Liver. Ed. by G. Csomos & Janos Feher. 1992. (Illus.). 192p. 84.00 (*0-387-54445-3*) Spr-Verlag.

Free Radicals, Cardiovascular Dysfunction & Protection Strategies. Rakesh C. Kukreja & Michael L. Hess. 1993. LC 93-41039. (Medical Intelligence Unit Ser.). 120p. 99.00 (*1-57059-012-5*) Landes Bioscience.

Free Radicals in Aging. Ed. by Byung P. Yu. 1993. 320p. 119.00 (*0-8493-4518-9*, RB170) CRC Pr.

Free Radicals in Biological Medicine, Vol. 3. J. V. Bannister et al. 1985. x, 266p. pap. text 252.00 (*3-7186-0285-7*) Gordon & Breach.

Free Radicals in Diagnostic Medicine: A Systems Approach to Laboratory Technology, Clinical Correlations & Antioxidant Therapy, Vol. 366. Ed. by Donald Armstrong. 1995. LC 95-3634. (Advances in Experimental Medicine & Biology Ser.: Vol. 366). 480p. (C). text 125.00 (*0-306-44981-1*, Kluwer Plenum) Kluwer Academic.

Free Radicals in Exercise & Aging. Zsolt Radak. 2000. LC 00-44938. (Illus.). xiii, 265p. 47.00 (*0-88011-881-4*) Human Kinetics.

Free Radicals in Medicine. Ed. by T. F. Slater & K. H. Cheeseman. 1993. (Illus.). 320p. text (*0-443-04926-2*) Church.

Free Radicals in Medicine: International Symposium, Vienna, Nov. 1988, Vol. 7, Nos. 3-6. Ed. by T. F. Slater. 1989. (Free Radical Research Communications Ser.: Vol. 4). iv, 272p. pap. text 421.00 (*3-7186-5010-X*) Gordon & Breach.

Free Radicals in the Pathogenesis of Liver Injury: Proceedings of the Second Congress on Free Radicals in Liver Injury, Turin, Italy, 9-11 June 1988. Ed. by P. A. Poli et al. 1989. (Advances in the Biosciences Ser.: No. 76). (Illus.). 330p. 100.50 (*0-08-037382-8*, Pergamon Pr) Elsevier.

Free Radicals in Tropical Diseases. Ed. by Okezie I. Aruoma. 1993. LC 92-48845. xxii, 281p. text 114.00 (*3-7186-5261-7*) Gordon & Breach.

Free Radicals, Oxidative Stress & Antioxidants: Pathological & Physiological Significance. Ed. by Tomris Özben. 1998. LC 98-18042. (NATO Advanced Science Institutes Ser.: No. 296). (Illus.). 406p. (C). text 129.50 (*0-306-45813-6*, Kluwer Plenum) Kluwer Academic.

Free-Standing & Office-Based Ambulatory Care: Surgicenters, Emergency Clinics, Occupational Clinics, & Office-Based Surgery. Ed. by Peter Allen. 2nd ed. 1984. 208p. pap. 795.00 (*0-931634-33-4*) FIND-SVP.

Free Time Boredom: Manual & Testing Tool. Mounir Ragheb et al. 1995. 68p. (Orig.). (C). pap. 20.00 (*1-882883-19-5*, 114) Idyll Arbor.

Free to Be Fit, an Exercise Book for People with Type II Diabetes. Janine Holloway & Debra Jarvis. Ed. by Faye Hoffman. 1989. LC 89-3766. 72p. pap. text 9.95 (*0-939838-27-3*) Pritchett & Hull.

Free to Grieve: Coping with the Trauma of Miscarriage. Maureen Rank. 1985. LC 85-11273. 176p. pap. 8.99 (*0-87123-806-3*) Bethany Hse.

Free to Lead: The Doctor's Guide to Profitable Leadership Performance. Betty A. Derricott. Ed. by Martha Khoury & Ellen Campbell. 1994. LC 93-74929. (Illus.). 200p. pap. 29.95 (*0-9640156-0-9*) Derricott Dental.

Free Your Body of Tumors & Cysts. 1997. 77p. pap. text 7.00 (*1-883713-18-8*) Hanna Kroeger.

Free Your Self from Harmful Stress. Trevor Powell. 1997. LC 96-12655. (Eyewitness Garden Handbks.). (Illus.). 144p. pap. 19.95 (*0-7894-1475-9*) DK Pub Inc.

Free Yourself from Headaches: The Natural, Drug-Free Program for Prevention & Relief. Jan Stromfeld & Anita Weil. 2nd ed. 1995. LC 95-16567. 223p. (C). pap. 14.95 (*1-883319-31-5*) Frog Ltd CA.

Free Yourself from Neck Pain & Headache. David F. Fardon. 1983. 190p. pap. 6.95 (*0-13-330712-3*) P-H.

Free Yourself from Tranquilizers & Sleeping Pills: A Natural Approach. Shirley Trickett. 1997. LC 97-60061. 192p. pap. text 9.95 (*1-56975-074-2*) Ulysses Pr.

Freedom & Control of Biomedical Research - The Planned Revision of the Declaration of Helsinki see Forschungsfreiheit und Forschungskontrolle in der Medizin - Zur Geplanten Revision der Deklaration von Helsinki

Freedom from Abuse in Organized Care Settings for the Elderly & Handicapped: Lessons from Human Service Administration. Roger D. MacNamara. 1988. 104p. (C). text 37.95 (*0-398-05493-2*) C C Thomas.

Freedom from AIDS: Messmate to Helpmeet. Leale G. Anderson. Ed. by Mary E. Anderson. 1993. 236p. (Orig.). pap. 15.00 (*0-9636771-0-1*) White Dove Ent.

Freedom from Arthritis Through Nutrition: A Guide to Pain-Free Living, with Original Recipes. Philip J. Welsh & Bianca Leonardo. 6th rev. ed. 1992. LC 92-9274. (Illus.). 255p. pap. text 14.95 (*0-930852-15-X*) Tree Life Pubns.

Freedom from Backaches. Lawrence W. Friedman. 1987. pap. 5.50 (*0-671-66331-3*) PB.

Freedom from Chronic Pain: The Breakthrough Program that Brings Relief to Chronic Sufferers. Norman J. Marcus & Jean S. Arbeiter. 1994. 240p. 19.50 (*0-671-79892-8*) S&S Trade.

Freedom from Depression Workbook. Les Carter & Frank Minirth. 1995. LC 96-121330. (Minirth-Meier Ser.). 256p. pap. 15.99 (*0-8407-6207-0*) Nelson.

Freedom from Digestive Distress: Medicine-Free Relief from Heartburn, Gas, Bloating & Irritable Bowel Syndrome. Gary L. Gitnick & Karen Cooksey. 2000. LC 00-37724. (Illus.). 256p. pap. 14.00 (*0-8129-3262-5*, Three Riv Pr) Crown Pub Group.

Freedom from Fear. 1985. (Pocket Power Ser.). 16p. (Orig.). pap. 1.25 (*0-89486-257-X*, 1282B) Hazelden.

Freedom from Fear Forever. James V. Durlacher. Ed. by Guy McGill. 1995. LC 94-62181. (Illus.). 245p. pap. 18.95 (*0-9645713-1-5*) Van Ness Pub.

Freedom from Fibromyalgia: The 5-Week Proven Program to Conquer Pain & Banish the Demon. Nancy Selfridge & Franklynn Peterson. 2001. LC 00-46668. 272p. pap. 14.00 (*0-8129-3375-3*, Three Riv Pr) Harmony Bks.

Freedom from Headaches. Joel R. Saper & Kenneth R. Maggee. rev. ed. 1986. LC 79-26364. (Fireside Book Ser.). (Illus.). 234p. pap. 12.00 (*0-671-25404-9*, Fireside) S&S Trade Pap.

Freedom from Memory, Desire, & Understanding: Psychoanalysis & Gestalt Psychology. Marvin Lifschitz. 1995. LC 93-20971. (Frontiers of Consciousness Ser.). (Illus.). 260p. (C). text 34.95 (*0-8290-2452-2*) Ardent Media.

Freedom from Stress. Edward E. Ford. 1989. (Illus.). 184p. (Orig.). pap. 10.00 (*0-9616716-1-0*) Brandt Pub.

Freedom from Stress: A Holistic Approach. Phil Nuernberger. 1981. LC 80-80542. (Illus.). 261p. (C). pap. 14.95 (*0-89389-064-2*) Himalayan Inst.

Freedom from Teeth Clenching & Night Grinding. Leonard G. Horowitz. 1989. (Freedom from Ser.). 32p. audio 14.95 (*0-9609386-8-0*) Tetrahedron Pub.

Freedom from the Self: Sufism, Meditation, & Psychotherapy. Mohammad Shafii. 1988. 261p. (C). 32.95 (*0-89885-231-5*); pap. 19.95 (*0-89885-395-8*) Kluwer Academic (Kluwer Acad Hman Sci).

Freedom from TMJ Pain Syndrome. Leonard G. Horowitz. unabr. ed. 1988. (Freedom from Ser.). (Illus.). 72p. 29.95 incl. audio (*0-9609386-3-X*) Tetrahedron Pub.

Freedom of Choice in Health Insurance. John C. Goodman & Gerald L. Musgrave. 1988. pap. 10.00 (*0-943802-38-5*, 134) Natl Ctr Pol.

Freedom of Choice in the Healing Arts. Harold E. Buttram. 1971. 52p. (Orig.). pap. 2.00 (*0-916285-28-6*) Humanitarian.

Freedom Through Health. Terry S. Friedmann. 1993. 200p. pap. 11.95 (*0-9638366-2-5*) Harvest.

Freedom to Inquire: Self Psychological Perspectives on Women's Issues, Masochism, & the Therapeutic Relationship. Esther Menaker. 1995. LC 94-49182. 360p. 50.00 (*1-56821-475-8*) Aronson.

Freeing Ourselves from Our Family of Origins: The Houdini Experience. Gary Embelton et al. 1996. LC 96-7604. 261p. 40.00 (*1-56821-852-4*) Aronson.

Freeing Your Child from Obsessive-Compulsive Disorder: A Powerful, Practical Program for Parents of Children & Adolescents. Tamar E. Chansky. 2001. 368p. pap. 14.95 (*0-8129-3117-3*, Three Riv Pr) Harmony Bks.

Freizeit in der Schule-Schulbau fuer die Freizeit: Eine Empirische Untersuchung an Ganztags-Schulen. Ed. by W. Kroner & K. Opperman. 1977. (Psychologische Praxis Ser.: Band 51). (Illus.). 21.00 (*3-8055-2686-5*) S Karger.

Fremantle Hospital: A Social History to 1987. Phyl Garrick & Chris Jeffery. 35.00 (*0-7316-1196-9*); pap. 25.00 (*0-7316-1212-4*) Intl Spec Bk.

Fremdblutsparende Massnahmen in der Operativen Medizin. G. Singbartl. Ed. by W. Schleinzer et al. 1993. (Beitraege zur Infusionstherapie und Klinische Ernaehrung Ser.: Vol. 29). (Illus.). viii, 300p. 98.50 (*3-8055-5541-5*) S Karger.

French Connections: Hemingway & Fitzgerald Abroad. Bryer Kennedy. 1999. LC 96-49632. 370p. pap. 18.95 (*0-312-22450-8*) St Martin.

French Dictionary of Medicine & Biology: Dictionnaire Francais de Medicine et de Biologie Alexandre Manuila. 1981. (FRE.). 450.00 (*0-8288-1817-7*, M15579) Fr & Eur.

French DNA: Trouble in Purgatory. Paul Rabinow. 1999. LC 99-12162. 200p. 25.00 (*0-226-70150-6*) U Ch Pr.

French-English - English-French Dictionary of Medical & Biological Terms. Pierre Lepine. 2nd ed. 1991. (ENG & FRE.). 162.50 (*0-7859-8938-2*) Fr & Eur.

French-English-French Dictionary of Medical Sciences. J. Delamare & Delamare-Riche. 3rd ed. 1992. (ENG & FRE.). 542p. 225.00 (*0-8288-0564-4*, M6107) Fr & Eur.

French Lexicon of Internal Medicine Symbols & Siglas: Lexique Francais des Symboles et des Sigles en Medecine Interne. Maurice A. Touati. 1994. (ENG & FRE.). 548p. 125.00 (*0-8288-0567-9*, M7853) Fr & Eur.

French Medicine. Maxime Laignel-Lavastine. LC 75-23666. (Clio Medica Ser.: 15). (Illus.). reprint ed. 37.50 (*0-404-58915-4*) AMS Pr.

French Paracelsians: The Chemical Challenge to Medical & Scientific Tradition in Early Modern France. Allen G. Debus. 1991. (Illus.). 265p. (C). text 74.95 (*0-521-40049-X*) Cambridge U Pr.

French Physician Desk's Reference see Dictionnaire Vidal

French Physician's Desk Reference see Dictionnaire Vidal: 1995 Edition

French-Polish Medical Dictionary. Nezunan. 1990. (FRE & POL.). 150.00 (*0-8288-7273-2*) Fr & Eur.

French's Index of Differential Diagnosis. Ed. by Ian A. D. Bouchier et al. 13th ed. 1996. LC 97-189034. (An Arnold Publication). (Illus.). 832p. pap. (*0-7506-1434-X*) E A GBR. *Dist:* OUP.

French's Index of Surgical Differential Diagnosis. Harold Ellis & Herbert French. 1999. LC 99-201843. (Illus.). 448p. pap. (*0-7506-2763-8*) E A GBR. *Dist:* OUP.

Frequency of the Rheumatic Diseases. Sidney Cobb. 1971. LC 72-158427. (Vital & Health Statistics Monographs, American Public Health Association). (Illus.). 171p. 22.00 (*0-674-32325-4*) HUP.

Frequency of the Rheumatic Diseases. Sidney Cobb. 1999. 174p. lib. bdg. 24.95 (*0-7351-0184-1*) Replica Bks.

Fresh Look at Psychoanalysis: The View from Self Psychology. Arnold Goldberg. 1992. 296p. reprint ed. pap. 29.95 (*0-88163-156-6*) Analytic Pr.

Fresh Perspectives on Anxiety Disorders. Ed. by Paul M. Emmelkamp et al. 1989. viii, 300p. (*90-265-1016-0*) Swets.

Freshwater Snails of Africa & Their Medical Importance. David S. Brown. 2nd ed. 1994. 550p. (*0-7484-0026-5*) Tay Francis Ltd GBR. *Dist:* Taylor & Francis.

Freud: Conflict & Culture. Ed. by Michael Roth. 2000. 304p. pap. 14.00 (*0-679-77292-8*) Vin Bks.

Freud: Darkness in the Midst of Vision. Louis Breger. 2001. LC 99-59994. (Illus.). 480p. 30.00 (*0-471-31628-8*) Wiley.

Freud: Dictionary of Psychoanalysis. Sigmund Freud. Ed. by Nandor Fodor & Frank Gaynor. 1969. LC 73-90510. 208p. reprint ed. lib. bdg. 62.50 (*0-8371-2135-3*, FRP, Greenwood Pr) Greenwood.

Freud: General Psychological Theory. Sigmund Freud. 1963. 224p. pap. 6.95 (*0-02-076350-6*) Macmillan.

Freud: Living & Dying. Max Schur. 1972. LC 71-143379. 587p. 95.00 (*0-8236-2025-5*); pap. 24.95 (*0-8236-8052-5*, 22025) Intl Univs Pr.

Freud: The Mind of the Moralist. Philip Rieff. 3rd ed. 1979. LC 78-69967. 464p. pap. text 25.00 (*0-226-71639-2*, P777) U Ch Pr.

Freud, Adler, & Jung. Walter Kaufmann. 1992. (Discovering the Mind Ser.: Vol. 3). 397p. (C). pap. text 24.95 (*0-88738-395-5*) Transaction Pubs.

Freud among the Philosophers: The Psychoanalytic Unconscious & Its Philosophical Critics. Donald Levy. 1996. LC 96-2169. 200p. 30.00 (*0-300-06632-5*) Yale U Pr.

Freud & Anthropology: A History & Reappraisal. Edwin R. Wallace, IV. 1984. LC 83-193. (Psychological Issues Monographs: No. 55). xi, 306p. 45.00 (*0-8236-2012-3*) Intl Univs Pr.

Freud & Beyond. Stephen A. Mitchell. 2000. 320p. pap. 17.00 (*0-465-01405-4*) HarperCollins Pubs.

Freud & Cezanne: Psychotherapy As Modern Art. Alexander Jasnow. 1993. LC 93-14278. (Frontiers in Psychotherapy Ser.). 197p. 77.00 (*0-89391-920-9*); pap. 39.50 (*1-56750-064-1*) Greenwood (Ablex).

Freud & Contemporary Culture. New York Academy of Medicine Staff. Ed. by Iago Galdston. 1977. LC 77-142674. (Essay Index Reprint Ser.). 14.95 (*0-8369-2112-7*) Ayer.

Freud & His Aphasia Book: Language & the Sources of Psychoanalysis. Valerie D. Greenberg. 1997. LC 97-18277. (Cornell Studies in the History of Psychiatry). (Illus.). 240p. 35.00 (*0-8014-3284-7*) Cornell U Pr.

Freud & His Critics. Paul W. Robinson. 1993. LC 92-12935. 281p. (C). text 35.00 (*0-520-08029-7*) U CA Pr.

Freud & His Followers. Paul Roazen. 1992. (Da Capo Series in Science Ser.). (Illus.). 643p. reprint ed. pap. 17.95 (*0-306-80472-7*) Da Capo.

Freud & His Mother: Preoedipal Aspects of Freud's Personality. Deborah P. Margolis. 1996. LC 94-44328. 472p. 40.00 (*1-56821-448-0*) Aronson.

Freud & His Patients. Ed. by Mark Kanzer & Jules Glenn. 1979. LC 79-51909. (Downstate Psychoanalytic Institute Twenty-Fifth Anniversary Ser.: Vol. II). 376p. 40.00 (*0-87668-367-7*) Aronson.

Freud & His Self Analysis. Ed. by Mark Kanzer & Jules Glenn. 1983. LC 84-45087. (Downstate Psychoanalytic Institute Twenty-Fifth Anniversary Ser.: Vol. I). 320p. 50.00 (*0-87668-712-5*) Aronson.

Freud & Judaism. David Meghnagi. 1993. 200p. pap. text (*1-85575-002-3*) Karnac Bks GBR. *Dist:* Other Pr LLC.

Freud & Jung: Conflicts of Interpretation. Robert S. Steele. 1982. 300p. 35.00 (*0-7100-9067-6*, Routledge Thoemms) Routledge.

Freud & Jung: Patterns in Conflict. Terence Duniho. Date not set. pap. (*1-878287-29-X*) Type & Temperament.

Freud & Man's Soul. Bruno Bettelheim. 1983. LC 83-47809. 128p. mass mkt. 9.00 (*0-394-71036-3*) Vin Bks.

Freud & Modern Psychology Vol. 2: The Emotional Basis of Human Behavior. Helen B. Lewis. 1983. (Emotions, Personality, & Psychotherapy Ser.). (Illus.). 246p. (C). 72.00 (*0-306-41329-9*, Plenum Trade) Perseus Pubng.

Freud & Modern Psychology, Vol. 1: The Emotional Basis of Mental Illness. Helen B. Lewis. 1981. LC 80-20937. (Emotions, Personality, & Psychotherapy Ser.). 258p. 49.50 (*0-306-40525-3*, Plenum Trade) Perseus Pubng.

Freud & Moses: The Long Journey Home. Emanuel Rice. 1990. LC 89-77695. 266p. (C). text 22.50 (*0-7914-0453-6*) State U NY Pr.

Freud & Oedipus. Peter L. Rudnytsky. 1992. (Psychoanalysis & Culture Ser.). 416p. (C). pap. 20.50 (*0-231-06353-9*) Col U Pr.

Freud & Religious Belief. Howard L. Philp. 1974. LC 72-12635. 140p. reprint ed. lib. bdg. 38.50 (*0-8371-6682-9*, PHFR, Greenwood Pr) Greenwood.

Freud & the Bolsheviks: Psychoanalysis in Imperial Russia & the Soviet Union. Martin A. Miller. 1998. LC 98-3630. 256p. 35.00 (*0-300-06810-7*) Yale U Pr.

Freud & the Child Woman: The Memoirs of Fritz Wittels. Ed. & Comment by Edward Timms. 1995. LC 95-21047. 188p. (C). 35.00 (*0-300-06485-3*) Yale U Pr.

Freud & the History of Psychoanalysis. Ed. by Toby Gelfand & John Kerr. 1992. LC 92-7019. 416p. text 49.95 (*0-88163-136-1*) Analytic Pr.

Freud & the Legacy of Moses. Richard J. Bernstein. 1998. LC 98-14400. (Cambridge Studies in Religion & Critical Thought: No. 4). 168p. (C). text 59.95 (*0-521-63096-7*); pap. text 21.95 (*0-521-63877-1*) Cambridge U Pr.

Freud & the Neurosciences: From Brain Research to the Unconscious. Giselher Guttman. 1999. (Illus.). 116p. pap. text (*3-7001-2740-5*) Verlag Osterreich.

Freud & the Question of Pseudoscience. Frank Cioffi. 1998. LC 98-26764. 340p. pap. 26.95 (*0-8126-9385-X*) Open Court.

Freud & the Scientific Method. Paul Rosenfels. 1980. LC 80-118217. (Ninth Street Center Monographs). (Orig.). pap. 3.95 (*0-932961-06-1*) Ninth St Ctr.

Freud & the Twentieth Century. Ed. by Benjamin Nelson. 1990. 18.75 (*0-8446-2097-1*) Peter Smith.

Freud As a Writer. Patrick J. Mahony. 1981. LC 81-14306. 227p. 35.00 (*0-8236-2018-2*) Intl Univs Pr.

Freud at the Crossroads. Alexander Grinstein. 1990. LC 89-27738. 600p. 90.00 (*0-8236-2015-8*) Intl Univs Pr.

Freud, Biologist of the Mind: Beyond the Psychoanalytic Legend. Frank J. Sulloway. 1992. LC 92-16180. (Illus.). 640p. pap. 24.95 (*0-674-32335-1*) HUP.

Freud, Dora & Vienna, 1900. Hannah S. Decker. 1992. 320p. pap. 14.95 (*0-02-907212-3*) Free Pr.

Freud Evaluated: The Completed Arc. Malcolm Macmillan. 1991. (Advances in Psychology Ser.: No. 75). 688p. 185.00 (*0-444-88717-2*, North Holland) Elsevier.

Freud in Germany: Revolution & Reaction in Science, 1893-1907. Hannah Decker. 1977. LC 77-20062. (Psychological Issues Monographs: No. 41). 360p. (Orig.). 52.50 (*0-8236-2023-9*); pap. 42.50 (*0-8236-2022-0*) Intl Univs Pr.

Freud, Jung & Christianity. James Forsyth. 1989. 300p. pap. 20.00 (*0-7766-0212-8*) Paul & Co Pubs.

Freud, Jung & Hall the King-Maker: The Expedition to America, 1909. Saul Rosenzweig. 2000. 477p. reprint ed. text 27.00 (*0-7881-6864-9*) DIANE Pub.

Freud, Jung & Hall the Kingmaker: The Historic Expedition to America (1909) Saul Rosenzweig. 1992. (Illus.). 400p. 27.50 (*0-88937-110-5*) Hogrefe & Huber Pubs.

Freud-Jung Letters: The Correspondence Between Sigmund Freud & C. G. Jung. Sigmund Freud & Carl Gustav Jung. Ed. by William McGuire. Tr. by R. F. C. Hull & Ralph Manheim. 1974. LC 76-166373. (Bollingen Ser.: No. 94). 650p. 99.50 (*0-691-09890-5*) Princeton U Pr.

Freud-Jung Letters: The Correspondence Between Sigmund Freud & C. G. Jung. Sigmund Freud. Ed. by William McGuire. Tr. by Ralph Manheim & R. F. C. Hull. abr. ed. 1994. LC 93-46096. 320p. (C). pap. 17.95 (*0-691-03643-8*) Princeton U Pr.

Freud-Jung Letters: The Correspondence Between Sigmund Freud & C. G. Jung. Sigmund Freud & Carl Gustav Jung. Ed. by William McGuire. Tr. by Ralph Manheim & R. F. C. Hull from GER. 1988. LC 87-33916. (Illus.). 692p. reprint ed. pap. text 18.00 (*0-674-32330-0*) HUP.

Freud-Klein Controversies. Ed. by Pearl King & Riccardo Steiner. 1992. (New Library of Psychoanalysis). 1000p. (C). pap. 68.95 (*0-415-08274-9*, A9695) Routledge.

Freud, Master & Friend. Hanns Sachs. 1977. LC 78-133531. (Select Bibliographies Reprint Ser.). 19.95 (*0-8369-5563-3*) Ayer.

Freud on Schreber: Psychoanalytic Theory & the Critical Act. C. Barry Chabot. 1982. LC 81-16476. 192p. lib. bdg. 27.50 (*0-87023-348-3*) U of Mass Pr.

Freud on Women: A Reader. Intro. by Elizabeth Young-Bruehl. 1992. 416p. pap. 14.95 (*0-393-30870-7*) Norton.

Freud or Jung. Edward Glover. 1990. LC 91-3303. 208p. pap. 14.95 (*0-8101-0904-2*) Northwestern U Pr.

Freud, Proust & Perversion. Hendrika Halberstadt-Freud. 1991. 220p. (*90-265-1111-6*) Swets.

Freud Reappraised: A Fresh Look at Psychoanalytic Theory. Robert R. Holt. 1989. LC 88-35623. 433p. 49.95 (*0-89862-387-1*) Guilford Pubns.

Freud Scenario. Jean-Paul Sartre. Tr. by Quinton Hoare. 1994. LC 86-11243. xviii, 550p. (C). pap. 14.95 (*0-226-73514-1*); 24.95 (*0-226-73513-3*) U Ch Pr.

Freud, Surgery & the Surgeons. Paul E. Stepansky. 1999. LC 99-13483. 280p. 42.50 (*0-88163-289-9*) Analytic Pr.

Freud: The Fusion of Science & Humanism: The Intellectual History of Psychoanalysis. Ed. by John E. Gedo & George H. Pollock. 1975. LC 75-792. (Psychological Issues Monographs: No. 34-35, Vol. 9, No. 2-3). 447p. (C). 65.00 (*0-8236-2031-X*); pap. 47.50 (*0-8236-2030-1*) Intl Univs Pr.

Freud 2000. Anthony Elliott. 1999. LC 98-29061. 320p. pap. 22.95 (*0-415-92253-4*) Routledge.

Freud under Analysis: History, Theory, Practice - Essays in Honor of Paul Roazeu. Todd Dufresne & Paul Roazen. 1997. LC 96-49860. 344p. 60.00 (*0-7657-0057-3*) Aronson.

Freud Without Hindsight: Reviews of His Work, 1893-1939. Norman Kiell. 1988. 776p. 80.00 (*0-8236-2055-7*) Intl Univs Pr.

Freud, Women & Society. J. O. Wisdom. 1991. 120p. (C). text 32.95 (*0-88738-444-7*) Transaction Pubs.

Freudian Body: Psychoanalysis & Art. Leo Bersani. 1990. LC 85-22334. (Illus.). 126p. pap. text 18.00 (*0-231-06219-2*, King's Crown Paperbacks) Col U Pr.

Freudian Mystique: Freud, Women & Feminism. Samuel Slipp. 1993. LC 92-35872. 288p. (C). text 45.00 (*0-8147-7968-9*) NYU Pr.

Freudian Psychology & Veblen's Social Theory. Louis Schneider. 1974. LC 73-19119. 270p. reprint ed. lib. bdg. 35.00 (*0-8371-7308-6*, SCFP, Greenwood Pr) Greenwood.

Freudian Reading: Analytical & Fictional Constructions. Lis Moller. 1991. LC 91-22539. 184p. (Orig.). (C). text 32.50 (*0-8122-3126-0*); pap. text 14.95 (*0-8122-1381-5*) U of Pa Pr.

Freudian Subject. Mikkel Borch-Jacobsen. Tr. by Catherine Porter from FRE. 1988. LC 87-30548.Tr. of Sujet Freudien. 288p. 51.00 (*0-8047-1440-1*) Stanford U Pr.

Freudians: A Comparative Perspective. Edith Kurzweil. 1998. LC 97-2269. (Psychiatry & Social Psychology Ser.). 380p. pap. text 29.95 (*1-56000-956-X*) Transaction Pubs.

Freud's Brain: Neuropsychodynamic Foundations of Psychoanalysis. Laurence Miller. 1991. LC 91-16480. 276p. 35.00 (*0-89862-762-1*) Guilford Pubns.

Freud's Case Studies: Self-Psychological Perspectives. Barry Magid. 1993. 216p. text 39.95 (*0-88163-132-9*) Analytic Pr.

Freud's Concept of Passivity. Russell H. Davis. 1993. LC 91-3036. (Psychological Issues Monographs: No. 60). 250p. 37.50 (*0-8236-2032-8*) Intl Univs Pr.

Freud's Dora: A Psychoanalytic, Historical, & Textual Study. Patrick J. Mahony. 1996. LC 96-10372. 192p. 30.00 (*0-300-06622-8*) Yale U Pr.

Freud's Dream: A Complete Interdisciplinary Science of Mind. Patricia Kitcher. (Illus.). 1992. 255p. 32.50 (*0-262-11172-1*); 1995. 256p. reprint ed. pap. 18.95 (*0-262-61115-5*) MIT Pr (Bradford Bks).

Freud's Dream of Interpretation. Ken Frieden. 1990. LC 89-4597. (SUNY Series in Modern Jewish Literature & Culture). 159p. (C). text 20.50 (*0-7914-0124-3*) State U NY Pr.

Freud's Models of the Mind: An Introduction. Joseph Sandler. 1997. 224p. pap. (*1-85575-167-4*) Karnac Bks GBR. *Dist:* Other Pr LLC.

Freud's Neurological Education & Its Influence on Psychoanalytic Theory. Peter Amacher. 1966. LC 65-19461. (Psychological Issues Monographs: No. 16, Vol. 4, No. 4). 93p. (Orig.). 27.50 (*0-8236-2040-9*) Intl Univs Pr.

Freud's Paranoid Quest: Psychoanalysis & Modern Suspicion. John Farrell. LC 95-50156. 276p. (C). 1998. pap. text 18.50 (*0-8147-2650-X*); 1996. text 55.00 (*0-8147-2649-6*) NYU Pr.

Freud's Russia: National Identity in the Evolution of Psychoanalysis. James L. Rice. 1993. LC 92-31244. 210p. (C). text 39.95 (*1-56000-091-0*) Transaction Pubs.

Freud's Self-Analysis. Didier Anzieu. 1986. LC 86-14924. 92.50 (*0-8236-2045-X*) Intl Univs Pr.

Freud's Wishful Dream Book. Alexander Welsh. 1994. LC 94-10758. 160p. 28.95 (*0-691-03718-3*) Princeton U Pr.

***Friendgrief: An Absence Called Presence.** Harold Ivan Smith. 2001. LC 2001-25406. (Death, Value & Meaning Ser.). (Illus.). 263 p. 49.95 (*0-89503-258-9*) Baywood Pub.

***Friends in Low Places.** James Willis. 2001. 232p. pap. (*1-85775-404-2*) Radcliffe Med Pr GBR. *Dist:* Balogh.

Friendship in Childhood & Adolescence. Phil Erwin. 1998. LC 97-39543. (Psychology Focus Ser.). 176p. (C). 50.00 (*0-415-16232-7*); pap. 15.95 (*0-415-16233-5*) Routledge.

***Frightful Stages: From the Primitive to the Therapeutic.** Ed. by Robert B. Marchesani & E. Mark Stern. 2001. LC 2001-24215. 238p. pap. 34.95 (*0-7890-1366-5*); 69.95 (*0-7890-1365-7*) Haworth Pr.

Frigidity in Woman in Relation to Her Love Life Wilhelm Stekel. 1943. (C). 14.40 (*0-87140-843-0*) Liveright.

Fritz Perls. Petruska Clarkson. 1993. (Key Figures in Counselling & Psychotherapy Ser.). (Illus.). 160p. (C). pap. 24.95 (*0-8039-8453-7*, 9660) Sage.

Fritz Perls, Here & Now: An Oral Biography of the Father of Gestalt Therapy. 2nd ed. 1979. LC 77-90020. (Illus.). 440p. reprint ed. 23.95 (*0-9610310-0-X*); pap. 17.50 (*0-9610310-1-8*) Integrated Pr.

Fritz Spiegl's Sick Notes: An Alphabetical Browsing - Book of Derivatives, Abbreviations, Mnemonics, & Slang for the Amusement & Edification of Medics, Nurses, Patients, & Hypochondriacs. Fritz Spiegl. 1996. LC 95-41861. (Illus.). 184p. lib. bdg. 20.95 (*1-85070-627-1*, Parthenon Pbng) CRC Pr.

From a Different Viewpoint: The Lives & Experiences of Visually Impaired People. Sally French & John Swain. 1997. 224p. pap. text (*1-85302-551-8*) Jessica Kingsley GBR. *Dist:* Taylor & Francis.

From a Surgeon's Diary. Clifford Ashdown. 1977. 10.00 (*1-880418-07-X*) D M Grant.

From Abortion to Reproductive Freedom: Transforming a Movement. Ed. by Marlene G. Fried. 1990. 300p. (C). 35.00 (*0-89608-388-8*); pap. 18.00 (*0-89608-387-X*) South End Pr.

From Acorn to Oak: A History of the Healthcare Financial Management Association. Robert M. Shelton. 1991. 171p. 39.95 (*0-930228-84-7*) Hlthcare Fin Mgmt.

From Acupressure to Zen: An Encyclopedia of Natural Therapies. Barbara Nash. 1998. 266p. pap. text 16.00 (*0-7881-5698-5*) DIANE Pub.

From Advocacy to Intervention: Steps for Successful Establishment of Universal Infant Hearing Detection Programs. Terese Finitzo et al. 1998. 38.00 incl. audio (*1-58041-008-1*, 0112080) Am Speech Lang Hearing.

From AI to Zeitgeist: A Philosophical Guide for the Skeptical Psychologist, 11. N. H. Pronko. 1988. LC 87-14921. (Contributions in Psychology Ser.: No. 11). 281p. lib. bdg. 68.00 (*0-313-25888-0*, PPT/, Greenwood Pr) Greenwood.

From Allergy to Immunology: Anniversary Symposium in Honour of Professor Dr. Alain de Weck. Ed. by B. M. Stadler & W. J. Pichler. 1988. LC 88-21230. 164p. 29.00 (*0-920887-40-6*) Hogrefe & Huber Pubs.

From Alveoli Back to Bronchi: Contribution of Bronchoalveolar, BAL & Bronchial, BL Lavage to the Understanding of Bronchial Disease. Ed. by C. F. Donner et al. 1952. (Journal: Vol. 59, Suppl. 1, 1992). (Illus.). vi, 54p. pap. 26.25 (*3-8055-5575-X*) S Karger.

From Antarctica to Outer Space: Life in Isolation & Confinement. Ed. by A. A. Harrison et al. 1990. (Illus.). 410p. 87.95 (*0-387-97310-9*) Spr-Verlag.

From Antigen Presentation to Immunity & Allergy: Abstracts. Ed. by P. H. Lambert et al. 1987. (Journal: Vol. 83, Suppl. 1). iv, 44p. pap. 19.25 (*3-8055-4602-5*) S Karger.

From Asthma to Thalassaemia: Medical Conditions in Childhood. Ed. by S. Curtis. 1989. (C). (*0-903534-69-X*) Brit Ag for Adopt & Fost GBR. *Dist:* St Mut.

From Basic Cancer Research to Clinical Application: International Society for Oncodevelopmental Biology & Medicine, 25th Anniversary Meeting, Montreux, September 1997: Abstracts. Ed. by Jean-Pierre Mach. 1997. (Tumor Biology Ser.: Vol. 18, Suppl. 2, 1997). 138p. pap. 41.75 (*3-8055-6596-8*) S Karger.

From Bedlam to Shalom: Towards a Practical Theology of Human Nature, Interpersonal Relationships & Mental Health Care. John Swinton. 2000. LC 98-53526. (Pastoral Theology Ser.: Vol. 1). xiv, 176p. (C). 47.95 (*0-8204-4425-1*) P Lang Pubng.

From Behavior Theory to Behavior Therapy. Ed. by Joseph J. Plaud & Georg H. Eifert. 1998. LC 97-23806. 352p. (C). 63.00 (*0-205-17477-9*) Allyn.

From Borderline Adolescent to Functioning Adult: The Test of Time. James F. Masterson & Jacinta L. Costello. 3rd ed. 1986. LC 80-14270. 320p. text 38.95 (*0-87630-234-7*) Brunner-Routledge.

From Boy to Man, from Delinquency to Crime. Marvin E. Wolfgang et al. 1996. LC 87-10776. (Studies in Crime & Justice). (Illus.). 236p. 35.95 (*0-226-90555-1*) U Ch Pr.

From Brains to Behavior. Ed. by James W. Kalat & Thomas J. Norton. 1973. 47.50 (*0-8422-5115-4*) Irvington.

From Brains to Consciousness? Essays on the New Science of the Mind. Steven P. Rose. 1999. LC 98-24383. (Illus.). 278p. 35.00 (*0-691-00469-2*) Princeton U Pr.

From Cell to Brain: The Cytoskeleton - Intra & Inter-Cellular Communication - The Central Nervous System; Proceedings of the Les Houches Summer School, Session LXV, July 8th to 26th, 1996. Ed. by G. Zaccai et al. 1998. 310p. 131.50 (*0-444-50086-3*, North Holland) Elsevier.

From Chance to Choice: Genetics & Justice. Allen Buchanan et al. 2000. LC 99-24025. (Illus.). 412p. text 29.95 (*0-521-66001-7*) Cambridge U Pr.

From Clinic to Classroom: Medical Ethics & Moral Education. Contrib. by Howard B. Radest. 2000. LC 99-37525. 224p. 62.50 (*0-275-96194-X*, Praeger Pubs) Greenwood.

From Clinician to Manager: An Introduction to Hospital & Health Services Management. James Lawson & A. Rotem. 1995. (Illus.). 256p. text 44.00 (*0-07-470153-3*) McGraw-Hill Med Pub.

From Clone to Clinic. Ed. by D. J. Crommelin & H. Schellekens. 1990. (Developments in Biotherapy Ser.). (C). text 221.50 (*0-7923-0945-6*) Kluwer Academic.

From Cognitive-Behavior Therapy to Psychotherapy Integration. Marvin R. Goldfried. 1995. LC 94-39953. 304p. 42.95 (*0-8261-8780-3*) Springer Pub.

From Colored Water till Now: The True Story of One Woman's Struggle for Equality. Mattie Lawson. 1994. 176p. mass mkt. 3.95 (*0-87067-394-7*) Holloway.

From Conception to Birth: Our Most Important Journey. Tony Lipson. 1994. (Illus.). 168p. (Orig.). pap. 12.95 (*1-86429-006-4*) Morehouse Pub.

From Conflict to Resolution: Skills & Strategies for Individual, Couple & Family Theraphy. Susan M. Heitler. 1993. 368p. pap. 16.95 (*0-393-31093-0*) Norton.

From Consumption to Tuberculosis: A Documentary History. Ed. by Barbara G. Rosencrantz. 1994. LC 93-23171. (Disease, Epidemics & Medicine Ser.: Vol. 1). 648p. text 109.00 (*0-8153-0608-3*, SS808) Garland.

From Crime to Choice: The Transformation of Abortion in America, 60. Nanette J. Davis. 1985. LC 85-8018. (Contributions in Women's Studies: No. 60). (Illus.). 290p. 55.00 (*0-313-24929-6*, DCC/, Greenwood Pr) Greenwood.

From Custodial to Therapeutic Patient Care in Mental Hospitals. Milton Greenblatt et al. Ed. by Gerald N. Grob. 1980. LC 78-22562. (Historical Issues in Mental Health Ser.). reprint ed. lib. bdg. 40.95 (*0-405-11916-X*) Ayer.

From Death to Birth: Mortality Decline & Reproductive Change. Committee on Population, National Research Council. Ed. by Mark R. Montgomery & Barney Cohen. 1997. LC 97-33802. 450p. pap. text 59.00 (*0-309-05896-1*) Natl Acad Pr.

From Democedes to Harvey: Studies in the History of Medicine. Vivian Nutton. 1990. (Collected Studies: No. CS277). (Illus.). 332p. (C). reprint ed. text (*0-86078-225-5*) Variorum GBR. *Dist:* Ashgate Pub Co.

From DNA to Diversity: Molecular Genetics & the Evolution of Animal Design. Sean B. Carroll et al. 2001. LC 00-62165. (Illus.). 192p. pap. 47.95 (*0-632-04511-6*) Blackwell Sci.

***From DNA to the Community: International Conference on Community Genetics, Jonquiere, Quebec, June 2000.** Ed. by B. Modell et al. 2001. (Community Genetics 2000 Ser.: Vol. 3, No. 3). (Illus.). 64p. 25.25 (*3-8055-7209-3*) S Karger.

From Doctor to Healer: The Transformative Journey. Robbie Davis-Floyd & Gloria St. John. 1998. LC 97-39343. (Illus.). 293p. (C). text 50.00 (*0-8135-2519-5*); pap. text 20.00 (*0-8135-2520-9*) Rutgers U Pr.

From Downsizing to Recovery: Strategic Transition Options for Organizations & Individuals. Richard L. Knowdell et al. 1994. LC 94-8909. 264p. 24.95 (*0-89106-067-7*, 7185, Davies-Black Pub) Consulting Psychol.

From Fasting Saints to Anorexic Girls: The History of Self-Starvation. Walter Vandereycken & Ron Van Deth. 1994. LC 94-2859. 280p. (C). text 42.50 (*0-8147-8783-5*); pap. text 18.50 (*0-8147-8784-3*) NYU Pr.

From Fatigued to Fantastic! A Manual for Moving Beyond Chronic Fatigue & Fibromyalgia. Jacob Teitelbaum. 1996. LC 95-79047. (Illus.). 195p. pap. 18.95 (*0-9637599-7-3*) Mateel Pr.

From Fetus to Child: An Observational & Psychoanalytic Study. Alessandra Piontelli. 1992. LC 91-5236. (New Library of Psychoanalysis). 272p. (C). pap. 29.99 (*0-415-07437-1*, A7373) Routledge.

From Foal to Full-Grown. Janet Lorch. 1993. (Illus.). 192p. 29.95 (*0 7153 9976 4*) Trafalgar.

From Fragmentation to Wholeness: The Black South African Family under Seige. Keith U. Appolis. 1995. 198p. (Orig.). (C). pap. text 32.50 (*0-7618-0132-4*); lib. bdg. 60.50 (*0-7618-0131-6*) U Pr of Amer.

From Freud's Consulting Room: The Unconscious in a Scientific Age. Judith M. Hughes. 1994. LC 93-47172. 249p. 27.95 (*0-674-32452-8*, HUGFRO) HUP.

From G. Prochaska to J. E. Purkinje. Karel B. Absolon. 1987. (Illus.). 130p. (Orig.). pap. 39.50 (*0-930329-15-5*) Kabel Pubs.

From Genetics to Quality of Life - The Optimal Treatment & Management of Asthma: Proceedings of the XVth World Congress of Asthmology - Montpellier, France, April 24-27, 1996. Ed. by P. Chanez et al. 1996. (Illus.). 240p. text 58.00 (*0-88937-169-5*) Hogrefe & Huber Pubs.

From Genome to Therapy: Integrating New Technologies with Drug Development - No. 229. Novartis staff. 2000. LC 00-43348. (CIBA Foundation Symposia Ser.: Vol. 229). (Illus.). 174p. 125.00 (*0-471-62744-5*) Wiley.

From Health Care to Health: A New Approach to Resource Allocation. Jack A. Meyer et al. 1993. 44p. (Orig.). pap. (*0-9629870-4-2*) Milbank Memorial.

From Health Dollars to Health Services: New York City, 1965-1985. Ed. by Conservation of Human Resources Project Staff & Eli Ginzberg. 1986. (Conservation of Human Resources Ser.: No. 25). 176p. text 52.50 (*0-8476-7440-1*) Rowman.

From Hegel to a Definitive Clinical Psychology: Therapy, Self-Understanding, Education. Kipling Forbes. 1995. LC 93-46823. 225p. text 37.50 (*0-89341-743-2*) Hollowbrook.

From Here to Maternity: Confessions of a First-Time Mother. Carol Weston. 1991. 15.95 (*0-316-93163-2*, Little Brwn Med Div) Lppncott W & W.

From High School to High-Skilled Health Careers: New Models of Work-&-Learning in Health Care. 1992. 82p. pap. 20.00 (*1-887410-75-9*) Jobs for Future.

From Hippocrates to Virchow: Reflections on Human Disease. James M. Byers. 1987. LC 87-18835. (Illus.). 160p. text 20.00 (*0-89189-257-5*) Am Soc Clinical.

From Home to Hospital: Jewish & Italian American Women & Childbirth, 1920-1940. Angela D. Danzi. 1997. LC 97-33580. 244p. (C). 43.50 (*0-7618-0911-2*) U Pr of Amer.

From Human Being to Psycho-Therapist. D. Thomas. Ed. by Ronale McClure. 1993. 67p. (Orig.). pap. 6.95 (*0-9637770-1-7*) DJT Pub.

From Humors to Medical Science: A History of American Medicine. John Duffy. 2nd ed. 1993. LC 92-48760. (C). 432p. 42.50 (*0-252-01736-6*); 418p. pap. 17.95 (*0-252-06300-7*) U of Ill Pr.

From Hypertension to Heart Failure. Ed. by M. Bohm et al. 1998. LC 98-17988. (Illus.). 271p. pap. 60.00 (*3-540-63542-4*) Spr-Verlag.

E
F
G

From Image to Action: Reflection in Nursing Practice. Annette F. Street. 1995. (C). pap. (*0-7300-1250-6*, NPR300) Deakin Univ AUS. *Dist:* St Mut.

From Inner Sources: New Directions in Object Relations Psychotherapy. Ed. by N. Gregory Hamilton. 1992. LC 92-6967. 336p. 45.00 (*0-87668-540-8*) Aronson.

From Instinct to Self: Selected Papers of W. R. D. Fairbairn, Set. Ed. by David E. Scharff & Ellinor F. Birtles. 1995. LC 94-6784. 720p. 80.00 (*1-56821-366-2*) Aronson.

From Instinct to Self: Selected Papers of W. R. D. Fairbairn: Vol. II: Applications & Early Contributions. Ed. by E. Fairbairn Birtles. 1995. LC 94-6784. 20p. 45.00 (*1-56821-251-8*) Aronson.

From Klein to Kristeva: Psychoanalytic Feminism & the Search for the "Good Enough" Mother. Janice Doane & Devon Hodges. 1993. LC 92-36505. (Critical Perspectives on Women & Gender Ser.). 112p. (C). pap. 14.95 (*0-472-06433-9*, 06433) U of Mich Pr.

From Luigi Galvani to Contemporary Neurobiology: Contributions to the Celebration of the IX Centenary of the University of Bologna, Bologna, 27-28 September, 1988. Ed. by A. Baruzzi et al. 1990. (FIDIA Research Ser.: Vol. 22). 192p. 106.00 (*0-387-97229-3*) Spr-Verlag.

From Management to Leadership: Interpersonal Skills for Success in Health Care. Jo Manion. 1998. LC 98-9873. 232p. 40.00 (*1-55648-233-7*) AHPI.

From Mastery to Analysis: Theories of Gender in Psychoanalytic Feminism. Patricia Elliot. 1991. LC 91-14406. (Reading Women Writing Ser.). 256p. 47.50 (*0-8014-2546-8*); pap. 17.95 (*0-8014-9780-9*) Cornell U Pr.

From Medical School to Residency: How to Complete Successfully in the Residency Match Program. Roger P. Smith. 2000. LC 00-24951. (Illus.). 192p. pap. 29.95 incl. cd-rom (*0-387-95003-6*) Spr-Verlag.

From Medication to Meditation. Osho. Date not set. pap. 29.95 (*0-8464-4390-2*) Beekman Pubs.

From Medication to Meditation. Osho. 1994. LC 97-208522. 184p. pap. (*0-85207-280-5*) C W Daniel GBR. *Dist:* Natl Bk Netwk.

From Medicine to Mysticism. William S. Eidelman. 1998. (Illus.). 198p. pap. 13.95 (*1-890693-13-8*) Earthpulse Pr.

From Memories to Mental Illness: A Conceptual Journey. William M. Hall. 1996. LC 96-25549. (Emotions, Personality, & Psychotherapy Ser.). (Illus.). 288p. (C). 47.50 (*0-306-45244-8*, Plenum Trade) Perseus Pubng.

From Menarche to Menopause: Reproductive Lives of Peasant Women in Two Cultures. Yewoubdar Beyene. 1989. LC 88-2244. (SUNY Series in Medical Anthropology). 169p. (C). pap. text 22.95 (*0-88706-867-7*) State U NY Pr.

***From Mesmer to Freud: Magnetic Sleep & the Roots of Psychological Healing.** Adam Crabtree. 2001. 413p. (C). reprint ed. 30.00 (*0-7881-9765-7*) DIANE Pub.

From Midwives to Medicine: The Birth of American Gynecology. Deborah K. McGregor. 1998. LC 98-6811. (Illus.). 272p. (C). text 55.00 (*0-8135-2571-3*); pap. text 23.00 (*0-8135-2572-1*) Rutgers U Pr.

From Models to Modules: Studies in Cognitive Science from the McGill Workshops. Ed. by I. Gopnik et al. 1986. LC 85-20952. (Theoretical Issues in Cognitive Science Ser.: Vol. 2). 304p. (C). 85.00 (*0-89391-355-3*, Ablex) Greenwood.

From Molecular Biology to Therapeutics. Ed. by B. A. Bernard & B. Shroot. 1993. (Pharmacology & the Skin Ser.: Vol. 5). (Illus.). viii, 196p. 216.75 (*3-8055-5776-0*) S Karger.

From Molecule to Men: Molecular Basis of Congenital Cardiovascular Disorders. M. Zehender et al. 2000. (Illus.). 190p. (C). (*3-7985-1168-3*) D Steinkopff DEU. *Dist:* Spr-Verlag.

From Neuron to Action: An Appraisal of Fundamental & Clinical Research. Ed. by L. Deecke & V. B. Mountcastle. 1991. (Illus.). 677p. 118.00 (*0-387-52072-4*) Spr-Verlag.

From Neuron to Brain: A Cellular & Molecular Approach to the Function of the Nervous System. John G. Nicholls et al. 4th ed. 2000. LC 00-36529. (Illus.). text 75.95 (*0-87893-439-1*) Sinauer Assocs.

From Neuropsychology to Mental Structure. Tim Shallice. 1988. (Illus.). 480p. text 90.00 (*0-521-30874-7*); 478p. pap. text 32.95 (*0-521-31360-0*) Cambridge U Pr.

From Normal to Healthy: Paths to the Liberation of Consciousness. Georg Kuhlewind. Tr. by Michael Lipson from GER. 1988.Tr. of Von Normalen zum Gesunden. 232p. pap. 16.95 (*0-940262-10-X*, Lindisfarne) Anthroposophic.

From Novice to Expert: Excellence & Power in Clinical Nursing Practice. Patricia E. Benner. 1984. 336p. (C). pap. text 39.93 (*0-201-00299-X*, Health Sci) Addison-Wesley.

From Nursing Assistant to Clinical Care: Associate Workbook. H. S. Miele. 1998. 272p. pap. text, wbk. ed. 23.60 (*0-8359-5117-0*) P-H.

From Nursing Assistant to Clinical Care Associate. 1998. 208p. text 24.80 (*0-8359-5299-1*) S&S Trade.

From Nursing Assistant to Clinical Care Associate. Carole Miele. 1998. LC 98-23249. 512p. pap. text 47.00 (*0-8359-5108-1*) Allyn.

From Nursing Assistant to Patient Care Technician: New Roles, New Knowledge, New Skills. Donna J. Brust & Joyce A. Foster. 1997. (Illus.). pap., tchr. ed. (*0-7216-7087-3*) Saunders.

From Nursing Assistant to Patient Care Technician: New Roles, New Knowledge, New Skills. Donna J. Brust & Joyce A. Foster. Ed. by Lisa Biello. 1996. 432p. pap. text 41.95 (*0-7216-6046-0*) Saunders.

From Obstetrics & Gynecology to Women's Health: The Road Ahead. Mahmoud F. Fathalla. 1997. LC 97-25463. (Illus.). 302p. pap. 25.00 (*1-85070-993-9*, Parthenon Pbng) CRC Pr.

From One to Another. Norma Jacob. 1959. LC 59-8917. (Orig.). pap. 4.00 (*0-87574-102-9*) Pendle Hill.

From Pain to Violence: The Traumatic Roots of Destructiveness. Felicity De Zulueta. 1993. 342p. pap. 56.00 (*1-56593-253-6*, 0549) Singular Publishing.

From Panic to Peace of Mind: Overcoming Panic & Agoraphobia. C. B. Scrignar. 1991. (Illus.). 304p. 19.95 (*0-945032-02-1*) Bruno Pr.

From Paralysis to Fatigue: A History of Psychosomatic Illness in the Modern Era. Edward Shorter. 1993. LC 91-24912. 420p. pap. 14.95 (*0-02-928667-0*); 1991. 400p. text 29.95 (*0-02-928665-4*) Free Pr.

From Parasitic Infection to Parasitic Disease. Ed. by P. L. Gigase & E. E. Van Marck. 1982. (Contributions to Microbiology & Immunology Ser.: Vol. 7). (Illus.). x, 270p. 156.75 (*3-8055-3543-0*) S Karger.

From Pathology to Politics: Public Health in America. James T. Bennett & Thomas J. DiLorenzo. 2000. LC 00-30270. 160p. text 29.95 (*0-7658-0023-3*) Transaction Pubs.

From Patient to Payment: Insurance Procedures for the Medical Office. Rhonda Collins. 2nd ed. 1997. LC 97-28931. pap. (*0-02-801988-1*) Glencoe.

From Patient to Person - First Steps: A Workbook for People with Chronic Pain. Penney Covan. Ed. by Edward Carington & Darna Lan. 2000. Orig. Title: ACPA Workbook Manual. (Illus.). 195p. pap. 25.00 (*0-9673878-3-3*, 13300) Amer Chronic.

From Patients to Persons: The Psychiatric Critiques of Thomas Szasz, Peter Sedgwick & R. D. Laing. Janet Vice. 1993. LC 91-18621. (American University Studies: Ser. V, Vol. 128). 191p. (C). text 38.95 (*0-8204-1659-2*) P Lang Pubng.

From Physician Bonding to Alliances. 1995. 39.00 (*0-937925-98-5*, FPBA) Capitol Publns.

From Pigments to Perception: Advances in Understanding the Visual Processes. A. Valberg & B. B. Lee. 1991. (NATO Advanced Science Institutes Ser.: Vol. 203). (Illus.). 498p. (C). text 149.50 (*0-306-43905-0*, Kluwer Plenum) Kluwer Academic.

From PMS to Menopause: Female Hormones in Context. Raymond Peat. 2001. LC 00-191565. 190p. pap. 12.00 (*0-9702913-2-9*, 300) R Peat.

From Pragmatism to Vision: Leadership & Values in Academic Health Centers. Ed. by Clayton Rich et al. 1991. 150p. (Orig.). pap. 14.95 (*1-879694-02-6*) AAH Ctrs.

***From Premature Gray Hair to Helicase-Werner Syndrome: Implications for Aging & Cancer.** Ed. by M. Goto & R. W. Miller. 2001. (Gann Monographs on Cancer Research: No. 49). 243.50 (*3-8055-7158-5*) S Karger.

From Prevention to Wellness Through Group Work. Ed. by Joan K. Parry. 1997. LC 96-48820. 180p. 49.95 (*0-7890-0164-0*) Haworth Pr.

From Proposal to Publication: An Informal Guide to Writing about Nursing Research. Elizabeth M. Tornquist. 1986. 215p. (C). pap. text 38.00 (*0-201-08012-5*) Addison-Wesley.

From "Quantity of Radiation" & "Dose" to "Exposure" & "Absorbed Dose" An Historical Review. Harold O. Wyckoff. 1980. LC 80-83036. (Taylor Lectures: No. 4). pap. 20.00 (*0-913392-53-7*) NCRP Pubns.

From Reading to Neurons. Ed. by Albert M. Galaburda. 1989. (Issues in the Biology of Language & Cognition Ser.). 608p. 75.00 (*0-262-07115-0*) MIT Pr.

From Research to Clinical Practice: The Implications of Social & Developmental Research for Psychotherapy. Ed. by George Stricker & Robert H. Keisner. 1985. LC 84-24881. 476p. 90.00 (*0-306-41758-8*, Plenum Trade) Perseus Pubng.

From Residency to Reality. Patricia A. Hoffmeir & Jean A. Bohner. 1988. LC 87-26160. 208p. pap. 24.00 (*0-07-029212-4*) McGraw-Hill Prof.

From Rhetoric to Reality: Comparative Health Policy & the New Right. Ed. by Christa Altenstetter & Stuart C. Haywood. 1991. LC 90-44165. 366p. text 65.00 (*0-312-05343-6*) St Martin.

From Safety to Superego: Selected Papers of Joseph Sandler. Joseph Sandler. 1987. LC 86-26990. (Guilford Psychoanalysis Ser.). 348p. text 50.00 (*0-89862-327-8*) Guilford Pubns.

From Scarcity to Surfeit: A History of Food & Nutrition in New South Wales. Robin Walker & Dave Roberts. 1988. pap. (*0-86840-011-4*) New South Wales Univ Pr AUS. *Dist:* Intl Spec Bk.

From Shell Shock to Combat Stress: A Comparative History of Military Psychiatry. Hans Binneveld. 1998. LC 98-170762. 224p. pap. text (*90-5356-270-2*) Amsterdam U Pr NLD. *Dist:* U of Mich Pr.

From Soul to Mind: The Emergence of Psychology, from Erasmus Darwin to William James. Edward S. Reed. 1997. LC 96-49051. 288p. 35.00 (*0-300-06967-7*) Yale U Pr.

From Soup to Nuts: Finding & Keeping Healthcare Employees. Steven Benson. rev. ed. 1999. 22.50 (*0-929442-40-7*, 2147PP) Prof Prnting & Pub.

From Stress to Wellbeing: Guidelines for Psychospiritual Counseling. Craig W. Ellison. 1994. LC 94-1699. (Resources for Christian Counseling Ser.: Vol. 9). 216p. 22.99 (*0-8499-0875-2*) Nelson Ref & Elec Pub.

From Subjects to Subjectivities: A Handbook of Interpretive & Participatory Methods. Ed. by Deborah L. Tolman et al. 2000. LC 00-10743. (Qualitative Studies in Psychology). x, 340p. pap. 22.50 (*0-8147-8259-0*) NYU Pr.

From Survival to Fulfillment: A Framework for the Life-Trauma Dialectic. Paul Valent. 1998. LC 97-48882. (Series in Trauma & Loss). 54.00 (*0-87630-921-X*); pap. 26.95 (*0-87630-922-8*) Brunner-Routledge.

From Surviving to Thriving: A Therapist's Guide to Stage II Recovery for Survivors of Childhood Abuse. Mary Bratton. 1998. LC 98-39341. 282p. 39.95 (*0-7890-0255-8*); 302p. pap. 24.95 (*0-7890-0256-6*) Haworth Pr.

From Surviving to Thriving: Incest, Feminism, & Recovery. Christine Dinsmore. 1991. LC 90-40378. (SUNY Series in the Psychology of Women). 204p. (C). text 26.50 (*0-7914-0628-8*); pap. text 25.95 (*0-7914-0629-6*) State U NY Pr.

From Surviving to Thriving: Promoting Mental Health in Young People. Andrew R. Fuller. 1998. pap. (*0-86431-277-6*) Aust Council Educ Res AUS. *Dist:* St Mut, Stylus Pub VA.

From Test Tube to Patient: New Drug Development in the U. S. 2nd ed. 1995. (Illus.). 67p. (C). pap. text 25.00 (*0-7881-1923-0*) DIANE Pub.

From Test Tube to Patient: New Drug Development in the United States. 1995. (Illus.). 68p. pap. text 30.00 (*1-57979-035-6*) DIANE Pub.

From Test Tube to Patient: New Drug Devevlopment in the U. S. rev. ed. 1994. (Illus.). 67p. (C). pap. text 30.00 (*0-7881-1285-6*) DIANE Pub.

From the Ashes: A Head Injury Self-Advocacy Guide. Constance Miller & Kay Campbell. 1987. (Illus.). 107p. (Orig.). stu. ed. 23.00 (*0-9636594-0-5*) Phoenix Seattle.

From the Brain to the Mouth: Acquired Dysarthria & Dysfluency in Adults. Ed. by Yvan Lebrun. 1997. LC 96-6578. (Neuropsychology & Cognition Ser.). 196p. (C). text 93.50 (*0-7923-4427-8*) Kluwer Academic.

From the Couch to the Jungle: The Story of My Life As a Multicultural Psychiatrist. Thomas L. Chiv. 1998. (Illus.). 180p. pap. 29.95 (*1-884092-04-7*) R Altschuler.

From the Dawn of One Century to the Promise of the Next: Our Story...Charlton Health System. David Eskes. 1997. 168p. 30.00 (*0-929690-37-0*) Herit Pubs AZ.

From the Earth to Beyond the Sky: Native American Medicine. Evelyn Wolfson. 1993. LC 92-46035. (Illus.). 112p. (gr. 4-7). 16.00 (*0-395-55009-2*) HM.

From the Fat of Our Souls: Social Change, Political Process, & Medical Pluralism in Bolivia. Libbet Crandon-Malamud. 1991. LC 90-37178. (Comparative Studies of Health Systems & Medical Care: Vol. 26). (Illus.). 308p. text 55.00 (*0-520-07011-9*); pap. text 19.95 (*0-520-08430-6*) U CA Pr.

From the Greenwich Hulks to Old St. Pancras: A History of Tropical Disease in London. G. C. Cook. 1992. LC 92-10542. 400p. (C). text (*0-485-11411-9*) Athlone Pr GBR. *Dist:* Transaction Pubs, Humanities.

From the Horse's Mouth Vol. 1: The Horseman's Guide to Equine Dental Health & Aging. Len Lookingbill. 139p. text 18.95 (*0-9644682-0-4*) Diamond L Pub.

From the Inside Out: A Self-Teaching & Laboratory Manual for Biofeedback. E. Peper & E. A. Williams. 1981. LC 80-20551. (Illus.). 446p. (C). spiral bd. 49.50 (*0-306-40535-0*, Plenum Trade) Perseus Pubng.

From the Lab into the World: A Pill for People, Pets & Bugs. Carl Djerassi. 1994. LC 94-17603. 230p. text 29.95 (*0-8412-2808-6*) Am Chemical.

From the Life & Work of C. G. Jung. Aniela Jaffe. 1995. 213p. pap. 16.95 (*3-85630-515-7*) Continuum.

From the Listening Place: The Languages of Intuition. Ed. by Margaret Blanchard. 1997. LC 96-39490. (Illus.). (Orig.). pap. 19.95 (*1-885349-05-X*) Astarte Shell Pr.

From the Mind into the Body: The Cultural Origins of Psychosomatic Symptoms. Edward Shorter. 1993. LC 93-5430. 250p. 24.95 (*0-02-928666-2*) Free Pr.

From the Other Side of the Couch: Candid Conversations with Psychiatrists & Psychologists, 23. Chris E. Stout. 1993. LC 93-7716. (Contributions in Psychology Ser.: No. 23). 192p. 67.00 (*0-313-27765-6*, SYX/, Greenwood Pr) Greenwood.

From the Source: A Guide for Implementing Perinatal Addiction Prevention & Treatment Programs. Marjorie Rosenweig et al. 1998. (Illus.). 196p. (C). pap. text 35.00 (*0-7881-4876-1*) DIANE Pub.

From the Watching of Shadows: The Origins of Radiological Tomography. Steve Webb. 1990. LC 89-26820. (Illus.). 368p. 95.00 (*0-85274-305-X*) Inst of Physics Pubng.

From the Words of My Mouth: Tradition in Psychotherapy. Ed. by Laurence Spurling. 1992. LC 92-5063. 272p. (C). text 85.00 (*0-415-06256-X*, A7791) Routledge.

From Theoretical Physics to Biology: Proceedings of the International Conference, 3rd, Versailles, 1971. Ed. by M. Marois. 1973. 102.75 (*3-8055-1578-2*) S Karger.

***From This Moment On: A Guide for Those Recently Diagnosed with Cancer.** Arlene Cotter. 2002. (Illus.). 453p. reprint ed. 20.00 (*0-7567-5263-9*) DIANE Pub.

From Thoughts to Obsessions: Obsessive Compulsive Disorder in Children & Adolescents. Hove Thomsen. 1998. LC 98-41229. 144p. pap. (*1-85302-721-9*) Jessica Kingsley.

From Tumor Biology to Clinical Oncology: 26th Meeting of the International Society for Oncodevelopmental Biology & Medicine (ISOBM) 1998, Umea' August/September 1998:Abstracts, No. 19 Ed. by Torgny Stigbrand. 1998. (Tumor Biology Ser.: No. 2). ii, 114p. pap. 36.50 (*3-8055-6774-X*) S Karger.

From Tumor Biology to Clinical Oncology: 28th Meeting of the International Society for Oncodevelopmental Biology & Medicine, ISOBM, Munich, September 2000: Abstracts. Ed. by R. Lamerz & P. Stieber. 2000. (Tumor Biology Ser.: Vol. 21, Suppl. 1 (2000)). ii, 116p. pap. 45.25 (*3-8055-7146-1*) S Karger.

From Uptight to All Right: A Twelve Step Program for Stress Prevention. Jerome Murray. 1987. LC 87-7762. 187p. (Orig.). pap. 12.95 (*0-942383-06-0*) Manor Hse Pub.

From Victim to Victor see Wellness Community Guide to Fighting for Recovery from Cancer

From Victims to Survivors: Reclaimed Voices of Women Sexually Abused in Childhood by Females. Juliann Whetsell-Mitchell & Jill Morse. 1997. LC 97-33606. 298p. (*1-56032-569-0*) Hemisp Pub.

From Victims to Survivors: Reclaimed Voices of Women Sexually Abused in Childhood by Females. Juliann Whetsell-Mitchell et al. 1997. LC 97-33606. 200p. pap. 26.95 (*1-56032-570-4*) Hemisp Pub.

From War Babies to Grandmothers: Forty-Eight Years in Psychoanalysis. Ilse Hellman. 1990. 272p. pap. text (*0-946439-66-4*) Karnac Bks GBR. *Dist:* Brunner-Routledge.

Front Office Skills for Medical Assistants. De A. Eggers & Anne M. Conway. 1999. LC 99-23139. (Illus.). 576p. (gr. 13). text 35.95 (*0-8151-2386-8*, 28881) Mosby Inc.

Frontal Dementias: Ethiological, Clinical, Therapeutical & Pathological Aspects, 3rd International Conference, Lund, August 1998. L. Gustafson & A. Brun. 1999. (Dementia & Geriatric Cognitive Disorders Ser.: Vol. 10, Suppl. 1, 1999). (Illus.). iv, 102p. pap. 25.25 (*3-8055-6920-3*) S Karger.

Frontal Lobe Function & Dysfunction. Ed. by Harvey S. Levin et al. 1991. (Illus.). 448p. (C). text 58.00 (*0-19-506284-1*) OUP.

Frontal Lobes & Neuropsychiatric Illness. Ed. by Stephen P. Salloway et al. 2001. LC 00-46472. (Illus.). x, 264p. 59.00 (*0-88048-800-X*, 8800) Am Psychiatric.

Frontal Lobes Revisited. Ed. by Ellen Perecman. 1988. 312p. 79.95 (*0-8058-0288-6*) L Erlbaum Assocs.

Frontal Sinus. Nikhil J. Bhatt. 2001. (Illus.). 200p. 141.95 (*0-7693-0154-1*) Singular Publishing.

Frontier Nursing Service Oral History Project: An Annotated Guide. Ed. by Susan E. Allen & Terry L. Birdwhistell. 1987. LC 85-51419. (University of Kentucky Libraries Occasional Papers: No. 9). (Illus.). 125p. (Orig.). pap. 15.00 (*0-917519-05-1*) U of KY Libs.

Frontier of Brief Psychotherapy: An Example of the Convergence of Research & Clinical Practice. D. H. Malan. 1976. LC 76-9646. (Topics in General Psychiatry Ser.). (Illus.). 388p. (C). 49.50 (*0-306-30895-9*, Plenum Trade) Perseus Pubng.

Frontiers in Arterial Chemoreception: Proceedings of the XIIIth International Symposium Held in Santiago, Chile, March 25-29, 1996. Ed. by Patricio Zapata et al. 1997. LC 96-49626. (Advances in Experimental Medicine & Biology Ser.: Vol. 410). 494p. 125.00 (*0-306-45490-4*, Kluwer Plenum) Kluwer Academic.

Frontiers in Bioethics: Essays Dedicated to John C. Fletcher. Ed. by Franklin G. Miller. 2000. 224p. pap. 19.95 (*1-55572-075-7*) Univ Pub Group.

Frontiers in Biomedical Polymer Applications, Vol. 1. Ed. by Raphael M. Ottenbrite. 1998. LC 97-62207. 317p. 169.95 (*1-56676-577-3*) CRC Pr.

Frontiers in Biomedical Research. Ed. by D. Hartmann et al. 1993. (Clinical Pharmacology Ser.: Vol. 9). (Illus.). 190p. text (*3-88603-464-X*) W Zuckschwerdt DEU. *Dist:* Scholium Intl.

Frontiers in Brain & Dream Research. William P. Frost. 1991. LC 91-46330. 172p. lib. bdg. 79.95 (*0-88946-229-1*) E Mellen.

Frontiers in Cellular Surface Research: Boehringer Ingelheim Symposium. 1981. 39.95 (*0-915340-09-7*) PJD Pubns.

Frontiers in Cerebral Vascular Biology: Transport & Its Regulation. L. R. Drewes & A. L. Betz. 1993. LC 93-16860. (Advances in Experimental Medicine & Biology Ser.: Vol. 331). (Illus.). 306p. (C). text 95.00 (*0-306-44416-X*, Kluwer Plenum) Kluwer Academic.

Frontiers in Cerebrovascular Disease: Mechanisms, Diagnosis, & Treatment. Ed. by James T. Robertson & Thaddeus S. Nowak, Jr. 1997. LC 97-26376. (American

Heart Association Monograph Ser.). (Illus.). 384p. 98.00 (*0-87993-674-6*) Futura Pub.

Frontiers in Cognitive Neuroscience. Ed. by Stephen M. Kosslyn & Richard A. Andersen. 1995. 736p. pap. 50.00 (*0-262-61110-4*); 1992. LC 91-36146. 729p. 85.00 (*0-262-11163-2*) MIT Pr (Bradford Bks).

Frontiers in European Radiology, Book 9. Ed. by A. L. Baert & F. H. Heuck. 1993. (Illus.). 250p. 137.00 (*0-387-55280-4*) Spr-Verlag.

Frontiers in European Radiology, Vol. 3. C. Muhr et al. 1983. (Illus.). 136p. 79.95 (*0-387-11446-7*) Spr-Verlag.

Frontiers in European Radiology, Vol. 4. Ed. by Pierre L. Lasjaunias et al. 1984. (Illus.). 158p. 69.95 (*0-387-13410-7*) Spr-Verlag.

Frontiers in European Radiology, Vol. 6. Ed. by A. L. Baert et al. 1989. (Illus.). 87p. 95.00 (*0-387-50466-4*) Spr-Verlag.

Frontiers in European Radiology, Vol. 8. Ed. by A. L. Baert & F. H. Heuck. 1991. (Illus.). 117p. 118.00 (*0-387-53189-0*) Spr-Verlag.

Frontiers in General Hospital Psychiatry. Ed. by Louis Linn. 1961. LC 61-10147. 508p. 72.50 (*0-8236-2080-8*, BN 02080) Intl Univs Pr.

Frontiers in Head & Neck Trauma: Clinical & Biomechanical. Ed. by A. Sances et al. 1998. LC 97-75190. (Biomedical & Health Research Ser.: Vol. 21). 743p. 98.00 (*90-5199-369-2*, 369-2) IOS Press.

Frontiers in Health Policy Research. Ed. by Alan M. Garber. 2001. (Frontiers in Health Policy Research Ser.: Vol. 4). 224p. pap. 24.00 (*0-262-57150-1*) MIT Pr.

Frontiers in Health Policy Research. Alan M. Garber. 3rd ed. 2000. LC 99-110956. (Frontiers in Health Policy Research Ser.). 200p. pap. 20.00 (*0-262-57141-2*); (Illus.). 40.00 (*0-262-07212-2*) MIT Pr.

Frontiers in Health Policy Research. Ed. by Alan M. Garber. (NBER Frontiers in Health Policy Ser.). (Illus.). 200p. Vol. 1. 1998. 35.00 (*0-262-07187-8*); Vol. 2. 1999. pap. 15.00 (*0-262-57129-3*) MIT Pr.

Frontiers in Health Policy Research, Vol. 4. Alan M. Garber. 2001. 224p. 55.00 (*0-262-07218-1*) MIT Pr.

Frontiers in Health Policy Research: 1998, Vol. 1. Ed. by Alan M. Garber. 1998. (NBER Frontiers in Health Policy Ser.). (Illus.). 200p. pap. text 15.00 (*0-262-57120-X*) MIT Pr.

Frontiers in Histamine Research - A Tribute to Heinz Schild: Based on an International Symposium Held at Jouy-en-Josas (near Paris), France, 25-27 July 1984. Ed. by C. R. Ganellin & J. C. Schwartz. 1985. (Illus.). 464p. 83.50 (*0-08-031989-0*, Pergamon Pr) Elsevier.

Frontiers in Hypertension Research. Ed. by John H. Laragh. 1981. (Illus.). 628p. 94.00 (*0-387-90557-X*) Spr-Verlag.

Frontiers in Interventional Cardiology. Rafael Beyar et al. 1998. 480p. (C). text (*1-85317-487-4*) Mosby Inc.

Frontiers in Medicine. New York Academy of Medicine Staff. 1977. LC 70-142675. (Essay Index Reprint Ser.). 19.95 (*0-8369-2113-5*) Ayer.

Frontiers in Medicine: Implications for the Future. Ed. by Robert J. Morin & Richard J. Bing. 1984. 272p. 45.95 (*0-89885-209-9*, Kluwer Acad Hman Sci) Kluwer Academic.

Frontiers in Microbiology. Ed. by Erik de Clercq. 1987. (New Perspectives in Clinical Microbiology Ser.). text 218.00 (*0-89838-959-3*) Kluwer Academic.

Frontiers in Multiple Sclerosis. Oded Abramsky. 1997. 320p. (*1-85317-384-3*) Martin Dunitz GBR. *Dist:* Mosby Inc.

Frontiers in Multiple Sclerosis, Vol. 2. Ed. by Aksel Siva et al. 1999. 281p. (*1-85317-506-4*) Martin Dunitz.

Frontiers in Pediatric Neuroendocrinology. Ed. by M. O. Savage et al. Date not set. LC 94-1693. (Illus.). 192p. pap. (*0-86542-837-9*) Blackwell Sci.

Frontiers in Self Psychology. Arnold Goldberg. 1987. (Progress in Self Psychology Ser.: Vol. 3). 312p. text 45.00 (*0-88163-066-7*) Analytic Pr.

Frontiers in the Chemical Sciences. Ed. by William Spindel & Robert M. Simon. 1986. LC 86-14038. 624p. 29.85 (*0-87168-312-1*, 85-10S) AAAS.

Frontiers in Thyroidology. Ed. by Eduardo Gaitan & Geraldo A. Medeiros-Neto. 1987. LC 86-30538. 1684p. 225.00 (*0-306-42490-8*, Plenum Trade) Perseus Pubng.

Frontiers in Tissue Engineering. Charles W. Patrick, Jr. et al. 1998. LC 97-50321. 716p. 155.50 (*0-08-042689-1*, Pergamon Pr) Elsevier.

Frontiers in Vestibular & Oculo-Motor Research. Ed. by Jan Stahle. 1979. (Advances in OtoRhinoLaryngology Ser.: Vol. 25). (Illus.). 86.25 (*3-8055-2988-0*) S Karger.

Frontiers in Virology: In Honour of Joseph L. Melnick on the Occasion of His 60th Birthday. Ed. by Fred Rapp. 1976. (Progress in Medical Virology Ser.: Vol. 21). (Illus.). 250p. 86.25 (*3-8055-2202-9*) S Karger.

Frontiers of Cardiac Electrophysiology. Ed. by M. Rosenbaum & M. Elizari. 1983. text 475.50 (*90-247-2663-8*) Kluwer Academic.

Frontiers of Cognitive Therapy. Ed. by Paul M. Salkovskis. 1997. 553p. pap. 28.00 (*1-57230-113-9*) Guilford Pubns.

Frontiers of Cognitive Therapy. Paul M. Salkovskis. 1996. LC 96-22618. 553p. 50.00 (*1-57230-112-0*) Guilford Pubns.

Frontiers of Developmental Psychopathology. Ed. by Jeffery J. Haugaard & Mark F. Lenzenweger. 1996. LC 94-23362. (Illus.). 256p. text 45.00 (*0-19-509001-2*) OUP.

Frontiers of Gastrointestinal Research, Vol. 15-16. Ed. by G. Dinari et al. 1989. (Illus.). xvi, 628p. 443.50 (*3-8055-4973-3*) S Karger.

Frontiers of Health: From Healing to Wholeness. Christine R. Page. 256p. pap. 29.95 (*0-8464-4180-2*); 2000. 248p. pap. 29.95 (*0-8464-5204-9*) Beekman Pubs.

Frontiers of Internal Medicine, 1974: Proceedings of the International Congress of Internal Medicine, 12th, Tel Aviv, 1974. International Congress of Internal Medicine Staff. Ed. by S. H. Blondheim. 1976. xxii, 450p. 167.00 (*3-8055-2205-3*) S Karger.

Frontiers of Mathematical Psychology: Essays in Honor of Clyde Coombs. Ed. by D. R. Brown & J. E. Keith-Smith. 1990. (Recent Research in Psychology Ser.). (Illus.). 202p. 71.95 (*0-387-97451-2*) Spr-Verlag.

Frontiers of Medical Information Sciences. Ed. by Robert L. Kuhn. 1988. LC 87-32682. 246p. 68.00 (*0-275-92750-4*, C2750, Praeger Pubs) Greenwood.

Frontiers of Medicine in the Anglo-Egyptian Sudan, 1899-1940. Heather Bell. 1999. LC 98-40976. (Illus.). 278p. text 78.00 (*0-19-820749-2*) OUP.

Frontiers of Motivational Psychology. Ed. by D. R. Brown & J. Veroff. 1986. (Recent Research in Psychology Ser.). 194p. 38.00 (*0-387-96444-4*) Spr-Verlag.

Frontiers of Neurology. Ed. by Donald J. Reis & Jerome B. Posner. 1998. LC 97-32679. (Annals of the New York Academy of Sciences Ser.: No. 835). 421p. 90.00 (*1-57331-096-4*) NY Acad Sci.

Frontiers of Neurology: A Symposium in Honor of Fred Plum. Ed. by Donald J. Reis & Jerome B. Posner. 1998. LC 97-32679. (Annals of the New York Academy of Sciences Ser.: No. 835). 421p. pap. 90.00 (*1-57331-097-2*) NY Acad Sci.

Frontiers of Osteosarcoma Research. Ed. by Josef F. Novak & James H. McMaster. 1993. LC 92-49083. (Illus.). 592p. 138.00 (*0-88937-113-X*) Hogrefe & Huber Pubs.

Frontiers of Reactive Oxygen Species in Biology & Medicine: Proceedings of the 6th International Conference on Superoxide & Superoxide Dismutase, Kyoto, Japan, 11-15 October 1993. Sixth International Conference on Superoxide and Sup. Ed. by K. Asada & T. Yoshikawa. 1994. (International Congress Ser.: Vol. 1058). 602p. text 253.50 (*0-444-81778-6*, Excerpta Medica) Elsevier.

Frontiers of Sex Research. Ed. by Vern Bullough. 1979. LC 79-2462. 198p. (C). pap. 22.00 (*0-87975-113-4*) Prometheus Bks.

Frontiers of Stress Research. Ed. by Henry Weiner et al. 1989. LC 88-13142. (Neuronal Control of Bodily Function Ser.: Vol. 4). 550p. 79.00 (*0-920887-39-2*) Hogrefe & Huber Pubs.

Frontrunners' Q&A Review for the Internal Medicine Boards: 1234 Questions & Answers to Prepare You. Bradley D. Mittman. 2001. (Illus.). 228p. per. 149.00 (*0-9677025-4-2*) Frontrunners.

Frostbite & Other Cold Injuries. Deborah Mercy. 2nd ed. 1990. (Fisheries Safety & Survival Ser.: No. 7). 19p. reprint ed. pap., stu. ed. 4.00 (*1-56612-008-X*) AK Sea Grant CP.

Frozen Human Semen: A Royal College of Obstetricians & Gynaecologists Workshop in the Cryobiology of Human Semen & Its Role on Artificial Insemination by Donor, March 22 & 23, 1979. Ed. by David W. Richardson et al. 1980. (Developments in Obstetrics & Gynecology Ser.: No. 4). 280p. text 148.50 (*90-247-2370-1*) Kluwer Academic.

Fructose-One, Six-Diphosphates & Its Role in Gluconeogenesis. Ed. by R. W. McGilvery & B. M. Pogell. 1964. 12.50 (*0-934454-40-X*) Lubrecht & Cramer.

Fruition of an Idea: Fifty Years of Psychoanalysis in New York. Ed. by Martin Wangh et al. 1962. LC 62-17380. 124p. 27.50 (*0-8236-2100-6*) Intl Univs Pr.

Frustration & Aggression. John Dollard et al. 1980. LC 79-26458. 209p. reprint ed. lib. bdg. 35.00 (*0-313-22201-0*, DOFR, Greenwood Pr) Greenwood.

Frustration & Conflict. Aubrey J. Yates. 1982. LC 81-20086. 236p. reprint ed. lib. bdg. 62.50 (*0-313-23247-4*, YAFC, Greenwood Pr) Greenwood.

Frustration & Regression: An Experiment with Young Children. Roger Barker et al. 1976. LC 75-34765. (Studies in Play & Games). (Illus.). reprint ed. 28.95 (*0-405-07934-6*) Ayer.

Frustration Theory: An Analysis of Dispositional Learning & Memory. Abram Amsel. 1992. (Problems in the Behavioral Sciences Ser.: No. 11). (Illus.). 294p. (C). text 80.00 (*0-521-24784-5*) Cambridge U Pr.

Frye's Nursing Bullets for NCLEX-RN. Charles M. Frye. 3rd ed. 1994. LC 93-44756. 192p. 16.95 (*0-87434-699-1*) Springhouse Corp.

Frye's 2500 Nursing Bullets for NCLEX-PN. Charles M. Frye. 2nd ed. 1999. LC 99-40688. 176p. pap. 19.95 (*1-58255-007-7*) Springhouse Corp.

Frye's 2500 Nursing Bullets for NCLEX-RN. Charles M. Frye. 4th ed. 1999. LC 99-38477. 240p. pap. 19.95 (*0-87434-985-0*) Springhouse Corp.

Frye's 2000 Nursing Bullets NCLEX-PN. Charles M. Frye. 1995. LC 95-25055. 144p. 15.95 (*0-87434-819-6*) Springhouse Corp.

FSH Action & Intraovarian Regulation: Proceedings of the 6th Reinier De Graaf Symposium, Noordwijk, The Netherlands, September 26-28, 1996. M. Fauser. Ed. by Bart C. Fauser. 1997. LC 97-2670. (Studies in Profertility: Vol. 6). (Illus.). 270p. lib. bdg. 74.95 (*1-85070-957-2*, Parthenon Pbng) CRC Pr.

Fu Qing-Zhu's Gynecology. Fu Qing-Zhu. Tr. by Yang Shou-Zhong & Liu Da-Wei from CHI. 1992. LC 92-71293. 267p. (Orig.). pap. 23.95 (*0-936185-35-X*) Blue Poppy Pr.

Fuchs's Radiographic Exposure, Processing & Quality Control. Quinn B. Carroll & Arthur W. Fuchs. 6th ed. 1998. LC 97-36977. (Illus.). 588p. text 59.95 (*0-398-06830-5*) C C Thomas.

Fuel Homeostasis & the Nervous System. Ed. by Mladen Vranic et al. 1991. (Advances in Experimental Medicine & Biology Ser.: Vol. 291). (Illus.). 288p. (C). text 114.00 (*0-306-43907-7*, Kluwer Plenum) Kluwer Academic.

Fulfilling the Essence: A Handbook of Traditional & Contemporary Chinese Treatments for Female Infertility. Bob Flaws. Ed. by Honora L. Wolfe. 1993. 290p. (Orig.). (C). pap. text 21.95 (*0-936185-48-1*) Blue Poppy Pr.

Fulfilling the Promises: Desyrel - A Five-Year Review. Ed. by Robert E. Rakel & Marc A. Schuckit. 1987. (Journal: Vol. 20, Suppl. 1, 1987). (Illus.). vi, 146p. pap. 47.00 (*3-8055-4653-X*) S Karger.

Full Battery Codebook: A Guide to Psychological Test Interpretation. Ken R. Vincent. Ed. by Glenn R. Caddy. 1987. LC 87-1759. (Developments in Clinical Psychology Ser.). 252p. 77.00 (*0-89391-395-2*, Ablex) Greenwood.

Full Disclosure: The Truth about the AIDS Epidemic. Gary L. Glum. 1994. 215p. 165.00 (*0-9620364-1-2*) Silent Walker Pub.

Full Face: A Correspondence about Becoming Deaf in Mid-Life. Clare Blatchford. 1997. LC 97-179598. pap. 9.95 (*1-884362-21-4*) Butte Pubns.

Full of Life: How to Achieve & Maintain Peak Immunity. Luc De Schepper. 1991. (Illus.). 221p. pap. 12.95 (*0-942139-12-7*) Full of Life.

Full Scope of Retinoscopy. Ed. by Sally M. Corngold. rev. ed. (Introduction to Behavioral Optometry Ser.). 64p. reprint ed. pap. text 18.00 (*0-943599-07-5*) OEPF.

Full-time Earnings in the United States, 1999 Edition. Kurt V. Krueger. 2001. spiral bd. 129.00 (*0-9667944-3-5*) Expectancy Data.

***Fuller Breasts: A Woman's Guide to Breast Augmentation.** R. Scott Smith & Kathy Alba. 2001. (Illus.). xi, 210p. pap. 13.95 (*0-9709909-1-X*) Thatch Tree.

Fullness of Time: Short Stories of Women & Aging. Martha W. Hickman. 1990. pap. 8.95 (*0-687-60391-9*) Abingdon.

Fully Halogenated Chlorofluorocarbons. 1990. (Environmental Health Criteria Ser.: No. 113). 164p. pap. text 32.00 (*92-4-157113-6*, 1160113) World Health.

Fumonisins in Food. Ed. by Lauren S. Jackson et al. 1996. (Advances in Experimental Medicine & Biology Ser.: Vol. 392). (Illus.). 412p. (C). 120.00 (*0-306-45216-2*, Kluwer Plenum) Kluwer Academic.

Function & Dysfunction in the Basal Ganglia. Ed. by A. J. Franks et al. 1992. LC 92-23208. (Studies in Neurosciences: No. 1). 290p. 185.00 (*0-08-041982-8*, Pergamon Pr) Elsevier.

Function & Dysfunction in the Basal Ganglia. William Winlow et al. 1990. LC 89-12808. (Studies in Neuroscience). 304p. (*0-7190-2620-2*) Manchester Univ Pr GBR. *Dist:* St Martin.

Function & Dysfunction in the Nervous System. 1997. (Symposia on Quantitative Biology Ser.: No. LXI). (Illus.). 876p. text 161.00 (*0-87969-071-2*); pap. text 69.00 (*0-87969-072-0*) Cold Spring Harbor.

Function & Specificity of T Cells: International Workshop Schloss Elmau, Bavaria, FRG, October 14-16, 1990. Ed. by K. Pfeffer et al. 1991. (Current Topics in Microbiology & Immunology Ser.: Vol. 173). (Illus.). 296p. 118.00 (*0-387-53781-3*) Spr-Verlag.

Function of Somatic Cells in the Testis. Ed. by Andrzej Bartke. 1994. LC 93-39374. (Illus.). 466p. 162.00 (*0-387-94196-7*) Spr-Verlag.

Functional AAC Intervention: A Team Approach. Cynthia Cottier et al. Ed. by Cindy Drolet. 1997. (Illus.). 152p. spiral bd. 41.00 (*1-883315-22-0*, 7203) Imaginart Intl.

Functional Abnormalities of the Aorta. Ed. by Harisios Boudoulas et al. 1996. (Illus.). 416p. 85.00 (*0-87993-619-3*) Futura Pub.

Functional Accounts of Emotion. James J. Gross. 1999. 160p. pap. 39.95 (*0-86377-644-2*) L Erlbaum Assocs.

Functional Analysis in Clinical Psychology. Peter Sturmey. 1996. LC 95-31822. (Clinical Psychology & Personality Ser.). 270p. 225.00 (*0-471-95848-4*); pap. 60.00 (*0-471-96170-1*) Wiley.

Functional Analysis of Problem Behavior: A Practical Assessment Guide. Robert O'Neill et al. Ed. by Alan C. Repp & Nirbhay N. Singh. 1990. 85p. (C). pap. text 21.95 (*0-9625233-2-1*) Sycamore Pub.

Functional Analysis of the Human Genome. F. Farzaneh & D. N. Cooper. 1995. (Human Molecular Genetics Ser.). 300p. (*1-872748-46-5*) Bios Sci GBR. *Dist:* Coronet Bks.

Functional Analytic Psychotherapy: Creating Intense & Curative Therapeutic Relationships. R. J. Kohlenberg & M. Tsai. 1991. (Illus.). 232p. (C). 49.50 (*0-306-43857-7*, Plenum Trade) Perseus Pubng.

Functional Anatomy & Physiology for Emergency Care in the Streets. Joshua S. Yamamoto & Stephen A. Brada. 1995. LC 95-22329. 224p. pap. text 34.95 (*0-316-96726-2*, Little Brwn Med Div) Lppncott W & W.

Functional Anatomy of Craniofacial Arteries. Pierre L. Lasjaunias & Alejandro Berenstein. 1987. (Surgical Neuroangiography Ser.: Vol. 1). 426p. 199.00 (*3-540-16534-7*) Spr-Verlag.

Functional Anatomy of Speech, Language & Hearing: A Primer. William H. Perkins & Raymond D. Kent. 1991. 512p. (C). pap. text 92.00 (*0-205-13572-2*) Allyn.

Functional Anatomy of the Digestive System. R. M. McMinn & M. H. Hobdell. 1974. (Illus.). 282p. pap. text 45.00 (*0-272-00123-6*) St Mut.

Functional Anatomy of the Digestive System. R. M. McMinn & M. H. Hobdell. 1974. pap. 16.95 (*0-8464-0434-6*) Beekman Pubs.

Functional Anatomy of the Neuroendocrine Hypothalamus - Symposium No. 168. Ed. by Derek J. Chadwick & Joan Marsh. 1992. LC 92-5731. (CIBA Foundation Symposia Ser.: Vol. 168). 310p. 128.00 (*0-471-93440-2*) Wiley.

Functional Anatomy of the Olfactory System in 23 Orders of Birds. Betsy G. Bang. 1971. (Acta Anatomica Ser.: Suppl. 58, Vol. 79). pap. 19.25 (*3-8055-1193-0*) S Karger.

Functional Anatomy of the Spine. Jean Oliver & Alison Middleditch. (Illus.). 1991. 336p. text 52.50 (*0-7506-0052-7*); 2nd ed. 2002. 224p. pap. 50.00 (*0-7506-2717-4*) Buttrwrth-Heinemann.

Functional Anatomy of the Urogenital System. David Bulmer. 1974. (Illus.). 184p. pap. 27.95 (*0-8464-0444-3*) Beekman Pubs.

Functional Anatomy of the Visual System. Ruskell. 1995. 264p. pap. text (*0-7506-1467-6*) Buttrwrth-Heinemann.

Functional & Stereotactic Neurosurgery. E. I. Kandel. rev. ed. 1989. (Illus.). 724p. text 175.00 (*0-306-42701-X*, Kluwer Plenum) Kluwer Academic.

Functional Appliances: Atlas of Clinical Prescription & Laboratory Construction. Andrew Orton. 1990. (Illus.). 373p. text 72.00 (*1-85097-012-2*) Quint Pub Co.

Functional Approach to Child Language. Annette Karmiloff-Smith. 1981. LC 78-15450. (Studies in Linguistics: No. 24). (Illus.). 266p. pap. text 27.95 (*0-521-28549-6*) Cambridge U Pr.

Functional Approach to Group Work in Occupational Therapy. Margot C. Howe & Sharan L. Schwartzberg. 3rd ed. 2001. LC 00-53505. (Illus.). 288p. text 38.00 (*0-7817-2109-1*) Lppncott W & W.

Functional Aspects of Energy Metabolism in Neural Tissue. Ed. by J. Edmon & J. B. Clark. 1994. (Journal: Vol. 15, Nos. 3-5, 1993). (Illus.). 236p. pap. 83.50 (*3-8055-6033-8*) S Karger.

Functional Aspects of Mononuclear Phagocytes: Proceedings, Set. Conference on Mononuclear Phagocytes, Third, Noorw. Ed. by Ralph Van Furth. 1980. text 565.50 (*90-247-2211-X*) Kluwer Academic.

Functional Aspects of the Normal, Hypertrophied, & Failing Heart. Ed. by Francis L. Abel & Walter H. Newman. 1984. (Developments in Cardiovascular Medicine Ser.). text 146.50 (*0-89838-665-9*) Kluwer Academic.

Functional Assessment & Intervention in Geriatric Physical Therapy. Jackson-Wyatt. 1996. (*0-443-07645-6*, J0331) Church.

Functional Assessment & Outcome Measures for the Rehabilitation Health Professional. Sharon S. Dittmar & Glen E. Gresham. 1998. LC 97-7201. 224p. 55.00 (*0-8342-0929-2*, 20929) PRO-ED.

Functional Assessment & Program Development for Problem Behavior: A Practical Handbook. Horner et al. 2nd ed. 1996. LC 96-41160. (Special Education Ser.). 123p. pap. text 46.95 (*0-534-26022-5*) Brooks-Cole.

Functional Assessment in Massage Therapy. Whitney Lowe. 3rd rev. ed. 1995. (Illus.). 181p. pap. text 29.95 (*0-9661196-0-6*) OMERI.

Functional Assessment in Transition & Rehabilitation for Adolescents & Adults with Learning Disorders. Michael Bullis & Cheryl Davis. 1999. LC 98-30835. (*0-89079-803-6*) PRO-ED.

Functional Assessment of Low Vision. Roy Cole. Ed. by Bruce P. Rosenthal. 1995. (Illus.). 192p. (C). (gr. 13). pap. text 37.95 (*0-8151-7347-4*, 24266) Mosby Inc.

Functional Assessment Scale. Estelle Breines. 1983. tchr. ed. 21.00 (*0-941930-02-5*) Geri-Rehab.

Functional Behavior of Orthopedic Biomaterials. Ed. by Paul Ducheyne & Garth W. Hastings. 1984. Vol. I. 176p. 105.00 (*0-8493-6265-2*, RD755); Vol. II. LC 83-3737. 224p. 129.00 (*0-8493-6266-0*, RD755) Franklin (CRC Reprint).

Functional Behavioral Assessment: A Systematic Process for Assessment & Intervention in General & Special Education Classroom. Mary E. McConnell. 2000. LC 00-104333. 112p. (C). pap. text 24.95 (*0-89108-277-8*) Love Pub Co.

Functional Behavioral Assessment: An Interactive Training Module. Carl J. Liaupsin et al. 2nd rev. ed. 2000. 105p. per. 79.00 incl. cd-rom (*1-57035-274-7*, 140FBA) Sopris.

***Functional Biomaterials.** Ed. by N. Katsube et al. 2001. 324p. (*0-87849-871-0*) Trans T Pub CHE. *Dist:* Enfield Pubs NH.

Functional Biomechanics. Roger Soames. 1999. 264p. pap. 18.95 (*0-7506-0181-7*) Buttrwrth-Heinemann.

Functional Brain Imaging. William W. Orrison et al. 1994. (Illus.). 496p. (C). (gr. 13). text 98.00 (*0-8151-6509-9*, 24274) Mosby Inc.

Functional Brain Imaging. Ed. by G. Pfurtscheller & F. H. Lopes da Silva. 1988. LC 88-19071. 276p. (C). text 98.00 (*0-920887-28-7*) Hogrefe & Huber Pubs.

Functional Capillary Density: Active & Passive Determinants. Ed. by Marcos Intaglietta & P. C. Johnson. 1996. (International Journal of Microcirculation Ser.: Vol. 15, No. 5, 1995). (Illus.). 64p. pap. 51.50 (*3-8055-6288-8*) S Karger.

Functional Chordate Anatomy. Ronald G. Wolff. 2000. LC 90-82265. 710p. (C). text 73.16 (*0-669-21895-2*) HM Trade Div.

Functional Communication: Analyzing the Non-Linguistic Skills of Individuals with Severe or Profound Handicaps. L. Sternberg. Ed. by R. L. Taylor. 1990. (Disorders of Human Learning, Behavior, & Communication Ser.). (Illus.). 129p. 79.95 (*0-387-97261-7*) Spr-Verlag.

Functional Diagnostics of the Lower Urinary Tract. Attila Tanko. 1990. (Illus.). 204p. (*963-05-5327-9*) Akade Kiado HUN. *Dist:* Intl Spec Bk, St Mut.

Functional Disorders of the Gut. Ed. by S. F. Phillips & D. L. Wingate. 1995. (Illus.). 384p. (*0-443-05420-7*) Church.

Functional Documentation. Marcia H. Stamer. 1998. (C). pap. text 41.00 (*0-12-784589-5*) Acad Pr.

Functional Dyspepsia & Irritable Bowel Syndrome: Concepts & Controversies. Ed. by H. Goebell et al. 1998. (Falk Symposium Ser.). 256p. 98.00 (*0-7923-8735-X*) Kluwer Academic.

Functional Electrical Rehabilitation: Technological Restoration after Spinal Cord Injury. C. A. Phillips. 1991. (Illus.). 209p. 170.00 (*0-387-97459-8*) Spr-Verlag.

Functional Electrical Stimulation: Standing & Walking after Spinal Cord Injury. Alojz R. Kralj & Tadej Bajd. 1989. 208p. 179.00 (*0-8493-4529-4*, RD594) CRC Pr.

Functional Electrical Stimulation (FES) Resource Guide for Persons with Spinal Cord Injury or Multiple Sclerosis. Jeanne O. Teeter et al. 1995. 224p. pap. text 13.35 (*1-888470-03-8*) FES Info Ctr.

Functional Electrical Stimulation for Ambulation by Paraplegics: Twelve Years of Clinical Observations & Design Considerations & System Studies. Daniel Graupe & Kate H. Kohn. 1994. LC 93-4568. 210p. (C). lib. bdg. 39.50 (*0-89464-845-4*) Krieger.

Functional Endocrine Pathology. Kalman Kovacs & Sylvia L. Asa. 2nd ed. 1998. LC 97-36793. (Illus.). 904p. 269.95 (*0-86542-522-1*) Blackwell Sci.

Functional Endoscopic Sinus Surgery. Stammberger. 1991. (Illus.). 576p. (C). text 314.00 (*0-941158-96-9*) Mosby Inc.

Functional Evaluation & Outcomes in Sports & Orthopedic Physical Therapy: Evaluation, Treatment & Outcomes. Bruce Brownstein & Shaw Bronner. 1996. LC 96-36811. text (*0-443-07530-1*) Church.

Functional Evaluation of Stroke Patients. Ed. by N. Chino & J. L. Melvin. 1996. (Illus.). 140p. 84.00 (*4-431-70156-7*) Spr-Verlag.

Functional Foods: The Consumer, the Products & the Evidence. Ed. by M. Sadler & M. Saltmarsh. 1998. (Special Publications: Vol. 215). 234p. 124.95 (*0-85404-792-1*) Spr-Verlag.

Functional Foods for Disease Prevention. Ed. by Takayuki Shibamoto et al. 1998. LC 98-6978. (ACS Symposium Ser.: No. 702). (Illus.). 298p. text 95.00 (*0-8412-3573-2*) OUP.

Functional Foot Orthosis. J. W. Philps. 1990. (Illus.). 180p. pap. text (*0-443-04058-3*); 2nd ed. 1995. text (*0-443-04991-2*) Church.

Functional Fracture Bracing: Tibia, Humerus, & Ulna. Augusto Sarmiento & Loren L. Latta. 2nd rev. ed. 1995. (*3-540-55356-8*); (Illus.). 290p. 260.00 (*0-387-55356-8*) Spr-Verlag.

Functional Gastrointestinal Disorders see Rome II: The Functional Gastrointestinal Disorders: Diagnosis, Pathophysiology & Treatment - A Multinational Consensus

Functional Gastrointestinal Disorders: Diagnosis Pathophysiology & Treatment - a Multinational Consensus. Ed. by Douglas A. Drossman et al. 1994. 370p. pap. 49.95 (*0-9656837-0-2*, 00971) Degnon Assocs.

Functional Heterogeneity of Liver Tissue. Fernando Vidal-Vanaclocha. 1996. (Medical Intelligence Unit Ser.). 242p. (C). pap. 89.95 (*0-412-10861-5*) Chapman & Hall.

Functional Histology. Myrin Borysenko & Theodore Beringer. 2nd ed. 1984. 400p. pap. text 23.00 (*0-316-10304-7*) Lppncott W & W.

***Functional Human Anatomy.** Lane. 1996. (Illus.). (C). 70.00 (*0-8087-7536-7*) Pearson Custom.

Functional Human Anatomy. Lindsay. 1995. (C). text 283.12 (*0-8016-6472-1*) Mosby Inc.

Functional Human Anatomy. David T. Lindsay. 1995. (Illus.). 976p. (C). text 104.06 (*0-8016-6471-3*) McGrw-H Hghr Educ.

Functional Human Anatomy. David T. Lindsay & Deloris Wenzel. 1996. 448p. (C). pap., stu. ed. 32.19 (*0-8151-5448-8*) McGrw-H Hghr Educ.

Functional Human Anatomy. David T. Lindsay et al. 1996. 400p. (C). pap., lab manual ed. 47.19 (*0-8151-5449-6*) McGrw-H Hghr Educ.

Functional Human Anatomy. James E. Crouch. 4th ed. 1985. LC 83-24862. (Illus.). 645p. text 47.50 (*0-8121-0930-9*) Lppncott W & W.

Functional Human Anatomy. Olson. 5th ed. 1999. pap. text, lab manual ed. 22.00 (*0-536-02786-2*) Pearson Custom.

Functional Imaging: Principles & Methods. Ed. by Gustav K. Von Schulthess & Jurgen Hennig. 1997. LC 97-27805. (Illus.). 496p. text 175.00 (*0-397-51606-1*) Lppncott W & W.

Functional Imaging in Movement Disorders. Ed. by Martin W. R. Wayne. 1990. 256p. 190.00 (*0-8493-5837-X*, RM) CRC Pr.

Functional Imaging in the Epilepsies, Vol. 83. Thomas R. Henry et al. 2000. 352p. text 169.00 (*0-7817-2266-7*) Lppncott W & W.

Functional Implications of the Design of Skeletal Muscles. Ed. by Roland R. Roy & Akihiko Ishihara. 1998. (Acta Anatomica Ser.: Vol. 159, No. 2-3, 1997). (Illus.). 98p. pap. 83.50 (*3-8055-6682-4*) S Karger.

Functional Insulin Treatment: Principles, Teaching Approach & Practice. K. Howorka. Tr. by K. M. Nelson. 2nd ed. 1996. (Illus.). 218p. 31.95 (*3-540-60352-2*) Spr-Verlag.

Functional Job Analysis: A Foundation for Human Resources Management. Sidney A. Fine & Steven F. Cronshaw. 1999. LC 99-20566. (Applied Psychology Ser.). 250p. 69.95 (*0-8058-1274-1*) L Erlbaum Assocs.

Functional Kinetics. Susanne Klein-Vogelbach. 1989. (Illus.). 337p. 52.00 (*0-387-15350-0*) Spr-Verlag.

Functional Laws of Psychodynamics. E. Szekely. 1979. (Illus.). 353p. 108.00 (*0-387-90371-2*) Spr-Verlag.

***Functional Magnetic Resonance Imaging: An Introduction to Methods.** Ed. by Peter Jezzard et al. 2001. LC 2001-35793. (Illus.). 368p. text 195.95 (*0-19-263071-7*) OUP.

***Functional Magnetic Resonance Imaging Studies of Visual Motion Processing in the Human Brain.** Stefan Sunaert. 2001. (Acta Biomedical Lovaniensia Ser.: No. 226). (Illus.). 142p. pap. (*90-5867-100-3*) Leuven Univ BEL. *Dist:* Coronet Bks.

Functional Mapping in Biology & Medicine: Computer Assisted Autoradiography. Ed. by D. L. McEachron. 1986. (Experimental Biology & Medicine Ser.: Vol. 11). (Illus.). viii, 280p. 225.25 (*3-8055-4325-5*) S Karger.

***Functional Materials Studies by Mossbauer Spectroscopy.** Erik Nordstrom. 2001. (Comprehensive Summaries of Uppsala Dissertations from the Faculty of Science & Technology Ser.: No. 630). (Illus.). 52p. (*91-554-5031-8*) Uppsala Universitet SWE. *Dist:* Coronet Bks.

Functional Medicine: The Origin & Treatment of Chronic Diseases, Vol. 1. Helmut W. Schimmel. Tr. by Victor Penzer from GER. unabr. ed. 1997. (Illus.). 357p. (Orig.). (C). pap. text (*3-7760-1635-3*) Edits Haug Intl BEL. *Dist:* Medicina Bio.

Functional Methods: A Manual for Palpatory Skill Development in Osteopathic Examination & Manipulation of Motor Function. William L. Johnston & Harry D. Friedman. 1995. (Illus.). (C). 45.00 (*0-940668-02-5*); pap. 35.00 (*0-940668-03-3*) Am Acad Osteopathy.

Functional Morphology of Forelimb Joints in the Wooly Monkey Lagothrix Lagothricha. L. K. Ziemer. Ed. by F. S. Szalay. 1978. (Contributions to Primatology Ser.: Vol. 14). (Illus.). 68.00 (*3-8055-2821-3*) S Karger.

Functional Morphology of Neuroendocrine Systems. Berta Scharrer et al. 1988. (Illus.). 229p. 118.00 (*0-387-18155-5*) Spr-Verlag.

Functional Morphology of the Heart. Ed. by E. Bajusz & G. Jasmin. 1971. (Methods & Achievements in Experimental Pathology Ser.: Vol. 5). 172.25 (*3-8055-1209-0*) S Karger.

Functional Morphology of the Hepatic Vascular System. Gy Ungvary. 1977. 226p. (C). (*963-05-1074-X*) Akade Kiado HUN. *Dist:* St Mut.

Functional Morphology of the Hip & Thigh of the Lorisiformes. J. McArdle. 1981. (Contributions to Primatology Ser.: Vol. 17). (Illus.). viii, 132p. pap. 28.00 (*3-8055-1767-X*) S Karger.

Functional Morphology of the Human Endometrium & Decidua. U. M. Spornitz. Ed. by F. Beck et al. 1992. (Advances in Anatomy, Embryology & Cell Biology Ser.: Vol. 124). (Illus.). 99p. 105.00 (*0-387-54519-0*) Spr-Verlag.

Functional Morphology of Vertebrates. Ed. by H. R. Duncker & G. Fleischer. 1985. LC 85-17538. 752p. (*0-89574-207-1*) Gustav Fischer DEU. *Dist:* Lubrecht & Cramer, Balogh.

Functional Movement Development Across the Life Span. Donna Cech & Suzanne T. Martin. 1994. LC 93-37402. text 39.00 (*0-7216-3174-6*) Saunders.

Functional Neuroanatomy: Text & Atlas. Adel K. Afifi et al. 1997. LC 97-45690. (Illus.). 744p. pap. 59.95 (*0-07-001589-9*) McGraw-Hill Prof.

Functional Neuroimaging. Ed. by Roger E. Kelley. 1994. LC 94-6179. (Illus.). 560p. 98.00 (*0-87993-590-1*) Futura Pub.

Functional Neuroimaging: Technical Foundations. Ed. by Robert W. Thatcher et al. 1994. LC 93-37671. (Illus.). 303p. text 170.00 (*0-12-685845-4*) Acad Pr.

Functional Neuroscience. C. Barber et al. 1996. LC 96-48525. (Electroencephalography & Clinical Neurophysiology Ser.). 380p. 196.50 (*0-444-82430-8*) Elsevier.

Functional Neuroscience. Oswald Steward. 2000. LC 98-21387. (Illus.). 640p. pap. 49.95 (*0-387-98543-3*) Spr-Verlag.

Functional Neuroscience: Evoked Potentials & Magnetic Fields. Ed. by C. Barber et al. 1999. LC 99-37657. (Supplements to Electroencephalography & Clinical Neurophysiology Ser.: Vol. 49). 350p. 187.00 (*0-444-50062-6*) Elsevier.

Functional Neuroscience: Neurometric Assessment of Brain Disfunction in Neurological Patients, Vol. 3. Thalia Harmony. 1984. 600p. text 99.95 (*0-89859-044-2*) L Erlbaum Assocs.

Functional Organization & Plasticity of the Auditory Cortex. Ed. by R. V. Harrison et al. 1998. (Audiology & Neuro-Otology Ser.: Vol. 3, No. 2-3, 1998). (Illus.). 162p. pap. 54.00 (*3-8055-6683-2*) S Karger.

Functional Orthodontic Appliances. C. D. Stephens et al. 2nd ed. 2002. (Illus.). 144p. 125.00 (*0-7236-1058-4*) Buttrwrth-Heinemann.

Functional Osteology & Myology of the Shoulder in the Chiroptera. Timothy L. Strickler. 1977. (Contributions to Vertebrate Evolution Ser.: Vol. 4). (Illus.). 75.00 (*3-8055-2699-7*) S Karger.

Functional Partial Laryngectomy: Conservation Surgery for Carcinoma of the Larynx. Ed. by M. E. Wigand et al. 1984. (Illus.). 328p. 103.00 (*0-387-13175-2*) Spr-Verlag.

Functional Pathology of the Endometrium & Cervical Biopsy Specimens. H. Jellinek & F. Toth. 1976. 388p. (C). (*963-05-0687-4*) Akade Kiado HUN. *Dist:* St Mut.

Functional Performance in Older Adults. Bette R. Bonder & Marilyn B. Wagner. 2nd ed. 2000. LC 00-64402. (Illus.). 425p. text 49.00 (*0-8036-0543-9*) Davis Co.

Functional Progressions for Sport Rehabilitation. Steven R. Tippett & Michael L. Voight. 1995. LC 93-46409. (Illus.). 128p. (Orig.). pap. text 28.00 (*0-87322-660-7*, BTIP0660) Human Kinetics.

Functional Psychiatric Disorders of the Elderly. Ed. by Edmond Chiu & David Ames. 1994. LC 93-33740. (Illus.). 649p. (C). text 130.00 (*0-521-43160-3*) Cambridge U Pr.

Functional Psychoses: Classification & Prognosis. Ed. by Nils Retterstol & A. Dahl. 1986. (Journal: Vpl. 29, No. 1-2, 1986). (Illus.). 92p. pap. 68.00 (*3-8055-4317-4*) S Karger.

Functional Psychoses: Recent Follow-up Studies, 1991 - Psychopathology Journal, Vol. 24, No. 5. Nils Retterstol et al. 1991. (Illus.). 92p. pap. 38.50 (*3-8055-5534-2*) S Karger.

***Functional Reconstruction of The Female Genito-Urinary Tract.** R. Turner-Warwick. 2001. LC 2001-52781. (Illus.). 1550p. 450.00 (*0-86542-695-3*) Blackwell Sci.

Functional Rehabilitation in Orthopaedics. Trudy S. Goldstein. 1994. (Illus.). 276p. 75.00 (*0-8342-0556-4*, 20556) PRO-ED.

Functional Rehabilitation of Sports & Musculoskeletal Injuries. Ed. by W. Ben Kibler et al. 1996. LC 97-41935. (Rehabilitation Institute of Chicago Publication Ser.). 300p. 86.00 (*0-8342-0612-9*) PRO-ED.

Functional Roles of Glial Cells in Health & Disease: Dialogue Between Glia & Neurons. Ed. by Rebecca Matsas & Marco Tsacopoulos. 1999. LC 99-42891. (Advances in Experimental Medicine & Biology Ser.: Vol. 468). (Illus.). x, 389p. pap. (*0-306-46205-2*, Kluwer Plenum) Kluwer Academic.

Functional Skills Program. Wamboldt. 1998. 170p. (C). pap. text 51.00 (*0-12-784585-2*) Acad Pr.

Functional Soft-Tissue Examination & Treatment by Manual Methods: New Perspectives. Warren I. Hammer. 2nd rev. ed. 1999. LC 98-36103. (Illus.). 640p. 119.00 (*0-8342-0630-7*) Aspen Pub.

Functional Somatic Syndromes: Etiology, Diagnosis & Treatment. Ed. by Peter Manu. 1999. LC 98-24733. (Illus.). (C). 320p. text 105.00 (*0-521-59130-9*); 314p. pap. text 46.95 (*0-521-63491-1*) Cambridge U Pr.

Functional Status Measurement in Primary Care. Ed. by J. Froom & W. E. Fabb. 1990. (Frontiers of Primary Care Ser.). (Illus.). 267p. 115.00 (*0-387-97198-X*) Spr-Verlag.

***Functional Studies of Calcein Acetoxymethyl Ester in Human Tumor Cells.** Gunnar Liminga. 1999. (Comprehensive Summaries of Uppsala Dissertations from the Faculty of Medicine Ser.: No. 867). (Illus.). 59p. pap. (*91-554-4547-0*) Uppsala Universitet SWE. *Dist:* Coronet Bks.

Functional Surgery of the Larynx & Pharynx. Ed. by Waryam Singh & David S. Soutar. 1993. LC 92-49424. (Illus.). 224p. text (*0-7506-0612-6*) E A GBR. *Dist:* OUP.

Functional Theory of Cognition. Norman H. Anderson. 1996. 512p. 69.95 (*0-8058-2244-5*) L Erlbaum Assocs.

Functional Urology Towards the Next Millenium: Proceedings of the 4th International Congress of the Dutch Urological Association (DUA-IV), Maastricht, November 1997. Ed. by Ruud A. Janknegt & Philip E. Van Kerrebroeck. 1998. (European Urology Ser.: Vol. 34, Supplement 1, 1998). (Illus.). iv, 58p. pap., suppl. ed. 25.25 (*3-8055-6758-8*) S Karger.

Functional Vascular Anatomy of Brain, Spinal Cord & Spine. Pierre L. Lasjaunias & Alejandro Berenstein. 1990. (Surgical Neuroangiography Ser.: Vol. 3). 337p. 198.00 (*3-540-17501-6*) Spr-Verlag.

Functional Visual Behavior: A Therapist's Guide to Evaluation & Treatment Options. Ed. by Michele Gentile. 1997. LC 97-196348. 551p. pap. text 55.00 (*1-56900-071-9*, 1206) Am Occup Therapy.

Functionality & Protein Structure. Ed. by Akiva Pour-El. 1979. LC 78-31964. (ACS Symposium Ser.: No. 92). 32.95 (*0-8412-0478-0*) Am Chemical.

Functions of the Aging Brain from Physiological Ageing to Dementia. Ed. by M. Le Poncin Lafitte et al. 1986. (Journal: Vol. 32, Suppl. 1, 1986). (Illus.). iv, 128p. pap. 41.75 (*3-8055-4386-7*) S Karger.

Functions of the Brain, 3. David Ferrier. 1978. LC 77-72191. (Contributions to the History of Psychology Ser.: Pt. E, Vol. III, Physiological Psychology). 498p. reprint ed. lib. bdg. 89.50 (*0-313-26951-3*, U6951, Greenwood Pr) Greenwood.

Functions of the Cortico-Basal Ganglia Loop. Ed. by M. Kimura & A. M. Graybiel. 1995. LC 95-12417. 107.00 (*4-431-70148-6*); (Illus.). 224p. 98.00 (*0-387-70148-6*) Spr-Verlag.

Functions of the Natural Immune System. C. W. Reynolds & R. H. Wiltrout. 1989. LC 88-22488. (Illus.). 506p. (C). text 145.00 (*0-306-42951-9*, Kluwer Plenum) Kluwer Academic.

Functions of the Proteoglycans. CIBA Foundation Staff. 1986. LC 86-18886. (CIBA Foundation Symposia Ser.: No. 124). 310p. 128.00 (*0-471-91090-2*) Wiley.

Functions of Vitamins Beyond Recommended Dietary Allowances: Proceedings of the European Academy of Nutritional Sciences Workshop, Nice, October 1997. Ed. by P. Walter et al. 2001. LC 00-43435. (Bibliotheca Nutritio et Dieta Ser.: Vol. 55). x, 214p. 198.25 (*3-8055-7073-2*) S Karger.

Fundamental Anatomy for Operative Orthopaedic Surgery, Vol. 2. S. T. Donell & A. W. Lettin. 1991. (Fundamental Anatomy Ser.). (Illus.). 90p. 30.00 (*0-387-19669-2*) Spr-Verlag.

Fundamental Approaches to the Diagnosis & Treatment for Prostate Cancer & BPH: Proceedings of the Fifth Tokyo Symposium on Prostate Cancer, December 16-17, 1993, Keidanren-Kaikan, Tokyo, Japan. Kyoichi Imai et al. 1994. 95.00 (*0-940030-45-4*) Adenine Pr.

Fundamental Aspects of Biocompatibility D. F. Williams. 1981. (Biocompatability Ser.: Vol. 1). 240p. 135.00 (*0-8493-6611-9*, R857);Vol. 2. 328p. 179.00 (*0-8493-6612-7*) Franklin (CRC Reprint).

Fundamental Aspects of Cancer. Ed. by Ronald H. Goldfarb. 1988. (Cancer Growth & Progression Ser.). (C). text 211.50 (*0-89838-990-9*) Kluwer Academic.

Fundamental Conceptions of Psychoanalysis. Abraham Arden Brill. 1973. LC 73-2390. (Mental Illness & Social Policy; the American Experience Ser.). reprint ed. 24.95 (*0-405-05198-0*) Ayer.

Fundamental Concepts of Fitness & Wellness. Charles Corbin et al. 2000. LC 00-105433. (Illus.). 352p. (C). pap. 22.81 (*0-07-240990-8*) McGrw-H Hghr Educ.

Fundamental Fault in Hypertension. Mohinder P. Sambhi. 1984. (Developments in Cardiovascular Medicine Ser.). text 219.50 (*0-89838-638-1*) Kluwer Academic.

Fundamental Immunology. Robert M. Coleman et al. 2nd ed. 1992. 624p. (C). text 67.00 net. (*0-697-11310-8*); text, stu. ed. 24.37 (*0-697-16329-6*) McGrw-H Hghr Educ (WCB McGr Hill).

Fundamental Immunology. Mary F. Lombard & Raymond Sicard. 2nd ed. 1999. 632p. (C). pap. 90.31 (*0-07-235747-9*) McGrw-H Primis Cstm.

Fundamental Immunology. William E. Paul. 4th ed. 1998. LC 98-3611. (Illus.). 1,616p. text 149.00 (*0-7817-1412-5*) Lppncott W & W.

Fundamental Mathematics for Health Careers. Jerome D. Hayden & Howard Davis. 2nd ed. 1990. (Applied Mathematics Ser.). 280p. (gr. 11-12). pap., tchr. ed. 16.00 (*0-8273-3793-0*); pap. text 25.95 (*0-8273-3792-2*) Delmar.

Fundamental Mathematics for Health Careers. Jerome D. Hayden & Howard T. Davis. 3rd rev. ed. 1996. LC 95-14206. 96p. 12.00 (*0-8273-6689-2*) Delmar.

Fundamental Neuroscience. Ed. by Duane E. Haines & M. D. Ard. 1996. LC 96-18576. 498p. text (*0-443-08874-8*) Church.

Fundamental Neuroscience. Ed. by Michael J. Zigmond et al. 1998. LC 98-86877. (Illus.). 1600p. (C). 89.95 (*0-12-780870-1*) Acad Pr.

***Fundamental Neuroscience.** M. D. Ard. Ed. by Duane E. Haines. 2nd ed. 2001. LC 2001-28830. (*0-443-06603-5*) Church.

Fundamental Nursing Concepts & Skills. Grace Cole. 2nd ed. 1996. (Illus.). 912p. tchr. ed. (*0-8151-1816-3*);Set. (C). text (*0-8151-1926-7*) Mosby Inc.

Fundamental Nursing Concepts & Skills: Checklists. Grace Cole. 2nd ed. 1996. (*0-8151-1925-9*) Mosby Inc.

Fundamental Nursing Procedures. Rita Tobler. 1991. LC 91-4843. (Notes Ser.). 176p. pap. 18.95 (*0-87434-369-0*) Springhouse Corp.

Fundamental of Biochemistry. D. Deb. 4th ed. 1990. (C). (*0-7855-4671-5*) Current Dist IND. *Dist:* St Mut.

Fundamental Orthopedic Management For The Physical Therapist Assistant. Gary A. Shankman. 1996. (Illus.). 352p. (C). (gr. 13). text 37.00 (*0-8151-7541-8*, 24394) Mosby Inc.

Fundamental Orthopedic Management for the Physical Therapist Assistant. Gary A. Shankman. 1996. (Illus.). 96p. (C). (gr. 13). pap. text, wbk. ed. 9.95 (*0-8151-7542-6*, 24395) Mosby Inc.

Fundamental Physical Constants & the Frontiers of Medicine. B. W. Petley. rev. ed. 1984. 356p. 81.00 (*0-85274-427-7*) Taylor & Francis.

Fundamental Quantities & Units for Ionizing Radiation. International Commission on Radiation Units & Meas. 1998. LC 98-42758. (ICRU Report Ser.: Vol. 60). 18p. 30.00 (*0-913394-59-9*) Intl Comm Rad Meas.

Fundamental Research in Ultra High Dilution & Homoeopathy. J. Schulte & P. C. Endler. 1998. LC 98-16258. 276p. 119.00 (*0-7923-5051-0*) Kluwer Academic.

Fundamental Skills & Concepts in Patient Care. Barbara Kuhn Timby. 7th ed. 2000. LC 00-25008. (Illus.). 896p. pap. text 41.95 (*0-7817-1878-3*) Lppncott W & W.

Fundamental Skills for the Clinical Laboratory Professional. Jacquelyn R. Marshall. 1993. LC 92-49234. 698p. (C). mass mkt. 50.95 (*0-8273-4823-1*) Delmar.

Fundamental Skills for the Clinical Laboratory Professional Instructor's Guide. Jacquelyn R. Marshall. 1993. 79p. pap., tchr. ed. 14.00 (*0-8273-4825-8*) Delmar.

Fundamental Skills in Physical Education. Phyllis C. Jacobson & Ann Valentine. 1977. LC 76-51371. (Illus.). xviii, 221p. (C). pap. text 5.95 (*0-8425-0113-4*, Friends of the Library) Brigham.

Fundamental Skills in Surgery. Thomas F. Nealon, Jr. & William H. Nealon. 4th ed. 1994. LC 93-32194. (Illus.). 480p. text 49.95 (*0-7216-6460-1*) Saunders.

Fundamental Statistics for the Behavioral Sciences. David C. Howell. 3rd ed. 1994. LC 94-15870. (Business Statistics-Softside). 368p. pap. 57.75 net. (*0-534-23976-5*) Wadsworth Pub.

Fundamental Statistics for the Behavioral Sciences. Robert B. McCall. 5th ed. 1990. 464p. (C). text 67.00 (*0-15-529476-8*); pap. text, stu. ed. 23.50 (*0-15-529477-6*) Harcourt Coll Pubs.

Fundamental System: Bad Feet - Bad Spine. Roy S. Ashton. 2nd ed. 1996. 130p. reprint ed. spiral bd. 15.50 (*0-7873-0045-4*) Hlth Research.

Fundamental Techniques in Veterinary Surgery. Charles B. Knecht et al. 3rd ed. 1987. LC 87-4935. (Illus.). 368p. text 65.00 (*0-7216-1397-7*) Saunders.

***Fundamental Techniques of Plastic Surgery: And Their Surgical Applications.** Alan D. McGregor & Ian A. McGregor. 10th ed. 2001. (Illus.). 221p. pap. (*0-443-06372-9*) Church GBR. *Dist:* Saunders.

Fundamental Techniques of Plastic Surgery & Their Surgical Applications. Ian A. McGregor. 8th ed. 1989. (Illus.). 235p. pap. text (*0-443-03353-6*) Church.

Fundamental Techniques of Plastic Surgery & Their Surgical Applications. McGregor. 9th ed. 1995. pap. text (*0-443-05028-7*, M3572) Church.

Fundamental Themes in Clinical Supervision. John R. Cutcliffe et al. 2001. LC 00-45951. 304p. pap. 27.95 (*0-415-22887-5*) Routledge.

Fundamental Themes in Clinical Supery. John Cutcliffe et al. 2001. LC 00-45951. 304p. lib. bdg. 85.00 (*0-415-22886-7*) Routledge.

Fundamental Toxicology & Risk Assessment. National Environment on Health Staff. 1991. 259p. lib. bdg. 495.00 (*0-87371-641-8*) Lewis Pubs.

Fundamental Virology. Ed. by Bernard N. Fields et al. 3rd ed. 1995. (Illus.). 1,360p. text 99.00 (*0-7817-0284-4*) Lppncott W & W.

***Fundamental Virology.** Ed. by David M. Knipe et al. 4th ed. 2001. (Illus.). 1344p. text 99.95 (*0-7817-1833-3*) Lppncott W & W.

Fundamentals, No. 1. Ann Ehrlich. 2nd ed. 1993. 18.95 (*0-940012-37-5*) Colwell Syst.

Fundamentals for Ophthalmic Technical Personnel. Barbara Cassin. Ed. by Latif M. Hamed. 1995. (Illus.). 464p. text 54.00 (*0-7216-4931-9*) Saunders.

Fundamentals in Cancer Chemotherapy: Application of Cancer Chemotherapy, Proceedings, Set. Ed. by F. M. Schabel, Jr. 1978. (Antibiotics & Chemotherapy Ser.: Vol. 23 & 24). (Illus.). 120.00 (*3-8055-2893-0*) S Karger.

Fundamentals in Cancer Chemotherapy: Proceedings of the 10th International Congress, Zurich, September 1977. Anticancer-Symposium Staff et al. 1978. (Antibiotics & Chemotherapy Ser.: Vol. 23). (Illus.). 76.75 (*3-8055-2830-2*) S Karger.

Fundamentals in Musculoskeletal Radiology. Quillen. 1997. pap. text (*0-7216-6087-8*) Saunders.

Fundamentals of Abnormal Psychology. Ronald J. Comer. Date not set. (C). pap., tchr. ed. 16.00 (*0-7167-2963-6*) W H Freeman.

Fundamentals of Aerospace Medicine. Roy L. DeHart. 2nd ed. 1996. LC 96-3274. (Illus.). 1008p. 139.00 (*0-683-02396-9*) Lppncott W & W.

Fundamentals of an Integrated Model of Psychotherapy. Hector Fernandez-Alvarez. 2001. LC 98-42259. (Illus.). xxii, 326p. 35.00 (*0-7657-0189-8*) Aronson.

Fundamentals of Anatomy & Physiology. Frederic H. Martini. 2nd ed. 1992. LC 91-31947. 1120p. (C). text 97.00 (*0-13-334590-4*) P-H.

Fundamentals of Anatomy & Physiology. Martini. 5th ed. 2000. 1246p. stu. ed. 99.96 (*0-13-032479-5*) PH School.

Fundamentals of Anorectal Surgery. Ed. by David E. Beck & Steven D. Wexner. 1992. LC 92-2983. 509p. text 99.00 (*0-07-105436-7*, RD544) McGraw-Hill Educ Grp.

Fundamentals of Applied Psychiatry for Non-Medical Physicians. Thomas T. Lake. 1996. 102p. reprint ed. spiral bd. 16.50 (*0-7873-0520-0*) Hlth Research.

Fundamentals of Artistic Therapy: The Nature & Tasks of Painting Therapy. Margarethe Hauschka. Tr. by Vera Taberner et al from GER. 1986.Tr. of Kuenstlerische Therapie. (Illus.). 80p. pap. (*0-85440-434-1*) R Steiner Pr GBR. *Dist:* Anthroposophic.

Fundamentals of Ayurvedic Medicine. Vaidya B. Dash. 1984. 245p. text 20.00 (*0-89744-052-8*) Auromere.

Fundamentals of Ayurvedic Medicine. Baidya B. Dash. 1996. (C). reprint ed. (*81-220-0026-6*) Konark Pubs IND. *Dist:* S Asia.

Fundamentals of Ayurvedic Medicine. Vaidya B. Dash. 2nd ed. 1987. 246p. (C). text 21.95 (*0-940500-05-1*) Asia Bk Corp.

Fundamentals of Ayurvedic Medicine. Vaidya B. Dash. 7th rev. ed. 1990. 200p. text (*81-220-0117-3*) Konark Pubs Pvt Ltd IND. *Dist:* Advent Bks Div.

Fundamentals of Basic Surgery. John Niederhuber. 1999. (Illus.). 836p. (C). pap. text 49.95 (*0-8385-0509-0*, A-0509-8, Apple Lange Med) McGraw.

Fundamentals of Behavior Analytic Research. Alan D. Poling et al. 1995. (Applied Clinical Psychology Ser.). (Illus.). 236p. (C). 51.00 (*0-306-45056-9*, Plenum Trade) Perseus Pubng.

Fundamentals of Behavioral Research. Badla. 1998. 36.25 net. (*0-07-229965-7*) McGraw.

Fundamentals of Behavioral Statistics. Richard P. Runyon & Audrey Haber. 1985. LC 83-6327. 480p. (C). 10.00 (*0-394-35068-5*); 5th ed. text (*0-394-35018-9*) Random.

Fundamentals of Biochemistry. Ed. by A. C. Deb. 1989. (C). (*0-89771-370-2*) Current Dist IND. *Dist:* St Mut.

Fundamentals of Body CT. W. Richard Webb et al. Ed. by Lisette Bralow. 2nd ed. 1997. LC 97-5450. (Illus.). 352p. pap. text 49.00 (*0-7216-6862-3*) Saunders.

Fundamentals of Body Mechanics & Conditioning: An Illustrated Teaching Manual. Mabel Lee & Miriam M. Wagner. 1969. LC 75-91765. 377p. reprint ed. lib. bdg. 65.00 (*0-8371-2417-4*, LEBM, Greenwood Pr) Greenwood.

Fundamentals of Cancer Epidemiology. Philip C. Nasca & Harris Pastides. 2001. LC 2001-16068. (Illus.). 368p. 68.00 (*0-8342-1776-7*) Aspen Pub.

Fundamentals of Cardiac Surgery. Charles Marks & Peter H. Marks. 1993. LC 93-12008. 256p. (gr. 13). pap. 56.95 (*0-412-54310-9*, Chap & Hall NY) Chapman & Hall.

Fundamentals of Case Management: Guidelines for Practicing Case Managers. Judith M. Siefker. 1997. LC 97-16816. (Illus.). 272p. (C). (gr. 13). pap. text 33.95 (*0-8151-2498-8*, 31049) Mosby Inc.

Fundamentals of Chest Radiology. Andrew Meholic et al. Ed. by Sandra Valkoff. 1996. LC 95-43902. 288p. pap. text 39.95 (*0-7216-5400-2*) Saunders.

Fundamentals of Chinese Acupuncture. Andrew W. Ellis et al. Ed. by Richard Feit. rev. ed. 1993. (Illus.). 500p. (Orig.). pap. text 39.95 (*0-912111-33-X*) Paradigm Publns.

Fundamentals of Chinese Medicine. Tr. by Nigel A. Wiseman & Andrew Ellis. 1996. 532p. text 55.00 (*0-912111-52-6*) Paradigm Publns.

Fundamentals of Chinese Medicine. Nigel A. Wiseman. rev. ed. 1995. LC 94-18576. 600p. (C). pap. text 58.00 (*0-912111-44-5*) Paradigm Publns.

Fundamentals of Chiropractic Diagnosis & Management. Dana J. Lawrence. 1990. (Illus.). 608p. 89.00 (*0-683-04902-X*) Lppncott W & W.

Fundamentals of Clinical Endocrinology. Reginald L. Hall & Michael Besser. 4th ed. 1989. (Illus.). 492p. text (*0-443-03649-7*) Church.

Fundamentals of Clinical Hematology. Marcella L. Stevens. Ed. by Selma Kaszczuk. 1996. LC 96-16711. (Illus.). 368p. text 47.00 (*0-7216-4177-6*) Saunders.

Fundamentals of Clinical Nutrition. Sarah L. Morgan & Roland L. Weinsier. 2nd ed. 1998. (Illus.). 288p. pap. (*84-8174-466-2*) Mosby-Doyma Libros ESP. *Dist:* Mosby Inc.

Fundamentals of Clinical Nutrition. Roland L. Weinsier. Ed. by Sarah L. Morgan. 2nd ed. 1997. LC 97-19137. (Illus.). 288p. (C). (gr. 13). pap. text 24.95 (*0-8151-9669-5*, 29127) Mosby Inc.

***Fundamentals of Clinical Ophthalmology Scleritis.** Ed. by Peter McCluskey & Susan Lightman. 2001. (Fundamentals of Clinical Ophthalmology Ser.). (Illus.). 144p. text (*0-7279-1586-X*) BMJ Pub GBR. *Dist:* AIDC.

Fundamentals of Clinical Practice: A Textbook on the Patient, Doctor & Society. Ed. by Mark B. Mengel & Warren L. Holleman. 1996. LC 96-46673. (Illus.). 517p. (C). text 71.00 (*0-306-45348-7*, Kluwer Plenum) Kluwer Academic.

Fundamentals of Clinical Trials. L. M. Friedman et al. 3rd ed. 1998. LC 98-26138. 379p. pap. 47.95 (*0-387-98586-7*) Spr-Verlag.

Fundamentals of Co-Counseling Manual. Harvey Jackins. Tr. by Sami Kaskkainen from FIN. 1992.Tr. of Manuel Elementaire Pour Coconseillers. pap. 6.00 (*0-913937-68-1*) Rational Isl.

Fundamentals of Co-Counseling Manual: Croatian Translation. Harvey Jackins. Tr. by Branka Drascic. 1979. pap. 6.00 (*0-913937-57-6*) Rational Isl.

Fundamentals of Co-Counseling Manual: Greek Translation. Harvey Jackins. Tr. by Ersi Zarangali. 1983. pap. 6.00 (*0-911214-71-2*) Rational Isl.

Fundamentals of Co-Counseling Manual: Hebrew Translation. Harvey Jackins. 1979. (Orig.). pap. 6.00 (*0-911214-70-4*) Rational Isl.

Fundamentals of Co-Counseling Manual: Indonesian Translation. Harvey Jackins. Tr. by Jenny Toisuta. 1987. pap. 6.00 (*0-913937-29-0*) Rational Isl.

Fundamentals of Co-Counseling Manual: Kannada Translation. Harvey Jackins. Tr. by Shamrad Kulkarni from ENG. 1982. (Orig.). pap. 6.00 (*0-911214-79-8*) Rational Isl.

Fundamentals of Co-Counseling Manual: Kiswahili Translation. Harvey Jackins. 1993. pap. 6.00 (*0-913937-79-7*) Rational Isl.

Fundamentals of Co-Counseling Manual: Romanian Translation. Harvey Jackins. Tr. by Violeta Vajda. 1992. pap. 6.00 (*0-913937-58-4*) Rational Isl.

Fundamentals of Co-Counseling Manual: Tamil Translation. Harvey Jackins. 1986. pap. 6.00 (*0-913937-16-9*) Rational Isl.

Fundamentals of Co-Counseling Manual: Telugu Translation. Harvey Jackins. Tr. by Goteti Krishnamurty. 1979. pap. 6.00 (*0-911214-69-0*) Rational Isl.

Fundamentals of Cognitive-Behavior Therapy: From Both Sides of the Desk. Bill Borcherdt. 1996. LC 96-5122. 249p. (C). 49.95 (*0-7890-6030-2*) Haworth Pr.

Fundamentals of Cognitive Psychology. Henry C. Ellis & R. Reed Hunt. 5th ed. 1992. 432p. (C). text 36.00 net. (*0-697-10543-1*) Brown & Benchmark.

Fundamentals of Cognitive Psychology. R. Reed Hunt & Henry C. Ellis. 6th ed. 1998. LC 98-9559. 408p. pap. 47.50 (*0-697-20174-0*, WCB McGr Hill) McGrw-H Hghr Educ.

Fundamentals of Colon Hydrotherapy Vol. 1: An Independent Learning Program. Eddy H. Pevovar. 1997. (Illus.). 180p. ring bd. 98.00 (*0-9660627-0-1*) Dotolo Inst.

Fundamentals of Comparative & Alternative Medicine. Micozzi. 2000. pap. text (*0-323-01192-6*) Mosby Inc.

Fundamentals of Comparative Vertebrate Endocrinology. I. Chester-Jones et al. 1987. LC 86-22703. (Illus.). 682p. (C). text 145.00 (*0-306-42314-6*, Kluwer Plenum) Kluwer Academic.

Fundamentals of Complementary & Alternative Medicine. Ed. by Marc S. Micozzi. 1995. LC 95-39128. (Complementary & Alternative Medicine Ser.). 303p. pap. text (*0-443-05355-3*) Church.

Fundamentals of Complementary & Alternative Medicine. Marc S. Micozzi. 2nd ed. 2000. LC 00-52332. 430p. 49.00 (*0-443-06576-4*) Mosby Inc.

Fundamentals of Contemporary Nursing Practice. Carol A. Lindeman & Marylou McAthie. Ed. by Thomas Eoyang. 1999. LC 98-36263. (Illus.). 1020p. text (*0-7216-3527-X*) Saunders.

Fundamentals of Craniofacial Growth. Andrew D. Dixon et al. 1997. LC 96-38685. 512p. 149.95 (*0-8493-4575-8*) CRC Pr.

Fundamentals of Dental Hygiene Instrumentation. Jill S. Nield & Ginger A. Houseman. 2nd ed. 1988. LC 87-25975. (Illus.). 521p. pap. text 37.00 (*0-8121-1130-3*) Lppncott W & W.

Fundamentals of Dental Radiography. Lincoln R. Manson-Hing. 3rd ed. 1989. LC 89-7971. (Illus.). 269p. pap. text 39.50 (*0-8121-1253-9*) Lppncott W & W.

Fundamentals of Dermatology. Franklin S. Glickman & Alan R. Shalita. 1990. (Basic & Clinical Dermatology Ser.: Vol. 3). (Illus.). 224p. text, stu. ed. 89.75 (*0-8247-8338-7*) Dekker.

Fundamentals of Diagnostic Mycology. Fran Fisher & Norma B. Cook. Ed. by Selma Kaszczuk. 1998. LC 97-29245. (Illus.). 304p. (C). pap. text 39.95 (*0-7216-5006-6*) Saunders.

Fundamentals of Diagnostic Radiology. Ed. by William E. Brant & Clyde A. Helms. 1994. LC 93-34269. (Illus.). 1312p. 139.00 (*0-683-01011-5*) Lppncott W & W.

Fundamentals of Diagnostic Radiology. William E. Brant & Clyde A. Helms. 1993. (Illus.). 1136p. 135.00 (*0-683-01105-7*) Lppncott W & W.

Fundamentals of Diagnostic Radiology. Ed. by William E. Brant & Clyde A. Helms. 2nd ed. 1999. LC 97-51178. 1,600p. text 159.00 (*0-683-30093-8*) Lppncott W & W.

Fundamentals of E. N. T. K. Des. 45th ed. 1990. (C). (*0-7855-4659-6*) Current Dist IND. *Dist:* St Mut.

Fundamentals of Ear Acupuncture. Helmut Kropej. 4th ed. 1991. (Illus.). 105p. pap. (*3-7760-0777-X*) K F Haug Pubs DEU. *Dist:* Medicina Bio.

Fundamentals of Ear, Nose & Throat Diseases. S. K. De. 1985. (*0-7855-0730-2*) Current Dist IND. *Dist:* St Mut.

Fundamentals of EEG Technology. Richard Burgess. 2nd ed. 1998. text (*0-397-51858-7*) Lppncott W & W.

Fundamentals of EEG Technology Vol. 1: Basic Concepts & Methods, Vol. 1. Fay S. Tyner et al. 1983. (Illus.). 332p. spiral bd. 115.00 (*0-89004-385-X*) Lppncott W & W.

Fundamentals of EEG Technology Vol. 2: Clinical Correlates, No. 2. Fay S. Tyner et al. 1989. 302p. pap. text 115.00 (*0-89004-909-2*) Lppncott W & W.

Fundamentals of Electroacupuncture According to Voll. H. Leonhardt. Tr. by Helga Sarkisyanz from GER. 1980. (Illus.). 284p. text (*3-88136-081-6*) ML-Verlag DEU. *Dist:* Medicina Bio.

Fundamentals of Electrocardiography. R. W. Jelliffe. 1989. (Illus.). 214p. 105.00 (*0-387-97185-8*) Spr-Verlag.

Fundamentals of Emergency Care. Richard W. O. Beebe & Deborah L. Funk. 2001. LC 00-50889. (Illus.). 928p. 52.95 (*0-7668-1498-X*) Delmar.

***Fundamentals of Emergency Care Flash.** 2001. audio compact disk 29.95 (*0-7668-4321-1*) Delmar.

Fundamentals of Emergency Radiology. Philip W. Wiest & Paul B. Roth. Ed. by Sandra Valkoff. 1996. LC 95-41651. (Illus.). 224p. pap. text 39.95 (*0-7216-5182-8*) Saunders.

Fundamentals of ENT Radiology. Spar. 1996. (C). pap. text (*0-7216-5383-9*) Saunders.

Fundamentals of Enzymology. Nicholas C. Price & Lewis Stevens. 2nd ed. 1989. (Illus.). 544p. (C). pap. text 44.95 (*0-19-855296-3*) OUP.

Fundamentals of Esthetics. Claude Rufenacht. 1990. (Illus.). 372p. text 156.00 (*0-86715-230-3*) Quint Pub Co.

Fundamentals of Exercise Testing. K. Lange Andersen et al. 1970. 116p. pap. text 21.60 (*92-4-156001-0*, 1150046) World Health.

Fundamentals of Family Mediation. John M. Haynes. 1994. LC 93-38027. (Series in Transpersonal & Humanistic Psychology). 245p. (C). pap. text 20.95 (*0-7914-2036-1*) State U NY Pr.

Fundamentals of Family Medicine: The Family Medicine Clerkship Textbook. Ed. by R. B. Taylor et al. 2nd ed. 1998. LC 98-2746. (Illus.). 619p. pap. 42.95 (*0-387-98445-3*) Spr-Verlag.

Fundamentals of Fitness. Judd Biasiotto & Ed Ritter. 1983. 100p. (Orig.). pap. 7.00 (*0-933079-02-8*) World Class Enterprises.

Fundamentals of Fixed Prosthodontics. Herbert T. Shillingburg. 3rd ed. 1997. LC 96-24703. (Illus.). 592p. text 58.00 (*0-86715-201-X*) Quint Pub Co.

Fundamentals of Functional Brain Imaging: A Guide to the Methods & Their Applications to Psychology & Behavioral Neuroscience. A. C. Papanicolaou. 1998. LC 98-30131. (Studies on Neuropsychology, Development & Cognition: Vol. 1). (Illus.). 156p. (*90-265-1528-6*) Swets.

Fundamentals of Gastroenterology. Michael Davis & Jeffrey D. Houston. 1999. LC 2001-31369. (Illus.). 179p. pap. text (*0-7216-5203-4*) Saunders.

Fundamentals of Gastroenterology. L. Powell & D. Piper. 5th ed. 1991. 288p. pap. 39.00 (*0-07-050617-5*) McGraw-Hill Prof.

Fundamentals of Gastroenterology. Ed. by Lawrie W. Powell & Douglas W. Piper. 6th ed. 1995. (Illus.). 292p. 54.95 (*0-07-470192-4*) McGraw-Hill Med Pub.

Fundamentals of Genetic Epidemiology. Muin J. Khoury et al. 1993. LC 92-16492. (Illus.). 400p. text 59.50 (*0-19-505288-9*) OUP.

Fundamentals of Geriatrics for Health Professionals: An Annotated Bibliography, 11. Compiled by Jodi L. Teitelman & Iris A. Parham. 1990. LC 89-28653. (Bibliographies & Indexes in Gerontology Ser.: No. 11). 255p. lib. bdg. 72.95 (*0-313-26225-X*, TFD/, Greenwood Pr) Greenwood.

Fundamentals of Head & Neck Reconstruction Vol. I: The Angiosome Concept & Pedicled Myocutaneous Flaps. Jonathan E. Aviv & Andrew Blitzer. 1998. LC 97-42867. (Self-Instructional Package Ser.). (Illus.). 47p. pap. text 25.00 (*1-56772-058-7*, 5506315) AAO-HNS.

Fundamentals of Health Assisting. Richards. (Home Care Aide Ser.). Date not set. pap., tchr. ed. 14.00 (*0-8273-6145-9*); 1997. pap. 28.95 (*0-8273-6143-2*); 1997. pap., wbk. ed. 16.95 (*0-8273-6144-0*) Delmar.

Fundamentals of Health Assisting CTB. Richards. 1997. (Home Care Aide Ser.). 64.95 (*0-8273-6146-7*) Delmar.

Fundamentals of Health Care Quality Management. Patrice L. Spath. 2000. 168p. 30.00 (*1-929955-08-1*) Brown Spath.

Fundamentals of Health Insurance, Pt. A. Ed. by Jane J. Stein. 1997. LC 97-186574. 257p. pap. text 30.00 (*1-879143-36-4*) Health Ins Assn Am.

Fundamentals of Health Insurance, Pt. B. Ed. by Jane Stein. 1997. LC 97-186574. 273p. pap. text 30.00 (*1-879143-38-0*) Health Ins Assn Am.

Fundamentals of Health Insurance Study Manual. HIAA Staff. 1997. Pt. A. 58p. pap., stu. ed. 10.00 (*1-879143-37-2*); Pt. B. 52p. pap. 10.00 (*1-879143-39-9*) Health Ins Assn Am.

Fundamentals of Health Law. Douglas A. Hastings et al. 1995. (Orig.). pap. (*0-918945-18-6*) Am Hlth Lawyers.

Fundamentals of Human Behavior: Beyond the Mind - Body Dichotomy. Henry D. Hill. 1993. LC 93-71910. 146p. (C). pap. 30.00 (*0-9637136-1-2*); lib. bdg. 45.00 (*0-9637136-0-4*) CNC of Naprapathy.

Fundamentals of Human Neuropsychology: Printed Test Bank. Kolb. 1996. (C). 16.00 (*0-7167-2727-7*) W H Freeman.

Fundamentals of Human Relations. Ralph D. Wray. 1996. (General Business & Business Education Ser.). stu. ed. 14.95 (*0-8273-6801-1*) Delmar.

E F G

Fundamentals of Human Relations: Applications for Life & Work. Ralph D. Wray et al. 1995. LC 95-42284. (Career Development Ser.). mass mkt. 60.95 (*0-538-71396-8*) S-W Thomson.

Fundamentals of Immunohematology. Mary L. Turgeon. 2nd ed. 1995. 48.50 (*0-8121-1769-7*) Lppncott W & W.

Fundamentals of Immunology. O. G. Bier et al. 1986. (Illus.). 442p. 20.00 (*0-387-90529-4*) Spr-Verlag.

Fundamentals of Immunology & Allergy. Richard F. Lockey & Samuel C. Bukantz. 1987. (Illus.). 352p. pap. text 41.00 (*0-7216-2054-X*) Saunders.

Fundamentals of Industrial Hygiene. H. Plogg. Ed. by Barbara A. Plog. 4th rev. ed. 1995. (Illus.). 1011p. 124.95 (*0-87912-171-8*, 15134-0000) Natl Safety Coun.

Fundamentals of Laparoscopic Surgery. Ed. by Lawrence W. Way et al. 1995. LC 95-10714. (Illus.). pap. text (*0-443-08991-4*) Church.

Fundamentals of Mammography. Lee. 1995. pap. text 57.95 (*0-7020-1797-3*) Saunders.

Fundamentals of Manual Therapy: Physiology, Neurology & Psychology. Eyal Lederman. 1997. LC 97-705. text (*0-443-05275-1*) Church.

Fundamentals of Marital Therapy. D. Russell Crane. 1996. LC 96-34763. (Basic Principles into Practice Ser.: Vol. 14). 192p. pap. 31.95 (*0-87630-801-9*) Brunner-Routledge.

Fundamentals of Mathematics for Health Careers. Jerome D. Hayden & Howard T. Davis. 3rd ed. 1995. (Health Occupations Ser.). 288p. (C). pap. text 46.95 (*0-8273-6688-4*) Delmar.

Fundamentals of Maxillofacial Surgery. James W. Ferraro. 1997. LC 96-1685. 347p. 170.00 (*0-387-94737-X*) Spr-Verlag.

Fundamentals of Medical Cell Biology Vol. 1: Evolutionary Biology. E. Edward Bittar. 1991. 344p. 90.00 (*1-55938-303-8*) Jai Pr.

Fundamentals of Medical Cell Biology Vol. 8: Cumulative Index, Vols. 1-7, 1991-1992, Vol. 8. Ed. & Intro. by E. Edward Bittar. 1993. 220p. 90.00 (*1-55938-308-9*) Jai Pr.

Fundamentals of Medical Management: A Guide for the New Physician Executive. Ed. by Jerry L. Hammon. 1993. LC 92-72278. 260p. (C). text 50.00 (*0-924674-17-2*) Am Coll Phys Execs.

Fundamentals of Memory Formation: Neuronal Plasticity & Brain Function. Ed. by Heinrich Rahmann. 1990. (Progress in Zoology/Fortschritte der Zoologie Ser.: Vol. 37). 431p. (*0-89574-297-7*) Gustav Fischer DEU. *Dist:* Lubrecht & Cramer, Balogh.

Fundamentals of Mental Health Nursing. Kathryn C. Neeb. (Illus.). 1997. LC 96-37436. 411p. (C). pap. text 27.95 (*0-8036-0205-7*); 2nd ed. 2001. LC 2001-17381. 416p. per. 29.95 (*0-8036-0728-8*) Davis Co.

Fundamentals of Microbiology. I. Edward Alcamo. 4th ed. 1994. LC 93-46618. (C). pap. text, stu. ed. 18.75 (*0-8053-0327-8*) Benjamin-Cummings.

Fundamentals of Microbiology. I. Edward Alcamo. 6th ed. 2000. LC 00-24358. (Illus.). 928p. (C). text 84.95 (*0-7637-1067-9*, 1067-9) Jones & Bartlett.

Fundamentals of Monitoring Psychoactive Drug Therapy. Lindsay DeVane. 1989. (Illus.). 298p. 31.00 (*0-683-02452-3*) Lppncott W & W.

Fundamentals of Mortality Risks During the Perinatal Period & Infancy. Ed. by Frank Falkner. 1977. (Monographs in Pediatrics: Vol. 9). (Illus.). 190p. 74.00 (*3-8055-2651-2*) S Karger.

Fundamentals of MRI. Donald W. Chakeres. 1991. (Illus.). 320p. 70.00 (*0-683-01666-0*) Lppncott W & W.

Fundamentals of Musculoskeletal Assessment Techniques. M. Lynn Palmer et al. 2nd ed. 1998. LC 97-48521. 432p. spiral bd. 49.95 (*0-7817-1007-3*) Lppncott W & W.

Fundamentals of Musculoskeletal Imaging. George L. Spaeth. 1999. pap. text (*0-7216-4198-9*) Saunders.

Fundamentals of Neuroimaging. Blaine Hart et al. Ed. by Sandra Valkoff. 1996. (Fundamentals of Radiology Ser.). 192p. pap. text 39.00 (*0-7216-5163-1*) Saunders.

Fundamentals of Neuroimaging. William W. Woodruff. 1992. LC 92-13388. (Illus.). 588p. text 120.00 (*0-7216-3717-5*) Saunders.

Fundamentals of Neuropathology. Haruo Okazaki. 2nd ed. 1989. LC 89-2048. (Illus.). 328p. 79.00 (*0-89640-156-1*) Igaku-Shoin.

Fundamentals of Neurophysiology. Ed. by Richard F. Schmidt. Tr. by M. A. Biedermann-Thorson from GER. 3rd rev. ed. 1985. (Illus.). 346p. 79.95 (*0-387-96147-X*) Spr-Verlag.

Fundamentals of Nonverbal Behavior. Ed. by Robert S. Feldman & Bernard Rime. 1991. (Studies in Emotion & Social Interaction). (Illus.). 527p. (C). pap. text 34.95 (*0-521-36700-X*) Cambridge U Pr.

Fundamentals of Normal & Clinical Nutrition. Corinne B. Cataldo et al. 1996. LC 95-3813. 700p. (C). pap. 60.95 (*0-314-04449-3*) West Pub.

Fundamentals of Nuclear Pharmacy. Gopal B. Saha, Jr. 4th ed. 1998. LC 97-34137. (Illus.). 375p. 54.95 (*0-387-98341-4*) Spr-Verlag.

Fundamentals of Nursing. Helen Chandler Harkreader. 2000. LC 99-17270. li, 1716p. text 66.00 (*0-7216-8669-9*) Harcrt Hlth Sci Grp.

Fundamentals of Nursing. June L. Olsen. 1991. LC 90-9636. (Nursetest: A Review Ser.). 336p. (Orig.). pap. 21.95 (*0-87434-302-X*) Springhouse Corp.

Fundamentals of Nursing. Jack Rudman. (Regents College Proficiency Examination Ser.: Vol. 12). 43.95 (*0-8373-5462-5*); (College Level Examination Ser.: Vol. 30). 47.95 (*0-8373-5380-7*); 1994. (Regents College Proficiency Examination Ser.: CPEP-12). pap. 23.95 (*0-8373-5412-9*); 1994. (College Level Examination Ser.: Vol. CLEP-30). pap. 27.95 (*0-8373-5330-0*); 1994. (ACT Proficiency Examination Program Ser.: Vol. PEP-36). pap. 23.95 (*0-8373-5536-2*) Natl Learn.

Fundamentals of Nursing. Karen Berger. 2nd ed. 1998. LC 97-37909. 1700p. pap. text 63.95 (*0-8385-2594-6*) Appleton & Lange.

Fundamentals of Nursing. Mary C. Sundberg. 2nd ed. 1989. 1632p. 67.50 (*0-86720-422-2*) Jones & Bartlett.

***Fundamentals of Nursing.** Patricia A. Potter & Anne G. Perry. 5th ed. 2001. stu. ed. 19.95 (*0-323-01210-8*) Mosby Inc.

Fundamentals of Nursing. Patricia A. Potter & Anne G. Perry. 5th ed. 2000. (Illus.). 1000p. text 68.00 incl. cd-rom (*0-323-01141-1*) Mosby Inc.

Fundamentals of Nursing. 6th ed. 2000. (*0-8053-8363-8*) Addison-Wesley.

Fundamentals of Nursing. Barbara Kozier. 6th ed. 1999. 392p. (C). pap. text 22.80 (*0-8053-8342-5*) Benjamin-Cummings.

***Fundamentals of Nursing.** Kozier & Erb. 6th ed. 2000. suppl. ed. 142.33 (*0-13-055923-7*) P-H.

Fundamentals of Nursing, No. 3. Potter. 1992. (*0-8016-6958-8*) Mosby Inc.

Fundamentals of Nursing: A Canadian Perspective. Patricia A. Potter et al. 4th ed. 1997. LC 96-37669. (Illus.). 1568p. (C). (gr. 13). text 65.75 (*0-8151-8901-X*, 28983) Mosby Inc.

Fundamentals of Nursing: Collaborating for Optimal Health. Karen J. Berger & Marilyn A. Williams. 1992. LC 91-33329. (Illus.). 1632p. (C). 63.95 (*0-8385-1213-5*, A1213-6) P-H.

***Fundamentals of Nursing: Computerized Testbank.** Patricia A. Potter & Anne G. Perry. 5th ed. 2001. 500.00 (*0-323-01143-8*) Mosby Inc.

Fundamentals of Nursing: Concepts & Procedures. Barbara Kozier et al. 2nd ed. 1983. 38.95 (*0-201-11711-8*, Health Sci); stu. ed. (*0-201-11714-2*) Addison-Wesley.

Fundamentals of Nursing: Concepts, Process & Practice. Patricia A. Potter. 3rd ed. 1992. LC 92-49926. 1808p. (C). (gr. 13). text 31.50 (*0-8016-7204-X*, 07204) Mosby Inc.

Fundamentals of Nursing: Concepts, Process & Practice. Patricia A. Potter & Anne G. Perry. 4th ed. (Illus.). stu. ed. (*0-8151-9369-6*); 1997. 1568p. (*0-323-00498-9*); 1997. 1568p. (*0-8151-8502-2*) Mosby Inc.

Fundamentals of Nursing: Concepts, Process & Practice. Patricia A. Potter et al. 4th ed. 1997. (Illus.). 400p. (C). pap. text, stu. ed. (*0-8151-4656-6*, 28985) Mosby Inc.

Fundamentals of Nursing: Concepts, Process & Practice. Barbara Kozier. 5th rev. ed. 1997. LC 97-26045. 1536p. (C). text 76.88 (*0-8053-7472-8*) Addison-Wesley.

Fundamentals of Nursing: Concepts, Process & Practice: Checklists. Patricia A. Potter & Anne G. Perry. 4th ed. 1997. (C). pap. text (*0-8151-8501-4*, 28445) Mosby Inc.

Fundamentals of Nursing: Critical Thinking Activities. Patricia Potter. 3rd ed. 1994. 80p. (C). (gr. 13). text, suppl. ed. 9.95 (*0-8151-6403-3*) Mosby Inc.

Fundamentals of Nursing: Instructors Manual with Disk. Berger. 1998. 250p. incl. disk (*0-8385-2640-3*, A2640-9) Appleton & Lange.

Fundamentals of Nursing: Media Edition. Berger & Williams. 2nd ed. 2000. 1584p. pap. 82.00 incl. disk (*0-13-054947-9*) P-H.

Fundamentals of Nursing: Review & Study Guide. Zimbler. rev. ed. 1998. pap. text, stu. ed. 21.95 (*0-8385-2773-6*) P-H.

Fundamentals of Nursing: Standards & Practice. Sue C. Delaune & Patricia K. Ladner. 1997. LC 97-22117. (Nursing Education Ser.). 1332p. (C). 80.95 (*0-8273-6378-8*) Delmar.

Fundamentals of Nursing: Standards & Practice Annotated Instructors Edition. Sue C. Delaune et al. annot. ed. 1998. LC 97-52692. 1364p. text, tchr. ed. 250.00 (*0-8273-9096-3*) Delmar.

***Fundamentals of Nursing: Standards & Practices.** Sue C. Delaune & Patricia K. Ladner. 2nd ed. 2002. LC 2001-53867. 320p. text 68.95 (*0-7668-2452-7*) Delmar.

Fundamentals of Nursing: The Art & Science of Nursing Care. Carol Taylor et al. 4th ed. 2001. LC 00-57589. 1,424p. text 67.95 (*0-7817-2273-X*) Lppncott W & W.

Fundamentals of Nursing - Standards & Practice Classroom Manager. Delaune. 1998. 208p. text 250.00 (*0-8273-9091-2*) Delmar.

Fundamentals of Nursing & Practice Skills Checklist. Delaune & Campbell. 1998. (C). pap. 9.00 (*0-7668-0899-8*) Delmar.

Fundamentals of Nursing Practice. Barbara W. Narrow & Kay Buschl. 2nd ed. 1989. 1024p. 14.95 (*0-8273-4322-1*) Delmar.

Fundamentals of Nursing Research. Dorothy Brockopp. 1993. (Nursing-Health Science Ser.). (Illus.). 416p. (C). pap. text 33.75 (*0-86720-689-6*, 689-6) Jones & Bartlett.

Fundamentals of Nursing Research. Dorothy Young Brockopp & Marie H. Tolsma. 2nd ed. 1994. (Nursing-Health Science Ser.). (Illus.). 376p. (C). pap. text 46.95 (*0-86720-687-X*, 687-X) Jones & Bartlett.

Fundamentals of Nursing Research. Dorothy Young Brockopp & Marie T. Hastings-Tolsma. 3rd ed. 2002. (Illus.). 384p. (C). pap. text 44.95 (*0-7637-1567-0*, 1567-0) Jones & Bartlett.

Fundamentals of Nursing Standards & Practice: Student Study Guide. Delaune. 1998. 192p. stu. ed. 18.95 (*0-8273-9093-9*) Delmar.

Fundamentals of Obstetric & Gynecologic Ultrasound. E. Albert Reece et al. 1994. (Illus.). 272p. (C). pap. text 95.00 (*0-8385-9247-3*, A9247-6, Apple Lange Med) McGraw.

Fundamentals of Obstetric & Gynecological Radiology. Rosenberg. 1999. pap. text (*0-7216-5157-7*) Saunders.

***Fundamentals of Obstetrics & Gynaecology: Obstetricia y Ginecologia.** Derek Llewellyn-Jones. 7th ed. 1999. (Illus.). 368p. pap. (*84-8174-447-6*) Mosby-Doyma Libros ESP. *Dist:* Mosby Inc.

Fundamentals of Obstetrics & Gynecology. Derek Llewellyn-Jones. 6th ed. 1994. text 36.00 (*0-7234-2000-9*) Mosby Inc.

Fundamentals of Oncology. Henry C. Pitot. 3rd rev. ed. 1985. (Illus.). 544p. text 55.00 (*0-8247-7457-4*) Dekker.

***Fundamentals of Operating Department Practice.** Colin Ince. 1999. (Illus.). 400p. pap. text (*1-900151-18-9*) Greenwich Med GBR. *Dist:* JAMCO Dist.

Fundamentals of Operative Dentistry: Contemporary Concepts. Richard S. Schwartz et al. 1996. LC 96-20651. (Illus.). 432p. pap. text 68.00 (*0-86715-311-3*) Quint Pub Co.

Fundamentals of Operative Techniques in Neurosurgery. E. Sander Connolly et al. 2001. (Illus.). 800p. 79.00 (*0-86577-836-1*) Thieme Med Pubs.

Fundamentals of Ophthalmic Practice. Kamenetzky. 1993. 220p. (C). (gr. 13). (*1-56375-158-5*) Gower-Mosby.

Fundamentals of Oral Medicine: A Practical Guide. Crispian Scully. 2001. (Illus.). 192p. pap. 54.00 (*0-7236-1074-6*) Buttrwrth-Heinemann.

Fundamentals of Orofacial Myology. Marvin L. Hanson & Richard H. Barrett. 1989. (Illus.). 380p. 75.95 (*0-398-05518-1*) C C Thomas.

Fundamentals of Orthognathic Surgery. Harris. 1991. pap. text 79.00 (*0-7020-1511-3*) Saunders.

Fundamentals of Orthopedic Radiology. Lynn McKinnis. 1996. LC 96-33387. (Contemporary Perspectives in Rehabilitation Ser.). (Illus.). 429p. (C). text 56.00 (*0-8036-0139-5*) Davis Co.

Fundamentals of Orthopedics. John J. Gartland. 4th ed. 1986. (Illus.). 440p. text 45.00 (*0-7216-1413-2*) Saunders.

Fundamentals of Pediatric Dentistry. Richard J. Mathewson & Robert E. Primosch. 3rd ed. 1995. LC 94-43277. (Illus.). 400p. (Orig.). pap. text 58.00 (*0-86715-262-1*, B2621) Quint Pub Co.

Fundamentals of Pediatric Orthopedics. Lynn T. Staheli. 2nd ed. 1998. LC 98-23006. 168p. text 95.00 (*0-7817-1632-2*) Lppncott W & W.

Fundamentals of Pediatric Radiology. Williamson. 2000. LC 2001-34482. (Illus.). xv, 246p. pap. text (*0-7216-4180-6*) Saunders.

Fundamentals of Perinatal Social Work: A Guide for Clinical Practice with Women, Infants & Families. Ed. by Regina F. Lind & Debra H. Bachman. 1997. LC 97-6350. (Social Work in Health Care Ser.: Vol. 24, Nos. 3-4). 224p. (C). 44.95 (*0-7890-0043-1*); pap. text 24.95 (*0-7890-0049-0*) Haworth Pr.

Fundamentals of Periodontal Instrumentation. Jill S. Nield-Gehrig. 4th ed. 2000. 576p. spiral bd. 48.00 (*0-7817-2860-6*) Lppncott W & W.

Fundamentals of Periodontics. Ed. by Thomas G. Wilson, Jr. & Kenneth S. Kornman. 1996. LC 96-4579. (Illus.). 576p. pap. text 74.00 (*0-86715-303-2*) Quint Pub Co.

Fundamentals of Physiology. Lauralee Sherwood. 2nd ed. 1994. LC 94-20836. 689p. (C). 105.95 (*0-314-04272-5*) West Pub.

Fundamentals of Plastic Surgery. Malcolm W. Marks & Charles Marks. Ed. by Larry McGrew. 1997. LC 96-8868. 400p. text 78.00 (*0-7216-6449-0*) Saunders.

Fundamentals of Psychiatric Nursing. Theresa G. Muller. 1974. (Quality Paperback Ser.: No. 308). 226p. reprint ed. pap. 11.00 (*0-8226-0308-X*) Littlefield.

Fundamentals of Psychiatric Treatment Planning. James A. Kennedy. 1992. LC 91-22231. 224p. spiral bd. 38.50 (*0-88048-407-1*, 8407) Am Psychiatric.

Fundamentals of Psychology. Culkin. 1995. (General Business & Business Education Ser.). stu. ed. 14.95 (*0-8273-6802-X*) Delmar.

Fundamentals of Psychology. Edward J. Smith et al. 2000. LC 00-104764. (Illus.). 624p. (C). pap. text 73.95 (*0-15-501225-8*) Wadsworth Pub.

Fundamentals of Psychology. Audrey Haber & Richard P. Runyon. 4th ed. (C). 1987. pap. text 20.00 net. (*0-07-553721-4*); 1986. 600p. pap. text 48.25 net. (*0-07-555259-0*) McGraw.

Fundamentals of Psychology: Applications for Life & Work. Culkin. 1995. (CA - Career Development Ser.). mass mkt. 44.95 (*0-538-65048-6*) S-W Thomson.

Fundamentals of Psychology: Applications for Life & Work. Joseph Culkin & Richard S. Perrotto. 1995. LC 94-6813. text 37.95 (*0-8273-6293-5*) Delmar.

Fundamentals of Psychoneuroimmunology. Cai Song & Brian E. Leonard. 2000. LC 99-59485. 294p. 90.00 (*0-471-98671-2*) Wiley.

Fundamentals of Psychopharmacology. Brian Leonard. 1997. LC 96-49182. 408p. pap. 59.95 (*0-471-96115-9*) Wiley.

Fundamentals of Radiologic Urology. Anthony Y. Smith & Michael R. Williamson. 1999. LC 99-44545. vii, 152p. (C). pap. text (*0-7216-5399-5*) Saunders.

Fundamentals of Radiology. Lucy F. Squire & Robert A. Novelline. 4th ed. 1988. LC 87-33875. (Illus.). 372p. text 45.00 (*0-674-32926-0*) HUP.

***Fundamentals of Removable Partial Dentures.** 1998. (Illus.). pap. (*1-919713-23-9*) U Cape Town.

Fundamentals of Research Methodology for Health Care Professionals. Hilla Brink. 1996. 232p. pap. (*0-7021-3719-7*) Juta & Co ZAF. *Dist:* Intl Spec Bk, Gaunt.

Fundamentals of Sensory Physiology. Robert F. Schmidt. 3rd ed. 1986. 300p. 49.00 (*3-540-15870-7*) Spr-Verlag.

Fundamentals of Sensory Physiology: Springer Study Edition. Ed. by Richard F. Schmidt. Tr. by M. A. Biederman-Thorson from GER. 3rd enl. rev. ed. 1986. (Illus.). 300p. 53.95 (*0-387-15870-7*) Spr-Verlag.

Fundamentals of Skeletal Radiology. Clyde A. Helms. 2nd ed. 1994. 256p. pap. text 41.00 (*0-7216-4680-8*) Saunders.

Fundamentals of Social Psychology. Emory S. Bogardus. 1974. LC 73-2963. (Classics in Psychology Ser.). reprint ed. 29.95 (*0-405-05136-0*) Ayer.

***Fundamentals of Social Work Research: A Guide for Students & Beginning Practitioners.** pap. (*0-7021-3432-5*) Juta & Co ZAF. *Dist:* Intl Spec Bk.

Fundamentals of Special Radiographic Procedures. Albert M. Snopek. 3rd ed. 1992. (Illus.). 426p. text 50.00 (*0-7216-3441-9*) Saunders.

Fundamentals of Special Radiographic Procedures. Albert M. Snopek. Ed. by Andrew Allen. 4th ed. 1999. LC 98-32246. (Illus.). 430p. (C). text 45.00 (*0-7216-7314-7*) Saunders.

Fundamentals of Sports Injury Management. Marcia K. Anderson. 1997. wbk. ed. 49.95 (*0-683-30345-7*) Lppncott W & W.

Fundamentals of Sports Injury Management. Marcia K. Anderson et al. 1997. LC 96-46312. (Illus.). 689p. 43.95 (*0-683-30001-6*) Lppncott W & W.

Fundamentals of Strategic Planning for Healthcare Organizations. Stan Williamson et al. 1996. LC 95-43398. 260p. 49.95 (*0-7890-0060-1*) Haworth Pr.

Fundamentals of Successful Wound Healing: An Educational Program for the Quality Caregiver. Cathy T. Hess. 1992. (Video Ser.: No. 1). (Illus.). 46p. (Orig.). (C). stu. ed. 99.95 (*0-9628084-1-5*) Hlth Mngmnt Pubns.

Fundamentals of Tooth Preparations: For Cast Metal & Porcelain Restorations. Herbert T. Shillingburg et al. rev. ed. 1987. (Illus.). 376p. text 82.00 (*0-86715-157-9*, 1579) Quint Pub Co.

Fundamentals of Tumor Metastasis. B. Zetter & R. Kerbel. Date not set. (Basic & Clinical Oncology Ser.). (*0-8247-9520-2*) Dekker.

Fundamentals of Urine & Body Fluid Analysis. Nancy A. Brunzel. 1994. LC 92-48472. (Illus.). 544p. pap. text 41.00 (*0-7216-3976-3*) Saunders.

Fundamentals of Veterinary Ophthamology. Douglas H. Slatter. 3rd ed. 1997. LC 00-49255. (Illus.). xiv, 640p. text 79.00 (*0-7216-2705-6*) Saunders.

Fundamentals of Visual Psychophysics. Thomas T. Norton et al. 2001. LC 2001-52908. (Illus.). 256p. 55.00 (*0-7506-9935-3*) Buttrwrth-Heinemann.

***Fundamentos de Enfermeria en Salud Mental (Foundations of Mental Health Nursing)** Michelle Morrison-Valfre. 1997. (Illus.). 592p. pap. (*84-8174-349-6*) Mosby-Doyma Libros ESP. *Dist:* Mosby Inc.

Funding Health Sciences Research: A Strategy to Restore Balance. Ed. by Institute of Medicine Staff. 1990. 276p. text 27.95 (*0-309-04343-3*) Natl Acad Pr.

Funding of Young Investigators in the Biological & Biomedical Sciences. National Research Council Staff. 1994. 128p. (Orig.). (C). pap. text 24.00 (*0-309-05077-4*) Natl Acad Pr.

Funding Sources: A Guide for Future Audiologists, Speech-Language Pathologists, & Speech, Language, & Hearing Scientists. Patricia A. Cole et al. 1996. LC 98-116508. pap. 20.00 (*0-910329-85-0*, 0112018) Am Speech Lang Hearing.

Fundraising for Health & Social Service Executives. Joyce J. Fitzpatrick & Sandra S. Deller. 2000. LC 00-58829. (Illus.). ix, 193p. (*0-8261-1367-2*) Springer Pub.

Fundus Fluorescein Angiography. Amresh Chopdar. 1995. LC 95-14151. (Illus.). 192p. text 100.00 (*0-7506-1885-X*) Buttrwrth-Heinemann.

Fundus Periphery. Pierre Bec. Tr. by Frederick C. Blodi. 1986. (Illus.). 484p. (C). (gr. 13). text 113.50 (*0-89352-211-2*) Mosby Inc.

Fungal Antigens: Isolation, Purification, & Detection. Ed. by J. P. Latge et al. 1989. (Illus.). 486p. 125.00 (*0-306-43115-7*, Plenum Trade) Perseus Pubng.

Fungal Cell Wall & Immune Response. Ed. by J. P. Latge & D. Boucias. 1991. (NATO ASI Ser.: Vol. 53). (Illus.). 472p. 218.00 (*0-387-53147-5*) Spr-Verlag.

Fungal Community: Its Organization & Role in the Ecosystem. Ed. by Carroll & Donald T. Wicklow. 2nd ed. 1992. (Mycology Ser.: Vol. 9). (Illus.). 952p. text 295.00 (*0-8247-8605-X*) Dekker.

Fungal Dimorphism: With Emphasis on Fungi Pathogenic for Humans. Ed. by Paul J. Szaniszlo. 1985. LC 85-12412. 414p. 105.00 (*0-306-42020-1*, Plenum Trade) Perseus Pubng.

Fungal Disease. Ed. by Paul H. Jacobs & Lexie Nall. 1996. LC 96-18673. (Basic & Clinical Dermatology Ser.: Vol. 12). (Illus.). 600p. text 230.00 (*0-8247-9402-8*) Dekker.

Fungal Diseases of Amenity of Turf Grasses. J. Drew-Smith et al. 1989. 416p. 160.00 (*0-419-11530-7*, A2404, Spon) Routledge.

Fungal Diseases of the Lung. George A. Sarosi & Scott F. Davies. 3rd ed. 2000. LC 99-51562. (Illus.). xii, 322p. text 139.00 (*0-7817-1758-2*) Lppncott W & W.

Fungal Infection: Diagnosis & Management. Malcolm D. Richardson & David W. Warnock. 1993. LC 93-1576. (Pocket Consultant Ser.). 232p. pap. 38.95 (*0-632-03514-5*) Blackwell Sci.

Fungal Infection: Diagnosis & Management. Malcolm D. Richardson & D. W. Warnock. 2nd ed. 1997. LC 97-5802. (Illus.). 256p. pap. 58.95 (*0-86542-724-0*) Blackwell Sci.

Fungal Infections & Immune Responses. J. W. Murphy et al. 1993. (Infectious Agents & Pathogenesis Ser.). (Illus.). 596p. (C). text 135.00 (*0-306-44075-X*, Kluwer Plenum) Kluwer Academic.

Fungal Nutrition & Physiology. Michael O. Garraway & Robert C. Evans. 1992. LC 91-4011. 412p. reprint ed. text 59.95 (*0-89464-631-1*) Krieger.

***Fungal Pathogenesis.** Calderone & Cihlar. 2001. LC 2001-53342. (Mycology Ser.: Vol. 14). (*0-8247-0568-8*) Dekker.

Fungal Spore & Disease Initiation in Plants & Animals. G. T. Cole & H. C. Hoch. 1991. (Illus.). 578p. (C). text 135.00 (*0-306-43454-7*, Kluwer Plenum) Kluwer Academic.

Fungi & Allergic Disease: Diagnosis & Treatment. H. A. Burge & W. Solomon. Date not set. (Clinical Allergy & Immunology Ser.). (Illus.). text (*0-8247-9482-6*) Dekker.

Fungi Pathogenic for Humans & Animals, Vol. A. Ed. by Dexter H. Howard. 1983. (Mycology Ser.: Vol. 3). (Illus.). 672p. text 250.00 (*0-8247-1875-5*) Dekker.

Fungicolous, Lichenicolous & Myxomyceticolous Species of Hypocreopsis, Nectriopsis, Nectria, Peristomialis & Trichonectria. Gary J. Samuels. 1988. LC 88-28896. (Memoirs Ser.: No. 48). (Illus.). 78p. pap. text 14.00 (*0-89327-330-9*) NY Botanical.

Funny Thing Happened at the Doctor's Office. Thomas Briggs. Ed. by Milton Adams. 1998. (Illus.). 80p. pap. 6.95 (*1-890676-07-1*) Beavers Pond.

Funny, You Don't Look Crazy: Life with Obsessive-Compulsive Disorder. Constance H. Foster. 1995. LC 93-74548. 128p. (YA). pap. 14.00 (*0-9639070-0-X*) ebooksonthe.

Funny, You Don't Look Like a Diabetic! Janet Waterston. 1997. 173p. pap. (*1-85398-070-6*) Ashgrove Pr GBR. *Dist:* Words Distrib.

Further Contributions to the Theory & Technique of Psycho-Analysis. S. Ferenczi. 1994. 480p. (*1-85575-086-4*) Karnac Bks GBR. *Dist:* Other Pr LLC.

Further Dimensions of Healing Addictions. Donna Cunningham & Andrew Ramer. 1988. (Illus.). 168p. (Orig.). pap. 9.95 (*0-945946-00-7*) Cassandra Pr.

Further MRCP, Pt. I. Norman Johnson & Chris Bunker. 1995. LC 94-38013. (Brainscan MCQs Ser.). 29.00 (*0-387-19781-8*) Spr-Verlag.

Further Programming in Prolog: Writing Application Programs. P. H. Hepburn. 1987. LC 87-21345. (Computers & Their Applications Ser.). 259p. pap. 47.95 (*0-470-20928-3*) P-H.

Further Reflections on Hazelden's Spiritual Odyssey. Damian McElrath. 1999. LC 98-35227. xiv, 134p. 19.95 (*1-56838-308-8*) Hazelden.

Further Studies on the Etiology & Significance of Congenital Cranial Osteoporosis. Elena Boder. 1948. (SRCD M Ser.: Vol. 13, No. 2). pap. 25.00 (*0-527-01544-X*) Periodicals Srv.

Further Training of Community Pharmacists. 1992. (*92-871-2174-5*) Council of Europe FRA. *Dist:* Manhattan Pub Co.

***Furthur Advances in Surfactant Replacement: 16th International Workshop on Surfactant Replacement, Edinburgh, June 2001: Proceedings.** Ed. by I. A. Laing et al. 2001. (Biology of the Neonate Ser.: Vol. 80). (Illus.). iv, 42p. pap. 25.25 (*3-8055-7246-8*) S Karger.

Fusion Nuclear por Medio del Laser. Vicente Aboites. (Ciencia para Todos Ser.). (SPA.). pap. 6.99 (*968-16-4615-0*) Fondo CA.

Fusion of Cultural Horizons: Cultural Influences on the Assessment of Psychopathology in Children & Adolescents, Vol. 1, No. 3. Ed. by Kimberly Hoagwood et al. 1997. 58p. pap. 20.00 (*0-8058-9861-1*) L Erlbaum Assocs.

Fussy Baby: How to Bring Out the Best in Your High Need Child. William M. Sears. 1985. LC 85-80904. (Growing Family Ser.). (Illus.). 192p. mass mkt. 5.99 (*0-912500-20-4*) La Leche.

Fuszard's Innovative Teaching Strategies in Nursing. Arlene J. Lowenstein & Martha J. Bradshaw. 3rd ed. 2000. LC 00-40127. (Illus.). 400p. 54.00 (*0-8342-1668-X*, 1668x) Aspen Pub.

Future Care: New Directions in Planning Health & Care Environments. Ed. by Martin S. Valins & Derek Salter. 1996. LC 96-33854. (Illus.). 176p. pap. 36.95 (*0-632-03577-3*) Blackwell Sci.

Future Developments in Blood Banking. Ed. by Smith C. Sibinga et al. 1986. (Developments in Hematology & Immunology Ser.). text 92.00 (*0-89838-824-4*) Kluwer Academic.

Future Directions in the Management of Cardiac Disease: Proceedings of the Cardiovascular Disease Conference, 7th, Snowmass at Aspen, Colorado, 1976. Cardiovascular Disease Conference Staff. Ed. by H. K. Vogel. 1977. (Advances in Cardiology Ser.: Vol. 20). 65.25 (*3-8055-2412-9*) S Karger.

Future Environment for Health & Health Care in the United States. 1995. lib. bdg. 260.95 (*0-8490-8361-3*) Gordon Pr.

Future for Palliative Care: Issues of Policy & Practice. Ed. by David Clark. 1993. LC 92-49440. pap. (*0-335-15764-5*) OpUniv Pr.

Future for the NHS? Health Care in the 1990s. Wendy Ranade. 1994. LC 93-14037. pap. text (*0-582-05978-X*) Longman.

Future Health: Computers & Medicine in the 21st Century. Ed. by Clifford A. Pickover. 1995. LC 95-34799. (Illus.). 224p. 25.95 (*0-312-12602-6*) St Martin.

Future in Medicine: The March of Medicine, 1949, Laity Lectures, No. 14. New York Academy of Medicine Staff. 1977. LC 74-167391. (Essay Index Reprint Ser.). reprint ed. 19.95 (*0-8369-2465-7*) Ayer.

Future Medical Research Without the Use of Animals: Facing the Challenge - May 15-16, 1990, Tel Aviv, Israel. Ed. by Nina Natelson. 1991. (Illus.). (Orig.). pap. (*0-9631596-0-7*) CFH Animals IS.

Future Medicare Payment Alternatives. Healthcare Financial Management Association Staff. 1988. 20p. (C). pap. 10.00 (*0-930228-60-X*) Hlthcare Fin Mgmt.

Future of Biomedical Research. Ed. by Claude E. Barfield & Bruce L. Smith. 1997. LC 97-34604. 100p. 29.95 (*0-8447-4036-5*); 125p. pap. 14.95 (*0-8447-4037-3*) Am Enterprise.

Future of Counselling & Psychotherapy. Stephen Palmer & Ved Varma. 1997. LC 97-65038. 240p. 69.95 (*0-7619-5106-7*, 2075); pap. 27.95 (*0-7619-5107-5*, 2076) Sage.

Future of Disease. Matt Ridley. 1999. LC 99-206565. (Predictions Ser.). 58p. pap. (*0-297-84065-7*) Weidenfeld & Nicolson GBR. *Dist:* Trafalgar.

Future of Folk Psychology: Intentionality & Cognitive Science. Ed. by John D. Greenwood. 1991. (Illus.). 303p. (C). text 59.95 (*0-521-40335-9*); pap. text 21.95 (*0-521-40898-9*) Cambridge U Pr.

Future of General Practice. 1992. (Illus.). 116p. pap. text (*0-7279-0316-0*) BMJ Pub GBR. *Dist:* AIDC.

Future of Healing: Exploring the Parallels of Eastern & Western Medicine. Michael P. Milburn. 2001. LC 2001-17462. (Illus.). 370p. pap. 16.95 (*1-58091-065-3*) Crossing Pr.

Future of Health & Health Care Systems in the Industrialized Societies. Ed. by Dang H. Bui. 1988. LC 87-7292. 304p. 77.00 (*0-275-92491-2*, C2491, Praeger Pubs) Greenwood.

Future of Health Care. 1992. (Illus.). 104p. pap. text (*0-7279-0742-5*) BMJ Pub GBR. *Dist:* AIDC.

Future of Health Care Governance: Redesigning Boards for a New Era. James E. Orlikoff & Mary K. Totten. 1996. LC 96-852. 143p. pap. 40.00 (*1-55648-160-8*, 196112) AHPI.

Future of Health Policy. Victor R. Fuchs. 1993. LC 93-14894. (Illus.). 256p. text 37.95 (*0-674-33825-1*) HUP.

Future of Hospitals: Transactions & Studies of the College of Physicians of Philadelphia. United Hospital Fund Staff. 1990. 192p. 10.00 (*0-934459-70-3*) United Hosp Fund.

Future of Long-Term Care: Social & Policy Issues. Ed. by Robert H. Binstock et al. 1996. LC 96-2146. 288p. 42.95 (*0-8018-5320-6*) Johns Hopkins.

Future of Medicines in Health Care: Scenario Report. Steering Committee on Future Health Scenarios Staff & Scenario Committee on Medicine in Health Care. 1995. LC 95-30328. 312p. pap. text 106.00 (*0-7923-3624-0*) Kluwer Academic.

Future of Piagetian Theory: The Neo-Piagetians. Ed. by Valerie L. Shulman et al. 1985. (Illus.). 248p. (C). 66.00 (*0-306-41940-8*, Plenum Trade) Perseus Pubng.

Future of Play Theory: A Multidisciplinary Inquiry into the Contributions of Brian Sutton-Smith. Ed. by Anthony D. Pellegrini. 1995. LC 94-41396. (SUNY Series, Children's Play in Society). 306p. (C). text 26.50 (*0-7914-2641-6*); pap. text 25.95 (*0-7914-2642-4*) State U NY Pr.

Future of Public Health. Institute of Medicine Staff. 1988. 240p. pap. text 24.95 (*0-309-03830-8*) Natl Acad Pr.

Future of Social Psychology: Defining the Relationship Between Sociology & Psychology. Ed. by C. W. Stephan et al. 1991. (Recent Research in Psychology Ser.). (Illus.). 121p. 29.50 (*0-387-97487-3*) Spr-Verlag.

Future of the Cognitive Revolution. Ed. by David Johnson & Christina Erneling. 1997. LC 96-23813. (Illus.). 416p. pap. text 35.00 (*0-19-510334-3*) OUP.

Future of the Internet in Health Care: Five Year Forcast. Robert Mittman & Mary Cain. Ed. by Charles Grosel. unabr. ed. 1999. 41p. pap. (*1-929008-03-1*) CA HlthCare Fnd.

Future of Work & Health. Rick J. Carlson et al. 1985. LC 85-18627. (Illus.). 215p. (Orig.). 49.95 (*0-86569-088-X*, Auburn Hse) Greenwood.

Future Options for General Practice: Primary Care Development. Ed. by Geoff Meads. 1995. (*1-85775-079-9*) Radcliffe Med Pr GBR. *Dist:* Balogh.

Future Perspectives in Behavior Therapy. Ed. by Samuel M. Turner et al. 1981. LC 81-10689. (Applied Clinical Psychology Ser.). 366p. 59.50 (*0-306-40680-2*, Plenum Trade) Perseus Pubng.

Future Perspectives in Gastroenterology: International Congress, Leipzig, June 1996. Ed. by Frieder Berr et al. 1997. (Digestion Ser.: Vol. 58, Suppl. 1, 1997). iv, 116p. pap. 50.50 (*3-8055-6503-8*) S Karger.

Future Practice Alternatives in Medicine. Ed. by David B. Nash. 2nd ed. 1993. LC 93-14635. (Illus.). 432p. pap. 25.00 (*0-89640-236-3*) Igaku-Shoin.

Future Scenarios on Dental Health Care: A Reconnaissance of the Period 1990-2020. A. M. Nelissen et al. 1994. LC 94-636. (Scenario Report Ser.). pap. text 136.00 (*0-7923-2694-6*) Kluwer Academic.

Future Strategies for Drug Delivery with Particulate Systems. J. E. Diederichs & Rainer H. Muller. 1998. LC 97-46682. 194p. per. 79.95 (*0-8493-3941-3*) CRC Pr.

Future Time Perspective & Motivation: Theory & Research Method. W. Lens & J. M. Nuttin. 1984. 235p. (Orig.). pap. (*90-6186-172-1*) Leuven Univ BEL. *Dist:* Coronet Bks.

Future Time Perspective & Motivation: Theory & Research Method. Joseph R. Nuttin. 1985. (Louvain Psychology Ser.: Studia Psychologica). 238p. 49.95 (*0-89859-611-4*) L Erlbaum Assocs.

Future Trends in Juvenile Diabetes. Ed. by Z. Laron & M. Karp. 1986. (Pediatric & Adolescent Endocrinology Ser.: Vol. 15). (Illus.). xiv, 410p. 304.50 (*3-8055-3958-4*) S Karger.

Future Trends in Research on AIDS, Cancer & Therapies. Ed. by Eva Lotzova & B. Sredni. 1988. (Journal: Vol. 7, No. 3, 1988). (Illus.). 68p. pap. 34.00 (*3-8055-4859-1*) S Karger.

Future U. S. Healthcare System: Who Will Care for the Poor & Uninsured? Ed. by Stuart H. Altman et al. 1997. LC 97-23221. 426p. pap. text 50.00 (*1-56793-067-0*, PUSHS-1009) Health Admin Pr.

Futurescan 2000: A Millennium Forecast of Healthcare Trends 2000-2004. Russell C. Coile, Jr. 2000. 32p. (Orig.). pap. 45.00 (*0-9676441-1-9*) Soc Healthcare Strategy.

***Fuzzy Logic in Medicine.** Ed. by S. Barrow & R. Marin. 2002. (Studies in Fuzziness & Soft Computing: Vol. 83). (Illus.). 320p. 84.00 (*3-7908-1429-6*) Spr-Verlag.

Fuzzy Mathematics in Medicine. John N. Mordeson et al. 2000. LC 00-45668. (Studies in Fuzziness & Soft Computing: Vol. 55). (Illus.). xii, 256p. (*3-7908-1325-7*) Physica-Verlag DEU. *Dist:* Spr-Verlag.

Fuzzy Set Analysis for Behavioral & Social Sciences. M. Smithson. 1986. (Recent Research in Psychology Ser.). 327p. 47.00 (*0-387-96431-2*) Spr-Verlag.

G

G. I. Nightingales: The Army Nurse Corps in World War II. Barbara Tomblin. 1996. LC 96-1018. (Illus.). 272p. text 29.95 (*0-8131-1951-0*) U Pr of KY.

***G. I./General Surgery Words & Phrases.** Health Professions Institute Staff. 2001. pap. 56.00 (*0-13-094085-2*) P-H.

G Protein-Coupled Receptors: New Opportunities for Commercial Development. Ed. by Nancy Mulford. 1996. (Biomedical Library). 312p. pap. 895.00 (*1-57936-005-X*) Drug & Market Dev.

G Protein Linked Receptor FactsBook. Ed. by Steve Watson & Steve Arkinstall. 1994. (Factsbook Ser.). (Illus.). 427p. pap. text 61.00 (*0-12-738440-5*) Acad Pr.

G Protein Methods & Protocols: Role of G Proteins in Psychiatric & Neurological Disorders. Ed. by Ram K. Mishra et al. 1997. (Neuromethods Ser.: Vol. 31). (Illus.). 448p. 135.00 (*0-89603-490-9*) Humana.

G Proteins: Signal Transduction & Disease. Ed. by Graeme Milligan & Michael Wakelam. 1992. (Illus.). 247p. text 104.00 (*0-12-497515-1*) Acad Pr.

G Proteins, Cytoskeleton, & Cancer. Hiroshi Maruta et al. 1998. LC 98-20518. (Molecular Biology Intelligence Unit Ser.). 99.00 (*1-57059-551-8*) Landes Bioscience.

G Proteins, Receptors & Disease. Ed. by Allen M. Spiegel. 1998. (Contemporary Endocrinology Ser.: Vol. 6). (Illus.). 336p. 155.00 (*0-89603-430-5*) Humana.

G Spot. Alice K. Ladas et al. 1983. 256p. mass mkt. 6.99 (*0-440-13040-9*) Dell.

G. Stanley Hall: The Psychologist As Prophet. Dorothy Ross. 1998. LC 75-165180. 502p. lib. bdg. 30.00 (*0-226-72821-8*) U Ch Pr.

GABA & Benzodiazepine Receptor. Squires. 1987. Vol. I. 3p. 90.00 (*0-8493-5875-2*); Vol. II. 144p. 84.00 (*0-8493-5876-0*) Franklin (CRC Reprint).

GABA & Benzodiazepine Receptors, Set, Vols. 1 & 2. Ed. by Richard F. Squires. 1987. LC 87-18374. 173.00 (*0-8493-5874-4*, QP364, CRC Reprint) Franklin.

GABA & Neuropeptides in the CNS: Handbook of Chemical Neuroanatomy, Vol. 4, Pt. 1. Ed. by Anders T. Bjorklund & Tomas B. Hokfelt. 1985. 652p. 383.00 (*0-444-90353-4*) Elsevier.

GABA & the Brain: Health Uses. 1996. lib. bdg. 250.95 (*0-8490-5900-3*) Gordon Pr.

GABA-Benzodiazepine Receptor As a Target. Adam Doble. 1996. (Medicine Ser.). (Illus.). 274p. pap. 89.95 (*0-412-10091-6*, VNR) Wiley.

GABA Benzodiazepine Receptor As a Target for Psychoactive Drugs. Adam Doble & Ian L. Martin. 1996. LC 95-37910. 248p. 89.95 (*1-57059-305-1*) Landes Bioscience.

Gaba in the Nervous System: 50 Years of Progress. David L. Martin & Richard W. Olsen. 2000. LC 00-39133. (Illus.). xiii, 510p. text 149.00 (*0-7817-2267-5*) Lppncott W & W.

GABA in the Retina & Central Visual System. R. E. Marc et al. 1992. LC 91-46934. (Progress in Brain Research Ser.: Vol. 90). 546p. 274.75 (*0-444-81446-9*) Elsevier.

GABA Outside the CNS: Proceedings of the International Symposium on Peripheral GABAergic Mechanisms, Rome, July 19-21, 1991. Ed. by Sandor L. Erdo. 1992. (Illus.). 312p. 136.00 (*0-387-54532-8*) Spr-Verlag.

***GABAA/Benzodiazepine Receptor as a Target for Psychoactive Drugs.** Adam Doble & Ian L. Martin. 1997. LC 97-3313. (Neuroscience Intelligence Unit Ser.). (Illus.). 274p. (C). 100.00 (*3-540-60565-7*) Spr-Verlag.

Gabrovo Health Services Model in the People's Republic of Bulgaria: Report on a Study. D. K. Sokolov & J. E. Asvall. 1980. (EURO Reports & Studies: No. 27). 94p. 7.00 (*92-9020-166-5*, 1330027) World Health.

Gahart IV Medications. Betty L. Gahart. 15th ed. 1998. LC 99-185174. 976p. (C). (gr. 13). spiral bd. 28.95 (*0-8151-2988-2*, 31786) Mosby Inc.

Gahart IV Medications. Betty L. Gahart & Adrienne R. Nazareno. 16th ed. 1999. LC 99-16510. 976p. spiral bd. 28.95 (*0-8151-2729-4*, 31785) Mosby Inc.

Gait Vol. 1: Basic Research. 1993. 369p. pap. 42.00 (*0-912452-88-9*, P-93) Am Phys Therapy Assn.

Gait Vol. 2: Clinical Issues. 1993. 268p. pap. 42.00 (*0-912452-90-0*, P-96) Am Phys Therapy Assn.

Gait Analysis. S. Giannini et al. 1994. LC 94-7639. 285p. 77.00 (*90-5199-170-3*) IOS Press.

Gait Analysis. Michael W. Whittle. 2nd ed. 1996. LC 96-206860. 248p. pap. text 42.50 (*0-7506-2222-9*, Focal) Buttrwrth-Heinemann.

Gait Analysis: Normal & Pathological Function. Jacquelin Perry. 1992. LC 90-50830. 556p. 55.00 (*1-55642-192-3*) SLACK Inc.

Gait Analysis: Theory & Application. Rebecca L. Craik & Carol A. Oatis. 1994. (Illus.). 432p. (C). (gr. 13). text 53.95 (*0-8016-6964-2*, 06964) Mosby Inc.

Gait Analysis in Cerebral Palsy. James R. Gage. 1991. (Clinics in Developmental Medicine Ser.: No. 121). (Illus.). 206p. (C). text 64.95 (*0-521-41277-3*) Cambridge U Pr.

Gait Disturbances in the Elderly. Ed. by Joseph Masdeu et al. 1997. LC 97-4217. (Illus.). 464p. text 110.00 (*0-316-54915-0*, Little Brwn Med Div) Lppncott W & W.

Gait in Rehabilitation. Ed. by Gary L. Smidt. 1990. (Illus.). 329p. text (*0-443-08663-X*) Church.

Gait Workbook: A Practical Guide to Clinical Gait Analysis. Jan Bruckner. 1997. (Illus.). 208p. (Orig.). pap. text 30.00 (*1-55642-344-6*, 43446) SLACK Inc.

Galactography & Galactophorectomy. F. Grosso et al. 1982. 82p. text (*1-57235-062-8*) Piccin Nuova.

Galaxies of Life: The Human Aura in Acupuncture & Kirlian Photography. Ed. by Stanley Krippner & Daniel Rubin. 1973. (Social Change Ser.). xxviii, 182p. text 147.00 (*0-677-15480-1*) Gordon & Breach.

Galbraith Fundamentals of Pharmacoology. Alan Galbraith. 1998. (C). pap. text (*0-201-33127-6*) Addison-Wesley.

Gale Encyclopedia of Alternative Medicine Ed. by Kristine M. Krapp & Jacqueline L. Longe. 2000. LC 00-61013. (Illus.). 1937p. 350.00 (*0-7876-5000-5*); (*0-7876-5001-3*); (*0-7876-5002-1*) Gale.

Gale Encyclopedia of Alternative Medicine, 4 vols. Kristine M. Krapp & Jacqueline L. Longe. 2000. LC 00-61013. (Illus.). (*0-7876-5003-X*) Gale.

Gale Encyclopedia of Alternative Medicine, Set. Gale Group Staff. 2001. LC 00-61013. (Illus.). 1600p. 350.00 (*0-7876-4999-6*) Gale.

Gale Encyclopedia of Cancer Ellen Thackery. Incl. Vol. 1. (*0-7876-5610-0*); Vol. 2. (*0-7876-5611-9*); 2001. LC 2001-46015. (Illus.). 1000p. 2001. 275.00 net. (*0-7876-5609-7*) Gale.

***Gale Encyclopedia of Cancer.** Ellen Thackery. 2001. LC 2001-46015. Vol. 1. (*0-7876-5610-0*); Vol. 2. (*0-7876-5611-9*) Gale.

***Gale Encyclopedia of Genetic Disorders.** Ed. by Stacey Blachford. 2001. LC 2001-40100. (*0-7876-5613-5*) Gale.

Gale Encyclopedia of Genetic Disorders Ed. by Stacey Blachford. 2001. LC 2001-40100. (Illus.). 1200p. 275.00 net. (*0-7876-5612-7*) Gale.

E
F
G

Gale Encyclopedia of Medicine Ed. by Karen Boyden et al. 1998. LC 98-37918. (Illus.). 3442p. 499.00 (*0-7876-1868-3*, GML14099-111288) Gale.

Gale Encyclopedia of Medicine Donna Olendorf et al. 1998. LC 98-37918. (Illus.). 3442p. (*0-7876-1869-1*); (*0-7876-1870-5*); (*0-7876-1871-3*); (*0-7876-1872-1*); (*0-7876-1873-X*) Gale.

Gale Encyclopedia of Medicine 2nd ed. Ed. by Jacqueline L. Longe & Deirdre S. Blanchfield. Incl. Vol. 1. (*0-7876-5490-6*); Vol. 3. (*0-7876-5492-2*); LC 2001-51245. 2001. 525.00 net. (*0-7876-5489-2*) Gale.

***Gale Encyclopedia of Medicine.** Ed. by Jacqueline L. Longe & Deirdre S. Blanchfield. 2nd ed. 2001. LC 2001-51245. Vol. 1. (*0-7876-5490-6*); Vol. 3. (*0-7876-5492-2*) Gale.

***Gale Encyclopedia of Nursing & Allied Health** Ed. by Kristine M. Krapp. 2001. LC 2001-40910. (*0-7876-4939-2*) Gale.

Gale Encyclopedia of Nursing & Allied Health Ed. by Kristine M. Krapp. Incl. (*0-7876-4939-2*); Vol. 1. (*0-7876-4935-X*); Vol. 2. (*0-7876-4936-8*); Vol. 3. (*0-7876-4937-6*); Vol. 4. (*0-7876-4938-4*); 2001. LC 2001-40910. (Illus.). 1600p. 2001. 850.00 net. (*0-7876-4934-1*) Gale.

***Gale Encyclopedia of Nursing & Allied Health.** Ed. by Kristine M. Krapp. 2001. LC 2001-40910. Vol. 1. (*0-7876-4935-X*); Vol. 2. (*0-7876-4936-8*); Vol. 3. (*0-7876-4937-6*); Vol. 4. (*0-7876-4938-4*) Gale.

Gale Encyclopedia of Psychology. Bonnie B. Strickland. 2nd ed. 2000. LC 00-34736. (Illus.). xiii, 701p. 135.00 (*0-7876-4786-1*) Gale.

***Galen & Galenism: Theory & Medical Practice from Antiquity to the European Renaissance.** Luis Garcia-Ballester. 2002. (Variorum Collected Studies: Vol. CS710). (ENG & SPA.). 350p. (*0-86078-846-6*) Ashgate Pub GBR. *Dist:* Ashgate Pub Co.

Galen on Psychology, Psychopathology & Function & Disease of the Nervous System: An Analysis of His Doctrines Observations & Experiments. R. E. Siegel. 1973. 300p. 102.75 (*3-8055-1479-4*) S Karger.

Galen on Sense Perception: His Doctrines, Observation & Experiments on Vision, Hearing, Smell, Touch & Pain, & Their Historical Sources. R. E. Siegel. 1970. (Illus.). 67.00 (*3-8055-1022-5*) S Karger.

Galen on the Affected Parts: Translation from the Greek Text with Explanatory Footnotes. R. E. Siegel. 1976. pap. 78.50 (*3-8055-2201-0*) S Karger.

Galenics of Insulin. J. Brange. 1987. (Illus.). 103p. 30.00 (*0-387-17673-X*) Spr-Verlag.

Galen's Exzerpte aus Aelteren Pharmakologen. Cajus Fabricius. 1972. (Ars Medica, Abt. 2, Griechisch Lateinische Medizin Ser.: Vol. 2). x, 266p. 119.25 (*3-11-001802-0*) De Gruyter.

Galen's Method of Healing: Proceedings of the 1982 Galen Symposium. Ed. by Fridolf Kudlien & Richard J. Durling. 1991. LC 90-27138. (Studies in Ancient Medicine: No. 1). (ENG & GER.). viii, 205p. 82.50 (*90-04-09272-2*) Brill Academic Pubs.

Galenus Latinus I. Ed. by R. J. Durling. 1976. (Ars Medica Ser.: Vol. 6). (C). text 184.65 (*3-11-005759-X*) De Gruyter.

Gall Bladder & Bile Ducts. Ed. by Nicholas F. Larusso. 1997. LC 96-43739. (Gastroenterology & Hepatology Ser.: Vol. 6). (Illus.). 219p. text (*0-443-07858-0*) Church GBR. *Dist:* Saunders.

Gallaudet Encyclopedia of Deaf People & Deafness Ed. by John V. Van Cleve. 1987. LC 86-15396. (Illus.). 1400p. text 355.00 (*0-07-079229-1*) McGraw-Hill Prof.

Gallaudet Survival Guide to Signing. Leonard G. Lane. rev. ed. 1987. LC 89-25686. (Illus.). 220p. pap. 6.95 (*0-930323-67-X*) Gallaudet Univ Pr.

Gallbladder, Bile Ducts, Pancreas, Vol. II. Ed. by K. Kremer et al. Tr. by Gerhard S. Sharon. 1992. LC 92-405. (Illus.). 169.00 (*0-86577-434-X*) Thieme Med Pubs.

Gallenblasensteine. C. Wolpers. 1987. (Illus.). x, 202p. 138.50 (*3-8055-4522-3*) S Karger.

Gallensteine im Roentgenbild. C. Wolpers. 1981. (Illus.). 66p. pap. 24.50 (*3-8055-2031-X*) S Karger.

Gallstone Disease & Its Management. Ed. by M. C. Bateson. 1986. text 167.00 (*0-85200-979-8*) Kluwer Academic.

Gallstones & Their Treatment: A Guide for Patients. James Norman. Ed. by Larry Carey. 1995. (Surgical Ser.). (Illus.). 24p. (Orig.). pap. 2.95 (*1-885274-21-1*) Health InfoNet Inc.

Game of Childhood Diseases. Frank Bialosiewicz & Julie Burns. 1983. (Technical Notes Ser.: No. 23). (Illus.). 30p. (Orig.). pap. text 2.00 (*0-932288-70-7*) Ctr Intl Ed U of MA.

Games Alcoholics Play. Claude M. Steiner. 1984. 224p. mass mkt. 6.99 (*0-345-32383-1*) Ballantine Pub Grp.

Games of Poetics: Ludic Criticism & Postmodern Fiction. Ruth E. Burke. 1993. LC 92-20765. (American University Studies: Ser. III, Vol. 47). XIV, 149p. (C). text 38.95 (*0-8204-1943-5*) P Lang Pubng.

Games to Enhance Social & Emotional Skills: Games That Teach Children, Adolescents, & Adults Skills Critical to Success in Life. John Malouff & Nicola S. Schutte. 1998. LC 97-41232. (Illus.). 218p. spiral bd. 35.95 (*0-398-06836-4*) C C Thomas.

Gamete & Embryo Micromanipulation in Human Reproduction. Fishel. 240p. (*0-340-57370-8*) E A GBR. *Dist:* Routldge.

Gamete & Embryo Quality: The Proceedings of the Fourth Organon Round Table Conference, Thessaloniki, Greece, 24-25 June 1993. Ed. by Luigi Mastroianni, Jr. et al. 1994. LC 93-40905. 248p. lib. bdg. 107.95 (*1-85070-543-7*, Parthenon Pbng) CRC Pr.

Gametes - the Oocyte. Ed. by J. Gedes Grudzinskas & J. Yovich. 1995. (Cambridge Reviews in Human Reproduction Ser.). (Illus.). 455p. (C). pap. text 39.95 (*0-521-47995-9*) Cambridge U Pr.

Gametes - the Spermatozoon. Ed. by J. Gedes Grudzinskas & J. Yovich. 1995. (Reviews in Human Reproduction Ser.). (Illus.). 328p. (C). pap. text 31.95 (*0-521-47996-7*) Cambridge U Pr.

Gamma-Aminobutyric Acid in the Regulation of Hormone Secretion, 6. Alan N. Elias. 1985. LC 85-565. (Endocrinology & Metabolism Ser.: Vol. 6). 142p. 60.00 (*0-275-91312-0*, C1312, Praeger Pubs) Greenwood.

***Gamma-Delta T Cells.** Ed. by P. R. Bergstresser & A. Takashima. 2001. (Chemical Immunology Ser.: Vol. 79). (Illus.). viii, 142p. 155.00 (*3-8055-7205-0*) S Karger.

Gamma Images in Benign & Metabolic Bone Diseases Wilfrido M. Sy. 1981. Vol. 1. 288p. 165.00 (*0-8493-5361-0*, RC930); Vol. 2. 296p. 166.00 (*0-8493-5362-9*) Franklin (CRC Reprint).

Gamma Interferon: A Pleiotropic Cytokine with Antiviral Activity. Gunasegaran Karupiah. 1997. (Medical Intelligence Unit Ser.). 250p. pap. 89.95 (*0-412-13041-6*) Chapman & Hall.

Gamma Knife Brain Surgery. Ed. by L. D. Lunsford et al. 1998. LC 98-12266. (Progress in Neurological Surgery Ser.: Vol. 14, 1998). (Illus.). viii, 228p. 188.00 (*3-8055-6637-9*) S Karger.

Gamma Knife Surgery. Jeremy C. Ganz. 2nd rev. ed. 1997. LC 97-14849. (Illus.). 216p. 73.00 (*3-211-82840-0*) Spr-Verlag.

Gamma Knife Surgery: A Guide for Referring Physicians. Jeremy C. Ganz. 1993. (Illus.). 150p. pap. (*3-211-82476-6*) Spr-Verlag.

Gamma Particle: A Study of Cell-Organelle Interactions in the Development of the Water Mold Blastocladiella Emersonii. R. B. Myers & E. C. Cantino. 1974. (Monographs in Developmental Biology: Vol. 8). 150p. 58.50 (*3-8055-1735-1*) S Karger.

Gamut Index of Skeletal Dysplasias: An Aid to Radiodiagnosis. Kazimierz Kozlowski & Peter H. Beighton. 2nd ed. 1995. LC 95-7047. 232p. 58.95 (*3-540-19941-1*) Spr-Verlag.

Gamut Index of Skeletal Dysplasias: An Aid to Radiodiagnosis. Kazimierz Kozlowski & Peter Beighton. 3rd ed. 2001. LC 00-63760. 280p. pap. 95.95 (*1-85233-365-0*) Spr-Verlag.

Gamuts in Nuclear Medicine. Frederick L. Datz. 3rd ed. 1994. LC 94-231304. 512p. (C). (gr. 13). pap. text 46.95 (*0-8016-8097-2*, 08097) Mosby Inc.

Ganciclovir Therapy for Cytomegalovirus Infection. Ed. by Stephen A. Spector. 1991. (Illus.). 270p. text 115.00 (*0-8247-8572-X*) Dekker.

Gangliosides & Modulation of Neuronal Functions. Ed. by H. Rahmann. 1987. (NATO ASI Ser.: Vol. 7). 647p. 153.00 (*0-387-17587-3*) Spr-Verlag.

Gangliosides & Neuronal Plasticity: Proceedings of the Symposium "Neuronal Plasticity & Gangliosides" Held at Mantova, Italy, May 29-31, 1985. Ed. by Gino Toffano et al. 1987. (FIDIA Research Ser.). 483p. 204.00 (*0-387-96457-6*) Spr-Verlag.

Gangrene & Glory: Medical Care During the American Civil War. Frank R. Freemon. 1998. LC 97-42816. (Illus.). 256p. 52.50 (*0-8386-3753-1*) Fairleigh Dickinson.

Ganja in Jamaica. Vera Rubin & Lambros Comitas. 1975. (New Babylon Studies in the Social Sciences: No.26). 206p. text (*90-279-7731-3*) Mouton.

Ganodermataceae in China. Ji-Ding Zhao. 1989. (Bibliotheca Mycologica: Vol. 132). (GER., Illus.). 176p. (*3-443-59033-0*) Gebruder Borntraeger DEU. *Dist:* Balogh.

Ganzk Orper-Computertomographie see Whole-Body Computed Tomography

Gap Junctions: Basic Principles & Clinical Implications. Ed. by Renato Rozental. 2000. 99.95 (*0-12-601081-1*) Acad Pr.

Gap Junctions in the Nervous System. David C. Spray & Rolf Dermietzel. 1996. LC 96-28050. (Neuroscience Intelligence Unit Ser.). 253p. 99.00 (*1-57059-384-1*) Landes Bioscience.

Garcinis Cambogia: Weight Loss Wonder. Deanne Tenney. 1997. (Woodland Health Ser.). 32p. pap. text 3.95 (*1-885670-75-3*) Woodland UT.

Garden in the Machine: The Emerging Science of Artificial Life. Claus Emmeche. Tr. by Steven Sampson. 1994. LC 93-39101.Tr. of Det Levende Spil. 216p. 40.00 (*0-691-03330-7*) Princeton U Pr.

Garden of Herbal Remedies. W. Craig Dodd. 1997. LC 97-156489. (Gift of Health Ser.). (Illus.). 96p. pap. text (*1-85368-670-0*) New Holland Pubs GBR. *Dist:* Sterling.

Garden of Orthodontics. Giuseppe Cozzani. 2000. LC 00-27503. (Illus.). 423p. 158.00 (*0-86715-388-1*) Quint Pub Co.

Garden Within: Acidophilus-Candida Connection. Keith W. Sehnert. 1989. 32p. 2.00 (*0-9624780-0-8*) HealthWorld.

Gardner Social Maturity Developmental Scale. Morrison F. Gardner. 1994. 11.95 (*0-931421-69-1*) Psychol Educ Pubns.

Garf Assessment Sourcebook: Using the DSM-IV Global Assessment of Relational Functioning. Yingling. 1998. LC 97-22610. 184p. 29.95 (*0-87630-864-7*) Brunner-Routledge.

Garhart's Intravenous Medications. 13th ed. 1997. 49.95 (*1-56712-381-3*) Franklin Elect.

Garland Studies on the Elderly in America, Set. Ed. by Stuart Bruchey. 1992. 1763.00 (*0-8153-0505-2*) Garland.

Garlic: Nature's Healer. Morton Walker. 3rd rev. ed. 1984. (Dr. Morton Walker Good Health Guides Ser.). (Illus.). 56p. (Orig.). pap. 4.95 (*0-8159-5623-1*) Devin.

Garlic: Nature's Original Remedy. Stephen Fulder & John Blackwood. 2000. LC 2001-516034. (Illus.). 144p. pap. 6.95 (*0-89281-725-9*, Heal Arts VT) Inner Tradit.

Garlic: Review & Recommendations Cancer & Heart Disease. Orville C. Green, III & Nicholas Polydoris. 1993. 90p. pap. text 9.95 (*0-9637713-0-2*) Real Est News.

Garlic - Medical & Health Qualities: Index of Modern Authors & Subjects for Rapid Research. Richard C. Trovatto. rev. ed. 1994. 57.50 (*0-7883-0186-1*); pap. 47.50 (*0-7883-0187-X*) ABBE Pubs Assn.

Garlic in Biology & Medicine: Proceedings Of The First World Congress On The Health Significance of Garlic & Garlic Constituents. Ed. by Robert I. Lin. 1995. (Illus.). 275p. (Orig.). pap. text 150.00 (*0-9640678-0-3*) Nutrit Intl.

Garlic, Medical & Health Qualities: Index of Modern Authors & Subjects for Rapid Research. Richard C. Trovatto. 1996. LC 96-6363. 57.50 (*0-7883-1072-0*); pap. 47.50 (*0-7883-1073-9*) ABBE Pubs Assn.

Garlic Research: The Miracle Food in Action. 1994. (Alternative Medicine Ser.). lib. bdg. 254.95 (*0-8490-8944-1*) Gordon Pr.

Garrison's History of Neurology. Lawrence C. McHenry, Jr. 1969. (Illus.). 568p. 96.95 (*0-398-01261-X*) C C Thomas.

Garrod's Inborn Factors in Disease. Ed. by Charles R. Scriver & Barton Childs. 1989. (Oxford Monographs on Medical Genetics: No. 16). (Illus.). 264p. 53.00 (*0-19-261574-2*) OUP.

Garum & Salsamenta: Production & Commerce in Materia Medica. Robert I. Curtis. 1991. LC 91-16000. (Studies in Ancient Medicine: No. 3). (Illus.). xv, 226p. 82.00 (*90-04-09423-7*) Brill Academic Pubs.

Garzanti Medical Encyclopedia: Enciclopedia Medica Garzanti, Set. Garzanti. 4th ed. 1982. (ITA.). 1296p. 95.00 (*0-8288-1845-2*, M14439) Fr & Eur.

Gas & Liquid Chromatography Abstracts: Cumulative Indexes 1969-73. Ed. by C. E. Knapman. 1976. 381p. 68.50 (*0-85334-643-7*) Elsevier.

Gas Chromatographic Retention Indices of Toxicologically Relevant Substances on Packed or Capillary Columns with Dimthylsilicone Stationary Phase: Report Xviii of the DFG Commission for Clinical-Toxicological Analysis. Rokus A. De Zeeuw et al. Ed. by International Association of Forensic Toxicologist. 3rd enl. rev. ed. 1992. LC 92-49393. (Commission Reports of the Deutsche Forschungsgmeinschaft). (Illus.). 408p. 165.00 (*3-527-27396-4*, 0930-7958, Wiley-VCH) Wiley.

Gas Chromatography: Biochemical, Biomedical & Clinical Applications. Ray E. Clement. 1990. LC 90-12799. (Chemical Analysis Monographs). 393p. 198.00 (*0-471-01048-0*) Wiley.

Gas Chromatography Abstracts: 1963. Institute of Petroleum Staff. 1963. 286p. 30.75 (*0-444-39990-9*) Elsevier.

Gas Chromatography Abstracts: 1964-67 & 1969-72. Institute of Petroleum Staff. 1972. 43.25 (*0-85334-472-8*); 1971. 45.00 (*0-85334-478-7*); 1970. 43.25 (*0-85334-497-3*); 1969. 30.75 (*0-444-39930-5*); 1967. 30.75 (*0-444-39947-X*); 1966. 30.75 (*0-444-39954-2*); 1965. 30.75 (*0-444-39960-7*); 1964. 30.75 (*0-444-39976-3*) Elsevier.

Gas Chromatography Symposia. Institute of Petroleum Staff et al. 1972. 54.00 (*0-85334-479-5*); 1970. 63.00 (*0-85334-492-2*); 1966. 65.00 (*0-444-39957-7*) Elsevier.

Gas Exchange Function of Normal & Diseased Lungs. Ed. by J. Piiper & P. Scheid. 1981. (Progress in Respiratory Research Ser.: Vol. 16). (Illus.). xvi, 320p. 172.25 (*3-8055-1638-X*) S Karger.

Gas Mixing & Distribution in the Lung. L. A. Engel. 1985. (Lung Biology in Health & Disease Ser.: Vol. 25). (Illus.). 432p. text 199.00 (*0-8247-7284-9*) Dekker.

***Gaschromatographie in Bildern.** 1999. 244p. pap. 49.00 (*3-527-29880-0*) Wiley.

Gases in Medicine. Ed. by E. B. Smith & S. Daniels. 1999. 190p. 120.00 (*0-85404-718-2*) Spr-Verlag.

Gasless Laparoscopy in General Surgery & Gynecology: Diagnostic-Operative Procedures. Ed. by V. Paolucci & B. Schaeff. 1996. LC 96-4646. (Illus.). 176p. pap. text 89.00 (*0-86577-604-0*) Thieme Med Pubs.

Gasless Laparoscopy with Conventional Instruments: The Next Phase in Minimally Invasive Surgery. Claude H. Organ, Jr. & R. Stephen Smith. 1993. LC 93-26738. (Illus.). 153p. 98.00 (*0-930405-61-7*) Norman SF.

Gassed in the Gulf: The Insider Story of the Pentagon-CIA Cover-Up of Gulf War Syndrome. Patrick G. Eddington. 1997. LC 97-160334. (Illus.). 388p. 23.95 (*0-9652400-3-7*) Insignia Publng.

Gasteromycetes: Morphological & Developmental Features. Hope H. Miller & Orson K. Miller, Jr. 1987. 150p. pap. 16.95 (*0-916422-74-7*) Mad River.

Gastric & Gastroduodenal Motility, 4. Ed. by Louis M. Akkermans et al. 1984. LC 84-16090. (Surgical Science Ser.: Vol. 4). 244p. 72.50 (*0-275-91420-8*, C1420, Praeger Pubs) Greenwood.

Gastric Cancer. Ed. by Harold O. Douglass, Jr. 1988. (Contemporary Issues in Clinical Oncology Ser.: Vol. 8). (Illus.). 244p. text (*0-443-08536-6*) Church.

Gastric Cancer. Ed. by M. Nishi et al. 1994. LC 93-31369. (Illus.). 528p. 304.00 (*0-387-70127-3*) Spr-Verlag.

Gastric Cancer. Ed. by T. Sugimura & M. Sasako. 1997. LC 97-187538. (Illus.). 324p. (C). text 115.00 (*0-19-262620-5*) OUP.

Gastric Cancer: Proceedings of the International Symposium on Gastric Cancer, Birmingham, 22-23 Sept. 1980. Ed. by J. W. Fielding et al. 1981. (Advances in the Biosciences Ser.: Vol. 32). (Illus.). 247p. 50.00 (*0-08-026398-4*, Pergamon Pr) Elsevier.

Gastric Carcinoma. Ed. by J. Hotz et al. 1989. (Illus.). 194p. 93.00 (*0-387-96955-1*) Spr-Verlag.

Gastric Cytoprotection: A Clinician's Guide. D. Hollander & A. Tarnawski. 1989. (Illus.). 214p. (C). text 54.50 (*0-306-43266-8*, Kluwer Plenum) Kluwer Academic.

Gastric Secretion. M. Plebani & F. Di Mario. 1992. (Advances in Gastroenterology Ser.: No. 5). 160p. text (*1-57235-021-0*) Piccin Nuova.

Gastritis. David Y. Graham et al. 1998. LC 98-32439. (Illus.). 272p. text 199.00 (*0-397-51675-4*) Lppncott W & W.

Gastritis. Robert A. Kozol. 1992. 240p. 119.00 (*0-8493-5497-8*, RC831) CRC Pr.

Gastro-Entero-Pancreatic Tumors, Proceedings of Somatostatin Analogues - Peptide Therapy in Action Symposium, Session I, January 1989 & Perspectives in Gastroenterology, Proceedings of Somatostatin Analogues - Peptide Therapy in Action Symposium, Session II, January 1989, Vol. 45, Suppl. 1, 1990. Ed. by S. R. Bloom & M. J. Farthing. 1990. (Illus.). 88p. pap. 38.50 (*3-8055-5202-5*) S Karger.

Gastro-Esophageal Cytology. M. Drake. 1985. (Monographs in Clinical Cytology Ser.: Vol. 10). (Illus.). xii, 268p. 107.00 (*3-8055-3931-2*) S Karger.

Gastro-Esophageal Reflux. Glyn G. Jamieson & Andre Duranceau. 1988. (Illus.). 256p. text 90.00 (*0-7216-2319-0*) Saunders.

Gastro-Intestinal Diseases: Directory of Authors of New Medical & Scientific Reviews with Subject Index. Science and Life Consultants Association Staff. 1995. 160p. 57.50 (*0-7883-0578-6*); 1995. 160p. pap. 47.50 (*0-7883-0579-4*); 1998. 169p. 57.50 (*0-7883-2076-9*); 1998. 169p. pap. 47.50 (*0-7883-2077-7*) ABBE Pubs Assn.

Gastroduodenal Disease & Helicobacter Pylori: Pathophysiology, Diagnosis & Treatment. Ed. by T. Ulf Westblom et al. 1998. (Current Topics in Microbiology & Immunology Ser.: Vol. 241). (Illus.). 319p. 189.00 (*3-540-65084-9*) Spr-Verlag.

Gastroenteritis Viruses, No. 238. Novartis Foundation Symposium. 2001. LC 2001-17866. (CIBA Foundation Symposia Ser.: Vol. 238). (Illus.). 334p. 125.00 (*0-471-49663-4*) Wiley.

Gastroenterologic Endoscopy Michael V. Sivak, Jr. Ed. by Richard Zorab. 2nd ed. 1999. LC 96-4868. (Illus.). 1340p. (C). cd-rom 250.00 (*0-7216-6633-7*) Saunders.

***Gastroenterologic Endoscopy**, Set. Michael V. Sivak, Jr. 2nd ed. 2000. (Illus.). 1776p. 260.00 (*0-7216-9001-7*) Saunders.

Gastroenterological Problems from the Tropics. Ed. by G. C. Cook. 1995. 152p. (C). pap. text (*0-7279-0902-9*) BMJ Pub GBR. *Dist:* AIDC.

Gastroenterology. L. K. Harding & Philip J. Robinson. 1991. (Clinician's Guide to Nuclear Medicine Ser.). (Illus.). 144p. text (*0-443-04418-X*) Church.

Gastroenterology. Douglas M. Heuman et al. Ed. by William Schmitt. 1996. LC 96-41122. (Illus.). 368p. pap. text 36.95 (*0-7216-5864-4*) Saunders.

Gastroenterology. M. Lancaster-Smith. 1985. (Management of Common Diseases in Family Practice Ser.). 22.00 (*0-88416-529-9*) Mosby Inc.

Gastroenterology. David Sachar & Jerome Wayne. 1989. (House Officer Ser.). (Illus.). 353p. (Orig.). pap. text 20.00 (*0-683-07488-1*) Lppncott W & W.

Gastroenterology. 2nd ed. 1984. (Medical Ser.). (Illus.). 68p. (C). 12.95 (*0-935920-18-8*, Ntl Pubs Blck) P-H.

Gastroenterology. S. P. L. Travis et al. 2nd ed. 1998. LC 98-15947. (Pocket Consultant Ser.). (Illus.). 505p. pap. 69.95 (*0-632-04887-5*) Blackwell Sci.

Gastroenterology. Elizabeth K. White. 3rd ed. 1993. LC 92-48839. (Regents - Prentice-Hall Medical Assistant Kit Ser.). 112p. pap. 16.40 (*0-13-105958-0*) P-H.

Gastroenterology: An Essential Slide Collection. N. Ian McNeil. 1987. 83p. (gr. 13). (*0-397-46363-4*, GM0138) Gower-Mosby.

Gastroenterology: Quick Reference Guides for Family Physicians. Martin S. Lipsky. 2000. LC 00-30963. (Academy Collection). 208p. pap. text 29.95 (*0-7817-2054-0*) Lppncott W & W.

Gastroenterology & Hepatology. Ed. by Gabrielle B. Porro et al. 1999. (Clinical Medicine Ser.). (Illus.). 768p. pap. text 79.95 (*0-07-709519-7*) McGraw-Hill Med Pub.

E
F
G

***Gastroenterology & Hepatology**, Set. Ed. by Mark Feldman. 1996. (Illus.). 1910p. (0-443-07794-0) Church GBR. *Dist:* Saunders.

***Gastroenterology & Hepatology Set: Including CD-ROMs & Slides**, Set Ed. by Mark Feldman et al. 1999. incl. cd-rom (0-443-07841-6) Church GBR. *Dist:* Saunders.

Gastroenterology & Liver Disease. Peter C. Hayes. 1995. LC 94-30145. (Colour Guide Ser.). (Illus.). pap. text 16.95 (0-443-04955-6) Harcrt Hlth Sci Grp.

Gastroenterology & Liver Disease. Gregory Holdstock & Ralph Wright. 1989. (Colour Aids Ser.). (Illus.). 160p. pap. text (0-443-03033-2) Church.

Gastroenterology Assistant: A Laboratory Manual. Melvin Schapiro & Joel Kuritsky. 2nd ed. 1981. LC 81-50268. (Illus.). 150p. 25.00 (0-9605718-3-3) Valley Presbyterian.

Gastroenterology Assistant: A Laboratory Manual. Melvin Schapiro & Joel Kuritsky. 1990. (Illus.). 230p. tchr. ed. 40.00 (0-9621879-3-3) Zephyr Med Enter.

Gastroenterology in Primary Care: An Evidence Based Guide to Management. Pali Hungin & Greg Rubin. 2000. LC 99-54485. (Illus.). xi, 108p. pap. 41.95 (0-632-05191-4) Blackwell Sci.

Gastroenterology Nursing: A Core Curriculum. Society of Gastroenterology Nurses and Associates Staff. 2nd ed. 1998. LC 98-15852. (Illus.). 544p. (C). text 54.95 (0-8151-3693-5, 31035) Mosby Inc.

Gastroenterology Practice Management. Ed. by William D. Carey & Thomas F. Fise. 1993. LC 93-14755. 280p. 70.00 (0-89640-237-1) Igaku-Shoin.

Gastroenterology 2000: An Internet Resource Guide. Ed. by Dan Goldenson. 2000. pap. 24.95 (0-9700525-4-5) eMedguides.

Gastroesophageal Reflux Disease & Airway Disease. Ed. by Mark R. Stein. 1999. LC 98-56649. (Lung Biology in Health & Disease Ser.: No. 129). (Illus.). 376p. text 175.00 (0-8247-0230-1) Dekker.

Gastroesophageal Reflux Disease (GERD): Back to Surgery? International Meeting, Bern, May 1996. Ed. by M. W. Buechler et al. 1997. LC 97-7704. (Progress in Surgery Ser.: Vol. 23, 1997). (Illus.). viii, 248p. 184.50 (3-8055-6476-7) S Karger.

Gastro/Hepatlogy, Set. Feldman. 1995. text 790.00 (0-443-07798-3) Saunders.

Gastrointestinal & Hepatic Immunology. Ed. by Richard V. Heatley. 1995. (Cambridge Reviews in Clinical Immunology Ser.). (Illus.). 408p. (C). text 100.00 (0-521-44509-4) Cambridge U Pr.

Gastrointestinal & Hepatic Infections. Ed. by Christina Surawicz & Robert Owen. 1994. LC 93-15671. (Illus.). 651p. text 115.00 (0-7216-4062-1) Saunders.

Gastrointestinal & Hepatobiliary Pathophysiology. S. Rose. 1997. (Pathophysiology Ser.). 475p. (C). pap. 30.95 (1-889325-01-5) Blackwell Sci.

Gastrointestinal & Hepatobiliary Surgery: The Requisites. Ashley Brooks & Hodin Matthews. 2000. (Illus.). 544p. text 65.00 (0-8151-4386-9, 31680) Mosby Inc.

Gastrointestinal & Oesophageal Pathology. Ed. by Richard Whitehead. 1989. (Illus.). 850p. text (0-443-03589-X) Church.

Gastrointestinal & Oesophageal Pathology. Ed. by R. Whitehead. 2nd ed. 1995. LC 94-43498. 1007p. text (0-443-04764-2) Church.

Gastrointestinal Bleeding. Ed. by Neville Krasner. 1996. 368p. (0-7279-1008-6) BMJ Pub GBR. *Dist:* AIDC.

Gastrointestinal Cancer: Advances in Basic Sciences. Ed. by P. Rozen et al. 1979. (Frontiers of Gastrointestinal Research Ser.: Vol. 4). (Illus.). 82.75 (3-8055-2903-1) S Karger.

Gastrointestinal Cancer: Advances in Diagnostics Techniques & Therapy. Ed. by P. Rozen et al. 1979. (Frontiers of Gastrointestinal Research Ser.: Vol. 5). (Illus.). 82.75 (3-8055-2905-8) S Karger.

Gastrointestinal Cancer I. Paul Sherlock. Ed. by Jerome J. DeCosse. 1981. 544p. text 239.50 (90-247-2461-9) Kluwer Academic.

Gastrointestinal Cancers: Biology, Diagnosis, & Therapy. Ed. by Anil K. Rustgi. 1995. LC 95-2641. (Illus.). 688p. text 199.00 (0-7817-0276-3) Lppncott W & W.

Gastrointestinal Cancers: Biology, Diagnosis, & Therapy. Anil K. Rustgi. 2001. text (0-7216-8963-9) Saunders.

Gastrointestinal Disease: An Endoscopic Approach Ed. by Anthony J. DiMarino, Jr. & Stanley B. Benjamin. 1997. LC 97-678. (Illus.). 1504p. 414.95 (0-86542-501-9) Blackwell Sci.

Gastrointestinal Disease: An Endoscopic Approach. Anthony J. DiMarino, Jr. & Stanley B. Benjamin. 2nd ed. 2001. 1200p. text 295.00 (1-55642-511-2) SLACK Inc.

Gastrointestinal Disease Book. Anthony J. DiMarino, Jr. & Stanley B. Benjamin. 1998. (Illus.). 499.95 incl. cd-rom (0-632-04355-5) Blackwell Sci.

Gastrointestinal Disease (Fifth Series) Test & Syllabus. Dennis M. Balfe et al. 1995. (Profession Self-Evaluation Program Ser.: Vol. 39). (Illus.). 750p. 220.00 (1-55903-039-9) Am Coll Radiology.

Gastrointestinal Disease (Fourth Series) Test & Syllabus. David H. Stephens et al. 1990. (Professional Self-Evaluation & Continuing Education Program Ser.: Vol. 29). (Illus.). 600p. 190.00 (1-55903-029-1) Am Coll Radiology.

Gastrointestinal Disease in Primary Care. Lyman E. Bilhartz & Carol Lynn Croft. 2000. LC 99-55265. 224p. pap. text 49.95 (0-683-30444-5) Lppncott W & W.

Gastrointestinal Diseases. Ed. by B. B. Dahms & S. Qualman. 1997. (Perspectives in Pediatric Pathology Ser.: Vol. 20). (Illus.). x, 176p. 189.75 (3-8055-6343-4) S Karger.

Gastrointestinal Diseases & Disorders Sourcebook: Basic Information about Gastroesophageal Reflex Disease, Ulcers, Diverticulosis & More. Ed. by Linda M. Ross. 1996. LC 96-26198. (Health Reference Ser.: Vol. 16). lib. bdg. 78.00 (0-7808-0078-8) Omnigraphics Inc.

Gastrointestinal Disorders. Dorothy B. Doughty. 1993. (Illus.). 368p. (C). (gr. 13). text 37.00 (0-8016-2096-1, 02096) Mosby Inc.

Gastrointestinal Disorders in Diabetes Mellitus. S. Forgacs. Tr. by E. Farkas from HUN. 1985. (Illus.). 104p. (963-05-3948-9) Akade Kiado HUN. *Dist:* St Mut.

Gastrointestinal Drug Therapy in the Elderly. Ed. by James W. Cooper & William E. Wade. 1998. LC 97-42595. (Journal of Geriatric Drug Therapy Ser.: Vol. 12). 144p. 29.95 (0-7890-0395-3, Pharmctl Prods) Haworth Pr.

Gastrointestinal Emergencies. Tony C. K. Tham & John S. A. Collins. 2001. (Illus.). 264p. pap. text (0-7279-1485-5) BMJ Pub GBR. *Dist:* AIDC.

Gastrointestinal Emergencies. Mark B. Taylor et al. 2nd ed. 1997. LC 96-3276. (Illus.). 800p. text 155.00 (0-683-08108-X) Lppncott W & W.

Gastrointestinal Emergencies Two: Proceedings of the 2nd International Symposium on Gastrointestinal Emergencies, Rome, 7-8 June 1979. Ed. by Franz R. Barany et al. 1980. (Advances in the Biosciences Ser.: Vol. 27). (Illus.). 184p. 32.50 (0-08-024927-2, Pergamon Pr) Elsevier.

Gastrointestinal Endocrinology. George H. Greeley, Jr. 1999. LC 98-33918. (Contemporary Endocrinology Ser.: Vol. 8). 592p. 160.00 (0-89603-506-9) Humana.

Gastrointestinal Endoscopy. John Baillie. 1997. LC 96-50473. (Illus.). 158p. text (0-7506-9555-2) E A GBR. *Dist:* OUP.

Gastrointestinal Endoscopy. Jacques Van Dam. 2000. (Vademecum Ser.). spiral bd. 45.00 (1-57059-572-0) Landes Bioscience.

Gastrointestinal Endoscopy: Old Problems, New Techniques, 4. Ed. by Michael V. Sivak, Jr. & John Petrini. 1985. LC 85-16997. 299p. 95.00 (0-275-91299-X, C1299, Praeger Pubs) Greenwood.

Gastrointestinal Endoscopy for Surgeons. Russell K. Pearl. 1984. 225p. 58.00 (0-316-69615-3, Little Brwn Med Div) Lppncott W & W.

Gastrointestinal Endosonography. Jacques Van Dam & Michael V. Sivak. Ed. by Richard Zorab. 1998. LC 98-20110. (Illus.). 330p. (C). text (0-7216-7989-7) Saunders.

Gastrointestinal Health, rev ed: Completely New & Revised. Steven Peiken. rev. ed. 1999. LC 98-54416. (Illus.). 368p. pap. 15.00 (0-06-095318-7) HarperCollins Pubs.

Gastrointestinal Infections: Diagnosis & Management. J. Thomas Lamont. 1997. LC 97-18585. (Gastroenterology Ser.). (Illus.). 504p. text 150.00 (0-8247-0055-4) Dekker.

Gastrointestinal Infections in the Tropics. Ed. by V. K. Rustgi. 1990. (Illus.). viii, 248p. 208.75 (3-8055-5211-4) S Karger.

Gastrointestinal Lymphoma: Future Perspectives. Ed. by Wolfgang Fischbach. 2000. LC 99-43214. (Recent Results in Cancer Research Ser.: Vol. 156). (Illus.). 160p. 109.00 (3-540-65324-4) Spr-Verlag.

Gastrointestinal Microcirculation. Ed. by K. Messmer & F. Hammersen. 1991. (Progress in Applied Microcirculation Ser.: Vol. 17). (Illus.). x, 222p. 195.00 (3-8055-5176-2) S Karger.

Gastrointestinal Motility: Tests & Problem-Oriented Approach. Ed. by Satish S. Rao. 1999. LC 99-16121. (0-306-46129-3) Kluwer Academic.

Gastrointestinal Motility Disorders for the Clinician: Practical Guidelines for Patient Care. Ed. by Sidney Phillips et al. 1998. (Illus.). v, 25p. pap. text 24.95 (0-934205-13-2) Academy Prof Inform.

Gastrointestinal Mucosal Biopsy. Harvey Goldman. 1995. (Contemporary Issues in Surgical Pathology Ser.: Vol. 20). 592p. text (0-443-08990-6) Church.

***Gastrointestinal Mucosal Protective Mechanisms: Modulatory Effects of Helicobacter Pylori on the Gastric Mucus Gel Barrier & Mucosal Blood Flow in Vivo.** Christer Atuma. 2000. (Comprehensive Summaries of Uppsala Dissertations from the Faculty of Medicine Ser.: No. 972). (Illus.). 60p. pap. (91-554-4851-8) Uppsala Universitet SWE. *Dist:* Coronet Bks.

Gastrointestinal Oncology. Al Benson. 1998. LC 98-22563. (Cancer Treatment & Research Ser.). 17p. (0-7923-8205-6) Kluwer Academic.

Gastrointestinal Oncology. Ed. by John S. MacDonald. 1987. (Cancer Treatment & Research Ser.). text 241.50 (0-89838-829-5) Kluwer Academic.

Gastrointestinal Pathology. Para Chandrasoma. 1998. LC 98-25826. 640p. (C). 225.00 (0-8385-3093-1, Apple Lange Med) McGraw.

Gastrointestinal Pathology. Christopher S. Foster. 1993. (C). text 250.00 incl. disk (1-56815-016-4) Mosby Inc.

Gastrointestinal Pathology. Ed. by G. T. Williams. 1990. (Current Topics in Pathology Ser.: Vol. 81). (Illus.). 358p. 157.00 (0-387-51016-8) Spr-Verlag.

Gastrointestinal Pathology: An Atlas & Text. Cecilia M. Fenoglio-Preiser et al. 1989. (Illus.). 903p. text 259.50 (0-88167-459-1) Lppncott W & W.

Gastrointestinal Pathology: An Atlas & Text. Fenoglio-Preiser et al. 2nd ed. 1998. LC 97-39423. (Illus.). 1,312p. text 299.00 (0-397-51640-1) Lppncott W & W.

Gastrointestinal Pathology & Its Clinical Implications, Set. Klaus J. Lewin et al. 1992. LC 88-28473. (Illus.). 1488p. 345.00 (0-89640-153-7) Igaku-Shoin.

Gastrointestinal Pharmacology. Richard W. McCallum. 1996. LC 96-41245. 832p. text 199.00 (0-397-51625-8, Lippnctt) Lppncott W & W.

Gastrointestinal Pharmacology, Vol. 1. James Lewis & Andre Dubois. 1997. (Illus.). 342p. 75.00 (0-86542-521-3) Blackwell Sci.

Gastrointestinal Pharmacotherapy. Ed. by M. Michael Wolfe. 1993. LC 92-48474. (Illus.). 384p. text 75.00 (0-7216-3190-8) Saunders.

Gastrointestinal Physiology. Ed. by Leonard R. Johnson. 5th ed. 1996. (Illus.). 208p. (C). (gr. 13). pap. text 29.95 (0-8151-4934-4, 28158) Mosby Inc.

Gastrointestinal Physiology. Leonard R. Johnson. 6th ed. 2000. LC 00-33876. (Mosby Physiology Monograph Ser.). (Illus.). xi, 206p. (0-323-01239-6) Mosby Inc.

Gastrointestinal Polyps. N. Y. Haboubi et al. 2002. (Medical Media Ser.). (Illus.). 256p. text (1-900151-21-9) Greenwich Med GBR. *Dist:* JAMCO Dist.

Gastrointestinal Problems in General Practice. Ed. by Roger Jones. 1993. (Oxford General Practice Ser.: No. 26). (Illus.). 258p. (C). pap. text 39.95 (0-19-262227-7) OUP.

Gastrointestinal Radiology. Jack Farman. 1991. (Illus.). 208p. (gr. 13). text (1-56375-004-X, GM0194) Gower-Mosby.

Gastrointestinal Radiology: A Concise Text. Branko M. Plavsic et al. 1991. 640p. (0-08-040685-8) PPI GBR. *Dist:* McGraw.

Gastrointestinal Radiology: A Pattern Approach. Ronald L. Eisenberg. 3rd ed. 1995. LC 95-8381. 1,216p. text 250.00 (0-397-51480-8) Lppncott W & W.

Gastrointestinal Radiology: Performing & Interpreting the Fluroscopic Examinations. David W. Gelfand. 1984. (Illus.). 354p. pap. text (0-443-08096-8) Church.

Gastrointestinal Radiology: The Requisites. Robert D. Halpert & Peter J. Feczko. 2nd ed. 1999. LC 99-10221. (Illus.). 416p. text 80.00 (0-8151-4370-2, 31225) Mosby Inc.

Gastrointestinal Radiology Companion: Imaging Fundamentals. Ronald L. Eisenberg. 1998. LC 98-29513. 320p. pap. text 65.00 (0-7817-1946-1) Lppncott W & W.

Gastrointestinal Regulatory Peptides. Ed. by David R. Brown. 1993. LC 92-49563. (Handbook of Experimental Pharmacology Ser.: Vol. 106). (Illus.). 446p. 485.00 (0-387-55970-1) Spr-Verlag.

Gastrointestinal Sourcebook. M Sara Rosenthal. abr. ed. 1999. LC 99-461916. (Illus.). 272p. pap. 16.95 (0-7373-0081-7) NTC Contemp Pub Co.

Gastrointestinal Surgical Patient: Preoperative & Postoperative Care. Eamonn M. Quigley & Michael F. Sorrell. 1994. (Illus.). 583p. 89.00 (0-683-07001-0) Lppncott W & W.

***Gastrointestinal System at a Glance.** Satish Keshav. 2001. (At a Glance Ser.). 96p. pap. 19.95 (0-632-05472-7) Blackwell Sci.

Gastrointestinal System Course. Competence Assurance Systems Staff. 1981. (Illus.). pap. text 50.00 (0-89147-065-4) CAS.

Gastrointestinal Transit: Pathophysiology & Pharmacology. Ed. by Michael A. Kamm & John E. Lennard-Jones. 1991. 272p. (1-871816-11-4) Wrightson Biomed GBR. *Dist:* Taylor & Francis.

Gastrointestinal Ultrasonography. Ed. by Alfred B. Kurtz & Barry B. Goldberg. 1988. (Clinics in Diagnostic Ultrasound Ser.: Vol. 23). (Illus.). 312p. text (0-443-08574-9) Church.

Gastrokamera- und Roentgendiagnostik: Ein Atlas der kombinierten Magenuntersuchung mit histologischer Dokumentation. H. Oshima et al. 1972. (Illus.). xii, 140p. (C). 226.95 (3-11-001687-7) De Gruyter.

Gastronintestinal Tract & Endocrine System. Ed. by M. V. Singer. 1995. LC 95-20106. (Falk Symposium Ser.). 640p. (C). text 276.00 (0-7923-8877-1) Kluwer Academic.

Gastronomic Bibliography. Katherine Bitting. 1994. 718p. reprint ed. 75.00 (1-888262-38-9) Martino Pubng.

Gatekeeper: A Guide to Capitation for the Primary Care Physician. John F. McCally. 1995. 200p. 40.00 (1-55738-634-X, Irwn Prfssnl) McGraw-Hill Educ Grp.

Gatekeeping in the Intensive Care Unit. Martin A. Stosberg & Daniel Teres. 1997. LC 97-7169. pap. 20.00 (1-56793-055-7) Health Admin Pr.

Gates of the Dream. Geza Roheim. 1969. reprint ed. pap. 24.95 (0-8236-8060-6, 22110) Intl Univs Pr.

Gateways to Improving Lesbian Health & Health Care: Opening Doors. Ed. by Christy M. Ponticelli. 1997. LC 97-30299. 114p. 29.95 (0-7890-0350-3); pap. 14.95 (1-56023-103-3) Haworth Pr (Harrington Park).

Gay & Lesbian Issues: Abstracts of the Psychological & Behavioral Literature 1985-1996. Ed. by Clinton W. Anderson & Amanda R. Adley. 1997. LC 97-12944. (Bibliographies in Psychology Ser.: Vol. 17). 227p. pap. text 27.50 (1-55798-445-X) Am Psychol.

Gay & Sober: Directions for Counseling & Therapy. Ed. by Thomas O. Ziebold & John E. Mongeon. 1985. LC 84-22466. 107p. pap. text 9.95 (0-918393-10-8, Harrington Park) Haworth Pr.

Gay, Lesbian, & Heterosexual Teachers: An Investigation of Acceptance of Self, Acceptance of Others, Affectional & Lifestyle Orientation: Their Rightful Place. Martin P. Mayer. 1993. LC 93-26785. 196p. text 79.95 (0-7734-2236-6) E Mellen.

Gay Men's Wellness Guide. Robert E. Penn. 1998. 624p. pap. 19.95 (0-8050-4772-7); LC 97-27009. (Illus.). 35.00 (0-8050-4771-9) St Martin.

Gay Personality & Sexual Labeling. Ed. by John P. De Cecco. 1985. LC 84-22578. 106p. pap. text 9.95 (0-918393-01-9, Harrington Park) Haworth Pr.

Gay, Straight & In-Between: The Sexology of Erotic Orientation. John Money. 1988. (Illus.). 304p. text 29.95 (0-19-505407-5) OUP.

Gays, AIDS & You. Enrique T. Rueda & Michael Schwartz. 1987. LC 87-24527. (Illus.). 118p. 7.95 (0-8159-5624-X) Devin.

Gays & Acquired Immune Deficiency Syndrome (AIDS) A Bibliography. 1986. (Medical Bibliography Ser.). lib. bdg. 79.95 (0-87700-875-2) Revisionist Pr.

Gays, Lesbians, & Their Therapists. Charles Silverstein. 1991. 274p. 34.95 (0-393-70116-6) Norton.

Gazing into the Oracle: The Delphi Method & Its Application to Social Policy & Public Health. Ed. by Michael Adler & Erio Ziglio. 1994. 252p. pap. 39.95 (1-85302-104-0) Taylor & Francis.

GC/MS in Clinical Chemistry. Petra Gerhards. 1999. LC 99-189304. 258p. 98.00 (3-527-29623-9) Wiley.

GCP Harmonization Handbook. Donald Maynard & Robert De Woskin. 1996. 476p. ring bd. 197.00 (1-57491-013-2) IHS Health Grp.

GCP Quality Audit Manual. James E. Sayre, Jr. 2nd ed. 1994. (Illus.). 151p. ring bd. 234.00 (0-935184-56-2) IHS Health Grp.

Gecris Endoscopy Dictionary. George Cristino & Donna M. Cristino. 2nd ed. 1996. 172p. (C). text 85.00 (1-886974-09-8) Inst Knowledge.

Gefahren, Fehler & Erfolge in der Vaskulaeren Chirurgie & Ihre Wirklichkeit. Ed. by M. Sperling. 1991. (Illus.). vi, 206p. 64.50 (3-8055-5533-4) S Karger.

Gellis & Kagan's Current Pediatric Therapy. Fredric D. Burg et al. 15th ed. 1995. (Illus.). 976p. (C). text 83.00 (0-7216-5016-3) Saunders.

Gellis & Kagan's Current Pediatric Therapy. Fredric D. Burg et al. Ed. by Judy Fletcher. 16th ed. 1998. (Illus.). 928p. (C). text 98.00 (0-7216-6998-0) Saunders.

GEM Pharmacy: Nature's Mineral Supports. Dorothee L. Mella & Michelle Lusson. 1992. 56p. pap. 4.95 (0-9636345-1-8) Domel.

Gemeinsame Jahrestagung der Deutschen und der Osterreichischen Gesellschaft Fur Hamatologie und Onkologie (dgho/ogho) 1999. vi, 210p. 58.25 (3-8055-6939-4) S Karger.

Gemini: Gifted Education Manual for Individualizing Networks of Instruction. Christine L. Lewis et al. 1980. 50p. pap., tchr. ed. 15.00 (0-89824-015-8) Trillium Pr.

Gender Ed. by Carol N. Jacklin. 1992. (International Library of Critical Writings in Business History). 2000p. (C). 1. lib. bdg. 150.00 (0-8147-4185-1); 2. lib. bdg. 150.00 (0-8147-4186-X); 3. lib. bdg. 150.00 (0-8147-4187-8); 4. lib. bdg. 150.00 (0-8147-4188-6); Set. lib. bdg. 575.00 (0-8147-4184-3) NYU Pr.

Gender: Psychological Perspectives. Linda Brannon. 2nd ed. 1998. LC 98-3200. 528p. pap. text 59.00 (0-205-27589-3) Allyn.

Gender & Addictions: Men & Women in Treatment. Shulamith Lala Ashenberg Straussner. Ed. by Elizabeth Zelvin. 1997. LC 97-5148. (LSAAT Ser.). 528p. text 65.00 (0-7657-0070-0) Aronson.

Gender & Desire: Uncursing Pandora. Polly Young-Eisendrath. 1997. LC 96-39207. (Carolyn & Ernest Fay Series in Analytical Psychology: Vol. 6). 160p. (C). text 19.95 (0-89096-746-6) Tex A&M Univ Pr.

Gender & Envy. Nancy Burke. 1998. LC 98-2534. 448p. (C). 95.00 (0-415-91627-5); pap. 26.95 (0-415-91628-3) Routledge.

Gender & Family Therapy. Charlotte Burck & Gwyn Daniel. 1995. 176p. pap. text (1-85575-072-4) Karnac Bks GBR. *Dist:* Other Pr LLC.

Gender & Health: International Perspective. Ed. by Carolyn F. Sargent & Caroline B. Brettell. 1995. LC 95-37457. 370p. pap. 41.00 (0-13-079427-9) P-H.

Gender & Health Issues: A Resource Handbook. American Speech, Language and Hearing Foundation Staff et al. 1996. 250p. pap. 23.00 (0-910329-87-7, 0112014) Am Speech Lang Hearing.

Gender & Nonverbal Behavior. Ed. by C. Mayo & N. H. Henley. 1981. (Social Psychology Ser.). (Illus.). 284p. 64.00 (0-387-90601-0) Spr-Verlag.

Gender & Personality: Current Perspectives on Theory & Research. Ed. by Abigail J. Stewart & Brinton M. Lykes. 1985. LC 85-16240. v, 325p. (Orig.). pap. text 20.95 (0-8223-0262-4) Duke.

Gender & Psychoanalytic Treatment. Ed. by Morton Kissen. 1992. LC 92-17460. (Current Issues in

E F G

Psychoanalytic Practice Ser.: No. 5). 128p. text 31.95 (*0-87630-687-3*) Brunner-Routledge.

Gender & Psychology. Karen Trew & John Kremer. 1998. (Arnold Publication). (Illus.). 256p. pap. text 28.00 (*0-340-69179-4*) OUP.

Gender & Psychopathology. Ed. by Mary V. Seeman. 1995. LC 95-4161. 432p. text 54.00 (*0-88048-564-7*, 8564) Am Psychiatric.

Gender & Social Psychology. Vivien Burr. 1998. LC 97-37617. (Psychology Focus Ser.). (Illus.). 184p. (C). 52.95 (*0-415-15814-1*); pap. 15.95 (*0-415-15815-X*) Routledge.

Gender & Stress. Ed. by Rosalind Barnett et al. 1987. LC 87-12053. 400p. 50.00 (*0-02-901380-1*) Free Pr.

Gender & the Life Course. Ed. by Alice S. Rossi. 1985. LC 84-12335. (Illus.). 389p. pap. text 27.95 (*0-202-30312-8*) Aldine de Gruyter.

Gender & the Professional Predicament in Nursing. Celia Davies. 1995. LC 94-40172. 240p. pap. (*0-335-19402-8*) OpUniv Pr.

Gender & the Social Construction of Illness. Judith Lorber. 1997. LC 97-4588. (Gender Lens Ser.). 204p. pap. (*0-8039-5814-5*); 160p. (*0-8039-5813-7*) AltaMira Pr.

Gender Conundrum: Psychoanalytic Perspectives on Masculinity & Femininity. Ed. by Dana Birksted-Breen. 1993. LC 92-37650. (New Library of Psychoanalysis : No. 18). 664p. (C). pap. 31.95 (*0-415-09164-0*, B0875) Routledge.

Gender Development. Susan Golombok & Robyn Fivush. 1994. (Illus.). 287p. (C). text 54.95 (*0-521-40304-9*); pap. text 19.95 (*0-521-40862-8*) Cambridge U Pr.

Gender Differences in Human Cognition. John T. Richardson. 1997. LC 96-44115. (Counterpoints Ser.). (Illus.). 192p. pap. text 19.95 (*0-19-511291-1*) OUP.

Gender Differences in Metabolism: Practical & Nutritional Implications. Mark Tarnopolsky. 1998. LC 98-32080. (Nutrition in Exercise & Sport Ser.). 368p. 94.95 (*0-8493-8194-0*, 8194) CRC Pr.

Gender Differences in Mood & Anxiety Disorders: From Bench to Bedside. Ellen Leibenluft. 1999. LC 99-10440. (Review of Psychiatry Ser.: Vol. 18). 224p. 27.50 (*0-88048-958-8*) Am Psychiatric.

E
F
G

Gender Discrimination in X-Ray Technology: The Diminishing Role of the Male X-Ray Technologist. Ricardo Scott. 1999. (Ras Cardo Truths : Ras Cardo Speaks on Health). 85p. pap. (*1-883427-99-1*, RAS1999) Crnerstone GA.

Gender Disorders & the Paraphilias. William B. Arndt, Jr. 1991. 500p. 62.50 (*0-8236-2150-2*) Intl Univs Pr.

Gender Dysphoria: Development, Research & Management. B. W. Steiner. 1985. LC 84-18144. (Perspectives in Sexuality Ser.). (Illus.). 448p. (C). text 100.00 (*0-306-41694-8*, Kluwer Plenum) Kluwer Academic.

Gender Dysphoria: Interdisciplinary Approaches in Clinical Management. Ed. by Eli Coleman. 1993. LC 93-20482. (Journal of Psychology & Human Sexuality: Vol. 5, No. 4). (Illus.). 174p. pap. text 19.95 (*1-56024-473-9*); lib. bdg. 39.95 (*1-56024-459-3*) Haworth Pr.

Gender, Ethnicity & Health Research. Sana Loue. 1999. LC 99-33678. xiii, 195p. (C). text (*0-306-46172-2*, Kluwer Plenum) Kluwer Academic.

Gender Gap in Psychotherapy. Ed. by Patricia P. Rieker & Elaine H. Carmen. 1984. LC 84-11511. (Illus.). 392p. (C). 90.00 (*0-306-41657-3*, Plenum Trade) Perseus Pubng.

Gender, Health & Illness: A Case of Nerves. Ed. by Dona L. Davis & Setha M. Low. 1989. 175p. 63.95 (*0-89116-903-2*) Hemisp Pub.

Gender, Health & Longevity: Multidisciplinary Perspectives. Ed. by Marcia G. Ory & Huber R. Warner. 1990. LC 90-35541. 208p. 39.95 (*0-8261-7140-0*) Springer Pub.

Gender Identity Disorder & Psychosexual Problems in Children & Adolescents. Kenneth J. Zucker & Susan J. Bradley. 1995. LC 95-21764. 440p. 55.00 (*0-89862-266-2*, 2266) Guilford Pubns.

Gender in Early Childhood. Nicola Yelland. 1998. LC 97-49215. 288p. (C). 80.00 (*0-415-15408-1*); pap. 26.95 (*0-415-15409-X*) Routledge.

Gender in Psychoanalytic Space. Ed. by Muriel Dimen & Virginia Goldner. 1999. (C). (gr. 13). 55.00 (*0-415-91230-X*) Routledge.

Gender in Transition: A New Frontier. J. Offerman-Zuckerberg. 1989. (Illus.). 326p. (C). 59.50 (*0-306-43132-7*, Kluwer Plenum) Kluwer Academic.

***Gender Inequalities in Health: A Swedish Perspective.** Ed. by Piroska Ostlin. 2002. LC 2001-16628. 328p. pap. 15.00 (*0-674-00528-7*) HUP.

Gender Issues Across the Life Cycle. Ed. by Barbara R. Wainrib. 1992. LC 91-5141. 224p. 32.95 (*0-8261-7680-1*) Springer Pub.

Gender Issues in AIDS. Lorraine Sherr et al. 1997. LC 96-18071. (Social Aspects of AIDS Ser.). 283p. 89.95 (*0-7484-0231-4*); 208p. pap. 29.95 (*0-7484-0232-2*) Taylor & Francis.

Gender Issues in Clinical Psychology. Ed. by Paula Nicolson & Jane M. Ussher. 1992. LC 91-25284. 240p. (C). pap. 25.99 (*0-415-05486-9*) Routledge.

Gender Issues in Health Projects & Programmes. Sundari Ravindran. 1995. (Oxfam Research Discussion Papers). 28p. (C). pap. (*0-85598-295-0*) Oxfam Pub GBR. *Dist:* Stylus Pub VA.

Gender Issues in the Workplace: A Guide for Physician Executives. Ed. by J. Sim Tan. 1991. LC 97-72113. (Orig.). pap. text 25.95 (*0-924674-09-1*) Am Coll Phys Execs.

Gender Justice & the Health Care System. Karen L. Baird. 1998. LC 97-35313. (Health Care Policy in the United States Ser.). 286p. text 63.00 (*0-8153-3056-1*) Garland.

Gender of Sexuality: Exploring Sexual Possibilities. Pepper Schwartz & Virginia Rutter. 1998. LC 97-33723. (Gender Lens Ser.). 254p. (C). pap. (*0-8039-9042-1*) AltaMira Pr.

Gender Outlaw: On Men, Women & the Rest of Us. Kate Bornstein. 1994. LC 93-46979. (Illus.). 224p. (C). (gr. 13). 32.95 (*0-415-90897-3*) Routledge.

Gender Outlaw: On Men, Women & the Rest of Us. Kate Bornstein. 1995. LC 94-23477. (Illus.). 272p. pap. 13.00 (*0-679-75701-5*) Vin Bks.

Gender Power & Change in Health Institutions of the European Union. 1997. (*92-828-1362-2*, CE-07-97-507ENC) Comm Europ Commun BEL. *Dist:* Bernan Associates.

Gender, Power & Organization: A Psychological Perspective. Paula Nicolson. 1996. 192p. (C). pap. 24.95 (*0-415-10403-3*) Routledge.

Gender, Power & Relationships. Ed. by Charlotte Burck & Bebe Speed. 1994. LC 94-13591. 225p. (C). pap. 25.99 (*0-415-10637-0*, B4169) Routledge.

Gender-Specific Aspects of Human Biology for the Practicing Physician. Marianne J. Legato. 1996. LC 96-32122. 160p. 19.95 (*0-87993-648-7*) Futura Pub.

Gender, Work & Medicine: Women & the Medical Division of Labour. Elianne Riska & Katarina Wegar. 1993. LC 93-83603. (International Sociology Ser.: Vol. 44). (Illus.). 224p. (C). 69.95 (*0-8039-8902-4*, 9445); pap. 25.95 (*0-8039-8903-2*, 9446) Sage.

Gendercide: The Implications of Sex Selection. Mary E. Warren. 1985. LC 85-14452. (New Feminist Perspectives Ser.). 224p. (C). pap. 25.50 (*0-8476-7334-0*) Rowman.

Gendered Moods: Psychotropics & Society. Elizabeth Ettorre & Elianne Riska. 1995. LC 94-44550. 240p. (C). pap. 27.95 (*0-415-08214-5*); (gr. 13). 90.00 (*0-415-08213-7*) Routledge.

Gendered Object. Pat Kirkham. 1996. LC 95-40183. (Illus.). 272p. text (*0-7190-4474-X*); text (*0-7190-4475-8*) Manchester Univ Pr GBR. *Dist:* St Martin.

Gendering of Melancholia: Feminism, Psychoanalysis & the Symbolics of Loss in Renaissance Literature. Juliana Schiesari. 1992. LC 91-55529. 264p. 47.50 (*0-8014-2686-3*); pap. 18.95 (*0-8014-9971-2*) Cornell U Pr.

Gene: Its Structure, Function & Evolution. L. S. Dillon. 1987. LC 86-25291. (Illus.). 908p. (C). text 186.00 (*0-306-42319-7*, Kluwer Plenum) Kluwer Academic.

Gene Bomb: Does Higher Education & Advanced Technology Accelerate the Selection of Genes for Learning Disorders, ADHD, Addictive & Disruptive Behaviors. David E. Comings. 1996. LC 96-8110. 300p. pap. 25.95 (*1-878267-39-6*) Hope Pr CA.

Gene Engineering in Endocrinology. Ed. by Margaret A. Shupnik. 2000. LC 99-31872. (Contemporary Endocrinology Ser.: Vol. 22). (Illus.). 444p. 135.00 (*0-89603-718-5*) Humana.

Gene Expression & Its Control. Ed. by Kay E. Davies & Shirley M. Tilghman. 1991. (Genome Analysis Ser.: Vol. 2). (Illus.). 118p. (C). text 49.00 (*0-87969-359-2*) Cold Spring Harbor.

Gene Expression in Algae & Fungi Including Yeast: Bibliography January 1991-November 1992. Robert D. Warmbrodt. Ed. by Janet Saunders. 2001. 59p. (C). reprint ed. pap. 20.00 (*0-7881-2167-7*) DIANE Pub.

Gene Expression Technology. Ed. by John N. Abelson et al. 1990. (Methods in Enzymology Ser.: Vol. 185). 681p. text 121.00 (*0-12-182086-6*) Acad Pr.

Gene Future: The Promise & Perils of the New Biology. Thomas F. Lee. 1993. LC 93-27834. (Illus.). 350p. (C). 24.95 (*0-306-44509-3*) Da Capo.

Gene Interactions in Development. L. I. Korochkin. 1981. (Monographs in Theoretical & Applied Genetics: Vol. 4). (Illus.). 318p. 78.95 (*0-387-10112-8*) Spr-Verlag.

Gene-Mapping Techniques & Applications. Ed. by Lawrence B. Schook et al. 1991. (Illus.). 352p. text 199.00 (*0-8247-8535-5*) Dekker.

Gene Quantification. Ed. by Francois Ferre. 1997. LC 97-21838. (Advanced Biomedical Technologies Ser.). (*3-7643-3945-4*); (Illus.). 400p. 125.00 (*0-8176-3945-4*) Birkhauser.

Gene Regulation: A Eukaryotic Perspective. David S. Latchman. 3rd ed. 1998. 336p. pap. 49.95 (*0-412-81790-X*) Thomson Learn.

Gene Regulation by Steroid Hormones. Ed. by A. K. Roy & J. H. Clark. 1980. (Illus.). 316p. 175.00 (*0-387-90464-6*) Spr-Verlag.

Gene Regulation by Steroid Hormones II. Ed. by A. K. Roy & J. H. Clark. 1983. (Illus.). 384p. 205.00 (*0-387-90784-X*) Spr-Verlag.

Gene Regulation by Steroid Hormones III. Ed. by A. K. Roy & J. H. Clark. 1987. (Illus.). 302p. 223.00 (*0-387-96436-3*) Spr-Verlag.

Gene Splicing Wars: Reflections on the Recombinant DNA Controversy. Ed. by Raymond A. Zilinskas & Burke K. Zimmerman. 1986. 320p. (C). 27.95 (*0-02-948560-6*) Free Pr.

Gene Targeting. Manuel A. Vega. 1994. 256p. per. 83.95 (*0-8493-8950-X*) CRC Pr.

Gene Technology: Stem Cell & Leukemia Research. Ed. by Axel R. Zander et al. 1996. LC 96-4657. (NATO ASI Ser.: Vol. 94). 560p. 260.00 (*3-540-60743-9*) Spr-Verlag.

Gene Therapeutics: Methods & Applications of Direct Gene Transfer. Ed. by Jon A. Wolff. 1995. LC 93-42919. (Illus.). 417p. 89.00 (*0-8176-3650-1*) Birkhauser.

Gene Therapy. N. Lemoine & D. N. Cooper. 1996. (Human Molecular Genetics Ser.). 320p. text (*1-85996-205-X*) Bios Sci GBR. *Dist:* Bks Intl VA.

Gene Therapy. Ed. by K. Zanthopoulos. 1998. LC 98-2583. (NATO ASI Ser.: Series H, Vol. 105). (Illus.). 231p. 99.00 (*3-540-64112-2*) Spr-Verlag.

Gene Therapy: A Handbook for Physicians. Kenneth W. Culver. 1994. (Illus.). 128p. lib. bdg. 44.95 (*0-913113-63-8*) M Liebert.

Gene Therapy: Application of Molecular Biology. J. W. Larrick & K. B. Burck. 3rd ed. 1992. 575p. (C). pap. text 45.00 (*0-8385-3104-0*, A3104-5, Apple Lange Med) McGraw.

Gene Therapy: From Laboratory to the Clinic. K. M. Hui. 1994. LC 94-33830. 288p. pap. text 43.00 (*981-02-1655-6*) World Scientific Pub.

Gene Therapy: From Laboratory to the Clinic. Ed. by K. M. Hui. 1994. 600p. text 86.00 (*981-02-1654-8*) World Scientific Pub.

***Gene Therapy: Is There Oversight for Patient Safety: Congressional Hearing.** Ed. by Bill Frist. 2001. 126p. (C). pap. text 30.00 (*0-7567-1081-2*) DIANE Pub.

Gene Therapy: Principles & Applications. Ed. by T. Blankenstein. 1999. LC 98-37011. 400p. 132.00 (*3-7643-5972-2*) Birkhauser.

Gene Therapy & Molecular Biology Vol. 1: From Basic Mechanisms to Clinical Applications. Teni Boulikas. 1998. (Illus.). 832p. 127.00 (*1-892245-00-0*) Gene Therapy.

Gene Therapy & Neurological Diseases. Gary Weisinger & Jacques Mallet. 1999. 450p. 125.00 (*0-89603-558-1*) Humana.

Gene Therapy & Tissue Engineering in Orthopaedic & Sports Medicine. Ed. by Johnny Huard & Freddie H. Fu. 2000. LC 99-58338. (Methods in Bioengineering Ser.). (Illus.). xvi, 286p. 94.00 (*0-8176-4071-1*) Birkhauser.

Gene Therapy for Diseases of the Lung. Kenneth L. Brigham. 1997. LC 97-7151. (Lung Biology in Health & Disease Ser.: Vol. 104). (Illus.). 416p. text 195.00 (*0-8247-0060-0*) Dekker.

Gene Therapy for HIV Infection. Clay Smith. 1998. LC 98-23834. (Biotechnology Intelligence Unit Ser.). (*1-57059-540-2*) Landes Bioscience.

Gene Therapy for Neurological Disorders & Brain Tumors. Ed. by E. Antonio Chiocca & Xandra O. Breakefield. 1997. LC 97-42613. (Contemporary Neuroscience Ser.). (Illus.). 464p. 175.00 (*0-89603-507-7*) Humana.

Gene Therapy in Cancer. Ed. by Malcolm K. Breener & Robert C. Moen. 1996. (Basic & Clinical Oncology Ser.: Vol. 10). (Illus.). 256p. text 165.00 (*0-8247-9481-8*) Dekker.

Gene Therapy in Inflammatory Diseases. Ed. by C. H. Evans & P. D. Robbins. 2000. (Progress in Inflammation Research Ser.). (Illus.). 350p. 145.00 (*3-7643-5855-6*) Birkhauser.

Gene Therapy in the Treatment of Cancer: Progress & Prospects. Ed. by Brian E. Huber & Ian Magrath. 1999. LC 97-24818. (Cancer Ser.). (Illus.). 228p. (C). text 80.00 (*0-521-44436-5*) Cambridge U Pr.

Gene Therapy of Cancer: Methods & Protocols. Ed. by P. Walden et al. 1998. (Advances in Experimental Medicine & Biology Ser.: 451). (Illus.). 584p. (C). text 165.00 (*0-306-46027-0*, Kluwer Plenum) Kluwer Academic.

Gene Therapy of Cancer: Methods & Protocols. Ed. by Wolfgang Walther & Ulrike Stein. 2000. LC 99-38474. (Methods in Molecular Medicine Ser.: Vol. 35). (Illus.). 664p. 129.50 (*0-89603-714-2*); 99.50 (*0-89603-843-2*) Humana.

Gene Therapy of Cancer: Translational Approaches from Preclinical Studies to Clinical Implementation. Ed. by Edmund C. Lattime & Stanton L. Gerson. 1998. LC 98-85115. (Illus.). 406p. (C). 119.95 (*0-12-437190-6*) Acad Pr.

***Gene Therapy of Cancer: Translational Approaches from Preclinical Studies to Clinical Implementation.** Ed. by Edmund C. Lattime & Stanton L. Gerson. 2nd ed. 2001. 149.95 (*0-12-437551-0*) Acad Pr.

Gene Therapy Protocols. Ed. by Paul D. Robbins. 1996. LC 96-42147. (Methods in Molecular Medicine Ser.: Vol. 7). (Illus.). 448p. 140.00 (*0-89603-484-4*) Humana.

Gene Therapy Technologies & Regulations: From Laboratory to Clinic. Anthony Meager. 1999. LC 99-15301. (Illus.). 438p. 150.00 (*0-471-96709-2*) Wiley.

Gene Transcription. Robert J. White. 2001. LC 00-40330. (Illus.). 256p. pap. 39.95 (*0-632-04888-3*) Blackwell Sci.

Gene Transfer & Therapy in the Nervous System. Ed. by F. Gage & Yves Christen. 1992. LC 92-49569. (Research & Perspectives in Neurosciences Ser.). (*3-540-55889-6*); (Illus.). 268p. 91.00 (*0-387-55889-6*) Spr-Verlag.

Gene Transfer in the Cardiovascular System: Experimental Approaches & Therapeutic Implications. Ed. by Keith L. March. 1997. LC 96-29740. (Developments in Cardiovascular Medicine Ser.). 536p. (C). text 185.00 (*0-7923-9859-9*) Kluwer Academic.

Gene Vaccination: Theory & Practice. Ed. by E. Raz. 1998. LC 98-22471. (Principles & Practice Ser.). (Illus.). 192p. 129.00 (*3-540-64428-8*) Spr-Verlag.

Gene Wars: Science, Politics & the Human Genome. Robert Cook-Deegan. 1996. 416p. pap. 14.95 (*0-393-31399-9*, Norton Paperbks) Norton.

Genealogy of Psychoanalysis. Michel Henry. Tr. by Douglas Brick. 1993. LC 92-49101. 384p. (C). 61.00 (*0-8047-1604-8*) Stanford U Pr.

Genealogy of Trauma. Ruth Leys. 1999. LC 99-52681. x, 318p. lib. bdg. 55.00 (*0-226-47765-7*) U Ch Pr.

General Anatomy. D. Datta. 3rd ed. 1987. (C). (*0-7855-4655-3*) Current Dist IND. *Dist:* St Mut.

General & Emergency Surgery. Ed. by Simon Paterson-Brown. 1997. (Companion Guide to Specialist Surgical Practice Ser.: Vol. 1). (Illus.). 415p. text (*0-7020-2140-7*) W B Saunders GBR. *Dist:* Saunders.

General & Oral Pathology for the Dental Hygienist. Lynch & Pickett. 1991. (Illus.). 500p. 35.00 (*0-8016-3101-7*) Mosby Inc.

General & Oral Pathology for the Dental Hygienist. Miller. 1995. (C). (gr. 13). tchr. ed. (*0-8151-6952-3*) Mosby Inc.

General & Oral Pathology for the Dental Hygienist. Richard L. Miller et al. 1995. (Illus.). 400p. (C). (gr. 13). pap. text 43.00 (*0-8016-7024-1*, 07024) Mosby Inc.

General & Plastic Surgery Devices Panel Breast Implants Transcript of the FDA Panel Meeting on November 12, 13 & 14, 1991. Ed. by Bernard D. Reams. 1992. LC 92-49827. (Federal Health Law Ser.: Part 7). 1294p. reprint ed. 135.00 (*0-89941-806-6*, 307590) W S Hein.

General & Plastic Surgery Devices Panel Transcript of the FDA Meeting on Silicone Gel-Filled Breast Implants on February 18, 19 & 20, 1992. Ed. by Bernard D. Reams. 1992. LC 92-49830. (Federal Health Law Ser.: Part 6). 1390p. reprint ed. 135.00 (*0-89941-805-8*, 307600) W S Hein.

General & Systematic Pathology. J. C. Underwood. 3rd ed. 1999. LC 99-36745. (Illus.). 833p. text (*0-443-06285-4*) Church.

General & Vascular Ultrasound: Case Review. Middleton. 2000. (Illus.). 224p. pap. 39.95 (*0-323-00736-8*) Mosby Inc.

General Biology. Jack Rudman. 1994. (College Level Examination Ser.: CLEP-5). pap. 27.95 (*0-8373-5305-X*) Nat Learn.

General Book's Hardbound Hurts. (*0-201-62682-9*) Addison-Wesley.

General Chemistry Pearls of Wisdom. Clark. 1999. (Pearls of Wisdom Ser.). pap. 18.00 (*1-890369-22-5*) Boston Medical.

General Considerations, Vol. 1. Helen B. Taussig. 2nd ed. 1960. (Commonwealth Fund Publications). (Illus.). 232p. 29.50 (*0-674-16150-5*) HUP.

General Energetics: Energy in the Biosphere & Civilization. Vaclav Smil. 1991. LC 90-42106. (Environmental Science & Technology Ser.). 369p. 175.00 (*0-471-62905-7*) Wiley.

General Hematology. 1994. 250.00 (*1-56238-216-0*, SC7-B) NCCLS.

General Histology of the Mammal. R. V. Krstic. Tr. by S. Forster from GER. 1985. (Illus.). 404p. 116.00 (*0-387-15346-2*) Spr-Verlag.

General Histology of the Mammal: An Atlas for Students of Medicine & Biology. Radivoj V. Krstic. 1985. 404p. 98.95 (*3-540-15346-2*) Spr-Verlag.

General Human Pathology, Vol. 1. Davy Hovsky. 1969. 802p. 30.00 (*0-8464-1255-1*) Beekman Pubs.

General Immunology. E. L. Cooper. 1982. LC 80-42218. (Illus.). 300p. (*0-08-026368-2*) Pergamon Repr GBR. *Dist:* Franklin.

General Intensive Care. Goodland. 1978. 112p. pap. text (*0-7236-0503-3*) John Wright.

General Medical Knowledge for Eyecare Paraprofessionals. Marvin L. Bittinger. 1998. LC 98-21940. (Basic Bookshelf for Eyecare Professionals Ser.). (Illus.). 112p. pap. text 30.00 (*1-55642-334-9*, 63349) SLACK Inc.

General Microbiology: Study Guide. Wright. 1984. pap. text, stu. ed. 10.95 (*0-8016-5691-5*) Mosby Inc.

General Ophthamology: A Lange Medical Book. Daniel G. Vaughan et al. 15th ed. 1998. (Illus.). 500p. pap. 49.95 (*0-8385-3137-7*) McGraw-Hill Prof.

General, Organic & Biochemistry. Charles H. Henrickson & Larry C. Byrd. 2nd ed. 1996. 400p. (C). text, lab manual ed. 27.50 net. (*0-697-29399-8*, WCB McGr Hill) McGrw-H Hghr Educ.

General, Organic & Biological Chemistry. Michael S. Matta & Antony C. Wilbraham. 2nd ed. 1986. LC 85-15765. (Illus.). 800p. (C). text 47.50 (*0-8053-9630-6*) Benjamin-Cummings.

General, Organic & Biological Chemistry: A Brief Introduction. M. Lynn James & James O. Schreck. 1982. 480p. (C). text 63.96 (*0-669-03862-8*) HM Trade Div.

General, Organic & Biological Chemistry: Chemistry for the Living System. M. Lynn James et al. 1980. 752p. (C). tchr. ed. 2.66 *(0-669-01330-7)*; stu. ed. 25.96 *(0-669-01331-5)* HM Trade Div.

General Orthopaedics. Ed. by Frank C. Wilson & Patrick P. Lin. 1996. LC 96-35345. (Illus.). 558p. text 69.00 *(0-07-070757-X)* McGraw-Hill Prof.

General Pain Control in Dentistry. Norman Trieger. 2nd ed. 1993. LC 93-39375. (C). (gr. 13). text 52.00 *(1-55664-284-9)* Mosby Inc.

General Pathobiology. Paris Constantinides. 1994. LC 92-48537. (Illus.). 307p. (C). pap. text 44.95 *(0-8385-3119-9*, A3119-3, Apple Lange Med) McGraw.

General Pathology. Ian A. More & Ian L. Brown. 1991. (Colour Aids Ser.). (Illus.). 130p. (Orig.). pap. text *(0-443-04057-5)* Church.

General Pathology. Ian A. More & Ian L. Brown. 1994. LC 93-29877. (Colour Guide Ser.). (Orig.). pap. text 16.95 *(0-443-04949-1)* Harcrt Hlth Sci Grp.

General Pathology. J. B. Walter & M. S. Israel. 6th ed. 1987. (Illus.). 752p. text *(0-443-03089-8)* Church.

General Pathology: A Programmed Text. Thomas H. Kent. 1975. 33.50 *(0-316-48920-4*, Little Brwn Med Div) Lppncott W & W.

General Pathology, Microbiology, & Immunolgy for Health Care Students. J. H. Playfair et al. 1997. LC 97-49686. 229p. pap. text *(0-443-05722-2)* Church.

***General Pathology Vivas: Key Questions in Basic Pathology.** David Lowe. 2001. (Illus.). 226p. pap. incl. cd-rom *(1-84110-059-5)* Greenwich Med GBR. *Dist:* JAMCO Dist.

General Pharmacology. A. J. Clark. 1970. LC 75-105699. (Handbook of Experimental Pharmacology Ser.: Vol. 4). (Illus.). reprint ed. 76.95 *(0-387-04845-6)* Spr-Verlag.

General Physics Pearls of Wisdom. Amstutz. 1999. (Pearls of Wisdom Ser.). pap. 18.00 *(1-890369-23-3)* Boston Medical.

General Practice. 1964. (Technical Report Ser.: No. 267). 24p. pap. text 3.00 *(92-4-120267-X)* World Health.

General Practice. Nigel Ineson. 1996. (Medico-Legal Practitioner Ser.). 505p. *(1-85941-218-1)* Cavendish Pubng GBR. *Dist:* Gaunt.

General Practice. John Murtagh. 1994. 750p. text 79.00 *(0-07-452807-6)* McGraw-Hill Med Pub.

General Practice. R. J. Taylor et al. 1998. (Illus.). 128p. pap. *(0-443-06045-2)* Church.

General Practice. John Murtagh. 2nd ed. 1999. (Illus.). 1208p. text 129.00 *(0-07-470436-2)* McGraw-Hill Prof.

***General Practice: Companion Handbook.** John Murtagh. 2nd ed. 1999. (Companion Handbooks Ser.). (Illus.). 450p. 35.00 *(0-07-470722-1*, Apple Lange Med) McGraw.

***General Practice: Essential Facts.** Richard Jones & Scott Menzies. 1999. 128p. pap. *(1-85775-250-3)* Radcliffe Med Pr GBR. *Dist:* Balogh.

General Practice & Ethics. Christopher Dowrick & Lucy Frith. 1999. LC 98-38318. (Professional Ethics Ser.). (Illus.). x, 196p. 80.00 *(0-415-16498-2)*; pap. 26.95 *(0-415-16499-0)* Routledge.

General Practice Management Handbook: A Volume in The Management Of Health Care. Ed. by Peter Orton & Claire Hill. 1998. (Illus.). 270p. pap. *(0-7020-2204-7)* W B Saunders.

General Practitioner Education: U. K. & Nordic Perspectives. Ed. by M. Lawrence & L. Pritchard. 1992. 192p. 24.95 *(0-387-19741-9)* Spr-Verlag.

General Practitioner His Patient & Their Feelings: Exploring the Emotions Behind the Physical Symptoms. Sotiris Zalidis. 2000. 260p. pap. *(1-85343-527-9)* Free Assoc Bks GBR. *Dist:* Intl Spec Bk.

General Practitioner's Guide to Genitourinary Medicine & Sexual Health. Chris Sonnex. 1996. (Illus.). 121p. (C). pap. text 31.95 *(0-521-55656-2)* Cambridge U Pr.

General Practitioners' Update. 1999. 99.00 incl. audio PA Bar Inst.

General Principles in the Basic Sciences. National Medical School Review Staff. 1996. LC 96-22034. (Board Simulator Ser.). 263p. pap. 24.95 *(0-683-06330-8)* Lppncott W & W.

General Principles in the Basic Sciences: A Body Systems-Based Review for USMLE Step 1. National Medical School Review Staff. 2nd ed. 1997. LC 97-6903. (Board Simulator Ser.). 375p. pap. text 25.95 *(0-683-30296-5)* Lppncott W & W.

General Principles of Human Reflexology: An Introduction to the Objective Study of Personality. Vladimir M. Bechterev. 1976. LC 73-2961. (Classics in Psychology Ser.). reprint ed. 30.95 *(0-405-05134-4)* Ayer.

General Processes of Radiotracer Localization. Leopold J. Anghileri & L. Colombetti. 1982. LC 81-18063. (Radiotracers Biology & Medicine Ser.). 272p. 153.00 *(0-8493-6027-7*, CRC Reprint) Franklin.

General Processes of Radiotracer Localization, Vol. II. Ed. by Leopold J. Anghileri. 1982. 272p. 152.00 *(0-8493-6028-5*, QP519, CRC Reprint) Franklin.

General Psychology. Jack Rudman. (College Level Examination Ser.: Vol. 14). 47.95 *(0-8373-5364-5)* Nat Learn.

General Psychopathology. Karl Jaspers. Tr. by J. Hoenig & Marian W. Hamilton. 1997. LC 97-18291. (General Psychopathology Ser.: Vol. 1). 594p. Vol. 1. pap. text 26.00 *(0-8018-5775-9)*; Vol. 2. pap. text 26.00 *(0-8018-5815-1)* Johns Hopkins.

General Psychopathology. Karl Jaspers. 7th ed. 1963. LC 63-9736. lib. bdg. 55.00 *(0-226-39487-5)* U Ch Pr.

General Relief-Medical: Last Resort for the Uninsured. Catherine L. Gaylord & David Schaefer. 1989. 181p. (Orig.). pap. 20.00 *(0-932622-16-X)* Ctr Public Rep.

General Sonography: A Clinical Guide. Beth Anderhub. 1994. (Illus.). 416p. (C). (gr. 13). text 53.00 *(0-8016-7421-2*, 00031) Mosby Inc.

General Surgery. Alex M. Jacocks. 2nd ed. 1996. LC 96-13502. (Oklahoma Notes). 189p. pap. text 24.95 *(0-387-94637-3)* Spr-Verlag.

General Surgery at the District Hospital. Ed. by J. Cook et al. 1988. (ENG, FRE, RUS & SPA., Illus.). 230p. pap. text 27.00 *(92-4-154235-7*, 1150300) World Health.

General Surgery Board Review. Ed. by Michael S. Gold et al. 3rd ed. 1998. LC 98-29424. (Illus.). 544p. pap. text 59.95 *(0-397-51851-X)* Lppncott W & W.

General Surgery Module. Ed. by American Association for Medical Transcription Staff. 2nd ed. 1996. (Exploring Transcription Practices Ser.). 93p. (C). wbk. ed. 225.00 incl. audio *(0-935229-29-9)* Am Assoc Med.

General Surgery MS Pearls of Wisdom: Over 3000 Questions. Breckler & Maull. 1999. (Pearls of Wisdom Ser.). pap. 32.00 *(1-890369-19-5)* Boston Medical.

General Surgery Pearls of Wisdom. Breckler & Maull. 1998. (Pearls of Wisdom Ser.). pap. 88.00 *(1-890369-11-X)* Boston Medical.

***General Surgical Anatomy & Examination: An Illustrated Color Test.** Alastair Thompson. 2001. (Illus.). 107p. pap. *(0-443-06376-1)* Church GBR. *Dist:* Saunders.

General Surgical Operations. Ed. by R. M. Kirk & R. C. Williamson. 3rd ed. 1994. LC 93-9078. text *(0-443-04715-4)* Church.

General Surgical Operations. R. M. Kirk. 4th ed. 2000. (Illus.). 775p. text 135.00 *(0-443-06396-6)* Saunders.

General Surgical Outpatient Decisions. 2000. (Illus.). 384p. pap. *(0-7506-4124-X)* E A GBR. *Dist:* OUP.

General Symptoms, Vol. 2. H. Barthel. 1987. 491p. 130.00 *(3-7760-0560-2)* Medicina Bio.

General Systems Theory & Psychiatry. Ed. by W. Gray et al. 1982. (Systems Inquiry Ser.). 450p. (Orig.). (C). reprint ed. pap. text 17.95 *(0-914105-07-8)* Intersystems Pubns.

General Systems Theory Applied to Nursing. Arlene M. Putt. 1978. 14.00 *(0-316-72300-2*, Little Brwn Med Div) Lppncott W & W.

General Techniques of Hypnotism. Andre M. Weitzenhoffer. 1967. (Illus.). 476p. text 78.00 *(0-8089-0523-6*, 794785, Grune & Strat) Harcrt Hlth Sci Grp.

General Thoracic Surgical Anatomy & Procedures. Jonathan C. Nesbitt & Gary G. Wind. 1998. 500p. *(0-683-06429-0)* Lppncott W & W.

General Ultrasound. Ed. by Carol A. Mittelstaedt. 1992. (Illus.). 1231p. text *(0-443-08735-0)* Church.

General Zoology. Tracy I. Storer et al. 6th ed. 1979. 928p. (C). 54.69 *(0-07-061780-5)* McGraw.

General Zoology of the Invertebrates. G. S. Carter. 1965. (Illus.). (C). 35.00 *(0-8464-1166-0)* Beekman Pubs.

Generalization for Students with Severe Handicaps: Strategies & Solutions. Ed. by Norris G. Haring. 1989. (Illus.). 224p. pap. 20.00 *(0-295-96807-9)* U of Wash Pr.

Generalized Epilepsy. M. Avoli et al. 1990. 500p. 140.50 *(0-8176-3445-2)* Birkhauser.

Generalized Nets in General & Internal Medicine. A. Shannon et al. 1998. (Illus.). 223p. pap. *(954-430-542-4)* Akadem izdatelstvo BGR. *Dist:* Coronet Bks.

Generalized Nets in Medicine. A. G. Shannon et al. 1997. (Illus.). 186p. pap. *(954-430-501-7)* Akadem izdatelstvo BGR. *Dist:* Intl Scholars.

Generalized Nets in Neurology. K. Atanasov et al. 1997. (Illus.). 359p. pap. *(954-430-522-X)* Akadem izdatelstvo BGR. *Dist:* Intl Scholars.

Generalized Non-Convulsive Epilepsy: Focus on GABA-B Receptors. Ed. by C. Marescaux et al. 1992. LC 92-2422. (Journals of Neural Transmission: Suppl. 35). (Illus.). 160p. 111.00 *(0-387-82340-9)* Spr-Verlag.

Generating Fluent Speech: A Comprehensive Speech Processing Approach: Program. 1997. LC 96-47774. pap. 159.00 *(0-930599-48-9)* Thinking Pubns.

Generation of Antibodies by Cell & Gene Immortalization. Ed. by C. P. Terhorst et al. 1993. (Year in Immunology Ser.: Vol. 7). (Illus.). x, 246p. 239.25 *(3-8055-5714-0)* S Karger.

Generation of Diversity: Clonal Selection Theory & the Rise of Molecular Immunology. Scott H. Podolsky & Alfred I. Tauber. 1998. LC 97-22942. (Illus.). 512p. 78.95 *(0-674-77181-8)* HUP.

Generation on Hold: Coming of Age in the Late Twentieth Century. James E. Cote & Anton L. Allahar. 1995. 220p. (C). text 45.00 *(0-8147-1531-1)*; LC 95-18151. pap. text 18.50 *(0-8147-1532-X)* NYU Pr.

Generativity & Adult Development: How & Why We Care for the Next Generation. Ed. by Dan P. McAdams & Ed de St. Aubin. 1998. LC 97-32831. 511p. 49.95 *(1-55798-470-0)* Am Psychol.

Generic & Innovator Drugs: A Guide to FDA Approval Requirements. Donald O. Beers. 3rd ed. 1992. 1280p. ring bd. 136.00 *(0-13-225111-6)* Aspen Law.

Generic & Innovator Drugs: A Guide to FDA Approval Requirements. Donald O. Beers. 5th ed. 1995. LC 98-37519. 1992p. 215.00 *(0-7355-0281-1)* Panel Pubs.

Generic Drug Identification Guide. J. R. Swim. 3rd ed. 1990. LC 90-81369. 330p. pap. text 21.95 *(0-9626339-0-9)* Drug Info Serv Co.

Generic Prescription Pharmaceutical Markets: Patent Expirations Breathe New Life into Generic Competitors. Market Intelligence Staff. 1993. 314p. 1995.00 *(1-56753-480-5)* Frost & Sullivan.

Genero y la Reforma del Sector Salud. Hilary Standing. 2000. (SPA.). pap. 14.00 *(92-75-32283-X)* PAHO.

Generous Confidence see Art of Asylum-Keeping: Thomas Story Kirkbride & the Origins of American Psychiatry

Genes & Aging. M. S. Kanungo. 1994. LC 93-2766. (Illus.). 336p. (C). text 90.00 *(0-521-38299-8)* Cambridge U Pr.

Genes & Antigenes in Cancer Cells: The Monocolonal Antibody Approach. Ed. by Hilary Koprowski et al. 1984. (Beitraege Zur Onkologie, Contributions to Oncology Ser.: Vol. 19). (Illus.). x, 192p. 55.00 *(3-8055-3843-X)* S Karger.

Genes & Environment in Cancer. Ed. by M. Schwab et al. 1998. LC 98-21384. (Recent Results in Cancer Research Ser.: Vol. 154). (Illus.). 382p. 129.00 *(3-540-64430-X)* Spr-Verlag.

Genes & Gender: On Hereditarianism & Women, Vol. I. Ed. by Ethel Tobach & Betty Rosoff. 1978. LC 78-50640. 96p. pap. 12.50 *(0-87752-215-4)* Gordian.

Genes & Gender Four: The Second X & Women's Health. Ed. by Myra Fooden et al. 1983. LC 83-5552. 203p. (C). pap. 15.00 *(0-87752-223-5)* Gordian.

Genes & Gender Two: Pitfalls in Research on Sex & Gender. Ed. by Ruth Hubbard et al. 1979. LC 78-50640. 160p. pap. text 12.50 *(0-87752-219-7)* Gordian.

Genes & Genetics of Autoimmunity. Ed. by Argyrios N. Theofilopoulos. 2nd ed. 1999. LC 99-19308. (Current Directions in Autoimmunity Ser.). (Illus.). x, 340p. pap. 200.00 *(3-8055-6814-2)* S Karger.

Genes & Mechanisms in Vertebrate Sex Determination. G. William Scherer & M. Schmidt. 2001. LC 00-48566. (Milestones in Drug Therapy Ser.: Vol. 91). (Illus.). xii, 205p. 109.00 *(3-7643-6168-9)* Birkhauser.

Genes & Phenotypes. Ed. by Kay E. Davies & Shirley M. Tilghman. 1991. (Genome Analysis Ser.: Vol. 3). 174p. (C). text 49.00 *(0-87969-402-5)* Cold Spring Harbor.

Genes & Proteins Underlying Microbial Urinary Tract Virulence: Basic Aspects & Applications. Ed. by Levente Emody et al. 2000. LC 00-42249. (Advances in Experimental Medicine & Biology Ser.: Vol. 485). (Illus.). 382p. 110.00 *(0-306-46455-1*, Kluwer Plenum) Kluwer Academic.

***Genes & Viruses in Multiple Sclerosis.** Ed. by O. R. Hommes et al. 2001. 276p. 125.00 *(0-444-50694-2)* Elsevier.

Genes & Your Fate: Understanding Your Genetic Heritage. Philip R. Reilly. 1994. text 24.95 *(0-02-926045-0)* Free Pr.

Genes, Blood & Courage: A Boy Called Immortal Sword. David G. Nathan. 1995. LC 95-6080. (Illus.). 288p. (C). 24.95 *(0-674-34473-1*, Belknap) HUP.

Genes, Brains & Politics: Self Selection & Social Life. Elliott White. 1993. LC 92-28548. (Human Evolution, Behavior, & Intelligence Ser.). 208p. 60.00 *(0-275-94468-9*, C4468, Praeger Pubs) Greenwood.

Genes, Cancer, & Ethics in the Work Environment. Ed. by Sheldon W. Samuels & Arthur C. Upton. 1998. LC 98-226374. 184p. text 49.00 *(1-883595-18-5*, 23045, OEM Pr) OEM Health.

Genes, Cancer & Radiation Protection. Ed. by Mortimer Mendelsohn. 1992. LC 92-49792. (Annual Meeting Proceedings Ser.: No. 13). 350p. (Orig.). pap. text 40.00 *(0-929600-24-X)* NCRP Pubns.

Genes, Culture & Personality: An Empirical Approach. L. J. Eaves et al. 1989. 750p. text 100.00 *(0-12-228290-6)* Acad Pr.

Genes in Medicine: Molecular Biology & Human Genetic Disorders. Istvan Rasko & C. Stephen Downes. 1994. LC 94-72640. (Illus.). 419p. (C). (gr. 13). pap. text 53.95 *(0-412-37340-8)* Chapman & Hall.

Genes Involved in the Metastatic Process. Ed. by R. S. Kerbek. 1989. (Journal: Vol. 9, No. 6, 1989). (Illus.). 84p. pap. 35.75 *(3-8055-5118-5)* S Karger.

Genes on the Couch: Explorations in Evolutionary Psychology. Paul Gilbert & Kent G. Bailey. 2000. LC 00-59072. 384p. 44.95 *(1-58391-102-2)* Brunner-Routledge.

Genes, Oncogenes & Hormones: Advances in Cellular & Molecular Biology of Breast Cancer. Ed. by Robert B. Dickson & Marc E. Lipman. 1992. LC 92-15491. (Cancer Treatment & Research Ser.: Vol. 61). 464p. text 257.50 *(0-7923-1748-3)* Kluwer Academic.

Genesis of Glaucoma. Ed. by H. J. Merte. 1978. (Documenta Ophthalmologica Proceedings Ser.: No. 16). text 171.00 *(90-6193-156-8)* Kluwer Academic.

Genesis of Hand Preference. Minnie Giesecke. 1936. (SRCD M Ser.: Vol. 1, No. 5). 25.00 *(0-527-01490-7)* Periodicals Srv.

Genethics: Moral Issues in the Creation of People. David Heyd. 1992. LC 91-30300. 276p. (C). text 55.00 *(0-520-07714-8)* U CA Pr.

GenEthics: Technological Intervention in Human Reproduction As a Philosophical Problem. Kurt Bayertz. 1995. 362p. (C). text 90.00 *(0-521-41693-0)* Cambridge U Pr.

Genetic Alchemy: The Social History of the Recombinant DNA Controversy. Sheldon Krimsky. 1984. (Illus.). 440p. pap. 25.00 *(0-262-61038-8)* MIT Pr.

Genetic Analysis of Autoimmune Diseases Using Animal Models: Mapping Susceptivility Genes for Multiple Sclerosis & Rheumatoid Arthritis. Hai-Tao Yang. 2000. (Comprehensive Summaries of Uppsala Dissertations from the Faculty of Medicine Ser.: No. 927). (Illus.). 44p. pap. *(91-554-4717-1)* Uppsala Universitet SWE. *Dist:* Coronet Bks.

Genetic Analysis of Tumour Suppression - Symposium No. 142. CIBA Foundation Staff. 1989. (CIBA Foundation Symposia Ser.: No. 142). 268p. 128.00 *(0-471-92299-4)* Wiley.

Genetic Analysis Workshop Seven: Issues in Gene Mapping & Detection of Major Genes Held at Bergamo Conference Center, Dayton, Ohio, October 1990. Ed. by David R. Cox et al. 1992. (Journal: Vol. 59, No. 2-3, 1992). (Illus.). 176p. pap. 62.75 *(3-8055-5578-4)* S Karger.

Genetic & Biochemical Aspects of the Development of Datura. Marie E. Conklin. Ed. by A. Wolsky. 1976. (Monographs in Developmental Biology: Vol. 12). (Illus.). 170p. 65.25 *(3-8055-2307-6)* S Karger.

Genetic & Chemical Causes of Mental Disorders. 1991. lib. bdg. 77.95 *(0-8490-4614-9)* Gordon Pr.

***Genetic & Environmental Risk Factors for Cervical Carcinoma in Situ.** Agnetha Josefsson. 2000. (Comprehensive Summaries of Uppsala Dissertations from the Faculty of Medicine Ser.: No. 917). (Illus.). 45p. pap. *(91-554-4688-4)* Uppsala Universitet SWE. *Dist:* Coronet Bks.

Genetic & Environmental Risk Factors of Major Cardiovascular Malformations: The Baltimore-Washington Infant Study - 1981-1989. Ed. by Charlotte Ferencz et al. 1997. (Perspectives in Pediatric Cardiology Ser.: No. 5). (Illus.). 496p. 95.00 *(0-87993-675-4)* Futura Pub.

Genetic & Physical Mapping. Ed. by Kay E. Davies & Shirley M. Tilghman. 1991. (Genome Analysis Ser.: Vol. 1). (Illus.). 250p. (C). text 49.00 *(0-87969-358-4)* Cold Spring Harbor.

Genetic & Therapeutic Aspects of Lipids & Purine Metabolism. Ed. by G. Wolfram. 1989. (Illus.). 162p. 79.95 *(0-387-50408-7)* Spr-Verlag.

Genetic Approaches in the Prevention of Mental Disorders. Ed. by V. Bulyzhenkov et al. 1990. (Illus.). 119p. 66.95 *(0-387-52244-1)* Spr-Verlag.

Genetic Approaches of Coronary Heart Disease & Hypertension. Ed. by Kare Berg et al. 1991. (Illus.). 150p. 109.00 *(0-387-54476-3)* Spr-Verlag.

Genetic Approaches to Development Neurobiology. Ed. by Y. Tsukada. 1982. (Illus.). 269p. 69.95 *(0-387-11872-1)* Spr-Verlag.

Genetic Approaches to Mental Disorders. Ed. by Elliot S. Gershon & C. Robert Cloninger. 1994. LC 93-3019. (American Psychopathological Association Ser.). 320p. text 19.95 *(0-88048-951-0*, 8951) Am Psychiatric.

Genetic Approaches to Noncummunicable Diseases. Ed. by Kare Berg et al. 1995. (Illus.). 155p. 89.95 *(3-540-60289-5)* Spr-Verlag.

Genetic Aspects Anaphylactoid Reactions. Ed. by P. Dukor et al. 1980. (Par Pseudo-Allergic Reactions, Involvement of Drugs & Chemicals Ser.: Vol. 1). (Illus.). xiv, 310p. 113.25 *(3-8055-0537-X)* S Karger.

Genetic Aspects of Alcoholism. Ed. by K. Kiianmaa et al. 1989. (Finnish Foundation for Alcohol Studies: Vol. 37). pap. 30.00 *(951-9192-40-9)* Rutgers Ctr Alcohol.

Genetic Basis at Spontaneous Activity in the Albino Rat. Elizabeth G. Brody. 1942. (Comparative Psychology Monographs). pap. 40.00 *(0-527-24924-6)* Periodicals Srv.

Genetic Basis for Carcinogenesis: Tumor Suppressor Genes & Oncogenes. Ed. by Alfred Knudson, Jr. et al. 1990. (Princess Takamatsu Symposia Ser.: No. 20). 336p. *(0-7484-0017-6)* Tay Francis Ltd GBR. *Dist:* Taylor & Francis.

Genetic Basis of Abnormal Human Behavior. Charles D. Mellon. 1997. LC 96-77828. (Illus.). 260p. pap. 19.95 *(0-9653362-4-7)* Genetics Heritage.

Genetic Basis of Alcohol & Drug Actions. J. C. Crabbe, Jr. & R. A. Harris. 1991. (Illus.). 400p. (C). text 110.00 *(0-306-43868-2*, Kluwer Plenum) Kluwer Academic.

Genetic Basis of Autoimmune Disease: Cellular & Genetic Basis. Ed. by Julius M. Cruse & R. E. Lewis. 1988. (Concepts in Immunopathology Ser.: Vol. 5). (Illus.). vi, 202p. 148.00 *(3-8055-4635-1)* S Karger.

Genetic Basis of Common Diseases. Ed. by Richard A. King et al. 1992. (Oxford Monographs on Medical Genetics: No. 20). (Illus.). 992p. text 150.00 *(0-19-505482-2)* OUP.

Genetic Basis of Human Cancer. Bert Vogelstein & Kenneth W. Kinzler. 1997. LC 97-26598. (Illus.). 744p. text 99.00 *(0-07-067596-1)* McGraw-Hill Prof.

Genetic Connections: A Guide to Documenting Your Individual & Family Health History. Danette L. Nelson-Anderson & Cynthia V. Waters. 1995. LC 94-67892. (Illus.). 335p. pap. 34.95 *(0-9639154-3-6)*; text 39.95 *(0-9639154-2-8)* Sonters Pubng.

E F G

Genetic Counseling. W. Fuhrmann & F. Vogel. Tr. by S. Kurth-Scherer from GER. 3rd ed. 1982. (Illus.). 188p. 82.95 (*0-387-90715-7*) Spr-Verlag.

Genetic Counseling: Psychological Dimensions. Ed. by Seymour Kessler. 1979. LC 78-87879. text 85.00 (*0-12-405650-4*) Acad Pr.

Genetic Counselling: Practice & Principles. Ed. by Angus Clarke. 1994. LC 93-5884. (Professional Ethics Ser.). (Illus.). (C). 280p. 90.00 (*0-415-08257-9*, B3413); 272p. pap. 29.95 (*0-415-08258-7*, B3417) Routledge.

Genetic Destiny: Scientific Controversy & Social Conflict, No. 11. Ed. by Harold M. Proshansky. LC 76-5964. (Studies in Modern Society: Political & Social Issues). 32.50 (*0-404-10130-5*) AMS Pr.

Genetic Determinants of Pulmonary Disease. Litwin. 1978. (Lung Biology in Health & Disease Ser.: Vol. 11). (Illus.). 304p. text 165.00 (*0-8247-6608-3*) Dekker.

Genetic Differences in Chemical Carcinogenesis. R. E. Kouri. 1980. 240p. 135.00 (*0-8493-5285-1*, RC268, CRC Reprint) Franklin.

Genetic Disease: The Unwanted Inheritance. Ed. by John D. Rainer et al. 1989. LC 89-20100. (Loss, Grief & Care Ser.: Vol. 3, Nos. 3 & 4). (Illus.). 213p. text 6.95 (*0-86656-953-7*) Haworth Pr.

Genetic Disease in Dogs: A Guide to Diagnosis & Control. Patterson. 1999. 288p. (C). (gr. 13). pap. text 44.95 (*0-8151-4380-X*, 31126) Mosby Inc.

***Genetic Diseases of Dogs: A Guide to Diagnosis & Control - Information Package.** Donald F. Patterson. 2001. 150.00 (*0-323-01241-8*) Mosby Inc.

Genetic Diseases of the Eye Ed. by Elias I. Traboulsi. 1999. LC 97-34011. (Oxford Monographs on Medical Genetics: No. 36). (Illus.). 916p. text 198.50 (*0-19-509676-2*) OUP.

Genetic Diseases of the Skin. V. M. Der Kaloustian & A. K. Kurban. 1979. LC 78-25740. (Illus.). 339p. 195.00 (*0-387-09151-3*) Spr-Verlag.

Genetic Disorders among Arab Populations. Ed. by Ahmad S. Teebi & T. I. Farag. 1996. (Oxford Monographs on Medical Genetics: No. 30). (Illus.). 520p. text 98.50 (*0-19-509305-4*) OUP.

Genetic Disorders & Pregnancy Outcome. Ed. by Lawrence D. Platt. 1997. LC 96-39335. 156p. 93.95 (*1-85070-721-9*, Parthenon Pbng) CRC Pr.

Genetic Disorders & the Fetus: Diagnosis, Prevention & Treatment. A. Milunsky. 2nd ed. 1986. LC 86-20477. (Illus.). 924p. (C). text 155.00 (*0-306-42301-4*, Kluwer Plenum) Kluwer Academic.

Genetic Disorders & the Fetus: Diagnosis, Prevention, & Treatment. Ed. by Aubrey Milunsky. 4th ed. 1998. LC 97-41341. 1,198p. 175.00 (*0-8018-5801-1*) Johns Hopkins.

Genetic Disorders of Endocrine Neoplasia. Ed. by P. L. M. Dahia & C. Eng. 2001. (Frontiers of Hormone Research Ser.: Vol. 28). (Illus.). viii, 218p. 239.25 (*3-8055-7203-4*) S Karger.

Genetic Disorders-Prevention, Treatment & Rehabilitation: Proceedings of the WHO Scientific Group, Geneva, 1968. WHO Staff. 1972. (Technical Reports: No. 497). pap. text 6.00 (*92-4-120497-4*, 1100497) World Health.

Genetic Disorders Sourcebook: Basic Information about Heritable Diseases & Disorders & Including Source Listings for Further Help & Information. Ed. by Karen Bellenir. 1996. LC 95-44907. (Health Reference Ser.: Vol. 13). xi, 642p. lib. bdg. 78.00 (*0-7808-0034-6*) Omnigraphics Inc.

Genetic Effects on Aging. Ed. by David E. Hamson. 1990. (Illus.). 400p. 83.00 (*0-936923-31-8*, QP86) CRC Pr.

Genetic Engineering: Principles & Methods. Ed. by Jane K. Setlow & Alexander Hollaender. LC 79-644807. Vol. 1. 1979. 278p. 69.50 (*0-306-40154-1*); Vol. 2. 1980. 294p. 69.50 (*0-306-40447-8*); Vol. 3. 1981. 356p. 69.50 (*0-306-40729-9*); Vol 6. 1984. 356p. 69.50 (*0-306-41710-3*); Vol. 7. 1985. 370p. 69.50 (*0-306-42004-X*) Perseus Pubng (Plenum Trade).

Genetic Engineering: Principles & Methods, Vol. 9. Ed. by Jane K. Setlow. 1987. LC 79-644807. (Illus.). 300p. 69.50 (*0-306-42663-3*, Plenum Trade) Perseus Pubng.

Genetic Engineering: The Ethical Issues. J. K. Anderson. 1982. 128p. (Orig.). pap. 4.95 (*0-310-45051-9*, 12707P) Zondervan.

Genetic Engineering & Biotechnology Related Firms Worldwide Directory 1994-95. 13th ed. 1994. 599.00 (*1-880866-08-0*) Intl Pubns Serv.

Genetic Engineering Benefits & Biohazards. Ananda M. Chakrabarty. 1978. (Uniscience Ser.). 208p. 75.00 (*0-8493-5259-2*, QH442, CRC Reprint) Franklin.

Genetic Engineering, DNA & Cloning: A Bibliography in the Future of Genetics. Joseph Menditto & Debbie Kirsch. 1983. LC 82-50417. xiv, 783p. 65.00 (*0-87875-241-2*) Whitston Pub.

Genetic Engineering of Plants & Micro-Organisms Important for Agriculture. Ed. by E. Magnien & D. De Nettancourt. 1985. (Advances in Agricultural Biotechnology Ser.). text 145.50 (*90-247-3131-3*) Kluwer Academic.

Genetic Epidemiology of Cancer. Ed. by Henry T. Lynch & Takeshi Hirayama. 1989. 376p. 249.00 (*0-8493-6756-5*, RC268) CRC Pr.

Genetic Errors of Glycoprotein Metabolism. Ed. by P. Durand & J. S. O'Brien. 1983. (Illus.). 220p. 68.95 (*0-387-12066-1*) Spr-Verlag.

Genetic Factors in Atherosclerosis: Approaches & Model Systems. Ed. by Robert S. Sparkes & A. J. Lusis. 1989. (Monographs in Human Genetics: Vol. 12). (Illus.). x, 227p. 172.25 (*3-8055-4890-7*) S Karger.

Genetic Factors in Congenital Malformations: Proceedings of the WHO Scientific Group, Geneva, 1968. WHO Staff. 1970. (Technical Reports: No. 438). pap. text 5.00 (*92-4-120438-9*, 1100438) World Health.

Genetic Factors in Coronary Heart Disease. Ed. by Uri Goldbourt et al. 1994. LC 94-4615. 480p. text 276.00 (*0-7923-2752-7*) Kluwer Academic.

Genetic Factors in Drug Therapy: Clinical & Molecular Pharmacogenetics. Evans D. Price. 1994. (Illus.). 681p. (C). text 140.00 (*0-521-41296-X*) Cambridge U Pr.

Genetic Field Theory of Ego Formation: Its Implications for Pathology. Rene A. Spitz. 1962. LC 58-9230. (New York Psychoanalytic Institute Freud Anniversary Lecture Ser.). (Illus.). 123p. 27.50 (*0-8236-2180-4*) Intl Univs Pr.

Genetic Immune & Molecular Predisposition to Hypertension. Ed. by P. M. Frossard et al. 1999. (Illus.). 276p. (*90-6764-311-4*) Uppsala Universitet SWE. *Dist:* Coronet Bks.

***Genetic Information & Health Care: Congressional Hearing.** Ed. by James M. Jeffords. 2001. 72p. (C). reprint ed. pap. text 25.00 (*0-7567-0285-2*) DIANE Pub.

Genetic Instabilities & Hereditary Neurological Diseases. Ed. by Robert D. Wells et al. 1998. LC 98-84947. (Illus.). 829p. (C). 159.95 (*0-12-742935-2*) Acad Pr.

Genetic Instability & Tumorigenesis. Ed. by M. B. Kastan et al. 1996. LC 97-108052. (Current Topics in Microbiology & Immunology Ser.: Vol. 221). (Illus.). 180p. 140.00 (*3-540-61518-0*) Spr-Verlag.

Genetic Issues for Perinatal Nurses. Lynn G. Wellman et al. 1996. LC 96-20007. (*0-86525-071-5*) March of Dimes.

Genetic Manipulation. J. Grange et al. 1990. 135.00 (*0-632-02926-9*) Blackwell Sci.

Genetic Manipulation: Impact on Man & Society. Werner Arber et al. 1984. LC 83-26166. 304p. text 85.00 (*0-521-26417-0*) Cambridge U Pr.

Genetic Manipulation of the Kidney. Ed. by Masanori Kitamura. 1997. (Journal: Vol. 5, No. 2, 1997). (Illus.). 78p. pap. 39.25 (*3-8055-6480-5*) S Karger.

Genetic Mapping of Disease Genes. Ed. by I. H. Pawlowitzki et al. 1997. LC 97-11844. (Illus.). 288p. text 75.00 (*0-12-232735-7*) Acad Pr.

Genetic Markers of Haematological Malignancy: Journal: Tumor Biology 1990, Vol 2, Suppl. 1. Ed. by P. H. Pinkerton & M. D. Reis. 1990. (Illus.). iv, 94p. pap. 30.50 (*3-8055-5312-9*) S Karger.

Genetic Mechanisms in Multiple Endocrine Neoplasia Type 2A. Barry D. Nelkin. 1996. (Medical Intelligence Unit Ser.). 200p. (C). pap. 89.95 (*0-412-10771-6*) Chapman & Hall.

Genetic Mechanisms in Multiple Endocrine Neoplasia Type 2A. Barry D. Nelkin. 1996. LC 96-30948. (Medical Intelligence Unit Ser.). 202p. 99.00 (*1-57059-402-3*) Landes Bioscience.

Genetic Medicine. Karl H. Muench. 1992. (Illus.). 399p. (C). pap. text 45.00 (*0-8385-3121-0*, A3121-9, Apple Lange Med) McGraw.

Genetic Medicine: A Logic of Disease. Barton Childs. 1999. LC 99-12783. (Illus.). 376p. 59.95 (*0-8018-6130-6*) Johns Hopkins.

Genetic Metabolic Diseases. Ed. by B. H. Landing et al. 1993. (Perspectives in Pediatric Pathology Ser.: Vol. 17). (Illus.). xiv, 190p. 208.75 (*3-8055-5581-4*) S Karger.

Genetic Models of Immune & Inflammatory Diseases. Ed. by Abdul K. Abbas & R. Flavell. 1996. LC 95-46669. (Serono Symposia Ser.). (Illus.). 177p. 110.00 (*0-387-94649-7*) Spr-Verlag.

Genetic Origins of Tumor Cells. Ed. by F. J. Cleton & J. W. Simons. 1980. (Developments in Oncology Ser.: Vol. 1). xv, 125p. text 88.00 (*90-247-2272-1*) Kluwer Academic.

Genetic Predisposition to Cancer. Ed. by R. Eeles et al. 1996. (Illus.). 432p. (*0-412-56580-3*) E A GBR. *Dist:* OUP.

Genetic Profile of Marginal Zone B-Cell Lymphoma. Judith Dierlamm. 1999. (Acta Biomedica Lovaniensia Ser.: Vol. 200). (Illus.). 120p. pap. (*90-6186-965-X*) Leuven Univ BEL. *Dist:* Coronet Bks.

Genetic Programming: On the Programming of Computers by Means of Natural Selection. John R. Koza. 1992. LC 92-25785. (Complex Adaptive Systems Ser.). (Illus.). 800p. 75.00 (*0-262-11170-5*, Bradford Bks) MIT Pr.

Genetic Recombination. D. Leach. 1996. LC 95-21294. (Illus.). 256p. pap. 52.95 (*0-632-03861-6*) Blackwell Sci.

Genetic Regulation of Placental Development, & Immunology. Donald Morrish & Richard K. Miller. 1998. LC 98-2599. (Trophoblast Research Ser.: Vol. 11). (Illus.). 408p. 120.00 (*1-58046-032-1*) U of Rochester.

Genetic Research in Psychiatry: C.I.N.P. President's Workshop, 2nd, Munchner Genetikgesprache, September 12-15, 1991. Ed. by Julien Mendlewicz & H. Hippius. 1992. (Illus.). 280p. 118.00 (*0-387-54827-0*) Spr-Verlag.

Genetic Research Strategies in Psychobiology & Psychiatry. Ed. by Eliot S. Gershon et al. 1981. (Psychobiology & Psychopathology Ser.: Vol. 1). 38.50 (*0-910286-84-1*) Boxwood.

Genetic Screening: Index of Modern Authors & Subjects with Guide for Rapid Research. Mark W. Hallcrest. 1991. LC 90-56283. 160p. 47.50 (*1-55914-348-7*); pap. 44.50 (*1-55914-349-5*) ABBE Pubs Assn.

Genetic Services in Europe: A Comparative Study of 31 Countries by the Concerted Action on Genetic Services in Europe. Ed. by Rodney Harris. 1997. (European Journal of Human Genetics Ser.: Vol. 5, Suppl. 2, 1997). vi, 220p. pap. 66.25 (*3-8055-6629-8*) S Karger.

***Genetic Studies of Endocrine Abdominal Tumors.** Ola Hessman. 2001. (Comprehensive Summaries of Uppsala Dissertations from the Faculty of Medicine Ser.: No. 1038). (Illus.). 64p. (*91-554-5026-1*) Uppsala Universitet SWE. *Dist:* Coronet Bks.

***Genetic Studies of Rheumatoid Arthritis Using Animal Models.** Niklas Nordquist. 2001. (Comprehensive Summaries of Uppsala Dissertations from the Faculty of Medicine Ser.: No. 1074). (Illus.). 48p. pap. (*91-554-5117-9*) Acta Univ SWE. *Dist:* Coronet Bks.

***Genetic Studies of Schizophrenia.** Eva Lindholm. 2001. (Comprehensive Summaries of Uppsala Dissertations from the Faculty of Medicine Ser.: Vol. 991). (Illus.). 54p. pap. (*91-554-4918-2*) Uppsala Universitet SWE. *Dist:* Coronet Bks.

Genetic Studies of the Cystic Fibrosis Transmembrane Conductance Regulator Gene in Belgian CF Patients. Harry Cuppens. 1995. (Acta Biomedica Lovaniensia Ser.: Vol. 110). (Illus.). 138p. (Orig.). pap. (*90-6186-682-0*) Leuven Univ BEL. *Dist:* Coronet Bks.

***Genetic Studies of Two Inherited Human Phenotypes: Hearing Loss & Monoamine Oxidase Activity.** Jorune Balciuniene. 2001. (Comprehensive Summaries of Uppsala Dissertatons from the Faculty of Medicine: No. 90). (Illus.). 54p. (Orig.). pap. (*91-554-4917-4*) Uppsala Universitet SWE. *Dist:* Coronet Bks.

Genetic Susceptibility to Cancer. ICRP Staff. 1999. (International Commission on Radiological Protection Ser.: Vol. 79). 168p. pap. 121.50 (*0-08-042752-9*, Pergamon Pr) Elsevier.

***Genetic Susceptibility to Cervical & Gastric Cancer.** Patrik Magnusson. 2000. (Comprehensive Summaries of Uppsala Dissertations from the Faculty of Medicine Ser.: No. 911). (Illus.). 61p. pap. (*91-554-4665-5*) Uppsala Universitet SWE. *Dist:* Coronet Bks.

Genetic Susceptibility to Environmental Factors - A Challenge for Public Intervention. Ed. by Ulf Smith et al. 1988. (First Intl Symposium, Malmo, Sweden, May 1987). (Illus.). 169p. 106.00 (*91-22-01262-1*) Coronet Bks.

Genetic Switch. Mark Ptashne. 2nd ed. 1992. (Illus.). 192p. (Orig.). pap. 52.95 (*0-86542-209-5*) Blackwell Sci.

Genetic Syndromes in Communication Disorders. Jack H. Jung. 1989. LC 90-50383. (Illus.). 285p. (C). text 38.00 (*0-89079-280-1*, 1703) PRO-ED.

Genetic Takeover & the Mineral Origins of Life. A. G. Cairns-Smith. 1987. LC 81-17070. (Illus.). 488p. pap. text 44.95 (*0-521-34682-7*) Cambridge U Pr.

Genetic Testing & Screening for Health-Care Purposes. 1993. (Bioethics Ser.). (*92-871-2291-1*) Council of Europe FRA. *Dist:* Manhattan Pub Co.

Genetic Testing for Alzheimer Disease: Ethical & Clinical Issues. Stephen G. Post & Peter J. Whitehouse. 1998. LC 97-42661. (Illus.). 512p. 50.00 (*0-8018-5840-2*) Johns Hopkins.

Genetic Testing of Children. Ed. by A. Clarke. 1997. 300p. (*1-85996-181-9*) Bios Sci GBR. *Dist:* Coronet Bks.

Genetic Tests & Health Insurance: Results of a Survey. 1993. (Illus.). 78p. (Orig.). (C). pap. text 30.00 (*1-56806-637-6*) DIANE Pub.

Genetic Toxicology. Albert P. Li & Robert H. Heflich. 1991. 504p. 139.00 (*0-8493-8815-5*, RA1224) CRC Pr.

Genetic Vaccines & Immunotherapeutic Strategies. Ed. by Cathy Thibeault. 1997. (Biomedical Library). pap. (*1-57936-027-0*) Drug & Market Dev.

Genetic Variation & Dietary Response. Ed. by A. P. Simopoulos & P. J. Nestel. 1997. LC 96-44582. (World Review of Nutrition & Dietetics Ser.: Vol. 80, 1997). (Illus.). xvi, 172p. 172.25 (*3-8055-6347-7*) S Karger.

Genetic Variation & Human Disease: Principles & Evolutionary Approaches. Kenneth M. Weiss. 1995. (Studies in Biological Anthropology: No. 11). (Illus.). 378p. (C). pap. text 29.95 (*0-521-33660-0*) Cambridge U Pr.

Genetic Variation & Nutrition. Ed. by Artemis P. Simopoulos & Barton Childs. 1990. (World Review of Nutrition & Dietetics Ser.: Vol. 63). xii, 300p. 211.50 (*3-8055-5126-6*) S Karger.

Genetic Variation in Hormone Systems John G. Shire. 1979. Vol. 1. 208p. 121.00 (*0-8493-5283-5*, QP187); Vol. 2. 192p. 111.00 (*0-8493-5284-3*) Franklin (CRC Reprint).

Genetic Witness: Forensic Uses of DNA Tests. 1993. (Illus.). 196p. (C). pap. text 25.00 (*1-56806-842-5*) DIANE Pub.

Genetica y la Revolucion en las Ciencias Biologicas. rev. ed. 1975. (Serie de Biologia: No. 1). (SPA.). pap. 3.50 (*0-8270-6045-9*) OAS.

Genetical, Functional & Physical Studies of Hemoglobins: Proceedings of the Hemoglobin Symposium, 1st Inter-American, Caracas, 1969. Hemoglobin Symposium Staff. Ed. by T. Arends et al. 1971. 69.75 (*3-8055-1255-4*) S Karger.

Genetically Altered Viruses & the Environment. Ed. by B. Fields et al. 1985. LC 85-21294. (Banbury Reports: No. 22). 362p. 65.00 (*0-87969-222-7*) Cold Spring Harbor.

Genetically Defined Animal Models of Neurobehavioral Dysfunctions. Ed. by P. Driscoll. 1992. xx, 304p. 120.00 (*0-8176-3460-6*) Birkhauser.

Genetically Engineered Vaccines. J. E. Ciardi et al. 1993. LC 92-48784. (Advances in Experimental Medicine & Biology Ser.: Vol. 327). (Illus.). 336p. (C). text 105.00 (*0-306-44349-X*, Kluwer Plenum) Kluwer Academic.

Genetics. Bell. 2000. (Quick Look Veterinary Ser.). 23.95 (*1-889325-15-5*) Fence Crk Pubng.

Genetics. Gerald D. Elseth & D. Baugardner. 1984. (Illus.). 720p. (*0-201-03953-2*) Addison-Wesley.

Genetics. John Fincham. 1983. (Illus.). 643p. text 78.95 (*0-86720-026-X*, 026-X) Jones & Bartlett.

Genetics. Ed. by David C. Glass. 1968. LC 68-24635. (Illus.). 270p. 13.00 (*0-87470-008-6*) Rockefeller.

Genetics. Olf. 1994. pap. text 36.00 (*0-443-05273-5*) Saunders.

Genetics. Jan M. Friedman et al. 2nd ed. 1996. (National Medical Series for Independent Study). 304p. pap. text 29.00 (*0-683-06217-4*) Lppncott W & W.

Genetics. N. A. McNiel & C. W. Magill. 2nd ed. 1977. (Illus.). 225p. pap. text 14.95 (*0-89641-004-8*) American Pr.

Genetics: A Study Manual. Gerald D. Elseth & D. Baugardner. 1984. (Illus.). 720p. stu. ed. 8.00 net. (*0-201-03482-4*) Addison-Wesley.

Genetics: Rheumatic Disease. David M. Grennan. 1989. text 53.00 (*0-7020-1307-2*) Saunders.

Genetics & Aging. F. A. Lints. 1978. (Interdisciplinary Topics in Gerontology Ser.: Vol. 14). (Illus.). pap. 51.50 (*3-8055-2891-4*) S Karger.

Genetics & Biology of Alcoholism. Ed. by C. Robert Cloninger & Henri Begleiter. 1991. (Banbury Reports: No. 33). (Illus.). 430p. (C). text 85.00 (*0-87969-233-2*) Cold Spring Harbor.

Genetics & Birth Defects in Clinical Practice. Murray Feingold & Hermione Pashayan. 1983. 64.95 (*0-316-27715-0*, Little Brwn Med Div) Lppncott W & W.

Genetics & Cancer: A Second Look. Ed. by B. A. Ponder et al. 1995. LC 96-185636. (Cancer Surveys Ser.: Vol. 25). (Illus.). 425p. (C). 75.00 (*0-87969-469-6*) Cold Spring Harbor.

Genetics & Criminal Behavior. David Wasserman & Robert Wachbroit. 2001. LC 00-37821. (Studies in Philosophy & Public Policy). (Illus.). 348p. text 64.95 (*0-521-62214-X*) Cambridge U Pr.

Genetics & Criminal Behavior. Ed. by David Wasserman & Robert Wachbroit. 2001. LC 00-37821. (Studies in Philosophy & Public Policy). (Illus.). 348p. (C). pap. text 22.95 (*0-521-62728-1*) Cambridge U Pr.

Genetics & Criminality: The Potential Misuse of Scientific Information in Court. Ed. by Jeffrey R. Botkin et al. 1999. LC 99-20607. 277p. 39.95 (*1-55798-580-4*, 431-728A) Am Psychol.

Genetics & Epidemiology of Inflammatory Bowel Disease. Ed. by R. McConnell et al. 1986. (Frontiers of Gastrointestinal Research Ser.: Vol. 11). (Illus.). viii, 180p. 123.50 (*3-8055-4265-8*) S Karger.

Genetics & Evolution of Aging. Ed. by Michael R. Rose & Caleb E. Finch. 1994. LC 94-16569. (Contemporary Issues in Genetics & Evolution Ser.: Vol. 3). 312p. (C). text 213.00 (*0-7923-2902-3*) Kluwer Academic.

Genetics & Hearing Impairment. Ed. by Allessandro Martini. 1996. (Illus.). 348p. (Orig.). pap. 59.95 (*1-56593-792-9*, 1546) Singular Publishing.

Genetics & Hearing Loss. Ed. by Charles I. Berlin & Bronya J. B. Keats. 2000. LC 99-45186. 180p. text 71.95 (*0-7693-0103-7*) Singular Publishing.

Genetics & Medicine in the United States, 1800 to 1922. Alan R. Rushton. 1994. LC 93-35943. 224p. 49.00 (*0-8018-4781-8*) Johns Hopkins.

Genetics & Mental Illness: Evolving Issues for Research & Society. Ed. by Laura L. Hall. 1996. (Illus.). 240p. (C). text 59.00 (*0-306-45166-2*, Kluwer Plenum) Kluwer Academic.

Genetics & Molecular Biology. Robert F. Schleif. 1986. 800p. (C). text 49.50 (*0-201-07418-4*) Benjamin-Cummings.

Genetics & Product Formation in Streptomyces. Ed. by S. Baumberg et al. 1991. (FEMS Symposium Ser.: No. 55). (Illus.). 340p. (C). text 138.00 (*0-306-43885-2*, Kluwer Plenum) Kluwer Academic.

Genetics & Psychiatric Disorders. Ed. by Jan Wahlstrom. 1998. 340p. 164.50 (*0-08-042746-4*) Elsevier.

Genetics & Psychopharmacology. Ed. by Julien Mendlewicz. 1975. (Modern Problems of Pharmacopsychiatry Ser.: Vol. 10). viii, 132p. 50.50 (*3-8055-2117-0*) S Karger.

Genetics & Public Health in the 21st Century: Using Genetic Information to Improve Health & Prevent Disease. Ed. by Muin J. Khoury et al. 2000. LC 99-49548. (Oxford Monographs on Medical Genetics: 40). (Illus.). 664p. text 65.00 (*0-19-512830-3*) OUP.

Genetics & Society. Ed. by Barry Holland & Charalambos Kyriacou. 1993. LC 93-13618. 123p. (C). pap. text 35.00 (*0-201-56515-3*) Addison-Wesley.

Genetics & the Origin of Species. Theodosius Dobzhansky & Niles Eldridge. Ed. by Stephen Jay Gould. 1982. LC 82-4278. (Classics of Modern Evolution Ser.). 416p. reprint ed. pap. text 27.50 (*0-231-05475-0*) Col U Pr.

Genetics & the Social Behavior of the Dog: The Classic Study. Ed. by John P. Scott & John L. Fuller. 1998. LC 64-23429. (Illus.). 468p. reprint ed. pap. text 20.00 (*0-226-74338-1*) U Ch Pr.

Genetics & Your Health: A Guide for the 21st Century Family. Raye Lynn Alford. 1999. LC 98-31950. (Illus.). 270p. pap. 19.95 (*0-9666748-1-2*, Medford Press) Plexus Pub.

Genetics, Development, & Evolution. Ed. by J. Perry Gustafson et al. 1986. LC 79-635774. (Stadler Genetics Symposia Ser.). 374p. 85.00 (*0-306-42268-9*, Plenum Trade) Perseus Pubng.

Genetics in Anesthesiology: Syndromes & Science. Guy L. Weinberg. 1996. 222p. text 89.99 (*0-7506-9479-3*) Buttrwrth-Heinemann.

Genetics in Clinical Practice: New Directions for Nursing & Health Care. Dale H. Lea et al. 1998. LC 98-10873. (Nursing Ser.). (Illus.). 352p. (C). pap. text 44.95 (*0-7637-0542-X*, 0542-X) Jones & Bartlett.

Genetics in Obstetrics & Gynecology. Joe L. Simpson & Mitchell S. Golbus. 2nd ed. 1992. (Illus.). 362p. text 65.00 (*0-7216-3510-5*) Saunders.

Genetics in Obstetrics & Gynecology. 3rd ed. 2000. text (*0-7216-4164-4*) Saunders.

Genetics in Otorhinolaryngology. Ed. by K. Kitamua & K. P. Steel. 2000. LC 99-88947. (Advances in OtoRhinoLaryngology Ser.: Vol. 56). (Illus.). x, 298p. 224.50 (*3-8055-6956-4*) S Karger.

Genetics in Primary Care & Clinical Medicine. Margretta Seashore. 1996. 334p. (C). pap. text 34.95 (*0-8385-3128-8*, A3128-4, Apple Lange Med) McGraw.

Genetics in the Clinic. Ed. by Mary B. Mahowald. 2001. LC 00-135004. 256p. pap. text 39.95 (*0-323-01203-5*) Mosby Inc.

Genetics in the Courts. Henry M. Butzel. 1986. LC 86-21725. (Studies in Health & Human Services: Vol. 9). 802p. lib. bdg. 149.95 (*0-88946-134-1*) E Mellen.

Genetics in Wild Mice: Its Application to Biomedical Research. Ed. by M. Kazuo et al. 1994. (Illus.). x, 334p. 259.25 (*3-8055-6054-0*) S Karger.

Genetics of Alcoholism. Ed. by Henri Begleiter & Benjamin Kissin. 1995. LC 93-35497. (Alcohol & Alcoholism Ser.: No. 1). (Illus.). 416p. text 79.50 (*0-19-508877-8*) OUP.

Genetics of Allergy & Asthma: Methods for Investigative Studies. Malcolm N. Blumenthal & Bengt Bjorksten. 1997. LC 96-40953. (Clinical Allergy & Immunology Ser.: Vol. 10). (Illus.). 384p. text 175.00 (*0-8247-9480-X*) Dekker.

Genetics of Asthma & Atopy. Ed. by I. P. Hall. 1996. LC 96-31775. (Monographs in Allergy: Vol. 33). (Illus.). vi, 174p. 158.25 (*3-8055-6333-7*) S Karger.

Genetics of Bacteria. Ed. by John Scaife et al. 1986. pap. text 52.00 (*0-12-621181-7*) Acad Pr.

Genetics of Cancer. Michael J. Waring & B. A. Ponder. 1995. (Cancer Biology & Medicine Ser.: Vol. CABM 04). 240p. (C). text 129.00 (*0-7923-8886-0*) Kluwer Academic.

Genetics of Cancer: Genes Associated with Cancer Invasion, Metastasis & Cell Proliferation. G. V. Sherbet & M. S. Lakshmi. 1997. LC 97-11843. (Illus.). 360p. text 85.00 (*0-12-639875-5*) Morgan Kaufmann.

Genetics of Candida. Ed. by Donald R. Kirsch et al. 1990. 224p. 110.00 (*0-8493-5570-2*, QR201) CRC Pr.

Genetics of Cardiovascular Disease. Ed. by Mary E. Pierpont. 1986. text 254.00 (*0-89838-790-6*) Kluwer Academic.

Genetics of Cellular, Individual, Family & Population Variability. Ed. by Charles F. Sing & Craig L. Harris. 1993. LC 92-20412. (Illus.). 320p. (C). text 75.00 (*0-19-506625-1*) OUP.

Genetics of Cerebrovascular Disease. Mark J. Alberts. 1998. LC 98-18758. (Illus.). 500p. 120.00 (*0-87993-584-7*) Futura Pub.

Genetics of Colorectal Cancer for Clinical Practice. No. 72. Fred H. Menko. 1993. LC 92-48226. (Developments in Oncology Ser.: Vol. 72). 196p. (C). text 155.50 (*0-7923-2100-6*) Kluwer Academic.

Genetics of Common Diseases: Future Therapeutic & Diagnostic Possibilities. Ed. by I. Day & S. Humphries. 1997. (UCL Molecular Pathology Ser.). 300p. (*1-85996-041-3*) Bios Sci.

Genetics of Complement. Ed. by Matteo Adinolfi. 1988. (Journal: Vol. 5, No. 2-3, 1988). (Illus.). 100p. pap. 31.50 (*3-8055-4860-5*) S Karger.

Genetics of Criminal & Antisocial Behaviour. Michael Rutter. 1996. (CIBA Foundation Symposia Ser.: Vol. 194). 292p. 134.95 (*0-471-95719-4*) Wiley.

Genetics of Focal Epilepsies. S. F. Berkovic. 1999. 296p. (*0-86196-569-8*) J Libbey Med GBR. *Dist:* Buttrwrth-Heinemann.

Genetics of Hearing Loss & Genetic Counseling: What the Practicing Audiologist Needs to Know. Edward Cohn et al. 1998. 44p. 48.00 incl. audio (*1-58041-025-1*, 0112146) Am Speech Lang Hearing.

Genetics of Hematological Disorders. Ed. by Christos S. Bartsocas & Dimitris Loukopoulos. 1991. 256p. 140.00 (*1-56032-205-5*) Hemisp Pub.

Genetics of Human Mentality. Jon L. Karisson. 1991. LC 90-14194. 208p. 62.50 (*0-275-93808-5*, C3808, Praeger Pubs) Greenwood.

Genetics of Human Populations. Albert Jacquard. Tr. by D. M. Yermanos from FRE. 1978. LC 77-83065.Tr. of Genetique des Populations humaines. (Illus.). 36.25 (*0-87735-421-9*) Jones & Bartlett.

Genetics of Influenza Viruses. Peter Palese. 1983. (Illus.). 340p. 112.00 (*0-387-81743-3*) Spr-Verlag.

Genetics of Mental Disorders: A Guide for Students, Clinicians & Researchers. Stephen V. Faraone et al. 1999. LC 99-13077. 272p. 33.00 (*1-57230-479-0*, C0479) Guilford Pubns.

Genetics of Mental Retardation: Biomedical, Psychosocial & Ethical Issues. Ed. by E. K. Hicks & Joseph M. Berg. 1988. 225p. (C). lib. bdg. (*1-55608-062-X*) Kluwer Academic NLD. *Dist:* Kluwer Academic.

Genetics of Neurological Disorders. Michael Baraitser. (Oxford Monographs on Medical Genetics: No. 18). (Illus.). 2nd ed. 1990. 744p. text 125.00 (*0-19-261814-8*); 3rd ed. 1997. LC 97-8304. 450p. text 89.50 (*0-19-262814-3*) OUP.

Genetics of Neurological Disorders, Vol. 6. Ed. by Alexander G. Bearn et al. 1985. LC 85-508. (Progress in Medical Genetics: Vol. VI). 320p. 82.50 (*0-275-91331-7*, C13311, Praeger Pubs) Greenwood.

Genetics of Neuropsychiatric Disorders: Basic & Clinical Aspects. P. Gejman & E. S. Gershon. Date not set. (Medical Psychiatry Ser.). (*0-8247-9417-6*) Dekker.

Genetics of Obesity. Claude Bouchard. 1994. 256p. lib. bdg. 179.00 (*0-8493-4880-3*, RC628) CRC Pr.

Genetics of Ocular Disease: Acute Retinal Necrosis Syndrome, Phthisis Bulbi. W. Straub. 1985. (Developments in Ophthalmology Ser.: Vol. 10). (Illus.). viii, 164p. 112.25 (*3-8055-3933-9*) S Karger.

Genetics of Osteoporosis & Metabolic Bone Disease. Ed. by Michael J. Econs. 2000. LC 99-58332. (Illus.). 474p. 145.00 (*0-89603-702-9*) Humana.

Genetics of Populations. Philip W. Hedrick. 1983. 629p. 53.75 (*0-86720-011-1*) Jones & Bartlett.

Genetics of Primary Immunodeficiency Diseases: A Molecular & Genetic Approach. Ed. by Hans D. Ochs et al. 1998. LC 97-46505. (Illus.). 544p. text 139.50 (*0-19-510486-2*) OUP.

Genetics of Speciation: Collisions & Aftershocks. Hope Hollocher. 2000. 69.95 (*0-12-352760-0*) Acad Pr.

Genetics of the Cell Surface. Compiled by W. F. Bodmer. 1978. LC 79-670277. (Proceedings of the Royal Society Ser.). text 25.00 (*0-85403-101-4*) Scholium Intl.

Genetics of the Epilepsies. Ed. by G. Beck-Managetta et al. 1989. (Illus.). 215p. 118.00 (*0-387-18421-X*) Spr-Verlag.

Genetics of the Evolutionary Process. Theodosius Dobzhansky. 1972. LC 72-127363. 505p. pap. text 32.50 (*0-231-08306-8*) Col U Pr.

Genetics of the Human Blood Groups. Geoff Daniels. 1995. LC 95-5792. 735p. 215.00 (*0-86542-914-6*) Blackwell Sci.

Genetics of the Hungarian Population: Ethnic Aspects, Genetic Markers, Ecogenetics & Disease Spectrum. Ed. by A. Czeizel et al. Tr. by K. Sankaranarayanan. 1991. (Illus.). 350p. 71.95 (*0-387-53580-2*) Spr-Verlag.

Genetics of the Immune Response: Proceedings of the WHO Scientific Group, Geneva, 1967. WHO Staff. 1968. (Technical Reports: No. 402). 52p. pap. text 5.00 (*92-4-120402-8*, 1100402) World Health.

Genetics of the Skeleton: Animal Models of Skeletal Development. D. R. Johnson. 1986. (Illus.). 350p. 90.00 (*0-19-854163-5*) OUP.

Genetics of Vectors & Insecticide Resistance. 1964. (Technical Report Ser.: No. 268). 40p. pap. text 3.00 (*92-4-120268-8*) World Health.

Genetics Problem Solver. Research and Education Association Staff. rev. ed. 1999. LC 85-62730. (REA Problem Solvers Ser.). (Illus.). 640p. pap. text 23.95 (*0-87891-560-5*) Res & Educ.

Genetics, Society & Clinical Practice. Peter S. Harper & Angus J. Clarke. 1997. 253p. (*1-85996-206-8*) Bios Sci GBR. *Dist:* Bks Intl VA.

Genetics, Syndromes & Communication Disorders. Robert J. Shprintzen. 1997. LC 97-20621. (Illus.). 324p. text 68.95 (*1-56593-620-5*, 1288) Thomson Learn.

Genetics Testing in the New Millennium: Advances, Standards & Implications: Congressional Hearing. Ed. by Constance A. Morella. 2001. 123p. (C). reprint ed. pap. text 30.00 (*0-7567-0548-7*) DIANE Pub.

Genetics, the Fetus & Our Future. Carmel Bagness. 1998. 112p. pap. text 29.99 (*1-898507-65-1*, RJ131) Buttrwrth-Heinemann.

Genetics with a Computer. Thomas G. Luce. pap. 16.95 (*0-87567-076-8*) Entelek.

Genetique des Populations humaines see Genetics of Human Populations

Genetische Grundlagen der Artbildung in der Gattung Polyporus. P. Hoffman. 1978. (Bibliotheca Mycologica Ser.: No. 65). (Illus.). pap. text 18.00 (*3-7682-1210-6*) Lubrecht & Cramer.

Genioplasty. Bahman Guyuron. 1992. LC 92-49148. (Illus.). 176p. 199.95 (*0-316-33226-7*, Little Brwn Med Div) Lppncott W & W.

Genital & Neonatal Herpes. Ed. by Lawrence R. Stanberry. 1997. LC 96-14628. 256p. 159.95 (*0-471-96713-0*) Wiley.

Genital Dermatology. Peter J. Lynch. 1994. LC 94-19068. 292p. text (*0-443-08885-3*) Church.

Genital Herpes. 1984. lib. bdg. 250.00 (*0-87700-542-7*) Revisionist Pr.

***Genital Herpes.** Hunter Handsfield. 2001. 45p. pap. 29.95 (*0-07-137971-1*) McGraw-Hill Prof.

Genital Human Papillomavirus Disease: Diagnosis, Management & Prevention. Task Force on Human Papillomavirus Disease, Americ & Henry W. Buck. 2nd rev. ed. 1997. (Illus.). 19p. (Orig.). pap. text 10.00 (*1-877918-00-8*) Am Coll Hlth.

Genital Skin Disorders: A Guide to Non-Sexually Transmitted Conditions. R. Cerio. 1995. (Illus.). 104p. (*0-412-55020-2*) E A GBR. *Dist:* OUP.

Genital System. Ed. by Thomas C. Jones et al. 1987. (Monographs in Pathology of Laboratory Animals). (Illus.). 304p. 316.00 (*0-387-17604-7*) Spr-Verlag.

Genital Warts: Human Papilloma Virus Infection. Ed. by Adrian Mindel. 1995. 304p. (*0-340-57924-2*) E A GBR. *Dist:* OUP.

Genitalendometriose. Ed. by M. Litschgi. 1985. (Illus.). viii, 112p. 51.50 (*3-8055-3984-3*) S Karger.

Genitourinary Cancer. Ed. by Timothy L. Ratliff & William J. Catalona. 1987. (Cancer Treatment & Research Ser.). text 219.00 (*0-89838-830-9*) Kluwer Academic.

Genitourinary Cancer I. David F. Paulson. 1982. text 199.50 (*90-247-2480-5*) Kluwer Academic.

Genitourinary Disorders. Mikel Gray. 1992. LC 92-16487. (Clinical Nursing Ser.). (Illus.). 331p. (C). (gr. 13). text 36.00 (*0-8016-6876-X*, 06876) Mosby Inc.

Genitourinary Medicine Services: Health Care Needs Assessment: The Epidemiologically Based Needs Assessment Reviews, Second Series. Wessex Institute for Health Research and Development et al. Ed. by Andrew Stevens & James Raftery. 1997. LC 97-24978. (*1-85775-221-X*) Radcliffe Med Pr GBR. *Dist:* Balogh.

Genitourinary Radiology: Diagnostic & Therapeutic. Syed Z. Jafri et al. 1997. LC 96-3329. 578p. 214.00 (*0-387-94706-X*) Spr-Verlag.

Genitourinary Radiology: The Requisites. Rondal J. Zagoria & Glenn A. Tung. 1997. (Illus.). 432p. (C). (gr. 13). text 82.00 (*0-8016-7482-4*, 03630) Mosby Inc.

Genitourinary Surgery. James J. Nagle. 1997. (Perioperative Nursing Ser.). (Illus.). 400p. (C). (gr. 13). text 54.95 (*0-8151-7029-7*, 27474) Mosby Inc.

Genitourinary Tract Set: Endoscopic Procedures Hugh N. Whitfield. Ed. by David C. Carter et al. 5th ed. 1993. LC 92-22884. (Illus.). 200p. (C). 228.95 (*0-7506-1240-1*) Chapman & Hall.

Genitourinary Tract Disease (Fourth Series) Test & Syllabus. Harold A. Mitty et al. 1992. LC 92-21930. (Professional Self-Evaluation & Continuing Education Program Ser.: Vol. 33). (Illus.). 650p. 190.00 (*1-55903-033-X*) Am Coll Radiology.

Genitourinary Tract Pathology. Mark A. Weiss. 1992. (C). (gr. 13). text (*1-56375-026-0*) Gower-Mosby.

Genius & Eminence. Ed. by Robert S. Albert. 2nd ed. 2001. LC 92-12055. (International Series in Experimental Social Psychology: Vol. 22). 428p. pap. 34.95 (*0-08-037765-3*, Prgamon Press) Buttrwrth-Heinemann.

Genius & Eminence. Ed. by Robert S. Albert. 2nd ed. 1998. LC 92-12055. (Experimental Social Psychology Ser.: Vol. 22). 428p. lib. bdg. 68.95 (*0-08-037764-5*) Routledge.

Genodermatoses: A Full-Color Clinical Guide to Genetic Skin Disorders. Joel L. Spitz. 1996. LC 95-2987. (Illus.). 304p. 139.00 (*0-683-07904-2*) Lppncott W & W.

Genomanalyse Bei Claviceps Purpurea. Uta Jungehuelsing. 1995. (Bibliotheca Mycologica: Vol. 161). (GER., Illus.). viii, 136p. (*3-443-59063-2*) Gebruder Borntraeger DEU. *Dist:* Balogh.

***Genome Mapping in the Horse.** Gabriella Lindgren. 2001. (Comprehensive Summaries of Uppsala Dissertations from the Faculty of Science & Technology Ser.: No. 632). (Illus.). 33p. (*91-554-5036-9*) Uppsala Universitet SWE. *Dist:* Coronet Bks.

Genomic & Non-Genomic Effects of Aldosterone. Ed. by Martin Wheling. 1994. LC 94-12406. (Pharmacology & Toxicology Ser.). 176p. lib. bdg. 110.00 (*0-8493-8385-4*) CRC Pr.

Genomic Imprinting: Causes & Consequences. Ed. by R. Ohlsson et al. 1996. (Illus.). 392p. (C). text 95.00 (*0-521-47243-1*) Cambridge U Pr.

Genomic Imprinting: Methods & Protocols. Ed. by Andrew Ward. 2001. LC 2001-24456. (Methods in Molecular Biology Ser.: Vol. 181). 400p. 99.50 (*0-89603-741-X*) Humana.

Genomic Instability & Immortality in Cancer: Proceedings of the Eighth Annual Pezcoller Symposium Held in Trento, Italy, June 17-19, 1996. Ed. by Enrico Mihich & Leland Hartwell. 1998. LC 97-29967. (Pezcoller Foundation Symposia Ser.). 262p. 89.50 (*0-306-45700-8*, Kluwer Plenum) Kluwer Academic.

***Genomic Rearrangements at the Cause of Three Genetic Disorders in Man.** Kristina Lagerstedt. 2001. (Comprehensive Summaries of Uppsala Dissertations from the Faculty of Medicine Ser.: No. 1032). (Illus.). 48p. (*91-554-5013-X*) Uppsala Universitet SWE. *Dist:* Coronet Bks.

Genomics & Human Therapeutic Development. James W. Hawkins. Ed. by Susan C. DiClemente. 1997. LC 98-229268. (Illus.). 375p. spiral bd. (*1-57936-061-0*, 938) Drug & Market Dev.

Gentamicin-PMMA-Chains in Bone & Soft-Tissue Infections. Ed. by H. Eberle. 1988. (Reconstruction Surgery & Traumatology Ser.: Vol. 20). (Illus.). vi, 122p. 95.75 (*3-8055-4603-3*) S Karger.

Gentians. Wilkie. 1977. LC 76-46559. (Illus.). reprint ed. 12.50 (*0-913728-19-5*) Theophrastus.

Gentle Annie: The True Story of a Civil War Nurse. Mary Francis Shura. 1994. LC 90-39251. 192p. (J). (gr. 4-7). pap. 4.50 (*0-590-43500-0*) Scholastic Inc.

Gentle Birth Choices: A Guide to Making Informed Decisions. Barbara Harper. 1994. LC 93-20959. (Illus.). 224p. pap. 16.95 (*0-89281-480-2*, Heal Arts VT) Inner Tradit.

Gentle Giant: The Inspiring Story of an Autistic Child. Wendy Robinson. 1999. LC 98-42682. 192p. pap. 16.95 (*1-86204-304-3*) Element MA.

Gentle Healing for Baby & Child: A Parent's Guide to Child-Friendly Herbs & Other Natural Remedies for Common Ailments & Injuries. Andrea Candee & David Andrusia. 2001. LC 00-60657. 288p. pap. 13.95 (*0-671-03622-X*) PB.

Gentle Healing with Homeopathy: A Practical Primer to Self-Treatment of Common Ailments. Ariel Winters. 1978. LC 97-7715. 240p. pap. 9.95 (*0-8069-8112-1*) Sterling.

Gentle Is the Way. Josephine Shoemaker. 1981. LC 81-65527. (Illus.). 68p. (Orig.). pap. 6.50 (*0-87516-444-7*) DeVorss.

Gentle Legions: National Voluntary Health Organizations in America. Richard Carter. 1992. 332p. (C). text 39.95 (*1-56000-053-8*) Transaction Pubs.

Gentle Path Through the Twelve Steps: The Classic Guide for All People in the Process of Recovery. Patrick J. Carnes. rev. ed. 1994. (Illus.). 310p. pap. 16.00 (*1-56838-058-5*) Hazelden.

Gentle Roads to Survival: Making Self-Healing Choices in Difficult Circumstances. Andre Auw. 1991. LC 90-48311. 160p. (Orig.). pap. 10.95 (*0-944031-18-8*) Aslan Pub.

Gentle Surgery: A Manual on How to Operate Without Tissue Damage or Blood Loss. Charles V. Perrill. Ed. by Bertha C. Perrill. 2000. 144p. lab manual ed. 89.95 (*0-9701415-0-5*) C V Perrill.

Genuine Works of Hippocrates. Francis Adams. 1972. 384p. reprint ed. 42.50 (*0-88275-002-X*) Krieger.

Genus Nysius & Its Allies in the Hawaiian Islands. Robert L. Usinger. 1969. (BMB Ser.: No. 173). reprint ed. 25.00 (*0-527-02281-0*) Periodicals Srv.

Genus Psilocybe: Revision of the Known Species (Hallucinogenic Species) Gaston Guzman. 1983. (Beiheft zur Nova Hedwigia Ser.: No. 74). (Illus.). 650p. lib. bdg. 140.00 (*3-7682-1319-6*) Lubrecht & Cramer.

Genus Schistocerca. Dirsch. 1974. (Sent Ser.). text 148.50 (*90-6193-120-7*) Kluwer Academic.

Genus Yersinia: Epidemiology, Molecular Biology & Pathogenesis. Ed. by K. J Prpic & B. R. Davey. 1987. (Contributions to Microbiology & Immunology Ser.: Vol. 9). (Illus.). x, 346p. 243.50 (*3-8055-4482-0*) S Karger.

Geographic Aspects of Health. Ed. by Neil McGlashan & John R. Blunden. 1983. text 132.00 (*0-12-483780-8*) Acad Pr.

Geographic Information Systems in Public Health. Morgan. 2000. 63.00 (*0-8342-1813-5*) Aspen Pub.

Geographic Medicine for the Practitioner. K. S. Warren & Adel A. Mahmoud. 2nd ed. 1985. LC 85-9983. (Illus.). 212p. reprint ed. 98.00 (*0-387-96143-7*) Spr-Verlag.

Geographic Medicine for the Practitioner: Algorithms in the Diagnosis & Management of Exotic Diseases. Ed. by Kenneth S. Warren et al. 1978. LC 77-17007. (Studies in Infectious Disease Research). 148p. lib. bdg. 30.00 (*0-226-87386-2*) U Ch Pr.

Geographic Methods for Health Services Research: A Focus on the Rural-Urban Continuum. Ed. by Thomas C. Ricketts et al. 396p. 2001. 72.50 (*0-8191-9532-4*); 1994. pap. 45.00 (*0-8191-9533-2*) U Pr of Amer.

Geographical Structure of Epidemics. Peter Haggett. 2000. LC 00-31359. (Clarendon Lectures in Geography & Environmental Studies). (Illus.). 166p. pap. 24.95 (*0-19-924145-7*) OUP.

Geographics of Women's Health. Isabel Dyck et al. 2001. LC 00-45838. (Illus.). lib. bdg. 110.00 (*0-415-23607-X*) Routledge.

Geography Is Destiny: California Variations in Medical Practice. Katherine W. Herbst. 2000. (Illus.). 31p. pap. (*1-929008-26-0*) CA HlthCare Fnd.

Geography of AIDS. Gary W. Shannon et al. 1990. LC 90-14112. 192p. 35.00 (*0-89862-445-2*) Guilford Pubns.

Geography of Health. Ed. by Andrew Learmonth. 1981. (Social Science & Medicine Ser.: No. 15). (Illus.). 268p. 30.00 (*0-08-027434-X*, Pergamon Pr) Elsevier.

Geography of Health Services in Britain. Robin Haynes. 1986. 272p. (*0-7099-3766-0*) C Helm GBR. *Dist:* Routldge.

Geography of National Health: An Essay in Welfare Geography. John Eyles. 1987. 256p. (C). (*0-7099-0928-4*) C Helm GBR. *Dist:* Routldge.

Geological Evidence of the Antiquity of Man. Charles Lyell. 4th ed. LC 72-1728. (Illus.). reprint ed. 72.50 (*0-404-08138-X*) AMS Pr.

Geomedicine. Ed. by Jul Lag. 1990. 256p. lib. bdg. 184.95 (*0-8493-6755-7*, RA792) CRC Pr.

E F G

Geomedizinische Ergometrie bei Jugendlichen: Vergleichende Ergometrie & Spirographie bei Stadt-, Land- & Hochgebirgskindern. K. Biener. Ed. by G. Ritzel. 1976. (Sozialmedizinische und Paedagogische Jugendkunde Ser.: Band 11). 21.00 (*3-8055-2281-9*) S Karger.

Geometric, Physical & Visual Optics. Michael P. Keating. 1988. LC 87-25699. (Illus.). 577p. pap. text 89.00 (*0-409-90106-7*) Buttrwrth-Heinemann.

Geometrical & Positional Fatty Acid Isomers. Ed. by Edward A. Emken & H. J. Dutton. 1979. 356p. 40.00 (*0-935315-03-9*) Am Oil Chemists.

Geometrical Optics Workbook. David S. Loshin. 1991. LC 91-3279. 224p. pap. text 44.99 (*0-7506-9052-6*) Buttrwrth-Heinemann.

Geometrical Optics Workbook. David S. Loshin. 2nd ed. 2001. 266p. pap. 35.00 (*0-7506-9796-2*) Buttrwrth-Heinemann.

Geopolitics of Drugs 1996 Edition: Observatoire Geopolitique des Drogues. Tr. by Deke Dusinberre et al. 1996. (Illus.). 224p. text 65.00 (*1-55553-262-4*) NE U Pr.

George Bottini: Painter of Montmartre. Edna C. Southard. 1984. LC 83-62982. (Illus.). 119p. (Orig.). pap. 15.00 (*0-940784-06-8*) Miami Univ Art.

George Dock, M.D. A Bibliography of His Writings. Ed. by Alison K. Mauer & Edgar F. Mauer. 2nd ed. 1991. (Illus.). 36p. pap. text 20.00 (*0-9631270-0-4*) Fr Lib LA Cty Med.

Georgia. Robert B. Remar & Richard N. Hubert. 1996. LC 96-19783. (Law & Mental Health Professionals Ser.). 510p. (C). text 59.95 (*1-55798-364-X*, 431-5090) Am Psychol.

Georgia Health Care in Perspective 2000. Ed. by Kathleen O'Leary Morgan & Scott E. Morgan. 2000. 21p. spiral bd. 19.00 (*0-7401-0209-5*) Morgan Quitno Corp.

Georgia Health Care Perspective, 1998. Ed. by Kathleen O'Leary Morgan & Scott E. Morgan. 1998. 20p. pap. 19.00 (*1-56692-809-5*) Morgan Quitno Corp.

Georgia Mental Health Sourcebook: A Resource Guide for Consumers & Professionals. Carla S. Rogg & Oskar H. Rogg. 1994. 177p. (Orig.). pap. 19.95 (*0-9631939-6-1*); spiral bd. 24.95 (*0-9631939-8-8*) Care Solutions.

Georgia Senior Resource Guide: A Guide for Older Adults, Caregivers & Eldercare Professionals. Carla S. Rogg & Oskar H. Rogg. 1995. 258p. (Orig.). pap. 19.95 (*0-9631939-9-6*) Care Solutions.

Georgiade Plastic, Maxillofacial & Reconstructive Surgery. Ed. by Nicholas G. Georgiade et al. 3rd ed. 1997. LC 96-14580. (Illus.). 1,312p. text 249.00 (*0-683-03455-3*) Lppncott W & W.

Georgi's Parasitology for Veterinarians. Dwight D. Bowman. 6th ed. 1994. (Illus.). 432p. (C). text 62.00 (*0-7216-5589-0*) Saunders.

Georgis' Parasitology for Veterinarians. Dwight D. Bowman. Ed. by Ray Kersey. 7th ed. 1998. LC 98-17175. (Illus.). 415p. (C). text 55.00 (*0-7216-7097-0*) Saunders.

Geraghty's Care for Children. O'Hagan. 3rd ed. 1996. pap. text 30.50 (*0-7020-1918-6*) Saunders.

Geragogics: European Research in Gerontological Education & Educational Gerontology. Ed. by Celia Berdes et al. 1993. LC 92-40000. (Gerontology & Geriatrics Education Ser.: Vol. 13, Nos. 1 & 2). (Illus.). 180p. 39.95 (*1-56024-397-X*) Haworth Pr.

Geraniums for the Iroquois: A Field Guide to American Indian Medicinal Plants. Daniel E. Moerman. Ed. by Keith Irvine. 1982. LC 81-52514. (Illus.). 29.00 (*0-917256-15-8*) Ref Pubns.

GERD: Current Issues & Controversies. Ed. by J. E. Richter. 2000. (Digestive Diseases Ser.: Vol. 18, No. 1 (2000)). (Illus.). 48p. pap. 25.25 (*3-8055-7079-1*) S Karger.

Geriatics: A Study of Maturity. Barbara R. Hegner. 5th ed. 1991. 480p. (C). mass mkt. 51.95 (*0-8273-4531-3*) Delmar.

Geriatric Aide. Jane H. Stolten. 1973. (Illus.). 17.00 (*0-316-81741-4*, Little Brwn Med Div) Lppncott W & W.

Geriatric Assessment. Ed. by Dan Osterweil et al. 2000. LC 99-87542. 838p. text 75.00 (*0-07-134725-9*) McGraw-Hill Prof.

Geriatric Assessment & the Twenty Minute Visit: Instructional Manual for Residents & Attending Physicians. Joshua Chodosh et al. 1997. 24p. 80.00 (*1-892273-02-0*) U Rchstr Med & Dntstry.

Geriatric Assessments in Health & Disease Including Life-Styles & Happiness Quality. Robert O. Coons. 1996. 150p. pap. 47.50 (*0-7883-1285-5*) ABBE Pubs Assn.

Geriatric Assessments in Health & Disease Including Life-Styles & Happiness Quality: Index of New Information. Robert O. Coons. rev. ed. 1997. 129p. 57.50 (*0-7883-1848-9*); pap. 47.50 (*0-7883-1849-7*) ABBE Pubs Assn.

Geriatric Assessments in Health & Disease Including Life-Styles & Happiness Quality: Index of New Information for Reference & Research. Robert O. Coons. 1996. 150p. 57.50 (*0-7883-1284-7*) ABBE Pubs Assn.

Geriatric Audiology. Barbara E. Weinstein. 2000. LC 00-25383. (Illus.). 332p. 59.00 (*0-86577-701-2*, W1544) Thieme Med Pubs.

Geriatric Cardiology: Principles & Practice. Ed. by Anthony Martin & A. John Camm. 1994. LC 93-40107. 832p. 355.00 (*0-471-94064-X*) Wiley.

Geriatric Care Plans. Diane K. Newman et al. 1990. LC 90-9856. 352p. pap. 39.95 (*0-87434-263-5*) Springhouse Corp.

Geriatric Case Practice in the Nursing Home. Susan O. Mercer et al. 1991. (Geriatric Case Practice Training Ser.: Vol. 1). (Illus.). 280p. 76.95 (*0-8039-2916-1*, 6719); pap. 31.95 (*0-8039-2917-X*, 6720) Sage.

Geriatric Clinical Chemistry: Reference Values. Ed. by Willard R. Faulkner & Samuel Meites. 1993. 672p. pap. text 26.00 (*0-915274-65-5*, 623, AACC Pr) Am Assn Clinical Chem.

***Geriatric Consultation Liaison Psychiatry.** Ed. by Pamela Melding & Brian Draper. 2001. LC 2001-32141. (Oxford Medical Publications). 336p. text 68.00 (*0-19-263084-9*) OUP.

Geriatric Dentistry. Pederson Holm. 1988. 423p. (gr. 13). 49.95 (*87-16-09660-6*) Mosby Inc.

Geriatric Dentistry in Eastern Europe Countries. Walter Kunzel. 1991. (Illus.). 148p. pap. text 34.00 (*0-86715-223-0*) Quint Pub Co.

Geriatric Dermatology: Chronic Care & Rehabilitation. Robert A. Norman. 2001. LC 00-52879. (Illus.). 174p. 78.95 (*1-85070-311-6*, Parthenon Pbng) CRC Pr.

Geriatric Dermatology: Color Atlas & Practitioner's Guide. Edward Young et al. 1992. (Illus.). 250p. text 129.50 (*0-8121-1486-8*) Lppncott W & W.

Geriatric Drug Handbook for Long-Term Care. Jack D. McCue et al. 1992. LC 92-23440. (Illus.). 216p. pap. 29.00 (*0-683-05793-6*) Lppncott W & W.

Geriatric Drug Therapy Interventions. Ed. by James W. Cooper. 1998. LC 97-46982. 90p. 29.95 (*0-7890-0394-5*) Haworth Pr.

***Geriatric Education for Emergency Medical.** American Geriatrics Society Staff. 37.95 (*0-7637-2086-0*) Jones & Bartlett.

Geriatric Gastroenterology. Thomas M. Sodeman et al. 1989. 224p. text 62.00 (*0-7216-2799-4*) Saunders.

Geriatric Home Health Care: The Collaboration of Physicians, Nurses & Social Workers. Ed. by Philip W. Brickner et al. 1996. LC 96-26154. (Illus.). 320p. 49.95 (*0-8261-9450-8*) Springer Pub.

Geriatric Interdisciplinary Team Training. Ed. by Eugenia L. Siegler et al. 1998. LC 98-10334. (Illus.). 304p. 53.95 (*0-8261-1210-2*) Springer Pub.

Geriatric Long-Term Procedures & Treatments: A Problem-Solving Approach. Marie Jaffe. 2nd ed. 1999. LC 99-226704. 344p. (C). pap. text 37.95 (*1-56930-072-0*) Delmar.

Geriatric Medicine. K. M. Kafetz. 1986. (Clinical Tests Ser.). (Illus.). 80p. text (*0-7234-0855-6*) Wolfe Publishing.

Geriatric Medicine. Michael S. Katz. 1991. (Contemporary Management in Internal Medicine Ser.: Vol. 1, No. 6). (Illus.). 188p. text (*0-443-08825-X*) Church.

Geriatric Medicine. Ed. by M. S. Pathy & Paul Finucane. 1989. (Illus.). 383p. 121.00 (*0-387-19525-4*) Spr-Verlag.

Geriatric Medicine. Robert W. Schrier. 1990. (Illus.). 528p. text 104.00 (*0-7216-3031-6*) Saunders.

Geriatric Medicine. Dennis W. Jahnigen et al. 2nd ed. 1996. LC 97-162980. 752p. 175.00 (*0-86542-394-6*) Blackwell Sci.

Geriatric Medicine. John W. Rowe & Richard W. Besdine. 2nd ed. 1988. (Illus.). 750p. 115.00 (*0-316-75969-4*, Little Brwn Med Div) Lppncott W & W.

Geriatric Medicine. Ed. by C. K. Cassel et al. 3rd ed. 1998. LC 96-13736. (Illus.). 1070p. 145.00 (*0-387-94692-6*) Spr-Verlag.

Geriatric Medicine Annual-1986. Ed. by Richard J. Ham. 1986. 276p. 25.00 (*0-87489-390-9*) Soc Tchrs Fam Med.

Geriatric Medicine in the United States & Great Britain, 1. David K. Carboni. 1982. LC 82-9245. (Contributions to the Study of Aging Ser.: No. 1). (Illus.). 159p. 55.00 (*0-313-23437-X*, CAO/, Greenwood Pr) Greenwood.

Geriatric Mental Health. Ed. by Joel P. Abrahams & Valerie C. Crooks. 1984. 304p. text 43.95 (*0-8089-1657-2*, 790005, Grune & Strat) Harcrt Hlth Sci Grp.

Geriatric Mental Health Care: A Treatment Guide for Health Professionals. Gary J. Kennedy. 2000. LC 00-42231. 347p. 40.00 (*1-57230-592-4*, 8R0592) Guilford Pubns.

Geriatric Nephrology. Ed. by Dimitrious G. Oreopoulos. 1986. (Developments in Nephrology Ser.). text 232.00 (*0-89838-781-7*) Kluwer Academic.

Geriatric Nephrology. Harry Preuss. 2nd ed. 1996. (*0-938607-34-0*) Field & Wood Inc Medical.

Geriatric Neuropsychology. Ed. by Marilyn S. Albert & Mark B. Moss. 1988. LC 88-10004. 316p. 45.00 (*0-89862-722-2*, 2722) Guilford Pubns.

Geriatric Neuropsychology: An Assessment Guide. Holly Tuokko & Thomas Hadjistavropoulos. 1998. LC 97-34403. 350p. (*0-8058-1991-6*) L Erlbaum Assocs.

Geriatric Nurse Practitioner Certification Review. JoAnn Zerwekh & Jo C. Clayborn. Ed. by Robin Carter. 1999. LC 98-34771. 220p. (C). pap. text 35.00 (*0-7216-7742-8*) Saunders.

Geriatric Nursing. Sidney B. Voss-Morice. 1996. LC 98-111019. (Outline Ser.). (Illus.). 300p. (Orig.). (C). per. 22.95 (*0-944132-90-1*) Delmar.

Geriatric Nursing Assistants: An Annotated Bibliography with Models to Enhance Practice, 12. George H. Weber. 1990. LC 90-3858. (Bibliographies & Indexes in Gerontology Ser.: No. 12). 144p. lib. bdg. 52.50 (*0-313-26665-4*, WGN, Greenwood Pr) Greenwood.

Geriatric Nursing Protocols for Best Practice. Melissa M. Bottrell et al. Ed. by Ivo Abraham. 1999. LC 98-52113. (Series on Geriatric Nursing). 33.95 (*0-8261-1251-X*) Springer Pub.

Geriatric Nursing Research Digest. Ed. by Joyce J. Fitzpatrick & Terry Fulmer. 2000. 464p. text 52.95 (*0-8261-1332-X*) Springer Pub.

Geriatric Nutrition: The Health Professional's Handbook. Ronnie Chernoff. 2nd ed. 1999. LC 99-14492. 518p. 79.00 (*0-8342-1082-7*, 10827) Aspen Pub.

Geriatric Nutrition Handbook, Vol. 5. Mary Marian et al. 1995. LC 97-16251. 175p. spiral bd. 22.00 (*0-412-13641-4*) Aspen Pub.

Geriatric Orthopaedics: Rehabilitative Management of Common Problems. Trudy Sandler Goldstein. 2nd rev. ed. 1995. LC 98-46715. (Illus.). 320p. 58.00 (*0-8342-1076-2*, 10762) PRO-ED.

Geriatric Patient: Common Problems & Approaches to Rehabilitation Management. Mary C. Singleton & Eleanor F. Branch. 1989. LC 88-24742. (Physical Therapy in Health Care Ser.: Vol. 2, Nos. 3-4). (Illus.). 105p. text 39.95 (*0-86656-875-1*) Haworth Pr.

Geriatric Pearls. Moira Fordyce. 1999. LC 99-13819. (Illus.). 264p. (C). pap. text 21.95 (*0-8036-0434-3*) Davis Co.

Geriatric Pharmacology. Ed. by Rubin Bressler & Michael D. Katz. 1992. LC 92-19631. (Illus.). 689p. pap. 55.00 (*0-07-007660-X*) McGraw-Hill Prof.

Geriatric Pharmacology. Rubin Bressler & Michael Katz. 2nd ed. 2001. (Illus.). 792p. pap. 55.00 (*0-07-007662-6*) McGraw-Hill Educ Grp.

Geriatric Physical Therapy. Ed. by Andrew A. Guccione. 1992. (Illus.). 456p. (C). (gr. 13). text 65.00 (*0-8016-7452-2*, 01960) Mosby Inc.

Geriatric Physical Therapy. 2nd ed. 1999. (C). pap. text 60.00 (*0-8385-3138-5*) Appleton & Lange.

Geriatric Physical Therapy. Andrew A. Guccione. 2nd ed. 1999. LC 00-701556. (Illus.). xiv, 507p. (C). text 74.50 (*0-323-00172-6*) Mosby Inc.

Geriatric Physical Therapy: A Clinical Approach. Carole B. Lewis & Jennifer M. Bottomley. 1993. LC 93-5965. (Illus.). 672p. (C). 73.00 (*0-8385-8875-1*, A8875-5) P-H.

Geriatric Physical Therapy: Principles & Practices. Ed. by Andrew Buccione. 1992. LC 92-49977. (*0-8016-1960-2*) Mosby Inc.

Geriatric Practice for the Occupational Therapy Assistant. Ed. by Helene Goldstein-Lohman et al. 1997. LC 97-18554. (Illus.). 336p. (C). (gr. 13). text 39.95 (*0-8151-3724-9*, 29916) Mosby Inc.

Geriatric Problems in Immunology & Immunogenetics. Ed. by F. Gotthard Schettler. 1993. (Journal: Vol. 9, No. 4, 1992). (Illus.). vi, 68p. pap. 47.00 (*3-8055-5761-2*) S Karger.

Geriatric Psychiatry. 1999. 550p. text 65.95 (*0-8151-2622-0*) Mosby Inc.

Geriatric Psychiatry: A Handbook for Psychiatrists & Primary Care Physicians. Ed. by Leopold Bellak & Byram Karasu. 1976. LC 76-26287. (Illus.). 320p. text 59.00 (*0-8089-0967-3*, 790509, Grune & Strat) Harcrt Hlth Sci Grp.

Geriatric Psychiatry: Grief, Loss & Emotional Disorders in the Aging Process. Ed. by Martin A. Berezin & Stanley H. Cath. 1965. 380p. 55.00 (*0-8236-2120-0*) Intl Univs Pr.

Geriatric Psychiatry: Key Research Topics for Clinicians. Ed. by Elaine Murphy et al. 1995. LC 94-21812. 338p. 196.00 (*0-471-95168-4*) Wiley.

Geriatric Psychiatry & the Law. Richard Rosner. 1987. (Critical Issues in American Psychiatry & the Law Ser.: Vol. 3). (Illus.). 386p. (C). 90.00 (*0-306-42522-X*, Plenum Trade) Perseus Pubng.

Geriatric Psychopathology: Directions in Geriatric Psychopharmacology. David A. Smith. 1999. 90p. pap. 97.00 (*1-884937-60-8*) Manisses Communs.

Geriatric Psychopharmacology. J Craig Nelson. 1997. LC 97-42394. (Medical Psychiatry Ser.). (Illus.). 488p. text 195.00 (*0-8247-9851-1*) Dekker.

Geriatric Psychotherapy. Terry L. Brink. 1979. LC 78-26232. 318p. 45.95 (*0-87705-344-8*); pap. 24.95 (*0-87705-346-4*) Kluwer Academic (Kluwer Acad Hman Sci).

Geriatric Rehabilitation. David X. Cifu. 2000. 224p. pap. 39.95 (*0-7506-9608-7*) Buttrwrth-Heinemann.

Geriatric Rehabilitation. Jackson. 2000. (C). pap. text (*0-443-06538-1*) Church.

Geriatric Rehabilitation Manual. Timothy L. Kauffman. Ed. by Andrew Allen. 1999. LC 99-19075. (Illus.). 415p. pap. text (*0-443-07651-0*) Church.

Geriatric Resource Manual. Patricia Yee & Deborah G. Ross-Swain. 1998. LC 97-43044. 39.00 (*0-89079-774-9*) PRO-ED.

Geriatric Respiratory Care. Sorenson et al. 1998. LC 97-9709. (Respiratory Care Ser.). 208p. (C). pap. text 30.95 (*0-8273-7054-7*) Delmar.

Geriatric Secrets. Ed. by Mary A. Forciea & Rise J. Lavizzo-Mourey. 2nd ed. 2000. LC 00-22109. (Secrets Ser.). (Illus.). 364p. pap. 39.00 (*1-56053-162-2*) Hanley & Belfus.

Geriatric Survival Handbook. Barbara Acello. 1998. LC 98-117874. (Nurse's Survival Guide Ser.). 380p. (C). pap. 38.95 (*1-56930-061-5*) Delmar.

Geriatric Symptom Assessment & Management Kathy Fletcher. 1997. 32p. incl. VHS (*0-8151-1227-0*) Mosby Inc.

Geriatric Symptom Assessment & Management Module 1. Kathy Fletcher. 1998. (Illus.). 32p. wbk. ed. (*0-8151-2696-4*) Mosby Inc.

Geriatric Symptom Assessment & Management Module 1: Symptom Assessment Framework Video & Workbook Package. Kathy Fletcher. 1998. (Illus.). wbk. ed. incl. VHS (*0-8151-2692-1*) Mosby Inc.

Geriatric Symptom Assessment & Management Module 2. Kathy Fletcher. 1998. (Illus.). 32p. wbk. ed. (*0-8151-2697-2*) Mosby Inc.

Geriatric Symptom Assessment & Management Module 2: Cardiopulmonary Video & Workbook Package. Kathy Fletcher. 1998. (Illus.). 32p. wbk. ed. incl. VHS (*0-8151-2693-X*) Mosby Inc.

Geriatric Symptom Assessment & Management Module 3. Kathy Fletcher. 1998. (Illus.). 32p. wbk. ed. (*0-8151-2698-0*) Mosby Inc.

Geriatric Symptom Assessment & Management Module 3: Gastrointestinal Video & Workbook Package. Kathy Fletcher. 1997. (Illus.). 32p. wbk. ed. incl. VHS (*0-8151-2694-8*) Mosby Inc.

Geriatric Symptom Assessment & Management Module 4. Kathy Fletcher. 1998. (Illus.). 32p. wbk. ed. (*0-8151-2699-9*) Mosby Inc.

Geriatric Symptom Assessment & Management Module 4: Neuromuscular & Urinary Video & Workbook Package. Kathy Fletcher. 1997. (Illus.). 32p. wbk. ed. incl. VHS (*0-8151-2695-6*) Mosby Inc.

Geriatric Treatment Manual: Practical Tasks & Activities for Stimulating Information Processing Skills. Deborah G. Ross-Swain & Patricia Yee. 1998. pap. text 38.00 (*0-89079-733-1*, 8513) PRO-ED.

Geriatrics: The Diseases of Old Age & Their Treatment. Ignatz L. Nascher. Ed. by Robert J. Kastenbaum. 1979. LC 78-22212. (Aging & Old Age Ser.). (Illus.). reprint ed. lib. bdg. 42.95 (*0-405-11825-2*) Ayer.

Geriatrics & Gerontology of the Dog & Cat. Richard T. Goldston & Johnny D. Hoskins. 1995. (Illus.). 544p. text 69.00 (*0-7216-4584-4*) Saunders.

Geriatrics & Thanatology, 1. Elizabeth R. Prichard et al. 1984. LC 84-3286. 224p. 57.75 (*0-275-91447-X*, C1447, Praeger Pubs) Greenwood.

Geriatrics & the Law: Understanding Patient Rights & Professional Responsibilities. Marshall B. Kapp. 3rd ed. 1999. LC 98-54241. (Illus.). 328p. 54.95 (*0-8261-4532-9*) Springer Pub.

Geriatrics Case Conference Curriculum: Ambulatory Care Settings. Gail Sullivan et al. 1998. 75p. ring bd. 80.00 (*1-891509-01-2*) Univ CT Hlth.

Geriatrics for Everyday Practice. Ed. by J. Andrews & H. P. Von Hahn. 1981. (Illus.). viii, 220p. pap. 34.00 (*3-8055-1803-X*) S Karger.

Geriatrics for the Primary Care Physician. Thomas T. Yoshikawa et al. 2nd ed. 1997. LC 97-19320. (Illus.). 552p. (C). (gr. 13). pap. text 39.95 (*0-8151-2449-X*, 31011) Mosby Inc.

Geriatrics Review Syllabus. AGS Staff. 4th ed. 1999. pap. text 395.00 (*0-7872-5541-6*, 41554101) Kendall-Hunt.

Geriatrische Tumorpatient. Ed. by M. Neises et al. 1994. (Beitraege Zur Onkologie, Contributions to Oncology Ser.: Vol. 45). (Illus.). viii, 234p. 100.00 (*3-8055-5808-2*) S Karger.

Geriopharmacotherapy in Home Health Care: New Frontiers in Pharmaceutical Care. Intro. by Steven R. Moore. 1993. LC 93-6677. (Journal of Geriatric Drug Therapy Ser.: Vol. 7, No. 3). (Illus.). 71p. lib. bdg. 29.95 (*1-56024-415-1*) Haworth Pr.

Geripause: Medical Management During the Late Menopause. B. A. Eskin & B. Troen. 2002. (Illus.). 250p. 86.95 (*1-84214-037-X*, Parthenon Pbng) CRC Pr.

Germ Cell Tumors, No. IV. Jones. 1998. 350p. (*0-86196-567-1*) J Libbey Med GBR. *Dist:* Buttrwrth-Heinemann.

Germ Cell Tumours II: Proceedings of the 2nd Conference on Germ Cell Tumours, Leeds, 15-19 April 1985. Ed. by W. J. Jones et al. 1985. (Illus.). 480p. 96.00 (*0-08-031997-1*, Pergamon Pr) Elsevier.

Germ Cell Tumours III. Ed. by W. G. Jones et al. 1994. 480p. 155.00 (*0-08-042198-9*, Pergamon Pr) Elsevier.

Germ-Line Intervention & Our Responsibilities to Future Generations, Vol. 55. Ed. by Emmanuel Agius et al. 1997. LC 97-31693. (Philosophy & Medicine Ser.: No. 5). 344p. text 152.50 (*0-7923-4828-1*) Kluwer Academic.

Germ of Laziness: Rockefeller Philanthropy & Public Health in the New South. John Ettling. 1981. LC 81-4174. (Illus.). 275p. (C). 37.95 (*0-674-34990-3*) HUP.

Germ Plasm: A Theory of Heredity. August Weismann et al. LC 72-1659. reprint ed. 55.00 (*0-404-08191-6*) AMS Pr.

Germ Theory & Its Application to Medicine & on the Antiseptic Principle of the Practice. Louis Pasteur & Joseph Lister. 1996. LC 96-15710. (Great Minds Ser.). 144p. pap. text 8.00 (*1-57392-065-7*) Prometheus Bks.

German Aviation Medicine, World War II, Set. Surgeon General, USAF Staff. Tr. by Aero Medical Center Staff from GER. 1971. LC 77-168949. (Illus.). 1302p. reprint ed. lib. bdg. 125.00 (*0-87936-000-3*) Scholium Intl.

German-English - English-German Medical Dictionary. Dieter W. Unseld. 10th ed. 1991. (ENG & GER.). 91.00 (*0-7859-8939-0*) Fr & Eur.

German-English - English-German Medical Dictionary. D. W. Unseld. 10th enl. rev. ed. 1982. (ENG & GER.). 697p. 88.00 (*3-8047-1175-8*) Adlers Foreign Bks.

German-English Glossary of Psychiatric Terms. G. Blythe. 1987. (ENG & GER.). 95p. lib. bdg. 95.00 (*0-8288-3409-1*, F79921) Fr & Eur.

German-English Medical & Pharmaceutical Dictionary. Werner E. Bunjes. 3rd ed. 1981. 574p. 185.00 (*0-8288-1833-9*, M8736) Fr & Eur.

German Essays on Psychology. Wolfgang Schirmacher. 2000. LC 00-31401. (German Library: Vol. 62). xvii, 333p. pap. text 19.95 (*0-8264-1238-6*) Continuum.

German Health Reforms in 1993: New Cost Control Initiatives. 1994. (Illus.). 55p. (Orig.). (C). pap. text 30.00 (*0-7881-0199-4*) DIANE Pub.

German-Hungarian Medical Dictionary. P. Veghelyi & M. Kuntner. 1981. 736p. 49.95 (*0-8288-1883-5*) Fr & Eur.

German Medicine. Wilhelm Haberling. LC 75-23664. (Clio Medica Ser.: 13). (Illus.). reprint ed. 39.50 (*0-404-58913-8*) AMS Pr.

German Physician's Desk Reference see Rote List 1999

German Psychological Warfare. Ed. by Ladislas Farago. 1978. LC 72-4666. (International Propaganda & Communications Ser.). 302p. reprint ed. 26.95 (*0-405-04747-9*) Ayer.

German Psychology of To-Day. Theodule A. Ribot. 333p. 90.00 (*1-85506-667-X*) Thoemmes Pr.

German Standard Methods/Analysis of Fats & Other Lipids, Section 1. German Society of Fat Sciences Staff. 1989. 98.00 (*3-8047-0977-X*) CRC Pr.

German to Russian Dictionary Veterinary Medicine. Beschlebnov. 1996. (ENG & GER.). 464p. 105.00 (*0-320-00526-7*) Fr & Eur.

German Warfare: Breakthroughs in Immunology. Alan G. Baxter. 2000. 240p. pap. (*1-86508-070-5*) Allen & Unwin Pty AUS. *Dist:* IPG Chicago.

German/English Dictionary of Medicine & Veterinary Medicine. Fritz-Jurgen Nohring. 1997. (ENG & GER.). 850p. 295.00 (*0-7859-9346-0*) Fr & Eur.

German/English Medical Dictionary. Peter Reuter. 1995. (ENG & GER.). 837p. 295.00 (*0-7859-9983-3*) Fr & Eur.

Geroanesthesia: Principles for Management of the Elderly Patient. Stanley Muravchick. 1996. (Illus.). 320p. (C). (gr. 13). text 66.95 (*0-8016-7238-4*, 07238) Mosby Inc.

Gerocounseling: Counseling Elders & Their Families. Virginia S. Burlingame. 1995. LC 94-43090. (Life Styles & Issues in Aging Ser.). 232p. 36.95 (*0-8261-8820-6*) Springer Pub.

Gerontechnology: A Sustainable Investment in the Future. J. Graafmans. Ed. by V. Taipale & N. Charness. 1998. LC 97-77023. (Studies in Health Technology & Informatics: Vol. 48). 470p. 108.00 (*90-5199-367-6*, 367-6) IOS Press.

Gerontechnology: Proceedings of the 1st International Conference on Technology & Aging, Eindhoven, Aug. 26-29, 1991. Ed. by Herman Bouma & Jan A. M. Graafmans. 1992. LC 92-53266. (Studies in Health Technology & Informatics: Vol. 3). 449p. 95.00 (*90-5199-072-3*) IOS Press.

Gerontologic Nursing. Annette Lueckenotte. 1996. tchr. ed. (*0-8151-5599-9*) Mosby Inc.

Gerontologic Nursing. Ed. by Annette G. Lueckenotte. 2nd ed. 2000. LC 2001-268946. (Illus.). xxix, 846p. text 58.00 (*0-323-00757-0*) Mosby Inc.

Gerontologic Nursing: Wholistic Care of the Older Adult. Mary Burke & Mary Walsh. 2nd ed. 1996. (Illus.). 640p. (C). (gr. 13). pap. text 36.00 (*0-8151-1331-5*, 28200) Mosby Inc.

Gerontologic Nursing: Wholistic Care of the Older Adult. Mickie Burke & Mary Walsh. 2nd ed. 1997. (Illus.). tchr. ed. (*0-8151-1332-3*) Mosby Inc.

Gerontological Aspects of Eye Research: Selected Papers. Association for Eye Research Staff. 1978. (Interdisciplinary Topics in Gerontology Ser.: Vol. 13). (Illus.). 112.25 (*3-8055-2877-9*) S Karger.

Gerontological Nurse. Jack Rudman. 1994. (Certified Nurse Examination Ser.: CN-5). pap. 27.95 (*0-8373-6105-2*) Nat Learn.

Gerontological Nurse Practitioner. Jack Rudman. 1994. (Certified Nurse Examination Ser.: CN-6). pap. 27.95 (*0-8373-6106-0*) Nat Learn.

***Gerontological Nurse Practitioner Review & Resource Manual (GNP)** Nurse Practitioner Alternatives in Education, Inc. Staff. 2001. 450p. (C). pap. text 90.00 (*1-55810-169-1*) Am Nurses Pub.

Gerontological Nursing. Mickey Stanley & Patricia G. Beare. 2nd ed. 1999. LC 98-45217. (Illus.). 374p. pap. 35.95 (*0-8036-0369-X*) Davis Co.

Gerontological Nursing. Charlotte Eliopoulos. 5th ed. 2001. LC 00-61150. (Illus.). xvii, 493p. pap. text 36.95 (*0-7817-2362-0*) Lppncott W & W.

Gerontological Nursing: A Primary Care Clinical Guide. Ed. by Sheila L. Molony et al. 1999. LC 98-45637. (Illus.). 720p. pap. 50.00 (*0-8385-3131-8*) P-H.

Gerontological Nursing: Concepts & Practice. Mary A. Matteson et al. Ed. by Ilze Rader. 2nd ed. 1996. (Illus.). 1024p. text 58.00 (*0-7216-3785-X*) Saunders.

Gerontological Nursing: Current Practice & Research. Virginia Burggraf & Richard Barry. 1996. 336p. pap. 35.00 (*1-55642-284-9*, 32849) SLACK Inc.

Gerontological Nursing: Current Practice & Research Faculty Guide. Virginia Burggraf & Richard Barry, Sr. 1997. (Illus.). 64p. pap. text, tchr. ed. Price not set. (*1-55642-359-4*, 33594) SLACK Inc.

Gerontological Nursing: Issues & Opportunities for the Twenty-First Century. Ed. by Mary Burke & S. Sherman. 1993. 98p. (C). pap. text 32.95 (*0-88737-572-3*, 14-2510) Natl League Nurse.

Gerontological Nursing Care. Shirley R. Tyson. 1998. LC 98-7041. (Illus.). 512p. pap. text 32.95 (*0-7216-5009-0*) Saunders.

Gerontological Nursing Certification Review Guide for the Generalist, Clinical Specialist, & Nurse Practitioner. Ed. by Catharine Kopac et al. rev. ed. 1996. LC 95-31660. 541p. (C). pap. text 26.00 (*1-878028-15-4*) Hlth Lead Assoc.

Gerontological Protocols for Nurse Practitioners. Jerilyn B. Brown & Nancy K. Bedford. 1998. LC 99-24355. 592p. spiral bd. 41.95 (*0-7817-1567-9*) Lppncott W & W.

Gerontological Rehabilitation Nursing. Kristen L. Easton. 1999. LC 98-37373. 415p. text (*0-7216-6344-3*) Saunders.

Gerontological Social Work Practice in Long-Term Care. Ed. by George S. Getzel & M. Joanna Mellor. 1983. LC 82-21371. (Journal of Gerontological Social Work Ser.: Vol. 5, Nos. 1-2). 191p. text 49.95 (*0-86656-146-3*) Haworth Pr.

Gerontological Social Work Practice in the Community. Ed. by George S. Getzel & M. Joanna Mellor. 1985. LC 85-2767. (Journal of Gerontological Social Work Ser.: Vol. 8, Nos. 3-4). 274p. pap. 19.95 (*0-86656-256-7*); text 49.95 (*0-86656-145-5*) Haworth Pr.

Gerontological Social Work Supervision. Ann Burack-Weiss & Frances C. Brennan. 1991. LC 91-339. 148p. (Orig.). lib. bdg. 39.95 (*0-86656-827-1*); pap. text 14.95 (*1-56024-182-9*) Haworth Pr.

Gerontology. Ed. by D. Platt. 1990. (Illus.). 316p. 95.00 (*0-387-51544-5*) Spr-Verlag.

Gerontology: Leadership Skills for Nurses. Mary K. Ringsven. 2nd ed. 1997. (LPN/LVN Nursing Ser.). 13.50 (*0-8273-6779-1*) Delmar.

Gerontology: Nursing Care of the Older Adult. Mildred O. Hogstel. 2001. LC 00-50898. (Illus.). xxiv, 616p. text 64.95 (*0-7668-0729-0*) Delmar.

Gerontology: Responding to an Aging Society. Ed. by Kevin Morgan. 1992. 200p. 29.95 (*1-85302-117-2*) Taylor & Francis.

Gerontology & Geriatrics Collections. Ed. by Prisca Von Dorotka Bagnell. 1982. LC 82-11697. (Special Collections: Vol. 1, No. 3-4). 171p. 49.95 (*0-917724-53-4*) Haworth Pr.

Gerontology & Geriatrics Libraries & Collections in the United States & Canada: A History, Description & Directory. Joyce A. Post. 1992. LC 91-46862. 224p. lib. bdg. 62.50 (*0-313-28443-1*, PGG, Greenwood Pr) Greenwood.

Gerontology & Leadership for Nurses: Instructor's Guide. Mary K. Ringsven & Donna Bond. 1991. 13.50 (*0-8273-3451-6*) Delmar.

Gerontology & Leadership Skills - Nurses. Mary K. Ringsven. 1991. pap. 32.95 (*0-8273-3450-8*) Delmar.

Gerontology & Leadership Skills for Nurses. Bond Ringsven. 2nd ed. 1996. LC 96-18183. (LPN/LVN Nursing Ser.). 434p. (C). pap. text 54.95 (*0-8273-6778-3*) Delmar.

Gerontology & the Construction of Old Age: A Study in Discourse Analysis. Bryan S. Green. 1993. LC 92-39626. (Communication & Social Order Ser.). 241p. lib. bdg. 51.95 (*0-202-30450-7*) Aldine de Gruyter.

Gerontology Clinical Companion. Hogstel. 2001. (C). pap. 24.95 (*0-7668-0730-4*) Delmar.

Gerontology for the Health Care Professional. Walter Chop & Regula H. Robnett. 1999. LC 99-10900. (Illus.). 355p. (C). pap. text 23.95 (*0-8036-0398-3*) Davis Co.

Gerontology in Theological Education: Local Program Development. Ed. by Earl D. Brewer. 1989. LC 89-37874. (Journal of Religion & Aging: Vol. 6, Nos. 3-4). (Illus.). 162p. text 4.95 (*0-86656-958-8*) Haworth Pr.

Gerontology One: Experimental Studies Reprinted Selected Top Articles Published 1976-1978. Ed. by H. P. Von Hahn. 1979. (Gerontology Ser.). (Illus.). pap. 13.25 (*3-8055-3008-0*) S Karger.

Gerontology Review Guide for Nurses. Elizabeth C. Shaid & Kay Huber. rev. ed. 1996. LC 95-53081. 288p. 39.95 (*0-8261-9120-7*) Springer Pub.

Geropsychiatric Nursing. Ed. by Mildred O. Hogstel. 2nd ed. 1995. (Illus.). 448p. (C). (gr. 13). pap. text 36.95 (*0-8016-7811-0*, 07811) Mosby Inc.

Geruestprothetik. T. Brunner & M. Kundert. 2nd rev. ed. 1988. (Illus.). x, 82p. pap. 34.00 (*3-8055-4553-3*) S Karger.

Geschichte der Arabischen Arzte und Naturforscher. Ferdinand Wustenfeld. 1978. xvi, 183p. reprint ed. (*3-487-00402-X*) G Olms Pubs.

Geschichte der Herzhythmusst Orungen see History of the Disorders of Cardiac Rhythm

Geschichte der Medizin in Japan see Japanese Medicine

Geschichte der Physiologie see History of Physiology

Geschlecht & Charakter see Sex & Character

Geschwuelste - Tumors Two. D. Bierwolf et al. 1975. LC 56-2297. (Handbuch der Allgemeinen Pathologie Ser.: Vol. 6, Pt. 6). (Illus.). 908p. 368.00 (*0-387-06820-1*) Spr-Verlag.

Gesellschaft Fur Nephrologie: Deutsche Arbeitsgemeinschaft Fur Klinische Nephrologie, Nederlandse Vereniging Voor Nefrologie: Joint Scientific Meeting, Aachen, September 1997: Invited Papers. Ed. by J. H. Berden et al. 1997. (Kidney & Blood Pressure Research Ser.: Vol. 20, No. 3, 1997). (Illus.). 74p. pap. 55.75 (*3-8055-6568-2*) S Karger.

Gesichtsmuskeln. R. Seiler. Ed. by H. Hofer et al. 1976. (Primatologia Ser.: Vol. 4, Lieferung 6). 290p. 134.00 (*3-8055-2324-6*) S Karger.

Gestalt Approach. Neil Clark & Tony Fraser. 2nd ed. 1991. (Illus.). 56p. (C). reprint ed. pap. text 8.00 (*0-939266-12-1*) Gestalt Journal.

Gestalt Approach & Eyewitness to Therapy. Fritz Perls. 1973. 206p. pap. 13.95 (*0-8314-0034-X*) Sci & Behavior.

Gestalt Approaches in Counseling. W. Passons. 1975. LC 74-22223. (C). pap. text 39.50 (*0-03-089421-2*) Harcourt Coll Pubs.

Gestalt Art Experience: Patterns that Connect. Janie Rhyne. 2nd ed. 1995. LC 94-72915. (Illus.). 230p. (C). pap. text 26.95 (*0-9613309-6-1*) Magnolia St Pub.

Gestalt in Pastoral Care & Counseling: A Holistic Approach, Incl. Instructor's Manual. Jeffrey D. Hamilton. 1997. LC 96-52302. (Illus.). 175p. (C). 39.95 (*0-7890-0148-9*); pap. 19.95 (*0-7890-0238-8*) Haworth Pr (Haworth Pastrl).

Gestalt Psychology. Wolfgang Kohler. 1992. LC 72-114375. (Illus.). 384p. reprint ed. pap. 14.95 (*0-87140-218-1*) Norton.

Gestalt Psychology: A Survey of Facts & Principles. George W. Hartmann. 1974. LC 73-16649. (Illus.). 325p. reprint ed. lib. bdg. 72.50 (*0-8371-7213-6*, HAGE, Greenwood Pr) Greenwood.

Gestalt Psychology: Its Nature & Significance. David Katz. Tr. by Robert Tyson. 1979. LC 79-12343. 175p. reprint ed. lib. bdg. 38.50 (*0-313-20896-4*, KAGE, Greenwood Pr) Greenwood.

Gestalt Psychology in German Culture, 1890-1967: Holism & the Quest for Objectivity. Mitchell G. Ash. 1998. (Cambridge Studies in the History of Psychology). (Illus.). 528p. (C). pap. text 27.95 (*0-521-64627-8*) Cambridge U Pr.

Gestalt Therapy: An Introduction. Vernon Van De Riet et al. 1980. (General Psychology Ser.). 200p. 31.00 (*0-08-025587-6*); pap. 13.95 (*0-08-025586-8*) Elsevier (Pergamon Pr).

Gestalt Therapy: Practice & Theory. Margaret P. Korb et al. 2nd ed. 1989. (Psychology Practitioner Guidebooks). 192p. text 30.00 (*0-08-036435-7*); pap. text 15.95 (*0-08-036434-9*) Elsevier.

Gestalt Therapy: Theory, Practice & Research. Eleanor O'Leary. 1992. LC 92-17085. 148p. 44.75 (*1-56593-036-3*, 0284) Singular Publishing.

Gestalt Therapy Book. Joel Latner. rev. ed. 1984. LC 73-82442. 240p. reprint ed. pap. 20.00 (*0-939266-04-0*) Gestalt Journal.

Gestalt Therapy Discussions with the Masters. Ed. by Robert L. Harman. 1990. 198p. (C). text 41.95 (*0-398-05664-1*) C C Thomas.

Gestalt Therapy Integrated: Contours of Theory & Practice. Irving Polster et al. 1974. LC 74-3424. 352p. mass mkt. 12.00 (*0-394-71006-1*, V-6) Vin Bks.

Gestalt Therapy Mini-Lectures. James Simkin. 1990. 124p. reprint ed. pap. 15.00 (*0-939266-09-1*) Gestalt Journal.

Gestalt Therapy Verbatim. Frederick Perls. Ed. by Joe Wysong. rev. ed. 1992. 304p. pap. 25.00 (*0-939266-16-4*) Gestalt Journal.

Gestalt Voices. Ed. by Edward W. Smith & Edward Tick. 1992. (Frontiers in Psychotherapy Ser.). 352p. (C). 85.00 (*0-89391-802-4*); pap. 42.50 (*0-89391-803-2*) Greenwood (Ablex).

Gestalting Addiction: The Addiction-Focused Group Therapy of Dr. Richard Louis Miller. Angela Browne-Miller. 1993. LC 93-12291. (Frontiers in Psychotherapy Ser.). 142p. 77.00 (*0-89391-904-7*); pap. 39.50 (*0-89391-905-5*) Greenwood (Ablex).

Gestational Diabetes. Lois Jovanovic-Peterson et al. 1994. 144p. pap. 9.95 (*0-471-34684-5*) Wiley.

Gestational Diabetes. Ed. by P. A. Weiss & Donald R. Coustan. 1988. (Illus.). 240p. 119.00 (*0-387-82007-8*) Spr-Verlag.

Gestational Diabetes. American Diabetes Association Staff. 3rd ed. 1997. LC 97-7990. 80p. pap. 9.95 (*0-945448-90-2*, 4902-01) Am Diabetes.

Gestational Trophoblastic Disease. B. W. Hancock et al. 1996. LC 96-86255. (Illus.). 280p. (*0-412-63100-8*) E A GBR. *Dist:* OUP.

Gestational Trophoblastic Disease. A. E. Szulman & Herbert J. Buchsbaum. 1987. (Clinical Perspectives in Obstetrics & Gynecology Ser.). (Illus.). 192p. 84.50 (*0-387-96443-6*) Spr-Verlag.

Gesture & Aphasia. Petra Lott. 1999. LC 99-50313. (Illus.). vi, 200p. 36.95 (*3-906763-43-9*) P Lang Pubng.

Gesundheit! Bringing Good Health to You, the Medical System, & Society Through Physician Service, Complementary Therapies, Humor, & Joy. Patch Adams & Maureen Mylander. rev. ed. 1998. LC 99-187488. (Illus.). 248p. pap. 14.95 (*0-89281-781-X*, Heal Arts VT) Inner Tradit.

Gesundheits - Brockhaus. 4th ed. 1990. (GER.). 848p. 110.00 (*0-7859-3736-6*) Fr & Eur.

Get a Good Nights Sleep. Katherine A. Albert. 1996. LC 96-21034. 208p. 21.50 (*0-684-80428-X*) S&S Trade.

Get into Medical School! A Guide for the Perplexed. Kenneth V. Iserson. 1997. LC 96-31926. 450p. (Orig.). pap. 34.95 (*1-883620-23-6*) Galen AZ.

Get into the PA School of Your Choice. Andrew J. Rodican. 1998. LC 97-29065. 125p. (C). pap. 44.95 (*0-8385-3132-6*, A-3132-6) McGraw-Hill Prof.

Get It Up! Revealing the Simple Surprising Lifestyle That Causes Migraines, Alzheimer's, Stroke, Glaucoma, Sleep Apnea, Impotence & More. Sydney Ross Singer & Soma Grismaijer. 2001. LC 00-190973. xviii, 202p. pap. 15.95 (*1-930858-00-0*) ISCD.

Get off Your Butt. Lauren D. Chouinard. 1989. LC 89-92242. (Illus.). 71p. pap. 9.95 (*0-945744-01-3*) Provideo Ent.

Get on Track Fitness & Nutrition Training Log. David DePasquale. 1993. (Illus.). 55p. reprint ed. spiral bd. 12.95 (*0-9640918-0-1*) D DiPasquale.

Get Ready, Get Set... Prepare to Make Psychotherapy a Successful Experience for You. Harvey L. Saxton. Ed. by Paula N. Carroll. 1993. LC 93-23778. 198p. (C). 58.00 (*0-8191-9190-6*); pap. 32.50 (*0-8191-9191-4*) U Pr of Amer.

Get Ready-Get Set-Go-Go-Go! A Marketing Primer for Home Health Care Professionals. Jerry Rosenstrach et al. Ed. by Nancy Borgstadt. 1997. (Orig.). pap. 39.95 (*0-9658572-0-4*) Vis Nurse Amer.

Get Rid of Your Butt: Tighter Buns, Thinner Thighs in 75 Minutes a Week. Jeanette Micelotta et al. 1998. (Illus.). 60p. reprint ed. pap. text 5.00 (*0-7881-5207-6*) DIANE Pub.

Get the Rubber Habit! The Sisters of Perpetual Indulgence. Photos by Denis Doran. 1994. LC 93-42119. (Cassell AIDS Awareness Ser.). (Illus.). (*0-304-32847-2*) Cassell GBR. *Dist:* Sterling.

Get Well at Home. Richard A. Hansen. 2nd rev. ed. 1995. LC 81-117423. (Illus.). 464p. pap. 19.95 (*0-9643914-1-4*) Shiloh Med.

Get Well Care: Guidelines for Programs Serving Mildly Ill Children. Ed. by Ellen O. Montanari. 1989. 30p. reprint ed. pap. 10.95 (*1-882149-40-8*) CPG Pub.

Get Well Naturally. Linda Clark. 1974. reprint ed. 19.95 (*0-8159-5605-3*) Devin.

Get Well Stay Well. Sherwood & Haggard. 2001. pap. (*0-00-710395-6*) Thorsons GBR. *Dist:* Natl Bk Netwk.

Getting a Job in Health Care. Robert H. Zedlitz. 2nd ed. 1997. tchr. ed. (*0-538-70405-5*); 1991. (C). mass mkt. 19.75 (*0-538-70685-6*) S-W Thomson.

Getting Beyond Sobriety: Clinical Approaches to Long-Term Recovery. Michael C. Clemmens. 1997. LC 96-47105. (Jossey-Bass Psychology Ser.). 198p. 40.00 (*0-7879-0840-1*) Jossey-Bass.

Getting Care: Poor Children & New York City Hospitals. Beth Weitzman. 1987. (Papers: No. 7). 28p. 5.00 (*0-934459-39-8*) United Hosp Fund.

Getting Control: Overcoming Your Obsessions & Compulsions. Lee Baer. 1992. 256p. pap. 12.95 (*0-452-26889-3*, Plume) Dutton Plume.

Getting Doctors to Listen: Ethics & Outcomes Data in Context. Ed. by Philip J. Boyle. 1998. LC 97-9533. (Hastings Center Studies in Ethics). 248p. 45.00 (*0-87840-654-9*) Georgetown U Pr.

Getting Fit Your Way: A Self-Paced Fitness Guide. 1995. lib. bdg. 253.75 (*0-8490-6731-6*) Gordon Pr.

Getting Healthy & Staying Healthy. Globe-Fearon Staff. pap. text, instr.'s gde. ed. 5.50 (*0-8359-0690-6*); 1996. pap. text 12.50 (*0-8359-0684-1*) Globe Fearon.

Getting Help: Treatments for Drug Abuse. Sidney Schnoll. 1987. LC 86-1284. (Encyclopedia of Psychoactive Drugs Ser.: No. 1). (Illus.). 124p. (YA). (gr. 7-12). lib. bdg. 19.95 (*0-87754-775-0*) Chelsea Hse.

Getting Help with Legionella Problems: Guidance for Good Decisions. Matthew R. Freije. 1998. LC 98-96024. 18p. pap. 14.00 (*0-9649926-7-1*, 307) HC Info Res.

Getting HIV-Positive Youth into Care: Issues & Opportunities: A Study of the Special Projects of National Significance Program Adolescent Care Projects, 1997. Ed. by Barry Leonard. 2000. 90p. (C). reprint ed. pap. text 20.00 (*0-7881-8482-2*) DIANE Pub.

Getting Horses Fit: Improve Your Horse's Performance. Sarah Pilliner & Zoe Davies. 3rd ed. 2000. LC 00-29789. (Illus.). 288p. pap. 36.95 (*0-632-04811-5*) Blackwell Sci.

Getting In: A Step-by-Step Plan for Gaining Admission to Graduate School in Psychology. American Psychological Association Staff. 1993. LC 93-33069. (Illus.). 221p. pap. text 14.95 (*1-55798-219-8*) Am Psychol.

Getting in: How Not to Apply to Medical School. Paul Jung. 1999. LC 99-6519. 141p. pap. 21.95 (*0-7619-1757-8*) Sage.

Getting in Touch: The Guide to New Body-Centered Therapies. Ed. by Christine Caldwell. 1997. LC 97-17060. 288p. (Orig.). pap. 14.00 (*0-8356-0761-5*, Quest) Theos Pub Hse.

Getting in Touch & Staying in Touch: A Numerical Quick Guide to Compatibility & Communication. Maryanna

Korwitts & Jim Gash. 1994. 59p. pap. 12.95 (*1-887270-01-9*) Spiritpoint Pr.

Getting into American Medical-Veterinary Schools: A Practical "How to" Guide. Rosalie Gottfried. 1978. LC 77-93397. (YA). (gr. 10 up). pap. text 5.50 (*0-931084-01-6*) Argee Pub.

Getting into Medical School. Sanford J. Brown. 8th rev. ed. 1997. LC 96-35971. 256p. pap. 11.95 (*0-8120-9647-9*) Barron.

Getting into Medical School Today. Scott H. Plantz & Antonio Acosta. 3rd ed. 1996. 688p. pap. 12.95 (*0-02-861064-4*, Arc) Hungry Minds.

Getting into Medical School Today. Scott H. Plantz. 4th ed. 1998. LC 97-81127. 176p. pap. text 14.95 (*0-02-862500-5*, Arc) Hungry Minds.

Getting into Overtime. Edmond C. Hallberg et al. 1984. (Illus.). 185p. (Orig.). (C). pap. 12.95 (*0-930175-00-X*) Omb.

Getting into the System: Living with Serious Mental Illness. Gwen Howe. 1997. LC 98-132001. (Living with Serious Mental Illness Ser.: Vol. 1). 160p. pap. (*1-85302-457-0*) Jessica Kingsley GBR. *Dist:* Taylor & Francis.

Getting It Together: Promoting Drug-Free Communities: A Resource Guide for Developing Effective Youth Coalitions. 1994. (Illus.). 71p. (Orig.). (C). pap. text 25.00 (*0-7881-0575-2*) DIANE Pub.

Getting It Together! Your Personal Fitness Program for Maximum Results. John E. Ireland. 1986. LC 85-31706. (Illus.). 160p. (Orig.). pap. 8.95 (*0-913581-05-4*) Publitec.

Getting off Cocaine, Thirty Days to Freedom: The Step-by-Step Program of Nutrition & Exercise. Michael Weiner. 1984. 160p. (Orig.). pap. 8.95 (*0-380-67900-0*, Avon Bks) Morrow Avon.

Getting Off the Pain Roller Coaster: Psychological Aspects of Pain & Pain Management. Barry W. Weiss & Lillie Weiss. 1995. LC 95-7614. (Illus.). 14.95 (*0-9645528-0-9*) Golden Psych.

Getting Paid for What You Do: Coding for Optimal Reimbursement. Gary M. Knaus. 4th ed. 1997. (Illus.). 370p. pap. text 49.95 (*1-57066-067-0*, ME120) Practice Mgmt Info.

Getting Past Resistance with the Out-of-Control Adolescent. Vance R. Sherwood. 1998. LC 97-41460. 232p. 45.00 (*0-7657-0149-9*) Aronson.

Getting Pregnant! Over 1,000 of the Most Important Questions & Answers about Fertility Problems. Melvin J. Frisch. 1989. pap. 14.00 (*0-399-51711-1*, Perigee Bks) Berkley Pub.

Getting Pregnant & Staying Pregnant: A Guide to Infertility & High-Risk Pregnancy. Diana Raab. Ed. by Kathe Roth. 1989. (Illus.). 308p. pap. 14.95 (*0-921240-01-5*) Bookpeople.

Getting Pregnant the Natural Way. Deborah Gordon & D. S. Feingold. 2000. LC 00-35908. (Women's Natural Health Ser.). (Illus.). 272p. pap. 14.95 (*0-471-37959-X*) Wiley.

Getting Pregnant When You Thought You Couldn't. Helane S. Rosenberg & Yakov M. Epstein. 1993. 377p. pap. 13.99 (*0-446-39388-6*) Warner Bks.

***Getting Pregnant When You Thought You Couldn't: The Interactive Guide That Helps You Beat the Odds.** Helane S. Rosenberg & Yakov M. Epstein. rev. ed. 2001. LC 2001-26246. (Illus.). 512p. pap. (*0-446-67683-7*) Warner.

Getting Ready for Childbirth: A Guide for Expectant Parents. N. Fenlon et al. 1979. LC 79-13442. pap. 7.95 (*0-13-354795-7*) P-H.

Getting Research Fundings into Practice. Ed. by Andrew Haines & Anna Donald. 1998. 160p. pap. (*0-7279-1257-7*) BMJ Pub GBR. *Dist:* AIDC.

Getting Rid of Anxiety & Stress. Toby R. Drews. 1983. LC 82-61228. 167p. pap. 9.99 (*0-88270-537-7*) Bridge-Logos.

Getting Started: An Introduction to Dynamic Psychotherapy. Joel Kotin. 1995. LC 94-45157. 312p. 50.00 (*1-56821-451-0*) Aronson.

Getting Stronger. Bill Pearl. 1988. pap. 14.95 (*0-679-73948-3*) Random.

Getting the Best from Your Doctor: What You Don't Know Can Hurt You. Alan N. Schwartz et al. 1998. LC 98-231238. 340p. 23.95 (*1-56561-155-1*) Wiley.

Getting the Lead Out: The Complete Resource on How to Prevent & Cope with Lead Poisoning. Irene Kessel & John T. O'Connor. 1997. LC 96-50951. (Illus.). 264p. (C). 28.95 (*0-306-45525-0*) Da Capo.

Getting the Most for Your Medical Dollar: A Consumer's Guide to Affordable Health Care. Charles B. Inlander & Karla Morales. 1997. (Illus.). 467p. reprint ed. 10.00 (*0-7881-5121-5*) DIANE Pub.

***Getting the Most Out of Medicare & Medicare Supplement Insurance.** Contrib. by Aal Qualitylife Resources. 2000. LC 00-104657. (Illus.). 82p. pap. 12.95 (*0-9701509-3-8*) AAL QualityLife.

Getting Them Sober: A Guide for Those Living with Alcoholism, Vol. 1. Toby R. Drews. 1980. LC 80-82751. 203p. (Orig.). mass mkt. 5.99 (*0-88270-460-5*) Bridge-Logos.

Getting Through: Communicating When Someone You Care for Has Alzheimer's Disease. Mary J. Santo Pietro & Elizabeth E. Ostuni. rev. ed. 1991. LC 86-61472. (Illus.). 100p. (Orig.). pap. 18.95 (*0-937857-01-7*, 1331) Speech Bin.

Getting to Dry: How to Help Your Child Overcome Bedwetting. Max Maizels et al. 1999. LC 97-36913. (Illus.). xxix, 240 p. 27.95 (*1-55832-130-6*); 176p. pap. 14.95 (*1-55832-131-4*) Harvard Common Pr.

Getting to the Point: HIV, Drug Abuse & Syringe Exchange in the United States. Tracey A. Hooker. 1992. (State Legislative Reports: Vol. 17, No. 14). 21p. pap. text 15.00 (*1-55516-286-X*, 7302-1714) Natl Conf State Legis.

Getting Tough on Gateway Drugs: A Guide for the Family. Robert L. DuPont, Jr. 1984. LC 84-14595. 332p. pap. 12.95 (*0-88048-046-7*, 8046) Am Psychiatric.

Getting up When You're Feeling Down: A Woman's Guide to Overcoming & Preventing Depression. Harriet B. Braiker. 1990. 320p. mass mkt. 5.99 (*0-671-68327-6*) PB.

Getting Well. Herbert M. Shelton. 1993. 248p. reprint ed. spiral bd. 18.50 (*0-7873-0778-5*) Hlth Research.

Getting Your Boss's Number: And Many Other Ways to Use the Enneagram at Work. Michael J. Goldberg. 1996. LC 96-20586. pap. 12.00 (*0-06-251325-7*) Harper SF.

Getting Your Children Sober. Toby R. Drews. 1987. LC 87-71392. 163p. (Orig.). pap. 9.99 (*0-88270-637-3*) Bridge-Logos.

Gewebsdifferenzierung mit Ultraschall. H. G. Trier. 1977. (Bibliotheca Ophthalmologica Ser.: No. 86). 42.75 (*3-8055-2404-8*) S Karger.

Ghosts in the Bedroom: A Guide for Partners of Incest Survivors. Ken Graber. 1991. 152p. pap. 8.95 (*1-55874-116-X*) Health Comm.

Ghostwatching: The Ghosthunter's Handbook. Tony Wells & John Spencer. 1996. (Illus.). 288p. pap. (*0-86369-719-4*) Virgin Bks GBR. *Dist:* London Brdge.

GHRH, GH, & IGF-1: Basic & Clincial Advances. Ed. by Marc R. Blackman. 1995. (Illus.). 319p. 162.00 (*0-387-94404-4*) Spr-Verlag.

GI Words & Phrases: A Quick-Reference Guide. 1989. 146p. pap. 23.00 (*0-934385-14-9*) Hlth Prof Inst.

Giant vs. Pygmy Plus Thots Vol. VII: Chiropractic Metaphysical Concepts. Frederick H. Barge. 1995. LC 94-94214. 136p. text 38.95 (*1-885408-06-8*) Barge Chiropract.

Giardia: From Molecules to Disease. Ed. by R. C. A. Thompson et al. 1994. (Illus.). 416p. text 120.00 (*0-85198-840-7*) OUP.

Giardia & Cryptosporidium Handbook: A Practical Guide. Joan B. Rose & Huw V. Smith. Date not set. 79.95 (*0-87371-220-X*) Lewis Pubs.

Giardia & Cryptosporidium in Water Supplies. 1991. 118p. pap. 38.00 (*0-89867-569-3*, 90583) Am Water Wks Assn.

Giddiness & Vestibulo-Spinal Investigations, Combined Audio-Vestibular Investigations, & Experimental Neurootology: Proceedings of the XXIII Scientific Meeting of the Neurootological & Equilibriometric Society Reg. (N.E.S.), Bad Kissingen, 22-24 March 1996, Vol. 100. Neurootological and Equilibriometric Society Staff et al. 1996. LC 96-29489. (International Congress Ser.: 1133). 456p. 168.00 (*0-444-82493-6*) Elsevier.

Gift. Phil Borges. 2000. LC 00-130137. (Illus.). 120p. 24.99 (*0-9703998-0-4*) Interplast.

Gift: Journey to the Self Through Psychotherapy. Kathleen B. Mountain. 1998. LC 98-70642. 288p. 24.95 (*0-9663271-0-1*) Inner Passages.

Gift from Self to Self. Herbert L. Beierle. 1981. pap. 9.95 (*0-940480-12-3*) UNIPress.

***Gift of ADD: Shattering Labels & Changing Expectations for Parents & Teachers.** Mary Ellen Jirak. 2001. 500p. pap. 24.95 (*0-9708893-2-1*) Great Begin CA.

Gift of an Aching Back. Kathryn Christie. 1999. LC 98-73945. (Illus.). 240p. pap. 13.95 (*1-883697-16-6*) Hara Pub.

Gift of Dyslexia: Why Some of the Smartest People Can't Read & How They Can Learn. Ronald D. Davis. 1994. LC 94-17275. (Illus.). 232p. 14.95 (*0-929551-23-0*) Ability Workshop Pr.

Gift of Healing. Olga N. Worrall & Ambrose Worrall. 1985. 264p. reprint ed. pap. 14.99 (*0-89804-142-2*) Ariel GA.

Gift of Life: A Page from the Life of a Living Organ Donor. Lynn Chabot-Long. Ed. by Paul Jenkins. 1996. (Illus.). 184p. per. 9.99 (*0-9650555-5-8*) Je-Lynn Pubns.

***Gift of Life: Increasing Bone Marrow Donation & Transplantation: Congressional Hearing.** Ed. by Bill Frist. 2001. 62p. (C). reprint ed. pap. text 25.00 (*0-7567-0710-2*) DIANE Pub.

Gift of Life: Organ & Tissue Transplantation - An Introduction to Issues & Information Sources. Ed. by Cecilia Scnmitz & Richard A. Gray. 1993. 112p. pap. 12.95 (*0-87650-309-1*) Pierian.

Gift of Life: The Effect of Organ Transplantation on Individual, Family & Societal Dynamics. Robert Simmons et al. 1987. 526p. pap. text 29.95 (*0-88738-684-9*) Transaction Pubs.

Gift of Pain: The Inspiring Story of a Surgeon Who Discovers Why We Hurt & What We Can Do about It. Paul W. Brand & Philip Yancey. 1997. LC 97-22699. pap. 12.99 (*0-310-22144-7*) Zondervan.

Gift of Stories: Realising How to Deal with Mental Illness. Ed. by Julie Leibrich. 1999. (Illus.). 160p. pap. (*1-877133-83-3*) Univ Otago Pr NZL. *Dist:* Intl Spec Bk.

***Gift of Therapy: An Open Letter to a New Generation of Therapists & Their Patients.** Irvin D. Yalom. 2001. LC 2001-39319. 288p. 23.95 (*0-06-621440-8*) HarperCollins Pubs.

Gift of Touch see Touch Therapy

Gift of Touch: Comfort Touch: Massage for the Elderly & the Chronically & Terminally Ill. Mary Rose. 1996. 60p. (Orig.). pap. 10.00 (*0-9655182-0-5*) Hospice of Bldr Cty.

Gifted Child Grows Up: Twenty-Five Years' Follow-up of a Superior Group. Lewis M. Terman & Melita H. Oden. 1947. (Genetic Studies of Genius: Vol. N). xiv, 448p. 66.00 (*0-8047-0012-5*) Stanford U Pr.

Gifted Children in the Regular Classroom: The Complete Guide for Teachers & Administrators. Kathryn T. Hegeman. 1980. (Illus.). 189p. pap., tchr. ed. 15.00 (*0-89824-023-9*) Trillium Pr.

Gifted Group at Mid-Life: Thirty-Five Years' Follow-up of the Superior Child. Lewis M. Terman & Melita H. Oden. 1959. (Genetic Studies of Genius: Vol. V). xiii, 187p. 61.00 (*0-8047-0013-3*) Stanford U Pr.

Gifted IQ: Early Developmental Aspects - The Fullerton Longitudinal Study. A. W. Gottfried et al. 1994. LC 94-26562. (Illus.). 220p. (C). 39.50 (*0-306-44683-9*, Kluwer Plenum) Kluwer Academic.

Gifted Parent Groups: The SENG Model. James T. Webb & Arlene R. DeVries. 1998. LC 98-21448. Orig. Title: Training Manual for SENG Guided Discussion Groups. (Illus.). 146p. (gr. k-12). pap. 26.00 (*0-910707-29-4*) Great Potential Pr.

Gifted Student: An Annotated Bibliography, 1. Jean M. Laubenfels. 1977. LC 77-82696. (Contemporary Problems of Childhood Ser.: No. 1). 220p. lib. bdg. 70.00 (*0-8371-9760-0*, LGC/, Greenwood Pr) Greenwood.

Giftedness in Every Child: Unlocking Your Child's Unique Talents, Strengths & Potential. Rita S. Dunn et al. 1992. (Science Editions Ser.). 224p. 22.95 (*0-471-52803-X*) Wiley.

Giggle Belly. Page Sakelaris. 2000. (Rookie Readers Ser.). (Illus.). 32p. (J). (gr. 1-2). pap. 4.95 (*0-516-27047-8*) Childrens.

Gilda's Disease: Sharing Personal Experiences & a Medical Perspective on Ovarian Cancer. Gene Wilder & M. Steven Piver. 1996. LC 96-22847. (Illus.). 184p. 28.00 (*1-57392-089-4*) Prometheus Bks.

Gili's Book: A Readjustment Model of Parental Bereavement. Henya Kagan. 1998. LC 98-17902. 192p. 42.00 (*0-8077-3747-X*) Tchrs Coll.

Gili's Book: A Therapist Confronts the Death of Her Daughter. Henya Kagan. 1998. LC 98-17902. (Counseling & Development Ser.). 250p. pap. 19.95 (*0-8077-3746-1*) Tchrs Coll.

GI/Liver Secrets: Questions You Will Be Asked on Rounds, in the Clinic, & on Oral Exams. Ed. by Peter R. McNally. 1996. LC 95-47442. (Secrets Ser.). (Illus.). 675p. (Orig.). pap. 45.95 (*1-56053-150-9*) Hanley & Belfus.

Gilomas. Mitchel S. Berger & Byron Wilson. Ed. by Richard Zorab. 1998. LC 95-42774. (Illus.). xxii, 796p. (C). text 235.00 (*0-7216-4825-8*) Saunders.

Ginduri Secunde: Lucrari Selectate de Psihanaliza. Wilfred R. Bion. Ed. & Tr. by Florin V. Vladescu. Tr. by Carmen Bujdei et al. 1993. (Illus.). 240p. (Orig.). pap. text 19.95 (*1-883881-00-5*) S Freud RT&PF.

Gingko Biloba Extract (EGb 761) Pharmacological Activities & Clinical Applications. F. V. DeFeudis. 204p. pap. 57.00 (*2-906077-21-6*) Elsevier.

Ginkgo Biloba - A Global Treasure: From Biology to Medicine. Ed. by T. Hori et al. 1997. LC 97-27106. (Illus.). 430p. 106.00 (*4-431-70204-0*) Spr-Verlag.

Ginkgo biloba Extract (EGb 761) As a Free-Radical Scavenger. C. Ferradini et al. 1993. 200p. pap. 58.00 (*2-906077-36-4*) Elsevier.

Ginny: A Love Remembered. Bob Artley. 1993. LC 93-1485. (Illus.). 278p. 24.95 (*0-8138-2104-5*) Iowa U Pr.

Ginseng - In Life & Health: Index of Modern Authors & Subjects with Guide for Rapid Research. Stanley X. Garrett. 1991. LC 90-56300. 160p. 47.50 (*1-55914-408-4*); pap. 44.50 (*1-55914-409-2*) ABBE Pubs Assn.

Ginseng & Other Medicinal Plants. A. R. Harding. rev. ed. 1972. 386p. pap. 6.00 (*0-936622-09-1*, A399155) A R Harding Pub.

Girl Who Died Twice: Every Patient's Nightmare - The Libby Zion Case & the Hidden Hazards of Hospitals. Natalie Robins. 1999. (Illus.). 350p. reprint ed. text 23.00 (*0-7881-6599-2*) DIANE Pub.

Girl Who Gave Birth to Rabbits: A True Medical Mystery. Clifford A. Pickover. 2000. LC 99-56193. (Illus.). 232p. pap. 19.00 (*1-57392-794-5*) Prometheus Bks.

Girlfriends' Guide to Pregnancy: Or Everything Your Doctor Won't Tell You. Vicki Iovine. Ed. by Dona Chernoff. 1995. LC 95-21981. 288p. pap. 14.00 (*0-671-52431-3*, PB Trade Paper) PB.

Girls at Puberty: Biological & Psychosocial Perspectives. J. Brooks-Gunn & A. C. Peterson. 1983. (Illus.). 370p. (C). 75.00 (*0-306-41144-X*, Plenum Trade) Perseus Pubng.

Girls on the City Streets: A Study of 1400 Cases of Rape. Jacob A. Goldberg & Rosamond W. Goldberg. 1977. LC 74-3952. (Women in America Ser.). 384p. reprint ed. 33.95 (*0-405-06099-8*) Ayer.

Gitsch, E., Festschrift. Ed. by E. Reinold. 1991. (Journal: Vol. 30, No. 4, 1990). (Illus.). xiv, 64p. pap. 32.25 (*3-8055-5393-5*) S Karger.

Give Me a Child Until He Is Seven: Brain Studies & Early Childhood Education. John Brierley. 2nd ed. 1994. LC 94-16346. 24.95 (*0-7507-0319-9*, Falmer Pr) Taylor & Francis.

Give Me Liberty. Matthews Gallin. 1999. 384p. pap. 14.95 (*0-312-24563-7*) St Martin.

Give This Man a Hand: A True Story of Losing a Hand & Regaining It. Earl Harrell & Cassandra Harrell. Ed. by Chris Roerden. 1990. LC 89-82137. (Illus.). 157p. (Orig.). pap. text 13.95 (*0-9625203-0-6*) E T Pub Co.

Give up False Expectations & "Disappointment" Harvey Jackins. Tr. by Francisco Lopez-Bustos from ENG. 1999.Tr. of Renunciemos a Falsas Expectativas y "Desilusiones". (SPA.). 12p. pap. 2.00 (*1-58429-044-7*) Rational Isl.

Give Your ADD Teen a Chance: A Guide for Parents of Teenagers with Attention Deficit Disorder. Lynn Weiss. 1996. LC 96-8057. 304p. pap. 15.00 (*0-89109-977-8*) Pinon Press.

Give Yourself Health: Thoughts, Attitudes & Your Health. Ed. by Scott Miners. 1990. 160p. (Orig.). pap. 7.95 (*0-9625720-0-4*) Turning Pt WA.

Giving Birth. Mary M. Kalergis. 1997. (Illus.). 93p. 19.95 (*0-9659646-1-2*, 00197); pap. 12.95 (*0-9659646-2-0*, 00197) Sugarday Bks.

Giving Comfort: What You Can Do When Someone You Love Is Ill. Linda B. Milstein. 1994. LC 93-32169. 128p. pap. 11.00 (*0-14-023538-8*, Penguin Bks) Penguin Putnam.

Glandular Mechanisms of Salivary Secretion. Ed. by John R. Garrett et al. 1998. LC 98-21627. (Frontiers of Oral Biology Ser.: Vol. 10). (Illus.). x, 226p. 167.00 (*3-8055-6630-1*) S Karger.

Glare & Contrast Sensitivity for Clinicians. Ed. by M. P. Nadler et al. 1989. (Illus.). 150p. 148.00 (*0-387-97009-6*) Spr-Verlag.

Glass Full of Tears: Dementia Day-by-Day. June L. Shiplett. Ed. by Lavern Hall. 1996. LC 96-60203. (Illus.). 200p. (Orig.). pap. text 14.95 (*0-9631441-2-X*) Writers Wrld.

Glass-Ionomer Cement. Alan D. Wilson & McLean. 1989. (Illus.). 274p. text 98.00 (*0-86715-200-1*, 2001) Quint Pub Co.

Glass of Heaven: The Faith of the Dramatherapist. Roger Grainger. 1995. 200p. pap. 29.95 (*1-85302-284-5*) Taylor & Francis.

Glass's Office Gynecology. Michele G. Curtis et al. 5th ed. 1998. LC 98-3829. (Illus.). 562p. 99.00 (*0-683-30201-9*) Lppncott W & W.

Glaucoma. Bennett. 2000. (Optometric Procedure Ser.). 112p. pap. text 34.95 (*0-7506-9625-7*) Buttrwrth-Heinemann.

Glaucoma: A Clinician's Guide. Barton Hodes. 1993. 275p. (C). (gr. 13). pap. 51.95 (*0-412-05681-X*) Chapman & Hall.

Glaucoma: A Color Manual of Diagnosis & Treatment. Jack J. Kanski et al. 2nd ed. 1996. (Illus.). 192p. text 110.00 (*0-7506-1820-5*, Focal) Buttrwrth-Heinemann.

Glaucoma: A Guide for Patients. Henry Jampel. Ed. by Morton Goldberg. 1997. (Opthalmology Ser.: Vol. 0801). (Illus.). 32p. (Orig.). pap. 2.95 (*1-885274-48-3*) Health InfoNet Inc.

Glaucoma: A Patient's Guide to the Disease. Graham E. Trope. 1996. (Illus.). 108p. pap. 8.95 (*0-8020-7847-8*) U of Toronto Pr.

Glaucoma: Decision Making in Therapy. M. G. Bucci. 1996. LC 96-25619. 690p. pap. 180.00 (*3-540-75021-5*) Spr-Verlag.

Glaucoma - Concepts in Evolution: Morphometric & Functional Parameters in the Diagnosis & Follow-Up of Management Glaucoma. Ed. by L. Bonomi & N. Orzalesi. 1991. LC 91-35342. (Illus.). 160p. lib. bdg. (*90-6299-081-9*) Kugler NLD. *Dist:* Lib Res.

Glaucoma - Diagnosis & Therapy: Transactions of the New Orleans Academy of Ophthalmology. Ed. by Stuart F. Ball & Rudolph M. Franklin. 1993. 216p. pap. text (*90-6299-105-X*) Kugler NLD. *Dist:* Lib Res.

Glaucoma Co-Management. 2002. 144p. pap. 55.00 (*0-7506-3782-X*) Buttrwrth-Heinemann.

Glaucoma Handbook. Anthony B. Litwak. 2000. LC 00-31220. 384p. text 95.00 (*0-7506-9776-8*) Buttrwrth-Heinemann.

Glaucoma Surgery. Maurice H. Luntz & R. Harrison. 1994. LC 95-122876. 228p. text 159.00 (*981-02-1418-9*) World Scientific Pub.

Glaucoma Surgery: Principles & Techniques. Robert N. Weinreb & Richard P. Mills. 2nd ed. 1998. LC 98-5579. (Opthalmology Monographs Ser.). xix, 240 p. (*1-56055-046-5*) Am Acad Ophthal.

Glaucoma Surgery: Principles & Techniques. Robert N. Weinreb & Richard P. Mills. 2nd ed. 1998. LC 98-5579. (Ophthalmology Monographs ;). pap. (*1-56066-046-5*) American Academic Assn for Peace in the Middle East.

Glaucoma Symposium Amsterdam: Diagnosis & Therapy. Ed. by Erik L. Greve. 1980. (Documenta Ophthalmologica Proceedings Ser.: No. 22). 419p. text 261.50 (*90-6193-164-9*) Kluwer Academic.

Glaucoma Therapy: Effective Pharmacological Approaches. Ed. by Xavier D. Martin. 1996. LC 96-77158. (Illus.). 134p. text 49.00 (*0-88937-176-8*) Hogrefe & Huber Pubs.

Glaucoma Update IV: Glaucoma Society of the International Congress of Ophthalmology, Bali, March 1990. Ed. by Gunter K. Krieglstein. 1991. (Illus.). 265p. 159.00 (*0-387-53176-9*) Spr-Verlag.

Glaucoma Update VI. Ed. by G. K. Krieglstein. 1999. LC 99-47506. (Illus.). xxiv, 267p. 112.00 (*3-540-65364-3*) Spr-Verlag.

Glaucomas, Vol. 2. M. Bruce Shields et al. 2nd ed. 1995. (Illus.). 1976p. (C). (gr. 13). text 330.00 (*0-8016-7702-5*, 07702) Mosby Inc.

Glaxo: A History to Nineteen Sixty-Two. R. P. Davenport-Hines & Judy Slinn. 1993. 422p. (C). text 100.00 (*0-521-41539-X*) Cambridge U Pr.

Glencoe Basic Medical Terminology. J. Patrick Fisher. 5th ed. 1998. LC 97-42695. pap. 30.00 (*0-02-801003-5*) McGraw.

***Glencoe Basic Medical Terminology: Microcomputer Test Bank.** J. Patrick Fisher. 5th ed. 1998. (*0-02-801006-X*) Glencoe.

***Glencoe Basic Medical Terminology Lab.** J. Patrick Fisher. 5th ed. 1998. 43.28 (*0-02-801005-1*) Glencoe.

Glencoe Computers in the Medical Office Using MediSoft for Windows. 1999. tchr. ed. 13.08 (*0-02-801991-1*) Glencoe.

Glencoe Medical Keyboarding. 1999. tchr. ed. 15.00 incl. disk (*0-02-804817-2*) Glencoe.

Glencoe Medical Keyboarding. (*0-02-804816-4*) McGraw-Hill Med Pub.

Glencoe Medical Laboratory Procedures. Tom Palko & Hilda Palko. 1997. LC 97-46117. (Allied Health Ser.). pap. 14.00 (*0-02-802015-4*); 2nd ed. 30.00 (*0-02-802014-6*) Glencoe.

Glencoe Nursing Assistant Fundamentals: A Patient Centered Approach. June Eastmond et al. 1998. LC 96-37169. 640p. text 29.75 (*0-02-802424-9*) Glencoe.

***Glencoe Nursing Assistant Fundamentals: A Patient-Centered Approach - Microcomputer Test Bank.** June Eastmond et al. (*0-02-802427-3*) Glencoe.

Glencoe's Medical Terminology: Language for Health Care. Joanne Becker. 2000. LC 00-45469. (Illus.). xxlv, 720p. (*0-02-801289-5*) Glencoe.

Glenn's Thoracic & Cardiovascular Surgery, Set, Vols. 1 & 2. Arthur Baue. 6th ed. 1996. (Illus.). 3276p. (C). pap. text 350.00 (*0-8385-3134-2*, A3134-2, Apple Lange Med) McGraw.

Glial Cells: Their Role in Behaviour. Ed. by Peter R. Laming et al. 1998. LC 98-10902. (Illus.). 440p. (C). text 160.00 (*0-521-57368-8*) Cambridge U Pr.

Glimpse. Joyce MacIver. 1983. LC 82-90994. 160p. 12.95 (*0-87212-174-7*) Libra.

Glimpses into the Psychology of Yoga. I. K. Taimni. 1976. 10.95 (*0-8356-7290-5*) Theos Pub Hse.

Glioma: Principles & Practice in Neuro-Oncology. Ed. by A. B. Karim & E. R. Laws. 1991. (Illus.). 289p. 163.00 (*0-387-52286-7*) Spr-Verlag.

Global Agenda for Caring. Ed. by Delores A. Gaut. 1993. (International Association for Human Caring Ser.). 394p. (C). pap. text 33.95 (*0-88737-578-2*, 15-2518) Natl League Nurse.

Global AIDS Policy. Ed. by Douglas A. Feldman. 1994. LC 94-2850. 264p. 72.50 (*0-89789-282-8*); pap. 22.00 (*0-89789-412-X*) Greenwood (Bergin & Garvey).

Global AIDS Strategy. 1992. (WHO AIDS Ser.: No. 11). (ENG, FRE & SPA.). v, 23p. pap. text 9.00 (*92-4-121011-7*, 1870011) World Health.

Global Alliances in Tourism & Hospitality Management. Ed. by John C. Crotts et al. 1999. LC 99-38667. 166p. pap. text 24.95 (*0-7890-0818-1*) Haworth Pr.

Global Atmospheric Change & Public Health: Papers Presented at a Meeting in Washington, D. C., Sponsored by the Air Resources Information Clearinghouse (ARIC), December 1989. Ed. by J. C. White et al. 1990. 280p. pap. 275.95 (*0-444-01565-5*) Elsevier.

Global Biotechnology Product Registration: E. U., U. S., & Japan. Mark M. Struck et al. 1997. LC 98-148383. 392 p. (*1-882615-32-8*) Parexel Intl.

Global Budgets vs. Competitive Cost-Control Strategies. Patricia M. Danzon. 1994. (Studies in Health Reform). 200p. (Orig.). pap. 9.95 (*0-8447-7023-X*, AEI Pr) Am Enterprise.

Global Challenge of AIDS: Ten Years of HIV-AIDS Research: Proceedings of the Tenth International Conference on AIDS-International Conference on STD, Yokohama, August 7-12, 1994. Ed. by Yuichi Shiokawa & Takashi Kitamura. 1995. LC 95-24766. (*4-06-207359-5*) Kodansha Ltd JPN. *Dist:* Bks Nippan.

Global Comparative Assessments in the Health Sector: Disease Burden, Expenditures & Intervention Packages. Ed. by C. J. Murray & A. D. Lopez. 1994. LC 96-211984. (Bulletin of WHO Ser.). viii, 196p. pap. text 18.00 (*92-4-156175-0*, 1150420) World Health.

Global Competitiveness in the Pharmaceutical Industry: The Effect of National Regulatory, Economic & Market Factors. Madhu Agrawal. 1999. LC 99-13600. 188p. lib. bdg. 69.95 (*0-7890-0715-0*, Pharmctl Prods) Haworth Pr.

Global Dermatology: Diagnosis & Management According to Geography, Climate, & Culture. Ed. by Lawrence C. Parish & Larry E. Millikan. 1994. LC 93-26905. (Illus.). 359p. 236.00 (*0-387-94140-1*) Spr-Verlag.

Global Epidemiology of Infectious Diseases. Christopher J. Murray & Alan D. Lopez. 1998. (Global Burden of Disease & Injury Ser.: Vol. 4). 600p. 49.95 (*0-674-35446-X*) HUP.

***Global Health: Joint U. N. Programme on HIV/AIDS Needs to Strengthen Country-Level Efforts & Measure Results.** John Hutton. 2001. 64p. (C). pap. 20.00 (*0-7567-1675-6*) DIANE Pub.

***Global Health: U. S. Agency for International Development Fights AIDS in Africa, but Better Data Needed to Measure Impact.** John P. Hutton. 2001. 51p. (C). pap. text 20.00 (*0-7567-1357-9*) DIANE Pub.

Global Health: U.S. Response to Infectious Diseases : Hearing Before the Subcommittee on Public Health & Safety of the Committee on Labor & Human Resources, United States Senate, One Hundred Fifth Congress, Second Session ... March 3, 1998. USGPO Staff. 1998. LC 98-190707. iii, 97 p. (*0-16-057073-5*) USGPO.

Global Health Care Markets: A Comprehensive Guide to Regions, Trends & Opportunities Shaping the International Health Arena. Walter W. Wieners. 2000. LC 00-60179. (Jossey-Bass Health Ser.). (Illus.). 448p. 75.00 (*0-7879-5307-5*) Jossey-Bass.

Global Health Jurisprudence: Materials & Analysis on International Law & Public Health. Ed. by David P. Fidler. 2000. LC 00-61541. (Illus.). xxiii, 645p. 145.00 (*1-57105-123-6*) Transnatl Pubs.

Global Health Policy, Local Realities: The Fallacy of the Level Playing Field. Ed. by Linda M. Whiteford & Lenore Manderson. 2000. LC 99-56616. (Directions in Applied Anthropology Ser.). vi, 333p. lib. bdg. 59.95 (*1-55587-874-1*) L Rienner.

Global Health Statistics. Ed. by Christopher J. Murray & Alan D. Lopez. 1996. LC 96-26652. (Global Burden of Disease & Injury Ser.: No. 2). (Illus.). 1010p. 45.00 (*0-674-35449-4*) HUP.

Global Healthcare Grid: Medicine Meets Virtual Reality. Ed. by Karen S. Morgan et al. 1997. LC 96-79462. (Studies in Health Technology & Informatics: Vol. 39). 632p. 98.00 (*90-5199-299-8*, 299-8) IOS Press.

Global Human Genome Programme. OECD Staff. 1995. 76p. (Orig.). pap. (*92-64-14575-3*) Org for Econ FRA. *Dist:* OECD.

Global Infectious Diseases: Prevention, Control & Eradication. Ed. by D. H. Walker. 1992. (Illus.). 240p. 120.00 (*0-387-82329-8*) Spr-Verlag.

Global Positioning System: Gold Code Balance-Run-Autocorrelation Properties Reference. Steven Callaghan. 1994. 200p. 50.00 (*0-925395-98-6*) SGC Biomedical.

Global Programme on AIDS, 1992-1993 Progress Report. 1995. viii, 178p. (C). pap. text 32.00 (*92-4-156177-7*, 1150425) World Health.

Global Report on Student Well-Being: Employment, Finances, Housing & Transportation. Alex C. Michalos. 1992. (Recent Research in Psychology Ser.: Vol. 3). 306p. 97.00 (*0-387-97948-4*) Spr-Verlag.

Global Report on Student Well-Being, Vol. One: Life Satisfaction & Happiness. Alex C. Michalos. 1991. (Recent Research in Psychology Ser.). (Illus.). 253p. 72.95 (*0-387-97460-1*) Spr-Verlag.

Global Strategy for Asthma Management & Prevention. 1996. (Illus.). 176p. (C). reprint ed. pap. text 40.00 (*0-7881-3401-9*) DIANE Pub.

Global Strategy for Health for All by the Year 2000. Date not set. text (*92-4-180003-8*) World Health.

Global Strategy for Malaria Control. Ed. by World Health Organization Staff. 1993. (ENG, FRE & SPA.). x, 30p. pap. text 11.00 (*92-4-156161-0*, 1150405) World Health.

Global Surgery Formula for the Casson-Walker Invariant. Christine Lescop. 1995. (Annals of Mathematics Studies: Vol. 140). 150p. 77.50 (*0-691-02133-3*); pap. 25.95 (*0-691-02132-5*) Princeton U Pr.

Global Village of Dentistry: Internet, Intranet, Online Services for Dental Professionals. Titus K. Schleyer et al. 1998. LC 97-47142. 164p. pap. text 32.00 (*0-86715-345-8*) Quint Pub Co.

Global Visions of Women Pharmacists: Speeches from an International Forum. Agathe Wehrli et al. 1998. LC 98-86033. (Illus.). 100p. (*0-9665347-0-0*) Ldrship Intl.

Globalization & Global Governance: Medical Ethics in Conflict with Religious Freedom. Ed. by Raimo Vayrynen. 1999. LC 98-48273. 304p. 82.00 (*0-8476-9154-3*); pap. 29.95 (*0-8476-9155-1*) Rowman.

Glomerular Basement Membrane. Ed. by G. Lubec. 1981. (Illus.). vii, 434p. 135.75 (*3-8055-2952-X*) S Karger.

Glomerulonephritis. Graeme R. Catto. 1990. 176p. text 107.00 (*0-7462-0109-5*) Kluwer Academic.

Glomerulonephritis: Proceedings of the Nephrology Symposium, 3rd, Hannover, June 1975. Nephrology Symposium Staff. Ed. by R. B. Sterzel. 1976. (Contributions to Nephrology Ser.: Vol. 2). (Illus.). 200p. 29.75 (*3-8055-2318-1*) S Karger.

Glomerulonephritis & Vasculitis/Tubolointerstitial Disease Ed. by Robert W. Schrier et al. 1998. LC 98-29127. (Atlas of Diseases of the Kidney Ser.: Vol. 2). (Illus.). 131.95 (*0-632-04387-3*) Blackwell Sci.

Glomerulonephritis in the Elderly. Ed. by M. Meroni et al. 1993. (Contributions to Nephrology Ser.: Vol. 105). (Illus.). viii, 184p. 49.75 (*3-8055-5752-3*) S Karger.

Gloria Lorings Guide to Health & Beauty. Gloria Loring. 1985. (Illus.). 128p. (Orig.). pap. (*0-932565-00-X*) Camex.

Glorious Victory of Truth: The Tiszaeszlar Blood Libel Trial, 1882-3: A Historical-Legal-Medical Research. Edith Stern. 1998. LC 98-180353. (Illus.). 176p. (*965-09-0079-9*, 99550) R Mass Ltd ISR. *Dist:* Lambda Pubs.

Glossaire de Psychiatrie: Glossary of Psychiatry. Pierre Marchais. 1970. (FRE.). 238p. 79.95 (*0-8288-6537-X*, M-6398) Fr & Eur.

Glossarium - Drugs of Abuse. European Communities Staff. 1995. LC 96-122904. 168p. pap. text (*92-826-8045-2*) Comm Europ Commun BEL. *Dist:* Bernan Associates.

Glossarium - Toxicology. European Communities Staff. 1995. 225p. pap. text (*92-826-8050-9*) Comm Europ Commun BEL. *Dist:* Bernan Associates.

Glossary & Bibliography of Rational-Emotive Therapy Concepts. Ben Neal Ard, Jr. 1993. LC 93-16905. 152p. 39.95 (*1-880921-30-8*); pap. 25.95 (*1-880921-19-7*) Austin & Winfield.

Glossary & Guidelines for Immunodiagnostic Procedures, Reagents & Reference Materials: Approved Guideline (1992) Contrib. by Robert M. Nakamura. 1992. 75.00 (*1-56238-140-7*, D11-A2) NCCLS.

Glossary for Radiologic Technologists. Patricia A. Myers. 1981. LC 80-20917. 194p. 59.95 (*0-275-91351-1*, C1351, Praeger Pubs) Greenwood.

Glossary of an Evolving Health Care Marketplace. Ed. by Kenneth R. Cohen et al. 2000. ii, 186p. pap. 12.95 (*0-9702957-1-5*); 1999. ii, 184p. pap. 12.95 (*0-9702957-0-7*) Logical Hlth.

Glossary of Anesthesia & Related Terminology. Sanford L. Klein. 2nd ed. 1993. LC 92-2223. (*3-540-97831-3*); (Illus.). 641p. 99.00 (*0-387-97831-3*) Spr-Verlag.

Glossary of Ayurveda, Tibetan, & Unani Medicines. 1999. LC 98-908931. (Indian Medical Science Ser.). 293 p. (*81-7030-598-5*) Sri Satguru Pubns.

Glossary of Genetics & Cytogenetics. R. Rieger et al. 4th rev. ed. 1976. LC 76-16183. (Illus.). pap. 25.00 (*3-540-07668-9*) Spr-Verlag.

Glossary of Health Care Terminology. J. Hogarth. 1978. (Public Health in Europe Ser.: No. 4). 434p. 25.00 (*92-9020-123-1*, 1320004) World Health.

Glossary of Health Services. Canada Communication Group Staff. 1992. (Glossary Ser.: No. 205). (ENG & FRE.). 39.95 (*0-8288-7372-0*, 660565331) Fr & Eur.

Glossary of HIV/AIDS - Related Terms. Ed. by Barry Leonard. 1999. 110p. reprint ed. pap. text 25.00 (*0-7881-7014-7*) DIANE Pub.

Glossary of Indian Medicinal Plants. R. N. Chopra. 1988. (C). (*0-7855-2287-5*) Scientific GBR. *Dist:* St Mut.

Glossary of Lay Language Synonyms for Common Terms Used in Informed Consent Documents for Clinical Studies: A Handbook for Clinical Researchers. Deborrah Norris. 1996. 69p. pap. 39.95 (*0-9631310-3-6*) Plexus Pub.

Glossary of Managed Care Medical Terms, Abbreviations & Acronyms. Margaret D. Bischel. 1997. 97p. ring bd. 25.00 (*1-893826-08-2*) Apollo Managed.

Glossary of Mycology. Walter Snell & Esther A. Dick. 2nd ed. 1971. LC 77-134946. (Illus.). 215p. 25.00 (*0-674-35451-6*) HUP.

Glossary of Neuroanatomy. Stephen Wertheim. 1990. 200p. 30.00 (*0-8176-3432-0*) Birkhauser.

Glossary of Periodontic Terms 1992. American Academy of Periodontology Staff. 1992. 52p. pap. 35.00 (*0-9624699-3-9*) Amer Acad Periodontology.

Glossary of Preventive Toxicology. P. Elster & P. Luderitz. 1985. (ENG, GER & RUS.). 120p. 35.00 (*0-8288-0942-9*, M6741) Fr & Eur.

Glossary of Psychiatric Terminology: Spanish-English, English-Spanish. Gallardo. 1989. (ENG & SPA.). 316p. pap. 55.00 (*0-7859-7490-3*, 8487189148) Fr & Eur.

Glossary of Psychiatry: Glossaire de Psychiatrie. Lise Moor. 1986. (FRE.). 196p. 75.00 (*0-8288-1819-3*, M6417) Fr & Eur.

Glossary on Air Pollution. 1980. (WHO Regional Publications, European Ser.: No. 9). 114p. 12.00 (*92-9020-109-6*, 1310009) World Health.

Glowing Health Through Diet & Posture. J. Lawson-Wood & Denis Lawson-Wood. 1980. 35.00 (*0-85032-190-5*) St Mut.

GLP Applications for Test Substance Control, Formulation, & Analysis. Richard Halliday et al. 1996. 60p. (Orig.). pap. 69.00 (*1-57491-021-3*) IHS Health Grp.

GLP Quality Audit Manual. Milton A. Anderson. 2nd ed. 1992. 408p. ring bd. 169.00 (*0-935184-33-3*) IHS Health Grp.

Glucagon. Ed. by Piero P. Foa et al. 1977. LC 77-13657. (Role in Physiology & Clinical Medicine Ser.). 132.00 (*0-387-90297-X*) Spr-Verlag.

Glucagon in Acute Medicine: Pharmacological, Clinical, & Therapeutic Implications. Ed. by J. Picazo. 1993. LC 93-24960. text 58.00 (*0-7923-8832-1*) Kluwer Academic.

Glucagon in Gastroenterology & Hepatology: Pharmacological, Clinical & Therapeutic Implications. Ed. by J. Picazo. 1982. 160p. text 101.50 (*0-85200-447-8*) Kluwer Academic.

Glucagon in Nineteen Eighty-Seven: Gastronintestinal & Hepatobiliaty Physiology, Diagnosis & Treatment. Ed. by J. Picazo. 1987. (C). lib. bdg. (*0-7462-0055-2*) Kluwer Academic NLD. *Dist:* Kluwer Academic.

***Glucocorticoid-Induced Osteoporosis.** Ed. by A. Giustina et al. 2001. (Frontiers of Hormone Research Ser.: Vol. 30). (Illus.). x, 200p. 170.50 (*3-8055-7296-4*) S Karger.

Glucocorticoid Receptors in Leukemic Cell Responses. Bahiru Gametchu. 1995. LC 95-7531. (Molecular Biology Intelligence Unit Ser.). 176p. 89.00 (*1-57059-252-7*) Landes Bioscience.

Glucocorticoid Therapy in Chronic Inflammatory Bowel Disease: From Basic Principles to Rational Therapy. Ed. by H. W. Mollmann. 1996. (Falk Symposium Ser.). 160p. (C). text 88.00 (*0-7923-8708-2*) Kluwer Academic.

Glucose Nonfermenting Gramnegative Bacteria in Clinical Microbiology. Gerald L. Gilardi. 1978. 256p. 145.00 (*0-8493-5331-9*, QR67, CRC Reprint) Franklin.

Glucose Revolution Pocket Guide to the Glycemic Index & Your Child. Jennie Brand Miller et al. 2001. LC 2001-30144. (Illus.). 128p. pap. 4.95 (*1-56924-588-6*) Marlowe & Co.

Glucose Revolution Pocket Guide to Type-1 Diabetes. Jennie Brand Miller et al. 2001. LC 2001-22218. (Illus.). 128p. pap. 4.95 (*1-56924-638-6*) Marlowe & Co.

Glucose Syrups & Related Carbohydrates. Ed. by Gordon G. Birch et al. 1971. (Illus.). 118p. 38.00 (*0-444-20103-3*) Elsevier.

Glucuronidation of Drugs & Other Compounds. G. J. Dutton. 1980. 288p. 129.95 (*0-8493-5295-9*, RM301) CRC Pr.

Glue Sniffing & Volatile Substance Abuse: Case Studies of Children & Young Adults. Denis O'Connor. 1983. LC 83-16464. 103p. text (*0-566-00641-3*) Avebry GBR. *Dist:* Ashgate Pub Co.

Glutamate, Cell Death & Memory. Ed. by P. Ascher et al. 1991. (Research & Perspectives in Neurosciences Ser.: Vol. 1). (Illus.). 160p. 56.95 (*0-387-54134-9*) Spr-Verlag.

Glutamate, Glutamine, Glutathione, & Related Compounds, Vol. 113. Ed. by Sidney P. Colowick & Anthan O. Kaplan. 1985. (Methods in Enzymology Ser.). text 179.00 (*0-12-182013-0*) Acad Pr.

Glutamate Synapse As a Therapeutical Target: Molecular Organization & Pathology of the Glutamate Synapse. O. P. Ottersen et al. 1998. LC 98 29333. (Progress in Brain Research Ser.). 500p. 184.50 (*0-444-82754-4*) Elsevier.

Glutamate-Transmitter & Toxin, Vol. 36. Ed. by O. Kempski. 1993. (Clinical Nutrition Ser.). (Illus.). 150p. text (*3-88603-481-X*) W Zuckschwerdt DEU. *Dist:* Scholium Intl.

Glutamine & Glutamate in Mammals. Ed. by Elling Kvamme. 1988. Vol. I. 272p. 159.00 (*0-8493-6856-1*, QP562); Vol. II. 208p. 115.00 (*0-8493-6857-X*, QP562) Franklin (CRC Reprint).

Glutamine Metabolism in Mammalian Tissues. Ed. by Helmut Sies & Dieter Haussinger. 1984. (Illus.). 298p. 104.00 (*0-387-13454-9*) Spr-Verlag.

Glutathione in the Nervous System. Christopher A. Shaw. 1997. LC 97-22575. 389p. 99.95 (*1-56032-643-3*) Hemisp Pub.

Gluten-Sensitive Enteropathy. Ed. by D. Branski et al. 1991. (Frontiers of Gastrointestinal Research Ser.: Vol. 19). (Illus.). viii, 218p. 205.25 (*3-8055-5331-5*) S Karger.

Gluthathione: Metabolism & Physiological Functions. Ed. by Jose Vina. 1990. 892p. lib. bdg. 239.00 (*0-8493-3274-5*, QP552) CRC Pr.

Glycation Hypothesis of Atherosclerosis. Camilo Colaco. 1997. (Medical Intelligence Unit Ser.). 224p. 99.00 (*1-57059-444-9*) Landes Bioscience.

Glycobiology & the Brain. Ed. by Marino Nicolini & R. F. Zatta. 1994. LC 93-21168. (Studies in Neurosciences). 304p. 188.00 (*0-08-042283-7*, Pergamon Pr) Elsevier.

Glycobiology of Fertilization. Ed. by E. Topfer-Peterson & F. Sinowatz. 2001. (Cells Tissues Organs Ser.: Vol. 168). 124p. 39.25 (*3-8055-7172-0*) S Karger.

Glycoenzymes. Ed. by M. Ohnishi. 2000. (Illus.). x, 264p. 231.50 (*3-8055-7076-7*) S Karger.

Glycoimmunology: Proceedings of the Third Jenner International Glycoimmunology Meeting Held in Il Ciocco, Tuscany, Italy, October 11-14, 1994, Vol. 1. A. Alavi & J. S. Axford. 1995. (Advances in Experimental Medicine & Biology Ser.: Vol. 376). (Illus.). 306p. 105.00 (*0-306-45102-6*, Kluwer Plenum) Kluwer Academic.

Glycoimmunology 2: Proceedings of the Fourth Jenner International Glycoimmunology Meeting Held in Loutraki, Greece, November 12-15, 1996. Ed. by John S. Axford. 1998. LC 97-50383. (Advances in Experimental Medicine & Biology Ser.: Vol. 435). (Illus.). 280p. 95.00 (*0-306-45777-6*, Kluwer Plenum) Kluwer Academic.

Glycopeptide Antibiotics. Ed. by Ramakrishnan Nagarajan. 1994. LC 94-585. (Drugs & the Pharmaceutical Sciences Ser.: Vol. 63). (Illus.). 448p. text 215.00 (*0-8247-9193-2*) Dekker.

Glycoprotein Hormone. Joyce W. Lustbader et al. 1994. LC 93-33014. (Illus.). 381p. 162.00 (*0-387-94165-7*) Spr-Verlag.

Glycoprotein Hormones: Structure, Synthesis & Biologic Function. Ed. by William W. Chin & Irving Boime. 1990. (Serono Symposia, U. S. A. Ser.). (Illus.). 462p. (C). text 75.00 (1-878601-01-6) Serono Symposia USA.

Glycoprotein Methods & Protocols: The Mucins. Ed. by Anthony P. Corfield. 2000. LC 99-25785. (Methods in Molecular Biology Ser.: Vol. 125). (Illus.). xvii, 506p. 119.50 (0-89603-720-7) Humana.

Glycoproteins & Disease. Jean Montreuil et al. 1996. LC 96-33252. (New Comprehensive Biochemistry Ser.). 512p. 188.00 (0-444-82396-4) Elsevier.

Glycoproteins & Human Disease. Inka Brockhausen & William Kuhns. 1997. (Medical Intelligence Unit Ser.). 242p. (C). pap. 89.95 (0-412-10741-4) Chapman & Hall.

Glycoproteins & Human Disease. Inka Brockhausen & William Kuhns. 1996. LC 97-11132. (Medical Intelligence Unit Ser.). (Illus.). 204p. 99.00 (1-57059-412-0) Landes Bioscience.

Glycoproteins II. Ed. by Jean Montreuil et al. 1997. LC 97-40500. (New Comprehensive Biochemistry Ser.: Vol. 29B). 678p. 243.00 (0-444-82393-X) Elsevier.

Glycosaminoglycans & Arterial Diseases. Ed. by R. W. Robinson et al. 1975. (Monographs on Atherosclerosis: Vol. 5). (Illus.). viii, 134p. 60.00 (3-8055-2089-1) S Karger.

Glycosaminoglycans & Proteoglycans in Physiological & Pathological Processes of Body Systems. Ed. by R. S. Varma. 1982. (Illus.). xii, 520p. 286.25 (3-8055-3440-X) S Karger.

Glycosciences, Vol.161. Ed. by H. J. Gabius & F. Sinowath. 1998. (Acta Anatomica Ser.: Vol. 161, No. 1-4 (1998)). (Illus.). 278p. pap. 125.25 (3-8055-6775-8) S Karger.

Glyphosate. 1994. (Environmental Health Criteria Ser.: No. 159). (ENG, FRE & SPA.). 177p. pap. text 36.00 (92-4-157159-4, 1160159) World Health.

GMC Apprentice Program Battery Tests (GMC) Jack Rudman. 1994. (Admission Test Ser.: ATS-94). pap. 29.95 (0-8373-5094-8) Nat Learn.

GMP "How to" Essentials: How to Apply Quality Assurance Principles. Michael Cutter. 1995. (GMP Training Ser.). (Illus.). 150p. tchr. ed., ring bd. 175.00 (0-935184-93-7) IHS Health Grp.

GMP "How to" Essentials: How to Organize a Validation File. Michael Cutter. 1995. (GMP Training Ser.). (Illus.). 150p. tchr. ed., ring bd. 175.00 (0-935184-95-3) IHS Health Grp.

GMP "How to" Essentials: How to Perform Retrospective Validation. Michael Cutter. 1995. (GMP Training Ser.). (Illus.). 150p. tchr. ed., ring bd. 175.00 (0-935184-97-X) IHS Health Grp.

GMP "How to" Essentials: How to Prepare for an FDA Inspection. Michael Cutter. 1995. (GMP Training Ser.). (Illus.). 150p. tchr. ed., ring bd. 175.00 (0-935184-89-9) IHS Health Grp.

GMP "How to" Essentials: How to Review & Redesign SOP Systems. Michael Cutter. 1995. (GMP Training Ser.). (Illus.). 150p. tchr. ed., ring bd. 175.00 (0-935184-99-6) IHS Health Grp.

GMP "How to" Essentials: How to Write Policies & Procedures. Michael Cutter. 1995. (GMP Training Ser.). (Illus.). 150p. tchr. ed., ring bd. 175.00 (0-935184-91-0) IHS Health Grp.

GMP in Practice: Regulatory Expectations for the Pharmaceutical Industry. James Vesper. 2000. 224p. 69.50 (1-930114-17-6) Davis Horwood Intl.

GMP/ISO-9000 Quality Audit Manual for Healthcare Manufacturers & Their Suppliers see GMP/ISO/EN Quality Audit Manual for Healthcare Manufacturers & Their Suppliers

GMP/ISO/EN Quality Audit Manual for Healthcare Manufacturers & Their Suppliers. Leonard Steinborn. 5th ed. Orig. Title: GMP/ISO-9000 Quality Audit Manual for Healthcare Manufacturers & Their Suppliers. Vol. 1. 1997. 410p. ring bd. 249.00 (1-57491-058-2); Vol. 2. 1998. 400p. ring bd. 289.00 (1-57491-074-4) IHS Health Grp.

Gnathologic Tooth Preparation. Charles E. Stuart. 1985. LC 85-12039. (Illus.). 164p. text 82.00 (0-86715-121-8, 1218) Quint Pub Co.

Gnathosonic Diagnosis & Occlusal Dynamics. David M. Watt. 1981. 224p. 77.00 (0-275-91356-2, C1356, Praeger Pubs) Greenwood.

GnRH Analogues: The State of the Art 1993. Ed. by B. Lunenfeld & V. Insler. 1993. (Illus.). 156p. lib. bdg. 60.95 (1-85070-526-7, Parthenon Pbng) CRC Pr.

GnRH Analogues: The State of the Art 1996. Ed. by Bruno Lunenfeld & V. Insler. 1996. (Illus.). 190p. 60.95 (1-85070-759-6, Parthenon Pbng) CRC Pr.

GnRH Analogues in Cancer & Human Reproduction: Basic Sciences. Ed. by B. H. Vickers & Bruno Lunenfeld. 1990. (C). lib. bdg. 113.50 (0-7923-8927-1) Kluwer Academic.

GnRH Analogues in Cancer & Human Reproduction: GnRH Analogues in Reproduction & Gynecology. Ed. by B. H. Vickery & Bruno Lunenfeld. 1990. (C). lib. bdg. 102.00 (0-7923-8929-8) Kluwer Academic.

GnRH Analogues in Prostatic Cancer: The Way Forward: 4th International Symposium on GnRH Analogues in Cancer & Human Reproduction, Geneva, February, 1996. Ed. by D. Jocham. 1996. (Journal: Vol. 30, Suppl. 1). (Illus.). iv, 52p. pap. 26.25 (3-8055-6368-X) S Karger.

Go Ahead, Kill Yourself! Save Your Family the Trouble. Thomas M. Saunders. 1990. LC 90-44102. 144p. (C). pap. 14.95 (0-942963-06-7) Distinctive Pub.

Go & Learn: The International Story of Jews & Medicine in Scotland. K. Collins. 1988. (Illus.). 240p. (0-08-036408-X) Aberdeen U Pr GBR. *Dist:* Macmillan.

Go Natural! Mark Virkler & Patti Virkler. 1994. LC 95-158515. 300p. (Orig.). pap. 13.99 (1-56043-138-5) Destiny Image Pubs.

Go Not Gently: Letters from a Patient with Amyotrophic Lateral Sclerosis. Frances McGill. Ed. by Lillian G. Kutscher. 1980. LC 79-48047. (Foundation of Thanatology Ser.). lib. bdg. 20.95 (0-405-12643-3) Ayer.

Go See the Movie in Your Head: Imagery: The Key to Awareness. Joseph E. Shorr. 1983. 234p. pap. 9.95 (0-915520-65-6) Inst for Psycho-Imag.

***Go with the Flow: A Systems Approach to Healthcare Planning.** 1996. 138p. pap. (1-85315-277-3) Royal Soc of Medicine Pr Ltd GBR. *Dist:* Balogh.

Goal Attainment Scaling: Applications, Theory & Measurement. Ed. by Thomas Kiresuk et al. 1994. 328p. text 69.95 (0-89859-889-3) L Erlbaum Assocs.

Goal Concepts in Personality & Social Psychology. Ed. by Lawrence A. Pervin. 1989. 520p. pap. 45.00 (0-8058-0383-1) L Erlbaum Assocs.

Goal-Directed Action. Mario Von Cranach. 1983. (European Monographs in Social Psychology: No. 30). text 151.00 (0-12-724760-2) Acad Pr.

Goal-Directed Behaviour. Michael Weir. 1984. (Studies in Cybernetics: Vol. 6). xvi, 290p. text 158.00 (0-677-06570-1) Gordon & Breach.

Goal of B. F. Skinner & Behavior Analysis. R. W. Proctor & D. J. Weeks. 1991. (Recent Research in Psychology Ser.). (Illus.). 223p. 39.95 (0-387-97236-6) Spr-Verlag.

Goals & Limits of Medicine. Ed. by Lennart Nordenfelt & Per-Anders Tengland. 1996. 239p. (Orig.). pap. 52.50 (91-22-01713-5) Coronet Bks.

Goals of Medicine: The Forgotten Issue in Health Care Reform. Ed. by Mark J. Hanson & Daniel Callahan. 2001. LC 98-44650. (Hastings Center Studies in Ethics). 256p. text 55.00 (0-87840-707-3) Georgetown U Pr.

Goals of Psychoanalysis: Identification, Identity & Supervision. Leon Grinberg. 1992. 416p. pap. text (0-946439-83-4) Karnac Bks GBR. *Dist:* Other Pr LLC.

Goat Medicine. Smith. Ed. by Carroll C. Cann. 1994. (Illus.). 620p. 80.00 (0-8121-1478-7) Lppncott W & W.

Goat Milk Magic: One of Life's Greatest Healing Foods. Bernard Jensen. 1994. (Dr. Jensen's Health Handbooks Ser.: Vol. 6). (Illus.). 112p. pap. text 12.99 (0-932615-32-5, P-0296) B Jensen.

Goatkeeper's Veterinary Book. Peter Dunn. 3rd ed. 1994. (Illus.). 198p. (0-85236-279-X) Farming Pr GBR. *Dist:* Diamond Farm Bk.

Goats: Homoeopathic Remedies. George MacLeod. 192p. (Orig.). pap. 29.95 (0-8464-4178-0); pap. 29.95 (0-8464-4217-5) Beekman Pubs.

Goats: Homoeopathic Remedies. George MacLeod. 1991. 128p. (Orig.). pap. (0-85207-244-9) C W Daniel GBR. *Dist:* Natl Bk Netwk.

God & Golem, Inc. A Comment on Certain Points Where Cybernetics Impinges on Religion. Norbert Wiener. 1966. pap. 14.95 (0-262-73011-1) MIT Pr.

God Did Not Create Sickness or Disease. Joe M. Parkhill. 1983. 160p. (Orig.). pap. text 6.95 (0-936744-05-7) Country Bazaar.

God Given Herbs. Ed. by William R. McGrath. 1988. 97p. 6.99 (0-9617405-9-0) S Schupp.

God, Medicine, & Suffering. Stanley M. Hauerwas. 1994. 168p. pap. 13.00 (0-8028-0896-4) Eerdmans.

God Speaks His Heart: A Spiritual Message. Helen R. McClellan. 1996. LC 96-61138. 130p. (Orig.). pap. 15.95 (0-9653155-3-3, 84333) Stuart Victor.

God, the Substance of All Form. Joel S. Goldsmith & Lorraine Sinkler. 1998. LC 98-11315. 134p. reprint ed. pap. 12.95 (1-889051-30-6, I Lvl) Acrpls Bks GA.

***God Wants You Well: How to Obtain Freedom from Illness & Health Problems.** Beth M. Ley. 2001. LC 2001-334. 257p. pap. 14.95 (1-890766-19-4) B L Pubns.

God, Where Is Love? Break Free from the Pain of Codependency. Claire W. 1989. 120p. (Orig.). pap. 13.95 (0-9619383-6-6) Books West CA.

God, Why Me? Cancer. Clyde C. Cone and Associates Staff. 1989. LC 88-92761. 137p. (Orig.). pap. 7.95 (0-9621961-0-X) C C Cone.

Goddess, Mother of the Trinity: A Jungian Implication. John P. Dourley. 1990. LC 90-37579. (Studies in the Psychology of Religion: Vol. 4). 112p. lib. bdg. 59.95 (0-88946-244-5) E Mellen.

Godless Jew: Atheism, & the Making of Psychoanalysis. Peter Gay. 1989. 182p. (C). reprint ed. pap. 16.00 (0-300-04608-1) Yale U Pr.

Godless Jew: Freud, Atheism, & the Making of Psychoanalysis. Peter Gay. 1987. LC 87-8267. 208p. 27.50 (0-300-04008-3) Yale U Pr.

God's Celestial Rays: A Source of Pain Relief, Healing & Rejuvenation. Wilton Kullmann. 1992. (Illus.). 74p. pap. (3-85068-362-1) Ennsthaler AUT. *Dist:* Am Educ Systs.

God's Healing Leaves. Robert McClintock. 1998. 102p. pap. 9.95 (1-883012-82-1) Remnant Pubns.

Gods In Everyman Reissue: New Psychology of Men's Lives & Loves, A. Jean S. Bolen. 1993. LC 88-45663. 352p. reprint ed. pap. 14.00 (0-06-097280-7, Perennial) HarperTrade.

God's Medicine Bottle. Derek Prince. 1995. 62p. mass mkt. 4.99 (0-88368-332-6) Whitaker Hse.

God's Plan Included Lupus. O. D. Rodgers. 1998. LC 98-85906. 152p. text 18.95 (1-56167-443-5) Noble House.

God's Touch: Faith, Wholeness & the Healing Miracles of Jesus. Bruce G. Epperly. 2001. LC 00-63402. xiv, 236p. pap. 19.95 (0-664-22281-1) Westminster John Knox.

Going for the Cure. Francesca M. Thompson. 1992. 295p. reprint ed. pap. 11.50 (0-9633186-0-8) Intl Myeloma.

Going Home: A Family Facing AIDS. AIDS Committee. 1993. 87.25 net. (0-697-24332-X, WCB McGr Hill) McGrw-H Hghr Educ.

***Going into Medical Practice.** Rebecca B. Campen. 2001. LC 2001-3589. pap. (0-632-04621-X) Blackwell Sci.

***Going Paperless: A Guide to Computerization in Primary Care.** Nicola Shaw. 2001. 216p. pap. (1-85775-519-7) Radcliffe Med Pr GBR. *Dist:* Balogh.

Going Private: Changing Expectations about Health Care? Michael W. Calnan et al. 1993. LC 92-40057. (State of Health Ser.). x, 113p. 80.00 (0-335-09981-5); pap. 23.00 (0-335-09980-7) OUP.

Going to the Doctor Kid Kit. EDC Publishing Staff. 2001. 16p. (ps-3). 13.95 (1-58086-173-3, Usborne) EDC Pubng.

Going to the Dog: Therapy Stories for Grown-Ups. Paul De Mielche. 2nd ed. 1994. (Illus.). 148p. (Orig.). pap. 14.95 (1-883785-02-2) Paw Print Pub.

Going Under: Preparing Yourself for Anesthesia. Monica W. Furlong & Elliot T. Essman. 1994. LC 93-72364. 190p. (Orig.). pap. 14.95 (0-9636451-6-1) Autonomy Pub.

Gold Counselling: A Practical Psychology with NLP. Georges Philips & Lyn Buncher. 1997. 221p. pap. (1-899836-06-3) Crown Hse GBR. *Dist:* LPC Group.

Goldberg's Genetic & Metabolic Eye Disease. William A. Renie. 2nd ed. 1986. 608p. 142.00 (0-316-74016-0, Little Brwn Med Div) Lppncott W & W.

Golden Anniversary Anatomic Pathology Slide Seminar: Proceedings of the Forty Ninth Annual Anatomic Pathology Slide Seminar of the ASCP. Ed. by William M. Christopherson et al. 1985. 155p. 35.00 (0-89189-191-9) Am Soc Clinical.

Golden Cage. Shancastel Ltd. Staff. 1999. 20.01 (0-375-50172-X) Random.

Golden Cage: The Enigma of Anorexia Nervosa. Hilde Bruch. 1978. 168p. text 24.95 (0-674-35650-0) HUP.

Golden Era of Preventive Medicine. Robert K. Stevenson. 1982. LC 82-99906. 120p. (Orig.). pap. 10.00 (0-9606252-2-4) R Stevenson Conslt.

Golden Hour: The Handbook of Advanced Pediatric Life Support. David G. Nichols. 2nd ed. 1995. (Illus.). 560p. (C). (gr. 13). pap. text 37.95 (0-8151-6394-0, 24726) Mosby Inc.

Golden Hour: The Handbook of Advanced Pediatric Life Support. David G. Nichols. Ed. by Dorothy G. Lappe et al. 1996. (Volume in the Year Book Handbooks Ser.). (Illus.). 560p. pap. (84-8174-182-5) Mosby-Doyma Libros ESP. *Dist:* Mosby Inc.

Golden Needle. Bertsching. 1996. text 67.00 (0-443-04390-6) Saunders.

Golden Seal - Etc. A Phamacognosy of Wild Herbs. Louise Veninga & Benjamin R. Zaricor. 1976. (Illus.). 193p. (Orig.). (C). pap. 10.00 (0-915178-03-6) Ruka Pubns.

Golden Transition: Menopause Made Easy with Maharishi Vedic Medicine. Kumuda Reddy & Sandra Willbanks. 2001. (Illus.). 300p. pap. 18.95 (1-929297-16-5) Samhita Prodns.

Golden Wand of Medicine: A History of the Caduceus Symbol in Medicine, 35. Walter J. Friedlander. 1992. LC 91-28356. (Contributions in Medical Studies Ser.: No. 35). 200p. 60.00 (0-313-28023-1, FGW/, Greenwood Pr) Greenwood.

Golden Years: A Resource Guide for Caregivers of Aging Adults. Catherine L. Collins. Ed. by Janice Ward. 1990. 180p. (Orig.). pap. (0-923109-02-1); pap. text (0-923109-01-3) Hlth Care Creat.

Goldenseal. Rita Elkins. 1997. (Woodland Health Ser.). 32p. pap. text 3.95 (1-885670-39-7) Woodland UT.

Goldensohn's EEG Interpretation: Problems of Overreading & Underreading. Ed. by Eli S. Goldensohn et al. 2nd rev. ed. 1998. LC 98-234796. (Illus.). 300p. 175.00 (0-87993-086-1) Futura Pub.

Goldfrank's Toxicological Emergencies. Lewis R. Goldfrank. 6th ed. 1998. LC 97-42664. 1589p. text 199.00 (0-8385-3148-2) McGraw-Hill Prof.

Goldfrank's Toxicological Emergencies. Lewis R. Goldfrank & Flomenbaum. 6th ed. 1998. 368p. (C). pap., stu. ed. 55.00 (0-8385-3149-0) McGraw-Hill Prof.

Gold's Gym Nutrition Bible. Bill Reynolds et al. 1986. 224p. (Orig.). pap. 16.95 (0-8092-5188-4, 518840, Contemporary) McGraw-Hill Trade.

Golf Injury Handbook: Professional Advice for Amature Athletes. Allan M. Levy & Mark L. Fuerst. 1999. LC 98-24885. (Illus.). 171p. pap. 14.95 (0-471-24853-3) Wiley.

Golgi Apparatus. W. G. Whaley. 1975. LC 75-20055. (Cell Biology Monographs: Vol. 2). (Illus.). 200p. 71.00 (0-387-81315-2) Spr-Verlag.

Golgi Atlas of the Postnatal Mouse Brain. F. Valverde. 1998. LC 98-10813. (Illus.). 158p. 129.00 (3-211-83063-4) Spr-Verlag.

Gonadal Proteins & Peptides & Their Biological Significance: Proceedings of the International Symposium Held at Le Chateau, Montebello, Quebec, June 1984. Ed. by M. R. Sairam & L. E. Atkinson. 1985. 416p. 98.00 (9971-966-85-9) World Scientific Pub.

Gonadotrophins: Current Research, Vol. 1. J. P. Hearn et al. 1974. text 24.50 (0-8422-7204-6) Irvington.

Gonioscopy & the Glaucomas. Barry M. Fisch. 1993. (Illus.). 205p. text 80.00 (0-7506-9049-6) Buttrwrth-Heinemann.

Gonococci & Meningococci. Ed. by J. T. Poolman et al. 1988. (C). text 542.00 (90-247-3607-2) Kluwer Academic.

Gonorrhea & Syphilis: A Drugless Treatment of Veneral Diseases (1912) J. H. Tilden. 1996. 188p. reprint ed. pap. 14.95 (1-56459-875-6) Kessinger Pub.

Gonorrhea Transmission Dynamics & Control. Herbert W. Hethcote & J. A. Yorke. 1984. (Lecture Notes in Biomathematics: Vol. 56). 105p. 31.95 (0-387-13870-6) Spr-Verlag.

Good Beginnings: Parenting in the Early Years. Judith Evans & Ellen M. Ilfeld. 1982. LC 82-885. (Illus.). 200p. (Orig.). pap. 15.95 (0-931114-15-2, SU-F1000) High-Scope.

Good Birth, a Safe Birth: Choosing & Having the Childbirth Experience You Want. Diana Korte & Roberta Scaer. Ed. by Leslie A. Baker. 3rd rev. ed. 1992. LC 92-9757. 400p. 21.95 (1-55832-042-3); pap. 15.95 (1-55832-041-5) Harvard Common Pr.

Good Body: Ascetism in Contemporary Culture. Ed. by Mary G. Winkler & Letha B. Cole. 1994. LC 93-48225. 247p. 40.00 (0-300-05628-1) Yale U Pr.

Good Bye Back Pain! Leonard J. Faye. 1990. (Illus.). 250p. pap. 14.95 (0-942139-01-1) Tale Weaver.

Good-Bye Diet Demon: You Can Become Sophisticated at Permanent Weight Control! Scarlett Mack. 1989. LC 88-50008. 176p. pap. 14.95 (0-945654-00-6) Aroc Pub.

Good-Bye, Glasses see Complete Guide to Refractive Surgery: Nearsightedness, Farsightedness, & Astigmatism

Good-Bye, Glasses: A Comprehensive Guide to Radial Keratotomy, A Microsurgical Procedure to Permanently Correct Nearsightedness. Susan Abbas. 1990. (Illus.). 133p. (Orig.). pap. 14.95 (0-9628886-0-5) Patton Pub.

Good-Bye to Bad Backs: Simple Stretching & Strengthening Exercises for Alignment & Freedom from Lower Back Pain. Judith Scott. 2nd ed. 1992. LC 92-34672. (Illus.). 269p. pap. 16.95 (0-87127-186-9) Princeton Bk Co.

Good Care Management. Jenyth Wirsley. 1991. (C). (0-86242-104-7) Age Concern Eng GBR. *Dist:* St Mut.

Good Care, Painful Choices: Medical Ethics of Ordinary People. Richard J. Devine. 2nd ed. 2000. LC 99-48585. 272p. pap. 18.95 (0-8091-3924-3) Paulist Pr.

Good Cholesterol, Bad Cholesterol: What You Need to Know to Reduce Your Risk of Heart Disease. Eli M. Roth & Sandra Streicher. 1989. 192p. reprint ed. pap. 9.95 (1-55958-025-9) Prima Pub.

Good Clinical Practice, Vol. 2. 1993. 58.95 (0-387-55239-1) Spr-Verlag.

Good Clinical Practice: Standard Operating Procedures for Clinical Researchers. Paul Meng et al. 1998. LC 97-41919. 210p. pap. 72.95 (0-471-96936-2) Wiley.

Good Clinical Practice & Ethics in European Drug Research. Ed. by Peter Bennett. 1994. (0-86197-121-3) Bath Univ Pr GBR. *Dist:* Intl Spec Bk.

Good Computer Validation Practices: Common Sense Implementation. C. Branning et al. Ed. by Teri Stokes. 1994. (Illus.). 324p. 249.00 (0-935184-55-4) IHS Health Grp.

Good Days, Bad Days: The Self in Chronic Illness & Time. Kathleen C. Charmaz. 1993. LC 90-28864. 311p. pap. 16.00 (0-8135-1967-5) Rutgers U Pr.

Good Death: Conversations with East Londoners. Michael Young & Lesley Cullen. 1996. LC 95-25968. 272p. (C). 90.00 (0-415-13796-9); 1301st ed. pap. 27.95 (0-415-13797-7) Routledge.

Good Doctors. Ray Thompson. 1986. LC 85-62562. 256p. text 27.95 (0-9615658-0-2) MD Vet Med Assn.

Good Doctors, Good Patients: Partners in HIV Treatment. Judith G. Rabkin et al. 1995. 212p. pap. 15.00 (0-9643884-0-5) NCM Pubs.

Good Drug Regulatory Practices: A Regulatory Affairs Quality Manual. Helene Dumitriu. 1997. LC 97-26489. (Good Drug Development Ser.: Vol. 1). (Illus.). 300p. ring bd. 169.00 (1-57491-051-5) IHS Health Grp.

Good Dying: Shaping Health Care for the Last Months of Life. Ed. by Joan K. Harrold & Joanne Lynn. 1998. LC 98-10051. (Illus.). 188p. pap. 19.95 (0-7890-0502-6) Haworth Pr.

Good Dying: Shaping Health Care for the Last Months of Life. Joanne Lynn. Ed. by Joan K. Harrold. 1998. LC 98-10051. 188p. 49.95 (0-7890-0399-6) Haworth Pr.

Good Enough: When Losing Is Winning, Perfection Becomes Obsession, & Thin Enough Can Never Be Achieved. Cynthia N. Bitter. 1998. LC 97-93354. 285p. pap. 14.95 (0-9657755-6-9) HopeLines.

Good Fight: Medicine in Colonial Pennsylvania. Larry L. Burkhart. 1989. (Studies in Historical Demography). 360p. reprint ed. text 25.00 (*0-8240-3395-7*) Garland.

Good Food for Diabetes. Ruby M. Brown. 1998. pap. text (*1-86351-216-0*) Sally Milner AUS. *Dist:* Sterling.

Good Food Game. Merilyn Cummings. 1989. 112p. (Orig.). pap. 19.95 (*0-9617195-0-8*) Abrahamson Pub.

Good for You: A Handbook on Lesbian Health & Wellbeing. Tamsin Wilton. 1997. LC 97-6628. (Sexual Politics Ser.). 256p. pap. 18.95 (*0-304-33632-7*) Continuum.

Good for You: Eating Right for a Better Life. Mary L. Hogenson. Ed. by Jane H. Combs. 1991. (Success Ser.). (Illus.). 32p. (Orig.). pap. text 3.25 (*0-9625440-2-7*) Longmuir Jones Pub.

Good Health Directory. Naomi Craft et al. 2000. LC 00-101044. (Illus.). 208p. spiral bd. 18.95 (*0-7641-5314-5*) Barron.

***Good Health for African Americans: The 24-Week Sankofa Program.** Barbara M. Dixon & Josleen Wilson. 2001. 414p. reprint ed. 26.00 (*0-7881-9641-3*) DIANE Pub.

Good Health Handbook: 100s of Tips to Improve Your Health. Bobbie Hasselbring et al. Ed. by American College of Preventive Medicine Staff. 1997. LC 97-141226. (Illus.). 576p. (*0-7853-2411-9*) Pubns Intl Ltd.

Good Health Journal. Deborah Riney. 1993. 112p. pap. 10.95 (*0-9635454-0-X*) DER Prods.

Good Herbs(Latino Folk Medicine) see Yerbas Buenas

Good Hospital Practice: Ethylene Oxide Gas-Ventilation Recommendations & Safe Use. 3rd ed. 1993. (AAMI Technical Information Report Ser.). 42p. pap. 90.00 (*1-57020-006-8*, ST43-209) Assn Adv Med Instrn.

Good Hospital Practice: Flash Sterilization - Steam Sterilization of Patient-Care Items for Immediate Use. 3rd ed. 1996. 14p. pap. 70.00 (*0-910275-67-X*, ST37-209) Assn Adv Med Instrn.

Good Hospital Practice: Guidelines for the Selection & Use of Reusable Rigid Sterilization Container Systems for EO & Steam Sterilization. 1990. 16p. pap. 82.00 (*0-910275-97-1*, ST33-209) Assn Adv Med Instrn.

Good Hospital Practice: Safe Handling & Biological Decontamination of Reusable Medical Devices in H.C. Facilities & In Non-Clinical Settings. 2nd ed. 1991. 14p. pap. 90.00 (*0-910275-55-6*, ST35-209) Assn Adv Med Instrn.

Good Hospital Practice: Steam Sterilization & Sterility Assurance. 3rd ed. 1993. (AAMI Technical Information Report Ser.). 51p. pap. 90.00 (*1-57020-010-6*, ST46-209) Assn Adv Med Instrn.

Good Hospital Practice: Table-Top Dry Heat (Heated Air) Sterilization & Sterility Assurance in Dental & Medical Facilities. AAMI Staff. 1992. (Illus.). 27p. (Orig.). pap. 82.00 (*0-910275-16-5*, ST40-209) Assn Adv Med Instrn.

Good Housekeeping Family First Aid Book. Good Housekeeping Editors. 2000. LC 99-58359. (Illus.). 288p. pap. 18.00 (*0-688-17894-4*, Wm Morrow) Morrow Avon.

Good Housekeeping Family Health & Medical Guide. Good Housekeeping Editors. 1988. 788p. 24.95 (*0-688-06164-8*) Hearst Bks.

Good If Not Great Living with Lung Disease. Phil Petersen. 4th ed. 1999. 124p. pap. 14.50 (*0-9621726-4-2*) Raven Pubs.

Good If Not Great Travel with Oxygen. Phil Petersen. Ed. by Mary Lee & Pam Paisley. 3rd rev. ed. 1996. 64p. (Orig.). pap. 5.95 (*0-9621726-3-4*) Raven Pubs.

Good Laboratory & Clinical Practices: Techniques for the Quality Assurance Professional. Ed. by Philip A. Carson & Nigel J. Dent. 1994. 416p. reprint ed. pap. (*0-7506-1957-0*) E A GBR. *Dist:* OUP.

Good Laboratory Practice Regulations. Ed. by Sandy Weinberg. 2nd exp. rev. ed. 1995. LC 95-10741. (Drugs & the Pharmaceutical Sciences Ser.: Vol. 69). (Illus.). 312p. text 135.00 (*0-8247-9377-3*) Dekker.

Good Life: A Return to Simple Principles of Healthy Living. Ruth McGinnis. 1998. LC 98-122583. 256p. pap. 12.99 (*0-7852-7150-3*, J Thoma Bks) Nelson.

Good Looking, Easy Swallowing: Creative Catering for Modified Texture Diets. Janet Martin & Jane Backhouse. 1994. (Illus.). 389p. text 65.00 (*1-875412-02-6*) Buttrwrth-Heinemann.

Good Manufacturing Practice: Philosophy & Applications. John Sharp. 1991. 155p. 69.00 (*0-935184-25-2*) IHS Health Grp.

Good Manufacturing Practices for Pharmaceuticals: A Plan for Total Quality Control. Sidney H. Willig & James R. Stoker. 4th ed. 1996. LC 96-31653. (Drugs & the Pharmaceutical Sciences Ser.: Vol. 78). (Illus.). 512p. text 125.00 (*0-8247-9770-1*) Dekker.

Good Manufacturing Practices for Pharmaceuticals: A Plan for Total Quality from Manufacturer to Consumer. Sidney H. Willig. 5th exp. rev. ed. 2000. LC 00-60188. (Drugs & the Pharmaceutical Sciences Ser.: Vol. 109). (Illus.). xii, 732p. text 135.00 (*0-8247-0425-8*) Dekker.

Good Medicine. Bruce Robinson. 1998. LC 98-96761. (Illus.). 132p. pap. 8.95 (*0-9666956-0-7*) Berco Pubng.

Good Medicine: Four Las Vegas Doctors & the Golden Age of Medicine. Annie Blachley. Ed. by Anton P. Sohn. 1999. LC 99-88657. (Illus.). xvii, 202p. 35.00 (*0-9649759-7-1*) Greasewood.

Good Monitoring Practices. Nancy J. Stark. 3rd ed. 1999. 320p. ring bd. 225.00 (*1-889160-06-7*) Clinical Design.

Good Mood: The New Psychology of Overcoming Depression. Julian L. Simon. 1993. LC 93-14946. 327p. 52.95 (*0-8126-9097-4*); pap. 18.95 (*0-8126-9098-2*) Open Court.

Good News about High Blood Pressure. Thomas Pickering. 1997. LC 95-45136. 336p. per. 13.00 (*0-684-83211-9*, Fireside) S&S Trade Pap.

Good News about High Blood Pressure: Everything You Need to Know to Take Control of Hypertension...& Your Life. Thomas Pickering. 1996. LC 95-45136. 336p. 23.00 (*0-684-81396-3*) S&S Trade.

Good News about Women's Hormones: Complete Information & Proven Solutions for the Most Common Hormonal Problems. Geoffrey P. Redmond. 1995. LC 94-18095. 528p. pap. 13.99 (*0-446-39454-8*) Warner Bks.

Good News Eating Plan for Type II Diabetes. Elaine Magee. 1997. LC 97-38639. (Illus.). 240p. pap. 15.95 (*0-471-17624-9*) Wiley.

Good News for Bad Backs. Robert L. Swezey & Annette M. Swezey. (Good News Ser.). (Illus.). 304p. rev. ed. 1992. 19.95 (*1-881206-00-9*); 3rd rev. ed. 1994. pap. 12.95 (*1-881206-01-7*) Cequal.

Good Night & God Bless You Love, Jane: Cancer Challenged Our Faith, Our Family, & Our Lives. Jane Shafiroff & Paul G. Shafiroff. Ed. by Barbara Swann. 1996. (Illus.). 175p. (Orig.). pap. text 12.00 (*0-9648228-4-9*) Elysium Pubng.

Good Pharmaceutical Freeze-Drying Practice. Peter Cameron. 1996. LC 96-39290. 350p. 195.00 (*1-57491-031-0*) IHS Health Grp.

Good Practice of Clinical Drug Trials. A. Spriet & T. Dupin-Spriet. 1992. (Illus.). viii, 280p. pap. 129.75 (*3-8055-5367-6*) S Karger.

Good Practice of Clinical Drug Trials. Alain Spriet & Therese Dupin-Spriet. Tr. by Robert Coluzzi & John Young. 2nd exp. rev. ed. 1997. (Illus.). viii, 288p. 148.00 (*3-8055-6448-1*) S Karger.

Good Practices in Palliative Care: A Psychosocial Perspective. David Oliviere. Ed. by Rosalind Hargreaves & Barbara Monroe. 1998. LC 98-12751. 210p. pap. (*1-85742-396-8*, R726.8.O45) Ashgate Pub GBR. *Dist:* Ashgate Pub Co.

Good Practices in Palliative Care (H) A Psychosocial Perspective. David Oliviere et al. 1998. LC 98-12751. 210p. text (*1-85742-395-X*, R726.8.O45) Ashgate Pub GBR. *Dist:* Ashgate Pub Co.

Good Samaritan: Helping in an Emergency. National Safety Council Staff. 1996. LC 95-41959. (Illus.). 50p. (C). pap. text 99.95 (*0-86720-544-X*, 544-X) Jones & Bartlett.

Good Skin Doctor: A Leading Dermatologist's Guide to Beating Acne. Tony Chu & Anne Lovell. 1999. pap. (*0-7225-3675-5*) Thorsons GBR. *Dist:* Natl Bk Netwk.

Good Sleep Without Drugs. Cyril Scott. 1982. pap. 2.95 (*0-87904-012-2*) Lust.

Good Society & the Inner World. Michael Rustin. 1991. 300p. (gr. 13). pap. 20.00 (*0-86091-544-1*, A5355) Verso.

Good Therapy - Bad Therapy: Choosing the Right Therapy That Works for You. Michael J. Hurd. 1996. pap. text 14.95 (*0-935016-38-4*) Arrowood Pr.

Good Thinking: Test-Taking, Problem Solving & Study Skills for Nursing Students. Poorman W. Molcan. 1994. (Illus.). 300p. (C). pap. text 27.00 (*0-9640556-0-0*) Stat Nursing.

Goodbye Pain! Two Dozen Ways You Can Prevent & Relieve Pain. Ronald M. Lawrence. 1988. LC 88-28001. (Illus.). 112p. pap. 5.95 (*0-88007-169-9*) Woodbridge Pr.

Goodbye to the White Lady: Cocaine Addiction & Recovery. C. C. Nuckols. 1992. 154p. 17.95 (*0-8306-3388-X*); pap. 7.95 (*0-8306-3385-5*) McGraw-Hill Educ Grp.

Goodman & Gilman's Essentials of Pharmacology. Theodore W. Rall. 8th ed. 1994. (Illus.). 800p. pap. 37.00 (*0-07-105430-8*) McGraw.

Goodman & Gilman's the Pharmacological Basis of Therapeutics. Alfred G. Gilman et al. 8th ed. 1990. (Illus.). 1840p. (*0-08-040296-8*) PPI GBR. *Dist:* McGraw.

Goodman & Gilman's the Pharmacological Basis of Therapeutics. Ed. by Joel G. Hardman et al. 9th ed. 1992. LC 95-36658. (Illus.). 1905p. text 125.00 (*0-07-026266-7*) McGraw-Hill Educ Grp.

Goodness! Eating Healthily. Christine Mulliss. 1977. 63p. (C). pap. 9.95 (*0-8464-1014-1*) Beekman Pubs.

Gordon Diagnostic System Interpretive Guide. Michael Gordon et al. 3rd ed. 1996. 128p. ring bd. 40.00 (*1-887306-01-3*) GSI Pubns.

Gordon's Guide to the Surgical Morbidity & Mortality Conference. Leo A. Gordon. 1994. LC 93-79226. 88p. pap. 22.95 (*1-56053-103-7*) Hanley & Belfus.

Gorney-Moreno: Introduction to Home Health Nursing. Mary Jo Gorney-Moreno. 1999. text 199.00 (*0-323-00422-9*) Saunders.

Gospel of Germs: Men, Women, & the Microbe in American Life. Nancy Tomes. 1998. LC 97-28734. (Illus.). 336p. 32.50 (*0-674-35707-8*) HUP.

Gospel of Life & the Vision of Health Care: Proceedings of the Fifteenth Bishops' Workshop, Dallas, Texas. Bishops of the United States and Canada Staff. Ed. by Russell E. Smith. 1996. LC 96-46483. 212p. (Orig.). pap. 19.95 (*0-935372-40-7*) NCBC.

Gossypol: A Potential Contraceptive for Men. Ed. by Sheldon J. Segal. 1984. LC 84-18230. 286p. 75.00 (*0-306-41884-3*, Plenum Trade) Perseus Pubng.

Gould Chiampo Encyclopedia of Medicine: Il Gould Chiampo Dizionario Enciclopedico di Medicina Inglese-Italiano: Italiano-Inglese. Luigi Chiampo. 1988. (ENG & ITA.). 2304p. lib. bdg. 295.00 (*0-8288-3359-1*, F39060) Fr & Eur.

Gout: The Patrician Malady. Roy Porter & G. S. Rousseau. (Illus.). 2000. 408p. pap. 16.95 (*0-300-08274-6*); 1998. LC 98-16881. 352p. pap. 40.00 (*0-300-07386-0*) Yale U Pr.

Gout, Hyperuricemia & Other Crystal-Associated Arthropathies. Ed. by Charley J. Smyth & V. Michael Holers. 1998. LC 98-42977. (Illus.). 448p. text 185.00 (*0-8247-0210-7*) Dekker.

Governaunce of Good Helthe, Erasmus Beynge Interpretoure. Plutarch. 1968. LC 68-54657. (English Experience Ser.: No. 16). 32p. reprint ed. 20.00 (*90-221-0016-2*) Walter J Johnson.

Governing Health: The Politics of Health Policy. Carol S. Weissert & William G. Weissert. 1996. LC 95-44487. (Illus.). 392p. (C). pap. text 26.95 (*0-8018-5266-8*) Johns Hopkins.

Governing Health Systems: Ten Stories. Frwd. by Daniel M. Fox & Mary A. Pittman. 1997. LC 97-212606. 96p. (Orig.). pap. (*1-887748-08-3*) Milbank Memorial.

Governing Policies Manual for Medical Practices. Alys Novak. 1996. 464p. (Orig.). pap. 148.50 (*1-56829-079-9*, 4929) M G M A.

Government Affairs Handbook. American Academy of Pediatrics Staff. 1998. LC 98-70032. 172p. pap. 40.00 (*1-58110-004-3*) Am Acad Pediat.

Government & Health Services: Government's Role in the Development of U. S. Health Services, 1930-1980. William Shonick. 1995. (Illus.). 536p. text 75.00 (*0-19-506968-4*) OUP.

Government Policy & Women's Health Care: The Swedish Alternative. Ed. by Gunnela Westlander. 1988. LC 88-2927. (Women & Health Ser.: Vol. 13, Nos. 3-4). (Illus.). 180p. text 49.95 (*0-86656-706-2*) Haworth Pr.

Government Response to the Reports of the Health Committee on Health Services of Command Paper 3792. 1997. (Command Papers: No. 81011068). (*0-10-137932-3*, HM79323) Statnry Office GBR. *Dist:* Bernan Associates.

Governmental Inspection of the Baby Factory. Scott H. Isaacman. 2nd ed. 1991. LC 91-92148. (Illus.). 106p. pap. 9.95 (*0-9631469-9-8*); text 29.95 (*0-9631469-8-X*) Harvard Terrace HC.

Governments & Agencies: Index of Activities & Information. American Health Research Institute Staff. 1990. LC 88-47565. 150p. 47.50 (*1-55914-204-9*); pap. 47.50 (*1-55914-205-7*) ABBE Pubs Assn.

Governments & Health Systems: Implications of Differing Involvements. David P. Chinitz et al. 1998. LC 97-45912. 646p. 175.00 (*0-471-98199-0*) Wiley.

Governor's Policy Guide on AIDS. Mona Rowe & Caitlin Ryan. Ed. by Karen Glass. 1989. 40p. (Orig.). pap. text 35.00 (*1-55877-049-6*) Natl Governor.

Governors' Proposal on Welfare & Medicaid: Hearings Before the Committee on Finance, United States Senate, One Hundred Fourth Congress, Second Session, on the National Governors' Association Policy on Welfare Reform & Medicaid (with Administration & Public Views), February 22, 28, & 29, 1996. U. S. Congress, Senate Committee on Finance. 1997. LC 97-174300. (Illus.). (*0-16-054203-0*) USGPO.

GP & the Primary Health Care Team. N. D. Mackichan. 1976. (Illus.). pap. 29.00 (*0-8464-0453-2*) Beekman Pubs.

GP Commissioning & Evidence-Based Healthcare. Ron Singer & Angela Coulter. 1997. LC 96-29998. (*1-85775-184-1*) Radcliffe Med Pr GBR. *Dist:* Balogh.

GP Consultation: A Registrar's Guide. Peter G. Livesey. 1997. LC 96-290. 160p. pap. text 37.50 (*0-7506-3130-9*) Buttrwrth-Heinemann.

***GP Guide to Secondary Care Investigations.** Ed. by Keith Hopcoft. 2000. 216p. pap. (*1-85775-398-4*) Radcliffe Med Pr GBR. *Dist:* Balogh.

***GP Quiz Book,** No. 2. A. Munro. 1999. 200p. pap. (*1-85775-383-6*) Radcliffe Med Pr GBR. *Dist:* Balogh.

***GP Quiz Book Bk. 1: Detection & Management of Physical Disease.** Alick Munro. 1999. 200p. pap. (*1-85775-229-5*) Radcliffe Med Pr GBR. *Dist:* Balogh.

GP Training Handbook. M. Hall et al. 3rd ed. 1999. LC 98-40497. pap. 52.95 (*0-632-05039-X*) Blackwell Sci.

Grabb & Smith's Plastic Surgery. Sherrell J. Aston et al. 5th ed. 1997. LC 97-16691. 1,184p. text 159.00 (*0-316-32255-5*) Lppncott W & W.

Grabb's Encyclopedia of Flaps: Head & Neck, Vol. 1. Berish Strauch & Luis O. Vasconez. 2nd ed. 1997. LC 98-136539. 944p. text 225.00 (*0-7817-1464-8*) Lppncott W & W.

Grabb's Encyclopedia of Flaps: Torso, Pelvis & Lower Extremities, Vol.III. Berish Strauch & Luis O. Vasconez. 2nd ed. 1997. LC 98-136539. 784p. text 225.00 (*0-7817-1466-4*) Lppncott W & W.

Grabb's Encyclopedia of Flaps: Upper Extremities, Vol. II. Berish Strauch & Luis O. Vasconez. 2nd ed. 1997. LC 98-136539. 544p. text 225.00 (*0-7817-1465-6*) Lppncott W & W.

***Gracefully Insane: The Rise & Fall of America's Premier Mental Hospital.** Alex Beam. 2001. LC 2001-48339. (Illus.). 288p. text 26.00 (*1-891620-75-4*) PublicAffairs NY.

Grading Health Care: The Science & Art of Developing Consumer Scorecards. Pamela P. Hanes & Merwyn R. Greenlick. 1998. LC 98-4892. 166p. 45.00 (*0-7879-4027-5*) Jossey-Bass.

Graduate Education in Internal Medicine: A Resource Document. Jack Ende et al. 1997. LC 97-3199. 224p. pap. text 24.00 (*0-943126-60-6*) Amer Coll Phys.

Graduate Education in Nursing - Advanced Practice Nursing, Vol. 2. 1997. (Nursing DataSource, 1997 Ser.: Vol. II). 80p. 35.00 (*0-88737-752-1*, 19-7521, NLN Pr) Natl League Nurse.

Graduate Medical Education Directory, 1999-2000. American Medical Association Staff. 1999. 64.95 (*0-89970-984-2*) AMA.

Graduate Medical Education in the European Region. 1983. (Euro Reports & Studies Ser.: No. 77). 151p. pap. text 12.00 (*92-890-1243-9*) World Health.

Graduate Studies in Biology, Health, & Agricultural Sciences, 1998. Date not set. (Compact Guides to Graduate Studies in . . . Ser.). 1129p. pap. 24.95 incl. cd-rom (*0-7689-0000-X*) Petersons.

Graduate Study in Psychology 2000. Ed. by American Physiological Society Staff. 33rd ed. 2000. (Graduate Study in Psychology Ser.). 568p. pap. 21.95 (*1-55798-660-6*) Am Psychol.

Graduate Therapeutics: A Primer for MRCP & Specialist Training. Derek G. Waller. 2001. 410p. pap. text 28.00 (*0-7506-4293-9*) Buttrwrth-Heinemann.

Graft vs. Host-Disease. Nelson J. Chao. 2nd ed. 1999. LC 98-53442. (Medical Intelligence Unit Ser.). 204p. 99.00 (*1-57059-534-8*) Landes Bioscience.

Graft vs Host Disease. Ed. by James L. Ferrara et al. 2nd ed. 1996. LC 96-31581. (Illus.). 848p. text 230.00 (*0-8247-9728-0*) Dekker.

Graft vs. Leukemia in Man & Animal Models. Ed. by James P. O'Kunewick & Ruby F. Meredith. 1981. 288p. 157.00 (*0-8493-5745-4*, RC643) CRC Pr.

Grainger & Allison's Diagnostic Radiology: A Textbook of Imaging Ronald G. Grainger. 3rd ed. 1996. text (*0-443-05167-4*, G6455) Church.

Grains & Greens see Wright Diet - Food for Humans - The First Lesson in Medicine for Everyone

Gram-Positive Bacteria: Vaccine Vehicles for Mucosal Immunization. Gianni Pozzi. Ed. by Jeremy M. Wells. 1997. LC 97-2675. (Biotechnology Intelligence Unit Ser.). 175p. 95.00 (*1-57059-439-2*) Landes Bioscience.

Gram-Positive Bacteria: Vaccine Vehicles for Mucosal Immunization. Ed. by Gianni Pozzi & Jeremy M. Wells. 1997. LC 97-2675. (Biotechnology Intelligence Unit Ser.). (Illus.). 180p. 99.00 (*3-540-62776-6*) Spr-Verlag.

Gram-Positive Pathogens. Ed. by Vincent A. Fischetti et al. 1999. LC 99-35911. (Illus.). xiii, 735p. 115.95 (*1-55581-166-3*) ASM Pr.

Gramatical Categories & Cognition. John A. Lucy. 1996. 270p. pap. 17.95 (*0-521-56536-7*) Cambridge U Pr.

Grammar & Writing Skills for the Health Professional. Browning Staff. 2001. LC 00-60154. (Allied Health Ser.). (Illus.). 256p. (C). pap. text 30.95 (*0-7668-1259-6*) Delmar.

Grammar of Attic Inscriptions Vol. 2: Morphology. Leslie Threatte. 1996. xxv, 839p. (C). lib. bdg. 437.00 (*3-11-014363-1*) De Gruyter.

Grammar of the Unconscious: The Conceptual Foundations of Psychoanalysis. Charles R. Elder. 1994. LC 93-35531. (C). 452p. pap. 23.95 (*0-271-01311-7*); 248p. text 49.50 (*0-271-01310-9*) Pa St U Pr.

Grammatical Analysis of Language Disability. David Crystal et al. 2nd ed. 1990. (Illus.). 200p. (C). pap. text 39.95 (*1-879105-00-4*, A018) Singular Publishing.

Gran Dilema Humano: La Vida, Complicada e Incomprendida. Iraida Negroni. 1988. (SPA., Illus.). 372p. (Orig.). (C). pap. 12.00 (*0-9620054-0-1*) I Negroni.

Grand Design: A Manic Depressive's True Story. Randall G. Buerkle. 225p. (Orig.). (C). pap. 10.95 (*1-885397-02-X*) Flagship Pubns.

Grand Dictionnaire Larousse de la Psychologie. Henriette Bloch. 1991. (FRE.). 862p. 175.00 (*0-7859-7664-7*, 2035010306) Fr & Eur.

Grand Priory of the Order of the Hospital of St. John of Jerusalem in England: A Short History. Edwin J. King. LC 76-29826. reprint ed. 39.50 (*0-404-15420-4*) AMS Pr.

Grand Rounds in Surgery 1994: Hot Issues & Recent Advances in Surgery. Ed. by Samuel P. Kwok. 1995. (Illus.). 226p. (C). text 72.50 (*962-201-661-8*) Coronet Bks.

Grand Rounds in Transplantation. Harold J. Helderman & William H. Frist. 1994. LC 94-22642. (Illus.). 248p. (*0-412-04271-1*) E A GBR. *Dist:* OUP.

Grande Encyclopedie Atlas de la Medecine, Set. Gerard Bordes. 1976. (FRE.). 320p. 995.00 (*0-8288-5701-6*, M6291) Fr & Eur.

Grandma Called It Roughage: Fiber Facts & Fallacies. Robert L. Ory. 1991. LC 91-24259. (Illus.). 170p. text 30.00 (*0-8412-1749-1*); pap. text 19.95 (*0-8412-1764-5*) Am Chemical.

Grandma's Home Remedies. Myles Bader. 1999. 14.95 (*0-688-16217-7*) Hearst Bks.

Grandma's Remedies: A Compendium of Old Time Remedies. 1991. lib. bdg. 75.00 (*0-87700-966-X*) Revisionist Pr.

Grandma's Remedies - Old Time Remedies. 1997. pap. 9.50 (*0-7873-0987-7*) Hlth Research.

Grandparents as Carers of Children with Disabilities: Facing the Challenges. Ed. by Philip McCallion & Matthew P. Janicki. 2000. LC 00-57551. (Journal of Gerontological Social Work Ser.: Vol. 33, No. 3). xix, 127p. (C). 49.95 (*0-7890-1192-1*); pap. 24.95 (*0-7890-1193-X*) Haworth Pr.

Grant Application Writers Handbook. Liane Reif-Lehrer. 3rd ed. 1995. (Illus.). 496p. (C). pap. text 42.95 (*0-86720-874-0*, 874-0) Jones & Bartlett.

Grant's Atlas of Anatomy. Anne M.R. Agur & Ming J. Lee. 10th ed. 1999. 784p. LC 99-25481. (Illus.). pap. text 60.95 (*0-683-30264-7*); text 95.00 (*0-7817-2260-8*) Lppncott W & W.

Grants Dissector. Eberhardt K. Sauerland. 10th ed. 1991. 192p. pap. text 29.00 (*0-683-03707-2*) Lppncott W & W.

Grants for at-risk Youth. Ed. by HADG Staff. 2001. 212p. pap. 145.00 (*0-8342-2007-5*) Aspen Pub.

***Grants for at-Risk Youth.** Aspen Health and Administration Development Group. 3rd ed. 2000. 220p. 145.00 (*0-8342-1895-X*) Aspen Pub.

***Granulocyte Adhesion to Matrix Proteins & the Effect on the Release of Granule Proteins: Development of a Simple Method & Its Application in Experimental & Clinical Studies.** Xiaoyan Xu. 2001. (Comprehensive Summaries of Uppsala Dissertations from the Faculty of Medicine Ser.: No. 1071). (Illus.). 46p. pap. (*91-554-5112-8*) Acta Univ SWE. *Dist:* Coronet Bks.

Granulomatous Disorders. Ed. by D. Geraint James & A. Zumla. 1999. LC 98-35107. (Illus.). 628p. (C). text 240.00 (*0-521-59221-6*) Cambridge U Pr.

Granville Sharp Pattison: Anatomist & Antagonist, 1791-1851. F. L. Pattison. 1987. LC 87-10835. (History of American Science & Technology Ser.). (Illus.). 304p. text 32.00 (*0-8173-0375-8*) U of Ala Pr.

Graphics of Motion: The Electromyography of Muscular Dynamics. Gabriel E. Sella. 2000. LC 00-92686. (Illus.). 350p. text 120.00 (*1-884325-13-0*) G E Sella.

Graphs & Genes. S. N. Rodin. Tr. by B. G. Mirkin & H. L. Beus. 1984. (Biomathematics Ser.: Vol. II). (Illus.). 197p. 75.95 (*0-387-12657-0*) Spr-Verlag.

Graphs & Tables for Use in Radiology. F. Wachsmann & G. Drexler. 2nd enl. rev. ed. 1976. 238p. 53.95 (*0-387-07809-6*) Spr-Verlag.

Grasping Hand. Christine L. MacKenzie & Thea Iberall. 1994. LC 93-47171. 500p. 137.50 (*0-444-81746-8*, North Holland) Elsevier.

Grasping the Wind. Andrew W. Ellis et al. Ed. by Robert L. Felt. 1993. LC 89-2984. 250p. pap. text 27.00 (*0-912111-19-4*) Paradigm Publns.

Grass Is Green in Suburbia: A Sociological Study of Adolescent Usage of Illicit Drugs. Nechama Tec. 1974. LC 73-91302. 15.00 (*0-87212-030-9*) Libra.

Gratte ou Ciguatera (Ciguatera Poisoning) Ses Remedes Traditionnels dans le Pacifique Sud (Traditional Remedies in the South Pacific) D. Laurent et al. 1993.Tr. of Ciguatera Poisoning - Traditional Remedies in the South Pacific.. (FRE., Illus.). 152p. pap. (*2-7099-1171-X*) LInstitut Francais FRA. *Dist:* Balogh.

Gravel (Urinary Stone) Materia Medica Relating to Gravel. 2000. LC 99-97766. 90p. pap. 6.95 (*1-929410-05-0*) dttm.

Graves' Ophthalmopathy. Ed. by C. R. Picardt. 1989. (Developments in Ophthalmology Ser.: Vol. 20). (Illus.). 230p. 169.75 (*3-8055-5040-5*) S Karger.

Graves' Ophthalmopathy. Ed. by Jack R. Wall & Jacques How. 1990. (Illus.). 208p. 49.95 (*0-86542-106-4*) Mosby Inc.

Gravest Show on Earth. Elinor Burkett. 1999. pap. 23.95 (*0-670-85230-9*) Viking Penguin.

***Gray Matters: Dementia Research Has Unexpected Consequences.** Alfred Berutti. 2001. pap. 16.00 (*0-7388-5095-0*) Xlibris Corp.

Graying of the World: Who Will Care for the Frail Elderly? Ed. by Laura K. Olson. 1994. LC 92-1661. (Illus.). 320p. lib. bdg. 69.95 (*1-56024-363-5*) Haworth Pr.

Gray's Anatomy. Henry Gray. 1992. 10.98 (*1-55521-784-2*) Bk Sales Inc.

Gray's Anatomy. Henry Gray. 1999. pap. 14.99 (*0-517-20904-7*); 1988. LC 76-52804. (Illus.). 1248p. 14.99 (*0-517-22365-1*) Random Hse Value.

Gray's Anatomy. Henry Gray. (Illus.). 1248p. 1999. 18.98 (*0-7624-0673-9*); 1974. LC 74-19510. pap. 12.95 (*0-914294-08-3*) Running Pr.

Gray's Anatomy: The Anatomical Basis of Medicine & Surgery. Ed. by Peter L. Williams et al. 38th ed. 1995. LC 95-5806. (Illus.). 2092p. text (*0-443-04560-7*) Church.

Gray's Anatomy Deluxe. Peter Williams. 38th deluxe ed. 1995. text 450.00 (*0-443-05327-8*) Saunders.

Gray's Anatomy of the Human Body. Ed. by Carmine D. Clemente. 30th ed. 1985. LC 84-5741. (Illus.). 1,676p. 96.00 (*0-8121-0644-X*) Lppncott W & W.

Gray's Pocket Medical Dictionary. Ed. by Nancy Roper. 2nd rev. ed. 1995. pap. text (*0-443-07683-9*) Church.

Grayson's Disease of the Cornea. Robert C. Arffa. 4th ed. 1998. (Illus.). 784p. (*84-8174-343-7*) Mosby-Doyma Libros ESP. *Dist:* Mosby Inc.

Grayson's Diseases of the Cornea. Robert C. Arffa. 4th ed. 1997. LC 97-18628. (Illus.). 784p. (C). (gr. 13). text 199.00 (*0-8151-3654-4*, 30969) Mosby Inc.

GRE Psychology Test Prep. Ronald T. Kellogg. 2000. pap. 31.95 incl. disk (*0-87891-336-X*) Res & Educ.

GRE Subject Test Practice Books: Psychology Test. Educational Testing Service Staff. 1986. mass mkt. 6.95 (*0-446-38469-0*) Warner Bks.

Great American Fraud: A Series of Articles on the Patent Medicine Evil. Samuel H. Adams. 1976. reprint ed. 49.00 (*0-403-05771-X*, Regency) Scholarly.

Great & Growing Evil? The Medical Consequences of Alcohol Abuse. Royal College of Physicians Staff. 1987. 144p. (C). text (*0-422-61140-9*) Tavistock GBR. *Dist:* Routldge.

Great Billion Dollar Medical Swindle. Keith Alan Lasko. 1980. 10.95 (*0-672-52625-5*) Sams.

Great Biologists. John A. Thompson. 1977. LC 67-23272. (Essay Index Reprint Ser.). 19.95 (*0-8369-0935-6*) Ayer.

Great Book of Hemp: The Complete Guide to the Environmental, Commercial, & Medicinal Uses of the World's Most Extraordinary Plant. Rowan Robinson. 1995. LC 95-33699. (Illus.). 256p. pap. 19.95 (*0-89281-541-8*, Heal Arts VT) Inner Tradit.

Great Break: A Short History of the Separation of Medical Science from Religion. Joseph Mauceri. 1987. 156p. pap. 9.95 (*0-940170-13-2*) Station Hill Pr.

Great Cases in Psychoanalysis. Ed. by Harold Greenwald. rev. ed. 1973. LC 73-81210. 256p. 45.00 (*0-87668-786-9*) Aronson.

Great Catalog of the C. H. Stoelting Company, 1930-1937: A Facsimile Reproduction. Stoelting, C. H., Co. Staff. 1997. LC 97-36171. 334p. 75.00 (*0-8201-1504-5*) Schol Facsimiles.

Great Communication, Great Production. Cathy Jameson. 1994. LC 94-32276. 44.95 (*0-87814-427-7*) PennWell Corp.

Great Deal! . . . Compensation Negotiation for Nurse Practitioners & Physician Assistants. Heidi L. Bourne. Ed. by Carol Sweig & Don Banducci. 3rd rev. ed. 1998. 72p. pap. 29.95 (*0-9654977-1-2*) Open Spaces.

Great Debate on Population Policy: An Instructive Entertainment. Bernard Berelson. 1975. LC 75-22229. 32p. (Orig.). pap. text 2.95 (*0-87834-050-5*) Population Coun.

Great Doctors: A Biographical History of Medicine. Henry E. Sigerist. Tr. by Eden Paul & Cedar Paul. 1977. LC 74-156716. (Essay Index Reprint Ser.). reprint ed. 40.95 (*0-8369-2297-2*) Ayer.

Great Doctors of the Nineteenth Century. William Hale-White. 1977. LC 74-108639. (Essay Index Reprint Ser.). 25.95 (*0-8369-1575-5*) Ayer.

Great Expectations. Green. 1998. 300p. pap. text 49.99 (*1-898507-58-9*) Buttrwrth-Heinemann.

Great Feuds in Medicine: 10 of the Livliest Disputes Ever. Hal Hellman. 2001. LC 00-63349. 256p. 24.95 (*0-471-34757-4*) Wiley.

Great Ideas in Psychotherapy. Richard D. Chessick. 1988. LC 76-22868. 462p. reprint ed. 60.00 (*0-87668-787-7*) Aronson.

Great Ideas in the History of Surgery. Leo Zimmerman & Ilza Veith. 1993. (Illus.). 608p. reprint ed. 95.00 (*0-930405-53-6*) Norman SF.

Great Issues for Medicine in the Twenty-First Century: A Consideration of the Ethical & Social Issues Arising Out of Advances in the Biomedical Sciences. Ed. by Joseph L. Goldstein & Michael S. Brown. LC 99-30118. (Annals of the New York Academy of Sciences Ser.: Vol. 882). (Illus.). xix, 277p. 1999. pap. text 60.00 (*1-57331-143-X*); 1998. pap. 60.00 (*1-57331-144-8*) NY Acad Sci.

Great Lakes Human Health Effects Research Program. Ed. by Barry L. Johnson. 2000. (Illus.). 60p. (C). reprint ed. pap. text 20.00 (*0-7567-0012-4*) DIANE Pub.

Great Medical Milestones. Betty Lou Kratoville. 1996. (Illus.). 64p. (gr. 5-12). pap. 12.00 (*1-57128-020-0*) High Noon Bks.

Great Plague in London in 1665. Walter G. Bell. LC 75-23682. (Illus.). reprint ed. 47.50 (*0-404-13235-9*) AMS Pr.

Great Pox: The French Disease in Renaissance Europe. Jon Arrizabalaga et al. 1997. LC 96-23453. 368p. 45.00 (*0-300-06934-0*) Yale U Pr.

Great Psychologists. Evans & Robert Irving Watson. 5th ed. 1997. LC 90-39371. 750p. (C). lib. bdg. 96.00 (*0-06-041919-9*) Addson-Wesley Educ.

Great Supplement Hoax: The Dangers in Synthetic Vitamins & Supplements. 1992. lib. bdg. 77.95 (*0-8490-8810-0*) Gordon Pr.

Greater Omentum: Anatomy, Physiology, Pathology, Surgery. Ed. by D. Liebermann-Meffert et al. 1983. (Illus.). 369p. 348.00 (*0-387-11882-9*) Spr-Verlag.

Greater than the Parts: Holism in Biomedicine, 1920-1950. Ed. by Christopher Lawrence & George Weisz. 1998. (Illus.). 384p. text 55.00 (*0-19-510904-X*) OUP.

Greater Vision: A Comprehensive Program for Physical, Emotional & Spiritual Clarity. Marc Grossman & Vinton McCabe. 2001. LC 00-67784. (Illus.). 336p. pap. 16.95 (*0-658-00643-6*) McGraw-Hill Prof.

Greatest Benefit to Mankind: A Medical History of Humanity. Roy Porter. 1999. LC 98-10219. (Illus.). 872p. pap. 17.95 (*0-393-31980-6*, Norton Paperbks) Norton.

Greatest Benefit to Mankind: A Medical History of Humanity from Antiquity to the Present. Roy Porter. 1998. LC 98-10219. (Illus.). 800p. 35.00 (*0-393-04634-6*) Norton.

Greatest Good to the Greatest Number: Penicillin Rationing on the American Home Front, 1940-1945. David P. Adams. 1991. LC 90-6081. (American University Studies: Ser. IX, Vol. 93). (Illus.). VII, 228p. (C). text 38.95 (*0-8204-1284-8*) P Lang Pubng.

Greek & Interbehavioral Psychology: Selected & Revised Papers of Noel W. Smith. Noel W. Smith. rev. ed. 1993. 424p. (C). pap. 55.50 (*0-8191-9331-3*) U Pr of Amer.

Greek & Latin in Scientific Terminology. Oscar E. Nybakken. 1985. LC 59-5992. (ENG, GRE & LAT.). 322p. pap. text 29.95 (*0-8138-0721-2*) Iowa U Pr.

Greek Biology & Greek Medicine. Charles J. Singer. LC 75-23760. reprint ed. 34.50 (*0-404-13366-5*) AMS Pr.

Greek-English, English-Greek Medical Dictionary. D. N. Gelis. (ENG & GRE.). 585p. 175.00 (*0-7859-7492-X*) Fr & Eur.

Greek Medicine. Fred B. Lund. LC 75-23668. (Clio Medica Ser.: 18). (Illus.). reprint ed. 37.50 (*0-404-58918-9*) AMS Pr.

Greek Medicine: From the Heroic to the Hellenistic Age: A Source Book. Ed. by James Longrigg. 1998. LC 98-15593. 272p. (C). pap. 27.95 (*0-415-92087-6*, D5784) Routledge.

Greek Medicine, Being Extracts Illustrative of Medical Writing from Hippocrates to Galen. Ed. by Arthur J. Brock. LC 76-179302. (Library of Greek Thought: No. 8). reprint ed. 36.50 (*0-404-07806-0*) AMS Pr.

Greek Medicine in Rome. T. C. Allbutt. 1977. LC 69-13230. reprint ed. (*0-405-08201-0*) Blom Pubns GBR. *Dist:* Ayer.

Greek Rational Medicine: Philosophy & Medicine from Alcmaeon to the Alexandrians. James Longrigg. 1993. LC 92-28865. (Illus.). 296p. (C). 80.00 (*0-415-02594-X*, B0350) Routledge.

Greeley Guide to Managed Care Credentialing. Hugh Greeley. 1998. LC 00-501956. (Illus.). 180p. pap. text 127.00 (*1-57839-032-X*) Opus Communs.

Greeley Guide to Medical Staff Credentialing. Hugh Greeley. 1998. 180p. pap. text 127.00 (*1-57839-031-1*) Opus Communs.

Green Barley Essence. Yoshihide Hagiwara. 1986. (Good Health Guides). 32p. pap. 3.95 (*0-87983-423-4*, 34234K, Keats Pubng) McGraw-Hill Trade.

***Green Fluorescent Protein: Applications & Protocols.** Ed. by Barry W. Hicks. 2002. (Methods in Molecular Biology Ser.: Vol. 183). 385p. 99.50 (*0-89603-905-6*) Humana.

Green Medicine: Traditional Mexican American Herbal Remedies. Eliseo Torres. 1983. (Illus.). 64p. (Orig.). pap. 4.95 (*0-9612008-0-4*) Nieves Pr.

Green Pharmacy. James A. Duke. 1997. LC 97-6175. 528p. 29.95 (*0-87596-316-1*) Rodale Pr Inc.

Green Pharmacy: New Discoveries in Herbal Remedies for Common Diseases & Conditions from the World's Foremost Authority on Healing Herbs. James A. Duke. 1999. LC 97-6175. (Illus.). 507p. pap. 17.95 (*1-57954-124-0*) Rodale Pr Inc.

Green Pharmacy: The History & Evolution of Western Herbal Medicine. Barbara Griggs. 1997. LC 96-1660. 416p. pap. 19.95 (*0-89281-727-5*, Heal Arts VT) Inner Tradit.

Green Pharmacy: The Ultimate Compendium of Natural Remedies from the World's Foremost Authority on Healing Herbs. James A. Duke. 1998. LC 97-6175. (Green Pharmacy Ser.: Vol. 1). (Illus.). 617p. mass mkt. 6.99 (*0-312-96648-2*, Tor Books) T Doherty Assocs.

Green Pharmacy Anti-Aging Prescriptions. James A. Duke. 2001. LC 00-12885. (Illus.). xiii, 546p. 29.95 (*1-57954-198-4*) Rodale Pr Inc.

***Green Pharmacy Herbal Handbook.** 2002. mass mkt. (*0-312-98151-1*) St Martin.

Green Psychology: Transforming Our Relationship to the Earth. Ralph Metzner. 1999. LC 99-20490. 240p. 14.95 (*0-89281-798-4*, Park St Pr) Inner Tradit.

Green Tea: Health Benefits & Applications. Yukihiko Hara. 2000. LC 00-47597. (Food Science & Technology Ser.). (Illus.). xvi, 252p. text 125.00 (*0-8247-0470-3*) Dekker.

Green Witch Herbal: Restoring Nature's Magic in Home, Health, & Beauty Care. Barbara Griggs. 1994. LC 94-6533. (Illus.). 168p. pap. 14.95 (*0-89281-496-9*, Heal Arts VT) Inner Tradit.

Greenfield's Neuropathology. 5th ed. (*0-340-54629-8*) E A GBR. *Dist:* Routldge.

Greenfield's Neuropathology David I. Graham & Peter L. Lanton. 6th ed. 1996. LC 96-48860. (Illus.). 2288p. (*0-340-59809-3*) E A GBR. *Dist:* OUP, Routldge.

***Greenfield's Neuropathology** Ed. by David I. Graham & Peter L. Lantos. 7th ed. 2001. (Arnold Publication). (Illus.). 2400p. text (*0-340-74231-3*) E A GBR. *Dist:* OUP.

***Greenfield's Neuropathology** Ed. by David I. Graham & Peter L. Lantos. 7th ed. 2002. (Arnold Publication). text 599.00 incl. cd-rom (*0-340-80661-3*) OUP.

Greenhouse for the Mind. Jacquelyn S. Sanders. 1989. LC 88-23346. 172p. 23.95 (*0-226-73464-1*) U Ch Pr.

Green's Gynecology. Daniel Clarke-Pearson & M. Yusoff Dawood. 4th ed. 1990. (Illus.). 650p. pap. text 54.95 (*0-316-14490-8*, Little Brwn Med Div) Lppncott W & W.

Green's Operative Hand Surgery 4th ed. Ed. by David P. Green et al. Incl. Vol. 1. (*0-443-06500-4*); Vol. 2. (*0-443-06501-2*); 1999. LC 97-51666. (Illus.). 1855p. 1998. text (*0-443-07955-2*) Church.

***Green's Operative Hand Surgery** Ed. by David P. Green et al. 4th ed. 1999. LC 97-51666. (Illus.). Vol. 1. (*0-443-06500-4*); Vol. 2. (*0-443-06501-2*) Church.

Grenzbereiche der Anaesthesie und Intensivmedizin. Ed. by U. Nordmeyer et al. 1991. (Beitraege zur Intensiv und Notfallmedizin Ser.: Vol. 7). (GER., Illus.). viii, 190p. pap. 50.50 (*3-8055-5413-3*) S Karger.

Grey Cases for Paediatric Examinations. Field. 1995. pap. text 34.00 (*0-443-05011-2*) Saunders.

Grief: A Basic Reaction to Alcoholism. Joseph L. Kellermann. 1987. 28p. (Orig.). pap. 2.50 (*0-89486-037-2*, 1297B) Hazelden.

Grief & the Healing Arts: Creativity As Therapy. Ed. by Sandra L. Bertman. 1998. (Death, Value & Meaning Ser.). (Illus.). 438p. LC 97-48681. 58.95 (*0-89503-189-2*); pap. 29.95 (*0-89503-198-1*) Baywood Pub.

Grief as a Family Process: A Developmental Approach to Clinical Practice. Ester R. Shapiro. 1994. LC 94-18297. 307p. 36.00 (*0-89862-196-8*, 2196) Guilford Pubns.

Grief Counseling & Grief Therapy: A Handbook for the Mental Health Practitioner. J. William Worden. 2nd ed. 1991. LC 90-10422. 200p. 28.95 (*0-8261-4161-7*) Springer Pub.

***Grief Counseling & Grief Therapy: A Handbook for the Mental Health Professional.** J. William Worden. 3rd ed. 2001. LC 2001-49001. (*0-8261-4162-5*) Springer Pub.

Grief Counselling Casebook: A Student's Guide to Unresolved Grief. John C. Gunzburg & William Stewart. 1994. LC 93-40110. (*0-412-57080-7*) Chapman & Hall.

Grief Counselling Casebook: A Student's Guide to Unresolved Grief. John C. Gunzburg & William Stewart. 1994. LC 93-40110. 328p. pap. 47.75 (*1-56593-313-3*, 0636) Singular Publishing.

Grief in Children: A Handbook for Adults. Atle Dyregrov. 1991. 144p. pap. 19.95 (*1-85302-113-X*) Taylor & Francis.

Grieve's Modern Manual Therapy: The Vertebral Column. Ed. by Jeffrey D. Boyling & Nigel Palastanga. 2nd ed. 1994. (Illus.). 924p. text (*0-443-04348-5*) Church.

Grieving: COPE Program for Depression. John H. Greist et al. 1999. (Illus.). 32p. pap. (*0-9702974-6-7*) Healthcare Sys.

***Grieving... Heroism... Daring... Igniting Your Goodness Within!** Ted Borgeas. 2002. LC 2001-119484. 100p. pap. 15.95 (*0-9666110-1-2*) Cameltrotters.

Grieving Mental Illness: A Guide for Patients & Their Caregivers. Virginia Lafond. 1994. LC 95-120664. 96p. text 30.00 (*0-8020-0614-0*); 190p. pap. text 12.95 (*0-8020-7578-9*) U of Toronto Pr.

Griffith's 5 Minute Clinical Consult 1998. Mark R. Dambro. 1997. 54.95 (*0-683-30405-4*) Lppncott W & W.

Griffith's 5 Minute Clinical Consult, 1998. Mark R. Dambro. 1997. (*0-683-23136-7*) Lppncott W & W.

Griffith's 5-Minute Clinical Consult, 2001. Ed. by Mark R. Dambro. 2000. 1408p. text 59.95 (*0-7817-2565-8*) Lppncott W & W.

Griffith's 5-Minute Clinical Consultant, 1996. Mark C. Dambro. 1995. 54.95 (*0-683-02320-9*) Lppncott W & W.

Griffith's Instructions for Patients. Stephen W. Moore. Ed. by Ray Kersey. 6th ed. 1998. (Illus.). LC 98-3258. 624p. (C). pap. text 55.00 (*0-7216-7375-9*); 9624p. pap. text 55.00 (*0-7521-6737-5*) Saunders.

Grit Behind the Miracle. Alice E. Sink. 1998. LC 98-5976. (Illus.). 240p. (C). 41.50 (*0-7618-1086-2*) U Pr of Amer.

Gross Anatomy. W. J. Felts. 1991. (Oklahoma Notes). (Illus.). xiii, 199p. (C). pap. 16.95 (*0-387-96337-5*) Spr-Verlag.

Gross Anatomy. Larsen. 1999. pap. text 29.95 (*0-7216-4646-8*) Saunders.

Gross Anatomy. Richard S. Snell. 1990. pap. 28.95 (*0-316-80197-6*, Little Brwn Med Div) Lppncott W & W.

Gross Anatomy. Kyung W. Chung. 2nd ed. 1991. (Board Review Ser.). (Illus.). 368p. 19.95 (*0-683-01565-6*) Lppncott W & W.

Gross Anatomy. W. J. Felts. 2nd ed. 1992. (Oklahoma Notes). (Illus.). 192p. 16.95 (*0-387-97295-1*) Spr-Verlag.

Gross Anatomy & Embryology: 2000 Multiple-Choice Questions & Answers. 1999. 294p. spiral bd. 25.95 (*1-893720-00-4*) Biotest.

Gross Anatomy Lab. Ed. by Brynmill Press Limited Staff. 1989. (C). (*0-907839-18-5*) Brynmill Pr Ltd GBR. *Dist:* St Mut.

Gross & Microscopic Pathology of the Skin, Set. Milton R. Okun et al. 2nd ed. 1988. LC 87-71751. (Illus.). 375.00 (*0-9618536-0-3*) Derma Found Pr.

Gross Motor Skills in Children with Down Syndrome: A Guide for Parents & Professionals. Patricia C. Winders. 1997. LC 97-19243. (Topics in Down Syndrome Ser.). (Illus.). 236p. (Orig.). pap. 16.95 (*0-933149-81-6*) Woodbine House.

Gross Pathology. David Blomberg. 1994. text 400.00 (*1-56815-027-X*) Mosby Inc.

Grossman's Cardiac Catheterization, Angiography, & Intervention. Donald S. Baim & William Grossman. 6th ed. 2000. LC 00-27379. (Illus.). xv, 943p. text 125.00 (*0-683-30741-X*) Lppncott W & W.

Grothendieck Spaces in Approximation Theory. Joerg Blatter. 1972. LC 52-42839. (Memoirs Ser.: No. 1/120). 121p. pap. 16.00 (*0-8218-1820-1*, MEMO/1/120) Am Math.

Ground Rules in Psychotherapy & Counselling. Robert J. Langs. 1998. 232p. pap. (*1-85575-171-2*) Karnac Bks GBR. *Dist:* Other Pr LLC.

Grounded Theory in Medical Research: From Theory to Practice. Ed. by C. L. Weiner & W. M. Wijsmans. 1990. (Publications of the Helen Dowling Institute for Biopsychosocial Medicine: Vol. 2). 96p. pap. (*90-265-1122-1*) Swets.

Grounded Theory in Practice. Anselm L. Strauss & Juliet M. Corbin. 1997. LC 96-45918. 280p. (C). 74.95 (*0-7619-0747-5*, 80819) Sage.

Grounded Theory in Practice: A Collection of Readings. Anselm L. Strauss & Juliet M. Corbin. 1997. LC 96-45918. 160p. (C). pap. 37.95 (*0-7619-0748-3*, 80820) Sage.

Groundworks: Narratives of Embodiment, Vol. 2. Don Johnson. 1997. LC 96-43807. (Groundworks Ser.: Vol. 2). 200p. pap. text 14.95 (*1-55643-235-6*) North Atlantic.

Group Activities for Adults at Risk for Chemical Dependence: A Guide for Counselors, Therapists, & Other Professionals. Martin Fleming. 1994. LC 94-41744. 118p. pap. 39.95 (*1-56246-099-4*, 3268, HazeldenJohnson Inst) Hazelden.

Group Activities for Adults with Brain Injury. Elaine Ziol & Susan Caputo. Ed. by Cindy Drolet. rev. ed. 1998. 192p. spiral bd. 42.00 (*1-883315-33-6*, 8502) Imaginart Intl.

Group Analytic Psychotherapy: Methods & Principles. S. H. Foulkes. 1975. LC 73-88415. xii, 178p. text 106.00 (*0-677-05120-4*) Gordon & Breach.

Group Analytic Psychotherapy: Methods & Principles. S. H. Foulkes. 1991. (Illus.). 177p. reprint ed. pap. text (*0-946439-22-2*) Karnac Bks GBR. *Dist:* Other Pr LLC.

Group Beliefs. Daniel Bar-Tal. 1989. (Social Psychology Ser.). 140p. 104.00 (*0-387-97085-1*) Spr-Verlag.

Group Care Practice with Children. Ed. by Leon C. Fulcher & Frank Ainsworth. 1985. 300p. (Orig.). pap. text 14.95 (*0-422-78200-9*, 9631) Routledge.

Group Cognitive Therapy: A Treatment Approach for Depressed Older Adults. Elizabeth B. Yost et al. 1986. LC 85-28366. (Psychology Practitioner Guidebooks). 160p. text 30.00 (*0-08-031919-X*, J115); pap. text 15.95 (*0-08-031918-1*) Elsevier (Pergamon Pr).

Group Cohesion: Theoretical & Clinical Perspectives. Ed. by Henry Kellerman. 1981. 465p. text 61.00 (*0-8089-1330-1*, 792273, Grune & Strat) Harcrt Hlth Sci Grp.

Group Cohesiveness in the Industrial Work Group. Stanley E. Seashore. Ed. by Leon Stein. 1977. LC 77-70531. reprint ed. lib. bdg. 19.95 (*0-405-10199-6*) Ayer.

Group Counseling: A Sourcebook of Theory & Practice. Ed. by Robert C. Berg & James A. Johnson. 1975. 19.95 (*0-405-18853-6*, 113) Ayer.

Group Counseling: Concepts & Procedures. Robert C. Berg & Garry L. Landreth. 2nd ed. 1990. LC 89-81013. xvi, 352p. (C). 31.95 (*1-55959-008-4*) Accel Devel.

Group Counseling: Strategies & Skills. Edward E. Jacobs et al. Ed. by Riley L. Harvill & Robert L. Masson. 1987. LC 87-7984. 314p. (C). pap. 28.50 (*0-534-08070-7*) Brooks-Cole.

Group Counseling: Strategies & Skills. Edward E. Jacobs et al. 3rd ed. 1997. LC 97-8769. (Counseling Ser.). 416p. pap. text 49.95 (*0-534-34486-0*) Brooks-Cole.

Group Counseling: Theory & Practice. Rickey L. George & Dick Dustin. 1988. (Illus.). 256p. text 38.00 (*0-13-365156-8*) P-H.

Group Counseling & Psychotherapy with Adolescents. Beryce W. MacLennan & Kathryn R. Dies. 2nd ed. 1992. LC 92-13564. 224p. text 40.50 (*0-231-07834-X*); pap. text 17.50 (*0-231-07835-8*) Col U Pr.

Group Counseling for Elementary & Middle School Children. Nina W. Brown. 1994. LC 93-5396. 168p. 60.00 (*0-275-94651-7*, Praeger Pubs) Greenwood.

Group Counseling with Juvenile Delinquents: The Limit & Lead Approach. Matthew L. Ferrara. 1991. LC 91-7627. (Human Services Guides Ser.: Vol. 65). (Illus.). 235p. pap. 34.95 (*0-8039-3885-3*, 8996) Sage.

Group Drug Counseling: Participant Recovery Workbook. Dennis Daley. 1998. 32p. pap. 11.95 (*1-55691-136-X*) Learning Pubns.

Group Drug Counseling Manual. Dennis Daley. 1998. 128p. pap. 21.95 (*1-55691-137-8*) Learning Pubns.

Group Dynamics. Forsyth. 3rd ed. 1998. (Psychology Ser.). 640p. spiral bd. 83.95 (*0-534-26148-5*) Brooks-Cole.

Group Dynamics in Occupational Therapy: Instructor's Manual. Marilyn B. Cole. 1998. (Illus.). 80p. pap., tchr. ed. Price not set. (*1-55642-410-8*, 34108) SLACK Inc.

Group Encounters in Speech & Language Therapy. Margaret Fawcus. 1992. 162p. pap. 34.95 (*1-56593-567-5*, 0487) Singular Publishing.

Group Exercises for Adolescents: A Manual for Therapists. Susan Carrell. 1993. LC 93-28206. (Illus.). pap. 37.95 (*0-8039-5292-9*, 7514); 2nd ed. 2000. LC 99-6772. 188p. pap. 28.95 (*0-7619-1953-8*, 85132) Sage.

Group Facilitation Handbook. Bertie Ryan Synowiec, M.S. & Carla Chenoweth, M.A. 1996. 55p. pap. 20.00 (*1-885335-05-9*) Positive Support.

Group Field Dynamics: Finding the Fulcrum in Face to Face Groups. Richard B. Polley. 1992. LC 92-4870. 224p. (C). text 38.00 (*0-8039-4434-9*); pap. text 18.95 (*0-8039-4435-7*) Sage.

Group Homes: Staffed & Unstaffed. British Institute of Mental Handicap Staff. 1985. 28p. 45.00 (*0-906054-51-6*) St Mut.

Group in Depth. Helen Durkin. 1966. LC 64-7550. 378p. (Orig.). 57.50 (*0-8236-2240-1*) Intl Univs Pr.

Group Interaction As Therapy, 13. Richard Stephenson & Frank R. Scarpitti. 1974. LC 72-830. (Contributions in Sociology Ser.: No. 13). 235p. 67.00 (*0-8371-6399-4*, SCG/, Greenwood Pr) Greenwood.

Group Interactive Art Therapy: Its Use in Training & Treatment. Diane Waller. 1993. LC 92-49164. 176p. (C). pap. 27.95 (*0-415-04844-3*) Routledge.

Group Interventions with Children, Adolescents & Parents: An Ego & Self Psychological Approach. Ed. by Ester S. Buchholz & Judith M. Mishne. 1994. LC 94-70251. (Master Work Ser.). 286p. pap. 50.00 (*1-56821-243-7*) Aronson.

Group Involvement Training: A Step-by-Step Program to Help Chronic Mentally Ill Patients. Catherine H. Chambliss. 1993. 160p. pap. text 24.95 (*0-934986-65-7*) New Harbinger.

Group Medical Insurance Large Claims Data Base Collection & Analysis. Kyle L. Grazier. 1997. LC 97-220809. (SOA Monographs: No. M-HB96-2). pap. 35.00 (*0-938959-45-X*) Soc Actuaries.

Group Mind. William McDougall. 2nd ed. 1976. LC 73-2976. (Classics in Psychology Ser.). reprint ed. 29.95 (*0-405-05148-4*) Ayer.

Group Practice Personnel Policies Manual. Courtney Price. rev. ed. 1997. 785p. pap. 150.00 incl. disk (*1-56829-081-0*, 4987) M G M A.

Group Process & Family Therapy: Extensions & Applications of Basic Principles. S. M. Thompson & J. H. Kahn. 1987. 246p. pap. text 33.00 (*0-08-034786-X*); 2nd ed. text 87.75 (*0-08-034787-8*) Elsevier (Pergamon Pr).

Group Process & Structure in Psychosocial Occupational Therapy. Ed. by Diane Gibson. 1989. LC 88-15325. (Occupational Therapy in Mental Health Ser.: Vol. 8, No. 3). (Illus.). 164p. text 39.95 (*0-86656-829-8*) Haworth Pr.

Group Processes & Personal Change. Peter B. Smith. 1980. 272p. pap. (*0-335-09807-X*) OpUniv Pr.

Group Protocols: A Psychosocial Compendium. Ed. by Susan Haiman. 1990. LC 89-71711. (Occupational Therapy in Mental Health Ser.: Vol. 9, No. 4). 136p. (C). text 39.95 (*0-86656-969-3*) Haworth Pr.

Group Psychology & Political Theory. C. Fred Alford. 1994. LC 94-6774. 248p. 35.00 (*0-300-05958-2*) Yale U Pr.

Group Psychotherapist's Handbook: Contemporary Theory & Technique. Irwin L. Kutash & Alexander Wolf. 1990. text 46.00 (*0-231-06840-9*) Col U Pr.

Group Psychotherapy. Gabriel. 1997. 27.95 (*0-02-911043-2*) Free Pr.

Group Psychotherapy. Martha A. Gabriel. 1996. LC 92-2932. 224p. 29.95 (*0-684-82786-7*) Free Pr.

Group Psychotherapy: A Peer Focused Approach. Richard A. Hogan. 1980. LC 80-13569. 287p. 70.00 (*0-275-90496-2*, C0496, Praeger Pubs) Greenwood.

Group Psychotherapy & Managed Mental Health Care: A Clinical Guide for Providers, Vol. 2. Henry I. Spitz. 1995. LC 95-36970. (Mental Health Practice under Managed Care Ser.: No. 2). 224p. pap. text 23.95 (*0-87630-791-8*) Brunner-Routledge.

Group Psychotherapy & Personality: Intersecting Structures. Henry Kellerman. 1979. 368p. text 44.00 (*0-8089-1182-1*, 792272, Grune & Strat) Harcrt Hlth Sci Grp.

Group Psychotherapy & Political Reality: A Two-Way Mirror. Ed. by Bertram Cohen et al. 2000. LC 2001-24194. 312p. pap. 26.90 (*0-8236-2228-2*, 02228) Intl Univs Pr.

Group Psychotherapy for Eating Disorders. Ed. by Heather Harper-Giuffre & K. Roy MacKenzie. 1992. LC 91-25958. 353p. text 48.00 (*0-88048-419-5*, 8419) Am Psychiatric.

Group Psychotherapy for People with Chronic Mental Illness. Walter N. Stone. 1996. LC 95-41586. 220p. text 34.00 (*1-57230-076-0*, 0076) Guilford Pubns.

Group Psychotherapy for Psychological Trauma. Ed. by Robert H. Klein & Victor L. Schermer. 2000. LC 00-27240. (Illus.). 364p. 45.00 (*1-57230-557-6*, 8R0557) Guilford Pubns.

Group Psychotherapy of the Psychoses: Concepts, Interventions & Contexts. Victor C. Schermer. 1999. LC 00-265884. (International Library of Group Analysis: Vol. 2). (Illus.). 430p. (*1-85302-583-6*) Jessica Kingsley.

Group Psychotherapy, Studies in Methodology of Research & Therapy. Florence B. Powdermaker & Jerome D. Frank. 1973. LC 72-6188. (Illus.). 615p. reprint ed. lib. bdg. 100.00 (*0-8371-6450-8*, POGP, Greenwood Pr) Greenwood.

Group Psychotherapy with Addicted Populations. Philip J. Flores. 1988. LC 87-7596. (Addiction Treatment Ser.: No. 1). 563p. text 69.95 (*0-86656-664-3*); pap. text 24.95 (*0-86656-757-7*) Haworth Pr.

Group Psychotherapy with Addicted Populations: An Integration of Twelve-Step & Psychodynamic Theory. Philip J. Flores. 2nd ed. 1996. LC 96-358. (Illus.). 657p. (C). pap. 49.95 (*0-7890-6000-0*); pap. 29.95 (*0-7890-6001-9*) Haworth Pr.

Group Psychotherapy with Adult Children of Alcoholics: Treatment Techniques & Countertransference Considerations. Marsha Vannicelli. LC 89-7551. (Substance Abuse Ser.). 222p. 1993. pap. 23.00 (*0-89862-533-5*, 2533); 1989. 39.95 (*0-89862-167-4*) Guilford Pubns.

Group Psychotherapy with Children: The Theory & Practice of Play-Therapy. Haim G. Ginott. 1994. LC 94-71461. (Master Work Ser.). 224p. pap. 40.00 (*1-56821-291-7*) Aronson.

Group Sequential Methods with Applications to Clinical Trials. Chris Jennison. 1999. LC 99-43218. (Interdisciplinary Statistics Ser.). 416p. (C). 64.95 (*0-8493-0316-8*, Chap & Hall CRC) CRC Pr.

Group Sessions Designed to Improve Self-Concept: Guidebook. Maurice E. Wagner. 1981. 103p. (Orig.). 2.95 (*0-940445-01-8*) Christ Growth Pubs.

Group System: The Therapeutic Activity Group in Occupational Therapy. Barbara Borg & Mary A. Bruce. 1990. LC 89-43517. 275p. pap. 29.00 (*1-55642-065-X*) SLACK Inc.

Group Techniques. Gerald Corey et al. rev. ed. 1987. LC 87-15129. 181p. (C). pap. 18.50 (*0-534-08586-5*) Brooks-Cole.

Group Techniques. Marianne Schneider Corey et al. 2nd ed. 1991. LC 91-10852. 198p. (C). mass mkt. 30.95 (*0-534-16248-7*) Brooks-Cole.

Group Techniques for Aging Adults: Putting Geriatric Skills Enhancement into Practice. Kathie T. Erwin. 1996. LC 96-7905. 200p. pap. (*1-56032-440-6*) Tay Francis Ltd GBR. *Dist:* Taylor & Francis.

Group Therapy. Shelby Hearon. 1984. LC 83-45500. 288p. 14.95 (*0-689-11444-3*) Atheneum Yung Read.

Group Therapy. Shelby Hearon. 1990. reprint ed. mass mkt. 4.95 (*0-446-36063-5*) Warner Bks.

Group Therapy: Thematic Activities Adults & Adolescents with Language Impairment. Stephanie Meek. 1993. LC 92-38672. (Illus.). (C). spiral bd. 39.00 (*0-89079-577-0*, 6592) PRO-ED.

Group Therapy Experience: From Theory to Practice. Louis Ormont. 5th ed. 1991. 256p. 24.95 (*0-312-07036-5*) St Martin.

Group Therapy for Adolescents: A Practical List of Group Ideas. Mark Halebsky. 1991. LC 91-66470. 144p. pap. 8.95 (*1-880793-00-8*) Pers & Prof Growth.

Group Therapy for Medically Ill Patients. Ed. by James L. Spira. 1997. LC 96-27736. 335p. text 40.00 (*1-57230-168-6*, 0168) Guilford Pubns.

Group Therapy for Schizophrenic Patients. Nick Kanas. 1996. (Clinical Practice in Psychiatry Ser.: No. 39). 192p. text 32.00 (*0-88048-172-2*, 8172) Am Psychiatric.

Group Therapy in Clinical Practice. Ed. by Anne Alonso & Hillel I. Swiller. 1993. LC 92-10416. 581p. text 61.95 (*0-88048-323-7*, 8323) Am Psychiatric.

Group Therapy in Independent Practice. Ed. by Scott Simon Fehr. LC 99-17706. (Journal of Psychotherapy in Independent Practice Ser.: 1No. 2). 93p. 2000. pap. 17.95 (*0-7890-1034-8*); 2nd ed. 1999. (C). 29.95 (*0-7890-0758-4*) Haworth Pr.

Group Therapy with Alcoholics: Outpatient & Inpatient Approaches. Baruch Levine & Virginia Gallogly. 1985. (Human Services Guides Ser.: Vol. 40). 136p. (C). pap. 34.95 (*0-8039-2504-2*, 5848) Sage.

Group Therapy with Children & Adolescents. Ed. by Paul Kymissis & David A. Halperin. 1995. LC 95-19715. 400p. text 54.00 (*0-88048-654-6*, 8654) Am Psychiatric.

Group Therapy with Troubled Youth: A Cognitive Behavioral Interactive Approach. Sheldon D. Rose. 1998. LC 97-33797. 512p. 91.95 (*0-7619-0927-3*, 81031); pap. 46.95 (*0-7619-0928-1*, 81032) Sage.

Group Treatment for Adult Survivors: A Handbook for Practitioners. Laura P. Webb & James Leehan. 1996. (Interpersonal Violence Ser.: Vol. 14). 196p. 79.95 (*0-8039-5171-X*, 4883) Sage.

Group Treatment for Sexually Abused Children. Joan G. Mandell et al. 1989. LC 89-7462. 170p. pap. 30.00 (*0-89862-516-5*) Guilford Pubns.

Group Treatment Manual. Johnston & Roseby. 1996. pap. 35.00 (*0-02-874129-3*) Free Pr.

***Group Treatment of Adolescents.** Aronson. 2001. 140p. pap. 24.95 (*0-8236-2258-4*) Intl Univs Pr.

Group Treatment of Adult Incest Survivors. Mary A. Donaldson. 1994. LC 94-6852. (Interpersonal Violence Ser.: Vol. 5). 79.95 (*0-8039-6165-0*, 7583); pap. 31.95 (*0-8039-6166-9*, 7582) Sage.

Group Treatment of Human Problems: A Social Learning Approach. Ed. by Gloria G. Harris. 1977. LC 77-22371. 274p. text 70.00 (*0-8089-1023-X*, 791915, Grune & Strat) Harcrt Hlth Sci Grp.

Group Treatment of Neurogenic Communication Disorders. Roberta J. Elman. 1998. 200p. text 39.99 (*0-7506-9084-4*) Buttrwrth-Heinemann.

Group Work: A Counseling Specialty. Gladding. 3rd ed. 1998. LC 98-19446. 544p. (C). 72.00 (*0-13-875543-4*) P-H.

Group Work: Cybernetic, Constructivist, & Social Constructionist Perspectives. Raphael J. Becvar et al. 1997. 168p. (C). pap. text 29.95 (*0-89108-252-2*, 9703) Love Pub Co.

Group Work in Occupational Therapy. Finlay. 1993. 251p. pap. 49.95 (*1-56593-124-6*, 0436) Thomson Learn.

Group Work in Professional Nursing. Brackley. 1998. pap. text (*0-7216-4184-9*) Saunders.

Group Work with Children & Adolescents. Kedar N. Dwivedi. 1993. LC 93-240496. 350p. pap. 29.95 (*1-85302-157-1*) Taylor & Francis.

Group Work with Elders: 50 Therapeutic Exercises for Reminiscence, Validation, & Remotivation. Ann L. Link. 1997. LC 97-11591. (Illus.). 142p. (Orig.). otabind 29.45 (*1-56887-030-2*, GWWBP, Prof Resc Pr) Pro Resource.

Group Work with Overwhelmed Clients: How the Power of Groups Can Help People Transform Their Lives. June G. Hopps & Elaine Pinderhughes. 1999. LC 98-34825. 224p. 29.95 (*0-684-82772-7*) Free Pr.

Group Work with the Aged. Susan H. Kubie & Gertrude Landau. 1969. reprint ed. pap. 24.95 (*0-8236-8065-7*, 22260) Intl Univs Pr.

Group Work with the Elderly. Ronald W. Toseland. 1995. LC 94-48382. (Illus.). 288p. 41.95 (*0-8261-8910-5*) Springer Pub.

Group Work with the Emotionally Disabled. Baruch Levine. 1990. LC 90-4281. (Social Work with Groups Ser.: Vol. 13, No. 1). 133p. text 39.95 (*0-86656-994-4*) Haworth Pr.

Group Work with the Poor & Oppressed. Judith A. Lee. 1989. LC 88-32009. (Social Work with Groups Ser.: Vol. 11, No. 4). (Illus.). 138p. text 39.95 (*0-86656-884-0*) Haworth Pr.

Groups: A Manual for Chemical Dependency & Psychotic Treatment. Mark et al. 1994. (Illus.). 405p. (Orig.). (C). pap. text (*1-887398-00-7*) CL Prodns.

Groups: Process & Practice. Gerald Corey & Marianne Schneider Corey. 2nd ed. 1982. LC 82-4117. (Psychology Ser.). 352p. (C). pap. 19.50 (*0-534-01174-8*) Brooks-Cole.

Groups: Process & Practice. Marianne Schneider Corey & Gerald Corey. (Counseling Ser.). (C). 3rd ed. 1986. LC 86-2595. 381p. pap. 26.75 (*0-534-06540-6*); 4th ed. 1992. LC 90-26069. 464p. pap. 29.50 (*0-534-16122-7*) Brooks-Cole.

Groups: Process & Practice. Marianne Schneider Corey. 5th ed. 1996. LC 95-49750. (Counseling Ser.). 454p. (C). pap. text 60.95 (*0-534-34224-8*) Brooks-Cole.

Groups in Health Care Settings. Ed. by Janice H. Schopler & Maeda J. Galinsky. 1990. LC 90-4018. (Social Work with Groups Ser.: Vol. 12, No. 4). 194p. text 49.95 (*0-86656-972-3*); 184p. pap. 19.95 (*0-86656-973-1*) Haworth Pr.

Groups under Stress: Psychological Research in Sealab 2. Roland Radloff & Robert Helmreich. 1968. LC 68-19962. (Century Psychology Ser.). (Illus.). (C). 30.50 (*0-89197-191-2*) Irvington.

Groupwork in Occupational Therapy. Linda Finlay. 1993. LC 92-47360. (Therapy in Practice Ser.: No. 38). (*0-412-35220-6*) Chapman & Hall.

Grow Old Gracefully. Albert J. Nimeth. 1989. 88p. reprint ed. pap. 1.95 (*0-8199-0509-7*, Frncscn Herld) Franciscan Pr.

Growers Guide to Medicinal Plants. Kara M. Dinda & Lyle E. Cranker. 1999. (Illus.). spiral bd. (*0-9629868-4-4*) HSMP Pr.

Grower's Reference on Gamebird Health. L. Dwight Schwartz. Ed. by Glenn D. Bengtson. 1995. 360p. (Orig.). pap. 29.95 (*0-9644732-0-8*) Avicon.

Growing a Therapist. Jeffrey A. Kottler. 1995. LC 94-32447. (Social & Behavioral Sciences Ser.). 215p. 32.00 (*0-7879-0049-4*) Jossey-Bass.

Growing Beyond Abuse: A Workbook for Survivors of Sexual Exploitation or Childhood Sexual Abuse. Signe L. Nestingen & Laurel Lewis. 1991. 192p. wbk. ed. 18.95 (*0-9628703-0-7*) Omni Recovery.

Growing Child. Helen L. Bee. 1997. LC 94-37748. 511p. (C). 86.00 (*0-673-99359-0*) Addson-Wesley Educ.

Growing Critical: Alternatives to Developmental Psychology. John R. Morss. 1995. LC 95-8132. (Critical Psychology Ser.). 184p. (C). 80.00 (*0-415-06108-3*); pap. 27.95 (*0-415-06109-1*) Routledge.

Growing Free: A Manual for Survivors of Domestic Violence. Ed. by Wendy Susan Deaton & Michael Hertica. 2001. LC 00-47212. (Illus.). 75p. (C). pap. text 14.95 (*0-7890-1280-4*) Haworth Pr.

Growing from Infancy to Adulthood: A Summary of the Changing Characteristics of Children & Youth. Edward C. Britton & J. Merritt Winans. 1958. LC 58-7149. (Illus.). (Orig.). pap. text 7.95 (*0-89197-193-9*) Irvington.

Growing Old: The Process of Disengagement. Elaine Cumming & William E. Henry. Ed. by Robert J. Kastenbaum. 1979. LC 78-22197. (Aging & Old Age Ser.). (Illus.). reprint ed. lib. bdg. 30.95 (*0-405-11814-7*) Ayer.

Growing Older & Wiser: Coping with Expectations, Challenges & Change in the Later Years. Nathan Billig. 1992. LC 92-24310. 230p. 29.95 (*0-669-27678-2*) Lxngtn Bks.

Growing Older, Getting Better: A Handbook for Women in the Second Half of Life. Jane Porcino. 1983. LC 82-24438. (Illus.). 366p. pap. 12.95 (*0-201-05592-9*) Addison-Wesley.

Growing Sane: Psychological Disturbances Accompanying the Growth of Consciousness. James Stallone & Sy Migdal. 1991. LC 91-75033. 150p. (Orig.). pap. 11.95 (*0-912975-06-7*) Upshur Pr.

Growing Through Pain & Suffering, Set. Cornelius J. Van der Poel. 1995. LC 94-61812. 128p. pap. 9.95 (*0-89622-636-0*) Twenty-Third.

Growing up Feeling Good: A Child's Introduction to Sexuality. Stephanie Waxman. 1979. 64p. (C). 10.95 (*0-915572-41-9*); pap. 5.95 (*0-915572-35-4*) Panjandrum.

Growing up in Smoke. Michell. 1990. 147p. (C). pap. (*0-7453-0446-X*) Pluto GBR GBR. *Dist:* Stylus Pub VA.

Growing up Observed: Tales from Analysts' Children. Ed. by Herbert S. Strean. 1987. LC 87-21080. (Current Issues in Psychoanalytic Practice Ser.: Vol. 4, Nos. 1-2). 90p. 3.95 (*0-86656-634-1*) Haworth Pr.

Growing up Small: A Handbook for Short People. Kate G. Phifer. 1979. LC 78-11290. (Illus.). 9.95 (*0-8397-3136-1*) Eriksson.

Growing up to Be Violent: A Longitudinal Study of the Development of Aggression. M. M. Lefkowitz et al. 1977. (*0-08-019515-6*) Pergamon Repr GBR. *Dist:* Franklin.

Growing up Tobacco Free: Preventing Nicotine Addiction in Children & Youths. Institute of Medicine Staff. Ed. by Barbara S. Lynch & Richard J. Bonnie. 1994. LC 94-31455. 320p. (Orig.). (C). pap. 24.95 (*0-309-05129-0*) Natl Acad Pr.

Growing up with Bach Flower Remedies. Judy Howard. Date not set. pap. 23.95 (*0-8464-4338-4*) Beekman Pubs.

Growing up with Bach Flower Remedies. Judy Howard. 1994. 106p. pap. (*0-85207-273-2*) C W Daniel GBR. *Dist:* Natl Bk Netwk.

Growing up with Diabetes: What Kids with Diabetes Want Their Parents to Know. McAuliffe. 1998. 128p. pap. 12.95 (*0-471-34731-0*) Wiley.

Growing up with Diabetes: What Kids with Diabetes Want Their Parents to Know. Alicia McAuliffe. 1998. LC 98-230248. 128p. pap. 10.95 (*1-56561-150-0*) Wiley.

Growing Your Family Medical Tree. Fran Carlson. l.t. ed. 1997. LC 97-94338. 60p. 14.95 (*0-9660319-0-3*, 001) KISS.

Growth: A Study of Johnny & Jimmie. Myrtle B. McGraw. 1975. LC 74-21422. (Classics in Child Development Ser.). 372p. reprint ed. 37.95 (*0-405-06471-3*) Ayer.

Growth & Development. Theis & Travers. 2000. (Quick Look Nursing Ser.). 18.95 (*1-889325-21-X*) Fence Crk Pubng.

Growth & Endocrine Aspects in Children & Adolescents with Chronic Renal Failure. Ed. by K. Schaerer. 1989. (Pediatric & Adolescent Endocrinology Ser.: Vol. 20). (Illus.). 188p. 155.00 (*3-8055-4990-3*) S Karger.

Growth & Growth Disorders: An Update: Diagnostic & Therapeutic Aspects. Ed. by G. Saggese. 1995. (Journal: Vol. 44, Suppl. 3, 1995). (Illus.). iv, 80p. pap. 36.50 (*3-8055-6258-6*) S Karger.

Growth & Growth Hormone Treatment of Children Born SGA, Body Composition: 2nd KIGS Expert Meeting on Growth & Growth Disorder, Lake Como, November 1996. Ed. by M. B. Ranke & M. A. Preece. 1997. (Journal: Vol. 48, Suppl. 1, 1997). (Illus.). iv, 76p. pap. 35.00 (*3-8055-6505-4*) S Karger.

Growth & Guilt: Psychology & the Limits of Development. Luigi Zoja. 1995. LC 94-16332. 272p. (C). (gr. 13). pap. 29.95 (*0-415-11661-9*, B4187) Routledge.

Growth & Hyperplasia of Cardiac Muscle Cells, 3. P. P. Rumyantsev. 1991. (Soviet Medical Reviews Supplement Ser.). 376p. text 283.00 (*3-7186-4958-6*, Harwood Acad Pubs) Gordon & Breach.

Growth & Regeneration of Axons in the Nervous System. Ed. by M. Berry. 1982. (Bibliotheca Anatomica Ser.: No. 23). (Illus.). vi, 126p. pap. 99.25 (*3-8055-3528-7*) S Karger.

Growth & Sexual Development. Ed. by Christopher T. Cowell. 1993. 288p. text 92.00 (*3-7186-5403-2*, Harwood Acad Pubs) Gordon & Breach.

Growth, Cancer & the Cell Cycle: The Molecular, Cellular & Developmental Biology. Ed. by Philip Skehan & Susan J. Friedman. 1984. LC 84-22468. (Experimental Biology & Medicine Ser.: Vol. 5). 353p. 129.50 (*0-89603-071-7*) Humana.

Growth Chart: A Tool for Use in Infant & Child Health Care. 1986. (ARA, FRE & SPA.). 33p. pap. text 12.00 (*92-4-154208-X*, 1150252) World Health.

Growth Disorders: Physiology & Treatment. Ed. by Christopher J. Kelnar et al. 1999. (Illus.). 844p. text (*0-412-73700-0*) E A GBR. *Dist:* OUP.

Growth Factor: Its Relevance to Aging & Illnesses. Sharwar Kakar. 1994. LC 94-77877. (Illus.). 86p. (Orig.). (C). pap. 12.50 (*0-9638976-1-6*) S K Kakar.

***Growth Factor Receptor Signalling in Thyrocytes of Normal & Neoplastic Origin.** Daniel Bergstrom. 2000. (Comprehensive Summaries of Uppsala Dissertations from the Faculty of Medicine Ser.: No. 902). (Illus.). 47p. pap. (*91-554-4644-2*) Uppsala Universitet SWE. *Dist:* Coronet Bks.

Growth Factors. Waterfield. 1989. text 99.00 (*0-443-04198-9*) Saunders.

Growth Factors: Cell Growth, Morphogenesis & Transformation. Ed. by Toshikazu Nakamura & Kunio Matsumoto. 1994. LC 94-7003. (Gann Monographs on Cancer Research: No. 42). 94.95 (*0-8493-7775-7*) CRC Pr.

Growth Factors & Alzheimer's Disease. Ed. by F. Hefti et al. 1991. (Research & Perspectives in Alzheimer's Disease Ser.). (Illus.). 272p. 98.00 (*0-387-53325-7*) Spr-Verlag.

Growth Factors & the Cardiovascular System. Ed. by Peter Cummins. 1993. LC 93-11507. (Developments in Cardiovascular Medicine Ser.: Vol. 147). 400p. (C). text 191.00 (*0-7923-2401-3*) Kluwer Academic.

Growth Factors & Wound Health: Basic Science & Potential Clinical Applications. Thomas R. Ziegler & Glenn F. Pierce. 1997. LC 97-9561. (Illus.). 365p. 162.00 (*0-387-94968-2*) Spr-Verlag.

Growth Factors As Drugs for Neurological & Sensory Disorders. Ed. by Gregory R. Bock & Jamie A. Goode. 1996. LC 95-48131. (CIBA Foundation Symposia Ser.: Vol. 196). 264p. 128.00 (*0-471-95721-6*) Wiley.

Growth Factors in Biology & Medicine. CIBA Foundation Staff. 1985. (CIBA Foundation Symposia Ser.: No. 116). 320p. 128.00 (*0-471-91085-6*) Wiley.

Growth Factors in Clinical Applications: Manual of GM-CSF. Michael Marty. 1995. 259p. pap. 89.95 (*0-86542-818-2*) Blackwell Sci.

Growth Factors in Endocrinology: Recent Advances, Therapeutic Prospects, 36th International Henri-Pierre Klotz Days of Clinical Therapeutic Prospects, Paris, May 1993, No. 42. Ed. by J. M. Saez. 1994. (Journal: No. 1-2, 1994). (Illus.). 80p. pap. 94.00 (*3-8055-6037-0*) S Karger.

Growth Factors in Fertility Regulation. Ed. by Florence P. Haseltine & Jock K. Findlay. 1991. (Scientific Basis of Fertility Regulation Ser.). (Illus.). 400p. (C). text 95.00 (*0-521-39026-5*) Cambridge U Pr.

Growth Factors in Neural Crest Cell Differentiation. Maya Sieber-Blum. 1998. LC 98-15840. 288p. lib. bdg. 169.95 (*0-8493-4004-7*) CRC Pr.

Growth Factors of the Vascular & Nervous Systems: Functional Characterization & Biotechnology. Ed. by C. L. Lenfant et al. 1992. (Illus.). viii, 132p. 108.00 (*3-8055-5475-3*) S Karger.

Growth, Health & Fitness of Teenagers. Ed. by Han C. Kemper. 1985. (Medicine & Sport Science Ser.: Vol. 20). (Illus.). xii, 204p. 101.00 (*3-8055-4042-6*) S Karger.

Growth Hormone. Stephen Harvey. 1994. 544p. 141.95 (*0-8493-8697-7*) CRC Pr.

Growth Hormone & Somatomedins During Lifespan. Ed. by E. E. Miller et al. 1993. LC 93-19508. (Illus.). 260p. (*3-540-56690-2*) Spr-Verlag.

Growth Hormone & Somatomedins During Lifespan. Ed. by Eugenio E. Muller et al. 1993. LC 93-19508. (Illus.). 358p. 174.00 (*0-387-56690-2*) Spr-Verlag.

Growth Hormone Deficiency in Childhood: Evaluation of Diagnostic Procedures. E. E. Joss. 1975. (Monographs in Pediatrics: Vol. 5). (Illus.). 100p. 42.75 (*3-8055-2159-6*) S Karger.

Growth Hormone in Critical Illness. Michael H. Torosian. 1996. (Medicine Ser.). 249p. pap. 89.95 (*0-412-09971-3*) Chapman & Hall.

Growth Hormone in Critical Illness: Research & Clinical Studies. Michael H. Torosian. 1996. LC 95-34053. (Medical Intelligence Unit Ser.). 225p. 99.00 (*1-57059-285-3*) Landes Bioscience.

Growth Hormone Secretagogues. Ed. by Barry B. Bercu & R. F. Walker. 1996. LC 96-632. (Proceedings of the Serono Symposia Ser.). (Illus.). 460p. 159.00 (*0-387-94707-8*) Spr-Verlag.

Growth Hormone Secretagogues. Carlos Dieguez. 1999. LC 99-36529. 340p. 94.00 (*0-444-82933-4*) Elsevier.

Growth Hormone Secretagogues in Clinical Practice. Barry B. Bercu & Richard F. Walker. 1998. LC 98-13319. (Illus.). 504p. text 195.00 (*0-8247-9832-5*) Dekker.

Growth Hormone Therapy in Turner Syndrome. Ed. by R.G. Thompson. 1993. (Journal: Vol. 39, Suppl. 2, 1993). (Illus.). iv, 72p. pap. 33.25 (*3-8055-5795-7*) S Karger.

Growth Hormone Two: Basic & Clinical Aspects. Ed. by Barry B. Bercu & Richard F. Walker. 1994. LC 93-28882. (Illus.). 379p. 156.00 (*0-387-94133-9*) Spr-Verlag.

Growth Hormones: Research & Therapy: Asian Pacific Symposium, Kobe, September 1996. Ed. by Nobutake Matsuo. 1998. (Hormone Research Ser.: Vol. 49, Suppl. 1, 1998). (Illus.). iv, 58p. pap. 27.00 (*3-8055-6600-X*) S Karger.

Growth Hypothesis in Psychology: The Humanistic Psychology of Abraham Maslow & Carl Rogers. Roy J. DeCarvalho. 1991. LC 91-17536. 180p. pap. 59.95 (*0-7734-9908-3*) E Mellen.

Growth in Childhood. Ed. by T. J. Wilkin. 1989. x, 124p. text 110.00 (*3-7186-4941-1*) Gordon & Breach.

Growth in Children. John Brierley. Ed. by C. E. Wragg. 1992. (Education Matters Ser.). 192p. pap. 29.95 (*0-304-32581-3*); text 90.00 (*0-304-32601-1*) Continuum.

Growth in the Aging Craniofacial Skeleton. Behrents. 1985. (Craniofacial Growth Ser.: Vol. 17). (Illus.). 145p. 45.00 (*0-929921-13-5*) UM CHGD.

Growth, Maturation, & Body Composition: The Fels Longitudinal Study, 1929-1991. Alex F. Roche. 1992. (Studies in Biological Anthropology: No. 9). (Illus.). 296p. (C). text 80.00 (*0-521-37449-9*) Cambridge U Pr.

Growth Modification: What Works, What Doesn't & Why. H. C. Slavkin et al. Ed. by J. A. McNamara, Jr. 1999. (Craniofacial Growth Series: Vol. 35). (Illus.). 388p. 79.00 (*0-929921-31-3*) UM CHGD.

Growth Monitoring & Promotion in Young Children: Guidelines for the Selection of Methods & Training Techniques. Derrick B. Jelliffe & E. F. Jelliffe. 1990. (Illus.). 144p. pap. text 19.95 (*0-19-505623-X*) OUP.

Growth of Bone, Muscle & Overlying Tissues. Harold C. Stuart. 1940. (SRCD M Ser.: Vol. 5, No. 3). 25.00 (*0-527-01515-6*) Periodicals Srv.

Growth of Children in Hawaii: Based on Observations by Louis R. Sullivan. C. Wissler. 1930. (BMB Ser.). (Orig.). 45.00 (*0-527-01667-5*) Periodicals Srv.

Growth of Farm Animals. T. L. Lawrence & V. R. Fowler. 1997. LC 96-48880. 344p. pap. text 45.00 (*0-85198-849-0*) OUP.

Growth of Gastroenterologic Knowledge During the 20th Century. Joseph B. Kirsner. 1994. (Illus.). 522p. text 75.00 (*0-8121-1592-9*) Lppncott W & W.

Growth of Hospitals 1850-1939: An Economic History in Baltimore. Ed. by Jon M. Kingsdale. 1989. (Medical Care in the United States Ser.). 410p. text 25.00 (*0-8240-8336-9*) Garland.

Growth of Medical Knowledge. Ed. by Henk ten Have. 1990. 922p. (C). lib. bdg. (*0-7923-0736-4*) Kluwer Academic NLD. *Dist:* Kluwer Academic.

Growth of Medicine from the Earliest Times to About 1800. Albert H. Buck. LC 75-23688. reprint ed. 67.50 (*0-404-13241-3*) AMS Pr.

Growth of Scientific Physiology. G. J. Goodfield. 1975. LC 74-26265. (History, Philosophy, & Sociology of Science Ser.). reprint ed. 19.95 (*0-405-06593-0*) Ayer.

Growth of the Gastrointestinal Test. Ed. by Jean Morisset. 1990. 240p. 149.00 (*0-8493-4617-7*, R) CRC Pr.

Growth of the Mind. Kurt Koffka. 1980. LC 80-50103. (Social Science Classics Ser.). 383p. reprint ed. text 44.95 (*0-87855-360-6*); pap. text 29.95 (*0-87855-784-9*) Transaction Pubs.

Growth of the Surface Area of the Human Body, Vol. 10. Edith Boyd. 1970. LC 75-14249. (University of Minnesota Institute of Child Welfare Monographs: No. 10). (Illus.). 145p. reprint ed. lib. bdg. 48.00 (*0-8371-8069-4*, CWBS, Greenwood Pr) Greenwood.

Growth Opportunities in Biomedical Devices: Key Development with Near-Term Commercial Potential. unabr. ed. 1997. LC 98-118622. 432p. spiral bd. 2250.00 (*1-56217-029-5*) Tech Insights.

Growth Regulation & Carcinogenesis, Vol. 1. Ed. by Walter Paukovits. 1990. 328p. 217.00 (*0-8493-5960-0*, QH604) CRC Pr.

Growth Regulation & Carcinogenesis, Vol. 2. Ed. by Walter R. Paukovits. 1990. 368p. 239.00 (*0-8493-5961-9*, QH604) CRC Pr.

Growth Regulation of Thyroid Gland & Thyroid Tumors. Ed. by P. E. Goretzki & H. D. Roher. 1989. (Frontiers of Hormone Research Ser.: Vol. 18). (Illus.). 164p. 143.50 (*3-8055-4984-9*) S Karger.

Growth, Stature, & Psychosocial Well-Being. Urs Eiholzer et al. 1999. LC 98-16774. (Illus.). xii, 201p. 39.00 (*0-88937-197-0*) Hogrefe & Huber Pubs.

Growth Substances: Directory of Authors of New Medical & Scientific Reviews with Subject Index. Science and Life Consultants Association Staff. Ed. by Science and Life Consultants Association Staff. 1995. 160p. 57.50 (*0-7883-0584-0*); pap. 47.50 (*0-7883-0585-9*) ABBE Pubs Assn.

Growth Through Choice. Saccuzzo. 2nd ed. 1998. (C). pap. text 33.00 (*0-15-502300-4*) Harcourt Coll Pubs.

Grunderna I Epidemiologi see Introduction to Modern Epidemiology

Grundfragen der Palontologie: Geologische Zeitmessung, Organische Stammesentwicklung, Biologische Systematick (Basic Question of Paleontology: Geologic Chronology, Organic Phylogeny, Biologic Systematics. Otto H. Schindewolf. Ed. by Stephen Jay Gould. 1980. LC 79-8347. (GER., Illus.). reprint ed. lib. bdg. 50.95 (*0-405-12741-3*) Ayer.

Grundlagen und Technik der Infusionstherapie und Klinischen Ernaehrung. E. Roth et al. 1985. (Handbuch der Infusionstherapie und Klinischen Ernaehrung Ser.: Band 2). (GER.). x, 278p. 108.75 (*3-8055-3746-8*) S Karger.

Grundriss der Perinatalmedizin. Willibald Pschyrembel & J. W. Dudenhausen. 1972. (GER., Illus.). 336p. (C). 29.25 (*3-11-003694-0*) De Gruyter.

GSH Phenomenon: Nature's Most Powerful Antioxidant & Healing Agent. Alan H. Pressman & Sheila Buff. 1997. LC 96-17980. 256p. 23.95 (*0-312-15135-7*) St Martin.

Gua Sha: Traditional Technique for Modern Practice. Arya Nielsen. 1995. LC 95-7286. pap. text (*0-443-05181-X*) Church.

Guanidines Vol. 2: Further Explorations of the Biological & Clinical Significance. Akitane Mori et al. 1989. (Illus.). 380p. 105.00 (*0-306-43223-4*, Plenum Trade) Perseus Pubng.

Guanidino Compounds in Biology & Medicine. Deyn. 450p. (*0-86196-330-X*) J Libbey Med GBR. *Dist:* Bks Intl VA.

Guanidino Compounds in Biology & Medicine - II, No. II. Deyn. 1997. 450p. (*0-86196-543-4*) J Libbey Med GBR. *Dist:* Buttrwrth-Heinemann.

Guarana: The Energy Seeds & Herbs of the Amazon Rainforest. Michael Van Straten. Date not set. pap. 14.95 (*0-8464-4339-2*) Beekman Pubs.

Guaranteeing Health Care! How to Get Medical Assistance for Pennsylvania's Uninsured. Ruth Groff. 1994. (Illus.). 53p. (Orig.). (C). pap. text 15.00 (*0-7881-0861-1*) DIANE Pub.

Guarding Against Drug & Alcohol Abuse: Building Public - Private Partnerships. Susan C. Biemesderfer. 1992. 48p. pap. text 10.00 (*1-55516-697-0*, 6635) Natl Conf State Legis.

Guarding Your Gold: A Consumer's Guide to Protect Your Assets by Insuring Against the High Costs of Long Term Care, Short Term Care, Home Health Care, Medicare. Ronald J. Iverson. l.t. ed. 1999. 240p. pap. 19.95 (*0-9673193-0-7*) MAS Mktg.

Guattari Reader. Ed. & Tr. by Gary Genosko. 1996. (Blackwell Readers Ser.). 232p. (C). text 65.95 (*0-631-19707-9*); pap. text 29.95 (*0-631-19708-7*) Blackwell Pubs.

Guia de Bolsillo para los Proveedores de Servicios de Planificacion Familiar. Paul D. Blumenthal & Noel McIntosh. 1995. (SPA., Illus.). (Orig.). pap. text 15.00 (*0-929817-13-3*) JHPIEGO.

Guia de Bolso para Proveedores de Servicos de Planejamento Familiar. Paul D. Blumenthal & Noel McIntosh. 1995. (POR., Illus.). (Orig.). pap. text 15.00 (*0-929817-12-5*) JHPIEGO.

Guia Farmacologica en Psiquiatria. S. Lopez Galan. 2nd ed. 1995. (SPA.). 412p. pap. (*84-7978-162-9*) Ediciones Diaz ESP. *Dist:* IBD Ltd.

Guia Ilustrada del Medico para el Auto-Tratamiento Emocional. Maxie C. Maultsby, Jr. Tr. by Gabriela Munoz & Rossnilda O. Maultsby from ENG. 1977.Tr. of You & Your Emotions. (ENG & SPA., Illus.). 109p. reprint ed. pap. 8.95 (*0-932838-06-5*) Tangrm Bks.

Guia Laem para Oir Mejor: Respuestas a Sus Preguntas sobre Audicion. Wayne J. Staab. 1992. LC 90-90428. (SPA., Illus.). 135p. pap. 15.00 (*1-881148-05-X*) W J Staab.

Guia Para Dejar de Fumar Por Su Salud y Su Familia. 1995. (SPA., Illus.). 36p. (Orig.). (C). pap. text 15.00 (*0-7881-2317-3*) DIANE Pub.

Guia Para Vivir con la Infeccion VIH: Desarrollado por la Clinica Johns Hopkins del SIDA. John G. Bartlett & Ann K. Finkbeiner. 3rd ed. 1996. LC 96-32867. (SPA.). 464p. pap. 18.95 (*0-8018-5420-2*) Johns Hopkins.

Guia Practica. Gatell. 1995. (SPA.). (*84-458-0240-2*) Ediciones Cientificas ESP. *Dist:* P H Brookes.

Guias para Efectuar el Examen de Ultrasonido Abdominal y Retroperitoneal. 1994.Tr. of Standards for Performance of the Abdominal & Retroperitoneal Ultrasound Examination. (SPA.). 8p. pap. 10.00 (*1-930047-06-1*, GAS) Am Inst Ultrasound.

Guidance Manual in the Evaluation of Rating Manuals & Filings Concerning Small Employer Health Insurance. 1994. 140p. (C). pap. 25.00 (*0-89382-292-2*) Nat Assn Insurance.

Guidance on Our Journeys. Edward C. Sellner. 1983. 24p. pap. 2.00 (*0-89486-216-2*, 1298B) Hazelden.

Guide for Adult Immunization. American College of Physicians Task Force on Adult. 3rd ed. 1994. LC 94-3075. 240p. pap. 24.00 (*0-943126-23-1*) Amer Coll Phys.

Guide for Beginning Psychotherapists. Joan S. Zaro. 1977. LC 77-76080. 256p. pap. text 32.95 (*0-521-29230-1*) Cambridge U Pr.

Guide for Clinical Social Work in Health Care: New Biopsychosocial Approaches. Stephen R. Wallace et al. 1984. LC 83-13744. 242p. 45.00 (*0-275-91338-4*, C1338, Praeger Pubs) Greenwood.

Guide for Epidemiological Studies of Oral Manifestations of HIV Infection. S. L. Melnick et al. 1993. (ENG, FRE & SPA.). ix, 27p. pap. text 9.00 (*92-4-154453-8*, 1150399) World Health.

Guide for Food & Nutrition in the Later Years. rev. ed. 1980. 16p. pap. 2.00 (*0-910869-04-9*) Soc Nutrition Ed.

Guide for General Practitioners K. Kapoor. 1989. (C). (*0-7855-4675-8*) Current Dist IND. *Dist:* St Mut.

Guide for Interventional Radiology Coding. Rogers & HADG Staff. 2000. pap. 89.00 (*0-8342-1723-6*) Aspen Pub.

Guide for Introducing Visiting Animal Programs. Jody Gammonty et al. 2000. pap. 35.00 (*1-889785-06-7*) Delta Soc.

Guide for New Principles. Mike Pringle et al. 1996. (Oxford General Practice Ser.). (Illus.). 222p. pap. text 39.50 (*0-19-262536-5*) OUP.

Guide for Piano Instruction for the Educationally Blind. Dorothy Simpson. 1968. LC 78-57770. 3.95 (*0-8497-6099-2*, GP23B) Kjos.

Guide for Senior Citizens: Social Security, Medicare, Legal & Tax Assistance Including an Address & Phone Number Directory That Help the Elderly. 1991. lib. bdg. 75.00 (*0-8490-4140-6*) Gordon Pr.

Guide for Starting a Medical Office. American Academy of Pediatrics Staff. 1997. pap. text 44.95 (*0-910761-86-8*) Coker Publishing.

Guide for State Planning for the Prevention of Mental Retardation & Related Disabilities. Raymond M. Peterson & James O. Cleveland. 1987. 32p. (*1-55672-020-3*) US HHS.

Guide for Testing Ventilation Systems. 1991. (Illus.). (C). pap. text 8.00 (*0-936712-93-7*) Am Conf Govt Indus Hygienist.

Guide for the Beginning Therapist: Relationship Between Diagnosis & Treatment. Amy Lamson. 2nd ed. 1986. LC 78-4061. 130p. 32.95 (*0-89885-293-5*); pap. 19.95 (*0-89885-295-1*) Kluwer Academic (Kluwer Acad Hman Sci).

Guide for the Care of Infants in Groups. Sally Provence. 1967. LC 67-26025. 104p. (C). pap. 12.95 (*0-87868-061-6*) Child Welfare.

Guide for the Development & Management of Nursing Libraries & Information Resources. Dorothy L. Moore. 1997. LC 97-14566. 356p. pap. 31.95 (*0-88737-729-7*) Natl League Nurse.

Guide for the Family of the Alcoholic. Joseph L. Kellermann. 1987. 10p. (Orig.). pap. 1.55 (*0-89486-057-7*, 1300B) Hazelden.

Guide for the Family Therapist. Patricia A. Boyer & Ronnald J. Jeffrey. 1994. LC 83-3799. 190p. pap. 35.00 (*1-56821-285-2*) Aronson.

Guide for Training American Red Cross Emergency Response Instructors. Jose V. Salazar et al. 1997. LC 98-129218. vi, 121 p. (*0-8151-1274-2*) Mosby Inc.

Guide Pratique de Psycho-Geriatrie. J. C. Monfort et al. (FRE.). Vol. 1. 1992. 174p. pap. 38.00 (*2-906077-32-1*); Vol. 2. 1994. 176p. pap. 38.00 (*2-906077-49-6*) Elsevier.

Guide Pratique des Medicaments. P. Dorosz. 19th ed. 1998. (FRE.). 1800p. 125.00 (*0-320-00696-4*) Fr & Eur.

Guide Pratique d'Homeopathie Dictionnaire des Malades et Traitements. Jacques Hodler. 1983. (FRE.). 532p. 75.00 (*0-7859-7939-5*, 2712600320) Fr & Eur.

Guide to a Better Back. Dee Massengale. Ed. by Phyllis Mueller. 1988. LC 87-31104. (Illus.). 104p. (Orig.). pap. 13.95 (*0-932419-12-7*) Cherokee.

Guide to Adult Neuropsychological Diagnosis. Anthony Y. Stringer. 1996. LC 95-41972. (Illus.). 528p. (C). pap. 49.95 (*0-8036-0072-0*) OUP.

Guide to Alzheimer's Disease: For Families, Spouses & Friends. Barry Reisberg. 1984. LC 80-69717. 216p. (C). pap. 13.95 (*0-02-926370-0*) Free Pr.

Guide to America's Top Dentists. 2000. 304p. 29.95 (*0-9676546-0-2*) Consumer Research.

Guide to Audiologic Interpretation. Jacobson. 2002. 30.75 net. (*1-56593-627-2*) Thomson Learn.

Guide to Bach Flower Remedies. 1996. pap. 8.95 (*0-8464-1202-0*) Beekman Pubs.

Guide to Basic & 12-Lead ECG Interpretation. Sharron Daggett. 2000. (Illus.). ii, 93p. pap. 29.95 (*0-9701171-1-6*, 2702) Natl Inst Nurse.

Guide to Basic Electrocardiography. J. W. Beasley & E. W. Grogan. 1990. LC 90-7327. (Illus.). 180p. (C). spiral bd. 47.00 (*0-306-43296-X*, Kluwer Plenum) Kluwer Academic.

Guide to Benchmarking in Healthcare: Practical Lessons from the Field. Arthur G. Tweet et al. 1998. LC 97-34887. 273p. 45.00 (*0-527-76337-3*) Product Pr.

Guide to Better Hearing. Wayne J. Staab. rev. ed. 1995. LC 90-90428. (Illus.). 138p. pap. 15.00 (*1-881148-08-4*) W J Staab.

Guide to Bone Marrow Transplantation. H. J. Deeg et al. 1988. (Illus.). 192p. 76.50 (*0-387-18802-9*) Spr-Verlag.

Guide to Books on AIDS. Ed. & Compiled by R. P. Russel. 1994. (Illus.). 107p. text 95.00 (*1-56072-179-0*) Nova Sci Pubs.

Guide to Brand Name & Generic Prescription Drugs: Fast, Authoritative Reference Guide. Gary A. Holt et al. 1994. LC 94-67792. 183p. pap. 19.95 (*0-944496-41-5*) Precept Pr.

Guide to Buying Physician Practices. George W. Bodenger et al. 2nd rev. ed. 1998. 158p. pap. 93.00 (*0-929156-24-2*) Atlantic Info Services Inc.

Guide to Capitation Contracting, Monograph 3. 1993. (Cardiovascular Specialist's Guide to Managed Care Ser.). 44p. (Orig.). pap. text (*1-882764-06-4*) Am Coll Cardiology.

Guide to Cardiology. Ed. by Robert A. Kloner. 2nd ed. 1990. (Illus.). 500p. pap. 44.00 (*0-9626020-0-0*) Le Jacq Commns.

Guide to Cardiology. Robert A. Kloner. 3rd unabr. ed. 1995. (Illus.). 752p. pap. text 68.00 (*0-9626020-1-9*) Le Jacq Commns.

Guide to Centralized Credentialing: Evaluating Current Issues & Trends. Christina W. Black & Beverly E. Pybus. 1997. (Illus.). 180p. ring bd. 157.00 (*1-57839-005-2*) Opus Communs.

Guide to Choosing a Good Plastic Surgeon: How to Avoid Becoming a Victim of Malpractice & Protect Your Health, Appearance, Money & Time. Mark Sugar. 1992. (Orig.). pap. 4.95 (*0-9632757-2-0*) Mark Sugar.

Guide to Clinical Drug Research. Ed. by Adam Cohen & John Posner. 1996. LC 95-8825. 212p. (C). text 99.50 (*0-7923-3508-2*) Kluwer Academic.

Guide to Clinical Drug Research. John Posner. Ed. by Adam Cohen. 2nd ed. 2000. LC 99-89541. 224p. 115.00 (*0-7923-6171-7*, Kluwer Plenum) Kluwer Academic.

Guide to Clinical Drug Reserach. John Posner. Ed. by Adam Cohen. 2nd ed. 2000. LC 99-89541. 224p. pap. 50.00 (*0-7923-6172-5*, Kluwer Plenum) Kluwer Academic.

Guide to Clinical Neurology. Ed. by J. P. Mohr & J. C. Gautier. 1995. LC 95-8195. (Illus.). text (*0-443-08927-2*) Church.

Guide to Clinical Nursing Practice. Elizabeth M. Jamieson. 3rd ed. 1996. 335p. pap. text (*0-443-05290-5*) Church.

Guide to Clinical Preventive Services. U. S. Preventive Services Task Force. 1993. (Illus.). 295p. (Orig.). (C). pap. text 30.00 (*1-56806-297-4*) DIANE Pub.

Guide to Clinical Preventive Services: Report of the U. S. Preventive Services Task Force. U. S. Preventive Services Task Force. 1989. 488p. 30.00 (*0-683-08507-7*) Lppncott W & W.

Guide to Clinical Preventive Services: Report of the U. S. Preventive Services Task Force. 2nd ed. 1997. 933p. (C). pap. text 60.00 (*0-7881-3827-8*) DIANE Pub.

Guide to Clinical Preventive Services: Report of the U. S. Preventive Services Task Force. U. S. Preventive Services Task Force. 2nd ed. 1996. 933p. pap. 24.00 (*1-883205-13-1*) Intl Med Pub.

Guide to Clinical Preventive Services: Report of the U. S. Preventive Services Task Force. U. S. Preventive Services Task Force. 2nd ed. 1996. LC 95-23165. (Illus.). 504p. pap. 32.95 (*0-683-08508-5*) Lppncott W & W.

Guide to Clinical Trials. Bert Spilker. 1991. 1,184p. text 189.00 (*0-88167-767-1*) Lppncott W & W.

Guide to Coding & Reimbursement. Wanda L. Adams. 1994. LC 94-229708. 256p. (C). (gr. 13). pap. text 37.95 (*0-8151-0136-8*, 24217) Mosby Inc.

Guide to Collections in the Archives & Special Collections on Women in Medicine at the Medical College of Pennsylvania. Erika T. Miller. 1987. 69p. (Orig.). (C). 10.00 (*0-944542-00-X*) Med Coll PA ASCWM.

Guide to Computerized Patient Accounting Systems. Ed. by Michael S. Geffen. 1989. LC 88-3558. 153p. text 49.95 (*0-86656-651-1*) Haworth Pr.

Guide to Conducting Art Therapy Research. Ed. by Harriet Wadeson. 1992. 272p. (Orig.). (C). pap. text 35.00 (*1-882147-03-0*) Am Art Therapy.

Guide to Conducting Healthcare Facility Visits. Craig Zimring. 1994. 80p. (C). pap. 27.00 (*0-9638938-1-5*) Ctr for Hlth.

Guide to Consulting Services for Emerging Healthcare Organizations. Robert J. Cimasi. 1999. LC 98-52741. (Illus.). 501p. 95.00 (*0-471-31625-3*) Wiley.

Guide to Contented Hearts. D. Charles Van Fulpen. 1995. (Illus.). 112p. (Orig.). pap. 19.95 (*0-9637562-0-6*) Contented Hrts.

Guide to Contracting & Negotiation, Monograph 4. 1993. (Cardiovascular Specialist's Guide to Managed Care Ser.). 63p. (Orig.). (C). pap. text (*1-882764-05-6*) Am Coll Cardiology.

Guide to Coronary Angioplasty & Stenting. Peter J. B. Hubner. 1998. 292p. text 60.00 (*90-5702-278-8*, Harwood Acad Pubs) Gordon & Breach.

Guide to Coverage of Complementary & Alternative Medicine. Ed. by David Strickland & Luci Koizumi. 1999. 539p. pap. 265.00 (*1-57987-111-9*) Faulkner & Gray.

Guide to Creative Group Programming in the Psychiatric Day Hospital. Lois E. Passi. 1998. LC 43-9237. (Illus.). 244p. lib. bdg. 39.95 (*0-7890-0406-2*) Haworth Pr.

Guide to Crisis Intervention. Kristi Kanel. 1998. LC 97-52343. (Counseling Ser.). 200p. pap. text 27.95 (*0-534-35521-8*) Brooks-Cole.

Guide to Curriculum Planning in Health Education. 1986. 203p. 30.00 (*1-57337-074-6*) WI Dept Pub Instruct.

Guide to Curriculum Review for Basic Nursing Education: Orientation to Primary Health Care & Community Health. WHO Staff. 1985. 53p. 15.00 (*92-4-154202-0*) World Health.

Guide to Dangerous Drugs. Mark A. De Bernardo. 1995. (Illus.). 16p. pap. 2.40 (*1-889437-08-5*) Inst Drug-Free Wrkpl.

Guide to Dental Radiography. Rita A. Mason & Sarah Bourne. 4th ed. 1998. (Illus.). 272p. pap. text 69.50 (*0-19-262671-X*); LC 97-28365. (*0-01-926272-8*); LC 97-28365. pap. (*0-01-926271-X*) OUP.

Guide to Developing & Managing an Emergency Service: Infection Control Program. 1996. 190p. (Orig.). pap. text 40.00 (*0-7881-2815-9*) DIANE Pub.

Guide to Diagnostic Clinical Chemistry. R. N. Walmsley & G. H. White. 3rd ed. (Illus.). 672p. Date not set. pap. (*0-86793-289-9*); 1994. LC 93-2152. 115.00 (*0-632-03735-0*) Blackwell Sci.

Guide to Dietary Management of Small Animals. Lon D. Lewis et al. rev. ed. 1989. 37p. (C). pap. text 1.50 (*0-945837-02-X*) M Morris Assocs.

Guide to Dynamics of Feminist Therapy. Doris Howard. 2nd ed. 1987. LC 86-33616. (Women & Therapy Ser.: Vol. 5, No. 2-3). 341p. pap. 19.95 (*0-918393-37-X*, Harrington Park) Haworth Pr.

Guide to Eating Right During Pregnancy. Susan K. Podell. 1993. LC 92-42111. 48p. pap. 2.99 (*0-385-46775-3*) Doubleday.

Guide to ECG Analysis. Robert A. Catalano. 1993. 430p. pap. text 34.00 (*0-397-55015-4*) Lppncott W & W.

***Guide to Education & Training for Primary Care.** Ed. by Yvonne Carter & Neil Jackson. 2002. 224p. (Orig.). pap. text 37.50 (*0-19-263293-0*) OUP.

Guide to Effective Care in Pregnancy & Childbirth. Murray Enkin et al. 3rd ed. 2000. LC 00-21832. (Oxford Medical Publications). (Illus.). xiii, 525p. pap. 37.50 (*0-19-263173-X*) OUP.

Guide to EKG Interpretation. John Brose et al. 2nd rev. ed. 2000. LC 00-22811. (White Coat Pocket Guide Ser.). (Illus.). 230p. 20.00 (*0-8214-1328-7*) Ohio U Pr.

Guide to Enterprise-Wide Networks in Health Care. Ed. by Luci Koizumi. 1999. (Illus.). 320p. pap. 275.00 (*1-57987-160-7*) Faulkner & Gray.

Guide to Equine Acute Laminitis. James N. Moore & Douglas Allen. 1994. 40p. pap. text 21.00 (*1-884254-17-9*) Vet Lrn Syst.

Guide to Equine Field Radiography. Barbara J. Watrous. 1995. 64p. pap. text 18.00 (*1-884254-21-7*) Vet Lrn Syst.

Guide to Family-Centered Circle Drawings (F-C-C-D) with Symbol Probes & Visual Free Association. Robert C. Burns. 1990. LC 90-1935. (Illus.). 160p. text 30.95 (*0-87630-587-7*) Brunner-Routledge.

Guide to Feminist Family Therapy. Ed. by Lois Braverman. 1988. LC 87-35180. (Journal of Psychotherapy & the Family Ser.: Vol. 3, No. 4). 180p. text 19.95 (*0-918393-48-5*, Harrington Park) Haworth Pr.

Guide to Fitness after Fifty. R. Harris & L. J. Frankel. 1977. LC 77-2296. (Illus.). 374p. (C). text 55.00 (*0-306-30995-5*, Kluwer Plenum) Kluwer Academic.

Guide to Florida Poisonous Snakes. Robert Anderson. 1984. (Illus.). 60p. (Orig.). reprint ed. pap. 4.95 (*0-932855-04-0*) Winner Enter.

Guide to Forensic Pathology. Jay Dix. 1998. LC 99-21246. (Illus.). v, 257p. per. 34.95 (*0-8493-0267-6*) CRC Pr.

Guide to Forensic Pathology. Jay Dix & Robert Calaluce. unabr. ed. 1998. (Illus.). 257p. pap. 30.00 (*0-9663422-0-8*) Acad Info Systs.

Guide to Forming Physician-Directed Managed Care Networks. American Medical Association Staff. 1995. 48.95 (*0-89970-730-0*, OP601595WE) AMA.

Guide to Forming Physician Networks. Thomas A. Mayer & Albert E. Barnett. 1997. 95p. pap. 93.00 (*0-929156-30-7*) Atlantic Info Services Inc.

Guide to Formulation for Safety Testing. Richard Halliday & Catherine Johnson. 1996. 44p. pap. 69.00 (*1-57491-011-6*) IHS Health Grp.

Guide to General Toxicology. Ed. by Judith K. Marquis. 2nd rev. ed. 1989. (Continuing Education Ser.: Vol. 5). (Illus.). x, 294p. 59.25 (*3-8055-4924-5*) S Karger.

Guide to Genetic Counseling. Diane L. Baker et al. 1998. LC 98-5906. 433p. 94.95 (*0-471-18541-8*); pap. 62.50 (*0-471-18867-0*) Wiley.

Guide to Good Nutrition During & after Chemotherapy & Radiation. Saundra N. Aker & Polly Lenssen. 3rd rev. ed. 1988. LC 87-83467. (Illus.). 147p. pap. 5.00 (*0-945278-00-4*) Hutchinson Cancer Res Ctr.

Guide to Governance for Hospital Trustees. American Hospital Association Staff et al. 1990. (Illus.). 110p. (Orig.). pap. 54.95 (*0-87258-546-8*, 196600) Am Hospital.

Guide to Grammar & Usage for Psychology & Related Fields. John E. Bellquist. 1994. 120.00 (*1-56321-141-6*); 25.00 (*1-56321-142-4*) L Erlbaum Assocs.

Guide to Growing Up. Ed. by John Robson. 1982. (Illus.). 45p. (Orig.). (gr. 4-6). pap. 2.50 (*0-936098-32-5*) Intl Marriage.

Guide to Health. Benjamin Colby. enl. rev. ed. 1985. 9.95 (*0-913923-53-2*) Woodland UT.

Guide to Health & Hygiene in Agricultural Work. 1980. (Illus.). xii, 309p. pap. 24.75 (*92-2-101974-8*) Intl Labour Office.

Guide to Health Care Consulting. Kenneth A. Koskay et al. 1998. Vol. 1. ring bd. (*0-7646-0592-5*); Vol. 2. ring bd. (*0-7646-0593-3*) Prctnrs Pub Co.

Guide to Health Care Coverage for the Child with a Chronic Illness or Disability. Catherine L. Gaylord & Alice M. Leonard. 2nd ed. 1988. 134p. reprint ed. pap. 20.00 (*0-932622-14-3*) Ctr Public Rep.

Guide to Health Claims Examinations. Insurance Career Development Center Staff & Caitlind L. Alexander. Ed. by Caitlind L. Alexander & Sharon E. Brown. 4th rev. ed. 1995. (Illus.). 421p. (C). pap. text 35.95 (*0-8151-4813-5*, 26045-4) ICDC Pubng.

Guide to Health Claims Examining. Insurance Career Development Center Staff & Caitlind L. Alexander. Ed. by Caitlind L. Alexander & Sharon E. Brown. (Illus.). (C). 4th rev. ed. 1995. 475p. pap. text, tchr. ed. 14.95 (*0-8151-4801-1*, 26045-4); 5th rev. ed. 1999. 420p. pap. text 35.95 (*1-881159-16-7*, 26045-5) ICDC Pubng.

Guide to Health Insurance Billing. Marie A. Moisio. 2000. LC 00-60328. (Allied Health Ser.). (Illus.). 496p. pap. text 46.95 (*0-7668-1207-3*) Thomson Learn.

Guide to Health Insurance for People with Medicare. rev. ed. 1995. (Illus.). 35p. (C). pap. text 15.00 (*0-7881-2204-5*) DIANE Pub.

Guide to Health Insurance for People with Medicare. 1984. lib. bdg. 250.00 (*0-87700-536-2*) Revisionist Pr.

***Guide to Healthcare Resources on the Internet.** Ed. by Robert Kiley. 2001. 116p. pap. (*1-85315-473-3*) Royal Soc of Medicine Pr Ltd GBR. *Dist:* Balogh.

Guide to Healthcare Resources on the Internet, 2000 Edition. John W. Hoben & Paul Engstrom. Ed. by Luci Kozzumi. rev. ed. 1999. 606p. pap. text 285.00 (*1-57987-123-2*) Faulkner & Gray.

Guide to Heart Sounds: Normal & Abnormal. Donald W. Novey et al. 1988. 104p. audio 62.95 (*0-8493-0153-X*, RC683) CRC Pr.

Guide to Heritage Assessment & Health Traditions. Rachel E. Spector. 1996. (Illus.). 48p. (*0-8385-1484-7*, A1484-3) Appleton & Lange.

Guide to HMO Billing. Caitlind L. Alexander. Ed. by Sharon E. Brown. unabr. ed. 1999. 135p. pap. (*1-881159-28-0*) ICDC Pubng.

***Guide to Holistic Healing: In the New Millennium.** Ingfried Hobert. 2002. 107p. pap. 12.95 (*0-8464-5195-6*) Beekman Pubs.

Guide to Home-Based Psychological Services. Nancy A. Newton & Kadi Sprengle. 2000. LC 99-87587. xv, 296p. (*0-8261-1339-7*) Springer Pub.

Guide to Home Health Care & The Marketing of Home Health Care Services, Set. 1992. lib. bdg. 620.95 (*0-8490-8897-6*) Gordon Pr.

***Guide to Homoeopathic Remedies: The Complete Modern Handbook for Home Use.** Paul Houghton. 2001. 248p. pap. (*0-285-63557-3*) Souvenir Pr Ltd GBR. *Dist:* IPG Chicago.

Guide to Homoeopathy. 1998. 188p. reprint ed. text 15.00 (*0-7881-5169-X*) DIANE Pub.

Guide to Hospital Security. John E. Nichols. 1983. 176p. text (*0-566-02359-8*) Gower GBR. *Dist:* Ashgate Pub Co.

Guide to Human Genome Computing. Ed. by Martin Bishop. 2nd ed. 1998. LC 98-14458. (Illus.). 320p. 69.95 (*0-12-102051-7*) Morgan Kaufmann.

Guide to Human Helminths. Isabel Coombs & David W. Crompton. 1991. 203p. (*0-85066-807-7*) Tay Francis Ltd GBR. *Dist:* Taylor & Francis.

Guide to Human Relations in Business & Industry. Martin M. Bruce. 1969. LC 73-6907. pap. 20.35 (*0-935198-00-8*) M M Bruce.

Guide to Independence for the Visually Impaired & Their Families. Vivian Younger & Jill Sardegna. 1994. LC 94-26012. 248p. pap. 29.95 (*0-939957-61-2*) Demos Medical.

Guide to Indian Herbs. Raymond Stark. Ed. by Margaret Campbell. 1984. (Illus.). 48p. (Orig.). reprint ed. pap. 7.95 (*0-88839-077-7*) Hancock House.

Guide to Infection Control in the Hospital. Richard P. Wenzel et al. 1998. 182p. pap. (*1-55009-059-3*) DEKR.

Guide to Information Sources in Alternative Therapy. Barbara Allan. 1988. 216p. text (*0-566-05611-9*) Gower GBR. *Dist:* Ashgate Pub Co.

Guide to Internal Medicine. Douglas S. Paauw et al. 1999. LC 99-14131. xvi, 302p. 29.00 (*0-323-00921-2*) Mosby Inc.

Guide to Interpretation of Hemodynamic Data in the Coronary Care Unit. 1997. LC 96-44088. 224p. pap. text 49.95 (*0-397-58782-1*) Lppncott W & W.

Guide to Journals in Psychology & Education. Wing H. Loke. 1990. LC 90-33603. 415p. 47.50 (*0-8108-2327-6*) Scarecrow.

***Guide to Laboratory Investigations.** Michael McGhee. 3rd ed. 2000. 176p. pap. (*1-85775-357-7*) Radcliffe Med Pr GBR. *Dist:* Balogh.

Guide to Laboratory Test Selection. Michael Laposata et al. 1998. LC 96-45495. pap. text (*0-443-07610-3*) Church.

Guide to Laparoscopic Surgery. Azad Najmaldin & Pierre J. Guillou. 1998. LC 98-5987. (Illus.). 169p. pap. 57.95 (*0-86542-649-X*) Blackwell Sci.

Guide to Lasers in the OR. Judith I. Pfister & Julia A. Kneedler. 1983. (Illus.). (*0-9613138-0-3*) ED Inc.

Guide to Legal Rights for People with Disabilities. Marc D. Stolman. 1994. 152p. pap. 24.95 (*0-939957-59-0*) Demos Medical.

Guide to Leprosy Control. WHO Staff. 2nd ed. 1988. 129p. 23.00 (*92-4-154223-3*) World Health.

Guide to Libraries & Information Sources in Medicine & Health Care. Compiled by Peter Dale. 1995. (Key Resources Ser.). 162p. pap. 69.95 (*0-7123-0823-7*) L Erlbaum Assocs.

Guide to Libraries & Information Sources in Medicine & Health Care. Peter Dale. 2nd ed. 1997. LC 96-147051. (Key Resources Ser.). 656p. pap. (*0-7123-0839-3*) SRIS GBR. *Dist:* L Erlbaum Assocs.

Guide to Living with Bladder Cancer. Mark P. Schoenberg. 2000. LC 00-9271. (Johns Hopkins Press Health Bks.). (Illus.). 192p. 42.50 (*0-8018-6405-4*) Johns Hopkins.

Guide to Living with Bladder Cancer. Mark P. Schoenberg & Johns Hopkins Genitourinary Oncology Group. 2000. LC 00-9271. (Johns Hopkins Press Health Bks.). (Illus.). 184p. pap. 15.95 (*0-8018-6406-2*) Johns Hopkins.

Guide to Living with Bladder Cancer. Mark P. Schoenberg. l.t. ed. 2001. (Illus.). 320p. pap. 19.95 (*0-8018-6519-0*) Johns Hopkins.

Guide to Living with HIV Infection: Developed at the Johns Hopkins AIDS Clinic. John G. Bartlett et al. 4th rev. ed. 1998. LC 97-36903. (Johns Hopkins Press Health Bks.). 440p. 49.95 (*0-8018-5853-4*); pap. 15.95 (*0-8018-5854-2*) Johns Hopkins.

E
F
G

Guide to Managed Care Medicine. William N. Tindall & W. C. Williams, III. 2000. LC 99-57558. 208p. pap. 45.00 (*0-8342-1765-1*) Aspen Pub.

Guide to Managed Care Strategies, 1998: An Annual Report on the Latest Practices & Policies in the New Managed Care Environment. Ed. by Joseph Burns et al. 1997. (Illus.). 342p. pap. 225.00 (*1-57987-029-5*) Faulkner & Gray.

Guide to Managed Care Strategies, 1999. Ed. by Luci Koizumi & Joseph Burns. 1998. 368p. pap. 245.00 (*1-57987-083-X*) Faulkner & Gray.

Guide to Mechanical Ventilation & Intensive Respiratory Care. Lynelle N. Pierce. 1995. (Illus.). 400p. spiral bd. 28.00 (*0-7216-6478-4*) Saunders.

Guide to Medi-Cal Programs: A Description of Medi-Cal Programs, Aid Codes & Eligibility Groups. Claudia Page & Susan Ruiz. unabr. ed. 1999. (Illus.). 42p. spiral bd. (*1-929008-17-1*) CA HlthCare Fnd.

Guide to Medical Cures & Treatments. Reader's Digest Editorial Staff. 1996. LC 95-39005. (Illus.). 480p. 30.00 (*0-89577-846-7*) RD Assn.

Guide to Medical Laboratory Instruments. Clifford D. Ferris. 1980. LC 80-80585. 260p. 20.00 (*0-316-28127-1*, Little Brwn Med Div) Lppncott W & W.

Guide to Medical Practice Management Software: And The Requirements Analyst Ronald B. Sterling & Sheldon Needle. rev. ed. 1997. 180p. ring bd. 495.00 incl. disk (*0-917429-19-2*) CTS.

***Guide to Medical Practice Software.** Ronald R. Sterling. 1999. 175.00 incl. cd-rom (*0-15-606994-6*) Harcourt Prof.

Guide to Medical School Admission: A Straight Forward Guide to Getting into Medical School. W. G. Byrd. 1997. (Illus.). 122p. lib. bdg. 18.95 (*1-85070-796-0*, Parthenon Pbng) CRC Pr.

Guide to Medical School & the MCAT. David A. Hacker & Kenneth Ibsen. 1997. LC 96-20389. (Illus.). 304p. 19.95 (*0-683-00679-7*) Lppncott W & W.

Guide to Medical School Preparation: Developing a System for Successful Admission. Andrew Goliszek. 1984. LC 84-70246. 104p. 4.95 (*0-916833-00-3*) Bio-Pub.

Guide to Medicinal Wild Fruits & Berries. Julie Gomez. 1999. (Illus.). 64p. 7.95 (*0-88839-445-4*) Hancock House.

Guide to Middle Ear Infection. Tim Peters. 1998. (Humanatomy Board Bks.). (Illus.). 12p. bds. 9.95 (*1-879874-11-3*) T Peters & Co.

***Guide to Myofascial Therapy & Clinical Neuromuscular Re-Education.** 2001. (*1-884325-17-3*) G E Sella.

Guide to Natural Therapies: Choosing & Using Natural Methods for Physical & Mental Well-Being. Mark Evans. 1998. (Illus.). 128p. text 27.00 (*0-7881-5881-3*) DIANE Pub.

Guide to Neurological & Neurosurgical Nursing. Ed. by Mariahm Snyder. 2nd ed. 1991. 609p. pap. 45.00 (*0-8273-4381-7*) Delmar.

Guide to NIH Grant Programs. Samuel M. Schwartz & Mischa E. Friedman. 1992. LC 92-6084. (Illus.). 320p. text 39.95 (*0-19-506934-X*) OUP.

Guide to Nursing Management & Leadership. Ann Marriner-Tomey. (Illus.). 5th ed. 1996. 544p. tchr. ed. (*0-8151-6293-6*); 5th ed. 1995. 544p. (C). (gr. 13). pap. text 38.00 (*0-8151-6401-7*, 25500); 6th ed. 2000. LC 00-22918. 590p. pap. 39.00 (*0-323-01066-0*) Mosby Inc.

***Guide to Nursing Management & Leadership.** Ann Marriner-Tomey. 6th ed. 2000. (Illus.). pap. (*0-323-01076-8*) Mosby Inc.

Guide to Nutritional Assessment. I. Beghin et al. 1988. (Nonserial Publication). 80p. pap. text 17.00 (*92-4-154221-7*, 1150286) World Health.

Guide to Ocular Leprosy for Health Workers. Paul Courtright & Susan Lewallen. 1993. 52p. pap. text 33.00 (*981-02-1328-X*) World Scientific Pub.

Guide to over-the-Counter Drugs, Vitamins, & Natural Medicines: More Than 100 of the Most Common Traditional & Alternative Medications, Including. Ed. by Time-Life Books Editors. 1999. LC 98-3426. (Time-Life Medical Guides). (Illus.). 144p. pap. 6.95 (*0-7370-1103-3*, Time Life) Henninger Prod.

Guide to Patient Evaluation: History Taking, Physical Examination & the Nursing Process. Jacques L. Sherman, Jr. & Sylvia K. Fields. 5th ed. 1987. 649p. pap. 39.50 (*0-444-01158-7*) Elsevier.

Guide to Pediatric Cardiovascular Physical Examination. Colin K. Phoon & Paul Stanger. 1998. LC 98-5745. 160p. pap. text 34.95 (*0-7817-1042-1*) Lppncott W & W.

Guide to Pediatric Tracheotomy Care. Pat Adamo-Tumminelli. 2nd ed. 1993. LC 93-24350. (Illus.). 90p. (C). pap. 31.95 (*0-398-05887-3*) C C Thomas.

Guide to Personnel Monitoring for Radiation in the Hospital Environment. Landauer, Inc. Staff & Man-Sung Yim. 1994. LC 93-80627. (Illus.). 60p. (Orig.). pap. text 40.00 (*0-9639768-0-X*) Landauer.

Guide to Pharmacologic Effects. Dermarders. 1998. text (*0-7216-6236-6*) Saunders.

Guide to Physicians & Other Health Care Professionals, Set. William J. Cole et al. Incl. Vol. 1. ring bd. (*0-7646-0875-4*); Vol. 2. ring bd. (*0-7646-0876-2*); Vol. 3. ring bd. (*0-7646-0877-0*); 1999. Set ring bd. 155.00 (*0-7646-0874-6*);Vol. 1. ring bd. (*0-7646-0875-4*);Vol. 2. ring bd. (*0-7646-0876-2*);Vol. 3. ring bd. (*0-7646-0877-0*) Prctnrs Pub Co.

Guide to Planning Alcoholism Treatment Programs. 1994. (Illus.). 90p. (Orig.). (C). pap. text 30.00 (*0-7881-0652-X*) DIANE Pub.

Guide to Planning & Evaluating Inmate Medical - Mental Health Services. 1993. (Illus.). 79p. (Orig.). (C). pap. text 25.00 (*1-56806-825-5*) DIANE Pub.

Guide to Planning Health Promotion for AIDS Prevention & Control. 1989. (WHO AIDS Ser.: No. 5). (CHI, ENG & SPA.). iv, 71p. pap. text 14.00 (*92-4-121005-2*, 1870005) World Health.

Guide to Poisonous Plants. Keith Allison & Christopher Day. 1997. pap. (*0-85131-698-0*) J A Allen GBR. *Dist:* Trafalgar, St Mut.

Guide to Poliovirus Isolation & Serological Techniques for Poliomyelitis Surveillance. D. Magrath. 1979. (WHO Offset Publications: No. 45). 26p. 4.00 (*92-4-170046-7*) World Health.

Guide to Population-Family Planning Information Sources. Ed. by Judith M. Wilkinson. 1979. LC 79-19047. 50p. (Orig.). pap. 8.00 (*0-933438-03-6*, SP 2) APLIC Intl.

Guide to Postgraduate Medical Education. Brian Keighley & Stuart Murray. 1996. 157p. pap. text (*0-7279-1072-8*, 340300160) BMJ Pub GBR. *Dist:* AIDC.

Guide to Practice Management, Monograph 5. 1993. (Cardiovascular Specialist's Guide to Managed Care Ser.). 68p. (Orig.). pap. text (*1-882764-04-8*) Am Coll Cardiology.

Guide to Prevention of Transmission of Human Immunodeficiency Virus & Hepatitis B Virus to Health-Care & Public-Safety Workers. 1991. lib. bdg. 75.00 (*0-8490-5043-X*) Gordon Pr.

Guide to Principles & Applications. Nancy J. Brent. Ed. by Thomas Eoyang. 1997. LC 96-30633. (Illus.). 525p. pap. text 28.50 (*0-7216-3463-X*) Saunders.

Guide to Program Evaluation for Physical Therapy & Occupational Therapy Services. Ed. by Evelyn M. Andamo. 1984. LC 84-8962. 151p. (C). text 4.95 (*0-86656-261-3*) Haworth Pr.

Guide to Prosthetic Cardiac Valves. Ed. by D. Morse et al. 1985. (Illus.). 362p. 240.00 (*0-387-96123-2*) Spr-Verlag.

Guide to Psychiatric Disorders II. Ed. by Hatherleigh Editorial Board. 7th ed. 1999. LC 00-33885. (Guides to Mental Health Ser.: Vol. 13). (Illus.). 280p. pap. 29.95 (*1-57826-023-X*, Five Star Pub) Hatherleigh.

Guide to Psychiatry in Primary Care. Patricia R. Casey. 2nd rev. ed. 1997. LC 97-7979. 320p. (*1-871816-33-5*) Wrightson Biomed GBR. *Dist:* Taylor & Francis.

Guide to Psychoactive Drugs: An Up-to-the-Minute Reference to Mind-Altering Substances. Richard Seymour & David E. Smith. 1987. LC 87-12062. 186p. (Orig.). pap. text 14.95 (*0-918393-43-4*, Harrington Park) Haworth Pr.

Guide to Psychological Practice in Geriatric Long-Term Care. Peter A. Lichtenberg. 1993. LC 92-48389. (Illus.). 210p. pap. 19.95 (*1-56024-411-9*); lib. bdg. 49.95 (*1-56024-410-0*) Haworth Pr.

Guide to Psychotherapy & Aging: Effective Clinical Interventions in a Life-Stage Context. Ed. by Steven H. Zarit & Bob G. Knight. 1996. LC 96-20258. 294p. text 29.95 (*1-55798-373-9*) Am Psychol.

Guide to Psychotherapy with Gay & Lesbian Clients. Ed. by John C. Gonsiorek. 1985. LC 84-19275. (Journal of Homosexuality Ser.: Vol. 7, Nos. 2 & 3). 212p. pap. text 14.95 (*0-918393-03-5*, Harrington Park) Haworth Pr.

Guide to Radiological Procedures. Ed. by Stephen Chapman & Richard Nakielny. 3rd ed. 1993. (Illus.). 448p. pap. text (*0-7020-1678-0*) W B Saunders GBR. *Dist:* Saunders.

***Guide to Radiological Procedures.** S. Chapman & R. Nakielney. 4th ed. 2001. (Illus.). 445p. pap. (*0-7020-2565-8*) W B Saunders GBR. *Dist:* Saunders.

Guide to Rational Living. Albert Ellis & Robert A. Harper. 3rd rev. ed. 1975. LC 75-4961. 283p. reprint ed. pap. 15.00 (*0-87980-042-9*) Wilshire.

Guide to Reasonable Accommodation for OT Practitioners with Disabilities: Fieldwork to Employment. Shirley A. Wells & Sandy Hanebrink. 1998. LC 98-234060. 179 p. 25.00 (*1-56900-088-3*) Am Occup Therapy.

Guide to Reference & Resources in Child Abuse & Neglect. Ed. by Jerry G. Jones & Carolyn J. Levitt. 2nd ed. 1998. LC 97-74709. 292p. pap. 34.95 (*0-910761-93-0*) Am Acad Pediat.

Guide to Rehabilitation, Set. Paul Deutsch & Horace W. Sawyer. 1985. 3000p. text 180.00 (*1-887515-02-X*) AHAB Press.

Guide to Reproduction: Social Issues & Human Concerns. Irina Pollard. 1994. (Illus.). 426p. (C). text 80.00 (*0-521-41862-3*); pap. text 29.95 (*0-521-42925-0*) Cambridge U Pr.

Guide to Research in Gerontology: Strategies & Resources. Dorothea R. Zito & George V. Zito. 1988. LC 88-17773. 144p. lib. bdg. 47.50 (*0-313-25904-6*, ZGG/, Greenwood Pr) Greenwood.

Guide to Rotational Atherectomy. Mark Beisman. Date not set. (Illus.). 317p. (C). pap. text 59.95 (*1-890114-02-2*) Physicians Pr.

Guide to Safety & Health in Dock Work. 1988. x, 287p. pap. 29.25 (*92-2-101081-3*) Intl Labour Office.

Guide to Sanitation in Natural Disasters. M. M. Assar. 1971. (Illus.). 135p. pap. text 16.00 (*92-4-154011-7*, 1150054) World Health.

Guide to Selected HIV- & AIDS-Related Information Services in the U. S. 1994. 50p. (Orig.). (C). pap. text 20.00 (*0-7881-1468-9*) DIANE Pub.

Guide to Selecting a Computerized Patient Record System for Your Office. Gil L. Solomon et al. 1998. pap. 99.00 (*0-9637397-9-4*) Hlthcare Comput.

Guide to Short-Term Tests for Detecting Mutagenic & Carcinogenic Chemicals. 1985. (Environmental Health Criteria Ser.: No. 51). 208p. pap. text 26.00 (*92-4-154191-1*, 1160051) World Health.

Guide to Simple Sanitary Measures for the Control of Enteric Diseases. S. Rajagopalan. 1974. pap. text 32.00 (*92-4-154047-8*, 1150058) World Health.

Guide to Skin & Haircoat Problems in Dogs. Lowell J. Ackerman. 1994. LC 93-37070. (Illus.). 192p. pap. 27.95 (*0-931866-65-0*) Alpine Pubns.

Guide to State & Federal Drug-Testing Laws. Mark A. De Bernardo & Nancy N. Delogu. 7th ed. 1998. pap. 225.00 (*1-889437-20-4*) Inst Drug-Free Wrkpl.

Guide to State & Federal Drug-Testing Laws. Mark A. De Bernardo et al. 9th ed. 2000. pap. 295.00 (*1-889437-22-0*) Inst Drug-Free Wrkpl.

Guide to State Medicaid Managed Care Laws & Rules: 1996-97 Edition. Jane Anderson. Ed. by Ashli Towler. 2nd ed. 1996. 85p. pap. 134.00 (*1-56925-053-7*, SMM2) Capitol Publns.

Guide to Stress Reduction. L. John Mason. rev. ed. 1986. LC 79-2577. (Illus.). 192p. text 12.95 (*0-89087-452-2*) Celestial Arts.

Guide to Substance Abuse Services for Primary Care Physicians. Ed. by Eleanor Sullivan & Michael Fleming. 1998. (Illus.). 168p. (C). pap. text 30.00 (*0-7881-7346-4*) DIANE Pub.

Guide to Success: Physical Therapist Assistant's Review for Licensure. Scott M. Giles. Ed. by Therese C. Giles. rev. ed. 2002. 360p. stu. ed., per. 39.95 (*1-890989-13-4*) Mainely Phys.

Guide to Success: Review for Licensure in Physical Therapy. Scott M. Giles. Ed. by Therese C. Giles. rev. ed. 2002. 385p. stu. ed., per. 39.95 (*1-890989-12-6*) Mainely Phys.

Guide to Success in American Medical Boards. Zafar Y. Ibrahim. Ed. by Deborah D. Richards. 2nd rev. ed. 1991. 64p. spiral bd. 15.00 (*0-9626615-1-1*) Overseas Pub.

Guide to Successful Private Practice in Speech-Language Pathology. 1996. ring bd. 38.00 (*0-910329-90-7*, 0112026) Am Speech Lang Hearing.

Guide to Surgical Principles & Practice. Ed. by Iain E. Gillespie et al. 1992. (Illus.). 560p. (Orig.). pap. text (*0-443-04430-9*) Church.

Guide to Surviving Nursing School. Joan M. Regan. 2nd ed. 1995. LC 95-9126. (Springhouse Notes Ser.). 144p. pap. 16.95 (*0-87434-816-1*) Springhouse Corp.

Guide to Symptom Relief in Advanced Cancer. Peter J. Ravenscroft & John Cavanaugh. 1994. 160p. pap. text 19.95 (*0-07-470134-7*) McGraw-Hill Med Pub.

Guide to Symptom Relief in Advanced Disease. Claud F. B. Regnard & Sue Tempest. 4th ed. 1998. LC 98-155044. 152p. pap. (*1-898507-38-4*) Books For Midwives Pr GBR. *Dist:* Balogh.

Guide to Teaching Managed Care. Marcie Weinstein. 1999. (Illus.). pap. text 35.00 (*1-56900-116-2*) Am Occup Therapy.

Guide to Tertiary Package Contracting, Monograph 2. 1993. (Cardiovascular Specialist's Guide to Managed Care Ser.). (Illus.). 60p. (Orig.). (C). pap. text (*1-882764-03-X*) Am Coll Cardiology.

Guide to the Bach Flower Remedies. Julian Barnard. 8th ed. 52p. pap. 8.95 (*0-8464-4221-3*) Beekman Pubs.

Guide to the Big Book's Design for Living see Programa para Ti: Una Guia Disenada del Libro Grande

Guide to the Clinical Use of the 16 PF. Samuel Karson & Jerry W. O'Dell. 1976. LC 76-23339. pap. 15.00 (*0-918296-09-9*) Inst Personality & Ability.

Guide to the Extrapyramidal Side Effects of Antipsychotic Drugs. D. G. Owens. 1999. LC 98-7142. (Illus.). 362p. (C). pap. text 49.95 (*0-521-63353-2*) Cambridge U Pr.

Guide to the Family Medicine Clerkship. Susan L. Montauk. 2001. 432p. pap. text 25.95 (*0-7817-2349-3*) Lppncott W & W.

Guide to the Guidelines: Disease Management Made Simple. Peter Smith. 2nd ed. 1996. LC 96-13771. (*1-85775-102-7*); 3rd ed. 1997. LC 97-20952. (*1-85775-286-4*) Radcliffe Med Pr GBR. *Dist:* Balogh.

Guide to the Handling of Patients. E. N. Corlett et al. 4th ed. 1994. (Illus.). 134p. (C). reprint ed. pap. text 27.95 (*1-879864-01-0*) IMPACC USA.

Guide to the Herbal Remedies. Mark Evans. 96p. (Orig.). pap. 20.95 (*0-8464-4222-1*) Beekman Pubs.

Guide to the History of Psychology. John D. Lawry. 1990. LC 90-41777. 128p. (C). reprint ed. pap. 20.50 (*0-8191-7851-9*) U Pr of Amer.

Guide to the Human Eye. Tim Peters. 1993. (Humanatomy Board Bks.). (Illus.). 12p. bds. 9.95 (*1-879874-16-4*) T Peters & Co.

Guide to the Laboratory Diagnosis of Trachoma. 1975. pap. text 12.00 (*92-4-154048-6*, 1150059) World Health.

Guide to the Language of Psychoanalysis: An Empirical Study of the Relationships among Psychoanalytic Terms & Concepts. George H. Klumpner. 1994. LC 93-40943. 200p. (C). spiral bd. 40.00 (*0-8236-2277-0*) Intl Univs Pr.

Guide to the Managed Care Industry. 1996. (*1-57372-023-2*); 1995. (*1-880678-65-9*) Solucient.

Guide to the Managed Care Industry, 1997. 1997. pap. 245.00 (*1-57372-056-9*) Solucient.

Guide to the MRCP Part Two Written Paper. Anthony N. Warrens et al. 1993. LC 93-23428. (Illus.). 288p. pap. text (*0-412-43470-9*) Chapman & Hall.

Guide to the NTE Audiology Specialty Area Test. Educational Testing Service Staff. 1995. 128p. pap. 16.00 (*0-446-39602-8*) Warner Bks.

Guide to the NTE Speech-Language Pathology Specialty Area Test. Educational Testing Service Staff. 1995. (Praxis Ser.). 128p. pap. 16.00 (*0-446-39604-4*) Warner Bks.

Guide to the Nursing Home Industry, 1997. Arthur Anderson. 1997. pap. 249.00 (*1-57372-098-4*) Solucient.

Guide to the Optometric Training of Myopia Control. Sonja Collier-Vanhimbeeck. 1997. LC 97-37728. (Illus.). 54p. 20.00 (*0-943599-94-6*) OEPF.

Guide to the Practice of Paediatric Endocrinology. Charles G. Brook. 1993. (Illus.). 191p. (C). text 59.95 (*0-521-43179-4*) Cambridge U Pr.

Guide to the Psycho-Motor Development of the Child. Jacqueline Gassier. 1985. (Illus.). 149p. text (*0-443-02969-5*) Church.

Guide to the Sodium Contents of Your Food. U. S. Department of Agriculture Staff. 1985. (Cookery Ser.). 48p. reprint ed. pap. 1.95 (*0-486-24829-1*) Dover.

Guide to the Texas Medical Center. Clyde W. Burleson & Suzy W. Burleson. 1987. (Illus.). 160p. pap. 7.95 (*0-292-72727-5*) U of Tex Pr.

Guide to Total Nutrient Admixtures. Penny Wells. 1992. LC 91-67485. 112p. pap. 39.95 (*0-944496-28-8*) Precept Pr.

Guide to Training Resources in Mental Handicap. Linda Averill et al. 1989. (C). 65.00 (*0-906054-68-0*) St Mut.

***Guide to Treatments That Work.** Ed. by Peter Nathan & Jack M. Gorman. 2nd ed. 2002. (Illus.). 732p. text 85.00 (*0-19-514072-9*) OUP.

Guide to Treatments That Work: A Review of the Outcome Studies on Psychotherapies & Drugs. Peter E. Nathan & Jack M. Gorman. 1997. LC 97-36492. (Illus.). 624p. text 75.00 (*0-19-510227-4*) OUP.

Guide to Ultrasound Examination of the Abdomen. M. Leon Skolnick. 1986. (Illus.). 240p. 143.00 (*0-387-96225-5*) Spr-Verlag.

Guide to Undergraduate RN Education. D. Louden. 5th ed. 1997. 200p. pap. 34.95 (*0-88737-737-8*, 19-7378, NLN Pr) Natl League Nurse.

Guide to Understanding & Living with Epilepsy. Orrin Devinsky. 1994. LC 94-10823. (Illus.). 347p. (C). pap. text 19.95 (*0-8036-2556-1*) Davis Co.

Guide to United Nations Information Sources on Health (ACCIS) 227p. 36.00 (*92-1-100363-6*, E.GV.91.0.11) UN.

Guide to Urban Arterial Systems. Compiled by American Society of Civil Engineers Staff. 1981. LC 81-69231. 344p. pap. 28.00 (*0-87262-280-0*) Am Soc Civil Eng.

Guide to Veterinary Medical Terminology. Phillip E. Cochran. 1991. LC 90-85893. (Illus.). 300p. pap. text 31.95 (*0-939674-31-9*) Am Vet Pubns.

Guide to Wheelchair Selection: How to Use the ANSI-RESNA Wheelchair Standards to Buy a Wheelchair. Peter Axelson et al. 1994. (Illus.). (Orig.). pap. (*0-929819-06-3*) Paralyzed Vets.

Guide to Women Physicians in the Washington D. C. Area. Judy Grande. 1993. 232p. pap. 12.95 (*0-9636565-0-3*) Rocky Run.

Guide to Your Cat's Symptoms. Elizabeth Randolph. 1999. (*0-375-50078-2*) Villard Books.

Guide to Your Dog's Symptoms. Elizabeth Randolph. 1999. (*0-375-50079-0*) Villard Books.

Guidebook for Clinical Psychology Interns. Ed. by Gary K. Zammit & James W. Hull. 1995. LC 94-49186. (Applied Clinical Psychology Ser.). 242p. pap. 37.50 (*0-306-44859-9*, Plenum Trade) Perseus Pubng.

Guidebook for Developing Individualized Educational Programs for Gifted & Talented Students. Joseph S. Renzulli & Linda H. Smith. 1979. 56p. (gr. k-12). pap. 12.95 (*0-936386-13-4*, 670) Creative Learning.

Guidebook for Patient Counseling. Harvey M. Rappaport et al. 1993. LC 93-79389. 108p. 31.95 (*1-56676-089-5*) CRC Pr.

Guidebook of Gastrointestinal Problem. Date not set. pap. (*1-884350-66-6*) Alpha Pubng.

Guidebook on Molecular Modeling in Drug Design. Ed. by N. Claude Cohen. 1996. LC 95-21396. (Illus.). 361p. text 59.95 (*0-12-178245-X*) Acad Pr.

Guidebook to Better Medical Writing. Robert L. Iles. 1997. (Illus.). vi, 197p. pap. 27.95 (*0-9661831-0-X*) Island Pr KS.

Guidebook to Endovascular Coronary Diagnostic Techniques. Ed. by Herbert J. Geschwind & Morton J. Kern. 1997. LC 96-33341. (Illus.). 576p. 125.00 (*0-87993-641-X*) Futura Pub.

Guidebook to Managed Care & Practice Management Terminology. Norman Winegar & L. Michelle Hayter. 1998. LC 98-12222. 86p. (C). 39.95 (*0-7890-0447-X*) Haworth Pr.

Guidebook to Protein Toxins & Their Use in Cell Biology. Ed. by Rino Rappuoli & Cesare Montecucco. 1997. LC 96-29554. (Guidebook Ser.). (Illus.). 274p. pap. text 50.00 (*0-19-859954-4*) OUP.

Guidebook to Re-Evaluation Counseling: Kannada Translation. Harvey Jackins. 1983. pap. 3.00 (*0-913937-00-2*) Rational Isl.

Guided Bone Regeneration in Implant Dentistry. Daniel Buser et al. 1994. LC 94-242. (Illus.). 270p. text 120.00 (*0-86715-249-4*) Quint Pub Co.

Guided Brain Operations. E. A. Spiegel. 1982. (Illus.). x, 246p. 55.00 (*3-8055-3451-5*) S Karger.

Guided Change of the American Health System: Where the Levers Are. Pamela Doty. 1980. LC 80-12484. (Center for Policy Research Monographs: Vol. II). 299p. 43.95 (*0-87705-472-X*, Kluwer Acad Hman Sci) Kluwer Academic.

Guided Imagery for Healing Children & Teens: Wellness Through Visualization. Ellen Curran. 2001. LC 00-45493. (Illus.). xvi, 171p. pap. 14.95 (*1-58270-041-9*) Beyond Words Pub.

Guided Imagery for Self-Healing: An Essential Resource for Anyone Seeking Wellness. Martin L. Rossman. 2nd ed. 2000. LC 00-55924. (Illus.). xxi, 280p. pap. 14.95 (*0-915811-88-X*) H J Kramer Inc.

Guided Tour of Veterinary Anatomy: Domestic Ungulates. James E. Smallwood. 1999. (Illus.). ix, 359p. (C). pap. 42.50 (*0-9702165-0-5*) J E Smallwood.

Guided Tour of Veterinary Anatomy: Domestic Ungulates & Laboratory Mammals. James E. Smallwood. 1991. LC 91-3647. (Illus.). 400p. text 46.00 (*0-7216-3731-0*) Saunders.

Guideline for Establishing & Administering Medical Instrumentation Maintenance Programs. 2nd ed. 1992. (Illus.). 48p. pap. text 55.00 (*0-910275-10-6*, MIR2-209) Assn Adv Med Instrn.

Guideline for Facilities Treating Chemically Dependent Patients at Risk for AIDS Or Infected by HIV. Larry Siegel et al. rev. ed. 1991. 34p. reprint ed. pap. 3.00 (*1-880425-00-9*) Am Soc Addict Med.

Guideline for Isolation Precautions in Hospitals & Guideline for Infection Control in Hospital Personnel. 1992. lib. bdg. 250.00 (*0-8490-5329-3*) Gordon Pr.

Guideline for the Format & Content: The Summary for New Drug & Antibiotic Applications. 1987. 28p. pap. text 25.00 (*1-57979-161-1*, 2086) DIANE Pub.

Guideline on Formatting, Assembling, & Submitting New Drug & Antibiotic Applications. (Illus.). 1998. 66p. pap. text 20.00 (*0-7881-4784-6*); 1987. 40p. pap. text 25.00 (*1-57979-160-3*, 2085) DIANE Pub.

Guidelines & Documentation for Social Workers in Home Health Care. Leah Blanchard et al. 1991. 25p. pap. 9.95 (*0-87101-181-6*) Natl Assn Soc Wkrs.

Guidelines & Gamuts in Musculoskeletal Ultrasound. Ed. by Rethy Chhem & Etienne Cardinal. 1998. LC 98-21528. (Illus.). 408p. 127.00 (*0-471-19755-6*, Wiley-Liss) Wiley.

Guidelines & Procedures for Meeting the Specialized Physical Health Care Needs of Pupils. California Department of Education Staff. 1990. (Illus.). 212p. pap. 11.00 (*0-8011-0902-7*) Calif Education.

Guidelines & Self-Assessments for Clinical Education. 2000. 75p. pap. 6.00 (*1-887759-68-9*) Am Phys Therapy Assn.

Guidelines for a National Programme for the Control of Iodine Deficiency Disorders in the Eastern Mediterranean Region. 1988. (EMRO Technical Publication Ser.: No. 12). pap. text 9.90 (*92-9021-036-2*) World Health.

Guidelines for Administration of Intravenous Medications to Pediatric Patients. Stephanie J. Phelps & Emily B. Cochran. 4th ed. 1993. 136p. pap. text 35.00 (*1-879907-28-3*) Am Soc Hlth-Syst.

Guidelines for Administration of Intravenous Medications to Pediatric Patients. Stephanie J. Phelps & Emily B. Hak. 5th ed. 1996. 50.00 (*1-879907-63-1*) Am Soc Hlth-Syst.

Guidelines for Adolescent Preventive Services (gaps) Clinical Evaluation & Management Handbook. Patricia B. Levenberg et al. 1995. LC 98-147764. 152 p. (*0-89970-745-9*) AMA.

Guidelines for Air & Ground Transport of Neonatal & Pediatric Patients. American Academy of Pediatrics Staff. 1993. 153p. pap. 24.95 (*0-910761-44-2*) Am Acad Pediat.

Guidelines for Antimicrobial Resistance Surveillance. 1996. (WHO Regional Publications, European Mediterranean Ser.: No. 15). 34p. pap. 9.00 (*92-9021-213-6*, 1440015) World Health.

Guidelines for Antimicrobial Therapy. WHO Staff. 1989. (Western Pacific Education in Action Ser.: No. 3). 96p. 8.00 (*92-9061-133-2*) World Health.

Guidelines for Audiologic Screening. American Speech, Language and Hearing Foundation Staff. 1997. LC 98-114043. spiral bd. 10.00 (*0-910329-96-6*, 0112060) Am Speech Lang Hearing.

Guidelines for Authors. 1997. 18p. pap. 8.00 (*0-9655310-1-5*) Jannetti Pubns.

Guidelines for Blood Utilization Review. 2000. pap. text (*1-56395-133-9*) Am Assn Blood.

***Guidelines for Blood Utilization Review.** Ed. by James P. Aubuchon. 2001. (*1-56395-148-7*) Am Assn Blood.

Guidelines for Care of Migrant Farmworkers' Children. 2000. 200p. pap. 44.95 (*1-58110-044-2*) Am Acad Pediat.

Guidelines for Chiropractic Quality Assurance & Practice Parameters: Proceedings of the Mercy Center Consensus Conference. Ed. by Scott Haldeman et al. 1992. LC 92-26844. 264p. pap. 56.00 (*0-8342-0388-X*) Aspen Pub.

Guidelines for Cholera Control. 1993. (CHI, ENG, FRE & SPA.). vi, 61p. pap. text 15.00 (*92-4-154449-X*, 1150398) World Health.

Guidelines for Clinical Nursing Practices. Elizabeth Jamieson. 2nd ed. 1992. (Illus.). 325p. (Orig.). pap. text (*0-443-04440-6*) Church.

Guidelines for Clinical Research on Acupuncture. WHO Staff. 1995. (WHO Regional Publications, Western Pacific Ser.: No. 15). 62p. 6.80 (*92-9061-114-6*) World Health.

Guidelines for Clinical Testing, Lens Prescribing & Vision Care: A Field Manual for Behavioral Optometry. Earl P. Schmitt. Ed. by Willard Bleything. rev. ed. 1995. 82p. (C). reprint ed. lib. bdg. 18.00 (*0-943599-81-4*) OEPF.

Guidelines for Counselling about HIV Infection & Disease. 1990. (AIDS Ser.: No. 8). (ARA, ENG, FRE, RUS & SPA.). v, 48p. pap. text 11.00 (*92-4-121008-7*, 1870008) World Health.

Guidelines for Critical Care Nursing. Nancie Urban et al. 1995. LC 94-48566. (Illus.). 832p. (C). (gr. 13). pap. text 46.95 (*0-8016-7840-4*, 07840) Mosby Inc.

Guidelines for Curriculum Development on End-of-Life & Palliative Care in Nursing Education. Nancy English & Cindy Yocum. 1998. LC 99-175933. 28p. (*0-931207-55-X*) Natl Hospice.

Guidelines for Design & Construction of Hospital & Health Care Facilities: 1996-97. American Institute of Architects, Academy of Architecture Staff & U. S. Department of Health & Human Services Staff. 1996. (Illus.). 146p. pap. 60.00 (*1-55835-151-5*, J189-96) AIA Press.

Guidelines for Developing a Specialty Practice in Diabetes Care. Condit S. Steil. 1995. 37p. (Orig.). (C). pap. 20.00 (*0-910769-31-1*) Am Coll Apothecaries.

Guidelines for Drinking-Water Quality Vol. 2: Health Criteria & Other Supporting Information. 2nd ed. 1996. (FRE & SPA.). 973p. (Orig.). (C). 260.00 (*92-4-154480-5*, 1152404) World Health.

Guidelines for Drinking-Water Quality, Vol. 3: Drinking-Water Quality Control in Small-Community Supplies. 1985. 121p. pap. text 17.00 (*92-4-154170-9*, 1153219) World Health.

Guidelines for Employee Health Promotion Programs. Association for Worksite Health Promotion Staff. 1991. LC 92-29747. (Illus.). 152p. pap. text 34.00 (*0-87322-351-9*, BAFB0351) Human Kinetics.

Guidelines for Evaluating a Training Programme for Health Personnel. F. Katz. 1978. (WHO Offset Publications: No. 38). 35p. 6.00 (*92-4-170038-6*) World Health.

Guidelines for Evaluation of Drugs for Use in Man: Proceedings of the WHO Scientific Group, Geneva, 1974. WHO Staff. 1975. (Technical Reports: No. 563). pap. text 7.00 (*92-4-120563-6*, 1100563) World Health.

Guidelines for Health & Safety in Metal Finishing. Ed M. Roper. 1991. 80p. (*0-904477-06-1*) FMJ Intl GBR. *Dist:* St Mut.

Guidelines for Health Manpower Planning: A Course Book. P. Hornby et al. 1980. (Nonserial Publication). 368p. pap. text 26.00 (*92-4-154156-3*, 1150065) World Health.

Guidelines for Health Supervision III, Cue Cards. American Academy of Pediatrics Staff. 3rd ed. 1997. LC 96-79630. 257p. pap. 44.95 (*0-910761-83-3*) Am Acad Pediat.

Guidelines for Improving Communications in Pharmacy Practice. Matthew Perri. 2nd ed. 1995. 24p. 20.00 (*0-910769-29-X*) Am Coll Apothecaries.

Guidelines for K-12 Substance Abuse Prevention Education: Curriculum Development. 1994. 141p. (Orig.). (C). (gr. k-12). pap. text 30.00 (*0-7881-0427-6*) DIANE Pub.

Guidelines for Laboratory Quality Auditing. Donald C. Singer & Ronald P. Upton. 1992. LC 92-29093. (Quality & Reliability Ser.: Vol. 39). (Illus.). 432p. text 75.00 (*0-8247-8784-6*) Dekker.

Guidelines for Marketing a Community Pharmacy. Quentin M. Srnka. 2nd ed. 1995. 75p. pap. 20.00 (*0-910769-30-3*) Am Coll Apothecaries.

Guidelines for Neuroleptic Relapse Prevention in Schizophrenia: Proceedings of a Consensus Conference Held April 19-20, 1989 in Bruges, Belgium. Ed. by W. Kissling. 1991. (Illus.). 166p. 58.95 (*0-387-53985-9*) Spr-Verlag.

Guidelines for Nursing Management of People Infected with Human Immunodeficiency Virus (HIV) 1988. (WHO AIDS Ser.: No. 3). (ARA, ENG, FRE, RUS & SPA.). iv, 42p. pap. text 9.00 (*92-4-121003-6*, 187003) World Health.

Guidelines for Occupational Therapy Practice in Home Health. American Occupational Therapy Association Staff. 1995. LC 95-171546. 150p. (C). pap. text 25.00 (*1-56900-023-9*) Am Occup Therapy.

Guidelines for Oncology Nursing Practice. Oncology Nursing Society Staff. 2nd ed. 1991. (Illus.). 476p. pap. text 58.00 (*0-7216-3419-2*) Saunders.

Guidelines for Orthopaedic Nursing: Adult Trauma. Sharon G. Childs & Sue Baird-Holmes. 1998. (Illus.). 40p. pap. 25.00 (*1-892665-01-8*) Natl Assn Ortho Nurse.

Guidelines for Patient Outcome-Oriented Documentation. Mary Hartnett & Alexis A. Wilson. 1995. LC 94-60640. 163p. (Orig.). text 59.95 (*0-9633599-1-6*) Wilson & Assocs.

Guidelines for Perinatal Care. American Academy of Pediatrics Staff & American College of Obstetricians and Gynecologists Staff. 4th ed. 1997. LC 97-19319. 472p. 60.00 (*0-915473-35-6*) Am Coll Obstetric.

Guidelines for Planning & Design of Biomedical Research Laboratory Facilities. American Institute of Architects Staff et al. 1999. (Illus.). 100p. pap. 50.00 (*1-879304-95-3*) AIA DC.

Guidelines for Preparing Core Clinical-Safety Information on Drugs: Report of CIOMS Working Group III. 1995. 69p. (C). pap. text 15.00 (*92-9036-062-3*, 1840018) World Health.

Guidelines for Preventing the Transmission of Mycobaterium Tuberculosis in Health-Care Facilities (1994) 1995. 132p. (Orig.). (C). pap. text 40.00 (*0-7881-1992-3*) DIANE Pub.

Guidelines for Preventing the Transmission of Tuberculosis in Health-Care Facilities. 1995. lib. bdg. 251.75 (*0-8490-7526-2*) Gordon Pr.

Guidelines for Preventing Workplace Violence for Health Care & Social Services Workers. 1997. lib. bdg. 250.95 (*0-8490-6219-5*) Gordon Pr.

Guidelines for Prevention of Transmission of Human Immunodeficiency Virus & Hepatitis Virus to Health-Care & Public-Safety Workers. 1996. 46p. (C). reprint ed. pap. text 25.00 (*0-7881-3622-4*) DIANE Pub.

Guidelines for Protecting the Safety & Health of Health Care Workers. 1992. (Orig.). lib. bdg. 250.00 (*0-8490-5328-5*) Gordon Pr.

Guidelines for Pulmonary Rehabilitation Programs. American Academy of Cardiovascular and Pulmonary Rehabilitation Staff. 2nd rev. ed. 1998. LC 97-46467. (Illus.). 264p. pap. text 39.00 (*0-88011-863-6*, BAAC0863) Human Kinetics.

Guidelines for Quality Assurance Programmes for Blood Transfusion Services. 1993. (ENG, FRE & SPA.). iv, 50p. pap. text 12.00 (*92-4-154448-1*, 1150392) World Health.

Guidelines for Surviving Heat & Cold: A Question-&-Answer Introduction to Protecting Yourself & Others from the Discomforts & Dangers of Summer & Winter. Thomas Adams. 1992. 143p. (C). pap. text 14.80 (*0-87563-403-6*) Stipes.

Guidelines for the Blood Transfusion Service in the United Kingdom. National Blood Service Staff. 4th ed. 2000. 296p. (*0-11-322313-7*) Statnry Office GBR. *Dist:* Balogh.

***Guidelines for the Blood Transfusion Services in the U. K.** National Blood Service Staff. 5th ed. 2001. 368p. pap. (*0-11-702555-0*) Statnry Office GBR. *Dist:* Balogh.

Guidelines for the Clinical Management of HIV Infection in Children. 1994. (Illus.). 88p. (Orig.). (C). pap. text 30.00 (*0-7881-1012-8*) DIANE Pub.

Guidelines for the Development of a Food & Nutrition Surveillance System for Countries in the Eastern Mediterranean Region: Based on the Deliberations of a WHO/FAO Intercountry Meeting on Nutrition Surveillance. 1989. (EMRO Technical Publications Ser.: No. 13). pap. text 10.00 (*92-9021-070-2*) World Health.

Guidelines for the Development of a Simplified Dietary Assessment to Identify Groups at Risk for Inadequate Intake of Vitamin A. Ed. by Barbara A. Underwood et al. 1989. LC 89-84854. 64p. ring bd. 3.50 (*0-944398-03-0*) ILSI.

Guidelines for the Development of Health Management Information Systems. R. Van Konkelenberg & I. Ring. 1993. ix, 127p. pap. text 18.00 (*92-9061-106-5*, 1520002) World Health.

Guidelines for the Diagnosis & Management of Asthma. 1996. (Illus.). 44p. (Orig.). (C). pap. text 25.00 (*0-7881-2738-1*) DIANE Pub.

Guidelines for the Diagnosis & Management of Asthma. 1997. (Orig.). lib. bdg. 250.95 (*0-8490-8136-X*) Gordon Pr.

Guidelines for the Management of Acute Head Injuries. Richard Ashpole et al. 2nd ed. 1995. LC 96-147002. pap. text 29.99 (*1-898507-30-9*) Buttrwrth-Heinemann.

Guidelines for the Management of Nutrition Programmes: A Manual for Nutrition Officers. K. Bagchi. 1990. (WHO EMRO Technical Publications: No. 15). xi, 165p. pap. text 20.00 (*92-9021-099-0*, 1450015) World Health.

Guidelines for the Organization of a Blood Transfusion Service. Ed. by W. N. Gibbs & A. F. Britten. 1992. (ENG, FRE & SPA.). x, 150p. pap. text 25.00 (*92-4-154445-7*, 1150376) World Health.

Guidelines for the Preparation of Tables of Food Composition. Ed. by D. A. Southgate. 1974. 80p. pap. 16.75 (*3-8055-1780-7*) S Karger.

Guidelines for the Security & Safety of Health Care & Community Service Workers. Joyce A. Simonowitz. 1994. 46p. (Orig.). (C). pap. text 25.00 (*0-7881-0815-8*) DIANE Pub.

Guidelines for the Selection & Training of Sensory Panel Members - STP 758. Ed. by American Society for Testing and Materials Staff. 1981. 35p. pap. 13.00 (*0-8031-0783-8*, STP758) ASTM.

Guidelines for the Treatment, Investigation, & Control of Animal Bites. 1993. (Illus.). 74p. (Orig.). (C). pap. text 25.00 (*0-7881-0135-8*) DIANE Pub.

Guidelines for the Treatment of Alcohol & Other Drugs-Abusing Adolescents: A Treatment Improvement Protocol. 1994. (Illus.). 188p. (Orig.). (C). pap. text 40.00 (*0-7881-1164-7*) DIANE Pub.

Guidelines for the Use of ILO International Classification of Radiographs of Pneumoconioses. 7th ed. 1995. (Occupational Safety & Health Ser.: No. 22). reprint ed. pap. 6.75 (*92-2-102463-6*) Intl Labour Office.

Guidelines for the Use of Psychotropic Drugs: A Clinical Handbook. Ed. by Harvey C. Stancer et al. 1984. LC 83-14592. (Illus.). 472p. text 59.95 (*0-88331-147-X*) R B Luce.

Guidelines for Training Community Health Workers in Nutrition. 2nd ed. 1986. (FRE & SPA.). viii, 121p. pap. text 16.00 (*92-4-154210-1*, 1150256) World Health.

Guidelines for Treatment of Cancer Pain. 1993. (Illus.). 67p. (Orig.). (C). pap. text 15.00 (*1-56806-202-8*) DIANE Pub.

Guidelines in Patient Care in Radiography. Christine Gunn & Christine S. Jackson. 2nd ed. 1991. (Illus.). 240p. pap. text (*0-443-04391-4*) Church.

Guidelines in Psychiatry. L. S. Gillis. 3rd ed. 1986. 299p. (C). reprint ed. pap. text (*0-7021-1759-5*) Juta & Co ZAF. *Dist:* Intl Spec Bk.

Guidelines of AIDS & First Aid in the Workplace. 1990. (WHO AIDS Ser.: No. 7). (ARA, ENG, FRE & SPA.). iii, 12p. pap. text 4.00 (*92-4-121007-9*, 1870007) World Health.

Guidelines to Authenticity Stepping Stones to Health. Bernard M. Bane. 1977. LC 77-87980. 60p. pap. 3.00 (*0-9600164-6-5*) BMB Pub Co.

Guidelines to Handling. R. York-Moore & P. Steward. 1985. (Management of the Physically Handicapped Child Ser.: No. 1). 20p. (*0-906054-19-2*) Brit Inst Lrning GBR. *Dist:* Taylor & Francis.

Guidelines to Lifting, Carrying, & Seating. R. York-Moore & P. Stewart. 1985. (Management of the Physically Handicapped Child Ser.: No. 2). 20p. 20.00 (*0-906054-24-9*) St Mut.

Guides Casebook: Cases to Accompany Guides to the Evaluation of Permanent Impairment. American Medical Association Staff. 4th ed. 1999. LC 00-500900. 59.95 (*0-89970-970-2*) AMA.

Guides des Soins Oculaires Primaires pour le Personnel de Sante see Simple Eye Care for Health Care Workers

Guides to Clinical Aspiration Biopsy: Flow Cytometry. Phillippe Vielh. 1991. LC 90-15654. (Illus.). 192p. 66.00 (*0-89640-204-5*) Igaku-Shoin.

Guides to Clinical Aspiration Biopsy: Head & Neck. Vicky S. Chen et al. 2nd ed. 1996. LC 95-22621. (Guides to Clinical Aspiration Biopsy Ser.). (Illus.). 432p. 98.50 (*0-89640-286-X*) Igaku-Shoin.

Guides to Clinical Aspiration Biopsy: Pediatrics. Phillippe Vielh & Lydia Howell. 1996. LC 93-20498. (Guides to Clinical Aspiration Biopsy Ser.). (Illus.). 264p. 95.00 (*0-89640-239-8*) Igaku-Shoin.

Guides to the Evaluation of Permanent Impairment. AMA Staff et al. 5th ed. 2000. LC 2001-271657. (Illus.). xxii, 613p. 139.00 (*1-57947-085-8*) AMA.

Guiding Autobiography Groups for Older Adults: Exploring the Fabric of Life. James E. Birren & Donna E. Deutchman. 1991. LC 90-15625. (Series in Contemporary Medicine & Public Ser.). 160p. pap. text 19.95 (*0-8018-4213-1*) Johns Hopkins.

Guiding Strabismus Therapy. Lora G. McGraw. Ed. by Sally M. Corngold. 1991. (Illus.). 90p. (C). lib. bdg. 15.00 (*0-929780-02-7*) VisionExtension.

Guiding the Process of Therapeutic Change. Frederick H. Kanfer & Bruce K. Schefft. 1988. LC 87-62115. 496p. pap. text 24.95 (*0-87822-285-5*, 2855) Res Press.

Guigonis de Caulhiaco: Inventarium sive Chirurgia Magna, Vol. 2: Commentary. Ed. by Michael R. McVaugh & Margaret Ogden. 1997. (Studies in Ancient Medicine: No. 14.2). vi, 438p. 170.50 (*90-04-10784-3*) Brill Academic Pubs.

Guilford-Zimmerman Temperament Survey Handbook. Joan S. Guilford et al. 1976. LC 76-17988. 22.75 (*0-912736-19-4*) EDITS Pubs.

Guillain-Barre Syndrome. R. A. Hughes. Ed. by John P. Conomy & Michael Swash. 1990. (Clinical Medicine & the Nervous System Ser.). (Illus.). 308p. 155.00 (*0-387-19634-X*) Spr-Verlag.

Guilt. Gerhard Ockel. 1951. (C). pap. 4.00 (*0-87574-061-8*) Pendle Hill.

Guilt. Caryll Houselander. 1971. LC 76-131251. (Illus.). 296p. (C). reprint ed. 35.00 (*0-87752-053-4*) Gordian.

Guilt & Children. Jane Bybee. 1997. LC 97-80321. (Illus.). 296p. text 59.95 (*0-12-148610-9*) Morgan Kaufmann.

Guilt & Depression. Leon Grinberg. 1993. 336p. pap. text (*1-85575-006-6*) Karnac Bks GBR. *Dist:* Other Pr LLC.

Guilt Free Gourmet: Food That Tastes "Too Good" to Be "Good for You" over 1,200 Recipes, Vol. 1. Sam Miles. 1997. 422p. 49.95 (*0-9641843-0-3*) Wellness.

Gulf War & Mental Health: A Comprehensive Guide. Ed. by James A. Martin et al. 1996. LC 96-2200. 232p. 60.00 (*0-275-95631-8*, Praeger Pubs) Greenwood.

Gulf War Illnesses: Improved Monitoring of Clinical Progress & Reexamination of Research Emphasis Are Needed. Sushil K. Sharma. 1998. (Illus.). 140p. (C). pap. text 35.00 (*0-7881-4189-9*) DIANE Pub.

E F G

Gulf War Syndrome: To Examine New Studies Suggesting Links Between Gulf Service & Higher Rates of Illnesses. Ed. by Christopher Shays. 1998. (Illus.). 332p. (C). pap. text 50.00 (*0-7881-7083-X*) DIANE Pub.

Gulls & Plovers: The Ecology of Mixed-Species Feeding Groups. C. J. Barnard & D. B. Thompson. 1985. LC 85-12581. 320p. text 62.50 (*0-231-06262-1*) Col U Pr.

Gunshot Wounds: Practical Aspects of Firearms, Ballistics, & Forensic Techniques. Vincent J. Di Maio. 1992. LC 93-13497. 352p. reprint ed. 78.95 (*0-8493-9504-6*, RA1121); 2nd ed. 1998. LC 99-187476. 424p. 84.95 (*0-8493-8163-0*) CRC Pr.

Gunshot Wounds: Practical Aspects of Firearms, Ballistics, Evidence & Forensic Techniques. Vincent J. Di Maio. 1985. (Series in Practical Aspects of Criminal & Forensic Investigations: Vol. 3). 454p. 43.00 (*0-444-00928-0*) CRC Pr.

Gunshot Wounds & Other Injuries of Nerves. S. Weir Mitchell et al. 1989. (American Civil War Surgery Ser.: No. 3). 164p. reprint ed. 75.00 (*0-930405-13-7*) Norman SF.

Guru Papers: Masks of Authoritarian Power. Joel Kramer et al. 1993. LC 93-18494. 385p. (Orig.). pap. 16.95 (*1-883319-00-5*) Frog Ltd CA.

Guru, Psychotherapist & Self: A Comparative Study of the Guru-Disciple Relationship & the Jungian Analytic Process. Peter P. Coukoulis. 1977. 96p. 14.00 (*0-87516-222-3*); pap. 8.90 (*0-87516-221-5*) DeVorss.

Gustave Dore's Primer on the Medical Profession. George M. Hall. 1991. (Illus.). 164p. (C). pap. 17.50 (*0-87527-298-3*) Green.

Gut & Liver. Ed. by H. E. Blum et al. 1998. LC 98-146171. (Falk Symposium Ser.). 448p. 225.00 (*0-7923-8736-8*) Kluwer Academic.

Gut & Nutrition: Proceedings of the European Nutritionist, 12th Symposium, Cambridge, July, 1973. European Nutritionists Staff. Ed. by J. C. Somogyi & Ian Macdonald. 1975. (Bibliotheca Nutritio et Dieta Ser.: No. 22). 200p. pap. 62.75 (*3-8055-1738-6*) S Karger.

Gut As a Model in Cell & Molecular Biology. Ed. by F. Halter et al. 1998. LC 98-122774. (Falk Symposium Ser.). 352p. text 191.00 (*0-7923-8726-0*) Kluwer Academic.

Gut-Derived Infectious-Toxic Shock (GITS) A Major Variant of Septic Shock. Ed. by H. Cottier & R. Kraft. 1991. (Current Studies in Hematology & Blood Transfusion: No. 59). (Illus.). x, 370p. 301.00 (*3-8055-5435-4*) S Karger.

Gut Dysfunction in Critically Ill Patients, No. 26. John L. Rombeau & J. Takala. 1996. LC 96-27697. (Update in Intensive Care & Emergency Medicine Ser.). (Illus.). 416p. 139.50 (*3-540-61127-4*) Spr-Verlag.

***Gut Reactions: A Radical New 4-Step Program for Treating Chronic Stomach Distress & Unlocking the Secret to Total Body Wellness.** Raphael Kellman & Carol Colman. 2002. LC 2001-52843. 256p. pap. 14.95 (*0-7679-0736-1*) Broadway BDD.

Gut Regulatory Peptides: Their Role in Health & Disease. Ed. by E. Blazquez. 1988. (Frontiers of Hormone Research Ser.: Vol. 16). (Illus.). viii, 236p. 161.00 (*3-8055-4520-7*) S Karger.

Gutta Podagrica: A Treatise of the Gout, Perused by P. H. Dr. in Physick. 1971. LC 72-25642. (English Experience Ser.: No. 319). reprint ed. 25.00 (*90-221-0319-6*) Walter J Johnson.

Guy Patin & the Medical Profession in Paris in the XVIIth Century. Francis R. Packard. 1970. LC 78-95624. (Illus.). xxii, 344p. reprint ed. 45.00 (*0-678-03759-0*) Kelley.

Guydos Questions Newly Corrected. De Cauliaco Guido. 1968. LC 68-54627. (English Experience Ser.: No. 35). 390p. reprint ed. 50.00 (*90-221-0035-9*) Walter J Johnson.

Guyton Physiology Review. Hall. 2000. (C). pap. text (*0-7216-8307-X*) Saunders.

Gymnastic Skills. Roger Mace & Barry Benn. 1982. (Illus.). 144p. 18.50 (*0-7134-4307-3*) Trafalgar.

Gymnastics & Variations: Index of New Information Including Practices Injury, Theory & Medical Applications. Hugo H. Bronsen. 1995. 145p. 57.60 (*0-7883-0640-5*); pap. 47.50 (*0-7883-0641-3*) ABBE Pubs Assn.

Gyn Akolgische Vitalcytologie in der Praxis see Gynecological Vital Cytology in Practice: An Atlas of Phase-Contrast Microscopy

GYN Exam Handbook. Maria Taylor. 1991. (Orig.). (YA). (gr. 7 up). pap. 129.00 incl. VHS (*1-56304-033-6*) J Stanfield.

Gynaecologic Rapid Revision. Sidney Hirschowitz. 1986. (Illus.). 128p. (C). text 29.95 (*0-409-10366-7*) Buttrwrth-Heinemann.

Gynaecological Oncology. Ed. by Hannah E. Lambert & Peter R. Blake. 1992. (Illus.). 248p. pap. 39.50 (*0-19-262203-X*) OUP.

Gynaecological Oncology: A Guide to Clinical Management. P. Blake. Ed. by H. Lambert & R. Crawford. 1998. (Illus.). 284p. text 79.50 (*0-19-262798-8*) OUP.

Gynaecology. Janice Rymer. 1992. (Colour Guide Ser.). (Illus.). 122p. pap. text 19.95 (*0-443-04513-5*) Harcrt Hlth Sci Grp.

Gynaecology. Ed. by R. W. Shaw et al. 1992. (Illus.). 871p. text (*0-443-04139-3*) Church.

Gynaecology. Janice Rymer et al. 2nd ed. 1997. LC 97-16821. (Colour Guide Ser.). (*0-443-05775-3*) Harcrt Hlth Sci Grp.

Gynaecology. Shaw. 2nd ed. 1997. text 150.00 (*0-443-05231-X*) Saunders.

Gynaecology: Health Care Needs Assessment: The Epidemiologically Based Needs Assessment Reviews, Second Series. Andrew Stevens et al. 1997. LC 97-13353. (*1-85775-226-0*) Radcliffe Med Pr GBR. *Dist:* Balogh.

Gynaecology by Ten Teachers. Ed. by Geoffrey V. P. Chamberlain. 16th ed. 1995. 320p. pap. text (*0-340-57315-5*) E A GBR. *Dist:* OUP.

Gynaecology by Ten Teachers. Ed. by Stuart Campbell & Ash Monga. 17th ed. 2001. LC 2001-273808. (Arnold Publication). (Illus.). 320p. (Orig.). pap. text 35.00 (*0-340-71987-7*) OUP.

Gynaecology Color Guide. Rymer. 2nd ed. 1998. (Illus.). 114p. (C). pap. text (*0-443-05878-4*) Church.

Gynaecology Illustrated. A. D. Govan et al. 3rd ed. 1985. (Illus.). 490p. pap. text (*0-443-03293-9*) Church.

Gynaecology Illustrated. Alasdair D. Govan et al. 4th ed. 1994. LC 93-11193. (Illus.). 502p. pap. text (*0-443-04799-5*) Church.

***Gynaecology Nursing: A Practical Guide.** Elizabeth A. Gangar. 2001. 370p. (*0-443-06202-1*) Church GBR. *Dist:* Saunders.

Gynaekologie. E. Bernoth et al. 1984. (Illus.). 656p. 180.00 (*3-8055-3861-8*) S Karger.

Gynaekologie: Proceedings of the Schweizerische Gesellschaft, Lyon, June 19-21, 1975. Schweizerische Gesellschaft Staff. Ed. by H. Erb. 1976. (Journal: Vol. 15, Suppl. 1). (Illus.). 128p. 35.00 (*3-8055-2313-0*) S Karger.

Gynaekologische Urologie: Journal: Gynaekologische Rundschau, Vol. 31, Suppl. 1. Ed. by J. Eberhard. 1991. (Illus.). iv, 52p. pap. 17.50 (*3-8055-5455-9*) S Karger.

Gynecologic & Obstetric Surgery. David H. Nichols. 1993. (Illus.). 1200p. (C). (gr. 13). text 170.00 (*0-8016-6245-1*, 06245) Mosby Inc.

Gynecologic & Obstetric Surgery. Ed. by David H. Nichols & Daniel L. Clarke-Pearson. 2nd ed. 1999. LC 99-27194. (Illus.). xv, 1248p. (C). text 159.00 (*0-8151-3670-6*, 31391) Mosby Inc.

Gynecologic & Obstetric Urology. Herbert J. Buchsbaum & Joseph D. Schmidt. 3rd ed. 1992. (Illus.). 752p. text 156.00 (*0-7216-3051-0*) Saunders.

Gynecologic & Obstetrical Disorders, Vol. 1. Ed. by W. Dwayne Lawrence & Fadi W. Abdul-Karim. 1998. (Differential Diagnosis in Pathology Ser.). (Illus.). 192p. (*0-89640-304-1*) Igaku-Shoin.

Gynecologic Cancer Surgery. C. Paul Morrow & John P. Curtin. 1995. LC 96-17074. (Illus.). 824p. text (*0-443-08970-1*) Church.

Gynecologic Consideration of the Sexual Act. Denslow Lewis. Ed. by Marc H. Hollender. 1970. 20.00 (*0-87730-002-X*) M & S Pr.

Gynecologic Cytopathology. Ed. by Thomas a. Bonfiglio & Yener S. Erozan. 1996. LC 96-15640. 240p. text 159.00 (*0-397-51501-4*) Lppncott W & W.

Gynecologic Decision Making. Roger P. Smith. 2001. (Illus.). LC 00-49268. viii, 257p. 49.00 (*0-7216-8761-X*); 2nd ed. LC 00-68798. 350p. text 89.00 (*0-7216-8716-4*) Saunders.

Gynecologic Endocrinology. Ed. by Jay J. Gold & John B. Josimovich. 4th ed. 1986. LC 86-22666. (Illus.). 716p. (C). text 180.00 (*0-306-42189-5*, Kluwer Plenum) Kluwer Academic.

Gynecologic Endoscopy: Principles in Practice. Ed. by Michael J. Sammarco et al. 1996. (Illus.). 256p. 75.00 (*0-683-07509-8*) Lppncott W & W.

***Gynecologic Hysteroscopy, Resectoscopy & Endometrial Ablation.** E. Bieber. 2002. 250p. 79.95 (*1-84214-117-1*, Parthenon Pbng) CRC Pr.

Gynecologic, Obstetric & Breast Radiology: A Text & Atlas of Imaging in Women. Amy Thurmond et al. 1996. LC 97-133987. (Illus.). 749p. 245.00 (*0-86542-407-1*) Blackwell Sci.

Gynecologic Oncology. C. Thomas Griffiths. 1996. text (*0-7234-2032-7*) Wolfe Publishing GBR. *Dist:* Mosby Inc.

Gynecologic Oncology. C. Thomas Griffiths & Arlan F. Fuller, Jr. 1983. text 233.00 (*0-89838-555-5*) Kluwer Academic.

Gynecologic Oncology. Ed. by Robert F. Ozols. 1998. LC 97-41948. (Cancer Treatment & Research Ser.). 387p. 365.00 (*0-7923-8070-3*) Kluwer Academic.

Gynecologic Oncology. Ed. by Malcolm Coppleson et al. 2nd ed. 1991. (Illus.). 1052p. text (*0-443-04114-8*) Church.

Gynecologic Oncology: Controversies & New Developments. Ed. by Mace L. Rothenberg. 1994. LC 93-41309. (Cancer Treatment & Research Ser.). 144p. (C). text 169.00 (*0-7923-2634-2*) Kluwer Academic.

Gynecologic Oncology: Current Diagnosis. Hugh M. Shingleton. 1996. (C). text 120.00 (*0-7020-1839-2*) Harcourt.

Gynecologic Oncology: Treatment Rationale & Techniques. B. Greer & Jonathan S. Berek. 1991. (Current Topics Ser.). (Illus.). 320p. (C). (gr. 13). pap. 93.95 (*0-412-04571-0*) Chapman & Hall.

Gynecologic Pathology. Goff. 1998. pap. text 129.00 (*0-8385-3535-6*, Apple Lange Med) McGraw.

Gynecologic Resectoscope. Eric Bieber & F. Loffer. 1995. (Minimally Invasive Gynecology Ser.). (Illus.). 256p. 75.00 (*0-86542-349-0*) Blackwell Sci.

Gynecologic Surgery. Ed. by William J. Mann & Thomas G. Stovall. 1996. LC 96-17726. 884p. text (*0-443-08958-2*) Church.

Gynecologic Surgery. Luis E. Sanz. 2nd ed. 1995. (Illus.). 352p. 125.00 (*0-86542-341-5*) Blackwell Sci.

Gynecologic Ultrasound Course Syllabus. A. C. Fleischer. 1993. (Illus.). pap. (*1-930047-39-8*, GYS) Am Inst Ultrasound.

Gynecological Care Manual for HIV Positive Women. Risa Denenberg. 1993. 173p. (Orig.). pap. 12.95 (*0-929240-58-8*) EMIS.

Gynecological Endocrinology. Ed. by Andrea R. Genazzani et al. 1987. (Illus.). 702p. 95.00 (*1-85070-107-5*, Parthenon Pbng) CRC Pr.

Gynecological Endocrinology & Reproductive Medicine B. Runnebaum & T. Rabe. 1997. LC 96-36079. (Illus.). 1096p. 479.00 (*3-540-60930-X*) Spr-Verlag.

Gynecological Endoscopic Surgery. C. Sutton. 1997. (Illus.). 168p. 55.00 (*0-412-58040-3*) OUP.

Gynecological Endoscopy. Alan G. Gordon & B. Victor Lewis. 1988. LC 65-40132. (Gower Bk.). (Illus.). 200p. (*0-397-44570-9*, GM0042) Gower-Mosby.

Gynecological Endoscopy Manual Series, Set. R. F. Valle et al. 1998. LC 97-23447. (Illus.). 3p. lib. bdg. 253.95 (*1-85070-638-7*, Parthenon Pbng) CRC Pr.

Gynecological Imaging. John C. Anderson. 1998. (C). text (*0-443-05239-5*) Church.

Gynecological Sourcebook. M Sara Rosenthal. 3rd rev. ed. 1999. LC 99-14428. (Illus.). 448p. pap. 21.95 (*0-7373-0086-8*) McGraw-Hill Prof.

Gynecological Sourcebook. M Sara Rosenthal. 1997. LC 94-6010. 480p. 15.00 (*1-56565-634-2*) NTC Contemp Pub Co.

Gynecological Sourcebook: Everything You Need to Know. M Sara Rosenthal. 1995. 480p. pap. 17.00 (*1-56565-331-9*) Lowell Hse.

Gynecological Sourcebook: Everything You Need to Know. M Sara Rosenthal. 1994. 300p. 25.00 (*1-56565-123-5*) Lowell Hse.

Gynecological Symptoms in Primary Care. Robert H. Hammond & Michael McGhee. 1996. LC 95-51671. 160p. (Orig.). pap. 36.95 (*0-86542-679-1*) Blackwell Sci.

Gynecological Vital Cytology in Practice: An Atlas of Phase-Contrast Microscopy. Peter Stoll & Gisela Dallenbach-Hellweg. 2nd rev. ed. 1993. LC 92-48209.Tr. of Gyn Akolgische Vitalcytologie in der Praxis. (Illus.). 126p. 132.00 (*0-387-54515-8*) Spr-Verlag.

***Gynecologist Secrets.** Thomas J. Bader. 3rd ed. 2002. LC 2001-39726. (Secrets Ser.). 375p. pap. 39.95 (*1-56053-475-3*) Hanley & Belfus.

Gynecologist's Second Opinion: The Questions & Answers You Need to Take Charge of Your Health. William Parker et al. 2nd ed. 1996. LC 95-50766. 432p. pap. 13.95 (*0-452-27674-8*, Plume) Dutton Plume.

Gynecology. Ed. by Susan E. Davis. 1995. LC 95-7923. (New York City Resource Guide Ser.). (*0-9643861-0-0*) Wom Hlth Educ.

Gynecology. Trevor P. Dutt. Ed. by Walter Scott. 1996. (Medico-Legal Practitioner Ser.). 300p. (*1-85941-215-7*) Cavendish Pubng GBR. *Dist:* Gaunt.

Gynecology Langdon Parsons & Sheldon C. Sommers. 2nd ed. 1978. LC 75-8184. (Illus.). 1660p. text 180.00 (*0-7216-7081-4*) Saunders.

Gynecology: A Practical Approach. Victor Gomel & Malcolm G. Munro. 1990. 352p. pap. 35.00 (*0-683-03631-9*) Lppncott W & W.

Gynecology: Essentials of Clinical Practice. Thomas H. Green, Jr. 3rd ed. 1977. 32.50 (*0-316-32632-1*, Little Brwn Med Div) Lppncott W & W.

Gynecology: Principles & Practice. Robert W. Kistners & Ryan. 6th ed. 1995. (Illus.). 944p. (C). (gr. 13). text 110.00 (*0-8151-7479-9*, 24380) Mosby Inc.

Gyn/Ecology: The Metaethics of Radical Feminism. Mary Daly. 1990. LC 90-52596. 517p. pap. 19.00 (*0-8070-1413-3*) Beacon Pr.

Gynecology: Well-Woman Care. Ronnie Lichtman & Susan Papera. 1989. (Illus.). 512p. (C). pap. text 94.51 (*0-8385-9682-7*, A9682-4) Appleton & Lange.

Gynecology: Well-Woman Care. Ronnie Lichtman. 2nd ed. 1999. (C). text 84.95 (*0-8385-3514-3*) Appleton & Lange.

Gynecology & Obstetrics: 1999-2000 Edition. Paul D. Chan & Christopher R. Winkle. rev. ed. 1999. (Current Clinical Strategies Ser.). 149p. pap. 30.95 incl. cd-rom (*1-881528-70-7*) Current Clin Strat.

Gynecology & Obstetrics: A Longitudinal Approach. Ed. by Thomas R. Moore et al. 1993. (Illus.). 984p. text (*0-443-08811-X*) Church.

Gynecology & Obstetrics: Loose Leaf: New Page Service, Set. Loose Leaf Reference Services Staff et al. Ed. by Herbert J. Buchsbaum et al. ring bd. 495.00 (*0-06-148008-8*) Lppncott W & W.

Gynecology & Obstetrics. Ed. by Gunther O. Schlag et al. 1994. LC 94-3787. (Fibrin Sealing in Surgical & Nonsurgical Fields Ser.: Vol. 7). (Illus.). 129p. 74.95 (*0-387-58227-4*) Spr-Verlag.

Gynecology & Textuality: Popular Representations of Reproductive Technology. Chloe Diepenbrook. 1998. LC 98-41890. (Garland Studies in American Popular History & Culture). 200p. 50.00 (*0-8153-3222-X*) Garland.

Gynecology for the Primary Care Physician. Thomas G. Stovall & Frank W. Ling. 1999. LC 98-50638. 79.95 (*1-57340-126-9*) Current Med.

Gynecology for the Primary Care Provider. Scott Ransom & Gene McNeeley. Ed. by William Schmitt. 1997. LC 96-37235. (Illus.). 288p. text 49.00 (*0-7216-6433-4*) Saunders.

***Gynecology Highlights 2000-2001.** Stones. 2001. (Fast Facts Ser.). (Illus.). 68p. pap. (*1-899541-89-6*, 1) Health Pr GBR. *Dist:* JAMCO Dist.

Gynecology in Primary Care. Roger P. Smith. 1996. LC 96-13603. (Primary Care Ser.: Vol. 1). 400p. 56.95 (*0-683-07779-1*) Lppncott W & W.

Gynecology in Primary Care: A Step-by-Step Approach. Robert L. Barbieri et al. 1999. LC 99-26450. (Illus.). 100p. pap. 39.95 (*0-89454-032-7*) WebMD.

Gynecology, Obstetrics, & the Female Urinary Tract. 1984. (Medical Ser.). (Illus.). 76p. pap. text 12.95 (*0-935920-16-1*, Ntl Pubs Blck) P-H.

Gynesis: Configurations of Woman & Modernity. Alice Jardine. 1986. LC 84-45806. 288p. (C). pap. 18.95 (*0-8014-9396-X*) Cornell U Pr.

H

H & P: A Nonphysicians Guide to the Medical History & Physical Examination. John H. Dirckx. rev. ed. 1991. 152p. pap. 28.00 (*0-934385-04-1*) Hlth Prof Inst.

H C F A: Three Largest Medicare Overpayment Settlemens Were Improper. Robert H. Hastings. 2000. 55p. (C). pap. text 25.00 (*0-7567-0483-9*) DIANE Pub.

H. I. S. Desk Reference. 1996. 495.00 (*1-57372-065-8*, DR-9701) Solucient.

H. I. S. Desk Reference. 1996. (*1-57372-033-X*) Solucient.

H I V/ AIDS. Janet Heinrich. 2000. (Illus.). 51p. (C). pap. text 25.00 (*0-7567-0491-X*) DIANE Pub.

H. P. Blavatsky & the Secret Doctrine. Max Heindel. Ed. by R. I. Robb. 1991. LC 90-71844. 96p. reprint ed. pap. 6.00 (*0-913510-60-2*) Wizards.

H. Pylori: Techniques for Clinical Diagnosis. Lee. 1995. text 55.00 (*0-7020-1999-2*) Saunders.

H. R. Giger's Biomechanics. H. R. Giger. Tr. by Clara H. Frame from GER. 1990. (Illus.). 96p. 69.50 (*0-9623447-1-0*) Morpheus Intl.

H. R. 956, Drug-Free Communities Act of 1997: Hearing Before the Subcommittee on National Security, International Affairs & Criminal Justice of the Committee on Government Reform & Oversight, House of Representatives, One Hundred Fifth Congress, First Session, on H. R. 956, to Amend the National Narcotics Leadership Act of 1988... to Reduce Substance Abuse among Youth... March 13, 1997. Contrib. by U. S. Congress, House Committee on Government Reform and Oversight, Subcommittee on National Security, International Affairs and Criminal Justice. 1997. LC 98-115570. (*0-16-055425-X*) USGPO.

H. V. O. The Life & Letters of Dr. Henry Vining Ogden, 1857-1931. Leonard Weistrop. 1986. (Illus.). 260p. lib. bdg. 35.00 (*0-9617070-0-3*) Milw Acad Med.

Ha Ha & Aha: The Role of Humor in Psychotherapy. Harold Mosak. 1987. LC 87-70349. viii, 152p. text 23.95 (*0-915202-65-4*) Accel Devel.

Haa Tuwunaagu Yis, for Healing Our Spirit. Ed. by Nora M. Dauenhauer & Richard Dauenhauer. 1990. (Classics of Tlingit Oral Literature Ser.: Vol. II). (Illus.). 664p. pap. 22.50 (*0-295-96850-8*) U of Wash Pr.

Haas Ischaemic Heart Disease. 1970. text 155.50 (*90-6021-012-3*) Kluwer Academic.

Habermas, Critical Theory & Health. Graham Scambler. 2001. LC 00-51776. pap. 85.00 (*0-415-19181-5*) Routledge.

Habermas, Critical Theory & Health. Ed. by Graham Scambler. 2001. LC 00-51776. pap. 25.95 (*0-415-19182-3*) Routledge.

Habilidades de Capacitacion Clinica para Professionales en Salud Reproduction. Rick Sullivan et al. 2nd ed. 1999. (SPA., Illus.). pap. text 15.00 (*0-929817-71-0*) JHPIEGO.

Habilidades de Treinamento Clinico para Professionais de Saude em Saude Reprodutiva. Rick Sullivan et al. 1996. (POR.). 208p. pap. text 15.00 (*0-929817-28-1*) JHPIEGO.

Habilitation Planning for Adults with Disabilities. Robert L. Schalock et al. Ed. by R. L. Taylor & L. Sternberg. 1990. (Disorders of Human Learning, Behavior, & Communication Ser.). (Illus.). 233p. 86.95 (*0-387-97209-9*) Spr-Verlag.

Habit & Instinct. Conwy L. Morgan. 361p. 100.00 (*1-85506-684-X*) Thoemmes Pr.

Habit & Instinct. C. Lloyd Morgan. 1977. LC 73-2978. (Classics in Psychology Ser.). reprint ed. 25.95 (*0-405-05150-6*) Ayer.

Habits: Their Making & Unmaking. Knight Dunlap. 1949. LC 77-184102. 336p. pap. 3.95 (*0-87140-267-X*) Liveright.

H I

Habits & Virtues: A Philosophical Analysis. George P. Klubertanz. 1965. LC 65-23606. 46.50 (*0-89197-196-3*) Irvington.

Habits Not Diets: The Secret to Lifetime Weight Control. James M. Ferguson & Cassandra Ferguson. 3rd rev. ed. 1997. LC 97-25169. (Illus.). 350p. pap. 18.95 (*0-923521-41-0*) Bull Pub.

***Habits of Mind: The Power & Limits of Rational Thought.** Laszlo Mero. 2001. (Illus.). 320p. 27.50 (*0-387-95077-X*) Spr-Verlag.

Habits That Handicap: The Menace of Opium, Alcohol, & Tobacco, & the Remedy. Charles B. Towns. Ed. by Gerald N. Grob. 1981. LC 80-1249. (Addiction in America Ser.). reprint ed. lib. bdg. 29.95 (*0-405-13619-6*) Ayer.

Habitual Physical Activity & Health. K. Lange Andersen et al. 1978. (WHO Regional Publications, European Ser.: No. 6). 188p. 25.00 (*92-9020-106-1*, 1310006) World Health.

Hadrontherapy in Oncology: Proceedings of the First International Symposium on Hadrontherapy, Como, Italy, October 1993. Ed. by Ugo Amaldi & Borje Larrson. 1994. LC 94-36767. (International Congress Ser.: No. 1077). 782p. 314.00 (*0-444-81918-5*) Elsevier.

Haematological Pathology. Newland. 1998. (C). text 150.00 (*0-443-04792-8*) Saunders.

Haematology. David Linch & A. P. Yates. 1986. LC 85-16585. (Colour Aids Ser.). (Illus.). 124p. (Orig.). (C). pap. (*0-443-02842-7*) Church.

Haematology. Chris Pallister. 1999. LC 99-13003. 272p. pap. (*0-7506-2457-4*) E A GBR. *Dist:* OUP.

Haematology: An Illustrated Colour Text. Martin R. Howard & Peter J. Hamilton. 1997. LC 97-3872. pap. text (*0-443-05276-X*) Church.

Haematology at a Glance. A. Victor Hoffbrand & Atul B. Mehta. 2000. LC 99-40674. (At a Glance Ser.). (Illus.). 122p. pap. 24.95 (*0-632-04793-3*) Blackwell Sci.

Haematology for MRCP. Galvani. 1995. pap. text 32.00 (*0-7020-1883-X*) Saunders.

Haematology in the Newborn. 1997. 250p. text 33.00 (*1-86094-049-8*) World Scientific Pub.

Haematology in the Newborn. I. A. Roberts & N. A. Murray. 1997. 250p. 48.00 (*981-02-3098-2*) World Scientific Pub.

Haematology Practical Laboratory. O. W. Van Assendelft. 2000. (Illus.). 256p. (*0-7506-3414-6*) E A GBR. *Dist:* OUP.

Haematopoietic Growth Factors: Biology & Clinical Use - Journal: Acta Haematologica, Vol. 86, No. 3, 1991. Ed. by E. E. Polli. 1992. (Illus.). 52p. pap. 57.50 (*3-8055-5557-1*) S Karger.

Haematopoietic System. Ed. by Ulrich Mohr et al. 1994. LC 93-178961. (Illus.). 40p. pap. text 30.00 (*92-832-0124-8*) OUP.

Haemodialysis. Ed. by Graeme R. Catto. 1989. (New Clinical Applications in Nephrology Ser.). (C). text 95.50 (*0-7462-0100-1*) Kluwer Academic.

Haemodynamic Effects of Nitric Oxide. Ed. by Robert T. Mathie & Tudor M. Griffith. 1998. 400p. (*1-86094-081-1*) Imperial College GBR. *Dist:* World Scientific Pub.

Haemodynamic Monitoring of the Critical Care Patient: A Practical Handbook. C. A. Dillon et al. 1996. (Illus.). 100p. (Orig.). pap. text (*1-85996-230-0*) Bios Sci GBR. *Dist:* Bks Intl VA.

Haemoglobin: Research & Applications. Ed. by A. D. Stephens. 1987. (Acta Haematologica Ser.: Vol. 78, No. 2-3). (Illus.). 160p. pap. 100.00 (*3-8055-4679-3*) S Karger.

Haemoglobinopathies & Allied Disorders: Report of a WHO Scientific Group, 1996. WHO Staff. 1966. (Technical Report Ser.: No. 38). 40p. 5.00 (*92-4-120338-2*) World Health.

Haemoglobinopathy Diagnosis. Barbara J. Bain. 2001. LC 00-34309. (Illus.). 240p. 99.00 (*0-632-05577-4*) Blackwell Sci.

Haemolytic Anaemias Vol. 4: Secondary or Symptomatic Haemolytic Anaemias, Vol. 4. John Vivian Dacie. 3rd ed. 1995. 434p. text (*0-443-03503-2*, 68660) Church.

Haemolytic Anaemias - Three: The Haemolytic Anemicas of Immune Origin. John Vivian Dacie. 3rd ed. 1992. (Illus.). 528p. text (*0-443-03502-4*) Church.

Haemolytic Anemias, Vol. 5. Dacie. 3rd ed. 1999. (C). text (*0-443-06269-2*) Church.

Haemophiliac in the Eighties. Ed. by H. Egli & M. J. Inwood. 1981. (Haemostasis Ser.: Vol. 10, Suppl. 1,1981). (Illus.). xii, 310p. pap. 83.50 (*3-8055-2885-X*) S Karger.

Haemophilus, Actinobacillus & Pasteurella: Proceedings of the Third International Conference Held in Edinburgh, Scotland, July 31-August 4, 1994. Ed. by W. Donachie et al. 1995. LC 95-35588. (Illus.). 254p. 95.00 (*0-306-45104-2*, Plenum Trade) Perseus Pubng.

Haemostasis & Thrombosis. Ed. by Arthur L. Bloom & Duncan P. Thomas. 2nd ed. 1987. (Illus.). 1040p. (*0-443-03190-8*) Church.

Haemostasis & Thrombosis Ed. by Arthur L. Bloom et al. 3rd ed. 1993. LC 93-10621. (Illus.). 1152p. text (*0-443-04521-6*) Church.

Haemostasis & Thrombosis Abstracts: New Developments in Hemostaseology. Ed. by H. K. Breddin et al. 1988. (Journal: Vol. 18, Suppl. 2, 1988). (Illus.). iv, 196p. pap. 59.25 (*3-8055-4796-X*) S Karger.

Haemostasis & Thrombosis in Obstetrics & Gynaecology. Ed. by Greer et al. 1991. LC 95-24612. (Illus.). 592p. (C). (gr. 13). pap. 209.95 (*0-412-30920-3*) Chapman & Hall.

Haemostasis & Thrombosis in Obstetrics & Gynaecology. Ed. by I. A. Greer et al. 1992. (Illus.). 592p. 109.95 (*0-442-31560-0*) Chapman & Hall.

Haemostasis in Cerebrospinal Fluid. P. Hindersin et al. 1985. (Acta Neurochirurgica Ser.: Supplementum 34). (Illus.). 100p. 43.95 (*0-387-81839-1*) Spr-Verlag.

Haemostatic Drugs. Marc Verstraete. 1977. pap. text 85.50 (*90-247-2020-6*) Kluwer Academic.

Haemotological Effect of Systemic Diseases. Delamore. 1990. text 133.00 (*0-7020-1408-7*) Saunders.

Hagan & Bruner's Microbiology & Infectious Diseases of Domestic Animals. John F. Timoney et al. 8th ed. 1988. LC 87-47848. (Illus.). 912p. 69.50 (*0-8014-1896-8*) Cornell U Pr.

Hague Workshop: Short-Term Dynamic Psychotherapy, II. Ed. by J. H. Van Birglen & J. Y. Hartzuiker. 1981. (Journal: Vol. 35, No. 4). (Illus.). 64p. pap. 34.00 (*3-8055-3449-3*) S Karger.

Haimovici's Vascular Surgery. Ed. by Henry Haimovici et al. 3rd ed. 1992. (Illus.). 1080p. (C). pap. text 225.00 (*0-8385-9382-8*, A9382-1, Apple Lange Med) McGraw.

Haimovici's Vascular Surgery. Henry Haimovici et al. 4th ed. 1995. LC 95-32072. 1600p. 262.95 (*0-86542-344-X*) Blackwell Sci.

Haines & Taylor Obstetrical & Gynaecological Pathology H. Fox. 4th ed. 1995. text (*0-443-04537-2*, F0267) Church.

Hair & Hair Diseases. Ed. by C. E. Orfanos & R. Happle. 1990. (Illus.). 1057p. 318.00 (*0-387-50960-7*) Spr-Verlag.

Hair & Scalp Disorders: Common Presenting Signs, Differential Diagnosis & Treatment. Rodney Dawber & Dominique Van Neste. 1995. (Illus.). 208p. text 95.00 (*0-397-51421-2*) Lppncott W & W.

Hair Cell Micromechanics & Hearing. Ed. by Charles I. Berlin & Richard P. Bobbin. 2000. LC 00-61212. 160p. pap. 57.50 net. (*0-7693-0125-8*) Singular Publishing.

Hair, or, the Ligurinus Shock: On a Narcissistic Crisis in Puberty & Its Recurrence in the Man of Fifty. Gunter Mecke. 1975. LC 74-82753. 10.00 (*0-87212-044-9*) Libra.

Hair Replacement: Surgical & Medical. Ed. by Dow B. Stough & Robert S. Haber. 1995. (Illus.). 688p. (C). (gr. 13). text 210.00 (*0-8151-7543-4*, 24432) Mosby Inc.

Hair Replacement Surgery: Micrografts & Flaps. C. O. Uebel. 2000. (Illus.). 376p. 185.00 (*0-387-98693-6*) Spr-Verlag.

Hair Replacement Surgery: Textbook & Atlas, Vol. VIII. F. Bouhanna et al. 1996. LC 95-31817. (Hair Replacement Surgery Ser.: Vol. VIII). (Illus.). 236p. 165.00 (*3-540-59030-7*) Spr-Verlag.

Hair Research. Ed. by U. Blume. 1993. (Journal: Vol. 7, No. 1-2, 1994). (Illus.). 108p. pap. 94.00 (*3-8055-5858-9*) S Karger.

Hair Structure & Chemistry Simplified. A. H. Powitt. 1977. (Illus.). 320p. (gr. 9-12). pap. 31.95 (*0-87350-080-6*) Milady Pub.

Hair Transplant Surgery. O'Tar T. Norwood & Richard C. Shiell. 2nd ed. 1984. (Illus.). 356p. (C). 83.95 (*0-398-04946-7*) C C Thomas.

Hairy Cell Leukemia. J. Burthem & J. C. Cawley. 1996. (Illus.). 128p. 125.00 (*3-540-76028-8*) Spr-Verlag.

Haitian Creole (Kreyol) - English Pocket Medical Translator. Marcus Harding. 1996. (CRP.). 128p. (Orig.). pap. 9.95 (*0-9649425-1-8*) Intl Med Volntrs.

Halacha & Medicine Today. Mordechai Koenigsberg. 1997. 19.95 (*0-87306-796-7*) Feldheim.

Halcion: An Independent Assessment of Safety & Efficacy Data. Institute of Medicine Staff. 1997. LC 98-119250. 176p. (C). pap. text 36.00 (*0-309-05976-3*) Natl Acad Pr.

Hale Clinic Guide to Good Health: How to Choose the Right Complementary Therapy. Teresa Hale. 1998. LC 97-7942. (Illus.). 256p. 34.95 (*0-87951-805-7*) Overlook Pr.

Half Century of Public Health: Jubilee Historical Volume of the American Public Health Association in Commemoration of the Fiftieth Anniversary Celebration of Its Foundation, New York City, Vol. 14. Ed. by Mazyck P. Ravenel. 1976. LC 74-112569. (Rise of Urban America Ser.). (Illus.). reprint ed. 35.95 (*0-405-02472-X*) Ayer.

Half Century with Juvenile Delinquents: Or, the New York House of Refuge & Its Times. Bradford K. Peirce. 1969. LC 69-16242. (Criminology, Law Enforcement, & Social Problems Ser.: No. 91). (Illus.). reprint ed. 25.00 (*0-87585-091-X*) Patterson Smith.

Halfway House Movement: A Search for Sanity. Harold L. Raush & Charlotte L. Raush. 1968. LC 68-18037. (Century Psychology Ser.). (C). 30.50 (*0-89197-197-1*) Irvington.

***Halgin Abnormal Psychology: Mind Map.** 3rd ed. 2000. 78.44 incl. cd-rom (*0-07-241171-6*) McGrw-H Hghr Educ.

Hall & Colman's Diseases of the Ear, Nose & Throat. Martin N. Burton et al. 15th ed. 1999. LC 99-23406. 224p. (*0-443-06190-4*) Church.

Hall Jackson & the Purple Foxglove: Medical Practice & Research in Revolutionary America, 1760-1820. J. Worth Estes. 1979. LC 79-63083. (Illus.). xvii, 291p. 20.00 (*0-88135-173-3*, Sci Hist) Watson Pub Intl.

Hallas' the Care of People with Intellectual Disabilities. Charles H. Hallas et al. 9th ed. 1998. LC 97-26657. 320p. pap. (*0-7506-2653-4*) E A GBR. *Dist:* OUP.

Hallucinations. Manfred Spitzer. 1991. (Psychiatry Ser.). 600p. 65.00 (*0-471-53072-7*) Wiley.

Hallucinations. Alexandre-Jacques-Francois Brierre De Boismont. 1976. LC 75-16689. (Classics in Psychiatry Ser.). reprint ed. 48.95 (*0-405-07419-0*) Ayer.

Hallucinations in Clinical Psychiatry: A Guide for Mental Health Professionals. Ghazi Asaad. 1990. LC 90-2125. (Clinical Psychiatry Monographs: No. 2). 160p. text 29.95 (*0-87630-592-3*) Brunner-Routledge.

Hallucinogens & Culture. Peter T. Furst. 1976. LC 75-25442. (Cross-Cultural Themes Ser.). (Illus.). 208p. pap. text 14.95 (*0-88316-517-1*) Chandler & Sharp.

Hallux Valgus & Forefoot Surgery. Vincent J. Hetherington. 1994. (Illus.). text (*0-443-08775-X*) Church.

Halo in the Sky: Observations on Anality & Defense. Leonard Shengold. 1992. 208p. (C). reprint ed. pap. 18.00 (*0-300-05710-5*) Yale U Pr.

Halstead-Reitan Neuropsychological Test Battery: Theory & Clinical Interpretation. Ralph M. Reitan & Deborah Wolfson. 1985. LC 85-71561. 486p. tchr. ed. (*0-934515-04-2*); text 39.95 (*0-934515-02-6*) Neuropsych Pr.

Haltungsschwaeche, Lungenfunktion, & Freizeitverhalten bei Schulkindern. B. N. Trost. 1976. (Sozialmedizinische und Paedagogische Jugendkunde Ser.: Band 13). 17.50 (*3-8055-2359-9*) S Karger.

Hamburg Short Psychotherapy Comparison Experiment. Ed. by A.E. Meyer. 1981. (Psychotherapy & Psychosomatics Ser.: Vol. 35, Nos. 2-3, 1981). (Illus.). 136p. 34.00 (*3-8055-3435-3*) S Karger.

Hamilton & Hardy's Industrial Toxicology. Stoeckle. 1991. (*0-8151-8341-0*) Mosby Inc.

Hamilton & Whitney's Nutrition: Concepts & Controversies. Frances S. Sizer & Eleanor N. Whitney. Ed. by Marshall. 6th ed. 1993. LC 93-33543. 550p. (C). mass mkt. 45.75 (*0-314-02692-4*) West Pub.

Hamilton & Whitney's Nutrition: Concepts & Controversies. Sizer & Whitney. 7th ed. 1997. 600p. pap. (*0-314-20336-2*) West Pub.

Hamilton Bailey's Demonstrations of Physical Signs: Picture Tests. J. S. P. Lumley. 2000. LC 99-30121. (Illus.). 208p. pap. (*0-7506-4339-0*) E A GBR. *Dist:* OUP.

Hamilton Bailey's Emergency Surgery. Ed. by Brian W. Ellis & Simon Paterson-Brown. 12th ed. 1995. LC 94-32582. (Illus.). 866p. text 210.00 (*0-7506-1484-6*) Buttrwrth-Heinemann.

Hamilton Bailey's Emergency Surgery. Brian W. Ellis & Simon Paterson-Brown. 12th ed. 2000. (Illus.). 880p. text (*0-7506-4253-X*) E A GBR. *Dist:* OUP.

Hamilton Bailey's Physical Signs: Demonstration of Physical Signs in Clinical Surgery. Hamilton Bailey's. Ed. by John S. P. Lumley. 18th ed. 1997. (An Arnold Publication). (Illus.). 528p. pap. (*0-7506-1621-0*) E A GBR. *Dist:* OUP.

Hamlyn Encyclopedia of Family Health: Diagnosis & Treatments for More Than 2000 Ailments, Using Orthodox & Complimentary Medicine. Michael Apple. 2000. LC 00-690791. (Illus.). 384p. (*0-600-59254-5*) Hamlyn Pub GBR. *Dist:* Sterling.

Hamster: Reproduction & Behavior. H. I. Siegel. 1985. LC 84-24860. (Illus.). 458p. (C). text 115.00 (*0-306-41791-X*, Kluwer Plenum) Kluwer Academic.

Hand. Ed. by James W. Strickland. 1997. LC 97-20951. (Master Techniques in Orthopaedic Surgery Ser.). 608p. text 199.00 (*0-7817-0038-8*) Lppncott W & W.

Hand, Vol. III. Raoul Tubiana. 1988. (Illus.). 1296p. text 379.00 (*0-7216-8909-4*) Saunders.

Hand, Vol. 4. Ed. by Raoul Tubiana. 1993. (Illus.). 960p. text 350.00 (*0-7216-8910-8*) Saunders.

Hand, Vol. V. Ed. by Raoul Tubiana & Richard Lampert. 5th ed. 1999. (Illus.). 1076p. (C). text 379.00 (*0-7216-5915-2*) Saunders.

Hand: Examination & Diagnosis. American Society for Surgery of the Hand Staff. 3rd ed. 1990. (Illus.). 136p. pap. text (*0-443-08715-6*) Church.

Hand: Fundamentals of Therapy. Judith Boscheinen-Morrin et al. 3rd ed. 2001. LC 00-51928. (Illus.). 243p. pap. text 54.99 (*0-7506-4577-6*) Buttrwrth-Heinemann.

Hand: How Its Use Shapes the Brain, Language & Human Culture. Frank R. Wilson. 1998. LC 97-46427. (Illus.). 396p. 30.00 (*0-679-41249-2*) Pantheon.

Hand: MRI Atlas. Trager. 2000. text (*0-7216-5670-6*) Saunders.

Hand: Primary Care of Common Problems. American Society for Surgery of the Hand Staff. 2nd ed. 1990. (Illus.). 173p. pap. text (*0-443-08584-6*) Church.

Hand: Techniques in Reconstruction. G. Lister. 1998. (Illus.). 400p. (*0-443-04544-5*) Church.

Hand & Foot Reflexology. Kevin Kunz & Barbara Kunz. 1984. 224p. pap. 14.00 (*0-671-76319-9*, Fireside) S&S Trade Pap.

Hand & Wrist Injuries. Akelman. 2000. 270p. Price not set. (*0-7216-6966-2*) Saunders.

Hand & Wrist Pain. John P. Adams et al. 1987. (Illus.). 523p. 85.00 (*0-87473-302-2*, 62010-10, MICHIE) LEXIS Pub.

Hand-Arm Vibration: A Comprehensive Guide for Occupational Health Professionals. Ed. by P. L. Pelmear & D. E. Wasserman. 2nd ed. 1998. LC 98-66605. 272p. text 80.00 (*1-883595-22-3*, 23049, OEM Pr) OEM Health.

Hand-Book of Hygienic Practice Intended As a Practical Guide for the Sick-Room (1864) R. T. Trall. 1996. 300p. reprint ed. pap. 24.95 (*1-56459-807-1*) Kessinger Pub.

Hand Book of Ophthalmology. G. N. Seal. 2nd ed. 1981. 313p. (*0-7855-0732-9*) Current Dist IND. *Dist:* St Mut.

Hand, Diagnosis & Indications. Graham Lister. 3rd ed. 1993. LC 92-49326. 593p. text (*0-443-04545-3*) Church.

Hand Eczema. Ed. by Torkil Menne & Howard I. Maibach. 1993. LC 93-19124. (Series in Dermatology: Clinical & Basic Science). 352p. 141.95 (*0-8493-7355-7*, RL251) CRC Pr.

Hand Eczema. Torkil Menne & Howard I. Maibach. 2nd ed. 2000. (Dermatology: Clinical & Basic Science Ser.). 448p. 99.95 (*0-8493-7362-X*) CRC Pr.

Hand Fractures. Alan E. Freeland. 2000. LC 00-22469. 100p. (C). text (*0-443-07419-4*) Saunders.

Hand in Hand: A Trainer's Manual. Jeanne G. Prickett et al. 1995. LC 95-8265. pap., tchr. ed. 29.95 (*0-89128-940-2*) Am Foun Blind.

Hand in Hand: Selected Reprints on Working with Students Who Are Deaf-Blind. Therese R. Welch et al. Ed. by Kathleen M. Huebner. 1995. LC 94-32864. pap. 29.95 (*0-89128-938-0*) Am Foun Blind.

Hand Injuries: A Therapeutic Approach. Maureen I. Salter. 1987. LC 87-756. (Illus.). 214p. (Orig.). pap. text (*0-443-02984-9*) Church.

Hand Injuries in Athletes. Strickland & Rettig. 1991. (Illus.). 288p. text 92.00 (*0-7216-2779-X*) Saunders.

Hand Pain & Impairment. Rene Cailliet. 4th ed. 1994. LC 93-46466. (Pain Ser.). (Illus.). 311p. pap. 24.95 (*0-8036-1619-8*) Davis Co.

Hand Recovery after Stroke: Exercises & Results Measurements. Johannes G. Smits & Else Boone-Smits. 2000. (Illus.). 176p. pap. text 29.99 (*0-7506-7272-2*) Buttrwrth-Heinemann.

Hand Reflexology. Jungen Kaiser. 2000. LC 00-28507. (Illus.). 192p. pap. 14.95 (*0-8069-5535-X*) Sterling.

Hand Reflexology Instructor Manual. Barbara Kunz & Kevin Kunz. 1999. (Illus.). 202p. pap. (*0-9606070-5-6*) Reflex Res Proj.

Hand Reflexology Workbook. Kevin Kunz & Barbara Kunz. 1995. (Illus.). pap. 10.95 (*0-9606070-2-1*) Reflex Res Proj.

Hand Reflexology Workbook. Barbara Kunz & Kevin Kunz. rev. ed. 2001. (Illus.). 208p. per. 9.95 (*0-9606070-4-8*) Reflex Res Proj.

Hand Rehabilitation. Ed. by Christine A. Moran. 1986. (Clinics in Physical Therapy Ser.: Vol. 9). (Illus.). 232p. text (*0-443-08353-3*) Church.

Hand Rehabilitation: A Practical Guide. Ed. by Gaylord L. Clark. 2nd ed. 1996. LC 96-48429. pap. text (*0-443-07642-1*) Church.

Hand Rehabilitation: A Quick Reference Guide & Review. Nancy Falkenstein. 1999. LC 98-44802. (Illus.). (*0-323-00251-X*) Mosby Inc.

Hand Rehabilitation in Occupational Therapy. Ed. by Florence S. Cromwell & Jane Bear-Lehman. 1988. LC 87-32518. (Occupational Therapy in Health Care Ser.: Vol. 4, Nos. 3 & 4). (Illus.). 194p. text 49.95 (*0-86656-698-8*) Haworth Pr.

Hand Secrets: Questions You Will Be Asked, on Rounds, in the Clinic, on Oral Exams. Peter J. Jebson & Morton L. Kasdan. 1998. LC 97-46650. 275p. pap. 39.95 (*1-56053-217-3*) Hanley & Belfus.

Hand Splinting: Principles & Methods. Elaine Fess & Philips. 2nd ed. 1987. (Illus.). 608p. (C). (gr. 13). text 63.95 (*0-8016-1578-X*, 01578) Mosby Inc.

Hand Splinting: Principles & Methods. Elaine Fess et al. 3rd ed. 2000. (Illus.). 675p. (C). (gr. 13). text 65.00 (*0-8016-7522-7*, 07522) Mosby Inc.

Hand Surgery. Roger A. Daley. 2000. (Vademecum Ser.). spiral bd. 45.00 (*1-57059-573-9*) Landes Bioscience.

***Hand Surgery.** John Ford & Jones. 2001. text 149.95 (*0-7234-2644-9*) Mosby Inc.

Hand Surgery: A Clinical Atlas. Vincent R. Hentz & Robert A. Chase. 1999. LC 2001-20951. (Illus.). x, 852p. text (*0-7216-5532-7*) Saunders.

Hand Surgery - A Current Concepts Review: Proceedings of the Frankfurt International Hand Surgery Conference, November, 1996. Ed. by S. Rehart & R. Zichner. rev. ed. 1997. (Illus.). 100p. pap. 55.00 (*0-86577-723-3*) Thieme Med Pubs.

Hand Surgery Board Review. Anthony A. Smith & Stephen H. Lacey. 1996. (Illus.). 260p. (C). (gr. 13). text 69.95 (*0-8151-7872-7*, 25276) Mosby Inc.

Hand Surgery Review. Roy A. Meals. 4th ed. 1995. 153p. pap. text 28.95 (*0-942219-82-1*) Quality Med Pub.

Hand Surgery Study Guide. Steven F. Viegas. 1996. LC 96-13742. (Illus.). 179p. 68.00 (*0-387-94749-3*) Spr-Verlag.

Hand Surgery Update. Ed. by American Society for Surgery of the Hand Staff. 1996. (Illus.). 454p. pap. 50.00 (*0-89203-150-6*) Amer Acad Ortho Surg.

Hand Surgery Update 2. American Society for Surgery of the Hand Staff. Ed. by Terry R. Light. 2nd ed. 1999. LC 99-42929. 444p. pap. 115.00 (*0-89203-233-2*) Amer Acad Ortho Surg.

Hand Trembling, Frenzy Witchcraft, & Moth Madness: A Study of Navajo Seizure Disorders. Jerrold Levy et al. 1995. LC 87-19445. 196p. pap. 18.95 (*0-8165-1572-7*) U of Ariz Pr.

Handbook: Living Life's Emergencies. Patrick LaValla. 1981. (Illus.). 72p. pap. 4.00 (*0-913724-25-4*) Emerg Response Inst.

Handbook & Atlas of Gastrointestinal Exfoliative Cytology. Joao C. Prolla & Joseph B. Kirsner. 1994. LC 72-80621. (Illus.). 152p. (C). lib. bdg. 25.00 (*0-226-68451-2*) U Ch Pr.

Handbook Antibiotic Compounds. Janos Berdy. 1981. (CRC Handbook of Antibiotic Compounds Ser.: Vol. 5). 576p. 307.00 (*0-8493-3456-X*, QV350, CRC Reprint) Franklin.

Handbook Antibiotic Compounds. Ed. by Janos Berdy. 1985. Vol. XI, Pt. I. 704p. lib. bdg. 271.00 (*0-8493-3463-2*, QV250); Vol. XI, Pt. II. 408p. lib. bdg. 242.00 (*0-8493-3464-0*) Franklin (CRC Reprint).

Handbook Comparative Pharmacokinetics & Residues: Pesticides & Environmental Contaminants - Animals. Jim Edmond Riviere. 1995. 592p. 224.95 (*0-8493-3213-3*) CRC Pr.

Handbook for Action Research in Health & Social Care. Richard Winter & Carol Munn-Giddings. 2001. LC 00-47058. (Illus.). 280p. pap. 25.95 (*0-415-22484-5*) Routledge.

***Handbook for Action Research in Health & Social Care.** Richard Winter & Carol Munn-Giddings. 2001. LC 00-47058. (Illus.). 304p. (C). (gr. 13). lib. bdg. 85.00 (*0-415-22483-7*) Routledge.

Handbook for Anesthesia & Co-Existing Disease. Robert K. Stoelting & Stephen F. Dierdorf. 1993. (Illus.). 424p. pap. text (*0-443-08893-4*) Church.

Handbook for Assessing & Treating Addictive Disorders. Ed. by Chris E. Stout et al. 1992. LC 91-35117. 392p. lib. bdg. 87.50 (*0-313-27634-X*, SGV/, Greenwood Pr) Greenwood.

Handbook for Avoiding Drug Side Effects. Ed. by Solomon Huriash. 2nd ed. 1997. LC 2001-268117. 258p. (Orig.). pap. 9.99 (*0-9618098-1-7*) Land Pub FL.

Handbook for Beginning Medical-Dental Assistants & Receptionists. Carl W. Salser et al. 1988. 260p. (Orig.). pap. 19.95 (*0-89420-258-8*, 422105) Natl Book.

Handbook for Beginning Mental Health Researchers. Peter J. Hauri et al. 1988. LC 87-35377. 148p. text 39.95 (*0-86656-719-4*) Haworth Pr.

Handbook for Clinical Investigators. Christopher T. Kirkpatrick. 1999. 100p. 26.95 (*0-7484-0712-X*) Taylor & Francis.

Handbook for Clinical Teachers. David I. Newble. 1983. 148p. text (*0-85200-728-0*) Kluwer Academic.

Handbook for Communication & Problem Solving: Skills Training: A Cognitive-Behavioral Approach. Jeffrey R. Bedell & Shelley S. Lennox. 1996. LC 96-24667. (Einstein Psychiatry Publication Ser.). 288p. 110.00 (*0-471-08250-3*) Wiley.

Handbook for Computing the Cost of an Hour of Direct Homemaker/HomeCare Aide Service. Eugene B. Shinn. 2nd rev. ed. 1999. (Illus.). vi, 32p. pap. (*1-930304-04-8*) Home Care Univ.

Handbook for Curing the Common Cold: The Zinc Lozenge Story. George A. Eby. 1994. LC 93-90841. (Illus.). 140p. (Orig.). pap. 25.00 (*0-9638967-0-9*) G Eby Research.

Handbook for Data Analysis in the Behavioral Sciences. Ed. by Gideon Keren & Charles Lewis. 1992. 584p. pap. 55.00 (*0-8058-1037-4*); LC 92-49442. 552p. pap. 49.95 (*0-8058-1093-5*); 584p. text 125.00 (*0-8058-1036-6*); LC 92-49442. 552p. text 125.00 (*0-8058-1092-7*);Set. 1136p. pap. 85.00 (*0-8058-1314-4*) L Erlbaum Assocs.

Handbook for Dental Hygienists. W. J. Collins & T. W. Walsh. 3rd ed. 1992. (Illus.). 336p. pap. text 60.00 (*0-7236-0980-2*) Buttrwrth-Heinemann.

Handbook for Dental Hygienists. W. J. Collins. 4th ed. 1999. LC 99-198085. 284p. (*0-7236-1740-6*) John Wright GBR. *Dist:* Buttrwrth-Heinemann.

Handbook for Differential Diagnosis of Infectious Diseases. David L. Schlossberg & Jonas A. Shulman. 2nd ed. 1996. LC 95-4784. (Illus.). 260p. pap. 39.95 (*0-683-07659-0*) Lppncott W & W.

Handbook for Directors of Nursing in Long-Term Care. Ethel L. Mitty. 1997. LC 96-4649. (Professional Reference - Nursing Ser.). 367p. pap. text 33.95 (*0-8273-6777-5*) Delmar.

Handbook for Enhancing Undergraduate Education in Psychology. Ed. by Thomas V. McGovern. 1993. LC 93-7081. 273p. pap. text 19.95 (*1-55798-196-5*) Am Psychol.

Handbook for Family Planning Operations Research Design see Manuel de Recherche Operationnele en Matiere de Planification Familiale

Handbook for Group Discussion Leaders: Alternatives to Lecturing Medical Students to Death. Neal A. Whitman & Thomas L. Schwenk. 1983. 38p. (C). reprint ed. pap. text 10.00 (*0-940193-01-9*) Univ UT Sch Med.

Handbook for Health Directors. C. M. Buttery. 1991. (Illus.). 224p. text 35.00 (*0-19-506449-6*) OUP.

Handbook for Health Records in LTC. Janice Copeland. 1986. 259p. (C). 52.00 (*0-929442-00-8*, 2205pp) Prof Prnting & Pub.

Handbook for Home Care Aide. Ed. by Marcie L. Barnette. 3rd rev. ed. 1999. (Illus.). vii, 135p. pap. (*1-930304-00-5*) Home Care Univ.

Handbook for Housemen. D. Baldwin & K. I. Hopcroft. 2nd ed. 1993. (Illus.). 208p. pap. 29.95 (*0-632-03334-7*) Blackwell Sci.

Handbook for Managing Change in Health Care. Ed. by Chip Caldwell. 1998. LC 97-2861. (Illus.). 735p. 75.00 (*0-87389-403-0*, H0943) ASQ Qual Pr.

Handbook for Medical Teachers. David I. Newble. (C). 2nd ed. 1987. 160p. text 42.50 (*0-85200-673-X*); 3rd ed. 1994. LC 94-22258. (Illus.). 185p. text 42.50 (*0-7923-8850-X*) Kluwer Academic.

Handbook for Pharmacy Educators: Contemporary Teaching Principles & Strategies. Ed. by Noel E. Wilkin. 2000. LC 00-28035. 171p. 39.95 (*0-7890-1005-4*); pap. 24.95 (*0-7890-1006-2*) Haworth Pr (Pharmctl Prods).

Handbook for Prescribing Medications During Pregnancy. Donald R. Coustan & Tara K. Mochizuki. 3rd ed. 1998. LC 98-17363. 528p. pap. text 39.95 (*0-316-15826-7*) Lppncott W & W.

Handbook for Primary Care Options. Amos. 1999. text (*0-7216-5921-7*) Saunders.

Handbook for Sexual Abuser Assessment & Treatment. Ed. by Mark S. Carich & Steven E. Mussack. 2000. LC 00-55375. 249p. pap. 28.00 (*1-884444-58-X*, WP083) Safer Soc.

Handbook for Staging of Cancer: From the Manual For Staging Cancer. Fleming. 5th ed. 1998. 288p. pap. text 45.00 (*0-397-58419-9*) Lppncott W & W.

Handbook for Teaching Introductory Psychology. Ed. by Ludy T. Benjamin et al. 1985. 240p. pap. 27.50 (*0-89859-561-4*) L Erlbaum Assocs.

Handbook for the Assessment of Dissociation: A Clinical Guide. Marlene Stein. 1995. LC 94-24448. 448p. text 56.00 (*0-88048-682-1*, 8682) Am Psychiatric.

Handbook for the Care of Infants, Toddlers & Young Children with Disabilities & Chronic Conditions. Ed. by Marilyn J. Krajicek et al. 1997. LC 96-49479. 488p. tchr. ed., spiral bd. 59.00 (*0-89079-708-0*, 8377) PRO-ED.

Handbook for the Disabled. Susanne Lunt. 1984. (Illus.). 288p. pap. 9.95 (*0-684-18030-8*, Macmillan Ref) Gale.

Handbook for the Hospital Medical Secretary. Joan Griffiths. 1993. LC 93-13007. 256p. pap. 30.95 (*0-632-03584-6*) Blackwell Sci.

Handbook for the Military Surgeon. Charles S. Tripler & George C. Blackman. 1989. (American Civil War Surgery Ser.: No. 7). 121p. reprint ed. 60.00 (*0-930405-06-4*) Norman SF.

***Handbook for the New Health Care Manager.** Donald N. Lombardi. 2nd ed. 2001. LC 2001-637. (Jossey-Bass/AHA Press Ser.). (Illus.). 512p. pap. 55.00 (*0-7879-5560-4*) Jossey-Bass.

Handbook for the New Health Care Manager: Practical Strategies for Challenging Times. Donald N. Lombardi. 1993. LC 93-26300. 484p. pap. 52.00 (*1-55648-109-8*, 001121) AHPI.

Handbook for the Operation & Maintenance of Hospital Medical Waste Incinerators. 1994. (Illus.). 97p. (Orig.). (C). pap. text 35.00 (*1-56806-155-2*) DIANE Pub.

Handbook for the Ophthalmic Practice: Documentation & Record Keeping Made Easy. Pamela J. Miller. 1997. LC 97-20888. 124p. (Orig.). pap. 25.00 (*0-943599-91-1*) OEPF.

Handbook for the Personal Orientation Inventory (POI) Robert R. Knapp. 1990. LC 75-17256. pap. text 23.00 (*0-912736-17-8*) EDITS Pubs.

Handbook for the Recovering Alcoholic-Addict. Mary P. Degroodt. Ed. by Bonnie J. Rayha. 1989. (Illus.). 85p. (Orig.). pap. text 6.95 (*0-9625297-0-2*) Dunbar Bks.

Handbook for the Special Education Administrator: Organization & Procedures for Special Education. Arthur R. Crowell, Jr. 1990. LC 89-48346. (Studies in Education: Vol. 9). 96p. lib. bdg. 49.95 (*0-88946-922-9*) E Mellen.

Handbook for the Study of Mental Health: Social Contexts, Theories, & Systems. Ed. by Allan V. Horwitz & Teresa L. Scheid. 1999. LC 98-11638. (Illus.). 694p. (C). text 85.00 (*0-521-56133-7*) Cambridge U Pr.

Handbook for the Traveling Free-Lance Physician: A Guide for Free-Lancers, Part-time Physicians, & Moonlighters. Gary L. Monroe. Ed. by James Streetman. 1990. LC 90-92170. (Illus.). 154p. 75.00 (*0-9628241-0-0*) Magellan Pub.

Handbook for Treatment of Attachment-Trauma Problems in Children. Beverly James. 1994. LC 94-21395. 290p. 34.95 (*0-02-916005-7*) Free Pr.

Handbook in Zoonoses: Viral Zoonoses, Sect B: Vol. 1. George W. Beran. 1981. 544p. 287.00 (*0-8493-2911-6*, RC113, CRC Reprint) Franklin.

Handbook in Zoonoses: Viral Zoonoses, Sect. B: Vol. 2. Ed. by George W. Beran. 1981. 528p. 275.00 (*0-8493-2912-4*, RC113, CRC Reprint) Franklin.

Handbook in Zoonoses, CRC, Section A: Bacterial, Rickettsial & Mycotic Diseases, Vol. 1. Ed. by Herbert Stoenner. 1979. (Handbook Series in Zoonoses). 672p. 357.00 (*0-8493-2906-X*, RC113, CRC Reprint) Franklin.

Handbook of Abusable Drugs. Kenneth Blum. 1996. pap. text 79.95 (*0-89876-227-8*); (Illus.). 721p. pap. text, suppl. ed. 69.95 (*0-89876-196-4*) Gardner Pr.

Handbook of Acute Critical Care Neurology. Ed. by Robert J. Henning & David L. Jackson. 1985. LC 84-18092. 300p. 72.50 (*0-275-91316-3*, C1316, Praeger Pubs) Greenwood.

Handbook of Adhesives & Sealants. Edward M Petrie. 1999. LC 99-35410. (McGraw-Hill Handbooks). (Illus.). 896p. text 99.95 (*0-07-049888-1*) McGraw-Hill Prof.

Handbook of Adolescent Death & Bereavement. Ed. by Charles A. Corr & David E. Balk. 1996. LC 95-42074. (Illus.). 438p. 52.95 (*0-8261-9240-8*) Springer Pub.

Handbook of Adolescent Health Risk Behavior. Ed. by Ralph J. DiClemente et al. 1996. LC 95-43464. (Clinical Child Psychology Library). (Illus.). 464p. 90.00 (*0-306-45147-6*, Kluwer Plenum) Kluwer Academic.

Handbook of Adolescent Inpatient Psychiatric Treatment. Ed. by Harinder S. Ghuman & Richard M. Sarles. 1994. LC 93-42921. 336p. text 45.95 (*0-87630-731-4*) Brunner-Routledge.

Handbook of Adolescent Psychology. Ed. by Vincent B. Van Hasselt & Michel Hersen. 1987. (General Psychology Ser.: No. 142). 516p. 95.00 (*0-08-031923-8*, J115, Pergamon Pr) Elsevier.

Handbook of Adolescent Psychopathology. Vincent B. Van Hassel. 1995. 49.95 (*0-669-27677-4*) Free Pr.

Handbook of Adult & Pediatric Respiratory Home Care. Joan Turner et al. 1993. (Illus.). 429p. (C). (gr. 13). text 40.95 (*0-8016-5163-8*, 05163) Mosby Inc.

Handbook of Adult Primary Care. Carla Greene. 1989. LC 86-24577. 1117p. text 53.50 (*0-8273-4250-0*) Delmar.

Handbook of Affective Disorders. Ed. by Eugene S. Paykel. 2nd ed. 1992. (Illus.). 700p. text (*0-443-04302-7*) Church.

Handbook of Affective Disorders. Ed. by E. S. Paykel. 2nd ed. 1992. LC 92-1553. 699p. reprint ed. 85.00 (*0-89862-674-9*) Guilford Pubns.

Handbook of African Medicinal Plants. Maurice M. Iwu. 1993. 464p. 189.95 (*0-8493-4266-X*, RS164) CRC Pr.

Handbook of Aggressive & Destructive Behavior in Psychiatric Patients. Ed. by M. Hersen et al. 1994. (Illus.). 550p. (C). 95.00 (*0-306-44549-2*, Plenum Trade) Perseus Pubng.

Handbook of Aging & Mental Health: An Integrative Approach. J. Lomranz. 1998. LC 98-29824. (Series in Adult Development & Aging). (Illus.). 502p. 85.00 (*0-306-45750-4*, Kluwer Plenum) Kluwer Academic.

Handbook of Alcoholism Treatment Approaches: Effective Alternatives. R. K. Hester & W. R. Miller. 1989. (General Psychology Ser.). 344p. text 35.00 (*0-08-036428-4*, Pergamon Pr) Elsevier.

Handbook of Alcoholism Treatment Approaches: Effective Alternatives. Ed. by Reid K. Hester & William R. Miller. 2nd ed. 1995. LC 94-35263. 480p. 74.00 (*0-205-16376-9*, Longwood Div) Allyn.

***Handbook of Allergy & Allergic Diseases.** A. Barry Kay. 2001. (Illus.). 1872p. 99.00 (*0-632-05449-2*) Blackwell Sci.

Handbook of Allergy & Rhinitis. Robert K. Bush. 1997. LC 96-42504. (Illus.). 304p. pap. 38.95 (*0-86542-433-0*) Blackwell Sci.

Handbook of Alternatives to Chemical Medicine. Mildred Jackson & Terri Teague. Ed. by Alexandra Macdonald. 1975. LC 77-155218. (Illus.). pap. 7.95 (*0-932516-01-7*) Lawton-Teague.

Handbook of Alternatives to Chemical Medicine. Mildred Jackson & Terri Teague. 1997. LC 97-11846. (Illus.). 256p. reprint ed. pap. 14.95 (*1-57731-059-4*) New Wrld Lib.

Handbook of Ambulatory Anesthesia. V. M. Khosla. 1991. (*0-8151-5039-3*) Mosby Inc.

Handbook of Ambulatory Cardiology. Victor F. Froelicher & Susan Quaglietti. 1997. LC 96-39468. 416p. pap. text 39.95 (*0-316-29447-0*) Lppncott W & W.

Handbook of American Aging Programs. Ed. by Lorin S. Baumhover & Joan D. Jones. 1977. LC 76-28641. 188p. lib. bdg. 59.00 (*0-8371-9287-0*, BAA/, Greenwood Pr) Greenwood.

Handbook of Amyotrophic Lateral Sclerosis. Ed. by Richard Alan Smith. 1992. (Neurological Disease & Therapy Ser.: Vol. 12). (Illus.). 808p. text 295.00 (*0-8247-8610-6*) Dekker.

Handbook of Anal Endosonography. Clive Bartram & Andrea Frudinger. 1997. LC 97-9522. 128p. pap. (*1-871816-35-1*) Wrightson Biomed GBR. *Dist:* Taylor & Francis.

Handbook of Analytical Derivatization Reactions. Daniel R. Knapp. 1979. LC 78-12944. 768p. 210.00 (*0-471-03469-X*) Wiley.

Handbook of Analytical Therapeutic Drug Monitoring & Toxicology. Steven H. Wong & Irving Sunshine. 1996. LC 96-20670. 368p. 94.95 (*0-8493-2648-6*) CRC Pr.

Handbook of Analytical Toxicology, CRC. Ed. by Irving Sunshine. 1969. LC 69-20046. (Handbook Ser.). 85.00 (*0-8493-3551-5*, RA1221, CRC Reprint) Franklin.

Handbook of Anatomy & Physiology for Students of Medical Radiation Technology. Marshall Mallett. 3rd ed. 1995. (Illus.). 280p. (C). reprint ed. text 30.00 (*0-916973-00-X*) Burnell Co.

Handbook of Anesthetics & Perioper. Ponte. 1994. (Illus.). 412p. pap. text 30.50 (*0-7020-1689-6*) Saunders.

Handbook of Animal Diseases in the Tropics. M. M. Sewell & D. W. Brocklesby. 4th ed. 1990. (Illus.). 397p. (*0-7020-1502-4*) W B Saunders GBR. *Dist:* Saunders.

Handbook of Animal Models for the Rheumatic Diseases Ed. by Robert A. Greenwald & Herbert S. Diamond. 1988. Vol. I. 256p. lib. bdg. 195.00 (*0-8493-2988-4*, RC927); Vol. II. 240p. lib. bdg. 169.00 (*0-8493-2989-2*, RC927) CRC Pr.

Handbook of Animal Models in Transplantation Research. Ed. by Leonard Makowka. 1993. 368p. 250.95 (*0-8493-3629-5*, RD120) CRC Pr.

Handbook of Animal Models of Pulmonary Disease Ed. by Jerome O. Cantor. 1989. Vol. I. 256p. 220.00 (*0-8493-2978-7*, RC756); Vol. II. 264p. 220.00 (*0-8493-2979-5*) CRC Pr.

Handbook of Animal Models of Renal Failure. Ed. by Stephen R. Ash & Jerry A. Thornhill. 1985. 232p. lib. bdg. 203.00 (*0-8493-2975-2*, RC918, CRC Reprint) Franklin.

Handbook of Antibiotic Compounds, Vol. XII. Ed. by Janos Berdy. 1985. 720p. lib. bdg. 271.00 (*0-8493-3465-9*, QV250) CRC Pr.

Handbook of Antibiotic Compounds. Janos Berdy. 1987. Vol. XIV, Pt. 1. 464p. lib. bdg. 200.00 (*0-8493-3435-7*); Vol. XIV, Pt. 2. 344p. lib. bdg. 200.00 (*0-8493-3436-5*) CRC Pr.

Handbook of Antibiotic Compounds. Ed. by Janos Berdy. (Miscellaneous Antibiotics with Unknown Chemical Structure Ser.). Vol. 7. 1981. 272p. 153.00 (*0-8493-3458-6*, QV250); Vol. X. 1982. 560p. 308.00 (*0-8493-3462-4*, QV250) Franklin (CRC Reprint).

Handbook of Antibiotic Compounds: Alicyclic, Aromatic & Aliphatic Antibiotics, Vol. 6. Ed. by Janos Berdy. 1981. (CRC Handbook of Antibiotic Compounds Ser.). 384p. 260.00 (*0-8493-3457-8*, QV250, CRC Reprint) Franklin.

Handbook of Antibiotic Compounds: Antibiotics from Higher Forms of Life: Higher Plants, Vol. VIII, Pt. I. Ed. by Janos Berdy. 1982. 424p. 234.00 (*0-8493-3459-4*, QV250, CRC Reprint) Franklin.

Handbook of Antibiotic Compounds: Antibiotics from Higher Forms of Life: Higher Plants, Vol. VIII, Pt. II. Janos Berdy. 1982. 448p. 244.00 (*0-8493-3460-8*, QV250, CRC Reprint) Franklin.

Handbook of Antibiotic Compounds: Antibiotics from Higher Forms of Life: Lichens, Algae, & Animal Organisms, Vol. IX. Ed. by Janos Berdy. 1982. (CRC Handbook of Antibiotic Compounds Ser.). 248p. 137.00 (*0-8493-3461-6*, QV250, CRC Reprint) Franklin.

Handbook of Antibiotic Compounds: Vol. XIII: Microbial Metabolites, Pts. 1, 2, 3 Ed. by Janos Berdy et al. 1987. 485.00 (*0-8493-3430-6*, RS431) CRC Pr.

Handbook of Antimicrobial Therapy: Revised Edition, 1998. Ed. by Mark Abramowicz. rev. ed. 1998. 209p. 14.00 (*0-9660510-2-5*) Med Letter.

Handbook of Antimicrobial Therapy for Infections of the Eye. Khalid Tabbara & Robert A. Hyndiuk. 1996. 128p. pap. 30.00 (*0-7506-9638-9*) Buttrwrth-Heinemann.

Handbook of Antisocial Behavior. Ed. by Jack D. Maser et al. 1997. LC 96-53445. 600p. 175.00 (*0-471-12452-4*) Wiley.

Handbook of Anxiety Disorders. Ed. by Cynthia G. Last & Michel Hersen. 1988. (General Psychology Ser.: No. 151). 600p. 110.00 (*0-08-032766-4*); 75.00 (*0-08-035564-1*) Elsevier (Pergamon Pr).

Handbook of Applied Dog Behavior & Training Vol. 2: Etiology & Assessment of Behavior Problems. Steven Lindsay. 2001. (Illus.). 304p. 44.95 (*0-8138-2868-6*) Iowa U Pr.

Handbook of Applied Gerontology. Gari Lesnoff-Caravaglia. 1987. LC 86-20811. 460p. 54.95 (*0-89885-314-1*, Kluwer Acad Hman Sci) Kluwer Academic.

Handbook of Applied Mycology Vol. 2: Humans, Animals & Insects. Ed. by Dilip K. Arora et al. 1991. (Illus.). 800p. text 250.00 (*0-8247-8435-9*) Dekker.

Handbook of Applied Mycology Vol. 3: Foods & Feeds. Ed. by Dilip K. Arora et al. 1991. (Illus.). 640p. text 250.00 (*0-8247-8491-X*) Dekker.

Handbook of Applied Mycology Vol. 4: Fungal Biotechnology. Ed. by Dilip K. Arora et al. 1991. (Illus.). 1144p. text 250.00 (*0-8247-8501-0*) Dekker.

Handbook of Applied Psycholinguistics: Major Thrusts of Research & Theory. Ed. by Sheldon Rosenberg. 1982. LC 81-9891. (Illus.). 608p. text 120.00 (*0-89859-173-2*) L Erlbaum Assocs.

Handbook of Applied Therapeutics. Lloyd Y. Young et al. 6th ed. 1996. LC 95-75489. 936p. pap. 50.00 (*0-915486-24-5*) Applied Therapeutics.

Handbook of Art Therapy. Tessa Dalley & Caroline Case. 1992. LC 91-36908. (Illus.). 272p. (C). pap. 31.95 (*0-415-04381-6*, A7102) Routledge.

Handbook of Arterial Blood Gas Interpretation & Ventilator Management. Sharron Daggett. 1999. iii, 69p. pap. 29.95 (*0-970117l-0-8*, 2701) Natl Inst Nurse.

Handbook of Asian American Psychology. Lee C. Lee & Nolan W. Zane. 1998. LC 98-8967. 101.95 (*0-8039-4963-4*, 4537) Sage.

***Handbook of Assessment & Treatment Planning for Psychological Disorders.** Ed. by Martin M. Antony & David H. Barlow. 2001. LC 2001-40518. 589p. 65.00 (*1-57230-703-X*) Guilford Pubns.

Handbook of Assessment in Childhood Psychopathology: Applied Issues in Differential Diagnosis & Treatment Evaluation. C. L. Frame & J. L. Matson. 1987. LC 87-18565. (Applied Clinical Psychology Ser.). (Illus.). 704p. (C). 125.00 (*0-306-42436-3*, Plenum Trade) Perseus Pubng.

Handbook of Assessment Methods for Eating Behaviors & Weight Related Problems: Measures, Theory & Research. Ed. by David B. Allison. 1995. LC 94-33567. 550p. 106.95 (*0-8039-4791-7*, 4207) Sage.

Handbook of Assistive Devices for the Handicapped Elderly: New Help for Independent Living. Joseph M. Breuer. 1982. LC 81-20270. (Physical & Occupational Therapy in Geriatrics Ser.: Vol. 1, No. 2). (Illus.). 77p. text 29.95 (*0-86656-152-8*) Haworth Pr.

Handbook of Assistive Technology. Gregory Church. Ed. by Sharon L. Glennen. 1991. (Illus.). 394p. (Orig.). (C). pap. text 45.00 (*1-879105-53-5*, 0234) Thomson Learn.

Handbook of Atopic Eczema. Ed. by T. Ruzicka et al. 1991. (Illus.). 484p. 185.00 (*0-387-52992-6*) Spr-Verlag.

Handbook of Autism: A Guide for Parents & Professionals. Maureen Aarons & Tessa Gittens. 1991. 144p. (C). pap. 24.99 (*0-415-05566-0*, A5984) Routledge.

Handbook of Autonomic Drugs & Autacoids. Matthew Verderame. 1986. 288p. 149.00 (*0-8493-3289-3*, RM323, CRC Reprint) Franklin.

Handbook of Autonomic Nervous System Dysfunction. Ed. by Amos D. Korczyn. 1995. LC 94-42250. (Neurological Disease & Therapy Ser.: Vol. 38). (Illus.). 560p. text 215.00 (*0-8247-9246-7*) Dekker.

Handbook of Avian Medicine. Glenn H. Olsen & Susan E. Orosz. 1999. (Illus.). 512p. (C). (gr. 13). pap. text 49.95 (*0-8151-8466-2*, 28825) Mosby Inc.

Handbook of Ayurveda. Vaidya B. Dash & Acarya M. Junius. 1983. 221p. (Orig.). text 10.95 (*0-89744-053-6*) Auromere.

Handbook of Ayurveda. Bhagwan Dass. 1988. (C). (*0-7855-2282-4*) Scientific GBR. *Dist:* St Mut.

Handbook of Ayurveda. Shantha Godagama. 1998. (Illus.). 128p. pap. 14.95 (*1-885203-59-4*) Jrny Editions.

Handbook of Ayurvedic Medicinal Plants. Ed. by L. D. Kapoor. 1989. 424p. 330.95 (*0-8493-0559-4*, RS164) CRC Pr.

Handbook of Ayurvedic Medicinal Plants. L. D. Kapoor. 999th ed. 2000. LC 00-49360. (Herbal Reference Library). (Illus.). 416p. 124.95 (*0-8493-2929-9*) CRC Pr.

Handbook of Bacterial Adhesion: Principles, Methods & Applications. Ed. by Yuehuei H. An & Richard J. Friedman. 2000. 672p. 150.00 (*0-89603-794-0*) Humana.

Handbook of Basic Clinical Manipulation. Donald L. McCabe. 1996. LC 95-23661. (Clinical Handbook Ser.). (Illus.). 240p. 49.95 (*1-85070-670-0*, M1439, Parthenon Pbng) CRC Pr.

Handbook of Basic Pharmacokinetics: Including Clinical Applications. Wolfgang A. Ritschel & Gregory L. Kearns. 5th rev. ed. 1998. (Illus.). 563p. pap. text 49.00 (*0-917330-73-0*, T222) Am Pharm Assn.

Handbook of Basic Vascular & Interventional Radiology. Ed. by Raymond B. Dyer. 1992. (Illus.). 275p. text (*0-443-08840-3*) Church.

Handbook of Behavior Modification with the Mentally Retarded. J. L. Matson. 2nd ed. 1990. LC 89-23235. (Applied Clinical Psychology Ser.). (Illus.). 544p. (C). 100.00 (*0-306-43309-5*, Plenum Trade) Perseus Pubng.

Handbook of Behavior Therapy & Pharmacotherapy for Children: A Comparative Analysis. Ed. by Vincent B. Van Hasselt & Michel Hersen. 1993. LC 92-49851. 400p. (C). 94.00 (*0-205-13949-3*, Longwood Div) Allyn.

Handbook of Behavior Therapy & Psychological Science: An Integrative Approach. Ed. by P. R. Martin. 1991. (General Psychology Ser.). 608p. (*0-08-036129-3*); pap. (*0-08-040629-7*) PPI GBR. *Dist:* Elsevier.

Handbook of Behavior Therapy in Education. J. C. Witt et al. 1988. LC 88-4191. (Illus.). 856p. (C). 130.00 (*0-306-42633-1*, Plenum Trade) Perseus Pubng.

Handbook of Behavior Therapy in the Psychiatric Setting. Ed. by Alan S. Bellack & Michel Hersen. 1993. (Critical Issues in Psychiatry Ser.). (Illus.). 672p. (C). 95.00 (*0-306-44275-2*, Plenum Trade) Perseus Pubng.

Handbook of Behavior Therapy with Children & Adults: A Developmental & Longitudinal Perspective. Ed. by Robert T. Ammerman & Michel Hersen. 1991. (General Psychology Ser.). 552p. (*0-08-037902-8*); (*0-08-041243-2*) PPI GBR. *Dist:* Elsevier.

Handbook of Behavioral Assessment. Anthony R. Ciminero et al. 2nd ed. 1986. LC 86-11010. (Personality Processes Ser.). 789p. 280.00 (*0-471-88849-4*) Wiley.

Handbook of Behavioral Group Therapy. Ed. by Dennis Upper & Steven M. Ross. 1985. LC 85-20496. (Applied Clinical Psychology Ser.). (Illus.). 526p. (C). 120.00 (*0-306-41989-0*, Plenum Trade) Perseus Pubng.

Handbook of Behavioral Medicine for Women. Ed. by Elaine A. Blechman & Kelly D. Brownell. 1988. (General Psychology Ser.: No. 149). 518p. 90.00 (*0-08-032383-9*, Pergamon Pr) Elsevier.

Handbook of Behavioral Teratology. E. P. Riley & C. V. Vorhees. 1986. LC 86-20517. (Illus.). 542p. (C). 110.00 (*0-306-42246-8*, Plenum Trade) Perseus Pubng.

Handbook of Behavioural Problems of the Dog & Cat. Gary M. Landsberg et al. 1997. LC 96-15793. (Veterinary Handbook Ser.). (Illus.). 220p. pap. text 60.00 (*0-7506-3060-4*) Buttrwrth-Heinemann.

Handbook of Biochemistry & Molecular Biology: Section A: Proteins Ed. by Gerald D. Fasman. 3rd ed. 1976. (Handbook Ser.). Vol. I. 448p. 189.00 (*0-87819-504-1*, QP514); Vol. II. 790p. lib. bdg. 175.00 (*0-87819-505-X*, QP514); Vol. III. 633p. 196.00 (*0-87819-510-6*, QP514) CRC Pr.

Handbook of Biochemistry & Molecular Biology: Section B: Nucleic Acids Ed. by Gerald D. Fasman. 3rd ed. 1976. (Handbook Ser.). Vol. I. 637p. 129.95 (*0-87819-506-8*, QP514); Vol. II. 923p. lib. bdg. 184.00 (*0-87819-507-6*, QP514) CRC Pr.

Handbook of Biochemistry & Molecular Biology: Section C: Lipids, Carbohydrates & Steroids, Vol. I. Ed. by Gerald D. Fasman. 3rd ed. 1975. (Handbook Ser.). 570p. lib. bdg. 163.00 (*0-87819-508-4*, QP514) CRC Pr.

Handbook of Biochemistry in Aging. Richard C. Adelman. Ed. by James R. Florini. 1981. LC 80-23060. (Series in Aging). 320p. 175.00 (*0-8493-3141-2*, QP86, CRC Reprint) Franklin.

Handbook of Biodegradable Polymers. Ed. by Abraham J. Domb et al. 1997. (Drug Targeting & Delivery Ser.: Vol. 7). 512p. text 155.00 (*90-5702-153-6*, Harwood Acad Pubs) Gordon & Breach.

Handbook of Biomaterial Properties. Black & Hastings. 1998. (Illus.). 336p. pap. 159.95 (*0-412-60330-6*, Chap & Hall NY) Chapman & Hall.

Handbook of Biomaterials Evaluation: Scientific, Technical & Clinical Testing of Implant Materials. Andreas Von Recum. 2nd ed. 1998. LC 98-36552. (Illus.). xix, 915p. text 210.00 (*1-56032-479-1*) Hemisp Pub.

Handbook of Biostatistics: A Review & Text. C. P. Carvounis. 2000. LC 98-44804. (Illus.). 118p. 25.95 (*1-85070-749-9*, Parthenon Pbng) CRC Pr.

Handbook of Black American Health: The Mosaic of Conditions, Issues, Policies, & Prospects. Ed. by Ivor L. Livingston. 1994. LC 93-4852. 496p. lib. bdg. 105.00 (*0-313-28640-X*, LHB/, Greenwood Pr) Greenwood.

Handbook of Blood Gases Analysis. Jenkins. 1995. (Respiratory Care Ser.). pap. 19.95 (*0-8273-5687-0*) Delmar.

Handbook of Blood Pressure Measurement. Leslie A. Geddes. 1991. LC 90-15638. (Illus.). 176p. 99.50 (*0-89603-194-2*) Humana.

Handbook of Borderline Disorders. Ed. by Daniel Silver & Michael Rosenbluth. 1992. LC 91-20814. 750p. 85.00 (*0-8236-2290-8*) Intl Univs Pr.

Handbook of Botulinum Toxin Treatment. Ed. by Peter Moore. 1995. LC 95-184. 320p. 110.00 (*0-632-03616-8*) Blackwell Sci.

Handbook of Brain Theory & Neural Networks. Ed. by Michael A. Arbib. 1995. LC 94-44408. 185.00 (*0-262-01148-4*, Bradford Bks) MIT Pr.

Handbook of Breast Imaging. Mary E. Peters et al. Ed. by Dawn R. Voegeli & Kathleen A. Scanlan. 1989. (Handbooks of Diagnostic Imaging Ser.: Vol. 4). (Illus.). 344p. text (*0-443-08620-6*) Church.

Handbook of Cancer Chemotherapy. Roland T. Skeel. 2nd ed. 1987. (Spiral Manual Ser.). spiral bd. 24.00 (*0-316-79573-9*, Little Brwn Med Div) Lppncott W & W.

***Handbook of Cancer Risk-Assessment & Prevention.** Graham Colditz & DeVita. 2002. (Illus.). (C). text 39.95 (*0-7637-1883-1*, 1883-1) Jones & Bartlett.

Handbook of Carcinogen Testing. Ed. by Harry A. Milman & Elizabeth K. Weisburger. 2nd ed. 1994. LC 94-15231. (Illus.). 856p. 145.00 (*0-8155-1356-9*) Noyes.

Handbook of Cardiac Anesthesia & Critical Care: A Demythologized Approach. John D. Wasnick. 1997. LC 97-26004. (Illus.). 388p. pap. text 49.99 (*0-7506-9748-2*) Buttrwrth-Heinemann.

Handbook of Cardiac Arrhythmia. Ed. by Philip J. Podrid & Peter R. Kowey. 1996. (Illus.). 512p. pap. 29.95 (*0-683-06909-8*) Lppncott W & W.

Handbook of Cardiac Drugs. Ralph E. Purdy & Mark Jr. Boucek. 2nd ed. 1994. LC 94-22278. 400p. pap. text 39.95 (*0-316-72246-4*) Lppncott W & W.

***Handbook of Cardiac Emergencies.** Ian McConachie & David Hesketh Roberts. 2000. (Greenwich Medical Media Ser.). 250p. pap. (*1-84110-041-2*) Greenwich Med GBR. *Dist:* JAMCO Dist.

Handbook of Cardiac Relab. Linda Hojnacki & Marsha Halfman. 1982. pap. text 18.95 (*0-8359-0673-6*) P-H.

Handbook of Cardiac Transplantation. Ed. by Robert W. Emery & Leslie Miller. 1995. 289p. (Orig.). pap. 40.00 (*1-56053-157-6*) Hanley & Belfus.

Handbook of Cardiothoracic Surgery. F. Baumgartner & Bassam Omari. 1996. (Medical Intelligence Unit Ser.). 200p. (C). pap. 49.95 (*0-412-12121-2*) Chapman & Hall.

Handbook of Cardiovascular & Anti-Inflammatory Agents. Ed. by Matthew Verderame. 1986. 336p. lib. bdg. 175.95 (*0-8493-3290-7*, RM345, CRC Reprint) Franklin.

Handbook of Cardiovascular Clinical Trials. Shilpesh S. Patel et al. 1996. LC 96-43506. pap. text (*0-443-07925-0*) Church.

Handbook of Cardiovascular Emergencies. James W. Hoekstra. 1996. LC 96-28913. 694p. pap. text 39.95 (*0-316-36760-5*) Lppncott W & W.

Handbook of Cardiovascular Interventions. Ed. by M. Bertrand et al. 1996. LC 96-16865. 948p. pap. text (*0-443-07970-6*) Church.

Handbook of Carotid Artery Surgery: Facts & Figures. Norman Rosenberg. 1989. 328p. lib. bdg. 175.00 (*0-8493-2957-4*, RD598); 2nd ed. 1994. LC 93-29684. 368p. reprint ed. 179.00 (*0-8493-3252-4*, RD598) CRC Pr.

Handbook of CDER Staffing & Review. Ed. by Mark Mathieu. 1996. 213p. (Orig.). pap. 125.00 (*1-882615-28-X*) Parexel Intl.

Handbook of Cell Biology of Aging. V. Cristofalo & Richard C. Adelman. 1985. LC 84-14312. (Series in Aging). 608p. lib. bdg. 279.95 (*0-8493-3142-0*, CRC Reprint) Franklin.

Handbook of Census Methods for Terrestrial Vertebrates. Ed. by David E. Davis. 1982. 424p. 261.95 (*0-8493-2970-1*, QL752) CRC Pr.

Handbook of Central Auditory Processing Disorders in Children. Jack A. Willeford & Joan M. Burleigh. 1985. 206p. text 29.00 (*0-8089-1727-7*, Grune & Strat) Harcrt Hlth Sci Grp.

Handbook of Cerebellar Diseases. Richard Lechtenberg. 1993. (Neurological Disease & Therapy Ser.: Vol. 16). (Illus.). 592p. text 245.00 (*0-8247-8776-5*) Dekker.

Handbook of Cerebrovascular Diseases. Harold P. Adams, Jr. 1993. (Neurological Disease & Therapy Ser.: Vol. 17). (Illus.). 728p. text 275.00 (*0-8247-8820-6*) Dekker.

Handbook of Challenging Behavior: Mental Health Aspects of Mental Retardation. Steven Reiss. 1994. LC 94-77561. 301p. (C). text 29.95 (*0-9642598-1-8*) IDS Pubng.

Handbook of Character Studies: Psychoanalytic Explorations. Ed. by Manfred F. Kets de Vries & Sidney Perzow. 1991. LC 91-7878. 656p. 95.00 (*0-8236-2295-9*) Intl Univs Pr.

Handbook of Chemical & Pharmacological Restraint. Ed. by Kari Blaho & Stephen Winbery. 2001. (Forensic Science & Medicine Ser.). 450p. 125.00 (*0-89603-600-6*) Humana.

Handbook of Chemical Toxicity Profiles Biological Species Vol. 2: Avian, Vol. 2. Sub Ramamoorthy. 1995. LC 94-41896. 416p. 139.95 (*1-56670-014-0*, L1014) Lewis Pubs.

Handbook of Chemotherapeutic Agents, Vol. I. Ed. by Matthew Verderame. 1986. 352p. 163.00 (*0-8493-3286-9*, RM262, CRC Reprint) Franklin.

Handbook of Chemotherapeutic Agents, Vol. II. Ed. by Mathew Verderame. 1986. 376p. 204.00 (*0-8493-3287-7*, CRC Reprint) Franklin.

Handbook of Chemotherapy Regimens. Ed. by Ishmael A. Jaiyesimi & Richard Pazdur. 2000. 105p. pap. (*1-891483-06-4*) PRR.

Handbook of Chemotherapy Regimens for Gynecologic Cancers: An Indispensable Quick Reference Guide. Maurie Markman. 1999. 108p. pap. text 39.95 (*1-56625-136-2*) Bonus Books.

Handbook of Chest Radiology, Vol. 2. Groskin. 2nd ed. 1999. (Illus.). 512p. (C). (gr. 13). pap. text 45.00 (*0-8151-3848-2*, 29326) Mosby Inc.

Handbook of Child Abuse Research & Treatment. Ed. by John R. Lutzker. 1997. LC 97-39967. (Issues in Clinical Child Psychology Ser.). 612p. (C). 95.00 (*0-306-45659-1*, Plenum Trade) Perseus Pubng.

Handbook of Child & Adolescent Assessment. Ed. by M. Hersen & Thomas H. Ollendick. 1991. (General Psychology Ser.: PGP 167). 564p. (*0-08-036804-2*); (*0-08-040642-4*) PPI GBR. *Dist:* Elsevier.

Handbook of Child & Adolescent Clinical Psychology: A Contextual Approach. Alan Carr. 1999. LC 98-25289. 150.00 (*0-415-19491-1*); pap. 50.00 (*0-415-19492-X*) Routledge.

Handbook of Child & Adolescent Outpatient, Day Treatment & Community Psychiatry. Harinder S. Ghuman & Richard M. Sarles. 1998. LC 98-18544. 69.95 (*0-87630-874-4*) Brunner-Routledge.

Handbook of Child & Adolescent Psychiatry Joseph D. Noshpitz. 1998. 1800p. 750.00 (*0-471-19329-1*) Wiley.

Handbook of Child & Adolescent Psychiatry: The Grade-School Child. Ed. by Paulina F. Kernberg et al. 1997. LC 96-17210. (Child & Adolescent Mental Health Ser.: Vol. 2). 720p. 250.00 (*0-471-55075-2*) Wiley.

Handbook of Child & Adolescent Psychiatry Vol. 4: Varieties of Development. Ed. by Norman E. Alessi & Joseph D. Noshpitz. 1997. (Child & Adolescent Mental Health Ser.: Vol. 4). 704p. 250.00 (*0-471-55078-7*) Wiley.

Handbook of Child & Adolescent Psychiatry Vol. 7: Advances & New Directions, Vol. 7, Advances and New Directions. Ed. by Joseph D. Noshpitz et al. 1998. (Handbook of Child & Adolescent Psychiatry Ser.: Vol. 7). 581p. 250.00 (*0-471-19332-1*) Wiley.

Handbook of Child & Adolescent Psychiatry, 4 Vol. Set, Vol. 4. Ed. by Joseph D. Noshpitz. 1997. 2828p. 1000.00 (*0-471-17640-0*) Wiley.

Handbook of Child & Adolescent Psychotherapy. Monica Lanyado. 1999. LC 98-48880. xv, 475p. 85.00 (*0-415-17258-6*); 400p. pap. 29.95 (*0-415-17259-4*) Routledge.

Handbook of Child & Adolescent Sexual Problems. George A. Rekers. 1995. LC 94-40653. (Series in Scientific Foundations of Clinical & Counseling Psychology). 500p. 45.00 (*0-02-926317-4*) Hungry Minds.

Handbook of Child & Adolescent Treatment Manuals. Craig W. LeCroy. 1994. LC 93-40136. 432p. 40.00 (*0-02-918485-1*) Free Pr.

Handbook of Child & Adolesent Psychiatry, Set. Ed. by Joseph D. Noshpitz. Incl. Handbook of Child & Adolescent Psychiatry: The Grade-School Child. Ed. by Paulina F. Kernberg & Jules R. Bemporad. LC 96-17210. 720p. 1997. 250.00 (*0-471-55075-2*); Handbook of Child & Adolescent Psychiatry Vol. 4: Varieties of Development. Ed. by Norman E. Alessi. 704p. 1997. 250.00 (*0-471-55078-7*); Infancy & Preschoolers. LC 96-17210. 624p. 1997. 250.00 (*0-471-55079-5*); Vol. 5, Clinical Assessment and Intervention Plann. Clinical Assessment & Intervention Planning. Ed. by Saul Harrison & Spencer Eth. 848p. 1998. 250.00 (*0-471-19330-5*); Vol. 6, Basic Psychiatric Science and Treatment. Basic Psychiatric Science & Treatment. Ed. by Norman E. Alessi. 640p. 1998. 250.00 (*0-471-19331-3*); Vol. 7, Advances and New Directions. Handbook of Child & Adolescent Psychiatry Vol. 7: Advances & New Directions. Ed. by Paul L. Adams & Efrain Bleiberg. 581p. 1998. 250.00 (*0-471-19332-1*); LC 96-17210. (Child & Adolescent Mental Health Ser.). 4300p. 1998. 1750.00 (*0-471-19328-3*) Wiley.

Handbook of Child & Adult Psychology: A Longitudinal Perspective. Hersen. 1992. 496p. (C). 165.00 (*0-205-14361-X*, H4361, Longwood Div) Allyn.

Handbook of Child & Adult Psychopathology: A Longitudinal Perspective. Michel Hersen & Cynthia G. Last. 1990. (General Psychology Ser.). (Illus.). 500p. (*0-08-036101-3*) PPI GBR. *Dist:* Elsevier.

***Handbook of Child Behavior Therapy in the Psychiatric Setting.** Ammerman. 2001. 528p. pap. 55.00 (*0-471-11393-X*) Wiley.

Handbook of Child Behavior Therapy in the Psychiatric Setting. Ed. by Robert T. Ammerman & Michel Hersen. 1994. LC 93-50916. (Personality Processes Ser.). 512p. 200.00 (*0-471-57844-4*) Wiley.

Handbook of Child Health Nursing. Sandra R. Mott. 1986. pap. text 15.96 (*0-201-13699-6*) Addison-Wesley.

Handbook of Child Nutrition. Leonard Taitz & Bridget Wardley. 1989. (Illus.). 192p. text 45.00 (*0-19-261759-1*) OUP.

Handbook of Child Nutrition. B. L. Wardley et al. 2nd ed. 1998. LC 97-12677. (Illus.). 268p. pap. text 39.50 (*0-19-262786-4*) OUP.

Handbook of Child Psychiatry for Primary Care. Brian Robertson. 1997. LC 98-145634. (Illus.). 376p. pap. 34.50 (*0-19-571372-9*) OUP.

Handbook of Child Psychoanalysis: Research, Theory, & Practice. Ed. by Benjamin B. Wolman. 1995. LC 95-20758. (Master Work Ser.). 660p. pap. text 70.00 (*1-56821-722-6*) Aronson.

Handbook of Child Psychology 4th ed. Ed. by Paul H. Mussen & Ellen M. Markman. Incl. Vol. 3. Cognitive Development. Ed. by John H. Flavell. LC 83-3468. 942p. 94.95 (*0-471-09064-6*); Vol. 4. Handbook of Child Psychology: Socialization, Personality & Social Development. Ed. by E. Mavis Hetherington. LC 83-6552. 1043p. 94.95 (*0-471-09065-4*); 1983. 3819p. 1983. Set text 379.80 (*0-471-05194-2*) Wiley.

Handbook of Child Psychology: Socialization, Personality & Social Development, Vol. 4. Ed. by Paul H. Mussen et al. 4th ed. 1983. LC 83-6552. 1043p. 94.95 (*0-471-09065-4*) Wiley.

Handbook of Child Psychology Vol. 2: Cognition, Perception & Language. Ed. by Deanna Kuhn et al. 5th ed. 1997. (Handbook of Child Psychology Ser.: Vol. 2). 1030p. 285.00 (*0-471-05730-4*) Wiley.

Handbook of Child Psychology Vol. 3: Social, Emotional, & Personality Development. Ed. by William Damon & Nancy Eisenberg. 5th ed. 1997. (Handbook of Child Psychology Ser.: Vol. 3). 1232p. 285.00 (*0-471-07668-6*) Wiley.

Handbook of Child Psychology Vol. 4. Ed. by William Damon et al. 5th ed. 1997. (Handbook of Child Psychology Ser.: Vol. 4). 1188p. 285.00 (*0-471-07663-5*) Wiley.

Handbook of Child Psychopathology. Ed. by Thomas H. Ollendick & Michael Hersen. 2nd ed. 1989. (Illus.). 570p. 85.00 (*0-306-42975-6*, Plenum Trade) Perseus Pubng.

Handbook of Child Psychopathology. Ed. by Thomas H. Ollendick et al. 3rd ed. 1997. LC 97-40923. 694p. 97.50 (*0-306-45321-5*, Kluwer Plenum) Kluwer Academic.

Handbook of Childhood Impulse Disorders & ADHD: Theory & Practice. Ed. by Leonard F. Koziol et al. 1993. LC 92-48239. (Illus.). 252p. 61.95 (*0-398-05844-X*) C C Thomas.

Handbook of Chinese Healing Herbs. Daniel Reid. 1995. LC 94-44220. 336p. pap. 15.95 (*1-57062-093-8*) Shambhala Pubns.

Handbook of Chinese Hematology. Simon Beeker. 2000. Orig. Title: The Treatment of Blood Diseases with Chinese Medicine. 240p. pap. text 39.95 (*1-891845-16-0*) Blue Poppy Pr.

Handbook of Chinese Herbal Formulas. Him-che Yeung. 2nd rev. ed. 1995. (CHI & ENG.). 455p. pap. text 35.00 (*0-9639715-1-4*) Inst Chinese Med.

Handbook of Chinese Herbs. Him-che Yeung. 2nd rev. ed. 1996. (CHI & ENG., Illus.). 736p. pap. text 55.00 (*0-9639715-2-2*) Inst Chinese Med.

Handbook of Chinese Massage: Tuina Techniques to Awaken Body & Mind. Maria Mercati. 1997. LC 97-17132. (Illus.). 144p. pap. 19.95 (*0-89281-745-3*, Heal Arts VT) Inner Tradit.

Handbook of Chinese Psychology. Ed. by Michael H. Bond. 1996. (Illus.). 608p. text 90.00 (*0-19-586598-7*) OUP.

Handbook of Chromatography: Drugs, Vol. I. Ed. by Ram N. Gupta & Irving Sunshine. 1981. LC 81-10157. (Series in Chromatography). 352p. 197.00 (*0-8493-3031-9*, RS189, CRC Reprint) Franklin.

Handbook of Chromatography: General Data & Principles, Vol. II. Ed. by Gunter Zweig & Joseph Sherma. 1973. 343p. 154.00 (*0-8493-3003-3*, QD305) CRC Pr.

Handbook of Chromatography: General Data & Principles, Vol. I. Ed. by Gunter Zweig & Joseph Sherma. 1973. LC 76-163067. (Series in Chromatography). 784p. 432.00 (*0-8493-3002-5*, QD117, CRC Reprint) Franklin.

Handbook of Chromatography: Steroids, Vol. I. Ed. by Joseph C. Touchstone. 1986. LC 85-17066. (Series in Chromatography). 272p. 153.00 (*0-8493-3014-9*, QP572, CRC Reprint) Franklin.

Handbook of Clinical Adult Psychology. Ed. by Stan Lindsay & Graham Powell. 2nd ed. 1994. LC 93-33181. 832p. (C). pap. 52.95 (*0-415-07216-6*, B3734) Routledge.

Handbook of Clinical & Experimental Neuropsychology. Denes Gianfranco. 1998. LC 99-187204. 1120p. 150.00 (*0-86377-542-X*) Taylor & Francis.

Handbook of Clinical Anesthesia. Goldstone. 1996. pap. text (*0-443-04984-X*, G0518) Church.

Handbook of Clinical Anesthesia. Paul G. Barash et al. 4th ed. 2001. LC 00-44812. 976p. pap. text 39.95 (*0-7817-2918-1*) Lppncott W & W.

Handbook of Clinical Assessment of Children & Adolescents Ed. by Clarice J. Kestenbaum & Daniel T. Williams. 608p. (C). 1992. pap. text 75.00 (*0-8147-4628-4*); 1988. text 170.00 (*0-8147-4590-3*) NYU Pr.

Handbook of Clinical Audiology. Ed. by Jack Katz. 4th ed. 1994. LC 93-3629. (Illus.). 864p. 70.00 (*0-683-04548-2*) Lppncott W & W.

Handbook of Clinical Behavior Therapy. Samuel M. Turner et al. 2nd ed. 1992. LC 91-44490. (Personality Processes Ser.: No. 1341). 496p. 200.00 (*0-471-63563-4*) Wiley.

Handbook of Clinical Behavior Therapy with Adults. M. Hersen & A. S. Bellack. 1985. LC 85-9503. (Illus.). 750p. (C). 130.00 (*0-306-41875-4*, Plenum Trade) Perseus Pubng.

Handbook of Clinical Behavior Therapy with the Elderly Client. A. M. Gross & R. S. Drabman. 1990. LC 89-22927. (Applied Clinical Psychology Ser.). (Illus.). 442p. (C). 95.00 (*0-306-43180-7*, Plenum Trade) Perseus Pubng.

Handbook of Clinical Behavior Therapy with the Elderly Client. Ed. by P. A. Wisocki. 1991. LC 91-1962. (Applied Clinical Psychology Ser.). (Illus.). 528p. (C). 95.00 (*0-306-43756-2*, Plenum Trade) Perseus Pubng.

Handbook of Clinical Child Neuropsychology. Ed. by Cecil R. Reynolds & Elaine Fletcher-Janzen. 2nd ed. 1997. LC 96-52991. (Critical Issues in Neuropsychology Ser.). 762p. (C). 95.00 (*0-306-45257-X*, Kluwer Plenum) Kluwer Academic.

Handbook of Clinical Chiropractic. Lawrence H. Wyatt. 1991. LC 91-22352. (Illus.). 264p. pap. 61.00 (*0-8342-0250-6*) Aspen Pub.

Handbook of Clinical Dental Assisting. Gregory M. Schuster et al. Ed. by Shirley Kuhn. 1998. LC 98-24847. (Illus.). 224p. (C). pap. text 22.50 (*0-7216-4536-4*) Saunders.

Handbook of Clinical Dietetics. American Dietetic Association Staff. 1981. LC 80-11317. 480p. 65.00 (*0-300-02256-5*) Yale U Pr.

***Handbook of Clinical Drug Data.** Philip O. Anderson et al. 10th ed. 2001. 1104p. pap. 44.95 (*0-07-136362-9*) McGraw-Hill Prof.

Handbook of Clinical Endocrinology. Ed. by Paul A. Fitzgerald. 1986. LC 86-80635. (Illus.). 480p. pap. text 19.95 (*0-930010-12-4*) Jones Med.

Handbook of Clinical Engineering, Vol. 1. Ed. by Barry N. Feinberg. 1980. 384p. 214.00 (*0-8493-0244-7*, R856, CRC Reprint) Franklin.

Handbook of Clinical Gerontology. Laura L. Carstensen & Barry A. Edelstein. 1987. (General Psychology Ser.: No. 146). 600p. 90.00 (*0-08-031947-5*, Pergamon Pr) Elsevier.

Handbook of Clinical Geropsychology. M. Hersen & V. B. Van Hasselt. 1998. LC 98-21527. (Plenum Series in Adult Development & Aging). (Illus.). 562p. (C). text 90.00 (*0-306-45661-3*, Kluwer Plenum) Kluwer Academic.

Handbook of Clinical Health Psychology. T. Millon et al. 1982. LC 82-11236. (Illus.). 632p. (C). 100.00 (*0-306-40932-1*, Plenum Trade) Perseus Pubng.

Handbook of Clinical Hypnosis. Ed. by Judith W. Rhue et al. 1993. 765p. pap. 49.95 (*1-55798-440-9*) Am Psychol.

Handbook of Clinical Interventions in Child Sexual Abuse. Suzanne M. Sgroi. 1981. LC 81-47707. (Illus.). 400p. pap. 27.95 (*0-669-05213-2*) Free Pr.

Handbook of Clinical Lab Science, Section A-Nuclear Med., Vol. II. David Seligson. 1982. 592p. 322.00 (*0-8493-7072-8*, RB37, CRC Reprint) Franklin.

Handbook of Clinical Nursing Procedures for Community Nurses. Ed. by Maria Kenrick & Karen A. Luker. 1995. LC 95-213931. (Illus.). 213p. pap. 38.95 (*0-632-03858-6*, RT98) Blackwell Sci.

Handbook of Clinical Nursing Research. Ada Sue Hinshaw et al. 1999. LC 99-6034. 99.95 (*0-8039-5784-X*, 8197) Sage.

Handbook of Clinical Nursing Research. Ed. by J. Robertson. 1994. (Illus.). 200p. pap. (*0-443-04866-5*) Church.

Handbook of Clinical Nutrition. Roland L. Weinsier. 3rd ed. 1996. LC 96-20199. (Illus.). 624p. (C). (gr. 13). spiral bd. 35.95 (*0-8151-9274-6*, 28570) Mosby Inc.

Handbook of Clinical Opthalmology for Eyecare Professionals. Janice K. Ledford. 2000. LC 00-57412. 384p. (C). pap. text 33.00 (*1-55642-464-7*) SLACK Inc.

Handbook of Clinical Pathology. Julianne Sandstad et al. 1992. 270p. 40.00 (*0-89189-314-8*) Am Soc Clinical.

Handbook of Clinical Pathology. American Society of Clinical Pathologists Staff. 2nd ed. 1999. LC 99-24739. 60.00 (*0-89189-376-8*) Am Soc Clinical.

Handbook of Clinical Pharmacokinetics. Ed. by L. F. Prescott & M. Gibaldi. 1200p. text (*0-86792-004-1*) Mosby Inc.

Handbook of Clinical Pharmacology. Felix Bochner et al. 2nd ed. 1983. 352p. 30.95 (*0-316-10064-1*, Little Brwn Med Div) Lppncott W & W.

Handbook of Clinical Psychology: Theory, Research & Practice. Ed. by C. E. Walker. 1983. (Professional Bks.). (C). Vol. I. LC 82-73409. 556p. text 71.95 (*0-534-10448-7*); Vol. II. 912p. text 71.95 (*0-534-10449-5*) Brooks-Cole.

Handbook of Clinical Psychology in Medical Settings. Ed. by J. J. Sweet et al. 1991. (Illus.). 662p. (C). 100.00 (*0-306-43550-0*, Plenum Trade) Perseus Pubng.

Handbook of Clinical Psychoneuroendocrinology. Ed. by Charles B. Nemeroff & Peter T. Loosen. 1987. LC 86-31837. 502p. 80.95 (*0-89862-698-6*) Guilford Pubns.

Handbook of Clinical Psychopharmacology. Ed. by Joe P. Tupin et al. LC 87-33442. 1988. 486p. 70.00 (*0-87668-997-7*); 2nd ed. 1993. 496p. reprint ed. pap. 60.00 (*0-87668-523-8*) Aronson.

Handbook of Clinical Psychopharmacology for Therapists. John D. Preston et al. 2nd rev. ed. 1997. LC 97-69492. (Illus.). 264p. text 49.95 (*1-57224-094-6*) New Harbinger.

Handbook of Clinical Research & Practice with Adolescents. Ed. by Patrick H. Tolan & Bertram J. Cohler. 1992. LC 92-5603. (Personality Processes Ser.). 592p. 250.00 (*0-471-61333-9*) Wiley.

Handbook of Clinical Skills. Ed. by Patricia Schull. 1996. LC 96-28896. (Illus.). 960p. (Orig.). spiral bd. 39.95 (*0-87434-870-6*) Springhouse Corp.

Handbook of Clinical Teaching: Exercises & Guidelines for Health Professionals Who Teach Patients, Train Staff or Supervise Students. Nancy T. Watts. 1990. (Illus.). 276p. (Orig.). pap. text (*0-443-03604-7*) Church.

Handbook of Clinical Techniques in the Management of Chronic Pain. J. R. Wedley & C. A. Gauci. 1994. 98p. text 77.00 (*3-7186-5399-0*, Harwood Acad Pubs) Gordon & Breach.

Handbook of Clinical Toxicology of Animal Venoms & Poisons. Ed. by Jurg Meier & Julian White. 1995. LC 95-17705. 768p. 139.95 (*0-8493-4489-1*, 4489) CRC Pr.

Handbook of Clinical Trials: The Neurobehavioral Approach. Ed. by E. Mohr & P. Brouwers. 1991. 388p. (*90-265-1028-4*) Swets.

Handbook of CNS Agents & Local Anesthetics. Matthew Verderame. 1986. LC 85-22390. (Medicinal Chemistry Ser.). 392p. 217.00 (*0-8493-3288-5*, CRC Reprint) Franklin.

Handbook of Cognitive-Behavioral Therapies. Ed. by Keith S. Dobson. 1987. LC 87-27. 426p. text 65.00 (*0-89862-704-4*); 1990. LC 87-27. 426p. reprint ed. pap. 26.95 (*0-89862-524-6*); 2nd ed. 2000. LC 00-64027. 446p. text 45.00 (*1-57230-601-7*, C0601) Guilford Pubns.

Handbook of Cognitive Neuropsychology: What Deficits Reveal about the Human Mind. Brenda Rapp. 2001. LC 00-42545. 592p. (*0-86377-592-6*) Psychol Pr GBR. *Dist:* Taylor & Francis.

Handbook of Cognitive Neuropsychology: What Deficits Reveal about the Human Mind. Brenda Rapp. 2000. LC 00-42545. pap. (*1-84169-044-9*) Psychol Pr GBR. *Dist:* Taylor & Francis.

Handbook of Cognitive Neuroscience. Michael S. Gazzaniga. 1984. LC 83-21317. (Illus.). 428p. (C). text 90.00 (*0-306-41290-X*, Kluwer Plenum) Kluwer Academic.

Handbook of Cognitive, Social, & Neuropsychological Aspects of Learning Disabilities Ed. by S. J. Ceci. 1986. (C). 1. 555p. text 99.95 (*0-89859-682-3*); Vol. 2. 432p. text 99.95 (*0-89859-797-8*) L Erlbaum Assocs.

Handbook of Cognitive Therapy Techniques. Rian E. McMullin. 1986. (Professional Bks.). 356p. 34.95 (*0-393-70035-6*) Norton.

Handbook of Colorectal Surgery. Ed. by David E. Beck. 1996. (Illus.). 485p. text 39.00 (*1-57626-012-7*) Quality Med Pub.

Handbook of Colorimetry. Ed. by Arthur C. Hardy. 1936. (Illus.). 95p. 45.00 (*0-262-08001-X*) MIT Pr.

Handbook of Colposcopy. Ed. by David Luesley et al. 1996. LC 96-86086. (Illus.). 176p. pap. (*0-412-71550-3*) E A GBR. *Dist:* OUP.

Handbook of Commercial & Home Health Nursing: Tools for Assessment, Intervention & Education. Marcia Stanhope & Ruth N. Knollmueller. 3rd ed. 1999. LC 00-267319. (Illus.). xviii, 668p. pap. 33.95 (*0-323-00875-5*) Mosby Inc.

Handbook of Common Foot Problems. Ed. by Lawrence B. Harkless & Steven M. Krych. 1990. (Illus.). 105p. pap. text (*0-443-08622-2*) Church.

Handbook of Common Ocular Drugs. G. John DiGregorio et al. 1991. 153p. pap. 13.00 (*0-942447-07-7*) Med Surveill.

Handbook of Common Orthopaedic Fractures. Scott H. Kozin & Anthony C. Berlet. 4th ed. 2000. (Illus.). 300p. pap. 18.95 (*0-942447-36-0*) Med Surveill.

Handbook of Common Poisonings in Children. American Academy of Pediatrics Staff. 3rd ed. 1994. LC 94-71471. 280p. pap. 44.95 (*0-910761-58-2*) Am Acad Pediat.

Handbook of Commonly Prescribed Drugs. G. John DiGregorio. 11th ed. 1996. pap. 15.50 (*0-942447-21-2*, D5668); 13th ed. 1998. pap. 18.00 (*0-942447-25-5*) Med Surveill.

Handbook of Commonly Prescribed Drugs. G. John DiGregorio & E. Barbieri. 15th ed. 2000. 300p. pap. 18.95 (*0-942447-35-2*) Med Surveill.

Handbook of Commonly Prescribed Pediatric Drugs. Edward J. Barbieri et al. 6th ed. 1998. 250p. 18.50 (*0-942447-27-1*) Med Surveill.

***Handbook of Commonly Prescribed Prescribed Drugs.** John G. Diregorio. 16th ed. 2001. pap. 18.95 (*0-942447-41-7*) Med Surveill.

Handbook of Commonly Rx Geriatric Drugs. G. John DiGregorio et al. 1993. 334p. pap. 15.00 (*0-942447-01-8*) Med Surveill.

Handbook of Commonly Used Chemotherapy Regimens: A Quick Reference Guide to More Than 100 Currennt Cytotoxic Therapies. Ed. by F. Anthony Greco. 1996. LC 96-68385. 168p. (Orig.). pap. 39.95 (*0-944496-49-0*) Precept Pr.

Handbook of Communication & Aging Research. Ed. by Jon F. Nussbaum & Justine Coupland. 1995. (Communication Ser.). 536p. text 89.95 (*0-8058-1453-1*) L Erlbaum Assocs.

Handbook of Communication & People with Disabilities: Research & Application. Ed. by Dawn O. Braithwaite & Teresa L. Thompson. 1999. LC 99-29094. (LEA's Communication Ser.). (Illus.). xviii, 555p. (*0-8058-3059-6*) L Erlbaum Assocs.

Handbook of Community & Home Health Nursing: Tools for Assessment. Marcia Stanhope & Ruth N. Knollmueller. 2nd ed. 1995. LC 95-44620. (Illus.). 608p. (C). (gr. 13). spiral bd. 32.95 (*0-8151-8150-7*, 25623) Mosby Inc.

***Handbook of Community Cancer Care.** Mark N. Gaze & Isobel M. Wilson. 2002. (Illus.). 140p. pap. (*1-84110-001-3*) Greenwich Med GBR. *Dist:* JAMCO Dist.

Handbook of Community Cancer Care. Mark N. Gaze & Isobel M. Wilson. 2000. (Greenwich Medical Media Ser.). (Illus.). 120p. pap. text 32.50 (*1-900151-91-X*) OUP.

Handbook of Comparative Opioid & Related Neuropeptide Mechanism. George B. Stefano. 1986. LC 85-16225. Vol. 1. 116.00 (*0-8493-3257-5*); Vol. 2. 304p. 170.00 (*0-8493-3258-3*) Franklin (CRC Reprint).

Handbook of Conferences on Teaching Skills for Residents, 1989. 1989. 95.00 (*1-56321-079-7*); 95.00 (*1-56321-016-9*) L Erlbaum Assocs.

Handbook of Congenital & Early Onset Hearing Loss. Michael H. Fritsch & Annemarie Sommer. 1991. LC 90-4227. (Illus.). 184p. 70.00 (*0-89640-184-7*) Igaku-Shoin.

Handbook of Constructive Therapies: Innovative Techniques from Leading Practitioners. Michael F. Hoyt. 1998. LC 98-6859. 500p. 45.60 (*0-7879-4044-5*) Jossey-Bass.

Handbook of Contact Dermatitis. Howard I. Maibach et al. 1995. 350p. 69.95 (*0-8493-7351-4*) CRC Pr.

Handbook of Contemporary Group Psychotherapy: Contributions from Object Relations, Self Psychology, & Social Systems Theories. Ed. by Robert H. Klein et al. 1992. LC 91-35400. 445p. (C). 65.00 (*0-8236-2285-1*) Intl Univs Pr.

Handbook of Contraception & Abortion. Ronald Burkman. 1989. 32.95 (*0-316-09167-7*, Little Brwn Med Div) Lppncott W & W.

Handbook of Contrast Echocardiography: Left Ventricle Function & Myocardial Perfusion. Harald Becher & Peter N. Burns. 2000. LC 00-26586. (Illus.). 150p. 54.00 (*3-540-67083-1*) Spr-Verlag.

Handbook of Coronary Care. Joseph S. Alpert & Gary S. Francis. 6th ed. 2000. LC 00-22471. 240p. pap. text 39.95 (*0-7817-1958-5*) Lppncott W & W.

Handbook of Counseling & Psychotherapy with Men. Murray Scher et al. 1993. 440p. pap. 51.95 (*0-8039-5355-0*, 4984) Sage.

Handbook of Counseling Psychology. Ray Woolfe & Windy Dryden. 1996. (C). pap. 32.95 (*0-8039-8992-X*, 2260) Sage.

Handbook of Couples & Family Forensics: A Sourcebook for Mental & Legal Professionals. Ed. by Florence W. Kaslow. 1999. LC 98-53730. (Couples & Family Dynamics & Treatment Ser.). 554p. 105.00 (*0-471-19129-9*) Wiley.

Handbook of Creativity: Assessment, Research, & Theory. J. A. Glover et al. 1989. (Perspectives on Individual Differences Ser.). (Illus.). 470p. (C). 90.00 (*0-306-43160-2*, Plenum Trade) Perseus Pubng.

Handbook of Critical Care. James L. Berk & James F. Sampliner. 2nd ed. 1982. 39.50 (*0-316-09171-5*, Little Brwn Med Div) Lppncott W & W.

Handbook of Critical Care. Robert R. Kirby. 2nd ed. 1996. 850p. pap. text (*0-397-51790-4*) Lppncott W & W.

Handbook of Critical Care. Robert R. Kirby et al. 2nd ed. 1996. LC 96-39112. 960p. spiral bd. 49.95 (*0-397-51597-9*) Lppncott W & W.

Handbook of Critical Care Drug Therapy. Gregory M. Susla et al. 1994. LC 94-15739. pap. text (*0-443-08936-1*) Church.

Handbook of Critical Care Drug Therapy. Gregory M. Susla et al. 2nd ed. 1997. LC 97-30273. 436p. pap. 32.95 (*0-683-30293-0*) Lppncott W & W.

Handbook of Critical Care Nursing. David Moreau & Springhouse Publishing Company Staff. 1996. LC 95-41588. (Illus.). 736p. pap. 38.95 (*0-87434-774-2*) Springhouse Corp.

Handbook of Critical Care Obstetrics. Steven L. Clark et al. 1994. (Illus.). 504p. pap. 46.95 (*0-86542-351-2*) Blackwell Sci.

Handbook of Cross-Cultural & Multicultural Personality Assessment. Ed. by Richard Dana. 1999. LC 99-30954. (Personality & Clinical Psychology Ser.). (Illus.). xviii, 719p. (*0-8058-2789-7*) L Erlbaum Assocs.

Handbook of Cross-Cultural Counseling & Therapy. Ed. by Paul B. Pedersen. 376p. 1987. LC 87-9337. pap. 24.95 (*0-275-92713-X*, B2713, Praeger Pubs); 1985. LC 84-12832. lib. bdg. 59.95 (*0-313-23914-2*, PRH/, Greenwood Pr) Greenwood.

Handbook of Cross-Cultural Psychology: Basic Processes & Human Development, Vol. 2. Ed. by John W. Berry et al. 2nd ed. 1997. LC 96-16261. (Handbook of Cross-Cultural Psychology Ser.: Vol. 2). 439p. (C). 70.00 (*0-205-16075-1*) Allyn.

Handbook of Cross-Cultural Psychology: Theory & Method. Ed. by John W. Berry et al. 2nd ed. 1996. LC 96-16261. (Handbook of Cross-Cultural Psychology Ser.: Vol. 1). 406p. (C). 70.00 (*0-205-16074-3*) Allyn.

***Handbook of Cultural Psychiatry.** Wen-Shing Tseng. 2001. (Illus.). 864p. 149.95 (*0-12-701632-5*) Acad Pr.

Handbook of Culture & Mental Illness: An International Perspective. Ed. by Ihsan Al-Issa. 1995. 391p. 57.50 (*0-8236-2288-6*) Intl Univs Pr.

Handbook of Current Diagnosis & Treatment. Pounder. 1996. pap. text 28.00 (*0-443-05599-8*) Saunders.

Handbook of Current Diagnosis & Treatment: Quick A-Z Reference. Pounder. 2000. pap. text 28.00 (*0-443-05600-5*) Saunders.

Handbook of Data Recording, Maintenance, & Management for the Biomedical Sciences. Shayne C. Gad & Stephanie Taulbee. 1996. LC 96-3960. 96p. otabind 54.95 (*0-8493-0137-8*) CRC Pr.

Handbook of Dementia Care. Jean M. Stehman et al. 1996. LC 95-44909. (Illus.). 152p. (Orig.). (C). pap. text 21.50 (*0-8018-5277-3*) Johns Hopkins.

Handbook of Dementing Illnesses. Ed. by John C. Morris. 1993. LC 93-38090. (Neurological Disease & Therapy Ser.: Vol. 22). (Illus.). 688p. text 215.00 (*0-8247-8837-0*) Dekker.

Handbook of Demonstrations & Activities in Teaching of Psychology, Set. Ed. by Mark E. Ware & David E. Johnson. 1996. pap. 99.95 (*0-8058-1793-X*) L Erlbaum Assocs.

Handbook of Demonstrations & Activities in Teaching of Psychology Vol. 1: Introductory, Statistics, Research Methods, & History. Ed. by Mark E. Ware & David E. Johnson. 1996. 288p. pap. 45.00 (*0-8058-1790-5*) L Erlbaum Assocs.

Handbook of Demonstrations & Activities in Teaching of Psychology Vol. 2: Physiological-Comparative, Perception, Learning, Cognition, & Developmental - Child, Adolescent, Adult/Aging, & Lifespan. Ed. by Mark E. Ware & David E. Johnson. 1996. 352p. pap. 49.95 (*0-8058-1791-3*) L Erlbaum Assocs.

Handbook of Demonstrations & Activities in Teaching of Psychology Vol. 3: Personality, Abnormal, Clinical-Counseling, & Social. Ed. by Mark E. Ware & David E. Johnson. 1996. 320p. pap. 49.95 (*0-8058-1792-1*) L Erlbaum Assocs.

Handbook of Dental Local Anaesthesia. Hans Evers. 1981. (C). (*0-907789-00-5*) A H S Ltd GBR. *Dist:* St Mut.

Handbook of Dental Marketing: Ideas & Techniques That Work. Richard E. Stallard et al. 1986. 199p. 10.00 (*0-87814-310-6*) PennWell Corp.

Handbook of Depression. Ed. by E. Edward Beckham & William R. Leber. 2nd ed. LC 94-49600. 628p. 1997. pap. 37.00 (*1-57230-224-0*, 0224); 1995. text 65.00 (*0-89862-841-5*) Guilford Pubns.

Handbook of Depression & Anxiety: A Biological Approach. Ed. by Den Boer & J. M. Sitsen. 1994. (Medical Psychiatry Ser.: Vol. 1). (Illus.). 712p. text 195.00 (*0-8247-8858-3*) Dekker.

Handbook of Depression in Children & Adolescents. Ed. by W. M. Reynolds & H. F. Johnston. 1994. (Issues in Clinical Child Psychology Ser.). (Illus.). 632p. (C). text 95.00 (*0-306-44742-8*, Kluwer Plenum) Kluwer Academic.

Handbook of Dermatologic Treatment. R. Kenneth Landow. 1986. LC 83-80541. 219p. pap. text 19.95 (*0-930010-09-4*) Jones Med.

Handbook of Dermatology for Primary Care. Norma Saxe et al. 1997. (Illus.). 230p. pap. 34.50 (*0-19-571129-7*) OUP.

Handbook of Developmental & Physical Disabilities. Ed. by Vincent B. Van Hasselt et al. 1988. (General Psychology Ser.: No. 148). 584p. 95.00 (0-08-031595-X); 65.00 (0-08-033627-2) Elsevier (Pergamon Pr).

Handbook of Developmental Disabilities: Resources for Interdisciplinary Care. Ed. by Lisa A. Kurtz et al. 2000. 576p. 70.00 (0-8342-0786-9) PRO-ED.

Handbook of Developmental Neurotoxicology. Ed. by William Slikker & Louis W. Chang. 1998. LC 98-85622. (Illus.). 748p. text 159.95 (0-12-648860-6) Acad Pr.

Handbook of Developmental Psychopathology. Ed. by Michael Lewis & Suzanne M. Miller. 1990. LC 89-23243. (Illus.). 556p. (C). 90.00 (0-306-43190-4, Plenum Trade) Perseus Pubng.

Handbook of Developmental Psychopathology. Ed. by Arnold J. Sameroff et al. 2nd ed. 2000. LC 00-28722. (Illus.). xxxi, 813p. 95.00 (0-306-46275-3) Kluwer Academic.

Handbook of Developmental Toxicology. Ed. by Ronald D. Hood. 1996. LC 96-11629. 784p. 159.95 (0-8493-0135-1) CRC Pr.

Handbook of Diabetes. G. Williams & J. C. Pickup. 1992. (Illus.). 128p. pap. 39.95 (0-632-02888-2) Blackwell Sci.

Handbook of Diabetes Medical Nutrition Therapy. Margaret A. Powers. 2nd ed. 1996. 544p. 110.00 (0-8342-0631-5) Aspen Pub.

Handbook of Diagnosis & Treatment of the DSM-IV Personality Disorders. Len Sperry. 1995. LC 94-44790. 551p. text 29.95 (0-87630-780-2) Brunner-Routledge.

Handbook of Diagnostic Biochemistry & Hematology. Gillian Lockitch. 1992. 256p. 145.95 (0-8493-3518-3, RG558) CRC Pr.

Handbook of Diagnostic Electron Microscopy for Pathologist-in-Training. Society for Ultrastructural Pathology Handbook Committee & Irving Dardick. 1996. (Illus.). 200p. 62.50 (0-89640-307-6) Igaku-Shoin.

Handbook of Diagnostic Endocrinology. Ed. by Ishwarlal Jialal et al. 1999. 250p. pap. 43.00 (1-890883-08-5, 246) Am Assn Clinical Chem.

Handbook of Diagnostic Tests. Springhouse Publishing Company Staff. 2nd ed. 1999. LC 98-51301. (Illus.). 768p. spiral bd. 37.95 (0-87434-982-6) Springhouse Corp.

Handbook of Dialysis Access. David Eisenbud. 1996. (Illus.). 125p. pap. 22.95 (0-9646891-7-0) Anadem Pubng.

Handbook of Diet Therapy. Dorothea Turner. 5th ed. 1993. LC 65-24984. lib. bdg. 17.50 (0-226-81718-0) U Ch Pr.

Handbook of Dietary Fiber: An Applied Approach. Mark L. Dreher. 1987. (Food Science & Technology Ser.: Vol. 25). (Illus.). 488p. text 175.00 (0-8247-7655-0) Dekker.

Handbook of Dietary Fiber in Human Nutrition. Gene F. Spiller. 1986. 464p. 272.00 (0-8493-3530-2, QP141, CRC Reprint) Franklin.

Handbook of Dietary Fiber in Human Nutrition. Gene A. Spiller. 2nd ed. 1992. 672p. 136.95 (0-8493-4249-X, QP141) CRC Pr.

Handbook of Dietary Supplements, Vitamins, & Other Health Supplements. Pamela M. Mason. 1995. LC 95-202231. 240p. pap. 50.95 (0-632-03923-X) Blackwell Sci.

Handbook of Differential Diagnosis in Internal Medicine. Norton J. Greenberger et al. 5th ed. 1998. 347p. pap. 24.95 (0-323-00131-9) Mosby Inc.

Handbook of Differential Diagnosis in Internal Medicine: Medical Book of Lists. Norton J. Greenberger et al. 5th ed. 1998. 416p. pap. (84-8174-096-9) Mosby-Doyma Libros ESP. *Dist:* Mosby Inc.

Handbook of Differential Diagnosis in Neurology. Nicholas P. Poolos. 2001. LC 00-51904. (Illus.). 288p. pap. text 39.99 (0-7506-7002-9) Buttrwrth-Heinemann.

Handbook of Difficult Airway Management. Cain A. Hagberg. Ed. by Allan Ross. 1999. LC 98-31197. (Illus.). xix, 411p. pap. text 25.00 (0-443-07788-6) Saunders.

Handbook of Disaster Medicine. Ed. by J. De Boer & M. Dubouloz. 2000. (Illus.). 550p. (90-6764-316-5) VSP NLD. *Dist:* Coronet Bks.

Handbook of Diseases. Springhouse Publishing Company Staff. 1995. LC 95-4485. (Illus.). 928p. 32.95 (0-87434-838-2) Springhouse Corp.

Handbook of Diseases of Sugar Beet, Set. A. N. Mukhopadhyay. 1987. 467p. 240.00 (0-8493-3130-7, SB608) CRC Pr.

Handbook of Diseases of the Breast. J. M. Dixon & J. R. Sainsbury. 2nd ed. 1998. (Illus.). 208p. pap. (0-443-06185-8) Church.

Handbook of Diseases of the Hair & Scalp. Rodney Sinclair et al. 1999. LC 98-29004. (Illus.). 224p. pap. 68.95 (0-86542-928-6) Blackwell Sci.

Handbook of Diseases of the Nails & Their Management. D. A. De Berker et al. 1995. LC 94-46339. 177p. pap. 78.95 (0-86542-907-3) Blackwell Sci.

Handbook of Dissociation: Theoretical, Empirical, & Clinical Perspectives. Ed. by Larry K. Michelson & William J. Ray. 1996. (Illus.). 615p. (C). 110.00 (0-306-45150-6, Plenum Trade) Perseus Pubng.

Handbook of Diversity Issues in Health Psychology: Issues of Age, Gender & Orientation, & Ethnicity. Ed. by Pamela M. Kato & Traci Mann. 1996. LC 96-3256. (Plenum Series in Culture & Health: Vol. 1). (Illus.). 467p. (C). 83.00 (0-306-45325-8, Plenum Trade) Perseus Pubng.

Handbook of Dosimetry Data for Radiotherapy. Sharish K. Jani. 1993. 208p. 106.95 (0-8493-3263-X, RM849) CRC Pr.

Handbook of Dramatherapy. Sue Jennings et al. 1994. LC 93-1457. 240p. (C). pap. 29.95 (0-415-09056-3) Routledge.

Handbook of Dream Analysis. Emil A. Gutheil. 1970. LC 78-114371. pap. 17.95 (0-87140-219-X) Liveright.

Handbook of Drug Analysis: Applications in Forensic & Clinical Laboratories. Ray H. Liu & Daniel E. Gadzala. 1997. LC 96-38029. 385p. text 135.00 (0-8412-3448-5) Am Chemical.

Handbook of Drug & Alcohol Abuse. F. Hofman et al. 3rd ed. 1992. (Illus.). 240p. pap. text 27.95 (0-19-506397-X) OUP.

Handbook of Drug Interactions. L. D. Karalleidde. LC 99-159353. 960p. pap. (0-340-66204-2) E A GBR. *Dist:* OUP.

Handbook of Drug Therapy in Liver & Kidney Diseases. Robert W. Schrier. 1991. 45.00 (0-316-77485-5, Little Brwn Med Div) Lppncott W & W.

Handbook of Drug Therapy in Psychiatry. Jerrold G. Bernstein. 3rd ed. 1995. LC 95-17730. 576p. (C). (gr. 13). text 49.95 (0-8016-8101-4) Mosby Multi-Media.

Handbook of Drugs & Chemicals Used in the Treatment of Fish Diseases: A Manual of Fish Pharmacology & Materia Medica. Nelson Herwig. 1979. (Illus.). 288p. 51.95 (0-398-03852-X) C C Thomas.

Handbook of Drugs for Nursing Practice. Virginia B. Karb et al. 2nd ed. 1995. LC 95-39930. (Illus.). 1360p. (C). (gr. 13). text 34.95 (0-8151-5240-X, 24507) Mosby Inc.

Handbook of Drugs for Tropical Parasitic Infections. Yakoub A. Abdi et al. 2nd ed. 1995. LC 96-128933. 208p. (0-7484-0167-9); pap. (0-7484-0168-7) Tay Francis Ltd GBR. *Dist:* Taylor & Francis.

Handbook of Drugs in Primary Eyecare. D. Reid Woodard. 2nd rev. ed. 1997. LC 96-29702. 477p. (C). pap. 41.95 (0-8385-3603-4, A-3603-6) McGraw-Hill Prof.

Handbook of Dual Diagnosis, Vol. 1. JoAnne Nugent. 2nd rev. ed. 1997. 150p. pap. 27.95 (0-9662099-0-7) Mariah Manage.

Handbook of Dystonia. Ed. by Joseph King Ching Tsui & Donald B. Calne. 1995. (Neurological Disease & Therapy Ser.: Vol. 39). (Illus.). 496p. text 195.00 (0-8247-9515-6) Dekker.

Handbook of Ear, Nose & Throat. Dulal K. Basu. 1985. 300p. (0-7855-0733-7) Current Dist IND. *Dist:* St Mut.

Handbook of Ear, Nose & Throat for Primary Care. Christopher Prescott. 1999. (Illus.). 228p. (Orig.). pap. text 29.95 (0-19-571585-3) OUP.

Handbook of Early Childhood Intervention. Ed. by Samuel J. Meisels & Jack P. Shonkoff. 1990. (Illus.). 784p. (C). pap. text 36.95 (0-521-38777-9) Cambridge U Pr.

Handbook of Early Language Impairment in Children. Linda R. Watson et al. 1999. LC 99-50328. (Early Childhood Education Ser.). 320p. pap. text 44.95 (0-8273-7524-7) Delmar.

Handbook of Early Language Impairment in Children: Nature. Ed. by Thomas L. Layton et al. 1999. LC 99-52108. (Early Childhood Education Ser.). (Illus.). 425p. pap. text 44.95 (0-8273-7523-9) Delmar.

Handbook of Eating Disorders: Physiology, Psychology & Treatment. Ed. by Kelly D. Brownell & John P. Foreyt. 1986. LC 85-48021. 528p. pap. 55.00 (0-465-02862-4) Basic.

Handbook of Echo-Doppler Interpretation. Edmund K. Kerut et al. 1996. LC 95-45488. (Illus.). 288p. 39.00 (0-87993-636-3) Futura Pub.

Handbook of Ecotoxicology, Vols. 1 & 2. Peter Calow. 1994. 295.00 (0-86542-849-2) Blackwell Sci.

Handbook of Ecotoxicology Vol. 2, Vol. 2. Peter Calow. 1994. LC 92-39663. (Illus.). 500p. (0-632-02989-7) Blckwell Science.

Handbook of ECT. Charles H. Kellner et al. 1997. LC 96-29955. 122p. spiral bd. 23.50 (0-88048-683-X, 8683) Am Psychiatric.

Handbook of Edible Weeds. James A. Duke. 999th ed. 2000. LC 00-49385. (Herbal Reference Library). (Illus.). 256p. 69.95 (0-8493-2946-9) CRC Pr.

Handbook of Effective Psychotherapy. Ed. by Thomas R. Giles. 1993. LC 93-23996. (Plenum Behavior Therapy Ser.). (Illus.). 524p. (C). 90.00 (0-306-44428-3, Plenum Trade) Perseus Pubng.

Handbook of Eicosanoids. Willis. 1987. Vol. I, Pt. A. 328p. 245.00 (0-8493-3221-4); Vol. IB. 288p. 245.00 (0-8493-3222-2) CRC Pr.

Handbook of Electrosurgery in Endoscopy. Arnaud Wattiez. 1995. LC 94-32504. 288p. 99.95 (0-86542-918-9) Blackwell Sci.

Handbook of Emergencies in General Practice. Ed. by Norman Lawrence et al. 2nd ed. 1996. (Illus.). 390p. pap. 39.95 (0-19-262545-4) OUP.

Handbook of Emergency. G. Golwalla. 2nd ed. 1983. (C). (0-7855-4672-3) Current Dist IND. *Dist:* St Mut.

Handbook of Emergency Laboratory Tests. L. I. Worthley. 1996. (Illus.). 202p. pap. (0-443-05313-8) Church.

Handbook of Emergency Psychiatry for Clinical Administrators. Ed. by Gail Barton & Rohn Friedman. 1986. LC 86-12090. (Emergency Health Services Review Ser.: Vol. 3, Nos. 2-3). 390p. 59.95 (0-86656-532-9) Haworth Pr.

Handbook of Emergency Toxicology. Ed. by Peter Viccellio. 2nd ed. 1998. LC 98-15949. 1,312p. pap. text 99.00 (0-316-90237-3, Little Brwn Med Div) Lppncott W & W.

Handbook of Emergency Toxicology: A Guide for the Identification, Diagnosis & Treatment of Poisoning. Sidney Kaye. 5th ed. 1988. (Illus.). 586p. 126.95 (0-398-05403-7) C C Thomas.

Handbook of Emotion, Adult Development, & Aging. Ed. by Carol Magai & Susan H. McFadden. 1996. LC 96-22522. (Illus.). 470p. text 75.00 (0-12-464995-5) Acad Pr.

Handbook of Emotions. Ed. by Michael Lewis & Jeannette M. Haviland-Jones. 2nd ed. 2000. LC 99-86558. (Illus.). 720p. 75.00 (1-57230-529-0, 8R0529) Guilford Pubns.

Handbook of Empirical Social Work Practice, Set. Ed. by Bruce A. Thyer & John S. Wodarski. Incl. Mental Disorders. LC 97-15312. 528p. 1998. 99.95 (0-471-15361-3); LC 97-15312. 1200p. 1998. 190.00 (0-471-15363-X) Wiley.

Handbook of Endocrinology, Vol. 1. Ed. by George H. Gass & Harold M. Kaplan. 2nd rev. ed. 1996. LC 96-13983. (Handbook of Endocrinology Ser.: Vol. 1). 368p. 159.95 (0-8493-9429-5) CRC Pr.

Handbook of Endocrinology, Set. Ed. by George H. Gass & Harold M. Kaplan. 1982. 368p. 146.95 (0-8493-3239-7, QP187, CRC Reprint) Franklin.

Handbook of Endoglycosidases & Glycoamidases. Ed. by Takashi Muramatsu. 1992. 362p. lib. bdg. 199.00 (0-8493-3618-X, QP 609) CRC Pr.

Handbook of Endovascular Surgery: Vademecum. S. S. Ahn. Ed. by D. I. Obrand. 1997. LC 97-31215. (Systems Publications). (Illus.). viii, 194p. 98.00 (3-8055-6598-4) S Karger.

Handbook of Engineering in Medicine & Biology, CRC, Vol. 1: General Date. Ed. by David G. Fleming & Barry N. Feinberg. 1976. (Handbook Ser.). 432p. 247.00 (0-87819-285-9, R856, CRC Reprint) Franklin.

Handbook of Engineering in Medicine & Biology, CRC: Section B-Instruments & Measurements, Vol. 2. David G. Fleming & Barry N. Feinberg. 1978. (Engineering in Medicine & Biology Ser.). 446p. 75.00 (0-8493-0242-0, R856) CRC Pr.

Handbook of Environmental Control, Vol. 5: Hospital & Health Care Facilities. C. Straub. 1975. LC 72-92118. 242.00 (0-87819-275-1, CRC Reprint) Franklin.

Handbook of Environmental Health & Safety, Vol. I. Herman Koren. 2nd ed. 1991. 632p. lib. bdg. 87.00 (0-87371-272-2, L272) Lewis Pubs.

Handbook of Environmental Health & Safety: Principles & Practices, Vol. II. Herman Koren. 2nd ed. 1991. 696p. lib. bdg. 87.00 (0-87371-414-8, L414) Lewis Pubs.

Handbook of Environmental Psychology Ed. by Daniel Stokols & Irwin Altman. 1991. LC 91-11177. 1684p. reprint ed. 225.00 (0-89464-609-5) Krieger.

Handbook of Environmental Radiation. Ed. by Alfred W. Klement, Jr. 1982. 496p. 268.00 (0-8493-3761-5, QC795, CRC Reprint) Franklin.

Handbook of Enzyme Biotechnology. Alan Wiseman. 2nd ed. 1985. LC 84-25167. (Baker Lectures). 457p. 115.00 (0-470-20153-3) P-H.

Handbook of Epilepsy Treatment. Simon D. Shorvon. 2000. (Illus.). 240p. pap. 67.95 (0-632-04849-2) Blackwell Sci.

Handbook of Equine Colic. N. A. White & Barrie Edwards. 1999. LC 99-35352. (Illus.). 146p. pap. text 52.50 (0-7506-3587-8) Buttrwrth-Heinemann.

Handbook of Equine Colic. N. A. White et al. Date not set. (Pergamon Veterinary Handbook Ser.). text (0-08-042521-6, Pergamon Pr) Elsevier.

Handbook of Equine Colic. White et al. Date not set. (Pergamon Veterinary Handbook Ser.). pap. text (0-08-042520-8, Pergamon Pr) Elsevier.

Handbook of Ericksonian Psychotherapy. Ed. by Brent Geary & Jeffrey K. Zeig. 2000. 356p. text 48.95 (1-891944-40-1) Zeig Tucker Theisen.

Handbook of Essential Drugs & Regimens in Hematological Oncology. Aaron Polliack. 1991. xii, 165p. text 96.00 (3-7186-5096-7); 165p. pap. text 43.00 (3-7186-5097-5) Gordon & Breach (Harwood Acad Pubs).

Handbook of Essential Psychopharmacology. Ronald W. Pies. 1998. LC 97-24581. 416p. 42.95 (0-88048-765-8, 8765) Am Psychiatric.

Handbook of Evolutionary Psychology: Ideas, Issues, & Applications. Charles Crawford & Dennis Krebs. 1997. LC 97-16301. 150.00 (0-8058-1666-6) L Erlbaum Assocs.

Handbook of Exercise Testing. Victor F. Froelicher & Susan Quaglietti. 1995. LC 95-21519. 176p. pap. text 39.95 (0-316-29429-2, Little Brwn Med Div) Lppncott W & W.

Handbook of Exercises for Eliminating Headaches. Errol Lader. 1983. (Illus.). 65p. pap. 2.95 (0-9610782-6-X) Vadare.

Handbook of Experiential Psychotherapy. Ed. by Leslie S. Greenberg et al. 1998. LC 98-35433. (Guilford Family Therapy Ser.). 477p. 57.00 (1-57230-374-3) Guilford Pubns.

Handbook of Experimental Pharmacology. Born. 1993. (Illus.). 658p. 380.00 (0-387-56937-5) Spr-Verlag.

Handbook of Experimental Stomatology. Barnet M. Levy & S. Dreizen. 1982. LC 81-7734. (Experimental Oral Biology Ser.). 224p. 131.00 (0-8493-3161-7, RC815, CRC Reprint) Franklin.

Handbook of Eye Emergencies: New England Eye Center. Bradford J. Shingleton et al. 1998. LC 98-22559. (Illus.). 144p. pap. text 49.00 (1-55642-385-3, 63853) SLACK Inc.

Handbook of Family Development & Intervention. William C. Nichols et al. 2000. LC 99-37989. (Couples & Family Dynamics & Treatment Ser.). (Illus.). 482p. 80.00 (0-471-29967-7) Wiley.

***Handbook of Family Planning & Reproductive Health Care.** Anna Glasier et al. 2001. (Illus.). 441p. pap. (0-443-06450-4) Church GBR. *Dist:* Saunders.

Handbook of Family Planning & Reproductive Health Care. Ed. by Nancy Loudon et al. 3rd ed. 1995. LC 96-179935. (Illus.). 462p. (C). pap. (0-443-05157-7) Church.

Handbook of Family Psychology & Therapy, I. Luciano L'Abate. 1985. LC 84-71293. (Professional Bks.). (C). text 79.95 (0-534-10443-6) Brooks-Cole.

Handbook of Family Therapy, Vol. I. Alan S. Gurman & David P. Kniskern. 1987. LC 80-20357. 800p. text 83.95 (0-87630-242-8) Brunner-Routledge.

Handbook of Family Therapy, Vol. II. Ed. by Alan S. Gurman & David P. Kniskern. 1991. LC 80-20357. 832p. text 78.95 (0-87630-642-3) Brunner-Routledge.

Handbook of Family Therapy Training & Supervision. Ed. by Howard A. Liddle et al. 1988. LC 87-24848. (Family Therapy Ser.). 432p. 55.00 (0-89862-073-2, 2073) Guilford Pubns.

Handbook of Feline Medicine. Ed. by Jo Wills & Alice Wolf. 1993. LC 92-31279. (Veterinary Handbook Ser.). text 110.00 (0-08-040829-X, Pergamon Pr) Elsevier.

Handbook of Feminist Therapy: Women's Issues in Psychotherapy. Lynne B. Rosewater & Lenore E. Walker. 1985. 384p. 44.95 (0-8261-4970-7) Springer Pub.

Handbook of Fetal Heart Rate Monitoring. Julian T. Parer. Ed. by William Schmitt. 2nd ed. 1997. LC 96-37238. 304p. pap. text 33.00 (0-7216-3639-X) Saunders.

Handbook of Feynman Path Integrals. C. Grosche & F. Steiner. 1998. LC 98-25806. (Tracts in Modern Physics Ser.: Vol. 145). x, 459p. 189.00 (3-540-57135-3) Spr-Verlag.

Handbook of Fine Needle Aspiration Biopsy Cytology. Tilde S. Kline. 2nd ed. 1988. (Illus.). 492p. text (0-443-08466-1) Church.

Handbook of Fish Diseases. Dieter Untergasser. Ed. by Herbert R. Axelrod. Tr. by Howard Hirschhorn from GER. 1988. (Illus.). 160p. (C). lib. bdg. 35.95 (0-86622-703-2, TS-123) TFH Pubns.

Handbook of Fluid, Electrolyte & Acid-Based Disorders. Leonard G. Feld. 2001. (Illus.). 272p. pap. 35.00 (0-7506-9957-4) Buttrwrth-Heinemann.

Handbook of Food Additives. Chism. 3rd ed. 1994. (0-8493-0544-6) CRC Pr.

Handbook of Food Allergies. James C. Breneman. 1986. (Immunology Ser.: Vol. 29). (Illus.). 320p. text 175.00 (0-8247-7558-9) Dekker.

Handbook of Foodborne Diseases of Biological Origin. Ed. by Miloslav Rechcigl, Jr. 1983. 535p. lib. bdg. 163.00 (0-8493-3964-2, RA1258, CRC Reprint) Franklin.

Handbook of Forensic Psychology. Ed. by Allen K. Hess & Irving B. Weiner. 2nd ed. 1998. LC 98-23732. (Illus.). 768p. 130.00 (0-471-17771-7) Wiley.

Handbook of Forensic Rehabilitation. William H. Burke. 1995. LC 94-41909. 304p. (Orig.). pap. 34.50 (1-882855-31-0) HDI Pubs.

Handbook of Forensic Science. 1997. lib. bdg. 250.95 (0-8490-8229-3) Gordon Pr.

Handbook of Forensic Services. rev. ed. 2000. (Illus.). 150p. pap. (0-932115-16-0) FBI Lab.

Handbook of Forensic Sexology: Biomedical & Criminological Perspectives. Ed. by James J. Krivacska & John Money. 1994. LC 94-8451. 594p. (C). 130.00 (0-87975-883-X) Prometheus Bks.

Handbook of Fractures. Clayton R. Perry et al. 2nd ed. 1999. LC 99-38946. (Illus.). 399p. pap. 39.95 (0-07-048624-7) McGraw-Hill Prof.

Handbook of Free Radicals & Antioxidants in Biomedicine. Ed. by Jaime Miquel et al. 1988. Vol. I. 352p. 203.00 (0-8493-3268-0, RB170); Vol. II. 384p. lib. bdg. 229.00 (0-8493-3269-9, RB170); Vol. III. 328p. lib. bdg. 229.00 (0-8493-3270-2, RB170) CRC Pr.

Handbook of Functional Gastrointestinal Disorders, No. 4. Ed. by Kevin W. Olden. 1996. (Medical Psychiatry Ser.: Vol. 4). (Illus.). 436p. text 165.00 (0-8247-9409-5) Dekker.

Handbook of Functional Neuroimaging of Cognition. Ed. by Roberto Cabeza & Alan Kingstone. 2000. LC 00-22253. (Illus.). viii, 410p. (C). 59.95 (0-262-03280-5, Bradford Bks) MIT Pr.

Handbook of Gastro-Esophageal Disease. A. I. Morris & J. Bancewicz. 1998. (Illus.). 288p. pap. (0-443-05387-1) Church.

Handbook of Gastroenterology. David S. Cantor. 1991. (0-8151-1423-0) Mosby Inc.

Handbook of Gastroenterology. Ed. by Peter G. Traber et al. 1998. LC 98-12187. 528p. spiral bd. 49.95 (0-397-51427-1) Lppncott W & W.

Handbook of Gender, Culture & Health. Ed. by Richard M. Eisler & Michel Hersen. 1999. LC 99-30953. x, 531p. (*0-8058-2638-6*) L Erlbaum Assocs.

Handbook of Gene Level Diagnostics in Clinical Practice. Victor A. Bernstam. 1992. 672p. lib. bdg. 125.00 (*0-8493-6824-3*, RB155) CRC Pr.

Handbook of General Hospital Psychiatry. Massachusetts General Hospital Staff. Ed. by Ned H. Cassem. 4th ed. 1997. LC 97-20147. (Illus.). 688p. (C). (gr. 13). pap. text 44.95 (*0-8151-1478-8*, 25731) Mosby Inc.

Handbook of General Surgery. P. Gilroy Bevan & I. A. Donovan. 1992. (Illus.). 576p. pap. 38.95 (*0-632-01111-4*) Blackwell Sci.

Handbook of Genetic Influences on the Nervous System. Donald W. Pfaff. 1999. LC 99-21820. (Illus.). 504p. 99.95 (*0-8493-2688-5*) CRC Pr.

Handbook of Genetic Skin Disorders. Fred M. Novice et al. 1994. LC 93-25389. (Illus.). 704p. text 115.00 (*0-7216-3803-1*) Saunders.

Handbook of Geriatric Assessment. Joseph J. Gallo et al. 3rd ed. 1999. LC 99-36370. 384p. pap. 55.00 (*0-8342-1248-X*, 1248X) Aspen Pub.

Handbook of Geriatric Care Management. Cathy Cress. 2000. LC 00-48088. 336p. 55.00 (*0-8342-1667-1*, 16671) Aspen Pub.

Handbook of Geriatric Communication Disorders. Ed. by Danielle N. Ripich. 1991. LC 90-74311. 494p. text 41.00 (*0-89079-423-5*, 1944) PRO-ED.

Handbook of Geriatric Drug Therapy. Frwd. by Kathleen Fletcher. 2000. LC 99-58888. 1024p. spiral bd. 38.95 (*0-87434-998-2*) Springhouse Corp.

Handbook of Geriatric Drugs. Michael A. Jenike. 1991. (*0-8151-4893-3*) Mosby Inc.

Handbook of Geriatric Nursing Care. Springhouse Publishing Company Staff. 1998. LC 98-11712. (Illus.). 640p. spiral bd. 38.95 (*0-87434-940-0*) Springhouse Corp.

Handbook of Geriatrics. S. R. Gambert. 1987. LC 86-25355. (Illus.). 420p. (C). spiral bd. 65.00 (*0-306-42336-7*, Kluwer Plenum) Kluwer Academic.

Handbook of Gerontological Services. Ed. by Abraham Monk. 2nd ed. 1990. 656p. text 76.00 (*0-231-06902-2*) Col U Pr.

Handbook of Group Activities for Impaired Older Adults. Elsbeth M. Hegelson & Scott C. Willis. 1987. LC 87-274. (Activities, Adaptation & Aging Ser.: Vol. 9, No. 2). 107p. text 24.95 (*0-86656-628-7*) Haworth Pr.

Handbook of Group Psychotherapy: An Empirical & Clinical Synthesis. Ed. by Addie Fuhriman & Gary M. Burlingame. 1994. LC 94-8476. (Personality Processes Ser.). 588p. 160.00 (*0-471-55592-4*) Wiley.

Handbook of Growth Factors Pimentel. 1994. 628.80 (*0-8493-2508-0*) CRC Pr.

Handbook of Growth Factors. Enrique Pimentel. 1994. LC 93-40108. 384p. 1. 146.95 (*0-8493-2505-6*); Vol. 3. 146.95 (*0-8493-2507-2*) CRC Pr.

***Handbook of Gyn Oncology.** Joseph T. Santoso. 2001. (Illus.). 150p. pap. 35.00 (*0-8385-3532-1*) McGraw-Hill Prof.

***Handbook of Gynaecological Management.** Ed. by Sylvia Rosevear & Mrcog Frnzcog. 2001. (Illus.). 320p. pap. 38.95 (*0-632-05588-X*) Blackwell Sci.

***Handbook of Gynaecological Oncology.** Mahmood Shafi et al. 2001. (Illus.). 320p. pap. (*0-443-06397-4*) Church GBR. *Dist:* Saunders.

Handbook of Gynaecology. Bikash C. Basu. 1981. 490p. (*0-7855-0734-5*) Current Dist IND. *Dist:* St Mut.

Handbook of Gynecologic Oncology. Ed. by M. Steven Piver. 2nd rev. ed. 1995. LC 95-331. 450p. pap. text 39.95 (*0-316-70939-5*, Little Brwn Med Div) Lppncott W & W.

Handbook of Gynecology & Obstetrics. Jeanette Brown & William Crombleholme. 1996. (Illus.). 626p. (C). pap. text 39.95 (*0-8385-3608-5*, A3608-5, Apple Lange Med) McGraw.

Handbook of Haematological Investigations in Children. R. F. Stevens. 1989. (Illus.). 117p. pap. text 75.00 (*0-7236-1307-9*) Buttrwrth-Heinemann.

Handbook of Hazard Communication & OSHA Requirements. George G. Lowry & Robert C. Lowry. 1985. LC 85-6982. (Illus.). 300p. lib. bdg. 68.00 (*0-87371-022-3*, L022) Lewis Pubs.

Handbook of Head & Neck Imaging. June M. Unger. 1987. (Handbooks of Diagnostic Imaging Ser.: Vol. 2). (Illus.). 232p. text (*0-443-08471-8*) Church.

Handbook of Head & Neck Imaging. H. Ric Harnsberger. 2nd rev. ed. 1994. LC 94-35225. (Handbooks in Radiology Ser.). (Illus.). 576p. (C). (gr. 13). pap. text 50.95 (*0-8151-4233-1*, 24206) Mosby Inc.

Handbook of Head & Spine Trauma. Jonathan Greenberg. 1993. (Neurological Disease & Therapy Ser.: Vol. 19). (Illus.). 784p. text 275.00 (*0-8247-9051-0*) Dekker.

Handbook of Head Trauma: Acute Care to Recovery. Ed. by C. J. Long et al. 1992. (Critical Issues in Neuropsychology Ser.). (Illus.). 466p. (C). text 85.00 (*0-306-43947-6*, Kluwer Plenum) Kluwer Academic.

Handbook of Headache. Randolph W. Evans & Ninan T. Mathew. 2000. 352p. pap. text 39.95 (*0-7817-1877-5*) Lppncott W & W.

Handbook of Headache Disorders. Arthur H. Elkind. 2nd ed. 1994. 171p. (Orig.). (C). pap. 14.95 (*0-929240-62-6*) EMIS.

Handbook of Headache Management: A Practical Guide to Diagnosis & Treatment of Head, Neck, & Facial Pain. Joel R. Saper et al. 1992. LC 92-23747. (Illus.). 224p. 29.00 (*0-683-05801-0*) Lppncott W & W.

Handbook of Headache Management: A Practical Guide to Diagnosis & Treatment of Head, Neck & Facial Pain. Joel R. Saper et al. 2nd ed. 1999. LC 00-269707. (Illus.). 344p. pap. text 42.00 (*0-7817-2048-6*) Lppncott W & W.

Handbook of Health Administration & Policy. Ed. by Anne O. Kilpatrick et al. 1998. LC 98-37296. (Illus.). 1120p. text 250.00 (*0-8247-0221-2*) Dekker.

Handbook of Health & Rehabilitation Psychology. Ed. by Anthony J. Goreczny. 1995. LC 95-40862. (Rehabilitation & Health Ser.). (Illus.). 718p. (C). 100.00 (*0-306-44970-6*, Plenum Trade) Perseus Pubng.

Handbook of Health Assessment. Ellen B. Rudy & V. Ruth Gray. 2nd ed. 1985. 304p. pap. text 13.95 (*0-89303-493-2*, Appleton-Century-Crofts); 3rd ed. 1991. (Illus.). 320p. (C). pap. 30.40 (*0-8385-3602-6*, A3602-8) P-H.

Handbook of Health Care Accounting & Finance William O. Cleverley. 2nd ed. 1989. 1043p. 299.00 (*0-8342-0056-2*) Aspen Pub.

Handbook of Health Care Management. Ed. by W. Jack Duncan et al. 1997. LC 97-13926. 610p. text 89.95 (*1-55786-833-6*) Blackwell Pubs.

Handbook of Health Careers: A Guide to Employment Opportunities. Janet Z. Nassif. 1980. LC 79-23027. 354p. 49.95 (*0-87705-489-4*, Kluwer Acad Hman Sci) Kluwer Academic.

Handbook of Health Economics Ed. by A. J. Culyer & J. P. Newhouse. 2000. LC 2001-275530. (Handbooks in Economics). (Illus.). 1096p. 224.50 (*0-444-82290-9*, North Holland) Elsevier.

Handbook of Hearing Aid Amplification Vol. I: Theoretical & Technical Considerations, Vol. 1. Ed. by Robert E. Sandlin. 1995. (Illus.). 336p. (C). reprint ed. pap. 55.00 (*1-56593-399-0*, 0171) Thomson Learn.

Handbook of Hearing Aid Amplification Vol. II: Clinical Considerations & Fitting Practices, Vol. 2. Ed. by Robert E. Sandlin. 1995. (Illus.). 312p. (C). reprint ed. pap. text 55.00 (*1-56593-400-8*, 0172) Thomson Learn.

Handbook of Hematologic & Oncologic Emergencies. J. P. Dutcher & P. H. Wiernik. 1988. LC 87-7374. (Illus.). 372p. (C). text 85.00 (*0-306-42646-3*, Kluwer Plenum) Kluwer Academic.

Handbook of Hematological Pathology. Ed. by Sanford A. Stass & Harold R. Schumacher. Date not set. (Illus.). 792p. text 225.00 (*0-8247-0170-4*) Dekker.

Handbook of Hemodynamic Monitoring. Gloria Obdlouk Darovic & Cory M. Franklin. Ed. by Robin Carter. 1999. LC 99-11311. (Illus.). 445p. pap. text 24.00 (*0-7216-7370-8*) Saunders.

Handbook of Hemostasis & Thrombosis. Jack E. Ansell. 1986. (Illus.). 130p. 28.95 (*0-316-04331-1*, Little Brwn Med Div) Lppncott W & W.

Handbook of High-Risk Perinatal Home Care. Health Care Resources Staff & Carolyn B. Mitchell. 1996. 208p. (C). (gr. 13). spiral bd. 27.95 (*0-8151-2865-7*, 30525) Mosby Inc.

Handbook of Hip Fracture Management. Martyn Parker et al. 1997. LC 96-40887. 160p. pap. text (*0-7506-2179-6*) E A GBR. *Dist:* OUP.

Handbook of Histology Methods for Bone & Cartilage. Ed. by Yuehuei H. An & Kylie L. Martin. 2001. 500p. 135.00 (*0-89603-960-9*) Humana.

Handbook of HIV Prevention. Ed. by John L. Peterson & Ralph J. DiClemente. 2000. LC 99-53994. (AIDS Prevention & Mental Health Ser.). 340p. 115.00 (*0-306-46223-0*, Kluwer Plenum) Kluwer Academic.

Handbook of HIV Prevention Policy Analysis. D. R. Holtgrave. 1998. LC 98-39090. (AIDS Prevention & Mental Health Ser.). (Illus.). 304p. 69.50 (*0-306-45749-0*, Kluwer Plenum) Kluwer Academic.

Handbook of Home Health Care Administration. Ed. by Marilyn D. Harris. 2nd ed. 1997. LC 97-6069. 800p. 95.00 (*0-8342-0918-7*, 20918) Aspen Pub.

Handbook of Home Health Nursing Procedures. Rice. 2nd ed. 1999. (Illus.). (C). text 31.95 (*0-323-00911-5*) Mosby Inc.

Handbook of Home Health Standards & Documentation: Guidelines for Reimbursement, Vol. 3. Tina M. Marrelli. 3rd ed. 1997. LC 98-139539. (Illus.). 688p. spiral bd. 29.95 (*0-8151-2399-X*, 31044) Mosby Inc.

Handbook of Homeopathy. Gerhard Koehler. 1989. LC 92-48302. 240p. pap. 16.95 (*0-89281-345-8*, Heal Arts VT) Inner Tradit.

Handbook of Hormones, Vitamins & Radiopaques: CRC Series in Medicinal Chemistry. Matthew Verderame. 1986. (Medicinal Chemistry Ser.). 320p. 190.00 (*0-8493-3291-5*, QP571, CRC Reprint) Franklin.

Handbook of Hospice Care. Robert W. Buckingham. 1996. LC 96-11357. (Illus.). 262p. pap. 21.00 (*1-57392-060-6*) Prometheus Bks.

Handbook of Hospital Based Substance Abuse Treatment. William D. Lerner & Marjorie A. Barr. 1990. (Illus.). 256p. (*0-08-036077-7*); pap. (*0-08-036076-9*) PPI GBR. *Dist:* McGraw.

Handbook of Hospital Infection. Philpott. 1994. pap. text 41.00 (*0-7020-1658-6*) Saunders.

Handbook of Hospital Psychiatry: A Practical Guide to Therapy. Louis Linn. 1955. LC 55-8237. pap. 24.95 (*0-8236-8069-X*, 22300) Intl Univs Pr.

Handbook of Hospital Safety. Ed. by Paul E. Stanley. 1981. 416p. 227.00 (*0-8493-0751-1*, RA969, CRC Reprint) Franklin.

Handbook of Hospital Security & Safety. James T. Turner. 1987. 272p. pap. 110.00 (*0-87189-887-X*) Aspen Pub.

Handbook of HPLC in Pharmaceutical Analysis, Vol. I: General Considerations. Ed. by Gabor Szepesi. 1990. 328p. 249.00 (*0-8493-6998-3*, RS189) CRC Pr.

Handbook of HPLC in Pharmaceutical Analysis: Practical Applications, Vol. 2. Ed. by Gabor Szepesi. 1990. 360p. 249.00 (*0-8493-6999-1*, RS189) CRC Pr.

Handbook of Human Blood Constituent. Richard W. Richardson. 1994. 357p. lib. bdg. 210.00 (*0-8493-8664-0*) CRC Pr.

Handbook of Human Growth & Development, Vol. I: Neural, Sensory, Motor & Integrative Development, Vol. 1. Ed. by Esmail Meisami & Paola S. Timiras. 1988. 216p. 199.00 (*0-8493-3181-1*, RJ131); 184p. 150.00 (*0-8493-3183-8*, RJ131); 320p. lib. bdg. 215.00 (*0-8493-3182-X*, RJ131) CRC Pr.

Handbook of Human Performance: Health & Performance, Vol. 2. Ed. by Andy Smith & Dyland Jones. 1992. (Illus.). text 95.00 (*0-12-650352-4*) Acad Pr.

Handbook of Human Services for Older Persons. Ed. by Monica B. Holmes & Douglas Holmes. 1979. LC 78-27668. 300p. 42.95 (*0-87705-381-2*, Kluwer Acad Hman Sci) Kluwer Academic.

Handbook of Human Stress & Immunity. Ed. by Ronald Glaser et al. 1994. LC 94-20811. 414p. text 84.95 (*0-12-285960-X*) Acad Pr.

Handbook of Human Toxicology. Edward J. Massaro. 1997. LC 97-721. 1136p. 149.95 (*0-8493-4493-X*) CRC Pr.

Handbook of Human Vibration. Michael J. Griffin. 1990. 1008p. text 262.00 (*0-12-303040-4*) Acad Pr.

Handbook of Human Vibration. Michael J. Griffin. 1996. (Illus.). 1008p. (C). pap. text 59.95 (*0-12-303041-2*) Morgan Kaufmann.

Handbook of Hydropathy: A Popular Account of the Treatment & Prevention of Disease by Means of Water. Ed. by Joel Shew. 1997. 145p. reprint ed. pap. 15.00 (*0-7873-0787-4*) Hlth Research.

Handbook of Hydropathy: The Treatment & Prevention of Diseases by Means of Water. Joel Shew. 1991. lib. bdg. 75.00 (*0-87700-935-X*) Revisionist Pr.

Handbook of Hygienic Practice: Intended for a Practical Guide for the Sickroom. R. T. Trall. 1996. 300p. reprint ed. spiral bd. 23.00 (*0-7873-0893-5*) Hlth Research.

Handbook of Hyperbaric Oxygen Therapy. B. Fischer et al. 1988. (Illus.). 359p. 115.00 (*0-387-18344-2*) Spr-Verlag.

Handbook of Hypnosis for Professionals. Roy Udolf. 2nd ed. 1995. LC 92-27304. 532p. pap. 70.00 (*1-56821-727-7*) Aronson.

Handbook of Hypnotic Phenomena in Psychotherapy. John H. Edgette & Janet S. Edgette. 1995. LC 94-35103. 318p. text 36.95 (*0-87630-750-0*) Brunner-Routledge.

Handbook of Hypnotic Suggestions & Metaphors. Ed. by D. Corydon Hammond. 1990. 618p. (C). 70.00 (*0-393-70095-X*) Norton.

Handbook of Imaging for Neonatal Care. Haresh Kirpalani et al. 1999. 173p. pap. text 39.00 (*0-443-05544-0*) Saunders.

Handbook of Immediate Care. Greaves. 1995. pap. text 41.00 (*0-7020-1881-3*) Saunders.

Handbook of Immigrant Health. Ed. by S. Loue. 1998. LC 98-34164. (Illus.). 668p. 115.00 (*0-306-45959-0*, Kluwer Plenum) Kluwer Academic.

Handbook of Immune Response Genes. Tak W. Mak. 1998. LC 97-48244. (Illus.). 408p. (C). text 95.00 (*0-306-45647-8*, Kluwer Plenum) Kluwer Academic.

Handbook of Immunoblotting of Proteins Ed. by Ole J. Bjerrum & Niels H. Heegaard. 1988. Vol. I. 280p. 260.00 (*0-8493-0549-7*, QP519); Vol. 2. 224p. 273.95 (*0-8493-0550-0*, QP519) CRC Pr.

Handbook of Immunology of Aging. Ed. by Takashi Makinodan & Marguerite M. Kay. 1981. LC 80-24315. (Series in Aging). 328p. 181.00 (*0-8493-3144-7*, QP86, CRC Reprint) Franklin.

Handbook of In Vitro Fertilization. Alan O. Trounson. 1993. 336p. 119.00 (*0-8493-2922-1*, R6135) CRC Pr.

Handbook of in Vitro Fertilization. Alan O. Trounson & David K. Gardner. 2nd ed. 1999. LC 99-27298. (Illus.). 576p. 125.00 (*0-8493-4002-0*) CRC Pr.

Handbook of Individual Therapy. Windy Dryden. 1996. 416p. 82.00 (*0-8039-7842-1*, 9729); pap. 29.95 (*0-8039-7843-X*, 9730) Sage.

Handbook of Industrial Toxicology & Hazardous Materials. Nicholas P. Cheremisinoff. 1999. LC 98-55662. (Illus.). 928p. text 259.00 (*0-8247-1935-2*) Dekker.

Handbook of Infant, Child & Adolescent Psychotherapy Vol. I: A Guide to Diagnosis & Treatment. Ed. by Bonnie S. Mark & James A. Incorvaia. 1995. LC 94-44248. 464p. 60.00 (*1-56821-444-8*) Aronson.

Handbook of Infant, Child & Adolescent Psychotherapy Vol. 2: New Directions in Integrative Treatment. Ed. by Bonnie S. Mark & James A. Incorvaia. 1997. LC 94-44248. 528p. 60.00 (*0-7657-0044-1*) Aronson.

Handbook of Infant Development. Ed. by Joy D. Osofsky. 2nd ed. 1987. LC 86-28906. (Personality Processes Ser.). 1424p. 385.00 (*0-471-88565-7*) Wiley.

Handbook of Infant Mental Health. Ed. by Charles H. Zeanah, Jr. 2nd rev. ed. 1999. LC 99-51343. 588p. text, instr.'s hndbk. ed. 63.00 (*1-57230-515-0*, CO515) Guilford Pubns.

Handbook of Infant Mental Health, Set. Ed. by Joy D. Osofsky & Hiram E. Fitzgerald. Incl. Early Intervention, Evaluation, & Assessment. 575p. 220.00 (*0-471-18944-8*); Infant Mental Health Groups at High Risk. 617p. 220.00 (*0-471-18947-2*); Parenting & Child Care. 425p. 220.00 (*0-471-18946-4*); Perspectives on Infant Mental Health. 403p. 220.00 (*0-471-18941-3*); 1999. LC 99-11893. (Parenting & Child Care Ser.). (Illus.). 2432p. 2000. 880.00 (*0-471-18988-X*) Wiley.

Handbook of Infectious Diseases. Stewart M. Brooks et al. 1980. 14.00 (*0-316-10968-1*, Little Brwn Med Div) Lppncott W & W.

***Handbook of Infertility.** S. Bayer & M. Alper. 2001. 200p. 77.95 (*1-84214-102-3*, Parthenon Pbng) CRC Pr.

Handbook of Informatics for Nurses & Health Care Professionals. Toni Lee Hebda et al. 2nd ed. 2000. LC 00-52408. (Illus.). 416p. pap. 29.95 (*0-13-031102-2*) P-H.

Handbook of Infusion Therapy. Springhouse Publishing Company Staff. 1998. LC 98-42250. (Illus.). 512p. 38.95 (*0-87434-941-9*) Springhouse Corp.

Handbook of Innovative Programs for the Impaired Elderly. Ed. by Eloise H. Killeffer et al. 1985. LC 84-22502. (Physical & Occupational Therapy in Geriatrics Ser.: Vol. 3, No. 3). 126p. text 29.95 (*0-86656-381-4*) Haworth Pr.

Handbook of Institutional Pharmacy Practice. Pref. by Thomas R. Brown. 3rd ed. 1992. (C). text 60.00 (*1-879907-21-6*) Am Soc Hlth-Syst.

***Handbook of Integrated Short-Term Psychotherapy.** Arnold Winston & Beverly Winston. 2001. LC 2001-22960. 288p. pap. 37.95 (*0-88048-814-X*, 8814) Am Psychiatric.

Handbook of Integrative Psychotherapies for Children & Adolescents. Sebastiano Santostefano. 1998. LC 97-10315. 608p. 60.00 (*0-7657-0083-2*) Aronson.

Handbook of Intensive Brief & Emergency Psychotherapy. Leopold Bellak et al. 2nd rev. ed. 1992. 257p. pap. 24.95 (*0-918863-04-X*) CPS Inc.

Handbook of Intensive Brief & Emergency Psychotherapy (B. E. P.) Leopold Bellak. 1987. LC 83-20947. 170p. (Orig.). reprint ed. pap. 14.95 (*0-918863-00-7*) CPS Inc.

Handbook of Interpersonal Competence Research. Brian H. Spitzberg & W. R. Cupach. 1988. (Recent Research in Psychology Ser.). 352p. 46.00 (*0-387-96866-0*) Spr-Verlag.

Handbook of Interpersonal Psychotherapy. Ed. by Jack C. Anchin & Donald J. Kiesler. 1981. (General Psychology Ser.). 368p. 65.00 (*0-08-025959-6*, Pergamon Pr) Elsevier.

Handbook of Interpretation of Diagnostic Tests. Jacques Wallach. 1998. LC 97-51668. (Illus.). 576p. pap. text 29.95 (*0-7817-1221-1*) Lppncott W & W.

Handbook of Interpretations for the Comrey Personality Scales. Andrew Comrey. 1980. LC 80-67424. pap. 25.75 (*0-912736-23-2*) EDITS Pubs.

Handbook of Interventional Radiologic Procedures. Krishna Kandarpa. 3rd ed. 2001. pap. text 49.95 (*0-7817-2358-2*) Lppncott W & W.

Handbook of Interventional Radiology & Angiography. Myron Wojtowycz. 2nd ed. 1995. LC 95-172. (Handbooks in Radiology Ser.). (Illus.). 448p. (C). (gr. 13). pap. text 49.00 (*0-8151-9440-4*, 23909) Mosby Inc.

Handbook of Intrauterine Insemination. Ed. by Godwin I. Meniru et al. 1997. (Illus.). 261p. (C). pap. text 52.95 (*0-521-58676-3*) Cambridge U Pr.

Handbook of Iridiagnosis & Rational Therapy. Robert Wilborn et al. 1996. 155p. reprint ed. 37.50 (*0-7873-0970-2*) Hlth Research.

Handbook of IV Medications. Betty L. Gahart. 17th ed. 2000. (Intravenous Medications Ser.). (Illus.). 960p. 29.95 (*0-323-00984-0*) Mosby Inc.

Handbook of IV Medications, 1991. Phyllis F. Nentwich. 1991. (Illus.). 544p. (C). pap. text 34.95 (*0-86720-441-9*, 441-9) Jones & Bartlett.

Handbook of Kidney Transplantation. Gabriel M. Danovitch. 3rd ed. 2000. LC 00-32255. 464p. pap. text 49.95 (*0-7817-2066-4*) Lppncott W & W.

Handbook of Laboratory & Diagnostic Tests with Nursing Implications. Joyce LeFever Kee. 4th ed. 2000. 508p. pap. 31.93 (*0-13-030517-0*) P-H.

Handbook of Laboratory Animal Science. Ed. by Per Svendsen & Jann Hau. 1994. Vol. 1. 448p. 146.95 (*0-8493-4378-X*); Vol. 2. 224p. 129.95 (*0-8493-4390-9*) CRC Pr.

Handbook of Laboratory Diagnosis & Treatment of Infertility. Brooks A. Keel. 1990. 448p. 157.95 (*0-8493-3549-3*) CRC Pr.

Handbook of Laboratory Health & Safety Measurement. Ed. by S. B. Pal. 2nd rev. ed. 1991. 600p. text 267.50 (*0-7462-0077-3*) Kluwer Academic.

Handbook of Lasik Surgery. Rasik B. Vajpayee et al. 2000. 102p. (C). text (*81-7179-726-1*) Jaypee Brothers IND. *Dist:* SLACK Inc.

Handbook of Learning & Cognitive Processes Vol. 1: Introduction to Concepts & Issues. Ed. by William K. Estes. 1975. 303p. (C). text 59.95 (*0-89859-145-7*) L Erlbaum Assocs.

Handbook of Learning Disabilities: A Multisystem Approach. Jack C. Westman. 1990. LC 89-28184. 870p. (C). 80.00 (*0-205-12120-9*, H21207, Longwood Div) Allyn.

Handbook of Lipids in Human Nutrition. Ed. by Gene F. Spiller. 1995. LC 95-17919. 256p. 144.95 (*0-8493-4248-1*, 4248) CRC Pr.

Handbook of Liver Disease. Lawrence S. Friedman & Emmet B. Keeffe. 1998. LC 97-38311. (C). pap. text (*0-443-05520-3*) Church.

Handbook of Local Anesthesia. Stanley F. Malamed. 4th ed. 1996. (Illus.). 352p. (C). (gr. 13). pap. text 48.00 (*0-8151-6423-8*, 26260) Mosby Inc.

Handbook of Longitudinal Research Vol. 1: Birth & Childhood Cohorts Ed. by Sarnoff A. Mednick et al. 1981. LC 83-24723. 740p. 140.00 (*0-275-90681-7*, C06811, Praeger Pubs) Greenwood.

Handbook of Longitudinal Research Vol. 2: Teenage & Adult Cohorts Ed. by Sarnoff A. Mednick et al. 1984. LC 83-24723. 608p. 105.00 (*0-275-91228-0*, C12282, Praeger Pubs) Greenwood.

Handbook of Lower Extremity Infections. Warren S. Joseph. 1990. 236p. pap. text (*0-443-08690-7*) Church.

Handbook of Managed Behavioral Health Care: A Complete & Up-to-Date Guide for Students & Practitioners. Gayle L. Zieman. 1998. LC 98-8922. (Psychology Ser.). 240p. pap. 40.00 (*0-7879-4153-0*) Jossey-Bass.

Handbook of Management for Primary Health Care Centre Personnel. L. Ramachandran. 1993. (*0-7069-6820-4*) Vikas IND. *Dist:* S Asia.

Handbook of Marine Mammal Medicine: Health, Disease, & Rehabilitation. Ed. by Leslie A. M. D. Dierhauf. 1990. LC 89-38878. 784p. 125.95 (*0-8493-2990-6*, SF997) CRC Pr.

Handbook of Marital Interventions. Ed. by Luciano L'Abate & Sherry McHenry. 1983. 404p. text 66.00 (*0-8089-1502-9*, 792421, Grune & Strat) Harcrt Hlth Sci Grp.

Handbook of Marital Therapy: A Positive Approach to Helping Troubled Relationships. R. P. Liberman et al. 1980. LC 79-9103. (Applied Clinical Psychology Ser.). (Illus.). 278p. (C). 45.00 (*0-306-40235-1*, Plenum Trade) Perseus Pubng.

Handbook of Mass Spectra of Drugs. Ed. by Irving Sunshine. 1981. 472p. 259.00 (*0-8493-3572-8*, RS189, CRC Reprint) Franklin.

Handbook of Maternal Newborn Nursing. Kathleen A. Buckley. 2nd ed. 1989. (Nursing Education Ser.). 29.95 (*0-8273-4214-4*) Delmar.

***Handbook of Measurement & Evaluation in Rehabilitation.** James A. Blackman. 3rd ed. 1995. tchr. ed. (*0-8342-1919-0*) PRO-ED.

Handbook of Measurement & Evaluation in Rehabilitation. Brian F. Bolton. 3rd ed. 1997. LC 00-40126. xiv, 482p. 55.00 (*0-8342-1819-4*, 18194) PRO-ED.

Handbook of Measurements for Marriage & Family Therapy. Norman Fredman & Robert Sherman. 1987. LC 87-9417. 240p. text 41.95 (*0-87630-466-8*) Brunner-Routledge.

Handbook of Mechanical Ventilatory Support. Azriel Perel & M. Christine Stock. 1991. (Illus.). 328p. 40.00 (*0-683-06856-3*) Lppncott W & W.

Handbook of Mechanical Ventilatory Support. M. Christine Stock & Azriel Perel. 2nd ed. 1997. LC 97-3786. (Illus.). 387p. pap. 49.95 (*0-683-30261-2*) Lppncott W & W.

Handbook of Media for Clinical Microbiology. James W. Snyder & Ronald M. Atlas. 1995. LC 95-17855. 320p. 149.95 (*0-8493-9497-X*, 9497) CRC Pr.

Handbook of Medical & Orthopedic Gymnastics. Anders Wide. (Physical Education Reprint Ser.). (Illus.). reprint ed. lib. bdg. 42.50 (*0-697-00106-7*) Irvington.

Handbook of Medical Anthropology: Contemporary Theory & Method. Ed. by Carolyn F. Sargent & Thomas M. Johnson. rev. ed. 1996. LC 95-40052. 584p. lib. bdg. 140.00 (*0-313-29658-8*, Greenwood Pr) Greenwood.

***Handbook of Medical Care in Hostile Environments.** James M. Ryan. 2002. LC 2001-34160. (*1-85233-348-0*); (*1-85233-347-2*) Springer Pub.

Handbook of Medical Image Processing. Issac Bankman. 2000. LC 00-101315. (Biomedical Engineering Ser.). (Illus.). xvi, 901p. 119.00 (*0-12-077790-8*) Acad Pr.

Handbook of Medical Imaging Richard L. Van Metter et al. Ed. by Jacob Beutel. 2000. LC 99-54487. (Illus.). 949p. 110.00 (*0-8194-3621-6*) SPIE.

Handbook of Medical Imaging. 2. Ed. by Jacob Beutel. 2000. LC 99-54487. 130.00 (*0-8194-3622-4*) SPIE.

Handbook of Medical Informatics. Contrib. by Jan H. van Bemmel et al. LC 97-205519. (Illus.). (*90-313-2294-6*) Wolters Kluwer.

Handbook of Medical Information. Ed. by J. Van Bemmel. 1997. LC 97-205519. (Illus.). 655p. 64.00 (*3-540-63351-0*) Spr-Verlag.

Handbook of Medical Library Practice Vol. III: Health Science Librarianship & Administration. Ed. by Louise Darling et al. 4th ed. 1988. 35.00 (*0-8108-2426-4*) Scarecrow.

Handbook of Medical Malacology. Thomas M. Sodeman, Jr. 1992. (*0-8493-3638-4*, CRC Reprint) Franklin.

Handbook of Medical Parasitology. S. K. Sarkar. 1989. (C). (*0-89771-359-1*) Current Dist IND. *Dist:* St Mut.

Handbook of Medical Parasitology & Clinical Pathology. S. K. Sarkar. 1978. 337p. (*0-7855-0792-2*) Current Dist IND. *Dist:* St Mut.

Handbook of Medical Physics, Vol. I. Robert G. Waggener. 1982. 336p. 190.00 (*0-8493-0526-8*, R895, CRC Reprint) Franklin.

Handbook of Medical Physics, Vol. II. Ed. by Robert G. Waggener et al. 1984. 576p. lib. bdg. 158.00 (*0-8493-0527-6*, R895, CRC Reprint) Franklin.

Handbook of Medical Psychiatry. David P. Moore & James W. Jefferson. 1996. LC 96-15602. (Illus.). 560p. (C). (gr. 13). text 49.95 (*0-8151-6484-X*, 26343) Mosby Inc.

Handbook of Medical Psychotherapy: Cost-Effective Strategies in Mental Health. Ed. by K. N. Anchor. 1991. LC 90-5007. (Illus.). 429p. 64.00 (*0-920887-67-8*) Hogrefe & Huber Pubs.

Handbook of Medical Specialties. Henry Wechsler. 1976. LC 74-19051. 315p. 45.95 (*0-87705-232-8*); pap. text 24.95 (*0-87705-292-1*) Kluwer Academic (Kluwer Acad Hman Sci).

Handbook of Medical Supportive Care of AIDS Patients. N. Clumeck & G. Friedland. Date not set. (Basic & Clinical Oncology Ser.). (*0-8247-9299-8*) Dekker.

Handbook of Medical-Surgical Nursing. SPC Staff. Ed. by David Moreau. 2nd ed. 1997. LC 97-20429. (Illus.). 992p. spiral bd. 37.95 (*0-87434-877-3*) Springhouse Corp.

Handbook of Medical Treatment. David Watts. 17th ed. 1983. LC 62-13251. 478p. pap. text 12.95 (*0-930010-07-8*) Jones Med.

Handbook of Medical Treatment. Ed. by H. David Watts. 18th ed. 1988. 500p. (gr. 13). 17.95 (*0-930010-14-0*, HSM-18) Mosby Inc.

Handbook of Medicinal Herbs. James A. Duke. 1987. 696p. 393.95 (*0-8493-3630-9*, QP93); 2nd ed. Date not set. 125.00 (*0-8493-3631-7*); 999th ed. 2000. LC 00-49386. (Illus.). 696p. 124.95 (*0-8493-2928-0*) CRC Pr.

Handbook of Medicinal Mints (Aromathematics) Phytochemicals & Biological Activities. Stephen M. Beckstrom-Sternberg & James A. Duke. 999th ed. 2000. LC 00-49387. (Herbal Reference Library). (Illus.). 480p. 124.95 (*0-8493-2724-5*) CRC Pr.

Handbook of Medicine of the Fetus & Mother. Albert E. Reece et al. 1994. LC 94-30432. (Illus.). 704p. spiral bd. 57.95 (*0-397-51347-X*) Lppncott W & W.

Handbook of Memory Disorders. Alan D. Baddeley. 1999. LC 99-204415. 668p. pap. 125.00 (*0-471-96704-1*) Wiley.

Handbook of Memory Disorders. Ed. by Alan D. Baddeley et al. 1995. LC 94-28317. 668p. 375.00 (*0-471-95078-5*) Wiley.

Handbook of Mental Health & Aging. Ed. by James E. Birren et al. 2nd ed. 1992. LC 91-41083. (Illus.). 996p. text 69.95 (*0-12-101277-8*) Acad Pr.

Handbook of Mental Health & Mental Disorder among Black Americans. Ed. by Dorothy S. Ruiz. 1990. LC 89-71401. 352p. lib. bdg. 65.00 (*0-313-26330-2*, SRZ/, Greenwood Pr) Greenwood.

Handbook of Mental Health Economics & Health Policy, Vol. 1, Schizophrenia, Vol. 1, Schizophrenia. Norman Sartorius et al. 1996. LC 95-24232. (Handbook of Mental Health Economics & Health Policies Ser.: Vol. 1). 570p. 275.00 (*0-471-96108-6*) Wiley.

Handbook of Mental Health Policy in the United States. Ed. by David A. Rochefort. 1989. LC 88-32052. 563p. lib. bdg. 99.50 (*0-313-25009-X*, RHM, Greenwood Pr) Greenwood.

Handbook of Mental Illness in the Mentally Retarded. Ed. by Frank J. Menolascino & Jack A. Stark. 1984. LC 84-13263. (Illus.). 472p. (C). 114.00 (*0-306-41648-4*, Plenum Trade) Perseus Pubng.

Handbook of Mental Retardation. Ed. by Johnny L. Matson & James A. Mulick. 1983. (General Psychology Ser.: No. 121). (Illus.). 650p. 100.00 (*0-08-028060-9*, Pergamon Pr) Elsevier.

Handbook of Mental Retardation. Ed. by J. L. Matson. 2nd ed. 1991. (General Psychology Ser.: No. 121). 800p. (*0-08-035862-4*); pap. (*0-08-035863-2*) PPI GBR. *Dist:* Elsevier.

Handbook of Mental Retardation & Development. Ed. by Jacob A. Burack et al. 1998. (Illus.). (C). 764p. text 80.00 (*0-521-44123-4*); 782p. pap. text 29.95 (*0-521-44668-6*) Cambridge U Pr.

Handbook of Metal-Ligand Interactions in Biological Fluid: Bioinorganic Chemistry. Ed. by Guy Berthon. 1995. LC 95-32797. (Illus.). 630p. text 545.00 (*0-8247-9636-5*) Dekker.

Handbook of Metal-Ligand Interactions in Biological Fluids: Bioinorganic Medicine. Ed. by Guy Berthon. 1995. LC 95-32798. (Illus.). 1632p. text 495.00 (*0-8247-9638-1*);Vol. 1. 692p. text 495.00 (*0-8247-9637-3*) Dekker.

Handbook of Microbiological Investigations for Laboratory Animal Health. J. R. Needman. 1979. text 104.00 (*0-12-515950-1*) Acad Pr.

Handbook of Microbiological Quality Control in Pharmaceuticals & Medical Devices. Ed. by Stephen Denyer et al. 2000. (Illus.). 252p. (*0-7484-0614-X*) Tay Francis Ltd GBR. *Dist:* Taylor & Francis.

Handbook of Microbiology, Vol. V. Ed. by Allen I. Laskin & Hubert A. Lechevalier. 2nd ed. 1984. 936p. lib. bdg. 197.00 (*0-8493-7205-4*, QR6, CRC Reprint) Franklin.

Handbook of Microbiology: Bacteria, Vol. I. Ed. by Allen I. Laskin & Hubert A. Lechevalier. 2nd ed. 1977. 770p. 418.00 (*0-8493-7201-1*, QR6, CRC Reprint) Franklin.

Handbook of Microbiology: Fungi, Algae, Protozoa & Viruses, Vol. II. Allen I. Laskin & Hubert Lechevalier. 2nd ed. 1979. 888p. lib. bdg. 175.00 (*0-8493-7202-X*, QR6, CRC Reprint) Franklin.

Handbook of Microbiology: Microbial Composition: Carbohydrates, Lipids & Minerals, Vol. IV. Ed. by Allen I. Laskin & Hubert A. Lechevalier. 2nd ed. 1982. 744p. 403.00 (*0-8493-7204-6*, QR6, CRC Reprint) Franklin.

Handbook of Microbiology, CRC, Vol. 3: Microbial Metabolism, Genetics & Immunology. Ed. by Allen I. Laskin & Hubert A. Lechevalier. 1974. LC 72-88766. (Handbook Ser.). 800p. 53.95 (*0-87819-584-X*, CRC Reprint) Franklin.

Handbook of Microsurgery. Waldemar L. Olszewski. 1984. Vol. 1. LC 83-15087. lib. bdg. 182.00 (*0-8493-3920-0*); Vol. 2. LC 82-15087. lib. bdg. 182.00 (*0-8493-3921-9*) Franklin (CRC Reprint).

Handbook of Military Psychology, Vol. 1. Ed. by Reuven Gal & David Mangelsdorff. 1991. LC 90-49615. (Handbook of Military Psychology Ser.: Vol. 1). 812p. 900.00 (*0-471-92045-2*) Wiley.

Handbook of Modern Hospital Safety. William Charney. 1999. LC 98-37222. 11p. 125.00 (*1-56670-256-9*) Lewis Pubs.

Handbook of Modern Item Response Theory. Wim J. Van der Linden & Ronald K. Hambleton. 1996. LC 95-49217. (Illus.). 510p. 89.95 (*0-387-94661-6*) Spr-Verlag.

Handbook of Molecular & Cellular Methods in Biology & Medicine. Peter B. Kaufman et al. 1995. LC 94-22515. 496p. spiral bd. 104.95 (*0-8493-2511-0*) CRC Pr.

Handbook of Molecular Descriptors. Roberto Todeschini & Viviana Consonni. 2000. (Methods & Principles in Medicinal Chemistry Ser.). 690p. 245.00 (*3-527-29913-0*) Wiley.

Handbook of Monochromatic XPS Spectra, Set. B. Vincent Crist. 2000. LC 00-32484. (Illus.). 568p. 535.00 (*0-471-49266-3*) Wiley.

Handbook of Monochromatic Xps Spectra, Set. B. Vincent Crist. 2000. LC 00-32484. (Illus.). 548p. 535.00 (*0-471-49265-5*); 2nd ed. 454p. 535.00 (*0-471-49267-1*) Wiley.

Handbook of Motivation & Cognition Vol. 2: Foundations of Social Behavior. Ed. by E. Tory Higgins & Richard M. Sorrentino. 1990. LC 85-24916. 621p. 79.95 (*0-89862-432-0*) Guilford Pubns.

Handbook of Motivation & Congnition Vol. 3: The Interpersonal Context. Ed. by Richard M. Sorrentino & E. Tony Higgins. 1996. LC 85-24916. (Handbook of Motivation & Cognition Ser.: Vol. 3). 646p. text 79.95 (*1-57230-052-3*, 0052) Guilford Pubns.

Handbook of Mouse Mutations with Skin & Hair Abnormalities: Animal Models & Biomedical Tools. Ed. by John P. Sundberg. 1994. LC 93-41187. (CRC Series in Dermatology). 560p. 209.95 (*0-8493-8372-2*) CRC Pr.

Handbook of Movement Disorders. Stanley Fahn. 1997. LC 97-31216. (Illus.). 175p. 56.95 (*1-57340-110-2*) Current Med.

Handbook of Movement Disorders. P. A. Lewitt. Date not set. (Neurological Disease & Therapy Ser.). (*0-8247-9495-8*) Dekker.

Handbook of MRI Technique. Catherine Westbrook. 1994. (Illus.). 224p. pap. (*0-632-03884-5*) Blckwell Science.

Handbook of MRI Techniques. Catherine Westbrook. 2nd ed. 1999. LC 98-40986. (Illus.). 438p. pap. 50.95 (*0-632-05264-3*) Blackwell Sci.

Handbook of Mucosal Immunology. Ed. by Warren Strober et al. 1994. LC 93-11197. (Illus.). 766p. text 199.00 (*0-12-524730-3*) Acad Pr.

Handbook of Multiple Sclerosis. Stuart D. Cook. 2nd ed. 1996. LC 96-24682. (Neurological Disease & Therapy Ser.: Vol. 43). (Illus.). 640p. text 199.00 (*0-8247-9726-4*) Dekker.

Handbook of Multivariate Experimental Psychology. J. R. Nesselroade & R. B. Cattell. 2nd ed. 1988. LC 88-9806. (Perspectives on Individual Differences Ser.). (Illus.). 996p. (C). 150.00 (*0-306-42526-2*, Plenum Trade) Perseus Pubng.

Handbook of Muscle Disease. Russell J. Lane. 1996. LC 96-21848. (Neurological Disease & Therapy Ser.: Vol. 42). (Illus.). 768p. text 235.00 (*0-8247-9494-X*) Dekker.

Handbook of Mushroom Poisoning. Barry H. Rumack. 1994. 464p. 178.95 (*0-8493-0194-7*) CRC Pr.

Handbook of Myasthenia Gravis & Myasthenic Syndromes. Robert P. Lisak. 1994. (Neurological Disease & Therapy Ser.: Vol. 23). (Illus.). 448p. text 210.00 (*0-8247-8825-7*) Dekker.

Handbook of Natural Folk Remedies. Elena Oumano. 1997. LC 96-96920. 256p. (Orig.). mass mkt. 5.99 (*0-380-78448-3*, Avon Bks) Morrow Avon.

Handbook of Natural Remedies for Common Ailments. Linda Clark. 1976. LC 75-13349. 292p. 19.95 (*0-8159-5710-6*) Devin.

Handbook of Natural Therapies: Exploring the Spiral of Healing. Marcia Starck. 1998. LC 98-4962. (Illus.). 192p. pap. 16.95 (*0-89594-869-9*) Crossing Pr.

Handbook of Natural Toxins, Vol. 5: Reptile Venoms & Toxins. Anthony T. Tu. 1991. (Illus.). 832p. text 275.00 (*0-8247-8376-X*) Dekker.

Handbook of Natural Toxins, Vol. 6: Toxicology of Plant & Fungal Compounds. Richard F. Keeler. 1991. (Illus.). 672p. text 250.00 (*0-8247-8375-1*) Dekker.

Handbook of Naturally Occurring Food Toxicants. Ed. by Miloslav Rechcigl, Jr. 1983. 360p. lib. bdg. 176.00 (*0-8493-3965-0*, TX531, CRC Reprint) Franklin.

Handbook of Nausea & Vomiting. Ed. by Marvin H. Sleisenger. 1994. (Illus.). 173p. (C). lib. bdg. 42.95 (*1-85070-528-3*, Parthenon Pbng) CRC Pr.

Handbook of Neonatal Anaesthesia. Hughes. 1995. pap. text 44.00 (*0-7020-1829-5*) Saunders.

***Handbook of Neonatal Intensive Care.** Henry Halliday et al. Ed. by Angela Bell & Richard Tubman. 4th ed. 1998. (Illus.). 445p. pap. text (*0-7020-1772-8*) W B Saunders GBR. *Dist:* Saunders.

Handbook of Neonatal Intensive Care. Gerald B. Merenstein. 4th ed. 1997. LC 97-20146. (Illus.). 792p. (C). (gr. 13). pap. text 45.95 (*0-8151-3696-X*, 31038) Mosby Inc.

Handbook of Neuro-Oncology. R. J. Wiley. Date not set. (Neurological Disease & Therapy Ser.). (Illus.). (*0-8247-9518-0*, 9518-0) Dekker.

Handbook of Neuro-Opthalmology: Diagnosis & Treatment. Robert L. Tomsak. 1996. LC 96-43030. 175p. pap. text 29.99 (*0-7506-9715-6*) Buttrwrth-Heinemann.

Handbook of Neuro-Urology. Ed. by David N. Rushton. 1994. LC 94-12979. (Neurological Disease & Therapy Ser.: Vol. 28). (Illus.). 424p. text 195.00 (*0-8247-9248-3*) Dekker.

Handbook of Neuroanesthesia: Clinical & Physiologic Essentials. Phillippa Newfield & James E. Cottrell. 1983. 437p. 29.50 (*0-316-60470-4*, Little Brwn Med Div) Lppncott W & W.

Handbook of Neurochemistry, Vol. 1: Chemical & Cellular Architecture. Ed. by Abel Lajtha. 2nd ed. 1982. LC 82-493. 516p. 120.00 (*0-306-40861-9*, Plenum Trade) Perseus Pubng.

Handbook of Neurochemistry, Vol. 2: Experimental Neurochemistry. Ed. by Abel Lajtha. 2nd ed. 1983. LC 82-493. 498p. 120.00 (*0-306-40972-0*, Plenum Trade) Perseus Pubng.

Handbook of Neurochemistry, Vol. 3: Metabolism in the Nervous System. Ed. by Abel Lajtha. 2nd ed. 1983. LC 82-493. 724p. 130.00 (*0-306-41153-9*, Plenum Trade) Perseus Pubng.

Handbook of Neurochemistry, Vol. 4: Enzymes in the Nervous System. Ed. by Abel Lajtha. 1983. LC 82-493. 572p. 120.00 (*0-306-41210-1*, Plenum Trade) Perseus Pubng.

Handbook of Neurochemistry, Vol. 5: Metabolic Turnover in the Nervous System. Ed. by Abel Lajtha. 2nd ed. 1983. LC 82-493. 518p. 120.00 (*0-306-41323-X*, Plenum Trade) Perseus Pubng.

Handbook of Neurochemistry, Vol. 8: Neurochemical Systems. Ed. by Abel Lajtha. 2nd ed. 1985. LC 82-493. 700p. 140.00 (*0-306-41579-8*, Plenum Trade) Perseus Pubng.

Handbook of Neurodevelopmental & Genetic Disorders in Children. Ed. by Sam Goldstein & Cecil R. Reynolds. 1999. LC 99-21821. (Illus.). xvi, 602p. text, instr.'s hndbk. ed. 70.00 (*1-57230-448-0*, C0448) Guilford Pubns.

Handbook of Neuroepidemiology. Ed. by Philip B. Gorelick & Milton Alter. 1994. (Neurological Disease & Therapy Ser.: Vol. 29). (Illus.). 640p. text 235.00 (*0-8247-9242-4*) Dekker.

Handbook of Neurohypophyseal Hormone Analogs, Pt. 1. Ed. by K. Jost et al. 1987. 280p. lib. bdg. 48.95 (*0-8493-3293-1*) CRC Pr.

Handbook of Neurolinguistics. Ed. by Brigitte Stemmer & Harry A. Whitaker. 1997. LC 97-80297. (Illus.). 788p. text 149.95 (*0-12-666055-7*) Morgan Kaufmann.

Handbook of Neurologic Rating Scales. Ed. by Robert M. Herndon. 1997. LC 97-23208. (Illus.). 280p. 135.00 (*1-888799-07-2*) Demos Medical.

Handbook of Neurological Emergencies. M. Sharief & M. Swash. 1997. 150p. pap. 39.00 (*3-540-76056-3*) Spr-Verlag.

Handbook of Neurological Examination & Case Recording. Derek Denny-Brown et al. 3rd ed. 1982. LC 81-13315. (Illus.). 104p. pap. 18.50 (*0-674-37101-1*) HUP.

Handbook of Neurological Lists. Lawrence M. Brass & Peter K. Stys. 1991. (Illus.). 397p. pap. text (*0-443-08696-6*) Church.

Handbook of Neurological Speech & Language Disorders. Ed. by Howard S. Kirshner. 1994. (Neurological Disease & Therapy Ser.: Vol. 33). (Illus.). 552p. text 215.00 (*0-8247-9282-3*) Dekker.

Handbook of Neurology. 1997. 400p. LC 97-159594. 60.00 (*981-02-3037-0*); 32.00 (*981-02-3063-X*) World Scientific Pub.

Handbook of Neuropsychological Assessment. Alex Gilandas et al. 1985. 304p. text 59.00 (*0-8089-1645-9*, 791553); pap. text 32.95 (*0-8089-1778-1*, 791556) Harcrt Hlth Sci Grp (Grune & Strat).

Handbook of Neuropsychological Assessment: A Biopsychosocial Perspective. Ed. by Robert J. McCaffrey & Antonio E. Puente. 1991. (Critical Issues in Neuropsychology Ser.). (Illus.). 488p. (C). text 90.00 (*0-306-43940-9*, Kluwer Plenum) Kluwer Academic.

Handbook of Neuropsychology. F. Boller et al. 2nd ed. 2000. 544p. 227.00 (*0-444-50358-7*) Elsevier.

Handbook of Neuropsychology, Vol. 1. Ed. by F. Boller et al. 1988. (Handbook of Neuropsychology Ser.: 1). 436p. reprint ed. pap. 91.50 (*0-444-81215-6*) Elsevier.

Handbook of Neuropsychology, Vol. 3. Ed. by G. Gianotti & Larry R. Squire. 1999. 502p. pap. 106.50 (*0-444-89168-4*, HON 3) Elsevier.

Handbook of Neuropsychology, Vol. 4. Ed. by R. D. Nebes & S. Corkin. 384p. 1991. pap. 73.00 (*0-444-89169-2*); 1990. 284.00 (*0-444-81234-2*) Elsevier.

Handbook of Neuropsychology, Vol. 5. S. Corkin et al. 396p. 1993. pap. 96.00 (*0-444-81501-5*); 1991. 246.50 (*0-444-81233-4*) Elsevier.

Handbook of Neuropsychology, Vol. 7. Isabelle Rapin & Sidney J. Segalowitz. 1992. 478p. 299.50 (*0-444-81209-1*) Elsevier.

Handbook of Neuropsychology, Vol. 8. H. Spinnier & F. Boller. 1997. 456p. pap. 76.00 (*0-444-82764-1*, North Holland) Elsevier.

Handbook of Neuropsychology, Vol. 9. F. Boller et al. 448p. 1997. pap. 76.00 (*0-444-82765-X*, North Holland); 1994. (Handbook of Neuropsychology Ser.: 9). 259.50 (*0-444-89966-9*) Elsevier.

Handbook of Neuropsychology, Vol. 10. F. Boller & J. Grafman. 1997. 510p. pap. 80.50 (*0-444-82766-8*, North Holland) Elsevier.

Handbook of Neuropsychology, Vol. 10. Ed. by F. Boller & Jordan Grafman. 1995. 510p. 219.00 (*0-444-89979-0*) Elsevier.

Handbook of Neuropsychology: Child Neuropsychology (Part 1), Vol. 6. Ed. by Isabelle Rapin & Sidney J. Segalowitz. 1994. 504p. pap. 94.00 (*0-444-82060-4*) Elsevier.

Handbook of Neuropsychology: Child Neuropsychology (Part 2), Vol. 7. Ed. by Isabelle Rapin & Sidney J. Segalowitz. 1994. 478p. pap. 94.00 (*0-444-82059-0*) Elsevier.

Handbook of Neuropsychology Section 10, Pt. 1: Child Neuropsychology, Vol. 6. Isabelle Rapin & Sidney J. Segalowitz. 1992. 520p. 299.50 (*0-444-81192-3*) Elsevier.

Handbook of Neuropsychology Sections 3 & 4, Pt. 2: Language, Aphasia & Related Disorders - Disorders of Visual Behavior, Vol. 2. Ed. by H. Goodglass & Antonio R. Damasio. 1990. 452p. reprint ed. pap. 69.50 (*0-444-81310-1*) Elsevier.

Handbook of Neuropsychology & Aging. Ed. by P. D. Nussbaum. 1997. LC 97-12001. (Critical Issues in Neuropsychology Ser.). (Illus.). 580p. (C). 85.00 (*0-306-45460-2*, Plenum Trade) Perseus Pubng.

Handbook of Neuroradiology: Brain & Skull. Anne G. Osborn & Karen A. Tong. 2nd ed. 1995. LC 95-25936. (Illus.). 736p. (C). (gr. 13). pap. text 46.95 (*0-8151-6593-5*, 25690) Mosby Inc.

Handbook of Neurorehabilitation. Ed. by David C. Good & James R. Couch, Jr. 1994. LC 93-42706. (Neurological Disease & Therapy Ser.: Vol. 24). (Illus.). 704p. text 235.00 (*0-8247-8822-2*) Dekker.

Handbook of Neurosurgery. Mark S. Greenberg. 5th rev. ed. 2000. (Illus.). 900p. pap. 65.95 (*0-86577-909-0*) Thieme Med Pubs.

Handbook of Neurotological Diagnosis. John W. House et al. 1986. (Science & Practice of Surgery Ser.: Vol. 7). (Illus.). 432p. text 165.00 (*0-8247-7511-2*) Dekker.

Handbook of Neurotoxicology, Vol. 2. Ed. by Louis W. Chang & Robert A. Dyer. 1995. (Neurological Disease & Therapy Ser.: Vol. 36). (Illus.). 1136p. text 235.00 (*0-8247-8873-7*) Dekker.

Handbook of Neurotoxicology, Vol. 2. Ed. by Edward J. Massaro. 2002. 684p. 175.00 (*0-89603-796-7*) Humana.

Handbook of Neurovirology. Ed. by Robert R. McKendall & William Stroop. 1994. (Neurological Disease & Therapy Ser.: Vol. 27). (Illus.). 832p. text 235.00 (*0-8247-8870-2*) Dekker.

Handbook of Nitrous Oxide & Oxygen Sedation. Morris S. Clark & Ann L. Brunick. 1998. LC 98-27413. (Illus.). 224p. pap. text 34.95 (*0-8151-8393-3*, 31693) Mosby Inc.

Handbook of Non-Invasive Methods & the Skin. Jorgen Serup & Gregor B. Jemec. 1994. 720p. 209.95 (*0-8493-4453-0*, 4453) CRC Pr.

Handbook of Nonprescription Drugs. Ed. by Linda L. Young. 12th ed. 2000. (Illus.). 900p. 120.00 (*0-917330-97-8*) Am Pharm Assn.

Handbook of Normal Physical Measurements. Judith G. Hall et al. 1990. (Illus.). 512p. pap. text 59.50 (*0-19-261696-X*) OUP.

Handbook of Normative Data for Neuropsychological Assessment. Maura Mitrushina et al. 1998. (Illus.). 560p. text 68.50 (*0-19-505675-2*) OUP.

Handbook of Northeastern Indian Medicinal Plants. James A. Duke. 1986. LC 85-62814. (Bioactive Plants Ser.: Vol. 3). (Illus.). 212p. lib. bdg. 30.00 (*0-88000-142-9*) Quarterman.

Handbook of Nuclear Medical Instruments. B. R. Bairi. 1994. pap. 12.95 (*0-07-462026-6*) McGraw-Hill Educ Grp.

Handbook of Nuclear Medicine. Frederick L. Datz. 2nd rev. ed. 1993. LC 93-14365. (Handbooks in Radiology Ser.). Orig. Title: Nuclear Medicine. (Illus.). 294p. (C). (gr. 13). reprint ed. pap. text 49.95 (*0-8016-7700-9*, 07700) Mosby Inc.

Handbook of Nuclear Medicine Vol. 3: Kidney. Ed. by Gustav Hor & H. W. Pabst. 1996. (Illus.). 290p. 300.00 (*3-437-11013-6*, Wiley-VCH) Wiley.

Handbook of Nuclear Reactors Calculations, Vol. I. Ed. by Yigal Ronen. 1986. 448p. 268.00 (*0-8493-2925-6*, TK9153, CRC Reprint) Franklin.

Handbook of Nursing & Health Research: Design. Abraham. 1996. 700p. 46.95 (*0-8016-7778-5*) Mosby Inc.

***Handbook of Nursing Procedures.** Springhouse Corporation Staff. 2001. LC 00-68776. (Illus.). v, 953p. 38.95 (*1-58255-139-1*) Springhouse Corp.

Handbook of Nutrition & Diet. B. B. Desai. 2000. LC 00-40479. (Food Science & Technology Ser.). (Illus.). viii, 797p. text 195.00 (*0-8247-0375-8*) Dekker.

Handbook of Nutrition & Food. Carolyn D. Berdanier. 2001. LC 2001-35595. 1600p. 249.00 (*0-8493-2705-9*) CRC Pr.

Handbook of Nutrition & Food. Ed. by Miloslav Rechcigl, Jr. 1977. (Comparative & Qualitative Requirements Ser.). (Illus.). 576p. 99.00 (*0-8493-2721-0*, QH519, CRC Reprint) Franklin.

Handbook of Nutrition & the Kidney. Ed. by William E. Mitch & Saulo Klahr. 3rd ed. 1998. LC 97-51461. (Illus.). 392p. pap. text 39.95 (*0-7817-1534-2*) Lppncott W & W.

Handbook of Nutrition in the Aged. Ed. by Ronald R. Watson. 1985. 368p. lib. bdg. 196.00 (*0-8493-2933-7*, QP86); 2nd ed. 1993. LC 93-7314. 464p. 187.95 (*0-8493-8645-4*, QP86) CRC Pr.

Handbook of Nutritional Requirements in a Functional Context. Ed. by Miloslav Rechcigl. 1981. Vol. I. 560p. 304.00 (*0-8493-3956-1*, QP82); Vol. II. 616p. 331.00 (*0-8493-3958-8*, QP82) Franklin (CRC Reprint).

Handbook of Nutritional Supplements Ed. by Miloslav Rechcigl, Jr. Vol. I: Human Use. 1983. 576p. lib. bdg. 214.00 (*0-8493-3969-3*, TX553); Vol. II: Agricultural Use. 1984. 424p. lib. bdg. 192.00 (*0-8493-3970-7*) Franklin (CRC Reprint).

Handbook of Nutritionally Essential Minerals. Boyd L. O'Dell & Roger A. Sunde. 1997. LC 97-55. (Clinical Nutrition in Health & Disease Ser.: Vol. 2). (Illus.). 712p. text 225.00 (*0-8247-9312-9*) Dekker.

Handbook of Nutritive Value of Processed Food: Food for Human Use, Vol. I. Ed. by Miloslav Rechcigl, Jr. 1982. 696p. 376.00 (*0-8493-3951-0*, TX551, CRC Reprint) Franklin.

***Handbook of Obesity Treatment.** Ed. by Thomas A. Wadden & Albert J. Stunkard. 2001. LC 2001-40507. 624p. 65.00 (*1-57230-722-6*) Guilford Pubns.

***Handbook of Obstetric Anesthesia.** Ed. by C. M. Palmer et al. 2001. (Clinical References Ser.). 300p. pap. (*1-85996-232-7*) Bios Sci GBR. *Dist:* Spr-Verlag.

Handbook of Obstetric Management. Sylvia Rosevear. 1996. LC 95-21394. 192p. pap. 29.95 (*0-632-03555-2*) Blackwell Sci.

Handbook of Obstetrical Emergencies. Constance Sinclair. Ed. by Barbara Nelson-Cullen. 1996. (Illus.). 152p. pap. text 22.50 (*0-7216-6431-8*) Saunders.

Handbook of Obstetrics. Ed. by Bikash C. Basu. 1986. (C). (*0-89771-338-9*) Current Dist IND. *Dist:* St Mut.

Handbook of Obstetrics & Gynaecology. M. Bennett et al. 4th ed. 1995. LC 95-74635. 496p. pap. (*0-412-58530-8*) E A GBR. *Dist:* OUP.

Handbook of Obstetrics/Gynecology & Primary Care. Frederick P. Zuspan et al. 1997. LC 97-27522. (Illus.). 704p. (C). (gr. 13). pap. text 39.95 (*0-8151-9931-7*, 27487) Mosby Inc.

Handbook of Occupational Dermatology. Ed. by L. Kanerva et al. 2000. (Illus.). 1600p. 295.00 (*3-540-64046-0*) Spr-Verlag.

Handbook of Occupational Health & Safety Software: Version 10.0. Kent W. Peterson. 10th ed. 1997. 500p. pap. 85.00 (*1-885190-04-2*) Amer Col Occ.

Handbook of Occupational Medicine see Practical Approach to Occupational & Environmental Medicine

Handbook of Occupational Safety & Health. Louis J. Diberardinis. 2nd ed. 1998. LC 97-49069. (Illus.). 1224p. 155.00 (*0-471-16017-2*) Wiley.

Handbook of Ocular Drug Therapy & Ocular Side Effects of Systemic Drugs. Deborah Pavan-Langston. 1990. 42.95 (*0-316-69545-9*, Little Brwn Med Div) Lppncott W & W.

Handbook of Ocular Infections, Inflammation & External Diseases. George M. Bohigian & Shailaja Valluri. 2000. LC 00-26584. 208p. (C). pap. text 33.00 (*1-55642-436-1*) SLACK Inc.

Handbook of Office Gynecology. Martin. 1994. 185.00 (*0-07-105450-2*) McGraw.

Handbook of Olfaction & Gustation. Ed. by Richard L. Doty. 1994. LC 94-33916. (Neurological Disease & Therapy Ser.: Vol. 32). (Illus.). 906p. text 275.00 (*0-8247-9252-1*) Dekker.

Handbook of Oncology Nursing. Bonny Libbey Johnson & Jody Gross. 1992. pap. 24.95 (*0-86720-630-6*) Jones & Bartlett.

Handbook of Oncology Nursing. Jody Gross. 2nd ed. 1994. (Nursing-Health Science Ser.). 816p. (C). pap. text 39.95 (*0-86720-309-9*) Jones & Bartlett.

Handbook of Oncology Nursing. Jody Gross & Bonny Libbey Johnson. 3rd ed. 1998. LC 98-14512. (Nursing Ser.). (Illus.). 832p. (C). pap. text 47.95 (*0-7637-0624-8*, 0624-8) Jones & Bartlett.

Handbook of Ophthalmology. M. L. Agarwal. 1990. 240p. (C). (*81-85017-53-0*) Interprint IND. *Dist:* St Mut.

Handbook of Ophthalmology. G. N. Seal. 1988. (C). (*0-89771-362-1*) Current Dist IND. *Dist:* St Mut.

Handbook of Organic Analytical Reagents. Ed. by K. L. Cheng et al. 1982. 544p. lib. bdg. 123.00 (*0-8493-0771-6*, QD77) CRC Pr.

Handbook of Organic Electrochemistry, Vol. 5. Louis Meites & Petr Zuman. 1982. 472p. 259.00 (*0-8493-7225-9*, QD272, CRC Reprint) Franklin.

Handbook of Organizational Behavior. Ed. by Robert T. Golembiewski. 1993. LC 93-2237. (Public Administration & Public Policy Ser.: Vol. 51). (Illus.). 528p. text 189.00 (*0-8247-9058-8*) Dekker.

Handbook of Organizational Health Psychology: Programs to Make the Workplace Healthier. Ed. & Intro. by Samuel H. Klarreich. 1998. LC 98-22824. 296p. 49.95 (*1-887841-17-2*, Psychosocial) Intl Univs Pr.

Handbook of Organizational Stress Coping Strategies. Ed. by Randall S. Schuler & Amarjit S. Sethi. 1984. LC 84-3082. 336p. text 32.00 (*0-88410-745-0*, HarpBusn) HarpInfo.

Handbook of Orthopaedic Emergencies. Raymond G. Hart & T. J. Rittenberry. 1998. LC 98-4109. 528p. pap. text 39.95 (*0-7817-1610-1*) Lppncott W & W.

Handbook of Orthopaedic Rehabilitation. Ed. by S. Brent Brotzman. abr. ed. 1996. LC 95-42301. (Illus.). 400p. (C). (gr. 13). text 44.95 (*0-8151-1102-9*, 24215) Mosby Inc.

***Handbook of Orthopaedic Rehabilitation.** Steven B. Brotzman. 2nd ed. 2001. (*0-323-01187-X*) Mosby Inc.

Handbook of Orthopaedic Surgery. H. Robert Brashear, Jr. & Richard B. Raney. 10th ed. 1986. (Illus.). 560p. (C). (gr. 13). text 57.95 (*0-8016-4080-6*, 04080) Mosby Inc.

Handbook of Orthopaedic Terminology. Ed. by R. F. Kilcoyne. 2nd ed. 1990. 160p. per. 69.95 (*0-8493-3537-X*, RD734) CRC Pr.

Handbook of Orthopedic Tests. Young. 236p. (*0-8151-9818-3*) Mosby Inc.

Handbook of Otoacoustic Emissions. James W. Hall, III. 1999. 350p. pap. 65.00 (*1-56593-873-9*, 1706) Thomson Learn.

Handbook of Outcomes Measurement in Audiology. Carol E. Johnson & Jeffrey L. Danhauer. 2001. LC 2001-16080. 350p. pap. 65.00 (*0-7693-0102-9*) Singular Publishing.

Handbook of Outpatient Treatment of Adults: Nonpsychotic Mental Disorders. Michael E. Thase et al. 1990. (Illus.). 700p. (C). 120.00 (*0-306-43267-6*, Plenum Trade) Perseus Pubng.

Handbook of Paediatric Accidents & Emergencies: A Symptom-Based Approach. Ed. by A. Capehorn et al. 1998. (Illus.). 305p. (C). pap. text (*0-7020-2168-7*) W B Saunders GBR. *Dist:* Saunders.

Handbook of Paediatric Dermatology. John I. Harper. 2nd ed. 1990. 228p. text (*0-7506-1027-1*) E A GBR. *Dist:* OUP.

***Handbook of Paediatric Investigations.** J. Stroobant. 2001. (Illus.). 380p. pap. (*0-443-05143-7*) Church GBR. *Dist:* Saunders.

Handbook of Pain Management. Ruth T. Kingdon et al. Ed. by Barbara N. Cullen. 1997. LC 97-16690. (Illus.). 352p. pap. text 24.95 (*0-7216-6329-X*) Saunders.

Handbook of Pain Syndromes: Biopsychosocial Perspectives. Ed. by Andrew R. Block et al. 1998. LC 98-36687. 705p. 175.00 (*0-8058-2680-7*) L Erlbaum Assocs.

Handbook of Palliative Care. Christina Faull et al. 1998. LC 98-9866. (Illus.). pap. 45.95 (*0-632-04779-8*) Blackwell Sci.

Handbook of Palliative Care in Cancer. Alexander Waller & Nancy L. Caroline. 2nd ed. 2000. LC 00-25392. (Illus.). 600p. pap. text 49.99 (*0-7506-7204-8*) Buttrwrth-Heinemann.

Handbook of Parenteral Nutrition: Hospital & Home Applications. H. A. Lee & G. Venkat Raman. 1990. 180p. pap. 25.50 (*0-412-28030-2*, A4435) Chapman & Hall.

Handbook of Parkinson's Disease. William C. Koller. 2nd rev. ed. 1992. (Neurological Disease & Therapy Ser.: Vol. 13). (Illus.). 648p. text 199.00 (*0-8247-8675-0*, 8675-0) Dekker.

Handbook of Parvoviruses. Ed. by Peter Tijssen. 1989. Vol. I. 320p. 240.00 (*0-8493-3217-6*, QR408); Vol. 2. 328p. 240.00 (*0-8493-3218-4*, QR408) CRC Pr.

Handbook of Pathological Gambling. Ed. by Thomas Galski. 1987. (Illus.). 228p. (C). 47.95 (*0-398-05268-9*) C C Thomas.

Handbook of Pathology B. Biswas. 1984. (C). (*0-7855-6119-6*) Current Dist IND. *Dist:* St Mut.

Handbook of Pathophysiology. Elizabeth J. Corwin. 2nd ed. 1999. LC 99-37060. (Illus.). xxx, 770p. spiral bd. 29.95 (*0-7817-1938-0*) Lppncott W & W.

Handbook of Patient Teaching. Mary M. Canobbio. 2nd ed. 2000. LC 00-699595. (Illus.). xxiv, 822p. pap. text 29.95 (*0-323-01103-9*) Mosby Inc.

***Handbook of Patient Transportation.** Martin. 2001. (Illus.). 192p. pap. (*1-84110-071-4*) Greenwich Med GBR. *Dist:* JAMCO Dist.

Handbook of Pediatric & Adolescent Health Psychology. Ed. by Anthony J. Goreczny & Michel Hersen. 1998. LC 97-36968. (Illus.). 477p. 91.00 (*0-205-15624-X*) Allyn.

Handbook of Pediatric & Neonatal Transport Medicine. David G. Jaimovich & Dharmapuri Vidyasagar. 1996. (Illus.). 520p. (Orig.). pap. 42.95 (*1-56053-060-X*) Hanley & Belfus.

Handbook of Pediatric Audiology. Ed. by Sanford E. Gerber. 1996. LC 95-44871. (Illus.). 470p. text 75.00 (*1-56368-037-8*) Gallaudet Univ Pr.

Handbook of Pediatric Cancer Pain. G. A. Finley et al. 350p. 39.95 (*0-471-59851-8*) Wiley.

Handbook of Pediatric Dermatology. S. B. Mallory & P. A. Treadwell. 2nd ed. 2002. (Illus.). 200p. 88.00 (*1-85070-753-7*, Parthenon Pbng) CRC Pr.

Handbook of Pediatric Drug Therapy. Ed. by Springhouse Publishing Company Staff. 2nd ed. 2000. LC 99-88084. (Illus.). 852p. pap. 42.95 (*1-58255-023-9*) Springhouse Corp.

Handbook of Pediatric Emergencies. Gregory A. Baldwin. 3rd ed. 2000. 736p. pap. text 39.95 (*0-7817-2236-5*) Lppncott W & W.

Handbook of Pediatric HIV Care. Steven L. Zeichner & Jennifer S. Read. 1999. LC 98-47946. 688p. pap. text 45.00 (*0-7817-1771-X*) Lppncott W & W.

Handbook of Pediatric Imaging. Ed. by Lori L. Barr. 1991. (Handbooks of Diagnostic Imaging Ser.). (Illus.). 492p. text (*0-443-08697-4*) Church.

Handbook of Pediatric Infection. Paul J. Edelson. 1992. 34.95 (*0-316-21074-9*, Little Brwn Med Div) Lppncott W & W.

Handbook of Pediatric Infectious Disease & Antimicrobial Therapy. Stanford T. Shulman et al. 1992. LC 92-49179. 448p. (C). (gr. 13). pap. text 35.00 (*0-8151-7805-0*, 21165) Mosby Inc.

***Handbook of Pediatric Intensive Care.** Gale Pearson. 2001. (Illus.). 395p. (*0-7020-2346-9*) W B Saunders GBR. *Dist:* Saunders.

Handbook of Pediatric Intensive Care. Ed. by Mark C. Rogers & Mark A. Helfaer. 3rd ed. 1998. LC 98-23780. 700p. pap. 69.95 (*0-683-30571-9*) Lppncott W & W.

Handbook of Pediatric Mock Codes. Mark G. Roback. 1998. LC 97-37730. pap. text 25.00 (*1-55664-452-3*) Mosby Inc.

Handbook of Pediatric Mock Codes. Mark G. Roback et al. 1998. (Illus.). 248p. pap. (*84-8174-399-2*) Mosby-Doyma Libros ESP. *Dist:* Mosby Inc.

Handbook of Pediatric Nutrition. Patricia Queen Samour & Kathy King Helm. 2nd ed. 1999. LC 99-37336. (Illus.). xv, 719p. 75.00 (*0-8342-1199-8*) Aspen Pub.

Handbook of Pediatric Oncology. Robert A. Gottlieb. 1989. 36.95 (*0-316-32169-9*, Little Brwn Med Div) Lppncott W & W.

Handbook of Pediatric Orthopedics. Paul D. Sponseller. 1996. LC 96-6386. 368p. pap. text 39.95 (*0-316-80872-5*) Lppncott W & W.

Handbook of Pediatric Physical Diagnosis. Lewis A. Barness. 7th ed. 1998. LC 97-50212. (Illus.). 224p. pap. text 39.95 (*0-7817-1682-9*) Lppncott W & W.

Handbook of Pediatric Physical Therapy. Toby M. Long & Holly M. Cintas. 1995. LC 94-38122. (Illus.). 304p. pap. 31.00 (*0-683-05155-5*) Lppncott W & W.

Handbook of Pediatric Primary Care. Ed. by Raymond C. Baker. 1995. LC 95-20030. 376p. pap. text 34.95 (*0-316-07825-5*) Lppncott W & W.

Handbook of Pediatric Primary Care. Marilyn P. Chow et al. 2nd ed. 1990. LC 83-26038. 1304p. text 62.95 (*0-8273-4224-1*) Delmar.

Handbook of Pediatric Psychology. Ed. by Michael C. Roberts. 2nd ed. LC 95-8536. 1998. 738p. pap. 42.00 (*1-57230-366-2*, C0366); 1995. 814p. 75.00 (*0-89862-156-9*) Guilford Pubns.

Handbook of Pediatric Psychology & Psychiatry: Disease, Injury, & Illness, Vol. 2. Ed. by Robert T. Ammerman & John V. Campo. 1998. LC 97-42736. (Handbook of Pediatric Psychology & Psychiatry Ser.). 400p. (C). 78.00 (*0-205-27601-6*) Allyn.

Handbook of Pediatric Radiology. Vesna Martich Kriss. 1997. LC 97-29968. (Illus.). 456p. (C). (gr. 13). pap. text 39.95 (*0-8151-3749-4*, 30602) Mosby Inc.

Handbook of Pediatric Urology. Larry Baskin et al. 1997. LC 97-5381. (Illus.). 368p. pap. text 39.95 (*0-316-08352-6*) Lppncott W & W.

Handbook of Pediatrics. Gerald B. Merenstein et al. 18th rev. ed. 1996. LC 63-10679. 1029p. (C). pap. text 36.95 (*0-8385-3625-5*, A3625-9, Apple Lange Med) McGraw.

Handbook of Pedodontics. Ed. by N. Das. (C). 1985. (*0-89771-345-1*); 2nd ed. 1980. (*0-7855-4652-9*) Current Dist IND. *Dist:* St Mut.

Handbook of Perception & Action Vol. 1: Perception, Vol. 1. Ed. by Wolfgang Prinz & Bruce Bridgeman. 1996. (Handbook of Perception & Action Ser.: Vol. 1). (Illus.). 456p. text 99.95 (*0-12-516161-1*) Acad Pr.

Handbook of Perception & Action Vol. 3: Attention, Vol. 3. Ed. by Odmar Neumann & Andries F. Sanders. 1996. (Handbook of Perception & Action Ser.: Vol. 3). (Illus.). 448p. text 99.95 (*0-12-516163-8*) Acad Pr.

Handbook of Percutaneous Central Venous Catheterisation. Ed. by Michael Rosen et al. 2nd ed. 1992. (Illus.). 264p. text (*0-7020-1539-3*) W B Saunders GBR. *Dist:* Saunders.

Handbook of Perinatal Infections. John L. Sever et al. 2nd ed. 1988. 35.95 (*0-316-78171-1*, Little Brwn Med Div) Lppncott W & W.

Handbook of Peripheral Nerve Entrapments. Ed. by Oscar A. Turner et al. 1990. LC 90-4085. (Illus.). 240p. 109.50 (*0-89603-146-2*) Humana.

Handbook of Peripheral Neuropathies. J. Mendell. Date not set. (Neurological Disease & Therapy Ser.). (*0-8247-8827-3*) Dekker.

Handbook of Personality: Theory & Research. Ed. by Lawrence A. Pervin. 1990. LC 90-37936. 738p. text 79.95 (*0-89862-430-4*) Guilford Pubns.

Handbook of Personality Psychology. Ed. by Robert Hogan et al. 1997. LC 94-39181. (Illus.). 987p. text 150.00 (*0-12-134645-5*) Morgan Kaufmann.

Handbook of Pesticide Toxicology. Hayes. 1990. text 188.00 (*0-12-334162-0*); text 188.00 (*0-12-334163-9*) Acad Pr.

Handbook of Pesticide Toxicology. Wayland J. Hayes. Ed. by Edward R. Laws. 1990. text 188.00 (*0-12-334161-2*) Acad Pr.

Handbook of Pharmaceutical Additives. Compiled by Michael Ash & Irene Ash. 1996. LC 95-37911. 1132p. (*0-566-07596-2*) Gower GBR. *Dist:* Ashgate Pub Co.

Handbook of Pharmaceutical & Clinical Measurement & Analysis. Harry E. Thomas. 1977. text 29.95 (*0-87909-335-8*) P-H.

Handbook of Pharmaceutical Controlled Release Technology. Donald L. Wise. 2000. LC 00-40474. (Illus.). 904p. text 225.00 (*0-8247-0369-3*) Dekker.

Handbook of Pharmaceutical Excipients. Ed. by Arthur H. Kibbe. 3rd rev. ed. 1999. (Illus.). 665p. 295.00 (*0-917330-96-X*) Am Pharm Assn.

***Handbook of Pharmaceutical Excipients.** Arthur H. Kibbe. 3rd ed. 2000. audio compact disk (*0-85369-468-0*); (Illus.). 686p. incl. cd-rom (*0-85369-469-9*) Pharmaceutical Pr GBR. *Dist:* Rittenhouse.

Handbook of Pharmacokinetic/Pharmacodynamic Correlation. Ed. by Hartmutt Derendorf & Gunther Hochhaus. 1995. LC 94-22365. (Handbook of Pharmacology & Toxicology Ser.). 496p. 179.95 (*0-8493-8303-X*) CRC Pr.

Handbook of Pharmacologic Methodologies for the Study of the Neuroendocrine System. Ed. by Richard W. Steger & Anthony Johns. 1985. 448p. 247.00 (*0-8493-2965-5*, QP356, CRC Reprint) Franklin.

Handbook of Pharmacologic Therapeutics: A Disease-Oriented Review. Phyllis Bogner. 1987. (Illus.). 379p. pap. 30.95 (*0-316-10088-9*, Little Brwn Med Div) Lppncott W & W.

Handbook of Pharmacology & Physiology in Anesthetic Practice. Robert K. Stoelting. 1995. LC 95-14253. 704p. spiral bd. 49.95 (*0-397-51498-0*) Lppncott W & W.

Handbook of Pharmacology of Aging. Ed. by David L. Snyder & Jay Roberts, Jr. 2nd rev. ed. 1996. LC 96-14773. (Pharmacology & Toxicology Ser.). Orig. Title: CRC Handbook of Pharmacology of Aging. 400p. 209.95 (*0-8493-8306-4*) CRC Pr.

Handbook of Phase I-II Clinical Drug Trials. Ed. by John O'Grady & Pieter H. Joubert. 1997. LC 96-23811. 576p. lib. bdg. (*0-8493-9230-6*) BMJ Pub GBR. *Dist:* AIDC.

Handbook of Phlebotomy. Garland E. Pendergraph. 3rd ed. 1992. (Illus.). 126p. pap. text 25.95 (*0-8121-1564-3*) Lppncott W & W.

Handbook of Phlebotomy & Patient Service Techniques. Garland E. Pendergraph & Cynthia B. Pendergraph. 4th ed. 1998. LC 98-13761. 175p. pap. 25.95 (*0-683-30556-5*) Lppncott W & W.

Handbook of Physical Medicine & Rehabilitation Basics. Susan J. Garrison. 1994. (Illus.). 480p. spiral bd. 49.95 (*0-397-51336-4*, Lippncttl) Lppncott W & W.

Handbook of Physician Health: The Essential Guide to Understanding the Health Care Needs of Physicians. American Medical Association Staff. Ed. by Larry S. Goldman et al. 2000. (Illus.). 225p. 42.95 (*1-57947-004-1*) AMA.

Handbook of Physiology: Section 1, The Nervous System Ed. by Ian Darian-Smith. 1988. (American Physiological Society Book). (Illus.). 1244p. text 275.00 (*0-19-520660-6*) OUP.

Handbook of Physiology: Section 1, The Nervous System, Vol. IV: Intrinsic Regulatory Systems of the Brain. Ed. by Floyd E. Bloom. 1988. (American Physiological Society Book). (Illus.). 850p. text 258.00 (*0-19-520661-4*) OUP.

Handbook of Physiology: Section 2, The Cardiovascular System, Vol. IV, Pts. 1 & 2: Microcirculation. Ed. by Eugene M. Renkin & C. Charles Michel. 1988. (American Physiological Society Book). (Illus.). 1124p. text 275.00 (*0-19-520666-5*) OUP.

Handbook of Physiology: Section 3, The Respiratory System, Vol. II, Pts. 1 & 2: Control of Breathing. Ed. by Neil S. Cherniack & John G. Widdicombe. 1988. (American Physiological Society Book). (Illus.). 972p. text 245.00 (*0-19-520668-1*) OUP.

Handbook of Physiology: Section 3, The Respiratory System, Vol. III, Pts. 1 & 2: Mechanics of Breathing. Jere Mead. Ed. by Peter T. Macklem. 1988. (American Physiological Society Book). (Illus.). 834p. text 245.00 (*0-19-520669-X*) OUP.

Handbook of Physiology: Section 8: Renal Physiology, Vols. I & II. Ed. by Erich E. Windhager. rev. ed. 1992. (Handbook of Physiology Ser.). (Illus.). 2544p. text 395.00 (*0-19-506006-7*) OUP.

Handbook of Physiology Sect. 6, Vol. I: Gastrointestinal System: Motility & Circulation, Pts. 1 & 2, Pts. 1 & 2. Ed. by Jackie D. Wood & Stanley G. Schultz. 1989. (American Physiological Society Book). (Illus.). 1906p. text 295.00 (*0-19-520791-2*) OUP.

Handbook of Physiology Sect. 6, Vol. II: The Gastrointestinal System: Neural & Endocrine Biology. Ed. by Gabriel M. Makhlouf & Stanley G. Schultz. 1989. (American Physiological Society Book). (Illus.). 736p. text 195.00 (*0-19-520795-5*) OUP.

Handbook of Physiology Sect. 6, Vol. III: The Gastrointestinal System: Salivary, Gastric, Pancreatic, & Hepatobiliary Secretion. Ed. by John G. Forte & Stanley G. Schultz. 1989. (American Physiological Society Book). (Illus.). 788p. text 195.00 (*0-19-520816-1*) OUP.

Handbook of Physiology Sect. 6, Vol. IV: The Gastrointestinal System: Intestinal Absorption & Secretion. Michael Field & Raymond A. Frizzell. Ed. by Stanley G. Schultz. 1991. (American Physiological Society Book). (Illus.). 672p. text 195.00 (*0-19-520817-X*) OUP.

Handbook of Physiology Sect. 7/2: Endocrinology: Endocrine Pancreas & Regu. Ed. by Leonard S. Jefferson & Alan D. Cherrington. 2000. (Handbook of Physiology Ser.). (Illus.). 1284p. text 295.00 (*0-19-511326-8*) OUP.

Handbook of Physiology in Aging. Ed. by Edward J. Masoro. 1981. LC 80-19983. (Series in Clinical Laboratory Science). 520p. 282.00 (*0-8493-3143-9*, QP86, CRC Reprint) Franklin.

Handbook of Physiology, Section 7, the Endocrine System Vol. III: Endocrine Regulation of Water & Electrolyte Balance. Ed. by John C. S. Fray. 1999. LC 98-12003. (Handbook of Physiology Ser.). (Illus.). 752p. text 225.00 (*0-19-511044-7*) OUP.

Handbook of Phytochemical Constituents of GRAS Herbs & Other Economic Plants. James A. Duke. 999th ed. 2000. LC 00-49359. (Herbal Reference Library). (Illus.). 680p. 159.95 (*0-8493-3865-4*) CRC Pr.

Handbook of Phytochemical Constituents of Grass Herbs & Other Economic Plants. Compiled by James A. Duke. 1992. 688p. 273.95 (*0-8493-3672-4*, SB351) CRC Pr.

Handbook of Placental Pathology. Vijay V. Joshi. 1994. LC 93-46480. (Illus.). 144p. 45.00 (*0-89640-254-1*) Igaku-Shoin.

Handbook of Plant & Fungal Toxicants. J. P. D'Mello. 1997. LC 96-27516. (Handbooks of Pharmacology & Toxicology Ser.). 368p. 110.00 (*0-8493-8551-2*) CRC Pr.

Handbook of Plastic Surgery. Mason. 2001. pap. text (*0-323-01181-0*) Mosby Inc.

Handbook of Play Therapy. Linnet McMahon. 1992. LC 91-37179. 304p. (Orig.). (C). text 99.95 (*0-415-07923-3*, A6909); (Illus.). pap. 29.95 (*0-415-05986-0*, A6913) Routledge.

Handbook of Play Therapy, Vol. 1. Charles E. Schaefer & Kevin J. O'Connor. 1983. LC 82-21818. (Personality Processes Ser.). 512p. 130.00 (*0-471-09462-5*) Wiley.

Handbook of Play Therapy Vol. 2: Advances & Innovations. Ed. by Charles E. Schaefer et al. 1994. (Handbook of Play Therapy Ser.: Vol. 2). 447p. 120.00 (*0-471-58463-0*) Wiley.

Handbook of Poisoning in Dogs & Cats. Alexander Campbell & Michael Chapman. 2000. LC 99-54108. 272p. pap. text (*0-632-05029-2*) Blckwell Science GBR. *Dist:* Iowa U Pr.

Handbook of Polysomnographic Technology. Wendi M. Nugent. 1995. (Illus.). 256p. pap. 50.00 (*0-7506-9513-7*) Buttrwrth-Heinemann.

Handbook of Post-Traumatic Therapy. Mary B. Williams. 1994. LC 93-14437. 656p. lib. bdg. 140.00 (*0-313-28143-2*, Greenwood Pr) Greenwood.

Handbook of Poultry Parasitology. Larry R. McDougald. Ed. by Peter L. Long. 1985. LC 83-2141. 250p. 29.50 (*0-03-062489-4*, Praeger Pubs) Greenwood.

Handbook of Practical Critical Care Medicine. Joseph Varon & Robert E. Fromm. 2001. LC 2001-20052. (Illus.). 504p. 39.95 (*0-387-95165-2*) Spr-Verlag.

Handbook of Practical Medical Terms. William Wei & Anthony Ng. 3rd ed. 1998. LC 98-192038. (CHI & ENG.). 192p. pap. (*962-209-455-4*) HK Univ Pr HKG. *Dist:* Intl Spec Bk, Coronet Bks.

Handbook of Practical Medicine & Treatment. K. Majumdar. 1989. (C). (*0-89771-353-2*) Current Dist IND. *Dist:* St Mut.

Handbook of Practice Management. John C. Hasler et al. 1991. (Illus.). 288p. (C). text (*0-443-04576-3*) Church.

Handbook of Practice Nursing. M. Fletcher et al. 1992. (Illus.). 272p. text (*0-443-04781-2*) Church.

Handbook of Pre-Clinical Continuous Intravenous Infusion. Guy Healing & David Smith. 2000. LC 00-37718. (Illus.). 352p. (*0-7484-0867-3*) Tay Francis Ltd GBR. *Dist:* Taylor & Francis.

Handbook of Pregnancy & Perinatal Care in Family Practice. Ed. by Stephen Ratcliffe et al. 1996. LC 95-39444. (Illus.). 500p. pap. 50.95 (*1-56053-113-4*) Hanley & Belfus.

Handbook of Prehospital Medications. Nancy L. Caroline. 1995. LC 94-32684. 144p. pap. text 17.00 (*0-316-55447-2*) Lppncott W & W.

Handbook of Prenatal Diagnosis. Ed. by Ronald J. Trent. 1995. (Illus.). 300p. (C). pap. text 28.95 (*0-521-46613-X*) Cambridge U Pr.

Handbook of Prescribing Medications for Geriatric Patients. Judith C. Ahronheim. 1992. pap. 34.95 (*0-316-02042-7*, A2305) Lppncott W & W.

Handbook of Prescriptive Treatment for Adults. Ed. by M. Hersen & R. T. Ammerman. 1994. (Illus.). 536p. (C). 95.00 (*0-306-44682-0*, Plenum Trade) Perseus Pubng.

Handbook of Prescriptive Treatments for Children & Adolescents. Ed. by Robert T. Ammerman et al. 2nd ed. 1999. LC 98-39961. 426p. 91.00 (*0-205-26836-6*) Allyn.

***Handbook of Prevention & Treatment with Children & Adolescents: Intervention in the Real World Context.** Ammerman. 2001. 672p. pap. 55.00 (*0-471-11455-3*) Wiley.

Handbook of Prevention & Treatment with Children & Adolescents: Intervention in the Real World Context. Robert T. Ammerman et al. 1997. LC 96-51877. 656p. 135.00 (*0-471-12163-0*) Wiley.

Handbook of Preventive & Social Medicine. S. C. Basu. 1977. 420p. (*0-7855-0817-1*) Current Dist IND. *Dist:* St Mut.

Handbook of Preventive & Therapeutic Nutrition. James A. Gerber. 1992. 436p. pap. 56.00 (*0-8342-0318-9*, 20318) Aspen Pub.

Handbook of Primary Care Medicine. Dale D. Berg. 2nd ed. 1998. LC 97-48991. 768p. pap. text 45.00 (*0-7817-1431-1*) Lppncott W & W.

Handbook of Problem-Oriented Psychotherapy: A Guide for Psychologists, Social Workers, Psychiatrists & Other Mental Health Professionals. A. H. Chapman & Miriam Chapman-Santana. 1997. LC 95-52522. 232p. 40.00 (*1-56821-682-3*) Aronson.

Handbook of Properties of Condensed Phases of Hydrogen & Oxygen. Ed. by B. I. Verkin. 1991. LC 66-56185. 250p. 132.00 (*0-89116-714-5*) Hemisp Pub.

Handbook of Proprietary Medicines: Bottle Collecting. James S. White. 1974. LC 74-25847. (Illus.). 96p. pap. 4.95 (*0-8323-0278-3*) Binford Mort.

Handbook of Protoctista. Lynn Margulis et al. 1989. (C). 225.00 (*0-86720-052-9*) Jones & Bartlett.

Handbook of Psoriasis. Charles Camisa. 1999. LC 97-45689. (Illus.). 321p. pap. 47.95 (*0-86542-558-2*) Blackwell Sci.

Handbook of Psychiatric Consultation with Children & Youth. Ed. by Norman Bernstein & James N. Sussex. 1984. LC 84-3376. 416p. text 44.95 (*0-88331-148-8*) R B Luce.

Handbook of Psychiatric Diagnostic Procedures, Volume 1. Ed. by R. C. Hall & Thomas P. Beresford. 1987. 343p. 45.00 (*0-08-034962-5*, Pergamon Pr) Elsevier.

Handbook of Psychiatric Diagnostic Procedures, Volume 2. Ed. by R. C. Hall & Thomas P. Beresford. 1986. 376p. 45.00 (*0-08-035167-0*, Pergamon Pr) Elsevier.

Handbook of Psychiatric Drug Therapy. Steven E. Hyman & George W. Arana. 1986. 173p. pap. 19.50 (*0-316-38718-5*, Little Brwn Med Div) Lppncott W & W.

Handbook of Psychiatric Drug Therapy. George W. Arana et al. 4th ed. 2000. LC 00-25396. (Illus.). 272p. pap. text 39.95 (*0-7817-1609-8*) Lppncott W & W.

Handbook of Psychiatric Drug Therapy for Children & Adolescents. Ed. by Karen A. Theesen. LC 95-8194. 297p. (C). 1997. pap. 19.95 (*0-7890-0206-X*); 1995. (Illus.). 49.95 (*1-56024-929-3*) Haworth Pr (Pharmctl Prods).

Handbook of Psychiatric Drugs for PDAs & Desktops: 2002. Lawrence J. Albers, MD et al. rev. ed. 2001. (Current Clinical Strategies Ser.). 109p. pap. 28.95 incl. cd-rom (*1-881528-95-2*) Current Clin Strat.

Handbook of Psychiatric Drugs, 1998-99 Edition: Current Clinical Strategies. Lawrence Albers. 1998. 102p. pap. 8.75 (*1-881528-54-5*) Current Clin Strat.

Handbook of Psychiatric Drugs. Lawrence J. Albers et al. rev. ed. 2000. (Current Clinical Strategies Ser.). 109p. pap. text 12.95 (*1-881528-94-4*) Current Clin Strat.

Handbook of Psychiatric Education & Faculty Development. Ed. by Jerald Kay et al. 1999. LC 98-32453. 496p. 52.00 (*0-88048-780-1*, 8780) Am Psychiatric.

Handbook of Psychiatric Genetics. Ed. by Kenneth Blum et al. 1996. LC 96-19053. 512p. 139.95 (*0-8493-4486-7*) CRC Pr.

Handbook of Psychiatric Measures. American Psychiatric Association Staff. 2000. LC 00-24851. xxviii, 820p. 129.00 incl. audio compact disk (*0-89042-415-2*, 2415) Am Psychiatric.

Handbook of Psychiatric Practice in the Juvenile Court. Ed. by American Psychiatric Association Staff. 1992. LC 91-23403. 198p. pap. text 12.95 (*0-89042-233-8*, 2233) Am Psychiatric.

Handbook of Psychiatric Rehabilitation. Ed. by Robert P. Liberman. 1991. (General Psychology Ser.). 364p. (*0-08-040631-9*); (*0-08-040632-7*) PPI GBR. *Dist:* Elsevier.

Handbook of Psychiatry for Primary Care. Ed. by C. W. Allwood & C. A. Gagiano. 1998. LC 98-146717. (Medical Handbook Ser.). (Illus.). 336p. pap. 32.50 (*0-19-571182-3*) OUP.

Handbook of Psychoanalysis. Hand Herma & Gertrud M. Kurth. 1990. 17.75 (*0-8446-2244-3*) Peter Smith.

Handbook of Psychodiagnostic Testing: Personality Analysis & Report Writing. Henry Kellerman & Anthony Burry. 1981. LC 81-6935. 222p. (C). text 37.95 (*0-8089-1403-0*, 792274, Grune & Strat) Harcrt Hlth Sci Grp.

Handbook of Psychodrama. Marcia Karp et al. 1998. LC 97-50005. (Illus.). 328p. (C). pap. 27.95 (*0-415-14846-4*); 89.95 (*0-415-14845-6*) Routledge.

Handbook of Psycholinguistics. Ed. by Morton A. Gernsbacher. 1994. LC 93-23396. (Illus.). 1174p. text 139.95 (*0-12-280890-8*) Acad Pr.

Handbook of Psychological & Educational Assessment of Children: Personality, Behavior & Context. Ed. by Cecil R. Reynolds & Randy W. Kamphaus. 1990. LC 89-38018. 618p. 75.00 (*0-89862-392-8*, 2392) Guilford Pubns.

Handbook of Psychological Approaches with Violent Offenders: Contemporary Strategies & Issues. V. B. Van Hasselt & M. Hersen. 1999. LC 98-40748. (Series in Crime & Justice). (Illus.). 508p. (C). text 110.00 (*0-306-45845-4*, Kluwer Plenum) Kluwer Academic.

Handbook of Psychological Assessment. Ed. by Gerald Goldstein & Michel Hersen. 1984. LC 84-3092. (General Psychology Ser.: No. 131). 500p. 88.00 (*0-08-029401-4*, Pergamon Pr) Elsevier.

Handbook of Psychological Assessment. Gerald Goldstein & Michel Hersen. 3rd ed. 1999. LC 99-51936. 612p. 93.50 (*0-08-043645-5*, Pergamon Pr) Elsevier.

Handbook of Psychological Assessment. Ed. by Gerald Goldstein & Michel Hersen. 2nd ed. 1990. (General Psychology Ser.: No. 131). 650p. (*0-08-035866-7*); stu. ed. (*0-08-040635-1*) PPI GBR. *Dist:* Elsevier.

Handbook of Psychological Assessment. Gary Groth-Marnat. 3rd ed. 1996. LC 96-23803. 848p. 99.55 (*0-471-05220-5*) Wiley.

Handbook of Psychological Assessment in Business. Ed. by Curtiss P. Hansen & Kelley A. Conrad. 1991. LC 91-6822. 368p. 69.95 (*0-89930-565-2*, HPA/, Quorum Bks) Greenwood.

Handbook of Psychological Change: Psychotherapy Processes & Practices for the 21st Century. C. R. Snyder & Rick E. Ingram. 2000. LC 99-51907. 784p. (C). 84.76 (*0-471-24191-1*) Wiley.

Handbook of Psychological Law. Norman Hetland. 1996. 23p. reprint ed. spiral bd. 10.00 (*0-7873-1168-5*) Hlth Research.

Handbook of Psychological Signs, Symptoms, & Syndromes. Donald P. Ogdon. 1981. LC 81-52961. (Professional Handbook Ser.). 102p. pap. 38.50 (*0-87424-173-1*, W-173) Western Psych.

Handbook of Psychological Testing. Paul Kline. 1993. LC 92-12226. 656p. (C). pap. 55.00 (*0-415-05481-8*, B0631); 2nd ed. 1999. LC 98-53738. vii, 744p. text 150.00 (*0-415-21157-3*); 2nd ed. 1999. LC 98-53738. (Illus.). vii, 744p. pap. 60.00 (*0-415-21158-1*) Routledge.

Handbook of Psychological Treatment Protocols for Children & Adolescents. Ed. by Vincent B. Van Hasselt & Michel Hersen. 1997. LC 97-25173. (Personality & Clinical Psychology Ser.). 600p. text (*0-8058-1782-4*) L Erlbaum Assocs.

Handbook of Psychology & Diabetes: A Guide to Psychological Measurement in Diabetes Research & Management. Ed. by Claire Bradley. 1994. LC 94-4391. pap. (*3-7186-5563-2*); 437p. text 63.00 (*3-7186-5562-4*) Gordon & Breach.

Handbook of Psychology & Law. Ed. by D. Kagehiro & William S. Laufer. 1991. (Illus.). 628p. 119.00 (*0-387-97568-3*) Spr-Verlag.

Handbook of Psychology for Forensic Practitioners. Graham J. Towl & David A. Crighton. 1996. LC 96-7563. 240p. (C). 89.95 (*0-415-12887-0*); pap. 27.95 (*0-415-12888-9*) Routledge.

Handbook of Psychopharmacology Vol. 20: Psychopharmacology of the Aging Nervous System. L. Iversen et al. 1988. LC 88-5929. (Illus.). 500p. (C). text 125.00 (*0-306-42744-3*, Kluwer Plenum) Kluwer Academic.

Handbook of Psychopharmacology Trials: An Overview of Scientific, Political, & Ethical Concerns. Ed. by Marc Hertzman & Douglas E. Feltner. 1997. LC 96-45902. 450p. (C). text 85.00 (*0-8147-3532-0*) NYU Pr.

Handbook of Psychopharmacology, Vol. 15: New Techniques in Psychopharmacology. Ed. by Leslie L. Iversen et al. 1982. LC 82-16506. 442p. 95.00 (*0-306-40975-5*, Plenum Trade) Perseus Pubng.

Handbook of Psychopharmacology, Vol. 16: Neuropeptides. Ed. by Leslie L. Iversen et al. 1983. LC 75-6851. 592p. 110.00 (*0-306-41048-6*, Plenum Trade) Perseus Pubng.

Handbook of Psychopharmacology, Vol. 17: Biochemical Studies of CNS Receptors. Ed. by Leslie L. Iversen et al. 1983. LC 82-22376. 450p. 95.00 (*0-306-41145-8*, Plenum Trade) Perseus Pubng.

Handbook of Psychopharmacology, Vol. 18: Drugs, Neurotransmitters & Behavior. Ed. by Leslie L. Iversen et al. 1984. LC 83-19187. 548p. 95.00 (*0-306-41415-5*, Plenum Trade) Perseus Pubng.

Handbook of Psychopharmacology, Vol. 19: New Directions in Behavioral Pharmacology. Ed. by Leslie L. Iversen et al. 1987. LC 87-2551. 638p. 110.00 (*0-306-42447-9*, Plenum Trade) Perseus Pubng.

Handbook of Psychosocial Nursing Care. Holly S. Wilson & Carol R. Kneisl. 1984. 384p. pap. text 11.96 (*0-201-11705-3*, Health Sci) Addison-Wesley.

Handbook of Psychosomatic Medicine. Ed. by Giovanni A. Fava & Hellmuth Freyberger. 1998. LC 97-27749. (Stress & Health Ser.: Vol. 9). 780p. 85.00 (*0-8236-2302-5*) Intl Univs Pr.

Handbook of Psychotherapy. Ed. by Petruska Clarkson & Michael Pokorny. 1994. LC 93-32583. 496p. (C). text 69.95 (*0-415-07722-2*) Routledge.

Handbook of Psychotherapy & Behavior Change. Ed. by Allen E. Bergin & Sol L. Garfield. 4th ed. 1994. pap. text 21.95 (*0-471-01023-5*); 1993. LC 93-23313. 880p. 111.95 (*0-471-54513-9*) Wiley.

Handbook of Psychotherapy Case Formulation. Ed. by Tracy D. Eells. 1997. LC 97-3394. 442p. 48.00 (*1-57230-216-X*, C0216) Guilford Pubns.

Handbook of Psychotherapy for Anorexia Nervosa & Bulimia. Ed. by David M. Garner & Paul E. Garfinkel. 1984. LC 84-19332. 592p. text 55.00 (*0-89862-642-0*) Guilford Pubns.

Handbook of Psychotherapy Integration. Ed. by John C. Norcross & Marvin R. Goldfried. 1992. LC 92-52740. 416p. 60.00 (*0-465-02879-9*) Basic.

Handbook of Psychotherapy Supervision. C. Edward Watkins, Jr. 1997. LC 96-35571. (Clinical Psychology & Personality Ser.). 672p. 110.00 (*0-471-11219-4*) Wiley.

Handbook of Psychotherapy with Children & Adolescents. Ed. by Thomas R. Kratochwill & Richard J. Morris. 1993. LC 92-49065. 656p. (C). pap. text 109.95 (*0-205-14804-2*, H48044, Longwood Div) Allyn.

Handbook of Public & Community Health Nursing Practice: A Health Promotion Guide. Marcia Stanhope & Ruth N. Knollmueller. 2nd ed. 2001. LC 00-46540. (Illus.). xix, 932p. 35.95 (*0-323-01332-5*) Mosby Inc.

Handbook of Pulmonary Drug Therapy. Ed. by Samuel V. Spagnolo et al. 1993. (Handbook Ser.). 368p. pap. 34.95 (*0-316-80474-6*, Little Brwn Med Div) Lppncott W & W.

Handbook of Quality Assurance in Mental Health. G. Stricker & A. R. Rodriguez. 1988. LC 87-29101. (Illus.). 526p. (C). 75.00 (*0-306-42435-5*, Plenum Trade) Perseus Pubng.

Handbook of Quality Management in Behavioral Health. Ed. by George Stricker et al. 1999. LC 99-47994. (Issues in the Practice of Psychology Ser.). (Illus.). xiv, 410p. 125.00 (*0-306-46149-8*) Plenum.

Handbook of Radiation Effects. Andrew Holmes-Siedle & Len Adams. 1993. LC 92-22567. (Illus.). 502p. (C). text 89.00 (*0-19-856347-7*) OUP.

***Handbook of Radiation Effects.** Andrew Holmes-Siedle & Len Adams. 2nd ed. 2001. LC 2001-53096. (Illus.). 500p. 110.00 (*0-19-850733-X*) OUP.

Handbook of Radiobiology. Kedar N. Prasad. 2nd ed. 1995. LC 94-30433. (Illus.). 352p. 149.95 (*0-8493-2501-3*) CRC Pr.

Handbook of Radiopharmaceuticals. Azuwuike Owunwanne et al. 1994. 256p. (gr. 13). pap. 104.95 (*0-412-54880-1*) Chapman & Hall.

Handbook of Regional Cerebral Blood Flow. Ed. by Stevo Knezevic et al. 1987. (Neuropsychology & Neurolinguistics Ser.). 312p. text 59.95 (*0-89859-558-4*) L Erlbaum Assocs.

Handbook of Rehabilitation Psychology. Robert G. Frank & Timothy R. Elliott. 2000. LC 99-87407. (Illus.). xiv, 727p. 59.95 (*1-55798-644-4*, 431-742A) Am Psychol.

Handbook of Relational Diagnosis & Dysfunctional Family Patterns. Ed. by Florence W. Kaslow. 1996. LC 95-30113. (Couples & Family Dynamics & Treatment Ser.). 592p. 100.00 (*0-471-08078-0*) Wiley.

Handbook of Religion & Mental Health. Harold George Koenig. 1998. LC 98-84981. (Illus.). 408p. 79.95 (*0-12-417645-3*) Acad Pr.

***Handbook of Renal Biopsy Pathology.** Alexander J. Howie. 2001. 240p. pap. 89.00 (*0-7923-6894-0*) Kluwer Academic.

Handbook of Research & Quantitative Methods in Psychology. Ed. by R. M. Yaremko et al. 1986. 336p. (C). reprint ed. pap. 32.50 (*0-89859-867-2*) L Erlbaum Assocs.

Handbook of Research Methods in Cardiovascular Behavioral Medicine. N. Schneiderman et al. 1989. (Behavioral Psychophysiology Ser.). (Illus.). 736p. (C). text 130.00 (*0-306-42960-8*, Kluwer Plenum) Kluwer Academic.

Handbook of Research Methods in Clinical Psychology. Ed. by Philip C. Kendall et al. 2nd ed. 1999. LC 98-33853. (Illus.). 768p. 100.00 (*0-471-29509-4*) Wiley.

Handbook of Research on Face Processing. Ed. by A. W. Young, Jr. & Hadyn D. Ellis. 1989. 606p. 278.00 (*0-444-87143-8*, North Holland) Elsevier.

Handbook of Residential Care. John Burton. 1993. LC 93-14836. (Illus.). 240p. pap. (*0-415-08636-1*); (C). 90.00 (*0-415-08635-3*, B2231) Routledge.

Handbook of Rodent & Rabbit Medicine. Ed. by Kathy Laber-Laird et al. 1996. LC 94-45569. (Pergamon Veterinary Handbook Ser.). 300p. pap. 59.99 (*0-08-042504-6*, Pergamon Pr) Elsevier.

Handbook of Rorschach Research Scales. Ed. by Paul M. Lerner. 1974. LC 73-7022. 523p. 77.50 (*0-8236-2305-X*) Intl Univs Pr.

Handbook of Routine Urinalysis. Laurine Graff. 1983. (Illus.). 284 / 250 Fullp. spiral bd. 40.95 (*0-397-52111-1*, Lippncott) Lppncott W & W.

Handbook of Rural Community Mental Health. Ed. by Peter A. Keller & Dennis J. Murray. 1982. LC 81-7048. (Illus.). 262p. 45.95 (*0-89885-065-7*, Kluwer Acad Hman Sci) Kluwer Academic.

Handbook of Rural Health. Ed. by Sana Loue & Beth E. Quill. 2001. LC 00-62191. (Illus.). 353p. 85.00 (*0-306-46479-9*, Kluwer Plenum) Kluwer Academic.

Handbook of Safety & Accident Prevention. F. G. Lange. 1991. lib. bdg. 125.95 (*0-8490-4526-6*) Gordon Pr.

Handbook of Sample Size Guidelines for Clinical Trials. Ed. by Jonathan J. Shuster. 1990. 221p. 314.95 (*0-8493-3542-6*, RM301) CRC Pr.

Handbook of School Art Therapy: Introducing Art Therapy into a School System. Janet Bush. 1997. LC 96-48444. (Illus.). 206p. text 50.95 (*0-398-06740-6*); pap. text 37.95 (*0-398-06741-4*) C C Thomas.

Handbook of School-Based Interventions: Resolving Student Problems & Promoting Healthy Educational Environments. Jeffrey J. Cohen & Marian C. Fish. 1993. LC 93-3619. (Social & Behavioral Science Ser.). 544p. 60.00 (*1-55542-549-6*, C965-Y3H) Jossey-Bass.

Handbook of School Psychology. Terry B. Gutkin & Cecil R. Reynolds. 2nd ed. 1990. LC 89-39299. 1120p. 97.95 (*0-471-01181-9*) Wiley.

Handbook of Self-Concept: Developmental, Social, & Clinical Considerations. Ed. by Bruce A. Bracken. 1995. LC 95-15681. (Personality Processes Ser.). 539p. 200.00 (*0-471-59939-5*, Wiley-Interscience) Wiley.

Handbook of Sensory Physiology: Vestibular System, Psychophysics, Applied Aspects & General Interpretations, Vol. 6, Pt. 2. Ed. by H. H. Kornhuber. 1975. (Illus.). 680p. 220.00 (*0-387-06864-3*) Spr-Verlag.

Handbook of Severe Disability: A Text for Rehabilitation Counselors, Other Vocational Practitioners & Allied Health Professionals 1997. lib. bdg. 600.99 (*0-8490-8215-3*) Gordon Pr.

Handbook of Severe Disability: A Text for Rehabilitation Counselors, Other Vocational Practitioners, & Allied Health Professionals. Ed. by Walter C. Stolov & Michael R. Clowers. 2000. (Illus.). 445p. (C). reprint ed. text 45.00 (*0-7567-0024-8*) DIANE Pub.

Handbook of Sex Therapy. J. LoPiccolo & L. LoPiccolo. 1978. LC 77-18818. (Perspectives in Sexuality Ser.). (Illus.). 552p. (C). 65.00 (*0-306-31074-0*, Plenum Trade) Perseus Pubng.

Handbook of Sexual Assault: Issues, Theories, & Treatment of the Offender. Ed. by William L. Marshall et al. 1990. LC 89-23174. (Applied Clinical Psychology Ser.). (Illus.). 424p. (C). 75.00 (*0-306-43272-2*, Plenum Trade) Perseus Pubng.

Handbook of Sexuality-Related Measures. Clive M. Davis et al. 1998. LC 98-19732. 920p. 149.95 (*0-8039-7111-7*, 4129) Sage.

Handbook of Sexually Transmitted Diseases: A Clinical Approach. Marc C. Robin. 1995. LC 94-78412. (Illus.). 240p. pap. text 34.95 (*0-929894-15-4*) K-W Pubns.

Handbook of Short-Term Dynamic Psychotherapy. Ed. by Paul Crits-Christoph & Jacques P. Barber. 1991. LC 91-70846. 368p. (C). pap. 50.00 (*0-465-02875-6*) Basic.

Handbook of Short-Term Therapy Groups. Ed. by Max Rosenbaum. 1996. LC 96-35207. (Master Works). 448p. pap. 65.00 (*0-7657-0045-X*) Aronson.

Handbook of Signs & Symptoms. Springhouse Publishing Company Staff. 1998. LC 97-51521. (Illus.). 672p. spiral bd. 38.95 (*0-87434-893-5*) Springhouse Corp.

Handbook of Skin Clues of Systemic Disease. Paul H. Jacobs & Todd S. Anhalt. 2nd ed. 1991. LC 91-15499. 150p. pap. 19.95 (*0-8121-1464-7*) Lppncott W & W.

Handbook of Sleep Disorders. Ed. by Michael J. Thorpy. 1990. (Neurological Disease & Therapy Ser.: Vol. 6). 920p. 275.00 (*0-8247-8295-X*) Dekker.

Handbook of Sleep Medicine. John M. Shneerson. 2000. LC 00-23876. (Illus.). 240p. 110.95 (*0-632-05135-3*) Blackwell Sci.

Handbook of Small Animal Dermatology. K. A. Moriello & I. S. Mason. 1995. LC 94-18014. (Pergamon Veterinary Handbook Ser.: No. 11). 80.00 (*0-08-042281-0*); pap. 60.00 (*0-08-042280-2*) Elsevier (Pergamon Pr).

***Handbook of Small Animal Gastroenterology.** Todd R. Tams. 2001. (Illus.). 565p. pap. (*0-7216-8676-1*) Saunders.

Handbook of Small Animal Gastroenterology. Todd R. Tams. 1995. LC 95-14622. (Illus.). 464p. pap. text, tchr. ed. 49.00 (*0-7216-2478-2*) Saunders.

Handbook of Small Animal Ophthalmic Surgery Vol. 1: Extraocular Procedures. Kirk N. Gelatt & Janice P. Gelatt. 1994. (Pergolesi Studies: No. 7). 200p. text 105.00 (*0-08-042292-6*);Vol. 1. pap. text 60.00 (*0-08-042269-1*) Elsevier (Pergamon Pr).

Handbook of Small Animal Ophthalmic Surgery Vol. 2: Corneal & Intraocular Procedures. Gelatt. 1995. (Pergamon Veterinary Handbook Ser.: No. 8). 300p. text 120.00 (*0-08-042293-4*, Pergamon Pr) Elsevier.

Handbook of Small Animal Ophthalmic Surgery Vol. 2: Corneal & Intraocular Procedures. Kirk N. Gelatt & J. P. Gelatt. 1995. 300p. pap. (*0-08-042271-3*) Elsevier NLD. *Dist:* Elsevier.

Handbook of Small Animal Oral Emergencies. Ed. by Peter Emily et al. 1993. LC 93-9460. (Veterinary Handbook Ser.). pap. text 40.00 (*0-08-042270-5*, Pergamon Pr) Elsevier.

Handbook of Small Animal Orthopedics & Fracture Repair. Donald L. Piermattei & Gretchen L. Flo. Ed. by Ray Kersey. 3rd ed. 1997. LC 96-39430. (Illus.). 736p. pap. text 60.00 (*0-7216-5689-7*) Saunders.

Handbook of Small Animal Practice. Rhea V. Morgan. 3rd ed. 1997. LC 96-45945. (Illus.). 1210p. (C). text 155.00 (*0-7216-3329-3*) Harcourt.

Handbook of Small Animal Toxicology & Poisonings. Gfeller et al. 1997. LC 97-42301. 416p. (gr. 13). pap. text 49.95 (*0-8151-6454-8*, 26581) Mosby Inc.

Handbook of Snake Bites. P. Banerji. 1985. 430p. pap. (*0-7855-0365-X*) Intl Bks & Periodicals IND. *Dist:* St Mut.

Handbook of Social & Clinical Psychology: The Health Perspective. C. R. Snyder & Donelson R. Forsyth. 1991. (General Psychology Ser.: No. 162). 896p. (*0-08-036128-5*); (*0-08-040617-3*) PPI GBR. *Dist:* Elsevier.

Handbook of Social & Evaluation Anxiety. H. Leitenberg. 1990. LC 90-6853. (Illus.). 570p. (C). 100.00 (*0-306-43438-5*, Kluwer Plenum) Kluwer Academic.

Handbook of Social Gerontology: Societal Aspects of Aging. Clark Tibbitts. 1999. LC 60-5469. (Illus.). 789p. lib. bdg. 32.50 (*0-226-80221-3*) U Ch Pr.

Handbook of Social Psychology, Set. Ed. by Gardner Lindzey & Elliot Aronson. 3rd ed. 1985. (C). text 150.00 (*0-89859-720-X*) L Erlbaum Assocs.

Handbook of Social Psychology Vol. I: Theory & Methods. Ed. by Gardner Lindzey & Elliot Aronson. 3rd ed. 1985. 832p. (C). text 70.00 (*0-89859-718-8*) L Erlbaum Assocs.

Handbook of Social Support & the Family. Ed. by I. G. Sarason et al. 1996. LC 96-17181. (Plenum Series on Stress & Coping). (Illus.). 545p. (C). 102.00 (*0-306-45232-4*, Plenum Trade) Perseus Pubng.

Handbook of Solution-Focused Brief Therapy. Ed. by Scott D. Miller et al. 1996. LC 95-48252. (Psychology Ser.). 732p. 50.00 (*0-7879-0217-9*) Jossey-Bass.

Handbook of SOPs for Good Clinical Practice. Donald Maynard & B. Joyce Baird. 1996. 271p. ring bd. 229.00 (*1-57491-009-4*) IHS Health Grp.

Handbook of Spectrophotometric Data of Drugs. Ed. by Irving Sunshine. 1981. 496p. 270.00 (*0-8493-3571-X*, RS189, CRC Reprint) Franklin.

Handbook of Spina Bifida. Singh. 1998. 26.00 net. (*1-56593-204-8*) Singular Publishing.

Handbook of Spinal Anaesthesia & Analgesia. Benjamin G. Covino et al. 1994. (Illus.). 168p. text 94.50 (*0-7216-5606-4*) Saunders.

Handbook of Spinal Cord Monitoring: Proceedings of the Fifth International Symposium, London, June 2-5, 1992. Ed. by S. J. Jones et al. 1994. LC 93-31307. text 178.50 (*0-7923-8833-X*) Kluwer Academic.

Handbook of Sport Psychology. Ed. by Robert N. Singer et al. 2nd ed. 2000. LC 00-42291. 896p. 95.00 (*0-471-37995-6*) Wiley.

Handbook of Sports Epidemiology. Barry Jordan. 1999. 125.00 (*0-8493-2504-8*) CRC Pr.

Handbook of Sports Injuries. R. Charles Bull. 1998. LC 98-36208. (Illus.). 430p. pap. 39.95 (*0-07-008993-0*) McGraw-Hill Prof.

Handbook of Sports Medicine. Jason L. Dragoo. 1993. LC 93-92722. (Illus.). 192p. (Orig.). pap. 14.95 (*0-9637144-0-6*) Renaiss AZ.

Handbook of Sports Medicine: A Symptom-Oriented Approach. Ed. by Wade A. Lillegard & Karen S. Rucker. 1993. (Illus.). 298p. text 70.00 (*1-56372-052-3*) Buttrwrth-Heinemann.

Handbook of Sports Medicine: A Symptom-Oriented Approach. Wade A. Lillegard et al. 2nd ed. 1998. LC 98-26931. 448p. text 74.99 (*0-7506-9041-0*) Buttrwrth-Heinemann.

Handbook of Staff Development. Horner. 1995. pap. text 34.00 (*0-443-05145-3*) Saunders.

Handbook of Statistical Methods in Biological & Medical Sciences. Ed. by C. R. Rao & Ranajit Chakraborty. 1991. (Handbooks of Statistics: No. 8). 554p. 176.00 (*0-444-88095-X*, North Holland) Elsevier.

Handbook of Stereoisomers: Drugs in Psychopharmacology. Ed. by Donald F. Smith. 1983. 504p. 165.00 (*0-8493-2940-X*, RM315) CRC Pr.

Handbook of Stereoisomers: Therapeutic Drugs. Ed. by Donald F. Smith. 1989. 416p. 310.00 (*0-8493-3421-7*, RM301) CRC Pr.

Handbook of Stress: Theoretical & Clinical Aspects. Ed. by Leo Goldberger & Shlomo Breznitz. 2nd ed. 1993. LC 92-23125. 819p. pap. 40.00 (*0-02-912036-5*) Free Pr.

Handbook of Stress, Coping, & Health: Implications for Nursing Research, Theory, & Practice. Virginia Hill Rice. 1999. LC 99-50741. (Nursing Ser.). (Illus.). 590p. pap. 59.95 (*0-7619-1821-3*, 83566) Sage.

Handbook of Stress Medicine: An Organ System Approach. J. R. Hubbard & Edward A. Workman. 1997. LC 97-15758. 448p. 110.00 (*0-8493-2515-3*) CRC Pr.

Handbook of Stress, Medicine, & Health. Ed. by Cary L. Cooper. 1995. LC 95-7307. 400p. 139.95 (*0-8493-2908-6*, 2908C2W) CRC Pr.

Handbook of Stroke. David O. Wiebers et al. 1997. LC 96-44188. (Little, Brown Handbook Ser.). (Illus.). 448p. pap. text 49.95 (*0-316-94760-1*, Little Brwn Med Div) Lppncott W & W.

Handbook of Structured Techniques in Marriage & Family Therapy. Robert Sherman & Norman Fredman. 10th ed. 1986. LC 85-32064. 264p. text 41.95 (*0-87630-424-2*) Brunner-Routledge.

Handbook of Studies on Preventive Psychiatry. Ed. by Beverly Raphael & Graham D. Burrows. 1995. 716p. 219.00 (*0-444-81836-7*) Elsevier.

Handbook of Subacute Health Care. Kathleen Griffin. 1995. 368p. 108.00 (*0-8342-0661-7*, 20661) Aspen Pub.

Handbook of Substance Abuse: Neurobehavioral Pharmacology. Ed. by R. E. Tarter et al. 1999. LC 98-36286. (Illus.). 602p. (C). text 110.00 (*0-306-45884-5*, Kluwer Plenum) Kluwer Academic.

Handbook of Supportive Care in Cancer. Ed. by Jean Klastersky et al. 1994. LC 94-41531. (Basic & Clinical Oncology Ser.: Vol. 7). (Illus.). 616p. text 115.00 (*0-8247-9272-6*) Dekker.

Handbook of Surgery. F. R. C. S. Staff & Subash Ch. Bose. 1985. (*0-7855-0818-X*) Current Dist IND. *Dist:* St Mut.

Handbook of Surgery. Theodore Schrock. 8th ed. 1985. LC 84-62416. (Illus.). 586p. pap. text 15.95 (*0-930010-10-8*) Jones Med.

Handbook of Surgery. Ed. by Theodore Schrock. 10th ed. 1993. LC 93-15748. (Illus.). 1024p. (C). (gr. 13). pap. text 39.95 (*0-8016-7637-1*, 07637) Mosby Inc.

Handbook of Surgery Rep. S. C. Basu. 1990. (C). (*0-89771-336-2*) Current Dist IND. *Dist:* St Mut.

Handbook of Surgical Intensive Care. Thomas A. D'Amico. Ed. by Scott K. Pruitt. 4th ed. 1995. (Illus.). 592p. (C). (gr. 13). pap. text 47.95 (*0-8151-2249-7*, 24275) Mosby Inc.

Handbook of Surgical Intensive Care: Practices of the Surgical Residents at Duke University Medical Center. Bryan M. Clary & Camelo A. Milano. 5th ed. 2000. LC 00-33874. (Illus.). xii, 482p. pap. text (*0-323-01106-3*) Mosby Inc.

Handbook of Surgical Knot Tying see Surgical Knots & Suturing Techniques: A Handbook for Students of Surgery

Handbook of Surgical Oncology. E. George Elias. 1988. 288p. 215.00 (*0-8493-3277-X*, RD651) CRC Pr.

Handbook of Surgical Operations. Stephen Smith. 1990. LC 88-60671. (American Civil War Surgery Ser.: No. 8). (Illus.). 279p. reprint ed. 45.00 (*0-930405-07-2*) Norman SF.

Handbook of Surgical Pathology. Susan C. Lester. 1998. LC 00-25390. (Illus.). 336p. text (*0-443-07918-8*) Church.

Handbook of Symptom Oriented Neurology. William H. Olson et al. 2nd ed. 1993. (Illus.). 632p. (C). (gr. 13). pap. text 37.95 (*0-8016-7779-3*, 07779) Mosby Inc.

Handbook of Synthetic Antioxidants. Ed. by Lester Packer & Enrique Cadenas. 1997. LC 96-53380. (Antioxidants in Health & Disease Ser.). (Illus.). 464p. text 175.00 (*0-8247-9810-4*) Dekker.

Handbook of Synthetic Substrates. E. C. Hemker. 1983. text 141.50 (*0-89838-556-3*) Kluwer Academic.

Handbook of Tapeworm Identification. Gerald D. Schmidt. 1986. (Illus.). 688p. 374.00 (*0-8493-3280-X*, QL391, CRC Reprint) Franklin.

Handbook of TCM Patterns & Treatments. Bob Flaws & Daniel Finney. Ed. by Honora L. Wolfe & Rose Crescenz. 1996. LC 95-83250. 220p. text 29.95 (*0-936185-70-8*) Blue Poppy Pr.

Handbook of TCM Pediatrics: A Practitioner's Guide to the Care & Treatment of Common Childhood Diseases. Bob Flaws. Ed. by Honora L. Wolfe. 1996. LC 96-84825. (Illus.). 380p. 49.95 (*0-936185-72-4*) Blue Poppy Pr.

Handbook of TCM Urology & Male Sexual Dysfunction. Anna Lin. Ed. by Bob Flaws. 1992. LC 92-73392. 240p. (Orig.). pap. 19.95 (*0-936185-36-8*) Blue Poppy Pr.

Handbook of Teaching for Physical Therapists. Katherine F. Shepard & Gail M. Jensen. 1997. LC 96-50472. 406p. text 39.99 (*0-7506-9596-X*) Buttrwrth-Heinemann.

Handbook of Teaching for Physical Therapists. Shepard & Jensen. 2nd ed. 2001. LC 2001-52648. 432p. pap. 39.99 (*0-7506-7309-5*) Buttrwrth-Heinemann.

Handbook of the Aging Brain. Ed. by Eugenia Wang & D. Stephen Snyder. 1998. LC 98-84430. (Illus.). 263p. (C). 79.95 (*0-12-734610-4*) Acad Pr.

Handbook of the Assisted Reproduction Laboratory. Brooks A. Keel et al. 2000. LC 99-86572. (Illus.). 416p. 99.95 (*0-8493-1677-4*) CRC Pr.

Handbook of the Biology of Aging. Ed. by Edward L. Schneider et al. 4th ed. 1996. (Handbooks of Aging). (Illus.). 507p. pap. text 49.95 (*0-12-627873-3*) Acad Pr.

Handbook of the Brief Psychotherapies. Ed. by R. A. Wells & V. J. Gianetti. 1990. (Applied Clinical Psychology Ser.). (Illus.). 624p. (C). 105.00 (*0-306-43270-6*, Plenum Trade) Perseus Pubng.

Handbook of the Clinical Psychology of Aging. Ed. by Robert T. Woods. 1996. LC 96-1474. 694p. 275.00 (*0-471-96136-1*) Wiley.

Handbook of the Hemopoietic Microenvironment. Ed. by Mehdi Tavassoli. 1989. LC 89-15497. (Contemporary Biomedicine Ser.: Vol. 9). (Illus.). 472p. 145.00 (*0-89603-147-0*) Humana.

***Handbook of the Medical Care of Catastrophes.** J. S. P. Lumley et al. 1996. 223p. pap. (*1-85315-296-X*) Royal Soc of Medicine Pr Ltd GBR. *Dist:* Balogh.

Handbook of the Nutritional Contents of Foods. U. S. Department of Agriculture Staff. 1975. LC 75-2616. (Illus.). 192p. reprint ed. pap. 13.95 (*0-486-21342-0*) Dover.

Handbook of the Psychology of Aging Ed. by James E. Biren et al. 4th ed. 1996. pap. 112.00 (*0-12-044520-4*) Acad Pr.

Handbook of the Psychology of Aging. Ed. by James E. Birren et al. 4th ed. 1996. LC 95-19905. (Handbooks of Aging). (Illus.). 416p. pap. text 49.95 (*0-12-101261-1*) Acad Pr.

Handbook of the Radiology of Syndromes & Metabolic Disorders. Hooshang Taybi. 1997. LC 97-8264. 504p. (C). (gr. 13). pap. text 39.95 (*0-8151-2721-9*, 31334) Mosby Inc.

Handbook of the Skin & Systemic Disease. M. Lebwohl. 1997. (Illus.). 288p. pap. (0-443-05793-1) Church.

Handbook of the Treatment of the Anxiety Disorders. Ed. by Carol Lindemann. 2nd exp. ed. 1996. LC 95-51105. 296p. 65.00 (1-56821-805-2) Aronson.

Handbook of Theoretical Models in Biomedical Research. David B. Jack. 1999. (Pharmacology & Toxicology Ser.). 95.00 (0-8493-8301-3) CRC Pr.

***Handbook of Third Molar Surgery.** George Dimitroulis. 2001. 168p. pap. text 35.00 (0-7236-1084-3) Buttrwrth-Heinemann.

Handbook of Tourette's Syndrome & Related Tic & Behavioral Disorders. Roger Kurlan. 1992. (Neurological Disease & Therapy Ser.: Vol. 15). (Illus.). 560p. text 215.00 (0-8247-8787-0) Dekker.

Handbook of Toxic & Hazardous Chemicals & Carcinogens, Set. Marshall Sittig. 3rd ed. 1992. LC 91-16020. 1685p. 249.00 (0-8155-1286-4) Noyes.

Handbook of Toxicologic Pathology. Ed. by Wanda M. Haschek & Colin G. Rousseaux. 1991. LC 91-4604. (Illus.). 1080p. text 209.00 (0-12-330220-X) Acad Pr.

Handbook of Toxicology, Vol. 2. Thomas J. Haley & William O. Berndt. Date not set. (0-89116-863-X) Hemisp Pub.

Handbook of Toxicology of Controlled Substances. Gabriel G. Nahas. 1995. (0-8493-7939-3) CRC Pr.

Handbook of Toxinology. W. Thomas Shier & Gudrun Mebs. 1990. (Illus.). 872p. text 250.00 (0-8247-8374-3) Dekker.

Handbook of Traditional Chinese Dermatology. Liang Jian-hui. Tr. by Zhang Ting-liang from CHI. 1993. 176p. pap. 17.95 (0-936185-46-5) Blue Poppy Pr.

Handbook of Traditional Chinese Gynecology. Zhejiang College og Traditional Chinese Medicine S. Ed. by Bob Flaws. Tr. by Zhang Ting-liang from CHI. 1987.Tr. of Zhong Yi Fuke Shou Ce. 267p. (Orig.). pap. 22.95 (0-936185-06-6) Blue Poppy Pr.

Handbook of Transcranial Doppler. J. P. McCartney et al. 1996. LC 96-13737. (Illus.). 99p. pap. 46.95 (0-387-94693-4) Spr-Verlag.

***Handbook of Transfusion Medicine.** Ed. by Christopher D. Hillyer et al. 2001. 369p. 79.95 (0-12-348775-7) Acad Pr.

Handbook of Treatment Approaches in Childhood Psychopathology. J. L. Matson. 1988. LC 88-19648. (Applied Clinical Psychology Ser.). (Illus.). 612p. (C). 110.00 (0-306-42844-X, Plenum Trade) Perseus Pubng.

Handbook of Treatment for Eating Disorders. Ed. by David M. Garner & Paul E. Garfinkel. 2nd ed. 1997. LC 97-3395. 528p. text 60.00 (1-57230-186-4, 0186) Guilford Pubns.

Handbook of Tremor Disorders. Ed. by Lesley J. Findley & William C. Koller. 1994. (Neurological Disease & Therapy Ser.: Vol. 30). (Illus.). 600p. text 235.00 (0-8247-8859-1) Dekker.

Handbook of Trout & Salmon Diseases. Ronald J. Roberts & C. Jonathan Shepherd. 2nd ed. 1989. (Illus.). 232p. 54.95 (0-85238-138-7) Blackwell Sci.

Handbook of Trout & Salmon Diseases. Ronald J. Roberts & C. Jonathan Shepherd. 1978. 90.00 (0-7855-6929-4) St Mut.

***Handbook of Tumor Pathology Nomenclature.** Ed. by P. H. McKee & C. J. M. de Wolf. 2001. LC 00-68054. 384p. pap. 79.95 (0-471-18485-3) Wiley.

Handbook of Ultrasound & Gynecology, II. Ed. by A. Kurjak. 1990. 328p. lib. bdg. 195.00 (0-8493-3254-0) CRC Pr.

Handbook of Ultrasound in Obstetrics & Gynecology, Vol. 1. Ed. by A. Kurjak. 1990. 376p. 210.00 (0-8493-3253-2, AG527) CRC Pr.

Handbook of Venous Diseases. Belcaro. 1995. pap. text 39.00 (0-7020-2016-8) Saunders.

***Handbook of Venous Disorders.** Ed. by Peter Gloviczki & James S. T. Yao. 2nd ed. 2001. (Arnold Publication). 448p. text 129.95 (0-340-76130-X) OUP.

Handbook of Venous Disorders: Guidelines of the American Venous Forum. Ed. by James S. T. Yao & Peter Gloviczki. 1995. LC 95-71379. (Illus.). 704p. (0-412-72730-7) E A GBR. *Dist:* OUP.

Handbook of Vertebrate Immunology. Ed. by Paul-Pierre Pastoret et al. 1998. LC 97-45873. (Illus.). 704p. 150.00 (0-12-546401-0) Acad Pr.

Handbook of Vestibular Rehabilitation. Ed. by Rosalyn A. Davies & Linda M. Luxon. 1997. LC 97-8265. (Illus.). 200p. (Orig.). pap. 49.95 (1-56593-847-X, 1654) Thomson Learn.

Handbook of Veterinary Anesthesia. W. M. Muir & John T. Hubbell. 2nd ed. 1994. LC 94-24404. (Illus.). 496p. (C). (gr. 13). text 54.00 (0-8016-7656-8, 07656) Mosby Inc.

Handbook of Veterinary Drugs. Dana G. Allen. 2nd ed. 1998. LC 98-9454. 896p. pap. text 46.95 (0-397-58435-0) Lppncott W & W.

Handbook of Veterinary Drugs. Dana G. Allen & John K. Pringle. 2nd ed. 1998. 688p. pap. text (0-7817-1443-5) Lppncott W & W.

Handbook of Veterinary Neurology. John E. Oliver, Jr. 3rd ed. 1997. LC 96-38603. (Illus.). x, 453p. (C). pap. text 58.00 (0-7216-7140-3) Harcourt.

Handbook of Veterinary Nuclear Medicine. Ed. by Clifford R. Berry & Gregory B. Daniel. 1996. (Illus.). 184p. (Orig.). pap. text 35.00 (0-9651794-0-0) N C State Univ.

***Handbook of Veterinary Nursing.** H. Orpet & P. Welsh. 2001. LC 2001-43327. (0-632-05258-9) Blackwell Sci.

Handbook of Veterinary Obstetrics. Jackson. 1995. text 52.00 (0-7020-1796-5) Saunders.

Handbook of Veterinary Procedures & Emergency Treatment. Ed. by Stephen I. Bistner et al. 7th ed. 2000. LC 99-41999. (Illus.). 1020p. text 59.00 (0-7216-7166-7) Saunders.

Handbook of Viral & Rickettsial Hemorrhagic Fever. Ed. by James H. Gear. 1988. 288p. 229.95 (0-8493-3517-5, RC147) CRC Pr.

Handbook of Vitamins, No. 40. Lawrence J. Machlin. 2nd rev. ed. 1990. (Food Science & Technology Ser.). (Illus.). 616p. text 65.00 (0-8247-8351-4) Dekker.

Handbook of Vocational Psychology: Theory, Research, & Practice. Ed. by W. Bruce Walsh & Samuel H. Osipow. 2nd ed. 1995. 480p. text 79.95 (0-8058-1374-8) L Erlbaum Assocs.

Handbook of Voice Quality Measurement. Ed. by Raymond D. Dent & Martin J. Ball. 1999. LC 99-19664. (Illus.). 475p. pap. 65.00 (1-56593-991-3, 1960) Thomson Learn.

Handbook of Work & Health Psychology. Ed. by Marc H. Schabracq et al. 1996. LC 95-31233. 512p. 300.00 (0-471-95789-5) Wiley.

***Handbook of Work & Organizational Psychology.** Ed. by Pieter J. D. Drenth & C. J. De Wolff. 2nd ed. 2001. (Handbook of Work & Organizational Psychology Ser.: Vol. 2). Vol. 2. 304p. pap. (0-86377-523-3); Vol. 3. 432p. pap. (0-86377-525-X) Psychol Pr GBR. *Dist:* Taylor & Francis.

***Handbook of Work & Organizational Psychology,** Vol. 4. Ed. by Pieter J. D. Drenth & C. J. De Wolff. 2nd ed. 2001. (Handbook of Work & Organizational Psychology Ser.). 512p. pap. (0-86377-527-6) Psychol Pr GBR. *Dist:* Taylor & Francis.

Handbook of Workplace Drug Testing. Ed. by Ray H. Liu & Bruce A. Goldberger. 2nd ed. 1995. 380p. reprint ed. pap. 24.00 (0-915274-77-9, 202638, AACC Pr) Am Assn Clinical Chem.

Handbook on Adoption: A Psychoanalytic View. Herbert Wieder. 1995. 112p. pap. 14.00 (1-887478-01-9, WiseAcre) Red Sea NY.

Handbook on AIDS, IV Drug Users, & Sexual Behavior in the United States. Ed. by Barry S. Brown. 1993. LC 92-35550. 632p. lib. bdg. 120.00 (0-313-28374-5, BKL, Greenwood Pr) Greenwood.

Handbook on Antibiotic Compounds. Janos Berdy. 1987. Vol. XIII, Pt. 1. 344p. lib. bdg. 225.00 (0-8493-3431-4); Vol. XIII, Pt. 2. 416p. lib. bdg. 225.00 (0-8493-3432-2); Vol. XIII, Pt. 3. 376p. lib. bdg. 225.00 (0 8493 3433-0) CRC Pr.

Handbook on Critical Life Issues. Ed. by John A. Leies et al. 6th rev. ed. 1988. LC 88-38958. 218p. pap. 9.95 (0-935372-24-5) NCBC.

Handbook on Critical Sexual Issues. Ed. by Edward J. Bayer et al. rev. ed. 1989. LC 89-16252. 220p. pap. 9.95 (0-935372-25-3) NCBC.

Handbook on Dementia Caregiving: Evidence-Based Interventions for Family Caregivers. Ed. by Richard Schulz. 2000. LC 99-53867. (Illus.). 272p. 49.95 (0-8261-1312-5) Springer Pub.

Handbook on Drug & Nutrient Interactions: A Problem-Oriented Reference Guide. Daphne A. Roe. 4th ed. 1989. LC 89-17781. 150p. spiral bd. 21.95 (0-88091-046-1, 0102) Am Dietetic Assn.

Handbook on Drug & Nutrient Interactions: A Reference & Study Guide. Daphne A. Roe. 5th ed. 1994. LC 94-35993. (Illus.). spiral bd. 29.95 (0-88091-135-2) Am Dietetic Assn.

Handbook on Endocrinology, Vol. IIA. George H. Gass. Ed. by Harold M. Kaplan. 1987. 184p. lib. bdg. 148.95 (0-8493-3236-2) CRC Pr.

Handbook on Endocrinology, Vol. IIB. George H. Gass & Kaplan Staff. 1987. 216p. lib. bdg. 148.95 (0-8493-3237-0) CRC Pr.

Handbook on Ethnicity, Aging & Mental Health. Ed. by Deborah K. Padgett. 1995. LC 94-11220. 376p. lib. bdg. 99.50 (0-313-28204-8, Greenwood Pr) Greenwood.

Handbook on Human Resources Management for Health Care Professionals. Ed. by Eucharia E. Nnadi-Okolo. 1997. LC 96-44092. 200p. (Orig.). (C). pap. text 17.95 (0-88258-195-3, OKHHP) Howard U Pr.

Handbook on Hyperbaric Medicine. Ed. by G. Oriani et al. 1996. 900p. 198.00 (3-540-75016-9) Spr-Verlag.

Handbook on Injectable Drugs. Lawrence A. Trissel. 8th ed. 1994. (Illus.). 1192p. text 100.00 (1-879907-42-9); 9th ed. 1996. (C). 138.00 (1-879907-64-X) Am Soc Hlth-Syst.

Handbook on Motor Unit Number Estimation for Nerve & Muscular Disorders: Methods, Cautions, Clinical, & Research Uses. Mark B. Bromberg. 1999. 99.00 (0-89603-559-X) Humana.

Handbook on Nursing Homes. Scott Blankenship. 2000. 153p. 43.00 (1-56072-383-1) Nova Sci Pubs.

Handbook on Pharmacology of Aging. P. Goldberg & J. Roberts. Ed. by Brody. 1983. LC 82-17829. (Series in Aging). 288p. 153.00 (0-8493-3145-5, RC953, CRC Reprint) Franklin.

Handbook on Running: Olympic Handbook of Sports Medicine. John A. Hawley. 2000. LC 99-47560. (Handbook of Sports Medicine & Science Ser.). (Illus.). ix, 96p. pap. 29.95 (0-632-05391-7) Blackwell Sci.

Handbook on Stuttering. Oliver Bloodstein. 4th rev. ed. 1987. (Illus.). 531p. pap. 17.95 (0-933851-04-9, G-19313) Natl Easter Seal.

Handbook on the Aged in the United States. Ed. by Erdman B. Palmore. 1984. LC 84-4463. (Illus.). 458p. lib. bdg. 110.00 (0-313-23721-2, PHA/, Greenwood Pr) Greenwood.

Handbook on the Assessment of Learning Disabilities: Theory, Research, & Practice. Ed. by H. Lee Swanson. 1991. LC 89-13458. (Illus.). 438p. (Orig.). pap. text 37.00 (0-89079-406-5, 1589) PRO-ED.

Handbook on the Bach Flower Remedies. Phillip Chancellor. 1980. LC 79-93435. 252p. (Orig.). pap. 11.95 (0-87983-196-0, 31960K, Keats Pubng) McGraw-Hill Trade.

Handbook on the Late Effects of Poliomyelitis for Physicians & Survivors. Ed. by G. Laurie et al. 1984. 48p. (Orig.). pap. 6.75 (0-931301-00-9) Gazette Intl.

Handbook on the Medical Aspects of Nuclear, Biological, & Chemical Defense Operations. 1991. lib. bdg. 79.95 (0-8490-4066-3) Gordon Pr.

Handbook on the Physics & Chemistry of Rare Earths. Ed. by K. A. Gschneidner, Jr. & L. Eyring. 1999. 576p. 220.50 (0-444-50185-1, North Holland) Elsevier.

Handbook Pharmacy Health Care. Ed. by Robin Harman. 1990. 587p. (0-85369-230-0) Pharmaceutical Pr GBR. *Dist:* Rittenhouse.

Handbook Pharmacy Health Education. Martin. 1991. (0-85369-263-7) Pharmaceutical Pr GBR. *Dist:* Rittenhouse.

Handbook Series in Zoonoses, Vol. I, Section D. Ed. by James H. Steele. 1984. 464p. lib. bdg. 185.00 (0-8493-2921-3, RC113, CRC Reprint) Franklin.

Handbook Series in Zoonoses, CRR, Section A: Bacterial, Rickettsial & Mycotic Diseases, Vol. 2. Ed. by Herbert Stoenner et al. 1980. 608p. 317.00 (0-8493-2907-8, RC113, CRC Reprint) Franklin.

Handbook to Patient Education. Susan B. Bastable. 2001. (Illus.). 416p. (C). pap. text 46.95 (0-7637-1442-9) Jones & Bartlett.

Handbook to Saunders Paramedic. Thomas. 2000. pap. text (0-7216-6312-5) Harcrt Hlth Sci Grp.

Handbuch der Infusionstherapie und Klinischen Ernaehrung: Band 1-6. 1988. 1674p. 523.50 (3-8055-3747-6) S Karger.

Handbuch der Intensivmedizin. Ed. by James L. Berk & J. E. Sampliner. 3rd enl. rev. ed. 1986. (Illus.). xiv, 650p. pap. 77.50 (3-8055-3766-2) S Karger.

Handedness & Developmental Disorder. D. V. Bishop. 1991. (Clinics in Developmental Medicine Ser.: No. 110). (Illus.). 208p. (C). text (0-521-41195-5) Mc Keith Pr GBR. *Dist:* Cambridge U Pr.

Handholder's Handbook: A Guide for Caregivers of People with Alzheimer's or Other Dementias. Rosette Teitel. 2001. LC 00-45680. (Illus.). xiv, 192p. (C). pap. 17.00 (0-8135-2940-9); text 40.00 (0-8135-2939-5) Rutgers U Pr.

Handicapped & the Disabled: Index of Modern Authors & Subjects with Guide for Rapid Research. Science and Life Consultants Association Staff. 1991. LC 90-56328. 160p. 47.50 (1-55914-446-7); pap. 44.50 (1-55914-447-5) ABBE Pubs Assn.

Handicapped Child in the Family: A Guide for Parents. Verda Heisler. 1972. LC 71-168847. 176p. text 45.00 (0-8089-0734-4, 791960, Grune & Strat) Harcrt Hlth Sci Grp.

Handicapped Children in Britain: Their Problems & Education & Index Catalogue of a Library of Rehabilitation of the Disabled Wendy A. Axford & Douglas C. McMurtrie. Ed. by William R. Phillips & Janet Rosenberg. 1980. LC 79-6894. (Physically Handicapped in Society Ser.). reprint ed. lib. bdg. 19.95 (0-405-13105-4) Ayer.

Handicapped Community: The Relation Between Primary Health Care & Community Based Rehabilitation. Ed. by H. Finkenflugel. 1994. (Primary Health Care Publications: Vol. 7). 140p. (Orig.). pap. (90-5383-211-4) VU Univ Pr NLD. *Dist:* Paul & Co Pubs.

Handicapped Service Aide. Jack Rudman. 1994. (Career Examination Ser.: C-3305). pap. 27.95 (0-8373-3305-9) Nat Learn.

Handicapping the Handicapped: Decision Making in Students' Educational Careers. Hugh Mehan et al. 1986. LC 85-22084. (Illus.). xvi, 193p. 46.00 (0-8047-1304-9) Stanford U Pr.

Handicaps in Childhood. Ed. by M. Manciaux. 1981. (Child Health & Development Ser.: Vol. 1). (Illus.). x, 182p. 72.25 (3-8055-2935-X) S Karger.

Handing Over: Developing Consistency Across Shifts in Residential & Health Settings. Barry Mason. 1992. 96p. pap. text (1-85575-018-X) Karnac Bks GBR. *Dist:* Other Pr LLC.

Handle with Care: A Question of Alzheimer's. Dorothy S. Brown. 1984. LC 84-61253. 120p. pap. 21.00 (0-87975-272-6) Prometheus Bks.

Handle with Care: Helping Children Prenatally Exposed to Drugs & Alcohol. Sylvia Villarreal. 1992. pap. 17.95 (1-56071-077-2) ETR Assocs.

***Handle with Care: Serving the Mental Health Needs of Youth Offenders.** Ed. by Kenneth Schatz. 2001. 112p. (C). pap. text 30.00 (0-7567-0886-9) DIANE Pub.

Handle with Care: Understanding Fragile X Syndrome. Marcia Braden. 3rd rev. ed. 2000. 228p. pap. 25.00 (0-915667-26-6) Spectra Pub Co.

Handling Conflict in Hospital Management: Conflict Among Peers (Game I) Erwin Rausch & Wallace Wohlking. 1973. (Simulation Game Ser.). pap. 26.25 (0-89401-036-0) Didactic Syst.

Handling Conflict in Hospital Management: Superior - Subordinate Conflict (Game III) Erwin Rausch & Wallace Wohlking. 1974. (Simulation Game Ser.). pap. 26.25 (0-89401-043-3) Didactic Syst.

Handling It: You & Your Long Term Disease. Susan Molloy. 1995. 142p. (Orig.). pap. (0-85572-261-4) Hill Content Pubng AUS. *Dist:* Seven Hills Bk.

Handling of Radiation Accident Patients by Para-Hospital Personnel. Thomas Carder. 2nd ed. 1993. 240p. 79.95 (0-8493-8696-9, RC93) CRC Pr.

Handling of Radiation Accidents. Incl. Handling of Radiation Accidents: 1977. (Illus.). 593p. 1977. pap. 130.00 (92-0-020077-X, ISP463, IAEA); (Proceedings Ser.). (ENG, FRE & RUS.). Illus.). 710p. (Orig.). 1969. Set pap. 85.00 (92-0-020269-1, ISP229) Bernan Associates.

Handling of Radiation Accidents: 1977. 1977. (Proceedings Ser.: No. 2). (Illus.). 593p. pap. 130.00 (92-0-020077-X, ISP463, IAEA) Bernan Associates.

Handling Soft Tissue Injury Cases, Set. Stanley E. Preiser et al. 1985. 240.00 (0-930273-13-3, 65910-10, MICHIE) LEXIS Pub.

Handling Stress with Humor. Charles W. Winkler. Ed. by Grace Shaffer. 1988. (Illus.). 172p. pap. 6.95 (0-9610522-0-1) Winkler Pub.

Handlist of Arabic Medical Manuscripts in the Research Library, UCLA. Nancy E. Gallagher. 1983. LC 82-50985. (Aids & Research Tools in the Middle East Studies: Vol. 1). (Illus.). xx, 24p. pap. 9.00 (0-89003-128-2) Undena Pubns.

Handmade Medicines: Simple Recipes for Herbal Health. Christopher Hobbs. 1998. LC 97-51397. (Illus.). 120p. pap. 12.95 (1-883010-50-0) Interweave.

Hands Feel It: Healing & Spirit Presence among a Northern Alaskan People. Edith Turner. 1996. LC 95-26638. (Illus.). 240p. pap. 20.00 (0-87580-573-6) N Ill U Pr.

Hands Heal: Documentation for Massage Therapy: A Guide to S.O.A.P. Charting. Diana L. Thompson. Ed. by Phoenix. 1993. (Illus.). 88p. (Orig.). (C). pap. text 17.95 (0-9638347-0-3) D L Thompson.

Hands of the Living God: An Account of a Psychoanalytic Treatment. Marion Milner. 1969. LC 78-85201. (Illus.). 444p. text 75.00 (0-8236-2320-3) Intl Univs Pr.

Hands on Feet: The New System That Makes Reflexology a Snap. Michelle R. Kluck. 2001. (Illus.). 160p. pap. 19.95 (0-7624-0961-4) Running Pr.

Hands-on Guide for House Officers. Anna Donald & Michael Stein. 1996. LC 95-50825. (Illus.). 160p. pap. 31.95 (0-86542-921-9) Blackwell Sci.

Hands-on Guide to Clinical Pharmacology. Sukhdev Chatu et al. 2000. LC 99-8908. 176p. pap. 29.95 (0-632-05518-9) Blackwell Sci.

Hands-on Healing: A Practical Guide to Channeling Your Healing Energy. Jack Angelo. 1997. LC 97-1080. (Illus.). 256p. pap. 16.95 (0-89281-734-8, Heal Arts VT) Inner Tradit.

Hands-On Healing: Massage for Total Health - The Shaman's Way. Lewis Harrison. 1998. LC 00-500403. 320p. pap. 12.95 (1-57566-361-9) Kensgtn Pub Corp.

Hands on Health. Reader's Digest Editorial Staff. 1999. LC 98-50504. (Health & Healing the Natural Way Ser.). (Illus.). 19.95 (0-7621-0146-6) RD Assn.

Hands-on Horse Care: The Complete Book of Equine First-Aid. Karen E. Hayes. Ed. by Thomas C. Bohanon & Sue M. Copeland. 1998. (Illus.). 400p. 29.95 (0-86573-861-0) Creat Pub Intl.

Hands-On, No-Nonsense, Need-to-Know Guide to Office Management. Andrew R. Peters. 2000. ring bd. 39.95 (0-9702725-5-3) A Peters Consult.

Handy Charting Guidelines for Nursing Facilities. Ed. by Ann G. Uniack. 1998. 142p. (Orig.). pap. text 22.95 (1-881671-18-6) S N A P.

Handy Medical Guide for Seafarers, Fisherman, Trawlermen & Yachtsmen. R. W. Scott. 1978. 40.00 (0-7855-6930-8) St Mut.

Hanging on & Letting Go: Understanding the Onset, Progression & Remission of Depression. T. Pyszczynski & J. Greenberg. 1992. (Illus.). 169p. 139.00 (0-387-97756-2) Spr-Verlag.

Hans Krebs Vol. 2: Architect of Intermediary Metabolism, 1933-1937, Vol. 2. Frederic L. Holmes. 1993. (Monographs on the History & Philosophy of Biology). (Illus.). 504p. text 70.00 (0-19-507657-5) OUP.

***Hansen's Disease: The Shared Paradigm.** M. J. De Mallac. 2001. 124p. (1-85776-597-4) Book Guild Ltd GBR. *Dist:* Trans-Atl Phila.

Hansten & Horn's Managing Clinically Important Drug Interactions. Philip D. Hansten & John R. Horn. Ed. by Lloyd Y. Young & Mary A. Koda-Kimble. 1998. 553p. (C). pap. 79.95 (0-915486-30-X) Applied Therapeutics.

Hantavirus in the Americas: Guidelines for Diagnosis, Treatment, Prevention & Control. 1999. (Technical Publications: No. 47). 63p. 14.00 (92-75-13047-7, TP 47) PAHO.

Hantavirus Infection in the United States & California. Marsha Devine. 1993. 4p. pap. (1-58703-014-4) CA Res Bureau.

H
I

Hantaviruses: Emerging Viral Diseases. Ed. by J. S. Mackenzie. 1999. (Illus.). 67p. pap. text 20.00 (*0-7881-8078-9*) DIANE Pub.

Happiness Is a Healthy Life. London H. Smith. 1991. 192p. pap. 10.95 (*0-87983-547-8*, 35478K, Keats Pubng) McGraw-Hill Trade.

Happiness, Pleasure, & Judgment: The Contextual Theory & Its Applications. Allen Parducci. 1995. LC 95-14486. 232p. text 45.00 (*0-8058-1891-X*) L Erlbaum Assocs.

Happy Birth Days: Personal Accounts of Birth at Home the Intimate, Husband/Wife Way. Ed. by Marilyn A. Moran. 1986. (Illus.). 134p. (Orig.). pap. 12.95 (*0-940128-02-0*) Terra Publng.

Happy Health Organizer: A Personal Medical Journal. Carol C. Knight. 1993. 143p. (Orig.). pap. text 12.95 (*0-937866-41-5*) Atlantic Pub Co.

Happy-Healthy Way to Live. Paul Smallie. 1985. LC 85-50570. 144p. text 20.00 (*0-9614296-4-X*) Wrld-Wide Bks.

Happy Heart Cookbook. Grace M. Kurasz. 1990. LC 90-90397. (Illus.). 160p. spiral bd. 10.95 (*0-9628432-0-2*) G Kurasz.

Happy Hours: Alcohol in a Woman's Life. Devon Jersild. 2001. LC 00-35880. 400p. 25.00 (*0-06-019268-2*, Cliff Street) HarperTrade.

Harassment Therapy: A Case Study of Psychiatric Violence. Don Stannard-Friel. 1981. 183p. pap. text 13.95 (*0-87073-160-2*) Schenkman Bks Inc.

Hard Capsules: Development - Technology. Ridgway. 1987. (*0-85369-159-2*) Pharmaceutical Pr GBR. *Dist:* Rittenhouse.

Hard Choices in Health Care. Ed. by Jo Lenaghan. 1996. LC 97-151067. 204p. pap. text (*0-7279-1081-7*, 340300260) BMJ Pub GBR. *Dist:* AIDC.

Hard-Earned Lessons from Counselling in Action. Windy Dryden. 1992. (Counselling in Action Ser.: Vol. 15). 160p. (C). 49.95 (*0-8039-8668-8*); pap. 24.95 (*0-8039-8669-6*, 9150) Sage.

Hard Facts in Orthopaedics. Robert C. Schenck, Jr. 1993. LC 92-48563. (Illus.). 100p. pap. 28.00 (*0-942219-46-5*) Quality Med Pub.

Hard Labor. Susan L. Diamond. 1998. 416p. pap. 17.95 (*0-312-85308-4*, Forge Bks) T Doherty Assocs.

Hard Labor: Reflections of an Obstetrical Nurse. Susan L. Diamond. 1996. LC 96-1555. 384p. 25.95 (*0-312-85682-2*, Tor Books) T Doherty Assocs.

Hard of Hearing Child. Ed. by Frederick S. Berg & Samuel Fletcher. 1970. LC 70-110449. 368p. text 47.50 (*0-8089-0642-9*, 790554, Grune & Strat) Harcrt Hlth Sci Grp.

Hard Pharmacopoeia of Easter Medicine. Ed. by Hakim M. Said. 1997. (C). (*81-7030-520-9*) Sri Satguru Pubns IND. *Dist:* S Asia.

Hard-Pressed Researcher: A Research Handbook for the Caring Professions. Anne Edwards & Robin Talbot. 1994. LC 94-68. pap. text (*0-582-09993-5*) Addison-Wesley GBR. *Dist:* Trans-Atl Phila.

Hardcore Bodybuilding: The Blood, Sweat & Tears of Pumping Iron. Robert Kennedy. 1982. LC 82-50549. (Illus.). 192p. pap. 12.95 (*0-8069-7646-2*) Sterling.

Harderian Glands: Porphyrin Metabolism, Behavioral, & Endocrine Effects. Ed. by R. A. Hoffman et al. 1992. (Illus.). 325p. 152.00 (*0-387-54113-6*) Spr-Verlag.

Hardest Choice: Selecting a Nursing Home for an Alzheimer's Patient. 1994. (Illus.). 24p. pap. 2.00 (*1-930181-03-5*) A H A F.

Hardest Drug: Heroin & Public Policy. John Kaplan. 1994. LC 82-17514. (Studies in Crime & Justice). xii, 248p. reprint ed. pap. text 10.95 (*0-226-42428-6*) U Ch Pr.

Hare Brain, Tortoise Mind: Why Intelligence Increases When You Think Less. Guy Claxton. 1999. LC 98-16001. (Illus.). 259p. reprint ed. 25.95 (*0-88001-622-1*) HarperCollins Pubs.

Hare's Bacteriology & Immunity for Nurses. E. Mary Cooke. 7th ed. 1991. (Illus.). 240p. pap. text (*0-443-04140-7*) Church.

Harlem Hospital Story: One Hundred Years of Struggle Against Illness, Racism, & Genocide. A. Peter Bailey. 1991. LC 90-63874. 100p. (Orig.). pap. 11.98 (*0-9625169-7-X*) Native Sun Pubs.

Harley's Pediatric Opthalmology. Leonard B. Nelson. Ed. by Richard Lampert. 4th ed. 1998. LC 97-13498. (Illus.). 576p. text 185.00 (*0-7216-6842-9*) Saunders.

***Harm Reduction: The New Paradigm for Treating Drug & Acohol Problems.** Andrew Tatarsky. 2002. LC 2001-46079. (*0-7657-0352-1*) Aronson.

Harm Reduction in Prison/Risikominderung im Gefangnis: Strategies Against Drugs, AIDS & Risk Behaviour/Strategien Gegen Drogen, AIDS und Risikoverhalten. Ed. by Joachim Nelles & Andreas Fuhrer. 1997. LC 96-52165. 264p. (C). pap. text (*0-8204-3402-7*) P Lang CHE. *Dist:* P Lang Pubng.

Harm We Do: A Catholic Doctor Confronts Church, Moral, & Medical Teaching. Joyce Poole. 1993. LC 92-82673. 168p. (Orig.). pap. 12.95 (*0-89622-543-7*) Twenty-Third.

Harmful Effects of Allopathic (Western) Medicine: Drugs Degenerate the Body. Arthur M. Baker. 1994. LC 93-93558. 42p. (Orig.). pap. 8.95 (*1-883989-29-9*) Self Hlth Care.

Harmonics of Sound, Color & Vibration. Elias DeMohan. 1980. (Illus.). 160p. (Orig.). pap. 11.95 (*0-87516-411-0*) DeVorss.

Harmony: A Psychoacoustical Approach. R. Parncutt. 1989. (Information Sciences Ser.: Vol. 19). (Illus.). 206p. 79.95 (*0-387-51279-9*) Spr-Verlag.

Harmony of the Soul: Mental Health & Moral Virtue Reconsidered. Neal O. Weiner. 1993. LC 93-20449. (SUNY Series in the Philosophy of Psychology). 196p. (C). text 20.50 (*0-7914-1731-X*) State U NY Pr.

Harney's Medical Malpractice. Richard Patterson. 4th ed. 1999. LC 99-67534. xvii, 689p. 125.00 (*0-327-04982-0*, 6272011) LEXIS Pub.

Harold Glendon Scheie, MD: Ophthalmic Surgery & the Scheie Eye Institute. Harold G. Scheie. 1989. (Ophthalmology Oral History Ser.). (Illus.). 355p. (C). lib. bdg. 45.00 (*0-926866-02-8*) FAAO.

Harp Full of Stars: The Journey of a Music Healer. Joel Andrews. 1989. LC 89-80782. (Illus.). 264p. (Orig.). pap. 14.95 (*0-9623165-4-7*) Golden Harp.

HarperCollins Illustrated Medical Dictionary. Ida G. Dox et al. 1993. LC 92-53299. 592p. 40.00 (*0-06-271548-8*, Harper Ref); (Illus.). pap. 27.50 (*0-06-273142-4*) HarperCollins Pubs.

HarperCollins Illustrated Medical Dictionary. Ida G. Dox et al. 4th ed. 2001. LC 00-54200. (Illus.). 800p. pap. 35.00 (*0-06-273646-9*) HarperCollins Pubs.

Harriet Lane Handbook. Johns Hopkins Hospital Staff. Ed. by Michael A. Barone. 14th ed. 1996. (Illus.). 800p. (C). (gr. 13). pap. text 34.95 (*0-8151-4944-1*, 28698) Mosby Inc.

Harriet Lane Handbook. Johns Hopkins Hospital, Dept Pediatrics Staff. 15th ed. 1999. (C). text 35.95 (*0-323-00812-7*) Mosby Inc.

Harriet Lane Handbook. Johns Hopkins Hospital Staff et al. 15th ed. 2000. (Illus.). 1046p. pap. (*84-8174-274-0*) Mosby-Doyma Libros ESP. *Dist:* Mosby Inc.

Harriet Roth's Cholesterol Control Cookbook. Harriet Roth. 1991. LC 90-28736. (Illus.). 432p. reprint ed. pap. 15.95 (*0-452-26612-2*, Plume) Dutton Plume.

***Harrison's Manual of Medicine.** Eugene Braunwald et al. 15th ed. 2001. (Internal Medicine Ser.). (Illus.). 1000p. pap. 39.95 (*0-07-137377-2*) McGraw-Hill Prof.

Harrison's Principles of Internal Medicine. Ed. by Anthony S. Fauci et al. 14th ed. 1998. LC 97-14184. (Harrison's Principles of Internal Medicine Ser.). (Illus.). 2784p. text 125.00 (*0-07-020291-5*) McGraw-Hill Educ Grp.

Harrison's Principles of Internal Medicine. Tinsley R. Harrison & Anthony S. Fauci. 14th ed. 1997. LC 97-14184. (*0-07-020292-3*); (*0-07-020293-1*) McGraw.

Harrison's Principles of Internal Medicine Eugene Braunwald. 15th ed. 2001. LC 00-63809. (Illus.). (*0-07-007273-6*) McGraw.

Harrison's Principles of Internal Medicine Eugene Braunwald. 15th ed. 2001. LC 00-63809. (Illus.). (*0-07-007274-4*) McGraw-Hill Med Pub.

***Harrison's Principles of Internal Medicine.** Eugene Braunwald et al. 15th ed. 2001. 2780p. 272.00 incl. cd-rom (*0-07-139100-2*) McGraw-Hill Prof.

Harrison's Principles of Internal Medicine. Set. Ed. by Anthony S. Fauci et al. 14th ed. 1997. LC 97-14184. (Illus.). 2688p. text 149.00 (*0-07-912013-X*) McGraw-Hill Educ Grp.

Harrison's Principles of Internal Medicine: Self-Assessment & Board Review. Richard M. Stone. 14th ed. 1998. LC 97-35730. (Illus.). 384p. pap. 45.00 (*0-07-052537-4*) McGraw-Hill Educ Grp.

***Harrison's Principles of Internal Medicine: Self-Assessment & Board Review.** Richard M. Stone. 15th ed. 2001. LC 2001-30947. (Illus.). 400p. pap. 55.00 (*0-07-137375-6*) McGraw-Hill Prof.

***Harrison's Principles of Internal Medicine: Textbook, Self-Assessment & Board Review.** Eugene Braunwald et al. 15th ed. 2001. (Illus.). text 153.00 (*0-07-139102-9*) McGraw-Hill Prof.

Harry Stack Sullivan: Interpersonal Theory & Psychotherapy. F. Barton Evans. 1996. LC 96-16169. (Makers of Modern Psychotherapy Ser.). 256p. (C). 84.95 (*0-415-11972-3*); pap. 27.95 (*0-415-11973-1*) Routledge.

Hartland's Medical & Dental Hypnosis. David Waxman. 3rd ed. 1989. 520p. pap. text (*0-7020-1323-4*) W B Saunders GBR. *Dist:* Saunders.

Hartrampf's Breast Reconstruction with Living Tissue. Carl R. Hartrampf, Jr. & Bryan J. Michelow. 1990. 384p. text 215.00 (*0-88167-618-7*) Lppncott W & W.

Harvard Guide to Women's Health. Karen J. Carlson et al. 1996. (Harvard University Press Reference Library). (Illus.). 704p. LC 95-50876. pap. 24.95 (*0-674-36769-3*); pap. 39.95 incl. cd-rom (*0-674-36771-5*); LC 95-50876. 39.95 (*0-674-36768-5*) HUP.

Harvard Lectures. Anna Freud. Ed. & Anno. by Joseph Sandler. 1992. LC 92-1531. 154p. 30.00 (*0-8236-2310-6*) Intl Univs Pr.

Harvard List of Books in Psychology. Harvard University Psychologists Staff. 4th ed. 1990. LC 71-152700. 108p. pap. 8.95 (*0-674-37601-3*) HUP.

Harvard Med: The Story Behind America's Premier Medical School & the Making of America's Doctors. John Langone. 1996. LC 95-51744. 400p. pap. 14.00 (*1-55850-610-1*) Adams Media.

Harvard Medical School Family Health Guide. Anthony L. Komaroff. 1999. LC 99-27223. (Illus.). 1248p. 40.00 (*0-684-84703-5*) Free Pr.

Harvard Medical School Family Health Guide. Anthony L. Komaroff. 2000. 34.95 (*0-13-018960-X*) P-H.

***Harvard Medical School Guide to Men's Health: Insights from the Harvard Study of 90,000 Men.** Simon. Date not set. (*0-684-87181-5*) Free Pr.

Harvard Medical School Guide to Suicide Assessment & Intervention. Ed. by Douglas Jacobs. 1998. LC 98-25332. (Health & Psychology Ser.). (Illus.). 720p. 70.00 (*0-7879-4303-7*) Jossey-Bass.

Harvest of Hope: The Pilgrimage of a Mexican-American Physician. Jorge Prieto. 1989. LC 89-40024. 168p. (C). text 24.50 (*0-268-01087-0*) U of Notre Dame Pr.

Harvey A. K. Whitney Award Lectures: 1950-1997. rev. ed. 1997. LC 98-145919. (Illus.). 472p. pap. 25.00 (*1-879907-77-1*) Am Soc Hlth-Syst.

Harvey A. K. Whitney Award Lectures, 1950-1995. rev. ed. 1995. (Illus.). 440p. pap. 25.00 (*1-879907-59-3*) Am Soc Hlth-Syst.

Harvey A. K. Whitney Award Lectures, 1950-1999. annuals rev. ed. 1999. 400p. pap. text (*1-58528-009-7*) Am Soc Hlth-Syst.

Harvey A.K. Whitney Award Lectures: 1950-2000. 2000. (Illus.). 410p. pap. 25.00 (*1-58528-022-4*) Am Soc Hlth-Syst.

Harvey Cushing: A Biography. John F. Fulton. Ed. by I. Bernard Cohen. 1980. LC 79-7961. (Three Centuries of Science in America Ser.). (Illus.). reprint ed. lib. bdg. 78.95 (*0-405-12542-9*) Ayer.

Hashemite Kingdom of Jordan: Health Sector Study. Contrib. by World Bank Staff. 1997. LC 97-1137. (Illus.). (*0-8213-3894-3*) World Bank.

Haskell F. Norman Library of Science of Medicine 1998. (Illus.). 250.00 (*1-57898-142-5*) Martino Pubng.

Hastings Center's Bibliography of Ethics, Biomedicine & Professional Responsibility. Ed. by Hastings Center Staff. 1984. LC 84-7297. 109p. pap. 26.95 (*0-313-27091-0*, P7091); lib. bdg. 59.95 (*0-313-27045-7*, U7045) Greenwood.

Hatha Yoga Manual II. Samskriti & Judith Franks. 1978. 176p. spiral bd. 14.95 (*0-89389-043-X*) Himalayan Inst.

Hatherleigh Guide to Child & Adolescent Therapy. Ed. by Hatherleigh Editorial Board. 1996. LC 96-21525. (Hatherleigh Guides to Mental Health Ser.: Vol. 5). 336p. (Orig.). (C). pap. 29.95 (*1-886330-46-8*) Hatherleigh.

Hatherleigh Guide to Psychiatric Disorders. Hatherleigh Editorial Board. 1996. LC 95-52213. (Hatherleigh Guides to Mental Health Ser.: Vol. 1). 304p. pap. 29.95 (*1-886330-05-0*) Hatherleigh.

Hatherleigh Guide to Psychopharmacology. Ed. by Hatherleigh Editorial Board. 1998. LC 99-11869. (Guides to Mental Health Ser.: Vol. 11). (Illus.). xvi, 384p. pap. 29.95 (*1-57826-022-1*, Five Star Pub) Hatherleigh.

Hatherleigh Guide to Psychotherapy. Hatherleigh Editorial Board. 1995. LC 95-51373. (Guides to Mental Health Care Ser.: Vol. 2). 300p. pap. 29.95 (*1-886330-04-2*) Hatherleigh.

Hatherleigh Guide to Substance Abuse II. Ed. by Hatherleigh Editorial Board. 1996. LC 96-26093. (Guides to Mental Health Care Ser.: Vol. 8). 328p. (C). pap. 29.95 (*1-886330-49-2*) Hatherleigh.

Hatherleigh Guide to Treating Substance Abuse I. Ed. by Hatherleigh Editorial Board. 1996. LC 96-26093. (Hatherleigh Guides to Mental Health Ser.: Vol. 7). 304p. (Orig.). (C). pap. 29.95 (*1-886330-48-4*) Hatherleigh.

Hatherleigh Guides to Mental Health Practice Vol. 11: Master Index. Ed. by Hatherleigh Editorial Board. 1998. LC 97-25688. 200p. pap. 29.95 (*1-886330-52-2*) Hatherleigh.

Haunted Children: Rethinking Medication of Common Psychological Disorders. Arthur F. Roemmelt. 1998. LC 97-40869. (Series in Transpersonal & Humanistic Psychology). 224p. (C). text 54.50 (*0-7914-3885-6*); pap. text 17.95 (*0-7914-3886-4*) State U NY Pr.

Have a Healthy Baby: The March of Dimes Complete Guide to Pregnancy & Childbirth. Richard Johnston & Gray Williams. 1996. 480p. pap. 15.00 (*0-02-077335-8*) Macmillan.

Have We Become Surrogates for Failure? Proposing a New Nutrition Education. Richard K. Manoff. 1993. LC 93-27281. (Martin J. Forman Memorial Lectures: Vol. 6). (Illus.). 32p. (Orig.). pap. 7.50 (*0-915173-25-5*) Helen Keller Intl.

Have You Hugged a Monster Today? Alan Cohen. 2nd ed. 1983. (Illus.). 64p. (Orig.). reprint ed. pap. 5.00 (*0-942494-73-3*) Coleman Pub.

Having a Baby. 1997. LC 96-29521. (For Your Information Ser.). pap. 9.50 (*1-56853-032-3*) New Readers.

Having a Baby in Europe: Report on a Study. 1985. (Public Health in Europe Ser.: No. 26). 157p. pap. text 13.00 (*92-890-1162-9*, 1320026) World Health.

Having a First Baby - Experiences in 1951 & 1985 Compared: Two Social, Obstetric & Dietary Studies of Married Primigravidae in Aberdeen. B. Thompson et al. 1989. pap. text (*0-08-036596-5*) Aberdeen U Pr GBR. *Dist:* Macmillan.

Having Epilepsy: The Experience & Control of Illness. Joseph W. Schneider & Peter Conrad. 1985. 240p. pap. 22.95 (*0-87722-398-X*) Temple U Pr.

Having Leukemia Isn't So Bad. Of Course It Wouldn't Be My First Choice: A Story of Hope for Families of Children with Cancer. Cynthia A. Krumme. 1993. 149p. pap. 9.95 (*0-9635554-4-8*) Sargasso Ent.

Having Twins: A Parents Guide to Pregnancy, Birth & Early Childhood. Elizabeth Noble. 2nd ed. 1991. 430p. pap. 18.00 (*0-395-49338-2*) HM.

Having Your Baby: The Complete Illustrated Guide. Gill Thorn. 1997. LC 97-3675. (Illus.). 208p. pap. 15.95 (*1-55561-133-8*) Fisher Bks.

Having Your Baby & What You Need to Know When You're Pregnant: A Guide for African American Women. H. Hutcherson. 1997. LC 96-46919. 432p. pap. 12.95 (*0-345-39403-8*) Ballantine Pub Grp.

Having Your Baby by Donor Insemination: A Complete Resource Guide. Elizabeth Noble. 1988. 352p. pap. 15.95 (*0-395-45395-X*) HM.

Hawaii Health Care in Perspective 2000. Ed. by Kathleen O'Leary Morgan & Scott E. Morgan. 2000. 21p. spiral bd. 19.00 (*0-7401-0210-9*) Morgan Quitno Corp.

Hawaii Health Care Perspective, 1998. Ed. by Kathleen O'Leary Morgan & Scott E. Morgan. 1998. 20p. pap. 19.00 (*1-56692-810-9*) Morgan Quitno Corp.

Hawaiian Fungi. F. L. Stevens. 1969. (BMB Ser.). reprint ed. 30.00 (*0-527-02122-9*) Periodicals Srv.

Hawley's Condensed Chemical Dictionary & the VNR Dictionary of Environmental Health & Safety & Sax's Dangerous Properties of Industrial Materials. Richard J. Lewis & Frank S. Lisella. 8th ed. 1995. 150.00 (*0-442-02044-9*, VNR) Wiley.

Hay Fever. Catherine Steven. 1999. (Natural Way Ser.). 128p. pap. 5.95 (*1-86204-309-4*) Element MA.

Hazard Assessment Ethylene Oxide. L. Golberg. 1986. LC 86-4186. 120.00 (*0-8493-6525-2*, CRC Reprint) Franklin.

Hazard Communication - Right-to-Know for Health Care Facilities. Robert C. Brandys. 1991. LC 90-14463. (Management & Compliance Ser.: Vol. 6). (Illus.). 150p. ring bd. 110.00 (*0-87258-532-8*, 055205) Am Hospital.

Hazard Communication Guide. Keller, J. J., and Associates, Inc. Staff. rev. ed. 2000. LC 85-80596. 1100p. ring bd. 189.00 (*0-934674-54-X*, 32-G) J J Keller.

Hazardous & Industrial Waste Management & Testing: Third Symposium - STP 851. Ed. by Larry P. Jackson et al. 1985. 400p. 46.00 (*0-8031-0405-7*, STP851) ASTM.

Hazardous Materials: Medical Response, Practices & Procedures. Phillip L. Currance & Alvin C. Bronstein. 1999. LC 98-56388. (Illus.). 231p. (C). (gr. 13). pap. text 34.95 (*0-8151-1984-4*, 28068) Mosby Inc.

Hazardous Materials Exposure: Emergency Response & Patient Care. Jonathan Borak et al. 1990. LC 90-1307. (Continuing Education Ser.). 304p. pap. text 53.00 (*0-89303-722-2*) P-H.

Hazardous Materials in the Histopathology Laboratory: Regulations, Risks, Handling & Disposal. Janet C. Dapson & Richard W. Dapson. 3rd ed. 1995. (Illus.). (Orig.). pap. 75.00 (*0-9645197-0-4*) Anatech MI.

Hazardous Materials Injuries: A Handbook for Pre-Hospital Care. Douglas R. Stutz & Scott Ulin. 4th ed. 1997. (Illus.). 560p. pap. text 34.95 (*0-913019-05-4*) BRADCOMM.

Hazardous Solid Waste Testing: First Conference - STP 760. Ed. by Conway & Malloy Conway. 1983. 352p. 39.00 (*0-8031-0795-1*, STP760) ASTM.

Hazardous to Our Health: FDA Regulation of Health Care Products. Paul H. Rubin & Ronald W. Hansen. Ed. by Robert Higgs. 1995. LC 95-41675. (Independent Studies in Political Economy). 130p. (C). pap. 14.95 (*0-945999-41-0*) Independent Inst.

Hazardous Waste: The Scarlet Letter A for AIDS. 1996. (Illus.). 25p. pap. 10.00 (*0-942561-25-2*) Bone Hollow.

Hazardous Waste Incineration & Human Health. Curtis C. Travis & S. Chrystal Cook. 1989. 168p. 184.95 (*0-8493-6754-9*, RA578) CRC Pr.

Hazards of Deafness. Roy K. Holcomb. Ed. by John Joyce. 1977. LC 77-93545. (Illus.). pap. 14.95 (*0-917002-14-8*, 457) Joyce Media.

Hazards of Life & All That. J. Bond. 1996. LC 96-28766. (Illus.). 244p. 32.00 (*0-7503-0360-3*) Inst of Physics Pubng.

Hazmat Emergency: Leader's Guide. Lee Richmond. Ed. by Gordon Massingham. 2nd ed. 1992. pap. 20.00 (*0-945790-04-X*) Detrick Lawrence.

Haztox: EMS Response to Hazardous Materials Incidents. Douglas Stutz & Scott Ulin. 1993. 460p. pap. 32.95 (*0-9638425-0-1*) GDS Communs.

Hazwoper Compliance System Ed. by Erik M. Roy. 1992. 199.00 (*0-931690-49-8*); 332p. tchr. ed. (*0-931690-50-1*) Genium Pub.

HBS Antigen Subtypes: Proceedings of the International Workshop, 1st, Paris, April, 1975. International Workshop on HBS Antigen Subtypes Staff. Ed. by J. P. Soulier et al. 1976. (Current Studies in Hematology & Blood Transfusion: No. 42). (Illus.). 140p. 65.25 (*3-8055-2293-2*) S Karger.

HCO Abnormal Psychol. Timothy W. Costello & Joseph T. Costello. 2nd ed. 1992. LC 90-56016. (HarperCollins College Outline Ser.). (Illus.). 448p. (C). pap. 18.00 (*0-06-467121-6*, Harper Ref) HarperCollins Pubs.

HCO Intro to Psychol. Ann L. Weber. 1991. LC 90-56019. (HarperCollins College Outline Ser.). (Illus.). 304p. pap. 16.95 (*0-06-467103-8*, Harper Ref) HarperCollins Pubs.

HCP Directory of Medical Office Management Computer System Vendors with Satisfaction Ratings. Vinson J. Hudson. rev. ed. 1999. 300p. pap. 150.00 (*0-9637397-7-8*) Hlthcare Comput.

HCP Directory of Medical Office Management Computer System Vendors with Satisfaction Ratings 1997/1998. Vinson J. Hudson. 1997. 300p. (Orig.). pap. 150.00 (*0-9637397-6-X*) Hlthcare Comput.

HCP Directory of Medical Software, 1999/2000. Ed. by Bruce H. Frisch. rev. ed. 1999. 300p. pap. 233.95 (*0-9672843-0-9*) Hlthcare Comput.

HCPCS 1997: Medicare Level II National Codes. Context Software Systems, Inc., Staff. 1996. pap. 29.95 (*0-07-600824-X*) McGraw.

HCPCS Level II Code Book, 1999. Yale Wasserman, D.M.D. Medical Publishers, Limited. 10th ed. 1999. per. 49.00 (*1-881072-36-3*) Y W DMD Med.

HCPCS 1999 Coder's Choice. HCFA Staff. Ed. by James B. Davis & Kathryn M. Swanson. 1999. pap. 44.95 (*1-57066-099-9*, 9937) Practice Mgmt Info.

HCPCS 1999 Codes on Disk. 1999. pap. 99.95 incl. disk (*1-57066-126-X*, 9939) Practice Mgmt Info.

HCPCS, 2000. 1999. (Illus.). text 49.95 (*0-89970-999-0*) AMA.

HCPCS 2000 Coder's Choice. HCFA Staff. Ed. by James B. Davis & Kathryn Swanson. 2000. pap. text 44.95 (*1-57066-161-8*, 20037) Practice Mgmt Info.

HCPCS 2000 Codes on Disk. HCFA Staff. Ed. by James B. Davis & Kathryn Swanson. 2000. 99.95 incl. disk (*1-57066-163-4*, 20039) Practice Mgmt Info.

***HCPCS 2001.** Ingenix, Inc. Staff. pap. 59.95 (*1-56337-354-8*) Ingenix Inc.

***HCPCS 2001: Procedure Codes.** annuals 2000. (Illus.). 575p. pap. text 49.95 (*1-57066-194-4*, 21037); ring bd. 59.95 (*1-57066-195-2*, 21038) Practice Mgmt Info.

HCPCS 2000 TimeSaver Binder. HCFA Staff. Ed. by James B. Davis & Kathryn Swanson. 2000. ring bd. 54.95 (*1-57066-162-6*, 20038) Practice Mgmt Info.

HCV & Related Liver Diseases. Ed. by K. Okita. 1999. (Illus.). 136p. 79.00 (*4-431-70235-0*) Spr-Verlag.

HDI Coping Series 1989. (Orig.). pap. 45.00 (*1-882855-54-X*) HDI Pubs.

HDI Professional Series on Traumatic Brain Injury Rehabilitation, Vols. 1-20. Ed. by William H. Burke. 1995. (Orig.). pap. 175.00 (*1-882855-29-9*) HDI Pubs.

HDL Deficiency & Atherosclerosis, No. 174. Ed. by G. Assmann. 1996. (Developments in Cardiovascular Medicine Ser.: Vol. 174). 96p. text 48.00 (*0-7923-8888-7*) Kluwer Academic.

He: Understanding Masculine Psychology. Robert A. Johnson. rev. ed. 1989. LC 89-45097. 96p. reprint ed. pap. 10.00 (*0-06-096396-4*) HarperTrade.

He Ayurveda: The Ancient Indian Healing Art. Scott Gerson. 1997. (Health Essentials Ser.). 128p. pap. 9.95 (*1-86204-096-6*) Element MA.

He Used to Be Somebody: A Journey into Alzheimer's Disease Through the Eyes of a Caregiver. Beverly B. Murphy. 1995. 348p. (Orig.). pap. 16.95 (*0-943909-14-7*) Gibbs Assocs.

He Will Never Remember: Caring for the Victims of Child Abuse. A. Jane Purdy. Ed. by Phyllis Mueller. 1989. LC 89-31362. 180p. (Orig.). pap. 13.95 (*0-932419-22-4*) Cherokee.

Head - Neck Sensory Motor System. Alain Berthoz et al. 1992. (Illus.). 784p. text 150.00 (*0-19-506820-3*) OUP.

Head & Brain: Volumes 8, 8a & 8b, Set. Loring F. Chapman & John W. Evans. 1972. (Courtroom Medicine Ser.). ring bd. 760.00 (*0-8205-1251-6*) Bender.

Head & Brain Injuries. Elaine Landau. 2002. LC 00-12074. (Diseases & People Ser.). (Illus.). 112p. (J). (gr. 6 up). lib. bdg. 20.95 (*0-7660-1473-8*) Enslow Pubs.

Head & Face Pain Syndromes. Rene Cailliet. 1992. (Pain Ser.). (Illus.). 229p. (C). pap. text 19.95 (*0-8036-1625-2*) Davis Co.

***Head & Neck Anatomy: A Clinical Reference.** B. K. Berkovitz & B. J. Moxham. 2001. (Illus.). 464p. (*1-899066-75-6*) Isis Med GBR. *Dist:* Bks Intl VA.

***Head & Neck Anatomy for Dental Assisting.** Marjorie J. Short. 3rd ed. 2002. 416p. text 44.95 (*0-7668-1889-6*) Delmar.

Head & Neck Cancer. Ed. by Steven E. Vogl. 1987. (Contemporary Issues in Clinical Oncology Ser.: Vol. 7). (Illus.). 156p. text (*0-443-08401-7*) Church.

Head & Neck Cancer: Basic & Clinical Aspects. Ed. by Waun Ki Hong & Randall S. Weber. 1995. LC 94-27497. (Cancer Treatment & Research Ser.: Vol. 74). text 272.50 (*0-7923-3015-3*) Kluwer Academic.

Head & Neck Cancer: Organ Preservation, Function, & Rehabilitation. K. Thomas Robbins & Thomas Murry. 1998. (Illus.). 140p. pap. 75.00 (*1-56593-972-7*, 1924) Thomson Learn.

Head & Neck Cancer - Advances in Basic Research: Proceedings of the International Symposium on Advances in Head & Neck Cancer, Kiel, Germany, 18-20 January 1996. J. A. Werner et al. 1996. LC 96-29394. (International Congress Ser.). 724p. 222.50 (*0-444-82374-3*) Elsevier.

Head & Neck Cancers: Directory of Authors of New Medical & Scientific Reviews with Subject Index. Science and Life Consultants Association Staff. 1995. 160p. 57.50 (*0-7883-0580-8*); 1995. 160p. pap. 47.50 (*0-7883-0581-6*); 1998. 141p. 57.50 (*0-7883-2116-1*); 1998. 141p. pap. 47.50 (*0-7883-2117-X*) ABBE Pubs Assn.

Head & Neck Disorders (Fourth Series) Test & Syllabus. Peter M. Som et al. 1992. LC 92-48821. (Professional Self-Evaluation & Continuing Education Program Ser.: Vol. 34). (Illus.). 750p. 190.00 (*1-55903-034-8*) Am Coll Radiology.

Head & Neck, Eye, & Central Nervous System, Vol. 3. Arnold J. Rudolph. 1997. (Atlas of the Newborn Ser.: Vol. 3). (Illus.). incl. cd-rom (*1-55009-033-X*) DEKR.

Head & Neck Histology & Anatomy: A Self-Instructional Program. Sara K. Smith. 1999. LC 98-32396. (Illus.). 816p. (C). pap. 59.00 (*0-8385-3652-2*) P-H.

Head & Neck Imaging. annuals Ed. by Lalitha Shankar et al. 1997. LC 97-30021. (Illus.). 560p. text 89.00 (*0-07-057999-7*) McGraw-Hill Prof.

Head & Neck Imaging. Ed. by Peter M. Som & Hugh D. Curtin. 3rd ed. 1995. (Illus.). 1710p. (C). (gr. 13). text 325.00 (*0-8151-7718-6*, 23907) Mosby Inc.

Head & Neck Imaging: A Teaching File. Anthony A. Mancuso & Ronald G. Quisling. 1998. LC 2001-50231. (Illus.). text 99.00 (*0-683-30144-6*) Lppncott W & W.

Head & Neck Imaging: Case Review. David M. Yousem. 1998. LC 98-10654. (Case Review Ser.). 39.95 (*0-323-00019-3*) Mosby Consmer Hlth.

Head & Neck Injuries in Sporting, STP 1229. Ed. by Earl F. Hoerner. 1994. LC 94-42668. (Special Technical Publications: Vol. 1229). 370p. pap. 59.00 (*0-8031-1886-4*, STP1229) ASTM.

Head & Neck Injury. 1994. (Proceedings Ser.). 262p. pap. 55.00 (*1-56091-499-8*, P-276) Soc Auto Engineers.

Head & Neck Management of the Cancer Patient. Ed. by Douglas E. Peterson et al. 1986. (Developments in Oncology Ser.). text 226.00 (*0-89838-747-7*) Kluwer Academic.

Head & Neck Manifestations of Gastroesophageal Reflux. Ricardo L. Carrau et al. 2nd ed. 1998. LC 98-4058. (Self-Instructional Package Ser.). (Illus.). 60p. reprint ed. pap. text 25.00 (*1-56772-065-X*, 5506245) AAO-HNS.

Head & Neck Medicine & Surgery in Small Animal Practice - The Compendium Collection. 1996. pap. text 54.00 (*1-884254-24-1*) Vet Lrn Syst.

Head & Neck Nursing. Michael J. Hahn & Anne Jones. 2000. LC 99-34394. text (*0-443-05854-7*) Church.

Head & Neck Oncology. Ed. by Gregory T. Wolf. 1984. (Cancer Treatment & Research Ser.). text 240.00 (*0-89838-657-8*) Kluwer Academic.

Head & Neck Oncology: Clinical Management. A. Robert Kagan & John Miles. 1989. (Illus.). 192p. 67.00 (*0-08-034479-8*, Pergamon Pr) Elsevier.

Head & Neck Oncology: Diagnosis, Treatment, & Rehabilitation. E. M. Myers. 1991. 115.00 (*0-316-59317-6*, Little Brwn Med Div) Lppncott W & W.

Head & Neck Oncology for the General Surgeon. Ed. by Paul E. Preece et al. 1991. (Illus.). text (*0-7020-1551-2*) W B Saunders GBR. *Dist:* Saunders.

Head & Neck Oncology Research. Ed. by Gregory T. Wolf & Thomas E. Carey. 1989. LC 88-22982. (Illus.). 517p. lib. bdg. (*90-6299-049-5*) Kugler NLD. *Dist:* Lib Res.

Head & Neck Radiology. Mafee. 2000. 700p. Price not set. (*0-7216-5863-6*) Saunders.

Head & Neck Radiology. Arnold M. Noyek. 1991. (Illus.). 128p. (gr. 13). text (*1-56375-002-3*, GM0192) Gower-Mosby.

Head & Neck Reconstruction: A Defect-Oriented Approach. Mark L. Urken. 1998. text 275.00 (*0-397-51835-8*) Lppncott W & W.

Head & Neck Surgery Incl. Vol. 1. Face, Nose & Facial Skull. Ed. by Hans H. Naumann & J. Helms. LC 95-11552. 1995. 299.00 (*0-86577-586-9*); Vol. 2. Ear. J. A. Jahrsdoerfer. Ed. by Hans H. Naumann. (Illus.). 500p. 1996. text 189.00 (*0-86577-660-1*); Vol. 3. Neck. Ed. by Hahns H. Naumann. (Illus.). 450p. 1997. 199.00 (*0-86577-624-5*); 2nd ed. 599.00 (*0-86577-792-6*) Thieme Med Pubs.

***Head & Neck Surgery: Otolaryngology.** Ed. by Byron J. Bailey et al. 3rd ed. 2001. (Illus.). 2640p. 499.00 (*0-7817-3273-5*); 2624p. text 339.00 (*0-7817-2908-4*) Lppncott W & W.

Head & Neck Surgery — Otolaryngology. Byron J. Bailey. 2nd ed. 1998. LC 98-6115. 3,136p. text 325.00 (*0-397-51805-6*) Lppncott W & W.

Head & Neck Surgery — Otolaryngology: Study Guide. Byron J. Bailey. 2nd ed. 1998. 384p. pap. text 49.95 (*0-397-51846-3*) Lppncott W & W.

Head & Neck Surgery - Otolarnygology Ed. by Byron J. Bailey et al. 1993. LC 92-49766. (Illus.). 1. (*0-397-51334-8*); 2. (*0-397-51335-6*); Set. 350.00 (*0-397-51333-X*) Lppncott W & W.

Head & Neck Surgery 2. Shah. 2nd ed. 1997. 654.00 (*0-8151-4274-9*, 29976) Mosby Inc.

Head & Neck Surgical Pathology. Ben Z. Pilch. 2000. LC 00-42837. (Illus.). xiii, 721p. text 279.00 (*0-397-51727-0*) Lppncott W & W.

Head Injured Children: Who Cares? Ed. by David Johnson et al. 1989. 200p. 42.00 (*1-85000-378-5*); pap. 20.00 (*1-85000-379-3*) Taylor & Francis (Falmer Pr).

Head Injuries. Ed. by R. A. Frowein et al. 1989. (Advances in Neurosurgery Ser.: Vol. 17). (Illus.). 369p. 103.00 (*0-387-50550-4*) Spr-Verlag.

Head Injuries: Frontlines. Conrad Williams. 1998. LC 98-205269. (Frontlines Ser.). 206 p. pap. (*1-899344-36-5*) Do-Not Pr GBR. *Dist:* Dufour.

Head Injuries in the Newborn & Infant. Ed. by Anthony J. Raimondi et al. 1986. (Principles of Pediatric Neurosurgery Ser.). (Illus.). 292p. 136.00 (*0-387-96208-5*) Spr-Verlag.

Head Injury. Ed. by Pierre J. Vinken et al. rev. ed. 1990. 526p. 228.00 (*0-444-81276-8*) Elsevier.

Head Injury: A Guide to Functional Outcomes in Occupational Therapy. Karen M. Kovich & Diane E. Bermann. 1997. LC 88-2181. 236p. (C). spiral bd. 89.00 (*0-87189-762-8*) PRO-ED.

Head Injury: Pathophysiology & Management of Severe Closed Injury. Ed. by Peter Reilly & Ross Bullock. 1997. LC 97-66517. (Illus.). 500p. (*0-412-58540-5*) E A GBR. *Dist:* OUP.

Head Injury: The Facts. Dorothy Gronwall et al. 2nd ed. 1998. LC 97-18414. (Facts Ser.). (Illus.). 184p. pap. 19.95 (*0-19-262713-9*) OUP.

Head Injury & Postconcussive Syndrome. Ed. by Matthew Rizzo & Daniel Tranel. 1995. 533p. text (*0-443-08964-7*) Church.

Head Injury & the Family: A Life & Living Perspective. Arthur E. Dell Orto & Paul W. Power. 1994. LC 93-85847. 256p. per. 39.95 (*1-878205-61-7*) St Lucie Pr.

Head Injury Guide for Survivors, Families, & Caregivers. Ed. by Delores M. John. 1993. (Illus.). 71p. (Orig.). (C). pap. text 20.00 (*1-56806-185-4*) DIANE Pub.

Head Injury Rehabilitation: An Overview. Ed. by William H. Burke. 1996. (Professional Series on Traumatic Brain Injury: Vol. 1). 48p. pap. 9.50 (*1-882855-08-6*) HDI Pubs.

Head Injury Rehabilitation: Children & Adolescents. Ed. by Mark Ylvisaker. 1985. LC 90-9182. (Illus.). 463p. (C). 42.50 (*0-7506-9720-2*, 1573) Buttrwrth-Heinemann.

Head Lice. Allison Lassieur. 2000. LC 98-53649. (My Health Ser.). (Illus.). 48p. (YA). (gr. 3-5). pap. 6.95 (*0-531-16450-0*) F Watts.

Head Lice. Alvin Silverstein et al. 2000. LC 98-53649. (My Health Ser.). (Illus.). 48p. (J). (gr. 3-5). lib. bdg. 23.00 (*0-531-11624-7*) F Watts.

Head, Neck & Dental Anatomy. Marjorie J. Short. 2nd ed. 1994. LC 93-47377. 364p. (C). mass mkt. 48.95 (*0-8273-5713-3*) Delmar.

Head, Neck & Trunk. John H. Warfel. 6th ed. 1993. LC 92-17320. (Illus.). 140p. pap. text 19.95 (*0-8121-1583-X*) Lppncott W & W.

Head Nurse. Jack Rudman. 1994. (Career Examination Ser.: C-321). pap. 39.95 (*0-8373-0321-4*) Nat Learn.

Head Nurse: Her Leadership Role. Ed. by Jean Berrett. 1987. 468p. (C). (*81-7002-054-9*) Himalayan Bks IND. *Dist:* St Mut.

Head Space Analysis & Related Methods in Gas Chromatography. B. V. Ioffe & A. G. Vitenberg. 1984. LC 83-10632. 304p. 198.00 (*0-471-06507-2*) Wiley.

Head Trauma: Strategies for Educational Reintegration. Joan P. Gerring & Joan M. Carney. 2nd ed. 1992. LC 92-11621. (Illus.). 177p. (C). pap. 39.95 (*1-879105-74-8*, 0337) Thomson Learn.

Head Trauma Cases: Law & Medicine. Arthur C. Roberts. 2nd ed. 2000. pap. text, suppl. ed. 112.00 (*0-7355-1426-7*) Aspen Pub.

Head Trauma Cases 1999: Law & Medicine. Arthur C. Roberts. 2nd ed. 1998. pap. text 82.00 (*0-7355-0104-1*) Aspen Pub.

Head Trauma Cases Vol. 2: Law & Medicine. Arthur C. Roberts. 2nd ed. 1996. LC 96-14331. (Personal Injury Library). 816p. 260.00 (*0-471-12182-7*) Wiley.

Head Trauma Sourcebook: Basic Information about Open-Head & Closed-Head Injuries, Treatment Advances, Recovery & Rehabilitation. Ed. by Karen Bellenir. 1997. LC 97-1008. (Health Reference Ser.: Vol. 23). 424p. 78.00 (*0-7808-0208-X*) Omnigraphics Inc.

Headache. Ed. by T. Fowler. 1987. (Practical Clinical Medicine Ser.). 240p. (C). pap. text 106.00 (*0-7462-0037-4*) Kluwer Academic.

Headache. Peter J. Goadsby et al. 1997. LC 96-50464. (Blue Books of Practical Neurology Ser.: Vol. 17). 411p. text 99.00 incl. audio compact disk (*0-7506-9871-3*) Buttrwrth-Heinemann.

Headache, No. 4. Ed. by Pierre J. Vinken et al. 1985. (Revised Ser.: Vol. 4). 556p. 327.50 (*0-444-90393-3*) Elsevier.

Headache: Material Medica Relating to Headache. 2000. LC 99-96161. 81p. pap. 6.95 (*1-929410-03-4*) dttm.

Headache: Most Common Complaints. Egiluis L. Spierings. 1998. LC 98-3398. (Most Common Complaints Ser.). 236p. pap. text 29.99 (*0-7506-7128-9*) Buttrwrth-Heinemann.

Headache: Problems in Diagnosis & Management. Anthony Hopkins. 1988. (Major Problems in Neurology Ser.: Vol. 15). (Illus.). 398p. text 126.00 (*0-03-919016-1*) H Holt & Co.

Headache & Diet: Tyramine-Free Recipes. Seymour Diamond et al. 1990. LC 89-26854. 280p. spiral bd. 27.50 (*0-8236-2315-7*) Intl Univs Pr.

Headache & Facial Pain. Franco Mongini. 1999. LC 99-25746. 99.00 (*0-86577-852-3*) Thieme Med Pubs.

Headache & Neck Pain Workbook: An Integrated Mind & Body Program. Douglas Earl DeGood et al. 1997. LC 97-66083. (Illus.). 184p. pap. 14.95 (*1-57224-086-5*) New Harbinger.

Headache & Your Child: The Complete Guide to Understanding & Treating Migraines & Other Headaches in Children. Seymour Diamond & Amy Diamond. 2001. LC 2001-31306. (Illus.). 256p. pap. 13.00 (*0-684-87309-5*, Fireside) S&S Trade Pap.

Headache Free. Roger Cady & Kathleen Farmer. 1993. (Illus.). 110p. pap. text (*0-9636528-0-X*) Moray Pr.

Headache Handbook: Diagnosis & Treatment. Gary W. Jay. 1998. LC 98-24219. 192p. 69.95 (*1-57444-221-X*) St Lucie Pr.

Headache Help: A Complete Guide to Understanding Headaches & the Medications That Relieve Them. Lawrence Robbins. rev. ed. 2000. LC 00-36940. (Illus.). xv, 332p. pap. 15.00 (*0-618-04436-1*) HM.

***Headache in Clinical Practice.** Ed. by Stephen D. Silberstein et al. 2nd ed. 2001. (Illus.). 250p. (*1-899066-55-1*) Isis Med.

Headache Pack. Journey Editions Staff. 1997. (Cures for Modern Times Ser.). (Illus.). 64p. 16.95 (*1-885203-44-6*) Jrny Editions.

Headache Relief for Women: How You Can Manage & Prevent Pain. Alan M. Rapoport & Fred D. Sheftell. 2000. 242p. reprint ed. 25.00 (*0-7881-9237-X*) DIANE Pub.

Headache Sourcebook. Joel Paulino & Ceabert J. Griffith. 2001. LC 2001-28223. 320p. pap. 17.95 (*0-7373-0545-2*) McGraw-Hill Prof.

Headache Today - An Update by 21 Experts. Ed. by A. P. Friedman et al. 1978. (Pain & Headache Ser.: Vol. 6). (Illus.). 56.75 (*3-8055-2924-4*) S Karger.

Headaches. Mary Kittredge. 2001. LC 00-27516. (Twenty-First Century Health & Wellness Ser.). 103p. (J). (gr. 7-12). 24.95 (*0-7910-5981-2*) Chelsea Hse.

Headaches. Jes Olesen et al. 2nd ed. 1999. LC 99-21427. (Illus.). 1,056p. text 199.00 (*0-7817-1597-0*) Lppncott W & W.

Headaches: A People's Medical Society Book. Charles B. Inlander & Porter Shimer. 1995. 96p. 16.95 (*0-8027-1314-9*); LC 95-20541. 86p. pap. 8.95 (*0-8027-7473-3*) Walker & Co.

Headaches? Eyesight? Hearing? Breathing? TMJ? Can Head Bones "Move"? Be "Adjusted"? Influence Health? Memorial Version of Cranial Adjusting Step by Step. 1997. 250p. 30.00 (*0-917628-17-9*) Coraco.

Headaches & Cranial Neuralgias. Ed. by Pierre J. Vinken & George W. Bruyn. 1969. 166.25 (*0-444-10302-3*) Elsevier.

Headaches & Migraine. Maggie Jones. 1999. LC 98-56503. (Your Child Ser.). 128p. pap. 9.95 (*1 86204 397-3*) Element MA.

Headaches & Migraines in Childhood. Charles F. Barlow. 1991. (Clinics in Developmental Medicine Ser.: No. 91). (Illus.). 288p. (C). text (*0-521-41211-0*) Mc Keith Pr GBR. *Dist:* Cambridge U Pr.

Headaches & Their Origin. 1996. lib. bdg. 252.95 (*0-8490-5873-2*) Gordon Pr.

Headaches Aren't Forever. Gerald H. Smith. Ed. by Gloria Brown. 1986. (Illus.). 212p. (Orig.). 11.95 (*0-9617838-0-X*) ICNR Newtown.

Headaches in Children: Practical Informative Guide for Parents, Teachers & Paramedical Personnel. Leonardo Garcia-Mendez. 1996. LC 95-81048. (Pediatric Neurology Ser.). (Illus.). 220p. (Orig.). (C). pap. text 13.99 (*0-9639269-1-8*) Lemar Pubs.

***Heading to the Hospital: 77 Tips for Getting the Most Out of Your Adventure.** Katherine M. Konzen. 2001. LC 2001-131381. (Illus.). 120p. pap. 9.99 (*0-9707950-2-5*) Healing Place CA.

Headline News, Science Views II. National Research Council Staff. Ed. by David Jarmul. 1993. LC 93-16471. 256p. pap. 19.95 (*0-309-04834-6*) Natl Acad Pr.

Heal Abuse & Trauma Through Art: Increasing Self-Worth, Healing of Initial Wounds & Creating a Sense of Connectivity. Linda B. Spencer. 1997. LC 96-41715. (Illus.). 250p. text 62.95 (*0-398-06729-5*); pap. text 41.95 (*0-398-06730-9*) C C Thomas.

Heal Arthritis: Physically, Mentally, Spiritually - The Edgar Cayce Approach. William A. McGarey. 1998. LC 97-31083. 168p. pap. 12.95 (*0-87604-399-6*, 513) ARE Pr.

Heal Environmental Illness... And Reclaim Your Life. Lorraine D. Smith. Ed. by Erika Hetzner. 1999. LC 99-96135. (Illus.). 256p. pap. (*0-9675624-0-6*) Diveena Pubns.

***Heal the Pain, Comfort the Spirit: The Hows & Whys of Modern Pain Treatment.** Dorene O'Hara. 2001. LC 2001-48035. pap. 19.95 (*0-8122-1795-0*) U of Pa Pr.

Heal Thyself. Edward Bach. 1993. pap. (*0-85207-301-1*) C W Daniel GBR. *Dist:* Natl Bk Netwk.

Heal Thyself: An Explanation of the Real Cause & Cure of Disease. Edward Bach. 1985. 52p. pap. 4.50 (*0-89540-152-5*, SB-152) Sun Pub.

Heal with Your Heart: A New Vision for Holistic Nursing. Joan Alfano. 1996. (Illus.). 256p. (Orig.). pap. 11.95 (*1-885610-04-1*) European Amer.

Heal Your Body A-Z: The Mental Causes for Physical Illness & the Way to Overcome Them. Louise L. Hay. (Illus.). 1998. LC 98-3261. 122p. spiral bd. 19.95 (*1-56170-490-3*, 553, Hay Hse Lifestyles); 2001. 156p. reprint ed. pap. 11.95 (*1-56170-792-9*, 553T) Hay House.

Heal Your Body A-Z: The Mental Causes for Physical Illness & the Way to Overcome Them. Louise L. Hay. 1999. (Illus.). (*84-7953-327-7*) Urano.

Heal Your Heart: How You Can Prevent or Reverse Heart Disease. K. Lance Gould. 1998. LC 97-39172. (Illus.). 256p. 25.00 (*0-8135-2523-3*) Rutgers U Pr.

Heal Your Mind, Heal Your Body: A Practical Guide to Wellness of Body, Mind & Spirit. Evan Porter. 1994. LC 94-65441. 290p. reprint ed. pap. 14.95 (*0-940683-21-0*) Sync Society Pubng.

Heal Your Self, Heal Your World: Turn Illness & Suffering into Health & Peace Through Scientifically Proven Methods. Brian Rees. 1997. LC 96-8994. (Illus.). 350p. 27.50 (*0-9652319-3-3*) Manu Pub.

Heal Your Self of Anything: (Example - Glaucoma) Mary M. Harris. unabr. ed. 1995. (Heal Your Self Ser.). 28p. pap. 5.00 (*0-9636781-2-4*, 292) BBCS.

Heal Yourself: A Practical Self-Help Manual of Natural Healing. Walter Last. 1988. LC 88-1685. 14.95 (*0-943920-56-6*) Metamorphous Pr.

Heal Yourself: A Step-by-Step Guide to Self-Healing Through Affirmations. Shereen Noon. 1990. 154p. (Orig.). pap. 9.95 (*0-9624690-0-9*) Welcome Home.

Heal Yourself Home Handbook of Unusual Remedies. Lionel Rolfe & Nigey Lennon. 1982. LC 82-14274. 205p. pap. 4.95 (*0-13-384677-6*, Parker Publishing Co) P-H.

Healed of Cancer. D. Osteen. 1986. 96p. mass mkt. 4.00 (*0-912631-33-3*) J O Pubns.

Healer: The Story of Francis Schlatter. Norman Cleveland. 1989. LC 89-19679. (Illus.). 120p. pap. 14.95 (*0-86534-139-7*) Sunstone Pr.

Healer Within: Using Traditional Chinese Techniques To Release Your Body's Own Medicine. Roger Jahnke. 1998. LC 96-38129. (Illus.). 288p. pap. 14.00 (*0-06-251477-6*) HarperCollins Pubs.

Healers. Deanne Durrett. 1996. LC 96-23072. (American Indian Lives Ser.). (Illus.). 144p. (YA). (gr. 5-12). 25.00 (*0-8160-3406-0*) Facts on File.

Healers: A History of American Medicine. John Duffy. 1979. LC 78-27222. 385p. (gr. 9-12). reprint ed. pap. 12.95 (*0-252-00743-3*) U of Ill Pr.

Healers & Alternative Medicine: A Sociological Examination of Alternative Medicine. Gary Easthope. 1986. 152p. text (*0-566-05098-6*) Avebry GBR. *Dist:* Ashgate Pub Co.

Healers & Healing in Early Modern Europe. David Gentilcore. 1998. (Social & Cultural Values in Early Modern Europe Ser.). (Illus.). (*0-7190-4199-6*) Manchester Univ Pr GBR. *Dist:* St Martin.

Healer's Art. Eric J. Cassell. 1985. 240p. pap. 20.00 (*0-262-53062-7*) MIT Pr.

Healers at Work: Firsthand Accounts of the Difference Alternative Healing Makes. Peter Downie. 1996. LC 96-910434. (Illus.). 224p. (*1-55145-080-1*) NStone Publ.

Healer's Handbook: A Holistic Guide to Wellness in the New Age. Patricia Telesco. 1997. LC 97-17739. 296p. pap. 15.95 (*1-57863-018-5*) Red Wheel ME.

Healer's Manual: A Beginner's Guide to Energy Therapies. Ted Andrews. 1999. LC 93-34270. (Health & Healing Ser.). (Illus.). 256p. pap. 12.95 (*0-87542-007-9*) Llewellyn Pubns.

Healers of Arnhem Land. John Cawte. 1996. LC 97-145841. 160p. pap. (*0-86840-351-2*) New South Wales Univ Pr AUS. *Dist:* Intl Spec Bk.

Healers on Healing. Ed. by Richard Carlson & Benjamin Shield. 1989. (New Consciousness Reader Ser.). 224p. (Orig.). pap. 14.95 (*0-87477-494-2*, Tarcher Putnam) Putnam Pub Group.

Healers on Horseback. Ed. by R. H. Smythe. 1990. 134p. pap. (*0-85131-282-9*) J A Allen GBR. *Dist:* St Mut.

Healer's Power. Howard Brody. 1993. 324p. (C). pap. 20.00 (*0-300-05783-0*) Yale U Pr.

Healer's Tale: Transforming Medicine & Culture. Sharon R. Kaufman. LC 92-34798. (Life Course Studies). 368p. 1995. pap. text 15.95 (*0-299-13554-3*); 1994. (C). text 29.00 (*0-299-13550-0*) U of Wis Pr.

Healing. Ronald D. Tucker. 1985. LC 84-81179. (Illus.). 57p. (Orig.). pap. 4.00 (*0-933643-27-6*) Grace Ch-St Louis.

Healing: A Woman's Guide to Recovery after Mastectomy. Rosalind Benedet. 1993. 108p. pap. 10.00 (*0-9637917-0-2*) Benedet Pbng.

Healing: A Women's Guide to Lumpectomy & Radiation Therapy. Rosalind Benedet. 1996. 120p. pap. 10.00 (*0-9637917-1-0*) Benedet Pbng.

Healing: Pagan & Christian. George G. Dawson. LC 75-23704. reprint ed. 42.50 (*0-404-13256-1*) AMS Pr.

Healing: The Emerging Holistic Paradigm. L. Bauer-Freitag. 1999. (Illus.). 148p. per. 16.00 (*0-615-11458-X*) HARKEN!.

Healing: Unorthodox Therapies. Lomas St. Aubyn. 1984. (Illus.). 162p. 16.95 (*0-434-03500-9*); pap. 9.95 (*0-434-03501-7*) Trafalgar.

Healing - the Pain That Binds You. Jacqueline Grenier. 1996. (Orig.). pap. 8.95 (*0-533-12077-2*) Vantage.

Healing ADD. Thom Hartmann. 1998. LC 98-9476. 240p. (Orig.). pap. 10.00 (*1-887424-37-7*) Underwood Bks.

Healing ADD: The Breakthrough Program That Allows You to See & Heal the 6 Types of ADD. Daniel G. Amen. 2001. LC 00-62677. (Illus.). 432p. 27.95 (*0-399-14644-X*) Penguin Putnam.

Healing AIDS Naturally: Natural Therapies for the Immune System. Laurence E. Badgley. 1990. LC 86-83290. (Illus.). 410p. pap. 14.95 (*0-941523-00-4*) Human Energy Pr.

Healing & Herbal Medicine. 1992. (Alternative Medicine Ser.). lib. bdg. 88.00 (*0-8490-5369-2*) Gordon Pr.

Healing & History: Essays for George Rosen. Ed. by Charles E. Rosenberg. 1979. lib. bdg. 27.00 (*0-88202-180-X*) Watson Pub Intl.

Healing & Religion. Ed. by Marion Bowman. 1996. pap. (*1-874312-29-X*) Hisarlik Pr GBR. *Dist:* Intl Spec Bk.

Healing & Restoring: Health & Medicine in the World's Religious Tradition. Ed. by Lawrence E. Sullivan. 1989. 468p. 35.00 (*0-02-923791-2*) Free Pr.

Healing & Society in Medieval England: A Middle English Translation of the Pharmaceutical Writings of Gilbertus Anglicus. Faye M. Getz. 1991. LC 90-50643. (Wisconsin Publications in the History of Science & Medicine: Vol. 8). 456p. 24.95 (*0-299-12930-6*) U of Wis Pr.

Healing & The Grief Process. Sally S. Roach & Beatriz C. Nieto. 1996. LC 96-576. (Nurse as Healer Ser.). 208p. pap. text 23.95 (*0-8273-6968-9*) Delmar.

Healing & the Mind. Bill Moyers. Ed. by Betty Sue Flowers. 1993. LC 92-31074. 384p. 25.00 (*0-385-46870-9*) Doubleday.

Healing & Transformation in Sandplay: Creative Processes Become Visible. Ruth Ammann. 1991. LC 91-18685. (Illus.). 160p. 37.95 (*0-8126-9140-7*); pap. 18.95 (*0-8126-9141-5*) Open Court.

Healing & Treatment of Skin Defects. J. Moserova & E. Houskova. 1989. (Illus.). viii, 163p. 65.25 (*3-8055-4704-8*) S Karger.

Healing Art of Sports Massage. Joan Johnson. 1995. LC 94-45679. (Illus.). 192p. (Orig.). pap. 16.95 (*0-87596-186-X*) Rodale Pr Inc.

Healing Arthritis Naturally. Doctors' Prescription Staff. 2000. 156p. pap. 6.95 (*1-893910-10-5*, 904-009) Freedom Pr Inc.

Healing Arthritis the Natural Way: The Breakthrough Program for Reversing Arthritis Using Nutrition & Supplements. Luke Bucci. 1997. LC 97-21101. 288p. (Orig.). pap. 16.99 (*1-56530-277-X*) Summit TX.

Healing Arts. Ishwar C. Puri. Ed. by Marta Crothers. 1988. 37p. (Orig.). pap. 3.00 (*0-937067-10-5*) Insti Study Aware.

Healing Arts in Dialogue: Medicine & Literature. Ed. by Joanne Trautmann. 1982. LC 81-8964. (Medical Humanities Ser.). 195p. 21.95 (*0-8093-1028-7*) S Ill U Pr.

Healing at a Distance. Fenwicke L. Holmes & Ernest S. Holmes. 1997. 50p. pap. 3.00 (*0-89540-341-2*, SB-341) Sun Pub.

Healing at Your Fingertips. Jack Forem. 1999. LC 98-39481. (Illus.). 352p. pap. text 15.00 (*0-7352-0006-8*) PH Pr.

Healing Awareness: The Feldenkrais Method Explained with Exercises. Stephen Shafarman. 2000. LC 96-41924. 224p. pap. 16.00 (*0-201-69469-7*) Perseus Bks Grp.

Healing Back Pain: The Mind-Body Connection. John E. Sarno. 1991. LC 90-44949. (Illus.). 193p. reprint ed. pap. 13.99 (*0-446-39230-8*) Warner Bks.

Healing Back Pain Naturally: The Mind-Body Program Proven to Work. Art Brownstein. 2001. (Illus.). 320p. reprint ed. pap. 14.95 (*0-7434-2464-6*, PB Trade Paper) PB.

Healing Between: A Clinical Guide to Dialogical Psychotherapy. William G. Heard. 2nd rev. ed. 2000. 235p. (C). pap. text (*0-9641576-2-4*) Soulprint Pubng.

***Healing Beyond the Body: Medicine & the Infinite Reach of the Mind.** Larry Dossey. 2001. LC 2001-31060. 320p. 24.95 (*1-57062-860-2*) Shambhala Pubns.

Healing Blade: A Tale of Neurosurgery. Edward J. Sylvester. rev. ed. 1997. (Illus.). 250p. pap. 13.95 (*0-9660972-0-3*) Beck Pr.

Healing Body & Soul: The Meaning of Illness in the New Testament & in Psychotherapy. John A. Sanford. 1992. 144p. (Orig.). pap. 15.95 (*0-664-25351-2*) Westminster John Knox.

Healing Bond: The Patient-Practitioner Relationship & Therapeutic Responsibility. Ursala Sharma & Susan Budd. 1994. LC 94-990. 224p. (C). pap. 29.95 (*0-415-09052-0*, B4196) Routledge.

Healing Bond: Treating Addictions in Groups. Ronald L. Rogers & C. Scott McMillan. 1989. (C). pap. 13.95 (*0-393-70088-7*) Norton.

Healing Brain: A Scientific Reader. Ed. by Robert Ornstein & Charles Swencionis. 1991. LC 89-16968. 262p. reprint ed. pap. 25.00 (*0-89862-463-0*, 2463) Guilford Pubns.

Healing Brain: Breakthrough Discoveries about How the Brain Keeps Us Healthy. Robert Ornstein & David Sobel. 1988. 304p. pap. 12.00 (*0-671-66236-8*, Touchstone) S&S Trade Pap.

Healing Brain: Breakthrough Discoveries about How the Brain Keeps Us Healthy. Robert Ornstein et al. 1999. LC 98-52480. 301p. reprint ed. pap. 16.00 (*1-883536-17-0*) ISHK.

Healing Celebrations: Miraculous Recoveries Through Ancient Scriptures, Natural Medicine & Modern Science. Leonard G. Horowitz. unabr. ed. 2000. LC 00-90697. (Illus.). 220p. 22.95 (*0-923550-08-9*, 08-9) Tetrahedron Pub.

Healing Ceremonies: Bridging Native American Medicine & Spirituality with the Modern Worlds Frontiers & Consciousness. Lewis E. Mehl. 250p. (*0-8290-5205-4*) Irvington.

Healing Ceremonies: Creating Personal Rituals for Spiritual, Emotional, Physical, & Mental Health. Carl A. Hammerschlag & Howard D. Silverman. 1997. LC 96-46201. 224p. pap. 13.00 (*0-399-52303-0*, Perigee Bks) Berkley Pub.

Healing Childhood Ear Infections: Prevention, Home Care, & Alternative Treatment. Michael Schmidt. 2nd rev. ed. 1996. LC 95-53679. Orig. Title: Childhood Ear Infections. (Illus.). 313p. reprint ed. pap. 16.95 (*1-55643-216-X*) North Atlantic.

Healing Children Naturally. Michael A. Weiner. 1993. 300p. pap. 12.95 (*0-912845-10-4*) Quantum Bks.

Healing Choice: Your Guide to Emotional Recovery After an Abortion. Candace De Puy & Dana Dovitch. 1997. LC 96-47484. 256p. per. 13.00 (*0-684-83196-1*, Fireside) S&S Trade Pap.

Healing Community: Dynamics of the Therapeutic Milieu. Richard Almond. 1974. LC 73-17733. 464p. 40.00 (*0-87668-111-9*) Aronson.

Healing Crisis. Bruce Fife. unabr. ed. 1997. LC 97-14626. 96p. pap. 15.00 (*0-941599-33-7*, HlthWise Pubns) Piccadilly Bks.

Healing Diet: How to Reduce Your Risk & Live a Longer & Healthier Life. Rtemis P. Simopoulos et al. 1995. LC 96-119828. (Illus.). 352p. (J). (gr. 1-9). pap. 14.95 (*0-02-860442-3*) Hungry Minds.

Healing Digestive Disorders: Natural Treatments for Gastrointestinal Conditions. Andrew Gaeddert. 1998. LC 98-17745. (Illus.). 220p. pap. 15.95 (*1-55643-281-X*) North Atlantic.

Healing Drama: Psychodrama & Drama Therapy with Abused Children. Anne Bannister. 1997. LC 98-129945. pap. (*1-85343-383-7*) Free Assoc Bks GBR. *Dist:* Intl Spec Bk, NYU Pr.

Healing Dramas & Clinical Plots: The Narrative Structure of Experience. Cheryl Mattingly. 1998. LC 97-38627. (C). 208p. text 59.95 (*0-521-63004-5*); 206p. pap. text 22.95 (*0-521-63994-8*) Cambridge U Pr.

Healing Drum: African Wisdom Teachings. Yaya Diallo & Mitchell Hall. 1989. 222p. pap. 14.95 (*0-89281-256-7*, Destiny Bks) Inner Tradit.

Healing Ear: Intermediate Auricular Therapy. Dennis L. Greenlee. Ed. by Carolyn W. Greenlee. 1995. (Illus.). 107p. spiral bd. 32.50 (*1-887400-09-5*) Earthen Vessel Prodns.

Healing Energies of Heat & Light: A Quantum Leap in Health Care. Charles T. McGee. 2000. LC 00-191385. (Illus.). 224p. pap. 20.00 (*0-9636979-6-X*) MediPress.

Healing Energies of Light. Roger Coghill. 2000. (Illus.). 160p. pap. 17.95 (*1-58290-012-4*) Jrny Editions.

Healing Energies of Music. Hal A. Lingerman. 2nd ed. 1995. LC 94-36151. 300p. pap. 16.00 (*0-8356-0722-4*, Quest) Theos Pub Hse.

Healing Essence: A Cancer Doctor's Program for Hope & Recovery. Mitchell L. Gaynor. 1995. LC 95-18162. 236p. 22.00 (*1-56836-079-7*) Kodansha.

Healing Essence: The Proven Path to Wellness. Mitchell L. Gaynor. 2000. 240p. reprint ed. pap. 14.00 (*1-57566-585-9*, Knsington) Kensgtn Pub Corp.

Healing Everything with Magnets. Gary Null. 1998. LC 00-267550. 224p. pap. 11.95 (*0-7867-0530-2*) Carroll & Graf.

***Healing Fibroids: A Doctor's Guide to a Natural Cure.** Allan Warshowsky. 2002. (Illus.). 288p. pap. 14.00 (*0-7434-1824-7*) PB.

Healing Fiction. James Hillman. 1994. LC 94-9422. 246p. reprint ed. pap. 15.00 (*0-88214-363-8*) Spring Pubns.

Healing Foods. Patricia Hausman. 1992. 480p. mass mkt. 6.99 (*0-440-21440-8*) Dell.

Healing Forest: Medicinal & Toxic Plants of the Northwest Amazonia. Richard E. Schultes & Robert F. Raffauf. 1990. LC 89-34261. (Historical, Ethno-and Economic Botany Ser.). (Illus.). 500p. 69.95 (*0-931146-14-3*, Dioscorides) Timber.

Healing, Forever-Settled. Kenneth Hagin, Jr. 1989. pap. 3.95 (*0-89276-723-5*) Faith Lib Pubns.

Healing from Allergy (Hay Fever & Perennial Rhinitis) & Vasomotor Rhinitis. William C. Uy. 2000. (Illus.). 192p. per. 12.95 (*0-9704843-0-5*) W C Uy.

Healing from Cancer: A Call to Freedom. Antonia G. Milo. 1999. LC 98-94872. (Illus.). 132p. pap. 9.95 (*0-9653664-2-1*) Balanced Way.

Healing from Childhood Abuse Vol. 1: We Have a Voice Now! My Sides & Their Journey Back to Life. Julie Martin. unabr. ed. 2000. LC 00-92018. (Illus.). 130p. pap. 20.00 (*0-9702723-0-8*) J Martin.

Healing from the Inside Out. Sheri Perl. 1997. LC 96-49827. 15.95 (*1-889828-03-3*) SethNet Pub.

Healing Garden: Nature's Restorative Powers. Marjorie Harris. (Illus.). 128p. 1998. text 16.00 (*0-7881-5943-7*); 2000. reprint ed. pap. 10.00 (*0-7881-9414-3*) DIANE Pub.

Healing Hands. Allegra Taylor. 1993. LC 93-60273. (Tuttle Alternative Health Ser.). (Illus.). 56p. pap. 12.95 (*0-8048-1832-0*) Tuttle Pubng.

Healing Hands: The Natural Healing Arts. Walter G. Bazan. 1998. 104p. reprint ed. pap. 11.00 (*0-7873-0082-9*) Hlth Research.

Healing Hands: The Story of the Palmer Family - Discoverers & Developers of Chiropractic. Joseph E. Maynard. 4th ed. 1992. LC 59-14319. 432p. 34.95 (*0-9630413-0-4*) Jonorm Pubs.

Healing Hands, Healing Words: Positive Suggestion & Loving Touch for Family & Friends. Ray Cullis. 1998. LC 97-28383. (Illus.). 177p. pap. 12.95 (*0-87604-394-5*, 490) ARE Pr.

Healing, Health & Transformation: New Frontiers in Medicine. Elaine R. Ferguson. 1990. 266p. 19.95 (*1-878743-17-1*) LaVonne Pr.

Healing Hepatitis Naturally: How Clinically Validated Natural Medicines Can Enhance the Healing Response. Doctor's Prescription for Healing Medicines Staff. 2000. 124p. pap. 5.95 (*1-893910-15-6*) Freedom Pr Inc.

Healing Herbs: Energy, Health & Great Looks - Right Here, Right Now. Leslie Kenton. 2001. (Illus.). 224p. (*0-09-186838-6*) Ebury Pr GBR. *Dist:* Trafalgar.

Healing Herbs Spanish Edition. Michael Castleman. 1995. LC 94-44615. (SPA.). 448p. 26.95 (*0-87596-267-X*) Rodale Pr Inc.

Healing Herbs of the Upper Curtin. Leonora S. Curtin. 1976. (Illus.). 281p. 25.95 (*0-405-09499-X*) Arno Press.

Healing Hip, Joint, & Knee Pain: A Mind-Body Guide to Recovery from Surgery & Injuries. Kate S. O'Shea. 1998. LC 97-38017. Orig. Title: Finding Your Balance. (Illus.). 154p. reprint ed. pap. 14.95 (*1-55643-258-5*) North Atlantic.

Healing HIV: How to Rebuild Your Immune System. Jon D. Kaiser. 1999. LC 98-35964. 372p. pap. 19.95 (*0-9666373-0-5*) HealthFirst Pr.

Healing Imagination: The Meeting of Psyche & Soul. Ann Ulanov & Barry Ulanov. 2000. 192p. pap. (*3-85630-591-2*) Daimon Pubs CHE. *Dist:* Cassell & Continuum.

Healing in Community: Medicine, Contested Terrains, & Cultural Encounters Among the Tuareg. Susan Rasmussen. 2001. LC 00-48605. 272p. 64.95 (*0-89789-761-7*, H761, Bergin & Garvey) Greenwood.

Healing in Hypnosis. Milton H. Erickson. Ed. by Ernest L. Rossi et al. 1989. (Seminars, Workshops & Lectures of Milton H. Erickson). (Illus.). 311p. 18.95 (*0-8290-3154-5*); pap. 20.00 (*0-8290-3159-6*) Irvington.

Healing in Psychotherapy: The Path & Process of Inner Change. Diane Shainberg. 2nd ed. 1993. LC 93-7872. (Perspectives in Psychotherapy: A Series of Monographs: Vol. 2). 162p. text 40.00 (*2-88124-573-0*); pap. text 25.00 (*2-88124-574-9*) Gordon & Breach.

Healing in Psychotherapy: The Process of Holistic Change. Diane Shainberg. 1983. LC 82-24247. (Perspectives in Psychotherapy: A Series of Monographs: Vol. 1). XVI, 126p. pap. text 28.00 (*0-677-21880-X*) Gordon & Breach.

Healing in the Relational Paradigm: The Image Relationship Therapy Casebook. Ed. by Wade Luquet & Mo T. Hannah. 1997. LC 97-45130. 225p. 37.95 (*0-87630-861-2*) Brunner-Routledge.

Healing into Immortality: A New Spiritual Medicine of Healing Stories & Imagery. Gerald Epstein. 1994. LC 94-17700. 304p. pap. 14.95 (*1-883148-04-9*) ACMI Pr.

Healing into Life & Death. Stephen Levine. 1989. 312p. pap. 12.95 (*0-385-26219-1*) Doubleday.

Healing Journey: Overcoming the Crisis of Cancer. Alastair J. Cunningham. 2nd rev. ed. 2000. (Illus.). 158p. pap. (*1-55263-107-9*) Key Porter CAN. *Dist:* Firefly Bks Limited.

Healing Life's Crises: A Guide for Nurses. Noreen C. Frisch & Jane Kelley. 1995. LC 94-48614. (Nurse as Healer Ser.). 208p. pap. text 23.95 (*0-8273-6399-0*) Delmar.

Healing Magnetism: The Transference of Vital Force. Heinz Schiegl. 1987. LC 86-50197. (Illus.). 200p. (Orig.). pap. 10.95 (*0-87728-644-2*) Red Wheel ME.

Healing Makes Our Hearts Happy: Spirituality & Cultural Transformation among the Kalahari Ju/'hoansi. Richard Katz et al. 1997. LC 96-938. (Illus.). 240p. pap. 29.95 (*0-89281-557-4*) Inner Tradit.

Healing Mandalas. Edwin V. Sylvester. 1989. (Illus.). 84p. (Orig.). pap. 9.50 (*0-925634-01-8*) Hickory Corners.

Healing Massage: A Practical Guide to Relaxation & Well-Being. Susan Mumford. 1998. (Illus.). 128p. pap. 18.00 (*0-452-27994-1*, Plume) Dutton Plume.

Healing Meditation: Nurse as Healer Series. Mary G. Umlauf. 1996. LC 96-14002. (Nurse as Healer Ser.). (Illus.). 208p. pap. text 23.95 (*0-8273-6395-8*) Delmar.

Healing Mind. Martin. 1999. 384p. pap. 16.95 (*0-312-24300-6*) St Martin.

Healing Mind, Healthy Woman: Using the Mind-Body Connection. Alice D. Domar & Henry Dreher. 1997. 448p. pap. 14.95 (*0-385-31894-4*) Doubleday.

Healing Miracles. William A. McGarey. 1996. 212p. mass mkt. 5.99 (*0-312-95948-6*) St Martin.

Healing, Miracles & the Bite of the Gray Dog. Majid Ali. 1997. 550p. (Orig.). pap. 19.00 (*1-879131-11-0*) Inst of Prev Med.

***Healing Moves: How to Cure, Prevent & Relieve Common Ailments with Exercise.** Carol Krucoff & Mitchell Krucoff. 2001. (Illus.). 336p. pap. 14.00 (*0-609-80795-1*, Three Riv Pr) Harmony Bks.

Healing Moves with Power Therapies: Finding the Energy to Heal. Maggie Phillips. 2000. LC 00-56858. (Illus.). 272p. 35.00 (*0-393-70326-6*) Norton.

Healing Muscle Pain: Tools, Techniques & Tips to Bring Your Muscles Back to Health. Elisabeth Aaslid & Kate A. Schultz. 2001. LC 00-36842. (Illus.). 304p. pap. 16.95 (*0-471-37891-7*) Wiley.

Healing Nutrients Within. Eric R. Braverman et al. 2nd rev. ed. 1997. LC 96-53006. 536p. pap. 19.95 (*0-87983-706-3*, 37063K, Keats Pubng) McGraw-Hill Trade.

Healing Nutrition. Keegan. 2nd ed. 2001. LC 2001-53762. 240p. (C). text 20.95 (*0-7668-2571-X*) Delmar.

Healing Nutrition: Nurse as Healer Series. Lynn Keegan. 1995. LC 94-44097. (Nurse as Healer Ser.). 208p. pap. text 23.95 (*0-8273-6868-2*) Delmar.

Healing of Cancer: The Cures, the Cover-ups & the Solution Now! Barry Lynes. 1989. 211p. (Orig.). pap. 12.95 (*0-919951-44-9*) New Leaf Dist.

Healing of Memories. David A. Seamands. 1986. LC 2001-5535. 156p. pap. text 10.99 (*0-89693-169-2*, 6-2169) Cook Communs Minist.

Healing on the Edge of Now: A Practical Guide for the Use of Psychoneuroimmunology. Carl Brahe. Ed. by Jack Hofer. 1992. LC 92-80669. 208p. (Orig.). pap. 11.95 (*0-9615743-2-1*) SunShine CO.

***Healing Options: A Report on Graves' Disease Treatments.** 2nd rev. ed. 2001. (Illus.). 226p. pap. 21.95 (*0-9665981-1-3*) S Breer.

Healing Others: A Practical Guide. Walter L. Weston. 1998. LC 98-72217. (Healing Ser.). 200p. pap. text 11.95 (*1-57174-090-2*) Hampton Roads Pub Co.

Healing Ourself: Growing Beyond the True Cause of Disease. Kathy Oddenino. 1994. (Illus.). 600p. (Orig.). pap. 24.95 (*0-923081-04-6*) Joy Pubns MD.

***Healing Outside the Margins: A Cancer Survivor's Guide to Complementary Therapy.** Carole O'Toole & Carolyn B. Hendricks. 2002. 364p. 21.95 (*0-89526-193-6*, LifeLine Press) Regnery Pub.

Healing Pain: Attachment, Loss & Grief Therapy. Nini Leick & Marianne Davidsen-Nielsen. 1991. LC 90-8509. 224p. (C). pap. 24.95 (*0-415-04795-1*, A5419) Routledge.

Healing Past: Pharmaceuticals in the Biblical & Rabbinic World. Ed. by Irene Jacob & Walter Jacob. 1993. LC 93-13693. (Studies in Ancient Medicine: Vol. 7). xv, 126p. 64.50 (*90-04-09643-4*) Brill Academic Pubs.

Healing Path: Practical Guide to the Holistic Traditions of China, India, Tibet & Japan. Jacqueline Young. 2001. (Illus.). 180p. (*0-00-761263-X*) Thorsons GBR. *Dist:* Natl Bk Netwk.

Healing Path of Prayer: A Modern Mystic's Guide to Spiritual Power. Ron Roth & Peter Occhiogrosso. 1998. 256p. pap. 13.00 (*0-609-80226-7*) Harmony Bks.

Healing Paw: Not All Angels Have Wings. Billy Roberts. 2001. 140p. pap. (*0-00-710949-0*) Thorsons GBR. *Dist:* Natl Bk Netwk.

Healing Photons: The Science & Art of Blood Irradiation Therapy. Kenneth J. Dillon. 1998. LC 97-62342. (Illus.). 180p. pap. 19.95 (*0-9642976-5-5*) Spectrum Biosci.

Healing Plants. Mannfried Pahlow. 1993. (Illus.). 224p. pap. 18.95 (*0-8120-1498-7*) Barron.

Healing Plants: A Medicinal Guide to Native North American Plants & Herbs. Ana N. Heatherley. 1998. LC 97-28531. (Illus.). 288p. pap. 16.95 (*1-55821-509-3*, Lyons) Globe Pequot.

Healing Plants: Medicine of the Florida Seminole Indians. Alice Micco Snow & Susan Enns Stans. 2001. LC 00-69078. (Illus.). xv, 134p. 24.95 (*0-8130-2062-X*) U Press Fla.

Healing Power of Balanced Emotions. Frederick W. Bailes. 1972. 77p. pap. 8.95 (*0-87516-124-3*) DeVorss.

Healing Power of Breath: An Introduction to Wholistic Breath Therapy. Jonathon Daemion. 1989. 256p. (Orig.). pap. (*1-85327-015-6*) Prism Pr GBR. *Dist:* Assoc Pubs Grp.

Healing Power of Foods: Nutrition Secrets for Vibrant Health & Long Life. Michael T. Murray. 1993. LC 93-16251. 448p. (Orig.). pap. 18.95 (*1-55958-317-7*, Prima Health) Prima Pub.

Healing Power of Grapefruit Seed: The Practical Handbook for Using Grapefruit Seed Extract to Heal Infections, Allergies & Much More. Shalila Sharamon & Bodo J. Baginsky. 1996. 144p. (Orig.). pap. 12.95 (*0-914955-27-6*) Lotus Pr.

Healing Power of Herbs. May Bethel. 1980. 164p. pap. 5.00 (*0-87980-047-X*) Wilshire.

Healing Power of Herbs: The Enlightened Person's Guide to the Wonders of Medicinal Plants. Michael T. Murray. 2nd exp. rev. ed. 1995. (Illus.). 432p. pap. 16.95 (*1-55958-700-8*) Prima Pub.

Healing Power of Minerals, Special Nutrients & Trace Elements. Paul Bergner. 1997. LC 97-20545. 320p. pap. 15.00 (*0-7615-1021-4*) Prima Pub.

***Healing Power of Movement: How too Benefit from Physical Activity During Your Cancer Treatment.** Lisa Hoffman & Alison Freeland. 2002. 112p. pap. text 15.00 (*0-7382-0540-0*) Perseus Bks Grp.

Healing Power of Natural Foods. May Bethel. 1978. 207p. pap. 7.00 (*0-87980-363-0*) Wilshire.

Healing Power of the Mind: Practical Techniques for Health & Empowerment. Rolf Alexander. 1997. LC 97-644. 128p. pap. 10.95 (*0-89281-729-1*, Heal Arts VT) Inner Tradit.

Healing Powers: Alternative Medicine, Spiritual Communities, & the State. Fred M. Frohock. 1992. LC 91-36941. (Morality & Society Ser.). (Illus.). 350p. 29.95 (*0-226-26584-6*) U Ch Pr.

Healing Powers & Modernity: Traditional Medicine, Shamanism, & Science in Asian Societies. Ed. by Linda H. Connor & Geoffrey Samuel. 2001. LC 00-29256. 296p. 69.95 (*0-89789-715-3*, H715, Bergin & Garvey) Greenwood.

Healing Powers of Plants: A Beginner's Guide. Kristyna Arcarti. 1998. (Beginner's Guide Ser.). (Illus.). 96p. pap. (*0-340-71148-5*) Hodder & Stought Ltd GBR. *Dist:* Lubrecht & Cramer, Trafalgar.

Healing Powers of Vinegar: A Complete Guide to Nature's Most Remarkable Remedy. Cal Orey. 2000. LC 2001-274863. (Illus.). viii, 263p. pap. 12.00 (*1-57566-609-X*, Knsington) Kensgtn Pub Corp.

Healing Practices in the South Pacific. Claire D. Parsons. 1995. LC 85-14191. (Illus.). 266p. (C). reprint ed. pap. 19.00 (*0-939154-56-0*) Inst Polynesian.

Healing Psoriasis: The Natural Alternative. John O. Pagano. 1991. (Illus.). (Orig.). pap. 24.95 (*0-9628847-0-7*) Pagano Organization.

Healing Remedies: Herbal Medicine, Homeopathy, Chinese Herbal Medicine 1998. (In a Nutshell Ser.). (Illus.). 24.00 (*1-86204-365-5*) Element MA.

Healing Remedies That Really Work. Health Advisory Board. 1999. 352p. pap. 24.95 (*1-893910-05-9*) Freedom Pr Inc.

Healing Repetitive Stress Injuries. William Wong. 2000. 128p. pap. 9.95 (*1-893910-14-8*, 904-007) Freedom Pr Inc.

Healing Ritual: Studies in the Technique & Tradition of the Southern Slavs. Phyllis Kemp. LC 75-23731. reprint ed. 40.00 (*0-404-13289-8*) AMS Pr.

Healing Runes: Tools for the Recovery of Body, Mind, Heart, & Soul. Ralph H. Blum & Susan Loughan. 1995. LC 95-24221. 160p. 29.95 (*0-312-13507-6*) St Martin.

Healing Secrets from the Bible. Patrick Quillin. 1996. pap. text 14.95 (*0-9638372-1-4*) Nutrit Times.

Healing Secrets of Ancient China. Pier Tsui-Po. 1994. (Illus.). 164p. (Orig.). pap. 14.95 (*0-85572-245-2*) Seven Hills Bk.

Healing Secrets of the Ages. Catherine Ponder. rev. ed. 1985. LC 67-26503. 278p. reprint ed. pap. 16.95 (*0-87516-550-8*) DeVorss.

Healing Secrets of the Animals. Carol C. Garey. 2000. (*0-688-17698-4*) Hearst Bks.

***Healing Secrets of the East.** Josh Holzer. 2000. (Illus.). 155p. pap. 39.95 (*1-893479-08-0*) Agora Financl.

Healing Shattered Reality: Understanding Contactee Trauma. Alice Bryant & Linda Seebach. 1991. 296p. pap. 13.00 (*0-926524-16-X*) Granite Pub.

Healing Sounds: Fundamentals of Chirophonetics. Alfred Baur. 1993. 42.95 (*0-945803-24-9*) R Steiner Col.

Healing Sounds from the Malaysian Rainforest: Temiar Music & Medicine. Marina Roseman. 1991. LC 90-11253. (Comparative Studies of Health Systems & Medical Care: Vol. 28). (Illus.). 278p. pap. text 18.95 (*0-520-08281-8*) U CA Pr.

Healing Spirit: Explorations in Religion & Psychotherapy. Paul R. Fleischman. 1994. LC 90-35390. 288p. pap. 13.95 (*1-55778-334-9*) Bonne Chance.

Healing Stories: Giving, Receiving, Teaching, Learning Energy-Based Therapy. Mary Jo Bulbrook. 2000. pap. text 25.00 (*1-889293-09-1*) NC Ctr Healing.

Healing Stories: Narrative in Psychiatry & Psychotherapy. Ed. by Glenn Roberts & Jeremy Holmes. 1999. LC 98-19457. (Illus.). 248p. text 89.95 (*0-19-262827-5*) OUP.

Healing Sylvia: Childhood Sexual Abuse & the Construction of Identity. Michele Davies. 1995. 176p. pap. 24.95 (*0-7484-0176-8*) Taylor & Francis.

Healing Techniques of the Holy East. Sant Keshavadas. 1980. LC 80-50447. (Illus.). 116p. (Orig.). pap. 10.00 (*0-931290-30-9*) Vishwa.

Healing Technology: Feminist Perspectives. Ed. by Kathryn S. Ratcliff. 1989. 436p. pap. text 19.95 (*0-472-06395-2*, 06395) U of Mich Pr.

Healing the Addictive Mind: Freeing Yourself from Addictive Patterns & Relationships. Lee L. Jampolsky. 1995. LC 90-2171. 172p. text 12.95 (*0-89087-623-1*) Celestial Arts.

Healing the Anxiety Diseases. T. L. Leaman. 1992. LC 91-45635. (Illus.). 304p. (C). 23.95 (*0-306-44128-4*) Da Capo.

Healing the Blues: A Personal Account by a Patient & Her Therapist. Dorothea Nudelman & David Willingham. 1997. LC 98-102904. 202p. pap. 12.95 (*1-885987-10-2*, ME082, Health Info Pr) Practice Mgmt Info.

Healing the Blues: Drug-Free Psychotherapy of Depression. Ed. by Dorothea Nudelman & David Willingham. 1994. LC 94-12688. 235p. 22.00 (*0-940168-31-6*) Boxwood.

Healing the Body Naturally with Cell Salts. Skye Weintraub. 1993. 147p. pap. 20.00 (*0-9638267-0-0*) Complement Med.

Healing the Child: A Mother's Story. Nancy Cain. 1997. 288p. per. 14.00 (*0-671-01001-8*) PB.

Healing the Child: A Mother's Story. Nancy Cain. 1996. LC 96-3568. 288p. 21.50 (*0-684-80169-8*) S&S Trade.

Healing the Child Within: Discovery & Recovery for Adult Children of Dysfunctional Families. Charles L. Whitfield. 1987. LC 87-137. (Illus.). 150p. (Orig.). pap. 8.95 (*0-932194-40-0*) Health Comm.

Healing the Children of War. Ed. by Phyllis Kilbourn. 1995. LC 95-167516. 330p. 21.95 (*0-912552-87-5*, MARC Pubns) World Vision Intl.

Healing the Divided Self: Clinical & Ericksonian Hypnotherapy for Post-Traumatic & Dissociative Conditions. Maggie Phillips & Claire Frederick. 1995. LC 94-40282. 384p. 40.00 (*0-393-70184-0*) Norton.

Healing the Dying. Melodie Olson. 2nd ed. 2001. (C). pap. text 22.95 (*0-7668-2572-8*) Delmar.

Healing the Dying: Nurse as Healer Series. Melodie Olson. 1996. LC 95-45489. (Nurse as Healer Ser.). (Illus.). 208p. pap. text 23.95 (*0-8273-6603-5*) Delmar.

Healing the Emerging Holistic Paradigm. Lilo Bauer-Freitag. 1998. 160p. pap. 16.00 (*1-880710-30-7*) Monterey Pacific.

Healing the Eye the Natural Way: Alternative Medicine & Macular Degeneration. Edward Kondrot. 2001. LC 2001-16265. 204p. pap. 18.95 (*1-55643-402-2*) North Atlantic.

Healing the Eye the Natural Way: Alternative Medicine & Macular Degeneration. Edward C. Kondrut. 2000. LC 99-69770. xviii, 204p. per. 19.95 (*0-9672346-1-1*) Nutrit Res.

Healing the Female Heart: A Holistic Approach to Prevention & Recovery from Heart Disease. Elizabeth Ross & Judith Sachs. Ed. by Julie Rubenstein. 1996. LC 95-9494. 288p. (Orig.). per. 12.00 (*0-671-89470-6*, PB Trade Paper) PB.

Healing the Forgotten Child: Support & Recovery for the Adult Children of Alcoholics (& Other Children of Dysfunctional Families) Karen Martin. 1989. 60p. (Orig.). (C). pap., stu. ed. 79.95 (*0-9623925-0-2*) Resource Dynamics.

Healing the Fractured Self. John F. Walters. 1985. 122p. (Orig.). pap. 10.95 (*0-86683-883-X*) Harper SF.

Healing the Gender Wars: Object Relations Therapy with Men. Samuel Slipp. 1996. LC 95-46925. 248p. 50.00 (*1-56821-773-0*) Aronson.

Healing the Generations: A History of Physical Therapy & the American Physical Therapy Association. Wendy B. Murphy. Date not set. (Illus.). 256p. 105.00 (*0-944641-13-X*, APTA-20) Greenwich Pub Group.

Healing the Greatest Hurt: Healing Grief & the Family Tree. Dennis Linn et al. 1985. LC 85-60407. 258p. (Orig.). pap. 12.95 (*0-8091-2714-8*) Paulist Pr.

***Healing the Healer: The Addicted Physician.** Daniel H. Angres et al. 2001. xx, 252p. reprint ed. pap. text 29.95 (*1-887841-49-0*, 62318, Psychosocial) Intl Univs Pr.

Healing the Healer: Treating the Addicted Physician. Daniel H. Angres et al. 1998. LC 98-15857. (Illus.). 231p. 32.50 (*1-887841-15-6*, Psychosocial) Intl Univs Pr.

Healing the Heart: A Therapeutic Approach to Disturbed Children in Group Care. Alvin Rosenfeld & Saul Wasserman. 1990. 96p. pap. 15.95 (*0-87868-391-7*) Child Welfare.

Healing the Hospital Environment: Design, Maintenance & Management of Healthcare Premises. Sarah Hosking & Liz Haggard. 1999. LC 98-42212. (Illus.). xviii, 193p. pap. 55.00 (*0-419-23170-6*, Spon) Routledge.

Healing the Hungry Heart: The Link Between Eating Disorders & Sexual Abuse. Karin J. Gubin & Richard K. Thomas. 1994. 128p. (Orig.). per. 11.95 (*0-9643336-0-0*) Medical Srvs.

Healing the Hurt: Rebuilding Relationships with Your Children; a Self-Help Guide for Parents in Recovery. Rosalie C. Jesse. 1990. 170p. pap. text 12.95 (*0-935908-54-4*, 3210, HazeldenJohnson Inst) Hazelden.

Healing the Hurt Child: A Developmental-Contextual Approach. Denis M. Donovan & Deborah McIntyre. 1990. (C). 34.95 (*0-393-70093-3*) Norton.

Healing the Incest Wound: Adult Survivors in Therapy. Christine A. Courtois. 1996. 416p. pap. 21.95 (*0-393-31356-5*); 1988. 396p. 34.95 (*0-393-70051-8*) Norton.

Healing the Infertile Family: Strengthening Your Relationship in the Search for Parenthood. Gaylene Becker. 1997. LC 97-8565. 327p. pap. 18.95 (*0-520-21180-4*) U CA Pr.

Healing the Masses: Cuban Health Politics at Home & Abroad. Julie M. Feinsilver. 1993. LC 92-31124. text 50.00 (*0-520-08218-4*); pap. text 19.95 (*0-520-08298-2*) U CA Pr.

Healing the Mind: A History of Pyschiatry from Antiquity to the Present. Michael Stone. 1997. LC 96-28209. (Illus.). 448p. 49.00 (*0-393-70222-7*) Norton.

Healing the Pain: Medical, Alternative & Self-Help Options for Pain Relief. Consumer Guide Editors. 1998. 256p. pap. 5.99 (*0-451-19419-5*, Sig) NAL.

Healing the Schism: Epidemiology, Medicine, & the Public's Health. K. L. White. Ed. by M. Lipkin, Jr. 1991. (Frontiers of Primary Care Ser.). 304p. 49.00 (*0-387-97574-8*) Spr-Verlag.

Healing the Sick. T. L. Osborn. 1981. 420p. pap. 14.99 (*0-89274-187-2*, HH-187) Harrison Hse.

Healing the Social Body: A Holistic Approach to Public Health Policy. Elizabeth R. Mackenzie. 1998. LC 97-11610. (Health Care Policy in the United States Ser.). 256p. text 67.00 (*0-8153-2909-1*) Garland.

Healing the Soul in the Age of the Brain: Becoming Conscious in an Unconscious World. Elio Frattaroli. 2001. LC 2001-23996. 512p. 25.95 (*0-670-86189-8*, Viking) Viking Penguin.

Healing the Trauma of Mind, Body & Spirit. M. A. Flaherty. 1997. (C). pap. text 24.95 (*0-8273-6965-4*) Delmar.

Healing the Unaffirmed: Recognizing the Deprivation Neurosis. Conrad W. Baars & Anna A. Terruwe. 1979. LC 76-7897. 214p. reprint ed. pap. 6.95 (*0-8189-0393-7*) Alba.

Healing the Whole Person. Jonathon D. Miller. Date not set. (Orig.). pap. 9.98 (*0-935815-04-X*) Lifecircle.

Healing the Wounds: A Physician Looks at His Work. David Hilfiker. 2nd rev. ed. 1997. LC 96-47942. xx, 209p. pap. 14.95 (*1-881871-23-1*) Creighton U Pr.

Healing Their Wounds: Psychotherapy with Holocaust Survivors & Their Families. Ed. by Paul Marcus & Alan Rosenberg. 1989. LC 89-8638. 324p. 55.00 (*0-275-92948-5*, C2948, Praeger Pubs) Greenwood.

Healing Through Communication: The Practice of Caring. Carol L. Montgomery. 1993. (Illus.). 180p. (C). pap. 29.95 (*0-8039-5121-3*, 3270) Sage.

Healing Through Movement & Body Therapy: Nurse as Healer Series. B. Kazanis & C. McClain. 2001. (Professional Reference - Nursing Ser). 208p. pap. 21.95 (*0-8273-7412-7*) Thomson Learn.

Healing Through the Power of Prayer: What the Bible Says about Healing. Consumer Guide Editors. 1998. 256p. pap. 5.99 (*0-451-19421-7*, Sig) NAL.

***Healing Through the Senses: Cosmo-Therapy.** Dietrich Gumbel. Ed. by Veronica M. Sauter. Tr. by Marianne Greene. 2001. Orig. Title: Heilen Durch die Sinne: Die-Cosmo-Therapie. (Illus.). pap. 29.00 (*0-9714327-0-8*, 6005) Cosmo Therapy.

***Healing Touch.** Southwater Staff. 2001. 96p. text (*1-84215-406-0*, Swater) Ann3ess GBR. *Dist:* Natl Bk Netwk.

Healing Touch: A Resource for Health Care Professionals. Dorothea Hover-Kramer. 2nd ed. 2001. LC 2001-42337. (Illus.). 256p. pap. 20.95 (*0-7668-2519-1*) Delmar.

Healing Touch: An Introduction to Organismic Psychotherapy. Malcolm Brown. 1990. (Illus.). 325p. reprint ed. pap. 20.00 (*0-940795-01-9*) LifeRhythm.

Healing Touch: Keeping the Doctor-Patient Relationship Alive under Managed Care. David L. Cram. Ed. by Rod Colvin. 1997. LC 97-17574. 127p. (Orig.). pap. 9.95 (*1-886039-31-3*) Addicus Bks.

***Healing Touch: Level I Notebook.** Janet Mentgen & Mary Jo Bulbrook. 2001. 98p. pap. text 20.00 (*1-889293-10-5*) NC Ctr Healing.

Healing Touch: Level I Notebook. Janet Mentgen & Mary Jo Bulbrook. 100p. 2000. pap. text 15.00 (*1-889293-08-3*); 1994. pap. text 12.00 (*1-889293-01-6*) NC Ctr Healing.

Healing Touch: Level II Notebook. Janet Mentgen & Mary Jo Bulbrook. 2000. 175p. pap. text 20.00 (*1-889293-07-5*); 1995. 206p. pap. text 20.00 (*1-889293-02-4*) NC Ctr Healing.

Healing Traditions: Alternative Medicine & the Health Professions. Bonnie B. O'Connor. 1995. (Studies in Health, Illness, & Caregiving). (Illus.). (Orig.). (C). 288p. text 39.95 (*0-8122-3184-8*); 287p. pap. text 17.95 (*0-8122-1398-X*) U of Pa Pr.

Healing Tuberculosis in the Woods: Medicine & Science at the End of the Nineteenth Century, 41. David L. Ellison. 1994. LC 94-13689. (Contributions in Medical Studies Ser.: No. 41). 216p. 62.50 (*0-313-29005-9*, Greenwood Pr) Greenwood.

Healing 2000: Western Medicine & Beyond. Graham S. Palmer. 2000. 275p. pap. text 40.00 (*1-55605-308-8*) Wyndham Hall.

Healing Victims of Sexual Abuse. Paula Sandford. 1988. 192p. (Orig.). pap. 9.99 (*0-932081-21-5*) Victory Hse.

Healing Waters: Fifty Original European Water Cures. Edmond B. Szekely. 1976. (Illus.). 64p. pap. 3.50 (*0-89564-049-X*) IBS Intl.

Healing Wisdom of Doctor P. P. Quimby. Ed. by Mason A. Clark. 1982. LC 82-24232. (Illus.). 128p. (Orig.). pap. text 8.95 (*0-931400-02-3*) Frontal Lobe.

Healing Wise. Susun S. Weed. 1989. LC 89-84619. (Wise Woman Herbal Ser.: No. 2). (Illus.). 312p. (Orig.). (C). pap. 12.95 (*0-9614620-2-7*) Ash Tree.

***Healing with Acupressure.** Helen Saul. 2nd ed. 2001. LC 2001-47705. (Healing Wisdom Ser.). (Illus.). 160p. pap. 11.95 (*0-658-01239-8*) McGraw-Hill Prof.

Healing with Aloe - Tissue Therapy, Aloe Therapy, Agave Healing System: The Turning Point for Many Ailments. Wolfgang Wirth. 2nd ed. 1996. (Illus.). 80p. pap. (*3-85068-213-7*) Ennsthaler AUT. *Dist:* Am Educ Systs.

***Healing with Aromatherapy: A Concise Guide to Using Essential Oils to Enhance Your Life.** 2001. (Essentials for Health & Harmony... Ser.). (Illus.). 64p. (*1-84215-380-3*, Swater) Ann3ess GBR. *Dist:* Natl Bk Netwk.

Healing with Chinese Herbs. Richard Hyatt. 1990. LC 90-30392. 160p. pap. 12.95 (*0-89281-277-X*, Heal Arts VT) Inner Tradit.

Healing with Chinese Herbs. Lesley Tierra. 1997. LC 97-11515. (Healing Ser.). 160p. pap. 14.95 (*0-89594-829-X*) Crossing Pr.

H
I

*Healing with Colour: A Complete Guide to Restoring Balance & Natural Health. 2001. (Essentials for Health & Harmony... Ser.). (Illus.). 64p. (1-84215-382-X, Swater) Ann3ess GBR. Dist: Natl Bk Netwk.
Healing with Complementary & Alternative Therapies. Lynn Keegan. 2000. LC 00-63858. (Illus.). xxi, 520p. (C). text 28.95 (0-7668-1890-X) Delmar.
Healing with Crystals & Gemstones. Daya S. Chocron. 1986. LC 86-4072. (Illus.). 144p. pap. 12.95 (0-87728-646-9) Red Wheel ME.
*Healing with Flowers. Southwater Staff & Jessica Houdret. 2001. (Essentials for Health & Harmony... Ser.). 64p. text (1-84215-440-0, Swater) Ann3ess GBR. Dist: Natl Bk Netwk.
Healing with Herbal Juices: A Practical Guide to Herbal Juice Therapy: Nature's Preventative Medicine. Siegfried Gursche. 2nd ed. 1993. LC 93-915151. (Illus.). 252p. pap. 16.95 (0-920470-34-3) Alive Bks.
*Healing with Herbs. Southwater Staff & Jessica Houdret. 2001. (Essentials for Health & Harmony... Ser.). 64p. text (1-84215-392-7, Swater) Ann3ess GBR. Dist: Natl Bk Netwk.
Healing with Herbs & Home Remedies A-Z: How to Heal Your Mind & Body with Herbs, Home Remedies & Minerals. Hanna Kroeger. 1998. LC 97-51592. (Lifestyles Ser.). (Illus.). 156p. (C). text 19.95 (1-56170-488-1, 551) Hay House.
Healing with Homeopathy: The Doctor's Guide. Wayne B. Jonas & Jennifer Jacobs. 1998. LC 98-2761. (Illus.). 368p. pap. (0-446-67342-0) Warner.
Healing with Love: A Breakthrough Mind/Body Medical Program for Healing Yourself & Others. Leonard Laskow. 2nd ed. 1998. LC 98-61230. (Illus.). 341p. reprint ed. pap. 18.00 (0-9665195-0-7) Wholeness Pr.
Healing with Osteopathy see Discover Osteopathy: A First-Step Handbook to Better Health
Healing with Plants in the American & Mexican West. Margarita A. Kay. 1996. LC 96-10101. 315p. (Illus.). 19.95 (0-8165-1646-4); pap. 19.95 (0-8165-1647-2) U of Ariz Pr.
*Healing with Reflexology: A Concise Guide to Massaging Reflex Points to Enhance Health & Wellbeing. 2001. (Essentials for Health & Harmony... Ser.). (Illus.). 64p. (1-84215-381-1, Swater) Ann3ess GBR. Dist: Natl Bk Netwk.
Healing with Vitamins. Prevention Magazine Editors. 1996. 95.85 (0-87596-381-1) St Martin.
Healing with Vitamins: The Most Effective Vitamin & Mineral Treatments for Everyday Health Problems & Serious Disease. Prevention Magazine Editors. Ed. by Alice Feinstein. 1998. LC 97-46593. (Illus.). 608p. pap. 17.95 (1-57954-018-X) Rodale Pr Inc.
Healing with Words. Rob McNeilly & Jenny Brown. 1994. 108p. (Orig.). pap. 14.95 (0-85572-246-0) Seven Hills Bk.
Healing Within: Medicine, Health & Wholeness. Robin Price. 1986. 19p. pap. (0-904674-11-8) Octagon Pr GBR. Dist: ISHK.
Healing Within: The Complete Guide to Colon Health. Stanley Weinberger. 1996. 320p. pap. text 15.95 (0-9616184-7-7) Healing Within Prods.
Healing Within: The Complete Guide to Colon Health. Stanley Weinberger. Ed. by Beth Kuper. 3rd rev. ed. (Illus.). 250p. reprint ed. pap. 12.95 (0-9616184-2-6) Healing Within Prods.
Healing Words: The Power of Prayer & the Practice of Medicine. Larry Dossey. 1995. LC 92-56132. 320p. pap. 14.00 (0-06-250252-2) Harper SF.
Healing Your Body Naturally: Alternative Treatments to Illness. Gary Null. 3rd rev. ed. 1997. LC 96-39683. (Illus.). 336p. pap. 16.95 (1-888363-46-0) Seven Stories.
Healing Your Child: An A-Z Guide to Using Natural Remedies. Francis Darragh & Louise Darragh Law. 2000. LC 00-56853. (Illus.). 224p. pap. 13.95 (1-56924-614-9) Marlowe & Co.
Healing Your Child: Natural Care for Children with Chronic Illnesses. Barry Gillespie. 1999. (Illus.). 150p. text 24.95 (0-9678523-0-7) Pubns Chldrn.
Healing Your Emotions: Discover Your Element Type & Change Your Life. Angela Hicks & John Hicks. 1999. pap. (0-7225-3728-X) Thorsons GBR. Dist: Natl Bk Netwk.
Healing Your Insecurities. Roy Hicks. 1982. 122p. (Orig.). mass mkt. 5.99 (0-89274-249-6, HH-249) Harrison Hse.
Healing Your Prostate: Natural Cures That Work. Eva Urbaniak. 1998. LC 98-6573. (Health Ser.). (Illus.). 120p. pap. 14.95 (0-936197-35-8) Harbor Pr.
Healing Yourself: A Nurse's Guide to Self-Care & Renewal. Sherry Kahn et al. 1993. LC 93-26360. (Real Nursing Ser.). 221p. (C). mass mkt. 28.95 (0-8273-6150-5) Delmar.
Healing Yourself: A Practical Guide. Walter L. Weston. 1998. LC 98-72218. (Healing Ser.). 200p. pap. text 11.95 (1-57174-091-0) Hampton Roads Pub Co.
Healing Yourself with Homeopathy: How to Use the Hidden Key to Homeopathy: Get Great Results! Martha M. Christy. 1994. LC 94-62058. (Natural Health at Home Ser.). (Illus.). 254p. (Orig.). pap. 15.95 (0-9632091-2-4) Wishland Inc.
Healing Yourself with Self-Hypnosis. Frank Caprio et al. 2nd exp. rev. ed. 1998. LC 97-53295. 288p. (C). 30.00 (0-13-906678-0) P-H.
Healtcare Records Management, Disclosure & Retention: The Complete Legal Guide. Timothy Carse et al. 2nd rev. ed. 1993. 665p. (C). text 75.00 (0-07-413117-6, Irwn McGrw-H) McGrw-H Hghr Educ.
Health. 18.97 (0-673-21547-4) Addson-Wesley Educ.
Health. Judy Baker. 1998. LC 97-75315. xxi, 196p. (C). pap. text 16.36 (0-395-90247-9) HM.
Health. Joseph J. Bevelacqua. 1995. LC 94-19851. 456p. 105.00 (0-471-01801-5) Wiley.
Health. Marjorie Ford & Jon Ford. 1997. LC 97-72470. (Ford Reader Ser.). (C). pap. text 9.16 (0-395-86799-1) HM.
Health. Gold. 1994. text 67.80 (0-03-075324-4) Holt R&W.
Health. Michael H. Hamrick et al. 1986. 576p. (C). pap. 42.00 (0-675-20320-1, Merrill Coll) P-H.
Health: 1994. Gold. 1994. text, tchr. ed. 92.00 (0-03-075326-0) Holt R&W.
Health: Basics. 4th ed. 2000. 480p. (C). (0-205-32410-X) Allyn.
Health: Basics: Instructors Manual. 4th ed. 2000. (0-205-32580-7) Allyn.
Health: Basics:Take Charge. 4th ed. 2000. wbk. ed. 11.00 (0-205-32583-1) Allyn.
Health: Health, Mental Health, Food & Substance Abuse. 2000. (Enduring Issues Ser.). ring bd. 100.00 (0-89777-221-0) SIRS Pubng.
Health: Nutrition Concern Quarterly, 5. CBS Staff. 1995. (C). text 67.00 (0-03-016413-3) Harcourt.
Health: The Basic. 2nd ed. 2000. 200p. (0-205-31818-5) Allyn.
Health: The Family Planning Factor. Erik P. Eckholm. 1977. pap. (0-916468-09-7) Worldwatch Inst.
Health - Dangers, Risks & Assessments: Index of Modern Authors & Subjects with Guide for Rapid Research. Mary B. Schneply. 1991. LC 90-56252. 200p. 47.50 (1-55914-290-1); pap. 44.50 (1-55914-291-X) ABBE Pubs Assn.
Health - How Americans Behave to Improve, Ignore or Ruin Their Best Planet Connection: Index of New Information with Authors, Subjects & References. David K. Delgrado. 1996. (Illus.). 150p. 57.50 (0-7883-1338-X); pap. 47.50 (0-7883-1339-8) ABBE Pubs Assn.
Health - Personal Influences, Attitudes, Behavior & Self-Care: Index of New Information. John C. Bartone. 1998. (Illus.). 150p. 57.50 (0-7883-2034-3); pap. 47.50 (0-7883-2035-1) ABBE Pubs Assn.
Health - Problems & Progress. Samuel J. Huang & Paul Roby. 1989. (Illus.). 340p. (C). pap. text 29.95 (0-89863-135-1) Star Pub CA.
Health - The World's Most Important & Valuable Venture & Its Blatant Neglect: Index of New Information for Homo Sapiens on Planet Earth. John C. Bartone. 1998. (Illus.). 180p. 57.50 (0-7883-2012-2); pap. 47.50 (0-7883-2013-0) ABBE Pubs Assn.
Health—Dangers, Risks & Assessments: Index of Modern Authors & Subjects with Guide for Rapid Research. Mary B. Schneply. rev. ed. 1997. 177p. 57.50 (0-7883-1534-X); pap. 47.50 (0-7883-1535-8) ABBE Pubs Assn.
*Health Address Book: A Directory of Health Support Groups. Royal Society of Medicine Staff. 3rd ed. 2000. 226p. pap. (1-85315-455-5) Royal Soc of Medicine Pr Ltd GBR. Dist: Balogh.
Health Against Wealth. George Anders. 1998. LC 96-24869. 304p. pap. 15.00 (0-395-82282-3) HM.
Health Against Wealth: HMOs & the Breakdown of Medical Trust. George Anders. l.t. ed. 1997. LC 96-49737. 523p. 26.95 (0-7838-8054-5, Macmillan Ref) Gale.
Health Aide. Jack Rudman. 1994. (Career Examination Ser.: C-1301). pap. 23.95 (0-8373-1301-5) Nat Learn.
Health America. Tom McDevitt. 1992. 615p. pap., tchr. ed. 37.56 (0-933046-06-5); Chapter 26 Supplement. 1995. pap. 8.95 (0-933046-07-3) Little Red Hen.
Health & Access to Health Care: The Special Challenge of Older Women. 1994. 52p. (Orig.). (C). pap. text 25.00 (0-7881-1087-X) DIANE Pub.
Health & Aging. Tom Hickey. 1980. LC 79-25033. (Social Gerontology Ser.). 192p. (C). pap. 19.95 (0-8185-0374-2) Brooks-Cole.
Health & Biomedical Information in Europe. Paul Weiss. 1986. (Public Health in Europe Ser.: No. 27). 111p. pap. text 10.00 (92-890-1163-7, 1320027) World Health.
Health & British Magazines in the 19th Century: An Annotated Bibliography. E. M. Palmegiano. 1998. LC 98-3909. 296p. 65.00 (0-8108-3486-3) Scarecrow.
Health & Canadian Society: Sociological Perspectives. David Coburn. 3rd rev. ed. 1998. LC 98-218123. 1406p. text 60.00 (0-8020-4192-2); 1170p. pap. text 34.95 (0-8020-8052-9) U of Toronto Pr.
Health & Change in the Subarctic. T. Kue Young. 1988. (Illus.). 312p. pap. 16.95 (0-8020-6697-6); 168p. text 30.00 (0-8020-5784-5) U of Toronto Pr.
Health & Culture: Beyond the Western Paradigm. Collins O. Airhihenbuwa. 1995. LC 95-2551. (Illus.). 176p. 66.95 (0-8039-7156-7, 2673); pap. 32.95 (0-8039-7157-5, 2672) Sage.
Health & Cultures: Exploring the Relationships: Policy, Practices, & Education, Vol. I. Ed. by Ralph Masi et al. 1995. 300p. reprint ed. pap. 21.95 (0-88962-549-2) Mosaic.
Health & Cultures: Exploring the Relationships: Programs, Services & Care, Vol. II. Ed. by Ralph Masi et al. 1995. 300p. reprint ed. pap. 21.95 (0-88962-550-6) Mosaic.
Health & Deprivation: Inequality & the North. Peter Townsend et al. 1988. 192p. lib. bdg. (0-7099-4351-2) C Helm GBR. Dist: Routldge.
Health & Development. Ed. by David R. Phillips & Yola Verhasselt. 1994. LC 93-13465. (Illus.). 304p. (C). pap. 29.95 (0-415-08529-2) Routledge.
Health & Disease: A Reader. Ed. by Basiro Davey et al. 2nd ed. 1995. LC 94-2470. 384p. pap. (0-335-19209-2) OpUniv Pr.
Health & Disease: A Reader. Ed. by Basiro Davey et al. 2nd ed. 1995. LC 94-2470. 384p. 112.00 (0-335-19326-9) Taylor & Francis.
Health & Disease - Special Edition. Gary A. Thibodeau & Kevin T. Patton. 1991. (Illus.). 720p. (C). (gr. 13). text 32.95 (0-8016-6413-6, 06413) Mosby Inc.
Health & Disease among Women: Biological & Environmental Influences. Ed. by Roberta B. Ness & Lewis H. Kuller. 1998. (Illus.). 488p. text 65.00 (0-19-511396-9) OUP.
Health & Disease in Farm Animals. W. H. Parker. 3rd ed. 1980. text 86.00 (0-08-025900-6); pap. text 21.00 (0-08-025899-9) Elsevier (Pergamon Pr).
Health & Disease in Human History: A Journal of Interdisciplinary History Reader. Ed. by Robert I. Rotberg. 2000. LC 00-35135. (Journal of Interdisciplinary History Ser.). (Illus.). 345p. pap. 25.00 (0-262-68122-6); (C). 60.00 (0-262-18207-6) MIT Pr.
Health & Disease in the Holy Land: Studies in the History & Sociology of Medicine from Ancient Times to the Present. Ed. by Manfred Waserman & Samuel S. Kottek. 1996. LC 96-18883. 500p. text 109.95 (0-7734-8764-6) E Mellen.
Health & Diseases of Woman. R. T. Trall. 1991. lib. bdg. 74.95 (0-8490-4997-0) Gordon Pr.
Health & Ecological Assessment of Polynuclear Aromatic Hydrocarbons. Ed. by Si Duk Lee & Lester Grant. 1981. LC 80-83656. 378p. 57.00 (0-930376-20-X) Chem-Orbital.
Health & Ecological Implications of Radioactively Contaminated Environments. Ed. by C. R. Richmond. 1991. LC 91-10034. (Annual Meeting Proceedings Ser.: No. 12). 233p. (Orig.). pap. text 40.00 (0-929600-14-2) NCRP Pubns.
Health & Economics. Alan Williams. 1987. 256p. (0-333-43734-9) Intl Spec Bk.
Health & Efficiency: A Sociology of Health Economics. Malcolm Ashmore et al. 1989. 224p. (0-335-09913-0); pap. (0-335-09912-2) OpUniv Pr.
Health & Environment. Edgar Sydenstricker. 1972. LC 75-180593. (Medicine & Society in America Ser.). 234p. reprint ed. 20.95 (0-405-03975-1) Ayer.
Health & Environmental Hazards from Toxic Chemicals in Air: U. S.-Dutch Export Workshop. Ed. by T. Schneider et al. 1990. (Toxicology & Industrial Health Ser.: Vol. 6, No. 5). 65.00 (0-911131-22-1) Specialist Journals.
Health & Environmental Research on Complex Organic Mixtures. Ed. by Robert H. Gray. 1987. (Twenty-Fourth Hanford Symposium on Health & the Environment Ser.). 772p. 57.50 (0-935470-35-2) Battelle.
Health & Environmental Risk Assessment. Ricci & Rowe. 1985. 60.00 (0-08-031579-8, Pergamon Pr) Elsevier.
*Health & Ethnicity. Ed. by Helen Macbeth & Shetty Prakash. 2001. LC 00-46676. (Illus.). 256p. (C). (gr. 13). pap. 32.95 (0-415-24167-7) Routledge.
Health & Ethnicity. Helen Macbeth & Prakash S. Shetty. 2001. LC 00-46676. (Society for the Study of Human Biology Symposium Ser.: Vol. 41). (Illus.). 256p. 84.95 (0-415-24166-9) Routledge.
Health & Exclusion: Policy & Practice in Health Provision. Michael Purdy & David Banks. 1999. LC 98-51639. 224p. pap. 29.95 (0-415-18017-1) Routledge.
Health & Faith: Medical, Psychological & Religious Dimensions. Ed. by John T. Chirban. 1991. 152p. (C). pap. text 23.00 (0-8191-8285-0); lib. bdg. 44.50 (0-8191-8284-2) U Pr of Amer.
Health & Fitness. Ed. by Scott Barbour & Karin L. Swisher. 1996. LC 96-7203. (Opposing Viewpoints Ser.). 188p. 26.20 (1-56510-403-X); pap. 16.20 (1-56510-402-1) Gale (Greenhaven Pr).
Health & Fitness: Essentials for Men - Get Fit, Feel Great, Be Well. 2000. (Illus.). 192p. (1-84000-319-7, HEA015000) Mitchell Beazley GBR. Dist: Sterling, Sterling.
Health & Fitness Excellence: The Scientific Action Plan. Robert K. Cooper. 1990. 544p. pap. 16.00 (0-395-54453-X) HM.
Health & Fitness for Older Persons: Answers to Important Questions. James H. Humphrey. 1992. LC 90-49752. (Studies in Education: No. 9). 18.00 (0-404-61679-8) AMS Pr.
Health & Fitness in Modern Society, Vols. 1-5. Ed. by James H. Humphrey. (0-404-64150-4) AMS Pr.
Health & Fitness in Plain English. Jolie Bookspan. 1998. LC 98-201787. (Illus.). x, 357p. pap. 14.00 (1-57566-288-4, Knsington) Kensgtn Pub Corp.
Health & Fitness in the Workplace: Health Education in Business Organizations. Ed. by Samuel H. Klarreich. 1987. LC 87-18262. 428p. 88.00 (0-275-92359-2, C2359, Praeger Pubs) Greenwood.
Health & Free Radicals-Growing Importance of Research & Results: Index of New Information. Roscoe Y. Stoy. Date not set. (Illus.). 160p. 57.50 (0-7883-1868-3); pap. 47.50 (0-7883-1869-1) ABBE Pubs Assn.
Health & Global Environment. Ross H. Hall. 1990. 220p. (C). text 52.95 (0-7456-0559-1) Blackwell Pubs.
Health & Happiness: How You Can Be Healthier with Little Effort. Sara M. Jordan. 1998. 12.95 (0-8159-5702-5) Devin.
Health & Happiness: Simple, Safe & Sound Systems & Solutions. Emanuel Cheraskin. 1989. LC 88-62803. 250p. (Orig.). pap. 14.95 (0-942333-05-5) Bio-Comns Pr.
Health & Happiness Are Twins. Ethel Foresman. 1961. 10.00 (0-8315-0034-4) Speller.
Health & Healing: With a New Preface by the Author. Andrew Weil. 1998. LC 83-10845. 296p. pap. 13.00 (0-395-91153-2) HM.
Health & Healing in Early Modern England: Studies in Social & Intellectual History. Andrew Wear. 1998. LC 98-6523. (Variorum Collected Studies: Vol. 613). (Illus.). 332p. text (0-86078-690-0) Ashgate Pub GBR. Dist: Ashgate Pub Co.
Health & Health Behavior among Elderly Americans: An Age-Stratification Perspective. Fredric D. Wolinsky. 1990. LC 90-9417. 264p. 37.95 (0-8261-7410-8) Springer Pub.
Health & Health Care 3rd World. David Phillips. 1990. pap. 55.95 (0-582-01418-2, Drumbeat) Longman.
Health & Health Care in Britain. Rob Baggott. 1994. LC 93-43781. 49.95 (0-312-12109-1) St Martin.
Health & Health Care in Developing Countries: Sociological Perspectives. Ed. by Peter Conrad & Eugene B. Gallagher. 1993. LC 92-49629. 352p. (C). 59.95 (1-56639-027-3) Temple U Pr.
Health & Health Care in Israel: Studies of Israeli Society, Vol. 5. Ed. by Aaron Antonovsky. 1990. 400p. text 44.95 (0-88738-308-4); pap. text 24.95 (0-88738-824-8) Transaction Pubs.
Health & Health Care in Later Life. Christina R. Victor. 1991. 192p. pap. (0-335-09283-7) OpUniv Pr.
Health & Health Care in Latin America During the Lost Decade: Insights for the 1900s. Ed. by Connie Weil & Joseph L. Scarpaci. (Minnesota Latin American Series - Iowa International Papers: No. 3, Nos. 5-8). (Illus.). 359p. (Orig.). pap. 14.95 (0-910235-36-8) Prisma Bks.
Health & Health Care in New York City: Local, State, & National Perspectives. Compiled by Division of Research, Analysis, and Planning Staff. 1985. LC 85-8598. 136p. 25.00 (0-934459-04-5) United Hosp Fund.
Health & Health Care in New York City: Local, State, & National Perspectives. Melvin I. Krasner. 1988. 94p. 30.00 (0-934459-48-7) United Hosp Fund.
Health & Health Care in New York City: Local, State, & National Perspectives. United Hospital Fund Staff. 1987. 132p. 30.00 (0-934459-46-0) United Hosp Fund.
Health & Health Care in Transition: The Example of Vietnam. Ed. by Eric Naterop & Ivan Wolffers. 1996. LC 96-127627. (Primary Health Care Publications: No. 10). 114p. pap. (90-5383-406-0) VUB Univ Pr BEL. Dist: Paul & Co Pubs.
Health & Health Care Profile of New York City's New School Admissions, 1990-1991. Minh L. Griffin. 1993. 106p. 10.00 (0-88156-156-8) Comm Serv Soc NY.
*Health & Health Care 2010. 2nd ed. 2002. 300p. pap. 35.00 (0-7879-5974-X) Jossey-Bass.
Health & Health Care 2010: The Forecast, the Challenge. Contrib. by Institute for the Future Staff et al. 2000. LC 99-88438. (Illus.). 224p. pap. 28.00 (0-7879-5348-2) Jossey-Bass.
Health & Health Care Utilization in Later Life. Ed. by Jon Hendricks. 1995. LC 94-20403. (Perspectives on Aging & Human Development Ser.). 228p. pap. 28.95 (0-89503-168-X) Baywood Pub.
Health & Health Services: An Introduction to Health Care in Britain. John R. Butler & Michael S. Vaile. 1984. LC 83-27031. 256p. (Orig.). 15.95 (0-7100-9902-9, Routledge Thoemms) Routledge.
Health & Healthcare in the United States. Michael J. Long. 1988. LC 98-12438. 175p. 42.00 (1-56793-086-7) Health Admin Pr.
*Health & HIV/AIDS. Commonwealth Secretariat Staff. 2001. (Gender Management System Ser.). 72p. pap. (0-85092-655-6) Comm Sec GBR. Dist: Stylus Pub VA.
Health & Human Behavior. Robert E. Kaplan et al. 1993. (C). pap. text, tchr. ed. 35.00 (0-07-033567-2) McGraw.
Health & Human Behavior. Robert E. Kaplan et al. 1993. 576p. (C). text 65.00 (0-07-033566-4) McGrw-H Hghr Educ.
Health & Human Nature. Paul Snyder. 1980. LC 78-14627. 256p. pap. 10.95 (0-8019-6798-8) NP-Chilton.
Health & Human Rights: A Reader. Jonathan M. Mann. 1999. LC 98-20899. 448p. (C). 90.00 (0-415-92101-5) Routledge.
Health & Human Rights: A Reader. Ed. by Jonathan M. Mann et al. 1999. LC 98-20899. 448p. pap. 30.95 (0-415-92102-3, D5779) Routledge.
Health & Human Rights in Burma. Howard Hu et al. 1991. 14p. pap. 3.00 (1-879707-04-7) Phy Human Rights.
Health & Humanitarian Concerns: Principles & Ethics. Henryk L. Zielinski. 1994. LC 94-3631. (Nijhoff Law Specials Ser.). 140p. (C). pap. text (0-7923-2963-5) M Nijhoff NLD. Dist: Kluwer Academic.

Health & Hygiene: Skills for Life. Couch et al. 1996. pap. 24.00 net. (*0-314-20343-5*) Thomson Learn.

Health & Illness: The Lay Perspective. Michael W. Calnan. 1987. LC 87-1534. 192p. pap. (*0-422-79420-1*) Tavistock GBR. *Dist:* Routldge.

Health & Illness in a Changing Japanese Society. Kyoichi Sonoda. 1988. 200p. (*0-86008-424-8*) U of Tokyo JPN. *Dist:* Col U Pr.

Health & Illness in a Changing Society. Michael Bury & Mary Ann Elston. 1997. LC 97-199904. (Illus.). 240p. (C). 85.00 (*0-415-11514-0*); pap. 29.95 (*0-415-11515-9*) Routledge.

Health & Lifestyle Survey: Seven Years On. Ed. by Brian D. Cox. 1993. 412p. (*1-85521-410-5*) Dartmth Pub GBR. *Dist:* Ashgate Pub Co.

Health & Light. John N. Ott. 1990. LC 72-85334. 232p. pap. 10.95 (*0-89804-098-1*) Ariel GA.

Health & Light. John N. Ott. 1988. (Illus.). 225p. 12.95 (*0-8159-5703-3*) Devin.

Health & Low-Frequency Electromagnetic Fields. William R. Bennett, Jr. 1994. LC 93-40340. (Illus.). 208p. (C). 30.00 (*0-300-05763-6*) Yale U Pr.

Health & Medical Aspects of Disaster Preparedness. Ed. by J. C. Duffy. 1990. (NATO Challenges of Modern Society Ser.: Vol. 14). (Illus.). 200p. (C). text 107.00 (*0-306-43495-4*, Kluwer Plenum) Kluwer Academic.

Health & Medical Care in the U. S. A Critical Analysis. Ed. by Vicente Navarro. 1977. LC 77-70380. (Policy, Politics, Health & Medicine Ser.: Vol. 1). 162p. pap. 25.00 (*0-89503-000-4*) Baywood Pub.

Health & Medical Care of African-Americans. Ed. by Wornie L. Reed. 1993. LC 92-30000. 184p. 55.00 (*0-86569-217-3*, T217); pap. 18.95 (*0-86569-218-1*, R218) Greenwood (Auburn Hse).

Health & Medical Care of African-Americans, Vol. V. Ed. by Wornie L. Reed. 1990. (Assessment of the Status of African-Americans Ser.). 150p. (C). pap. 8.95 (*1-878358-01-4*) U MA W M Trotter Inst.

Health & Medical Concerns on Infections. Albert E. Jones. 1992. (Health Concerns Ser.). (Illus.). 131p. pap. text 18.95 (*1-883883-00-8*) A E Jones Sci.

Health & Medical Diagnostic Errors in Human Therapy & Treatments: Index of New Information. Elgin S. Witzleban. 1994. 150p. 57.50 (*0-7883-0002-4*); pap. 47.50 (*0-7883-0003-2*) ABBE Pubs Assn.

Health & Medical Year Book, 1993. Colliers. 1993. 45.00 (*0-02-942578-6*) Free Pr.

Health & Medicine in Britain since 1860. Anne Hardy. 2000. LC 00-30890. (Social History in Perspective Ser.). xi, 220p. (*0-312-23738-3*) St Martin.

Health & Medicine in Medieval Southern Italy. Patricia Skinner. 1997. LC 96-45334. (Illus.). 192p. 65.50 (*90-04-10394-5*) Brill Academic Pubs.

Health & Medicine in the Eastern Orthodox Tradition: Faith, Liturgy & Wholeness. Stanley Samuel Harakas. 2nd ed. 1990. LC 89-9998. (Health & Medicine in Faith Tradition Ser.). 190p. reprint ed. pap. 15.95 (*0-8245-0934-X*) Light&Life Pub Co MN.

Health & Medicine in the Islamic Tradition: Change & Identity. Fazlur Rahman. 1997. LC 99-216697. 156p. (C). pap. 15.95 (*1-871031-64-8*) Kazi Pubns.

Health & Medicine on the Internet: An Annual Guide to the World Wide Web for Health Care Professionals. Ed. by James Davis et al. 1998. (Illus.). 600p. (Orig.). pap. text 29.95 (*1-57066-065-4*, ME121) Practice Mgmt Info.

Health & Medicine on the Internet: Annual Guide to the World Wide Web. annuals Ed. by James Davis. 1998. LC 96-78922. (Illus.). 622p. (Orig.). pap. 19.95 (*1-885987-03-X*, ME078, Health Info Pr) Practice Mgmt Info.

***Health & Medicine on the Internet 2001.** annuals Ed. by Maureen Lynch. 2001. (Illus.). 1500p. pap. text 29.95 (*1-57066-207-X*, 21090) Practice Mgmt Info.

Health & Medicine on the Internet, 2000: Annual Guide to the World Wide Web for Consumers. Ed. by Maureen Lynch et al. 2nd rev. ed. 2000. (Illus.). 950p. pap. 19.95 (*1-885987-18-8*, ME093, Health Info Pr) Practice Mgmt Info.

Health & Medicine on the Internet, 2000: Annual Guide to the World Wide Web for Health Care Professionals. Ed. by James B. Davis et al. 2nd rev. ed. 1999. (Illus.). 950p. pap. 29.95 (*1-57066-144-8*) Practice Mgmt Info.

Health & Mental Health: Directory of Key Legislators & Legislative Staff. 1991. 83p. 10.00 (*1-55516-695-4*, 6632) Natl Conf State Legis.

Health & National Reconstruction in Nationalist China: The Development of Modern Health Services, 1928-1937. Ka-che Yip. 1996. LC 95-32271. (Monograph & Occasional Papers: No. 50). 34.00 (*0-924304-28-6*) Assn Asian Studies.

Health & Numbers: Basic Biostatistical Methods. Chap T. Le. 1994. LC 94-25553. 260p. pap. 62.50 (*0-471-01248-3*) Wiley.

Health & Physical Assessment. Violet H. Barkauskas et al. (Illus.). tchr. ed. (*0-8151-0407-3*) Mosby Inc.

Health & Physical Assessment. Ed. by Violet H. Barkauskas. 2nd ed. 1997. LC 97-14864. (Illus.). 816p. (C). (gr. 12). text 56.00 (*0-8151-2776-6*, 31045) Mosby Inc.

Health & Physical Assessment. Violet H. Barkauskas et al. 2nd ed. 1998. (Illus.). 816p. stu. ed. (*0-323-00032-0*) Mosby Inc.

Health & Physical Assessment. Violet Barkauskas et al. 3rd ed. 2001. (Illus.). 745p. pap. text (*0-323-01214-0*) Mosby Inc.

Health & Physical Assessment: Includes Testbank. Violet Barkauskas et al. 2nd ed. 1998. (Illus.). 816p. tchr. ed. (*0-8151-2802-9*) Mosby Inc.

***Health & Physical Assessment: Instructor's Resource Manual.** Violet Barkauskas et al. 3rd ed. 2001. (Illus.). (*0-323-01231-0*) Mosby Inc.

Health & Physical Education 2001. Dianne R. Hales. Ed. by Charlene Zart. 2000. LC 00-43976. pap. 31.00 net. (*0-534-58203-6*) Wadsworth Pub.

Health & Population Information As APLIC Comes of Age: APLIC Proceedings of the 21st Annual Conference. Ed. by Jane Vanderlin & William Barrows. 1989. 112p. (Orig.). pap. text 16.00 (*0-933438-14-1*) APLIC Intl.

Health & Poverty. Ed. by Michael J. Holosko & Marvin D. Feit. 1997. LC 97-9585. (Illus.). 252p. (C). 49.95 (*0-7890-0149-7*); pap. 24.95 (*0-7890-0228-0*) Haworth Pr.

Health & Safety. NEBS Management Staff. 1986. (Open Learning for Supervisory Management Ser.). pap. text 19.50 (*0-08-033961-1*, Pergamon Pr) Elsevier.

Health & Safety. 2nd ed. 1991. (Open Learning Super Ser.). pap. text 26.00 (*0-08-041644-6*, Pergamon Pr) Elsevier.

Health & Safety Audits. John W. Spencer. 1992. 325p. pap. text 85.00 (*0-86587-297-X*) Gov Insts.

Health & Safety Beyond the Workplace. Ed. by Lester V. Cralley et al. 1990. 336p. 350.00 (*0-471-50452-1*) Wiley.

Health & Safety Book. 1986. (Open Learning for Supervisory Management Ser.). pap. text 19.50 (*0-08-070109-4*, Pergamon Pr) Elsevier.

Health & Safety for Nurses. Chard. 1993. 250p. pap. 41.50 (*1-56593-142-4*, 0454) Singular Publishing.

Health & Safety Guidelines for the Laboratory. Lynn Montgomery. 1995. LC 94-8501. 20.00 (*0-89189-382-2*) Am Soc Clinical.

Health & Safety in Schools. David Brierley. 1991. (Administration & Leadership Ser.). 240p. pap. (*1-85396-130-2*, 83738) P Chapman GBR. *Dist:* Sage.

Health & Safety in Small Industry: A Practical Guide for Managers. University of Medicine and Dentistry of New Jersey Staff. 1989. (Illus.). 224p. lib. bdg. 79.95 (*0-87371-195-5*, L195) Lewis Pubs.

Health & Safety Management for Medical Practices 2000. Linda F. Chaff. 2000. 200p. pap. 70.00 (*1-57947-083-1*) AMA.

Health & Safety of Workers: Case Studies in the Politics of Professional Responsibility. Ed. by Ronald Bayer. 1988. 318p. text 45.00 (*0-19-505365-6*) OUP.

Health & Science Majors. Peterson's Guides Staff. 6th ed. 1998. (Peterson's Job Opportunities for Health Ser.). 216p. pap. text 21.95 (*0-7689-0025-5*) Petersons.

Health & Selected Socioeconomic Characteristics of the Family: United States, 1988-1990. 1996. LC 96-50051. (Vital & Health Statistics Ser.: Series 10, No. 195). (*0-8406-0523-4*) Natl Ctr Health Stats.

Health & Social Change in International Perspective. Ed. by Lincoln C. Chen et al. 1994. LC 93-1755. (Series on Population & International Health). (Illus.). 420p. pap. text 17.95 (*0-674-38562-4*) HUP.

Health & Social Change in Russia & Eastern Europe. William C. Cockerham. 1999. LC 98-29877. 288p. (C). pap. 24.95 (*0-415-92081-7*, D5647); (gr. 13). 80.00 (*0-415-92080-9*, D5643) Routledge.

Health & Social Class in Imperial Germany. Richrad Spree. 1988. LC 87-22397. 208p. 19.95 (*0-85496-527-0*) Berg Pubs.

Health & Social Needs of Young Adults with Physical Disabilities. Ed. by Andrew Thomas et al. 1991. (Clinics in Developmental Medicine Ser.: No. 106). (Illus.). 161p. (C). text (*0-521-41222-6*) Mc Keith Pr GBR. *Dist:* Cambridge U Pr.

Health & Social Organization: Towards a Health Policy for the Twenty-First Century. Ed. by David Blane et al. 1996. LC 96-222385. 344p. (C). pap. 27.95 (*0-415-13070-0*) Routledge.

Health & Social Policy. Marvin D. Feit & Stanley F. Battle. 1995. LC 93-6093. (Illus.). 292p. lib. bdg. 49.95 (*1-56024-342-2*); pap. 19.95 (*1-56024-343-0*) Haworth Pr.

Health & Social Science in Latin America. Ugalde. 1985. (Social Science & Medicine Ser.). pap. 28.00 (*0-08-033374-5*, Pergamon Pr) Elsevier.

Health & Social Support of the Elderly. K. Raube. 1994. 124p. (Orig.). (C). pap. text 40.00 (*0-7881-1056-X*) DIANE Pub.

Health & Social Welfare. Ed. by Edgard Pisani. 1990. (Journal of Contemporary European Affairs Ser.: No. 2). 182p. pap. 13.00 (*0-08-040234-8*, 2701; 2902; 3002, Pergamon Pr) Elsevier.

Health & Societies. 256p. (*0-340-62512-0*) E A GBR. *Dist:* Routldge.

Health & Societies: Changing Perspectives. Sarah Curtis & Ann Taket. 1995. (Arnold Publication). (Illus.). 384p. pap. 35.00 (*0-340-62513-9*) OUP.

Health & Society: A Collection of Articles 131. Jan Marquard. 1998. text 15.95 (*1-56870-326-0*) RonJon Pub.

Health & Society in 20th Century Britain. Helen Jones. 1994. LC 93-25751. (Themes in British Social History Ser.). (C). pap. text 32.50 (*0-582-00459-4*) Longman.

Health & Society in Britain since 1939. Virginia Berridge. 1999. LC 98-43280. (New Studies in Economic & Social History: No. 38). (Illus.). 144p. (C). text 39.95 (*0-521-57230-4*); pap. text 11.95 (*0-521-57641-5*) Cambridge U Pr.

Health & Society in Revolutionary Russia. Ed. by Susan G. Solomon & John F. Hutchinson. 1990. LC 89-45410. (Indiana-Michigan Series in Russian & East European Studies). (Illus.). 270p. 29.95 (*0-253-35332-7*) Ind U Pr.

Health & Sugar Substitutes. Ed. by B. Guggenheim. 1979. pap. 83.50 (*3-8055-2961-9*) S Karger.

Health & the American Indian. Ed. by Priscilla A. Day & Hilary N. Weaver. 1999. LC 99-12963. 88p. 49.95 (*0-7890-0658-8*) Haworth Pr.

Health & the Environment. 1979. (Public Health in Europe Ser.: No. 8). 161p. 18.00 (*92-9020-127-4*, 1320008) World Health.

Health & the Environment. Fiona Godlee & Alison Walker. 1992. (Illus.). 126p. pap. text (*0-7279-0318-7*) BMJ Pub GBR. *Dist:* AIDC.

Health & the Environment: One Lung to Go. Leonard F. Pax. 2000. 240p. 22.95 (*1-58244-085-9*) Rutledge Bks.

Health & the Female Adolescent. Ed. by Sharon Golub. 1985. LC 84-19772. (Women & Politics Ser.: Vol. 9, Nos. 2 & 3). 141p. pap. text 14.95 (*0-918393-05-1*, Harrington Park) Haworth Pr.

***Health & the Food-Chain.** Ed. by David I. Thurnham & Terry A. Roberts. 2000. (British Medical Bulletin Ser.: Vol. 56, No. 1). 274p. pap. (*1-85315-453-9*) Royal Soc of Medicine Pr Ltd GBR. *Dist:* Balogh.

Health & the Hunter-Gatherer. G. T. Nurse & T. Jenkins. 1976. (Monographs in Human Genetics: Vol. 8). 44.50 (*3-8055-2401-3*) S Karger.

Health & the Law: A Handbook for Health Professionals. Tom Christoffel. 1985. LC 82-70808. 450p. pap. 19.95 (*0-02-905960-7*) Free Pr.

Health & the National Health Service. John Carrier & Ian Kendall. LC 97-18611. 420p. (C). 1998. (*0-485-80007-1*); 1997. pap. (*0-485-80107-8*) Athlone Pr GBR. *Dist:* Transaction Pubs.

Health & the New Civilization. Mokichi Okada. 1991. LC 91-60112. 96p. (Orig.). pap. 3.75 (*0-9629183-0-X*) Johrei Fellow.

Health & the New Media: Technologies Transforming Personal & Public Health. Ed. by Linda M. Harris. 1995. (Communication Ser.). 280p. text 69.95 (*0-8058-1569-4*); LC 95-7208. (Illus.). pap. 29.95 (*0-8058-1954-1*) L Erlbaum Assocs.

Health & the Rise of Civilization. Mark N. Cohen. 1991. 295p. (C). reprint ed. pap. 18.00 (*0-300-05023-2*) Yale U Pr.

Health & the Sociology of Emotions. Veronica James & Jonathan Gabe. 1997. LC 96-47977. pap. 22.95 (*0-631-20351-6*) Blackwell Pubs.

Health & Toxicology. Nicholas P. Cheremisinoff. 1997. LC 96-40506. 768p. 150.00 (*0-88415-386-X*) Buttrwrth-Heinemann.

Health & Wealth from Within. William E. Towne. 1981. 175p. pap. 7.50 (*0-89540-081-2*, SB-081) Sun Pub.

***Health & Welfare for Families in the 21st Century.** Helen Wallace et al. 2nd ed. 2002. (Illus.). (C). pap. text 59.95 (*0-7637-1859-9*, 1859-9) Jones & Bartlett.

Health & Well-Being. Michele MacDonnell. 2000. 64p. pap. (*1-84215-123-1*, Swater) Ann3ess GBR. *Dist:* AOL Time Warner.

Health & Well-Being: Ayurveda. Sally Morningstar. 2000. 64p. pap. 6.95 (*1-84215-171-1*) Anness Pub.

Health & Well-Being: Color. Lilian Verner-Bonds. 2000. 64p. pap. (*1-84215-092-8*, Swater) Ann3ess GBR. *Dist:* AOL Time Warner.

Health & Wellness. Questech Staff. 1997. (Illus.). 120p. text 99.95 (*1-58100-022-7*) Beckley Cardy.

Health & Wellness. Gordon Edlin & Eric Golanty. 2nd ed. 1985. (Illus.). 667p. (C). pap. text 22.50 (*0-86720-055-3*, 055-3) Jones & Bartlett.

Health & Wellness. Gordon Edlin & Eric Golanty. 4th ed. 1992. (Illus.). (C). pap. text 195.00 (*0-86720-764-7*, 764-7) Jones & Bartlett.

Health & Wellness. Gordon Edlin et al. 5th ed. (Illus.). (C). 1998. LC 97-52084. 312p. pap. text 47.50 (*0-7637-0718-X*, 0718-X); 1996. 544p. pap. text 48.95 (*0-86720-994-1*, 994-1) Jones & Bartlett.

Health & Wellness Reference Guide. Prod. by McGowan Publications Staff. 1998. (Illus.). 568p. pap. 59.95 (*1-928752-20-9*) Mc Gowan Pubns.

Health & Wholeness. Bart Resta. 1994. (Lifesearch Ser.). 64p. (Orig.). pap. text 6.00 (*0-687-77869-7*) Abingdon.

Health & Work: Critical Perspectives. Norma Daykin. 1999. LC 99-19219. 272p. 55.00 (*0-312-22342-0*) St Martin.

Health & Work under Capitalism: An International Perspective. Ed. by Vicente Navarro & Daniel Berman. 1983. (Policy, Politics, Health & Medicine Ser.: Vol. 5). 311p. pap. text 31.00 (*0-89503-035-7*) Baywood Pub.

Health as Expanding Consciousness. Margaret A. Newman. 2nd ed. 1994. 174p. pap. 36.95 (*0-88737-620-7*, 14-2626) Natl League Nurse.

Health As Liberation: Medicine, Theology & the Quest for Justice. Alastair V. Campbell. 1995. LC 94-40930. 112p. (Orig.). 14.95 (*0-8298-1022-6*) Pilgrim OH.

Health Aspects of Aging: The Experience of Growing Old. Gari Lesnoff-Caravaglia. 1999. LC 99-44461. vii, 206p. text 41.95 (*0-398-07011-3*); pap. text 29.95 (*0-398-07012-1*) C C Thomas.

Health Aspects of Chemical & Biological Weapons: Report of a WHO Group of Consultants. 1970. 132p. pap. text 12.00 (*92-4-156034-7*, 1150068) World Health.

Health Aspects of Endurance Training. Ed. by O. Appenzeller. 1978. (Medicine & Sport Science Ser.: Vol. 12). 41.75 (*3-8055-2960-0*) S Karger.

Health Aspects of Environmental Pollution Control-Planning & Implementation of Nationnal Programmes: Proceedings of the WHO Expert Committee, Geneva, 1973. WHO Staff. 1974. (Technical Reports: No. 554). pap. text 6.00 (*92-4-120554-7*, 1100554) World Health.

Health Aspects of Family Planning: A Guide to Resources in the United States. Allison G. Stettner & Anita P. Cowan. 1982. LC 81-1651. 247p. (C). 43.95 (*0-89885-005-3*, Kluwer Acad Hman Sci) Kluwer Academic.

Health Aspects of Human Settlements: A Review Base on the Technical Discussions Held During 29th WHA, 1976. A. Martin. 1977. (Public Health Papers: No. 66). 57p. pap. text 8.00 (*92-4-130066-3*, 1110066) World Health.

Health Aspects of Nitrates & Its Metabolites (Particularly Nitrite) Proceedings - International Workshop - Bilthoven (Netherlands), 8-10 November, 1994. 1995. (*92-871-2792-1*) Council of Europe FRA. *Dist:* Manhattan Pub Co.

Health Aspects of Pregnancy & Childbirth, United States, 1982-88. Anjani Chandra. 1995. LC 95-32301. (Vital & Health Statistics Ser.: Series 23, No. 18). (*0-8406-0509-9*) Natl Ctr Health Stats.

Health Aspects of Residues of Anabolics in Meat: Report on a WHO Working Group. 1982. (Euro Reports & Studies Ser.: No. 59). 38p. pap. text 4.00 (*92-890-1225-0*) World Health.

Health Aspects of Supply & Use of Non-Human Primates for Biomedical Purposes: Proceedings of the WHO Scientific Group, Geneva, 1970. WHO Staff. 1971. (Technical Reports: No. 470). pap. text 5.00 (*92-4-120470-2*, 1100470) World Health.

Health Aspects of Using Smoke Flavours As Food Ingredients. 1992. (*92-871-2189-3*) Council of Europe FRA. *Dist:* Manhattan Pub Co.

Health Assessment. Melcher. Date not set. text (*0-7216-1913-4*) Saunders.

Health Assessment: An Illustrated Pocket Guide. June M. Thompson. 3rd ed. 1991. (Illus.). 96p. (C). (gr. 13). pap. text 8.95 (*0-8016-6577-9*, 06577) Mosby Inc.

Health Assessment: Spanish-English Version. Diana V. Sanchez. Ed. by Gloria Picariello. 1995. LC 94-61759. (ENG & SPA., Illus.). 128p. pap. 24.95 (*1-880254-23-9*) Vista.

Health Assessment No. 2. Susan F. Wilson & Jean Foret. 2nd ed. 2000. (Illus.). 845p. text 58.00 (*0-323-00876-3*) Mosby Inc.

Health Assessment & Physical Examination. Estes. 1997. LC 97-13500. (Nursing Education Ser.). 880p. (C). 75.95 (*0-8273-7147-0*) Delmar.

Health Assessment & Physical Examination: Student Lab Manual. Estes & Schaefer. 1998. 240p. stu. ed., lab manual ed. 18.95 (*0-7668-0911-0*) Delmar.

Health Assessment & Promotion Strategies Through the Life Span. Ruth B. Murray & Judith P. Zentner. 6th ed. 1997. 136p. tchr. ed. (*0-8385-6990-0*, A6990-4) Appleton & Lange.

Health Assessment for Nursing Practice. Jean Giddens. 1998. (Illus.). 352p. stu. ed., wbk. ed. (*1-55664-502-3*) Mosby Inc.

Health Assessment for Nursing Practice. June M. Thompson & Susan F. Wilson. 1996. (Illus.). 864p. (C). (gr. 13). text 55.00 (*0-8151-8774-2*, 27168) Mosby Inc.

***Health Assessment for Nursing Practice: Computerized Test Bank.** Susan F. Wilson & Jean F. Giddens. 2nd ed. 2001. 500.00 (*0-323-00988-3*) Mosby Inc.

***Health Assessment for Nursing Practice: Instructor's Resource Manual.** Susan F. Wilson & Jean F. Giddens. 2nd ed. 2001. 250.00 (*0-323-00987-5*) Mosby Inc.

Health Assessment in Nursing. Lina K. Sims et al. 1994. LC 94-38953. 800p. (C). 70.99 (*0-8053-7347-0*) Addison-Wesley.

Health Assessment in Nursing: Clinical Handbook. Lina K. Sims et al. 1995. LC 94-45761. (C). pap. text 27.19 (*0-8053-7349-7*) Addison-Wesley.

Health Assessment in Nursing: Includes Free Asses. Tools. Janet Weber. 1997. LC 97-24815. 1,232p. text 58.95 (*0-397-55325-0*) Lppncott W & W.

Health Assessment Manual. Dorothy A. Jones. 1991. 17.95 (*0-8016-6052-1*) Mosby Inc.

Health Assessment Nursing Handbook. Sims. 1995. pap. text 90.13 (*0-8053-7354-3*) Benjamin-Cummings.

Health Assessment of the Older Individual, Vol. 2. Mathy D. Mezey et al. 2nd rev. ed. 1993. LC 92-49574. (Geriatric Nursing Ser.). 256p. 29.95 (*0-8261-2902-1*) Springer Pub.

Health at Home: Your Complete Guide to Symptoms, Solutions, & Self-Care. American Institute for Preventive Medicine Staff & Don R. Powell. 6th ed. 2000. LC 97-169384. (Illus.). 384p. (Orig.). pap. 17.95 (*0-9635612-8-6*) Am Inst Prevent.

H I

Health at the Crossroads: Exploring the Conflict Between Natural Healing & Conventional Medicine. Dean Black. 1988. 168p. pap. 8.95 (*0-929283-07-4*) Tapestry Pr.

Health at the Crossroads: Transport Policy & Urban Health. Ed. by Tony McMichael & Anthony C. Fletcher. 1997. LC 96-4969. 354p. 117.95 (*0-471-96272-4*) Wiley.

Health Basics. M. Thorson. 1995. (Illus.). 100p. (Orig.). 23.00 (*1-56216-160-1*); pap. 14.00 (*1-56216-161-X*) Systems Co.

Health Behavior: Emerging Research Perspectives. D. S. Gochman. 1988. LC 88-19672. (Illus.). 464p. (C). text 75.00 (*0-306-42874-1*, Kluwer Plenum) Kluwer Academic.

Health, Behavior & the Community: An Ecological Perspective. Ralph Catalano. 1979. LC 78-23714. (General Psychology Ser.: Vol. 76). (Illus.). 55.00 (*0-08-022972-7*); pap. 19.95 (*0-08-022971-9*) Elsevier (Pergamon Pr).

Health Behaviors. Rosalind Reed & Thomas A. Lang. 1986. LC 85-26551. (Illus.). 602p. (C). pap. text, tchr. ed. (*0-314-96653-6*); 2nd ed. mass mkt. 42.00 (*0-314-93409-X*) West Pub.

Health Benefits at Work: An Economic & Political Analysis of Employment-Based Health Insurance. Mark V. Pauly. 1997. LC 97-18341. 200p. (C). text 44.50 (*0-472-10857-3*, 10857) U of Mich Pr.

Health Benefits Clerk. Jack Rudman. 1994. (Career Examination Ser.: C-3558). pap. 27.95 (*0-8373-3558-2*) Nat Learn.

Health Benefits Guide for Seniors see Long-Term Care Planning Guide

Health Benefits of Cayenne. John Heinerman. 1998. LC 98-204450. (Keats Good Health Guides). 48p. pap. 3.95 (*0-87983-703-9*, 37039K, Keats Pubng) McGraw-Hill Trade.

Health Benefits of FOS (Fructooligosaccharides) Robert Crayhon. Ed. by Don R. Bensen. 1995. (Good Health Guides). 48p. pap. 3.95 (*0-87983-693-8*, 36938K, Keats Pubng) McGraw-Hill Trade.

Health Benefits of HGH. Aftab J. Ahmed. 1998. (Good Health Guides). 48p. pap. 3.95 (*0-87983-817-5*, 38175K, Keats Pubng) McGraw-Hill Trade.

Health Benefits of Smoking Cessation. Set. 1995. lib. bdg. 599.95 (*0-8490-7572-6*) Gordon Pr.

Health Benefits of Smoking Cessation: A Report of the Surgeon General. 1995. (Illus.). 628p. (Orig.). (C). pap. text 50.00 (*0-7881-2315-7*) DIANE Pub.

Health Cards '97. Ed. by L. Van den Broek & A. J. Sikkel. 1997. LC 97-77028. (Studies in Health Technology & Informatics: Vol. 49). 250p. 86.00 (*90-5199-379-X*) IOS Press.

Health-Care. Ed. by Gordon Gebert. 1981. 40p. pap. 20.00 (*0-08-028091-9*, Pergamon Pr) Elsevier.

Health Care. Ed. by James D. Torr. 2000. LC 98-55105. (Opposing Viewpoints Ser.). 221p. (YA). (gr. 9 up). 21.96 (*0-7377-0129-3*, Greenhaven Pr) Gale.

Health Care: An International Perspective. Ed. by John M. Virgo. 1984. LC 83-82337. 325p. (Orig.). pap. 25.00 (*0-914943-00-6*) IHEMI.

Health Care: Conflicting Opinions, Tough Decisions. William Weiss. 1992. 330p. (Orig.). pap. (*1-55021-071-8*) NC Ltd CAN. *Dist:* U of Toronto Pr.

Health Care: Employers Urge Hospitals to Battle Costs Using Performance Data Systems. 1995. (Illus.). 47p. (Orig.). (C). pap. text 20.00 (*0-7881-1775-0*) DIANE Pub.

Health Care: Federal & State Antitrust Actions Concerning the Health Care Industry. 1995. 60p. (Orig.). (C). pap. text 30.00 (*0-7881-1860-9*) DIANE Pub.

Health Care: History, Hype, & Help. Edward Annis et al. 1994. 61p. 10.00 (*1-886306-11-7*) Nevada Policy.

Health Care Across the Border: The Experience of U. S. Citizens in Mexico. David C. Warner & Kevin J. Reed. 1993. (U. S. - Mexican Policy Report Ser.: No. 4). 252p. pap. 15.00 (*0-89940-319-0*) LBJ Sch Pub Aff.

Health Care Administration: Planning, Implementing, & Managing Organized Delivery Systems. Lawrence F. Wolper. 3rd ed. 1999. LC 98-45196. 736p. 79.00 (*0-8342-1066-5*, 10665) Aspen Pub.

Health Care Administrative Costs: State of Minnesota. James Nobles. 1998. (Illus.). 96p. reprint ed. pap. text 20.00 (*0-7881-4210-0*) DIANE Pub.

Health Care Administrator's Managed Care Manual. Ed. by David B. Nash. 1997. (Illus.). 250p. (Orig.). spiral bd. 54.95 (*1-890045-05-5*) T L C Med Pub.

Health Care after Retirement: Who Will Pay the Cost? John C. Goodman & Gerald L. Musgrave. 1989. 38p. pap. 10.00 (*0-943802-42-3*, 139) Natl Ctr Pol.

Health Care Agenda for the States. Ed. by Louise Arnheim & Lee Webb. 1985. 150p. 10.95 (*0-89788-083-8*) CPA Washington.

Health Care Alliances & Conversions: A Handbook for Nonprofit Trustees. James Schwartz & H. Chester Horn, Jr. 1998. LC 98-40155. (Business & Management Ser.). (Illus.). 198p. 70.00 (*0-7879-4177-8*) Jossey-Bass.

Health Care Almanac: A Resource Guide to the Medical Field. American Medical Association Staff. 1999. (Illus.). 410p. pap. 29.95 (*0-89970-707-6*, OP311795WE) AMA.

Health Care Alternative Dispute Resolution. AHLCC Staff. 2000. LC 00-61070. (Illus.). 486p. ring bd. 199.00 (*0-8342-1794-5*) Aspen Pub.

Health Care Alternatives: A Report. Center for Self-Sufficiency Staff. rev. ed. 1993. 90p. ring bd. 27.95 (*0-910811-37-7*) Ctr Self Suff.

Health Care & Antitrust Law. Set. John J. Miles. 1992. LC 92-5626. (Health Law Ser.). ring bd. 475.00 (*0-87632-831-1*) West Group.

Health Care & Cost Containment in the European Union. Ed. by Elias Mossialos & Julian Le Grand. 1999. LC 98-44661. 600p. text (*1-84014-403-3*) Ashgate Pub GBR. *Dist:* Ashgate Pub Co.

Health Care & Disability Case Management. Ed. by Michael J. Leahy & Fong Chan Onn. unabr. ed. 1999. LC 98-60530. (Illus.). 715p. pap. text 60.00 (*0-9664026-0-X*) Vocat Consult.

Health Care & Freedom: An American Dilemma. James H. Parker. 1993. 88p. (Orig.). (C). 45.50 (*0-8191-9302-X*); pap. 19.50 (*0-8191-9303-8*) U Pr of Amer.

Health Care & Gender. Charlotte F. Muller. 1992. (Illus.). 258p. pap. 14.95 (*0-87154-611-6*); 1990. LC 90-8383. 272p. text 45.00 (*0-87154-610-8*) Russell Sage.

Health Care & Human Values. Ed. by Gary E. McCuen. 1993. (Ideas in Conflict Ser.). (Illus.). 180p. (YA). (gr. 7-12). lib. bdg. 15.95 (*0-86596-088-7*) G E M.

Health Care & Industrial Relations: Costs, Conflicts & Controversy. Ed. by Rosalind M. Schwartz. 1981. (Monograph & Research Ser.: No. 28). 90p. 7.50 (*0-89215-112-9*) U Cal LA Indus Rel.

Health Care & Information Ethics: Protecting Fundamental Human Rights. Ed. by Audrey Chapman. 1997. LC 97-772. 480p. (Orig.). pap. 29.95 (*1-55612-922-X*, LL1922) Sheed & Ward WI.

Health Care & Its Costs. Ed. by Carl J. Schramm. 1987. LC 87-7710. (American Assembly Ser.). (Illus.). 301p. (C). pap. text 8.50 (*0-393-95671-7*) Norton.

Health Care & Its Costs: A Challenge for the Church. Ed. by Walter E. Wiest. 1988. LC 88-21540. (Illus.). 356p. (C). pap. text 37.00 (*0-8191-7130-1*); lib. bdg. 63.00 (*0-8191-7129-8*) U Pr of Amer.

Health Care & Its Financing in the Single European Market. Ed. by R. Leidl. 1997. LC 97-75044. (Biomedical & Health Research Ser.: Vol. 18). 35p. 92.00 (*90-5199-359-5*, 359-5) IOS Press.

Health Care & Medicine on the Internet. Mary J. Cronin. 1997. 400p. text 49.95 (*0-442-02560-2*, VNR) Wiley.

Health Care & Peer Review: Index of New Information & Bibliography. Paula H. Campbell. 1996. 150p. 57.50 (*0-7883-0994-3*); pap. 47.50 (*0-7883-0995-1*) ABBE Pubs Assn.

Health Care & Poor Relief in Protestant Europe 1500-1700. Ed. by Peter Grell & Andrew Cunningham. 1997. (Studies in the Social History of Medicine). 272p. (C). 90.00 (*0-415-12130-2*) Routledge.

Health Care & Public Policy: An Australian Analysis. George R. Palmer & Stephanie D. Short. 2nd ed. 1994. LC 94-118799. 350p. (*0-7329-2008-6*); pap. (*0-7329-2007-8*) Macmill Educ AUS. *Dist:* Paul & Co Pubs.

Health Care & Public Policy: An Australian Analysis. George Palmer & Stephanie Short. 3rd ed. 2000. LC 2001-326477. (Illus.). 400p. pap. (*0-7329-6340-0*) Macmill Educ AUS. *Dist:* Paul & Co Pubs.

Health Care & Public Policy: The Australian Experience. George R. Palmer. 1989. 320p. pap. (*0-333-50334-1*) Intl Spec Bk.

Health Care & Reform in Industrialized Countries. Ed. by Marshall W. Raffel. 1997. (Illus.). LC 96-13824. 696p. pap. 24.50 (*0-271-01644-2*); LC 97-16895. 912p. text 55.00 (*0-271-01620-5*) Pa St U Pr.

Health Care & Spirituality: Listening, Assessing, Caring. Ed. by Richard B. Gilbert & John D. Morgan. 2001. LC 00-63056. (Death, Value & Meaning Ser.). xix, 336p. pap. 36.95 (*0-89503-250-3*) Baywood Pub.

Health Care & the Law. Meg Wallace. 2nd ed. 1995. LC 95-194987. 400p. pap. (*0-455-21293-7*) LawBk Co AUS. *Dist:* Gaunt.

Health Care & the Law. Vol. I. Michael E. Carbine. 1988. (Papers of the Roscoe Pound Foundation Ser.). 50p. pap. 20.00 (*0-933067-07-0*) Roscoe Pound Inst.

Health Care & the Law. Vol. II. John Guinther. 1988. (Papers of the Roscoe Pound Foundation). 17p. (Orig.). pap. 20.00 (*0-933067-08-9*) Roscoe Pound Inst.

Health Care & the Law: A Guide for Nurses. Meg Wallace. 1991. 300p. pap. (*0-455-21038-1*) LawBk Co AUS. *Dist:* Gaunt.

Health Care & the Law: Reports on Three Roundtable Discussions. Vol. III. Michael E. Carbine. 1990. 68p. pap. 20.00 (*0-933067-10-0*) Roscoe Pound Inst.

Health Care & the Rise of Christianity. Hector Avalos. 1999. LC 99-11023. (Illus.). 176p. pap. 12.95 (*1-56563-337-7*) Hendrickson MA.

Health Care & the Social Services. Richard J. Estes. 1984. (Allied Health Professions Monograph). (Illus.). 424p. (C). 42.50 (*0-87527-266-5*) Green.

Health Care Annual: An Update on Trends & Facilities in New York. Division of Research, Analysis, and Planning Staff. 1991. 128p. 40.00 (*0-934459-91-6*) United Hosp Fund.

Health Care Annual: An Update on Trends & Facilities in New York. Compiled by Division of Research, Analysis, and Planning Staff. 1990. 114p. 40.00 (*0-934459-69-X*) United Hosp Fund.

Health Care Annual, 1992: An Update on Trends & Facilities in New York. 1992. 144p. 40.00 (*0-934459-98-3*) United Hosp Fund.

Health Care Annual, 1993 Update: Data on Hospitals in New York. 1993. 34p. 20.00 (*1-881277-15-1*) United Hosp Fund.

Health Care Annual, 1994 Update: Data on Hospitals in New York. 1994. 44p. 20.00 (*1-881277-07-0*) United Hosp Fund.

Health Care Annual, 1995 Update: Data on Hospitals in New York. 1995. 64p. pap. 20.00 (*1-881277-23-2*) United Hosp Fund.

Health Care Annual, 1996 Update: Data on Hospitals in New York. 1996. 62p. pap. 20.00 (*1-881277-28-3*) United Hosp Fund.

Health Care As Social History: The Glasgow Case. O. Checkland & M. Lamb. 1982. (Illus.). 308p. 105.00 (*0-08-028444-2*, R130, Pergamon Pr) Elsevier.

Health Care Assistant. Esther Caldwell & Barbara R. Hegner. 4th ed. 1985. LC 84-26021. 352p. (C). tchr. ed. 13.95 (*0-8273-2454-5*) Delmar.

Health Care at the Abyss: Managed Care vs. the Goals of Medicine. Erin Williams & Leo Van der Reis. 1997. LC 96-50374. (Illus.). 222p. 48.95 (*1-57588-201-9*, 310690) W S Hein.

Health Care Basics Mac Cd-Rom Multiple Site License. Lifeline Staff. 1996. 352p. pap. text (*0-8151-4559-4*) Mosby Inc.

Health Care Basics Mac Cd-Rom Singlesite License. Lifeline Staff. 1996. 352p. pap. text 195.00 (*0-8151-4558-6*) Mosby Inc.

Health Care Budgeting & Financial Management for Non-Financial Managers. William J. Ward. 1993. LC 93-24757. 280p. 65.00 (*0-86569-211-4*, R231); pap. 31.95 (*0-86569-231-9*, T211) Greenwood (Auburn Hse).

Health Care Businesses: Telemarketing Update Script Presentations. 1997. 100p. (C). ring bd. 69.95 (*1-890928-10-0*) Frieda Carrol.

***Health Care Challenge: Acnowledging Disparity, Confronting Discrimination & Ensuring Equality.** Ed. by Mary Frances Berry. 2001. (Illus.). 287p. (C). reprint ed. pap. text 40.00 (*0-7567-1068-5*) DIANE Pub.

Health Care Chaplaincy in Oncology. Ed. by Laurel A. Burton & George Handzo. 1993. LC 92-25898. (Journal of Health Care Chaplaincy Ser.: Vol. 4, Nos. 1/2). (Illus.). 151p. 39.95 (*1-56024-200-0*) Haworth Pr.

Health Care Choice for Today's Consumer: Families U. S. A. Guide to Quality & Cost. Marc S. Miller & Families United for Senior Action Foundation Staff. exp. rev. ed. 1997. LC 96-35919. (Robert L. Bernstein Bks.). (Illus.). 480p. pap. 17.95 (*0-471-17090-9*) Wiley.

Health Care Choices: Private Contracts As Instruments of Health Reform. Clark C. Havighurst. 1994. LC 94-26932. 150p. pap. 17.95 (*0-8447-3867-0*) Am Enterprise.

Health Care Choices for Today's Consumer: The Families U. S. A. Guide to Quality & Cost. Families U. S. A. Staff. Ed. by Marc S. Miller. 1995. (Families U. S. A. Guide to Quality & Cost Ser.). (Illus.). 352p. (Orig.). pap. 14.95 (*1-879326-23-X*) Living Planet Pr.

Health Care Choices in the Boston Area: Families U. S. A. Guide to Quality & Cost. Marc S. Miller & Martha S. Grover. 1995. (Illus.). 212p. (Orig.). pap. 10.95 (*1-879326-24-8*) Fam USA Found.

Health Care Choices in the Washington Area: Families U. S. A. Guide to Quality & Cost. Martha S. Grover. Ed. by Marc S. Miller. 1995. (Illus.). 224p. (Orig.). pap. 10.95 (*1-879326-25-6*) Living Planet Pr.

Health Care Collector Training Guide. Aspen Health and Administration Development Group. 2000. 150p. 65.00 (*0-8342-1883-6*, 18836) Aspen Pub.

Health Care Communication Using Personality Type: Patients Are Different! Judy Allen & Susan A. Brock. 2000. LC 99-55354. 176p. 59.95 (*0-415-21373-8*) Routledge.

Health Care Compliance Professional's Manual. Roy Snell & Aspen Health Law and Compliance Center Staff. 1999. LC 99-47708. ring bd. 209.00 (*0-8342-1742-2*) Aspen Pub.

Health Care Computing: A Survival Guide for PC Users. Philip Burnard. 1994. 212p. pap. 29.95 (*1-56593-414-8*, 1080) Singular Publishing.

Health Care Constitutions. Diane Longley. Ed. by Vivienne Harpwood. 1995. LC 96-157186. (Medico-Legal Practitioner Ser.). 193p. pap. (*1-85941-020-0*) Cavendish Pubng GBR. *Dist:* Gaunt.

Health Care Consumers in the 1990s: A Handbook of Trends, Techniques, & Information Sources for Health Care Executives. 1993. LC 92-55060. 180p. 42.50 (*0-936889-18-7*); pap. 29.95 (*0-936889-19-5*) Intertec Pub Bks.

Health Care Corporate Law: Facilities & Transactions. William S. Brewbaker, III & Mark A. Hall. 1995. LC 95-80384. 942p. ring bd. 209.00 (*0-316-34036-7*) Aspen Pub.

Health Care Corporate Law: Formation & Regulation Hall. Set. 1994. 249.00 (*0-316-34049-9*); Vol. 1. 1993. 960p. 145.00 (*0-316-34003-0*) Aspen Law.

Health Care Corporate Law: Formation & Regulation. Vol. 2. Hall. 1994. LC 93-79759. 145.00 (*0-316-34032-4*) Aspen Pub.

Health Care Cost-Containment Policy: An Econometric Study. Manas Chatterji. 1983. lib. bdg. 169.00 (*0-89838-119-3*) Kluwer Academic.

Health Care Cost Containment Strategies: A Bibliography. Robert J. Juster & Joyce A. Lanning. 1982. (CPL Bibliographies Ser.: No. 85). 52p. 10.00 (*0-86602-085-3*, Sage Prdcls Pr) Sage.

Health Care Cost Controls: A BNA PLUS Resource Guide. 1991. 195.00 (*1-55871-217-8*, BSP 179) BNA PLUS.

Health Care Cost Explosion. National Issues Forum Institute Staff. 1993. 32p. 3.25 (*0-8403-8656-7*); 3.25 (*0-8403-8657-5*) Kendall-Hunt.

Health Care Cost Management: A Basic Guide. Madelon L. Finkel. Ed. by Judith A. Sankey. 3rd ed. 1996. LC 96-76749. 204p. pap. 15.00 (*0-89154-498-4*) Intl Found Employ.

Health Care Crisis: Containing Costs, Expanding Coverage. National Issues Forum Institute Staff. abr. ed. 1992. 32p. pap. text 3.25 (*0-8403-7433-X*) Kendall-Hunt.

Health Care Crisis in America. Linda B. Ropes. 1991. LC 92-31474. (Contemporary World Issues Ser.). lib. bdg. 39.50 (*0-87436-616-X*) ABC-CLIO.

Health Care Crisis in the United States: A Bibliography. Ed. & Compiled by Joan Nordquist. 1997. LC 98-110993. (Contemporary Social Issues: Vol. 46). 72p. (Orig.). pap. 20.00 (*0-937855-90-1*) Ref Rsch Serv.

Health Care Criteria for Performance Excellence: Baldrige National Quality Program 2000. Ed. by Harry S. Hertz. 2000. (Illus.). 58p. (C). pap. text 20.00 (*0-7567-0005-1*) DIANE Pub.

***Health Care Criteria for Performance Excellence: Baldrige National Quality Program, 2000.** Ed. by Harry S. Hertz. 2001. (Illus.). 58p. (C). pap. 25.00 (*0-7567-0937-7*) DIANE Pub.

***Health Care Criteria for Performance Excellence: Baldrige National Quality Program (2002)** Ed. by Harry S. Hertz. 2002. (Illus.). 61p. (C). pap. text 25.00 (*0-7567-1950-X*) DIANE Pub.

Health Care Data Source Book: Finding the Right Information & Making the Most of It. John D. Fry et al. 2nd ed. 1995. LC 95-16417. pap. 50.00 (*1-55648-141-1*, 127151) AHPI.

Health Care Defined: A Glossary of Current Terms. Bruce Goldfarb. 1996. LC 96-31716. 347p. pap. 34.95 (*0-683-03615-7*) Lppncott W & W.

Health Care Delivery: Current Issues & the Public Policy Debate. Ronald Kaufman et al. 1991. (Health Policy Annual Ser.: Vol. I). (Orig.). pap. 19.95 (*1-879694-01-8*) AAH Ctrs.

Health Care Delivery in the U. S. Anthony R. Kovner. 5th ed. 1994. (Illus.). 600p. (C). pap. 32.95 (*0-8261-2078-4*) Springer Pub.

Health Care Delivery in the U. S. Ed. by Anthony R. Kovner. 5th ed. 1994. LC 90-9449. (Illus.). 600p. (C). 49.95 (*0-8261-2079-2*) Springer Pub.

Health Care Delivery Planning. Vol. 2. A. Reisman & M. Kiley. 1973. (Studies in Operations Research). x, 374p. text 171.00 (*0-677-04570-0*) Gordon & Breach.

Health Care Delivery to Hearing Impaired Patients: An Instructional Guide for Hospitals on Developing Policies & Procedures. Metro Deaf Senior Citizens, Inc. Staff. Ed. by Margaret R. Thomas & Jocelyn Ancheta. 1984. 112p. 70.00 (*0-9613623-0-8*) Metro Deaf Senior.

Health Care Dilemma. J. H. Brown. 1978. LC 78-3891. 183p. 32.95 (*0-87705-360-X*, Kluwer Acad Hman Sci) Kluwer Academic.

Health Care Divided: Race & Healing a Nation. David B. Smith. 1999. LC 98-40200. 400p. text 42.50 (*0-472-10991-X*, 10991) U of Mich Pr.

Health Care Economics. Paul J. Feldstein. 5th ed. 1998. LC 98-15358. 608p. 87.95 (*0-7668-0699-5*) Delmar.

Health Care Economics, Policies & Issues in Singapore. Toh M. Heng & Linda Low. 1991. (Centre for Advanced Studies Occasional Papers: No. 7). 56p. pap. (*981-210-001-6*) Times Academic SGP. *Dist:* Intl Spec Bk.

Health Care Environment: The User's Viewpoint. Ed. by William C. Beck & Ralph Meyer. 1982. 272p. 154.00 (*0-8493-6150-8*, RA967, CRC Reprint) Franklin.

Health Care Environmental Services: Staffing the Department - Key Considerations & Options. Ed. by Pamela L. Blyth. 1993. LC 93-1311. (Illus.). 96p. (Orig.). pap. 75.00 (*0-87258-640-5*, 057015) Am Hospital.

Health Care Ethics: A Theological Analysis. Benedict M. Ashley & Kevin D. O'Rourke. 4th ed. 1997. LC 96-46599. 544p. pap. 36.00 (*0-87840-644-1*) Georgetown U Pr.

Health Care Ethics: An Introduction. Ed. by Donald VanDeVeer & Tom Regan. 1986. LC 85-22048. 480p. pap. 24.95 (*0-87722-441-2*) Temple U Pr.

Health Care Ethics: Critical Issues for the 21st Century. John F. Monagle & David C. Thomasma. 2nd ed. 1997. LC 97-23734. 640p. 73.00 (*0-8342-0911-X*, 20911) Aspen Pub.

Health Care Ethics: Principles & Problems. Thomas M. Garrett & Harold W Baillie. 4th ed. 2000. LC 00-28573. (Illus.). 358p. pap. 33.60 (*0-13-019448-4*) P-H.

Health Care, Ethics & Insurance. Tom Sorell. 1998. LC 98-13842. (Professional Ethics Ser.). 208p. (C). 80.00 (*0-415-16284-X*); pap. 26.95 (*0-415-16285-8*) Routledge.

Health Care Ethics Committees: The Next Generation. Judith W. Ross et al. 1993. LC 93-17509. 198p. 45.00 (*1-55648-104-7*, 058300) AHPI.

Health Care Ethics Consultant. Ed. by Francoise C. Baylis. 1994. LC 94-13467. (Contemporary Issues in Biomedicine, Ethics & Society Ser.). 224p. text 49.50 (*0-89603-278-7*) Humana.

Health Care Executives Guides' to Fraud & Abuse. Paul R. Demuro & Russell Hayman. 1998. 144p. pap. 93.00 (*0-929156-37-4*) Atlantic Info Services Inc.

Health Care Exploration. Deem. 1998. (C). LC 98-26921. 416p. pap. text 38.95 (*0-8273-8004-6*); pap. text, tchr. ed. 15.00 (*0-8273-8005-4*); pap. text, wbk. ed. 21.95 (*0-8273-8007-0*) Delmar.

Health Care Facilities Law. Anne M. Dellinger. 1991. 110.00 (*0-316-18040-8*) Aspen Law.

Health Care Facilities Risk Management Forms, Checklists & Guidelines. Ed. by Sara N. Di Lima & Simon B. Weavers. 1995. LC 98-42526. ring bd. 209.00 (*0-8342-1099-1*) Aspen Pub.

Health Care Facilities Standard & Handbook. Burton Klein. 1996. 778p. 98.50 (*0-87765-407-7*, 99HB96) Natl Fire Prot.

Health Care Facility Projects in Developing Areas: Planning, Implementation & Operation. B. Kleczkowski & N. Nilsson. 1984. (Public Health Papers: No. 79). 87p. pap. text 9.00 (*92-4-130079-5*, 1110079) World Health.

Health Care Finance: Basic Tools for Nonfinancial Managers. Judith J. Baker & R. W. Baker. 1999. LC 99-38261. 263p. pap. 62.00 (*0-8342-1206-4*) Aspen Pub.

Health Care Finance: Cost, Productivity, & Strategic Design. Steven R. Eastaugh. 1998. LC 98-23192. 272p. pap. 47.00 (*0-8342-1181-5*, 11815) Aspen Pub.

Health Care Finance: Economic Incentives & Productivity Enhancement. Steven R. Eastaugh. 1992. LC 91-26255. 560p. 85.00 (*0-86569-044-8*, T044); pap. 34.95 (*0-86569-049-9*, R049) Greenwood (Auburn Hse).

Health Care Financial Management. Ed. by Montague Brown. 1992. (HCMR Ser.). 222p. pap. 55.00 (*0-8342-0303-0*, 20303) Aspen Pub.

Health Care Financial Transactions Manual: A Seven Step Analysis Thomas C. Fox et al. 1993. LC 93-6471. (Health Law Ser.). 130.00 (*0-87632-908-3*) West Group.

Health Care Financing. 1991. lib. bdg. 247.95 (*0-8490-5091-X*); Set. 1992. lib. bdg. 955.95 (*0-8490-5327-7*) Gordon Pr.

Health Care Financing Administration Financial Report: Fiscal Year 1998. Nancy-Ann M. DeParle. 2000. (Illus.). 141p. (C). pap. text 30.00 (*0-7567-0212-7*) DIANE Pub.

Health Care Financing for Severe Developmental Disabilities. Herbert J. Cohen et al. 1990. pap. 18.00 (*0-940898-24-1*) Am Assn Mental.

Health Care Financing in Mainland Tanzania. Manuel Gottlieb. 1975. (Foreign & Comparative Studies Program, African Ser.: No. 20). 104p. (Orig.). pap. text 5.50 (*0-915984-17-2*) Syracuse U Foreign Comp.

Health Care Financing in New York State: A Blueprint for Change. 1993. 56p. pap. 25.00 (*0-934459-97-5*) United Hosp Fund.

Health Care Financing in the United States: Index of New Information with Authors & Subjects. Samuel M. Morris. rev. ed. 1996. LC 96-3652. 133p. 57.50 (*0-7883-1064-X*); pap. 47.50 (*0-7883-1065-8*) ABBE Pubs Assn.

Health Care Financing Review: Medicare & Medicaid Statistical Supplement (1995) 1996. (Illus.). 388p. (Orig.). (C). pap. text 55.00 (*0-7881-2654-7*) DIANE Pub.

Health Care Financing Status Report: Research & Demonstrations in Health Care Financing. 1992. lib. bdg. 90.00 (*0-8490-5508-3*) Gordon Pr.

Health Care Finishes: Problems & Solutions - an Environmental Services Perspective. Ed. by Pamela L. Blyth. 1993. 92p. (Orig.). pap. 60.00 (*0-87258-643-X*, 057016) Am Hospital.

Health Care Fiscal Analyst. Jack Rudman. 1994. (Career Examination Ser.: C-3620). pap. 34.95 (*0-8373-3620-1*) Nat Learn.

Health Care for Adolescents: Developing Comprehensive Services. Karyn L. Feiden. 1993. LC 92-48518. (Papers: Vol. 22). pap. 10.00 (*1-881277-04-6*) United Hosp Fund.

Health Care for an Aging Society: Cost-Conscious Community Care & Self-Care Approaches. David Haber. 1989. (Death Education, Aging & Health Care Ser.). 189p. pap. 30.95 (*1-56032-227-6*) Hemisp Pub.

Health Care for Beginners. David Brizer. 1994. (Illus.). 192p. pap. 9.95 (*0-86316-170-7*) Writers & Readers.

Health Care for Children: What's Right, What's Wrong, What's Next. Ruth E. Stein. 1997. LC 97-12033. (*1-881277-31-3*) United Hosp Fund.

Health Care for Lesbians & Gay Men: Confronting Homophobia & Heterosexism. Ed. by K. Jean Peterson. 1996. LC 96-23147. (Journal of Gay & Lesbian Social Services Ser.: Vol. 5, No. 1). 121p. 29.95 (*1-56024-772-X*, Haworth Pastrl); pap. 12.95 (*1-56023-079-7*, Harrington Park) Haworth Pr.

Health Care for Older Women. Ed. by Julie George & Shah B. Ebrahim. 1992. 288p. 59.50 (*0-19-262068-1*) OUP.

Health Care for the Elderly: A Manual for Primary Health Care Workers. Ed. by G. Hafez & K. Bagchi. 1994. (WHO Regional Publications: No. 10). 57p. pap. text 9.00 (*92-9021-186-5*, 1440010) World Health.

Health Care for the Elderly: Regional Responses for National Policy Issues. Ed. by Kathleen G. Andreoli et al. 1987. LC 86-14869. (Home Health Care Services Quarterly Ser.: Vol. 7, Nos. 3 & 4). 363p. text 11.95 (*0-86656-607-4*) Haworth Pr.

Health Care for the Medically Indigent. Sally Coughlin. 1986. (Orig.). pap. text 1.00 (*0-915757-10-9*) League Women Voters TX.

Health Care for the Older Woman. Ed. by Morton A. Stechever. 2nd ed. 1995. LC 95-21175. 416p. (gr. 13). 104.95 (*0-412-05401-9*) Chapman & Hall.

Health Care for the Poor & Elderly: Meeting the Challenge. Ed. by Duncan Yaggy & William G Anylan. 1984. LC 83-25312. (Duke Press Policy Studies). xiv, 146p. text 35.00 (*0-8223-0508-9*) Duke.

Health Care for the Poor & Uninsured: Strategies That Work. Ed. by Nellie P. Tate. 1992. LC 92-1696. (Journal of Health & Social Policy: Nos. 3 & 4). (Illus.). 151p. text 29.95 (*1-56024-315-5*) Haworth Pr.

Health Care for the Poor in Latin America & the Caribbean. Carmelo Mesa-Lago. 1992. (PAHO Scientific Publications: No. 539). (ENG & SPA.). v, 234p. pap. text 56.00 (*92-75-11539-7*, 1610539) World Health.

Health Care for the Poor in Omaha-Douglas County: Problems & Policy Options. David DiMartino et al. 1985. 136p. (Orig.). pap. 9.50 (*1-55719-108-5*) U NE CPAR.

***Health Care for the Uninsured: The Role of Safety Net Providers: Hearing Before the Commite on Health, Education, Labor & Pensions, U. S. Senate.** Ed. by Bill Frist. 2001. (Illus.). 84p. pap. text 25.00 (*0-7567-1662-4*) DIANE Pub.

Health Care for Women: Access, Utilization, Outcomes. 1994. lib. bdg. 250.00 (*0-8490-8609-4*) Gordon Pr.

Health Care for Women: Access, Utilization, Outcomes: Bibliography-1990-1993. Ed. by Loretta D. Ulincy & Susan J. Simmons. 1994. 51p. (Orig.). (C). pap. text 25.00 (*0-7881-1369-0*) DIANE Pub.

Health Care Fraud: Enforcement & Compliance, 00636. Robert Fabrikant et al. rev. ed. 1996. 525p. ring bd. 149.00 (*1-58852-073-0*, Law Journal Pr) Amer Lawyer Media.

Health Care Fraud: Information-Sharing Proposals to Improve Enforcement Efforts. David P. Alexander & Pamela V. Williams. 1996. (Illus.). 96p. (Orig.). (C). pap. text 25.00 (*0-7881-3665-8*) DIANE Pub.

Health Care Fraud & Abuse. Aspen Health Law and Compliance Center Staff. 1998. LC 98-9393. (Current Issue Ser.). 144p. pap. 48.00 (*0-8342-1159-9*, 11599) Aspen Pub.

Health Care Fraud & Abuse: A Guide to Federal Sanctions Paul P. Cacioppo. 1991. LC 90-23174. (Health Law Ser.). ring bd. 210.00 (*0-87632-806-0*) West Group.

Health Care Fraud & Abuse: A Physician's Guide to Compliance. American Medical Association Staff. 2000. 224p. pap. 59.95 (*0-89970-978-8*, OP083599) AMA.

Health Care Fraud & Abuse: Aspen Health Law Center Current Issues. Aspen Health Law Center Staff. 1998. LC 98-9393. 144p. pap. 39.00 (*0-8342-1123-8*) Aspen Pub.

Health Care Fraud & Abuse: Enforcement & Compliance. John J. Meyer et al. 1997. (Health Law & Business Ser.: No. 2600). 125.00 (*1-55871-356-5*) BNA.

Health Care Fraud & Abuse Compliance Manual. Aspen Health Law and Compliance Center Staff. 1997. LC 96-46731. 388p. ring bd. 219.00 (*0-8342-0899-7*, 5451) Aspen Pub.

Health Care Fraud & Finance Conference (1995) 1995. 139p. 50.00 (*1-56986-253-2*) Federal Bar.

Health Care Future Vol. 1: Defining the Argument, Healing the Debate. James J. Pattee & Orlo J. Otteson. 1998. 227p. 27.50 (*0-9629614-1-8*) North Ridge Pr.

Health Care Guide. Ed. by Jeffrey D. Momorsky. 1995. LC 94-186078. 297.00 (*0-7913-1968-7*) Warren Gorham & Lamont.

Health Care in California State Prisons. Marcus Nieto. 1998. 69p. pap. (*1-58703-087-X*, CRB-98-009) CA Res Bureau.

Health Care in Crisis: Preparing the Eye Care Practitioner's Office for the Year 2000. Diana Driscoll et al. 1998. (Illus.). 79p. pap. 89.95 (*0-9667727-0-9*) Priority Consult.

Health Care in Crisis: Preparing the Medical Office for the Year 2000. Diana Driscoll et al. 1998. (Illus.). 79p. pap. 89.95 (*0-9667727-1-7*) Priority Consult.

Health Care in Hawaii: Implications for National Reform. 1994. (Illus.). 56p. (Orig.). (C). pap. text 25.00 (*0-7881-1513-8*) DIANE Pub.

Health Care in Jamaica: Quality, Outcomes, & Labor Supply. Victor Lavy et al. 1995. LC 95-17080. (LSMS Working Papers: No. 116). 40p. pap. 22.00 (*0-8213-3243-0*, 13243) World Bank.

Health Care in Java, Past & Present. Ed. by Peter Boomgaard et al. 1996. LC 97-145593. (KITLV Proceedings Ser.). vi, 197p. pap. (*90-6718-104-8*) KITLV Pr NLD. *Dist:* Book Bin.

Health Care in Muslim Asia: Development & Disorder in Wartime Afghanistan. Ronald W. O'Connor. 1994. LC 94-2655. (Illus.). 312p. (C). 72.50 (*0-8191-9444-1*); pap. 30.50 (*0-8191-9445-X*) U Pr of Amer.

Health Care in Nicaragua: Primary Care in Changing Regimes. Richard Garfield & Glen Williams. 1992. LC 91-32069. (Illus.). 320p. text 39.95 (*0-19-506753-3*) OUP.

Health Care in Oklahoma: Prescription for Reform: A Common Sense Alternative to National Health Insurance. Joseph L. Bast et al. Ed. by Terry Tanner. 1993. 172p. (Orig.). pap. 12.95 (*0-913507-47-4*) New Forums.

Health Care in South-East Asia. 1989. (WHO Regional Publications, South-East Ser.: No. 14). 210p. pap. text 30.00 (*92-9022-114-3*, 1560014) World Health.

Health Care in Texas: A Data Book. William P. Hobby & David C. Warner. 1993. (Special Project Reports: Vol. SP-HCT). 162p. pap. 12.50 (*0-89940-900-8*) LBJ Sch Pub Aff.

Health Care in the Black Community: Empowerment, Knowledge, Skills & Collectivism. Ed. by Sadye Louise Logan & Edith M. Freeman. 2000. LC 00-38882. (C). 300p. 69.95 (*0-7890-0456-9*); (Illus.). xix, 276p. pap. text 34.95 (*0-7890-0457-7*) Haworth Pr.

Health Care in the New Millennium: Vision, Values & Leadership. Ian Morrison. 2000. LC 99-44361. 288p. 42.00 (*0-7879-5115-3*) Jossey-Bass.

Health Care in the United States: What We Should Keep & What We Should Change. Rita Ricardo-Campbell et al. 1994. LC 94-10295. (Essays in Public Policy Ser.: No. 50). pap. 5.00 (*0-8179-5552-6*) Hoover Inst Pr.

Health Care in Transition: Technology Assessment in the Private Sector. Richard A. Rettig. 1997. LC 96-41468. (Illus.). 156p. pap. 15.00 (*0-8330-2444-2*, MR-754-DHHS/ASP) Rand Corp.

Health Care in Uganda: Selected Issues. Paul Hutchinson. 1999. LC 99-32550. (Discussion Paper Ser.: No. 404). 224p. pap. 30.00 (*0-8213-4531-1*, 14531) World Bank.

Health Care Information Management Forms, Checklists, Guidelines, Policies & Procedures. Aspen Reference Group Staff. Ed. by Joan Liebler. 1998. ring bd. 189.00 (*0-8342-1101-7*, S467) Aspen Pub.

Health Care Information Series Compiled by Division of Research, Analysis, and Planning Staff. 1985. 45.00 (*0-934459-05-3*) United Hosp Fund.

Health Care Innovations & Venture Trends. Courtney Price. 1992. pap. 41.95 (*0-8273-4964-5*) Delmar.

Health Care Inservice Curriculum Resource Manual. Aspen Reference Group Staff. 1997. LC 97-16280. 400p. ring bd. 199.00 (*0-8342-0879-2*, S446) Aspen Pub.

Health Care Inservice Program: An Interdisciplinary Approach. Andrew Gruen & Kathleen Coffrey. 1995. spiral bd. 179.00 (*0-8342-0749-4*, 5446) Aspen Pub.

Health Care Insurance Reform in the United States: A Market Approach with Application from the Federal Republic of Germany. Frankie P. Albritton, Jr. 1993. LC 92-31546. 108p. (C). 46.00 (*0-8191-8896-4*) U Pr of Amer.

Health Care Integration: Structural & Legal Issues. Andrew J. Demetriou & Thomas E. Dutton. 1996. (Health Law & Business Ser.: No. 1300). 125.00 (*1-55871-338-7*) BNA.

Health Care Issues in Black America: Policies, Problems & Prospects, 100. Ed. by Woodrow Jones, Jr. & Mitchell F. Rice. 1987. LC 86-14233. (Contributions in Afro-American & African Studies Ser.: No. 100). 269p. 39.95 (*0-313-24886-9*, JHE/) Greenwood.

Health Care Joint Ventures: Drafting to Meet Objectives. James L. Hall, Jr. et al. 1996. (Health Law & Business Ser.: No. 2200). 95.00 (*1-55871-343-3*) BNA.

Health Care Labor Manual, Set. 1995. LC 74-24672. ring bd. 950.00 (*0-912862-11-4*) Aspen Pub.

Health Care Law. Jonathan Montgomery. 1997. LC 96-36931. 532p. text 95.00 (*0-19-876260-7*); pap. text 42.00 (*0-19-876259-3*) OUP.

Health Care Law: A Practical Guide. Scott Becker. 1985. ring bd. 235.00 (*0-8205-1398-9*) Bender.

Health Care Law: Text, Cases, & Materials. Jean V. McHale et al. 1997. LC 97-135153. 963 p. (*0-421-51180-X*) Sweet & Maxwell.

Health Care Law & Ethics. Cody. 2000. (Allied Health Ser.). (C). pap. 28.00 net. (*0-7668-0649-9*) Delmar.

Health Care Law & Ethics. American Association of Medical Assistants Staff. rev. ed. 1995. v, 320p. pap. 20.00 (*0-942732-02-2*) Am Med Assts.

Health Care Law & Ethics. William J. Curran. 5th ed. 1998. LC 97-42574. 1512p. 66.00 (*1-56706-809-X*) Panel Pubs.

Health Care Law & Ethics in a Nutshell. Mark A. Hall et al. (Nutshell Ser.). (C). 1989. 401p. reprint ed. text 18.50 (*0-314-67645-7*); 2nd ed. 1991. 461p. pap. text 33.50 (*0-314-89868-9*) West Pub.

Health Care Law & Policy. Clark C. Havighurst. 1990. (University Casebook Ser.). 110p. reprint ed. pap. text (*0-88277-717-3*) Foundation Pr.

Health Care Law & Policy. Clark C. Havighurst et al. 2nd ed. 1998. LC 98-8152. (University Casebook Ser.). 1200p. text 65.00 (*1-56662-617-X*) Foundation Pr.

Health Care Law & Policy: Readings, Notes, & Questions. Clark C. Havighurst. 1990. (University Casebook Ser.). 1299p. reprint ed. text 45.00 (*0-88277-638-X*) Foundation Pr.

Health Care Law & Policy, 1992 Supplement to (Readings, Notes & Questions) Clark C. Havighurst. 1992. (University Casebook Ser.). 125p. (C). pap. text 6.95 (*1-56662-043-0*) Foundation Pr.

Health Care Law Sourcebook: Compendium of Federal Laws, Regulations & Documents Related to Health Care Weissburg and Aronson Inc. Staff. 1989. 476.00 (*0-8205-1299-0*) Bender.

Health Care Law Treatise (Treatise on Health Care Law), Vol. 4. Irwin M. Birnbaum. Ed. by Alexander M. Capron et al. 1991. 696.00 (*0-8205-1407-1*) Bender.

Health Care Legislation, 1989. 1991. 238p. 20.00 (*1-55516-692-X*, 6630) Natl Conf State Legis.

Health Care Legislation, 1995. Compiled by NCSL Health Care Program Staff. 1996. 150p. 25.00 (*1-55516-606-7*, 6655) Natl Conf State Legis.

Health Care Legislation,1997. NCSL Health Care Program Staff. 1998. 25.00 (*1-55516-826-4*) Natl Conf State Legis.

Health Care M & A: How to Structure the Transaction. Irwin M. Birnbaum et al. 1997. LC 97-153504. (Corporate Law & Practice Course Handbook Ser.). 384p. 129.00 (*0-87224-323-0*) PLI.

Health Care Made Better by Disease Prevention Using Health Promotion: Index of New Information with Authors, Subjects & References. Francis C. Doty. 1997. (Illus.). 183p. 57.50 (*0-7883-1294-4*); pap. 47.50 (*0-7883-1295-2*) ABBE Pubs Assn.

Health Care Malpractice: A Primer on Legal Issues for Professionals. Ron Scott. 2nd ed. 1998. LC 98-30161. (Illus.). 264p. pap. 34.95 (*0-07-054145-0*) McGraw-Hill Prof.

Health Care Management: A Text in Organization Theory & Behavior. Stephen M. Shortell & Arnold D. Kaluzny. 2nd ed. 1989. LC 87-14786. (Health Services Ser.). 542p. text 42.95 (*0-8273-4362-0*) Delmar.

Health Care Management: Issues in Corrections. Kenneth L. Faiver. 1998. LC 97-17919. 301p. 44.95 (*1-56991-070-7*) Am Correctional.

Health Care Management: Organization Design & Behavior. Stephen M. Shortell & Arnold D. Kaluzny. (Delmar Series in Health Services Administration Ser.). 3rd ed. 1994. LC 93-35863. 424p. (C). pap. 79.95 (*0-8273-5675-7*); 4th ed. 1999. LC 99-31968. 448p. 87.95 (*0-7668-1072-0*) Delmar.

Health Care Management: Strategy, Structure, & Process. Ed. by Montague Brown. 1992. (HCMR Ser.). 232p. pap. 55.00 (*0-8342-0299-9*, 20299) Aspen Pub.

Health Care Management in Mind: Eight Careers. Contrib. by Anthony R. Kovner et al. 2000. LC 99-57678. xii, 156p. (*0-8261-1315-X*) Springer Pub.

Health Care Management Policy. Chatterji. 78.95 (*1-85972-606-2*) Ashgate Pub Co.

Health Care Management Review Series, Set. Ed. by Montague Brown. 1992. pap. 347.00 (*0-8342-0337-5*) Aspen Pub.

Health Care Managers in Transition: Shifting Roles & Changing Organizations. Wendy Leebov & Gail Scott. 1990. LC 90-38789. (Health Management Ser.). 232p. 45.00 (*1-55542-248-9*) Jossey-Bass.

Health Care M&A Report 1-4 Quarters, 1999 Irving Levin Associates, Inc. Staff. 1999. (Illus.). per. 1495.00 (*1-930625-15-4*) I Levin.

Health Care M&A Year in Review: March 2000. annuals Irving Levin Associates, Inc. Staff. 6th ed. 2000. (Illus.). iii, 16p. pap. 79.00 (*1-930625-00-6*) I Levin.

Health Care Marketing: A Foundation for Managed Quality. Ed. by Philip D. Cooper. 3rd ed. 1994. 544p. 59.00 (*0-8342-0527-0*) Aspen Pub.

Health Care Marketing Management. Ed. by Montague Brown. 1992. (HCMR Ser.). 224p. pap. 55.00 (*0-8342-0302-2*, 20302) Aspen Pub.

Health Care Marketing Management: A Case Approach. Philip D. Cooper & Larry M. Robinson. 1982. LC 82-3904. 368p. (C). 98.00 (*0-89443-394-6*) Aspen Pub.

Health Care Marketing Plans: From Strategy to Action. Steven G. Hillestad & Eric N. Berkowitz. 2nd ed. 1991. (Health Care Administration Ser.). 270p. 83.00 (*0-8342-0188-7*) Aspen Pub.

Health Care Mergers & Acquisitions: The Antitrust Perspective. David A. Ettinger & Stanford P. Berenbaum. 1996. (Health Law & Business Ser.: No. 1400). 125.00 (*1-55871-330-1*) BNA.

Health Care Mergers & Acquisitions: The Transactional Perspective. Paul R. DeMuro & Marilee C. Unruh. 1996. (Health Law & Business Ser.: No. 2100). 125.00 (*1-55871-344-1*) BNA.

Health Care Needs: Meaning & Measurement. Per-Erik Liss. 1993. 147p. (*1-85628-453-0*) Avebry GBR. *Dist:* Ashgate Pub Co.

Health Care Needs Assessment, Set. Ed. by Andrew Stevens & James Raftery. 1995. (*1-85775-047-0*) Radcliffe Med Pr GBR. *Dist:* Balogh.

Health Care Needs Assessment: The Epidemiologically Based Needs Assessment Reviews. Andrew Stevens et al. 1996. LC 96-47140. (*1-85775-199-X*) Radcliffe Med Pr GBR. *Dist:* Balogh.

Health Care Networks & Managed Care: Antitrust Aspect of Integration & Exclusion. Phillip A. Proger et al. 1996. (Health Law & Business Ser.: No. 2500). 125.00 (*1-55871-331-X*) BNA.

Health Care of Children in Out-of-House Care: A Survey of State Child Welfare Commissioners. Ellen S. Battistelli & Child Welfare League of America Staff. 1998. LC 98-3391. 32p. pap. 9.95 (*0-87868-706-8*, 7068, CWLA Pr) Child Welfare.

HI

Health Care of the Aged: Needs, Policies & Services. Ed. by Abraham Monk. 1990. LC 90-4941. (Journal of Gerontological Social Work Ser.: Vol. 15, Nos. 3-4). 185p. text 39.95 (*1-56024-065-2*) Haworth Pr.

Health Care of the Elderly: Strategies for Prevention & Intervention. Ed. by Gari Lesnoff-Caravaglia. 1980. LC 79-19192. (Frontiers in Aging Ser.: Vol. I). 232p. 42.95 (*0-87705-417-7*, Kluwer Acad Hman Sci) Kluwer Academic.

Health Care of the Female Adolescent. Ed. by Sharon Golub. LC 84-4560. (Women & Health Ser.: Vol. 9, Nos. 2-3). 156p. 1985. pap. text 2.95 (*0-86656-434-9*); 1984. text 39.95 (*0-86656-298-2*) Haworth Pr.

Health Care of Women: Gynecological Assessment. J. W. Hawkins & L. P. Higgins. 1982. LC 81-16245. (Nursing-Health Science Ser.). (Illus.). 150p. (C). text 42.95 (*0-8185-0505-2*, 505-2) Jones & Bartlett.

Health Care of Women: Labor. J. W. Hawkins et al. 1982. LC 81-16202. (Illus.). 150p. (C). text 38.95 (*0-8185-0510-9*, 510-9) Jones & Bartlett.

Health Care of Women & Children in Developing Countries. Ed. by Helen M. Wallace et al. 2nd ed. 1995. (Illus.). 888p. pap. text 34.95 (*0-89914-043-2*, 0432) Third Party Pub.

Health Care Organization & Administration for Emerging Nations. Edward Khiwa-Kiwuwa. Ed. by Curtis Battles & Soas. 152p. (C). pap. text 37.65 (*0-9643899-0-8*) E K Kiwuwa.

Health Care Organization & Finance. Barry R. Furrow et al. 2nd ed. 1991. (American Casebook Ser.). 550p. (C). pap. text 35.50 (*0-314-89870-0*) West Pub.

Health Care Outcomes: Collaborative, Path-Based Approaches. Suzanne Smith Blancett & Dominick L. Flarey. 1998. LC 98-9760. xviii, 403p. pap. 72.00 (*0-8342-1137-8*, 11378) Aspen Pub.

Health Care Outcomes & Cardiovascular Outcomes. Suzanne Smith Blancett & Dominick L. Flarey. 1995. 400p. pap. 121.00 (*0-8342-1048-7*, 10487) Aspen Pub.

Health Care Patterns & Planning in Developing Countries, 29. Ed. by Rais Akhtar. 1991. LC 89-25941. (Contributions in Medical Studies Ser.: No. 29). 360p. 75.00 (*0-313-26745-6*, AHC/, Greenwood Pr) Greenwood.

Health Care Policies & Europe: The Implications for Practice. Carole Ludvigsen et al. 1997. LC 96-13094. 288p. pap. text 45.00 (*0-7506-2485-X*) Buttrwrth-Heinemann.

Health Care Policy & Politics: Lessons from Four Countries. Helms. 1993. LC 93-29700. 50p. (Orig.). pap. 7.75 (*0-8447-3838-7*, AEI Pr) Am Enterprise.

Health Care Policy & Regulation. Ed. by Thomas A. Abbott, 3rd. 1995. (Topics in Regulatory Economics & Policy Ser.: 20). 272p. (C). lib. bdg. 107.50 (*0-7923-9540-9*) Kluwer Academic.

Health Care Policy Explained. Ed. by Rushika Fernandopulle & Bradley Marino. 1995. LC 94-45372. pap. 39.95 (*0-86542-447-0*) Blackwell Sci.

Health Care Policy in Contemporary America. Ed. by Alan I. Marcus & Hamilton Cravens. 1997. LC 97-13457. (Issues in Policy History Ser.: Vol. 7). 156p. pap. 19.95 (*0-271-01740-6*) Pa St U Pr.

Health Care Policy Process. Carol Barker. 1996. 176p. LC 96-68056. 74.50 (*0-8039-7627-5*, 1579); pap. 25.95 (*0-8039-7628-3*, 1580) Sage.

Health Care Politics & Policy in America. Kant Patel & Mark E. Rushefsky. 1995. LC 95-4603. (Illus.). 312p. text 86.95 (*1-56324-558-2*) M E Sharpe.

Health Care Politics & Policy in America. Kant Patel et al. 1995. LC 95-4603. (Illus.). 312p. (C). pap. text 40.95 (*1-56324-559-0*) M E Sharpe.

Health Care Politics & Policy in America. Kant Patel & Mark E. Rushefsky. 2nd ed. 1999. LC 98-56200. 480p. pap. text 32.95 (*0-7656-0390-X*); (Illus.). (gr. 13). text 86.95 (*0-7656-0389-6*) M E Sharpe.

Health Care Politics, Policy, & Distributive Justice: The Ironic Triumph. Robert P. Rhodes. LC 90-10364. (SUNY Series in Health Care Politics & Policy). 339p. (C). 1992. text 64.50 (*0-7914-0777-2*); 1991. pap. text 21.95 (*0-7914-0778-0*) State U NY Pr.

Health Care Professional's Guide to Disease Management: Patient-Centered Care for the 21st Century. James B. Couch. 1995. LC 98-27918. 368p. pap. 57.00 (*0-8342-1166-1*, 11661) Aspen Pub.

Health Care Professional's Guide to Spinal Rehabilitation. Ed. by David E. Stude. 1999. LC 99-17146. (Illus.). 581p. (C). text 89.00 (*0-8385-3685-9*) McGraw-Hill Prof.

Health Care Professional's Guide to Successful Computerization. David B. Freeman. Ed. by Joyce Freeman. 1989. 224p. (Orig.). (C). pap. 10.00 (*0-944372-04-X*) Nissi Pubns.

***Health Care Professionals Who Are Blind or Visually Impaired.** Deborah Kendrick. 2001. LC 2001-56151. (*0-89128-388-9*) Am Foun Blind.

Health Care Protocols: A Handbook for DD Nurses. Mc Gowan Consultants Staff. 1998. (Illus.). 486p. pap. 49.95 (*1-928752-02-0*) Mc Gowan Pubns.

Health Care Provision: Past, Present & Future. Audrey Leathard. 2nd ed. 2000. LC 2001-278270. (Illus.). 320p. pap. (*0-7487-3354-X*) Nelson Thornes GBR. *Dist:* Intl Spec Bk, Trans-Atl Phila.

Health Care Quality: Grievance Procedures: Congressional Heargin. Ed. by James M. Jeffords. 2000. 134p. (C). reprint ed. pap. text 30.00 (*0-7567-0344-1*) DIANE Pub.

Health Care Quality: Grievance Procedures: Hearing of the Committee on Labor & Human Resources, United States Senate, One Hundred Fifth Congress, Second Session on Examining How to Implement Improved Health Claim Grievance Procedures, Focusing on the Employee Retirement Income Security Act (ERISA) Requirements Regarding Internal Review of Health Benefit Claims & the Need for Independent External Review, & S. 1712. Contrib. by U. S. Congress, Senate Committee on Labor and Human Resources. 1998. LC 98-209653. (*0-16-057297-5*) USGPO.

Health Care Quality & Outcomes Management. Jo Gulledge et al. 1999. LC 99-27113. ring bd. 209.00 (*0-8342-1709-0*) Aspen Pub.

Health Care Quality Improvement Act of 1986: A Legislative History of Pub. Law No. 99-660. Ed. by Bernard D. Reams. 1990. LC 89-83918. (Federal Health Law Ser.: Part 3). 721p. lib. bdg. 75.00 (*0-89941-693-4*, 306000) W S Hein.

Health Care Quality in California: A Primer. David B. Hansen. 2000. (Illus.). 36p. pap. (*1-929008-25-2*) CA HlthCare Fnd.

Health Care Quality Management. Vincent K. Omachonu. 1998. LC 98-31216. 49.95 (*0-89806-187-3*, OMACH) Eng Mgmt Pr.

Health Care Quality Management. Patrice L. Spath. 2000. 166p. tchr. ed. 39.00 (*1-929955-09-X*); 111p. stu. ed., wbk. ed. 16.00 (*1-929955-10-3*) Brown Spath.

Health Care Quality Management 1998/99 Resources Directory. Peter G. Goldschmidt & Jenny Liao. 1998. pap. 12.95 (*0-9666866-0-8*) World Development.

Health Care Quality Toolkit: Leader's Guide. 1999. 150p. ring bd. 99.95 (*0-9640405-1-4*) Hlth Interact.

Health Care Recipak see Quick Reference Health Care Guide: For Busy Families, Young Adults & Seniors: Professional Medical Advice in Clear Easy Steps

Health Care Recipak: The Self-Care & Wellness Guide: Clear Recipe-Style Advice on 140+ Ailments & Injuries. Health Education Resources Staff. 2nd rev. ed. 1996. LC 96-77753. (Illus.). 310p. reprint ed. pap. 11.95 (*0-9653928-3-X*, HCR-2) Hlth Educ Res.

Health Care Reform: A Human Rights Approach. Ed. by Audrey R. Chapman. 1994. LC 94-2311. 326p. pap. 14.95 (*0-87840-555-0*); 37.50 (*0-87840-554-2*) Georgetown U Pr.

Health Care Reform: Ensuring Quality at an Affordable Price. Ed. by Alexander T. Hunt. 1995. LC 94-23961. (CSIS Panel Report Ser.). 35p. (C). pap. 9.95 (*0-89206-313-0*) CSIS.

Health Care Reform: Essential Mental Health Services. Judith B. Krauss. 1993. (Illus.). 69p. (C). pap. text 17.95 (*1-55810-089-X*, CH-24) Am Nurses Pub.

Health Care Reform: Index of New Information with Authors, Subjects & References. Carl J. Dobbins. 1997. 157p. 57.50 (*0-7883-1514-5*); pap. 47.50 (*0-7883-1515-3*) ABBE Pubs Assn.

Health Care Reform: Learning from International Experience. Christopher Ham. 1997. LC 96-52124. (State of Health Ser.). (*0-335-19890-2*) OpUniv Pr.

Health Care Reform: Learning from International Experience. P. Hammersley. 1997. LC 96-52124. (State of Health Ser.). pap. (*0-335-19889-9*) OpUniv Pr.

Health Care Reform & Child Welfare: Meeting the Needs of Abused & Neglected Children. Madelyn DeWoody. 1994. pap. 12.95 (*0-87868-507-3*) Child Welfare.

Health Care Reform As Social Change. Richard E. Thompson. 1993. LC 93-79321. 179p. (Orig.). pap. text 34.00 (*0-924674-24-5*) Am Coll Phys Execs.

Health Care Reform in Hawaii. 1994. (Illus.). 48p. (Orig.). (C). pap. text 30.00 (*0-7881-1464-6*) DIANE Pub.

Health Care Reform in the Nineties. Ed. by Pauline V. Rosenau. LC 94-6009. 268p. (C). 1995. 69.95 (*0-8039-5729-7*, 4095); 1994. pap. 34.95 (*0-8039-5730-0*, 4096) Sage.

Health Care Reform: Specifics, Economics & Legislative Actions & Philosophy of Health Care: Index of Progress, 1994-1995. American Health Research Institute Staff. 1995. 322p. 57.50 (*0-7883-0650-2*); pap. 47.50 (*0-7883-0651-0*) ABBE Pubs Assn.

Health Care Registration Forms, Checklists & Guidelines. Aspen Health and Administration Development Group. 1997. LC 97-11746. ring bd. 199.00 (*0-8342-0876-8*, S445) Aspen Pub.

Health Care Report Cards, 1998-99. Ed. by Beth Melville & Susan Namovicz-Peat. 4th rev. ed. 1998. 158p. pap. 93.00 (*0-929156-41-2*) Atlantic Info Services Inc.

Health Care Research by Degrees. Norma Reid. 1993. LC 92-28523. (Illus.). 224p. pap. 36.95 (*0-632-03466-1*) Blackwell Sci.

Health Care Resource Book. 1994. (Illus.). 127p. (C). pap. text 30.00 (*1-56806-164-1*) DIANE Pub.

Health Care Resource Book. 1994. lib. bdg. 250.95 (*0-8490-5628-4*); lib. bdg. 254.95 (*0-8490-9031-8*) Gordon Pr.

Health Care Resources on the Internet: A Guide for Librarians & Health Care Consumers. Ed. by M. Sandra Wood. 1999. LC 99-37569. xxi, 205p. 39.95 (*0-7890-0632-4*); pap. text 24.95 (*0-7890-0911-0*) Haworth Pr.

Health Care Rights. Nancy Levitin. 1996. LC 95-49196. (Orig.). pap. 14.00 (*0-380-78025-9*, Avon Bks) Morrow Avon.

Health Care Series 1991. (*0-8273-3985-2*); tchr. ed. 10.00 (*0-8273-3984-4*);Bk. 1: Learning about Health Care. (*0-8273-3979-8*);Bk. 2: Preparing for a Job in Health Care. (*0-8273-3980-1*);Bk. 3: Getting Ready to Be a Nursing Assistant. (*0-8273-3982-8*);Bk. 4: Working as a Nursing Assistant. (*0-8273-3983-6*) Delmar.

Health Care Services in Prisons: Index of New Information with Authors, Subjects, & Bibliography. Kermit L. Zussman. 1996. LC 96-186. 57.50 (*0-7883-1132-8*); pap. 47.50 (*0-7883-1133-6*) ABBE Pubs Assn.

Health Care Services in the Nineteen Nineties: A Consumer's Guide. Stephen J. Williams & Sandra J. Guerra. 1991. LC 90-19591. 408p. 80.00 (*0-275-93867-0*, C3867); pap. 22.95 (*0-275-93909-X*, B3909) Greenwood (Praeger Pubs).

Health Care Shortage Areas: Designations Not a Useful Tool for Directing Resources to the Underserved. 1996. (Illus.). 55p. (Orig.). (C). pap. text 20.00 (*0-7881-3026-9*) DIANE Pub.

Health Care Social Work Practice. 1999. (C). pap. text 34.67 (*0-205-28734-4*, Macmillan Coll) P-H.

***Health Care Spending.** Ed. by Kathleen O'Leary Morgan & Scott E. Morgan. 2001. (State Statistical Trends Ser.). 100p. per. 50.00 (*0-7401-0703-8*) Morgan Quitno Corp.

Health Care Spending Control: The Experiences of France, Germany & Japan. 1994. (Illus.). 78p. (Orig.). (C). pap. text 25.00 (*0-7881-0574-4*) DIANE Pub.

Health Care State Rankings 1996. Ed. by Kathleen O'Leary Morgan et al. 1996. 540p. 49.95 (*1-56692-312-3*) Morgan Quitno Corp.

Health Care State Rankings 1997. Ed. by Kathleen O'Leary Morgan & Scott E. Morgan. 1997. 540p. 49.95 (*1-56692-317-4*) Morgan Quitno Corp.

***Health Care State Rankings 2002.** Ed. by Kathleen O'Leary Morgan & Scott E. Morgan. 2002. 540p. per. 54.95 (*0-7401-0039-4*) Morgan Quitno Corp.

Health Care State Rankings, 1998. Ed. by Kathleen O'Leary Morgan & Scott E. Morgan. 1998. 540p. pap. 49.95 (*1-56692-330-1*) Morgan Quitno Corp.

Health Care State Rankings 2000: Health Care in the 50 United States. Ed. by Kathleen O'Leary Morgan & Scott E. Morgan. 2000. 540p. per. 52.95 (*0-7401-0001-7*) Morgan Quitno Corp.

Health Care Strategic Plans. Steven G. Hillestad & Eric N. Berkowitz. 3rd ed. 2000. 250p. 59.00 (*0-8342-0989-6*, 09896) Aspen Pub.

Health Care Study for Older Americans: A Staff Report for the Federal Council on Aging. 1987. 70p. (*1-55672-019-X*) US HHS.

Health Care Supervisor on Career Development. Ed. by Charles R. McConnell. 1993. LC 93-195. (Health Care Supervisor Ser.). 238p. pap. 53.00 (*0-8342-0364-2*) Aspen Pub.

Health Care Supervisor on Effective Communication. Ed. by Charles R. McConnell. 1993. (Health Care Supervisor Ser.). 228p. pap. 53.00 (*0-8342-0365-0*) Aspen Pub.

Health Care Supervisor on Effective Employee Relations. Ed. by Charles R. McConnell. 1993. (Health Care Supervisor Ser.). 240p. pap. 53.00 (*0-8342-0366-9*) Aspen Pub.

Health Care Supervisor on Law. Ed. by Charles R. McConnell. 1993. (Health Care Supervisor Ser.). 238p. pap. 53.00 (*0-8342-0367-7*) Aspen Pub.

Health Care Supervisor on Productivity. Ed. by Charles R. McConnell. 1993. LC 93-9324. (Health Care Supervisor Ser.). 240p. pap. 53.00 (*0-8342-0368-5*) Aspen Pub.

Health Care Supervisor on Professional Nursing Management. Charles R. McConnel. 1993. (Health Care Supervisor Ser.). 236p. pap. 53.00 (*0-8342-0369-3*) Aspen Pub.

Health Care Surveyor. Jack Rudman. 1994. (Career Examination Ser.: C-3361). pap. 34.95 (*0-8373-3361-X*) Nat Learn.

Health Care Systems: Moral Conflicts in European & American Public Policy. Ed. by Martin Scrivener. 1988. 388p. (C). text 183.00 (*1-55608-045-X*) Kluwer Academic.

Health Care Systems Around the World: Characteristics, Issues, Reforms. William R. Lassey. 1996. LC 96-10745. 370p. (C). pap. 62.00 (*0-13-104233-5*) P-H.

Health Care Systems Conference, Nov. 21-22, 1972, Dallas, TX. Ed. by Eugene B. Konecci. 1974. (Science & Technology Ser.: Vol. 32). (Illus.). 265p. 25.00 (*0-87703-067-7*, Am Astronaut Soc) Univelt Inc.

Health Care Systems in Liberal Democracies. Ed. by Ann Wall. 1996. LC 96-11329. 224p. (C). 90.00 (*0-415-11806-9*); pap. 27.95 (*0-415-11807-7*) Routledge.

Health Care Systems in Transition: An International Perspective. Francis D. Powell & Albert F. Wessen. LC 98-19744. 1999. 428p. 84.95 (*0-7619-1081-6*, 81681); 1998. pap. 53.95 (*0-7619-1082-4*, 81682) Sage.

Health Care Teambook. Tim Porter-O'Grady & Cathleen Krueger Wilson. 1998. LC 99-181996. 384p. pap. text 29.95 (*1-55664-504-X*) Mosby Inc.

Health Care Teamwork: Interdisciplinary Practice & Teaching. Theresa J. K. Drinka & Phillip G. Clark. 2000. LC 00-20903. (Illus.). 224p. 68.00 (*0-86569-297-1*); pap. 24.95 (*0-86569-298-X*, R298, Aburn Hse Paperback) Greenwood.

Health Care Technology & Its Assessment in Eight Countries. Ed. by H. David Banta et al. 1995. (Illus.). 368p. (Orig.). (C). pap. text 65.00 (*0-7881-2501-X*) DIANE Pub.

Health Care, Technology, & the Competitive Environment. Ed. by Henry P. Brehm & Ross M. Mullner. 1989. LC 89-3961. 290p. 72.95 (*0-275-93033-5*, C3033, Praeger Pubs) Greenwood.

Health Care Twenty Ten: Health Care Delivery, Therapies, & Pharmaceutical Industries. Ed. by C. Bezold & K. Knabner. 1994. LC 93-43683. (Schering Foundation Workshop Ser.: Vol. 8). (Illus.). 117p. 49.00 (*0-387-57373-9*) Spr-Verlag.

***Health Care 2000 - Do Health Care Markets Require a New Model? Proceedings of a Conference Held May 4-5, 2000 at Stanford University.** Contrib. by Alain C. Enthoven et al. unabr. ed. 2001. (Comparative Health Care Policy Research Project Division Papers Ser.). 72p. 10.00 (*1-931368-01-5*) Asia-Pacific Res.

Health Care U. S. A. Understanding Its Organization & Delivery. Harry A. Sultz & Kristina M. Young. 3rd ed. 2001. LC 00-67398. xviii, 461p. pap. 57.00 (*0-8342-1912-3*) Aspen Pub.

Health Care Without Medicare: A New Practice Manual for Community-Based Care Management. Joseph A. Jackson. unabr. ed. 2000. LC 00-191374. 325p. pap. 29.95 (*0-9702208-0-4*, 001, Socarean Pr) Jos A Jackson.

Health Care Work Redesign. Kathleen Kelly. 1995. (Series on Nursing Administration: 7). 256p. 78.95 (*0-8039-7164-8*, 7928) Sage.

Health Care Work Redesign, Series on Nursing Ad. Kelly. 1995. 256p. 35.95 (*0-8016-8034-4*) Mosby Inc.

Health Care Worker: An Introduction to Health Occupations. Shirley A. Badasch & Doreen S. Chesebro. 1984. (Illus.). 288p. tchr. ed. 11.95 (*0-89303-502-5*); text 23.95 (*0-89303-514-9*) P-H.

Health Care Worker's Primer on Professionalism. 1999. 144p. text 29.27 (*0-13-021416-7*) P-H.

Health Care Worker's Primer on Professionalism. Sherry Makely. 2nd ed. 1999. LC 99-17379. (Illus.). 170p. pap. text 27.80 (*0-8359-5483-8*, Prentice Hall) P-H.

Health Care, You Wouldn't Live Without. H. N. Fowler. 1996. LC 96-95007. 160p. (Orig.). pap. text 9.95 (*0-9648173-0-6*) Lafayette NH.

Health Career Planning: A Realistic Guide. Ellen Lederman. 1988. 224p. 35.95 (*0-89885-397-4*); pap. 18.95 (*0-89885-401-6*) Kluwer Academic (Kluwer Acad Hman Sci).

Health Careers: A Guidebook. 1984. lib. bdg. 275.00 (*0-87700-530-3*) Revisionist Pr.

Health Careers & Medical Sciences. George Milles. 1975. LC 74-79837. (Allied Health Ser.). (gr. 11-12). pap. 7.87 (*0-672-61384-0*) Macmillan.

Health Careers Today. Judith A. Gerdin. 1990. (Illus.). 544p. (C). (gr. 13). text 31.95 (*0-8016-2469-X*, 02469) Mosby Inc.

Health Careers Today. Judith Gerdin. 2nd ed. 1997. (Illus.). 224p. wbk. ed. (*0-8151-9830-2*); 1996. 12.95 (*0-8151-3459-2*, G1707); 1996. LC 96-10791. (Illus.). 528p. (C). 39.00 (*0-8151-9829-9*, 24694); 1996. (Illus.). 528p. tchr. ed. (*0-8151-9831-0*) Mosby Inc.

Health Careers Today, Resource Kit. Marshall. 1991. 192p. 55.00 (*0-8016-3282-X*) Mosby Inc.

Health Care's Forgotten Majority: Nurses & Their Frayed White Collars. Jacqueline Goodman-Draper. 1995. LC 95-3751. 192p. 58.00 (*0-86569-248-3*, Auburn Hse) Greenwood.

Health Centre Concept in Primary Health Care. R. Kohn. 1983. (Public Health in Europe Ser.: No. 22). 236p. pap. text 20.00 (*92-890-1158-0*) World Health.

Health Characteristics of Large Metropolitan Statistical Areas: United States, 1988-1989. Public Health Service Staff et al. 1993. LC 93-7390. (Vital & Health Statistics Ser. 10: Data from the National Health Interview Survey: No. 187). (*0-8406-0479-3*) Natl Ctr Health Stats.

Health, Civilization & the State: A History of Public Health from Ancient to Modern Times. Dorothy Porter. 1999. LC 98-21836. 376p. pap. 27.95 (*0-415-20036-9*) Routledge.

Health Communication: Lessons from Family Planning & Reproductive Health. Phyllis T. Piotrow et al. 1997. LC 97-19235. 328p. 65.00 (*0-275-95577-X*); pap. 25.95 (*0-275-95578-8*) Greenwood (Praeger Pubs).

Health Communication: Strategies for Health Professionals. Northouse. 3rd ed. 1997. LC 97-14846. 350p. (C). pap. 47.00 (*0-8385-3680-8*, A-3680-4) P-H.

Health Communication: Theory & Practice. Gary Kreps & Barbara Thornton. 2nd ed. 1992. 233p. (C). pap. text 20.95 (*0-88133-643-2*) Waveland Pr.

Health Communication Research: A Guide to Developments & Directions. Ed. by Lorraine D. Jackson & Bernard K. Duffy. 1998. LC 98-14240. 264p. lib. bdg. 75.00 (*0-313-29925-0*, Greenwood Pr) Greenwood.

Health Communications in China: A Special Issue of Health Communication. Ed. by David H. Smith. 1999. 104p. pap. 20.00 (*0-8058-9785-2*) L Erlbaum Assocs.

Health Concerns of Hispanics in New York City. Jacob J. Lindenthal & Mareleyn Schneider. 1991. LC 91-21072. 256p. lib. bdg. 89.95 (*0-7734-9852-4*) E Mellen.

Health Concerns Quarterly. Saundersco. 1993. (C). pap. text, tchr. ed. 14.00 (*0-03-009229-9*) Harcourt Coll Pubs.

Health Concerns Quarterly: Fall 1994. Saundersco. 5th ed. 1994. (C). pap. text, tchr. ed. (*0-03-009237-X*) Harcourt Coll Pubs.

Health Concerns Quarterly: Summer 1994. Saundersco. 4th ed. 1994. (C). pap. text, tchr. ed. (*0-03-009234-5*) Harcourt Coll Pubs.

Health Conditions among the Currently Employed: United States, 1988. 1993. LC 93-21793. (Vital & Health Statistics Ser.: Series 10, No. 186). 67p. 5.00 (*0-8406-0478-5*) Natl Ctr Health Stats.

Health Conditions in Cambodia's Prisons. Physicians for Human Rights Staff & American Refugee Committee. 1995. 91p. pap. 7.00 (*1-879707-18-7*) Phy Human Rights.

Health Conditions in Haiti's Prisons. Physicians for Human Rights Staff. 1992. 40p. pap. text 3.00 (*1-879707-08-X*) Phy Human Rights.

Health Conditions in the Americas Vol. 1 & 2: 1994 Edition, Set. 1994. (PAHO Scientific Publications: No. 549). (ENG & SPA.). 905p. pap. text 100.00 (*92-75-11549-4*, 1610549) World Health.

Health Consequences of Service During the Persian Gulf War: Initial Findings & Recommendations for Immediate Action. Institute of Medicine Staff. 1995. LC 94-74965. 104p. (Orig.). (C). pap. text 25.00 (*0-309-05241-6*) Natl Acad Pr.

Health Consequences of Smoking: Cancer & Chronic Lung Disease in the Workplace: A Report of the Surgeon General. 1995. (Illus.). 542p. (Orig.). (C). pap. text 50.00 (*0-7881-2311-4*) DIANE Pub.

Health Consequences of Smoking: Cardiovascular Disease: A Report of the Surgeon General (1983) 1995. (Illus.). 384p. (Orig.). (C). pap. text 50.00 (*0-7881-2312-2*) DIANE Pub.

Health Consequences of Smoking: Nicotine Addiction: A Report of the Surgeon General (1988) 1995. (Illus.). 639p. (Orig.). (C). pap. text 50.00 (*0-7881-2314-9*) DIANE Pub.

Health Consequences of Smoking for Women: A Report of the Surgeon General (1985) 1995. (Illus.). 359p. (Orig.). (C). pap. text 50.00 (*0-7881-2316-5*) DIANE Pub.

Health Consequences of the Chernobyl Accident: Results of the IPHECA Pilot Projects & Related National Programmes Summary Report. 1995. LC 96-149706. (FRE & SPA.). 38p. (C). pap. 11.00 (*92-4-156181-5*, 1150440) World Health.

Health Counseling. Judith A. Lewis et al. 1993. LC 92-37322. 291p. text 41.00 (*0-534-13446-7*) Brooks-Cole.

Health Counts: A Fat & Calorie Guide. Kaiser Permanente. 1991. LC 90-38128. 272p. pap. 16.95 (*0-471-52949-4*) Wiley.

Health Crisis 2000. Peter O'Neil. 1983. pap. text 25.00 (*92-890-1009-6*) World Health.

Health, Culture & Community: Case Studies of Public Reactions to Health Programs. Ed. by Benjamin D. Paul. 1955. LC 55-10583. 494p. pap. 22.50 (*0-87154-653-1*) Russell Sage.

Health Dangers in Our Drinking Water: Index of New Information & Research Bible. Jay Klingenhagen et al. 1995. LC 95-19728. 167p. 57.50 (*0-7883-0500-X*); pap. 47.50 (*0-7883-0501-8*) ABBE Pubs Assn.

***Health Dangers of Free Radical Chemistry: Index of New Information & Guide-Book for Consumers, Reference & Research.** Alfred H. Towson. 2002. (Illus.). 180p. 57.50 (*0-7883-2552-3*); pap. 47.50 (*0-7883-2553-1*) ABBE Pubs Assn.

Health Dangers, Risks & Damages in Medication Errors: Index of New Information with Authors, Subjects & References. Marie S. Zampiello. 1997. 150p. 57.50 (*0-7883-1388-6*); pap. 47.50 (*0-7883-1389-4*) ABBE Pubs Assn.

***Health Dangers Without Disease - By Nutrition Deficiencies & Nutritional Disorders: Index of New Information for Consumers, Reference & Research.** Ed. by Research and Development Division Staff & John C. Bartone. 2001. (Illus.). 180p. 47.50 (*0-7883-2436-5*); pap. 44.50 (*0-7883-2437-3*) ABBE Pubs Assn.

Health Data Directory, 1997. Ed. by Alice McCart. 1996. 424p. pap. 365.00 (*1-881393-83-6*) Faulkner & Gray.

Health Data in the Information Age: Use, Disclosure, & Privacy. Institute of Medicine, Committee on Regional Health. Ed. by Kathleen N. Lohr & Molla S. Donaldson. 1994. LC 94-2613. 272p. (C). text 39.95 (*0-309-04995-4*) Natl Acad Pr.

Health Data on Older Americans. 1997. lib. bdg. 250.99 (*0-8490-8208-0*) Gordon Pr.

Health Data on Older Americans: U. S., 1992. 1994. (Illus.). 309p. (Orig.). (C). pap. text 60.00 (*0-7881-1008-X*) DIANE Pub.

Health Data on Older Americans: United States, 1992. 1992. LC 92-48880. (Vital & Health Statistics Ser. 3: Analytical & Epidemiological Studies: No. 27). (*0-8406-0470-X*) Natl Ctr Health Stats.

Health Decision Support Systems. Tan. 1998. tchr. ed. 59.00 (*0-8342-1154-8*) Aspen Pub.

Health Decision Support Systems. Joseph K. H. Tan & Samuel Sheps. 1998. LC 97-42745. 432p. 65.00 (*0-8342-1065-7*, 10657) Aspen Pub.

Health Department Investigator. Jack Rudman. 1994. (Career Examination Ser.: C-3074). pap. 29.95 (*0-8373-3074-2*) Nat Learn.

Health Department Volunteer Services Guide. Harold E. Knight, III. 1988. 60p. (Orig.). pap. 24.95 (*0-945253-02-8*) Thornsbury Bailey Brown.

Health-Development Link. Rosalia Rodriguez-Garcia et al. 1993. 164p. pap. text (*0-9636369-0-1*) PAHO.

Health Diary: Myself, My Baby. 1994. (Illus.). 85p. (Orig.). (C). pap. text 20.00 (*0-7881-0333-4*) DIANE Pub.

Health Diary for Women of Color: Your Personal Log. Melody T. McCloud. 1999. 66p. pap. 9.95 (*0-9643554-1-8*) New Life GA.

Health Dimensions of Economic Reform. 1992. ix, 68p. pap. text 15.00 (*92-4-156146-7*, 1150384) World Health.

Health Discoveries Advanced from the 21st Century: A Special Report for Health Care Professionals & Patients. Tracy W. Humble. Ed. by Sheila A. Nicholson. 1993. 132p. (Orig.). 14.95 (*1-882799-01-1*); pap. 14.95 (*1-882799-03-8*) Edutainment.

Health, Disease, & Causal Explanations in Medicine. Ed. by Lennart Nordenfelt & Ingemar B. Lindahl. 1984. 286p. text 109.00 (*90-277-1660-9*) Kluwer Academic.

Health, Disease & Society: An Introduction to Medical Geography. Graham Moon & Kelvyn Jones. 1988. (Illus.). 256p. pap. text 19.95 (*0-7102-1219-4*, Routledge Thoemms) Routledge.

Health, Disease & Survival: A Biomedical & Genetic Analysis of the Orang Asli of Malaysia. A. Baer. 1999. LC 98-945286. (Illus.). pap. text (*983-40042-0-6*) Ctr Orang Asli MYS. *Dist:* OR St Zoology.

Health Disease & the Environment. Harold D. Foster. 1992. LC 92-3951. xvii, 516p. 71.00 (*0-8493-7737-4*, RB152) CRC Pr.

Health Disease in Tropical Africa: Geographical & Medical Viewpoints. Ed. by Rais Akhtar. 1987. xii, 520p. text 312.00 (*3-7186-0300-4*) Gordon & Breach.

Health, Disease, Medicine & Famine in Ethiopia: A Bibliography, 13. Ed. by Zein A. Zein. 1991. LC 90-22698. (African Special Bibliographic Ser.: No. 13). 424p. lib. bdg. 95.00 (*0-313-27488-6*, KHJ, Greenwood Pr) Greenwood.

Health Doctors-Their Views, Interviews, Writings, Rights, Codes & Criticisms: Index of New Information. Charles L. Karney. 1994. 150p. 57.50 (*0-7883-0008-3*); pap. 47.50 (*0-7883-0009-1*) ABBE Pubs Assn.

Health Doctors with Impairments, AIDS, Decline & Decadence, Burn-out & Abuse of Drugs & Substances: Index of New Information. Jeffery R. Sutton. 1994. 150p. 57.50 (*0-7883-0000-8*); pap. 47.50 (*0-7883-0001-6*) ABBE Pubs Assn.

Health Economics. Peter Zweifel & Friedrich Breyer. Tr. by Peter Zweifel. 1997. LC 96-8384. (Illus.). 400p. text 62.95 (*0-19-510813-2*) OUP.

Health Economics. Charles E. Phelps. 2nd ed. 1997. LC 96-47469. (Addison-Wesley Series in Economics Ser.). 687p. (C). 105.00 (*0-673-99398-1*) Addison-Wesley.

Health Economics: Efficiency, Quality, & Equity. Steven R. Eastaugh. 1992. LC 91-26275. 480p. 69.50 (*0-86569-196-7*, T196); pap. 32.95 (*0-86569-197-5*, R197) Greenwood (Auburn Hse).

Health Economics: Fundamentals & Flow of Funds. Thomas E. Getzen. 1998. LC 96-21162. 480p. text 73.95 (*0-471-58648-X*) Wiley.

Health Economics: Latin American Perspectives. 1989. (PAHO Scientific Publication Ser.: No. 517). 198p. text 36.00 (*92-75-11517-6*) World Health.

Health Economics: Prospects for the Future. George Teeling-Smith. 1987. LC 87-8998. 288p. lib. bdg. (*0-7099-1958-1*) C Helm GBR. *Dist:* Routldge.

Health Economics: Theories, Applications, & Industry Studies. Stephen P. Neun & Rexford E. Santerre. 1995. 420p. (C). text 67.50 (*0-256-15113-X*, Irwn McGrw-H) McGrw-H Hghr Educ.

Health Economics: Theories, Insights & Industry Studies. Rexford E. Santerre. 1999. LC 98-89949. (Dryden Press Series in Economics). 672p. (C). text 107.00 (*0-03-025629-1*) Harcourt.

Health Economics & Development. Stuart Wells & Steven Klees. 1980. LC 79-24821. 165p. 55.00 (*0-275-90566-7*, C0566, Praeger Pubs) Greenwood.

Health Economics & Health Policy in the 1990s: Surprises from the Past, Forecasts for the Future, Vol. 11. Pref. by Louis F. Rossiter. 1990. (Advances in Health Economics & Health Services Research Ser.). 250p. 73.25 (*1-55938-137-X*) Jai Pr.

Health Economics & Policy. James W. Henderson. 1998. LC 98-17410. (Miscellaneous/Catalogs Ser.). 400p. text 94.95 (*0-538-87484-8*) S-W Thomson.

Health Economics for Nurses: An Introductory Guide. Stephen Morris. 1997. LC 97-41281. (Prentice Hall Nursing Ser.). 296p. pap. 57.00 (*0-13-255993-5*) P-H.

Health Economics for the Uninitiated. Tony Lockett. 1996. LC 95-52776. (*1-85775-069-1*) Radcliffe Med Pr GBR. *Dist:* Balogh.

Health Economics of Dementia. Ed. by Anders Wimo. 1998. LC 98-16101. 592p. 295.00 (*0-471-98376-4*) Wiley.

Health Economics of Depression, Vol. 4. Ed. by B. Jonsson & J. F. Rosenbaum. 1993. LC 93-8864. (Perspectives in Psychiatry Ser.: Vol. 4). 164p. 245.00 (*0-471-93746-0*) Wiley.

Health Economics of Japan: Patients, Doctors, & Hospitals under a Universal Health Insurance Program. Aki Yoshikawa et al. 1996. LC 96-222134. 300p. (*0-86008-518-X*) U of Tokyo JPN. *Dist:* Col U Pr.

Health Economics Research in Developing Countries. Ed. by Anne Mills & Kenneth Lee. 1993. LC 92-49379. (Oxford Medical Publications). (C). pap. (*0-19-262320-6*) OUP.

Health Economics Worldwide. Ed. by Peter Zweifel & H. E. Frech, III. 1991. (Developments in Health Economics & Public Policy Ser.). 368p. (C). lib. bdg. 149.50 (*0-7923-1219-8*) Kluwer Academic.

Health Economy. Victor R. Fuchs. 1986. LC 85-16442. (Illus.). 411p. reprint ed. pap. 16.95 (*0-674-38341-9*) HUP.

***Health Education.** 2001. pap. 39.95 (*0-412-55110-1*) Chapman & Hall.

Health Education: A Cognitive Behavioral Approach. Donald A. Read. 1996. LC 96-22262. (Series in Health Sciences). (Illus.). 336p. (C). pap. text 43.95 (*0-7637-0147-5*, 0147-5) Jones & Bartlett.

Health Education: A Programmes Review. 1974. (Offset Publications: No. 7). pap. text 17.00 (*92-4-170007-6*, 1120007) World Health.

Health Education: A Source Book for Teaching. Beryl I. Ford. 1978. text 33.00 (*0-08-021327-8*); pap. text 22.00 (*0-08-021326-X*) Elsevier (Pergamon Pr).

Health Education: An Annotated Bibliography on Lifestyle, Behavior, & Health. Marion C. Chafetz. 1981. 272p. 65.00 (*0-306-40754-X*, Plenum Trade) Perseus Pubng.

Health Education: Cognitive Behavior. Patricia A. Read & Houston. 1996. (Health Science Ser.). (Illus.). 112p. (C). pap. text, tchr. ed. 13.95 (*0-7637-0351-6*, 0351-6) Jones & Bartlett.

Health Education: Creating Strategies for School & Community Health. Glen G. Gilbert & Robin G. Sawyer. (Illus.). (C). 1995. LC 94-22602. 400p. pap. text 46.25 (*0-86720-812-0*, 812-0); 2nd ed. 2000. LC 00-24685. 368p. pap. text 47.50 (*0-7637-1334-1*, 1334-1) Jones & Bartlett.

Health Education: Effectiveness & Efficiency. Keith Tones et al. 1990. 320p. 82.50 (*0-412-32980-8*, A4223) Chapman & Hall.

Health Education & Health Promotion. Randall R. Cottrell et al. 1998. LC 98-38235. 306p. pap. text 45.00 (*0-205-27365-3*) Allyn.

Health Education & the Media. D. S. Leathar. 1985. pap. 22.75 (*0-08-031996-3*, Pergamon Pr) Elsevier.

Health Education in Health Aspects of Family Planning: Proceedings of the WHO Scientific Group, Geneva, 1970. WHO Staff. 1971. (Technical Reports: No. 483). pap. text 6.00 (*92-4-120483-4*, 1100483) World Health.

Health Education in Primary Health Care: A Perspective. A. B. Hiramani. 1992. (C). (*81-7018-700-1*) BR Pub IND. *Dist:* S Asia.

Health Education in Senior High Schools. Dorothy N. Ruef. LC 79-177219. (Columbia University, Teachers College - Contributions to Education Ser.: No. 636). reprint ed. 37.50 (*0-404-55636-1*) AMS Pr.

Health Education in the Control of Schistosomiasis. 1990. (CHI, ENG, FRE & SPA.). 61p. pap. text 11.00 (*92-4-154407-4*, 1150342) World Health.

Health Education in the Elementary School. Dean F. Miller et al. 3rd ed. 2000. LC 00-20991. (Illus.). xii, 338p. pap. 50.31 (*0-697-29433-1*) McGraw.

Health Education (K-12) A Maryland Curricular Framework. Ed. by Russell Henke & Janet Pabst. 1994. (Illus.). 49p. (Orig.). (C). pap. text 30.00 (*0-7881-0368-7*) DIANE Pub.

Health Education, Principles, Preparation & Practice. Ed. by Karen M. Lorentzen & Robert D. Neal. 1990. (Illus.). 124p. pap. 18.75 (*0-87527-473-0*) Green.

Health Effect Assessments of the Basic Acrylates. Ed. by Tipton R. Tyler et al. 1993. LC 93-14268. 144p. 154.95 (*0-8493-4721-1*, RA1242) CRC Pr.

Health Effects Models for Nuclear Power Plant Accident Consequence Analysis: Introduction, Integration & Summary. 1994. lib. bdg. 250.00 (*0-8490-8422-9*) Gordon Pr.

Health Effects of Asbestos & of Other Minerals & Fibres: An Annotated Compilation of the Worlds' Literature on Asbestos 1906-1986, Set. Premysl V. Pelnar. Ed. by George H. Scherr. 1988. 2400p. 362.00 (*0-930376-46-3*) Chem-Orbital.

Health Effects of Combined Exposures in the Work Environment. 1981. (Technical Report Ser.: No. 662). 76p. pap. text 4.00 (*92-4-120662-4*) World Health.

Health Effects of Disinfectants & Disinfection By-Products. 1991. 208p. 63.00 (*0-89867-566-9*, 90577) Am Water Wks Assn.

Health Effects of Exposure to Low Levels of Ionizing Radiation: Beir V. National Research Council Staff. 1990. LC 89-64118. (Beir Ser.: Vol. 5). 436p. pap. text 39.95 (*0-309-03995-9*) Natl Acad Pr.

Health Effects of Exposure to Radon: BEIR VI. National Research Council Staff. 1998. 350p. text 54.95 (*0-309-05645-4*, Joseph Henry Pr) Natl Acad Pr.

Health Effects of Exposure to Radon: Time for Reassessment? National Research Council Staff. 1994. LC 94-66478. (Beir Ser.: Vol. 6). 114p. (Orig.). (C). pap. text 24.00 (*0-309-05087-1*) Natl Acad Pr.

Health Effects of Hazardous Materials. Neal K. Ostler. 1996. LC 96-17137. (Prentice Hall's Environmental Technology Ser.: Vol. 3). 256p. (C). pap. 81.00 (*0-02-389551-9*, Macmillan Coll) P-H.

Health Effects of Ingested Fluoride. National Research Council Staff. 1993. LC 93-85306. 206p. (Orig.). (C). pap. text 35.00 (*0-309-04975-X*) Natl Acad Pr.

Health Effects of Internally Deposited Radionuclides Emphasis on Radium & Thorium. G. Van Kaick et al. 1995. 360p. text 106.00 (*981-02-2015-4*) World Scientific Pub.

Health Effects of Low Frequency Electric & Magnetic Fields. 1995. lib. bdg. 604.99 (*0-8490-6719-7*) Gordon Pr.

Health Effects of Low-Frequency Electric & Magnetic Fields. 1995. lib. bdg. 263.99 (*0-8490-8376-1*) Gordon Pr.

Health Effects of Low-Level Radiation. Sohei Kondo. 1993. (Illus.). 211p. (Orig.). pap. text 33.95 (*0-944838-43-X*) Med Physics Pub.

Health Effects of Synthetic Silica Particulates-STP 732. Ed. by D. Dunnom. 1981. 223p. 24.00 (*0-8031-0734-X*, STP732) ASTM.

Health Effects of W3 Polyunsaturated Fatty Acids in Seafoods. Ed. by Artemis P. Simopoulos et al. 1991. (World Review of Nutrition & Dietetics Ser.: Vol. 66). (Illus.). xxiv, 592p. 433.25 (*3-8055-5244-0*) S Karger.

Health Enhancement Handbook. Glenn Richardson & Michael Felts. 1990. 310p. (Orig.). (C). pap. text 19.95 (*0-89641-196-6*) American Pr.

Health, Environment & Development. Rabindra N. Pati. 1992. (C). (*81-7024-460-9*) Ashish Pub Hse IND. *Dist:* S Asia.

Health Evaluation of Heavy Metals in Infant Formula & Junior Food, Berlin: 1981, Proceedings. Ed. by E. H. Schmidt & A. Hildebrandt. 1982. (Illus.). 192p. 38.00 (*0-387-11823-3*) Spr-Verlag.

Health Expenditures in New York City 1983. Willine Carr. 1985. (Papers: No. 1). 32p. 5.00 (*0-934459-09-6*) United Hosp Fund.

Health Facilities in Southern New York: A Guide to Inpatient, Outpatient, & Long-Term Care. Division of Research, Analysis, and Planning Staff. 1988. 70p. 20.00 (*0-934459-49-5*) United Hosp Fund.

Health Facilities in Southern New York: A Guide to Inpatient, Outpatient, & Long-Term Care. United Hospital Fund Staff. 1989. 88p. 20.00 (*0-934459-55-X*); 1987. 70p. 20.00 (*0-934459-38-X*) United Hosp Fund.

Health Facilities in Southern New York: A Guide to Inpatient, Outpatient, & Long-Term Care, Vol. I. Compiled by Division of Research, Analysis, and Planning Staff. 1985. 70p. 15.00 (*0-934459-06-1*) United Hosp Fund.

Health Facilities in Southern New York: A Guide to Inpatient, Outpatient, & Long-Term Care, 1983 Edition. Compiled by Division of Planning, Distribution and Development S. 1983. (Health Care Information Ser.). 72p. 15.00 (*0-934459-82-7*) United Hosp Fund.

Health Facilities Manager. Jack Rudman. (Career Examination Ser.: C-3634). pap. 34.95 (*0-8373-3634-1*) Nat Learn.

Health Facilities Planner. Jack Rudman. 1994. (Career Examination Ser.: No. C-3531). pap. 34.95 (*0-8373-3531-0*) Nat Learn.

Health Facilities Review, Vol. 2. Ed. by AIA Committee on Architecture for Health. 1988. 128p. (Orig.). pap. 10.00 (*1-55835-017-9*) AIA Press.

Health Facilities Review, 1992-93. American Institute of Architects Staff. 1993. (Illus.). 176p. pap. 20.00 (*1-55835-090-X*) AIA Press.

Health Facility Malpractice Cases: A Management Prevention Guide. W. A. Rothman & Monroe M. Title. 1995. LC 95-8061. 187p. lib. bdg. 145.00 (*1-56072-227-4*) Nova Sci Pubs.

Health Facility Management Assistant. Jack Rudman. 1994. (Career Examination Ser.: C-3387). pap. 29.95 (*0-8373-3387-3*) Nat Learn.

Health Factors Involved in Working under Conditions of Heat Stress: Proceedings of the WHO Scientific Group, Geneva, 1967. WHO Staff. 1969. (Technical Reports: No. 412). pap. text 5.00 (*92-4-120412-5*, 1100412) World Health.

Health Facts: A Critical Evaluation of the Major Problems, Treatments & Alternatives Facing Medical Consumers. Maryann Napoli. 1984. LC 81-2127. 400p. 22.95 (*0-87951-132-X*); pap. 8.95 (*0-87951-196-6*) Overlook Pr.

Health, Food, & Nutrition in Third World Development, 6. Ed. by Pradip K. Ghosh. 1984. LC 83-26504. (International Development Resource Bks.: No. 6). (Illus.). 617p. lib. bdg. 125.00 (*0-313-24142-2*, GHF/, Greenwood Pr) Greenwood.

Health Food Book. Robert Berkley. 1982. (Runner's World Ser.). pap. 9.95 (*0-02-499520-7*, Macmillan Coll) P-H.

Health Foods: A Source Guide. 1991. lib. bdg. 77.95 (*0-8490-4846-X*) Gordon Pr.

Health Foods & Disease Avoidance: Index of New Information with References. Dolly M. Callahan. 1999. (Illus.). 150p. 57.50 (*0-7883-2224-9*); pap. 47.50 (*0-7883-2225-7*) ABBE Pubs Assn.

Health for All. Herbert M. Shelton. 1993. 216p. reprint ed. spiral bd. 15.50 (*0-7873-0780-7*) Hlth Research.

Health for All - A Challenge to Research in Health Manpower Development: Highlights of the Ibadan Conference. 1983. (CIOMS Publication Ser.). pap. text 15.00 (*92-9036-012-7*) World Health.

H I

Health for All - A Challenge to Research in Health Manpower Development: Proceedings of the Ibadan Conference. 1983. (CIOMS Round Table Proceedings Ser.: No. 16). pap. text 20.00 (*92-9036-014-3*) World Health.

Health for All Targets: The Health Policy for Europe. 1993. (European Health for All Ser.: No. 4). (ENG, FRE, GER & RUS.). xi, 228p. pap. text 36.00 (*92-890-1311-7*, 1360004) World Health.

Health for Our Times. Matha Halperin. 2000. (Science for Our Times Ser.). (Illus.). 164p. (gr. 5-12). pap. text, wbk. ed. 10.95 (*0-87594-347-0*, 3500) Book-Lab.

Health for the Farmer. C. F. Stanford. 1991. (*0-85236-221-8*) Farming Pr GBR. *Dist:* Diamond Farm Bk.

Health for the Millions. Herbert M. Shelton. 2nd ed. 1996. LC 96-86835. 328p. reprint ed. pap. 9.95 (*0-914532-41-3*, 242) Amer Natural Hygiene.

Health for the Whole Person: A Complete Guide to Holistic Medicine. Ed. by Arthur C. Hastings et al. 1980. 529p. text 42.50 (*0-89158-883-3*); pap. text 25.00 (*0-89158-884-1*) Westview.

Health Framework for California Public Schools, K-12. California Department of Education Staff. 1994. (Illus.). 244p. pap. 10.00 (*0-8011-1064-5*) Calif Education.

Health Freedom: Preventive Medicine Can Save Your Life & Fortune. Ed. by N. V. Peterson. 1994. LC 93-74785. 66p. (Orig.). pap. 9.00 (*1-57000-028-X*); pap. 2.00 (*1-57000-029-8*) W S Dawson.

Health from Space Research: Austrian Accomplishments. Ed. by Austrian Society for Aerospace Medicine Staff. 1992. LC 92-31166. 40.95 (*0-387-82413-8*) Spr-Verlag.

Health from the Hedgerow: Encyclopedia of Medicinal Plants. Dennis Furnell. 1985. (Illus.). 192p. 20.95 (*0-7134-4712-5*) Trafalgar.

Health from the Inside Out Vol. 1. John-Roger. 1995. 112p. 24.95 (*0-914829-32-7*) Mandeville LA.

Health Funds Grants Resources Yearbook. Ed. by Beth-Ann Kerber. 7th ed. 1996. (Illus.). 522p. spiral bd. 152.00 (*1-882364-07-4*); 8th ed. 1999. 564p. per. 165.00 (*1-882364-30-9*, Amer Busn Pub) Hlth Res Pub.

***Health Funds Grants Resources Yearbook.** Beth-Ann Kerber. Ed. by Beth-Ann Kerber. 9th ed. 2001. 500p. pap. 165.00 (*1-882364-58-9*) Hlth Res Pub.

Health Gap see Droit a la Sante: Au-Dela de la Grossesse et de la Reproduction

Health Goals & Health Indicators: Policy, Planning & Evaluation. Ed. by Jack Elinson et al. 1978. LC 77-14044. (AAAS Selected Symposium Ser.: No. 2). text 34.00 (*0-89158-429-3*) Westview.

Health Groups in Washington: A Directory. 10th rev. ed. 1989. 170p. 15.00 (*0-929852-01-X*); 11th ed. 1991. (*0-929852-03-6*) Natl Health Coun.

***Health Handbook.** Louise Tenney. 1994. 331p. pap. 7.95 (*0-913932-58-2*) Woodland UT.

Health Handbook: A Guide to Family Health. Louise Tenney. l.t. ed. 1987. 331p. pap. 11.95 (*0-913923-71-0*) Woodland UT.

Health, Happiness & Hormones: One Woman's Journey Towards Health after a Hysterectomy. Arlene Swaney. 1996. LC 95-69734. 192p. pap. 9.95 (*0-914984-72-1*) Starburst.

Health, Happiness & Human Needs: An Introduction to Symbolization. Marge Reddington. 1994. LC 94-60127. 254p. pap. 19.95 (*0-9640594-0-1*) TDC Pubng.

Health Hazards - Skin Problems & Disorders Caused by Employment Sites & Occupational Diversity: Index of New Information with Authors, Subjects, & References. American Health Research Institute Staff. 1996. LC 96-12482. 57.50 (*0-7883-1044-5*); pap. 47.50 (*0-7883-1045-3*) ABBE Pubs Assn.

Health Hazards, Gender, & Society. Ed. by Indu Mathur & Sanjay Sharma. 1995. (C). (*81-7033-239-7*) Rawat Pubns IND. *Dist:* S Asia.

Health Hazards in Adolescence. Ed. by Klaus Hurrelmann & Friedrich Losel. 1990. (Prevention & Intervention in Childhood & Adolescence Ser.: No. 8). (Illus.). x, 528p. (C). lib. bdg. 69.95 (*3-11-012448-3*) De Gruyter.

Health Hazards in Occupations: Index of Modern Information. Mary B. Schneply. 1990. LC 88-47993. 150p. 47.50 (*1-55914-156-5*); pap. 44.50 (*1-55914-157-3*) ABBE Pubs Assn.

Health Hazards Manual for Artists. Michael McCann. 4th ed. 1990. LC 93-46519. (Illus.). 144p. pap. 11.95 (*1-55821-306-6*, Lyons) Globe Pequot.

Health Hazards of Electromagnetic Radiation. Bruce Fife. 2000. LC 98-34136. (Illus.). 64p. (YA). (gr. 8-12). reprint ed. pap. 10.00 (*0-941599-42-6*, HlthWise Pubns) Piccadilly Bks.

Health Hazards of the Human Environment. 1973. pap. text 44.00 (*92-4-156037-1*, 1150069) World Health.

Health Hazards of Video Display Terminals: A Comprehensive Bibliography on a Critical Issue of Workplace Health & Safety. 3rd ed. 1987. (Information Alert Ser.: No. 4). 62p. 9.95 (*0-942158-04-0*) Ryan Research.

***Health, Healing & Beyond: The Living Tradition of Krishnamacharya.** T. K. V. Desikachar & R. H. Cravens. 2001. (Illus.). 256p. pap. 24.95 (*0-89381-941-7*) Aperture.

Health, Healing, & Healers in Conventional & Alternative Medicine: What You Need to Know to Safeguard the Life Force Within You. Edward Zebrowski. 1998. LC 98-60452. 266p. pap. 17.95 (*0-9640096-3-3*) Woodstock Books.

Health, Healing & Religion: A Cross-Cultural Perspective. David R. Kinsley. 1995. LC 95-25271. 212p. pap. text 45.00 (*0-13-212771-7*) P-H.

Health, Health Care & Health Economics: Perspectives on Distribution. M. L. Barer et al. 1998. LC 98-19860. 576p. 145.00 (*0-471-97879-5*) Wiley.

Health Hints for Hikers. Albert P. Rosen. 1994. LC 94-31690. (Illus.). 131p. pap. 5.95 (*1-880775-02-6*) NY-NJ Trail Confer.

Health, Hope & Healing. David A. Tate. 1991. LC 89-23833. 252p. pap. 9.95 (*0-87131-658-7*) M Evans.

Health, Hope, & Healing: A Survivor of Cancer & Heart Attack Tells How He Used Holistic Techniques & a Spiritual Perspective As Well As Traditional Search for Wellness. David A. Tate. 1998. 234p. reprint ed. text 18.00 (*0-7881-5574-1*) DIANE Pub.

Health I. Jack Rudman. 1994. (Regents College Proficiency Examination Ser.: CPEP-17). pap. 23.95 (*0-8373-5417-X*) Nat Learn.

Health I: Personal Health, Physical Aspects. Jack Rudman. 1994. (ACT Proficiency Examination Program Ser.: PEP-33). pap. 23.95 (*0-8373-5533-8*) Nat Learn.

Health II. Jack Rudman. 1994. (Regents College Proficiency Examination Ser.: No. CPEP-18). pap. 23.95 (*0-8373-5418-8*) Nat Learn.

Health II: Personal Health, Emotional-Social Aspects. Jack Rudman. 1994. (ACT Proficiency Examination Program Ser.: No. PEP-34). pap. 23.95 (*0-8373-5534-6*) Nat Learn.

Health III. Jack Rudman. 1994. (Regents College Proficiency Examination Ser.: CPEP-19). pap. 23.95 (*0-8373-5419-6*) Nat Learn.

Health III: Public & Environmental Health. Jack Rudman. 1994. (ACT Proficiency Examination Program Ser.: PEP-35). pap. 23.95 (*0-8373-5535-4*) Nat Learn.

Health, Illness & Healing: Society, Social Context & Self : An Anthology. Ed. by Kathleen Charmaz & Debora A. Paterniti. 1999. (Illus.). 600p. (C). pap. text (*0-935732-98-5*) Roxbury Pub Co.

Health, Illness, & the Social Body: A Critical Sociology. Peter E. Freund & Meredith B. McGuire. 3rd ed. 1998. LC 97-39102. 418p. (C). pap. text 53.33 (*0-13-897075-0*) P-H.

Health Impact of Different Energy Source: A Challenge for the End of the Century. 1986. (WHO Regional Publications, European Ser.: No. 19). 71p. pap. text 13.00 (*92-890-1110-6*, 1310019) World Health.

Health Impacts of Large Releases of Radionuclides - Symposium No. 203. Herwig Paretzke. 1997. LC 97-294. (CIBA Foundation Symposia Ser.: Vol. 203). 256p. 170.00 (*0-471-96510-3*) Wiley.

Health Implications of Exercise & Sports in the School Aged Child & Adolescent. Oded Bar-Or. 1986. (Journal: Vol.13, No. 1). (Illus.). 60p. pap. 35.75 (*3-8055-4469-3*) S Karger.

Health Implications of Fungi in Indoor Environments. Ed. by R. A. Samson. 1994. LC 95-129638. (Air Quality Monographs: Vol. 2). 622p. 237.00 (*0-444-81866-9*) Elsevier.

***Health Improvement Programmes.** Ed. by Salman Rawaf & Peter Orton. 2000. 175p. pap. (*1-85315-388-5*) Royal Soc of Medicine Pr Ltd GBR. *Dist:* Balogh.

Health in Aging: Sociological Issues & Policy Directions. Ed. by Russell A. Ward & Sheldon S. Tobin. 1987. 320p. (C). 38.95 (*0-8261-6130-8*) Springer Pub.

Health in America: A Multicultural Perspective. Nakamura. 1998. LC 98-26179. 272p. pap. text 42.00 (*0-205-29012-4*) Allyn.

Health in Colonial Ghana: Disease, Medicine, & Socio-Economic Change, 1900-1955. K. David Patterson. 1981. 187p. 20.00 (*0-918456-42-8*) African Studies Assn.

Health in Day Care: A Manual for Health Professionals. American Academy of Pediatrics Staff. 1987. 243p. pap. 42.95 (*0-910761-13-2*) Am Acad Pediat.

Health in Europe: The 1993-1994 Health for All Monitoring Report. 1994. (WHO Regional Publications: No. 56). xii, 58p. pap. text 17.00 (*92-890-1320-6*, 1310056) World Health.

Health in Rural North America: The Geography of Health Care & Services & Delivery. Ed. by Wilbert M. Gesler & Thomas C. Ricketts, III. 1992. LC 91-17840. 280p. (C). text 40.00 (*0-8135-1759-1*); pap. text 18.00 (*0-8135-1760-5*) Rutgers U Pr.

Health in Scotland, 1995. HMSO Staff. 1996. 142p. pap. (*0-11-495817-3*, HM958173) Statnry Office GBR. *Dist:* Bernan Associates.

Health in Stress - Actions, Reactions & the General Adaptation Syndrome: Index of New Information & Bibliography. Nelson L. Nies. 1996. 150p. 57.50 (*0-7883-0980-3*); pap. 47.50 (*0-7883-0981-1*) ABBE Pubs Assn.

Health in the 21st Century: Will Doctors Survive? see Saludo en el Siglo: Sobreviviran los Medicas?

Health in the Headlines: The Stories Behind the Stories. Stephen Klaidman. 1991. 264p. 30.00 (*0-19-505298-6*) OUP.

Health in the Later Years. Ferrini. 4th ed. Date not set. pap. text 27.00 (*0-697-29445-5*) McGraw.

Health in the New Communications Age. Ed. by M. J. Ladeira et al. 1995. LC 95-7959. (Studies in Health Technology & Informatics: Vol. 24). 733p. 120.00 (*90-5199-224-6*) IOS Press.

Health in the Southern United States: An Original Anthology. Ed. by Barbara G. Rosenkrantz. 1977. LC 76-40667. (Public Health in America Ser.). (Illus.). reprint ed. lib. bdg. 29.95 (*0-405-09875-8*) Ayer.

Health in the Twentieth Century: An Original Anthology. Ed. by Barbara G. Rosenkrantz. 1977. LC 76-40666. (Public Health in America Ser.). reprint ed. lib. bdg. 39.95 (*0-405-09874-X*) Ayer.

Health in the 21st Century: Will Doctors Survive? Francisco Contreras. Ed. by Pamela M. Lowe. Tr. by Luisa Ruiz from SPA. 1997.Tr. of Salud en el Siglo XXI, "Sobreviviran Los Medicos?. (Illus.). 392p. (Orig.). mass mkt. 19.95 (*1-57946-000-3*) Interpacific Pr.

Health in Your Hands: How to Gain a Detailed Picture of Your State of Health from Your Hands. Lori Reid. 1993. 256p. (*1-85538-182-6*) Aqrn Pr GBR. *Dist:* Harper SF.

Health Industry QuickSource: A Complete Descriptive Reference to Health Care Information Resources. Ed. by Mary J. Cilurzo. 1995. 1100p. (Orig.). pap. 225.00 (*1-886515-08-5*) QuickSource Pr.

Health Informatics: An Overview. Hovenga. 1998. pap. text 36.00 (*0-443-05236-0*) Saunders.

Health Informatics Directory, 1996. Tim Kieschnick. 1996. 304p. 21.00 (*0-683-04566-0*, K0712) Lppncott W & W.

Health Information: Management of a Strategic Resource. Ed. by Mervat Abdelhak et al. 1996. (Illus.). 784p. tchr. ed. (*0-7216-5151-8*) Saunders.

Health Information: Management of a Strategic Resource. Mervat Abdelhak et al. 1996. (Illus.). 752p. text 52.50 (*0-7216-5132-1*) Saunders.

Health Information: Management of a Strategic Resource, Textbook & Workbook Package. Ed. by Mervat Abdelhak et al. 1996. (Illus.). 784p. text, wbk. ed. 69.00 (*0-7216-5114-3*) Saunders.

***Health Information: Management of a Strategic Resource - ExaMaster.** Mervat Abdelhak et al. 2001. (*0-7216-8649-4*) Saunders.

Health Information: New Possibilities. Ed. by Tony McSean. 1995. LC 95-21647. 281p. (C). text 114.50 (*0-7923-3584-8*) Kluwer Academic.

Health Information for International Travel. 1994. lib. bdg. 250.00 (*0-8490-6473-2*) Gordon Pr.

Health Information for International Travel 1996-97. CDC Staff & DHHS Staff. 1997. (Illus.). 220p. pap. 14.95 (*1-883205-33-6*) Intl Med Pub.

Health Information for International Travel (1996-97) Ed. by Rosamond R. Dewart. 1997. (Illus.). 210p. (Orig.). pap. text 35.00 (*0-7881-4498-7*) DIANE Pub.

Health Information for International Travel, 1999-2000. Ed. by Rosamond R. Dewart. 1999. (Illus.). 225p. pap. text 40.00 (*0-7881-8395-8*) DIANE Pub.

Health Information Management. Ed. by Joseph Mangano & Melani C. Karaffa. 1993. 260p. 49.95 (*1-878487-54-X*, ME051) Practice Mgmt Info.

Health Information Management. Edna K. Huffman. Ed. by Jennifer Cofer. 10th rev. ed. 1994. LC 94-67623. Orig. Title: Medical Record Management. (Illus.). 800p. (C). 41.00 (*0-917036-17-4*) Physicians Rec.

Health Information Management: Medical Records Process in Group Practice. Lynn Kuehn & Jeanine Barlow. 1997. (Illus.). 166p. (Orig.). pap. 39.00 (*1-56829-016-0*, 4950) M G M A.

Health Information Management: What Strategies? Ed. by Suzanne Bakker. 1997. LC 97-13932. 364p. text 184.00 (*0-7923-4546-0*) Kluwer Academic.

Health Information Management Compliance: A Model Program for Healthcare Organizations. Sue Prophet. 1998. (Illus.). 86p. pap. text 40.00 (*1-58426-012-2*, AB102198) Am Hlth Info.

Health Information Management Exams. Mervat Abdelhak. 1996. 250.00 (*0-7216-5149-6*) Saunders.

Health Information Management in Hospitals: Principles & Organization for Health Record Services. Margaret F. Skurka. 1994. LC 93-41464. 180p. pap. 36.00 (*1-55648-113-6*, 148153) AHPI.

Health Information Management Manual. Joan Gratto Liebler. 1998. LC 97-43786. ring bd. 219.00 incl. disk (*0-8342-0944-6*, S467) Aspen Pub.

Health Information Practice Standards: Tools for Assessing Your Organization. 1998. (Illus.). 212p. pap. text 42.00 (*1-58426-014-9*, AB102398) Am Hlth Info.

Health Information Resources in the Federal Government. 1992. lib. bdg. 79.95 (*0-8490-5331-5*) Gordon Pr.

Health Information Systems. Ed. by Paul E. Leaverton & Louis Masse. 1984. LC 84-3480. 220p. 45.00 (*0-275-91440-2*, C1440, Praeger Pubs) Greenwood.

Health Information Systems: A Bibliography. Ed. by Donald B. Ziegenfuss & James T. Ziegenfuss. 1984. LC 83-24719. (IFI Data Base Library). 256p. 95.00 (*0-306-65208-0*, Kluwer Plenum) Kluwer Academic.

Health Information Systems: Design Issues & Analytic Applications. Elizabeth A. McGlynn et al. 1999. LC 98-44204. (Health Information Systems Ser.: Vol. 1). (Illus.). 500p. 55.00 (*0-8330-2599-6*, MR-967-HF); 350p. pap. 40.00 (*0-8330-2630-5*, MR-967-HF) Rand Corp.

Health Inform's Resource Guide to Alternative Health: An Annual Directory of Information Sources on Alternative & Complementary Therapies. Ed. by Kate Page & Janet Gotkin. 1997. 325p. pap. 79.95 (*0-9659104-0-7*) Infolink New York.

Health Inspector. Jack Rudman. 1994. (Career Examination Ser.: C-322). pap. 29.95 (*0-8373-0322-2*) Nat Learn.

Health Instruction: Theory & Application. John T. Fodor & Gus T. Dalis. 4th ed. 1989. LC 88-13741. (Illus.). 171p. pap. text 27.00 (*0-8121-1209-1*) Lppncott W & W.

Health Instruction: Theory & Application. John T. Fodor et al. 5th ed. 1994. LC 93-39568. 202p. 27.95 (*0-683-03301-8*) Lppncott W & W.

Health Insurance: A Guide for Artists, Consultants, Entrepreneurs & Other Self-Employed. Lenore Janecek. 1993. LC 93-23270. 232p. pap. 15.95 (*1-879903-11-3*) Am for the Arts.

Health Insurance: How to Get It, Keep It, or Improve What You've Got. Robert Enteen. 2nd rev. ed. 1996. LC 96-10530. 308p. pap. 29.95 (*1-888799-01-3*) Demos Medical.

Health Insurance: Management Strategies Used by Large Employers to Control Costs. Michael Gutowski. 1998. (Illus.). 86p. pap. text 25.00 (*0-7881-4754-4*) DIANE Pub.

Health Insurance Administrator. Jack Rudman. 1994. (Career Examination Ser.: C-2687). pap. 39.95 (*0-8373-2687-7*) Nat Learn.

Health Insurance among Children of Unemployed Parents. Jacob A. Klerman. 1997. LC 97-22407. ix, 25p. pap. text 9.00 (*0-8330-2520-1*, MR-883) Rand Corp.

Health Insurance & Access to Medical Services: A Secondary Analysis of Three Years of NCHS Health Interview Surveys. Howard E. Freeman & Christopher R. Corey. 1994. (Illus.). 73p. (Orig.). (C). pap. text 30.00 (*0-7881-1054-3*) DIANE Pub.

Health Insurance & Canadian Public Policy: The Seven Decisions that Created the Canadian Health Insurance System & Their Outcomes. Malcolm G. Taylor. rev. ed. 1987. (Canadian Public Administration Ser.). 584p. text (*0-7735-0628-4*) McG-Queens Univ Pr CAN. *Dist:* CUP Services.

Health Insurance & Public Policy: Risk, Allocation, & Equity, 299. Ed. by Miriam K. Mills & Robert H. Blank. 1992. LC 91-43370. (Contributions in Political Science Ser.: No. 299). 252p. 67.00 (*0-313-28465-2*, MHX/, Greenwood Pr) Greenwood.

Health Insurance Answer Book. Charles E. Vadakin & Zelda Lipton. 1986. LC 86-18648. 79.00 (*0-916592-67-7*) Panel Pubs.

***Health Insurance Carrier Directory 2001: Coder's Choice.** annuals Ed. by Maureen Lynch & Kathryn Swanson. rev. ed. 2000. 430p. pap. text 54.95 (*1-57066-187-1*, 21041) Practice Mgmt Info.

***Health Insurance Carrier Directory 2001: Timesaver Binder.** annuals Ed. by Maureen Lynch & Kathryn Swanson. 2000. 430p. ring bd. 59.95 (*1-57066-188-X*, 21042) Practice Mgmt Info.

Health Insurance Carrier Directory 2000 TimeSaver Binder. Ed. by Kathryn Swanson & Maureen Lynch. 1999. ring bd. 59.95 (*1-57066-166-9*, 20042) Practice Mgmt Info.

Health Insurance Carrier Directory 2000 Coder' Choice. Ed. by Kathryn Swanson & Maureen Lynch. 1999. pap. text 49.95 (*1-57066-165-0*, 20041) Practice Mgmt Info.

Health Insurance Coverage for 55- to 64-Year-Olds: Congressional Hearing. Ed. by James M. Jeffords. 2000. (Illus.). 76p. (C). pap. text 25.00 (*0-7567-0374-3*) DIANE Pub.

Health Insurance for Children: Many Remained Uninsured Despite Medicaid Expansion. 1996. 44p. (Orig.). (C). pap. text 20.00 (*0-7881-2935-X*) DIANE Pub.

Health Insurance for Children: Private Insurance Coverage Continues to Deteriorate. 1996. (Illus.). 28p. (Orig.). (C). pap. text 15.00 (*0-7881-3391-8*) DIANE Pub.

Health Insurance Portability & Accountability Act: Hearing Before the U. S. Senate. Ed. by James M. Jeffords. 1998. 124p. (C). pap. text 30.00 (*0-7881-7082-1*) DIANE Pub.

Health Insurance Primer: An Introduction to How Health Insurance Works. Ed. by Terry R. Lowe. 2000. 188p. pap. 30.00 (*1-879143-49-6*) Health Ins Assn Am.

Health Insurance Primer: Werbel's Sickness & Accident. Raymond A. D'Amico et al. rev. ed. 2000. 172p. (C). pap. text 19.95 (*1-884803-02-4*) Werbel Pub.

Health Insurance Status of the Civilian Noninstitutionalized Population, 1998. Jeffrey A. Rhoades et al. 2000. (MEPS Research Findings Ser.: Vol. 11). pap. (*1-58763-003-6*) Agency Healthcare.

Health Interview Survey, 1975. National Center for Health Statistics Staff. 1982. LC 82-80685. (*0-89138-926-1*, ICPSR 7672) ICPSR.

Health into Mathematics. Gibbs & Mutunga. 1991. pap. text (*0-582-05839-2*) Addison-Wesley GBR. *Dist:* Trans-Atl Phila.

Health Is a Community Affair: Report. National Commission on Community Health Services. 1966. LC 66-27415. (Illus.). 266p. pap. 15.95 (*0-674-38451-2*) HUP.

Health Is a Question of Balance. Paul Brenner. 2nd ed. 1992. pap. 12.95 (*0-9633554-0-6*) Continuum Pr.

H I

Health Issues & Adolescents: Growing up, Speaking Out. Janet Shucksmith & Leo B. Hendry. 1998. LC 97-46525. (Adolescence & Society Ser.). 176p. (C). 68.95 (*0-415-16848-1*); pap. 22.95 (*0-415-16849-X*) Routledge.

Health Issues for Minority Adolescents. Marjorie Kagawa-Singer et al. 1996. LC 95-41942. (Child, Youth, & Family Services Ser.). 273p. text 45.00 (*0-8032-2732-9*) U of Nebr Pr.

Health Issues in Rural America. National Governors' Association Staff. 1988. (New Alliances for Rural America Ser.). 120p. (Orig.). pap. text 6.00 (*1-55877-015-1*) Natl Governor.

Health Issues in the Black Community. Ed. by Ronald L. Braithwaite & Sandra E. Taylor. 1992. LC 92-20174. (Health Management Ser.). 371p. pap. 52.00 (*1-55542-477-5*) Jossey-Bass.

***Health Issues in the Latino Community.** Marilyn Aguirre-Molina et al. 2001. LC 2001-29048. (Jossey Bass Health Ser.). (Illus.). 528p. 60.00 (*0-7879-5315-6*) Jossey-Bass.

Health Issues Related to Alcohol Consumption. Ed. by Paulus M. Verschuren. 1993. 329p. pap. 40.00 (*0-944398-17-0*, 398170) ILSI.

Health Laboratory Facilities in Emergency & Disaster Situations. Ed. by M. M. El-Nageh & C. Heuck. 1994. LC 96-108724. (WHO Regional Publications: No. 6). 169p. pap. text 16.00 (*92-9021-182-2*, 1440006) World Health.

Health Laboratory Services in Support of Primary Health Care in Developing Countries. Ed. by K. B. Sharma. 1994. (WHO Regional Publications: No. 24). xv, 145p. pap. text 13.50 (*92-9022-167-4*, 1560024) World Health.

Health Law: 1994. Hall. 1994. suppl. ed. 60.00 (*0-316-33942-3*) Aspen Law.

Health Law: Cases, Materials & Problems. Barry R. Furrow et al. 2nd ed. 1991. (American Casebook Ser.). 174p. (C). pap. text (*0-314-92864-2*); 1236p. reprint ed. 56.50 (*0-314-83133-9*) West Pub.

Health Law: Commentary & Materials. Peter MacFarlane. 1993. 240p. pap. (*1-86287-098-5*); 3rd ed. 2000. LC 00-303427. xviii, 318p. pap. (*1-86287-357-7*) Federation Pr AUS. *Dist:* Gaunt.

Health Law Vol. 1. Timothy Stoltzfus Jost et al. 1994. LC 94-19536. (Practitioner Treatise Ser.). 1500p. text (*0-314-04151-6*) West Pub.

Health Law Vol. 2. Timothy Stoltzfus Jost et al. 1994. LC 94-19536. (Practitioner Treatise Ser.). 1500p. text (*0-314-04152-4*) West Pub.

Health Law Adaptable to Courses Utilizing Furrow, Johnson, Jost & Schwartz's Casebook on Health Law. Ed. by Norman S. Goldenberg & Peter Tenen. 1997. (Legal Briefs Ser.). (C). pap. 20.50 (*0-87457-192-8*, 1650) Casenotes Pub.

Health Law Handbook, 1992. Ed. by Alice G. Gosfield. 1992. pap. 75.00 (*0-87632-840-0*) West Group.

Health Law in Canada Ed. by Gilbert S. Sharpe et al. 1993. 120.00 (*0-409-90781-2*, MICHIE) LEXIS Pub.

Health Law Practice Guide National Health Lawyers Association Staff. Ed. by Marylou King. 1993. LC 93-17568. (Health Law Ser.). 450.00 (*0-87632-912-1*) West Group.

Health Law Reader: An Interdisciplinary Approach. annuals John H. Robinson et al. 1998. LC 98-28630. 848p. pap. 60.00 (*0-89089-907-X*) Carolina Acad Pr.

Health, Life & Disease - Or Why Research Should Be of Great Importance to All Governments, Consumers, Community Leaders, Military Chiefs, Civic & Civilian Pioneers, Cosmopolitans & Librarians: A Philosophy of Progress Made Simple. John C. Bartone. 1997. 120p. 57.50 (*0-7883-1424-6*); pap. 47.50 (*0-7883-1425-4*) ABBE Pubs Assn.

Health, Lifestyles & Services for the Elderly. Ed. by Eino Heikkinen et al. 1989. (Public Health in Europe Ser.: No. 29). xx, 222p. pap. text 18.00 (*92-890-1165-3*, 1320029) World Health.

Health Literature Services by the Year 2000. WHO Staff. 1990. (Western Pacific Education in Action Ser.: No. 4). 46p. 6.50 (*92-9061-134-0*) World Health.

Health Magazine: The Essential Women's Health Guide 2001. Health Magazine Editors. 2000. LC 00-37423. (Illus.). 224p. (*0-7370-1621-3*) Time-Life Bks GBR. *Dist:* AOL Time Warner.

Health Maintenance & Microbial Diseases of Culture Fish. John A. Plumb. 1994. 272p. lib. bdg. 99.95 (*0-8493-4614-2*) CRC Pr.

Health Maintenance Organizations: Dimensions of Performance. Harold S. Luft. 1987. 468p. pap. text 29.95 (*0-88738-681-4*) Transaction Pubs.

Health Management Information Systems: A Handbook for Decision Makers. Jack Smith. 1999. LC 99-39514. pap. (*0-335-20566-6*) OpUniv Pr.

Health Management Information Systems: Methods & Practical Applications. Joseph K. H. Tan. 2nd ed. 2000. LC 00-40602. (Illus.). xx, 380p. 65.00 (*0-8342-1777-5*, 17775) Aspen Pub.

Health Manpower: Planning, Production & Management. Ed. by Andrew F. Long et al. 1987. 300p. lib. bdg. (*0-7099-4172-2*) C Helm GBR. *Dist:* Routldge.

Health Manpower & Health Policy. Eli Ginzberg. 1978. LC 78-62203. (Conservation of Human Resources Ser.: No. 10). 244p. text 34.50 (*0-916672-19-0*) Rowman.

Health Manpower Out of Balance: Conflicts & Prospects, Proceedings of the 20th CIOMS Round Table Conference, Acapulco, Mexico, 7-12 Sept. 1987. Ed. by Z. Bankowski & A. Mijia. 1987. 210p. pap. text 20.00 (*92-9036-030-5*, 1830020) World Health.

Health Manpower Planning. Ed. by P. C. Jaspers et al. 1983. text 155.50 (*0-89838-557-1*) Kluwer Academic.

Health Marketing & Consumer Behavior: A Guide to Basic Linkages. Ed. by William J. Winston. 1985. LC 85-14082. (Health Marketing Quarterly Ser.: Vol. 3, No. 1). 101p. text 32.95 (*0-86656-462-4*); pap. text 2.95 (*0-86656-463-2*) Haworth Pr.

Health Matters: A Sociology of Illness, Prevention & Care. Ed. by Alan Petersen & Charles Waddell. 1998. LC 98-194038. 384p. (*1-86448-564-7*) Allen & Unwin Pty AUS. *Dist:* Paul & Co Pubs.

Health Measurments Scales: A Practical Guide to Their Development & Use. David L. Streiner & Geoffrey R. Norman. 2nd ed. 1995. (Illus.). 240p. (C). pap. text 42.50 (*0-19-262670-1*) OUP.

Health Media Review Index, 1984-1986: A Guide to Reviews & Descriptions of Commercially Available Nonprint Material for the Medical, Mental, Allied Healthy Human Service, & Related Counseling Professions. Ed. by Deborah J. McCalpin et al. 1988. LC 88-18452. 771p. 60.00 (*0-8108-2172-9*) Scarecrow.

Health, Medicine, Society. Ed. by M. Sokolowska et al. 1976. LC 76-7916. text 176.50 (*90-277-0552-6*) Kluwer Academic.

Health Movement in America: Promoting Fitness. Michael S. Goldstein. 1992. LC 91-28694. (Social Movements Past & Present Ser.). 250p. (C). 15.95 (*0-8057-9725-4*) Macmillan.

Health Needs & Health Services in Rural Ghana. Conference on Blood Viscosity in Heart Disease, Th. Ed. by E. De Kadt et al. 1981. 140p. pap. 18.00 (*0-08-028136-2*, Pergamon Pr) Elsevier.

Health Needs Assessment: Theory & Practice. Jane Robinson & Ruth Elkan. 1996. LC 96-5331. 250p. pap. text (*0-443-05233-6*) Church.

Health Needs Assessment in Practice. Ed. by John Wright. 1998. (Illus.). 99p. pap. text (*0-7279-1270-4*) BMJ Pub GBR. *Dist:* AIDC.

Health Needs of Adolescents: Report of a WHO Expert Committee, 1977. 1977. (Technical Report Ser.: No, 609). 49p. pap. text 7.00 (*92-4-120609-8*, 1100609) World Health.

***Health Needs of People with Learning Disability: The Public Health Agenda.** Jeanette Thompson & Sharon Pickering. 2001. (Illus.). 315p. pap. (*0-7020-2532-1*) W B Saunders GBR. *Dist:* Saunders.

Health Needs of Women As They Age. Ed. by Sharon Golub & Rita J. Freedman. 1985. (Women & Health Ser.: Vol. 10, Nos. 2-3). 122p. LC 85-947. text 4.95 (*0-86656-413-6*); LC 85-947. pap. text 2.95 (*0-86656-414-4*); LC 85-7642. reprint ed. pap. 14.95 (*0-918393-23-X*, Harrington Park) Haworth Pr.

Health Network Innovations: How 20 Communities Are Improving Their Systems Through Collaboration. Richard J. Bogue & Claude H. Hall. 1997. LC 97-6224. 419p. pap. 60.00 (*1-55648-198-5*) AHPI.

Health Networks: Can They Be the Solution? Thomas P. Weil. 2001. LC 00-11174. (Illus.). 392p. (C). text 50.00 (*0-472-11193-0*, 11193) U of Mich Pr.

Health, 1999-2000. Richard Yarian. 20th ed. 1999. (Annual Editions Ser.). pap., stu. ed. 17.50 (*0-07-039799-6*) McGrw-H Hghr Educ.

Health 1996/97. Richard Yarian. 17th annot. ed. 1996. tchr. ed. (*0-697-31597-5*, WCB McGr Hill) McGrw-H Hghr Educ.

Health Nutrient Biblie: The Complete Encyclopedia of Food as Medicine. Lynn Sonberg. Ed. by Maureen Callahan. 1995. LC 95-25139. 560p. pap. 16.00 (*0-684-81071-9*, Fireside) S&S Trade Pap.

Health, Nutrition & Population Strategy for the East Asia & Pacific Region. Fadia Saadah & James Knowles. 2000. LC 00-42280. (Health, Nutrition, & Population Ser.). (Illus.). ix, 57p. (*0-8213-4739-X*) World Bank.

Health Occupations: Explorations & Career Planning. Joan M. Birchenall & Mary E. Streight. 1990. (Illus.). 400p. tchr. ed. (*0-8151-2689-1*) Mosby Inc.

Health Occupations: Explorations & Career Planning. Joan M. Birchenall & Mary Eileen Streight. 1989. (Illus.). 400p. (C). (gr. 13). text 22.95 (*0-8016-0477-X*, 00477) Mosby Inc.

Health Occupations Aptitude Examination (HOAE) Jack Rudman. (Admission Test Ser.: Vol. 98). 49.95 (*0-8373-5198-7*); 1994. pap. 29.95 (*0-8373-5098-0*) Nat Learn.

Health Occupations Workplace Readiness. Bruce J. Colbert. 1998. LC 98-22220. (Health Occupations Ser.). 150p. 27.95 (*0-8273-7781-9*) Delmar.

Health of Adults in the Developing World. Ed. by Richard G. Feachem et al. 1992. (Illus.). 368p. text 49.95 (*0-19-520879-X*, 60879) OUP.

Health of Americans. Ed. by Boisfeuillet Jones. 1970. LC 70-120793. 5.95 (*0-13-385070-6*) Am Assembly.

Health of Black Americans from Post-Reconstruction to Integration, 1871-1960: An Annotated Bibliography of Contemporary Sources, 26. Compiled by Mitchell F. Rice & Woodrow Jones, Jr. 1990. LC 89-78161. (Bibliographies & Indexes in Afro-American & African Studies: No. 26). 256p. lib. bdg. 70.00 (*0-313-26314-0*, RHB/, Greenwood Pr) Greenwood.

Health of Britain's Ethnic Minorities: Findings from a National Survey. James Y. Nazroo. 1997. LC 98-161210. (PSI Report Ser.). x, 219p. (*0-85374-709-1*) Pol Studies Inst.

Health of Dairy Cattle. A. H. Andrews. 2000. (Illus.). 320p. text (*0-632-04103-X*) Blckwell Science GBR. *Dist:* Iowa U Pr.

Health of Former Prisoners of War: Results from the Medical Examination Survey of Former POWs of World War II & the Korean Conflict. Institute of Medicine Staff & William F. Page. 1992. 176p. (C). pap. text 31.00 (*0-309-04791-9*) Natl Acad Pr.

***Health of Municipal Sewage Workers: Studies of Cancer Incidence, Biomarkers of Carcinogenicity & Genotoxicity, & Self-Reported Symptoms.** Lennart Friis. 2001. (Comprehensive Summaries of Uppsala Dissertations from the Faculty of Medicine Ser.: No. 1015). (Illus.). 67p. (*91-554-4980-8*) Uppsala Universitet SWE. *Dist:* Coronet Bks.

Health of Nations: An International Perspective on U. S. Health Care Reform. Laurene A. Graig. 2nd ed. 1993. LC 93-7666. 215p. (YA). (gr. 11). pap. text 31.95 (*0-87187-871-2*) Congr Quarterly.

Health of Nations: An International Perspective on U. S. Health Care Reform. Laurene A. Graig. 1991. LC 91-66011. pap. (*0-9630189-0-6*) Wyatt Co.

Health of Nations: Disease, Medicine & Development in the Third World. B. Folasade Iyune et al. 1995. 320p. (*1-85628-922-2*) Avebry GBR. *Dist:* Ashgate Pub Co.

Health of Nations: Public Opinion & the Making of American & British Health Policy. Lawrence R. Jacobs. 1993. LC 92-54967. 280p. 45.00 (*0-8014-2761-4*) Cornell U Pr.

Health of Native Americans: Towards a Biocultural Epidemiology. T. Kue Young. 1994. LC 93-20705. (Illus.). 288p. text 49.95 (*0-19-507339-8*) OUP.

Health of Native People of North America: A Bibliography & Guide to Resources, 1970 to 1994. Sharon A. Gray. 1996. LC 96-11844. (Native American Bibliography Ser.: No. 20). (Illus.). 400p. 65.00 (*0-8108-3170-8*) Scarecrow.

Health of Older People: A Social Survey. Ethel Shanas. Ed. by Leon Stein. 1980. LC 79-8685. (Growing Old Ser.). (Illus.). reprint ed. lib. bdg. 26.95 (*0-405-12802-9*) Ayer.

Health of Our Nation's Children: United States, 1988. Mary J. Coiro. 1994. LC 94-33533. (Vital & Health Statistics. Series 10, Data from the National Health Survey: No. 191). 4.75 (*0-8406-0500-5*) Natl Ctr Health Stats.

Health of Pigs: Nutrition, Housing & Disease Prevention. Ed. by John Hill & David Sainsbury. 1996. (Illus.). 392p. (*0-582-06100-8*) Addison-Wesley GBR. *Dist:* Trans-Atl Phila, Longman.

Health of Populations: An Introduction. Andrew C. Harper & Laurie J. Lambert. 2nd ed. 1993. LC 93-37157. 296p. pap. text 37.95 (*0-8261-5511-1*) Springer Pub.

Health of Seamen. C. C. Lloyd. 1987. (*0-7855-1134-2*) St Mut.

Health of the Elderly: Report of a WHO Expert Commitee, 1987. WHO Staff. 1989. (Technical Report Ser.: No. 779). 98p. 12.00 (*92-4-120779-5*) World Health.

Health of the Elderly in Hong Kong. Ed. by Shiu-Kum Lam. 1997. LC 98-170579. 232p. (Orig.). pap. (*962-209-431-7*) HK Univ Pr HKG. *Dist:* Intl Spec Bk, Coronet Bks.

Health of the Industrial Worker. Edgar L. Collis & Major Greenwood. Ed. by Leon Stein. 1977. LC 77-70489. (Illus.). reprint ed. lib. bdg. 42.95 (*0-405-10161-9*) Ayer.

Health of the Nation. Ed. by Richard Smith. 1991. (Illus.). 237p. pap. text (*0-7279-0314-4*) BMJ Pub GBR. *Dist:* AIDC.

Health of the Nation: Solutions That Make Everyone a Winner. Vincent Anku. 1995. (Illus.). 144p. pap. text 9.95 (*0-9647741-0-0*) Achilles Pub.

Health of the Republic: Epidemics, Medicine, & Moralism As Challenges to Democracy. Dan E. Beauchamp. 1988. LC 87-35335. (Health, Society, & Policy Ser.). 312p. (C). 34.95 (*0-87722-558-3*) Temple U Pr.

Health of the Schoolchild: A History of the School Medical Service in England & Wales, 1908-1974. Bernard Harris. 1995. LC 94-48785. 260p. (*0-335-09995-5*); 272p. pap. (*0-335-09994-7*) OpUniv Pr.

Health of the State. Paul Adams. Ed. by Neil Gilbert & Harry Specht. 1982. LC 81-22647. (Studies in Social Welfare Policies & Programs). 198p. 55.50 (*0-275-90749-X*, C0749, Praeger Pubs) Greenwood.

Health of Women: A Global Perspective. Ed. by Marge Koblinsky et al. 1992. 312p. (C). pap. text 32.00 (*0-8133-1608-1*) Westview.

***Health of Women of Reproductive Age: A Survey in Rural Zimbabwe.** Carin Nilses. 2000. (Comprehensive Summaries of Uppsala Disertations from the Faculty of Medicine: No. 981). (Illus.). 65p. (Orig.). pap. (*91-554-4893-3*) Uppsala Universitet SWE. *Dist:* Coronet Bks.

Health of Young People: A Challenge & A Promise. WHO Staff. 1993. (ENG, FRE & SPA.). x, 109p. pap. text 23.00 (*92-4-156154-8*, 1150394) World Health.

Health of Youth: A Cross-National Survey. 1996. (WHO Regional Publications, European Ser.: No. 69). (Illus.). 232p. (Orig.). pap. text 53.10 (*92-890-1333-8*, 1310069) World Health.

***Health on File.** Victoria Chapman and Associates Staff. 2nd ed. 2001. LC 2001-55596. (Illus.). 288p. ring bd. 185.00 (*0-8160-4345-0*) Facts on File.

Health on the Internet. Denis Anthony. 1996. LC 96-15920. 240p. (Orig.). pap. 40.95 (*0-632-04072-6*) Blackwell Sci.

Health Outcome Measures in Primary & Out-Patient Care. Ed. by Allen Hutchinson et al. 1996. 216p. text 70.00 (*3-7186-5899-2*); pap. text 27.00 (*3-7186-5900-X*) Gordon & Breach.

Health Outcomes: Biological, Social & Economic Perspectives. Ed. by Helen Macbeth. 1996. (Biosocial Society Ser.: No. 8). (Illus.). 176p. text 98.50 (*0-19-854879-6*) OUP.

Health Outcomes & Pharmaceutical Care: Measurement, Applications, & Initiatives. Ed. by Alan Escovitz & Dev S. Pathak. LC 96-26209. (Journal of Research in Pharmaceutical Care: Vol. 7, No. 4 & Vol. 8, No. 1). 227p. (C). 1997. pap. 19.95 (*0-7890-0203-5*); 1996. 49.95 (*0-7890-0008-3*) Haworth Pr (Pharmctl Prods).

Health Pass: An Evaluation of a Managed Care Program for Certain Philadelphia Recipients. 1993. 77p. (Orig.). (C). pap. text 25.00 (*0-7881-0050-5*) DIANE Pub.

Health Performance Measurement in the Public Sector: Principles & Policies for Implementing an Information Network. National Research Council Staff. Ed. by Edward B. Perrin et al. 1999. LC 99-6159. 192p. pap. 32.00 (*0-309-06436-8*, Joseph Henry Pr) Natl Acad Pr.

***Health Physics.** Alexander Elliott & Andrew McCormick. 2001. 96p. pap. text (*0-521-78726-2*) Cambridge U Pr.

Health Physics & Radiological Health Handbook. Ed. by Bernard Shleien. rev. ed. 1992. (Illus.). 734p. (C). text 95.00 (*0-917251-05-9*) Scinta.

Health Planner. Jack Rudman. 1994. (Career Examination Ser.: C-3027). pap. 34.95 (*0-8373-3027-0*) Nat Learn.

Health Planner Trainee. Jack Rudman. 1994. (Career Examination Ser.: C-3026). pap. 29.95 (*0-8373-3026-2*) Nat Learn.

Health Planning: A Systematic Approach. Herbert H. Hyman. 2nd ed. 1982. LC 81-12780. 606p. (C). text 89.00 (*0-89443-379-2*) Aspen Pub.

Health Planning: Qualitative Aspects & Quantitative Techniques. Ed. by William A. Reinke & Kathleen N. Williams. 1972. LC 79-189139. (Illus.). 360p. 12.00 (*0-912888-00-8*) Dept Intl Health.

Health Planning & Organization of Medical Care. 1972. (Public Health in Europe Ser.: No. 1). 131p. 15.00 (*92-9020-120-7*, 1320001) World Health.

Health Planning & Social Change. Leonard J. Duhl. 1986. 320p. 44.95 (*0-89885-301-X*, Kluwer Acad Hman Sci) Kluwer Academic.

Health Planning for Effective Management. Ed. by William A. Reinke. 1988. (Illus.). 304p. text 35.00 (*0-19-505337-0*) OUP.

Health Planning in India. Ed. by G. Ramachandrudu. 1997. LC 97-905307. (Illus.). xiv, 178p. (C). (*81-7024-876-0*) APH Pubng IND. *Dist:* Nataraj Bks.

Health Planning in Transition: Structure & Performance in Arkansas, Oklahoma & Texas, No. 29. David C. Warner. 1978. (Policy Research Project Report Ser.). 90p. pap. 4.00 (*0-89940-625-4*) LBJ Sch Pub Aff.

Health Planning Predicament: France, Quebec, England & the United States. Victor G. Rodwin. Ed. by Charles M. Leslie. 1984. LC 82-45910. (Comparative Studies of Health Systems & Medical Care: Vol. 8). 160p. (C). pap. text (*0-520-04446-0*) U CA Pr.

Health Policies & Black Americans. David P. Willis. 1988. 532p. (C). pap. text 29.95 (*0-88738-249-5*) Transaction Pubs.

Health Policy. Ed. by James W. Bjorkman & Christa Altenstetter. 1998. LC 97-44515. (International Library of Comparative Public Policy: No. 7). 800p. 300.00 (*1-85898-587-0*) E Elgar.

Health Policy: Development, Implementation & Evaluation in Australia. Ed. by Heather Gardner. 1992. (Illus.). 328p. (Orig.). pap. text (*0-443-04394-9*) Church.

Health Policy: Understanding Our Choices from National Reform to Market Forces. Ed. by Marilynn M. Rosenthal & Max Heirich. 1998. LC 97-14374. 352p. (C). text 88.00 (*0-8133-9023-0*) Westview.

Health Policy & Administration: Study Guide. Deakin University Press Staff. 1990. 193p. (C). pap. (*0-7300-0714-6*, SSS220) Deakin Univ AUS. *Dist:* St Mut.

***Health Policy & Economics: Strategic Issues in Health Care Management.** 2001. 308p. text 69.95 (*0-7546-1612-6*) Ashgate Pub Co.

Health Policy & Management: The Healthcare Agenda in a British Political Context. C. R. Paton. 1995. 400p. pap. 63.75 (*1-56593-285-4*, 0609) Singular Publishing.

Health Policy & Nursing: Crisis & Reform in the U. S. Health Care Delivery System. Ed. by Charlene Harrington & Carroll L. Estes. 1994. LC 93-14285. (Illus.). 535p. pap. text 44.95 (*0-86720-813-9*, 813-9) Jones & Bartlett.

Health Policy & Nursing: Crisis & Reform in the U. S. Health Care Delivery System. Charlene Harrington & Carroll L. Estes. 2nd ed. 1997. LC 97-12192. (Nursing Ser.). (Illus.). 544p. (C). pap. text 48.95 (*0-7637-0404-0*, 0404-0) Jones & Bartlett.

Health Policy & Politics: A Nurse's Guide. Jeri A. Milstead. 1999. LC 98-37498. 300p. 50.00 (*0-8342-1055-X*, 1055X) Aspen Pub.

Health Policy & Technological Innovation. Ed. by J. M. Newsom-Davis & David Weatherall. 1993. LC 93-21164. 192p. (gr. 13). pap. 120.95 (*0-412-54250-1*, Chap & Hall NY) Chapman & Hall.

Health Policy & the Disadvantaged. Ed. by Lawrence D. Brown. 1991. LC 91-21831. 222p. text 39.95 (*0-8223-1138-0*); pap. text 17.95 (*0-8223-1142-9*) Duke.

Health Policy & the NHS. Judith Allsop. 2nd ed. 1995. LC 94-28346. (Social Policy in Britain Ser.). (*0-582-04279-8*) Longman.

Health Policy, Ethics & Human Values: Proceedings of the CIOMS Round Table Coference, an International Dialogue, XVIIIth. Ed. by Z. Bankowski & J. H. Bryant. 1985. 336p. pap. text 25.00 (*92-9036-023-2*, 1830018) World Health.

Health Policy, Ethics & Human Values - An International Dialogue: Highlights of the XVIIIth CIOMS Round Table Conference. Z. Bankowski & J. H. Bryant. 1985. (CIOMS Publication Ser.). pap. text 10.00 (*92-9036-021-6*) World Health.

Health Policy, Ethics & Human Values: An Islamic Perspective: Reflections on the Cairo Seminar. 1989. pap. text 6.00 (*92-9036-038-0*) World Health.

Health Policy, Ethics & Human Values: European & North American Perspectives: Conference Highlights, Papers & Conclusions, XXIst CIOMS Conference. Z. Bankowski & J. H. Bryant. 1988. (CIOMS Round Table Proceedings Ser.: No. 21). pap. text 20.00 (*92-9036-034-8*) World Health.

Health Policy, Federalism, & the American States. Robert F. Rich & William D. White. 1996. LC 96-33521. (Illus.). 350p. pap. 28.50 (*0-87766-660-1*) Urban Inst.

Health Policy, Federalism & the American States. Robert F. Rich & William D. White. 1996. LC 96-33521. (Illus.). 350p. 69.50 (*0-87766-659-8*) Urban Inst.

Health Policy for HIV Infection & AIDS: New Information with Authors & Subjects. Science and Life Consultants Association Staff. 1992. LC 92-54205. 180p. 47.50 (*1-55914-562-5*); pap. 44.50 (*1-55914-563-3*) ABBE Pubs Assn.

Health Policy Implications of Unemployment. 1985. 409p. pap. text 40.00 (*92-890-1029-0*, 1340024) World Health.

Health Policy in Australia. Heather Gardner. 1997. LC 97-183590. 240p. pap. text 39.50 (*0-19-553968-0*) OUP.

Health Policy in Britain. Christopher Ham. 1982. 224p. (C). text 37.95 (*0-89503-046-2*) Baywood Pub.

Health Policy in Transition: A Decade of Health Politics, Policy, & Law. Ed. by Lawrence D. Brown. 1987. LC 87-13714. viii, 176p. (C). pap. text 16.95 (*0-8223-0790-1*) Duke.

Health Policy Issues: An Economic Perspective. Paul J. Feldstein. 2nd ed. 1999. LC 99-28614. 373p. pap. 48.00 (*1-56793-109-X*) Health Admin Pr.

Health Policy Issues Affecting Medical Education. Ed. by Donald G. Langsley. 1990. lib. bdg. 44.95 (*0-934277-13-3*) Am Bd Med Spec.

H
I

Health Policy Reform: Competition & Controls. Robert B. Helms. 1993. LC 93-36870. 250p. 19.95 (*0-8447-3844-1*, AEI Pr) Am Enterprise.

Health Policy Reform in America: Innovations from the States. Ed. by Howard M. Leichter. (C). (gr. 13). 1992. LC 92-22293. 240p. 73.95 (*1-56324-053-X*); 1992. LC 92-22293. 240p. pap. 38.95 (*1-56324-054-8*); 2nd ed. 1997. LC 96-43276. 280p. pap. text 30.95 (*1-56324-900-6*) M E Sharpe.

Health Policy Reform, National Variations & Globalization. Ed. by Christa Altenstetter & James W. Bjorkman. 1997. LC 96-10820. (Advances in Political Science Ser.). 405p. text 65.00 (*0-312-16101-8*) St Martin.

Health Policymaking in the United States. Beaufort B. Longest. 2nd ed. 1998. LC 97-34809. xxiv, 315p. 52.00 (*1-56793-072-7*) Health Admin Pr.

***Health Policymaking in the United States.** Beaufort B. Longest. 3rd ed. 2002. LC 2001-51689. (*1-56793-173-1*) Health Admin Pr.

Health Politics: Interest & Institutions in Western Europe. Ellen M. Immergut. 1992. (Studies in Comparative Politics). (Illus.). 362p. (C). text 90.00 (*0-521-41335-4*) Cambridge U Pr.

Health Politics & Policy. Theodor J. Litman & Leonard S. Robins. 1989. LC 83-26042. (Health Services Ser.: No. 1-456). 403p. (C). text 46.25 (*0-8273-4289-6*) Delmar.

Health Politics & Policy. Theodor J. Litman. 2nd ed. 1991. text 48.50 (*0-8273-4555-0*); 3rd ed. 1997. LC 96-39278. 672p. 81.95 (*0-8273-6776-7*) Delmar.

Health Practitioner's Guide to the Behavioral & Social Sciences. Michael V. Angrosino. 1986. LC 86-14642. 222p. 57.95 (*0-86569-157-6*, Auburn Hse) Greenwood.

***Health Practitioners in Ontario.** Patricia O'Reilly. 2000. LC 00-364662. xiv, 389p. text (*0-8020-4420-4*) U of Toronto Pr.

Health Priorities in the U. S. A: Index of New Information. Courtney H. Hannaford. 1994. (Illus.). 150p. 57.50 (*0-7883-0004-0*); pap. 47.50 (*0-7883-0005-9*) ABBE Pubs Assn.

Health Problem Sources. Marion O. Lerrigo. LC 76-176989. (Columbia University. Teachers College. Contributions to Education Ser.: No. 224). reprint ed. 37.50 (*0-404-55224-2*) AMS Pr.

Health Problems in Australia & New Zealand. Ed. by N. D. McGlashan. 1980. 180p. pap. 24.00 (*0-08-026103-5*, Pergamon Pr) Elsevier.

Health Problems of the Empire, Past, Present & Future. Vol. 5. A. Balfour & H. H. Scott. Ed. by Hugh Gunn. 17.50 (*0-404-54305-7*) AMS Pr.

Health Professional & Patient Interaction. Ruth B. Purtilo & Amy Haddad. Ed. by Margaret Biblis. 5th ed. 1996. 416p. pap. text 30.00 (*0-7216-6048-7*) Saunders.

Health Professionals Abroad. Tim Ryder. 1997. pap. (*1-85458-172-4*) Vac Wrk Pubns GBR. *Dist:* Petersons.

Health Professionals' Communications Guide: An Effective Performance Tool for the Health Care Provider. Joseph R. Sullivan & Fred Leafgren. Ed. by Bill Hettler & Joeli Hettler. 2nd rev. ed. 1999. 109p. pap. 99.00 (*1-929112-01-7*) Personality Res.

Health Professional's Drug Guide 2001. Margaret T. Shannon et al. 2000. 1616p. 32.95 (*0-13-028293-6*) P-H.

Health Professional's Guide to Diabetes & Exercise. Ed. by American Diabetes Association Staff. 1995. LC 95-31497. (Illus.). 352p. pap. 49.95 (*0-945448-52-X*) Am Diabetes.

Health Professional's Guide to Popular Dietary Supplements. Allison Sarubin. 1999. LC 99-52827. (Illus.). xi, 452p. (*0-88091-180-8*) Am Dietetic Assn.

Health Professionals in Management. Beaufort B. Longest, Jr. 1995. LC 94-43677. 318p. (C). pap. text 31.95 (*0-8385-3679-4*, A3679-6, Apple Lange Med) McGraw.

Health Professionals in Management. Composed by Longest. 2nd ed. 1999. (C). pap. text 29.95 (*0-8385-3682-4*) Appleton & Lange.

Health Professionals Stylebook: Putting Your Language to Work. Shirley H. Fondiller & Barbara J. Nerone. 1993. 152p. 15.95 (*0-88737-603-7*, 14-2551, NLN Pr) Natl League Nurse.

Health Professions Career & Education Directory. American Medical Association Staff. 28th ed. 2000. 450p. pap. text 60.00 (*1-57947-063-7*); 1997. pap. text 60.00 (*0-89970-834-X*) AMA.

Health Professions Education Directory. American Medical Association Staff. 1999. LC 98-642439. 54.95 (*0-89970-987-7*) AMA.

Health Program Administrator. Jack Rudman. 1994. (Career Examination Ser.: C-3601). pap. 39.95 (*0-8373-3601-5*) Nat Learn.

Health Program Aide. Jack Rudman. 1994. (Career Examination Ser.: C-3588). pap. 27.95 (*0-8373-3588-4*) Nat Learn.

Health Program for the Children of a County. Thomas G. Bennett. LC 77-176555. (Columbia University. Teachers College. Contributions to Education Ser.: No. 584). reprint ed. 37.50 (*0-404-55584-5*) AMS Pr.

Health Program Investigations Specialist. Jack Rudman. 1994. (Career Examination Ser.: C-3388). pap. 34.95 (*0-8373-3388-1*) Nat Learn.

Health Programme Evaluation Guiding Principles. 1981. text (*92-4-180006-2*) World Health.

Health Programs - Scope, Strategies, Criticisms & Practices: Index of New Information. American Health Research Institute Staff. 1995. LC 95-18253. 153p. 57.50 (*0-7883-0694-4*); pap. 47.50 (*0-7883-0695-2*) ABBE Pubs Assn.

***Health Project Book: A Handbook for New Researchers in the Field of Health.** Neil Wood. 2001. LC 00-56012. (Illus.). 224p. (C). (gr. 13). 24.95 (*0-415-24321-1*) Routledge.

Health-Promoting & Health-Compromising Behaviors among Minority Adolescents. Ed. by Dawn K. Wilson et al. 1996. LC 96-34967. (Application & Practice in Health Psychology Ser.: Vol. 3). 388p. 29.95 (*1-55798-397-6*, 431 7830) Am Psychol.

Health-Promoting Palliative Care. Allan Kellerhear. 1999. LC 99-234220. 207p. text 49.95 (*0-19-550785-1*) OUP.

Health Promotion. Michael L. Teague et al. 3rd ed. 1997. LC 97-127061. 400p. (C). pap. 45.10 (*0-697-26268-5*, WCB McGr Hill) McGrw-H Hghr Educ.

Health Promotion: An Anthology. 1996. LC 96-160109. (PAHO Scientific Publication Ser.: No. 557). 371p. text 64.00 (*92-75-11557-5*, 1610557) World Health.

Health Promotion: Concepts & Practice. Alan Cribb. Ed. by Alison Dines. 1993. LC 93-1873. 192p. pap. 36.95 (*0-632-03543-9*) Blackwell Sci.

***Health Promotion: Effectiveness, Efficiency & Equity.** Keith Tones & Sylvia Tilford. 3rd ed. 2001. 384p. pap. (*0-7487-4527-0*) Nelson Thornes GBR. *Dist:* Intl Spec Bk.

Health Promotion: Foundations for Practice. Jennie Naidoo & Jane Wills. 1995. (Illus.). 314p. pap. text (*0-7020-1680-2*); 2nd ed. 2000. LC 99-17031. xii, 400p. text (*0-7020-2448-1*) W B Saunders GBR. *Dist:* Saunders.

Health Promotion: Models & Values. R. S. Downie et al. 2nd ed. 1996. (Illus.). 232p. (C). text 75.00 (*0-19-262592-6*); pap. text 39.95 (*0-19-262591-8*) OUP.

Health Promotion: Philosophy, Practice, & Prejudice. David Seedhouse. 1997. LC 96-2928. 212p. pap. 42.95 (*0-471-93910-2*) Wiley.

Health Promotion: Principles & Practice. Marylou O'Connor & Elizabeth Parker. 1996. LC 96-146977. 310p. pap. (*1-86373-897-5*) Allen & Unwin Pty AUS. *Dist:* Paul & Co Pubs.

Health Promotion & Aging: Implications for the Health Professions. David Haber. 2nd ed. 1999. LC 98-42976. 368p. 46.95 (*0-8261-8461-8*) Springer Pub.

Health Promotion & Chronic Illness: Discovering a New Quality of Health. Ed. by A. Kaplun. 1992. (WHO Regional Publications, European Ser.: No. 44). xviii, 461p. pap. text 61.20 (*92-890-1307-9*, 1310044) World Health.

Health Promotion & Community Action for Health in Developing Countries. H. S. Dhillon & L. Philip. 1994. LC 95-129771. (ENG, FRE & SPA.). vii, 122p. pap. text 25.00 (*92-4-156167-X*, 1150411) World Health.

Health Promotion & Disease Prevention in Clinical Practice. Ed. by Steven H. Woolf et al. 1996. LC 95-1212. (Illus.). 488p. 45.00 (*0-683-09270-7*) Lppncott W & W.

Health Promotion & Disease Prevention, United States, 1990. Andrea L. Piani & Charlotte A. Schoenborn. 1992. LC 92-48186. (Vital & Health Statistics Ser.: No. 185). (*0-8406-0474-2*) Natl Ctr Health Stats.

Health Promotion & Exercise for Older Adults: An Instructor's Guide. Carole B. Lewis & Linda Campanelli. 1996. LC 90-739. 192p. pap. 65.00 (*0-8342-0169-0*) PRO-ED.

Health Promotion & Interactive Technology: Theoretical Applications & Future Directions. Ed. by Richard L. Street, Jr. et al. 1997. LC 96-37803. (LEA's Communication Ser.). 224p. pap. 29.95 (*0-8058-2205-4*) L Erlbaum Assocs.

Health Promotion & Patient Education: A Professional's Guide. Ed. by Patricia Webb. 1994. LC 93-31643. 41.50 (*1-56593-020-7*, 0263) Singular Publishing.

Health Promotion & Preventive Programs: Models of Occupational Therapy Practice. Ed. by Jerry A. Johnson & Evelyn Jaffe. 1989. LC 89-19767. (Occupational Therapy in Health Care Ser.: Vol. 6, No. 1). (Illus.). 135p. text 4.95 (*0-86656-957-X*) Haworth Pr.

***Health Promotion & Professional Ethics.** Alan Cribb & Peter Duncan. 2001. LC 2001-43512. (*0-632-05603-7*) Blackwell Sci.

Health Promotion at the Community Level. Neil Bracht. 1990. (Sourcebooks for the Human Services: Vol. 15). (Illus.). 320p. (C). pap. 39.95 (*0-8039-3859-4*, 7512) Sage.

Health Promotion At the Community Level: New Advances. Neil F. Bracht. 2nd ed. 1999. LC 98-40267. 384p. pap. 34.95 (*0-7619-1304-1*, 82152) Sage.

Health Promotion Evaluation: Measuring the Organizational Impact. Ed. by Joseph P. Opatz. 1987. (Illus.). (Orig.). pap. 22.95 (*0-940981-00-9*) Natl Wellness Inst.

Health Promotion for All: Strategies for Reaching Diverse Populations at the Workplace. Stephen Ramirez. 1994. LC 94-232169. 128p. (Orig.). pap. 25.00 (*0-9628334-3-6*) WELCOA.

Health Promotion for Working Populations: Report of a WHO Expert Committee. 1988. (Technical Report Ser.: No. 765). 49p. pap. text 8.00 (*92-4-120765-5*, 1100765) World Health.

Health Promotion Goes to Work: Programs with an Impact. 1994. 61p. (Orig.). (C). pap. text 30.00 (*0-7881-0701-1*) DIANE Pub.

Health Promotion Handbook. Sherri Sheinfeld Gorin et al. 1998. LC 97-52568. (Illus.). 416p. (C). (gr. 13). pap. text 29.95 (*0-8151-3611-0*, 30311) Mosby Inc.

Health Promotion Ideas That Work. Timothy E. Glaros. 1997. LC 97-9584. (Illus.). 152p. (Orig.). pap. text 21.00 (*0-87322-888-X*, BGLA0888) Human Kinetics.

Health Promotion in Communities: Holistic & Wellness Approaches. Ed. by Carolyn Chambers Clark. 2001. LC 00-67911. (Illus.). 496p. 69.95 (*0-8261-1407-5*) Springer Pub.

Health Promotion in Diverse Cultural Communities. Virginia M. Gonzalez et al. 1991. 58p. (Orig.). pap. 14.00 (*1-879552-14-0*) SCRDP.

Health Promotion in Midwifery. 288p. pap. (*0-340-61473-0*) E A GBR. *Dist:* Routldge.

Health Promotion in Midwifery. Jacqueline Dunkley. 2000. (Illus.). 280p. pap. text (*0-7020-2424-4*) W B Saunders GBR. *Dist:* Saunders.

Health Promotion in Nursing. Doherty & Mavil. 1996. (Professional Reference - Nursing Ser.). (C). pap. text, tchr. ed. 10.00 (*0-8273-8009-7*) Delmar.

Health Promotion in Nursing. Janice A. Maville & Carolina G. Huerta. 2001. LC 2001-28467. (Professional Reference - Nursing Ser.). (Illus.). xviii, 453p. (C). pap. text 39.95 (*0-8273-8008-9*) Delmar.

Health Promotion in Nursing Practice. Nola J. Pender. 3rd ed. 1996. LC 96-143912. 320p. (C). pap. 52.00 (*0-8385-3659-X*, A3659-8) P-H.

Health Promotion in the Schools: Innovative Approaches to Facilitating Physical & Emotional Well-Being. Ed. by Joseph E. Zins et al. 1985. LC 84-25227. (Special Services in the Schools Ser.: Vol. 1, No. 3). 134p. text 39.95 (*0-86656-303-2*); pap. text 19.95 (*0-86656-428-4*) Haworth Pr.

Health Promotion in the Workplace. Michael P. O'Donnell & Jeffrey S. Harris. 2nd ed. 1993. LC 93-676. 554p. (C). pap. 75.95 (*0-8273-4940-8*) Delmar.

Health Promotion In The Workplace. Michael P. O'Donnell. 3rd ed. 2001. LC 00-60290. (Illus.). 614p. text 65.95 (*0-7668-2866-2*) Delmar.

Health Promotion Planning: An Educational & Environmental Approach. Lawrence W. Green & Marshall W. Krueter. 2nd ed. 1991. LC 90-20500. 506p. (C). text 60.95 (*0-87484-779-6*, 779) Mayfield Pub.

Health Promotion Research: Towards a New Social Epidemiology. Ed. by B. Badura & Ilona Kickbusch. 1991. (WHO Regional Publications, European Ser.: No. 37). x, 496p. pap. text 78.00 (*92-890-1128-9*, 1310037) World Health.

Health Promotion Strategies & Methods. Garry Egger et al. 1991. (Illus.). 131p. pap. text 19.50 (*0-07-452782-7*) McGraw-Hill Med Pub.

Health Promotion Strategies & Methods. Garry Egger et al. 2nd ed. 1999. (Illus.). 199p. pap. 39.95 (*0-07-470483-4*) McGraw-Hill Prof.

Health Promotion Throughout the Lifespan. Carole Lium Edelman. 4th ed. 1997. LC 97-36797. (Illus.). 720p. (C). (gr. 13). pap. text 44.00 (*0-8151-2389-2*, 31042) Mosby Inc.

Health Protection Against Sickness & Disease by Using Preventive Medicine: Index of New Information with Authors, Subjects & References. Francis C. Doty. 1996. (Illus.). 150p. 57.50 (*0-7883-1292-8*); pap. 47.50 (*0-7883-1293-6*) ABBE Pubs Assn.

Health Protection & Improvements by Advice, Teachings, Preventive Medicine & Philosophy: Index of New Information with Authors, Subjects & Bibliography. Terry H. Grasberger. 1993. 180p. 47.50 (*1-55914-812-8*); pap. 44.50 (*1-55914-813-6*) ABBE Pubs Assn.

Health Protection & Promotion Against Sickness & Disease: Index of New Information with Authors, Subjects & References. Amy C. Maynard. 1997. 150p. 57.50 (*0-7883-1376-2*) ABBE Pubs Assn.

Health Psychology. Bernard. 1993. (C). pap. text, tchr. ed. 35.00 (*0-03-098881-0*) Harcourt Coll Pubs.

Health Psychology. Larry Bernard & Edward Krupat. 1994. LC 93-78967. (Illus.). 600p. (C). text 93.50 (*0-03-074417-2*) Harcourt Coll Pubs.

Health Psychology. Anthony J. Curtis. 1999. LC 99-32420. (Modular Psychology Ser.). (Illus.). xvi, 190p. pap. 12.99 (*0-415-19273-0*) Routledge.

Health Psychology. Harvey. 1989. pap. text (*0-582-29623-4*) Addison-Wesley GBR. *Dist:* Trans-Atl Phila.

Health Psychology. Neil Niven. 1989. 396p. pap. text (*0-443-03665-9*) Church.

Health Psychology. Philip L. Rice. 1997. LC 97-11794. (Psychology Ser.). 580p. spiral bd. 80.95 (*0-534-33915-8*) Wadsworth Pub.

Health Psychology. Straub. 2001. LC 2001-46904. text 61.00 (*1-57259-786-0*) Worth.

Health Psychology. Linda Brannon & Jess Feist. 2nd ed. 1992. (Psychology Ser.). pap., stu. ed. 14.50 (*0-534-16538-9*) Brooks-Cole.

Health Psychology. Shelley E. Taylor. 3rd ed. 1994. LC 94-31017. (C). text 54.25 net. (*0-07-063259-6*) McGraw.

Health Psychology. Shelley E. Taylor. 4th ed. 1998. LC 97-47345. 656p. (C). text 78.44 (*0-07-292746-1*) McGrw-H Hghr Educ.

Health Psychology: A Discipline & a Profession. Ed. by George C. Stone et al. 1987. LC 86-27254. xii, 562p. (C). 42.00 (*0-226-77557-7*) U Ch Pr.

Health Psychology: A Textbook. Jane Ogden. 1996. LC 95-24922. 192p. (*0-335-19544-X*) OpUniv Pr.

Health Psychology: A Textbook. Contrib. by Jane Ogden. 2nd ed. 2000. LC 99-56965. 384p. (*0-335-20596-8*) OpUniv Pr GBR. *Dist:* Taylor & Francis.

Health Psychology: An Introduction for Nurses & Other Health Care Professionals. Neil Niven. 2nd ed. 1994. LC 94-8465. pap. text (*0-443-04810-X*) Church.

Health Psychology: An Introduction to Behavior & Health. Jess Feist & Linda Brannon. 1987. 434p. (C). mass mkt. 44.00 (*0-534-08274-2*) Brooks-Cole.

Health Psychology: An Introduction to Behavior & Health. Linda Brannon & Jess Feist. (C). 2nd ed. 1992. 544p. text 43.25 (*0-534-16536-2*); 3rd ed. 1996. 560p. mass mkt. 49.75 (*0-534-34306-6*) Brooks-Cole.

Health Psychology: An Introduction to Behavior & Health. Linda Brannon & Jess Feist. 4th ed. 1999. LC 99-25890. 592p. spiral bd. 87.95 (*0-534-36850-6*) Thomson Learn.

Health Psychology: An Introduction to Behavior & Health Study Guide. Linda Brannon & Jess Feist. 3rd ed. 1996. (Psychology Ser.). (C). mass mkt., stu. ed. 14.75 (*0-534-34307-4*) Brooks-Cole.

Health Psychology: Biopsychosocial Interactions. Edward P. Sarafino. 3rd ed. 1997. LC 97-20461. 608p. 73.95 (*0-471-16917-X*) Wiley.

Health Psychology: Challenging the Biomedical Model. Charles L. Sheridan & Sally A. Radmacher. 1991. LC 91-10347. 416p. (C). 71.95 (*0-471-50852-7*) Wiley.

Health Psychology: Processes & Applications. Annabel K. Broome. 1990. (Illus.). 440p. pap. 47.50 (*0-412-33210-8*, A4057) Chapman & Hall.

Health Psychology & Public Health: An Integrative Approach. R. A. Winett et al. 1989. (General Psychology Ser.). 448p. (Orig.). (C). text 49.50 (*0-08-033641-8*); pap. text 22.50 (*0-08-033640-X*) Elsevier (Pergamon Pr).

Health Psychology for Health Care Professionals. Neil Niven. 3rd ed. 2000. LC 99-31875. (*0-443-05989-6*) Church.

Health Psychology in Global Perspective. Frances E. Aboud. 1998. LC 97-33937. (Cross-Cultural Psychology Ser.). 342p. 96.95 (*0-7619-0940-0*, 81035); pap. 37.95 (*0-7619-0941-9*, 81036) Sage.

Health Psychology of Women. Ed. by Catherine A. Niven & Douglas Carroll. 1993. LC 92-49332. 214p. text 51.00 (*3-7186-5335-4*) Gordon & Breach.

Health Psychology Through the Life Span: Practice & Research Opportunities. Ed. by Robert J. Resnick & Ronald H. Rozensky. 1996. LC 96-41438. 464p. 39.95 (*1-55798-378-X*, 431-7780); pap. 34.95 (*1-55798-391-7*) Am Psychol.

Health Psychology with InfoTrac. Rice. 1998. (Psychology Ser.). 48.50 incl. cd-rom (*0-534-36359-8*) Brooks-Cole.

Health Purifiers & Their Enemies: A Study of the Natural Health Movement in the United States with a Comparison to Its Counterpart in Germany. Julius A. Roth. 1977. LC 77-2210. 15.00 (*0-88202-117-6*) Watson Pub Intl.

Health Quality & Choice. OECD Staff. 1994. (Health Policy Studies: No. 4). 140p. (Orig.). pap. 28.00 (*92-64-14213-4*) OECD.

***Health Question & Answer Review for E.K.G.** Karen Ellis. 2001. 272p. pap. 44.00 (*0-13-019748-3*) P-H.

Health Question & Answer Review for Phlebotomy & Blood Collection. Kathleen Becan-McBride & Diana Garza. 5th ed. 2000. LC 00-59861. 254p. pap. 43.33 (*0-13-088715-3*) P-H.

Health, Race & German Politics Between National Unification & Nazism, 1870-1945. Paul Weindling. (History of Medicine Ser.). 656p. (C). 1993. (Illus.). pap. text 52.95 (*0-521-42397-X*); 1989. text 90.00 (*0-521-36381-0*) Cambridge U Pr.

Health Rational for Family Planning: Timing of Births & Child Survival. LC 95-121987. (Population Studies: No. 141). 128p. pap. 17.50 (*92-1-151275-1*, E.95.XIII.3) UN.

Health Reference Series Cumulative Index: A Comprehensive Index to All Volumes of the Health Reference Series, 1990-1998. Ed. by Edward Prucha. 1999. LC 99-52056. (Health Reference Ser.). xvii, 989p. lib. bdg. 78.00 (*0-7808-0382-5*) Omnigraphics Inc.

Health Reform for Communities: Financing Substance Abuse Services. Frwd. by Calvin Hill. 1996. (Illus.). 27p. (Orig.). (C). pap. text 15.00 (*0-7881-2553-2*) DIANE Pub.

Health Reform in Africa: Lessons from Sierra Leone. Bruce Siegel et al. 1996. (Discussion Paper Ser.: No. 347). 50p. pap. 22.00 (*0-8213-3825-0*, 13825) World Bank.

Health Reform in Australia & New Zealand. Abby Bloom. 2000. LC 00-708677. (Illus.). 320p. pap. text 39.95 (*0-19-550860-2*) OUP.

Health-Related Disorders in Children & Adolescents: A Guidebook for Understanding & Educating. Ed. by LeAdelle Phelps. 1998. LC 98-13919. (School Psychology Ser.). 743p. 59.95 (*1-55798-485-9*) Am Psychol.

Health-Related Effects of Phyllosilicates. Ed. by J. Bignon. 1990. (NATO ASI Ser.: Vol. 21). (Illus.). 449p. 183.00 (*0-387-51765-0*) Spr-Verlag.

Health-Related Fitness for Grades 5-6. Chris Hopper et al. 1996. LC 96-33878. (Illus.). 160p. (Orig.). pap., tchr. ed. 18.00 (*0-88011-480-0*, BHOP0480) Human Kinetics.

Health-Related Fitness for Grades 1-2. Chris Hopper et al. 1996. LC 96-12408. (Illus.). 128p. (Orig.). pap., tchr. ed. 29.95 (*0-87322-498-1*, BHOP0498) Human Kinetics.

Health-Related Fitness for Grades 3-4. Chris Hopper et al. 1996. LC 96-11314. (Illus.). 136p. (Orig.). pap., tchr. ed. 17.00 (*0-87322-499-X*, BHOP0499) Human Kinetics.

Health-Related Water Microbiology 1986: Proceedings of An IAWPRC Seminar Held in Rio de Janeiro, Brazil, 20-22 August 1986. Ed. by W. O. Grabow. 1987. LC 82-645900. (Water Science & Technology Ser.: No. 18). (Illus.). 278p. pap. 57.00 (*0-08-035580-3*, Pergamon Pr) Elsevier.

Health Related Water Microbiology, 1988: Proceedings of a Seminar Organized by the IAWPRC Specialist Group on Health-Related Water Microbiology As Part of the IAWPRC 14th Biennial Conference, Brighton, UK, July 19-21, 1988. Ed. by W. O. Grabow et al. 1989. (Water Science & Technology Ser.). 330p. pap. 139.00 (*0-08-037380-1*) Elsevier.

Health-Related Water Microbiology 1992. Ed. by R. W. Morris et al. 1993. (Water Science & Technology Ser.: Vol. 27). 500p. pap. 258.00 (*0-08-042207-1*, Pergamon Pr) Elsevier.

Health-Related Water Microbiology 1994: Selected Proceedings of the International Symposium Organized by the IAWQ Specialist Group on Health-Related Water Microbiology as Part of Water Quality International 1994, 17th Biennial Conference of the IAWQ, Budapest, Hungary, Held July 24-30, 1994. Ed. by R. Morris et al. 1995. (Water Science & Technology Ser.). (Illus.). 488p. pap. 230.50 (*0-08-042655-7*, Pergamon Pr) Elsevier.

Health Research: Essential Link to Equity in Development. Commission on Health Research for Development Staf. 1990. (Illus.). 160p. pap. text 17.95 (*0-19-520838-2*) OUP.

Health Research: Index of New Information with Authors & Subjects. Science and Life Consultants Association Staff. 1992. LC 92-54204. 180p. 47.50 (*1-55914-560-9*); pap. 44.50 (*1-55914-561-7*) ABBE Pubs Assn.

Health Research & Design. Ed. by Eucharia Nnadi Okolo. 1990. 272p. lib. bdg. 159.00 (*0-8493-4627-4*, R850) CRC Pr.

Health Research in Practice: Political, Ethical & Methodological Issues. Colquhoun. 1993. 160p. pap. 47.75 (*1-56593-143-2*, 0455) Singular Publishing.

Health Research in Practice Vol. 2: Personal Experiences, Public Issues, 2. Ed. by D. Colquhoun & Allan Kellehear. 1995. 224p. (Orig.). pap. 42.95 (*1-56593-608-6*, 1262) Singular Publishing.

Health Research Methodology: A Guide for Training in Research Methods. 1992. (WHO Regional Publications: No. 5). v, 282p. pap. text 50.00 (*92-9061-135-9*, 1500005) World Health.

Health Research on Military Personnel: Index of New Information. Erin E. Fallon. 1998. 57.50 (*0-7883-1824-1*); pap. 47.50 (*0-7883-1825-X*) ABBE Pubs Assn.

Health Resources & the Law. Alexander M. Smith. 1994. (Medico-Legal Issues Ser.: Vol. 10). text (*1-85521-033-9*) Dartmth Pub GBR. *Dist:* Ashgate Pub Co.

Health Resources Online: A Guide for Mental Health & Addiction Specialists. Ed. by John Grohol et al. 1997. (Illus.). 115p. (Orig.). pap. 39.95 (*1-884937-42-X*) Manisses Communs.

Health Resources Sourcebook: Basic Consumer Health Information about Sources of Medical Assistance... Ed. by Dawn D. Matthews. 2002. (Health Reference Ser.). 500p. lib. bdg. 78.00 (*0-7808-0328-0*) Omnigraphics Inc.

Health Restoration: Area I. Jack Rudman. (Regents External Degree Ser.: Vol. 31). 43.95 (*0-8373-5681-4*); (ACT Proficiency Examination Program Ser.: Vol. 51). 43.95 (*0-8373-5926-0*); 1994. (ACT Proficiency Examination Program Ser.: PEP-51). pap. 23.95 (*0-8373-5901-5*); 1994. (Regents External Degree Ser.: Vol. REDP-31). pap. 23.95 (*0-8373-5631-8*) Nat Learn.

Health Restoration: Area II. Jack Rudman. (Regents External Degree Ser.: Vol. 32). 43.95 (*0-8373-5682-2*); (ACT Proficiency Examination Program Ser.: Vol. 52). 43.95 (*0-8373-5927-9*); 1994. (ACT Proficiency Examination Program Ser.: PEP-52). pap. 23.95 (*0-8373-5902-3*); 1994. (Regents External Degree Ser.: Vol. REDP-32). pap. 23.95 (*0-8373-5632-6*) Nat Learn.

Health Revolution in Cuba. Sergio Diaz-Briquets. 1983. LC 82-10865. (Special Publication / Institute of Latin American Studies, U). 245p. text 19.95 (*0-292-75071-4*) U of Tex Pr.

Health Risk Assessment Through Dermal & Inhalation Exposure. Wang. 1992. 544p. 199.00 (*0-8493-7357-3*, RL803) CRC Pr.

Health Risk Behaviors among Our Nation's Youth: United States, 1992. P. F. Adams et al. 1995. LC 95-8593. (Vital & Health Statistics Ser.: Series 10, No. 192). (*0-08-406050-6*) Natl Ctr Health Stats.

Health Risks Analysis for Toxic Air Pollutants. Dydek. Date not set. 69.95 (*0-87371-567-5*, L567) Lewis Pubs.

Health Risks & Developmental Transitions During Adolescence. Ed. by John Schulenberg et al. 1997. (Illus.). 600p. (C). text 74.95 (*0-521-48053-1*) Cambridge U Pr.

Health Risks & Hazardous Substances at Work. Roach. 1992. 558p. text 173.00 (*0-08-040837-0*, Pergamon Pr) Elsevier.

Health Risks of Obesity. Frances M. Berg. 1993. (Illus.). 192p. pap. 29.95 (*0-918532-41-8*, Hlthy Weight Jrnl) Hlthy Wght Network.

Health Risks of Weight Loss. Frances M. Berg. 3rd rev. ed. 1995. (Illus.). 160p. (C). pap. text 19.95 (*0-918532-44-2*, Hlthy Weight Jrnl) Hlthy Wght Network.

Health Risks, Risk-Taking Behavior, Assessments & Management: Index of New Information with Authors, Subjects & References. Henry B. Rysso. 1996. 150p. 57.50 (*0-7883-1290-1*); pap. 47.50 (*0-7883-1291-X*) ABBE Pubs Assn.

Health Robbers: A Close Look at Quackery in America. Steven Barrett & William Jarvis. rev. ed. 1993. LC 93-25357. (Consumer Health Library). (Illus.). 544p. 35.00 (*0-87975-855-4*) Prometheus Bks.

Health, Safety, & Nutrition for the Young Child. Marie Cross et al. 3rd ed. 1993. LC 92-18290. (Illus.). 545p. pap. 35.50 (*0-8273-4932-7*) Delmar.

Health, Safety & Nutrition for the Young Child. Lynn R. Marotz & Edna Hill. 4th ed. 1997. LC 96-28773. (Early Childhood Education Ser.). 528p. pap. 42.95 (*0-8273-7273-6*) Delmar.

Health, Safety, & Nutrition for the Young Child. Lynn R. Marotz et al. 5th ed. 2000. LC 00-30718. (Illus.). 512p. (C). pap. text 67.95 (*0-7668-0946-3*) Delmar.

Health Science & Publication Bias: Index of New Information & Bibliography. Stanley T. Hollis. 1996. 150p. 57.50 (*0-7883-1002-X*); 1996. 150p. pap. 47.50 (*0-7883-1003-8*); 1999. 151p. pap. 47.50 (*0-7883-1991-4*) ABBE Pubs Assn.

Health Science Documentations: Survey, Methods & Standards : Index of New Information with Authors & Subjects. Arnold R. Fredericks. rev. ed. 1994. LC 94-32482. 179p. 57.50 (*0-7883-0230-2*); pap. 47.50 (*0-7883-0231-0*) ABBE Pubs Assn.

Health Science in Ancient India. B. L. Raina. 1990. (C). 44.00 (*81-7169-089-0*, Commonwealth) S Asia.

Health Sciences Literature Review Made Easy: The Matrix Method. Judith Garrard. 1999. LC 98-49815. 224p. pap. 25.00 (*0-8342-1223-4*) Aspen Pub.

Health Sciences Simulation. Ed. by James G. Anderson & Meyer Katzper. 1999. 216p. pap. 80.00 (*1-56555-160-5*) Soc Computer Sim.

Health Scientists Bible of Bibliography with Index of Authors & Subjects. Arnold R. Fredericks. 1993. 180p. 47.50 (*1-55914-854-3*); pap. 44.50 (*1-55914-855-1*) ABBE Pubs Assn.

Health Scientists' Bible of Bibliography with Index of Authors & Subjects. American Health Research Institute Staff. rev. ed. 1995. 193p. 57.50 (*0-7883-0626-X*); 1995. 193p. pap. 47.50 (*0-7883-0627-8*); 1994. 57.50 (*0-7883-0194-2*); 1994. pap. 47.50 (*0-7883-0195-0*) ABBE Pubs Assn.

Health Secrets From the Ancient World. John Heinerman. 1991. (Illus.). 170p. (Orig.). pap. 9.95 (*0-945946-11-2*) Cassandra Pr.

Health Secrets You Were Never Suppose to Have. David G. Williams. 1989. 60p. pap. 14.95 (*0-944649-05-X*) Mtn Home Pub.

Health Sector Reform in Developing Countries: Making Health Development Sustainable. Ed. by Peter A. Berman. 1996. LC 95-20671. (Series on Population & International Health). 416p. pap. 15.00 (*0-674-38525-X*) HUP.

Health Sector Strategy for the Europe & Central Asia Region. Verdon S. Staines. 1999. LC 99-24418. (Human Development Network Ser.). 96p. 25.00 (*0-8213-4481-1*, 14481) World Bank.

Health Security: The President's Report to the American People. White House Domestic Policy Council Staff. 1993. (Illus.). 136p. (Orig.). (C). pap. text 30.00 (*0-7881-0190-0*) DIANE Pub.

Health Security Act: A Section-by-Section Analysis. 1994. lib. bdg. 258.75 (*0-8490-5822-8*) Gordon Pr.

Health Security Act: Analysis of Veterans' Health Care Provisions. 1995. 56p. (Orig.). (C). pap. text 20.00 (*0-7881-2082-4*) DIANE Pub.

Health Sense: The Cancer Manual - Deal from Strength. Dee Maria. 2nd rev. ed. 1998. Orig. Title: Back to Health. 60p. pap. 7.95 (*0-9660414-1-0*) Dee Maria Pub.

Health Service. AIT Staff. 1997. pap. 120.00 net. (*0-538-68005-9*) Thomson Learn.

Health Service: Past, Present & Future. George Godber. 1975. (Heath Clark Lectures). 48p. (C). text (*0-485-26324-6*) Athlone Pr GBR. *Dist:* Humanities.

Health Service Finance & Accounting in Britain. Maurice S. Rigden. 1983. (Illus.). 272p. pap. 24.95 (*0-434-91730-3*) Trafalgar.

Health Service Nurse. Jack Rudman. 1994. (Career Examination Ser.: C-350). pap. 27.95 (*0-8373-0350-8*) Nat Learn.

Health Service Quality. John Ovretveit. 1991. (Illus.). 200p. pap. 40.95 (*0-632-03279-0*) Blackwell Sci.

Health Services: Concepts & Information for Planning & Management. K. White et al. 1977. (Public Health Papers: No. 67). 117p. pap. text 10.00 (*92-4-130067-1*, 1110067) World Health.

Health Services Administration: Policy Cases & the Case Method. Ed. by Roy Penchansky. 1968. LC 68-15640. 475p. 45.95 (*0-674-38550-0*) HUP.

Health Services Administration Handbook: Education & Practice. Karen M. Lorentzen & Linda Roemer. 1988. 128p. pap. 19.50 (*0-87527-353-X*) Green.

Health Services & Health Hazards: The Employee's Need to Know. Ed. by R. H. Egdahl & Diana C. Walsh. 1978. LC 78-18241. (Springer Series in Industry & Health Care: Vol. 4). (Illus.). 184p. 42.00 (*0-387-90335-6*) Spr-Verlag.

Health Services Cyclopedic Dictionary. Thomas C. Timmreck. 3rd ed. 1997. LC 96-46403. (Health Science Ser.). (Illus.). 872p. (C). text 71.95 (*0-86720-515-6*, 515-6) Jones & Bartlett.

Health Services in the People's Republic of China. Rhoada L. Sun. 1980. 124p. pap. text 13.95 (*0-87073-897-6*) Schenkman Bks Inc.

Health Services in the U. S. S. R. WHO Staff. 1960. (Public Health Papers: No. 3). 58p. 2.00 (*92-4-130003-5*) World Health.

Health Services Management: A Book of Cases. Anthony R. Kovner. 5th ed. 1997. LC 97-16063. pap. 45.00 (*1-56793-059-X*) Health Admin Pr.

Health Services Management: A Book of Cases. Anthony R. Kovner & Duncan Neuhauser. 6th ed. 2000. LC 00-59694. (Illus.). xxiii, 237p. (*1-56793-146-4*) Health Admin Pr.

Health Services Management: Readings & Commentary. Anthony R. Kovner & Duncan Neuhauser. 6th ed. 1997. LC 97-20194. 63.00 (*1-56793-065-4*); 7th ed. 2000. LC 00-59714. (Illus.). ix, 492p. (*1-56793-145-6*) Health Admin Pr.

Health Services Manager. Jack Rudman. 1994. (Career Examination Ser.: C-3178). pap. 39.95 (*0-8373-3178-1*) Nat Learn.

Health Services Organization in the Event of Disaster. 1983. (Technical Publications: Vol. 443). 112p. 8.00 (*92-75-11443-9*) PAHO.

Health Services Privatization in Industrial Societies. Ed. by Joseph L. Scarpaci. 1991. 260p. (*1-85302-064-8*) Jessica Kingsley GBR. *Dist:* Taylor & Francis.

Health Services Privitization in Industrial Societies. Ed. by Joseph L. Scarpaci. 1989. LC 88-36764. 260p. (C). text 45.00 (*0-8135-1437-1*); pap. text 18.95 (*0-8135-1438-X*) Rutgers U Pr.

Health Services Research. Ed. by G. N. Fracchia & M. Theofilatou. 1993. LC 93-78259. (Biomedical & Health Research Ser.: Vol. 1). 429p. (*90-5199-136-3*) IOS Pr NLD. *Dist:* IOS Press.

Health Services Research: An Anthology. B. Starfield & C. Ordonez. 1992. (PAHO Scientific Publications: No. 534). (ENG & SPA.). xxiv, 1082p. pap. text (*92-75-11534-6*, 1610534) World Health.

Health Services Research: Key to Health Policy. Eli Ginzberg. 1991. (Illus.). 416p. pap. 24.95 (*0-674-38576-4*) HUP.

Health Services Research: Key to Health Policy. Ed. by Eli Ginzberg. 1991. LC 90-4955. (Illus.). 416p. 47.00 (*0-674-38575-6*, GINHEA) HUP.

Health Services Research Methods. Leiyu Shi. 1996. LC 96-16768. (Delmar Series in Health Services Administration Ser.). 368p. 91.95 (*0-8273-7133-0*) Delmar.

Health Services Sources of Information for Research. 1995. lib. bdg. 251.95 (*0-8490-8360-5*) Gordon Pr.

Health Services Survey of Residents of Lexington, Nebraska. Curtis R. Winkle. 1986. 120p. (Orig.). pap. 8.50 (*1-55719-050-X*) U NE CPAR.

Health, Solar UV Radiation & Environmental Change. A. Kricker et al. 1993. (IARC Scientific Publications Ser.: No. 13). 212p. pap. text 27.00 (*92-832-1427-7*, 1770013) World Health.

Health South Spinal Cord Injury Handbook for Patients & Their Families. Richard C. Senelick & Karla Dougherty. 1998. (Illus.). 170p. pap. 12.95 (*1-891525-01-8*, HealthSouth Pr) HealthSouth.

Health Statistics: An Annotated Bibliographic Guide to Information Resources. Ed. by Freida Weise. 2nd ed. 1996. LC 96-44016. 184p. 48.00 (*0-8108-3056-6*) Scarecrow.

Health Statistics for the Americas. Haeduck Lee & Jose Luis Bobadilla. 1994. LC 94-36261. (Technical Papers: No. 262). 64p. pap. 22.00 (*0-8213-3037-3*, 13037) World Bank.

Health Status & Health Policy: Quality of Life in Health Care Evaluation & Resource Allocation. Donald L. Patrick & Pennifer Erickson. 1993. LC 92-6173. (Illus.). 504p. text 69.50 (*0-19-505027-4*) OUP.

Health Status & Well-Being of the Elderly: National Health & Nutrition Examination, No. I: Epidemiologic Follow-up Survey. Joan Cornoni-Huntley et al. 1990. LC 89-9212. (Illus.). 320p. text 55.00 (*0-19-504962-4*) OUP.

Health Status Measurement: A Brief but Critical Introduction. Crispin Jenkinson & Hannah M. McGee. 1998. LC 99-171270. 104p. pap. (*1-85775-228-7*) Radcliffe Med Pr GBR. *Dist:* Balogh.

Health Status of Minorities & Low-Income Groups. 3rd ed. 1995. (Illus.). 376p. (C). reprint ed. pap. text 45.00 (*0-7881-1872-2*) DIANE Pub.

Health Styles: Decisions for Life. B. E. Pruitt. rev. ed. Date not set. (C). pap. text (*0-03-005917-8*) Harcourt Coll Pubs.

Health Subject Matter in Natural Sciences. Claude S. Chappelear. LC 78-176637. (Columbia University. Teachers College. Contributions to Education Ser.: No. 341). reprint ed. 37.50 (*0-404-55341-9*) AMS Pr.

Health Support: Area I. Jack Rudman. 1994. (ACT Proficiency Examination Program Ser.: PEP-48). pap. 23.95 (*0-8373-5548-6*); (Regents External Degree Ser.: Vol. REDP-24). pap. 23.95 (*0-8373-5624-5*) Nat Learn.

Health Support: Area II. Jack Rudman. 1994. (ACT Proficiency Examination Program Ser.: PEP-49). pap. 23.95 (*0-8373-5549-4*); (Regents External Degree Ser.: Vol. REDP-25). pap. 23.95 (*0-8373-5625-3*) Nat Learn.

Health Surveillance at Work. S. Deacon. 1996. pap. (*1-85953-000-1*) Tech Comm GBR. *Dist:* St Mut.

Health Survey for England, 1991. 1993. (Series HS: No. 1). 359p. pap. (*0-11-691532-3*, HM15323) Statnry Office GBR. *Dist:* Bernan Associates.

Health Survey for England 1992. 1994. (Series HS 1). 359p. pap. (*0-11-691569-2*, HM15692) Statnry Office GBR. *Dist:* Bernan Associates.

Health Survey for England, 1994. HMSO Staff. 1996. (Series HS: Vol. 4). 352p. pap. (*0-11-321895-8*, HM18958) Statnry Office GBR. *Dist:* Bernan Associates.

Health Survey for England, No. 6, 1996, No. 6. 1998. (OPCS Reference Ser. - All Publications Ser.: No. 81020274). 352p. pap. (*0-11-322091-X*, HM2091X) Statnry Office GBR. *Dist:* Bernan Associates.

Health Syllabus & Tests. 1999. 10p. ring bd. 2.50 (*1-57896-065-7*, 2317, Hewitt Homeschl Res) Hewitt Res Fnd.

Health System Decentralization: Concepts, Issues, & Country Experience. Ed. by A. Mills et al. 1990. (ENG, FRE & SPA.). 151p. pap. text 23.40 (*92-4-156137-8*, 1150340) World Health.

Health System Support for Primary Health Care. B. Kleczkowski et al. 1984. (Public Health Papers: No. 80). 104p. pap. text 10.00 (*92-4-130080-9*, 1110080) World Health.

Health System's Role in Abortion Care: The Need for a Pro-Active Approach. Katie E. McLaurin et al. 1991. (Issues in Abortion Care Ser.). 34p. pap. 7.50 (*1-882220-00-5*) IPAS.

Health Teachers Book of Lists. Patricia Rizzo Toner & Marian D. Milliken. 1999. LC 98-50233. 304p. spiral bd. 29.95 (*0-87628-476-4*) Ctr Appl Res.

Health Teaching in Nursing Practice: A Professional Model. Marlyn Boyd. 3rd ed. 1997. LC 96-53077. 350p. (C). pap. 47.00 (*0-8385-3681-6*, A3681-2) P-H.

Health Teaching in Secondary Schools. Carl E. Willgoose. 3rd ed. 1982. (C). text 25.75 (*0-03-058493-0*) SCP.

Health Technologists & Technicians. 1996. 19p. pap. 1.50 (*0-16-048473-1*) USGPO.

Health Technology Assessment: A Needs-Based Approach. Ed. by Yves Bergevin. 1996. LC 97-700149. xviii, 156p. pap. (*0-88936-752-3*) IDRC-CRDI CAN. *Dist:* Stylus Pub VA.

Health Technology Assessment Methodologies for Developing Countries. 1989. 117p. pap. text 28.00 (*92-75-12023-4*) World Health.

Health Technology Transfer: Whose Responsibility? Ed. by Z. Bankowski & Gordon L. Ada. 1990. (Proceedings of the XXIIIrd CIOMS Round Table Conference Ser.). 165p. pap. text 20.00 (*92-9036-043-7*, 1830023) World Health.

Health Telematics Education. Ed. by J. Mantas. 1997. LC 97-70264. (Studies in Health Technology & Informatics: Vol. 41). 398p. 91.00 (*90-5199-329-3*) IOS Press.

Health Telematics for Clinical Guidelines & Protocols. Ed. by C. Gordon & J. P. Christensen. 1995. LC 94-7335. (Studies in Health Technology & Informatics: Vol. 16). 235p. 90.00 (*90-5199-199-1*) IOS Press.

Health, the Bible & the Church. Daniel E. Fountain. 1989. (BGC Monograph). (Illus.). 215p. pap. 7.00 (*1-879089-02-5*) Evangelism & Missions.

Health, the Medical Profession & Regulation. Ed. by Peter Zweifel. 1998. LC 97-43550. (Developments in Health Economics & Public Policy Ser.). 261p. lib. bdg. 140.00 (*0-7923-8101-7*) Kluwer Academic.

Health Through Balance: An Introduction to Tibetan Medicine. Yeshi Donden. Ed. by Jeffrey Hopkins. Tr. by Lobsang Rabgay & Alan Wallace. 1986. LC 86-1879. (TIB., Illus.). 252p. (C). pap. 14.95 (*0-937938-25-4*) Snow Lion Pubns.

Health Through God's Pharmacy: Advice & Experiences with Medicinal Herbs. Maria Treben. 26th ed. 1998. (Illus.). 92p. pap. (*3-85068-124-6*) Ennsthaler AUT. *Dist:* Am Educ Systs.

Health Through God's Pharmacy/French: French Edition. Maria Treben. 1998. (FRE.). 112p. pap. (*3-85068-123-8*) Ennsthaler AUT. *Dist:* Am Educ Systs.

Health Through Inner Body Cleansing: The Famous MAYR Intestinal Therapy From Europe. Erich Rauch. Tr. by Mollie C. Peters from GER. 3rd ed. 1990. (Illus.). 89p. pap. (*3-7760-1179-3*) K F Haug Pubs DEU. *Dist:* Medicina Bio.

Health Through Oral Health. World Health Organization Staff. 1989. (Illus.). 77p. pap. text 28.00 (*1-85097-008-4*) Quint Pub Co.

***Health, 2001-2002.** annuals Richard Yarian. 22nd ed. 2001. 240p. pap. 18.44 (*0-07-243364-7*) McGrw-H Hghr Educ.

Health 2000-2001. Richard Yarian. 21st ed. 2000. (Annual Editions Ser.). 240p. (C). pap. 17.50 (*0-07-236587-0*) McGrw-H Hghr Educ.

Health U. S., 1999: Health & Aging Chartbook. Ed. by Ellen A. Kramarow & Harold R. Lentzner. 23rd ed. 2000. (Illus.). 166p. pap. text 35.00 (*0-7881-8783-X*) DIANE Pub.

Health, U. S., 1993: The Annual National Report on Health. 1994. (Illus.). 225p. (Orig.). (YA). (gr. 12 up). pap. text 45.00 (*0-7881-0839-5*) DIANE Pub.

Health Unit Coordinating. Ed. by Myrna LaFleur Brooks. 3rd ed. 1993. (Illus.). 541p. pap., tchr. ed. (*0-7216-4304-3*) Saunders.

Health Unit Coordinating. Myrna LaFleur Brooks. Ed. by Selma Kaszczuk. 4th ed. 1998. LC 97-36857. (Illus.). 560p. (C). text 39.95 (*0-7216-7186-1*) Saunders.

Health Unit Coordinating. Ed. by Myrna LaFleur Brooks. 4th ed. 1998. (Illus.). 555p. pap. (*0-7216-7187-X*) Saunders.

Health Unit Coordinating: Expanding the Scope of Practice. Madeline A. Clark & Virginia S. Mazza. Ed. by Maureen Pfeiffer. 1999. LC 98-24850. (Illus.). 655p. pap. text (*0-7216-7036-9*) Saunders.

Health Unit Coordinating: Principles & Practices. Velma L. Kerschner. 1992. pap. 33.95 (*0-8273-2745-5*) Delmar.

Health Unit Coordinator Instructor's Guide. Velma L. Kerschner. 1988. pap., tchr. ed. 14.00 (*0-8273-2746-3*) Delmar.

Health United States 1995. 20th ed. 1996. (Illus.). x, 328p. pap. 40.00 (*0-9656560-5-5*) DIANE Pub.

Health United States 1996-97 & Injury Chart Book. Ed. by Kate Prager et al. 1999. (Illus.). 341p. (C). reprint ed. pap. text 45.00 (*0-7881-8248-X*) DIANE Pub.

Health United States 2000 & Injury Chartbook. 2000. 300p. per. 45.00 (*0-16-050401-5*, GPO14882) USGPO.

Health Units for Nonreaders. Joy Cole et al. 1995. (Illus.). 143p. spiral bd. 24.00 (*1-884135-17-X*) Mayer-Johnson.

Health U. S. 1994: The Annual National Report on Health. 1996. (Illus.). 307p. (Orig.). (C). pap. text 45.00 (*0-7881-2697-0*) DIANE Pub.

Health Visiting: Specialist & Higher Level Practice. Anne Robotham & Doreen Sheldrake. 2000. LC 99-53179. (Illus.). x, 447p. text (*0-443-06203-X*) Harcrt Hlth Sci Grp.

Health Visiting: Towards Community Health Nursing. Karen A. Luker & Jean Orr. 2nd ed. 1992. (Illus.). 272p. pap. 34.95 (*0-632-03324-X*) Blackwell Sci.

Health Visiting & the Elderly People. Mary McClymont et al. 2nd ed. 1991. (Illus.). 340p. pap. text (*0-443-04228-4*) Church.

Health Visiting in Practice. Carol Robertson. 2nd ed. 1991. (Illus.). 1991p. pap. text (*0-443-04137-7*) Church.

Health, Weather & Climate. Felix G. Sulman. 1976. (Perspectives in Medicine Ser.: Vol. 7). (Illus.). 160p. 22.75 (*3-8055-2350-5*) S Karger.

Health, Welfare & Practice: Reflecting on Roles & Relationships. Jan Walmsley et al. 256p. (C). 1993. 83.00 (*0-8039-8794-3*, 9419); 1992. pap. 27.95 (*0-8039-8795-1*, 9420) Sage.

Health, Wellness & Restoration: The Complete Guide for Restoring Your Health the Natural Way. Denise Davis. 1998. (Illus.). 175p. 23.60 (*0-9668415-0-6*) Denise D.

Health Wise: A Handbook on Healthy Aging. Christina Dye. rev. ed. 1992. pap. 3.50 (*0-89230-232-1*) Do It Now.

Health, Work, & the Workplace: A Special Issue of the International Journal of Behavioral Medicine. Ed. by Brian Oldenburg. 1999. 88p. pap. 20.00 (*0-8058-9797-6*) L Erlbaum Assocs.

Health Work with the Poor: A Practical Guide. Christie W. Kiefer. 2000. LC 99-45961. xiv, 239p. (C). text 49.00 (*0-8135-2776-7*) Rutgers U Pr.

Health Workers & AIDS: Research, Intervention & Current Issues in Burnout & Response. Lydia Bennett & David Miller. 1995. LC 96-139391. 419p. text 60.00 (*3-7186-5659-0*, Harwood Acad Pubs) Gordon & Breach.

Health Workers & AIDS: Research, Intervention & Current Issues in Burnout & Response. Lydia Bennett et al. 1995. LC 96-139391. 419p. pap. text 30.00 (*3-7186-5660-4*, Harwood Acad Pubs) Gordon & Breach.

Health Workforce Issues for the Twenty-First Century. Ed. by Paul F. Larson et al. 1994. LC 94-15952. (Health Policy Annual Ser.: No. 4). 206p. pap. 20.00 (*1-879694-08-5*) AAH Ctrs.

Healthcare Advertising: Consumer Responses & Attitudes. Robert J. Van Dellen. 1989. LC 89-84008. 290p. (Orig.). pap. text 325.00 (*0-9622718-0-2*) Hlthcare Mktg & Comns.

Healthcare Advertising & Marketing: A Practical Approach to Effective Communications. Patricia S. Meade. 1998. LC 98-31110. (Illus.). 225p. 55.00 (*0-07-041236-7*) McGraw.

Healthcare Almanac & Yearbook, 2000 Edition. Ed. by Luci Kozzumi & Dan Moskowitz. 1999. 656p. pap. text 225.00 (*1-57987-162-3*) Faulkner & Gray.

Healthcare Basics Cd-Rom for Windows Single Site License. Mosby Lifeline Staff. 1996. 400p. pap. text 195.00 (*0-8151-5561-1*) Mosby Inc.

Healthcare Book of Lists. Ed. by Richard K. Thomas et al. 1994. LC 93-85846. (Illus.). 752p. per. 115.95 (*1-878205-25-0*) St Lucie Pr.

Healthcare Business Strategy: Lessons from the Management Masters for Today's Healthcare Professional. Ira Studin. 1995. LC 96-106482. 200p. text 35.00 (*1-55738-631-5*, Irwn Prfssnl) McGraw-Hill Educ Grp.

Healthcare Call Centers: Improving Patient Service, Satisfaction & Retention, Vol. 12, No. 2. 1998. pap. 28.00 (*0-7879-4243-X*) Jossey-Bass.

Healthcare Card Systems: Eurocards Concerted Action Results & Recommendations. Ed. by H. Doare et al. 1995. LC 95-7970. (Studies in Health Technology & Informatics: Vol. 22). 218p. 70.00 (*90-5199-225-4*) IOS Press.

Healthcare Communication Using Personality Type: Patients Are Different! Judy Allen & Susan A. Brock. 2000. LC 99-55354. 176p. pap. 27.95 (*0-415-21374-6*) Routledge.

Healthcare Compendium: A Demographic & Statistical Analysis Beyond Government Sources. Market Intelligence Staff. 1992. 240p. (Orig.). 695.00 (*1-56753-052-4*) Frost & Sullivan.

Healthcare Compendium 1997. Frost & Sullivan. 1996. 159p. spiral bd. 995.00 (*0-7889-0639-9*, 5539-59) Frost & Sullivan.

Healthcare Computing. Benson. 1995. pap. text (*0-582-22978-2*) Addison-Wesley GBR. *Dist:* Trans-Atl Phila, Longman.

Healthcare Cost Accounting: Practice & Applications. Jeffrey A. Gottlieb. 1989. 59p. per. 40.00 (*0-930228-67-7*) Hlthcare Fin Mgmt.

Healthcare Cost Containment Reference: HCCR. Jonathan Epher. 1992. 2600p. 99.00 (*1-880891-00-X*) Work-Loss Data.

Healthcare Design. Ed. by Sara O. Mayberry. 1996. LC 96-12446. (Healthcare & Senior Living Design Ser.). 340p. 90.00 (*0-471-13349-3*) Wiley.

Healthcare Economics: Text, Cases, Readings. Ed. by K. Choudhury & Tahamina Zaman. 1997. 250p. 39.95 (*1-884015-84-0*) St Lucie Pr.

Healthcare Enterprise Liability. Alan D. Lieberson. 1997. 110.00 (*1-55834-548-5*, 80979) LEXIS Pub.

Healthcare Enterprise Liability: 1997 Edition. Allan Lieberson. 1997. LC 97-73504. 1146p. text 110.00 (*1-55834-559-0*, 80979-10, MICHIE) LEXIS Pub.

Healthcare Enterprise Liability, 1998 Supplement. Alan D. Lieberson. 1998. 320p. suppl. ed. (*0-327-00559-9*, 8098010) LEXIS Pub.

Healthcare Environments for Children & Their Families. ACCH Staff. 1998. LC 97-69788. 320p. per. 39.95 (*0-7872-4336-1*) Kendall-Hunt.

Healthcare Equipment International: Market Trends, Companies, Statistics. Derrick A. Patient. 1989. 342p. pap. text (*0-582-03683-6*) Church.

***Healthcare Ethics & Human Values: An Introductory Text with Readings & Case Studies.** William Fulford et al. 2002. LC 2001-58123. 584p. 69.95 (*0-631-20223-4*); pap. 34.95 (*0-631-20224-2*) Blackwell Pubs.

Healthcare Ethics Committee Experience: Selected Readings from HEC Forum. Ed. by Stuart F. Spicker. 1998. LC 97-36976. 472p. (C). 59.50 (*1-57524-024-6*) Krieger.

Healthcare Facilities Law, Set. Dellinger. 1997. 864p. 159.00 (*0-316-18028-9*) Lppncott W & W.

Healthcare Finance: An Introduction to Accounting & Financial Management. Louis C. Gapenski. 1998. LC 98-8639. x, 556p. 75.00 (*1-56793-090-5*) Health Admin Pr.

***Healthcare Finance: An Introduction to Accounting & Financial Management.** Louis C. Gapenski. 2nd ed. 2001. LC 2001-39229. (*1-56793-165-0*) Health Admin Pr.

Healthcare Finance for the Non-Financial Manager: Basic Guide to Financial Analysis, Control. Louis C. Gapenski. 1994. (C). text 47.50 (*1-55738-610-2*, Irwn Prfssnl) McGraw-Hill Educ Grp.

Healthcare Fraud, Waste, Abuse & Safe Harbors: The Complete Legal Guide. Jonathan P. Tomes. 1993. 264p. (C). text 60.00 (*1-55738-601-3*) Hlthcare Fin Mgmt.

Healthcare Hiring & Staffing. David Debatto. 1996. 200p. 35.00 (*0-7863-1076-6*, Irwn Prfssnl) McGraw-Hill Educ Grp.

Healthcare Industry Market Yearbook. Ed. by Melanie Jenkins. 1996. (Illus.). 829p. pap. (*1-882364-11-2*) Hlth Res Pub.

Healthcare Industry Market Yearbook. Ed. by Melanie A. Matthews. 2nd ed. 1999. 715p. per. 545.50 (*1-882364-29-5*, Amer Busn Pub) Hlth Res Pub.

***Healthcare Informatics.** 2001. (General Methods & Instrumentation Ser.: Vol. 14.01). 1244p. pap. 189.00 (*0-8031-3024-4*) ASTM.

Healthcare Information Management. Medical Records Staff. 1994. text 70.00 (*0-7602-0047-5*, Irwn Prfssnl) McGraw-Hill Educ Grp.

Healthcare Information Management Systems: A Practical Guide. Ed. by M. J. Ball et al. 2nd ed. 1997. LC 95-6682. (Computers in Health Care Ser.). (Illus.). 358p. 59.00 (*0-387-94477-X*) Spr-Verlag.

Healthcare Information Systems: Challenges of the New Millennium. Ed. by Adi Armoni. 2000. LC 99-52784. (Illus.). 243p. (C). pap. 69.95 (*1-878289-62-4*) Idea Group Pub.

Healthcare Infostructures: The Development of Information-Based Infrastructures for the Healthcare Industry. Diebold Institute for Public Policy Studies, Inc.,. 1995. LC 95-34413. 60.00 (*0-275-95157-X*); pap. 18.95 (*0-275-95158-8*) Greenwood (Praeger Pubs).

Healthcare Integration: A Legal Manual for Constructing Integrated Organizations. Ed. by Gerald R. Peters. 1995. 615p. 75.00 (*0-918945-17-8*) Am Hlth Lawyers.

Healthcare IPO Report, 1999 Edition. 1999. 40p. pap. 99.00 (*1-887986-09-X*) Strafford Pubns.

Healthcare IS/IT Market Yearbook. Ed. by Edward H. Miles. 1999. 498p. per. 433.50 (*1-882364-36-8*, Amer Busn Pub) Hlth Res Pub.

***Healthcare IS/IT Market Yearbook.** Ed. by Jodi L. Kastel. 2nd ed. 2001. 658p. pap. 425.00 (*1-882364-60-0*, Amer Busn Pub) Hlth Res Pub.

Healthcare Joint Ventures: The Next Generation. Ed. by Gerald R. Peters. 1991. 369p. 45.00 (*0-918945-12-7*) Am Hlth Lawyers.

Healthcare Law & Ethics: Issues for the Age of Managed Care. Dean M. Harris. 1999. LC 99-24357. xv, 317p. 52.00 (*1-56793-107-3*) Health Admin Pr.

Healthcare Leaders Guide to Integrated Delivery Systems. Ed. by Meg Matheny. 1996. 423p. ring bd. 195.00 (*1-56925-061-8*, HIDS) Capitol Publns.

Healthcare Market Engineering. Market Intelligence Staff. 1994. (Orig.). 95.00 (*0-7889-0053-6*) Frost & Sullivan.

Healthcare Market Research. Date not set. 655p. (*0-7889-0350-0*) Frost & Sullivan.

Healthcare Marketing Plans That Work. David Marlowe. 1999. 115p. pap. 50.00 (*0-9676441-0-0*) Soc Healthcare Strategy.

Healthcare Marketing Research. Eric Berkowitz & Louis G. Pol. 1996. LC 96-38962. 264p. (C). text 45.00 (*1-55738-642-0*, Irwn Prfssnl) McGraw-Hill Educ Grp.

Healthcare Marketing, Sales & Service: An Executive Companion. John F. O'Malley. 2000. LC 00-47292. (Illus.). xi, 167p. (*1-56793-150-2*) Health Admin Pr.

***Healthcare Media Planning Guide.** Medical Economics Co. Staff & Joann Kirchner. 2001. 200p. pap. (*1-56363-400-7*) Med Econ.

***Healthcare Mergers & Acquisitions.** Ed. by Richard O. Jacobs. 2001. LC 2001-53446. (*0-7355-2523-4*) Aspen Law.

Healthcare Online for Dummies. Howard Wolinsky & Judi Wolinsky. 2001. LC 99-69389. (For Dummies Ser.). (Illus.). 360p. pap. 24.99 incl. cd-rom (*0-7645-0684-6*, Dummies Tech) Hungry Minds.

Healthcare Planning & Marketing. California College for Health Sciences Staff. 1994. 246p. (C). spiral bd. Price not set. (*0-933195-13-3*) CA College Health Sci.

Healthcare Practitioner's Handbook of Management. Larry D. Grieshaber. 1997. LC 97-181148. (Illus.). 344p. 69.95 (*1-57444-096-9*) St Lucie Pr.

Healthcare Privacy & Confidentiality: The Complete Legal Guide. Jonathan P. Tomes. 1994. LC 96-116687. 225p. (C). text 60.00 (*1-55738-611-0*, Irwn Prfssnl) McGraw-Hill Educ Grp.

Healthcare Product Comparison System: Clinical Laboratory Edition 1994. Ed. by Linda Weir. 1994. ring bd. 975.00 (*0-941417-03-4*) ECRI.

Healthcare Product Comparison System: Diagnostic Imaging & Radiology Edition 1994, Set. Ed. by Linda Weir. 1994. ring bd. 975.00 (*0-941417-06-9*) ECRI.

Healthcare Product Comparison System: Hospital Edition, 1994 Ed. by Linda Weii. 1994. ring bd. 975.00 (*0-941417-07-7*) ECRI.

Healthcare Professional as Friend & Healer: Building on the Work of Edmund D. Pellegrino. Ed. by David C. Thomasma & Judith Lee Kissell. 2000. LC 00-26362. xv, 303p. text 65.00 (*0-87840-809-6*); pap. text 24.95 (*0-87840-810-X*) Georgetown U Pr.

***Healthcare Professionals as Witnesses to the Court.** Mark Solon et al. 2000. 160p. (*1-900151-22-7*) Greenwich Med GBR. *Dist:* JAMCO Dist.

Healthcare Receivables Management: A Workflow-Based Approach to Operational Policies & Procedures. Bobette M. Gustafso & Sandra J. Wolfskill. 1996. 250p. (C). per. 80.00 (*1-55738-629-3*, Irwn Prfssnl) McGraw-Hill Educ Grp.

Healthcare Records Management, Disclosure & Retention: The Complete Legal Guide. Jonathan P. Tomes. 2nd ed. 1993. 600p. (C). text 75.00 (*1-882198-04-2*) Hlthcare Fin Mgmt.

Healthcare Reform D. O. A. Why Politics Will Destroy Healthcare & How One Physician's Plan Can Prevent It. Gene R. Moss. 1994. 206p. pap. 14.95 (*0-9639747-0-X*) Behav Med Assocs.

Healthcare Resource Directory: National Edition. Gary Nichols. Ed. by Mark L. Reed. 1993. 224p. (Orig.). pap. 25.00 (*0-933745-13-3*) Med Prod.

Healthcare Safety Sourcebook. Ray Moughalian. 2000. Orig. Title: MOHR's Guide. (Illus.). 202p. pap. text 99.00 (*1-57839-069-9*) Opus Communs.

Healthcare Scenarios in the Year 2000: A Common Sense Look at Four Alternatives to Get Us There. Market Intelligence Staff. 1993. 279p. 95.00 (*1-56753-421-X*) Frost & Sullivan.

Healthcare Standards 2001: Official Directory. rev. ed. 2000. ix, 3000p. 425.00 (*0-941417-08-5*) ECRI.

Healthcare Strategic Planning: Approaches for the 21st Century. Alan M. Zuckerman. 1998. LC 97-29506. viii, 122p. 44.00 (*1-56793-068-9*) Health Admin Pr.

Healthcare Teams: Building Continuous Quality Improvement. Peter Mears. 1994. (Illus.). 200p. stu. ed., per. 36.95 (*1-884015-41-7*) St Lucie Pr.

Healthcare Teams: Building Continuous Quality Improvement Facilitator's Guide. Peter Mears. 1994. (Illus.). 120p. tchr. ed., per. 57.95 (*1-884015-43-3*) St Lucie Pr.

Healthcare.com: Rx for Reform. David Friend. 1999. LC 99-40268. 112p. per. 24.95 (*1-57444-274-0*) St Lucie Pr.

Healthful Eating Through the Seasons. Christine Stone Tarantino. 1991. 118p. pap. 5.00 (*1-887480-43-9*) Wrds Lght Intl.

Healthiest City: Milwaukee & the Politics of Health Reform. Judith W. Leavitt. rev. ed. 1996. LC 96-5117. (Illus.). 318p. pap. 19.95 (*0-299-15164-6*) U of Wis Pr.

Healthline: Using Medline Efficiently in a Busy Clinical Practice. S. Thomas Deahl. 1998. (Informatics Ser.: No. 1). 115p. pap. 15.00 (*1-893549-04-6*) Biomed Genl.

HealthMate Medical Planner: A Practical Guide for Taking Control of Your Health & Having Your Medical Records Always Available...Even When Your Doctor Isn't. Kathleen R. DeRemer. 1997. LC 97-65096. ring bd. 29.95 (*0-9656350-5-8*) Six Ponies Pr.

Healthnet: Your Essential Resource for the Most Up-to-Date Medical Information Online. Jeanne C. Ryer. 1997. LC 96-9503. 240p. pap. 16.95 (*0-471-13769-3*) Wiley.

Healthquest: Staying Strong:Reclaiming The Wisdom Of African-American Healing. Ed. by Sara L. Reese et al. 1999. LC 99-94878. (Illus.). x, 341p. pap. 14.00 (*0-380-79402-0*, Avon Bks) Morrow Avon.

Healthquest for Windows. Gold. 1999. pap. text 27.02 net. (*0-07-239347-5*) McGraw.

Healthsaver's Guide to Keeping Fit after Bypass Surgery. Arline Frecker & Harold Frecker. 1990. 110p. (Orig.). pap. (*0-927839-14-8*) HlthSavers Pr.

Healthsmarts: How to Spot the Quacks, Avoid the Nonsense & Get the Facts that Affect Your Health. John H. Renner. Ed. by Lewis Vaughn. 1990. 160p. (Orig.). pap. 12.95 (*0-9626145-0-5*) Health Facts Pub.

Healthspan: A Holistic Guide to Discovering & Following Your Path of Health & Happiness from Here to 100. Jack Woodard & Genevieve J. Woodard. 1999. LC 99-95248. (Illus.). 360p. pap. 19.95 (*0-9671247-0-0*) Healthspirit Pr.

Healthspeak: A Complete Dictionary of America's Health Care System. Ellen Freudenheim. 1996. LC 95-10965. 288p. 35.00 (*0-8160-3210-6*) Facts on File.

HealthStyles: Decisions for Living Well. B. E. Pruitt et al. 2nd ed. 1998. LC 98-14502. 600p. pap. text 71.00 (*0-205-27229-0*) Allyn.

HealthTrip: Take the Trip of a Lifetime. Wellness Councils of America Staff. Ed. by Sandra Wendel. 1996. (Illus.). 60p. (Orig.). pap. 89.00 (*0-9628334-6-0*) WELCOA.

Healthwise: The Recipe & Reference Book for Health-Conscious Individuals & People on Special Diets. Billie J. English & Sharon C. Calhoun. 1994. 328p. spiral bd. (*0-9638533-0-9*) Cooper Ent.

Healthwise Handbook: A Self-Care Manual for You. Donald W. Kemper & Healthwise Staff. Ed. by Terry Smith. 13th rev. ed. 1997. (Illus.). 340p. pap. text 9.95 (*1-877930-63-6*) Healthwise.

Healthy Aging. Priscilla Ebersole & Patricia Hess. 2000. (Illus.). 512p. 34.95 (*0-323-01062-8*) Mosby Inc.

Healthy Aging: Challenges & Solutions. Ken Dychtwald. 1998. LC 98-39726. 448p. pap. 51.00 (*0-8342-1363-X*) Aspen Pub.

Healthy Aging Breakthrough: Amazing Supplements for Ideal Weight & Disease Prevention. Nick R. Delgado. Ed. by Shawna Kendell. 1999. LC 98-94176. (Illus.). 288p. pap. 15.95 (*1-879084-05-8*, Health Wellness Studios) Delgado.

***Healthy Aging for Functional Longevity: Molecular & Cellular Interactions in Senescence.** Sang Chul Park & Hyun-Sook Kim. 2001. (Annals of the New York Academy of Sciences Ser.). 400p. pap. text 29.50 (*0-8018-6832-7*) NY Acad Sci.

Healthy Aging, Healthy Treatment: The Impact of Telling Stories. Thomas H. Peake. 1998. LC 97-33704. 168p. 55.00 (*0-275-95922-8*, Praeger Pubs) Greenwood.

Healthy Aging Sourcebook: Basic Consumer Health Information about Maintaining Health Throughout the Aging Process. Ed. by Jenifer Swanson. 1999. LC 99-24387. (Health Reference Ser.). (Illus.). xii, 537p. 78.00 (*0-7808-0390-6*) Omnigraphics Inc.

Healthy America: The Challenge for States. Ed. by Karen Glass. 1991. 200p. (Orig.). pap. text 18.75 (*1-55877-125-5*) Natl Governor.

Healthy at Last: Solutions to Chronic Ill Health, Allergies & Environmental Illness. Cynthia Clinkscales. 1991. LC 89-81991. (Orig.). (C). pap. 11.95 (*0-9624764-1-2*) CECOM Pub.

Healthy Babies: State Initiatives for Pregnant Women at Risk. Susan C. Biemesderfer. 1993. 40p. pap. text 15.00 (*1-55516-703-9*, 6643) Natl Conf State Legis.

Healthy Babies, Healthy Business: An Employer's Guidebook on Improving Maternal & Infant Health. 1993. LC 93-5947. (*0-86525-056-1*) March of Dimes.

Healthy Back Book: Simple Exercises for an Active, Pain-Free Back. Elizabeth Sharp. 1994. LC 93-41013. (Illus.). pap. 14.95 (*1-85230-444-8*) Element MA.

Healthy Balance: A Qualitative Study of Men's Health Beliefs. Kenneth Mullen. 1993. 200p. (*1-85628-548-0*) Avebry GBR. *Dist:* Ashgate Pub Co.

Healthy Body & Victorian Culture. Bruce Haley. 1978. LC 78-6933. 312p. 37.95 (*0-674-38610-8*) HUP.

Healthy Breasts: Every Woman's Birthright! Iris A. Michael. 1991. (Illus.). 151p. (Orig.). pap. text 16.95 (*0-9627883-0-9*) Clarke Pub.

Healthy Cat, Happy Cat: A Complete Guide to Cat Diseases & Their Treatment. Ulrike Muller et al. Tr. by Kranke Katze. 1995. LC 95-9792. (ENG & GER., Illus.). 128p. pap. 8.95 (*0-8120-9136-1*) Barron.

Healthy Child. Edelstein. Date not set. tchr. ed. (*0-314-04881-2*) West Pub.

Healthy Child: His Physical, Psychological, & Social Development. Ed. by Harold C. Stuart & Dane G. Prugh. 1960. LC 60-8004. 523p. 51.95 (*0-674-38600-0*) HUP.

Healthy Children—Toxic Environments: Acting on the Unique Vulnerability of Children Who Dwell Near Hazardous Waste Sites. Ed. by Theresa Ramsey. 1998. 39p. pap. text 15.00 (*0-7881-7534-3*) DIANE Pub.

Healthy Children 2000. U. S. Department of Health & Human Services Staff. 1992. (Health Science Ser.). (Illus.). 232p. (C). pap. text 36.95 (*0-86720-756-6*, 756-6) Jones & Bartlett.

Healthy Children 2010: Establishing Preventive Services. Roger P. Weissberg et al. Ed. by Gerald A. Adams. 1997. LC 97-4687. (Issues in Children's & Families' Lives Ser.: Vol. 9). 300p. 86.95 (*0-7619-1089-1*, 81593) Sage.

Healthy Cities. Ed. by John Ashton. 1991. 192p. pap. (*0-335-09476-7*) OpUniv Pr.

Healthy Communities Two Thousand: Model Standards. APHA Project Task Force Staff. 3rd ed. 1991. 470p. 35.00 (*0-87553-204-7*) Am Pub Health.

Healthy Decisions. Clint E. Bruess & Glenn Richardson. 96p. (C). 1994. text, stu. ed. 10.00 (*0-697-25867-X*); 1993. (gr. 10-12). text, stu. ed. 19.20 net. (*0-697-17043-8*) Brown & Benchmark.

Healthy Decisions: Black & White Edition. Clint E. Bruess & Glenn Richardson. 1993. 432p. (C). pap. 30.31 (*0-697-21449-4*) McGrw-H Hghr Educ.

Healthy Dog, Happy Dog: A Complete Guide to Dog Diseases & Their Treatments. Uwe Streitferdt. 1994. 128p. pap. 9.95 (*0-8120-1842-7*) Barron.

Healthy Dying. Rob George & Peter Houghton. 1997. LC 96-48681. text (*1-85302-436-8*) Jessica Kingsley GBR. *Dist:* Taylor & Francis.

Healthy Eating. U. S. Department of Agriculture Staff. 1996. 160p. pap. 6.95 (*1-879582-26-0*) Platinum Pr.

Healthy Eating on a Renal Diet: A Cookbook for People with Kidney Disease. Renal Resource Center Staff. 1991. 183p. pap. 33.00 (*0-8036-9887-9*) Davis Co.

Healthy Eyes Without Glasses: Increasing the Strength of the Eyes & the Eye Muscles Without the Aid of Glasses. R. A. Richardson. 1996. reprint ed. pap. 16.00 (*0-7873-0715-7*) Hlth Research.

Healthy for Life. Williams. 1993. (Health Sciences Ser.). tchr. ed. 41.25 (*0-534-15499-9*) Brooks-Cole.

Healthy for Life: Brief Version. Brian K. Williams & Sharon M. Knight. 1995. LC 94-35242. (Psychology Ser.). 488p. mass mkt. 32.75 (*0-534-24354-1*) Brooks-Cole.

Healthy for Life: Health & the Art of Living. Brian Williams & Sharon M. Knight. 1993. (C). mass mkt. 44.75 (*0-534-15498-0*) Brooks-Cole.

Healthy for Life: Study Guide. Brain K. Williams & Sharon M. Knight. exp. ed. (Health Sciences Ser.). 1994. stu. ed. 15.50 (*0-534-15505-7*); 1994. stu. ed. 15.50 (*0-534-15506-5*); 1993. stu. ed. 15.50 (*0-534-15507-3*) Brooks-Cole.

Healthy Habits: Twenty Simple Things to Improve Your Health. Anne E. Frahm & David J. Frahm. 1993. LC 93-34570. 205p. pap. 14.00 (*0-89109-754-6*) Pinon Press.

Healthy Healing: A Guide to Self-Healing for Everyone. Linda R. Page. 10th rev. ed. 1997. (Illus.). 480p. pap. 28.95 (*1-884334-85-7*) Hlthy Healing.

Healthy Heart. Reader's Digest Editorial Staff. 2000. LC 99-54731. (Health & Healing the Natural Way Ser.). (*0-7621-0263-2*) RD Assn.

Healthy Heart Cafe: Forget Fat Forever. Frederica Jackson & John Jackson. 1996. 143p. 14.95 (*0-9651216-0-7*) Source Pubng.

Healthy Heart Handbook. Neal Pinckney. 1996. 306p. pap. 11.95 (*1-55874-384-7*, 3847) Health Comm.

Healthy Heart Handbook for Women. 1995. lib. bdg. 250.99 (*0-8490-6690-5*) Gordon Pr.

Healthy Heart Handbook for Women. Marian Sandmaier. 1993. (Illus.). 90p. (Orig.). pap. text 20.00 (*1-56806-422-5*) DIANE Pub.

Healthy Heart Sourcebook for Women: Consumer Health Information about Cardiac Issues Specific to Women. Ed. by Dawn D. Matthews. 2000. LC 00-21143. (Health Reference Ser.). (Illus.). xii, 336p. 48.00 (*0-7808-0329-9*) Omnigraphics Inc.

***Healthy High-Tech Body.** Garcia Oz & Sharyn Kohlberg. 2001. LC 2001-31961. 368p. 26.00 (*0-06-039408-0*, ReganBooks) HarperCollins Pubs.

Healthy Homes in a Toxic World: Preventing, Identifying & Eliminating Hidden Health Hazards in Your Home. Maury M. Breecher & Shirley M. Linde. 1992. LC 91-40600. 256p. pap. 14.95 (*0-471-54024-2*) Wiley.

Healthy House Answer Book: Answers to the 133 Most Commonly Asked Questions. John Bower & Lynn M. Bower. 1998. LC 97-94365. 192p. pap. 8.95 (*0-9637156-4-X*) Hlthy Hse.

Healthy House Catalog: National Directory of Indoor Pollution Resources, 1990 Edition. Ed. by Stuart Greenberg & Robert Staib. 1989. 208p. (Orig.). pap. 19.95 (*0-9624845-0-4*) Environ Hlth Watch & H C R Ctr.

Healthy Humor... Stat! Contrib. by Gene Machamer. 2000. LC 00-91671. (Illus.). 112p. pap. 7.00 (*0-9627369-7-X*) Carlisle Pr.

Healthy Immune System. 1996. lib. bdg. 251.95 (*0-8490-5889-9*) Gordon Pr.

Healthy Kids: State Initiatives to Improve Children's Health. Martha P. King. 1993. 58p. 15.00 (*1-55516-698-9*, 6634) Natl Conf State Legis.

Healthy Living Caroline M. Levchuck & Michele Ingber Drohan. 2000. LC 99-53258. (J). (*0-7876-3921-4*) Gale.

Healthy Living Contrib. by Caroline M. Levchuck & Michele Ingber Drohan. 2000. LC 99-53258. (J). (*0-7876-3920-6*) Gale.

Healthy Living. Eileen Murphy. 1992. (Skills for Caring Ser.). (Illus.). 40p. (Orig.). pap. text (*0-443-04529-1*) Church.

Healthy Living: An Active Approach to Wellness. Ed. by William M. Kane et al. 1985. (*0-672-61611-4*); pap. text (*0-672-61610-6*) Macmillan.

Healthy Living in Wisconsin. Susan J. Montgomery et al. 1988. (Orig.). pap. 12.95 (*0-929807-00-6*) Montgomery Media.

Healthy Living with Diabetes: A Behavioral & Cognitive Protocol for the Treatment of OCD. Margot J. Fromer. 1998. LC 97-95483. (Illus.). 251p. pap. 13.95 (*1-57224-112-8*) New Harbinger.

Healthy Markets? The New Competition in Medical Care. Mark A. Peterson. LC 98-29193. 464p. 1999. 64.95 (*0-8223-2236-6*); 1998. pap. 22.95 (*0-8223-2138-6*) Duke.

Healthy Medicine: Challenges Facing Australia's Health Services. Stephen R. Leeder. 2000. LC 99-487746. (Illus.). xv, 155p. pap. (*1-86508-054-3*) Allen & Unwin Pty AUS. *Dist:* Paul & Co Pubs.

Healthy Mind, Healthy Body: Five Hundred Easy Methods! Joy M. Johnson. 1993. LC 91-77996. (Illus.). 300p. (Orig.). 23.95 (*1-880782-78-2*); pap. 17.95 (*1-880782-77-4*) Spirit Dance.

Healthy Mind Healthy Body Handbook. David S. Sobel & Robert Ornstein. 2nd ed. 1996. 284p. pap. 14.95 (*1-57577-032-6*) DRx.

Healthy Moms & Healthy Babies: Your Role in the Prenatal Care Initiative. rev. ed. 1994. (Illus.). 65p. (Orig.). (C). pap. text 20.00 (*0-7881-0225-7*) DIANE Pub.

Healthy Mouth, Healthy Body: The Natural Dental Program for Total Wellness. Victor Zeines. 2000. LC 00-127486. (Illus.). 304p. pap. 15.00 (*1-57566-589-1*, Knsington) Kensgtn Pub Corp.

Healthy Nutrition: Preventing Nutrition-Related Diseases in Europe. James & Ferro-Luzzi. 1988. (WHO Regional Publications, European Ser.: No. 24). 150p. pap. text 20.00 (*92-890-1115-7*) World Health.

Healthy Parents, Better Babies: A Couple's Guide to Pre-Conception Health Care. Francesca Naish & Janette Roberts. 1999. LC 98-55113. Orig. Title: Natural Way to Better Babies. 396p. pap. 18.95 (*0-89594-955-5*) Crossing Pr.

Healthy People: The Surgeon General's Report on Health Promotion & Disease Prevention (1979) 1995. (Illus.). 177p. (C). reprint ed. pap. text 35.00 (*0-7881-2132-4*) DIANE Pub.

Healthy People for the Year 2000: National Health Promotion & Disease Prevention Objectives 1992. lib. bdg. 555.95 (*0-8490-5509-1*) Gordon Pr.

Healthy People 2000. U. S. Department of Health & Human Services Staff. 1991. (Illus.). 712p. text 59.95 (*0-86720-179-7*, 179-7) Jones & Bartlett.

Healthy People 2000: 1991 Summary. 1995. (Illus.). 153p. (Orig.). (C). pap. text 25.00 (*0-7881-2107-3*) DIANE Pub.

Healthy People 2000: Midcourse Review & 1995 Revisions. U. S. Department of Health and Human Services Staff. 1996. (Illus.). 304p. (C). pap. text 36.95 (*0-7637-0041-X*, 0041-X) Jones & Bartlett.

Healthy People 2000: National Health Promotion & Disease Prevention Objectives 1997. lib. bdg. 600.25 (*0-8490-6229-2*) Gordon Pr.

Healthy People 2000: National Health Promotion & Disease Prevention Objectives (1991) (Full Report) 1994. (Illus.). 692p. (Orig.). (C). reprint ed. pap. text 35.00 (*0-7881-1196-5*) DIANE Pub.

Healthy People 2000: Summary Report. U. S. Department of Health & Human Services Staff. 1991. (Illus.). 172p. (C). pap. text 36.95 (*0-86720-180-0*, 180-0) Jones & Bartlett.

Healthy People 2000 Review, (1994) 1998. (Illus.). 149p. reprint ed. pap. text 25.00 (*0-7881-3248-2*) DIANE Pub.

Healthy People 2000, Review, 1997: National Health Promotion & Disease Prevention. Kathleen M. Turczyn & Richard J. Klein. 5th ed. 1998. (Illus.). 223p. (C). pap. text 35.00 (*0-7881-7559-9*) DIANE Pub.

Healthy People 2000 Review, 1995-96: National Health Promotion & Disease Prevention Objectives. Kathleen M. Turczyn & Richard J. Klein. 1998. (Illus.). 208p. (C). reprint ed. pap. text 40.00 (*0-7881-3928-2*) DIANE Pub.

***Healthy People 2010** U. S. Department of Health & Human Services Staff. 2001. 1200p. pap. 49.50 (*1-58808-110-9*) Intl Med Pub.

Healthy People 2010 U. S. Department of Health & Human Services Staff. 2000. 1000p. 75.00 (*1-883205-75-1*) Intl Med Pub.

Healthy People, 2010: Conference Edition, Vol. I & II. Pref. by Donna E. Shalala. 2000. (Illus.). 1100p. (C). pap. text 60.00 (*0-7881-8923-9*) DIANE Pub.

***Healthy People 2010: Tracking Healthy People 2010.** Ed. by Diane K. Wagener & Richard J. Klein. 2001. 800p. pap. text 90.00 (*0-7567-1514-8*) DIANE Pub.

Healthy People 2010: Understanding & Improving Health. 2000. (Illus.). 63p. pap. text 25.00 (*0-7567-0008-6*) DIANE Pub.

***Healthy People 2010: Understanding & Improving Health.** 2000. 70p. pap. 10.00 (*0-16-050528-3*, Hlth & Human) USGPO.

Healthy Pregnancy. Deni Bown. 1997. (101 Essential Tips Ser.). (Illus.). 72p. pap. 4.95 (*0-7894-1078-8*) DK Pub Inc.

Healthy Pregnancy. Miriam Stoppard. 1998. LC 97-48455. (DK Healthcare Ser.). (Illus.). 80p. pap. 7.95 (*0-7894-3089-4*) DK Pub Inc.

Healthy Pregnancy-Healthy Baby. American Red Cross Staff. 1995. 208p. pap. text, wbk. ed. 8.75 (*0-86536-196-7*) Mosby Inc.

Healthy Prostate Program: A Doctor's Guide to Prevention & Treatment of Prostate Problems. Arnold Fox & Barry Fox. 1996. LC 95-24189. 256p. pap. 14.95 (*0-471-11982-2*) Wiley.

Healthy Public Policy at the Local Level. Ed. by Adalbert Evers et al. 1990. 242p. (C). pap. text 33.50 (*0-8133-7957-1*) Westview.

Healthy Respect: Ethics in Health Care. R. S. Downie & Kenneth C. Calman. 2nd ed. 1994. 310p. (Orig.). pap. text 31.95 (*0-19-262408-3*) OUP.

Healthy Rhode Islanders 2000. Barbara A. DeBuono. 1995. (Illus.). 77p. (Orig.). (C). pap. text 30.00 (*0-7881-1560-X*) DIANE Pub.

Healthy Runner's Handbook. Lyle J. Micheli & Mark Jenkins. 1996. LC 95-26222. (Illus.). 264p. pap. 16.95 (*0-88011-524-6*, PMIC0524) Human Kinetics.

Healthy Senior Workbook: Your Personal Health Management Planner. Ed. by Barbara Lambesis. 1991. 160p. pap. 11.95 (*0-9624798-1-0*) Mktg Methods Pr.

Healthy Start Initiative Vol. III: A Community Driven Approach to Infant Mortality Reduction. Thurma McCann et al. 1995. LC 95-72697. 120p. pap. (*1-57285-024-8*) Nat Ctr Educ.

Healthy Steps Interactive Multimedia Training & Resource Kit User Manual. Toby Kleban Levine. Ed. by Kelley McDonald & Joan Seidman Welsh. 2000. (Illus.). 48p. pap. (*1-930783-11-6*) Independ Prod.

Healthy Teens: Success in High School & Beyond. Alice R. McCarthy. Ed. by James McCarthy et al. 2nd rev. ed. 1997. LC 97-213198. 130p. (Orig.). pap. 5.95 (*0-9621645-4-2*, HT-2D) Bridge Commns Inc.

Healthy Ten: Reference Guide for Gymnasts & Other Athletes. Jack E. Jensen et al. 1992. (Illus.). 185p. (Orig.). pap. 16.95 (*0-9633870-8-1*) J E Jensen.

Healthy Water. Martin Fox. rev. ed. 1998. 32p. pap. 4.95 (*0-9617432-3-9*) Health Water Res.

Healthy, Wealthy & Wise: Fundamentals of Workplace Health Promotion. Ed. by Sandra Wendel. 3rd ed. 1993. (Illus.). 288p. stu. ed. 95.00 (*0-9628334-2-8*) WELCOA.

Healthy, Wealthy, or Wise? Issues in American Health Care Policy. Charles T. Stewart, Jr. 1995. LC 95-6892. (Illus.). 270p. (C). (gr. 13). 86.95 (*1-56324-504-3*); pap. 39.95 (*1-56324-505-1*) M E Sharpe.

Healthy Weigh: A Practical Food Guide. Maureen Callahan. 1991. 33p. pap. text 6.25 (*0-88091-085-2*, 0808) Am Dietetic Assn.

Healthy Weight Loss. Miriam Stoppard. 1999. LC 98-25876. (DK Healthcare Ser.). (Illus.). 96p. pap. 7.95 (*0-7894-3757-0*) DK Pub Inc.

Healthy Woman: Menopause & Other Things We Don't Talk About. Susan Davis. 1996. LC 96-6777. 160p. pap. 13.95 (*0-87630-806-X*) Brunner-Routledge.

Healthy Women, Healthy Lives, Set. Lucia Beck Weiss & Sandra P. Levison. Ed. by Ana E. Nunez. 2000. (C). text, tchr. ed. 375.00 (*0-9658774-1-8*) MCP Hahn Schl.

Healthy Women, Healthy Lives: A Guide to Preventing Disease from the Landmark Nurses' Health Study. Ed. by Susan E. Hankinson et al. 2001. LC 2001-34154. (Illus.). xxviii, 416p. 26.00 (*0-684-85519-4*) Free Pr.

Healthy Work: Stress, Productivity, & the Reconstruction of Working Life. Robert A. Karasek & Torres Theorell. 1992. LC 89-42514. 381p. pap. 18.00 (*0-465-02897-7*) Basic.

Healthy Worker - Healthy Workplace: The Productivity Connection. Phillip L. Polakoff & Paul F. O'Rourke. 1994. (Illus.). 65p. (Orig.). (C). pap. text 25.00 (*0-7881-0348-2*) DIANE Pub.

***Healthy Young Child.** Houghton. 2001. 342p. (C). 41.00 (*0-536-63572-2*) Pearson Custom.

HealthyLife Self-Care Guide. American Institute for Preventive Medicine Staff & Don R. Powell. 1997. 96p. pap. 4.95 (*0-9635612-2-7*) Am Inst Prevent.

Hear: A Four-Letter Word. Ciwa Griffiths. 1992. 263p. pap. 12.95 (*0-9630709-0-8*) Wide Range.

Hear Well Again: A Step by Step Program to Better Hearing. Michael F. Craine. 1994. 144p. (Orig.). pap. 19.00 (*1-880365-76-6*) Prof Pr NC.

Hearcare: An Instructional Guide for Long Term Care Facilities on Developing Policies & Procedures. Metro Deaf Senior Citizens, Inc. Staff et al. 1985. 112p. 47.50 (*0-9613623-1-6*) Metro Deaf Senior.

Hearing. Robert M. Ogden. 1977. LC 75-124248. (Select Bibliographies Reprint Ser.). 33.95 (*0-8369-5137-9*) Ayer.

Hearing: An Introduction to Psychological & Physiologic Acoustics. Stanley A. Gelfand. 3rd ed. 1998. LC 97-44121. (Illus.). 496p. text 75.00 (*0-8247-0143-7*) Dekker.

Hearing: Its Function & Dysfunction. E. D. Schubert. 1980. (Disorders of Human Communication Ser.: Vol. 1). (Illus.). 200p. 39.00 (*0-387-81579-1*) Spr-Verlag.

Hearing: Its Psychology & Physiology. Stanley S. Stevens & Hallowell Davis. 1983. LC 88-371701. 512p. pap. 26.00 (*0-88318-426-5*) Acoustical Soc Am.

Hearing: Physiological Acoustics, Neural Coding, & Psychoacoustics. W. Lawrence Gulick et al. 2nd ed. 1989. (Illus.). 430p. (C). text 62.95 (*0-19-504307-3*) OUP.

Hearing - The Brain & Auditory Communication in Marsupials. Lindsay Aitkin. 1998. LC 97-36128. (Zoophysiology & Ecology Ser.: Vol. 36). (Illus.). 128p. 109.00 (*3-540-62946-7*) Spr-Verlag.

Hearing Abyss: A National Epidemic. William P. Stearns. 1985. LC 85-70510. (Illus.). 43p. (Orig.). pap. 5.00 (*0-9614656-0-3*) Clinical Hearing Consults.

Hearing Aid Dispensing for Audiologists: A Guide for Clinical Service. Ed. by Angela M. Loavenbruck & Jane R. Madell. 1980. (Illus.). 203p. text 28.00 (*0-8089-1323-9*, 792581, Grune & Strat) Harcrt Hlth Sci Grp.

Hearing-Aid Handbook: Clinician's Guide to Client Orientation. Donna S. Wayner. 1990. LC 90-3010. (Illus.). 206p. (Orig.). pap. text 34.95 (*0-930323-56-4*, Clerc Bks) Gallaudet Univ Pr.

Hearing-Aid Handbook: User's Guide for Adults. Donna S. Wayner. 1990. LC 90-3009. (Illus.). 56p. (Orig.). pap. text 7.95 (*0-930323-70-X*, Clerc Bks) Gallaudet Univ Pr.

Hearing-Aid Handbook: User's Guide for Children. Donna S. Wayner. 1990. LC 90-3017. (Illus.). 54p. (Orig.). pap. text 7.95 (*0-930323-73-4*, Clerc Bks) Gallaudet Univ Pr.

Hearing Aids. Maurice Miller. 1972. LC 72-190707. (Studies in Communicative Disorders). (C). pap. (*0-672-61284-4*, Bobbs) Macmillan.

Hearing Aids: A Manual for Clinicians. Robert A. Goldenberg. 1996. LC 96-23365. 320p. text 85.00 (*0-397-51687-8*) Lppncott W & W.

Hearing Aids: A User's Guide. Wayne J. Staab. 1991. LC 90-90428. (Illus.). 135p. pap. 15.00 (*1-881148-02-5*) W J Staab.

Hearing Aids: Standards, Options, & Limitations. Michael Valente. 1996. LC 95-32782. (Illus.). 416p. 49.00 (*0-86577-576-1*) Thieme Med Pubs.

Hearing Aids - Who Needs Them? What They Can Do for You, Where to Buy Them, How to Use Them. David P. Pascoe. Ed. by Muriel S. Pascoe. 1991. LC 90-86318. (Illus.). 176p. (Orig.). pap. 10.50 (*0-9628963-0-6*) Muriel S Pascoe.

Hearing & Hearing Impairment. Ed. by Larry J. Bradford & William G. Hardy. 1979. 672p. text 84.00 (*0-8089-1145-7*, 790652, Grune & Strat) Harcrt Hlth Sci Grp.

Hearing Assessment with the Acoustic Reflex. Ed. by Gerald R. Popelka. 1981. (Illus.). 168p. text 25.00 (*0-8089-1361-1*, 793342, Grune & Strat) Harcrt Hlth Sci Grp.

Hearing Care for the Older Adult: Audiologic Rehabilitation. Patricia B. Kricos et al. 1995. LC 95-1130. (Communication Disorders Ser.). (Illus.). 282p. text 54.99 (*0-7506-9531-5*) Buttrwrth-Heinemann.

Hearing Conservation Program. Mark M. Moran. 1992. (OSHA Written Compliance Programs Ser.: No. 15). (Illus.). 59p. ring bd. 169.00 (*1-890966-10-X*) SafetyCertified.

Hearing Conservation Programs: Practical Guidelines for Success. Julia D. Royster & Larry H. Royster. 1990. (Illus.). 136p. 85.00 (*0-87371-307-9*, L307) Lewis Pubs.

Hearing Examiner. Jack Rudman. 1994. (Career Examination Ser.: C-351). pap. 34.95 (*0-8373-0351-6*) Nat Learn.

Hearing for the Speech Language Pathologist & the Healthcare Professional. Lida G. Wall. 1995. LC 95-15261. (Communication Disorders Ser.). (Illus.). 456p. text 54.99 (*0-7506-9526-9*) Buttrwrth-Heinemann.

***Hearing Healthcare Practitioner's Handbook: A Guide to the Successful Treatment of Hearing Loss with Auditory Prosthetics.** Paul Popp & Gregg Hackett. 2002. LC 2001-96996. 256p. 75.00 (*0-9715385-0-6*) N Amricn Inst Audtry.

Hearing Impaired Child in School. Ed. by Raymond H. Hull & Karen L. Dilka. 1984. 208p. text 36.50 (*0-8089-1663-7*, 792081, Grune & Strat) Harcrt Hlth Sci Grp.

Hearing-Impaired Children in the Mainstream. Ed. by Mark Ross. 1990. LC 90-71342. (Illus.). 336p. (Orig.). (C). pap. text 31.50 (*0-912752-22-X*) York Pr.

Hearing Impairment. John Bamford & Elaine Saunders. 2nd ed. 1991. (Illus.). 304p. (C). pap. text 41.50 (*1-879105-07-1*, A007) Thomson Learn.

Hearing Impairment & Language Disorders: Assessment & Intervention. Ed. by Katharine G. Butler. 2000. LC 93-31105. 244p. pap. 44.00 (*0-8342-0588-2*) PRO-ED.

Hearing Impairment & the Labyrinthine Perilymphatic System. E. Miriszlai. 1983. 134p. (C). 30.00 (*963-05-3153-4*) St Mut.

Hearing in Aging. Raymond H. Hull. 1995. (Illus.). 302p. (C). pap. text 47.95 (*1-56593-385-0*, 0753) Thomson Learn.

Hearing in Children. Jerry L. Northern & Marion P. Downs. 4th ed. 1991. (Illus.). 432p. 58.00 (*0-683-06574-2*) Lppncott W & W.

Hearing in Children. Jerry Northern. 5th ed. 2001. LC 2001-38193. 450p. text 60.00 (*0-683-30764-9*) Lppncott W & W.

Hearing Loss. William L. Meyerhoff & Peter Roland. 1996. (Illus.). 288p. text 69.00 (*0-86577-623-7*) Thieme Med Pubs.

Hearing Loss. Robert Thayer Sataloff. 3rd ed. 1993. (Illus.). 544p. text 95.00 (*0-8247-9041-3*) Dekker.

Hearing Loss: Questions You Have...Answers You Need. Jennifer Hay. 1994. LC 94-30069. (Illus.). 192p. (Orig.). pap. 10.95 (*1-882606-15-9*) Peoples Med Soc.

Hearing of School Children. A. Ciocco. 1941. (SRCD M Ser.: Vol. 6, No. 3). pap. 25.00 (*0-527-01519-9*) Periodicals Srv.

Hearing on Prostate Cancer : The Silent Killer: Hearing Before the Special Committee on Aging, United States Senate, One Hundred Fifth Congress, First Session, Washington, DC, September 23, 1997. U. S. Government Staff. 1997. LC 98-133158. (S. Hrg. Ser.). iii, 66 p. (*0-16-055990-1*) USGPO.

Hearing Science & Hearing Disorders. Ed. by M. E. Lutman & M. P. Haggard. 1983. text 99.95 (*0-12-460440-4*) Acad Pr.

Hearing the Internal Trauma: Working with Children & Adolescents Who Have Been Sexually Abused. Sandra Wieland. 1996. LC 96-10127. (Interpersonal Violence Ser.: Vol. 17). 216p. pap. 31.95 (*0-7619-0366-6*, 2604); (Illus.). 79.95 (*0-7619-0365-8*, 2603) Sage.

Hearing Therapy for Children. Alice Streng et al. 2nd rev. ed. 1958. LC 58-11706. (Illus.). 360p. text 52.50 (*0-8089-0489-2*, 794410, Grune & Strat) Harcrt Hlth Sci Grp.

Heart see Hurst's the Heart: Update 1

Heart, Vol. 2. Ed. by W. E. Adam. 1993. (Handbook of Nuclear Medicine Ser.). 466p. 315.00 (*1-56081-301-6*, Wiley-VCH) Wiley.

Heart: Fundamentals of Electrocardiography, Exercise Physiology, & Exercise Stress Testing. David R. Adamovich. 1984. LC 83-50971. (Illus.). 414p. (Orig.). pap. 35.00 (*0-914363-00-X*) Sports Med Bks Inc.

Heart: Physiology & Metabolism. Lionel H. Opie. 2nd ed. 1991. (Illus.). 528p. 89.50 (*0-88167-751-5*) Lppncott W & W.

Heart: Physiology, from Cell to Circulation. Lionel H. Opie. 3rd ed. 1998. LC 97-41380. (Illus.). 656p. text 99.00 (*0-7817-1560-1*) Lppncott W & W.

***Heart Section 2.** Ed. by Ernest Page et al. 2001. (Handbook of Physiology Ser.). (Illus.). 832p. text 195.00 (*0-19-509886-2*) OUP.

Heart-Aches: Heart Disease & the Psychology of the Broken Heart. Rudiger Dahlke. 1996. LC 95-48174. (Illus.). 320p. (Orig.). pap. 14.50 (*1-885394-14-4*) Bluestar Communs.

Heart & Essence of Dan-xi's Methods of Treatment: A Translation of Zhu Dan-xi's Dan Xi Zhi Fa Xin Yao. Zhu Dan-xi. Ed. by Bob Flaws. Tr. & Intro. by Yang Shou-zhong. 1993. LC 93-72799. 450p. pap. text 29.95 (*0-936185-50-3*) Blue Poppy Pr.

Heart & Exercise: A Practical Guide for the Clinician. Ed. by Randal J. Thomas. 1996. LC 95-32008. (Illus.). 160p. pap. 29.95 (*0-89640-302-5*) Igaku-Shoin.

Heart & Heart-Lung Transplantation. Fritz Baumgartner & Reitz. 1989. (Illus.). 442p. text 210.00 (*0-7216-2101-5*) Saunders.

Heart & Heart-Lung Transplantation. John Wallwork. 1989. text 170.00 (*0-7216-2787-0*) Saunders.

Heart & Heart-Lung Transplantation. William Baumgartner et al. 2nd ed. Date not set. LC 2001-42969. 575p. text (*0-7216-7363-5*) Saunders.

Heart & Its Action: Roentgenkymographic Studies. Gilbert H. Alexander. 1971. LC 78-96979. (Illus.). 272p. 32.50 (*0-87527-001-8*) Green.

Heart & Lung in Obesity. Martin A. Alpert & James K. Alexander. 1998. LC 97-30470. (Illus.). 264p. 81.00 (*0-87993-685-1*) Futura Pub.

Heart & Mind: The Practice of Cardiac Psychology, A1412. Ed. by Robert Allan & Stephen Scheidt. 1996. LC 96-10543. 510p. 49.95 (*1-55798-356-9*) Am Psychol.

Heart & Soul: The Therapeutic Face of Philosophy. Chris Mace. 1999. LC 98-34501. 85.00 (*0-415-17000-1*); xiv, 286 p. pap. 29.95 (*0-415-17001-X*) Routledge.

Heart Attack. Edward J. Speedling. 1982. 177p. pap. (*0-422-77800-1*, NO. 3687) Tavistock GBR. *Dist:* Routldge.

***Heart Attack: Advice for Patients by Patients.** Kathleen Berra et al. 2001. LC 2001-33256. 224p. 30.00 (*0-300-08980-5*); pap. 14.95 (*0-300-09190-7*) Yale U Pr.

Heart Attack: Bouncing Back. Julia A. Purcell et al. 1997. LC 96-50006. (Illus.). 48p. (Orig.). pap. 5.75 (*0-939838-45-1*) Pritchett & Hull.

Heart Attack: What's Ahead? Julia A. Purcell et al. Ed. by Nancy R. Hull. rev. ed. 1993. LC 80-25793. (Illus.). 64p. reprint ed. pap. text 9.95 (*0-939838-02-8*) Pritchett & Hull.

Heart Attack Prevention: Lowering Your Risk for Heart Disease: A Special Report from the Editors of Heart Advisor. Holly Strawbridge. Ed. by Dennis L. Sprecher & Jean Rothman. 2000. 50p. pap. 24.95 (*1-929942-05-2*) Torstar.

Heart Attack Recovery Book: A Look at the Emotional & Practical Problems Encountered During Rehabilitation, for Patients & Their Families. Elizabeth W. McCormick. 1991. pap. 9.95 (*0-904575-37-3*) Sigo Pr.

Heart Attack Recovery Handbook. Harvey Wolinsky & Gary Ferguson. 1988. 128p. (Orig.). pap. 6.95 (*0-446-38582-4*) Warner Bks.

Heart Attacks. Tom Smith. 2000. pap. (*0-85969-737-1*) Sheldon Pr GBR. *Dist:* Intl Pubs Mktg.

Heart Attacks & Rehabilitation: Index of New Information. Pearline A. Dignan. 1994. 150p. 57.50 (*0-7883-0042-3*); pap. 47.50 (*0-7883-0043-1*) ABBE Pubs Assn.

Heart Attacks-Real, Imagined & Suspicious: Index of New Information. Pearline A. Dignan. 1994. 150p. 57.50 (*0-7883-0040-7*); pap. 47.50 (*0-7883-0041-5*) ABBE Pubs Assn.

Heart-Brain Interactions. Ed. by Giuseppe Di Pasquale & Giuseppe Pinelli. 1992. LC 92-2301. (Illus.). xiii, 228p. (*3-540-54052-0*) Spr-Verlag.

Heart Cell Communication in Health & Disease. Ed. by Walmor C. De Mello & Michael J. Janse. 1998. LC 97-40862. (Developments in Cardiovascular Medicine Ser.). 312p. text 153.00 (*0-7923-8052-5*) Kluwer Academic.

Heart Cell in Culture, Vol. I. Arie Pinson. 1987. 208p. 117.00 (*0-8493-4697-5*, CRC Reprint) Franklin.

Heart Defects in Children: What Every Parent Should Know. Cheryl Wild. 1998. 160p. pap. 14.95 (*0-471-34735-3*); LC 98-230648. (Illus.). pap. 14.95 (*1-56561-166-7*) Wiley.

Heart Development. Ed. by Richard P. Harvey & Nadio Rosenthal. 1998. LC 98-86437. (Illus.). 530p. (C). 159.95 (*0-12-329860-1*) Acad Pr.

Heart Disease. 1996. lib. bdg. 250.75 (*0-8490-5888-0*) Gordon Pr.

Heart Disease. Eugene Braunwald. 1989. pap. text (*0-7216-2803-6*) Saunders.

Heart Disease. Douglas Wetherill et al. 2000. LC 00-699792. (What You Should Know Ser.). (Illus.). viii, 136p. pap. 6.99 (*1-55870-550-3*, Betrwy Bks) F & W Pubns Inc.

Heart Disease Eugene Braunwald et al. 2nd ed. 2000. LC 00-25391. (Illus.). xx, 2297p. text 165.00 (*0-7216-8561-7*) Saunders.

***Heart Disease.** Douglas L. Wetherill & Dean J. Kereiakes. 2nd ed. 2001. (What You Should Know Ser.). (Illus.). 136p. pap. 8.99 (*0-632-04529-9*) Blackwell Sci.

Heart Disease: A Textbook of Cardiovascular Medicine. Ed. by Eugene Braunwald. 5th ed. 1996. LC 95-24767. text 130.00 (*0-7216-5666-8*);Set. text 145.00 (*0-7216-5663-3*) Saunders.

Heart Disease Vol. 1: A Textbook of Cardiovascular Medicine, Vol. 1. Ed. by Eugene Braunwald. 5th ed. 1996. LC 95-24767. (*0-7216-5664-1*) Saunders.

Heart Disease Vol. 2: A Textbook of Cardiovascular Medicine, Vol. 2. Ed. by Eugene Braunwald. 5th ed. 1996. LC 95-24767. (*0-7216-5665-X*) Saunders.

Heart Disease & Rehabilitation. Ed. by Michael L. Pollock & Donald H. Schmidt. 3rd ed. 1994. LC 94-12879. 488p. text 65.00 (*0-87322-588-0*, BPOL0588) Human Kinetics.

Heart Disease Breakthrough: What Even Your Doctor Doesn't Know about Preventing a Heart Attack. Thomas A. Yannios. 1999. LC 98-38925. (Illus.). 256p. 24.95 (*0-471-25533-5*) Wiley.

Heart Disease Diagnosis & Therapy: A Practical Approach. M. Gabriel Khan et al. 1996. LC 95-48872. (Illus.). 680p. pap. 49.95 (*0-683-04614-4*) Lppncott W & W.

Heart Disease, Environment, Stress & Gender. 90.00 (*1-58603-082-5*) IOS Press.

Heart Disease in Pregnancy. Ed. by Celia Oakley. 1996. 442p. text (*0-7279-1065-5*, 340300360) BMJ Pub GBR. *Dist:* AIDC.

Heart Disease in Primary Care. Michael L. Hess & Andrea Hastillo. 1998. LC 98-3520. (Primary Care Ser.). 400p. pap. 44.95 (*0-683-03988-1*) Lppncott W & W.

Heart Disease in the Adolescent. Ed. by H. M. Sondheimer. 1987. (Journal: Vol. 13, No. 4, 1986). (Illus.). iv, 80p. pap. 49.75 (*3-8055-4572-X*) S Karger.

Heart Disease in Women. Wilansky. 1998. text (*0-443-07546-8*) Church.

Heart Disease Prevention: Everything You Need to Know about Heart Disease. Richard Harkness. 2000. LC 98-53498. (Natural Pharmacist Ser.). 208p. pap. 6.99 (*0-7615-1731-6*) Prima Pub.

Heart Disease Sourcebook. Roger Cicala. 1997. LC 97-38624. 336p. reprint ed. 25.00 (*1-56565-635-0*, 06350W, Anodyne) Lowell Hse.

Heart Disease Sourcebook: A Complete Guide from Preconception to Postdelivery. Roger Cicala. 1998. LC 97-38624. (Illus.). 336p. reprint ed. pap. 18.00 (*0-7373-0020-5*, 00205W) NTC Contemp Pub Co.

Heart Diseases & Disorders Sourcebook: Basic Consumer Health Information about Heart Attacks, Angina, Rhythm Disorders, Heart Failure & More. Ed. by Karen Bellenir. 2nd ed. 1999. LC 99-58043. (Health Reference Ser.). (Illus.). xiii, 612p. lib. bdg. 78.00 (*0-7808-0238-1*) Omnigraphics Inc.

Heart Dysfunction in Diabetes. Grant N. Pierce et al. 1988. 256p. 146.00 (*0-8493-6887-1*, RC682, CRC Reprint) Franklin.

Heart Failure. Horacio J. Androgue & Donald E. Wesson. 1994. (Basics in Medicine Ser.). 320p. pap. 24.95 (*0-86542-429-2*) Blackwell Sci.

Heart Failure. Ed. by R. Shabetai. 1989. (Journal: Vol. 76, No. 5, 1989). (Illus.). 80p. pap. 48.75 (*3-8055-5110-X*) S Karger.

Heart Failure. Springhouse Publishing Company Staff. 1999. LC 99-25002. (Incredibly Easy Miniguide Ser.). (Illus.). viii, 144p. pap. 18.95 (*1-58255-011-5*) Springhouse Corp.

Heart Failure. Adam D. Timmis & Simon W. Davies. 1992. LC 92-1543. (Pocket Picture Guides Ser.). (*1-56375-581-5*) Gower-Mosby.

Heart Failure: A Guide for Patients. Harvey Kemp. Ed. by Elliott Rapaport. 1996. (Cardiology Ser.). (Illus.). 32p. (Orig.). pap. 2.95 (*1-885274-40-8*) Health InfoNet Inc.

Heart Failure: Basic Science & Clinical Aspects. Ed. by Judith K. Gwathmey et al. 1993. LC 93-15908. (Fundamental & Clinical Cardiology Ser.: Vol. 15). (Illus.). 744p. text 255.00 (*0-8247-8772-2*) Dekker.

Heart Failure: Cardiac Function & Dysfunction. Wilson Colucci. 1995. LC 94-41113. (Atlas of Heart Diseases Ser.: No. 4). (Illus.). 272p. text 134.00 (*1-878132-27-X*) Current Med.

Heart Failure: Evaluation & Care of Patients with Left-Ventricular Systolic Dysfunction. 1997. lib. bdg. 252.95 (*0-8490-8149-1*) Gordon Pr.

Heart Failure: Evaluation & Care of Patients with Left-Ventricular Systolic Dysfunction - Commentary on the Agency for Health Care Policy & Research Clinical Practice Guidelines. Edward K. Kasper. 1996. LC 96-9561. 200p. pap. (*0-412-11261-2*) E A GBR. *Dist:* OUP.

Heart Failure: Frontiers in Cardiology. Akira Kitabatake et al. 2000. LC 00-21752. (Illus.). 300p. 109.00 (*4-431-70239-3*) Spr-Verlag.

Heart Failure: Management of Patients with Left Ventricular Systolic Dysfunction. 1995. lib. bdg. 605.75 (*0-8490-6705-7*) Gordon Pr.

Heart Failure: Management of Patients with Left-Ventricular Systolic Dysfunction. 1995. lib. bdg. 251.95 (*0-8490-6849-5*) Gordon Pr.

Heart Failure: Scientific Principles & Clinical Practice. Philip A. Poole-Wilson. 1996. LC 96-46029. text (*0-443-07501-8*) Church.

Heart Failure: The Promise & Practice of Dopaminergic Agonists. Ed. by S. H. Taylor et al. 1991. (Illus.). iv, 42p. pap. 21.00 (*3-8055-5384-6*) S Karger.

Heart Failure in Clinical Practice. John J. McMurray & John G. Cleland. 1996. 318p. (*1-85317-225-1*) Martin Dunitz GBR. *Dist:* Mosby Inc.

***Heart Failure in Practice.** Gregory Y. H. Lip et al. 2001. (In Practice Ser.). 76p. pap. (*1-85315-487-3*) Royal Soc of Medicine Pr Ltd GBR. *Dist:* Balogh.

Heart-Failure Mechanisms & Management. Ed. by B. S. Lewis & A. Kimchi. 1991. (Illus.). 480p. 125.00 (*0-387-53145-9*) Spr-Verlag.

Heart Failure Renin System. Gorlin. 50.00 (*0-7216-1949-5*) Harcourt.

Heart Failure Today. Ed. by Lionel H. Opie & F. Sabino. 1988. (Journal: Vol. 75, Suppl. 1, 1988). (Illus.). iv, 160p. pap. 48.75 (*3-8055-4929-6*) S Karger.

Heart Family Handbook: A Complete Guide for the Entire Family of Anyone with Any Heart Condition - To Help Make It the Speediest, Most Complete Recovery Possible. Jane Schoenberg & JoAnn Stichman. 1990. LC 89-81864. (Illus.). 232p. 16.95 (*0-932883-23-0*) Hanley & Belfus.

Heart Fitness for Life: The Essential Guide for Preventing & Reversing Heart Disease. Mary P. McGowan. 1999. (Illus.). 336p. pap. 13.95 (*0-19-512909-1*) OUP.

Heart Fitness for Life: The Essential Guide for Preventing & Reversing Heart Disease. Mary P. McGowan & J. McGowan Chopra. 1997. LC 97-29834. (Illus.). 336p. 25.00 (*0-19-511624-0*) OUP.

Heart Function & Metabolism. Ed. by Naranjan S. Dhalla et al. 1987. (Developments in Cardiovascular Medicine Ser.). text 186.00 (*0-89838-865-1*) Kluwer Academic.

Heart Function in Health & Disease: Proceedings of the Cardiovascular Program Sponsored by the Council of Cardiac Metabolism of the International Society & Federation of Cardiology During the Regional Meeting of the International Union of Physiological Sciences, Prague, Czechoslovakia, June 30 - July 5, 1991. Ed. by Bohuslav Ostadal & Naranjan S. Dhalla. 1993. LC 92-48911. (Developments in Cardiovascular Medicine Ser.: Vol. DICM 140). 352p. (C). text 172.50 (*0-7923-2052-2*) Kluwer Academic.

Heart Function Tests: Directory of Authors of New Medical & Scientific Reviews with Subject Index. Science and Life Consultants Association Staff. 1995. 160p. 57.50 (*0-7883-0586-7*); pap. 47.50 (*0-7883-0587-5*) ABBE Pubs Assn.

Heart Health: An American Yoga Association Guide. Alice Christensen. 2001. (Illus.). 144p. pap. 12.00 (*1-57566-662-6*, Twin Streams) Kensgtn Pub Corp.

Heart Health for Black Women: Simple Steps to Healing Your Health & Soul Naturally. Beverly Yates. 2000. LC 99-51304. (Illus.). 256p. pap. text 15.95 (*1-56261-428-2*) Marlowe & Co.

Heart Hypertrophy & Failure, Vol. 169. Ed. by Naranjan S. Dhalla et al. 1996. LC 95-23370. (Developments in Cardiovascular Medicine Ser.). 560p. (C). text 284.50 (*0-7923-3572-4*) Kluwer Academic.

Heart in Diabetes. Ed. by John C. Chatham et al. 1996. (Developments in Cardiovascular Medicine Ser.: Vol. 185). 272p. (C). text 140.50 (*0-7923-4052-3*) Kluwer Academic.

Heart in Distress. Dipak K. Das & New York Academy of Sciences Staff. 1999. LC 99-34749. (Annals of the New York Academy of Sciences Ser.: Vol. 874). (Illus.). x, 438p. (*1-57331-165-0*) NY Acad Sci.

Heart in End-Stage Renal Failure. Ed. by V. Wizemann et al. 1987. (Contributions to Nephrology Ser.: Vol. 52). (Illus.). viii, 150p. 29.75 (*3-8055-4358-1*) S Karger.

Heart in Hypertension: A Tribute to Robert Tarazi Developments in Cardiovascular Medicine. Ed. by Michel E. Safar & F. Fouad-Tarazi. 1990. (C). text 303.50 (*0-7923-0197-8*) Kluwer Academic.

Heart in Stress. Ed. by Dipak K. Das. 1999. LC 99-34749. (Annals of the New York Academy of Sciences Ser.: Vol. 874). (Illus.). x, 438p. text 140.00 (*1-57331-164-2*) NY Acad Sci.

Heart-Lung Interactions in Health & Disease. Cassidy. Ed. by Steven M. Scharf. 1989. (Lung Biology in Health & Disease Ser.: Vol. 42). (Illus.). 1168p. text 295.00 (*0-8247-7986-X*) Dekker.

Heart Lung Machine & Related Technologies of Open Heart Surgery. Jon W. Austin. Ed. by David L. Harner. 1985. (Illus.). 235p. (C). text (*0-938633-00-7*) Phoenix Medical.

Heart Monitor Training for the Complete Idiot. John L. Parker. 2nd ed. 1998. 212p. pap. 14.95 (*0-915297-25-6*) Cedarwinds.

Heart Muscle Disease. Ed. by J. F. Goodwin. 1985. (Current Status of Clinical Cardiology Ser.). text 171.50 (*0-85200-722-1*) Kluwer Academic.

Heart of a Child: What Families Need to Know about Heart Disease in Children. Catherine A. Neill et al. 2nd ed. 2001. LC 00-48797. (Health Bks.). (Illus.). 352p. pap. 17.95 (*0-8018-6636-7*) Johns Hopkins.

Heart of a Child: What Families Need to Know about Heart Disorders in Children. Catherine A. Neill et al. 1992. 352p. 45.00 (*0-8018-4234-4*) Johns Hopkins.

Heart of Being Helpful: Empathy & the Creation of a Healing Presence. Peter Breggin. 1997. LC 97-2442. 200p. 42.95 (*0-8261-9680-2*) Springer Pub.

Heart of History: Individuality in Evolution. John W. Perry. 1987. LC 86-14428. (Series in Transpersonal & Humanistic Psychology). 249p. (C). pap. text 20.95 (*0-88706-400-0*) State U NY Pr.

Heart of Listening: A Visionary Approach to Craniosacral Work, Vol. I. Hugh Milne. 2nd ed. 1998. LC 98-15082. (Illus.). 240p. pap. text 25.00 (*1-55643-279-8*) North Atlantic.

Heart of Listening Vol. 2: Anatomy, Technique, Transcendence, Vol. II. Hugh Milne. 2nd ed. 1998. LC 98-15082. (Heart of Listening Ser.: Vol. II). (Illus.). 344p. (Orig.). pap. text 35.00 (*1-55643-280-1*) North Atlantic.

Heart of Long-Term Care. Rosalie A. Kane et al. 1998. LC 98-5831. (Illus.). 344p. text 39.95 (*0-19-512238-0*) OUP.

Heart of Psychotherapy. George Weinberg. 1996. LC 95-26018. 320p. pap. 12.95 (*0-312-14110-6*) St Martin.

Heart of the Matter: An African-American Guide to Heart Disease, Heart Treatment, & Heart Wellness. Hilton M. Hudson, II & Herbert J. Stern. 2000. LC 00-710680. (Illus.). ix, 299p. 24.95 (*0-9675258-0-2*) Hilton Pubg.

Heart of the Matter: The African American's Guide to Heart Disease, Heart Treatment & Heart Wellness. Hilton M. Hudson, II & Herbert Stern. 2001. (Illus.). 312p. pap. 16.95 (*0-9675258-3-7*) Hilton Pubg.

Heart of the Mind: Engaging Your Inner Power to Change with Neuro-Linguistic Programming. Steve Andreas & Connirae Andreas. 1989. 288p. 14.00 (*0-911226-30-3*); pap. 10.50 (*0-911226-31-1*) Real People.

Heart of Yoga: Developing a Personal Practice. T. K. Desikachar. rev. ed. 1999. LC 99-462597. (Illus.). 272p. 19.95 (*0-89281-764-X*, Heal Arts VT) Inner Tradit.

Heart Owner's Handbook: Live Longer & Feel Better. Texas Heart Institute Staff. 1995. LC 95-33694. 396p. pap. 16.95 (*0-471-04420-2*); (Illus.). 416p. 40.00 (*0-471-05982-X*) Wiley.

Heart Patient Recovers: Social & Psychological Factors. Sydney Croog & Sol Levine. 1977. LC 77-608112. 432p. 45.95 (*0-87705-247-6*, Kluwer Acad Hman Sci) Kluwer Academic.

Heart Physiology & Pathophysiology. Ed. by Nicholas Sperelakis et al. 4th ed. 2000. LC 00-106896. (Illus.). xxi, 1261p. 199.95 (*0-12-656975-4*) Acad Pr.

Heart Rate as a Determinant of Cardiac Function - Basic Mechanisms & Clinical Significance. Ed. by G. Hasenfuss & H. Just. 2000. 256p. (C). (*3-7985-1073-3*) D Steinkopff DEU. *Dist:* Spr-Verlag.

Heart Rate Variability. Ed. by Marek Malik & A. John Camm. 1995. LC 94-45665. (Illus.). 400p. 98.00 (*0-87993-607-X*) Futura Pub.

***Heart Replacement No. 7: Artificial Heart.** T. Akutsu & H. Koyanagi. 7th ed. 2001. (Illus.). 256p. (*1-901865-36-3*) Isis Med GBR. *Dist:* Bks Intl VA.

Heart Revolution: The B Vitamin Breakthrough That Lowers Homocysteine, Cuts Your Risk of Heart Disease & Protects Your Health. Kilmer S. McCully & Martha McCully. 2000. 234p. text 24.00 (*0-7881-6865-7*) DIANE Pub.

***Heart Sense for Women: Your Plan for Natural Prevention & Treatment.** Stephen T. Sinatra. 2001. 448p. pap. 15.00 (*0-452-28271-3*, Plume) Dutton Plume.

Heart Sense for Women: Your Plan for Natural Prevention & Treatment. Stephen Sinatra et al. 2000. LC 00-38063. 250p. 21.95 (*0-89526-285-1*, LifeLine Press) Regnery Pub.

Heart Smart. Becker. 1984. pap. 3.50 (*0-671-30924-2*) PB.

Heart Sounds: New Facts & Their Clinical Implications. Aldo A. Luisada & Francesco Portaluppi. 1982. LC 81-19240. 246p. 59.95 (*0-275-91372-4*, C1372, Praeger Pubs) Greenwood.

Heart Sounds & Murmurs: A Practical Guide. Barbara Erickson. 3rd ed. (Illus.). 152p. (C). (gr. 13). 1997. 46.95 incl. audio compact disk (*0-8151-3659-5*, 31279); 1996. LC 96-29333. pap. text 36.95 (*0-8151-3146-1*, 28261) Mosby Inc.

Heart Spirit: Transforming Work Stress. Will Masters. 1997. 25p. (Orig.). (C). pap. text (*1-886112-08-8*) Antares.

Heart Surgeon's Little Instruction Book. Daniel J. Waters. 1995. 145p. pap. text 10.00 (*0-942219-97-X*) Quality Med Pub.

Heart Surgery Trap: Why Most Invasive Procedures Are Unnecessary & How to Avoid Them. Julian M. Whitaker. 1992. 336p. 21.00 (*0-671-74333-3*) S&S Trade.

Heart Talk: Understanding Cardiovascular Diseases. Mark V. Barrow. 1992. (Illus.). 500p. (Orig.). pap. 30.00 (*0-9630510-0-8*) Cor-Ed Pub.

Heart Therapy: Regaining Your Cardiac Health. Anita Maximin et al. 1998. LC 97-75473. 272p. pap. 13.95 (*1-57224-104-7*) New Harbinger.

Heart to Heart: A Guide to the Psychological Aspects of Heart Disease. Herbert N. Budnick. 1995. (Illus.). 117p. reprint ed. pap. 8.95 (*0-929173-15-5*) Health Press.

Heart to Heart: A Holistic Approach to Heartcare. H. S. Wasir. 1990. 176p. text (*0-7069-4932-3*) Vikas IND. *Dist:* S Asia.

Heart Transplantation. Ed. by D. K. Cooper & R. P. Lanza. 1984. text 193.50 (*0-85200-862-7*) Kluwer Academic.

Heart Transplantation. Mudge. 2000. text 135.00 (*0-7216-7786-X*) Saunders.

Heart Trouble Encyclopedia. Henry J. L. Marriott & M. Gabriel Khan. 1996. LC 99-192855. 368p. pap. (*0-7737-5744-9*) Stoddart Publ CAN. *Dist:* General Distrib Services.

Heart Valve Surgery. Lawrence H. Patzelt & Nancy L. Berends. Ed. by Oliver D. Grin & Dorothy L. Bouwman. 1991. (Patient Education Ser.). (Illus.). 30p. (Orig.). pap. text 4.00 (*0-929689-42-9*) Ludann Co.

Heartbeat: A Complete Guide to Understanding & Preventing Heart Disease. Emmanuel Horovitz. 1988. LC 87-82715. (Illus.). 360p. (Orig.). pap. 14.95 (*0-9619329-6-1*) Health Trend.

Heartburn: Extinguishing the Fire Inside. Thomas J. Nesi & M. Michael Wolfe. 1997. LC 96-35815. 192p. pap. 12.95 (*0-393-31634-3*) Norton.

***Heartburn (Gastro-Esophageal Reflex, Acid Reflex) Index of New Information & Guide-Book for Consumers, Reference & Research.** Ed. by Research and Development Division Staff & John C. Bartone. 2001. 47.50 (*0-7883-2516-7*); pap. 44.50 (*0-7883-2517-5*) ABBE Pubs Assn.

Heartmates: A Guide for the Spouse & Family of the Heart Patient. Rhoda F. Levin. rev. ed. LC 87-11392. 1995. 368p. pap. 18.95 (*0-9637795-1-6*); 1998. audio 24.95 (*0-9637795-4-0*) MinervaPress.

Heartmates Meditation Journal: A Companion for Partners of People with Heart Disease. Rhoda F. Levin. 1995. 256p. (Orig.). otabind 15.00 (*0-9637795-2-4*) MinervaPress.

***Heartmath Solution: The Revolutionary Program for Engaging the Power of the Heart's Intelligence.** Doc Childre & Howard Martin. 2001. (Illus.). 281p. reprint ed. 24.00 (*0-7567-5105-5*) DIANE Pub.

HeartPower! A Teacher Resource Book. American Heart Association Staff. 1996. (HeartPower! American Heart Association Schoolsite Program Ser.). (Illus.). 104p. pap. (*0-87493-304-8*); 104p. pap. (*0-87493-306-4*); (SPA., 88p. pap. (*0-87493-308-0*) Am Heart.

Hearts & Arteries: What Scientists Are Learning about Age & the Cardiovascular System. Caroline McNeil. 1996. (Illus.). 35p. reprint ed. pap. text 15.00 (*0-7881-2838-8*) DIANE Pub.

Heart's Eye: Emotional Influences in Perception & Attention. Ed. by Paula M. Niedenthal & Shinobu Kitayama. 1994. LC 93-23395. (Illus.). 289p. text 65.00 (*0-12-410560-2*) Acad Pr.

Hearts Open Wide: Stories of Midwives & Births. Ed. by Pam Wellish & Susan Root. 1987. LC 86-32600. (Illus.). 224p. (Orig.). pap. 9.95 (*0-914728-54-7*) Wingbow Pr.

Heartsave AED for the Lay Rescuer & First Responder, Vol. 70-2006. Ed. by Tom P. Aufderheide et al. 1998. (Illus.). 104p. pap. text 10.00 (*0-87493-690-X*) Am Heart.

Heartsaver Facts. AHA, American Society for Healthcare Materials Management & NSC Staff. 1998. (Illus.). 104p. (C). pap. text, tchr. ed. 30.00 (*0-7637-0994-8*, 0994-8) Jones & Bartlett.

Heartsaver Guide. Subcommittee on Basic Life Support Staff. 1993. LC 98-203727. (Illus.). 78p. (Orig.). pap. text (*0-87493-614-4*) Am Heart.

Heartsaver Plus, 1997-99. 1997. (Emergency Cardiovascular Care Programs Ser.). (Illus.). 84p. pap. 5.00 (*0-87493-631-4*) Am Heart.

Heartsearch: Toward Healing Lupus. Donna H. Talman. 1990. LC 90-21860. 260p. (Orig.). pap. 12.95 (*1-55643-072-8*) North Atlantic.

Heat Shock. Ed. by Bruno Maresca & S. Lindquist. 1991. (Illus.). 320p. 110.00 (*0-387-54111-X*) Spr-Verlag.

Heat Shock & Development. Ed. by W. Hennig et al. 1991. (Results & Problems in Cell Differentiation Ser.: Vol. 17). (Illus.). 229p. 208.00 (*0-387-53119-X*) Spr-Verlag.

Heat Shock in Organ Preservation. George Perdrizet. 1997. (Medical Intelligence Unit Ser.). 200p. (C). pap. 89.95 (*0-412-10831-3*) Chapman & Hall.

Heat Shock Proteins & Gamma-Delta T Cells. Ed. by C. F. Brosnan. 1992. (Chemical Immunology Ser.: Vol. 53). (Illus.). viii, 132p. 108.00 (*3-8055-5508-3*) S Karger.

Heat Shock Proteins & the Cardiovascular System. Ed. by A. A. Knowlton. 1997. LC 97-7938. 248p. text 142.00 (*0-7923-9910-2*) Kluwer Academic.

Heat Shock Proteins & the Ischemic Myocardial. Rakesh C. Kukreja & Michael L. Hess. 2000. (Medical Intelligence Unit Ser.). 184p. 99.00 (*1-58706-021-3*) Eurekah.

Heat Shock Proteins in the Nervous System. Ed. by R. John Mayer & I. R. Brown. 1994. (Neuroscience Perspectives Ser.). (Illus.). 297p. text 83.00 (*0-12-480960-X*) Acad Pr.

Heat Shock Response. Lutz Nover. 1991. (Illus.). 866p. lib. bdg. 259.00 (*0-8493-4912-5*, QP552) CRC Pr.

Heat Stress & Heat Disorders. 1984. 33p. pap. 6.95 (*0-939874-62-8*) ASSE.

Heat Transfer in Medicine & Biology: Analysis & Applications Ed. by Avraham Shitzer & Robert C. Eberhart. 1985. (Illus.). (C). Vol. 1. 454p. text 150.00 (*0-306-41597-6*); Vol. 2. 462p. text 150.00 (*0-306-41695-6*) Kluwer Academic (Kluwer Plenum).

Heave Ho! My Little Green Book of Seasickness. Charles Mazel. 1996. (Illus.). xii, 116p. reprint ed. pap. 9.95 (*0-9641887-1-6*) Bernel Bks.

Heavenly Hurts: Surviving AIDS-Related Deaths & Losses. Sandra J. Klein. 1997. LC 97-20522. (Death, Value & Meaning Ser.). 166p. text 32.95 (*0-89503-181-7*) Baywood Pub.

Heaven's Banquet: Vegetarian Cooking for Lifelong Health the Ayurveda Way. Miriam K. Hospodar. 1999. LC 98-41308. (Illus.). 600p. 39.95 (*0-525-94383-8*, Dutt) Dutton Plume.

Heavy Drinking: The Myth of Alcoholism As a Disease. Herbert Fingarette. 1988. 195p. pap. 15.95 (*0-520-06754-1*) U CA Pr.

Heavy Menstrual Flow & Anemia: Self Help Book. Susan M. Lark. 3rd rev. ed. 1996. LC 95-22254. 184p. text 16.95 (*0-89087-774-2*) Celestial Arts.

***Hedge's Pocket Guide to Treatment in Speech-Language Pathology.** M. N. Hedge & M. N. Hegde. 2nd ed. 2001. LC 00-49225. (Illus.). xii, 576p. pap. 49.95 (*0-7693-0159-2*) Singular Publishing.

Hegde's Pocketguide to Assessment in Speech-Language Pathology. M. N. Hegde. 2nd ed. 2001. LC 00-49225. (Illus.). 552p. pap. 49.95 (*0-7693-0158-4*) Singular Publishing.

Hegel & Whitehead: Contemporary Perspectives on Systematic Philosophy. Ed. by George R. Lucas, Jr. 1986. LC 85-9745. (SUNY Series in Hegelian Studies). 325p. (C). text 20.50 (*0-88706-144-3*) State U NY Pr.

Hegel's Theory of Madness. Daniel Berthold-Bond. 1995. LC 94-32809. (SUNY Series in Hegelian Studies). 309p. (C). text 21.50 (*0-7914-2505-3*) State U NY Pr.

Heidelberg External Fixation: Unilateral Fixation Techniques in Limb Deformity Corrections. Pfeil. 1998. pap. 75.00 (*0-86577-756-X*) Thieme Med Pubs.

Heider "Notebooks", Vol. Five: Attribution & Interpersonal Evaluation. 1989. 577p. 139.00 (*0-387-91299-1*) Spr-Verlag.

Heider "Notebooks", Vol. Four: Balance Theory. 1989. 436p. 199.00 (*0-387-91298-3*) Spr-Verlag.

Heider "Notebooks", Vol. Six: Units & Coinciding Units. 1990. 138.00 (*0-387-91300-9*) Spr-Verlag.

Heider "Notebooks", Vol. Three: Motivation. 1988. 152.00 (*0-387-91297-5*) Spr-Verlag.

Heider "Notebooks", Vol. Two: Perception. 1988. 152.00 (*0-387-91296-7*) Spr-Verlag.

Height, Health & History: Nutritional Status in the United Kingdom, 1750-1980. Roderick Floud et al. 1990. (Cambridge Studies in Population, Economy & Society in Past Time: No. 9). (Illus.). 378p. (C). text 95.00 (*0-521-30314-1*) Cambridge U Pr.

Heilen Durch die Sinne: Die-Cosmo-Therapie see Healing Through the Senses: Cosmo-Therapy

Heilverfahren Aller Krebsarten (The Cure for All Cancers) Mit Uber 100 Fallgeschichten Geheilter Personen. Hulda Regehr Clark. 3rd ed. 1993. (GER., Illus.). 589p. reprint ed. 19.95 (*1-890035-03-3*) New Century Pr.

Heinemann Modern Dictionary for Dental Students. Jennifer Fowler. 1973. (ENG & FRE.). 184p. 29.95 (*0-8288-6299-0*, M-6257) Fr & Eur.

Heinemann New Family Medical Encyclopedia. Paul Paxton et al. 1984. (Illus.). 304p. 32.95 (*0-434-65410-8*) Trafalgar.

Heinerman's Encyclopedia of Anti-Aging Remedies. John Heinerman. 1996. LC 96-28173. 352p. (C). text 27.95 (*0-13-272816-8*) P-H.

Heinerman's Encyclopedia of Healing Herbs & Spices. John Heinerman. 1995. LC 95-34371. 516p. (C). pap. 13.95 (*0-13-310210-6*) PH Pr.

Heinerman's New Encyclopedia of Fruits & Vegetables. John Heinerman. rev. ed. 1995. LC 95-19016. 352p. pap. 15.00 (*0-13-209230-1*) PH Pr.

Heinrich Warner Stiftung: The Operable Renal Cell Carcinoma Progress in Basic Research Diagnosis, Surgical & Medical Therapy - European Urology Journal, Vol. 18, Suppl. 2. Ed. by H. Huland & H. Klosterhalfen. 1990. (Journal). (Illus.). vi, 58p. pap. 20.00 (*3-8055-5253-X*) S Karger.

Heinz Kohut: The Making of a Psychoanalyst. Charles B. Strozier. 2001. LC 00-45459. (Illus.). xiii, 495p. 35.00 (*0-374-16880-6*) FS&G.

Heinz Kohut & the Psychology of the Self. Allen M. Siegel. 1996. LC 96-7012. (Makers of Modern Psychotherapy Ser.). 240p. (C). pap. 26.95 (*0-415-08638-8*); (Illus.). 84.95 (*0-415-08637-X*) Routledge.

Heinz Werner, Eighteen Ninety to Nineteen Sixty-Four: Papers in Memoriam. Ed. by Seymour Wapner & Bernard Kaplan. 1966. LC 73-2147. (Monographs in Psychology & Related Disciplines: No. 3). 94p. pap. 6.00 (*0-914206-04-4*) Clark U Pr.

Held by an Angel's Wings: A Survival Guide for Women with Breast Cancer. Raeia Hinson. 1997. LC 95-81640. 208p. (Orig.). pap. 10.99 (*1-56384-114-2*, Vital Issue Pr) Huntington Hse.

Helene Deutsch: A Psychoanalyst's Life. Paul Roazen. 1985. 384p. 19.95 (*0-671-25028-0*) S&S Trade.

Helene Deutsch: A Psychoanalyst's Life. Paul Roazen. 1991. 384p. (C). pap. text 24.95 (*1-56000-552-1*) Transaction Pubs.

Helical & Incremental CT: Technical Manual. Ruedi F. Thoeni. 1998. 304p. (*0-89640-346-7*) Lppncott W & W.

Helical-Spiral CT: A Practical Approach. Robert K. Zeman et al. 1994. (Illus.). 332p. text 99.00 (*0-07-072653-1*) McGraw-Hill Med Pub.

Helicobacter in Ulcer Disease. 1994. lib. bdg. 272.95 (*0-8490-5788-4*) Gordon Pr.

***Helicobacter Infectio.** Ed. by M. J. G. Farthing & S. E. Patchett. 1998. (British Medical Bulletin Ser.: Vol. 54, No. 1). 263p. (*1-85315-342-7*) Royal Soc of Medicine Pr Ltd GBR. *Dist:* Balogh.

Helicobacter Pylori. J. J. Misiewicz & A. W. Harris. 1996. LC 96-42936. (Illus.). 66p. (Orig.). pap. 34.95 (*0-86542-639-2*) Blackwell Sci.

Helicobacter Pylori: Basic Mechanisms to Clinical Cure 1996, Proceedings. Ed. by Richard H. Hunt & Guido N. Tytgat. 1996. LC 96-42936. 419p. text 213.50 (*0-7923-8717-1*) Kluwer Academic.

Helicobacter Pylori: Basic Mechanisms to Clinical Cure, 1998. Ed. by R. H. Hunt & Guido N. Tytgat. 1998. LC 98-195920. 507p. 240.00 (*0-7923-8739-2*) Kluwer Academic.

Helicobacter Pylori: Basic Research to Clinical Cure. Ed. by R. H. Hunt & Guido N. Tytgat. 1994. LC 94-5793. 640p. (C). text 259.00 (*0-7923-8838-0*) Kluwer Academic.

Helicobacter Pylori: Biology & Clinical Practice. Ed. by C. Stewart Goodwin & Bryan W. Worsley. 1993. 480p. 249.00 (*0-8493-6451-5*, QR201) CRC Pr.

Helicobacter Pylori: Implications & Practice. Ed. by C. A. O'Morain & H. O'Connor. 1994. LC 94-66536. pap. 25.00 (*0-926592-14-9*) Normed Verlag.

***Helicobacter Pylori: Molecular & Cellular Biology.** Ed. by Mark Achtman & Sebastian Suerbaum. 2001. LC 2001-411778. (Illus.). 344p. (*1-898486-25-5*) Horizon Sci GBR. *Dist:* Intl Spec Bk, Spr-Verlag.

Helicobacter Pylori: Pathophysiology, Epidemiology, & Management. Ed. by T. C. Northfield. 1993. LC 93-38532. text 89.00 (*0-7923-8825-9*) Kluwer Academic.

Helicobacter Pylori & Gastroduodenal Disease. B. J. Rathbone & Richard V. Heatley. 2nd ed. 1992. (Illus.). 312p. 150.00 (*0-632-03346-0*) Blackwell Sci.

Helicobacter Pylori & Gastroduodenal Pathology. Ed. by J. M. Pajares et al. 1993. LC 92-30270. (Illus.). 400p. 217.00 (*0-387-55432-7*) Spr-Verlag.

Helicobacter Pylori Handbook. Richard V. Heatley. 1995. LC 95-21040. 56p. pap. 9.95 (*0-86542-659-7*); 2nd ed. 1999. LC 98-24769. (Illus.). 64p. pap. 31.95 (*0-632-05176-0*) Blackwell Sci.

Helicobacter Pylori Protocols. Ed. by Christopher L. Clayton & Harry L. T. Mobley. 1997. LC 97-9080. (Methods in Molecular Medicine Ser.: Vol. 8). (Illus.). 288p. 120.00 (*0-89603-381-3*) Humana.

Hell of Al - The Way of Schizophrenia. Maria Kuman. pap. 20.00 (*1-893637-21-2*) Hlth & Hap.

Hellenistic Treatise on Poisonous Animals (The "Theriaca" of Nicander of Colophon) A Contribution to the History of Toxicology. Peter K. Knoefel & Madeline C. Covi. 1991. LC 91-29285. (Illus.). 188p. lib. bdg. 79.95 (*0-7734-9674-2*) E Mellen.

Helmholtz's Treatise on Physiological Optics, Set. Tr. by James Southall. 5th ed. 2000. (History of Science Ser.). 1555p. 385.00 (*1-85506-831-1*) Thoemmes Pr.

Helminth Zoonoses. Ed. by S. Geerts et al. 1987. (Current Topics in Veterinary Medicine & Animal Science Ser.). (C). text 161.50 (*0-89838-896-1*) Kluwer Academic.

Helminths of Fish Eating Birds of the Palaeartic Region: Volume 1, Nematoda. Ed. by B. Rysavy & K. M. Ryzhikov. 1978. (Illus.). text 155.50 (*90-6193-551-2*) Kluwer Academic.

Help! The Quick Guide to First Aid for Your Dog. Michelle Bamberger. 1993. (Illus.). 160p. pap. 9.95 (*0-87605-557-9*, Howell) Hungry Minds.

Help Against Coronary Heart Disease. 1995. 22p. pap. 2.00 (*1-930181-09-4*) A H A F.

Help! & Homeopathy: Using Homeopathy in First Aid Crisis. 1997. 190p. (Orig.). pap. 16.95 (*0-9634662-6-7*) Blue Turtle.

Help at Last: A Complete Guide to Coping with Chemically Dependent Men. Edward Kaufman. 1991. LC 89-23285. 226p. 29.95 (*0-89876-166-2*) Gardner Pr.

Help, Comfort & Hope after Losing Your Baby in Pregnancy or the First Year. Hannah Lothrop. 1997. LC 96-48501. 296p. pap. 15.00 (*1-55561-120-6*) Fisher Bks.

Help Desk Practitioner's Handbook. Barbara Czegel. 1998. LC 98-31159. (Illus.). 432p. pap. 44.99 (*0-471-31992-9*) Wiley.

Help for Dyslexic Children. T. R. Miles & Elaine Miles. 1983. 116p. pap. 9.95 (*0-416-33740-6*, NO. 3829) Routledge.

Help for the Depressed. Samuel H. Kraines & Eloise S. Thetford. 1979. (Illus.). 272p. spiral bd. 47.95 (*0-398-02335-2*) C C Thomas.

Help for the Hyperactive Child. William G. Crook. 1991. (Illus.). 248p. (Orig.). pap. 14.95 (*0-933478-18-6*) Prof Bks Future Health.

Help, She's Having a Baby. Nancy Crowley. 1994. (Illus.). 64p. (Orig.). pap. (*0-9640358-0-4*) N Crowley.

Help She's Having a Baby: Emergency Childbirth. Nancy Crowley. rev. ed. 1994. LC 94-220147. (Illus.). 88p. pap. 8.95 (*0-9640358-1-2*) N Crowley.

H I

Help System. G. J. Kuperman et al. Ed. by Bruce I. Blum. 1991. (Computers & Medicine Ser.). (Illus.). 334p. 69.00 (*0-387-97431-8*) Spr-Verlag.

Help! The Quick Guide to First Aid for Your Cat: The Quick Guide to First Aid for Your Cat. Michelle Bamberger. 1995. LC 94-37313. (Illus.). 160p. pap. 9.95 (*0-87605-794-6*, Howell) Hungry Minds.

Help with Your Project. Diane Owen & Moya Davis. 2nd rev. ed. 1996. (Illus.). 80p. pap. text 24.95 (*1-56593-801-1*, 1566) Thomson Learn.

Help Your Child Avoid Multiple Sclerosis: A Parenting Decision. Joseph V. Goldbach & Dorothy M. Goldbach. 1999. LC 94-12045. (Illus.). 255p. pap. 23.00 (*0-9669096-6-6*) Herit Global.

Help Your Child to Perfect Eyesight Without Glasses. Janet Goodrich. 1998. (Illus.). 264p. text 17.95 (*0-89087-870-6*) Celestial Arts.

Help Your Child to Perfect Eyesight Without Glasses. Janet Goodrich. 1997. (Illus.). 258p. pap. (*1-86351-194-6*) Sally Milner AUS. *Dist:* Seven Hills Bk.

Help Yourself: A Guide to Organizing a Phobia Self-Help Group. Meg McGarrah. 1990. 100p. pap. (*0-935943-01-3*) Anxiety Disorders.

Help Yourself: A Treatment for Migraine Headaches. Patrick J. McGrath et al. 1990. 110p. pap., tchr. ed. 10.00 (*0-7766-0249-7*); 490p. pap., stu. ed. 20.00 (*0-7766-0248-9*) Paul & Co Pubs.

Help Yourself: Problem Solving for the Disabled. Douglas R. Bucy. 1996. LC 96-16206. 192p. pap. 14.95 (*0-02-861059-8*) Macmillan.

Help Yourself: The Beginner's Guide to Natural Medicine. Karolyn A. Gazella. 1995. LC 95-95161. (Help Yourself Ser.). (Illus.). 132p. (Orig.). pap. 8.95 (*0-9647489-1-6*) IMPAKT Communs.

Help Yourself to Better Sight. Margaret D. Corbett. 1980. pap. 10.00 (*0-87980-048-8*) Wilshire.

Help Yourself to Chronic Pain Relief: The Patient's Point of View. Gloria J. Epstein. 1981. LC 81-80224. 104p. (Orig.). pap. 4.95 (*0-9605792-0-6*) Manchester Group.

Help Yourself to Health. Linda Clark. 2nd rev. ed. 1990. 268p. reprint ed. pap. 12.95 (*0-8159-5722-X*) Devin.

Helpers in Case-Managed Community Care. Hazel Qureshi et al. 1989. (Illus.). 245p. text (*0-566-05809-X*) Arena GBR. *Dist:* Ashgate Pub Co.

Helpflanzen-Lexikon fur Arzte und Apotheker: Lexicon for Doctors & Pharmacists. Hans Bruan. 5th ed. 1987. (GER.). 315p. 85.00 (*0-7859-8361-9*, 3437110713) Fr & Eur.

Helping Adolescents with ADHD & Learning Disabilities: Ready-to-Use Tips, Techniques & Checklists for School Success. Judith Greenbaum & Geraldine Markel. 2001. LC 00-50765. (Illus.). xxi, 321p. pap. 28.95 (*0-13-016778-9*) P-H.

Helping & Healing: Religious Commitment in Health Care. Edmund D. Pellegrino & David C. Thomasma. 1997. LC 96-46598. 176p. pap. 15.95 (*0-87840-643-3*) Georgetown U Pr.

Helping Bereaved Children: A Handbook for Practitioners. Ed. by Nancy B. Webb. 1993. LC 93-3506. 304p. 32.50 (*0-89862-130-5*) Guilford Pubns.

Helping Cancer Patients Cope: A Problem-Solving Approach. Arthur M. Nezu et al. 1999. LC 98-36683. 314p. 39.95 (*1-55798-533-2*, 431-721A) Am Psychol.

Helping Children Cope with Grief. Alan D. Wolfelt. 1983. LC 83-70222. xv, 176p. pap. text 16.95 (*0-915202-39-5*) Accel Devel.

Helping Children Cope with Separation & Loss. Claudia J. Jarratt. Ed. by Dan Rosenberg. rev. ed. 1994. LC 93-33178. 240p. pap. 12.95 (*1-55832-051-2*) Harvard Common Pr.

Helping Children Cope with Stress. Avis Brenner. 1997. LC 97-19819. 208p. pap. 22.00 (*0-7879-3864-5*, F225-E2F) Jossey-Bass.

Helping Children Manage Loss. Brenda Mallon. 1998. LC 98-204421. 184p. pap. (*1-85302-605-0*) Jessica Kingsley GBR. *Dist:* Taylor & Francis.

Helping Children Manage Stress: A Guide for Adults. James H. Humphrey. 1998. LC 98-25980. 112p. 18.95 (*0-87868-668-1*, 6681) Child Welfare.

Helping Children Take Healthy Steps: Abstracts of Selected Articles on Early Childhood Interventions. Ed. by Jeanne Brooks-Gunn. 1999. 147p. (C). reprint ed. pap. text 30.00 (*0-7881-7662-5*) DIANE Pub.

Helping Children to Like Themselves: Activities for Building Self-Esteem. James E. Carothers & Ruth S. Gasten. 1978. pap. 4.95 (*0-9602090-1-8*) RJ Assocs.

Helping Children Who Are Blind: Family & Community Support for Children with Vision Problems. Sandy Niemann & Namita Jacob. 2000. LC 00-58209. (Early Assistance Series for Children with Disabilities). (Illus.). 192p. pap. 12.00 (*0-942364-34-1*) Hesperian Found.

Helping Clients Forgive: An Empirical Guide for Resolving Anger & Restoring Hope. Robert D. Enright & Richard P. Fitzgibbons. 2000. LC 00-26160. xiii, 376p. 39.95 (*1-55798-689-4*, 431-750A) Am Psychol.

Helping Families Through Divorce: An Eclectic Approach. Ellen Bogolub. 1995. LC 95-18572. 272p. 39.95 (*0-8261-9060-X*) Springer Pub.

Helping Families with Special Problems. Ed. by Martin R. Textor. 1983. LC 82-24471. (Helping Families Special Problem CL Ser.). 250p. 50.00 (*0-87668-635-8*) Aronson.

Helping Hands for Dental Hygienists: 101 Timeless Treasures for a Successful Career. Linda Harvey. 2000. LC 00-100804. 128p. 12.95 (*0-9678758-0-3*) Horizon Consltng.

Helping Health Workers Learn: A Book of Methods, Aids, & Ideas for Instructors at the Village Level. Bill Bower & David B. Werner. 1982. LC 81-85010. (Illus.). 640p. (C). pap. 20.00 (*0-942364-10-4*) Hesperian Found.

Helping Health Workers Learn: A Book of Methods, Aids & ideas for instructors at the Village Level see Aprendiendo a Promover la Salud: Un Libro de Metodos, Materiales e Ideas para Instructores que Trabajan en la Comunidad

Helping Low Birth Weight, Premature Babies: The Infant Health & Development Program. Ed. by Ruth T. Gross et al. 1997. LC 96-1368. 77.00 (*0-8047-2612-4*) Stanford U Pr.

Helping Mentally Ill Homeless People: A Manual for Shelter Workers. Ed. by Mary E. Stefl. 1989. 64p. 10.00 (*0-87553-158-X*) Am Pub Health.

Helping Our Peers Effectively: A Skills Development Manual. Janet Molina. 1992. 220p. pap. text 19.95 (*0-9634612-0-6*) Metamorphic.

Helping Parents Help Their Kids: A Clinical Guide to Six Child Problem Behaviors. Ennio Cipani. 1998. LC 98-28099. 62.95 (*0-87630-951-1*); 204p. pap. 31.95 (*0-87630-952-X*) Brunner-Routledge.

Helping Parents Solve Their Children's Behavior Problems. Ed. by Charles E. Schaefer & Andrew R. Eisen. 1998. LC 97-38469. (Child Therapy Ser.). 432p. 60.00 (*0-7657-0148-0*) Aronson.

Helping Parents, Youth, & Teachers Understanding Medications for Behavioral & Emotional Problems: A Resource Book of Medication Information Handouts. Ed. by Mina K. Dulcan. 1998. LC 98-16698. (Illus.). xvi, 178p. spiral bd. 39.95 (*0-88048-794-1*, 8794) Am Psychiatric.

Helping People Change: A Textbook of Methods. Ed. by Frederick H. Kanfer & Arnold P. Goldstein. 560p. 2nd ed. 1980. LC 79-17929. text 46.00 (*0-08-025098-X*); 2nd ed. 1980. LC 79-17929. pap. text 17.50 (*0-08-025097-1*); 3rd ed. 1985. (General Psychology Ser.: No. 52). 65.00 (*0-08-031601-8*); 3rd ed. 1985. (General Psychology Ser.: No. 52). pap. 19.50 (*0-08-031600-X*) Elsevier (Pergamon Pr).

Helping People Change: A Textbook of Methods. Frederick H. Kanfer & A. P. Goldstein. 4th ed. 1991. (General Psychology Ser.). 576p. text (*0-08-037893-5*); pap. text (*0-08-037892-7*) PPI GBR. *Dist:* Elsevier.

Helping People in Crisis: A Practical, Family-Oriented Approach to Effective Crisis Intervention. Douglas A. Puryear. 1979. LC 79-88108. (Social & Behavioral Science Ser.). 225p. 42.00 (*0-87589-421-6*) Jossey-Bass.

Helping People to Help Themselves: Self-Help & Prevention. Ed. by Leonard D. Borman et al. 1982. LC 82-924. (Prevention in Human Services Ser.: Vol. 1, No. 3). 129p. text 39.95 (*0-917724-67-4*) Haworth Pr.

Helping People with Incontinence. 1997. lib. bdg. 250.95 (*0-8490-7763-X*) Gordon Pr.

Helping Relationship: Process & Skills. Lawrence W. Brammer & Ginger MacDonald. 7th ed. 1998. LC 98-20672. 198p. (C). pap. text 51.00 (*0-205-29042-6*) Allyn.

Helping Relationships Through Self-Love: A Creative Nondirective Approach to Psychotherapy & Education. Collette Portelance. 1995. LC 96-748. (ENG & FRE.). 420p. pap. (*2-9801489-4-6*) Cram Pubs CAN. *Dist:* Seven Hills Bk.

Helping Skills II: Life Development Intervention. Steven J. Danish et al. 1983. (C). 160p. stu. ed. 20.95 (*0-89885-146-7*); 18.95 (*0-89885-145-9*) Kluwer Academic (Kluwer Acad Hman Sci).

Helping Strategies in Child Sexual Abuse. Celia Doyle. 1996. LC 95-218955. 224p. pap. text (*1-871177-39-1*) Whiting & Birch GBR. *Dist:* Paul & Co Pubs.

Helping Teens Work Through Grief. Mary K. Perschy. 1997. LC 96-48297. 150p. pap. 19.95 (*1-56032-558-5*) Hemisp Pub.

Helping the Aging Family: A Guide for Professionals. Victoria E. Bumagin & Kathryn F. Hirn. 1990. 320p. reprint ed. 38.95 (*0-8261-7530-9*) Springer Pub.

Helping the Bereaved: Therapeutic Interventions for Children, Adolescents, & Adults. Alicia S. Cook & Daniel S. Dworkin. 1992. LC 91-57905. (Illus.). 193p. 45.00 (*0-465-02717-2*) Basic.

Helping the Cancer Victim: Patient Rights, Medical Freedom & the Need for New Laws. Barry Lynes. 1990. 58p. (Orig.). pap. text (*0-919951-05-8*) New Leaf Dist.

Helping the Child of Exceptional Ability. Susan Leyden. l.t. ed. 1985. LC 85-4137. (Special Education Ser.). 102p. (Orig.). pap. (*0-7099-1635-3*) C Helm GBR. *Dist:* Routldge.

Helping the Child Who Doesn't Fit In: Clinical Psychologists Decipher the Hidden Dimensions of Social Rejection. Stephen Nowicki, Jr. & Marshall Duke. 1992. (Illus.). 192p. pap. 14.95 (*1-56145-025-1*) Peachtree Pubs.

Helping the Handicapped: Problems & Prospects. Arvindrai N. Desai. 1990. (*81-7024-261-4*) Ashish Pub Hse IND. *Dist:* S Asia.

Helping the Hard-Core Smoker: A Clinician's Guide. Ed. by Daniel F. Seldman & Lirio S. Covey. 1999. LC 98-22971. xvii, 320 p. 32.00 (*0-8058-2755-2*) L Erlbaum Assocs.

Helping the Noncompliant Child: A Clinician's Guide to Parent Training. Rex L. Forehand & Robert J. McMahon. 1981. LC 81-6629. 253p. (C). 35.00 (*0-89862-611-0*, 2611) Guilford Pubns.

Helping the Retarded: A Systematic Behavioural Approach. E. A. Perkins et al. 1985. 105p. 40.00 (*0-906054-18-4*); pap. 30.00 (*0-906054-40-0*) St Mut.

Helping the Retarded: Developmental Checklist. E. A. Perkins et al. 1985. 16p. 30.00 (*0-906054-25-7*) St Mut.

Helping the Struggling Adolescent: A Counseling Guide. Leslie Parrott, III. 1993. 144p. pap. 12.99 (*0-310-61511-9*) Zondervan.

Helping the Troubled Child: Interprofessional Case Studies. Ed. by Stephen Murgatroyd. 1980. 196p. pap. (*0-335-09818-5*) OpUniv Pr GBR. *Dist:* Taylor & Francis.

Helping the Woman You Love Recover from Breast Cancer. Andy Murcia. 1991. 220p. mass mkt. 4.99 (*0-312-92191-8*) St Martin.

Helping Troubled Children. M. Rutter. 1975. LC 76-25475. (Illus.). 376p. (C). 55.00 (*0-306-30969-6*, Plenum Trade) Perseus Pubng.

Helping Victims of Sexual Abuse. Lynn Heitritter & Jeanette Vought. 1989. LC 89-15153. 272p. (Orig.). pap. 9.99 (*0-87123-930-2*) Bethany Hse.

Helping Women Cope with Grief. Phyllis R. Silverman. 1981. (Human Services Guides Ser.: Vol. 25). 111p. pap. 34.95 (*0-8039-1735-X*, 5019) Sage.

Helping Women Keep Well: A Guide to Health Promotion & Illness Prevention for the Health Professional. Richard Blum & LeRoy Heinrichs. 1988. LC 88-2752. 487p. text 52.50 (*0-8290-1793-3*) Irvington.

Helping Women Recover from Abortion. Nancy Michaels. 1988. LC 88-10447. 192p. (Orig.). pap. 8.99 (*0-87123-621-4*) Bethany Hse.

Helping Young Children at Risk: A Psychoeducational Approach. Agnes M. Plenk. 1993. LC 93-20303. 232p. 62.95 (*0-275-94591-X*, C4591); pap. 22.95 (*0-275-94592-8*) Greenwood (Praeger Pubs).

Helping Your Chemically Dependent Teenager Recover: A Guide for Parents & Other Concerned Adults. Peter R. Cohen. 1991. pap. 12.00 (*1-56246-015-3*, 3178, HazeldenJohnson Inst) Hazelden.

Helping Your Child Sleep Through the Night. Joanne Cuthbertson & Susanna Schevill. 1985. LC 84-18807. (Illus.). 256p. pap. 12.95 (*0-385-19250-9*) Doubleday.

*__Helping Your Children Cope With Your Cancer: A Guide for Parents.__ Peter Van Dernoot. 2002. 240p. pap. 15.95 (*1-57826-105-8*) Hatherleigh.

Helping Your Dyslexic Child: A Guide to Improving Your Child's Reading, Writing, Spelling, Comprehension & Self-Esteem. Eileen Cronin. 1997. LC 97-223137. 208p. pap. 14.95 (*0-7615-1004-4*) Prima Pub.

Helping Your Health Through Handwriting. Phyllis Harrison. 2nd expurg. rev. ed. 1985. LC 85-10082. (Illus.). 208p. pap. 9.95 (*0-89407-069-X*) Strawberry Hill.

*__Helping Your Heart: A Handbook for Patients & Their Families.__ 2001. (Illus.). 142p. 29.95 (*1-931876-02-9*) Allina Health Pr.

Helping Your Mate Face Breast Cancer: Tips for Becoming an Effective Support Partner. Judy C. Kneece. 3rd rev. ed. 1999. LC 99-93958. (Illus.). 136p. pap. 12.95 (*1-886665-11-7*) EduCare Pub.

Helping Yourself with Autogenics. Sidney Petrie & Robert B. Stone. 1983. LC 82-14488. 205p. pap. 4.95 (*0-13-387399-4*, Parker Publishing Co) P-H.

Helping Yourself with Psycho-Cosmic Power. Al G. Manning. 1983. LC 68-12433. pap. 6.95 (*0-941698-06-8*) Pan Ishtar.

Helpmates: Support in Times of Critical Illness. Harry A. Cole. 1991. 144p. pap. 12.00 (*0-664-25141-2*) Westminster John Knox.

Hemangiomas & Vascular Malformations of the Head & Neck. Milton Waner & James Y. Suen. 1999. LC 98-10332. (Illus.). 396p. 210.00 (*0-471-17597-8*) Wiley.

Hemato-Oncology & Hemato-Immunology: Sicilian International Conference, Catania, Italy, 2nd, November 1986. Ed. by E. Cacciola. 1988. (Acta Haematologica Ser.: Vol. 78, Suppl. 1). (Illus.). iv, 220p. pap. 68.00 (*3-8055-4727-7*) S Karger.

Hematologic & Oncologic Emergencies. Ed. by William R. Bell. 1993. 254p. text (*0-443-08871-3*) Church.

Hematologic Disorders in Maternal-Fetal Medicine. Ed. by Murray M. Bern & Fredric D. Frigoletto. 1990. LC 89-12460. 706p. 367.00 (*0-471-56213-0*) Wiley.

Hematologic Malignancies. Ed. by B. Hoogstraten. 1986. (Current Treatment of Cancer Ser.). (Illus.). 111p. 43.95 (*0-387-16293-3*) Spr-Verlag.

Hematologic Malignancies: Methods & Techniques. Ed. by Guy B. Faguet. 2001. LC 00-40789. (Methods in Molecular Medicine Ser.: Vol. 55). (Illus.). xv, 360p. 99.50 (*0-89603-543-3*) Humana.

Hematologic Pathophysiology. R. Rubin & L. Leopold. 1997. (Pathophysiology Ser.). (C). pap. 30.95 (*1-889325-04-X*) Blackwell Sci.

Hematologic Pathophysiology. Fred Schiffman. 1998. LC 97-46468. 400p. pap. text 34.95 (*0-397-51536-7*) Lppncott W & W.

Hematologic Problems in the Neonate. Robert D. Christensen. Ed. by Judy Fletcher. 1999. LC 98-52044. (Illus.). x, 453p. text (*0-7216-7727-4*) Saunders.

Hematologic Stress Syndrome: The Biological Response to Disease. Peter Reizenstein. 1983. LC 83-4023. 190p. 59.95 (*0-275-91408-9*, C1408, Praeger Pubs) Greenwood.

Hematologie. B. Dreyfus. 1984. (FRE., Illus.). 950p. lib. bdg. 99.00 (*2-257-12526-6*) S M P F Inc.

Hematology. E. Besa et al. 1993. LC 91-21620. (National Medical Series for Independent Study). (Illus.). 335p. pap. text 29.00 (*0-683-06222-0*) Lppncott W & W.

Hematology. Burns. 1999. pap. text (*0-7216-4693-X*) Saunders.

Hematology. Cotter. 2000. (Quick Look Veterinary Ser.). 23.95 (*1-889325-46-5*) Fence Crk Pubng.

Hematology. Richert E. Goyette. Ed. by Gregg Rogers. 1997. (Illus.). 1100p. text 69.95 (*1-57066-008-5*, ME225) Practice Mgmt Info.

Hematology. Mobley. 1995. (Medical Lab Technician Ser.). pap., lab manual ed. 32.95 (*0-8273-5950-0*) Delmar.

Hematology. Jack Rudman. 1994. (College Level Examination Ser.: CLEP-33). pap. 27.95 (*0-8373-5333-5*) Nat Learn.

Hematology. Larry Waterbury. (House Officer Ser.). (Illus.). 3rd ed. 1988. 176p. pap. 21.95 (*0-683-08853-X*); 4th ed. 1996. LC 96-9114. 179p. pap. 29.95 (*0-683-08854-8*) Lppncott W & W.

Hematology. Ed. by William S. Beck. 5th ed. 1991. (Illus.). 664p. 60.00 (*0-262-02316-4*); LC 90-13588. pap. 42.95 (*0-262-52157-1*) MIT Pr.

Hematology: A Combined Theoretical & Practical Approach. Simmons. 2nd ed. 1996. LC 96-47476. 507p. pap. text (*0-7506-9848-9*) E A GBR. *Dist:* OUP.

Hematology: A Combined Theoretical & Technical Approach. Simmons. 1989. 464p. text 59.95 (*0-7216-1716-6*) Saunders.

Hematology: A Pathophysiological Approach. Bernard M. Babior & Thomas P. Stossel. 3rd ed. 1994. (Illus.). pap. text (*0-443-08939-6*) Church.

Hematology: Basic Principles & Practice. Ronald Hoffman et al. Ed. by Marc Strauss. 3rd ed. 1999. LC 98-43923. (Illus.). xxxi, 25840p. text (*0-443-07954-4*) Church.

Hematology: Physiopathologic Basis for Clinical Practice. Paul R. Reich. 2nd ed. 1984. 528p. 31.00 (*0-316-73863-8*, Little Brwn Med Div) Lppncott W & W.

Hematology: Principles & Procedures. Barbara Brown. 6th ed. 1993. (Illus.). 453p. text 49.95 (*0-8121-1643-7*) Lppncott W & W.

Hematology & Heart Surgery. Michael D'Ambra & Theodore A. Alston. 1999. 125.00 (*0-89603-723-1*) Humana.

*__Hematology & Oncology: Certification Review.__ Chu & DeVita. 2002. (Illus.). (C). pap. text 39.95 (*0-7637-1882-3*, 1882-3) Jones & Bartlett.

*__Hematology & Oncology: Clinical Diagnosis & Practice.__ Bruce Furie et al. 2001. (Illus.). 955p. (*0-443-06556-X*) Church GBR. *Dist:* Saunders.

Hematology in Clinical Practice. Robert S. Hillman & Ken A. Ault. 2nd ed. 1998. LC 98-4646. (Illus.). 600p. pap. 54.95 (*0-07-029023-7*) McGraw-Hill Prof.

*__Hematology in Clinical Practice: A Guide to Diagnosis & Management.__ Robert Hillman & Kenneth A. Ault. 3rd ed. 2001. 624p. pap. 59.95 (*0-07-137502-3*) McGraw-Hill Prof.

Hematology Laboratory Management & Practice. Ed. by S. M. Lewis & John A. Koepke. 1995. LC 94-35300. (Illus.). 256p. text (*0-7506-0964-8*) E A GBR. *Dist:* OUP.

Hematology Reviews: Cellular Mechanisms of the System Regulating the Aggregate State of Blood, Vol. 3. S. V. Andreev et al. 1990. (Soviet Medical Reviews Ser.: Vol. 3, Pt. 3). 76p. pap. text 82.00 (*3-7186-4961-6*) Gordon & Breach.

Hematology Reviews: Hemoglobinopathies, Enzymopathies & Methods of Diagnosing Hemopoietic Disturbances, Vol. 2. O. K. Gavrilov. 1990. (Soviet Medical Reviews Ser.: Vol. 2, Pt. B). xii, 244p. text 544.00 (*3-7186-4964-0*) Gordon & Breach.

Hematology Reviews: Immune Mechanisms of the System Regulating the Aggregate State of Blood, Vol. 3. E. V. Barkovsky et al. 1990. (Soviet Medical Reviews Ser.: Vol. 3, Pt. 2). iv, 60p. pap. text 75.00 (*3-7186-4962-4*) Gordon & Breach.

Hematology Reviews: Regulation of Hemopoiesis, Vol. 2. O. K. Gavrilov. 1990. (Soviet Medical Reviews Ser.: Vol. 2, Pt. A). xiv, 214p. text 390.00 (*3-7186-4939-X*) Gordon & Breach.

Hematology Reviews Vol. 3, Pt. 1: Biochemical Mechanisms of the System Regulating the Aggregate State of Blood, Vol. 3. S. V. Andreev. 1990. (Soviet Medical Reviews Ser.: Section C). iv, 126p. pap. text 142.00 (*3-7186-4963-2*, Harwood Acad Pubs) Gordon & Breach.

Hematology Reviews Vol. 3, Pt. 4: Clinical Disorders of the System Regulating the Aggregate State of Blood & Methods for Their Management, Vol. 3. M. K. Alliev. 1990. (Soviet Medical Reviews Ser.: Section C). v, 111p. text 121.00 (*3-7186-4960-8*, Harwood Acad Pubs) Gordon & Breach.

HI

Hematology Reviews Vol. 3, Pt. 5: Problems in Molecular Biology & Hemostasiology, Vol. 3. O. K. Gavrilov. 1991. (Soviet Medical Reviews Ser.: Section C). 60p. pap. text 63.00 (*3-7186-5153-X*, Harwood Acad Pubs) Gordon & Breach.

Hematology Reviews Vol. 4, Pt. 1: The Mechanisms of the Effects of Extracorporeal Regulation of the Aggregate State of the Blood & Recent Developments, Vol. 4. O. K. Gavrilov. 1991. (Soviet Medical Reviews Ser.: Section C). 86p. pap. text 118.00 (*3-7186-5152-1*, Harwood Acad Pubs) Gordon & Breach.

Hematology Reviews Vol. 4, Pt. 2: The Mechanisms of the Effects of Extracorporeal Regulation of the Aggregate State of the Blood & Recent Developments, Vol. 4. O. K. Gavrilov. 1991. (Soviet Medical Reviews Ser.: Section C). 83p. pap. text 106.00 (*3-7186-5241-2*, Harwood Acad Pubs) Gordon & Breach.

Hematology Reviews Vol. 4, Pt. 3: The Regulation of Hemopoisis & Hemostasis, Vol. 4. O. K. Gavrilov. 1992. (Soviet Medical Reviews Ser.: Section C). 138p. pap. text 131.00 (*3-7186-5242-0*, Harwood Acad Pubs) Gordon & Breach.

Hematology Reviews Vol. 4, Pt. 4: Myelodysplasia: Hematological Genetics, Vol. 4. O. K. Gavrilov. 1992. (Soviet Medical Reviews Ser.: Section C). 82p. pap. text 83.00 (*3-7186-5252-8*, Harwood Acad Pubs) Gordon & Breach.

Hematology Reviews Vol. 5, Pt. 1: Intensive Cytoplasmapheresis & Endovascular Surgery in Hematological Practice, Vol. 5. F. E. Fainshtein. 1992. (Soviet Medical Reviews Ser.: Section C). 76p. pap. text 84.00 (*3-7186-5253-6*, Harwood Acad Pubs) Gordon & Breach.

Hematology Reviews Vol. 5, Pt. 2: Intensive Cytoplasmapheresis & Endovascular Surgery in Hematological Practice, Vol. 5. L. G. Kovaleva. 1992. (Soviet Medical Reviews Ser.: Section C). 73p. pap. text 77.00 (*3-7186-5254-4*, Harwood Acad Pubs) Gordon & Breach.

Hematology Reviews Vol. 5, Pt. 3: Intensive Cytoplasmapheresis & Endovascular Surgery in Hematological Practice, Vol. 5. O. K. Gavrilov. 1992. (Soviet Medical Reviews Ser.: Section C). 68p. pap. text 77.00 (*3-7186-5255-2*, Harwood Acad Pubs) Gordon & Breach.

Hematology Reviews Vol. 5, Pt. 4: Hormones & Hemostasis, Vol. 5. Y. I. Sokolov. 1992. (Soviet Medical Reviews Ser.: Section C). 106p. pap. text 174.00 (*3-7186-5355-9*, Harwood Acad Pubs) Gordon & Breach.

Hematology Reviews Vol. 6, Pt. 2: Hormones & Hemostasis in Hemorrhagic Hemostasiopathies, Vol. 6. V. A. Germanov. 1993. (Soviet Medical Reviews Ser.: Section C). 78p. pap. text 114.00 (*3-7186-5462-8*, Harwood Acad Pubs) Gordon & Breach.

Hematology Reviews & Communications, Vol. 3, No. 1. Ed. by M. Corn & Stuart Roath. 1989. 88p. pap. text 182.00 (*3-7186-4935-7*) Gordon & Breach.

Hematology Reviews 1: Blood Coagulation, Embolism & Thrombosis, Vol. 1. O. K. Gavrilov. 1987. (Soviet Medical Reviews Ser.). xii, 426p. text 468.00 (*3-7186-0352-7*) Gordon & Breach.

Hematology Techniques & Concepts for Veterinary Technicians. Gregg L. Voigt. 2000. LC 99-56719. (Illus.). 160p. 39.95 (*0-8138-0491-4*) Iowa U Pr.

Hematology, the Lymphatic System, & the Immune System: The Lymphatic System, & the Immune System. Elizabeth K. White. 3rd ed. 1993. LC 92-48846. (Regents/Prentice Hall Medical Assistant Kit Ser.). 74p. pap. 19.47 (*0-13-036690-0*) P-H.

Hematology/Oncology Secrets. Marie E. Wood. 2nd rev. ed. 1999. LC 99-11380. (Secrets Ser.). (Illus.). 400p. pap. 39.95 (*1-56053-313-7*) Hanley & Belfus.

Hematolymphatic & Neoplastic Disorders. Anne E. Belcher. 1992. (Illus.). 288p. (C). (gr. 13). text 36.00 (*0-8016-1809-6*, 01809) Mosby Inc.

Hematopoiesis: Long-Term Effects of Chemotherapy & Radiation. Gale & Bernard Testa. 1988. (Hematology Ser.: Vol. 8). (Illus.). 440p. text 210.00 (*0-8247-7938-X*) Dekker.

Hematopoietic Cell Transplantation. Stephen J. Forman et al. 2nd ed. 1998. LC 98-25820. (Illus.). 1260p. 314.95 (*0-632-04371-7*) Blackwell Sci.

Hematopoietic Growth Factors in Clinical Applications. Roland Mertelsmann & S. Gillis. Date not set. (*0-8247-9400-1*) Dekker.

Hematopoietic Growth Factors in Clinical Applications. Ed. by Roland Mertelsmann & Friedhelm Herrmann. 2nd exp. rev. ed. 1994. LC 94-22881. (Illus.). 424p. text 195.00 (*0-8247-9268-8*) Dekker.

Hematopoietic Lineages in Health & Disease. Nydia G. Testa et al. 1997. LC 97-5698. (Illus.). 384p. text 150.00 (*0-8247-9512-1*) Dekker.

Hematopoietic Progenitor Cells: A Primer for Medical Professionals. Ed. by N. Rebecca Haley & Edward L. Snyder. 2000. text (*1-56395-112-6*) Am Assn Blood.

Hematopoietic Progenitor Cells: Processing, Standards & Practice. Ed. by Mark E. Brecher et al. 1995. (Illus.). 205p. (C). 50.00 (*1-56395-050-2*) Am Assn Blood.

Hematopoietic Stem Cell Transplantation. R Hass. Ed. by Anthony Ho & Richard Champlin. 2000. LC 00-31599. (Illus.). 624p. text 185.00 (*0-8247-0273-5*) Dekker.

Hematopoietic Stem Cells, Vol. 15, Supplement 1. T. A. Bock et al. 1997. LC 97-73748. 308p. text 69.00 (*1-880854-23-6*) AlphaMed Pr.

Hematopoietic Stem Cells: Biology & Therapeutic Applications. Levitt & R. Mertelsmann. 1995. (Illus.). 681p. text 195.00 (*0-8247-9305-6*) Dekker.

Hematopoietic Stem Cells: Their Assay, Ontogeny, Isolation & Molecular Functions. Suzanne M. Watt. 1997. (Medical Intelligence Unit Ser.). 200p. 89.95 (*0-412-11421-6*) Chapman & Hall.

Heme Oxygenase: Clinical Applications & Functions. Mahin D. Maines. 1992. 288p. 225.00 (*0-8493-5408-0*, QP603) CRC Pr.

Hemifacial Spasm: A Multidisciplinary Approach. Marc Sindou & Yves Keravel. 1997. LC 96-48002. (Illus.). 200p. 190.00 (*3-211-82792-7*) Spr-Verlag.

Hemispheric Communication: Mechanisms & Models. Ed. by Frederick L. Kitterle. 1995. 392p. text 79.95 (*0-8058-1144-3*) L Erlbaum Assocs.

Hemispheric Specialisation in Animals & Humans: A Special Issue of Laterality. Barbara Bulman-Fleming. 1998. 64.95 (*0-86377-964-6*) L Erlbaum Assocs.

Hemodialysis: High Efficiency Treatments. Ed. by Juan P. Bosch. 1993. (Illus.). 360p. text (*0-443-08848-9*) Church.

Hemodialysis Systems. 2nd ed. 1992. 33p. pap. 90.00 (*0-910275-70-X*, RD5-209) Assn Adv Med Instrn.

Hemodialyzer Reuse: Issues & Solutions. 1985. 73p. pap. 90.00 (*0-910275-51-3*, TAR10-209) Assn Adv Med Instrn.

Hemodialyzer Reuse in the 1990s: Practice, Regulation, & Patient Safety. 1995. (Orig.). pap. 145.00 (*1-57020-052-1*, HEM094-209) Assn Adv Med Instrn.

Hemodilution: New Aspects in the Management of Circulatory Blood Flow Improvement of Macro- & Microcirculation. J. Koscielny et al. Ed. by H. Kiesewetter et al. 1992. LC 92-2267. (Illus.). 296p. 73.95 (*0-387-55352-5*) Spr-Verlag.

Hemodilution & Flow Improvement: Bibliotheca Haematologica, No. 47. Ed. by K. Messmer et al. 1982. (Illus.). viii, 356p. pap. 164.50 (*3-8055-2899-X*) S Karger.

Hemodynamic Aspects of Cerebral Angiomas. W. Hassler. 1987. (Acta Neurochirurgica Ser.: Supplementum 37). (Illus.). 150p. 120.00 (*0-387-81970-3*) Spr-Verlag.

Hemodynamic Basis of Atherosclerosis: With Critique of the Cholesterol-Heart Disease Hypothesis. Meyer Texon. 2nd exp. ed. 1996. 150p. 87.50 (*1-56700-029-0*) Begell Hse.

Hemodynamic Monitoring. Marilyn Schactman et al. 1995. (Outline Ser.). (Illus.). 200p. (Orig.). (C). per. 22.95 (*1-56930-034-8*) Delmar.

Hemodynamic Monitoring: A Bedside Reference Manual. Dana Oakes. 1995. (Illus.). 320p. ring bd. 19.95 (*0-932887-07-4*) Health Ed Pubns.

***Hemodynamic Monitoring: Invasive & Noninvasive Clinical Application.** Gloria Oblouk Darovic & Robert J. Henning. 2001. (Illus.). 910p. (*0-7216-8266-9*) Saunders.

Hemodynamic Monitoring: Invasive & Noninvasive Clinical Application. Gloria O. Darovic. 2nd ed. 1995. LC 94-21276. (Illus.). 905p. pap. text 47.00 (*0-7216-4901-7*) Saunders.

Hemodynamic Monitoring of the Critically Ill Obstetric Patient. Mildred G. Harvey. Ed. by Karla Damus & Margaret C. Freda. 1994. LC 94-37838. (*0-86525-060-X*) March of Dimes.

Hemodynamic Monitoring Study Guide. Dana Oakes. 1995. 98p. 10.95 (*0-932887-10-4*) Health Ed Pubns.

Hemodynamic Waveform Recognition. Thomas S. Ahrens. 1993. (Illus.). 224p. pap. text 23.00 (*0-7216-4313-2*) Saunders.

Hemodynamics in Cardiology: Calculations & Interpretations. Franklin B. Saksena. 1983. LC 82-5290. (Illus.). 475p. 75.00 (*0-275-91410-0*, C1410, Praeger Pubs) Greenwood.

Hemodynamics in Daily Practice. Ed. by E. Andries & R. Stroobandt. 1991. (DICM Ser.). (C). text 144.00 (*0-7923-0725-9*) Kluwer Academic.

Hemofiltration. Ed. by K. Schaefer. 1982. (Contributions to Nephrology Ser.: Vol. 32). (Illus.). viii, 228p. pap. 29.75 (*3-8055-3515-5*) S Karger.

Hemoglobins. Ed. by Sidney P. Colowick & Eraldo Antonini. 1981. (Methods in Enzymology Ser.: Vol. 76). text 188.00 (*0-12-181976-0*) Acad Pr.

Hemoglobins Pt. C: Biophysical Methods. Ed. by John N. Abelson et al. 1994. (Methods in Enzymology Ser.: Vol. 232). (Illus.). 725p. text 115.00 (*0-12-182133-1*) Acad Pr.

Hemoglobins Pt. B: Biochemical & Analytical Methods. Ed. by John N. Abelson et al. 1994. (Methods in Enzymology Ser.: Vol. 231). (Illus.). 743p. text 125.00 (*0-12-182132-3*) Acad Pr.

Hemogram Interpretation for Dogs & Cats. A. H. Rebar et al. 1999. (Illus.). 108p. (*0-9678005-1-X*) Gloyd Grp Inc.

Hemolytic Uremic Syndrome & Thrombotic Thrombocytopenic Purpura. Ed. by Bernard S. Kaplan et al. 1992. LC 92-18548. (Kidney Disease Ser.: Vol. 10). (Illus.). 608p. text 235.00 (*0-8247-8663-7*) Dekker.

Hemoperfusion. Ed. by V. Bonomini & T. M. Chang. 1982. (Contributions to Nephrology Ser.: Vol. 29). (Illus.). vi, 150p. pap. 71.25 (*3-8055-3421-3*) S Karger.

***Hemophilia.** 2002. (Diseases & Disorders Ser.). 27.45 (*1-56006-906-6*, Lucent Books) Gale.

Hemophilia. Ed. by C. D. Forbes et al. 1997. LC 96-86288. (Illus.). 392p. (*0-412-63820-7*) E A GBR. *Dist:* OUP.

Hemophilia B: Treatment Issues & Options. Ed. by Geoffrey F. Savidge. 1995. (Acta Haematologica Ser.: Vol. 94, Suppl. 1, 1995). (Illus.). iv, 60p. pap. 29.75 (*3-8055-6148-2*) S Karger.

***Hemophilia Care in the New Millennium.** Ed. by Monroe McDougald. 2001. LC 00-54579. (Advances in Experimental Medicine & Biology Ser.: Vol. 489). (Illus.). 173p. 90.00 (*0-306-46521-3*, Kluwer Plenum) Kluwer Academic.

Hemopoietic Colony-Stimulating Factors: From Biology to Clinical Applications. Donald Metcalf & Nicos A. Nicola. 1995. (Illus.). 352p. (C). text 90.00 (*0-521-46158-8*) Cambridge U Pr.

Hemopoietic Growth Factors & Mononuclear Phagocytes. Ed. by Ralph Van Furth. 1993. (Illus.). x, 222p. 172.25 (*3-8055-5678-0*) S Karger.

Hemopoietic Growth Factors, Oncogenes & Cytokines in Clinical Hematology: Current Aspects & Future Directions. Ed. by E. Cacciola et al. 1994. LC 93-40874. (Illus.). viii, 306p. 216.75 (*3-8055-5842-2*) S Karger.

Hemopoietic Growth Factors Symposium. Alexander S. Spiers. 1992. (Hematology Reviews & Communications Ser.). 128p. pap. text 231.00 (*3-7186-5270-6*, Harwood Acad Pubs) Gordon & Breach.

Hemopoietic System. Ed. by Thomas C. Jones et al. 1990. (Monographs in Pathology of Laboratory Animals). (Illus.). 336p. 347.00 (*0-387-52212-3*) Spr-Verlag.

Hemorphins & Ednomorphins: Experimental Studies on Novel Opioid Peptides with Emphasis on Procesing & Modulation of Pain & Inflammation. Katarina Sanderson Nydahl. 2000. (Comprehensive Summaries of Uppsala Dissertations from the Faculty of Pharmacy Ser.: 219). (Illus.). 70p. (Orig.). pap. (*91-554-4626-4*) Uppsala Universitet SWE. *Dist:* Coronet Bks.

Hemorrhagic Fever with Renal Syndrome, Tick- & Mosquito-Borne Viruses, Supplementum 1: Archives of Virology. C. H. Calisher. 1991. (Illus.). 347p. 206.00 (*0-387-82217-8*) Spr-Verlag.

Hemorrhoids: A Book for Silent Sufferers. Jager Rama. 1990. 164p. pap. 8.95 (*0-9625295-0-8*) Colon & Rectal Care.

Hemorrhoids: A Cure & Preventative. Michael Mitchell. 4th ed. 1997. LC 77-86391. (Illus.). 196p. reprint ed. 19.95 (*0-930926-25-0*) Calif Fin Pubns.

Hemostasis: A Case Oriented Approach. Douglas A. Triplett. 1985. LC 83-2654. (Illus.). 331p. 45.00 (*0-89640-099-9*) Igaku-Shoin.

Hemostasis & Animal Venoms. Hubert Pirkle. Ed. by Francis S. Markland, Jr. 1988. (Hematology Ser.: Vol. 7). (Illus.). 658p. text 275.00 (*0-8247-7806-5*) Dekker.

Hemostasis & Cancer. Ed. by Laszo Muzbek. 1987. 280p. 159.00 (*0-8493-5754-3*, RC262, CRC Reprint) Franklin.

Hemostasis & Circulation. Ed. by Akikazy Takada & A. Z. Budzynski. 1992. LC 92-2218. (Illus.). 224p. 64.95 (*0-387-70096-X*) Spr-Verlag.

Hemostasis & Stroke. Ed. by Christof M. Kessler & Axel Rosengart. 1994. LC 94-5153. 176p. 102.00 (*0-8493-7650-5*) CRC Pr.

Hemostasis & Thrombosis: A Conceptual Approach. Jack Hirsh & Elizabeth A. Brain. 2nd ed. 1983. LC 82-19726. (Illus.). 164p. pap. text (*0-443-08220-0*) Church.

Hemostasis & Thrombosis: Basic Principles & Clinical Practice. Robert W. Colman et al. 4th ed. 2000. LC 99-86649. (Illus.). xix, 1578p. text 299.00 (*0-7817-1455-9*) Lppncott W & W.

Hemostasis & Thrombosis Protocols. Ed. by David J. Perry & K. John Pasi. 1999. LC 99-10466. (Methods in Molecular Medicine Ser.: Vol. 31). (Illus.). 384p. 99.50 (*0-89603-419-4*) Humana.

Hemostasis in Cardiac Surgery. Ed. by Safuh Attar. 1999. LC 98-31869. (Illus.). 13p. 59.00 (*0-87993-410-7*) Futura Pub.

Hemostatic Mechanisms & Metastasis. Ed. by Kenneth V. Honn & Bonnie F. Sloane. 1984. (Developments in Oncology Ser.). text 159.50 (*0-89838-667-5*) Kluwer Academic.

Hemp for Health: The Nutritional & Medicinal Uses of the World's Most Extraordinary Plant. Chris Conrad. 1997. LC 96-51628. (Illus.). 160p. pap. 14.95 (*0-89281-539-6*, Heal Arts VT) Inner Tradit.

Hendrick, E. B., Festschrift: Journal: Pediatric Neurosurgery, Vol. 16, Nos. 4-5, 1990-1991. Ed. by R. P. Humphreys. 1992. (Illus.). 96p. pap. 45.25 (*3-8055-5580-6*) S Karger.

Henkes History of Ophthalmology, Vol. 6. Harold E. Henkes. 1994. pap. text 85.50 (*0-7923-3101-X*) Kluwer Academic.

Henry Ford Hospital: The First 75 Years. Patricia S. Painter. 1997. 20.00 (*0-9659494-0-0*) H F Hlth Syst.

Hep-Cats, Narcs, & Pipe Dreams: A History of America's Romance with Illegal Drugs. Jill Jonnes. 1999. LC 99-17266. (Illus.). 520p. pap. 18.95 (*0-8018-6165-9*) Johns Hopkins.

Hepadnaviruses: Molecular Biololgy & Pathogenesis. Ed. by Michael B. Oldstone et al. 1991. (Current Topics in Microbiology & Immunology Ser.: Vol. 168). (Illus.). 206p. 138.00 (*0-387-53060-6*) Spr-Verlag.

Heparan Sulfate Proteoglycans in Malignant Cells. Kris Nackaerts. 1998. (Acta Biomedica Lovaniensia Ser.). (Illus.). 127p. pap. (*90-6186-891-2*) Leuven Univ BEL. *Dist:* Coronet Bks.

Heparin. David A. Lane. 1989. 143.00 (*0-8493-7100-7*, R) CRC Pr.

Heparin: New Biochemical & Medical Aspects: Proceedings. Deutsche Gesellschaft fur Klinishe Chemie Symposiu. Ed. by Irene Witt. 1983. xvi, 372p. 119.25 (*3-11-008637-9*) De Gruyter.

Heparin - Present & Future. Ed. by Neri Serneri. 1990. (Journal: Vol. 20, Suppl. 2, 1990). vi, 226p. pap. 69.75 (*3-8055-5277-7*) S Karger.

***Hepatic & Peritoneal Colorectal Metastases: Aspects of Prognosis & Treatment.** Haile Mahteme. 2001. (Comprehensive Summaries of Uppsala Dissertations from the Faculty of Medicine Ser.: No. 987). (Illus.). 70p. pap. (*91-554-4912-3*) Uppsala Universitet SWE. *Dist:* Coronet Bks.

Hepatic Encephalopathy. Ed. by K. Mullen & Peter Ferenci. 1996. (Illus.). iv, 64p. pap. 21.75 (*3-8055-6358-2*) S Karger.

Hepatic Encephalopathy: Pathophysiology & Treatment. Ed. by Roger F. Butterworth et al. 1989. LC 89-20039. (Experimental Biology & Medicine Ser.: Vol. 22). 640p. 146.50 (*0-89603-164-0*) Humana.

Hepatic Encephalopathy: Syndromes & Therapies. Ed. by Harold O. Conn & Johannes Bircher. 1994. LC 93-36530. 430p. text 63.95 (*0-936741-04-X*) Medi-Ed Pr.

Hepatic Encephalopathy, Hyperammonemia & Ammonia Toxicity. Ed. by Vicente Felipo & Santiago Grisolia. 1995. (Advances in Experimental Medicine & Biology Ser.: Vol. 368). (Illus.). 228p. (C). text 85.00 (*0-306-44985-4*, Kluwer Plenum) Kluwer Academic.

Hepatic Metabolism & Disposition of Endo- & Xenobiotics. Ed. by K. W. Bock et al. 1991. (Falk Symposium Ser.). xii, 324 p. (C). text 225.50 (*0-7923-8953-0*) Kluwer Academic.

Hepatic Metastases: Diagnosis & Management. D. L. Morris et al. Ed. by Gary M. Onik. 1996. LC 95-7176. (Illus.). 224p. text 115.00 (*0-7506-0879-X*) Buttrwrth-Heinemann.

Hepatic Non-Parenchymal Cells & Their Role in Disease. P. Thomas. 1997. (Medical Intelligence Unit Ser.). 200p. (C). 89.95 (*0-412-10851-8*) Chapman & Hall.

Hepatic Transplantation. Williams. 1989. 256p. text 155.00 (*0-7216-2502-9*) Saunders.

Hepatic Transplantation: Anesthetic & Perioperative Management. Ed. by Peter M. Winter & Yoo G. Kang. 1986. LC 85-28319. 279p. 75.00 (*0-275 92129-8*, C2129, Praeger Pubs) Greenwood.

Hepatic Transport of Organic Substances. Ed. by E. Petzinger et al. 1989. (Illus.). 435p. 112.00 (*0-387-50494-X*) Spr-Verlag.

Hepatitis A. Ed. by Ian D. Gust & Stephen M. Feinstone. 1988. 256p. 143.00 (*0-8493-5767-5*, QR201, CRC Reprint) Franklin.

Hepatitis A to G: The Facts You Need to Know about All Forms of This Dangerous Disease. Alan Berkman & Nicholas Bakalar. 2000. LC 00-700025. (Illus.). 224p. mass mkt. (*0-446-60832-7*) Warner.

***Hepatitis A to G: The Facts You Need to Know about All the Forms of This Dangerous Disease.** Alan Berkman & Nicholas Bakalar. 2001. LC 2001-17543. 214p. pap. (*0-446-67723-X*) Warner.

Hepatitis A Virus Transmission by Blood Products. Ed. by C. Prowse et al. 1994. (Vox Sanguinis: Vol. 67, Supplement 1, 1994). (Illus.). iv, 86p. pap. 39.25 (*3-8055-6006-0*) S Karger.

Hepatitis B Vaccines in Clinical Practice. Ronald W. Ellis. 1992. (Infectious Disease & Therapy Ser.: Vol. 7). (Illus.). 440p. text 225.00 (*0-8247-8780-3*) Dekker.

Hepatitis B Virus: Molecular Mechanisms in Disease & Novel Strategies for Therapy. Ed. by Rajen Koshy & Wolfgang H. Caselmann. 1998. LC 98-23905. 340p. reprint ed. (*1-86094-007-2*) Imperial College GBR. *Dist:* World Scientific Pub.

Hepatitis B Virus Vol. 38, No. 1-2: Selected Topics. Ed. by Wolfram H. Gerlich. 1995. (Journal: Vol. 38, Nos. 1 & 2, 1995). (Illus.). 120p. pap. 76.50 (*3-8055-6252-7*) S Karger.

Hepatitis B Virus & Primary Liver Cancer. Ed. by Joseph L. Melnick & P. Maupas. 1981. (Progress in Medical Virology Ser.: Vol. 27). (Illus.). viii, 212p. 108.75 (*3-8055-1784-X*) S Karger.

Hepatitis C. John Gallin. 2000. LC 00-102552. (Biomedical Research Reports: Vol. 2). (Illus.). xxi, 493p. 99.95 (*0-12-447870-0*) Morgan Kaufmann.

Hepatitis C: A Personal Guide to Good Health. Beth A. Petro Roybal. 2nd ed. 1999. LC 00-500854. (Illus.). 168p. pap. 13.95 (*1-56975-183-8*) Ulysses Pr.

Hepatitis C: Directory of New Medical & Scientific Reviews with Subject Index. Science and Life Consultants Association Staff. 1997. 151p. 57.50 (*0-7883-1620-6*); 1997. 151p. pap. 47.50 (*0-7883-1621-4*); 1995. 160p. 49.50 (*0-7883-0570-0*); 1995. 160p. pap. 34.50 (*0-7883-0571-9*) ABBE Pubs Assn.

Hepatitis C: Practical, Medical & Spiritual Guidelines for Daily Living with HCV. Mark Jenkins. 2000. LC 99-58532. (Hazelden Pocket Health Guides). xxiii, 151p. pap. 12.00 (*1-56838-368-1*) Hazelden.

Hepatitis C Handbook. Matthew Dolan. rev. ed. 1999. LC 98-52148. 400p. pap. 25.00 (*1-55643-313-1*) Frog Ltd CA.

Hepatitis C Protocols. Johnson Y. N. Lau. 1998. LC 98-24896. (Methods in Molecular Medicine Ser.: Vol. 19). 648p. 109.50 (*0-89603-521-2*) Humana.

Hepatitis C Virus. Ed. by H. W. Reesink. (Current Studies in Hematology & Blood Transfusion: No. 61). (Illus.). 1994. viii, 212p. 210.50 (*3-8055-5866-X*); 2nd rev. ed. 1998. LC 97-41314. x, 270p. 172.25 (*3-8055-6542-9*) S Karger.

Hepatitis C Virus & Its Involvement in the Development of Heptocellar Carcinoma: 25th International Symposium. Ed. by Kenichi Kobayashi et al. 1996. (Proceedings of the Princess Takamatsu Cancer Research Fund Ser.). (Illus.). 282p. text 75.00 (*0-911131-60-4*) Specialist Journals.

Hepatitis C Viruses. Ed. by C. H. Hagedorn & C. M. Rice. 1999. (Current Topics in Microbiology & Immunology Ser.: Vol. 242). (Illus.). 220p. 239.00 (*3-540-65358-9*) Spr-Verlag.

Hepatitis Delta Virus. Ed. by Gail Dinter-Gottlieb. 1995. (Medical Intelligence Unit Ser.). 140p. text 79.00 (*1-57059-144-X*) Landes Bioscience.

Hepatitis E: Index of New Information. Marcus Stevenson. Date not set. 160p. 57.50 (*0-7883-1930-2*); pap. 47.50 (*0-7883-1931-0*) ABBE Pubs Assn.

Hepatitis Viruses. 1994. (IARC Scientific Publications Ser.: Vol. 59). 286p. pap. text 65.00 (*92-832-1259-2*, 1720059) World Health.

Hepatitis Viruses. Ed. by David E. Bernstein & Maria D. De Medina. 7th rev. ed. 1998. (Illus.). 79p. pap. text 25.00 (*1-879772-11-6*) Health Studies.

***Hepatobiliary & Pancreatic Surgery.** Ed. by Leslie H. Blumgart & Graeme J. Poston. 2001. (Illus.). 608p. (*1-899066-97-7*) Isis Med.

Hepatobiliary & Pancreatic Surgery. Ed. by O. James Garden. 1997. (Companion Guide to Specialist Surgical Practice Ser.: Vol. 3). (Illus.). 380p. text (*0-7020-2142-3*) W B Saunders GBR. *Dist:* Saunders.

Hepatobiliary & Pancreatic Surgery. David Carter. 5th ed. 1996. 688p. (*0-412-61930-X*) E A GBR. *Dist:* OUP.

***Hepatobiliary & Pancreatic Surgery: A Companion to Specialist Surgical Practice.** O. James Garden. 2nd ed. 2001. (Illus.). 415p. pap. (*0-7020-2592-5*) W B Saunders GBR. *Dist:* Saunders.

Hepatobiliary & Pancreatic Surgery: Imaging Strategies & Surgical Decision-Making. Stephen R. Evans & Susan M. Ascher. 1997. LC 97-37513. 589p. 170.00 (*0-471-14755-9*, Wiley-Liss) Wiley.

Hepatobiliary Cancer. Leslie H. Blumgart et al. 2000. (ACS Atlas of Clinical Oncology Ser.). 300p. incl. cd-rom (*1-55009-132-8*) DEKR.

Hepatobiliary Cancer. Ed. by Paul H. Sugarbaker. 1994. LC 93-33050. (Cancer Treatment & Research Ser.: No. 69). 352p. (C). text 290.00 (*0-7923-2501-X*) Kluwer Academic.

Hepatobiliary Diseases. Ed. by J. Prieto et al. 1992. LC 91-5205. (Illus.). 1128p. 207.00 (*0-387-54326-0*) Spr-Verlag.

Hepatobiliary Imaging & Pancreatic Radiology: Imaging & Intervention. G. Scott Gazelle et al. 1997. LC 97-30186. (Illus.). 752p. 169.00 (*0-86577-716-0*) Thieme Med Pubs.

Hepatobiliary Malignancy: Its Multidisciplinary Management. Ed. by John Terblanch. 1994. (An Arnold Publication). (Illus.). 690p. (*0-340-58898-5*) E A GBR. *Dist:* OUP.

Hepatobiliary, Pancreatic & Splenic Disease in Children: Medical & Surgical Management. Ed. by W. F. Balistreri et al. 1997. LC 97-901. 632p. 225.00 (*0-444-82052-3*) Elsevier.

Hepatocelluar Carcinoma: Proceedings of the "Takahashi Memorial Forum", Held in Tokyo, Japan, 2 November, 1996, Vol. 3. Masami L. Yamanaka et al. 1997. LC 97-43447. (Progress in Hepatology Ser.). 156p. 137.50 (*0-444-82678-5*) Elsevier.

Hepatocellular Carcinoma. T. Nakashima & M. Kojiro. 1987. (Illus.). 267p. 312.00 (*0-387-70018-8*) Spr-Verlag.

Hepatocellular Carcinoma. Ed. by J. Y. Wong & S. T. Fan. 1995. (Journal: Vol. 12, No. 1, 1995). (Illus.). 86p. pap. 50.50 (*3-8055-6190-3*) S Karger.

Hepatocellular Carcinoma: Diagnosis Investigation & Management. Anthony S. Leong et al. 1999. LC 99-24540. (An Arnold Publication). (Illus.). 304p. (*0-340-74096-5*) E A GBR. *Dist:* OUP.

Hepatocellular Carcinoma: Methods & Protocols. Ed. by Nagy A. Habib. 2000. (Methods in Molecular Medicine Ser.: Vol. 45). 350p. 110.00 (*0-89603-785-1*) Humana.

Hepatocellular Carcinoma & Liver Metastases Diagnosis & Treatment. Henri-Marcel Hoogewoud. 1993. LC 92-48503. (Illus.). 111p. 69.95 (*0-387-56272-9*) Spr-Verlag.

Hepatocellular Proliferative Process. Ed. by L. Pollice. 1988. (Journal: Vol. 6, No. 2, 1988). (Illus.). 88p. pap. 50.50 (*3-8055-4788-9*) S Karger.

Hepatocyte: Kupfer Cell Interactions. Timothy R. Billiar. 1992. 320p. lib. bdg. 225.00 (*0-8493-6109-5*, RC846) CRC Pr.

Hepatocyte Transplantation: Tissue Engineering. Ed. by M. Mito & M. Sawa. 1998. LC 97-41357. (Systems Publications). (Illus.). xiv, 348p. 139.00 (*3-8055-6603-4*) S Karger.

Hepatology: A Textbook of Liver Disease, Set. David Zakim & Thomas D. Boyer. Ed. by Richard Zorab. 3rd ed. 1996. LC 95-37079. (Illus.). 1664p. text 320.00 (*0-7216-4836-3*) Saunders.

Hepatopancreatoduodenectomy. F. Hanyu. 1997. LC 96-23897. (Illus.). 192p. 115.00 (*4-431-70157-5*) Spr-Verlag.

Hepatotoxicity: The Adverse Effects of Drugs & Other Chemicals on the Liver. Hyman J. Zimmerman. 2nd ed. 1999. LC 99-24990. (Illus.). 800p. text 169.00 (*0-7817-1952-6*) Lppncott W & W.

Hepatoxicology. Ed. by Robert G. Meeks. 1991. 712p. 159.00 (*0-8493-8810-4*, R) CRC Pr.

Heptinstall's Pathology of the Kidney, In Two Volumes. J. Charles Jennette & Jean L. Olson. 5th ed. 1998. LC 97-45779. 1,704p. text 349.00 (*0-7817-1533-4*) Lppncott W & W.

Her Father's Daughter: The Work of Anna Freud. Raymond Dyer. 1983. LC 82-11334. (Her Fathers Daug Wks Anna Freud, CL. Ser.). 352p. 45.00 (*0-87668-627-7*) Aronson.

Her Healthy Heart: A Woman's Guide to Preventing & Reversing Heart Disease Naturally. Linda Ojeda. 1998. LC 98-35412. (Illus.). 352p. 24.95 (*0-89793-226-9*); pap. 14.95 (*0-89793-225-0*) Hunter Hse.

***Her-2: The Making of Herceptin, a Revolutionary Treatment for Breast Cancer.** Robert Bazell. 2001. 214p. 24.00 (*0-7567-5019-9*) DIANE Pub.

Herb Book. John B. Lust. 1974. LC 74-75368. (Illus.). 640p. pap. 8.95 (*0-87904-055-6*, Beneficial Bks) Lust.

Herb Bounty! see Herbal Renaissance

Herb Contraindications & Drug Interactions. Ed. by Kathryn Rosson. 2nd ed. 1998. 260p. reprint ed. pap. 19.95 (*1-888483-07-5*) Eclectic Med.

***Herb Contraindications & Drug Interactions.** Francis Brinker. 3rd expurg. ed. 2001. LC 2001-132481. (Illus.). 440p. pap. 25.95 (*1-888483-11-3*) Eclectic Med.

Herb Contraindications & Drug Interactions: With Appendices Addressing Certain Conditions & Medicines. Francis Brinker. Ed. by Nancy Stodart. 1997. LC 97-61558. 148p. pap. 14.95 (*0-9659135-0-3*) Eclectic Inst.

Herb-Doctors & Physicians in the Ancient World: The Divine Origin of the Craft of the Herbalist. E.A. Wallis Budge. 1978. xii, 96p. pap. 10.00 (*0-89005-252-2*) Ares.

Herb-Drug & Supplement-Drug Interactions Handbook. John Tomera et al. 2000. 400p. pap. 29.95 (*1-930256-00-0*) Integratv Med Commn.

Herb Walk Medicinal Guide: Holistic Medical Procedures, Herbal First-Aid, Comparative Healing Methods & Information on Body Systems & Organs. Mary A. Chai. 1992. (Illus.). 127p. per. 8.95 (*0-935596-01-1*) LM Pubns.

Herbal & Folk Medicine of Louisiana & the South. Samuel J. Touchstone. rev. ed. 1993. 195p. pap. text 8.95 (*0-914917-13-7*) Folk-Life.

Herbal & Magical Medicine: Traditional Healing Today. Ed. by James Kirkland et al. 1992. LC 91-25003. 252p. text 54.95 (*0-8223-1208-5*); pap. text 19.95 (*0-8223-1217-4*) Duke.

Herbal Antibiotics. Stephen Harrod Buhner. 1999. LC 99-33056. (Storey Medicinal Herb Guide Ser.). (Illus.). 144p. pap. 12.95 (*1-58017-148-6*) Storey Bks.

Herbal Birth Control: A Brief History with Ancient & Modern Herbal Recipes. R. R. McGregor. 1993. (Illus.). 64p. (Orig.). pap. 10.00 (*0-9636602-0-9*) Cloud Chief.

Herbal Companion to AHFS DI 2001. 2000. 188p. pap. 39.95 (*1-58528-017-8*) Am Soc Hlth-Syst.

Herbal Connection. Dan Ostrander. 1996. 145p. (Orig.). pap. 9.95 (*0-9653302-0-6*) D Ostrander.

Herbal Defense: Positioning Yourself to Truimph over Illness & Aging. Ed. by Robyn Landis & Karta P. Khalsa. 1997. LC 97-1817. 562p. pap. (*0-446-67242-4*) Warner.

Herbal Drugs & Phytopharmaceuticals. Ed. by Max Wichtl & Norman G. Bisset. Tr. by Norman G. Bisset from GER. 1994. 568p. 190.00 (*0-8493-7192-9*, V7192) CRC Pr.

Herbal Elixirs of Life. Raymond Bernard. 1996. 31p. reprint ed. spiral bd. 8.50 (*0-7873-0096-9*) Hlth Research.

Herbal Emissaries: Bringing Chinese Herbs to the West. Steven Foster & Yue Chongxi. 1992. LC 92-1054. 336p. pap. 16.95 (*0-89281-349-0*, Heal Arts VT) Inner Tradit.

Herbal Guide to Stress Relief: Gentle Remedies & Techniques for Healing & Calming the Nervous System. David Hoffmann. 1991. 192p. reprint ed. pap. 12.95 (*0-89281-426-8*, Heal Arts VT) Inner Tradit.

Herbal Handbook: A User's Guide to Medical Herbalism. David Hoffmann. rev. ed. 1998. 240p. pap. 14.95 (*0-89281-782-8*, Heal Arts VT) Inner Tradit.

Herbal Healing for Women: Simple Home Remedies for Women of All Ages. Rosemary Gladstar. 1993. LC 94-186091. 304p. pap. 13.00 (*0-671-76767-4*, Fireside) S&S Trade Pap.

Herbal Healing Rapid Reference. Brent Davis. 2001. 158p. per. 12.95 (*1-890612-21-9*) Vital Health.

Herbal Healing Secrets of the Orient. Darlena L'Orange. 1998. LC 97-41799. (Illus.). 352p. (C). text 26.95 (*0-13-849324-3*) P-H.

Herbal Health. Dorothy Decorso. 1995. (Home Herbalist Ser.). (Illus.). 64p. (*0-85091-649-6*) Lothian Pub AUS. *Dist:* Seven Hills Bk.

Herbal Home Companion. Theresa Loe. 1996. LC 96-213928. 256p. pap. 14.00 (*1-57566-085-7*, Knsington) Kensgtn Pub Corp.

Herbal Home Health Care. John R. Christopher. 2nd ed. 1976. LC 90-205302. (Illus.). 196p. per. 12.95 (*1-879436-03-5*, 99103) Christopher Pubns.

***Herbal Internet Companion: Herbs & Herbal Medicine Online.** David J. Owen. 2001. LC 2001-39562. 194p. (C). pap. 19.95 (*0-7890-1052-6*, Haworth Info Pr) Haworth Pr.

Herbal Knowledge. Clive Buchanan. 1996. 14.95 (*1-885670-05-2*) Woodland UT.

Herbal Medicinals: A Clinician's Guide. Ed. by Lucinda G. Miller & Wallace J. Murray. 1998. LC 98-12043. 383p. pap. 39.95 (*0-7890-0467-4*, Pharmctl Prods); (Illus.). 59.95 (*0-7890-0466-6*, Hawrth Medical) Haworth Pr.

Herbal Medicine. Anne McIntyre. 1993. (Alternative Health Ser.). (Illus.). 128p. pap. 12.95 (*0-8048-1837-1*) Tuttle Pubng.

Herbal Medicine. Rudolf F. Weiss. 1988.Tr. of Lehrbuch der Phytotherapie. (Illus.). 386p. pap. (*0-906584-19-1*) Beaconsfield GBR. *Dist:* Medicina Bio.

Herbal Medicine. R. F. Weiss & V. Fintelmann. 2nd ed.Tr. of Lehrbuch der Phytotherapie. (Illus.). 500p. 2001. pap. 29.00 (*0-86577-933-3*); 2000. 59.00 (*0-86577-970-8*) Thieme Med Pubs.

Herbal Medicine: A Concise Overview for Professionals. Ed. by Edzard Ernst. 2000. LC 99-56378. (Illus.). 120p. pap. text 36.00 (*0-7506-4540-7*) Buttrwrth-Heinemann.

Herbal Medicine: Documents, Proceedings & Recommendations of the International Symposium on Herbal Medicine. San Diego State University Staff & University of Hawaii Staff. 1998. 45.00 (*1-879167-05-0*); pap. 25.00 (*1-879167-06-9*) SDSU Coll Hlth Hum Servs.

Herbal Medicine: Expanded Commission E Monographs. Alicia Goldberg. Ed. by Mark Blumenthal & Josef Brinckmann. 1999. (Illus.). 519p. 51.95 (*0-9670772-1-4*) Integratv Med Commn.

Herbal Medicine: Principles & Practice. Christopher Robbins. 2001. 256p. pap. 63.00 (*0-7506-4541-5*) Buttrwrth-Heinemann.

Herbal Medicine: Safe & Effective Treatment of Children. Anne McIntyre. 2002. 192p. pap. 29.95 (*0-7506-5174-1*) Buttrwrth-Heinemann.

Herbal Medicine: The Use of Herbs for Health & Healing. Vicki Pitman. 1995. LC 94-23421. (Health Essentials Ser.). 128p. pap. 9.95 (*1-85230-591-6*) Element MA.

Herbal Medicine for Human Health. R. R. Chaudhury. 1992. (WHO Regional Publications: No. 20). ix, 87p. pap. text 8.00 (*92-9022-162-3*, 1560020) World Health.

Herbal Medicine for the Primary Health Care Team. Sue Eldin et al. 1999. LC 99-13063. 180p. pap. text 39.95 (*0-7506-4053-7*) Buttrwrth-Heinemann.

Herbal Medicine from the Heart of the Earth. Sharol Tilgner. 1999. LC 99-91002. (Illus.). 384p. pap. (*1-881517-02-0*) Wise Acres.

Herbal Medicine Maker's Handbook: A Home Manual. James Green. 2000. LC 00-30708. (Illus.). 384p. pap. 18.95 (*0-89594-990-3*) Crossing Pr.

Herbal Medicine Past & Present: A Reference Guide to Medicinal Plants, 2. John K. Crellin & Jane Philpott. 1989. LC 97-17089. 560p. (Orig.). text 69.95 (*0-8223-0879-7*) Duke.

Herbal Medicine Past & Present, Vol. 1: Trying to Give Ease. John K. Crellin & Jane Philpott. 1989. LC 97-15490. 347p. text 39.95 (*0-8223-0877-0*) Duke.

Herbal Medicines. 1996. 296p. (*0-85369-289-0*) Pharmaceutical Pr GBR. *Dist:* Rittenhouse.

***Herbal Medicines: A Guide for Health-Care Professionals.** 2nd ed. 2002. cd-rom (*0-85369-500-8*) Pharmaceutical Pr GBR. *Dist:* Rittenhouse.

Herbal Medicines Biodiversity & Conservation Strategies. M. K. Rai & Rajak. 1996. pap. (*81-7089-221-X*) Intl Bk Distr IND. *Dist:* St Mut.

Herbal Medicines for Neuropsychiatric Diseases: Current Developments & Research. Kanba Shigenobu. 1999. LC 98-45054. 29.95 (*0-87630-804-3*) Brunner-Routledge.

Herbal Menopause Book: Herbs, Nutrition & Other Natural Therapies. Amanda M. Crawford. 1996. (Illus.). 224p. (Orig.). pap. 16.95 (*0-89594-799-4*) Crossing Pr.

Herbal Poetry Book of Medicinal Uses, Bk. 1. Alpha Pyramis Research Division Staff. 1992. 11p. pap. text 7.95 (*0-913597-54-6*) Prosperity & Profits.

Herbal Preparations & Natural Therapies: Creating & Using a Home Herbal Medicine Chest. Debra N. St. Claire. 1989. (Illus.). 140p. (Orig.). pap., stu. ed. 149.00 incl. VHS (*0-9623812-0-9*) Mrngstar Pubns.

Herbal Prescriptions for Better Health: Your Up-to-Date Guide to the Most Effective Herbal Treatments. Donald J. Brown. 1997. (Illus.). 368p. pap. 16.00 (*0-7615-1001-X*) Prima Pub.

Herbal Prescriptions for Health & Healing: Your Everyday Guide to Using Herbs Safely & Effectively. Donald J. Brown. 8th ed. 2000. LC 00-45287. (Illus.). 464p. pap. 24.95 (*0-7615-2410-X*, Prima Health) Prima Pub.

Herbal Remedies. Ed. by Peter Albright. 1996. LC 95-37892. (Naturally Better Bks.). (Illus.). 64p. pap. 12.95 (*0-02-860834-8*) Hungry Minds.

Herbal Remedies. Andrew Weil. 1998. mass mkt. 2.99 (*0-8041-1811-6*) Ivy Books.

Herbal Remedies: An Introductory Guide to Herbs for Health & Well-Being. Vicki Pitman. 2000. (New Perspectives Ser.). (Illus.). 128p. pap. (*1-86204-767-7*) Oneworld.

Herbal Remedies: Chinese. 1992. lib. bdg. 78.95 (*0-8490-5397-8*) Gordon Pr.

Herbal Remedies: Harmful & Beneficial Effects. S. Talalaj & A. S. Czechowicz. 1994. 387p. (Orig.). pap. (*0-85572-189-8*) Hill Content Pubng AUS. *Dist:* Seven Hills Bk.

Herbal Remedies: The Complete Guide to Natural Healing. Jill Nice. 1996. pap. text (*0-7499-1090-9*) Piatkus Bks GBR. *Dist:* London Brdge.

Herbal Remedies Approved for Modern Uses of Cure. William Thomas Fernie. 1977. lib. bdg. 59.95 (*0-8490-1940-0*) Gordon Pr.

Herbal Remedies for Dummies. Christopher Hobbs. 1998. LC 98-88386. (For Dummies Ser.). (Illus.). 384p. pap. 19.99 (*0-7645-5127-2*) Hungry Minds.

Herbal Remedies for Healing: A Complete A-Z of Ailments & Treatments. Jill Nice. 1999. (Illus.). 256p. pap. (*0-7499-1840-3*) Piatkus Bks GBR. *Dist:* London Brdge.

Herbal Remedies for Insomnia. 1996. lib. bdg. 250.95 (*0-8490-5907-0*) Gordon Pr.

Herbal Remedies for Women: Discover Nature's Wonderful Secrets Just for Women. Amanda M. Crawford. 1997. LC 97-7653. 304p. pap. 19.95 (*0-7615-0980-1*, Prima Health) Prima Pub.

Herbal Remedies Handbook: Essential Tips. Andrew Chevallier. 2001. LC 00-45195. (Healing Handbooks Ser.). (Illus.). 128p. pap. 12.95 (*0-7894-7177-9*) DK Pub Inc.

Herbal Remedies in Pots. Effie Romain & Sue Hawkey. 1996. LC 95-44392. (Illus.). 96p. pap. 16.95 (*0-7894-0431-1*) DK Pub Inc.

Herbal Remedy for Prostate Cancer. James Lewis. 2000. LC 99-37184. 216p. pap. 18.95 (*1-883257-02-6*) Hlth Edu Lit.

Herbal Renaissance. Steven Foster. rev. ed. 1993. Orig. Title: Herb Bounty!. (Illus.). 240p. reprint ed. pap. 21.95 (*0-87905-523-5*) Gibbs Smith Pub.

Herbal Rituals. Judith Berger. 1999. (Illus.). 256p. pap. 12.95 (*0-312-24301-4*) St Martin.

Herbal Teas. C. J. Puotinen. Ed. by Phyllis Herman. 1996. (Good Health Guides). 48p. pap. 3.95 (*0-87983-707-1*, 37071K, Keats Pubng) McGraw-Hill Trade.

Herbal Teas for Health & Pleasure. D. Law. 1980. 40.00 (*0-85032-020-8*) St Mut.

Herbal Therapy for Women. Elisabeth Brooke. 1993. 160p. (*0-7225-2722-5*) Thorsons.

Herbal Tonic Therapies. Daniel B. Mowrey. 1993. LC 93-3022. (Illus.). 400p. pap. 14.95 (*0-87983-565-6*, 35656K, Keats Pubng) McGraw-Hill Trade.

Herbal Tonic Therapies. Daniel B. Mowrey. 1996. LC 96-14551. 416p. 10.99 (*0-517-18241-6*) Random Hse Value.

Herbalism: The Healing Power of Plants - Regional Traditions, Remedies & Recipes. Frank J. Lipp. 2000. (Illus.). 184p. (*1-900131-04-8*) D Baird Pubs GBR. *Dist:* Trafalgar.

Herbalist. Michael J. Katz. 1992. 288p. (C). pap. 38.50 (*0-8191-8553-1*) U Pr of Amer.

Herbalist. J. E. Mayer. 1992. (Alternative Medicine Ser.). lib. bdg. 79.99 (*0-8490-5409-5*) Gordon Pr.

***Herbert Rosenfeld at Work: The Italian Seminars.** Herbert Rosenfeld. 2001. 264p. pap. (*1-85575-252-2*) Karnac Bks GBR. *Dist:* Other Pr LLC.

Herbicides: Chemistry, Degradation, & Mode of Action, Vol. 3. Philip C. Kearney. Ed. by Donald D. Kaufman. 1988. (Illus.). 405p. text 185.00 (*0-8247-7804-9*) Dekker.

Herbicides & Plant Growth Regulators Pt. 1. Ed. by T. Roberts. 1998. 864p. (*0-85404-494-9*) Royal Soc Chem GBR. *Dist:* Spr-Verlag.

Herbs. Lesley Bremness. LC 93-26815. (Eyewitness Handbooks Ser.). (Illus.). 304p. (Orig.). 2000. pap. 18.95 (*1-56458-496-8*); 1994. pap. 29.95 (*1-56458-497-6*) DK Pub Inc.

Herbs: Foods, Medicines Or Poisons? 1992. lib. bdg. 79.95 (*0-8490-8804-6*) Gordon Pr.

Herbs Against Cancer. Ralph W. Moss. 1998. LC 98-26261. 216p. pap. text 16.95 (*1-881025-40-3*) Equinox Pr.

Herbs & Aromatherapy for the Reproductive System. Jeanne Rose. 1994. LC 94-19980. 128p. (Orig.). (C). pap. 7.95 (*1-883319-17-X*) Frog Ltd CA.

Herbs & Herbal Medicine. William H. Lee. Ed. by Richard A. Passwater & Earl R. Mindell. 1982. (Good Health Guides). 31p. pap. 3.95 (*0-87983-294-0*, 32940K, Keats Pubng) McGraw-Hill Trade.

Herbs & Old Time Remedies. Joseph VanSeters. 1999. LC 99-93555. 366p. pap. 14.95 (*0-7392-0391-6*, PO3616) Morris Pubng.

Herbs & Weeds. Joh Kuenzle. 1996. 58p. reprint ed. spiral bd. 8.50 (*0-7873-0514-6*) Hlth Research.

Herbs for a Healthy Heart: Strengthen Your Cadiovascular System & Ease Symptoms of Hypertension, Congestive Heart Failure & Angina. David Hoffmann. 2000. LC 00-38793. (Medicinal Herb Guide Ser.). (Illus.). 121p. pap. 12.95 (*1-58017-251-2*) Storey Bks.

Herbs for Children. Rita Elkins. 1997. (Woodland Health Ser.). pap. text 3.95 (*1-885670-42-7*) Woodland UT.

Herbs for Chronic Fatigue. Kathi Keville. 1998. LC 97-43371. (Good Herb Guides). 96p. pap. 4.95 (*0-87983-809-4*, 38094K, Keats Pubng) McGraw-Hill Trade.

Herbs for Common Ailments. Anne McIntyre. 1992. (Illus.). 96p. (Orig.). pap. 12.00 (*0-671-74632-4*, Fireside) S&S Trade Pap.

Herbs for Detoxification. Karen Bradstreet. 1997. (Woodland Health Ser.). 32p. pap. 3.95 (*1-885670-68-0*) Woodland UT.

Herbs for Digestion. Rita Elkins. 1997. (Woodland Health Ser.). 32p. pap. 3.95 (*1-885670-69-9*) Woodland UT.

Herbs for Easy Breathing: Natural Treatments for Asthma, Colds, Flu, Coughs, Allergies & Sinusitus. David Hoffmann. 2000. LC 00-38792. (Medicinal Herb Guide Ser.). (Illus.). 123p. pap. 12.95 (*1-58017-252-0*) Storey Bks.

Herbs for Health. Otto Mausert. 1991. (Longevity Ser.). lib. bdg. 75.00 (*0-8490-4195-3*) Gordon Pr.

Herbs for Health. Otto Mausert. 1996. 200p. reprint ed. spiral bd. 19.00 (*0-7873-0590-1*) Hlth Research.

Herbs for Health: How to Grow & Use Them. Louise E. Doole. 1979. pap. 7.00 (*0-87980-052-6*) Wilshire.

Herbs for Health & Healing. Storey Publishing Staff. pap. 14.95 (*0-676-57352-5*) Random.

Herbs for Healthy Bones & Joints: A Natural Approach to Treating Arthritis, Osteoporosis, Tendinitis, Myalgia & Bursitis. David Hoffmann. 2000. LC 00-38791. (Medicinal Herb Guide Ser.). (Illus.). 121p. pap. 12.95 (*1-58017-253-9*) Storey Bks.

***Herbs for Pets: All You Ever Wanted to Know.** Gregory L. Tilford & Mary Wulff-Tilford. 2001. (Illus.). 384p. pap. 29.95 (*1-889540-64-1*) Bowtie Press.

Herbs for the Reproductive System, with Charts: Herbs for Men & Women, for Health, for Reproduction, Menstrual Regularity & Abortives. Jeanne Rose. 1988. (Illus.). stu. ed. 7.95 (*0-9620838-9-5*, J R Herb Pubns) Herb Studies Library.

Herbs for the Urinary Tract. Michael Moore. 1998. LC 98-15966. (Keats Good Herb Guides). 96p. pap. 4.95 (*0-87983-815-9*, 38159K, Keats Pubng) McGraw-Hill Trade.

Herbs, Helps & Pressure Points for Pregnancy & Childbirth. Katherine Tarr. 4th rev. ed. 1994. (Illus.). 96p. pap. 7.95 (*1-885653-05-0*) W W Whitman.

Herbs in Medicine: Index of New Information. Todd W. Cocchiola. 1998. 57.50 (*0-7883-1812-8*); pap. 47.50 (*0-7883-1813-6*) ABBE Pubs Assn.

Herbs Northwest: A Medicinal Plant Networking Journal. Ed. by Krista Thie. unabr. ed. 1996. (Illus.). 34p. (Orig.). mass mkt. 4.00 (*0-9624868-2-5*) Longevity Herb Pr.

Herbs of Choice: The Therapeutic Use of Phytomedicinals. Varro E. Tyler. 1994. LC 93-41977. 209p. 39.95 (*1-56024-894-7*); pap. 14.95 (*1-56024-895-5*) Haworth Pr.

Herbs of Grace: Becoming Independently Healthy. Farida Sharan. 1994. LC 94-76390. (Illus.). 200p. (Orig.). pap. 23.95 (*1-57093-003-1*) Schl Nat Med.

Herbs of the Rain Forest: Uncovering the Miraculous Medicinal Uses of Rain Forest Herbs. Rita Elkins. 1997. 160p. pap. text 10.95 (*1-885670-65-6*) Woodland UT.

Herbs of Yesterday for Today - Charts: Medicinal Herbs of Yesterday for Today Frank J. Hurd & Rosalie Hurd. 1992. pap. 6.95 (*0-9603532-8-3*) Ten Talents.

Herbs, Spices & Medicinal Plants: Recent Advances in Botany, Horticulture & Pharmacology, Vol. 1. Ed. by Lyle E. Craker & James E. Simon. 1986. LC 85-11551. (Illus.). 368p. lib. bdg. (*0-89774-143-9*) Haworth Pr.

Herbs, Spices & Medicinal Plants: Recent Advances in Botany, Horticulture, & Pharmacology, Vol. 2. Ed. by Lyle E. Craker & James E. Simon. 1987. (Illus.). 272p. (*0-89774-332-6*) Haworth Pr.

Herbs, Spices, & Medicinal Plants: Recent Advances in Botany, Horticulture, & Pharmacology, Vol. 4. Lyle E. Craker & James E. Simon. 1990. 280p. (*0-89774-363-6*) Haworth Pr.

Herbs That Heal. Janet A. Weiner & Michael A. Weiner. 1994. 400p. pap. 18.95 (*0-912845-11-2*) Quantum Bks.

Herbs to Relieve Arthritis. CJ Puotinen. 1996. LC 96-27547. (Keats Good Herb Guides). 96p. (Orig.). mass mkt. 4.95 (*0-87983-743-8*, Keats Pubng) McGraw-Hill Trade.

Herd Health. Hoard's Dairyman Staff. rev. ed. 1993. (Illus.). 100p. (C). pap. text 7.00 (*0-932147-18-6*, Hoards Dairyman) Hoard & Sons Co.

Herd Health: Food, Animal, Production, Medicine. O. M. Radostits et al. 2nd ed. 1993. LC 92-43548. (Illus.). 640p. text 110.00 (*0-7216-3655-1*) Saunders.

Herder-Lexikon Medizin. D. Oeter. 35.00 (*0-8288-7921-4*, M7446) Fr & Eur.

Herder-Lexikon Psychologie. Blumenbrg & Kury. 2nd ed. 1976. (GER.). 239p. pap. 35.00 (*0-8288-5705-9*, M7451) Fr & Eur.

***Here & Now: Inspirational Stories of Cancer Survivors.** Elena Dorfman & Heidi Schultz Adams. 2001. (Illus.). 160p. pap. 22.95 (*1-56924-603-3*) Marlowe & Co.

Here Comes Doctor Ward: A Climb to Glory. Howard E. Cartwright. 1995. (Illus.). 238p. 25.00 (*1-886094-06-3*) Chicago Spectrum.

Here I Stand: Former U. S. Surgeon General on HIV - School-Based Health Care - Adolescent Self-Esteem - Health Care Reform - What Concerned Citizens Can Do. Chester R. Jones. 1997. 125p. pap. 10.00 (*0-9653996-1-3*) Dncng Bear AR.

Hereditary & Acquired Complement Deficiencies in Animals & Man. Ed. by K. Rother & U. Rother. 1987. (Progress in Allergy Ser.: Vol. 39). (Illus.). vi, 406p. 248.75 (*3-8055-4378-6*) S Karger.

Hereditary Bone & Joint Diseases in the Dog: Osteochondroses, Hip Dysplasia, Elbow Dysplasia. Joe Morgan et al. 1997. (Illus.). 300p. text (*3-87706-548-1*) Schlutersche Verlags DEU. *Dist:* Iowa U Pr.

Hereditary Cancer: Second International Research Conference on Familial Cancer, Approaches to Familial Cancer in the 21st Century, Basel, September, 1995. Ed. by H. Muller et al. 1996. LC 96-30501. (Illus.). xii, 234p. 137.50 (*3-8055-6329-9*) S Karger.

Hereditary Cancer & Preventive Surgery. Ed. by W. Weber et al. 1990. (Illus.). x, 118p. 85.25 (*3-8055-5186-X*) S Karger.

Hereditary Diseases & Blood Transfusion: Proceedings of the Nineteenth Annual International Symposium on Blood Transfusion, Groningen, 1994. Ed. by P. C. Das et al. 1995. (Developments in Hematology & Immunology Ser.: Vol. 30). 256p. (C). text 104.50 (*0-7923-3694-1*) Kluwer Academic.

Hereditary Hearing Loss & Its Syndromes. Ed. by Robert J. Gorlin et al. 1995. (Oxford Monographs on Medical Genetics: No. 28). (Illus.). 488p. text 195.00 (*0-19-506552-2*) OUP.

Hereditary Kidney Diseases: Vimercate, September 1996. Ed. by Adalberto Sessa et al. 1997. LC 97-33564. (Contributions to Nephrology Ser.: Vol. 122, 1997). (Illus.). xii, 218p. 199.25 (*3-8055-6551-8*) S Karger.

Hereditary Madness: The Evolution of Psychiatric Genetic Thought. Charles D. Mellon. 1996. LC 96-77792. 172p. (C). 24.95 (*0-9653362-5-5*) Genetics Heritage.

Hereditary Malignant Melanoma. Ed. by Henry T. Lynch. 1991. 128p. 223.00 (*0-8493-6051-X*, RC280, CRC Reprint) Franklin.

Hereditary Nephritis. Ed. by M. Meroni et al. 1990. (Contributions to Nephrology Ser.: Vol. 80). (Illus.). x, 168p. 29.75 (*3-8055-5172-X*) S Karger.

Hereditary Neuropathies & Spinocerebellar Atrophies. Pierre J. Vinken et al. 1992. (Handbooks of Clinical Neurology: Vol. 60(16)). 850p. 349.50 (*0-444-81279-2*) Elsevier.

Hereditary Retinal Degeneration. Ed. by E. Lutejen-Drecoll & E. Zrenner. 1998. (Acta Anatomica Ser.: Vol. 162, No. 2-3 (1998)). (Illus.). 124p. pap. 151.50 (*3-8055-6810-X*) S Karger.

Hereditary Vitreoretinal Degeneration. W. Lisch. 1983. (Developments in Ophthalmology Ser.: Vol. 8). (Illus.). viii, 92p. 56.75 (*3-8055-3615-1*) S Karger.

Heredity: A Psychological Study of Its Phenomena, Laws, Causes, & Consequences. Theodule A. Ribot. LC 78-72821. (Brainedness, Handedness, & Mental Abilities Ser.). reprint ed. 40.00 (*0-404-60890-6*) AMS Pr.

Heredity & Visual Development. Ed. by J. B. Sheffield & S. R. Hilfer. 1985. LC 85-12569. (Cell & Developmental Biology of the Eye Ser.). (Illus.). 214p. 151.00 (*0-387-96180-1*) Spr-Verlag.

Heredity, Environment & Personality: A Study of 850 Sets of Twins. John C. Loehlin & Robert C. Nichols. 1976. LC 75-33794. 214p. (C). 17.50 (*0-292-73003-9*) U of Tex Pr.

Heredity in Relation to Eugenics. Charles B. Davenport. 1972. LC 73-180571. (Medicine & Society in America Ser.). (Illus.). 320p. reprint ed. 24.95 (*0-405-03946-8*) Ayer.

Heredity of Behavior Disorders in Adults & Children. Steven G. Vandenberg et al. 1986. LC 86-15095. (Illus.). 316p. (C). text 90.00 (*0-306-42191-7*, Kluwer Plenum) Kluwer Academic.

Here's How: Health Education by Extension. Ronald S. Seaton & Edith B. Seaton. 1976. LC 76-40599. 123p. pap. 7.99 (*0-87808-150-X*) William Carey Lib.

Heresy: Sandor Rado & the Psychoanalytic Movement. Paul Roazen & Bluma Swerdloff. 1995. LC 94-21882. 232p. 50.00 (*1-56821-321-2*) Aronson.

Heritage. Judy Miller. 1997. LC 98-126346. 260p. pap. 10.95 (*0-942341-13-9*) Dawn Pubns TX.

Heritage Answers for Women: A Guide to Their Menstruation. Elga Stoddard & Nancy Cihylik. 1997. LC 98-92712. (Illus.). 75p. 19.99 (*0-9663791-0-1*) H A W M.

Heritage of Healing: The Story of Baptist Hospital, Nashville, Tennessee, 1918-1998. Ed. by Dimples Kellogg. 1998. LC 98-75321. (Illus.). 160p. 39.95 (*1-57736-124-5*) Providence Hse.

Hermaphrodites & the Medical Invention of Sex. Alice D. Dreger. 1999. LC 97-40487. 320p. text 37.00 (*0-674-08927-8*) HUP.

Hermeneutics & Psychological Theory, Vol. 2: Interpretative Perspectives on Personality, Psychotherapy, & Psychopathology. Ed. by Stanley B. Messer et al. 1988. (Rutgers Symposia on Applied Psychology Ser.). 500p. (C). pap. text 20.00 (*0-8135-1292-1*) Rutgers U Pr.

Hermeneutics of Medicine & the Phenomenology of Health: Steps Towards a Philosophy of Medical Practice. Fredrik Svenaeus. 2001. LC 00-52051. (International Library of Ethics, Law, & the New Medicine: Vol. 5). xi, 201p. (*0-7923-6757-X*) Kluwer Academic.

Hermippus Redivivus. Johann H. Cohausen. Ed. by Robert J. Kastenbaum. 1979. LC 78-22194. (Aging & Old Age Ser.). reprint ed. lib. bdg. 23.95 (*0-405-11811-2*) Ayer.

Hernia. Lloyd M. Nyhus & Robert E. Condon. 4th ed. 1994. (Illus.). 640p. (C). text 179.00 (*0-397-51286-4*, Lippncttt) Lppncott W & W.

Hernia & Surgery of the Abdominal Wall. Ed. by J. P. Chevrel. Tr. by E. Goldstein & N. Marston from FRE. 2nd ed. 1997. LC 97-41300. (Illus.). 300p. 160.00 (*3-540-62749-9*) Spr-Verlag.

Hernia Repair: Open vs. Laparoscopic Approaches. Guy J. Maddern et al. 1997. LC 97-133. text (*0-443-05523-8*) Church.

Hernia-Simple & Complex: Index of New Information & Medical Research Bible. Salvatore L. Leeds. 1994. 150p. 57.50 (*0-7883-0136-5*); pap. 47.50 (*0-7883-0137-3*) ABBE Pubs Assn.

Heroes, Rogues & Lovers: Testosterone & Behavior. James M. Dabbs et al. 2000. LC 00-55888. (Illus.). 256p. text 24.95 (*0-07-135739-4*) McGraw-Hill Prof.

Heroic Self: Sociological Dimensions of Clinical Practice. C. Margaret Hall. 1998. LC 98-11405. 168p. text 41.95 (*0-398-06864-X*); pap. text 28.95 (*0-398-06865-8*) C C Thomas.

Heroin: The Junk Equation. Jim Parker. rev. ed. 2000. pap. 0.50 (*0-89230-164-3*) Do It Now.

Heroin: The Street Narcotic. Fred Zackon & William E. McAulyfe. 1987. LC 85-31440. (Encyclopedia of Psychoactive Drugs Ser.: No. 1). (Illus.). 124p. (YA). (gr. 7-11). lib. bdg. 19.95 (*0-87754-769-6*) Chelsea Hse.

Heroin Addiction: Theory, Research & Treatment, Vol. 1. Jerome J. Platt. 2nd ed. 1989. LC 88-13253. 464p. (C). reprint ed. lib. bdg. 46.50 (*0-89464-325-8*) Krieger.

Heroin Addiction Vol. 2: Theory, Research & Treatment: The Addict, the Treatment Process, & Social Control. Jerome J. Platt. 1995. LC 83-19584. 288p. (C). 37.50 (*0-89464-267-7*) Krieger.

Heroin Addiction & Drug Policy: The British System. Ed. by John Strang & Michael Gossop. 1994. LC 93-42495. (Illus.). 384p. 95.00 (*0-19-262046-0*) OUP.

Heroin in the Age of Crack-Cocaine. James A. Inciardi & Lana D. Harrison. 1998. LC 97-21226. (Drugs, Health, & Social Policy Ser.). 63.95 (*0-7619-0423-9*, 2617); pap. 31.95 (*0-7619-0424-7*, 2618) Sage.

Herophilus: The Art of Medicine in Early Alexandria. Heinrich Von Staden. 1989. 712p. text 150.00 (*0-521-23646-0*) Cambridge U Pr.

Herpes. Jennifer James. 1999. pap. 0.50 (*0-89230-189-9*) Do It Now.

Herpes: A Nutritional Approach. Louise Tenney. 1987. (Woodland Health Ser.: No. 7). 30p. pap. 3.95 (*0-913923-60-5*) Woodland UT.

Herpes Controlled: New Drugs, New Strategies, New Solutions. Jerry O. Stern et al. Ed. by Michael V. Reitano & Lawrence Corey. 1999. (Sexual Health Home Library). (Illus.). 160p. pap. 19.95 (*0-9666416-0-4*) Sexual Health Mag.

Herpes Hoax. 1992. lib. bdg. 69.00 (*0-8490-8809-7*) Gordon Pr.

Herpes Simplex. T. Natasha Posner. 1998. LC 97-17152. (Experience of Illness Ser.). (Illus.). 160p. (C). pap. 26.95 (*0-415-10744-X*) Routledge.

Herpes Simplex & Pseudorabies Viruses. A. S. Kaplan. 1969. (Virology Monographs: Vol. 5). (Illus.). 35.00 (*0-387-80932-5*) Spr-Verlag.

Herpes Simplex Virus Protocols. Ed. by S. Moira Brown & Alasdair R. MacLean. 1997. LC 97-35999. (Methods in Molecular Medicine Ser.: Vol. 10). (Illus.). 432p. 109.50 (*0-89603-347-3*) Humana.

Herpes Virus of Man & Animal: Standardization of Immunological Procedures. Ed. by M. Bonneau & W. Hennessen. 1983. (Developments in Biological Standardization Ser.: Vol. 52). (Illus.). x, 574p. pap. 61.00 (*3-8055-3636-4*) S Karger.

Herpes Viruses, Vol. 5. I. Barinsky & S. Cheshik. 1993. (Soviet Medical Reviews Series, Section E: Virology Review: Vol. 5, Pt. 2). 165p. pap. text 239.00 (*3-7186-5394-X*) Gordon & Breach.

Herpes Zoster & Postherpetic Neuralgia. Ed. by C. Peter Watson. 1993. LC 93-4246. (Pain Research & Clinical Management Ser.: Vol. 8). 286p. 224.00 (*0-444-89271-0*) Elsevier.

Herpesvirus: Recent Studies, Vol. 1. Joseph A. Bellanti et al. 1974. LC 73-13558. 156p. (C). text 25.50 (*0-8422-7164-3*) Irvington.

Herpesvirus: Recent Studies, Vol. 2. Daniel M. Albert et al. 1974. LC 73-13558. 25.50 (*0-8422-7169-4*) Irvington.

Herpesvirus: Recent Studies, Vol. 3. Lajos Gergely et al. 1974. LC 73-13558. 201p. (C). text 25.50 (*0-8422-7176-7*) Irvington.

Herpesvirus Diseases of Cattle, Horses, & Pigs. Ed. by G. Wittman & Yechiel Becker. 1989. (Developments in Veterinary Virology Ser.). (C). text 199.50 (*0-7923-0118-8*) Kluwer Academic.

Herpesvirus DNA. Ed. by Yechiel Becker. 1981. text 206.50 (*90-247-2512-7*) Kluwer Academic.

Herpesvirus Infections. Ed. by Ronald Glaser & James F. Jones. 1994. (Infectious Disease & Therapy Ser.: Vol. 13). (Illus.). 296p. text 137.50 (*0-8247-8867-2*) Dekker.

Herpesvirus Transcription & Its Regulation. Ed. by Edward K. Wagner. 1991. 400p. 242.00 (*0-8493-6097-8*, QR400) CRC Pr.

Herpesviruses. Ed. by Bernard Roizman. LC 82-15034. (Viruses Ser.). (Illus.). (C). Vol. 1. 1982. 460p. 132.00 (*0-306-40922-4*); Vol. 3. 1985. 432p. text 132.00 (*0-306-41778-2*) Kluwer Academic (Kluwer Plenum).

Herpesviruses: Immunobiology & Prophylaxis of Human Herpesvirus Infections, Vol. 4. Ed. by Bernard Roizman & Carlos Lopez. 1985. LC 82-15034. (Viruses Ser.). (Illus.). 458p. (C). text 132.00 (*0-306-41793-6*, Kluwer Plenum) Kluwer Academic.

Herpesviruses & Immunity. Ed. by P. G. Medveczky et al. 1998. (Infectious Agents & Pathogenesis Ser.). (Illus.). 340p. (C). text 115.00 (*0-306-45890-X*, Kluwer Plenum) Kluwer Academic.

Herpesviruses, the Immune System & AIDS. Ed. by Laure Aurelian. 1990. (Developments in Medical Virology Ser.). (C). text 199.00 (*0-7923-0803-4*) Kluwer Academic.

Herpetic Eye Disease: International Symposium. Ed. by R. Sundmacher. 1981. (Illus.). 560p. 93.95 (*0-387-00324-X*) Spr-Verlag.

Herpetic Eye Diseases. Ed. by P. C. Maudgal & L. Missotten. 1985. (Documenta Ophthalmologica Proceedings Ser.). text 247.50 (*90-6193-527-X*) Kluwer Academic.

Herpetology. F. H. Pough & Robin M. Andrews. 2nd ed. 2000. LC 00-33615. (Illus.). xi, 612p. pap. 86.67 (*0-13-030795-5*) P-H.

Herpetology in Australia. Ed. by Surrey Beatty Staff. 1999. 414p. pap. (*0-9599951-8-8*) Surrey Beatty & Sons AUS. *Dist:* St Mut.

Herpin's Contribution to the Knowledge of Epilepsy: A Translation of an Early French Epileptologist's 19th Century. Herpin. 2001. 99p. (*0-86196-609-0*) John Libby GBR. *Dist:* Buttrwrth-Heinemann.

Hershey Board Certification Review Outline Study Notes. Jonathan M. Singer & Samuel L. Deitch. Ed. by James Lawton. 1996. 755p. 350.00 (*0-9639030-0-4*) PA Podiatric.

HER2/neu Overexpression in Breast Cancer: The Role of Emerging Therapies (Audioconference Workbook) 1998. (*1-57130-038-4*) Medicine Grp USA.

Herzkrankheiten. 1996. 263.00 (*3-540-58461-7*) Spr-Verlag.

Herzl, King of the Jews: A Psychoanalytic Biography of Theodor Herzl. Avner Falk. 1993. LC 92-33938. 700p. (C). 87.00 (*0-8191-8925-1*) U Pr of Amer.

Hesitation: Impulsivity & Reflection, 15. Leonard William Doob. 1990. LC 90-32107. (Contributions in Psychology Ser.: No. 15). 224p. 57.95 (*0-313-27446-0*, DOH, Greenwood Pr) Greenwood.

Heterocyclische Verbindungen. Beilstein Institut fur Literatur der Organischen Chemie. Ed. by H. G. Boit. 1975. (Beilstein's Handbuch der Organischen Chemie Ser.: Vol. 17, Pt. 6). 868p. 1165.00 (*0-387-07359-0*) Spr-Verlag.

Heterocyclische Verbindungen. Beilstein Institut fur Literatur der Organischen Chemie. 1975. (Beilstein's Handbuch der Organischen Chemie Ser.: Vol. 17, Pts. 3-5). Pt. 3. 1210.00 (*0-387-07084-2*); Pt. 4. 1675.00 (*0-387-07220-9*); Pt. 5. 1055.00 (*0-387-07310-8*) Spr-Verlag.

Heterogeneity in Cross-Culture Psychology. Ed. by Daphne M. Keats et al. 1990. viii, 584p. pap. (*90-265-1018-7*) Swets.

Heterogeneity of Alzheimer's Disease. Ed. by F. Boller et al. 1992. LC 92-48751. (Research & Perspectives in Alzheimer's Disease Ser.). (*3-540-55918-3*); (Illus.). 189p. 99.00 (*0-387-55918-3*) Spr-Verlag.

Heterosexual AIDS: Myth or Fact? Kenneth Matsumura. 1988. LC 88-70310. pap. 9.95 (*0-9606924-3-6*) Alin Found Pr.

Heterosexual Transmission of AIDS in Africa. Ed. by Dieter Koch-Weser & Hannelore Vanderschmidt. 1988. (Illus.). 320p. 40.00 (*0-89011-603-2*); pap. 30.00 (*0-89011-604-0*) Abt Bks.

Heterosis. Ed. by R. Frankel. 1983. (Monographs in Theoretical & Applied Genetics: Vol. 6). (Illus.). 290p. 145.00 (*0-387-12125-0*) Spr-Verlag.

Heterotrimeric G Proteins. Ed. by Ravi Iyengar et al. 1994. (Methods in Enzymology Ser.: Vol. 257). (Illus.). 561p. text 104.00 (*0-12-182138-2*) Acad Pr.

Hexachlorobutadiene. Ed. by World Health Organization Staff. 1994. (Environmental Health Criteria Ser.: No. 156). (ENG, FRE & SPA.). 136p. pap. text 29.00 (*92-4-157156-X*, 1160156) World Health.

Hexachlorocyclopentadiene. 1991. (Environmental Health Criteria Ser.: No. 120). (ENG, FRE & SPA.). 126p. pap. text 21.60 (*92-4-157120-9*, 1160120) World Health.

Hexal Medical Dictionary, English-German/German-English. R. Walburga. 1995. (ENG & GER.). 36.00 (*0-7859-9694-X*) Fr & Eur.

Hexal Medical Dictionary German-English - English-German: Englisch-Deutsch/Deutsch-Englisch (English-German/German-English) R. B. Walburga. 1995. (ENG & GER.). 764p. pap. (*3-541-13781-9*) Urban & Schwarz AUT. *Dist:* IBD Ltd.

Hexal Medical Dictionary German/English-English/German. R. Walburga. 1995. (ENG & GER.). 36.00 (*0-7859-9706-7*) Fr & Eur.

H I

Hiatal Hernia: The Natural Approach to Overcoming Hiatal Hernia & Other Gastrointestinal ... Jack Ritchason. 1997. pap. text 11.95 (*1-885670-34-6*) Woodland UT.

Hiatal Hernia Syndrome: Insidious Link to Major Illness. Theodore A. Baroody, Jr. 1987. (Illus.). 150p. (Orig.). pap. text 9.95 (*0-9619595-2-5*) Holographic Hlth.

Hickey Multi-Sensory Language Course. Augur. 2nd ed. 1992. 300p. pap. 143.75 (*1-56593-556-X*, 0240) Singular Publishing.

Hidden Affects in Somatic Disorders: Psychoanalytic Perspectives on Asthma, Psoriasis, Diabetes, Cerebrovascular Disease, & Other Disorders. Luis A. Chiozza. 1998. LC 98-15126. 200p. 35.00 (*1-887841-16-4*, Psychosocial) Intl Univs Pr.

Hidden Arguments: Political Ideology & Disease Prevention Policy. Sylvia N. Tesh. 1988. 210p. (C). text 37.00 (*0-8135-1269-7*); pap. text 16.00 (*0-8135-1315-4*) Rutgers U Pr.

Hidden Bedroom Partners: Needs & Motives That Destroy Sexual Pleasure. Frank Hajcak & Patricia Garwood. 1987. LC 84-62865. (Illus.). 256p. (C). 17.95 (*0-87212-190-9*) Libra.

Hidden Child: The Linwood Method for Reaching the Autistic Child. Jeanne Simons & Sabine Oishi. 1987. LC 86-50459. (Illus.). 251p. (Orig.). pap. 17.95 (*0-933149-06-9*) Woodbine House.

Hidden Cost of AIDS: The Challenge of HIV to Development, 001. 1994. (Panos Dossier Ser.: No. 6). (Illus.). 176p. pap. (*1-870670-29-9*) Panos Pubns GBR. *Dist:* Paul & Co Pubs.

Hidden Dangers in Our Diet, Vol. 1. Clive Emsley. Date not set. (*0-7167-4555-0*) W H Freeman.

Hidden Dangers in Polio Vaccine. Elanor McBean. 1993. 86p. reprint ed. spiral bd. 9.00 (*0-7873-0593-6*) Hlth Research.

Hidden Dangers of Reflexology. Cathy Burns. 1997. 16p. pap. 0.50 (*1-891117-08-4*) Sharing.

Hidden Dimension: Psychodynamics of Compulsive Drug Use. Leon Wurmser. 1995. LC 95-16673. (Master Work Ser.). 676p. pap. 65.00 (*1-56821-591-6*) Aronson.

Hidden Dimension of Illness: Human Suffering. Ed. by Patricia Starck & John McGovern. 1992. 320p. (Orig.). (C). 35.95 (*0-88737-544-8*) Natl League Nurse.

Hidden Disorder: A Clinician's Guide to Attention Deficit Hyperactivity Disorder in Adults. Robert J. Resnick. 2000. LC 00-32283. 250p. 39.95 (*1-55798-724-6*, 431-761A) Am Psychol.

Hidden Epidemic: A Story about Manic Depression. Vernon White. 1996. 200p. (Orig.). pap. (*1-57502-112-9*) Morris Pubng.

Hidden Epidemic: Confronting Sexually Transmitted Disease. Institute of Medicine Staff. Ed. by Thomas R. Eng & William T. Butler. 1997. LC 97-4218. (Illus.). 448p. (C). 39.95 (*0-309-05495-8*) Natl Acad Pr.

Hidden in the Blood: A Personal Investigation of AIDS in the Yucatan. Carter Wilson. 1996. 192p. pap. 15.50 (*0-231-10191-0*) Col U Pr.

Hidden Library of Tanith Lee: Themes & Subtexts from Dionysos to the Immortal Gene. Mavis Haut. 2001. LC 2001-30516. (Illus.). 224p. per. 32.00 (*0-7864-1085-X*) McFarland & Co.

Hidden Meaning of Illness: Disease As a Symbol & Metaphor. Bob Trowbridge. 1996. LC 95-46753. 279p. pap. 12.95 (*0-87604-358-9*, 454) ARE Pr.

Hidden Mind: Psychology, Psychotherapy & Unconscious Processes. Orbach. 1995. 228p. pap. 65.00 (*0-471-95864-6*) Wiley.

Hidden Questions, Clinical Musings. M. Robert Gardner. 1995. LC 95-41685. 208p. 29.95 (*0-88163-212-0*) Analytic Pr.

Hidden Secret of Ayurveda. Robert E. Svoboda. 2nd ed. 1996. LC 94-71731. pap. 5.95 (*1-883725-04-6*) Ayurvedic Pr.

Hidden Selves: Between Theory & Practice in Psychoanalysis. R. Khan & M. Masud. 1983. 204p. (C). 30.00 (*0-8236-2323-8*) Intl Univs Pr.

Hidden Skills: A Dynamic Systems Analysis of Treadmill Stepping During the First Year. Esther Thelen & Beverly D. Ulrich. 1991. (Monographs of the Society for Research in Child Development: No. 223, Vol. 56, No. 1). 100p. pap. text 15.00 (*0-226-79476-8*) U Ch Pr.

Hidden Society. Vilhelm Aubert. 1982. LC 80-18939. (Social Science Classics Ser.). 359p. reprint ed. pap. text 24.95 (*0-87855-730-X*) Transaction Pubs.

Hidden Spring: A Buddhist Woman Confronts Cancer. Sandy Boucher. 2000. LC 00-32066. 224p. pap. 16.95 (*0-86171-171-8*) Wisdom MA.

Hidden Truth of Cancer. Morishita. 1984. pap. 3.50 (*0-916508-28-5*) Happiness Pr.

Hidden Victims - Hidden Healers: An Eight Stage Healing Process for Family & Friends of the Mentally Ill. Julie T. Johnson. 2nd rev. ed. 1994. LC 94-65648. 214p. pap. 12.95 (*0-9640430-0-9*) PEMA Pubns.

Hideous Idiocy: Forth Years of Psychiatric Slander by the U. S. Government. Fletcher Bartholomew. 1996. LC 96-94052. 212p. (Orig.). pap. 13.95 (*0-939823-03-9*) Info Inst.

Hiding, Hurting, Healing. Mary F. Clark. 1985. 176p. (Orig.). mass mkt. 3.95 (*0-310-30551-9*, 11612P) Zondervan.

Hidrocefalia y Comunicacion Ventriculo-Peritoneal. Oliver D. Grin & Dorothy L. Bouwman. 1992. (Patient Education Ser.). (SPA., Illus.). 20p. (Orig.). pap. text 4.00 (*0-929689-56-9*) Ludann Co.

Hierarchical Concepts in Psychoanalysis: Theory, Research, & Clinical Practice. Ed. by Arnold Wilson & John E. Gedo. 1993. LC 93-12380. 333p. text 45.00 (*0-89862-987-X*) Guilford Pubns.

Hierarchically Structured Materials. Ed. by I. A. Askay et al. 1992. (Symposium Proceedings Ser.: Vol. 255). 445p. text 19.50 (*1-55899-149-2*) Materials Res.

Hierbas Milagrosas (Miracle Herbs) La Guia de las 50 Hierbas Mas Poderosas del Mundo (The Guide to the World's 50 Most Powerful Herbs) Michael Castleman. 1998. LC 98-22475. (SPA., Illus.). 192p. pap. 12.95 (*1-57954-031-7*) Rodale Pr Inc.

High Acuity Nursing. Pamela Kidd. 2nd ed. 1997. tchr. ed. (*0-8385-3744-8*, A3744-8) Appleton & Lange.

High Acuity Nursing. Pamela A. Kidd & Kathleen D. Wagner. 3rd ed. 2000. LC 00-34017. (Illus.). 1042p. pap. 55.00 (*0-8385-3745-6*) P-H.

High Altitude & Lung. Ed. by Luigi Allegra & Annalisa Cogo. 1997. (Respiration Ser.: Vol. 64, No. 6, 1997). (Illus.). 68p. pap. 50.50 (*3-8055-6609-3*) S Karger.

High Altitude & Man. Ed. by John B. West & Sukhamay Lahiri. 1988. (American Physiological Society Book). (Illus.). 207p. text 39.00 (*0-19-520690-8*) OUP.

High Altitude Deterioration. Ed. by P. Cerretelli et al. 1985. (Medicine & Sport Science Ser.: Vol. 19). (Illus.). xvi, 228p. 126.25 (*3-8055-3972-X*) S Karger.

High Altitude Illness & Wellness: Beyond the Basics. Charles S. Houston. 1993. LC 92-47107. (Illus.). 80p. (Orig.). pap. 6.99 (*0-934802-72-6*) Globe Pequot.

High Altitude Medicine, No. 1. Herbert N. Hultgren. 1997. LC 97-93140. (Illus.). 550p. (Orig.). pap. 59.95 (*0-9655183-0-2*) Hultgren Pubns.

High-Altitude Medicine & Pathology. Donald Heath & David R. Williams. 4th ed. 1995. (Illus.). 462p. text 145.00 (*0-19-262504-7*) OUP.

High Altitude Medicine & Physiology. Michael P. Ward et al. 1989. LC 88-26133. (Illus.). 534p. (C). text 112.95 (*0-8122-8172-1*) U of Pa Pr.

High Altitude Medicine & Physiology. Michael P. Ward. 2nd ed. 1994. LC 94-71202. 640p. (C). (gr. 13). 181.95 (*0-412-54610-8*) Chapman & Hall.

High Altitude Medicine Handbook. Andrew J. Pollard & David R. Murdoch. 2nd ed. 1998. LC 98-27326. (*1-85775-214-7*) Radcliffe Med Pr GBR. *Dist:* Balogh.

High Altitude Physiology & Medicine I: Physiology of Adaptation. Ed. by W. Brendel & R. A. Zink. 1982. (Topics in Environmental Physiology & Medicine Ser.). (Illus.). 316p. 145.00 (*0-387-90482-4*) Spr-Verlag.

High Angle Rescue Techniques. Tom Vines. 2nd ed. 1998. (Illus.). 296p. (gr. 13). pap. text 34.95 (*0-8151-9500-1*, 29430) Mosby Inc.

High Blood Pressure. Sarah Brewer. 1997. pap. (*0-7225-3390-X*) Thorsons GBR. *Dist:* Natl Bk Netwk.

High Blood Pressure. Caroline Shreeve. l.t. ed. (*1-85695-053-0*) ISIS Lrg Prnt GBR. *Dist:* Transaction Pubs.

High Blood Pressure. Caroline Shreeve. 1998. 128p. pap. (*0-7225-3041-2*) Thorsons GBR. *Dist:* Natl Bk Netwk.

High Blood Pressure: Treat It for Life. 1995. (Illus.). 52p. (Orig.). (C). pap. text 15.00 (*0-7881-2168-5*) DIANE Pub.

High Blood Pressure: What You Need to Know. Mark Giuliucci. 1999. LC 99-26954. (Johns Hopkins Health Ser.). 192p. (YA). (gr. 9-12). pap. 9.95 (*0-7370-1610-8*) Time-Life Educ.

High Blood Pressure: What Your Doctor Doesn't Tell You. Richard Burns. 1995. pap. (*0-949142-40-9*) Stirling Pr AUS. *Dist:* Intl Spec Bk.

High Bloodpressures, Heart Attack, Diagrams. Dyob Re'lem, pseud. rev. ed. 1989. LC 89-92415. (Illus.). 90p. pap. (*0-9622463-2-8*) B Melger.

High Bloodpressures, Infarction, Diagrams. Boyd A. Melger, pseud. 1988. LC 88-92898. (Illus.). 63p. (Orig.). pap. (*0-9622463-0-1*) B Melger.

High Conflict, Violent & Separating Families: A Group Treatment Manual for School Age Children. Janet Johnston & Vivienne Roseby. 1997. LC 97-10284. 160p. pap. 34.95 (*0-684-82769-7*) Free Pr.

High Cost of Healing: Physicians & the Health Care System. J. H. Brown. 1985. 213p. 35.95 (*0-89885-222-6*, Kluwer Acad Hman Sci) Kluwer Academic.

High Density Lipoproteins & Atherosclerosis: Proceedings of the 3rd Argenteuil Symposium Held Under the Auspices of the Foundation Cardiologique Princesse Liliane in Waterloo, Belgium, Nov., 1977. Ed. by Antonio M. Gotto, Jr. et al. 1978. (Argenteuil Symposia Ser.: Vol. 3). 147.50 (*0-444-80047-6*) Elsevier.

High-Dose Cancer Therapy: Pharmacology, Hematopoietins, Stem Cells. James O. Armitage & Karen H. Antman. 1992. (Illus.). 840p. 160.00 (*0-683-00254-6*) Lppncott W & W.

High-Dose Cancer Therapy: Pharmacology, Hematopoietins, Stem Cells. Ed. by James O. Armitage & Karen H. Antman. 2nd ed. 1995. LC 94-46701. 150.00 (*0-683-02627-5*) Lppncott W & W.

High Dose Cancer Therapy: Pharmacology, Hematopoietins, Stem Cells. James O. Armitage & Karen H. Antman. 3rd ed. 1999. LC 99-33655. (Illus.). 976p. text 149.00 (*0-683-30654-5*) Lppncott W & W.

High Dose Rate Afterloading in the Treatment of Cancer of the Uterus. Thelma D. Bates & R. J. Berry. 1980. (British Institute of Radiology Report Series Special Report: No. 17). pap. (*0-905749-07-3*) Med Physics Pub.

High Dose Therapy & Transplantation of Haematopoietic Stem Cells. Wolfgang Schultze. 2000. 189p. pap. 67.95 (*0-632-05598-7*) Blackwell Sci.

High Fantasy. Jeffrey Dillow. 1981. 14.95 (*0-8359-2827-6*); pap. 12.95 (*0-8359-2826-8*) P-H.

High-Frequency Jet Ventilation: Experimental & Clinical Studies. M. Chiaranda & G. P. Giron. 1985. 182p. text (*1-57235-045-8*) Piccin Nuova.

High Frequency Ventilation. Lyle H. Hamilton et al. 1986. 192p. 102.00 (*0-8493-6739-5*, RC87, CRC Reprint) Franklin.

High-Functioning Individuals with Autism. Ed. by Eric Schopler & Gary B. Mesibov. 1992. (Current Issues in Autism Ser.). (Illus.). 336p. (C). 59.00 (*0-306-44064-4*, Plenum Trade) Perseus Pubng.

High Level Wellness. Donald B. Ardell. 1986. LC 77-10993. 384p. reprint ed. pap. 9.95 (*0-89815-162-7*) Ten Speed Pr.

High Levels of Natural Radiation, 1996: Radiation Dose & Health Effects: Proceedings of the 4th International Conference on High Levels of Natural Radiation, Held in Beijing, China on October 21 to 25, 1996. Wei, Luxin, Conference on High Levels of Natural R et al. 1997. LC 97-10754. (International Congress Ser.). 456p. 166.00 (*0-444-82630-0*) Elsevier.

High Life: A History of High-Altitude Physiology & Medicine. John B. West & Irving B. Weiner. 1998. LC 97-45875. (People & Ideas Ser.). (Illus.). 512p. text 79.50 (*0-19-512194-5*) OUP.

High Mist Training Center: Role Play Peacegames. David W. Felder. 1996. 48p. pap. text 8.95 (*0-910959-66-8*, B&G 13B) Wellington Pr.

High Performance Capillary Electrophoresis: Theory, Techniques, & Applications. Morteza G. Khaledi. 1998. LC 97-35765. (Chemical Analysis Monographs). 1047p. 180.00 (*0-471-14851-2*, Wiley-Interscience) Wiley.

High Performance Computing in Biomedical Research. Theo Pilkington et al. 1992. 544p. 125.00 (*0-8493-4474-3*, R853) CRC Pr.

High Performance Health. John Yiamouyiannis. 1987. (Illus.). 300p. 14.95 (*0-913571-02-4*) Health Act Pr.

High Performance Liquid Chromatography. John H. Knox. 1981. 205p. pap. (*0-85224-383-9*) Edinburgh U Pr GBR. *Dist:* Col U Pr.

High Performance Liquid Chromatography in Medical Microbiology, Vol. 2. Ed. by David S. Reeves & Uwe Ullmann. 1986. 272p. (Orig.). pap. text (*0-89574-215-2*) Gustav Fischer DEU. *Dist:* Lubrecht & Cramer, Balogh.

High Performance Liquid Chromatography in Protein & Peptide Chemistry. Ed. by F. Lottspeich et al. 1982. (Illus.). 123.10 (*3-11-008542-9*) De Gruyter.

High-Performance Medical Libraries: Advances in Information Management for the Virtual Era. Ed. by Naomi Broering. 1993. LC 93-11527. (Medical Information Management & Libraries: No. 68). 175p. pap. 39.50 (*0-88736-878-6*) Mecklermedia.

High-Power Gradient MR-Imaging: Advances in MRI II. M. Oudkerk. 1997. (Illus.). 159.00 (*0-632-04861-1*) Blackwell Sci.

High-Power Laser Radiation in Atmospheric Aerosols. A. A. Zemlyanov et al. 1985. text 203.00 (*90-277-1736-2*) Kluwer Academic.

High Pressure Biology & Medicine: Essays Presented to the Fifth International Meeting on High Pressure Biology. Ed. by Peter B. Bennett et al. 1998. LC 98-18397. 418p. 75.00 (*1-58046-033-X*) Univ Rochester Pr.

High Pressure Bioscience & Biotechnology: Proceedings of the International Conference on High Pressure Bioscience & Biotechnology, Kyoto, Japan, November 5-9, 1995. Rikimaru Hayashi & Claude Balny. 1996. LC 96-42331. (Progress in Biotechnology Ser.). 544p. 265.75 (*0-444-82555-X*) Elsevier.

High Pressure Food Science, Bioscience & Chemistry. Ed. by N. S. Issacs. 1998. 528p. 175.00 (*0-85404-728-X*) Spr-Verlag.

High Resolution Atlas of Cranial Neuroanatomy. Charles L. Truwit & Todd E. Lempert. 1994. (Illus.). 624p. text 199.00 (*0-683-08401-1*) Lppncott W & W.

High Resolution CT of the Chest: A Comprehensive Atlas. Eric J. Stern et al. 2nd ed. 2000. LC 00-30467. (Illus.). 384p. text 169.00 (*0-7817-2037-0*) Lppncott W & W.

High-Resolution Electrophoresis & Immunofixation: Techniques & Interpretation. David F. Keren. 2nd ed. 1994. LC 94-25021. (Illus.). 416p. (*0-7506-9469-6*) E A GBR. *Dist:* OUP.

High Risk & Critical Care: Intrapartum Nursing. Lisa K. Mandeville & Nan H. Troiano. 2nd ed. 1998. LC 98-21938. 496p. pap. text 42.95 (*0-397-55467-2*) Lppncott W & W.

High Risk & High Stakes: Health Professionals, Politics, & Policy, 100. Earl Wysong. 1992. LC 91-47158. (Contributions in Sociology Ser.: No. 100). 192p. 67.00 (*0-313-28475-X*, WHN, Greenwood Pr) Greenwood.

High-Risk Breast Cancer: Therapy. Ed. by J. Ragaz & Irving M. Ariel. 1991. (Illus.). 517p. 218.00 (*0-387-51092-3*) Spr-Verlag.

High-Risk Fetus: Pathophysiology, Diagnosis, & Management. Ed. by Chin-Chu Lin et al. 1992. LC 92-2378. (Illus.). 708p. 176.00 (*0-387-97836-4*) Spr-Verlag.

High Risk Foot in Diabetes Mellitus. R. G. Frykberg et al. 2nd ed. 1998. (Illus.). 640p. text (*0-443-07792-4*) Church.

High-Risk Infants: Identification, Assessment & Intervention. Louis M. Rossetti. 1986. LC 90-9220. 238p. (C). pap. text 29.00 (*0-89079-367-0*, 1783) PRO-ED.

High-Risk Infants: Identification, Assessment & Intervention. Louis Michael Rossetti. 1986. LC 86-17139. (*0-316-75757-8*) Little.

High-Risk Newborn Home Care Manual. Mary A. Chestnut. 1997. LC 97-25844. 224p. pap. text 42.50 (*0-397-55477-X*) Lppncott W & W.

High-Risk Perinatal Home Care Manual. Mary A. Chestnut. 1997. LC 97-11184. 224p. pap. text 42.50 (*0-397-55478-8*) Lppncott W & W.

High Risk Perinatal Nurse. Jack Rudman. 1994. (Certified Nurse Examination Ser.: CN-10). pap. 27.95 (*0-8373-6110-9*) Nat Learn.

High-Risk Pregnancy: A Team Approach. Robert A. Knuppel & Drukker. 2nd ed. 1993. (Illus.). 790p. text 70.00 (*0-7216-3455-9*) Saunders.

High Risk Pregnancy: Chronic Medical Conditions. Patricia M. Sauer et al. 1997. LC 97-42662. (*0-86525-080-4*) March of Dimes.

High Risk Pregnancy: Management Options. D. K. James et al. 1994. 1088p. text (*0-7216-1575-9*) Saunders.

High Risk Pregnancy & Child. Ed. by Z. Stembera et al. Tr. by M. Schierlova from CZE. 1976. (Illus.). 308p. (*90-247-1924-0*) Kluwer Academic NLD. *Dist:* Kluwer Academic.

High-Risk Pregnancy Sourcebook. Denise Chism. 1998. LC 97-9345. 304p. pap. 16.00 (*1-56565-858-2*, 08582W) Lowell Hse.

High-Risk Sexual Behavior: Interventions with Vulnerable Populations. Evvie Becker et al. 1998. LC 98-28252. (Prevention in Practice Library). (Illus.). 180p. (C). pap. text 22.50 (*0-306-45858-6*, Kluwer Plenum) Kluwer Academic.

High-Risk Sexual Behavior: Interventions with Vulnerable Populations. Evvie Becker et al. 1998. LC 98-28252. (Prevention in Practice Library). (Illus.). 180p. (C). 39.50 (*0-306-45857-8*, Plenum Trade) Perseus Pubng.

High School Vol. 1: A Teenager's Drug Addiction, Treatment & Lasting Recovery. Craig E. Fraser. 2nd rev. ed. 1998. LC 97-93835. Orig. Title: Burnt - A Teenage Addict's Road to Recovery. (Illus.). 306p. pap. 13.95 (*0-9658466-9-5*) AYNI Pr.

High Speed Healing: The Fastest, Safest & Most Effective Shortcuts to Lasting Relief. Prevention Magazine Health Book Staff. 1993. 656p. mass mkt. 6.99 (*0-553-56476-5*) Bantam.

High-Tech Conception: A Comprehensive Handbook for Consumers. Brian Kearney. 1998. LC 97-44172. 384p. pap. 14.95 (*0-553-37899-6*) Bantam.

High-Tech Cycling. Ed. by Edmund R. Burke. 1995. LC 95-81020. (Illus.). 312p. pap. 19.95 (*0-87322-535-X*, PBUR0535) Human Kinetics.

High Tech Home Care. Lisa Gorski. 2nd ed. 1999. 370p. ring bd. 149.00 (*0-8342-1148-3*, 11483) Aspen Pub.

High-Tech Practice: Thriving in Dentistry's Computer Age. Cheryl Farr. 1996. LC 95-42552. 213p. 59.95 (*0-87814-472-2*) PennWell Corp.

High Tech Urology: Technologic Innovations & Their Clinical Applications. Joseph A. Smith. 1992. (Illus.). 432p. text 105.00 (*0-7216-3053-7*) Saunders.

High Technology Medicine: Benefits & Burdens. Bryan J. Jennett. 1986. 318p. pap. 15.95 (*0-19-261588-2*) OUP.

High Throughput Screening: The Discovery of Bioactive Substances. John P. Devlin. 1997. LC 97-9333. (Illus.). 704p. text 250.00 (*0-8247-0067-8*) Dekker.

High Time: Life & Times of Howard Marks. David Leigh. 1985. 272p. 24.95 (*0-434-41339-9*) Trafalgar.

High Tops: Therapist's Guide. Phyllis Spinal-Robinson & Randi E. Wickham. 1993. (Illus.). 22p. (Orig.). pap. 4.95 (*0-9627375-6-9*) Jalice Pubs.

High Wire Angel: The Angel Wallenda Story. Paul W. Heimel. 1993. LC 92-32467. (Illus.). 192p. pap. 11.00 (*0-941599-15-9*) Piccadilly Bks.

High-Yield Acid Base. J. Craig Longenecker. 1998. LC 97-44427. 100p. pap. text 19.95 (*0-683-30393-7*) Lppncott W & W.

High-Yield Embryology. Ronald W. Dudek. 2nd ed. 2000. LC 00-59359. 192p. pap. text 17.95 (*0-7817-2132-6*) Lppncott W & W.

High-Yield General Surgery. R. Nirula. 2000. LC 00-30506. (Science of Review Ser.). (Illus.). 160p. pap. text 19.95 (*0-683-30691-X*) Lppncott W & W.

High-Yield Gross Anatomy. Ronald W. Dudek. 1997. LC 97-6715. (Illus.). 144p. pap. text 17.95 (*0-683-18215-3*) Lppncott W & W.

***High-Yield Gross Anatomy.** Ronald W. Dudek. 2nd ed. 2001. LC 2001-38572. 200p. pap. text 17.95 (*0-7817-3043-0*) Lppncott W & W.

High-Yield Histology. Ronald W. Dudek. 2nd ed. 2000. LC 99-57932. 232p. pap. text 17.95 (*0-7817-2134-2*) Lppncott W & W.

High-Yield Inpatient Medicine: A Practical Approach. Sanjay Saint & Craig Frances. 1997. LC 96-29151. (Illus.). 533p. pap. text 25.95 (*0-683-07547-0*) Lppncott W & W.

High-Yield Internal Medicine. R. Nirula. 1997. LC 97-7043. 197p. pap. text 19.95 (*0-683-18044-4*) Lppncott W & W.

High Yield MCAT. Chirag Amin. 1997. (Illus.). 217p. pap. 14.95 (*0-683-18058-4*) Lppncott W & W.

High-Yield Microbiology & Infectious Diseases. Contrib. by Louise B. Hawley. 2000. LC 99-59026. 208p. pap. text 17.95 (*0-683-30277-9*) Lppncott W & W.

***High-Yield Obstetrics & Gynecology.** Elmar P. Sakala. 2001. LC 00-140209. (Illus.). xiii, 184p. pap. text 19.95 (*0-7817-2394-9*) Lppncott W & W.

High-Yield Pathology. Ivan Damjanov. 2000. LC 00-32737. 160p. pap. text 17.95 (*0-7817-2367-1*) Lppncott W & W.

High-Yield Psychiatry. Barbara Fadem & Steven S. Simring. 1998. LC 98-12980. 100p. pap. text 18.95 (*0-683-30203-5*) Lppncott W & W.

Higher Cortical Functions in Man. A. R. Luria. 2nd ed. 1980. LC 77-20421. (Illus.). 656p. 54.50 (*0-306-10966-2*, Kluwer Plenum) Kluwer Academic.

Higher Ground. Joseph B. Strauss. 1996. 245p. 26.00 (*1-890419-07-9*) Fnd Chiropractic Educ.

Higher Ground: Biomedical Ethics & the Physician Executive. Ed. by Donald H. Hofreuter. 1991. LC 91-71673. 86p. (C). pap. text 25.95 (*0-924674-07-5*) Am Coll Phys Execs.

Higher Integrative Systems of the Brain. A. S. Batuev. 1987. xvi, 296p. text 220.00 (*2-88124-143-3*) Gordon & Breach.

Higher-Order Processing in the Visual System, No. 29-6. Ed. by Gregory R. Bock & Jamie A. Goode. 1994. LC 94-13268. (CIBA Foundation Symposia Ser.: Vol. 184). 256p. 150.00 (*0-471-94412-2*) Wiley.

Higher Stages of Human Development: Perspectives on Adult Growth. Ed. by Charles N. Alexander & Ellen J. Langer. 1990. (Illus.). 416p. text 68.00 (*0-19-503483-X*) OUP.

***Higher Surgical Training in General Surgery.** Alfred Cuschieri et al. 4th ed. 2001. (Arnold Publication). 880p. text 187.50 (*0-340-80638-9*) OUP.

Highlights, Set. Benjamin F. Boyd. 1993. (ENG & SPA.). (C). text (*958-95544-1-5*) Highlights Opthal PAN. *Dist:* SLACK Inc.

Highlights in Coloproctology. P. F. Schoefield et al. 1993. 165p. (*3-540-19779-6*) Spr-Verlag.

Highlights in Coloproctology. Philip F. Schofield et al. 1993. LC 93-17623. 163p. 101.00 (*0-387-19779-6*) Spr-Verlag.

Highlights in Food Allergy: 6th International Symposium on Immunological & Clinical Problems of Food Allergy, Lugano, September, 1995. Ed. by B. Wuethrich & C. Ortolani. 1996. (Monographs in Allergy: Vol. 32, 1996). (Illus.). x, 260p. 141.00 (*3-8055-6224-1*) S Karger.

Highlights in Immunology. Ed. by J. M. Cruse. 1991. (Journal: Vol. 10, No. 1, 1991). (Illus.). 88p. pap. 33.25 (*3-8055-5394-3*) S Karger.

Highlights in the History of the Army Nurse Corps. 1995. lib. bdg. 250.00 (*0-8490-6580-1*) Gordon Pr.

Highly Dispersed Metals. C. V. Vishveshwara et al. 1987. (Physical Chemistry Ser.). 208p. 129.00 (*0-470-20185-1*) P-H.

Highly Selective Neurotoxins: Basic & Clinical Applications. Ed. by Richard M. Kostrzewa. 1997. LC 98-100022. (Contemporary Neuroscience Ser.). (Illus.). 416p. 145.00 (*0-89603-465-8*) Humana.

High/Scope Child Observation Record. 1992. (J). (ps-1). pap. 90.95 (*0-929816-40-4*, SU-P1084SET) High-Scope.

Highway to Health: Transforming U. S. Health Care in the Information Age. 1996. (Illus.). x, 85p. (Orig.). pap. 25.00 (*1-889866-16-4*) Coun on Competitiveness.

Highway to Health: Transforming U. S. Health Care in the Information Age. 1996. (Illus.). 85p. (Orig.). pap. text 35.00 (*0-7881-3339-X*) DIANE Pub.

Hildegarde E. Peplau: Interpersonal Nursing Theory. Cheryl Forchuk. 1993. LC 93-28310. (Notes on Nursing Theories Ser.: Vol. 10). pap. 14.95 (*0-8039-4858-1*, 4348) Sage.

Hillcrest Medical Center. Novak & Ireland. 5th ed. 1998. 208p. tchr. ed. 25.95 (*0-7668-0324-4*) Delmar.

Hillcrest Medical Center: Beginning Medical Transcription Course. Mary A. Novak & Patricia A. Ireland. 4th ed. 1995. 240p. pap., tchr. ed. incl. disk (*0-538-71210-4*) S-W Thomson.

Hillcrest Medical Center - Beginning Medical Transcription Course. Novak & Ireland. 5th ed. 1998. LC 98-16973. (Allied Health Ser.). 272p. (C). pap. text 57.95 (*0-7668-0322-8*) Delmar.

Hills of Sidon: Journal of an American Doctor in Lebanon. Leila Richards. 1988. 224p. 17.95 (*1-55774-015-1*) Lambda Pubs.

Hilton Head Over-35 Diet. Peter M. Miller. 1990. mass mkt. 6.99 (*0-446-35861-4*) Warner Bks.

Hindu Medicine. Heinrich R. Zimmer. 1979. 25.95 (*0-405-10640-8*) Ayer.

Hindu-Yogi Practical Water Cure. Yogi Ramacharaka. reprint ed. pap. text 7.50 (*0-911662-12-X*) Yoga.

Hints for a Healthier Liver. A. Vogel. 1990. (Swiss Nature Doctor Ser.). 24p. (Orig.). pap. 2.95 (*0-87983-525-7*, Keats Pubng) McGraw-Hill Trade.

Hints for Success in Medical School & the Match. Eric Giza. 2000. (Illus.). 153p. pap. 15.00 (*0-8036-0758-X*) Davis Co.

Hints for Success in Medical School & the Match. Eric Giza. 2000. pap. 15.00 (*1-888308-07-9*) J & S Pub VA.

Hints on the Preservation of Health in Armies: Bound with: Manual of Instructions for Military Surgeons. John Ordronaux. 1990. (American Civil War Medical Ser.: No. 1). 238p. reprint ed. 45.00 (*0-930405-34-X*) Norman SF.

Hinweise Zur Konservativen Behandlung des Akuten Nierenversagens. Gudrun Spaeth. 1977. (Illus.). 10.50 (*3-8055-2749-7*) S Karger.

Hip. Ed. by Richard A. Balderston et al. 1991. (Illus.). 544p. 149.50 (*0-8121-1302-0*) Lppncott W & W.

Hip. Ed. by Clement B. Sledge. 1998. LC 97-24104. (Master Techniques in Orthopaedic Surgery Ser.). 384p. text 199.00 (*0-7817-0034-5*) Lppncott W & W.

Hip: Proceedings of the Thirteenth Open Scientific Meeting of the Hip Society 1985. Hip Society Staff. 1986. 72.00 (*0-8016-2249-2*) Mosby Inc.

Hip & Its Disorders. Steinberg. 1990. (Illus.). 1184p. text 240.00 (*0-7216-1812-X*) Saunders.

Hip & Thigh: Volumes 7 & 7a. Jules R. Kalisch & Harold Williams. 1972. (Courtroom Medicine Ser.). ring bd. 417.00 (*0-8205-1248-6*) Bender.

Hip Arthroplasty. Harlan C. Amstutz. 1991. (Illus.). 1001p. text (*0-443-08505-6*) Church.

Hip Arthroscopy. Glick. 2000. (C). text (*0-443-06536-5*) Church.

Hip Biomechanics. Ed. by Shinichi Imura et al. 1993. LC 93-5020. (Illus.). 348p. 290.00 (*0-387-70118-4*) Spr-Verlag.

Hip Fracture: Setting Priorities for Effectiveness Research. Committee of the Institute of Medicine Division of. Ed. by Kim Heithoff & Kathleen N. Lohr. 1990. 72p. pap. text 15.00 (*0-309-04299-2*) Natl Acad Pr.

Hip Fracture Management. Parker. 1994. pap. 230.00 (*0-8151-6051-8*) Mosby Inc.

Hip Fracture Management. Martyn J. Parker & Glyn Pryor. 1993. LC 92-49128. 304p. 150.00 (*0-632-03263-4*) Blackwell Sci.

Hip Fracture Outcomes in People Age Fifty & Over. Katie Maslow. 1994. (Illus.). 95p. (Orig.). (C). pap. text 35.00 (*0-7881-1414-X*) DIANE Pub.

HIP Handbook. Timothy L. Fagerson. 1998. LC 97-34807. 366p. pap. text 49.99 (*0-7506-9689-3*) Buttrwrth-Heinemann.

Hip Hop Rhymes of Tough Love to Addicts Out of Control: A Seven Minute Treatment. incl. audio (*0-9638949-1-9*) Winning Artist.

Hip Replacements: What You Need to Know. M. T. Simon, pseud. 2000. LC 98-39491. 277p. pap. 18.95 (*1-56072-474-9*, Nova Kroshka Bks) Nova Sci Pubs.

Hip Surgery. Laurent Sedel & Miguel E. Cabanela. 1998. 424p. (*1-85317-237-5*) Martin Dunitz GBR. *Dist:* Mosby Inc.

***HIPAA Compliance Handbook: Electronic Transactions & Privacy Standards.** Aspen Health Law and Compliance Center Staff. 2001. 143p. per. 59.00 (*0-8342-2034-2*) Aspen Pub.

***HIPAA Compliance Handbook: Final Rule on Standards for Privacy.** Clay Countryman et al. 2001. LC 2001-22550. (*0-8342-2061-X*) Aspen Pub.

Hippocampus. R. L. Isaacson & K. H. Pribram. 1986. LC 75-28121. (Illus.). Vol. 3. 456p. 95.00 (*0-306-42156-9*); Vol. 4. 398p. 95.00 (*0-306-42198-4*) Kluwer Academic (Kluwer Plenum).

Hippocampus: Functions & Clinical Relevance: Proceedings of the Satellite Symposium of the Fourth IBRO World Congress of Neuroscience, Kyoto, Japan, 15-16 July 1995. Ed. by Nobumasa Kato. 1996. LC 96-2451. (Developments in Neurology Ser.: No. 11). 510p. 182.25 (*0-444-82271-2*) Elsevier.

***Hippocrates.** Jacques Jouanna. 2001. (Medicine & Culture Ser.). 536p. pap. text 24.95 (*0-8018-6818-1*) Johns Hopkins.

Hippocrates. Jacques Jouanna. 1999. LC 98-6999. (Medicine & Culture Ser.). 536p. 52.95 (*0-8018-5907-7*) Johns Hopkins.

Hippocrates. Tr. by Paul Potter from GRE. 1989. (Loeb Classical Library: No. 472). Vol. V. 349p. text 18.95 (*0-674-99520-1*); Vol. VI. 377p. text 18.95 (*0-674-99522-8*) HUP.

Hippocrates, Vol. VIII. Ed. & Tr. by Paul Potter. 1995. LC 23-12030. (Hippocrates Ser.: Vol. 482). (Illus.). 432p. (C). text 18.95 (*0-674-99531-7*) HUP.

Hippocrates: Places in Man. Hippocrates. Ed. & Tr. by Elizabeth M. Craik. 1998. (Illus.). 288p. text 85.00 (*0-19-815227-2*) OUP.

Hippocrates: Pseudepigraphic Writings: Letters-Embassy-Speech from the Altar-Decree. Ed. & Tr. by Wesley D. Smith from GRE. 1990. LC 90-42993. (Studies in Ancient Medicine: Vol. 2). x, 133p. 62.50 (*90-04-09290-0*) Brill Academic Pubs.

Hippocrates: The Natural Regimen. Robert Van de Weyer. 1997. pap. (*0-85305-411-8*, 1928) Arthur James GBR. *Dist:* Morehouse Pub.

Hippocrates: Volume 7, Epidemics 2, 4-7. Ed. by Wesley Smith. 1994. LC 93-19601. (Loeb Classical Library: No. 477). 440p. text 18.95 (*0-674-99526-0*) HUP.

Hippocrates - Concordantia in Corpus Hippocraticum Ed. by Gilles Maloney & Winnie Frohn. 1986. (Alpha Omega, Reihe A Ser.: No. LXXV). (GER.). Set. xxiii, 4869p. lib. bdg. 1025.70 (*3-487-07740-X*); Vol. 6. vi, 487p. lib. bdg. (*3-487-09130-5*) G Olms Pubs.

Hippocrates & His Successors in Relation to the Philosophy of Their Time. Robert O. Moon. LC 75-23745. reprint ed. 37.50 (*0-404-13351-7*) AMS Pr.

Hippocrates' Handmaidens: Women Married to Physicians. Esther M. Nitzberg. 1991. (Women Ser.: Vol. 4). 238p. LC 90-41947. text 59.95 (*0-86656-880-8*); LC 90-41946. pap. 22.95 (*0-918393-81-7*, Harrington Park) Haworth Pr.

Hippocrates Health Program: A Proven Guide to Healthful Living. Brian R. Clement. Ed. by Trish Miller & Alix Weill. 1989. (Illus.). 88p. (Orig.). pap. 5.95 (*0-9622373-0-2*) Hippocrates Pubns.

Hippocrates' Latin American Legacy: Humoral Medicine in the New World, Vol. 1. George M. Foster. 1993. LC 93-17985. (Theory & Practice in Medical Anthropology & International Health Ser.). 256p. text 49.00 (*2-88124-610-9*); pap. text 22.00 (*2-88124-611-7*) Gordon & Breach.

Hippocrates Now! Is Your Doctor Ethical? Particia Parsons & Arthur Parsons. 1995. 480p. text 35.00 (*0-8020-0526-8*) U of Toronto Pr.

Hippocrates Now! Is Your Doctor Ethical? Patricia Parsons & Arthur Parsons. 1995. LC 95-149491. 370p. pap. 14.95 (*0-8020-6963-0*) U of Toronto Pr.

Hippocrates' Woman: Reading the Female Body in Ancient Greece. Helen King. LC 98-3728. (C). 1999. 320p. 90.00 (*0-415-13894-9*, D6165); 1998. 13p. pap. 29.95 (*0-415-13895-7*, D6169) Routledge.

Hippocratic Lives & Legends. Jody R. Pinault. 1992. LC 91-43634. (Studies in Ancient Medicine: No. 4). x, 160p. 74.50 (*90-04-09574-8*) Brill Academic Pubs.

Hippocratic Medicine. William A. Heidel. Ed. by I. Bernard Cohen. 1981. LC 80-2129. (Development of Science Ser.). (Illus.). lib. bdg. 19.95 (*0-405-13878-4*) Ayer.

Hippocratic Oath. L. Edelstein. 1979. 90p. 15.00 (*0-89005-272-7*) Ares.

Hippokratische Medizin und Antike Philosophie. Renate Wittern & Pierre Pellegrin. 1995. (Medizin der Antike Ser.: Vol. 1). (GER.). 650p. (*3-487-10037-1*) G Olms Pubs.

Hippokratische Schrift De Morbis I. Renate Wittern. 1974. (Altertumswissenschaftliche Texte und Studien: Bd. 3). cxxii, 249p. (*3-487-05592-9*) G Olms Pubs.

Hippokratische Untersuchungen. Carl Fredrich. 1976. LC 75-13264. (History of Ideas in Ancient Greece Ser.). (GER.). reprint ed. 19.95 (*0-405-07306-2*) Ayer.

Hiring the Head Injured: What to Expect. Tampa General Rehabilitation Center Staff. 1989. (Coping Ser.: Vol. 3). 64p. (Orig.). pap. 9.50 (*1-882855-02-7*) HDI Pubs.

Hirsutism. Alan N. Elias & Grant Gwinup. 1983. LC 83-2428. 139p. 52.50 (*0-275-91390-2*, C1390, Praeger Pubs) Greenwood.

His Brother's Keeper: A Psychobiography of Samuel Taylor Coleridge. Stephen M. Weissman. 1990. (Applied Psychoanalysis Monographs: No. 1). 370p. 52.50 (*0-8236-2342-4*) Intl Univs Pr.

Hispanic Aged Mental Health. Ed. by T. L. Brink. 1992. LC 92-1473. 207p. pap. 19.95 (*1-56024-217-5*) Haworth Pr.

Hispanic Children & Adults with Communication Disorders: Assessment & Intervention. Henrette W. Langdon. 1991. LC 91-42491. (Excellence in Practice Ser.). 450p. 72.00 (*0-8342-0288-3*) PRO-ED.

Hispanic Psychology: Critical Issues in Theory & Research. Ed. by Amado M. Padilla. 1995. LC 94-33265. 336p. 86.95 (*0-8039-5552-9*, 4665); pap. 39.95 (*0-8039-5553-7*, 4666) Sage.

Hispanic Voices: Hispanic Health Educators Speak Out. Sara Torres & NLN Staff. 1999. (Illus.). 256p. (C). pap. text 34.95 (*0-7637-1109-8*, 1109-8, N L N Bart) Jones & Bartlett.

Hispanics in the United States: Abstracts of the Psychological & Behavioral Literature, 1980-1989. Ed. by Esteban L. Olmedo & Verna R. Walker. 1990. LC 90-1218. (PsycINFO Bibliographies in Psychology Ser.: No. 8). 307p. pap. 19.95 (*1-55798-103-5*) Am Psychol.

Hist & Cell Bio Review. Burns. 2001. text (*0-323-00834-8*) Mosby Inc.

Histamine: Its Role in Physiological & Pathological Processes. M. A. Beaven. 1978. (Monographs in Allergy: Vol. 13). (Illus.). pap. 33.25 (*3-8055-2887-6*) S Karger.

Histamine & H1-Receptor Antagonists in Allergic Disease. F. Estelle Simons. 1996. (Clinical Allergy & Immunology Ser.: Vol. 7). (Illus.). 448p. text 115.00 (*0-8247-9509-1*) Dekker.

Histamine & Histamine Antagonists. Ed. by B. Uvnas et al. 1991. (Handbook of Experimental Pharmacology Ser.: No. 97). (Illus.). 796p. 445.00 (*0-387-52803-2*) Spr-Verlag.

Histamine H3 Receptor: A Target for New Drugs. Robert Leurs & Henk Timmerman. 1998. LC 98-48712. 304p. 197.00 (*0-444-82936-9*) Elsevier.

Histamine in Marine Products: Production by Bacteria, Measurement & Prediction of Formation. 1985. 67p. (*92-5-102244-5*, F2792) FAO ITA. *Dist:* Bernan Associates.

Histamine in Normal & Cancer Cell Proliferation. Ed. by M. Garcia-Caballero et al. 1993. (Advances in the Biosciences Ser.: Vol. 89). 416p. 181.50 (*0-08-042202-0*, Pergamon Pr) Elsevier.

Histochemical & Immunohistochemical Techniques: Applications to Pharmacology & Toxicology. Peter H. Bach & John R. Baker. 1991. (Illus.). 256p. (C). (gr. 13). text 104.00 (*0-412-35100-5*, A5576) Chapman & Hall.

Histochemistry: Theoretical & Applied, Vols. 1-3. Peter J. Stoward. 4th ed. 1992. 728p. text (*0-443-02996-2*) Church.

Histochemistry in Pathology. Ed. by M. Isabel Filipe & Brian D. Lake. 2nd ed. 1990. (Illus.). 496p. text (*0-443-04019-2*) Church.

Histochemistry, Vol. 1: Theoretical & Applied. A. G. Pearse. 4th ed. 1993. (Illus.). 456p. text (*0-443-01998-3*) Church.

Histochemistry, Vol 2: Theoretical & Applied. A. G. Pearse. 4th ed. 1985. (Illus.). 624p. text (*0-443-02997-0*) Church.

Histocompatibility Testing Nineteen Eighty. Paul I. Terasaki & Walter F. Bodmer. 1980. LC 80-36737. (Illus.). 10.00 (*0-9604606-0-8*) UCLA Tissue.

Histoire de la Douleur see History of Pain

Histoire de la Medecine et des Medecins. Jean-Charles Sournia. 1991. (FRE.). 592p. 395.00 (*0-7859-9890-X*) Fr & Eur.

Histoire des Sciences Medicales. Comprenant l'Anatomie, la Physiologie, la Medicine, la Chirurgie et les Doctrines de Pathologie Generale Charles Daremberg. fac. ed. 1974. (FRE., Illus.). 1336p. reprint ed. (*3-201-00907-5*) Akademische Druck-und AUT. *Dist:* Balogh.

Histoires, Disputes et Discours des Illusions et Impostures des Diables, des Magiciens Infames, Sorcieres et Empoisonneurs Jean Weyer Wier. 1976. LC 75-16738. (Classics in Psychiatry Ser.). (FRE.). reprint ed. 52.95 (*0-405-07461-1*);Set. 104.95 (*0-405-07460-3*) Ayer.

Histologic Diagnosis of Inflammatory Skin Diseases: An Algorithmic Method Based on Pattern Analysis. A. Bernard Ackerman et al. 2nd ed. 1997. LC 96-2903. 943p. 250.00 (*0-683-00010-1*) Lppncott W & W.

Histologic Diagnosis of Inflammatory Skin Diseases: An Algorithmic Method Based on Pattern Analysis. Bruce Bennin et al. 2nd ed. 1997. LC 96-29038. (Illus.). 1,200p. text 325.00 (*0-683-30376-7*) Lppncott W & W.

Histologic Differential Diagnosis of Skeletal Lesions. Harry A. Schwamm & Carl L. Millward. 1995. LC 94-30600. (Illus.). 136p. 118.50 (*0-89640-271-1*) Igaku-Shoin.

Histological & Histochemical Methods: Theory & Practice. K. A. Kiernan. 1981. (Illus.). 400p. text 115.00 (*0-08-024936-1*); pap. text 35.00 (*0-08-024935-3*) Elsevier (Pergamon Pr).

Histological & Histochemical Methods: Theory & Practice. J. A. Kiernan. 3rd ed. 2000. (An Arnold Publication). (Illus.). 512p. pap. (*0-7506-4936-4*) E A GBR. *Dist:* OUP.

Histological & Histopathological Evaluation of the Testis. Lonnie D. Russell & Robert A. Ettlin. Ed. by Amiya P. Hikim & Eric D. Clegy. 1990. (Illus.). 286p. (C). 62.50 (*0-9627422-0-1*) Cache River Pr.

Histological Classification of Bone & Joint Tumors in Domestic Animals. Slayter et al. 1994. (Illus.). 50p. pap. text 20.00 (*1-881041-12-3*) Am Registry Path.

Histological Color Atlas of the Human Larynx. Monoru Hirano & Kiminori Sato. 1993. LC 92-49696. (Illus.). 120p. (C). pap. 145.00 (*1-56593-077-0*, 0383) Thomson Learn.

Histological Diagnosis of Tumours by Pattern Analysis: An A-Z Guide. Awatif I. Al-Nafussi & David E. Hughes. 1997. LC 97-160230. (Illus.). 752p. (*0-340-58606-0*) E A GBR. *Dist:* OUP, Routldge.

Histological Typing of Bone Tumors. Fritz Schajowicz. 2nd ed. 1996. LC 93-17622. (International Histological Classification of Tumors Ser.). (Illus.). 128p. 78.00 (*0-387-56460-8*) Spr-Verlag.

Histological Typing of Cancer & Precancer of the Oral Mucosa. J. J. Pindborg & P. N. Wahi. 2nd ed. 1997. LC 97-8019. (International Histological Classification of Tumors Ser.). (Illus.). 57p. pap. 68.00 (*3-540-61848-1*) Spr-Verlag.

Histological Typing of Endocrine Tumours. Enrico Solcia et al. 2nd ed. 2000. LC 99-49865. (International Histological Classification of Tumors Ser.). (Illus.). 176p. pap. 76.00 (*3-540-66169-7*) Spr-Verlag.

Histological Typing of Female Genital Tract Tumours. Ed. by R. E. Scully et al. 2nd ed. 1994. (Illus.). 202p. 72.00 (*0-387-57157-4*) Spr-Verlag.

Histological Typing of Intestinal Tumours. J. R. Jass & Leslie H. Sobin. 2nd ed. 1993. (World Health Organization Ser.). (Illus.). 145p. 74.00 (*0-387-50711-6*) Spr-Verlag.

Histological Typing of Kidney Tumours. F. K. Mostofi et al. 2nd ed. 1997. LC 97-30425. (International Histological Classification of Tumors Ser.). (Illus.). 117p. pap. 73.00 (*3-540-63199-2*) Spr-Verlag.

Histological Typing of Lung & Pleural Tumours. William D. Travis et al. 3rd ed. 1999. LC 99-20160. (International Histological Classification of Tumors Ser.: No. 1). (Illus.). 169p. pap. 81.00 (*3-540-65219-1*) Spr-Verlag.

Histological Typing of Odontogenic Tumours. Jens J. Pindborg et al. Ed. by Leslie H. Sobin. 2nd ed. 1997. (World Health Organization Ser.). (Illus.). 118p. reprint ed. 63.00 (*0-387-54142-X*) Spr-Verlag.

Histological Typing of Oesophageal & Gastric Tumours. H. Watanabe & Jass. 1989. (International Histological Classification of Tumours Ser.: No. 18). text (*3-540-51629-8*) World Health.

Histological Typing of Oesophageal & Gastric Tumours. H. Watanabe et al. 2nd ed. 1998. (World Health Organization Ser.). (Illus.). 2109p. 59.00 (*0-387-51629-8*) Spr-Verlag.

Histological Typing of Ovarian Tumours. Robert Scully et al. 2nd ed. 1999. LC 99-10480. (World Health Organization Ser.). (Illus.). 146p. pap. 82.00 (*3-540-64059-2*) Spr-Verlag.

Histological Typing of Salivary Gland Tumours: WHO International Histological Classification of Tumours. G. Seifert. 2nd ed. 1996. (Illus.). 113p. reprint ed. 63.00 (*0-387-54031-8*) Spr-Verlag.

Histological Typing of Skin Tumours. P. J. Heenan et al. 2nd ed. 1996. LC 96-13284. (Illus.). 120p. pap. 72.00 (*3-540-60850-8*) Spr-Verlag.

Histological Typing of Soft Tissue Tumours. S. W. Weiss. 2nd ed. 1996. LC 93-21300. (International Histological Classification of Tumors Ser.). (Illus.). 142p. 92.00 (*0-387-56794-1*) Spr-Verlag.

Histological Typing of Testis Tumours. F. K. Mostofi et al. 2nd ed. 1997. LC 97-30424. (International Histological Classification of Tumors Ser.). (Illus.). 132p. pap. 74.00 (*3-540-63374-X*) Spr-Verlag.

Histological Typing of Thryoid Tumours. C. Hedinger. 2nd ed. 1995. (International Histological Classification of Tumors Ser.). (Illus.). 67p. pap. 62.00 (*3-540-19244-1*) Spr-Verlag.

Histological Typing of Thyroid Tumours. E. D. Williams et al. 2nd ed. 1995. (World Health Organization Ser.). (Illus.). xii, 67p. reprint ed. 60.00 (*0-387-19244-1*) Spr-Verlag.

Histological Typing of Tumours of the Central Nervous System. Paul Kleihues et al. 2nd ed. (Illus.). 1993. 130p. pap. (*3-540-56971-5*); 1996. LC 93-25312. 112p. reprint ed. 92.00 (*0-387-56971-5*) Spr-Verlag.

Histological Typing of Tumours of the Exocring Pancreas. G. Kloppel et al. 2nd ed. 1996. (World Health Organization Ser.). (Illus.). 61p. reprint ed. 72.00 (*3-540-60280-1*) Spr-Verlag.

Histological Typing of Tumours of the Gallbladder & Extrahepatic Bile Ducts: In Collaboration with Pathologists in 5 Countries. Jorge Albores-Saavedra et al. 2nd ed. 1994. (Illus.). 96p. 48.00 (*0-387-52838-5*) Spr-Verlag.

Histological Typing of Tumours of the Thymus. Juan Rosai. 2nd ed. 1999. LC 99-36794. (World Health Organization Ser.). (Illus.). 80p. pap. 70.00 (*3-540-65731-2*) Spr-Verlag.

Histological Typing of Tumours of the Upper Respiratory Tract & Ear: In Collaboration with L. H. Sobin & Pathologists in Eight Countries. K. Shanmugaratnam. 2nd ed. 1996. (Illus.). 201p. reprint ed. 83.00 (*0-387-53880-1*) Spr-Verlag.

Histological Typing of Urinary Bladder Tumours. F. K. Mostofi et al. 2nd ed. 1999. LC 99-36795. (World Health Organization Ser.). 130p. pap. 76.00 (*3-540-64063-0*) Spr-Verlag.

Histology. Ronald A. Bergman et al. 1996. (Illus.). 384p. text 31.95 (*0-7216-3089-8*) Saunders.

Histology. D. L. Feeback. 1991. (Oklahoma Notes). (Illus.). 193p. 14.95 (*0-387-96339-1*) Spr-Verlag.

Histology. A. Stevens & J. Lowe. 1991. (Illus.). 392p. (gr. 13). (*0-397-44633-0*) Gower-Mosby.

Histology. D. L. Feeback. 2nd ed. 1992. (Oklahoma Notes). (Illus.). 192p. 13.95 (*0-387-97294-3*) Spr-Verlag.

Histology: A Color Atlas of Microscopic Anatomy. Johannes Sobotta. Ed. by Frithjof Hammersen. 3rd ed. 1985. LC 84-29084. (Illus.). 272p. 39.95 (*0-683-07828-3*) Lppncott W & W.

Histology: A Photographic Atlas. Stephen Downing. 1992. (Illus.). (C). 500.00 incl. disk (*1-56815-002-4*) Mosby Inc.

Histology: A Text & Atlas. Michael H. Ross et al. (Illus.). 2nd ed. 1989. 815p. text 52.00 (*0-683-07368-0*); 3rd ed. 1994. 704p. 57.95 (*0-683-07369-9*) Lppncott W & W.

Histology: From Normal Microanatomy to Pathology. P. S. Amenta. 6th ed. 1991. 660p. (C). text (*1-57235-000-8*) Piccin Nuova.

Histology & Histopathology of the Aging Brain. Ed. by J. Ulrich. 1988. (Interdisciplinary Topics in Gerontology Ser.: Vol. 25). (Illus.). x, 182p. 148.00 (*3-8055-4771-4*) S Karger.

Histology & Neural Anatomy: 2000 Multiple-Choice Questions & Answers. 1999. 322p. spiral bd. 25.95 (*1-893720-01-2*) Biotest.

Histology for Pathologists. Stephen S. Sternberg. 2nd ed. 1997. LC 96-41470. 1,216p. text 225.00 (*0-397-51718-1*) Lppncott W & W.

Histology Image Review. Frank J. Wilson. 1999. pap. 54.95 incl. cd-rom (*0-8385-3748-0*) McGraw-Hill Prof.

Histology of Borderline Cancer. W. W. Park & J. W. Corkhill. 1980. LC 79-26151. (Illus.). 480p. 93.00 (*3-540-09792-9*) Spr-Verlag.

***Histology Picture Tests.** B. Young. 2001. (Illus.). 155p. pap. (*0-443-06020-7*) Church GBR. *Dist:* Saunders.

Histology Technician. Jack Rudman. 1994. (Career Examination Ser.: C-2837). pap. 29.95 (*0-8373-2837-3*) Nat Learn.

Histopathologic Methods & Color Atlas of Special Stains & Tissue Artifacts. Lee G. Luna. 1992. LC 92-70140. (Illus.). 767p. 80.00 (*0-9649737-0-7*) Am HistoLabs.

Histopathology. Paul J. Scheuer & B. T. Chalk. 1986. (Clinical Tests Ser.). (Illus.). 128p. text (*0-7234-0885-8*) Wolfe Publishing.

Histopathology. Gisela Dallenbach-Hellweg. 4th ed. 1987. (Illus.). 416p. 177.00 (*0-387-18156-3*) Spr-Verlag.

Histopathology: A Step-by-Step-Approach. Martin G. Lewis & Geoffrey Rowden. 1984. 250p. 40.95 (*0-316-52340-2*, Little Brwn Med Div) Lppncott W & W.

Histopathology: Color Atlas & Textbook. Ivan Damjanov. 1996. LC 94-47026. (Illus.). 304p. pap. 47.00 (*0-683-02334-9*) Lppncott W & W.

Histopathology Atlas for S. I. D. S. Valdez-Depena et al. 1993. (Illus.). 339p. pap. text 40.00 (*1-881041-05-0*) Am Registry Path.

Histopathology of Chemically Induced Tumors: Electronic Color Atlas. Nobuyuki Ito & Yuzo Hayashi. Tr. by Naoki Yoshime. 2000. (Illus.). (C). 120.00 incl. audio compact disk (*0-9701785-1-4*); cd-rom 85.00 (*0-9701785-0-6*) Texas Histopages.

Histopathology of Disease. Jay H. Lefkowitch. 1989. (Illus.). 234p. text (*0-443-08566-8*) Church.

Histopathology of Infectious Diseases. Marty. 1997. 165.00 (*0-397-51309-7*, M2964) Lppncott W & W.

Histopathology of Non-Hodgkin Lymphomas: Kiel Classification. K. Lennert. 1981. (Illus.). 135p. 48.00 (*0-387-10445-3*) Spr-Verlag.

Histopathology of Non-Hodgkin's Lymphomas: Based on the Updated Kiel Classification. K. Lennert & A. C. Feller. 2nd rev. ed. 1994. (Illus.). 312p. 176.00 (*0-387-51270-5*) Spr-Verlag.

Histopathology of Preclinical Toxicity Studies: Interpretation & Relevance in Drug Safety Evaluation. Ed. by P. Greaves. 1991. 824p. 404.50 (*0-444-81311-X*) Elsevier.

Histopathology of the Endometrium. G. Dallenbach-Hellweg. Tr. by F. B. Dallenbach from GER. 3rd rev. ed. 1981. (Illus.). 359p. 86.00 (*0-387-10658-8*) Spr-Verlag.

Histopathology of the Liver, Set. Gerald Klatskin & Harold O. Conn. 1993. (Illus.). 768p. text 250.00 (*0-19-504393-6*) OUP.

Histopathology Reporting: Guidelines for Surgical Cancer. Derek C. Allen. 2000. LC 99-54065. (Illus.). xxix, 384p. 79.00 (*1-85233-185-2*) Spr-Verlag.

Histophysiology Immunology of Lymphoid Tissues. Eric Claassen & Suzan H. Jeurissen. 1999. 80.00 (*0-8493-9220-9*) CRC Pr.

Histophysiology of the Circulating Platelet. L. J. Wurzinger. 1990. (Advances in Anatomy, Embryology & Cell Biology Ser.: Vol. 120). (Illus.). 104p. 44.00 (*0-387-52258-1*) Spr-Verlag.

Histophysiology of the Immune System: The Life History, Organization, & Interactions of Its Cell Populations. Ed. by S. Fossum & Bent Rolstad. 1988. (Advances in Experimental Medicine & Biology Ser.: Vol. 237). (Illus.). 926p. 165.00 (*0-306-42981-0*, Plenum Trade) Perseus Pubng.

Histophysiology of the Obesity-Diabetes Syndrome in Sand Rats. Herwig H. Von Dorsche et al. 1994. LC 94-13303. (Advances in Anatomy, Embryology & Cell Biology Ser.: Vol. 130). (Illus.). 103p. 78.95 (*0-387-57913-3*) Spr-Verlag.

Histoplasmosis. Jan Schwarz. 1981. LC 80-21673. (Life Science Ser.). 472p. 115.00 (*0-275-91353-8*, C1353, Praeger Pubs) Greenwood.

Historia de la Medicina en Cuba II: Ejercicios y Ensenanza de las Ciencias Medicas en la Epoca Colonial. Cesar A. Mena. 1993. LC 91-76473. (Coleccion Cuba y sus Jueces). (SPA., Illus.). 380p. (Orig.). pap. 39.00 (*0-89729-646-X*) Ediciones.

Historia de la Medicina en Cuba, Vol. 1: Hospitales y Centros Beneficos en Cuba Colonial. Cesar A. Mena & Armando F. Cobelo. 1992. LC 91-76473. (Coleccion Cuba y sus Jueces). (SPA., Illus.). 717p. (Orig.). pap. 49.00 (*0-89729-624-9*) Ediciones.

Historia de la Odontologia en Cuba: Cuba Comunista y en el Exilio 1959-1983, Vol. IV. Cesar A. Mena. 1984. LC 81-652235. (Coleccion Cuba y sus Jueces). (SPA., Illus.). 752p. (Orig.). pap. 33.00 (*0-89729-344-4*) Ediciones.

Historia de la Odontologia en Cuba: Vol. 1, Periodo Colonial(1492-1898), Vol. I. Cesar A. Mena. 1981. LC 81-65235. (Coleccion Cuba y sus Jueces). (SPA., Illus.). 394p. (Orig.). pap. 29.00 (*0-89729-293-6*) Ediciones.

Historic Expedition to America (1909) Freud, Jung & Hall the King-Maker. Saul Rosenzweig. 2000. 477p. reprint ed. pap. 17.00 (*0-7881-9424-0*) DIANE Pub.

Historical Account of the Climates & Diseases of the U. S. A. & of the Remedies & Methods of Treatment. William Currie. 1972. LC 70-180570. (Medicine & Society in America Ser.). 428p. reprint ed. 25.95 (*0-405-03945-X*) Ayer.

Historical & Contemporary Perspectives on Philosophy of Science in Nursing: An Anthology. E. Carol Polifroni & Marylouise Welch. 1998. LC 98-15842. 560p. pap. text 47.95 (*0-7817-1201-7*) Lppncott W & W.

Historical & Geographical Influences on Psychopathology. Ed. by Patricia Cohen et al. 1998. LC 98-7194. 408p. 99.95 (*0-8058-2426-X*); pap. 45.00 (*0-8058-2427-8*) L Erlbaum Assocs.

Historical Aspects of American Trypanosomiasis (Chagas' Disease) Matthias Perleth. LC 98-51844. (Medizin in Entwicklungslandern, Schriftenreihe zur Medizin und zu Gesundheitsproblemen in Landern der Dritten Welt Ser.: Bd. 43). (Illus.). 171p. 1997. pap. 35.95 (*3-631-31063-3*); 1996. pap. 35.95 (*0-8204-3232-6*) P Lang Pubng.

***Historical Atlas of Dermatology & Dermatologists.** J. T. Crissey & L. C. Parish. 2002. LC 2001-56031. (Illus.). 200p. 89.95 (*1-84214-100-7*, Parthenon Pbng) CRC Pr.

Historical Development of British Psychiatry, Vol. 1: Eighteenth & Nineteenth Century. D. Leigh. 1961. LC 61-14243. (*0-08-009537-2*) Pergamon Repr GBR. *Dist:* Franklin.

Historical Dimensions of Psychological Discourse. Ed. by Carl F. Graumann & Kenneth J. Gergen. 1996. 291p. (C). text 49.95 (*0-521-48021-3*) Cambridge U Pr.

Historical Landmarks in Head & Neck Cancer Surgery. Donald P. Shedd. 2000. LC 99-96559. (Illus.). 107p. pap. (*0-9675702-0-4*) Head & Neck.

Historical Perspectives & the International Status of Comparative Psychology. Ed. by Ethel Tobach. 1987. 264p. (C). text 59.95 (*0-89859-651-3*) L Erlbaum Assocs.

Historical Perspectives on Homosexuality. Ed. by Salvatore J. Licata & Robert P. Petersen. LC 80-6262. (Journal of Homosexuality Ser.: Vol. 6, Nos. 1-2). 224p. 1985. pap. 2.95 (*0-86656-436-5*); 1982. text 39.95 (*0-917724-27-5*) Haworth Pr.

Historical Reflections: The Community & the Afro-American Pioneer Physicians of Columbus, Ohio. William K. Allen. 1990. LC 89-85838. (Illus.). 60p. 17.00 (*0-9624897-0-0*) W K Allen.

Historical Relations of Medicine & Surgery to the End of the 16th Century. Thomas C. Allbutt. LC 75-23672. reprint ed. 36.00 (*0-404-13225-1*) AMS Pr.

Historical Review of the Department of Surgery of Case Western Reserve University 1843-1986. Elden C. Weckesser. 1986. (Illus.). 180p. 38.00 (*0-9616613-0-5*) CWRU Dept Surgery.

Historical Scientific & Practical Essay on Milk, As an Article of Human Sustenance: Consideration of the Effects Consequent upon the Unnatural Methods of Producing It for the Supply of Large Cities. Robert M. Hartley. Ed. by Barbara G. Rosenkrantz. 1977. LC 76-40629. (Public Health in America Ser.). (Illus.). reprint ed. lib. bdg. 29.95 (*0-405-09822-7*) Ayer.

Historical Typing of Tumors of the Liver: International Histological Classification of Tumors. K. G. Ishak et al. 2nd ed. 1994. (Surgery, Pathology, & Hepatology Ser.). (Illus.). 125p. 72.00 (*0-387-58154-5*) Spr-Verlag.

Historie of Life & Death: Observations Naturall & Experimentall for the Prolonging of Life. Francis Bacon. Ed. by Robert J. Kastenbaum. 1977. LC 76-19558. (Death & Dying Ser.). reprint ed. lib. bdg. 33.95 (*0-405-09554-6*) Ayer.

Historie of Life & Death: With Observations Naturall & Experimentall. Francis Bacon. 1968. LC 68-54613. (English Experience Ser.: No. 20). 324p. reprint ed. 35.00 (*90-221-0020-0*) Walter J Johnson.

Historie of Man. John Banister. 1969. LC 74-26164. (English Experience Ser.: No. 122). (Illus.). 250p. reprint ed. 60.00 (*90-221-0122-3*) Walter J Johnson.

Histories: A Journal of Archetype & Culture, No. 64. Bianca Garufi et al. Ed. by Charles Boer & Jay Livernois. 2000. (Spring Journal Ser.: Vol. 64). 308p. (C). pap. 17.50 (*1-882670-14-0*) Spring Jrnl.

Histories of Sexually Transmitted Diseases & HIV/AIDS in Sub-Saharan Africa, 44. Maryinez Lyons. Ed. by Philip Setel & Milton Lewis. 1999. LC 98-38207. (Contributions in Medical Studies Ser.: Vol. 44). 280p. 78.00 (*0-313-29715-0*, Greenwood Pr) Greenwood.

Historiography & Causation in Psychoanalysis. Edwin R. Wallace. 1984. (Psychoanalytic Monographs: Vol. 2). 285p. text 39.95 (*0-88163-015-2*) Analytic Pr.

Historiography of Psychoanalysis. Paul Roazen. 2000. LC 00-64757. (Illus.). xiii, 480p. text 39.95 (*0-7658-0019-5*) Transaction Pubs.

History & Bibliography of Anatomic Illustration. Ludwig Choulant. Tr. by Mortimer Frank from GER. 1993. (Illus.). 462p. reprint ed. 85.00 (*1-888262-41-9*) Martino Pubng.

History & Epidemiology of Syphilis. William A. Pusey. LC 75-23753. reprint ed. 32.50 (*0-404-13359-2*) AMS Pr.

History & Evolution of Surgical Instruments. C. J. S. Thomson. 2000. (Illus.). 114p. reprint ed. 50.00 (*1-57898-219-7*) Martino Pubng.

History & Function of the Target Cities Management Information Systems. Matthew G. Hile. 1998. LC 98-9784. 39.95 (*0-7890-0520-4*) Haworth Pr.

History & Geography of Human Genes. Luigi L. Cavalli-Sforza et al. 1994. LC 93-19339. (Illus.). 522p. 195.00 (*0-691-08750-4*) Princeton U Pr.

History & Iconography of Endemic Goitre & Cretinism. F. Merke. 1984. 330p. 68.00 (*3-456-81189-6*) Hogrefe & Huber Pubs.

History & Influence of the American Psychiatric Association. Walter E. Barton. 1987. LC 86-17250. 400p. text 29.95 (*0-88048-231-1*, 8231) Am Psychiatric.

History & Literature of Surgery. John S. Billings. 1970. reprint ed. 20.00 (*0-87266-038-9*) Argosy.

History & Pathology of Vaccination Edgar M. Crookshank. LC 75-23702. reprint ed. (*0-404-13330-4*) AMS Pr.

History & Perspectives of Cardiology: Catheterization, Angiography, Surgery, Concepts of Circular Control. Ed. by H. A. Snellen et al. 1981. xii, 204p. text 99.50 (*90-6021-480-3*) Kluwer Academic.

History & Philosophy of Ayurveda. Vasant Lad. 2001. LC 00-9373. (Textbook of Ayurveda Ser.: Bk. 1). (Illus.). xix, 275p. (*1-883725-07-0*) Ayurvedic Pr.

History & Physical Exam Casebook. Diane L. Eliot & Linn Goldberg. 1997. LC 97-5555. 400p. pap. text 29.95 (*0-316-23339-0*, Little Brwn Med Div) Lppncott W & W.

History & Physical Examination for PDAs & Desktops: 2001-2002. Paul D. Chan. rev. ed. 1999. (Current Clinical Strategies Ser.). 89p. pap. 28.95 incl. cd-rom (*1-881528-82-0*) Current Clin Strat.

History & Physical Examination, 2001- 2002 Edition: Current Clinical Strategies. Paul D. Chan. rev. ed. 1999. (Current Clinical Strategies Ser.). 100p. pap. 9.95 (*1-881528-81-2*) Current Clin Strat.

History & Politics of Mental Health. Murray Levine. 1981. 232p. pap. text 19.95 (*0-19-502956-9*) OUP.

History & Present State of Discoveries Relating to Vision, Light, & Colours. Joseph Priestley. Ed. by I. Bernard Cohen. 1981. LC 80-2142. (Development of Science Ser.). (Illus.). lib. bdg. 77.95 (*0-405-13897-0*) Ayer.

History & Psychoanalysis. Saul Friedlander. Tr. by Susan Suleiman from FRE. 1978. LC 77-18524. 175p. (C). pap. 18.95 (*0-8419-0611-4*) Holmes & Meier.

History & Psychology: Main Current Psychological Thought. Ed. by Prentice-Hall Staff. 5th ed. 2000. (C). text (*0-13-040236-2*) P-H.

History & Systems of Psychology. James F. Brennan. 5th ed. 1997. LC 97-7922. 374p. 77.00 (*0-13-857418-9*) P-H.

History & Theory of Informed Consent. Ruth R. Faden et al. 1986. LC 85-13858. (Illus.). 432p. (C). text 49.95 (*0-19-503686-7*) OUP.

History, Language & Literacy in the Byzantine World. Robert Browning. 1989. (Collected Studies: No. CS299). (Illus.). 276p. (C). reprint ed. text (*0-86078-247-6*) Variorum GBR. *Dist:* Ashgate Pub Co.

***History of a Genetic Disease.** Alan E. H. Emery & Marcia L. H. Emery. 1997. (History of Medicine Ser.). (*1-85315-249-8*) Royal Soc of Medicine Pr Ltd GBR. *Dist:* Balogh.

History of Academic Psychology in Canada. Ed. by Mary J. Wright & C. Roger Myers. 1995. (Illus.). 270p. (C). pap. text 22.00 (*0-88937-004-4*) Hogrefe & Huber Pubs.

History of Addenbrooke's Hospital, Cambridge. Arthur Rook et al. 1992. (Illus.). 535p. (C). text 120.00 (*0-521-40529-7*) Cambridge U Pr.

History of Aggression in Freud Psychological Issues. Paul E. Stepansky. 1977. LC 76-53907. (Psychological Issues Monographs: No. 39). 212p. 40.00 (*0-8236-2326-2*); pap. 35.00 (*0-8236-2325-4*) Intl Univs Pr.

History of American Pediatrics. Thomas E. Cone, Jr. 1980. 27.00 (*0-316-15289-7*, Little Brwn Med Div) Lppncott W & W.

History of Anaesthesia. Ed. by R. S. Atkinson & T. B. Boulton. 1989. (History of Medicine Ser.). (Illus.). 649p. 118.00 (*1-85070-276-4*, Parthenon Pbng) CRC Pr.

History of Anatomy: The Post-Vesalian Era. T. V. Persaud. 1997. LC 97-3002. (Illus.). 372p. text 96.95 (*0-398-06772-4*); pap. text 79.95 (*0-398-06773-2*) C C Thomas.

History of Ancient Psychiatry, 16. Giuseppe Roccatagliata. 1986. LC 84-15721. (Contributions in Medical Studies Ser.: No. 16). 304p. 78.00 (*0-313-24419-7*, RHI/, Greenwood Pr) Greenwood.

History of Behavioral Psychology. Mills. 2000. LC 98-19699. 256p. pap. text 20.00 (*0-8147-5612-3*) NYU Pr.

History of Bethlem. Jonathan Andrews. 1997. LC 96-52471. (Illus.). 768p. (C). 265.00 (*0-415-01773-4*) Routledge.

History of Blood Gases, Acids & Bases. Poul Astrup & John W. Severinghaus. 1986. (Illus.). 332p. text 72.50 (*91-1-606496-8*) Coronet Bks.

History of Breast Cancer. Olson. 1997. 25.00 (*0-02-923836-6*); 25.00 (*0-684-82806-5*) Free Pr.

History of British Mammals Gerald E. Barrett-Hamilton & Martin A. Hinton. Ed. by Keir B. Sterling. 1978. LC 77-81081. (Biologists & Their World Ser.). (Illus.). reprint ed. Set. lib. bdg. 101.95 (*0-405-10648-3*); Vol. 1. lib. bdg. 50.95 (*0-405-10649-1*); Vol. 2. lib. bdg. 50.95 (*0-405-10650-5*) Ayer.

History of British Midwifery from 1650 to 1800. Herbert R. Spencer. LC 75-23761. reprint ed. 39.50 (*0-404-13367-3*) AMS Pr.

History of Cancer: An Annotated Bibliography, 3. James S. Olson. 1989. LC 89-2174. (Bibliographies & Indexes in Medical Studies: No. 3). 434p. lib. bdg. 104.50 (*0-313-25889-9*, OHY/, Greenwood Pr) Greenwood.

History of Carcinology, Vol. 8. Ed. by F. M. Truesdale & Frederick R. Schramm. 1993. (Crustacean Issues Ser.). (Illus.). 482p. (C). text (*90-5410-137-7*) A A Balkema NLD. *Dist:* Ashgate Pub Co.

History of Cardiology. Louis J. Acierno. 2001. (Illus.). 758p. pap. 55.00 (*1-85070-049-4*, Parthenon Pbng) CRC Pr.

HI

History of Cardiology: Men, Ideas & Contributions. Louis J. Acierno. 1994. (History of Medicine Ser.). (Illus.). 758p. (C). lib. bdg. 107.95 (*1-85070-339-6*, Parthenon Pbng) CRC Pr.

History of Cardiothoracic Surgery from Early Times. Raymond Hurt. 1996. LC 95-41860. 532p. lib. bdg. 107.95 (*1-85070-681-6*, Parthenon Pbng) CRC Pr.

History of Child Psychoanalysis. Claudine Geissmann-Chambon & Pierre Geissmann. 1998. LC 97-12477. 368p. (C). 100.00 (*0-415-11020-3*); pap. 39.99 (*0-415-11296-6*) Routledge.

History of Chinese Medicine K. C. Wong & Wu Lien-Teh. 1976. lib. bdg. 500.00 (*0-8490-3062-5*) Gordon Pr.

History of Chinese Medicine, Being a Chronicle of Medical Happenings in China from Ancient Times to the Present Period. Chi-Min Wong & Wu Lien-Teh. LC 73-38570. reprint ed. 237.50 (*0-404-07990-3*) AMS Pr.

History of Chiropractic Education in North America. Joseph C. Keating, Jr. et al. 1998. LC 98-72099. (Illus.). 516p. 79.95 (*0-9659131-1-2*) Assn Hist Chiro.

History of Circumcision, from the Earliest Times to the Present. Peter C. Remondino. LC 72-9675. (Physicians' & Students' Ready Reference Ser.). reprint ed. 47.50 (*0-404-57492-0*) AMS Pr.

History of Clinical Chemistry. Ed. by J. Buttner. 1983. LC 83-1968. (Illus.). 91p. 89.25 (*3-11-008912-2*) De Gruyter.

History of Clinical Endocrinology: A Comprehensive Account of Endocrinology from Earliest Times to the Present Day. V. C. Medvei. 1993. (History of Medicine Ser.). (Illus.). 451p. lib. bdg. 140.95 (*1-85070-427-9*, Parthenon Pbng) CRC Pr.

History of Clinical Psychiatry: The Origin & History of Psychiatric Diseases. Ed. by German E. Berrios & Roy Porter. 1995. LC 95-31496. 480p. (C). text 65.00 (*0-8147-1259-2*) NYU Pr.

History of Clinical Psychiatry: The Origin & History of Psychiatric Disorders. German E. Berrios & Roy Porter. 1999. LC 98-52022. 15p. pap. (*0-485-24211-7*) Athlone Pr GBR. *Dist:* Transaction Pubs.

History of Clinical Psychology. John M. Reisman. 2nd ed. 1991. 424p. 99.95 (*1-56032-041-9*); pap. 36.95 (*1-56032-188-1*) Hemisp Pub.

History of Contraception: From Antiquity to the Present Day. Angus McLaren. 1992. pap. 27.95 (*0-631-18729-4*) Blackwell Pubs.

History of Dentistry. Walter A. Hoffmann-Axthelm. 1981. (Illus.). 436p. text 126.00 (*3-87652-161-0*) Quint Pub Co.

History of Dermatology. William A. Pusey. LC 75-23754. reprint ed. 55.00 (*0-404-13360-6*) AMS Pr.

History of Dermatology: A Global Perspective. G. G. Russo & J. L. Parish. 2001. 600p. 98.00 (*1-84214-053-1*, Parthenon Pbng) CRC Pr.

History of Drug Containers & Their Labels. George Griffen Hagen & Mary Bogard. Ed. by Gregory J. Higby & Elaine Stroud. rev. ed. 1999. (New Ser.: No. 17). (Illus.). 150 p. pap. 19.95 (*0-931292-26-3*) Am Inst Hist Pharm.

History of Electrocardiography. George E. Burch & Nicholas DePasquale. 1990. (Illus.). 309p. reprint ed. 125.00 (*0-930405-21-8*) Norman SF.

History of Embryology. Joseph Needham. 2nd ed. 1979. LC 74-26280. (History, Philosophy, & Sociology of Science Ser.). reprint ed. 33.95 (*0-405-06607-4*) Ayer.

History of Endocrine Surgery. Richard B. Welbourn et al. 1990. LC 89-16118. 410p. 105.00 (*0-275-92586-2*, C2586, Praeger Pubs) Greenwood.

History of Endocrinology. V. C. Medvei. 1982. (Illus.). 900p. text 286.50 (*0-85200-245-9*) Kluwer Academic.

History of Epileptic Therapy: An Account of How Medication Was Developed. D. F. Scott. 1993. (History of Medicine Ser.). (Illus.). 180p. (C). lib. bdg. 74.95 (*1-85070-391-4*, Parthenon Pbng) CRC Pr.

History of Experimental Virology. A. Grafe. 1991. (Illus.). 343p. 86.95 (*0-387-51925-4*) Spr-Verlag.

History of Free Skin Crafting. Knowledge or Empiricism? H. J. Klason. 1981. (Illus.). 190p. 63.95 (*0-387-10802-5*) Spr-Verlag.

History of Gastric Secretion & Digestion: Experimental Studies to 1975. Horace W. Davenport. 1992. (Illus.). 432p. text 79.00 (*0-19-507393-2*) OUP.

History of Gastroenterology. T. S. Chen & P. S. Chen. 1995. (History of Medicine Ser.). (Illus.). 328p. lib. bdg. 96.95 (*1-85070-365-5*, Parthenon Pbng) CRC Pr.

History of Healing, a Future of Care: Saint Mary of Nazareth Hospital Center, Celebrating a Century of Catholic Hospitality. Charles W. Sanford, Jr. Ed. by Phyllis Pavese & Rodney Nelson. 1994. 150p. (C). 35.00 (*0-929690-24-9*) Herit Pubs AZ.

History of Health & Medicine in Queensland 1824-1960. Ross Patrick. 1988. LC 86-27250. (Illus.). 561p. text (*0-7022-2078-7*) Univ Queensland Pr AUS. *Dist:* Intl Spec Bk.

History of Health, & the Art of Preserving It. James MacKenzie. Ed. by Robert J. Kastenbaum. 1979. LC 78-22208. (Aging & Old Age Ser.). reprint ed. lib. bdg. 39.95 (*0-405-11822-8*) Ayer.

History of Health Services in Missouri. John C. Crighton. 1993. (Illus.). 278p. text 34.95 (*0-9639699-0-0*) J C Crighton Pub.

History of HLA: Ten Recollections. Ed. by Paul I. Terasaki. 1990. 15.00 (*0-9604606-6-7*) UCLA Tissue.

History of Hospital Point - La Historia de Punta Hospital: Pioneer Medical Center, 1899-1920. Clyde S. Stephens. 1997. LC 97-66141. (ENG & SPA., Illus.). 56p. (Orig.). pap. 10.00 (*0-9625049-1-2*) Banana Bk.

History of Hypnotism. Alan Gauld. 1992. (Illus.). 756p. (C). text 130.00 (*0-521-30675-2*) Cambridge U Pr.

History of Ideas about the Prolongation of Life: The Evolution of Prolongevity Hypotheses to 1800. Gerald J. Gruman. Ed. by Robert J. Kastenbaum. 1977. LC 76-19574. (Death & Dying Ser.). (Illus.). reprint ed. lib. bdg. 19.95 (*0-405-09572-4*) Ayer.

History of Immunology. Arthur M. Silverstein. 1989. LC 88-14538. 746p. text 73.00 (*0-12-643770-X*) Acad Pr.

History of Malaria in the Roman Campagna from Ancient Times. Angelo Celli. Ed. by Anna Celli-Fraentzel. LC 75-23694. reprint ed. 39.50 (*0-404-13243-X*) AMS Pr.

History of Medi-Cal Physician Payment Rates. Michele Prestowitz & Lucy Streett. 2000. (Illus.). 24p. pap. (*1-929008-27-9*) CA HlthCare Fnd.

History of Medical Care in New York City: The Principal Founders of Cornell University Medical College with Articles on the Development of Medical Education & Care in the U. S. Carl A. Berntsen. Ed. by Elise B. Stanbury. 1998. 323p. text 100.00 (*0-9668386-0-2*) E B Stanbury.

History of Medical Informatics. Bruce I. Blum & Karen Duncan. 1990. LC 89-17960. (ACM Press History Ser.). (Illus.). 496p. (C). 59.99 (*0-201-50128-7*) Addison-Wesley.

History of Medical Informatics in the United States: 1950 to 1990. Morris F. Collen. 1995. LC 95-34109. 489p. 40.00 (*0-9647743-0-5*) Am Med Info Assn.

History of Medical Mycology in the United States: Development of the Discipline. Anna Espiel-Ingroff. 2000. LC 98-18319. (Illus.). 340p. 39.95 (*0-89863-204-8*) Star Pub CA.

History of Medications for Women: Materia Medica Woman. Michael J. O'Dowd. 2001. LC 00-38506. (Illus.). 570p. lib. bdg. 84.95 (*1-85070-002-8*, Parthenon Pbng) CRC Pr.

History of Medicine. Ed. by Rebecca Greene. 1988. LC 88-2793. (Trends in History Ser.: Vol. 4, Nos. 2-3). 133p. text 39.95 (*0-86656-309-1*) Haworth Pr.

History of Medicine. Ed. by Lois N. Magner. 1992. (Illus.). 400p. text 65.00 (*0-8247-8673-4*) Dekker.

History of Medicine: A Scandalously Short Introduction. Jacalyn Duffin. 1999. (Illus.). 838p. pap. text 24.95 (*0-8020-7912-1*) U of Toronto Pr.

History of Medicine Vol. 1: Primitive & Ancient Medicine, 1. Plinio Prioreschi. 2nd enl. rev. ed. 1996. LC 95-81354. 587p. lib. bdg. 115.00 (*1-888456-01-9*) Horatius Pr.

History of Medicine Vol. 1: Primitive & Archaic Medicine, Vol. 1. Henry E. Sigerist. 1987. (Illus.). 586p. pap. text 26.95 (*0-19-500739-5*) OUP.

History of Medicine Vol. 2: Early Greek, Hindu & Persian Medicine, Vol. 2. Henry E. Sigerist. 1987. (Illus.). 368p. pap. text 24.95 (*0-19-505079-7*) OUP.

History of Medicine Vol. 2: Greek Medicine, 2. Plinio Prioreschi. 2nd enl. rev. ed. 1996. 695p. lib. bdg. 135.00 (*1-888456-02-7*) Horatius Pr.

History of Medicine Vol. 3: Roman Medicine, 3. Plinio Prioreschi. 1998. LC 91-29934. 822p. lib. bdg. 150.00 (*1-888456-03-5*) Horatius Pr.

History of Medicine in Butler County. Jean Purvis. 2000. 80p. 30.00 (*0-929690-52-4*) Herit Pubs AZ.

History of Medicine in New York: Three Centuries of Medical Progress James J. Walsh. LC 75-23765. reprint ed. 300.00 (*0-404-13440-8*) AMS Pr.

History of Medicine in the Americas. L. N. Magner. Date not set. (*0-8247-9905-4*) Dekker.

History of Medieval Jewish Gynaecological Texts. Ron Barkai. 1998. LC 97-52122. (Jewish Studies). 87.50 (*90-04-10995-1*) Brill Academic Pubs.

History of Mental Health & Industry. Ed. by Pasquale A. Carone et al. 1985. (Problems of Industrial Psychiatric Medicine Ser.: Vol. 10). 128p. 30.95 (*0-89885-207-2*, Kluwer Acad Hman Sci) Kluwer Academic.

History of Mental Symptoms: Descriptive Psychopathology since the Nineteenth Century. German E. Berrios. 1996. (Illus.). 581p. (C). text 225.00 (*0-521-43135-2*); pap. text 80.00 (*0-521-43736-9*) Cambridge U Pr.

History of Military Medicine, 124. Richard A. Gabriel & Karen S. Metz. 1992. LC 91-32404. (Contributions in Military Studies Ser.: No. 124). 600p. 130.00 (*0-313-27746-X*, GHM/, Greenwood Pr) Greenwood.

History of Military Medicine Vol. I: From Ancient Times to the Middle Ages, Vol. 1. Richard A. Gabriel & Karen S. Metz. 1992. LC 91-32404. (Contributions in Military Studies Ser.: No. 124). 272p. 75.00 (*0-313-28402-4*, GHM01, Greenwood Pr) Greenwood.

History of Military Medicine Vol. II: From the Renaissance Through Modern Times, Vol. 2. Richard A. Gabriel & Karen S. Metz. 1992. LC 91-32404. (Contributions in Military Studies Ser.). 328p. 75.00 (*0-313-28403-2*, GHM02, Greenwood Pr) Greenwood.

History of Modern Cataract Surgery. Ed. by Marvin L. Kwitko & Charles D. Kelman. 1998. (Illus.). x, 297p. (*90-6299-154-8*) Kugler NLD. *Dist:* Lib Res.

History of Modern Psychology. C. James Goodwin. 1998. LC 98-5650. (Illus.). 512p. pap. 59.95 (*0-471-12805-8*) Wiley.

History of Modern Psychology: Test Bank. Schultz. 6th ed. 1995. (C). pap. text, tchr. ed. 42.00 (*0-15-503524-X*) Harcourt Coll Pubs.

History of Natural Hygiene & Principles of Natural Hygiene Being the Teachings of Doctors Jennings, Graham, Trall & Tilden. Herbert M. Shelton. 1996. 95p. reprint ed. pap. 9.95 (*1-56459-734-2*) Kessinger Pub.

History of Nephrology 1: Reports from the First Congress on the International Association for the History of Nephrology, Kos, October 1996. Ed. by N. G. De Santo et al. 1994. LC 95-101529. (Journal: Vol. 14, No. 4-6, 1994). (Illus.). vi, 244p. 64.50 (*3-8055-6072-9*) S Karger.

History of Nephrology 3: Reports from the 2nd Congress of the International Association for the History of Nephrology, Padova, October 1998. Ed. by G. Eknoyan et al. 1999. LC 99-232404. (American Journal of Nephrology: Vol. 19, No. 2). (Illus.). iv, 180p. reprint ed. 64.50 (*3-8055-6855-X*) S Karger.

History of Nerve & Muscle Physiology. C. Ladd Prosser. 2000. (People & Ideas Ser.). (Illus.). 450p. 75.00 (*0-19-511354-3*) OUP.

History of Neuroscience in Autobiography. Ed. by Larry R. Squire. 1996. LC 96-70950. (Illus.). 604p. 49.00 (*0-916110-51-6*) Society for Neuroscience.

History of Neurosurgery. Ed. by Samuel H. Greenblatt et al. 1997. (Illus.). 600p. 95.00 (*1-879284-17-0*) Am Assn Neuro.

History of Nursing: An Index to the Microfiche Collection Set. 150.00 (*0-8357-0607-9*); Vol. 1. 1983. 90.00 (*0-8357-0608-7*); Vol. 2. 1985. 90.00 (*0-8357-0609-5*); Vol. 3. 1988. 90.00 (*0-8357-0751-2*) Univ Microfilms.

History of Nursing in the Field of Mental Retardation & Development Disabilities. Wendy M. Nehring. 1999. LC 99-41728. (Illus.). xiv, 205p. 39.95 (*0-940898-68-3*) Am Assn Mental.

History of Obstetrics & Gynecology. M. J. O'Dowd & E. E. Philipp. 2000. (Illus.). 720p. lib. bdg. 60.95 (*1-85070-040-0*) CRC Pr.

History of Obstetrics & Gynecology. Ed. by M. J. O'Dowd & E. E. Philipp. 1994. (History of Medicine Ser.). (Illus.). 710p. 125.00 (*1-85070-224-1*, Parthenon Pbng) CRC Pr.

History of Ophthalmology. Daniel M. Albert. 1996. LC 96-9847. (Illus.). 350p. 138.95 (*0-86542-378-4*) Blackwell Sci.

History of Ophthalmology. H. E. Henkes. 1988. (Documenta Ophthalmologica Proceedings Ser.: Vol. 68 1-2). (C). text 177.50 (*0-89838-366-8*) Kluwer Academic.

History of Ophthalmology. Ed. by H. E. Henkes. (C). Vol. 2. 1989. pap. text 85.50 (*0-7923-0273-7*); Vol. 3. 1990. pap. text 171.00 (*0-7923-0826-3*); Vol. 4. 1992. pap. text 92.50 (*0-7923-1545-6*) Kluwer Academic.

History of Ophthalmology, Vol. 7. Albert. 1995. pap. text 125.00 (*0-7923-3401-9*) Kluwer Academic.

History of Orthopedics. David Le Vay. 1990. (History of Medicine Ser.). (Illus.). 693p. 125.00 (*1-85070-145-8*, Parthenon Pbng) CRC Pr.

History of Pain. Roselyne Rey. Tr. by Louise E. Wallace et al from FRE. 1995. LC 94-31948.Tr. of Histoire de la Douleur. 394p. text 47.50 (*0-674-39967-6*, REYHIS) HUP.

History of Paratuberculosis, Johne's Disease: A Review of the Literature 1985-1992. Compiled by Rodrick J. Chiodini. 1993. LC 93-12657. 125.00 (*0-9633043-1-3*) Intl Assn Paratuber.

History of Physics: From the Time of Galen to the Beginning of the Sixteenth Century John Freind. 4th ed. reprint ed. 75.00 (*0-404-07987-3*) AMS Pr.

History of Physiology. Karl E. Rothschuh. Tr. by Gunter B. Risse from GER. LC 74-158126. Orig. Title: Geschichte der Physiologie. (Illus.). 400p. 1973. 43.50 (*0-88275-069-0*); 1980. reprint ed. pap. 28.50 (*0-89874-254-4*) Krieger.

History of Psychiatry: An Evaluation of Psychiatric Thought & Practice from Prehistoric Times to the Present. Franz Gabriel Alexander et al. 1995. LC 95-20598. 494p. pap. 60.00 (*1-56821-754-4*) Aronson.

History of Psychiatry: From the Era of the Asylum to the Age of Prozac. Edward Shorter. (Illus.). 448p. 1996. LC 96-15292. 30.00 (*0-471-15749-X*); 2nd ed. 1998. pap. 24.95 (*0-471-24531-3*) Wiley.

History of Psychoanalysis: From Healing Magic to Encounter. Reuben Fine. 1990. LC 89-49692. 784p. reprint ed. 75.00 (*0-87668-791-5*) Aronson.

History of Psycholgy in Letters. Ludy T. Benjamin, Jr. 1992. 240p. (C). pap. 37.50 (*0-697-12980-2*, WCB McGr Hill) McGrw-H Hghr Educ.

History of Psychology. Rice. 1999. pap. text (*0-582-30375-3*) Addison-Wesley.

History of Psychology: Original Sources & Contemporary Research. Ludy T. Benjamin, Jr. 1988. 576p. (C). pap. text 37.74 net. (*0-07-004561-5*) McGraw.

History of Psychology in Autobiography, Vol. VIII. Ed. by Gardner Lindzey. 1989. LC 30-20129. (Illus.). 504p. 66.00 (*0-8047-1492-4*) Stanford U Pr.

History of Psychotherapy. Ed. by Jan Ehrenwald. 1991. LC 76-25782. (History of Psychotherapy Encore CL Ser.). 592p. reprint ed. 55.00 (*0-87668-280-8*) Aronson.

History of Psychotherapy: A Century of Change. Ed. by Donald K. Freedheim et al. 1992. (Illus.). 964p. text 79.95 (*1-55798-149-3*) Am Psychol.

History of Public Health. George Rosen. 1993. LC 93-9821. 632p. reprint ed. pap. text 20.95 (*0-8018-4645-5*) Johns Hopkins.

History of Public Health in New York City, 1625 - 1866,, Vol. 1. John Duffy. 1968. LC 68-25852. 620p. lib. bdg. 55.00 (*0-87154-212-9*) Russell Sage.

History of Regional Medical Programs: The Life & Death of a Small Initiative of the Great Society. Stephen P. Strickland. 2000. LC 00-44330. 138p. 37.50 (*0-7618-1775-1*) U Pr of Amer.

History of Sanitation. J. J. Cosgrove. 1977. lib. bdg. 59.95 (*0-8490-1985-0*) Gordon Pr.

History of Sexuality, Vol. 1. Michel Foucault. 1990. LC 79-7460. (History of Sexuality Ser.: Vol. 1). pap. 11.00 (*0-679-72469-9*) Vin Bks.

History of Shock Treatment. Ed. by Leonard R. Frank. 1978. LC 78-13550. (Illus.). 206p. pap. 14.00 (*0-9601376-1-0*) L R Frank.

History of Stroke: Its Recognition & Treatment. William S. Fields & Noreen A. Lemak. 1989. (Illus.). 224p. text 35.00 (*0-19-505755-4*) OUP.

History of Surgery: With Emphasis on the Netherlands. Daniel De Moulin. 1987. (C). lib. bdg. 225.50 (*0-89838-968-2*) Kluwer Academic.

History of Surgery in Houston. Ed. by Kenneth L. Mattox. ltd. ed. 1998. LC 98-28964. (Illus.). 488p. lthr. 100.00 (*1-57168-258-9*) Eakin Press.

History of Surgery in Houston: Fifty Year Anniversary of the Hauston Surgical Society. Ed. by Joseph S. Coselli et al. 1998. LC 98-28964. 424p. 39.95 (*1-57168-254-6*) Eakin Press.

History of Surgery in the United States 1775-1900 Vol. II: Periodical & Pamphlet Literature. Ira M. Rutkow. 1992. (Bibliography & Surgery Ser.: Nos. 5 & 4). (Illus.). 434p. 175.00 (*0-930405-48-X*) Norman SF.

History of Surgery in the United States 1775-1990 Vol. I: Textbooks, Monographs, & Treatises. Ira M. Rutkow. 1988. LC 87-62662. (Bibliography & Surgery Ser.: No. 2). (Illus.). 514p. 145.00 (*0-930405-02-1*) Norman SF.

History of Syphilis. Claude Quetel. Tr. by Judith Braddock & Brian Pike from FRE. 1992. (Illus.). 342p. reprint ed. pap. text 18.95 (*0-8018-4392-8*) Johns Hopkins.

History of the American Academy of Periodontology 1945-1989. Maynard K. Hine. 1989. (Illus.). 103p. (Orig.). 15.00 (*0-9624699-0-4*) Amer Acad Periodontology.

History of the American Board of Ophthalmology, 1916-1991. Robert N. Shaffer. 1992. 25.00 (*0-9632791-0-6*) Am Bd Ophthal.

History of the American Council of Otolaryngology, 1968-1981. John E. Bordley. 1993. (Illus.). 89p. (Orig.). pap. text 30.00 (*1-56772-000-5*, 4763015) AAO-HNS.

History of the American Lung Association. Frances Ogasawara. 172p. 12.50 (*0-915116-19-7*) Am Lung Assn.

History of the American Physiological Society: The First Century, 1887-1987. Ed. by John R. Brobeck et al. 1988. (American Physiological Society Book). (Illus.). 542p. text 45.00 (*0-19-520697-5*) OUP.

History of the British Medical Administration of East Africa, 1900-1950. Ann Beck. 1970. LC 70-115472. (Commonwealth Fund Publications). 277p. 29.95 (*0-674-40170-0*) HUP.

History of the British Veterinary Profession, 1791-1948. Iain Pattison. 1990. 222p. (*0-85131-379-5*) J A Allen GBR. *Dist:* St Mut.

History of the Cabell County Medical Society in West Virginia 1890-1985. Charles H. Moffat. 1986. 336p. 76.00 (*0-9616839-0-2*) Cabell Cty Med Soc.

History of the Department of Anesthesiology, 1942-1997: Wake Forest University School of Medicine. Wilson Somerville & Wake Forest University Staff. 1998. LC 98-60628. (*0-9644070-1-9*) Wake Forest Univ.

History of the Disorders of Cardiac Rhythm. Berndt Luderitz. rev. ed. 1997. LC 94-26949.Tr. of Geschichte der Herzhythmusst Orungen. (GER., Illus.). 188p. 60.00 (*0-87993-606-1*) Futura Pub.

History of the Division of Psychoanalysis of the American Psychological Association. Ed. by Robert C. Lane & Murray Meisels. 1994. 384p. pap. text 49.95 (*0-8058-1323-3*) L Erlbaum Assocs.

History of the First Inebriate Asylum in the World by Its Founder. J. E. Turner. Ed. by Gerald N. Grob. 1981. LC 80-1250. (Addiction in America Ser.). (Illus.). reprint ed. lib. bdg. 49.95 (*0-405-13621-8*) Ayer.

History of the Howe Laboratory. David G. Cogan. 1993. LC 93-12361. 55.00 (*0-86542-337-7*) Blackwell Sci.

History of the Imperial Cancer Research Fund 1902-1986. Joan Austoker. 1988. (Illus.). 398p. 84.00 (*0-19-723075-X*) OUP.

History of the International Union of Psychological Science. Mark R. Rozenzweig et al. 2000. 256p. (*1-84169-197-6*) Psychol Pr GBR. *Dist:* Taylor & Francis.

History of the Management of Pain: From Early Principles to Present Practice. Ed. by R. D. Mann. 1988. (History of Medicine Ser.). (Illus.). 204p. 58.00 (*1-85070-183-0*, Parthenon Pbng) CRC Pr.

History of the Massachusetts General Hospital to August 5, 1851. Nathaniel Bowditch. 2nd ed. 1972. LC 74-180558. (Medicine & Society in America Ser.). (Illus.). 768p. reprint ed. 50.95 (*0-405-03938-7*) Ayer.

H
I

History of the Medical Department of the United States Army. Percy M. Ashburn. LC 75-23675. reprint ed. 49.50 (*0-404-13228-6*) AMS Pr.

History of the Midwest Association of Plastic Surgeons. Reid Hansen. 1996. LC 97-184155. (Illus.). 80p. pap. (*1-886094-50-0*) Chicago Spectrum.

History of the Pennsylvania Hospital, 1751-1895. Thomas G. Morton. 1973. LC 73-2408. (Mental Illness & Social Policy; the American Experience Ser.). reprint ed. 48.95 (*0-405-05218-9*) Ayer.

History of the Primates. W. E. Clark. 5th ed. 1966. (Illus.). pap. text 1.25 (*0-226-10936-4*, P227) U Ch Pr.

History of the Psychopathic Hospital, Boston, Massachusetts. L. Vernon Briggs et al. 1973. LC 73-2386. (Mental Illness & Social Policy; the American Experience Ser.). reprint ed. 23.95 (*0-405-05194-8*) Ayer.

History of the Radiologic Sciences: Radiation Oncology. Ed. by Raymond Gagliardi & J. Frank Wilson. 1997. (Illus.). 334p. 60.00 (*1-890705-02-0*) Am Roentgen.

History of the RAVC, 1919-1961. J. Clabby. 1990. (Illus.). 244p. (*0-85131-082-6*) J A Allen GBR. *Dist:* St Mut.

History of the Royal Dental Hospital of London & School of Dental Surgery, 1858-1985. Ernest Smith & Beryl Cottell. 1997. LC 97-11096. 178p. (*0-485-11517-4*) Athlone Pr GBR. *Dist:* Humanities.

***History of the Royal Society of Medicine.** Penelope Hunting. 2001. 400p. (*1-85315-497-0*) Royal Soc of Medicine Pr Ltd GBR. *Dist:* Balogh.

History of the Society of Apothecaries of London. Charles R. Barrett. LC 75-23680. (Illus.). reprint ed. 49.50 (*0-404-13233-2*) AMS Pr.

History of the Study of Medicine in the British Isles. Norman Moore. LC 75-23746. reprint ed. 32.50 (*0-404-13352-5*) AMS Pr.

History of the University Founded by Johns Hopkins. John C. French. 1979. 32.95 (*0-405-10601-7*) Ayer.

History of the Western General Hospital. Ed. by M. Eastwood & A. Jenkinson. 1996. 300p. pap. (*0-85976-423-0*) J Donald GBR. *Dist:* St Mut.

History of Traditional Medicine & Health Care in Pre-Colonial East-Central Africa. Gloria M. Waite. 1993. LC 92-49071. 200p. text 79.95 (*0-7734-9707-2*) E Mellen.

History of Transplantation. Ed. by Paul I. Terasaki. 1991. 20.00 (*0-9604606-7-5*) UCLA Tissue.

History of Transplantation Immunology. Leslie Brent. 1996. LC 96-36685. (Illus.). 488p. text 54.95 (*0-12-131770-6*) Morgan Kaufmann.

History of Tropical Medicine, Set. Henry H. Scott. LC 75-23759. reprint ed. 140.00 (*0-404-13430-0*) AMS Pr.

History of Tropical Medicine. Henry H. Scott. 1976. lib. bdg. 75.00 (*0-8490-2010-7*) Gordon Pr.

History of Urology. Leonard J. Murphy. 1972. (Illus.). 548p. 95.95 (*0-398-02366-2*) C C Thomas.

History of Urology American Urological Association Staff. Ed. by Edgard G. Ballanger et al. LC 75-23674. reprint ed. 90.00 (*0-404-13300-2*) AMS Pr.

History of War: Index of Foreign Medical Literature. Tony A. Pellicano. rev. ed. 1998. 153p. 57.50 (*0-7883-2112-9*); pap. 47.50 (*0-7883-2113-7*) ABBE Pubs Assn.

History of Western Medicine in Zimbabwe. R. T. Mossop. 1998. LC 97-43750. (Studies in African Health & Medicine: Vol. 9). (Illus.). 624p. text 129.95 (*0-7734-8536-8*) E Mellen.

History of Women in Medicine from the Earliest Times to the Beginning of the 19th Century. Kate C. Mead. LC 75-23739. (Illus.). reprint ed. 72.50 (*0-404-13296-0*) AMS Pr.

History of Women's Contribution to World Health. Theodora P. Dakin. 1992. LC 91-46383. (Studies in Health & Human Services: Vol. 21). 128p. lib. bdg. 59.95 (*0-7734-9624-6*) E Mellen.

History Repeats Itself: Tuberculosis. Charles A. Illian. 1995. (In Service Sourcebook Ser.). 72p. pap. text 29.95 (*1-888343-00-1*) Hartman Pub.

History Taking, Examination, & Record Keeping in Emergency Medicine. Henry R. Guly. 1996. LC 95-20108. (Oxford Handbooks in Emergency Medicine Ser.: No. 12). (Illus.). 240p. (C). text 79.50 (*0-19-262462-8*); pap. text 45.00 (*0-19-262461-X*) OUP.

Histotechnology: A Self Assessment Workbook. Freida L. Carson. 2nd ed. 1997. 97p. 40.00 (*0-89189-412-8*) Am Soc Clinical.

Histotechnology: A Self-Instructional Text, Set. Freida L. Carson. 1990. sl. 250.00 (*0-89189-356-3*) Am Soc Clinical.

Hit Below the Belt: Facing up to Prostate Cancer. F. Ralph Berberich. 2001. LC 2001-17164. 224p. pap. 14.95 (*1-58761-077-9*) Celestial Arts.

Hitchhiker's Guide to Effective Time Management. Christopher S. Frings. 1997. 107p. pap. 20.00 (*0-915274-95-7*, 202737, AACC Pr) Am Assn Clinical Chem.

Hitchhiker's Guide to Point-of-Care Testing. Karen Bourlier. 1998. 88p. pap. 20.00 (*1-890883-06-9*, 202026) Am Assn Clinical Chem.

Hite Report: A Study of Male Sexuality. Shere Hite. 1987. 1088p. mass mkt. 7.99 (*0-345-35248-3*) Ballantine Pub Grp.

Hitler: Diagnosis of a Destructive Prophet. Fritz Redlich. 1998. LC 97-48888. (Illus.). 466p. 35.00 (*0-19-505782-1*) OUP.

***Hitting the Wall: Memoir of a Cancer Journey.** Barbara P. Glacel. 2001. 250p. pap. 19.95 (*1-883697-73-5*) Hara Pub.

Hitti's Dictionary of Medical Terms: English-Arabic. Yusuf K. Hitti. 1989. (ARA & ENG., Illus.). 913p. 65.00 (*0-86685-067-8*, LDL0678) Intl Bk Ctr.

Hitti's English-Arabic Medical Dictionary. Yusuf K. Hitti. 4th ed. 1980. (ARA & ENG.). 925p. 150.00 (*0-8288-0556-3*, M9979) Fr & Eur.

Hitti's Pocket Medical Dictionary: Arabic - English. Yusuf K. Hitti & Ahmed Khatib. 1988. (ARA & ENG.). 281p. pap. 18.95 (*0-86685-506-8*, LDL5068) Intl Bk Ctr.

HIV. Ed. by Howard Libman & Harvey Makadon. 2000. LC 99-57890. (Key Diseases Ser.). (Illus.). 250p. pap. text 35.00 (*0-943126-84-3*, 330300890) Amer Coll Phys.

HIV - AIDS & Hepatitis: Everything You Need to Know to Protect Yourself & Others. Douglas D. Schoon. 1993. LC 93-27797. (Career Development Ser.). 144p. pap. 16.95 (*1-56253-175-1*) Thomson Learn.

HIV - AIDS & Sexuality. Michael W. Ross. 1995. LC 95-21375. (Journal of Psychology & Human Sexuality: Vol. 7, Nos. 1 & 2). 222p. pap. 19.95 (*1-56023-068-1*, Harrington Park) Haworth Pr.

HIV - AIDS & Sexuality. Ed. by Michael W. Ross. 1995. LC 95-21375. (Journal of Psychology & Human Sexuality: Vol. 7, Nos. 1 & 2). 222p. 49.95 (*1-56024-730-4*) Haworth Pr.

HIV - AIDS & the Drug Culture: Picking up the Pieces. Elizabeth Hagan & Joan Gormley. 1998. 212p. pap. text 19.95 (*1-56023-933-6*, Harrington Park) Haworth Pr.

HIV-AIDS: A 2 Hour Overview. Lori A. DeLorenzo. 2nd ed. 1998. (Illus.). 78p. pap. 19.95 (*1-57801-026-8*) Western Schls.

HIV-AIDS: A Special Issue of Families in Society. FIS Staff. 1994. 72p. pap. 8.95 (*0-87304-274-3*) Manticore Pubs.

HIV-AIDS: An 1 Hour Overview. Lori A. DeLorenzo. Tr. by Kathy Johnson. 2nd ed. 1998. (Illus.). 61p. pap. 12.95 (*1-57801-027-6*) Western Schls.

HIV-AIDS: Instructional Guide for Teachers, Grades 4 Through 5. 1994. (Illus.). 75p. (Orig.). pap. text 15.00 (*1-56806-138-2*) DIANE Pub.

HIV-AIDS & Child Care: Fact Book & Facilitator's Guide. Barbara Kaiser & Judy S. Rasminsky. 1995. 20p. pap. (*0-9696697-1-2*, 708) Natl Assn Child Ed.

HIV, AIDS & Childbearing: Public Policy, Private Lives. Ed. by Ruth R. Faden & Nancy Kass. 1996. LC 95-50070. (Illus.). 512p. (C). text 39.95 (*0-19-509958-3*) OUP.

HIV, AIDS & Children: A Cause for Concern. Naomi Honigsbaum. 1994. 188p. pap. (*0-902817-63-9*) Natl Childrens Bur GBR. *Dist:* Paul & Co Pubs.

HIV-AIDS & the Older Adult. Ed. by Kathleen M. Nokes. 1996. 264p. 59.95 (*1-56032-429-5*); pap. 29.95 (*1-56032-430-9*) Hemisp Pub.

HIV-AIDS Education for Nurses: Practice Issues & Curriculum Guidelines. 1994. 145p. (Orig.). (C). pap. text 35.00 (*0-7881-1408-5*) DIANE Pub.

HIV-AIDS Fact Finder. NCSL Staff. 1993. 125p. pap. 25.00 (*1-55516-702-0*, 6640) Natl Conf State Legis.

HIV-AIDS Facts to Consider: November 1994 Update. Tracey A. Hooker. 1994. LC 97-195320. 20p. 10.00 (*1-55516-705-5*, 6649) Natl Conf State Legis.

HIV AIDS Information for Children: A Guide to Issues & Resources. Virginia A. Walter & Melissa Gross. 1996. LC 96-28416. 261p. 35.00 (*0-8242-0902-8*) Wilson.

HIV AIDS Internet Information Sources & Resources. Jeffrey T. Huber. 1998. LC 98-8526. 165p. 34.95 (*0-7890-0544-1*, Hawrth Medical); 19.95 (*1-56023-117-3*, Harrington Park) Haworth Pr.

HIV-AIDS Prevention Education Curriculum & Guide for Ages 2 to 20 Plus. African Methodist Episcopal Church, First Episcopa. Ed. by Catherine W. Wilson & Margaret J. Cousin. 1993. (Illus.). 62p. pap. text 35.00 (*0-9638634-0-1*) Home Mgmt.

HIV-AIDS Reference Library for Nurses: Developing the Nursing Component in a National AIDS Prevention & Control Program, 2. 1993. vi, 34p. pap. text 6.00 (*92-9061-108-1*, 1522004) World Health.

HIV-AIDS Reference Library for Nurses Vol. 1: Basic Information on AIDS. 1993. vi, 26p. pap. text 6.00 (*92-9061-111-1*, 1521004) World Health.

HIV-AIDS Reference Library for Nurses Vol. 3. 1993. vi, 48p. pap. text 6.00 (*92-9061-112-X*, 1523004) World Health.

HIV-AIDS Reference Library for Nurses Vol. 4: HIV Infection & AIDS: Guidelines for Nursing Care. 1993. viii, 79p. pap. text 10.00 (*92-9061-107-3*, 1524004) World Health.

HIV-AIDS Reference Library for Nurses Vol. 5: Training Modules for Basic Nursing & Midwifery Education in the Prevention & Control of AIDS. 1993. x, 204p. pap. text 10.00 (*92-9061-113-8*, 1525004) World Health.

HIV-AIDS Reference Library for Nurses Vol. 6: Integrating HIV-Related Content into a Competency-Based Curriculum. 1993. vi, 26p. pap. text 6.00 (*92-9061-109-X*, 1526004) World Health.

HIV-AIDS Resources: The National Directory of Resources on HIV Infection-AIDS. Marion L. Peterson. 1994. 600p. pap. text 110.00 (*1-885461-00-3*) National Direct.

HIV-AIDS Resources the National Directory of Resources on HIV Infection - AIDS. Marion L. Peterson. 2nd rev. ed. 650p. pap. text 116.00 (*1-885461-02-X*) National Direct.

HIV-AIDS Work Group on Health Care Access Issues for African Americans. Ed. by G. Stephen Bowen. 1998. (Illus.). 46p. (C). reprint ed. pap. text 20.00 (*0-7881-7054-6*) DIANE Pub.

HIV & AIDS. K. E. Nye & J. M. Parkin. 1994. (Medical Perspectives Ser.). 160p. (Orig.). pap. (*1-872748-96-1*) Bios Sci GBR. *Dist:* Coronet Bks.

HIV & AIDS: A Strategy for Nursing Care. Robert J. Pratt. 3rd ed. 1992. 486p. pap. 35.25 (*1-56593-544-6*, 0516) Singular Publishing.

HIV & AIDS: A Strategy for Nursing Care. Robert J. Pratt. 3rd ed. 1991. 28.25 net. (*0-340-54841-X*) Thomson Learn.

HIV & AIDS: A Strategy for Nursing Care. Robert J. Pratt. 4th ed. LC 95-223579. 488p. pap. (*0-340-59233-8*) E A GBR. *Dist:* Routldge.

HIV & AIDS: Management by the Primary Care Team. Adrian Moss. 1992. (Practical Guides for General Practice Ser.: No. 16). 112p. pap. text 21.95 (*0-19-262216-1*) OUP.

HIV & AIDS: Testing, Screening & Confidentiality. Ed. by Rebecca Bennett & Charles A. Erin. 2001. (Issues in Biomedical Ethics Ser.). 302p. pap. text 19.95 (*0-19-924314-X*) OUP.

HIV & AIDS: The Last Stand : the Total Strategy for the Annihilation of HIV & AIDS in Zimbabwe & the Rest of the World. David Chiweza. 1997. LC 99-892434. (Illus.). (*0-7974-1658-7*) S African Res & Doc.

HIV & AIDS: Your Questions. Barter. 1994. pap. text 25.00 (*0-443-04752-9*) Saunders.

HIV & AIDS in Africa. Douglas Webb. 1997. LC 97-7776. 268p. (*0-7453-1125-3*) Pluto GBR GBR. *Dist:* Stylus Pub VA.

HIV & Communication Disorders: What Speech & Hearing Professionals Need to Know. Connie R. Larsen. 1998. LC 98-3471. (Illus.). 192p. pap. 35.00 (*1-56593-968-9*, 1916) Thomson Learn.

HIV & Community Mental Healthcare. Ed. by Michael D. Knox & Caroline H. Sparks. 1997. LC 97-24462. 316p. pap. text 27.95 (*0-8018-5804-6*) Johns Hopkins.

HIV & Confidentiality: Guidelines for Managing Health Information Relating to HIV Infection. Mary D. Brandt. 1997. 68p. pap. text 32.00 (*1-58426-004-1*, AB100997) Am Hlth Info.

HIV & Dementia: Proceedings of the NIMH-Sponsored Conference "Pathogenesis of HIV Infection of the Brain: Impact on Function & Behavior", No. 202. Ed. by Michael B. Oldstone & L. Vitkovic. 1995. LC 15-12910. (Current Topics in Microbiology & Immunology Ser.: Vol. 202). (Illus.). 279p. 170.00 (*3-540-59117-6*) Spr-Verlag.

***HIV & Depression: Context & Care.** Francisco Jose Gonzales. Ed. by Robert Marks & James W. Dilley. 2000. 100p. (C). pap. 12.95 (*1-879168-05-7*) AIDS Hlth Project.

HIV & Learning Disability. Ed. by Paul Cambridge & Hilary Brown. 1996. 250p. pap. (*1-873791-91-7*) Brit Inst Lrning GBR. *Dist:* Taylor & Francis.

HIV & Membrane Receptors. Dimiter S. Dimitrov & Christopher C. Broder. 1997. LC 97-22035. (Medical Intelligence Unit Ser.). text 99.00 (*1-57059-464-3*) Landes Bioscience.

HIV & Molecular Immunity: Prospects for the AIDS Vaccine. Omar Bagasra. 1999. LC 99-10473. (Illus.). 216p. text 42.95 (*1-881299-10-4*, BioTechniques) Eaton Pub Co.

HIV & Social Work: A Practitioner's Guide. Ed. by David M. Aronstein & Bruce J. Thompson. 1998. LC 97-21867. (Haworth Psychosocial Issues of HIV/AIDS Ser.). (Illus.). 586p. 69.95 (*0-7890-0180-2*); (C). pap. 24.95 (*1-56023-906-9*) Haworth Pr (Harrington Park).

HIV & Surgery. Ed. by G. Champault & A. Bourgeon. 1994. (Monographs of the French Surgical Association). (Illus.). 69.00 (*0-387-59607-0*) Spr-Verlag.

HIV & the Blood Supply: An Analysis of Crisis Decision Making. Institute of Medicine Staff. Ed. by Lauren B. Leveton et al. 1995. LC 95-20469. 352p. text 47.95 (*0-309-05329-3*) Natl Acad Pr.

HIV & the Eye. Ed. by Susan Lightman. 1998. LC 99-29629. (Illus.). 270p. (*1-86094-084-6*) Imperial College GBR. *Dist:* World Scientific Pub.

HIV & the Immune System. Ed. by R. B. Gallagher. viii,130p. pap. 51.25 (*1-85166-564-1*) Elsevier.

HIV & the Nervous System. Ed. by Stanislaw Kubicki et al. 1988. LC 88-21162. 227p. pap. text (*0-89574-265-9*) Gustav Fischer DEU. *Dist:* Lubrecht & Cramer, Balogh.

HIV & the Pathogenesis of AIDS. Jay A. Levy. 2nd rev. ed. 1997. LC 97-42731. (Illus.). 600p. (C). pap. 79.95 (*1-55581-122-1*) ASM Pr.

***HIV Associated Cardiovascular Disease: Clinical & Biological Insights.** 2001. 300p. 130.00 (*1-57331-354-8*) NY Acad Sci.

HIV Care: A Comprehensive Handbook for Providers. Laurie J. Andrews & Laurie B. Novick. 1995. LC 94-40645. 250p. 71.95 (*0-8039-7083-8*, 7586); pap. 36.95 (*0-8039-7150-8*, 8246) Sage.

HIV Disease: Lesbians, Gays, & the Social Services. Ed. by Gary A. Lloyd & Mary A. Kuszelewicz. 1995. LC 95-22564. 194p. 39.95 (*1-56024-749-5*) Haworth Pr.

HIV Drug Book. Project Inform Staff & Carolyn B. Mitchell. 2nd rev. ed. 1998. LC 99-180938. 704p. per. 18.00 (*0-671-01490-0*, PB Trade Paper) PB.

***HIV Epidemic in the United States Continues: Index of New Information & Guide-Book for Consumers, Reference & Research.** Silvester V. Polanta. 2002. 57.50 (*0-7883-2442-X*) ABBE Pubs Assn.

HIV, Health & Your Community: A Guide for Action. Reuben Granich & Jonathan Mermin. 1999. LC 99-12967. (Illus.). 245p. pap. 15.95 (*0-8047-3351-1*) Stanford U Pr.

***HIV in Obstetrics & Gynaecology.** Barron et al. 2001. (Fast Facts Ser.). (Illus.). 64p. pap. (*1-899541-61-6*) Health Pr GBR. *Dist:* JAMCO Dist.

HIV-Infected Health Workers: Debating the Issues. Rebecca T. Craig & Lucinda L. Bryant. 1992. (State Legislative Reports: Vol. 17, No. 18). 11p. pap. text 15.00 (*1-55516-290-8*, 7302-1718) Natl Conf State Legis.

HIV Infection: A Clinical Approach. Mary M. Fanning. Ed. by Ray Kersey. 2nd ed. 1996. LC 96-22874. 304p. pap. text 29.00 (*0-7216-2792-7*) Saunders.

HIV Infection: A Primary Care Approach: Adapted from Articles Published in AIDS Clinical Care Newsletter. Frederick M. Hecht & Bruce Soloway. Ed. by Deborah J. Cotton & Gerald H. Friedland. 2nd ed. 1994. LC 93-25777. (Illus.). 64p. pap. text 9.95 (*0-910133-39-5*) Mass Med Pub Div.

HIV Infection & AIDS. Martin A. Birchall & Siobhan M. Murphy. 1992. LC 92-12583. (Colour Guide Ser.). 121p. pap. text 17.95 (*0-443-04578-X*) Harcrt Hlth Sci Grp.

HIV Infection & AIDS. Siobhan M. Murphy & Gary Brook. 2000. LC 99-89461. (*0-443-06168-8*) Harcrt Hlth Sci Grp.

HIV Infection & AIDS: Surgeon General's Report to the American Public. 1993. (Illus.). 26p. (Orig.). (C). pap. text 15.00 (*1-56806-589-2*) DIANE Pub.

HIV Infection & Intravenous Drug Use. Gennaro Ottomanelli. 1992. LC 92-3260. 160p. 55.00 (*0-275-94301-1*, C4301, Praeger Pubs) Greenwood.

HIV Infection in Children: A Guide to Practical Management. Ed. by Jacqueline Mok & Marie-Louise Newell. 1995. (Illus.). 327p. (C). text 90.00 (*0-521-45421-2*) Cambridge U Pr.

***HIV Infection in Primary Care.** R. Michael Buckley. 2001. (Illus.). 380p. (*0-7216-8601-X*) Saunders.

HIV Infection in Women Conference '95: Program & Abstracts. Ed. by J. Lasker et al. 1995. 157p. (Orig.). pap. text 25.00 (*0-924236-09-4*) Phila Scis Group.

HIV Infections - Who, How & Why: Index of New Information. Andrew B. Kemp. Date not set. 160p. 57.50 (*0-7883-1932-9*); pap. 47.50 (*0-7883-1933-7*) ABBE Pubs Assn.

HIV Manual: A Guide to Diagnosis & Treatment. Ed. by David H. Spach & Thomas M. Hooton. 1996. (Illus.). 480p. text 55.00 (*0-19-510036-0*) OUP.

HIV Manual for Health Care Professionals. Richard D. Muma et al. 2nd rev. ed. 1997. LC 96-41640. 501p. (C). pap. 29.95 (*0-8385-3773-1*, A3773-7) McGraw-Hill Prof.

HIV Medicine Handbook: A Manual for Clinicians Working with HIV Infection. Francis Bowden et al. 1996. LC 96-158585. 264p. pap. (*0-522-84613-0*) Melbourne Univ Pr AUS. *Dist:* Paul & Co Pubs.

HIV Nursing & Symptom Management. Mary Ropka & Ann Williams. 1998. LC 98-13527. (Nursing Ser.). (Illus.). 832p. (C). pap. text 42.95 (*0-7637-0544-6*, 0544-6) Jones & Bartlett.

HIV Positive. Debra Jarvis. 1990. 48p. pap. 2.99 (*0-7459-1820-4*) Lion USA.

HIV, Prenatal Infections & Therapy: The Role of the Placenta. Ed. by Richard K. Miller & Henry A. Thiede. 1995. (Trophoblast Research Ser.: Vol. 8). (Illus.). 632p. 135.00 (*1-878822-45-4*) Univ Rochester Pr.

HIV Prevention: Health Facts. Jill Schettler et al. 1994. LC 93-43137. 12.95 (*1-56071-184-1*, H304) ETR Assocs.

HIV Prevention Education for Physical Educators, Coaches, & Athletic Trainers. 1995. 87p. (Orig.). pap. 8.00 (*0-88314-602-9*, 301-10031) AAHPERD.

HIV Protocols. Ed. by Nelson Michael & Jerome H. Kim. 1999. LC 98-27244. (Methods in Molecular Medicine Ser.: Vol. 17). (Illus.). 432p. 110.00 (*0-89603-369-4*) Humana.

HIV Resident Pocket Survival Guide. Kirk Miller & Michael Polis. 1999. 100p. (C). pap. 9.95 (*1-883205-35-2*) Intl Med Pub.

HIV Seropositivity & AIDS Prevention & Control: Report on a WHO Meeting. 1989. 39p. pap. text 10.00 (*92-890-1060-6*) World Health.

HIV Surveillance, Reporting & Testing Policies: Controversial Issues for Women. Leslie R. Wolfe. 1995. 12p. pap. 8.00 (*1-877966-25-8*) Ctr Women Policy.

HIV Test: What You Need to Know to Make an Informed Decision. Marc Vargo. Ed. by Claire Zion. 1992. 160p. reprint ed. per. 9.00 (*0-671-77950-8*) PB.

HIV Tracing & Transmission in People in Working, Sports & Professional Populations: Index of New Information. Emma L. Dubrowski. rev. ed. 1997. 147p. 57.50 (*0-7883-1524-2*); pap. 47.50 (*0-7883-1525-0*) ABBE Pubs Assn.

H I

HIV Tracing & Transmission in People in Working, Sports, Business, & Professional Populations. Emma L. Dubrowski. 1996. 150p. 57.50 (0-7883-0786-X) ABBE Pubs Assn.

HIV Treatment: Mental Health Aspects of Antiviral Therapy. Michael Shernoff & Raymond Smith. 2000. LC 00-23461. (UCSF AIDS Health Project Monograph Ser.: No. 4). vi, 98p. (C). pap. 10.95 (1-879168-04-9) AIDS Hlth Project.

HIV Vaccines: Adverse Reactions & Compensation. 1996. lib. bdg. 255.75 (0-8490-6391-4) Gordon Pr.

HIV Wellness Sourcebook: The East/West Guide to Living Well. Misha Cohen. 1998. LC 97-31830. 256p. pap. 14.95 (0-8050-5117-1) H Holt & Co.

HIV/AIDS: A Guide to Primary Care Management. Peter J. Ungavarski & Jacqueline H. Flaskerud. Ed. by Thomas Eoyang. 4th ed. 1998. LC 98-20112. (Illus.). 576p. (C). pap. text 45.00 (0-7216-7322-8) Saunders.

HIV/AIDS: Loss, Grief, Challenge & Hope. Mary O'Donnell. 1996. LC 95-45406. 200p. 69.95 (1-56032-329-9); pap. 29.95 (1-56032-330-2) Taylor & Francis.

HIV/AIDS: Practical, Medical & Spiritual Guidelines for Daily Living When You're HIV-Positive. Mark Jenkins. 2000. LC 00-20074. (Hazelden Pocket Health Guide Ser.). xxv, 171p. pap. 12.00 (1-56838-369-X) Hazelden.

HIV/AIDS: U. S. Aid & U. N. Response to the Epidemic in the Developing World. Jess T. Ford. 1999. (Illus.). 72p. pap. text 20.00 (0-7881-7962-4) DIANE Pub.

HIV/AIDS: Understanding Your Responsibility. Satya Krishnan. 1995. LC 95-33634. (1-56796-133-9) WRS Group.

HIV/AIDS & HIV/AIDS-Related Terminology: A Means of Organizing the Body of Knowledge. Jeffrey T. Huber & Mary L. Gillaspy. 1996. LC 96-1981. (Haworth Medical Information Sources Ser.). 107p. 24.95 (1-56024-970-6) Haworth Pr.

HIV/AIDS & Prisons. Ed. by J. Norberry et al. 1991. (Australian Institute Conference Proceedings Ser.: Vol. 4). 300p. pap. (0-642-16202-6) Aust Inst Criminology AUS. *Dist:* Advent Bks Div.

HIV/AIDS & the Drug Culture: Shattered Lives. Elizabeth Hagan & Joan Gormley. 1998. LC 98-6097. 219p. 39.95 (0-7890-0465-8, Harrington Park); pap. 14.95 (0-7890-0554-9) Haworth Pr.

HIV/AIDS Community Information Services: Experiences in Serving Both At-Risk & HIV-Infected Populations. Jeffrey T. Huber. 1996. LC 95-51653. 144p. 39.95 (1-56024-910-4) Haworth Pr.

HIV/AIDS Education for Students with Special Needs: A Guide for Teachers. David Birch & Rebecca Marte. 1995. 44p. pap. 8.00 (0-88314-601-0, 301-10030) AAHPERD.

HIV/AIDS Handbook for Personal Service Providers. Noella Charest-Papagno. l.t. ed. 1999. LC 97-93938. (Illus.). 58p. spiral bd. 8.95 (0-9604610-9-4, JJPLB) JJ Pub FL.

HIV/AIDS in Correctional Facilities. 1994. (Illus.). 104p. pap. text 30.00 (1-57979-191-3) DIANE Pub.

HIV/AIDS in Prisons: Background Materials - Canada. Ralf Jurgens. 1995. (Illus.). 188p. (Orig.). (C). pap. text 45.00 (0-7881-2432-3) DIANE Pub.

HIV/AIDS in Prisons: Final Report of the Expert Committee on AIDS & Prisons - Canada. 1995. 144p. (Orig.). (C). pap. text 40.00 (0-7881-2246-0) DIANE Pub.

HIV/AIDS in Prisons: Summary Report & Recommendations of the Expert Committee on AIDS & Prisons - Canada. Ralf Jurgens. 1995. 44p. (Orig.). (C). pap. text 40.00 (0-7881-2431-5) DIANE Pub.

***HIV/AIDS in the Caribbean: Issues & Options.** Contrib. by World Bank Staff. 2001. LC 2001-17897. (Country Study Ser.). (Illus.). xvii, 88p. 22.00 (0-8213-4921-X, 14921) World Bank.

HIV/AIDS Nursing Care Plans. Lucy Bradley-Springer. 2nd rev. ed. 1999. LC 99-235965. (Nursing Care Plans Ser.). 230p. (C). per. 39.95 (1-56930-097-6) Delmar.

HIV/AIDS Nursing Care Summit Proceedings: Nursing Care Summit Proceedings. American Academy of Nursing Staff. Ed. by William L. Holzemer & Carmen F. Portillo. 1994. 272p. (Orig.). pap. 22.50 (1-55810-102-0, G-186) Am Nurses Pub.

HIV/AIDS Nursing Handbook. Carl Kirton et al. 1999. LC 2001-274850. (Illus.). xxiii, 535p. (C). text 24.95 (0-323-00336-2) Mosby Inc.

HIV/AIDS Prevention: Current Issues in Community Practice. Joseph R. Ferrari & Doreen D. Salina. 1999. LC 99-47991. 82p. (0-7890-0694-4) Haworth Pr.

HIV/AIDS Primary Care Handbook. Cynthia G. Carmichael. 1995. LC 95-122385. 228p. (C). spiral bd. 19.95 (0-8385-3557-7, A3557-4, Apple Lange Med) McGraw.

***HIV/AIDS Surveillance Report: U. S. HIV & AIDS Cases Reported Through December 2000.** W. Meade Morgan. 2001. (Illus.). 51p. (C). pap. text 20.00 (0-7567-1684-5) DIANE Pub.

Hives of Sickness: Public Health & Epidemics in New York City. Ed. by David Rosner. 1995. LC 94-29784. (Illus.). 230p. (C). text 35.00 (0-8135-2158-0) Rutgers U Pr.

HLA & Allergy. Ed. by A. L. De Weck. 1977. (Monographs in Allergy: Vol. 11). (Illus.). 41.75 (3-8055-2639-3) S Karger.

HLA & Disease. Robert Lechler. 1994. (Illus.). 320p. (C). text 39.95 (0-12-440320-4) Acad Pr.

HLA & Disease: A Comprehensive Review. William E. Braun. 1979. 160p. 89.00 (0-8493-5795-0, QR184, CRC Reprint) Franklin.

HLA & Disease Associations. J. Tiwari & Paul I. Terasaki. 1985. (Illus.). 472p. 173.00 (0-387-96081-3) Spr-Verlag.

HLA & the Maternal-Fetal Relationship. Ed. by J. Hunt. 1996. (Medical Intelligence Unit Ser.). (Illus.). 207p. (C). pap. 89.95 (0-412-11311-2) Chapman & Hall.

HLA & the Maternal-Fetal Relationship. Joan S. Hunt. 1996. LC 96-16528. (Medical Intelligence Unit Ser.). 207p. 99.00 (1-57059-240-3) Landes Bioscience.

HLA Beyond Tears. Glenn Rodey. 1991. 190p. pap. text 24.95 (0-9631020-0-1) De Novo TX.

HLA System: A New Approach. Ed. by Holland, Jerome H., Laboratory Staff & J. Lee. 1990. (Illus.). 236p. 87.95 (0-387-97441-5) Spr-Verlag.

HLA System: An Introductory Survey. A. Svejgaard et al. 2nd ed. 1979. (Monographs in Human Genetics: Vol. 7). (Illus.). pap. 31.50 (3-8055-3049-8) S Karger.

HLA System in Clinical Transplantation: Basic Concepts & Importance. Ed. by Soldano Ferrone et al. 1992. LC 92-48813. (Illus.). 350p. 179.00 (0-387-55456-4) Spr-Verlag.

HLA Typing: Methodology & Clinical Aspects Ed. by Soldano Ferrone & Bjarte G. Solheim. 1982. Vol. I. 208p. 117.00 (0-8493-6410-8, QR184); Vol. II. 200p. 114.00 (0-8493-6411-6) Franklin (CRC Reprint).

HMG Coa Reductase Inhibitors: New Horizons in the Management of Hypercholesterolemia - Journal: Cardiology, 1990, Vol. 77, Suppl. 4. Ed. by J. L. DeGennes. 1991. (Illus.). iv, 72p. pap. 23.50 (3-8055-5278-5) S Karger.

HMO 101: Introduction to HMOs. Rhys W. Jones. 2nd ed. 1997. (Illus.). pap. 14.95 (0-9635819-3-7) TTM Pub.

HMO-PPO Directory 1987. Ed. by William J. Feinberg. 1987. 225p. pap. text 75.00 (0-938184-19-9) Whole World.

HMO/PPO Directory, 2001. Medical Economics Staff. 2000. (HMO/PPO Directory Ser.). (Illus.). 350p. 215.00 (1-56363-389-2, PDR) Med Econ.

HMOs & the Patient's Bill of Rights. Molly Shapiro. 1999. LC 99-36402. (Vital Information Ser.). 159p. pap. 11.95 (1-58091-024-6) Crossing Pr.

Hoax of Freudism: A Study of Brainwashing the American Professionals & Laymen. Ratibor-Ray M. Jurjevich. 1985. 528p. reprint ed. pap. 18.95 (0-930711-02-5) Ichthys Bks.

Hoax of Medicine: Reducing Medical Expenses to Zero. 1992. lib. bdg. 85.85 (0-8490-8802-X) Gordon Pr.

Hodgkin's Disease. Peter M. Mauch. 1999. LC 98-55677. 832p. 199.00 (0-7817-1502-4) Lppncott W & W.

Hodgkin's Disease. Henry S. Kaplan. 2nd rev. ed. 1980. LC 79-16054. (Commonwealth Fund Publications). (Illus.). 703p. 102.00 (0-674-40485-8) HUP.

Hodgkin's Disease I: Basic Research. David H. Katz et al. 1974. LC 73-23030. (Hodgkin's Disease Ser.: Vol. 1). 168p. text 24.00 (0-8422-7193-7) Irvington.

Hodgkin's Disease II: Pathological Considerations. Ed. by Richard S. Neiman et al. 1974. LC 73-23030. (Hodgkin's Disease Ser.: Vol. 2). 141p. text 24.00 (0-8422-7194-5) Irvington.

Hodgkin's Disease III: Occurrence & Diagnosis. Ed. by M. R. Alderson et al. 1974. LC 73-23030. (Hodgkin's Disease Ser.: Vol. 3). 155p. text 24.00 (0-8422-7195-3) Irvington.

Hodgkin's Disease in Children: Controversies & Current Practice. Ed. by W. A. Kamps et al. 1988. (C). text 219.50 (0-89838-372-2) Kluwer Academic.

Hoekelman's Handbook: Primary Pediatric Care Companion. Robert A. Hoekelman et al. 1997. (Illus.). 320p. (C). (gr. 13). text 29.00 (0-8151-4485-7, 27884) Mosby Inc.

Hoge Bloeddruk, Hart Infarct, Grafieken. Dyob Re'lem, pseud. rev. ed. 1989. (DUT., Illus.). 90p. pap. (0-9622463-3-6) B Melger.

Hoge Bloeddruk, Myocardiale Infarct, Grafieken. Dyob Re'lem, pseud & Boyd A. Melger. 1989. (DUT., Illus.). 69p. (Orig.). pap. (0-9622463-1-X) B Melger.

Hold the Fat, Sugar & Salt. Jacqueline B. Williams & Goldie Silverman. 1984. (Illus.). 160p. pap. 10.00 (0-399-51073-7, Perigee Bks) Berkley Pub.

Holding the Hope: A Parent's Guide to Living with Dystonia. Karen K. Ross. 2nd ed. 1996. reprint ed. pap. (0-9659941-2-0) Natl Spasmodic Dysphonia.

Holding the Hope: A Parent's Guide to Living with Dystonia. Karen K. Ross. Ed. by Valerie F. Levitan. 2nd rev. ed. 1996. 54p. pap. 10.00 (0-9659941-0-4) Natl Spasmodic Dysphonia.

***Hole's Human Anatomy & Physiology.** David N. Shier et al. 8th ed. (C). 106.25 (0-07-241844-3) McGrw-H Hghr Educ.

Holisitc Medicine: A Meeting of East & West. Henry E. Altenberg. 1998. 192p. pap. 19.95 (0-87040-902-6) Japan Pubns USA.

Holistic & Metaphysical Resource Book for Maryland, Virginia & Washington D. C., 1997-1998. Karen L. Meengs & Deborah R. Eby. 1997. (Illus.). x, 362p. 19.95 (0-9661147-0-1) Over Cliff.

Holistic Approach to Cancer. Ian Pearce. 1989. 106p. pap. (0-85207-211-2) C W Daniel GBR. *Dist:* Natl Bk Netwk.

Holistic Approach to Cancer. Ian Pierce. 152p. (Orig.). pap. 14.95 (0-8464-4225-6) Beekman Pubs.

Holistic Approach to Health & Happiness (HAHAH) Maria Kuman & Stan Kuman Narten. pap. 20.00 (1-893637-38-7) Hlth & Hap.

Holistic Approach to Human Ecology. Maria Kuman. pap. 20.00 (1-893637-37-9) Hlth & Hap.

Holistic Approach to Stress Management. Maria Kuman. pap. 20.00 (1-893637-16-6) Hlth & Hap.

Holistic Approaches to Stress Relief & Pain Management. Mary Jo Bulbrook. 1991. pap. text 22.00 (1-889293-00-8) NC Ctr Healing.

Holistic Aromatherapy. Christine Wildwood. 1993. 176p. pap. (0-7225-2825-6) Thorsons.

Holistic Care for Birds: Effective Care for Birds. Pamela L. Higdon et al. 1999. LC 00-502660. (Illus.). 320p. pap. 24.95 (0-87605-566-8, Howell) Hungry Minds.

Holistic Conceptualization of Stress & Disease. Benjamin H. Newberry et al. 1991. LC 86-82021. (Stress in Modern Society Ser.: No. 7). 32.50 (0-404-63258-0) AMS Pr.

Holistic Foot Care: Methods, Treatments & Cures. Morton Walker & Denis F. Augustine. 1985. (Dr. Morton Walker Good Health Guides Ser.). (Illus.). 56p. (Orig.). pap. 4.95 (0-8159-5521-9) Devin.

Holistic Guide for a Healthy Dog. Wendy Volhard & Kerry L. Brown. 1995. LC 94-45507. (Illus.). 304p. per. 27.95 (0-87605-560-9, Howell) Hungry Minds.

Holistic Healing. Hildegard of Bingen. 1994. LC 94-1902. 236p. (Orig.). pap. 17.95 (0-8146-2224-0) Liturgical Pr.

Holistic Healing. Rachel Lewin. 1998. (Healing Ser.). (Illus.). 160p. pap. (965-494-042-6) Astrolog Pub ISR. *Dist:* Assoc Pubs Grp, IPG Chicago.

Holistic Healing & the Edgar Cayce Readings. Raymond Ouellette. 1980. LC 80-80446. 384p. 11.95 (0-936450-07-X); pap. 7.75 (0-936450-08-8) Aero Pr.

Holistic Health: High Level Wellness & Menopause. Judith Bergman. pap. 6.95 (1-884570-13-5) Research Triangle.

Holistic Health & Biomedical Medicine: A Countersystem Analysis. Stephen Lyng. 1990. LC 89-11531. (SUNY Series in the Political Economy of Health Care). 268p. (C). text 64.50 (0-7914-0255-X); pap. text 21.95 (0-7914-0256-8) State U NY Pr.

Holistic Health & Yoga, Herbs, Hypnosis & Body Movement. 1992. lib. bdg. 254.95 (0-8490-5613-6) Gordon Pr.

***Holistic Health Handbook: A Personalized Guide to Holistic Health Practitioners & Products.** Ed. by C'esca Lawrence & Nadine Cutright. 2000. 98p. pap. 9.95 (0-9701223-0-6) Anew View.

Holistic Health Lifebook. Compiled by Berkeley Holistic Health Center Staff. 1981. LC 81-2846. (Illus.). 430p. pap. 12.95 (0-915904-53-5) And-Or Bks.

Holistic Health Promotion & Complementary Therapies: A Resource for Integrated Practice. Aspen Reference Group Staff. 1998. LC 98-29791. 410p. ring bd. 179.00 (0-8342-1005-3, S488) Aspen Pub.

Holistic Health Resource Directory of New Jersey & Pennsylvania. David Destiny. 7th ed. 1997. 160p. pap. 9.95 (0-9651767-1-1) Hlistic Hlth Assn.

Holistic Health Through Macrobiotics: A Complete Guide to Mind-Body Healing. Michio Kushi & Edward Esko. 1993. (Illus.). 320p. (Orig.). pap. 19.00 (0-87040-895-X) Japan Pubns USA.

Holistic Interpretation of Autism: A Theoretical Framework. Cheryl D. Seifert. 1990. 84p. (Orig.). (C). 35.50 (0-8191-7739-3); pap. 14.00 (0-8191-7740-7) U Pr of Amer.

Holistic Living: The Millenium Guide for a Healthy & Joyous Life. Ed. by Luise Light. 1999. 400p. pap. 19.95 (0-87983-973-2, Keats Pubng) McGraw-Hill Trade.

Holistic Management: A New framework for Decision-Making. Allan Savory & Jody Butterfield. 2nd ed. 1999. LC 98-42237. (Illus.). 616p. text 50.00 (1-55963-487-1); pap. text 30.00 (1-55963-488-X) Island Pr.

Holistic Management of Dogs. Keith Allison & Christopher Day. 1999. (Illus.). 168p. (0-85131-693-X) J A Allen GBR. *Dist:* Trafalgar.

Holistic Medicine: A Meeting of Easy & West. Henry E. Altenberg. 1992. (Illus.). 192p. (Orig.). pap. 22.00 (0-87040-876-3) Japan Pubns USA.

Holistic Medicine: From Stress to Optimum Health. Kenneth R. Pelletier. 1984. 25.00 (0-8446-6092-2) Peter Smith.

Holistic Menopause. Judy Hall & Robert Jacobs. 1998. (Illus.). 220p. (Orig.). pap. (1-899171-32-0) Findhorn Pr GBR. *Dist:* Lantern Books.

Holistic Midwifery - A Comprehension Textbook for Midwives in Homebirth Practice Vol. I: Care During Pregnancy. Anne Frye. rev. ed. 1998. (Illus.). 1199p. reprint ed. pap. 69.00 (1-891145-55-X) Labrys Pr.

Holistic Nursing: A Handbook for Practice. Barbara Montgomery Dossey et al. 3rd ed. 1999. LC 99-27912. 848p. pap. 49.00 (0-8342-1629-9) Aspen Pub.

Holistic Parenting: Raising Children to a New Physical, Emotional, & Spiritual Well-Being. Lynn Wiese Sneyd. 2000. LC 00-63438. xxii, 313p. pap. 17.95 (0-658-00306-2) NTC Contemp Pub Co.

Holistic Pediatrician: Pediatrician's Comprehensive Guide to Safe & Effective Therapies for Common Pr. Kathi J. Kemper. 1996. LC 95-48456. 432p. pap. 18.00 (0-06-095177-X) HarperCollins Pubs.

Holistic Pregnancy & Childbirth. James Marti & Heather Burton. 1999. LC 98-27943. 304p. pap. 16.95 (0-471-18509-4) Wiley.

***Holistic Protocol for the Immune System: A Manual for HIV-ARC-AIDS & Other Opportunistic Infections.** Scott J. Gregory. Ed. by Bianca Leonardo. 7th deluxe l.t. ed. 2001. (Illus.). 126p. reprint ed. pap. 17.00 (0-9602850-5-9) Leaves of Healing.

Holistic Protocol for the Immune System: A Manual for HIV-ARC-AIDS & Other Opportunistic Infections. Scott J. Gregory. Ed. by Bianca Leonardo. 6th rev. ed. 1995. LC 89-20310. (Illus.). 126p. pap. 16.95 (0-930852-29-X) Tree Life Pubns.

Holistic Self-Health Care: The Theory & Practical Application of Natural Hygiene. Arthur M. Baker. 1994. LC 93-93557. 67p. (Orig.). pap. 8.95 (1-883989-36-1) Self Hlth Care.

Holistic Veterinary Handbook: Safe, Effective Treatment Plans for the Companion Animal Practitioner. William G. Winter. 1997. LC 96-38140. 240p. (Orig.). pap. 39.95 (1-880090-47-3) Galde Pr.

Holistic Way to Health, Happiness & Harmony. V. K. Subramanian. 1996. (81-7017-323-X) Abhinav IND. *Dist:* S Asia.

Holistic Woman's Herbal: How to Achieve Health & Well-Being at Any Age. Kitty Campion. 1996. LC 96-18750. 256p. pap. 16.95 (1-885203-37-3) Jrny Editions.

Hollinshead's Textbook of Anatomy. Cornelius Rosse & Penelope Gaddum-Rosse. 5th ed. 1997. LC 96-8005. 912p. text 52.50 (0-397-51256-2) Lppncott W & W.

Hollywood Facelift: Facelifting, Cosmetic Surgery & the New You. Nola Rocco. 1995. pap. 19.95 (0-935016-32-5) Zinn Pub Grp.

Hollywood Shot by Shot: Alcoholism in American Cinema. Norman K. Denzin. 1991. (Communication & Social Order Ser.). 309p. (C). lib. bdg. 49.95 (0-202-30344-6) Aldine de Gruyter.

Holocaust Survivors' Mental Health. Intro. by T. L. Brink. 1994. LC 94-4500. (Clinical Gerontologist Ser.). (Illus.). 117p. lib. bdg. 39.95 (1-56024-669-3) Haworth Pr.

Holotropic Breathwork Workshop: A Manual for Trained Facilitators. Kylea Taylor. 1991. 113p. (Orig.). pap. text 26.95 (0-9643158-2-3) Hanford Mead.

Holy Anorexia. Rudolph M. Bell. 1985. LC 85-8460. (Illus.). xii, 248p. 22.50 (0-226-04204-9) U Ch Pr.

Holyistic Attitudes: God's Prescription for Your Good Health. Harold P. Adolph & Dave Bourne. 1991. pap. 7.95 (0-929292-16-2) Hannibal Bks.

Hombre Humanizador: Un Estudio sobre la Adiccion a Drogas. Alberto D. Tristani. 1986. LC 85-26331. 415p. 12.00 (0-8477-2910-9) U of PR Pr.

***Hombre y Sus Simolos (Man & His Symbols)** Carl Gustav Jung. (SPA.). (84-217-4208-6) Noguer Edit ESP. *Dist:* AIMS Intl.

Home & Community Care for Chronically Ill Children. James M. Perrin et al. 1993. 176p. (C). text 39.50 (0-19-507120-4) OUP.

Home Aromatherapy Kit. Lawless. (1-85626-205-7) Cathie Kyle GBR. *Dist:* Trafalgar.

Home Back Program by Post Rehabilitation Fitness. David Dallmeyer et al. 1998. (Illus.). 25p. 40.00 (1-930241-04-6) F I Intl.

Home-Based Care for a New Century. Ed. by Daniel M. Fox & Carol Raphael. 1997. 318p. (C). 66.95 (1-57718-040-2) Blackwell Pubs.

Home-Based Maternal Records: Guidelines for Development, Adaptation & Evaluation. 1994. viii, 85p. pap. text 20.00 (92-4-154464-3, 1150408) World Health.

Home Birth: An Invitation & A Guide. Alice Gilgoff. 1988. LC 88-27611. (Illus.). 192p. 45.00 (0-89789-179-1); pap. 14.95 (0-89789-178-3) Greenwood (Bergin & Garvey).

Home Birth: Step-by-Step Instructions for Natural & Emergency Childbirth. Edwin W. Flatto. Ed. by Carol L. Flatto. 12th rev. ed. 2001. LC 97-69560. Orig. Title: Manual for Midwives. (Illus.). 148p. pap. 19.95 (0-935540-02-4) Plymouth Pr.

Home Birth Advantage: A Time Honored Tradition for the New Millennium. Mayer Eisenstein. 2nd rev. ed. 2000. Orig. Title: The Home Court Advantage. 304p. pap. 16.95 (0-9670444-0-5) CMI.

Home Care: A Technical Manual for the Professional. Rovinski & Zastocki. 1989. 459p. pap. text 47.00 (0-7216-2449-9) Saunders.

Home Care: Patient & Family Instructions. Deborah K. Zastocki & Rovinski Wagner. 2nd ed. 2000. LC 99-44465. (Illus.). 395p. pap. text 64.95 (0-7216-8442-4) Saunders.

Home Care Aide. Joan M. Birchenall & Eileen Steight. 1996. LC 97-118486. (Illus.). 496p. (C). (gr. 13). pap. text 31.00 (0-8151-0726-9, 24172) Mosby Inc.

Home Care Aide. Perspective Press Inc. Staff. 1995. 304p. (gr. 13). pap. text 24.95 (0-8151-4748-1, 24903) Mosby Inc.

Home Care & Clinical Paths: Effective Care Planning Across the Continuum 97-98. Marrelli. 1997. 48p. (C). (gr. 13). text 19.95 (0-8151-3419-3, 31839) Mosby Inc.

Home Care & Clinical Paths: Effective Care Planning Across the Continuum. T. M. Marrelli. 1995. LC 95-24640. (Illus.). 256p. (C). (gr. 13). text 62.95 (0-8151-5853-X, 26256) Mosby Inc.

H I

Home Care & Extended Care in a Comprehensive Prepayment Plan. Arnold V. Hurtado et al. 1972. LC 72-85388. (Illus.). 127p. 10.00 (*0-87914-019-4*, 567151) Hosp Res & Educ.

Home Care & Hospice Law: A Handbook for Executives. William A. Dombi & Betsy J. Houchen. 2000. LC 00-130300. 508p. 250.00 (*1-886450-10-2*) Caring Pub.

Home Care & Managed Care: Strategies for the Future. Ed. by Eric B. Linne. 1995. LC 95-24529. 264p. pap. 55.00 (*1-55648-145-4*, 079201) AHPI.

Home Care Companion's Quick Tips for Caregivers. Marion Karpinski. l.t. ed. 2000. (Illus.). pap. 24.95 (*0-9653873-9-9*) Healing Arts Comns.

Home Care Compliance Manual: Accreditation & Legal Requirements. Aspen Health Law and Compliance Center Staff et al. Ed. by Carol Clarke. 1999. LC 99-19054. (Health Law Ser.). (Illus.). pap. 95.00 (*0-8342-1145-9*) Aspen Pub.

Home Care Corporate Compliance Program. Marian Heyinck & Carol Schaffer. 1998. 208p. spiral bd. 69.00 (*0-8342-1108-4*, 11084) Aspen Pub.

Home Care for People with Alzheimer's Disease Video Series Incl. Activities for Daily Living. 17.00 (*0-8342-0721-4*); Activities for Daily Living. VHS 94.00 (*0-8342-0722-2*); Communication. 17.00 (*0-8342-0719-2*); Communication. VHS 94.00 (*0-8342-0720-6*); Home Safety. 17.00 (*0-8342-0723-0*); Home Safety. VHS 94.00 (*0-8342-0724-9*); 1995. 199.00 (*0-8342-0718-4*) Aspen Pub.

Home Care for Seriously Ill Children: A Manual for Parents. D. Gay Moldow & Ida M. Martinson. 2nd ed. 1991. 92p. reprint ed. pap. 7.95 (*0-932321-00-3*) Child Hospice VA.

Home Care for the Client Living with HIV/AIDS. Jetta Lee Fuzy. 1999. LC 99-14434. (Home Care Aide Ser.). 192p. (C). pap. text 22.95 (*0-7668-0210-8*) Delmar.

Home Care for the Client Needing Rehabilitation. Fuzy. abr. rev. ed. 1998. LC 97-45220. 224p. (C). pap. text 25.95 (*0-8273-7931-5*) Delmar.

Home Care for the Client Who Has Had a Cerebrovascular Accident. Jetta Lee Fuzy. 1999. LC 99-26841. (Home Care Aide Ser.). 192p. (C). pap. text 22.95 (*0-7668-0209-4*) Delmar.

Home Care for the Client with Alzheimer's. Fuzy. abr. rev. ed. 1998. LC 98-20363. 224p. (C). pap. text 25.95 (*0-8273-7933-1*) Delmar.

Home Care for the Client with Diabetes. Fuzy. 1998. LC 98-18759. 224p. (C). pap. text 25.95 (*0-8273-7935-8*) Delmar.

Home Care for the Client with Diabetes - IML. Fuzy. 1998. 36p. (C). tchr. ed. 12.00 (*0-8273-7936-6*) Delmar.

Home Care for the Elderly: An International Perspective. Abraham Monk & Carole Cox. 1991. LC 90-1280. 184p. 58.00 (*0-86569-005-7*, T005, Auburn Hse) Greenwood.

Home Care for the High Risk Infant: A Family-Centered Approach. Ed. by Elizabeth Ahmann. 2nd rev. ed. 1996. LC 96-7422. 256p. 70.00 (*0-8342-0750-8*) Aspen Pub.

Home Care for the Stroke Patient. Johnstone. 3rd ed. 1996. text 32.00 (*0-443-05660-9*) Saunders.

Home Care for the Stroke Patient: Living in a Pattern. Margaret Johnstone. 2nd ed. 1987. LC 86-9553. (Illus.). 218p. (Orig.). pap. text (*0-443-03399-4*) Church.

Home Care Guide for Cancer: How to Care for Family & Friends at Home. Ed. by Peter S. Houts. 1996. LC 94-5995. (American College of Physicians Homecare Guides Ser.). 272p. pap. 29.95 (*0-943126-30-4*) Amer Coll Phys.

Home Care Helper: A Guide to Personal & Medical Information. Mary R. Barringer & Cindy L. Womack. 1995. pap. 6.50 (*0-9641671-0-7*) MarCin Enter.

Home Care Human Resources Manual. Barbara Stover Gingerich & Deborah Anne Ondeck. 1997. LC 97-19838. 340p. ring bd. 99.00 (*0-8342-0940-3*) Aspen Pub.

Home Care I. V. Therapy. Cora Spencer et al. 2nd ed. 1996. LC 96-24187. ring bd. 175.00 (*0-8342-0836-9*, 20836) Aspen Pub.

Home Care in New York City: Providers, Payers, Clients. Dale Bell. 1987. (Papers: No. 6). 48p. 5.00 (*0-934459-11-8*) United Hosp Fund.

Home Care Management of the Blood Cell Transplant Patient. Cathy H. Kelley et al. 3rd ed. 1997. LC 97-18410. (Nursing Ser.). (Illus.). 176p. (C). pap. text 42.95 (*0-7637-0612-4*, 0612-4) Jones & Bartlett.

Home Care Manual: Making the Transition. Sheryl Zang. 1997. LC 96-26199. 587p. spiral bd. 32.50 (*0-397-55401-X*) Lppncott W & W.

Home Care Nursing Delegation Skills: A Handbook for Practice. Ruth I. Hansten et al. 1999. 348p. pap. 40.00 (*0-8342-1233-1*, 12331) Aspen Pub.

Home Care Nursing Handbook. Carolyn J. Humphrey. 3rd ed. 1998. LC 98-4346. (Illus.). 512p. spiral bd. 44.00 (*0-8342-1017-7*, 10177) Aspen Pub.

Home Care Nursing Practice. Robyn Rice. 3rd ed. 2000. LC 00-45242. (Illus.). xviii, 538p. pap. text 36.95 (*0-323-01107-1*) Mosby Inc.

Home Care of Older People in Europe: A Comparison of Policies & Practices. Ed. by Anne Jamieson. 1991. (CEC Health Services Research Ser.: No. 7). (Illus.). 368p. text 95.00 (*0-19-262050-9*) OUP.

Home Care Redesign: A Proactive Approach to Managed Care. Barbara Stover Gingerich et al. 1996. LC 96-19464. 250p. 79.00 (*0-8342-0781-8*, 20781) Aspen Pub.

Home Care Resource Book: A Compilation from IPA Medication Teaching Manual, & Practice Standards of ASHP. 1993. 520p. pap. 56.00 (*1-879907-41-0*) Am Soc Hlth-Syst.

Home Care Salary & Benefits Report, 1993-94. 1994. pap. 250.00 (*0-939326-78-7*) Hosp & Hlthcare.

Home Care Services. Elaine Roberts & Betty Templeton. 1992. (Skills for Caring Ser.). (Illus.). 48p. pap. (*0-443-04623-9*) Church.

Home Care Services: Index of New Information. Eldridge P. Falatasa. 1998. 57.50 (*0-7883-1820-9*); pap. 47.50 (*0-7883-1821-7*) ABBE Pubs Assn.

Home Care Survival Guide. Green. 1998. LC 97-42737. 416p. pap. text 32.95 (*0-397-55275-0*) Lppncott W & W.

Home Care Therapy: Quality, Documentation & Reimbursement - A Handbook for Physical Therapists, Speech-Language Pathologists, & Occupational Therapists. Tina M. Marrelli & Linda H. Krulish. 1999. 400p. 34.95 (*0-9647801-2-7*) Marrelli.

Home Child Care: The Tender Business. Ellie R. Peters. 1990. LC 90-82384. 105p. (Orig.). pap. 5.95 (*0-937779-16-4*) Greenlawn Pr.

Home Chiropractic Handbook. Karl V. Holmquist. 1985. (Illus.). 194p. (Orig.). pap. 24.00 (*0-935081-00-3*) One Eight Inc.

Home Course in Nutrition. Eric F. Powell. 1980. 106p. pap. (*0-85032-158-1*) C W Daniel GBR. *Dist:* Natl Bk Netwk.

Home Court Advantage see Home Birth Advantage: A Time Honored Tradition for the New Millennium

Home Diagnostic & Monitoring Markets: FDA & Distribution Issues Characterize a Changing Marketplace. Market Intelligence Staff. 1992. 230p. 1895.00 (*1-56753-405-8*) Frost & Sullivan.

Home Drug Infusion Therapy under Medicare. 1992. (Illus.). 208p. (Orig.). (C). pap. text 40.00 (*1-56806-100-5*) DIANE Pub.

Home Emergency Guide. HarperCollins Staff. 1998. (Gem Ser.). 256p. (YA). pap. 8.00 (*0-00-472178-0*) Collins SF.

Home Exercise Guide for Lower Extremity Amputees. Robert S. Gailey et al. 1995. (Rehabilitation Series for Lower Extremity Amputees: Vol. 4). (Illus.). 59p. (C). pap. text 7.00 (*1-888131-03-9*) Adv Rehab Therapy.

Home from Seven North. Millard Thomas. 1984. LC 81-83739. 15.00 (*0-87212-158-5*) Libra.

Home Health Administation. Jean Syer. 2000. LC 99-48215. 304p. text 115.00 (*0-323-00771-6*) Mosby Inc.

Home Health Aide. Jack Rudman. (Career Examination Ser.: C-3635). pap. 27.95 (*0-8373-3635-X*) Nat Learn.

Home Health Aide - Guidelines for Care: A Handbook for Caregiving at Home. Tina M. Marrelli & Sandra M. Whittier. 1996. 225p. spiral bd. 24.95 (*0-9647801-0-0*) Marrelli.

Home Health Aide - Guidelines for Care: A Resource Guide to Accompany "Home Health Aide: Guidelines for Care" Tina M. Marrelli & Laura Friend. 1996. (Illus.). 125p. tchr. ed., ring bd. 89.95 (*0-9647801-1-9*) Marrelli.

Home Health Aide Handbook. Jetta Fuzy. 2000. LC 2001-268524. (Illus.). 224p. pap. 18.25 (*1-888343-37-0*) Hartman Pub.

Home Health Aide Training Manual. Kay Green. 1996. 352p. ring bd. 121.00 (*0-8342-0746-X*) Aspen Pub.

Home Health & Rehabilitation: Concepts of Care. Bella J. May. 2nd ed. 1998. LC 98-17364. (Illus.). 368p. 65.00 (*0-8036-0382-7*) Davis Co.

Home Health Care: An Annotated Bibliography, 16. Compiled by Ada R. Davis et al. 1992. LC 91-46848. (Bibliographies & Indexes in Gerontology Ser.: No. 16). 168p. lib. bdg. 55.00 (*0-313-28334-6*, DHH, Greenwood Pr) Greenwood.

Home Health Care: Can Agencies Survive New Regulations? Congressional Hearing. Ed. by Christopher S. Bond. 2000. (Illus.). 228p. reprint ed. pap. text 45.00 (*0-7567-0443-X*) DIANE Pub.

Home Health Care: Its Role in the Changing Health Services Market. Eli Ginzberg et al. 1984. LC 84-3468. (Conservation of Human Resources Ser.: No. 18). (Illus.). 196p. (C). text 52.50 (*0-916672-65-4*) Rowman.

***Home Health Care: Will the New Payment System & Regulatory Overkill Hurt Our Seniors?: Congressional Hearing.** Ed. by Susan M. Collins. 2001. 218p. (C). pap. text 35.00 (*0-7567-0955-5*) DIANE Pub.

Home Health Care Administration. Susan C. Schulmerich et al. 1995. LC 95-21975. (Professional Reference - Nursing Ser.). 295p. pap. 84.95 (*0-8273-6508-X*) Delmar.

Home Health Care & National Health Policy. Brahna Trager. 1980. LC 80-15988. (Home Health Care Services Quarterly Ser.: Vol. 1, No. 2). 103p. text 39.95 (*0-917724-20-8*) Haworth Pr.

Home Health Care Corporate Compliance Manual. Carol L. Schaffer. 139.00 (*0-8342-1215-3*) Aspen Pub.

Home Health Care Equipment: A Consumer Guidebook. Patricia R. Peterson. 1989. LC 89-62034. (Illus.). 156p. (Orig.). 16.95 (*0-944871-34-8*); pap. 9.95 (*0-944871-35-6*) Riegel Pub.

Home Health Care Forms, Checklists & Guidelines. Aspen Reference Group Staff. 1989. ring bd. 199.00 (*0-8342-1052-5*) Aspen Pub.

Home Health Care Law Parts 1-3: Liability & Risk Management. Fay Rozovsky. 1993. 125.00 (*0-316-76076-5*) Aspen Law.

Home Health Care Law Parts 1-3: Liability & Risk Management, Set. Fay Rozovsky & Lorne E. Rozovsky. 1994. 340p. 125.00 (*0-316-76100-1*, Little Brwn Med Div) Lppncott W & W.

Home Health Care Law Manual. Martha D. Nathanson. 1996. 780p. ring bd. 99.00 (*0-8342-0807-5*, S290) Aspen Pub.

Home Health Care Management. Lazelle E. Benefield. 1988. (Illus.). 416p. text 50.00 (*0-89303-682-X*) P-H.

Home Health Care Nursing. Martinson. 2nd ed. 2000. LC 2001-57695. pap. text (*0-7216-7766-5*) Saunders.

Home Health Care Patient Education Manual. Aspen Reference Group Staff. 1994. LC 94-17353. ring bd. 229.00 (*0-8342-0565-3*, S124) Aspen Pub.

Home Health Care Practice. Ed. by Patrick Catania & Martin M. Rosner. 2nd ed. 1994. LC 93-79105. (Illus.). 352p. (C). pap. 60.00 (*0-9627640-4-3*) Hlth Mrkts Res.

Home Health Care Signaling Equipment, UL 1637. 1998. (C). pap. text 330.00 (*0-7629-0303-1*) Underwrtrs Labs.

Home Health Care the Easy Way: A Step-by-Step Guide to Caring for a Patient in Your Home. Diane M. Burgan & Lois V. Seamans. 1998. LC 97-92465. (Illus.). 112p. pap. 9.95 (*0-9660704-0-2*) Creat Opportunities.

Home Health Client. Karen Martin. (Illus.). (C). (gr. 13). 1998. 170p. text, tchr. ed. 26.00 (*0-8151-8592-8*, 28844); 1996. LC 97-122274. 480p. text 68.00 (*0-8151-8593-6*, 28845) Mosby Inc.

Home Health Guide to Poisons & Antidotes. Carol Turkington. 1995. (Illus.). 372p. pap. 12.95 (*0-8160-3316-1*) Facts on File.

Home Health Handbook. 1989. (Illus.). (*1-886614-02-4*) Intl Masters Pub.

Home Health Handbook of Pediatric Procedures. Rice. 1998. (Illus.). 462p. (C). (gr. 13). text 28.95 (*0-8151-3819-9*, 31842) Mosby Inc.

Home Health Nurse. Jack Rudman. (Certified Nurse Examination Ser.: Vol. 26). 27.95 (*0-8373-6176-1*); 1997. pap. 27.95 (*0-8373-6126-5*, CN26) Nat Learn.

Home Health Nursing: Assessment & Careplanning. Linda Skidmore-Roth & Marie Jaffe. 3rd ed. 1996. LC 96-23053. 480p. (C). (gr. 13). spiral bd. 29.95 (*0-8151-4877-1*, 28203) Mosby Inc.

Home Health Nursing: Nursing Diagnosis & Care Plans. Carol A. Bedrosian. 1989. LC 88-16788. 640p. (C). pap. 42.61 (*0-8385-3842-8*, A3842-0) Appleton & Lange.

Home Health Nursing Practice: Concepts & Application. Robyn Rice. 2nd rev. ed. 1995. LC 95-39774. (Illus.). 512p. (C). (gr. 13). pap. text 36.95 (*0-8151-7240-0*, 26255) Mosby Inc.

Home Health Orientation Manual. Tina M. Marrelli & Lynda Hilliard. 1997. LC 99-173195. (Illus.). 304p. (C). (gr. 13). text 99.95 (*0-8151-4650-7*, 29745) Mosby Inc.

Home Health Practice: A Guide for the Occupational Therapist. Ed. by Catherine Verrier Piersol & Phyllis L. Ehrlich. 2000. LC 00-39559. (Illus.). 208p. spiral bd. 51.50 (*1-883315-50-6*) Imaginart Intl.

Home Healthcare: Wired & Ready for Telemedicine. Audrey Kinsella et al. 1997. (Illus.). 236p. (Orig.). pap. text 295.00 (*0-9657674-0-X*) Info Tomorrow.

Home Healthcare: Wired & Ready for Telemedicine: The Second Generation. Audrey Kinsella et al. 1998. (Illus.). 250p. pap. (*0-9657674-7-7*) Info Tomorrow.

Home Healthcare - Wired & Ready for Telemedicine: The Nurses' & Nursing Students' Edition. Audrey Kinsella. 1997. (Illus.). 118p. (C). pap. 95.00 (*0-9657674-1-8*) Info Tomorrow.

Home Healthcare Nurse on Hospice & Palliative Care. Carolyn J. Humphrey. 2000. pap. text 10.95 (*0-7817-2864-9*) Lppncott W & W.

Home Hemodialysis Training. Regional Kidney Disease Program, Interstate Divisi. 1980. 194p. ring bd. 25.00 (*1-56488-007-9*) Dialyrn.

Home Hospice after Your Home: A Michigan Law Case. Ed. by Thomas J. Rundquist. 1998. (Illus.). 130p. (C). pap. 29.95 (*1-884239-24-2*) Nova Media.

Home Infusion Therapy Current Status & Future Trends. Ed. by Ronald B. Conners & Robert W. Winters. 1995. LC 95-36061. 276p. pap. 72.00 (*1-55648-146-2*, 079202) AHPI.

Home Is Where the Art Is: An Art Therapy Approach to Family Therapy. Doris Banowsky Arrington. 2001. LC 00-66658. (Illus.). xxviii, 265p. pap. 42.95 (*0-398-07161-6*) C C Thomas.

***Home Is Where the Art Is: An Art Therapy Approach to Family Therapy.** Doris Banowsky Arrington. 2001. LC 00-66658. (Illus.). xxviii, 265p. 61.95 (*0-398-07160-8*) C C Thomas.

Home Is Where We Start From: Essays from a Psychoanalyst. Donald Woods Winnicott. 1990. pap. 14.95 (*0-393-30667-4*) Norton.

Home Leg Program by Post Rehabilitation Fitness. David Dallmeyer et al. 1998. (Illus.). 25p. 40.00 incl. VHS (*1-930241-05-4*) F I Intl.

Home Made Health: A Family Guide to Nutrition, Exercise, Stress Control & Preventive Medicine. Raymond S. Moore & Dorothy N. Moore. 5th ed. 1996. LC 86-15874. 233p. reprint ed. pap. 11.95 (*0-8499-3172-X*) Moore Fnd.

Home Medical Advisor: The New Self Help Guide to Symptoms, Diseases & Medical Emergencies. American Medical Association Staff. 1988. 320p. 24.95 (*0-394-56523-1*) Random.

Home Medical Dictionary. 1994. 256p. pap. (*1-884907-08-3*) Paradise Pr FL.

Home Medical Dictionary. R. F. Patterson. 1989. 256p. (Orig.). pap. 5.95 (*0-938261-99-1*) PSI & Assocs.

Home Medicine: The Newfoundland Experience. John K. Crellin. 1994. (McGill-Queen's Studies in the History of Religion Ser.). (Illus.). 288p. (*0-7735-1196-2*); LC 95-165979. pap. (*0-7735-1197-0*) McG-Queens Univ Pr CAN. *Dist:* CUP Services.

Home or Nursing Home: Making the Right Choices. Michael J. Salamon & Gloria Rosenthal. 1990. LC 89-21910. (Adulthood & Aging Ser.: Vol. 25). 128p. 26.95 (*0-8261-6680-6*) Springer Pub.

Home Rehabilitation Exercises: Hand. Kay Lee & Shirley Marcus. 1990. (Illus.). 16p. (Orig.). (C). pap. text 6.00 (*0-910317-58-5*) Am Occup Therapy.

Home Rehabilitation Exercises: Shoulder, Elbow, Forearm, Wrist. Kay Lee & Shirley Marcus. 1990. (Illus.). 16p. (Orig.). (C). pap. text 6.00 (*0-910317-57-7*) Am Occup Therapy.

Home Rehabilitation Guide. Wendy Anemaet. 1999. LC 99-40803. xvi, 718p. spiral bd. 32.95 (*0-323-00285-4*) Mosby Inc.

Home Rehabilitation Program Guide. Paul A. Roggow et al. rev. ed. 1993. LC 89-43335. (Illus.). 184p. pap. 29.00 (*1-55642-231-8*) SLACK Inc.

Home Remedies: A Handbook of Herbal Cures for Common Ailments. T. V. Sairam & Lena Weyer. 1998. LC 98-909145. xxiii, 333 p. (*0-14-027709-9*) Viking Penguin.

Home Remedies: Herbal & Homeopathic Treatments for Use at Home. Otto Wolff. Tr. by J. Collis & Anna R. Meuss from GER. 2nd ed. 2000.Tr. of Naturgemasse Hausapotheke. 124p. pap. 10.95 (*0-88010-362-0*) Anthroposophic.

Home Remedies: Hydrotherapy, Massage, Charcoal, & Other Simple Treatments. Agatha Thrash & Calvin L. Thrash, Jr. 1981. (Illus.). 174p. pap. 17.95 (*0-942658-02-7*) NLB.

Home Remedies & the Black Elderly: A Reference Manual for Health Care Providers. Eddie L. Boyd et al. 1991. 26p. (C). reprint ed. pap. 9.95 (*0-9631310-0-1*) Pharm Info.

Home Remedies from the Country Doctor: Oatmeal, Cucumbers, Ammonia, Lemon, Gin-Soaked Raisins - Timeless Solutions to More Than 200 Common Aches, Pains & Illnesses. Jay Heinrichs et al. 1999. LC 99-10121. (Illus.). xii, 500p. 29.95 (*1-57954-065-1*) Rodale Pr Inc.

Home Remedies Handbook. Consumer Guide Editors. 1993. (Illus.). 400p. 19.98 (*1-56173-747-X*, 3211000) Pubns Intl Ltd.

Home Safety. 1995. 17.00 (*0-8342-0723-0*); VHS 94.00 (*0-8342-0724-9*) Aspen Pub.

Home Shoulder Program by Post Rehabilitation Fitness. David Dallmeyer et al. 1998. (Illus.). 28p. 40.00 incl. VHS (*1-930241-03-8*) F I Intl.

Home "Tele-Infusion" Directions in Infusion Therapies Delivered Via Telecommunication. Audrey Kinsella. 1998. (Illus.). 200p. pap. (*0-9657674-9-3*) Info Tomorrow.

Home Telehealth in the 21st Century: A Resource Book about Improved Care Services That Work. Audrey Kinsella & Ronald K. Goodenow. 2000. 195.00 (*0-9657674-4-2*) Info Tomorrow.

Home Wellness Center. Bernard Jensen. 1988. pap. 12.99 (*0-932615-11-2*) B Jensen.

Homecare Management of the Bone Marrow Transplant Patient. Jean N. Lonergan et al. 2nd ed. 1995. (Illus.). 160p. pap. text 33.75 (*0-86720-744-2*, 744-2) Jones & Bartlett.

Homecare Salary & Benefits Report, 1991-92. Hospital Compensation Service Staff. 1992. pap. 250.00 (*0-939326-67-1*) Hosp & Hlthcare.

Homehealth Guides. 1997. spiral bd. 114.00 (*0-8151-9694-6*, 29974) Mosby Inc.

Homeless People & Health Care: An Unrelenting Challenge. Susan Neibacher. 1990. (Papers: No. 14). 32p. 5.00 (*0-934459-62-2*) United Hosp Fund.

Homeless Women & Homeless Women with Mental Illnesses. annot. ed. 1995. 28p. (Orig.). (C). pap. text 15.00 (*0-7881-2584-2*) DIANE Pub.

Homelessness: Abstracts of the Psychological & Behavioral Literature 1967-1990. Ed. by Mary B. Shinn et al. 1990. (Bibliographies in Psychology Ser.: No. 7). 80p. pap. text 19.95 (*1-55798-052-7*) Am Psychol.

Homelessness & Drinking: A Study of a Street Population. Ed. by Bernard Segal. 1992. LC 91-25836. (Drugs & Society Ser.: Vol. 5, Nos. 3-4). (Illus.). 150p. 39.95 (*1-56024-210-8*) Haworth Pr.

Homelessness, Health Care, & Welfare Provision. Ed. by Kevin Fisher & John Collins. 1993. LC 92-40458. pap. (*0-415-05000-6*); 208p. (C). (gr. 13). 85.00 (*0-415-04999-7*, A7819) Routledge.

Homelessness Prevention in Treatment of Substance Abuse & Mental Illness: Logic Models & Implementation of Eight American Projects. Ed. by Kendon J. Conrad et al. 1999. LC 99-32742. xxii, 220p. 49.95 (*0-7890-0750-9*) Haworth Pr.

Homemaker: Home Health Aide. Helen Huber & Audree Spatz. (C). 4th ed. 1993. LC 92-40574. 450p. mass mkt. 50.95 (*0-8273-5270-0*); 5th ed. 1997. 176p. wbk. ed. 14.50 (*0-8273-8086-0*) Delmar.

Homemaker: Home Health Aide Workbook. Julie K. Wernig. 1989. (Illus.). 176p. pap. text, wbk. ed. 7.95 (*0-8016-5529-3*) Mosby Inc.

Homemaker - Home Health Aide - IML. Helen Huber. 5th ed. 1997. 224p. tchr. ed. 17.95 (*0-8273-8085-2*) Delmar.

Homemaker-Home Health Aide. Sheila A. Sorrentino & Julie K. Wernig. 1988. (Illus.). 432p. (gr. 13). pap. text 27.95 (*0-8016-5390-8*, 05390) Mosby Inc.

Homemaker Home Health Aide. Helen Huber & Audree Spatz. Ed. by Carole Coviello. 3rd ed. 304p. (gr. 11-12). 1990. pap. 29.95 (*0-8273-3436-2*); 1989. pap., tchr. ed. 15.75 (*0-8273-3437-0*); 1989. pap., stu. ed. 14.95 (*0-8273-3438-9*) Delmar.

Homemaker/Home Health Aide. Helen Huber & Audree Spatz. 5th ed. 1997. LC 97-12232. (Allied Health Ser.). 528p. (C). pap. text 49.95 (*0-8273-8084-4*) Delmar.

Homeopathic Aide-Memoire. Peter Coats. 1984. 106p. (*0-85032-165-4*) C W Daniel GBR. *Dist:* Natl Bk Netwk.

Homeopathic Aide-Memoire. Peter Coats. 2nd ed. 96p. 11.95 (*0-8464-4227-2*) Beekman Pubs.

Homeopathic Care for Cats & Dogs: Small Doses for Small Animals. Donald Hamilton. 1999. LC 98-41291. (Illus.). xxi, 482p. pap. text 25.00 (*1-55643-295-X*) North Atlantic.

Homeopathic Childbirth Manual: A Practical Guide for Labor, Birth & the Immediate Postpartum Period. Betty Idarius. 1996. (Orig.). pap. 14.95 (*0-9649304-9-8*) Idarius Pr.

Homeopathic Color Remedies. Ambika Wauters. 1999. LC 98-55114. 133p. pap. 12.95 (*0-89594-997-0*) Crossing Pr.

Homeopathic Correspondence Course: Advanced Level. Noel Puddephatt. 1996. 92p. reprint ed. spiral bd. 14.00 (*0-7873-1076-X*) Hlth Research.

Homeopathic Drug Pictures. Margaret L. Tyler. 1952. 885p. (C). 65.95 (*0-8464-1020-6*) Beekman Pubs.

Homeopathic Emergency Guide: A Quick Reference Handbook to Effective Homeopathic Care. Thomas A. Kruzel. 1992. 366p. (Orig.). pap. 22.95 (*1-55643-123-6*) North Atlantic.

Homeopathic Guide to Stress: Safe & Effective Natural Ways to Alleviate. Miranda Castro. 1999. 399p. reprint ed. pap. text 19.00 (*0-7881-6798-7*) DIANE Pub.

***Homeopathic Handbook of Natural Remedies: Safe & Effective Treatment of Common Ailments & Injuries.** Laura Josephson. 2002. LC 2001-51106. pap. 15.00 (*0-8129-9188-5*) Random Trade.

Homeopathic Materia Medica for Nurses. B. C. Woodbury. Ed. by Jay Yasgur. 1991. (C). pap. text 23.95 (*1-886149-02-X*) Van Hoy Pubs.

Homeopathic Medicine: A Doctor's Guide to Remedies for Common Ailments. Trevor Smith. 1989. 256p. pap. 10.95 (*0-89281-293-1*, Heal Arts VT) Inner Tradit.

Homeopathic Medicine: First Aid & Emergency Care. Lyle Morgan. 1989. 144p. pap. 12.95 (*0-89281-249-4*, Heal Arts VT) Inner Tradit.

Homeopathic Medicine at Home: Natural Remedies for Everyday Ailments & Minor Injuries. Maesimund B. Panos & Jane Himlich. 1981. LC 79-63802. 288p. 12.95 (*0-87477-195-1*, Tarcher Putnam) Putnam Pub Group.

Homeopathic Medicine for Children & Infants. Dana Ullman. 1992. 256p. 13.95 (*0-87477-692-9*, Tarcher Putnam) Putnam Pub Group.

Homeopathic Medicine for Mental Health. Trevor Smith. 1989. Orig. Title: Homeopathic Treatment of Emotional Illness. 208p. pap. 12.95 (*0-89281-291-5*, Heal Arts VT) Inner Tradit.

Homeopathic Medicine for Women: An Alternative Approach to Gynecological Health Care. Trevor Smith. 1988. 176p. pap. 12.95 (*0-89281-236-2*, Heal Arts VT) Inner Tradit.

Homeopathic Medicine in the Home: A Correspondence Study Course. Jonathan Breslow. 1992. LC 88-71470. (Illus.). 155p. (C). pap. 29.95 (*0-9620939-0-4*) Ashwin Pubns.

Homeopathic Method: Implications for Clinical Practice & Medical Science. Jeremy Swayne. 1998. LC 97-24464. pap. text (*0-443-05926-8*) Church.

Homeopathic Methodology: Repertory, Case Taking, & Case Analysis: An Introductory Homeopathic Workbook. Todd Rowe. 1998. LC 98-17727. 175p. 18.95 (*1-55643-277-1*) North Atlantic.

Homeopathic Pediatrics: Assessment & Case Management. Randall Neustaedter. 1991. LC 91-37458. 337p. 39.95 (*1-55643-120-1*) North Atlantic.

Homeopathic Pharmacy. Kayne. 1997. text 44.95 (*0-443-05018-X*) Saunders.

Homeopathic Remedies: For Health Professionals & Laypeople. Dale Buegal et al. rev. ed. 2000. (Illus.). 250p. pap. 15.95 (*0-89389-177-0*) Himalayan Inst.

Homeopathic Remedies for Children. Phyllis Speight. 1990. 99p. (Orig.). pap. 15.95 (*0-8464-1336-1*) Beekman Pubs.

Homeopathic Remedies for Dogs. Geoffrey Llewellyn. 1998. (Illus.). 128p. 19.95 (*1-85279-086-5*, GB046) TFH Pubns.

Homeopathic Remedies for Ears, Nose & Throat. Phyllis Speight. 76p. (Orig.). pap. 9.95 (*0-8464-4228-0*) Beekman Pubs.

Homeopathic Remedies for Ears, Nose & Throat. Phyllis Speight. 1990. 107p. (Orig.). pap. (*0-85207-217-1*) C W Daniel GBR. *Dist:* Natl Bk Netwk.

Homeopathic Remedies for 100 Children's Common Ailments. Carolyn Dean. Ed. by Phyllis Herman. 1995. (Good Health Guides). 56p. pap. 3.95 (*0-87983-668-7*, 36687K, Keats Pubng) McGraw-Hill Trade.

Homeopathic Remedies for Women's Ailments. Phyllis Speight. 3rd ed. 152p. pap. 17.95 (*0-8464-4229-9*) Beekman Pubs.

Homeopathic Self-Care: The Quick & Easy Guide for the Whole Family. Robert Ullman. 1997. LC 97-1079. 448p. pap. 19.95 (*0-7615-0706-X*, Prima Health) Prima Pub.

Homeopathic Teachings from a Master. Cotter. 1987. 107p. pap. (*0-85207-183-3*) C W Daniel GBR. *Dist:* Natl Bk Netwk.

Homeopathic Teachings from a Master. Edward Cottier. 88p. (Orig.). pap. 11.95 (*0-8464-4230-2*) Beekman Pubs.

Homeopathic Treatment for Birds. Beryl M. Chapman. 68p. (Orig.). pap. 11.95 (*0-8464-4231-0*) Beekman Pubs.

Homeopathic Treatment for Birds. Beryl M. Chapman. 1991. 129p. (Orig.). pap. (*0-85207-235-X*) C W Daniel GBR. *Dist:* Natl Bk Netwk.

Homeopathic Treatment of Children: Pediatric Constitutional Types. Paul N. Herscu. 1991. LC 91-2390. 374p. (Orig.). pap. 22.50 (*1-55643-090-6*) North Atlantic.

Homeopathic Treatment of Emotional Illness see Homeopathic Medicine for Mental Health

Homeopathic Treatment of Small Animals. Christopher Day. 1990. 129p. pap. (*0-85207-216-3*) C W Daniel GBR. *Dist:* Natl Bk Netwk.

Homeopathic Treatment of Small Animals. Christopher E. Day. 224p. (Orig.). pap. 29.95 (*0-8464-4232-9*) Beekman Pubs.

Homeopathic Treatment of Sports Injuries. Lyle W. Morgan. 1987. LC 87-10161. 144p. pap. 9.95 (*0-89281-227-3*, Heal Arts VT) Inner Tradit.

Homeopathy. Ilana Dannheisser & Penny Edwards. 1998. LC 98-22373. (Illustrated Guides Ser.). (Illus.). 144p. pap. 19.95 (*1-86204-168-7*) Element MA.

Homeopathy: A Critical Appraisal. Ed. by Edzard Ernst & Eckhart G. Hahn. 1998. LC 98-143075. 256p. pap. text 47.50 (*0-7506-3564-9*, 105838) Buttrwrth-Heinemann.

Homeopathy: A Guide. 1994. lib. bdg. 250.95 (*0-8490-5661-6*) Gordon Pr.

Homeopathy: A Home Prescriber. Phyllis Speight. 224p. (Orig.). pap. 26.95 (*0-8464-4234-5*) Beekman Pubs.

Homeopathy: A Step-by-Step Guide. Ed. by Caro Ness. 1997. LC 98-188286. (In a Nutshell Ser.). (Illus.). 64p. pap. 7.95 (*1-86204-007-9*) Element MA.

Homeopathy: Beyond Flat Earth Medicine: An Essential Guide for the Homeopathic Patient. Timothy R. Dooley. 1995. LC 95-60000. 128p. (Orig.). pap. 9.00 (*1-886893-00-4*) Timing CA.

Homeopathy: For Health & Well Being. Robin Hayfield. 2000. (Health & Well-Being Ser.). (Illus.). 64p. pap. (*1-84215-002-2*, Swater) Ann3ess GBR. *Dist:* AOL Time Warner.

Homeopathy: From Alchemy to Medicine. Elizabeth Danciger. 1989. 118p. pap. 5.95 (*0-89281-290-7*, Heal Arts VT) Inner Tradit.

Homeopathy: Heart & Soul. Keith Souter. 1993. 288p. (Orig.). pap. 23.95 (*0-8464-4172-1*) Beekman Pubs.

Homeopathy: Index of Modern Information. Arthur S. Glocks. 1990. LC 89-78056. 150p. 47.50 (*1-55914-184-0*); pap. 44.50 (*1-55914-185-9*) ABBE Pubs Assn.

Homeopathy: Natural Medicine for the Whole Person. Peter Adams. 1996. LC 96-34074. (Health Essentials Ser.). 128p. pap. 9.95 (*1-85230-879-6*) Element MA.

Homeopathy: Nature's Healing Law. M. L. Scott. 1996. 19p. reprint ed. spiral bd. 8.00 (*0-7873-0753-X*) Hlth Research.

Homeopathy: Science or Myth? Bill Gray. 2000. LC 99-53966. (Illus.). xxi, 190p. pap. text 14.95 (*1-55643-332-8*) North Atlantic.

Homeopathy: The Great Riddle. Richard Grossinger. 2nd rev. ed. 1998. LC 98-6345. (Illus.). 180p. pap. 14.95 (*1-55643-290-9*) North Atlantic.

Homeopathy: Twenty-First Century Medicine. Dana Ullman. 1987. 256p. (Orig.). pap. 16.95 (*1-55643-015-9*) North Atlantic.

Homeopathy A-Z. Dana Ullman. 2001. (Illus.). 156p. pap. 11.95 (*1-56170-798-8*, L483) Hay House.

Homeopathy & Immunization. James G. Speight. 1982. 107p. pap. (*0-85032-199-9*) C W Daniel GBR. *Dist:* Natl Bk Netwk.

Homeopathy & Immunization. Leslie J. Speight. 16p. pap. 4.95 (*0-8464-4235-3*) Beekman Pubs.

Homeopathy & the Medical Profession. Phillip Nichols. 1988. 250p. lib. bdg. (*0-7099-1836-4*) C Helm GBR. *Dist:* Routldge.

Homeopathy for Animals: Tales & Techniques from a Country Practitioner. Kaetheryn Walker. 1997. LC 97-18370. (Illus.). 240p. pap. 14.95 (*0-89281-737-2*, Heal Arts VT) Inner Tradit.

Homeopathy for Back & Neck Pain Ursula Stone. 1999. LC 00-701459. (Illus.). 159p. mass mkt. 4.99 (*1-57566-443-7*) Kensgtn Pub Corp.

Homeopathy for Birthing: A Simplied Guide for Mothers Midwives & Other Health Professionals. Jana Shiloh. rev. ed. 1991. (Illus.). 58p. pap. text 10.95 (*0-9619203-1-9*) Rocky Mtn Homeopathics.

Homeopathy for Birthing: A Simplified Guide for Mothers, Midwives & Other Health Care Professionals. Jana Shiloh. 2nd ed. 1990. 60p. (Orig.). pap. text (*0-9619203-2-7*) Rocky Mtn Homeopathics.

Homeopathy for Children: A Parent's Guide to the Treatment of Common Childhood Illnesses. Gabrielle Pinto & Murray Feldman. 2000. 280p. pap. (*0-85207-337-2*) C W Daniel GBR. *Dist:* Natl Bk Netwk.

Homeopathy for Common Ailments. Robin Hayfield. 1993. LC 93-46857. (Illus.). 95p. (C). reprint ed. pap. 14.95 (*1-883319-14-5*) Frog Ltd CA.

Homeopathy for Emergencies. Phyllis Speight. 64p. (Orig.). pap. 7.95 (*0-8464-4233-7*) Beekman Pubs.

Homeopathy for Headaches. Ursula Stone. 1999. LC 00-500193. 183p. mass mkt. 4.99 (*1-57566-417-8*) Kensington Hse Publishing Ltd.

Homeopathy for Menopause. Beth MacEoin. 1997. LC 97-6962. 256p. pap. 14.95 (*0-89281-648-1*, Heal Arts VT) Inner Tradit.

Homeopathy for Midwives. Barbara Geraghty. 1997. LC 97-4293. pap. text (*0-443-05708-7*) Church.

Homeopathy for Musculoskeletal Healing. Asa Hershoff. 1996. LC 96-38435. (Illus.). 250p. pap. 20.00 (*1-55643-237-2*) North Atlantic.

Homeopathy for Pets. Shawn Messonnier. 1998. (Pet Care Naturally Ser.). 64p. pap. 4.95 (*0-87983-925-2*, Keats Pubng) McGraw-Hill Trade.

Homeopathy for Pregnancy, Birth, & Your Baby's First Year. Miranda Castro. 1993. LC 92-28880. pap. 16.95 (*0-312-08809-4*) St Martin.

Homeopathy for the First Aider. Dorothy Sheperd. 1980. (C). pap. 9.95 (*0-8464-1021-4*) Beekman Pubs.

Homeopathy for the Modern Pregnant Woman & Her Infant: A Therapeutic Practice Guidebook for Midwives, Physicians & Practitioners. Sandra J. Perko. 1997. LC 96-96765. xiv, 460p. 59.95 (*0-9653187-0-2*) Benchmark Homeopathic.

Homeopathy for the Soul. Cassandra Marks & Cassandra Lorius. 2001. (*0-00-711335-8*) Thorsons GBR. *Dist:* Natl Bk Netwk.

Homeopathy for the Third Age. Keith Souter. 1993. 107p. pap. (*0-85207-268-6*) C W Daniel GBR. *Dist:* Natl Bk Netwk.

Homeopathy for Women: A Comprehensive, Easy-to-Use Guide for Women of All Ages. Barry Rose & Christina Scott-Moncrieff. 1999. (Illus.). 176p. pap. 19.95 (*1-55209-303-4*) Firefly Bks Limited.

Homeopathy Handbook. Andrew Lockie. 2001. LC 00-45196. (Healing Handbooks Ser.). (Illus.). 128p. pap. 12.95 (*0-7894-7178-7*) DK Pub Inc.

Homeopathy in Primary Care. Bob Leckridge. 1997. LC 96-37984. 281p. pap. text (*0-443-05521-1*) Church.

Homeopathy in Veterinary Practice. K. J. Biddis. 86p. (Orig.). pap. 11.95 (*0-8464-4236-1*) Beekman Pubs.

Homeopathy Made Simple: A Quick Reference Guide. R. Donald Papon. 1998. LC 98-71592. 264p. pap. 11.95 (*1-57174-110-0*) Hampton Roads Pub Co.

Homeopathy: Medicine for the 21st Century see Discovering Homeopathy: Your Introduction to the Science & Art of Homeopathic Medicine

Homeopathy, Medicine That Works! Who It Can Help, What It Can Cure, How It Works, Where to Find It. Robert S. Wood. 1990. LC 90-45190. (Orig.). pap. 9.95 (*0-913238-04-X*) Condor UT.

Homeopathy 911: What to Do in an Emergency Before Help Arrives. Eileen Nauman & Gail Derin-Kellogg. 2000. LC 2001-267407. xxii, 310p. pap. 14.00 (*1-57566-694-4*, Knsington) Kensgtn Pub Corp.

Homeopathy Simplified: Domestic Practice Made Easy. John A. Tarbell. rev. ed. 1996. 372p. reprint ed. spiral bd. 20.00 (*0-7873-0853-6*) Hlth Research.

Homeopathy Unveiled: An Explanation of How It Really Works. Giri D. Wescott. 1995. (Illus.). 80p. (Orig.). pap. 9.00 (*0-9641323-1-1*) Satyam Pub.

Homeopathy Workshop. Cook. pap. (*1-86126-246-9*) Crowood Pr GBR. *Dist:* Trafalgar.

Homeostasis & Thermal Stress: International Symposium on Pharmacology of Thermoregulation, 6th, Jasper, Alta, August 1985. Ed. by K. Cooper et al. 1986. (Illus.). xiv, 210p. 101.00 (*3-8055-4228-3*) S Karger.

Homeothermia of the Brain Cerebral Blood Flow, Metabolic Rate & Brain Temperature in the Cold: The Possible Role of Neurolgia. S. Z. Donhoffer. 1980. 140p. (C). pap. (*963-05-2405-8*) Akade Kiado HUN. *Dist:* St Mut.

Homes & Health: How Housing & Health Interact. B. Ineichen. 1993. LC 92-45673. 153.95 (*0-419-17100-2*, Spon) Routledge.

Homes for the Mad: Life Inside Two Nineteenth-Century Asylums. Ellen Dwyer. 1987. 281p. text 40.00 (*0-8135-1182-8*) Rutgers U Pr.

Homes of Their Own: A Community Care Initiative for Children with Learning Difficulties. Anne Leonard. 1991. (Studies in Cash & Care). 161p. text (*1-85628-156-6*) Avebry GBR. *Dist:* Ashgate Pub Co.

Homestasis, Nephrotoxicity & Renal Anomalies in the Newborn. Ed. by Jose Strauss. 1985. text 141.00 (*0-89838-766-3*) Kluwer Academic.

Homestead Doctor. Joe Hoadley. 1995. (Illus.). 200p. (Orig.). 27.95 (*0-9649106-0-8*); pap. 18.95 (*0-9649106-3-2*) Image Ad Vantage.

Hometown Hero: An Action Guide for the Solo Practice. Joseph M. O'Donnell. 1995. LC 94-48595. 44.95 (*0-87814-435-8*) PennWell Corp.

Homicide Investigation: Practical Information for Coroners, Police Officers, & Other Investigators. LeMoyne Snyder. 3rd ed. 1977. (Illus.). 416p. 74.95 (*0-398-03632-2*) C C Thomas.

Homme aux Loups. Sigmund Freud. 1990. (FRE.). pap. 16.95 (*0-7859-3014-0*) Fr & Eur.

Homo Schizo I: Human & Cultural Hologenesis. Alfred De Grazia. 1983. (Quantavolution Ser.). 278p. pap. 16.00 (*0-940268-01-9*) Metron Pubns.

Homo Schizo II: Human Nature & Behavior. Alfred De Grazia. 1983. (Quantavolution Ser.). 240p. pap. 15.00 (*0-940268-02-7*) Metron Pubns.

Homocysteine Metabolism: From Basic Science to Clinical Medicine. Ed. by Ian Graham et al. 1998. LC 97-22535. (Developments in Cardiovascular Medicine Ser.). 296p. text 165.00 (*0-7923-9983-8*) Kluwer Academic.

Homocystinuria: A Risk Factor of Premature Vascular Disease. G. H. Boers. 1986. (Clinical Research Ser.: No. 3). vii, 166p. (Orig.). (C). pap. text (*3-11-013366-0*) Mouton.

Homoeopathic Aide Memoire. Coats. Date not set. 11.95 (*0-8464-1203-9*) Beekman Pubs.

Homoeopathic Drug Pictures. 1980. 30.00 (*0-85032-184-0*) St Mut.

Homoeopathic Drug Pictures. M. L. Tyler. 1952. 162p. (*0-85032-021-6*) C W Daniel GBR. *Dist:* Natl Bk Netwk.

Homoeopathic Medicine. Harris L. Coulter. 1972. LC 74-190020. pap. 2.50 (*0-89378-072-3*) Formur Intl.

Homoeopathic Medicine for Dogs. 1998. pap. 26.95 (*0-8464-4565-4*) Beekman Pubs.

Homoeopathic Remedies for Children. Phyllis Speight. 1983. 61p. pap. (*0-85207-158-2*) C W Daniel GBR. *Dist:* Natl Bk Netwk.

Homoeopathic Remedies for Women's Ailments. Phyllis Speight. 1985. pap. (*0-85032-200-6*) C W Daniel GBR. *Dist:* Natl Bk Netwk.

Homoeopathy: A Home Prescriber. Phyllis Speight. 1992. 107p. pap. (*0-85207-262-7*) C W Daniel GBR. *Dist:* Natl Bk Netwk.

Homoeopathy for the First Aider. Dorothy Shepherd. 1953. 107p. pap. (*0-85032-091-7*) C W Daniel GBR. *Dist:* Natl Bk Netwk.

Homoeopathy for the First Aider. Dorothy Shepherd. 1980. 30.00 (*0-85032-182-4*) St Mut.

Homoeopathy for the Primary Health Care Team. Paul Downey. 1997. LC 97-29166. 224p. pap. text 37.50 (*0-7506-2999-1*) Buttrwrth-Heinemann.

Homoeopathy for the Third Age. Keith Souter. (Orig.). pap. 24.95 (*0-8464-4214-0*) Beekman Pubs.

Homoeopathy in Epidemic Diseases. Dorothy Shepherd. 1995. 100p. (*0-85032-185-9*); 1967. pap. (*0-85207-305-4*) C W Daniel GBR. *Dist:* Natl Bk Netwk.

Homoeopathy in Paediatric Practice: Experiences From My Practice. Hedwig Imhauser. Tr. by Sigrid Penrod from GER. 1988. 280p. pap. text (*3-7760-0944-6*) K F Haug Pubs DEU. *Dist:* Medicina Bio.

Homoeopathy in the United States: A Bibliography of Homoeopathic Medical Imprints, 1825-1925. Francesco Cordasco. 1991. (Illus.). 230p. 54.00 (*0-940198-07-X*) St Aedans Pr & Bk.

Homoeopathy in Veterinary Practice. K. J. Biddis. 1987. 86p. pap. (*0-85207-196-5*) C W Daniel GBR. *Dist:* Natl Bk Netwk.

Homogenized Milk May Cause Your Heart Attack: The XO Factor. Kurt A. Oster et al. 1983. (Advances in Preventive Health Ser.). (Illus.). 312p. 14.95 (*0-943550-01-7*); pap. 10.95 (*0-943550-02-5*) Park City Pr.

Homologous Artificial Insemination. Ed. by J. C. Emperaire & A. Audebert. 1980. (Clinics in Andrology Ser.: Vol. 1). (Illus.). x, 234p. text 141.50 (*90-247-2269-1*) Kluwer Academic.

Homosexualities: Reality, Fantasy, & the Arts. Ed. by Charles W. Socarides & Vamik D. Volkan. 1991. LC 90-4937. 400p. 57.50 (*0-8236-2347-5*) Intl Univs Pr.

Homosexualities & the Therapeutic Process. Ed. by Charles W. Socarides & Vamik D. Volkan. 1991. LC 91-20827. 340p. (C). 47.50 (*0-8236-2348-3*) Intl Univs Pr.

Homosexuality: Psychoanalytic Therapy. Charles W. Socarides. 1989. LC 89-17913. 664p. 60.00 (*0-87668-883-0*) Aronson.

Homosexuality & Creative Genius. Hendrik M. Ruitenbeek. 1965. 25.00 (*0-8392-1149-X*) Astor-Honor.

Homosexuality & Medicine, Health & Science. Ed. by Wayne R. Dynes & Stephen Donaldson. 1992. LC 92-13993. (Studies in Homosexuality: Vol. 9). 360p. text 88.00 (*0-8153-0554-0*) Garland.

Homosexuality & Psychotherapy: A Practitioner's Handbook of Affirmative Models. Ed. by John C. Gonsiorek. LC 82-3072. (Journal of Homosexuality Ser.: Vol. 7, Nos. 2-3). 212p. 1985. pap. 14.95 (*0-86656-435-7*); 1982. text 49.95 (*0-917724-63-1*) Haworth Pr.

H I

Homosexuality & the Family. Frederick Bozett. 1989. pap. 19.95 (*0-918393-57-4*, Harrington Park) Haworth Pr.

Homosexuality, Masculinity, & Femininity. Ed. by Michael Ross. 1985. LC 84-19778. (Journal of Homosexuality Ser.: Vol. 9, No. 1). 107p. pap. text 9.95 (*0-918393-04-3*, Harrington Park) Haworth Pr.

Homosexuals Anonymous: A Psychoanalytic & Theological Analysis of Colin Cook & His Cure for Homosexuality. Arthur F. Ide. 1987. LC 87-6487. (Illus.). xvi, 76p. (Orig.). pap. 6.00 (*0-934667-06-3*) Tangelwuld.

Honduras: Toward Better Health Care for All. World Bank Staff. 1998. LC 98-11111. (Country Study Ser.). 76p. pap. 22.00 (*0-8213-4190-1*, 14190) World Bank.

Honest Answers for the Recently Diagnosed Alzheimer's Patient. 1998. (Illus.). 43p. pap. 5.00 (*1-930181-00-0*) A H A F.

Honest Herbal. Varro E. Tyler. 2nd ed. 1987. 18.95 (*0-397-53081-1*) Lppncott W & W.

Honest Herbal: A Sensible Guide to the Use of Herbs & Related Remedies. Varro E. Tyler. 3rd ed. 1993. (Illus.). 375p. lib. bdg. 49.95 (*1-56024-286-8*) Haworth Pr.

Honest Medicine: Shattering the Myths about Aging & Health Care. Donald J. Murphy. 1996. LC 94-27801. 336p. pap. 12.00 (*0-87113-658-9*, Atlntc Mnthly) Grove-Atltic.

Honest Talk about Eating Disorders. Sharon Kutz-Mellem. 2000. LC 00-46831. 28p. (YA). (*1-57895-096-1*) Bridge Resources.

Honest Truth about Lying with Statistics. Cooper B. Holmes. 1990. (Illus.). 92p. (C). text 30.95 (*0-398-05673-0*) C C Thomas.

Honesty. 1985. (Pocket Power Ser.). 16p. pap. 1.25 (*0-89486-255-3*, 1336B) Hazelden.

Honey, Mud, Maggots & Other Medical Marvels: The Science Behind Folk Remedies & Old Wives' Tales. Robert Bernstein et al. 1998. 288p. pap. 13.00 (*0-395-92492-8*) HM.

Honolulu Heart Program: An Epidemiological Study of Coronary Heart Disease & Stroke. Ed. by Abraham Kagan. 1996. 206p. text 90.00 (*3-7186-5802-X*); pap. text 33.00 (*3-7186-5803-8*) Gordon & Breach (Harwood Acad Pubs).

Honoring Patient Preferences: A Guide to Complying with Multicultural Patient Requirements. Anne Rundle. 1999. LC 99-66011. (Jossey-Bass Health Ser.). 300p. 260.00 (*0-7879-4650-8*) Jossey-Bass.

***Honoring Patient Preferences: A Guide to Complying with Multicultural Patient Requirements.** Ed. by Anne K Rundle et al. 2002. pap. (*0-7879-6221-X*) Jossey-Bass.

Hooked - But Not Hopeless: Kicking Nicotine Addiction. Patricia Allison & Jack Yost. 1996. (Illus.). 192p. pap. 14.95 (*0-9623683-3-4*) BridgeCity Bks.

Hookworm Infection & Anaemia: Approaches to Prevention & Control. Z. S. Pawlowski et al. 1991. (ENG, FRE & SPA.). vi, 96p. pap. text 17.10 (*92-4-154415-5*, 1150360) World Health.

Hoosier Home Remedies. Varro E. Tyler. 1985. LC 85-9515. 228p. 18.95 (*0-911198-77-6*) Purdue U Pr.

Hope. 1985. (Packet Power Ser.). 16p. (Orig.). pap. 1.25 (*0-89486-256-1*, 1337B) Hazelden.

Hope: A Shield in the Economy of Borderline States. Anna Potamaniou. 1997. LC 95-50977. 128p. (C). 84.95 (*0-415-12176-0*); pap. 29.95 (*0-415-12177-9*) Routledge.

Hope: An International Human Becoming Perspective. Rosemarie Rizzo Parse & NLN Staff. 1999. (National League for Nursing Ser.). (Illus.). 256p. (C). LC 98-43151. text 42.95 (*0-7637-0958-1*, 0958-1); pap. text 33.95 (*0-7637-0976-X*, 0976-X) Jones & Bartlett (N L N Bart).

Hope - At Last - In Cancer Treatment. Vincent Anku. 1999. (Illus.). 243p. pap. 14.95 (*0-9647741-1-9*) Achilles Pub.

Hope & Mortality: Psychodynamic Approaches to AIDS & HIV. Ed. by Mark J. Blechner. 1997. LC 97-13637. 288p. 45.00 (*0-88163-223-6*) Analytic Pr.

Hope for Healing: New Holistic Approaches to AIDS & Other Immune Disorders. Jason Serinus. 1992. pap. 12.95 (*0-8290-3164-2*) Irvington.

Hope for Hepatitis: A Personal Guide for Healing & Empowerment: Nutritional & Natural Solutions. Michael Wald. Ed. by Robin Wald. 2000. LC 00-91037. (Illus.). pap. 21.00 (*0-9671597-0-9*, 01) Optimal Hlth Pr.

Hope for the Families: New Directions for Parents of Persons with Retardation or Other Disabilities. Robert Perske. 1981. LC 81-5700. (Illus.). 112p. (Orig.). pap. text 14.00 (*0-687-17380-9*) Abingdon.

Hope for the Future: A Career Development Guide for Physician Executives. Barbara J. Linney. 1996. LC 96-86461. 142p. (Orig.). pap. 48.00 (*0-924674-47-4*) Am Coll Phys Execs.

Hope Homes Dietary Training Manual. David I. Eatmon. 1990. (Illus.). 101p. (Orig.). pap., stu. ed. (*1-878228-01-3*) Hope Homes Pubs.

Hope in Long-Term Care. Marylou Hughes. 1998. 23.50 (*0-929442-33-4*, 2144PP) Prof Prnting & Pub.

Hope Lives! The After Breast Cancer Treatment Survival Handbook. Margit Esser Porter. 2000. LC 00-104204. (Illus.). 189p. pap. 12.00 (*0-9700443-0-5*) hic pubng.

Hope Scrapie Model Human Neuro. 1988. lib. bdg. (*0-7462-0073-0*) Kluwer Academic.

Hope Springs Eternal: Surviving a Chronic Illness. David R. Arkinson. 1999. LC 98-10631. 200p. pap. 12.95 (*0-87604-408-9*, 502) ARE Pr.

Hope Under Siege: Terror & Family Support in Chile. Michelle K. Ritterman. Ed. by Edward Tick. 1991. (Frontiers in Psychotherapy Ser.). 304p. 77.00 (*0-89391-758-3*); pap. 39.50 (*0-89391-801-6*) Greenwood (Ablex).

Horizons in Medicine, Vol. 5. Seymour & Weetman. 1994. (Illus.). 456p. 99.95 (*0-86542-815-8*) Blackwell Sci.

Horizons in Medicine, Vol. 7. Stafford L. Lightman. 1996. (Illus.). 608p. 99.95 (*0-86542-756-9*) Blackwell Sci.

Horizons of Health. Ed. by Henry Wechsler et al. 1978. (Illus.). 448p. pap. 20.50 (*0-674-40631-1*) HUP.

Horizons of Pediatric Neuroimaging: Journal: Pediatric Neurosurgery, Vol. 18, No. 2, 1992. Ed. by R. A. Zimmerman. 1992. (Illus.). 64p. pap. 48.00 (*3-8055-5694-2*) S Karger.

Hormesis with Ionizing Radiation. T. D. Luckey. 1980. 232p. 134.00 (*0-8493-5841-8*, QP82, CRC Reprint) Franklin.

Hormonal Binding Proteins: Physiology & Clinical Implications - International Henri-Pierre Klotz Days of Clinical Endocrinology 38th International Symposium. Ed. by M. G. Forest. 1996. (Journal: Vol. 45, Nos. 3-5, 1996). (Illus.). 146p. pap. 133.25 (*3-8055-6290-X*) S Karger.

Hormonal Carcinogenesis: Proceedings of the First International Symposia, March 19-21, 1991. Ed. by J. J. Li et al. 1992. (Illus.). 340p. 115.00 (*0-387-97797-X*) Spr-Verlag.

Hormonal Carcinogenesis II: Proceedings of the Second International Symposium on Hormonal Carcinogenesis, No. II. Ed. by J. J. Li et al. 1995. (Illus.). 500p. 137.00 (*0-387-94469-9*) Spr-Verlag.

Hormonal Carciogenesis III: Proceedings of the Third International Symposium. Ed. by J. J. Li et al. 2000. (Illus.). 584p. 195.00 (*0-387-95127-X*) Spr-Verlag.

Hormonal Control Gluconeogenesis, Vol. II. Naomi Kraus-Friedmann. 1986. 248p. 334.00 (*0-8493-5060-3*, QP702) CRC Pr.

Hormonal Control of Gluconeogenesis, Vol. 2: Signal Transmission. Friedmann N. Kraus. 1986. LC 86-6315. 248p. 138.00 (*0-8493-5068-9*, CRC Reprint) Franklin.

Hormonal Control of Gluconeogenesis, Vol. 3: Hormonal Effects Mitochondrial & Protein Phosphorylation. Friedmann N. Kraus. 1986. LC 86-6315. 163.00 (*0-8493-5069-7*, CRC Reprint) Franklin.

Hormonal Control of Reproduction. Ed. by C. R. Austin & R. V. Short. 2nd ed. 1984. LC 81-18060. (Reproduction of Mammals Ser.: Bk. 3). 252p. pap. text 29.95 (*0-521-27594-6*) Cambridge U Pr.

Hormonal Manipulation: A New Era of Monstrous Athletes. William N. Taylor. 1985. LC 85-42523. (Illus.). 144p. per. 29.95 (*0-89950-166-4*) McFarland & Co.

Hormonal, Metabolic, & Cellular Influences on Cardiovascular Disease in Women. Ed. by Trudy M. Forte. 1997. LC 97-12112. (American Heart Association Monograph Ser.). (Illus.). 384p. 85.00 (*0-87993-668-1*) Futura Pub.

Hormonal Metabolic Derangements in Renal Failure. Ed. by A. Heidland et al. 1986. (Contributions to Nephrology Ser.: Vol. 50). (Illus.). viii, 216p. 29.75 (*3-8055-4336-0*) S Karger.

Hormonal Regulation of Bone Mineral Metabolism. Ed. by Daniel E. Bikle & Andres Negro-Vilar. 1995. (Endocrine Reviews Monographs: Vol. 4). 400p. pap. 15.00 (*1-879225-19-0*) Endocrine Soc.

Hormonal Regulation of Gene Expression: Proceedings of the 24th Gunma Symposium on Endocrinology, Japan, 1986. Ed. by H. Hayaishi. 1987. 200p. lib. bdg. (*90-6764-112-X*) VSP NLD. *Dist:* Coronet Bks.

Hormonal Regulation of Testicular Descent. U. F. Habenicht & F. Neumann. 1983. (Advances in Anatomy, Embryology & Cell Biology Ser.: Vol. 81). (Illus.). 70p. 34.95 (*0-387-12439-X*) Spr-Verlag.

Hormonal Regulation of the Menstrual Cycle: The Evolution of Concepts. J. G. Gruhn & R. R. Kazer. 1989. (Illus.). 256p. (C). text 59.50 (*0-306-43077-0*, Kluwer Plenum) Kluwer Academic.

Hormonal Resistance Syndromes. Ed. by P. Jaquet & P. Vague. 1993. (Journal: Vol. 38, Nos. 1-2, 1992). (Illus.). 100p. pap. 89.75 (*3-8055-5784-1*) S Karger.

Hormonal Restructuring of the Adult Brain: Basic & Clinical Perspectives, 743. Ed. by Victoria Luine & Cheryl F. Harding. 1994. LC 94-24685. (Annals Ser.: Vol. 743). pap. text 75.00 (*0-89766-920-7*); (Illus.). 273p. 75.00 (*0-89766-919-3*) NY Acad Sci.

Hormonal Steroids in Contraception: Report of a WHO Scientific Group, 1968. 1968. (Technical Report Ser.: No. 386). 28p. pap. text 3.00 (*92-4-120386-2*, 1100386) World Health.

Hormonal Therapy: Will It Benefit Me? Donald F. Kaltenbach. 1997. 36p. pap. 5.00 (*0-9651827-3-8*) Proste Cancer.

Hormonal Therapy - A Growing Role in Early Prostate Cancer. Ed. by F. H. Schroder. 1999. (European Urology Ser.). iv, 30p. 25.25 (*3-8055-6978-5*) S Karger.

Hormonale Kontrazeption: Eine Standortbestimmung. Ed. by Marianne Mall-Haefeli. 1983. (Illus.). viii, 148p. 51.50 (*3-8055-3767-0*) S Karger.

Hormonally Active Brain Peptides: Stucture & Function. Ed. by Kenneth W. McKerns & Vladmir Pantic. 1982. LC 82-9147. (Biochemical Endocrinology Ser.). 652p. 110.00 (*0-306-40865-1*, Plenum Trade) Perseus Pubng.

Hormonally Induced Changes in Mind & Brain. Ed. by Jay Schulkin. 1993. LC 93-9947. (Illus.). 407p. text 74.95 (*0-12-631330-X*) Acad Pr.

Hormone Action Pt. I: Peptide Hormones. Ed. by Sidney P. Colowick & Nathan O. Kaplan. 1985. (Methods in Enzymology Ser.: Vol. 109). text 188.00 (*0-12-182009-2*) Acad Pr.

Hormone Action Pt. C: Cyclic Nucleotides. Bert W. O'Malley. 1974. (Methods in Enzymology Ser.: Vol. 38). text 199.00 (*0-12-181938-8*) Acad Pr.

Hormone Action Pt. D: Isolated Cells, Tissues, & Organ Systems. Ed. by J. G. Hardman & Bert W. O'Malley. 1975. (Methods in Enzymology Ser.: Vol. 39). text 199.00 (*0-12-181939-6*) Acad Pr.

Hormone Action Pt. A: Steroid Hormones. Ed. by J. G. Hardman & Bert W. O'Malley. 1975. (Methods in Enzymology Ser.: Vol. 36). text 199.00 (*0-12-181936-1*) Acad Pr.

Hormone Action Pt. B: Peptide Hormones. Ed. by J. G. Hardman & Bert W. O'Mallely. 1975. (Methods in Enzymology Ser.: Vol. 37). text 199.00 (*0-12-181937-X*) Acad Pr.

Hormone Action Pt. E: Nuclear Structure & Function. Ed. by J. G. Hardman & Bert W. O'Malley. 1975. (Methods in Enzymology Ser.: Vol. 40). text 199.00 (*0-12-181940-X*) Acad Pr.

Hormone Action Pt. G: Calmodulin & Calcium-Binding Proteins. Anthony R. Means & Bert W. O'Malley. 1983. (Methods in Enzymology Ser.: Vol. 102). text 188.00 (*0-12-182002-5*) Acad Pr.

Hormone Action Pt. J: Neuroendocrine Peptides. Ed. by Sidney P. Colowick & Nathan O. Kaplan. 1986. (Methods in Enzymology Ser.: Vol. 124). text 178.00 (*0-12-182024-6*) Acad Pr.

Hormone Analysis: Methodology & Clinical Intrepretation G. W. Pennington & Sandra Naik. 1981. 320p. I. 174.00 (*0-8493-5539-7*, RD48); II. 163.00 (*0-8493-5540-0*, RB48) Franklin (CRC Reprint).

Hormone Antagonists. Ed. by M. K. Agarwal. 1982. (Illus.). 734p. 138.50 (*3-11-008613-1*) De Gruyter.

Hormone Assays in Reproductive Medicine. Ed. by E. Nieschlag. 1978. (Journal: Vol. 9, No. 6). (Illus.). pap. 27.00 (*3-8055-2975-9*) S Karger.

***Hormone Connection: Revolutionary Discoveries Linking Hormones & Women's Health Problems.** Gale Maleskey et al. 2001. LC 2001-4510. 544p. pap. 18.95 (*1-57954-401-0*) Rodale Pr Inc.

Hormone-Dependent Cancer. Ed. by Benita S. Katzenellenbogen. 1996. (Illus.). 602p. text 199.50 (*0-8247-9697-7*) Dekker.

Hormone Depletion & Urogenital Tract. Ed. by F. Fabris. 1994. (Journal: Vol. 40, Suppl. 3, 1994). vi, 18p. pap. 21.75 (*3-8055-6084-2*) S Karger.

Hormone Heresy: What Women Must Know about Their Hormones. Sherrill Sellman. 1998. (Illus.). 256p. pap. (*0-9587252-0-9*) Get Well Intl.

Hormone Physiology: Index of Modern Information. Martha G. Gorman. 1989. LC 88-48001. 150p. 47.50 (*1-55914-074-7*); pap. 44.50 (*1-55914-075-5*) ABBE Pubs Assn.

Hormone-Related Malignant Tumors. Ed. by L. Beck et al. 1990. (Recent Results in Cancer Research Ser.: Vol. 118). (Illus.). 269p. 137.00 (*0-387-51258-6*) Spr-Verlag.

Hormone-Related Tumors. Ed. by Hiroshi Nagasawa & K. Abe. 1981. 320p. 95.00 (*0-387-10925-0*) Spr-Verlag.

Hormone Replacement Therapy. Khaw. 1992. text 107.00 (*0-443-04717-0*) Saunders.

Hormone Replacement Therapy. Ed. by A. Wayne Meikle. 1999. LC 99-13398. (Contemporary Endocrinology Ser.: Vol. 13). (Illus.). 439p. 135.00 (*0-89603-601-4*) Humana.

Hormone Replacement Therapy. Donald P. Swartz. 1992. (Illus.). 288p. 57.00 (*0-683-08035-0*) Lppncott W & W.

Hormone Replacement Therapy. Whitehead. 2nd ed. 1998. (C). pap. text (*0-443-05044-9*) Church.

Hormone Replacement Therapy. R. Don Gambrell, Jr. 5th ed. 1997. (Illus.). 167p. (C). pap. 14.95 (*0-929240-81-2*) EMIS.

Hormone Replacement Therapy: An Option for Women at Menopause. William N. Spellacy & David Sturdes. 1996. (Women's Health Ser.). (Illus.). 32p. pap. 2.95 (*1-885274-18-1*) Health InfoNet Inc.

Hormone Replacement Therapy: Conventional Medicine & Natural Alternatives Your Guide to Menopause. Linda Laucella. 2nd ed. 1999. LC 99-39388. 256p. pap. 16.95 (*0-7373-0251-8*, 02518W) NTC Contemp Pub Co.

Hormone Replacement Therapy: Standardized or Individually Adapted Doses? Ed. by B. Von Schoultz. 1994. (Illus.). 72p. lib. bdg. 20.95 (*1-85070-545-3*, Parthenon Pbng) CRC Pr.

Hormone Replacement Therapy: Yes or No? How to Make an Informed Decision. Betty Kamen. 4th rev. ed. 1997. (Illus.). 276p. pap. 14.95 (*0-944501-10-9*) Nutrition Encounter.

Hormone Replacement Therapy & Breast Cancer. G. Marsden. 2002. 200p. 85.00 (*1-84214-039-6*, Parthenon Pbng) CRC Pr.

Hormone Replacement Therapy & Breast Cancer Risk. Ronald D. Mann. 1992. LC 92-14083. (Illus.). 321p. lib. bdg. 85.95 (*1-85070-399-X*, Parthenon Pbng) CRC Pr.

Hormone Replacement Therapy & Cancer. A. R. Genazzani. 2001. LC 2001-56032. (Controversial Issues in Climacteric Medicine Ser.). (Illus.). 300p. 77.95 (*1-84214-079-5*, Parthenon Pbng) CRC Pr.

Hormone Replacement Therapy & Cardiovascular Disease. Andrea R. Genazzani. 2001. LC 2001-21760. (Controversial Issues in Climacteric Medicine Ser.). (Illus.). 200p. lib. bdg. 77.95 (*1-84214-038-8*, Parthenon Pbng) CRC Pr.

Hormone Replacement Therapy & Osteoporosis. Ed. by Junzo Kato et al. 2000. LC 99-88036. (Ernst Schering Research Foundation Ser.: Suppl. 4). (Illus.). 224p. 69.95 (*3-540-66480-7*) Spr-Verlag.

Hormone Replacement Therapy & Osteoporosis. M. Kleerekoper. 2002. 200p. 76.95 (*1-84214-030-2*, Parthenon Pbng) CRC Pr.

Hormone Replacement Therapy & Quality of Life. H. P. G. Schneider. 2002. 250p. 74.95 (*1-84214-014-0*, Parthenon Pbng) CRC Pr.

Hormone Replacement Therapy & the Endometrium. Farook Al-Azzawi. 2001. (Illus.). 182p. 74.95 (*1-85070-092-3*, Parthenon Pbng) CRC Pr.

Hormone Replacement Therapy & the Skin. M. Brincat. 2001. (Illus.). 192p. 74.95 (*1-85070-810-X*, Parthenon Pbng) CRC Pr.

Hormone Replacement Therapy & Urogenital Aging. L. Cardozo & D. Robinson. 2002. 200p. 74.95 (*1-84214-029-9*, Parthenon Pbng) CRC Pr.

Hormone Replacement Therapy in the Male. L. Tenover. 2001. 250p. 98.00 (*1-84214-042-6*, Parthenon Pbng) CRC Pr.

Hormone Resistance & Other Endocrine Paradoxes. 1987. (Endocrinology & Metabolism Ser.: Vol. 1). (Illus.). 271p. 108.00 (*0-387-96517-3*) Spr-Verlag.

Hormone Resistance Syndromes. J. Larry Jameson. 1999. LC 98-41146. (Contemporary Endocrinology Ser.: Vol. 14). (Illus.). 300p. 125.00 (*0-89603-652-9*) Humana.

Hormone Therapy & the Brain: A Clinical Perspective on the Role of Estrogen. V. W. Henderson. 1999. LC 99-40685. (Illus.). 120p. lib. bdg. 60.95 (*1-85070-078-8*) CRC Pr.

Hormone Therapy in Breast & Prostate Cancer. Ed. by V. Craig Jordan & Barrington J. A. Furr. 2002. (Cancer Drug Discovery & Development Ser.). 420p. 135.00 (*0-89603-673-1*) Humana.

Hormone Treatment Today & in the Future: Conference on the Treatment of Hormone Dependent Tumors, Tokyo, January 2000. Ed. by Y. Lino. 2000. (Oncology Ser.: Vol. 59, Suppl. 1). (Illus.). iv, 48p. 25.25 (*3-8055-7154-2*) S Karger.

Hormones. Anthony W. Norman & Gerald Litwack. 2nd ed. 1997. LC 97-80235. (Illus.). 558p. text 79.95 (*0-12-521441-3*) Acad Pr.

Hormones, Adaptation & Evolution: International Symposium. Ed. by Susumu Ishii. 1980. (Illus.). 343p. 71.95 (*0-387-10033-4*) Spr-Verlag.

Hormones & Aggressive Behavior. Ed. by Bruce B. Svare. 1983. LC 83-4020. 610p. 110.00 (*0-306-41055-9*, Plenum Trade) Perseus Pubng.

Hormones & Aging. Ed. by Paola S. Timiras et al. 1995. LC 94-35653. 448p. 149.95 (*0-8493-2446-7*) CRC Pr.

Hormones & Antagonists: Proceedings of the International Seminar on Reproductive Physiology & Sexual Endocrinology, 4th, Brussels, May, 1972. International Seminar on Reproductive Physiology &. Ed. by P. O. Hubinont et al. 1973. (Gynecologic & Obstetric Investigation Ser.: Vol. 2, Nos. 1-6; Vol. 3, Nos. 1-4). (Illus.). 97.50 (*3-8055-1446-8*) S Karger.

Hormones & Behavior in Higher Vertebrates. Ed. by J. Balthazart et al. 1983. (Proceedings in Life Sciences Ser.). (Illus.). 489p. 129.00 (*0-387-12576-0*) Spr-Verlag.

Hormones & Calcium Metabolism. Ed. by H. Corvilain & M. Fuss. 1984. (Journal: Vol. 20, No. 1). 92p. pap. 34.00 (*3-8055-3888-X*) S Karger.

Hormones & Cancer. Ed. by Wayne V. Vedeckis. 1996. LC 96-4653. (Hormones in Health & Disease Ser.). (Illus.). 612p. 109.00 (*0-8176-3797-4*) Birkhauser.

Hormones & Carcinogenesis. Aurel Lupulescu. 1983. LC 82-15110. 357p. 84.00 (*0-275-91402-X*, C1402, Praeger Pubs) Greenwood.

Hormones & Fetal Pathophysiology. Scholler. 1992. (Illus.). 808p. text 250.00 (*0-8247-8651-3*) Dekker.

Hormones & Growth Factors in Development & Neoplasia. Ed. by Robert B. Dickson & David S. Salomon. 1998. LC 97-17442. 461p. 162.00 (*0-471-16899-8*, Wiley-Liss) Wiley.

Hormones & Hyacinths. Martic C. Rosner. 1980. LC 79-82087. 5.95 (*0-87212-126-7*) Libra.

Hormones & Immunity. Ed. by Istvan Berczi & Kalman Kovacs. 1987. text 242.50 (*0-85200-848-1*) Kluwer Academic.

Hormones & Inflammation. Ed. by J. Garcia Leme. 1988. 248p. 143.00 (*0-8493-5928-7*, RB131, CRC Reprint) Franklin.

Hormones & Metabolic Control: A Medical Student's Guide to Control of Various Aspects of Normal & Abnormal Metabolism. David A. White & Michael Baxter. 2nd ed. 1994. (Illus.). 192p. pap. text, stu. ed. (*0-340-56355-9*) E A GBR. *Dist:* OUP.

Hormones & Nutrition in Obesity & Cachexia. Ed. by M. J. Muller et al. 1990. (Illus.). 176p. 47.95 (*0-387-51637-9*) Spr-Verlag.

Hormones & the Fetus. Kincl. 1986. 125.00 (*0-08-032005-8*, Pergamon Pr) Elsevier.

Hormones & the Fetus, Vol. 2. F. A. Kincl et al. 1991. LC 84-344. (Illus.). 300p. (*0-08-035720-2*) Pergamon Repr GBR. *Dist:* Franklin.

Hormones & the Heart in Health & Disease. Ed. by Leonard Share. 1999. (Contemporary Endocrinology Ser.: Vol. 21). (Illus.). 266p. 135.00 (*0-89603-726-6*) Humana.

Hormones & the Kidney. Ed. by G. S. Stokes & J. H. Mahony. 1981. (Progress in Biochemical Pharmacology Ser.: Vol. 17). (Illus.). viii, 268p. 142.75 (*3-8055-1090-X*) S Karger.

Hormones & Vitamins in Cancer Treatment. Aurel Lupulescu. 1990. (Illus.). 336p. lib. bdg. 229.00 (*0-8493-5973-2*, 5973) CRC Pr.

Hormones, Autacoids & the Kidney. Ed. by Stanley Goldfarb & Fuad N. Ziyadeh. 1991. (Contemporary Issues in Nephrology Ser.: Vol. 23). (Illus.). 422p. text (*0-443-08737-7*) Church.

***Hormones, Brain, & Behavior**, Set. Ed. by Donald W. Pfaff. 2001. 3000p. 850.00 (*0-12-532104-X*) Acad Pr.

Hormones, Gender & the Aging Brain: The Endocrine Basis of Geriatric Psychiatry. Ed. by Mary F. Morrison. 2000. LC 99-45853. (Illus.). 378p. (C). text 95.00 (*0-521-65304-5*) Cambridge U Pr.

Hormones, Health & Behavior: A Socio-Ecological & Lifespan Perspective. Ed. by C. Panter-Brick & C. M. Worthman. 1999. LC 98-15373. (Illus.). 304p. (C). text 69.95 (*0-521-57332-7*) Cambridge U Pr.

Hormones Hot Flashes. Clark Gillespie. rev. ed. 1994. LC 93-39092. 256p. pap. 13.00 (*0-06-095017-X*, Perennial) HarperTrade.

Hormones in Development & Aging. A. Vernadakis. 1981. 718p. (C). text 80.00 (*0-88331-150-X*) R B Luce.

Hormones in Human Blood: Detection & Assay. Ed. by Harry N. Antoniades. 1976. 811p. 85.00 (*0-674-40635-4*, ANHH) HUP.

Hormones in Lipoprotein Metabolism. Ed. by A. Steinmetz et al. 1993. LC 92-34028. (Illus.). 192p. 82.95 (*0-387-55995-7*) Spr-Verlag.

Hormones in Muscular Activity: Adaptive Effect of Hormones in Exercise, Vol. II. Ed. by Atko Viru. 1985. 200p. lib. bdg. 165.95 (*0-8493-5494-3*, QP301) CRC Pr.

Hormones in Muscular Activity: Hormonal Ensemble in Exercise, Vol. I. Ed. by Atko Viru. 1985. 208p. lib. bdg. 165.95 (*0-8493-5493-5*, QP301) CRC Pr.

Hormones in Normal & Abnormal Human Tissues, Vol. 1. Ed. by K. Fotherby & S. B. Pal. 1980. (C). 111.55 (*3-11-008031-1*) De Gruyter.

Hormones in Normal & Abnormal Human Tissues, Vol. 3. Ed. by K. Fotherby. 1983. 297p. 115.40 (*3-11-008616-6*) De Gruyter.

Hormones, Receptors, & Breast Cancer. Ed. by William L. McGuire. 1978. LC 77-90595. (Progress in Cancer Research & Therapy Ser.: Vol. 10). 383p. 82.50 (*0-89004-261-6*) Lppncott W & W.

Hormones, Sex & Society: The Science of Physicology. Helmuth Nyborg. 1994. LC 94-8640. (Human Evolution, Behavior, & Intelligence Ser.). 256p. 72.50 (*0-275-94608-8*, Praeger Pubs) Greenwood.

Hornbook on Health Law. Barry R. Furrow et al. 1995. LC 95-22221. (Hornbook Ser.). 962p. (C). 44.00 (*0-314-06457-5*) West Pub.

Horns & Halos: Towards the Blessing of Darkness. Michael DeMaria. 1992. LC 91-37962. (Reshaping of Psychoanalysis Ser.: Vol. 2). 180p. (C). text 29.95 (*0-8204-1737-8*) P Lang Pubng.

Horrendous Death & Health: Towards Action. Ed. by Daniel Leviton. 1991. (Death Education, Aging & Health Care Ser.). 408p. 99.95 (*1-56032-186-5*) Hemisp Pub.

Horrific Traumata: A Pastoral Response to the Post-Traumatic Stress Disorder. N. Duncan Sinclair. 1994. 120p. pap. 12.95 (*1-56024-294-9*); 1993. LC 92-4194. 146p. lib. bdg. 39.95 (*1-56024-293-0*) Haworth Pr.

Horse: Physiology. Julie Brega. 1993. (Open College Ser.: Bk. 4). pap. text (*0-85131-607-7*) J A Allen GBR. *Dist:* Trafalgar, St Mut.

Horse: Structure & Movement. R. H. Smythe. 1992. pap. 20.00 (*0-87556-321-X*) Saifer.

Horse Anatomy. Peter C. Goody. 1978. pap. 25.00 (*0-87556-610-3*) Saifer.

Horse & Buggy Doctor. Arthur E. Hertzler. 1991. (American Biography Ser.). 322p. reprint ed. lib. bdg. 79.00 (*0-7812-8179-2*) Rprt Serv.

Horse & Buggy Doctor. Arthur E. Hertzler. 1970. LC 78-105646. 322p. reprint ed. pap. 14.95 (*0-8032-5717-1*, Bison Books) U of Nebr Pr.

Horse & Pony Ailments: Recognition & Treatment of Common Horse & Pony Ailments. 9th ed. 1993. (T. V. Vet Ser.). (*0-85236-213-7*) Farming Pr GBR. *Dist:* Diamond Farm Bk.

Horse & Stable Management: Incorporating Horse Care. Jeremy H. Brown et al. 3rd ed. 1996. LC 96-24285. 470p. (Orig.). pap. 39.95 (*0-632-04152-8*) Blackwell Sci.

Horse Foot Care. Doug Butler. rev. ed. 1999. LC 93-248306. (Illus.). pap. text 7.95 (*0-916992-15-2*) Btler Pub.

Horse Genetics. Ann T. Bowling. 1996. (CAB International Publication). 224p. pap. text 37.50 (*0-85199-101-7*) OUP.

Horse Health Care: A Step-by-Step Photographic Guide to Mastering Over 100 Horsekeeping Skills. Cherry Hill. 1997. LC 96-34003. (Horsekeeping Skills Library). (Illus.). 160p. (Orig.). pap. 18.95 (*0-88266-955-9*) Storey Bks.

***Horse in Motion.** Sarah Pilliner & Samantha Elmhurst. 2002. LC 2001-52688. 256p. pap. 29.95 (*0-632-05137-X*) Blackwell Sci.

Horse Nutrition & Feeding. Sarah Pilliner. 1992. pap. 32.95 (*0-632-03239-1*); 2nd ed. 1999. LC 99-32651. pap. 29.95 (*0-632-05016-0*) Blackwell Sci.

Horse Owner's Field Guide to Toxic Plants. Sandra Burger & A. P. Knight. 1996. LC 95-83901. (Illus.). 200p. pap. text 26.50 (*0-914327-62-3*) Breakthrgh NY.

Horse Owner's Guide to Holistic Medicine. Sara Wyche. 1997. (Illus.). 160p. (*1-85223-942-5*) Crowood Pr GBR. *Dist:* Trafalgar.

Horse Owners Home Veterinary Handbook. James Giffin. 2nd ed. 1997. LC 97-26490. (Illus.). 560p. pap. 39.95 (*0-87605-606-0*, Howell) Hungry Minds.

Horse Owner's Veterinary Handbook. James M. Griffin & Tom Gore. 1989. (Illus.). 424p. pap. 29.95 (*0-87605-880-2*, Howell) Hungry Minds.

Horse Owner's Veterinary Handbook. Pavord & Fisk. (*1-85223-682-5*) Crowood Pr GBR. *Dist:* Trafalgar.

Horse Psychology. Moira Williams. 1978. pap. 25.00 (*0-87556-616-2*) Saifer.

Horse Psychology. Moyra Williams. 1990. 208p. pap. (*0-85131-238-1*) J A Allen GBR. *Dist:* Trafalgar, St Mut.

Horse Source 1998-99: Your Guide to Equine Supplies, Equipment, & Services, 1998. Horse Editors. Ed. by Kimberly S. Herbert. 1998. (Illus.). 250p. pap. 19.95 (*0-939049-99-6*) Blood-Horse.

Horse Veterinary Materia Medica & Theapeutics. C. Greig. 1987. (*0-7855-3056-8*) Intl Bk Distr IND. *Dist:* St Mut.

Horseowner's Guide to Lameness. Ted S. Stashak & Cherry Hill. 1996. LC 94-30066. (Illus.). 460p. 37.95 (*0-683-07985-9*) Lppncott W & W.

Horse's Health from A to Z: An Equine Veterinary Dictionary. Peter D. Rossdale & Susan M. Wreford. 1990. (Illus.). 472p. (*0-7153-9266-2*) Trafalgar.

Horticultural Therapy & the Older Adult Population. Ed. by Suzanne E. Wells. 1997. LC 97-6431. 210p. 39.95 (*0-7890-0036-9*) Haworth Pr.

Horticultural Therapy at a Physical Rehabilitation Facility. Eugene A. Rothert & James R. Daubert. 1981. (Illus.). 130p. (Orig.). (C). pap. 10.00 (*0-939914-02-6*) Chi Horticult.

Horticultural Therapy for Nursing Homes, Senior Centers, Retirement Living. Eugene A. Rothert & James R. Daubert. 1981. (Illus.). 130p. (Orig.). pap. 10.00 (*0-939914-01-8*) Chi Horticult.

Horticultural Therapy for the Mentally Handicapped. James R. Daubert & Eugene A. Rothert, Jr. 1981. (Illus.). 118p. (C). pap. 10.00 (*0-939914-04-2*) Chi Horticult.

Hosken Report: Genital & Sexual Mutilation of Females. Fran P. Hosken. 4th enl. rev. ed. 1994. (Illus.). 448p. pap. text 45.00 (*0-942096-09-6*) WINNEWS.

Hospice: Development & Administration. Ed. by Glen Davidson. 2nd ed. 1985. LC 84-19211. (Death Education, Aging & Health Care Ser.). (Illus.). 300p. (C). 59.95 (*0-89116-370-0*) Hemisp Pub.

Hospice: Practice, Pitfalls, & Promise. Stephen R. Connor. 1997. LC 97-28959. pap. (*1-56032-513-5*) Hemisp Pub.

Hospice: Practice, Pitfalls & Promise. Stephen R. Connor. 1997. LC 97-28959. (*1-56032-512-7*) Hemisp Pub.

Hospice & Palliative Care: Concepts & Practice. 128p. pap. (*0-340-54462-7*) E A GBR. *Dist:* Routldge.

Hospice & Palliative Care: Concepts & Practice. Denice Sheehan & Walter Forman. 1996. LC 96-3660. (Nursing Ser.). (Illus.). 216p. (C). pap. text 39.95 (*0-86720-737-X*, 737-X) Jones & Bartlett.

Hospice & Palliative Care: Concepts & Practice. Denice C. Sheehan & Walter B. Forman. 2nd ed. 2002. (Illus.). 224p. (C). pap. text 37.95 (*0-7637-1566-2*, 1566-2) Jones & Bartlett.

Hospice & Palliative Care: Questions & Answers. Virginia F. Sendor et al. 1997. LC 97-10620. 272p. 45.00 (*0-8108-3308-5*) Scarecrow.

Hospice & Palliative Care Handbook: Quality, Compliance & Reimbursement. Fred F. Ferri & T. M. Marrelli. 3rd ed. 1998. LC 98-35982. (Illus.). 544p. (C). (gr. 12). spiral bd. 29.95 (*0-8151-3557-2*, 31841) Mosby Inc.

Hospice Bibliography. National Hospice Organization Staff. 1993. 185p. 26.25 (*0-931207-29-0*) Natl Hospice.

Hospice Care: Principles & Practice. Ed. by Charles A. Corr & Donna M. Corr. 1983. (Death & Suicide Ser.: Vol. 5). 384p. (C). 34.95 (*0-8261-3540-4*) Springer Pub.

Hospice Care - A Physician's Guide. National Hospice Organization. 2nd ed. 1998. LC 98-196850. 96p. pap. 5.95 (*0-931207-54-1*) Natl Hospice.

Hospice Care & Cultural Diversity. Ed. by Donna L. Infeld et al. 1995. LC 95-38319. 101p. 24.95 (*1-56024-766-5*) Haworth Pr.

Hospice Care & Culture: A Comparison of the Hospice Movement in the West & Japan. Teresa C. Maruyama. 1999. (Avebury Series in Philosophy). 204p. (C). text (*1-84014-866-7*) Ashgate Pub GBR. *Dist:* Ashgate Pub Co.

***Hospice Care for Children.** Ann Armstrong-Dailey. 2nd ed. 2001. LC 00-64972. (Illus.). 432p. text 45.00 (*0-19-513330-7*) OUP.

Hospice Care for Patients with Advanced Progressive Dementia. Ed. by Ladislav Volicer & Ann Hurley. 1998. LC 97-32680. (Series on Ethics, Law, & Aging). (Illus.). 360p. 48.95 (*0-8261-1162-9*) Springer Pub.

Hospice Care on the International Scene. Ed. by Dame C. Saunders & Robert J. Kastenbaum. 1997. LC 96-40364. (Series on Death & Suicide). (Illus.). 320p. 48.95 (*0-8261-9580-6*) Springer Pub.

Hospice Care Planning: An Interdisciplinary Guide. Cynthia L. Frozena & Maryann Hurtt. 1999. LC 99-25475. ring bd. 149.00 (*0-8342-1625-6*) Aspen Pub.

Hospice Code of Ethics. National Hospice Organization Ethics Committee. 1995. 7p. (Orig.). pap. 8.30 (*0-931207-43-6*, 713024) Natl Hospice.

Hospice Concepts: A Guide to Palliative Care in Terminal Illnesses. Shirley Ann Smith. 2000. LC 00-133931. 272p. pap. text 19.95 (*0-87822-453-X*) Res Press.

Hospice Coordinator. Jack Rudman. 1994. (Career Examination Ser.: C-3034). pap. 29.95 (*0-8373-3034-3*) Nat Learn.

Hospice Legislation: 1977-1994. National Hospice Organization Staff. 1995. 252p. (C). ring bd. 60.00 (*0-931207-34-7*) Natl Hospice.

Hospice Means Hope. Kenneth B. Wentzel. 1991. 109p. (Orig.). pap. (*1-879601-05-2*) Semaphore Bks.

Hospice Movement: Easing Death's Pains. Cathy Siebold. 1992. LC 92-18052. (Social Movements Past & Present Ser.). 200p. pap. 15.95 (*0-8057-3868-1*) Macmillan.

Hospice Salary & Benefits Report, 1993-94. 1993. pap. 195.00 (*0-939326-79-5*) Hosp & Hlthcare.

Hospice Services Guidelines & Definitions. National Hospice Organization Staff. Ed. by Katherine Brandt. 1995. 8p. (Orig.). pap. 7.35 (*0-931207-31-2*) Natl Hospice.

Hospice Way of Death. Paul DuBois. 1980. LC 79-12326. 223p. 35.95 (*0-87705-415-0*, Kluwer Acad Hman Sci) Kluwer Academic.

Hospices: An Annotated Bibliography of Journal Articles, 1980-1988. Helen M. Wilkinson & Nelly E. Doll. 1991. LC 91-9726. 276p. text 10.00 (*0-8240-7229-4*, 91-9726) Garland.

Hospital: 90th Anniversary of the Founding of Rideout Memorial Hospital. Terald A. Zall. Ed. by James McClatchy. 1998. (Illus.). 64p. 10.00 (*0-9667500-0-4*) Fremont Rideout Found.

Hospital: An Oral History of Cook County Hospital. Sydney Lewis. 1994. LC 94-21775. xviii, 350p. text 25.00 (*1-56584-138-7*) New Press NY.

Hospital: From Center of Excellence to Community Support. N. Vetter. 1995. (Illus.). 288p. pap. 65.00 (*1-56593-417-2*, 1083) Singular Publishing.

Hospital-Acquired Infection. G. A. J. Ayliffe et al. 2nd ed. 1990. (Illus.). 152p. pap. text 50.00 (*0-7506-1560-5*) Buttrwrth-Heinemann.

Hospital-Acquired Infection: Principles & Prevention. G. A. Ayliffe et al. 3rd ed. 1999. LC 98-53304. (Illus.). 224p. pap. (*0-7506-2105-2*) E A GBR. *Dist:* OUP.

Hospital-Acquired Infections: Guidelines to Laboratory Methods. M. T. Parker. 1978. (WHO Regional Publications, European Ser.: No. 4). 63p. 8.00 (*92-9020-104-5*, 1310004) World Health.

Hospital Acquisition Report, 2000. Irving Levin Associates, Inc. Staff. 2000. (Illus.). v, 84p. pap. 395.00 (*1-930625-04-9*) I Levin.

Hospital Administration Consultant. Jack Rudman. 1994. (Career Examination Ser.: C-2768). pap. 39.95 (*0-8373-2768-7*) Nat Learn.

Hospital Administration for Veterinary Staff. T. H. Pettit. 1994. LC 93-74972. 200p. pap. text 29.95 (*0-939674-53-X*) Am Vet Pubns.

Hospital Administration Intern. Jack Rudman. 1994. (Career Examination Ser.: C-1967). pap. 29.95 (*0-8373-1967-6*) Nat Learn.

Hospital Administrator. Jack Rudman. 1994. (Career Examination Ser.: C-1654). pap. 34.95 (*0-8373-1654-5*) Nat Learn.

Hospital Affiliated IDS Vol. 2: Formation, Operation, & Contracts Handbook. 1995. 291p. 50.00 (*0-87258-684-7*) Am Hlth Lawyers.

Hospital & Physician Liability: A Legal & Risk Management Overview. Ed. by Myra C. Selby et al. 1992. 149p. 50.00 (*0-918945-14-3*) Am Hlth Lawyers.

Hospital & Physician Rate Setting Systems. Jerry Cromwell. 1996. LC 96-35121. (HFMA Healthcare Financial Management Ser.). 224p. text 65.00 (*0-7863-1084-7*, Irwn Prfssnl) McGraw-Hill Educ Grp.

Hospital & Rehospitalization Data by Geographic Area for Aged Medicare Beneficiaries, Set. 1991. lib. bdg. 450.75 (*0-8490-5081-2*) Gordon Pr.

Hospital As Employer. Stephen Allred. rev. ed. 1992. (Hospital Law in North Carolina Ser.). 36p. pap. 10.50 (*1-56011-224-7*, 85.03P) Institute Government.

Hospital Attendant. Jack Rudman. 1994. (Career Examination Ser.: C-325). pap. 23.95 (*0-8373-0325-7*) Nat Learn.

***Hospital Autopsy.** Ed. by Julian L. Burton & Guy N. Rutty. 2nd ed. 2001. (Arnold Publication). 224p. text (*0-340-76420-1*) OUP.

Hospital-Based Essential Community Providers: Challenges for Public Hospitals, Teaching Hospitals, & Academic Health Science Centers in Medicaid Managed Care. Maureen A. Milligan. 1995. (Working Papers Ser.: Vol. 83). 39p. pap. 5.50 (*0-89940-564-9*) LBJ Sch Pub Aff.

Hospital-Based Palliative Care Teams: The Hosptial-Hospice Interface. Robert Dunlop & Jo Hockley. 2nd ed. 1998. LC 98-22223. (Illus.). 174p. pap. text 34.50 (*0-19-262980-8*) OUP.

Hospital Builder: Quincy E. Fortier, A Nevada Physician. Quincy E. Fortier. Ed. by Anton P. Sohn. Date not set. LC 96-76755. (Biographies of Medical Practitioners Ser.). 200p. (C). (*0-9649759-1-2*) Greasewood.

Hospital Care for Schizophrenia in California in 1984. Laurie Crumpton et al. 1989. (Working Papers Ser.: No. 54). 18p. pap. 5.00 (*0-89940-535-5*) LBJ Sch Pub Aff.

Hospital Care Investigator. Jack Rudman. 1994. (Career Examination Ser.: C-326). pap. 27.95 (*0-8373-0326-5*) Nat Learn.

Hospital Care Investigator Trainee. Jack Rudman. 1994. (Career Examination Ser.: C-327). pap. 23.95 (*0-8373-0327-3*) Nat Learn.

***Hospital Chargemaster Guide 2001.** Ingenix, Inc. Staff. per. 199.95 (*1-56329-722-1*) Ingenix Inc.

Hospital Clerk. Jack Rudman. 1994. (Career Examination Ser.: C-328). pap. 23.95 (*0-8373-0328-1*) Nat Learn.

Hospital Closures in New York City: Proceedings of the Health Policy Forum on Hospital Closures in New York City. United Hospital Fund Staff. 1980. 158p. 10.00 (*0-934459-02-9*) United Hosp Fund.

Hospital Consultation Neurology. Ed. by Martin A. Samuels. 1999. LC 98-46555. (Blue Books of Practical Neurology: No. 19). 768p. text 99.00 (*0-7506-9779-2*) Buttrwrth-Heinemann.

Hospital Contracts Manual, Set. Baker and Hostetler, McCutchen Black, Staff. 1982. LC 82-16344. 1500p. ring bd. 529.00 (*0-89443-828-X*) Aspen Pub.

Hospital Controller. Jack Rudman. 1994. (Career Examination Ser.: C-1760). reprint ed. pap. 34.95 (*0-8373-1760-6*) Nat Learn.

Hospital Cost Analysis. James R. Butler. 1995. LC 94-41366. (Developments in Health Economics & Public Policy Ser.: Vol. 3). xxii, 393p. lib. bdg. 118.00 (*0-7923-3247-4*) Kluwer Academic.

Hospital Costs: Adoption of Technologies Drives Cost Growth. 1993. (Illus.). 40p. (Orig.). (C). pap. text 30.00 (*1-56806-680-5*) DIANE Pub.

Hospital Costs in Massachusetts: An Econometric Study. Mary L. Ingbar & Lester D. Taylor. 1968. LC 68-14258. (Wertheim Publications in Industrial Relations). (Illus.). 252p. 24.00 (*0-674-40700-8*) HUP.

Hospital Dentistry. Harold A. Black & Raymond F. Zambito. 1996. (Illus.). 448p. (C). (gr. 13). pap. text 42.00 (*0-8151-9855-8*, 25547) Mosby Inc.

Hospital Employee Health: Practical Solutions to Current & Potential Problems. Ed. by Byron Breedlove et al. 1982. 502p. text 49.00 (*0-9603332-2-3*) Am Health Consults.

Hospital Epidemiology & Infection Control. C. Glen Mayhall. 2nd ed. 1999. LC 99-19467. 1,600p. text 179.00 (*0-683-30608-1*) Lppncott W & W.

Hospital Experience: A Complete Guide to Understanding & Participating in Your Own Care. Judith Nierenberg & Florence Janovic. 1978. LC 78-55658. (Illus.). 12.95 (*0-672-52372-8*); pap. 9.95 (*0-672-52373-6*) Macmillan (Bobbs).

Hospital Financial Accounting Theory & Practice. L. Vann Seawell. 1987. LC 74-27241. (Illus.). 569p. (C). tchr. ed. 56.25 (*0-930228-34-0*); LC 74-27241. (Illus.). 569p. (C). text 23.60 (*0-930228-00-6*, 1454); 2nd ed. 722p. 55.00 (*0-8403-4062-1*) Hlthcare Fin Mgmt.

Hospital Financial Reports: A Survey. Price Waterhouse Staff. 1987. 150p. (C). per. 35.00 (*0-930228-52-9*) Hlthcare Fin Mgmt.

Hospital for Sick Children Handbook of Pediatrics 9. Hospital for Sick Children Staff. 9th ed. 1997. LC 97-10. (Illus.). 688p. (C). (gr. 13). pap. text 39.95 (*0-8151-4664-7*, 29278) Mosby Inc.

Hospital Handbook on Multiculturalism & Religion. Neville A. Kirkwood. 1998. LC 98-33924. 128p. pap. 6.95 (*0-8192-1793-X*) Morehouse Pub.

Hospital Health Physics: Proceedings of the 1993 Health Physics Society Summer School. Ed. by Joseph J. Shonka. 1993. (Illus.). viii, 305p. (C). 45.00 (*1-883021-10-3*) Research Ent.

Hospital Home Care: Strategic Management for Integrated Care Delivery. Ed. by Dan Lerman & Eric B. Linne. 1993. LC 93-16411. 328p. pap. 60.00 (*1-55648-096-2*, 079200) AHPI.

Hospital-Hospice Mangement Models: Integration & Collaboration. Ed. by Dan Lerman & Claire Tehan. 1995. LC 95-14333. pap. 32.00 (*1-55648-137-3*) AHPI.

Hospital in Rural & Urban Districts: Report of a WHO Study Group on the Functions of Hospitals at the First Referral Level. 1992. (WHO Technical Reports: No. 819). (ENG, FRE & SPA.). vii, 74p. pap. text 12.00 (*92-4-120819-8*, 1100819) World Health.

Hospital Infection Control: Principles & Practice. Mary Castle & Elizabeth Ajemian. 2nd ed. 1989. text 33.10 (*0-8273-4222-5*) Delmar.

Hospital Infection Control: Setting Up a Cost-Effective Resources. Shaheen Mehtar. 1992. LC 92-49489. (Illus.). 208p. (C). 45.00 (*0-19-262266-8*); 29.50 (*0-19-262033-9*) OUP.

Hospital Infection Control Equipment & Supply Markets: Human & Monetary Costs Shape Sterilization & Disinfection Industries. Market Intelligence Staff. 1993. 213p. 1995.00 (*1-56753-443-0*) Frost & Sullivan.

H
I

Hospital Infection Control for Nurses. Peter Meers et al. 1992. LC 92-49510. 41.50 (*1-56593-060-6*, 0366) Singular Publishing.

Hospital Infections. Ed. by John V. Bennett & Philip S. Brachman. 4th ed. 1997. LC 97-28724. (Illus.). 800p. text 179.00 (*0-316-08902-8*) Lppncott W & W.

Hospital Infections - Prevention & Control: Index of New Information with References. Patricia P. Poole. 1996. 150p. 57.50 (*0-7883-0794-0*); 1996. 150p. pap. 47.50 (*0-7883-0795-9*); 1997. 169p. 57.50 (*0-7883-1552-8*); 1997. 169p. pap. 47.50 (*0-7883-1553-6*) ABBE Pubs Assn.

Hospital Infections & Patient Complications: Index of New Information with References. Patricia P. Poole. 1996. 150p. 57.50 (*0-7883-0792-4*); 1996. 150p. pap. 47.50 (*0-7883-0793-2*); 1997. 167p. 57.50 (*0-7883-1550-1*); 1997. 167p. pap. 47.50 (*0-7883-1551-X*) ABBE Pubs Assn.

Hospital Information Systems: Design & Development Characteristics, Impact & Future Architecture. Ed. by H. U. Prokosch & J. Dudeck. 1995. LC 95-20592. (Medical Artificial Intelligence Ser.: Vol. 2). 414p. 217.50 (*0-444-82129-5*, R858) Elsevier.

Hospital Inpatient Statistics (1996) A. Elixhauser. 2000. 69p. (C). pap. text 20.00 (*0-7881-8701-5*) DIANE Pub.

Hospital Integrated Picture Archiving & Communication Systems: A Second Generation PACS Concept. Ed. by M. Osteaux et al. 1992. (Illus.). 384p. 255.00 (*0-387-54592-1*) Spr-Verlag.

Hospital Is a Uterus: Western Discourses of a Childbirth in Late Modernity - A Case Study from Northern Italy. Tove Holmqvist. 2000. 316p. pap. (*91-7265-096-6*) Almqvist & Wiksell SWE. *Dist:* Coronet Bks.

Hospital Jobs. Fearon Staff. 1997. 64p. (gr. 6-12). pap. text 8.25 (*0-8224-1310-8*) Globe Fearon.

Hospital Law. Ed. by A. Carmi & Stephen H. Schneider. 1988. (Medicolegal Library: Vol. 7). (Illus.). 220p. 118.00 (*0-387-18642-5*) Spr-Verlag.

Hospital Law in North Carolina, Chapters 1-14. Ed. by Anne M. Dellinger. 1985. LC 85-622120. (C). ring bd. 72.00 (*1-56011-072-4*) Institute Government.

Hospital Law Manual: Administrator Set, Set. Health Law Center Staff. LC 74-80713. 699.00 (*0-912862-06-8*) Aspen Pub.

Hospital Law Manual: Administrator's & Attorney's Set Health Law Center Staff. LC 74-80713. 875.00 (*0-912862-07-6*) Aspen Pub.

Hospital Law Manual: Attorney Set, Set. Health Law Center Staff. 1995. LC 74-80713. 2000p. ring bd. 1200.00 (*0-912862-05-X*) Aspen Pub.

Hospital Legal Forms, Checklists & Guidelines Howard S. Rowland et al. 1986. LC 86-17391. ring bd. 499.00 (*0-87189-053-4*) Aspen Pub.

Hospital Legislation & Hospital Systems. R. F. Bridgman & M. I. Roemer. 1973. (Public Health Papers: No. 50). pap. text 12.00 (*92-4-130050-7*, 1110050) World Health.

Hospital Liability Law. Margaret C. Jasper. 1999. LC 00-265915. (Legal Almanac Ser.). 194p. text 25.50 (*0-379-11333-3*) Oceana.

Hospital Literature Index: 1992 Annual Cumulative. American Hospital Association Staff. 1993. 604p. 260.00 (*0-87258-598-0*, 121480) Am Hospital.

Hospital Literature Index: 1993 Cumulative Annual. American Hospital Association Staff. 1993. 600p. 290.00 (*0-87258-656-1*, 121490) Am Hospital.

Hospital Material Management Forms, Checklists, & Guidelines. Aspen Reference Group Staff. 1992. 500p. ring bd. 199.00 (*0-8342-0266-2*) Aspen Pub.

Hospital Medicine. Robert M. Wachter et al. 2000. LC 99-52579. (Illus.). 1,120p. text 79.00 (*0-683-30482-8*) Lppncott W & W.

Hospital Patient Services Clerk. Jack Rudman. 1994. (Career Examination Ser.: C-3610). pap. 27.95 (*0-8373-3610-4*) Nat Learn.

Hospital Pediatrics. Anthony D. Milner. 3rd ed. 1998. (Orig.). (C). pap. text 49.95 (*0-443-05392-8*) Saunders.

Hospital Pharmacy Management Forms, Checklists, & Guidelines 1995. ring bd. 236.00 (*0-8342-0269-7*) Aspen Pub.

Hospital Phone Book, 2001. annuals Ed. by Keith Cavedo & Patrick Snyder. rev. ed. 2001. 850p. 175.00 (*0-87228-155-8*) Douglas Pubns.

Hospital-Physician Integration: Strategies for Success. Terence Murphy & C. Thompson Hardy. 1994. LC 94-27666. 223p. pap. 57.50 (*1-55648-124-1*, 145159) AHPI.

Hospital Planning & Administration. R. Llewelyn-Davies & H. M. Macaulay. 1966. (Monographs: No. 54). (ENG, FRE, RUS & SPA., Illus.). 215p. pap. text 32.00 (*92-4-140054-4*, 1140054) World Health.

Hospital Plans in Case of Disaster: For Latin America & the Caribbean Countries. Norberto T. Manzo et al. 1996. (Illus.). 124p. (Orig.). (C). pap. text 35.00 (*0-7881-3377-2*) DIANE Pub.

Hospital Policy in the United Kingdom: Its Development, Its Future. Sally Prentice & Anthony Harrison. 1997. LC 97-230. 229p. pap. 22.95 (*1-56000-978-0*) Transaction Pubs.

Hospital Privileges & Specialty Medicine. Ed. by Donald G. Langsley & Mona Signer. 1986. LC 86-70590. (Illus.). 352p. lib. bdg. 34.95 (*0-934277-08-7*) Am Bd Med Spec.

Hospital Privileges & Specialty Medicine. Ed. by Donald G. Langsley & Beauregard Stubblefield. 2nd ed. 1992. LC 92-73099. 537p. lib. bdg. 44.95 (*0-934277-17-6*) Am Bd Med Spec.

Hospital Rate Directory of Southern New York, Vol. III. United Hospital Fund Staff. 1985. 85p. 15.00 (*0-934459-08-8*) United Hosp Fund.

Hospital Records Aide. Jack Rudman. 1994. (Career Examination Ser.: C-3451). pap. 23.95 (*0-8373-3451-9*) Nat Learn.

Hospital Referrals. Ed. by Martin Roland & Angela Coulter. 1993. LC 92-19067. (Oxford General Practice Ser.: No. 22). (Illus.). 234p. pap. text 35.00 (*0-19-262174-2*) OUP.

Hospital Reform: Innovations in Health Care. Ed. by Alexander S. Preker & April Harding. 2000. LC 00-39852. (*0-8213-4494-3*) World Bank.

Hospital Relative Value Method As An Alternative for Recalibrating DRG Relative Weights. Grace M. Carter & Jeannette A. Rogowski. 1993. LC 92-48505. pap. text 13.00 (*0-8330-1323-8*, MR-156-HCFA) Rand Corp.

Hospital Safety Officer. Jack Rudman. 1994. (Career Examination Ser.: C-118). pap. 29.95 (*0-8373-0118-1*) Nat Learn.

Hospital Safety Officer Trainee. Jack Rudman. 1994. (Career Examination Ser.: C-119). pap. 23.95 (*0-8373-0119-X*) Nat Learn.

Hospital Salary & Benefits Report, 1993-94. 1993. pap. 250.00 (*0-939326-77-9*) Hosp & Hlthcare.

Hospital Salary Survey Report, 1992-93. Hospital Compensation Service Staff. 1992. pap. 250.00 (*0-939326-70-1*) Hosp & Hlthcare.

Hospital Salary Survey Report, 1991-92. Zabka, John R., Associates Inc. Staff. 21st ed. 1991. pap. 250.00 (*0-939326-66-3*) Hosp & Hlthcare.

Hospital Security Officer. Jack Rudman. 1994. (Career Examination Ser.: C-353). pap. 27.95 (*0-8373-0353-2*) Nat Learn.

Hospital Ships. Rupert Goodman. 1990. 170p. (C). (*0-86439-139-0*) Boolarong Pubns AUS. *Dist:* St Mut.

Hospital Smarts. Theodore Tyberg & Kenneth Rothaus. 1997. LC 97-224785. 256p. pap. text 13.95 (*0-13-894866-6*) P-H.

Hospital Smarts: The Insider's Survival Guide to Your Hospital, Your Doctor, the Nursing Staff - & Your Bill! Theodore Tyberg & Kenneth Rothaus. 1997. 240p. pap. 13.95 (*1-56561-119-5*) Wiley.

Hospital Space Programming: Guidelines for Departmental Space Requirements. Kenneth N. Dickerman. 1992. Set. 257p. ring bd. 350.00 (*1-881556-00-X*); Vol. 1. 149p. (*1-881556-01-8*); Vol. 2. 108p. (*1-881556-02-6*) Hlth Facility.

Hospital Staff Privileges: What Every Health Care Practitioner & Lawyer Needs to Know. Marcia J. Pollard & Grace J. Wigal. 1995. LC 95-40425. 210p. pap. 19.50 (*1-56793-037-9*, 0972) Health Admin Pr.

Hospital Steam Sterilizers. AAMI Staff. 1994. (Illus.). 16p. pap. 70.00 (*1-57020-016-5*, ST8-209) Assn Adv Med Instrn.

Hospital Steward's Manual. Joseph Woodward. 1991. (American Civil War Medical Ser.: No. 2). 324p. reprint ed. 50.00 (*0-930405-35-8*) Norman SF.

Hospital Strategies in Managed Care: Survival Tactics & Success Strategies for the Age of Managed Care. Ed. by Joseph Burns & Martin Sipkoff. 1997. (Illus.). 320p. (Orig.). pap. 195.00 (*1-57987-003-1*) Faulkner & Gray.

Hospital Strategies in Managed Care, 1999. Ed. by Luci Koizumi. 1998. 352p. pap. 225.00 (*1-57987-048-1*) Faulkner & Gray.

Hospital Strategies in Managed Care, 2000 Edition: Survival Tactics & Success Strategies for the Age of Managed Care. Ed. by Joseph Burns et al. 1999. (Illus.). 368p. pap. 225.00 (*1-57987-109-7*) Faulkner & Gray.

Hospital Time. Amy Hoffman. 1997. LC 96-35144. 144p. pap. 12.95 (*0-8223-1920-9*); 168p. lib. bdg. 34.95 (*0-8223-1927-6*) Duke.

Hospital Trusteeship in an Era of Health Reform. Susan S. Tyler. 1994. 12p. pap. text (*0-9629870-5-0*) Milbank Memorial.

Hospital Visitation Manual. Perry H. Biddle, Jr. rev. ed. 1994. LC 94-10496. 208p. pap. 16.00 (*0-8028-0698-8*) Eerdmans.

Hospital-Wide Quality Assurance: Model for Implementation & Development - A Canadian Perspective. Christopher R. Wilson. 1987. 135p. pap. 39.00 (*0-920513-04-2*) Saunders.

Hospital with a Heart: Women Doctors & the Paradox of Separatism at the New England Hospital, 1862-1969. Virginia G. Drachman. 1984. LC 83-45930. (Illus.). 256p. 38.50 (*0-8014-1624-8*) Cornell U Pr.

Hospital Words. Fearon Staff. 1997. 64p. (gr. 6-12). pap. text 8.25 (*0-8224-1312-4*) Globe Fearon.

Hospitalization in the United States, 1997. Anne Elixhauser et al. 2000. iv, 40p. pap. (*1-58763-005-2*) Agency Healthcare.

Hospitalized Children & Books: A Guide for Librarians, Families & Caregivers. Marcella F. Anderson. 2nd ed. 1992. LC 91-41698. (Illus.). 154p. reprint ed. 30.00 (*0-8108-2519-8*) Scarecrow.

Hospitalized Children Play & Play Activities. Sara M. Derrick et al. 1983. (Illus.). 106p. (Orig.). pap. (*0-89279-049-0*) S M Derrick.

Hospitalized Schizophrenics: Their Socio Sexual Life & Rehabilitation. R. K. Upadhyay. 1987. (*81-7099-018-1*) Mittal Pubs Dist IND. *Dist:* S Asia.

Hospitals. Diane Barnet. 1998. LC 98-26924. (Vital Information Ser.). 112p. pap. 11.95 (*0-89594-908-3*) Crossing Pr.

Hospitals: What They Are & How They Work. I. Donald Snook. 2nd ed. 1991. 288p. (C). 70.00 (*0-8342-0247-6*) Aspen Pub.

Hospitals & Children. Ed. by James Robertson. 1963. 160p. 27.50 (*0-8236-2360-2*) Intl Univs Pr.

Hospitals & Health for All. 1987. (Technical Reports: No. 744). 82p. pap. text 12.00 (*92-4-120744-2*, 1100744) World Health.

Hospitals & Health Networks Leadership Report: Key Issues Shaping the Future of Health Care. Alden T. Solovy. 1998. LC 97-46585. 220p. 149.00 (*1-55648-216-7*) Am Hospital.

Hospitals & the Long-Stay Patient. D. Norton. 1967. pap. (*0-08-011052-5*) Pergamon Repr GBR. *Dist:* Franklin.

Hospitals & the Poor: Strategies for Primary Care. 1991. (Papers: No. 16). 28p. 10.00 (*0-934459-65-7*) United Hosp Fund.

Hospitals & the Uninsured Poor: Measuring & Paying for Uncompensated Care. Ed. by Sally J. Rogers et al. 1985. 192p. 30.00 (*0-934459-00-2*) United Hosp Fund.

Hospitals, Homes & Community: Public, Private, Voluntary & Domestic Care Provision. N. James. 1998. (Illus.). 224p. (Orig.). pap. 39.95 (*1-56593-430-X*, 1097) Singular Publishing.

Hospitals in History. Ed. by Lindsay Granshaw & Roy Porter. 1989. (Wellcome Institute Series in the History of Medicine). 300p. 35.00 (*0-415-00375-X*) Routledge.

Hospitals, Paternalism & the Role of the Nurse. Jo Ann Ashley. 1976. LC 76-7908. 158p. pap. 16.95 (*0-8077-2470-X*) Tchrs Coll.

Hospitalwide Approach to AIDS see Management of HIV Infection in the Hospital

Hospitalwide Education & Training. Robert J. Munk & Marc Lovett. 1977. LC 77-13675. (Illus.). 12.00 (*0-87914-045-3*, 549615) Hosp Res & Educ.

Host Defense & Infection. M. T. Labro. 1994. (Illus.). 72p. text 35.00 (*0-8247-9218-1*) Dekker.

Host Defense & the Role of Surfactant in the Lung, Amsterdam, September 1987. Lung Defensive System: Damages & Treatment, Milan, September, 1987: Journal: Respiration, Vol. 55, Supplement 1. Ed. by M. T. Lopez-Vidriero. 1989. (Illus.). 100p. pap. 30.50 (*3-8055-5071-5*) S Karger.

Host Defense Dysfunctions in Trauma, Shock, & Sepsis: Mechanisms & Therapeutic Approaches. Ed. by Eugen Faist et al. 1993. LC 92-2333. 1200p. 248.00 (*0-387-55329-0*) Spr-Verlag.

Host Defenses & Immunomodulation to Intracellular Pathogens. Toby K. Eisenstein. 1988. LC 88-25164. (Advances in Experimental Medicine & Biology Ser.: Vol. 239). (Illus.). 404p. 105.00 (*0-306-43026-6*, Plenum Trade) Perseus Pubng.

Host Factors in Infection & Tropical Diseases. Cook. 1999. (Illus.). 240p. (Orig.). pap. 35.95 (*0-412-48150-2*, Chap & Hall NY) Chapman & Hall.

Host-Parasite Interactions in Urinary Tract Infections. Ed. by Catharina S. Eden. 1989. LC 86-50118. (Studies in Infectious Diseases Research). 488p. lib. bdg. 82.00 (*0-226-18443-9*) U Ch Pr.

Host Response to International Parasitic Zoonoses. Ed. by H. Ishikura et al. 1998. LC 98-21933. (Illus.). 136p. 110.00 (*4-431-70217-2*) Spr-Verlag.

Host Response to Intracellular Pathogens. Stefan H. Kaufmann. 1996. LC 96-30888. (Medical Intelligence Unit Ser.). 324p. 99.00 (*1-57059-389-2*) Landes Bioscience.

Hostage. Murray S. Miron & Arnold P. Goldstein. rev. ed. 1979. LC 77-16554. (General Psychology Ser.: No. 79). 170p. pap. text 16.95 (*0-08-023876-9*, Pergamon Pr) Elsevier.

Hostage Brain. Bruce S. McEwen & Harold M. Schmeck, Jr. LC 94-67849. (Illus.). 323p. pap. 19.95 (*0-87470-056-6*); 1994. text 39.95 (*0-87470-054-X*) Rockefeller.

Hostility & Aggression. Dolf Zillmann. 1979. 432p. 89.95 (*0-89859-501-0*) L Erlbaum Assocs.

Hostility, Coping, & Health. Ed. by Howard S. Friedman. 1992. 263p. pap. 19.95 (*1-55798-467-0*) Am Psychol.

Hot Flashes, Warm Bottles: First-Time Mothers over Forty. Nancy London. 2001. LC 2001-28128. xi, 204p. text 14.95 (*0-89087-971-0*) Celestial Arts.

Hot Legs: Shaping a Tight & Trim Lower Body. Robert Kennedy & Dwayne Hines, II. 1998. LC 97-901234. (Illus.). 64p. pap. (*1-55210-009-X*) MuscleMag Intl CAN. *Dist:* BookWorld.

Hot Stuff to Help Kids Chill Out: The Anger Management Book. Jerry Wilde. 1997. (Illus.). 64p. (YA). (gr. 4-12). pap. 9.95 (*0-9657610-0-2*) LGR Pubg Inc.

Hot Topics in General Practice. E. Stacey. 1996. 304p. pap. (*1-85996-210-6*) Bios Sci GBR. *Dist:* Coronet Bks.

Hot Zone. Richard Preston. l.t. ed. 1995. LC 95-3710. (Large Print Bks.). 26.95 (*1-56895-205-8*) Wheeler Pub.

Hot Zone: A Terrifying True Story. Richard Preston. 1995. LC 95-5751. (Illus.). 448p. reprint ed. mass mkt. 7.99 (*0-385-47956-5*, Anchor NY) Vintage Anchor.

Hotline Handbook. Mark J. Pastin. Ed. by Christina M. Brecto & Elisa M. Goldberg. 1996. LC 96-72260. 55p. (Orig.). pap. 125.00 (*0-9656061-0-4*) Coun of Ethical.

Hotspots: The Legacy of Hiroshima & Nagasaki. Sue R. Roff. 1995. LC 95-15514. pap. 24.95 (*0-304-33438-3*) Continuum.

House As a Mirror of Self: Exploring the Deeper Meaning of Home. Clare C. Marcus. 1995. LC 95-9232. (Illus.). 352p. 24.95 (*0-943233-92-5*) Conari Press.

House Calls: Life of a Country Doctor. Eugene L. Vickery. 1993. (Illus.). 300p. pap. 15.00 (*0-937775-12-6*) Stonehaven Pubs.

House of Cards. Robyn M. Dawes. 1996. LC 96-12597. 352p. 17.95 (*0-684-83091-4*) S&S Trade.

House of Cards: Psychology & Psychotherapy Built on Myth. Robyn Dawes. 1994. 338p. 22.95 (*0-02-907205-0*) Free Pr.

House of Make-Believe: Children's Play & the Developing Imagination. Dorothy G. Singer & Jerome L. Singer. (Illus.). 1992. 352p. pap. 17.50 (*0-674-40875-6*); 1990. 360p. 45.95 (*0-674-40874-8*) HUP.

House Officer: Becoming a Medical Specialist. R. L. Cohen. 1988. LC 88-17930. (Illus.). 272p. (C). text 36.50 (*0-306-42942-X*, Kluwer Plenum) Kluwer Academic.

House Staff & Thanatology. Ed. by Robert DeBellis et al. 1982. 19.95 (*0-405-14211-0*) Ayer.

House-Tree-Person & Draw-a-Person as Measures of Abuse in Children: A Quantitative Scoring System. Valerie Van Hutton. 1994. LC 94-20965. 140p. 47.00 (*0-911907-17-3*) Psych Assess.

House-Tree-Person Drawings: An Illustrated Diagnostic Handbook. Stanley L. Wenck. 1977. LC 76-62733. (Illus.). 108p. pap. 39.50 (*0-87424-147-2*, W-147) Western Psych.

Housecall Veterinarian's Manual. Carin A. Smith. rev. ed. 1999. 100p. ring bd., wbk. ed. 79.00 (*1-885780-10-9*) Smith Vet Srvs.

Household Chemicals & Emergency First Aid. Charles R. Foden & Jack L. Weddell. 1992. 448p. lib. bdg. 110.00 (*0-87371-901-8*, L901) Lewis Pubs.

Household Products & Labels - Their Effects on Life & Health Including Cancer Invitations: Index of New Information. Cindy A. Faye & Chester B. Faye. 1998. (Illus.). 160p. 57.50 (*0-7883-2040-8*); pap. 47.50 (*0-7883-2041-6*) ABBE Pubs Assn.

Housestaff Book of Forms. Thomas M. Masterson. 1993. 50p. (Orig.). (C). pap. text 7.50 (*0-9634063-7-X*) Intl Med Pub.

Housing & Health: APHA-CDC Recommended Minimum Housing Standards. Ed. by Eric W. Mood. 1986. LC 86-10884. 8.50 (*0-87553-138-5*) Am Pub Health.

Housing, Care & Psychological Well-Being of Captive & Laboratory Primates. Ed. by Evalyn F. Segal. 1989. LC 89-30309. (Noyes Series in Animal Behavior, Ecology, Conservation, & Ser.). (Illus.). 544p. 89.00 (*0-8155-1201-5*) Noyes.

Housing Frail Elders: International Policies, Perspectives, & Prospects. Ed. by Jon Pynoos & Phoebe S. Liebig. 1995. LC 94-30037. (Illus.). 304p. 46.00 (*0-8018-4980-2*) Johns Hopkins.

Houston Eldercare Directory: A Resource Guide for Older Adults, Caregivers, & Eldercare Professionals. Carla S. Rogg & Oskar H. Rogg. 1992. (Orig.). pap. 24.95 (*0-9631939-1-0*) Care Solutions.

Houston Medical Directory, 1990. Ed. by Shari Liken. 1990. 700p. 34.95 (*0-933745-06-0*) Med Prod.

Houston Medical Directory, 1991. Ed. by Shari Liken. 1990. 710p. 39.95 (*0-933745-07-9*) Med Prod.

Houston Medical Directory, 1993. Gary Nichols. Ed. by Shirley Schellhous & Mark L. Reed. 10th ed. 1993. 850p. 54.95 (*0-933745-11-7*) Med Prod.

Houston Medical Directory 1994. Gary Nichols. Ed. by Shirley Schellhous. 11th ed. 1994. 750p. pap. 59.95 (*0-933745-14-1*) Med Prod.

Houston Referral Directory 1994. Gary Nichols. Ed. by Shirley Schellhous. 4th ed. 1994. 150p. pap. 19.95 (*0-933745-15-X*) Med Prod.

Hovels, Haciendas & House Calls: The Life of Carl H. Gellenthien, M.D. Dorothy S. Beimer. 1986. LC 85-14881. (Illus.). 320p. (Orig.). pap. 16.95 (*0-86534-074-9*) Sunstone Pr.

How? N. Y. S. Workers' Compensation Board & State Insurance Fund Maliciously Compromised our Mother's Health Mentally, Physically & Financially! Todd Dante et al. 1994. 156p. (Orig.). pap. text 24.95 (*1-885899-00-9*) One Plus One.

***How Accurate Is the FDA's Monitoring of Supplements Like Ephedra? Congressional Hearing.** Ed. by Dan Burton. 2001. (Illus.). 214p. (C). reprint ed. pap. text 40.00 (*0-7567-1189-4*) DIANE Pub.

How Americans Use Time: A Social-Psychological Analysis of Everyday Behavior. John Robinson. 1977. LC 76-58838. (Special Studies). 209p. 40.95 (*0-275-90273-0*, C0273, Praeger Pubs) Greenwood.

How & How Much Can Intelligence Be Increased. Ed. by Douglas K. Detterman & Robert J. Sternberg. 1982. LC 82-1787. 256p. 77.00 (*0-89391-117-8*, Ablex) Greenwood.

How & Why Children Hate: A Study of Conscious & Unconscious Sources. Ed. by Ved P. Varma. 1993. 250p. pap. 24.95 (*1-85302-185-7*) Taylor & Francis.

How Animals Work. Knut Schmidt-Nielsen. 1972. LC 77-174262. (Illus.). 120p. pap. text 18.95 (*0-521-09692-8*) Cambridge U Pr.

How are Affordances Related to Events? An Exchange of Views, A Special Issue of Ecological Psychology. Ed. by William Mace. 2000. 103p. pap. (*0-8058-9766-6*) L Erlbaum Assocs.

How Behavior Means. Albert E. Scheflen. 1975. LC 74-18605. 240p. 25.00 (*0-87668-188-7*) Aronson.

How Brain-Like Is the Spinal Cord? U. Windhorst. 1988. (Studies of Brain Function: Vol. 15). (Illus.). 334p. 159.00 (*0-387-18405-8*) Spr-Verlag.

How Brains Think: Evolving Intelligences, Then & Now. William H. Calvin. 1997. 192p. pap. 13.00 (*0-465-07278-X*); Vol. 7. 1996. LC 96-21086. (Illus.). 176p. 20.00 (*0-465-07277-1*) Basic.

How Can I Find Healing? Guidelines for Sick & Worried People. Jim Glennon. 1984. LC 84-73039. 140p. mass mkt. 5.99 (*0-88270-580-6*) Bridge-Logos.

How Can Talking Help? An Introduction to the Technique of Analytic Therapy. Roy M. Mendelsohn. 1992. LC 91-35243. 328p. 50.00 (*0-87668-503-3*) Aronson.

How Clean Is Clean? How Safe Is Safe? A Review of Environmental Priorities. Merril Eisenbud. 1993. LC 93-8948. (Focus on Science Ser.). pap. 9.95 (*0-944838-33-2*, Cogito Bks) Med Physics Pub.

How Clients Make Therapy Work: The Process of Active Self-Healing. Arthur C. Bohart & Karen Tallman. 1999. LC 98-48623. (Illus.). 347p. 39.95 (*1-55798-571-5*) Am Psychol.

How Dentistry Can Be a Joyous Path to Financial Freedom: A Master Plan for Personal, Professional, & Financial Triumph. John A. Wilde. 1995. 240p. pap. 46.90 (*0-9648511-9-9*) Novel Pen.

How Do Brains Work? Papers of a Comparative Neurophysiologist. Theodore H. Bullock. 1993. LC 93-17434. (Contemporary Neuroscientists Ser.). (Illus.). 656p. 194.00 (*0-8176-3535-1*) Birkhauser.

How Do Families Cope with Chronic Illness? Ed. by Robert Cole & David Reiss. 1993. (Advances in Family Research Ser.). 240p. text 49.95 (*0-8058-1111-7*) L Erlbaum Assocs.

How Do I Do This When I Can't See What I'm Doing: Information Processing for the Visually Disabled. 1996. lib. bdg. 252.75 (*0-8490-5927-5*) Gordon Pr.

How Do I Pay for My Long Term Health Care. Maya Altman et al. 1988. (Illus.). 120p. pap. 12.95 (*0-9620825-0-3*) Berkeley Planning Assocs.

How Do You Feel? Koj Puas Xis Nyob (English-Hmong Medical Handbook) Jean Leyman. Tr. by Xeng Ly. 1983. LC 82-91138. (Illus.). 36p. pap. 6.50 (*0-9610684-0-X*) Mulberry Tree.

How Do You Talk to a Doctor in German, French, Italian, Spanish & English? Wie Sagt's der Arzt Auf Deutsch, Franzoesisch, Italienisch, Spanisch, & Englisch? Pia M. Guardiola & U. F. Gruber. 2nd ed. 1985. (ENG, FRE, GER, ITA & SPA.). 71p. pap. 39.95 (*0-7859-4746-9*) Fr & Eur.

How Does Analysis Cure? Contributions to the Psychology of the Self. Heinz Kohut. Ed. by Arnold I. Goldberg & Paul Stepansky. 1984. LC 83-24090. 254p. (C). 30.00 (*0-226-45034-1*) U Ch Pr.

How Does Treatment Help? On the Modes of Therapeutic Action of Psychoanalytic Psychotherapy. Ed. by Arnold Rothstein. 1988. LC 88-13604. (Workshop Series of the American Psychoanalytic Association: Monograph 4). 242p. 35.00 (*0-8236-2362-9*) Intl Univs Pr.

How Does Your Engine Run? Leader's Guide to the Alert Program for Self-Regulation. Mary Sue Williams & Sherry Shellenberger. 1994. 130p. spiral bd. 40.00 (*0-9643041-0-4*) Therapy Wrks.

How Drugs Work. Gesina L. Longenecker. 1994. LC 95-109267. (How It Works Ser.). (Illus.). 256p. (Orig.). pap. 19.95 (*1-56276-241-9*, Ziff-Davis Pr) Que.

How Fast is Fertility Declining in Botswana & Zimbabwe. Thomas Duncan & Ityai Muvandi. 1994. LC 94-29584. (Discussion Papers, 258, Africa Technical Department Ser.). 44p. pap. 22.00 (*0-8213-2993-6*, 12993) World Bank.

How Freud Worked: First-Hand Accounts of Patients. Paul Roazen. 1995. LC 95-11733. 328p. 40.00 (*1-56821-556-8*) Aronson.

How Health Care Reform Affects Pharmaceutical Research & Development. Anna Cook & Philip Webre. 1994. (Illus.). 65p. (Orig.). (C). pap. text 40.00 (*0-7881-1092-6*) DIANE Pub.

How Health Care Reform Affects Small Business. 34.95 (*1-56706-040-4*) Aspen Pub.

***How Healthy are the Government's Medicare Fraud Fighters? Congressional Hearing.** Ed. by Fred Upton. 2001. 166p. reprint ed. pap. 35.00 (*0-7567-1159-2*) DIANE Pub.

How Heavy Smokers Can Become Nonsmokers Using a Comprehensive Behavioral Smoking-Cessation Program with Nicoderm. Thomas M. Cooper & Richard R. Clayton. 1992. (Illus.). 160p. (Orig.). pap. text 12.00 (*0-9621398-1-5*) SBC SBC.

How Human the Animals. Jean Pommery. 1981. LC 78-24613. 224p. (C). pap. 6.95 (*0-8128-6086-1*, Scrbrough Hse) Madison Bks UPA.

How Humans Relate: A New Interpersonal Theory. John Birtchnell. 1993. LC 93-20296. 320p. 70.00 (*0-275-94405-0*, C4405, Praeger Pubs) Greenwood.

How I Became a Nurse Entrepreneur: Tales from 50 Nurses in Business. 1991. 300p. (*0-9629419-0-5*) Ntl Nurses Bus.

How I Became a Nurse Entrepreneur: Tales from 50 Nurses in Business. Ed. by Power Publications Staff. 1998. pap. 19.95 (*1-888315-03-2*) Power NY.

How I Conquered Cancer: A Naturopathic Alternative. Eric Gardiner. 1997. LC 97-21002. (Illus.). 128p. pap. 9.95 (*1-885373-11-2*) Emerald Ink.

How I Cured My Allergies to Cats & Dogs & You Can, Too. Lori Prokop. 1998. (Illus.). 100p. (Orig.). pap. 9.95 (*0-9651842-6-9*) Who You Are.

How I Lost Weight. A. D. Printup, II et al. 1985. LC 84-71480. 84p. pap. 5.25 (*0-932365-00-0*) DeWitt & Sheppard.

***How I Overcame Psoriasis.** Kent Trussell. 2001. 208p. pap. (*1-86351-283-7*) Sally Milner AUS. *Dist:* Sterling.

***How I Survived Nursing School: And Lived to Tell About It.** Darlene Haskell. 2001. pap. 7.95 (*0-533-13969-4*) Vantage.

How I Survived Prostate Cancer, & So Can You: A Guide for Diagnosing & Treating Prostate Cancer. James Lewis. 1994. LC 94-10168. (Illus.). 274p. pap. 18.95 (*1-883257-06-9*) Hlth Edu Lit.

How Implicit Is Implicit Learning? Debates in Psychology. Ed. by Dianne C. Berry. 1998. LC 97-37706. (Debates in Psychology Ser.). (Illus.). 254p. text 85.00 (*0-19-852352-1*) OUP.

How in the World? A Fascinating Journey Through the World of Human Ingenuity. Reader's Digest Editorial Staff. 1990. LC 90-30663. (Illus.). 448p. 32.00 (*0-89577-353-8*) RD Assn.

How Increased Competition from Generic Drugs Has Affected Prices & Returns in the Pharmaceutical Industry. Anna Cook. 1998. (Illus.). 75p. (C). pap. text 20.00 (*0-7881-7351-0*) DIANE Pub.

How Indians Use Wild Plants for Food, Medicine & Crafts. Frances Densmore. 1974. (Illus.). 155p. reprint ed. pap. 6.95 (*0-486-23019-8*) Dover.

How Long? A Sixteen-Year Chronicle from Breast Cancer Discovery to Death. Earl Ditmars. Ed. by Dave Frailey. 1993. 152p. (Orig.). pap. 10.00 (*0-89824-419-6*) Trillium Pr.

How Many Doctors Do We Need? Ed. by Duncan Yaggy & Patricia Hodgson. 1986. LC 85-31097. (Duke Press Policy Studies). (Illus.). xii, 164p. text 39.95 (*0-8223-0577-1*) Duke.

How Medicines Work. 1995. 19.95 (*1-56276-290-7*, Ziff-Davis Pr) Que.

How Men Can Live As Long As Women: Seven Steps to a Longer & Better Life. Ken Goldberg. Ed. by Chris Tucker & Mike Towle. 1993. LC 93-38419. (Illus.). 242p. 22.95 (*1-56530-025-4*) Summit TX.

How Not to Catch a Cold. Hadayat Dehesh. 1996. 88p. 16.95 (*0-9649707-0-8*) Global MI.

How Nutrition Works. Kristine M. Napier. 1995. (How It Works Ser.). (Illus.). 169p. (Orig.). pap. 19.95 (*1-56276-254-0*, Ziff-Davis Pr) Que.

How People Change: Inside & Outside Therapy. R. C. Curtis & G. Stricker. 1991. (Social-Clinical Psychology Ser.). (Illus.). 234p. (C). 49.50 (*0-306-43784-8*, Plenum Trade) Perseus Pubng.

How Prayer Heals: A Scientific Approach. Walter L. Weston. 1998. LC 98-72216. (Healing Ser.). 328p. pap. text 12.95 (*1-57174-092-9*) Hampton Roads Pub Co.

How Psychiatrists Look at Aging, Vol. II. Ed. by George H. Pollock. 1994. (Mental Health Library Ser.: Monograph 3). 300p. 42.00 (*0-8236-2367-X*) Intl Univs Pr.

How Psychotherapy Heals. Richard D. Chessick. 1987. LC 77-91953. reprint ed. 45.00 (*0-87668-821-0*) Aronson.

How Psychotherapy Works: Process & Technique. Joseph Weiss. 1993. LC 93-25473. 224p. 34.00 (*0-89862-548-3*, 2548) Guilford Pubns.

***How Safe Is Our Food?** 2000. (J). pap., tchr. ed. 59.95 incl. VHS (*1-55933-282-4*, 5550VD) Know Unltd.

How Scientists Explain Disease. Paul Thagard. (Illus.). 2000. 268p. pap. 17.95 (*0-691-05083-X*); 1999. LC 98-34717. xviii, 263p. 45.00 (*0-691-00261-4*) Princeton U Pr.

How Should Health Services Be Financed? A Patient's View. Allan Massie. 1988. (David Hume Papers). 58p. pap. text (*0-08-036585-X*) Aberdeen U Pr GBR. *Dist:* Macmillan.

How Should I Feed My Child: From Pregnancy to Preschool. Sandra K. Nissenberg et al. 1993. LC 93-21042. 192p. pap. 12.95 (*1-56561-035-0*) Wiley.

How the Basic Human Needs of Patients Are Met: Analysis, Testing, & Application of Maslow's Motivation Theory for Patient Care. I. E. Heidenborg. 1981. 290p. (Orig.). pap. text 33.50 (*91-554-1235-1*) Coronet Bks.

How the Blood Works. Stanley O. Williford. 1996. LC 96-60911. 128p. 14.95 (*0-9651783-0-7*) Vision Publng.

How the Body Works. John Lenihan. 1995. LC 94-42774. 200p. pap. 17.95 (*0-944838-48-0*, Cogito Bks) Med Physics Pub.

How the Body Works: 100 Ways Parents & Kids Can Share the Miracles of the Human Body. Steve Parker. 1994. LC 93-31689. (Illus.). 192p. 24.00 (*0-89577-575-1*) RD Assn.

How the Brain Keeps Us Healthy. 1991. lib. bdg. 75.95 (*0-8490-4666-1*) Gordon Pr.

How The Brain Learns. Ed. by Fred R. Volkmar. 2000. 160p. (*0-88210-301-6*, 0301) S&S Trade.

How the Brain Talks to Itself: A Clinical Primer of Psychotherapeutic Neuroscience. Jay E. Harris. 1998. LC 97-20703. (Advances in Psychology & Mental Health Ser.). (Illus.). (C). 428p. pap. text 39.95 (*0-7890-0409-7*); 420p. lib. bdg. 69.95 (*0-7890-0408-9*) Haworth Pr (Hawrth Medical).

***How the Brain Works.** Mark Wm Dubin. 2001. LC 2001-1882. (How It Works Ser.). (Illus.). 112p. pap. 19.95 (*0-632-04441-1*) Blackwell Sci.

How the Circulatory System Works. Robert E. Mehler. Ed. by Lauren M. Sompayrac. 2000. LC 00-39753. (How It Works Ser.). (Illus.). vii, 85p. (C). pap. 20.95 (*0-86542-548-5*) Blackwell Sci.

***How the Endocrine System Works.** Matthew J. Neal. 2001. LC 2001-1141. (How It Works Ser.). (Illus.). vii, 104p. pap. 19.95 (*0-632-04556-6*) Blackwell Sci.

How the Immune System Works. Lauren M. Sompayrac. 1998. LC 99-162566. (Illus.). 120p. pap. 22.95 (*0-632-04413-6*) Blackwell Sci.

How the Mind Works. Ed. by Cyril L. Burt. 1977. LC 78-105000. (Essay Index Reprint Ser.). 23.95 (*0-8369-1454-6*) Ayer.

How the Science of Psychology Gets Done. Bruce B. Svore. 1998. (Illus.). 60p. (C). pap. text 14.00 (*0-9666323-0-3*, 100-1) Bordalice.

How Therapists ACT: Combining Major Approaches to Psychotherapy & the Adaptive Counseling & Therapy Model. Don W. Nance. 1995. 232p. 69.95 (*1-56032-410-4*); LC 94-49231. pap. 29.95 (*1-56032-390-6*) Taylor & Francis.

How Therapists Diagnose: Seeing Through the Psychiatric Eye. Bruce Hamstra. 1995. LC 95-17383. pap. 15.95 (*0-312-13087-2*) St Martin.

How to Achieve Quality of Life & Care in a Nursing Home. Elizabeth Yeh. 1995. 216p. (Orig.). pap. text 14.95 (*0-932495-10-9*) Student Coll.

How to Add Sparkle & Pizzazz to Your Health Promotion Program: Powerful Programming Tips to Attract & Motivate Participants. Kathy K. Cash. 1998. LC 98-8965. pap. 29.95 (*1-57025-168-1*) Whole Person.

How to Address Common Compliance Issues in Ambulatory Care. Joint Commission on Accreditation of Healthcare Organizations. 1999. (Illus.). 200p. pap. 45.00 (*0-86688-633-8*, CCI-300) Joint Comm Hlthcare.

How to Address Common Compliance Issues in Long Term Care, Subacute Programs & Dementia Special Care Units. Joint Commission on Accreditation of Healthcare Organizations. 1999. (Illus.). 194p. pap. 45.00 (*0-86688-609-5*, CCI-200) Joint Comm Hlthcare.

How to Assess for Rehabilitation of the Pulmonary Patient, Vol. 6 No. 1. Gerilynn A. Connors. 1987. (Master Module Ser.). 14.99 (*0-931263-35-2*) Educ Res Consortium.

How to Assess the Pulmonary Patient at the Bedside, Vol I. Robert L. Wilkins. 1986. (Master Module Ser.). 14.99 (*0-931263-34-4*) Educ Res Consortium.

How to Avoid Back Surgery: Chiropractic - The Proven Method for Back Pain. J.C. Smith. 1996. (Illus.). 140p. (Orig.). pap. 7.95 (*0-9646206-0-X*) James C Smith.

How to Avoid Old Age. Stanley L. Robinson. 1990. LC 90-91721. (Illus.). 152p. (*0-9626830-0-0*) Remington NJ.

How to Be a Truly Excellent Junior Medical Student. Lederman. 1997. pap. 12.00 (*1-883205-18-2*) Intl Med Pub.

How to Be a Truly Excellent Junior Medical Student 6th ed. Robert J. Lederman. 6th rev. ed. 2000. 128p. pap. 9.95 (*1-882742-12-5*) Tarascon Pub.

How to Be Happy with Yourself: A Guide to Overcome Depression & Failure. Tom Yarbrough. 1975. LC 74-24607. 10.00 (*0-87212-038-4*) Libra.

How to Be Your Own Herbal Pharmacist: Herbal Traditions, Expert Formulations. Linda R. Page. 2nd rev. ed. 1998. (Illus.). 264p. pap. 18.95 (*1-884334-78-4*) Hlthy Healing.

How to Be Your Own Nutritionist. Stuart M. Berger. 1988. 384p. mass mkt. 6.99 (*0-380-70318-1*, Avon Bks) Morrow Avon.

How to Be Your Own Psychologist: The Art of Irresistible Influence—Compossibility! Peter G. Cranford. 1981. 223p. 14.95 (*0-9605822-0-7*) Great Pyramid.

How to Be Your Own Thin Self. Maxine T. Vaneven. 1981. LC 81-52960. pap. 4.95 (*0-916774-03-1*) Tolvan Co.

How to Be Your Own Veterinarian (Sometimes) A Do-It-Yourself Guide for the Horseman. Ruth B. James. 1990. (Illus.). 360p. pap. 19.95 (*0-9615114-0-0*) Alpine Pr.

How to Become a Medical Transcriptionist: A Career for the 21st Century. George Morton. 1998. LC 98-96009. 150p. pap. 12.95 (*0-9663470-0-5*) Med Lang Dev.

How to Become a Physical Therapist. Skip Hunter & Lori Whitlow. 1996. LC 95-95046. 115p. (Orig.). (C). pap. 19.95 (*0-9649873-0-9*) S Hunter.

How to Become a Schizophrenic: The Case Against Biological Psychiatry. John Modrow. Ed. by Caroline Klumpar. 2nd rev. ed. 1996. LC 92-71410. 295p. (Orig.). pap. 14.95 (*0-9632626-7-X*) Apollyon Pr.

How to Become Dentally Self-Sufficient. Robert O. Nara & Steven A. Mariner. 1979. LC 79-90865. pap. (*0-933420-01-3*) Oramedics Intl.

How to Become Forever Thin. Byron L. Wilt. 1993. (Be Free Ser.). 83p. stu. ed. 23.97 incl. audio (*0-9637814-0-5*) Prof Human Being.

How to Become Your Own Best Infertility Counselor: Helping You Understand Your Struggle; Deciding What's Best for You & Educating Others to Accept Your Choice. Joyce S. Friedeman. 1995. (Illus.). 106p. (Orig.). pap. 8.95 (*0-9645952-0-6*) Jolance Pr.

How to Begin a Psychotherapy Group: Six Approaches. Ed. by H. M. Rabin & Max Rosenbaum. 1976. iv, 140p. text 80.00 (*0-677-15800-9*) Gordon & Breach.

How to Begin in Re-Evaluation Counseling. Tr. by Ibtisam Basakat from ENG. 1999. (ARA.). 16p. pap. 1.00 (*1-58429-050-1*) Rational Isl.

How to Begin "Re-Evaluation Counseling" see Comment Debuter "La Re-Evaluation par la Co-Ecoute"

How to Begin "Re-Evaluation Counseling" Tr. by Margie Doyle-Papadopoulou from GRE. 1999. 16p. pap. 1.00 (*1-58429-046-3*) Rational Isl.

How to Benefit from Stress. Nicola M. Tauraso & L. Richard Batzler. 1979. LC 79-3843. 15.95 (*0-935710-00-0*) Hid Valley MD.

How to Break Bad News: A Guide for Health Care Professionals. Robert Buckman. 1992. LC 92-10298. 240p. pap. text 18.95 (*0-8018-4491-6*) Johns Hopkins.

How to Break Bad News: A Guide for Health Care Professionals. Robert Buckman & Yvonne Kason. 1992. 370p. pap. text 17.95 (*0-8020-6790-5*) U of Toronto Pr.

How to Build & Market Your Mental Health Practice. Linda L. Lawless. 1999. LC 96-35437. 224p. pap. 44.95 (*0-471-14760-5*) Wiley.

How to Build Special Furniture & Equipment for Handicapped Children. Ruth B. Hofmann. fac. ed. 1974. (Illus.). 100p. spiral bd. 21.95 (*0-398-00854-X*) C C Thomas.

How to Build-up a Successful Acupuncture Practice. Acupuncture News Staff. 1976. 37.50 (*0-914322-04-4*) Chans Corp.

How to Buy Almost Any Drug Legally Without a Prescription. James H. Johnson. 1990. (Orig.). pap. 5.99 (*0-380-76033-9*, Avon Bks) Morrow Avon.

How to Care for Aging Parents: A Complete Guide. Virginia Morris. 1996. LC 94-19321. (Illus.). 544p. (Orig.). pap. 15.95 (*1-56305-435-3*, 3435) Workman Pub.

How to Choose? A Comparison of the U. S. & Canadian Health Care Systems. Ed. by Robert J. Chernomas & Ardeshir Sepehri. 1998. LC 97-14841. (Policy, Politics, Health & Medicine Ser.). 296p. text 51.00 (*0-89503-180-9*) Baywood Pub.

How to Choose a Medical Specialty. Anita D. Taylor. 2nd ed. 1992. LC 92-49819. 287p. pap. text 24.95 (*0-7216-4375-2*) Saunders.

How to Choose a Nursing Home: A Guide to Quality Caring. Joanne Meshinsky. 1991. pap. 7.95 (*0-380-76078-9*, Avon Bks) Morrow Avon.

How to Choose the Sex of Your Baby. Landrum B. Shettles & David M. Rorvik. rev. ed. 1989. 264p. pap. 9.95 (*0-385-24442-8*) Doubleday.

How to Choose the Sex of Your Baby: The Method Best Supported by Scientific Evidence. Landrum B. Shettles & David M. Rorvik. rev. ed. 1996. LC 96-17524. 240p. pap. 12.95 (*0-385-48562-X*) Doubleday.

How to Comfort the Sick & Dying. Joseph A. Koebs. 1994. 304p. text 17.95 (*0-912141-11-5*) Roman Cath Bks.

How to Comply with OSHA in Health Care Facilities. Ed. by David Epstein. 1996. 500p. ring bd. 395.00 (*0-929321-32-4*) WEKA Pub.

How to Conduct a One-Day Conference on Death Education. Ellen Zinner & Jan McMahon. 1980. LC 79-90047. (Thanatology Service Ser.). 70p. pap. 8.95 (*0-930194-04-7*) Ctr Thanatology.

How to Conquer Depression. Earl Paulk. 1989. (Orig.). mass mkt. 2.50 (*0-917595-30-0*) Cathedral Holy Spirit.

How to Conquer Physical Death. Friend Stuart. 1980. 212p. vinyl bd. 29.95 (*0-912132-02-7*) Dominion Pr.

How to Conquer Your Fears, Phobias & Anxieties: Stop Running Scared. Herbert Fensterheim & Jean Baer. 1977. LC 95-33152. 326p. pap. text 14.95 (*0-941968-05-7*) Wildcat Pubs.

How to Consciously Overcome Mental Illness. Mary M. Harris. unabr. ed. 1997. (Heal Your Self Ser.). (Illus.). 61p. 9.95 incl. audio (*0-9636781-6-7*, 594) BBCS.

How to Control Diabetes. Seymour Alterman. 1997. 304p. mass mkt. 6.99 (*0-345-42158-2*) Ballantine Pub Grp.

How to Control Diabetes: A Complete Guide & Meal Planner to Live a Longer, Healthier & Happier Life. Seymour L. Alterman. Ed. by Donald A. Kullman. 2000. (Illus.). 266p. reprint ed. pap. text 15.00 (*0-7881-6897-5*) DIANE Pub.

How to Control High Blood Pressure Without Drugs. Robert L. Rowan. 1987. 320p. mass mkt. 5.99 (*0-8041-0144-2*) Ivy Books.

How to Cope with a Fatal Illness: The Rational Management of Death & Dying. Albert Ellis & Michael Abrams. 1994. LC 93-45551. 284p. pap. 14.95 (*1-56980-005-7*) Barricade Bks.

How to Cope With Anemia. Joan Gomez. 1998. LC 99-494984. (Overcoming Common Problems Ser.). 112p. pap. (*0-85969-788-6*) Sheldon Pr GBR. *Dist:* Intl Pubs Mktg.

How to Cope with Arthritis. 1991. lib. bdg. 75.00 (*0-8490-5142-8*) Gordon Pr.

HI

How to Cope with Chronic Pain. Nelson H. Hendler & Judith A. Fenton. rev. ed. 1986. 192p. pap. 9.95 (*0-89709-145-0*) Liberty Pub.

How to Cope with Depression: A Complete Guide for You & Your Family. J. Raymond DePaulo & Keith Russell Ablow. 1989. 240p. text 19.95 (*0-07-016409-6*) McGraw.

How to Cope with Menstrual Problems: A Wholistic Approach. Nikki Goldbeck. Ed. by Richard A. Passwater & Earl R. Mindell. 1983. (Good Health Guides). 32p. pap. 2.95 (*0-87983-300-9*, 33009K, Keats Pubng) McGraw-Hill Trade.

How to Cope with Your Medical Costs: A Survival Guide to Analyzing the Bills & Making the Most of Your Medical Experience. Alan Kolz. 1994. 134p. (Orig.). pap. 19.95 (*0-88100-081-7*) Natl Writ Pr.

How to Create the Dental Practice of Your Dreams: Guidelines to Achieving Joy & Success in Dentistry & Life. John A. Wilde. 1996. (Illus.). 300p. (Orig.). pap. 46.90 (*0-9648511-8-0*) Novel Pen.

How to Cure Toenail Fungus. Max. 1997. (Illus.). 50p. pap. 40.00 (*0-922070-55-5*) M Tecton Pub.

How to Cut Your Company's Health Care Costs. George Halvorson. 1987. 187p. pap. 27.50 (*0-13-404526-2*, Busn) P-H.

How to Deal with Back Pain & Rheumatoid Joint Pain. F. Batmanghelidj. 1991. (Illus.). 100p. pap. 14.95 (*0-9629942-0-0*) Global Hlth.

How to Define & Determine Reference Intervals in the Clinical Laboratory: Approved Guideline (1995) Contrib. by Edward A. Sasse. 1995. 75.00 (*1-56238-269-1*, C28-A) NCCLS.

How to Design a Problem-Based Curriculum for the Preclinical Years, Pt. 8. Howard S. Barrows. 1985. (Medical Education Ser.: Vol. 8). 160p. 32.95 (*0-8261-4900-6*) Springer Pub.

How to Design an Infectious Material & Hazardous Chemicals Exposure Control Plan for Your Medical Practice: The Complete OSHA Manual for Chemical Storage, Waste Disposal, MSDS, Safety, Blood Borne Pathogens & More. Ed. by Thayer Group Staff. 1993. 125p. (Orig.). (C). pap. text 79.95 (*1-56806-356-3*) DIANE Pub.

How to Design & Use a Patient Teaching Module. Myrna R. Spicer. Ed. by Sue Pritchett. rev. ed. 1991. LC 86-12325. (Illus.). 52p. 9.95 (*0-939838-21-4*) Pritchett & Hull.

How to Design, Develop, & Market Health Care Seminars. Ronald J. Friedman & Penny Altman. 1997. LC 97-16166. 224p. pap. 29.45 (*1-56887-029-9*, HDDBP, Prof Resc Pr) Pro Resource.

How to Detect, Reduce & Eliminate Lead in School Drinking Water: A Manual for School Officials. 1989. 69p. (Orig.). pap. text, stu. ed. 25.00 (*0-941375-14-5*) DIANE Pub.

How to Develop a Policy & Procedure Manual for a Midwifery Service. Katherine C. Carr. 1988. 15p. (Orig.). pap. 3.95 (*0-937604-09-7*, Pennypr) Intl Childbirth.

How to Develop an Exceptional Memory. Morris N. Young & Walter B. Gibson. 1976. pap. 10.00 (*0-87980-058-5*) Wilshire.

How to Develop & Implement Therapist Driven Protocols: A Clinician's Manual. J. Volpe. 1994. 150p. (C). 69.95 (*0-933195-72-9*) CA College Health Sci.

How to Develop & Manage Qualification Protocols for FDA Compliance. Phillip A. Cloud. 1999. LC 99-28537. (Illus.). x, 375p. 229.00 (*1-57491-098-1*) IHS Health Grp.

How to Direct the Life Force to Dispel Mild Aches & Pains. Robert H. Hover. 1979. LC 79-88460. 96p. (Orig.). pap. 15.00 (*0-934414-01-7*) Hover.

How to Do Experiential Psychotherapy: A Manual for Practitioners. Alvin R. Mahrer. 1989. 284p. pap. 13.00 (*0-7766-0242-X*) Paul & Co Pubs.

How to Do Groups. William H. Friedman. 1983. LC 84-45117. 284p. 25.00 (*0-87668-718-4*) Aronson.

How to Do Groups. W. Friedman. 2nd ed. 1995. 288p. pap. text 50.00 (*1-56821-793-5*) Aronson.

How to Do It. D. Reece. 3rd ed. 1995. 240p. pap. text (*0-7279-0895-2*) BMJ Pub GBR. *Dist:* AIDC.

How to Do It. Ed. by D. Reece. 3rd ed. 1995. 264p. pap. text (*0-7279-0896-0*);Vol. 1. 272p. pap. text (*0-7279-0848-0*) BMJ Pub GBR. *Dist:* AIDC.

How to Do Self-Analysis & Other Self-Psychotherapies. Louis A. Gottschalk. 1989. LC 89-30781. 216p. 40.00 (*0-87668-847-4*) Aronson.

How to Do Your Own NCLEX-RN Review. Rose Strohmann. 1987. 594p. (C). pap. 53.00 (*0-929136-00-4*); ring bd. 53.00 (*0-929136-01-2*) Health Ed Res Intl.

How to Eat Away Arthritis. Lauri M. Aesoph. 2nd exp. rev. ed. 1996. LC 96-23887. 320p. (C). text 26.95 (*0-13-242900-4*) P-H.

How to Eat Away Arthritis. Lauri M. Aesoph. 2nd exp. rev. ed. 1996. LC 96-23887. 320p. (C). pap. 13.95 (*0-13-242892-X*) PH Pr.

***How to Eat Away Diabetes: Win the Blood-Sugar Battle & Beat Type 2 Diabetes.** Kristine M. Napier & Byron J. Hoogwerf. 2001. 320p. pap. 14.00 (*0-7352-0251-6*) PH Pr.

How to Enjoy Better Health: A Self Help Guide to Health & Healing. Dana Britton. 2nd ed. 1990. LC 89-71428. 98p. pap. 12.95 (*0-944478-10-7*) Dock Pub Co.

How to Enjoy Your Surgery: A Lighthearted Look at Health & Medicine. John Davis. 2000. 128p. pap. 7.95 (*0-9635865-5-6*) Pinegrove Publishing.

How to Evaluate & Select a Nursing Home. Charles B. Inlander et al. 1988. LC 87-30636. pap. 7.64 (*0-201-07263-7*) Addison-Wesley.

How to Evaluate Progressive Pharmaceutical Services. Alan B. McKay et al. 1987. 159p. (Orig.). pap. text 31.00 (*0-930530-81-0*) Am Soc Hlth-Syst.

How to Evaluate Residents. Ed. by John S. Lloyd. 1986. LC 86-72620. 400p. lib. bdg. 39.95 (*0-934277-09-5*) Am Bd Med Spec.

How to Examine the Nervous System. R. T. Ross. 3rd ed. 1998. LC 98-215433. (Illus.). 256p. pap. 22.00 (*0-8385-3852-5*) McGraw-Hill Prof.

How to Excel in Medical School. Norma S. Saks et al. 1998. 185p. pap. 15.00 (*0-8036-0725-3*) Davis Co.

How to Excel in Medical School. Norma S. Saks et al. 1998. LC 98-65380. (Illus.). 187p. pap. 15.00 (*1-888308-04-4*) J & S Pub VA.

How to Face the Faces of Cardiac Pacing. Ed. by E. Andries. 1992. (Developments in Cardiovascular Medicine Ser.). 296p. (C). text 213.50 (*0-7923-1528-6*) Kluwer Academic.

How to Fall Out of Love. Debora Phillips & Robert Judd. 1994. 192p. mass mkt. 5.99 (*0-446-31408-0*) Warner Bks.

How to Fight Cancer & Win. William L. Fischer. Ed. by Juilene McKnight-Osborne. 1987. LC 86-82612. (Illus.). 298p. pap. 14.95 (*0-915421-07-0*) Fischer Pub.

How to Fight Cancer & Win. William L. Fischer. Ed. by Rebekah Schreffler. rev. ed. 1994. (Illus.). 360p. 29.97 (*0-915421-18-6*) Fischer Pub.

How to Fight Osteoporosis & Win! The Miracle of Microcrystalline Hydroxyapitite (MCHC) Beth M. Ley. 1996. LC 96-27467. (Health Learning Handbook Ser.). (Illus.). 80p. (Orig.). pap. 6.95 (*0-9642703-5-8*) B L Pubns.

How to Find a Good Psychotherapist: A Consumer Guide. Judi Striano. 1987. LC 87-61143. 142p. (Orig.). (C). pap. 7.95 (*0-943659-00-0*) J Striano Bks.

***How to Find & Secure Clinical Grants.** David Ginsberg. 2001. pap. 15.99 (*1-930624-23-9*) CenterWatch.

How to Find Information - Medicine & Biology: A Guide to Searching in Published Sources. Rupert Lee. 1996. (How to Find Ser.). 56p. pap. (*0-7123-0837-7*) SRIS GBR. *Dist:* L Erlbaum Assocs.

How to Find Information About AIDS. Ed. by Jeffrey T. Huber. 2nd ed. LC 91-7966. 288p. 1994. pap. 19.95 (*0-918393-99-X*); 1992. lib. bdg. 49.95 (*1-56024-140-3*) Haworth Pr.

How to Find Medical Information on the Internet: A Print & Online Tutorial for the Healthcare Professional & Consumer. Diane K. Kovacs & Ann L. Carlson. 2000. LC 00-702360. (Internet Workshop Ser.: Vol. 10). (Illus.). xii, 128p. pap. text 60.00 (*1-882208-27-7*) Library Solns.

How to Find Out in Psychology: A Guide to the Literature & Methods of Research. D. H. Borchardt & R. D. Francis. 1984. LC 84-2827. (How to Find Out Ser.). 155p. (*0-08-031280-2*) Pergamon Repr GBR. *Dist:* Franklin.

How to Find Source Materials: British Library Collections on the History & Culture of Science, Technology & Medicine. Anne Summers. 1996. (How to Find Ser.). 92p. pap. (*0-7123-0835-0*) SRIS GBR. *Dist:* L Erlbaum Assocs.

How to Find the Best Doctors: Chicago Metropolitan Area. Intro. by John J. Connolly. 1999. LC 99-70719. (How to Find the Best Doctors Ser.). 485p. pap. 19.99 (*1-883769-11-6*) Castle Connolly Med.

How to Find the Best Doctors: Florida. Intro. by John J. Connolly. 1999. 500p. pap. 24.95 (*1-883769-25-6*) Castle Connolly Med.

How to Find the Best Doctors: New York Metro Area. John J. Connolly. 3rd rev. ed. 1998. LC 98-92928. vii, 1326p. pap. 19.95 (*1-883769-07-8*) Castle Connolly Med.

How to Find the Best Doctors: New York Metro Area. Ed. by John J. Connolly. 4th rev. ed. 1999. 1375p. pap. 24.95 (*1-883769-66-3*) Castle Connolly Med.

How to Find the Best Doctors, Hospitals & HMOs for You & Your Family **see Buyer's Guide to Choosing the Best Healthcare**

How to Find the Best Doctors, Hospitals, & HMOs for You & Your Family: Castle Connolly Pocket Guide. John J. Connolly. Ed. by Sue Berkman. 1994. LC 94-92449. 457p. (Orig.). pap. 9.95 (*1-883769-70-1*) Castle Connolly Med.

How to Find Your Perfect Job in Nursing. Shelly Burke & Martha Whited. 1997. 220p. pap. (*1-57579-052-1*) Pine Hill Pr.

How to Get Along with Big Brother **see Psychotherapists' Guide to Managed Care in the 21st Century: Surviving Big Brother**

How to Get Families More Involved in the Nursing Home: Four Programs That Work & Why. Ed. by Tammy LaBrake. 1996. LC 96-20595. (Illus.). 103p. (C). 29.95 (*0-7890-0056-3*) Haworth Pr.

How to Get Free Health Care. 1992. lib. bdg. 254.95 (*0-8490-5619-5*) Gordon Pr.

How to Get Free Health Care Anywhere in America: A Report on Hill-Burton Hospitals & Their Obligations. Michael E. Samonek. 1992. LC 92-81346. 102p. pap. 19.95 (*0-9632877-1-0*) MES FX Pub.

How to Get into Medical School: The Insider's Guide - All of the Questions - All of the Answers. Ronald A. Shugar et al. 4th ed. 1997. 132p. pap. 24.95 (*1-891671-00-6*) G J Shugar.

How to Get into the Right Nursing Program. Carla S. Rogers. 1998. LC 97-51235. (How to Get Into...Ser.). (Illus.). 160p. pap. 14.95 (*0-8442-4192-X*, 4192X, VGM Career Bks) McGraw-Hill Trade.

How to Get More Private Practice Referrals: A Practical Marketing Guide for Mental Health Professionals. Philip J. Diehm. 1996. LC 96-69005. (Illus.). 187p. (Orig.). pap. 24.88 (*1-889423-00-9*) SMC Publng.

How to Get Out of the Hospital Alive: A Guide to Patient Power. Sheldon P. Blau. 2000. (Illus.). 226p. 21.95 (*0-7858-1209-1*) Bk Sales Inc.

How to Get Out of the Hospital Alive: A Guide to Patient Power. Sheldon P. Blau et al. 1998. LC 98-22861. 256p. pap. 14.95 (*0-02-862363-0*) Hungry Minds.

How to Get Out of the Hospital Alive: A Guide to Patient Power. Sheldon P. Blau & Elaine F. Shimberg. 1999. 226p. reprint ed. text 22.00 (*0-7881-6661-1*) DIANE Pub.

How to Get Pregnant. Sherman J. Silber. 1989. 336p. reprint ed. pap. 14.95 (*0-446-38642-1*) Warner Bks.

How to Get Pregnant with the New Technology. Sherman J. Silber. 1991. pap. 15.99 (*0-446-39322-3*) Warner Bks.

How to Get Pregnant with the New Technology: A World-Renowned Fertility Expert Tells You What Really Works, What Doesn't & Why. Sherman J. Silber. rev. ed. 1998. LC 98-18543. 416p. pap. (*0-446-67405-2*) Warner.

How to Get Well: Dr. Airola's Handbook of Natural Healing. Paavo O. Airola. 1984. 304p. 14.95 (*0-932090-03-6*) Health Plus.

How to Give Treatments & Cure Disease Permanently. F. W. Sears. 1991. lib. bdg. 69.95 (*0-8490-4520-7*) Gordon Pr.

How to Go on Living When Someone You Love Dies. Therese A. Rando. 1991. LC 91-7380. 352p. pap. 14.95 (*0-553-35269-5*) Bantam.

How to Grow Marijuana Indoors for Medicinal Use. G. W. Carver. 1997. (Illus.). 128p. (Orig.). pap. 19.95 (*0-930180-15-1*, Sun Magic) Homestead Bk.

How to Grow Ten Years Younger. Barry Stier. Ed. by Eunice Tatum. 1989. LC 89-90807. (Illus.). 204p. (Orig.). pap. 12.95 (*0-9622584-0-7*) Oceanco Ltd.

How to Handle a Hard-to-Handle Kid: A Parents' Guide to Understanding & Changing Problem Behaviors. C. Drew Edwards. 1998. LC 98-34589. (Illus.). 218p. (J). (ps-7). pap. 15.95 (*1-57542-046-5*) Free Spirit Pub.

How to Have a Boy: A Step-by-Step Guide to Scientifically Maximize Your Chances of Conceiving a Son. J. Martin Young. 1995. (Illus.). 172p. pap. 19.95 (*0-9643420-1-4*) Yng Ideas.

How to Have a Girl: A Step by Step Guide to Scientifically Maximize Your Chances of Conceiving a Daughter. J. Martin Young. 1995. (Illus.). 160p. pap. 19.95 (*0-9643420-2-2*) Yng Ideas.

How to Heal the Sick. Stuart Gramenz. 1989. 208p. (C). pap. text 7.99 (*1-85240-010-2*) Omega Pubns OR.

How to Heal the Sick. Charles Hunter & Frances Hunter. 1981. 208p. pap. 6.95 (*0-917726-40-5*) Hunter Bks.

How to Hear Better in 77 Steps: A Step-Wise Method to Help You Hear. Michael D. Riley. 1997. (Illus.). 24p. pap. 2.95 (*0-9635378-1-4*) Listening Inst.

How to Help & Understand the Alcoholic or Drug Addict. Arthur Pratt. 1981. LC 80-82964. 127p. pap. 4.95 (*0-915216-63-9*) Marathon Intl Bk.

How to Help Children Through a Parent's Serious Illness: Supportive, Practical Advice. Kathleen McCue. 3rd ed. 1996. LC 96-22605. (Illus.). 240p. pap. 12.95 (*0-312-14619-1*) St Martin.

How to Help Children with Common Problems. Charles E. Schaefer & Howard L. Millman. 2000. LC 94-71313. (Master Work Ser.). 448p. 50.00 (*1-56821-272-0*) Aronson.

How to Help Your Patients Stop Smoking: A Manual for Physicians. Thomas J. Glynn & Marc W. Manley. 1992. 88p. (Orig.). (C). pap. text 25.00 (*1-56806-110-2*) DIANE Pub.

How to Help Your Patients Stop Using Tobacco: A Manual for the Oral Health Team. 1992. 60p. (Orig.). (C). pap. text 30.00 (*1-56806-111-0*) DIANE Pub.

How to Integrate Autistic & Other Severely Handicapped Children into a Classroom. Robert L. Koegel. 1982. (Teaching the Autistic Ser.). 30p. pap. text 8.00 (*0-89079-064-7*, 1034) PRO-ED.

How to Interpret Your Dreams: Practical Techniques Based on the Edgar Cayce Readings. Mark Thurston. 1978. 192p. pap. 12.95 (*0-87604-107-1*, 292) ARE Pr.

How to Interview Sexual Abuse Victims: Including the Use of Anatomical Dolls. Marcia K. Morgan. 1994. (Interpersonal Violence Ser.). pap. 31.95 (*0-8039-5289-9*, 4298); 79.95 (*0-8039-5288-0*, 4299) Sage.

How to Join, Buy or Merge a Physician's Practice. Yvonne M. Fox. 1997. LC 97-218220. 424p. (C). (gr. 13). pap. text 29.95 (*0-8151-2878-9*, 31053) Mosby Inc.

How to Keep a Clinical Confidence: A Summary of Law & Guidance. 1994. 130p. pap. (*0-11-701832-5*, HM18325) Statnry Office GBR. *Dist:* Bernan Associates.

How to Keep Well While Traveling in the Tropics. Douglas Keshishian. 1974. LC 74-15723. (Illus.). pap. 3.00 (*0-930422-02-3*) Dennis-Landman.

How to Keep Your Brain Alive: 89 Neurobic Exercises. Lawrence Katz & Manning Rubin. 1998. LC 98-18888. (Illus.). 160p. pap. 8.95 (*0-7611-1052-6*) Workman Pub.

How to Keep Your Family Fit & Healthy. Bonnie Prudden. 1975. (Illus.). 10.00 (*0-88349-041-2*) Bonnie Prudden.

How to Keep Your Feet & Legs Healthy for a Lifetime: The Complete Guide to Foot & Leg Care. Gary Null & Howard Robins. 1990. LC 89-71438. (Illus.). 288p. (Orig.). pap. 14.95 (*1-888363-30-4*) Seven Stories.

How to Keep Your Hair On. 1980. 30.00 (*0-85032-191-3*) St Mut.

How to Keep Your Healing. Kenneth E. Hagin. 1980. pap. 1.00 (*0-89276-059-1*) Faith Lib Pubns.

How to Keep Your Kids Drug Free. Robert A. Morey. 1989. 128p. (Orig.). pap. (*0-925703-01-X*) Crown MA.

How to Know If It's Medical Malpractice. Robert S. Sigman. 1991. (Law for the Layman Ser.). 90p. (C). pap. text (*1-878135-07-4*) Legovac.

How to Know the Protozoa. Theodore L. Jahn et al. 2nd ed. 1978. (Pictured Key Nature Ser.). 304p. (C). spiral bd. 33.75 (*0-697-04759-8*, WCB McGr Hill) McGrw-H Hghr Educ.

How to Learn & Teach in Medical School: A Learner-Centered Approach. Mark E. Quirk. 1994. LC 94-21620. (Illus.). 224p. (C). text 54.95 (*0-398-05925-X*) C C Thomas.

How to Live a Long Life. Betty Yulin Ho. 2001. LC 00-69479. (System of Government in the Living Body Ser.: Vol. 17). (Illus.). 300p. (J). pap. 22.00 (*1-884996-01-9*) Juvenescent.

How to Live Between Office Visits: A Guide to Life, Love & Health. Bernie S. Siegel. 1994. LC 92-54736. 256p. reprint ed. pap. 13.95 (*0-06-092467-5*, Perennial) HarperTrade.

How to Live Longer. Linus Pauling. 1987. 416p. pap. 6.99 (*0-380-70289-4*, Avon Bks) Morrow Avon.

How to Live with a Mentally Ill Person: A Handbook of Day-to-Day Strategies. Christine A. Adamec. 1996. LC 95-42076. 256p. pap. 15.95 (*0-471-11419-7*) Wiley.

How to Live with a Neurotic. Albert Ellis. 1986. pap. 10.00 (*0-87980-404-1*) Wilshire.

How to Live with a Spinal Cord Injury. Elle Becker. 1989. LC 89-85624. (Illus.). 96p. (Orig.). pap. 6.95 (*0-915708-27-2*) Cheever Pub.

How to Live with Cancer. Richard M. Cromie. 5th rev. ed. 1992. LC 84-72666. 24p. reprint ed. pap. 2.95 (*0-914733-01-X*) Desert Min.

How to Lose Seventy-Five Pounds by Your (Next) Birthday: Happy Birthday to the New Thin You. Greg Shelton. 1987. LC 86-90595. (Orig.). pap. 19.95 (*0-9617594-0-2*) Shelton Pubns.

How to Love a PMSing Woman: When Timing Is Everything. Jay S. Stuller. 1996. LC 96-20942. 160p. (Orig.). pap. 11.95 (*1-888843-88-8*) Bridgeline Pr.

How to Love Yourself When You Don't Know How: Healing All Your Inner Children. Jacqui Bishop & Mary Grate. 1991. 165p. pap. 12.95 (*0-88268-131-1*) Station Hill Pr.

How to Lower Health Care Costs by Improving Health Care Quality: Results-Based Continuous Quality Improvement. M. Daniel Sloan. 1994. LC 93-43790. 247p. pap. 28.00 (*0-87389-250-X*, H0804) ASQ Qual Pr.

How to Lower Your Fat Thermostat: The No-Diet Reprogramming Plan for Lifelong Weight Control. Dennis W. Remington et al. 1983. LC 83-80794. (Illus.). 256p. pap. 9.95 (*0-912547-01-4*) Vitality Hse Int Inc.

***How to Make More Money & Do Better Dentistry Than You've Ever Dreamed Possible! A Priceless Collection of Gems from Dr. Tom Orent.** Tom Orent. 2001. pap. 197.00 (*0-9651544-3-2*) Gems Pubng.

How to Make Plumbing Systems Less Conducive to Legionella & Other Bacteria. Matthew R. Freije. 1998. LC 98-92507. 24p. pap. 19.00 (*0-9649926-1-2*, 302) HC Info Res.

How to Make Shift Work Safe & Effective. Timothy H. Monk. 1988. 58p. 23.00 (*0-939874-84-9*) ASSE.

How to Manage a Doctor's Office. Monty Campbell. 1989. 75p. (Orig.). (C). pap. 6.50 (*1-877718-02-5*) Archangel Pr.

How to Manage the Business Called Private Practice: What They Didn't Teach You in Medical School. Yvonne Mart Fox. 1994. (Illus.). 375p. reprint ed. pap. 54.00 (*0-9643703-0-1*) Y M Fox.

How to Market Medical Devices: An Effective, Economical, & Ethical Approach. Robert J. Fauteux et al. 1997. LC 97-61349. (*0-914176-75-7*) Wash Busn Info.

How to Master the Art of Personal Health: The Power of Attaining & Maintaining Your Health. Jack Schwarz. 1996. LC 95-92838. 210p. pap. 14.95 (*1-887417-00-1*) Schwarz Pub.

How to Measure & Improve Case Management Performance. Patrice L. Spath. 2000. (Illus.). 134p. 35.00 (*1-929955-06-5*) Brown Spath.

How to Measure Angles from Foot Radiographs. A. E. Oestreich. 1989. (Illus.). 65p. 36.00 (*0-387-97107-6*) Spr-Verlag.

How to Meet the Most Frequently Cited Hospital Standards. Joint Commission on Accreditation of Healthcare Organizations. 1999. LC 98-75816. (Illus.). 265p. pap. 55.00 (*0-86688-571-4*, FCS-100) Joint Comm Hlthcare.

How to Negotiate a Physician's Employment. American Medical Association Staff. 1998. (Managed Health Care Handbook Ser.). 43p. pap. 40.00 (*0-89970-703-3*, OP653795WE) AMA.

How to Negotiate Capitation for Laboratory Services. Philip L. Beard & E. Paul Kerens. 1996. 80p. pap. 39.00 (*0-915274-89-2*, 202686, AACC Pr) Am Assn Clinical Chem.

How to Nurse the Sick & Dyspepsia & Its Treatment, Combined with, Tea & Coffee, Their Physical, Intellectual, & Moral Effects on the. James C. Jackson et al. 1996. 87p. reprint ed. spiral bd. 12.00 (*0-7873-0466-2*) Hlth Research.

How to Obtain a Place in Medical School. Westall. 2nd ed. 1987. (Illus.). 80p. (Orig.). (C). (gr. 13). pap. text 24.50 (*0-412-29750-7*) Chapman & Hall.

How to Overcome Fear of Dentistry: Discover How Proven Methods Can Help You Overcome Barriers to Oral Health & a Beautiful Smile. Robert F. Kroeger. 1988. LC 87-82919. (Illus.). 191p. (Orig.). pap. 17.95 (*0-9618291-1-7*) Heritage Cinn.

How to Overcome Premature Ejaculation. Helen S. Kaplan. 1989. LC 88-35193. (Illus.). 126p. pap. 15.95 (*0-87630-542-7*) Brunner-Routledge.

How to Parent Carefully: A Handbook on Parenting & Self Care. A. Ambrose Netzer. 1985. LC 85-70262. (Illus.). 146p. (Orig.). pap. 9.95 (*0-9614588-0-1*) Center Creative Life.

How to Partner with Managed Care. Charles H. Browning & Beverley J. Browning. 1995. 358p. (Orig.). pap. text 29.95 (*0-8309-0714-9*) Herald Pub Hse.

How to Partner with Managed Care: A Do-It-Yourself-Kit for Building Working Relationships & Getting Steady Referrals. Charles H. Browning & Beverley J. Browning. exp. ed. 1997. LC 93-23447. 366p. (Orig.). pap. 34.95 (*0-911663-84-3*) Duncliffs Intl.

How to Pass Your Massage Therapy Exams see Massage Therapy Exam Questions

How to Pay for Health Care: Public & Private Alternatives. Ed. by David Gladstone. 1997. (Choice in Welfare Ser.: No. 37). 60p. pap. (*0-255-36397-4*) Inst Economic Affairs GBR. *Dist:* Coronet Bks.

How to Perform Your Own Urinalysis Without a Doctor for Under Fifty Cents. Richard Anthony. (Illus.). pap. 10.00 (*0-916976-00-9*) P I Industries.

How to Persuade Your Lover to Use a Condom: Complete Information & Advice, Including the New Female Condom. Patti Breitman et al. 2nd rev. ed. 1994. LC 93-23553. 96p. pap. 7.95 (*1-55958-437-8*, Prima Lifesty) Prima Pub.

How to Plan for Generalization. Donald M. Baer. 1999. LC 98-38350. (How to Manage Behavior Ser.). pap. (*0-89079-793-5*) PRO-ED.

How to Play HMO Hardball: The Patient's Self-Protection Manual. Robert D. Finney. 1998. LC 98-93384. pap. 19.95 (*0-9666067-0-1*, 2001) Countrpnt Commns.

How to Practice Brief Psychodynamic Psychotherapy: The Core Conflictual Relationship Theme Method. Howard Book. 1997. LC 97-35592. 181p. text 39.95 (*1-55798-465-4*) Am Psychol.

How to Prepare for & Respond to a Crisis. Robert Lichtenstein et al. 1995. LC 95-41771. pap. 7.95 (*0-87120-258-1*) ASCD.

How to Prepare for the GRE, Graduate Record Examination: Psychology. Edward L. Palmer. 4th ed. 1997. LC 97-7931. 272p. pap. text 14.95 (*0-8120-9656-8*) Barron.

How to Prepare for the Medical College Admission Test (MCAT) William R. Bishai et al. rev. ed. 1987. LC 86-3162. 484p. pap. 12.95 (*0-15-600933-1*) Harcourt.

How to Prepare for the N. E. S. P. A. National Examination in Speech Pathology & Audiology. K. T. Payne & Noma B. Anderson. 1991. LC 91-21685. (Illus.). 188p. (Orig.). (C). pap. 39.95 (*1-879105-33-0*, 0217) Thomson Learn.

How to Prepare for the NCLEX-PN with CAT. Vashti Curlin et al. 4th ed. 2000. (Illus.). 480p. pap. 29.95 incl. cd-rom (*0-7641-7237-9*) Barron.

How to Prepare for the Nursing School Entrance Exam. Corinne E. Grimes & Sandra S. Swick. 1998. LC 98-6193. 448p. pap. 14.95 (*0-7641-0338-5*) Barron.

How to Prepare for the Practical Nurse Licensure Examination (NCLEX-PN) Patricia Jenkins-Murphy et al. 1984. (Books for Professionals). 252p. pap. 7.95 (*0-15-600852-1*) Harcourt.

How to Prepare for the Praxis Exam in Audiology. Kay T. Payne. 2000. LC 00-37161. (Illus.). 160p. pap. text 49.95 (*0-7693-0161-4*) Singular Publishing.

How to Prepare for the Praxis Examination in Speech-Language Pathology. Kay T. Payne. 2nd ed. 2000. LC 00-37162. 240p. pap. text 49.95 (*0-7693-0160-6*) Singular Publishing.

How to Prepare for the Registered Nurse Licensure Examination (NCLEX-RN) Patricia Harward & Patricia O. Jana. 1985. 289p. pap. 7.95 (*0-15-601196-4*) Harcourt.

How to Prepare for the Step 1 Medical Exam. John R. Thornborough & Hilary J. Schmidt. 2nd ed. 1993. LC 92-48780. (Pretest Simulated Exam Ser.). (Illus.). 160p. text 12.95 (*0-07-064522-1*) McGraw-Hill Med Pub.

How to Prepare for the Step 1 Medical Exam. John R. Thronborough & Hilary J. Schmidt. 3rd ed. 1996. LC 95-20661. (Pretest Simulated Exam Ser.). (Illus.). 274p. pap. text 15.95 (*0-07-064524-8*) McGraw-Hill Med Pub.

How to Prevent Arthritis. Max. 1997. 50p. pap. 35.00 (*0-922070-37-7*) M Tecton Pub.

How to Prevent Breast Cancer. Ross Pelton et al. 1995. LC 95-35251. 384p. pap. 13.00 (*0-684-80022-5*, Fireside) S&S Trade Pap.

***How to Prevent, Cure & Control Diabetes.** Seymour L. Alterman. Ed. by Donald A. Kullman. 2001. pap. 16.95 (*0-88391-027-6*) F Fell Pubs Inc.

How to Prevent Headaches. Max. 1997. (Illus.). 50p. pap. 40.00 (*0-922070-90-3*) M Tecton Pub.

How to Prevent Home Accidents & Handle Emergencies Effectively. Boyce N. Berkel. 1979. LC 79-55195. (Illus.). pap. 7.50 (*0-9603184-0-2*) B Berkel.

How to Prevent Miscarriages & Other Crises of Pregnancy: A Leading High-Risk Doctor's Prescription for Carrying Your Baby to Term. Stefan Semchyshyn & Carol Colman. 1990. 256p. reprint ed. pap. 9.95 (*0-02-036855-0*) Hungry Minds.

How to Prevent Spills of Hazardous Substances. W. Unterberg et al. 1989. LC 88-17017. (Pollution Technology Review Ser.: No. 156). (Illus.). 185p. 39.00 (*0-8155-1177-9*) Noyes.

How to Prevent Unbundling: An Orthopedist's Guide: A Compendium of HCFA's Correct Coding Initiative. 1997. 449p. 149.00 (*1-889115-11-8*) Med Learn.

How to Prolong Life: An Inquiry into the Cause of Old Age & Natural Death Showing the Diet & Agents Best Adapted for a Lengthened Prolongation of Life. C. W. Evans. 1991. (Longevity Ser.). lib. bdg. 250.00 (*0-87700-985-6*) Revisionist Pr.

How to Protect Your Life Savings from Catastrophic Illness & Nursing Homes. Harley Gordon. 3rd ed. 1995. 225p. pap. 19.95 (*0-9642896-0-1*) Finan Strats Pr.

How to Quit Drinking Without A. A. A Complete Self-Help Guide. Jerry Dorsman. 2nd rev. ed. 1997. 336p. (Orig.). pap. 15.95 (*0-7615-1290-X*, Prima Lifesty) Prima Pub.

How to Raise a Healthy Child in Spite of Your Doctor. Robert S. Mendelsohn. 1987. 304p. mass mkt. 6.99 (*0-345-34276-3*) Ballantine Pub Grp.

***How to Read a Paper: The Basics of Evidence Based Medicine.** Trisha Greenhalgh. 2nd ed. 2001. 240p. pap. (*0-7279-1578-9*) BMJ Pub GBR. *Dist:* AIDC.

How to Read Pediatric ECGS. Myung K. Park & Warren G. Guntheroth. 3rd ed. 1992. (Illus.). 264p. (C). pap. text 52.00 (*0-8016-6834-4*, 06834) Mosby Inc.

How to Read Yourself Like an Open Book. Kathryn A. Valaske. 1986. (Illus.). 80p. (Orig.). pap. 5.95 (*0-9616601-0-4*) Valaske Pub.

How to Recognize & Classify Seizures & Epilepsy. Epilepsy Foundation of America Staff. 1992. 21p. pap. 2.95 (*0-916570-18-5*) Epilepsy Foundation of America.

How to Recognize & Overcome Depression: A Woman's Personal Experience. Janice Rector. 1994. LC 93-85051. 112p. (Orig.). pap. 10.95 (*0-9637222-0-4*) Sunrise Internat.

How to Recover from a Stroke & Make a Successful Comeback. Clarence E. Longenecker. 1977. LC 77-79690. 18.95 (*0-87949-105-1*) Ashley Bks.

How to Reduce Autistic & Severely Maladaptive Behaviors. Stephen C. Luce & Walter P. Christian. 1981. (Teaching the Autistic Ser.). 39p. pap. 8.00 (*0-89079-053-1*, 1032) PRO-ED.

How to Reduce Your Risk of Heart Disease. Farquhar. 1994. (Cardiology Ser.). pap. text 2.95 (*1-885274-03-3*) Health InfoNet Inc.

How to Relieve Cramps & Other Menstrual Problems. Marcia L. Storch & Carrie Carmichael. 1982. LC 81-40508. (Illus.). 128p. pap. 5.95 (*0-89480-191-0*, 464) Workman Pub.

How to Report Statistics in Medicine: A Guide for Authors, Editors & Reviewers. Thomas A. Lang & Michelle Secic. 1997. LC 96-30333. (Medical Writing & Communication Ser.). 376p. pap. 39.95 (*0-943126-44-4*) Amer Coll Phys.

How to Respond to Hazardous Chemical Spills. W. Unterberg et al. 1989. LC 88-17885. (Pollution Technology Review Ser.: No. 155). (Illus.). 274p. 39.00 (*0-8155-1176-0*) Noyes.

How to Reverse & Prevent Heart Disease & Cancer. Naras Bhat. 1995. LC 95-69189. (Illus.). 440p. pap. 19.95 (*0-9624780-8-3*) HealthWorld.

How to Reverse Immune Dysfunction. Mark Konlee. 8th ed. 2000. 148p. pap. 24.95 (*1-887831-06-1*) Keep Hope Alive.

How to Reverse Immune Dysfunction: A Nutritional Protocol for the Immune Compromised. Mark Konlee. 4th rev. ed. 1995. 124p. (Orig.). spiral bd. 19.95 (*1-887831-00-2*) Keep Hope Alive.

How to Reverse Immune Dysfunction: A Nutritional Protocol for the Immune Compromised. Mark Konlee. Ed. by Mark Konlee. 5th ed. 1997. 124p. (Orig.). pap. 19.95 (*1-887831-03-7*) Keep Hope Alive.

How to Run a Brain Bank. Ed. by F. F. Cruz-Sanchez & E. Tolosa. 1993. (Journals of Neural Transmission: Suppl. 39). (Illus.). 254p. 100.00 (*0-387-82426-X*) Spr-Verlag.

How to Save Big Bucks on Your Pet's Veterinary Bills. Alan W. MacCarthy, Jr. 1992. 128p. pap. 14.95 (*1-882822-00-5*) First-Care.

How to Save Money on Your Healthcare Costs: An Insider's Perspective. Steven J. Addonizio. 1995. 63p. (Orig.). pap. 15.00 (*1-882194-15-2*) TN Valley Pub.

How to Save Your Clients from Themselves: And Yourself from Them. Curtis Hills. 1988. LC 87-31316. (Illus.). 125p. 14.95 (*0-944861-77-6*) Olde & Oppenheim.

How to Save Your Teeth: Toxic-Free Preventive Denistry. David Kennedy. 1996. (Illus.). 200p. pap. 12.00 (*0-913571-06-7*) Health Act Pr.

***How to Score & Interpret Single-Hem Health Status Measures: A Manual for Users of the SF-8 Health Survey.** John E. Ware, Jr. et al. 2001. (Illus.). 133p. pap. text 89.95 (*1-891810-08-1*) Quality Metric.

How to Screen Any Property for Any Apparent Environmental Hazards: Harrison's Illustrated Guide. Henry S. Harrison. 1991. (Illus.). 150p. (Orig.). (C). pap. text 34.95 (*0-927054-11-6*) H Sq Co.

How to Search the Medical Sources. Barry Strickland-Hodge. 1989. 128p. text (*0-566-03533-2*) Gower GBR. *Dist:* Ashgate Pub Co.

How to See Like a Hawk When You're Blind as a Bat: A Patients' Guide to Lasik Laser Vision Correction. Matthew Ehrlich. unabr. ed. 1999. LC 99-61193. (Illus.). 176p. pap. 14.95 (*0-9669272-0-6*) Doctors Advice.

How to See Your Health: The Book of Oriental Diagnosis. Michio Kushi. 1980. LC 79-89346. (Illus.). 208p. (Orig.). pap. 19.00 (*0-87040-467-9*) Japan Pubns USA.

How to Select a Computerized Hospital Information System. Ed. by Marion J. Ball. 1972. (Data Processing in Medicine Ser.: Vol. 2). (Illus.). 51.50 (*3-8055-1465-4*) S Karger.

How to Select Reinforcers. R. Vance & Marilyn C. Hall. 1980. (How to Teach Ser.). 39p. pap. 8.00 (*0-89079-052-3*, 1001) PRO-ED.

How to Select Residents. Ed. by Donald G. Langsley. 1988. LC 87-73378. 300p. lib. bdg. 39.95 (*0-934277-11-7*) Am Bd Med Spec.

How to Sell Validatable Equipment to Pharmaceutical Manufacturers. Erik Kopp. 1999. LC 99-28568. (Illus.). xiv, 351p. 219.00 (*1-57491-097-3*) IHS Health Grp.

How to Sleep Better. 1992. lib. bdg. 69.95 (*0-8490-8813-5*) Gordon Pr.

How to Solve Your Stress & Aging Problems. Menicos A. Spartalis. 1994. LC 94-6113. (Illus.). 18.95 (*0-944957-44-7*) Rivercross Pub.

How to Spot & Handle Suppression in Medicine: Identical Medical & Religious Patterns of Suppression in the Late Twentieth Century. Anthony Di Fabio. 1997. LC 93-90267. 126p. pap. 12.00 (*0-9658941-0-X*) Confront Pubns.

How to Start a Private Practice. Yvonne Mart Fox. 2000. 149p. pap. 36.00 (*0-9643703-1-X*) Y M Fox.

How to Start & Maintain a Consulting Practice. Christopher S. Frings. 1999. 100p. pap. 20.00 (*1-890883-14-X*, AACC Pr) Am Assn Clinical Chem.

How to Stay Healthy a Lifetime Without Medicines. Betty Yulin Ho. 1979. LC 77-86248. (System of Government in the Living Body Ser.). 140p. pap. 25.00 (*0-9600148-3-7*) Juvenescent.

How to Stay Healthy & Fit on the Road: The Ultimate Health Guide for Road Warriors. Joanne V. Lichten. 2001. 208p. pap. 9.95 (*1-880347-53-9*) Nutrifit Pub.

How to Stay Out of the Doctor's Office: An Encyclopedia for Alternative Healing. Edward M. Wagner & Sylvia Goldfarb. 1993. LC 92-32307. 320p. 29.98 (*0-941683-18-4*) Instant Improve.

How to Stay Sober: Recovery Without Religion. James Christopher. 1988. LC 88-1139. 191p. pap. 22.00 (*0-87975-457-5*) Prometheus Bks.

How to Stay Young & Vibrant. 1986. (*0-918935-06-7*) Magnoart Pubns.

How to Stay Younger Longer Handbook. Charles F. Sexauer. 1980. 96p. pap. 4.95 (*0-9607148-0-4*) C F Sexauer.

How to Stop Heartburn: Simple Ways to Heal Heartburn & Acid Reflux. Anil Minocha & Christine A. Adamec. 2001. LC 2001-17916. (Illus.). 272p. pap. 14.95 (*0-471-39139-5*) Wiley.

How to Stop Overeating: Handbook to Stop Overeating, Using Tranquilizers, Diet Pills, Alcohol, Caffeine, Cigarettes & Being a Workaholic, People Pleaser, Hypochondriac, Anorexic or Having Bulimia. Jeanie Darnell & Buddy Piper. 1992. (Illus.). 128p. (Orig.). pap. 9.95 (*0-9633475-0-0*) Darnell & Piper.

How to Stop Smoking & Stay Stopped for Good. Gillian Riley. 1997. 160p. pap. 15.95 (*0-09-180969-X*) Trafalgar.

How to Stop Smoking Once & for All. Rhoda Nichter. Ed. by Debbie Hammond. 1980. LC 79-12134. 22.95 (*0-87949-173-6*) Ashley Bks.

How to Stop the Pain of Arthritis. Henry B. Rothblatt et al. 1985. LC 84-61541. 140p. (Orig.). pap. 4.95 (*0-936320-23-0*) Compact Books.

How to Succeed in the Practice of Medicine. Joseph M. Mathews. 1972. LC 74-180582. (Medicine & Society in America Ser.). (Illus.). 244p. reprint ed. 19.95 (*0-405-03959-X*) Ayer.

How to Survive ACLS. David Doernbach. 1998. LC 97-47792. (Illus.). 368p. pap. text 33.50 (*0-7817-1202-5*) Lppncott W & W.

How to Survive ACLS. David P. Doernbach. 1996. (Illus.). 350p. (Orig.). pap. text, wbk. ed. 30.00 (*0-9638043-3-2*) Vital Signs.

How to Survive as a Psychotherapist. Nina E. Coltart. LC 93-30192. 128p. pap. 25.00 (*1-56821-064-7*) Aronson.

How to Survive Hearing Loss. Charlotte Himber. l.t. ed. 1993. LC 93-14809. 378p. reprint ed. pap. 18.95 (*0-8161-5732-4*, Macmillan Ref) Gale.

How to Survive Hearing Loss. Charlotte Himber. 1989. (Illus.). 254p. pap. 13.95 (*1-56368-013-0*) Gallaudet Univ Pr.

How to Survive Hospital Care: Why They Keep Bedpans in the Freezer. William C. Anderson. Ed. by Jean Terra. 1996. LC 95-80408. (Illus.). 108p. pet. 6.95 (*1-887747-00-1*, 297-231-X) Legendary Pub.

How to Survive in Anaesthesia. Ed. by P. Neville Robinson & George M. Hall. 1997. 172p. pap. (*0-7279-1066-3*) BMJ Pub GBR. *Dist:* AIDC.

How to Survive in the Hospital. Joan Hass-Unger. Ed. by Juilene McKnight-Osborne. 1986. LC 86-82471. (Illus.). 170p. (Orig.). pap. 12.95 (*0-915421-06-2*) Fischer Pub.

How to Survive Medical Treatment. Stephen Fulder. Date not set. pap. 20.95 (*0-8464-4391-0*) Beekman Pubs.

How to Survive Menopause - Without Going Crazy. Leona Lipari Lee. 1998. 185p. pap. 10.00 (*1-888315-04-0*) Power NY.

How to Survive Your Clinical Rotations. Michael Steingard. 1998. (Illus.). pap. text 19.95 (*0-9669115-0-4*) Lar Pubg.

How to Survive Your Hospital Stay. Judy B. Crane. 1997. LC 97-26727. (Illus.). 128p. spiral bd. 11.95 (*1-889198-05-6*) Ctr Pr CA.

How to Survive Your Parents. Roy Master. 1982. LC 82-71162. 190p. pap. 15.95 (*0-933900-10-4*) Foun Human Under.

How to Take Care of Your Heart: Your Survival & Lifestyle Handbook. Mark Payne. 1989. (Illus.). 150p. pap. (*0-7463-0563-X*, H563) How To Bks GBR. *Dist:* Trans-Atl Phila.

How to Take Care of Yourself: Managing Your Own Medical Problems & Reduce Doctor Visits. 1992. (Alternative Medicine Ser.). lib. bdg. 92.95 (*0-8490-5399-4*) Gordon Pr.

How to Teach Autistic & Other Severely Handicapped Children. Robert L. Koegel & Laura Schreibman. 1981. (Teaching the Autistic Ser.). 54p. pap. 8.00 (*0-89079-065-5*, 1033) PRO-ED.

How to Teach Prevocational Skills to Severely Handicapped Persons. Dennis E. Mithaug. 1981. (Teaching the Autistic Ser.). 62p. pap. 8.00 (*0-89079-056-6*, 1037) PRO-ED.

How to Teach Your Children to Say No to Drugs: And Keep Their Friends. Leo Paur. 1992. 126p. 12.95 (*0-929753-00-3*) Paramount Bks.

How to Think Like a Psychologist: Critical Thinking in Psychology. Donald H. McBurney. 1995. LC 95-25246. 111p. (C). pap. 17.33 (*0-02-378392-3*, Macmillan Coll) P-H.

How to Think Like the Worlds Greatest High-Tech Titans. Erika Brown. 2000. LC 00-55010. (Leader's Edge Ser.). 216p. text 18.95 (*0-07-136068-9*) McGraw-Hill Prof.

How to Train Humans: A Behavior Modification Manual. Ronald A. Havens. 1974. LC 74-83123. (Illus.). 118p. pap. 5.00 (*0-87936-006-2*) Scholium Intl.

How to Treat Self-Injurious Behavior. Judith E. Favell & James W. Greene. 1980. (Teaching the Autistic Ser.). 46p. pap. 8.00 (*0-89079-055-8*, 1031) PRO-ED.

How to Treat the Sick Without Medicine. James C. Jackson. 1996. 537p. reprint ed. pap. 28.50 (*0-7873-0467-0*) Hlth Research.

How to Treat Yourself with Chinese Herbs. Hong-Yen Hsu. rev. ed. 1993. LC 78-26617. (Illus.). 296p. reprint ed. pap. 12.95 (*0-87983-603-2*, 36032K, Keats Pubng) McGraw-Hill Trade.

How to Turn Your Healthcare Experience Into Cash. M. Wade Curl. 1992. LC 91-92499. (Illus.). 108p. (C). pap. text 35.99 (*1-880610-00-0*) PRO-ACT Pub.

How to Understand & Analyze Your Own Dreams. Louis A. Gottschalk. 1983. LC 84-45110. 112p. reprint ed. 15.00 (*0-87668-714-1*) Aronson.

How to Understand People: An Introduction to Personality & Character. Sidney Vernon. 1982. (Illus.). 100p. (Orig.). pap. 6.95 (*0-943150-01-9*) Rovern Pr.

How to Use Computers & Cyberspace in the Clinical Practice of Psychotherapy. Jeri Fink. 1998. LC 98-6846. (Horizons in World Physics Ser.). (Illus.). xxii, 336p. pap. 40.00 (*0-7657-0173-1*) Aronson.

How to Use Food & Vitamin Supplements Safely & Sensibly. 1994. lib. bdg. 250.00 (*0-8490-5669-1*) Gordon Pr.

How to Use Herbs Safely. 1994. lib. bdg. 250.00 (*0-8490-5671-3*) Gordon Pr.

How to Use Homoeopathy. Christopher Hammond. 1992. 192p. pap. 14.95 (*1-85230-208-9*) Element MA.

How To Use Index Medicus Psychological Abstracts & Excerpta Medica. Barry Strickland-Hodge. 2nd ed. 1994. 150p. pap. (*0-566-07555-5*) Gower GBR. *Dist:* Ashgate Pub Co.

How to Use Leg Wraps, Bandages & Boots: Supportive Leg Care for Your Horse. Sue A. Allen. Ed. by Betty J. McKinney. 1996. LC 96-962. (Illus.). 112p. pap. 13.95 (*0-931866-72-3*) Alpine Pubns.

H I

How to Use Reprimands. Ron Van Houten. 1980. (How to Teach Ser.). 37p. pap. 8.00 (*0-89079-051-5*, 1008) PRO-ED.

How to Use Self-Control. Karen Esveldt-Dawson & Alan E. Kazdin. 1982. (How to Teach Ser.). 30p. pap. text 8.00 (*0-89079-067-1*, 1013) PRO-ED.

How to Use Sensory Extinction. Arnold Rincover. 1981. (Teaching the Autistic Ser.). 34p. pap. 8.00 (*0-89079-062-0*, 1036) PRO-ED.

How to Use the American College of Sports Medicine Metabolic Equations. Sheryl T. Zigon. 1990. 98p. (Orig.). pap. text 11.95 (*0-944183-06-9*) PRC Pub.

How to Use the HKI Food Frequency Method to Assess Community Risk of Vitamin A Deficiency. Helen Keller International Staff. 1994. (Orig.). pap. 10.00 (*0-915173-30-1*) Helen Keller Intl.

How to Use the Repertory. Glen I. Bidwell. 128p. pap. 8.95 (*0-8464-4237-X*) Beekman Pubs.

How to Use Token Economy & Point Systems. Teodoro Ayllon. 2nd ed. 1999. LC 98-35124. pap. (*0-89079-794-3*) PRO-ED.

How to Value a Medical Practice. 10th ed. 2000. 200p. pap. text 45.00 (*1-58383-158-4*, VALUE1) Robert D Keene.

How to Weigh & Measure Children. 94p. 25.00 (*92-1-130127-0*, 88.IV.2) UN.

How to Win at the Healthcare Sales Game: A Successful Approach for Medical Salespeople & Buyers. John Jascoll. 1994. (Illus.). 56p. pap. 10.00 (*0-9643012-1-0*) Hazelwood Pr.

How to Win at Weight Loss see Solved - The Riddle of Weight Loss: Restore Healthy Body Chemistry & Lose Weight Naturally

How to Win over Impotence-Frigidity. Salem Kirban. 1981. 199p. 12.95 (*0-912582-42-1*) Second Comng Inc.

How to Win over Worry. Ed. by John Haggai. l.t. ed. 1987. 11.95 (*0-8027-2576-7*) Walker & Co.

How to Work & Communicate in a Hospital or Convalescent Home. 1987. (How to Ser.). (ENG & SPA., Illus.). pap. text 6.95 (*0-918050-46-4*) Newhouse Pr.

***How to Work with Sex Offenders: A Handbook for Criminal Justice, Human Service & Mental Health Professionals.** Rudy Flora. 2001. LC 00-69717. (Haworth Marriage & the Family Ser.). 256p. (C). pap. 22.95 (*0-7890-1499-8*, Haworth Clinical) Haworth Pr.

How to Write a Marketing Plan for Health Care Organizations. William J. Winston. 1985. LC 85-10037. (Health Marketing Quarterly Ser.: No. 2). 170p. text 39.95 (*0-86656-450-0*) Haworth Pr.

How to Write a Paper. Ed. by G. M. Hall. 1994. 128p. pap. text (*0-7279-0822-7*) BMJ Pub GBR. *Dist:* AIDC.

How to Write a TCM Herbal Formula: A Rational Methodology for the Step-by-Step Formulation & Administration of Chinese Herbal Medicine in Decoction. Bob Flaws. 1993. LC 93-72800. 90p. (Orig.). (C). pap. 4.95 (*0-936185-49-X*) Blue Poppy Pr.

How to Write a Winning Workers' Compensation Report: A Programmed Textbook. Gregory L. Smith. 1995. 137p. pap. 39.95 (*1-883595-03-7*, 23029, OEM Pr) OEM Health.

How to Write an I. E. P. 2001. John Arena. 1989. 128p. pap. text 15.00 (*0-87879-072-1*) Acad Therapy.

How to Write & Publish Articles in Nursing. Donna R. Sheridan & Donna L. Dowdney. 2nd ed. 1997. LC 96-49183. (Illus.). 296p. 39.95 (*0-8261-4981-2*) Springer Pub.

How to Write Health Science Papers, Dissertations & Theses. Shane A. Thomas. 2000. LC 99-86909. 152p. 24.95 (*0-443-06283-8*) Harcrt Hlth Sci Grp.

How to Write Meaningful Nursing Standards. Elizabeth J. Mason. 1989. LC 84-13005. 261p. (C). pap. text 39.95 (*0-8273-4300-0*) Delmar.

How to Write Psychology. Leslie Parrott, III. 1997. LC 93-3171. 144p. (C). pap. 14.00 (*0-06-501798-6*) Addson-Wesley Educ.

How to Write Psychology Papers. Parrot. 2nd ed. 1999. (C). pap. text 12.00 (*0-321-03111-3*) Addson-Wesley Educ.

How We Feel: An Insight into the Emotional World of Teenagers. Jacki Gordon & Gillian Grant. 1997. LC 96-38788. 250p. pap. (*1-85302-439-2*) Jessica Kingsley GBR. *Dist:* Taylor & Francis.

How We Grieve: Relearning the World. Thomas A. Attig. 1996. LC 95-31907. 224p. pap. 19.95 (*0-19-507456-4*) OUP.

How We Learn, How We Remember - Toward an Understanding of the Brain & Neural Systems: Selected Papers. Leon N. Cooper. 1995. LC 95-37677. 400p. text 99.00 (*981-02-1814-1*); pap. text 53.00 (*981-02-1815-X*) World Scientific Pub.

How We Live. Sherwin B. Nuland. 1998. 432p. pap. 14.00 (*0-679-78140-4*) Vin Bks.

How Well Are You Willing to Bee? Beginners Auto Fix-It Guide. Pat Wagner. 2nd rev. ed. 1994. LC 94-96615. 80p. (Orig.). pap. 27.00 (*0-9644344-4-X*) JBS Pub.

How Well Can We Assess Genetic Risk? Not Very. James F. Crow. 1981. (Taylor Lectures: No. 5). pap. 20.00 (*0-913392-56-1*) NCRP Pubns.

How You Can Achieve Happiness, Health & Wealth. Lawrence R. Horn. Ed. by Lawrence R. Horn. 1995. 224p. pap. 19.50 (*0-9643340-9-7*) Sage Pubng.

How You Can Achieve Total Success Through Self-Hypnosis. C. J. Barker. 1997. 32p. pap. 7.95 (*0-934650-05-5*) Sunnyside.

How Your Baby Is Born. Amy B. Tuteur. 1994. LC 95-109310. (How It Works Ser.). (Illus.). 240p. (Orig.). pap. 19.95 (*1-56276-239-7*, Ziff-Davis Pr) Que.

How Your Brain Works. Anne Novitt-Moreno. 1995. (How It Works Ser.). (Illus.). 192p. (Orig.). pap. 19.95 (*1-56276-255-9*, Ziff-Davis Pr) Que.

How Your Mind Can Keep You Well. Roy Masters. Ed. by Dorothy Baker. 15th ed. 1978. 201p. pap. 15.95 (*0-933900-09-0*) Foun Human Under.

Howard Florey: Penicillin & After. Trevor I. Williams. 1984. (Illus.). 420p. 35.00 (*0-19-858173-4*) OUP.

How's Your Marriage? A Book for Men & Women. Michael F. Myers. 1998. LC 97-25511. 240p. 24.95 (*0-88048-695-3*, 8695) Am Psychiatric.

HPLC in Nucleic Acid Research: Methods & Applications. Phyllis R. Brown. 1984. (Chromatographic Science Ser.: Vol. 28). (Illus.). 424p. text 190.00 (*0-8247-7236-9*) Dekker.

HPLC in the Pharmaceutical Industry. Goodwin W. Fong & Stanley K. Lam. 1991. (Drugs & the Pharmaceutical Sciences Ser.: Vol. 47). (Illus.). 328p. text 155.00 (*0-8247-8499-5*) Dekker.

HPLC Methods for Pharmaceutical Analysis. George Lunn & Norman R. Schmuff. 1997. LC 96-29417. 1632p. 495.00 (*0-471-13078-8*); 295.00 (*0-471-18176-5*) Wiley.

HPLC Methods for Pharmaceutical Analysis, Set. George Lunn. 2000. 7009p. 995.00 incl. cd-rom (*0-471-33297-6*) Wiley.

HPLC Methods on Drug Analysis. M. K. Ghosh. 1995. (Illus.). 585p. 152.00 (*0-387-53824-0*) Spr-Verlag.

HPLC of Proteins, Peptides & Polynucleotides. Ed. by Milton T. Hearn. 1991. (Analytical Techniques in Clinical Chemistry & Laboratory Medicine Ser.). 776p. text 125.00 (*0-89573-295-5*, Wiley-VCH) Wiley.

H.R. 2976, the "Patient Right to Know Act of 1996" Hearing Before the Subcommittee on Health of the Committee on Ways & Means, House of Representatives, One Hundred Fourth Congress, Second Session, July 30, 1996. USGPO Staff. 1998. LC 98-190827. xi, 139p. (*0-16-057039-5*) USGPO.

HRT & Osteoporosis. Ed. by J. O. Drife & John W. Studd. 1990. (Illus.). 394p. 136.00 (*0-387-19628-5*) Spr-Verlag.

Hsiung's Diagnostic Virology: As Illustrated by Light & Electron Microscopy. Gueh-Djen Hsiung et al. 4th ed. 1994. LC 93-6338. (Illus.). 416p. 75.00 (*0-300-05845-4*) Yale U Pr.

H2O: Healing Water for Mind & Body. Anna Selby. 2000. LC 00-701491. (Illus.). 144p. pap. (*1-85585-744-8*) Collins & Br.

Huf und Klauenkunde mit Hufbeschlaglehre. G. Prietz. 1985. (GER., Illus.). 166p. 43.50 (*3-8055-4003-5*) S Karger.

Huffman Psychology in Action. Huffman. 4th ed. 1996. 432p. pap., stu. ed. 25.95 (*0-471-16094-6*) Wiley.

Hugh Cairns: First Nuffield Professor of Surgery, University of Oxford. G. J. Frankel. 1991. (Illus.). 314p. text 85.00 (*0-19-262095-9*) OUP.

Hughes' Outline of Modern Psychiatry. Jennifer Barraclough & David Gill. 4th rev. ed. 1996. LC 95-50016. 312p. pap. 55.00 (*0-471-96358-5*) Wiley.

Hughston Clinic Sports Medicine Field Manual. Champ L. Baker, Jr. 1996. (Illus.). 400p. 29.95 (*0-683-00310-0*) Lppncott W & W.

Hughston Clinic Sports Medicine Field Manual. Ed. by Champ L. Baker, Jr. et al. 1996. LC 95-25585. (*0-683-00031-4*) Lppncott W & W.

Hum Your Way to Health. Martin J. Fritz. 1996. 9p. reprint ed. spiral bd. 8.00 (*0-7873-0337-2*) Hlth Research.

Human Abilities in Cultural Contexts. Ed. by Sidney H. Irvine & John W. Berry. 1988. (Illus.). 640p. text 130.00 (*0-521-34482-4*) Cambridge U Pr.

Human Abnormalities Caused by Chemicals, Drugs & Substances: Index of New Information with References. American Health Research Institute Staff. rev. ed. 1998. 157p. 57.50 (*0-7883-1894-2*); 1998. 157p. pap. 47.50 (*0-7883-1895-0*); 1995. LC 95-17182. 147p. 57.50 (*0-7883-0654-5*); 1995. LC 95-17182. 147p. pap. 47.50 (*0-7883-0655-3*) ABBE Pubs Assn.

Human Achondroplasia: A Multidisciplinary Approach. B. Nicoletti et al. 1988. LC 88-25288. (Basic Life Sciences Ser.: Vol. 48). (Illus.). 514p. (C). text 130.00 (*0-306-43006-1*, Kluwer Plenum) Kluwer Academic.

Human Acid-Base Physiology. Oliver Wendell Holmes. 1993. LC 92-41400. 208p. (gr. 13). pap., stu. ed. 37.95 (*0-412-47610-X*) Chapman & Hall.

Human Adaptability: A Historical & Compendium of Research for the International Biological Programme. Ed. by J. S. Weiner et al. 1989. 368p. 45.00 (*0-85066-087-4*) Taylor & Francis.

Human Adaptation & Population Growth: A Non-Malthusian Perspective. David S. Kleinman. 1981. LC 78-59176. 296p. text 41.00 (*0-916672-18-2*, R3380) Rowman.

Human Adjustment. Jane S. Halonen & John W. Santrock. 2nd ed. 1996. LC 95-83923. 544p. (C). pap. 69.38 (*0-697-23571-8*, WCB McGr Hill) McGrw-H Hghr Educ.

Human Adjustment. Jane S. Halonen et al. 2nd ed. 1996. (C). pap., stu. ed. 28.13 (*0-697-23573-4*, WCB McGr Hill) McGrw-H Hghr Educ.

Human Adult Odontometrics. Julius A. Kieser. 1990. (Cambridge Studies in Biological Anthropology: No. 4). (Illus.). 206p. (C). text 64.95 (*0-521-35390-4*) Cambridge U Pr.

Human Ageing & Later Life. Anthony M. Warnes. 1990. 240p. pap. 25.00 (*0-340-42953-4*) Trafalgar.

Human Aggression. Robert A. Baron & D. R. Richardson. 2nd ed. 1994. (Perspectives in Social Psychology Ser.). 440p. 39.50 (*0-306-44458-5*, Plenum Trade) Perseus Pubng.

Human Aggression: Naturalistic Approaches. Ed. by Kevin D. Browne & John Archer. 1989. 240p. pap. 16.95 (*0-415-03037-4*); lib. bdg. 49.95 (*0-415-03036-6*) Routledge.

Human Aggression: Theories, Research, & Implications for Social Policy. Ed. by Russell G. Geen & Edward Donnerstein. 1998. LC 98-84364. (Illus.). 309p. (C). text 69.95 (*0-12-278805-2*) Morgan Kaufmann.

Human Aging. Ed. by James E. Birren et al. 1980. LC 79-8658. (Growing Old Ser.). (Illus.). reprint ed. lib. bdg. 33.95 (*0-405-12776-6*) Ayer.

Human Aging: Biological Perspectives. Augustine Gaspar DiGiovanna. 1994. LC 93-16897. 336p. (C). pap. text 38.25 net. (*0-07-016915-2*) McGraw.

Human Aging & Chronic Disease. Cary S. Kart & Eileen M. Metress. 1992. (Life Science Ser.). (Illus.). 352p. (C). text 48.95 (*0-86720-315-3*, 315-3) Jones & Bartlett.

Human Airway Inflammation: Sampling Techniques & Analytical Protocols. Ed. by Duncan F. Rodgers & Louise E. Donnelly. 2001. (Methods in Molecular Medicine Ser.: Vol. 56). 456p. 135.00 (*0-89603-923-4*) Humana.

Human Anatomy. Robert Carola et al. 1991. (C). text 75.25 net. (*0-07-010527-8*); pap. text, stu. ed. 25.00 (*0-07-010547-2*) McGraw.

Human Anatomy. Anthony J. Gaudin. 1994. (C). pap. text, tchr. ed., suppl. ed. (*0-03-096854-2*) Harcourt Coll Pubs.

Human Anatomy. Edward A. Joy. pap. 6.00 (*0-89741-006-8*) Gila River.

Human Anatomy. Hole. 2nd ed. 1994. text 74.50 net. (*0-697-26061-5*, WCB McGr Hill) McGrw-H Hghr Educ.

Human Anatomy. John W. Hole, Jr. & Karen Koos. 2nd ed. 1993. (Illus.). 688p. (C). text 63.50 net. (*0-697-12252-2*, WCB McGr Hill) McGrw-H Hghr Educ.

Human Anatomy. 3rd ed. 2000. tchr. ed. (*0-8053-4931-6*) Benjamin-Cummings.

Human Anatomy. Elaine Nicpon Marieb & Jon Mallatt. 3rd ed. 2000. LC 00-34063. (Illus.). xxxi, 844p. (*0-8053-4925-1*); (C). text 118.00 (*0-8053-4920-0*) Benjamin-Cummings.

Human Anatomy. Martini & Timmons. 3rd ed. 1999. suppl. ed. (*0-13-018810-7*) P-H.

Human Anatomy. Kent M. Van De Graaff. 4th ed. (C). 1995. 320p. text, stu. ed. 36.50 net. (*0-697-16068-8*); 1994. 128p. text, stu. ed. 16.00 net. (*0-697-24167-X*); 1994. text, stu. ed. 68.00 net. (*0-697-25531-X*); 1994. 448p. text, stu. ed. 26.87 (*0-697-21100-2*); Vol. 1. 1994. 832p. text (*0-697-16065-3*) McGrw-H Hghr Educ (WCB McGr Hill).

Human Anatomy: A Text & Colour Atlas. J. A. Gosling et al. 2nd ed. 1991. (Illus.). 348p. (gr. 13). text (*0-397-44767-1*, GM0000) Gower-Mosby.

Human Anatomy: An Illustrated Reference to Drawing Humans. Gottfried Bammes. 1994. 14.98 (*0-7858-0054-9*) Bk Sales Inc.

***Human Anatomy: Pelvis.** Nielsen. 1995. (Illus.). (C). stu. ed. 36.60 (*0-8087-1473-2*) Pearson Custom.

Human Anatomy: Synoptic Approach. N. J. Mizeres. 1992. (Synoptic Approach Ser.). 342p. (C). pap. text 45.00 (*0-8385-3902-5*, A3902-2, Apple Lange Med) McGraw.

Human Anatomy & Physiology. Robert Carola et al. 1992. (C). pap. text, stu. ed. 27.25 net. (*0-07-010972-9*) McGraw.

Human Anatomy & Physiology. Anthony J. Gaudin & Kenneth C. Jones. 1989. 219p. (C). pap. text, tchr. ed. 34.00 (*0-15-539707-9*) SCP.

Human Anatomy & Physiology. Robert Bauman, Jr. & Steve Dutton. 2nd ed. 1992. (Illus.). 200p. (Orig.). (C). pap. text, stu. ed. 22.50 (*1-878045-06-7*) Whittier Pubns.

Human Anatomy & Physiology. Robert Carola et al. 2nd ed. 1992. (C). text 273.12 (*0-07-010978-8*); pap. text, stu. ed. 25.50 net. (*0-07-010971-0*) McGraw.

Human Anatomy & Physiology. Joan G. Creager. 2nd ed. 1991. 960p. (C). text, stu. ed. 48.50 net. (*0-697-12844-X*, WCB McGr Hill) McGrw-H Hghr Educ.

Human Anatomy & Physiology. Elaine N. Marieb. Ed. by Melinda Adams. 2nd ed. 1104p. (C). 1994. tchr. ed. 28.33 (*0-8053-4128-5*); 1994. trans. 470.33 (*0-8053-4124-2*); 1992. disk 268.95 (*0-8053-4125-0*) Addison-Wesley.

Human Anatomy & Physiology. Elaine N. Marieb. 2nd ed. 1985. pap. text 29.25 (*0-8053-6727-6*); pap. text 34.50 (*0-8053-6726-8*) Benjamin-Cummings.

Human Anatomy & Physiology. Eldra P. Solomon. 2nd ed. 1990. (C). pap. text, tchr. ed., lab manual ed. 34.00 (*0-03-032642-7*); pap. text, tchr. ed. 34.00 (*0-03-032652-4*) Harcourt Coll Pubs.

Human Anatomy & Physiology. Shirley R. Burke. 3rd ed. 1991. (C). mass mkt. 48.95 (*0-8273-4853-3*) Delmar.

Human Anatomy & Physiology. Rovert Carola et al. 3rd ed. 1994. 1120p. (C). 95.94 (*0-07-011171-5*) McGraw.

Human Anatomy & Physiology. Elaine Marieb. 5th ed. 2000. pap. 16.00 (*0-8053-4984-7*); 384p. instr.'s training gde. ed. 25.29 (*0-8053-4969-3*) Benjamin-Cummings.

Human Anatomy & Physiology. Elaine N. Marieb. 5th ed. 2000. pap., stu. ed. 27.00 (*0-8053-4974-X*) Benjamin-Cummings.

Human Anatomy & Physiology. Elaine Nicpon Marieb. 5th ed. 2000. LC 00-39805. (Illus.). xxii, 1249p. 90.00 (*0-8053-4950-2*) Benjamin-Cummings.

Human Anatomy & Physiology. John W. Hole, Jr. 6th ed. 1008p. (C). 1993. text, stu. ed. 16.00 net. (*0-697-22787-1*); 1992. (Illus.). (gr. 11-12). text 69.00 net. (*0-697-12271-9*); 1992. text, stu. ed. 25.62 (*0-697-12280-8*) Brown & Benchmark.

Human Anatomy & Physiology. Hole. 7th ed. 1995. pap. text 541.87 (*0-697-20964-4*, WCB McGr Hill) McGrw-H Hghr Educ.

Human Anatomy & Physiology. John W. Hole, Jr. & Nancy Ann Sickles Corbett. 7th ed. 1995. 288p. (C). text, stu. ed. 25.62 (*0-697-20963-6*, WCB McGr Hill) McGrw-H Hghr Educ.

Human Anatomy & Physiology. John W. Hole, Jr. & Terry Martin. 7th ed. 1995. 464p. (C). text, lab manual ed. 38.50 net. (*0-697-20961-X*, WCB McGr Hill) McGrw-H Hghr Educ.

Human Anatomy & Physiology. David G. Gantt. Ed. by Denson K. McLain. 1996. LC 95-83836. (Illus.). 160p. (Orig.). (C). Pt. I. pap. 12.99 (*1-884612-05-9*); Pt. II. pap. 12.99 (*1-884612-07-5*) AudioText.

Human Anatomy & Physiology: A Laboratory Manual of, Vol. 1. Donald R. Ferruzzi. 5th ed. 1994. (Illus.). 248p. pap. text 32.95 (*0-9609098-1-8*) Biomat Pub Co.

Human Anatomy & Physiology: BIO 110. Kathleen Horton. 1985. 189p. (C). stu. ed., ring bd. (*0-933195-41-9*) CA College Health Sci.

Human Anatomy & Physiology: Cat Manual. Elaine Marieb. 5th ed. 1995. (C). pap. text, lab manual ed. 67.00 incl. disk (*0-8053-4055-6*) Addison-Wesley.

Human Anatomy & Physiology: Lab Manual - Cat Version. Elaine N. Marieb. 6th ed. 1998. LC 98-26986. 804p. 76.00 incl. cd-rom (*0-8053-4345-8*) Benjamin-Cummings.

Human Anatomy & Physiology: Lab Manual - Main Version. Elaine N. Marieb. 5th ed. 1999. LC 98-26985. (C). spiral bd., lab manual ed. 52.50 incl. cd-rom (*0-8053-4347-4*) Benjamin-Cummings.

Human Anatomy & Physiology: Lab Manual - Pig Version. Elaine N. Marieb. 3rd ed. 1989. (Illus.). 700p. (C). (gr. 10-12). pap. text 36.75 (*0-8053-0111-9*) Benjamin-Cummings.

Human Anatomy & Physiology: The Integrated Approach. Burggren. 1996. (C). text (*0-03-000564-7*) Harcourt Coll Pubs.

Human Anatomy & Physiology Coloring Workbook & Study Guide. Paul D. Anderson. 1990. 304p. pap., stu. ed., wbk. ed. 28.75 (*0-86720-145-2*) Jones & Bartlett.

Human Anatomy & Physiology Instructor's Guide. Shirley R. Burke. 3rd ed. 1992. pap., tchr. ed. 16.00 (*0-8273-4854-1*) Delmar.

Human Anatomy & Physiology Workbook. Maura T. Scali-Sheahan. 1994. LC 93-45428. 195p. 17.95 (*1-56253-157-3*) Milady Pub.

Human Anatomy & Physiology Workbook. Shirley R. Burke. 3rd ed. 1993. pap., lab manual ed. 18.95 (*0-8273-5047-3*) Delmar.

Human Anatomy Coloring Atlas. Stephen W. Langjahr & Robert D. Brister. 2nd ed. 1992. 202p. (C). pap. text 35.40 (*0-8053-4020-3*) Benjamin-Cummings.

Human Anatomy Colouring. Gosling. 1996. (*0-7234-2919-7*) Wolfe Publishing GBR. *Dist:* Mosby Inc.

Human Anatomy Laboratory Textbook. Harold J. Benson & Kathleen P. Talaro. 4th ed. 1992. 368p. (C). text 38.50 net. (*0-697-15020-8*, WCB McGr Hill) McGrw-H Hghr Educ.

Human Anatomy, Physiology & Pathophysiology. G. E. Thews et al. 1985. 784p. pap. 101.50 (*0-444-80704-7*) Elsevier.

Human Anatomy Picture Tests. J. A. Gosling et al. 1992. (Illus.). 176p. (gr. 13). (*1-56375-542-4*, GM0279) Gower-Mosby.

Human Anatomy with Cat Dissection. Elaine E. Marieb. 3rd ed. 2000. LC 00-50866. 554p. spiral bd., lab manual ed. 59.00 (*0-8053-4968-5*) Benjamin-Cummings.

***Human Anatomy with Over-Use Syndromes & Cumulative Trauma Disorders: Index of New Information & Guide-Book for Consumers, Reference & Research.** Jean Gray Yodell. 2002. 180p. pap. 47.50 (*0-7883-2447-0*) ABBE Pubs Assn.

***Human Anatomyphysiology.** Elaine Marieb. 5th ed. 2001. (Illus.). suppl. ed. 86.00 (*0-8053-5332-1*) Benjamin-Cummings.

Human & Animal Nutrition. Ed. by Geoffrey H. Bourne. 1978. (World Review of Nutrition & Dietetics Ser.: Vol. 32). (Illus.). 128.75 (*3-8055-2855-8*) S Karger.

Human & Animal Relationships: A Comprehensive Treatise on Fungi as Experimental System for Basic & Applied Research. Ed. by D. H. Howard & J. D. Miller. 1996. (Mycota Ser.: Vol. 6). (Illus.). 399p. 251.00 (*0-387-58007-7*) Spr-Verlag.

Human & Artificial Intelligence. Ed. by Frederick J. Crosson. 1970. LC 78-131431. (Orig.). (C). pap. text 12.95 (*0-89197-220-X*) Irvington.

Human & Machine Vision: Analogies & Divergencies. V. Cantoni. 1994. LC 94-43083. (Illus.). 410p. (C). text 125.00 (*0-306-44902-1*, Kluwer Plenum) Kluwer Academic.

Human & Mammalian Cytogenetics: A Historical Perspective. T. C. Hsu. 1979. (Heidelberg Science Library). (Illus.). 45.00 (*0-387-90364-X*) Spr-Verlag.

Human & Veterinary Nutrition, Biochemical Aspects of Nutrients. Ed. by Geoffrey H. Bourne. 1978. (World Review of Nutrition & Dietetics Ser.: Vol. 30). (Illus.). 128.75 (*3-8055-2789-6*) S Karger.

Human Animal. Weston La Barre. 1993. LC 54-12371. pap. 2.25 (*0-226-46706-6*, P45) U Ch Pr.

Human Apolipoprotein Mutants III: In Diagnosis & Treatment. Cesare R. Sirtori. 1993. LC 93-20507. (NATO ASI Ser.). 291p. 212.00 (*0-387-54613-8*) Spr-Verlag.

Human Apolipoprotein Mutants, Vol. 2: From Gene Structure to Phenotypic Expression. Cesare R. Sirtori et al. 1989. (NATO ASI Series A, Life Sciences: Vol. 167). (Illus.). 268p. 79.50 (*0-306-43213-7*, Plenum Trade) Perseus Pubng.

Human Artificial Procreation. Council of Europe Staff. 1989. (Bioethics Ser.). (*92-871-1676-8*) Council of Europe FRA. *Dist:* Manhattan Pub Co.

Human Aspects of Biomedical Innovation. Ed. by Everett I. Mendelsohn et al. 1971. LC 74-160027. (Harvard Studies in Technology & Society). (Illus.). 246p. 47.50 (*0-674-41331-8*) HUP.

Human Associative Memory. John R. Anderson & Gordon H. Bower. 1980. LC 79-28349. 538p. 89.95 (*0-89859-108-2*); 288p. pap. 29.95 (*0-89859-020-5*) L Erlbaum Assocs.

Human Atmosphere: Bridging the Gap Between Religious Tradition, Occult Tradition & Medicine, the Human Aura. Walter J. Kilner. 1991. lib. bdg. 86.95 (*0-8490-4492-8*) Gordon Pr.

Human Attachment. Virginia L. Colin. 1995. (Series in Developmental Psychology). 448p. (C). pap. 29.38 (*0-07-011839-6*) McGrw-H Hghr Educ.

Human Attachment. Virginia L. Colin. 1996. 448p. (C). lib. bdg. 69.95 (*1-56639-459-7*) Temple U Pr.

Human Aura. Swami Panchadasi. reprint ed. pap. 3.00 (*0-911662-37-5*) Yoga.

Human Autoerotic Practices. Ed. by Manfred DeMartino. 1979. LC 78-8766. 378p. 43.95 (*0-87705-373-1*); pap. 24.95 (*0-87705-403-7*) Kluwer Academic (Kluwer Acad Hman Sci).

Human B Cell Populations. Ed. by Manlio Ferrarini & Federico Caligaris-Cappio. 1997. (Chemical Immunology Ser.: Vol. 67, 1997). (Illus.). x, 138p. 139.25 (*3-8055-6460-0*) S Karger.

Human Basophils & Mast Cells, Set. Ed. by Gianni Marone. 1995. (Chemical Immunology Ser.: Vols. 61 & 62). (Illus.). 470p. 419.25 (*3-8055-6129-6*) S Karger.

Human Basophils & Mast Cells: Biological Aspects. Ed. by Gianni Marone. 1995. (Chemical Immunology Ser.: Vol. 61). (Illus.). xiv, 242p. 228.00 (*3-8055-6127-X*) S Karger.

Human Basophils & Mast Cells: Clinical Aspects. Ed. by Gianni Marone. 1995. (Chemical Immunology Ser.: Vol. 62). (Illus.). x, 240p. 237.50 (*3-8055-6128-8*) S Karger.

Human Becoming School of Thought. Rosemarie Rizzo Parse. 1998. LC 98-8893. 130p. 79.95 (*0-7619-0582-0*, 80547); pap. 39.95 (*0-7619-0583-9*, 80548) Sage.

Human Behavior & Public Policy - Political Psychology. Marshall H. Segall. 1977. text 60.00 (*0-08-017087-0*); pap. text 25.00 (*0-08-017853-7*) Elsevier (Pergamon Pr).

Human Behavior & the Developing Brain. Ed. by Geraldine Dawson & Kurt W. Fischer. 1994. LC 93-36030. 568p. 66.00 (*0-89862-092-9*, 2092) Guilford Pubns.

Human Behavior in Global Perspective: An Introduction to Cross-Cultural Psychology. Marshall H. Segall et al. 1990. (General Psychology Ser.). 450p. text (*0-08-036814-X*); pap. text (*0-08-036813-1*) PPI GBR. *Dist:* Elsevier.

Human Behavior in the Caring Context. Ed. by Neil Moonie et al. 1999. 200p. pap. (*0-7487-1769-2*) Nelson Thornes GBR. *Dist:* Trans-Atl Phila.

Human Behavior in the Concentration Camp. Elie A. Cohen. 1984. LC 84-544. 295p. reprint ed. lib. bdg. 38.50 (*0-313-24417-0*, CHBE/, Greenwood Pr) Greenwood.

Human Behavior in the Social Environment. Carel B. Germain. 1991. text 53.50 (*0-231-05404-1*) Col U Pr.

Human Behavior in the Social Environment: Families, Groups, Organizations, & Communities. Vimala Pillari & Moses Newsome. 1997. LC 97-26559. 228p. pap. text 40.95 (*0-534-35029-1*) Brooks-Cole.

Human Behavior in the Social Environment: The Developing Person in a Holistic Context. Pillari. 2nd ed. 1997. LC 97-26560. 350p. pap. text 49.95 (*0-534-35028-3*) Brooks-Cole.

Human Behavior in Today's World. Ed. by Waris Ishaq. 1991. LC 90-48698. 328p. 70.00 (*0-275-93588-4*, C3588, Praeger Pubs) Greenwood.

Human Biology. 2000. (Illus.). 794p. (C). 64.00 (*0-536-61205-6*) Pearson Custom.

Human Biology. Sandra M. Alters-Gottfried. 1993. (Illus.). 523p. (C). pap. 80.63 (*0-8016-7972-9*) McGrw-H Hghr Educ.

Human Biology. Clinton L. Benjamin et al. 1996. LC 95-45014. (*0-07-022896-5*) McGraw.

Human Biology. Corrigan. 1999. (C). pap. text, lab manual ed. 23.00 (*0-03-005798-1*) Harcourt Coll Pubs.

Human Biology. Mannino. 1995. (*0-8151-5980-3*) Mosby Inc.

Human Biology. Joseph Mannino. 1994. LC 96-222594. (Illus.). 420p. pap. 80.63 (*0-8016-5850-0*) McGrw-H Hghr Educ.

Human Biology. Joseph Mannino & Carl Thurman. 1995. 136p. (C). pap., stu. ed. 25.63 (*0-8151-6353-3*) McGrw-H Hghr Educ.

Human Biology. Starr. (Adaptable Courseware Ser.). Date not set. mass mkt. 20.00 (*0-534-56570-0*); 1994. mass mkt., tchr. ed. 58.50 (*0-534-20211-X*) Wadsworth Pub.

Human Biology. Cecie Starr & Beverly McMillan. 1994. 527p. mass mkt. 42.75 (*0-534-20208-X*) Wadsworth Pub.

Human Biology. Sandy Alters. 2nd ed. 2004. (Illus.). 608p. (C). text 56.25 (*0-7637-0836-4*, 0836-4) Jones & Bartlett.

Human Biology. Daniel D. Chiras. 2nd ed. 1995. (Life Science Ser.). (Illus.). 195p. (C). pap. text 19.95 (*0-314-04954-1*, 04954-1) Jones & Bartlett.

Human Biology. Sylvia S. Mader. 2nd ed. 1989. 576p. (C). text, stu. ed. 30.50 net. (*0-697-10194-0*, WCB McGr Hill) McGrw-H Hghr Educ.

Human Biology: An Evolutionary & Biocultural Approach. Sara Stinson et al. 2000. 639p. 75.00 (*0-471-13746-4*) Wiley.

Human Biology: An Introduction to Human Evolution, Variation, Growth, & Ecology. G. Ainsworth Harrison et al. 2nd ed. 1977. (Illus.). (C). text 36.50 (*0-19-857164-X*) OUP.

Human Biology: Answers to End of Chapter Questions. Starr & McMillan. 2nd ed. 1996. (Biology). mass mkt. 2.50 (*0-534-50910-X*) Wadsworth Pub.

Human Biology: Biology of AIDS, Set. Donald J. Farish et al. 1993. text 68.75 (*0-86720-867-8*) Jones & Bartlett.

Human Biology: Health. Daniel Chiras. 2nd ed. 1995. (Life Science Ser.). (Illus.). 361p. pap. text, stu. ed. 26.25 (*0-314-04749-2*, 04749-2) Jones & Bartlett.

Human Biology: Health & Environment. Daniel D. Chiras. Ed. by Westby. 1991. (Life Science Ser.). (Illus.). 610p. (C). pap. text 46.25 (*0-314-79498-0*, 79498-0) Jones & Bartlett.

Human Biology: Health, Homeostasis & the Environment. Daniel D. Chiras. 2nd ed. 1995. LC 94-12440. (Life Science Ser.). (Illus.). 720p. (C). pap. text 53.95 (*0-314-03921-X*, 03921-X) Jones & Bartlett.

Human Biology: Health, Test Bank. Daniel D. Chiras. 2nd ed. 1995. (Life Science Ser.). (Illus.). 344p. pap. text, tchr. ed. 10.00 (*0-314-05093-0*, 05093-0) Jones & Bartlett.

Human Biology & Health: An Evolutionary Approach. Ed. by Basiro Davey & Tim Halliday. 2nd rev. ed. 1994. LC 93-49558. (Health & Disease Ser.: Bk. 4). 192p. pap. (*0-335-19253-X*) OpUniv Pr.

Human Biology & Social Inequality. Ed. by S. S. Strickland & P. S. Shetty. 1998. LC 97-23261. (Society for the Study of Human Biology Symposium Ser.: No. 39). (Illus.). 358p. (C). text 80.00 (*0-521-57043-3*) Cambridge U Pr.

Human Biology-Recent Advances: Proceedings of the International Symposium on Human Growth, Vol. 1. I. J. Bansal. 1982. 307p. (*0-88065-249-7*) Today Tomorrow IND. *Dist:* Lubrecht & Cramer, Scholarly Pubns.

Human Biology with Environmental Topics. Clinton L. Benjamin et al. 1996. LC 95-45015. 688p. (C). pap. 78.13 (*0-07-022907-4*) McGrw-H Hghr Educ.

Human Biorhythms & the Moon. A. P. Dubrov. 1994. (Illus.). 147p. (C). lib. bdg. 95.00 (*1-56072-145-6*) Nova Sci Pubs.

Human Birth: An Evolutionary Perspective. Wenda R. Trevathan. 1987. (Evolutionary Foundations of Human Behavior Ser.). (Illus.). 280p. (C). lib. bdg. 47.95 (*0-202-02029-0*) Aldine de Gruyter.

Human Blastogenesis. H. Voegler. 1987. (Bibliotheca Anatomica Ser.: No. 30). (Illus.). xii, 152p. 113.25 (*3-8055-4628-9*) S Karger.

***Human Blood Cells: Consequences of Genetic Polymorphisms & Variations.** Ed. by May-Jean King. 2000. LC 00-39672. 407p. (*1-86094-196-6*) Imperial College.

Human Blood Groups: Chemical & Biochemical Basis of Antigen Specificity. Helmut Schenkel-Brunner. 2nd rev. ed. 2000. (Illus.). 652p. 99.00 (*3-211-83471-0*) Spr-Verlag.

Human Blood Groups: Proceedings of the International Convocation on Immunology, 5th, Buffalo, New York, 1976. International Convocation on Immunology Staff. Ed. by J. F. Mohn et al. 1977. (Illus.). 85.25 (*3-8055-2422-6*) S Karger.

Human Body. Parramon Studios Staff & Eduard Arnau. 1998. LC 98-17944. (Illus.). 96p. 19.95 (*0-7641-5078-2*) Barron.

Human Body. Bruce D. Wingerd. 1994. LC 93-85932. 46p. (C). text 119.50 (*0-03-055507-8*) Harcourt Coll Pubs.

Human Body. Wingerd. 2nd ed. 1998. (C). text 60.50 (*0-03-011258-3*) Harcourt Coll Pubs.

Human Body: An Illustrated Guide to Its Structure, Function, & Disorders. Ed. by Charles B. Clayman. 1995. LC 94-37165. (Illus.). 240p. 29.95 (*1-56458-992-7*) DK Pub Inc.

Human Body: Health & Disease. Thibode. 2nd ed. 1997. 250.00 (*0-8151-2127-X*); 250.00 (*0-8151-2128-8*) Mosby Inc.

Human Body & the Law. David W. Meyers. 2nd ed. 1991. LC 90-71394. 368p. 56.00 (*0-8047-1885-7*) Stanford U Pr.

Human Body as Symbol: Psychotherapy of Schizophrenia Through Existential Dialectics. Thorsten Herner. 1990. 150p. 79.00 (*91-22-01323-7*) Coronet Bks.

Human Body Composition. G. B. Forbes. 1987. (Illus.). 350p. 141.00 (*0-387-96394-4*) Spr-Verlag.

Human Body Composition: In Vivo Methods, Models & Assessment. K. J. Ellis & J. D. Eastman. 1993. (Basic Life Sciences Ser.: Vol. 60). (Illus.). 416p. (C). text 120.00 (*0-306-44569-7*, Kluwer Plenum) Kluwer Academic.

Human Body Dynamics: Impact, Occupational & Athletic Aspects. Ed. by Dhanjoo N. Ghista. 1982. (Oxford Medical Engineering Ser.). (Illus.). 562p. 89.00 (*0-19-857548-3*) OUP.

Human Body Explained: An Owner's Guide to the Incredible Living Maching. Ed. by Philip Whitfield. 1995. LC 95-86. (Reference Bks.). (Illus.). 192p. 40.00 (*0-8050-3752-7*) H Holt & Co.

Human Body in Health & Disease. 2000. tchr. ed. (*0-13-017265-0*) P-H.

Human Body in Health & Disease. Edwin F. Bartholomew et al. 1999. LC 99-58973. (Illus.). 596p. pap. text 52.00 (*0-13-856816-2*) P-H.

Human Body in Health & Disease. Linda Swisher. 2nd ed. 1997. (Illus.). 384p. pap. text, stu. ed. 17.95 (*0-8151-8872-2*) Mosby Inc.

Human Body in Health & Disease. Thibodeau. 2nd ed. 1997. (C). 34.95 (*0-323-01104-7*) Mosby Inc.

Human Body in Health & Disease. Gary A. Thibodeau & Kevin T. Paton. 2nd ed. 1997. (Illus.). 736p. (C). text, stu. ed. 36.95 (*0-8151-8870-6*, 28299) Mosby Inc.

Human Body in Health & Disease. Gary Thibodeau & Kevin T. Patton. 2nd ed. 1997. tchr. ed. (*0-8151-8871-4*) Mosby Inc.

Human Body in Health & Disease. Gary A. Thibodeau & Kevin T. Patton. 3rd ed. 2001. LC 00-57877. (Illus.). 736p. pap. 35.95 (*0-323-01338-4*) Mosby Inc.

***Human Body in Health & Disease: Computerized Test Bank.** Gary A. Thibodeau & Kevin T. Patton. 3rd ed. 2001. (*0-323-01350-3*) Mosby Inc.

***Human Body in Health & Disease: Electronic Instructor's Curriculum.** Gary A. Thibodeau & Kevin T. Patton. 3rd ed. 2001. (*0-323-01351-1*) Mosby Inc.

***Human Body in Health & Disease: Instructor's Resource Manual.** Gary A. Thibodeau & Kevin T. Patton. 3rd ed. 2001. (*0-323-01348-1*) Mosby Inc.

Human Body in Health & Illness. Barbara Herlihy. 2000. 575p. pap. text, stu. ed. 17.95 (*0-7216-6108-4*) Harcrt Hlth Sci Grp.

***Human Body in Health & Illness.** Barbara Herlihy & Nancy K. Maebius. 2000. 500.00 (*0-7216-8629-X*) Saunders.

Human Body in Health & Illness. Barbara Herlihy & Nancy K. Maebius. Ed. by Terri Wood. 1999. LC 99-26386. (Illus.). 590p. pap. 34.95 (*0-7216-6107-6*) Saunders.

Human Body Odor: Etiology, Treatment, & Related Factors. M. Inaba & Y. Inaba. 1992. LC 92-49858. (Illus.). 280p. 187.00 (*0-387-70098-6*) Spr-Verlag.

Human Body Temperature: Its Measurement & Regulation. Ed. by Y. Houdas et al. 1982. LC 82-9856. 256p. 69.50 (*0-306-40872-4*, Plenum Trade) Perseus Pubng.

Human Bone Marrow: Anatomy Physiology & Pathophysiology. Ed. by Sidney Trubowitz & Stephen Davis. 1982. Vol. I. 272p. 154.00 (*0-8493-6105-2*, RC645); Vol. II. 296p. 167.00 (*0-8493-6106-0*) Franklin (CRC Reprint).

Human Brain. Paul Glees. 1988. (Illus.). 224p. text 64.95 (*0-521-24974-0*) Cambridge U Pr.

Human Brain: A Guided Tour. Susan A. Greenfield. 1998. LC 97-5131. (Science Masters Ser.). 176p. pap. text 13.00 (*0-465-00726-0*) Basic.

Human Brain: An Introduction to Its Functional Anatomy. John Nolte. 4th ed. 1998. (Illus.). (C). 224p. pap. text, stu. ed. 21.95 (*0-8151-8993-1*, 29043); LC 98-17069. xi, 606p. (gr. 13). pap. text 43.95 (*0-8151-8911-7*, 29042) Mosby Inc.

***Human Brain: An Introduction to Its Functional Anatomy, Including Study Guide.** John Nolte. 4th ed. 1999. (Illus.). 704p. pap. 60.00 (*0-323-00474-1*) Mosby Inc.

Human Brain: Surface, Three-Dimensional Sectional Anatomy with MRI & Vascularization. Henri M. Duvernoy & Emmanuel A. Cabanis. 1999. LC 99-22443. (*3-211-82260-7*) Spr-Verlag.

Human Brain Anatomy in Computerized Images. Hanna Damasio. 1995. LC 94-14527. (Illus.). 320p. text 95.00 (*0-19-508204-4*) OUP.

Human Brain & Spinal Cord: A Historical Study Illustrated by Writings from Antiquity to the 20th Century. Edwin Clarke & C. D. O'Malley. 2nd ed. 1995. (Illus.). 973p. 225.00 (*0-930405-25-0*) Norman SF.

Human Brain & Spinal Cord: Functional Neuroanatomy & Dissection Guide. Lennart Heimer. (Illus.). 1993. 402p. pap. 54.95 (*0-387-90740-8*); 1983. 402p. 40.00 (*0-387-90741-6*); 2nd ed. 1994. LC 94-241. 506p. 68.95 (*0-387-94227-0*) Spr-Verlag.

Human Brain Circulation: Functional Changes in Disease. Ed. by Rosemary D. Bevan & John A. Bevan. 1994. LC 94-15788. (Vascular Biomedicine Ser.). (Illus.). 470p. text 145.00 (*0-89603-271-X*) Humana.

Human Brain Coloring Book. Marian C. Diamond et al. 1986. LC 86-126855. (Cos Ser.: Vol. 306). (Illus.). 320p. (Orig.). pap. 19.95 (*0-06-460306-7*, CO 306, Harper Ref) HarperCollins Pubs.

Human Brain Function: An Introduction to Clinical Neurophysiology. Ed. by Robert Lavine. 1996. 264p. (C). pap. text 51.00 (*0-536-59822-3*) Pearson Custom.

Human Brain in Dissection. Donald G. Montemurro & J. Edward Bruni. 2nd ed. 1988. (Illus.). 208p. pap. text 29.95 (*0-19-504926-8*) OUP.

Human Brain in Photographs & Diagrams. John Nolte & Jay B. Angevine. 1995. (Illus.). 208p. (C). (gr. 13). spiral bd. 36.00 (*0-8016-8125-1*, 08125) Mosby Inc.

Human Brain in Photographs & Diagrams. John Nolte & Jay B. Angevine, Jr. 2nd ed. 2000. LC 00-31875. (Illus.). ix, 212p. text (*0-323-01126-8*) Mosby Inc.

Human Brain Stem & Cerebellum: Surface, Structure, Vascularization & Three-Dimensional Sectional Anatomy with MRI. Henri M. Duvernoy. 1995. LC 94-46338. (Radiology, Neurosurgery Anatomy Ser.). (Illus.). 480p. 235.00 (*0-387-82503-7*) Spr-Verlag.

Human Brain Stem & Cerebellum: Surface, Structure, Vascularization, Three Dimensional Sectional Anatomy, & MRI. Henri M. Duvernoy. 1995. (Illus.). 480p. 260.00 (*3-211-82503-7*) Spr-Verlag.

Human Brain Stem Vessels: Including the Pineal Gland & Information on Brain Stem Infarction. Illus. by J. L. Vannson. 2nd expurg. rev. ed. 1999. LC 99-10481. 271p. 269.00 (*3-540-64349-4*) Spr-Verlag.

Human Calorimeters, Vol. 7. Paul Webb. 1985. LC 85-3530. 176p. 60.00 (*0-275-91328-7*, C1328, Praeger Pubs) Greenwood.

Human Cancer: Epidemiology & Environmental Causes. John Higginson et al. 1992. (Cambridge Monographs on Cancer Research). (Illus.). 603p. (C). text 150.00 (*0-521-41288-9*) Cambridge U Pr.

Human Cancer in Primary Culture. Ed. by John R. Masters. 1991. (C). text 181.00 (*0-7923-1088-8*) Kluwer Academic.

Human Cancer Markers. Ed. by Stewart Sell & Britta Wahren. 1982. LC 81-80902. (Contemporary Biomedicine Ser.: Vol. 2). (Illus.). 428p. 119.50 (*0-89603-029-6*) Humana.

Human Carcinogens: Index of New Information with Authors, Subjects & References. John C. Bartone. 1997. 150p. 57.50 (*0-7883-1358-4*); pap. 47.50 (*0-7883-1359-2*) ABBE Pubs Assn.

Human Cardiovascular Control. Loring B. Rowell. 1993. LC 92-16434. (Illus.). 520p. text 69.50 (*0-19-507362-2*) OUP.

Human Care Services Directory of Metropolitan Chicago: Of Metropolitan Chicago. Ed. by Carol Southern & Taia K. Butterworth. 37th ed. 1996. 700p. (Orig.). pap. 54.90 (*0-925133-02-7*) Volt Directory.

Human CD38 & Related Molecules. Ed. by K. Mehta. 1999. LC 00-267829. (Chemical Immunology Ser.: Vol. 75). (Illus.). xii, 281p. 238.25 (*3-8055-6923-8*) S Karger.

Human Cell Culture Vol. III: Cancer Continuous Cell Lines: Leukaemias & Lymphomas. John R. W. Masters. Ed. by Bernhard O. Palsson. 2000. LC 99-164711. (Human Cell Culture Ser.). (Illus.). 384p. 210.00 (*0-7923-6225-X*, Kluwer Plenum) Kluwer Academic.

Human Cells in In-Vitro Pharmaco-Toxicology: Present Status Within Europe, 001. Ed. by Vera Rogiers et al. 1994. (Illus.). 328p. (*90-5487-041-9*) VUB Univ Pr BEL. *Dist:* Paul & Co Pubs.

Human Central Nervous System. Hanaway. 1998. (Illus.). 195p. pap. text (*0-7216-4746-4*) Saunders.

Human Central Nervous System. 3rd ed. 1996. (Illus.). 437p. text 85.00 (*3-540-13441-7*) Spr-Verlag.

Human Central Nervous System. R. Nieuwenhuys et al. 3rd ed. 1996. (Illus.). 440p. 74.95 (*0-387-13441-7*) Spr-Verlag.

Human Chromosome Preparation: Essential Techniques. D. E. Rooney & B. H. Czepulkowski. 1997. LC 96-38485. 154p. pap. 49.95 (*0-471-96299-6*) Wiley.

Human Chromosomes: A Manual of Basic Techniques. Ram S. Verma & Arvind Babu. 1989. 256p. 64.00 (*0-08-035774-1*); pap. 31.95 (*0-08-036839-5*) Elsevier (Pergamon Pr).

Human Circulating Tumor Markers: Current Concepts & Clinical Applications. James T. Wu & Robert M. Nakamura. 1997. LC 97-10403. 45.00 (*0-89189-419-5*) Am Soc Clinical.

Human Cloning. James M. Humber & Robert F. Almeder. 1998. (Biomedical Ethics Reviews Ser.). 224p. 49.50 (*0-89603-565-4*) Humana.

Human Communication & Its Disorders. Harris Winitz. 1. 1987. 272p. 77.00 (*0-89391-270-0*); 3. 1990. (Human Communication & Its Disorders Ser.: Vol. 3). 248p. (C). 77.00 (*0-89391-583-1*) Greenwood (Ablex).

Human Complement System in Health & Disease. Ed. by Volanakis & Frank. 1998. LC 97-47602. (Illus.). 672p. text 225.00 (*0-8247-9898-8*) Dekker.

Human Conception In Vitro. R. G. Edwards & J. M. Purdy. 1982. LC 82-71006. text 136.00 (*0-12-232740-3*) Acad Pr.

Human Core: The Intrapsychic Base of Behavior. Leo Rangell. 1990. Vol. 1. x, 468p. 70.00 (*0-8236-2365-3*); Vol. 2. 500p. 72.50 (*0-8236-2366-1*) Intl Univs Pr.

Human Cross-Sectional Anatomy: A Pocket Atlas. Ed. by Harold Ellis. 1994. 256p. pap. (*0-7506-2028-5*) E A GBR. *Dist:* OUP.

H I

Human Cytogenetic Cancer Markers. Ed. by Sandra R. Wolman & Stewart Sell. 1997. LC 97-7392. (Contemporary Biomedicine Ser.: Vol. 13). (Illus.). 512p. 150.00 (*0-89603-357-0*) Humana.

Human Cytogenetics: Essential Data. Ed. by D. E. Rooney & B. H. Czepulkowski. 1995. LC 94-30736. (Essential Data Ser.). 128p. pap. 39.95 (*0-471-95076-9*) Wiley.

Human Cytogenetics: Malignancy & Acquired Abnormalities, Vol. 2. Ed. by Barbara Czepulkowski & D. E. Rooney. 3rd ed. 2000. LC 2001-276309. (Practical Approach Ser.). (Illus.). 306p. pap. text 55.00 (*0-19-963841-1*) OUP.

Human Cytokines Bharwat Aggarwal & Raj Puri. 1997. (Illus.). pap. 195.00 (*0-632-04333-4*) Blackwell Sci.

Human Cytokines Vol. 3: Handbook for Basic & Clinical Research. Bharat B. Aggarwal. 1997. (Illus.). pap. text 90.00 (*0-86542-533-7*) Blackwell Sci.

Human Cytokines & Cytokine Receptors. Reno Debets & Huub Savelkoul. 1999. (Methods in Molecular Biology Ser.: No. 99). (Illus.). 350p. 109.50 (*0-89603-486-0*); spiral bd. 69.50 (*0-89603-445-3*) Humana.

Human Decision Making & Manual Control. Ed. by H. P. Willumeit. 1986. 420p. 151.50 (*0-444-70030-7*, North Holland) Elsevier.

Human Development 1996/97. Freiberg. 24th annot. ed. 1996. tchr. ed. (*0-697-31667-X*, WCB McGr Hill) McGrw-H Hghr Educ.

Human Development. Robert V. Kail & John C. Cavanaugh. 1995. LC 95-2840. 680p. mass mkt. 49.75 (*0-534-22224-2*) Brooks-Cole.

Human Development. Margaret Miller et al. 1992. LC 92-13561. (Skills for Caring Ser.). (Illus.). 40p. (Orig.). pap. text (*0-443-04531-3*) Church.

Human Development. Trygve Steen. 1994. 37p. pap. text 5.00 (*0-9617645-3-8*) Oreg Mus Sci & Indus.

Human Development. Roberta Kestenbaum. 2nd ed. 1994. 288p. pap. text, stu. ed. 26.20 (*0-02-363155-4*, Macmillan Coll) P-H.

Human Development. Dacey & Travers. 3rd ed. 1995. tchr. ed. 23.12 (*0-697-21005-7*, WCB McGr Hill) McGrw-H Hghr Educ.

Human Development. James W. Vander Zanden. 3rd ed. 1985. pap. text, stu. ed. 10.50 (*0-394-34752-8*, KnopfC) Knopf.

Human Development. James W. Vander Zanden. 6th ed. 1996. LC 96-14320. 752p. (C). pap. 79.69 (*0-07-067044-7*) McGrw-H Hghr Educ.

Human Development. Meyer. 7th ed. 1996. pap. text, stu. ed. 27.40 (*0-13-233156-X*) P-H.

Human Development. Craig et al. 8th ed. 1998. LC 98-28291. 691p. (C). 90.00 (*0-13-922774-1*) P-H.

Human Development: A Lifespan Approach. Karen L. Freiberg. 4th ed. 1992. (Nursing-Health Science Ser.). (Illus.). (C). 144p. pap. text, stu. ed. 18.95 (*0-86720-634-9*, 634-9); 528p. text, stu. ed. 59.95 (*0-86720-323-4*, 323-4) Jones & Bartlett.

Human Development: A Lifespan Approach. John Golley. 4th ed. 1992. (Nursing-Health Science Ser.). (C). disk 195.00 (*0-86720-635-7*) Jones & Bartlett.

Human Development: Across the Life Span. Fergus P. Hughes. 1990. 640p. (C). text 62.20 (*0-675-21241-3*, Merrill Coll) P-H.

Human Development: Study Guide. Kail. 1995. (Psychology Ser.). pap., stu. ed. 18.25 (*0-534-33908-5*) Brooks-Cole.

Human Development & Homeostasis: The Science of Psychiatry. William E. Powles. 1992. LC 90-15604. 600p. (C). 80.00 (*0-8236-2363-7*) Intl Univs Pr.

Human Development & Public Health: Proceedings of the WHO Scientific Group, Geneva, 1971. WHO Staff. 1972. (Technical Reports: No. 485). pap. text 4.00 (*92-4-120485-0*, 1100485) World Health.

Human Development & the Life Course: Multidisciplinary Perspectives. Ed. by Aage B. Sorensen et al. 1986. 632p. (C). text 89.95 (*0-89859-664-5*) L Erlbaum Assocs.

Human Development for Occupational Therapists: Conception Through Adolescence. Margaret A. Short-DeGraff. 1988. 604p. (C). text 43.00 (*0-683-07703-1*) Lppncott W & W.

Human Development Hoax: Time to Tell the Truth. C. Ward Kischer & Dianne N. Irving. 2nd ed. 1997. LC 97-92690. x, 293p. pap. 10.00 (*0-9660344-0-6*) C W Kischer.

Human Development in Adulthood. L. R. Aiken. 1998. LC 97-51716. (Series in Adult Development & Aging). (Illus.). 416p. (C). 52.50 (*0-306-45734-2*, Plenum Trade) Perseus Pubng.

Human Development in Cultural Context: A Third World Perspective. A. Bame Nsamenang. 1992. (Cross-Cultural Research & Methodology Ser.: Vol. 16). 320p. (C). 96.95 (*0-8039-4636-8*, 3467) Sage.

Human Development Theories: Windows on Culture. Contrib. by R. Murray Thomas. 1999. LC 99-6589. (Developmental Ser.). 271p. 67.95 (*0-7619-2015-3*, 85461) Sage.

Human Diet & Nutrition: A Source Guide. 1991. lib. bdg. 77.90 (*0-8490-4831-1*) Gordon Pr.

Human Digestive System. H. P. Lazar. 1972. (Perspectives in Medicine Ser.: Vol. 4). (Illus.). pap. 16.75 (*3-8055-1429-8*) S Karger.

Human Dignity & Animal Well-Being: A Kantian Contribution to Biomedical Ethics. Mats G. Hansson. 1991. (Uppsala Studies in Social Ethics: No. 12). 210p. (Orig.). pap. 49.50 (*91-554-2681-6*) Coronet Bks.

Human Disease for Dental Students. Ed. by R. N. Baird et al. 1981. 340p. pap. 35.00 (*0-8464-1217-9*) Beekman Pubs.

***Human Disease for Dentists.** Gawkrodger. 2002. text 24.99 (*0-632-06453-6*) Blackwell Sci.

Human Diseases. John H. Dirckx. 1997. LC 98-234807. (Illus.). 350 p. (Orig.). pap. 28.00 (*0-934385-69-6*) Hlth Prof Inst.

***Human Diseases.** Health Professions Institute Staff. 2001. 350p. pap. 40.00 (*0-13-094084-4*) P-H.

Human Diseases. Ruth Tannehill-Jones. 1999. LC 98-55678. (Allied Health Ser.). 454p. (C). pap. text 35.95 (*0-7668-0214-0*) Delmar.

Human Diseases: A Systemic Approach. Mary Lou Mulvihill. 5th ed. 2000. LC 00-51491. (Illus.). 496p. pap. 40.00 (*0-8385-3930-0*) P-H.

Human Diseases: A Systemic Approach: Teachers Manual & Testbank. Pamela J. Carlton et al. 4th ed. 1995. (Illus.). 474p. tchr. ed. (*0-8385-3929-7*, A3929-5) Appleton & Lange.

Human Diseases: Systemic Approach. 5th ed. 2001. (C). 33.33 (*0-8385-3691-3*, Medical Exam) Appleton & Lange.

Human Diseases & Conditions Ed. by Neil Izenberg. 1999. LC 99-51442. (Illus.). (J). 3. 80.00 (*0-684-80621-5*, Macmillan Ref); Set. 912p. 250.00 (*0-684-80543-X*, C Scribners Sons) Gale.

Human Diseases & Conditions, Vol. 2. Contrib. by Gale Group Staff. 2001. suppl. ed. 85.00 net. (*0-684-80664-9*, C Scribners Sons) Gale.

Human Diseases & Conditions Supplement: Human Behavioral Health & Disorders. annuals Ed. by Neil Izenberg. 2000. (Illus.). 300p. suppl. ed. 75.00 (*0-684-80643-6*, C Scribners Sons) Gale.

Human Diseases & Disorders Ed. by Neil Izenberg. 1999. LC 99-51442. (Illus.). (J). Vol. 1. 125.00 (*0-684-80541-3*); Vol. 2. 125.00 (*0-684-80542-1*) S&S Trade.

Human Diseases for Medical Assistants. Jones Staff. 2000. (Medical Assisting Ser.). (Illus.). 352p. pap. 24.00 (*0-7668-1088-7*) Delmar.

Human Diversity: Perspectives on People in Context. Ed. by Edison J. Trickett et al. 1994. LC 94-17753. (Jossey-Bass Social & Behavioral Science Ser.). 512p. 55.00 (*0-7879-0029-X*) Jossey-Bass.

Human DNA: Law & Policy: International & Comparative Perspectives. Ed. by Bartha M. Knoppers et al. 1997. LC 97-25285. 476p. text 142.50 (*90-411-0361-9*) Kluwer Law Intl.

Human Ear Canal: Theoretical Implications & Clinical Considerations Including Cerumen Management. Bopanna B. Ballachanda. 1995. (Illus.). 276p. (C). 85.00 (*1-56593-169-6*, 0478) Thomson Learn.

Human Ecology Thomas S. Robertson. 1973. 560p. 600.00 (*0-87968-340-6*) Gordon Pr.

Human Ecology & Susceptibility to the Chemical Environment. Theron G. Randolph. 1981. (Illus.). 160p. 35.95 (*0-398-01548-1*) C C Thomas.

***Human Effect in Medicine: Theory, Research & Practice.** Michael Dixon & Kieran Sweeney. 2000. 176p. pap. (*1-85775-369-0*) Radcliffe Med Pr GBR. *Dist:* Balogh.

Human Embryo: Aristotle & the Arabic & European Traditions. Ed. by G. R. Dunstan. 1990. (Illus.). 248p. text (*0-85989-340-5*) Univ Exeter Pr GBR. *Dist:* David Brown.

Human Embryology. William J. Larsen. 2nd ed. 1997. LC 97-8214. pap. text (*0-443-07989-7*) Church.

Human Embryology. William J. Larsen. 3rd ed. 2001. (Illus.). 525p. pap. text (*0-443-06583-7*) Harcrt Hlth Sci Grp.

Human Embryology & Developmental Biology. Bruce M. Carlson. 2nd ed. 1999. LC 98-29769. (Illus.). 511p. pap. text 49.00 (*0-8151-1458-3*, 29128) Mosby Inc.

Human Embryology & Teratology. Ronan O'Rahilly & Fabiola Muller. 2nd ed. 1996. LC 95-48297. (Illus.). 480p. 295.00 (*0-471-13351-5*) Wiley.

***Human Embryonic Stem Cell Debate: Science, Ethics, & Public Policy.** Ed. by Suzanne Holland et al. 2001. LC 2001-30624. 70.00 (*0-262-08299-3*); pap. 24.95 (*0-262-58208-2*) MIT Pr.

Human Emotions. C. E. Izard. 1977. LC 77-1989. (Emotions, Personality, & Psychotherapy Ser.). (Illus.). 512p. (C). 55.00 (*0-306-30986-6*, Plenum Trade) Perseus Pubng.

Human Emotions: A Reader. Ed. by Jennifer M. Jenkins et al. 1998. LC 97-38756. (Illus.). 400p. pap. 36.95 (*0-631-20748-1*) Blackwell Pubs.

Human Endometrium. Ed. by Carlo Bulletti et al. 1994. LC 94-28726. (Annals Ser.: Vol. 734). (Illus.). 500p. pap. 155.00 (*0-89766-871-5*) NY Acad Sci.

Human Energy Requirements: A Manual for Planners & Nutritionists. W. P. James & E. C. Schofield. 1990. (Illus.). 182p. text 90.00 (*0-19-261891-1*) OUP.

Human Engineering: The Body Re-Examined. John Lenihan. 1975. LC 74-25318. 212p. 7.95 (*0-8076-0782-7*) Braziller.

Human Enterovirus Infections. Ed. by Harley A. Rotbart. 1994. LC 94-39792. xvi, 445p. 99.95 (*1-55581-092-6*) ASM Pr.

Human Error: Cause, Prediction & Reduction. Ed. by J. Senders & N. Moray. 1991. (Applied Psychology Ser.). 168p. (C). text 34.50 (*0-89859-598-3*) L Erlbaum Assocs.

Human Error in Medicine. Ed. by Marilyn S. Bogner. 1994. 424p. pap. 45.00 (*0-8058-1386-1*); text 89.95 (*0-8058-1385-3*) L Erlbaum Assocs.

Human Ethics in Pediatric Hematology-Oncology. Ed. by John T. Truman & Jan Van Eys. 1986. LC 86-20525. 188p. 60.00 (*0-275-92263-4*, C2263, Praeger Pubs) Greenwood.

Human Ethology. Irenaus Eibl-Eibesfeldt. 1989. (Evolutionary Foundations of Human Behavior Ser.).Tr. of Biologie des menschlichen Verhaltens: Grundriss der Humanethologie. (Illus.). 863p. lib. bdg. 79.95 (*0-202-02030-4*) Aldine de Gruyter.

Human Evolution. Ed. by M. H. Day. 1973. (Symposia of the Society for the Study of Human Biology Ser.: Vol. 11). 162p. 36.00 (*0-85066-061-0*) Taylor & Francis.

Human Exceptionality: School, Family & Society. Michael L. Hardman et al. 3rd ed. 1990. 576p. text 45.00 (*0-205-12372-4*, H23724) Allyn.

Human Experimentation: Index of Modern Authors & Subjects with Guide for Rapid Research. Douglas R. Conway. 1991. LC 90-56253. 200p. 47.50 (*1-55914-288-X*); pap. 44.50 (*1-55914-289-8*) ABBE Pubs Assn.

Human Experimentation: Methodologic Issues Fundamental to Clinical Trials. Ton J. Cleophas. 1999. LC 99-33163. (*0-7923-5827-9*) Kluwer Academic.

Human Experimentation: When Research is Evil. Ed. by Gary E. McCuen. 1998. (Ideas in Conflict Ser.). (Illus.). 176p. (YA). (gr. 7-12). lib. bdg. 15.95 (*0-86596-144-1*) G E M.

Human Experimentation & Medical Ethics: XVth CIOMS Round Table Conference. Z. Bankowski & N. Howard-Jones. 1982. (CIOMS Round Table Proceedings Ser.: No. 15). text 30.00 (*92-9036-009-7*) World Health.

Human Factor in Nursing Home Care. Ed. by David B. Oliver & Sally Tureman. 1988. LC 87-36625. (Activities, Adaptation & Aging Ser.: Vol. 10, Nos. 3 & 4). (Illus.). 202p. text 39.95 (*0-86656-715-1*); pap. text 14.95 (*0-86656-732-1*) Haworth Pr.

Human Factor in the Behavior of Peoples. Thorne Deuel. 1971. (Scientific Papers: Vol. XIII). (Illus.). 204p. pap. 5.75 (*0-89792-047-3*) Ill St Museum.

Human Factors & Safety. Jeremy Stranks. 1994. (Health & Safety in Practice Ser.). 192p. (Orig.). pap. (*0-273-60440-6*) Pitman Pub GBR. *Dist:* Trans-Atl Phila.

Human Factors, Engineering Guidelines, & Preferred Practices for the Design of Medical Devices. 1993. (American National Standard Ser.). 46p. pap. 90.00 (*1-57020-004-1*, HE48-209) Assn Adv Med Instrn.

Human Factors in Air Traffic Control. Ed. by Mark W. Smolensky & Earl S. Stein. 1998. LC 97-80792. (Illus.). 477p. text 75.00 (*0-12-653010-6*) Morgan Kaufmann.

Human Factors Research Needs for an Aging Population. National Research Council Staff. 1990. 110p. pap. text 15.00 (*0-309-04178-3*) Natl Acad Pr.

Human Factors Testing & Evaluation. David Meister. 1986. (Advances in Human Factors-Ergonomics Ser.: No. 5). 424p. 204.50 (*0-444-42701-5*) Elsevier.

Human Feelings: Explorations in Affect Development & Meaning. Ed. by Steven L. Ablon et al. 1993. LC 93-14309. 456p. text 59.95 (*0-88163-144-2*) Analytic Pr.

***Human Fertilisation & Embryology: Regulating the Reproductive Revolution.** Robert G. Lee & Derek Morgan. 2001. LC 2001-616084. (C). pap. (*1-84174-119-1*) Blackstone Pr GBR. *Dist:* Intl Spec Bk.

Human Fertility: Problems, Aids, Drugs & Reults: Index of New Information. Jerry J. Kerley. 1998. 57.50 (*0-7883-1842-X*); pap. 47.50 (*0-7883-1843-8*) ABBE Pubs Assn.

Human Fertility: The Basic Components. Henri Leridon. Tr. by Judith F. Helzner from FRE. 1977. LC 77-1913. 208p. lib. bdg. 25.50 (*0-226-47297-3*) U Ch Pr.

Human Fertility: The Modern Dilemma. Robert C. Cook. 1971. LC 72-156185. 380p. reprint ed. lib. bdg. 80.00 (*0-8371-6128-2*, COHU, Greenwood Pr) Greenwood.

***Human Fertility & Reproduction: The Oocyte, the Embryo, & the Uterus.** Ed. by Carlo Bulletti et al. 2001. 375p. 140.00 (*1-57331-332-7*) NY Acad Sci.

Human Fertility Behaviour in the Desert Margin. A. K. Tiwari. 1980. 86p. (C). (*0-7855-1969-6*) Scientific GBR. *Dist:* St Mut.

Human Figure Drawing Test, HFDT: An Illustrated Handbook for Clinical Interpretation & Standardized Assessment of Cognitive Impairment. Jerry Mitchell et al. 1993. (Illus.). 182p. pap. 49.50 (*0-87424-286-X*, W-286A) Western Psych.

Human Frontal Lobes: Functions & Disorders. Ed. by Bruce L. Miller & Jeffrey L. Cummings. 1998. LC 98-36944. (Science & Practice of Neuropsychology Ser.). 616p. 80.00 (*1-57230-390-5*, C0390) Guilford Pubns.

***Human Frontiers, Environments & Disease.** A. J. McMichael. 2001. LC 2001-273445. (Illus.). 430p. text 59.95 (*0-521-80311-X*) Cambridge U Pr.

Human Gait. W. Braune & O. Fischer. 1987. (Illus.). 440p. 234.00 (*0-387-15270-9*) Spr-Verlag.

Human Gene Mapping 6, Oslo 1981. Ed. by Kare Berg et al. 1982. (Journal: Vol. 32, No. 1-4). (Illus.). viii, 320p. pap. 94.00 (*3-8055-3559-7*) S Karger.

Human Gene Mapping 9-5: Ninth International Workshop, New Haven, Connecticut, August 1988. Ed. by K. K. Kidd et al. 1988. (Journal: Vol. 49, No. 1-3). (Illus.). viii, 260p. pap. 62.75 (*3-8055-4938-5*) S Karger.

Human Gene Mapping Eight: Eighth International Workshop on Human Gene Mapping, Helsinki, Finland, August 1985. Ed. by A. De la Chapelle. 1985. (Journal: Vol. 40, No. 1-4, 1985). (Illus.). vi, 824p. pap. 139.25 (*3-8055-4248-8*) S Karger.

Human Gene Mapping London Conference, No. 11: International Workshop on Human Gene Mapping, New Connaught Rooms, London, U. K., August 1991. Set. Ed. by E. Solomon & C. Rawlings. 1992. (Journal: Vol. 58, Nos. 1-4, 1991). (Illus.). viii, 2200p. pap. 519.25 (*3-8055-5572-5*) S Karger.

Human Gene Mapping Nine: Journal: Cytogenetics & Cell Genetics, Vol. 46, Nos. 1-4, 1987. Ed. by J. Frezal & H. P. Klinger. 1988. (Illus.). 272p. pap. 168.75 (*3-8055-4795-1*) S Karger.

Human Gene Mapping Seven: Seventh International Workshop, Los Angeles, August 1983. Ed. by H. P. Klinger et al. 1983. (Journal: Vol. 37, No. 1-4). (Illus.). vi, 666p. pap. 98.50 (*3-8055-3840-5*) S Karger.

Human Gene Mapping Three: Proceedings - Journal: Cytogenetics & Cell Genetics, Vol. 16, Nos. 1-5. Baltimore Conference Staff. Ed. by Daniel Bergsma. 1976. (Illus.). 420p. pap. 95.75 (*3-8055-2345-9*) S Karger.

Human Gene Mapping Two: Proceedings of the Rotterdam Conference, 1974 - Journal: Cytogenetics & Cell Genetics, Vol. 14, Nos. 3-6. Rotterdam Conference Staff. Ed. by Daniel Bergsma. 1975. (Illus.). 332p. pap. 68.75 (*3-8055-2251-7*) S Karger.

Human Gene Therapy. 1993. 219p. 2650.00 (*0-89336-955-1*, C-160) BCC.

Human Gene Therapy. James W. Hawkins. 1995. (Illus.). 474p. spiral bd. 2950.00 (*1-57936-049-1*, 906) Drug & Market Dev.

Human Gene Therapy. Eve K. Nichols & Institute of Medicine Staff. 1988. LC 88-574. 264p. pap. text 14.50 (*0-674-41480-2*) HUP.

***Human Gene Therapy.** James W. Hawkins. Ed. by Susan C. DiClemente. 2nd rev. ed. 1998. (Illus.). 754p. 4950.00 (*1-57936-122-6*, 937) International Business.

Human Genetic Information: Science, Law & Ethics. CIBA Foundation Staff. 1990. LC 89-70550. (CIBA Foundation Symposia Ser.: No. 149). 222p. 128.00 (*0-471-92624-8*) Wiley.

Human Genetics. 1996. LC 96-143232. pap. (*0-86153-208-2*) St Andrew Press GBR. *Dist:* St Mut.

Human Genetics. John B. Jenkins. 1983. 488p. text 43.25 (*0-8053-5010-1*) Benjamin-Cummings.

Human Genetics: A Problem Based Approach. Bruce R. Korf. (Illus.). 1996. LC 96-228925. 512p. pap. text 42.95 (*0-86542-353-9*); 2nd ed. 1999. LC 99-30762. pap. 50.95 (*0-632-04425-X*) Blackwell Sci.

Human Genetics: Choice & Responsibility. British Medical Association Staff. 1998. (Illus.). 250p. pap. text 26.50 (*0-19-288055-1*) OUP.

Human Genetics: Concepts & Applications. Ricki Lewis. (C). 1994. 416p. text, stu. ed. 20.62 (*0-697-20817-6*, WCB McGr Hill); 1993. 160p. spiral bd., wbk. ed. 28.44 (*0-697-22287-X*); 2nd ed. 1996. LC 96-85271. 427p. text 56.55 (*0-697-24030-4*, WCB McGr Hill) McGrw-H Hghr Educ.

Human Genetics: Problems & Approaches. F. Vogel & A. G. Motulsky. 3rd rev. ed. 1997. (Illus.). 900p. 105.00 (*3-540-60290-9*) Spr-Verlag.

Human Genetics & Public Health. 1964. (Technical Report Ser.: No. 282). 38p. pap. text 5.00 (*92-4-120282-3*) World Health.

Human Genome. Tom Strachan. 1992. (Medical Perspectives Ser.). 170p. (Orig.). pap. (*1-872748-80-5*) Bios Sci GBR. *Dist:* Coronet Bks.

Human Genome Project. Ed. by Marianne Postiglione. 1993. (Illus.). iv, 286p. (Orig.). pap. 15.95 (*0-9625431-6-0*) ITEST Faith.

Human Genome Project: How Private Sector Developments Affect the Government Program: Hearing Before the Subcommittee on Energy & Environment of the Committee on Science, U. S. House of Representatives, One Hundred Fifth Congress, Second Session, June 17, 1998. Contrib. by U. S. Congress, House Committee on Science, Subcommittee on Energy and Environment. 1998. LC 99-181549. (Illus.). (*0-16-057661-X*) USGPO.

Human Genome Project & the Future of Health Care. Ed. by Thomas H. Murray et al. 1996. LC 96-1718. (Medical Ethics Ser.). (Illus.). 264p. 29.95 (*0-253-33213-3*) Ind U Pr.

Human-Gentechnik, Naturteleologie und Ethik: Moralisch-Ethische Probleme von Reproduktionsmedizin und Human-Gentechnik. Freddy Zulicke. 1994. (Europaische Hochschulschriften Ser.: Bd. 433). (GER.). 196p. 37.95 (*3-631-47506-3*) P Lang Pubng.

Human Germ-Line Therapy: Scientific, Moral & Political Issues. David Resnik et al. 1999. LC 98-43505. (Medical Intelligence Unit Ser.: Vol. 9). 189p. 99.00 (*1-57059-586-0*) Landes Bioscience.

Human Growth & Development. Jack Rudman. 1994. (College Level Examination Ser.: CLEP-17). pap. 27.95 (*0-8373-5317-3*) Nat Learn.

Human Growth & Development: A Psychological Approach. Frank Wesley & Edith Sullivan. 2nd ed. 1986. LC 79-21929. 326p. 45.95 (0-89885-316-8); pap. 25.95 (0-89885-317-6) Kluwer Academic (Kluwer Acad Hman Sci).

Human Growth & Development Throughout Life: A Nursing Perspective. Patty M. Hill & Patricia Humphrey. 2nd ed. 1989. LC 81-16472. 496p. text 34.95 (0-8273-4257-8) Delmar.

Human Growth Hormone. Ed. by Salvatore Raiti & Robert A. Tolman. 1986. LC 86-3288. (Illus.). 676p. (C). text 174.00 (0-306-42053-8, Kluwer Plenum) Kluwer Academic.

Human Growth Hormone: Basic & Clinical Aspects. Ed. by Kathleen T. Shiverick & Arlan Rosenbloom. 1995. LC 94-30842. (Pharmacology & Toxicology: Basic & Clinical Aspects Ser.). 192p. 129.95 (0-8493-8384-6) CRC Pr.

Human Growth Hormone: Research & Clinical Practice. Roy G. Smith & Michael O. Thorner. 2000. LC 99-42873. (Contemporary Endocrinology Ser.: Vol. 19). (Illus.). 360p. 135.00 (0-89603-505-0) Humana.

Human Growth, Physical Fitness & Nutrition. Ed. by Roy J. Shephard & Jane Parizkova. 1991. (Medicine & Sport Science Ser.: Vol. 31). (Illus.). viii, 172p. 152.25 (3-8055-5275-0) S Karger.

Human Growth Variation. Graham. 1998. text (0-7216-3664-0) Saunders.

Human Health. Robley Dunglison. Ed. by Barbara G. Rosenkrantz. 1977. LC 76-25660. (Public Health in America Ser.). reprint ed. lib. bdg. 39.95 (0-405-09815-4) Ayer.

Human Health: The Contributions of Microorganisms. Ed. by S. A. W. Gibson. 1994. LC 93-49559. (Springer Series in Applied Biology). (Illus.). 191p. 124.00 (0-387-19871-7) Spr-Verlag.

Human Health & Environment, Vol. 1 & 2. Ed. by A. K. Sinha et al. 1997. ix, 615p. (81-7024-846-9) APH Pubng IND. *Dist:* Nataraj Bks.

Human Health & the Environment. Weir & Smith. 1991. (0-8151-9196-0) Mosby Inc.

Human Health Risk-Based Evaluation of Petroleum Contaminated Site: Implementation of the Working Group Approach. Wade Weisman & Donna Vorhees. 1998. (Total Petroleum Hydrocarbon Criteria Working Group Ser.: Vol. 5). (Illus.). 100p. pap. 19.95 (1-884940-20-X) Amherst Sci Pubs.

Human Health Risks from Chemical Exposure: Great Lakes Ecosystem. Warren R. Flint. 1991. 272p. lib. bdg. 119.00 (0-87371-435-0, L435) Lewis Pubs.

Human Heart: A Basic Guide to Heart Disease. Brendan Phibbs. 1997. LC 96-35094. (Illus.). 272p. pap. text 45.00 (0-316-70513-6, Little Brwn Med Div) Lppncott W & W.

Human Heart Replacement: A New Challenge for Physicians & Reporters. Ed. by Sandra Blakeslee & Dale E. Shaps. 1986. LC 86-82064. 99p. (Orig.). pap. 5.00 (0-910755-04-3) Foun Am Comm.

Human Hemoglobin Genetics. G. R. Honig & J. G. Adams, III. 1986. (Illus.). 467p. 135.00 (0-387-81872-3) Spr-Verlag.

Human Heredity: Principles & Issues. Michael R. Cummings. 3rd ed. 1993. LC 93-26154. 500p. (C). text 60.25 (0-314-02747-5) West Pub.

Human Hippocampus. Henri M. Duvernoy. 1988. (Illus.). 160p. 125.00 (0-387-00375-4) Spr-Verlag.

Human Hippocampus: Functional Anatomy, Vascularization & Serial Sections with MRI. Henri M. Duvernoy & P. Bourgouin. 2nd exp. rev. ed. 1997. LC 97-35996. (Illus.). 213p. 175.00 (3-540-63205-0) Spr-Verlag.

Human Histology. Alan Stevens & James S. Lowe. 2nd ed. 1996. 408p. pap. 46.00 (0-7234-2485-3) Mosby Inc.

Human Histology. Alan Stevens & James S. Lowe. 2nd ed. 1996. (Illus.). 416p. pap. (84-8174-282-1) Mosby-Doyma Libros ESP. *Dist:* Mosby Inc.

Human Histology, Cytology & Microanatomy. Helmut Leonhardt. 4th ed. 1977. (Illus.). pap. 20.95 (0-8151-5375-9) Mosby Inc.

Human Hybridomas & Monoclonal Antibodies. Ed. by Edgar G. Engleman et al. 1985. LC 85-12401. 550p. 115.00 (0-306-41982-3, Plenum Trade) Perseus Pubng.

Human Hypothalamus in Health & Disease: Proceedings of the 17th International Summer School of Brain Research, Held at the Auditorium of the University of Amsterdam, the Netherlands, 26-30 August 1991. Ed. by D. F. Swaab et al. 1992. LC 92-18423. (Progress in Brain Research Ser.: Vol. 93). 482p. 339.50 (0-444-89538-8) Elsevier.

Human Identification: Case Studies in Forensic Anthropology. Ed. by Ted A. Rathbun & Jane E. Buikstra. 1984. (Illus.). 456p. (C). 91.95 (0-398-04875-4) C C Thomas.

Human Ig Genetic Markers. Ed. by R. Grubb & Gerda G. De Lange. 1988. (Journal: Vol. 6, No. 1, 1989). (Illus.). 132p. pap. 76.75 (3-8055-4910-5) S Karger.

Human Immunodeficiency Virus: Innovative Techniques for Isolation & Identification of HIV & for Monitoring of AIDS Patients. Ed. by Joseph L. Melnick & N. C. Khan. 1990. (Monographs in Virology: Vol. 18). viii, 130p. 116.75 (3-8055-5182-7) S Karger.

Human Immunodeficiency Virus & the Lung. Ed. by Mark J. Rosen & James M. Beck. 1998. LC 98-7847. (Lung Biology in Health & Disease Ser.). (Illus.). 584p. text 215.00 (0-8247-9883-X) Dekker.

Human Immunodeficiency Virus Epidemic: A National Strategy to Slow Or Stop the Spread of the Virus, to Provide Care for Those Who Have Contracted the Virus & to Protect the Rights of Both Infected & Non-Infected Persons. 1992. lib. bdg. 88.00 (0-8490-5506-7) Gordon Pr.

Human Immunodeficiency Virus Type 1, Reference Material Specifications: Approved Guideline (1991) Contrib. by Thomas A. O'Brian. 1991. 95.00 (1-56238-134-2, I/LA13-A) NCCLS.

Human Immunodeficiency Viruses & Human T-Cell Lymphotropic Viruses: IARC Monographs on the Evaluation of Carcinogenic Risks to Humans. 1997. (IARC Scientific Publications Ser.: No. 67). 424p. pap. 72.00 (92-832-1267-3, 1720067) Am Soc Clinical.

Human Immunogenetics: Basic Principles & Clinical Relevance. Stephen D. Litwin. 1989. (Immunology Ser.: Vol. 43). (Illus.). 856p. text 250.00 (0-8247-7899-5) Dekker.

Human Immunogenetics: Principles & Clinical Applications. J. E. Bernal. Tr. by D. F. Roberts. 1986. LC 86-5677. 220p. 99.95 (0-85066-355-5); pap. 44.95 (0-85066-334-2) Taylor & Francis.

Human Implantation: Cell Biology & Immunology. Y. W. Loke & Ashley King. 1996. 313p. (C). text 85.00 (0-521-44193-5) Cambridge U Pr.

Human In Vitro Fertilization: A Case Study in the Regulation of Medical Innovation. Jennifer Gunning & Veronica English. 1993. LC 93-24213. (Medico-Legal Issues Ser.). 232p. (1-85521-347-8) Dartmth Pub GBR. *Dist:* Ashgate Pub Co.

Human in Vitro Fertilization & Embryo Transfer. Ed. by Don P. Wolf & Martin M. Quigley. 1984. LC 83-27133. 456p. 95.00 (0-306-41623-9, Plenum Trade) Perseus Pubng.

Human Insulin. D. R. Owens. 1986. text 206.50 (0-85200-951-8) Kluwer Academic.

Human Insulin by Tryptic Transpeptidations of Porcine Insulin & Biosynthetic Precursors. J. Markussen. 1987. text 144.00 (0-7462-0058-7) Kluwer Academic.

Human Intellect & Cognitive Science: Towards a General Unified Theory of Intelligence. Morton Wagman. 1996. LC 95-24233. 192p. 62.50 (0-275-95179-0, Praeger Pubs) Greenwood.

Human Intelligence: Perspectives on Its Theory & Measurement. Ed. by Robert J. Sternberg & Douglas K. Detterman. 1979. LC 79-17994. 272p. 77.00 (0-89391-030-9, Ablex) Greenwood.

Human Kinesiology: Applications to Physical Rehabilitation. Neumann. 2000. (Illus.). 496p. (gr. 13). text 42.95 (0-8151-6349-5, 23746) Mosby Inc.

Human Lactation, Vol. 2: Maternal & Environmental Factors. Ed. by Margit Hamosh & Armond S. Goldman. 1986. LC 86-20537. 672p. 120.00 (0-306-42389-8, Plenum Trade) Perseus Pubng.

Human Lead Exposure. Herbert L. Needleman. 1991. 290p. lib. bdg. 199.00 (0-8493-6034-X, RC347) CRC Pr.

Human Learned Helplessness: A Coping Perspective. M. Mikulincer. 1994. (Series in Social/Clinical Psychology). (Illus.). 324p. (C). 49.50 (0-306-44743-6, Plenum Trade) Perseus Pubng.

Human Leukemia. Dion & Aaron Polliack. 1984. text 307.50 (0-89838-585-7) Kluwer Academic.

Human Leukemias. Aaron Polliack. 1984. (Developments in Oncology Ser.). lib. bdg. 115.00 (90-247-2338-8) Kluwer Academic.

Human Life: Considered in Its Present Condition & Future Developments. William Sweetser. Ed. by Robert J. Kastenbaum. 1979. LC 78-22219. (Aging & Old Age Ser.). reprint ed. lib. bdg. 30.95 (0-405-11832-5) Ayer.

Human Life & Health Care Ethics. Ed. by James Bopp, Jr. 1985. LC 84-29133. 320p. lib. bdg. 55.00 (0-313-27064-3, U7064, Greenwood Pr) Greenwood.

Human Life & Medical Practice. J. K. Mason. 1990. pap. text (0-85224-584-X) Edinburgh U Pr GBR. *Dist:* Col U Pr.

Human Life Expectancy - Experiences & Analyses: Index of New Information with Authors, Subjects & References. Science and Life Consultants Association Staff. rev. ed. 1995. LC 95-15407. 199p. 57.60 (0-7883-0648-0); pap. 47.50 (0-7883-0649-9) ABBE Pubs Assn.

Human Longevity. David W. Smith. 1993. LC 92-49136. (Illus.). 192p. (C). text 37.50 (0-19-508313-X) OUP.

Human Longevity: Its Fact & Its Fiction. William J. Thomas. Ed. by Robert J. Kastenbaum. 1979. LC 78-22220. (Aging & Old Age Ser.). reprint ed. lib. bdg. 27.95 (0-405-11833-3) Ayer.

Human Longevity - Analysis, Influences, Measures, Risks, Varieties & Maintenance: Index of New Information with Authors & Subjects. Rosemary H. Booker. rev. ed. 1997. 164p. 57.50 (0-7883-1512-9); 1997. 164p. pap. 47.50 (0-7883-1513-7); 1996. 180p. pap. 47.50 (0-7883-0953-6) ABBE Pubs Assn.

Human Lymphoma: Clinical Implications of the Real Classification. D. Y. Mason & Nancy L. Harris. 1999. LC 98-49714. 352p. 275.00 (1-85233-129-1) Spr-Verlag.

Human Machine. R. McNeill Alexander. 1992. LC 92-10517. (Illus.). 224p. (C). 41.00 (0-231-08066-2) Col U Pr.

Human Machine: How It Breaks Down. Acierno. 1989. 390p. (C). pap. text 85.00 (0-536-57360-3) Pearson Custom.

Human Macrophage-System Activity & Functional Morphology. Horst Michna. 1988. (Bibliotheca Anatomica Ser.: No. 31). (Illus.). xii, 84p. 81.75 (3-8055-4641-6) S Karger.

Human Malformations, Set. Ed. by Roger E. Stevenson et al. 1993. (Illus.). 1800p. text 295.00 (0-19-506232-9) OUP.

Human Malignancies. Ed. by D. Drahovsky & B. Kornhuber. 1989. (Illus.). 160p. 35.95 (0-387-19219-0) Spr-Verlag.

Human Mechanisms. Gerald Etra. 1994. (Illus.). 200p. (Orig.). (C). pap. text, stu. ed. 17.00 (1-878045-27-X) Whittier Pubns.

Human Medicinal Agents from Plants. Ed. by A. Douglas Kinghorn & Manuel F. Balandrin. 1993. LC 93-22180. (ACS Symposium Ser.: Vol. 534). (Illus.). 359p. 100.00 (0-8412-2705-5) Am Chemical.

Human Medicine: Ethical Perspective on Today's Medical Issues. James B. Nelson & Jo A. Rohricht. exp. rev. ed. 1984. LC 84-12411. 224p. (Orig.). pap. 18.99 (0-8066-2086-2, 10-3187, Augsburg) Augsburg Fortress.

Human Memory: A Multi-Modal Approach. Johannes EngelKamp & Hubert D. Zimmer. 1994. LC 93-36825. (Illus.). 532p. (C). text 54.00 (0-88937-116-4) Hogrefe & Huber Pubs.

Human Memory: An Introduction to Research, Data, & Theory. Ian Neath. 1997. LC 97-24356. (Psychology Ser.). 450p. pap. text 71.95 (0-534-34197-7) Brooks-Cole.

Human Memory: Exploration & Application. Karl Haberlandt. 1998. LC 98-16954. 373p. pap. 63.00 (0-205-18992-X) Allyn.

Human Memory: The Processing of Information. Geoffrey R. Loftus & Elizabeth F. Loftus. 1976. 192p. pap. text 27.50 (0-89859-135-X) L Erlbaum Assocs.

Human Memory: Theory, Research & Individual Differences, Vol. 22. Michael W. Eysenck. 1977. (0-08-020405-8) Pergamon Repr GBR. *Dist:* Franklin.

Human Memory & Cognition. Mark H. Ashcraft. 2nd ed. 1997. LC 93-32908. 650p. (C). pap. 98.00 (0-673-46789-9) Addson-Wesley Educ.

Human Metabolism of Alcohol Ed. by Crow. 1989. I. 224p. lib. bdg. 159.00 (0-8493-4521-9, QP801); Vol. 2. 280p. 195.00 (0-8493-4522-7, QP801); Vol. 3. 248p. 195.00 (0-8493-4523-5) CRC Pr.

Human Microbial Ecology. Ed. by Michael J. Hill & Philip D. Marsh. 1989. 162p. 159.00 (0-8493-4201-5, QR171) CRC Pr.

Human Milk & Infant Development. Ed. by Margit Hamosh. 1998. (Biology of the Neonate Ser.: Vol. 74, No. 2). (Illus.). 118p. pap. 59.25 (3-8055-6738-3) S Karger.

Human Milk Fat Globule Membrane Antigens as Diagnostic Markers for Ovarian Carcinoma. P. Ashorn. 1987. 117p. (Orig.). pap. 38.50 (951-44-2127-2) Coronet Bks.

Human Mind in Its Relations with the Brain & Nervous System. Daniel Noble. LC 78-72817. (Brainedness, Handedness, & Mental Abilities Ser.). reprint ed. 37.50 (0-404-60886-8) AMS Pr.

Human Mind Revisited: Essays in Honor of Karl A. Menninger. Ed. by Sidney Smith. 1978. LC 77-92363. 503p. 75.00 (0-8236-2370-X) Intl Univs Pr.

Human Monkeypox. Z. Jezek & Frank Fenner. 1988. (Monographs in Virology: Vol. 17). (Illus.). x, 142p. 108.75 (3-8055-4818-4) S Karger.

Human Monocytes. Ed. by M. Zembala & G. L. Asherson. 1989. 553p. text 146.00 (0-12-779440-9) Acad Pr.

Human Motion Analysis: Current Applications & Future Directions. Gerald F. Harris & Peter A. Smith. 1996. LC 95-41085. (Tab-IEEE Press Book Ser.). 480p. 89.95 (0-7803-1111-6, PC4648) Inst Electrical.

Human Motivation. Yoshio Kondo. 1991. 200p. pap. text (4-906224-64-4, 224644) Three A JPN. *Dist:* Qual Resc.

Human Motivation. Bernard Weiner. 1989. 480p. reprint ed. 79.95 (0-8058-0711-X) L Erlbaum Assocs.

Human Motivation. Robert E. Franken. 2nd ed. 1988. LC 87-29959. 545p. (C). mass mkt. 47.25 (0-534-08988-7); 3rd ed. 1993. LC 93-30440. mass mkt. 57.75 (0-534-15612-6) Brooks-Cole.

Human Motivation & Emotion. Ross W. Buck. 2nd ed. 1988. LC 87-31636. 704p. 62.95 (0-471-89705-1) Wiley.

Human Motivation & the Dynamic Calculus. Raymond B. Cattell. 1985. LC 84-15153. 164p. 49.95 (0-275-90071-1, C0071, Praeger Pubs) Greenwood.

Human Motives. James J. Putnam. 1973. LC 73-2413. (Mental Illness & Social Policy; the American Experience Ser.). reprint ed. 19.95 (0-405-05223-5) Ayer.

Human Motor Behavior: An Introduction. Ed. by J. A. Kelso. 1982. (Illus.). 320p. text 45.00 (0-89859-188-0) L Erlbaum Assocs.

Human Motor Control. David A. Rosenbaum. 1990. LC 90-1063. 411p. (C). text 49.95 (0-12-597030-4) Acad Pr.

Human Motor Development: A Lifespan Approach. V. Gregory Payne & Larry D. Isaacs. 4th ed. 1998. LC 98-13523. xxii, 474p. pap. text 51.95 (0-7674-0523-4, 0523-4) Mayfield Pub.

***Human Movement: An Introductory Text.** Marion Trew & Tony S. Everett. 2001. (Illus.). 323p. pap. (0-443-07068-7) Church GBR. *Dist:* Saunders.

Human Muscular Function During Dynamic Exercise. Ed. by J. Poortmans et al. 1996. (Medicine & Sport Science Ser.: Vol. 41, 1996). (Illus.). viii, 152p. pap. 159.25 (3-8055-6274-8) S Karger.

Human Nature Pt. 1: The Unwritten Law. Ken Zenka. unabr. ed. 1996. 301p. (YA). (gr. 12-13). 24.95 (0-9654901-0-6, 1) Galaxy IN.

Human Nature & Management: Application of Psychology to Executive Leadership. Ordway Tead. Ed. by Leon Stein. 1977. LC 77-70537. reprint ed. lib. bdg. 31.95 (0-405-10207-0) Ayer.

Human Nature & Natural Knowledge. Ed. by Alan Donagan et al. 1985. 396p. text 191.50 (90-277-1974-8) Kluwer Academic.

Human Nature & Public Policy: Scientific Views of Women, Children, & Families. Ed. by Lynette Friedrich-Cofer. 1986. LC 86-18210. 359p. 77.00 (0-275-92344-4, C2344, Praeger Pubs) Greenwood.

Human Needs & Behavior. Frederick Samuels. 1984. LC 84-5337. 240p. 19.95 (0-87073-697-3); pap. 15.95 (0-87073-698-1) Schenkman Bks Inc.

Human Nervous System. Ed. by George T. Paxinos. 1990. 1195p. text 99.00 (0-12-547625-6) Acad Pr.

Human Nervous System: Introduction & Review. Charles R. Noback et al. 4th ed. 1991. LC 90-5882. (Illus.). 448p. text 39.00 (0-8121-1343-8) Lppncott W & W.

Human Neuroblastoma: Recent Advances in Clinical & Genetic Analysis. Ed. by Manfred Schwab et al. 1993. LC 92-48891. 270p. text 105.00 (3-7186-5353-2) Gordon & Breach.

Human Neurophysiology. Oliver Wendell Holmes. 2nd ed. 1996. (Illus.). 504p. pap. (0-412-48920-1) E A GBR. *Dist:* OUP.

Human Neurophysiology. Oliver Wendell Holmes. 1990. (Illus.). 350p. (C). text 80.00 (0-04-612041-6); pap. text 34.95 (0-04-612042-4) Routledge.

Human Neuropsychology. G. Neil Martin. 1998. LC 97-11667. 514p. pap. text 71.00 (0-13-802331-X) P-H.

Human Nonverbal Behavior: An Annotated Bibliography. Compiled by Constance E. Obudho. 1979. LC 79-7586. 196p. lib. bdg. 59.95 (0-313-21094-2, OBH/, Greenwood Pr) Greenwood.

Human Nutrition. Guthrie. 1995. tchr. ed. 14.06 (0-8151-4046-0) Mosby Inc.

Human Nutrition. Helen A. Guthrie & Mary F. Picciano. 1994. LC 94-38703. (Illus.). 800p. (C). text 84.06 (0-8151-4043-6) McGrw-H Hghr Educ.

Human Nutrition. Benjamin T. Burton. 3rd ed. 1975. (Illus.). text 39.95 (0-07-009282-6) McGraw.

Human Nutrition. R. F. Mottram. 3rd ed. 1979. 179p. pap. 30.00 (0-917678-09-5) Food & Nut Pr.

Human Nutrition: A Health Perspective. Mary E. Barisi. 1997. LC 97-218916. (Arnold Publication). (Illus.). 336p. pap. text 34.50 (0-340-64567-9) OUP.

Human Nutrition & Animal Feeding. Ed. by Geoffrey H. Bourne. 1981. (World Review of Nutrition & Dietetics Ser.: Vol. 37). (Illus.). xii, 292p. 215.00 (3-8055-2143-X) S Karger.

Human Nutrition & Diet. Ed. by Geoffrey H. Bourne. 1981. (World Review of Nutrition & Dietetics Ser.: Vol. 36). (Illus.). x, 226p. 167.00 (3-8055-1347-X) S Karger.

Human Nutrition & Metabolism. Sara M. Hunt & James L. Groff. Ed. by Marshall. 1990. 517p. (C). text 68.50 (0-314-57936-2) West Pub.

Human Nutrition & Nutrition & Pesticides in Cattle. Ed. by Geoffrey H. Bourne. 1980. (World Review of Nutrition & Dietetics Ser.: Vol. 35). (Illus.). 238p. 167.00 (3-8055-0442-X) S Karger.

Human Nutrition & Obesity. Ed. by Stanley G. Korenman & David Heber. 1999. LC 99-33358. (Atlas of Clinical Endocrinology Ser.: Vol. 5). (Illus.). xiii, 226p. 125.00 (0-632-04401-2) Blackwell Sci.

Human Nutrition in the Developing World. FAO Staff. 1997. LC 98-103490. (Food & Nutrition Ser.: No. 29). 508p. pap. (92-5-103818-X, F3818X) FAO ITA. *Dist:* Bernan Associates.

Human Nutrition, Report No. 2: Benefits from Nutrition Research. U. S. Department of Agriculture Staff. 1992. 129p. (Orig.). pap. 9.95 (0-9634791-8-0) Blue Danube Pub.

Human Nutrition Research. Ed. by Gary R. Beecher. 1981. LC 79-91006. (Beltsville Symposia in Agricultural Research Ser.: No. 4). (Illus.). 318p. text 56.50 (0-916672-48-4) Rowman.

Human Obesity - Treatment & Therapy: Index of Authors & Subjects. Georgette R. Darvonne. rev. ed. 1995. LC 95-15284. 177p. 57.50 (0-7883-0670-7) ABBE Pubs Assn.

Human Odyssey: Life-Span Development. Paul S. Kaplan. Ed. by Marshall. 2nd ed. 1992. LC 92-9148. 575p. (C). mass mkt. 44.00 (0-314-00843-8) West Pub.

Human Odyssey: Life-Span Development. Kaplan Staff. 3rd ed. 1997. LC 97-19669. (Psychology Ser.). 603p. (C). spiral bd. 80.95 (0-534-34951-X) Brooks-Cole.

Human Oncogenic Viruses: Molecular Analysis & Diagnosis. Ed. by Albert A. Luderer & Howard H. Weetall. 1986. LC 86-7518. (Oncogenes Ser.). (Illus.). 281p. 145.00 (0-89603-088-1) Humana.

Human Organ Transplantation: A Report on Developments under the Auspices of Who (1987-1991) 1991. (ENG & FRE.). 28p. reprint ed. pap. text 8.00 (92-4-169304-5, 1959101) World Health.

Human Organic Memory Disorders. Andrew R. Mayes. 1988. (Problems in the Behavioral Sciences Ser.: No. 7).

H I

(Illus.). 312p. text 85.00 (*0-521-34418-2*); pap. text 29.95 (*0-521-34879-X*) Cambridge U Pr.

Human Osteology. Tim D. White. 2nd ed. 1999. LC 99-61961. (Illus.). xxiii, 563p. 69.95 (*0-12-746612-6*) Acad Pr.

Human Osteology: A Laboratory & Field Manual. William M. Bass. 4th rev. ed. 1995. (Special Publications: No.2). (Illus.). 361p. (C). spiral bd. 25.00 (*0-943414-81-4*, 140240) MO Arch Soc.

Human Paleopsychology: Applications to Aggression & Pathological Processes. Kent G. Bailey. 1986. 568p. (C). text 115.00 (*0-89859-810-9*) L Erlbaum Assocs.

Human Papillomavirus Infection in Dermatovenerology. Gerd Gross & Geo Von Krough. 1996. LC 96-8779. (Dermatology Ser.). 464p. 119.95 (*0-8493-7356-5*) CRC Pr.

Human Papillomaviruses. 1995. 409p. (Orig.). pap. text (*92-832-1264-9*, 1720064) IARC FRA. *Dist:* OUP.

Human Parasitology. Bogitsh. 1990. (C). text (*0-15-540381-8*) Harcourt Coll Pubs.

Human Parasitology. Burt J. Bogitsch & Thomas C. Cheng. 2nd ed. 1999. LC 98-84421. (Illus.). 496p. (C). text 59.95 (*0-12-110870-8*) Morgan Kaufmann.

Human Parturition: New Concepts & Developments. Ed. by Marc J. Keirse et al. 1979. (Boerhaave Series for Postgraduate Medical Education: No. 15). text 126.50 (*90-6021-445-5*) Kluwer Academic.

Human Parvovirus B19. Ed. by L. J. Anderson & N. S. Young. Tr. by S. Neal. 1997. LC 96-50380. (Monographs in Virology: Vol. 20, 1996). (Illus.). viii, 154p. 139.25 (*3-8055-6353-1*) S Karger.

Human Pathogenic Papillomaviruses. Ed. by H. Zur Hausen. 1994. LC 15-12910. (Current Topics in Microbiology & Immunology Ser.: Vol. 186). (Illus.). 287p. 139.95 (*0-387-57193-0*) Spr-Verlag.

Human Pathogenic Protozoa: Atlas of Electron-Microscopy. E. G. Rondanelli et al. 1987. 356p. text (*1-57235-027-X*) Piccin Nuova.

Human Performance in the Undersea Environment: An Annotated Bibliography. Raymond E. Reilly. 1970. LC 76-135084. 90p. 15.00 (*0-403-04530-4*) Scholarly.

Human Pharmacology: Molecular to Clinical. Harold J. Brody et al. Ed. by Joseph Larner. 3rd ed. 1997. LC 97-22474. (Illus.). 1024p. (C). (gr. 13). pap. text 52.95 (*0-8151-2456-2*, 31204) Mosby Inc.

Human Physiology. 2000. 140p. (C). lab manual ed. 14.80 (*0-536-60676-5*) Pearson Custom.

Human Physiology. B. K. Chakraborty. 1985. (*0-7855-0737-X*) Current Dist IND. *Dist:* St Mut.

Human Physiology C. Chatterjee. 1987. (C). (*0-7855-4649-9*) Current Dist IND. *Dist:* St Mut.

***Human Physiology.** A. Davies et al. 2001. 980p. (*0-443-04559-3*) Church GBR. *Dist:* Saunders.

Human Physiology. Sheila Jennett. 1989. (Illus.). 460p. pap. text (*0-443-03696-9*) Church.

Human Physiology. Elliott B. Mason. 1983. 575p. text 52.75 (*0-8053-6885-X*) Benjamin-Cummings.

Human Physiology. Ed. by Richard F. Schmidt & G. E. Thews. 2nd ed. 1989. (Illus.). 825p. 116.00 (*0-387-19432-0*) Spr-Verlag.

Human Physiology. Robert F. Schmidt & Gerhard Thews. 2nd ed. 1989. 825p. 99.00 (*3-540-19432-0*) Spr-Verlag.

Human Physiology. Rhoades. 3rd ed. 1995. (C). pap. text, stu. ed. 32.50 (*0-03-015863-X*) Harcourt.

Human Physiology. Stuart Ira Fox & Laurence G. Thouin, Jr. 5th ed. 1995. 288p. (C). text, stu. ed. 18.12 (*0-697-20987-3*, WCB McGr Hill) McGrw-H Hghr Educ.

Human Physiology: A Course Manual. Anthony V. DeFina. 1991. (Illus.). 287p. tchr. ed. 25.00 (*0-916209-08-3*); (YA). (gr. 11 up). reprint ed. pap., stu. ed. 20.00 (*0-916209-00-8*) Owlet Pubns.

Human Physiology: Foundations & Frontiers. Kevin T. Patton & Ann B. Vernon. 2nd ed. 1993. (Illus.). 368p. (C). pap., stu. ed. 65.00 (*0-8016-7126-4*) McGrw-H Hghr Educ.

Human Physiology: From Cells to Systems. Lauralee Sherwood. 4th ed. 2000. LC 00-36011. (Biology Ser.). (Illus.). xx, 766p. mass mkt. 69.75 (*0-534-56826-2*) Wadsworth Pub.

Human Physiology: From Cells to Systems. Lauralee Sherwood. Ed. by Westby. 2nd ed. 1993. LC 92-48672. 760p. (C). text 75.25 (*0-314-01225-7*) West Pub.

Human Physiology: Mechanisms of Disease. Arthur C. Guyton & John E. Hall. Ed. by William Schmitt. 6th ed. 1996. 768p. text 55.00 (*0-7216-3299-8*) Saunders.

Human Physiology: Statical & Dynamical. John W. Draper. 1992. (Notable American Authors Ser.). reprint ed. lib. bdg. 90.00 (*0-7812-2699-6*) Rprt Serv.

Human Physiology: The Mechanics of Body Function. Arthur J. Vander et al. 7th ed. 1997. LC 97-28929. 848p. 95.94 (*0-07-067065-X*) McGraw.

Human Physiology: The Mechanisms of Body Function. Donna Van Wynsberghe. 6th ed. 1994. (C). pap. text, stu. ed. 23.75 (*0-07-066993-7*) McGraw.

Human Physiology & Health in the Caring Context. Sue Ford et al. 1999. 150p. pap. (*0-7487-1770-6*) Nelson Thornes GBR. *Dist:* Trans-Atl Phila.

Human Physiology & Mechanisms of Disease. Arthur C. Guyton. 5th ed. 1992. (Illus.). 700p. (*0-7216-3961-5*) Saunders.

Human Physiology Exercises with Cat Dissections. Gerard J. Tortora & Hope H. Adams. 1989. 650p. (C). pap. text, lab manual ed. 39.00 (*0-02-421203-2*, Macmillan Coll) P-H.

Human Physiology Laboratory Experiments. George B. Cline. 1992. spiral bd. 14.65 (*0-88252-152-7*) Paladin Hse.

Human Physiology with Infotrac. Sherwood. 3rd ed. 1997. (Biology Ser.). mass mkt. 69.75 (*0-534-54095-3*) Wadsworth Pub.

Human Pituitary Hormones: Circadian & Episodic Variations. Ed. by E. Van Cauter & G. Copinschi. 1981. 359p. text 191.50 (*90-247-2481-3*) Kluwer Academic.

Human Placenta. C. W. Redman et al. 1992. (Illus.). 608p. 199.95 (*0-632-02721-5*) Blackwell Sci.

Human Population Genetics: A Centennial Tribute to J. B. S. Haldane. P. P. Majumder. 1993. LC 93-32262. (Illus.). 358p. (C). text 110.00 (*0-306-44572-7*, Kluwer Plenum) Kluwer Academic.

Human Posture: The Nature of Inquiry. John A. Schumacher. 1989. LC 88-38268. (SUNY Series in Science, Technology, & Society). 259p. (C). text 22.50 (*0-7914-0120-0*); pap. text 22.95 (*0-7914-0121-9*) State U NY Pr.

Human Prenatal Diagnosis. Filkins & Russo. 2nd rev. ed. 1990. (Illus.). 624p. text 250.00 (*0-8247-8314-X*) Dekker.

Human Problems of a State Mental Hospital. Ivan Belknap. Ed. by Gerald N. Grob. 1980. LC 78-22548. (Historical Issues in Mental Health Ser.). (Illus.). reprint ed. lib. bdg. 23.95 (*0-405-11902-X*) Ayer.

Human Procreation & Its Natural Regulation. Hermann Knaus. 1965. (Illus.). 14.95 (*0-8392-1138-4*) Astor-Honor.

Human Psyche. John C. Eccles. 1980. (Illus.). 279p. 46.00 (*0-387-09954-9*) Spr-Verlag.

Human Psychology of the Single Person: Index of New Information with Authors, Subjects & Bibliography. Louis A. Lesniak. rev. ed. 1996. 180p. pap. 47.50 (*0-7883-1193-X*) ABBE Pubs Assn.

Human Psychopharmacology: Measures & Methods, Vol. 5. Ed. by I. Stonier Hindmarch & P. D. Stonier. 1995. LC 86-19125. 302p. 225.00 (*0-471-95040-8*) Wiley.

Human Psychopharmacology - Measures & Methods. Vol. 6. I. Stonier Hindmarch. 1999. 250p. 81.00 (*0-471-95042-4*) Wiley.

Human Psychopharmacology V 6, Vol. 6. Ed. by I. Stonier Hindmarch & P. D. Stonier. 1998. 258p. 245.00 (*0-471-95041-6*) Wiley.

Human Psychophysics. Ed. by William A. Yost et al. 1996. LC 93-4695. (Handbook of Auditory Research Ser.: Vol. 3). (Illus.). 243p. 98.00 (*0-387-97840-2*) Spr-Verlag.

Human Radiation Experiments: Final Report of the President's Advisory Committee. Final Report of the Advisory Committee on Human Ra. Ed. by Ruth R. Faden. 1996. (Illus.). 656p. (C). text 42.50 (*0-19-510792-6*) OUP.

Human Radiation Experiments: Hearing Before the Committee on Governmental Affairs, U. S. Senate. 1998. (Illus.). 434p. (C). pap. text 50.00 (*0-7881-4869-9*) DIANE Pub.

Human Radiological Anatomy. B. K. Omar. 1989. (C). (*0-89771-358-3*) Current Dist IND. *Dist:* St Mut.

Human Relations: Principles & Practices Barry L. Reece & Rhonda Brandt. 1993. (C). pap. 27.96 (*0-395-52996-4*) HM.

Human Relations & Interpersonal Effective. Michael G. Aamodt. 2000. LC 00-36339. (Psychology). (Illus.). xxi, 530p. (C). pap. 40.95 (*0-534-35508-0*) Brooks-Cole.

Human Relations in Modern Industry. Roger F. Tredgold. 2nd rev. ed. 1963. LC 74-135212. 192p. 30.00 (*0-8236-2390-4*) Intl Univs Pr.

Human Relationship with Nature: Development & Culture. Peter H. Kahn, Jr. 1999. LC 98-47085. (Illus.). xiv, 281p. 34.95 (*0-262-11240-X*) MIT Pr.

Human Reliability: Analysis, Prediction, & Prevention of Human Errors. K. S. Parks. 1987. (Advances in Human Factors-Ergonomics Ser.: No. 7). 340p. 191.50 (*0-444-42727-9*) Elsevier.

Human Reproduction, Emerging Technologies & Conflicting Rights. Robert Blank & Janna C. Merrick. 1995. LC 95-10455. 269p. pap. 29.95 (*0-87187-938-7*, CQ Pr Coll) CQ Pr.

Human Reproductive Biology. Richard E. Jones. 2nd ed. 1997. LC 96-47585. (Illus.). 581p. text 64.95 (*0-12-389775-0*) Morgan Kaufmann.

Human Reproductive Biology. Sylvia S. Mader. 2nd ed. 1991. 224p. (C). pap. 58.75 (*0-697-11805-3*, WCB McGr Hill) McGrw-H Hghr Educ.

Human Reproductive Decisions: Biological & Social Perspectives: Proceedings of the Thirteenth Annual Symposium of the Galton Institute, London, 1993. Ed. by Robin Dunbar. 1995. LC 94-32721. 320p. 79.95 (*0-312-12436-8*) St Martin.

Human Reproductive Ecology: Interactions of Environment, Fertility, & Behavior. Ed. by Kenneth L. Campbell & James W. Wood. 1994. LC 94-697. (Annals Ser.: Vol. 709). 429p. pap. 115.00 (*0-89766-842-1*) NY Acad Sci.

Human Resource Management in Health Care. Ed. by Montague Brown. 1992. (HCMR Ser.). 256p. pap. 55.00 (*0-8342-0340-5*, 20340) Aspen Pub.

Human Resource Management in the Health Care Sector: A Guide for Administrators & Professionals. Ed. by Amarjit S. Sethi & Randall S. Schuler. 1989. LC 88-18313. 369p. 69.50 (*0-89930-201-7*, SHJ/, Quorum Bks) Greenwood.

Human Resources & Organizational Behavior: Cases in Health Services Management. Anne O. Kilpatrick & James A. Johnson. 1999. LC 98-56539. xviii, 133p. 34.00 (*1-56793-104-9*) Health Admin Pr.

Human Resources for Primary Health Care in the Middle East. 1981. 24.95 (*0-8156-6056-1*) Syracuse U Pr.

Human Resources in Health Care: A Manager's Guide. Anthony Strike. 1995. LC 95-233934. 192p. pap. 35.95 (*0-632-03974-4*) Blackwell Sci.

Human Resources in Patient Financial Services. Dianne P. Barry. 1993. 160p. text 40.00 (*1-882198-13-1*) Hlthcare Fin Mgmt.

Human Resources Specialist. Jack Rudman. 1994. (Career Examination Ser.: C-356). pap. 27.95 (*0-8373-0356-7*) Nat Learn.

Human Responses to Neurologic Dysfunction. AANN Staff. 2nd ed. 1999. LC 99-57047. (Illus.). 700p. text 69.95 (*0-7216-2288-7*) Saunders.

Human Retrovirology. J. Schuepbach. 1989. (Current Topics in Microbiology & Immunology Ser.: Vol. 142). (Illus.). 115p. 59.00 (*0-387-50455-9*) Spr-Verlag.

Human Retrovirology. J. Schupbach. 1990. (Illus.). 115p. 69.95 (*0-387-51850-9*) Spr-Verlag.

Human Rights & Disabled Persons. (Human Rights Study Ser.: No. 6). 43p. 20.00 (*92-1-154090-9*, E.92.XIV.4) UN.

Human Rights & Public Health in the AIDS Pandemic. Lawrence O. Gostin & Zita Lazzarini. 1997. LC 96-33501. 232p. 29.95 (*0-19-511442-6*) OUP.

Human Rights, Ethical & Moral Dimensions of Health Care: 120 Practical Case Studies. Council of European Publishing Staff. 1998. 485p. pap. (*92-871-3055-8*) Statnry Office GBR. *Dist:* Balogh.

Human Rights on Hold: A Report on Emergency Measures & Access to Health Care in the Occupied Territories. Physicians for Human Rights Staff. 1992. LC 93-83144. 87p. pap. 10.00 (*1-879707-09-8*) Phy Human Rights.

Human Saliva: Clinical Chemistry & Microbiology Ed. by Jorma O. Tenovuo. 1989. Vol. 1. 216p. 159.00 (*0-8493-6391-8*, RB52); Vol. 2. 264p. 210.00 (*0-8493-6392-6*, RB52) CRC Pr.

Human Schistosomiasis. Ed. by P. Jordan et al. 1993. (Illus.). 480p. text 150.00 (*0-85198-844-X*) OUP.

Human Sectional Anatomy: Atlas of Body Sections, CT & MRI Images. Harold Ellis et al. 2nd ed. 1999. LC 00-265450. (Illus.). 256p. pap. (*0-7506-3367-0*) E A GBR. *Dist:* OUP.

***Human Sectional Anatomy: Pocket Atlas of Body Sections, CT & MRI Images.** Harold Ellis et al. 2nd ed. 2001. (Arnold Publication). 256p. (Orig.). pap. text 29.95 (*0-340-80764-4*) OUP.

Human Sense of Smell. Ed. by D. G. Laing et al. 1991. (Illus.). 395p. 175.00 (*0-387-53355-9*) Spr-Verlag.

Human Services for Older Adults: Concepts & Skills. Leon H. Ginsberg & Anita S. Harbert. 2nd rev. ed. 1990. LC 89-24900. 249p. pap. text 19.95 (*0-87249-682-1*) U of SC Pr.

Human Services Today. Karin Eriksen. 1977. text 12.95 (*0-87909-336-6*) P-H.

Human Sex-Role Behavior. Alfred B. Heilbrun, Jr. 1981. LC 80-26415. (General Psychology Ser.: No. 96). 224p. 55.00 (*0-08-025974-X*, Pergamon Pr) Elsevier.

Human Sexual Behavior: History, Sociology, Psychology, Ethics & Ethnology, Set. (AMS Press Reprint Ser.). reprint ed. (*0-404-57400-9*) AMS Pr.

Human Sexual Response. William H. Masters & Virginia E. Johnson. 1966. 366p. text 79.95 (*0-316-54987-8*, Little Brwn Med Div) Lppncott W & W.

Human Sexuality. Ed. by C. R. Austin & R. V. Short. 1980. LC 78-18959. (Reproduction in Mammals Ser.: Bk. 8). (Illus.). 192p. text 59.95 (*0-521-22361-X*); pap. text 21.95 (*0-521-29461-4*) Cambridge U Pr.

Human Sexuality. Davis. (C). 2000. pap. text, stu. ed. 22.00 (*0-15-503603-5*); 1998. pap. text, tchr. ed., suppl. ed. 28.00 (*0-15-503605-X*) Harcourt Coll Pubs.

Human Sexuality. Patricia Koch. 1995. 448p. (C). pap. text 50.95 (*0-8403-9472-1*, 40947201) Kendall-Hunt.

Human Sexuality. Pruitt. 1999. (C). pap. text, stu. ed. 19.50 (*0-03-007607-2*) Harcourt Coll Pubs.

Human Sexuality. Buzz E. Pruitt. 1998. 704p. (C). text 68.00 (*0-03-007603-X*) SCP.

Human Sexuality. Wade. 2nd ed. 1991. (C). pap. text, stu. ed. 31.00 (*0-15-540433-4*) Harcourt Coll Pubs.

Human Sexuality: A Bibliography & Critical Evaluation of Recent Texts. Mervyn L. Mason. 1983. LC 83-12688. 207p. lib. bdg. 62.50 (*0-313-23932-0*, MHU/, Greenwood Pr) Greenwood.

Human Sexuality: A Text with Readings. Sam Wilson et al. 1980. 499p. tchr. ed. (*0-8299-0584-7*) West Pub.

Human Sexuality: HP 615 Course. Crenshaw. 1991. 100p. (C). 69.95 incl. audio (*0-933195-65-6*) CA College Health Sci.

Human Sexuality: Test Bank. Davis. 2000. (C). pap. text, tchr. ed., suppl. ed. 31.00 (*0-15-503604-1*) Harcourt Coll Pubs.

Human Sexuality: The Search for Understanding. David Knox. 1984. (Illus.). 635p. (C). text 56.00 (*0-314-77999-X*); (*0-314-82417-0*) West Pub.

Human Sexuality & Its Problems. John D. Bancroft. 2nd ed. 1989. (Illus.). 748p. pap. text (*0-443-03455-9*) Church.

Human Sexuality & the Developmentally Handicapped: A Guidebook for Health Care Professionals. William Rowe et al. 1987. LC 86-28463. (Studies in Health & Human Services: Vol. 7). 245p. lib. bdg. 89.95 (*0-88946-132-5*) E Mellen.

Human Sexuality & the Family Physician: A Special Journal Issue of Family Practice Research. Eli Coleman. 1988. 66p. pap. 14.95 (*0-89885-426-1*, Kluwer Acad Hman Sci) Kluwer Academic.

Human Sexuality CEU Course: 30 CEUs. Crenshaw. 1991. 100p. (C). stu. ed. 49.95 incl. audio (*0-933195-79-6*) CA College Health Sci.

Human Sexuality, Ethnoculture & Social Work. Ed. by Larry Lister. 1987. LC 86-14899. (Journal of Social Work & Human Sexuality: Vol. 4, No. 3). 163p. text 39.95 (*0-86656-609-0*) Haworth Pr.

Human Sexuality in Biocultural Perspective: A Special Issue of the Journal of Medical Anthropology. Ed. by Frances E. Mascia-Less. 1989. 103p. pap. text 36.00 (*2-88124-347-9*) Gordon & Breach.

Human Sexuality in Medical Social Work. Ed. by Larry Lister & David A. Shore. 1984. LC 83-26449. (Journal of Social Work & Human Sexuality: Vol. 2, No. 1). 130p. text 39.95 (*0-86656-254-0*) Haworth Pr.

Human Sexuality, 1996-1997. Susan Bunting. 21st annot. ed. 1996. tchr. ed. (*0-697-31602-5*, WCB McGr Hill) McGrw-H Hghr Educ.

Human Sexuality & Its Problems. Bancroft. 3rd ed. 1999. text 83.00 (*0-443-05161-5*) Saunders.

Human Side of Diabetes: Beyond Doctors, Diets & Drugs. Mike Raymond. 1991. LC 91-50644. 288p. (Orig.). pap. 13.95 (*1-879360-09-8*) Noble Pr.

Human Side of Human Beings. Harvey Jackins. Tr. by June MacKay. 1980. (ITA.). pap. 4.00 (*0-911214-73-9*) Rational Isl.

Human Side of Human Beings. Harvey Jackins. Tr. by Aquiles Cordeiro from ENG. 1979. (POR.). pap. 4.00 (*0-911214-66-6*) Rational Isl.

Human Side of Human Beings: Chinese Translation. Harvey Jackins. Tr. by Li Mei-Ge. 1982. pap. 4.00 (*0-911214-84-4*) Rational Isl.

Human Situation. Harvey Jackins. Tr. by Ileana Vajda. 2000. (RUM.). pap. 4.00 (*1-58429-069-2*) Rational Isl.

Human Skeleton. Robert M. McMinn et al. 1986. 30p. (C). (gr. 13). 41.95 (*0-8151-5795-9*, 09417) Mosby Inc.

Human Skeleton. Pat Shipman et al. 1985. (Illus.). 360p. text 54.00 (*0-674-41610-4*) HUP.

Human Skeleton: Functional Model. Leon Schlossberg. 1961. tchr. ed. 99.50 (*0-8018-0577-5*) Johns Hopkins.

Human Skeleton in Forensic Medicine. Wilton M. Krogman & M. Yasar Iscan. 2nd ed. 1986. (Illus.). 568p. (C). 140.95 (*0-398-05224-7*) C C Thomas.

Human Skull: Its Mechanics, Measurements & Variations. Spencer L. Rogers. 1984. (Illus.). 118p. (C). 29.95 (*0-398-04955-6*) C C Thomas.

Human Sleep: Research & Clinical Care. W. B. Mendelson. 1987. LC 87-7372. (Illus.). 456p. (C). text 80.00 (*0-306-42627-7*, Kluwer Plenum) Kluwer Academic.

Human Spatial Abilities: Sources of Sex Difference. Mark McGee. 1979. 145p. 60.00 (*0-275-90391-5*, C0391, Praeger Pubs) Greenwood.

Human Species: The Biology of Man. S. A. Barnett. 1990. (Illus.). 18.75 (*0-8446-0477-1*) Peter Smith.

Human Sperm Competition: Copulation, Masturbation & Infidelity. R. Robin Baker. 1994. 376p. (C). (gr. 13). pap. text 119.95 (*0-412-45430-0*) Chapman & Hall.

Human Spermatozoa in Assisted Reproduction. Ed. by Anibal A. Acosta & Thinus F. Kruger. 2nd ed. 1996. LC 95-39885. 536p. lib. bdg. 137.95 (*1-85070-590-9*, Parthenon Pbng) CRC Pr.

Human Stress & the Environment: Health Aspects, Vol.5. Ed. by J. Rose. 1994. LC 94-2603. (Environmental Topics Ser.: Vol. 5). 240p. text 179.00 (*2-88124-851-9*) Gordon & Breach.

Human Stress, Work & Job Satisfaction: A Critical Approach. T. M. Fraser. 1987. (Occupational Safety & Health Ser.: No. 50). 72p. (Orig.). pap. 13.50 (*92-2-103042-3*) Intl Labour Office.

Human Subjects Research: A Handbook for Institutional Review Boards. Ed. by Robert A. Greenwald & James E. Mulvihill. 1982. 316p. 65.00 (*0-306-40920-8*, Plenum Trade) Perseus Pubng.

Human Submission. Morrison I. Swift. 1977. lib. bdg. 59.95 (*0-8490-2027-1*) Gordon Pr.

Human Substantia Nigra & Ventral Tegmental Area, Vol. 121: A Neuroanatomical Study with Notes on Aging & Aging Diseases. P. H. Van Domburg & H. J. Ten Donkelaar. Ed. by F. Beck et al. 1991. (Advances in Anatomy, Embryology & Cell Biology Ser.). (Illus.). 132p. 79.95 (*0-387-52823-7*) Spr-Verlag.

Human T-Cell Leukemia - Lymphoma Virus: The Family of Human T-Lymphotropic Retroviruses: Their Role in Malignancies & Association with AIDS. Ed. by Robert,C. Gallo et al. 1984. LC 84-1757. (Illus.). 375p. 65.00 (*0-87969-170-0*) Cold Spring Harbor.

Human T-Cell Lymphotropic Virus Type I. Ed. by Per Hollsberg. 1996. LC 96-4960. 338p. 166.95 (*0-471-96676-2*) Wiley.

Human T-Cell Receptor Repertoire & Transplantation. P. Van den Elsen. 1995. LC 95-14122. (Molecular Biology Intelligence Unit Ser.). 166p. 89.00 (*1-57059-279-9*) Landes Bioscience.

Human T-Lymphocyte Activation Deficiencies. Jose R. Regueiro et al. 1994. LC 93-39483. (Medical Intelligence Unit Ser.). 208p. 99.00 (*1-57059-020-6*) Landes Bioscience.

Human Tendons: Anatomy, Physiology, & Pathology. Laszlo Jozsa et al. 1997. LC 96-31551. (Illus.). 584p. text 88.00 (*0-87322-484-1*, BJOZ0484) Human Kinetics.

Human Teratomas: Experimental & Clinical Biology. Ed. by Ivan Damjanov et al. 1983. LC 82-48865. (Contemporary Biomedicine Ser.: Vol. 3). 374p. 119.50 (*0-89603-040-7*) Humana.

***Human Thermal Environments.** Kenneth C. Parsons. 2nd ed. 2001. 480p. (C). (gr. 13). text 115.00 (*0-415-23792-0*) Routledge.

Human Thermal Environments. Kenneth C. Parsons. 1993. LC 93-20570. 450p. (*0-7484-0040-0*); pap. (*0-7484-0041-9*) Tay Francis Ltd GBR. *Dist:* Taylor & Francis.

Human Touch in High Tech: Proceedings of the West Virginia Nurses' Association, 1987 Research Symposium. Ed. by Janet F. Wang & Patricia S. Simoni. 1987. (Illus.). 97p. (*0-930284-32-1*) Morgantown Print & Bind.

Human Toxicology. Jacques G. Descotes. 1996. LC 96-26766. (Illus.). 858p. 232.50 (*0-444-81557-0*) Elsevier.

Human Toxicology of Pesticides. Fina P. Kaloyanova & M. A. El Batawi. 1991. (Illus.). 232p. lib. bdg. 149.00 (*0-8493-5192-8*, RA1270) CRC Pr.

Human Toxoplasmosis. Ed. by Darrel O. Ho-Yen & Alex W. Joss. 1992. (Illus.). 278p. text 69.50 (*0-19-854750-1*) OUP.

Human Tumor Cloning. Ed. by Sydney E. Salmon & Jeffrey M. Trent. 1984. 720p. text 115.00 (*0-8089-1671-8*, 793750, Grune & Strat) Harcrt Hlth Sci Grp.

Human Tumor Markers: Proceedings of the International Conference Lacco Ameno d'Ischia, 3rd, Napoli, Italy, April 23-26, 1986. F. Cimino et al. 1987. xiv, 922p. (C). lib. bdg. 292.35 (*3-11-010935-2*) De Gruyter.

Human Tumor Viruses. Dennis J. McCance. 1998. LC 98-12185. (Illus.). 375p. 99.95 (*1-55581-130-2*) ASM Pr.

Human Types. Raymond W. Firth. rev. ed. 1983. LC 83-13026. (Illus.). 184p. reprint ed. lib. bdg. 60.00 (*0-313-24176-7*, FIHU, Greenwood Pr) Greenwood.

Human Vaccines & Vaccination. M. MacKett & J. Williamson. 1994. (Medical Perspectives Ser.). 160p. pap. (*1-872748-77-5*) Bios Sci GBR. *Dist:* Coronet Bks.

Human Values in Critical Care Medicine. Ed. by Stuart J. Youngner. 1986. LC 86-22569. 197p. 59.00 (*0-275-92264-2*, C2264, Praeger Pubs) Greenwood.

Human Variability in Response to Chemical Exposures: Measures, Modeling & Risk Assessment. David A. Neumann et al. 1998. LC 98-3610. 272p. 104.95 (*0-8493-2805-5*, 2805); 257p. (*1-57881-000-0*) CRC Pr.

Human Variation: Causes & Consequences. Jim Asher. 1993. (C). stu. ed. 15.00 (*1-881592-18-9*) Hayden-McNeil.

Human Variation & Natural Selection. Ed. by D. F. Roberts. 1975. (Symposia of the Society for the Study of Human Biology Ser.: Vol. 13). 220p. 36.00 (*0-85066-080-7*) Taylor & Francis.

Human Viral & Rickettsial Vaccines: Proceedings of the WHO Scientific Group, Geneva, 1965. WHO Staff. 1966. (Technical Reports: No. 325). (ENG, FRE, RUS & SPA.). 79p. pap. text 5.00 (*92-4-120325-0*, 1100325) World Health.

Human Viruses in Sediments, Sludges, & Soils. Ed. by V. Shalapati Ras & Joseph L. Melnick. 1987. LC 87-20942. 272p. 144.00 (*0-8493-6572-4*, RA644, CRC Reprint) Franklin.

Human Viruses in Water, Wastewater & Soil: Report of a Scientific Group, 1979. 1979. (Technical Report Ser.: No. 639). 50p. pap. text 4.00 (*92-4-120639-X*, 1100639) World Health.

Human Voice: Its Anatomy, Physiology, Pathology, Therapeutics, & Training (1872) R. T. Trall. 1996. 107p. reprint ed. pap. 11.95 (*1-56459-811-X*) Kessinger Pub.

Human Yolk Sac & Yolk Sac Tumors. Ed. by Francisco Nogales. 1993. LC 92-48512. (Illus.). 367p. 327.00 (*0-387-56031-9*) Spr-Verlag.

Humane Managed Care? Providers Respond. Gerald Schamess & Anita Lightburn. 1998. LC 98-8336. 1146p. pap. 29.95 (*0-87101-294-4*) Natl Assn Soc Wkrs.

Humane Medicine. Miles Little. 1995. (Illus.). 207p. (C). pap. text 17.95 (*0-521-49863-5*) Cambridge U Pr.

Humane Medicine: A Leading Surgeon Examines What Doctors Do, What Patients Expect of Them, & How the Expectations of Both Are Not Being Met. Miles Little. 1995. (Illus.). 207p. (C). text 49.95 (*0-521-49513-X*) Cambridge U Pr.

Humane Medicine: A New Paradigm in Medical Education & Health Care Delivery. Richard A. Williams. 1998. LC 98-43507. (*0-7817-2030-3*) Lppncott W & W.

Humane Movement in the United States, 1910-1922. William J. Shultz. LC 68-57581. (Columbia University. Studies in the Social Sciences: No. 252). reprint ed. 21.00 (*0-404-51252-6*) AMS Pr.

Humanetics Testing Procedure. Edgar Brown & Kaye Behrens. 1985. (Illus.). 12p. (Orig.). pap. 2.95 (*0-9613697-2-8*) Madison Ave Pub.

Humanhood: Essays in Biomedical Ethics. Joseph Fletcher. 1979. LC 79-1756. 216p. (C). 34.00 (*0-87975-112-6*) Prometheus Bks.

Humanism & Environmentalism Vol. 24: Philosophical Perspectives in Counseling. James E. Nowlin & J. Vernon Blackburn. 1995. LC 93-44078. (American University Studies: Ser. XIV, Vol. 24). 178p. (C). 41.95 (*0-8204-1109-4*) P Lang Pubng.

Humanistic Nursing. Loretta T. Zderad & Josephine G. Paterson. 1988. 136p. pap. 21.95 (*0-88737-398-4*, 41-2218) Natl League Nurse.

Humanistic Psychology. John B. Shaffer. 1978. LC 77-15044. (Foundations of Modern Psychology Ser.). (Illus.). (C). pap. text 18.80 (*0-13-447680-8*) P-H.

Humanistic Psychology: Concepts & Criticisms. Ed. by Joseph R. Royce & Leendert P. Mos. 1981. (PATH in Psychology Ser.). 332p. 49.50 (*0-306-40596-2*, Plenum Trade) Perseus Pubng.

Humanistic Psychosomatic Medicine. Hiroshi Takashima. 1984. (Illus.). 100p. (Orig.). pap. 9.95 (*0-917867-00-9*) V Frankl Inst.

Humanizing Brain: Where Religion & Neuroscience Meet. James B. Ashbrook & Carol R. Albright. 1997. LC 97-25730. (Illus.). 272p. (Orig.). pap. 20.95 (*0-8298-1200-8*) Pilgrim OH.

Humanizing Maternity Services Through Family-Centered Care. Susan McKay. 1982. 52p. 2.00 (*0-934024-07-3*) Intl Childbirth.

Humans As Guinea Pigs in Clinical Experiments: Index of New Information. Roger L. Samuels. 1997. 160p. 57.50 (*0-7883-1548-X*); pap. 47.50 (*0-7883-1549-8*) ABBE Pubs Assn.

Humans As Self-Constructing Living Systems: A Developmental Perspective on Behavior & Personality. Donald H. Ford. 2nd ed. 1994. (Illus.). 787p. (C). text 30.00 (*0-932990-06-1*) IDEALS PA.

Humans As Self Constructing Systems: Putting the Framework to Work. Martin E. Ford. Ed. by Donald H. Ford. 1987. 424p. (C). 79.95 (*0-89859-667-X*) L Erlbaum Assocs.

Humans in Spaceflight. Ed. by Carolyn L. Huntoon. 1995. (Space Biology & Medicine Ser.: Vol. III). (Illus.). 600p. 129.95 (*1-56347-180-9*) AIAA.

Humerus: Musculoskeletal Trauma Series. Evan L. Flatow & Christoph Ulrich. 1996. LC 96-17376. (Musculoskeletal Trauma Ser.). 304p. text 130.00 (*0-7506-0840-4*) Buttrwrth-Heinemann.

Humility. 1985. (Pocket Power Ser.). 16p. pap. 1.25 (*0-89486-254-5*, 1338B) Hazelden.

Humor & Psychotherapy. Thomas L. Kuhlman. 1994. LC 94-72084. (Master Work Ser.). 140p. pap. 25.00 (*1-56821-317-4*) Aronson.

Humor & the Healing Arts: A Multimethod Analysis of Humor Use in Healthcare. Athena Du Pre. 1998. LC 97-17943. (Communication Ser.). 250p. (*0-8058-2647-5*); pap. (*0-8058-2648-3*) L Erlbaum Assocs.

Humor & the Health Professions: The Therapeutic Use of Humor in Health Care. Vera M. Robinson. 2nd ed. 1990. LC 89-43106. 256p. pap. 25.00 (*1-55642-141-9*) SLACK Inc.

Humor & Wellness in Clinical Intervention. Ed. by Waleed A. Salameh & William F. Fry. 2001. LC 00-52428. (Illus.). 280p. 70.00 (*0-275-96155-9*, Praeger Pubs) Greenwood.

Humor, Irony, & the Realm of Madness: Psychological Studies in Dickens, Butler, & Others. Margaret Ganz. 1990. LC 87-45801. (Studies in the Nineteenth Century: No. 9). 39.50 (*0-404-61489-2*) AMS Pr.

Humoral Factors in the Regulation of Tissue Growth: Blood, Blood Vessels, Skeletal System, & Teeth. Ed. by Piero P. Foa & M. P. Cohen. 1992. LC 92-20284. (Endocrinology & Metabolism Ser.: Vols. 5-6). (Illus.). 312p. 258.00 (*0-387-97879-8*) Spr-Verlag.

Hunan Hand & Other Ailments: Letters to the New England Journal of Medicine. Ed. by Shirley B. Moskow. 1987. 15.95 (*0-316-58533-5*, Little Brwn Med Div) Lppncott W & W.

Hundesprog see Dog Language: An Encyclopedia of Canine Behavior

100 Mitos de la Salud. Vivas. 1997. pap. text (*84-7880-677-6*) E Temas de Hoy ESP. *Dist:* Planeta.

Hungarian-English Medical Dictionary. P. Veghelyi & M. Kuntner. 2nd ed. 1986. 942p. 39.95 (*0-8288-1882-7*, F96910) Fr & Eur.

Hungarian-English Medical Dictionary. Ed. by P. Veghelyi & T. Csink. 3rd ed. 1991. 942p. (*963-205-257-9*) Akade Kiado HUN. *Dist:* IBD Ltd.

Hungarian-German Dictionary of Medical Terms. I. Hera. 1993. 800p. (*963-05-5985-4*) Akade Kiado HUN. *Dist:* St Mut.

Hunger Diseases. Raymond Battegay. 1991. (Illus.). 160p. text 34.50 (*0-88937-054-0*) Hogrefe & Huber Pubs.

Hunger So Wide & So Deep: A Multicultural View of Women's Eating Problems. Becky W. Thompson. 1994. LC 93-43613. 161p. text 37.95 (*0-8166-2434-8*) U of Minn Pr.

Hunger So Wide & So Deep: American Women Speak Out on Eating Problems. Becky W. Thompson. 1996. LC 93-43613. 176p. (C). pap. 14.95 (*0-8166-2435-6*) U of Minn Pr.

Hunger Strike: The Anorectic's Struggle as a Metaphor for Our Age. Susie Orbach. 1988. 272p. mass mkt. 4.50 (*0-380-70393-9*, Avon Bks) Morrow Avon.

Hungers & Compulsions: The Psychodynamic Treatment of Eating Disorders & Addictions. Ed. by Jean Petrucelli & Catherine Stuart. 2001. LC 00-67596. 50.00 (*0-7657-0318-1*) Aronson.

Hunnius Pharmazeutisches Woerterbuch. Curt Hunnius. 7th ed. 1993. (GER.). 1556p. 250.00 (*0-7859-8276-0*, 3110126990) Fr & Eur.

Hunter Holmes McQuire: Stonewall Jackson Doctor. John W. Schildt. 2001. LC 2001-57513. (Illus.). 160p. 17.95 (*1-57249-258-9*) White Mane Pub.

Hunterian Lectures in Comparative Anatomy. Richard Owen. Ed. by Phillip R. Sloan. 1992. (Illus.). 356p. lib. bdg. 48.50 (*0-226-64189-9*); LC 91-21017. pap. text 18.95 (*0-226-64190-2*) U Ch Pr.

Hunter's Diseases of Occupations. Donald Hunter. Ed. by Andrew Raffle et al. 8th ed. 1994. 818p. (*0-340-55173-9*) E A GBR. *Dist:* OUP.

Hunter's Diseases of Occupations, Bk. 1. Ed. by P. A. Raffle et al. 8th ed. 1994. LC 93-46316. (*0-340-57173-X*) E A GBR. *Dist:* Routldge.

Hunter's Rehabilitation Handbook. Mackin. 45th ed. 2001. LC 2001-55842. pap. 225.00 (*0-323-01094-6*) Mosby Inc.

Hunter's Tropical Medicine. G. Thomas Strickland. 7th ed. 1991. (Illus.). 1056p. text 220.00 (*0-7216-2970-9*) Saunders.

Hunter's Tropical Medicine. G. Thomas Strickland. Ed. by Ray Kersey. 8th ed. 1999. LC 98-13361. (Illus.). xxviii, 1192p. text (*0-7216-6223-4*) Saunders.

Huntington Sexual Behavior Scale. Vince Huntington. 1998. (Perspectives in Psychotherapy Ser.: Vol. 1). 400p. pap. text 49.95 (*0-938198-03-3*) Weidner & Sons.

Huntington's Disease. Peter S. Harper. 2nd ed. 1996. (C). text 105.00 (*0-7020-2153-9*) Harcourt.

Huntington's Disease. Ed. by Peter S. Harper. 1991. (Major Problems in Neurology Ser.: Vol. 22). (Illus.). 454p. (*0-7020-1538-5*) W B Saunders GBR. *Dist:* Saunders.

Hurst's The Heart. Robert A. O'Rourke. 8th ed. 1995. pap. text 45.00 (*0-07-048157-1*) McGraw.

Hurst's the Heart. R. Wayne Alexander et al. 10th ed. 2000. LC 00-61611. (Illus.). 2256p. text 150.00 (*0-07-135694-0*) McGraw-Hill Prof.

Hurst's The Heart. R. Wayne Alexander. 10th ed. 2000. Vol. 2, Bk. 1. (*0-07-135695-9*); Vol. 2, BK. 2. (*0-07-135696-7*) McGraw.

Hurst's the Heart: Arteries & Veins. Ed. by Wayne Alexander et al. 9th ed. 1998. LC 97-19289. (Illus.). 2480p. text 150.00 (*0-07-057717-X*); 2344p. text 165.00 (*0-07-912951-X*) McGraw-Hill Educ Grp.

Hurst's The Heart: Companion Handbook. Ed. by Robert C. Schlant & R. Wayne Alexander. 8th ed. 1994. (Illus.). 538p. pap. text 29.50 (*0-07-055469-2*) McGraw-Hill Med Pub.

***Hurst's The Heart: Manual of Cardiology.** Valentin Fuster et al. 10th ed. 2001. (Cardiology Ser.). (Illus.). 798p. pap. 39.95 (*0-07-135415-8*) McGraw-Hill Prof.

Hurst's the Heart: Pre-Test Self-Assessment & Review. Ed. by Jerre Lutz. 9th ed. 1998. LC 98-2988. (Illus.). 275p. pap. 45.00 (*0-07-039142-4*) McGraw-Hill Prof.

***Hurst's the Heart: Self-Assessment & Board Review.** Lutz. 10th ed. 2001. (Specialty Board Review & Health Related Professions Ser.). (Illus.). 300p. pap. 59.95 (*0-07-137469-8*) McGraw-Hill Prof.

Hurst's the Heart: Update 1. Ed. by Robert A. O'Rourke. 8th ed. 1995. Orig. Title: The Heart. (Illus.). 192p. pap., suppl. ed. 45.00 (*0-07-048207-1*) McGraw-Hill Prof.

Hurt? Medical Phrases in Arabic/English/French/German/Greek/Italian/Persian/Polish/Portuguese/Romanian/Russian/Serbian/Spanish/Turkish. Kelland & Jordan. 1995. (ARA, ENG, FRE, GER & GRE.). 215p. 79.95 (*0-320-00551-8*) Fr & Eur.

Hurting & Healing: How to Overcome the Trauma of Sexual Abuse & Rape. Gloria Wade. 2000. 160p. pap. 13.95 (*1-86204-560-7*) Element MA.

Hurting for Love: Munchausen by Proxy Syndrome. Herbert A. Schreier & Judith A. Libow. 1993. LC 92-48483. 265p. 35.00 (*0-89862-121-6*, 2121) Guilford Pubns.

Husband-Focused Marital Therapy: An Approach to Dealing with Marital Distress. Robert P. Rugel. 1997. LC 97-20409. (Illus.). 230p. text 51.95 (*0-398-06792-9*); pap. text 37.95 (*0-398-06793-7*) C C Thomas.

Hutchison's Clinical Methods. Michael Swash. 20th ed. 1995. pap. text 30.00 (*0-7020-1675-6*) Saunders.

Hutt Adaptation of the Bender Gestalt Test. Max L. Hutt. 4th ed. 1985. 256p. text 36.00 (*0-8089-1718-8*, 792091, Grune & Strat) Harcrt Hlth Sci Grp.

***Hyaluronan & Renal Fluid Handling: Studies During Normal & Pathological Conditions of Renal Function.** Viktoria Goransson. 2001. (Comprehensive Summaries of Uppsala Dissertations from the Faculty of Medicine Ser.: No. 1090). (Illus.). 62p. pap. (*91-554-5146-2*) Acta Univ SWE. *Dist:* Coronet Bks.

Hybridization of Dental Hard Tissues. Nobuo Nakabayashi & David H. Pashley. 2000. (Illus.). 135p. pap. (*4-87417-575-9*) QPC JPN. *Dist:* Quint Pub Co.

Hybridoma Technology in Agricultural & Veterinary Research. Ed. by Norman J. Stern & H. Ray Gamble. 1984. LC 84-17795. (Illus.). 354p. 84.00 (*0-8476-7362-6*) Rowman.

Hybridoma Technology in the Biosciences & Medicine. Ed. by Timothy A. Springer. 1985. LC 85-12083. 628p. 135.00 (*0-306-41996-3*, Plenum Trade) Perseus Pubng.

Hydergine: Pharmacologic & Clinical Facts. C. Weil. 2nd ed. 1988. (Illus.). 130p. 54.95 (*0-387-19282-4*) Spr-Verlag.

Hydrazines & Cancer: A Guidebook on the Carcinogenic Activities of Hydrazines, Related Chemicals & Hydrazine Containing Natural Products. Bela Toth. 2000. 264p. 95.00 (*90-5702-631-7*, G & B Science) Gordon & Breach.

Hydrocele in the Temperate & Tropical Countries, II. Ed. by Fortunato Fasana. 1983. LC 82-7242. 100.00 (*0-8493-6077-3*, RC898, CRC Reprint) Franklin.

Hydrocephalus. Ed. by Peter H. Schurr & C. E. Polkey. 1993. LC 92-49516. (Illus.). 268p. text 89.50 (*0-19-261863-6*) OUP.

Hydrocephalus: A Guide for Patients, Families & Friends. Chuck Toporek & Kellie Robinson. Ed. by Linda Lamb. 1999. LC 98-52974. (Patient-Centered Guides Ser.). (Illus.). 382p. pap. 19.95 (*1-56592-410-X*) OReilly & Assocs.

Hydrocephalus: Pathogenesis & Treatment. Ed. by Shoichi Matsumoto & N. Tamaki. 1992. (Illus.). 720p. 292.00 (*0-387-70080-3*) Spr-Verlag.

Hydrogels for Medical & Related Applications. Ed. by Joseph D. Andrade. 1976. LC 76-28170. (ACS Symposium Ser.: No. 31). 32.95 (*0-8412-0338-5*) Am Chemical.

Hydrogels in Medicine & Pharmacy. Ed. by Nikolaos A. Peppas. Vol. I: Fundamentals. 1986. 192p. 112.00 (*0-8493-5546-X*, R857, CRC Reprint); Vol. II: Polymers. 1987. LC 86-4195. 184p. 107.00 (*0-8493-5547-8*, R857); Vol. III: Properties & Applications. 1987. 240p. 120.00 (*0-8493-5548-6*, CRC Reprint) Franklin.

Hydronephrosis in Childhood: An Experimental & Clinical Study. Nils Wahlin. 2000. (Comprehensive Summaries of Uppsala Dissertations from the Faculty of Medicine Ser.: No. 934). (Illus.). 56p. pap. (*91-554-4732-5*) Uppsala Universitet SWE. *Dist:* Coronet Bks.

Hydropathic Highway to Health: Women & Water-Cure in Antebellum America, 17. Jane B. Donegan. 1986. LC 85-10083. (Contributions in Medical Studies Ser.: No. 17). (Illus.). 249p. 55.00 (*0-313-23816-2*, DWH/, Greenwood Pr) Greenwood.

Hydrophilic Polymer Coatings for Medical Devices: Structure/Properties, Development, Manufacture & Applications. Richard J. LaPorte. 1997. LC 96-62021. 186p. 174.95 (*1-56676-504-8*) CRC Pr.

Hydroquinone. Ed. by World Health Organization Staff. 1994. (Environmental Health Criteria Ser.: No. 157). (ENG, FRE & SPA.). 178p. pap. text 36.00 (*92-4-157157-8*, 1160157) World Health.

Hydrotherapy & Heliotherapy: Natural Healing with Water, Herbs, & Sunlight. Maureen O'Rourke. 1995. 88p. (C). pap. text 14.95 (*0-9649356-0-0*) Educ Hands.

Hydrotherapy & Massage. Ed. by Health Research Staff. 1996. 95p. reprint ed. spiral bd. 8.00 (*0-7873-0400-X*) Hlth Research.

Hydrotherapy in Practice. Bridget C. Davis & Ronald H. Harrison. 1988. (Illus.). 183p. pap. text (*0-443-03062-6*) Church.

Hydrothermal Experimental Techniques. Ed. by Gene C. Ulmer & Hubert L. Barnes. 1987. LC 86-32416. 544p. 199.00 (*0-471-82145-4*) Wiley.

Hydroxyapatite & Related Materials. Ed. by Paul W. Brown & Brent Constantz. 1994. LC 93-47252. 368p. 159.00 (*0-8493-4750-5*) CRC Pr.

Hydroxybenzoic Acids—Index of New Information & Medical Research Bible. Benard J. Miles. 1994. 150p. pap. 44.50 (*0-7883-0095-4*) ABBE Pubs Assn.

Hydroxyl Radicals: Index of New Information for Health & Disease Research. Salvatore D. Sisson. 1997. 150p. pap. 47.50 (*0-7883-1355-X*) ABBE Pubs Assn.

Hydroxylapatite Implants. H. Dennissen et al. 1985. 168p. text (*1-57235-076-8*) Piccin Nuova.

Hygieia: A Woman's Herbal. Jeannine Parvati. 1979. LC 78-67918. (Illus.). 52p. pap. 15.00 (*0-913512-54-0*) Freestone Pub Co.

***Hygiene: In the Early Modern Medical Tradition.** Heikki Mikkeli. 1999. (Illus.). pap. (*951-41-0869-8*) Finnish Acad FIN. *Dist:* Intl Spec Bk.

Hygiene for Care. Marion Stewart. 1992. (Skills for Caring Ser.). (Illus.). 40p. (Orig.). pap. text (*0-443-04620-4*) Church.

Hygiene of the Brain & Nerves & the Cure of Nervousness. Martin L. Holbrook. LC 78-72799. reprint ed. 27.50 (*0-404-60862-0*) AMS Pr.

Hyla Doc: Surgeon in China Through War & Revolution, 1924-1949. Elsie H. Landstrom & Hyla S. Watters. 1990. LC 90-40637. (Illus.). 312p. (Orig.). pap. 12.95 (*0-936609-19-2*) QED Ft Bragg.

Hyla Doc in Africa: 1950-1961. Ed. by Elsie H. Landstrom. 1994. LC 93-6280. (Illus.). 104p. (Orig.). pap. 10.50 (*0-936609-32-X*) QED Ft Bragg.

Hyman's Comparative Vertebrate Anatomy. Ed. by Marvalee H. Wake. 3rd ed. 1993. LC 79-731. (Illus.). lib. bdg. 36.00 (*0-226-87011-1*) U Ch Pr.

Hyper Kids Workbook. Lendon H. Smith. 1990. (Illus.). 104p. (Orig.). 9.95 (*0-9626972-0-6*) Shaw Spelling.

Hyperactive Child, Adolescent, & Adult: Attention Deficit Disorder Through the Lifespan. Paul H. Wender. 1987. 172p. pap. 8.95 (*0-19-504952-7*); text 24.95 (*0-19-504291-3*) OUP.

Hyperactive Child with Minimal Brain Dysfunction. J. Gordon Millicap. 1975. (Illus.). 31.00 (*0-8151-5911-0*) Mosby Inc.

Hyperactive Children Grown Up: ADHD in Children, Adolescents & Adults. Gabrielle Weiss & Lily T. Hechtman. 2nd ed. 1993. LC 93-6950. 473p. pap. 26.00 (*0-89862-596-3*, 2596) Guilford Pubns.

Hyperactivity: Why Won't My Child Pay Attention? Sam Goldstein & Michael Goldstein. 1993. 224p. LC 91-24325. pap. 17.95 (*0-471-53307-6*); text 59.90 incl. audio (*0-471-30323-2*) Wiley.

Hyperactivity: Why Won't My Child Pay Attention. Sam Goldstein & Michael Goldstein. 1992. LC 91-24325. 224p. 27.95 (*0-471-53077-8*) Wiley.

Hyperactivity & Attention Disorders in Children. Martin Baren. 2000. (Pediatrics Ser.). 32p. pap. text 2.95 (*1-885274-01-7*) Health InfoNet Inc.

Hyperactivity Disorders of Childhood. Ed. by Seija Sandberg. 1996. (Monographs on Child & Adolescent Psychiatry: No. 2). (Illus.). 541p. (C). text 130.00 (*0-521-43250-2*) Cambridge U Pr.

Hyperactivity, the So-Called Attention-Deficit Disorder, & the Group of MBD Syndromes. Richard A. Gardner. 1987. LC 87-13499. (Illus.). 199p. 20.00 (*0-933812-15-9*) Creative Therapeutics.

*__Hyperacute Stroke: Imaging & Intervention.__ Gonzalez et al. 2001. (Illus.). 224p. (*1-901865-32-0*) Isis Med GBR. *Dist:* Bks Intl VA.

Hyperbaric Facility Safety: A Practical Guide. Ed. by Wilbur T. Workman. 1999. LC 99-61588. (Illus.). 754p. 128.00 (*0-941332-76-4*, B0997) Best Pub Co.

Hyperbaric Medicine: Proceedings of the 8th International Congress. Ed. by Eric P. Kindwall & George B. Hart. 1987. 335p. (C). text 44.00 (*0-941332-07-1*, D244) Best Pub Co.

Hyperbaric Medicine Practice. Ed. by Eric P. Kindwall & Harry T. Whelan. 2nd ed. 1999. LC 99-61376. (Illus.). 952p. 128.00 (*0-941332-78-0*, B0479) Best Pub Co.

Hyperbaric Oxygen Therapy Committee Report. Neil B. Hampson. rev. ed. 1999. 82p. pap. text 30.00 (*0-930406-14-1*) Undersea & Hyperbaric.

Hyperbaric Oxygen Therapy in Otorhinolaryngology. Ed. by Noriyuki Yanagita & Tsutomu Nakashima. 1998. LC 97-42559. (Advances in OtoRhinoLaryngology Ser.: Vol. 54, 1998). (Illus.). viii, 130p. 117.50 (*3-8055-6541-0*) S Karger.

Hyperbaric Physiology & Medicine. Ed. by Yu-Chong Lin & Alan K. Niu. 1988. (Illus.). 170p. (C). text 31.50 (*0-941332-11-X*, D272) Best Pub Co.

Hyperbrachycephaly As Influenced by Cultural Conditioning. J. Franklin Ewing. 1969. (Harvard University Peabody Museum of Archaeology & Ethnology Monographs). reprint ed. pap. 25.00 (*0-527-01257-2*) Periodicals Srv.

Hypercalcemia of Malignancy. Ed. by F. Raue. 1994. (Recent Results in Cancer Research Ser.: Vol. 137). (Illus.). 163p. 93.00 (*0-387-57631-2*) Spr-Verlag.

Hypercholesterolemia, Hypocholesterolemia & Hypertriglyceridemia in Vivo Kinetics. Ed. by C. L. Malmendier et al. 1991. LC 91-2557. (Advances in Experimental Medicine & Biology Ser.: Vol. 285). (Illus.). 454p. (C). text 150.00 (*0-306-43814-3*, Kluwer Plenum) Kluwer Academic.

Hyperglycemia, Diabetes & the Vascular Disease. Ed. by Neil Ruderman et al. 1992. (Clinical Physiology Ser.). (Illus.). 320p. text 90.00 (*0-19-506773-8*) OUP.

Hypericum & Depression. Peter McWilliams et al. 1997. LC 97-168746. 203p. pap. text 7.95 (*0-931580-36-6*) Mary Bks.

Hypericum Handbook: St. John's Wort, Nature's Antidepressant. Carol Turkington. 1998. LC 98-188410. 128p. pap. 9.95 (*0-87131-857-1*) M Evans.

Hyperinflation Therapy. Lonny J. Ashworth. 1998. (CPG Mentor - Patient Cases in Respiratory Care Ser.: Unit 1). (*0-8151-2277-2*) Mosby Inc.

Hyperkinetic Child. Carol A. Winchell. 1975. LC 74-28527. 182p. lib. bdg. 55.00 (*0-8371-7813-4*, WHC/, Greenwood Pr) Greenwood.

Hyperlipidaemia: Diagnosis & Management. Paul N. Durrington. 2nd ed. 1995. LC 94-33682. 352p. text (*0-7506-0876-5*) E A GBR. *Dist:* OUP.

Hyperlipidaemia Handbook. M. Godfrey. 1991. (C). text 59.00 (*0-7923-8960-3*) Kluwer Academic.

Hypermobility of Joints. Peter Beighton et al. 3rd ed. 1999. LC 99-10453. 192p. (C). (*1-85233-142-9*) Spr-Verlag GBR. *Dist:* Spr-Verlag, Spr-Verlag.

Hypersensitivity Pneumonitis: A Clinical Approach. O. P. Sharma. 1989. (Progress in Respiratory Research Ser.: Vol. 23). (Illus.). x, 186p. 151.50 (*3-8055-4974-1*) S Karger.

Hypertension. Bruce B. Brintnall & Ruth A. Brintnall. Ed. by Oliver D. Grin & Dorothy L. Bouwman. 1990. (Patient Education Ser.). (Illus.). 26p. pap. text 4.00 (*0-929689-00-3*) Ludann Co.

Hypertension. Frohlich. 1994. text (*0-397-51184-1*) Lppncott W & W.

Hypertension. Mary D. Litchford & Laura Yordy. 1995. (C). pap. 6.00 (*1-880989-54-9*) Case Sftware.

Hypertension. Ed. by Gerald Sandler. 1987. (Practical Clinical Medicine Ser.). (C). pap. text 73.50 (*0-7462-0041-2*) Kluwer Academic.

Hypertension. Albert Zanchetti. Ed. by Lennart Hansen et al. 2001. (Illus.). 400p. pap. 79.95 (*0-07-709523-5*) McGraw-Hill Med Pub.

*__Hypertension.__ MacGregor & Norman Kaplan. 2nd ed. 2001. (Fast Facts Ser.). (Illus.). 72p. pap. (*1-899541-39-X*) Health Pr GBR. *Dist:* JAMCO Dist.

Hypertension: A Companion to Brenner & Rector's the Kidney. Suzanne Oparil & Michael A. Weber. Ed. by Richard Zorab. 1999. LC 98-47451. (Illus.). 757p. text 95.00 (*0-7216-7764-9*) Saunders.

Hypertension: A Multidisciplinary Clinical Approach. Ed. by Robert L. Bloomfield et al. 1995. LC 93-72953. 398p. 85.00 (*0-89089-545-7*) Carolina Acad Pr.

Hypertension: A Policy Perspective. Milton C. Weinstein & William Stason. 1976. 240p. 25.50 (*0-674-43900-7*, WEHP) HUP.

Hypertension: Approach in Specialized Populations. Edward D. Frohlich. 1997. LC 98-14944. 300p. 55.00 (*0-683-30343-0*) Lppncott W & W.

Hypertension: Directory of Authors of New Medical & Scientific Reviews with Subject Index. Science and Life Consultants Association Staff. 1995. 160p. 57.50 (*0-7883-0590-5*); 1995. 160p. pap. 47.50 (*0-7883-0591-3*); 1997. 165p. 57.50 (*0-7883-1516-1*); 1997. 165p. pap. 47.50 (*0-7883-1517-X*) ABBE Pubs Assn.

Hypertension: Instructors Guide. Laura Yordy & Mary D. Litchford. 1990. (C). 3.5 hd 139.00 (*1-880989-07-7*); 3.5 hd 139.00 (*1-880989-05-0*); 5.25 hd 139.00 (*1-880989-06-9*); 5.25 hd 139.00 (*1-880989-04-2*) Case Sftware.

Hypertension: Mechanisms & Management. Ed. by T. Philip & A. Distler. 1980. 279p. 62.95 (*0-387-10171-3*) Spr-Verlag.

Hypertension: Mechanisms & Therapy. Norman K. Hollenberg. 2nd ed. 1998. LC 97-165613. (Atlas of Heart Diseases Ser.). 125.00 (*1-57340-111-0*) Current Med.

Hypertension: Pathophysiology & Clinical Implications of Early Structural Changes. Ed. by B. Folkow et al. 1985. (Illus.). 456p. (Orig.). pap. text 99.00 (*91-85520-37-3*) Coronet Bks.

Hypertension: Pathophysiology, Diagnosis, & Management John H. Laragh & Barry M. Brenner. 2nd ed. 1994. (Illus.). 3,344p. text 475.00 (*0-7817-0157-0*) Lppncott W & W.

Hypertension after Menopause. Ed. by M. Stimpel & A. Zanchetti. 1996. (Illus.). x, 123p. (Orig.). (C). pap. text 91.45 (*3-11-015518-4*) De Gruyter.

Hypertension & Co-Existing Disease. Francisco Leyva & Andrew J. Coats. 2000. LC 98-32240. (Illus.). 241p. pap. 99.00 (*0-632-05073-X*) Blackwell Sci.

Hypertension & Nutrition. Eric R. Braverman. Ed. by Don R. Bensen. 1996. LC 95-49091. 208p. pap. 12.95 (*0-87983-688-1*, 36881K, Keats Pubng) McGraw-Hill Trade.

Hypertension & Renal Disease. Ed. by G. Maschio et al. 1987. (Contributions to Nephrology Ser.: Vol. 54). (Illus.). viii, 232p. 29.75 (*3-8055-4372-7*) S Karger.

Hypertension & Stress: A Unified Concept. Alvin P. Shapiro. 1996. LC 95-52714. 128p. 29.95 (*0-8058-1904-5*) L Erlbaum Assocs.

Hypertension & Stroke Control in the Community: Proceedings of the WHO Expert Committee of Experts, Tokyo, March 11-13, 1974. WHO Staff. Ed. by S. Hatano et al. 1976. (ENG & FRE., Illus.). pap. text 30.00 (*92-4-156052-5*, 1150074) World Health.

Hypertension & the Heart: Proceedings of an International Conference Held As Part of the Menarini Series on Cardiovascular Diseases in Berlin, Germany, February 27-28, 1997. A. Zanchetti et al. 1998. LC 97-45693. (Advances in Experimental Medicine & Biology Ser.: Vol. 432). 300p. 95.00 (*0-306-45774-1*, Kluwer Plenum) Kluwer Academic.

Hypertension & the Kidney Ed. by Robert W. Schrier & Christopher S. Wilcox. 1999. LC 98-29127. (Atlas of Diseases of the Kidney Ser.: Vol. 3). (Illus.). 131.95 (*0-632-04389-X*) Blackwell Sci.

Hypertension Control: Report of a WHO Expert Committee. 1996. LC 97-132687. (Technical Reports: Vol. 862).Tr. of Lutte Contre L'Hypertension, Lucha Contra la Hypertension. (ENG, FRE & SPA.). 83p. (Orig.). pap. 16.00 (*92-4-120862-7*, 1100862) World Health.

Hypertension Education Course. Competence Assurance Systems Staff. 1982. (Illus.). pap. text 80.00 (*0-89147-056-5*) CAS.

Hypertension, Fluid-Electrolytes, & Tubulopathies in Pediatric Nephrology. Jose Strauss. 1982. text 141.50 (*90-247-2633-6*) Kluwer Academic.

Hypertension in Children. Leonard G. Feld. 1996. LC 96-9301. 233p. text (*0-7506-9678-8*) E A GBR. *Dist:* OUP.

*__Hypertension in Focus.__ Shankie. 2001. 152p. (*0-85369-456-7*) Pharmaceutical Pr GBR. *Dist:* Rittenhouse.

Hypertension in Kidney Disease. Ed. by Jhoong S. Cheich. 1986. (Developments in Nephrology Ser.). text 218.00 (*0-89838-797-3*) Kluwer Academic.

Hypertension in Postmenopausal Women. Ed. by Franz H. Messerli & Franz C. Aepfelbacher. 1995. LC 95-39859. (Illus.). 312p. text 135.00 (*0-8247-9652-7*, RC685) Dekker.

Hypertension in Postmenopausal Women. Ed. by Alberto Zanchetti et al. 1995. LC 94-29872. (Illus.). 95p. 42.95 (*0-387-58144-8*) Spr-Verlag.

Hypertension in Practice. D. G. Beevers & G. A. MacGregor. 3rd ed. 1999. 286p. (*1-85317-591-9*) Martin Dunitz.

Hypertension in Pregnancy. Ed. by J. J. Walker & N. Gant. 1997. LC 96-70877. (Illus.). 360p. (*0-412-30910-6*) E A GBR. *Dist:* OUP.

Hypertension in Primary Care. A and L New Media Staff. 1999. cd-rom 160.00 (*0-8385-3969-6*, Apple Lange Med) McGraw.

Hypertension in Primary Care: Pocketbook Edition. Henry L. Elliot. 2000. (Illus.). 72p. (*1-85317-628-1*) Martin Dunitz GBR. *Dist:* Blackwell Sci.

Hypertension in the Community. Ed. by T. Rosenthal & D. Silverberg. 1987. (Bibliotheca Cardiologica Ser.: No. 42). (Illus.). x, 178p. 148.00 (*3-8055-4521-5*) S Karger.

Hypertension in the Elderly, No. 157. Ed. by Gastone Leonetti & Cesare Cuspidi. 1994. LC 94-12005. (Developments in Cardiovascular Medicine Ser.: Vol. 157). 152p. text 98.00 (*0-7923-2852-3*) Kluwer Academic.

Hypertension in the Older Adult. Ed. by Andrew K. Scott. 1997. LC 97-171529. (An Arnold Publication). (Illus.). 208p. (*0-340-61475-7*) E A GBR. *Dist:* OUP.

Hypertension Management: Clinical Pathways, Guidelines & Patient Education. Jo Gulledge et al. 1995. LC 99-31851. (Chronic Disease Management Ser.). 212p. pap. 76.00 (*0-8342-1702-3*) Aspen Pub.

Hypertension Medicine. Ed. by Michael A. Weber. 2000. LC 00-33587. (Current Clinical Practice Ser.). (Illus.). 464p. 89.50 (*0-89603-788-6*) Humana.

Hypertension Primer. Ed. by Joseph L. Izzo, Jr. et al. 1993. LC 93-41432. 34.95 (*0-87493-201-7*) Am Heart.

Hypertension Sourcebook. Mary P. McGowan & Jo McGowan Chopra. 2001. LC 00-67785. 320p. pap. 17.95 (*0-7373-0539-8*) McGraw-Hill Prof.

Hypertension Treatment: User Guide. Norman M. Kaplan. 2nd ed. 1993. pap. 5.95 (*0-929240-53-7*) EMIS.

Hypertension User's Manual. Mary D. Litchford et al. rev. ed. 1995. (C). pap. 7.00 (*1-880989-22-0*) Case Sftware.

Hypertensive Cardiovascular Disease. A. Amery. 1982. text 482.00 (*90-247-2534-8*) Kluwer Academic.

Hypertensive Disorders in Women. Baha M. Sibai. 2000. LC 00-49272. (Illus.). x, 262p. (C). text 85.00 (*0-7216-7374-0*) Saunders.

Hypertensive Disorders of Pregnancy. Judith H. Poole et al. 1997. LC 97-20040. (*0-86525-077-4*) March of Dimes.

Hypertensive Heart Disease. B. E. Strauer. 1980. (Illus.). 105p. 34.95 (*0-387-10041-5*) Spr-Verlag.

Hypertensive Retinopathy. Ed. by S. S. Hayreh. 1989. (Journal: Vol. 198, No. 4). (Illus.). iv, 96p. pap. 56.75 (*3-8055-4996-2*) S Karger.

Hyperthermia & Cancer: Human Clinical Trail Experience, Vol. I. Ned B. Hornback & Robert E. Shupe. 1984. 160p. 119.00 (*0-8493-5675-X*, RC271) CRC Pr.

Hyperthermia & Cancer: Human Clinical Trail Experience, Vol. II. Ned B. Hornback & Robert E. Shupe. 1984. 176p. 101.00 (*0-8493-5676-8*, RC271, CRC Reprint) Franklin.

Hyperthermia & Oncology: Biology of Thermal Potentiation of Radiotherapy, Vol. II. Ed. by M. Urano & E. Douple. 1989. (Illus.). 175p. (*90-6764-119-7*) VSP NLD. *Dist:* Coronet Bks.

Hyperthermia & Radiation Therapy-Chemotherapy in the Treatment of Cancer. Ed. by J. M. Vaeth. 1984. (Frontiers of Radiation Therapy & Oncology Ser.: Vol. 18). (Illus.). viii, 196p. 142.75 (*3-8055-3725-5*) S Karger.

Hyperthermia & the Therapy of Malignant Tumors. Ed. by C. Streffer. 1987. (Recent Results in Cancer Research Ser.: Vol. 104). (Illus.). 207p. 113.00 (*0-387-17250-5*) Spr-Verlag.

Hyperthermia in Cancer Treatment. Ed. by Leopold J. Anghileri & Jacques Robert. 1986. Vol. I. 256p. 141.00 (*0-8493-6045-5*, RC271); Vol. II. 288p. 161.00 (*0-8493-6046-3*, RC271) Franklin (CRC Reprint).

Hyperthermic & Hypermetabolic Disorders: Exertional Heat Stroke, Malitgnant Hyperthermia & Related Syndromes. Ed. by Philip M. Hopkins & F. R. Ellis. 1996. (Illus.). 298p. (C). text 80.00 (*0-521-44381-4*) Cambridge U Pr.

Hyperthermic Oncology: Proceedings of the Fourth International Conference on Hyperthermic Oncology, 1984, Set. Ed. by Jens Overgaard. 1984. 1270p. 209.00 (*0-8002-3824-9*) Taylor & Francis.

Hyperthermic Oncology, Vol. 1: Summary Papers. Ed. by Jens Overgaard. 1984. 870p. 154.00 (*0-85066-273-7*) Taylor & Francis.

Hyperthermic Oncology, Vol. 2: Review Lectures, Symposium Summaries & Workshop Summaries. Ed. by Jens Overgaard. 1984. 400p. 88.00 (*0-85066-281-8*) Taylor & Francis.

Hyperthermie und Tumormikrozirkulation. B. Endrich. 1988. (Beitraege Zur Onkologie, Contributions to Oncology Ser.: Vol. 31). (Illus.). xii, 138p. 51.50 (*3-8055-4758-7*) S Karger.

Hypertrophic Response in Smooth Muscle. Henry M. Seidel. 1987. 208p. 122.00 (*0-8493-6299-7*, QP321, CRC Reprint) Franklin.

Hyperviscosity in Hypertension. Leopold Dintenfass. (Illus.). 192p. 1982. pap. text 31.00 (*0-08-024815-2*, Pergamon Pr); 1981. text 52.00 (*0-08-024816-0*) Elsevier.

Hypnoanalysis. Lewis R. Wolberg. 2nd ed. 1964. LC 64-20777. 446p. text 70.00 (*0-8089-0534-1*, 794867, Grune & Strat) Harcrt Hlth Sci Grp.

Hypnoanalysis for Individual & Marital Psychotherapy. John A. Scott, Sr. 1993. 256p. (C). pap. text 29.95 (*0-89876-202-2*) Gardner Pr.

Hypnoanalytic Techniques: Practice of Clinical Hypnosis, Vol. II John G. Watkins. 1989. (Illus.). 300p. (C). 14.00 (*0-8290-2306-2*) Irvington.

Hypnosis: A Jungian Perspective. James A. Hall. 1989. LC 88-37199. (Guilford Clinical & Experimental Hypnosis Ser.). 179p. 30.00 (*0-89862-382-0*, 2382) Guilford Pubns.

Hypnosis: A Scientific Approach. Theodore X. Barber. 1995. LC 95-37615. 298p. pap. 55.00 (*1-56821-740-4*) Aronson.

Hypnosis: New Tool in Nursing Practice. Ed. by Gil Boyne. 1982. 197p. (C). 25.00 (*0-930298-12-8*) Westwood Pub Co.

Hypnosis: The Application of Ideomotor Techniques. David B. Cheek. enl. rev. ed. 1993. LC 93-29853. 336p. 85.00 (*0-205-15595-2*, Longwood Div) Allyn.

Hypnosis: The Cognitive-Behavioral Perspective. Ed. by Nicholas P. Spanos & John F. Chaves. 1989. LC 88-43037. (Psychology Ser.). 511p. 55.00 (*0-87975-469-9*) Prometheus Bks.

Hypnosis: Trance As a Coping Mechanism. F. H. Frankel. 1976. LC 76-14856. (Topics in General Psychiatry Ser.). (Illus.). 196p. (C). 54.50 (*0-306-30932-7*, Plenum Trade) Perseus Pubng.

Hypnosis, Acupuncture & Pain. Maurice M. Tinterow & Jon Sward. 1989. LC 89-62007. (Illus.). 250p. (Orig.). pap. 10.95 (*0-942333-08-X*) Bio-Comns Pr.

Hypnosis & Behavioral Medicine. Daniel P. Brown & Erika Fromm. 1987. LC 86-19961. 296p. text 59.95 (*0-89859-925-3*) L Erlbaum Assocs.

Hypnosis & Hypnotherapy. David T. Rowley. 1986. LC 86-71023. 208p. 24.95 (*0-914783-13-0*); pap. 17.95 (*0-914783-15-7*) Charles.

Hypnosis & Hypnotherapy with Children. Karen Olness & Daniel P. Kohen. 3rd ed. 1996. LC 95-26800. (Illus.). 457p. 52.00 (*1-57230-054-X*, 0054) Guilford Pubns.

Hypnosis & Memory. Ed. by Helen M. Pettinati. 1988. LC 87-7597. (Clinical & Experimental Hypnosis Ser.). 301p. 45.00 (*0-89862-338-3*) Guilford Pubns.

Hypnosis & Suggestive Management of Pain: A Clinical Guide. Joseph Barber et al. 1996. LC 96-6382. 432p. 45.00 (*0-393-70216-2*) Norton.

Hypnosis & the Treatment of Depressions: Strategies for Change. Michael D. Yapko. 1992. LC 92-17478. 224p. text 32.95 (*0-87630-682-2*) Brunner-Routledge.

Hypnosis, Dissociation & Absorption: Theories, Assessment & Treatment. Marty Sapp. 2000. LC 99-86788. (Illus.). xv, 182p. 35.95 (*0-398-07054-7*) C C Thomas.

Hypnosis for Change. Josie Hadley & Carol Staudacher. 1987. 368p. mass mkt. 6.99 (*0-345-34293-3*) Ballantine Pub Grp.

Hypnosis for the Seriously Curious. Kenneth Bowers. 1983. 176p. (C). pap. 13.00 (*0-393-95339-4*) Norton.

Hypnosis, Imagination & Human Potentialities. Theodore X. Barber et al. 1974. LC 73-19539. pap. text 22.00 (*0-08-017931-2*, Pergamon Pr) Elsevier.

Hypnosis in the Relief of Pain. Ernest R. Hilgard & Josephine R. Hilgard. rev. ed. 1994. LC 93-49073. 312p. pap. text 29.95 (*0-87630-700-4*) Brunner-Routledge.

Hypnosis in Treatment. William Moodie. 1960. 16.95 (*0-87523-121-7*) Emerson.

Hypnosis Induction Technics. Myron Teitelbaum. 1980. 200p. text 40.95 (*0-398-01907-X*) C C Thomas.

Hypnosis, Memory & Behavior in Criminal Investigation. Kevin M. McConkey & Peter W. Sheehan. 1995. LC 95-14251. (Clinical & Experimental Hypnosis Ser.). 240p. 40.00 (*1-57230-008-6*, 0008) Guilford Pubns.

Hypnosis to End Anxiety & Panic Attacks. Josie Hadley & Carol Staudacher. 1982. (Hypnosis Tape Ser.). 11.95 incl. audio (*0-934986-56-8*) New Harbinger.

Hypnosis, Will & Memory: A Psycho-Legal History. Jean-Roch Laurence & Campbell Perry. 1988. LC 87-19672. (Clinical & Experimental Hypnosis Ser.). 432p. pap. 28.50 (*0-89862-504-1*) Guilford Pubns.

Hypnotheraphy & Hypnoanalysis. Daniel P. Brown & Erika Fromm. 1986. LC 86-19736. 392p. text 59.95 (*0-89859-783-8*) L Erlbaum Assocs.

Hypnotherapist's Creative Guide: A Collection of Scripts, Processes & Case Histories. Ed. by Katherine Zimmerman. 1999. 200p. pap. 29.00 (*1-929957-04-1*) TranceTime.

Hypnotherapy. Dave Elman. 1984. 336p. 34.95 (*0-930298-04-7*) Westwood Pub Co.

Hypnotherapy: A Guide to Improving Health & Well-Being with Hypnosis. Ursula Markham. 1997. (Illus.). 128p. pap. (*0-09-181519-3*) Random.

Hypnotherapy: A Handbook. Ed. by Michael Heap & Wendy Dryden. 1991. (Psychology Handbook Ser.). 224p. pap. (*0-335-09887-8*) OpUniv Pr.

Hypnotherapy: A Modern Approach. Golden. 1992. 176p. (C). pap. text 48.00 (*0-205-14334-2*, H4334) Allyn.

Hypnotherapy: A Modern Approach. William L. Golden et al. 1987. (Psychology Practitioner Guidebooks). 192p. text 30.00 (*0-08-034303-1*); pap. text 15.95 (*0-08-034302-3*) Elsevier (Pergamon Pr).

Hypnotherapy: A Survey of the Literature. Margaret Brenman & Merton M. Gill. 1971. (Menninger Foundation Monograph Ser.: No. 5). 303p. (Orig.). 40.00 (*0-8236-2420-X*); pap. 24.95 (*0-8236-8073-8*, 022420) Intl Univs Pr.

Hypnotherapy: An Exploratory Casebook. Milton H. Erickson & Ernest L. Rossi. 1980. LC 78-23839. 512p. text 49.95 incl. audio (*0-8290-0347-9*) Ardent Media.

Hypnotherapy for Healing the Mind & Body. Steven Mitchell & Karyn K. Mitchell. 1997. 200p. (Orig.). stu. ed., per. (*0-9640822-0-9*) Mind Rivers.

Hypnotherapy for Health, Harmony, & Peak Performance: Expanding the Goals of Psychotherapy. Set. Catherine Walters & Ronald A. Havens. 1993. LC 92-48326. 224p. text 43.95 incl. audio (*0-87630-690-3*) Brunner-Routledge.

Hypnotherapy for Troubled Children. Robert E. Duke. 1984. 220p. text 29.95 incl. audio (*0-8290-1030-0*) Irvington.

Hypnotherapy for Troubled Children. Robert E. Duke. 1994. 14.95 (*0-88282-007-9*) New Horizon NJ.

Hypnotherapy of Pain in Children with Cancer. Josephine R. Hilgard & Samuel LeBaron. 1991. LC 84-17160. 250p. reprint ed. text 25.95 (*0-86576-074-8*) Brunner-Routledge.

Hypnotherapy Scripts: A Neo-Ericksonian Approach to Persuasive Healing. Ronald A. Havens & Catherine R. Walters. 1989. LC 89-17356. 214p. text 32.95 (*0-87630-547-8*) Brunner-Routledge.

Hypnotic Alteration of Sensory, Perceptual & Psychophysiological Processes. Milton H. Erickson. Ed. by Ernest L. Rossi. 1980. (Collected Papers of Milton H. Erickson on Hypnosis: Vol. II). 368p. reprint ed. pap. 29.95 (*0-8290-1207-9*); text 49.95 (*0-8290-0543-9*) Ardent Media.

Hypnotic Brain: Hypnotherapy & Social Communication. Peter Brown. 1991. 335p. 22.50 (*0-300-05001-1*) Yale U Pr.

Hypnotic Investigation of Psychodynamic Processes. Milton H. Erickson. Ed. by Ernest L. Rossi. 1980. (Collected Papers of Milton H. Erickson on Hypnosis: Vol. III). 368p. (C). reprint ed. pap. 29.95 (*0-8290-1208-7*); text 49.95 (*0-8290-0544-7*) Ardent Media.

Hypnotic Methods in Nonhypnotic Therapies. Aaron N. Hoorwitz. 1989. 264p. text 42.95 (*0-8290-1802-6*) Irvington.

Hypnotic Realities: The Induction of Clinical Hypnosis & Forms of Indirect Suggestion. Milton H. Erickson et al. 1976. LC 76-20636. 39.95 incl. audio (*0-8290-0112-3*) Ardent Media.

Hypnotism & Meditation. Ormond McGill. Ed. by Diane L. England & Charles Mignosa. 1981. 99p. (C). pap. 14.95 (*0-930298-08-X*) Westwood Pub Co.

Hypnotism Today. Leslie M. LeCron & Jean Bordeaux. 1953. LC 47-1654. 287p. text 56.00 (*0-8089-0259-8*, 792490, Grune & Strat) Harcrt Hlth Sci Grp.

Hypnotize Me & Make Me Great. Judd Biasiotto. Ed. by Jim Trunzo & Tim McClellan. 1985. 100p. (Orig.). pap. 7.00 (*0-933079-00-1*) World Class Enterprises.

Hypochondriack James Boswell. Ed. by Margery Bailey. LC 78-39512. reprint ed. 85.00 (*0-404-07654-8*) AMS Pr.

Hypochondriac's Guide to Life: A Slightly Hysterical Guide to Life & Death. Gene Weingarten. 1998. LC 98-19532. 192p. 22.00 (*0-684-85280-2*) Simon & Schuster.

Hypochondriac's Handbook. Wendy Marston. 1998. LC 98-17271. (Illus.). 144p. 10.95 (*0-8118-2192-7*) Chronicle Bks.

Hypochondriasis: or Death's Hobby Horse: A Practical Treatise, etc. on the Nature & Cure of That Disorder Call'd the Hyp or Hypo. John Hill. 1969. LC 92-49673. (Augustan Reprints Ser.: No. 135). reprint ed. 14.50 (*0-404-70135-3*, RC552) AMS Pr.

Hypodermics. Stephen Oldroyd & Kenneth Stoffers. 1980. 48p. lthr. 45.00 (*0-88014-022-4*) Mosaic Pr OH.

Hypoglycaemic Tumors. J. Laurent et al. 1971. 30.50 (*90-219-2029-8*, Excerpta Medica) Elsevier.

Hypoglycemia. Ed. by Health Education Staff. 1988. 4p. pap. 1.00 (*0-937721-10-7*) Wiley.

Hypoglycemia. Marilyn H. Light. Ed. by Richard A. Passwater & Earl R. Mindell. 1983. (Good Health Guides). 31p. (Orig.). pap. 3.95 (*0-87983-302-5*, 33025K, Keats Pubng) McGraw-Hill Trade.

Hypoglycemia: A Better Approach. Paavo O. Airola. 1977. 192p. pap. 7.95 (*0-932090-01-X*) Health Plus.

Hypoglycemia: A Nutritional Approach. Louise Tenney. 1989. (Woodland Health Ser.: No. 9). 55p. pap. 3.95 (*0-913923-77-X*) Woodland UT.

Hypoglycemia: Directory of Authors of New Medical & Scientific Reviews with Subject Index. Science and Life Consultants Association Staff. 160p. 1995. 57.50 (*0-7883-0602-2*); 1995. pap. 47.50 (*0-7883-0603-0*); 1998. 57.50 (*0-7883-1940-X*); 1998. pap. 47.50 (*0-7883-1941-8*) ABBE Pubs Assn.

Hypoglycemia: Low Blood Sugar. 1997. lib. bdg. 250.75 (*0-8490-5884-8*) Gordon Pr.

Hypoglycemia: Pathophysiology, Diagnosis, & Treatment. Philip E. Cryer. 1997. LC 96-54723. (Illus.). 198p. (C). text 49.95 (*0-19-511325-X*) OUP.

Hypoglycemia: The Deadly Roller Coaster. David G. Williams. 1987. 65p. pap. 6.95 (*0-944649-02-5*) Mtn Home Pub.

Hypoglycemia: The Disease Your Doctor Won't Treat. Jeraldine Saunders & Harvey M. Ross. 1996. LC 96-213123. 240p. pap. 13.00 (*1-57566-064-4*, Knsington) Kensgtn Pub Corp.

Hypoglycemia & Diabetes. Brian Frier & Miles Fisher. 1993. 416p. (*0-340-55421-5*) E A GBR. *Dist:* OUP.

Hypoglycemia & Diabetes Cope Book see Hypoglycemia & Diabetes Wellness Guide

Hypoglycemia & Diabetes Wellness Guide. Freda Whalen & Gilbert Manso. Ed. by Charles Ingram. 1995. Orig. Title: Hypoglycemia & Diabetes Cope Book. 310p. pap. 19.95 (*0-9638201-1-7*) Body Care.

Hypoglycemia-Diabetes Cope Book: A Guide to Healthy Living. Freda Whalen & Gilbert Manso. 1993. 310p. per. (*0-9638201-0-9*) Body Care.

Hypokinesia & Weightlessness: Clinical & Physiological Aspects. Oleg Atkov & V. S. Bednenko. 1992. 561p. (C). 85.00 (*0-8236-2415-3*) Intl Univs Pr.

Hypoplastic Left Heart Syndrome: A Handbook for Parents. Anna Jaworski. 2nd rev. ed. 1997. (Illus.). 110p. reprint ed. pap. 20.00 (*0-9652508-6-5*) Baby Hearts.

Hypothalamic Peptides in Endocrinology: Morphological & Physiological Aspects: Proceedings of the 22nd Gunma Symposium on Endocrinology, Japan, 1984. Ed. by M. Suzuki. 1985. 220p. lib. bdg. (*90-6764-061-1*) VSP NLD. *Dist:* Coronet Bks.

Hypothalamic-Pituitary-Adrenocortical(HPA) Regulation: A Contribution to Its Assessment, Development, & Disorders in Infancy & Childhood with Special Reference to Plasma Cortisol Circadian Rhythm. R. P. Zurbruegg. 1976. (Monographs in Pediatrics: Vol. 7). (Illus.). 120p. 42.75 (*3-8055-2253-3*) S Karger.

***Hypothalamic-Pituitary Development: Genetic & Clinical Aspects.** Ed. by R. Rappaport & S. Amselem. 2001. (Endocrine Development Ser.: Vol. 4). (Illus.). viii, 192p. 163.50 (*3-8055-7239-5*) S Karger.

Hypothalamus. 1962. 415.00 (*0-387-02837-4*) Spr-Verlag.

Hypothermia. 1992. (Education Publication Ser.: No. 15). (Illus.). 20p. (Orig.). pap. 4.00 (*1-56612-006-3*) AK Sea Grant CP.

Hypothermia - Ashore & Afloat: Proceedings of 3rd International " Action for Disaster " Conference, Aberdeen 1979. James M. Adam. 1981. (Illus.). 216p. 48.00 (*0-08-025750-X*, Pergamon Pr) Elsevier.

Hypothermia & Cerebral Ischemia: Mechanisms & Clinical Applications. Ed. by Carolina M. Maier & Gary K. Steinberg. 2000. 350p. 145.00 (*0-89603-660-X*) Humana.

Hypothermia, Frostbite & Other Cold Injuries: Prevention, Recognition, Pre Hospital Treatment. Ed. by James A. Wilkerson et al. 1986. LC 86-690. (Illus.). 128p. (Orig.). pap. 12.95 (*0-89886-024-5*) Mountaineers.

Hypothesis & Evidence in Psychoanalysis. Marshall Edelson. LC 83-9281. 1985. 196p. pap. text 10.00 (*0-226-18436-6*); 1984. xiv, 180p. 27.00 (*0-226-18432-3*) U Ch Pr.

Hypothesis Testing Behavior. Fenna Poletiek. 2001. LC 00-59070. (Essays in Cognitive Psychology Ser.). 192p. (*1-84169-159-3*) Psychol Pr GBR. *Dist:* Taylor & Francis.

Hypothyroidism: The Unsuspected Illness. Broda Barnes & Lawrence Galton. 1976. LC 75-29251. 320p. 26.00 (*0-690-01029-X*) HarperTrade.

Hypovalemic Anemia of Trauma: The Missing Blood Syndrome. C. Robert Valeri & Mark D. Altschule. 1981. 192p. 109.00 (*0-8493-5389-0*, RC641, CRC Reprint) Franklin.

Hypoxia: Into the Next Millennium. Robert C. Roach et al. 1999. LC 99-47777. (Advances in Experimental Medicine & Biology Ser.). xvi, 456p. (*0-306-46289-3*, Kluwer Plenum) Kluwer Academic.

Hypoxia & Cold. Ed. by John R. Sutton. 1987. LC 85-25658. 560p. 140.00 (*0-275-92081-X*, C2081, Praeger Pubs) Greenwood.

Hypoxia & the Brain: Proceedings of the 8th International Hypoxia Symposium Held at Lake Louise, Canada, February 9-13, 1993. Ed. by John R. Sutton et al. 1993. (Illus.). 350p. (Orig.). pap. text 12.00 (*0-9612246-1-4*) C S Houston.

Hypoxia, High Altitude & the Heart: Proceedings of the Cardiovascular Disease Conference, 1st, Snowmass at Aspen, Colorado, 1970. Cardiovascular Disease Conference Staff. Ed. by J. H. Vogel. 1970. (Advances in Cardiology Ser.: Vol. 5). 61.75 (*3-8055-0728-3*) S Karger.

Hypoxia, Metabolic Acidosis & the Circulation. Ed. by Allen I. Arieff. 1992. (Clinical Physiology Ser.). (Illus.). 232p. text 59.50 (*0-19-506062-8*, 10045) OUP.

Hyssop Superior Healing Power: Twenty-First Century Herbs. Willie Southall. 1993. 160p. text 19.00 (*0-9639682-1-1*); pap. text 16.00 (*0-9639682-0-3*) Southall Res.

Hysterectomy. Ed. by Michael Diamond et al. 1994. (Illus.). 208p. 85.00 (*0-86542-355-5*) Blackwell Sci.

Hysterectomy. Ed. by Thomas G. Stovall. 1993. (Current Topics in Obstetrics & Gynecology Ser.). (Illus.). 224p. (gr. 13). 73.95 (*0-412-04681-4*) Chapman & Hall.

Hysterectomy: A Guide for Women. Michael S. Hoffman. Ed. by William N. Spellacy. 1996. (Women's Health Ser.). (Illus.). 24p. pap. 2.95 (*1-885274-19-X*) Health InfoNet Inc.

Hysterectomy: A Review of the Literature on Indications, Effectiveness, & Risks. Steven Bernstein et al. 1998. LC 95-48361. 109p. pap. 15.00 (*0-8330-2347-0*) Rand Corp.

Hysterectomy: Clinical Recommendations & Indications for Use. Ed. by Steven Bernstein et al. 1997. LC 97-47170. pap. 15.00 (*0-8330-2574-0*) Rand Corp.

Hysterectomy: Clinical Recommendations & Indications for Use. Lucian L. Leape et al. 1998. LC 97-11334. (Illus.). 34p. pap. 15.00 (*0-8330-2501-5*) Rand Corp.

Hysterectomy: Learning the Facts, Coping with the Feelings, Facing the Future. Wanda Wigfall-Williams. LC 86-7317. (Illus.). 152p. 1988. pap. 12.95 (*0-935576-15-0*); 1986. 17.95 (*0-935576-17-7*) Kesend Pub Ltd.

Hysterectomy: New Options & Advances. Lorraine Dennerstein et al. 2nd ed. 1999. (Illus.). 204p. pap. 22.95 (*0-19-551033-X*) OUP.

Hysterectomy: Ratings of Appropriateness. Steven J. Bernstein et al. 1998. LC 97-32738. (Illus.). 137p. pap. 15.00 (*0-8330-2571-6*, MR-592/3) Rand Corp.

Hysterectomy Before & After: A Comprehensive Guide to Preventing, Preparing for, & Maximizing Health after Hysterectomy. Winnifred B. Cutler. 1990. LC 87-46132. 464p. reprint ed. pap. 16.00 (*0-06-091629-X*, Perennial) HarperTrade.

Hysteria: The Elusive Neurosis. Alan Krohn. 1978. LC 76-45546. (Psychological Issues Monographs: Nos. 45/46). 345p. 50.00 (*0-8236-2426-9*); 38.00 (*0-8236-2425-0*) Intl Univs Pr.

Hysteria: The History of a Disease. Ilza Veith. 1992. LC 65-24429. (Illus.). pap. text 3.25 (*0-226-85253-9*, P351) U Ch Pr.

Hysteria & Other Cases: A Maine Doctor Looks Back. James E. Poulin. 1993. 88p. pap. 7.95 (*0-9635457-0-1*) Mtn Greenery.

Hysteria Beyond Freud. Sander L. Gilman et al. 1993. LC 92-30932. 478p. text 45.00 (*0-520-08064-5*) U CA Pr.

Hysteria from Freud to Lacan: Body & Language in Psychoanalysis. Monique David-Menard. Tr. by Catherine Porter from FRE. 1989. LC 89-42870. 240p. 45.00 (*0-8014-2100-4*) Cornell U Pr.

Hysteria from Freud to Lacan: The Splendid Child of Psychoanalysis. Juan-David Nasio. 1997. LC 98-39631. (Lacanian Clinical Field Ser.). 176p. reprint ed. pap. 17.95 (*1-892746-02-6*, 46026) Other Pr LLC.

Hysterical Psychosis: A Historical Survey. Katrien Libbrecht. 1995. LC 94-8720. 290p. (C). text 44.95 (*1-56000-181-X*) Transaction Pubs.

Hysterosalpingo-Contrast Sonography: An Atlas & Textbook. Ed. by Ulrich Deichert & Reinhard Schlief. 1995. LC 94-48294. (*0-7923-3335-7*) Kluwer Academic.

Hysterosalpingography: A Text & Atlas. David J. Ott & Jamil A. Fayez. 1991. (Illus.). 144p. text 82.00 (*0-683-06658-7*) Lppncott W & W.

Hysterosalpingography: A Text & Atlas. David J. Ott et al. 2nd ed. 1998. LC 98-10427. (Illus.). 162p. 129.00 (*0-683-30378-3*) Lppncott W & W.

Hysteroscopy. H. Van der Pas et al. 1983. 250p. text 164.00 (*0-85200-726-4*) Kluwer Academic.

Hysteroscopy: Textbook & Atlas. Klaus J. Neis & Hermann Hepp. 1994. (Illus.). 128p. text 89.00 (*0-86577-489-7*) Thieme Med Pubs.

Hysteroscopy & Microcolpohysteroscopy Text & Atlas. Jacques Hamou. 1992. (Illus.). 340p. (C). pap. 189.00 (*0-8385-3995-5*, A3995-9) McGraw-Hill Educ Grp.

Hystories: Hysterical Epidemics & Modern Culture. Elaine Showalter. 1997. LC 96-44108. 244p. 26.50 (*0-231-10458-8*) Col U Pr.

I

I Always Start My Diet on Monday: A Unique Program to Permanently Conquer Emotional Overeating. Janice Alpert. unabr. ed. 1997. 208p. (Orig.). pap. 13.95 (*0-9655023-0-9*) Pearl Pub IL.

I Am Not a Victim: One Man's Triumph over Fear & AIDS. Louie Nassaney et al. 1990. LC 88-84105. (Illus.). 128p. pap. 9.00 (*0-937611-47-6*, 111) Hay House.

I Amness: The Discovery of the Self Beyond the Ego. Ian Kent & William Nicholls. 1972. LC 78-161250. pap. 3.95 (*0-672-51620-9*, Bobbs) Macmillan.

I & the "Not-I" A Study in the Development of Consciousness. M. Esther Harding. 1974. LC 65-11535. (Bollingen Ser.: Vol. 79). (Illus.). 254p. pap. 17.95 (*0-691-01796-4*) Princeton U Pr.

I Awaken to Glory: Essays Celebrating the Sesquicentennial of The Discovery of Anesthesia by Horace Wells, December 11, 1844-December 11, 1994. Ed. by Richard J. Wolfe & Leonard F. Menczer. 1994. LC 95-113558. 442p. 28.95 (*0-88135-161-X*) Watson Pub Intl.

I Can Cope: Staying Healthy with Cancer. Judi Johnson & Linda Klein. 2nd enl. rev. ed. 1994. LC 93-23399. 352p. pap. 14.95 (*1-56561-039-3*, 004236) Wiley.

I Can Problem Solve: An Interpersonal Cognitive Problem-Solving Program for Children—Preschool. Myrna B. Shure. rev. ed. 2000. LC 00-133939. (Illus.). 336p. otabind 39.95 (*0-87822-457-2*) Res Press.

I Can't Wait until Tomorrow: Stories, Essays & Poems on Medicine. 2000. 160p. pap. 14.95 (*1-891576-01-1*) North Shore Pr.

I Ching: Images of Psychological Typology & Development. Richard Grant. 1990. (Illus.). 90p. (Orig.). pap. 10.95 (*1-878287-26-5*) Type & Temperament.

I Did It! So Can You! Larry Fournier. Ed. by Greta Bishop. 1988. LC 88-90657. (Illus.). 141p. (Orig.). pap. 9.95 (*0-934739-05-6*) Pussywillow Pub.

I Didn't Have Cancer for Nothing. Lyn Ellis. 1989. 177p. (C). text (*0-902662-75-9*); pap. text (*0-902662-76-7*) R K Pubns GBR. *Dist:* St Mut.

I Don't Know Who You Are Anymore: A Family's Struggle with Depression. Kellie Branson & Dale A. Babcock. Ed. by Jean Terra. 1992. LC 91-76568. 192p. (Orig.). pap. 12.95 (*0-9625040-3-3*, 297-231-X) Legendary Pub.

I Don't Remember Signing up for Cancer. Sherry K. Waldrip. 1996. (Illus.). 158p. pap. 10.00 (*0-939513-74-9*) Joy Pub SJC.

I Don't Want to Talk about It: Overcoming the Secret Legacy of Male Depression. Terrence Real. 1997. LC 96-41711. 384p. 24.00 (*0-684-83102-3*) Scribner.

I Got Pregnant, You Can Too! How Healing Yourself Physically, Mentally & Spiritually Leads to Fertility. Katie Boland. 1998. LC 98-9477. 185p. (Orig.). pap. 12.00 (*1-887424-38-5*) Underwood Bks.

I Have a Friend with Mental Illness: Basic Manuals for Friends of the Disabled. Hannah Carlson & Dale Carlson. 1996. LC 96-84060. (Basic Manuals for Friends of the Disabled Ser.: Vol. 6). (Illus.). 64p. (Orig.). pap. 9.95 (*1-884158-13-7*) Bick Pub Hse.

I Have a Hunch: The Autobiography of Jose Silva Jose Silva. (Illus.). 350p. (Orig.). 1. pap. 12.95 (*0-913343-01-3*); 2. pap. 12.95 (*0-913343-05-6*); Set. pap. 24.95 (*0-913343-10-2*) Inst Psych Inc.

I Have a Pain in My... A Child's Diary for Expressing Pain & Personal Feelings. Donna C. Grice. Ed. by MSW Publishing Co Staff. 1995. (Illus.). 130p. (Orig.). (J). (gr. 1-6). pap. text 9.95 (*0-9640903-3-3*) M S W Pubng.

I Just Lost Myself: Psychological Abuse of Women in Marriage. Valerie N. Chang. 1996. LC 95-30660. 184p. 58.00 (*0-275-95209-6*, Praeger Pubs) Greenwood.

I Know You Really Love Me: A Psychiatrist's Journal of Erotomania, Stalking & Obsessive Love. Doreen R. Orion. 1997. LC 97-14348. 312p. 23.95 (*0-02-861665-0*) Macmillan.

I Make a Difference: Making the Transition from Clinician to Educator. Ed. by Larry Hudson et al. 1992. LC 92-10180. 340p. (C). mass mkt. 27.25 (*0-8273-4990-4*) Delmar.

I Need Help: A Stroke Patient's Plea: Suggestions for Patients & Caregivers Including Simplified Medical Terminology. Helen Underwood. Ed. by Paul M. Clemens. 1992. LC 91-27780. 112p. (Orig.). pap. 8.95 (*0-931892-72-4*) B Dolphin Pub.

I Never Knew I Had a Choice. Gerald Corey. 3rd ed. 1985. LC 85-11306. (Psychology-Counseling Ser.). 520p. (C). pap. 30.50 (*0-534-05418-8*) Brooks-Cole.

I Never Knew I Had a Choice. Gerald Corey & Marianne Schneider Corey. (Psychology-Counseling Ser.). 4th ed. 1989. LC 89-32330. 464p. (C). pap. 38.50 (*0-534-11586-1*); 5th ed. 1993. LC 92-35589. 402p. pap. 33.75 (*0-534-20166-0*) Brooks-Cole.

I Never Told Anyone This Before: Managing the Initial Disclosure of Sexual Abuse Re-Collections. Janice A. Gasker. 1999. LC 98-39342. (Illus.). 176p. (C). lib. bdg. 29.95 (*0-7890-0461-5*, Maltreatment & Trauma Pr) Haworth Pr.

I Quit: Subliminal Audio Conditioning Helps You Stop Smoking. Eugene Eye. 1981. LC 81-81352. 35p. (Orig.). wbk. ed. 49.50 incl. audio (*0-939968-00-2*) R E Fellows.

I Rejected Bypass Surgery for a Better Life. Robert A. Gegan. 1981. LC 81-66843. (Illus.). 300p. (Orig.). pap. 7.95 (*0-940062-01-1*) Consumer Info Pubns.

I. S. M. Principles of Biostatistics. Pagano. 2nd ed. 1998. (Statistics Ser.). pap. (*0-534-22903-4*) Brooks-Cole.

I. V. Antibiotics Education Course. Competence Assurance Systems Staff. 1985. (Illus.). pap. text 85.00 (*0-89147-060-3*) CAS.

I. V. Therapy. Springhouse Publishing Company Staff. 1998. LC 98-21797. (Incredibly Easy Ser.). (Illus.). 292p. pap. 34.95 (*0-87434-958-3*) Springhouse Corp.

I Want More of Everything. Eda LeShan. 1994. LC 94-22544. 256p. 20.00 (*1-55704-211-X*) Newmarket.

I Want to Be a Veterinarian. Created & Prod. by Stephanie Maze. 1999. LC 96-215. (Illus.). 48p. (J). (gr. 3-9). pap. 9.00 (*0-15-201965-0*, Harcourt Pbk) Harcourt Childs Bks.

I Want to Remember: An Alzheimer Journey & Reflection. David D. Gray. 1990. (Illus.). 128p. (Orig.). pap. 14.95 (*0-934512-06-X*) Roundtable Pr.

I Want to See. Arthur S. M. Lim. 2nd ed. 2000. 216p. 50.00 (*981-02-4311-1*); pap. 25.00 (*981-02-4312-X*) World Scientific Pub.

H
I

I Wish... Dreams & Realities of Parenting a Special Needs Child. Kate D. McAnaney. 1992. 96p. (Orig.). pap. 8.95 (*0-9632338-0-7*) United Cereb Palsy.

I Wish I Were Thin - I Wish I Were Fat: The Real Reasons We Overeat & What We Can Do about It. Michelle Joy Levine. 1997. LC 97-60106. 240p. 23.95 (*0-9656686-4-9*) Vanderbilt Press.

IA Antigens. Soldano Ferrone & Chella S. David. 1982. LC 00-8493. Vol. I: Mice. 264p. 148.00 (*0-8493-6461-2*, QR184); Vol. II: Man & Other Species. 176p. 103.00 (*0-8493-6462-0*) Franklin (CRC Reprint).

IARC Annual Report 1982. 1982. (IARC Scientific Publications Ser.). 174p. 12.00 (*92-832-1082-4*, 1750082) World Health.

IARC Annual Report 1983. 1983. (IARC Scientific Publications Ser.). 194p. 12.00 (*92-832-1083-2*, 1750083) World Health.

IARC Annual Report 1984. 1984. (IARC Scientific Publications Ser.). 217p. 12.00 (*92-832-1084-0*, 1750084) World Health.

IARC Biennial Report 1986-1987: For the Period July 1, 1985 to June 30, 1987. 1988. (IARC Scientific Publications Ser.). 234p. 15.00 (*92-832-1087-5*, 1758687) World Health.

IARC Biennial Report 1988-1989: For the Period July 1, 1988 to June 30, 1989. 1989. (IARC Scientific Publications Ser.). 265p. 15.00 (*92-832-1089-1*, 1758889) World Health.

IARC Biennial Report 1990-1991: For the Period July 1, 1989 to June 30, 1991. 1991. (IARC Scientific Publications Ser.). 250p. 15.00 (*92-832-1091-3*, 1759091) World Health.

IARC Handbooks of Cancer Prevention: Non-Steroidal Anti-Inflammatory Drugs, Vol. 1. Ed. by IARC Working Group of the Evaluation of Cancer Pre. 1998. (IARC Scientific Publications Ser.). (Illus.). 224p. pap. text 135.00 (*92-832-3001-9*) OUP.

IARC Handbooks of Cancer Prevention Vol. 2: Carotenoids. IARC Working Group on the Evaluation of the Carcin. 1998. (IARC Scientific Publications Ser.). (Illus.). 344p. pap. text 135.00 (*92-832-3002-7*) OUP.

IARC Handbooks of Cancer Prevention Vol. 3: Vitamin A. Ed. by IARC Working Group on the Evaluation of the Carcinogenic Risk of Chemicals to Man 1976 Staff. 1999. (Illus.). 290p. pap. text 69.00 (*92-832-3003-5*) OUP.

IAT Guide to Hair Loss. David Salinger. 3rd rev. ed. 1982. 60p. pap. 10.00 (*0-9614548-0-6*) Intl Assn Trichologists.

Iatro-Chemistry of Ayurveda (Rasa Sastra) Vaidya B. Dash & Vaidya L. Kashyap. 1995. LC 94-907330. (C). (*81-7022-527-2*) Concept IND. *Dist:* S Asia.

Iatrogenic Diseases. L. Preger. 1986. LC 85-24300. 100.00 (*0-8493-5888-4*, CRC Reprint) Franklin.

Iatrogenic Diseases. R. R. Raje & P. D. Wong. 1999. LC 99-10525. (Textbooks for Students Ser.). 144p. 23.95 (*0-915340-22-4*) PJD Pubns.

Iatrogenic Diseases: Ultrasound of Iatrogenic Disease. Ed. by Leslie Preger. 1986. 208p. 298.00 (*0-8493-5879-5*, RC90) CRC Pr.

Iatrogenic Disorders of the Fetus, Infant, & Child. Ed. by E. G. Kassner. 1985. (Radiology of Iatrogenic Disorders Ser.: Vol. 1). (Illus.). 401p. 249.00 (*0-387-90930-3*);Vol. 2. LC 84-23530. 500p. 286.00 (*0-387-96005-8*) Spr-Verlag.

Iatrogenic Gastrointestinal Complications. Ed. by M. A. Meyers & G. G. Ghahremani. 1981. (Radiology of Iatrogenic Disorders Ser.). (Illus.). 307p. 172.00 (*0-387-90505-7*) Spr-Verlag.

Iatrogenic Multiple Pregnancy: Clinical Implications. Ed. by I. Blickstein & L. G. Keith. 2001. LC 00-56682. (Illus.). 330p. lib. bdg. 109.95 (*1-85070-726-X*, Parthenon Pbng) CRC Pr.

Iatrogenic Vascular Injuries. S. E. Bergentz & D. Bergqvist. 1989. (Illus.). 195p. 94.00 (*0-387-50308-0*) Spr-Verlag.

Iatrogenics in Professional Practice & Education: A Handbook - When Helping Hurts. Ed. by Robert F. Morgan. 1994. 466p. pap. 13.00 (*1-885679-11-4*) Morgan Fnd Pubs.

Iatromathematics in Islam. Felix Klein-Franke. 1984. (Texte und Studien Zur Orientalistik Ser.: Vol. 3). vi, 161p. (*3-487-07533-4*) G Olms Pubs.

IBD & Chronic Recurrent Abdominal Pain. Ed. by F. Hadziselimovic & B. Herzog. 1997. (Falk Symposium Ser.: No. 91). 256p. text 120.50 (*0-7923-8722-8*) Kluwer Academic.

***IBD at the End of Its First Century.** Ed. by G. Rogler. 2000. LC 00-699108. (Falk Symposium Ser.: Vol. 111). (Illus.). xiii, 321p. 132.00 (*0-7923-8756-2*, Kluwer Acad) Kluwer Academic.

IBD Nutrition Book. Jan K. Greenwood. 1992. LC 91-41117. 288p. pap. 17.95 (*0-471-54630-5*) Wiley.

IBM-PC in the Clinical Laboratory. Helen J. Cronenberger et al. 1985. 227p. 41.95 (*0-316-16146-2*, Little Brwn Med Div) Lppncott W & W.

Ibn Al-Jazzar on Fevers: A Critical Edition. Gerritt Bos. 2000. LC 96-42485. (Sir Henry Wellcome Asian Ser.). (ARA & ENG.). v, 217p. (*0-7103-0570-2*) Kegan Paul Intl GBR. *Dist:* Col U Pr.

Ibn Al-Jazzar on Sexual Diseases & Their Treatment Bk. 6: A Critical Edition of Zad Al-Musafir Wa-Gut Al-Hadir: Provisions for the Traveller & Nourishment for the Sedentary. Ibn Al-Jazzar. 1997. LC 96-36415. (Sir Henry Wellcome Asian Ser.). 417p. (*0-7103-0569-9*) Kegan Paul Intl GBR. *Dist:* Col U Pr.

Ibopamine in the Management of Congestive Heart Failure: Journal: Cardiology, Vol. 77, Suppl. 5, 1990. Ed. by J. P. Bounhoure & P. Magrassi. 1990. (Illus.). vi, 96p. pap. 30.50 (*3-8055-5309-9*) S Karger.

IBS: A Doctor's Plan for Chronic Digestive Troubles: The Definitive Guide to Prevention & Relief. Gerard L. Guillory. 2nd rev. ed. 1996. LC 96-16956. 206p. pap. 14.95 (*0-88179-130-X*); 3rd ed. 2001. LC 2001-24135. (Illus.). 256p. pap. 16.95 (*0-88179-179-2*) Hartley & Marks.

***IBS & Colitis: Symptoms, Causes, Orthodox Treatment.** Jill Wright. 2002. 128p. pap. (*1-85703-726-X*) How To Bks GBR. *Dist:* Midpt Trade.

***IBS Breakthrough: Healing Irritable Bowel Syndrome for Good with Ancient Chinese Medicine.** Leigh Fortson. 2001. pap. 15.95 (*1-931412-62-6*) Fair Winds Pr.

IBS Handbook: Learning to Live with Irritable Bowel Syndrome. Gerard L. Guillory & Mike Snipes. 1989. (Illus.). 96p. (Orig.). pap. text 5.95 (*0-9622533-0-8*) MTA Pub.

IBS Relief: A Doctor, a Dietitian & a Psychologist Provide a Team Approach to Managing Irritable Bowel Syndrome. Geoffrey Turnbull. 1998. 192p. pap. 14.95 (*0-471-34741-8*) Wiley.

IBS Relief: A Doctor, a Dietitian & a Psychologist Provide a Team Approach to Managing Irritable Bowel Syndrome. Geoffrey K. Turnbull & Dawn Burstall. 1998. LC 98-231230. 192p. pap. 13.95 (*1-56561-145-4*) Wiley.

Ibuprofen: A Critical Bibliographic Review. K. D. Rainsford. 1999. LC 00-500429. 575p. 165.00 (*0-7484-0694-8*) Taylor & Francis.

ICACI XV - EAACI '94 Abstracts: 15th International Congress of Allergology & Clinical Immunology & Annual Meeting of the European Academy of Allergology & Clinical Immunology. Ed. by S. G. O. Johansson. 1994. (ACI News Supplement, 1994 Ser.: 2). 550p. pap. 49.00 (*0-88937-129-6*) Hogrefe & Huber Pubs.

ICACI XVI No. 4: Allergy & Clinical Immunology International, 1997 Supplement. 1997. 326p. 49.00 (*0-88937-178-4*) Hogrefe & Huber Pubs.

ICD-10 Classification of Mental & Behavioural Disorders: Diagnostic Criteria for Research. WHO Staff. 1993. xiii, 248p. pap. text 50.00 (*92-4-154455-4*, 1151371) World Health.

ICD-10 Field Trials of the Diagnostic Criteria for Research in German-Speaking Countries. Ed. by H. J. Freyberger et al. 1996. (Journal: Vol. 29, No. 5). (Illus.). 60p. pap. 40.00 (*3-8055-6402-3*) S Karger.

ICD-9-CM 1998 Coder's Choice. annuals rev. ed. 1997. Vols. 1-3. 1700p. pap. text 59.95 (*1-57066-120-0*, 9822); Vols. 1 & 2. 1400p. pap. text 54.95 (*1-57066-119-7*, 9821) Practice Mgmt Info.

ICD-9-CM 1998 Deluxe, Vols. 1-3. annuals rev. ed. 1997. 1700p. 64.95 (*1-57066-122-7*, 9825) Practice Mgmt Info.

ICD-9-CM 1999 Coder's Choice, Vols. 1-2. Ed. by Kathryn M. Swanson & Maureen Lynch. 1998. 1366p. pap. text 54.95 (*1-57066-087-5*, 9921) Practice Mgmt Info.

ICD-9-CM 1999 Coder's Choice, Vols. 1-3. Ed. by Kathryn Swanson & Maureen Lynch. 1998. 1700p. pap. text 59.95 (*1-57066-088-3*, 9922) Practice Mgmt Info.

ICD-9-CM 1999 Deluxe. Ed. by Kathryn M. Swanson & Maureen Lynch. 1998. 1366p. text 64.95 (*1-57066-090-5*, 9925) Practice Mgmt Info.

ICD-9-CM Workbook for Beginning Coders: In Cooperation with the American Hospital Association's Central Office on ICD-9-CM. Ed. by Janatha R. Ashton. 1997. 79p. pap. text 26.25 (*1-55648-204-3*, 148178) AHPI.

ICD-Conversion Programs for Cancer. J. Ferlay. 1994. (IARC Scientific Publications Ser.: No. 21). 21p. pap. text 27.00 (*92-832-1435-8*, 1770021) World Health.

ICD-9 Cheat Sheet. Ed. by Jerry Gill. 9th rev. ed. 1998. 406p. 39.00 (*1-889823-04-X*) GLB Worldwide.

ICD-9-CM. 1992. Vol. 1. (*1-880678-12-8*); Vol. 2. (*1-880678-13-6*); Vol. 3. (*1-880678-14-4*) Solucient.

ICD-9-CM: Beyond the Basics. Sherri A. Mallett. 2000. (Illus.). 198p. pap. text 60.00 (*1-58426-039-4*); 1999. 128p. pap. text 50.00 (*1-58426-021-1*, AC400799) Am Hlth Info.

ICD-9-CM Code Book Marleeta K. Jones. Ed. by Karen M. Schmidt & Anita Hart. (Illus.). 1456p. (C). 195.00 (*1-56329-360-9*) Ingenix Inc.

ICD-9-CM Code Book: Color-Coded Softbound Edition. Marleeta K. Jones. Ed. by Karen M. Schmidt & Anita Hart. 1193p. (C). pap. 69.95 (*1-56329-359-5*) Ingenix Inc.

ICD-9-CM Code Book: Color-Coded Updatable Edition Marleeta K. Jones. Ed. by Karen M. Schmidt & Anita Hart. 1193p. (C). 139.00 (*1-56329-358-7*) Ingenix Inc.

ICD-9-CM Code Book: Standard Edition Marleeta K. Jones. Ed. by Karen M. Schmidt & Anita Hart. 1148p. (C). 49.95 (*1-56329-357-9*) Ingenix Inc.

ICD-9-CM Code Book Color-Coded for Outpatient Services. Marleeta K. Jones. Ed. by Karen M. Schmidt & Anita Hart. 1081p. (C). 139.00 (*1-56329-363-3*) Ingenix Inc.

***ICD-9-CM Code Book for Home Health Services, Nursing Facilities & Hospices 2001**, Vol. 1, 2 & 3. Ingenix, Inc. Staff. per. 119.95 (*1-56329-704-3*) Ingenix Inc.

ICD-9-CM Code Book for Home Health Services, Nursing Homes & Hospices. Marleeta K. Jones. Ed. by Karen M. Schmidt & Anita Hart. 1148p. (C). 115.00 (*1-56329-364-1*) Ingenix Inc.

ICD-9-CM Coding for Long-Term Care. Ed. by Reese Gottschalk. 2000. 240p. pap. text 60.00 (*1-58426-028-9*, AC200800) Am Hlth Info.

ICD-9-CM Coding for Physicians' Offices. Billie C. Bradford. 2nd ed. 1997. (Illus.). 250p. pap. 44.95 (*1-57066-068-9*, ME118) Practice Mgmt Info.

ICD-9-CM Coding Handbook: 1998 Edition. Faye Brown. rev. ed. 1998. LC 99-161776. pap. 58.00 (*1-55648-238-8*) AHPI.

ICD-9-CM Coding Handbook: Handbook Without Answers. Faye Brown. 1999. 408p. pap. (*1-55648-282-5*) AHPI.

ICD-9-CM Coding Handbook for Physician Practices. Therese M. Jorwic. 1992. LC 92-21894. 562p. ring bd. 155.00 (*0-8342-0347-2*) Aspen Pub.

ICD-9-CM Coding Handbook, with Answers. Ed. by Faye Brown. 1997th rev. ed. 1997. LC 97-13109. 428p. pap. text 55.00 (*1-55648-202-7*, 148182) AHPI.

ICD-9-CM Coding Handbook, Without Answers. Faye Brown. 1998. pap. 48.00 (*1-55648-239-6*) AHPI.

ICD-9-CM Coding Handbook, Without Answers. Ed. by Faye Brown. 1997th rev. ed. 1997. LC 97-10675. 418p. pap. text 46.00 (*1-55648-203-5*, 148183) AHPI.

***ICD-9-CM Coding Made Easy.** James B. Davis. 2nd ed. 2000. pap. text 39.95 (*1-57066-184-7*, ME132) Practice Mgmt Info.

***ICD-9-CM Diagnosis Coding Advisor 2001.** Ingenix, Inc. Staff. per. 89.95 (*1-56329-728-0*) Ingenix Inc.

ICD-9-CM in a Snap, 1999, Vol. 1999. Ed. by Ann G. Uniack. rev. ed. 1998. 66p. spiral bd. 24.95 (*1-881671-19-4*) S N A P.

ICD-9-CM 1998 Codes on Disk. annuals rev. ed. 1997. 1700p. pap. 129.95 incl. disk (*1-57066-123-5*, 9828) Practice Mgmt Info.

ICD-9-CM 1998 Timesaver Binder, Vols. 1-3. annuals rev. ed. 1997. 1700p. ring bd. 64.95 (*1-57066-121-9*, 9824) Practice Mgmt Info.

ICD-9-CM 1999 Codes on Disk. Ed. by Kathryn M. Swanson & Maureen Lynch. 1998. pap. 149.95 incl. disk (*1-57066-091-3*, 9928) Practice Mgmt Info.

ICD-9-CM 1999 Timesaver. Ed. by Kathryn M. Swanson & Maureen Lynch. 1998. 1366p. ring bd. 69.95 (*1-57066-089-1*, 9924) Practice Mgmt Info.

ICD-9-CM ,1999-2000, Vols. 1-2. St. Anthony's Publishing Staff. 1999. (C). pap. 48.00 (*1-56329-666-7*) Thomson Learn.

ICD-9-CM 1997 Coder's Choice Ed. by Kathryn Swanson. 1996. (C). Vols. 1, 2 & 3. 5th rev. ed. LC 96-222721. 1700p. pap. text 59.95 (*1-57066-059-X*, 9722); Vols. 1 & 2. rev. ed. 1400p. pap. text 54.95 (*1-57066-058-1*, 9721) Practice Mgmt Info.

ICD-9-CM, 1997: International Classification of Diseases. Context Software Systems, Inc., Staff. 9th rev. ed. 1996. Vols. 1-3. pap. 44.95 (*0-07-600826-6*); Vols. 1 & 2. pap. 39.95 (*0-07-600825-8*) McGraw.

ICD-9-CM 2000 Ed. by Kathryn Swanson & Maureen Lynch. 1999. (Illus.). 1800p. pap. text 59.95 (*1-57066-151-0*, 20022);Vols. 1 & 2. pap. 44.95 (*1-57066-154-5*, 20020) Practice Mgmt Info.

ICD-9-CM 2000 Coder's Choice Ed. by Kathryn Swanson & Maureen Lynch. 1999. pap. text 54.95 (*1-57066-150-2*, 20021) Practice Mgmt Info.

ICD-9-CM 2000 Deluxe. Ed. by Kathryn Swanson & Maureen Lynch. 1999. (Illus.). pap. text 64.95 (*1-57066-153-7*, 20025) Practice Mgmt Info.

***ICD-9-CM 2001: Diagnosis Codes.** annuals Ed. by Kathryn Swanson. rev. ed. 2000. (Illus.). 1490p. text 64.95 (*1-57066-179-0*, 21025) Practice Mgmt Info.

***ICD-9-CM 2001: Timesaver Binder.** annuals Ed. by Kathryn Swanson. rev. ed. 2000. (Illus.). 1800p. ring bd. 74.95 (*1-57066-178-2*, 21024) Practice Mgmt Info.

***ICD-9-CM 2001 Set: Coder's Choice** annuals Ed. by Kathryn Swanson. rev. ed. 2000. (Illus.). 1490p. pap. text 59.95 (*1-57066-176-6*, 21021); 1800p. pap. text 69.95 (*1-57066-177-4*, 21022) Practice Mgmt Info.

***ICD-9-CM 2001 Set: Diagnosis Codes, Non-Indexed "Plain"** annuals Ed. by Kathryn Swanson. 2000. (Illus.). 1490p. pap. text 49.95 (*1-57066-181-2*, 21020) Practice Mgmt Info.

***ICD-9-CM 2001 Set: Diagnosis Codes, Plain** annuals Ed. by Kathryn Swanson. rev. ed. 2000. (Illus.). 1800p. pap. text 54.95 (*1-57066-182-0*, 21023) Practice Mgmt Info.

ICD-9-CM 2000 TimeSaver Binder. Ed. by Kathryn Swanson & Maureen Lynch. 1999. (Illus.). 69.95 (*1-57066-152-9*, 20024) Practice Mgmt Info.

***ICD-9 Hospital & Payor**, Vols. 1-3. Ingenix, Inc. Staff. (Illus.). pap. 89.95 (*1-56337-351-3*) Ingenix Inc.

ICD-9, 1999. American Medical Association Staff. 1998. per. 66.95 (*0-89970-952-4*) AMA.

ICD-10 Vol. 1: International Statistical Classification of Diseases & Related Health Problems: Tabular List. WHO Staff. 10th rev. ed. 1992. LC 93-154168. (FRE & SPA.). iv, 1243p. (C). text 119.00 (*92-4-154419-8*, 1151331) World Health.

ICD-10 Vol. 2: International Statistical Classification of Diseases & Related Health Problems: Instruction Manual. WHO Staff. rev. ed. 1993. LC 93-154168. (ENG, FRE & SPA.). vii, 160p. (C). text 38.00 (*92-4-154420-1*, 1152331) World Health.

ICD-10 Casebook: The Many Faces of Mental Disorders—Adult Case Histories According to ICD-10. T. B. Ustun et al. 1996. LC 96-21767. 266p. 37.00 (*0-88048-989-8*, 8989) Am Psychiatric.

ICD-10 Checklists. W. Hiller et al. rev. ed. 1996. 148.00 (*0-88937-164-4*) Hogrefe & Huber Pubs.

ICD-10 Classification of Mental & Behavioural Disorders: Clinical Descriptions & Diagnostic Guidelines. WHO Staff. 1992. (ARA & ENG.). 370p. pap. text 47.00 (*92-4-154422-8*, 1150371) World Health.

ICD-10 Coding Fundamentals. Sue Meads & Faye Brown. 2nd ed. 1999. LC 99-19557. (Illus.). xvi, 238p. pap. 34.95 (*1-57066-134-0*) Practice Mgmt Info.

ICD-10 Coding Fundamentals: A Comprehensive Coding Guide for Healthcare Professionals. Sue Meads & Faye Brown. 1997. LC 97-20325. (Illus.). 250p. pap. text 44.95 (*1-57066-115-4*, ME081) Practice Mgmt Info.

1998 Icd-10 Made Easy. Medicode Staff. 1999. LC 00-502207. (Illus.). iv, 213p. (C). pap. 75.00 (*1-56337-237-1*) Thomson Learn.

ICD Therapy. Karl-Heinz Kuck et al. 1996. (Clinical Approaches to Tachyarrhythmias Ser.). (Illus.). 64p. 16.00 (*0-87993-634-7*) Futura Pub.

***Ice Bound: A Doctor's Incredible Battle for Survival at the South Pole.** Jerri Nielsen & Maryanne Vollers. 2001. 384p. pap. 14.95 (*0-7868-8699-4*) Talk Miramax Bks.

ICH in Clinical Medicine. MacWalter. 1994. (Illus.). 128p. (C). (gr. 13). pap. text 29.00 (*0-8151-5805-X*, 22958) Mosby Inc.

ICH in Gastroenterology. Anthony Morris & John Y. Yiannakou. 2nd ed. 1994. (C). 28.00 (*0-8151-6222-7*, 22884) Mosby Inc.

Ichiban: Radiation Dosimetry for the Survivors of the Bombings of Hiroshima & Nagasaki. John A. Auxier. 1977. LC 76-30780. (ERDA Critical Review Ser.). 131p. fiche 9.00 (*0-87079-244-X*, TID-27080) DOE.

ICLAS Manual for Genetic Monitoring of Inbred Mice. Tatsuji Nomura et al. 1985. 200p. pap. (*0-86008-366-7*) U of Tokyo JPN. *Dist:* Col U Pr.

ICNP in Europe: Telenurse. Ed. by R. A. Mortensen. 1997. LC 97-70208. (Studies in Health Technology & Informatics: Vol. 38). 240p. 90.00 (*90-5199-321-8*) IOS Press.

Icones Fungorum Maris J. E. Kohlmeyer. 1969. 130.00 (*3-7682-2000-1*) Lubrecht & Cramer.

Icones Fungorum Omnium Hucusque Cognitorum: Ad Usum Sylloges Saccardianae Accomodatae A. N. Berlese. 1968. pap. 216.00 (*3-7682-0575-4*) Lubrecht & Cramer.

Icones of Medicinal Fungi from China. Jian-Zhe Ying et al. Tr. by Yu-Chan Xu from CHI. 1987. 272p. (C). text 110.00 (*7-03-000195-8*) Lubrecht & Cramer.

Iconographia Gyniatrica see Obstetrics & Gynecology: A History & Iconography

ICP in Infancy & Childhood. Ed. by E. Paraicz. 1982. (Monographs in Pediatrics: Vol. 15). (Illus.). viii, 148p. pap. 85.25 (*3-8055-3475-2*) S Karger.

ICPC-2: International Classification of Primary Care. World Organization of Family Doctors Staff. 2nd ed. 1998. LC 97-46472. 200p. pap. text 79.50 (*0-19-262802-X*) OUP.

ICRP Publication 47. Ed. by M. C. Thorne. 1986. (International Commission of Radiological Protection Ser.: No. 47). 28p. pap. 32.00 (*0-08-034020-2*, Pergamon Pr) Elsevier.

ICRP Publication 71; Age Dependent Doses to Members of the Public from Intake of Radionuclides Pt. 4: Inhalation Dose Coefficients, a Report of a Task Group Committee 2 of the International Commission on Radiological Protection. Ed. by ICRP Staff. 1996. (International Commission on Radiological Protection Ser.: Vol. 25). 410p. pap. 113.50 (*0-08-042736-7*, Pergamon Pr) Elsevier.

ICRP Publication 73: Radiological Protection & Safety in Medicine. Ed. by ICRP Staff. 1996. (International Commission on Radiological Protection Ser.: Vol. 26). 50p. pap. 62.50 (*0-08-042738-3*, Pergamon Pr) Elsevier.

ICRP Publication 72; Age-Dependent Doses to the Members of the Public from Intake of Radionuclides Pt. 5: Compilation of Ingestion & Inhalation Coefficients. Ed. by ICRP Staff. 1996. (International Commission on Radiological Protection Ser.: No. 26). 94p. pap. 62.50 (*0-08-042737-5*, Pergamon Pr) Elsevier.

ICRP 66 Respiratory Tract Model AICRP, Vol. 24/1-3. ICRP Staff. 1995. (International Communication & Popular Culture Ser.: No. 66). 300p. pap. 167.00 (*0-08-041154-1*, Pergamon Pr) Elsevier.

ICU — A Cost Benefit Analysis. Ed. by D. R. Miranda & D. Langrehr. 1987. 236p. 148.25 (*0-444-80823-X*, Excerpta Medica) Elsevier.

ICU Book. Paul L. Marino. 1991. LC 90-5622. (Illus.). 713p. text 49.50 (*0-8121-1306-3*); 2nd ed. 1998. LC 96-48756. 972p. pap. 65.00 (*0-683-05565-8*) Lppncott W & W.

ICU Care. Mark A. Helfaer. 1998. LC 97-42672. (Illus.). 200p. 29.95 (*0-683-30079-2*) Lppncott W & W.

ICU Intern Pocket Survival Guide. Thomas M. Masterson et al. 1992. 78p. (Orig.). (C). pap. text 7.50 (*0-9634063-3-7*) Intl Med Pub.

ICU Pocket Professor. Jonni Cooper. 1991. (C). (gr. 13). text 16.95 (*0-944132-45-6*) Mosby Inc.

ICU Quick Reference. Sheree R. Comer. 2nd rev. ed. 1998. 435p. (Orig.). (C). pap. text 41.95 (*1-56930-071-2*) Delmar.

ICU Recall. Curtis G. Tribble & Jeffrey T. Cope. 1997. LC 96-49031. 336p. pap. text 29.95 (*0-683-08408-9*) Lppncott W & W.

***ICU Recall PDA.** Curtis G. Tribble & Jeffrey T. Cope. 2002. 29.95 (*0-7817-3338-3*) Lppncott W & W.

ICU Therapeutics Handbook. Paul E. Marik. 1996. (Illus.). 304p. (C). (gr. 13). pap. text 37.95 (*0-8151-5698-7*, 26662) Mosby Inc.

Id & the Regulatory Principles of Mental Functioning. Max Schur. 1966. LC 66-20144. (Journal of the American Psychoanalytic Association Monograph Ser.: No. 4). 220p. 32.50 (*0-8236-2440-4*) Intl Univs Pr.

Ida Jean Orlando: A Nursing Process Theory. Norma J. Schmieding. 1993. LC 93-5729. (Notes on Nursing Theories Ser.: Vol. 12). (Illus.). 61p. (C). 29.95 (*0-8039-4907-3*, 4741); pap. 14.95 (*0-8039-4908-1*, 4742) Sage.

Idaho Health Care in Perspective 2000. Ed. by Kathleen O'Leary Morgan & Scott E. Morgan. 2000. 21p. spiral bd. 19.00 (*0-7401-0211-7*) Morgan Quitno Corp.

Idaho Health Care Perspective, 1998. Ed. by Kathleen O'Leary Morgan & Scott E. Morgan. 1998. 20p. pap. 19.00 (*1-56692-811-7*) Morgan Quitno Corp.

Idea Book for Activity Programs. Robert Haacker & Bonnie Guillory. 1985. (Illus.). 212p. (C). 46.50 (*1-877735-08-6*, 2109PP) Prof Prnting & Pub.

Idea of Health: Implications for the Nursing Professional. Judith A. Smith. 1983. LC 83-839. (Nursing Education Ser.). 144p. (C). pap. text 14.95 (*0-8077-2735-0*) Tchrs Coll.

Idea of the Past: History, Science, & Practice in American Psychoanalysis. Leonard Jonathan Lamm. (Psychoanalytic Crosscurrents Ser.). 1997. 320p. pap. text 20.00 (*0-8147-5139-3*); 1993. LC 92-44651. 288p. (C). text 50.00 (*0-8147-5073-7*) NYU Pr.

Idea to Product: The Process. Ed. by Nancy J. Alexander & Anne C. Wentz. 1996. (Illus.). 199p. 130.00 (*0-387-94742-6*) Spr-Verlag.

Ideas & Identities: The Life & Work of Erik Erikson. Robert S. Wallerstein & Leo Goldberger. 1998. LC 97-30053. 65.00 (*0-8236-2445-5*) Intl Univs Pr.

Ident-a-Drug Reference. Therapeutic Research Faculty Staff. 1999. 533p. pap. 39.50 (*0-9676136-1-2*) Theraptc Res.

Identifiable Neurons in Invertebrates: From Invariant Cells to Dynamic Systems. Ed. by J. L. Leonard. 2000. (Brain, Behavior & Evolution Ser.: Vol. 55, No. 5). (Illus.). 50p. pap. 25.25 (*3-8055-7144-5*) S Karger.

Identification & Assessment in Early Intervention. Ed. by James A. Blackman. 1996. LC 94-24184. (Infants & Young Children Ser.). 298p. pap. 41.00 (*0-8342-0644-7*) PRO-ED.

Identification & Character: A Book on Psychological Development. Howard Kamler. 1994. LC 93-48109. (SUNY Series, Alternatives in Psychology). 350p. (C). text 59.50 (*0-7914-2211-9*); pap. text 20.95 (*0-7914-2212-7*) State U NY Pr.

Identification & Characterization of the Human Sarco/Endoplasmic Reticulum Ca2+ - ATPase 3 (SERCA3) Gene. Leonard Dode. 1998. (Acta Biomedica Lovaniensia Ser.). (Illus.). 145p. pap. (*90-6186-889-0*) Leuven Univ BEL. *Dist:* Coronet Bks.

Identification & Control of Environmental & Occupational Diseases Pt. 1: Asbestos & Cancers. Myron A. Mehlman. 1994. (Advances in Modern Environmental Toxicology Ser.: Vol. 22). (Illus.). 518p. 135.00 (*0-911131-50-7*) Specialist Journals.

Identification & Treatment of Attention Deficit Disorder. Nancy Nussbaum & Erin D. Bigler. Ed. by Maggie Coleman. 1990. (Child Guidance Mental Health Ser.). 69p. pap. text 9.00 (*0-89079-263-1*, 1506) PRO-ED.

Identification Evidence: A Psychological Evaluation. J. W. Shepherd et al. 1982. 164p. text 28.00 (*0-08-028441-8*, Pergamon Pr) Elsevier.

***Identification of At-Risk Drinking & Intervention with Women of Childbearing Age: A Guide for Primary-Care Providers.** Michael Fleming. Ed. by Dorothea De Zafra. 2001. (Illus.). 64p. (C). reprint ed. pap. text 25.00 (*0-7567-1036-7*) DIANE Pub.

Identification of Low Caries Risk Dietary Components. T. N. Imfeld. 1983. (Monographs in Oral Science: Vol. 11). (Illus.). viii, 200p. 110.50 (*3-8055-3634-8*) S Karger.

Identification of the CF (Cystic Fibrosis) Gene: Recent Progress & New Research Strategies. Ed. by L. C. Tsui et al. 1991. (Advances in Experimental Medicine & Biology Ser.: Vol. 290). (Illus.). 420p. (C). text 150.00 (*0-306-43909-3*, Kluwer Plenum) Kluwer Academic.

Identification of Transcribed Sequences. U. Hochgeschwender & K. Gardiner. 1994. (Illus.). 316p. (C). text 95.00 (*0-306-44835-1*, Kluwer Plenum) Kluwer Academic.

Identification of Unusual Pathogenic Gram-Negative Aerobic & Facultatively Anaerobic Bacteria. Robbin S. Weyant et al. 2nd ed. 1996. LC 95-12416. (Illus.). 400p. pap. 55.00 (*0-683-00615-0*) Lppncott W & W.

Identification Papers: Readings on Psychoanalysis, Sexuality, & Culture. Diana Fuss. 1995. LC 95-22215. 200p. (C). (gr. 13). pap. 22.95 (*0-415-90886-8*, B3091) Routledge.

Identifying & Responding to New Forms of Drug Abuse: Lessons Learned from "Crack" & "Ice" Marcia R. Chaiken. 1994. 62p. (Orig.). (C). pap. text 30.00 (*0-7881-1303-8*) DIANE Pub.

Identifying Filamentous Fungi: A Clinical Laboratory Handbook. Guy St. Germain. 1995. (Illus.). 320p. text 59.95 (*0-89863-177-7*) Star Pub CA.

Identifying Health Technologies That Work: Searching For Evidence. 1996. (Illus.). 308p. reprint ed. pap. text 45.00 (*0-7881-3341-1*) DIANE Pub.

Identifying Medical Malpractice: 1990 Edition. Jack Schroder. 1990. text (*0-87473-585-8*, 66885-10, MICHIE) LEXIS Pub.

Identifying the Intersection: Adolescent Unwanted Pregnancy, HIV/AIDS, & Unsafe Abortion. Aruna Radhakrishna et al. 1997. LC 97-36830. (Issues in Abortion Care Ser.). (*1-882220-12-9*) IPAS.

Identities in the Lesbian World: The Social Construction of Self, 28. Barbara Ponse. 1978. LC 77-84763. (Contributions in Sociology Ser.: No. 28). 228p. 38.50 (*0-8371-9889-5*, PLW/, Greenwood Pr) Greenwood.

Identity see Woman's Identity

Identity & Interpersonal Competence: A New Direction in Family Research. Nelson N. Foote & Leonard S. Cottrell, Jr. 1993. LC 56-11957. lib. bdg. 25.00 (*0-226-25685-5*) U Ch Pr.

Identity & Intimacy in Marriage. S. Krauss Whitbourne & J. B. Ebmeyer. 1989. 162p. 62.95 (*0-387-97012-6*) Spr-Verlag.

Identity & the Life Cycle: Selected Papers. Erik H. Erikson. 1967. (Psychological Issues Monographs: No. 1, Vol. 1, No. 1). 171p. (Orig.). 30.00 (*0-8236-2460-9*) Intl Univs Pr.

Identity, Character, & Morality: Essays in Moral Psychology. Ed. by Owen Flanagan. 1993. (Illus.). 650p. pap. 27.95 (*0-262-56074-7*, Bradford Bks) MIT Pr.

Identity, Consciousness & Value. Peter Unger. 1992. 368p. reprint ed. pap. text 26.00 (*0-19-507917-5*) OUP.

Identity Development: Adolescence Through Adulthood. Contrib. by Jane Kroger. 1999. LC 99-6591. pap. 34.95 (*0-8039-7187-7*, 1038) Sage.

Identity Group Psychotherapy with Adolescents. Arnold W. Rachman. 1995. LC 95-22840. (Master Work Ser.). 340p. 50.00 (*1-56821-658-0*) Aronson.

Identity in Adolescence: The Balance Between Self & Other. J. Roger. 1989. (Adolescence & Society Ser.). 200p. 47.50 (*0-415-01087-X*, A3362); pap. 15.95 (*0-415-01088-8*, A3366) Routledge.

Identity in Adolescence: The Balance Between Self & Other. Jane Kroger. 2nd ed. 1996. LC 95-9380. (Adolescence & Society Ser.). 256p. (C). pap. 26.95 (*0-415-10679-6*) Routledge.

Identity of the Psychoanalyst. Edward D. Joseph et al. Ed. by Daniel Widlocher. 1981. LC 83-12568. (International Psycho-Analytical Association Monography: No. 2). xviii, 291p. 45.00 (*0-8236-2470-6*) Intl Univs Pr.

Identity's Architect: A Biography of Erik H. Erikson. Lawrence J. Friedman. 1999. 592p. pap. (*1-85343-471-X*) Free Assoc Bks GBR. *Dist:* Intl Spec Bk.

Identity's Architect: A Biography of Erik H. Erikson. Lawrence J. Friedman. 2000. 600p. pap. 19.95 (*0-674-00437-X*) HUP.

Identity's Architect: A Biography of Erik H. Erikson. Lawrence J. Friedman. 1999. LC 98-50266. (Illus.). 592p. 35.00 (*0-684-19525-9*) S&S Trade.

Ideologies of Breast Cancer: Feminist Perspectives. Laura Potts. 2000. LC 99-37438. (Illus.). xiv, 213p. 49.95 (*0-312-22851-1*) St Martin.

Ideology & Insanity: Essays on the Psychiatric Dehumanization of Man. Thomas Szasz. 1991. 265p. reprint ed. pap. 17.95 (*0-8156-0256-1*) Syracuse U Pr.

Ideology & Opinions: Studies in Rhetorical Psychology. Michael Billig. 1991. 224p. (C). pap. 24.95 (*0-8039-8332-8*, 9758) Sage.

Ideology, Conflict, & Leadership in Groups & Organizations. Otto F. Kernberg. 1998. LC 97-32793. 384p. 50.00 (*0-300-07355-0*) Yale U Pr.

Idiopathic Anaphylaxis. Ray Patterson. 1997. LC 97-65405. 100p. 56.00 (*0-936587-10-5*) OceanSide Pubns.

Idiopathic & Food or Drug-Induced PAR. Ed. by P. Dukor et al. 1985. (Par Pseudo-Allergic Reactions, Involvement of Drugs & Chemicals Ser.: Vol. 4). (Illus.). viii, 196p. 104.50 (*3-8055-3798-0*) S Karger.

Idiopathic Dilated Cardiomyopathy: Cellular & Molecular Mechanisms, Clinical Consequences. H. R. Figulla et al. 1993. LC 92-49036. (Illus.). 405p. 210.00 (*0-387-56132-3*) Spr-Verlag.

Idiopathic Generalized Epilepsies, Clinical, Experimental & Genetic Aspects. Malafosse. 1994. 560p. (*0-86196-436-5*) J Libbey Med GBR. *Dist:* Bks Intl VA, Buttrwrth-Heinemann.

Idiota de Mente. Nicolas DeCusa. Tr. by Clyde L. Miller. 1979. LC 77-86244. (Janus Ser.).Tr. of Lay Man: About Mind. 122p. 25.00 (*0-913870-65-X*) Abaris Bks.

Idiotypes & Diseases. Ed. by M. Zanetti et al. 1987. (Monographs in Allergy: Vol. 22). (Illus.). viii, 244p. 187.00 (*3-8055-4600-9*) S Karger.

Idiotypes in Biology & Medicine. Ed. by D. A. Carson et al. 1989. (Chemical Immunology Ser.: Vol. 48). Orig. Title: Progress in Allergy. (Illus.). 214p. 154.00 (*3-8055-5000-6*) S Karger.

Idiotypes in Medicine: Autoimmunity, Infection & Cancer. Ed. by Yehuda Shoenfeld et al. 1997. LC 97-17578. 552p. 219.50 (*0-444-82807-9*) Elsevier.

Idiotypic Network & Diseases. Ed. by Jan Cerny & Jacques Hiernaux. 1990. (Illus.). 246p. 79.95 (*1-55581-025-X*) ASM Pr.

Idle Thoughts of a Surgical Fellow: Being An Account of Experimental Surgical Studies 1956-1966. Stacey B. Day. 1984. LC 68-31066. (Illus.). 344p. (C). 25.00 (*0-934314-99-3*) Intl Found Biosocial Dev.

Idyll Arbor's Glossary for Therapists. Joan Burlingame & Thomas K. Skalko. 1997. LC 97-19810. (Illus.). 294p. pap. 35.00 (*1-882883-14-4*, 320) Idyll Arbor.

Idyll Arbor's Medical Abbreviations for the Health Professions. Thomas K. Skalko. 1998. LC 98-3763. 60p. pap. text 10.00 (*1-882883-34-9*, 345) Idyll Arbor.

***Idyll Arbor's Therapy Dictionary.** Anne Battiste. Ed. by Joan Burlingame & Thomas M. Blaschko. 2nd ed. 2001. LC 2001-24759. (*1-882883-46-2*) Idyll Arbor.

IEBM Handbook of International Business. Rosalie Tung. 1998. LC 99-172615. 704p. pap. 139.95 (*1-86152-216-9*) Thomson Learn.

IEEE Engineering in Medicine & Biology 15th Annual Conference, 1993. IEEE, Engineering in Medicine and Biology Staff. Ed. by Institute of Electrical and Electronics Engineers, Inc. Staff. 1993. LC 93-79061. 2200p. pap. text (*0-7803-1377-1*, 93CH3339-9); lib. bdg. (*0-7803-1378-X*, 93CH3339-9); fiche (*0-7803-1379-8*, 93CH3339-9) Inst Electrical.

IEEE Engineering in Medicine & Biology 16th Annual Conference, 1994. IEEE, Engineering in Medicine and Biology Staff. 1994. LC 94-77567. 2100p. pap. text (*0-7803-2050-6*); lib. bdg. (*0-7803-2051-4*, 94CH3474-4) Inst Electrical.

IEEE Nonrigid & Articulated Motion: Proceedings of the IEEE Computer Society, San Juan, Puerto Rico, 1997. 1997. LC 97-72010. 250p. pap. 110.00 (*0-8186-8040-7*) IEEE Comp Soc.

IEEE Std 790-1989, IEEE Guide for Medical Ultrasound Field Parameter Measurements (ANSI) Institute of Electrical and Electronics Engineers, Inc. Staff. 1990. (Illus.). 96p. (Orig.). pap. 52.00 (*1-55937-034-3*) IEEE Standards.

IEEE Std 1073-4.1-1994, IEEE Standard for Medical Device Communications-Physical Layer Interface-Cable Connected. Institute of Electrical and Electronics Engineers, Inc. Staff. 1995. (MIB 1073 Standards Ser.). (Illus.). 80p. pap. (*1-55937-503-5*, SH94261) IEEE Standards.

IEEE Std 1073-3.1-1994, IEEE Standard for Medical Device Communications-Transport Profile-Connection Mode. Institute of Electrical and Electronics Engineers, Inc. Staff. 1995. (MIB 1073 Standards Ser.). (Illus.). 192p. (Orig.). pap. text (*1-55937-504-3*, SH94263) IEEE Standards.

IEP Companion: Communication Goals for Therapy In & Out of the Classroom. Carolyn C. Wilson et al. 1992. 105p. spiral bd. 37.95 (*1-55999-222-0*, 222-0A1) LinguiSystems.

If a Partner Has AIDS: Guide to Clinical Intervention for Relationships in Crisis. R. Dennis Shelby. 1992. LC 91-19169. 288p. pap. 14.95 (*1-56023-002-9*, Harrington Park); lib. bdg. 39.95 (*1-56024-145-4*) Haworth Pr.

If Blindness Strikes Don't Strike Out: A Lively Look at Living with a Visual Impairment. Margaret M. Smith. 1984. 316p. 54.95 (*0-398-04937-8*) C C Thomas.

If I Am Very Ill. W. W. Woodward. 1994. LC 94-77543. 112p. 19.95 (*0-932845-67-3*) Lowell Pr.

If I Grow Up: Talking with Teens about AIDS, Love & Staying Alive. Scott M. Fried. 1997. LC 97-90703. 86p. (Orig.). pap. 10.00 (*0-9659046-0-1*) TALKAIDS.

If I Were a Rich Man Could I Buy a Pancreas? And Other Essays on the Ethics of Health Care. Arthur L. Caplan. 1992. LC 91-32112. (Medical Ethics Ser.). (Illus.). 372p. text 15.95 (*0-253-31307-4*) Ind U Pr.

If Men Got Pregnant, Abortion Would be a Sacrament! Ed. by Helen Forelle. rev. ed. 1991. LC 82-90728. 128p. pap. 8.99 (*1-877649-12-0*) Tesseract SD.

If Only I Could Quit: Recovering from Nicotine Addiction. Karen Casey. 320p. pap. 10.95 (*0-89486-438-6*, 5031A) Hazelden.

If Only My Patients Could Speak - English, That Is! Dean E. Ewing & Shirley Herd. 1995. LC 95-4553. (Illus.). 282p. (Orig.). pap. 15.95 (*0-930006-04-6*) S Deal Assoc.

If Only They Could Talk. James Herriot. l.t. ed. 1991. (General Ser.). 337p. lib. bdg. 19.95 (*0-8161-5162-8*, Macmillan Ref) Gale.

If Symptoms Persist: Anecdotes from a Doctor. Theodore Dalrymple. l.t. ed. (*1-85695-058-1*) ISIS Lrg Prnt GBR. *Dist:* Transaction Pubs.

If the President Had Cancer: Cancer Care, How to Find & Get the Best There Is. Gary L. Schine. 1994. 172p. pap. 13.95 (*0-9635824-9-6*) Sandra Pubns.

If the President Had Cancer: Cancer Care: How to Find & Get the Best There Is. Gary L. Schine & Ellen B. Berlinsky. 1993. LC 93-92558. 160p. (Orig.). pap. 13.95 (*0-9635824-8-8*) Sandra Pubns.

If There's Anything I Can Do... A Practical Guide for Helping Others Cope with Grief. Carlene V. Eneroth. 2nd ed. 1990. 63p. reprint ed. pap. 3.95 (*1-879331-01-2*) Marciel Pub & Print.

If We Can Keep a Severed Head Alive... Discorporation & U. S. Patent 4,666,425. Chet Fleming. 1988. LC 87-90566. (Illus.). (Orig.). (C). 15.95 (*0-942287-03-7*) Polinym Pr.

If We Knew Then What We Know Now: Planning for People with AIDS. Shelagh A. Masline. 1991. (Papers: No. 15). 32p. 10.00 (*0-934459-64-9*) United Hosp Fund.

If Wishes Were Horses: The Education of a Veterinarian. Loretta Gage. 1994. 295p. mass mkt. 6.99 (*0-312-92877-7*) St Martin.

***If You Are Struggling: Struggles Through Manic Depression, Sexual Abuse, Marital Stress & Multiple Personality Disorder.** Beverly Ann Needham. 2001. pap. 16.00 (*0-7388-5045-4*) Xlibris Corp.

If You Don't Take Care of Your Body Where Are You Going to Live? Teaching Individuals How to Take Charge of Their Health. Jane Pentz. Ed. by Elaine Greenwood. unabr. ed. 1998. 214p. ring bd. 19.95 (*1-892426-01-3*) LMA Publishing.

If You Felt Like I Did...You'd Start Running. Ray Murphy. 1990. LC 89-91634. 109p. pap. (*0-9626835-1-5*) Stethophonics.

If You Really Want to Do It Right: Try It the Wholistic Way! Linda M. Georgian. Ed. by Jacqueline Janssen et al. 1985. (Illus.). 300p. (Orig.). pap. 12.95 (*0-9611392-5-0*) Georgian Intl.

If Your Child Is Overweight: A Guide for Parents. Susan M. Kosharek. 1992. pap. 4.95 (*0-88091-111-5*) Am Dietetic Assn.

If Your Child Stutters: A Guide for Parents, No. 11. Stanley Ainsworth & Jane Fraser. 3rd ed. 1988. 54p. pap. 1.00 (*0-933388-23-3*) Stuttering Fnd Am.

IFEEL Pictures: A New Instrument for Interpreting Emotions. Ed. by Robert N. Emde et al. 1993. LC 92-49134. (Clinical Infant Reports of the National Center for Clinical Infant Programs: Report No. 5). 350p. 50.00 (*0-8236-2453-6*) Intl Univs Pr.

***IFETherapy & Its Healing Poems.** Yemi D. Ogunyemi. 2002. (*0-9652860-3-7*) DIASPORA PR AM.

Ifosfamide in the Treatment of Lung Cancer. Ed. by D. K. Hossfeld. 1990. (Beitraege Zur Onkologie, Contributions to Oncology Ser.: Vol. 35). (Illus.). viii, 154p. 65.25 (*3-8055-5199-1*) S Karger.

Ifosfamide in Tumor Therapy. Ed. by W. P. Brade et al. 1987. (Beitraege Zur Onkologie, Contributions to Oncology Ser.: Vol. 26). (Illus.). x, 462p. 95.00 (*3-8055-4647-5*) S Karger.

IGA Mesangial Nephropathy. Ed. by G. D'Amico et al. 1984. (Contributions to Nephrology Ser.: Vol. 40). (Illus.). x, 310p. 29.75 (*3-8055-3877-4*) S Karger.

IgA Nephropathy. Ed. by A. R. Clarkson. 1987. (Topics in Renal Medicine Ser.). text 161.50 (*0-89838-839-2*) Kluwer Academic.

IgA Nephropathy: The Twenty-Fifth Year. Ed. by M. C. Bene et al. 1993. (Contributions to Nephrology Ser.: Vol. 104). (Illus.). viii, 222p. 49.75 (*3-8055-5720-5*) S Karger.

IgE, Mast Cells & the Allergic Response. CIBA Foundation Staff. 1990. LC 89-24895. (CIBA Foundation Symposia Ser.: No. 147). 292p. 128.00 (*0-471-92309-5*) Wiley.

IGF System: Molecular Biology, Physiology & Clinical Applications. Ed. by Ron G. Rosenfeld & Charles T. Roberts. 1999. LC 98-55264. (Contemporary Endocrinology Ser.: Vol. 17). (Illus.). 800p. 195.00 (*0-89603-692-8*) Humana.

IGFs in the Nervous System (Insulin-Like Growth Factors in the Nervous System: Proceedings. E. Myller & E. E. Muller. 1998. LC 97-41301. 169p. pap. 49.00 (*3-540-75042-8*) Spr-Verlag.

IgG-Subklassen der Menschlichen Immunglobuline: Immunochemische Genetische, Biologische und Klinische Aspekte. A. Morell et al. 1975. (Illus.). 88p. pap. 25.25 (*3-8055-2153-7*) S Karger.

IHC - Care of Patients with Alzheimer's Disease. Glen Caspers Doyle. 1989. (Home Care Aide Ser.). pap. 325.00 (*0-8273-3358-7*) Delmar.

IHC/Financial Management Unit. University of Missouri Staff. 1987. (Home Care Aide Ser.). 140.00 (*0-8273-2901-6*) Delmar.

IHC/Independence May Require Changes - SLI. University of Missouri Ser. 1987. (Home Care Aide Ser.). 150.00 (*0-8273-2850-8*) Delmar.

IHC/Legal Rights & Boundaries - Safety/SLI. Universtiy of Missouri Staff. 1987. (Home Care Aide Ser.). 100.00 (*0-8273-2852-4*) Delmar.

IHC/Nutrition-Medications. University of Missouri Ser. 1987. (Home Care Aide Ser.). 125.00 (*0-8273-2854-0*) Delmar.

IHC/Universal Frontmatter. University of Missouri Staff. 1987. (Home Care Aide Ser.). 25.00 (*0-8273-2816-8*) Delmar.

IL-Four: Structure & Function. Hergen Spits. 1992. 288p. lib. bdg. 172.00 (*0-8493-6519-8*, QR185) CRC Pr.

IL-Six: Structure, Function, & Clinical Considerations. Pravin B. Sehgal. 1995. (*0-8493-4911-7*) CRC Pr.

IL-12. Ed. by Luciano Adorini. 1997. (Chemical Immunology Ser.: Vol. 68, 1997). (Illus.). x, 204p. 194.00 (*3-8055-6526-7*) S Karger.

Ilizarov Technique. Paley. 1993. (*0-397-51086-1*) Lppncott W & W.

Ill, Not Insane. Bonnie S. Busick & Martha Gorman. 1986. (Illus.). 311p. (Orig.). pap. 12.95 (*0-9617099-0-1*) New Idea Pr.

I'll Quit Tomorrow: A Practical Guide to Alcoholism Treatment. Vernon E. Johnson. 1990. LC 74-3759. 192p. pap. 15.00 (*0-06-250433-9*) Harper SF.

***Illegal Drugs: A Sagebrush Medical Guide.** Paul M. Gahlinger. 2001. 550p. pap. 29.95 (*0-9703130-1-2*) Sagebrush UT.

Illinois Case History in Orthopaedics, '99. Jones Staff. 1997. mass mkt. (*0-7234-2476-4*) Wolfe Publishing GBR. *Dist:* Mosby Inc.

Illinois Health Care in Perspective 2000. Ed. by Kathleen O'Leary Morgan & Scott E. Morgan. 2000. 21p. spiral bd. 19.00 (*0-7401-0212-5*) Morgan Quitno Corp.

Illinois Health Care Perspective, 1998. Ed. by Kathleen O'Leary Morgan & Scott E. Morgan. 1998. 20p. pap. 19.00 (*1-56692-812-5*) Morgan Quitno Corp.

Illlustrated Handbook of Skin Disease in HIV Infection. M. C. Lipman et al. 1997. LC 97-12646. (Illus.). 64p. lib. bdg. 27.95 (*1-85070-976-9*, Parthenon Pbng) CRC Pr.

Illness & Culture in Contemporary Japan: An Anthropological View. Emiko Ohnuki-Tierney. 1984. LC 83-14415. 250p. pap. text 22.95 (*0-521-27786-8*) Cambridge U Pr.

Illness & Culture in the Postmodern Age. David B. Morris. LC 98-7092. 2000. (Illus.). 360p. pap. 17.95 (*0-520-22689-5*); 1998. (*0-520-21441-2*) U CA Pr.

Illness & Healing. Louis M. Chauvet & Miklos Tomka. 1998. 150p. pap. 15.00 (*1-57075-191-9*) Orbis Bks.

Illness & Healing: In the Context of Cosmic Evolution. Rita Leroi. 1988. 96p. pap. (*0-904693-15-5*) Temple Lodge GBR. *Dist:* Anthroposophic.

Illness & Healing Alternatives in Western Europe. Ed. by Marijke Gijswit-Hofstra & Hilary Marland. 1997. LC 97-205228. (Social History of Medicine Ser.). 304p. (C). 95.00 (*0-415-13581-8*) Routledge.

Illness & Power: Women's Mental Disorders & the Battle Between Sexes. Brant Wenegrat. 217p. (C). 1996. pap. text 19.50 (*0-8147-9310-X*); 1995. text 45.00 (*0-8147-9282-0*) NYU Pr.

Illness & Social Relations: Essays in the Sociology of Health Care. Evan Willis. 1994. 192p. pap. (*1-86373-486-4*) Allen & Unwin Pty AUS. *Dist:* Paul & Co Pubs.

Illness As a Work of Thought: A Foucauldian Perspective of Psychosomatics. Monica Greco. 1998. LC 97-32080. 200p. (C). 80.00 (*0-415-17849-5*) Routledge.

Illness Behavior: A Multidisciplinary Model. Ed. by Sean McHugh. 1987. LC 87-2530. 442p. 85.00 (*0-306-42486-X*, Plenum Trade) Perseus Pubng.

Illness in the Analyst: Implications for the Treatment Relationship. Ed. by Harvey J. Schwartz & Ann L. Silver. 1990. LC 90-4463. 350p. 52.50 (*0-8236-2495-1*) Intl Univs Pr.

Illness Narratives: Suffering, Healing & the Human Condition. Arthur Kelinman. 1989. LC 87-47772. 304p. pap. 21.00 (*0-465-03204-4*) Basic.

Illumination by Darkness: Freud & the Social Bond. Bernard J. Bergen. 1992. LC 91-33002. (Reshaping of Psychoanalysis Ser.: Vol. 1). 148p. (C). text 39.95 (*0-8204-1759-9*) P Lang Pubng.

Illuminations: The Human Becoming Theory in Practice & Research. Ed. by Rosemarie Rizzo Parse. 1995. 409p. pap. 38.95 (*0-88737-637-1*) Natl League Nurse.

Illusion in Loving: A Psychoanalytic Approach to the Evolution of Intimacy & Autonomy. Joel Shor & Jean Sanville. 1978. LC 77-85416. 192p. (C). 30.00 (*0-930578-00-7*) Brunner-Routledge.

Illusion of Attitude Change: Towards a Response Contagion Theory of Persuasion. J. M. Nuttin. 1975. 243p. (Orig.). pap. (*90-6186-227-2*) Leuven Univ BEL. *Dist:* Coronet Bks.

Illusion of Love: Why the Battered Woman Returns to Her Abuser. David P. Celani. 1995. LC 94-29717. 224p. 42.00 (*0-231-10036-1*) Col U Pr.

Illusion of Trust: Toward a Medical Theological Ethics in the Postmodern Age. Edwin R. DuBose. 1995. LC 94-34129. (Theology & Medicine Ser.: Vol. 5). 144p. lib. bdg. (*0-7923-3144-3*) Kluwer Academic NLD. *Dist:* Kluwer Academic.

Illusions: The Adventures of a Reluctant Messiah. Richard Bach. 1989. 192p. mass mkt. 6.99 (*0-440-20488-7*) Dell.

Illusions of Reality: A History of Deception in Social Psychology. James H. Korn. 1997. LC 96-25688. 204p. (C). text 59.50 (*0-7914-3307-2*); pap. text 20.95 (*0-7914-3308-0*) State U NY Pr.

Illustrated Anatomy of the Head & Neck. Margaret J. Fehrenbach & Susan W. Herring. 1995. LC 95-11491. (Illus.). 304p. pap. text 41.95 (*0-7216-4082-6*) Saunders.

Illustrated Atlas of the Techniques of Neural Therapy with Local Anesthetics. Mathias Dosch. 1985. (Illus.). 207p. (*3-7760-0849-0*) K F Haug Pubs DEU. *Dist:* Medicina Bio.

Illustrated Case Histories in Cardiovascular Medicine. William A. Littler et al. 1994. LC 93-15158. 128p. (C). (gr. 13). pap. text 29.00 (*0-8151-5484-4*, 23043) Mosby Inc.

Illustrated Case Histories in Respiratory Medicine. John E. Earis & Mike Pearson. 1995. (Illus.). 128p. 33.00 (*0-7234-2146-3*) Mosby Inc.

Illustrated Cases in Acute Clinical Medicine. K. C. McHardy et al. 1994. LC 93-14398. (Illus.). pap. text (*0-443-04697-2*) Church.

Illustrated Catalogue of the Slide Archive of Historical Medical Photographs at Stonybrook. Center for Photographic Images of Medicine and Healt. 1984. LC 83-22626. (Illus.). 442p. lib. bdg. 105.00 (*0-313-24169-4*, FCM/, Greenwood Pr) Greenwood.

Illustrated Chinese Materia Medica. Jing-Nuan Wu. 2001. LC 00-58472. (Illus.). 688p. text 195.00 (*0-19-514017-6*) OUP.

Illustrated Computer Tomography: A Practical Guide to CT Interpretations. Ed. by S. Takahashi. 1983. (Illus.). 306p. 213.00 (*0-387-11432-7*) Spr-Verlag.

Illustrated Cutaneous & Aesthetic Laser Surgery. Jefrey S. Dover et al. 2nd ed. 1999. (Illus.). 142p. pap. 199.00 (*0-8385-4257-3*) McGraw-Hill Prof.

Illustrated Cutaneous Laser Surgery. Jeffrey S. Dover et al. 1989. (Illus.). 142p. (C). pap. text 125.00 (*0-8385-1432-4*, A1432-2, Apple Lange Med) McGraw.

Illustrated Dental Embryology, Histology, & Anatomy. Mary Bath-Balogh & Margaret J. Fehrenbach. 1997. (Illus.). 415p. pap., tchr. ed. (*0-7216-6688-4*) Saunders.

Illustrated Dictionary of Dermatologic Syndromes. Susan B. Mallory & Susana Leal-Khouri. 1994. LC 94-15125. (Illus.). 258p. 60.95 (*1-85070-458-9*, Parthenon Pbng) CRC Pr.

Illustrated Dictionary of Immunology. Cruse. 1994. 352p. 83.95 (*0-8493-4557-X*) CRC Pr.

***Illustrated Dictionary of Immunology.** Julius M. Cruse & Robert E. Lewis. 2001. (Illus.). 600p. text 139.95 (*0-8493-1935-8*, 1935) CRC Pr.

Illustrated Dictionary of Medicine: Diccionario de Medicina Ilustrado. B. John Melloni. 1982. (SPA., Illus.). 650p. 75.00 (*0-8288-1868-1*, S29945) Fr & Eur.

Illustrated Dictionary of Pregnancy & Childbirth. Carl Jones. 1991. 9.95 (*0-671-68993-2*) S&S Trade.

Illustrated Encyclopedia of Body-Mind Disciplines. Ed. by Nancy Allison. 1998. LC 98-24969. (Illus.). 480p. lib. bdg. 79.95 (*0-8239-2546-3*, ENBOMI) Rosen Group.

Illustrated Encyclopedia of Healing Remedies: Over 1,000 Natural Remedies for the Prevention, Treatment, & Cure of Common Ailments & Conditions. C. Norman Shealy. 1999. LC 98-3516. (Illus.). 496p. pap. 29.95 (*1-86204-516-X*) Element MA.

Illustrated Encyclopedia of Human Histology. R. V. Krstic. 1984. (Illus.). 450p. 99.00 (*0-387-13142-6*) Spr-Verlag.

Illustrated Encyclopedia of Human Histology. Radivoj J. Krstic. 1984. (Illus.). 450p. 89.95 (*3-540-13142-6*) Spr-Verlag.

Illustrated Essentials in Orthopedic Physical Assessment. Ronald C. Evans. 2nd ed. 2000. LC 00-45578. (Illus.). 736p. 59.95 (*0-323-00509-8*) Mosby Inc.

Illustrated Glossary of Hand & Reconstructive Surgery. E. Vaubel & J. Hussman. 1990. LC 90-11904. 229p. 90.00 (*0-89573-965-8*, Wiley-VCH) Wiley.

Illustrated Guide for the Diabetic Clinic. Emyr W. Jones. 1998. LC 98-18405. (Illus.). 137p. pap. 40.95 (*0-632-05151-5*) Blackwell Sci.

Illustrated Guide to Better Sex for People with Chronic Pain. Robert W. Rothrock & Gabriella D'Amore. 1991. 19p. pap. 8.95 (*0-9632602-0-0*); 2nd ed. 1992. (Illus.). 50p. pap. 11.95 (*0-9632602-1-9*) Rothrock & DAmore.

Illustrated Guide to Bone Marrow Diagnosis. Kevin Gatter & David C. Brown. 1997. (Illus.). 160p. 147.95 (*0-632-04234-6*) Blackwell Sci.

Illustrated Guide to Dental Care for Patients with Impaired Health. J. R. Grundy. 1992. 128p. (C). (gr. 13). 30.00 (*0-8151-4022-3*, 22829) Mosby Inc.

Illustrated Guide to Diagnostic Tests. SPC Staff. Ed. by Patricia Schull. 2nd ed. 1997. LC 96-45274. (Illus.). 1184p. 44.95 (*0-87434-882-X*) Springhouse Corp.

Illustrated Guide to Gastrointestinal Motility. Ed. by Devinder Kumar & Sven Gustavsson. 1988. LC 88-2435. (Illus.). 480p. 488.50 (*0-471-91949-7*) Wiley.

Illustrated Guide to Human Reproduction & Fertility Control. Robert J. Demarest & Rita Charon. 1996. LC 95-23415. (Illus.). 96p. lib. bdg. 38.95 (*1-85070-697-2*, Parthenon Pbng) CRC Pr.

Illustrated Guide to Pregnancy & Birth. Tina Otte. 2000. LC 00-711150. (Illus.). 160p. pap. 16.95 (*0-7373-0413-8*, 04138W) Lowell Hse.

Illustrated Guide to Skin Lymphoma Diagnosis. Lorenzo Cerroni et al. 1998. (Illus.). 176p. 209.95 (*0-632-05082-9*) Blackwell Sci.

Illustrated Guide to Taping & Bandaging. Karin Austin et al. 1993. (Illus.). 120p. 24.95 (*0-8151-0347-6*) Mosby Inc.

Illustrated Guide to the Hip. A. J. Tria & K. S. Klein. 1998. (Illus.). 150p. (*0-443-08850-0*) Church.

Illustrated Guide to the Knee. Alfred J. Tria, Jr. & Kenneth S. Klein. 1991. (Illus.). 168p. text (*0-443-08794-6*) Church.

Illustrated Guide to Veterinary Care of Horses. Colin J. Vogel. 1996. (Illus.). 176p. text (*0-8138-2080-4*) Manson Pubng GBR. *Dist:* Iowa U Pr.

Illustrated Guide to Veterinary Medical Terminology. Janet Romich. 1999. LC 99-45427. (Agriculture Ser.). (Illus.). 576p. (C). pap. text 40.95 (*0-7668-0751-7*) Delmar.

Illustrated Handbook of Cardiac Surgery. Bradley J. Harlan et al. 1995. LC 95-179. (Illus.). 334p. 64.00 (*0-387-94447-8*) Spr-Verlag.

Illustrated Handbook of Medical Physiology. C. T. Kirkpatrick. 1993. LC 91-8312. (Illus.). 556p. 176.95 (*0-471-91455-X*, Wiley-Liss) Wiley.

Illustrated Handbook of Nursing Care. SPC Staff. Ed. by Patricia Schull. 1997. LC 97-17858. (Illus.). 1008p. spiral bd. 42.95 (*0-87434-920-6*) Springhouse Corp.

Illustrated Handbook of Ocular Disease in HIV Infection. P. L. Wilson & M. C. I. Lipman. 1999. LC 98-50049. (Illus.). 64p. lib. bdg. 27.95 (*1-85070-981-5*, Parthenon Pbng) CRC Pr.

Illustrated Handbook of the Bach Flower Remedies. Chancellor. 1996. (Illus.). 251p. pap. (*0-85207-002-0*) C W Daniel GBR. *Dist:* Natl Bk Netwk.

Illustrated Handbook of the Bach Flower Remedies. Philip Chancellor. 14th ed. (Illus.). 256p. pap. 26.95 (*0-8464-4239-6*) Beekman Pubs.

Illustrated History of Brain Function: Imaging the Brain from Antiquity to the Present. Edwin Clarke et al. 2nd enl. rev. ed. 1995. (Illus.). 188p. reprint ed. 150.00 (*0-930405-65-X*) Norman SF.

Illustrated History of Malaria. Charles M. Poser & G. W. Bruyn. 1999. LC 98-50048. (Illus.). 172p. 82.95 (*1-85070-068-0*) CRC Pr.

Illustrated History of Veterinary Medicine. Robert H. Dunlop & David J. Williams. 1995. LC 95-5238. (Illus.). 704p. (gr. 13). text 92.00 (*0-8016-3209-9*, 03209) Mosby Inc.

Illustrated Invertebrate Anatomy: A Laboratory Guide. S. K. Pierce & T. K. Maugel. 1989. (Illus.). 320p. (C). reprint ed. pap. text 39.95 (*0-19-504077-5*) OUP.

Illustrated Manual for HMO Executives. Ann E. Wicklow. 1996. LC 96-92717. (Illus.). pap. 12.95 (*0-9655003-2-2*) Pithy Parodies.

Illustrated Manual of Nursing Practice. Springhouse Publishing Company Staff. 2nd ed. 1994. LC 93-2451. (Illus.). 1472p. 52.95 (*0-87434-609-6*) Springhouse Corp.

Illustrated Manual of Operative Surgery & Surgical Anatomy. C. Bernard & C. Huette. 1991. (American Civil War Medical Ser.: No. 7). (Illus.). 513p. reprint ed. 125.00 (*0-930405-42-0*) Norman SF.

Illustrated Manual of Orthopaedic Tests. Ronald C. Evans. 1993. (Illus.). 640p. (C). (gr. 13). text 81.95 (*0-8016-6612-0*, 06612) Mosby Inc.

Illustrated Manual of Sex Therapy. Helen S. Kaplan. 2nd ed. 1988. LC 87-18189. (Illus.). 200p. pap. 27.95 (*0-87630-518-4*) Brunner-Routledge.

Illustrated Pathology of the Spleen. Bridget Wilkins & Dennis Wright. 2000. LC 99-33418. (Illus.). 204p. (C). text 100.00 (*0-521-62227-1*) Cambridge U Pr.

Illustrated Physiology. B. R. Mackenna & Robin Callander. 6th ed. 1996. LC 96-27920. (Illus.). (C). pap. text (*0-443-05060-0*) Church.

Illustrated Pocket Guide to Clinical Medicine. Charles D. Forbes & William F. Jackson. 1996. (Illus.). 184p. pap. 18.00 (*0-7234-2951-0*) Mosby Inc.

Illustrated Pocketbook of Alzheimer's Disease. M. J. De Leon. 2001. 100p. pap. 29.00 (*1-84214-058-2*, Parthenon Pbng) CRC Pr.

Illustrated Pocketbook of Contact Dermatitis. L. Fry. 2001. 100p. pap. 29.00 (*1-84214-059-0*, Parthenon Pbng) CRC Pr.

Illustrated Pocketbook of Hypertension. P. F. Semple. 2001. 100p. pap. 29.00 (*1-84214-057-4*, Parthenon Pbng) CRC Pr.

Illustrated Pocketbook of Prostatic Diseases. R. S. Kirby. 2002. (Illus.). 100p. pap. 29.95 (*1-84214-056-6*, Parthenon Pbng) CRC Pr.

Illustrated Principles of Exercise Physiology. Kenneth Axen & Kathleen Vermitsky Axen. 2000. LC 00-48365. (Illus.). 306p. pap. 26.67 (*0-13-040022-X*) P-H.

Illustrated Review of Anatomy & Physiology (Lymphatric/Immune) The Lymphatic/Immune System. Glenn F. Bastian. 1997. 128p. (C). pap., wbk. ed. 14.20 (*0-06-501708-0*) Addson-Wesley Educ.

***Illustrated Self Assessment in Pediatrics.** Tom Lissauer et al. 2001. LC 2001-42798. (Illus.). 123p. pap. (*0-7234-3177-9*) Mosby Inc.

Illustrated Signs in Clinical Medicine. K. C. McHardy et al. 1997. (Illus.). 168p. pap. (*0-443-05545-9*) Church.

Illustrated Signs in Clinical Paediatrics. Adrian Minford & R. Arumugam. 1997. LC 97-43448. (Illus.). 149p. pap. text (*0-443-05529-7*) Church.

Illustrated Skeletal Muscles Flash Cards. David Garrison. 1997. (Illus.). 200p. text 39.95 (*0-07-022916-3*) McGraw-Hill Prof.

Illustrated Terminology, Definitions & Diagnostic Criteria in Digestive Endoscopy: Atlas. Zdenek Maratka. rev. ed. 1992. (Illus.). 46.00 (*0-926592-09-2*) Normed Verlag.

Illustrated Textbook of Gynaecology. Eric V. Mackay et al. 2nd ed. 1992. (Illus.). 605p. pap. text (*0-7295-1211-8*) Bailliere Tindall.

***Illustrated Textbook of Pediatrics.** Tom Lissauer & Graham Clayden. 2nd ed. 2001. (Illus.). 355p. pap. (*0-7234-3178-7*) Mosby Inc.

***Illustrated Tutorials in Clinical Ophthalmology.** Jack J. Kanski & Anne Bolton. 2001. (Illus.). 416p. 95.00 incl. cd-rom (*0-7506-5272-1*) Buttrwrth-Heinemann.

Illustrated Veterinary Anatomical Nomenclature Latin-English. Oskar Schaller. 1992. (ENG & LAT., Illus.). 614p. 195.00 (*0-7859-8904-8*) Fr & Eur.

Illustrated Veterinary Anatomical Nomenclature Latin-English. Oskar Schaller. 1992. (Illus.). 614p. 175.00 (*3-432-99591-1*) IBD Ltd.

Illustrated Veterinary Encyclopedia for Horsemen. Equine Research, Inc. Research Staff. Ed. by Don M. Wagoner & M. M. Vale. 1975. (Illus.). 744p. (C). text 85.00 (*0-935842-03-9*) Equine Res.

Illustrated Veterinary Guide for Dogs, Cats, Birds & Exotic Pets. Christopher C. Pinney. 1992. 512p. 29.95 (*0-8306-1986-0*) McGraw-Hill Educ Grp.

Illustration Catalog of the Library of New York Academy of Medicine. New York Academy of Medicine Staff. 3rd ed. 1981. 175.00 (*0-8161-1328-9*, Macmillan Ref) Gale.

Illustrations & Proofs of the Principle of Population: Being the First Work on Population in the English Language Recommending Birth Control. Francis Place. 1967. LC 67-16338. (Reprints of Economic Classics Ser.). reprint ed. 49.50 (*0-678-00210-X*) Kelley.

Illustrations of Madness (1801) John Haslam. Ed. by Roy Porter. 1989. (Tavistock Classic Reprints in the History of Psychiatry Ser.). 144p. 39.95 (*0-415-00637-6*) Routledge.

Illustrations to Supplement a Pathophysicology Course. Pat Taylor. 1998. (Illus.). 134p. (C). spiral bd. 29.95 (*0-7872-5247-6*, 41524701) Kendall-Hunt.

I'm a Nursing Assistant: A Vocabulary Workbook. Sharon Elwell. 1991. (Working English Ser.). (Illus.). 52p. (Orig.). pap. text 8.95 (*0-9626210-2-1*) Rattle OK Pubns.

I'm Glad You're Not Dead: A Liver Transplant Story. Elizabeth Parr. unabr. ed. 1996. LC 96-94745. 172p. pap. 9.95 (*0-9654728-0-9*); 2nd unabr. ed. 2000. LC 00-90041. (Illus.). pap. 12.95 (*0-9654728-1-7*) Jrny Pub TX.

I'm Here to Help: A Guide for Caregivers, Hospice Workers & Volunteers. M. Catherine Ray. 2nd ed. 1997. LC 96-26981. (Illus.). 128p. pap. 11.95 (*0-553-37797-3*) Bantam.

I'm Here to Help: A Hospice Worker's Guide to Communicating with Dying People & Their Loved Ones. M. Catherine Ray. 1992. (Illus.). 72p. reprint ed. pap. 7.00 (*0-9636311-0-1*) McRay.

I'm Not Crazy, I Just Lost My Glasses. Lonny Shavelson. 1986. LC 86-72109. (Illus.). 96p. (Orig.). pap. 12.95 (*0-912357-01-0*) De Novo Pr.

I'm Not My Fault: The Why of Shame & Codependency. Don Haury. Ed. by Adele Kalas. 1990. (Illus.). 51p. (Orig.). pap. 3.95 (*0-9626323-0-9*) Safe Place Pub.

I'm Still Dancing! A Gay Man's Health Experience. A. Stephen Pieters. 1991. 96p. pap. 8.95 (*1-888493-04-6*) Chi Rho Pr.

Image Analysis in Histology: Conventional & Confocal Microscopy. Ed. by Richard Wootton et al. 1995. (Postgraduate Medical Science Ser.: No. 2). (Illus.). 441p. (C). text 100.00 (*0-521-43482-3*) Cambridge U Pr.

Image & Insight: Essays in Psychoanalysis & the Arts. Ellen H. Spitz. 1991. text 44.00 (*0-231-07296-1*) Col U Pr.

Image & Metaphor: The Practice & Profession of Art Therapy. 1991. (Conference Proceedings Ser.). 143p. (Orig.). pap. 15.00 (*1-882147-09-X*) Am Art Therapy.

Image & Mind. Stephen M. Kosslyn. 1980. LC 80-10329. (Illus.). 515p. 42.00 (*0-674-44365-9*) HUP.

***Image & Mirage: Art Therapy with Dissociative Clients.** Dee Spring. 2001. LC 2001-44299. (*0-398-07247-7*); pap. (*0-398-07248-5*) C C Thomas.

Image Formation Psychotherapy: Revised Edition of Image & Cognition. Mardi J. Horowitz. rev. ed. 1995. LC 83-2597. 340p. pap. text 50.00 (*1-56821-730-7*) Aronson.

Image-Guided Neurosurgery: Clinical Applications of Surgical Navigation. Ed. by Gene H. Barnett et al. 1998. LC 98-13928. (Illus.). 264p. 160.00 (*1-57626-083-6*, QMP) Quality Med Pub.

Image-Guided Pain Management. P. Sebastian Thomas. 1996. LC 96-31992. 208p. text 115.00 (*0-397-51743-2*) Lppncott W & W.

Image of Madness: The Public Facing Mental Illness & Psychiatric Treatment. Ed. by J. Guimon et al. 3rd ed. 1999. LC 99-40704. (Illus.). XIV, 246p. 128.75 (*3-8055-6846-0*) S Karger.

Image of Man: The Creation of Modern Masculinity. George L. Mosse. 1998. (Studies in the History of Sexuality). (Illus.). 240p. reprint ed. pap. 17.95 (*0-19-512660-2*) OUP.

Image Reconstruction in Radiology. J. Anthony Parker. 1990. 536p. 198.95 (*0-8493-0150-5*, RC78) CRC Pr.

Image Understanding: Advances in Computational Vision, Vol. 2. Ed. by Whitman Richards & Shimon Ullman. 1987. 368p. 78.50 (*0-89391-311-1*, Ablex) Greenwood.

Imagerie Anatomique des Nerfs Craniens see Cranial Nerves: Anatomy, Imaging, Vascularisation

Imagery. John T. E. Richardson. 1999. LC 99-187241. (Cognitive Psychology Ser.). (Illus.). 176p. 44.95 (*0-86377-842-9*); pap. text 22.95 (*0-86377-843-7*) Taylor & Francis.

Imagery & Cognition. Ed. by C. Cornoldi & M. A. McDaniel. 1990. (Illus.). 310p. 71.95 (*0-387-97410-5*) Spr-Verlag.

Imagery & Related Mnemonic Processes. Ed. by M. A. McDaniel & M. Pressley. 1987. (Illus.). 470p. 140.00 (*0-387-96427-4*) Spr-Verlag.

Imagery & Symbolism in Counselling. William Stewart. 1996. LC 96-219946. 350p. pap. (*1-85302-350-7*) Jessica Kingsley GBR. *Dist:* Taylor & Francis.

Imagery & Symbolism in Counselling: An A-Z. William Stewart. 1996. 350p. pap. (*1-85302-351-5*) Jessica Kingsley GBR. *Dist:* Taylor & Francis.

Imagery & Verbal Processes. Allan Paivio. 1971. LC 73-150787. 608p. text 99.95 (*0-89859-069-8*) L Erlbaum Assocs.

Imagery & Visual Expression in Therapy. V. B. Lusebrink. 1990. LC 90-6901. (Emotions, Personality, & Psychotherapy Ser.). (Illus.). 300p. (C). 49.50 (*0-306-43453-9*, Plenum Trade) Perseus Pubng.

Imagery for Getting Well: Clinical Applications of Behavioral Medicine. Deidre Davis Brigham. 1996. 464p. pap. 20.00 (*0-393-70225-1*) Norton.

***Imagery in Healing: Shamanism & Modern Medicine.** Jeanne Achterberg. 2002. 272p. pap. 15.95 (*1-57062-934-X*) Shambhala Pubns.

Imagery in Working Memory & in Mental Discovery. Tore Helstrup. 2000. 160p. 39.95 (*0-86377-630-2*) L Erlbaum Assocs.

Imagery, Memory & Cognition: Essays in Honor of Allan Paivio. Ed. by John C. Yuille. 1983. (Illus.). 352p. (C). text 69.95 (*0-89859-215-1*) L Erlbaum Assocs.

Imagery Paradigm: Imaginative Consciousness in the Experimental & Clinical Setting. Akhter Ahsen. 1993. LC 93-71037. 465p. (Orig.). pap. text 25.00 (*0-913412-49-X*) Brandon Hse.

Imagery, Vol. 1: Its Many Dimensions & Applications. Ed. by Joseph E. Shorr et al. 1980. LC 80-15723. (Illus.). 408p. 85.00 (*0-306-40456-7*, Plenum Trade) Perseus Pubng.

Imagery, Vol. 3: Theoretical & Clinical Applications. Ed. by Joseph E. Shorr et al. 1983. LC 83-13331. 446p. 85.00 (*0-306-41464-3*, Plenum Trade) Perseus Pubng.

Images: A Unified View of Diffraction & Image Formation. C. A. Taylor. 1978. 180p. 36.00 (*0-85109-630-1*); pap. 18.00 (*0-85109-620-4*) Taylor & Francis.

Images in Clinical Medicine: Selections from the New England Journal of Medicine. Ed. by Jerome P. Kassirer & Kim Eagle. 1997. LC 97-73446. 320p. pap. 30.00 (*0-910133-41-7*) Mass Med Pub Div.

Images in Psychiatry: Canada. Ed. by Quentin Rae-Grant. 1996. LC 96-22436. (Illus.). 317p. pap. text 29.95 (*0-88048-900-6*, 8900) Am Psychiatric.

Images into the Mind: A Radical New Look at Understanding & Changing Behavior. Daniel G. Amen. 1995. (Illus.). 252p. pap. text 49.95 (*1-886554-01-3*) MindWrks.

Images of Art Therapy: New Developments in Theory & Practice. Tessa Dalley et al. 1987. (Illus.). 264p. pap. 17.95 (*0-422-60400-3*) Routledge.

Images of Art Therapy: New Developments in Theory & Practice. Tessa Dalley et al. 1987. (Illus.). 264p. (C). lib. bdg. (*0-422-60390-2*) Tavistock GBR. *Dist:* Routldge.

Images of Arthritis & Related Conditions: With Clinical Perspectives. George B. Greenfield et al. 2000. LC 00-41244. (Illus.). xi, 338p. text 149.00 (*0-7817-1536-9*) Lppncott W & W.

Images of Childhood. Philip C. Hwang & Irving E. Sigel. 1996. 232p. text 55.00 (*0-8058-1701-8*) L Erlbaum Assocs.

Images of Childhood. Philip C. Hwang et al. 1996. LC 95-49699. 275p. pap. 24.50 (*0-8058-1702-6*) L Erlbaum Assocs.

Images of Hope: Imagination as Healer of the Hopeless. William F. Lynch. 1987. LC 73-20418. (C). reprint ed. pap. text 15.00 (*0-268-00537-0*) U of Notre Dame Pr.

Images of the Body in Trauma. Jean M. Goodwin. 2000. 288p. pap. 45.00 (*0-465-09544-5*) Basic.

Images of the Self: The Sandplay Therapy Process. Estelle Weinrib. 1983. LC 83-11974. (Illus.). 172p. 32.50 (*0-938434-19-5*); pap. 19.95 (*0-938434-16-0*) Sigo Pr.

Imaginary Social Worlds: A Cultural Approach. John L. Caughey. 1984. LC 83-6702. 280p. text 50.00 (*0-8032-1421-9*) U of Nebr Pr.

Imagination & Healing. Ed. by Anees A. Sheik. 1984. (Imagery & Human Development Ser.: Vol. 1). 291p. pap. 36.95 (*0-89503-037-3*) Baywood Pub.

Imagination & Phenomenological Psychology. Ed. by Edward L. Murray. 1987. LC 87-13437. 230p. text 27.00 (*0-8207-0195-5*) Duquesne.

Imagination, Identification & Catharsis in Theatre & Therapy. Mary Duggan & Roger Grainger. 1997. LC 97-197779. 176p. pap. (*1-85302-431-7*) Jessica Kingsley GBR. *Dist:* Taylor & Francis.

Imagination Is Reality. Roberts Avens. 2000. 152p. pap. 15.00 (*0-88214-382-4*) Spring Pubns.

Imaginative Behavior of Preschool Children. Frances V. Markey. 1976. LC 75-35075. (Studies in Play & Games). reprint ed. 16.95 (*0-405-07925-7*) Ayer.

Imaginative Body: Psychodynamic Therapy in Health Care. Ed. by Aleda Erskine & Dorothy Judd. 1995. LC 94-9014. 264p. 50.00 (*1-56821-257-7*) Aronson.

Imagine Having Epilepsy. Linda O'Neill. 2000. LC 00-29079. (Imagine Ser.). (Illus.). 32p. (J). (gr. 1-4). pap. 23.93 (*1-57103-381-5*) Rourke Pr.

Imagine That! Awareness Through Imagery Practice. Lane L. Waas. 2nd rev. ed. 2000. LC 90-63767. (Illus.). 144p. (gr. k-12). pap. 18.95 (*1-880396-60-2*, JP9660-2) Jalmar Pr.

Imagine Yourself: Using Imagery to Get Well. Helen B. Barry. Ed. by Gwen Costa. 1990. LC 91-4450. pap. 13.95 (*0-87949-336-4*) Ashley Bks.

Imagineering for Health: Self-Healing Through the Use of the Mind. Serge K. King. 1981. LC 80-53949. (Quest Book Ser.). 211p. pap. 9.95 (*0-8356-0546-9*, Quest) Theos Pub Hse.

Imaging. Jeremy Hughes & Michael Hughes. 1997. LC 96-37372. (Colour Guide Ser.). pap. text 15.95 (*0-443-05591-2*) Harcrt Hlth Sci Grp.

Imaging. D. N. Redhead & N. Chalmers. 1995. LC 94-11040. (Colour Guide Ser.). pap. text 16.95 (*0-443-05020-1*) Harcrt Hlth Sci Grp.

Imaging Anatomy of the Head & Spine: A Photographic Color Atlas of MRI, CT, Gross & Microscopic Anatomy in Axial, Coronal, & Sagittal Planes. F. Reed Murtagh & H. Norman Schnitzlein. 2nd ed. 1990. (Illus.). 480p. 200.00 (*0-683-07622-1*) Lppncott W & W.

Imaging & Correlative Physiochemical Techniques. Ed. by Alan A. Boulton et al. 1988. LC 88-9191. (Neuromethods Ser.: Vol. 8). 442p. (C). 159.50 (*0-89603-116-0*) Humana.

Imaging & Intervention in Cardiology, Vol. 173. Ed. by Christoph A. Nienaber & Udo Sechtem. 1995. LC 95-34054. (Developments in Cardiovascular Medicine Ser.). 548p. (C). text 313.00 (*0-7923-3649-6*) Kluwer Academic.

Imaging & Invasive Radiology in the Intensive Care Unit. Ed. by Carl E. Ravin. 1992. LC 92-49509. (Illus.). 181p. text (*0-443-08868-3*) Church.

Imaging & Labelling Techniques in the Critically Ill. Ed. by W. J. Kox et al. 1989. (Current Concepts in Critical Care Ser.). (Illus.). 188p. 216.00 (*0-387-17483-4*) Spr-Verlag.

Imaging Atlas of Human Anatomy. Weir. 1993. (SPA.). 200p. (gr. 13). text 60.00 (*84-8086-069-3*) Mosby Inc.

Imaging Atlas of Orthopedic Appliances & Prostheses. Ed. by Thomas H. Berquist. 1994. LC 94-20580. (Illus.). 1,008p. text 235.00 (*0-7817-0222-4*) Lppncott W & W.

Imaging Atlas of the Normal Gallbladder & Its Variants. Ed. by Jon W. Meilstrup. 1994. LC 93-44006. 128p. 139.00 (*0-8493-4788-2*) CRC Pr.

Imaging Atlas of the Temporomandibular Joint. Leslie B. Heffez et al. LC 94-7256. (Illus.). 1995. 250p. 75.00 (*0-683-03983-0*); 1994. (*0-8121-1449-3*) Lppncott W & W.

Imaging Atlas on Osteoporotic Bone Disease. A. Boyde. 2001. (Encyclopedia of Visual Medicine Ser.). (Illus.). 120p. 88.00 (*1 85070 483-X*, Parthenon Pbng) CRC Pr.

Imaging Brain Structure & Function: Emerging Technologies in the Neurosciences. David S. Lester et al. 1997. (Annals of the New York Academy of Sciences Ser.). LC 97-13820. pap. 130.00 (*1-57331-069-7*); 185p. 130.00 (*1-57331-068-9*) NY Acad Sci.

Imaging Cerebrovascular Disease. Babikian et al. 2001. 320p. 155.00 (*0-7506-7302-8*) Buttrwrth-Heinemann.

Imaging Children Ed. by Helen Carty et al. 1994. (Illus.). 2019p. text (*0-443-04260-8*) Church.

Imaging Drug Action in the Brain. London. 1992. 432p. 195.00 (*0-8493-8843-0*, RM301) CRC Pr.

Imaging Drug Reactions & Toxic Hazards. Ed. by George Ansell. 3rd ed. 1997. (Illus.). 392p. text (*0-412-55590-5*) E A GBR. *Dist:* OUP.

Imaging for Junior Doctors: A Survival Guide. Peter Kember. 2000. 255p. pap. text (*0-7020-2498-8*) W B Saunders GBR. *Dist:* Saunders.

Imaging for Surgeons. Lisle. 1993. 336p. (Orig.). (*0-340-55170-4*) E A GBR. *Dist:* Routldge.

Imaging for Surgeons: A Clinical Guide. Barry E. Kelly & Colin S. McArdle. 2001. 128p. pap. text Price not set. (*0-7020-2434-1*) W B Saunders.

Imaging for Surgeons: A Clinical Guide. David A. Lisle. 2nd ed. 1998. LC 98-27855. (Arnold Publication). (Illus.). 232p. pap. text 55.00 (*0-340-69267-7*) OUP.

Imaging for the Surgeon. Niederhube. 1998. (C). text (*0-443-05629-3*) Church.

Imaging Handbook for House Officers. Ed. by Paul M. Silverman & Douglas J. Quint. 1996. LC 96-20853. 455p. pap. 72.50 (*0-471-13767-7*) Wiley.

Imaging Hardware & Software for Nuclear Medicine: Proceedings of the Midwinter Meeting of the Society of Nuclear Medicine Computer & Instrumentation Councils Held in Phoenix, Arizona, February 15-26, 1988. Ed. by Michael A. King et al. 1988. (American Association of Physicists in Medicine Symposium Ser.: No. 6). 224p. 45.00 (*0-88318-556-3*) Am Inst Physics.

Imaging Human Anatomy. Weir. 1994. text (*0-7234-2054-8*) Wolfe Publishing GBR. *Dist:* Mosby Inc.

Imaging in AIDS. Reeders. 1998. (Illus.). 200p. text (*0-7020-1904-6*) Bailliere Tindall.

Imaging in Alcohol Research. Ed. by Dianne M. Welsh. 1998. (Illus.). 71p. (C). pap. text 25.00 (*0-7881-4659-9*) DIANE Pub.

***Imaging in Anesthesia & Critical Care.** Gregory Hobbs & Ravi Mahajan. 2000. (Illus.). 182p. (*0-443-05310-3*) Church GBR. *Dist:* Saunders.

Imaging in Cardiovascular Disease. Gerald M. Pohost et al. 2000. 992p. text 125.00 (*0-397-51591-X*) Lppncott W & W.

Imaging in Esthetic Dentistry. Cary Goldstein et al. 1998. LC 97-39481. (Illus.). 188p. text 72.00 (*0-86715-238-9*) Quint Pub Co.

Imaging in Glaucoma. Joel S. Schuman. 1996. (Illus.). 224p. 110.00 (*1-55642-319-5*, 63195) SLACK Inc.

Imaging in Hepatobiliary & Pancreatic Disease: A Practical Clinical Guide. Ed. by J. Reeders et al. 1999. (Illus.). 305p. text (*0-7020-1873-2*) W B Saunders.

Imaging in Infertility & Gynecology. Isabel Yoder. 1988. 350p. 110.00 (*0-316-96881-1*, Little Brwn Med Div) Lppncott W & W.

Imaging in Liver Disease: From Diagnosis to Treatment. K. Takayasu & K. Okuda. 1997. (Illus.). 576p. text 275.00 (*0-19-262634-5*) OUP.

Imaging in Musculoskeletal & Sports Medicine. Brian Halpern et al. 1997. LC 97-12111. (Illus.). 368p. 141.95 (*0-86542-418-7*) Blackwell Sci.

Imaging in Neurologic Rehabilitation. Ed. by James Toole. 1995. 198p. pap. 84.95 (*0-939957-80-9*) Demos Medical.

Imaging in Paediatrics: A Casebook. Kieran McHugh. 1997. (Illus.). 232p. text 69.50 (*0-19-262776-7*) OUP.

Imaging in Radiation Therapy: 1998 AAPM Summer School Proceedings. Ed. by John D. Hazlett & Arthur L. Boyle. 1998. LC 98-66296. (Monograph Ser.: No. 24). 512p. text (*1-888340-12-6*) AAPM.

Imaging in Trauma: How to Plan Investigations for the Injured Patient. Robert Cocks et al. 2000. LC 99-16260. (Illus.). viii, 254p. text 75.00 (*0-19-262509-8*) OUP.

Imaging in Trauma & Critical Care. Stuart E. Mirvis & Jeremy W. Young. 1992. (Illus.). 592p. 140.00 (*0-683-06075-9*) Lppncott W & W.

Imaging, Measurement & Analysis of the Heart. Ed. by Samuel Sideman & Rafael Beyar. 1991. 400p. 115.00 (*1-56032-058-3*) Hemisp Pub.

Imaging Modalities in Spinal Disorders. Morrie E. Kricun. 1988. (Illus.). 608p. text 140.00 (*0-7216-1587-2*) Saunders.

Imaging, Nineteen-Ninety. Fred A. Mettler, Jr. 1989. 125.00 (*0-316-56829-5*, Little Brwn Med Div) Lppncott W & W.

Imaging of Acquired Cardiac Disorders. Benigno Soto. 1991. (gr. 13). text (*1-56375-094-5*) Gower-Mosby.

Imaging of Athletic Injuries: Advanced Techniques. Joseph R. Martire & Mark E. Levinsohn. 1991. 300p. text 129.00 (*0-07-040728-2*) McGraw-Hill Prof.

Imaging of Bone Tumors. Morrie E. Kricun. 1992. (Illus.). 704p. text 175.00 (*0-7216-5518-1*) Saunders.

Imaging of Cardiac Disorders Benigno Soto et al. 1991. (Illus.). 816p. (gr. 13). text (*0-397-44678-0*, GM0085) Gower-Mosby.

Imaging of Congenital Cardiac Disorders. Benigno Soto. 1991. (gr. 13). text (*1-56375-093-7*) Gower-Mosby.

Imaging of Diffuse Lung Disease. David A. Lynch & John D. Newell. 1999. LC 00-421471. (Illus.). ix, 322p. incl. cd-rom (*1-55009-092-5*) DEKR.

Imaging of Head Trauma. Alisa D. Gean. 1993. LC 93-16862. 592p. text 159.00 (*0-7817-0025-6*) Lppncott W & W.

Imaging of Hyposia: Tracer Developments. Hans-Jhurgen Machulla. 1999. LC 98-49717. (Developments in Nuclear Medicine Ser.). 17p. (*0-7923-5529-6*) Kluwer Academic.

Imaging of Infection & Inflammation. Peter H. Cox & John R. Buscombe. 1998. LC 98-21151. (Developments in Nuclear Medicine Ser.). 240p. 146.00 (*0-7923-5087-1*) Kluwer Academic.

Imaging of Musculoskeletal Stress Injury. Keats Pope. 2nd ed. 1999. (Illus.). 352p. (C). text 95.00 (*0-8151-3665-X*, 31335) Mosby Inc.

Imaging of Non-Traumatic & Hemorrhagic Disorders of the Central Nervous System. Ed. by Mohammed Sarwar & Solomon Batnitzky. 1989. (C). text 246.50 (*0-89838-417-6*) Kluwer Academic.

Imaging of Orthopedic Trauma. Ed. by Thomas H. Berquist. 2nd ed. 1991. 928p. text 170.00 (*0-88167-805-8*) Lppncott W & W.

Imaging of Orthopedic Trauma & Surgery. Thomas H. Berquist. 1986. (Illus.). 799p. text 220.00 (*0-7216-1102-8*) Saunders.

Imaging of Small Intestinal Tumours. Ed. by N. C. Gourtsoyiannis & D. J. Nolan. 1997. 414p. 259.00 (*0-444-89997-9*) Elsevier.

Imaging of Soft Tissue Tumors. A. M. De Schepper et al. 1996. LC 96-27265. (Illus.). 390p. 222.00 (*3-540-61392-7*) Spr-Verlag.

Imaging of Soft Tissue Tumors. Mark Kransdorf & Mark D. Murphey. Ed. by Lisette Bralow. 1996. 480p. text 152.00 (*0-7216-6069-X*) Saunders.

Imaging of Spinal Trauma in Children. Lawrence R. Kuhns. 1998. 293p. incl. cd-rom (*1-55009-056-9*) DEKR.

Imaging of the Brain in Psychiatry & Related Fields. Ed. by Konrad Maurer. 1993. LC 92-49551. (Illus.). 336p. 159.00 (*0-387-54785-1*) Spr-Verlag.

***Imaging of the Cervical Spine in Children: Normal, Congenital & Traumatic Findings.** L. Swischuk. 2001. LC 2001-49833. (Illus.). 250p. 99.00 (*0-387-95290-X*) Spr-Verlag.

Imaging of the Chest: A Teaching File. Patricia Mergo. 2001. text 95.00 (*0-683-30473-9*) Lppncott W & W.

Imaging of the Foot & Ankle. Julia R. Crim et al. 1996. LC 95-33415. 252p. text 169.00 (*0-397-51463-8*) Lppncott W & W.

Imaging of the Globe & Orbit: A Guide to Differential Diagnosis. N. Hosten. Tr. by Peter Winter. 1998. LC 97-34736. (Illus.). 208p. 89.00 (*0-86577-714-4*) Thieme Med Pubs.

Imaging of the Hand & Wrist. Louis A. Gilula & Yuming Yin. 1995. LC 95-5453. (Illus.). text 135.00 (*0-7216-5125-9*) Saunders.

Imaging of the Head & Neck. Richard A. Buckingham et al. 2nd ed. 1994. (Illus.). 620p. 199.00 (*0-86577-549-4*) Thieme Med Pubs.

Imaging of the Nervous System. Ed. by P. J. Butler et al. 1990. (Clinical Medicine & the Nervous System Ser.). 288p. 225.00 (*0-387-19522-X*) Spr-Verlag.

Imaging of the Newborn, Infant & Young Child. Leonard E. Swischuk. 3rd ed. 1988. (Illus.). 1248p. 160.00 (*0-683-08050-4*) Lppncott W & W.

Imaging of the Newborn, Infant, & Young Child. Leonard E. Swischuk. 4th ed. 1997. LC 96-47825. (Illus.). 1,088p. text 199.00 (*0-683-08051-2*) Lppncott W & W.

Imaging of the Pediatric Head, Neck, & Spine. Mauricio Castillo & Suresh K. Mukherji. 1995. LC 95-44623. (Illus.). 768p. text 175.00 (*0-397-51577-4*) Lppncott W & W.

Imaging of the Pediatric Urinary Tract. T. L. Slovis et al. 1989. 288p. text 90.00 (*0-7216-1871-5*) Saunders.

Imaging of the Pelvis. Fishman. 1990. 115.00 (*0-316-28396-7*, Little Brwn Med Div) Lppncott W & W.

Imaging of the Scrotum. Ed. by Hedvig Hricak et al. 1995. (Illus.). 288p. text 189.00 (*0-7817-0153-8*) Lppncott W & W.

Imaging of the Skeleton, Chest, & Abdomen: Interpretation of Pattern. Marchiori & McLean. 1998. LC 98-23694. (Illus.). 1120p. (gr. 13). text 149.00 (*0-8151-8616-9*, 30549) Mosby Inc.

Imaging of the Spine. Adam Greenspan & Pasquale Montesano. 1993. LC 92-48322. (gr. 13). (*1-56375-014-7*) Gower-Mosby.

Imaging of the Spine: A Teaching File. Mauricio Castillo & John H. Harris, Jr. 1998. LC 97-44168. (Illus.). 400p. 89.00 (*0-683-30244-2*) Lppncott W & W.

Imaging of the Spine & Spinal Cord. Ed. by Claude Manelfe. rev. ed. 1992. 928p. text 235.00 (*0-88167-863-5*) Lppncott W & W.

Imaging of the Temporal Bone. Joel D. Swartz & H. Ric Harnsberger. 3rd rev. ed. 1997. LC 97-34507. (Illus.). 408p. 139.00 (*0-86577-700-4*) Thieme Med Pubs.

Imaging of the Thyroid & Parathyroid Glands: A Practical Guide. Ed. by Brian Eisenberg. 1990. (Illus.). 209p. text (*0-443-08762-8*) Church.

Imaging of Tropical Diseases: Epidemiological, Pathological & Clinical Correlation 2nd ed. Philip E. S. Palmer & Maurice M. Reeder. Incl. Imaging of Tropical Diseases Vol. 2: With Epidemiological, Pathological & Clinical Correlation. 2048p. 2000. 350.00 (*3-540-62471-6*); Vol. 1. Imaging of Tropical Diseases: With Epidemiological, Pathological & Clinical Correlation. xxiv, 776p. 2001. 350.00 (*3-540-56028-9*); LC 99-39417. (Illus.). 2000p. 2001. 589.00 (*3-540-66219-7*) Spr-Verlag.

Imaging of Tropical Diseases: With Epidemiological, Pathological & Clinical Correlation, Vol. 1. Philip E. S. Palmer & Maurice M. Reeder. 2nd rev. ed. 2001. LC 99-39417. (Illus.). xxiv, 776p. 350.00 (*3-540-56028-9*) Spr-Verlag.

Imaging of Tropical Diseases Vol. 2: With Epidemiological, Pathological & Clinical Correlation Philip E. S. Palmer & Maurice M. Reeder. 2nd rev. ed. 2000. LC 99-39417. (Illus.). 2048p. 350.00 (*3-540-62471-6*) Spr-Verlag.

***Imaging of Tuberculosis: With Epidemiological, Pathological & Clinical Correlation.** Philip E. S. Palmer. 2001. LC 2001-40050. 160p. 54.95 (*3-540-41821-0*) Springer Pub.

Imaging of Vertebral Trauma. Richard H. Daffner. 2nd ed. 1996. 304p. text 159.00 (*0-397-51680-0*) Lppncott W & W.

Imaging Physiological Functions: Experience with the Dynamic Spatial Reconstructor. Erik L. Ritman et al. 1985. LC 84-18247. 318p. 82.50 (*0-275-91322-8*, C1322, Praeger Pubs) Greenwood.

***Imaging Selective Attention in the Human Brain.** Ed. by Jon Driver & Richard S. J. Frackowiak. 2001. LC 2001-55567. 124p. 63.00 (*0-444-50920-8*) Elsevier.

Imaging Strategies in Oncology. Daniel Vanel & David Stark. 1993. LC 92-48264. 500p. 357.00 (*0-471-59069-X*, Wiley-Liss) Wiley.

Imaging Strategy: A Guide for Clinicians. Bob Bury & Richard Fowler. 1992. LC 92-22706. 176p. 55.00 (*0-19-262323-0*); (Illus.). 172p. pap. text 27.50 (*0-19-262063-0*) OUP.

Imaging Systems for Medical Diagnosis: Fundamentalsand& Technical Solutions - X-Ray Diagnostics - Computed Tomography - Nuclear Medical Diagnostics - Magnetic Resonance Imaging - Ultrasound Technology. Ed. by E. Krestel. 1990. 627p. 125.00 (*3-8009-1564-2*) Wiley.

Imaging Technician in Medications Development: Preclinical & Clinical Aspects. 1995. (Illus.). 204p. (Orig.). (C). pap. text 45.00 (*0-7881-1632-0*) DIANE Pub.

HI

Imaging Techniques in Biomaterials: Digital Image Processing Applied to Orthopaedic & Dental Implants. Ed. by M. A. Barbosa & A. Campilho. 1994. LC 94-13351. 402p. 187.50 (*0-444-89774-7*) Elsevier.

Imaging Techniques of the CNS of the Neonate. Ed. by J. Haddad et al. 1991. (Illus.). 185p. 189.00 (*0-387-53774-0*) Spr-Verlag.

***Imaging the Neonatal Brain.** Mary Rutherford & Graeme Bydder. 2001. (Illus.). 315p. (*0-7020-2534-8*) W B Saunders GBR. *Dist:* Saunders.

Imago Dei: A Study of C. G. Jung's Psychology of Religion. James W. Heisig. 1979. LC 77-74405. 256p. 34.50 (*0-8387-2076-5*) Bucknell U Pr.

Imbroglio: Rising to the Challenge of Borderline Personality Disorder. Janice M. Cauwels. 1992. 448p. 31.95 (*0-393-03349-X*) Norton.

Imhotep, the Vizier & Physician of King Zoser & Afterwards the Egyptian God of Medicine. Jamieson B. Hurry. 2nd rev. ed. LC 75-23727. reprint ed. 34.50 (*0-404-13285-5*) AMS Pr.

Imidazole & Benzimidazole Synthesis. M. R. Grimmett. 1997. LC 97-21743. (Best Synthetic Methods Ser.). (Illus.). 288p. text 99.00 (*0-12-303190-7*) Morgan Kaufmann.

Imidazoline Receptor: Pharmacology, Functions, Ligands, & Relevance to Biology & Medicine. Ed. by Donald J. Reis et al. 1995. (Annals of the New York Academy of Sciences Ser.: Vol. 763). 707p. 190.00 (*0-89766-935-5*); LC 95-316. pap. 190.00 (*0-89766-936-3*) NY Acad Sci.

Imidazoline Receptors Linking the Brain & the Cardiovascular System. Hans R. Brunner. 1997. text (*0-397-51818-8*) Lppncott W & W.

Imipenem - Cilastatin: Experience with a Long-Acting Intramuscular Formulation, 1991 - Journal: Chemotherapy, Vol. 37, Suppl. 2. Ed. by M. Sande. 1991. (Illus.). iv, 60p. pap. 20.00 (*3-8055-5427-3*) S Karger.

Imitation Chez L'enfant see Imitation in Children

Imitation in Children. Paul Guillaume. Tr. by Elaine P. Halperin from FRE. 1992. LC 77-135742.Tr. of Imitation Chez L'enfant. xviii, 214p. lib. bdg. 13.00 (*0-226-31045-0*) U Ch Pr.

Imitators of Epilepsy. Ed. by Robert S. Fisher. 1994. 384p. text 74.95 (*0-939957-56-6*) Demos Medical.

IML Ethics & Issues in Contemporary Nursing. Burkhardt-Nathaniel. 1998. (Home Care Aide Ser.). 64p. tchr. ed. 12.00 (*0-8273-7703-7*) Delmar.

Immediate & Early Prosthetic Management: Rehabilitation Aspects. Philip S. King & J. H. Zettl. Ed. by John J. Gerhardt et al. 2nd ed. 1986. LC 85-27320. (Illus.). 305p. pap. text 38.00 (*0-920887-02-3*) Hogrefe & Huber Pubs.

Immediate Breast Reconstruction. Seckel. 1998. text 110.00 (*0-7216-5076-7*) Saunders.

Immediate Early Genes in the Central Nervous System. Ed. by T. R. Tolle et al. 1995. LC 95-2186. (Illus.). 166p. 81.95 (*3-540-58962-7*) Spr-Verlag.

Immediate Effects of Interpolated Rest Periods on Learning & Performance. John R. Gentry. LC 78-176803. (Columbia University. Teachers College. Contributions to Education Ser.: No. 799). reprint ed. 37.50 (*0-404-55799-6*) AMS Pr.

Immediate Effects on Patients of Psychoanalytic Interpretations. Edith L. Garduk & Ernest A. Haggard. 1972. LC 79-186504. (Psychological Issues Monographs: No. 28, Vol. 7, No. 4). 86p. (Orig.). 27.50 (*0-8236-2530-3*) Intl Univs Pr.

Immediate Eye Care. Nicola Ragge. 1991. (Illus.). 208p. (C). (gr. 13). text 115.00 (*0-8151-7008-4*, 21260) Mosby Inc.

Immediate Hints to Health Problems. Betty Yulin Ho. 1991. LC 89-15630. (System of Government in the Living Body Ser.). 264p. pap. 40.00 (*0-9600148-5-3*) Juvenescent.

Immigrant Women & Their Health: An Olive Paper. Afaf Ibrahim Meleis et al. 1998. (Monographs). 59p. (C). pap. text 20.00 (*0-9656391-6-9*, 1057) Sigma Theta Tau.

Immigrants & Insanity: An Original Anthology. Ed. by Gerald N. Grob. 1980. LC 78-22566. (Historical Issues in Mental Health Ser.). (Illus.). lib. bdg. 23.95 (*0-405-11920-8*) Ayer.

Immobilized Affinity Ligand Techniques. Greg T. Hermanson et al. 1992. LC 92-6321. (Illus.). 454p. pap. 52.00 (*0-12-342330-9*) Acad Pr.

Immobilized Enzymes. Ed. by Klaus Mosbach. 1977. (Methods in Enzymology Ser.: Vol. 44). text 199.00 (*0-12-181944-2*) Acad Pr.

Immobilized Enzymes & Cells, Pt. C. Ed. by Sidney P. Colowick et al. 1987. (Methods in Enzymology Ser.: Vol. 136). 584p. text 159.00 (*0-12-182036-X*) Acad Pr.

Immobilized Microbial Cells. Ed. by K. Venkatsubramanian. 1979. LC 79-15794. (ACS Symposium Ser.: No. 106). 38.95 (*0-8412-0508-6*); pap. 24.95 (*0-8412-0644-9*) Am Chemical.

Immortality of Love (Eulis) Paschal B. Randolph. Ed. by Emerson M. Clymer et al. 1979. 290p. 9.95 (*0-932785-17-4*) Philos Pub.

***Immune Advantage: The Powerful, Natural Immune-Boosting Program to Help You Prevent Disease, Enhance Vitality, Live a Longer, Healthier Life.** Ellen Mazo et al. 2002. LC 2001-5266. (Illus.). 480p. pap. 29.95 (*1-57954-355-3*) Rodale Pr Inc.

Immune & Metabolic Aspects of Therapeutic Blood Purification Systems. Ed. by L. C. Smeby et al. 1986. (Illus.). xii, 402p. 116.75 (*3-8055-4224-0*) S Karger.

Immune Crossover: The Two Faces of Immunity. Enrique Rewald. 1998. (Illus.). 134p. lib. bdg. 27.95 (*1-85070-018-4*, Parthenon Pbng) CRC Pr.

Immune-Deficient Animals. Ed. by Z. Jie. 1989. (Illus.). xiv, 362p. 276.75 (*3-8055-4934-2*) S Karger.

Immune-Deficient Animals: International Workshop, 4th, Chexbres, Oct.-Nov. 1982. Ed. by B. Sordat. 1984. (Illus.). xiv, 446p. 169.75 (*3-8055-3741-7*) S Karger.

Immune-Deficient Animals in Biomedical Research. Ed. by J. Rygaard & M. Spang-Thomsen. 1987. (Illus.). xvi, 420p. 232.25 (*3-8055-4385-9*) S Karger.

Immune Disorders. Ed. by Leo Van der Reis. 1975. (Frontiers of Gastrointestinal Research Ser.: Vol. 1). 200p. 85.25 (*3-8055-1751-3*) S Karger.

Immune Dysfunction: Winning My Battle Against Toxins, Illness & the Medical Establishment. Judith Lopez. 2001. LC 00-41114. xvii, 256p. pap. 14.95 (*0-9701270-4-9*) Millpond Pr.

Immune Globulin: Proceedings of the Immune Globulin Workshop, Bethesda, MD., October 1982. 1985. (Vox Sanguinis: Vol. 49, Suppl. 1, 1985). (Illus.). iv, 52p. pap. 21.00 (*3-8055-4196-1*) S Karger.

***Immune Interferon: Properties & Clinical Applications.** R. G. TSanev & Ivan Ivanov. 2001. LC 2001-43329. (*0-8493-1148-9*) CRC Pr.

Immune Mechanisms in Atherogenesis. Madalene C. Heng. 2000. LC 97-43984. (Medical Intelligence Unit Ser.). 210p. 89.00 (*1-57059-523-2*) Landes Bioscience.

Immune Mechanisms in Atherogenesis. Ming K. Heng. 1997. (Medical Intelligence Unit Ser.). 250p. 89.95 (*0-412-13031-9*) Chapman & Hall.

***Immune Mechanisms in Atherogenesis.** Ming K. Heng & Madalene C. Y. Heng. 2002. LC 97-43984. (Medical Intelligence Unit Ser.: Vol. 28). (*1-58706-037-X*) Eurekah.

Immune Mechanisms in Cutaneous Disease. Ed. by David A. Norris. 1989. (Immunology Ser.: Vol. 46). (Illus.). 848p. text 260.00 (*0-8247-7919-3*) Dekker.

Immune Mechanisms in Cutaneous Disease. D. A. Norris. 2nd rev. ed. Date not set. (Illus.). text (*0-8247-9498-2*) Dekker.

Immune Mediated Heart Disease. Ed. by Noel R. Rose et al. 1992. LC 92-49773. (*0-387-55614-1*) Spr-Verlag.

Immune Modulating Agents. Ed. by Kresina. 1997. LC 97-31538. (Illus.). 576p. text 215.00 (*0-8247-0103-8*) Dekker.

Immune Modulation by Infectious Agents. Ed. by Wolfgang Zschiesche. 1989. 315p. 80.00 (*0-89573-287-4*, Wiley-VCH) Wiley.

Immune Power: A Comprehensive Healing Program for HIV. Jon D. Kaiser. 1995. LC 93-680. pap. 10.95 (*0-312-11831-7*) St Martin.

Immune Privilege: Sites, Tissues, Strategies & Diseases. J. Wayne Streilein. 1997. (Medical Intelligence Unit Ser.). 250p. 89.95 (*0-412-11581-6*) Chapman & Hall.

Immune Reaction in Liver Disease. Adrian Eddleston & Roger Williams. 1978. (Illus.). pap. 34.95 (*0-8464-0503-2*) Beekman Pubs.

Immune Reactions. Ed. by A. Studer & H. Cottier. 1970. (Handbuch der Allgemeinen Pathologie Ser.: Vol. 7/3). (Illus.). 304.00 (*0-387-05129-5*) Spr-Verlag.

Immune Reactions in Headlines, Overviews, Tables & Graphics. H. H. Sedlacek & T. Moroy. 1995. LC 96-105454. 581p. 116.00 (*3-540-58957-0*) Spr-Verlag.

Immune Regulation. Ed. by Marc Feldmann & N. Avrion Mitchison. 1985. LC 85-5786. (Experimental Biology & Medicine Ser.: Vol. 8). (Illus.). 406p. 135.00 (*0-89603-083-0*) Humana.

Immune Respiratory Parasitic Infections, Vol. IV. E. J. Soulsby. 1987. 352p. 277.00 (*0-8493-6174-5*) CRC Pr.

Immune Respiratory Parasitic Infections. E. J. Soulsby. 1987. LC 85-29918. Vol. 1. 352p. 194.00 (*0-8493-6171-0*, RC119); Vol. 2. 232p. 133.00 (*0-8493-6172-9*, RC119); Vol. 3. 360p. 201.00 (*0-8493-6173-7*, RC119) Franklin.

Immune Response & the Eye. Ed. by J. Wayne Streilein. 3rd ed. 1999. (Chemical Immunology Ser.: Vol. 73). (Illus.). xii, 226p. 197.50 (*3-8055-6893-2*) S Karger.

Immune Response in the Critically Ill. Ed. by J. Marshall et al. 1999. LC 99-40677. (Update in Intensive Care & Emergency Medicine Ser.: Vol. 31). (Illus.). 480p. 179.00 (*3-540-62583-6*) Spr-Verlag.

Immune Response to Structurally Defined Proteins: The Lysozyme Model. Ed. by S. Smith-Gill & Eli E. Sercarz. 1989. LC 89-6832. (Illus.). 425p. lib. bdg. 90.00 (*0-940030-27-6*) Adenine Pr.

Immune Response to Viral Infections. Ed. by B. A. Askonas et al. 1989. (AEMB Candidate Ser.). (Illus.). 316p. 85.00 (*0-306-43360-5*, Plenum Trade) Perseus Pubng.

Immune Responses in Parasitic Infections: Immunology, Immunopathology, & Immunoprophylaxis, Set. E. J. Soulsby. 1987. 900.00 (*0-8493-6170-2*, RC119) CRC Pr.

Immune Responses in the Nervous System. Ed. by Nancy J. Rothwell. 1998. (Molecular & Cellular Neurobiology Ser.). (Illus.). 250p. 78.50 (*1-872748-79-1*) OUP.

Immune Responses to Metastases. R. B. Herberman & Robert H. Wiltrout. 1987. LC 86-7878. Vol. 1. 82.00 (*0-8493-5847-7*, RC268); Vol. 2. 92.00 (*0-8493-5848-5*, RC268) Franklin (CRC Reprint).

Immune Responses to Metastases: Host Responses & Tumor Metastases, Set. Ed. by Ronald B. Herberman et al. 1987. LC 86-7878. 304p. 173.00 (*0-8493-5849-3*, RC268, CRC Reprint) Franklin.

Immune System. 1992. lib. bdg. 143.95 (*0-8490-5562-8*) Gordon Pr.

Immune System. Willard H. Dean. Ed. by Nancy Wood & Karen Embertson. 1997. (Holistic Health Ser.). (Illus.). 68p. pap. 9.95 (*0-9657169-0-2*) Pathways Pr NM.

Immune System. Peter Parkham. 2000. LC 99-42006. (Illus.). pap. 48.95 (*0-8153-3043-X*) Garland.

Immune System: A Nutritional Approach. Louise Tenney. 1988. (Woodland Health Ser.: No. 2). 32p. pap. 3.95 (*0-913923-29-X*) Woodland UT.

Immune System: Festschrift in Honor of Niels Kaj Jerne, on the Occasion of His 70th Birthday Ed. by C. M. Steinberg & Ivan Lefkovits. 1981. (Illus.). xv, 912p. 448.75 (*3-8055-3409-4*);Vol. 1. 440p. 215.75 (*3-8055-3407-8*);Vol. 2. 472p. 233.25 (*3-8055-3408-6*) S Karger.

Immune System: How It Works. Lydia W. Schindler. rev. ed. 1996. (Illus.). 25p. pap. text 15.00 (*0-7881-3006-4*) DIANE Pub.

Immune System: Why & How the Immune System Is Destroyed & How to Rebuild the Immune System with Herbs, Vitamins, Minerals & Good Food. 1991. lib. bdg. 79.95 (*0-8490-5106-1*) Gordon Pr.

Immune System Accessory Cells. Lubor Fornusek. 1992. 448p. lib. bdg. 229.00 (*0-8493-5982-1*, QR185) CRC Pr.

Immune System & Cancer Proceeding of the International Symposium of The Princess Takamatsu Cancer Research Fund, No. 19. 1989. (Princess Takamatsu Symposia Series on Cancer Research). 370p. 192.00 (*0-85066-853-0*) Taylor & Francis.

Immune System & Infectious Diseases: Proceedings of the International Convocation on Immunology, 4th, Buffalo, June, 1974. International Convocation on Immunology Staff. Ed. by Felix Milgrom & E. Neter. 1975. (Illus.). xii, 549p. 143.50 (*3-8055-2177-4*) S Karger.

Immune System Control: Colostrum & Lactoferrin. Beth M. Ley. 2000. LC 00-8192. (Illus.). 200p. pap. 12.95 (*1-890766-11-9*) B L Pubns.

Immune System Cure. Lorna R. Vanderhaeghe & Patrick J. Bouie. 2000. 272p. pap. 14.00 (*1-57566-486-0*, Knsington) Kensgtn Pub Corp.

Immune System Disorders Sourcebook: Basic Information about Lupus, Multiple Sclerosis, Guillain-Barre' Syndrome & More. Ed. by Allan R. Cook. 1997. LC 96-33469. (Health Reference Ser.: Vol. 18). xii, 608p. lib. bdg. 78.00 (*0-7808-0209-8*) Omnigraphics Inc.

Immune System Herbal Greetings to Duplicate & Use. Lamp Light Press Staff. 1993. (Illus.). 60p. stu. ed., ring bd. 29.95 (*0-917593-26-X*, Lamp Light Pr) Prosperity & Profits.

Immune System Herbals, Approaches, Folklore: A How to Find or Locate Workbook. Lamp Light Press Staff. 1993. (Illus.). 70p. ring bd. 25.95 (*0-917593-28-6*, Lamp Light Pr) Prosperity & Profits.

Immune System in Space & Other Extreme Conditions, Vol. 3. I. V. Konstantinova. 1991. (Soviet Medical Reviews Supplement Ser.). xi, 258p. text 303.00 (*3-7186-5127-0*, Harwood Acad Pubs) Gordon & Breach.

Immune System Makeover. Janet C. Maccaro. 2000. LC 00-102254. xix, 263p. pap. 12.99 (*0-88419-692-5*) Creation House.

Immune Tolerance & the Treatment of Hemophiliacs with an Inhibitor: Proceedings. Ed. by G. Mariani & H. H. Brackmann. 1996. (Vox Sanguinis: Vol. 70, Suppl. 1, 1996). (Illus.). iv, 80p. pap., suppl. ed. 36.50 (*3-8055-6297-7*) S Karger.

Immune Trio: Dangers of Immunization, How to Legally Avoid Immunization, & Vaccinations & Immune Malfunction. Harold E. Buttram. 1996. 192p. pap. 10.00 (*0-916285-38-3*) Humanitarian.

Immunglobulintherapie. Ed. by R. E. Schmidt & I. Strochmann. 1983. (Beitraege zur Infusionstherapie und Klinische Ernaehrung Ser.: Vol. 11). viii, 96p. pap. 21.75 (*3-8055-3660-7*) S Karger.

Immuniobiology Bookshelf: The Comparative Resource. 1996. 66.00 (*0-8153-2860-5*) Garland.

Immunity & Concomitant Immunity in Infectious Diseases. Ed. by P. Kallos. 1982. (Progress in Allergy Ser.: Vol. 31). (Illus.). xvi, 364p. 172.25 (*3-8055-3464-7*) S Karger.

Immunity & Survival: Keys to Immune System Health - Vital Facts on AIDS, Cancer, & Infection. Sylvia Greenberg. 1989. 152p. 29.95 (*0-89885-435-0*, Kluwer Acad Hman Sci) Kluwer Academic.

Immunity in Invertebrates. Ed. by M. Brehelin. 1986. (Proceedings in Life Sciences Ser.). (Illus.). 233p. 113.00 (*0-387-15871-5*) Spr-Verlag.

Immunity of the Foetus & Newborn Infant. I. Miler. 1983. text 135.00 (*90-247-2610-7*) Kluwer Academic.

Immunity Pleasure Connection. Carl Charnetski. 2001. LC 2001-2096. (Illus.). 240p. 21.95 (*1-57954-346-4*) Rodale Pr Inc.

Immunity to Mycobacteria. Ian M. Orme. 1995. LC 95-19371. (Medical Intelligence Unit Ser.). 165p. 89.00 (*1-57059-265-9*) Landes Bioscience.

Immunity to Parasites: How Parasitic Infections Are Controlled. Derek Wakelin. 2nd ed. 1996. (Illus.). 222p. (C). text 74.95 (*0-521-56245-7*); pap. text 21.95 (*0-521-43635-4*) Cambridge U Pr.

Immunization: Benefit Versus Risk Factors. Ed. by W. Hennessen & C. Huygelen. 1979. (Developments in Biological Standardization Ser.: Vol. 43). (Illus.). pap. 61.00 (*3-8055-2816-7*) S Karger.

Immunization: Childhood & Travel Health. George C. Kassianos. 3rd ed. 1998. (Illus.). 388p. pap. 44.95 (*0-632-05074-8*) Blackwell Sci.

Immunization: Everything You Need to Know about Vaccinations & Immune-Boosting Therapies for Your Child. Harriet Griffey. 2000. 160p. pap. 10.95 (*1-86204-541-0*) Element MA.

Immunization: The Reality Behind the Myth. Walene James. 2nd rev. ed. 1995. LC 94-36206. 312p. (Orig.). 75.00 (*0-89789-359-X*, Bergin & Garvey) Greenwood.

Immunization: The Reality Being the Myth. Walene James. 2nd rev. ed. 1995. LC 94-36206. 312p. pap. 26.95 (*0-89789-360-3*, Bergin & Garvey) Greenwood.

Immunization Decision see Vaccine Guide: Making an Informed Choice

Immunization Dice. Michael Brody. 1987. (Twentieth Century Fund Papers). 77p. (Orig.). (C). pap. text 10.00 (*0-87078-211-8*) Century Foundation.

Immunization of Adult Birds with Inactive Oil Adjuvant Vaccines. Ed. by W. Hennessen. 1982. (Developments in Biological Standardization Ser.: Vol. 51). (Illus.). 400p. pap. 61.00 (*3-8055-3473-6*) S Karger.

Immunization Resource Guide: Where to Find Answers to All Your Questions about Childhood Vaccinations. Diane Rozario. 4th ed. 2001. LC 00-91401. ii, 245p. pap. 13.95 (*0-9643366-5-0*) Patter Pubns.

Immunizing Children: A Practical Guide. Richard T. Mayon-White et al. 1997. LC 96-53160. (*1-85775-154-X*) Radcliffe Med Pr GBR. *Dist:* Balogh.

Immunizing Children: A Practical Guide. Judith Moreton et al. 2nd ed. 1998. LC 98-219624. 104p. pap. (*1-85775-219-8*) Radcliffe Med Pr GBR. *Dist:* Balogh.

Immunizing Health Care Workers: A Practical Approach. Gregory A. Poland et al. 2000. LC 99-48212. (Illus.). 544p. 109.00 (*1-55642-450-7*) SLACK Inc.

Immuno-Gold Electron Microscopy in Virus Diagnosis & Research. Alex D. Hyatt. 1992. 464p. lib. bdg. 239.00 (*0-8493-6759-X*, QR87) CRC Pr.

Immuno-Ophthalmology. Ed. by Uwe Pleyer et al. 3rd ed. 1999. (Developments in Ophthalmology Ser.: Vol. 30). (Illus.). vii, 200p. 174.00 (*3-8055-6863-0*) S Karger.

Immunoassay: A Practical Guide. Brian Law. 1996. LC 97-105539. 222p. 95.00 (*0-7484-0560-7*) Taylor & Francis.

Immunoassay: Laboratory Analysis & Clinical Application. James P. Gosling & Lawrence V. Basso. 1994. LC 94-7400. (Illus.). 360p. text (*0-7506-9256-1*) E A GBR. *Dist:* OUP.

Immunoassay Automation: A Practical Guide. Ed. by Daniel W. Chan. 1992. (Illus.). 367p. pap. 58.00 (*0-12-167632-3*) Acad Pr.

Immunoassay Automation: An Updated Guide to Systems. Ed. by Daniel W. Chan. 1995. LC 95-30894. (Illus.). 312p. (C). 34.95 (*0-12-167640-4*) Acad Pr.

Immunoassay Handbook. Ed. by David Wild. 2nd ed. 2000. 906p. lib. bdg. 185.00 (*1-56159-270-6*) Nature Pubg Grp.

Immunoassay Methods & Protocols. Ed. by Andrey L. Ghindilis et al. 2001. (Methods in Molecular Biology Ser.). 425p. 89.50 (*0-89603-748-7*) Humana.

Immunoassays. Jim Gosling. 2000. LC 00-21358. (Practical Approach Ser.: No. 228). (Illus.). xix, 304p. pap. text 55.00 (*0-19-963710-5*) OUP.

Immunoassays: A Practical Approach. Jim Gosling. 2000. LC 00-21358. (Practical Approach Ser.: No. 228). (Illus.). xix, 304p. text 110.00 (*0-19-963711-3*) OUP.

Immunoassays: Essential Data. Ed. by Ray Edwards. 1996. LC 95-49525. (Essential Data Ser.). 158p. pap. 39.95 (*0-471-95275-3*) Wiley.

Immunoassays for Veterinary & Food Analysis - 1: Based on the Proceedings of the 2nd International Symposium held at the University of Surrey, Guilford, UK 15-17 July 1986. Ed. by B. A. Morris et al. 1988. 384p. 106.25 (*1-85166-138-7*) Elsevier.

Immunoassays in Coagulation Testing. Z. Parvez. 1984. (Illus.). xvi, 173p. 74.00 (*0-387-90932-X*) Spr-Verlag.

***Immunobiology: The Immune System in Health & Disease.** C. A. Janeway et al. 2001. (Illus.). 595p. pap. (*0-443-07098-9*) Church GBR. *Dist:* Saunders.

Immunobiology: The Immune System in Health & Disease. Charles A. Janeway, Jr. & Paul Travers. (Illus.). 1994. LC 94-11058. 590p. text 66.00 (*0-8153-1497-3*); 2nd ed. 1996. LC 95-4956. 450p. pap. text 44.00 (*0-8153-2044-2*) Garland.

Immunobiology: The Immune System in Health & Disease. Charles Janeway & Paul Travers. 3rd ed. 1997. (Immunobiology Ser.). (Illus.). 540p. pap. text 46.95 (*0-8153-2818-4*) Garland.

Immunobiology: The Immune System in Health & Disease. Charles Janeway. 4th ed. 1999. LC 98-30316. 635 p. (*0-443-06274-9*) Church.

Immunobiology & Clinical Implications of the Complement Anaphylatoxins: Journal: Complement, Vol. 3, No. 9, 1986. Ed. by Tony E. Hugli. 1986. (Illus.). 84p. pap. 72.25 (*3-8055-4486-3*) S Karger.

Immunobiology & Immunopharmacology of Bacterial Endotoxins. Ed. by Andor Szentivanyi & Herman Friedman. 1986. LC 86-25372. (University of South Florida International Biomedical Symposia Ser.). 528p. 110.00 (*0-306-42476-2*, Plenum Trade) Perseus Pubng.

Immunobiology & Pathogenesis of Persistent Virus Infections. Ed. by Carlos Lopez. 1988. (Illus.). 318p. text 59.00 (*1-55581-000-4*) ASM Pr.

Immunobiology & Prophylaxis of Human Herpesvirus Infections. Ed. by Carlos Lopez et al. 1990. (Advances in Experimental Medicine & Biology Ser.: Vol. 278). (Illus.). 306p. (C). text 114.00 (*0-306-43696-5*, Kluwer Plenum) Kluwer Academic.

Immunobiology & Transplantation, Cancer & Pregnancy. Ed. by Prasanta K. Ray. 1983. 500p. 200.00 (*0-08-025994-4*, Pergamon Pr) Elsevier.

Immunobiology, Histophysiology, Tumor Immunology in Otorhinolaryngology. Ed. by Jan E. Veldman. 1987. LC 87-7176. (Illus.). 513p. lib. bdg. (*90-6299-029-0*) Kugler NLD. *Dist:* Lib Res.

Immunobiology in Otology, Rhinology & Laryngology. Ed. by Brian F. McCabe et al. 1992. LC 92-10311. (Illus.). 407p. lib. bdg. (*90-6299-083-5*) Kugler NLD. *Dist:* Lib Res.

Immunobiology in Otorhinolaryngology: Progress of a Decade. Ed. by Goro Mogi et al. 1994. LC 94-23510. (Illus.). xliv, 674p. text (*90-6299-114-9*) Kugler NLD. *Dist:* Lib Res.

Immunobiology of Bacterial CpG-DNA. Ed. by H. Wagner. 2000. (Current Topics in Microbiology & Immunology Ser.: Vol. 247). (Illus.). 272p. 159.95 (*3-540-66400-9*) Spr-Verlag.

Immunobiology of Herpes Simplex Virus Infection. Ed. by Barry T. Rouse & Carlos Lopez. 1984. 176p. 105.00 (*0-8493-6037-4*, RC147, CRC Reprint) Franklin.

Immunobiology of HLA, Vols. 1 & 2. Ed. by B. Dupont. 1989. (Illus.). 1701p. 632.00 (*0-387-96826-1*) Spr-Verlag.

Immunobiology of HLA-Class-II Molecules. Ed. by J. J. Van Rood & R. R. De Vries. 1984. (Progress in Allergy Ser.: Vol. 36). (Illus.). vi, 226p. 106.25 (*3-8055-3893-6*) S Karger.

Immunobiology of Human Immunodeficiency Virus (HIV) Infection. J. Antonen. 1987. 99p. (Orig.). pap. 36.00 (*951-44-2126-4*) Coronet Bks.

Immunobiology of Infection With Herpes Simplex Virus. H. Kirchner. 1982. (Monographs in Virology: Vol. 13). viii, 104p. 56.75 (*3-8055-3517-1*) S Karger.

Immunobiology of Natural Killer Cells, Vol. II. Ed. by Eva Lotzova & Ronald B. Herberman. 1986. 272p. 138.00 (*0-8493-6543-0*, QR185, CRC Reprint) Franklin.

Immunobiology of Proteins & Peptides: Human Immunodeficiency Virus, Antibody Immunoconjugates, Bacterial Vaccines, Immunomodulators, Vol. 6. Ed. by M. Z. Atassi. 1991. (Advances in Experimental Medicine & Biology Ser.: Vol. 303). (Illus.). 312p. (C). text 114.00 (*0-306-44038-5*, Kluwer Plenum) Kluwer Academic.

Immunobiology of Proteins & Peptides 7: Unwanted Immune Responses, Vol. 7. Ed. by M. Z. Atassi. 1994. (Advances in Experimental Medicine & Biology Ser.: Vol. 347). (Illus.). 244p. (C). text 95.00 (*0-306-44665-0*, Kluwer Plenum) Kluwer Academic.

Immunobiology of Proteins & Peptides IV: T-Cell Recognition & Antigen Presentation. Ed. by M. Z. Atassi. 1987. LC 87-29231. (Advances in Experimental Medicine & Biology Ser.: Vol. 225). (Illus.). 346p. 85.00 (*0-306-42769-9*, Plenum Trade) Perseus Pubng.

Immunobiology of Proteins & Peptides, V: Vaccines. Ed. by M. Z. Atassi. 1989. (Advances in Experimental Medicine & Biology Ser.: Vol. 251). (Illus.). 368p. 95.00 (*0-306-43239-0*, Plenum Trade) Perseus Pubng.

Immunobiology of Reproduction. Ed. by Joan S. Hunt. 1994. LC 94-8895. (Illus.). 351p. 162.00 (*0-387-94292-0*) Spr-Verlag.

Immunobiology of the Aging Brain: Alzheimer's Disease. Ed. by Marguerite M. Kay. 1996. (Journal: Vol. 43, Nos. 1-2, 1997). (Illus.). 150p. pap. 81.75 (*3-8055-6447-3*) S Karger.

Immunobiology of the Major Histocompatibility Complex. Ed. by M. B. Zaleski et al. 1981. (Illus.). xii, 396p. 172.25 (*3-8055-1896-X*) S Karger.

Immunobiology of Transfusion Medicine. Garratty. 1993. (Illus.). 728p. text 275.00 (*0-8247-9122-3*) Dekker.

Immunobiology 3 Bookshelf: The Comparative Resource. Charles Janeway et al. 1997. 66.00 (*0-8153-3019-7*) Garland.

Immunochemical Methods for Environmental Analysis. Ed. by Jeanette M. Von Emon & Ralph O. Mumma. 1990. LC 90-48309. (ACS Symposium Ser.: No. 442). (Illus.). 250p. 75.00 (*0-8412-1875-7*) Am Chemical.

Immunochemical Methods in Cell & Molecular Biology. Ed. by R. John Mayer & J. H. Walker. 1988. (Biological Techniques Ser.). 325p. text 83.00 (*0-12-480855-7*) Acad Pr.

Immunochemical Protocols. Ed. by John Pound. 2nd ed. 1998. LC 97-39695. (Methods in Molecular Biology Ser.: Vol. 80). (Illus.). 528p. 129.50 (*0-89603-493-3*); spiral bd. 99.50 (*0-89603-388-0*) Humana.

Immunochemical Techniques. Ed. by Sidney P. Colowick et al. (Methods in Enzymology Ser.: Vol. 70). Pt. A. 1980. text 188.00 (*0-12-181970-1*); Pt. B. 1981. text 188.00 (*0-12-181973-6*) Acad Pr.

Immunochemical Techniques, Vol. 74, Pt. C. Ed. by John J. Langone & Helen Van Vunakis. 1981. (Methods in Enzymology Ser.). text 179.00 (*0-12-181974-4*) Acad Pr.

Immunochemical Techniques Pt. D: Selected Immunoassays. Ed. by Sidney P. Colowick & John J. Langone. 1982. LC 82-1678. (Methods in Enzymology Ser.: Vol. 84). 736p. text 188.00 (*0-12-181984-1*) Acad Pr.

Immunochemical Techniques Pt. E: Monoclonal Antibodies & General Immunoassay Methods. Ed. by Sidney P. Colowick & Nathan O. Kaplan. 1983. (Methods in Enzymology Ser.: Vol. 92). text 188.00 (*0-12-181992-2*) Acad Pr.

Immunochemical Techniques Pt. F: Conventional Antibodies, Fc Receptors, & Cytotoxicity. Ed. by Sidney P. Colowick & Nathan O. Kaplan. 1983. (Methods in Enzymology Ser.: Vol. 93). 393p. text 188.00 (*0-12-181993-0*) Acad Pr.

Immunochemical Techniques Vol. 108, Pt. G: Separation & Characterization of Lymphoid Cells. Ed. by Giovanni Di Sabato et al. 1984. (Methods in Enzymology Ser.). text 179.00 (*0-12-182008-4*) Acad Pr.

Immunochemical Techniques Vol. 121, Pt. I: Hybridoma Technology & Monoclonal Antibodies. Ed. by Sidney P. Colowick & Nathan O. Kaplan. 1986. (Methods in Enzymology Ser.). text 179.00 (*0-12-182021-1*) Acad Pr.

Immunochemical Techniques Laboratory Manual. John Goers. 1992. LC 92-17632. (Illus.). 188p. (C). spiral bd., lab manual ed. 19.95 (*0-12-287048-4*) Acad Pr.

Immunochemistry & Biochemistry of Connective Tissue & Its Disease States. Ed. by C. D. Angevine et al. 1970. (Rheumatology Ser.: Vol. 3). 70.50 (*3-8055-0622-8*) S Karger.

Immunochemistry in Practice. Alan P. Johnstone et al. 3rd ed. 1996. LC 95-39026. 362p. pap. 78.95 (*0-86542-633-3*) Blackwell Sci.

Immunochemistry Labfax. Ed. by M. A. Kerr & R. Thorpe. 1994. (Labfax Ser.). (Illus.). 256p. (C). text 39.95 (*0-12-404940-0*) Acad Pr.

Immunochemistry of AIDS. Ed. by Erling Norrby. 1993. (Chemical Immunology Ser.: Vol. 56). (Illus.). x, 168p. 161.75 (*3-8055-5655-1*) S Karger.

Immunochemistry of Man. George Kwapinski. 1991. LC 88-13755. 514p. (C). lib. bdg. 74.50 (*0-89464-304-5*) Krieger.

Immunochemistry of Proteins Ed. by M. Z. Atassi. 1977. LC 76-2596. (Illus.). 79.50 (*0-306-36222-8*); 79.50 (*0-306-36221-X*) Perseus Pubng (Plenum Trade).

Immunochemistry of the Cell Membrane, Ravello, 1975. Immunochemistry of the Cell Membrane, Ravello, 197. Ed. by P. M. Comoglio et al. 1977. (Experimental Cell Biology Ser.: Vol. 44, Nos. 3-6). 65.25 (*3-8055-2754-3*) S Karger.

Immunochemistry of the Extracellular Matrix Ed. by Heinz Furthmayr. 1982. Vol. I. 288p. 156.00 (*0-8493-6196-6*, QP552); Vol. II. 208p. 121.00 (*0-8493-6197-4*) Franklin (CRC Reprint).

Immunochemotherapy: A Guide to Intravenous Immunoglobulin Therapy. Ed. by U. E. Nydegger. 1982. LC 81-68971. text 136.00 (*0-12-523280-2*) Acad Pr.

Immunoconjugate Therapy of Hematologic Malignancies. Ed. by Steven T. Rosen & Timothy M. Kuzel. 1993. LC 93-15382. (Cancer Treatment & Research Ser.: Vol. 68). 224p. (C). text 191.00 (*0-7923-2270-3*) Kluwer Academic.

Immunocytochemical Methods & Protocols. Lorette C. Javois. 2nd ed. 1999. (Methods in Molecular Biology Ser.: Vol. 115). 465p. LC 98-46930. 125.00 (*0-89603-813-0*); (Illus.). 89.50 (*0-89603-570-0*) Humana.

Immunocytochemical Techniques: Principles & Practice. Ed. by Barbara Beltz & D. Burd. 1989. (Illus.). 208p. (C). pap., stu. ed. 49.95 (*0-86542-065-3*) Blackwell Sci.

Immunocytochemistry for Steroid Receptors. Louis P. Pertschuk. 1990. 240p. lib. bdg. 179.00 (*0-8493-6943-6*, RC280) CRC Pr.

Immunocytochemistry in Tumor Diagnosis. Ed. by Jose Russo. 1985. (Developments in Oncology Ser.). text 152.50 (*0-89838-737-X*) Kluwer Academic.

Immunodeficiencies. Ed. by Fred S. Rosen & Maxime Seligmann. 1993. LC 92-48452. 765p. text 334.00 (*3-7186-5343-5*); pap. text 131.00 (*3-7186-5344-3*) Gordon & Breach.

Immunodeficiency: Report of a WHO Scientific Group, 1978. 1978. (Technical Report Ser.: No. 630). 80p. pap. text 7.00 (*92-4-120630-6*, 1100630) World Health.

Immunodeficiency & Disease. A. D. Webster. 1988. (Immunology & Medicine Ser.). (C). text 112.00 (*0-85200-688-8*) Kluwer Academic.

Immunodeficiency & Skin. Ed. by P. Fritsch et al. 1989. (Current Problems in Dermatology Ser.: Vol. 18). (Illus.). 308p. 221.00 (*3-8055-4888-5*) S Karger.

Immunodeficiency in HIV Infection & AIDS. Ed. by G. Janossy et al. 1992. (Illus.). xiv, 300p. 241.75 (*3-8055-5547-4*) S Karger.

Immunodeficient Animals: Models for Cancer Research. Ed. by W. Arnold et al. 1996. LC 96-4622. (Beitraege Zur Onkologie, Contributions to Oncology Ser.: Vol. 51, 1996). (Illus.). xiv, 230p. 160.00 (*3-8055-6270-5*) S Karger.

Immunodermatology. Ed. by Bijan Safai & Robert A. Good. 1981. LC 80-15102. (Comprehensive Immunology Ser.: Vol. 7). (Illus.). 760p. 120.00 (*0-306-40380-3*, Plenum Trade) Perseus Pubng.

Immunodiagnosis of Cancer. Ronald B. Herberman & Donald W. Mercer. 2nd exp. rev. ed. 1990. (Immunology Ser.: Vol. 53). (Illus.). 760p. text 245.00 (*0-8247-8299-2*) Dekker.

Immunodiagnostic Markets: Long-Term R & D Pays Off. Market Intelligence Staff. 1992. 213p. 1995.00 (*1-56753-408-2*) Frost & Sullivan.

Immunodiagnostics. 1991. 97p. 25.00 (*92-1-106252-7*, 91.III.E.2) UN.

Immunodiagnostics. Ed. by Raymond Edwards. 2000. LC 99-20407. (Practical Approach Ser.: No. 206). 304p. pap. text 55.00 (*0-19-963588-9*) OUP.

Immunoelectrophoresis Theory, Methods, Identification, Interpretation. P. C. Arquembourg. 2nd rev. ed. 1975. (Illus.). ix, 104p. 53.25 (*3-8055-2136-7*) S Karger.

ImmunoFacts: Vaccines & Immunologic Drugs. Facts and Comparisons Staff. Ed. by John D. Grabenstein. 2001. 1000p. ring bd. 145.00 (*0-932686-03-6*) Facts & Comparisons.

Immunogenetic Aspects of ANCA-Associated Vasculitides. Ed. by Wolfgang L. Gross & Elene Csernok. 1998. (Experiments & Clinical Immunogenetics Ser.: Vol. 14, No. 3). (Illus.). 62p. pap. 33.25 (*3-8055-6643-3*) S Karger.

Immunogenetic Risk Assessment in Human Disease Vol. 12, No. 3: Experimental & Clinical Immunogenetics, 1995. Ed. by J. P. Panday. 1995. (Journal: Vol. 12, No. 3, 1995). (Illus.). 108p. pap. 50.50 (*3-8055-6215-2*) S Karger.

Immunogenetics: Advances & Education the First Congress of the Slovak Foundation, No. 35. Madrigal. 1997. LC 97-17214. 292p. text 174.00 (*0-7923-4613-0*) Kluwer Academic.

Immunogenetics of Autoimmune Disease. Nadir R. Farid. 1990. (Illus.). Vol. 1. 224p. 211.00 (*0-8493-6897-9*, RC200); Vol. 2. 336p. 211.00 (*0-8493-6898-7*) CRC Pr.

Immunogenetics of Insulin-Dependent Diabetes. Ed. by A. H. Barnett. 1987. text 102.00 (*0-85200-840-6*) Kluwer Academic.

Immunogenetics of the H-2 System: Proceedings of the Symposium, Liblice Prague, 1970. Symposium, Liblice Prague Staff. Ed. by Alena Lengerova & Marta Vojtiskova. 1971. 95.75 (*3-8055-1236-8*) S Karger.

Immunogenetics of the Major Histocompatibility Complex. Ed. by Rakesh Srivastava et al. 1991. 419p. 190.00 (*0-89573-780-9*, Wiley-VCH) Wiley.

Immunogenicity of Protein Antigens Repertoire & Regulation. J. A. Berzofsky & Eli E. Sercarz. 1987. Vol. 1. LC 87-5129. 100.00 (*0-8493-4340-2*, QR186); Vol. 2. LC 87-21856. 92.00 (*0-8493-4341-0*, QR186) Franklin (CRC Reprint).

Immunogenicity of Protein Antigens Repertoire & Regulation: Repertoire & Regulation, Set. Ed. by Jay A. Berzofsky & Eli E. Sercarz. 1988. (Immunologists & Biochemists Ser.). 192.00 (*0-8493-4339-9*, QR186, CRC Reprint) Franklin.

Immunoglobulin & T-Cell Receptor Gene Rearrangement Assays: Approved Guideline (1995) Contrib. by Timothy J. O'Leary. 1995. 75.00 (*1-56238-289-6*, MM2-A) NCCLS.

***Immunoglobulin Factsbook.** Marie-Paule Lefranc & Gerard Lefranc. 2001. (Factsbook Ser.). 457p. pap. 65.00 (*0-12-441351-X*) Acad Pr.

Immunoglobulin Receptors & Their Physiological & Pathological Roles in Immunity. P. Mark Hogarth. Ed. by Jan G. Van de Winkel. 1998. 352p. 146.00 (*0-7923-5021-9*) Kluwer Academic.

Immunoglobulin Subclass Deficiencies. Ed. by L. A. Hanson et al. 1986. (Monographs in Allergy: Vol. 20). (Illus.). x, 250p. 191.50 (*3-8055-4286-0*) S Karger.

Immunoglobulins: Extending the Horizon. Ed. by M. D. Kazatchkine & A. Louwagie. 1994. 76p. lib. bdg. 38.95 (*1-85070-647-6*, Parthenon Pbng) CRC Pr.

Immunoglobulins: Structure & Function. Roald S. Nezlin. 1998. LC 98-4750. (Illus.). 269p. 69.95 (*0-12-517970-7*) Acad Pr.

Immunoglobulins in Health & Disease. Ed. by M. A. French. 1986. (Immunology & Medicine Ser.). text 119.00 (*0-85200-962-3*) Kluwer Academic.

Immunohematology: Principles & Practice. Eva D. Quinley. 2nd ed. 1998. LC 97-42728. 496p. text 49.95 (*0-397-55469-9*) Lppncott W & W.

Immunohematology & Blood Banking. Jack Rudman. 1994. (College Level Examination Ser.: CLEP-34). pap. 27.95 (*0-8373-5334-3*) Nat Learn.

Immunohistology & Electron Microscopy of Anaplastic & Pleomorphic Tumors. Anthony S. Leong et al. 1997. LC 96-47099. (Illus.). 303p. (C). text 140.00 (*0-521-44092-0*) Cambridge U Pr.

Immunohistology in Diagnostic Pathology. J. Charles Jennette. 1988. 320p. 228.95 (*0-8493-4987-7*, RB46) CRC Pr.

Immunohistopathology: A Practical Approach to Diagnosis. Jules M. Elias. 1990. LC 90-682. 544p. 65.00 (*0-89189-300-8*) Am Soc Clinical.

Immunohomeostatic Disorders: An Inquiry into the Origins of Human Lymphomas. Sergio DeCarvalho. 1982. LC 81-82445. 81p. 11.90 (*0-930376-36-6*) Chem-Orbital.

Immunointervention in Man: A Critique of Clinical Trial Methodology. K. H. Wallace & Ronald A. Thompson. 1991. (Illus.). 238p. 49.95 (*0-19-261918-7*) OUP.

Immunologic Approaches to the Classification & Management of Lymphomas & Leukemias. Ed. by John M. Bennett & Kenneth A. Foon. 1988. (Cancer Treatment & Research Ser.). (C). text 179.50 (*0-89838-355-2*) Kluwer Academic.

Immunologic Aspects of Infectious Diseases. Robert Lehrer et al. Ed. by Roy Steigbigel. (C). pap. text (*1-878294-06-7*) Health Dimensions.

Immunologic Considerations in Toxicology Ed. by R. P. Sharma. 1981. 184p. Vol. I. 109.00 (*0-8493-5271-1*, QR188); Vol. II. 110.00 (*0-8493-5272-X*, QR188) Franklin (CRC Reprint).

Immunologic Defects in Laboratory Animals Ed. by M. Eric Gershwin & B. Merchant. 1981. LC 80-28192. Vol. 1. 380p. 85.00 (*0-306-40668-3*); Vol. 2. 402p. 85.00 (*0-306-40673-X*) Perseus Pubng (Plenum Trade).

Immunologic Diseases of the Ear. Ed. by Joel M. Bernstein et al. 1997. LC 97-42727. (Annals of the New York Academy of Sciences Ser.: Vol. 830). 376p. 120.00 (*1-57331-100-6*) NY Acad Sci.

Immunologic Diseases of the Ear. New York Academy of Sciences Staff. Ed. by Joel M. Bernstein et al. 1997. LC 97-42727. (Annals of the New York Academy of Sciences Ser.: Vol. 830). 376p. pap. 120.00 (*1-57331-101-4*) NY Acad Sci.

Immunologic Disorders. Christine Mudge-Grout et al. 1992. (Illus.). 368p. (C). (gr. 13). text 36.00 (*0-8016-2775-3*, 02775) Mosby Inc.

Immunologic Disorders in Infants & Children. E.Richard Stiehm. 4th ed. 1995. LC 95-8333. (Illus.). 832p. text 280.00 (*0-7216-4948-3*) Saunders.

***Immunologic Disorders in Infants & Children.** E. Richard Stiehm et al. 5th ed. 2001. (*0-7216-8964-7*) Saunders.

Immunologic Perspectives in Chronic Renal Failure. Ed. by H. J. Gurland et al. 1990. (Contributions to Nephrology Ser.: Vol. 86). (Illus.). viii, 198p. 29.75 (*3-8055-5254-8*) S Karger.

Immunologic Revolution: Facts & Witnesses. Ed. by Andor Szentivanyi & Herman Friedman. 1993. LC 93-32559. 432p. 252.95 (*0-8493-4722-X*, QR181) CRC Pr.

Immunological Adjuvants & Vaccines. Ed. by Gregory Gregoriadis et al. 1989. LC 89-25561. (NATO ASI Series A, Life Sciences: Vol. 179). (Illus.). 252p. (C). text 114.00 (*0-306-43386-9*) Plenum.

Immunological Alterations in Psychiatric Diseases: International Symposium, Reisensburg, September 1995. Ed. by A. E. Henneberg & Wolfgang P. Kaschka. 1997. LC 96-49578. (Advances in Biological Psychiatry Ser.: Vol. 18, 1996). (Illus.). x, 118p. 98.25 (*3-8055-6384-1*) S Karger.

Immunological & Allergological Items in Pediatric Otorhinolaryngology. Ed. by P. Van Cauwenberge. 1991. LC 91-20813. (Illus.). 62p. pap. text (*90-6299-069-X*) Kugler NLD. *Dist:* Lib Res.

Immunological & Infectious Diseases of the Peripheral Nerves. Ed. by N. Latov et al. 1998. (Illus.). 455p. (C). text 145.00 (*0-521-46265-7*) Cambridge U Pr.

Immunological & Inflammatory Disorders of the Central Nervous System. Neil Scolding. 1999. LC 99-230206. 272p. text 85.00 (*0-7506-2357-8*) Buttrwrth-Heinemann.

Immunological & Molecular Aspects of Bacterial Virulence. S. Patrick & M. J. Larkin. 1995. LC 94-24433. 292p. pap. 79.95 (*0-471-95251-6*) Wiley.

Immunological & Molecular Diagnosis of Infectious Disease. Carel J. Van Oss & D. Amsterdam. Date not set. (*0-8247-9868-6*) Dekker.

Immunological & Molecular Diagnosis of Infectious Disease. Carel J. Van Oss et al. Ed. by Daniel Amsterdam & Roger K. Cunningham. 1997. LC 97-5015. (Illus.). 328p. text 150.00 (*0-8247-0092-9*) Dekker.

Immunological & Pharmacological Aspects of Atopic & Contact Eczema. Ed. by J. M. Czernielewski. 1992. (Pharmacology & the Skin Ser.: Vol. 4). (Illus.). x, 254p. 215.75 (*3-8055-5433-8*) S Karger.

Immunological Approaches to Contraception & Promotion of Fertility. Ed. by Gursaran P. Talwar. 1986. LC 86-8199. (Reproductive Biology Ser.). 452p. 95.00 (*0-306-42274-3*, Plenum Trade) Perseus Pubng.

Immunological Approaches to the Diagnosis & Therapy of Breast Cancer. Ed. by Roberto L. Ceriani. 1987. LC 87-15373. (Illus.). 282p. 69.50 (*0-306-42601-3*, Plenum Trade) Perseus Pubng.

Immunological Aspects of Aging: Frontiers. Ed. by Marguerite M. Kay. 1985. (Journal: Vol. 31, No. 4, 1985). (Illus.). 88p. pap. 41.75 (*3-8055-4074-4*) S Karger.

Immunological Aspects of Contact Sensitivity. L. S. Polak. 1979. (Monographs in Allergy: Vol. 15). (Illus.). pap. 84.50 (*3-8055-3050-1*) S Karger.

Immunological Aspects of Cystic Fibrosis. Ed. by Emmanuel Gottlieb & Gregory B. Wilson. 1984. 240p. 140.00 (*0-8493-6373-X*, RC858, CRC Reprint) Franklin.

Immunological Aspects of Human Reproduction. 1966. (Technical Report Ser.: No. 334). 21p. pap. text 3.00 (*92-4-120334-X*) World Health.

Immunological Aspects of Mammalian Reproduction. Peter J. Hogarth. 1985. LC 81-86329. 204p. 67.95 (*0-275-91367-8*, C1367, Praeger Pubs) Greenwood.

HI

Immunological Aspects of Neoplasia. Ed. by R. S. Schwartz. 1970. (Progress in Experimental Tumor Research Ser.: Vol. 13). 71.50 (*3-8055-0396-2*) S Karger.

Immunological Aspects of Neurological Diseases. J. A. Aarli & O. Toender. 1980. (Monographs in Neural Sciences: Vol. 6). (Illus.). xiv, 190p. pap. 42.75 (*3-8055-0814-X*) S Karger.

Immunological Aspects of Oral Diseases. Ed. by L. Ivanyi. 1986. (Immunology & Medicine Ser.). text 155.50 (*0-85200-961-5*) Kluwer Academic.

Immunological Aspects of Renal Disease. David B. Oliveira. 1992. (Reviews in Clinical Immunology Ser.: No. 2). 239p. (C). text 69.95 (*0-521-40174-7*) Cambridge U Pr.

Immunological Aspects of Rheumatoid Arthritis: Proceedings of the International Symposium, Montpellier, March, 1974. Ed. by J. Clot. 1975. (Rheumatology Ser.: Vol. 6). 250p. 121.75 (*3-8055-2116-2*) S Karger.

Immunological Aspects of the Vascular Endothelium. Ed. by Caroline O. Savage & Jeremy D. Pearson. 1995. (Reviews in Clinical Immunology Ser.). (Illus.). 273p. (C). text 74.95 (*0-521-45249-X*) Cambridge U Pr.

Immunological Diseases see Samter's Immunologic Diseases

Immunological Disorders in Mice. Blanka Rihova & Vaclav Vetvicka. 1990. 280p. lib. bdg. 195.00 (*0-8493-5635-0*, QR188) CRC Pr.

Immunological Effects of Blood Transfusion. Ed. by Dharam P. Singal. 1994. LC 94-16337. 204p. 139.00 (*0-8493-4790-4*) CRC Pr.

Immunological Mechanisms in Asthma & Allergic Diseases: Symposium Held on the Occasion of Prof. A. Barry Kay's 60th Birthday & 20th Year As Head of Department, London, June 1999. Ed. by D. Robinson. 2000. (Chemical Immunology Ser.: Vol. 78). (Illus.). xii, 214p. 222.75 (*3-8055-7112-7*) S Karger.

Immunological Methods in Brucellosis Research: Procedures, Pt. 2. A. Olitzki. 1970. (Bibliotheca Microbiologica Ser.: Vol 9). pap. 92.25 (*3-8055-0149-8*) S Karger.

Immunological Reagents & Solutions: A Laboratory Handbook. Bassam B. Damaj. 2000. LC 00-22980. (Molecular Laboratory Methods Ser.). xii, 142p. spiral bd. 34.95 (*1-881299-29-5*) Eaton Pub Co.

Immunological Recognition. 1990. (Symposia on Quantitative Biology Ser.: Vol. LIV). (Illus.). 1010p. (C). text 200.00 (*0-87969-057-7*); pap. text 95.00 (*0-87969-058-5*) Cold Spring Harbor.

Immunological Surveillance. Burnet. 1970. 15.00 (*0-08-017481-7*, Pergamon Pr) Elsevier.

Immunological Techniques Applied to Aging Research. William H. Alder & Albert A. Nordin. 1981. 256p. 141.00 (*0-8493-5809-4*, QP86, CRC Reprint) Franklin.

Immunological Techniques in Food Analysis. Morgan. 1997. 250p. 1.00 (*0-12-506860-3*) Acad Pr.

Immunological Techniques Made Easy. Jean-Luc Teillaud et al. 1998. LC 97-43923. 352p. pap. 110.00 (*0-471-97277-0*) Wiley.

Immunologically Active Peptides. Victor A. Najjar. 1982. text 176.50 (*90-6193-842-2*) Kluwer Academic.

Immunologische Bestimmung des Mycotoxins Cyclopiazonsaeure. Sabine Hahnau. 1993. (Bibliotheca Mycologica: Vol. 151). (GER., Illus.). xii, 170p. (*3-443-59052-7*) Gebruder Borntraeger DEU. *Dist:* Balogh.

Immunology. Blackwell Science Inc., Publishing Staff & Jane Decker. 1999. LC 99-46471. (Eleventh Hour Ser.). (Illus.). 225p. pap. 20.95 (*0-632-04415-2*) Blackwell Sci.

***Immunology.** Bernadette Hannigan. 2001. (Biomedical Sciences Explained Ser.). (Illus.). 256p. (Orig.). pap. text (*0-340-76381-7*) E A GBR. *Dist:* OUP.

Immunology. J. Klein & V. Horejsi. 1999. (Illus.). 722p. pap. 81.95 (*0-632-05468-9*) Blackwell Sci.

***Immunology.** George Pinchuk. 2001. LC 2001-52198. (Schaum's Outlines Ser.). (Illus.). 304p. pap. 15.95 (*0-07-137366-7*, Schaums Outline) McGraw-Hill Trade.

Immunology. Leroy E. Hood et al. 2nd ed. 1984. 560p. text 43.95 (*0-8053-4407-1*) Benjamin-Cummings.

Immunology. Jan Klein & Vaclav Horesji. 2nd ed. 1997. LC 96-17956. (Illus.). 784p. 246.95 (*0-632-04228-1*) Blackwell Sci.

Immunology. D. K. Male et al. 2nd ed. 1989. (Illus.). 360p. (*0-397-44696-9*, GM0093) Gower-Mosby.

Immunology. Richard L. Myers. 3rd ed. 1999. pap. text, lab manual ed. 24.00 (*0-697-28600-2*) McGraw.

Immunology. Roitt. 4th ed. 1995. (*0-7234-2586-8*) Wolfe Publishing GBR. *Dist:* Mosby Inc.

Immunology. Ivan Roitt et al. 5th ed. 1998. (Illus.). 423p. 40.95 (*0-7234-2918-9*) Mosby Inc.

Immunology. Ivan Roitt et al. 5th ed. 1998. (Illus.). 416p. pap. (*84-8174-180-9*) Mosby-Doyma Libros ESP. *Dist:* Mosby Inc.

Immunology. John Stewart & Donald M. Weir. 8th ed. 1997. LC 96-37671. pap. text (*0-443-05452-5*) Church.

Immunology. D. M. Weir & John Stewart. 8th ed. 1997. LC 96-37671. (*0-443-05563-7*) Church.

***Immunology: A Comprehensive Review.** Darla J. Wise & G. R. Carter. 2001. LC 2001-4465. (*0-8138-1599-1*) Iowa U Pr.

Immunology: A Laboratory Manual. Richard L. Myers. 2nd ed. 1994. 144p. (C). spiral bd. 57.50 (*0-697-11313-2*, WCB McGr Hill) McGrw-H Hghr Educ.

Immunology: A Modern Introduction. Klein. 1990. 94.95 (*0-632-02587-5*) Mosby Inc.

Immunology: A Programmed Text. Wayne J. Streilein & John D. Hughes. 1977. 18.00 (*0-316-81919-0*, Little Brwn Med Div) Lppncott W & W.

Immunology: A Self-Instructional Approach. Catherine E. Roesel. 1978. pap. text 26.95 (*0-07-053411-X*) McGraw.

Immunology: A Short Course. Eli Benjamini et al. 4th ed. 2000. 528p. pap. 49.95 (*0-471-34890-2*) Wiley.

Immunology: An Illustrated Outline. David Male. 3rd ed. 1998. pap. text 17.95 (*0-7234-2617-1*) Mosby Inc.

Immunology: An Introduction. Ian R. Tizard. 4th ed. 1994. LC 94-61384. (C). text 97.50 (*0-03-004198-8*) Harcourt Coll Pubs.

Immunology: Cell Interactions, Myelopeptides Artificial Immunogens. Ed. by Rem. V. Petrov. 1987. (Soviet Medical Reviews: Section D, Immunology Reviews Ser.: Vol. 1). xviii, 443p. text 613.00 (*3-7186-0315-2*) Gordon & Breach.

Immunology: Clinical, Fundamental & Therapeutic Aspects. Ed. by Bhanu P. Ram et al. 1990. LC 89-24846. (Immunology, Biochemistry & Biotechnology Ser.: Vol. 1). 364p. text 85.00 (*0-89573-763-9*, Wiley-VCH) Wiley.

Immunology: The Making of a Modern Science. Ed. by Richard Gallagher et al. 1995. (Illus.). 246p. text 42.00 (*0-12-274020-3*) Acad Pr.

Immunology: Understanding the Immune System. Klaus D. Elgert. 1996. LC 95-42454. 468p. 72.95 (*0-471-11680-7*) Wiley.

Immunology & Aging. Nicola Fabris. 1982. text 122.00 (*90-247-2640-9*) Kluwer Academic.

Immunology & Blood Transfusion: Proceedings of the Seventeenth Annual International Symposium on Blood Transfusion, Groningen 1992, Organized by the Red Cross Blook Bank, Groningen-Drenthe. Ed. by C. Th. Smit Sibinga. 1993. LC 93-5012. (Developments in Hematology & Immunology Ser.). 296p. (C). text 113.00 (*0-7923-2380-7*) Kluwer Academic.

Immunology & Chinese Herbal Medicine. Pi-Kwang Tsung & Hong-Yen Hsu. 1986. (Educational Series on Chinese Medicine: No. 1). pap. text 3.95 (*0-941942-23-6*) Orient Heal Arts.

Immunology & Clinical Management of Interstitial Lung Diseases: A Clinician's Guide. Ed. by E. H. Walters & Du Bois. 1995. (Illus.). 360p. (C). (gr. 13). 169.95 (*0-412-48740-3*, Chap & Hall NY) Chapman & Hall.

Immunology & Epidemology. Ed. by G. W. Hoffman & F. Hraba. 1986. (Lecture Notes in Biomathematics: Vol. 65). 242p. 46.95 (*0-387-16431-6*) Spr-Verlag.

Immunology & Genetics of Mammalian Reproduction: Some Controversial. Ed. by M. Adinolfi. 1993. (Journal: Vol. 10, No. 2, 1993). (Illus.). 62p. pap. 47.00 (*3-8055-5867-8*) S Karger.

Immunology & Immunization of Fish: Proceedings of the Conference Held June 22-24, 1981 in Wageningen, Netherlands. Ed. by W. B. Van Muiswinkel. 1982. (Developmental & Comparative Immunology Ser.). 256p. pap. 61.00 (*0-08-028831-6*, Pergamon Pr) Elsevier.

Immunology & Immunopathology: Basic Concepts. Hokama Yoshitsugi & Robert M. Nakamura. 1982. 496p. 38.95 (*0-316-36932-2*, Little Brwn Med Div) Lppncott W & W.

Immunology & Immunopathology of Domestic Animals. Olsen et al. 2nd ed. 1994. LC 95-106545. (Illus.). 208p. (C). (gr. 13). text 81.95 (*0-8016-6398-9*, 06398) Mosby Inc.

Immunology & Immunopathology of Reproduction. Ed. by V. Toder & A. E. Beer. 1985. (Contributions to Gynecology & Obstetrics Ser.: Vol. 14). (Illus.). x, 214p. 135.75 (*3-8055-4059-0*) S Karger.

Immunology & Its Impact on Infections in Surgery. Ed. by R. Engemann et al. 1995. LC 94-28825. (Illus.). 253p. 107.00 (*0-387-58145-6*) Spr-Verlag.

Immunology & Liver. Ed. by K. H. Buschenfelde. 1993. LC 93-23189. 480p. (C). text 164.50 (*0-7923-8830-5*) Kluwer Academic.

Immunology & Molecular Biology of Cardiovascular Diseases. Ed. by Christopher J. Spry. 1987. (Current Status of Clinical Cardiology Ser.). (C). text 217.50 (*0-85200-973-9*) Kluwer Academic.

Immunology & Molecular Biology of Parasitic Infections. K. S. Warren. 3rd ed. 1992. (Illus.). 624p. 195.00 (*0-86542-095-5*) Blackwell Sci.

Immunology & Pathogenesis of Trypanosomiasis. Ed. by Ian R. Tizard. 1985. 248p. 142.00 (*0-8493-5640-7*, RC186, CRC Reprint) Franklin.

Immunology & Pathogenicity of Persistent Virus Infections. Ed. by Brian W.J. Mahy & Richard W. Compans. 1996. LC 99-521808. 292p. text 68.00 (*3-7186-0607-0*); pap. text 34.00 (*3-7186-0622-4*) Gordon & Breach (Harwood Acad Pubs).

Immunology & Serology in Laboratory Medicine. Mary L. Turgeon. 2nd ed. 1996. 108p. pap. text, wbk. ed. 17.95 (*0-8151-8790-4*); 1995. LC 95-42304. (Illus.). 512p. (C). (gr. 13). text 48.00 (*0-8151-8787-4*, 24150) Mosby Inc.

Immunology at a Glance. John H. Playfair. 6th ed. 1996. LC 95-40124. (At a Glance Ser.). (Illus.). 96p. pap. 21.95 (*0-86542-677-5*) Blackwell Sci.

Immunology at a Glance, 7th Edition. John H. Playfair & Benjamin Chain. 7th ed. 2001. LC 00-44446. (At a Glance Ser.). (Illus.). 96p. (C). pap. 26.95 (*0-632-05406-9*) Blackwell Sci.

Immunology Case Studies. Jonathan Brostoff et al. 3rd ed. 1997. 17.00 (*0-7234-2945-6*) Mosby Inc.

Immunology Case Studies. Ivan Roitt et al. 3rd ed. 1998. (Illus.). 112p. pap. (*84-8174-179-5*) Mosby-Doyma Libros ESP. *Dist:* Mosby Inc.

Immunology Education Course. Competence Assurance Systems Staff. 1984. (Illus.). pap. text 80.00 (*0-89147-059-X*) CAS.

Immunology for Life Scientists: A Basic Introduction. Lesley-Jane Eales. 1997. LC 97-974. 312p. pap. text 59.95 incl. disk (*0-471-96225-2*) Wiley.

Immunology for Medical Students. Constantin A. Bona. 1990. x, 250p. text 147.00 (*3-7186-0507-4*); 250p. pap. text 64.00 (*3-7186-0508-2*) Gordon & Breach (Harwood Acad Pubs).

***Immunology for The Boards & Wards.** Carlos Ayala. 2001. LC 00-66773. (Boards & Wards Ser.). (Illus.). 80p. pap. 14.95 (*0-632-04574-4*) Blackwell Sci.

Immunology for the Health Sciences. Nicholas J. Vardaxis. 1996. 218p. pap. (*0-7329-3092-8*) Macmill Educ AUS. *Dist:* Paul & Co Pubs.

Immunology Highlights: Proceedings Reports from the IXth International Congress of Immunology. C. A. Janeway et al. 1995. (Illus.). 112p. pap. text 38.00 (*0-88937-165-2*) Hogrefe & Huber Pubs.

Immunology Highlights: Proceedings Reports from the Xth International Congress of Immunology. Ed. by Jacinta Kelly et al. 1999. (Illus.). 80p. pap. 29.00 (*0-88937-221-7*) Hogrefe & Huber Pubs.

Immunology, Immunopathology & Immunity. Stewart Sell. 6th ed. 2001. LC 00-45350. (Illus.). xx, 753p. 69.95 (*1-55581-202-3*) ASM Pr.

Immunology in Diabetes Mellitus. Robert M. Galbraith. 1979. 96p. 59.00 (*0-8493-5365-3*, RC666, CRC Reprint) Franklin.

***Immunology in Medicine: A Comprehensive Guide to Clinical Immunology.** Ed. by E. J. Holborow & W. G. Reeves. 1983. (Illus.). 655p. 198.00 (*0-8089-1573-8*, Grune & Strat) Saunders.

Immunology Investigations: A Laboratory Manual. Loreli A. Batina. 1997. (Illus.). 210p. (C). pap. text, lab manual ed. 32.95 (*0-89863-176-9*) Star Pub CA.

Immunology Methods Manual: The Comprehensive Sourcebook of Techniques Ed. by Ivan Lefkovits et al. 1997. 2495p. 269.95 incl. cd-rom (*0-12-442716-2*) Acad Pr.

Immunology Methods Manual: The Comprehensive Sourcebook of Techniques, Set. Ed. by Ivan Lefkovits. 1996. LC 96-44884. (Illus.). 2176p. 183.00 (*0-12-442710-3*) Morgan Kaufmann.

Immunology Nomenclature: The Immunologist, Supplement 1, 1998. Jacob B. Natvig & Malcolm W. Turner. 1998. LC 98-73937. (Illus.). x, 147p. pap. 29.50 (*0-88937-208-X*) Hogrefe & Huber Pubs.

Immunology of Anergy & Systemic Lupus Erythematosus. Ed. by R. S. Schwartz. 1984. (Progress in Allergy Ser.: Vol. 35). (Illus.). viii, 176p. 85.25 (*3-8055-3824-3*) S Karger.

Immunology of Cancer. Ed. by V. Richards. 1974. (Progress in Experimental Tumor Research Ser.: Vol. 19). 416p. 128.75 (*3-8055-1762-9*) S Karger.

Immunology of Connective Tissue Diseases. Ed. by G. S. Panayi. 1994. LC 93-39860. (Immunology & Medicine Ser.: Vol. 22). 416p. (C). text 191.50 (*0-7923-8988-3*) Kluwer Academic.

***Immunology of Diabetes: The Fifth Congress of the Immunology of Diabetes Society.** Ed. by Carani B. Sanjeevi. 2001. 500p. 145.00 (*1-57331-362-9*) NY Acad Sci.

Immunology of Endocrine Diseases. Ed. by A. M. McGregor. 1986. (Immunology & Medicine Ser.). text 127.50 (*0-85200-963-1*) Kluwer Academic.

Immunology of ENT Disorders. Ed. by G. K. Scadding. 1995. (Immunology & Medicine Ser.: Vol. 24). 240p. (C). text 135.00 (*0-7923-8914-X*) Kluwer Academic.

Immunology of Eye Diseases. Ed. by Susan Lightman. 1989. (Immunology & Medicine Ser.). (C). text 114.50 (*0-7923-8908-5*) Kluwer Academic.

Immunology of Gastrointestinal Diseases. Ed. by T. C. MacDonald. 1992. (Immunology & Medicine Ser.). (C). text 223.00 (*0-7923-8961-1*) Kluwer Academic.

Immunology of Heart & Lung Transplantation. Ed. by Marlene L. Rose & Magdi H. Yacoub. 1993. (Illus.). 324p. text (*0-340-56016-9*) E A GBR. *Dist:* OUP.

Immunology of HIV Infection. Ed. by A. Graham Bird. 1991. (Immunology & Medicine Ser.). 192p. (C). text 126.50 (*0-7923-8962-X*) Kluwer Academic.

Immunology of HIV Infection. Ed. by Sudhir Gupta. 1996. (Illus.). 594p. (C). text 114.00 (*0-306-45255-3*, Kluwer Plenum) Kluwer Academic.

Immunology of Host-Ectoparasitic Arthropod Relationships. Ed. by Stephen K. Wikel. 1997. LC 97-158286. (CAB International Publication). 344p. text 120.00 (*0-85199-125-4*) OUP.

Immunology of Human Melanoma: Tumor-Host Interaction & Immunotherapy. Ed. by M. Maio. LC 95-8175. (Biomedical & Health Research Ser.: Vol. 12). 250p. (YA). (gr. 12 up). 95.00 (*90-5199-253-X*) IOS Press.

Immunology of Human Papillomaviruses. M. A. Stanley. 1994. (Illus.). 344p. (C). text 105.00 (*0-306-44714-2*, Kluwer Plenum) Kluwer Academic.

Immunology of Human Pregnancy. Henry N. Claman. 1993. LC 92-49012. 232p. 95.00 (*0-89603-251-5*) Humana.

Immunology of Human Reproduction. Ed. by M. Kurpisz & Nelson Fernandez. 1995. 450p. (*1-872748-59-7*) Bios Sci GBR. *Dist:* Coronet Bks.

Immunology of Infection. Dougan et al. 1998. (Methods in Microbiology Ser.: Vol. 305). (Illus.). 705p. (C). 59.95 (*0-12-402305-3*) Harcourt.

Immunology of Infection. Ed. by J. G. Sissons et al. 1994. LC 94-27318. (Immunology & Medicine Ser.: 25). text 123.00 (*0-7923-8968-9*) Kluwer Academic.

***Immunology of Infectious Disease.** Stefan Kaufmann et al. 2001. LC 00-69980. (Illus.). 557p. 115.95 (*1-55581-214-7*) ASM Pr.

Immunology of Intracellular Parasitism. Ed. by Fee Yow Liew & Frank E. Cox. 1998. (Chemical Immunology Ser.: Vol. 70, 1998). (Illus.). xii, 204p. text 197.50 (*3-8055-6621-2*) S Karger.

Immunology of Liver Disease. Ed. by H. C. Thomas & J. A. Waters. 1994. LC 93-11905. (Immunology & Medicine Ser.: Vol. 21). 224p. (C). text 107.00 (*0-7923-8975-1*) Kluwer Academic.

Immunology of Liver Transplantation. Ed. by James Neuberger & David Adams. 1993. 320p. (*0-340-55310-3*) E A GBR. *Dist:* OUP.

Immunology of Malaria: Proceedings of the WHO Scientific Group, Geneva, 1967. WHO Staff. 1968. (Technical Reports: No. 396). 50p. pap. text 5.00 (*92-4-120396-X*, 1100396) World Health.

Immunology of Malaria: With Summary in French. 1979. (Bulletin Supplement Ser.: No. 57). 290p. text 30.00 (*92-4-068571-5*) World Health.

Immunology of Malignant Diseases. Ed. by Vera S. Byers & R. W. Baldwin. 1987. (Immunology & Medicine Ser.). (C). text 156.00 (*0-85200-964-X*) Kluwer Academic.

Immunology of Milk & the Neonate. J. Mestecky et al. 1992. (Advances in Experimental Medicine & Biology Ser.: Vol. 310). (Illus.). 504p. (C). text 145.00 (*0-306-44105-5*, Kluwer Plenum) Kluwer Academic.

Immunology of Neuromuscular Disease. Ed. by R. Hohlfeld. 1994. LC 94-15123. (Immunology & Medicine Ser.: Vol. 23). text 156.00 (*0-7923-8844-5*) Kluwer Academic.

Immunology of Nude Mice. Miroslav Holub. 1989. 176p. lib. bdg. 169.00 (*0-8493-6662-3*, QR182) CRC Pr.

Immunology of Obstetrics & Gynecology. I. T. Manyonda & F. C. Hay. 2002. (Illus.). 350p. 89.95 (*1-85070-791-X*, Parthenon Pbng) CRC Pr.

Immunology of Pregnancy. Ed. by Gerard Chaouat. 1992. 288p. lib. bdg. 169.00 (*0-8493-8868-6*, RG557) CRC Pr.

Immunology of Pregnancy & Cancer. V. I. Govallo. Tr. by L. Jacobson. 1993. (Illus.). 247p. (C). lib. bdg. 135.00 (*1-56072-096-4*) Nova Sci Pubs.

Immunology of Pregnancy & Its Disorders. Ed. by C. Stern. 1989. (Immunology & Medicine Ser.). (C). text 132.50 (*0-7462-0065-X*) Kluwer Academic.

Immunology of Renal Disease. Ed. by Charles D. Pusey. 1991. (Immunology & Medicine Ser.). (C). text 174.50 (*0-7923-8964-6*) Kluwer Academic.

Immunology of Renal Transplantation. Ed. by G. R. D. Catto & Angus W. Thomson. 1993. 336p. (*0-340-55162-3*) E A GBR. *Dist:* OUP.

Immunology of Reproduction. Ed. by Rajesh K. Naz. 1992. 336p. 198.95 (*0-8493-5191-X*, QP252) CRC Pr.

Immunology of Rheumatoid Diseases. Walport. 1995. text 105.00 (*0-443-05334-0*) Saunders.

Immunology of Sexually Transmitted Diseases. Ed. by D. J. Wright. 1988. (Immunology & Medicine Ser.). (C). text 171.50 (*0-7462-0087-0*) Kluwer Academic.

Immunology of Silicones, 210. Ed. by M. Potter & N. Rose. 1996. (Current Topics in Microbiology & Immunology Ser.: Vol. 210). (Illus.). 430p. 197.00 (*3-540-60272-0*) Spr-Verlag.

Immunology of the Cornea. I. Missotten. 1994. 74p. (Orig.). pap. (*90-6186-632-4*) Leuven Univ BEL. *Dist:* Coronet Bks.

Immunology of the Fetus. Ed. by Gerard Chaouat. 1989. 336p. lib. bdg. 208.00 (*0-8493-4568-5*, RG613) CRC Pr.

Immunology of the Fungal Diseases. Cox. 1989. 264p. 169.00 (*0-8493-6153-2*, QR245) CRC Pr.

Immunology of the Gastrointestinal Tract, Set. Ed. by Klara Miller & Stephen Nicklin. 1987. 336p. 259.90 (*0-8493-4310-0*, RC817) CRC Pr.

Immunology of the Human Placenta & Proteins: Supplement to the Quarterly Journal "Placenta", Vol. 4. Ed. by A. I. Klopper. 1982. 136p. 62.50 (*0-275-91368-6*, C1368, Praeger Pubs) Greenwood.

Immunology of the Lymphomas. Ed. by Gottlieb. 1985. LC 84-1776. 208p. 122.00 (*0-8493-6371-3*, RC286, CRC Reprint) Franklin.

Immunology of the Nervous System. Ed. by Robert W. Keane & William F. Hickey. 1997. LC 96-24678. (Illus.). 848p. text 98.50 (*0-19-507817-9*) OUP.

H I

Immunology of the Skin & Eye. M. Zierhut & H. J. Thiel. 1998. 332p. (*90-70430-27-4*) Swets.

Immunology Reviews: Acquired Immunodeficiency Syndrome, Vol. 2. R. M. Khaitov. Ed. by R. V. Petrov. 1989. (Soviet Medical Reviews Ser.: Vol. 2, Pt. 2). xii, 94p. pap. text 117.00 (*3-7186-4920-9*) Gordon & Breach.

Immunology Reviews: Chemiluminescent Analysis of Phagocytic Cells, Vol. 2. Ed. by V. M. Zemskov & R. V. Petrov. 1989. (Soviet Medical Reviews Ser.: Vol. 2, Pt. 3). viii, 108p. pap. text 135.00 (*3-7186-4929-2*) Gordon & Breach.

Immunology Reviews: Immune Monitoring: Its Principles & Application in Natural & Model Clinical Systems, Vol. 2. K. A. Lebedev et al. Ed. by R. V. Petrov. 1989. (Soviet Medical Reviews Ser.: Vol. 2, Pt. 1). x, 124p. pap. text 156.00 (*3-7186-4922-5*) Gordon & Breach.

Immunology Reviews: Immunodeficiency in Children: Experience of a Specialized Department, Vol. 2. L. N. Khakhalin. Ed. by R. V. Petrov. 1989. (Soviet Medical Reviews Ser.: Vol. 2, Pt. 4). viii, 76p. pap. text 92.00 (*3-7186-4934-9*) Gordon & Breach.

Immunology Reviews: Immunodeficiency in Patients with Chronic Lung Diseases: Approaches to Immunomodulation, Vol. 3. A. A. Borisova et al. Ed. by R. V. Petrov. 1989. (Soviet Medical Reviews Ser.: Vol. 3, Pt. 1). vi, 134p. pap. text 161.00 (*3-7186-4937-3*) Gordon & Breach.

Immunology Reviews Vol. 3, Pt. 2: Glycoconjugates As Modifiers of Anti-Tumor Immunity-Glycosphingolipids As Immunodulators, Vol. 3. B. Fuchs. 1992. (Soviet Medical Reviews Ser.: Section D). 149p. pap. text 143.00 (*3-7186-5204-8*, Harwood Acad Pubs) Gordon & Breach.

Immunology Reviews Vol. 3, Pt. 3: The Immunomodulating Effects of a Low Molecular Weight RNA, Vol. 3. V. Zemskov. 1992. (Soviet Medical Reviews Ser.: Section D). 113p. pap. text 112.00 (*3-7186-5203-X*, Harwood Acad Pubs) Gordon & Breach.

Immunology Reviews Vol. 4, Pt. 1: The Structure & Immunomodulating Function of Glucosaminylmuranyl Pepties - the Thymus- & a Bone Marrow-Derived Immuno, Vol. 4. T. Andronova. 1992. (Soviet Medical Reviews Ser.: Section D). 143p. pap. text 137.00 (*3-7186-5202-1*, Harwood Acad Pubs) Gordon & Breach.

Immunology Reviews Vol. 4, Pt. 2: Some Molecular Aspects of Immediate Allergy & Its Drug Control, Vol. 4. I. S. Gushchin. 1992. (Soviet Medical Reviews Ser.: Section D). 57p. pap. text 70.00 (*3-7186-5281-1*, Harwood Acad Pubs) Gordon & Breach.

Immunology Reviews Vol. 4, Pt. 3: Physico-Chemical Criteria for the Construction of Artificial Immunomodulators & Immunogens on the Basis of Polyelectro, Vol. 4. R. V. Petrov. 1992. (Soviet Medical Reviews Ser.: Section D). 116p. pap. text 137.00 (*3-7186-5288-9*, Harwood Acad Pubs) Gordon & Breach.

Immunology/Gastrointestinal Tract, Vol. II. Miller. 1987. 144p. 85.00 (*0-8493-4312-7*, CRC Reprint) Franklin.

Immunomicroscopy: A Diagnostic Tool for the Surgical Pathologist. Clive R. Taylor. 2nd ed. 1994. LC 93-19430. (Major Problems in Pathology Ser.: Vol. 19). (Illus.). 448p. text 95.00 (*0-7216-6462-8*) Saunders.

Immunomodulation in Respiratory Infection. Ed. by J. M. Bernstein & P. Van Cauwenberge. 1992. (Journal: Vol. 59, Suppl. 3, 1992). (Illus.). iv, 32p. pap. 15.75 (*3-8055-5672-1*) S Karger.

Immunomodulation of Neoplasia. Ed. by J. M. Cruse. 1988. (Progress in Experimental Tumor Research Ser.: Vol. 32). (Illus.). vi, 246p. 207.00 (*3-8055-4595-9*) S Karger.

Immunomodulatory Agents from Plants Hildebert H. Wagner. 1999. LC 98-46563. (Progress in Inflammation Research Ser.). ix, 365p. (*0-8176-5848-3*) Birkhauser.

Immunomodulatory & Cytotoxic Agents in Dermatology. Charles J. McDonald. 1997. LC 96-45655. (Basic & Clinical Dermatology Ser.: Vol. 13). (Illus.). 425p. text 199.00 (*0-8247-9406-0*) Dekker.

Immunomodulatory Effects of Blood Transfusion. American Association of Blood Banks Staff. Ed. by Eleftherios C. Vamvakas & Morris A. Blajchman. 1999. (Illus.). 296p. (*3-8055-7057-0*) S Karger.

Immunomorphological Analysis of the Human Inner Ear. Ed. by M. Anniko & W. Arnold. 1995. (Journal: Vol. 57, No. 2, 1995). (Illus.). 54p. pap. 60.00 (*3-8055-6140-7*) S Karger.

Immunomorphology & Immunopathology of the Lung. A. Eskenasy. 1978. xiv, 314p. text 106.00 (*0-85626-108-4*, Abacus) Gordon & Breach.

Immunoneurology. Ed. by Michel Chofflon & Lawrence Steinman. 1996. LC 96-30167. (Illus.). 272p. 135.00 (*3-540-61559-8*) Spr-Verlag.

Immunoparasitology: Principles & Methods in Malaria & Schistosomiasis Research. Thomas G. Strickland. Ed. by Kenneth W. Hunter. 1982. LC 82-626. 294p. 79.50 (*0-275-91382-1*, C1382, Praeger Pubs) Greenwood.

Immunopathogenesis of HIV Infection. Ed. by Anthony S. Fauci & G. Pantaleo. 1997. LC 97-18097. (Seminars in Immunopathology Ser.). (Illus.). 156p. 136.00 (*3-540-63254-9*) Spr-Verlag.

***Immunopathogenesis of Schistosomiasis Mansoni: Immunity & Pathology in a Primary & a Secondary Infection Following Chemotherapy in the Mouse & the Baboon Models.** Idle Omar Farah. 2000. (Comprehensive Summaries of Uppsala Dissertations from the Faculty of Medicine Ser.: No. 903). (Illus.). 66p. (Orig.). pap. (*91-554-4648-5*) Uppsala Universitet SWE. *Dist:* Coronet Bks.

Immunopathogenetic Aspects of Disease Induced by Helminth Parasites. Ed. by David O. Freedman. 1997. LC 96-52549. (Chemical Immunology Ser.: Vol. 66, 1997). (Illus.). xii, 236p. 247.00 (*3-8055-6400-7*) S Karger.

Immunopathogentic Mechanisms of Arthritis. Ed. by J. Goodacre & Carson Dick. 1988. (C). text 164.50 (*0-85200-980-1*) Kluwer Academic.

Immunopathology. David J. Dabbs. 2000. 704p. text (*0-443-06566-7*) Harcrt Hlth Sci Grp.

Immunopathology: Proceedings of the International Convocation on Immunology, 6th. International Convocation on Immunology Staff. Ed. by Felix Milgrom & B. Albini. 1980. (Illus.). 129.75 (*3-8055-2971-6*) S Karger.

Immunopathology & Immunopharmacology of the Lung. Ed. by M. Baggiolini. 1985. (Journal: Vol. 76, Suppl. 1). (Illus.). iv, 128p. pap. 39.25 (*3-8055-4057-4*) S Karger.

Immunopathology of Lung Disease. Richard Kradin & Bruce Robinson. 1996. (Illus.). 578p. text (*0-7506-9282-0*) E A GBR. *Dist:* OUP.

Immunopharmaceuticals. Ed. by Edward S. Kimball. 1995. LC 95-36999. (CRC Pharmacology & Toxicology: Basic & Clinical Aspects Ser.). 288p. 139.95 (*0-8493-8388-9*, 8388) CRC Pr.

Immunopharmacology. Steven C. Gilman & Thomas J. Rogers. 1989. 500p. 99.00 (*0-936923-22-9*); lib. bdg. 59.95 (*0-936923-21-0*, RA370) CRC Pr.

Immunopharmacology: Principles & Perspectives. J. Drews. 1990. (Illus.). 300p. 118.00 (*0-387-52370-7*) Spr-Verlag.

Immunopharmacology in Autoimmune Diseases & Transplantation. H. E. Rugstad et al. 1992. (Illus.). 446p. (C). text 115.00 (*0-306-43994-8*, Kluwer Plenum) Kluwer Academic.

Immunopharmacology of Allergic Diseases. Ed. by Robert Townley & Devendra K. Agrawal. 1996. LC 96-20570. (Clinical Allergy & Immunology Ser.: Vol. 8). (Illus.). 736p. text 235.00 (*0-8247-9513-X*) Dekker.

Immunopharmacology of Endotoxicosis: Proceedings of the 5th International Congress of Immunology Satellite Workshop. Kyoto, Japan, August 27, 1983. Ed. by M. K. Agarwal & M. Yoshida. 1984. LC 84 7650. (Illus.). xiv, 376p. 138.50 (*3 11 009887 3*) De Gruyter.

Immunopharmacology of Eosinophils. Ed. by Harry Smith & Richard Cook. 1993. LC 93-171495. (Handbook of Immunopharmacology Ser.). (Illus.). 250p. text 94.00 (*0-12-652270-7*) Acad Pr.

Immunopharmacology of Epithelial Barriers. Ed. by Roy Goldie. 1994. (Handbook of Immunopharmacology Ser.). (Illus.). 296p. text 79.00 (*0-12-288030-7*) Acad Pr.

Immunopharmacology of Free Radical Species. Ed. by David Blake & Paul G. Winyard. 1995. (Handbook of Immunopharmacology Ser.). (Illus.). 322p. text 63.00 (*0-12-103520-4*) Acad Pr.

Immunopharmacology of Joints & Connective Tissue. Ed. by Elisabeth Davies & John Dingle. 1994. (Illus.). 288p. text 79.00 (*0-12-206345-7*) Acad Pr.

Immunopharmacology of Lymphocytes. Ed. by Marek Rola-Pleszczynski. 1994. (Handbook of Immunopharmacology Ser.). (Illus.). 304p. (C). text 59.95 (*0-12-593390-8*) Acad Pr.

Immunopharmacology of Macrophages & Other Antigen-Presenting Cells. Ed. by C. A. Bruijnzeel-Koomen & F. C. Hoefsmit. 1994. (Handbook of Immunopharmacology Ser.). (Illus.). 208p. text 79.00 (*0-12-137800-4*) Acad Pr.

Immunopharmacology of Mast Cells & Basophils. Ed. by John C. Foreman. 1993. (Handbook of Immunopharmacology Ser.). (Illus.). 256p. text 83.00 (*0-12-262210-3*) Acad Pr.

Immunopharmacology of Neutrophils. Ed. by P. G. Hellewell & T. J. Williams. 1994. (Handbook of Immunopharmacology Ser.). (Illus.). 352p. text 78.00 (*0-12-339250-0*) Acad Pr.

Immunopharmacology of Platelets. Ed. by Michael Joseph. 1995. (Handbook of Immunopharmacology Ser.). (Illus.). 272p. text 74.00 (*0-12-390120-0*) Acad Pr.

Immunopharmacology of the Gastrointestinal System. Ed. by John L. Wallace. 1993. (Handbook of Immunopharmacology Ser.). (Illus.). 198p. text 94.00 (*0-12-732860-2*) Acad Pr.

Immunopharmacology of the Heart. Ed. by M. J. Curtis. 1993. (Handbook of Immunopharmacology Ser.). (Illus.). 162p. text 79.00 (*0-12-200245-8*) Acad Pr.

Immunopharmacology of the Microcirculation. Ed. by Susan Brain. 1994. (Handbook of Immunopharmacology Ser.). (Illus.). 256p. text 79.00 (*0-12-125010-5*) Acad Pr.

Immunopharmacology of the Renal System. Ed. by C. Tetta. 1993. (Handbook of Immunopharmacology Ser.). (Illus.). 258p. text 83.00 (*0-12-685530-7*) Acad Pr.

Immunopharmacology of the Respiratory System. Ed. by Stephen T. Holgate. 1995. (Handbook of Immunopharmacology Ser.). (Illus.). 320p. (C). text 59.95 (*0-12-352325-7*) Acad Pr.

Immunopharmacology Reviews, Vol. 1. J. W. Hadden & A. Szentivanyi. 1990. (Illus.). 432p. (C). text 120.00 (*0-306-43273-0*, Kluwer Plenum) Kluwer Academic.

Immunopharmacology Reviews, Vol. 2. Ed. by John W. Hadden & Andor Szentivanyi. 1996. (Illus.). 429p. 155.00 (*0-306-45239-1*, Kluwer Plenum) Kluwer Academic.

Immunophenotyping of Blood & Bone Marrow Leukocytes: Application to the Determination of Immune Status & Malignant Haematopathies Analysis. Ed. by Marie-Christine Bene & Eric Martini. 1997. 256p. text (*90-5702-008-4*) GBSP NLD. *Dist:* Gordon & Breach.

Immunophysiology: The Role of Cells & Cytokines in Immunity & Inflammation. Ed. by Joost J. Oppenheim & Ethan M. Shevach. 1991. (Illus.). 448p. reprint ed. pap. text 59.95 (*0-19-507064-X*) OUP.

Immunoprecipitin Analyses: Procedures for Evaluating the Performance of Materials; Approved Guideline 1993. Contrib. by Robert M. Nakamura. 1993. 75.00 (*1-56238-194-6*, D12-A2) NCCLS.

Immunoregulation & Autoimmunity. Ed. by J. M. Cruse & R. E. Lewis. 1986. (Concepts in Immunopathology Ser.: Vol. 3). (Illus.). vii, 340p. 161.75 (*3-8055-4076-0*) S Karger.

Immunoregulation in Health & Disease: Experimental & Clinical Aspects. Ed. by Miodrag L. Lukic et al. 1997. LC 97-6622. (Illus.). 480p. text 99.95 (*0-12-459460-3*) Morgan Kaufmann.

Immunoregulatory Role of Thymus. Marek P. Dabrowski & Barbara K. Dabrowska-Bernstein. 1989. 240p. lib. bdg. 190.00 (*0-8493-6178-8*, QR185) CRC Pr.

Immunoscintigraphy, Vol. 1. Ed. by L. Donato & K. Britton. 1985. (Monographs in Nuclear Medicine). xviii, 378p. text 161.00 (*2-88124-076-3*) Gordon & Breach.

Immunosorption Techniques: Fundamentals & Applications. Peter Mohr et al. 1992. 129p. (*3-05-501350-6*) Akademie Verlag DEU. *Dist:* Wiley.

Immunostimulation. Ed. by L. Chedid. 1980. (Illus.). 236p. 36.00 (*0-387-10354-6*) Spr-Verlag.

Immunostimulatory DNA Sequences. Ed. by E. Raz. 2000. LC 00-711345. (Illus.). 192p. 90.00 (*3-540-67749-6*) Spr-Verlag.

Immunosuppressant Analogues in Neuroprotection. Ed. by Cesario V. Borlongan et al. 2002. 425p. 150.00 (*0-89603-944-7*) Humana.

Immunosuppression & Human Malignancy. Ed. by David Naor et al. 1990. LC 89-7474. (Contemporary Immunology Ser.). 288p. 119.50 (*0-89603-149-7*) Humana.

Immunosuppression by Progesterone in Pregnancy. Julia Szekeres. 1992. 176p. lib. bdg. 139.00 (*0-8493-5396-3*, RC248) CRC Pr.

***Immunosuppression in Inflammatory Bowel Diseases: Standards, New Developments, Future Trends.** K. Fellermann et al. 2001. (Falk Symposium Ser.: Vol. 119). 272p. 131.00 (*0-7923-8767-8*) Kluwer Academic.

Immunosuppression in Transplantation. Leo C. Ginns et al. 1999. LC 99-24601. (Illus.). 140p. 96.00 (*0-632-04445-4*) Blackwell Sci.

Immunosuppression Systematic Lupus Erythematosus. Ed. by J. Rotstein. 1974. (Rheumatology Ser.: Vol. 5). (Illus.). 100.00 (*3-8055-1540-5*) S Karger.

Immunosuppression under Trial. Conference on Transplantation and Clinical Immunology Staff et al. 1999. LC 99-32565. (Transplantation & Clinical Immunology Ser.). (*0-7923-5804-X*) Kluwer Academic.

Immunosuppressive Drugs: Developments in Anti-Rejection Therapy. Ed. by Angus W. Thompson & Thomas E. Starzl. 1994. (Illus.). 256p. (*0-340-56951-4*) E A GBR. *Dist:* OUP.

Immunosuppressive Drugs in Organ Transplantation: Immunology & Clinical Experience. Ed. by Raman Venkataramanan & Thomas Starzl. 1999. (Illus.). 99.50 (*0-89603-370-8*) Humana.

Immunotechnology. Ed. by J. P. Gosling & D. J. Reen. 1993. (Portland Press Proceedings Ser.: Vol. 4). 164p. (C). text (*1-85578-035-6*) Portland Pr Ltd GBR. *Dist:* Ashgate Pub Co.

Immunotherapeutic Prospects of Infectious Diseases. Ed. by W. Lange & K. Noel Masihi. 1991. (Illus.). 401p. 97.00 (*0-387-53214-5*) Spr-Verlag.

Immunotherapy & Vaccines. Stanley Cryz. 1990. LC 90-13146. 150p. 90.00 (*0-89573-969-0*, Wiley-VCH) Wiley.

Immunotherapy for Infectious Diseases. Ed. by Jeffrey M. Jacobson. 2002. (Infectious Disease Ser.). 375p. 99.50 (*0-89603-669-3*) Humana.

Immunotherapy Immune-Related Disease. Metzger. 1997. 500p. (*0-12-492560-X*) Acad Pr.

Immunotherapy in Cancer. Ed. by Martin Gore & Pamela Riches. 1996. LC 96-7005. 302p. 215.00 (*0-471-96007-1*) Wiley.

Immunotherapy of Asthma. Ed. by Jean Bousquet & Hans Yssel. 1999. LC 99-37341. (Lung Biology in Health & Disease Ser.). (Illus.). 720p. text 225.00 (*0-8247-0176-3*) Dekker.

Immunotherapy of Cancer: Report of a WHO Scientific Group, 1966. 1966. (Technical Report Ser.: No. 344). 38p. pap. text 5.00 (*92-4-120344-7*, 1100344) World Health.

Immunotherapy of Cancer with Sensitized T Lymphocytes. Ed. by Alfred E. Chang & Suyu Shu. 1994. (Medical Intelligence Unit Ser.). 118p. 99.00 (*1-57059-049-4*, LN9049) Landes Bioscience.

Immunotherapy of Diabetes & Selected Autoimmune Diseases. George S. Eisenbarth. 1989. 240p. lib. bdg. 190.00 (*0-8493-4558-8*, RC661) CRC Pr.

Immunotherapy of Disease. Ed. by T. J. Hamblin. 1990. (C). text 148.50 (*0-7462-0045-5*) Kluwer Academic.

Immunotherapy of Infections. Ed. by K. Noel Masihi. 1994. LC 94-16950. (Infectious Disease & Therapy Ser.: Vol. 15). (Illus.). 528p. text 215.00 (*0-8247-9209-2*) Dekker.

Immunotherapy of Renal Cell Carcinoma: Clinical & Experimental Developments. Ed. by F. M. Debruyne et al. 1991. (Illus.). 141p. 71.95 (*0-387-52835-0*) Spr-Verlag.

Immunotherapy of Urological Tumours. Ed. by Jean B. DeKernion. 1990. (Illus.). 384p. text (*0-443-04262-4*) Church.

Immunotherapy of Vaginal Infections. Ed. by H. Ruettgers. 1985. (Journal: Vol. 24, Suppl. 3, 1984). (Illus.). iv, 92p. pap. 28.00 (*3-8055-4072-8*) S Karger.

Immunotherapy with Intravenous Immunoglobulins. Ed. by P. Imbach. 1991. 484p. text 125.00 (*0-12-370725-0*) Acad Pr.

***Immunotics.** Robert Rountree & Carol Colman. 2001. reprint ed. pap. 13.95 (*0-399-52706-0*, Perigee Bks) Berkley Pub.

Immunotoxicology & Risk Assessment. Dennis K. Flaherty. 1999. LC 99-17059. (*0-306-45971-X*, Kluwer Plenum) Kluwer Academic.

Immunotoxicology of Environmental & Occupational Metals. Ed. by Judith T. Zelicoff & Peter T. Thomas. 1998. LC 98-141059. 374p. (*0-7484-0390-6*) Tay Francis Ltd GBR. *Dist:* Taylor & Francis.

Immunotoxin Methods & Protocols. Ed. by Walter A. Hall. 2001. LC 00-33501. (Methods in Molecular Biology Ser.: Vol. 166). (Illus.). 302p. 89.50 (*0-89603-775-4*) Humana.

Immunotoxins. Ed. by Arthur E. Frankel. 1988. (Cancer Treatment & Research Ser.). (C). text 306.50 (*0-89838-984-4*) Kluwer Academic.

Immunucytochemistry in Diagnostic Histopathology. Bharat Jasani & Kurt Schmid. 1993. (Illus.). 224p. (Orig.). text (*0-443-04018-4*) Church.

Imogene King No. 2: A Conceptual Framework for Nursing. Christina L. Evans. 1991. (Notes on Nursing Theories Ser.: Vol. 2). 40p. (C). pap. 14.95 (*0-8039-4086-6*, 3002) Sage.

Impact: An Innovative Approach to Substance Abuse Pervention & Education. Steven Ungerleider et al. 1987. (Orig.). pap. (*0-943277-01-9*) Integrated Res Servs.

Impact of AIDS: Psychological & Social Aspects of HIV Infection. Ed. by Jose Catalan et al. 1997. 312p. pap. text (*90-5702-041-6*) GBSP NLD. *Dist:* Gordon & Breach.

Impact of Biotechnology on Autoimmunity. Ed. by A. G. Dalgleish et al. 1994. LC 94-971. (Medical Science Symposia Ser.: Vol. 6). 148p. (C). text 89.00 (*0-7923-2724-1*) Kluwer Academic.

Impact of Cardiac Surgery on the Quality of Life: Neurological & Psychological Aspects. A. E. Willner & G. Rodewald. 1990. LC 90-14215. (Illus.). 566p. (C). text 145.00 (*0-306-43689-2*, Kluwer Plenum) Kluwer Academic.

Impact of Development Policies on Health: A Review of the Literature. J. F. Wilson et al. 1990. ix, 165p. pap. text 27.90 (*92-4-156141-6*, 1150349) World Health.

Impact of Energy Production on Human Health: An Evaluation of Means for Assessment: Proceedings. Ed. by Ernest C. Anderson & Elizabeth M. Sullivan. 1976. LC 76-22540. (ERDA Symposium Ser.). 154p. pap. 11.75 (*0-87079-032-3*, CONF-751022); fiche 9.00 (*0-87079-245-8*, CONF-751022) DOE.

Impact of External Review on Health Care Quality: Congressional Hearing. Ed. by John A. Boehner. 2000. 108p. pap. text 25.00 (*0-7567-0155-4*) DIANE Pub.

Impact of Freudian Psychiatry. Ed. by Franz Gabriel Alexander & Helen Ross. 1961. x, 304p. pap. text 3.95 (*0-226-01355-3*, P62) U Ch Pr.

Impact of Functional Imaging in Neurology & Psychiatry. Wade et al. 1987. (Current Problems in Neurology Ser.: Vol. 5). 208p. (*0-86196-106-4*) J Libbey Med GBR. *Dist:* Bks Intl VA.

***Impact of Genomics on Health Care.** Ed. by George Poste et al. 1999. (British Medical Bulletin Ser.: Vol. 55, No. 2). 191p. pap. (*1-85315-393-1*) Royal Soc of Medicine Pr Ltd GBR. *Dist:* Balogh.

Impact of HIV-AIDS on World Population. Peter O. Way & Karen A. Stanecki. 1994. (Illus.). 39p. (C). pap. text 25.00 (*0-7881-1497-2*) DIANE Pub.

Impact of Homophobia & Other Social Biases on AIDS: A Special Report by Public Media Center. Public Media Center Staff. 1995. 40p. (Orig.). pap. text 5.00 (*0-915287-00-5*) Pub Media Ctr.

Impact of Land Use on Nutrition & Health: A Study of Kosi Basin, U. P. G. S. Bisnt. 1988. (C). (*81-202-0210-4*) Ajanta IND. *Dist:* S Asia.

Impact of Managed Care on Psychodynamic Treatment. James W. Barron & Harry Sands. 1996. LC 96-9118. 320p. 47.50 (*0-8236-2542-7*) Intl Univs Pr.

Impact of Managed Care on the Practice of Psychotherapy: Innovations, Implementation, & Controversy. Ed. by Richard M. Alperin & David G. Phillips. 1996. LC 96-41932. 256p. 31.95 (*0-87630-830-2*) Brunner-Routledge.

H I

Impact of Mandated Reporting on the Therapeutic Process: Picking up the Pieces. Murray Levine & Howard J. Doueck. 1995. (Practice Ser.). (C). LC 95-18434. 169p. 61.95 (*0-8039-5472-7*, 3721); 168p. pap. 31.95 (*0-8039-5473-5*, 3722) Sage.

Impact of Molecular Biology & New Technical Developments on Diagnostic Imaging. W. Semmler & Markus Schwaiger. 1997. LC 97-13420. (Ernst Schering Research Foundation Ser.). (*0-387-63111-9*) Spr-Verlag.

Impact of Molecular Biology & New Technical Developments on Diagnostic Imaging. Ed. by W. Semmler & Markus Schwaiger. 1997. LC 97-13420. (Ernst Schering Research Foundation Ser.: Vol. 22). (Illus.). 268p. 54.00 (*3-540-63111-9*) Spr-Verlag.

Impact of New Ideas. Ed. by Arnold Goldberg. 1995. (Progress in Self Psychology Ser.: Vol. 11). 336p. 45.00 (*0-88163-213-9*) Analytic Pr.

Impact of Nutrition on Health & Disease. Ed. by Geoffrey H. Bourne. 1989. (World Review of Nutrition & Dietetics Ser.: Vol. 59). (Illus.). 220p. 179.25 (*3-8055-4919-9*) S Karger.

Impact of Plague in Tudor & Stuart England. Paul A. Slack. 1985. 416p. 49.95 (*0-7102-0469-8*, Routledge Thoemms) Routledge.

Impact of Prenatal Teratogenic Exposure on Phenotype & Brain Function. Ed. by A. Schinzel. 1993. (Journal: Vol. 6, Nos. 4-5, 1993). (Illus.). 124p. pap. 52.25 (*3-8055-5791-4*) S Karger.

Impact of Prescription Drug Diversion Control Systems on Medical Practice & Patient Care. 1994. lib. bdg. 295.00 (*0-8490-5749-3*) Gordon Pr.

Impact of Psychological Factors on Human Immune Response: A Training Manual for Using the Mind to Heal the Body. Larry Feldman. 1993. 192p. pap. text 29.95 (*1-883855-01-2*) St Georges Pr.

Impact of Stereochemistry on Drug Development & Use. Hassan Y. Aboul-Enein & Irving W. Wainer. 1997. LC 96-33491. (Chemical Analysis Monographs). 728p. 120.00 (*0-471-59644-2*) Wiley.

Impact of Technology on Long-Term Care. John M. Grana & David B. McCallum. 1985. LC 85-28438. (*0-930177-02-9*) Ctr Hlth Affairs.

Impact of the Aids Epidemic on Health Care Services & Planning in Europe. Council of Europe Staff. 1992. (*92-871-2060-9*) Council of Europe FRA. *Dist:* Manhattan Pub Co.

***Impact of the Anthrax Vaccine Program on Reserve & National Guard Units: Congressional Hearing.** Ed. by Christopher Shays. 2001. 125p. reprint ed. pap. text 30.00 (*0-7567-1811-2*) DIANE Pub.

Impact of the Food Quality Protection Act Implementation on Public Health: Congressional Hearing. Ed. by Bob Goodlatte. 2001. 104p. (C). reprint ed. pap. text 25.00 (*0-7567-0562-2*) DIANE Pub.

Impact of the Quality of Health Care on Children's Nutrition & Survival in Ghana. Victor Lavy et al. 1995. LC 94-41226. (LSMS Working Papers: No. 106). 62p. pap. 22.00 (*0-8213-2997-9*, 12997) World Bank.

Impact of Third-Party Payors on Collective Bargaining in the Health Care Industry. George W. Bohlander. 1980. (Monograph & Research Ser.: No. 26). 106p. 6.50 (*0-89215-109-9*) U Cal LA Indus Rel.

Impact of Violence on the Family: Treatment Approaches for Therapists & Other Professionals. Dean M. Busby. 1996. LC 95-40081. 320p. (C). 66.00 (*0-205-17570-8*) Allyn.

Impact of Vision Loss in the Elderly. Julia J. Kleinschmidt. rev. ed. 1995. LC 94-39772. (Studies on the Elderly in America). (Illus.). 120p. text 48.00 (*0-8153-1931-2*) Garland.

Impact Therapy. Ed Jacobs. 1994. LC 94-32320. 256p. pap. 29.00 (*0-911907-18-1*) Psych Assess.

Impacted Teeth. Ed. by Charles C. Alling, III et al. 1993. LC 92-49774. (Illus.). 512p. text 110.00 (*0-7216-2968-7*) Saunders.

Impacts of Antibiotic-Resistant Bacteria. 1996. (Illus.). 183p. (Orig.). (C). pap. text 45.00 (*0-7881-3043-9*) DIANE Pub.

Impacts of Antibiotic-Resistant Bacteria. 1996. (Orig.). lib. bdg. 255.99 (*0-8490-6370-1*) Gordon Pr.

Impacts on Nutrition & Health. Ed. by A. P. Simopoulos. 1991. (World Review of Nutrition & Dietetics Ser.: Vol. 65). (Illus.). viii, 168p. 159.25 (*3-8055-5266-1*) S Karger.

Impaired Health: Its Cause & Cure, Vol. 1. J. H. Tilden. 1998. 417p. reprint ed. pap. 21.00 (*0-7873-0874-9*) Hlth Research.

Impaired Health: Its Cause & Cure (1921) J. H. Tilden. 1996. 366p. reprint ed. pap. 19.95 (*1-56459-954-X*) Kessinger Pub.

Impaired Physician. Ed. by Stephen C. Scheiber & Brian B. Doyle. 1983. LC 82-22296. 230p. 45.00 (*0-306-41081-8*, Plenum Trade) Perseus Pubng.

Impaired Vision in Childhood: Proceedings of the Jerusalem Conference, May 1977. Jersualem Conference on Impaired Vision In childho. Ed. by I. Nawratzki & Saul Merin. 1979. (Illus.). pap. 100.00 (*0-08-024416-5*, Pergamon Pr) Elsevier.

Impairment & Disability Ratings: A Guide to the Guides. Craig G. Price & Ronald W. Dennie. 1992. 186p. (*1-882678-00-1*) Meriah-Morgan.

Impairment Rating & Disability Evaluation. Robert D. Rondinelli & Richard T. Katz. Ed. by Richard Lampert. 2000. LC 99-26872. (Illus.). 323p. (C). text 61.00 (*0-7216-7772-X*) Saunders.

Impasse: Resistance & Addiction Treatment: Combining Brief, Strategic & Twelve Step Approaches. Raymond McGarty. 1993. 110p. (Orig.). (C). pap. text 10.00 (*0-9638389-0-3*) Addiction Therap.

Impasse & Innovation in Psychoanalysis: Clinical Case Seminars. Ed. by John E. Gedo & Mark J. Gehrie. 1993. LC 92-49405. 328p. 49.95 (*0-88163-142-6*) Analytic Pr.

Impasse & Interpretation: Therapeutic & Anti-therapeutic Factors in the Psyco-analytic Treatment of Psychotic, Boderline, & Neutrotic Patients. Herbert Rosenfeld. Ed. by David Tuckett. 1987. (New Library of Psychoanalysis). 250p. lib. bdg. (*0-422-61010-0*) Tavistock GBR. *Dist:* Routldge.

Impedance Screening for Middle Ear Diseases in Children. Ed. by Earl R. Harford et al. 1978. LC 78-57629. 320p. text 36.50 (*0-8089-1097-3*, 791895, Grune & Strat) Harcrt Hlth Sci Grp.

Imperative Aid: General Medicine-Spanish. Russell Dollinger & Carolyn Uyeda. 2nd ed. 1987. LC 87-83658. (Medical Interpreting Aid Ser.). 210p. 29.95 (*0-945585-00-4*) Booksmythe.

Imperative of Health: Public Health & the Regulated Body. Deborah Lupton. 1995. 192p. (C). 74.50 (*0-8039-7935-5*, 2883); pap. 25.95 (*0-8039-7936-3*, 2882) Sage.

Imperial College Handbook of Maternal Disease & Its Effect on the Newborn Infant. D. Acolet et al. 2000. 200p. (*1-86094-229-6*) Imperial College GBR. *Dist:* World Scientific Pub.

Imperial Medicaments: Medical Prescriptions Written for Empress Dowager Cixi & Emperor Guangxu with Commentary. Ed. by Chen Keji. 1996. 323p. (*7-119-01336-X*) Beijing Foreign Lang CHN. *Dist:* China Bks.

Imperial Secrets of Health & Longevity. Bob Flaws. 1994. LC 94-161708. (Illus.). 125p. pap. 9.95 (*0-936185-51-1*) Blue Poppy Pr.

Imperialism & Medicine in Bengal: A Socio-Historical Perspective. Poonam Bala. 1991. LC 91-22537. (Illus.). 172p. 28.00 (*0-8039-9100-2*, 7637) Sage.

Imperialism, Health, & Medicine. Ed. by Vicente Navarro. 1981. LC 80-67832. (Policy, Politics, Health & Medicine Ser.: Vol. 3). 285p. (C). pap. text 31.00 (*0-89503-019-5*) Baywood Pub.

Impersonal Intimacy: The Story of an Adolescent's Psychotherapy As Viewed by Both the Patient & the Therapist. Norma G. Norriss. 1997. LC 97-92519. iv, 247p. pap. 10.95 (*0-9660066-0-7*) Sahuaro Pr.

Implant Dentistry Today: A Multidisciplinary Approach. Set. Leonard I. Linkow. 1990. 1624p. text (*1-57235-001-6*) Piccin Nuova.

Implant Prosthodontics: Clinical & Laboratory. Edward J. Fredrickson. 1994. LC 93-46993. (Illus.). 182p. (C). (gr. 13). text 94.95 (*0-8016-1635-2*, 01635) Mosby Inc.

Implant Prosthodontics: Clinical & Laboratory Procedures. Patrick J. Stevens et al. 2nd ed. 1999. (Illus.). 224p. (C). (gr. 13). text 109.00 (*0-8151-3567-X*, 30604) Mosby Inc.

Implant Restorations: A Step by Step Guide for Dentists. Carl J. Drago. Ed. & Illus. by Implant Innovations, Inc. Staff. 1997. xiii, 200p. text 100.00 (*0-9655930-0-2*) C Drago.

Implant Retrieval & Analysis. Bloebaum. 1995. 234.00 (*0-8493-6940-1*, CRC Reprint) Franklin.

Implant-Supported Prostheses: Occlusion, Clinical Cases, & Laboratory Procedures. Vicente Jimenez-Lopez & Pedro T. Lavina. 1995. LC 94-34517. Orig. Title: Prostesis Sobre Implantes. (Illus.). 256p. text 140.00 (*0-86715-257-5*) Quint Pub Co.

Implant Therapy Vol. II: Clinical Approaches & Evidence of Success. Joseph P. Fiorellini. Ed. by Myron Nevins & James T. Mellonig. 1998. LC 98-4259. (Illus.). 257p. text 128.00 (*0-86715-341-5*) Quint Pub Co.

Implantable Cardioverter - Defibrillator. Ed. by E. U. Alt et al. 1992. (Illus.). 256p. 89.00 (*0-387-53927-1*) Spr-Verlag.

Implantable Cardioverter-Defibrillator: A Practical Manual. L. Bing Liem. 2001. LC 00-51405. (Illus.). 224p. 85.00 (*0-7923-6743-X*) Kluwer Academic.

Implantable Cardioverter Defibrillator: A Videotape & Manual. Steven L. Higgins. 1997. (Illus.). 112p. 95.00 incl. VHS (*0-87993-663-0*) Futura Pub.

Implantable Cardioverter Defibrillator Therapy: The Engineering-Clinical Interface. Ed. by Mark W. Kroll. 1996. LC 96-46028. (Developments in Cardiovascular Medicine Ser.). 608p. (C). text 139.00 (*0-7923-4300-X*) Kluwer Academic.

Implantable Cardioverter-Defibrillators: A Comprehensive Text, No. 21. Ed. by Estes et al. 1994. (Fundamental & Clinical Cardiology Ser.: Vol. 21). (Illus.). 960p. text 235.00 (*0-8247-9194-0*) Dekker.

Implantable Contact Lens & Other Phakic IOLs. Carlo Lovisolo & Paolo Pesando. 1999. 386p. text (*88-87333-12-2*) Fabiano ITA. *Dist:* SLACK Inc.

Implantable Defibrillator: From Concept to Clinical Reality. L. Jordaens. 1996. LC 96-30591. (Advances in Cardiology Ser.: Vol. 38). (Illus.). xii, 168p. 118.25 (*3-8055-6221-7*) S Karger.

Implantable Drug Delivery Systems. Ed. by U. Laffer et al. 1991. (Illus.). viii, 68p. pap. 35.00 (*3-8055-5434-6*) S Karger.

Implantable Peripheral Nerve Stimulators. 2nd ed. 1995. 8p. pap. 62.00 (*1-57020-039-4*, NS15-209) Assn Adv Med Instrn.

Implantable Spinal Cord Stimulators. 2nd ed. 1995. 10p. pap. 70.00 (*0-910275-45-9*, NS14-209) Assn Adv Med Instrn.

Implantable Telemetry Systems. Ed. by H. P. Kimmich. 1981. (Biotelemetry & Patient Monitoring Journal: Vol. 8, No. 3). (Illus.). 68p. pap. 30.50 (*3-8055-3456-6*) S Karger.

Implantation & Early Pregnancy in Humans: A Combined Research & Clinical Approach. Ed. by Eytan R. Barnea et al. 1993. LC 93-34659. 506p. lib. bdg. 82.95 (*1-85070-513-5*, Parthenon Pbng) CRC Pr.

Implantation of the Ovum. Ed. by Koji Yoshinaga et al. 1976. 154p. 36.50 (*0-674-44523-6*) HUP.

Implantology. Hubertus Spiekermann. Ed. by Klaus H. Rateitschak & Herbert F. Wolf. 1995. (Color Atlas of Dental Medicine Ser.). (Illus.). 385p. 199.00 (*0-86577-561-3*) Thieme Med Pubs.

Implants & Restorative Dentistry. Gerard M. Scortecci & Carl E. Misch. 2000. 300p. (*1-85317-703-2*) Martin Dunitz GBR. *Dist:* Thieme Med Pubs.

Implants in Dentistry. Michael S. Block et al. Ed. by Judy Fletcher. 1997. LC 96-50087. 336p. text 65.00 (*0-7216-2174-0*) Saunders.

Implementation Manual for the 835 Health Care Claim-Payment - Advice. James J. Moynihan. 1992. 175p. 74.95 (*0-930228-91-X*) Hlthcare Fin Mgmt.

Implementation Manual for the 835 Health Care Claim Payment-Advice Supplement. James J. Moynihan. 1992. 40p. 50.00 (*1-882198-12-3*) Hlthcare Fin Mgmt.

Implementation Manual for the Healthcare Claim Payment Advice: Guidelines For... James Moynihan. 2nd rev. ed. 1996. 200p. (C). ring bd. 95.00 (*1-55738-625-0*, Irwn Prfssnl) McGraw-Hill Educ Grp.

Implementation of the Global Malaria Control Strategy: Report of a WHO Study Group on the Implementation of the Global Plan of Action for Malaria Control 1993-2000. 1993. (Technical Reports: No. 839). (ENG, FRE & SPA.). v, 57p. pap. text 10.00 (*92-4-120839-2*, 1100839) World Health.

Implementation of the Global Strategy for Health for All by the Year 2000: Eighth Report on the World Health Situation : Eastern Mediterranean Region, 6. 1996. pap. text 9.00 (*92-4-160286-4*) World Health.

Implementation of the Global Strategy for Health for All by the Year 2000, Second Evaluation Vol. 2: African Region. 1994. (ENG & FRE.). x, 252p. pap. text 18.00 (*92-4-160282-1*, 1232008) World Health.

Implementation of the Global Strategy for Health for All by the Year 2000, Second Evaluation Vol. 3: Region of the Americas. 1993. (ENG, FRE & SPA.). v, 125p. pap. text 26.00 (*92-4-160283-X*, 1233008) World Health.

Implementation of the Global Strategy for Health for All by the Year 2000, Second Evaluation Vol. 4: South-East Asia Region. 1993. ix, 197p. pap. text 20.00 (*92-4-160284-8*, 1234008) World Health.

Implementation of the Global Strategy for Health for All by the Year 2000, Second Evaluation Vol. 5: European Region. 1994. (ENG & FRE.). vi, 289p. pap. text 55.00 (*92-4-160285-6*, 1235008) World Health.

Implementation of the Global Strategy for Health for All by the Year 2000, Second Evaluation Vol. 7: Western Pacific Region. 1993. vii, 204p. pap. text 22.00 (*92-4-160287-2*, 1237008) World Health.

Implementing a Physican Organization. American Medical Association Staff. 1996. LC 98-147772. 72p. pap. 68.95 (*0-89970-733-5*, OP601695WE) AMA.

Implementing an Effective Customer Relations Program. Eric Joseph. 1994. 86p. (Orig.). pap. text 20.00 (*0-916499-59-6*) Care Educ Grp.

Implementing Change in the NHS: A Practical Guide for General Managers. F. Barwell & Peter Spurgeon. 1990. (HSMC Health Service Management Ser.). 256p. (C). pap. text (*0-412-37640-7*, A5658) Chapman & Hall.

Implementing Change with Clinical Audit. Richard Baker. 1999. LC 98-35855. 200p. pap. 39.95 (*0-471-98257-1*) Wiley.

Implementing Clinical Practice Guidelines: Strategies for Effective Implementation. Carmi Z. Margolis. 1998. LC 98-19064. (Illus.). 223p. 48.00 (*1-55648-237-X*) AHPI.

***Implementing Community Oriented Teaching in Medical Education: A Case from Vietnam.** Ed. by D. Burck & T. Bach. 2001. 80p. pap. (*90-6832-837-9*) Royal Tropical NLD. *Dist:* Stylus Pub VA.

Implementing Continuous Eligibility: Costs & Considerations. unabr. ed. 1999. 20p. pap. (*1-929008-16-3*) CA HlthCare Fnd.

Implementing Differentiated Nursing Practice: Transformation by Design. JoEllen Koerner & Kathryn L. Karpiuk. 1994. LC 93-34421. 352p. 79.00 (*0-8342-0569-6*, 20569) Aspen Pub.

Implementing Early Intervention: From Research to Effective Practice. Ed. by Donna M. Bryant & Mimi A. Graham. 1993. LC 93-30813. 358p. 44.00 (*0-89862-247-6*) Guilford Pubns.

Implementing GP Fundholding: Wild Card or Winning Hand? Howard Glennerster et al. 1994. LC 94-27679. (State of Health Ser.). 160p. (*0-335-19334-X*); pap. (*0-335-19108-8*) OpUniv Pr.

Implementing Health Care Information. 1988. (Illus.). 438p. 87.00 (*0-387-96690-0*) Spr-Verlag.

Implementing Health Policy. Meera Chatterjee. 1988. 324p. (C). (*81-85054-36-3*) Manohar IND. *Dist:* S Asia.

Implementing International Drug, Device, & Diagnostic GMPs: A Practical Guide. Carol De Sain & Charmaine Vercimak. 1994. 273p. 139.00 (*0-935184-53-8*) IHS Health Grp.

Implementing International Good Practices: GAPs, GCPs, GLPs, & GMPs. Ed. by Nigel J. Dent. 1993. (Illus.). 273p. 169.00 (*0-935184-44-9*) IHS Health Grp.

Implementing Planned Markets in Health Care: Balancing Social & Economic Responsibilities. Ed. by Casten Von Otter & Richard B. Saltman. 1995. LC 94-44777. (State of Health Ser.). 272p. (*0-335-19426-5*) Univ Pr.

Implementing Problem-Based Medical Education: Lessons from Successful Innovations. Arthur Kaufman. 1985. 304p. 38.95 (*0-8261-4660-0*) Springer Pub.

Implementing Quality Assurance. Paul Bozzo. 1991. LC 90-42512. 180p. 35.00 (*0-89189-290-7*) Am Soc Clinical.

Implementing Quality Management Health Care. Koch. Date not set. text (*0-582-20903-X*) Addison-Wesley GBR. *Dist:* Trans-Atl Phila.

Implementing TQM in Primary Care: Paradigms & Piranhas. P. Townes & D. Benson. 1996. (Quality Primary Care Ser.). 400p. pap. 59.00 (*1-884742-03-3*) Clarian Hlth.

Implication of Individual & Small Group Learning Systems in Medical Education: Proceedings of the WHO Scientific Group, Geneva, 1971. WHO Staff. 1972. (Technical Reports: No. 489). pap. text 6.00 (*92-4-120489-3*, 1100489) World Health.

Implications for Effective Psychotherapy with African-American Families & Individuals. Jay T. Willis. 1990. LC 89-92511. 134p. (Orig.). pap. 15.95 (*0-9618486-2-6*) J T Willis.

Implications of AIDS for Children in Care. Ed. by D. Batty. 1989. (C). (*0-903534-72-X*) Brit Ag for Adopt & Fost GBR. *Dist:* St Mut.

Implications of Gag Proteins for the Life Cycle of the Immunodeficiency Virus. Ed. by A. G. Bukrinskaya. 1996. (Soviet Medical Reviews Series, Section E: Virology Review: Vol. 5, Pt. 4). 140p. pap. text 69.00 (*3-7186-5759-7*, Harwood Acad Pubs) Gordon & Breach.

Implications of Genetics for Health Professional Education. Ed. by Mary Hager. 1999. (*0-9614362-0-4*) J Macy Foun.

Implications of New Data on Radiation Cancer Risk: Proceedings of the Thirty-Second Annual Meeting, 3-4 April 1996, As Presented at the Crystal City Marriott, Arlington, Va. National Council on Radiation Protection and Measure & John D. Boice. 1997. LC 97-3044. (Proceedings Ser.: Vol. 18). (Illus.). 314p. (Orig.). pap. 45.00 (*0-929600-55-X*) NCRP Pubns.

Implications of Psychopharmacology to Psychiatry: Biological, Nosological, & Therapeutical Concepts. Ed. by M. Ackenheil et al. 1995. (Illus.). 208p. 86.95 (*3-540-60533-9*) Spr-Verlag.

Implications of the Americans with Disabilities Act for Psychology. Ed. by Susanne M. Bruyere & Janet O'Keefe. 1994. LC 93-39427. 256p. pap. text 33.95 (*0-8261-8450-2*) Springer Pub.

Implications of the Blood-Brain Barrier & Its Manipulation: Basic Science Aspects, Vol. 1. E. A. Neuwelt. 1989. (Illus.). 434p. (C). text 110.00 (*0-306-42628-5*, Kluwer Plenum) Kluwer Academic.

Implicit & Explicit Mental Processes. Ed. by Kim Kirsner et al. 1997. LC 97-7356. 400p. (*0-8058-1359-4*) L Erlbaum Assocs.

Implicit Memory: New Directions in Cognition, Development, & Neuropsychology. Ed. by Peter Graf & Michael E. Masson. 1993. 376p. pap. 45.00 (*0-8058-1116-8*); text 89.95 (*0-8058-1115-X*) L Erlbaum Assocs.

Implicit Review Method for Measuring the Quality of In-Hospital Nursing Care of Elderly Cerebrovascular Accident Patients. Marjorie L. Pearson et al. 1997. LC 98-110399. pap. 13.00 (*0-8330-2563-5*) Rand Corp.

Import of Medical Devices: A Workshop Manual. 1995. lib. bdg. 251.95 (*0-8490-7562-9*); 1994. lib. bdg. 295.00 (*0-8490-5748-5*) Gordon Pr.

Importance & Applications of Patient Origin Information in Health Planning. United Hospital Fund Staff. 1980. 50p. 10.00 (*0-934459-24-X*) United Hosp Fund.

Importance of Animal Experimentation for Safety & Biomedical Research. Ed. by Silvio Garattini. 1990. (C). text 160.00 (*0-7923-0514-0*) Kluwer Academic.

Importance of Disappointment. Ian Craib. 1994. LC 94-5593. 256p. (C). pap. 26.95 (*0-415-09383-X*, B4585) Routledge.

Importance of Good Nutrition for Your Health, Good Looks & Longevity. Getty T. Ambau. 1993. (Illus.). 432p. (Orig.). pap. 19.95 (*1-884459-00-5*) Falcon Pr Intl.

H I

Importance of Haemorheologic Aspects in the Diagnosis & Treatment of Ischaemic Cerebrovascular Disease. Ed. by H. Lechner. 1983. (Journal: Vol. 22, Suppl. 1). (Illus.). iv, 132p. pap. 34.00 (*3-8055-3731-X*) S Karger.

***Importance of Monocyte & Granulocyte Activation in Rheumatoid Arthritis & Primary Sjogren's Syndrome.** Ingunn Torsteindottir. 1999. (Comprehensive Summaries of Uppsala Dissertations from the Faculty of Medicine Ser.: No. 869). (Illus.). 60p. pap. (*91-554-4554-3*) Uppsala Universitet SWE. *Dist:* Coronet Bks.

Importance of Observation & Documentation. Jetta Fuzy. 1998. (Illus.). 65p. pap. 29.95 (*1-888343-13-3*) Hartman Pub.

Importance of Prostacyclin & Potassium Channels for the Regulation of Vascular Tone. Ed. by J. C. Frolich & U. Forestermann. 1990. (Clinical Pharmacology Ser.: Vol. 7). (Illus.). 168p. text (*3-88603-383-X*) W Zuckschwerdt DEU. *Dist:* Scholium Intl.

Importation into the United States of the Parasites of the Gypsy Moth & the Brown-Tail Moth: Report of Progress of Previous & Concurrent Efforts of This Kind. Leland O. Howard & William F. Fiske. Ed. by Frank N. Egerton, 3rd. 1978. LC 77-74230. (History of Ecology Ser.). (Illus.). reprint ed. lib. bdg. 35.95 (*0-405-10400-6*) Ayer.

Imported Virus Infections. Ed. by T. E. Schwarz & Gunter Siegl. 1996. (Illus.). 216p. 150.00 (*3-211-82870-2*) Spr-Verlag.

Imported Virus Infections. Tino F. Schwarz & Gunter Siegl. 1996. LC 96-8183. (Archives of Virology Ser.). 143.00 (*3-211-82829-X*) Spr-Verlag.

Impossible Child see Nino Insoportable

***Impotence: A Guide for Men of All Ages.** Philip Kell & Wallace Dinsmore. 2001. 68p. pap. (*1-85315-402-4*) Royal Soc of Medicine Pr Ltd GBR. *Dist:* Balogh.

Impotence: An Integrated Approach to Clinical Practice. Ed. by Alain Gregoire & John J. Pryor. 1993. LC 92-13582. (Illus.). 232p. text (*0-443-04369-8*) Church.

Impotence: Index of Modern Information. Alexander D. Farrell. rev. ed. 1991. 47.50 (*1-55914-354-1*); pap. 44.50 (*1-55914-355-X*) ABBE Pubs Assn.

Impotence: It's Curable. Steven K. Wilson & Neil Baum. 1998. (Illus.). 143p. 18.50 (*1-890018-29-5*) Anadem Pubng.

Impotence: Physiological, Psychological, & Surgical Diagnosis & Treatment. Gorm Wagner & Richard Green. 1981. LC 81-15688. (Perspectives in Sexuality Ser.). 192p. 35.00 (*0-306-40719-1*, Plenum Trade) Perseus Pubng.

Impotence & Infertility. Marc Goldstein & Tom F. Lue. 1999. LC 98-10894. (Atlas of Clinical Urology Ser.: Vol. 1). (Illus.). 124.95 (*1-57340-119-6*) Current Med.

Impotence in the Male Wilhelm Stekel. rev. ed. 1959. LC 78-149627. (C). reprint ed. 12.00 (*0-87140-842-2*) Liveright.

Impotence Sourcebook. Christopher P. Steidle. 1999. (Illus.). 192p. pap. 15.95 (*0-7373-0252-6*, 02526w) NTC Contemp Pub Co.

Imprisoned Pain & Its Transformation. Ed. by Joan Symington. 2000. 256p. pap. (*1-85575-243-3*) Karnac Bks GBR. *Dist:* Other Pr LLC.

Improvability: Its Intercorrelations & Its Relations to Initial Ability. Henrietta V. Race. LC 73-177176. (Columbia University. Teachers College. Contributions to Education Ser.: No. 124). reprint ed. 37.50 (*0-404-55124-6*) AMS Pr.

Improve, Perfect & Perpetuate: Dr. Nathan Smith & Early American Medical Education. Oliver S. Hayward & Constance E. Putnam. 1998. LC 97-47155. (Illus.). 387p. lib. bdg. 40.00 (*0-87451-860-1*) U Pr of New Eng.

Improve Your Eyesight: A Guide to the Bates Method for Better Eyesight Without Glasses. Jonathan Barnes. 2000. (Illus.). 120p. pap. (*0-285-63508-5*) Souvenir Pr Ltd GBR. *Dist:* IPG Chicago.

Improve Your Eyesight: Vision Therapy Eye Exercises-Updates Bates Method. 2000. 107p. per. 44.95 incl. VHS (*0-9700150-0-3*) Avid Reader.

Improve Your Odds Against Cancer: What Everyone Should Know. John Potter. 1992. mass mkt. 4.50 (*1-56171-076-8*) SPI.

Improve Your Vision Without Glasses or Contact Lenses. Steven M. Beresford et al. 1996. LC 96-22038. 128p. per. 11.00 (*0-684-81438-2*) S&S Trade.

Improvement of Myocardial Perfusion. Ed. by J. Meyer et al. 1985. (Developments in Cardiovascular Medicine Ser.). lib. bdg. 193.00 (*0-89838-748-5*) Kluwer Academic.

Improvements in Dialysis Therapy. Ed. by C. A. Baldamus et al. 1990. (Contributions to Nephrology Ser.: Vol. 74). (Illus.). viii, 242p. 29.75 (*3-8055-4981-4*) S Karger.

Improving Access to Health Care: What Can the States Do? Ed. by John H. Goddeeris & Andrew J. Hogan. 1992. LC 92-5205. 273p. pap. text 19.00 (*0-88099-118-6*) W E Upjohn.

Improving Access to Health Services for Children & Pregnant Women. Joshua M. Wiener & Jeannie Engel. 1991. (Dialogues on Public Policy Ser.). 90p. (C). pap. text 10.95 (*0-8157-9375-8*) Brookings.

Improving Accountability in Medicare Managed Care: The Consumer's Need for Better Information. Ed. by Charles E. Grassley. 1998. (Illus.). 135p. (C). pap. text 25.00 (*0-7881-7251-4*) DIANE Pub.

Improving America's Diet & Health: From Recommendations to Action. Institute of Medicine Staff. Ed. by Paul R. Thomas. 1991. 256p. 29.95 (*0-309-04139-2*) Natl Acad Pr.

Improving & Evaluating Board Performance. Barry S. Bader & Richard J. Umbdenstock. Ed. by Mellen Candage. 1986. (Illus.). 84p. (Orig.). pap. text 12.00 (*0-915963-01-9*) Bader Assoc Inc.

***Improving Care at the End of Life with Complete Mentary Medicine: Congressional Hearing.** Dan Burton. 2001. 194p. (C). pap. text 35.00 (*0-7567-1819-8*) DIANE Pub.

Improving Care in the Nursing Home: Comprehensive Reviews of Clinical Research. Ed. by Laurence Z. Rubenstein & Darryl Wieland. 1993. (Illus.). 296p. (C). 67.95 (*0-8039-4306-7*, 3433); pap. 34.95 (*0-8039-4307-5*, 3434) Sage.

Improving Children's Lives: Global Perspectives on Prevention. George W. Albee et al. 1992. (Primary Prevention of Psychopathology Ser.: Vol. 14). (Illus.). 416p. (C). 74.95 (*0-8039-4610-4*, 7396) Sage.

Improving Clinical Outcomes with New ABR & OPOAE Techniques. Michael Gorga & David Stapells. 1998. 126p. 48.00 incl. audio (*1-58041-023-5*, 0112144) Am Speech Lang Hearing.

Improving Consensus Development for Health Technology Assessment: An International Perspective. Council on Health Care Technology Institute of Med. Ed. by Clifford Goodman & Sharon R. Baratz. 1990. 176p. pap. text 15.00 (*0-309-04239-9*) Natl Acad Pr.

Improving Doctor Performance: A Study in the Use of Information & Organizational Change. Steven Kelman. 1980. LC 79-21211. (Center for Policy Research Monographs: Vol. 1). 349p. 45.95 (*0-87705-444-4*, Kluwer Acad Hman Sci) Kluwer Academic.

Improving Drug Safety: A Joint Responsibility. Ed. by R. Dinkel et al. 1991. (Health Systems Research Ser.). (Illus.). 338p. 79.95 (*0-387-53505-5*) Spr-Verlag.

Improving Family Planning Evaluation: A Step-by-Step Guide for Managers & Evaluators. Jose Garcia-Nunez. 1992. LC 92-8193. (Library of Management for Development). (Illus.). xvii, 187p. (Orig.). (C). pap. 18.95 (*1-56549-015-0*) Kumarian Pr.

Improving Function in Dementia & Other Cognitive-Linguistic Disorders: A Guide & Resource Book. Kathryn A. Bayles & Cheryl K. Tomoeda. 1997. (Illus.). (C). pap. text 79.00 (*0-9639381-3-4*) Canyonlnds Pubng.

Improving Genetic Disease Resistance in Farm Animals. Ed. by A. J. Van der Zijpp & Watse Sybesma. 1989. (Current Topics in Veterinary Medicine & Animal Science Ser.). (C). text 132.50 (*0-7923-0518-3*) Kluwer Academic.

Improving Health & Welfare Work with Families in Poverty, a Handbook. Clare Blackburn. 1992. LC 91-46006. 119p. pap. (*0-335-09732-4*, RA418) OpUniv Pr.

Improving Health Care for Veterans: 1997 Annual Report. Ed. by John R. Feussner. 1999. (Illus.). 49p. reprint ed. pap. text 20.00 (*0-7881-7870-9*) DIANE Pub.

Improving Health-Care Management in the Workplace. Jerome M. Rosow & Robert Zager. 1985. 162p. 19.25 (*0-08-032797-4*) Work in Amer.

Improving Health Care of the Poor: The New York City Experience. Eli Ginzberg et al. 1997. LC 96-41534. 167p. 32.95 (*1-56000-288-3*) Transaction Pubs.

Improving Health in the Community: A Role for Performance Monitoring. Institute of Medicine Staff. Ed. by Jane S. Durch et al. 1997. LC 97-6336. 496p. (C). text 49.95 (*0-309-05534-2*) Natl Acad Pr.

Improving Health Policy & Management: Nine Critical Research Issues for the 1990s. Ed. by Stephen M. Shortell & Uwe E. Reinhardt. 1992. LC 92-1436. 505p. pap. 42.00 (*1-56793-027-1*, 0898) Health Admin Pr.

Improving Mobility in Older Persons: A Manual for Geriatric Specialists. Carole B. Lewis. 1997. LC 88-24244. (Aspen Series in Physical Therapy Ser.). (Illus.). 172p. (C). spiral bd. 68.00 (*0-8342-0020-1*) PRO-ED.

Improving Newborn Health in Developing Countries. Anthony Costello. 1998. LC 99-30272. (Illus.). xxxii, 570p. (*1-86094-097-8*) Imperial College GBR. *Dist:* World Scientific Pub.

Improving Nursing Performance. Timothy P. Williams & Mary E. Geary. 1997. LC 97-23917. 106p. pap. 40.00 (*0-944496-56-3*) Precept Pr.

***Improving Outcomes in Chronic Heart Failure.** Stewart. 2001. 176p. pap. (*0-7279-1602-5*) BMJ Pub.

***Improving Outcomes in Chronic Heart Failure with Specialist Nurse Intervention: A Practical Guide.** Ed. by Simon Stewart & Lynda Blue. 2001. (Illus.). 150p. pap. text (*0-7279-1591-6*) BMJ Pub GBR. *Dist:* AIDC.

Improving Outcomes in Heart Failure: An Interdisciplinary Approch. Debra K. Moser & Barbara J. Riegel. 2000. LC 00-63958. 371p. 87.00 (*0-8342-1644-2*, 16442) Aspen Pub.

Improving Patient Adherence to Tuberculosis Treatment. Ed. by Barry Leonard. rev. ed. 2000. 55p. (C). reprint ed. pap. text 20.00 (*0-7567-0092-2*) DIANE Pub.

Improving Patient Satisfaction Now: How to Earn Patient & Payer Loyalty. Anne-Marie Nelson et al. 2nd ed. 1997. LC 97-7706. 336p. 72.00 (*0-8342-0922-5*, 20922) Aspen Pub.

Improving Productivity in Health Care. J. H. Brown & Jacqueline Comola. 1988. 208p. 132.00 (*0-8493-6911-8*, RA10, CRC Reprint) Franklin.

Improving Psychological Services for Children & Adolescents with Severe Mental Disorders: Clinical Training in Psychology. Ed. by Phyllis R. Magrab & Paul Wohlford. 1990. LC 89-82575. 200p. pap. text 19.95 (*1-55798-080-2*) Am Psychol.

***Improving Public Health.** 2002. (*0-85323-337-3*) Liverpool Univ Pr GBR. *Dist:* Intl Spec Bk.

Improving Quality: A Guide to Effective Programs. Claire G. Meisenheimer. 2nd ed. 1997. LC 97-5136. 752p. 79.00 (*0-8342-0910-1*) Aspen Pub.

Improving Residential Life for Disabled People. Keith Tully. 1987. (Illus.). 272p. pap. (*0-443-03525-3*) Church.

Improving Risk Communication. National Research Council Staff. 1989. 352p. (C). pap. text 29.95 (*0-309-03943-6*) Natl Acad Pr.

Improving Staff Effectiveness in Human Service Settings: Organizational Behavior Management Approaches. Ed. by Lee W. Frederiksen & Anne W. Riley. 1984. LC 84-722. (Journal of Organizational Behavior Management: Vol. 5, Nos. 3-4). 195p. text 49.95 (*0-86656-282-6*) Haworth Pr.

Improving Staff Motivation & Competence in the General Hospital, Pt. 2. Esther L. Brown. 1962. 194p. pap. 19.95 (*0-87154-184-X*) Russell Sage.

Improving State Law to Prevent & Treat Infectious Disease. Lawrence O. Gostin et al. 1998. LC 98-124740. pap. (*1-887748-17-2*) Milbank Memorial.

***Improving Substance Abuse Treatment: The National Treatment Plan Initiative.** Frwd. by Nelba R. Chavez & H. Westley Clark. 2001. 54p. (C). pap. 25.00 (*0-7567-0999-7*) DIANE Pub.

Improving the Doctor-Patient Relationship. Fernando Siles & Carmen Richards. 1995. pap. 11.95 (*0-933025-41-6*) Blue Bird Pub.

Improving the Long-Range Effects of Psychotherapy: Models of Durable Outcome. Ed. by Paul Karoly & John J. Steffen. 1980. text 39.95 (*0-89876-047-X*) Gardner Pr.

Improving the Long-Term Management of Obesity: Theory, Research, & Clinical Guidelines. Michael G. Perri et al. 1992. LC 92-92. (Health Psychology & Behavioral Medicine Ser.). 320p. 160.00 (*0-471-52899-4*) Wiley.

Improving the Medicare Market: Adding Choice & Protections. Institute of Medicine Staff. Ed. by Stanley B. Jones & Marion E. Lewin. 1996. LC 96-42908. 384p. (C). text 49.95 (*0-309-05535-0*) Natl Acad Pr.

Improving the Public's Health Through Research Partnerships: Building Bridges IV, 1998, Conference Proceedings. Ed. by Larry S. Stepnick et al. 1999. (Illus.). 145p. (C). pap. text 30.00 (*0-7881-8375-3*) DIANE Pub.

Improving the Quality of Patient Care. Alan Gillies. 1997. LC 96-25143. 230p. pap. 54.95 (*0-471-96647-9*) Wiley.

Improving the Quality of the Medication Use Process: Error Prevention & Reducing Adverse Drug Events. Alan Escovitz et al. 1998. LC 98-12035. (Illus.). 228p. lib. bdg. 49.95 (*0-7890-0458-5*) Haworth Pr.

Improving the Regulatory Review Process: Assessing Performance & Setting Targets. Ed. by Neil McAuslane & Stuart R. Walker. 1998. LC 98-147056. (Centre for Medicines Research Workshop Ser.). 392p. 97.00 (*0-7923-8731-7*) Kluwer Academic.

Improving Therapeutic Communication: A Guide for Developing Effective Techniques. D. Corydon Hammond et al. 1977. LC 76-50704. (Social & Behavioral Science Ser.). (Illus.). 400p. 70.00 (*0-87589-308-2*) Jossey-Bass.

Improving Transfusion Practice for Pediatric Patients. Susan M. Wilson et al. 1991. LC 91-31040. (Illus.). 93p. (C). text 7.00 (*1-56395-003-0*) Am Assn Blood.

Improving Treatment for Drug-Exposed Infants: A Treatment Improvement Protocol. 1994. (Illus.). 93p. (Orig.). (C). pap. text 35.00 (*0-7881-1163-9*) DIANE Pub.

Improving Upper Body Control. Boehme. 1998. (Illus.). 210p. (C). pap. text 58.00 (*0-12-784579-8*) Acad Pr.

Improving Vocational Rehabilitation Outcomes: Opportunities for Early Intervention. John A. Gardner. 1988. LC 88-14213. 35.00 (*0-935149-14-7*, WC-88-3) Workers Comp Res Inst.

Improving Women's Health Services in the Russian Federation: Results of a Pilot Program. Patricia Stephenson et al. 1998. LC 98-14708. (Technical Paper Ser.: No. 404). 50p. pap. 22.00 (*0-8213-4197-9*, 14197) World Bank.

Improving World Health: A Least-cost Strategy. William U. Chandler. 1984. LC 84-51598. (Worldwatch Papers). pap. 5.00 (*0-916468-59-3*) Worldwatch Inst.

Improvisational Models of Music Therapy. Kenneth E. Bruscia. 1987. (Illus.). 606p. (C). text 101.95 (*0-398-05272-7*) C C Thomas.

Improvisational Therapy: A Practical Guide for Creative Clinical Strategies. Bradford P. Keeney. 1991. LC 91-74164. 123p. reprint ed. pap. 20.00 (*0-89862-486-X*) Guilford Pubns.

Improvisational Therapy: A Practical Guide for Creative Clinical Strategies. Bradford P. Keeney. 1990. LC 90-70423. 123p. pap. text 18.00 (*0-9626461-0-5*) Systemic Therapy.

Impulsive Client: Theory, Research, & Treatment. Ed. by William G. McCown et al. 1993. LC 93-11911. (Illus.). 434p. text 49.95 (*1-55798-208-2*) Am Psychol.

Impulsive Personality: Understanding People with Destructive Character Disorders. Howard A. Wishnie. 1977. LC 77-23464. (Illus.). 226p. (C). 51.00 (*0-306-30973-4*, Plenum Trade) Perseus Pubng.

Impulsivity: Theory, Assessment & Treatment. Ed. by Christopher D. Webster & Margaret A. Jackson. 1997. LC 97-20961. 462p. text 53.00 (*1-57230-225-9*, C0225) Guilford Pubns.

Impulsivity & Agression. Ed. by E. Hollander et al. 1995. LC 94-27712. 382p. 195.00 (*0-471-95328-8*) Wiley.

Impulsivity & Compulsivity. Ed. by John M. Oldham et al. 1996. 306p. text 42.00 (*0-88048-676-7*, 8676) Am Psychiatric.

Impure Science: AIDS, Activism, & the Politics of Knowledge. Steven Epstein. 1996. LC 96-16805. (Medicine & Society Ser.: No. 7). (Illus.). 480p. text 40.00 (*0-520-20233-3*) U CA Pr.

Impurities Evaluation of Pharmaceuticals. Satinder Ahuja. 1998. LC 98-5185. (Illus.). 304p. text 150.00 (*0-8247-9884-8*) Dekker.

Imputation of Employer Information for the 1996 Medical Expenditure Panel Survey Insurance Component. John Paul Sommers. 2000. 12p. (*1-58763-004-4*) Agency Healthcare.

Imunne Tolerance. J. Banchereau et al. 1996. 264p. pap. 49.00 (*2-906077-92-5*) Elsevier.

In a Different Voice: Psychological Theory & Women's Development. Carol Gilligan. 1982. LC 81-13478. 240p. 29.95 (*0-674-44543-0*); 1993. LC 93-243596. 204p. pap. text 12.00 (*0-674-44544-9*) HUP.

In a House of Dreams & Glass. Robert Klitzman. 1995. LC 94-31801. 366p. 24.00 (*0-671-73450-4*) S&S Trade.

In a House of Dreams & Glass: Becoming a Psychiatrist. Robert Klitzman. 1996. LC 95-95318. 333p. mass mkt. 5.99 (*0-8041-1436-6*) Ivy Books.

In a Tangled Wood: An Alzheimer's Journey. Joyce Dyer. 1996. LC 96-11354. 184p. pap. 12.95 (*0-87074-397-X*) SMU Press.

In a Time of Fallen Heroes: The Re-Creation of Masculinity. R. William Betcher & William S. Pollack. 1995. 288p. pap. 16.95 (*0-89862-844-X*, C2844) Guilford Pubns.

In a World of Their Own: Experiencing Unconsciousness. Madelaine Lawrence. 1998. LC 96-25076. 200p. pap. 20.95 (*0-89789-650-5*, Bergin & Garvey) Greenwood.

In All Our Affairs: Making Crises Work for You. 1990. LC 90-84512. 256p. pap. 10.00 (*0-910034-73-7*) Al-Anon.

In & Out of Harm's Way: A History of the Navy Nurse Corps. Doris M. Sterner. 2nd ed. 1998. LC 96-72362. 390p. pap. text 24.95 (*0-89716-706-6*) P B Pubng.

In Changing Times: Gay Men & Lesbians Encounter HIV-AIDS. Ed. by Martin P. Levine. 1997. LC 97-3414. 248p. lib. bdg. 55.00 (*0-226-27856-5*); (Illus.). pap. text 17.95 (*0-226-27857-3*) U Ch Pr.

In Charge of the Ward. Arline Matthews & Janet Welan. 3rd ed. 1993. LC 93-25221. 288p. pap. 36.95 (*0-632-03448-3*) Blackwell Sci.

In Cold Pursuit: Medical Intelligence Investigates the Common Cold. J. Barnard Gilmore. 1999. 320p. 24.95 (*0-7737-3119-9*) General Distrib Services.

In Commemoration of William James, 1842-1942. William James. reprint ed. 20.00 (*0-404-03550-7*) AMS Pr.

In Control: A Cancer Victim Describes His Struggle to Gain Control of His Mind & Body. Frederick A. Hesketh. LC 95-46545. 177p. 1998. 34.00 (*1-56072-285-1*); 1996. pap. 17.45 (*1-56072-272-X*, Nova Kroshka Bks) Nova Sci Pubs.

In Control: A Guide for Teens with Diabetes. Jean Betschart. 1995. (Juvenile Diabetes Foundation Library). 128p. (gr. 7-13). pap. 10.95 (*0-471-34742-6*) Wiley.

In Darkness & in Light: A Physician's Journey into Spiritual Healing. Lesley B. Heafitz. 1994. 96p. 12.95 (*0-9635307-3-9*) First Prsn Pr.

In Defense of Heterosexuality. Stanley Keleman. 1982. LC 82-83644. 97p. pap. 6.95 (*0-934320-06-3*) Center Pr.

In Defense of Human Consciousness. Joseph F. Rychlak. 1997. LC 97-3877. (Illus.). 351p. text 29.95 (*1-55798-421-2*, 431-6880) Am Psychol.

In Defense of Life. Antonio R. Saqueton. 1981. LC 81-69801. 232p. 24.95 (*0-941616-01-0*) ARS Pub.

In Defense of Narcissism: The Creative Self in Search of Meaning. Carl Goldberg. 1980. LC 80-15385. 224p. text 29.95 (*0-89876-005-4*) Gardner Pr.

In Defense of Schreber: Soul Murder & Psychiatry. Zvi Lothane. 1992. LC 92-16302. 568p. text 65.00 (*0-88163-103-5*) Analytic Pr.

In Defense of the Brain: Immunopathogenesis of Infection of the CNS. Phillip K. Peterson & Jack S. Remington. 1997. LC 97-4121. (Illus.). 384p. 95.00 (*0-86542-555-8*) Blackwell Sci.

In Defense of the Psychological. John W. Miller. 1985. 192p. reprint ed. pap. 6.50 (*0-393-30226-1*) Norton.

In-Depth Look at the Medical Furniture Market: Special Needs of an Aging Population Spur Growth. 1992. 235p. 1495.00 (*1-56753-023-0*) Frost & Sullivan.

In Dora's Case. Charles Bernheimer & Claire Kahane. 2nd ed. 1990. LC 90-1460. (Gender & Culture Ser.). 344p. pap. text 19.50 (*0-231-07221-X*) Col U Pr.

H I

In God's Hand: One Woman's Experience with Breast Cancer. Becky L. Wecksler & Michael Wecksler. 1989. LC 88-35807. 112p. (Orig.). pap. 7.99 (*0-8361-3492-3*) Herald Press.

In God's Shadow: The Collaboration of Victor White & C. G. Jung. Ann C. Lammers. 1994. LC 94-15329. (Jung & Spirituality Ser.). 352p. pap. 19.95 (*0-8091-3489-6*) Paulist Pr.

In Good Conscience: Abortion & Moral Necessity. David Mall. 1982. LC 82-9918. xii, 212p. pap. 10.00 (*0-9608410-0-8*) Kairos Bks.

In Health & in Sickness: Pharmacy, Pharmacists & the Pharmaceutical Industry in Late Imperial, Early Soviet Russia. Mary S. Conroy. 1994. LC 94-70069. viii, 702p. 62.00 (*0-88033-283-2*, 386) East Eur Monographs.

In Her Lifetime: Female Morbidity & Mortality in Sub-Saharan Africa. Institute of Medicine Staff. Ed. by Christopher P. Howson et al. 1996. LC 95-72800. 320p. (Orig.). pap. text 37.00 (*0-309-05430-3*) Natl Acad Pr.

In Her Own Right: The Institute of Medicine's Guide to Women's Health Issues. Beryl L. Benderly & Institute of Medicine Staff. 1997. LC 96-26155. 232p. 29.95 (*0-309-05327-7*) Natl Acad Pr.

In Her Own Words: Oral Histories of Women Physicians, 8. Ed. by Regina M. Morantz et al. 1982. LC 81-13349. (Contributions in Medical History Ser.: No. 8.). (Illus.). 284p. 67.00 (*0-313-22686-5*, MHO/, Greenwood Pr) Greenwood.

In Her Prime: A New View of Middle-Aged Women. Ed. by Judith K. Brown & Virginia Kerns. 1985. (Illus.). 240p. (C). 39.95 (*0-89789-056-6*, Bergin & Garvey) Greenwood.

In-Home Alzheimer's Screening Test (I-HAST) Roe E. Markin. l.t. ed. 1999. (Illus.). 40p. 29.95 (*0-9615223-2-1*) Flaming Hooker Pr.

In-Home Assessment of Older Adults: An Interdisciplinary Approach. Charles A. Emlet et al. 1997. 224p. pap. 58.00 (*0-8342-0681-1*) PRO-ED.

***In-Home Assessment of Older Adults: Interdisciplinary Approach.** Condon. 2nd ed. 1998. 55.00 (*0-8342-1943-3*) PRO-ED.

In-Home Breastfeeding Support Program: Guide for Training Breastfeeding Counselors: Teaching Materials, Vols. 1 & 2. Susan S. Baker et al. l.t. ed. 1997. 168.00 (*0-9659498-0-X*); 168.00 (*0-9659498-1-8*) N C Coop Ext.

In Honor of Women: A Revolutionary Approach to Preventing Breast Cancer. Stella T. Crawley. 1998. LC 98-96011. (Illus.). 320p. pap. 13.95 (*0-345-42513-8*) Ballantine Pub Grp.

In Hospital & Camp: The Civil War Through the Eyes of Its Doctors & Nurses. Harold E. Straubing. 1993. LC 92-25328. 176p. 16.95 (*0-8117-1631-7*) Stackpole.

In Memorian Prof. Dr. Med. Werner Lierse. Ed. by J. Sievers. 1994. (Journal: Vol. 150, No. 1, 1994). (Illus.). 86p. pap. 97.50 (*3-8055-6024-9*) S Karger.

In No Time at All: Healing with Past Life Regression. Mona Feirson. vii, 200p. 1998. spiral bd. 14.99 (*0-9661982-2-0*); Vol. 1. Date not set. mass mkt. 19.95 (*0-9661982-1-2*) Ensoulment Educ.

In Our Own Hands: A Book of Self-Help Therapy. Sheila Ernst & Lucy Goodison. 1997. pap. (*0-7043-3841-6*) Womens Press GBR. *Dist:* Trafalgar.

In Our Own Words: Readings on the Psychology of Women & Gender. Mary Crawford & Rhoda K. Unger. 1996. LC 96-38653. 350p. (C). pap. 33.44 (*0-07-065929-X*) McGrw-H Hghr Educ.

In-Patient Physiotherapy: Management of Orthopaedic Surgery. Lucinda Chipchase & Scott A. Brumby. 2001. (Illus.). 176p. pap. text 29.95 (*0-7506-4459-1*) Buttrwrth-Heinemann.

In-Patient Treatment for Alcoholism. H. Kufner & W. Feuerlein. 1989. (Illus.). 381p. 99.00 (*0-387-50698-5*) Spr-Verlag.

In Pity & in Anger: A Study of the Use of Animals in Science. John Vyvyan. Ed. & Comment by Roberta Kalechofsky. 1988. LC 86-33231. (Illus.). 178p. reprint ed. pap. 10.00 (*0-916288-21-8*) Micah Pubns.

In-Plant Practices for Job Related Health Hazards Control Ed. by Lester V. Cralley et al. 1989. Set. 1510p. 400.00 (*0-471-51097-1*); Vol. 1, Production Processes. LC 88-17200. 938p. 235.00 (*0-471-61975-2*) Wiley.

In-Plant Practices for Job Related Health Hazards Control: Engineering Aspects, Vol. 2, Engineering Aspects. Ed. by Lester V. Cralley et al. 1989. LC 88-17200. 578p. 235.00 (*0-471-50121-2*) Wiley.

In Pursuit of Excellence: The College of American Pathologists, 1946-1996. Loyd R. Wagner. 1997. LC 97-77181. viii, 188 p. (*0-930304-67-5*) Coll Am Pathol.

In Pursuit of Fertility: A Fertility Expert Tells You How to Get Pregnant. Robert R. Franklin & Dorothy K. Brockman. 2nd ed. 1996. LC 95-24961. pap. 16.00 (*0-8050-4181-8*) H Holt & Co.

In Pursuit of the Wild Prostate. Edward W. Maupin. 1996. (Illus.). 128p. (Orig.). pap. 12.95 (*0-9654257-0-3*) Dawn Eve Prod.

In Quest of Tomorrow's Medicines. Juergen Drews. Tr. by D. Kramer from GER. 1999. LC 98-27801. (Illus.). 272p. 29.95 (*0-387-98547-6*) Spr-Verlag.

In Search of a Vaginal Delivery: The Handy Book for Women in Labor. B. Carol Smith. 1998. (Illus.). 72p. 19.95 (*0-9656066-7-8*) Three Copper.

In Search of Coronary-Prone Behavior: Beyond Type A. A. W. Siegman & S. A. Dembroski. 1988. 256p. 59.95 (*0-8058-0341-6*) L Erlbaum Assocs.

In Search of Dreams: Results of Experimental Dream Research. Inge Strauch & Barbara Meier. Tr. by Martin Ebon from GER. 1996. LC 95-8151. (SUNY Series in Dream Studies). 252p. (C). pap. text 17.95 (*0-7914-2760-9*) State U NY Pr.

In Search of Emotional & Mental Well-Being: How to Overcome Depression & Other Mental & Emotional Problems. 1992. lib. bdg. 75.95 (*0-8490-8803-8*) Gordon Pr.

In Search of Equity: Health Needs & the Health Care System. Ed. by Ronald Bayer et al. 1983. LC 83-4095. (Hastings Center Series in Ethics). 266p. 45.00 (*0-306-41212-8*, Plenum Trade) Perseus Pubng.

In Search of Good Form: Gestalt Therapy with Couples & Families. Joseph C. Zinker. 1998. (Gestalt Institute of Cleveland Book Ser.). 352p. pap. 27.50 (*0-88163-293-7*) Analytic Pr.

In Search of Madness: Schizophrenia & Neuroscience. R. Walter Heinrichs. 2001. LC 00-62335. (Illus.). 368p. 39.95 (*0-19-512219-4*) OUP.

In Search of My Husband's Mind. Winnie Hirsch. Ed. by Eugene D. Wheeler. 1997. LC 97-17592. 176p. text 22.00 (*0-934793-64-6*) Pathfinder CA.

In Search of Nursing Science. Anna Omery & Christine E. Kasper. 1995. 328p. pap. 37.95 (*0-8039-5094-2*, 4948) Sage.

In Search of Parenthood: Coping with Infertility & High-Tech Conception. Judith N. Lasker & Susan O. Borg. enl. rev. ed. 1994. LC 94-12494. lib. bdg. 69.95 (*1-56639-258-6*); 216p. pap. text 22.95 (*1-56639-259-4*) Temple U Pr.

In Search of Physician Leadership. Barbara Letourneau & Wesley Curry. 1998. LC 98-13927. 180p. 45.00 (*1-56793-082-4*) Health Admin Pr.

In Search of Safety: Chemicals & Cancer Risk. John D. Graham et al. 1991. 280p. pap. 20.50 (*0-674-44636-4*, GRASEX) HUP.

In Search of Safety: Chemicals & Cancer Risks. John D. Graham et al. 1988. LC 88-11011. (Illus.). 336p. 55.00 (*0-674-44635-6*) HUP.

In Search of Self, in the Service to Others: Reflections of a Retired Physician on Medicine, the Bible & the Jews. Heinz Hartmann. 1998. LC 98-29224. 225p. 32.00 (*1-57392-230-7*) Prometheus Bks.

In Search of Serenity: A Black Family's Struggle with the Threat of AIDS. Patti E. Rose. 1993. LC 92-60058. 200p. (Orig.). pap. 10.95 (*0-88378-069-0*) Third World.

In Search of Solutions: Creating a Context for Change. William H. O'Hanlon & Michele Weiner-Davis. 1988. 208p. 25.00 (*0-393-70061-5*) Norton.

In Search of Supervision. Ed. by Michael Jacobs. 1996. LC 95-51061. 160p. pap. (*0-335-19258-0*) OpUniv Pr.

In Search of the Human Mind. Sternberg. 1995. (C). pap. text, tchr. ed. 35.00 (*0-15-502485-X*) Harcourt Coll Pubs.

***In Search of the Lost Cord: Solving the Mystery of Spinal Cord Regeneration.** Luba Vikhanski. 2001. LC 2001-39846. (Illus.). 275p. 27.95 (*0-309-07437-1*, Joseph Henry Pr) Natl Acad Pr.

In Search of the Lost Mother of Infancy. Lawrence E. Hedges. 1995. LC 94-8092. 384p. 40.00 (*1-56821-274-7*) Aronson.

In Search of the Modern Hippocrates. Ed. by Roger J. Bulger. 1987. LC 86-24950. 268p. text 33.95 (*0-87745-160-5*) U of Iowa Pr.

In Search of the Person: Philosophical Explorations in Cognitive Science. Michael A. Arbib. 1986. LC 85-14152. 176p. pap. 15.95 (*0-87023-500-1*); lib. bdg. 25.00 (*0-87023-499-4*) U of Mass Pr.

In Search of the Promise Land: The Collected Papers of Burton Blatt. Burton Blatt et al. 1999. LC 99-21914. (Illus.). xxi, 181p. 34.95 (*0-940898-63-2*) Am Assn Mental.

In Search of 20-20: Everything You Need to Know about Laser Eye Surgery. Arun Lakra & Howard V. Gimbel. 1997. LC 97-910013. (Illus.). 262p. pap. (*0-9681756-0-0*, 738800Q) Gibbel Eye CAN. *Dist:* IPG Chicago.

In Search of Wings: A Journey Back from Traumatic Brain Injury. Beverley Bryant. 1992. 256p. pap. 14.95 (*1-882332-00-8*) Wings Pub.

In Search of Your True Self: 21 Incredible Insights That Will Revitalize Your Body, Mind & Spirit. Walter Doyle Staples. 1996. (Illus.). 384p. 19.95 (*1-56554-226-6*) Pelican.

In Sickness & in Health: Caring for a Loved One with Alzheimer's. William Grubbs. 1997. LC 94-61039. iv, 153 p. pap. 12.95 (*0-943873-12-6*) Elder Bks.

In Sickness & in Health—What Every Man Should Know about the Woman He Loves. Mary E. O'Brien. 1991. LC 90-4408. (Illus.). 208p. (Orig.). pap. 14.95 (*0-929173-05-8*) Health Press.

In Sickness & in Wealth: American Hospitals in the Twentieth Century. Rosemary Stevens. 1999. LC 98-38184. 480p. pap. text 21.50 (*0-8018-6049-0*) Johns Hopkins.

***In Situ Detection of DNA Damage: Methods & Protocols.** Ed. by Vladimir V. Didenko. 2002. (Methods in Molecular Biology Ser.: No. 203). 340p. 89.50 (*0-89603-952-8*) Humana.

In Situ Hybridization. A. R. Leitch et al. 1994. (Microscopy Handbooks Ser.: No. 27). (Illus.). 128p. pap. (*1-872748-48-1*) Bios Sci GBR. *Dist:* Bks Intl VA.

In Situ Hybridization. Ed. by Michael B. Oldstone & A. T. Haase. 1989. (Current Topics in Microbiology & Immunology Ser.: Vol. 143). (Illus.). 90p. 88.95 (*0-387-50761-2*) Spr-Verlag.

In Situ Hybridization: Medical Applications. Ed. by G. R. Coulton & J. De Belleroche. 1992. (C). text 90.50 (*0-7923-8989-1*) Kluwer Academic.

In Situ Hybridization for the Brain. Ed. by W. Wisden & B. J. Morris. 1994. LC 95-120344. (Biological Techniques Ser.). (Illus.). 144p. pap. 45.00 (*0-12-759920-7*); 130p. text 79.00 (*0-12-759919-3*) Acad Pr.

In Situ Hybridization in Brain. Ed. by George R. Uhl. 1986. LC 86-25332. 320p. 79.50 (*0-306-42480-0*, Plenum Trade) Perseus Pubng.

In Situ Hybridization in Neurobiology: Advances in Methodology. Ed. by James H. Eberwine et al. 1994. (Illus.). 222p. (C). text 46.50 (*0-19-507507-2*) OUP.

In Social Relationships: An Introduction to the Social Psychology of Membership & Intimacy. Alan Radley. 1991. 192p. (*0-335-15197-3*) OpUniv Pr.

In Social Relationships: An Introduction to the Social Psychology of Membership & Intimacy. Alan Radley. 1991. 192p. pap. (*0-335-15196-5*) OpUniv Pr GBR. *Dist:* Taylor & Francis.

***In the Arms of Morpheus: The Tragic History of Morphine, Laudanum & Patent Medicines.** Barbara Hodgson. 2001. (Illus.). 160p. 24.95 (*1-55297-538-X*) Firefly Bks Limited.

In the Best Interest of the Patient: Ethical & Legal Issues in the Practice of Psychotherapy. Barbara Lipinski. 1999. LC 99-90292. per. 23.95 (*1-928702-02-3*) Pacific Meridian.

In the Best Interests of the Child. Joseph Goldstein et al. 1986. 192p. (C). pap. 14.95 (*0-02-912380-1*) Free Pr.

In the Best of Health? The Status & Future of Health Care in the U. K. Beck. 1992. 376p. pap. 47.75 (*1-56593-039-8*, 0287) Thomson Learn.

In the Blood: Sickle Cell Anemia & the Politics of Race. Melbourne Tapper. 1998. LC 98-30061. (Critical Histories Ser.). 160p. 22.50 (*0-8122-3471-5*) U of Pa Pr.

In the Cavern of the Demon of the Black Mountain: A Meditation on Oppression, Betrayal & the Tyranny of Control. Jon Ossoff. 1995. LC 95-80219. 135p. (C). pap. text 12.00 (*0-9648850-6-9*) L Canyon Bks.

In the Company of Others: Understanding the Human Needs of Cancer Patients. Jory Graham. 1987. 192p. pap. 4.95 (*0-15-644960-9*, Harvest Bks) Harcourt.

In the Country of Hearts: Journeys in the Art of Medicine. John Stone. 1996. LC 90-31474. 224p. pap. 14.95 (*0-8071-2104-5*) La State U Pr.

In the Eye of the Beholder: Contemporary Issues in Stereotyping. Ed. by Arthur G. Miller. 1982. LC 81-11849. 531p. 49.95 (*0-275-90861-5*, C0861, Praeger Pubs) Greenwood.

In the Eye's Mind: Vision & the Helmholtz-Hering Controversy. R. Steven Turner. 1994. LC 93-37258. 360p. 65.00 (*0-691-03397-8*) Princeton U Pr.

In the Face of Suffering: The Philosophical-Anthropological Foundations of Clinical Ethics. Jos V. Welie. 1998. xv, 304p. 29.95 (*1-881871-26-6*); pap. 17.00 (*1-881871-27-4*) Creighton U Pr.

In the Footsteps of the Yellow Emperor: Tracing the History of Traditional Acupuncture. Peter Eckman. 1996. (Illus.). 252p. 35.00 (*0-8351-2580-7*) China Bks.

In the Gaze of Narcissus: Memory, Affects & Creativity. Mauro Mancia. 1993. 220p. pap. text (*1-85575-042-2*) Karnac Bks GBR. *Dist:* Other Pr LLC.

In the House of the Moon: Reclaiming the Feminine Spirit of Healing. Jason Elias & Katherine Ketcham. 1998. 378p. pap. text 21.00 (*0-7881-5807-4*) DIANE Pub.

In the Image of God: A Psychoanalyst's View. Stanley A. Leavy. 1997. 128p. reprint ed. pap. 24.95 (*0-88163-276-7*) Analytic Pr.

In the Long Run... Longitudinal Studies of Psychopathology in Children No. 143: GAP Report. 1999. 224p. 35.00 (*0-87318-212-X*) Am Psychiatric.

In the Making of a Profession: The National College of Chiropractic 1906-1981. Ronald P. Beideman. Ed. by Dana J. Lawrence. 1995. (Illus.). (C). text 49.95 (*0-9615849-2-0*) Natl Coll Chiro.

In the Matter of Certain Recombinantly Produced Human Growth Hormones: Temporary Relief Proceedings. 1997. (Illus.). 237p. (C). reprint ed. pap. text 50.00 (*0-7881-4251-8*) DIANE Pub.

In the Matter of Karen Quinlan Vol. 1: The Complete Legal Briefs, Court Proceedings, & Decision in the Superior Court of New Jersey. New Jersey Supreme Court Staff. 1975. LC 75-42525. 567p. lib. bdg. 65.00 (*0-313-26920-3*, U6920, Greenwood Pr) Greenwood.

In the Matter of Karen Quinlan Vol. 2: The Complete Briefs, Oral Arguments, & Opinion in the New Jersey Supreme Court, Vol. 2. New Jersey Supreme Court Staff et al. 1976. LC 76-14598. 324p. lib. bdg. 65.00 (*0-313-26921-1*, U6921, Greenwood Pr) Greenwood.

In the Midst of Winter: Systemic Therapy with Families, Couples, & Individuals with AIDS Infection. Gillian Walker. 1991. LC 91-15060. 362p. (C). 34.95 (*0-393-70087-9*); 1995. LC 95-18597. 384p. pap. 19.00 (*0-393-70204-9*, Norton Paperbks) Norton.

In the Name of Eugenics: Genetics & the Uses of Human Heredity. Daniel J. Kevles. 1995. LC 95-18034. 448p. (Orig.). (C). pap. 19.95 (*0-674-44557-0*) HUP.

In the Name of Science: Issues in Responsible Animal Experimentation. F. Barbara Orlans. (Illus.). 312p. 1993. LC 92-39344. text 39.95 (*0-19-507043-7*); 1996. reprint ed. pap. text 21.95 (*0-19-510871-X*) OUP.

In the Name of the Child. Johnston & Roseby. 1997. 30.00 (*0-02-874133-1*) Free Pr.

In the Nation's Interest: Equity in Access to Health Care: Summary Report. Marsha Lillie-Blanton & Ana Alfaro-Correa. 1999. (Illus.). 51p. (C). reprint ed. pap. text 20.00 (*0-7881-7660-9*) DIANE Pub.

In the Palaces of Memory: How We Build the Worlds Inside Our Heads. George Johnson. 1992. 255p. pap. 14.00 (*0-679-73759-6*) Vin Bks.

In the Patient's Interest: Access to Hospital Care. Ed. by Helen Rehr & Mildred D. Mailick. 1982. LC 81-15781. 171p. text 17.50 (*0-88202-136-2*) Watson Pub Intl.

. . .In the Practice of My Calling: Retired Nurses Tell Their Stories. Alana Press Staff. 2000. LC 00-91005. (Illus.). viii,116p. 12.95 (*0-9702258-1-4*) Alana Pr.

In the Shade of an Acacia Tree: Memoirs of a Health Officer in Africa: 1945-59. Frank L. Lambrecht. 1991. LC 90-56110. (Memoirs Ser.: Vol. 194). (Illus.). 420p. (C). 30.00 (*0-87169-194-9*, M194-LAF) Am Philos.

In the Shadow of Illness: Parents & Siblings of Ill Children. Myra Bluebond-Langner. 1996. LC 96-6800. 328p. 45.00 (*0-691-02783-8*) Princeton U Pr.

In the Shadow of Madness. Dolores Brandon. Ed. by Paul Herron. 2000. LC 99-76406. (Illus.). 170p. pap. 14.95 (*0-9652364-5-5*) Sky Blue Pr.

In the Shadow of Medicine: Remaking the Division of Labor in Health Care. Arnold Birenbaum. 1990. LC 90-80203. (Illus.). 184p. (Orig.). text 35.95 (*0-930390-28-8*) Gen Hall.

In the Shadow of Moloch. Martin S. Bergmann. 1992. LC 91-28781. 328p. text 49.50 (*0-231-07248-1*) Col U Pr.

In the Shadow of Polio. Kathryn Black. 2000. 320p. pap. 12.00 (*0-201-15490-0*) Perseus Bks Grp.

In the Shadow of the Epidemic: Being HIV-Negative in the Age of AIDS. Walt Odets. 1995. LC 95-1311. (Series Q). 328p. text 49.95 (*0-8223-1626-9*) Duke.

In the Shadow of the Past: Psychology Portrays the Sexes. Ed. by Miriam Lewin. 1986. LC 83-10072. (Path in Psychology Ser.). 338p. pap. 22.00 (*0-231-05303-7*) Col U Pr.

In the Shadows: Living & Coping with a Loved One's Chronic Illness. David Luterman. 1995. LC 95-94103. pap. 19.95 (*0-9644862-0-2*) Jade Pr.

In the Theater of Consciousness: The Workspace of the Mind. Bernard J. Baars. 1997. LC 96-10379. (Illus.). 210p. 27.50 (*0-19-510265-7*) OUP.

In the Therapist's Mirror: Reality in the Making. Marilyn Wedge. 1996. LC 96-8687. 176p. 25.00 (*0-393-70235-9*) Norton.

In the Tropics with Children. 1988. (*3-8236-1138-0*, VJM1380) Bernan Associates.

In the Wake of Contact: Biological Responses to Conquest. Ed. by Clark S. Larsen & George R. Milner. 1993. 206p. 155.00 (*0-471-30544-8*) Wiley.

In the Wake of Reich. Ed. by David Boadella. 1978. LC 77-75314. 424p. 24.95 (*0-87949-103-5*) Ashley Bks.

In the Wake of Suicide: Stories of the People Left Behind. Victoria Alexander. 1998. LC 97-37016. 238p. pap. 25.00 (*0-7879-4052-6*) Jossey-Bass.

In Their Own Words: A Sexual Abuse Workbook for Teenage Girls. Lulie Munson & Karen Riskin. 1995. (Orig.). pap. text 10.95 (*0-87868-596-0*) Child Welfare.

In This Tretyse That Is Cleped Governayle of Helthe. 1969. LC 72-200. (English Experience Ser.: No. 192). reprint ed. 25.00 (*90-221-0192-4*) Walter J Johnson.

In Time & with Love: Caring for the Special Needs Baby. Marilyn Segal. 1991. LC 87-34711. 208p. pap. 15.95 (*0-937858-96-X*); (Illus.). 191p. 21.95 (*0-937858-95-1*) Newmarket.

In Time of Plague: The History & Social Consequences of Lethal Epidemic Disease. Ed. by Arien Mack. 272p. (C). 1992. pap. text 18.50 (*0-8147-5485-6*); 1991. text 45.00 (*0-8147-5467-8*) NYU Pr.

In Utero Diagnosis of Skeletal Disorders: An Atlas of Prenatal Sonographic & Postnatal Radiologic Correlation. Israel Meizner & Jacob Bar-Ziv. 1993. LC 92-48449. 304p. lib. bdg. 179.00 (*0-8493-5130-8*, R6629) CRC Pr.

In Vitro Diagnostic Medical Devices: Law & Practice in Five EU Member States. Ed. by Bernhard Maassen & Robin Whaite. 1994. LC 94-3568. 140p. (C). text 119.00 (*0-7923-2996-1*) Kluwer Academic.

In Vitro Diagnostics Industry Directory 2000-2001. Ed. by CTB Directories Group Staff. 2000. 318p. spiral bd. 277.00 (*1-887566-17-1*) CTB Intl.

In Vitro Embryotoxicity & Teratogenicity Tests. Ed. by F. Homburger. 1985. (Concepts in Toxicology Ser.: Vol. 3). (Illus.). viii, 152p. 138.50 (*3-8055-4018-3*) S Karger.

In Vitro Fertilisation in the 1990s: Towards Medical, Social, & Ethical Evaluation. Elisabeth Hildt & Dietmar Mieth. 1998. 386p. text (*1-85972-685-2*) Ashgate Pub GBR. *Dist:* Ashgate Pub Co.

In Vitro Fertilization. Brian Dale & Kay Elder. 1997. (Illus.). 201p. (C). pap. text 46.95 (*0-521-57567-2*) Cambridge U Pr.

In Vitro Fertilization. Carl Wood & Robyn Riley. 1994. 134p. (Orig.). pap. (*0-85572-212-6*) Hill Content Pubng AUS. *Dist:* Seven Hills Bk.

In Vitro Fertilization. Kay Elder & Brian Dale. 2nd ed. 2000. LC 00-269753. (Illus.). 322p. (C). pap. text 59.95 (*0-521-77863-8*) Cambridge U Pr.

In Vitro Fertilization: Building Policy from Laboratories to Legislatures. Andrea L. Bonnicksen. 1991. pap. 18.50 (*0-231-06905-7*) Col U Pr.

In Vitro Fertilization: The A. R. T. of Making Babies. Geoffrey Sher et al. 1995. LC 95-2587. (Illus.). 208p. 22.95 (*0-8160-3269-6*) Facts on File.

In Vitro Fertilization & Embryo Transfer: A Manuel of Basic Techniques. D. P. Wolf et al. 1988. (Illus.). 408p. (C). text 110.00 (*0-306-42900-4*, Kluwer Plenum) Kluwer Academic.

In Vitro-In Vivo Correlations: Proceedings of a Workshop Held in Baltimore, Maryland, September 4-6, 1996. Ed. by David Young et al. 1997. LC 97-17156. (Advances in Experimental Medicine & Biology Ser.: Vol. 423). 310p. (C). text 95.00 (*0-306-45600-1*, Kluwer Plenum) Kluwer Academic.

In Vitro Methods in Developmental Toxicology: Use in Defining Mechanisms & Risk Parameters. Ed. by G. L. Kimmel et al. 1989. 192p. 179.00 (*0-8493-6919-3*, RA1224) CRC Pr.

In Vitro Methods in Pharmaceutical Research. Ed. by J. V. Castell et al. 1996. (Illus.). 480p. 80.00 (*0-12-163390-X*) Acad Pr.

In Vitro Methods of Toxicology. Ronald R. Watson. 1992. 320p. 139.00 (*0-8493-7298-4*, RA1199) CRC Pr.

In Vitro Models for Cancer Research: Carcinomas of the Bladder-Kidneys, Vol. IV. Mutka M. Webber & Lea I. Sekely. 1986. 312p. 175.00 (*0-8493-5584-2*, RC267, CRC Reprint) Franklin.

In Vitro Models for Cancer Research: Carcinomas of the Mammary Gland, Uterus, & Skin, Vol. III. Mutka M. Webber & Lea I. Sekely. 1986. 352p. 192.00 (*0-8493-5583-4*, RC267, CRC Reprint) Franklin.

In Vitro Models for Cancer Research, Vol. V: Carcinomas of the Prostate & Testis. Ed. by Mutka M. Webber & Lea I. Sekely. 1988. 272p. 138.00 (*0-8493-5585-0*, RC267, CRC Reprint) Franklin.

In Vitro Models for Cancer Research, Vol. VI: Carcinomas of the Bronchus & Endothelial Cell Models. Ed. by Mutka M. Webber & Lea I. Sekely. 1988. 192p. 108.00 (*0-8493-5586-9*, RC267, CRC Reprint) Franklin.

In Vitro Models of Respiratory Epithelium. Leonard J. Schiff. 1986. 216p. 125.00 (*0-8493-5187-1*, QP88, CRC Reprint) Franklin.

In Vitro Perfusion of Human Placental Tissue. Ed. by H. Schneider & J. Dancis. 1985. (Contributions to Gynecology & Obstetrics Ser.: Vol. 13). (Illus.). x, 190p. 113.25 (*3-8055-3986-X*) S Karger.

In Vitro Techniques in Research: Recent Advances. Ed. by J. W. Payne. 1989. 224p. 113.00 (*0-335-15885-4*) Wiley.

In Vitro Testing. Ivor A. Emanuel. Ed. by Jacquelynne P. Corey. 1994. LC 94-36576. (American Academy of Otoloaryngic Allergy Monograph Ser.). (Illus.). 104p. text 29.90 (*0-86577-521-4*) Thieme Med Pubs.

In-Vitro Testing of Biomaterials. Jones Staff. 1999. (Illus.). 340p. pap. 86.50 (*0-412-56480-7*, Chap & Hall NY) Chapman & Hall.

In-Vitro Toxicity Testing: Applications to Safety Evaluation. Ed. by John M. Frazier. 1992. (Illus.). 312p. text 155.00 (*0-8247-8614-9*) Dekker.

In Vitro Toxicity Testing Protocols. Ed. by Sheila O'Hare & Christopher K. Atterwill. 1995. LC 95-3384. (Methods in Molecular Biology Ser.: Vol. 43). (Illus.). 346p. spiral bd. 109.50 (*0-89603-282-5*) Humana.

In Vitro Toxicology. Ed. by Alan M. Goldberg. 1985. (Alternative Methods in Toxicology Ser.: Vol. 3). 722p. text 251.00 (*0-913113-05-0*) M Liebert.

In Vitro Toxicology. Charlene A. McQueen. 1989. 450p. lib. bdg. 88.00 (*0-936923-23-7*, RA1199) CRC Pr.

In Vitro Toxicology. Shayne Cox Gad. 2nd ed. 2000. (Illus.). 544p. (gr. 13). text 125.00 (*1-56032-769-3*) Taylor & Francis.

In Vitro Toxicology: Approaches to Validation. Ed. by Alan M. Goldberg. 1987. (Alternative Methods in Toxicology Ser.: Vol. 5). 500p. text 207.00 (*0-913113-10-7*) M Liebert.

In Vitro Toxicology, Vol. 7: New Directions. Ed. by Alan M. Goldberg. 1989. (Alternative Methods in Toxicology Ser.: Vol. 7). 350p. 199.00 (*0-913113-23-9*) M Liebert.

***In Vivo Atlas of Deep Brain Structures: With 3-D Reconstructions.** S. Lucerna. 2001. LC 2001-49700. pap. (*3-540-42561-6*) Springer Pub.

In-Vivo Body Composition Studies. Seiichi Yasumura et al. 2000. LC 00-25357. (Annals of the New York Academy of Sciences Ser.: Vol. 904). (Illus.). xvi, 637p. pap. (*1-57331-258-4*) NY Acad Sci.

In Vivo Body Composition Studies, Vol. 904. Ed. by Seiichi Yasumura et al. 2000. LC 00-25357. (Annals of the New York Academy of Sciences Ser.: Vol. 904). (Illus.). xvi, 637p. 190.00 (*1-57331-257-6*) NY Acad Sci.

In Vivo Immunology: Regulatory Processes During Lymphopoiesis & Immunopoiesis. E. Heinen et al. 1994. (Advances in Experimental Medicine & Biology Ser.: Vol. 355). (Illus.). 326p. (C). text 89.50 (*0-306-44726-6*, Kluwer Plenum) Kluwer Academic.

In Vivo Models of Inflammation. D. W. Morgan & L. A. Marshall. 1999. LC 99-11901. (Progress in Inflammatory Research Ser.). (Illus.). ix, 347p. 159.00 (*3-7643-5876-9*) Birkhauser.

In Vivo Neuromethods. Ed. by Alan A. Boulton et al. 1997. (Neuromethods Ser.: Vol. 32). (Illus.). 408p. 129.50 (*0-89603-511-5*) Humana.

In Vivo NMR Spectroscopy: Principles & Techniques. Robin A. De Graaf. 1998. LC 98-17777. 530p. 295.00 (*0-471-98365-9*) Wiley.

In Vivo Study of Drug Action. Ed. by C. J. Van Boxtel. 1992. LC 92-18590. 430p. 256.50 (*0-444-81370-5*) Elsevier.

In Women's Experience, Vol. II. Ed. by Patricia L. Munhall. 1995. 425p. pap. 37.95 (*0-88737-647-9*) Natl League Nurse.

Inadequate Care of the Elderly: A Health Care Perspective on Abuse & Neglect. Terry Fulmer & Terry O'Malley. 1987. 192p. (C). 33.95 (*0-8261-4770-4*) Springer Pub.

Inalienable Rights: The Limits of Consent in Medicine & the Law. Terrance C. McConnell. 2000. LC 99-41540. 192p. text 35.00 (*0-19-513462-1*) OUP.

Inattentional Blindness. Arien Mack & Irvin Rock. 1998. LC 97-28254. (Mit Press/Bradford Books Series in Cognitive Psychology). (Illus.). 296p. 50.00 (*0-262-13339-3*) MIT Pr.

Inborn Errors of Metabolism in Man: 1st International Symposium on Inborn Errors of Metabolism in Man, Tel Aviv, June 1977: Abstracts. International Symposium on Inborn Errors of Metabolism Staff. Ed. by O. Sperling. 1977. (Human Heredity Ser.: Vol. 27, No. 3). 32.25 (*3-8055-2710-1*) S Karger.

Inborn Metabolic Diseases: Diagnosis & Treatment. Ed. by J. Fernandes et al. 3rd rev. ed. 2000. LC 99-53887. (Illus.). 480p. 119.00 (*3-540-65626-X*) Spr-Verlag.

Inbred Strains in Biomedical Research. Michael F. Festing. 2nd ed. 1999. 125.00 (*0-8493-9221-7*) CRC Pr.

Incapacity Benefit & Severe Disablement Allowance Quarterly Summary of Statistics. Department of Social Security Staff. 1998. LC 98-220962. 26p. (*1-85197-859-3*) Dept for Work & Pensions.

Incentive Relativity. Charles F. Flaherty. 1996. (Problems in the Behavioral Sciences Ser.: No. 15). (Illus.). 239p. (C). text 69.95 (*0-521-38118-5*) Cambridge U Pr.

Incentives in Health Systems: Health Systems Research. Ed. by G. Lopez-Casasnovas & W. Van Eimeren. 1991. (Illus.). 224p. 103.00 (*0-387-53933-6*) Spr-Verlag.

Incest: Understanding & Treatment. Domeena C. Renshaw. 1982. 38.95 (*0-316-74031-4*, Little Brwn Med Div) Lppncott W & W.

Incest - Acts, Myths & Facts: Index of Modern Authors & Subjects with Guide for Rapid Research. Lottie F. Lydeen. 1991. LC 90-56269. 200p. 47.50 (*1-55914-312-6*); pap. 44.50 (*1-55914-313-4*) ABBE Pubs Assn.

Incest & Human Love: The Betrayal of the Soul in Psychotherapy. Robert Stein. 1973. LC 73-82641. 24.95 (*0-89388-090-6*) Okpaku Communications.

Incest & Sexuality: A Guide to Understanding & Healing. Wendy Maltz & Beverly Holman. 1997. 166p. pap. 14.95 (*0-669-14085-6*) Lxngtn Bks.

Incest, Work, & Women: Understanding the Consequences of Incest on Women's Careers, Work, & Dreams. Leslie B. Berger. 1998. LC 98-22657. 234p. 51.95 (*0-398-06882-8*); pap. 37.95 (*0-398-06883-6*) C C Thomas.

Incidence of Illness & the Receipt & Costs of Medical Care Among Representative Families: Experiences in Twelve Consecutive Months During 1928-1931. Isidore S. Falk et al. 1976. LC 75-17220. (Social Problems & Social Policy Ser.). (Illus.). reprint ed. 28.95 (*0-405-07491-3*) Ayer.

Incidental Carcinoma of the Prostate. Ed. by J. E. Altwein et al. 1991. (Illus.). 129p. 98.00 (*0-387-53225-0*) Spr-Verlag.

Incisional Hernia. Ed. by Volker Schumpelick & Andrew N. Kingsnorth. 1999. LC 99-25520. (Illus.). 536p. 94.00 (*3-540-65619-7*) Spr-Verlag.

Including All of Us: An Early Childhood Curriculum about Disability. Merle Froschl et al. 1985. LC 84-26022. pap. text 14.95 (*0-931629-00-4*) Educ Equity Con.

Inclusion - Body Myositis & Myopathies. Ed. by Valerie Askanas et al. 1998. (Illus.). 413p. (C). text 130.00 (*0-521-57105-7*) Cambridge U Pr.

Inclusion Practices with Special Needs: Education, Training & Application. Ed. by Steven I. Pfeiffer & Linda A. Reddy. 2000. LC 99-58741. (Special Services in the Schools Monographs: Vol. 15, Nos. 1-2). (Illus.). 210p. 39.95 (*0-7890-0843-2*) Haworth Pr.

Income & Health in a North Indian Village. Mike Shepperdson. 1995. 200p. text 101.95 (*1-85628-036-5*) Ashgate Pub Co.

Income Maintenance Supervisor. Jack Rudman. 1994. (Career Examination Ser.: C-3724). pap. 29.95 (*0-8373-3724-0*) Nat Learn.

Income Replacement for Long-Term Disability: The Role of Workers' Compensation & SSDI. Karen R. DeVol. 1986. (Illus.). 95p. 35.00 (*0-935149-04-X*, SP-86-2) Workers Comp Res Inst.

Incompetent Doctor: Behind Closed Doors. Marilynn Rosenthal. 1994. (State of Health Ser.). 160p. (*0-335-19110-X*); pap. (*0-335-19109-6*) OpUniv Pr.

Inconceivable: Winning the Fertility Game. Julia Indichova. 1998. 201p. 21.00 (*0-9660078-5-9*) Adell Pr.

Inconscient A-t-Il un Fondement Ethique? Ed. by J. R. Freymann & A. Michels. 1989. (Apertura Ser.: Vol. 3). 220p. 31.95 (*0-387-59505-8*) Spr-Verlag.

Inconsistent Picture: A Compilation of Analyses of Economic Impacts of Competing Approaches to Health Care Reform by Experts & Stakeholders. 1994. (Illus.). 144p. (Orig.). (C). pap. text 40.00 (*0-7881-0474-8*) DIANE Pub.

Inconsistent Picture: A Compilcation of the Analyses of Economic Impacts of Competing Approaches to Health Care Reform. 1995. lib. bdg. 252.95 (*0-8490-7548-3*) Gordon Pr.

Inconstant Gene. Lawrence S. Dillon. 1983. LC 82-20414. 590p. 125.00 (*0-306-41084-2*, Plenum Trade) Perseus Pubng.

Incontinence: A Pelvic Team Approach. Malcolm Lucas et al. 1999. LC 98-49186. (Illus.). 154.95 (*0-632-05003-9*) Blackwell Sci.

Incontinence & Its Management. Ed. by Dorothy Mandelstam. 2nd ed. 1986. LC 85-27001. 288p. pap. (*0-7099-3580-3*) C Helm GBR. *Dist:* Routldge.

Incontinence & Ostomy Product Markets: Aggressive Marketers Target Alternate Sites. Market Intelligence Staff. 1993. 340p. 1695.00 (*1-56753-457-0*) Frost & Sullivan.

Incontinence in the Elderly. Tobin. 1992. 112p. pap. 25.00 (*0-340-54558-5*) Trafalgar.

Incorporating Toxicological Mechanisms in Risk Assessment. Thomas B. Starr. Date not set. (*0-89116-585-1*) Hemisp Pub.

Increase Your Learning Power. Geoffrey Dudley. 1976. pap. 5.00 (*0-87980-085-2*) Wilshire.

Increasing & Decreasing Behaviors of Persons with Severe Retardation & Autism, Set. Richard M. Foxx. 1982. pap. text 28.95 (*0-87822-265-0*, 2650) Res Press.

Increasing Patient Satisfaction: A Guide for Nurses. Roberta L. Messner & Susan J. Lewis. 1996. LC 95-25628. (Illus.). 240p. 35.95 (*0-8261-9250-5*) Springer Pub.

Increasing Physician Involvement in Quality Improvement Programs. Ed. by Edward C. Geehr & Joan Pine. 1992. LC 92-70827. 66p. (Orig.). (C). pap. text 25.95 (*0-924674-13-X*) Am Coll Phys Execs.

Increasing Provider Participation: Strategies for Improving State Perinatal Programs. Deborah Lewis-Idema. 1988. 75p. (Orig.). pap. text 15.00 (*1-55877-026-7*) Natl Governor.

Increasing Self Awareness. Ed. by William H. Burke. 1988. (Professional Series on Traumatic Brain Injury: Vol. 15). 48p. (Orig.). pap. 9.50 (*1-882855-22-1*) HDI Pubs.

Increasing the Relevance of Education for Health Professionals: Report of a WHO Study Group on Problem-Solving Education for the Health Professions. 1993. (WHO Technical Reports: No. 838). (ENG, FRE & SPA.). iv, 29p. pap. text 8.00 (*92-4-120838-4*, 1100838) World Health.

Increasing the Supply of Transplant Organs: The Virtue of an Options Market. Lloyd R. Cohen. 1995. LC 95-18622. (Medical Intelligence Unit Ser.). 154p. 79.00 (*1-57059-259-4*) Landes Bioscience.

Increasing Variety in Adult Life: A General-Case Approach. Daniel E. Steere. 1997. LC 97-11675. (Innovations Ser.). 21.95 (*0-940898-46-2*) Am Assn Mental.

Increasingly Safe & Successful Pregnancies-Focus:EPH Gestosis: Proceedings of the 27th International Congress on Pathophysiology of Pregnancy, 5-7 November 1995. Ed. by C. Yabes-Almirante & M. De Luna. 1996. (International Congress Ser.: Vol. 1107). 432p. 199.50 (*0-444-82296-8*, Excerpta Medica) Elsevier.

Incredible Internet Guide to Diet & Nutrition. Marc Dauphinais. Ed. by James R. Flowers, Jr. 2000. LC 00-268225. (Incredible Internet Guide Ser.). (Illus.). 328p. pap. 15.95 (*1-889150-14-2*) Facts on Demand.

Incredible Organizing Power of the Human Body: Phenomenal Facts of Physiology. Arthur M. Baker. 1994. 18p. (Orig.). pap. 5.95 (*1-883989-17-5*) Self Hlth Care.

Inculturation & African Religion: Indigenous & Western Approaches to Medical Practice. Stephen Owoahene-Acheampong. 1998. LC 96-478. (American University Studies: Vol. 16). XV, 225p. (C). text 43.95 (*0-8204-3129-X*) P Lang Pubng.

Incunabula Medica: A Study of the Earliest Printed Medical Books 1467-1480. William Osler. 1994. (Illus.). 152p. reprint ed. 60.00 (*1-888262-56-7*) Martino Pubng.

***Incurable Cancer Patient at the End of Life: Medical Care Utilization, Quality of Life & the Additive Analgesic Effect of Paracetamol in Concurrent Morphine Therapy.** Bertil Axelsson. 2001. (Comprehensive Summaries of Uppsala Dissertations from the Faculty of Medicine Ser.: No. 1013). (Illus.). 87p. (*91-554-4968-9*) Uppsala Universitet SWE. *Dist:* Coronet Bks.

Independence Means Swim or Sink: But There Are All Those Creepie Crawlies in the Water. Neil B. Kimerer. Ed. by Susan L. Coatney. 1996. LC 95-71246. 215p. text 21.95 (*0-9648589-1-6*) Sagacity Pr.

Independent Living. Kate Munro & Jim Elder-Woodward. 1992. (Skills for Caring Ser.). (Illus.). 40p. (Orig.). pap. text (*0-443-04533-X*) Church.

Independent Medical Coding: The Comprehensive Guidebook for Career Success As a Medical Coder. Donna Avila-Weil & Rhonda Regan. 1999. LC 98-48122. (Illus.). 288p. pap. 34.95 (*1-877810-17-7*, IMC) Rayve Prodns.

Independent Medical Evaluation Report Vol. 1: A Step-by-Step Guide with Models. Christopher Brigham et al. 1996. (Illus.). x, 200p. (Orig.). pap. 99.00 (*0-9652197-0-4*) SEAK.

Independent Medical Examination. J. Dowdle. 1998. (Illus.). 256p. (*0-443-07650-2*) Church.

Independent Medical Transcriptionist: The Comprehensive Guidebook for Career Success in a Home-Based Medical Transcription Business. Donna Avila-Weil & Mary Glaccum. 3rd ed. 1997. LC 97-31753. 424p. pap. 34.95 (*1-877810-23-1*) Rayve Prodns.

Independent Midwife. Lesley Hobbs. 1998. LC 98-134904. 113p. pap. text 29.99 (*1-898507-59-7*) Buttrwrth-Heinemann.

Independent Mind in British Psychoanalysis. Eric Rayner. 1991. LC 91-6403. 360p. 45.00 (*0-87668-560-2*) Aronson.

Independent Nursing Interventions. Mariah Snyder. 1989. 340p. text 35.00 (*0-8273-4380-9*); 2nd ed. 1992. (C). pap. 37.50 (*0-8273-4845-2*) Delmar.

Independent Practice for the Mental Health Professional: Growing a Private Practice for the 21st Century. Ralph Earle. 1999. LC 98-48430. 141p. 24.95 (*0-87630-838-8*) Brunner-Routledge.

Independent Practitioner: Practice Management for the Allied Health Professional. Robert M. Pressman & Rodie Siegler. 1983. LC 82-73633. (Professional Bks.). 266p. (C). text 43.95 (*0-534-11281-1*) Brooks-Cole.

Index Alphabeticus Klotzschii & Rabenhorstii Herbarii Mycologici. J. E. Kohlmeyer. 1962. pap. 24.00 (*3-7682-5404-6*) Lubrecht & Cramer.

Index & Repertory to the Homeopathic Drug Pictures of Dr. M. L. Tyler. Jollyman. 1988. 162p. (*0-85207-201-5*) C W Daniel GBR. *Dist:* Natl Bk Netwk.

Index & Repertory to the Homeopathic Drug Pictures of Dr. M. L. Tyler. M. L. Tyler. 224p. (Orig.). 35.95 (*0-8464-4240-X*) Beekman Pubs.

Index Medicus for the WHO Eastern Mediterranean Region. 1996. viii, 643p. text 32.40 (*92-9021-204-7*) World Health.

Index of Childhood Immunization. David Lewis. 2000. 19.95 (*1-873413-02-5*, 8290) Merit Pub Intl.

Index of Psychoanalytic Writings. Ed. by Alexander Grinstein. LC 56-8932. 10. 1971. 32.00 (*0-8236-2570-2*); 11. 1971. 32.00 (*0-8236-2571-0*); 12. 1971. 32.00 (*0-8236-2572-9*); 13. 1971. 32.00 (*0-8236-2573-7*); 14. 1971. 32.00 (*0-8236-2574-5*); Set, Vols. 1-5. 1960. 160.00 (*0-8236-8400-8*); Set, Vols. 6-9. 1966. 160.00 (*0-8236-8401-6*); Set, Vols. 10-14. 1971. 160.00 (*0-8236-8402-4*) Intl Univs Pr.

Index of Synonyms & Trade Names in Volumes 1 to 36. 1985. (IARC Scientific Publications Ser.: Supplement No. 5). 259p. pap. text 41.40 (*92-832-1408-0*, 1721005) World Health.

Index of Variant Human Fibrinogens, 1991 Edition. Ray F. Ebert. 1991. 406p. 227.00 (*0-8493-4231-7*, QP93, CRC Reprint) Franklin.

Index Ophthalmologicus. 1974. pap. text 234.00 (*90-207-0401-X*) Kluwer Academic.

Index Psychopharmacorum. Walter Poldinger & Francois Wider. 7th exp. rev. ed. 1991. 334p. text 37.00 (*0-88937-072-9*) Hogrefe & Huber Pubs.

Index to Dental Literature. annuals American Dental Association, Bureau of Library and I. 1981. 100.00 (*0-934510-11-3*) Am Dental.

Index to the Journal of the American Psychoanalytic Association, 1975-1984, Vols. 23-32. 140p. text 102.50 (*0-8236-1112-4*, BN 01112) Intl Univs Pr.

Indexing Managed Care. Dennis J. Patterson. 1997. LC 97-29562. (HFMA Healthcare Financial Management Ser.). 225p. 50.00 (*0-7863-1067-7*, Irwn Prfssnl) McGraw-Hill Educ Grp.

***India-Absolute Zero Population.** Manhar K. Jadav. 2001. 115p. pap. 12.00 (*0-9709184-0-2*) M K Jadav.

Indian Healing: Shamanic Ceremonialism in the Pacific Northwest Today. Wolfgang G. Jilek. 1997. (Illus.). 182p. reprint ed. pap. 17.95 (*0-88839-120-X*) Hancock House.

Indian Health Service: Improvements Needed in Credentialing Temporary Physicians. 1996. (Illus.). 43p. (Orig.). (C). pap. text 25.00 (*0-7881-3444-2*) DIANE Pub.

Indian Herbalogy of North America. Alma R. Hutchens. 1992. 27.25 (*0-8446-6616-5*) Peter Smith.

Indian Herbalogy of North America. Alma R. Hutchens. 1991. LC 91-52521. (Illus.). 424p. reprint ed. pap. 19.95 (*0-87773-639-1*) Shambhala Pubns.

H I

Indian Household Medicine Guide. J. I. Lighthall. 1996. 152p. pap. 14.95 (0-9663702-0-1) Fly Eagle.

Indian Household Medicine Guide. J. I. Lighthall. 1991. lib. bdg. 79.95 (0-8490-4100-7) Gordon Pr.

Indian Household Medicine Guide. J. I. Lighthall. 2nd ed. 1996. 152p. reprint ed. pap. 12.50 (0-7873-0560-X) Hlth Research.

Indian Materia Medica, Set. Ed. by K. M. Nadkarni. 1989. (0-8364-2572-3) Popular Prakashan IND. *Dist:* S Asia.

Indian Medical Text in Central Asia. Kshanika Saha. 1986. 8.50 (0-8364-1593-0) S Asia.

Indian Medicinal Plants, Set. K.R. Kirtikar-Basu. 1988. (C). (0-7855-2591-2) Scientific GBR. *Dist:* St Mut.

Indian Medicinal Plants, Vols. 1-4. K. R. Basu Kirtikar. 1999. 2791p. reprint ed. pap. (81-7089-055-1) Intl Bk Distr IND. *Dist:* St Mut.

Indian Medicine Power. Brad Steiger. Ed. by Marah Ren. 1984. LC 84-61049. 256p. pap. 12.95 (0-914918-65-6, Whitford) Schiffer.

Indian Physician. Jonas Rishel. 1980. 132p. 7.00 (0-88215-048-0) Friends Ohio St U Lib.

Indian Uses of Native Plants. Edith Van Allen Murphey. 3rd ed. 1987. (Illus.). 96p. (Orig.). pap. text 6.95 (0-916638-15-4) Meyerbooks.

Indiana Health Care Perspective, 1998. Ed. by Kathleen O'Leary Morgan & Scott E. Morgan. 1998. 20p. pap. 19.00 (1-56692-813-3) Morgan Quitno Corp.

Indiana Poor Law: Its Development & Administration with Special Reference to the Provision of State Care for the Sick Poor. Alice Shaffer et al. 1976. LC 75-17242. (Social Problems & Social Policy Ser.). reprint ed. 33.95 (0-405-07513-8) Ayer.

Indications for Child Analysis & Other Papers. Anna Freud. 1968. LC 67-9514. (Writings of Anna Freud: Vol. 4). 706p. 85.00 (0-8236-6873-8) Intl Univs Pr.

Indications for Psychoanalysis: Place of the Dream in Clinical Psychoanalysis. Ed. by Bernard D. Fine et al. 1967. LC 65-18383. (Kris Study Group Monographs: No. 2). 106p. (C). text 27.50 (0-8236-2620-2) Intl Univs Pr.

Indications in Vascular Surgery. Roger M. Greenhalgh. 1988. 437p. text 159.00 (0-7216-2623-8) Saunders.

Indications of Insanity. John Conolly. 1964. reprint ed. 44.95 (0-8464-0507-5) Beekman Pubs.

Indicators & Trends in Health & Health Care. Ed. by D. Schwefel. 1986. (Health Systems Research Ser.). (Illus.). 131p. 53.95 (0-387-16998-9) Spr-Verlag.

Indicators of Chronic Health Conditions: Monitoring Community-Level Delivery Systems. Ed. by Robert J. Newcomer & A. E. Benjamin. 1997. LC 96-42207. (Illus.). 392p. 67.00 (0-8018-5491-1); pap. text 26.95 (0-8018-5494-6) Johns Hopkins.

Indicators of Genotoxic Exposure. Ed. by Bryn A. Bridges & I. Bernard Weinstein. 1982. LC 82-12972. (Banbury Reports: Vol. 13). 580p. 62.50 (0-87969-212-X) Cold Spring Harbor.

Indices of Quality in Long-Term Care: Research & Practice. Ed. by NLN Staff. 1989. 192p. 5.95 (0-88737-454-9) Natl League Nurse.

Indicted: Cancer Research: Fraud, Fear, Futility, & the 150,000 Dollar Mouse Exposed at Last. Tibor J. Hegedus. 1993. LC 92-97251. 371p. (Orig.). pap. 19.95 (0-9634721-9-4) Avondale Lab.

Indigenous Drugs of India. R. C. Chopra. 1988. (C). (0-7855-2256-5) Scientific GBR. *Dist:* St Mut.

Indigenous Drugs of India. K. L. Dey. 1984. (C). 187p. (81-7089-900-1); 1187p. (0-7855-6887-5) Intl Bk Distr IND. *Dist:* St Mut.

Indigenous Fermented Foods of the Sudan: A Study in African Food & Nutrition. A. F. Dirar. 1993. LC 94-111474. (Illus.). 576p. text 140.00 (0-85198-858-X) OUP.

Indigenous Healers & the African State: Policy Issues Concerning African Indigenous Healers in Mozambique & Southern Africa. Edward C. Green. 1996. 15.00 (1-888753-04-8) PACT Pubns.

Indigenous Theories of Contagious Disease. Edward C. Green. 1998. LC 98-40172. 288p. 65.00 (0-7619-9199-9); pap. 24.95 (0-7619-8941-2) AltaMira Pr.

Indigestion: Living Better with Upper Intestinal Problems from Heartburn to Ulcers & Gallstones. Henry D. Janowitz. 1994. 256p. (C). reprint ed. pap. 11.95 (0-19-508554-X) OUP.

Indirect Perception. Irvin Rock. 1997. LC 96-26924. (Mit Press/Bradford Books Series in Cognitive Psychology). (Illus.). 424p. (C). 60.00 (0-262-18177-0, Bradford Bks) MIT Pr.

Individual & Community Responses to Trauma & Disaster: The Structure of Human Chaos. Robert J. Ursano et al. 1995. (Illus.). 438p. pap. text 54.95 (0-521-55643-0) Cambridge U Pr.

Individual & Environment: Monzygotic Twins Reared Apart. Tr. by Niels Juel-Nielsen from DAN. rev. ed. 1980. LC 79-22347. 352p. 45.00 (0-8236-2630-X) Intl Univs Pr.

Individual & Family: Therapy Toward an Integration. Fred M. Sander. 1979. LC 79-91901. (Individual & Family Therapy Ser.). 242p. 45.00 (0-87668-400-2) Aronson.

Individual & Social Responsibility: Child Care, Education, Medical Care & Long-Term Care in America. Ed. by Victor R. Fuchs. 1995. LC 95-20983. 364p. 55.00 (0-226-26786-5) U Ch Pr.

Individual & the Group: Boundaries & Interrelations Ed. by Malcolm Pines & Lise Rafaelsen. 1982. LC 81-17924. Vol. 1: Theory. 378p. 65.00 (0-306-40837-6); Vol. 2: Practice. 700p. 95.00 (0-306-40838-4) Perseus Pubng (Plenum Trade).

Individual & the Social Self: Unpublished Work of George Herbert Mead. George Herbert Mead. Ed. by David L. Miller. LC 82-4885. (Chicago Original Paperback Ser.). 232p. (C). 1995. pap. text 16.00 (0-226-51674-1); 1992. lib. bdg. 26.00 (0-226-51673-3) U Ch Pr.

Individual Delinquent, A Text-Book of Diagnosis & Prognosis for All Concerned in Understanding Offenders. William Healy. 1969. LC 69-16238. (Criminology, Law Enforcement, & Social Problems Ser.: No. 85). (Illus.). reprint ed. 35.00 (0-87585-085-5) Patterson Smith.

Individual Differences. James P. Connell et al. 1998. LC 99-191725. pap. text 14.00 (0-226-76171-1) U Ch Pr.

Individual Differences. Colin Cooper. 1997. LC 97-12827. 368p. pap. (0-340-66274-3) E A GBR. *Dist:* OUP.

Individual Differences & Cognition. 3. Douglas K. Detterman. 1993. (Current Topics in Human Intelligence Ser.: Vol. 3). 336p. 85.00 (0-89391-860-1, Ablex) Greenwood.

Individual Differences in Cardiovascular Response to Stress. J. R. Turner et al. 1992. (Perspectives on Individual Differences Ser.). (Illus.). 320p. (C). 59.50 (0-306-44155-1, Plenum Trade) Perseus Pubng.

Individual Differences in Children & Adolescents. Donald H. Saklofske & Sybil B. Eysenck. 1997. LC 97-4510. (Illus.). 344p. pap. text 24.95 (1-56000-981-0) Transaction Pubs.

Individual Differences in Hemispheric Specialization. Ed. by A. Glass. 1987. LC 87-14055. (NATO ASI Series A, Life Sciences: Vol. 130). (Illus.). 416p. 95.00 (0-306-42586-6, Plenum Trade) Perseus Pubng.

Individual Differences in Imaging: Their Measurement, Origins, & Consequences. Alan Richardson. 1994. LC 93-28218. (Imagery & Human Development Ser.). 223p. pap. 30.00 (0-89503-117-5); text 38.95 (0-89503-116-7) Baywood Pub.

Individual Differences in Infancy: Reliability, Stability, & Prediction. Ed. by John Colombo & Jeffrey W. Fagen. 1990. 480p. (C). text 125.00 (0-8058-0369-6) L Erlbaum Assocs.

Individual Differences in Posttraumatic Response: Problems with the Adversity-Distress Connection. Marilyn L. Bowman. 1997. LC 97-1892. 175p. text (0-8058-2713-7) L Erlbaum Assocs.

Individual Differences in the Behavioral Etiology of Drug Abuse. Ed. by Harold W. Gordon & Meyer D. Glantz. 1997. (Illus.). 358p. (C). pap. text 40.00 (0-7881-4608-4) DIANE Pub.

Individual Differences, Stress, & Health Psychology. Ed. by M. P. Janisse. 1988. (Contributions to Psychology & Medicine Ser.). (Illus.). 191p. 87.95 (0-387-96669-2) Spr-Verlag.

Individual Drug Counseling Approach to Cocaine Addiction: The Collaborative Cocaine Treatment Study Model. Delinda E. Mercer & George E. Woody. 2000. 83p. pap. text 25.00 (0-7881-8850-X) DIANE Pub.

Individual Drug Counseling Approach to Treat Cocaine Addiction: The Collaborative Cocaine Treatment Study Model. Delinda E. Mercer. 1999. LC 99-489402. 91p. pap. 9.50 (0-16-050144-X) USGPO.

Individual Equilibrium-Seeking Behavior: A Definition & a Test. Mark D. Menchik. 1969. (Discussion Papers: No. 33). pap. 10.00 (1-55869-056-5) Regional Sci Res Inst.

Individual Liberty & Medical Control. Heta Hayry. 1998. LC 98-73764. (Avebury Series in Philosophy). 114p. text (1-84014-572-2) Ashgate Pub GBR. *Dist:* Ashgate Pub Co.

Individual, Marriage, & the Family. Lloyd Saxton. 6th ed. 1985. 554p. (C). mass mkt. 31.50 net. (0-534-05682-2) Wadsworth Pub.

Individual Processes in Organizational Behavior. Jak Jabes. Ed. by Kenneth D. MacKenzie. 1978. LC 77-86012. (Organizational Behavior Ser.). (C). pap. text 15.95 (0-88295-450-4) Harlan Davidson.

Individual Programme Planning: A Mechanism for Developing Plans to Meet the Specific Needs of Individuals with Mental Handicaps. Ed. by Judith Jenkins et al. 1988. (C). 39.00 (0-906054-64-8) St Mut.

Individual Psychology: Theory & Practice. Guy J. Manaster & Raymond J. Corsini. 1982. LC 81-82887. 322p. pap. 19.95 (0-87581-274-0) Adler Sch Prof Psy.

Individual Psychology of Alfred Adler: A Systematic Presentation in Selections from His Writings. Alfred Adler. Ed. by Heinz Ludwig Ansbacher & Rowena R. Ansbacher. 1964. 544p. pap. 17.00 (0-06-131154-5, TB1154, Torch) HarperCollins Pubs.

Individual Psychotherapy & the Science of Psychodynamics. David H. Malan. 2nd ed. 1995. LC 95-195666. (Illus.). 320p. (0-7506-2387-X) E A GBR. *Dist:* OUP.

Individual Psychotherapy in LTC Settings. Marylou Hughes. 1995. 280p. (C). 28.00 (1-877735-48-5, 2297PP) Prof Prnting & Pub.

Individual Subject & Scientific Psychology. J. Valsiner. 1986. LC 86-18698. (Perspectives on Individual Differences Ser.). (Illus.). 422p. (C). 80.00 (0-306-42250-6, Plenum Trade) Perseus Pubng.

Individual Therapy Handbook. Wendy Dryden. 1990. (0-335-09446-5) OpUniv Pr.

Individual Therapy Handbook. Wendy Dryden. 1990. pap. (0-335-09445-7) OpUniv Pr GBR. *Dist:* Taylor & Francis.

Individual Therapy in Britain. Ed. by Wendy Dryden. 1984. 448p. pap. (0-335-09810-X) OpUniv Pr GBR. *Dist:* Taylor & Francis.

Individual Uses of Positive Substitution & Problem Solutions, Set-IP. Russell E. Mason. 1975. pap. 35.00 incl. audio (0-89533-007-5) F I Comm.

Individualism & Collectivism. Harry C. Triandis. 1995. LC 94-46567. (New Directions in Social Psychology Ser.). 280p. (C). pap. text 32.00 (0-8133-1850-5) Westview.

Individuality in Pain & Suffering. Asenath Petrie. 2nd ed. 1993. LC 77-93608. (Illus.). reprint ed. pap. text 4.95 (0-226-66347-7, P739) U Ch Pr.

Individualization: Principles & Procedures in Criminalistics. Harold Tuthill. 1994. LC 94-79056. 134p. (C). pap. 19.95 (0-9622305-3-7) Lightning Powder.

Individualization in Childhood & Adolescence Ser. Ed. by Georg Neubauer & Klaus Hurrelmann. 1995. (Prevention & Intervention in Childhood & Adolescence: No. 15). vi, 348p. (C). lib. bdg. 54.95 (3-11-014681-9) De Gruyter.

Individualized Dementia Care: Creative, Compassionate Approaches. Ed. by Elizabeth M. Tornquist & Joanne Rader. 1995. LC 94-45714. 320p. 41.95 (0-8261-8730-7) Springer Pub.

Individualized Therapy of Hypertension. Ed. by Norman M. Kaplan & Venkata S. Ram. 1994. (Fundamental & Clinical Cardiology Ser.: Vol. 22). (Illus.). 296p. text 125.00 (0-8247-9262-9) Dekker.

Individualizing Psychological Assessment. Constance T. Fischer. 1994. 424p. text 36.00 (0-8058-1586-4) L Erlbaum Assocs.

Individuals & Environment: A Psychosocial Approach to Workspace. Gustave-Nicolas Fischer. Tr. by Ruth Atkin-Etienne from FRE. 1997. LC 96-47257. (Studies in Organization: Vol. 78). xii, 195p. (C). text 74.95 (3-11-013577-9) De Gruyter.

Individuation & Narcissism: The Psychology of Self in Jung & Kohut. Mario Jacoby. 1991. 288p. (C). pap. 27.95 (0-415-06464-3, A6253) Routledge.

Individuation & the Absolute: Hegel, Jung, & the Path Toward Wholeness. Sean M. Kelly. 1993. LC 93-9166. (Jung & Spirituality Ser.). 224p. pap. 14.95 (0-8091-3394-6) Paulist Pr.

Individuation in Contemporary Psychoanalysis: The Emergence of Individuality in Interpersonal & Rational Theory & Practice. Thomas Jordan. 1999. LC 99-16844. (Illus.). xii, 314p. pap. 41.95 (0-398-07000-8); 314p. text 57.95 (0-398-06999-9) C C Thomas.

Indocyanine Green Angiography. Lawrence A. Yannuzzi et al. 1997. (Illus.). 400p. text 200.00 (0-8151-9774-8, 25288) Mosby Inc.

Indole & Biogenetically Related Alkaloids. Ed. by J. D. Phillipson & M. H. Zenk. 1981. (Annual Proceedings of the Phytochemical Society of Europe: No. 17). text 209.00 (0-12-554450-2) Acad Pr.

Indoor Air & Human Health. Ed. by Richard B. Gammage & Barry A. Berven. 2nd ed. 1996. LC 95-43001. 384p. 94.95 (1-56670-144-9) CRC Pr.

Indoor Air & Human Health: Major Indoor Air Pollutants & Their Health Implications. Ed. by R. B. Gammage & S. V. Kaye. 1985. LC 85-13134. (Illus.). 429p. lib. bdg. 84.95 (0-87371-006-1) Lewis Pubs.

Indoor Air Pollution: An Introduction for Health Professionals. 1996. (Illus.). 25p. reprint ed. pap. text 15.00 (0-7881-3084-6) DIANE Pub.

Indoor Air Quality: Biological Contaminants: Report on a WHO Meeting. 1990. (WHO Regional Publications, European Ser.: No. 31). (ENG, FRE, GER & RUS.). 67p. pap. text 9.00 (92-890-1122-X, 1310031) World Health.

Indoor Air Quality: Organic Pollutants. 1989. (Euro Reports & Studies Ser.: No. 111). 70p. pap. text 8.00 (92-890-1277-3) World Health.

Indoor & Outdoor Air Pollution & Human Cancer. Ed. by L. Tomatis. 1993. LC 93-10623. (Monographs of the European School of Oncology). (Illus.). 162p. 149.00 (0-387-56645-7) Spr-Verlag.

Indoor Environment in Schools - Respiratory Effects & Air Quality. Greta Smedje. 2000. (Comprehensive Summaries of Uppsala Dissertations from the Faculty of Medicine Ser.: No. 925). (Illus.). 58p. pap. (91-554-4713-9) Uppsala Universitet SWE. *Dist:* Coronet Bks.

Indoor Radon & Lung Cancer: Reality or Myth?, Set. Ed. by Fredrick T. Cross. 1992. (Hanford Symposium on Health & the Environment Ser.: No. 29). 1200p. pap. 89.95 (0-935470-69-7) Battelle.

Indoor Radon Remedial Action: The Scientific Basis & the Practical Implications: Abstracts of First International Workshop. 1994. 116p. (Orig.). (C). pap. text 40.00 (0-7881-1086-1) DIANE Pub.

Induced Abortion: Report of a WHO Scientific Group, 1978. 1978. (Technical Report Ser.: No. 623). 65p. pap. text 7.00 (92-4-120623-3, 1100623) World Health.

Induced Effects of Genotoxic Agents in Eukaryotic Cells. Ed. by Toby G. Rossman. 1992. LC 92-19547. 85.00 (1-56032-272-1) Hemisp Pub.

Induced Rhythms in the Brain. Ed. by E. Basar & Theodore H. Bullock. 1992. (Brain Dynamics Ser.). (Illus.). 480p. 212.50 (0-8176-3537-8) Birkhauser.

Induced Skeletal Muscle Ischemia in Man. Ed. by D. H. Lewis. 1982. (Illus.). iv, 180p. pap. 100.00 (3-8055-3427-2) S Karger.

Induction & Expression of Brain Metallothionein: Journal: Biological Signals, Vol. 3, No. 3. Ed. by M. Ebadi. 1994. (Journal). (Illus.). 58p. pap. 30.50 (3-8055-6053-2) S Karger.

Induction & Modulation of Gastrointestinal Inflammation: Proceedings of the Falk Symposium 104 Held in Sarbrhucken, Germany, March 5-7, 1998. A. Stallmach. 1999. LC 99-184905. (Falk Symposium Ser.). 326 p. (0-7923-8747-3) Kluwer Academic.

Induction of Thyroid Cancer by Ionizing Radiation. Intro. by Warren K. Sinclair. 1985. LC 84-21441. (Report Ser.: No. 80). 94p. pap. text 35.00 (0-913392-72-3) NCRP Pubns.

Indulation Coordination. A. Hileman. 1999. LC 99-30734. (Illus.). 784p. text 195.00 (0-8247-9957-7) Dekker.

Industrial & Confined Space Rescue. Mike Roop & Richie Wright. 1998. LC 97-22071. (Illus.). 400p. (gr. 13). pap. text 35.95 (0-8151-7383-0, 27761) Mosby Inc.

Industrial & Environmental Xenobiotics. Ed. by I. Gut et al. 1981. (Proceedings in Life Sciences Ser.). (Illus.). 409p. 79.95 (0-387-10960-9) Spr-Verlag.

Industrial & Organizational Psychology. Krumm. 2001. pap. text, stu. ed. 17.50 (1-57259-975-8) Worth.

Industrial & Organized Psychology. Ed. by Hughes. 1999. (C). text (0-321-01340-9) Addson-Wesley Educ.

Industrial Back Pain in Europe. Ed. by Peter R. Davis. 1984. (Ergonomics Ser.: Vol. 28, No. 1). 416p. pap. 23.00 (0-85066-985-5) Taylor & Francis.

Industrial Behavior Modification: A Learning Based Approach to Industrial-Organizational Problems. Ed. by Richard M. O'Brien et al. 1982. LC 81-19877. (General Psychology Ser.). (Illus.). 480p. 78.00 (0-08-025558-2, J125, L120, Pergamon Pr) Elsevier.

Industrial Conflict: Psychological Interpretation. Ed. by George W. Hartmann et al. 1977. LC 77-182. (Illus.). reprint ed. lib. bdg. 56.95 (0-405-10173-2) Ayer.

Industrial Fatigue & Efficiency. Horace M. Vernon. Ed. by Leon Stein. 1977. LC 77-70543. (Illus.). reprint ed. lib. bdg. 26.95 (0-405-10212-7) Ayer.

Industrial Health. Ed. by Jack E. Peterson. 2nd ed. 1991. (Illus.). (C). text 73.00 (0-936712-91-0) Am Conf Govt Indus Hygienist.

Industrial Hygiene: Index of New Information. James Q. Batchelor. 1998. 160p. 57.50 (0-7883-1660-5); pap. 47.50 (0-7883-1661-3) ABBE Pubs Assn.

Industrial Hygiene Aspects of Plant Operations: Engineering Considerations in Equipment Selection, Layout, & Building Design, III. Lewis J. Cralley. Ed. by Lester V. Cralley. 1985. 800p. (C). 89.50 (0-02-949370-6) Free Pr.

Industrial Hygiene Aspects of Plant Operations: Engineering Considerations in Equipment Selection, Layout, & Building Design, II. Lewis J. Cralley. Ed. by Lester V. Cralley. 1986. 552p. (C). text 77.50 (0-471-62492-6) Krieger.

Industrial Hygiene Engineering: Recognition, Measurement, Evaluation & Control. Ed. by John T. Talty. 2nd ed. 1989. LC 88-17863. (Illus.). 831p. 139.00 (0-8155-1175-2) Noyes.

Industrial Hygiene Management. Ed. by Jack T. Garrett et al. 1988. LC 87-27032. 416p. 130.00 (0-471-85128-0) Wiley.

Industrial Hygiene Program Management. Ed. by American Conference of Governmental Industrial Hygenists Staff. 2nd ed. 2000. LC 2001-278549. 172p. pap. text 39.00 (1-882417-37-2) Am Conf Govt Indus Hygienist.

Industrial Hygiene Workbook. D. Jeff Burton. 1993. 340p. 45.00 (0-9623160-9-1) IVE Inc.

Industrial Hygienist. Jack Rudman. 1994. (Career Examination Ser.: C-381). pap. 39.95 (0-8373-0381-8) Nat Learn.

Industrial Injury Prevention & Education Programs. Ed. by Silent Partners, Inc. Staff. 1994. (Illus.). 12p. pap. (1-878353-35-7) Silent Partners.

Industrial Medicine Desk Reference. David F. Tver & Kenneth A. Anderson. 1986. (Advanced Industrial Technology Ser.). 400p. text 39.95 (0-412-01101-8, 9532, Chap & Hall NY) Chapman & Hall.

Industrial Organ Psychology. Ed. by Cary L. Cooper. 1992. (C). Vol. I. lib. bdg. 175.00 (0-8147-1455-2); Vol. 2. lib. bdg. 175.00 (0-8147-1456-0) NYU Pr.

Industrial Process & Waste Stream Management. 1998. (Environmental Engineering Ser.). (C). pap. 59.95 (0-442-02599-8, VNR) Wiley.

Industrial Psychology. Charles S. Myers. Ed. by Leon Stein. 1977. LC 77-70519. (Illus.). reprint ed. lib. bdg. 19.95 (0-405-10188-0) Ayer.

Industrial Rehabilitation: Techniques for Success. Robin Saunders. 1995. LC 95-92434. (Illus.). 162p. (Orig.). (C). spiral bd. 44.95 (1-879190-08-7) Saunders Grp.

Industrial Rehabilitation Services: Forms, Checklists & Guidelines. Aspen Publishers Staff et al. 1997. LC 96-33462. ring bd. 159.00 (0-8342-0873-3) Aspen Pub.

Industrial Respiratory Protection. Michael F. Teresinski & Paul N. Cheremisinoff. 1989. (Illus.). 350p. pap. text 39.95 (0-925760-01-3) SciTech Pubs.

Industrial Safety, Environmental Pollution, Health Hazards & Nuclear Accidents: A Global Survey. Attar Chand. 1989. (*81-7099-128-5*) Mittal Pubs Dist IND. *Dist:* S Asia.

Industrial Society: Emergence of the Human Problems of Automation. Georges Friedman. Ed. by Leon Stein. 1977. LC 77-70497. reprint ed. lib. bdg. 41.95 (*0-405-10167-8*) Ayer.

Industrial Sterilization: International Symposium. Ed. by G. Briggs Phillips & William S. Miller. 1973. LC 72-97473. (Illus.). x, 430p. text 49.95 (*0-8223-0299-3*) Duke.

Industrial Therapy. Glenda L. Key. 1994. LC 94-46875. (Illus.). 572p. (C). (gr. 13). text 73.00 (*0-8151-5046-6*, 23640) Mosby Inc.

Industrial Toxicology. Harbison. 5th ed. 1998. LC 97-43981. (Illus.). 704p. (C). (gr. 13). text 79.00 (*0-8151-4181-5*, 27914) Mosby Inc.

Industrial Ventilation Workbook. D. Jeff Burton. 2nd ed. 1992. 345p. stu. ed. 45.00 (*0-9623160-2-4*) IVE Inc.

Industry Analysis: The Health Care Industries. 1993. 30.00 (*1-879087-25-1*) Assn I M&R.

Industry & HMOs: A Natural Alliance. Ed. by R. H. Egdahl & Diana C. Walsh. 1978. (Springer Series in Industry & Health Care: Vol. 5). (Illus.). 117p. 38.00 (*0-387-90366-6*) Spr-Verlag.

***Industry in Evolution: A Source Book of Charts & Statistics Providing Analysis & Insight into the Clinical Trials Industry.** Ed. by Mary Jo Lamberti. 3rd rev. ed. 2001. (Illus.). 247p. pap. 550.00 (*1-930624-15-8*) CenterWatch.

Industry Regulation: A Guide for the Healthcare Professional. Jonathan P. Tomes. 1993. 110p. (Orig.). per. 24.95 (*1-882198-00-X*) Hlthcare Fin Mgmt.

Industry's Voice in Health Policy. W. B. Goldbeck. 1979. (Springer Series in Industry & Health Care: Vol. 7). 136p. 57.00 (*0-387-90429-8*) Spr-Verlag.

Indwelling & Implantable Pressure Transducers. Ed. by David Fleming & Wen H. Ko. 1977. (Uniscience Ser.). 224p. 128.00 (*0-8493-5195-2*, R857, CRC Reprint) Franklin.

Inebriety: A Clinical Treatise on the Etiology, Symptomotology, Neurosis, Psychosis & Treatment & Medico-Legal Relations. T. D. Crothers. Ed. by Gerald N. Grob. 1981. LC 80-1221. (Addiction in America Ser.). reprint ed. lib. bdg. 35.95 (*0-405-13576-9*) Ayer.

Inebriety: Its Causes, Its Results, Its Remedy. Franklin D. Clum. Ed. by Gerald N. Grob. 1981. LC 80-1217. (Addiction in America Ser.). reprint ed. lib. bdg. 25.95 (*0-405-13573-4*) Ayer.

Inebriety: Its Source, Prevention, & Cure. Charles F. Palmer. Ed. by Gerald N. Grob. 1981. LC 80-1242. (Addiction in America Ser.). reprint ed. lib. bdg. 16.95 (*0-405-13612-9*) Ayer.

Inebriety or Narcomania: Its Etiology, Pathology, Treatment & Jurispruben. Norman Kerr. Ed. by Gerald N. Grob. 1981. LC 80-1238. (Addiction in America Ser.). reprint ed. lib. bdg. 60.95 (*0-405-13598-X*) Ayer.

Inebriism, a Pathological & Psychological Study. T. L. Wright. Ed. by Gerald N. Grob. 1981. LC 80-1254. (Addiction in America Ser.). reprint ed. lib. bdg. 25.95 (*0-405-13624-2*) Ayer.

Ineffective Erythropoiesis: A Probability Phenomenon. E. D. Pietrantonj. 1987. pap. text (*1-57235-059-8*) Piccin Nuova.

***Inequality & the Politics of Health: How Politics Makes Americans Sick.** Morone. 2001. 330p. 40.00 (*0-8133-9846-0*) Westview.

Inequality of Man. Hans J. Eysenck. 1975. 17.00 (*0-912736-16-X*) EDITS Pubs.

***Inequity & Madness: Psychology & Human Rights Issues.** J. Guimon. 2001. LC 2001-38778. 75.00 (*0-306-46674-0*, Kluwer Plenum) Kluwer Academic.

Inescapable Decisions: The Imperatives of Health Reform. David Mechanic. 1994. LC 93-13425. 256p. (C). text 44.95 (*1-56000-121-6*) Transaction Pubs.

Inevitability: Determinism, Fatalism, & Destiny, 12. Leonard William Doob. 1988. LC 88-10256. (Contributions in Psychology Ser.: No. 12). 170p. 58.00 (*0-313-26398-1*, DVY/, Greenwood Pr) Greenwood.

Infancy. J. Gavin Bremner. 2nd ed. 1994. (Illus.). 368p. (C). pap. 31.95 (*0-631-18466-X*) Blackwell Pubs.

Infancy: A Guide to Research & Resources. Kathleen P. Watkins et al. 1988. 182p. (C). reprint ed. pap. 16.95 (*0-8077-2921-3*) Tchrs Coll.

Infancy: Its Place in Human Development. Jerome Kagan et al. 1978. LC 77-26970. (Harvard Paperbacks Ser.). (Illus.). 342p. pap. text 15.50 (*0-674-45261-5*) HUP.

Infancy & Early Childhood: The Practice of Clinical Assessment & Intervention with Emotional & Developmental Challenges. Stanley I. Greenspan. 1992. LC 91-35367. 776p. (C). 82.50 (*0-8236-2633-4*) Intl Univs Pr.

Infancy & Preschoolers. Ed. by Joseph D. Noshpitz. 1997. LC 96-17210. (Child & Adolescent Mental Health Ser.: Vol. 1). 624p. 250.00 (*0-471-55079-5*) Wiley.

Infancy, Childhood & Adolescence: Development in Context. Wendy Dunn. 1991. (C). text, stu. ed. 21.87 (*0-07-061215-3*) McGraw.

Infancy of Medicine: Influence of Folklore Upon Scientific Medicine. Dan McKenzie. 1977. lib. bdg. 50.00 (*0-8490-2057-3*) Gordon Pr.

Infancy Research: A Summative Evaluation & a Look to the Future. Ed. by Frances D. Horowitz & John Colombo. 1990. LC 90-35955. 186p. (C). pap. 19.95 (*0-8143-2333-2*) Wayne St U Pr.

Infant & Child Care Skills. Monica Bassett. 1996. 32p. tchr. ed. 10.95 (*0-8273-5508-4*) Delmar.

Infant & Child Care Skills. Monica M. Bassett. 1995. LC 94-23165. (Education Ser.). (Illus.). 292p. (C). mass mkt. 25.75 (*0-8273-5507-6*) Delmar.

Infant & Child CPR. American Red Cross Staff. 1992. LC 92-582. 94p. (gr. 13). pap. text 9.70 (*0-8016-7061-6*) Mosby Inc.

Infant & Child CPR. National Safety Council Staff. 1997. (Emergency Care Ser.). (Illus.). (C). 96p. pap. text, tchr. ed. 15.00 (*0-7637-0583-7*, 0583-7); 64p. pap. text 22.50 (*0-7637-0211-0*, 0211-0) Jones & Bartlett.

Infant & Early Childhood Neuropsychology. Glen P. Aylward. 1997. LC 97-30571. (Clinical Child Psychology Library). 120p. pap. 21.50 (*0-306-45673-7*); (Illus.). 140p. (C). 45.00 (*0-306-45672-9*) Kluwer Academic (Kluwer Plenum).

Infant & Family Health in Australia: A Textbook for Community Health Workers. Ed. by Anthony Clements. 2nd ed. 1992. (Illus.). 416p. (Orig.). pap. text (*0-443-04770-7*) Church.

Infant & Toddler Care. California College for Health Sciences Staff. 1993. 134p. (C). ring bd. Price not set. (*0-933195-06-0*) CA College Health Sci.

Infant & Toddler Health Sourcebook: Basic Consumer Health Information about the Mental & Physical Development of Infants & Toddles. Ed. by Jenifer Swanson. 2000. LC 00-42784. (Health Reference Ser.). (Illus.). xiii, 585p. lib. bdg. 78.00 (*0-7808-0246-2*) Omnigraphics Inc.

Infant & Toddler Programs: A Guide to Very Early Childhood Education. Christine Z. Cataldo. 1983. LC 82-11418. (Illus.). 240p. pap. text 15.95 (*0-201-11020-2*) Addison-Wesley.

Infant & Toddler Strabismus & Amblyopia Vol. 41, No. 2: Behavioral Aspects of Vision Care. Ed. by Anne Barber. 2000. (Behavioral Aspects of Vision Care Ser.). (Illus.). 64p. pap. text 21.00 (*0-943599-33-4*) OEPF.

Infant Assessment. M. Virginia Wyly. 1996. 224p. pap. text (*0-697-12804-0*) Brown & Benchmark.

Infant Assessment. M. Virginia Wyly. 1997. LC 97-510. (Developmental Psychology Ser.). 240p. (C). pap. text 29.00 (*0-8133-3088-2*) Westview.

Infant Asylums & Children's Hospital: Medical Dilemmas & Development, 1850-1920. Ed. by Janet Golden. 1989. (Medical Care in the United States Ser.). 250p. reprint ed. text 15.00 (*0-8240-8334-2*) Garland.

Infant Behavior: Its Genesis & Growth. Arnold L. Gesell & Helen Thompson. 1970. LC 71-95101. 343p. reprint ed. lib. bdg. 35.00 (*0-8371-2704-1*, GEIB, Greenwood Pr) Greenwood.

Infant Care. 1993. (Illus.). 109p. (Orig.). pap. text 20.00 (*1-56806-419-5*) DIANE Pub.

Infant Care & Feeding in the South Pacific, Vol. 3. Ed. by Leslie B. Marshall. 1985. LC 85-12648. (Food & Nutrition in History & Anthropology Ser.). xxii, 356p. text 160.00 (*2-88124-037-2*) Gordon & Breach.

Infant Caregiving: A Design for Training. Alice S. Honig & J. Ronald Lally. 1981. (Illus.). 234p. pap. 16.95 (*0-8156-0169-7*) Syracuse U Pr.

Infant Cognition: Predicting Later Intellectual Functioning. John Colombo. 1993. LC 93-16099. (Individual Differences & Development Ser.: Vol. 5). pap. 31.95 (*0-8039-4960-X*, 4264) Sage.

Infant Colic: What It Is & What You Can Do About It. Christopher Farran. 1984. 144p. pap. 5.95 (*0-684-18153-3*); 1983. 106p. 10.95 (*0-684-17779-X*) Gale (Macmillan Ref).

Infant Communication: Development Assessment & Intervention. Ed. by Dan P. McClowery et al. 1982. 214p. text 36.50 (*0-8089-1533-9*, 792849, Grune & Strat) Harcrt Hlth Sci Grp.

Infant Depression. Paul V. Trad. 1986. (Illus.). 375p. 81.00 (*0-387-96343-X*) Spr-Verlag.

Infant Development: A Multidisciplinary Introduction. John Mercer. 1997. LC 96-52400. (Psychology Ser.). 519p. spiral bd. 77.95 (*0-534-33977-8*) Brooks-Cole.

Infant Development: Perspectives from German-Speaking Countries. Ed. by Heidi Keller & Michael E. Lamb. 1991. 400p. text 79.95 (*0-8058-0666-0*) L Erlbaum Assocs.

Infant Development & Mental Health in Early Intervention. Ed. by James A. Blackman. 1998. LC 94-24186. (Infants & Young Children Ser.). 258p. pap. 41.00 (*0-8342-0647-1*) PRO-ED.

Infant Development with InfoTrac. Mercer. 1998. (Psychology Ser.). 46.50 (*0-534-36356-3*) Brooks-Cole.

Infant Education. Ed. by Bettye Caldwell & Donald Stedman. 1977. pap. 9.95 (*0-8027-7267-6*) Walker & Co.

Infant Feeding: The Physiological Basis. Ed. by J. Akre. 1990. (FRE & SPA.). 108p. pap. text 20.00 (*92-4-068670-3*, 0036701) World Health.

Infant-Feeding Triad: Infant, Mother, & Household. Barry M. Popkin et al. 1986. (Food & Nutrition in History & Anthropology Ser.: Vol. 5). xvi, 248p. text 181.00 (*2-88124-142-5*) Gordon & Breach.

Infant Massage: A Handbook for Loving Parents. Vimala McClure. 3rd rev. ed. 2000. LC 00-39754. (Illus.). 272p. pap. 14.95 (*0-553-38056-7*) Bantam.

Infant Memory: Its Relation to Normal & Pathological Memory in Humans & Other Animals. Ed. by Morris Moscovitch. 1984. LC 84-9844. (Advances in the Study of Communication & Affect Ser.: Vol. 9). 236p. 65.00 (*0-306-41588-7*, Plenum Trade) Perseus Pubng.

Infant Mental Health Groups at High Risk Ed. by Joy D. Osofsky & Hiram E. Fitzgerald. 1999. LC 99-11893. (World Association for Infant Mental Health Ser.: Vol. 4). (Illus.). 617p. 220.00 (*0-471-18947-2*) Wiley.

Infant Mortality among Black Americans. Feroz Ahmed. 1992. 110p. pap. text 10.00 (*1-56669-000-5*) Howard U Inst UAR.

Infant Mortality & Child Health in the Kwazulu-Natal Province: 1988/1992. J. P. H. Rossouw & A. J. Jordaan. 1997. LC 98-134516. (Illus.). (*0-7969-1836-8*) Human Sci Res.

Infant Mortality & the Health of Societies. Kathleen Newland. 1981. pap. (*0-916468-46-1*) Worldwatch Inst.

Infant Mortality by Hispanic Origin of Mother, 20 States, 1985-87 Birth Cohorts. Lisa M. Pastore & Marian F. MacDorman. 1995. LC 95-25370. (Vital & Health Statistics, Series 20, Data from the National Vital Statistics System: No. 27). (*0-8406-0510-2*) Natl Ctr Health Stats.

Infant Mortality in Rural India. M. S. Ashraf. 1990. 177p. (C). (*81-85009-35-X*) Print Hse IND. *Dist:* St Mut.

Infant Mortality of Indian Muslims: Determinants & Implications. Mohammed O. Bajkhaif. 1993. 14.00 (*81-7018-737-0*) S Asia.

Infant-Mother Attachment: The Origins & Developmental Significance of Individual Differences in Strange Situation Behavior. Ed. by William Gardner et al. 1985. 328p. (C). text 79.95 (*0-89859-654-8*) L Erlbaum Assocs.

Infant Nutrition. Samuel J. Fomon. 1993. 600p. (C). (gr. 13). text 108.00 (*1-55664-248-2*) Mosby Inc.

Infant, Perinatal, Maternal, & Childhood Mortality in the United States. Sam Shapiro et al. 1968. LC 68-29183. (Vital & Health Statistics Monographs, Am). (Illus.). 405p. 45.50 (*0-674-45301-8*) HUP.

Infant Previewing: Predicting & Sharing Interpersonal Outcome. Paul V. Trad. 1990. 286p. 97.00 (*0-387-97197-1*) Spr-Verlag.

Infant Respiratory Function Testing: A Practical Guide. Ed. by Janet Stocks et al. 1996. LC 95-31246. 624p. 152.00 (*0-471-07682-1*) Wiley.

Infant Social Cognition: Theoretical & Empirical Considerations. Ed. by Michael E. Lamb & Lonnie R. Sherrod. 1981. LC 80-21137. 448p. text 79.95 (*0-89859-058-2*) L Erlbaum Assocs.

Infant Speech: A Study of the Beginnings of Language. Morris M. Lewis. 1978. LC 74-21420. (Classics in Child Development Ser.). 350p. reprint ed. 35.95 (*0-405-06470-5*) Ayer.

Infant Stimulation: For Whom, What Kind, When, & How Much? Ed. by Nina Guzenhauser. 1987. (Pediatric Round Table Ser.: No. 13). (Illus.). 206p. (Orig.). (C). pap. text 10.00 (*0-931562-15-5*) J & J Consumer Prods.

Infant-Toddler Assessment: An Interdisciplinary Approach. Louis M. Rossetti. 1990. LC 90-9185. (Illus.). 294p. (C). pap. text 31.00 (*0-89079-312-3*, 1782) PRO-ED.

Infant-Toddler Health Record: Birth to 24 Months. Sandy Abrams & William S. Greer. Ed. by Bill Greer. 1995. (Illus.). 120p. (Orig.). pap. 9.95 (*0-9641332-4-5*) Jormax Pubng.

Infant Vision. Ed. by Francois Vital-Durand et al. 1996. LC 95-30844. (European Brain & Behavior Ser.: Ser. 2). (Illus.). 458p. text 95.00 (*0-19-852316-5*) OUP.

Infant Vision: Basic & Clinical Research. Ed. by Kurt Simons. 1993. LC 92-42966. (Illus.). 600p. (C). text 145.00 (*0-19-507721-0*) OUP.

Infanticide & the Value of Life. Ed. by Marvin Kohl. 1978. LC 77-26376. 252p. 34.00 (*0-87975-100-2*) Prometheus Bks.

Infantile Nutrition - an Update. Ed. by R. Di Toro. 1991. (Beitraege zur Infusionstherapie und Klinische Ernaehrung Ser.: Vol. 27). (Illus.). viii, 170p. 68.75 (*3-8055-5343-9*) S Karger.

Infantile Origins of Sexual Identity. Herman Roiphe & Eleanor Galenson. 1981. LC 81-14290. 301p. 47.50 (*0-8236-2368-8*) Intl Univs Pr.

Infantile Psychosis & Early Contribution Vol. 1: The Selected Papers of Margaret S. Mahler. Margaret S. Mahler. 1995. LC 79-51915. (Master Work Ser.: Vol. 1). 334p. pap. text 55.00 (*1-56821-421-9*) Aronson.

Infantile Psychotic Self & Its Fates: Understanding & Treating Schizophrenics & Other Difficult Patients. Vamik D. Volkan. 1995. LC 94-34516. 352p. pap. 50.00 (*1-56821-379-4*) Aronson.

Infantile Spasms & West Syndrome. Ed. by Olivier Dulac et al. 1994. 310p. text 86.00 (*0-7020-1777-9*) Saunders.

Infants & Children with Prenatal Alcohol & Drug Exposure: A Guide to Identification & Intervention. Keeta D. Lewis. 1995. LC 94-47669. 367p. pap. 44.95 (*0-9624814-2-4*) Sunrise River Pr.

Infants & Hearing. Deborah Hayes & Jerry L. Northern. 1996. LC 96-24942. (Illus.). 420p. (Orig.). 59.95 (*1-56593-191-2*, 0633) Thomson Learn.

Infants & Parents: Clinical Case Reports. Ed. by Sally Provence. 1983. LC 83-18441. (Clinical Infant Reports: No. 2). xix, 306p. (C). 47.50 (*0-8236-2636-9*) Intl Univs Pr.

Infants & Toddlers. Rick A. Caulfield. 2000. LC 00-46953. (Illus.). 346p. pap. 66.00 (*0-13-014583-1*) P-H.

Infants & Toddlers. Watson et al. 4th ed. 1998. LC 98-17079. (Early Childhood Education Ser.). 466p. (C). pap. text 61.95 (*0-8273-8418-1*) Delmar.

Infants & Toddlers: A Resource Guide for Practioners. Ed. by Michael Bender & Carol A. Baglin. 1992. LC 91-5184. (Illus.). 204p. (Orig.). (C). pap. 34.95 (*1-879105-36-5*, 0220) Thomson Learn.

Infants & Toddlers with Hearing Loss: Family Centered Assessment & Intervention. Ed. by Jackson Roush & Noel Matkin. 1994. 360p. 38.50 (*0-912752-28-9*) York Pr.

Infants at Risk. Ed. by Catherine C. Brown. 1981. (Pediatric Round Table Ser.: No. 5). 132p. (Orig.). pap. text 10.00 (*0-931562-06-6*) J & J Consumer Prods.

Infants Born at Risk: Physiological, Perceptual & Cognitive Processes. Tiffany M. Field & Anita M. Sostek. 1983. 368p. (C). text 40.95 (*0-8089-1563-0*, 791258, Grune & Strat) Harcrt Hlth Sci Grp.

Infants, Children & Adolescents. Berk. 3rd ed. 1998. LC 98-25280. 736p. 86.00 (*0-205-28504-X*) Allyn.

Infants in Crisis: How Parents Cope with Newborn Intensive Care & Its Aftermath. G. Affleck et al. Ed. by R. L. Taylor & L. Sternberg. 1990. (Disorders of Human Learning, Behavior, & Communication Ser.). (Illus.). 156p. 89.95 (*0-387-97392-3*) Spr-Verlag.

Infants in Institutions: A Comparison of Their Development During the First Year of Life with Family-Reared Infants. Sally Provence & Rose C. Lipton. 1967. LC 62-21560. 191p. 31.50 (*0-8236-2648-2*) Intl Univs Pr.

Infants in Multirisk Families: Case Studies in Preventive Intervention. Ed. by Stanley I. Greenspan. 1987. LC 86-84. (Clinical Infant Reports: No. 3). 472p. (C). 77.50 (*0-8236-2645-8*) Intl Univs Pr.

Infants, Parents & Wet Nurses: Medieval Islamic Views on Breastfeeding & Their Social Implications. Avner Giladi. 1999. LC 98-42894. (Islamic History & Civilization Ser.: Vol. 25). x, 191p. 76.50 (*90-04-11223-5*) Brill Academic Pubs.

Infant's Reaction to Strangers. Therese G. Decarie et al. Tr. by Joyce Diamanti from FRE. 1973. LC 73-8080. (Illus.). 238p. (Orig.). (C). 35.00 (*0-8236-2650-4*) Intl Univs Pr.

Infants Toddlers: Curriculum & Teaching. LaVisa C. Wilson. 2nd ed. 1990. 432p. pap. 28.50 (*0-8273-3967-4*); pap., stu. ed. 10.00 (*0-8273-3968-2*) Delmar.

Infants Without Families: Reports on the Hampstead Nurseries. Anna Freud & Dorothy T. Burlingham. 1973. LC 72-8788. (Writings of Anna Freud: Vol. 3). 680p. 85.00 (*0-8236-6872-X*) Intl Univs Pr.

Infecting Ourselves: How Environmental & Social Disruptions Trigger Disease. Anne E. Platt. 1996. 70p. (Orig.). pap. 5.00 (*1-878071-31-9*) Worldwatch Inst.

Infection. Lesley Southgate et al. 1997. LC 97-12090. (Oxford General Practice Ser.: No. 40). (Illus.). 476p. (Orig.). pap. text 54.00 (*0-19-262092-4*) OUP.

Infection & Arthritis. Kippel & Keat. 1994. (C). (gr. 13). 200.00 (*0-8151-5216-7*, 24340) Mosby Inc.

Infection & Environment. Colin Kaplan. 1997. LC 97-939. 160p. pap. (*0-7506-2740-9*) E A GBR. *Dist:* OUP.

Infection & Immunity. John H. Playfair. 1995. (Illus.). 160p. text 39.50 (*0-19-854926-1*); pap. text 21.50 (*0-19-854925-3*) OUP.

Infection & Immunity in Farm Animals. Ed. by R. Pandey. 1984. (Progress in Veterinary Microbiology & Immunology Ser.: Vol. 1). (Illus.). xiv, 258p. 142.75 (*3-8055-3925-8*) S Karger.

Infection & Nursing Practice: Prevention & Control. Barbara M. Soule et al. 1994. (Illus.). 384p. (C). (gr. 13). text 45.95 (*0-8016-6947-2*, 06947) Mosby Inc.

Infection & Nursing Practice: Prevention & Control. Barbara M. Soule et al. 1994. (Illus.). 384p. (*84-8174-138-8*) Mosby-Doyma Libros ESP. *Dist:* Mosby Inc.

Infection Control: A Quick Reference for Infection Control in the Home & Community. Carol J. Stanton. 1997. (Illus.). vi, 84p. spiral bd. (*1-891814-00-1*) Found Care Mgmt.

Infection Control: Dilemmas & Practical Solutions. Ed. by K. R. Cundy et al. 1990. LC 89-26613. (Illus.). 224p. (C). text 102.00 (*0-306-43397-4*, Kluwer Plenum) Kluwer Academic.

***Infection Control: Hospital & Community.** 1997. (Illus.). pap. (*0-7487-3319-1*) Nelson Thornes GBR. *Dist:* Intl Spec Bk.

Infection Control & Management of Hazardous Materials for the Dental Team. Chris H. Miller & Charles John Palenik. 2nd ed. 1998. LC 98-13526. (Illus.). 376p. (C). (gr. 13). pap. text 29.00 (*0-8151-5688-X*, 29798) Mosby Inc.

Infection Control & Management of Hazardous Materials for the Dental Team. Chris H. Miller & Charles John Palenik. 2nd ed. 1998. (Illus.). 376p. pap. (*84-8174-468-9*) Mosby-Doyma Libros ESP. *Dist:* Mosby Inc.

Infection Control & OSHA Essentials. Barbara S. Russell. 3rd ed. 1998. LC 99-161718. 111p. (Orig.). pap. text 23.00 (*1-879772-12-4*) Health Studies.

Infection Control for Prehospital Care Providers. Lynn Zimmerman et al. 2nd rev. ed. 1993. (Illus.). pap. (*0-9615819-1-3*) Amer Med Res.

Infection Control for the Health Care Worker. Leigh G. Donowitz. 1993. LC 93-27555. 12.00 (*0-683-02608-9*); 2nd ed. 1995. pap. (*0-683-02607-0*) Lppncott W & W.

Infection Control for the Professions of Audiology & Speech-Language Pathology. Robert J. Kemp et al. 1995. 126p. 26.95 (*1-56593-591-8*, 1200) Singular Publishing.

Infection Control in Clinical Practice. Jennie Wilson. 1995. (Illus.). 355p. pap. text (*0-7020-1722-1*) W B Saunders GBR. *Dist:* Saunders.

Infection Control in Home Care. Mary M. Friedman & Emily Rhinehart. 1999. LC 98-32394. 256p. pap. 65.00 (*0-8342-1143-2*, 11432) Aspen Pub.

Infection Control in Intensive Care Unit. Ed. by H. K. Van Saene et al. 1997. LC 97-37810. 357p. 129.00 (*3-540-75043-6*) Spr-Verlag.

Infection Control in Intensive Care Units by Selective Decontamination. Ed. by H. K. Saene et al. 1989. (Illus.). 256p. 43.00 (*0-387-51041-9*) Spr-Verlag.

Infection Control in Long-Term Care Facilities. Ed. by Philip W. Smith. 1989. LC 83-21756. 341p. text 41.95 (*0-8273-4369-8*) Delmar.

Infection Control in Long Term Care Facilities. Marguerite A. Bouvette. 2nd ed. 1987. 91p. (C). 14.00 (*1-877735-15-9*, 2128PP) Prof Prnting & Pub.

Infection Control in Long-Term Care Facilities. Philip W. Smith. 2nd ed. 1994. (Health & Life Science Ser.). 268p. pap. 46.50 (*0-8273-5686-2*) Delmar.

***Infection Control in the Community.** Jean Lawrence & Dee May. 2001. (Illus.). 315p. pap. (*0-443-06406-7*) Church GBR. *Dist:* Saunders.

Infection Control in the Former Wet Finger Environment. R. R. Runnells. (Illus.). 182p. (C). pap. text (*0-936751-09-6*) Infection Control.

Infection Control in the Former Wet Finger Environment. Robert R. Runnells. 3rd ed. 1994. (Illus.). 274p. pap., stu. ed. 29.95 (*0-936751-12-6*) Infection Control.

Infection Control in the Immunocompromised Host. Mattias Schrappe & Harald Seifert. 1997. (Illus.). 158p. 75.00 (*3-89412-200-5*) Blackwell Sci.

Infection Control Management Forms, Checklist & Guidelines. Martha J. Grimes. 1996. ring bd. 239.00 (*0-8342-0538-6*, S140) Aspen Pub.

Infection Control Manual for Respiratory Care. Arthur J. McLaughlin & Roberto Palermo. 2nd ed. 1995. LC 96-21362. 243p. pap. 51.00 (*0-8342-0787-7*) PRO-ED.

Infection Control Nurse. Jack Rudman. 1994. (Career Examination Ser.: C-3213). pap. 29.95 (*0-8373-3213-3*) Nat Learn.

Infection Control Policy & Procedure Manual. W. H. Heaton. 1992. 724p. ring bd. 149.95 (*1-881057-05-4*) Heaton Pubns.

Infection Control, Science, Management & Practice. Janet Mcculloch. 1999. 240p. pap. text 29.95 (*1-86156-053-2*) Singular Publishing.

Infection Control Update, 1996. Barbara Acello. 1997. LC 96-32156. (*0-8273-8381-9*) Delmar.

***Infection Highlights 2000-2001.** Wilcox. 2001. (Fast Facts Ser.). (Illus.). 98p. pap. (*1-899541-94-2*) Health Pr GBR. *Dist:* JAMCO Dist.

Infection in Cardiothoracic Intensive Care. R. Freeman & F. K. Gould. 1988. (Illus.). 128p. (C). (*0-683-13025-0*) E A GBR. *Dist:* Williams & Wilkins.

Infection in Surgical Practice. Ed. by Eric W. Taylor. 1992. (Illus.). 348p. 125.00 (*0-19-262023-1*) OUP.

Infection Prevention: Multimedia Package, Training CD-ROM & Reference Booklet. AVSC International Staff. 2000. (Illus.). 75p. pap. text 40.00 (*1-885063-24-5*) EngenderHlth.

Infection Prevention: A Reference Booklet for Health Care Providers see Prevention des Infections: Guide de Reference a l'Intention des Prestataires de Soins de Sante

Infection Prevention for Family Planning Service Professionals: A Problem-Solving Reference Manual. Linda Tietjen et al. 1995. (RUS., Illus.). 248p. pap. text 15.00 (*0-929817-68-0*) JHPIEGO.

Infection Prevention for Family Planning Service Programs: A Problem-Solving Reference Manual. Linda Tietjen et al. 1995. (Illus.). 254p. pap. text 15.00 (*0-929817-65-6*) JHPIEGO.

Infection Prevention for Family Planning Service Programs: A Problem Solving Reference Manual. Linda Tietjen et al. 1992. (Illus.). 272p. (Orig.). pap. 12.95 (*0-929240-50-2*) EMIS.

Infection Prevention for Family Planning Service Programs: A Problem-Solving Reference Manual. Ed. by Linda Tietjen et al. 2nd ed. Date not set. (Illus.). pap. text 15.00 (*0-929817-11-7*) JHPIEGO.

Infections. Williams. 1999. (Companion Series to Bailey & Love's Short Practice of Surgery). (Illus.). 448p. (C). pap. 110.50 (*0-412-64170-4*, Chap & Hall NY) Chapman & Hall.

Infections & Abortions. Sebastian Faro & Pearlman. 1992. (Current Topic in Obstetrics & Gynecology). (Illus.). 116p. (C). (gr. 13). 65.95 (*0-412-04551-6*) Chapman & Hall.

Infections & Arthritis. Ed. by John J. Calabro & W. Carson Dick. 1989. (New Clinical Applications Rheumatology Ser.). lib. bdg. (*0-7462-0052-8*) Kluwer Academic NLD. *Dist:* Kluwer Academic.

Infections & Immunologic Disorders in Pediatric Surgery. Eric W. Fonkalsrud & Thomas Krummel. 1992. (Illus.). 312p. text 120.00 (*0-7216-4278-0*) Saunders.

Infections Associated with Indwelling Medical Devices. Ed. by Francis Waldvogel & Alan L. Bisno. 3rd rev. ed. 2000. LC 00-44762. 400p. pap. 99.95 (*1-55581-177-9*) ASM Pr.

Infections Associated with Prosthetic Devices. Ed. by B. Sugarman & E. J. Young. 1984. 296p. 167.00 (*0-8493-6111-7*, RD130, CRC Reprint) Franklin.

Infections by Hookworms (Bunostomiasis) Index of New Information. Martha M. Fornalle. 1994. (Illus.). 150p. 57.50 (*0-7883-0036-9*) ABBE Pubs Assn.

Infections by Multiresistant Staphylococci. Ed. by F. H. Kayser & C. Carbon. 1996. (Journal: Vol. 4, Suppl. 2). (Illus.). iv, 60p. pap., suppl. ed. 21.75 (*3-8055-6313-2*) S Karger.

Infections in Bones & Joints. Carl Norden & Gillespie. 1994. (Illus.). 400p. 99.95 (*0-86542-273-7*) Blackwell Sci.

Infections in Childhood: Ear, Nose, & Throat Aspects. Ed. by Jacob Sade. 1994. LC 94-6373. (International Congress Ser.: Vol. 1040). 458p. 227.25 (*0-444-81629-1*) Elsevier.

Infections in Children. Richard Andersen et al. 2nd ed. 1997. 286p. pap. 51.00 (*0-8342-0387-1*, 20387) PRO-ED.

Infections in Elderly Patients. W. J. MacLennan et al. 1994. 176p. (*0-340-55933-0*) E A GBR. *Dist:* OUP.

Infections in Gynecology (Colour Guide) Richard Smith. 1994. pap. text (*0-443-04756-1*) Church.

Infections in Immunocompromised Infants & Children. Christian C. Patrick. 1992. (Illus.). 979p. text (*0-443-08857-8*) Church.

Infections in Intravenous Drug Abusers. Ed. by Donald P. Levine & Jack D. Sobel. 1990. (Illus.). 416p. text 75.00 (*0-19-506223-X*) OUP.

Infections in Nursing Homes & Long Term Care Facilities. Ed. by Abraham Verghese & S. L. Berk. 1990. (Illus.). xvi, 248p. 128.00 (*3-8055-5075-8*) S Karger.

Infections in Outpatient Practice: Recognition & Management. R. A. Gleckman et al. 1988. (Illus.). 240p. (C). text 59.50 (*0-306-42970-5*, Kluwer Plenum) Kluwer Academic.

Infections in Pregnancy. Larry C. Gilstrap & Sebastian Faro. 2nd ed. 1997. LC 96-44294. (Illus.). 345p. 137.00 (*0-471-11699-8*) Wiley.

Infections in the Elderly. Ed. by Joseph F. Albright & Julia W. Albright. 2001. (Infectious Disease Ser.). 450p. 125.00 (*0-89603-644-8*) Humana.

Infections in the Elderly. Ed. by M. J. Denham. 1986. (Modern Geriatric Medicine Ser.). text 155.50 (*0-85200-800-7*) Kluwer Academic.

Infections in the Elderly. Richard A. Gleckman & Nelson M. Gantz. 1983. 360p. 41.00 (*0-316-31587-7*, Little Brwn Med Div) Lppncott W & W.

Infections of Leisure. Ed. by David L. Schlossberg. 2nd rev. ed. 1999. LC 99-17154. (Illus.). 350p. pap. 49.95 (*1-55581-160-4*) ASM Pr.

Infections of Leisure. Ed. by David L. Schlossberg. LC 93-3831. (Illus.). 425p. (*3-540-94069-3*); 1993. 345p. 115.00 (*0-387-94069-3*) Spr-Verlag.

Infections of the Central Nervous System. Ed. by W. Michael Scheld et al. 2nd ed. 1996. LC 96-17370. 1,072p. text 235.00 (*0-397-51696-7*) Lppncott W & W.

Infections of the Central Nervous System: Diagnosis & Management. Richard Osenbach & Seth M. Zeidman. 1998. LC 98-29117. 432p. text 129.00 (*0-397-51837-4*) Lppncott W & W.

Infections of the Female Genital Tract. Richard L. Sweet & Ronald S. Gibbs. 2nd ed. 1990. (Illus.). 376p. 75.00 (*0-683-08039-3*) Lppncott W & W.

Infections of the Foot: Diagnosis & Management. David E. Marcinko. 1997. (Illus.). 288p. (gr. 13). text 85.00 (*0-8016-7018-7*, 07018) Mosby Inc.

Infections of the Gastrointestinal Tract. Ed. by Martin J. Blaser et al. 1995. LC 95-2610. (Illus.). 1,632p. text 299.00 (*0-7817-0226-7*) Lppncott W & W.

Infections of the Head & Neck. Ed. by David L. Schlossberg. 1986. (Clinical Topics in Infectious Disease Ser.). (Illus.). 197p. 96.00 (*0-387-96370-7*) Spr-Verlag.

Infections of the Kidney & Urinary Tract. Ed. by W. R. Cattell. 1996. (Oxford Clinical Nephrology Ser.). (Illus.). 360p. (C). text 99.00 (*0-19-262441-5*) OUP.

Infections of the Nervous System. Ed. by David L. Schlossberg. 1990. (Clinical Topics in Infectious Disease Ser.). (Illus.). 396p. 264.00 (*0-387-97332-X*) Spr-Verlag.

Infections of the Urinary Tract: Proceedings of the International Symposium on Pyelonephritis, 3rd. International Symposium on Pyelonephritis Staff. Ed. by Edward H. Kass & William Brumfitt. 1996. LC 78-18215. (Studies in Infectious Diseases Research). 288p. lib. bdg. 36.00 (*0-226-42566-5*) U Ch Pr.

Infectious AIDS: Have We Been Misled? Peter H. Duesberg. 1995. 582p. LC 95-329397. 27.50 (*1-55643-204-6*); LC 95-32937. pap. 18.95 (*1-55643-195-3*) North Atlantic.

Infectious Causes of Cancer: Targets for Intervention. Ed. by James J. Goedert. 2000. LC 00-24929. (Infectious Disease Ser.). (Illus.). xiv, 336p. 125.00 (*0-89603-772-X*) Humana.

Infectious Complications at a Cancer Clinic, Vol. 3. A. Z. Smolyanskaya. 1989. (Soviet Medical Reviews Ser.: Vol. 3, Pt. 2). 66, ivp. pap. text 47.00 (*3-7186-4914-4*) Gordon & Breach.

Infectious Complications in Bone Marrow Transplantation. Ed. by Stephen C. Schimpff & Jean Klastersky. 1993. LC 92-48504. (Recent Results in Cancer Research Ser.: Vol. 132). (Illus.). 284p. 119.00 (*0-387-56455-1*) Spr-Verlag.

Infectious Complications in Transplant Patients. Ed. by Nina Singh & Jose M. Aguado. 2000. LC 00-64624. (Perspectives on Critical Care Infectious Diseases Ser.: Vol. 1). 328p. 190.00 (*0-7923-7972-1*) Kluwer Academic.

Infectious Complications of Cancer. Ed. by Jean Klastersky. 1995. (Cancer Treatment & Research Ser.: No. CTAR 79). 304p. (C). text 266.00 (*0-7923-3598-8*) Kluwer Academic.

Infectious Disease. Barbara A. Bannister et al. (Illus.). 1996. LC 95-42226. 450p. pap. text 74.95 (*0-632-03251-0*); 2nd ed. 2000. LC 00-23121. vi, 506p. (C). pap. 60.95 (*0-632-05319-4*) Blackwell Sci.

Infectious Disease Color Guide. A. P. Ball et al. 2nd ed. 1999. LC 99-28873. (Illus.). (C). pap. text (*0-443-05883-0*) Church.

Infectious Disease Epidemiology: Theory & Practice. Kenrad E. Nelson et al. 2000. LC 99-86958. 600p. 86.00 (*0-8342-1766-X*, 1766x) Aspen Pub.

Infectious Disease Handbook for Emergency Care Personnel. Ed. by Katherine H. West. 2nd ed. 1994. (Illus.). (C). pap. text 15.00 (*1-882417-05-4*) Am Conf Govt Indus Hygienist.

Infectious Disease in Emergency Medicine. Ed. by Judith C. Brillman & Ronald W. Quenzer. 1992. LC 92-17541. 150.00 (*0-316-10838-3*, Little Brwn Med Div) Lppncott W & W.

Infectious Disease in Pregnancy & the Newborn Infant, Vol. 2. Gwendolyn L. Gilbert. 1991. (Monographs in Clinical Pediatrics). xiv, 618p. text 230.00 (*3-7186-5069-X*); 618, xivp. pap. text 121.00 (*3-7186-5174-2*) Gordon & Breach (Harwood Acad Pubs).

Infectious Disease in the Aging: A Clinical Handbook. Ed. by Thomas T. Yoshikawa & Dean C. Norman. 2000. LC 00-24929. (Infectious Disease Ser.). 352p. 99.50 (*0-89603-744-4*) Humana.

Infectious Disease Manual. David Wilks et al. 1995. LC 95-6330. pap. 44.95 (*0-86542-844-1*) Blackwell Sci.

Infectious Disease Ob & Gyn. Faro & Gilstrap. 1999. pap. text 110.00 (*0-8385-4288-3*, Medical Exam) Appleton & Lange.

Infectious Disease Pathology: Clinical Cases. Gail L. Woods et al. 1998. LC 99-27855. 320p. (*0-7506-9673-7*) E A GBR. *Dist:* OUP.

Infectious Disease Pearls. Ed. by Burke Cunha. 1998. (Pearls Ser.). (Illus.). 214p. pap. 45.00 (*1-56053-203-3*) Hanley & Belfus.

Infectious Disease Resource Manual. Ed. by Sara N. Di Lima & Dwayne E. Eutsey. 1999. LC 98-43499. (Illus.). ring bd. 209.00 (*0-8342-1051-7*) Aspen Pub.

Infectious Disease Secrets. Robert H. Gates. 1998. LC 97-42429. (Secrets Ser.). 400p. pap. 39.95 (*1-56053-266-1*) Hanley & Belfus.

Infectious Disease Testing for Blood Transfusions. 1997. lib. bdg. 250.99 (*0-8490-8153-X*); 1996. lib. bdg. 250.99 (*0-8490-5951-8*) Gordon Pr.

Infectious Diseases. A. P. Ball. 1992. (Color Guide Ser.). (Illus.). 120p. (Orig.). pap. text (*0-443-04594-1*) Church.

Infectious Diseases. David Brooks & Edward M. Dunbar. 1986. (Management of Common Diseases in Family Practice Ser.). text 82.00 (*0-85200-760-4*) Kluwer Academic.

Infectious Diseases. A. P. Ball. 2nd ed. 1998. LC 98-45256. (Colour Aids Ser.). (Orig.). pap. text (*0-443-05771-0*) Church.

Infectious Diseases. Sherwood L. Gorbach et al. Ed. by Richard Zorab. 2nd ed. 1997. LC 96-28575. (Illus.). 2400p. text 225.00 (*0-7216-6119-X*) Saunders.

Infectious Diseases. Donald Armstrong & Jonathan Cohen. 5th ed. 1999. (Illus.). 1920p. 250.00 (*0-7234-2328-8*) Mosby Inc.

Infectious Diseases. Bibhat K. Mandal et al. 5th ed. 1996. LC 95-8411. (Lecture Notes). (Illus.). 264p. pap. 38.95 (*0-632-03351-7*) Blackwell Sci.

Infectious Diseases: Beyond Antibiotics. Paul G. Quie et al. (C). pap. text (*1-878294-07-5*) Health Dimensions.

Infectious Diseases: Colonising the Pacific? John Miles. 1997. LC 97-198317. 112p. pap. (*1-877133-26-4*) Univ Otago Pr NZL. *Dist:* Intl Spec Bk.

Infectious Diseases: Diagnosis & Treatment. Howard Heller et al. 1999. (Current Clinical Practice Ser.). (Illus.). 89.50 (*0-89603-532-8*) Humana.

Infectious Diseases: Soundness of World Health Organization Estimates for Eradication or Elimination. Benjamin F. Nelson. 1999. (Illus.). 58p. pap. text 20.00 (*0-7881-7974-8*) DIANE Pub.

Infectious Diseases & Antimicrobial Therapy of the Ears, Nose & Throat. Jonas T. Johnson & Victor Y. Yu. Ed. by Larry McGrew. 1996. 528p. text 175.00 (*0-7216-6154-8*) Saunders.

Infectious Diseases & Immunology: An Internet Resource Guide. Ed. by Dan Goldenson. 2000. pap. 24.95 (*0-9676811-4-6*) eMedguides.

Infectious Diseases Diagnosis: Current Status & Future Trends. Ed. by H. V. Smith & W. H. Stimson. 2000. (Parasitology Ser.: Vol. 117). 218p. (C). pap. text 39.95 (*0-521-78507-3*) Cambridge U Pr.

Infectious Diseases in an Age of Change: The Impact of Human Ecology & Behavior on Disease Transmission. Ed. by Bernard Roizman. 1995. LC 94-31151. 272p. (Orig.). (C). text 44.95 (*0-309-05136-3*) Natl Acad Pr.

Infectious Diseases in Child Day Care: Management & Protection. Ed. by Michael Osterholm et al. 1996. viii, 185p. lib. bdg. 36.00 (*0-226-63947-9*) U Ch Pr.

Infectious Diseases in Critical Care Medicine. Ed. by Burke A. Cunha. 1998. LC 98-7036. (Infectious Disease & Therapy Ser.: 0). (Illus.). 872p. text 250.00 (*0-8247-0114-3*) Dekker.

Infectious Diseases in Europe: A Fresh Look. B. Velimirovic. 1984. text 35.00 (*92-890-1015-0*) World Health.

Infectious Diseases in Immunocompromised Hosts. Vassil St. Georgiev. 1997. LC 97-28644. (CRC Series on Pharmacology & Toxicology). 1201p. lib. bdg. 159.95 (*0-8493-8553-9*) CRC Pr.

Infectious Diseases in Obstetrics & Gynecology. Daniell et al. 3rd ed. 1994. LC 93-80109. (Illus.). 730p. text 89.95 (*1-880906-09-0*) IDI Pub.

Infectious Diseases in Obstetrics & Gynecology. Gilles R. Monif & David Baker. 4th ed. 1998. (Illus.). 912p. text 179.95 (*1-880906-57-0*) IDI Pub.

Infectious Diseases in the Female Patient. Ed. by R. P. Galask & B. Larsen. 1985. (Clinical Perspectives in Obstetrics & Gynecology Ser.). (Illus.). xiii, 264p. 148.00 (*0-387-96181-X*) Spr-Verlag.

Infectious Diseases in Twentieth-Century Africa: A Bibliography of Their Distribution & Consequences. K. David Patterson. 1979. (Archival & Bibliographic Ser.). 251p. (Orig.). pap. 25.00 (*0-918456-29-0*, Crossroads) African Studies Assn.

Infectious Diseases in Women. Mark G. Martens et al. 2000. LC 00-30110. 1020p. text 169.00 (*0-7216-7379-1*) Saunders.

Infectious Diseases of Children. Samuel L. Katz. 10th ed. 1998. (Illus.). 784p. (*84-8174-369-0*) Mosby-Doyma Libros ESP. *Dist:* Mosby Inc.

Infectious Diseases of Children. Samuel Katz et al. 10th ed. 1997. LC 97-34587. (Illus.). 784p. (C). (gr. 13). text 79.95 (*0-8151-5251-5*, 27524) Mosby Inc.

Infectious Diseases of Fish. Shuzo Egusa. Ed. by V. S. Kothekar. 1992. (Illus.). 720p. text (*90-6191-180-X*) A A Balkema NLD. *Dist:* Ashgate Pub Co.

Infectious Diseases of Mice & Rats. National Research Council Staff. 1998. 410p. reprint ed. text 49.95 (*0-309-06332-9*); Set. 1991. 415p. text 65.00 (*0-309-03794-8*) Natl Acad Pr.

Infectious Diseases of the Dog & Cat. Craig E. Greene. Ed. by Ray Kersey. 2nd ed. 1998. LC 97-30657. (Illus.). 688p. (C). text 125.00 (*0-7216-2737-4*) Saunders.

Infectious Diseases of the Fetus & Newborn Infant. Ed. by Jack S. Remington & Jerome O. Klein. 4th ed. 1994. LC 94-23372. (Illus.). 1373p. text 210.00 (*0-7216-6782-1*) Saunders.

Infectious Diseases of the Fetus & Newborn Infant. Jack S. Remington & Jerome O. Klein. 5th ed. 2000. LC 99-50228. (Illus.). xiv, 1507p. text 210.00 (*0-7216-7976-5*) Saunders.

Infectious Diseases of the Liver. L. Bianchi et al. 1990. (C). text 192.00 (*0-7923-8902-6*) Kluwer Academic.

Infectious Diseases of the Lower Extremity. Carl Abramson et al. 1991. (Illus.). 448p. 89.00 (*0-683-00040-3*) Lppncott W & W.

Infectious Diseases of the Nervous System. Larry E. Davis & Peter G. E. Kennedy. 2000. (Illus.). 552p. text 95.00 (*0-7506-4213-0*) Buttrwrth-Heinemann.

Infectious Diseases of the Respiratory Tract. Ed. by Michael Ellis. 1998. (Illus.). 615p. (C). text 225.00 (*0-521-40554-8*) Cambridge U Pr.

Infectious Diseases of Wild Mammals. Ed. by Elizabeth S. Williams & Ian Barker. 3rd ed. 2001. LC 00-47258. (Illus.). viii, 558p. 109.95 (*0-8138-2556-3*) Iowa U Pr.

Infectious Diseases Update. Wilma Bower et al. rev. ed. (Illus.). pap. text 4.95 (*0-9616270-2-6*) Alliance Schl Health.

Infectious Mononucleosis. Ed. by David L. Schlossberg. 2nd ed. 1989. (Clinical Topics in Infectious Disease Ser.). (Illus.). 203p. 96.00 (*0-387-96959-4*) Spr-Verlag.

Infective Endocarditis. Ed. by Louis Weinstein & John L. Brusch. 1996. (Illus.). 376p. text 75.00 (*0-19-507395-9*) OUP.

Infective Endocarditis of Heart Valves: Proceedings of the Second Scientific Meeting of the International Association for Cardiac Biologic Implants. Ed. by Shlomo Gabbay et al. 1992. (Illus.). 268p. (*1-878353-23-3*) Silent Partners.

Inferential Statistics in Nursing & Healthcare. Open Learning Foundation Staff. 1998. 143p. pap. (*0-443-05740-0*) Church.

Inferior Olivary Complex. Anastasia Bozhilova-Pastirova & Wladimir A. Ovtscharoff. 2000. LC 00-39472. (Advances in Anatomy, Embryology & Cell Biology Ser.: Vol. 155). (Illus.). 85p. pap. 54.95 (*3-540-67234-6*) Spr-Verlag.

Inferiority Feelings in the Individual & the Group. F. Oliver Brachfeld. Tr. by Marjorie Gabain from FRE. 1973. LC 70-169849. 301p. reprint ed. lib. bdg. 68.50 (*0-8371-6245-9*, OLIF, Greenwood Pr) Greenwood.

Infertile Male: The Clinician's Guide to Diagnosis & Treatment. R. F. Spark. 1988. LC 88-15175. (Illus.). 384p. (C). text 80.00 (*0-306-42859-8*, Kluwer Plenum) Kluwer Academic.

Infertility. Ed. by A. A. Templeton & J. O. Drife. 1993. LC 92-49701. (*3-540-19743-5*); (Illus.). 448p. 205.00 (*0-387-19743-5*) Spr-Verlag.

Infertility: A Clinician's Guide to Diagnosis & Treatment. M. L. Taymor. 1990. LC 90-7659. (Illus.). 310p. (C). text 75.00 (*0-306-43555-1*, Kluwer Plenum) Kluwer Academic.

Infertility: A Comprehensive Text. Machelle M. Seibel. 2nd rev. ed. 1998. LC 96-17607. 903p. (C). pap. text 169.00 (*0-8385-4258-1*, A-4258-8, Apple Lange Med) McGraw.

Infertility: A Guide for Patients. Luigi Mastroiann. 1997. (Urology & Gyn Ser.). 32p. pap. text 2.95 (*1-885274-61-0*) Health InfoNet Inc.

Infertility: A Woman Doctor's Guide: Essential Facts on How to Achieve Pregnancy. Susan Treiser & Robin K. Levinson. 2001. 208p. mass mkt. 6.99 (*1-57566-638-3*, Knsington) Kensgtn Pub Corp.

Infertility: All Your Questions Answered. Gab Kovacs. 1996. pap. text (*0-85572-263-0*) Hill Content Pubng AUS. *Dist:* Seven Hills Bk.

Infertility: Diagnosis & Management. Ed. by E. J. Aiman. 1984. (Clinical Perspectives in Obstetrics & Gynecology Ser.). (Illus.). 370p. 152.00 (*0-387-90940-0*) Spr-Verlag.

Infertility: Evaluation & Treatment. Ed. by William R. Keye, Jr. et al. 1994. LC 93-48748. (Illus.). 864p. text 170.00 (*0-7216-3970-4*) Saunders.

Infertility: Male & Female. Ed. by Vaclav Insler & Bruno Lunenfeld. 1986. LC 85-4116. (Illus.). 740p. text (*0-443-02595-9*); 2nd ed. 1993. LC 92-48779. 776p. text (*0-443-04514-3*) Church.

Infertility: Medical, Emotional & Social Considerations. Miriam Mazor & Harriet F. Simons. 1984. 264p. pap. 22.95 (*0-89885-177-7*, Kluwer Acad Hman Sci) Kluwer Academic.

Infertility: Medical, Emotional & Social Considerations. Harriet F. Simons & Miriam Mazor. 1984. 264p. 36.95 (*0-89885-140-8*, Kluwer Acad Hman Sci) Kluwer Academic.

Infertility: Old Myths, New Meanings. Jan Rehner. 1994. 198p. pap. (*0-929005-06-6*) Sec Story Pr CAN. *Dist:* LPC InBook.

Infertility: Perspectives from Stress & Copins Research. A. L. Stanton & C. Dunkel-Schetter. 1991. (Stress & Coping Ser.). (Illus.). 260p. (C). 45.00 (*0-306-43844-5*, Plenum Trade) Perseus Pubng.

Infertility: Psychological Issues & Counseling Strategies. Sandra R. Leiblum. 1996. LC 96-23253. (Couples & Family Dynamics & Treatment Ser.). 278p. 90.00 (*0-471-12684-5*) Wiley.

Infertility: The Last Secret. Anna McGrail. 1999. pap. (*0-7475-4396-8*) Blmsbury Pub GBR. *Dist:* Trafalgar.

Infertility: The Tapestry Guide. Laurie S. Wallmark. 1997. 32p. (Orig.). pap. 8.95 (*0-9653409-1-0*) Tapestry Bks.

Infertility Vol. 53: A Crossroad of Faith, Medicine, & Technology. Ed. by Kevin W. Wildes. 1997. LC 96-1649. (Philosophy & Medicine Ser.). 248p. (C). text 136.00 (*0-7923-4061-2*) Kluwer Academic.

Infertility & Adoption: A Guide for Social Work Practice. Ed. by Deborah Valentine. 1988. LC 87-36635. (Journal of Social Work & Human Sexuality: Vol. 6, No. 1). (Illus.). 189p. text 5.95 (*0-86656-721-6*) Haworth Pr.

Infertility & Birth Defects: Is Mercury from Silver Dental Fillings an Unsuspected Cause? Sam Ziff & Michael F. Ziff. 1988. LC 87-72238. 448p. (Orig.). pap. 14.95 (*0-941011-03-8*) Bio-Probe.

Infertility & Contraception: A Textbook for Clinical Practice. O. Rodriguez-Armas et al. 1998. LC 98-26809. 250p. lib. bdg. 53.95 (*1-85070-056-7*) CRC Pr.

Infertility & Identity: New Strategies for Treatment. Lara L. Deveraux & Ann J. Hammerman. 1998. LC 97-49290. 322p. 41.00 (*0-7879-3881-5*) Jossey-Bass.

Infertility & IVF. Jo Benson. 1997. pap. text (*1-85727-093-2*) Scarlet Pr GBR. *Dist:* LPC InBook.

Infertility Book: A Comprehensive Medical & Emotional Guide. Carla Harkness. 2nd exp. rev. ed. 1995. LC 91-38181. (Illus.). 433p. text 16.95 (*0-89087-664-9*) Celestial Arts.

Infertility in Practice. Adam H. Balen & Howard S. Jacobs. 1997. LC 97-7775. pap. text (*0-443-05356-1*) Church.

Infertility in the Male. Larry I. Lipshultz. Ed. by Stuarts Howards. 3rd ed. 1996. (Illus.). 576p. (C). (gr. 13). text 119.00 (*0-8151-5501-8*, 25776) Mosby Inc.

Infertility in the Modern World: Present & Future Prospects. Ed. by Gillian R. Bentley & C. G. Mascie-Taylor. 2001. LC 00-37916. (Biosocial Society Symposium Ser.: No. 12). (Illus.). 276p. (C). text 69.95 (*0-521-64364-3*) Cambridge U Pr.

Infertility Self-Help: What You Can Do to Regain Fertility. Suzannah C. Doyle. 1991. (Illus.). 55p. (Orig.). stu. ed. 15.00 (*0-9628284-3-2*) FA Services.

Infibulation: Female Mutilation in Islamic Northeastern Africa. Esther K. Hicks. 1996. LC 92-24753. 220p. (C). text 39.95 (*1-56000-077-5*) Transaction Pubs.

Infinitesimal Dose. Colin Lessell. 1994. 107p. pap. (*0-85207-276-7*) C W Daniel GBR. *Dist:* Natl Bk Netwk.

***Inflammation.** Ed. by Andrzej Gorski et al. 2001. LC 2001-50272. 230p. 80.00 (*1-4020-0086-3*) Kluwer Academic.

Inflammation: A Review of the Process. Henry O. Trowbridge & Robert C. Emling. 5th ed. 1997. LC 96-39904. 200p. pap. text 42.00 (*0-86715-310-5*) Quint Pub Co.

Inflammation: Mechanisms & Therapeutics. N. S. Doherty. 1995. LC 95-11482. (Agents & Actions Supplements Ser.: Vol. AAS 47). 87.50 (*0-8176-5129-2*) Birkhauser.

Inflammation: Mediators & Pathways. Ed. by Robert R. Ruffolo, Jr. & Mannfred A. Hollinger. 1995. LC 94-44223. 224p. 149.95 (*0-8493-9473-2*, 9473) CRC Pr.

***Inflammation & Stroke.** G. Z. Feuerstein. 2001. (Progress in Inflammation Research Ser.). (Illus.). 300p. 145.00 (*3-7643-6511-0*) Birkhauser.

Inflammation in Gut: Esophagitis, Duodenitis, Segmental Colitis. Ed. by Zdenek Maratka & R. Ottenjann. 1970. (Bibliotheca Gastroenterologica Ser.: No. 9). (Illus.). pap. 51.50 (*3-8055-0043-2*) S Karger.

Inflammation Mechanisms & Their Impact on Therapy. Ed. by I. L. Bonta et al. 1980. (Agents & Actions Supplements Ser.: No. 3). (Illus.). 192p. 117.50 (*0-8176-0913-X*) Birkhauser.

Inflammatory & Artresia-Inducing Disease of the Liver & Bile Ducts. A. Perez-Soler. 1976. (Monographs in Pediatrics: Vol. 8). (Illus.). 68.00 (*3-8055-2257-6*) S Karger.

Inflammatory Bowel Disease. Ed. by A. Anagnostides et al. 1991. (Illus.). 480p. pap. 184.95 (*0-412-35110-2*) Chapman & Hall.

Inflammatory Bowel Disease. Richard MacDermott. 1992. (Illus.). 658p. (C). pap. text 125.00 (*0-8385-4069-4*, A4069-9, Apple Lange Med) McGraw.

Inflammatory Bowel Disease. D. Rachmilewitz. 1982. text 155.50 (*90-247-2612-3*) Kluwer Academic.

***Inflammatory Bowel Disease.** Rampton & Shanahan. 2000. (Fast Facts Ser.). (Illus.). 106p. pap. (*1-899541-49-7*) Health Pr GBR. *Dist:* JAMCO Dist.

Inflammatory Bowel Disease. Joseph B. Kirsner. 5th ed. 1999. LC 98-50605. (Illus.). xvi, 800p. text (*0-7216-7616-2*) Saunders.

Inflammatory Bowel Disease Ed. by Hugh J. Freeman. 1989. (Illus.). Vol. I. LC 96-8171. 280p. 153.00 (*0-8493-5522-2*, RC862); Vol. II. 288p. 153.00 (*0-8493-5523-0*) CRC Pr.

Inflammatory Bowel Disease: A Clinical Approach. Henry D. Janowtiz. 2nd ed. 1994. LC 93 30353. (Illus.). 336p. text 39.50 (*0-19-507830-6*) OUP.

Inflammatory Bowel Disease: A Guide for Patients & Their Families. Stephen B. Hanauer. 2nd ed. 1998. LC 98-21442. 256p. pap. text 39.95 (*0-397-51771-8*) Lppncott W & W.

Inflammatory Bowel Disease: Basic Research & Clinical Implications. Ed. by H. Goebell et al. 1988. (Falk Symposium Ser.). (C). text 248.00 (*0-7462-0067-6*) Kluwer Academic.

Inflammatory Bowel Disease: Basic Research, Clinical Implications & Trends in Therapy. Ed. by L. R. Sutherland et al. 1995. text 132.00 (*0-7923-8871-2*) Kluwer Academic.

Inflammatory Bowel Disease: Diagnosis & Therapeutics. Ed. by Russell D. Cohen. 2001. (Clinical Gastroenterology Ser.). 300p. 99.50 (*0-89603-909-9*) Humana.

Inflammatory Bowel Disease: Diagnosis, Treatment, Management. Zonderman. 1920. 24.95 (*0-471-54595-3*) Wiley.

Inflammatory Bowel Disease: Some International Data & Reflections. Ed. by F. T. De Dombal et al. 2nd ed. 1994. (Illus.). 764p. (C). text 135.00 (*0-19-262401-6*, 2290) OUP.

Inflammatory Bowel Disease & Coeliac Disease. F. Hadziselimovic et al. 1990. (C). text 123.00 (*0-7462-0125-7*) Kluwer Academic.

Inflammatory Bowel Disease in Children & Adolescents. Michael Pettei & Jeremiah Levine. 1995. (Monographs in Clinical Pediatrics). 257p. text 50.00 (*3-7186-5656-6*, Harwood Acad Pubs) Gordon & Breach.

Inflammatory Bowel Diseases. Ed. by Robert N. Allan et al. 2nd ed. 1990. (Illus.). 656p. text (*0-443-03819-8*) Church.

Inflammatory Bowel Diseases. R. N. Allan. 3rd ed. 1996. LC 97-5557. text (*0-443-05067-8*) Church.

Inflammatory Bowel Diseases: From Bench to Bedside. Ed. by T. Andus et al. 1997. (Falk Symposium Ser.: No. 96). 480p. text 240.50 (*0-7923-8728-7*) Kluwer Academic.

Inflammatory Bowel Diseases: New Developments & Standards: Proceedings of the Falk Symposium No. 82, Held in Halle-Saale, Germany, November 18-19, 1994. Ed. by W. E. Fleig. 1995. (Falk Symposium Ser.). 336p. (C). text 136.00 (*0-7923-8890-9*) Kluwer Academic.

Inflammatory Bowel Diseases: New Insights into Mechanisms of Inflammation & Challenges in Diagnosis & Treatment. Ed. by Estela Monteiro & F. Tavarela Veloso. 1995. LC 95-20104. text 129.00 (*0-7923-8884-4*) Kluwer Academic.

Inflammatory Bowel Diseases - Pathophysiology As Basis of Treatment. Ed. by J. Scholmerich. 1993. LC 94-105021. (Falk Symposium Ser.). 584p. (C). text 209.50 (*0-7923-8996-4*) Kluwer Academic.

Inflammatory Bowel Diseases - Progress in Basic Research & Clinical Implications. Ed. by H. Goebell et al. 1991. (Falk Symposium Ser.). (C). text 276.50 (*0-7923-8956-5*) Kluwer Academic.

Inflammatory Bowel Diseases 1986. Ed. by D. Rachmilewitz. 1986. (Developments in Gastroenterology Ser.). lib. bdg. 179.50 (*0-89838-796-5*) Kluwer Academic.

Inflammatory Bowel Diseases, 1990: Proceedings of the Third International Symposium on Inflammatory Bowel Diseases. Ed. by D. Rachmilewitz & J. Zimmerman. 1990. (Developments in Gastroenterology Ser.). (C). text 175.00 (*0-7923-0657-0*) Kluwer Academic.

Inflammatory Bowel Diseases, 1994: Proceedings of the 72nd Falk Symposium Held in Strasbourg, France, September 6-8, 1993. Ed. by D. Rachmilewitz. 1994. LC 93-44397. 320p. (C). text 140.00 (*0-7923-8845-3*) Kluwer Academic.

Inflammatory Bowel Diseases & Morbus Hirschsprung: Proceedings of the 65th Falk Symposium (II - International Falk Symposium on Pediatric & Surgical Gastroenterolgy) Held in Basel, Switzerland, April 10 & 11, 1992. Ed. by F. Hadziselimovic & B. Herzog. 1992. LC 92-49754. 336p. text 149.50 (*0-7923-8995-6*) Kluwer Academic.

Inflammatory Cells & Lung Disease. Ed. by William S. Lynn. 1983. 120p. 74.00 (*0-8493-5792-6*, RC771, CRC Reprint) Franklin.

Inflammatory Cells & Mediators in Bronchial Asthma. Devendra K. Agrawal & Robert Townley. 1990. (Illus.). 280p. lib. bdg. 175.00 (*0-8493-7294-1*, RC591) CRC Pr.

Inflammatory Disease Therapy: Preclinical & Clinical Developments. Ed. by Robert J. Bonney. 1993. LC 93-17038. (Agents & Actions Supplements Ser.: Vol. 41). ix, 209p. 98.50 (*0-8176-2859-2*) Birkhauser.

Inflammatory Diseases & Copper. Ed. by John R. J. Sorenson. 1982. LC 82-80151. (Experimental Biology & Medicine Ser.: Vol. 2). (Illus.). 622p. 145.00 (*0-89603-037-7*) Humana.

***Inflammatory Diseases of Blood Vessels.** Ed. by Gary Hoffman & Cornelia M. Weyand. 2001. 815p. 225.00 (*0-8247-0269-7*) Dekker.

Inflammatory Diseases of the Orbit: Clinical Features, Radiology, Differential Diagnosis. R. Unsold & Gabriele Greeven. 1999. LC 99-41443. (Illus.). 208p. 116.00 (*3-540-65098-9*) Spr-Verlag.

Inflammatory Indices in Chronic Bronchitis. Ed. by C. G. Persson et al. 1990. (Agents & Actions Supplements Ser.: Vol. 30). 296p. 87.50 (*0-8176-2370-1*) Birkhauser.

***Inflammatory Mechanisms in Allergic Diseases.** Ed. by Burton Zweiman & Lawrence B. Schwartz. 2001. (Clinical Allergy & Immunology Ser.). 581p. 195.00 (*0-8247-0540-8*) Dekker.

Inflammatory Mechanisms in Asthma, Vol. 117. Stephen T. Holgate & W. W. Busse. 1998. LC 98-16880. (Lung Biology in Health & Disease Ser.). (Illus.). 1090p. text 250.00 (*0-8247-0122-4*) Dekker.

***Inflammatory Mechanisms in Experimental CNS Trauma.** Jonas Isaksson. 2000. (Comprehensive Summaries of Uppsala Dissertations from the Faculty of Medicine Ser.: No. 906). (Illus.). 45p. pap. (*91-554-4653-1*) Uppsala Universitet SWE. *Dist:* Coronet Bks.

Inflammatory Process: An Introduction to the Study of Cellular & Hormonal Mechanisms. Ed. by Per Venge & Annie Lindbom. 1981. (Illus.). 340p. text 62.00 (*91-22-00443-2*) Coronet Bks.

Inflammatory Processes: Molecular Mechanisms & Therapeutic Opportunities. Ed. by G. L. Letts. 2000. (Progress in Inflammation Research Ser.). (Illus.). 200p. 119.00 (*3-7643-6025-9*) Birkhauser.

Inflammatory Vascular Diseases-Endo-Myocardial Fibrosis-Pulmonary Hypertension: Proceedings - Conference of the International Society of Geographical Pathology, 12th, Zurich, September 1975. Ed. by J. R. Ruettner et al. 1976. (Pathologia et Microbiologica Ser.: Vol. 43, No. 1-2). (Illus.). 180p. 68.00 (*3-8055-2311-4*) S Karger.

Inflationary Cosmology. L. Abbott & S. Y. Pi. 1986. 712p. text 117.00 (*9971-978-64-4*) World Scientific Pub.

Influence & Autonomy in Psychoanalysis. Stephen A. Mitchell. 1997. LC 97-40014. (Relational Perspectives Bks.: Vol. 9). 304p. 45.00 (*0-88163-240-6*) Analytic Pr.

Influence of Antibiotics on the Host-Parasite Relationship, Vol. III. Ed. by G. Gillissen et al. 1989. (Illus.). 291p. 135.00 (*0-387-19223-9*) Spr-Verlag.

Influence of Dose & Its Distribution in Time on Dose - Response Relationships for Low - LET Radiations. 1980. LC 80-81304. (Report Ser.: No. 64). 216p. pap. text 45.00 (*0-913392-48-0*) NCRP Pubns.

Influence of Edmund D. Pellegrino's Philosophy of Medicine. Ed. by David C. Thomasma. 1997. LC 97-12152. 224p. text 80.00 (*0-7923-4412-X*) Kluwer Academic.

Influence of Ethyl Alcohol on the Development of the Chondrocranium of Gallus Gallus. M. Heyns. 1997. LC 96-43006. (Advances in Anatomy, Embryology & Cell Biology Ser.: Vol. 134). (Illus.). 124p. text 84.95 (*3-540-61709-4*) Spr-Verlag.

Influence of Freud on American Psychology. David Shakow & David Rapaport. 1964. LC 64-21456. (Psychological Issues Monographs: No. 13, Vol. 4, No. 1). 243p. (Orig.). 37.50 (*0-8236-2656-3*); pap. 28.50 (*0-8236-2652-0*) Intl Univs Pr.

Influence of Habit on the Faculty of Thinking. Pierre Maine De Biran. Tr. by Margaret D. Boehm. 1970. LC 79-98854. 227p. reprint ed. lib. bdg. 35.00 (*0-8371-3124-3*, MBTH, Greenwood Pr) Greenwood.

Influence of Hormones on the Nervous System: Proceedings of the International Society of Psychoneuroendocrinology, Brooklyn, 1970. International Society of Psychoneuroendocrinology. Ed. by D. H. Ford. 1971. (Illus.). 114.00 (*3-8055-1216-3*) S Karger.

Influence of Local Oxygen Deficiency: On Function & Integrity of Liver, Kidney & Heart. Jens Hoper. 1991. (Illus.). 86p. (Orig.). pap. (*1-56081-322-9*) Gustav Fischer DEU. *Dist:* Lubrecht & Cramer, Balogh.

Influence of Maternal Hormones on the Fetus & Newborn. Ed. by Menachem Nitzan. 1979. (Pediatric & Adolescent Endocrinology Ser.: Vol. 5). (Illus.). pap. 86.25 (*3-8055-2902-3*) S Karger.

Influence of Molecular Biology on Drug Discovery, Vol. 1. Ed. by K. Udaka et al. 1989. (Clinical Pharmacology Ser.). (Illus.). 152p. text (*3-88603-363-5*) W Zuckschwerdt DEU. *Dist:* Scholium Intl.

Influence of Old Age on the Effect of Drugs. 1982. (Journal: Vol. 28, Suppl. 1). (Illus.). vi, 138p. pap. 50.50 (*3-8055-3509-0*) S Karger.

Influence of Race & Racial Indentity in Psychotherapy: Toward a Racially Inclusive Model. Robert T. Carter. 1998. 312p. pap. 50.00 (*0-471-24533-X*); 1995. LC 95-5145. 320p. 105.00 (*0-471-57111-3*) Wiley.

Influence of Specialized Training on Tests of General Intelligence. Katharine B. Graves. LC 73-176818. (Columbia University. Teachers College. Contributions to Education Ser.: No. 143). reprint ed. 37.50 (*0-404-55143-2*) AMS Pr.

Influence of Subliminal Suggestion on the Response to Two Films. Gerry K. Veeder. 1980. LC 79-6689. (Dissertations on Film, 1980 Ser.). lib. bdg. 12.95 (*0-405-12921-1*) Ayer.

Influence of the Host on Tumor Development. Ed. by Ronald B. Herberman. 1988. (Cancer Growth & Progression Ser.). (C). text 211.50 (*0-89838-993-3*) Kluwer Academic.

Influence of Tumor Development on the Host. Ed. by Lance A. Liotta. 1988. (Cancer Growth & Progression Ser.). (C). text 211.50 (*0-89838-992-5*) Kluwer Academic.

Influence of Varying Amounts of Punishment on Mental Connections. Jacob Tuckman. LC 74-177692. (Columbia University. Teachers College. Contributions to Education Ser.: No. 590). reprint ed. 37.50 (*0-404-55590-X*) AMS Pr.

Influence upon Learning of the Quantitative Variation of After-Effects. Robert T. Rock. LC 79-177199. (Columbia University. Teachers College. Contributions to Education Ser.: No. 650). reprint ed. 37.50 (*0-404-55650-7*) AMS Pr.

Influences of Hormones in Tumor Development John A. Kellen & Russell Hilf. 1979. Vol. 1. 192p. 112.00 (*0-8493-5351-3*, RC268); Vol. 2. 224p. 130.00 (*0-8493-5352-1*) Franklin (CRC Reprint).

Influences on Human Development: A Longitudinal Perspective. Robert L. Baker & Birgitte R. Mednick. 1984. lib. bdg. 91.00 (*0-89838-130-4*) Kluwer Academic.

Influenza. E. D. Kilbourne. 1987. LC 87-2510. (Illus.). 382p. (C). text 85.00 (*0-306-42456-8*, Kluwer Plenum) Kluwer Academic.

Influenza. Pilet. 1981. (Comparative Immunology & Microbiology Ser.). pap. 39.00 (*0-08-026842-0*, Pergamon Pr) Elsevier.

Influenza: A Review of Current Research. C. Andrewes & M. Burnet. 1954. (WHO Monograph Ser.: No. 20). 223p. 12.00 (*92-4-140020-X*) World Health.

Influenza 1918: The Worst Epidemic in American History. Lynette Iezzoni. (Illus.). 256p. 2000. LC 00-41197. pap. 15.00 (*1-57500-183-7*); 1999. (American Experience Ser.: Vol. 2). 24.95 (*1-57500-108-X*); 1998. 24.95 (*1-57500-067-9*) TV Bks.

Influenza Vaccines for Men & Horses: Proceedings of the International Association of Biological Standardization 39th Symposium, Institute of Child Health, London, November 1972. International Association of Biological Standardiz. Ed. by R. H. Regamey & F. T. Perkins. 1973. (Immunobiological Standardization Symposia Ser.: Vol. 20). 406p. 33.25 (*3-8055-1674-6*) S Karger.

Influenza Virus Haemagglutinin. Ed. by W. G. Laver & H. Bachmayer. 1978. LC 77-17581. (Topics in Infectious Diseases Ser.: Vol. 3). (Illus.). 47.95 (*0-387-81459-0*) Spr-Verlag.

Influenza Viruses. L. Hoyle. 1969. (Virology Monographs: Vol. 4). (Illus.). 92.00 (*0-387-80892-2*) Spr-Verlag.

Influenza Viruses. R. M. Krug. 1989. (Viruses Ser.). (Illus.). 450p. (C). text 120.00 (*0-306-43191-2*, Kluwer Plenum) Kluwer Academic.

Informal Assessment of Developmental Skills for Visually Handicapped Students. Ed. by Rose-Marie Swallow et al. 1978. 160p. pap. 19.95 (*0-89128-964-X*) Am Foun Blind.

Informatics: The Infrastructure for Quality Assessment & Improvement in Nursing: Proceedings of the Fifth International Nursing Informatics Symposium Post-Conference. Suzanne B. Henry et al. 1995. 106p. (Orig.). pap. 25.00 (*0-943671-11-6*) UCSF Schl Nursing.

Informatics & Telematics in Health: Present & Potential Uses. WHO Staff. 1988. 108p. 16.00 (*92-4-156117-3*) World Health.

Informatics for Healthcare Professionals. Kathleen M. Young. 2000. LC 99-88883. (Illus.). 282p. pap. text 29.95 (*0-8036-0619-2*) Davis Co.

Information Access & Delivery in Health Sciences Libraries. Ed. by Carolyn E. Lipscomb & Alison Bunting. 1996. LC 95-42302. (Current Practice in Health Sciences Librarianship Ser.: No. 3). 280p. 45.00 (*0-8108-3050-7*) Scarecrow.

Information & Behavior, Vol. 2. Ed. by Brent D. Ruben. 1987. 600p. text 54.95 (*0-88738-106-5*) Transaction Pubs.

Information & Creation. German A. Golitsyn & Vladimir M. Petrov. 1995. LC 95-23349. (*3-7643-2933-5*) Birkhauser.

Information & Data Handling Developments in Medicine: Highlighting Opportunities for Hardware, Software & Services. Contrib. by Barbara Breindel. 1995. 202p. 2650.00 (*1-56965-071-3*, G-155) BCC.

Information & Education for Health in South-East Asia. 1988. (SEARO Regional Health Papers: No. 17). 100p. pap. text 5.00 (*92-9022-186-0*) World Health.

Information & Instructions for Pediatric Patients. H. Winter Griffith et al. 1980. LC 80-51712. 320p. 35.00 (*0-938372-00-9*) Winter Pub Co.

Information Bulletin on the Survey of Chemicals Being Tested for Carcinogenicity, No. 12. Ed. by M. J. Ghess et al. 1986. 385p. pap. 50.00 (*92-832-1312-2*, 1740012) World Health.

Information Dissemination to Health Care Practitioners & Policymakers: An Annotated Bibliography. 1995. lib. bdg. 251.95 (*0-8490-6782-0*) Gordon Pr.

Information for Women about Safety of Silicone Breast Implants. Martha L. Grigg et al. 2000. LC 99-58759. (Illus.). 30p. 5.00 (*0-309-06593-3*) Natl Acad Pr.

Information in the Brain: A Molecular Perspective. Ira B. Black. 1994. (Illus.). 240p. pap. 22.00 (*0-262-52188-1*, Bradford Bks) MIT Pr.

Information in the Brain: A Molecular Perspective. Ira R. Black. 1991. LC 90-13591. (Illus.). 261p. 32.50 (*0-262-02321-0*, Bradford Bks) MIT Pr.

Information Integration by Children. Ed. by Friedrich Wilkening et al. 1980. LC 79-24289. (Illus.). 320p. text 69.95 (*0-89859-015-9*) L Erlbaum Assocs.

Information Management: A Guide to the JCAHO Standards. Jennifer I. Cofer et al. 2nd ed. 1996. LC 97-126091. 144p. pap. text 67.00 (*1-885829-30-2*) Opus Communs.

Information Management: Questions & Answers for Hospitals. Joint Commission on Accreditation of Healthcare Organizations. 1998. (Illus.). 174p. pap. 55.00 (*0-86688-561-7*, IM-100) Joint Comm Hlthcare.

Information, Management & Participation: A New Approach from Public Health in Brazil. Francesco D. Villarosa. 1998. LC 97-19271. 176p. (C). pap. text (*0-7146-4353-X*) F Cass Pubs GBR. *Dist:* Intl Spec Bk.

Information Management for Environmental Health & Safety: A Practical Guide. K. Noah Vieira. 1999. 59.95 (*1-56670-264-X*) Lewis Pubs.

Information Management for Health Professionals. Merida Johns. 1997. 352p. tchr. ed. (*0-8273-8321-5*) Delmar.

Information Management for Health Professions. Merida L. Johns. 1996. LC 96-18463. (Allied Health Ser.). (Illus.). 352p. (C). 59.95 (*0-8273-5949-7*) Delmar.

*__Information Management for Health Professions.__ Merida L. Johns. 2nd ed. 2001. LC 2001-42159. (Health Information Management Ser.). 316p. text 52.95 (*0-7668-2516-7*) Delmar.

Information Management for Health Services: Index for New Information for Health Services. Selina R. Stasser. 1998. 57.50 (*0-7883-1800-4*); pap. 47.50 (*0-7883-1801-2*) ABBE Pubs Assn.

Information Management in Health Services. Ed. by Justin Keen. 1994. LC 93-24065. (Health Services Management Ser.). 224p. pap. (*0-335-19116-9*) OpUniv Pr.

Information Mangement in Health Care. Richard D. Marreel & Janet M. McLellan. 21st abr. rev. ed. 1999. LC 98-51743. 215p. (C). 58.95 (*0-7668-1255-3*) Delmar.

Information Networks for Community Health. Patricia F. Brennan et al. 1996. LC 96-21900. (Computers in Health Care Ser.). (Illus.). 342p. 69.95 (*0-387-94697-7*) Spr-Verlag.

Information Notices Diagnosis of Occupational Diseases: EUR 14768 Report. 1997. (*92-828-1144-1*, CE-NB-14768-ENR) Comm Europ Commun BEL. *Dist:* Bernan Associates.

Information Plus Compact Reference Health 2001. 2001. (Information Plus Compact Ser.). 22.00 net. (*0-7876-5515-5*) Gale.

Information Plus Health 2001. 2001. (Information Plus Reference Ser.). 32.00 net. (*0-7876-5395-0*) Gale.

Information Processing by the Brain: Views & Hypotheses from a Physiological-Cognitive Perspective. Ed. by Hans J. Markowitsch. 1988. LC 87-22542. 272p. 69.00 (*0-920887-15-5*) Hogrefe & Huber Pubs.

Information Processing in Animals: Conditioned Inhibition. Ed. by Ralph R. Miller, Sr. & Norman E. Spear. 1985. 480p. (C). text 89.95 (*0-89859-506-1*) L Erlbaum Assocs.

Information Processing in Animals: Memory Mechanisms. Ed. by Norman E. Spear & Ralph R. Miller, Sr. 1981. 432p. (C). text 89.95 (*0-89859-157-0*) L Erlbaum Assocs.

Information Processing in Medical Imaging. Ed. by Stephen L. Bacharach. 1986. text 273.50 (*0-89838-787-6*) Kluwer Academic.

Information Processing in Medical Imaging. Ed. by C. N. De Graaf & Max A. Viergever. 1988. LC 87-36058. (Illus.). 640p. 125.00 (*0-306-42807-5*, Plenum Trade) Perseus Pubng.

Information Processing in Medical Imaging. Ed. by F. Deconinck. 1984. LC 84-1121. text 282.00 (*0-89838-677-2*) Kluwer Academic.

Information Processing in Medical Imaging: Proceedings: International Conference on Information Processing in Medical Imaging (14th: 1995: Ile de Berder, France) Ed. by Yves Bizais et al. 1995. (Computational Imaging & Vision Ser.: Vol. 3). 408p. (C). text 197.00 (*0-7923-3593-7*) Kluwer Academic.

Information Processing in Medical Imaging: Proceedings of the 13th International Conference, IPMI '93, Flagstaff, Arizona, USA, June 14-18, 1993. Ed. by H. H. Barrett & A. F. Gmitro. 1993. (Lecture Notes in Computer Science: Vol. 687). 583p. 86.95 (*0-387-56800-X*) Spr-Verlag.

*__Information Processing in Medical Imaging: Proceedings of the 17th International Conference, IPMI 2001, Davis, June 18-22, 2001.__ Ed. by M. F. Insana & R. M. Leahy. 2001. (Lecture Notes in Computer Science: Vol. 2082). xvi, 537p. pap. 85.00 (*3-540-42245-5*) Spr-Verlag.

Information Processing in Medical Imaging: Proceedings of the International Conference, IPMI, Wye, U. K., 12th, July 7-12, 1991. Ed. by A. C. Colchester et al. 1991. (Lecture Notes in Computer Science: Vol. 511). 512p. 101.00 (*0-387-54246-9*) Spr-Verlag.

Information Processing Underlying Gaze Control. E. Godaux et al. 1994. LC 94-19381. (Pergamon Studies in Neuroscience: No. 12). 474p. 207.00 (*0-08-042506-2*, Pergamon Pr) Elsevier.

Information Resources in Toxicology Pt. I: Basic Sciences. P. Wexler. 2nd ed. 1987. 510p. text 115.00 (*0-8385-4034-1*) Appleton & Lange.

Information Retrieval: A Health Care Perspective. William R. Hersh. 1995. LC 95-34175. (Computers & Medicine Ser.). (Illus.). 320p. 69.95 (*0-387-94454-0*) Spr-Verlag.

Information RN: Searching the Literature for Lifelong Learning in Nursing. Marilyn P. Verhey et al. 1998. LC 98-42249. 35.00 (*0-910478-60-0*) Cum Index Nursing.

Information Seeking & Veterinary Medical Scientists (HVMS) in Africa: Case Study from Borno State, Nigeria. Ken M. Nweke. 1992. 30p. 5.00 (*0-941934-59-4*) Indiana Africa.

Information, Sensation, & Perception. Kenneth H. Norwich. 1993. LC 93-16692. 326p. text 49.95 (*0-12-521890-7*) Acad Pr.

Information Services for HIV/AIDS: Recommendations to the NIH. 1995. 76p. (Orig.). (C). pap. text 25.00 (*0-7881-2347-5*) DIANE Pub.

Information Services for People with Developmental Disabilities: The Library Manager's Handbook. Linda L. Walling & Marilyn M. Irwin. 1995. LC 94-22016. (Library Management Collection). 368p. lib. bdg. 80.00 (*0-313-28780-5*, Greenwood Pr) Greenwood.

Information Sourcebook of Herbal Medicine. Ed. by David Hoffman. 1994. LC 93-44206. (Illus.). 188p. 40.00 (*0-89594-671-8*) Crossing Pr.

Information Sourcebook of Herbal Medicine. David Hoffmann. 2000. 305p. text 30.00 (*0-7881-9092-X*) DIANE Pub.

Information Sources in Pharmaceuticals. Ed. by W. R. Pickering. 1990. (Guides to Information Sources Ser.). 528p. lib. bdg. (*0-408-02518-2*) Bowker.

Information Sources in Psycholinguistics: Biographical Handbook. Jan Prucha. 1972. pap. text (*90-279-2362-0*) Mouton.

Information Storage & Retrieval: Index of New Information for Health Sciences. Selina R. Stasser. 1998. 57.50 (*0-7883-1802-0*); pap. 47.50 (*0-7883-1803-9*) ABBE Pubs Assn.

Information Support for New Public Health Action at District Level: Report of a WHO Expert Committee. 1994. LC 95-130394. (WHO Technical Reports: No. 845). (ENG, FRE & SPA.). iv, 31p. pap. text 8.00 (*92-4-120845-7*, 1100845) World Health.

Information Support to Mental Health Programs: An International Perspective. Ed. by Eugene M. Laska et al. 1983. 301p. 40.95 (*0-89885-083-5*, Kluwer Acad Hman Sci) Kluwer Academic.

Information Systems: Index of New Information for Health Sciences. Selina R. Stasser. 1998. 57.50 (*0-7883-1804-7*); pap. 47.50 (*0-7883-1805-5*) ABBE Pubs Assn.

Information, Systems & Psychoanalysis. Emanuel Peterfreund. 1971. LC 71-141662. (Psychological Issues Monographs: No. 25-26, Vol. 8, No. 1-2). 397p. 57.50 (*0-8236-2658-X*); pap. 45.00 (*0-8236-2659-8*) Intl Univs Pr.

Information Systems for Health Services Administration. Charles J. Austin & Stuart B. Boxerman. 5th ed. 1997. LC 97-29106. xix, 459p. 60.00 (*1-56793-070-0*) Health Admin Pr.

Information Systems Innovations for Nursing: New Visions & Ventures. Sue Moorhead & Connie W. Delaney. 1998. LC 98-9026. (Series on Nursing Administration). 251p. 77.95 (*0-7619-1670-9*, 82839); pap. 36.95 (*0-7619-1671-7*, 82840) Sage.

Information Systems Supporting Integrated Delivery Networks, Vol. 12, No. 3. Julie Forema. 1998. pap. 28.00 (*0-7879-4244-8*) Jossey-Bass.

*__Information Technologies in Medicine__, Set. Metin Akay & Andy Marsh. 2001. 500p. 110.00 (*0-471-41493-X*) Wiley.

Information Technologies in Medicine, Rehabilitation & Treatment Vol. 2: Rehabilitation & Treatment Metin Akay & Andy Marsh. 2001. LC 00-42259. (Illus.). 216p. 64.95 (*0-471-41492-1*) Wiley.

Information Technology for Emergency Management: The Use of Computers & Telecommunications in Natural & Technological Disasters. 1986. lib. bdg. 82.95 (*0-8490-3795-6*) Gordon Pr.

Information Technology for Integrated Health Systems: Positioning for the Future. Ernst and Young Staff et al. Ed. by Kerry Kissinger & Sandra Borchardt. 1995. LC 95-30079. (Ernst & Young Information Technology Ser.). 272p. 65.00 (*0-471-11452-9*) Wiley.

Information Technology for the Caring Professions: A User's Handbook. Sydney S. Chellen. LC 94-18463. 1996. text 90.00 (*0-304-33162-7*); 1995. pap. 29.95 (*0-304-33164-3*) Continuum.

Information Technology for the Health Professions. Lillian Burke. 1999. LC 99-42918. (Illus.). 242p. (C). pap. 34.00 (*0-13-083199-9*) P-H.

Information Technology for the Practicing Physician. Joan M. Kiel. 2000. LC 00-40038. (Health Informatics Ser.). (Illus.). 304p. 55.00 (*0-387-98984-6*) Spr-Verlag.

*__Information Technology in Health Care: An Interdisciplinary Approach.__ Sheila Englebardt & Ramona Nelson. 2001. LC 2001-44852. (Illus.). 550p. (*0-323-01257-4*) Mosby Inc.

Information Trading: How Information Influence the Health Policy Process. Ed. by Marion E. Lewin & Elise Lipoff. 1997. LC 97-222095. 152p. (C). pap. text 28.50 (*0-309-05793-0*) Natl Acad Pr.

Information Transfer, New Age-New Ways: Proceedings of the Third European Conference of Medical Libraries, Montpellier, France, September 23-26, 1992. Third European Conference of Medical Libraries. Ed. by Suzanne Bakker et al. 1993. LC 93-16492. lib. bdg. 264.50 (*0-7923-2214-2*) Kluwer Academic.

Informational Guides for Groups, Communication, Living & Change: Guides for Groups & Personal Change, Set-GL. Russell E. Mason. 1975. pap. 35.00 incl. audio (*0-89533-019-9*) F I Comm.

Informatore Farmaceutico 1998: Italian Physician's Desk Reference. 58th ed. 1998. (ITA.). pap. 695.00 (*0-7859-9678-8*) Fr & Eur.

Informed Consent. John A. Byrne. 1997. 288p. pap. 12.95 (*0-07-011784-5*) McGraw-Hill Educ Grp.

Informed Consent: A Guide for the Healthcare Professional. Jonathan P. Tomes. 1993. LC 92-35485. 168p. per. 24.95 (*1-882198-08-5*) Hlthcare Fin Mgmt.

Informed Consent: A Study of Decisionmaking in Psychiatry. Charles W. Lidz et al. 1984. LC 83-8488. (Perspectives on Law & Behavior Ser.). 365p. 47.00 (*0-89862-275-1*) Guilford Pubns.

Informed Consent: A Survival Guide. Donald J. Palmisano & Herbert J. Mang, Jr. 1987. 47p. (C). 15.00 (*0-940019-00-0*); 15.00 (*0-940019-01-9*) Invictus LA.

Informed Consent: Patient Autonomy & Clinician Beneficence in Health Care. Stephen Wear. Ed. by H. Tristram Engelhardt & Kevin W. Wildes. 2nd ed. 1998. LC 98-15856. (Clinical Medical Ethics Ser.). 240p. pap. 19.95 (*0-87840-706-5*) Georgetown U Pr.

Informed Consent: Patient Autonomy & Physician Beneficence Within Clinical Medicine. Stephen Wear. 1993. LC 92-48748. (Clinical Medical Ethics Ser.: Vol. 4). 184p. (C). lib. bdg. (*0-7923-2029-8*) Kluwer Academic NLD. *Dist:* Kluwer Academic.

Informed Consent & Voluntary Sterilization: An Implementation Guide for Program Managers. Phyllis Butta. rev. ed. 1994. 26p. reprint ed. pap. text 5.00 (*1-885063-03-2*) EngenderHlth.

Informed Consent for Blood Transfusion. Ed. by Christopher P. Stowell. 1997. LC 97-23445. pap. text 70.00 (*1-56395-087-1*) Am Assn Blood.

Informed Consent in Medical Research. Ed. by Len Doyal et al. 2001. 208p. (*0-7279-1486-3*) BMJ Pub GBR. *Dist:* AIDC.

Informed Consent to Surgery: Everything You Always Wanted to Know about Your Operaton but Were Afraid to Ask. Simon Marinker. 1991. 114p. (Orig.). pap. 11.95 (*0-9694811-0-1*) Gordon Soules Bk.

Informed Decisions: The Complete Book of Cancer Diagnosis, Treatment & Recovery. American Cancer Society et al. 1997. LC 96-18319. (Illus.). 704p. 39.95 (*0-670-85370-4*, PuffinBks) Viking Penguin.

Informed Infection Control Practice. Rozila Horton & Lynn Parker. 1997. LC 97-33317. text (*0-443-05330-8*) Church.

Informed Touch: A Clinician's Guide to the Evaluation & Treatment of Myofascial Disorders. Donna Finando & Steven Finando. 1999. LC 99-25845. (Illus.). 224p. 30.00 (*0-89281-740-2*, Heal Arts VT) Inner Tradit.

Informed Treatment: Milieu Management in Psychiatric Hospitals & Residential Treatment Centers. Nancy B. Soth. 1997. LC 96-49627. (Medical Library Association). 528p. 55.00 (*0-8108-3202-X*) Scarecrow.

Informed Woman's Guide to Breast Health: Breast Changes That Are Not Cancer. Kerry A. McGinn. Ed. by David C. Bull. rev. ed. 1992. (Illus.). 200p. pap. 13.95 (*0-923521-24-0*) Bull Pub.

Informed Woman's Guide to Breast Health: Breast Changes That Are Not Cancer. Kerry A. McGinn. 3rd ed. 2001. LC 00-66805. (Illus.). 144p. 12.95 (*0-923521-61-5*) Bull Pub.

Informing the Board about Medical Staff Credentialing & Development. Barry S. Bader. Ed. by Reggi Veatch. 1991. (Keys to Better Governance Through Better Information Ser.: Vol. 3). (Illus.). (Orig.). pap. text 9.00 (*0-915963-08-6*, MSC) Capitol Publns.

*__Infrainguinal Percutaneous Transluminal Angioplasty in Limbs with Severe Lower Limb Ischaemia.__ Anne-Marie Lofberg. 2001. (Comprehensive Summaries of Uppsala Dissertations from the Faculty of Medicine Ser.: No. 1060). (Illus.). 58p. pap. (*91-554-5079-2*) Acta Univ SWE. *Dist:* Coronet Bks.

Infrared & Raman Spectroscopy of Biological Materials. Hans-Ulrich Gremlich & Bing Yan. 2000. LC 00-60107. (Practical Spectroscopy Ser.: Vol. 24). (Illus.). ix, 581p. text 195.00 (*0-8247-0409-6*) Dekker.

Infrared Spectroscopy Vol. 3257: New Tool in Medicine. Ed. by Henry H. Mantsch & Michael Jackson. 1998. LC 98-233144. 330p. 80.00 (*0-8194-2696-2*) SPIE.

*__Infratemporal Fossa.__ Langdon et al. 2001. (Illus.). 208p. (*1-899066-79-9*) Isis Med GBR. *Dist:* Bks Intl VA.

Infusing Occupation Into Practice: Comparison of Three Clinical Approaches in Occupational Therapy. Ed. by Patricia Crist & Charlotte B. Royeen. 1997. LC 97-174733. 112p. (Orig.). (C). pap. text 22.00 (*1-56900-077-8*) Am Occup Therapy.

Infusion Chemotherapy—Irradiation Interactions: Principles & Applications to Organ Salvage & Prevention of Secondprimary Neoplasms. C. Julian Rosenthal & Marvin Rotman. 1997. LC 97-43316. 476p. 251.00 (*0-444-82608-4*) Elsevier.

Infusion Devices. 1992. 29p. pap. 82.00 (*0-910275-04-1*, ID26-209) Assn Adv Med Instrn.

Infusion Technology: A Self-Instructional Approach. Celeste M. Lindley & Kimberly H. Deloatch. 1993. 120p. pap. 219.00 incl. VHS (*1-879907-40-2*) Am Soc Hlth-Syst.

Infusion Technology & Therapy, 1983: Clinical Applications, Government Policy, Current Technology, Safety & Performance. 1983. (AAMI Technical Information Report Ser.). 90p. pap. text 30.00 (*0-910275-18-1*, TAR5-209) Assn Adv Med Instrn.

Infusion Therapy: Techniques & Medications. Marilyn F. Booker & Donna D. Ignatavicius. 1996. LC 95-17700. (Illus.). 846p. pap. text 31.00 (*0-7216-4923-8*) Saunders.

Infusionstherapie bei Volumenmangel und bei rheologischen Indikationen. Ed. by H. Reissigl et al. 1979. (Beitraege zur Infusionstherapie und Klinische Ernaehrung Ser.: Band 2). pap. 15.00 (*3-8055-3014-5*) S Karger.

Infusionstherapie mit Dextranen. Ed. by K. Steinbereithner & W. F. List. 1981. (Beitraege zur Infusionstherapie und Klinische Ernaehrung Ser.: Vol. 8). viii, 114p. 18.50 (*3-8055-2840-X*) S Karger.

Infusionstherapie und klinische Ernaehrung in der Inneren Medizin, Neurologie und Psychiatrie. Ed. by H. P. Schuster & G. Kleinberger. 1985. (Handbuch der Infusionstherapie und Klinischen Ernaehrung Ser.: Band 5). x, 288p. 116.75 (*3-8055-3742-5*) S Karger.

Infusionstherapie und klinische Ernaehrung in der Kinderheilkunde. H. Boehles. 1983. (Handbuch der Infusionstherapie und Klinischen Ernaehrung Ser.: Band 6). (Illus.). x, 166p. 61.75 (*3-8055-3719-0*) S Karger.

Infusionstherapie und Transfusionsmedizin (Infusion Therapy & Transfusion Medicine) Vol. 26, Suppl. 2: Deutsche Gesselschaft fur Transfusionsmedizin und Immunhamatologie. American Association of Blood Banks Staff. Ed. by U. E. Nydegger et al. 2000. (GER., Illus.). 48p. pap. 28.75 (*3-8055-6996-3*) S Karger.

Ingalls & Salerno's Maternal & Child Health Nursing. A. Joy Ingalls & M. Constance Salerno. 6th ed. 1995. (Illus.). 366p. pap. text, stu. ed. 17.95 (*0-8151-4802-X*) Mosby Inc.

Ingalls & Salerno's Maternal & Child Health Nursing. Julie C. Novak & Betty L. Broom. 8th ed. 1995. tchr. ed., suppl. ed. (*0-8151-6432-7*); 9th ed. 1999. (Illus.). 364p. stu. ed. (*0-323-00325-7*); Includes Testbank. 9th ed. 1999. tchr. ed. (*0-323-00323-0*) Mosby Inc.

Inglewood Way to Health. Antoinette Moses. 1991. (Illus.). 128p. 29.95 (*0-7153-9388-X*) Trafalgar.

Ingratiation: A Social Psychological Analysis. Edward E. Jones. 1964. LC 64-25812. (Century Psychology Ser.). 32.50 (*0-89197-230-7*); pap. text 14.95 (*0-89197-795-3*) Irvington.

Inguinal Hernia Repair. Ed. by V. Schumpelick & George E. Wantz. 1995. LC 94-44631. (Illus.). xii, 448p. 323.50 (*3-8055-6031-1*) S Karger.

Inhalants: The Toxic Fumes. John R. Glowa. 1992. LC 85-32569. (Encyclopedia of Psychoactive Drugs Ser.). (Illus.). 124p. (YA). (gr. 7-11). lib. bdg. 19.95 (*0-87754-758-0*) Chelsea Hse.

Inhalation Aerosols: Physical & Biological Basis for Therapy. Ed. by Anthony J. Hickey. 1996. LC 96-15857. (Lung Biology in Health & Disease Ser.: Vol. 94). (Illus.). 536p. text 215.00 (*0-8247-9702-7*) Dekker.

Inhalation Carcinogenesis: Proceedings. Ed. by Paul Nettesheim et al. 1970. LC 76-605835. (AEC Symposium Ser.). 524p. pap. 21.00 (*0-87079-246-6*, CONF-691001); fiche 9.00 (*0-87079-247-4*, CONF-691001) DOE.

Inhalation Delivery of Therapeutic Peptides & Proteins. Akete L. Adjei & Pramod K. Gupta. 1997. LC 97-15722. (Lung Biology in Health & Disease Ser.). (Illus.). 952p. text 275.00 (*0-8247-9780-9*) Dekker.

Inhalation Studies: Foundations & Techniques. Robert F. Phalen. 1984. 288p. 163.00 (*0-8493-5469-2*, RA1270, CRC Reprint) Franklin.

Inhalation Therapy: Roche & Genentech Symposium European Cystic Fibrosis Conference, Paris, June 1994. Ed. by Charles Koch & E. Puchelle. 1995. (Journal: Vol. 62, Suppl. 1, 1995). (Illus.). iv, 32p. pap. 21.75 (*3-8055-6164-4*) S Karger.

Inhalation Toxicology of Air Pollution: Clinical Research Considerations - STP 872. Ed. by Robert Frank et al. 1985. LC 85-20164. (Illus.). 131p. text 19.00 (*0-8031-0406-5*, STP872) ASTM.

Inhaled Glucocorticoids in Asthma. Ed. by Robert P. Schleimer et al. 1996. LC 96-32804. (Lung Biology in Health & Disease Ser.: Vol. 97). (Illus.). 808p. text 225.00 (*0-8247-9730-2*) Dekker.

Inhaled Particles Fundamentals & Applications. Ted B. Martonen. 1999. 59.95 (*0-87371-744-9*) Lewis Pubs.

Inheritance of Digital Malformation in Man. W. C. Farabee. 1969. (Harvard University Peabody Museum of Archaeology & Ethnology Monographs). reprint ed. pap. 25.00 (*0-527-01194-0*) Periodicals Srv.

Inheritance of Drinking Behavior. J. Partanen et al. 1966. (Finnish Foundation for Alcohol Studies: Vol. 14). 5.50 (*951-9192-05-0*) Rutgers Ctr Alcohol.

Inheritance of Kidney & Urinary Tract Diseases. Adrian Spitzer & Ellis Avner. 1990. 464p. text 259.50 (*0-7923-0287-7*) Kluwer Academic.

Inheritance of Mental Diseases. Abraham Myerson. 1976. LC 75-16724. (Classics in Psychiatry Ser.). reprint ed. 30.95 (*0-405-07448-4*) Ayer.

Inherited & Acquired Colour Vision Deficiencies. Cronly & Mandava. 1991. 137.00 (*0-8493-7507-X*) CRC Pr.

Inherited Disease of the Lung. Jack Lieberman. 1988. text 69.00 (*0-7216-2763-3*) Saunders.

***Inherited Diseases of the Pancreas**, Vol. 1, No. 5. Ed. by David C. Whitcomb & John P. Neoptolemos. 2001. (Pancreatology Special Issue Ser.). 164p. 45.25 (*3-8055-7277-8*) S Karger.

Inherited Disorders of the Kidney: Investigation & Management. Ed. by Steven Morgan & Jean-Pierre Grunfeld. 1998. LC 98-21523. (Oxford Clinical Nephrology Ser.). (Illus.). 644p. text 198.50 (*0-19-262473-3*) OUP.

Inherited Disorders of the Thyroid System. John Brutonn Stanbury. 1994. 232p. lib. bdg. 179.00 (*0-8493-4860-9*) CRC Pr.

Inherited Eye Diseases: Diagnosis & Clinical Management. Saul Merin. 1991. (Illus.). 528p. text 250.00 (*0-8247-7410-8*) Dekker.

Inherited Metabolic Diseases. Ed. by John B. Holton. 1987. (Illus.). 480p. (*0-443-03195-9*) Church.

Inherited Metabolic Diseases. Ed. by John B. Holton. 2nd ed. 1994. LC 93-4001. text (*0-443-04497-X*) Church.

Inherited Metabolic Diseases, Vol. 16. Harkness. 1995. pap. text 54.00 (*0-7923-8837-2*) Kluwer Academic.

Inherited Skin Diseases: The Genodermatoses. Ed. by John Harper. 1996. LC 97-114035. (Illus.). 368p. text 190.00 (*0-7506-1416-1*, Focal) Buttrwrth-Heinemann.

Inherited Skin Disorders. Ed. by John Harper. 2nd ed. 2000. (Illus.). 368p. pap. (*0-7506-4628-4*) E A GBR. *Dist:* OUP.

Inherited Susceptibility to Cancer: Clinical, Predictive & Ethical Perspectives. Ed. by William D. Foulkes & S. V. Hodgson. 1998. LC 97-35998. (Illus.). 470p. (C). text 95.00 (*0-521-56340-2*) Cambridge U Pr.

Inheriting Madness: Professionalization & Psychiatric Knowledge in Nineteenth-Century France. Ian Dowbiggin. 1991. LC 90-10914. (Medicine & Society Ser.: No. 4). 227p. text 48.00 (*0-520-06937-4*) U CA Pr.

Inhibition: History & Meaning in the Sciences of Mind & Brain. Roger Smith. 1992. LC 91-37839. 344p. (C). text 50.00 (*0-520-07580-3*) U CA Pr.

Inhibition in the Brain. Ed. by Charles E. Ribak. 1987. LC 82-642121. 173p. pap. 24.00 (*0-930195-04-3*) Inst Mind Behavior.

Inhibition of Carcinogenesis. Ed. by B. L. Van Duuren & B. A. Rubin. 1971. (Progress in Experimental Tumor Research Ser.: Vol. 14). 62.75 (*3-8055-1220-1*) S Karger.

Inhibition of Folate Metabolism in Chemotherapy: The Origins & Uses Of Co-trixomazole. Ed. by G. H. Hitchings. 1982. (Handbook of Experimental Pharmacology Ser.: Vol. 64). (Illus.). 457p. 312.00 (*0-387-11782-2*) Spr-Verlag.

Inhibition of Tumor Induction & Development. Ed. by Morris S. Zedeck & Martin Lipkin. 1981. LC 81-7324. 248p. 65.00 (*0-306-40687-X*, Plenum Trade) Perseus Pubng.

Inhibitions in Work & Love: Psychoanalytic Approaches to Problems in Creativity. Ed. by Herbert S. Strean. 1984. LC 83-22757. (Current Issues in Psychoanalytic Practice Ser.: Vol. 1, No. 1). 88p. text 39.95 (*0-86656-276-1*) Haworth Pr.

Inhibitors of Monoamine Oxidase B: Pharmacology & Clinical Use in Neurodegenerative Disorders. Ed. by I. Szelenyi. 1993. LC 92-49598. (Milestones in Drug Therapy Ser.). 384p. 119.50 (*3-7643-2782-0*); 146.50 (*0-8176-2782-0*) Birkhauser.

Inhibitors of Protein Biosynthesis. D. Vazquez. 1979. (Molecular Biology, Biochemistry & Biophysics Ser.: Vol. 30). (Illus.). 312p. 47.00 (*0-387-09188-2*) Spr-Verlag.

Inhibitors of Reverse Transciptase & Viral Protease. Hiroaki Mitsuya. 1992. 112p. pap. text 194.00 (*3-7186-5267-6*, Harwood Acad Pubs) Gordon & Breach.

Inhibitors to Coagulation Factors. Ed. by Louis M. Aledort et al. 1996. (Advances in Experimental Medicine & Biology Ser.: Vol. 386). (Illus.). 324p. (C). text 107.00 (*0-306-45196-4*, Kluwer Plenum) Kluwer Academic.

Inhibitory Processes in Attention, Memory, & Language. Ed. by Dale Dagenbach & Thomas H. Carr. 1994. LC 93-31495. (Illus.). 461p. text 69.95 (*0-12-200410-8*) Acad Pr.

Inhospital Ethylene Oxide Sterilization, 1984. 1984. 119p. pap. text 30.00 (*0-910275-37-8*, TAR8-209) Assn Adv Med Instrn.

Inhospital Sterility Assurance: Current Perspectives, 1982. Association for the Advancement of Medical Instruments Staff. 1982. (Illus.). 73p. (Orig.). pap. 30.00 (*0-910275-14-9*, TAR4-209) Assn Adv Med Instrn.

***Initial Management of Injuries: An Evidence Based Approach.** Ronald F. Sing et al. 2001. 304p. pap. (*0-7279-1477-4*) BMJ Pub GBR. *Dist:* AIDC.

Initial Processing of Pain & Its Descending Control: Spinal & Trigeminal Systems. A. R. Light. 1992. (Pain & Headache Ser.: Vol. 12). (Illus.). xiv, 306p. 304.50 (*3-8055-5569-5*) S Karger.

Initiation a la Science de la Gestion, Edition 1995: FLMI 340. Ed. by Joel V. Basarich. (FLMI Insurance Education Program Ser.). (FRE.). 93p. pap. 20.00 (*0-939921-65-0*) Life Office.

Initiation & Promotion in Skin or Liver Neoplasia: A 65 Year Annotated Bibliography of International Literature. E. B. Ilgren. 1991. 928p. 350.00 (*0-8493-4407-7*, Z6664) CRC Pr.

Injectable Contraceptives: Their Role in Family Planning Care. 1990. (CHI, ENG, FRE & SPA.). x, 117p. pap. text 21.00 (*92-4-154402-3*, 1150339) World Health.

Injectable Drug Development: Techniques to Reduce Pain & Irritation. Ed. by Pramod Gupta & Gayle Brazeau. 1999. LC 99-26911. 229.00 (*1-57491-095-7*) IHS Health Grp.

Injections in Orthopaedics & Sports Medicine. Saunders & Cameron. 1997. 125p. pap. text (*0-7020-2197-0*) W B Saunders GBR. *Dist:* Saunders.

Injured Athlete. Daniel N. Kulund et al. 2nd ed. 1988. LC 65-9293. (Illus.). 592p. text 98.00 (*0-397-50765-8*, Lippnctt) Lppncott W & W.

Injured Athlete. David Perrin. 3rd ed. 1998. LC 98-26849. 512p. text 89.00 (*0-397-51534-0*) Lppncott W & W.

Injured Brains of Medical Minds: Views from Within. Narinder Kapur. 1997. LC 96-25724. (Illus.). 442p. text 57.50 (*0-19-852144-8*) OUP.

Injured Hand: A Handbook for General & Clinical Practice. H. R. Mittelbach. 1979. (Illus.). 245p. 84.00 (*0-387-90365-8*) Spr-Verlag.

Injured Index & Pathogenic Bacteria: Occurrence & Detection in Foods, Water, & Feeds. Ed. by Bibek Ray. 1989. 224p. lib. bdg. 210.00 (*0-8493-4928-1*, QR115) CRC Pr.

Injured Workers in California: The Injured Worker's Guidebook. Monty Campbell. 1989. 103p. (Orig.). (C). pap. 9.00 (*1-877718-00-9*) Archangel Pr.

Injuries & Disorders of the Head & Brain. Lorne S. Label. 1997. LC 98-222999. 59.95 (*0-8205-2763-7*) Bender.

Injuries in Baseball. Ed. by James R. Andrews. 1998. LC 97-29923. 656p. text 159.00 (*0-7817-0259-3*) Lppncott W & W.

Injuries of the Brain & Skull Ed. by Pierre J. Vinken & George W. Bruyn. 1976. Pt. 1. 292.00 (*0-444-10877-7*); Pt. 2. 307.75 (*0-444-10878-5*) Elsevier.

Injuries of the Spine & Spinal Cord Ed. by Pierre J. Vinken & George W. Bruyn. 1976. Pt. 1. 202.75 (*0-444-10926-9*); Pt. 2. 216.50 (*0-444-11016-X*) Elsevier.

Injury & Illness Prevention Program. Med-Facts, Inc. Staff. rev. ed. 1992. 122p. 199.95 (*1-884006-26-4*) Med-Facts.

Injury & Poisoning Episodes & Conditions: National Health Interview Survey, 1997. Margaret Warner. 2000. 42p. pap. 5.50 (*0-16-050406-6*) USGPO.

Injury & Repair of the Musculoskeletal Soft Tissues, No. 1. Ed. by Savio L.-Y. Woo & Joseph A. Buckwalter. 1988. LC 87-72970. (Illus.). 548p. pap. 45.00 (*0-89203-023-2*) Amer Acad Ortho Surg.

Injury & Tumor Implantation. Satya M. Murthy & Edward F. Scanlon. 1993. LC 93-37851. (Medical Intelligence Unit Ser.). 99.00 (*1-879702-82-7*) Landes Bioscience.

Injury & Violence Prevention: Health Facts. Lucas Stang & Kathleen R. Miner. 1994. LC 93-47658. 12.95 (*1-56071-188-4*) ETR Assocs.

Injury Causation Analyses: Cases Studies & Data Sources, Set. Arthur C. Damask et al. 1990. 381p. 150.00 (*0-87473-660-9*, 61159-10, MICHIE) LEXIS Pub.

Injury Control: A Global View. Ed. by Lawrence R. Berger & Dinesh Mohan. 1996. (Illus.). 292p. (C). text 39.50 (*0-19-563680-5*) OUP.

Injury Control: Research & Program Evaluation. Ed. by Frederick P. Rivara et al. 2000. LC 00-27894. (Illus.). 314p. (C). text 95.00 (*0-521-66152-8*) Cambridge U Pr.

Injury Epidemiology. Leon S. Robertson. 1992. LC 91-20964. (Illus.). 256p. text 38.50 (*0-19-506956-0*) OUP.

Injury Epidemiology: Research & Control Strategies. Leon S. Robertson. 2nd ed. 1998. LC 97-35804. (Illus.). 288p. text 48.50 (*0-19-512202-X*) OUP.

Injury Fact Book. Susan P. Baker et al. 2nd ed. 1991. (Illus.). 368p. text 39.95 (*0-19-506194-2*) OUP.

Injury in the Aging. Ed. by Michael A. Horan & Roderick A. Little. 1998. LC 97-14855. (Illus.). 377p. (C). text 100.00 (*0-521-62160-7*) Cambridge U Pr.

Injury in the Young. R. A. Little. Ed. by M. P. Platt. 1998. LC 97-11815. (Illus.). 329p. (C). text 100.00 (*0-521-48117-1*) Cambridge U Pr.

Injury Prevention: Health Facts. Lucas Stang & Kathleen R. Miner. 1994. LC 94-24589. 21.95 (*1-56071-475-1*, H413) ETR Assocs.

Injury Prevention: An International Perspective: Epidemiology, Surveillance, & Policy. Peter Barss et al. 1998. LC 97-45595. (Illus.). 398p. text 59.50 (*0-19-511982-7*) OUP.

Injury Prevention & Control for Children & Youth. Mark D. Widome. 3rd ed. 1998. LC 97-73556. pap. 44.95 (*0-910761-90-6*) Am Acad Pediat.

Injury Prevention & Public Health: Practical Knowledge, Skills & Strategies. Tom Christoffel & Susan S. Gallagher. 1999. LC 98-49329. 416p. pap. 55.00 (*0-8342-0840-7*, 08407) Aspen Pub.

Injury Prevention & Violence: A Public Health Perspective. 1995. 56p. (Orig.). (C). pap. text 20.00 (*0-7881-1927-3*) DIANE Pub.

***Injury Visits to Hospital Emergency Departments: United States, 1992-95.** Ed. by Catharine W. Burt & Lois A. Fingerhut. 2001. (Illus.). 76p. (C). pap. text 20.00 (*0-7567-1791-4*) DIANE Pub.

Injury Visits to Hospital Emergency Departments: United States, 1992-95. Catharine W. Burt et al. 1998. LC 97-42729. (Vital & Health Statistics Ser.: Series 13, No. 131). (*0-8406-0536-6*) Natl Ctr Health Stats.

Injury/Illness Prevention Program. Mark M. Moran. 1992. (OSHA Written Compliance Programs Ser.: No. 16). (Illus.). 37p. ring bd. 169.00 (*1-890966-09-6*) SafetyCertified.

Inner-City Alcoholism: An Ecological Analysis & Cross-Cultural Study. Geoffrey Kane. 1981. LC 80-29389. 263p. 42.95 (*0-89885-023-1*, Kluwer Acad Hman Sci) Kluwer Academic.

Inner Cleansing: How to Free Yourself from Joint-Muscle-Artery-Circulation Sludge. Carlson Wade. rev. ed. 1992. 264p. (C). text 27.95 (*0-13-474586-8*) P-H.

Inner Ear Biology, Selected Papers from the 22nd Workshop, Wuerzburg, September 1985: Journal: ORL, Vol. 48, No. 2. Ed. by W. Arnold et al. 1986. (Illus.). 80p. pap. 42.75 (*3-8055-4268-2*) S Karger.

Inner Ear Pathobiology. Ed. by M Ciges & A. Campos. 1990. (Advances in OtoRhinoLaryngology Ser.: Vol. 45). (Illus.). x, 224p. 198.50 (*3-8055-5203-3*) S Karger.

Inner Ear Surgery. Ed. by I. Kaufman-Arenberg. 1991. LC 91-20841. (Illus.). 540p. lib. bdg. (*90-6299-078-9*) Kugler NLD. *Dist:* Lib Res.

Inner Environment: Clinical Research, Health Care Delivery, Economics. Frwd. by Robert A. Brungs. 1990. 172p. (Orig.). pap. 15.95 (*0-9625431-2-8*) ITEST Faith.

Inner Healing for Broken Vessels: Seven Steps to Mending Childhood Wounds. Linda H. Hollies. 1990. 130p. (Orig.). pap. text (*0-938503-03-0*) Welstar Pubns.

Inner Insights - The Book of Charts: Alternative Medicine & Awareness Quick Reference Charts. Linda Mackenzie. 1997. LC 97-91455. (Illus.). 112p. pap. 18.95 (*0-9656432-1-2*) Creat Hlth & Spirit.

Inner Knowing: Consciousness, Creativity, Insight & Intuition. Ed. by Helen Palmer. 1998. LC 98-24871. (New Consciousness Reader Ser.). 304p. 15.95 (*0-87477-936-7*, Tarcher Putnam) Putnam Pub Group.

Inner Life of Children with Special Needs. Ved P. Varma. 1996. 208p. 45.00 (*1-56593-322-2*, 1252) Singular Publishing.

***Inner Reiki: A Practical Guide for Healing & Meditation.** Tanmaya Honervogt. 2001. LC 2001-24540. (Illus.). pap. 20.00 (*0-8050-6690-X*, Owl) H Holt & Co.

Inner Torment: Living Between Conflict & Fragmentation. Salman Akhtar. 1998. LC 97-50487. (Illus.). xvii, 318p. 45.00 (*0-7657-0159-6*) Aronson.

Inner World: A Psycho-Analytic Study of Childhood & Society in India. Sudhir Kakar. 2nd ed. 1983. (Illus.). 250p. pap. text 12.95 (*0-19-561508-5*) OUP.

Inner World in the Outer World: Psychoanalytic Perspectives. Edward R. Shapiro. 1997. LC 96-8261. 208p. 37.00 (*0-300-06528-0*) Yale U Pr.

Inner World of Childhood. Frances G. Wickes. 3rd ed. 1988. (Inner World Ser.). (C). reprint ed. 304p. 32.50 (*0-938434-52-7*); 326p. pap. 17.95 (*0-938434-33-0*) Sigo Pr.

Inner World of Choice. Frances G. Wickes. 3rd ed. 1988. (Inner World Ser.). 318p. (C). reprint ed. 32.50 (*0-938434-54-3*); pap. 16.95 (*0-938434-35-7*) Sigo Pr.

Inner World of Man. Frances G. Wickes. 3rd ed. 1988. (Inner World Ser.). (Illus.). 352p. (C). reprint ed. 32.50 (*0-938434-53-5*); pap. 17.95 (*0-938434-34-9*) Sigo Pr.

Inner World of Trauma: Archetypal Defenses of the Personal Spirit. Donald Kalsched. 1996. LC 96-13507. 240p. (C). pap. 27.95 (*0-415-12329-1*) Routledge.

Innervation of the Gut: Pathophysiological Implications. Ed. by Yvette Tache et al. 1993. LC 93-4468. 384p. lib. bdg. 219.00 (*0-8493-4718-1*, QP368) CRC Pr.

Innocent Casualities: The FDA's War Against Humanity. Elaine Feuer. 1995. LC 96-84493. (Illus.). 192p. text 18.00 (*0-8059-3819-2*) Dorrance.

Innovating in Community Mental Health: International Perspectives. Ed. by Rockwell R. Schulz & James R. Greenley. 1995. LC 95-14415. 216p. 58.00 (*0-275-94931-1*, Praeger Pubs) Greenwood.

Innovation & Tradition at the University of Pennsylvania School of Medicine: An Anecdotal Journey. David Y. Cooper & Marshall A. Ledger. 1990. LC 90-12050. (Illus.). 360p. (C). text 34.95 (*0-8122-8242-6*) U of Pa Pr.

Innovation in Chinese Medicine. Ed. by Elisabeth Hsu. 2001. LC 00-45442. (Needham Research Institute Studies: Vol. 3). (Illus.). 400p. text 80.00 (*0-521-80068-4*) Cambridge U Pr.

Innovation in Community Care & Primary Health: The Marylebone Experiment. Ed. by P. Pietroni & C. Pietroni. 1995. (Illus.). 304p. pap. (*0-443-05296-4*) Church.

Innovation Processes in Medical Education. Margaret N. Bussigel et al. 1988. LC 87-27391. 170p. 67.00 (*0-275-92369-X*, C2369, Praeger Pubs) Greenwood.

Innovations in Abdominal Ultrasound. Ed. by N. Heyder et al. 1992. LC 92-49974. (Illus.). 160p. 125.00 (*3-540-55650-8*); 145p. 139.00 (*0-387-55650-8*) Spr-Verlag.

Innovations in Activities for the Elderly: Proceedings of the National Association of Activity Professionals Convention. Ed. by Jane Cook. 1985. LC 84-28996. (Activities, Adaptation & Aging Ser.: Vol. 6, Nos. 3 & 4). 120p. text 39.95 (*0-86656-389-X*) Haworth Pr.

Innovations in Antiviral Development & the Detection of Virus Infection. T. Block et al. 1992. (Advances in Experimental Medicine & Biology Ser.: Vol. 312). (Illus.). 240p. (C). text 89.50 (*0-306-44209-4*, Kluwer Plenum) Kluwer Academic.

Innovations in Cancer Risk Assessment (ED01 Study) 1979. LC 79-3153. 246p. 36.00 (*0-930376-09-9*) Chem-Orbital.

Innovations in Clincial Practice Vol. 13: A Source Book. Ed. by Leon VandeCreek et al. 1994. LC 82-7614. 480p. 39.95 (*1-56887-002-7*, I13-H-BP); ring bd. 39.95 (*1-56887-001-9*, I13-B-BP) Pro Resource (Prof Resc Pr).

Innovations in Clinical Practice: A Source Book. Ed. by Peter A. Keller & Lawrence G. Ritt. LC 82-7614. Vol. 4. 1985. 504p. 39.95 (*0-943158-09-5*, I4-HBP); Vol. 4. 1985. 504p. ring bd. 39.95 (*0-943158-10-9*, I4-BBP); Vol. 5. 1986. 472p. 39.95 (*0-943158-16-8*, I5-HBP); Vol. 5. 1986. 472p. ring bd. 39.95 (*0-943158-17-6*, I5-BBP) Pro Resource.

Innovations in Clinical Practice: A Source Book. Ed. by Peter A. Keller & Steven R. Heyman. LC 82-7614. Vol. 7. 1988. 540p. 39.95 (*0-943158-25-7*, I7-HBP); Vol. 7. 1988. 540p. ring bd. 39.95 (*0-943158-26-5*, I7-BBP); Vol. 9. 1990. 450p. 39.95 (*0-943158-63-X*, I9-HBP); Vol. 9. 1990. 450p. ring bd. 39.95 (*0-943158-62-1*, I9-BBP); Vol. 10. 1991. 550p. 39.95 (*0-943158-72-9*, I10-HBP); Vol. 10. 1991. 550p. ring bd. 39.95 (*0-943158-71-0*, I10-BBP) Pro Resource.

Innovations in Clinical Practice: A Source Book. Ed. by Leon VandeCreek et al. Vol. 11. 1992. LC 82-7614. 576p. 39.95 (*0-943158-81-8*, I11-HBP); Vol. 11. 1992. LC 82-7614. 576p. ring bd. 39.95 (*0-943158-80-X*, I11-BBP); Vol. 12. 1993. LC 82-7614. 624p. 39.95 (*0-943158-98-2*, I12-BBP); Vol. 12. 1993. LC 82-7614. 624p. ring bd. 39.95 (*0-943158-97-4*, I12-BBP); Vol. 14. 1995. 520p. 39.95 (*1-56887-016-7*, I14-H-BP); Vol. 14. 1995. ring bd. 39.95 (*1-56887-015-9*, I14-B-BP); Vol. 15. 1997. LC 82-7614. 522p. 39.95 (*1-56887-026-4*, I15HBP); Vol. 15. 1997. LC 82-7614. 522p. ring bd. 39.95 (*1-56887-025-6*, I15-BBP); Vol. 16. 1998. LC 82-7614. 496p. 65.45 (*1-56887-033-7*, I16-HBP); Vol. 16. 1998. LC 82-7614. 496p. ring bd. 70.45 (*1-56887-032-9*, I16-BBP) Pro Resource (Prof Resc Pr).

Innovations in Clinical Practice: A Source Book, Vol. 17. Ed. by Leon VandeCreek & Thomas L. Jackson. 1999. 522p. 65.45 (*1-56887-049-3*, I17BP); ring bd. 70.45 (*1-56887-048-5*, I17BP) Pro Resource (Prof Resc Pr).

Innovations in Clinical Practice: A Source Book, Vol.6. Ed. by Peter A. Keller & Steven R. Heyman. 1987. LC 82-7614. 450p. 39.95 (*0-943158-21-4*, I6-HBP); ring bd. 39.95 (*0-943158-22-2*, I6-BBP) Pro Resource.

Innovations in Community Care Management: Minimising Vulnerability. Gerald Wistow et al. 1992. (Avebury Studies of Care in the Community). 160p. (*1-85628-120-5*) Avebry GBR. *Dist:* Ashgate Pub Co.

H
I

Innovations in Community Mental Health. Ed. by Saul Cooper & Timothy H. Lentner. 1992. LC 92-5819. 256p. pap. 29.45 (*0-943158-76-1*, ICMBP, Prof Resc Pr) Pro Resource.

Innovations in Cross Cultural Psychology: Selected Papers from the 10th International Conference. Saburo Iwawaki et al. 1992. viii, 484p. pap. (*90-265-1232-5*) Swets.

Innovations in Disaster & Trauma Psychology, Vol. I. Ed. by George S. Everly, Jr. 1995. LC 97-178493. pap. text 32.00 (*1-883581-03-6*) Chevron Pub.

Innovations in Fee-for-Service Financing & Delivery. Ed. by Linda F. Wolf. 1998. (Illus.). 160p. (C). pap. text 25.00 (*0-7881-7242-5*) DIANE Pub.

Innovations in Head Injury Rehabilitation. Martin McMorrow & Kathleen Fralish. 1988. 1500p. text 135.00 (*1-887515-03-8*) AHAB Press.

Innovations in Health Care Financing: Proceedings of a World Bank Conference, March 10-11, 1997. Ed. by George Schieber. 1997. (World Bank Discussion Paper Ser.: No. 365). 266p. pap. 22.00 (*0-8213-3964-8*, 13964) World Bank.

Innovations in Health Promotion & Disease Prevention: Award Winners (1992) 1995. (Illus.). 32p. (Orig.). (C). pap. text 20.00 (*0-7881-1844-7*) DIANE Pub.

Innovations in Healthcare Design. Sara O. Marberry. 1995. text 62.95 (*0-442-01867-3*, VNR) Wiley.

Innovations in Hospital Marketing. Ed. by William J. Winston. 1984. LC 84-15664. (Health Marketing Quarterly Ser.: Vol. 2, No. 1). 138p. text 39.95 (*0-86656-349-0*); pap. text 19.95 (*0-86656-379-2*) Haworth Pr.

Innovations in Nursing Education Administration. Ed. by Mabel A. Wandelt & Betty Thomas. 1990. 96p. 13.95 (*0-88737-492-1*) Natl League Nurse.

Innovations in Nursing Practice. Kendrick. 256p. pap. (*0-340-60765-3*) E A GBR. *Dist:* Routldge.

Innovations in Occupational Therapy Education (IOTE) Ed. by Patricia A. Crist. 1999. LC 00-500449. (Illus.). xvii, 181p. pap. 25.00 (*1-56900-119-7*) Am Occup Therapy.

Innovations in Pain Management: A Practical Guide for Clinicians Ed. by Richard S. Weiner. 1993. (Illus.). Set. LC 90-84153. 2520p. lib. bdg. 195.00 (*1-878205-13-7*); Vol. 3. 4th ed. 724p. ring bd. 190.00 (*1-878205-03-X*); Vols. 1-4. 2256p. 350.00 (*1-878205-57-9*) St Lucie Pr.

Innovations in Perinatal Transfusion & Transplantation. American Association of Blood Banks Staff. Ed. by S. D. Roseff. 1998. (Illus.). 36p. ring bd. (*3-8055-6901-7*) S Karger.

Innovations in Physiological Anaesthesia & Monitoring. Ed. by R. Droh & R. Spintge. 1989. (Illus.). 179p. 69.95 (*0-387-50331-5*) Spr-Verlag.

Innovations in Rational-Emotive Therapy. Windy Dryden & Larry K. Hill. LC 92-49498. (Illus.). 320p. (C). 1993. 68.95 (*0-8039-4300-8*, 3065); 1992. pap. 34.95 (*0-8039-4301-6*, 3066) Sage.

Innovations in Rural Community Mental Health. Ed. by J. Dennis Murray & Peter A. Keller. 1986. 285p. (Orig.). (C). pap. text 19.95 (*0-940299-00-3*) Manfld U Rural.

Innovations in Urologic Oncology. Ed. by Steven Rosen et al. 1991. LC 91-67426. 144p. 29.95 (*0-944496-25-3*) Precept Pr.

Innovative Antimetabolites in Solid Tumours. M. S. Aapro. 1994. LC 94-30057. (ESO Monographs). (Illus.). 59p. 54.95 (*3-540-58341-6*); (*0-387-58341-6*) Spr-Verlag.

Innovative Applications of Gestalt Therapy. Shraga Serok. 2000. LC 98-33874. 264p. (C). text 37.50 (*1-57524-090-4*, 230904) Krieger.

Innovative Approaches for Difficult-to-Treat Populations. Ed. by Scott W. Henggeler et al. 1997. LC 96-4744. 512p. text 67.00 (*0-88048-680-5*, 8680) Am Psychiatric.

Innovative Behavioral Healthcare for Older Adults: A Guidebook for Changing Times. Paula E. Hartman-Stein. 1997. LC 97-14981. 268p. 37.00 (*0-7879-0963-7*) Jossey-Bass.

Innovative Hypnotherapy. Milton H. Erickson. Ed. by Ernest L. Rossi. 1980. (Collected Papers of Milton H. Erickson on Hypnosis: Vol. IV). 570p. (C). pap. 39.95 (*0-8290-1209-5*); text 59.95 (*0-8290-0545-5*) Ardent Media.

***Innovative Mental Health Interventions for Children: Programs That Work.** Ed. by Steven I. Pfeiffer & Linda A. Reddy. 2001. LC 2001-24318. xvi, 114p. 39.95 (*0-7890-1363-0*); pap. text 22.95 (*0-7890-1364-9*) Haworth Pr.

Innovative Partnerships for Affordable Health Care: Conference Proceedings, September 23-24, 1990, Washington, D. C.: Rx for a Healthy America. Ed. by Karen Glass. 1991. 155p. (Orig.). pap. text 20.00 (*1-55877-084-4*) Natl Governor.

Innovative Programmes of Medical Education in South-East Asia. N. M. Mattock & P. Abeykoon. 1993. (WHO Regional Publications, South-East Asia Ser.: No. 21). viii, 119p. pap. text 20.00 (*92-9022-163-1*, 1560021) World Health.

Innovative Psychotherapy Techniques in Child & Adolescent Therapy. Charles E. Schaefer. 2nd ed. 1999. LC 98-55167. (Illus.). 528p. 85.00 (*0-471-24404-X*) Wiley.

Innovative Therapy: A Handbook. David Jones. 1994. LC 94-1682. (Open University Press Psychotherapy Handbook Ser.). 224p. (*0-335-19140-1*); pap. (*0-335-19139-8*) OpUniv Pr.

Innovative Trends in Psychogeriatrics. Ed. by J. Wertheimer et al. 1989. (Interdisciplinary Topics in Gerontology Ser.: Vol. 26). (Illus.). xii, 120p. 100.00 (*3-8055-4907-5*) S Karger.

Innovators in Physician Education: The Process & Pattern of Reform in North American Medical Schools. Robert H. Ross & Harvey V. Fineberg. 1996. (Series on Medical Education: Vol. 19, 1995). (Illus.). 304p. 46.95 (*0-8261-9200-9*) Springer Pub.

Inorganic Chemistry in Biology & Medicine. Arthur E. Martell. 1980. LC 80-23248. (ACS Symposium Ser.: No. 140). 49.95 (*0-8412-0588-4*) Am Chemical.

Inorganic Mass Spectrometry. Ed. by F. Adams et al. 1988. LC 87-21561. (Monographs on Analytical Chemistry & Its Applications). 404p. 210.00 (*0-471-82364-3*) Wiley.

Inorganic Mercury. 1991. (Environmental Health Criteria Ser.: No. 118). (ENG, FRE & SPA.). 168p. pap. text 32.00 (*92-4-157118-7*, 1160118) World Health.

Inorganics in Drinking Water & Cardiovascular Disease. Ed. by Edward J. Calabrese et al. 1985. LC 85-62107. (Advances in Modern Environmental Toxicology Ser.: Vol. 9). (Illus.). 340p. 65.00 (*0-911131-10-8*) Specialist Journals.

Inositol & Phosphoinositides: Metabolism & Regulation. Ed. by John E. Bleasdale et al. 1985. LC 84-131. (Experimental Biology & Medicine Ser.: Vol. 6). (Illus.). 698p. 145.00 (*0-89603-074-1*) Humana.

Inositol Lipids in Cell Signalling. Ed. by Robert H. Michell et al. 1989. 534p. text 157.00 (*0-12-493860-4*) Acad Pr.

Inotropic Stimulation & Myocardial Energetics. Christian Holubarsch et al. 1989. 400p. 65.00 (*0-387-91361-0*) Spr-Verlag.

Inpatient Behavior Therapy for Children & Adolescents. V. B. Van Hasselt & D. J. Kolko. 1992. (Illus.). 464p. (C). 85.00 (*0-306-44079-2*, Plenum Trade) Perseus Pubng.

Inpatient Case Studies Using ICD-9-CM Codes. Gail I. Smith & Sherri Mallett. 1998. 108p. (C). ring bd. 38.00 (*1-58426-020-3*, AC900198) Am Hlth Info.

Inpatient Case Studies Using ICD-9-CM Codes. Gail I. Smith & Sherri A. Mallett. rev. ed. 2000. 143p. pap. text 38.00 (*1-58426-054-8*, AC900100) Am Hlth Info.

Inpatient Child Psychiatry. Jonathan Green & Brian Jacobs. 1998. LC 98-2991. (Illus.). 384p. (C). 105.00 (*0-415-19439-3*); pap. 47.95 (*0-415-14525-2*) Routledge.

Inpatient Group Psychotherapy. Cecil A. Rice. 1987. 26.95 (*0-07-105351-4*) McGraw.

Inpatient Group Psychotherapy. Irvin D. Yalom. 1983. LC 82-72411. 372p. pap. 50.00 (*0-465-03298-2*) Basic.

Inpatient Hospital Use in New York City: Community Hospital Profiles, Set. Compiled by Division of Planning, Distribution and Development S. 1980. (POIS Reports). 80.00 (*0-934459-75-4*) United Hosp Fund.

Inpatient Hospital Use in New York City, 1982, Vol. One: Service Patterns & Insurance Coverage. United Hospital Fund Staff. 1985. 216p. 30.00 (*0-934459-21-5*) United Hosp Fund.

Inpatient Hospital Use in New York City, 1982, Vol. Two: Community Profiles: Utilization & Clinical Service. United Hospital Fund Staff. 1985. 364p. 50.00 (*0-934459-22-3*) United Hosp Fund.

Inpatient Hospital Use in New York City, 1985, Set. Compiled by Division of Research, Analysis, and Planning Staff. 1987. 125.00 (*0-934459-42-8*) United Hosp Fund.

Inpatient Hospital Use in New York City, 1985, Vol. One: Service Patterns & Insurance Coverage. Compiled by Division of Research, Analysis, and Planning Staff. 1987. 220p. 30.00 (*0-934459-43-6*) United Hosp Fund.

Inpatient Hospital Use in New York City, 1985, Vol. Three: Community Profiles: Utilization & Insurance Coverage. Compiled by Division of Research, Analysis, and Planning Staff. 1987. 370p. 50.00 (*0-934459-45-2*) United Hosp Fund.

Inpatient Hospital Use in New York City, 1985, Vol. Two: Community Profiles: Utilization & Clinical Service. Compiled by Division of Research, Analysis, and Planning Staff. 1987. 370p. 50.00 (*0-934459-44-4*) United Hosp Fund.

Inpatient Obstetric Nursing. Jack Rudman. (Certified Nurse Examination Ser.: CN-20). pap. 27.95 (*0-8373-6120-6*) Nat Learn.

Inpatient Physical Therapy Policy & Procedure Manual. JoAnne Whipple. 1993. 110.00 (*1-879575-28-0*) Acad Med Sys.

Inpatient Psychiatry: Diagnosis & Treatment. Lloyd I. Sederer. 3rd ed. 1991. (Illus.). 480p. 62.00 (*0-683-07629-9*) Lppncott W & W.

Inpatient Psychiatry: Toward Rapid Restoration of Function. Marc Hertzman. 1984. LC 83-22640. 224p. 38.95 (*0-89885-152-1*); pap. 24.95 (*0-89885-189-0*) Kluwer Academic (Kluwer Acad Hman Sci).

Input & Interaction in Language Acquisition. Ed. by Clare Gallaway & Brian J. Richards. 1994. LC 93-5482. 335p. (C). pap. text 22.95 (*0-521-43725-3*) Cambridge U Pr.

Inquinal Hernia: Advances or Controversies? Ed. by Maurice E. Arregui & Robert Nagan. 1994. LC 94-7987. (*1-85775-046-2*) Radcliffe Med Pr GBR. *Dist:* Balogh.

Inquiries in Bioethics. Stephen G. Post. 1993. LC 93-17564. 208p. 37.50 (*0-87840-538-0*); pap. 18.95 (*0-87840-539-9*) Georgetown U Pr.

Inquiries into Human Faculty & Its Development. Francis Galton. LC 72-1638. reprint ed. 38.50 (*0-404-08127-4*) AMS Pr.

Inquiry & the National Science Education Standards: A Guide for Teaching & Learning. Steve Olson & Susan Loucks-Horsley. 2000. LC 00-8103. (Illus.). xviii, 202p. pap. 21.95 (*0-309-06476-7*) Natl Acad Pr.

Inquiry Concerning the Diseases & Functions of the Brain, the Spinal Cord the Nerves. Amariah Brigham. 1973. LC 73-2388. (Mental Illness & Social Policy; the American Experience Ser.). reprint ed. 25.95 (*0-405-05196-4*) Ayer.

Inquiry into Schizophrenia & Depression. 1988. (Animal Models of Psychiatric Disorders Ser.: Vol. 2). (Illus.). vi, 214p. 164.50 (*3-8055-4757-9*) S Karger.

Inquiry into the Nature & Origin of Mental Derangement Alexander Crichton. LC 75-14763. (Language, Man & Society Ser.). reprint ed. 94.50 (*0-404-08212-2*) AMS Pr.

Inquitante Etrangete et Autres Essais. Sigmund Freud. 1991. (FRE.). pap. 14.95 (*0-7859-2812-X*, 2070324672) Fr & Eur.

INS Dictionary of Neuropsychology. Ed. by David W. Loring. 1998. LC 98-23696. 192p. text 55.00 (*0-19-506977-3*) OUP.

INS Dictionary of Neuropsychology. David W. Lorring. 1998. LC 98-23696. 192p. pap. text 24.95 (*0-19-506978-1*) OUP.

Insane in the United States & Canada. Daniel H. Tuke. 1973. LC 73-2424. (Mental Illness & Social Policy; the American Experience Ser.). reprint ed. 23.95 (*0-405-05233-2*) Ayer.

Insane Therapy: Portrait of a Psychotherapy Cult. Marybeth F. Ayella. 1998. LC 97-38146. 224p. (C). text 54.95 (*1-56639-600-X*); pap. text 19.95 (*1-56639-601-8*) Temple U Pr.

Insanity: Its Causes & Prevention. Henry P. Stearns. Ed. by Gerald N. Grob. 1980. LC 78-22591. (Historical Issues in Mental Health Ser.). reprint ed. lib. bdg. 19.95 (*0-405-11942-9*) Ayer.

Insanity: Its Classification, Diagnosis & Treatment. Edward C. Spitzka. 2nd ed. 1973. LC 73-2420. (Mental Illness & Social Policy; the American Experience Ser.). reprint ed. 31.95 (*0-405-05229-4*) Ayer.

Insanity: The Idea & Its Consequences. Thomas Szasz. 1997. LC 96-45524. 436p. reprint ed. pap. 19.95 (*0-8156-0460-2*) Syracuse U Pr.

Insanity & Its Treatment: Lectures on the Treatment, Medical & Legal, of Insane Patients. G. Fielding Blandford. 1976. LC 75-16684. (Classics in Psychiatry Ser.). reprint ed. 41.95 (*0-405-07416-6*) Ayer.

Insanity Defense. Abraham S. Goldstein. 1980. LC 79-26323. 289p. reprint ed. lib. bdg. 59.75 (*0-313-22202-9*, GOID, Greenwood Pr) Greenwood.

Insanity on Trial. Norman J. Finkel. 1988. LC 88-19701. (Perspectives in Law & Psychology Ser.: Vol. 8). (Illus.). 398p. (C). 57.50 (*0-306-42899-7*, Plenum Trade) Perseus Pubng.

Inscapes of the Child's World: Jungian Counseling in Schools & Clinics. John A. B. Allan. 1988. LC 88-27831. (Illus.). 400p. pap. 19.50 (*0-88214-338-7*) Spring Pubns.

Insearch: Psychology & Religion. James Hillman. 2nd rev. ed. 1994. LC 94-24835. (Jungian Classics Ser.: Vol. 2). 144p. pap. 15.00 (*0-88214-512-6*) Spring Pubns.

Insect & Rodent Control Through Environmental Management: A Community Action Programme. 1991. (ENG, FRE & SPA.). vii, 107p. pap. text 90.00 (*92-4-154411-2*, 1150358) World Health.

Insect Man: The Fight Against Malaria in Africa. Alec Smith. 1993. (Illus.). 192p. (C). text (*1-85043-597-9*) I B T GBR. *Dist:* St Martin.

Insect Neurochemistry & Neurophysiology - 1989. Ed. by A. B. Borkovec & Edward P. Masler. 1990. LC 90-4001. (Experimental & Clinical Neuroscience Ser.). (Illus.). 482p. 129.50 (*0-89603-168-3*) Humana.

Insecticide Resistance & Vector Control. 1963. (Technical Report Ser.: No. 265). 227p. pap. text 9.00 (*92-4-120265-3*) World Health.

Insecticides & Fungicides Pt. 2. T. Roberts. 1999. 1500p. (C). (*0-85404-499-X*) Royal Soc Chem GBR. *Dist:* Spr-Verlag.

Insects: An Outline of Entomology. P. J. Gullan & Peter S. Cranston. 2nd ed. 2000. LC 99-30846. (Illus.). xvi, 470p. pap. 69.95 (*0-632-05343-7*) Blackwell Sci.

Inservice Manual Continuing Education Program for LTC. Mattie Locke. 1986. (Illus.). 120p. (C). 34.50 (*1-877735-12-4*, 2115PP) Prof Prnting & Pub.

Inservices on Loss, Families, Aging & Staff Stress. Marylou Hughes. 1992. (Illus.). 361p. (C). 65.00 (*1-877735-38-8*, 2199PP) Prof Prnting & Pub.

Inside an Emotional Health Program: A Field Study of Workplace Assistance for Troubled Employees. William J. Sonnenstuhl. 1986. LC 86-7145. 196p. (Orig.). 35.00 (*0-87546-119-0*); pap. 14.95 (*0-87546-120-4*) Cornell U Pr (ILR Press).

Inside Clinical Psychology: A Handbook for Graduate Students & Interns. Herbert M. Potash. 1981. LC 81-82640. 135p. text 19.95 (*0-940524-00-7*); pap. text 9.95 (*0-940524-01-5*) G Handwerk.

Inside Dentistry. Henry J. Hoffmann. 2nd ed. 1984. (Illus.). 444p. (C). lib. bdg. 34.95 (*0-9614287-0-8*) J H Hoffmann.

Inside Dentistry: Everything You Need to Know Before Your Next Dental Visit. Randall Nozawa et al. Ed. by Laurel Strand. 2000. (Illus.). 208p. pap. 14.95 (*0-9679932-0-2*) Isa Mira.

Inside Doctoring: Stages & Outcomes in the Professional Development of Physicians. Ed. by Robert H. Coombs et al. 1986. 315p. LC 86-15683. 72.50 (*0-275-92172-7*, C2172); LC 86-15083. pap. 22.95 (*0-275-92173-5*, B2173) Greenwood (Praeger Pubs).

Inside Dope. George L. Manthe. 1984. (Illus.). 177p. pap. 9.95 (*0-911603-01-8*) Rube Pubns.

Inside Family Therapy: A Case Study in Family Healing. annuals Michael P. Nichols. 1998. LC 98-14393. 242p. pap. 45.00 (*0-205-28412-4*) Allyn.

Inside Lives: Psychoanalysis & the Growth of Personality. Margot Waddell. 1999. LC 98-41208. (Tavistock Clinic Ser.). 221p. pap. 25.95 (*0-415-92289-5*) Routledge.

Inside Managed Care: Family Therapy in a Changing Environment. Jodi Aronson. 1996. LC 96-28522. 160p. pap. 19.95 (*0-87630-818-3*) Brunner-Routledge.

Inside Nursing: A Critical Ethnography of Clinical Nursing Practice. Annette F. Street. 1992. LC 90-10420. (SUNY Series in Teacher Empowerment & School Reform). 316p. (C). text 64.50 (*0-7914-0803-5*); pap. text 22.95 (*0-7914-0804-3*) State U NY Pr.

Inside-Out: Lesbian Theories, Gay Theories. Ed. by Diana Fuss. 1991. 288p. (C). (gr. 13). pap. 24.95 (*0-415-90237-1*, A4298) Routledge.

Inside Out: Rebuilding Self & Personality Through Inner Child Therapy. Ann E. Potter. 1994. 70p. pap., tchr. ed. 8.95 (*1-55959-063-7*) Accel Devel.

Inside Out & Outside In: Psychodynamic Clinical Theory & Practice in Contemporary Multicultural Contexts. Joan N. Berzoff et al. 1996. LC 95-47146. 472p. 50.00 (*1-56821-777-3*) Aronson.

Inside Outcomes: The National Review of Behavioral Healthcare Outcomes Programs. Tom Trabin et al. 1995. (Managed Behavioral Healthcare Library). 204p. 45.00 (*1-887452-02-8*) CentraLink.

Inside Story: Self-Evaluations Reflecting Basic Rorschach Types. Ed. by Molly Harrower & Dawn Bowers. 1987. (Personality Assessment Ser.). 264p. (C). text 49.95 (*0-89859-990-3*) L Erlbaum Assocs.

Inside Story of Medicines: A Symposium. Ed. by Gregory J. Higby & Elaine C. Stroud. 1997. (AIHP Publications: No. 16). (Illus.). 304p. text 25.00 (*0-931292-31-X*); LC 98-117787. pap. text 15.00 (*0-931292-32-8*) Am Inst Hist Pharm.

Inside the Brain: Revolutionary Discoveries of How the Mind Works. Ronald Kotulak. 224p. 1996. LC 95-45884. (Illus.). 21.95 (*0-8362-1043-3*); 1997. reprint ed. pap. 12.95 (*0-8362-3289-5*) Andrews McMeel.

Inside the Caring Services. 2nd ed. 352p. pap. (*0-340-57604-9*) E A GBR. *Dist:* Routldge.

Inside the Cell: Light & Fluorescence Microscopy. Douglas W. Kline. 2000. 35.00 (*0-12-414960-X*) Acad Pr.

Inside the Criminal Mind. Stanton E. Samenow. 1984. LC 83-45039. 285p. 25.00 (*0-8129-1082-6*, Crown) Crown Pub Group.

Inside the New Temple: The High Cost of Mistaking Medicine for Religion. James H. Stacey. 1993. 208p. (Orig.). pap. 12.95 (*0-9634395-1-0*) Conversation Pr.

Inside the Physician Practice Management Companies. 1997. 130p. (Orig.). pap. 195.00 (*1-56925-088-X*, PPMC) Capitol VA.

Inside Therapy: Illuminating Writings about Therapists, Patients & Psychotherapy. Ilana Rabinowitz. 1998. LC 98-5922. xxv, 291p. 24.95 (*0-312-18671-1*) St Martin.

Insider's Guide to Graduate Programs in Clinical & Counseling Psychology: 1996-1997 Edition. John C. Norcross et al. 1996. 275p. pap. 19.95 (*1-57230-086-8*) Guilford Pubns.

Insider's Guide to Graduate Programs in Clinical & Counseling Psychology: 1998-1999 Edition. Michael A. Sayette et al. 1998. 322p. pap. 21.95 (*1-57230-274-7*) Guilford Pubns.

Insider's Guide to Graduate Programs in Clinical & Counseling Psychology: 2000-2001 Edition. Tracy J. Mayne et al. rev. ed. 2000. (Insider's Guide to Graduate Programs in Clinical & Counseling Psychology Ser.). (Illus.). 342p. pap. 22.95 (*1-57230-495-2*, CO495) Guilford Pubns.

Insider's Guide to Home Health Care. Tova Navarra & Margaret Ferrer. 1996. LC 96-3195. 208p. pap. 28.00 (*1-55642-287-3*, 42873) SLACK Inc.

***Insider's Guide to Internet Health Searches.** Joan Price. 2002. LC 2001-7485. 240p. pap. 14.95 (*1-57954-515-7*) Rodale Pr Inc.

Insider's Guide to Medical School Admissions. R. Stephen Toyos. 1995. (Orig.). pap. text 19.95 (*0-9632231-4-3*) Innovat Pub & Graph.

Insider's Guide to Medical School Admissions. R. Stephen Toyos. 2nd ed. 1997. LC 96-37945. (Insider's Guide to Medical School Admissions Ser.). 192p. pap. 16.99 (*1-56414-272-8*) Career Pr Inc.

Insider's Guide to Medical Schools: Medical Students Tell You What You Really Want to Know. Jay K. Varma. 1999. LC 99-23444. (Peterson's Insider's Guide to Medical Schools Ser.). 336p. pap. 21.95 (*0-7689-0203-7*) Petersons.

Insider's Guide to Mental Health Resources Online. John M. Grohol. 1997. LC 97-15533. (Clinician's Toolbox Ser.). 326p. pap. 21.95 (*1-57230-229-1*) Guilford Pubns.

Insider's Guide to the MCAT. Contrib. by Chirag Amin et al. 1999. LC 99-33185. 280p. pap. text 21.95 (*0-683-30698-7*) Lppncott W & W.

Insider's Guide to the Usmle Step 2. John M. Stang. 1999. LC 99-21516. (Illus.). 415p. pap. text (*0-7216-8279-0*) Saunders.

Insight & Industry: On the Dynamics of Technological Change in Medicine. Stuart S. Blume. 1991. LC 91-18801. (Inside Technology Ser.). (Illus.). 356p. 49.95 (*0-262-02332-6*) MIT Pr.

Insight & Psychosis. Ed. by Xavier F. Amador & Anthony S. David. 1998. LC 96-18781. (Illus.). 384p. text 60.00 (*0-19-508497-7*) OUP.

Insight & Responsibility: Lectures on the Ethical Implications of Psychoanalytical Insight. Erik H. Erilson. 1994. pap. 10.00 (*0-393-31214-3*, Norton Paperbks) Norton.

Insight-Imagination: The Emancipation of Thought & the Modern World, 24. Douglas Sloan. 1983. LC 83-1668. (Contributions in Philosophy Ser.: No. 24). 272p. 55.00 (*0-313-23919-3*, SLN/, Greenwood Pr) Greenwood.

Insight into Value: An Exploration of the Premises of a Phenomenological Psychology. Andrew R. Fuller. 1990. LC 89-39369. 295p. (C). text 64.50 (*0-7914-0329-7*); pap. text 21.95 (*0-7914-0330-0*) State U NY Pr.

Insights about Your Outsides. Michael C. Giammatteo. rev. ed. 1999. (Illus.). pap. 8.95 (*0-918428-00-9*) Sylvan Inst.

Insights & Innovations in Community Mental Health: Ten Erich Lindemann Memorial Lectures. Ed. by David G. Satin et al. 1994. LC 93-50077. 192p. pap. text 35.00 (*1-56821-211-9*) Aronson.

Insights in Biology: The Blueprints of Infection. Education Development Center, Inc. Staff. 1997. 192p. stu. ed., per. 11.99 (*0-7872-2207-0*) Kendall-Hunt.

Insights in the Eyes: An Introduction to Sclerology. Jack Tips. 1996. 70p. 44.95 incl. VHS (*0-929167-11-2*) Apple-a-Day.

Insights into the Reach to Grasp Movement. Ed. by Keree M. B. Bennett & Umberto Castiello. 1994. LC 93-47507. (Advances in Psychology Ser.). 418p. 131.50 (*0-444-89931-6*, North Holland) Elsevier.

Insights into Troubled Sexuality: A Case Profile Anthology. Tunnadine. 1991. 218p. pap. 41.50 (*1-56593-007-X*, 0248) Thomson Learn.

Insights of a Senior Acupuncturist: One Combination of Points Can Treat Many Diseases. Miriam Lee. Ed. by Bob Flaws. 1992. LC 92-70742. 140p. (Orig.). pap. 17.95 (*0-936185-33-3*) Blue Poppy Pr.

Insolubilized Enzymes. Ed. by M. Salmona et al. 1974. 28.75 (*0-7204-7527-9*) Elsevier.

***Insomnia.** Daniel Brooks & Guillermo Verdecchia. 1999. LC 00-303511. 63p. pap. (*1-896239-54-4*) J G Shillingford Pub.

Insomnia: Psychological Assessment & Management. Charles M. Morin. 1996. LC 93-6564. (Treatment Manuals for Practitioners Ser.). 238p. pap. 23.00 (*1-57230-120-1*, 0120) Guilford Pubns.

***Insomnia & Sleep Disorders: Index of New Information for Consumers, Reference & Research.** Ed. by Research and Development Division Staff & John C. Bartone. 2001. 180p. 47.50 (*0-7883-2586-8*); pap. 44.50 (*0-7883-2587-6*) ABBE Pubs Assn.

Insomnia Pack. Journey Editions Staff. 1997. (Cures for Modern Times Ser.). (Illus.). 64p. 16.95 (*1-885203-42-X*) Jrny Editions.

Insomnia Plus... The Answer to Sleeplessness. Willa V. Bowles & Carl G. Wirth. 1990. 141p. pap. 7.95 (*0-9625716-0-1*) Temple Treasures Pubns.

***Insomniac's Handbook: A Companion for the Nocturnally Challenged.** Photos by Ben Asen. 2001. (Illus.). 144p. pap. 19.95 (*0-7893-0588-7*) Universe.

Inspecting the Newborn Baby's Eyes. N. O'Doherty. 1986. (Atlases of Childhood Ser.). text 309.00 (*0-85200-857-0*) Kluwer Academic.

Inspection: Sexually Transmitted Diseases. Frank L. Clark & Sandra L. Warren-Clark. Ed. by Joel E. Koopman. 1988. (Illus.). 124p. (Orig.). pap. 14.95 (*0-923944-00-1*) Pub Partners.

Inspiration: Your Guide to Better Breathing. Margaret A. Varnell. 1998. (Illus.). 143p. pap. 16.95 (*0-937776-11-4*) Good Commun Inc.

Inspiration & Motivation. 1982. LC 81-23459. 14.00 (*0-9603174-6-5*) Bks of Value.

Inspired Medicine: Sathya Sai Baba's Influence in Medical Practice. Ed. by Judy Warner. 2000. LC 00-103911. 288p. pap. 14.00 (*1-887906-02-9*) Leela Pr.

Instant Access to Chiropractic Guidelines & Protocols. Lew Huff & David Brady. 1998. LC 98-33726. xxvi, 406p. 32.95 (*0-323-00535-7*) Mosby Inc.

Instant Allergy. Niels Mygind et al. 1997. LC 96-44629. (Illus.). 184p. pap. 36.95 (*0-632-04232-X*) Blackwell Sci.

Instant Anatomy. Robert H. Whitaker & Neil R. Borley. (Illus.). 1994. LC 94-6652. 208p. pap. 27.95 (*0-86542-822-0*); 2nd ed. 2000. LC 99-39812. pap. 28.95 (*0-632-05403-4*) Blackwell Sci.

Instant Baby Food. Linda McDonald. 1975. LC 75-27760. (Illus.). 113p. 8.95 (*0-916198-02-2*); pap. 6.95 (*0-916198-01-4*) Oaklawn Pr.

Instant Drug Index 1998. Patricia Aloisi. 1998. spiral bd. 29.95 (*0-632-04331-8*) Blackwell Sci.

Instant Drug Index 1999. Patricia Aloisi. 1999. LC 99-217807. spiral bd. 29.95 (*0-632-04447-0*) Blackwell Sci.

Instant Drug Index, 1997. Patricia Aloisi. 1996. spiral bd. 29.95 (*0-632-04302-4*) Blackwell Sci.

Instant Drug Index 2000. Patricia Aloisi. 2000. LC 2001-268451. pap. 33.95 (*0-632-04523-X*) Blackwell Sci.

Instant Exam Review USMLE: Step 3. Joel S. Goldberg. 2nd rev. ed. 1997. LC 96-46590. (Appleton & Lange's Review Ser.). 409p. (C). pap. 39.95 (*0-8385-4337-5*, A4337-0) McGraw-Hill Educ Grp.

Instant Guide to Drug-Herb Interactions. Chris D. Melitis. 2001. LC 00-64406. (Illus.). 160p. pap. 12.95 (*0-7894-7150-7*) DK Pub Inc.

Instant Medical Adviser: Instant Answers to Your Medical Questions. Jeanne Smith & Isadore Rossman. 1994. LC 77-137337. 320p. 6.95 (*0-911744-08-8*) Career Pub IL.

Instant Medical Spelling Dictionary: 20,000 Medical, Biological & Pharmaceutical Words. Ed. by Donald O. Bolander & Rita Bisdorf. 1986. 6.95 (*0-911744-35-5*) Career Pub IL.

***Instant Notes in Medicinal Chemistry.** G. Patrick. 2001. 320p. pap. 27.95 (*0-387-91622-9*) Spr-Verlag.

Instant Notes in Neuroscience. Alan Longstaff. 2000. LC 00-42902. (Instant Notes Ser.). (Illus.). 280p. pap. 27.95 (*0-387-91582-6*) Spr-Verlag.

Instant Nursing Assessment: Mental Health. Delmar Publishing Staff. 1995. (Nursing Education Ser.). 212p. (C). pap. text 34.95 (*0-8273-7104-7*) Delmar.

Instant Nursing Assessment: Neurologic. Delmar Publishing Staff & Judith A. Mauro. 1995. LC 95-24076. (Instant Nursing Assessment Ser.). 224p. (C). mass mkt. 21.50 (*0-8273-7103-9*) Delmar.

Instant Nursing Assessment: Respiratory. Bmr-Delmar Staff. 1995. LC 95-371. (Instant Nursing Assessment Ser.). 224p. (C). mass mkt. 21.50 (*0-8273-7099-7*) Delmar.

Instant Nursing Assessment: Women's Health. Bmr-Delmar Staff et al. 1995. LC 95-22344. (Instant Nursing Assessment Ser.). 224p. (C). mass mkt. 21.50 (*0-8273-7100-4*) Delmar.

Instant Ophthalmology. Hector Bryson Chawla. 2001. (Illus.). 288p. pap. 77.00 (*0-7506-4461-3*) Buttrwrth-Heinemann.

Instant Pain Relief: A Proven Method of Immediate Resolution of Pain & Dysfunction. William J. Faber & Morton Walker. 1991. LC 90-84565. (Illus.). 240p. (Orig.). pap. 12.95 (*1-879361-00-0*) Bio Pubns.

Instant Physiology. Neil R. Borley & Vinod Achan. 2000. LC 99-29385. (Illus.). 224p. (C). pap. 28.95 (*0-632-05004-7*) Blackwell Sci.

Instant Psychopharmacology: A Guide for the Non-Medical Mental Health Professional. Ronald J. Diamond. 1998. LC 98-9703. (Professional Book Ser.). 120p. pap. 17.00 (*0-393-70269-3*) Norton.

***Instant Reference Medicine.** 2001. (Teach Yourself Ser.). (Illus.). 224p. pap. 10.95 (*0-658-01615-6*, Tch Yourself) McGraw-Hill Prof.

Instant Spanish at Work: Medical Spanish for the Care of Workers. Suzanne L. Sergile. 1999. LC 98-35462. (SPA.). 20.00 (*1-883595-23-1*) OEM Health.

Instant Stress Relief: A Book & Reflexology Tool, Incl. reflexology tool. Carol Ladas-Gaskin. 1998. 96p. pap. text 10.95 (*0-8362-3669-6*) Andrews McMeel.

Instant Teaching Tools for Health Care Educators. Michele Deck. 1995. LC 94-48054. (Illus.). 288p. (C). (gr. 13). pap. text 38.95 (*0-8151-2379-5*, 25191) Mosby Inc.

Instant Teaching Tools for Health Care Teams. Julia B. Riley. 1997. (Illus.). 376p. (C). (gr. 13). pap. text 36.95 (*0-8151-5589-1*, 29945) Mosby Inc.

Instant Teaching Treasures for Patient Education. Gaye Ragland. 1996. LC 96-29271. (Illus.). 300p. (C). (gr. 13). pap. text 37.95 (*0-8151-4699-X*, 29697) Mosby Inc.

Instinct, Environment & Behavior. Stephen Lea. Ed. by Peter Herriot. 1984. LC 83-17308. (New Essential Psychology Ser.). 160p. pap. 8.95 (*0-416-33640-X*, NO. 4042) Routledge.

Instinctive Behavior: The Development of a Modern Concept. Ed. by Claire H. Schiller. 1964. LC 57-10590. (Illus.). 328p. 47.50 (*0-8236-2880-9*); pap. 24.95 (*0-8236-8084-3*, 22880) Intl Univs Pr.

Instinctual Stimulation of Children: From Common Practice to Child Abuse. John L. Weil. 1989. Vol. I: Clinical Findings. 40.00 (*0-8236-2885-X*); Vol. II: Clinical Cases. 67.50 (*0-8236-2886-8*) Intl Univs Pr.

Institute for Macro Living Home Study Program, Set. Thea Alexander. Incl. Vol. 1: 1-12: Macro Resource Person Training. 1984. 199.00 (*0-913080-13-6*); 550.00 (*0-913080-21-7*) Macro Bks.

***Institute of Healthcare Management Yearbook, 2000-2001.** IHM Staff. 2001. 650p. (*0-11-702751-0*) Statnry Office GBR. *Dist:* Balogh.

Institute on Religion & Psychiatry, Congregation Adath Israel, Boston, 1947. Ed. by Joshua Loth. 1977. 202p. 19.95 (*0-8369-2658-7*) Ayer.

Institute to University: A Seventy-Fifth Anniversary Colloquium. James T. Flexner et al. 1977. LC 77-24825. 116p. pap. 2.95 (*0-87470-025-6*) Rockefeller.

Institutional Abuse of Children & Youth. Ed. by Ranae Hanson. 1982. LC 81-7194. (Child & Youth Services Ser.: Vol. 4, Nos. 1 & 2). 156p. text 44.95 (*0-917724-97-6*) Haworth Pr.

Institutional Care of Mental Patients in the United States. John M. Grimes. Ed. by Gerald N. Grob. 1980. LC 78-22563. (Historical Issues in Mental Health Ser.). reprint ed. lib. bdg. 18.95 (*0-405-11917-8*) Ayer.

Institutional Care of the Insane in the United States & Canada Ed. by Henry M. Hurd. 1973. LC 73-2404. (Mental Illness & Social Policy; the American Experience Ser.). reprint ed. Vol. 1. 210.95 (*0-405-05210-3*); Vol. 2. 53.95 (*0-405-05211-1*); Vol. 3. 53.95 (*0-405-05212-X*); Vol. 4. 53.95 (*0-405-05213-8*) Ayer.

Institutional Change & Healthcare Organizations: From Professional Dominance to Managed Care. W. Richard Scott et al. 2000. LC 99-48850. (Illus.). 442p. pap. text 25.00 (*0-226-74310-1*) U Ch Pr.

Institutional Inspector. Jack Rudman. 1994. (Career Examination Ser.: C-382). pap. 29.95 (*0-8373-0382-6*) Nat Learn.

***Institutional Review Board: Management & Function.** Robert J. Amdur & Elizabeth A. Bankert. 2001. LC 2001-58168. (Illus.). (C). text 28.00 (*0-7637-1686-3*, 1686-3, N L N Bart) Jones & Bartlett.

Instruction: Theoretical & Applied Perspectives. Ed. by Ronna F. Dillon & James W. Pellegrino. 1991. LC 90-42679. 208p. 62.50 (*0-275-92735-0*, C2735, Praeger Pubs) Greenwood.

Instruction & the Development of Moral Judgment: The Differences Between Piaget & Kohlberg. Iordanis Kavathatzopoulos. 1988. 112p. pap. (*91-554-2244-6*) Uppsala Universitet SWE. *Dist:* Coronet Bks.

Instruction in Pharmacology: New Approaches & New Faces - Journal: Health Communications & Informatics, Vol. 5, No. 1. Ed. by M. C. Gerald & J. P. Long. 1979. (Illus.). pap. 16.75 (*3-8055-2992-9*) S Karger.

Instructional Course Lectures, Vol. 45. Ed. by Douglas J. Pritchard. 1996. (Illus.). 550p. 95.00 (*0-89203-145-X*) Amer Acad Ortho Surg.

Instructional Course Lectures, Vol. 46. Ed. by Dempsey Springfield. 1997. 550p. 100.00 (*0-89203-161-1*) Amer Acad Ortho Surg.

Instructional Design Skills for Reproductive Health Professionals see Competences en Conception de Programmes Pedagogiques pour les Professionnels en Sante de la Reproduction

Instructional Design Skills for Reproductive Health Professionals. Rick Sullivan & Lynne Gaffikin. Ed. by Ann Blouse & Dana Lewison. 1997. LC 98-152671. (Illus.). 207p. (Orig.). pap. text 15.00 (*0-929817-01-X*) JHPIEGO.

Instructional Methods in Emergency Services: A Resource Text Designed for EMS, Fire, & Rescue Instructors. William D. McClincy. 1994. LC 94-37817. 352p. pap. text 67.00 (*0-89303-541-6*) P-H.

Instructions for Equine Clients. Richard A. Mansmann. 1995. (Illus.). 352p. (C). (gr. 13). text 80.00 (*0-8151-6455-6*, 26582) Mosby Inc.

Instructions for Geriatric Patients. William A. Sodeman, Jr. 1995. LC 94-21928. (Illus.). 352p. pap. text 41.95 (*0-7216-4335-3*) Saunders.

Instructions for Geriatric Patients. William A. Sodeman, Jr. Ed. by Ray Kersey. 2nd ed. 1999. LC 98-38026. (Illus.). 350p. (C). pap. text 45.00 (*0-7216-7490-9*) Saunders.

Instructions for Obstetric & Gynecologic Patients. Hugh S. Miller et al. Ed. by William Schmitt. 2nd ed. 1997. LC 97-7620. 272p. pap. text 45.00 (*0-7216-7368-6*) Saunders.

Instructions for Patients. H. Winter Griffith. Ed. by Ray Kersey. 5th ed. 1997. (SPA., Illus.). 608p. pap. text 49.95 (*0-7216-6997-2*) Saunders.

Instructions for Rehabilitation. Hennessey. 1999. pap. text (*0-7216-7146-2*) Saunders.

Instructions for Sports Medicine. Safran. 1999. pap. text (*0-7216-7704-5*) Saunders.

Instructions for the Diabetic Patient. William J. Steenrod, Jr. 1978. LC 78-54471. 130p. 8.95 (*0-9601944-1-X*) V Mason Clinic.

Instructions for Using the Zoe Gynecologic Simulator. 1998. (FRE & RUS.). 58p. pap. 15.00 incl. Beta (*0-929817-62-1*) JHPIEGO.

Instructions for Veterinary Clients: Canine & Feline Behavior Problems. Stefanie Schwartz. 2nd ed. 1996. LC 96-46441. (Illus.). 152p. (C). (gr. 13). text 47.95 (*0-8151-8909-5*, 29036) Mosby Inc.

Instructions for Veterinary Clients: Canine & Feline Medical-Surgical Problems. David L. Erlewein & Eugene L. Kuhns. 3rd ed. 1996. LC 96-1362. (Illus.). 528p. (C). (gr. 13). text 110.00 (*0-8151-3161-5*, 26577) Mosby Inc.

Instructions to Jurors on Identification Testimony: U. S. vs. Busic. J. Bartels. 1976. (Monographs: No. CR-46). 3.00 (*1-55524-047-X*) Ctr Respon Psych.

Instructor Curriculum Guide for the Medical Assistant: Administrative & Clinical. Kinn & Woods. Ed. by Adrianne Williams. 8th ed. 2000. 1260p. (*0-7216-7301-5*) Saunders.

Instructor Guide for Exercises in Health Claims Examining. Insurance Career Development Center Staff & Caitlind L. Alexander. Ed. by Sharon E. Brown. unabr. ed. 1999. (Illus.). (C). pap. text 9.95 (*1-881159-23-X*, 21995) ICDC Pubng.

Instructor Guide for Guide to Health Claims Examining. Insurance Career Development Center Staff & Caitlind L. Alexander. Ed. by Caitlind L. Alexander & Sharon E. Brown. 5th rev. ed. 1999. (Illus.). 110p. (C). pap. text 6.95 (*1-881159-17-5*, 26045-5) ICDC Pubng.

Instructor of the Blind. Jack Rudman. 1994. (Career Examination Ser.: C-2838). pap. 29.95 (*0-8373-2838-1*) Nat Learn.

Instructor Recertification Kit. National Safety Council Staff. 1997. (Emergency Care Ser.). 19.95 (*0-7637-0554-3*) Jones & Bartlett.

Instructor's Electronic Resource CD-ROM for Pharmacology: A Nursinf Process Approch. Joyce L. Kee. 3rd ed. 2000. pap., tchr. ed. 75.00 incl. cd-rom (*0-7216-8300-2*) Saunders.

Instructor's Guide for Health, Safety & Nutrition for the Young Child. Lynn R. Marotz et al. 3rd ed. 1993. (Illus.). 85p. tchr. ed. 14.95 (*0-8273-4933-5*) Delmar.

Instructor's Guide for Medical Terminology: The Language of Health Care. Marjorie C. Willis. 1995. LC 95-47792. (Illus.). 130p. (Orig.). tchr. ed. (*0-683-18193-9*) Lppncott W & W.

Instructor's Guide for Nursing in the Community. Mary J. Clark. 2nd ed. 1995. (C). (*0-8385-7092-5*, A7902-8) Appleton & Lange.

Instructor's Guide for Providing Home Care: A Textbook for Home Care Aides. Jetta Fuzy. 1999. (Illus.). 426p. pap. text, tchr. ed. 69.95 (*1-888343-21-4*) Hartman Pub.

Instructor's Guide to Accompany Assisting in Long-Term Care. Barbara R. Hegner & Esther Caldwell. 2nd ed. 1994. 166p. pap. 18.00 (*0-8273-5002-3*) Delmar.

Instructor's Guide to Accompany Cardiopulmonary Anatomy & Physiology Essentials for Respiratory Care. Terry R. Des Jardins. 2nd ed. 1993. 205p. pap., tchr. ed. 16.00 (*0-8273-5008-2*) Delmar.

Instructor's Guide to Accompany Therapeutic Communications for Allied Health Professions. Carol D. Tamparo & Wilburta Q. Lindh. 1993. 62p. pap., tchr. ed. 16.00 (*0-8273-5668-4*) Delmar.

Instructor's Guide to Ethical Responsibility in Pharmacy Practice. Robert A. Buerki & Louis D. Vottero. 1997. 261p. (Orig.). (C). pap. text, tchr. ed. 25.00 (*0-931292-30-1*) Am Inst Hist Pharm.

Instructors Manual for Activity-Based Costing. Baker. 1998. tchr. ed. (*0-8342-1127-0*) Aspen Pub.

Instructor's Manual for Advanced Cardiac Life Support. 272p. pap. text, tchr. ed. (*0-87493-627-6*) Am Heart.

Instructor's Manual for Advanced Medical Life. Mistovich. 1999. pap. text, tchr. ed. 39.00 (*0-8359-5280-0*) P-H.

Instructor's Manual for Basic Life Support. (Illus.). 124p. pap. text (*0-87493-616-0*) Am Heart.

Instructor's Manual for Clinical Pharmacology & Nursing. Marlene Ciranowicz. 3rd ed. 1996. 240p. tchr. ed. (*0-87434-773-4*) Springhouse Corp.

Instructors Manual for Dietetics: Practice & Future Trends. Winterfeldt. 1998. text, tchr. ed. (*0-8342-1118-1*) Aspen Pub.

Instructor's Manual for Essentials of Cost Accounting for Health Care Organizations. 1999. (Illus.). (*0-8342-1708-2*, 16808) Aspen Pub.

Instructor's Manual for Fundamentals of Contemporary Nursing Practice. Carol Lindeman. Date not set. 255p. tchr. ed. (*0-7216-8234-0*) Saunders.

Instructor's Manual for Managing Health Services Organizations. Jonathon S. Rakich et al. 3rd ed. 1992. 176p. pap. text 22.00 (*1-878812-13-0*) Hlth Prof Pr.

Instructor's Manual for Neonatal Resuscitation. American Academy of Pediatrics Staff & American Heart Association Staff. rev. ed. 1995. 212p. ring bd. 35.00 (*0-910761-64-7*) Am Acad Pediat.

Instructor's Manual for Nursing & the Law. Korenchuk. 5th ed. 1998. tchr. ed. (*0-8342-1112-2*) Aspen Pub.

Instructor's Manual for Patient Accounts Management Handbook. Allan P. DeKaye. 1998. tchr. ed. (*0-8342-1119-X*) Aspen Pub.

Instructor's Manual for Pediatric Basic Life Support. Ed. by Leon Chameides & Mary Fran Hazinski. 1997. LC 99-175398. 64p. pap. text, tchr. ed. (*0-87493-621-7*) Am Heart.

Instructor's Manual for Physical Agents. Michelle H. Cameron. Ed. by Adrianne Williams. 1998. 135p. pap. text (*0-7216-6245-5*) Saunders.

Instructor's Manual for the Human Body in Health & Illness. Barbara Herlihy. 2000. 155p. tchr. ed. (*0-7216-6112-2*) Saunders.

Instructor's Manual Heartsaver AED, Vol. 70-2007. Ed. by Tom P. Aufderheide et al. 1998. (Illus.). 63p. pap. text, tchr. ed. 15.00 (*0-87493-691-8*) Am Heart.

Instructor's Manual to Accompany Administrative Medical Assisting. Marilyn Takahashi Fordney & Joan J. Follis. 3rd ed. 1993. 148p. pap. 16.00 (*0-8273-4943-2*) Delmar.

Instructor's Manual to Accompany Legal & Ethical Perspectives in Healthcare: An Integrated Approach. Raymond S. Edge. 1997. (Allied Health Ser.). 76p. tchr. ed. 12.00 (*0-8273-7685-5*) Delmar.

Instructor's Manual to Accompany Linne & Ringrud's Clinical Laboratory Science: The Basics & Routine Techniques. Joseph K. Semak. 4th ed. 2000. (Illus.). 97p. pap. (*0-323-00866-6*) Mosby Inc.

Instructor's Manual to Accompany Medical Terminology Made Easy. Jean T. Dennerll. 1993. 44p. text, tchr. ed. 14.00 (*0-8273-5909-8*) Delmar.

Instructor's Manual to Accompany Quick & Easy Medical Terminology. Peggy C. Leonard. 3rd ed. 2000. (Illus.). 362p. pap., tchr. ed. (*0-7216-8272-3*) Saunders.

Instructor's Manual to Accompany the Administrative Medical Assistant. Mary E. Kinn. 4th ed. 2000. (Illus.). 482p. tchr. ed. (*0-7216-7294-9*) Saunders.

Instructor's Manual to Accompany the Strengths Model: Case Management with People Suffering from Severe & Persistent Mental Illness. Linda Carlson. 1997. 54p. pap. text (*0-19-512141-4*) OUP.

Instructor's Manual to Accompany Understanding Nursing Research. Susan K. Grove & Nancy Burns. Ed. by Thomas Eoyang. 1999. cd-rom 75.00 (*0-7216-8107-7*) Saunders.

Instructor's Manual to Maternal, Neonatal & Women's Health Nursing. Carole A. Kenner et al. 1991. (Illus.). 304p. tchr. ed. (*0-87434-333-X*) Springhouse Corp.

Instructor's Resource Kit for Nurse Assistant in Long-Term Care: A Rehab Approach. Marshall. 1992. 352p. pap. text 32.00 (*0-8016-6298-2*) Mosby Inc.

Instructor's Resource Manual to Accompany Fundamentals of Nursing. Patricia A. Potter & Anne G. Perry. 5th ed. 2000. 280p. 250.00 (*0-323-01142-X*) Mosby Inc.

Instrument Development in Occupational Therapy. Janet H. Watts & Chestina Brollier. 1989. LC 88-24330. (Occupational Therapy in Mental Health Ser.: Vol. 8, No. 4). (Illus.). 97p. text 39.95 (*0-86656-857-3*) Haworth Pr.

Instrument Development in the Affective Domain. Robert K. Gable. 1986. lib. bdg. 80.50 (*0-89838-209-2*) Kluwer Academic.

Instrument Development in the Affective Domain: Measuring Attitudes & Values in Corporate & School Settings. Robert K. Gable. 2nd ed. 1993. LC 93-17662. (Evaluation in Education & Human Services Ser.). 296p. (C). lib. bdg. 99.00 (*0-7923-9369-4*) Kluwer Academic.

Instrumental Data for Drug Analysis Terry Mills, III. 2nd ed. 1992. 1. 120.00 (*0-444-01281-8*); 2. 120.00 (*0-444-01282-6*) CRC Pr.

Instrumental Data for Drug Analysis, Set. J. Conrad Roberson et al. 2nd ed. 1991. (Forensic & Police Science Ser.). 631p. 425.00 (*0-444-01630-9*) CRC Pr.

Instrumental Data for Drug Analysis, Vol. 1. Terry Mills, III & J. Conrad Roberson. 2nd ed. 1992. LC 93-13539. (Forensic & Police Science Ser.). 785p. reprint ed. 179.95 (*0-8493-9521-6*, RS189) CRC Pr.

Instrumental Data for Drug Analysis. Mills, 3rd. 2nd ed. 1992. Vol. 4. 282p. 179.95 (*0-8493-9524-0*); Vol. 5. 628p. 179.95 (*0-8493-9516-X*) CRC Pr.

Instrumental Data for Drug Analysis, Vol. 5. J. Conrad Roberson et al. 2nd ed. 1991. (Forensic & Police Science Ser.). 631p. 120.00 (*0-444-01626-0*) CRC Pr.

Instrumental Data for Drug Analysis: Cumulative Indices. Vol. 7. Terry Mills et al. 2nd ed. 1996. LC 96-31352. (CRC Series on Forensic & Police Science). 464p. 179.95 (*0-8493-8115-0*) CRC Pr.

Instrumental Examination of the Motor System. S. Z. Toth. 1986. 281p. (C). (*963-05-3927-6*) Akade Kiado HUN. *Dist:* St Mut.

Instrumental Insemination. E. S. Hafez. 1982. text 278.00 (*90-247-2530-5*) Kluwer Academic.

Instrumental Methods & Scoring in Extrapyramidal Disorders. Ed. by H. Przuntek et al. 1995. (Illus.). 268p. 86.95 (*0-387-57875-7*) Spr-Verlag.

Instrumental Methods & Scoring in Extrapyramidal Disorders. H. Przuntek et al. 1995. LC 95-40048. xiv, 368p. pap. (*3-540-57875-7*) Spr-Verlag.

Instrumentation. Shirley M. Brooks Tighe. 5th ed. 1999. LC 98-53249. (Illus.). 384p. spiral bd. 43.00 (*0-323-00350-8*) Mosby Inc.

Instrumentation & Monitoring Methods for Radiation Protection. 1978. LC 78-62094. (Report Ser.: No. 57). 177p. pap. text 40.00 (*0-913392-40-5*) NCRP Pubns.

Instrumentation for Eyecare Paraprofessionals. Michelle Herrin. 1998. LC 98-38796. (Basic Bookshelf for Eyecare Professionals Ser.). (Illus.). 128p. pap. 30.00 (*1-55642-399-3*, 63993) SLACK Inc.

Instrumentation in the Hearing Sciences. Ed. by David L. Mcpherson & John W. Thatcher. 1977. 181p. text 45.00 (*0-8089-1005-1*, 792855, Grune & Strat) Harcrt Hlth Sci Grp.

Instrumentation, Measurements & Electronic Dosimetry: Health Physics Society 2000 Midyear Proceedings. 2000. (Illus.). 312p. pap. text 35.95 (*0-944838-93-6*) Med Physics Pub.

Instrumentation Requirements of Diagnostic Radiological Physicists: Report of the AAPM Diagnostic X-Ray Committee Task Group #4. 1998. (Report Ser.: No. 60). pap. text 10.00 (*1-888340-15-0*) AAPM.

Instrumented Spinal Surgery: Principles & Technique. Jurgen Harms et al. 1998. LC 98-23695. 139.00 (*3-13-110761-8*) Thieme Med Pubs.

Instrumented Systems for Microbiological Analysis of Body Fluids. Lorraine S. Gall & William A. Curby. 1980. 192p. 106.00 (*0-8493-5681-4*, QR67, CRC Reprint) Franklin.

Instruments for Clinical Health-Care Research. Marilyn Frank-Stromborg & Sharon J. Olsen. 2nd ed. 1997. LC 97-3049. (Nursing Ser.). (Illus.). 640p. (C). text 54.95 (*0-7637-0316-8*, 0316-8) Jones & Bartlett.

Instruments for Use in Nursing Education Research. Gloria Clayton & Marion Broome. Ed. by Linda Moody & Moira Shannon. 1989. 64p. 8.50 (*0-88737-424-7*) Natl League Nurse.

Instruments of Psychiatric Research. Ed. by Christopher Thompson. 1989. 356p. 395.00 (*0-471-91794-X*) Wiley.

Instruments Used for Oral Surgery: A Self-Instructional Guide, Bk. 1. James R. Hooley & Robert J. Whitacre. 3rd rev. ed. 1983. (Illus.). 56p. pap. 6.95 (*0-89939-011-0*) Stoma Pr.

Insulin Action. Ashok K. Srivastava & Barry I. Posner. 1998. LC 97-49618. (Developments in Molecular & Cellular Biochemistry Ser.). 194p. 187.50 (*0-7923-8113-0*) Kluwer Academic.

Insulin & the Cell Membrane. Ed. by Iwar Klimes. 1990. xiii, 537p. text 337.00 (*3-7186-0503-1*, Harwood Acad Pubs) Gordon & Breach.

Insulin-Dependent Diabetes. 1996. (Illus.). 35p. reprint ed. pap. text 15.00 (*0-7881-3096-X*) DIANE Pub.

Insulin Dump Therapy Book: Insights from the Experts. Bruce W. Bode et al. 1995. 157p. (Orig.). pap. text 19.00 (*0-9647837-0-3*) MiniMed Tech.

Insulin, IGFs & Growth Hormone: From Basic Research to Novel Clinical Applications. Ed. by P. Saenger et al. 1994. (Journal: Vol. 41, Suppl. 2, 1994). (Illus.). iv, 122p. pap. 55.00 (*3-8055-6003-6*) S Karger.

Insulin, Insulin-Like Growth Factors, & Their Receptors in the Central Nervous System. Ed. by Mohan K. Raizada et al. 1987. LC 87-20337. (Illus.). 366p. 85.00 (*0-306-42666-8*, Plenum Trade) Perseus Pubng.

Insulin-Like Growth Factors & Their Regulatory Proteins: Proceedings of the Third International Symposium on Insulin-Like Growth Factors, Sydney, February 1994. Ed. by R. C. Baxter et al. 1994. LC 94-15908. (International Congress Ser.: No. 1056). 484p. 278.50 (*0-444-81756-5*, Excerpta Medica) Elsevier.

Insulin Pump Therapy: Indication-Method-Technology. E. Austenat & T. Stahl. 1990. (Illus.). xii, 187p. (C). pap. 98.50 (*3-11-012265-0*) De Gruyter.

Insulin Resistance. Ed. by David Moller. 1993. LC 93-18929. 440p. 290.00 (*0-471-93977-3*) Wiley.

Insulin Resistance: A Clinical Handbook. Andrew J. Krentz. 2001. LC 00-37824. (Illus.). 192p. pap. 29.95 (*0-632-05662-2*) Blackwell Sci.

Insulin Resistance: The Metabolic Syndrome X. Ed. by Gerald M. Reaven & Ami Laws. 1999. LC 98-36840. (Contemporary Endocrinology Ser.: Vol. 12). (Illus.). 384p. 145.00 (*0-89603-588-3*) Humana.

Insulin Resistance in Human Disease: Proceedings of the 7th Korea-Japan Symposium on Diabetes Mellitus, Seoul, Korea, 13-14 April 1993. Ed. by Bum H. Kap et al. LC 93-32438. (*0-444-81649-6*, Excerpta Medica) Elsevier.

Insulin Resistance, Metabolic Diseases & Diabetic Complications: Proceedings of the 7th European Symposium on Metabolism, Padova, September 30-October 3, 1998. European Symposium on Metabolism Staff. Ed. by Gaetano Crepaldi et al. 1999. LC 99-37081. (ICS Ser.). (Illus.). 286p. 125.00 (*0-444-50022-7*) Elsevier.

Insulin Suflonylharnstoff: Kombinationstherapie Bei Typ II-Diabetes. Ed. by W. Bachmann et al. 1988. (Illus.). viii, 168p. 43.50 (*3-8055-4601-7*) S Karger.

Insulin-Sulphonylurea: Combination Therapy in Type-II Diabetes. Ed. by W. Bachmann et al. 1988. (Illus.). viii, 160p. 36.75 (*3-8055-4862-1*) S Karger.

Insulinotropic Gut Hormone Glucagon-Like Peptide-1. Ed. by H. C. Fehmann & B. Goeke. 1997. LC 97-4323. (Frontiers in Diabetes Ser.: Vol. 13, 1997). (Illus.). viii, 240p. 195.00 (*3-8055-6165-2*) S Karger.

Insurance Directory: Largest Nationwide Health Insurance Billing Directory. Ingenix, Inc. Staff. 1999. vi, 406p. (C). pap. (*1-56337-329-7*) Thomson Learn.

***Insurance Directory 2001.** Ingenix, Inc. Staff. pap. 64.95 (*1-56337-318-1*) Ingenix Inc.

Insurance Handbook for Medical Offices. Marilyn Takahashi Fordney. 6th ed. 1999. LC 98-56061. (Illus.). 205p. (C). pap. text 43.95 (*0-7216-7886-6*) Saunders.

Insurance Handbook for the Medical Office. Marilyn Takahashi Fordney. (Illus.). 4th ed. 1995. pap., tchr. ed. (*0-7216-5672-2*); 5th ed. 1997. pap. text, wbk. ed. 21.50 (*0-7216-6991-3*); 5th ed. 1997. pap., tchr. ed. (*0-7216-6988-3*) Saunders.

Insurance Liability & Legal Complications: Index of New Information for Consumers & Professional Personnel. Science and Life Consultants Association Staff. 1995. LC 94-34894. 159p. 57.50 (*0-7883-0348-1*); pap. 47.50 (*0-7883-0349-X*) ABBE Pubs Assn.

Insurgents. Jean Vercors. Ed. by Robert J. Kastenbaum. Tr. by Rita Barisse. 1979. LC 78-22223. (Aging & Old Age Ser.). reprint ed. lib. bdg. 27.95 (*0-405-11836-8*) Ayer.

Insuring Medical Malpractice. Frank A. Sloan et al. 1991. (Illus.). 264p. text 65.00 (*0-19-506959-5*) OUP.

Insuring National Health Care: The Canadian Experience. Malcolm G. Taylor. 1990. LC 90-50014. xvi, 254p. (C). pap. 14.95 (*0-8078-4295-8*) U of NC Pr.

Integral Yoga Hatha Booklet & Tape. Integral Yoga Institutes Staff. 1979. 10.95 (*0-932040-23-3*) Integral Yoga Pubns.

Integrated Approach to Health Science. Colbert. 1996. (Health Occupations Ser.). 144p. (C). text, wbk. ed. 20.50 (*0-8273-6083-5*); (Allied Health Ser.: I). 72p. text, tchr. ed. 15.95 (*0-8273-6084-3*) Delmar.

Integrated Approach to Health Sciences. Colbert. 1996. disk 71.95 (*0-8273-7689-8*); 288p. tchr. ed., ring bd. 59.95 (*0-8273-7688-X*) Delmar.

Integrated Approach to Health Sciences: Anatomy & Physiology, Math, Physics, & Chemistry. Bruce J. Colbert et al. rev. ed. 1995. LC 95-15277. 352p. (C). 57.95 (*0-8273-6082-7*) Delmar.

Integrated Approach to Trauma Care: The First 24 Hours. Ed. by R. J. Goris & O. Trentz. 1995. LC 95-11756. (Update in Intensive Care & Emergency Medicine Ser.: No. 22). (Illus.). 352p. 134.00 (*3-540-58446-3*) Spr-Verlag.

***Integrated Aromatic Medicine, 1998: Proceedings from the Grasse, France, 1998 Symposium.** Essential Science Publishing Staff. 2000. (Illus.). 150p. pap. text 19.95 (*0-943685-27-3*) Essential Science.

***Integrated Aromatic Medicine, 2000: Proceedings from the Grasse, France, 2000 Symposium.** Essential Science Publishing Staff. 2001. 130p. pap. text 19.95 (*0-943685-31-1*) Essential Science.

Integrated Basic Surgical Sciences. Ed. by James Toouli. 2000. LC 99-37244. (Illus.). 1000p. 149.50 (*0-340-70091-2*) OUP.

***Integrated Behavioral Health Continuum: Theory & Practice.** Ed. by Laurel J. Kiser et al. 2001. LC 2001-22958. (Illus.). 368p. pap. 39.00 (*0-88048-945-6*, 8945) Am Psychiatric.

***Integrated Behavioral Healthcare: Prospects, Issues, & Opportunities.** Nicholas A. Cummings et al. 2001. 320p. 59.95 (*0-12-198761-2*) Acad Pr.

***Integrated Biomaterials Science.** Rolando Barbucci. 2001. LC 2001-38949. (*0-306-46678-3*, Kluwer Plenum) Kluwer Academic.

Integrated Cancer Management. Michael Torosian. 1999. LC 99-37339. (Basic & Clinical Oncology Ser.). (Illus.). 680p. text 195.00 (*0-8247-7195-8*) Dekker.

Integrated Care Pathways: A Practical Guide. Susan Middleton & Adrian C. Roberts. 2000. (Illus.). 168p. pap. text 35.00 (*0-7506-4087-1*) Buttrwrth-Heinemann.

Integrated Children's Mental Health System: Coordinating the Needs of Children with Multiple Problems. Gary C. Cox. 1994. (Illus.). 114p. (Orig.). (C). pap. text 35.00 (*0-7881-0747-X*) DIANE Pub.

Integrated Circuit Design Book: Papers on the VSLI Design Methodology from the ICD NELSIS Project. Ed. by P. Dewilde. 1986. 960p. (Orig.). pap. text (*90-6275-246-2*) Delft U Pr NLD. *Dist:* Coronet Bks.

***Integrated Colposcopy: For Colposcopists, Histopathologists & Cytologists.** M. C. Anderson et al. 2nd ed. 1996. 286p. text 179.00 (*0-412-70840-X*) Lppncott W & W.

Integrated Colposcopy: For Colposcopists, Histopathologists & Cytologists. Sharp et al. 2nd ed. 1996. (Illus.). 296p. 359.00 incl. cd-rom (*0-412-79220-6*) Lppncott W & W.

Integrated Communication: Synergy of Persuasive Voices. Ed. by Esther Thorson & Jeri Moore. 1995. LC 95-19673. (Advertising & Consumer Psychology Ser.). 392p. text 79.95 (*0-8058-1391-8*) L Erlbaum Assocs.

Integrated Delivery Systems: Creation, Management, & Governance. Douglas Conrad. 1997. LC 97-27721. 45.00 (*1-56793-069-7*) Health Admin Pr.

Integrated English-Japanese Medical Dictionary. K. Kato. 1986. 1718p. 195.00 (*0-8288-1851-7*, M8464) Fr & Eur.

Integrated Family Therapy. David Will & Robert Wrate. 1985. 224p. (*0-422-79750-2*, 9632); pap. (*0-422-79760-X*, 9633) Tavistock GBR. *Dist:* Routldge.

Integrated Health Care: Case Studies Dean C. Coddington & Barbara J. Bendrick. 1994. 216p. (Orig.). pap. 33.00 (*1-56829-004-7*, 4066) M G M A.

Integrated Health Care: Reorganizing the Physician, Hospital & Health Plan Relationship Dean C. Coddington et al. 1994. 252p. 44.00 (*1-56829-003-9*, 4065) M G M A.

Integrated Health Care Delivery: Theory, Practice, Evaluation & Prognosis. Montague Brown. 1996. LC 95-52251. (Health Care Management Review Ser.). 224p. pap. 55.00 (*0-8342-0814-8*, 20814) Aspen Pub.

Integrated Health Care 100 Directory. American Hospital Association Staff et al. 1999. LC 97-52243. 595.00 (*1-55648-234-5*) AHPI.

Integrated Identity for Gay Men & Lesbians: Psychotherapeutic Approaches for Emotional Well Being. John DeCecco & Eli Coleman. 1994. LC 87-342. (Journal of Homosexuality Ser.: Vol. 14, No. 1-2). 343p. pap. text 24.95 (*0-918393-38-8*, Harrington Park) Haworth Pr.

Integrated Interdisciplinary Learning Between the Health & Social Care Professions: A Feasibility Study. Rosemary Tope. 1996. LC 96-84621. 624p. (*1-85972-357-8*) Avebry GBR. *Dist:* Ashgate Pub Co.

Integrated Mathematics of Radiographic Exposure. Sandra Jones. 1994. (Illus.). 176p. (gr. 13). pap. text 23.00 (*0-8151-4834-8*, 24086) Mosby Inc.

Integrated Medical Library. Helis Miido. 1991. (Illus.). 280p. 99.95 (*0-8493-0182-3*, Z65) CRC Pr.

Integrated Medical-Surgical Care in Acute Coronary Artery Disease: Proceedings of the Cardiovascular Disease Conference, 5th, Snowmass at Aspen, Colorado, Jan. 1974. Cardiovascular Disease Conference Staff. Ed. by J. H. Vogel. 1975. (Advances in Cardiology Ser.: Vol. 15). x, 199p. 94.00 (*3-8055-2098-0*) S Karger.

Integrated Mental Health Care: A Comprehensive Community-Based Approach. Ian R. H. Falloon. 1995. 353p. pap. text 32.95 (*0-521-49972-0*) Cambridge U Pr.

Integrated Mental Health Services: Modern Community Psychiatry. Ed. by William R. Breakey. 1996. (Illus.). 448p. (C). text 55.00 (*0-19-507421-1*) OUP.

Integrated Mind. Michael S. Gazzaniga & Joseph E. LeDoux. 1978. LC 77-20101. (Illus.). 180p. 42.50 (*0-306-31085-6*, Plenum Trade) Perseus Pubng.

Integrated Motor Activities Screening: Screening Interpretation Guide. Margot C. Heiniger. 1994. (Illus.). 54p. pap. 20.00 (*0-9625040-6-8*, 297-231-X) Legendary Pub.

Integrated Patient Care for the Imaging Professional. Nina Kowalczyk & Kathleen A. Donnett. 1996. LC 95-49882. (Illus.). 304p. (C). tchr. ed. (*0-8151-2545-3*, 24123) Mosby Inc.

Integrated Patient Care for the Imaging Professional: Instructor's Manual. Nina Kowalczyk & Kathleen A. Donnett. 1996. (Illus.). 304p. tchr. ed. (*0-8151-4649-3*) Mosby Inc.

Integrated Pest & Disease Management. Ed. by Rajeev K. Upadhyay. 1998. (Illus.). xiv, 695p. (*81-7024-925-2*) APH Pubng IND. *Dist:* Nataraj Bks.

Integrated Pharmacology. Clive P. Page et al. 1997. 606p. pap. (*0-7234-2556-6*) Wolfe Publishing GBR. *Dist:* Mosby Inc.

Integrated Pharmacology. Clive Page et al. 1997. (Illus.). 616p. (*84-8174-340-2*) Mosby-Doyma Libros ESP. *Dist:* Mosby Inc.

Integrated Primary Care: The Future of Medical & Mental Health Collaboration. Ed. by Alexander Blount. 1998. LC 97-44806. 320p. 40.00 (*0-393-70253-7*) Norton.

Integrated Psychological Therapy for Schizophrenic Patients (IPT) B. Hodel et al. rev. ed. 1994. LC 93-30084. (Illus.). 176p. text 49.50 incl. disk (*0-88937-085-0*) Hogrefe & Huber Pubs.

Integrated Quality Management & the Scientific Method: Ethics, Principles, & Operational Tools. Mark Gusack. 1996. LC 97-92915. (Health Care Management Ser.: Vol. 1). (Illus.). ix, 125p. (Orig.). pap. 24.95 (*1-890215-01-5*) MBG Indust Inc.

Integrated Radiography Workbook. Robert DeAngelis & Mary F. Lloyd. 1996. (Illus.). 549p. (C). pap., wbk. ed. 44.95 (*0-943589-19-3*) Health & Allied.

Integrated Respiratory Care Services: Course Study Guide. William Wojiechowski. 1992. 276p. (C). ring bd. Price not set. (*0-933195-14-1*) CA College Health Sci.

Integrated Science for Health Students. T. Randall Lankford. 3rd ed. 1984. (C). tchr. ed. (*0-8359-3101-3*); pap. text 38.95 (*0-8359-3106-4*) P-H.

Integrated Systematic Nephrology. M. K. Chan. rev. ed. 1989. 344p. (C). pap. text (*962-209-180-6*) HK Univ Pr HKG. *Dist:* Intl Spec Bk, Coronet Bks.

Integrated Systems in Frontier Health Care Delivery: The Unique Needs of Wyoming. Ed. by Sheryl R. Fox & Alexander T. Hunt. 1995. LC 95-7228. (CSIS Panel Report Ser.). 39p. (C). pap. 9.95 (*0-89206-304-1*) CSIS.

Integrated Systems of the CNS, Pt.II. Anders T. Bjorklund & Larry W. Swanson. Ed. by Tomas B. Hokfelt. 1990. (Handbooks of Chemical Neuroanatomy: Vol. 7). 436p. 320.00 (*0-444-81232-6*) Elsevier.

Integrated Systems of the CNS: Cerebellum, Basal Ganglia, Olfactory System, Pt. III. Ed. by L. W. Swanson et al. 1996. 600p. 251.00 (*0-444-82451-0*) Elsevier.

Integrated Teams in Primary Care. Ed. by Glyn Elwyn & June Smail. 1999. LC 99-187704. (Illus.). 144p. pap. (*1-85775-288-0*) Radcliffe Med Pr GBR. *Dist:* Balogh.

Integrated Textbook of Anatomy for Undergraduates: Gross Anatomy, Embryology, Histology. S. G. Malwatkar. 2000. LC 2001-274518. (Illus.). 616p. text 45.00 (*0-19-564872-2*) OUP.

***Integrated Treatment for Psychiatric Disorders.** Jerald Kay. 2001. (Review of Psychiatry Ser.: Vol. 20). 208p. pap. 29.95 (*1-58562-027-0*, 62027) Am Psychiatric.

Integrated Treatment of Child Sexual Abuse. Henry Giaretto. 1992. LC 81-86712. 315p. pap. 25.00 (*0-8314-0061-7*) Sci & Behavior.

Integrated Women's Health: Holistic Approaches for Comprehensive Care. Ellen Olshansky. 2000. LC 00-20617. xvi, 496p. pap. 43.00 (*0-8342-1219-6*) Aspen Pub.

Integrating Behavioral & Social Sciences with Public Health. Ed. by Neil Schneiderman et al. 2000. LC 00-33179. (Illus.). xvi, 405p. 39.95 (*1-55798-721-1*, 431-644A) Am Psychol.

Integrating Behavioral Health Services with General Medical Care. Richard J. Goldberg. 1996. 55p. (Orig.). pap. 60.00 (*1-884937-25-7*) Manisses Communs.

Integrating Behavioral Therapies with Medications in the Treatment of Drug Dependence. 1995. (Illus.). 194p. pap. text 40.00 (*1-57979-078-X*) DIANE Pub.

Integrating Behavioral Therapies with Medications in the Treatment of Drug Dependence. Ed. by Lisa S. Onken et al. 1995. (Illus.). 190p. (Orig.). (C). pap. text 30.00 (*0-7881-2466-8*) DIANE Pub.

Integrating Chinese & Western Medicine: A Handbook for Practitioners. Zhang Junwen et al. 1996. 146p. 29.95 (*0-8351-2845-8*) China Bks.

Integrating Community Resources. Ed. by Linda J. Courtney. 1994. 284p. (Orig.). pap. 16.50 (*1-882855-30-2*) HDI Pubs.

Integrating Community Service into Nursing Education: A Guide to Service-Learning. Ed. by Patricia A. Bailey et al. 1999. LC 99-26341. (Series on the Teaching of Nursing). (Illus.). 144p. text 31.95 (*0-8261-1268-4*) Springer Pub.

H I

***Integrating Complementary Medicine in Primary Care: A Practical Guide for Healthcare Professionals.** David Peters, pseud & Leon Chaitow. 2000. (Illus.). 235p. pap. (*0-443-06345-1*) Church GBR. *Dist:* Saunders.

Integrating Exercise, Sports, Movement, & Mind: Therapeutic Unity. Kate F. Hays. 1998. LC 97-51665. 181p. 49.95 (*0-7890-0380-5*) Haworth Pr.

Integrating Healthcare Information Systems. 1995. 70.00 (*1-56925-033-2*, IHIS) Capitol Publns.

Integrating Individual & Family Therapy. Larry B. Feldman. 1992. LC 91-25268. (Integrative Psychotherapy Ser.: No. 4). 224p. text 30.95 (*0-87630-623-7*) Brunner-Routledge.

Integrating Long-Term Care, Acute Care & Housing: Guilding Success Through a Continuum of Care. Connie Evashwick & Timmothy J. Holt. 2000. 116p. pap. 26.00 (*0-87125-253-8*) Cath Health.

Integrating Managed Care & Ethics. Robbins. 1997. 59.00 (*0-8342-0954-3*) Aspen Pub.

Integrating Managed Care & Ethics: Transforming Challenges into Positive Outcomes. Dennis A. Robbins. 1998. LC 97-48804. (Illus.). 400p. 60.00 (*0-07-053083-1*) McGraw.

Integrating Marker Passing & Problem Solving: A Spreading Activation Approach to Improved Choice in Planning. James A. Hendler. 1987. 312p. text 59.95 (*0-89859-982-2*) L Erlbaum Assocs.

Integrating Maternal & Child Health Services with Primary Health Care: Practical Considerations. R. H. Hart et al. 1990. (ENG, FRE & SPA.). 92p. pap. text 16.00 (*92-4-156138-6*, 1150347) World Health.

Integrating Oasis for Home Health Organizations. Barbara Stover Gingerich & Deborah A. Ondeck. 1998. LC 98-5455. 149.00 (*0-8342-1110-6*) Aspen Pub.

Integrating Personality & Social Psychology. Ed. by John F. Kihlstrom. 1987. (Special Issue, Journal of Personality & Social Psychology Ser.: Vol. 53, No. 6). 239p. pap. 16.00 (*1-55798-009-8*) Am Psychol.

Integrating Perspectives on Health. Ed. by Neil Cooper et al. 1996. LC 95-47214. 192p. (C). (*0-335-19357-9*); pap. (*0-335-19356-0*) OpUniv Pr.

Integrating Pharmacotherapy & Psychotherapy. Ed. by Bernard D. Beitman & Gerald L. Klerman. 1991. LC 90-14510. 458p. text 58.00 (*0-88048-350-4*, 8350) Am Psychiatric.

Integrating Sex & Marital Therapy: A Clinical Guide. Ed. by Gerald R. Weeks & Larry Hof. 1987. LC 86-23283. 264p. text 47.95 (*0-87630-447-1*) Brunner-Routledge.

Integrating Social Support in Nursing. Miriam J. Stewart. 1993. (Illus.). 200p. (C). 61.95 (*0-8039-4273-7*, 3453); pap. 31.95 (*0-8039-4274-5*, 3454) Sage.

Integrating Spirituality into Treatment: Resources for Practitioners. Ed. by William R. Miller. 1999. LC 99-12572. xix, 293p. text 39.95 (*1-55798-581-2*, 431-726A) Am Psychol.

Integrating the City of Medicine: Blacks in Philadelphia Health Care, 1910-1965. David McBride. 1989. LC 88-15924. 320p. (C). 49.95 (*0-87722-546-X*) Temple U Pr.

Integrating the Individual & the Organization. Chris Argyris. 1990. 405p. pap. text 24.95 (*0-88738-803-5*) Transaction Pubs.

Integrating the Practice of Medicine: A Decision Maker's Guide to Organizing & Managing Physician Services. Ed. by Ronald B. Conners. 1997. LC 97-17762. 469p. 52.00 (*1-55648-206-X*) AHPI.

Integrating the Rorschach & the MMPI-2 in Personality Assessment. Ronald J. Ganellen. 1996. LC 96-2583. (Personality & Clinical Psychology Ser.). 264p. text 42.50 (*0-8058-1617-8*) L Erlbaum Assocs.

Integrating Theory & Practice in Clinical Neuropsychology. Ellen Perecman. 1989. 464p. 95.00 (*0-8058-0285-1*) L Erlbaum Assocs.

Integration: Myth or Reality? Ed. by Len Barton. 1989. 250p. pap. 33.00 (*1-85000-615-6*, Falmer Pr) Taylor & Francis.

Integration & Self-Healing: Affect, Trauma & Alexithymia. Henry Krystal. 1993. 408p. reprint ed. pap. 34.50 (*0-88163-180-9*) Analytic Pr.

Integration & Skin Color see Not by the Color of Their Skin: The Impact of Racial Differences on the Child's Development

Integration in Thought & Behavior: A Neuropsychological Theory. Laura M. Morrison. 1984. LC 81-83785. (Illus.). 357p. pap. 24.95 (*0-937638-00-5*) Harbor Pub.

Integration of Health Care Delivery: Report of a WHO Study Group. 1996. (Technical Reports: Vol. 861).Tr. of Integration Soins de Sanre, Integration Atencion de Slaud. (ENG, FRE & SPA.). 68p. (Orig.). pap. 12.60 (*92-4-120861-9*, 1100861) World Health.

Integration of Mass Campaigns Against Specific Diseases into General Health Services. 1965. (Technical Report Ser.: No. 294). 25p. pap. text 3.00 (*92-4-120294-7*) World Health.

Integration of Medical & Sports Sciences: Proceedings of the 8th International Biochemistry of Exercise Conference, Nagoya, September 24-28, 1991. Ed. by Y. Sato et al. 1992. LC 92-23694. (Medicine & Sport Science Ser.: Vol. 37). (Illus.). xiv, 446p. 346.25 (*3-8055-5579-2*) S Karger.

Integration of Pharmaceutical Discovery & Development: Case Histories. R. T. Borchardt et al. 1998. LC 98-27185. (Pharmaceutical Biotechnology Ser.: Vol. 11). (Illus.). 384p. (C). text 125.00 (*0-306-45743-1*, Kluwer Plenum) Kluwer Academic.

Integration of Pharmacokinetics, Pharmacodynamics & Toxicokinetics in Rational Drug Development. A. Yacobi et al. 1993. LC 92-48285. (Illus.). 286p. (C). text 89.50 (*0-306-44356-2*, Kluwer Plenum) Kluwer Academic.

Integration of Pharmacological & Nonpharmacological Treatments in Drug - Alcohol Addictions. Ed. by Norman S. Miller & Barry Stimmel. 1997. LC 97-31682. (Journal of Addictive Diseases Ser.: Vol. 16, No. 4). 122p. 39.95 (*0-7890-0375-9*, Pharmctl Prods) Haworth Pr.

Integration of Special Hospital Patients into the Community. Margaret Norris. 1984. LC 84-13733. 180p. text (*0-566-00728-2*) Avebry GBR. *Dist:* Ashgate Pub Co.

Integration Soins de Sanre, Integration Atencion de Slaud see Integration of Health Care Delivery: Report of a WHO Study Group

Integration Strategies for the Medical Practice: The Physician's Handbook to Integration Alternatives. American Medical Association Staff. 1996. (Practice Success Ser.). pap. 54.00 (*0-89970-789-0*, OP315096WE) AMA.

Integrations of Clinical & Social Psychology. Ed. by Gifford Weary & Herbert Mirels. 1982. (Illus.). 329p. (C). pap. text 22.95 (*0-19-503051-6*) OUP.

Integrations of Psychotherapies: A Guide for Practicing Therapists. Alvin R. Mahrer. 1989. LC 87-26091. 208p. 38.95 (*0-89885-412-1*, Kluwer Acad Hman Sci) Kluwer Academic.

Integrative Activity of the Nervous System. Charles Sherrington. 2nd ed. 1976. LC 73-2989. (Classics in Psychology Ser.). reprint ed. 31.95 (*0-405-05162-X*) Ayer.

Integrative & Molecular Approach to Brain Function: Proceedings of the Uehara Memorial Foundation Symposium on Integrative & Molecular Approach to Brain Function, Tokyo, 25-27 June 1996. 1996. LC 96-47690. (International Congress Ser.). 338p. 148.00 (*0-444-82380-8*) Elsevier.

Integrative Approach to Language Disorders in Children. Ed. by Elizabeth Carrow-Woolfolk. 1981. (Illus.). 512p. text 45.00 (*0-8089-1406-5*, 790799, Grune & Strat) Harcrt Hlth Sci Grp.

Integrative Approaches to Family Art Therapy. Shirley Riley & Cathy A. Malchiodi. 1994. LC 94-72843. (Illus.). 262p. (Orig.). (C). pap. text 29.95 (*0-9613309-5-3*) Magnolia St Pub.

Integrative Aspects of Calcium Signalling. Ed. by Alexej Verkhratsky & Emil C. Toescu. 1998. LC 98-39453. (Illus.). 428p. (C). text 125.00 (*0-306-46032-7*, Kluwer Plenum) Kluwer Academic.

Integrative Assessment of Adult Personality. Ed. by Larry E. Beutler & Michael R. Berren. 1994. LC 94-19183. 414p. 40.00 (*0-89862-281-6*, 2281) Guilford Pubns.

Integrative Biological Psychiatry. Ed. by H. Emrich & M. Wiegand. 1992. (Illus.). 312p. 82.95 (*0-387-54946-3*) Spr-Verlag.

Integrative Brief Therapy: Cognitive, Psychodynamic, Humanistic & Neurobehavioral Approaches. John D. Preston. 1998. LC 98-7498. (Practical Therapist Ser.: Vol. 1). 272p. 27.95 (*1-886230-09-9*) Impact Pubs CA.

Integrative Counselling Skills in Action. Sue Culley. (Counselling in Action Ser.: Vol. 12). 160p. 1991. 57.95 (*0-8039-8276-3*, 9299); 1990. pap. 22.95 (*0-8039-8277-1*, 9300) Sage.

Integrative Family Therapy. David C. Olsen. 1993. LC 92-44125. (Creative Pastoral Care & Counseling Ser.). 96p. pap. 15.00 (*0-8006-2638-9*, 1-2638, Fortress Pr) Augsburg Fortress.

Integrative Health Care: Complementary & Alternative Therapies for the Whole Person. Victor Sierpina. 2001. LC 00-43047. (Illus.). xxiv, 420p. 29.95 (*0-8036-0704-0*) Davis Co.

Integrative Hypnotherapy. Hammond Corydon. Date not set. (*0-393-70137-9*) Norton.

Integrative Manual Therapy for the Autonomic Nervous System & Related Disorders: Utilizing Advanced Strain & Counterstrain Technique. Thomas Giammatteo & Sharon Weiselfish-Giammatteo. 1998. LC 98-209490. (Illus.). 130p. text 65.00 (*1-55643-272-0*) North Atlantic.

Integrative Medicine: Achieving Wellness Through the Best of Eastern & Western Medical Practices. Kathleen F. Phalen. 1998. LC 98-8672. (Illus.). 208p. 21.95 (*1-885203-61-6*) Jrny Editions.

Integrative Medicine: The Patient's Essential Guide to Conventional & Complementary Treatments for More Than 300 Common Disorders. Alan H. Pressman & Donna Shelley. 2000. LC 00-27966. (Illus.). xv, 590p. 39.95 (*0-312-25379-6*) St Martin.

Integrative Medicine: Your Quick Reference Guide. Carol M. Coughlin & Ruth M. DeBusk. 1998. 292p. ring bd. 70.00 (*1-892014-00-9*) Integrative Med.

Integrative Medicine: Your Quick Reference Guide: Supplement, 1998. Carol M. Coughlin & Ruth M. DeBusk. 1998. 150p. suppl. ed. 45.00 (*1-892014-03-3*) Integrative Med.

Integrative Neurobiology of Affiliation: Proceedings of a New York Academy of Sciences Conference, March 14-17, 1996. C. Sue Carter et al. 1997. LC 97-4325. (Annals of the New York Academy of Sciences Ser.). pap. 110.00 (*1-57331-059-X*) NY Acad Sci.

Integrative Neurobiology of Affiliation: Proceedings of a New York Academy of Sciences Conference, March 14-17, 1996. Ed. by Justine Cassell et al. 1999. LC 98-36500. (Bradford Book Ser.). (Illus.). 300p. 40.00 (*0-262-53158-5*) MIT Pr.

Integrative Neurobiology of Affiliation: Proceedings of a New York Academy of Sciences Conference, March 14-17, 1996, Vol. 807. Ed. by C. Sue Carter et al. 1996. LC 97-4325. 110.00 (*1-57331-058-1*) NY Acad Sci.

Integrative Neuroendocrinology: Molecular, Cellular & Clinical Aspects. Ed. by S. M. McCann & R. I. Weiner. 1987. (Illus.). viii, 244p. 156.75 (*3-8055-4467-7*) S Karger.

Integrative Paradigms of Psychotherapy. Ted L. Orcutt & Jan R. Prell. 1993. LC 93-24551. 272p. (C). 78.00 (*0-205-14823-9*, Longwood Div) Allyn.

Integrative Power of Cognitive Therapy. Brad A. Alford & Aaron T. Beck. 1998. 197p. pap. 21.00 (*1-57230-396-4*, C0396) Guilford Pubns.

Integrative Problem-Centered Therapy: A Synthesis of Family, Individual, & Biological Therapies. William M. Pinsof. 1995. (Illus.). 304p. text 48.00 (*0-465-03328-8*) Basic.

Integrative Processes & Socialization: Early to Middle Childhood. Thomas D. Yawkey & James E. Johnson. 1988. 280p. (C). text 55.00 (*0-89859-604-1*) L Erlbaum Assocs.

Integrative Psychotherapy for Children & Adolescents with ADHD. Sebastiano Santostefano. 1995. LC 95-16994. (Master Work Ser.). 288p. pap. 45.00 (*1-56821-574-6*) Aronson.

Integrative Schizophrenietherapie. 1999. viii, 204p. 56.50 (*3-8055-6936-X*) S Karger.

Integrative Stress Counselling: A Humanistic Problem & Goal Focused Approach. Patricia Milner & Stephen Palmer. 1998. LC 98-221243. (Stress Counselling Ser.). 224p. 75.00 (*0-304-33491-X*); pap. 24.95 (*0-304-33492-8*) Continuum.

***Integrative Therapy: A Practitioner's Guide.** Maja O'Brien & Gaie Houston. 2000. LC 2001-265134. ix, 198p. 85.00 (*0-7619-5384-1*, 80511) Sage.

Integrative Treatment of Anxiety Disorders. Ed. by James M. Ellison. 1995. 320p. text 43.50 (*0-88048-715-1*, 8715) Am Psychiatric.

Integrins & ICAM-One in Immune Responses. Ed. by Nancy Hogg. 1991. (Chemical Immunology Ser.: Vol. 50). viii, 168p. 146.25 (*3-8055-5429-X*) S Karger.

Integrity & Change: Mental Health in the Marketplace. Eileen Smith. 1997. LC 96-1617. 216p. (C). 84.95 (*0-415-14139-7*); (Illus.). pap. 27.95 (*0-415-14140-0*) Routledge.

Integrity & Personhood: Looking at Patients from a Bio/Psycho/Social Perspective. Roberta Springer Loewy. 2000. LC 00-29632. xv, 109p. 79.00 (*0-306-46384-9*, Kluwer Plenum) Kluwer Academic.

Integrity in Depth. John Beebe. 1992. LC 91-27214. (Carolyn & Ernest Fay Series in Analytical Psychology: No. 2). 192p. 19.50 (*0-89096-493-9*) Tex A&M Univ Pr.

Integrity in Health Care Institutions: Humane Environments for Teaching, Inquiry, & Healing. Ed. by Ruth E. Bulger & Stanley J. Reiser. 1990. LC 90-11189. 188p. text 29.95 (*0-87745-300-4*) U of Iowa Pr.

Integrity of the Body: A Discussion of Modern Immunological Ideas. Frank M. Burnet. 1962. LC 62-8180. (Books in Biology: No. 3). (Illus.). 199p. 26.95 (*0-674-45650-5*) HUP.

Integument: Scanning Electron Microscopy in Skin Biology. Ed. by Bo Forslind et al. 1985. (Illus.). 304p. (Orig.). reprint ed. pap. text 34.00 (*0-931288-35-5*) Scanning Microscopy.

Integument & Mammary Glands. Ed. by Thomas C. Jones et al. 1989. (Monographs in Pathology of Laboratory Animals). (Illus.). 347p. 290.00 (*0-387-51025-7*) Spr-Verlag.

Integument System. Thomas Braem. 1994. (Organs of the Human Anatomy: Vol. 5). 88p. (C). spiral bd. 15.95 (*1-878576-30-5*) Flash Anatomy Inc.

Integumentary System. Ed. by Ulrich Mohr et al. 1994. (Illus.). 56p. pap. text 30.00 (*92-832-0125-6*) OUP.

Intelitool Supplement to Accompany Anatomy & Physiology Labs. Terry R. Martin. 1996. pap. 10.31 (*0-697-33368-X*, WCB McGr Hill) McGrw-H Hghr Educ.

Intellectual & Personality Characteristics of Children: Social Class & Ethnic-Group Differences. Edward F. Zigler et al. 1979. 144p. 29.95 (*0-89859-001-9*) L Erlbaum Assocs.

Intellectual Basis of Family Practice. G. Gayle Stephens. 1982. 239p. 18.95 (*0-938372-01-7*) Soc Tchrs Fam Med.

Intellectual Functions & the Brain: An Historical Perspective. Hans J. Markowitsch. 1992. LC 92-1482. (Illus.). 240p. text 78.00 (*0-88937-081-8*) Hogrefe & Huber Pubs.

Intellectual History of Psychology. Daniel N. Robinson. 3rd ed. 1995. LC 95-5697. 390p. pap. 21.95 (*0-299-14844-0*) U of Wis Pr.

Intellectual Impairment. Ed. by Alastair Heron & Mary Myers. 1983. text 94.00 (*0-12-342680-4*) Acad Pr.

Intellectual Property Rights & Biodiversity Conservation: An Interdisciplinary Analysis of the Values of Medicinal Plants. Ed. by Timothy M. Swanson. 1998. (Illus.). 285p. (C). reprint ed. pap. text 28.95 (*0-521-63580-2*) Cambridge U Pr.

Intellectually Gifted: An Overview. Ed. by Wayne Dennis & Margaret W. Dennis. 1976. LC 76-41850. (Illus.). 352p. text 68.00 (*0-8089-0962-2*, 791025, Grune & Strat) Harcrt Hlth Sci Grp.

Intelligence: Its Structure, Growth & Action. Raymond B. Cattell. 1987. (Advances in Psychology Ser.: No. 35). 694p. 269.50 (*0-444-87922-6*, North Holland) Elsevier.

Intelligence: Multiple Perspectives. Howard Gardner et al. 1995. LC 95-79342. 368p. (C). text 58.50 (*0-03-072629-8*) Harcourt Coll Pubs.

Intelligence: Reconceptualization & Measurement. Ed. by H. A. Rowe. 1991. 312p. (C). text 65.00 (*0-8058-0942-2*) L Erlbaum Assocs.

Intelligence: The Psychometric View. Paul Kline. 1990. LC 90-32231. (Illus.). 160p. (C). pap. 22.95 (*0-415-05512-1*, A4937) Routledge.

Intelligence & Adaptation. Stanley I. Greenspan. 1980. LC 78-13893. (Psychological Issues Monographs: No. 47-48). (Illus.). 412p. 60.00 (*0-8236-2718-7*, 002718) Intl Univs Pr.

Intelligence & Affectivity: Their Relationship During Child Development. Ed. by Jean Piaget. Tr. by T. A. Brown & C. E. Kaegi. 1981. (Illus.). text 8.00 (*0-8243-2901-5*) Annual Reviews.

Intelligence & Affectivity in Early Childhood: An Experimental Study of Jean Piaget's Object Concept & Object Relations. Therese G. Decarie. 1966. LC 65-28439. 230p. (Orig.). 35.00 (*0-8236-2720-9*) Intl Univs Pr.

Intelligence & Immigration. Clifford Kirkpatrick. 1970. LC 76-129405. (American Immigration Collection. Series 2). reprint ed. 16.95 (*0-405-00558-X*) Ayer.

Intelligence & Personality Factors Associated with Poliomyelitis Among School Age Children. E. L. Phillips et al. 1947. (SRCD M Ser.: Vol. 12, No. 2). pap. 25.00 (*0-527-01541-5*) Periodicals Srv.

Intelligence as Adaptive Behavior: An Experiment in Computational Neuroethology. Randall D. Beer. 1990. (Perspectives in Artificial Intelligence Ser.: Vol. 6). 213p. 58.00 (*0-12-084730-2*) Morgan Kaufmann.

Intelligence, Heredity & Environment. Ed. by Robert J. Sternberg & Elena L. Grigorenko. 1997. (Illus.). 628p. (C). pap. text 27.95 (*0-521-46904-X*) Cambridge U Pr.

Intelligence, Mind & Reasoning: Structure & Development. Ed. by Andreas Demetriou & Anastasia Efklides. 1994. LC 94-4456. (Advances in Psychology Ser.: Vol. 106). 250p. 130.00 (*0-444-89714-3*, North Holland) Elsevier.

Intelligent Control in Biomedicine. Ed. by Derek A. Linkens. 1994. LC 94-25293. 328p. 99.50 (*0-7484-0115-6*) Accel Devel.

Intelligent Data Analysis. Nada Lavrac et al. 1997. LC 97-27564. xxi, 310p. text 142.00 (*0-7923-8000-2*) Kluwer Academic.

Intelligent Dieting for Weight Loss & Prevention of Disease. D. Porter Price. 1982. LC 82-61578. (Illus.). 200p. (Orig.). pap. 13.95 (*0-9606246-2-7*); lib. bdg. 17.95 (*0-9606246-1-9*) SWI.

Intelligent Imitator: Towards an Exemplar Theory of Behavioral Choice. Reidar Kvadsheim. 1992. LC 92-36816. (Advances in Psychology Ser.: Vol. 95). 360p. 142.75 (*0-444-88360-6*, North Holland) Elsevier.

Intelligent Medicine: A Guide to Optimizing & Preventing Illness for the Baby Boom Generation. Ronald L. Hoffman. 1997. LC 97-23750. 448p. per. 16.00 (*0-684-81082-4*) S&S Trade.

Intelligent Patient Guide to Breast Cancer: All You Need to Know to Take an Active Part in Your Treatment. Karen Gelmon. 2nd ed. 1998. 280p. pap. 24.95 (*0-9696125-4-0*) Gordon Soules Bk.

Intelligent Patient's Guide to the Doctor-Patient Relationship: Learning How to Talk So Your Doctor Will Listen. Barbara Korsch & Caroline Harding. 1997. LC 97-373. 304p. 25.00 (*0-19-510264-9*) OUP.

Intelligent Software for Product Formulation. R. C. Rowe & R. J. Roberts. 1998. LC 98-159195. (Series in Pharmaceutical Sciences). 288p. (*0-7484-0732-4*) Tay Francis Ltd GBR. *Dist:* Taylor & Francis.

Intelligent Systems & Technologies in Rehabilitation Engineering. H. N. Teodorescu. 2000. (International Series on Computational Intelligence Ser.). 352p. 99.95 (*0-8493-0339-7*) CRC Pr.

Intelligibility in Speech Disorders: Theory, Measurement & Management. Ed. by Raymond D. Kent. 1992. LC 92-4811. (Studies in Speech Pathology & Clinical Linguistics: Vol. 1). vi, 365p. 113.00 (*1-55619-387-4*) J Benjamins Pubng Co.

Intensifying Care: The Hospital Industry, Professionalization & the Reorganization of the Nursing Labor Process. Robert L. Brannon. 1994. LC 94-11059. (Critical Approaches in the Health Social Sciences Ser.). 192p. 34.00 (*0-89503-161-2*); 180p. pap. 25.50 (*0-89503-162-0*) Baywood Pub.

Intensive Behavior Therapy: The Behavioral Treatment of Complex Emotional Disorders. John C. Papajohn. 1982. (General Psychology Ser.: No. 112). 176p. 32.50 (*0-08-025544-2*, J115, Pergamon Pr) Elsevier.

H
I

Intensive Care. J. Oldfield. 1997. (Animal Alert Ser.: Bk 1). (Illus.). (J). mass mkt. (*0-340-68169-1*) Hodder & Stought Ltd GBR. *Dist:* Lubrecht & Cramer, Trafalgar.

Intensive Care: A Concise Text. Hinds. 2nd ed. 1995. pap. text 51.00 (*0-7020-1541-5*) Saunders.

Intensive Care: A Doctor's Journal. John F. Murray. 2000. LC 99-56892. xiv, 296p. 27.50 (*0-520-22089-7*) U CA Pr.

Intensive Care: Counseling Teenagers in Crisis. Rich Van Pelt. 1988. 224p. 15.95 (*0-310-31840-8*, 18308) Zondervan.

Intensive Care: How Congress Shapes Health Policy. Thomas E. Mann. Ed. by Norman J. Ornstein. 1995. LC 95-4436. 316p. pap. text 18.95 (*0-8157-5463-9*) Brookings.

Intensive Care: How Congress Shapes Health Policy. Ed. by Thomas E. Mann & Norman J. Ornstein. 1995. LC 95-4436. (Renewing Congress Ser.). 316p. (C). text 42.95 (*0-8157-5464-7*) Brookings.

Intensive Care: Medical Ethics & the Medical Profession. Robert Zussman. LC 91-36919. (Illus.). 260p. 1997. 34.50 (*0-226-99634-4*); 1994. pap. text 16.95 (*0-226-99635-2*) U Ch Pr.

Intensive Care Aftercare. Richard Griffiths & Christina Jones. 2002. 224p. pap. 34.99 (*0-7506-4983-6*) Buttrwrth-Heinemann.

Intensive Care & Monitoring of the Neurosurgical Patient. Ed. by A. M. Landolt. 1987. (Progress in Neurological Surgery Ser.: Vol. 12). (Illus.). xiv, 202p. 115.75 (*3-8055-4414-6*) S Karger.

Intensive Care in Childhood: A Challenge to the Future. Ed. by D. Tibboel & E. Van der Voort. 1996. LC 96-19674. (Update in Intensive Care & Emergency Medicine Ser.). (Illus.). 464p. 147.00 (*3-540-61130-4*) Spr-Verlag.

Intensive Care Manual. Teik E. Oh. 4th ed. 1997. LC 96-38861. 1032p. pap. text 80.00 (*0-7506-2358-6*) Buttrwrth-Heinemann.

***Intensive Care Medicine.** Ed. by T. Evans et al. 1999. (British Medical Bulletin Ser.: Vol. 55, No. 1). 304p. pap. (*1-85315-410-5*) Royal Soc of Medicine Pr Ltd GBR. *Dist:* Balogh.

Intensive Care Nursing: A Framework for Practice. Philip Woodrow & Jane Roe. 2000. LC 99-33382. (Illus.). xvi, 576p. pap. 60.00 (*0-415-18456-8*) Routledge.

Intensive Care Nursing: Developing Competent Practice. Paul Fulbrook & Helen E. Ellis. 2000. 160p. pap. 45.00 (*0-7506-4308-0*) Buttrwrth-Heinemann.

Intensive Care of the Fetus & Neonate. Spitzer. 1995. 1264p. (C). (gr. 13). text 195.00 (*0-8016-7711-4*, 07711) Mosby Inc.

Intensive Care of the Newly Born: Physiological Principles & Practice. P. R. Swyer & Ann Llewellyn. 1975. (Monographs in Pediatrics: Vol. 6). (Illus.). 220p. 59.25 (*3-8055-2184-7*) S Karger.

Intensive Care Procedures. Ed. by Rifat Latifi. 2001. 45.00 (*1-57059-596-8*) Landes Bioscience.

Intensive Care Unit Handbook of Formulas & Laboratory Values. Joseph Varon & Robert E. Fromm, Jr. 1996. LC 96-30467. (Illus.). 160p. (C). (gr. 13). pap. text 25.95 (*0-8151-8978-8*, 28922) Mosby Inc.

Intensive Care Unit Manual. Paul N. Lanken. Ed. by Richard Zorab. 1999. LC 98-40583. (Illus.). xxxiv, 1147p. pap. text 47.50 (*0-7216-2197-X*) Saunders.

Intensive Coronary Care. M. F. Oliver et al. 1974. pap. text 10.80 (*92-4-154046-X*, 1150082) World Health.

Intensive Diabetes Management. Ruth Farkas-Hirsch. 2nd ed. 1998. LC 98-4106. (Clinical Education Ser.). (Illus.). 169p. pap. 39.95 (*1-58040-020-5*, 5406-01) Am Diabetes.

Intensive Family Therapy: Theoretical & Practical Aspects. Ed. by Ivan Boszormenyi-Nagy & James L. Framo. 2nd ed. 1985. LC 85-13270. 528p. text 59.95 (*0-87630-412-9*) Brunner-Routledge.

Intensive Outpatient Treatment for the Addictions. Ed. by Edward Gottheil. 1997. LC 97-3576. (Journal of Addictive Diseases Ser.: Vol. 16, No. 2). 100p. (C). 39.95 (*0-7890-0313-9*) Haworth Pr.

Intensive Outpatient Treatment of Sex & Love Addicts. Ed. by Eric Griffin-Shelley. 1993. LC 92-18876. 176p. 60.00 (*0-275-94316-X*, C4316, Praeger Pubs) Greenwood.

Intensive Psychotherapy of Alcoholism. Gary G. Forrest. 1994. LC 94-77918. 230p. pap. text 45.00 (*1-56821-360-3*) Aronson.

Intensive Psychotherapy of the Borderline Patient. Richard D. Chessick. 1977. LC 76-22867. 303p. 50.00 (*0-87668-254-9*) Aronson.

Intensive Respiratory Care. John M. Luce et al. 2nd ed. 1993. LC 92-48898. (Illus.). 400p. pap. text 29.00 (*0-7216-4270-5*) Saunders.

Intensive Short-Term Dynamic Psychotherapy: Theory & Technique. Patricia C. Della Selva. 1996. LC 95-38658. 272p. 85.00 (*0-471-04717-1*) Wiley.

Intensive Structural Therapy: Treating Families in Their Social Conflicts. H. Charles Fishman. 1993. LC 92-56170. 240p. 42.00 (*0-465-03350-4*) Basic.

Intensive Thinking: Pediatric Critical Care. Rashed A. Hasan & Michael D. Pappas. 2000. 250p. pap. 29.95 (*0-9704158-0-X*) R A Hasan.

Intensive Training of Bilingual Workers in Mental Health & Cross-Cultural Communication. Myrna A. Adkins & Charles Ray. 1987. 93p. stu. ed. 25.00 (*0-940723-02-6*) SIIS.

Intensivmedizin und Organversagen. W. Behrendt et al. 1985. (Beitraege zur Intensiv und Notfallmedizin Ser.: Vol. 3). (Illus.). viii, 188p. 58.50 (*3-8055-4016-7*) S Karger.

Intentional Forgetting: Interdisciplinary Approaches. Jonathan M. Golding & Colin M. MacLeod. 1997. LC 97-10293. (*0-8058-2211-9*); pap. (*0-8058-2212-7*) L Erlbaum Assocs.

Intentional Interviewing & Counseling: Facilitating Client Development. Allen E. Ivey. 2nd ed. 1987. LC 87-12076. 346p. (C). pap. 25.50 (*0-534-08796-5*); 3rd ed. 1993. LC 93-907. 384p. pap. 31.25 (*0-534-21168-2*) Brooks-Cole.

Intentional Interviewing & Counseling: Facilitating Client Development in a Multicultural Society. Allen E. Ivey & Mary B. Ivey. 4th ed. 1998. LC 98-9790. (Illus.). 432p. pap. text 46.95 (*0-534-35756-3*, 063) Brooks-Cole.

Intentionality: An Essay in the Philosophy of Mind. John R. Searle. 1983. LC 82-19849. 288p. pap. text 27.95 (*0-521-27302-1*) Cambridge U Pr.

Inter-Cultural Therapy, Themes, Interpretations & Practice. J. Kareem & R. Littlewood. 1992. (Illus.). 272p. pap. 42.95 (*0-632-02325-2*) Blackwell Sci.

Inter-Noise '86: Proceedings of the International Conference on Noise Control, Massachusetts Institute of Technology, Cambridge, MA, July 21-23, 1986, Vols. 1 & 2. Ed. by Robert Lotz. 1986. (Inter-Noise Ser.). 75.00 (*0-931784-15-8*) Noise Control.

Inter Views: Conversations with Laura Pozzo on Psychotherapy, Biography, Love, Soul, Dreams, Work, Imagination, & the State of the Culture. James Hillman & Laura Pozzo. 1983. LC 90-28280. 198p. reprint ed. pap. 18.50 (*0-88214-348-4*) Spring Pubns.

Interacting with Video. Marsha Kinder et al. Ed. by Patricia Greenfield et al. 1996. (Advances in Applied Developmental Psychology Ser.: Vol. 11). (Illus.). 218p. pap. 39.50 (*1-56750-152-4*);11. 73.25 (*1-56750-131-1*) Greenwood (Ablex).

Interaction Between Medium Energy Nucleons in Nuclei. H. O. Meyer. 1982. LC 83-70649. (Conference Proceedings Ser.: No. 97). 433p. (C). 38.00 (*0-88318-196-7*) Am Inst Physics.

Interaction Between Mental & Physical Illness. Ed. by R. Ohman et al. 1989. (Illus.). 161p. 95.00 (*0-387-50161-4*) Spr-Verlag.

Interaction in Human Development. Ed. by M. H. Bornstein & Jerome S. Bruner. 1989. (Crosscurrents in Contemporary Psychology Ser.). 320p. (C). text 69.95 (*0-8058-0035-2*) L Erlbaum Assocs.

Interaction of Catholic Bioethics & Secular Society: Proceedings of the Eleventh Bishops' Workshop, Dallas, Texas. Ed. by Russell E. Smith. 1992. LC 92-34697. 310p. pap. 19.95 (*0-935372-34-2*) NCBC.

Interaction of Radiation & Anti-Tumor Drugs: Proceedings of the Stanford Code Memorial Symposium, Royal Institute, London, Sept., 1976. Stanford Cade Memorial Symposium Staff. Ed. by Kurt Hellmann. 1978. (International Journal of Radiation Oncology, Biology, & Physics : Vol. 4). (Illus.). pap. 58.00 (*0-08-022666-3*, Pergamon Pr) Elsevier.

Interaction of Ultrasonic Waves & Tissues: Modeling, Simulations & Applications. Jan D'Hooge. 1999. (Illus.). 260p. (*90-6186-990-0*) Leuven Univ BEL. *Dist:* Coronet Bks.

Interaction Rhythms: Periodicity in Communicative Behavior. Ed. by Martha Davis. 1982. LC 81-2936. 372p. 45.95 (*0-89885-003-7*, Kluwer Acad Hman Sci) Kluwer Academic.

Interactional Nature of Depression: Advances in Interpersonal Approaches. Ed. by Thomas Joiner & James C. Coyne. 1999. LC 98-31115. 423p. text 39.95 (*1-55798-534-0*, 431-609A) Am Psychol.

Interactional Psychotherapy: Stages & Strategies in Behavioral Change. Sheldon Cashdan. 1973. LC 73-5764. (Illus.). 168p. text 45.00 (*0-8089-0809-X*, 790800, Grune & Strat) Harcrt Hlth Sci Grp.

Interactions among Aptitudes, Strategies, & Knowledge in Cognitive Performance. Ed. by W. Schneider & Franz E. Weinert. 1989. (Research in Criminology Ser.). (Illus.). 316p. 108.00 (*0-387-97052-5*) Spr-Verlag.

Interactions Between Drugs & Natural Medicines: What the Physician & Pharmacist Must Know about Vitamins, Minerals, Foods & Herbs. Chris D. Meletis & Thad Jacobs. 1999. LC 99-75715. 363p. 35.00 (*1-888483-10-5*) Eclectic Med.

Interactions Between Retroviruses & Herpesviruses. H-J Kung. 1994. 136p. text 53.00 (*981-02-1625-4*) World Scientific Pub.

Interactions by Design: The Positive Interactions Program for Persons with Alzheimer's Disease & Related Disorders. Sylvia Nissenboim & Christine Vroman. rev. ed. 1989. LC 89-85538. (Series in Nonprofit Management). 100p. pap. 27.95 (*0-9621846-1-6*) Geri-Active.

Interactions of Biomedical Communicators Within the Health Care System. Ed. by Gunter Grupp. 1976. (Biosciences Communications Ser.: Vol. 2, No. 4). (Illus.). 26.25 (*3-8055-2427-7*) S Karger.

Interactions of Drugs, Biologics, & Chemicals in U. S. Military Forces. Institute of Medicine Staff. Ed. by Robert G. Petersdorf et al. 1996. LC 97-101761. 88p. (C). pap. text 15.00 (*0-309-05593-8*) Natl Acad Pr.

Interactions of Magnesium & Potassium on Cardiac & Vascular Smooth Muscle. Ed. by B. M. Altura & F. Kruck. 1985. (Journal: Vol. 3, No. 4-6, 1984). (Illus.). iv, 192p. pap. 75.75 (*3-8055-4149-X*) S Karger.

Interactive Assessment. Ed. by H. C. Haywood & D. Tzuriel. 1991. (Disorders of Human Learning, Behavior, & Communication Ser.). (Illus.). 527p. 97.00 (*0-387-97587-X*) Spr-Verlag.

Interactive Atlas of Transesophageal Color Doppler Echocardiography. R. De Simone & G. Paolella. 1997. 24p. pap. 340.00 incl. cd-rom (*3-540-14532-X*) Spr-Verlag.

Interactive Case Studies for Blood Banks. 2000. pap. text (*1-56395-127-4*) Am Assn Blood.

Interactive Cases. O'Donnell. 1998. (C). pap. text, wbk. ed. 16.75 (*0-03-024429-3*) Harcourt.

Interactive Counseling, 2. Ed. by Mark B. Shoenberg & Charles F. Preston. 1983. LC 82-24261. (Contributions in Psychology Ser.: No. 2). 278p. 68.00 (*0-313-22592-3*, SIC/, Greenwood Pr) Greenwood.

Interactive Field in Analysis, Vol. 1. Ed. by Murray Stein. 1995. LC 94-41370. (Chiron Clinical Ser.). 168p. (Orig.). pap. 24.95 (*0-933029-77-2*) Chiron Pubns.

Interactive First Aid Workbook. National Safety Council Staff. 1996. (Emergency Care Ser.). (Illus.). 80p. (C). pap. text, wbk. ed. 16.95 (*0-7637-0358-3*, 0358-3) Jones & Bartlett.

Interactive Group Learning. Deborah L. Ulrich & Kellie J. Glendon. 1999. LC 98-31025. 160p. 33.95 (*0-8261-1238-2*) Springer Pub.

Interactive Hematology Imagebank. Barbara J. Bain. 1999. cd-rom 220.95 (*0-632-05321-6*) Blackwell Sci.

Interactive Phenomena in the Cardiac System. S. Sideman & R. Beyar. 1994. (Advances in Experimental Medicine & Biology Ser.: Vol. 346). (Illus.). 446p. (C). text 135.00 (*0-306-44637-5*, Kluwer Plenum) Kluwer Academic.

Interactive Psychology. 2000. tchr. ed. (*0-205-33055-X*) Allyn.

Interactive Psychology. Lester A. Lefton. 2000. LC 00-33194. (Illus.). 512p. pap. 45.00 (*0-205-32286-7*) Allyn.

Interactive Staff Training: Rehabilitation Teams That Work. Patrick W. Corrigan & Stanley G. McCracken. 1997. LC 97-13636. (Series in Rehabilitation & Health). (Illus.). 292p. (C). 47.50 (*0-306-45523-4*, Plenum Trade) Perseus Pubng.

Interactive Technology & the New Paradigm for Health Care. Ed. by Karen Morgan et al. 1995. LC 94-7335. (Studies in Health Technology & Informatics: Vol. 18). 459p. 80.00 (*90-5199-201-7*) IOS Press.

Interactive Video: Expanding Horizons in Nursing. Ed. by Mary A. Rizzolo. 1994. 200p. (C). 29.95 (*0-937126-27-6*) Am Journal Nurse.

Interconnections Between Human & Ecosystem Health. R. T. Digiulio. 1996. 256p. pap. 101.95 (*0-412-62400-1*) Chapman & Hall.

Interdependence: The Route to Community. Al Condeluci. 2nd ed. 1995. LC 91-72030. 272p. per. 45.00 (*1-878205-11-0*) St Lucie Pr.

Interdependence of Tumor Biology & Clinical Oncology: 24th Meeting of the International Society for Oncodevelopmental Biology & Medicine, San Diego, November 1996: Abstracts. Ed. by Sabine Von Kleist. 1997. (Tumor Biology Ser.: Vol. 18, Suppl. 1, 1997). ii, 136p. pap. 41.75 (*3-8055-6563-1*) S Karger.

Interdependence, Partnership & Equity in Health: Report of a WHO Bi-Regional Conference on Technology Transfer. WHO Staff. 1987. (Western Pacific Reports & Studies: No. 3). 107p. 6.00 (*92-9061-163-4*) World Health.

Interdisciplinary Approach to Accident Patterns in Children. I. M. Marcus et al. 1960. (SRCD M Ser.: Vol. 25, No. 2). pap. 25.00 (*0-527-01584-9*) Periodicals Srv.

Interdisciplinary Approaches to Gene Therapy: Legal, Ethical & Scientific Aspects. Stefan Muller et al. 1997. LC 97-23254. 292p. (C). pap. 91.00 (*3-540-63056-2*) Spr-Verlag.

Interdisciplinary Case Studies in Health Care Redesign. Mickey L. Parsons et al. 1997. LC 97-21500. (Strategies for Improving Patient Care Ser.). 384p. pap. 70.00 (*0-8342-0970-5*, 20970) Aspen Pub.

Interdisciplinary Casebook in Geriatric Communication. Barbara B. Dreher & Joseph D. Alter. 1992. 96p. pap. text 19.95 (*0-8261-8160-0*) Springer Pub.

Interdisciplinary Dentofacial Therapy: A Comprehensive Approach to Optimal Patient Care. Richard D. Roblee. 1995. LC 94-20093. (Illus.). 236p. text 128.00 (*0-86715-188-9*) Quint Pub Co.

Interdisciplinary Guide to the Literature on Human Caring. Janet Smerke. 1990. 80p. 8.50 (*0-88737-478-6*) Natl League Nurse.

Interdisciplinary Intervention Program for the Moderately to Profoundly Language-Retarded Child. Sol Adler et al. 1980. 120p. text 34.50 (*0-8089-1301-8*, 790029, Grune & Strat) Harcrt Hlth Sci Grp.

Interdisciplinary Neuroendocrinology. H. Hoefler & G. F. Walter. Ed. by M. Ratzenhofer et al. 1984. (Frontiers of Hormone Research Ser.: Vol. 12). (Illus.). x, 202p. 128.75 (*3-8055-3804-9*) S Karger.

Interdisciplinary Perspectives in Child Abuse & Neglect. Ed. by Faye F. Untalan & Crystal S. Mills. 1992. LC 91-32685. 208p. 62.50 (*0-275-94046-2*, C4046, Praeger Pubs) Greenwood.

Interdisciplinary Perspectives on Health Policy & Practice: Competing Interests Or Complementary Interpretations? Jane Robinson. 1999. LC 99-490227. ix, 220p. (*0-443-05992-6*) Harcrt Hlth Sci Grp.

Interdisciplinary Research in Legal Databases: Environmental Law Databases - Proceedings of the 9th Colloquy (Rome, 1991) 1992. (*92-871-2166-4*) Council of Europe FRA. *Dist:* Manhattan Pub Co.

Interdisciplinary Team Practice: Issues & Trends. Ed. by Pedro J. Lecca & John S. McNeill. 1985. LC 85-3612. 256p. 62.95 (*0-275-90134-3*, C0134, Praeger Pubs) Greenwood.

Interdisciplinary Topics in Gerontology, Set, Vols. 19 & 20. Ed. by F. Clifford Rose. 1985. (Illus.). xx, 432p. 292.25 (*3-8055-3982-7*) S Karger.

Interdisziplinare Schmerztherapie Bei Tumorpatienten: Strolegen der Akut-Langzeibehandlung. Ed. by Hans H. Bartsch & Wilhelm F. Von Hornstein. 1998. (Band Der Ser.). (Illus.). viii, 140p. pap. 56.50 (*3-8055-6594-1*) S Karger.

Interested Approach to the Management of Chronic Pelvic Pain. Deborah A. Metzger et al. 1996. LC 96-71489. 52p. (Orig.). pap. text 30.00 (*1-890076-00-7*, 96-001) Pharmedica Pr.

Interests, Ideas, & Deregulation: The Fate of Hospital Rate Setting. John E. McDonough. 1997. LC 97-32100. 296p. text 44.50 (*0-472-10888-3*, 10888) U of Mich Pr.

Interface of Psychoanalysis & Psychology. Ed. by James W. Barron et al. 1992. 666p. 69.95 (*1-55798-156-6*) Am Psychol.

Interfaces Between Alcoholism & Mental Health. Ed. by Earl X. Freed. 1982. LC 79-620039. (NIAAA-RUCAS Alcoholism Treatment Ser.: No. 4). pap. 15.00 (*0-911290-50-8*) Rutgers Ctr Alcohol.

Interfaces in Medicine & Mechanics: Proceedings of the First International Conference, Held at the University College, Swansea, 12-15 April, 1989, Organized by the Biomaterials Research Group. Ed. by K. R. Williams & T. H. Lesser. 1991. 398p. 96.00 (*1-85166-428-9*) Elsevier.

Interfaces in Medicine & Mechanics - 2: Proceedings of Interfaces 90, the Second International Conference Held at the Istituti Ortopedici Rizzoli, Bologna, Italy, 9-14 Sept. 1990. K. R. Williams et al. 1991. 516p. 150.00 (*1-85166-583-8*) Elsevier.

Interfaces of Medicine & Law: The Liability of Negligently Caused Psychiatric Injury (Nervous Shock) Danuta Mendelson. 1998. LC 98-18563. 319p. text (*1-85521-924-7*, K925.M46) Ashgate Pub GBR. *Dist:* Ashgate Pub Co.

Interfacial Phenomena in Drug Delivery & Targeting. Graham Buckton. 1995. (Drug Targeting & Delivery Ser.). 304p. text 105.00 (*3-7186-5633-7*, Harwood Acad Pubs) Gordon & Breach.

Interfacing the IBM-PC to Medical Equipment: The Art of Serial Communication. R. W. Nickalls & R. Ramasubramanian. 1995. (Illus.). 424p. (C). text 100.00 (*0-521-46280-0*) Cambridge U Pr.

Interference & Inhibition in Cognition. Ed. by Frank N. Dempster & Charles J. Brainerd. 1995. LC 94-5430. (Illus.). 423p. text 69.95 (*0-12-208930-8*) Acad Pr.

Interferon. 1988. (Journal: Vol. 11, No. 4, 1988). (Illus.). 50p. pap. 20.00 (*3-8055-4645-9*) S Karger.

Interferon. Jan Vilcek. 1969. (Virology Monographs: Vol. 6). 40.00 (*0-387-80933-3*) Spr-Verlag.

Interferon: Principles & Medical Applications. Ed. by Samuel Baron et al. 1992. LC 92-18104. 500p. pap. text 23.00 (*0-9631172-0-3*) U TX MB Microb.

Interferon Alpha-2: Pre-Clinical & Clinical Evaluation. Ed. by Daniel L. Kisner & J. F. Smyth. 1985. (Developments in Oncology Ser.). text 73.50 (*0-89838-701-9*) Kluwer Academic.

Interferon & Cancer. Ed. by Karol Sikora. 1983. LC 83-9626. 224p. 55.00 (*0-306-41379-5*, Plenum Trade) Perseus Pubng.

Interferon & Nonviral Pathogens. Gerard I. Byrne. Ed. by Jenifer Turco. 1988. (Immunology Ser.: Vol. 42). (Illus.). 336p. text 155.00 (*0-8247-7973-8*) Dekker.

Interferon Crusade. Sandra Panem. 1984. LC 84-17629. 109p. text 26.95 (*0-8157-6900-8*); pap. text 9.95 (*0-8157-6899-0*) Brookings.

Interferon Therapy. 1982. (Technical Report Ser.: No. 676). 28p. pap. text 3.00 (*92-4-120676-4*) World Health.

Interferon Therapy of Multiple Sclerosis. Ed. by Anthony T. Reder. 1997. LC 96-39953. (Illus.). 560p. text 215.00 (*0-8247-9764-7*) Dekker.

Interferon Therapy on Chronic Hepatitic C: Proceedings of the Takahashi Memorial Forum, Held in Tokyo, Japan on 25 November 1995. Masami Yamanaka et al. 1996. LC 96-36842. (International Congress Ser.). 116p. 112.50 (*0-444-82379-4*) Elsevier.

Interferons, Pt. C. Ed. by Sidney P. Colowick & Nathan O. Kaplan. 1986. (Methods in Enzymology Ser.: Vol. 119). text 188.00 (*0-12-182019-X*) Acad Pr.

Interferons. Ed. by Sidney P. Colowick & Sidney Pestka. 1981. (Methods in Enzymology Ser.: Vol. 78). Pt. A. text 188.00 (*0-12-181978-7*); Pt. B. text 188.00 (*0-12-181979-5*) Acad Pr.

Interferons: Basic Principles & Clinical Applications. Zeev Estrov et al. 1993. LC 93-23314. (Medical Intelligence Unit Ser.). 120p. 99.00 (*1-879702-86-X*) Landes Bioscience.

Interferons: Biological Activities & Clinical Efficacy. C. Aul & W. Schneider. 1997. LC 96-36491. (Illus.). 304p. pap. 62.95 (*3-540-61051-0*) Spr-Verlag.

Interferons: Mechanisms of Action & Role in Cancer Therapy. Ed. by D. Crowther & U. Veronesi. 1991. (ESO Monographs). (Illus.). 72p. 49.00 (*0-387-54302-3*) Spr-Verlag.

Interferons & Their Actions. William E. Stewart et al. 1977. 224p. 128.00 (*0-8493-5159-6*, QR187, CRC Reprint) Franklin.

Intergenerational Approaches in Aging: Implications for Education, Policy, & Practice. Ed. by Kevin Brabazon & Robert Disch. 1997. LC 97-39668. 276p. 49.95 (*0-7890-0356-2*) Haworth Pr.

Intergenerational Arts in the Nursing Home: A Handbook. Patch Clark. 1991. LC 91-138. 200p. lib. bdg. 62.50 (*0-313-25965-8*, CKI, Greenwood Pr) Greenwood.

***Intergrative Medicine.** Alan Pressman. 2001. pap. (*0-312-27024-0*) St Martin.

Intergroup Behavior. Ed. by John G. Turner & Howard Giles. 1995. LC 81-52768. 224p. 21.00 (*0-226-81726-1*) U Ch Pr.

Intergroup Cognition & Intergroup Behavior. Ed. by Constantine Sedikides et al. 1997. LC 97-1712. (Applied Social Research Ser.). 375p. pap. 59.95 (*0-8058-2056-6*); (*0-8058-2055-8*) L Erlbaum Assocs.

Intergroup Relations: Essential Readings. Ed. by Michael A. Hogg & Dominic Abrams. 2000. LC 00-65312. (Key Readings in Social Psychology Ser.). (Illus.). xiv, 439p. (*0-86377-678-7*) Psychol Pr GBR. *Dist:* Taylor & Francis.

Interleukin-2. J. H. Waxman & F. R. Balkwill. 1992. (Frontiers in Pharmacology & Therapeutics Ser.). (Illus.). 256p. 135.00 (*0-632-03042-9*) Blackwell Sci.

Interleukin-8(NAP-1) & Related Chemotactic Cytokines. Ed. by M. Baggiolini & C. Muenster Sorg. 1991. (Cytokines Ser.: Vol. 4). (Illus.). viii, 164p. 156.75 (*3-8055-5426-5*) S Karger.

Interleukin-5: From Molecule to Drug Target for Asthma (TBC) Ed. by Colin Sanderson. 1998. LC 98-44758. (Lung Biology in Health & Disease Ser.). (Illus.). 410p. text 185.00 (*0-8247-0190-9*) Dekker.

Interleukin-1 in the Brain. Ed. by Nancy Rothwell & Robert Dantzer. 1992. LC 92-48945. (Studies in Neurosciences: No. 5). 220p. 180.00 (*0-08-041996-8*, Pergamon Pr) Elsevier.

Interleukin Protocols. Ed. by Luke A. J. O'Neill & Andrew Bowie. 2001. LC 2001-16960. (Methods in Molecular Medicine Ser.: Vol. 60). (Illus.). 443p. 125.00 (*0-89603-738-X*) Humana.

Interleukin-6-Type Cytokines. Ed. by Andrzej Mackiewicz et al. 1995. LC 95-30188. (Annals of the New York Academy of Sciences Ser.: Vol. 762). 522p. pap. 150.00 (*0-89766-932-0*); (*0-89766-931-2*) NY Acad Sci.

Interleukin-10. Jan E. De Vries et al. 1995. LC 94-40332. (Molecular Biology Intelligence Unit Ser.). 160p. text 99.00 (*1-57059-092-3*) Landes Bioscience.

Interleukin-2 & Killer Cells in Cancer. Ed. by Eva Lotzova & Ronald B. Herberman. 1989. (Illus.). 384p. 254.00 (*0-8493-5388-2*, RC271) CRC Pr.

Interleukins: Molecular Biology & Immunology. Ed. by T. Kishimoto. 1992. (Chemical Immunology Ser.: Vol. 51). (Illus.). xii, 330p. 278.50 (*3-8055-5440-0*) S Karger.

Interlimb Coordination: Neural, Dynamical, & Cognitive Constraints. Ed. by S. P. Swinnen et al. 1994. LC 93-30641. (Illus.). 637p. text 59.95 (*0-12-679270-4*) Acad Pr.

Intermediary Organization Skeleton. H. Frost. 1986. LC 85-16595. 384p. 210.00 (*0-8493-5948-1*, CRC Reprint) Franklin.

Intermediary Organization Skeleton, Set. Harold M. Frost. 1986. 123.95 (*0-8493-5947-3*, RC930) CRC Pr.

Intermediary Organization Skeleton, Vol. 2. H. Frost. 1986. LC 85-16595. 352p. 192.00 (*0-8493-5949-X*, CRC Reprint) Franklin.

Intermediary Xenobiotic Metabolism. Ed. by D. H. Hutson et al. 1989. 350p. (*0-85066-764-X*) Tay Francis Ltd GBR. *Dist:* Taylor & Francis.

Intermediate CPT/HCPCS for Physician Office Coding: 2000 Edition. Donna Didier. rev. ed. 2000. 144p. pap. text 60.00 (*1-58426-036-X*, AC401100) Am Hlth Info.

Intermediate Emergency Care. Bryan E. Bledsoe. 1994. pap., wbk. ed. 16.67 (*0-89303-024-4*) Mosby Inc.

Intermediate Emergency Care. Bryan E. Bledsoe et al. 2nd ed. 1997. LC 97-41364. 480p. pap. 42.95 (*0-8359-5160-X*) P-H.

Intermediate Emergency Care Exam Review. Richard A. Cherry. 1995. LC 95-33565. 96p. pap. text 35.40 (*0-8359-4978-8*) P-H.

Intermediate Filament Structure. David A. Parry & Peter M. Steinert. 1995. (Molecular Biology Intelligence Unit Ser.). 140p. text 79.00 (*1-57059-120-2*, LN9120) Landes Bioscience.

Intermediate Health & Social Care. Liam Clarke et al. 1995. 336p. (Orig.). pap. (*0-7487-1771-4*) Nelson Thornes GBR. *Dist:* Trans-Atl Phila.

Intermediate Physics for Medicine & Biology. Russell K. Hobbie. 3rd ed. 1997. LC 97-34134. (Biological Physics Ser.). (Illus.). 592p. 89.95 (*1-56396-458-9*) Spr-Verlag.

Intermediate Sex: A Study of Some Transitional Types of Men & Women. Edward Carpenter. 2nd ed. LC 78-22294. (Gay Experience Ser.). reprint ed. 39.50 (*0-404-61524-4*) AMS Pr.

Intermediate Uveitis. Ed. by W. R. Boeke et al. 1991. (Developments in Ophthalmology Ser.: Vol. 23). (Illus.). viii, 290p. 248.00 (*3-8055-5436-2*) S Karger.

Intern Pocket Admission Book. Thomas M. Masterson. 1993. 78p. pap. text 4.50 (*0-9634063-4-5*) Intl Med Pub.

Intern Pocket Survival Guide. Thomas M. Masterson. 1992. 78p. (Orig.). (C). pap. text 7.50 (*0-9634063-0-2*) Intl Med Pub.

Internal Consultancy in the Public Sector: Case Studies. Ed. by Clare Huffington & Halina Brunning. 1994. 192p. pap. text (*1-85575-054-6*) Karnac Bks GBR. *Dist:* Other Pr LLC.

Internal Consultation in Health Care Settings. Robert Bor & Riva Miller. 1992. 102p. pap. (*1-85575-020-1*) Karnac Bks GBR. *Dist:* Other Pr LLC.

Internal Derangements of Joints. Donald Resnick. 1997. LC 96-20546. (C). text 265.00 (*0-7216-6760-0*) Harcourt.

Internal Environment & Alimentary Behavior, Vol. 2. Second Conference, 1962. 1963. 10.00 (*0-934454-18-3*) Lubrecht & Cramer.

Internal Family Systems Therapy. Richard C. Schwartz. 1997. LC 94-21393. (Guilford Family Therapy Ser.). 248p. pap. 22.00 (*1-57230-272-0*, C0272) Guilford Pubns.

Internal Fixation in Reconstructive & Trauma Surgery of the Foot & Ankle. Sigvard T. Hansen, Jr. 1995. 400p. 120.00 (*0-7817-0151-1*); LC 99-88343. 544p. text 189.00 (*0-397-51752-1*) Lppncott W & W.

Internal Fixation of Small Fractures. Urs F. A. Heim & K. M. Pfeiffer. 1995. (Illus.). 400p. 215.00 (*0-387-17728-0*) Spr-Verlag.

Internal Fixation of Small Fractures: Techniques Recommended by the AO/ASIF Group. Urs F. A. Heim & Karl M. Pfeiffer. 3rd ed. 1995. (Illus.). 393p. 265.00 (*3-540-17728-0*) Spr-Verlag.

Internal Fixation of the Mandible. B. Spiessl. 1988. (Illus.). 375p. 350.00 (*0-387-16282-8*) Spr-Verlag.

Internal Fixation of the Mandible: A Manual of AO/ASIF Principles. Bernd Spiessl. 1989. 375p. 350.00 (*3-540-16282-8*) Spr-Verlag.

Internal Intra-Abdominal Hernias. Roberto L. Estrada. 1994. LC 93-40872. (Medical Intelligence Unit Ser.). 288p. 135.00 (*1-879702-91-6*, R) Landes Bioscience.

Internal Landscapes & Foreign Bodies: Eating Disorders & Other Pathologies. Gianna P. Williams. 1998. LC 97-48336. (Tavistock Clinic Ser.). 304p. (C). 90.00 (*0-415-92078-7*, D5714) Routledge.

Internal Markets in the Making: Health Systems in Canada, Iceland & the United Kingdom. 1995. 73p. pap. (*92-64-14339-4*) Org for Econ FRA. *Dist:* OECD.

Internal Medicine Steven M. Mitchell. 1998. (Clerkship Ser.). pap. text 24.95 (*1-889325-74-0*) Fence Crk Pubng.

Internal Medicine. Siegle. 1986. 20.00 (*0-316-79011-7*, Little Brwn Med Div) Lppncott W & W.

Internal Medicine. Dala R. Jarolim. 2nd ed. 1996. LC 96-13503. (Oklahoma Notes). 424p. pap. 24.95 (*0-387-94636-5*) Spr-Verlag.

Internal Medicine. Ed. by Jay H. Stein. 2nd ed. 1986. (Illus.). 2338p. 85.00 (*0-316-81235-8*, Little Brwn Med Div) Lppncott W & W.

Internal Medicine. Jay H. Stein. 1990. 3rd ed. 115.50 (*0-316-81230-7*); Set. 148.50 (*0-316-81244-7*) Lppncott W & W (Little Brwn Med Div).

Internal Medicine. Jay H. Stein. 5th ed. 1998. LC 97-51786. (Illus.). 2512p. (C). (gr. 13). text 89.95 (*0-8151-8698-3*, 28991) Mosby Inc.

Internal Medicine: 1976 Topics: Proceedings of the International Congress, 13th, Helsinki, Aug., 1976. International Congress on Internal Medicine Staff. Ed. by A. Louhija & V. Valtonen. 1977. (Illus.). 191.50 (*3-8055-2641-5*) S Karger.

Internal Medicine: A Board Review, Vol. 8. Juha P. Kokko & Sidney F. Stein. Ed. by Terry Hillman. 1997. (Illus.). 600p. (*0-918473-16-0*) Sci-Thru-Media.

Internal Medicine: Diagnosis & Therapy. Jay H. Stein. 3rd ed. 1993. (Illus.). 688p. (C). pap. text 29.95 (*0-8385-1112-0*, A1112-0, Apple Lange Med) McGraw.

Internal Medicine: Handbook for Clinicians. Wilson H. Tang et al. 2000. (Resident Survival Guides Ser.). (Illus.). 300p. (C). pap. 14.95 (*0-9645467-5-2*) Scrub Hill.

Internal Medicine & Critical Care Pocketbook. Robert J. Lederman. 2nd rev. ed. 2001. 160p. (Orig.). pap. 11.95 (*1-882742-20-6*) Tarascon Pub.

Internal Medicine & the Structures of Modern Medical Science: The University of Iowa, 1870-1990. Lee Anderson. 1996. LC 95-26592. (Illus.). 296p. (C). text 54.95 (*0-8138-2332-3*) Iowa U Pr.

Internal Medicine Board Certification Review. D. Kanjilal. 1998. LC 98-24053. (Illus.). 1000p. text 149.00 (*1-58141-028-X*) Rivercross Pub.

***Internal Medicine Board Review.** 9th ed. 2001. 284p. stu. ed. 395.00 (*0-9640788-6-4*);Vol. 2. 240p. stu. ed. 395.00 (*0-9640788-7-2*) MedStudy.

Internal Medicine Casebook: Real Patients, Real Answers. Robert W. Schrier. 2nd ed. 1999. LC 99-31881. 480p. pap. text 39.95 (*0-7817-2029-X*) Lppncott W & W.

Internal Medicine Cd-Rom. 1994. text 99.00 incl. audio compact disk (*0-8151-7925-1*, 24378) Mosby Inc.

Internal Medicine in Vietnam 2 vols., Set. 1995. lib. bdg. 625.95 (*0-8490-6581-X*) Gordon Pr.

Internal Medicine ISE. Jay H. Stein. 2nd ed. 1986. 40.00 (*0-316-81236-6*, Little Brwn Med Div) Lppncott W & W.

Internal Medicine MS Pearls of Wisdom. Michael Zevitz et al. 1998. (Pearls of Wisdom Ser.). pap. 32.00 (*1-890369-21-7*) Boston Medical.

Internal Medicine on Call. Steven A. Haist et al. 2nd ed. 1997. (Illus.). 593p. (C). pap. 34.95 (*0-8385-4056-2*, A4056-6) McGraw-Hill Prof.

Internal Medicine on Call. 3rd ed. 2000. (C). 24.95 (*0-8385-4278-6*) Appleton & Lange.

***Internal Medicine P. R. E. P. P., 2001.** Diem Chang et al. Ed. by Raymond K. J. Chang et al. 2nd ed. 2001. 412p. pap. text 69.50 (*0-9678841-1-X*) Internal Med.

Internal Medicine Pearls. Clay B. Marsh & Ernest L. Mazzaferri. Ed. by Steven A. Sahn & John E. Heffner. 1992. (Illus.). 276p. (Orig.). pap. 49.95 (*1-56053-024-3*) Hanley & Belfus.

Internal Medicine Pearls of Wisdom. Michael Zevitz et al. 1998. (Pearls of Wisdom Ser.). pap. 92.00 (*1-890369-09-8*) Boston Medical.

Internal Medicine Quickie. Afshine Emrani. 1998. pap. 12.95 (*0-9654687-2-0*) Emrani Publns.

Internal Medicine Simulated Test & Review, Bk. 1. Mauricio L. Waintrub. 1998. (Internal Medicine Ser.). (Illus.). 120p. (C). pap. 21.00 (*1-884083-61-7*) Maval Pub.

Internal Medicine Simulated Test & Review. Mauricio L. Waintrub et al. Ed. by Maria Luder. 2000. (Internal Medicine Ser.). (Illus.). 120p. (C). Bk. 2. pap. text 21.00 (*1-884083-62-5*); Bk. 3. 21.00 (*1-884083-63-3*) Maval Pub.

Internal Medicine Simulated Test & Review, Bk. 4. Valentin Waintrub et al. Ed. by Maria Luder. 2000. (Internal Medicine Ser.). (Illus.). 120p. (C). 21.00 (*1-884083-64-1*) Maval Pub.

Internal Medicine 2000: An Internet Resource Guide. Ed. by Dan Goldenson. 2001. pap. 24.95 (*0-9700525-2-9*) eMedguides.

Internal Medicine Words: Over 8000 Words, Terms, & Quick Definitions. Ed. by Pat Bowen. 1997. 288p. pap. 29.95 (*1-877810-68-1*, IMW) Rayve Prodns.

Internal Objects Revisited. Joseph Sandler & A. M. Sandler. 1998. 192p. pap. (*1-85575-191-7*) Karnac Bks GBR. *Dist:* Other Pr LLC.

Internal Operations Audit Manual for Health Care Facilities. D. K. Everitt & E. E. Murphy. 2000. LC 00-61098. (Illus.). 259.00 (*0-8342-1885-2*) Aspen Pub.

Internal World & External Reality. Otto F. Kernberg. 1985. LC 84-45723. 376p. 50.00 (*0-87668-758-3*) Aronson.

Internalization in Psychoanalysis, No. 50. William W. Meissner. 1980. LC 80-13867. (Psychological Issues Monographs: No. 50). ix, 279p. 42.50 (*0-8236-2726-8*, BN02713) Intl Univs Pr.

Internalizing & Externalizing Expressions of Dysfunction: Rochester Symposium on Developmental Psychopathology, Vol. 2. Ed. by Dante Cicchetti. 1991. 328p. (C). text 79.95 (*0-8058-0933-3*) L Erlbaum Assocs.

Internalizing Disorders in Children & Adolescents. Ed. by William M. Reynolds. 1992. LC 91-40212. (Personality Processes Ser.: No. 1341). 352p. 195.00 (*0-471-50648-6*) Wiley.

International Administration of Nursing Services. Ed. by Beverly Henry et al. 1989. LC 89-17408. 304p. text 35.00 (*0-914783-35-1*) Charles.

International Agency for Research for Cancer: Biennial Report 1992-1993. 1993. (ENG & FRE.). xvii, 244p. pap. text 25.00 (*92-832-1093-X*, 1759293) World Health.

International Agency for Research for Cancer: Biennial Report 1994-1995. 1995. (ENG & FRE.). xvii, 262p. pap. text 22.50 (*92-832-1095-6*, 1759495) World Health.

International Agency for Research on Cancer Annual Report for the Period July 1, 1984 to June 30, 1985. 1985. 240p. pap. 15.00 (*92-832-1085-9*) World Health.

International Albert Schweitzer Lecture Series at Yale University. Ed. by David H. Darst. (Illus.). 60p. (Orig.). pap. text 3.50 (*1-885007-06-X*) A Schweitzer.

International Annals of Adolescent Psychiatry, Vol. 1. Aaron H. Esman. Ed. by Sherman C. Feinstein & Serge Lebovici. 1988. LC 88-214971. (International Annals of Adolescent Psychiatry Ser.: Vol. 1). 314p. lib. bdg. 42.00 (*0-226-21755-8*) U Ch Pr.

International Annals of Adolescent Psychiatry: Psychosis & Psychotic Functioning, Vol. 2. Ed. by Allan Z. Schwartzberg. 1992. 356p. lib. bdg. 44.00 (*0-226-74219-9*) U Ch Pr.

International Approaches to Prevention in Mental Health & Human Services. Ed. by Robert E. Hess & Wolfgang Stark. 1995. LC 95-13451. 39.95 (*1-56024-717-7*) Haworth Pr.

International Assessment of Health Care Financing: Lessons for Developing Countries. Ed. by David W. Dunlop & J. M. Martins. 1996. LC 95-8983. (EDI Seminar Ser.). 206p. pap. 22.00 (*0-8213-3253-8*, 13253) World Bank.

International Association for Applied Psychology Early Conference Proceedings, 1920-1958, Set. Ed. by With an Introduction by Horst Gundlach. 1998. LC 99-228339. 5700p. (C). 1643.00 (*0-415-17215-2*) Routledge.

International Association of Logopaedics & Phoniatrics, 19th Congress, Edinburgh 1983: Abstracts. Ed. by Carol J. Miller. 1983. (Journal: Vol. 35, No. 3-4). 96p. pap. 31.50 (*3-8055-3730-1*) S Karger.

International Association of Logopaedics & Phoniatrics, 19th Congress, Edinburgh 1983: Main Papers. Ed. by A. Muller. 1983. (Journal: Vol. 35, No. 1-2). 96p. pap. 31.50 (*3-8055-3729-8*) S Karger.

International Association of Logopedics & Phoniatrics: 17th Congress, Copenhagen, August 1977: Abstracts. International Congress of Logopedics and Phoniatrics. Ed. by E. Loebell et al. 1977. (Folia Phoniatrica et Logopaedica Ser.: Vol. 28, No. 4-5). 43.50 (*3-8055-2755-1*) S Karger.

International Association of Logopedics & Phoniatrics: 24th World Congress, Amsterdam, August, 1998 - Main Reports. World Congress Amsterdam Staff. 1998. (Folia Phoniatrica et Logopaedica Ser.: Vol. 50, No. 3). (Illus.). 78p. pap. 37.50 (*3-8055-6723-5*) S Karger.

***International Association of Logopedics & Phoniatrics: 25th World Congress, Montreal, August 2001: Main Reports.** Ed. by E. Soderpalm. 2001. (Illus.). 56p. pap. 25.25 (*3-8055-7291-3*) S Karger.

International Association of Logopedics & Phoniatrics, 21st Congress, Prague, August 1989: Main Reports. Ed. by M. Lastovka. 1989. (Illus.). 96p. pap. 53.25 (*3-8055-5053-7*) S Karger.

International Association of Logopedics & Phoniatrics. Abstracts: 21st Congress, Prague, August 1989. 1989. (Illus.). 96p. pap. 53.25 (*3-8055-5059-6*) S Karger.

International Association of Logopedics & Phoniatrics, Twentieth Congress, Tokyo, August 1986 Abstracts: Journal: Folia Phoniatrica, Vol. 38, No. 5-6, 1986. Ed. by M. Sawashima. 1986. 112p. pap. 51.50 (*3-8055-4363-8*) S Karger.

International Association of Logopedics & Phoniatrics, Twentieth Congress, Tokyo, August 1986 Main Reports: Journal: Folia Phoniatrica, Vol. 38, Nos. 2-4. 1986. 220p. pap. 103.50 (*3-8055-4444-8*) S Karger.

***International Book of Dyslexia.** Smythe. 2001. 250p. 135.00 (*0-471-49841-6*); pap. 75.00 (*0-471-49646-4*) Wiley.

International Cartographic Association, 1959-84: The First Twenty Years of the International Cartographic Association. Compiled by Ferdinand J. Ormeling, Jr. 1988. 138p. pap. 65.00 (*90-70310-11-2*) Elsevier.

International Cell Biology, 1976-1977. Ed. by B. R. Brinkley & Keith R. Porter. 1977. LC 77-79991. (Illus.). 694p. text 15.00 (*0-87470-027-2*) Rockefeller.

International Cell Biology, 1980-1981. Ed. by H. G. Schweiger. 1981. (Illus.). 1033p. 104.00 (*0-387-10475-5*) Spr-Verlag.

***International Child Health Care: A Practical Manual for Hospitals Worldwide.** Child Advocacy International Staff. 2001. (Illus.). 626p. pap. text (*0-7279-1476-6*) BMJ Pub GBR. *Dist:* AIDC.

International Classification in Psychiatry: Unity & Diversity. Ed. by Juan E. Mezzich & Michael Von Cranach. 1988. (Illus.). 411p. text 100.00 (*0-521-32754-7*) Cambridge U Pr.

International Classification of Childhood Cancer 1996. Ed. by E. Kramarova et al. 1996. (IARC Scientific Publications Ser.: Vol. 29). 48p. pap. 27.00 (*92-832-1443-9*, 1770029) Am Soc Clinical.

International Classification of Diseases, Set. 1984. lib. bdg. 1800.00 (*0-87700-608-3*) Revisionist Pr.

International Classification of Diseases for Oncology (ICD-O) Ed. by C. Percy et al. 2nd rev. ed. 1991. (CHI.). xlvii, 144p. text 50.00 (*92-4-154414-7*, 1150350) World Health.

International Classification of Impairments, Disabilities, & Handicaps: A Manual of Classification Relating to the Consequences of Disease. 1980. 205p. pap. text 18.00 (*92-4-154126-1*, 1150088) World Health.

International Classification of Primary Care in the European Community: With a Multi-Language Layer. Ed. by Henk Lamberts et al. 1993. (Illus.). 254p. text 95.00 (*0-19-262298-6*) OUP.

International Classification of Procedures in Medicine. 1978. (Nonserial Publication). Vol. 1. 319p. pap. text 18.00 (*92-4-154124-5*, 1150089); Vol. 2. 152p. pap. text 18.00 (*92-4-154125-3*, 1150090) World Health.

International Classification of Rodent Tumours: The Mouse. Ed. by Ulrich Mohr. 2000. LC 00-64092. (Illus.). xix, 474p. 299.00 (*3-540-64578-0*) Spr-Verlag.

International Classification of Sleep Disorders: Diagnostic & Coding Manual. Amer. Sleep Disorders Assn. Staff. rev. ed. 1997. (*0-9657220-0-7*); pap. (*0-9657220-1-5*) Am Sleep Disorders.

International Clinical Trails: A Guide Book & Compendium of National Drug Laws Ed. by Dominique P. Brunier & Gerhard R. Nahler. 1999. LC 99-22061. 500p. 229.00 (*1-57491-094-9*) IHS Health Grp.

International Code of Marketing of Breast-Milk Substitutes. WHO Staff. 1981. LC 81-217037. (CHI, FRE & SPA.). 35p. pap. text 4.00 (*92-4-154160-1*, 1150094) World Health.

International Collation of Traditional & Folk, 2. 1997. 230p. text 33.00 (*981-02-3130-X*) World Scientific Pub.

International Collation of Traditional & Folk Medicine Vol. 3, Pt. III: Northeast Asia. Ed. by C. K. Sung et al. 1998. 200p. 48.00 (*981-02-3639-5*) World Scientific Pub.

H I

International College of Psychosomatic Medicine Madrid, October 1989, Selected Papers from the 10th World Congress: Journal: Psychotherapy & Psychosomatics, Vol. 52, No. 1-3, 1989. Ed. by J. Lopez-Ibor. 1990. (Illus.). 172p. pap. 108.00 (*3-8055-5273-4*) S Karger.

International Colloquium of Developmental Pharmacology, 3rd, Nancy, June 1981, Journal: Developmental Pharmacology & Therapeutics, Vol. 4, Suppl. 1, 1982. Ed. by P. Vert & J. V. Aranda. 1982. 232p. pap. 62.75 (*3-8055-3476-0*) S Karger.

International Colloquium of Developmental Pharmacology, 4th, Paris, May 1983. Ed. by G. Olive et al. 1984. (Journal: Vol. 7, Suppl. 1). (Illus.). viii, 224p. pap. 61.00 (*3-8055-3997-5*) S Karger.

International Colloquium on Paratuberculosis: 4th, 1994: Cambridge, England; Proceedings of the Fourth International Colloquium on Paratuberculosis, July 17-July 21, 1994: A Meeting of the International Association for Paratuberculosis, St. John's College, Cambridge, U. K. Ed. by Rodrick J. Chiodini et al. 1994. LC 95-2324. (*0-9633043-2-1*) Intl Assn Paratuber.

International Commission on Radiation Units & Measurements: An International Neutron Dosimetry Intercomparison, No. 27. 1978. LC 77-90632. 35.00 (*0-913394-46-7*) Intl Comm Rad Meas.

International Commission on Radiation Units & Measurements: Basic Aspects of High Energy Particle Interactions & Radiation Dosimetry, No. 28. 1978. LC 78-62474. 45.00 (*0-913394-22-X*) Intl Comm Rad Meas.

International Commission on Radiation Units & Measurements: Methods of Assessment of Absorbed Dose in Clinical Use of Radionuclides, No. 32. 1979. LC 79-90172. 45.00 (*0-913394-26-2*) Intl Comm Rad Meas.

International Commission on Radiation Units & Measurements: Neutron Dosimetry for Biology & Medicine, No. 26. 1977. LC 76-53369. 50.00 (*0-913394-20-3*) Intl Comm Rad Meas.

International Commission on Radiation Units & Measurements: Tissue Substitutes in Radiation Dosimetry & Measurement. 1989. LC 88-25113. (ICRU Report Ser.: No. 44). 189p. pap. text 60.00 (*0-913394-38-6*) Intl Comm Rad Meas.

International Communication for Biomedical Research: Journal: Health Communications & Informatics, Vol. 6, Nos. 3-4. Ed. by H. E. Kennedy & W. Bevan. 1980. (Illus.). 112p. pap. 16.75 (*3-8055-0974-X*) S Karger.

International Comparisons of Administrative Costs in Health Care. Michael E. Gluck. 1997. (Illus.). 74p. (C). reprint ed. pap. text 25.00 (*0-7881-4589-4*) DIANE Pub.

International Complement Workshop, 11th, Miami, Fla., November 1985: Abstracts. Ed. by D. T. Fearon. 1985. (Journal: Vol. 2, No. 1, 1985). (Illus.). 96p. pap. 48.00 (*3-8055-4234-8*) S Karger.

International Complement Workshop, 12th Abstracts, Chamonix, September 1987. Ed. by G. Arlaud et al. 1987. (Journal: Vol. 4, No. 3-4). iv, 132p. pap. 77.50 (*3-8055-4674-2*) S Karger.

***International Conference on Emerging Infectious Diseases (2000)** Joseph W. McDade. 2001. (Illus.). 166p. (C). pap. text 30.00 (*0-7567-1457-5*) DIANE Pub.

International Conference on Experimental Ulcer, 7th, Berlin, October, 1991 Abstracts: Digestion Journal, Vol. 49, Suppl. 1. Ed. by K. F. Sewing. 1991. ii, 58p. pap. 18.50 (*3-8055-5530-X*) S Karger.

***International Conference on Minimal Intervention Approach for Dental Treatment: Kuwait, December 1999: Proceedings.** Ed. by J. Behbehani & E. Honkala. 2001. (Illus.). 52p. pap. 25.25 (*3-8055-7331-6*) S Karger.

International Conference on Social Science & Medicine, 6th, Amsterdam, 1979: Second Special Conference Issue. Ed. by Peter J. McEwan. 1981. 80p. pap. 17.25 (*0-08-026763-7*, Pergamon Pr) Elsevier.

International Conference on the CEA (Gene) Family, Freiburg i.Br., December 1993: From Basic Research to Clinical Application. Ed. by J. A. Thompson. 1995. (Tumor Biology Ser.: Vol. 16, No. 1, 1995). (Illus.). 74p. pap. 23.50 (*3-8055-6135-0*) S Karger.

International Conference on the Neurohypophysis, Key Biscayne, Fla., November, 1976. International Conference on the Neurohypophysis St. Ed. by A. M. Moses & L. Share. 1977. (Illus.). 104.50 (*3-8055-2664-4*) S Karger.

International Conference on Thrombolysis, Paris, March 1985. Ed. by A. Serradimigni. 1986. (Journal: Vol. 73, No. 4-5, 1986). (Illus.). 152p. pap. 48.75 (*3-8055-4374-3*) S Karger.

International Conference on Ulcer Research, 8th Meeting, Kyoto-Japan, November 1994: Abstracts. Ed. by S. Okabe & K. Takeuchi. 1994. (Journal: Vol. 55, Supplement 2, 1994). (Illus.). ii, 62p. pap. 28.00 (*3-8055-6069-9*) S Karger.

International Congress of Essential Oils, Fragrances & Flavours, 11th, New Delhi, India, 12-16 November, 1989, Set. 1989. (*81-204-0460-2*) Oxford IBH IND. *Dist:* S Asia.

International Congress of Microbiological Standardization, 12th, Annecy, 1971. International Congress of Microbiological Standard. Ed. by R. H. Regamey et al. 1973. (Progress in Immunobiological Standardization Ser.: Vol. 5). 81.00 (*3-8055-1404-2*) S Karger.

International Congress of Nephrology, 8th, Athens, June 1981. W. Zurukzoglu et al. Ed. by M. Pyroasopoulos et al. 1981. (Illus.). xxiv, 1240p. 282.75 (*3-8055-2532-X*) S Karger.

International Congress of Nephrology, 7th, Montreal, June 18-23, 1978. International Congress of Nephrology Staff. Ed. by Michael Bergerson. 1978. 129.75 (*3-8055-2915-5*) S Karger.

International Congress of Nutrition, Mexico, Sept., 1972, Set. International Congress of Nutrition Staff. 1975. 365.25 (*3-8055-1394-1*) S Karger.

International Congress of Psychology, 11th: Paris, 1937 (Rapports et Compte-Rendu) 1969. reprint ed. 60.00 (*0-8115-3542-8*) Periodicals Srv.

International Congress of Psychology, 12th: Edinburgh, 1948 (Proceedings & Papers) 1969. reprint ed. 30.00 (*0-8115-3553-3*) Periodicals Srv.

International Congress of Psychology, 13th: Stockholm, 1951 (Proceedings & Papers) 1969. reprint ed. 35.00 (*0-8115-3554-1*) Periodicals Srv.

International Congress of Psychology, 14th: Montreal, 1954 (Proceedings & Papers) 1969. reprint ed. 45.00 (*0-8115-3555-X*) Periodicals Srv.

International Congress of Psychology, 15th: Brussels, 1957, (Actes) 1969. reprint ed. 65.00 (*0-8115-3556-8*) Periodicals Srv.

International Congress of Psychology, 16th: Bonn, 1960, (Bericht) 1969. reprint ed. 85.00 (*0-8115-3557-6*) Periodicals Srv.

International Congress of Psychology, 19th, London, 1969: Proceedings. 1990. reprint ed. 45.00 (*0-8115-3558-4*) Periodicals Srv.

International Congress of Psychology, 4th: Paris, 1900 (Compte Rendu des Seances et Texte des Memoires) 1969. reprint ed. 75.00 (*0-8115-3545-2*) Periodicals Srv.

International Congress of Psychology, 5th: Rome, 1905 (Atti) 1969. reprint ed. 70.00 (*0-8115-3546-0*) Periodicals Srv.

International Congress of Psychology, 6th: Geneva, 1909 (Rapports et Comptes Rendus) 1969. reprint ed. 75.00 (*0-8115-3547-9*) Periodicals Srv.

International Congress of Psychology, 7th: Oxford, 1923, (Proceedings & Papers) 1969. reprint ed. 45.00 (*0-8115-3548-7*) Periodicals Srv.

International Congress of Psychology, 8th: Groningen, 1926 (Proceedings & Papers) 1969. reprint ed. 45.00 (*0-8115-3549-5*) Periodicals Srv.

International Congress of Psychology, 9th: New Haven, 1929 (Proceedings & Papers) 1969. reprint ed. 55.00 (*0-8115-3550-9*) Periodicals Srv.

International Congress on Clinical Enzymology, Hannover, 6th, Sept. 1987. Ed. by F. W. Schmidt & Ellen Schmidt. 1987. (Enzyme Ser.: Vol. 38, Suppl. 1). (Illus.). ii, 62p. pap. 20.00 (*3-8055-4691-2*) S Karger.

International Congress on Clinical Enzymology, Osaka, 7th, September 1988, Abstracts. Ed. by K. Okuda. 1988. (Journal: Vol. 40, Suppl. 1, 1988). ii, 66p. pap. 21.00 (*3-8055-4915-6*) S Karger.

International Congress on Fibrinolysis, 6th, Lausanne, July 1982: Abstracts. Ed. by F. Bachmann et al. 1982. (Journal: Vol. 11, Suppl. 1, 1982). iv, 108p. pap. 30.50 (*3-8055-3590-2*) S Karger.

International Congress on Fibrinolysis, 7th Abstracts: Venice, March 1984. Ed. by S. Coccheri & Maria B. Donati. 1984. (Journal: Vol. 14, No. 1). 156p. pap. 45.25 (*3-8055-3882-0*) S Karger.

International Congress on Renal Nutrition & Metabolism: 9th International Congress, Vienna, August 1998: Proceedings. Ed. by J. D. Kopple et al. 2000. (Mineral & Electrolyte Metabolism Ser.: Vol. 25, No. 4-6 (2000)). (Illus.). iv, 204p. 48.75 (*3-8055-7018-X*) S Karger.

International Congress on Thrombosis: Plenary Lectures, 13th Congress, Bilbao, 1994. Ed. by J. Monasterio et al. 1994. (Journal: Vol. 24, No. 2, 1994). (Illus.). 94p. pap. 20.00 (*3-8055-6019-2*) S Karger.

International Congress on Thrombosis - 14th Congress, Montpellier, October 1996: Abstracts. Ed. by S. Levy-Toledano et al. 1996. (Haemostasis Ser.: Vol. 26, Supplement 3, 1996). (Illus.). 344p. pap. 104.50 (*3-8055-6399-X*) S Karger.

International Congress on Thrombosis - 14th Congress, Montpellier, October 1996: State of the Art. Ed. by M. H. Horellou & C. Legrand. 1996. (Journal: Vol. 26, Supplement 4, 1996). (Illus.). viii, 392p. pap. 85.25 (*3-8055-6437-6*) S Karger.

International Congress on Thrombosis, 8th, Istanbul, June 1984, Defibrotide Symposium. Ed. by O. N. Ulutin. 1986. (Journal: Vol. 15, Suppl. 1, 1985). (Illus.). iv, 68p. pap. 24.50 (*3-8055-4220-8*) S Karger.

International Continence Society, Annual Meeting, 7th, Portoroz, 1977. Ed. by Georges Mayo. 1978. (Urologia Internationalis Ser.: Vol. 33, No. 5). (Illus.). pap. 34.00 (*3-8055-2974-0*) S Karger.

International Continence Society Conference, 5th, Glascow, Sept. 4-6, 1976: Proceedings of the International Continence Society Conference, 5th, Glascow, Sept. 4-6, 1976. International Continence Society Staff. Ed. by E. S. Glen. 1977. (Urologia Internationalis Ser.: Vol. 32, Nos. 2-3). 64.50 (*3-8055-2745-4*) S Karger.

International Convocation on Immunology. Ed. by Noel R. Rose et al. 1969. 104.50 (*3-8055-0888-3*) S Karger.

International Cooperation for Health: Problems, Prospects & Priorities. Ed. by Michael R. Reich & Eiji Marui. 1989. LC 88-35321. 416p. 75.00 (*0-86569-189-4*, Auburn Hse) Greenwood.

International Cooperation in Response to AIDS. Leon Gordenker et al. 1995. 224p. pap. (*1-85567-283-9*); LC 95-14663. text (*1-85567-282-0*) P P Pubs GBR. *Dist:* Continuum.

International Data on Anthropometry. H. Jurgens et al. Ed. by International Labour Office Staff. 1990. (Occupational Safety & Health Ser.: No. 65).Tr. of Internationaler Anthropometrischer Datenatlas. vii, 113p. pap. 15.75 (*92-2-106449-2*) Intl Labour Office.

International Development of Health Manpower Policy. T. Fulop & M. I. Roemer. 1982. (WHO Offset Publications: No.61). 168p. pap. text 15.00 (*92-4-170061-0*, 1120061) World Health.

International Dictionary of Medicine & Biology. Ed. by Sidney I. Landau. 1988. (Illus.). 3200p. (*0-471-01849-X*) Church.

International Dimensions of Organizational Behavior. Nancy J. Adler. 2nd ed. 1990. 313p. (C). mass mkt. 21.50 (*0-534-92274-0*) S-W Thomson.

International Directory of Bioethics Organizations. Ed. by Anita L. Nolen & Mary C. Coutts. 1993. pap. 20.00 (*1-883913-11-X*) Geo U Kennedy Inst.

International Directory of eHealth & Telemedicine, 2000-2001. 2000. 400p. incl. cd-rom (*0-11-702474-0*) Statnry Office GBR. *Dist:* Balogh.

International Directory of Emergency Response Centres. 1993. 77p. (Orig.). (C). pap. text 30.00 (*1-56806-215-X*) DIANE Pub.

International Directory of Importers - Medical, Hospital, Surgical Equipment & Supplies. Compiled by Interdata Staff. rev. ed. 2000. 388p. ring bd. 270.00 (*1-58239-010-X*) Interdata.

International Directory of Mental Retardation Resources. 1988. 68p. (*1-55672-051-3*) US HHS.

International Directory of Occupational Safety & Health Institutions. 1990. (Occupational Safety & Health Ser.: No. 66). xxix, 272p. (Orig.). pap. 31.50 (*92-2-106452-2*) Intl Labour Office.

International Directory of Organizations: Standards & Developments in the Creation of Electronic Health Records. Ed. by C. Peter Waegemann. 2nd ed. 1995. (Illus.). 122p. pap. 42.50 (*0-9640667-6-9*) Medical Recs.

International Directory of Specialized Cancer Research & Treatment Facilities. Compiled by International Union Against Cancer Staff. 4th ed. 1986. 756p. 370.00 (*0-89116-010-8*) Hemisp Pub.

International Drinking Water Supply & Sanitation Decade: Review of Regional & Global Data (As at Dec. 31, 1983) 1986. (WHO Offset Publications: No. 92). 30p. pap. text 6.00 (*92-4-170092-0*, 1120092) World Health.

International Drinking Water Supply & Sanitation Decade: The Review of National Baseline Data (As at 31 December 1980) WHO Staff. 1984. (WHO Offset Publications: No. 85). 169p. 15.00 (*92-4-170085-8*) World Health.

International Drug Benefit - Risk Assessment Handbook: Australia & New Zealand, Vol. V. Ed. by Judith K. Jones. 1993. LC 90-111751. 320.00 (*0-9632020-1-4*) Degge Grp.

International Drug Benefit - Risk Assessment Handbook Vol. IV: Japan. Ed. by Judith K. Jones. 1992. text 295.00 (*1-879733-03-X*) Degge Grp.

International Drug Control: A Study of International Administration by & Through the League of Nations. B. A. Renborg. 1941. (Studies in the Administration of International Law & Organization). reprint ed. 25.00 (*0-527-00885-0*) Periodicals Srv.

International Drug Monitoring - The Role of National Centres: Proceedings of the WHO Expert Committee, Geneva, 1971. WHO Staff. 1972. (Technical Reports: No. 498). pap. text 4.00 (*92-4-120498-2*, 1100498) World Health.

International Drug Monitoring - The Role of the Hospital: Proceedings of the WHO Expert Committee, Geneva, 1968. WHO Staff. 1969. (Technical Reports: No. 425). pap. text 3.00 (*92-4-120425-7*, 1100425) World Health.

International Encyclopedia of Development & Instructional Psychology. E. De Corte & F. Weinert. 1996. LC 96-17900. (Resources in Education Ser.: 6). (Illus.). 1002p. 169.50 (*0-08-042980-7*, Pergamon Pr) Elsevier.

International Encyclopedia of Development & Instructional Psychology. E. De Corte & Franz E. Weinert. 1996. (*0-08-042706-5*, Pergamon Pr) Elsevier.

International Ethical Guidelines for Biomedical Research Involving Human Subjects. 1993. 63p. pap. text 10.00 (*92-9036-056-9*, 1840016) World Health.

International Experience with Nitrates. Ed. by Adam Schneeweiss & Marija Weiss. 1991. (Journal: Vol. 79, Supplement 2, 1991). (Illus.). 92p. pap. 28.75 (*3-8055-5486-9*) S Karger.

International Federation of Clinical Chemistry: Recommendations & Related Documents, Volume 1, 1978-1983. Ed. by Nils-Erik Saris. 1984. LC 84-16994. 146p. pap. 73.85 (*3-11-008766-9*) De Gruyter.

International Forum on Advanced Techniques in Lens & Cataract Research: 7th Scheimpflug Club Meeting, Kanazawa, June 1995. Ed. by K. Sasaki & Otto Hockwin. 1996. (Journal: Vol. 28, Suppl. 2, 1996). (Illus.). viii, 142p. pap. 47.00 (*3-8055-6379-5*) S Karger.

International Fragile X Conference Proceedings, 1992. Spectra Publishing Co., Inc. Staff. Ed. by Randi J. Hagerman & Pamela McKenzie. 1992. (Illus.). pap. text 20.00 (*0-915667-22-3*) Spectra Pub Co.

International Good Clinical Practice: The GCP Compliance Handbook. Nigel J. Dent et al. 1995. (Illus.). 380p. ring bd. 249.00 (*0-935184-83-X*) IHS Health Grp.

International Guidelines for Ethical Review of Epidemiological Studies. 1991. 31p. pap. text 6.00 (*92-9036-049-6*, 1840013) World Health.

International Handbook of Adolescence. Ed. by Klaus Hurrelmann. 1994. LC 93-14124. 488p. lib. bdg. 100.00 (*0-313-28584-5*, HIJ/, Greenwood Pr) Greenwood.

International Handbook of Behavior Modification & Therapy. Ed. by Alan S. Bellack et al. 2nd ed. 1989. (Illus.). 908p. (C). 130.00 (*0-306-43348-6*, Plenum Trade) Perseus Pubng.

International Handbook of Behavior Modification & Therapy: Student Edition. A. S. Bellack et al. abr. ed. 1985. LC 84-226552. (Illus.). 484p. (C). 49.50 (*0-306-41876-2*, Plenum Trade) Perseus Pubng.

International Handbook of Cognitive & Behavioural Treatments for Psychological Disorders. V. E. Caballo. 1998. LC 98-42129. 712p. 106.00 (*0-08-043433-9*, Pergamon Pr) Elsevier.

International Handbook of Community Services for the Mentally Retarded. Jack A. Stark et al. 1984. 280p. (C). text 49.95 (*0-89859-385-9*) L Erlbaum Assocs.

International Handbook of Health Care Systems. Ed. by Richard B. Saltman. 1988. LC 87-17797. 409p. lib. bdg. 95.00 (*0-313-24111-2*, SHH/, Greenwood Pr) Greenwood.

International Handbook of Medical Education. Ed. by Abudl W. Sajid et al. 1994. LC 93-37854. 544p. lib. bdg. 120.00 (*0-313-28423-7*, Greenwood Pr) Greenwood.

International Handbook of Neuropsychological Rehabilitation. Barbara P. Uzzell. Ed. by Anne-Lise Christensen. 1999. LC 99-41442. (Critical Issues in Neuropsychology Ser.). 392p. 110.00 (*0-306-46174-9*) Kluwer Academic.

International Handbook of Pancreas Transplantation. Ed. by J. M. Dubernard & David E. Sutherland. 1989. (Developments in Surgery Ser.). (C). text 346.00 (*0-89838-399-4*) Kluwer Academic.

International Handbook of Personality & Intelligence. Ed. by Donald H. Saklofske & Moshe Zeidner. 1995. (Perspectives on Individual Differences Ser.). (Illus.). 800p. (C). 114.00 (*0-306-44749-5*, Plenum Trade) Perseus Pubng.

International Handbook of Phobic & Anxiety Disorders in Children & Adolescents. Ed. by Thomas H. Ollendick et al. 1994. (Illus.). 510p. (C). 85.00 (*0-306-44759-2*, Plenum Trade) Perseus Pubng.

International Handbook of Psychology. Ed. by Albert R. Gilgen & Carol K. Gilgen. 1987. LC 86-29457. 687p. lib. bdg. 100.00 (*0-313-23832-4*, GIP/, Greenwood Pr) Greenwood.

***International Handbook of Psychology.** Ed. by Kurt Pawlik & Mark R. Rosenzweig. 2000. LC 00-712694. (Illus.). xxxii, 629p. 99.95 (*0-7619-5329-9*) Sage.

International Handbook of Public Health. Ed. by Klaus Hurrelman & Ulrich Laaser. 1996. LC 95-46131. 496p. lib. bdg. 110.00 (*0-313-29500-X*, Greenwood Pr) Greenwood.

International Handbook of Traumatic Stress Syndromes. Ed. by J. P. Wilson & B. Raphael. 1993. (Stress & Coping Ser.). (Illus.). 1046p. 180.00 (*0-306-43795-3*, Kluwer Plenum) Kluwer Academic.

International Handbook on Abortion. Ed. by Paul Sachdev. 1988. LC 87-11994. 532p. lib. bdg. 110.00 (*0-313-23463-9*, SBO/, Greenwood Pr) Greenwood.

International Handbook on Drug Control. Ed. by Scott B. MacDonald & Bruce Zagaris. 1992. LC 91-35118. 463p. lib. bdg. 105.00 (*0-313-27375-8*, MHB/, Greenwood Pr) Greenwood.

International Handbook on Mental Health Policy. Ed. by Donna R. Kemp. 1993. LC 92-48399. 512p. lib. bdg. 130.00 (*0-313-27567-X*, KHM, Greenwood Pr) Greenwood.

International Health. Paul F. Basch. 1978. (Illus.). 392p. text 29.95 (*0-19-502328-5*) OUP.

International Health. E. William Ebomoyi. 1995. 344p. (*0-697-16909-X*) Brown & Benchmark.

International Health & Safety Regulations. Kenneth Kilimnik. 1994. LC 94-6107. 151.00 (*90-6544-891-8*) Kluwer Law Intl.

International Health Care Reform: Legal, Economic & Political Analysis. Colleen Flood. 2000. LC 00-700460. (Studies in the Modern World Economy: Vol. 24). (Illus.). viii, 315p. (C). text 100.00 (*0-415-20844-0*) Routledge.

International Health Data Reference Guide, 1993. Jacqueline P. Davis. 6th ed. 1994. (Illus.). 118p. (C). pap. text 40.00 (*0-7881-0691-0*) DIANE Pub.

International Health Data Reference Guide, 1995. Jacqueline P. Davis. 1996. (Illus.). 140p. (Orig.). pap. text 40.00 (*0-7881-3244-X*) DIANE Pub.

*__International Health Data Reference Guide (1999)__ Ed. by Edward J. Sondik. 2001. 157p. (C). pap. text 45.00 (*0-7567-0608-4*) DIANE Pub.

__International Health Electives for Medical Students__, Set. 5th rev. ed. 1993. pap. (*1-878642-00-6*) AMSA Pubns.

__International Health Organisations & Movements, 1918-1939.__ Ed. by Paul Weindling. 1995. (History of Medicine Ser.). 355p. (C). text 69.95 (*0-521-45012-8*) Cambridge U Pr.

__International Health Statistics: What the Numbers Mean for the U. S.__ 1995. (Illus.). 163p. (C). pap. text 35.00 (*0-7881-2507-9*) DIANE Pub.

__International Health Statistics: What the Numbers Mean for the U. S.__ 1995. lib. bdg. 251.95 (*0-8490-6689-1*); 1994. lib. bdg. 250.00 (*0-8490-8403-2*) Gordon Pr.

__International Incidence of Childhood Cancer.__ Ed. by D. M. Parkin et al. (IARC Scientific Publications Ser.: No. 87). 1988. (Illus.). 432p. 75.00 (*92-832-1187-1*); Vol. 2. 1999. LC 99-462609. 504p. (C). pap. text 69.00 (*92-832-2144-3*) OUP.

__International Journal of Psychoanalytic Psychotherapy__, Vol. 8. Ed. by Robert J. Langs. 1980. LC 75-648853. 705p. 35.00 (*0-87668-428-2*) Aronson.

__International Journal of Psychoanalytic Psychotherapy__, Vol. 11. Ed. by John M. Ross. 1986. LC 75-648853. 460p. 40.00 (*0-87668-896-2*) Aronson.

__International Law & Infectious Diseases.__ David P. Fidler. 1999. LC 98-50345. (Oxford Monographs in International Law). (Illus.). 412p. text 75.00 (*0-19-826851-3*) OUP.

__International Law of Pollution: Protecting the Global Environment in a World of Sovereign States.__ Allen L. Springer. 1983. LC 82-23194. 218p. 62.95 (*0-89930-052-9*, SPO/, Quorum Bks) Greenwood.

__International Massage & Bodywork Resource Guide.__ Robert Calvert & Noel Abildgaard. 1991. 114p. pap. 12.95 (*1-879933-03-9*) Noah Pub.

__International Medical Communication.__ John C. Maher. 1992. LC 91-36916. 200p. (C). pap. text 17.95 (*0-472-08174-8*, 08174) U of Mich Pr.

__International Medical Device & Diagnostic GMPs.__ Ed. by Michael H. Anisfeld. 3rd ed. 1995. 225p. ring bd. 262.00 (*0-935184-35-X*) IHS Health Grp.

__International Medical Device Clinical Investigations: A Practical Approach.__ Ed. by Herman Pieterse et al. 1997. LC 97-26007. (Illus.). 550p. 219.00 (*1-57491-054-X*) IHS Health Grp.

__International Medical Device Clinical Investigations: A Practical Approach.__ Ed. by Hermann Pieterse et al. 2nd ed. 1998. LC 99-19067. 562p. text 219.00 (*1-57491-085-X*) IHS Health Grp.

__International Medical Device Registration.__ Ed. by Maria Donawa. 1996. 488p. ring bd. 249.00 (*0-935184-85-6*) IHS Health Grp.

__International Medical Graduate's Guide to U. S. Medicine: Negotiating the Maze.__ Louise B. Ball. 1995. LC 95-13724. 220p. (Orig.). pap. 28.95 (*1-883620-16-3*) Galen AZ.

__International Medical Graduates Guide to U. S. Medicine: Negotiating the Maze.__ Gloria A. Goldman. 2nd ed. 2001. pap. (*1-883620-04-X*) Galen AZ.

__International Medical Graduates in the United States: Challenges & Opportunities.__ Syed A. Husain et al. 1997. LC 97-152. (Issues in Psychiatry Ser.). 138p. pap. text 22.50 (*0-88048-294-X*, 8294) Am Psychiatric.

__International Medical Graduates in U. S. Hospitals: A Guide for Program Directors.__ Ed. by Faroque A. Khan & Lawrence G. Smith. 1995. LC 95-1646. 100p. pap. 26.00 (*0-943126-41-X*) Amer Coll Phys.

__International Medical Guide for Ships: Including the Ship's Medicine Chest.__ Illus. by S. Smyth. 2nd ed. 1988. vi, 368p. text 60.00 (*92-4-154231-4*, 1152078) World Health.

__International Medical Malpractice Law: A Comparative Study of Civil Responsibility Arising from Medical Care.__ Dieter Giesen. 1988. 940p. lib. bdg. 328.00 (*90-247-3705-2*) Kluwer Academic.

__International Medicines Regulations: A Forward Look to 1992.__ Ed. by Stuart R. Walker & John P. Griffin. 1989. (C). text 223.00 (*0-7462-0120-6*) Kluwer Academic.

__International Meeting on Spinal Cord Stimulation, 3rd.__ Ed. by Philip L. Gildenberg. 1981. (Illus.). 176p. pap. 91.50 (*3-8055-3462-0*) S Karger.

__International Mortality Chartbook: Levels & Trends, 1955-91.__ Alvan O. Zarate. 1997. (Illus.). 191p. (C). reprint ed. pap. text 40.00 (*0-7881-4212-7*) DIANE Pub.

__International Narcotics Control.__ L. E. Eisenlohr. Ed. by Gerald N. Grob. 1981. LC 80-1226. (Addiction in America Ser.). reprint ed. lib. bdg. 29.95 (*0-405-13584-X*) Ayer.

__International Natural Killer Cell Workshop, 8th, & First Meeting of the Society for Natural Immunity, St. Petersburg Beach, October 1992: Abstracts.__ Ed. by Eva Lotzova et al. 1992. (Journal: Vol. 11, No. 5, 1992). 80p. pap. 41.00 (*3-8055-5690-X*) S Karger.

__International Neutron Therapy Workshop.__ Yosh Maruyama. 1991. (Nuclear Science Applications Ser.: Vol. 2). 280p. pap. text 501.00 (*3-7186-5124-6*);Pt. 1. xx, 228p. pap. text 448.00 (*3-7186-5123-8*) Gordon & Breach (Harwood Acad Pubs).

__International Nomenclature of Diseases Vol. II: Infectious Diseases Pt. 1: Bacterial Diseases.__ 1985. 158p. pap. 20.00 (*92-9036-022-4*) World Health.

__International Nonproprietary Names (INN) for Pharmaceutical Substances: Lists 1-65 of Proposed INN & Lists 1-31 of Recommended INN.__ WHO Staff. 1992. (Cumulative List Ser.: No. 8). (FRE.). xlvi, 692p. pap. text 126.00 (*92-4-056015-7*, 0150389) World Health.

__International Nonproprietary Names (INN) for Pharmaceutical Substances No. 9: Lists 1-73 of Proposed INN & Lists 1-35 of Recommended INN Cumulative List.__ 1996. LC 97-161267. 885p. (Orig.). pap. 225.00 (*92-4-056016-5*, 0150442) Am Soc Clinical.

__International Nutrition in Health & Disease.__ Ed. by Geoffrey H. Bourne. 1987. (World Review of Nutrition & Dietetics Ser.: Vol. 51). (Illus.). x, 240p. 182.75 (*3-8055-4581-9*) S Karger.

__International Occupational & Environmental Medicine.__ Herzstein et al. 1998. LC 98-14012. (Illus.). 752p. (C). (gr. 13). text 115.00 (*0-8151-4362-1*, 30225) Mosby Inc.

__International Occupational Safety & Health Resource Catalogue.__ Jane H. Ives. 1981. LC 81-13823. 311p. 82.50 (*0-275-90651-5*, C0651, Praeger Pubs) Greenwood.

__International Perspectives in Environment, Development, & Health: Toward a Sustainable World.__ Ed. by Gurinder Shahi et al. 1996. LC 95-33678. (Illus.). 744p. 79.95 (*0-8261-9190-8*) Springer Pub.

__International Perspectives in Health Economics: Selected Papers from the World Congress in Health Economics, Leiden, the Netherlands, September 1980.__ Gavin H. Mooney. 1981. (Journal of Social Science & Medicine Ser.: No. 15). 72p. pap. 18.00 (*0-08-028131-1*, Pergamon Pr) Elsevier.

__International Perspectives on Healthcare for the Elderly.__ Ed. by G. Harry Stopp, Jr. 1994. LC 93-36817. 326p. 59.95 (*0-8204-2319-X*) P Lang Pubng.

__International Perspectives on Long-Term Care.__ Ed. by Laura Reif & Brahna Trager. 1985. LC 85-8442. (Home Health Care Services Quarterly Ser.: Vol. 5, Nos. 3 & 4). 341p. text 79.95 (*0-86656-400-4*); pap. text 24.95 (*0-86656-445-4*) Haworth Pr.

__International Perspectives on Psychology in the Schools.__ Ed. by T. Oakland & Philip A. Saigh. 1989. (School Psychology Ser.). 296p. 59.95 (*0-8058-0110-3*) L Erlbaum Assocs.

__International Perspectives on Self-Regulation & Health.__ J. G. Carlson & A. R. Seifert. 1991. (Behavioral Psychophysiology Ser.). (Illus.). 310p. (C). text 60.00 (*0-306-43557-8*, Kluwer Plenum) Kluwer Academic.

__International Perspectives on Social Work in Health Care: Past, Present, & Future.__ Ed. by Gail K. Auslander. 1997. LC 97-10583. 272p. 39.95 (*0-7890-0325-2*) Haworth Pr.

__International Pharmaceutical Marketing.__ Suresh B. Pradhan. 1983. LC 82-15022. 281p. 59.95 (*0-89930-009-X*, PPH/, Quorum Bks) Greenwood.

__International Pharmaceutical Registration.__ Alan A. Chalmers. 2000. LC 99-86387. 249.00 (*1-57491-103-1*) IHS Health Grp.

__International Pharmaceutical Services: The Drug Industry & Pharmacy Practice in Twenty-Three Major Countries of the World.__ T. Donald Parker. Ed. by Richard N. Spivey et al. 1996. LC 91-6794. 675p. pap. 39.95 (*0-7890-0078-4*) Haworth Pr.

__International Pharmaceutical Services: The Drug Industry & Pharmacy Practice in Twenty-Three Major Countries of the World.__ T. Donald Parker & George Griffinhagen. Ed. by Richard N. Spivey et al. 1992. LC 91-6794. (Illus.). 675p. 89.95 (*0-86656-906-5*) Haworth Pr.

__International Pharmacopoeia.__ 3rd ed. Vol. 2. 1982. (*0-85369-054-5*); Vol. 3. 1988. pap. (*0-85369-213-0*) Pharmaceutical Pr GBR. *Dist:* Rittenhouse.

__International Pharmacopoeia: General Methods of Analysis__, Vol. 1. 3rd ed. 1979. (Nonserial Publication). 223p. 36.00 (*92-4-154150-4*, 1151091) World Health.

__International Pharmacopoeia Vol. 3: Quality Specifications.__ WHO Staff. 1988. 407p. 64.00 (*92-4-154215-2*, 1153091) World Health.

__International Pharmacopoeia Vol. 4: Tests, Methods, & General Requirements; Quality Specifications for Pharmaceutical Substances, Excipients, & Dosage Forms.__ WHO Staff. 3rd ed. 1994. (FRE & SPA.). xv, 343p. pap. text 85.00 (*92-4-154462-7*, 1154091) World Health.

*__International Pharmacopoeia Vol. 5: Tests & General Requirements for Dosage Forms - Quality Specifications for Pharmaceutical Substances & Dosage Forms - Quality Specifications for Pharmaceutical Substances & Dosage Forms.__ World Health Organisation Staff. 3rd ed. 2001. 400p. 94.00 (*92-4-154536-4*) World Health.

__International Pilot Study of Schizophrenia__, Vol. 1. 1973. (Offset Publications: No. 2). pap. text 56.00 (*92-4-170002-5*, 1120002) World Health.

__International Practice in Cardiothoracic Surgery.__ Ed. by Wu Ying-Kai & Richard M. Peters. 1986. text 461.50 (*0-89838-784-1*) Kluwer Academic.

__International Practice of Anaesthesia__ Ed. by Cedric Prys-Roberts & Burnell R. Brown, Jr. 6th ed. 1996. LC 97-104572. 1536p. text 265.00 (*0-7506-0240-6*) Buttrwrth-Heinemann.

__International Practice of Anaesthesia Update.__ Roberts. Date not set. 448p. pap. text 60.00 (*0-7506-4216-5*) Buttrwrth-Heinemann.

__International Psychiatric Directory.__ American Psychiatric Association Staff. 1993. 80p. pap. 35.00 (*0-89042-248-6*, 2248) Am Psychiatric.

__International Psychological Science: Progress, Problems, & Prospects.__ Ed. by Mark R. Rosenzweig. 1992. 306p. pap. text 14.95 (*1-55798-168-X*) Am Psychol.

__International Psychotherapy: Theories, Research & Cross-Cultural Implications.__ Ed. by Lynn Simek-Downing. 1989. LC 88-26578. 270p. 67.00 (*0-275-93096-3*, C3096, Praeger Pubs) Greenwood.

__International Quarantine.__ Oleg Schepin & Waldemar Ermakov. 1991. 350p. 50.00 (*0-8236-2725-X*, BN#02725) Intl Univs Pr.

__International Rare Book Prices: Science & Medicine, 1988.__ Ed. by Michael Cole. 1988. 248p. (*1-870773-04-7*) Spoon River.

__International Regulatory Aspects for Pesticide Chemicals__, Vol. II. Ed. by G. Vettorazzi. 1982. 256p. 146.00 (*0-8493-5608-3*, RA1270) CRC Pr.

__International Regulatory Aspects for Pesticide Chemicals.__ G. Vettorazzi. 1979. 232p. 82.00 (*0-8493-5607-5*, CRC Reprint) Franklin.

__International Rehabilitation: Approaches & Programs.__ Richard E. Hardy et al. 1989. 200p. text 26.50 (*0-8290-0399-1*); pap. text 12.95 (*0-8290-0247-2*) Irvington.

__International Research in Sexology: Selected Papers from the Fifth World Congress__, 1. Harold I. Lief & Zwi Hoch. 1984. LC 83-21146. 216p. 62.95 (*0-275-91442-9*, C1442, Praeger Pubs) Greenwood.

__International Resource Directory for Preoperative Nursing.__ 1996. LC 96-224742. 90p. (Orig.). (C). pap. text 25.00 (*0-939583-95-X*) AORN.

__International Responses to Traumatic Stress: Humanitarian, Human Rights, Justice, Peace, & Development Contributions, Collaborative Actions, & Future Initiatives.__ Ed. by Yael Danieli et al. 1995. 484p. 48.00 (*0-89503-132-9*) Baywood Pub.

__International Review of Child Neurology.__ Ed. by International Child Neurology Association Staff. Date not set. (C). (*0-521-49490-7*) Cambridge U Pr.

__International Review of Cytology: A Survey of Cell Biology__, Vol. 148. Ed. by Kwang W. Jeon & Jonathan W. Jarvik. 1994. (Illus.). 319p. text 94.00 (*0-12-364551-4*) Acad Pr.

__International Review of Cytology: A Survey of Cell Biology__, Vol. 156. Ed. by Kwang W. Jeon & Jonathan Jarvik. 1994. (Illus.). 387p. text 90.00 (*0-12-364559-X*) Acad Pr.

__International Review of Cytology Vol. 165: A Survey of Cell Biology.__ Ed. by Kwang W. Jeon. 1996. (Illus.). 305p. text 85.00 (*0-12-364569-7*) Acad Pr.

__International Review of Cytology Vol. 202: A Survey of Cell Biology.__ Ed. by Kwang W. Jeon. 2000. 129.95 (*0-12-364606-5*) Acad Pr.

__International Review of Cytology Vol. 203: Cell Lineage & Embryo Patterning.__ Kwang W. Jeon. 2000. 544p. pap. 70.00 (*0-12-384621-8*) Acad Pr.

*__International Review of Cytology Vol. 206: A Survey of Cell Biology.__ Ed. by Kwang W. Jeon. 2001. (Illus.). 315p. 129.95 (*0-12-364610-3*) Acad Pr.

__International Review of Cytology, Molecular Biology of Receptors & Transporters, Vol. 137A: A Survey of Cell Biology, Bacterial & Glucose Transporters.__ Ed. by Kwang W. Jeon & Martin Friedlander. 1992. (Illus.). 376p. text 94.00 (*0-12-364537-9*) Acad Pr.

__International Review of Experimental Pathology__, Vol. 35. Ed. by Kim Solez & Sibrand Poppema. 1994. (Illus.). 202p. (C). text 84.00 (*0-12-364936-6*) Acad Pr.

__International Review of Experimental Pathology: Cytokine-Induced Pathology, Inflammatory Cytokines, Receptors, & Disease__, Vol. 34, Pt. B. Ed. by Bernhard Ryffel et al. 1993. (Illus.). 232p. (C). text 94.00 (*0-12-364935-8*) Acad Pr.

__International Review of Experimental Pathology Vol. 33: Progress in Hodgkins Disease.__ Ed. by Goetz W. Richter et al. 1992. (Illus.). 368p. (C). text 104.00 (*0-12-366833-6*) Acad Pr.

__International Review of Experimental Pathology Vol. 34, Pt. A: Cytokine-Induced Pathology, Interleukins & Hemopoietic Growth Factors.__ Ed. by Bernhard Ryffel et al. 1993. (Illus.). 252p. (C). text 94.00 (*0-12-364934-X*) Acad Pr.

__International Review of Experimental Pathology Vol. 36: New In Vivo & In Vitro Imaging Techniques.__ Ed. by Virginia J. Savin & Thomas B. Wiegmann. 1996. (Illus.). 224p. (C). text 89.00 (*0-12-364937-4*) Acad Pr.

__International Review of Health Psychology__, Vol. 1. Ed. by Stan Maes et al. 1992. 240p. 500.00 (*0-471-92754-6*) Wiley.

__International Review of Health Psychology, Vol. 2__, Vol. 2. Ed. by Stan Maes et al. 1993. 246p. 500.00 (*0-471-93826-2*) Wiley.

__International Review of Industrial & Organizational Psychology__, Vol. 95. Ed. by Cary L. Cooper & Ivan T. Robertson. 1995. 384p. 300.00 (*0-471-95241-9*) Wiley.

__International Review of Industrial & Organizational Psychology, 1987__, Vol. 87. Cooper. 1987. LC 86-643874. 378p. 325.00 (*0-471-91352-9*) Wiley.

__International Review of Industrial & Organizational Psychology, 1991__, Vol. 6. Ed. by C. L. Cooper & Ivan T. Robertson. 1991. LC 86-643874. 412p. 325.00 (*0-471-92819-4*) Wiley.

__International Review of Mental Imagery__, Vol. 1. Ed. by Anees Sheikh. 1984. 256p. 43.95 (*0-89885-164-5*, Kluwer Acad Hman Sci) Kluwer Academic.

__International Review of Neurobiology__, Vol. 34. Ed. by Ronald J. Bradley. 1992. (Illus.). 410p. (C). text 104.00 (*0-12-366834-4*) Acad Pr.

__International Review of Neurobiology__, Vol. 35. Ed. by Ronald J. Bradley & Robert A. Harris. 1993. (Illus.). 442p. (C). text 110.00 (*0-12-366835-2*) Acad Pr.

__International Review of Neurobiology__, Vol. 36. Ed. by Ronald J. Bradley & R. Adron Harris. 1994. (Illus.). 444p. (C). text 104.00 (*0-12-366836-0*) Acad Pr.

__International Review of Neurobiology: Neuromuscular Junctions in Drosophila__, Vol. 43. Ed. by Vivian Budnik et al. 1999. LC 99-207390. (International Review of Neurobiology Ser.: Vol. 43). (Illus.). 289p. pap. 59.95 (*0-12-139370-4*) Acad Pr.

__International Review of Neurobiology: Selectionism & the Brain__, Vol. 37. Ed. by Olaf Sporns & Giulio Tononi. 1994. (Illus.). 386p. (C). text 100.00 (*0-12-366837-9*) Acad Pr.

__International Review of Neurobiology Vol. 40: Neuroprotective Agents & Cerebral Ischaemia.__ Ed. by Alan J. Cross & A. Richard Green. 1996. (Illus.). 416p. (C). text 95.00 (*0-12-366840-9*); (International Review of Neurobiology Ser.: Vol. 40). pap. text 55.00 (*0-12-197880-X*) Morgan Kaufmann.

__International Review of Neurobiology Vol. 41: The Cerebellum & Cognition.__ Ed. by Ronald J. Bradley, Jr. et al. 1997. LC 97-202511. (Illus.). 665p. (C). text 99.95 (*0-12-366841-7*);41. (International Review of Neurobiology Ser.: Vol. 41). pap. text 69.95 (*0-12-625660-8*) Morgan Kaufmann.

__International Review of Perinatology.__ E. Nunes de Morais. 2002. 250p. 67.95 (*1-84214-041-8*, Parthenon Pbng) CRC Pr.

__International Review of Psychiatry__, Vol. 2. Ed. by Felice L. Mak & Carol C. Nadelson. 1996. LC 96-13648. 494p. text 59.95 (*0-88048-992-8*, 8992) Am Psychiatric.

__International Review of Research in Mental Retardation__, Vol. 18. Ed. by Norman W. Bray. 1992. (Illus.). 309p. (C). text 105.00 (*0-12-366218-4*) Acad Pr.

__International Review of Research in Mental Retardation.__ Ed. by Norman W. Bray. 1997. (Illus.). (C). Vol. 20. (International Review of Research in Mental Retardation Ser.: Vol. 20). 263p. text 90.00 (*0-12-366220-6*); Vol. 21. 268p. text 95.00 (*0-12-366221-4*) Morgan Kaufmann.

__International Review of Research in Mental Retardation__, Vol. 22. Ed. by Larraine M. Glidden. 1999. (International Review of Research in Mental Retardation Ser.: Vol. 22). (Illus.). 328p. 99.95 (*0-12-366222-2*) Acad Pr.

__International Society for Oncodevelopmental Biology & Medicine, 15th Annual Meeting, Quebec, 15th August-Sept. 1987 Abstracts.__ 1988. (Tumor Biology Ser.: Vol. 8, No. 6). 102p. pap. 60.00 (*3-8055-4759-5*) S Karger.

__International Society for Prosthetics & Orthotics, Proceedings, 7th World Congress.__ 1992. 486p. pap. 35.00 (*0-9633698-0-6*) Int Soc Pros & Orth.

__International Society of Blood Purification.__ Ed. by H. B. Lee & H. C. Park. 1995. (Journal: Vol. 13, Suppl. 1, 1995). (Illus.). 70p. pap. 21.75 (*3-8055-6239-X*) S Karger.

__International Society of Blood Purification: 15th Annual Meeting, Florence, September 1997: Abstracts.__ Ed. by Quirino Maggiore & Francesco Pizzarelli. 1997. (Blood Purification Ser.: Vol. 15, Suppl. 2, 1997). (Illus.). xiv, 52p. pap. 39.25 (*3-8055-6592-5*) S Karger.

__International Society of Blood Purification, 10th Annual Meeting, Louisville, October, 1992: Abstracts.__ Ed. by R. Ward. 1992. (Journal: Vol. 10, No. 2, 1992). (Illus.). 48p. pap. 36.75 (*3-8055-5675-6*) S Karger.

__International Society of Blood Purification, 11th Annual Meeting, Trondheim-Norway, September, 1993, Abstracts.__ Ed. by S. Jorstad. 1993. (Journal: Vol. 11, No. 3, 1993). (Illus.). 68p. pap. 44.50 (*3-8055-5859-7*) S Karger.

__International Society of Blood Purification, 11th Annual Meeting, Trondheim, September 1993.__ Ed. by T. E. Widere & K. L. Leunissen. 1994. (Journal: Vol. 12, No. 4-5, 1994). (Illus.). 82p. pap. 47.00 (*3-8055-6070-2*) S Karger.

__International Society of Blood Purification 12th Annual Meeting, Maastricht, September 1994 Abstracts: Journal: Blood Purification__, Vol. 12, No. 3. Ed. by K. M. Leunissen. 1994. (Journal). (Illus.). 62p. pap. 47.00 (*3-8055-6052-4*) S Karger.

__International Society of Blood Purification, 9th Annual Meeting, Nagoya, June 1991: Journal: Blood Purification__, Vol. 9, No. 1, 1991. Ed. by A. Saito. 1991. 60p. pap. 42.75 (*3-8055-5438-9*) S Karger.

__International Society of Blood Transfusion: 24th Congress, Makuhari Messe/Japan, March/April 1996.__ Ed. by K. Ito. 1996. (Vox Sanguinis: Vol. 70, Suppl. 2, 1996). (Illus.). viii, 199p. pap. 90.50 (*3-8055-6320-5*) S Karger.

__International Society of Blood Transfusion: 25th Congress, Oslo, June-July 1998: Abstracts.__ Ed. by Bjorn M. Eggen. 1998. (Vox Sanguinis Ser.: Vol. 74, Supplement 1, 1998). (Illus.). 256p. pap. 111.50 (*3-8055-6730-8*) S Karger.

International Society of Blood Transfusion: 25th Congress, Oslo, June-July 1998: Plenary & State-of-the-Art Lectures. Ed. by Tom Kristensen. 1998. (Vox Sanguinis Ser.: Vol. 74, Supplement 2, 1998). (Illus.). vi, 538p. pap. 236.50 (*3-8055-6731-6*) S Karger.

International Society of Blood Transfusion: 26th Congress, Vienna, July 2000: Abstracts. Ed. by W. R. Mayr & D. W. M. Schwartz. 2000. (Vox Sanguinis Ser.: Vol. 78). 254p. pap. 48.75 (*3-8055-7114-3*) S Karger.

International Society of Blood Transfusion: 26th Congress, Vienna, July 2000: Pienary & State-of-the-Art Lectures. Ed. by W. R. Mayr & D. W. M. Schwartz. 2000. vi, 310p. 48.75 (*3-8055-7115-1*) S Karger.

International Society of Blood Transfusion, 18th Congress, Munich 1984: Abstracts. 1984. 240p. pap. 26.25 (*3-8055-3943-6*) S Karger.

International Society of Blood Transfusion, 23rd Congress, Amsterdam 1994: State of the Art Lectures, No. 67. Ed. by W. G. Van Aken et al. 1994. (Vox Sanguinis: Supplement 3, 1994). (Illus.). iv, 274p. pap. 82.75 (*3-8055-6018-4*) S Karger.

International Sports Medicine Directory. International Federation of Sports Medicine Staff. 2000. 280p. pap. text 50.00 (*0-7360-3376-9*) Human Kinetics.

International Statistical Classification of Diseases & Related Health Problems (ICD-10) Vol. 3: Alphabetical Index. WHO Staff. 10th ed. 1994. LC 93-154168. (ENG, FRE & SPA.). iii, 750p. text 119.00 (*92-4-154421-X*, 1153331) World Health.

International Summer School of Brain Research. University of Amsterdam & Academic Medical Center. 1994. LC 94-23440. (Progress in Brain Research Ser.). 462p. 237.00 (*0-444-81819-7*) Elsevier.

International Surgical Practice. Ed. by David J. Leaper & Frank J. Branicki. 1992. (Illus.). 432p. pap. 59.00 (*0-19-262252-8*) OUP.

International Symposium Dorsal Root Entry Zone (DREZ) Lesions, Durham, N. C., 2nd, April 1987. Ed. by P. L. Gildenberg et al. 1988. (Journal: Vol. 51, Nos. 2-5, 1988). (Illus.). 204p. pap. 156.75 (*3-8055-4747-1*) S Karger.

International Symposium on Advanced Techniques & Clinical Applications in Biomedical Thermology. Ed. by K. Mabuchi. 1995. 324p. pap. text 61.00 (*3-7186-5628-0*, Harwood Acad Pubs) Gordon & Breach.

International Symposium on AIDS & Cancer, Sao Paulo, Brazil, August 1988: Natural Immunity & Cell Growth Regulation Journal, Vol. 9, No. 3, 1990. Ed. by Eva Lotzova et al. 1990. (Illus.). 108p. pap. 68.00 (*3-8055-5225-4*) S Karger.

International Symposium on BCG Vaccine, 32nd, Frankfurt, 1972: Proceedings of the International Symposium on BCG Vaccine, 32nd, Frankfurt, 1972. International Symposium on BCG Vaccine Staff. Ed. by R. H. Regamey et al. 1971. (Immunobiological Standardization Symposia Ser.: Vol. 17). 26.25 (*3-8055-1256-2*) S Karger.

International Symposium on Biological Preparations in the Treatment of Cancer. Ed. by International Association of Biological Standardiz & R. H. Regamey. 1978. (Developments in Biological Standardization Ser.: Vol. 38). (Illus.). 61.00 (*3-8055-2785-3*) S Karger.

International Symposium on Biotelemetry, 5th, Sapporo, June 1980 & Kyoto, June 1980. Ed. by H. P. Kimmich. 1980. (Journal: Vol. 7, No. 1). 56p. 28.75 (*3-8055-1073-X*) S Karger.

International Symposium on Biotelemetry III: 4th Symposium, Garmisch-Partenkirchen, May/June 1978: Abstracts. International Symposium on Bio-Telelemetry Staff. Ed. by H. P. Kimmich. 1978. (Biotelemetry & Patient Monitoring Journal: Vol. 5, No. 1). pap. 30.50 (*3-8055-2911-2*) S Karger.

International Symposium on Brucellosis 2. Ed. by R. H. Regamey et al. 1976. (Developments in Biological Standardization Ser.: Vol. 31). (Illus.). 61.00 (*3-8055-2364-5*) S Karger.

International Symposium on Cancer Progression & Metastasis: Proceedings of the 8th Sapporo Cancer Seminar, Sapporo, July 1988. Ed. by H. Kobayashi. 1989. (Journal: Vol. 9, No. 2). (Illus.). 80p. pap. 35.75 (*3-8055-4991-1*) S Karger.

International Symposium on Cerebral Hemodynamics in Association with the 1st Meeting of the European Society of Neurosonology & Cerebral Hemodynamics: 10th Symposium & 1st Meeting, Munich, September 1996 - Abstracts. Ed. by J. Klingelhoefer. 1996. (Journal: Vol. 6, Suppl. 3, 1996). (Illus.). xxxiv, 74p. pap. 32.25 (*3-8055-6381-7*) S Karger.

International Symposium on Computer Restorations: State of the Art of the CEREC-Method. Ed. by W. H. Mormann. 1991. (Illus.). 632p. (Orig.). pap. text 54.00 (*0-86715-163-3*, B1633) Quint Pub Co.

International Symposium on Cosmetic Efficacy: 3rd Symposium, Cologne, May, 1998. Ed. by H. F. Merk & E. M. Jackson. 1999. (Skin Pharmacology & Applied Skin Physiology Ser.: Vol. 12, No. 3). (Illus.). 62p. pap. 25.25 (*3-8055-6929-7*) S Karger.

International Symposium on Endocrine Therapy, Proceedings of, Monaco, November, 1988. Basil A. Stoll. 1989. (Journal: Vol. 32, Suppl. 1, 1989). (Illus.). 274p. pap. 120.00 (*3-8055-5105-3*) S Karger.

International Symposium on Endocrinology & Development: 14th Symposium, Palma de Mallorca, November 1995. Ed. by J. Argente & A. Attanasio. 1996. (Journal: Vol. 45, Suppl. 1, 1996). (Illus.). iv, 74p. pap. 33.25 (*3-8055-6322-1*) S Karger.

International Symposium on Endocrinology & Development: 15th Symposium, Paris, November 1997. Ed. by A. Attanasio. 1997. (Hormone Research Ser.: Vol. 48, Suppl. 4, 1997). (Illus.). iv, 76p. pap. 35.00 (*3-8055-6582-8*) S Karger.

International Symposium on Endocrinology & Development: Basic & Clinical Aspects, Athens, October 1990. 1992. (Journal: Vol. 37, Suppl. 3, 1992). (Illus.). iv, 112p. pap. 50.50 (*3-8055-5670-5*) S Karger.

International Symposium on Fetal & Neonatal Neurology, Tours, October 1992. Ed. by E. Saliba. 1992. (Journal: Vol. 62, No. 4, 1992). (Illus.). 120p. pap. 44.50 (*3-8055-5700-0*) S Karger.

International Symposium on Glucagon-Like Peptide-1. Ed. by B. Goeke. 1994. (Journal: Vol. 54, Vol. 6, 1993). (Illus.). 88p. pap. 85.25 (*3-8055-5944-5*) S Karger.

International Symposium on Immunotoxicology. Ed. by Gordon Gibson et al. 1984. text 125.00 (*0-12-282180-7*) Acad Pr.

International Symposium on Inborn Errors of Metabolism in Humans, Third, Munich, March 1984: Abstracts. 1984. 126p. pap. 25.25 (*3-8055-3894-4*) S Karger.

International Symposium on Inborn Errors of Metabolism in Man, Tel Aviv, June, 1977. International Symposium on Inborn Errors of Metabo. Ed. by L. Beckman & M. Hauge. 1978. (Monographs in Human Genetics: Vol. 9). (Illus.). Pt. I. 77.50 (*3-8055-2836-1*); Pt. II. 63.25 (*3-8055-2835-3*) S Karger.

International Symposium on Infections in the Immunocompromised Host, Second. Ed. by Charles S. Easmon & Harold Gaya. 1983. text 104.00 (*0-12-228020-2*) Acad Pr.

International Symposium on Influenza Immunization: Proceedings of the International Association of Biological Standardization, 53rd, Geneva, 1977. International Association of Biological Standardiz. Ed. by F. T Perkins & R. H. Regamey. 1977. (Developments in Biological Standardization Ser.: Vol. 39). (Illus.). 61.00 (*3-8055-2786-1*) S Karger.

International Symposium on Nicotine: The Effects of Nicotine on Biological Systems II. P. B. S. Clarke et al. 1996. (Abstracts Ser.). 80p. 29.50 (*0-8176-5087-3*) Birkhauser.

International Symposium on Rabies, 40th, Lyon, December 9-11, 1972. International Symposium on Rabies Staff. 1975. (Immunobiological Standardization Symposia Ser.: Vol. 21). 336p. 39.25 (*3-8055-1649-5*) S Karger.

International Symposium on Rabies Vaccines for Human Use Produces in Tissue Culture, No. 3. International Association of Biological Standardiz. Ed. by R. H. Regamey. 1978. (Developments in Biological Standardization Ser.: Vol. 40). (Illus.). 61.00 (*3-8055-2788-8*) S Karger.

International Symposium on Radiofrequency Lesion Making Procedures, Nov. 19, 1976. International Symposium on Radiofrequency Lesion Making Procedures Staff. Ed. by Philip L. Gildenberg. 1978. (Applied Neurophysiology Ser.: Vol. 39). (Illus.). 16.75 (*3-8055-2770-5*) S Karger.

International Symposium on Resistance Arteries, 3rd, Rebild, Skrping, Denmark, May 1991 Abstracts. Ed. by M. J. Mulvany. 1991. (Journal: Vol. 28, No. 4, 1991). 80p. pap. 55.00 (*3-8055-5409-5*) S Karger.

International Symposium on Rifampicin, Davos, June, 1970. International Symposium on Rifampicin Staff. Ed. by Virchow. 1972. (Respiration Journal: Vol. 28). (Illus.). pap. 31.50 (*3-8055-1286-4*) S Karger.

International Symposium on Senna: Second Proceedings, Konstanz 1993. Ed. by K. Ewe et al. 1993. (Journal: Vol. 47, Suppl. 1, 1993). (Illus.). x, 262p. reprint ed. 85.25 (*3-8055-5872-4*) S Karger.

International Symposium on Smallpox Vaccine, 37th, Bilthoven, October, 1972. International Symposium on Smallpox Vaccine Staff. Ed. by R. H. Regamey et al. 1974. (Immunobiological Standardization Symposia Ser.: Vol. 19). 365p. 33.25 (*3-8055-1773-4*) S Karger.

International Symposium on Standardization & Use of Vaccines in the Developing Countries, Guadeloupe, 1978. International Symposium on Standardization and Use of Vaccines in the Developing Countries Staff. Ed. by R. H. Regamey. 1978. (Developments in Biological Standardization Ser.: Vol. 41). (FRE., Illus.). 61.00 (*3-8055-2811-6*) S Karger.

International Symposium on Stereoencephalotomy Research, 6th, Tokyo, Oct., 1973. International Symposium on Stereoencephalotomy Resesearch Staff. Ed. by Philip L. Gildenberg & H. Narabayashi. 1975. (Advances in Stereoencephalotomy Ser.: Vol. 7). 350p. pap. 161.75 (*3-8055-2186-3*) S Karger.

International Symposium on Vaccination of Man & Animals by the Non-Parenteral Route: Proceedings, Douglas 1975. Ed. by R. H. Regamey et al. 1976. (Developments in Biological Standardization Ser.: Vol. 33). (Illus.). 61.00 (*3-8055-2399-8*) S Karger.

International Symposium on Vascular Surgery: Proceedings. Ed. by Yingkai Wu et al. 1989. (International Academic Publishers Ser.). 400p. 105.00 (*0-08-036145-5*, Pergamon Pr) Elsevier.

International Symposium on Viral Hepatitis: Proceedings of the International Association of Biological Standardization, 44th. International Association of Biological Standardiz. Ed. by R. H. Regamey et al. 1975. (Developments in Biological Standardization Ser.: Vol. 30). (Illus.). x, 492p. 61.00 (*3-8055-2312-2*) S Karger.

International Textbook of Diabetes Mellitus, Set. Paul Z. Zimmet. Ed. by Ralph A. DeFronzo et al. 2nd ed. 1997. LC 95-415. 1930p. 510.00 (*0-471-93930-7*) Wiley.

International Travel see International Travel Guidelines: Travel Healthy

International Travel & Health: Vaccination Requirements & Health Advice. WHO Staff. 1994. 98p. pap. 15.00 (*92-4-158019-4*) World Health.

International Travel & Health: Vaccination Requirements & Health Advice - 1996. 1996. LC 96-174783.Tr. of Voyages Internationaux et Sante 1996. 104p. pap. text 13.50 (*92-4-158021-6*, 1189600) Am Soc Clinical.

International Travel & Health, 1992: Vaccination Requirements & Health Advice. WHO Staff. 1992. 96p. 15.00 (*92-4-158017-8*) World Health.

International Travel Guidelines: Travel Healthy. Richard C. Johnston. Ed. & Illus. by Mary C. Haas. rev. ed. 1998. Orig. Title: International Travel. 40p. reprint ed. spiral bd. 9.95 (*0-9670573-0-2*, TH90098003) Infinite Des.

International Travel Health Guide. Stuart R. Rose. 7th ed. 1996. pap. 17.95 (*0-923947-07-8*) Travel Med.

International Travel Health Guide, 1995. Stuart R. Rose. 6th ed. 1995. (Illus.). 454p. pap. 17.95 (*0-923947-05-1*) Travel Med.

International Trends in General Thoracic Surgery Vol. 1: Lung Cancer, Vol. 1. Norman C. Delarue & Henri Eschapasse. 1985. (Illus.). 315p. text 98.00 (*0-7216-1349-7*) Saunders.

International Trends in General Thoracic Surgery Vol. 2: Major Challenges for the Thoracic Surgeon, Vol. 2. Hermes C. Grillo & Henri Eschapasse. 1987. (Illus.). 528p. text 99.00 (*0-7216-1350-0*) Saunders.

International Version for Developmental Psychology: Childhood & Adolescence. Shaffer. 5th ed. 1998. (Psychology Ser.). 630p. spiral bd. 87.95 (*0-534-36361-X*) Brooks-Cole.

International Vibramycin Symposium, Paris, June, 1974. International Vibramycin Symposium Staff & H. Swarz. 1975. (Chemotherapy Ser.: Vol. 21, Supplement 1). (Illus.). vii, 149p. 26.25 (*3-8055-2142-1*) S Karger.

International Vinca Alkaloid Symposium: Vindesine. Ed. by S. Seeber et al. 1981. (Beitraege Zur Onkologie, Contributions to Oncology Ser.: Vol. 6). xii, 460p. 68.75 (*3-8055-2501-X*) S Karger.

International Virus Prevention Conference Proceedings (1996) Intro. by Peter S. Tippett. 5th ed. 1996. (Illus.). 320p. pap. text 125.00 (*0-7881-3312-8*) DIANE Pub.

International Visual Field Symposium, 2nd. Ed. by Erik L. Greve. 1977. (Documenta Ophthalmologica Proceedings Ser.: No. 14). (Illus.). text 234.00 (*90-6193-154-1*) Kluwer Academic.

International Visual Field Symposium, 3rd. Ed. by Erik L. Greve. 1979. (Documenta Ophthalmologica Proceedings Ser.: Vol. 19). pap. text 255.50 (*90-6193-160-6*) Kluwer Academic.

International Who's Who in Medicine. 1987. (*0-900332-86-7*) Melrose GBR. *Dist:* Taylor & Francis.

International Who's Who in Medicine, 1995-96. 2nd ed. 1995. 620p. 199.00 (*0-948875-91-7*) Intl Pubns Serv.

International Who's Who in Sexology. Ed. by Loretta Haroian et al. 1984. 500p. 60.00 (*0-930846-04-4*) Specific Pr.

International Workshop Laparoscopic Colorectal Surgery, Norderstedt, November 27-29, 1995. E. H. Farthmann et al. 1996. LC 96-38499. (Illus.). 320p. 127.00 (*3-540-60839-7*) Spr-Verlag.

International Workshop on Human Gene Mapping: Edinburgh Conference, 5th, July 1979. Ed. by Harold J. Evans et al. 1980. (Human Gene Mapping Ser.: No. 5). (Illus.). vi, 236p. pap. 56.75 (*3-8055-0649-X*) S Karger.

International Workshop on Immune-Deficient Animals in Experimental Research, 4th, Chexbres, October 1982. Ed. by B. Sordat. 1983. (Journal: Vol. 50, No. 6). 60p. pap. 33.25 (*3-8055-3647-X*) S Karger.

International Workshop on Natural Killer Cells: 7th, Stockholm (Lidingo), June 1991 - Journal: Natural Immunity & Cell Growth Regulation, Vol. 10, No. 3, 1991. Ed. by Eva Lotzova et al. 1991. 68p. pap. 38.50 (*3-8055-5447-8*) S Karger.

International Yearbook of Nephrology Dialysis Transplantation, 1994. Ed. by Vittorio E. Andreucci & Leon G. Fine. 1994. (Illus.). 196p. 90.00 (*0-19-262491-1*) OUP.

International Yearbook of Nephrology, 1989. Ed. by Vittorio E. Andreucci et al. 1988. (C). text 190.00 (*0-7923-0015-7*) Kluwer Academic.

International Yearbook of Nephrology, 1990. Ed. by Vittorio E. Andreucci et al. 1989. text 163.50 (*0-7923-0562-0*) Kluwer Academic.

International Yearbook of Nephrology, 1991. Ed. by Vittorio E. Andreucci & Leon G. Fine. 1990. (International Yearbooks of Nephrology Ser.). (C). text 191.00 (*0-7923-1002-0*) Kluwer Academic.

International Yearbook of Nephrology, 1992. Ed. by Vittorio E. Andreucci & Leon G. Fine. 1992. (Illus.). 360p. 122.00 (*0-387-19697-8*) Spr-Verlag.

International Yearbook of Nephrology, 1993. Ed. by Vittorio E. Andreucci & Leon G. Fine. 1993. (Illus.). 376p. 247.00 (*0-387-19729-X*) Spr-Verlag.

Internationaler Anthropometrischer Datenatlas see International Data on Anthropometry

Internationally Acceptable Minimum Standards of Medical Education. 1962. (Technical Report Ser.: No. 239). 59p. pap. text 3.00 (*92-4-120239-4*) World Health.

Internet Access to the National Library of Medicine's Toxicology & Environmental Health Databases. Catharyn T. Liverman. 1998. LC 99-169728. 35 p. (*0-309-06299-3*) Natl Acad Pr.

Internet & Healthcare. Louis Nicholson. 2nd ed. 1999. LC 98-48490. 125p. 35.00 (*1-56793-097-2*) Health Admin Pr.

Internet Book Gene Therapy. Robert E. Sobol & Kevin J. Scanlon. 1996. (C). pap. text 75.00 (*0-8385-3101-6*, A3101-1) Appleton & Lange.

Internet Compendium: Guide to Resources by Subject: Subject Guides to Health & Science Resources. Ed. by Joseph Janes et al. 1995. LC 95-2171. 529p. 82.50 (*1-55570-219-8*) Neal-Schuman.

Internet Enhanced Compulsive Syndrome: IECS: A New Form of Addiction. Fabian Krause. Ed. by Raymond Fernando. 2000. (Illus.). viii, 168p. pap. (*0-620-25682-6*) Internet Clinic.

Internet for Nurses & Allied Health Professionals. Margaret J. Edwards. 2nd ed. 1997. LC 96-53902. (Illus.). 191p. pap. 26.95 (*0-387-94888-0*) Spr-Verlag.

Internet for Physicians. Roger P. Smith & Margaret J. a. Edwards. 2nd ed. 1999. LC 98-54987. (Illus.). 216p. pap. 32.95 incl. audio compact disk (*0-387-98724-X*) Spr-Verlag.

***Internet for Physicians.** R. P. Smith. 3rd ed. 2001. (Illus.). 272p. audio compact disk 34.95 (*0-387-95312-4*) Spr-Verlag.

Internet for Radiologist. Ed. by Davide Caramella & Paolo Pavone. 1998. LC 98-41691. (Illus.). 204p. pap. 32.95 (*3-540-63151-8*) Spr-Verlag.

Internet Guide for Rehabilitation Professionals. Kathlyn L. Reed & Sandra Cunningham. 1997. (Illus.). 320p. pap. text 34.95 (*0-397-55463-X*) Lppncott W & W.

Internet Medical & Health, Searching & Sources Guidebook: For Healthcare Consumers & Professionals Who Want to Know More. Colleen Lindell. Ed. by Paulette DeRose. 1998. LC 98-92026. (Illus.). 100p. pap. 7.95 (*0-9667080-4-0*) KC Press.

Internet Medical & Health Searching & Sources Guidebook II: For Healthcare Consumers & Professionals Who Want to Know More. Colleen Lindell & William R. Hersh. Ed. by Paulette DuRose. 2nd rev. ed. 1999. (Illus.). 275p. 7.95 (*0-9667080-3-2*) KC Press.

***Internet Pharmacies: Adding Disclosure Requirements Would Aid State & Federal Oversight.** Gloria E. Taylor. 2001. 56p. (C). 20.00 (*0-7567-1744-2*) DIANE Pub.

Internet Resource Guide for Nurses & Allied Health Professionals. Cynthia M. Mascara et al. 2nd ed. 2000. LC 00-66910. (Illus.). 112p. pap. 16.95 (*0-13-031103-0*) P-H.

Internet, Telematics & Health. Ed. by C. A. Gamboa et al. 1997. LC 96-77818. (Studies in Health Technology & Informatics: Vol. 36). 536p. 84.00 (*90-5199-289-0*, 289-0) IOS Press.

Internistische Gutachten. Ed. by H. Doerfler. 1991. viii, 352p. pap. 42.75 (*3-8055-5320-X*) S Karger.

Internistische Probleme in der Anaesthesie. L. Kaufman & E. Sumner. 1983. (Illus.). viii, 204p. 42.75 (*3-8055-3581-3*) S Karger.

Internship Training in Professional Psychology. Ed. by Theodore W. May & Richard Dana. 1987. 527p. 79.95 (*0-89116-580-0*); pap. 38.95 (*0-89116-773-0*) Hemisp Pub.

Interpersonal Approach to Child Therapy: The Treatment of Children & Adolescents from an Interpersonal Point of View. Stanley Spiegel. 1989. LC 89-30772. (Personality, Psychopathology & Psychotherapy: Theoretical & Clinical Perspectives Ser.). 260p. text 46.00 (*0-231-06292-3*) Col U Pr.

Interpersonal Approach to Mental Functioning: Assessment & Treatment. Elsa Schmid-Kitsikis. 1990. (Contributions to Human Development Ser.: Vol. 20). (Illus.). vii, 104p. 31.50 (*3-8055-5114-2*) S Karger.

Interpersonal Behaviour: The Psychology of Social Interaction. Ed. by Joseph P. Forgas. 1986. (Illus.). 416p. text 42.00 (*0-08-029868-0*); pap. text 22.00 (*0-08-029854-0*) Elsevier.

Interpersonal Communication & Psychology for Health Care. Rungapadiachy. 1998. 304p. pap. text 37.50 (*0-7506-4080-4*) Buttrwrth-Heinemann.

Interpersonal Communication in Nursing: Theory & Practice. Ed. by R. B. Ellis et al. 1995. (Illus.). 145p. pap. (*0-443-04996-3*) Church.

H I

Interpersonal Communication in Pharmaceutical Care. Helen Meldrum. 1994. LC 93-31220. 154p. pap. 14.95 (*1-56024-867-X*); 180p. lib. bdg. 49.95 (*1-56024-866-1*) Haworth Pr.

Interpersonal Diagnosis & Treatment of Personality Disorders. Lorna S. Benjamin. 2nd ed. 1995. LC 95-41650. (Diagnosis & Treatment of Mental Disorders Ser.). 431p. text 46.00 (*1-57230-060-4*, 0060) Guilford Pubns.

Interpersonal Expectations: Theory, Research, & Applications. Ed. by Peter D. Blanck. 1993. LC 92-36925. (Studies in Emotion & Social Interaction). (Illus.). 521p. (C). text 90.00 (*0-521-41783-X*); pap. text 34.95 (*0-521-42832-7*) Cambridge U Pr.

Interpersonal Group Psychotherapy for Borderline Personality Disorder. Elsa Marziali & Heather Munroe-Blum. 1999. 216p. reprint ed. text 25.00 (*0-7881-6499-6*) DIANE Pub.

Interpersonal Living: A Skills - Contract Approach to Human Relations Training in Groups. Gerard Egan. 1976. LC 76-6651. 318p. (C). 28.09 (*0-8185-0189-8*) Brooks-Cole.

***Interpersonal Nursing for Mental Health.** Jan Horsfall et al. 2001. LC 2001-20175. (Illus.). x, 341p. (*0-8261-1415-6*) Springer Pub.

Interpersonal Perception: A Social Relations Analysis. David A. Kenny. 1994. LC 94-8552. (Distinguished Contributions in Psychology Ser.). 270p. 42.00 (*0-89862-114-3*, 2114) Guilford Pubns.

Interpersonal Process in Cognitive Therapy. Jeremy D. Safran & Zindel V. Segal. 1996. LC 96-35422. 312p. pap. 50.00 (*1-56821-858-3*) Aronson.

Interpersonal Process in Psychotherapy: A Guide for Clinical Training. Edward M. Teyber. 1989. 204p. pap. 31.50 (*0-534-10861-X*); 2nd ed. 1991. 288p. (C). text 45.25 (*0-534-16920-1*) Brooks-Cole.

Interpersonal Process in Psychotherapy: A Relational Approach. Edward M. Teyber. 3rd ed. 1997. tchr. ed. (*0-534-34792-4*); 4th ed. 1999. pap., wbk. ed. 16.00 net. (*0-534-36566-3*) Brooks-Cole.

Interpersonal Psychoanalysis. Earl G. Witenberg. 1978. 155p. 30.00 (*0-89876-048-8*) Gardner Pr.

Interpersonal Psychotherapy. Ed. by John C. Markowitz. 1998. LC 98-10859. (Review of Psychiatry Ser.). 156p. pap. text 32.00 (*0-88048-836-0*, 8836) Am Psychiatric.

Interpersonal Psychotherapy for Depressed Adolescents. Laura Mufson et al. 1993. LC 93-1429. 218p. 30.00 (*0-89862-686-2*) Guilford Pubns.

Interpersonal Psychotherapy for Dysthymic Disorder. John C. Markowitz. 1998. LC 97-25436. 176p. 33.50 (*0-88048-914-6*, 8914) Am Psychiatric.

Interpersonal Psychotherapy of Depression. Gerald L. Klerman et al. 1994. LC 94-72437. (Master Work Ser.). 272p. pap. text 40.00 (*1-56821-350-6*) Aronson.

Interpersonal Psychotherapy of Depression. Gerald L. Klerman et al. 1984. LC 82-72961. 272p. pap. 49.95 (*0-465-03396-2*) Basic.

Interpersonal Relatedness from Projective Drawings: Applicability in Diagnostic & Therapeutic Practice. Andrew L. Sopchak et al. 1993. LC 93-9386. (Illus.). 292p. (C). text 68.95 (*0-398-05855-5*) C C Thomas.

Interpersonal Relations in Nursing: A Conceptual Frame of Reference for Psychodynamic Nursing. Hildegard E. Peplau. 1991. LC 91-4846. 360p. 41.95 (*0-8261-7910-X*) Springer Pub.

Interpersonal Relationships: Professional Communication Skills for Nurses. Elizabeth Arnold & Kathleen Boggs. 2nd ed. 1994. LC 93-48584. (Illus.). 608p. pap. text 30.50 (*0-7216-6684-1*) Saunders.

Interpersonal Relationships: Professional Communication Skills for Nurses. Ed. by Elizabeth Arnold & Kathleen U. Boggs. 2nd ed. 1995. (Illus.). 608p. pap., tchr. ed. (*0-7216-6685-X*) Saunders.

Interpersonal Skills for Healthcare Professionals. Robert Wondrak. 1998. LC 98-25010. 224p. pap. 38.95 (*0-632-04144-7*) Blackwell Sci.

Interpersonal Theory in Nursing Practice: Selected Works of Hildegard E. Peplau. Anita W. O'Toole & Sheila R. Welt. 1989. 400p. 45.95 (*0-8261-6060-3*) Springer Pub.

Interpersonal Theory of Psychiatry. Harry Stack Sullivan. Ed. by Helen S. Perry & Mary L. Gawel. 1968. reprint ed. pap. 12.95 (*0-393-00138-5*) Norton.

Interpersonal World of the Infant: A View from Psychoanalysis & Development Psychology. Daniel N. Stern. 1985. LC 85-47553. 320p. pap. 42.00 (*0-465-03403-9*) Basic.

Interphalangeal Joints. Ed. by William H. Bowers. 1987. (Hand & Upper Limb Ser.: Vol. 1). (Illus.). 320p. text (*0-443-03216-5*) Church.

Interpharm Complaint Tracker Manual. Interpharm Press Staff. 1998. (*1-57491-093-0*) IHS Health Grp.

Interpharm Guide to FDA International Inspections Vol. I: 1990-1993. Ed. by Michael H. Anisfeld. 1995. ring bd. 179.00 (*1-57491-008-6*) IHS Health Grp.

Interpharm International Clinical Research Coordinator Handbook: GCP Tools & Techniques. Deborah Rosenbaum & Michelle Dresser. 1996. LC 96-27948. (Practical Clinical Trials Ser.: Vol. 1). 309p. ring bd. 145.00 (*1-57491-022-1*) IHS Health Grp.

Interpharm International Dictionary of Biotechnology & Pharmaceutical Manufacturing. Dean E. Snyder. 1992. 270p. 69.00 (*0-935184-31-7*) IHS Health Grp.

Interpharm Master Keyword Guide to Twenty-One CFR: 1997-1998 Edition. Ed. by Michael H. Anisfeld. 1996. 604p. pap. 99.00 (*1-57491-036-1*) IHS Health Grp.

Interpharm Master Keyword Guide to Twenty-One CFR: 1998-1999 Edition. Ed. by Michael H. Anisfeld. 1998. 610p. 99.00 (*1-57491-091-4*) IHS Health Grp.

Interpharm Pharmaceutical Manager's Compliance Guide. Ed. by Laura Pence. 3rd ed. 1997. 140p. pap. 39.00 (*1-57491-044-2*) IHS Health Grp.

Interpharm Training Tracker II Validation Resource Reference Guide. Contrib. by Interpharm Press Staff. 1997. 318p. 950.00 (*1-57491-035-3*) IHS Health Grp.

Interpress Dictionary of Biology & Medical Science: English-Japanese. Interpress Staff. 1988. (ENG & JPN.). 1082p. reprint ed. 495.00 (*0-8288-7209-0*, 487198205X) Fr & Eur.

Interpress Dictionary of Biology & Medical Science: Japanese-English. Interpress Staff. 1988. (ENG & JPN.). 1082p. reprint ed. 495.00 (*0-8288-7208-2*, 4871982068) Fr & Eur.

Interpress Dictionary of Genetics, Zoology, Botany & Dentistry. Interpress Staff. 1980. (ENG & JPN.). 214p. 95.00 (*0-8288-0640-3*, M3857) Fr & Eur.

Interpretation & Extrapolation of Reproductive Data to Establish Human Safety Standards. Ed. by K. Khera & D. J. Cleeg. 1989. (Current Issues in Toxicology Ser.). (Illus.). 133p. 64.95 (*0-387-96962-4*) Spr-Verlag.

Interpretation & Interaction: Psychoanalysis or Psychotherapy? Jerome D. Oremland. 1991. 192p. text 29.95 (*0-88163-127-2*) Analytic Pr.

Interpretation & Significance of the Embedded & Non-Embedded Syndromes on Behavioral Optometric Case Analysis. Earl P. Schmitt. Ed. by Willard Bleything. 1993. 80p. (Orig.). (C). lib. bdg. 18.00 (*0-943599-67-9*) OEPF.

Interpretation & the Problem of the Intention of the Author Vol. 5: H.-G. Gadamer vs. E. D. Hirsch. Burhanettin Tatar. 1998. LC 98-44459. (Cultural Heritage & Contemporary Change. Series IIA, Islam: Vol. 5). pap. 17.50 (*1-56518-121-2*) Coun Res Values.

Interpretation & Uses of Medical Statistics. Leslie E. Daly & Geoffrey J. Bourke. 5th ed. 2000. LC 99-45805. (Illus.). xiii, 568p. pap. 83.95 (*0-632-04763-1*) Blackwell Sci.

Interpretation of Ancient Hindu Medicine. Chandra Chakraberty. 1993. (C). reprint ed. (*81-85418-97-7*) Low Price IND. *Dist:* S Asia.

Interpretation of Ancient Hindu Medicine. Chandra Chakraberty. 1988. (C). (*0-7855-2286-7*) Scientific GBR. *Dist:* St Mut.

Interpretation of Audiometric Results. Irving Hochberg. 1973. LC 72-85146. (Studies in Communicative Disorders). 45p. pap. text 2.50 (*0-672-61285-2*, Bobbs) Macmillan.

Interpretation of Biochemical Multitest Profiles: An Analysis of 100 Important Conditions. Paul L. Wolf. 1977. LC 76-54053. (Illus.). 296p. (gr. 13). 38.50 (*0-89352-002-0*) Mosby Inc.

Interpretation of Canine & Feline Urinalysis. Dennis J. Chew & Stephen P. DiBartola. 2000. (Illus.). 84p. (*0-9678005-2-8*) Gloyd Grp Inc.

Interpretation of Development & Heredity: A Study in Biological Method. E. S. Russell. 1977. LC 70-39699. (Select Bibliographies Reprint Ser.). 312p. reprint ed. 19.95 (*0-8369-9943-6*) Ayer.

Interpretation of Diagnostic Testing, No. 5. Wallach. 1991. 39.95 (*0-316-92050-9*, Little Brwn Med Div) Lppncott W & W.

Interpretation of Diagnostic Tests. Jacques Wallach. 7th ed. 2000. LC 99-55267. 1,040p. pap. text 49.95 (*0-7817-1659-4*) Lppncott W & W.

Interpretation of Diagnostic Tests: A Handbook Synopsis of Laboratory Medicine. Jacques B. Wallach. 4th ed. 1986. LC 73-10612. 24.00 (*0-316-92046-0*, Little Brwn Med Div) Lppncott W & W.

Interpretation of Dreams. Sigmund Freud. 1983. 191p. reprint ed. lib. bdg. 31.95 (*0-89966-441-5*) Buccaneer Bks.

Interpretation of Dreams: Freud's Theories Revisited. Lawrence M. Porter. 1987. LC 87-11940. (Masterwork Studies: No. 9). 152p. 25.95 (*0-8057-7971-X*) Macmillan.

Interpretation of Dreams in Clinical Work. Ed. by Arnold Rothstein. 1987. (American Psychoanalytic Association Workshop Ser.: Monograph 3). 35.00 (*0-8236-2910-4*) Intl Univs Pr.

Interpretation of Dreams in the Ancient Near East. Leo Oppenheim. LC 78-72754. (Ancient Mesopotamian Texts & Studies). reprint ed. 40.00 (*0-404-18198-8*) AMS Pr.

Interpretation of Electrophoretic Patterns of Proteins & Isoenzymes: A Clinical Pathologic Guide. Paul L. Wolf. 1981. (gr. 13). 34.00 (*0-89352-035-7*) Mosby Inc.

Interpretation of ERCP: With Associated Digital Imaging Correlation. Andrew Taylor. 1996. LC 96-30133. 352p. text 129.00 (*0-397-51579-0*, Lippnctt) Lppncott W & W.

Interpretation of Illness. Frederic D. Homer. 1987. LC 87-7221. 240p. pap. 18.95 (*0-911198-88-1*) Purdue U Pr.

Interpretation of Laboratory Results for Small Animal Clinicians. B. M. Bush. 1991. (Illus.). 528p. 92.95 (*0-632-03259-6*) Blackwell Sci.

Interpretation of Pediatric Tests. Jacques B. Wallach. 1983. 764p. 24.00 (*0-316-92045-2*, Little Brwn Med Div) Lppncott W & W.

Interpretation of Psychological Tests. Joel Allison et al. 1968. LC 66-41476. 342p. 38.95 (*0-89116-326-3*) Hemisp Pub.

Interpretation of the Halstead-Reitan Neuropsychological Test Battery: A Casebook Approach. Charles A. Golden et al. 1980. (Illus.). 401p. text 51.00 (*0-8089-1298-4*, 791621, Grune & Strat) Harcrt Hlth Sci Grp.

Interpretation of the Luria-Nebraska, Vol. 1. Ed. by James A. Moses, Jr. et al. 1983. 294p. text 44.00 (*0-8089-1532-0*, 792986, Grune & Strat) Harcrt Hlth Sci Grp.

Interpretation of the Luria-Nebraska Neuropsychological Test Battery, Vol. 2. James A. Moses et al. 1983. 464p. text 67.00 (*0-8089-1537-1*, 792987, Grune & Strat) Harcrt Hlth Sci Grp.

Interpretation of Wet Mount Preparations. Gilles R. Monif. 1996. (Illus.). 46p. 9.95 (*1-880906-44-9*) IDI Pub.

Interpreted World: An Introduction to Phenomenological Psychology. Ernesto Spinelli. 1989. 208p. (C). pap. 25.95 (*0-8039-8115-5*, 7005) Sage.

Interpreters of Nature: Essays. George Newman. 1977. LC 68-20325. (Essay Index Reprint Ser.). 22.95 (*0-8369-0741-8*) Ayer.

Interpreter's RX: A Training Program for Spanish/English Medical Interpreting. Holly M. Mikkelson. 1994. (ENG & SPA., Illus.). 262p. (C). pap. 69.95 incl. audio (*1-880594-11-0*, ACE012) ACEBO.

Interpreting: An Introduction. Nancy Frishberg. Ed. by Donna Reiter-Brandwein. rev. ed. 1990. (Illus.). 249p. (Orig.). (C). pap. text 22.50 (*0-916883-07-8*) RID Pubns.

Interpreting & Holding: The Paternal & Maternal Functions of the Psychotherapist. Ed. by Jeffrey Seinfeld. 1993. LC 93-19992. 344p. 50.00 (*0-87668-501-7*) Aronson.

Interpreting CT Head Scans. Lynda Albertyn. 1996. pap. text 39.00 (*0-443-05029-5*) Saunders.

Interpreting Disability: A Qualitative Reader. Ed. by Philip Ferguson et al. 1991. (Special Education Ser.: No. 10). (C). 424p. pap. 24.95 (*0-8077-3121-8*); 328p. text 50.00 (*0-8077-3122-6*) Tchrs Coll.

Interpreting Illness, Vol. 2, No. 1. Ed. by Marc Auge. 1986. (History & Anthropology Ser.: Vol. 2, Pt. 1). ii, 206p. 168.00 (*3-7186-0295-4*) Gordon & Breach.

Interpreting Interpretation: The Limits of Hermeneutic Psychoanalysis. Elyn R. Saks. 1999. LC 98-35063. 272p. 37.00 (*0-300-07603-7*) Yale U Pr.

Interpreting Professional Self-Regulation: A History of the United Kingdom Central Council for Nursing. Celia Davis et al. 2000. LC 00-27211. xix, 249p. 49.99 (*0-415-23033-0*) Routledge.

Interpreting Signs of Illness: A Case Study in Medical Semiotics. Kathryn V. Staiano. 1986. (Approaches to Semiotics Ser.: No. 72). (Illus.). xvii, 284p. (*0-89925-155-2*) Mouton.

Interpreting the Countertransference. Lawrence E. Hedges. 1992. LC 91-15933. 440p. 60.00 (*0-87668-532-7*) Aronson.

Interpreting the Medical Literature. Stephen H. Gehlbach. 3rd ed. 1992. LC 92-49250. 288p. pap. 44.95 (*0-07-105451-0*) McGraw-Hill Prof.

***Interpreting X-Ray Swallow Studies & Planning Treatment.** Jeri A. Logemann. 2000. pap. 150.00 incl. VHS (*1-58041-055-3*, 0112258) Am Speech Lang Hearing.

Interpretive Approaches to Interpersonal Communication. Ed. by Kathryn Carter & Mick Presnell. 1994. LC 93-7710. (SUNY Series in Human Communication Processes). 272p. (C). text 64.50 (*0-7914-1847-2*); pap. text 21.95 (*0-7914-1848-0*) State U NY Pr.

Interpretive Guide to the Comprehensive Rorschach System. Stuart Wilson. 5th rev. ed. 1994. LC 94-90146. 80p. (C). pap. text 24.50 (*0-9626846-2-7*) S Wilson.

Interpretive Guide to the Millon Clinical Multiaxial Inventory. James P. Choca & Eric J. Van Denburg. 2nd ed. 1996. LC 96-28271. 355p. text 49.95 (*1-55798-383-6*) Am Psychol.

Interpretive Guide to the Personality Assessment Inventory. Leslie C. Morey. 1996. LC 96-8181. 308p. 56.00 (*0-911907-22-X*) Psych Assess.

Interpretive Reasoning & the Halstead-Reitan Tests. David T. Bradford. 1992. LC 91-72061. 340p. (Orig.). pap. text 34.95 (*0-88422-113-X*) Clinical Psych.

Interrelations of Odontons & Tonsils to Organs, Fields of Disturbance, & Tissue Systems. Reinhold Voll. Tr. by Hartwig Schuldt from GER. 1978. (Electro-Acupuncture According to Voll Ser.). (Illus.). 180p. text (*3-88136-064-6*) ML-Verlag DEU. *Dist:* Medicina Bio.

Interrelationship among Aging, Cancer & Differentiation. Ed. by Bernard Pullman et al. 1985. text 176.50 (*90-277-2117-3*) Kluwer Academic.

Intersection & Beyond, Vol. II. Elizabeth Boyden Howes. 1986. LC 86-3067. 200p. (Orig.). pap. 8.50 (*0-917479-07-6*) Guild Psy.

Intersections: Science, Theology & Ethics. James M. Gustafson. 1996. LC 96-28322. 196p. (Orig.). pap. 16.95 (*0-8298-1137-0*) Pilgrim OH.

Intersections between Particle & Nuclear Physics 1986. Ed. by Donald F. Geesaman. 1985. LC 86-72018. (Conference Proceedings Ser.: No. 150). 1312p. (C). 99.00 (*0-88318-349-8*) Am Inst Physics.

Intersections in Basic & Applied Memory Research. Ed. by David G. Payne & Frederick G. Conrad. 1996. 368p. text 69.95 (*0-8058-1973-8*) L Erlbaum Assocs.

Intersections in Psychology, Psychiatry & Law: Readings in Forensic Science, Vol. II. R. Edward Geiselman. 1997. 212p. pap. 30.00 (*0-935645-12-8*) AJFP.

Intersectoral Action for Health: The Role of Intersectoral Cooperation in National Strategies for Health for All. 1986. (Illus.). 150p. pap. 24.00 (*92-4-156096-7*) World Health.

Intersectoral Coordination & Health in Environmental Management: An Examination of National Experience. M. Schaefer. 1981. (Public Health Papers: No. 74). 122p. pap. text 9.00 (*92-4-130074-4*, 1110074) World Health.

Intersectoral Linkages & Health Development: Case Studies in India (Kerala State), Jamaica, Norway, Sri Lanka & Thailand. G. Gunatilleke. 1984. (WHO Offset Publications: No. 83). 53p. 5.00 (*92-4-170083-1*) World Health.

Intersensory Perception & Sensory Integration. Ed. by Richard D. Walk & Herbert L. Pick, Jr. 1981. LC 80-29204. (Perception & Perceptual Development Ser.: Vol. 2). 436p. 75.00 (*0-306-40610-1*, Plenum Trade) Perseus Pubng.

Intersex Child. Ed. by Nathalie Josso. 1981. (Pediatric & Adolescent Endocrinology Ser.: Vol. 8). viii, 272p. pap. 143.50 (*3-8055-0909-X*) S Karger.

Intersex in the Age of Ethics. Ed. by Alice Domurat Dreger. 1999. LC 00-266617. (Ethics in Clinical Medicine Ser.). (Illus.). x, 227p. lib. bdg. 45.00 (*1-55572-125-7*); (C). pap. 19.95 (*1-55572-100-1*) Univ Pub Group.

Interstital-Lymphatic & Solute Movement. Ed. by N. C. Staub et al. 1987. (Advances in Microcirculation Ser.: Vol. 13). (Illus.). x, 290p. 203.50 (*3-8055-4544-4*) S Karger.

Interstitial & Intracavitary Thermoradiotherapy. J. M. Ardist et al. Ed. by Michael H. Seegenschmiedt & Rolf Sauer. 1993. LC 93-13822. (Medical Radiology Ser.). (Illus.). 397p. 330.00 (*0-387-55670-2*) Spr-Verlag.

Interstitial Cystitis. Ed. by Philip M. Hanno et al. 1990. (Illus.). 218p. 102.00 (*0-387-19598-X*) Spr-Verlag.

Interstitial Cystitis. Ed. by Grannum R. Sant. 1997. LC 97-10327. (Illus.). 304p. text 110.00 (*0-397-51695-9*) Lppncott W & W.

Interstitial Cystitis Survival Guide. Robert M. Moldwin. 2000. 238p. pap. 14.95 (*1-57224-210-8*) New Harbinger.

Interstitial, Endocavitary & Perfusional Hyperthermia. J. M. Cosset et al. 1990. (Clincial Thermology Ser.: Vol. 5). (Illus.). 90p. 125.00 (*0-387-50983-6*) Spr-Verlag.

Interstitial Hyperthermia. Ed. by L. Handl-Zeller. 1992. 224p. 135.00 (*0-387-82280-1*) Spr-Verlag.

Interstitial Hyperthermia: Physics, Biology, & Clinical Aspects. Ed. by M. Urano & E. B. Douple. 1991. (Hyperthermia & Oncology Ser.: Vol. 3). 360p. 210.00 (*90-6764-138-3*) Coronet Bks.

Interstitial Lung Disease. Schwarz. 1987. 59.00 (*0-941158-66-7*) Mosby Inc.

Interstitial Lung Disease. Marvin I. Schwarz & Talmadge E. King, Jr. 3rd ed. 1998. LC 98-162491. (Illus.). 760p. incl. cd-rom (*1-55009-060-7*) DEKR.

Interstitial Lung Disease & Bronchial Hyperreactivity: Selected Papers from the Meeting of the Italian Chapter of ACCP, Parma, May 1987, Journal: Respiration, Vol. 54, Supplement 1. Ed. by D. Olivieri. 1988. iv, 122p. pap. 39.25 (*3-8055-4891-5*) S Karger.

Interstitial Lung Diseases in Children, Set. L. R. Laraya & W. T. Hughes. 1988. LC 87-18185. 357.00 (*0-8493-4300-3*, RJ436, CRC Reprint) Franklin.

Interstitial Lung Diseases in Children L. R. Laraya-Cuasay. Ed. by W. T. Hughes. 1988. LC 87-18185. Vol. I. 224p. 119.00 (*0-8493-4301-1*, RJ436); Vol. 2. 208p. 123.00 (*0-8493-4302-X*, RJ436); Vol. III. 224p. 116.00 (*0-8493-4303-8*, RJ436) Franklin (CRC Reprint).

Interstitial Nephropathies: Proceedings of the Nephrology Symposium, 6th, Hannover, May 1978. Nephrology Symposium Staff. Ed. by K. Kuhn. 1979. (Contributions to Nephrology Ser.: Vol. 16). (Illus.). pap. 29.75 (*3-8055-2979-1*) S Karger.

Interstitial Pulmonary Diseases: Selected Topics. Moises Selman & Roberto Barrios. 1991. (Illus.). 336p. 135.00 (*0-8493-6432-9*, RC776) CRC Pr.

Intersubjective Communication & Emotion in Early Ontogeny. Ed. by Stein Braten. 1999. LC 97-47525. (Studies in Emotion & Social Interaction: No. 3). (Illus.). 472p. (C). text 74.95 (*0-521-62257-3*) Cambridge U Pr.

Intersubjective Perspective. Ed. by Robert D. Stolorow et al. 1994. LC 93-25711. 224p. pap. 40.00 (*1-56821-053-1*) Aronson.

Intersubjectivity, Projective Identification & Otherness. Maurice Apprey & Howard F. Stein. 1993. LC 92-47242. 304p. 39.95 (*0-8207-0247-1*) Duquesne.

Intersystem Model: Integrating Theory & Practice. Barbara M. Artinian & Margaret M. Conger. 1997. LC 96-45795. 358p. 81.95 (*0-8039-5558-8*, 4849); pap. 39.95 (*0-8039-5559-6*, 4850) Sage.

Intertrochanteric Osteotomy. Joseph Schatzker. 1984. (Illus.). 205p. 187.00 (*0-387-10719-3*) Spr-Verlag.

Intertwinements of Law & Medicine. J. Broekman. 1996. LC 98-209285. (Law Ser.: Vol. 7). 248p. (Orig.). pap. (*90-6186-778-9*) Leuven Univ BEL. *Dist:* Coronet Bks.

H
I

Interval Training Workout: Build Muscle & Burn Fat with Anaerobic Exercise. Joseph T. Nitti & Kimberlie Nitti. 2001. LC 2001-16621. (Illus.). 224p. pap. 16.95 (*0-89793-327-3*) Hunter Hse.

Intervening with Drug-Involved Youth. Clyde B. McCoy et al. 1996. LC 96-10052. 272p. 61.95 (*0-8039-7371-3*, 13555) Sage.

Intervention & Reflection: Basic Issues in Medical Ethics. Ronald Munson. (C). 2nd ed. 1983. 608p. pap. 27.00 net. (*0-534-01289-2*); 3rd ed. 1987. 602p. pap. 32.00 net. (*0-534-08088-X*); 4th ed. 1991. 669p. mass mkt. 38.25 (*0-534-16326-2*) Wadsworth Pub.

Intervention & Reflection: Basic Issues in Medical Ethics. Selected by Ronald Munson & Christopher A. Hoffman. 5th ed. 1995. LC 95-15103. (C). 45.00 (*0-534-25488-8*) Wadsworth Pub.

Intervention & Reflection: Basic Issues in Medical Ethics. Ronald Munson. 6th ed. 1999. LC 99-19759. (Philosophy Ser.). 720p. spiral bd. 76.95 (*0-534-52039-1*) Wadsworth Pub.

Intervention in Child Nutrition: Evaluation Studies in Kenya. Jan Hoorweg & Rudo Neimeijer. 1988. (Monographs from the African Studies Centre). 200p. text 75.00 (*0-7103-0276-2*) Routledge.

Intervention in Occupational Stress: A Handbook of Counselling for Stress at Work. Randall R. Ross & Elizabeth M. Altmaier. 1994. LC 94-65025. 196p. pap. 24.95 (*0-8039-8673-4*, 9322) Sage.

Intervention Instruction Inc. Level 2M DUI Risk Reduction Education & Treatment Program: Program Description & Operations Procedures. Ignatius D. McDermott et al. 1995. 107p. (Orig.). pap. 9.95 (*0-9654994-0-5*) Intervention Instruct Inc.

Intervention Mapping: Designing Theory & Evidence-Based Health Programs. Kay Bartholomew. 2001. LC 00-23290. (Illus.). xxiii, 515p. text (*0-7674-1278-8*) Mayfield Pub.

Intervention Planning for Children with Communication Disorders: A Guide for Clinical Practicum & Professional Practice. Harriet B. Klein & Nelson Moses. 2nd ed. 1998. LC 98-34775. 331p. (C). 67.00 (*0-205-28747-6*, Macmillan Coll) P-H.

Intervention Research in Learning Disabilities. Ed. by Bernice Y. Wong & Thomas E. Scruggs. 1990. (Illus.). 347p. 53.95 (*0-387-97280-3*) Spr-Verlag.

Intervention Strategies for Children with Emotional or Behavioral Disorders. Marvin L. Dice. 1993. LC 93-22671. (Illus.). 276p. (Orig.). (C). pap. text 39.95 (*1-56593-166-1*, 0474) Thomson Learn.

Intervention Strategies for Emotional Problems in Later Life. Dan G. Blazer. 1994. LC 94-72729. (Master Work Ser.). 272p. pap. 50.00 (*1-56821-220-8*) Aronson.

Intervention Strategies for Infants & Toddlers with Special Needs: A Team Approach. Sharon A. Raver. 2nd ed. 1998. LC 98-16979. 447p. (C). pap. 59.00 (*0-13-674730-2*) P-H.

Intervention Trials of Cancer Prevention: Results & New Research Programmes. E. Buiatti. 1994. (IARC Scientific Publications Ser.: No. 18). v, 52p. pap. text 30.00 (*92-832-1432-3*, 1770018) World Health.

Interventional Breast Procedures. Ed. by D. David Dershaw. 1995. LC 95-41719. text (*0-443-07630-8*) Church.

Interventional Cardiology. Ed. by A. D. Kapoor. 1988. (Illus.). 415p. 189.00 (*0-387-96783-4*) Spr-Verlag.

Interventional Cardiology: New Techniques & Strategies for Diagnosis & Treatment. Ed. by Christopher J. White & Stephen R. Ramee. 1995. (Fundamental & Clinical Cardiology Ser.: Vol. 25). (Illus.). 376p. text 150.00 (*0-8247-9415-X*) Dekker.

Interventional Cardiology: Review & Self Assessment. King, III et al. 1998. (Illus.). 325p. (C). (gr. 13). pap. text 48.95 (*0-8151-4949-2*, 30378) Mosby Inc.

Interventional Cardiology: The Essentials for the Boards: Questions & Answers, Clinical Cases & Pearls. Cindy L. Grines et al. 1999. LC 99-27741. (Illus.). v, 291p. pap. 39.00 (*0-87993-443-3*) Futura Pub.

Interventional Cardiology Handbook. Ed. by Morton J. Kern. 1996. (Illus.). 624p. (C). (gr. 13). spiral bd. 47.95 (*0-8151-5032-6*, 24296) Mosby Inc.

Interventional Cardiology Self-Assessment & Review. Martin B. Leon et al. Date not set. 380p. (C). pap. text 45.00 (*1-890114-04-9*) Physicians Pr.

Interventional Cardiovascular Medicine: Principles & Practice. Ed. by Gary S. Roubin et al. 1993. (Illus.). 976p. text (*0-443-08834-9*) Church.

Interventional Cardiovascular Techniques: Principles & Practice. Richard S. Stack et al. 2nd ed. 2000. 895p. (*0-443-07979-X*) Harcrt Hlth Sci Grp.

Interventional Diagnostic & Therapeutic Procedures. Barry T. Katzen. 1980. (Comprehensive Manuals in Radiology Ser.). (Illus.). 155p. 63.00 (*0-387-90390-9*) Spr-Verlag.

Interventional Electrophysiology. Igor Singer. 1997. LC 96-17640. (Illus.). 1,133p. text 129.00 (*0-683-07734-1*) Lppncott W & W.

Interventional Electrophysiology: A Textbook. Ed. by Sanjeev Saksena & Berndt Luderitz. 2nd ed. 1996. LC 95-50681. (Illus.). 704p. 160.00 (*0-87993-613-4*) Futura Pub.

Interventional Endoscopic Ultrasonography. Ed. by Manoop S. Bhutani. 1999. 325p. text 98.00 (*90-5702-601-5*, Harwood Acad Pubs) Gordon & Breach.

Interventional Endoscopy in Hepatology. J. F. Riemann & H. Joachim Neuhaus. 2000. (Falk Symposium Ser.: Vol. 116). 176p. 74.00 (*0-7923-8761-9*) Kluwer Academic.

Interventional Fluroscopy: Physics, Technology & Safety. Stephen Balter. 2000. LC 00-43394. (Illus.). 304p. 99.95 (*0-471-39010-0*) Wiley.

Interventional Hepatobiliary Radiology. Kerlan. 1997. (Illus.). text (*0-316-48823-2*) Lppncott W & W.

Interventional Magnetic Resonance Imaging. Ed. by J. F. Debatin & Gerhard Adam. 1997. LC 97-21329. (Medical Radiology Ser.). (Illus.). 319p. 165.00 (*3-540-62587-9*) Spr-Verlag.

Interventional MRI. Robert B. Lufkin. 1998. LC 98-39428. (Illus.). 421p. (C). (gr. 13). text 129.00 (*0-8151-4545-4*, 30561) Mosby Inc.

Interventional MRI. Robert B. Lufkin. 1999. (Illus.). 421p. (*84-8174-467-0*) Mosby-Doyma Libros ESP. *Dist:* Mosby Inc.

Interventional Pain Management. Steven D. Waldman & Alon P. Winnie. Ed. by Lesley Day. 1996. (Illus.). 544p. text 145.00 (*0-7216-5874-1*) Saunders.

Interventional Physiology Rounds: Case Studies in Coronary Pressure & Flow for Clinical Practice. Morton J. Kern. 1998. 230p. pap. 74.95 (*0-471-25226-3*, Wiley-Liss) Wiley.

Interventional Pulmonology. Ed. by John F. Beamis, Jr. & Praveen N. Mathur. 1998. LC 98-15847. (Illus.). 400p. text 149.00 (*0-07-005207-7*) McGraw-Hill Educ Grp.

Interventional Radiology. Ed. by Robert Dondelinger et al. 1990. (Illus.). 800p. text 185.00 (*0-86577-286-X*) Thieme Med Pubs.

Interventional Radiology. Man Chung Han & Jae Hyung Park. 1998. 776p. text 189.00 (*89-337-0352-7*) Lppncott W & W.

Interventional Radiology. David Kessell & Iain Robertson. 2000. 255p. pap. text 49.95 (*0-443-06289-7*) Saunders.

Interventional Radiology Wilfrido R. Castaneda-Zuniga. 3rd ed. 1816p. (*0-7817-2117-2*) Lppncott W & W.

Interventional Radiology, In Two Volumes. Wilfrido R. Castaneda-Zuniga et al. 3rd ed. 1996. LC 95-51106. (Illus.). 1,816p. text 335.00 (*0-683-01477-3*) Lppncott W & W.

Interventional Radiology, Set. Wilfrido R. Castaneda-Zuniga & S. Murthy Tadavarthy. 2nd ed. 1991. (Illus.). 1568p. 250.00 (*0-683-01476-5*) Lppncott W & W.

Interventional Radiology: A Multimedia Approach Special Pre-Pub. John L. Nosher. 2000. LC 00-44414. (Illus.). 240p. 199.00 incl. cd-rom (*0-632-04404-7*) Blackwell Sci.

Interventional Radiology: A Practical Guide. Anthony Watkinson & Andreas Adam. 1996. LC 95-47010. 256p. (*1-85775-031-4*, RD33) Radcliffe Med Pr GBR. *Dist:* Balogh.

Interventional Radiology: Adjunktive (sic) Medication & Monitoring. Ed. by W. Steinbrich & W. Gross-Fengels. 1992. LC 92-48713. (Illus.). 205p. 75.00 (*0-387-56092-0*) Spr-Verlag.

Interventional Radiology Advisor. Steven V. Lossef. 1998. cd-rom 110.00 (*0-683-30221-3*) Lppncott W & W.

Interventional Radiology & Endovascular Therapy: A Teaching File, Volume 1. Uflacker. 2001. text 99.00 (*0-683-30402-X*) Lppncott W & W.

Interventional Radiology Coder. 1997. 48p. pap. 89.00 (*1-889115-17-7*) Med Learn.

Interventional Radiology in Bone & Joint. Ed. by M. Bard & J. D. Laredo. 1988. (Illus.). 300p. 213.00 (*0-387-82029-9*) Spr-Verlag.

***Interventional Radiology in Otolaryngology.** Fried & Ferenc A. Jolesz. 2001. (Illus.). 224p. (*1-901865-35-5*) Isis Med GBR. *Dist:* Bks Intl VA.

Interventional Radiology of the Gallbladder: Percutaneous Cholecystostomy. J. G. McNulty. 1990. (Illus.). 65p. 65.00 (*0-387-52905-5*) Spr-Verlag.

Interventional Radiology Procedure Manual. Michael A. Braun et al. 1997. LC 96-53121. text (*0-443-07921-8*) Church.

Interventional Radiology Review. Smith. 1998. text (*0-443-07787-8*, S2317) Church.

Interventional Techniques in Cardiovascular Medicine. Ed. by V. Hombach et al. 1991. (Developments in Cardiovascular Medicine Ser.). (C). text 243.00 (*0-7923-0956-1*) Kluwer Academic.

Interventional Therapy in Acute Stroke. Stephen M. Davis et al. 1997. LC 97-13106. (Illus.). 240p. 152.95 (*0-86542-377-6*) Blackwell Sci.

Interventional Ultrasound. Ed. by S. Weiner & A. Kurjak. 1999. (Progress in Obstetric & Gynecological Sonography Ser.). (Illus.). 190p. lib. bdg. 85.95 (*1-85070-923-8*, Parthenon Pbng) CRC Pr.

Interventional Ultrasound in Obstetrics, Gynecology & the Breast. D. Lemery & Joaquin Santolaya-Forgas. 1998. LC 98-12984. (Illus.). 384p. 168.95 (*0-632-03874-8*) Blackwell Sci.

Interventions for ADHD: Treatment in Developmental Context. Phyllis Anne Teeter. 378p. 2000. 22.00 (*1-57230-594-0*, 8R0594); 1998. LC 98-39158. pap. 40.00 (*1-57230-384-0*) Guilford Pubns.

Interventions for Alzheimer's Disease: A Caregiver's Complete Reference. Ruth M. Tappen. 1997. LC 97-1680. (Illus.). 35.00 (*1-878812-39-4*) Hlth Prof Pr.

Interventions for Children of Divorce: Custody, Access, & Psychotherapy. William F. Hodges. 2nd ed. 1991. LC 91-7468. (Personality Processes Ser.). 400p. 130.00 (*0-471-52255-4*) Wiley.

Interventions for Students with Learning Disabilities: A Meta-Analysis of Treatment Outcomes. H. Lee Swanson et al. 1999. LC 99-29679. (Illus.). 714p. text 77.00 (*1-57230-449-9*, C0449) Guilford Pubns.

Interventions in Dementia: Toward Improving Quality of Life. M. Powell Lawton & Robert L. Rubinstein. 2000. LC 99-59273. (Illus.). xx, 188p. text 38.95 (*0-8261-1325-7*) Springer Pub.

Interventions in the Acute Phase of Myocardial Infarction. Ed. by Joel Morganroth & E. Neil Moore. 1984. 320p. text 108.00 (*0-89838-659-4*) Kluwer Academic.

Interventions with Infants & Parents: The Theory & Practice of Previewing. Paul V. Trad. 1991. LC 91-3043. (Child & Adolescent Mental Health Ser.: No. 1561). 576p. 275.00 (*0-471-53229-0*) Wiley.

***Interviewer's Guide to Structured Clients.** Marlene Steinberg. 1994. 62.00 (*0-88048-862-X*) Am Psychiatric.

Interviewer's Guide to the Structured Clinical Interview for DSM-IV Dissociative Disorders (SCID-D) Marlene Stein. rev. ed. 1994. LC 94-40649. 154p. spiral bd. 45.95 (*0-88048-861-1*, 8861) Am Psychiatric.

Interviewing & Counseling in Communicative Disorders: Principles & Procedures. Kenneth G. Shipley. 2nd ed. 1996. LC 96-7010. 264p. pap. text 40.00 (*0-205-19892-9*) P-H.

Interviewing & Helping Skills for Health Professionals. L. Sherilyn Cormier et al. 1984. LC 83-14596. 352p. (C). pap. text 37.50 (*0-86720-363-3*) Jones & Bartlett.

Interviewing & Patient Care. Allen J. Enelow et al. 4th ed. 1996. (Illus.). 224p. (C). text 39.95 (*0-19-506443-7*); pap. text 19.95 (*0-19-506444-5*) OUP.

Interviewing Strategies for Helpers. William H. Cormier & Sherilyn Cormier. 2nd ed. 1985. LC 84-19837. (Family Studies Ser.). 640p. (C). pap. 40.00 (*0-534-04416-6*) Brooks-Cole.

Interviewing Strategies for Helpers - Fundamental Skills & Cognitive Behavioral Interventions. William H. Cormier & Sherilyn N. Cormier. 3rd ed. 1990. (Counseling Ser.). 670p. (C). mass mkt. 52.25 (*0-534-13824-1*) Brooks-Cole.

Interviewing the Sexually Abused Child: Investigation of Suspected Abuse. David Phillip Jones & Mary G. McQuiston. 4th ed. 1993. LC 94-148507. 80p. pap. text (*0-88048-612-0*, 8612) Royal Coll Psych GBR. *Dist:* Parkwest Pubns.

Interviews with Patients in Psychotherapy: The Client Speaks. Ursula A. Falk. 1995. LC 93-33233. (Studies in Health & Human Services: Vol. 20). 224p. text 89.95 (*0-7734-9402-2*) E Mellen.

Intestinal Absorption & Secretion, No. 36. E. Skadhauge & K. Heintze. 1983. (Falk Symposium Ser.). 576p. text 217.50 (*0-85200-765-5*) Kluwer Academic.

Intestinal Absorption of Macromolecules & Immune Transmission from Mother to Young. Karoly Baintner. 1986. 288p. 144.00 (*0-8493-5589-3*, RA1231, CRC Reprint) Franklin.

Intestinal Absorption of Minerals: Experimental & Clinical. Ed. by D. B. Lee. 1990. (Journal: Vol. 16, Nos. 2-3, 1990). (Illus.). 100p. pap. 156.75 (*3-8055-5212-2*) S Karger.

Intestinal Absorptive Surface in Mammals of Different Sizes. Robert L. Snipes. Ed. by F. Beck et al. 1997. LC 97-18871. (Advances in Anatomy, Embryology & Cell Biology Ser.: No. 138). (Illus.). 90p. pap. 72.00 (*3-540-62986-6*) Spr-Verlag.

Intestinal & Pancreatic Adaptation: Adaptational Response & Repair Mechanisms in the Entero Pancreatic System - Journal: Digestion, Vol. 46, Suppl. 2, 1990. Ed. by E. O. Riecken et al. 1990. (Illus.). vi, 478p. pap. 148.00 (*3-8055-5314-5*) S Karger.

Intestinal Calcium Absorption & Its Regulation. Ed. by Alexander D. Kenny. 1981. 176p. 97.00 (*0-8493-5701-2*, QP535, CRC Reprint) Franklin.

Intestinal Failure. Ed. by Jeremy Nightingale. 2001. (Greenwich Medical Media Ser.). (Illus.). 570p. text (*1-900151-93-6*) Greenwich Med GBR. *Dist:* JAMCO Dist.

Intestinal Flora, Immunity, Nutrition & Health. Ed. by A. P. Simopoulos et al. 1993. (World Review of Nutrition & Dietetics Ser.: Vol. 74). (Illus.). xii, 154p. 184.50 (*3-8055-5771-X*) S Karger.

Intestinal Inflammation (Colitis, Enteritis, Crohn's Disease)—Treatment & Therapy: Index of New Information. American Health Research Institute Staff. 1997. 157p. 57.50 (*0-7883-1602-8*); pap. 47.50 (*0-7883-1603-6*) ABBE Pubs Assn.

Intestinal Lipid Metabolism. Ed. by Charles M. Mansbach et al. 2000. LC 00-28732. (Illus.). xxii, 434p. 135.00 (*0-306-46241-9*, Kluwer Plenum) Kluwer Academic.

Intestinal Mucosal Damage & Repair: 5th Eisai Biwako Symposium, Lake Biwa, Shiga, Japan, November 1999. T. Bamba. 1999. (Illus.). x, 112p. 34.00 (*3-8055-7183-6*) S Karger.

Intestinal Obstruction, Vol. 13. Ed. by L. Peter Fielding & John P. Welch. 1987. LC 86-29866. (Clinical Surgery International Ser.). (Illus.). 177p. text (*0-443-03351-X*) Church.

Intestinal Parasites & Worms in Adults & Children: Index of New Information. Yoon S. Myung. 1998. 57.50 (*0-7883-1844-6*); pap. 47.50 (*0-7883-1845-4*) ABBE Pubs Assn.

Intestinal Plasticity in Health & Disease. Ed. by Bertram Wiedenmann et al. 1998. LC 98-38635. (Annals of the New York Academy of Sciences Ser.). 100.00 (*1-57331-151-0*); pap. 100.00 (*1-57331-152-9*) NY Acad Sci.

Intestinal Protozoan & Helminthic Infections. 1981. (Technical Report Ser.: No. 166). 152p. pap. text 10.00 (*92-4-120666-7*) World Health.

Intestinal Regeneration. Shailandra K. Saxena et al. 1993. LC 93-24096. (Medical Intelligence Unit Ser.). (Illus.). 128p. 99.00 (*1-879702-71-1*) Landes Bioscience.

Intestinal Spirochaetes in Domestic Animals & Humans. Ed. by D. J. Hampson & T. B. Stanton. 1997. LC 96-46784. (CAB International Publication). 392p. text 120.00 (*0-85199-140-8*) OUP.

Intestinal Stomas: Principles, Techniques, & Management. Ed. by John M. MacKeigan & Peter A. Cataldo. 1993. LC 93-7281. (Illus.). 484p. 85.00 (*0-942219-40-6*) Quality Med Pub.

Intestinal Toxicity & Inner Cleansing. Jeffrey S. Bland. 1989. 31p. pap. 3.95 (*0-87983-433-1*, 34331K, Keats Pubng) McGraw-Hill Trade.

Intima-Media Thickness & Atherosclerosis: Predicting the Risk. Ed. by Pierre-Jean Touboul & J. R. Crouse, III. 1997. LC 96-27304. (Illus.). 180p. lib. bdg. 97.95 (*1-85070-733-2*, Parthenon Pbng) CRC Pr.

Intimacy. Ed. by Martin Fisher & George Stricker. 1982. LC 82-12260. 488p. 75.00 (*0-306-40921-6*, Plenum Trade) Perseus Pubng.

Intimacy: Living As a Woman after Cancer. Jacquelyn E. Johnson. 1987. 192p. pap. (*1-55021-025-4*) NC Ltd CAN. *Dist:* U of Toronto Pr.

Intimate Adversaries: Cultural Conflict Between Doctors & Women Patients. Alexandra D. Todd. 1989. LC 88-27957. 168p. (C). text 39.95 (*0-8122-8152-7*); pap. text 20.95 (*0-8122-1277-0*) U of Pa Pr.

Intimate Attachments: Toward a New Self Psychology. Morton Shane et al. 1997. LC 97-37393. 242p. text 37.00 (*1-57230-270-4*, C2704) Guilford Pubns.

Intimate Autonomy: Autonomous Intimacy. Ed. by Barbara J. Brothers. 1991. LC 90-25177. (Journal of Couples Therapy Ser.). 146p. text 39.95 (*1-56024-089-X*) Haworth Pr.

Intimate Billroth: The Intimate Story of the Founder of Modern Surgery. Ed. by Karel B. Absolon. 1985. (Illus.). 240p. pap. 39.50 (*0-930329-05-8*) Kabel Pubs.

Intimate Death: How the Dying Teach Us How to Live. Marie De Hennezel. Tr. by Carol B. Janeway. 1998. LC 96-32774. 208p. pap. 12.00 (*0-679-76859-9*) Knopf.

Intimate Edge: Extending the Reach of Psychoanalytic Interaction. Darlene B. Ehrenberg. 1992. LC 92-12790. xi, 210p. (C). 24.95 (*0-393-70140-9*) Norton.

Intimate Environments: Sex, Intimacy & Gender in Families. Ed. by David Kantor & Barbara F. Okun. 1989. LC 88-35802. 390p. 49.00 (*0-89862-748-6*, 2748) Guilford Pubns.

Intimate Partner Violence. Sana Loue. 2001. LC 00-49772. (Women's Health Issues Ser.). 216p. 45.00 (*0-306-46519-1*, Kluwer Plenum) Kluwer Academic.

Intimate Relationships: Some Social Work Perspectives on Love. Ed. by Wendell Ricketts et al. 1987. LC 87-19729. (Journal of Social Work & Human Sexuality: Vol. 5, No. 2). 140p. text 39.95 (*0-86656-712-7*) Haworth Pr.

Intimate Worlds: How Families Thrive & Why They Fail. Maggie Scarf. 1997. LC 96-97085. 512p. pap. 14.00 (*0-345-40667-2*) Ballantine Pub Grp.

Intimates in Conflict: A Communication Perspective. Ed. by Dudley D. Cahn. 1990. (Communication Ser.). 272p. (C). pap. 39.95 (*0-8058-1169-9*) L Erlbaum Assocs.

Into Adolescence: Learning about AIDS. Jory Post & Carole McPherson. Ed. by Kathleen Middleton. 1988. (Contemporary Health Ser.). (Illus.). 231p. (Orig.). pap., tchr. ed. 23.50 (*0-941816-62-1*) ETR Assocs.

Into Teachers' Hands: Creating Classroom Success. Ed. by Meredith Reed. 11th ed. 1998. (SDE Sourcebook Ser.). (Illus.). 336p. (J). (gr. k-12). pap., tchr. ed. 24.95 (*1-884548-22-9*, 5533, Crystal Spgs) Staff Dev Educ.

Into the Community. Joan C. Stackhouse. 1998. LC 97-36822. 480p. pap. text 33.95 (*0-397-55475-3*) Lppncott W & W.

Into the Daylight: A Wholistic Approach to Healing. Calvin Morrisseau. 1998. (Illus.). LC 98-207584. 320p. text 40.00 (*0-8020-4341-0*); 192p. pap. text 14.95 (*0-8020-8162-2*) U of Toronto Pr.

Into the Lives of Others: Connecting with Nursing Home Patients. Athena Warren. 1994. pap. text 9.90 (*0-913292-03-6*) Tiresias Pr.

Into the Mother Tongue: Early Language Development. Painter. 1992. text (*0-86187-463-3*) P P Pubs GBR. *Dist:* Cassell & Continuum.

Intoxications of the Nervous System. Ed. by Pierre J. Vinken & F.A. De Wolff. 1994. 518p. 233.00 (*0-444-81283-0*) Elsevier.

Intoxification, Abreactions, Side Effects. Pamela E. Marcus. 1996. (Psychiatric Emergencies Video Ser.: Module 2). 96p. (*0-8151-7289-3*) Mosby Inc.

Intra-Abdominal Infections, Hepatitis & Gastroenteritis. Ed. by Gerald L. Mandell & Bennett Lorber. 1996. LC 96-13984. (Atlas of Infectious Diseases Ser.: Vol. 7). (Illus.). 243p. text (*0-443-07730-4*) Church GBR. *Dist:* Saunders.

Intra-Abdominal Organ Transplantation 2000. Ed. by Linda S. Sher & Leonard Makowka. 1994. LC 94-8547. (Medical Intelligence Unit Ser.). 99.00 (*1-879702-72-X*) Landes Bioscience.

Intra & Extracorporeal Cardiovascular Fluid Dynamics Ed. by P. Verdonck. Incl. Intra & Extracorporeal Cardiovascular Fluid Dynamics Vol. 1: General Principles in Application. 272p. 1998. text (*1-85312-547-4*, 5474); Intra & Extracorporeal Cardiovascular Fluid Dynamics Vol. 2: Computational Fluid-Structure Interaction in the Cardiovascular System. Ed. by K. Perktold. 376p. 2000. text (*1-85312-655-1*, 6551); LC 98-84744. (Advances in Fluid Mechanics Ser.). 648p. (*1-85312-656-X*, 656X) WIT Pr GBR. *Dist:* Computational Mech MA.

Intra & Extracorporeal Cardiovascular Fluid Dynamics Vol. 1: General Principles in Application. Ed. by P. Verdonck. 1998. LC 98-84744. (Advances in Fluid Mechanics Ser.: Vol. 22). 272p. text (*1-85312-547-4*, 5474) WIT Pr GBR. *Dist:* Computational Mech MA.

Intra & Extracorporeal Cardiovascular Fluid Dynamics Vol. 2: Computational Fluid-Structure Interaction in the Cardiovascular System. Ed. by K. Perktold & P. Verdonck. 2000. LC 98-84744. (Advances in Fluid Mechanics Ser.: Vol. 23). 376p. text (*1-85312-655-1*, 6551) WIT Pr GBR. *Dist:* Computational Mech MA.

Intra-Arterial & Intracavitary Cancer Chemotherapy. Ed. by Stephen B. Howell. 1984. (Developments in Oncology Ser.). text 102.00 (*0-89838-691-8*) Kluwer Academic.

Intra-Articular Reconstruction of the Anterior Cruciate Ligament. Ed. by Angus E. Strover. 1993. LC 93-9837. (Illus.). 288p. text (*0-7506-1385-8*) E A GBR. *Dist:* OUP.

Intra-Operative Diagnosis of CNS Tumors. Tim H. Moss et al. 1997. LC 97-9708. (Arnold Publication). (Illus.). 202p. text 145.00 (*0-340-67737-6*) OUP.

Intra-Uterine Devices: Physiological & Clinical Aspects: Report of a WHO Scientific Group, 1968. 1968. (Technical Report Ser.: No. 397). 32p. pap. text 3.00 (*92-4-120397-8*, 1100397) World Health.

Intracardiac Conductance: A Special Issue of the Journal Automedica. Ed. by M. E. Valentinuzzi. 1989. 92p. pap. text 316.00 (*0-677-25940-9*) Gordon & Breach.

Intracellular Antibodies: Ectopic Antibody Expression for Intracellular & Intercellular Immunization. Antonio Cattaneo & Silvia Biocca. 1997. LC 97-20286. (Biotechnology Intelligence Unit Ser.). 157p. text 99.95 (*1-57059-462-7*) Landes Bioscience.

Intracellular Antibodies: Research & Disease Applications. Wayne A. Marasco. 1998. LC 97-36323. (Molecular Biology Intelligence Unit Ser.). 172p. 159.00 (*1-57059-509-7*) Landes Bioscience.

Intracellular Bacterial Vaccine Vectors: Immunology Cell Biology & Genetics, Vol. 1. Yvonne Paterson. 1999. LC 98-47838. (Illus.). 267p. 92.50 (*0-471-17278-2*) Wiley.

Intracellular Calcium Regulation. Ed. by Felix Bronner. 1990. 486p. 490.00 (*0-471-56216-5*) Wiley.

Intracellular Messengers. Ed. by Alan A. Boulton et al. 1992. LC 91-20801. (Neuromethods Ser.: Vol. 20). (Illus.). 580p. 145.00 (*0-89603-207-8*) Humana.

Intracellular Messengers. Ed. by Colin W. Taylor. 1993. LC 93-3450. (International Encyclopedia of Pharmacology & Therapeutics Ser.: Section 139). 360.00 (*0-08-042184-9*, Pergamon Pr) Elsevier.

Intracerebral Hemorrhage. Carlos S. Kase & Louis R. Caplan. 1994. 516p. text 180.00 (*0-7506-9308-8*) Buttrwrth-Heinemann.

Intracranial & Inner Ear Physiology & Pathophysiology. Robert Marchbanks et al. 1998. LC 99-168871. (Illus.). (*1-86156-066-4*) Whurr Pub.

Intracranial & Intralabyrinthine Fluids: Basic Aspects & Clinical Applications. Arne Ernst et al. 1996. LC 96-18317. (Illus.). 316p. 106.00 (*3-540-60979-2*) Spr-Verlag.

Intracranial Aneurysms, Vol. 1. J. L. Fox. 1983. (Illus.). 644p. 290.00 (*0-387-90717-3*) Spr-Verlag.

Intracranial Aneurysms, Vol. 2. Ed. by J. L. Fox. 1983. (Illus.). 537p. 353.00 (*0-387-90863-3*) Spr-Verlag.

Intracranial Aneurysms, Vol. 3. J. L. Fox. 1983. 360p. 288.00 (*0-387-90864-1*) Spr-Verlag.

Intracranial Electroencephalography. Michael R. Sperling. 1999. LC 93-27906. (Atlas of Electroencephalography Ser.: Vol. 3). 328p. pap. 116.00 (*0-444-81268-7*) Elsevier.

Intracranial Germ Cell Tumors. Ed. by Y. Sawamura et al. 1998. LC 98-21794. (Illus.). 390p. 219.00 (*3-211-83127-4*) Spr-Verlag.

Intracranial Pressure. 9th ed. 1995. 188.00 (*4-431-70146-X*) Spr-Verlag.

Intracranial Pressure, Vol. 5. Ed. by Susumu Ishii et al. 1983. (Illus.). 914p. 100.00 (*0-387-12564-7*) Spr-Verlag.

Intracranial Pressure & Neuromonitoring in Brain Injury: Proceedings of the Tenth International ICP Symposium, Williamsburg, May 25-29, 1997. Ed. by Anthony Marmarou et al. 1998. LC 98-16255. (Acta Neurochirurgica Ser.: Vol. 71). (Illus.). 400p. 199.00 (*3-211-83094-4*) Spr-Verlag.

Intracranial Pressure VIII. Ed. by C. J. Avezaat et al. 1993. (Illus.). 931p. 336.00 (*0-387-55946-9*) Spr-Verlag.

Intracranial Pressure Monitoring Devices. 1988. 10p. pap. 70.00 (*0-910275-82-3*, NS28-209) Assn Adv Med Instrn.

Intracranial Pressure VII. Ed. by J. T. Hoff & L. Betz. 1989. (Illus.). 1050p. 285.00 (*0-387-50156-8*) Spr-Verlag.

Intractable Epilepsy. Ed. by Svein I. Johannessen et al. 1995. LC 95-18193. 304p. (*1-871816-28-9*) Wrightson Biomed GBR. *Dist:* Taylor & Francis.

Intramedullary Nailing & Other Intermedullary Osteosyntheses. R. Maatz et al. 1986. 230p. text 145.00 (*0-7216-1279-2*) Saunders.

Intramedullary Spinal Cord Tumors. Ed. by Jacques Brotchi & Georges Fischer. 1996. (Illus.). 128p. text 119.00 (*0-86577-593-1*) Thieme Med Pubs.

Intramembrane Charge Movements in Striated Muscle. Christopher L. Huang. 1993. LC 92-46621. (Monographs of the Physiological Society: No. 44). (Illus.). 302p. (C). text 75.00 (*0-19-857749-4*, 3595, Clarendon Pr) OUP.

Intraneural Injections for Rheumatoid Arthritis & Osteoarthritis & the Control of Pain in Arthritis in the Knee. Paul Notrik, pseud. 1984. LC 84-61283. 97p. (Orig.). pap. 9.95 (*0-931150-14-0*) Arthritis Trust.

Intraocular Lenses: Basics & Clinical Applications. Robert L. Stamper et al. 1993. LC 93-4283. (Ophthalmology Monographs: Vol. 7). (*1-56055-072-4*) Am Acad Ophthal.

Intraocular Lenses & Corneal Endothelium. Ed. by A. Neetens. 1983. (Journal: Vol. 187, No. 2). (Illus.). x, 68p. pap. 45.25 (*3-8055-3758-1*) S Karger.

Intraocular Tumors. Shields. 1991. text 210.00 (*0-7216-4268-3*) Saunders.

Intraoperative & Laparoscopic Ultrasonography. O. J. Garden. 1995. LC 95-14241. 224p. 150.00 (*0-632-03553-6*) Blackwell Sci.

Intraoperative Choledochoscopy. Aldo Leggeri et al. 1983. 116p. text (*1-57235-041-5*) Piccin Nuova.

***Intraoperative Graft Patency Verification in Cardiac & Vascular Surgery.** Ed. by Ginseppe D'Ancona et al. 2001. LC 2001-18934. (Illus.). xiv, 248p. 80.00 (*0-87993-488-3*) Futura Pub.

Intraoperative Irradiation: Techniques & Results. Leonard L. Gunderson et al. 1999. LC 98-50919. (Current Clinical Oncology Ser.: Vol. 1). (Illus.). 560p. 195.00 (*0-89603-523-9*) Humana.

Intraoperative, Laparoscopic & Endoluminal Ultrasound. Robert A. Kane. Ed. by Stephanie Donley. 1998. LC 98-38543. 260p. (C). text (*0-443-07998-6*) Church.

Intraoperative Monitoring: Questions/Answers/ References. Ronald C. Pearlman. 1998. (Illus.). 60p. pap. text 45.00 (*0-9664927-0-6*) Pearlman Pr.

Intraoperative Neurophysiologic Monitoring. Aage R. Moller. 1995. 346p. text 83.00 (*3-7186-0592-9*); 300p. pap. text 42.00 (*3-7186-0593-7*) Gordon & Breach (Harwood Acad Pubs).

Intraoperative Neurophysiologic Monitoring in Neurosurgery. Ed. by J. Schramm & Aage R. Moller. 1991. (Illus.). 303p. 162.00 (*0-387-52655-2*) Spr-Verlag.

Intraoperative Radiation Therapy. Ed. by Ralph R. Dobelbower, Jr. & Mitsuyuki Abe. 1989. 432p. 210.00 (*0-8493-6846-4*, RD652) CRC Pr.

Intraoperative Radiation Therapy: Proceedings of the Third International Symposium on Intraoperative Radiation Therapy, November 12-15, 1990, Kyoto, Japan. Ed. by Mitsuyuki Abe & Masaji Takahashi. 1991. (Illus.). 300p. 91.00 (*0-08-040702-1*) McGraw.

Intraoperative Radiation Therapy in the Treatment of Cancer: 6th International IORT Symposium & 31st San Francisco Cancer Symposium, San Francisco, Calif., September 1996. Ed. by Jerome M. Vaeth. 1997. LC 97-5478. (Frontiers of Radiation Therapy & Oncology Ser.: Vol. 31, 1997). (Illus.). xiv, 280p. 249.00 (*3-8055-6456-2*) S Karger.

Intraoperative Ultrasonography in Hepato-Biliary & Pancreatic Surgery: A Practical Guide. Ed. by L. Bolondi et al. 1989. (Series in Radiology). (C). text 191.50 (*0-7923-0261-3*) Kluwer Academic.

Intrapartum Care. Ed. by Jo Alexander et al. 1993. 300p. pap. text 16.95 (*0-8020-7451-0*) U of Toronto Pr.

Intrapartum Management Modules: A Perinatal Education Program (Including Implementation Guidelines) Ed. by Jean Martin. 2nd ed. 1996. (Illus.). 701p. pap. text 39.95 (*0-683-17195-X*) Lppncott W & W.

Intrapartum Obstetrics. Ed. by John T. Repke. 1995. LC 95-32785. 575p. text (*0-443-08949-3*) Church.

Intrapsychic & Interpersonal Dimensions of Treatment. Harold Searles & Robert J. Langs. 1980. LC 80-7480. 336p. 50.00 (*0-87668-404-5*) Aronson.

Intrathecal Drug Therapy for Spasticity & Pain: Practical Patient Management, Vol. VIII. Janet M. Gianino et al. 1996. (Illus.). 218p. 41.95 (*0-387-94552-0*) Spr-Verlag.

Intrathymic T-Cell Development. Ed. by Janko Nikolic-Zugic. 1994. LC 93-41387. (Molecular Biology Intelligence Unit Ser.). 110p. 99.00 (*1-57059-014-1*, LN9014) Landes Bioscience.

Intrauterine Devices: Technical & Managerial Guidelines for Services. WHO Staff. 1997. LC 98-141852. 54.00 (*92-4-154497-X*) World Health.

Intrauterine Devices: Their Role in Family Planning Care. WHO Staff. 1983. (WHO Offset Publications: No. 75). 53p. 5.00 (*92-4-170075-0*) World Health.

Intrauterine Growth Restriction: Aetiology & Management. John Kingdom & Philip Baker. 2000. LC 99-37272. (Illus.). 456p. 149.00 (*1-85233-191-7*) Spr-Verlag.

Intravascular Ultrasound. Raimund Erbel et al. 1998. 296p. (*1-85317-315-0*) Martin Dunitz GBR. *Dist:* Mosby Inc.

Intravascular Ultrasound. Ed. by Jos R. Roelandt et al. 1993. LC 93-1382. (Developments in Cardiovascular Medicine Ser.). 184p. (C). text 89.00 (*0-7923-2301-7*) Kluwer Academic.

Intravascular Ultrasound: Techniques, Developments, Clinical Perspectives. Ed. by N. Bom & Jos R. Roelandt. 1989. (C). text 106.00 (*0-7923-0387-3*) Kluwer Academic.

Intravascular Ultrasound Imaging. Tobis. 1992. text 190.00 (*0-443-08888-8*) Saunders.

Intravascular Ultrasound Imaging. Ed. by Jonathan M. Tobis & Paul G. Yock. 1992. (Illus.). 262p. text (*0-443-08809-8*) Church.

Intravascular Ultrasound Imaging in Coronary Artery Disease. Ed. by Robert J. Siegel. 1997. LC 97-42391. (Fundamental & Clinical Cardiology Ser.). (Illus.). 392p. text 175.00 (*0-8247-0091-0*) Dekker.

Intravenous Conscious Sedation. Donna S. Watson. 1997. LC 97-34261. (Illus.). 272p. (C). (gr. 13). pap. text 29.95 (*0-8151-9265-7*, 27471) Mosby Inc.

Intravenous Conscious Sedation: A Manual for Nurses. Michael Kost. Ed. by Maura Connor. 1997. LC 97-14401. 336p. pap. text 29.95 (*0-7216-7194-2*) Saunders.

Intravenous Feeding of the Neonate. Victor Y. Yu & Robert A. MacMahon. 1992. (Illus.). 290p. 110.00 (*0-340-55241-7*) Trafalgar.

Intravenous Immunoglobins in Clinical Practice. Ed. by Martin L. Lee & Vibeke Strand. 1997. LC 97-25515. (Illus.). 536p. text 185.00 (*0-8247-9881-3*) Dekker.

Intravenous Immunoglobulin Research & Therapy. Ed. by Michael D. Kazatchkine. 1996. LC 96-45759. (Illus.). 406p. lib. bdg. 93.95 (*1-85070-766-9*, Parthenon Pbng) CRC Pr.

Intravenous Immunoglobulins: Clinical Benefits & Future Prospects. Ed. by Michael D. Kazatchkine. 1994. (Illus.). 136p. lib. bdg. 38.95 (*1-85070-648-4*, Parthenon Pbng) CRC Pr.

Intravenous Infusion Therapy for Nurses: Principles & Practice. Dianne L. Josephson & Lynn Keegan. 1998. LC 98-39792. (Nursing Education Ser.). 608p. (C). 75.95 (*0-8273-6314-1*) Delmar.

Intravenous Medications for Critical Care. Robert Lester & Marie Dente-Cassidy. 2nd ed. 1995. LC 95-3557. (Illus.). 387p. pap. text 26.00 (*0-7216-4887-8*) Saunders.

Intravenous Therapy. Phyllis F. Nentwich. 1990. (Illus.). 512p. (C). text 54.95 (*0-86720-419-2*, 419-2) Jones & Bartlett.

Intravenous Therapy: A Guide to Quality Care. Connie White Delaney & A. R. Lauer. 1988. (Illus.). 348p. text 21.50 (*0-397-54617-3*, Lippnctt) Lppncott W & W.

Intravenous Therapy: Clinical Principles & Practice. Intravenous Nurses Society Staff. Ed. by Judy Terry. 1995. (Illus.). 611p. text 99.00 (*0-7216-4267-5*) Saunders.

Intravenous Therapy in Nursing Practice. Lisa Dougherty & Julien Lambert. 1999. LC 99-17032. (*0-443-05983-7*) Church.

Intravenous Therapy Products: Technology & Markets. 1992. 2750.00 (*0-89336-947-0*, GB-159) BCC.

Intravitreal Surgery. Gholam A. Peyman & Joel A. Schulman. 2nd ed. 1994. (Illus.). 480p. (C). pap. text 295.00 (*0-8385-4320-0*, A4320-6, Apple Lange Med) McGraw.

Intricate Engagements: The Collaborative Basis of Therapeutic Change. Steven A. Frankel. 1995. LC 95-14435. 288p. 50.00 (*1-56821-590-8*) Aronson.

Intrinsic & Extrinsic Motivation: The Search for Optimal Motivation & Performance. Ed. by Carol Sansone & Judith M. Harackiewicz. 2000. LC 00-102571. (Educational Psychology Ser.). (Illus.). xix, 489p. 85.00 (*0-12-619070-4*) Acad Pr.

Intrinsic Asthma: Proceedings of the 4th International Symposium Held at the Hochgelbigsklinik Davas from September 18-20, 1988. Michael Schmitz-Schumann. 1989. (Agents & Actions Supplements Ser.: No. 28). 350p. 96.50 (*0-8176-2289-6*) Birkhauser.

Intrinsic Diseases of Bones. Ed. by J. H. Kaufmann. 1973. (Progress in Pediatric Radiology Ser.: Vol. 4). 186.25 (*3-8055-1396-8*) S Karger.

Intrinsic Factors: William Bosworth Castle & the Development of Hematology & Clinical Investigation at Boston City Hospital. Anand B. Karnad. 1997. (Francis Countway Library of Medicine). (Illus.). 270p. 24.95 (*0-674-46080-4*) HUP.

Intrinsic Freedom: The Art of Stress-Free Living. Peter Fenner & Penny Fenner. 1994. (Illus.). 150p. (Orig.). pap. 9.95 (*1-86429-000-5*) Morehouse Pub.

Intrinsic Motivation & Self-Determination in Human Behavior. E. L. Deci & R. M. Ryan. 1985. LC 85-12413. (Perspectives in Social Psychology Ser.). (Illus.). 388p. (C). 44.50 (*0-306-42022-8*, Plenum Trade) Perseus Pubng.

Intro to Managed Care Instructor's Kit. Julia K. Wooley. Ed. by Kristen L. Falk. 2nd rev. ed. tchr. ed., ring bd. 55.00 (*0-939921-69-3*) Life Office.

Intro to Measurement in PE & Exercise Science. Terry M. Wood & Margaret J. Safrit. 3rd ed. 1993. (*0-8016-7850-1*) Mosby Inc.

Intro to Personality. E. Jerry Phares. 4th ed. 1997. LC 96-38681. 718p. (C). 99.00 (*0-673-99456-2*) Addison-Wesley.

Intro to Psychology. Miller-Rebec. 1999. 46.50 net. (*0-697-07840-X*) McGraw.

Intro to Psychology. Plotnik. 5th ed. 1998. (Psychology Ser.). pap. 29.95 (*0-534-36535-3*) Brooks-Cole.

Intro to Psychology: Exploration & Applications. Dennis L. Coon. 8th ed. 1997. LC 97-34738. (Psychology). 733p. (C). pap. 57.25 net. (*0-534-34966-8*) Brooks-Cole.

Introduccion A la Permacultura. Bill Mollison & Reny M. Slay. 1994. 202p. pap. text (*0-908228-09-0*) Tagari Pubns AUS. *Dist:* RDLE INST Bkstre.

Introduccion a la Psicopatologia. W. Wolff. (Breviarios Ser.). (SPA.). pap. 10.99 (*968-16-0943-3*) Fondo CA.

Introducing Anthroposophical Medicine. Rudolf Steiner. Tr. by Catherine Creeger from GER. 1999. LC 99-20149. (Foundations of Anthroposophical Medicine Ser.: Vol. 1). 320p. pap. 24.95 (*0-88010-463-5*) Anthroposophic.

Introducing Clinical Anaesthesia. Carl L. Gwinnutt. 1996. pap. 52.95 (*0-86542-749-6*) Blackwell Sci.

Introducing Evolutionary Psychology. Dylan Evans. 2000. (Introducing Ser.). (Illus.). 176p. pap. 11.95 (*1-84046-043-1*) Totem Bks.

Introducing New Treatments for Cancer: Practical, Ethical & Legal Problems. Ed. by C. J. Williams. 1992. 506p. pap. 155.00 (*0-471-93445-3*); LC 91-24553. 305.00 (*0-471-93113-6*, Wiley-Liss) Wiley.

Introducing Ophthalmology: A Primer for Office Staff. 1992. LC 92-49241. (*1-56055-024-4*) Am Acad Ophthal.

Introducing Palliative Care. Robert G. Twycross. 1995. LC 95-3744. pap. (*1-85775-039-X*); 2nd ed. 1997. LC 96-53159. (*1-85775-260-0*) Radcliffe Med Pr GBR. *Dist:* Balogh.

***Introducing Palliative Care.** Robert G. Twycross. 3rd ed. 2000. 200p. pap. (*1-85775-389-5*) Radcliffe Med Pr GBR. *Dist:* Balogh.

Introducing Psychological Research: Sixty Studies That Shape Psychology. Philip Banyard & Andrew Grayson. 1996. LC 95-42254. (Illus.). 528p. (C). text 55.00 (*0-8147-1275-4*) NYU Pr.

Introducing Research in Nursing. Holly S Wilson. 1987. 368p. (C). pap. text 26.95 (*0-201-08864-9*) Addison-Wesley.

Introducing Research in Nursing. Holly S. Wilson. Ed. by Mark McCormick. 2nd ed. 1992. 300p. (C). pap. text 59.00 (*0-8053-9405-2*) Benjamin-Cummings.

Introducing User-Friendly Family Therapy. Sigurd Reimers & Andrew Treacher. 1994. LC 94-10723. 240p. (C). 84.95 (*0-415-07430-4*, B4450); pap. 29.95 (*0-415-07431-2*, B4454) Routledge.

Introducing WHO. 1976. pap. text 10.00 (*92-4-156049-5*, 1150183) World Health.

Introduction - Benefits of the Bach Flower Remedies. Date not set. 4.95 (*0-8464-4566-2*) Beekman Pubs.

Introduction a la Psychanalyse. Sigmund Freud. 1989. (FRE.). pap. 29.95 (*0-7859-3041-8*) Fr & Eur.

Introduction Medical Immunology. Ed. by Gabriel Virella. 4th ed. 1997. LC 97-22373. (Illus.). 656p. text 75.00 (*0-8247-9897-X*) Dekker.

Introduction of Radiation Medicine into the Undergraduate Medical Curriculum. 1958. (Technical Report Ser.: No. 155). 24p. pap. text 3.00 (*92-4-120155-X*) World Health.

Introduction Psychology. James V. Zanden & Sandra W. Scarr. 1983. (C). stu. ed. 7.95 (*0-394-33785-9*); text 23.00 (*0-394-32884-1*) Random.

Introduction Psychology Tests & Scales. Loewenthal. 1996. LC 97-101115. 144p. pap. (*1-85728-405-4*) UCL Pr Ltd GBR. *Dist:* Taylor & Francis.

Introduction Study Guide Public Health: And Study Guide for Nurses. D. Unwin et al. 1996. LC 96-20503. 112p. (*0-335-15786-6*) OpUniv Pr.

Introduction to Abdominal Ultrasonography. Y. Higashi et al. 1995. (Illus.). 232p. 75.00 (*0-387-51889-4*) Spr-Verlag.

Introduction to Acupuncture, Vol. 1. Johannes Bischko. 2nd rev. ed. 1985. (Illus.). 135p. (*3-7760-0842-3*) K F Haug Pubs DEU. *Dist:* Medicina Bio.

Introduction to Alcoholism Counselling: A Bio-Psycho-Social Approach. Jerome D. Levin. 2nd ed. 1995. 225p. 79.95 (*1-56032-355-8*); pap. 29.95 (*1-56032-358-2*) Taylor & Francis.

Introduction to Alternative Delivery Mechanisms: HMO's, PPO's, CMP's. Ed. by Jeanie M. Johnson. 1986. 84p. 15.00 (*0-918945-02-X*) Am Hlth Lawyers.

Introduction to American Sign Language Harry W. Hoemann. 1986. LC 85-73497. (Illus.). (C). text 14.95 (*0-9614621-0-8*); pap. text 10.50 (*0-9614621-1-6*) Bowling Gr Pr.

Introduction to Anatomy & Physiology. Jack Rudman. 1994. (Regents College Proficiency Examination Ser.: CPEP-28). reprint ed. pap. 23.95 (*0-8373-5428-5*) Nat Learn.

Introduction to Anesthesiology. Competence Assurance Systems Staff. 1982. (Illus.). pap. text 45.00 (*0-89147-072-7*) CAS.

H I

Introduction to Anesthesiology. Keith Ruskin et al. 1999. (Illus.). 500p. pap. text 32.00 (*0-07-006304-4*) McGraw-Hill Med Pub.

Introduction to Animal Cytogenetics. H. C. Macgregor. 1993. LC 93-13470. 256p. (C). (gr. 13). pap. text 59.95 (*0-412-54600-0*) Chapman & Hall.

Introduction to Animal Parasitology. James D. Smyth. 3rd ed. 1995. LC 93-33961. (Illus.). 569p. (C). text 160.00 (*0-521-41770-8*); pap. text 47.95 (*0-521-42811-4*) Cambridge U Pr.

Introduction to Animal Virology. I. Halliburton. 1998. (C). (gr. 13). 2p. pap. 83.00 (*0-412-41360-4*); 200p. pap. 43.50 (*0-412-41370-1*) Chapman & Hall (Chap & Hall NY).

Introduction to Art Therapy: Faith in the Product. Bruce L. Moon. 1994. LC 93-36346. (Illus.). 222p. (C). text 50.95 (*0-398-05893-8*) C C Thomas.

Introduction to Art Therapy: Studies of the "Free" Art Expression of Behavior Problem Children & Adolescents As a Means of Diagnosis & Therapy. Margaret Naumburg. rev. ed. 1973. LC 73-78074. (Illus.). 390p. pap. 18.95 (*0-8077-2425-4*) Tchrs Coll.

Introduction to Basic Acupuncture: A Practical Guide for GPs & Other Medical Personnel. P. F. Pearson. 1987. 84p. (C). text 73.50 (*0-85200-686-1*) Kluwer Academic.

Introduction to Basic Cardiac Dysrhythmias. Sandra Atwood et al. 2nd ed. 1996. LC 96-8015. (Illus.). 288p. (C). (gr. 13). pap. text 26.00 (*0-8151-0123-6*, 24407) Mosby Inc.

Introduction to Behavioral Neuroscience. Kolb & Whishaw. 2000. (C). text 60.00 (*0-7167-3000-6*) W H Freeman.

Introduction to Behavioral Research Methods. Mark R. Leary. 1990. 360p. (C). text 50.95 (*0-534-13818-7*); 2nd ed. 1994. LC 94-32272. 422p. pap. 92.95 (*0-534-20490-2*) Brooks-Cole.

Introduction to Behavioral Science in Medicine. F. R. Hine et al. 1982. (Illus.). 350p. 90.00 (*0-387-90736-X*) Spr-Verlag.

Introduction to Bioethics. 2000. (C). text (*0-8053-4564-7*) Benjamin-Cummings.

Introduction to Bioinstrumentation: With Biological, Environmental & Medical Applications. Clifford D. Ferris. 1979. LC 78-70579. (Contemporary Hematology Ser.). 340p. pap. 109.50 (*0-89603-000-8*); 352p. pap. 79.00 (*0-89603-003-2*) Humana.

Introduction to Biological & Artificial Neural Networks for Pattern Recognition. Steven K. Rogers & Matthew Kabrisky. 1991. 220p. pap. 15.00 (*0-8194-0534-5*, VOL. TT04) SPIE.

Introduction to Biological Control. R. Van den Bosch et al. 1982. LC 81-21125. (Illus.). 262p. (C). text 39.50 (*0-306-40706-X*, Kluwer Plenum) Kluwer Academic.

Introduction to Biological Radiation Effects. U. L. Prenn. 2nd ed. 1994. LC 94-20439. (Illus.). 130p. pap. 80.00 (*1-56216-206-3*) Systems Co.

Introduction to Biomedical Engineering. Ed. by Susan M. Blanchard et al. 1999. LC 98-38976. 656p. (C). text 69.95 (*0-12-238660-4*) Harcourt Coll Pubs.

Introduction to Biomedical Engineering. Arthur B. Ritter & Stanley Reisman. Date not set. (Illus.). text (*0-8247-9616-0*) Dekker.

Introduction to Biomedical Equipment Technology. Joseph J. Carr & John M. Brown. 1981. LC 80-6218. (Electronic Technology Ser.). 430p. (C). pap. text 6.00 (*0-471-04144-0*) P-H.

Introduction to Biomedical Equipment Technology. Joseph J. Carr & John Brown. 4th ed. 2000. LC 00-38505. 743p. 115.00 (*0-13-010492-2*) P-H.

Introduction to Biophysics with Medical Orientation. Imre Tarjan. 1991. 443p. (C). 175.00 (*0-569-09002-4*) St Mut.

Introduction to Biophysics with Medical Orientation. Ed. by Gyorgyi Ronto & Imre Tarjan. 2nd enl. rev. ed. 1997. LC 94-220531. 442p. pap. (*963-05-6757-1*) Akade Kiado HUN. *Dist:* Intl Spec Bk, St Mut.

Introduction to Biophysics with Medical Orientation. Imre Tarjan & G. Ronto. 2nd rev. ed. 1991. 441p. (C). (*963-05-5907-2*) Akade Kiado HUN. *Dist:* Intl Spec Bk, St Mut.

Introduction to Bioprogressive Therapy. Nakajima. 1987. (Illus.). 166p. text 80.00 (*1-85097-007-6*) Quint Pub Co.

Introduction to Biopsy Interpretation & Surgical Pathology. J. C. Underwood. 1981. (Illus.). 149p. 37.50 (*0-387-10434-8*) Spr-Verlag.

Introduction to Biopsy Interpretation & Surgical Pathology. J. C Underwood. 2nd ed. 1987. (Illus.). 217p. 43.95 (*0-387-17495-8*) Spr-Verlag.

Introduction to Brain Topography. P. K. Wong. 1991. LC 90-14228. (Illus.). 270p. (C). text 65.00 (*0-306-43738-4*, Kluwer Plenum) Kluwer Academic.

Introduction to Buddhist Psychology. Padmasiri De Silva. 3rd ed. 2001. 176p. 75.00 (*0-7425-0856-0*); pap. 24.95 (*0-7425-0857-9*) Rowman.

Introduction to Cardiology. L. C. Gupta. 1990. 342p. (C). (*81-85017-52-2*) Interprint IND. *Dist:* St Mut.

Introduction to Cardiovascular Physiology. J. R. Levick. (Illus.). (Orig.). 2nd ed. 1995. LC 94-45631. 336p. pap. (*0-7506-2167-2*); 3rd ed. 2000. LC 2001-268342. 432p. pap. text (*0-340-76376-0*) E A GBR. *Dist:* OUP.

Introduction to Cardiovascular Physiology. J. R. Levick. 3rd ed. 2000. 432p. (Orig.). pap. (*0-7506-4593-8*) E A GBR. *Dist:* OUP.

Introduction to Chemical Dependency Counseling (A1) Jerome D. Levin. 2001. LC 00-38965. 60.00 (*0-7657-0289-4*) Aronson.

Introduction to Child Development. John P. Dworetzky. 6th ed. 1996. LC 96-12902. 550p. spiral bd. 87.95 (*0-314-06748-5*) Wadsworth Pub.

Introduction to Child Development. John P. Dworetzky. Ed. by Clyde Perlee. 5th ed. 1993. LC 92-39465. 550p. (C). text 45.50 (*0-314-01135-8*) West Pub.

Introduction to Child Psychiatry. Stella Chess. 2nd ed. 1969. LC 69-15085. 272p. text 44.95 (*0-8089-0098-6*, 790830, Grune & Strat) Harcrt Hlth Sci Grp.

Introduction to Children with Language Disorders. Vicki A. Reed. 2nd ed. 1993. LC 93-2404. 544p. (C). pap. 94.00 (*0-02-399150-X*, Macmillan Coll) P-H.

Introduction to Chinese Medical Chinese. Nigel Wiseman & Ye Feng. 2000. LC 00-52436. (*0-912111-65-8*) Paradigm Publns.

Introduction to Classical & Modern Test Theory. Linda Crocker & James Algina. 1986. LC 85-17647. 512p. (C). pap. 82.00 (*0-03-061634-4*) Harcourt Coll Pubs.

Introduction to Clinical Allied Healthcare. Debra L. Garber. 2nd ed. 1998. LC 98-70063. (Clinical Allied Healthcare Ser.). (Illus.). 576p. (C). pap. text 44.95 (*0-89262-551-1*) Career Pub.

Introduction to Clinical Allied Healthcare: Instructor's Guide. Debra Garber. Ed. by Kay Cox-Stevens. 1998. (Clinical Allied Healthcare Ser.). (Illus.). 762p. tchr. ed., ring bd. 99.95 (*0-89262-552-X*) Career Pub.

Introduction to Clinical Allied Healthcare: Workbook. Debra Garber. Ed. by Kay Cox-Stevens. 1998. (Clinical Allied Healthcare Ser.). (Illus.). 148p. spiral bd., wbk. ed. 19.95 (*0-89262-550-3*) Career Pub.

Introduction to Clinical Cardiology. Edward K. Chung & Lisa S. Chung. 1983. (Continuing Education Ser.: Vol. 4). (Illus.). xiv, 546p. 85.25 (*3-8055-2997-X*) S Karger.

Introduction to Clinical Child Psychology. Stan Lindsay & Graham Powell. 1988. text (*0-566-05103-6*) Avebury GBR. *Dist:* Ashgate Pub Co.

Introduction to Clinical Ethics. Ed. by John C. Fletcher et al. 2nd rev. ed. 1997. 356p. pap. 39.00 (*1-55572-050-1*) Univ Pub Group.

Introduction to Clinical Examination. Ed. by John F. Munro & Michael J. Ford. 6th ed. 1995. LC 92-48188. 144p. pap. text (*0-443-04787-1*) Church.

Introduction to Clinical Imaging. D. L. Dixon & L. M. Dugdale. 1988. (Illus.). 316p. pap. text (*0-443-03060-X*) Church.

Introduction to Clinical Immunology & Serology. Frances K. Widmann & Carole A. Itatani. 2nd ed. 1998. (Illus.). 473p. (C). pap. text 36.95 (*0-8036-0302-9*) Davis Co.

Introduction to Clinical Lab Science: International Edition. Mahon. 1998. (C). pap. text 22.00 (*0-8089-2063-4*, Grune & Strat) Harcrt Hlth Sci Grp.

Introduction to Clinical Laboratory Science. Jeanne M. Clerc. 1991. (Illus.). 144p. (gr. 13). text 33.95 (*0-8016-1392-2*, 01392) Mosby Inc.

Introduction to Clinical Laboratory Science. Connie Mahon. 1998. LC 97-36630. 334p. (C). pap. text 29.95 (*0-7216-4990-4*) Saunders.

Introduction to Clinical Medicine. Steinmenn. Date not set. pap. text (*0-7216-6002-9*) Saunders.

Introduction to Clinical Medicine: A Student-to-Student Manual. Roger M. Macklis et al. 3rd ed. 1994. LC 94-14222. 320p. spiral bd. 29.95 (*0-316-54243-1*, Little Brwn Med Div) Lppncott W & W.

Introduction to Clinical Neurology. Douglas J. Gelb. 2nd ed. 2000. (Illus.). 416p. pap. text 39.99 (*0-7506-7202-1*) Buttrwrth-Heinemann.

Introduction to Clinical Neuropsychology: A Casebook. Richard I. Naugle et al. 1998. LC 97-6565. (Illus.). 320p. text 38.00 (*0-89079-714-5*, 8339) PRO-ED.

Introduction to Clinical Nutrition. Vishwanath M. Sardesai. 1997. LC 97-42393. (Illus.). 488p. text 85.00 (*0-8247-9865-1*) Dekker.

Introduction to Clinical Optometry. A. M. Skeffington. Ed. by Sally M. Corngold. rev. ed. 1988. (Introduction to Behavioral Optometry Ser.). (Illus.). 64p. reprint ed. pap. text 18.00 (*0-943599-05-9*) OEPF.

Introduction to Clinical Pharmacology. Marilyn W. Edmunds. 2nd ed. 1995. 160p. (C). pap. text, stu. ed. (*0-8151-3037-6*, 23776); 2nd ed. 1994. 448p. (C). (gr. 13). pap. text 32.00 (*0-8016-7890-0*, 07890); 3rd ed. 2000. (Illus.). 487p. pap., tchr. ed. (*0-323-00848-8*); 3rd ed. 2000. (Illus.). 487p. pap., stu. ed. 16.95 (*0-323-00846-1*); 3rd ed. 1999. LC 99-42911. (Illus.). xiii, 487p. (C). pap. text 32.00 (*0-323-00845-3*) Mosby Inc.

***Introduction to Clinical Pharmacology: Including Student Learning Guide.** Marilyn W. Edmunds. 2000. (Illus.). 487p. pap. 44.00 (*0-323-00844-5*) Mosby Inc.

Introduction to Clinical Pharmacology: Instructor's Resource Manual with Testbank. Marilyn W. Edmunds. 2nd ed. 1995. 448p. tchr. ed. (*0-8151-3038-4*) Mosby Inc.

Introduction to Clinical Pharmacology: Text & Student Learning Guide Package. Marilyn W. Edmunds. 2nd ed. 1995. stu. ed. (*0-8151-3036-8*) Mosby Inc.

Introduction to Clinical Psychiatry. G. David Elkin. 1998. (Lange Medical Bks.). (Illus.). 450p. (C). pap. text 34.95 (*0-8385-4333-2*, A-4333-9, Apple Lange Med) McGraw.

Introduction to Clinical Psychiatry. Brian Davies & Graham Burrows. 4th ed. 1991. 200p. pap. (*0-522-84328-X*) Melbourne Univ Pr AUS. *Dist:* Paul & Co Pubs.

Introduction to Clinical Psychology. Ed. by Lynda A. Heiden & Michel Hersen. 1995. LC 95-17695. (Illus.). 428p. (C). 44.50 (*0-306-44877-7*, Kluwer Plenum) Kluwer Academic.

Introduction to Clinical Psychology: Scientific Foundations to Clinical Practice. Michael Wierzbicki. 1998. LC 98-15832. 432p. (C). 71.00 (*0-205-15517-0*) Allyn.

Introduction to Clinical Psychopharmacology. Paul Smith & Cynthia L. Darlington. 1996. 152p. text 34.50 (*0-8058-2096-5*); pap. text 17.50 (*0-8058-2097-3*) L Erlbaum Assocs.

Introduction to Clinical Radiation Oncology. Lawrence R. Coia & David J. Moylan. 3rd ed. 1998. LC 96-9113. (Illus.). 580p. pap. text 48.95 (*0-944838-70-7*) Med Physics Pub.

Introduction to Clinical Radiology. Wallace T. Miller. 1982. 291p. 43.95 (*0-07-105300-X*) McGraw.

Introduction to Clinical Reproductive Endocrinology. Gillian C. Lachelin. 1991. 216p. pap. text (*0-7506-1171-5*) E A GBR. *Dist:* OUP.

Introduction to Clinical Research. Ed. by Catherine DeAngelis. 1990. (Illus.). 192p. text 37.50 (*0-19-506249-3*) OUP.

Introduction to Clinical Research in Communication Disorders. Mary Pannbacker & Grace Middleton. 1994. (Illus.). 302p. (Orig.). (C). pap. text 34.95 (*1-56593-219-6*, 0579) Thomson Learn.

Introduction to Clinical Research in Psychiatry. Dan G. Blazer & Judith C. Hays. 1998. (Oxford Psychiatry Ser.). (Illus.). 248p. text 39.95 (*0-19-510213-4*) OUP.

Introduction to Clinical Skills: A Patient-Centered Textbook. Ed. by Mark B. Mengel & Scott A. Fields. 1997. LC 96-39432. (Illus.). 519p. (C). text 59.50 (*0-306-45350-9*, Kluwer Plenum) Kluwer Academic.

Introduction to Cognitive & Neural Modeling. D. S. Levine. 1991. 456p. (C). pap. 27.50 (*0-8058-0268-1*) L Erlbaum Assocs.

Introduction to Cognitive Rehabilitation: Theory & Practice. McKay M. Sohlberg & Catherine A. Mateer. 1989. LC 88-24415. 414p. text 50.00 (*0-89862-738-9*, 2738) Guilford Pubns.

Introduction to Communication Disorders. Diana Syder. 1992. LC 92-17226. 182p. pap. 42.50 (*1-56593-041-X*, 0289) Thomson Learn.

Introduction to Communication Disorders: A Multicultural Approach. Charlena M. Seymour et al. 1997. LC 97-26063. 313p. text 49.99 (*0-7506-9559-5*) Buttrwrth-Heinemann.

Introduction to Communication Sciences & Disorders. Fred D. Minifie. 1994. tchr. ed. 19.95 (*1-56593-378-8*, 0708) Singular Publishing.

Introduction to Communicative Disorders: Student's Coursebook. M. N. Hegde. 2nd ed. 1995. 203p. pap. 19.00 (*0-89079-614-9*, 6871) PRO-ED.

Introduction to Community Health. James F. McKenzie & Robert R. Pinger. (Health Science Ser.). 1995. LC 94-20883. (C). pap. text, tchr. ed. 10.00 (*0-06-500798-0*); 2nd ed. 1997. LC 97-21863. (Illus.). 720p. pap. text 54.95 (*0-7637-0584-5*, 0584-5); 2nd ed. 1995. LC 94-20883. (Illus.). 688p. (C). pap. text 50.00 (*0-06-500797-2*, 00797-2) Jones & Bartlett.

***Introduction to Community Health.** James F. McKenzie et al. 4th ed. 2001. LC 2001-50232. 57.95 (*0-7637-1679-0*) Jones & Bartlett.

Introduction to Community Health: Web Enhanced. James F. McKenzie et al. 3rd ed. 1998. LC 98-41087. (Illus.). 720p. (C). pap. text 56.95 (*0-7637-0872-0*, 0872-0) Jones & Bartlett.

Introduction to Comparative Psychology. 2. C. Lloyd Morgan. 1977. LC 77-72191. (Contributions to the History of Psychology Ser.: Pt. D, Vol. II, Comparative Psychology). 240p. reprint ed. lib. bdg. 69.50 (*0-313-26946-7*, U6946, Greenwood Pr) Greenwood.

Introduction to Complementary & Alternative Therapies. Ed. by Georgia M. Decker. 1999. LC 99-68395. (Illus.). x, 261p. pap. text 35.00 (*1-890504-14-9*) Oncology Nursing.

Introduction to Computed Tomography. Lois E. Romans. 1995. LC 94-43673. (Illus.). 225p. pap. 30.95 (*0-683-07353-2*) Lppncott W & W.

Introduction to Configural Frequency Analysis: The Search for Types & Antitypes in Cross-Classifications. Alexander V. Eye. 1990. (Illus.). 284p. (C). text 54.95 (*0-521-38090-1*) Cambridge U Pr.

Introduction to Connectionist Modelling of Cognitive Processes. Peter McLeod et al. 1998. (Illus.). 404p. pap. text 37.95 (*0-19-852426-9*) OUP.

Introduction to Contemporary Nutrition. L. Whittaker. 2nd ed. 1994. (C). pap. text 31.00 net. (*0-07-069955-0*) McGraw.

Introduction to Cranialsacral Therapy: Anatomy, Function & Treatment. Don Cohen. 1996. LC 95-48203. (Illus.). 114p. (Orig.). (C). pap. 18.95 (*1-55643-183-X*) North Atlantic.

***Introduction to Critical Care Nursing.** Mary Lou Sole et al. 2001. (Illus.). stu. ed. 17.95 (*0-7216-8691-5*) Saunders.

Introduction to Critical Care Nursing. Jeanette Hartshorn & Mary L. Sole. Ed. by Barbara N. Cullen. 2nd ed. 1997. LC 96-16723. (Illus.). 608p. text 49.95 (*0-7216-6218-8*) Saunders.

Introduction to Critical Care Nursing. Jeanette Hartshorn et al. 2nd rev. ed. 1997. (Illus.). 605p. tchr. ed. (*0-7216-6219-6*) Saunders.

Introduction to Critical Care Skills. Janet-Beth Flynn. 1993. LC 92-48815. (Illus.). 544p. (C). (gr. 13). pap. text 39.00 (*0-8016-2455-X*, 02455) Mosby Inc.

Introduction to Cybernetics. W. Ross Ashby. 1964. reprint ed. pap. 17.95 (*0-416-68300-2*, NO. 2064) Routledge.

Introduction to Dental Assisting. Andrews. 1995. (Dental Assisting Procedures Ser.). pap. 29.95 (*0-8273-6141-6*) Delmar.

Introduction to Dental Materials. Van Noort. 1994. 240p. text 37.50 (*0-7234-1963-9*) Mosby Inc.

Introduction to Dermatological Surgery. Clifford M. Lawrence & Gerard Panting. 1996. LC 96-8184. (Illus.). 160p. (Orig.). pap. text 39.95 (*0-86542-964-2*) Blackwell Sci.

Introduction to Developmental Disabilities: A Neurodevelopmental Perspective. Frank R. Brown & Nick Elksnin. 1994. LC 94-7358. (Illus.). 232p. (Orig.). (C). pap. text 39.95 (*1-56593-103-3*, 0406) Thomson Learn.

Introduction to Diagnostic Flow Cytometry. Ed. by S. David Hudnall. 2000. 400p. 79.50 (*0-89603-819-X*) Humana.

Introduction to Diagnostic Imaging. Isadore Meschan & David J. Ott. 1984. (Illus.). 416p. text 65.00 (*0-7216-6277-3*) Saunders.

Introduction to Diagnostic Imaging. Gary K. Stimac. 1992. (Illus.). 655p. text 102.00 (*0-7216-1305-5*) Saunders.

Introduction to Diagnostic Microbiology. Orten C. Skinner. 1975. LC 74-78591. (Allied Health Ser.). pap. 16.15 (*0-672-61391-3*, Bobbs) Macmillan.

Introduction to Diagnostic Microbiology: A Text & Workbook. Maria D. Delost. 1996. LC 95-48334. (Illus.). 592p. (C). (gr. 13). pap. text 48.00 (*0-8016-7853-6*, 07853) Mosby Inc.

Introduction to Dialysis. Ed. by Martin G. Cogan & Patricia Schoenfield. 2nd ed. 1991. (Illus.). 384p. text (*0-443-08720-2*) Church.

Introduction to Dispensing. Vol. I. William A. Borover. 1981. (Illus.). 259p. per. 48.00 (*0-9606398-0-2*) Gracie Ent.

Introduction to Dramatherapy: Ariadne's Ball of Thread. Sue Jennings. 1995. LC 98-114033. 200p. pap. 24.95 (*1-85302-115-6*) Taylor & Francis.

Introduction to Dream Interpretation. Manly P. Hall. pap. 4.95 (*0-89314-323-5*) Philos Res.

Introduction to Drug Metabolism. I. Gibson & P. Skett. 2nd ed. 1993. (Illus.). 280p. (Orig.). pap. (*0-7514-0042-4*) B Acad & Prof GBR. *Dist:* Routldge.

***Introduction to Drug Metabolism.** 3rd ed. 2001. pap. (*0-7487-6011-3*) Nelson Thornes GBR. *Dist:* Intl Spec Bk.

Introduction to Dysphagia Management. Michael E. Groher & Michael A. Crary. 2001. (Illus.). 250p. 40.00 (*0-7506-9995-7*) Buttrwrth-Heinemann.

Introduction to Ear Acupuncture: Microsystem of the Auricle. A. Rubach. 2001. LC 00-48873. (Illus.). 248p. 59.00 (*0-86577-937-6*) Thieme Med Pubs.

Introduction to Ecology & Population Biology. Thomas C. Emmel. 1973. (Illus.). 224p. (C). (gr. 11-12). pap. text 17.00 (*0-393-09371-9*) Norton.

Introduction to Educational Gerontology. Ronald H. Sherron & D. Barry Lumsden. 3rd ed. 1989. 34.95 (*1-56032-039-7*); 78.95 (*0-89116-057-4*) Hemisp Pub.

Introduction to Educational Psychology. Hershel D. Thornburg. 1984. (Illus.). 555p. (C). pap. text 52.00 (*0-314-77830-6*) West Pub.

Introduction to Efficacy in Diagnostic Radiology & Nuclear Medicine (Justification of Medical Radiation Exposure) Intro. by Charles B. Meinhold. 1995. LC 95-24596. (NCRP Commentaries Ser.: No. 13). 29p. pap. text 20.00 (*0-929600-45-2*) NCRP Pubns.

Introduction to Electrocardiography. J. P. Hamer. 1975. (Illus.). text 50.00 (*0-272-00219-4*) St Mut.

Introduction to Electrocardiography. John Hamer. 1975. (Illus.). 144p. pap. 17.00 (*0-8464-0523-7*) Beekman Pubs.

Introduction to Electrocardiography. Paul L. Huang. 1993. (Illus.). 208p. pap. text 24.00 (*0-7216-4856-8*) Saunders.

Introduction to Electromyography & Nerve Conduction Testing. John L. Echternach. 2nd ed. 2002. 170p. lab manual ed. 29.00 (*1-55642-529-5*) SLACK Inc.

Introduction to Electromyography & Nerve Conduction Testing: A Laboratory Manual. John L. Echternach. 1994. LC 90-52863. (Illus.). 160p. pap. 25.00 (*1-55642-188-5*, 41885) SLACK Inc.

Introduction to Electron Microscopy. Cecil E. Hall. 2nd ed. 1983. LC 80-39788. 410p. reprint ed. lib. bdg. 40.50 (*0-89874-302-8*) Krieger.

Introduction to Electron Microscopy. Saul Wischnitzer. 3rd ed. 1981. LC 80-15266. 320p. text 88.00 (*0-08-026298-8*); pap. text 54.00 (*0-08-028038-2*) Elsevier (Pergamon Pr).

Introduction to EMS Systems. Bruce J. Walz. 2001. LC 2001-28225. (Illus.). xxi, 364p. (C). pap. text 33.95 (*0-7668-1984-1*) Delmar.

Introduction to English Terminology of Chinese Medicine: American Edition. Nigel Wiseman & Ye Feng. 2000. LC 00-51045. (CHI & ENG.). (0-912111-64-X) Paradigm Publns.

Introduction to Environmental Epidemiology. Ed. by Evelyn O. Talbott & Gunther F. Craun. 1995. LC 95-2746. 240p. lib. bdg. 75.00 (0-87371-573-X, L573) Lewis Pubs.

Introduction to Environmental Health. Ed. by Daniel S. Blumenthal & James Ruttenber. 2nd rev. ed. 1995. 392p. (C). 43.95 (0-8261-3901-9) Springer Pub.

Introduction to Epidemiology. Donald B. Stone et al. 1995. 208p. (C). pap. 50.31 (0-697-12289-1) McGrw-H Hghr Educ.

Introduction to Epidemiology. Thomas C. Timmreck. (Health Science Ser.). 1994. 504p. pap. 45.00 (0-86720-822-8); 2nd ed. 1999. (Illus.). 64p. (C). pap. text, tchr. ed. 62.95 (0-7637-0927-1, 0927-1) Jones & Bartlett.

Introduction to Epidemiology & Biometrics. Ed. by M. Y. Heshmat & J. Herson. 1974. LC 74-11495. 184p. pap. text 9.00 (0-8422-0394-X) Irvington.

Introduction to Ergonomics. W. T. Singleton. 1972. 145p. pap. text 18.00 (92-4-156038-X, 1150081) World Health.

Introduction to Ethos of Nursing. J. M. Mellish. 1989. pap. text 32.50 (0-409-10007-2) Buttrwrth-Heinemann.

Introduction to Eye Care for the Local Health Worker. Michael A. Henningsen. 1990. (Illus.). 86p. (Orig.). pap. text 8.00 (0-9626292-0-0) Vision Care Intl.

Introduction to Facet Theory: Content Design & Intrinsic Data Analysis in Behavioral Research. Samuel Shye et al. 1994. LC 93-44776. (Applied Social Research Methods Ser.: Vol. 35). 184p. (C). 69.95 (0-8039-5670-3, 4021); pap. 26.95 (0-8039-5671-1, 4022) Sage.

Introduction to Family Therapy. Ed. by Vincent D. Foley. 2nd ed. 1986. 240p. text 21.95 (0-8089-1810-9, 791290, Grune & Strat) Harcrt Hlth Sci Grp.

Introduction to Fermentation Practices. S. Cave & D. R. Harper. 2nd ed. 1998. LC 97-49308. (Medical Perspectives Ser.). 160p. pap. 32.50 (0-387-91557-5) Spr-Verlag.

Introduction to Fluorescent In-Situ Hybridization: Principles & Clinical Applications. Ed. by Michael Andreeff & Daniel Pinkel. 1999. LC 98-37311. (Illus.). 472p. 235.00 (0-471-01345-5) Wiley.

Introduction to Food Science. Rick Parker. 2001. LC 00-52395. 672p. (C). pap. 50.95 (0-7668-1314-2) Delmar.

Introduction to Free Radical Chemistry. Andrew Parsons. 2000. LC 00-36114. (Illus.). 316p. pap. 41.95 (0-632-05292-9) Blackwell Sci.

Introduction to Functional Electrical Stimulation (FES) Jeanne O. Teeter. 1992. 5p. pap. text 5.00 (1-888470-00-3) FES Info Ctr.

Introduction to Functional Magnetic Resonance Imaging: Principles & Techniques. Richard B. Buxton. 2001. LC 00-50235. (Illus.). 320p. (C). text 100.00 (0-521-58113-3) Cambridge U Pr.

Introduction to Functional Voice Therapy. D. A. Weiss. 1971. (Illus.). v, 94p. 14.00 (3-8055-1222-8) S Karger.

Introduction to Gene Therapy & Molecular Medicine. Ed. by Thomas F. Kresina. 2000. (Illus.). 300p. (C). text 45.00 (1-891786-02-4) Fitzgerald Sci.

Introduction to General Pathology. W. G. Spector. 3rd ed. 1989. (Illus.). 352p. pap. text 34.00 (0-443-03932-1) Saunders.

Introduction to Genetics. George J. Brewer & Charles F. Sing. 1983. (Biology Ser.). (Illus.). 784p. tchr. ed. 8.00 net. (0-201-10139-4) Addison-Wesley.

Introduction to Genetics. Sandra Pennington. 1999. LC 99-25401. (Eleventh Hour Ser.). (Illus.). 225p. pap. 20.95 (0-632-04438-1) Blackwell Sci.

Introduction to Gerontology: Aging in American Society. Colbert Rhodes. 1998. (Illus.). 240p. (C). text 43.95 (0-398-05376-6) C C Thomas.

Introduction to Group Analytic Psychotherapy: Studies in the Social Integration of Individuals & Groups. S. H. Foulkes. 1991. 185p. reprint ed. pap. text (0-946439-00-1) Karnac Bks GBR. *Dist:* Other Pr LLC.

Introduction to Group Dynamics. Donelson R. Forsyth. 1983. LC 82-12783. (Psychology Ser.). 512p. (C). mass mkt. 35.00 (0-534-01225-6) Brooks-Cole.

Introduction to Group Therapy. S. R. Slavson. 1970. 352p. pap. 24.95 (0-8236-8095-9, 22780) Intl Univs Pr.

Introduction to Group Therapy: A Practical Guide. Scott Simon Fehr. 1999. LC 98-41557. 264p. lib. bdg. 49.95 (0-7890-0612-X) Haworth Pr.

Introduction to Group Treatment for Aphasia: Design & Management. Robert C. Marshall. 1998. LC 98-44096. 192p. pap. text 34.99 (0-7506-7013-4) Buttrwrth-Heinemann.

Introduction to Gynecologic Cytopathology: With Histologic & Clinical Correlations. Leopold G. Koss et al. 1998. LC 98-18541. 205p. 149.00 (0-683-30557-3) Lppncott W & W.

Introduction to Health: Policy, Planning, & Financing. Brian Abel-Smith. 1994. LC 94-7222. pap. text (0-582-23865-X) Longman.

Introduction to Health: Policy, Planning & Financing. Brian Abel-Smith. 1994. LC 94-7222. text (0-582-23866-8) Longman.

Introduction to Health Care. Helen Krewson & Diane Breckenridge. 2001. (Illus.). 635p. text (0-7216-7926-9) Saunders.

***Introduction to Health Care.** Helen Krewson & Diane Breckenridge. 2001. (Illus.). tchr. ed. (0-7216-7934-X); wbk. ed. (0-7216-7972-2) Saunders.

Introduction to Health Care Administration - New Century Edition. Winborn Davis. rev. ed. 1999. LC 99-184339. 83.00 (0-929442-41-5, 2201PP) Prof Prnting & Pub.

Introduction to Health Care Delivery & Radiology Administration. Stephen S. Hiss. Ed. by Lisa Biello. 1997. 400p. pap. text 26.00 (0-7216-5314-6) Saunders.

Introduction to Health Education & Health Promotion. Bruce G. Simons-Morton et al. 2nd rev. ed. 1995. 510p. (C). pap. text 32.95 (0-88133-845-1) Waveland Pr.

***Introduction to Health Information Technology.** Nadina Davis & Melissa LaCour. 2001. (Illus.). LC 2001-49542. 605p. (0-7216-8353-3); pap., tchr. ed. (0-7216-8403-3); pap., wbk. ed. (0-7216-8354-1) Saunders.

***Introduction to Health Information Technology: ExaMaster.** Nadina Davis & Melissa LaCour. 2001. (0-7216-8360-6) Saunders.

Introduction to Health Occupations. Badasch & Doreen S. Chesebro. abr. ed. 1994. 144p. pap., stu. ed. 17.40 (0-89303-174-7) P-H.

Introduction to Health Occupations. Shirley A. Badasch & Doreen S. Chesebro. 4th ed. 1996. LC 96-20448. 720p. 59.00 (0-8359-5010-7) P-H.

***Introduction to Health Occupations: Today's Health Care Worker.** Badasch. 5th ed. 1999. 576p. suppl. ed., wbk. ed. 34.60 (0-13-013247-0) P-H.

Introduction to Health Occupations: Today's Health Care Worker. Shirley A. Badasch. 5th ed. 1999. LC 99-38341. (Illus.). 724p. 66.00 (0-13-013147-4) P-H.

Introduction to Health Physics. Herman Cember. 2nd ed. 1983. (Illus.). text 150.00 (0-08-030129-0); pap. text 47.50 (0-08-030936-4) Elsevier (Pergamon Pr).

Introduction to Health Physics. H. Herbert Cember. 3rd ed. 1993. text 45.00 (0-07-105453-7) McGraw-Hill Med Pub.

Introduction to Health Physics. Herman H. Cember. 3rd ed. 1996. LC 95-25269. 731p. pap. 49.95 (0-07-105461-8) McGraw-Hill Prof.

Introduction to Health Planning. Philip N. Reeves & Russell C. Coile, Jr. 4th ed. 1990. LC 89-81230. (Illus.). xvii, 321p. reprint ed. pap. 32.50 (0-87815-059-5) Info Resources.

Introduction to Health Psychology. Robert J. Gatchel & Andrew Baum. 1983. 352p. (C). pap. text 21.95 (0-394-34800-1) Random.

Introduction to Health Psychology. Andrew Baum et al. 2nd ed. 1988. 432p. (C). pap. text 23.95 (0-394-37921-7) Random.

Introduction to Health Psychology. Robert J. Gatchel et al. 2nd ed. 1988. LC 93-21072. (C). pap. text 37.74 net. (0-07-553860-1) McGraw.

Introduction to Health Psychology. Andrew Baum et al. 3rd ed. 1997. LC 96-35210. 448p. (C). pap. 55.00 (0-07-022961-9) McGrw-H Hghr Educ.

Introduction to Health Sciences Librarianship: A Management Handbook. Frank R. Kellerman. 1997. LC 96-8427. (Greenwood Library Management Collection). 240p. lib. bdg. 67.50 (0-313-29761-4, Greenwood Pr) Greenwood.

Introduction To Health Services. Ed. by Stephen J. Williams & Paul R. Torrens. 5th abr. rev. ed. 1998. LC 98-22182. (Delmar Series in Health Services Administration Ser.). 450p. 87.95 (0-8273-7852-1) Delmar.

***Introduction to Health Services.** Ed. by Stephen J. Williams & Paul R. Torrens. 6th ed. 2001. LC 2001-37292. 475p. text 83.95 (0-7668-3611-8) Delmar.

Introduction to Healthcare Delivery Organizations: Functions & Management. Robert M. Sloane et al. 4th ed. 1999. LC 99-14524. x, 223p. 45.00 (1-56793-106-5) Health Admin Pr.

Introduction to Hematology. Samuel I. Rapaport. 2nd ed. 1987. LC 65-10036. (Illus.). 624p. pap. text 39.95 (0-397-50838-7, Lippnctt) Lppncott W & W.

***Introduction to Home Health Nursing: A Computerized Resource CD-ROM, Individual Version.** Mary Jo Gorney-Moreno & Bonnie Faherty. 1999. pap. 49.00 incl. cd-rom (0-323-00421-0) Mosby Inc.

Introduction to Homeopathic Medicine in Primary Care. Sidney E. Skinner. 2000. LC 00-40159. xxii, 473p. pap. 54.00 (0-8342-1676-0, 16760) Aspen Pub.

Introduction to Hospital Accounting. L. Vann Seawell. 3rd ed. 1992. LC 77-74543. (Illus.). 588p. (C). tchr. ed., per. 45.00 (0-930228-93-6); stu. ed., per. 60.00 (0-930228-94-4) Hlthcare Fin Mgmt.

Introduction to Hospital Management. Robert Reid. 1997. (Hospitality, Travel, & Tourism Ser.). text 34.95 (0-442-00856-2, VNR) Wiley.

Introduction to Human Anatomy & Physiology. Eldra P. Solomon. 1992. (Illus.). pap., stu. ed., wbk. ed. 17.95 (0-7216-3967-4); 320p. pap. text 28.50 (0-7216-3966-6) Saunders.

Introduction to Human Body: The Essentials of Anatomy & Physiology. Gerard J. Tortora. 4th ed. 1997. text 67.00 (0-673-97535-5) Addison-Wesley.

Introduction to Human Development & Health Issues. Lorraine B. Dennis & Joan Hassol. 1983. (Illus.). 320p. pap. text 39.00 (0-7216-3030-8) Saunders.

Introduction to Human Disease. Leonard V. Crowley. 1983. (Illus.). 700p. (C). reprint ed. text 35.00 (0-86720-393-5, 393-5) Jones & Bartlett.

Introduction to Human Disease. Crowley. 3rd ed. 1992. (Health Science Ser.). 848p. (C). pap., tchr. ed. 10.00 (0-86720-850-3) Jones & Bartlett.

Introduction to Human Disease. Leonard V. Crowley. (Health Science Ser.). (Illus.). (C). 3rd ed. 1992. 848p. text 52.95 (0-86720-333-1, 333-1); 4th ed. 1996. 896p. text 61.95 (0-86720-736-1, 736-1); 4th ed. 1996. 240p. pap. text, tchr. ed. 10.00 (0-7637-0330-3, 0330-3) Jones & Bartlett.

Introduction to Human Disease. Thomas H. Kent & Michael N. Hart. 4th ed. 1998. LC 97-48337. 675p. (C). 62.00 (0-8385-4070-8) P-H.

Introduction to Human Immunology. Teresa L. Huffer et al. 1986. 175p. (Orig.). (C). 37.50 (0-86720-067-7) Jones & Bartlett.

Introduction to Human Movement: The Sciences of Physical Education. Charles H. Shea & David L. Wright. 1997. (C). tchr. ed. (0-205-26495-6, T6495-0) Allyn.

Introduction to Human Nutrition. 4th ed. 1998. (C). 21.00 (0-536-02225-9) Pearson Custom.

Introduction to Human Physiology. Kevin T. Patton & Victoria Schauf. 736p. 53.95 (0-8016-6337-7) Mosby Inc.

Introduction to Immunohematology. Neville J. Bryant. 3rd ed. 1994. LC 93-36574. text 47.00 (0-7216-3883-X) Saunders.

Introduction to Immunotoxicology. Jacques G. Descotes & Claude Bernard. 1998. 250p. pap. (0-7484-0307-8) Tay Francis Ltd GBR. *Dist:* Taylor & Francis.

Introduction to In Vitro Toxicology. Frank A. Barile. 1994. 240p. 104.95 (0-8493-8659-4) CRC Pr.

Introduction to Iridology: The Beginner's Guide to Iris Study. Donald R. Bamer. 1997. pap. text 5.95 (1-885670-46-X) Woodland UT.

***Introduction to Jungian Psychotherapy: The Therapeutic Relationship.** David Sedgwick. 2001. LC 2001-37371. (0-415-18339-1); pap. (0-415-18340-5) Brunner-Routledge.

Introduction to Laboratory Chemistry: Organic & Biochemistry. Arthur L. Williams et al. 1978. LC 77-81204. (Chemistry Ser.). tchr. ed. (0-201-08457-0) Addison-Wesley.

Introduction to Language Pathology. David Crystal & Rosemary Varley. 3rd ed. 1993. (Illus.). 260p. (C). pap. text 45.00 (1-56593-242-0, 0564) Thomson Learn.

Introduction to Learning & Behavior. Russell A. Powell et al. 2001. LC 2001-35728. (Psychology Ser.). (Illus.). 480p. pap. text 57.95 (0-534-36585-X) Duxbury.

Introduction to Legal Nurse Consulting. Cynthia Weishapple. 2000. LC 00-49944. (Paralegal Ser.). (Illus.). 450p. (C). pap. text 48.95 (0-7668-1052-6) Delmar.

Introduction to Light Microscopy. S. Bradbury & B. Bracegirdle. 1997. (Microscopy Handbooks Ser.). (Illus.). 144p. (Orig.). pap. (1-85996-121-5) Bios Sci GBR. *Dist:* Coronet Bks.

Introduction to Long Term Care Nursing: Principles & Practice. Donna Ignatavicius. 1998. LC 97-42724. (Illus.). 258p. (C). pap. text 28.95 (0-8036-0099-2) Davis Co.

Introduction to Magnetic Resonance Imaging. William R. Hendee. 1985. pap. 31.95 (0-8016-2149-6) Mosby Inc.

Introduction to Malaria Problems in India: Prevedic Times to Early 1950's. B. L. Raina. 1991. (C). (81-7169-108-0) Commonwealth IND. *Dist:* S Asia.

Introduction to Managed Care: Health Maintenance Organizations, Preferred Provider Organizations, & Competitive Medical Plans. Robert G. Shouldice. 1991. LC 91-73438. xxv, 545p. (C). text 38.95 (0-87815-062-5) Info Resources.

Introduction to Management & Leadership: Clinical Nurses. Russell C. Swansburg,R.N. 1993. (Nursing-Health Science Ser.). 448p. (C). pap. text 42.50 (0-86720-338-2) Jones & Bartlett.

Introduction to Manual Medicine. H. D. Neumann. 1989. (Illus.). 109p. 38.95 (0-387-50612-8) Spr-Verlag.

Introduction to Marital Theory & Therapy. Leroy G. Baruth & Charles H. Huber. 1991. 332p. (C). reprint ed. pap. text 24.95 (0-88133-608-4) Waveland Pr.

Introduction to Maternal & Child Health Nursing. M. Christine Neff & Martha Spray. 1996. LC 95-45452. 800p. text 51.95 (0-397-55025-1) Lppncott W & W.

Introduction to Maternity & Pediatric Nursing. Ed. by Eleanor D. Thompson. 2nd ed. 1995. (Illus.). tchr. ed. (0-7216-4829-0) Saunders.

Introduction to Maternity & Pediatric Nursing. Eleanor D. Thompson. 2nd ed. 1995. LC 94-18065. (Illus.). 896p. text 43.95 (0-7216-4828-2) Saunders.

Introduction to Maternity & Pediatric Nursing. Ed. by Eleanor D. Thompson. 2nd ed. 1995. (Illus.). pap. text, stu. ed. 17.95 (0-7216-5753-2); 1005p. text, stu. ed. 56.00 (0-7216-6247-1) Saunders.

Introduction to Mathematical Immunobiology of Cancer. V. A. Kunznetsov. 1998. (Series on Advnaces in Mathematics for Applied Sciences). 300p. text 58.00 (981-02-2316-1) World Scientific Pub.

Introduction to Mathematics for Life Scientists. Edward Batschelet. 3rd ed. 1992. (Illus.). 643p. reprint ed. 49.95 (0-387-09648-5) Spr-Verlag.

Introduction to Measurement in PE & Exercise. Terry M. Wood & Margaret J. Safrit. 1993. (0-8016-7869-2) Mosby Inc.

Introduction to Measurement in Physical Education & Exercise Science. Margaret J. Safrit & Terry Wood. 3rd ed. 1995. (Illus.). 704p. (C). text 63.44 (0-8016-7849-8) McGrw-H Hghr Educ.

Introduction to Measurement Theory. Mary J. Allen & Wendy M. Yen. 1979. LC 78-25821. 810p. (C). mass mkt. 40.00 (0-8185-0283-5) Brooks-Cole.

Introduction to Medical Decision Analysis. Jonathan Javitt. 1991. text 13.95 (0-07-032364-X) McGraw.

Introduction to Medical Electronics: For Electronics & Medical Personnel. Burton R. Klein. 1984. LC 83-24860. 320p. reprint ed. lib. bdg. 24.50 (0-89874-729-5) Krieger.

Introduction to Medical Electronics Appliance. L. D. M. Nokes. 1995. (Electrical Engineering Ser.). pap. 59.99 (0-340-61457-9) Buttrwrth-Heinemann.

Introduction to Medical Genetics. J. A. Roberts & M. E. Pembrey. 8th ed. 1985. (Illus.). 400p. pap. 29.95 (0-19-261409-6) OUP.

Introduction to Medical Informatics. Patrice Degoulet. 1996. LC 96-18687. (Computers in Health Care Ser.). (Illus.). 242p. 54.95 (0-387-94641-1) Spr-Verlag.

Introduction to Medical Law. Peter Blondel Marquand. 2000. LC 00-36116. 144p. pap. (0-7506-4239-4) E A GBR. *Dist:* OUP.

Introduction to Medical Malpractice Law in the United States & Sweden: The Rights of Patients. Lotta Westerhall. 1992. 146p. (Orig.). pap. 53.50 (91-38-50113-9) Coronet Bks.

Introduction to Medical Manipulation. L. Burn. 1985. text 57.00 (0-85200-878-3) Kluwer Academic.

Introduction to Medical Microbiology: BIO 120. Louise Gresham & Linn Isbell. 1993. 362p. (C). stu. ed., ring bd. (0-933195-46-X) CA College Health Sci.

Introduction to Medical Molecular Biology: Theory & Techniques. Jules M. Elias. 1997. (Illus.). 216p. pap. text 40.00 (0-936735-03-1) Grove Educ Tech.

Introduction to Medical Neuroscience: Basic Science & Clinical Correlations. James A. Weyhenmeyer et al. unabr. ed. 2000. (Illus.). 500p. (C). pap. text 50.00 (1-891786-04-0) Fitzgerald Sci.

***Introduction to Medical Office Transcription.** Karonne J. Becklin & Edith M. Sunnarborg. 2nd ed. 2002. LC 2001-54316. (0-07-826260-7) Glencoe.

Introduction to Medical Radiesthesia & Radionics. Vernon D. Wethered. 1987. 108p. (0-85207-109-4) C W Daniel GBR. *Dist:* Natl Bk Netwk.

Introduction to Medical Rehabilitation: An Australian Perspective. Graeme Penington & Hugh C. Burry. 1990. 196p. pap. (0-522-84391-3) Melbourne Univ Pr AUS. *Dist:* Paul & Co Pubs.

Introduction to Medical Statistics. Martin Bland. 3rd ed. 2000. (Illus.). 424p. pap. text 35.00 (0-19-263269-8) OUP.

Introduction to Medical Terminology: A Self-Teaching Package. Andrew Hutton. 2nd ed. 1998. LC 97-49689. 279p. (C). pap. text (0-443-05965-9) Church.

Introduction to Medical Terminology: Workbook. David W. Chang & Susan M. Glover. 1994. LC 94-6427. pap., wbk. ed. 21.95 (0-683-16193-8) Lppncott W & W.

Introduction to Medicinal Chemistry: How Drugs Act & Why. Alex Gringauz. LC 95-49331. 1997. 736p. 99.95 (0-471-18545-0); 1996. (Illus.). 1100p. 75.00 (0-89573-325-0, Wiley-VCH) Wiley.

Introduction to Medicine ISE, No. 2. Roger M. Macklis. 1988. 15.95 (0-316-54249-0, Little Brwn Med Div) Lppncott W & W.

Introduction to Memory & Cognition. 1998. (0-673-98209-2, Good Year) Pearson Learn.

Introduction to Memory Development During Childhood & Adolescence. Michael Pressley & Wolfgang Schneider. 1997. LC 97-1849. 260p. (0-8058-2705-6); pap. (0-8058-2706-4) L Erlbaum Assocs.

Introduction to Mental Health Nursing: A Workbook. Ed. by Emmanuel R. Lodoiska & Susan E. Plummer. 1997. 144p. (Orig.). pap. text, wbk. ed. 24.95 (1-56593-763-5, 1484) Singular Publishing.

Introduction to Mental Health Nursing. (0-340-60481-6) E A GBR. *Dist:* Routldge.

Introduction to Mental Retardation & Developmental Disabilities. W. L. Williams. 1999. (High Tide Disability Ser.). 55p. spiral bd. 10.95 (1-892696-02-9) High Tide Pr.

Introduction to Metal Ceramic Technology. Patrick Naylor. 1992. (Illus.). 196p. text 72.00 (0-86715-237-0) Quint Pub Co.

Introduction to Microbiology. John L. Ingraham et al. 1994. LC 94-10832. (Wadsworth Biology Ser.). 752p. pap. 65.50 (0-534-16728-4) Wadsworth Pub.

Introduction to Minimal Access Surgery. Ed. by T. H. Brown & M. H. Irving. 1996. 100p. (Orig.). pap. text (0-7279-0885-5) BMJ Pub GBR. *Dist:* AIDC.

Introduction to Modeling in Physiology & Medicine. Carson & Cobelli. 1999. 75.00 (0-12-160240-0) Morgan Kaufmann.

Introduction to Modern Approaches in Visual Perception. Terry Caelli. 1981. LC 80-40167. (Illus.). 200p. (0-08-024420-3) Pergamon Repr GBR. *Dist:* Franklin.

Introduction to Modern Behaviorism. Howard Rachlin. 3rd ed. 1990. LC 90-13951. 302p. (C). pap. text 23.95 (*0-7167-2176-7*) W H Freeman.

Introduction to Modern Epidemiology. Kenneth J. Rothman & Staffen E. Norell. 2nd ed. 1990. LC 90-3243.Tr. of Grunderna I Epidemiologi. 102p. (C). pap. text 16.00 (*0-917227-06-9*) Epidemiology.

Introduction to Modern Psychology: The Control-Theory View. Ed. by Richard J. Robertson & William T. Powers. 1990. (Illus.). 238p. (Orig.). (C). pap. text 25.00 (*0-9624154-1-3*) Benchmark CT.

Introduction to Modern Psychology: The Control Theory View. Ed. by Richard J. Robertson & William T. Powers. 1990. 238p. (C). reprint ed. pap. text 25.00 (*0-9647121-6-4*) Benchmark CT.

Introduction to Modern Virology. N. J. Dimmock & S. B. Primrose. 4th ed. 1994. LC 94-5996. (Basic Microbiology Ser.: Vol. 2). (Illus.). 464p. pap. 59.95 (*0-632-03403-3*) Blackwell Sci.

Introduction to Molecular Medicine. Dennis W. Ross. 2nd ed. 1997. LC 95-36653. (Illus.). 190p. 36.00 (*0-387-94468-0*) Spr-Verlag.

Introduction to Molecular Neurobiology. Ed. by Zach W. Hall. 1992. LC 91-5138. (Illus.). 530p. (C). text 67.95 (*0-87893-307-7*) Sinauer Assocs.

Introduction to Motor Behavior: A Neuropsychological Approach. George H. Sage. 2nd ed. 1977. LC 76-14660. (A-W Physical Ed Ser.). (C). text 28.00 net. (*0-201-06766-8*) Addison-Wesley.

Introduction to Music Therapy: Theory & Practice. William B. Davis et al. 1995. 400p. (C). text 31.50 net. (*0-697-33997-1*) Brown & Benchmark.

Introduction to Natural Health. Deanne Tenney. 175p. 1995. pap. text 7.95 (*0-913923-99-0*); 1992. pap. 7.95 (*0-913923-82-6*) Woodland UT.

Introduction to Natural Hygiene. Herbert M. Shelton. 1996. 92p. reprint ed. spiral bd. 12.50 (*0-7873-0781-5*) Hlth Research.

Introduction to Neurobiology. Heinrich Reichert. 1993. (Illus.). 272p. (C). reprint ed. pap. text 42.95 (*0-19-521010-7*) OUP.

Introduction to Neuroendocrinology. Richard E. Brown. 1994. (Illus.). 430p. (C). pap. text 44.95 (*0-521-42665-0*) Cambridge U Pr.

Introduction to Neurogenic Communication Disorders. Robert H. Brookshire. 5th ed. (Illus.). 1998. LC 00-266636. 378p. text 79.95 (*0-8151-3609-9*, 31840); 1997. 512p. pap. text 48.00 (*0-8151-1014-6*, 29387) Mosby Inc.

Introduction to Neuroimaging. William W. Orrison. 1988. (Illus.). 384p. 88.00 (*0-316-66492-8*, Little Brwn Med Div) Lppncott W & W.

Introduction to Neurology. McLeod. 2nd ed. 1989. pap. 24.95 (*0-86793-017-9*) Blackwell Sci.

Introduction to Neuropathic Pain. Misha Backonja. 1998. VHS 195.00 (*0-8493-1645-6*) CRC Pr.

Introduction to Neuropathology. Hume Adams et al. 2nd ed. 1994. LC 93-4546. pap. text (*0-443-04495-3*) Church.

Introduction to Neuropsychology. J. Graham Beaumont. 1983. LC 83-24265. 314p. pap. 25.00 (*0-89862-515-7*, 2515) Guilford Pubns.

Introduction to Neuroscience. Gary G. Matthews. 1999. LC 99-23051. (Eleventh Hour Ser.). (Illus.). 225p. pap. 20.95 (*0-632-04414-4*) Blackwell Sci.

Introduction to Neurosurgery. Bryan J. Jennett & Kenneth W. Lindsay. 5th ed. 1994. 352p. pap. text 60.00 (*0-7506-1580-X*) Buttrwrth-Heinemann.

Introduction to Nuclear Physics with Applications in Medicine & Biology. N. A. Dyson. 1982. LC 81-6720. (Physics & Medicine in Biology Ser.). 260p. 79.95 (*0-470-27277-5*) P-H.

Introduction to Nurse Paralegalism. Mulkeen. 2001. (Paralegal Ser.). (C). text 42.75 net. (*0-7668-1909-4*) Delmar.

Introduction to Nursing: Concepts, Issues & Opportunities. Janice B. Lindberg. 3rd ed. 1998. LC 97-35556. 480p. pap. text 32.95 (*0-7817-9199-5*) Lppncott W & W.

Introduction to Nursing Assistant/NonEnglish Speaking. Frey. 1995. (Home Care Aide Ser.). 192p. wbk. ed. 14.95 (*0-8273-6236-6*) Delmar.

Introduction to Nursing Assistant/NonEnglish Speaking Non-English. Frey. 1996. (Home Care Aide Ser.). 208p. 37.95 (*0-8273-6235-8*) Delmar.

Introduction to Nursing Assisting: Building Language Skills. Rita Frey. 1995. (Home Care Aide Ser.). 480p. (C). pap. text 44.95 (*0-8273-6233-1*) Delmar.

Introduction to Nursing Assisting: Building Language Skills. Rita Frey & Lisa A. Shearer-Cooper. 1996. 480p. pap. 37.80 net. (*0-8273-8785-7*) Delmar.

Introduction to Nursing Assisting/NonEnglish Speaking. Frey. 1995. (Home Care Aide Ser.). 99.95 (*0-8273-7595-6*) Delmar.

Introduction to Nursing Care for Adults. Linton. 1995. 125.00 (*0-7216-6012-6*) Harcourt.

Introduction to Nursing Concepts. Wendy B. Young. 1987. 384p. (C). pap. 37.28 (*0-8385-4375-8*, A4375-0) P-H.

Introduction to Nursing Informatics. Kathryn J. Hannah et al. 2nd ed. 1998. LC 98-17983. (Health Informatics Ser.). (Illus.). 369p. 42.95 (*0-387-98451-8*) Spr-Verlag.

Introduction to Nursing Leadership & Management. Mary L. Holle & Mary E. Blatchley. 2nd ed. 1987. (Illus.). (C). pap. text 47.95 (*0-86720-380-3*, 380-3) Jones & Bartlett.

Introduction to Nursing Practice. Lillie M. Shortridge & Juanita E. Lee. 1980. (Illus.). text 32.00 (*0-07-057056-6*) McGraw.

Introduction to Nursing Theory & Clinical Reasoning. Betty M. Johnson & Pamela B. Webber. 2001. LC 00-49740. (Illus.). 272p. pap. text 26.95 (*0-7817-2153-9*) Lppncott W & W.

***Introduction to Nutrition & Health Research.** Eunsook T. Koh & Willis L. Owen. 2000. LC 00-61056. 384p. 127.00 (*0-7923-7983-7*, Kluwer Plenum) Kluwer Academic.

Introduction to Nutrition & Metabolism. David A. Bender. 1997. (Illus.). 300p. pap. (*0-7484-0781-2*) Tay Francis Ltd GBR. *Dist:* Taylor & Francis.

Introduction to Nutrition & Metabolism. Karen E. Bender. 1993. 256p. (*1-85728-078-4*); pap. (*1-85728-079-2*) UCL Pr Ltd GBR. *Dist:* Taylor & Francis.

Introduction to Nutrition & Metabolism. David A. Bender. 2nd ed. 1997. 300p. (*0-7484-0782-0*) Tay Francis Ltd GBR. *Dist:* Taylor & Francis.

Introduction to Nutrition, Exercise & Health. Katch. 4th ed. 1992. text 53.95 (*0-8121-1672-0*) Lppncott W & W.

Introduction to Nutrition, Exercise & Health. Frank I. Katch & William D. McArdle. 4th ed. LC 92-10386. (Illus.). 1994. 494p. pap. text 47.95 (*0-8121-1555-4*); 1993. 304p. pap. text, stu. ed. 19.50 (*0-8121-1669-0*) Lppncott W & W.

Introduction to Object Relations. Lavinia Gomez. 1997. LC 96-48446. 200p. (C). text 45.00 (*0-8147-3096-5*); pap. text 19.50 (*0-8147-3095-7*) NYU Pr.

Introduction to Occupational Psychiatry, Report 138. Group for the Advancement of Psychiatry Staff. 1993. LC 93-11640. 91p. 11.95 (*0-87318-206-5*, 7206) Am Psychiatric.

Introduction to Occupational Therapy. Barbara Sabonis-Chafee & Susan M. Hussey. 2nd ed. 1997. LC 98-234805. 304p. (C). (gr. 13). pap. text 29.00 (*0-8151-8251-1*, 28153) Mosby Inc.

Introduction to Ocular Pharmacology & Toxicology. Popat N. Patil & Allan M. Burkman. 1995. (Illus.). 320p. (C). pap. text 22.40 (*1-57074-294-4*) Greyden Pr.

Introduction to Oncogenes & Molecular Cancer Medicine. D. W. Ross. 1998. LC 98-4703. (Illus.). 180p. pap. 32.95 (*0-387-98392-9*) Spr-Verlag.

Introduction to Operating Room Techniques, Set. 1995. lib. bdg. 1505.95 (*0-8490-6677-8*); 1992. lib. bdg. 395.95 (*0-8490-8875-5*) Gordon Pr.

Introduction to Ophthalmology. John Parr. 1996. (Illus.). 244p. pap. (*0-908569-48-3*) Univ Otago Pr NZL. *Dist:* Intl Spec Bk.

Introduction to Organ Transplantation. Ed. by Nadey S. Hakim. 1997. 200p. 48.00 (*1-86094-025-0*) World Scientific Pub.

Introduction to Organic & Biochemistry. William H. Brown. 2nd ed. 1979. 18.25 (*0-87150-719-6*, WG 4191); 5.25 (*0-87150-720-X*, WG 4196) PWS Pubs.

Introduction to Organizational Behavior: A Situational Approach. Robin Stuart-Kotze. 1980. (Illus.). tchr. ed. (*0-8359-3260-5*); text 45.33 (*0-8359-3259-1*) P-H.

Introduction to Orthodontics. Laura Mitchell. 1996. (Illus.). 240p. (Orig.). (C). pap. text 69.50 (*0-19-262431-8*) OUP.

Introduction to Orthopaedic Nursing. Cathy M. Ceccio et al. 2nd ed. 1999. LC 99-462575. (Illus.). 148p. pap. 52.00 (*1-892665-03-4*) Natl Assn Ortho Nurse.

Introduction to Parapsychology in the Context of Science. R. A. McConnell. 1983. LC 82-99945. (Illus.). xiv, 337p. pap. 18.00 (*0-9610232-3-6*) McConnell.

Introduction to Pathology for Radiographers. Prime. 1987. (Illus.). 336p. (Orig.). (C). pap. text 29.50 (*0-06-318362-5*) HarperCollins Pubs.

Introduction to Perinatal Development & General Care: RCP 304 Course. Wojciechowski et al. 1994. 282p. ring bd. 49.95 (*0-933195-73-7*) CA College Health Sci.

Introduction to Personality. Ed. by E. Jerry Phares. 4th ed. 1997. (C). pap. text, stu. ed. (*0-673-99457-0*) Addison-Wesley.

Introduction to Personality. E. Jerry Phares. 3rd ed. 1997. LC 90-22710. 679p. (C). pap. 91.00 (*0-673-46424-5*) Addson-Wesley Educ.

Introduction to Personality. Walter Mischel. 5th ed. 1993. (C). pap. text, tchr. ed., suppl. ed. 35.00 (*0-03-033707-0*) Harcourt Coll Pubs.

Introduction to Personality & Psychotherapy Joseph F. Rychlak. 2nd ed. 1981. LC 80-68141. (Illus.). 800p. (C). text 83.56 (*0-395-29736-2*) HM.

Introduction to Pharmaceutical Engineering. Edwards. Date not set. (Pharmaceutical Engineering Ser.: No. 1). 170.00 (*0-7506-5140-7*) Buttrwrth-Heinemann.

Introduction to Pharmaceutical Formulation. A. Fishburn. 1965. LC 65-27360. (*0-08-011244-7*) Pergamon Repr GBR. *Dist:* Franklin.

Introduction to Pharmacoeconomics. Randy Vogenberg. 2000. LC 00-53283. 301p. pap. 44.95 (*0-07-134846-8*) McGraw-Hill Prof.

Introduction to Pharmacology. Mannfred A. Hollinger. 1997. LC 97-4328. 256p. 105.00 (*1-56032-574-7*); pap. 36.95 (*1-56032-575-5*) Taylor & Francis.

Introduction to Phlebotomy: Instructor's Guide. Davis. 1994. (Medical Lab Technician Ser.). tchr. ed. 12.00 (*0-8273-5564-5*) Delmar.

Introduction to Phycology. G. South & A. Whittick. 1987. LC 87-7146. (Illus.). 368p. pap. 59.95 (*0-632-01726-0*) Blackwell Sci.

Introduction to Physical Therapy. Pagliarulo. 1995. (Illus.). 320p. (gr. 13). pap. text 31.95 (*0-8151-6714-8*, 24738) Mosby Inc.

Introduction to Physical Therapy. Michael A. Pagliarulo. 1996. (Illus.). tchr. ed. (*0-8151-4323-0*) Mosby Inc.

Introduction to Physiological Psychology. Allen M. Schneider & Barry Tarshis. 2nd ed. 1980. 528p. stu. ed. 6.50 (*0-394-32149-9*); text 22.00 (*0-394-32157-X*) Random.

Introduction to Practical Animal Breeding. Clive Dalton. 3rd ed. 1991. (Illus.). 174p. pap. 20.95 (*0-632-03126-3*) Blackwell Sci.

Introduction to Project Management: A Guide for New Researchers. Usherwood. 1996. LC 96-17727. 160p. (*0-335-19708-6*); pap. (*0-335-19707-8*) OpUniv Pr.

Introduction to Psychiatry. Oliver S. English & Stuart M. Finch. 3rd ed. 1964. (C). text 17.50 (*0-393-09738-2*) Norton.

Introduction to Psychoanalysis: Contemporary Theory & Practice. Anthony Bateman & Jeremy Holmes. 1995. LC 95-7617. 304p. (C). 80.00 (*0-415-10738-5*); pap. 27.99 (*0-415-10739-3*) Routledge.

Introduction to Psychoanalysis: Lectures for Child Analysts & Teachers. Anna Freud. 1974. LC 73-16853. (Writings of Anna Freud: Vol. 1). 200p. 35.00 (*0-8236-6870-3*) Intl Univs Pr.

Introduction to Psychodynamic Psychotherapy Technique. Sarah F. Usher. 1993. 200p. 35.00 (*0-8236-2750-0*) Intl Univs Pr.

Introduction to Psychodynamics: A New Synthesis. Mardi J. Horowitz. 1996. pap. (*1-56821-869-9*) Aronson.

Introduction to Psychodynamics & Psychotherapy: Clinical Vignettes & Interpretations. Irving Soloman. 1978. LC 77-87464. 10.95 (*0-87212-088-0*) Libra.

Introduction to Psycholinguistics. Jean Caron. Tr. by Tim Pownall. 1992. 440p. text 40.00 (*0-8020-5026-3*) U of Toronto Pr.

Introduction to Psycholinguistics. Tatiana Slama-Cazacu. 1975. (Janua Linguarum, Ser. Major: No. 60). (Illus.). 418p. text (*90-279-3033-3*) Mouton.

Introduction to Psychological Research. Mary J. Allen. 1994. LC 93-84981. 267p. (C). pap. text 37.00 (*0-87581-378-X*, IPR) F E Peacock Pubs.

Introduction to Psychological Tests & Scales. Kate M. Loewenthal. 2nd ed. 2001. LC 00-62772. 208p. pap. (*1-84169-139-9*) Psychol Pr GBR. *Dist:* Taylor & Francis.

Introduction to Psychological Tests & Scales. Kate Miriam Loewenthal. 2nd ed. 2001. LC 00-62772. 208p. (*1-84169-106-2*) Psychol Pr GBR. *Dist:* Taylor & Francis.

Introduction to Psychology. 1992. 11.84 (*0-02-800144-3*) Glencoe.

Introduction to Psychology. Ed. by Bornstien. 1920. (C). pap. text, stu. ed. (*0-321-01384-0*) Addson-Wesley Educ.

Introduction to Psychology. Ed. by Bornstien. 1999. (C). text (*0-321-01383-2*) Addson-Wesley Educ.

Introduction to Psychology. Mark Garrison. 1992. 596p. text 50.03 (*0-02-800140-0*) Glencoe.

Introduction to Psychology. James W. Kalat. 1986. 672p. (C). mass mkt. 41.25 (*0-534-04035-7*) Brooks-Cole.

Introduction to Psychology. Schacter. 2004. text (*0-7167-5215-8*) Worth.

Introduction to Psychology. Robert J. Sternberg. 1996. LC 97-107998. (Harcourt Brace Jovanovich College Outline Ser.). 288p. (C). pap. text 15.75 (*0-15-502071-4*) Harcourt Coll Pubs.

Introduction to Psychology. Arno F. Wittig & Gary S. Belkin. 1990. LC 88-13070. (McGraw-Hill's College Review Bks.). 320p. (C). pap. 12.95 (*0-07-071212-3*) McGraw-Hill Educ Grp.

Introduction to Psychology. Wilhelm M. Wundt. 1976. LC 73-2999. (Classics in Psychology Ser.). reprint ed. 19.95 (*0-405-05173-5*) Ayer.

Introduction to Psychology. James W. Kalat. 2nd ed. 1990. 701p. (C). mass mkt. 49.75 (*0-534-12060-1*) Brooks-Cole.

Introduction to Psychology. Matlin. 2nd ed. 1994. (C). stu. ed. 100.00 (*0-15-503095-7*) Harcourt.

Introduction to Psychology. Morris & Larkin. 2nd ed. 1998. 112p. pap. text 34.60 (*0-536-01201-6*) S&S Trade.

Introduction to Psychology. Rod Plotnik. 2nd ed. 1989. 688p. (C). text 37.50 (*0-394-38336-2*); stu. ed. (*0-394-38665-5*) Random.

Introduction to Psychology. Linda L. Davidoff. 3rd ed. 1986. 736p. (C). (gr. 10-12). text 65.25 net. (*0-07-015570-4*) McGraw.

Introduction to Psychology. Rod Plotnik. 3rd ed. 1993. 770p. (C). mass mkt., stu. ed. 17.00 (*0-534-16448-X*); 1992. 770p. (C). 49.75 (*0-534-16446-3*); 1993. stu. ed. 14.30 (*0-534-16453-6*); 1993. stu. ed. 14.30 (*0-534-16451-X*) Brooks-Cole.

Introduction to Psychology. James W. Kalat. 4th ed. 1995. LC 95-23816. (Psychology Ser.). 791p. pap. 52.50 (*0-534-25014-9*) Brooks-Cole.

Introduction to Psychology. Rod Plotnik. 4th ed. 1995. (Psychology Ser.). 760p. pap. 52.50 (*0-534-26142-6*); pap. 44.25 (*0-534-34244-2*); mass mkt. 17.00 (*0-534-33846-1*) Brooks-Cole.

Introduction to Psychology. Patricia M. Wallace & Jeffrey H. Goldstein. 4th ed. 1996. LC 95-83924. 608p. (C). pap. 56.56 (*0-697-23564-5*, WCB McGr Hill) McGrw-H Hghr Educ.

Introduction to Psychology. Rod Plotnik. 5th ed. 1998. LC 98-37913. (Psychology Ser.). 768p. text 80.95 (*0-534-35611-7*) Brooks-Cole.

***Introduction to Psychology.** James W. Kalat. 6th ed. 2001. 800p. 81.95 (*0-534-53998-X*) Duxbury.

***Introduction to Psychology.** Rod Plotnik. 6th ed. 2001. 768p. pap. 60.95 (*0-534-58027-0*) Duxbury.

Introduction to Psychology. Fred Whitford. 8th ed. 2000. 210p. (C). spiral bd. 26.95 (*0-7872-7320-1*) Kendall-Hunt.

Introduction to Psychology. Rita L. Atkinson. 12th ed. 1996. (C). pap. text, tchr. ed. 35.00 (*0-15-503073-6*) Harcourt Coll Pubs.

Introduction to Psychology: Coursekit. Patricia M. Wallace et al. 4th ed. 1996. (C). text 42.00 net. incl. cd-rom (*0-697-38067-X*) Brown & Benchmark.

Introduction to Psychology: Exploration & Application. Dennis L. Coon. Ed. by Clyde Perlee. 6th ed. 1992. 726p. (C). text 57.50 (*0-314-92211-3*) West Pub.

Introduction to Psychology: PSY 101. California College for Health Sciences Staff. rev. ed. 1993. 178p. (C). stu. ed., ring bd. (*0-933195-31-1*) CA College Health Sci.

Introduction To Psychology: Science of Behavior. 3rd ed. 2000. 112p. (C). 27.80 (*0-536-02749-8*) Pearson Custom.

Introduction to Psychology: Study Guide. James W. Kalat. 4th ed. 1995. (Psychology Ser.). pap., stu. ed. 19.25 (*0-534-25020-3*) Brooks-Cole.

Introduction to Psychology: Test Bank. Rita L. Atkinson. 12th ed. 1996. (C). pap. text, tchr. ed., suppl. ed. 44.50 (*0-15-503075-2*) Harcourt Coll Pubs.

Introduction to Psychology & Applied Psychology. James W. Kalat. 3rd ed. 1993. (Psychology Ser.). 52.95 (*0-534-17237-7*); stu. ed. 19.95 (*0-534-17249-0*); stu. ed. 17.95 (*0-534-17255-5*) Brooks-Cole.

Introduction to Psychology & Counseling: Christian Perspectives & Applications. Paul Meier et al. 2nd ed. 1991. LC 91-9525. (Illus.). 368p. (gr. 13). 34.99 (*0-8010-6275-6*) Baker Bks.

Introduction to Psychopathology. Shervert Frazier & Arthur C. Carr. 1983. LC 84-45111. 184p. 35.00 (*0-87668-702-8*) Aronson.

Introduction to Psychopathology. Alessandra Lemma. 1996. LC 96-68912. 240p. 69.95 (*0-8039-7470-1*, 2419); pap. 22.95 (*0-8039-7471-X*, 2420) Sage.

Introduction to Psychosomatic Medicine. C. Alberto Seguin. 1970. 320p. 35.00 (*0-8236-2760-8*); pap. 24.95 (*0-8236-8090-8*, 22760) Intl Univs Pr.

Introduction to Psychotherapy. Sidney Tarachow. 1970. LC 63-13476. 375p. reprint ed. 55.00 (*0-8236-2740-3*) Intl Univs Pr.

Introduction to Psychotherapy: Common Clinical Wisdom. Randolph B. Pipes & Donna S. Davenport. 2nd ed. 1998. LC 98-22426. 400p. (C). 86.00 (*0-205-29252-6*, Longwood Div) Allyn.

Introduction to Quantitative EEG & Neurofeedback. James R. Evans. 1999. LC 98-89312. (Illus.). xxi, 406p. 79.95 (*0-12-243790-X*) Acad Pr.

Introduction to Radiation Therapy Technology. Charles M. Washington & Dennis T. Leaver. 1996. (Illus.). 384p. tchr. ed. (*0-8151-9251-7*) Mosby Inc.

Introduction to Radiation Therapy Technology Vol. 1: Introduction to Radiation Therapy. Charles M. Washington & Dennis T. Leaver. 1996. LC 96-4954. (Illus.). 384p. (gr. 13). tchr. ed. (*0-8151-9145-6*, 24513) Mosby Inc.

Introduction to Radiobiology. M. Tubiana et al. 1990. 350p. (*0-85066-745-3*); pap. (*0-85066-763-1*) Tay Francis Ltd GBR. *Dist:* Taylor & Francis.

Introduction to Radiobiology. A. H. Nias. 2nd ed. 1998. LC 97-42811. 400p. pap. 64.95 (*0-471-97590-7*) Wiley.

Introduction to Radiography & Patient Care. Ed. by Arlene Adler & Rick Carlton. 1993. LC 93-14806. (Illus.). 368p. pap. text 37.95 (*0-7216-3465-6*) Saunders.

Introduction to Radiography & Patient Care. Arlene M. Adler & Richard R. Carlton. Ed. by Andrew Allan. 2nd ed. 1998. LC 98-25697. (Illus.). 415p. (C). pap. text 35.00 (*0-7216-7662-6*) Saunders.

Introduction to Radiologic Technology. Ed. by LaVerne T. Gurley & William J. Callaway. 4th ed. 1996. (Illus.). 432p. (gr. 13). pap. text 34.00 (*0-8151-3984-5*, 27078) Mosby Inc.

***Introduction to Radiologic Technology: Text & Integrated Patient Care Package.** LaVerne Tolley Gurley & William J. Callaway. 4th ed. 1996. (Illus.). pap. 59.00 (*0-8151-3934-9*) Mosby Inc.

Introduction to Randomised Controlled Clinical Trials. J. N. S. Matthews. 2000. LC 00-709663. (Arnold Texts in Statistics Ser.). (Illus.). 208p. pap. (*0-340-76143-1*) E A GBR. *Dist:* OUP.

Introduction to Recombinant DNA in Medicine. Alan E. Emery & Sue Malcolm. 2nd ed. 1995. LC 95-3818. 216p. pap. 49.95 (*0-471-93984-6*) Wiley.

Introduction to Reference Sources in the Health Sciences. Ed. by Joanne Bookman. 3rd ed. 1995. LC 94-10708. 301p. 40.00 (*0-8108-2889-8*) Scarecrow.

Introduction to Reflexology. Lynn T. Nelson & Gail L. Nelson. 3rd ed. 1995. (Illus.). 70p. (Orig.). (C). pap. 19.95 (*1-884727-01-8*) Digits Intl.

Introduction to Regional Anesthesia. D. Bruce Scott. 1996. LC 88-10374. 96p. (C). pap. text 59.95 (*0-8385-4390-1*, A4390-9, Apple Lange Med) McGraw.

Introduction to Reiki: Healing Energy for Mind, Body & Spirit. Mary Lambert. 2000. LC 00-266808. (Illus.). 96p. pap. (*1-85585-747-2*) Collins & Br.

Introduction to Research: Multiple Strategies for Health & Human Services. Depoy Gitlin. 2nd ed. 1998. LC 98-23839. (Illus.). 348p. pap. text 34.95 (*0-8151-0979-2*, 31713) Mosby Inc.

Introduction to Research in Psychology. University North Carolina Staff. 1998. 152p. (C). pap. text 17.40 (*0-536-01164-8*) Pearson Custom.

Introduction to Research in the Health Sciences. Stephen Polgar & Shane A. Thomas. 2nd ed. 1991. (Illus.). 357p. pap. text (*0-443-04363-9*); 3rd ed. 1995. pap. text (*0-443-05039-2*) Church.

Introduction to Respiratory Care. Levitzky et al. 1990. (Illus.). 608p. text 67.00 (*0-7216-1090-0*) Saunders.

Introduction to Respiratory Care. Mosby Staff. 1995. (Respiratory Care Workbook Ser.: No. 1). (C). (*0-8151-6303-7*, 26022) Mosby Inc.

Introduction to Respiratory Physiology. Harold A. Braun et al. 2nd ed. 1980. pap. 17.00 (*0-316-10699-2*, Little Brwn Med Div) Lppncott W & W.

Introduction to Risk Prediction & Preventive Dentistry. Per Axelsson. 2000. LC 99-16511. (Axelsson Series on Preventive Dentistry : Vol. 1). 159p. pap. text 58.00 (*0-86715-361-X*) Quint Pub Co.

Introduction to Scanning Transmission Electron Microscopy. P. Goodhew et al. 1998. LC 97-31937. (Microscopy Handbooks). (Illus.). 144p. pap. 32.95 (*0-387-91517-6*) Spr-Verlag.

Introduction to Scientific Psychology. Henry D. Schlinger, Jr. & Alan D. Poling. 1998. LC 98-9986. (Applied Clinical Psychology Ser.). (Illus.). 418p. (C). 42.50 (*0-306-45728-8*, Plenum Trade) Perseus Pubng.

Introduction to Sectional Anatomy. Madden. (Radiographic Technology Ser.). 1998. tchr. ed. 16.00 (*0-8273-7000-8*); 1998. text 45.95 (*0-8273-6998-0*); 1997. wbk. ed. 17.95 (*0-8273-6999-9*) Delmar.

Introduction to Sectional Anatomy. Michael E. Madden. 2000. LC 00-61820. (Illus.). 600p. text 53.00 (*0-7817-2105-9*) Lppncott W & W.

Introduction to Sexual Counseling. Robert R. Wilson. 1974. 56p. pap. 2.50 (*0-89055-108-1*) Carolina Pop Ctr.

Introduction to Skin Toxicology. Sharon Hotchkiss. 1998. 350p. text (*0-7484-0662-X*) Tay Francis Ltd GBR. *Dist:* Taylor & Francis.

Introduction to Social Psychology. Richard A. Lippa. 1989. 643p. (C). mass mkt. 54.75 (*0-534-11772-4*) Brooks-Cole.

Introduction to Social Psychology. William McDougall. 451p. 100.00 (*1-85506-693-9*) Thoemmes Pr.

Introduction to Sound. Speaks. 3rd ed. 1999. pap. 22.50 net. (*1-56593-980-8*); pap., wbk. ed. 22.50 net. (*1-56593-981-6*) Thomson Learn.

Introduction to Splinting: A Critical Thinking & Problem-Solving Approach. Brenda M. Coppard & Helene Lohman. Ed. by Judy C. Colditz. 1996. LC 95-42842. (Illus.). 352p. (C). (gr. 13). spiral bd. 39.95 (*0-8151-7126-9*, 26607) Mosby Inc.

Introduction to Statistics for the Social & Behavioral Sciences. Larry B. Christensen & Charles M. Stoup. 1986. LC 86-2313. (Psychology Ser.). 566p. (C). mass mkt. 42.50 (*0-534-05610-5*) Brooks-Cole.

Introduction to Sterilization, Disinfection & Infection Control. Joan F. Gardner & Margaret M. Peel. 2nd ed. 1991. (Illus.). 270p. text (*0-443-04286-1*) Church.

Introduction to Stroke. Barbara Bond-Howdard. 1993. (Therapy Enhancement Ser.). (Illus.). 94p. (Orig.). (C). ring bd. 16.00 (*1-882883-04-7*, 275) Idyll Arbor.

Introduction to Surgery. David H. Levien. 2nd ed. 1993. LC 92-48894. (Illus.). 304p. pap. text 31.95 (*0-7216-6647-7*) Saunders.

Introduction to Surgery. David H. Levien. Ed. by Lisette Bralow. 3rd ed. 1999. LC 98-36803. (Illus.). 335p. pap. text (*0-7216-7652-9*) Saunders.

Introduction to Surgical Nursing. 320p. pap. (*0-340-63176-7*) E A GBR. *Dist:* Routldge.

Introduction to Surgical Nursing. Penelope M. Simpson. 1997. (Illus.). 200p. (Orig.). pap. 32.95 (*1-56593-752-X*, 1462) Singular Publishing.

Introduction to Surgical Nursing. Torrance. 12th ed. 1997. pap. text 25.00 (*0-7020-1969-0*) Saunders.

Introduction to Symbolic & Augmentative Communication. Stephen Von Tetzchner & Harald Martinsen. 1992. LC 92-32746. 266p. 55.00 (*1-56593-050-9*, 0425) Singular Publishing.

Introduction to Telemedicine. Steven F. Viegas & Kimberley Dunn. 1998. LC 98-3397. 416p. pap. text 59.95 (*0-397-51843-9*) Lppncott W & W.

***Introduction to Telemedicine.** Ed. by Richard Wootton & John Craig. 1999. 207p. pap. (*1-85315-425-3*) Royal Soc of Medicine Pr Ltd GBR. *Dist:* Balogh.

Introduction to the Benefits of the Bach Flower Remedies. Jane Evans. 7th ed. 20p. pap. 4.95 (*0-8464-4244-2*) Beekman Pubs.

Introduction to the Benefits of the Bach Flower Remedies. Jane Evans. 1974. 108p. pap. (*0-85207-125-6*) C W Daniel GBR. *Dist:* Natl Bk Netwk.

Introduction to the Biological Basis of Feeding: Essential Biological Ideas Necessary to a Study of Living Beings from the Evolutionary Standpoint. Faustino Cordon. 1980. LC 79-40933. (Illus.). 250p. pap. 41.00 (*0-08-025484-5*, Pergamon Pr) Elsevier.

Introduction to the Blood-Brain Barrier. Hugh Davson et al. 1992. LC 92-49384. 120.00 (*0-8493-7761-7*, QP375) CRC Pr.

Introduction to the Blood-Brain Barrier: Methodology, Biology & Pathology. Ed. by William M. Pardridge. 1998. LC 97-26483. (Illus.). 500p. (C). text 140.00 (*0-521-58124-9*) Cambridge U Pr.

Introduction to the Cellular & Molecular Biology of Cancer. Ed. by L. M. Franks & N. M. Teich. 3rd ed. 1997. LC 97-13068. (Illus.). 480p. pap. text 49.50 (*0-19-854854-0*) OUP.

Introduction to the Diagnosis & Treatment of Food Sensitivities. Elaine R. Radford & Gary D. Becker. 2nd ed. 1993. (Self-Instructional Package Ser.). (Illus.). 65p. (Orig.). pap. text 25.00 (*1-56772-005-6*) AAO-HNS.

Introduction to the Health Professions. Peggy S. Stanfield. 2nd ed. 1995. LC 94-21055. pap. 40.00 (*0-86720-928-3*) Jones & Bartlett.

Introduction to the Health Professions. Peggy Stanfield & Y. H. Hui. 3rd ed. 1998. LC 98-3359. (Illus.). 512p. (C). pap. text 43.95 (*0-7637-0643-4*, 0643-4) Jones & Bartlett.

Introduction to the History of Psychology. B. R. Hergenhahn. (C). 1986. 443p. mass mkt. 46.00 (*0-534-06072-2*); 2nd ed. 1992. 594p. text 45.50 (*0-534-16812-4*); 3rd ed. 1996. LC 96-13025. 656p. mass mkt. 80.95 (*0-534-26370-4*) Brooks-Cole.

Introduction to the Human Body. John H. Jameson. 1982. tchr. ed. 9.28 (*0-8013-0082-7*, 75746); stu. ed. 24.60 (*0-88334-158-1*, 76125); 9.00 (*0-88334-163-8*, 76130) Longman.

Introduction to the Human Body. Mary Kleinelp. 3rd ed. Date not set. (C). tchr. ed. (*0-06-501390-5*) Addson-Wesley Educ.

Introduction to the Human Body. Moses. 3rd ed. Date not set. (C). (*0-06-501394-8*) Addson-Wesley Educ.

Introduction to the Human Body: The Essentials of Anatomy & Physiology. Gerard J. Tortora. 4th ed. 1997. LC 96-27182. 608p. (C). text 64.69 (*0-673-98222-X*) Longman.

Introduction to the Human Body: The Essentials of Anatomy & the Physiology. Mary Kleinelp. 3rd ed. 1994. LC 93-25243. (C). pap., stu. ed. 34.69 (*0-06-502291-2*) Addson-Wesley Educ.

Introduction to the Human Body: The Essentials of Anatomy & the Physiology. Gerard J. Tortora. 3rd ed. 1994. LC 93-25243. 630p. (C). (gr. 7-12). pap. 72.19 (*0-06-501363-8*) Addson-Wesley Educ.

Introduction to the Human Body:Essentials of Anatomy & Physiology. Gerard J. Tortora. 4th ed. 1997. text 62.81 (*0-673-97536-3*) Addison-Wesley.

Introduction to the Literature of Vertebrate Zoology: Titles in the Blacker Library of Zoology, the Emma Shearer Wood Library of Ornithology, the Bibliotheca Osleria & Other Libraries of McGill University, Montreal. Ed. by Casey A. Wood. 1974. LC 73-17849. (Natural Sciences in America Ser.). 670p. reprint ed. 45.95 (*0-405-05772-5*) Ayer.

Introduction to the Logic of Psychological Measurement. J. Michell. 1990. 200p. (C). text 55.00 (*0-8058-0566-4*) L Erlbaum Assocs.

Introduction to the Medical History of Ethiopia. Richard Pankhurst. 1990. LC 90-50990. 340p. (C). 45.00 (*0-932415-44-X*); pap. 14.95 (*0-932415-45-8*) Red Sea Pr.

Introduction to the Molecular Genetics of Cancer. Richard G. Vile. 1992. LC 91-41675. (Molecular Medical Science Ser.: No. 1976). 218p. 190.00 (*0-471-93333-3*, Wiley-Liss) Wiley.

Introduction to the Neurologic Examination. Michael F. Nolan. 1995. LC 95-21837. (Illus.). 224p. (C). pap. text 23.95 (*0-8036-0017-8*) Davis Co.

Introduction to the Neurosciences. Elliott Marcus et al. 2nd ed. 1996. LC 93-43196. (Illus.). 750p. text, stu. ed. 69.50 (*0-683-05542-9*) Lppncott W & W.

Introduction to the Physiology of Hearing. James O. Pickles. 2nd ed. 1988. 567p. pap. text 54.95 (*0-12-554754-4*) Acad Pr.

Introduction to the Practical Applications of Otoacoustic Emissions. Brenda L. Lonsbury-Martin & Glen K. Martin. 2000. 264p. pap. 49.95 (*1-56593-709-0*, 1394) Singular Publishing.

Introduction to the Principles & Practice of Homoeopathy. Charles E. Wheeler. 1971. 12.95 (*0-85032-062-3*) Formur Intl.

Introduction to the Principles & Practice of Homoeopathy. Charles E. Wheeler & J. D. Kenyon. 1980. 25.00 (*0-85032-180-8*) St Mut.

Introduction to the Principles of Disease. John B. Walter. 3rd ed. 1992. (Illus.). 676p. text 50.00 (*0-7216-9082-3*) Saunders.

Introduction to the Principles of Medical Imaging. C. N. Guy & D. H. Ffytche. 1998. 300p. 38.00 (*981-02-3451-1*) World Scientific Pub.

Introduction to the Principles of Psychology. B. R. Bugelski. 2nd ed. 1973. LC 73-323. 640p. (C). pap. text (*0-672-61266-6*); (*0-672-61344-1*) Macmillan (Bobbs).

Introduction to the Psychology of Dreaming. Kelly Bulkeley. 1997. LC 96-53613. 144p. 60.00 (*0-275-95889-2*); pap. 18.95 (*0-275-95890-6*) Greenwood (Praeger Pubs).

Introduction to the Psychotherapies. Ed. by Sidney Bloch. 2nd ed. 1986. 250p. pap. 28.50 (*0-19-261469-X*) OUP.

Introduction to the Psychotherapies. Sidney Bloch. 3rd ed. 1996. (Illus.). (C). 361p. text 75.00 (*0-19-262710-4*); 376p. pap. text 39.50 (*0-19-262709-0*) OUP.

Introduction to the Reading of Lacan: The Unconscious Structured Like a Language. Joel Dor. 1998. (Lacanian Clinical Field Ser.). 296p. pap. 18.95 (*1-892746-04-2*, 46042) Other Pr LLC.

Introduction to the Reading of Lacan: The Unconscious Structured Like a Language. Joel Dor & Judith Feher Gurewich. 1997. LC 96-17924. pap. 27.00 (*0-7657-0020-4*) Aronson.

Introduction to the Sociology of Dentistry: A Comparative Perspective. Peter Davis. 1987. 108p. pap. (*0-908569-40-8*) Univ Otago Pr NZL. *Dist:* Intl Spec Bk.

Introduction to the Study of Experimental Medicine. Claude Bernard. Tr. by Henry C. Greene. 1957. 226p. (C). pap. 7.95 (*0-486-20400-6*) Dover.

Introduction to the Study of Language. Leonard Bloomfield. 1983. (Classics in Psycholinguistics Ser.: Vol. 3). reprint ed. pap. 38.95 (*90-272-1892-7*) J Benjamins Pubng Co.

Introduction to the Study of Language. Leonard Bloomfield. 1983. (Classics in Psycholinguistics: Vol. 3). x, 335p. reprint ed. (*90-272-1891-9*) J Benjamins Pubng NLD. *Dist:* J Benjamins Pubng Co.

Introduction to the Study of Mammals, Living & Extinct. William H. Flower & Richard Lydekker. Ed. by Keir B. Sterling. 1978. LC 77-81075. (Biologists & Their World Ser.). (Illus.). reprint ed. lib. bdg. 65.95 (*0-405-10644-0*) Ayer.

Introduction to the Symptoms & Signs of Surgical Disease. Norman L. Browse. 3rd ed. 1997. LC 96-49623. (Arnold Publication). (Illus.). 464p. pap. 39.95 (*0-340-66211-5*) OUP.

Introduction to the Technique of Child Analysis. Anna Freud. 1978. LC 74-21408. (Classics in Child Development Ser.). reprint ed. 19.95 (*0-405-06460-8*) Ayer.

Introduction to the Technique of Psychotherapy: Practice Guidelines for Psychotherapists. Samuel I. Greenberg. 1998. LC 98-27916. 122p. pap. text 21.95 (*0-398-06905-0*) C C Thomas.

Introduction to the U. S. Health Care System. Steven Jonas. 3rd ed. 1991. LC 91-15830. 224p. (C). pap. text 26.95 (*0-8261-3984-1*) Springer Pub.

Introduction to the Visual System. Martin J. Tovee. 1996. (Illus.). 218p. (C). text 69.95 (*0-521-48290-9*); pap. text 24.95 (*0-521-48339-5*) Cambridge U Pr.

Introduction to the Work of Melanie Klein. Hanna Segal. 2nd ed. 1980. LC 73-91077. 160p. pap. text 16.00 (*0-465-03584-1*) Basic.

Introduction to Theories of Personality. Robert B. Ewen. 4th ed. 1992. 112p. tchr. ed. (*0-8058-1123-0*); 632p. text 42.50 (*0-8058-1120-6*) L Erlbaum Assocs.

Introduction to Theories of Personality. B. R. Hergenhahn. 5th ed. 1998. LC 98-16767. 614p. 94.00 (*0-13-895509-3*) P-H.

Introduction to Therapeutic Counseling. Jeffrey A. Kottler & Robert W. Brown. (Counseling Ser.). 1985. LC 84-19838. 342p. (C). pap. 36.25 (*0-534-04698-3*); 2nd ed. 1992. 450p. (C). text 57.95 (*0-534-17286-5*); 3rd ed. 1995. 464p. mass mkt. 51.00 (*0-534-26382-8*) Brooks-Cole.

Introduction to Therapeutic Counseling: Student Workbook. Jeffrey A. Kottler. 2nd ed. 1992. 72p. (C). pap., wbk. ed. 17.95 (*0-534-17287-3*) Brooks-Cole.

Introduction to Therapeutic Play: Working Together with Children, Young People, & Their Families. J. Carroll. 1997. LC 96-40403. (Working Together for Children, Young People, & Their Famil Ser.). (Illus.). 192p. pap. 44.95 (*0-632-04148-X*) Blackwell Sci.

Introduction to Time-Limited Group Psychotherapy. K. Roy MacKenzie. 1990. LC 89-17508. 317p. text 44.00 (*0-88048-168-4*, 8168) Am Psychiatric.

Introduction to Transfusion Medicine: A Case Study Approach. Elaine K. Jeter & Mary A. Spivey. 1996. LC 97-141249. (Illus.). 191p. (Orig.). pap. text 69.00 (*1-56395-054-5*, PC97-PR9601) Am Assn Blood.

***Introduction to 12-Lead ECG: The Art of Interpretation.** Thomas B. Garcia. 2002. (C). pap. 37.95 (*0-7637-1961-7*, 1961-7) Jones & Bartlett.

***Introduction to U. S. Health Policy.** Donald Barr. 2001. LC 2001-43693. 245p. 40.00 (*0-205-32419-3*) Allyn.

Introduction to Ultrasonography & Patient Care. Marveen Craig. (Illus.). 229p. 1993. pap., tchr. ed. (*0-7216-3777-9*); 1992. pap. text 32.50 (*0-7216-4229-2*) Saunders.

Introduction to Vascular Biology: From Physiology to Pathophysiology. Ed. by Alison Halliday et al. 1998. LC 97-23258. (Illus.). 288p. (C). pap. text 45.95 (*0-521-58998-3*) Cambridge U Pr.

Introduction to Vascular Scanning: A Guide for the Complete Beginner. Donald P. Ridgway. 2nd ed. 1998. LC 97-29697. pap. 59.95 (*0-941022-39-0*) Davies Pubng.

Introduction to Vascular Ultrasonography. Ed. by William J. Zwiebel. 3rd ed. 1992. (Illus.). 639p. text 99.00 (*0-7216-3551-2*) Saunders.

Introduction to Vascular Ultrasonography. William J. Zwiebel. Ed. by Lisette Bralow. 4th ed. 1999. LC 98-31218. (Illus.). 460p. text (*0-7216-6949-2*) Saunders.

Introduction to Veterinary Anatomy & Physiology. A. R. Mitchell & P. E. Watkins. 1993. (Illus.). 216p. pap. (*0-905214-12-9*) BSAVA GBR. *Dist:* Iowa U Pr.

Introduction to Veterinary Entomology. D. E. Bay & R. L. Harris. 2nd ed. 1989. (Illus.). 111p. (C). pap. text 25.00 (*0-9624083-0-1*) Stonefly Pub.

Introduction to Veterinary Genetics. Frank W. Nicholas. 2000. (Illus.). 336p. reprint ed. pap. 49.95 (*0-632-05639-8*) Blackwell Sci.

Introduction to Veterinary Medical Ethics: Theory & Cases. Bernard Rollin. 1999. LC 99-24729. (Illus.). 430p. pap. 39.95 (*0-8138-1659-9*) Iowa U Pr.

Introduction to Veterinary Pathology. Norman F. Cheville. 2nd ed. 1999. LC 99-22664. (Illus.). 352p. text 74.95 (*0-8138-2496-6*) Iowa U Pr.

Introduction to Visual Optics. Alan Tunnacliffe. 1989. (C). (*0-900099-21-6*) Assn Brit Dispen Opticians GBR. *Dist:* St Mut.

Introduction to X-Ray Physics & Techniques. Bontrager. 1985. 90p. (C). (gr. 13). text, stu. ed. 23.95 (*0-8016-5721-0*, 05721) Mosby Inc.

Introductory Biophysics. M. Cerdonio et al. 1986. 224p. text 38.00 (*9971-966-33-6*) World Scientific Pub.

Introductory Biostatistics for the Health Sciences. Robert C. Duncan et al. 2nd ed. 1989. LC 82-23822. 249p. (C). mass mkt. 35.50 (*0-8273-4230-6*) Delmar.

Introductory Concepts in Developmental Biology. Aron A. Moscona & A. A. Moscona. 1994. LC 78-7946. (Illus.). lib. bdg. 25.00 (*0-226-53476-6*) U Ch Pr.

Introductory Dictionary of Lacanian Psychoanalysis. Dylan Evans. 1996. LC 95-40239. (Illus.). 264p. (C). 85.00 (*0-415-13522-2*); pap. 27.99 (*0-415-13523-0*) Routledge.

Introductory Genetics. George J. Brewer & Charles F. Sing. 1983. (Biology Ser.). (Illus.). 784p. text (*0-201-10138-6*) Addison-Wesley.

Introductory Gerontological Nursing. Sally S. Roach. 2000. LC 00-42804. (Illus.). 416p. pap. text 26.95 (*0-397-55479-6*) Lppncott W & W.

Introductory Handbook for the Contact Lens Assistant. Pamela J. Miller. Ed. by Sally M. Corngold. 1995. LC 95-13939. (Illus.). 114p. (C). lib. bdg. 19.50 (*0-929780-06-X*) VisionExtension.

Introductory Immunobiology. Huw Davies. 1997. LC 96-84895. 394p. pap. 44.95 (*0-412-37240-1*) Chapman & Hall.

Introductory Lecture & Discourse on the Connexion Between Chemistry & Medicine Thomas Cooper. Ed. by I. Bernard Cohen. 1980. LC 79-7956. (Three Centuries of Science in America Ser.). reprint ed. lib. bdg. 25.95 (*0-405-12537-2*) Ayer.

Introductory Lectures on Psychoanalysis. Sigmund Freud. 1989. LC 77-5779. 500p. reprint ed. pap. 16.95 (*0-87140-118-5*) Liveright.

Introductory Management & Leadership for Nurses. Russell Swansburg & Richard J. Swansburg. 2nd ed. 1998. LC 98-21155. (Nursing Ser.). (Illus.). 800p. (C). pap. text 48.95 (*0-7637-0640-X*, 0640-X) Jones & Bartlett.

***Introductory Management & Leadership for Nurses.** Russell Swansburg & Richard J. Swansburg. 3rd ed. 2001. (Illus.). 672p. (C). pap. text 56.95 (*0-7637-1644-8*, 1644-8) Jones & Bartlett.

Introductory Medical Statistics. R. F. Mould. 3rd exp. rev. ed. 1998. LC 98-176710. (Medical Science Ser.). (Illus.). 350p. pap. 49.00 (*0-7503-0513-4*) Inst of Physics Pubng.

Introductory Medical-Surgical Nursing. Jeanne C. Scherer. 4th ed. 1986. LC 64-4479. (Illus.). 767p. text 35.50 (*0-397-54508-8*); stu. ed. 15.95 (*0-397-54509-6*) Lppncott W & W (Lippnctt).

Introductory Medical-Surgical Nursing. Barbara K. Timby & Jeanne C. Scherer. 7th ed. 1998. 416p. pap. text, stu. ed. 19.95 (*0-7817-1651-9*); LC 98-30557. 1,300p. text 51.95 (*0-7817-1599-7*) Lppncott W & W.

Introductory Medicinal Chemistry. J. B. Taylor & P. D. Kennewell. 1984. LC 81-6703. 202p. pap. 39.95 (*0-470-20137-1*) P-H.

Introductory Module. Ed. by American Association for Medical Transcription Staff. 1993. (Exploring Transcription Practices Ser.). 60p. (C). pap., stu. ed. 495.00 incl. audio (*0-935229-16-7*) Am Assoc Med.

Introductory Module Handbook. American Association for Medical Transcription Staff. 1993. (Exploring Transcription Practices Ser.). 60p. (C). pap. text, stu. ed. 50.00 incl. audio (*0-935229-17-5*) Am Assoc Med.

Introductory Neurology. James McLeod et al. 3rd ed. 1995. 300p. pap. 38.95 (*0-86793-329-1*) Blackwell Sci.

Introductory Nursing Care. Linton. 1995. (C). pap. text, stu. ed. 19.95 (*0-7216-3318-8*) Harcourt.

Introductory Nursing Care of Adults. Ed. by Adrianne D. Linton et al. 1995. (Illus.). tchr. ed. (*0-7216-4752-9*); 1271p. text, stu. ed. 63.00 (*0-7216-6216-1*) Saunders.

Introductory Nursing Care of Adults. Mary A. Matteson et al. 1995. (Illus.). 1216p. text 49.00 (*0-7216-3319-6*) Saunders.

Introductory Nursing Care of Adults. Linton. 2nd ed. 2000. (Illus.). 315p. (C). pap., stu. ed. (*0-7216-8167-0*) Saunders.

***Introductory Nursing Care of Adults: Including Study Guide for Mosby Dictionary.** Adrianne Dill Linton et al. 2000. (Illus.). stu. ed. 91.95 (*0-7216-9244-3*) Saunders.

***Introductory Nursing Care of Adults: Text & Study Guide for Miller Dictionary.** Adrianne Dill Linton et al. 2nd rev. ed. 2000. (Illus.). 90.95 (*0-7216-9246-X*) Saunders.

Introductory Nutrition & Nutrition Therapy. Marian M. Eschleman. 3rd ed. 1995. LC 95-19854. 736p. pap. text 33.95 (*0-397-55108-8*) Lppncott W & W.

Introductory Pediatric Nursing. Violet Broadribb. 3rd ed. 1982. (Illus.). 392p. text 26.00 (*0-397-54330-1*, 64-02739, Lippnctt) Lppncott W & W.

Introductory Physics of Nuclear Medicine. Ramesh Chandra. 4th ed. 1992. (Illus.). 221p. text 32.95 (*0-8121-1442-6*) Lppncott W & W.

Introductory Psychology. R. B. Burns & C. B. Dobson. 1984. pap. text 58.00 (*0-85200-491-5*) Kluwer Academic.

Introductory Psychology: Psychology As a Social Science, Spring 1997. Marcia Kremer. 4th ed. 1998. 808p. pap. text 31.75 (*0-536-01399-3*) Pearson Custom.

Introductory Psychology: Psychology as Social Science. 5th ed. 2000. 808p. (C). 38.00 (*0-536-02070-1*) Pearson Custom.

Introductory Psychology Environment. Ed. by Wolfe. 1999. (C). text (*0-321-01397-2*) Addson-Wesley Educ.

Introductory Reader in Developmental Psychology. Ed. by James D. Demetre. 1996. LC 97-189286. 596p. (C). pap. (*1-874529-36-1*) Greenwich Univ Pr GBR. *Dist:* NYU Pr.

Introductory Readings in Cognitive Psychology. Ed. by Richard P. Honeck. 2nd rev. ed. 1994. LC 90-84859. (Illus.). 320p. (C). text 14.95 (*1-56134-296-3*, Dshkn McG-Hill) McGrw-H Hghr Educ.

Introductory Sociology for Nurses. Hardey. 1998. 25.50 (*1-56593-532-2*, 0542) Singular Publishing.

Introductory Statistics for the Behavioral Sciences. Joan Welkowitz et al. 4th ed. 1990. 416p. (C). pap. text, stu. ed. 31.00 (*0-15-545988-0*) Harcourt Coll Pubs.

Introductory Statistics for the Behavioral Sciences. Robert K. Young & Donald J. Veldman. 4th ed. 1981. LC 80-26006. 688p. (C). text 100.00 (*0-03-043051-8*) Harcourt Coll Pubs.

***Introductory Textbook of Psychiatry.** Nancy C. Andreasen & Donald W. Black. 2001. LC 00-67401. 912p. 72.95 (*0-88048-946-4*, 8946) Am Psychiatric.

Introductory Textbook of Psychiatry. Nancy C. Andreasen & Donald W. Black. 2nd ed. 1995. LC 94-44481. 768p. pap. text 49.95 (*0-88048-705-4*, 8705) Am Psychiatric.

***Introductory Textbook of Psychiatry.** Nancy C. Andreasen & Donald W. Black. 3rd ed. 2001. LC 00-67401. 912p. pap. 52.95 (*1-58562-036-X*, 62036) Am Psychiatric.

Intrusiveness & Intimacy in the Couple. Ed. by Stanley Ruszczynski & James Fisher. 1995. LC 96-9160. 175p. pap. text (*1-85575-114-3*) Karnac Bks GBR. *Dist:* Other Pr LLC.

Intuition in der Medizin, Bd. 2. Brigitte Ausfeld-Hafter. 1999. (Komplementare Medizin Im Interdisziplinaren Diskurs Ser.). 204p. 32.00 (*3-906760-47-2*) P Lang Pubng.

Intuition Is Not Enough: Matching Learning with Practice in Therapeutic Child Care. Linnet McMahon & Adrian Ward. 1998. LC 97-34706. 272p. (C). pap. 27.95 (*0-415-15662-9*); 89.95 (*0-415-15661-0*) Routledge.

Intuitive Eating: Everybody's Natural Guide to Total Health & Lifelong Vitality Through Food. Humbart Santillo. Ed. by Regina S. Ryan. 1993. LC 93-77511. (Illus.). 444p. (Orig.). pap. 16.95 (*0-934252-27-0*) Hohm Pr.

Intuitive Healing: A Woman's Guide to Finding the Healer Within. Beth Moran. 1998. LC 98-6451. 224p. 19.95 (*1-86204-376-0*) Element MA.

Intuitive Predictions & Professional Forecasts: Cognitive Processes & Social Consequences. Jurgen T. Rehm & V. Gadenne. 1990. LC 90-31507. (International Series of Monographs in the Sciences: Vol. 20). (Illus.). 210p. (*0-08-036763-1*) Pergamon Repr GBR. *Dist:* Franklin.

Intuitive Psychotherapy: The Role of Creative Therapeutic Intervention. William N. Confer. 1987. LC 86-27506. 188p. 34.95 (*0-89885-337-0*, Kluwer Acad Hman Sci) Kluwer Academic.

Intuitive Sources of Probabilistic Thinking in Children. Ed. by Efraim Fischbein. 1975. LC 75-22376. (Synthese Library: No.85). xiii, 201p. lib. bdg. 104.50 (*90-277-0626-3*) Kluwer Academic.

Invasion & Metastasis: News & Current Views. Ed. by Jean-Paul Thiery. 1995. (Journal: Vol. 14, No. 1-6, 1995). (Illus.). 412p. reprint ed. pap. 135.75 (*3-8055-6205-5*) S Karger.

Invasive & Non-Invasive Blood Gas Sampling & Analysis. Lonny J. Ashworth. 1998. (CPG Mentor - Patient Cases in Respiratory Care Ser.: Unit 5). (*0-8151-2287-X*) Mosby Inc.

Invasive Bladder Carcinoma, Progress in Basic Research, Diagnosis, Surgical & Medical Therapy: Heinrich-Warner Stiftung, 2. Symposium, Hamburg, November 1987. Ed. by H. Huland & H. Klosterhalfen. 1988. (Journal: Vol. 14, Suppl. 1, 1988). (Illus.). iv, 48p. pap. 15.75 (*3-8055-4899-0*) S Karger.

Invasive Cardiology: Current Diagnostic & Therapeutic Issues. Ed. by George W. Vetrovec & Blase A. Carabello. 1995. (American Heart Association Monograph Ser.). (Illus.). 632p. 115.00 (*0-87993-608-8*) Futura Pub.

Invasive Cardiovascular Therapy. Ed. by H. H. Hilger & V. Hombach. 1987. (Developments in Cardiovascular Medicine Ser.). lib. bdg. 323.50 (*0-89838-818-X*) Kluwer Academic.

Invasive Fetal Diagnosis & Management. Ed. by Christopher R. Harman. 1994. LC 94-15786. (Illus.). 448p. 99.95 (*0-86542-208-7*) Blackwell Sci.

Invasive Management of the Coronary Patient. Ed. by Nanette K. Wenger. 1986. (Journal: Vol. 73, No. 4-5, 1986). (Illus.). 152p. pap. 66.25 (*3-8055-4402-2*) S Karger.

Invasive Procedures in Critical Care. Ed. by Charles L. Sprung & Ake Grenvik. 1985. (Clinics in Critical Care Medicine Ser.: Vol. 7). (Illus.). 294p. text (*0-443-08337-1*) Church.

Invasive Ultrasound. A. Lees. 1996. (*1-85317-133-6*) Martin Dunitz GBR. *Dist:* Mosby Inc.

Invasives und Nichtinvasives Monitoring von Atmung, Beatmung, Kreislauf, und Stoffwechsel. Ed. by G. Melichar et al. 1986. (Beitraege zur Intensiv und Notfallmedizin Ser.: Vol. 4). (Illus.). viii, 260p. 65.25 (*3-8055-4267-4*) S Karger.

Inventarium Sive Chirurgia Magna, Vol. 1. Guigonis De Caulhiaco. Ed. by Michael R. McVaugh. 1996. (Studies in Ancient Medicine: Vol. 14, I). (Illus.). xviii, 486p. 207.00 (*90-04-10706-1*, NLG385) Brill Academic Pubs.

Invented Worlds: The Psychology of the Arts. Ellen Winner. 1982. (Illus.). 448p. 36.50 (*0-674-46360-9*) HUP.

Inventing Our Selves: Psychology, Power & Personhood. Nikolas Rose. 1996. LC 95-42608. (Cambridge Studies in the History of Psychology). 232p. (C). text 54.95 (*0-521-43414-9*) Cambridge U Pr.

Inventing Pain Medicine: From the Laboratory to the Clinic. Isabelle Baszanger. 1998. LC 97-30922. 352p. (C). text 50.00 (*0-8135-2501-2*); pap. text 22.00 (*0-8135-2502-0*) Rutgers U Pr.

Inventing RSI: The Social Construction of an Occupational Hazard. Yolande Lucire. 2000. 368p. pap. (*0-86840-778-X*) New South Wales Univ Pr AUS. *Dist:* Intl Spec Bk.

Inventing the AIDS Virus. Peter Duesberg. 1996. LC 95-25754. 721p. 29.95 (*0-89526-470-6*) Regnery Pub.

Inventing the AIDS Virus. Peter H. Duesberg. 1997. 722p. pap. 17.95 (*0-89526-399-8*) Regnery Pub.

Inventing the AIDS Virus: The Truth Behind the World's Greatest Miscalculation. Peter Duesberg. 1994. (*0-201-62466-4*) Addison-Wesley.

Inventing the Feeble Mind: A History of Mental Retardation in the United States. James W. Trent, Jr. LC 93-32239. (Medicine & Society Ser.: Vol. 6). 356p. 1995. (Illus.). pap. text 19.95 (*0-520-20357-7*); 1994. text 40.00 (*0-520-08243-5*) U CA Pr.

Inventing the Psychological: Toward a Cultural History of Emotional Life in America. Joel Pfister & Nancy Schnog. 1997. LC 96-23275. 4000p. 50.00 (*0-300-06809-3*); 304p. pap. 20.00 (*0-300-07006-3*) Yale U Pr.

Invention of the Modern Hospital: Boston, 1870-1930. Morris J. Vogel. 1992. LC 79-26052. (Illus.). 172p. pap. text 6.95 (*0-226-86241-0*) U Ch Pr.

Inventive Step: Its Evolution in Canada, the United Kingdom, & the United States. John Bochnovic. Ed. by Friedrich-Karl Beier et al. 1982. (IIC Studies Ser.). 90p. pap. 45.00 (*3-527-25699-7*, Wiley-VCH) Wiley.

Inventory Control for Rehabilitation Workshops. Christopher A. Smith. 1986. (Illus.). 80p. (Orig.). pap. (*0-916671-59-3*) TRR.

Inventory Control Systems for Laboratory Supplies: Approved Guideline, 1994. Contrib. by Robert E. Wenk. 1994. 75.00 (*1-56238-203-9*, GP6-A) NCCLS.

Inverse Anchorage Technique in Fixed Orthodontic Treatment. Jose Carriere. 1991. (Illus.). 238p. text 95.00 (*0-86715-245-1*) Quint Pub Co.

Inverse Problems in Medical Imaging & Nondestructive Testing. Heinz W. Engl & William Rundell. 1997. LC 97-20953. (Illus.). 232p. text 69.95 (*3-211-83015-4*) Spr-Verlag.

Inversions: A Study of Warped Consciousness. 2nd rev. ed. 1973. (Illus.). viii, 464p. pap. 20.00 (*0-9600642-2-2*) Alpert.

Invertebrate Blood Cells: Anthropods to Urchordates Invertebrates & Vertebrates Compared, Vol. 2. Ed. by N. A. Ratcliffe & A. F. Rowley. 1981. LC 80-41248. text 209.00 (*0-12-582102-6*) Acad Pr.

Invertebrate Blood Cells: General Aspects, Animals Without True Circulatory Systems to Cephalopods, Vol. 1. Ed. by N. A. Ratcliffe & A. F. Rowley. 1981. LC 80-41248. text 209.00 (*0-12-582101-8*) Acad Pr.

Invertebrate Immune Responses: Cells & Molecular Products. Ed. by E. L. Cooper. 1996. (Advances in Comparative & Environmental Physiology Ser.: Vol. 23). (Illus.). 216p. 169.00 (*3-540-59154-0*) Spr-Verlag.

Invertebrate Models: Cell Receptors & Cell Communication. Ed. by A. H. Greenberg. 1987. (Illus.). x, 270p. 309.75 (*3-8055-4350-6*) S Karger.

Invertebrate Nervous Systems, Their Significance for Mammalian Neurophysiology. Cornelius G. Wiersma. Ed. by California Institute of Technology Staff. 1995. LC 66-23704. (Illus.). 370p. lib. bdg. 30.00 (*0-226-89638-2*) U Ch Pr.

Invertebrate Zoology. Edward E. Ruppert & Robert D. Barnes. 6th ed. 1993. LC 93-85930. 1056p. (C). text 116.00 (*0-03-026668-8*) SCP.

Invertebrates: A Synthesis. R. S. K. Barnes. 3rd ed. 2001. LC 00-44516. (Illus.). 488p. pap. 54.95 (*0-632-04761-5*) Blackwell Sci.

Invertebrates: Directory of Authors of New Medical & Scientific Reviews with Subject Index. Science and Life Consultants Association Staff. 1995. 160p. 57.50 (*0-7883-0592-1*); pap. 47.50 (*0-7883-0593-X*) ABBE Pubs Assn.

Inverted Medical Dictionary. Mary J. Stanaszek et al. 2nd ed. 1991. LC 91-65013. 328p. 74.95 (*0-87762-825-4*) CRC Pr.

Investigating Disease Patterns: The Science of Epidemiology. Paul D. Stolley & Tamar Lasky. 1998. (Illus.). 242p. pap. text 19.95 (*0-7167-6024-X*) W H Freeman.

Investigating Environmental Disease Outbreaks: A Training Manual. Y. Hasegawa & T. Kjellstrom. 1998. (Illus.). 70p. (C). reprint ed. pap. text 20.00 (*0-7881-7226-3*) DIANE Pub.

Investigating Neurological Disease: Epidemiology for Clinical Neurology. Ed. by Albert Hofmann & Richard Mayeux. 2001. (Illus.). 328p. (C). pap. text 58.95 (*0-521-00009-2*) Cambridge U Pr.

Investigating Phenomenal Consciousness: Methodologies & Maps. Ed. by Max Velmans. 2000. LC 00-39749. (Advances in Consciousness Research Ser.: Vol. 13). (Illus.). xii, 381p. pap. 38.95 (*1-55619-193-6*) J Benjamins Pubng Co.

Investigating Practices in Health Manpower Planning. 1986. 41p. pap. text 8.00 (*92-890-1044-4*, 1340028) World Health.

Investigation & Management of Disease in Wild Animals. G. A. Wobeser. 1994. (Illus.). 284p. (C). text 65.00 (*0-306-44703-7*, Kluwer Plenum) Kluwer Academic.

Investigation in Esophageal Disease Functional. Ed. by C. Scarpignato & J. P. Galmiche. 1994. (Frontiers of Gastrointestinal Research Ser.: Vol. 22). (Illus.). xii, 372p. 259.25 (*3-8055-5609-8*) S Karger.

Investigation of Anorectal Functional Disorders: With Special Emphasis on Defaecography. Ed. by P. Buchmann & W. Bruhlmann. 1993. LC 92-26472. (Illus.). 212p. 230.00 (*0-387-55326-6*) Spr-Verlag.

***Investigation of Incompatibility Reactions Caused by Biomaterials in Contact with Whole Blood Using a New in Vitro Model.** Anette Hagberg. 2001. (Comprehensive Summaries of Uppsala Dissertations from the Faculty of Medicine Ser.: Vol. 1049). (Illus.). 44p. (*91-554-5054-7*) Uppsala Universitet SWE. *Dist:* Coronet Bks.

Investigation of Nonresponse Bias: Hispanic Health & Nutrition Examination Survey. Michael L. Rowland & Ronald N. Forthofer. LC 93-29686. (Vital & Health Statistics Ser. 2: Data Evaluation & Methods Research: No. 119). 5.50 (*0-8406-0485-8*) Natl Ctr Health Stats.

Investigational Techniques in Oncology. Ed. by Norman M. Bleehen. 1987. (Illus.). 222p. 98.00 (*0-387-17075-8*) Spr-Verlag.

Investigative Interviews of Children: A Guide for Helping Professionals. Debra A. Poole & Michael E. Lamb. 1998. LC 98-16385. 295p. 39.95 (*1-55798-500-6*, 431-710A) Am Psychol.

Investigative Pathology of the Odontogenic Cysts. Ed. by Roger M. Browne. 1990. 264p. 195.00 (*0-8493-5038-7*, RK307) CRC Pr.

Investigative Ultrasonology. Ed. by C. Alvisi & C. R. Hill. 1981. 200p. pap. 55.00 (*0-8464-1221-7*) Beekman Pubs.

Investigative Urology IV. Ed. by D. Jocham et al. 1991. (Illus.). 272p. 182.00 (*0-387-52997-7*) Spr-Verlag.

Investigator's Guide to Clinical Research: How to Conduct Successful Clinical Trials: A Step by Step Approach: A Quick Reference. David Ginsberg. 2nd ed. 1999. 281p. pap. 79.00 (*0-9673029-0-0*) CenterWatch.

Investing for Business Value: How to Maximize the Strategic Benefits of Health Care Information Technology. Joseph M. DeLuca & Rebecca E. Cagan. 1996. LC 96-42116. 175p. (Orig.). pap. 52.00 (*1-55648-170-5*, 093107) AHPI.

Investing in Children. William U. Chandler. 1985. LC 85-51252. (Worldwatch Papers). pap. 5.00 (*0-916468-64-X*) Worldwatch Inst.

Investing in Health: Development Effectiveness in the Health, Nutrition, & Population Sector. Timothy A. Johnston & Susan Stout. 1999. LC 99-52688. (Illus.). xix, 71p. (*0-8213-4310-6*) World Bank.

Investing in Women's Health: Central & Eastern Europe. WHO Regional Office for Europe Staff. 1995. LC 96-116551. (Regional Publications, European Ser.: Vol. 55). 44p. pap. 11.00 (*92-890-1319-2*, 1310055) World Health.

Invisible: Issues in Women's Occupational Health/La Sant'e des Travailleuses. Ed. by Karen Messing et al. 1995. LC 96-106063. (Illus.). 556p. pap. (*0-921881-37-1*) Ragweed CAN. *Dist:* U of Toronto Pr.

Invisible Currents: Nature's Lessons for the Mind & Heart. Wanda McGee. 1999. LC 99-50201. (Illus.). 96p. pap. 12.95 (*0-917917-13-8*) Miles River.

Invisible Guests: The Development of Imaginal Dialogues. Mary Watkins. 3rd ed. 2000. LC 00-29157. (Classics in Archetypal Psychology). ii, 202p. pap. 19.00 (*0-88214-380-8*) Spring Pubns.

Invisible Light: 100 Years of Medical Radiology. Ed. by A. M. Thomas et al. 1995. 109p. pap. 29.95 (*0-86542-627-9*) Blackwell Sci.

Invisible Masters: Compulsions & the Fear That Drives Them. George Weinberg. 1998. 385p. text 23.00 (*0-7881-5708-6*) DIANE Pub.

Invisible Web: Gender Patterns in Family Relationships. Marianne Walters et al. LC 88-30083. (Family Therapy Ser.). 422p. reprint ed. 1991. pap. 25.00 (*0-89862-482-7*, 2482); 1988. 42.00 (*0-89862-734-6*) Guilford Pubns.

Invitation Health. Dianne R. Hales. 6th ed. 1994. LC 93-29432. (C). pap. text 41.95 (*0-8053-5480-8*) Benjamin-Cummings.

Invitation to Cognitive Science Vol. 2: Visual Cognition. Ed. by Daniel N. Osherson & Stephen M. Kosslyn. 2nd ed. 1995. (Illus.). 400p. 50.00 (*0-262-15042-5*, Bradford Bks) MIT Pr.

Invitation to Cognitive Science Vol. 3: Thinking. Ed. by Daniel N. Osherson & Edward E. Smith. 2nd ed. 1995. (Illus.). 400p. 55.00 (*0-262-15043-3*, Bradford Bks) MIT Pr.

Invitation to Health. Hales. 6th ed. 1994. (Health Sciences Ser.). stu. ed. 41.00 (*0-534-32713-3*) Brooks-Cole.

Invitation to Health. Dianne Hales. (Health Sciences Ser.). 6th ed. 1994. pap. 39.00 (*0-534-33958-1*); 6th ed. 1994. pap., stu. ed. 4.50 (*0-534-33964-6*); 7th ed. 1996. LC 96-9184. 728p. (C). pap. 41.00 (*0-534-34067-9*) Brooks-Cole.

Invitation to Health. Hales. 8th ed. 1998. (Health Sciences Ser.). spiral bd. 29.95 (*0-534-36467-5*) Brooks-Cole.

***Invitation to Health: Brief Edition.** Dianne Hales. 2nd ed. 2001. 350p. pap. 45.95 (*0-534-58958-8*) Duxbury.

Invitation to Health: Dallas Telecourse. Hales. 2nd ed. 1998. (Health Sciences Ser.). pap., stu. ed. 15.25 (*0-534-36450-0*) Brooks-Cole.

Invitation to Health with InfoTrac. Hales. 8th ed. 1998. LC 98-22337. (Health Sciences Ser.). pap. 37.00 (*0-534-35733-4*) Brooks-Cole.

Invitation to Person Centered Psychology. T. Merry. 1994. 166p. 49.95 (*1-56593-510-1*, 1178) Singular Publishing.

Invitation to Personal Construct Psychology. Burr. 1992. 148p. pap. 27.50 (*1-56593-560-8*, 0312) Singular Publishing.

Invitation to Pharmacology. Higley. (Nursing Education Ser.). 1998. (C). text 48.95 (*0-8273-6368-0*); 1997. tchr. ed. 12.50 (*0-8273-6369-9*) Delmar.

Invitation to Possibility Land: An Intensive Teaching Seminar with Bill O'Hanlon. Bob Bertolino & William H. O'Hanlon. 1998. LC 98-20700. 39.95 (*0-87630-875-2*) Brunner-Routledge.

Invitation to Psychodynamic Psychology. Alessandra Lemma-Wright. 1995. 150p. pap. 24.95 (*1-56593-500-4*, 1158) Singular Publishing.

Invitation to Psychology. 2000. tchr. ed. (*0-13-027892-0*) P-H.

***Invitation to Psychology.** Contrib. by Addison-Wesley Publishing Company. 1999. pap. 64.00 incl. audio compact disk (*0-321-06046-6*) Addison-Wesley.

Invitation to Psychology. Wade. 1998. 288p. (C). pap. text, stu. ed. 21.00 (*0-321-03492-9*) Addson-Wesley Educ.

Invitation to Psychology. Carole Wade & Carol Tavris. 2000. 626p. pap. 86.60 (*0-13-027891-2*) P-H.

Invitation to Psychology. Ed. by John P. Houston et al. 2nd ed. 1983. 840p. stu. ed. 9.00 (*0-12-356871-4*) Harcourt.

Invitation to Social Psychology. Philipchal. 1994. (C). pap. text, tchr. ed. 70.00 (*0-15-502462-0*); pap. text, stu. ed. 28.00 (*0-15-502463-9*) Harcourt Coll Pubs.

Invitation to Social Psychology: Test Bank. Philipchal. 1994. (C). pap. text, tchr. ed., suppl. ed. 82.00 (*0-15-502464-7*) Harcourt Coll Pubs.

Invitation to the Psychology of Religion. Raymond F. Paloutzian. 2nd ed. 1996. LC 95-36563. 400p. pap. 48.00 (*0-205-14840-9*) Allyn.

Invitational Counseling: A Self-Concept Approach to Professional Practice. William W. Purkey & John J. Schmidt. 1995. LC 95-8766. 215p. pap. text 54.95 (*0-534-33902-6*) Brooks-Cole.

Involuntary Civil Commitment: A Manual for Lawyers & Judges. 1988. 100p. pap. 15.00 (*0-89707-444-0*, 344-0014-01) Amer Bar Assn.

Involuntary Movements. Ed. by J. Siegfried et al. 1981. (Applied Neurophysiology Ser.: Vol. 45, No. 3). (Illus.). iv, 132p. pap. 34.00 (*3-8055-3498-1*) S Karger.

Invulnerable Child. Ed. by E. James Anthony & Bertram J. Cohler. 1987. LC 86-27120. (Guilford Psychiatry Ser.). 432p. 49.00 (*0-89862-227-1*, 2227) Guilford Pubns.

Inward Eye: Psychoanalysts Reflect on Their Lives & Work. Laurie W. Raymond & Susan Rosbrow-Reich. 1997. LC 96-12694. 504p. 59.95 (*0-88163-252-X*) Analytic Pr.

Inwardness & Existence: Subjectivity in - & Hegel, Heidegger, Marx, & Freud. Walter A. Davis. 1989. LC 88-40428. 440p. (C). pap. text 24.95 (*0-299-12014-7*) U of Wis Pr.

Iodine & the Brain. Ed. by G. R. DeLong et al. 1989. (Illus.). 380p. 105.00 (*0-306-43103-3*, Plenum Trade) Perseus Pubng.

Iodine Deficiency Disorders: A Strategy for Control in the Eastern Mediterranean Region. 1990. (WHO EMRO Technical Publications: No. 16). ix, 24p. pap. text 2.00 (*92-9021-117-2*, 1450016) World Health.

Iodine Deficiency in Europe: A Continuing Concern. F. Delange et al. 1993. (NATO Advanced Science Institutes Ser.: Vol. 241). (Illus.). 510p. (C). text 139.50 (*0-306-44410-0*, Kluwer Plenum) Kluwer Academic.

Iodine-Labeled Plasma Proteins, Vol. I. Ed. by Erwin Regoeczi. 1984. LC 96-7564. (Illus.). 240p. 135.00 (*0-8493-6556-2*, QP99, CRC Reprint) Franklin.

Ion Adventure in the Heartland: Exploring the Heart's Ionic-Molecular Microcosm. Dale Dubin. 2001. (Illus.). 600p. text 99.00 (*0-912912-11-1*) Cover Pub.

Ion Channel Pharmacology. Ed. by Bernat Soria & Valentin Cena. 1998. LC 97-51378. (Illus.). 486p. text 159.50 (*0-19-852360-2*) OUP.

Ion Channels. Ed. by John N. Abelson et al. 1992. (Methods in Enzymology Ser.: Vol. 207). (Illus.). 917p. text 125.00 (*0-12-182108-0*) Acad Pr.

Ion Channels & Ion Pumps: Metabolic & Endocrine Relationships in Biology & Clinical Medicine. Piero P. Foa & Mary Walsh. 1993. LC 93-31926. (Endocrinology & Metabolism Ser.: Vol. 6). (Illus.). 587p. 302.00 (*0-387-94083-9*) Spr-Verlag.

Ion Channels in Renal Epithelia. Ed. by F. P. Lang. 1990. (Journal: Vol. 13, No. 1-2, 1990). (Illus.). 128p. pap. 113.25 (*3-8055-5163-0*) S Karger.

Ion Channels in the Cardiovascular System. Ed. by Peter M. Spooner et al. 1993. LC 93-37793. (*0-87168-522-1*) Futura Pub.

Ion Channels in the Cardiovascular System: Function & Dysfunction. Ed. by Peter M. Spooner et al. 1996. (Illus.). 616p. tchr. ed. 85.00 (*0-87993-591-X*) Futura Pub.

Ion Channels in Vascular Smooth Muscle. G. Bkaily. 1994. LC 94-43011. (Molecular Biology Intelligence Unit Ser.). 119p. 99.00 (*1-57059-137-7*, LN9137) Landes Bioscience.

Ion Effect: How Air Electricity Rules Your Life & Health. Fred Soyka & Alan Edmonds. 1991. LC 76-40956. 181p. mass mkt. 4.99 (*0-553-19686-3*) Bantam.

Ion Flux in Pulmonary Vascular Control. E. K. Weir et al. 1993. (NATO Advanced Science Institutes Ser.: Vol. 251). (Illus.). 358p. (C). text 125.00 (*0-306-44561-1*, Kluwer Plenum) Kluwer Academic.

Ionic Channels & Effect of Taurine on the Heart: Proceedings of the International Symposium on Cardiac Ion Channels & Effects of Taurine on the Heart, Seoul, Korea, 1992. Ed. by Denis Noble & Yung E. Earm. 1993. LC 93-9516. (Developments in Cardiovascular Medicine Ser.: Vol. 141). 192p. (C). text 127.00 (*0-7923-2199-5*) Kluwer Academic.

Ionic Regulation of the Microcirculation. Ed. by B. M. Altura. 1982. (Advances in Microcirculation Ser.: Vol. 11). (Illus.). x, 174p. 129.75 (*3-8055-3429-9*) S Karger.

Ionic Transport in Hypertension: New Perspectives. Ed. by Antonio Coca & Ricardo Garay. 1993. 352p. lib. bdg. 197.00 (*0-8493-5474-9*, RC685) CRC Pr.

Ionized Calcium Determinations: Precollection Variables, Specimen Choice, Collection, & Handling; Approved Guideline (1993) Contrib. by Gary A. Graham. 1995. 75.00 (*1-56238-287-X*, C31-A) NCCLS.

Ionizing Radiation, Veterans Health Care & Related Issues: Congressional Hearing. Ed. by Arlen Specter. 2001. 195p. (C). reprint ed. pap. text 40.00 (*0-7567-0573-8*) DIANE Pub.

Ionotropic Glutamate Receptors in the CNS. Ed. by G. Adelmann et al. 2000. LC 99-46477. (Handbook of Experimental Pharmacology Ser.: Vol. 141). (Illus.). 512p. 299.00 (*3-540-66120-4*) Spr-Verlag.

Ions for Breathing: Control Air Electrical Climate for Health. Pilcox Cons Svc Staff & C. Bach. 1967. LC 67-27480. (*0-08-012463-1*) Pergamon Repr GBR. *Dist:* Franklin.

Iowa Health Care in Perspective 2000. Ed. by Kathleen O'Leary Morgan & Scott E. Morgan. 2000. 21p. spiral bd. 19.00 (*0-7401-0214-1*) Morgan Quitno Corp.

Iowa Health Care Perspective, 1998. Ed. by Kathleen O'Leary Morgan & Scott E. Morgan. 1998. 20p. pap. 19.00 (*1-56692-814-1*) Morgan Quitno Corp.

Iowa Legal Forms: Personal Injury, 1983-1993. Max E. Kirk. (Iowa Legal Forms Ser.). 170p. suppl. ed. 35.00 (*0-88063-900-8*, 81020-10); 1995. ring bd. 60.00 (*0-86678-101-3*, 81019-10) LEXIS Pub (MICHIE).

***Iowa Medical Directory.** Jola Publications Staff. 2001. 128p. 18.00 (*1-878373-51-X*) Jola Pubns.

Iowa Pharmacy, 1880-1905: An Experiment in Professionalism. Lee Anderson. 1989. LC 89-5036. (Illus.). 190p. text 27.95 (*0-87745-249-0*) U of Iowa Pr.

Iowa University Studies in Psychology. Ed. by Christian A. Ruckwick. 1969. (Psychological Monographs General & Applied: Vol. 43). reprint ed. pap. 55.00 (*0-8115-1442-0*) Periodicals Srv.

Iowa University Studies in Psychology. Ed. by Carl E. Seashore. 1969. (Psychology Monographs General & Applied: Vol. 31). reprint ed. No. 8. pap. 55.00 (*0-8115-1430-7*); No. 9. pap. 55.00 (*0-8115-1435-8*) Periodicals Srv.

Iowa University Studies in Psychology, No. 13. Ed. by Christian A. Ruckwick. 1969. (Psychology Monographs General & Applied: Vol. 40). reprint ed. pap. 55.00 (*0-8115-1439-0*) Periodicals Srv.

IP-6: Nature's Revolutionary Cancer-Fighter. Abulkalam M. Shamsuddin. 1998. 192p. mass mkt. 5.99 (*1-57566-357-0*) Kensgtn Pub Corp.

IPA Management: Organizational Structure & Strategic Planning. Kay Stanley & J. Max Reiboldt. 1999. LC 99-12324. (*0-07-134303-2*) McGraw.

IPA Thesaurus & Frequency List. Ed. & Intro. by Dwight R. Tousignaut. 7th ed. 1995. 275p. (C). pap. text 55.00 (*1-879907-56-9*) Am Soc Hlth-Syst.

IPA Three-Year Cumulative Index, 84-85-86. Dwight R. Tousignaut. 1987. 1500p. pap. text 250.00 (*0-930530-76-4*) Am Soc Hlth-Syst.

IPD Guide to Occupational Health & Organisational Effectiveness. Institute of Personnel Management Staff. 1995. pap. 60.00 (*0-85292-626-X*) IPM Hse.

IPPF-WHR Caribbean Contraceptive Prevalence Survey-3: Grenada. Tirbani P. Jagdeo. Ed. by Rene Jaimes. 1987. 180p. pap. 18.00 (*0-916683-18-4*) Intl Plan Parent.

IQ & Human Intelligence. N. J. Mackintosh. 1998. (Illus.). 430p. text 98.00 (*0-19-852368-8*); pap. text 35.00 (*0-19-852367-X*) OUP.

IQ Tests for Children. Martin Lutterjohann. 1978. LC 77-1520. 192p. pap. 4.95 (*0-8128-2271-4*, Scrbrough Hse) Madison Bks UPA.

IQ Tests for School Children: How to Test Your Child's Intelligence. Martin Lutterjohann. 1980. (Illus.). pap. 5.95 (*0-8128-6026-8*, Scrbrough Hse) Madison Bks UPA.

IqA Nephropathy: Pathogenesis & Treatment. Ed. by A. R. Clarkson & A. J. Woodroffe. 1995. (Contributions to Nephrology Ser.: Vol. 111). (Illus.). x, 212p. 199.25 (*3-8055-6030-3*) S Karger.

IR Genes: Past, Present & Future. Ed. by Carl W. Pierce et al. 1983. LC 82-4291. (Experimental Biology & Medicine Ser.: Vol. 4). (Illus.). 621p. 119.50 (*0-89603-050-4*) Humana.

Iridology: Health Analysis & Treatments from the Iris of the Eye. James Colton & Sheelagh Colton. 1996. LC 96-43198. (Health Essentials Ser.). 128p. pap. 9.95 (*1-85230-880-X*) Element MA.

Iridology: How the Eyes Reveal Your Health & Personality. Dorothy Hall. 1981. LC 80-84439. (Illus.). 256p. (Orig.). pap. 14.95 (*0-87983-241-X*, Keats Pubng) McGraw-Hill Trade.

Iridology Simplified. Bernard Jensen. 1980. pap. 7.99 (*0-9608360-8-X*) B Jensen.

Iridology Simplified. Joe S. Riley. 1996. reprint ed. spiral bd. 8.00 (*0-7873-0722-X*) Hlth Research.

Irigaray Reader. Ed. by Margaret Whitford. Tr. by David Macey from FRE. 1991. (C). pap. 31.95 (*0-631-17043-X*) Blackwell Pubs.

Irinotecan - Campto: Clinical Overview. Ed. by D. K. Hossfeld. 2000. (Onkologie Ser.: Vol. 23). (Illus.). iv, 40p. pap. 28.75 (*3-8055-7089-9*) S Karger.

Irisdiagnosis Notes. Ralph R. Weiss. 1997. 20p. reprint ed. pap. 10.00 (*0-7873-0945-1*) Hlth Research.

Irish Country Cures. Patrick Logan. 1994. LC 93-43393. (Illus.). 160p. (Orig.). pap. 6.95 (*0-8069-0718-5*) Sterling.

Irish Health System in the 21st Century. Austin L. Leahy & Miriam M. Wiley. 1998. LC 98-230783. (Illus.). (*1-86076-103-8*) Oak Tr.

Iron & Human Disease. Ed. by Randall B. Lauffer. 1992. 534p. lib. bdg. 249.00 (*0-8493-6779-4*, RC632) CRC Pr.

Iron & Infection. Ed. by D. J. Bullen & E. Griffiths. 2nd ed. 1999. LC 98-37166. (Illus.). 526p. 245.00 (*0-471-93940-4*) Wiley.

Iron & Your Health: Facts & Fallacies. Thomas F. Emery. 1991. 128p. 59.95 (*0-8493-6763-8*, QP535) CRC Pr.

Iron, Anemia, & Old Age. Ed. by J. Andrews & E. Woodford Williams. 1970. (Gerontologia Clinica Ser.: Vol. 13, No. 1-2). reprint ed. pap. 19.25 (*3-8055-0889-1*) S Karger.

Iron Carriers & Iron Proteins, Vol. 5. Ed. by Thomas M. Loehr. 1989. LC 89-5667. (Physical Bioinorganic Chemistry Ser.). 533p. lib. bdg. 180.00 (*0-89573-298-X*, Wiley-VCH) Wiley.

Iron Chelators in Medicine. Ed. by Ch. Hershko. 1996. (Acta Haematologica Ser.: Vol. 95, No. 1, 1996). (Illus.). 94p. pap. 28.00 (*3-8055-6292-6*) S Karger.

Iron Deficiency Anemia: Recommended Guidelines for the Prevention, Detection, & Management among U. S. Children & Women of Childbearing Age. Ed. by Robert O. Earl et al. 1994. 140p. (C). pap. text 29.00 (*0-309-04987-3*) Natl Acad Pr.

Iron Deficiency in Infancy & Childhood. Peter R. Dallman et al. Ed. by Thomas H. Bothwell et al. 1979. (Illus.). 49p. (Orig.). pap. text 3.50 (*0-935368-08-6*) ILSI.

Iron Deficiency in Women. Thomas H. Bothwell & Robert W. Charlton. Ed. by James D. Cook et al. 1981. (Illus.). 68p. (Orig.). pap. text 3.50 (*0-935368-25-6*) ILSI.

Iron Elephant: What You Should Know about the Dangers of Excess Body Iron. Roberta Crawford. 1992. LC 92-60466. 172p. (Orig.). pap. 12.95 (*0-9632547-0-7*) Vida Pub.

Iron in Central Nervous System Disorders: With Contributions by Numerous Experts. Ed. by P. Riederer & M. B. Youdim. 1994. (Key Topics in Brain Research Ser.). (Illus.). 212p. 79.95 (*0-387-82520-7*) Spr-Verlag.

Iron Metabolism. Ed. by Ivan Bernat. Tr. by Eva Gosztonyi from HUN. 1983. 416p. 85.00 (*0-306-30829-0*, Plenum Trade) Perseus Pubng.

Iron Metabolism. Ugo Testa. 2001. LC 2001-2267. 608p. 199.95 (*0-8493-8676-4*) CRC Pr.

Iron Metabolism: In Health & Disease. Ed. by Jeremy H. Brock et al. 1994. (Illus.). 495p. text (*0-7020-1732-9*) W B Saunders GBR. *Dist:* Saunders.

Iron Metabolism, Anemias, Diagnosis & Therapy: Novel Concepts in the Anemias of Renal & Rheumatoid Disease. M. Wick et al. 4th enl. ed. 2000. (Illus.). x, 204p. pap. 25.00 (*3-211-83357-9*) Spr-Verlag.

Iron Metabolism in Infants. Ed. by Bo Lonnerdal. 1989. 176p. lib. bdg. 141.00 (*0-8493-5433-1*, RJ128) CRC Pr.

Irony Through Psychoanalysis. Giorgio Sacerdoti. 1992. 240p. pap. text (*1-85575-010-4*) Karnac Bks GBR. *Dist:* Other Pr LLC.

Iroquois Medical Botany. James W. Herrick. Ed. & Frwd. by Dean R. Snow. 1997. (Iroquois & Their Neighbors Ser.). (Illus.). 284p. pap. 22.50 (*0-8156-0464-5*) Syracuse U Pr.

Iroquois Medical Botany. James W. Herrick. Ed. by Dean R. Snow. 1994. LC 94-32760. (Iroquois & Their Neighbors Ser.). (Illus.). 240p. (C). 39.95 (*0-8156-0295-2*) Syracuse U Pr.

Irradiation of Blood Components. Ed. by Michael L. Baldwin & Leigh C. Jefferies. 1992. LC 92-49758. 78p. 43.00 (*1-56395-012-X*) Am Assn Blood.

Irreverent Feline Memoirs: A God Is a Cat. Harold Stearns et al. 2000. 8.95 (*0-924799-30-7*) Am Articulat.

Irritable Bladder & Incontinence: A Natural Approach. Jennifer Hunt. 1997. LC 97-61006. (Illus.). 93p. pap. 8.95 (*1-56975-089-0*) Ulysses Pr.

Irritable Bowel Syndrome. Sarah Brewer. 1997. pap. (*0-7225-3392-6*) Thorsons GBR. *Dist:* Natl Bk Netwk.

Irritable Bowel Syndrome. Geoff Watts. 1996. 250p. pap. 9.99 (*0-7493-2466-X*) Buttrwrth-Heinemann.

Irritable Bowel Syndrome: A Natural Approach. Rosemary Nicol. 2nd rev. ed. 1999. 248p. (Orig.). pap. 13.95 (*1-56975-188-9*) Ulysses Pr.

Irritable Bowel Syndrome: Psychosocial Assessment & Treatment. Edward B. Blanchard. 2000. LC 00-40583. xi, 373p. 39.95 (*1-55798-730-0*, 431763A) Am Psychol.

Irritable Bowel Syndrome & Diverticulosis: A Self-Help Plan. Shirley Trickett. rev. ed. 1999. 192p. pap. (*0-7225-3861-8*) Thorsons GBR. *Dist:* Natl Bk Netwk.

Irritable Bowel Syndrome & the Mind-Body/Brain-Gut Connection. William B. Salt, II. 1997. LC 97-66275. (Illus.). 304p. pap. 19.95 (*0-9657038-9-4*) Parkview Pub OH.

Irritable Bowel Syndrome (IBS) & Gastrointestinal Solutions Handbook. Chet Cunningham. 1997. LC 95-60171. 240p. pap. 14.95 (*0-9614924-9-X*) United Res CA.

***Irritable Heart of Soldiers: The U. S. Civil War to Soldier's Heart: World War I.** Charles F. Wooley. 2002. (History of Medicine in Context Ser.). (Illus.). 320p. (*0-7546-0595-7*) Ashgate Pub GBR. *Dist:* Ashgate Pub Co.

Irritant Contact Dermatitis. Edward M. Jackson & Ronald Goldner. 1989. (Basic & Clinical Dermatology Ser.: Vol. 2). (Illus.). 240p. text 180.00 (*0-8247-8288-7*) Dekker.

Irritant Contact Dermatitis Syndrome. Ed. by Pieter Van der Valk & Howard I. Maibach. 1995. LC 95-11260. (Dermatology: Clinical & Basic Science Ser.). 416p. 139.95 (*0-8493-7354-9*, 7354) CRC Pr.

Irritant Dermatitis: New Clinical & Experimental Aspects. Ed. by Howard I. Maibach & P. Elsner. 1995. LC 95-4159. (Current Problems in Dermatology Ser.: Vol. 23). (Illus.). x, 302p. 259.25 (*3-8055-6083-4*) S Karger.

Irwin & Rippe's Intensive Care Medicine. Richard S. Irwin & Frank B. Cerra. 4th ed. 1998. LC 98-15923. 2,720p. text 239.00 (*0-7817-1425-7*) Lppncott W & W.

Irwin Guide to Healthcare Benefits Management: A Seven-Step Program for Reducing Your Company's Costs. Amy J. Katzoff. 1996. LC 96-11868. 256p. text 35.00 (*0-7863-0890-7*, Irwn Prfssnl) McGraw-Hill Educ Grp.

Is Cancer Curable? Alternative Viewpoints. 1991. lib. bdg. 250.00 (*0-8490-5017-0*) Gordon Pr.

Is Counting the Dead Enough? Strategies for Monitoring Health Care Needs in New York City. Emily Friedman. 1986. (Papers: No. 3). 36p. 5.00 (*0-934459-34-7*) United Hosp Fund.

Is Crohn's Disease a Mycobacterial Disease? Ed. by Chris J. Mulder & N. J. Tytgat. 1992. text 81.00 (*0-7923-2026-3*) Kluwer Academic.

Is Endometriosis Potentially Malignant? Third Japan Conference on Endometriosis, Kanagawa, Japan, April 2000: Proceedings. Ed. by H. Hoshiai et al. 2000. (Gynecologic & Obstetric Investigation Ser.: Vol. 50, Suppl. 1 (2000)). iv, 52p. 25.25 (*3-8055-7162-3*) S Karger.

Is Health Improving? Information Gathering for Community-Based Health Care. Elkanah Odembo & Keith Wright. 1996. (Illus.). (Orig.). pap. (*0-942716-07-8*) World Neigh.

Is Heart Surgery Necessary? What Your Doctor Won't Tell You. Julian M. Whitaker. 1995. 288p. 22.95 (*0-89526-473-0*) Regnery Pub.

Is It Hot in Here or Is It Me? Mastering the Maze of Menopause. Lorraine Dabate & Nancy Kenyon. 2000. pap. 10.95 (*1-890838-03-9*) Indus Pub.

Is It Safe? Injury Prevention for Young Children. Becky J. Smith. 1994. LC 94-5196. 17.95 (*1-56071-089-6*) ETR Assocs.

Is Marijuana the Right Medicine for You? Bill Zimmerman et al. 1998. LC 98-23433. 178p. pap. 12.95 (*0-87983-906-6*, 39066K, Keats Pubng) McGraw-Hill Trade.

Is Mind Modular or Unitary? Vol. 2, 2. Douglas K. Detterman. 1992. (Current Topics in Human Intelligence Ser.). 282p. (C). 85.00 (*0-89391-703-6*, Ablex) Greenwood.

Is My Baby All Right? A Guide for Expectant Parents. Christine Gosden et al. 1994. LC 94-5994. (Illus.). 106p. pap. 14.95 (*0-19-262482-2*) OUP.

Is My Child Chemically Dependent? A Professional's Personal Experience. Nikki Babbit. 1988. 36p. (Orig.). pap. 3.95 (*0-945485-04-2*) Comm Intervention.

Is Prevention Better Than Cure? Louise B. Russell. 1986. LC 85-21250. (Studies in Social Economics). 134p. text 32.95 (*0-8157-7632-2*); pap. text 12.95 (*0-8157-7631-4*) Brookings.

Is Psychology for Them? A Guide to Undergraduate Advising. Ed. by Paul J. Woods. 1988. LC 88-3341. 197p. (Orig.). pap. 29.95 (*1-55798-019-5*) Am Psychol.

Is Psychology the Major for You? Planning for Your Undergraduate Years. Ed. by Paul J. Woods & Charles S. Wilkinson. 1987. LC 87-18740. 137p. (Orig.). pap. 9.95 (*0-912704-78-0*) Am Psychol.

Is Religion Good for Your Health? The Effects of Religion on Physical & Mental Health. Harold George Koenig. 1997. LC 96-48053. (Illus.). 137p. 49.95 (*0-7890-0166-7*); pap. 19.95 (*0-7890-0229-9*) Haworth Pr (Haworth Pastrl).

Is Science Sexist? And Other Problems in the Biomedical Sciences. Michael Ruse. 1981. (University of Western Ontario Series in Philosophy of Science: No. 17). 318p. pap. text 51.50 (*90-277-1250-6*) Kluwer Academic.

Is Shame the Central Affect of Disorders of the Self? Ed. by Carr. 1999. (Psychoanalytic Inquiry Ser.: Vol. 19, No. 3). 20.00 (*0-88163-924-9*) Analytic Pr.

Is There a Cure for Aplastic Anaemia? In Memoriam Bruno Speck (1934-1998) Ed. by C. Nissen. 2000. (Acta Haematologica Ser.: Vol. 103, No. 1). (Illus.). 66p. pap. 25.25 (*3-8055-7040-6*) S Karger.

Is There a Doctor in the Barn? A Day in the Life of Forrest F. Tenney, Veterinarian. Elizabeth Yates. 1994. (Illus.). 207p. pap. 10.95 (*0-945980-46-9*) Nrth Country Pr.

Is There a Duty to Die? Ed. by James M. Humber & Robert F. Almeder. 2000. LC 00-501827. (Biomedical Ethics Reviews Ser.: Vol. 17). 232p. 49.50 (*0-89603-783-5*) Humana.

Is There a Duty to Die? And Other Essays in Medical Ethics. John Hardwig & Nat Hentoff. 1999. LC 99-13222. (Reflective Bioethics Ser.). 224p. pap. 21.99 (*0-415-92242-9*) Routledge.

Is There a Shrink in the Lord's House? How Psychologists Can Help the Church. Ed. by H. Newton Malony. 1986. LC 86-81513. (Orig.). pap. 12.95 (*0-9609928-4-7*) Integ Pr.

Is There Duty to Die? And Other Essays in Bio-Ethics. John Hardwig & Nat Hentoff. 2000. LC 99-13222. (Reflective Bioethics Ser.). 224p. (C). text 85.00 (*0-415-92241-0*) Routledge.

Is There Sex after 50? Toni Goffe. 1996. (Illus.). 96p. (Orig.). pap. 5.95 (*1-889647-05-5*) Boston Am.

Is Vasectomy Worth the Risk? A Physician's Case Against Vasectomania. H. J. Roberts. 1993. LC 92-64348. (Illus.). 125p. pap. 16.95 (*0-9633260-2-3*) Sunshine Sentinel.

Is Your Prescription Killing You? Richard Coleman. Ed. by Carolyn Richards. 1981. LC 79-28294. 21.95 (*0-87949-164-7*) Ashley Bks.

ISCAMI: Integrated Systems for the Management & Manipulation of Medical Images. Ed. by J. Demongeot & A. Sousa-Pereira. 1991. (Illus.). 120p. 74.95 (*0-387-59557-0*) Spr-Verlag.

Ischaemia: Preconditioning & Adaptation. M. Marber & Derek M. Yellon. 1996. (UCL Molecular Pathology Ser.). (Illus.). 250p. text (*1-85996-160-6*) Bios Sci GBR. *Dist:* Bks Intl VA.

Ischaemia in Head Injury: Proceedings of a Special Symposium. Ed. by T. C. Smith. 1996. LC 96-12893. (Illus.). 48p. pap. 43.95 (*3-540-61002-2*) Spr-Verlag.

Ischaemia-Reperfusion Injury. Pierce A. Grace & Robert T. Mathie. 1999. LC 98-22342. (Illus.). 384p. 246.95 (*0-632-05021-7*) Blackwell Sci.

Ischaemic Colitis. Jacques W. Reeders et al. 1984. (Illus.). 200p. text 185.50 (*0-89838-645-4*) Kluwer Academic.

Ischaemic Heart Disease. Ed. by K. Fox. 1987. (Current Status of Clinical Cardiology Ser.). text 137.50 (*0-85200-871-6*) Kluwer Academic.

Ischemia & Reperfusion. Ed. by F. Hammersen & K. Messmer. 1989. (Progress in Applied Microcirculation Ser.: Vol. 13). (Illus.). x, 136p. pap. 58.50 (*3-8055-4977-6*) S Karger.

Ischemia-Reperfusion in Cardiac Surgery. Ed. by Hans M. Piper & Claus J. Preuse. 1993. LC 93-16723. (Developments in Cardiovascular Medicine Ser.: Vol. 142). text 264.50 (*0-7923-2241-X*) Kluwer Academic.

Ischemia-Reperfusion Injury in Cardiac Surgery. Ed. by Friedhelm Beyersdorf. 2000. LC 99-22059. (Medical Intelligence Unit Ser.). 304p. 99.00 (*1-58706-002-7*) Eurekah.

Ischemia-Reperfusion Injury in Cardiac Surgery. Friedhelm Beyersdorf. 2000. LC 99-22059. (Medical Intelligence Unit Ser.). 304p. 89.00 (*1-57059-588-7*) Landes Bioscience.

Ischemia-Reperfusion Injury of Skeletal Muscle. G. A. Fantini. 1994. (Medical Intelligence Unit Ser.). 156p. 99.00 (*1-57059-131-8*) Landes Bioscience.

Ischemic Blood Flow in the Brain. Y. Fukuuchi et al. 2000. (Kelo University Symposia for Life Science & Medicine Ser.: Vol. 6). 484p. 199.00 (*4-431-70292-X*) Spr-Verlag.

Ischemic Cerebrovascular Disease. Harold P. Adams, Jr. et al. 2001. LC 00-62432. (Contemporary Neurology Ser.: Vol. 62). (Illus.). 598p. text 120.00 (*0-19-513289-0*) OUP.

Ischemic Extremity: Advances in Treatment. James S. Yao & William H. Pearce. 1995. 614p. (C). pap. text 169.00 (*0-8385-4397-9*, A4397-4, Apple Lange Med) McGraw.

Ischemic Heart. Jonathan Abrams. 1991. 95.95 (*0-316-00471-5*, Little Brwn Med Div) Lppncott W & W.

Ischemic Heart. Seibu Mochizuki. Ed. by Nobuakira Takeda et al. 1998. LC 97-42813. (Progress in Experimental Cardiology Ser.). 624p. lib. bdg. 205.00 (*0-7923-8105-X*) Kluwer Academic.

Ischemic Heart Disease. Attilio Maseri. 1995. LC 95-17707. text (*0-443-07910-2*) Church.

Ischemic Heart Disease: Surgical Management. Ed. by Brian Buxton et al. 1999. LC 98-47023. (*0-7234-2911-1*) Mosby Inc.

Ischemic Mitral Incompetence. Ed. by H. O. Vetter et al. 1991. 180p. 60.00 (*0-387-91355-6*) Spr-Verlag.

Ischemic "Preconditioning" The Concept of Endogenous Cardioprotection. Ed. by Karin Przyklenk et al. 1993. LC 93-21904. (Developments in Cardiovascular Medicine Ser.). 224p. (C). text 141.50 (*0-7923-2410-2*) Kluwer Academic.

Ischemic Stroke: From Basic Mechanisms to New Drug Development. Ed. by Chung Y. Hsu. 1997. LC 97-41311. (Monographs in Clinical Neuroscience: Vol. 16, 1998). (Illus.). x, 166p. 138.25 (*3-8055-6560-7*) S Karger.

Ischemic Stroke: Recent Advances in Understanding & Therapy. Ed. by James Grotta et al. 1995. (Biomedical Library). 602p. pap. 995.00 (*1-57936-006-8*) Drug & Market Dev.

Ischemic Stroke Vol. II: Advances in Understanding & Therapy. Ed. by Lynn Savage. 1996. (Biomedical Library). 294p. pap. 795.00 (*1-57936-014-9*) Drug & Market Dev.

Ischemic Stroke III. Ed. by Wendy Mori. 1997. (Illus.). (Orig.). pap. (*1-57936-041-6*) Drug & Market Dev.

ISCN Guidelines for Cancer Cytogenetics, 1991: Supplement to an International System for Human Cytogenetic Nomenclature. Ed. by Felix Mitelman. 1992. vi, 58p. pap. 38.50 (*3-8055-5567-9*) S Karger.

ISDS 17th World Congress: Hamburg, September 2000: Abstracts. Ed. by C. A. Pellegrini et al. 2000. (Digestive Surgery Ser.: Vol. 17). viii, 138p. pap. 39.25 (*3-8055-7152-6*) S Karger.

Iserson's Getting into a Residency: A Guide for Medical Students. Kenneth V. Iserson. 5th rev. ed. 2000. LC 00-25401. 550p. pap. 36.95 (*1-883620-27-9*) Galen AZ.

Islam & Alcoholism. M. B. Badri. 1976. LC 76-42173. pap. 3.00 (*0-89259-005-X*) Am Trust Pubns.

Islam, Medicine, & Practitioners in Northern Nigeria. Ismail H. Abdalla. 1997. LC 97-1343. (Studies in African Health & Medicine: Vol. 6). 192p. text 79.95 (*0-7734-8655-0*) E Mellen.

Islamic Medicine. Manfred Ullmann. 1997. (Islamic Surveys Ser.). 136p. pap. (*0-7486-0907-5*) Edinburgh U Pr GBR. *Dist:* Col U Pr.

Islamic Ruling on Male & Female Circumcision: The Right Path to Health, Health Education Through Religion, 8. 1996. pap. text 9.00 (*92-9021-217-9*) World Health.

Islamic Ruling on Smoking: The Right Path to Health, Health Education Through Religion, 1. 1996. pap. text 9.00 (*92-9021-167-9*) World Health.

Island Constraints: Theory, Acquisition & Processing. Ed. by Helen Goodluck. 1992. (Studies in Theoretical Psycholinguistics). 480p. (C). text 235.50 (*0-7923-1689-4*) Kluwer Academic.

Islands of Healing: A Guide to Adventure Based Counseling. Jim Schoel et al. Ed. by Conrad Willeman. 1988. (Illus.). 301p. (Orig.). pap. 24.95 (*0-934387-00-1*) Project Advent.

Isler's Patient Guide to Medical Terms, Tests, & Procedures: A Comprehensive Guide for Translating the Confusing Language of "Medicalese" into Easy-to-Understand English. Charlotte Isler. Ed. by Gregg Rogers. 3rd rev. ed. 1994. LC 94-39738. 275p. pap. 12.95 (*1-57066-004-2*, ME068) Practice Mgmt Info.

Isobenzan. 1992. (Environmental Health Criteria Ser.: No. 129). (ENG, FRE & SPA.). 62p. pap. text 16.00 (*92-4-157129-2*, 1160129) World Health.

ISOBM TD-3 International Workshop on Monoclonal Antibodies Against Prostate-Specific Antigen. Ed. by Phil D. Rye et al. 1999. (Tumor Biology Ser.: Vol. 20, Suppl. 1). (Illus.). vi, 94p. pap. 34.00 (*3-8055-6983-1*) S Karger.

Isodose Atlas for Use in Radiotherapy. G. Nemeth & H. Kuttig. 1981. 272p. text 176.50 (*90-247-2476-7*) Kluwer Academic.

Isoelastic Hip Prosthesis: Manual of Surgical & Operative Techniques. Ed. by Robert Mathys, Sr. 1992. LC 92-1481. (Illus.). 110p. pap. text 56.00 (*0-88937-094-X*) Hogrefe & Huber Pubs.

Isoelectric Focusing: Theory, Methodology & Applications. P. G. Righetti. 1983. (Laboratory Techniques in Biochemistry & Molecular Biology Ser.: Vol. 11). 402p. pap. 57.50 (*0-444-80467-6*, I-104-83) Elsevier.

Isokinetics: Testing, Interpretation & Clinical Applications. Zeevi Dvir. 1994. (Illus.). 199p. text (*0-443-04794-4*) Church.

Isolated Adult Cardiomyocytes Ed. by Hans M. Piper & Gerrit Isenberg. 1989. Vol. 1. 336p. 217.00 (*0-8493-4741-6*, QP114); Vol. II. 304p. 230.00 (*0-8493-4742-4*) CRC Pr.

Isolated Heart-Lung Preparation. P. H. Huisman & J. J. Schipperheyn. 1978. (Illus.). pap. text 59.00 (*90-247-2107-5*) Kluwer Academic.

Isolated Hyperthermic Limb Perfusion. Georg Omlor. Ed. by Peter Vaupel & Cristof Alexander. 1995. LC 95-17288. (Medical Intelligence Unit Ser.). 120p. 69.00 (*1-57059-178-4*) Landes Bioscience.

Isolated Liver Perfusion in Hepatic Tumors. Ed. by K. J. Oldhafer et al. 1998. LC 97-36940. (Recent Results in Cancer Research Ser.: Vol. 147). (Illus.). 198p. 114.00 (*3-540-63336-7*) Spr-Verlag.

Isolated Liver Perfusion in Hepatic Tumors, Vol. 147. K. J. Oldhafer et al. 1997. LC 97-36940. (Recent Results in Cancer Research Ser.). (*0-354-06336-7*) Spr-Verlag.

Isolation, Characterization & Utilization of CNS Stem Cells. F. Gage & Yves Christen. 1996. LC 96-38498. (Research & Perspectives in Neurosciences Ser.). (Illus.). 170p. 100.00 (*3-540-61696-9*) Spr-Verlag.

Isolation, Migration & Health. Ed. by D. F. Roberts et al. 1992. (Society for the Study of Human Biology Symposium Ser.: No. 33). (Illus.). 279p. (C). text 80.00 (*0-521-41912-3*) Cambridge U Pr.

Isolation Precautions in Hospitals. 1997. lib. bdg. 250.00 (*0-8490-6069-9*) Gordon Pr.

Isolator Technology: Applications in the Pharmaceutical & Biotechnology Industries. Ed. by Carmen Wagner & James E. Akers. 1995. 384p. 189.00 (*0-935184-78-3*) IHS Health Grp.

Isolators for Sterility Testing Conference Proceedings. 2000. 150.00 (*1-930114-25-7*) Davis Horwood Intl.

Isophorone. 1995. (C). (Environmental Health Criteria Ser.: Vol. 174). 84p. pap. 24.00 (*92-4-157174-8*, 1160174); (Health & Safety Guides Ser.: No. 91). 24p. pap. text 5.00 (*92-4-151091-9*, 1860091) World Health.

Isotope & Related Techniques in Animal Production & Health. International Atomic Energy Agency Staff. 1991. 612p. pap. (*92-0-010491-6*, STI/PUB/876) IAEA AUT. *Dist:* Bernan Associates.

Isotopes for Medicine & the Life Sciences. Institute of Medicine Staff. Ed. by S. James Adelstein & Frederick J. Manning. 1995. LC 94-74964. 144p. (Orig.). (C). pap. text 30.00 (*0-309-05190-8*) Natl Acad Pr.

Isozymes: Biochemical & Genetic Studies. Peggy Clark et al. 1973. LC 73-10223. 242p. (C). text 30.50 (*0-8422-7126-0*) Irvington.

Israel - A Precarious Sanctuary: War, Death & the Jewish People. Eugene Weiner & Anita Weiner. 1989. LC 89-5669. (Studies in Judaism). 134p. (C). 43.50 (*0-8191-7441-6*) U Pr of Amer.

ISS Membership Book. Ed. by Morrie E. Kricun et al. 2nd ed. 1998. LC 98-9192. 290p. 80.00 (*3-540-64017-7*) Spr-Verlag.

Issue of Compulsory Health Insurance. George W. Bachman & Lewis Meriam. 1976. LC 75-17203. (Social Problems & Social Policy Ser.). (Illus.). reprint ed. 23.95 (*0-405-07475-1*) Ayer.

Issues & Answers: A Guide for Parents of Children with Seizures, Ages Six to Twelve. Epilepsy Foundation of America Staff. 1993. 102p. pap. 12.95 (*0-916570-12-6*) Epilepsy Foundation of America.

Issues & Answers: A Guide for Parents of Children with Seizures, Birth to Age Six. Epilepsy Foundation of America Staff. 1993. 105p. pap. 12.95 (*0-916570-11-8*) Epilepsy Foundation of America.

Issues & Answers for Occupational Exposure to Bloodborne Pathogens. Mark M. Moran. 1996. (OSHA Issues & Answers Ser.: No. 4). (Illus.). 37p. (Orig.). pap. 25.00 (*1-890966-22-3*) SafetyCertified.

Issues & Answers in Vascular Surgery. William H. Brown, III et al. (Orig.). Vol. 1. 1985. pap. 47.50 (*0-935717-00-5*); Vol. II. 1986. 200p. pap. 47.50 (*0-935717-01-3*) Mercury Pub.

Issues & Answers in Vascular Surgery, Vol. III. William H. Brown et al. 1988. 240p. (Orig.). pap. 52.50 (*0-935717-02-1*) Mercury Pub.

Issues & Challenges for Group Practitioners. Holly Forester-Miller & Jeffrey A. Kottler. 1997. 232p. (C). pap. text 34.95 (*0-89108-251-4*, 9702) Love Pub Co.

Issues & Controversies in Prevention & Control of VRE, Vancomycin-Resistant Enterococci. Gina Pugliese & Robert A. Weinstein. 1998. LC 98-35461. pap. (*0-9659973-1-6*) ETNA Communs.

Issues & Controversies in the Psychotherapy of Schizophrenia. John G. Gunderson & Loren R. Mosher. 1994. LC 94-31204. (Master Work Ser.). 488p. pap. text 50.00 (*1-56821-397-2*) Aronson.

Issues & Ethics in the Helping Professions. Gerald Corey et al. (Psychology-Counseling Ser.). (C). 2nd ed. 1984. LC 83-10119. 480p. pap. 19.75 (*0-534-02819-5*); 4th ed. 1993. LC 91-37997. 438p. pap. 36.95 (*0-534-18762-5*) Brooks-Cole.

Issues & Perspectives on Health Care in Contemporary Sub-Saharan Africa. Ed. by Ezekiel Kalipeni & Philip Thiuri. 1997. LC 97-42276. (Studies in African Health & Medicine: Vol. 8). 436p. 109.95 (*0-7734-8433-7*) E Mellen.

Issues & Resources for the Cancer Nurse. Susan L. Groenwald. 1991. (Illus.). (C). pap. text 24.95 (*0-86720-307-2*, 307-2) Jones & Bartlett.

Issues & Reviews in Teratology, Vol. 5. Harold Kalter. 1990. LC 83-6323. (Illus.). 338p. (C). text 110.00 (*0-306-43319-2*, Kluwer Plenum) Kluwer Academic.

Issues & Reviews in Teratology. Ed. by Harold Kalter. LC 83-6323. Vol. 2. 1984. 532p. 95.00 (*0-306-41652-2*); Vol. 3. 1985. 314p. 75.00 (*0-306-41988-2*) Perseus Pubng (Plenum Trade).

Issues & Reviews in Teratology, Vol. 6. H. Kalter. 1993. (Illus.). 248p. (C). text 110.00 (*0-306-44381-3*, Kluwer Plenum) Kluwer Academic.

Issues & Reviews in Teratology. Vol. 7. Ed. by Harold Kalter. 1995. (Illus.). 296p. (C). text 110.00 (*0-306-44889-0*, Kluwer Plenum) Kluwer Academic.

Issues & Skills in Relating Primary Medical Care to the Other Human Services, Vol. 3. pap. (*0-89970-108-6*, OP-118) AMA.

Issues & Strategies for Educating Children with Fragile X Syndrome. Philip Wilson et al. 1994. (Orig.). pap. text 25.00 (*0-915667-23-1*) Spectra Pub Co.

Issues & Strategies for Nursing Care Quality: The Encyclopedia of Nursing Care Quality, Vol. 1. Patricia Schroeder. 1991. 238p. 77.00 (*0-8342-0213-1*, 20213) Aspen Pub.

Issues & Trends in Nursing. Grace L. Deloughery. 3rd ed. 1997. LC 98-222026. (Illus.). 504p. (C). (gr. 13). pap. text 28.00 (*0-8151-2608-5*, 31078) Mosby Inc.

***Issues in Accident & Emergency Nursing.** Sbaih. 1994. pap. 34.95 (*0-412-49830-8*) Chapman & Hall.

Issues in Aging & Vision: A Curriculum. Alberta L. Orr. 1998. LC 98-6543. 264p. (Orig.). 27.95 (*0-89128-947-X*) Am Foun Blind.

Issues in Australian Nursing, No. 2. Ed. by Genevieve Gray & Rosalie Pratt. 1989. (Illus.). 424p. pap. text (*0-443-04033-8*) Church.

Issues in Australian Nursing - Three. Ed. by Genevieve Gray & Rosalie Pratt. 3rd ed. 1992. (Illus.). 368p. (Orig.). pap. text (*0-443-04437-6*) Church.

Issues in Child Health & Adolescent Health: Handbook of Psychology & Health, Vol. 2. Ed. by Andrew Baum & J. E. Singer. 1982. 304p. 69.95 (*0-89859-184-8*) L Erlbaum Assocs.

Issues in Clinical Psychology. Jodi A. Mindell. 1992. 352p. (C). text 24.50 net. (*0-697-16945-6*) Brown & Benchmark.

Issues in Community Mental Health: Research - New Findings & Future Directions. Ed. by Steven J. Friedman & Thomas M. Hughes. 1992. (Illus.). 110p. (Orig.). pap. text 6.95 (*0-88135-056-7*, Prodist) Watson Pub Intl.

Issues in Community Mental Health: Respective Diversity: Treatment in the Context of Family & Culture. Ed. by Steven J. Friedman & Robert S. Olko. 1998. (Issues in Community Mental Health Ser.). (Illus.). iv, 138p. pap. 8.95 (*0-88135-200-4*, Sci Hist) Watson Pub Intl.

Issues in Contemporary International Health. T. A. Lambo & S. B. Day. 1990. LC 89-72169. (Illus.). 360p. (C). text 90.00 (*0-306-43344-3*, Kluwer Plenum) Kluwer Academic.

Issues in Cost Accounting for Health Care Organizations. Steven A. Finkler. 2nd ed. 1999. LC 98-54116. 440p. pap. 45.00 (*0-8342-1010-X*, 21010) Aspen Pub.

Issues in Coverage: Financing of Prescription Drugs. Ed. by Linda F. Wolf. 1999. (Illus.). 123p. (C). pap. text 25.00 (*0-7881-8673-6*) DIANE Pub.

Issues in Death & Dying Nursing: CEU. California College for Health Sciences Staff. 1993. 84p. (C). 49.95 (*0-933195-55-9*) CA College Health Sci.

Issues in Diagnostic Research. C. G. Last & M. Hersen. 1987. LC 86-30575. (Illus.). 360p. (C). 75.00 (*0-306-42424-X*, Plenum Trade) Perseus Pubng.

Issues in Epilepsy. 212p. pap. text (*0-86471-054-2*) Adis Intl NZL. *Dist:* Lppncott W & W.

Issues in Fetal Medicine: Proceedings of the 29th Annual Symposium of the Galton Institute, London, 1992. Ed. by S. Leonard Barron & D. F. Roberts. 1995. LC 94-233. 208p. 69.95 (*0-312-12161-X*) St Martin.

Issues in Geriatric Psychiatry. Ed. by Nathan Billig & Peter V. Rabins. 1989. (Advances in Psychosomatic Medicine Ser.: Vol. 19). (Illus.). vii, 184p. 90.50 (*3-8055-4972-5*) S Karger.

Issues in Glomerulonephritis & Renin System. Ed. by Eberhard Ritz. 1984. (Contributions to Nephrology Ser.: Vol. 43). (Illus.). viii, 204p. 29.75 (*3-8055-3912-6*) S Karger.

Issues in Graduate Nursing Education. 1987. 160p. 19.95 (*0-88737-381-X*, 18-2196) Natl League Nurse.

Issues in Health: Readings from the Washington Post, Vol. 2. Rebecca J. Donatelle. 4th ed. 1995. (C). pap. (*0-205-19926-7*, H9926-0) Allyn.

***Issues in Health Policy: Selections from the CQ Researcher.** CQ Editors. 2001. LC 00-65982. (Illus.). xiv, 239p. pap. 26.95 (*1-56802-633-1*, CQ Pr Coll) CQ Pr.

Issues in Hemodialysis - Systems Performance, Water Purity, Reimbursement, & Regulation, 1981. 1981. (Illus.). 87p. pap. text 30.00 (*0-910275-11-4*, TAR2-209) Assn Adv Med Instrn.

Issues in HIV/AIDS in the Australian Prison Systems. Ed. by J. Fortuin. 1992. 120p. pap. (*0-642-18311-2*) Aust Inst Criminology AUS. *Dist:* Advent Bks Div.

Issues in Medical Ethics. Eileen P. Flynn. 1996. 256p. (Orig.). pap. 16.95 (*1-55612-917-3*, LL1917) Sheed & Ward WI.

Issues in Medical Liability. 1995. lib. bdg. 250.99 (*0-8490-7579-3*) Gordon Pr.

Issues in Midwifery. Ed. by Tricis M. Black. 1995. LC 94-29342. pap. text (*0-443-04864-9*) Church.

Issues in Negotiation. California College for Health Sciences Staff. 1993. 250p. (C). spiral bd. Price not set. (*0-933195-12-5*) CA College Health Sci.

Issues in Nursing: An Annotated Bibliography. Vern Bullough et al. 1985. LC 84-48758. 600p. text 25.00 (*0-8240-8768-2*) Garland.

Issues in Pharmacy Practice Management. Andrew L. Wilson. 1996. LC 96-30121. 416p. pap. 47.00 (*0-8342-0908-X*, 20908) Aspen Pub.

Issues in Problem Drug Use & the Addictions: Behavior, Policy & Practice. Ed. by Mike Bloor & Fiona Wood. 1997. 208p. pap. (*1-85302-594-1*) Jessica Kingsley GBR. *Dist:* Taylor & Francis.

Issues in Psychiatric Classification: Science, Practice & Social Policy. Ed. by Alfred Freedman et al. 1986. 268p. 35.95 (*0-89885-294-3*, Kluwer Acad Hman Sci) Kluwer Academic.

Issues in Psychobiology. C. R. Legg. 1989. 256p. 47.50 (*0-415-01405-0*, 1091); pap. 17.95 (*0-415-01406-9*, A3367) Routledge.

Issues in Psychotherapy Research. Ed. by Michel Hersen et al. 1984. LC 83-22938. (Applied Clinical Psychology Ser.). 436p. 75.00 (*0-306-41401-5*, Plenum Trade) Perseus Pubng.

Issues in Reproductive Technology: An Anthology. Ed. by Helen B. Holmes. 1994. 449p. (C). pap. text 20.00 (*0-8147-3516-9*) NYU Pr.

Issues in Reproductive Technology I: An Anthology. Helen B. Holmes. 1992. LC 92-9929. 472p. text 66.00 (*0-8153-0035-2*, 729) Garland.

Issues in Risk Assessment. National Research Council Staff. 1993. LC 92-61838. 374p. (Orig.). (C). pap. text 46.50 (*0-309-04786-2*) Natl Acad Pr.

Issues in Sexual & Medical Ethics. Charles E. Curran. 1979. LC 77-89767. pap. 14.00 (*0-268-01142-7*) U of Notre Dame Pr.

Issues in Supportive Care of Cancer Patients. Ed. by Donald J. Higby. 1986. (Cancer Treatment & Research Ser.). text 161.50 (*0-89838-816-3*) Kluwer Academic.

Issues in the Developmental Approach to Mental Retardation. Ed. by Robert M. Hodapp et al. 1990. (Illus.). 352p. (C). text 69.95 (*0-521-34619-3*) Cambridge U Pr.

Issues in the Developmental Approach to Mental Retardation. Ed. by Edward F. Zigler et al. 1995. (Illus.). 352p. (C). pap. text 24.95 (*0-521-46757-8*) Cambridge U Pr.

Issues in the Educational Placement: Students with Emotional or Behavioral Disorders. Ed. by James M. Kauffman et al. 1995. 416p. pap. 45.00 (*0-8058-1533-3*); text 79.95 (*0-8058-1532-5*) L Erlbaum Assocs.

Issues in the Management of Depression: Depression in the Elderly. Ed. by Chris Fellner. 1996. (Series of Slide Lecture Programs: Vol. 2). pap. (*1-57130-023-6*) Medicine Grp USA.

Issues in the Management of Depression: Depression in the Medically Ill: Prevalence, Diagnosis, & Treatment. Dwight L. Evans. Ed. by Chris Fellner. 1997. (Series of Slide Lecture Programs). (Orig.). pap. (*1-57130-018-X*) Medicine Grp USA.

Issues in the Management of Depression: Neuropharmacology of Depression. Alan F. Schatzberg. Ed. by Chris Fellner. 1997. (Series of Slide Lecture Programs: Vol. 4). (Orig.). pap. (*1-57130-025-2*) Medicine Grp USA.

Issues in the Management of Depression: The Importance of Antidepressant Pharmacokinetics for the Primary Care Physician. Jerold F. Rosenbaum. Ed. by Chris Fellner. 1997. (Series of Slide Lecture Programs: Vol. 3). (Orig.). pap. (*1-57130-024-4*) Medicine Grp USA.

Issues in the Political Economy of Health Care. Ed. by John McKinlay. 1984. 275p. 29.95 (*0-422-78040-5*, NO. 9330); pap. 14.95 (*0-422-78050-2*, NO. 9184) Routledge.

Issues in Therapy with Lesbian, Gay, Bisexual, & Transgendered Clients. Contrib. by Charles Neal & Dominic Davies. 2000. LC 99-56819. (*0-335-20332-9*) OpUniv Pr GBR. *Dist:* Taylor & Francis.

Issues in Women's Health. Ed. by Lammers Hardy & J. Randell. 1989. (Recent Advances in Nursing Ser.: No. 25). (Illus.). 200p. pap. text (*0-443-04202-0*) Church.

Issues Related to Medicare Payment Policies for Home Health Agency & Skilled Nursing Facility Services: Hearing Before the Subcommittee on Health of the Committee on Ways & Means, House of Representatives, One Hundred Fourth Congress, Second Session, July 23, 1996. U. S. Government Printing Office Staff. 1997. LC 98-110346. iii, 204 p. (*0-16-055313-X*) USGPO.

ISSX European Meeting on Foreign Compound Metabolism. Ed. by J. Caldwell et al. 1986. (Xenobiotica Ser.: Vol. 16, Nos. 10 & 11). 196p. 91.00 (*0-85066-937-5*) Taylor & Francis.

It Is As Simple As That & More Vol. 8: Chiropractic Philosophy. Frederick H. Barge & B. J. Palmer. 1996. LC 96-83297. 208p. 38.95 (*1-885048-08-4*) Barge Chiropract.

It Just Ain't Fair: The Ethics of Health Care for African Americans. Annette Dula & Sara Goering. 1994. LC 93-43780. pap. 19.95 (*0-275-95057-3*, Greenwood Pr) Greenwood.

It Just Ain't Fair: The Ethics of Health Care for African Americans. Ed. by Annette Dula & Sara Goering. 1994. LC 93-43780. 336p. 69.50 (*0-275-94494-8*, Praeger Pubs) Greenwood.

It Only Takes a Second: Preventing Childhood Traumatic Injuries. Children's Hospital of Los Angeles Staff. 2000. LC 00-64525. (Illus.). xiii, 97p. pap. text 16.95 (*0-7668-2386-5*) Delmar.

It Runs in My Family: Overcoming the Legacy of Family Illness. Joan C. Barth. 1993. LC 93-24660. (Frontiers in Couples & Family Therapy Ser.: No. 7). (Illus.). 224p. pap. 21.95 (*0-87630-712-8*) Brunner-Routledge.

It Shouldn't Happen to a Patient: A Survivor's Guide to Fighting Life-Threatening Illness. Pittu Laungan. 1992. 192p. text (*1-871177-14-6*) Whiting & Birch GBR. *Dist:* Paul & Co Pubs.

It Shouldn't Hurt to Be a Child. Dianne Vasi. Ed. by Richard W. Coffen. 1985. (Better Living Ser.). 32p. (Orig.). pap. 0.89 (*0-8280-0310-6*) Review & Herald.

It Was Probably Something You Ate: A Practical Guide to Avoiding & Surviving Food-Borne Illness. Nicols Fox. 1999. LC 98-52910. 208p. pap. 13.95 (*0-14-027799-4*) Penguin Putnam.

It Will Never Happen to Me: Children of Alcholics as Youngsters, Addescents, Adults. Claudia Black. 1982. LC 59-776. (Illus.). 183p. pap. 9.95 (*0-910223-00-9*) MAC Pub.

***It Works for Me! Celebrity Stories of Alternative Healing.** Heide Banks. 2001. (Illus.). 205p. pap. 20.00 (*0-7881-9951-X*) DIANE Pub.

Italian-English - English-Italian Encyclopedic Dictionary of Biological Sciences & Medicine. Giovanni Delfin et al. (ENG & ITA.). 1726p. 195.00 (*0-8288-9421-3*, M4783) Fr & Eur.

Italian-English - English-Italian Medical Dictionary. M. Luchessi. 1987. 1456p. 150.00 (*88-7078-037-6*) IBD Ltd.

Italian-English - English-Italian Medical Dictionary. M. Petrelli. 1993. (ENG & ITA.). 737p. 115.00 (*0-7859-7524-1*, 8871660714); 110.00 (*0-7859-8825-4*) Fr & Eur.

Italian-English - English-Italian Medical Dictionary. M. Petrelli. 1993. 737p. (*88-7166-071-4*) Le Lettere ITA. *Dist:* IBD Ltd.

Italian Labyrinth: Italy in the 1980's. John Haycraft. 1987. (Illus.). 320p. 30.95 (*0-436-19137-7*) Trafalgar.

Itch: Mechanisms & Management of Pruritus. Jeffrey D. Bernhard. 1994. LC 93-21008. (Illus.). 454p. pap. 59.00 (*0-07-004935-1*) McGraw-Hill Educ Grp.

Item Interpretation of the Luria-Nebraska Neuropsychological Battery. Charles J. Golden. 1982. LC 81-16393. 243p. text 75.00 (*0-8032-2105-3*) U of Nebr Pr.

It's a Gas: A Study of Flatulence. Eric S. Rabkin & Eugene M. Silverman. 1991. (Illus.). 164p. (Orig.). pap. 9.95 (*1-879378-03-5*) Rabkin-Silverman.

It's a Jungle Out There! An Insider's Outlook on Jobs in Health Care. Sherry Makely & Lana Christian. 1996. (Illus.). 55p. spiral bd. 14.95 (*0-9652954-0-0*) Pine Ridge Publns.

It's All Right to Get Old. June Stephenson. 1987. LC 82-71128. 62p. pap. 9.95 (*0-941138-06-2*); 3rd rev. ed. 2000. pap. 15.00 (*0-941138-17-8*) Diemer-Smith.

It's in the Mail: How to Collect Health Care Bills. David Zimmerman & Bruce Nelson. 1989. 295p. reprint ed. pap. text 39.50 (*1-882987-01-2*) EagleBooks WI.

It's Never the Same: A Priest's Struggle with Multiple Sclerosis. Jimmy Doherty. 1988. 93p. (Orig.). pap. (*1-85390-087-7*) Veritas Pubns IRL. *Dist:* Irish Bks Media.

It's Not a Tumor! The Patients Guide to Common Neurological Problems. Robert Wiedemeyer. 1996. LC 95-78076. 180p. (Orig.). pap. 14.95 (*0-9647407-9-6*) Boxweed Pubng.

It's Not All in Your Head: Now Women Can Discover the Real Causes of Their Most Commonly Misdiagnosed Health Problems. Susan Anderson Swedo & Henrietta L. Leonard. 1997. LC 95-26602. (Illus.). 336p. pap. 15.00 (*0-06-251287-0*) Harper SF.

It's Not Carpal Tunnel Syndrome: RSI Theory & Therapy for Computer Professionals. Suparna Damany & Jack Bellis. 2000. LC 00-90189. (Illus.). 234p. pap. 19.95 (*0-9655109-9-9*) SIMAX.

***It's Not in Your Head, It's Your Hormones.** Melinda Bonk. 2001. 232p. pap. 14.95 (*1-931412-59-6*) Fair Winds Pr.

It's Not Quite Like Home: Illness, Career Descent, & the Stigma of Living at a Multilevel Care Retirement Facility. Bradley J. Fisher. rev. ed. 1991. LC 91-22334. (Studies on the Elderly in America). 208p. text 25.00 (*0-8153-0519-2*) Garland.

It's Not Too Late for a Baby: For Men & Women over Thirty-Five. Sylvia P. Rubin. 1980. (Illus.). 272p. 14.95 (*0-13-507046-5*, Spectrm) Hungry Minds.

It's So Natural Health Book. Alan Hayes. 2000. 156p. pap. (*1-86254-493-X*) Wakefield Pr AUS. *Dist:* BHB Intl.

It's Your Body: A Woman's Guide to Gynecology. Niels H. Lauersen & Steven Whitney. 1986. LC 80-80994. (Illus.). 576p. pap. 7.99 (*0-425-09917-2*) Berkley Pub.

It's Your Life! A Gynecologist's Guide for Taking Control of It. James A. Schaller. 1997. LC 96-40108. 360p. 24.95 (*1-57733-018-8*); pap. 16.95 (*1-57733-004-8*) B Dolphin Pub.

It's Your Pregnancy: Questions You Ask Yourself & Are Afraid to Ask Your Obstetrician. Niels H. Lauersen & Judy Hendra. 1987. 480p. pap. 12.95 (*0-671-50211-5*, Fireside) S&S Trade Pap.

Iubire, Vinovatie Si Alte Lucrari, 1921-1945. Melanie Klein. Ed. by F. V. Vladescu. Tr. by L. Pavel et al. 1994. (Scrierile Melanie Klein in Patru Volume Ser.: Vol. 1).Tr. of Writings of Melanie Klein, I Love, Guilt & Reparation & Other Works, 1921-1945. (RUM., Illus.). 414p. pap. 34.00 (*1-883881-03-X*, 03X) S Freud RT&PF.

IV-C Mercury Tox Program: A Guide for the Doctor. H.L. Sam Queen & Betty A. Queen. 1991. (Doctor's Guide for Lifestyle Counseling Ser.). 76p. (Orig.). pap. text 25.00 (*0-9620479-0-2*) Inst for Health Real.

IV-C Mercury Tox Program: A Guide for the Patient. H.L. Sam Queen & Betty A. Queen. 1991. (Doctor's Guide for Lifestyle Counseling Ser.). 72p. (Orig.). pap. text 25.00 (*0-9620479-2-9*) Inst for Health Real.

IV Drug Guide for Nurses. Jacqueline D. Sutton et al. 1993. LC 92-49638. (Illus.). 656p. (C). pap. 32.95 (*0-8385-4054-6*, A4054-1) P-H.

IV Therapy Video-Workbook. Springhouse Publishing Company Staff. 1995. 144p. pap. text, stu. ed., wbk. ed. 39.95 incl. VHS (*0-87434-818-8*) Springhouse Corp.

I've Got It under Control? A Parent's Guide to the First Step. Judith Strom. 1989. (Adult Pamphlet Ser.). (Illus.). 32p. (Orig.). pap. 1.75 (*0-925190-18-7*) Fairview Press.

Ivermectin & Abanectin. Ed. by W. C. Campbell. 1994. (Illus.). 363p. 105.00 (*0-387-96944-6*) Spr-Verlag.

IVIG Therapy Today. Ed. by Mark Ballow. 1992. LC 91-20896. (Illus.). 160p. 119.50 (*0-89603-223-X*) Humana.

J

J-Mail: JCAHO Survey Prep E-Mails for the Whole Staff. Candace Hamner. 1999. (Illus.). 100p. pap. text 119.00 (*1-57839-070-2*) Opus Communs.

Jablonski's Dictionary of Dentistry. Stanley Jablonski. 1992. LC 90-4590. 906p. (C). reprint ed. lib. bdg. 119.50 (*0-89464-477-7*) Krieger.

Jablonski's Dictionary of Syndromes & Eponymic Diseases. Stanley Jablonski. 2nd ed. 1991. 680p. (C). lib. bdg. 110.00 (*0-89464-224-3*) Krieger.

Jack-Roller: A Delinquent Boy's Own Story. Clifford R. Shaw. 1966. LC 66-23698. 225p. reprint ed. pap. text 11.95 (*0-226-75126-0*, P241) U Ch Pr.

Jackpot: Gaming the Home Health Care System - Congressional Hearing. Ed. by Charles Grassley. 1999. (Illus.). 328p. (C). reprint ed. pap. text 40.00 (*0-7881-8219-6*) DIANE Pub.

Jackpot: Gaming the Home Health Care System : Hearing Before the Special Committee on Aging, United States Senate, One Hundred Fifth Congress, First Session, Washington, DC, July 28, 1997. Contrib. by U. S. Congress, Senate Special Committee on Aging. 1997. LC 98-114746. (Illus.). (*0-16-055733-X*) USGPO.

JACM on Ambulatory Surgery. Ed. by Seth B. Goldsmith & Norbert Goldfield. 1994. LC 94-34193. 248p. pap. 53.00 (*0-8342-0672-2*) Aspen Pub.

JACM on Hospital-Based Ambulatory Care. Ed. by Seth B. Goldsmith. 1994. LC 94-33614. 284p. pap. 53.00 (*0-8342-0673-0*) Aspen Pub.

JACM on Managed Care. Ed. by Seth B. Goldsmith. 1994. LC 94-36039. 316p. pap. 53.00 (*0-8342-0670-6*) Aspen Pub.

JACM on Marketing Ambulatory Care. Ed. by Seth B. Goldsmith. 1994. LC 94-33589. 280p. pap. 53.00 (*0-8342-0671-4*) Aspen Pub.

Jacques Joseph's Rhinoplasty & Facial Plastic Surgery with a Supplement on Mammaplasty. Tr. by Stanley Milstein from GER. ltd. ed. 1987.Tr. of Nasenplastik und Sonstige Gesichtsplastik nebst Mammaplastik. (Illus.). 855p. 395.00 (*0-9605972-1-2*) Columella Pr.

Jacques Lacan. Jonathan S. Lee. 1990. (Twayne's World Authors Ser.: No. 817). 272p. (C). 26.95 (*0-8057-8256-7*) Macmillan.

Jacques Lacan. Jonathan S. Lee. 1991. LC 90-21076. 264p. pap. 18.95 (*0-87023-737-3*) U of Mass Pr.

Jacques Lacan. Madan Sarup. 1992. (Modern Cultural Theorists Ser.). 160p. 45.00 (*0-8020-2893-4*); pap. text 16.95 (*0-8020-7400-6*) U of Toronto Pr.

Jacques Lacan. Anika Lemaire. Tr. by David Macey from FRE. 1979. reprint ed. pap. 14.95 (*0-7100-0350-1*, Routledge Thoemms) Routledge.

Jacques Lacan: A Bibliography. Ed. by Joan Nordquist. 1987. (Social Theory: A Bibliographic Ser.: No. 5). 50p. pap. 20.00 (*0-937855-08-1*) Ref Rsch Serv.

Jacques Lacan: A Feminist Introduction. Elizabeth Grosz. 1990. LC 89-11005. 232p. (C). (gr. 13). pap. 22.99 (*0-415-01400-X*) Routledge.

Jacques Lacan: An Annotated Bibliography. Michael Clark. 1988. LC 84-45394. (Modern Critics & Critical Schools Ser.). 400p. text 20.00 (*0-8240-8848-4*) Garland.

Jacques Lacan: His Life & Work. Elizabeth Roudinesco. Tr. by Barbara Bray. 1997. LC 96-30125. (European Perspectives; A Series in Social Thought & Culturall Criticism Ser.). 464p. 39.00 (*0-231-10146-5*) Col U Pr.

Jacques Lacan: The Death of an Intellectual Hero. Stuart Schneiderman. 1983. LC 82-21236. 192p. pap. text 15.50 (*0-674-47116-4*) HUP.

Jacques Lacan: The French Context. Marcelle Marini. Tr. by Anne Tomiche. 1993. LC 92-9652. (ENG & FRE.). 310p. (C). 45.00 (*0-8135-1851-2*); pap. 18.00 (*0-8135-1852-0*) Rutgers U Pr.

Jacques Lacan & Co. A History of Psychoanalysis in France, 1925-1985. Elisabeth Roudinesco. 1990. LC 89-78164. (Illus.). 788p. 45.00 (*0-226-72997-4*) U Ch Pr.

Jacques Lacan & the Adventure of Insight: Psychoanalysis in Contemporary Culture. Shoshana Felman. 1989. 208p. LC 86-19458. (Illus.). 33.95 (*0-674-47120-2*); reprint ed. pap. 16.50 (*0-674-47121-0*) HUP.

Jacques Lacan & the Philosophy of Psychoanalysis. Ellie Ragland-Sullivan. 1987. LC 84-16125. 384p. pap. text 16.95 (*0-252-01465-0*) U of Ill Pr.

Jacques Lacan's Return to Freud: The Real, the Symbolic, & the Imaginary. Philippe Julien. Tr. by Devra B. Simiu. 1994. LC 93-40773. (Psychoanalytic Crosscurrents Ser.). 220p. (C). text 45.00 (*0-8147-4198-3*) NYU Pr.

Jacques Lacan's Return to Freud: The Real, the Symbolic, & the Imaginary. Devra B. Simiu. 1995. (Psychoanalytic Crosscurrents Ser.). 220p. (C). pap. text 18.50 (*0-8147-4226-2*) NYU Pr.

Jade Remedies: A Chinese Herbal Reference for the West. Peter Holmes. 1997. LC 99-218570. (Illus.). (Orig.). Vol. 1. 442p. pap. 50.00 (*1-890029-28-9*); Vol. 2. 450p. pap. 50.00 (*1-890029-29-7*) Snow Lotus.

Jadelle: Two-Rod Levonorgestrel Contraceptive Implant. Noel McIntosh & Elizabeth Oliveras. 1997. pap. 15.00 (*0-929817-56-7*) JHPIEGO.

Jahrestagung der Bayerischen Gesellschaft Fuer Geburtshilfe und der Oesterreichischen Gesellschaft fuer Gynaekologie und Geburtshilfe, Muenchen, Juni 1981. Ed. by Eduard Gitsch & E. Reinold. 1981. (Gynaekologische Rundschau Journal: Vol. 21, Suppl. 2). (Illus.). vii, 234p. pap. 45.25 (*3-8055-3478-7*) S Karger.

Jahrestagung der Bayerischen Gesellschaft Fuer Geburtshilfe und Frauenheilkunde und der Oesterreichischen Gesellschaft fuer Gynaekologie und Geburtshilfe, Velden am Woerthersee, Juni 1983. Ed. by Eduard Gitsch & E. Reinold. 1984. (Journal: Vol. 23, Suppl. 3). (Illus.). viii, 244p. pap. 48.00 (*3-8055-3802-2*) S Karger.

Jahrestagung der Oesterreichischen Gesellschaft Fuer Gyaekologie und Geburtshilfe, Krems, June 1980. Ed. by E. Reinold. 1981. (Gynaekologische Rundschau Journal: Vol. 20, Suppl. 2, 1981). (Illus.). xviii, 294p. pap. 57.50 (*3-8055-2191-X*) S Karger.

Jahrestagung der Oesterreichischen Gesellschaft Fuer Gynaekologie und Geburtshilfe, Bad Ischl, Juni 1982. Ed. by Eduard Gitsch & E. Reinold. 1982. (Journal: Vol. 22, Suppl. 1). (Illus.). vi, 190p. 43.50 (*3-8055-3625-9*) S Karger.

Jahrestagung der Oesterreichischen Gesellschaft Fuer Gynaekologie und Geburtshilfe, Eisenstadt, Mai 1986. Ed. by Eduard Gitsch & E. Reinold. 1987. (Gynaekologische Rundschau Journal: Vol. 26, Supp. 2). (Illus.). xii, 328p. 104.50 (*3-8055-4558-4*) S Karger.

Jahrestagung der Oesterreichischen Gesellschaft fuer Gynaekologie und Mitterndorf, Juni 1984. Ed. by Eduard Gitsch & E. Reinold. 1985. (Illus.). vi, 190p. pap. 48.00 (*3-8055-4013-2*) S Karger.

Jahresversammlung der Schweizerischen Gesellschaft Fuer Dermatologie und Venereologie, 60: Journal: Dermatologica, Vol. 159, No. 5, 1979. Ed. by R. Schuppli. 1979. (Illus.). pap. 28.75 (*3-8055-0103-X*) S Karger.

James Cook & the Conquest of Scurvy, 40. Francis E. Cuppage. 1994. LC 94-3050. (Contributions in Medical Studies Ser.: No. 40). 192p. 62.50 (*0-313-29181-0*, Greenwood Pr) Greenwood.

James Dobson's Gospel of Self-Esteem & Psychology. Martin Bobgan & Deidre Bobgan. rev. ed. 1998. LC 98-93727. 248p. pap. 15.00 (*0-941717-16-X*) EastGate Pubs.

James Jackson Putnam & Psychoanalysis: Letters Between Putnam & Sigmund Freud, Ernest Jones, William James, Sandor Ferenczi & Morton Prince, 1877-1917. James J. Putnam. Ed. by Nathan G. Hale, Jr. Tr. by Judith B. Heller. 1971. LC 70-150010. (Commonwealth Fund Publications). (Illus.). 400p. 37.00 (*0-674-47170-9*) HUP.

James Joyce & the Burden of Disease. Kathleen R. Ferris. 1994. LC 94-19905. (Illus.). 184p. 27.50 (*0-8131-1893-X*) U Pr of KY.

James Miles Langstaff: A Nineteenth-Century Medical Life. Dacalyn Duffin. 1993. (Illus.). 604p. pap. text 17.95 (*0-8020-7414-6*) U of Toronto Pr.

James Parkinson: His Life & Times by A. D. Morris. F. Clifford Rose. 1989. 308p. 96.50 (*0-8176-3401-0*) Birkhauser.

***James Parkinson, 1755-1824: From Apothecary to General Practitioner.** Shirley Roberts. 1998. (History of Medicine Ser.). (Illus.). 128p. (*1-85315-340-0*) Royal Soc of Medicine Pr Ltd GBR. *Dist:* Balogh.

James Taylor Gwathmey - American Pioneer Anesthesiologist. Ed. by Charles B. Pittinger. 1989. LC 88-51678. 630p. (C). 55.00 (*0-9623307-0-1*) Anesthesia Pr.

Jamu: The Ancient Indonesian Art of Herbal Healing. Susan-Jane Beers. 2001. (Illus.). 208p. pap. (*962-593-503-7*) Periplus HKG. *Dist:* Tuttle Pubng.

Jan van Rymsdyk: Medical Illustrator of the Eighteenth Century. John L. Thornton. 1981. (Medical Bks.: Vol. 1). (Illus.). 106p. (*0-906672-02-3*) Oleander Pr.

Jane Austen & the Body: "The Picture of Health" John Wiltshire. 1992. (Illus.). 265p. (C). text 74.95 (*0-521-41476-8*) Cambridge U Pr.

Jane Brody's Allergy Fighter. Jane E. Brody. 1998. LC 96-34499. 128p. pap. 10.00 (*0-393-31635-1*) Norton.

Jane Brody's Allergy Fighter: Relieve the Misery of Nasal Allergies with the Help of America's Most Trusted Authority on Personal Health. Jane Brody. 2000. 127p. pap. 5.99 (*0-7858-1254-7*) Bk Sales Inc.

Jane Brody's Cold & Flu Fighter. Jane Brody. 1995. LC 95-10236. 88p. 10.95 (*0-393-03913-7*) Norton.

Jane Brody's Cold & Flu Fighter. Jane E. Brody. 1995. LC 95-10236. Orig. Title: Cold & Flu Fighter. 88p. pap. 5.95 (*0-393-31353-0*) Norton.

Jane Brody's Cold Flu Fighter. Jane Brody. 2000. 128p. 5.99 (*0-7858-1253-9*) Bk Sales Inc.

Jane Brody's Nutrition Book. Jane E. Brody. 1982. LC 80-25117. 576p. pap. 17.95 (*0-553-34721-7*) Bantam.

Jane Brody's Nutrition Book: A Lifetime Guide to Eating for Better Health & Weight Control. Jane E. Brody. 1981. LC 80-25117. (Illus.). 576p. 29.95 (*0-393-01429-0*) Norton.

Japan Health Handbook. Meredith E. Maruyama et al. 1995. 320p. pap. 20.00 (*4-7700-1838-X*) Kodansha.

Japan Health Handbook. Louise P. Shimizu et al. rev. ed. 1998. 352p. pap. (*4-7700-2356-1*) Kodansha Intl JPN. *Dist:* Kodansha.

Japan Pharmaceutical Reference. 4th ed. 1996. 1380p. pap. 395.00 (*0-7859-9646-X*) Fr & Eur.

Japanese Acupuncture: A Clinical Guide. Stephen Birch & Junko Ida. Ed. by Robert L. Felt & Jack Lincoln. 1998. LC 94-18574. (Illus.). 350p. (Orig.). (C). pap. 40.00 (*0-912111-42-9*) Paradigm Publns.

Japanese & Western Bioethics: Studies in Moral Diversity, Vol. 54. Ed. by Kazumasa Hoshino. 1996. LC 96-22746. (Philosophy & Medicine Ser.). 236p. (C). text 144.00 (*0-7923-4112-0*) Kluwer Academic.

Japanese-Chinese-English Medical Dictionary. (CHI, ENG & JPN.). 295.00 (*0-7859-9414-9*) Fr & Eur.

Japanese Classical Acupuncture: Introduction to Meridian Therapy. Denmei Shudo. Tr. by Stephen Brown from JPN. 1990. LC 90-82526. (Illus.). 251p. (C). text 38.00 (*0-939616-11-4*) Eastland.

Japanese-Latin-English-German-French Medical Terminology. Kanehara. 1984. (ENG, FRE, GER, JPN & LAT.). 1259p. 250.00 (*0-8288-0579-2*, M9350) Fr & Eur.

Japanese Medical Terminology, English-Japanese. (ENG & JPN.). 295.00 (*0-7859-9421-1*) Fr & Eur.

Japanese Medical Terminology, Japanese-English. (ENG & JPN.). 295.00 (*0-7859-9413-0*) Fr & Eur.

Japanese Medicine. Yu Fujikawa. LC 75-23663. (Clio Medica Ser.: 12). Orig. Title: Geschichte der Medizin in Japan. (Illus.). reprint ed. 32.50 (*0-404-58912-X*) AMS Pr.

Jarm-How to Jog with Your Arms to Live Longer. Joseph D. Wassersug. 1984. LC 81-10919. 13.95 (*0-87949-197-3*) Ashley Bks.

Jason Winters Story: Killing Cancer, in Search of the Perfect Cleanse, Breakthrough, the Ultimate Combination. Jason Winters. 2nd ed. 1991. LC 91-195973. 361p. pap. 14.95 (*0-9621388-0-0*) Vinton.

Jay Haley on Milton H. Erickson. Jay Haley. 1993. LC 93-5375. 214p. VHS 79.95 (*0-87630-726-8*); text 29.95 (*0-87630-728-4*) Brunner-Routledge.

JCAHO Home Health Mock Survey Made Simple. Marcia Bowers & Karen Williams. 1998. LC 99-203976. (Illus.). 150p. pap. text 67.00 (*1-57839-026-5*) Opus Communs.

JCAHO Sentinel Event Resource Guide. Eric Joseph & Nancy Webster. 1998. 40p. pap. 20.00 (*0-916499-73-1*) Care Educ Grp.

JCAHO Troubleshooter: Best Policies, Practices & Model Documents for Survey Success. Steven W. Bryant et al. 2000. (Illus.). 280p. pap. text 147.00 (*1-57839-073-7*) Opus Communs.

Jealous Potter. Claude Levi-Strauss. Tr. by Benedicte Chorier. LC 87-30076. (Illus.). 1996. viii, 252p. pap. 15.95 (*0-226-47482-8*); 1988. 264p. 23.95 (*0-226-47480-1*) U Ch Pr.

Jealousy: Theory, Research & Clinical Strategies. Gregory L. White & Paul E. Mullen. LC 89-7534. 340p. 1989. text 42.00 (*0-89862-385-5*); 1992. reprint ed. pap. 24.00 (*0-89862-532-7*, 2532) Guilford Pubns.

Jean de Vigo, le Mal Francais: Selections from Ancient Syphilographers. Wallace B. Hamby. Tr. by Alfred Fournier. 1980. LC 78-50191. 124p. 15.00 (*0-87527-191-X*) Green.

Jean Piaget: Consensus & Controversy. Sohan Modgil & Celia Modgil. 1982. LC 81-84205. 446p. 55.00 (*0-275-90862-3*, C0862, Praeger Pubs) Greenwood.

Jeanne Rose's Herbal Studies Course: A Complete Home Study Herb Course, Set. Jeanne Rose. 1988. (Herbal Studies). (Illus.). 1200p. ring bd. 375.00 (*0-9620838-1-X*, J R Herb Pubns) Herb Studies Library.

Jeanne Rose's Herbal Studies Course Pt. I: The Seasonal Herbal. Jeanne Rose. 1988. (Herbal Studies). (Illus.). 350p. 125.00 (*0-9620838-2-8*, J R Herb Pubns) Herb Studies Library.

Jeanne Rose's Herbal Studies Course Pt. II: The Medicinal Herbal. Jeanne Rose. 1988. (Herbal Studies). (Illus.). 1200p. 125.00 (*0-9620838-4-4*, J R Herb Pubns) Herb Studies Library.

Jeanne Rose's Herbal Studies Course Pt. III: The Reference Herbal. Jeanne Rose. 1988. (Herbal Studies). (Illus.). 1200p. 125.00 (*0-9620838-3-6*, J R Herb Pubns) Herb Studies Library.

Jeff Galloway's Training Journal. Jeff Galloway. 1998. 168p. spiral bd. 13.95 (*0-9647187-2-3*) Phidippides.

Jekyll - Hyde Syndrome: Controlling Inner Conflict Through Authentic Living. Mark R. McMinn. 1996. 116p. pap. 13.95 (*0-913342-79-3*) Barclay Pr.

Jelliffe: American Psychoanalyst & Physician. John C. Burnham. Ed. by William McGuire. 1983. LC 83-1076. (Illus.). 344p. 30.00 (*0-226-08114-1*) U Ch Pr.

Jems EMT-B Certification Preparation & Review. Daniel Mack. 2nd ed. 1995. LC 95-23166. (Illus.). 200p. (C). (gr. 13). pap. text 21.95 (*0-8151-6204-9*, 25664) Mosby Inc.

Jems Paramedic Certification Preparation & Review. Werfel. 1999. 275p. (gr. 13). pap. text 24.95 (*0-8151-8977-X*, 29166) Mosby Inc.

Jenner on Trial: An Ethical Examination of Vaccine Research in the Age of Smallpox & the Age of AIDS. Thomas A. Kerns. 1997. LC 97-1740. 116p. 49.00 (*0-7618-0718-7*); pap. 44.50 (*0-7618-0719-5*) U Pr of Amer.

Jenny Craig Cookbook: Cutting Through the Fat. Jenny Craig. 1997. (Illus.). 224p. 24.95 (*0-8487-1496-2*) Oxmoor Hse.

Jensen & Swift's Diseases of Sheep. Cleon V. Kimberling. 3rd ed. 1987. LC 87-3229. (Illus.). 394p. text 68.00 (*0-8121-1099-4*) Lppncott W & W.

Jericho Plan: Breaking down the Walls Which Prevent Post-Abortion Healing. David C. Reardon. 1996. LC 96-83667. 120p. (Orig.). pap. 8.95 (*0-9648957-5-7*) Acorn Books.

Jerusalem, 1983: Symbolic & Clinical Approaches in Theory & Practice. Luigi Zoja & Robert Hinshaw. 1995. 375p. pap. 35.00 (*3-85630-504-1*) Continuum.

Jesse E. Edwards' Synopsis of Congenital Heart Disease. Brooks S. Edwards & Jesse E. Edwards. 2000. LC 00-22743. (Illus.). 160p. 72.00 (*0-87993-453-0*) Futura Pub.

Jesus Manuscript: A Look at Healing Rays Through the Eyes of an Egyptian. Brian A. Johnson. Ed. by Brian A. Johnson. Ed. & Illus. by Glenny V. Johnson. Illus. by Kathleen A. Milner. 1995. LC 96-214595. 415p. lib. bdg. 19.95 (*0-9650204-0-1*) Neurotechtonics.

Jesus' Parables: Finding Our God Within. Robert Winterhalter. Ed. by George W. Fisk. 1994. LC 93-26774. (Jung & Spirituality Ser.). 240p. pap. 14.95 (*0-8091-3442-X*) Paulist Pr.

Jet Smarter: The Air Traveler's Rx. Diana Fairechild. l.t. ed. 1999. LC 99-94854. (Illus.). 400p. pap. 14.95 (*1-892997-49-5*) Flyana.

Jewish Answers to Medical Questions: Questions & Answers from the Medical Ethics Department of Chief Rabbi of Great Britain. Nisson E. Shulman. 1998. LC 98-5337. 40.00 (*0-7657-6016-9*) Aronson.

Jewish Healing Wisdom. Steven M. Rosman. 1997. LC 97-10003. 144p. 25.00 (*0-7657-9956-1*) Aronson.

Jewish Medical Ethics. Immanuel Jakobovits. rev. ed. 1975. LC 75-4125. 425p. pap. 18.95 (*0-8197-0100-9*); lib. bdg. 27.50 (*0-8197-0097-5*) Bloch.

Jewish Origins of the Psychoanalytic Movement. Dennis B. Klein. 1981. LC 80-27480. 198p. 62.50 (*0-275-90660-4*, C0660, Praeger Pubs) Greenwood.

Jewish Origins of the Psychoanalytic Movement: With a New Preface. Dennis B. Klein. 1985. LC 84-28083. 218p. pap. text 13.50 (*0-226-43960-7*) U Ch Pr.

Jewish Physicians: A Biographical Index. Ed. by Nathan Koren. 1973. 275p. text 39.95 (*0-87855-184-0*) Transaction Pubs.

Jewish Thought & Scientific Discovery in Early Modern Europe. David B. Ruderman. 1995. LC 94-30520. 45.00 (*0-300-06112-9*) Yale U Pr.

Jewish Values in Bioethics. Ed. by Levi Meier. 1986. 195p. 35.95 (*0-89885-299-4*, Kluwer Acad Hman Sci) Kluwer Academic.

Jewish Values in Health & Medicine. Levi Meier. 1991. 220p. (C). pap. text 30.50 (*0-8191-8174-9*); lib. bdg. 58.00 (*0-8191-8173-0*) U Pr of Amer.

Jewish Women in Therapy: Seen but Not Heard. Ed. by Rachel J. Siegel & Ellen Cole. (Women & Therapy Ser.). 122p. 1994. pap. text 10.95 (*0-918393-93-0*); 1991. text 39.95 (*1-56024-080-6*) Haworth Pr.

Jews & Medicine: Religion, Culture, Science. Natalia Berger. 1997. LC 97-26717. (Illus.). 275p. 50.00 (*0-8276-0644-3*) JPS Phila.

Jew's Body. Sander L. Gilman. 1991. (Illus.). 256p. (C). (gr. 13). pap. 25.95 (*0-415-90459-5*, A5904) Routledge.

Jews, Medicine, & Medieval Society. Joseph Shatzmiller. 1995. LC 93-2810. 241p. text 45.00 (*0-520-08059-9*) U CA Pr.

Jhala & Raju's Medical Jurisprudence. R. M. Jhala. 1988. (C). 130.00 (*0-7855-3319-2*) St Mut.

Jiaogulan - China's "Immortality Herb" Unlocking the Secret of Nature's Powerful Adaptogen & Antioxidant. Jialiu Liu & Michael Blumert. 1999. LC 98-51697. (Illus.). 80p. pap. 7.95 (*1-887089-16-0*) Torchlght Pub.

Jill Nice's Herbal Remedies & Home Comforts. Jill Nice. 1996. (Illus.). 200p. (Orig.). pap. text (*0-7499-1008-9*) Piatkus Bks GBR. *Dist:* London Brdge.

Jin Shin Acutouch Bk. 1: The Tai Chi of Healing Touch. Barbara Clark. rev. ed. 1989. (Illus.). 350p. (C). pap. text 42.00 (*0-9618179-4-1*) IPSB Pubns.

Jin Shin Acutouch Bk. 2: The Tai Chi of Healing Touch. Barbara Clark. rev. ed. 1995. (Illus.). 200p. (C). pap. text 42.00 (*0-9618179-9-2*) IPSB Pubns.

Jin Shin Acutouch - Self Help: The Tai Chi of Healing Touch. Barbara Clark. rev. ed. 1987. (Illus.). 100p. (C). pap. text 10.00 (*0-9618179-3-3*) IPSB Pubns.

Jitendra: Lost Connections. Ed. by Michael Jacobs. 1996. LC 95-51047. 160p. pap. (*0-335-19242-4*) OpUniv Pr.

Job Analysis of Speech-Language Pathology Assistants: A Study to Aid in Defining the Job of SLP Assistants. Michael Rosenfeld & Susan P. Leung. 2000. LC 00-112318. 30.00 (*1-58041-066-9*) Am Speech Lang Hearing.

Job Demands & Worker Health. Robert D. Caplan et al. 1980. 358p. (Orig.). pap. 20.00 (*0-87944-265-4*) Inst Soc Res.

Job Description Manual: ADA Workbook. 1992. 1000p. (Orig.). pap. 590.00 (*0-87258-595-6*, 088200) Am Hospital.

Job Description Manual for Medical Practices. Courtney Price & Alys Novak. 1999. 612p. pap. 125.00 (*1-56829-095-0*) M G M A.

Job Description Models for Health Care Facilities. Robert W. Haacker. 1993. 280p. stu. ed., ring bd. 54.00 (*0-929442-16-4*, 2231PP) Prof Prnting & Pub.

Job Descriptions for Healthcare, Vol. 1. Mary D. Litchford. 1997. 143p. spiral bd. 95.00 (*1-879575-67-1*) Acad Med Sys.

Job Descriptions for Nursing, Vol. 2. Mary D. Litchford. 1997. 175p. spiral bd. 95.00 (*1-879575-73-6*) Acad Med Sys.

Job Performance & Chemical Dependency: A Guide for Supervisors & Managers. Robert B. Maddux & Lynda Voorhees. Ed. by Michael G. Crisp. 1987. LC 86-73172. (Fifty-Minute Ser.). (Illus.). 79p. pap. 12.95 (*0-931961-27-0*) Crisp Pubns.

Job Stress Interventions. Ed. by Lawrence R. Murphy et al. 1995. LC 95-37647. 439p. pap. text 24.95 (*1-55798-281-3*, 431-8410) Am Psychol.

Job's Body: A Handbook for Bodywork. Dean Jahan. Ed. by George Quasha. 1991. LC 87-10076. (Illus.). 384p. (C). pap. text 28.95 (*0-88268-134-6*) Station Hill Pr.

Job's Body: A Handbook for Bodywork. Deane Juhan. 2nd rev. ed. 1998. LC 98-28525. (Illus.). 400p. pap. 34.95 (*1-58177-022-7*) Barrytown Ltd.

Job's Illness - Loss, Grief & Integration: A Psychological Interpretation. J. H. Kahn. 1986. 166p. pap. (*0-902241-17-6*) Royal Coll Psych GBR. *Dist:* Parkwest Pubns, Balogh.

Jocasta's Children. Christine Olivier. 1989. 192p. 39.95 (*0-415-01434-4*); pap. 13.95 (*0-415-01435-2*) Routledge.

Jock Doc's Body Repair Kit. Andrew Feldman. 2nd ed. 2000. LC 98-42071. (Illus.). viii, 198p. pap. 16.95 (*0-312-19905-8*) St Martin.

Joe Blanco's Survival Street Spanish for 911 Telecommunicators, Vol. 1. 2nd rev. ed. 1996. (ENG & SPA., Illus.). 52p. pap. text 29.00 (*0-9702555-0-0*) Blanco.

Jogging—Physical Health & Mental Effects & Improvements: Index of New Information with References. ABBE Research Department Staff. 1999. (Illus.). 150p. 57.50 (*0-7883-2204-4*); pap. 47.50 (*0-7883-2205-2*) ABBE Pubs Assn.

John Bowlby & Attachment Theory. Jeremy Holmes. 1993. LC 92-45842. (Makers of Modern Psychotherapy Ser.). (C). 264p. (gr. 13). pap. 29.95 (*0-415-07730-3*); 272p. text 62.95 (*0-415-07729-X*, B0880) Routledge.

John Bowly - His Early Life: A Biographical Journey into the Roots of Attachment Theory. Suzan Van Dijken. 1998. 250p. (*1-85343-392-6*) Free Assoc Bks GBR. *Dist:* Intl Spec Bk, NYU Pr.

John Call Dalton on Experimental Method: An Original Anthology. John C. Dalton. Ed. by I. Bernard Cohen. 1980. LC 79-7957. (Three Centuries of Science in America Ser.). lib. bdg. 19.95 (*0-405-12538-0*) Ayer.

John Charnley. W. Waugh. 1991. (Illus.). 268p. 69.95 (*0-387-19587-4*) Spr-Verlag.

John Charnley: The Man & the Hip. William Waugh. 1991. 268p. 58.95 (*3-540-19587-4*) Spr-Verlag.

John Dalton's Colour Vision Legacy. Ed. by Christine Dickinson et al. 1997. LC 97-139108. 784p. (*0-7484-0310-8*) Tay Francis Ltd GBR. *Dist:* Taylor & Francis.

John Gibbon & His Heart-Lung Machine. Ada Romaine-Davis. 1992. LC 91-40290. (Illus.). 278p. (C). text 39.95 (*0-8122-3073-6*) U of Pa Pr.

John Gregory & the Invention of Professional Medical Ethics & Profession of Medicine. Laurence B. McCullough. 1998. LC 97-49822. (Philosophy & Medicine Ser.). 347p. (*0-7923-4917-2*) Kluwer Academic.

John Gregory's Writings on Medical Ethics & Philosophy of Medicine. John Gregory & Laurence B. McCullough. 1998. LC 98-9425. (Philosophy & Medicine Ser.). 847p. (*0-7923-5000-6*) Kluwer Academic.

John Hall & His Patients: The Medical Practice of Shakespeare's Son-in-Law. Joan Lane. 1996. (Illus.). 416p. (*0-7509-1094-1*) Sutton Pub Ltd GBR. *Dist:* Intl Pubs Mktg.

John Hopkins University School of Medicine Curriculum for the Twenty-First Century. Catherine D. De Angelis. 1999. LC 98-41891. (Illus.). 264p. 59.95 (*0-8018-5977-8*) Johns Hopkins.

John Hughlings Jackson: Father of English Neurology. MacDonald Critchley & Eileen A. Critchley. 1998. LC 97-42711. (Illus.). 256p. text 59.50 (*0-19-512339-5*) OUP.

John Locke & Medicine. Patrick Romanell. 1984. LC 84-42846. (Illus.). 225p. 43.00 (*0-87975-250-5*) Prometheus Bks.

John McFadyean. Iain Pattison. 1990. 240p. (*0-85131-352-3*) J A Allen GBR. *Dist:* St Mut.

John Money: A Tribute. Ed. by Eli Coleman. 1991. LC 91-21841. (Journal of Psychology & Human Sexuality). (Illus.). 212p. lib. bdg. 6.95 (*1-56024-190-X*) Haworth Pr.

John P. Merrill Festschrift: Nephrological Research Papers by Past & Present Members of the Merrill School of Nephrology. Ed. by E. A. Friedman. 1978. (Nephron Ser.: Vol. 22, Nos. 1-3). (Illus.). pap. 56.75 (*3-8055-2981-3*) S Karger.

John 3:16. Stanley Barnes. 1999. 150p. pap. 8.99 (*1-84030-066-3*) Emerald House Group Inc.

John Uri Lloyd: The Great American Eclectic. Michael A. Flannery. 1998. LC 97-29242. (Illus.). 288p. 34.95 (*0-8093-2167-X*) S Ill U Pr.

Johns Hopkins Atlas of Human Functional Anatomy. Ed. by George D. Zuidema. 2nd rev. ed. 1986. LC 79-25191. (Illus.). 144p. sl. 87.00 (*0-8018-2002-2*) Johns Hopkins.

Johns Hopkins Atlas of Human Functional Anatomy. Ed. by George D. Zuidema. 4th ed. LC 97-6904. (Illus.). 184p. 1998. 49.95 (*0-8018-5651-5*); 1997. pap. text 22.95 (*0-8018-5652-3*) Johns Hopkins.

Johns Hopkins Cardiac Surgical Manual. William S. Baumgartner et al. 1994. (Illus.). 560p. (C). (gr. 13). spiral bd. 54.95 (*0-8016-2248-4*, 02248) Mosby Inc.

Johns Hopkins Children's Health Reference. Johns Hopkin. 704p. 35.00 (*0-06-270202-5*, Harper Ref) HarperCollins Pubs.

Johns Hopkins Complete Guide to Preventing & Reversing Heart Disease. Peter O. Kwiterovich, Jr. 1998. LC 92-39918. (Illus.). 416p. pap. 16.95 (*0-7615-1447-3*, Prima Health) Prima Pub.

Johns Hopkins Complete Home Encyclopedia of Drugs: Developed Especially for People over 50. Simeon Margolis. 2000. LC 00-28044. (Illus.). 831p. pap. (*0-929661-59-1*); 1999. LC 98-20364. 768p. 39.95 (*0-929661-43-5*) Rebus.

***Johns Hopkins Consumer Guide to Drugs & Supplements.** Johns Hopkins Hospital Staff. 2002. LC 2001-48754. (Illus.). 39.95 (*0-929661-66-4*) Rebus.

***Johns Hopkins Consumer Guide to Medical Tests: What You Can Expect, How You Should Prepare, What Your Results Mean.** Simeon Margolis & Johns Hopkins Medical School Faculty Staff. 2001. LC 2001-19980. (Illus.). 432p. 39.95 (*0-929661-63-X*) Rebus.

Johns Hopkins Family Health Book: The Essential Home Medical Reference To Help You And Your Family Promote Good Health And Manage Illnessl. Johns Hopkin. 1998. LC 98-38133. (Illus.). 1680p. 49.95 (*0-06-270149-5*, Harper Ref) HarperCollins Pubs.

Johns Hopkins Guide to Diabetes: For Today & Tomorrow. Christopher D. Saudek et al. (Health Bks.). (Illus.). 1997. LC 96-49161. 440p. 45.00 (*0-8018-5580-2*); 1997. LC 96-49161. 440p. pap. 16.95 (*0-8018-5581-0*); 2001. LC 00-54964. 696p. pap. 21.50 (*0-8018-6657-X*) Johns Hopkins.

Johns Hopkins Handbook of in Vitro Fertilization & Assisted Reproductive Technologies. Marian D. Damewood. 1990. 42.95 (*0-316-17194-8*, Little Brwn Med Div) Lppncott W & W.

Johns Hopkins Hospital 2000 Guide to Medical Care of Patients with Hiv Infection. John G. Bartlett. 9th ed. 2000. 254p. pap. text 19.95 (*0-7817-2342-6*) Lppncott W & W.

Johns Hopkins Hospital Guide to Medical Care of Patients with HIV Infection. John G. Bartlett. 4th ed. 1993. LC 93-41024. 10.00 (*0-683-00448-4*); 5th ed. 1995. LC 95-10374. 13.95 (*0-683-00449-2*) Lppncott W & W.

Johns Hopkins Manual of Gynecology & Obstetrics. Johns Hopkins University Department of Gynecology Staff & Edward E. Wallach. 1997. 480p. spiral bd. 39.95 (*0-316-46720-0*) Lppncott W & W.

Johns Hopkins Manual of Gynecology & Obstetrics. Ed. by Nicholas C. Lambrou et al. 1999. LC 98-47453. 453p. (*0-7817-1890-2*) Lppncott W & W.

Johns Hopkins Manual of Oncology Nursing. Brenda Shelton & Johns Hopkins Oncology Unit Nurses Staff. 1998. 400p. spiral bd. (*0-316-97168-5*) Lppncott W & W.

Johns Hopkins Medical Handbook. Johns Hopkins Medical Institutions. 1992. 39.95 (*0-679-41806-7*) Random.

Johns Hopkins Medical Handbook: The 100 Major Medical Disorders of People over the Age of 50 : Plus a Directory to the Leading Teaching Hospitals, Research Organizations, Treatment Centers, & Support Groups. Simeon Margolis. 1999. LC 99-14516. 652p. (*0-929661-51-6*) Rebus.

Johns Hopkins Medical Handbook: The 100 Major Medical Disorders of People over the Age of 50: Plus a Directory to the Leading Teaching Hospitals, Research Organizations, Treatment Centers & Support Groups. Simeon Margolis. 1999. LC 99-14516. 652p. (*0-929661-54-0*) Rebus.

Johns Hopkins Medical Handbook & Directory: The 100 Major Medical Disorders of People over the Age of 50. Illus. by Johns Hopkins University Staff. 1992. LC 92-15420. 638p. 39.95 (*0-929661-04-4*) Random.

Johns Hopkins Medical Handbook & Directory: The 100 Major Medical Disorders of People over the Age of 50. Ed. by Johns Hopkins Medical Institutions Staff et al. rev. ed. 1996. LC 95-24371. (Illus.). 640p. 39.95 (*0-929661-32-X*) Random.

Johns Hopkins Symptoms & Remedies: The Complete Home Medical Reference. Johns Hopkins Medical Letter Health after 50 Edito. 1995. (Illus.). 830p. 39.95 (*0-929661-19-2*) Random.

Johns Hopkins University Psychology Laboratories: Studies. Ed. by George M. Stanton. 1969. (Psychology Monographs General & Applied: Vol. 10). reprint ed. pap. 55.00 (*0-8115-1409-9*) Periodicals Srv.

Johns Hopkins Women's Health Reference. Johns Hopkin. 2000. 704p. 35.00 (*0-06-270200-9*, Harper Ref) HarperCollins Pubs.

Johnson & Johnson First Aid Book. Stephen N. Rosenberg. 1985. 176p. (Orig.). mass mkt. 16.95 (*0-446-38252-3*) Warner Bks.

Johnson & Kennedy Radiographic Skeletal Anatomy. Glenda J. Bryan. 2nd ed. 1992. LC 82-12971. (Illus.). 302p. text (*0-443-01627-5*) Church.

Johnson's Emotional First Aid: How to Increase Your Happiness, Peace & Joy. Victoria A. Johnson. 1997. LC 96-92765. (Illus.). 72p. pap. 15.95 (*1-57733-015-3*) B Dolphin Pub.

Johnston's Essays on the Physiological & Psychological Characteristics of the Homeopathic Materi Medica-Sepia. Linda Johnston. 1995. 164p. (Orig.). (C). pap. 20.00 (*1-877691-25-9*) C Kent Agency.

***Joint & Soft Tissue Injection.** Trevor Silver. 3rd exp. ed. 2001. 128p. pap. (*1-85775-564-2*) Radcliffe Med Pr GBR. *Dist:* Balogh.

Joint & Soft Tissue Injection: Injecting with Confidence. Trevor Silver. 1996. LC 95-50013. 90p. pap. (*1-85775-143-4*) Radcliffe Med Pr GBR. *Dist:* Balogh.

Joint Arthroplasty. Ed. by Shinichi Imura et al. 1999. LC 98-46409. (Illus.). 448p. 179.00 (*4-431-70241-5*) Spr-Verlag.

Joint Attention: Its Origin & Role in Development. Ed. by Chris Moore & Philip Dunham. 1995. LC 94-40160. 296p. text 59.95 (*0-8058-1437-X*) L Erlbaum Assocs.

Joint Cartilage Degradation: Basic & Clinical Aspects. J. F. Woessmer, Jr. & D. S. Howell. 1992. (Infectious Disease & Therapy Ser.: Vol. 12). (Illus.). 576p. text 215.00 (*0-8247-8768-4*) Dekker.

Joint Destruction in Arthritis & Osteoporosis. Ed. by W. B. Van den Berg et al. 1993. ix, 276p. 71.50 (*0-8176-2773-1*); pap. (*3-7643-2773-1*) Birkhauser.

Joint Disease in the Horse. C. Wayne McIlwraith & Gayle W. Trotter. Ed. by Sandra Valkhoff. 1996. 416p. text 132.00 (*0-7216-5135-6*) Saunders.

Joint FAO/WHO Expert Committee on Meat Hygiene. 1962. (Technical Report Ser.: No. 241). 82p. pap. text 5.00 (*92-4-120241-6*) World Health.

Joint FAO/WHO Expert Committee on Nutrition. 1962. (Technical Report Ser.: No. 245). 65p. pap. text 5.00 (*92-4-120245-9*) World Health.

Joint ILO/WHO Committee on Occupational Health: Fifth Report. 1967. (Technical Report Ser.: No. 354). 19p. pap. text 3.00 (*92-4-120354-4*, 1100354) World Health.

Joint ILO/WHO Committee on the Hygiene of Seafarers. 1961. (Technical Report Ser.: No. 224). 14p. pap. text 3.00 (*92-4-120224-6*) World Health.

***Joint Motion: Clinical Measurement & Evaluation.** Roger W. Soames. 2001. (Illus.). 155p. pap. (*0-443-05808-3*) Church GBR. *Dist:* Saunders.

Joint Motion, Method of Measuring & Recording. American Academy of Orthopaedic Surgeons Staff. 1976. (Illus.). 88p. (Orig.). pap. text (*0-443-00270-3*) Church.

Joint OIE-IABS Symposium on Clostridial Products in Veterinary Medicine. Ed. by R. H. Regamey et al. 1976. (Developments in Biological Standardization Ser.: Vol. 32). 61.00 (*3-8055-2435-8*) S Karger.

Joint Pain: Diagnosis & Treatment Using Manipulative Techniques. John M. Mennell. 1964. 178p. 44.95 (*0-316-56668-3*, Little Brwn Med Div) Lppncott W & W.

Joint Pain Prescription. James M. Rippe. 2001. LC 2001-417. (Illus.). xi, 195p. 22.95 (*1-57954-456-8*) Rodale Pr Inc.

Joint Preserving Procedures of the Lower Extremities. Ed. by U. H. Weil. 1980. (Progress in Orthopedic Surgery Ser.: Vol. 4). (Illus.). 121p. 58.95 (*0-387-09856-9*) Spr-Verlag.

Joint Replacement Arthroplasty see Reconstructive Surgery of the Joints

Joint Replacement Arthroplasty. Ed. by Bernard F. Morrey. 1991. (Illus.). 1252p. text (*0-443-08725-3*) Church.

Joint Replacement in the Shoulder & Elbow. W. Angus Wallace. 1998. LC 97-30915. (Illus.). 176p. (*0-7506-1367-X*) E A GBR. *Dist:* OUP.

Joint Stiffness of the Upper Limb. Stephen A. Copeland et al. 9th ed. 1997. 400p. (*1-85317-414-9*) Martin Dunitz GBR. *Dist:* Mosby Inc.

Joint Structure & Function: A Comprehensive Analysis. Pamela K. Levangle & Cynthia C. Norkin. 3rd rev. ed. 2000. LC 00-60203. (Illus.). 495p. pap. text 45.95 (*0-8036-0710-5*) Davis Co.

Joint Surgery up to Date. Ed. by Kazushi Hirohata et al. 1990. (Illus.). 137p. 95.00 (*0-387-70048-X*) Spr-Verlag.

Joints & Bones of Humans-Afflictions, Conditions & Treatments: Index of New Information. Sylvester L. Catz. Date not set. 160p. 57.50 (*0-7883-1936-1*); pap. 47.50 (*0-7883-1937-X*) ABBE Pubs Assn.

Joints & Glands Exercises: As Taught by Sri Swami Rama of the Himalayas. Himalayan International Institute Staff. Ed. by Rudolph M. Ballentine. 2nd ed. 1982. (Illus.). 90p. spiral bd. 8.95 (*0-89389-083-9*) Himalayan Inst.

Joints of Pain: Living My Life with Rheumatoid Arthritis. Laura Pietro. 2000. 101p. pap. (*0-9704186-0-4*) L Pietro.

Jokes: Their Purpose & Meaning. Herbert S. Strean. 1994. LC 93-17050. 240p. 40.00 (*1-56821-070-1*) Aronson.

Jolla Cancer Research Foundation: The Miracle on Torrey Pines Mesa. W. J. Mcgill. 1995. LC 95-81189. (Illus.). 224p. (*0-9647206-0-4*) La Jolla Cancer Res.

Jon Lilypond: The Story of a Unique Person. Kitty Kurti. 1981. (Illus.). 206p. text 25.00 (*0-935886-00-1*, TXU 28-589) East & West Pubns.

Jonah: The Anatomy of the Soul. Stephen Goldberg. 1990. 96p. (Orig.). 9.95 (*0-940780-12-7*) MedMaster.

Jonas & Kovner's Healthcare Delivery in the U.S. Ed. by Anthony R. Kovner & Steven Jonas. 6th ed. 1998. LC 98-27316. pap. 34.95 (*0-8261-2082-2*); (Illus.). 600p. 56.95 (*0-8261-2083-0*) Springer Pub.

Jones' Clinical Paediatric Surgery. J. M. Hutson. 4th ed. 1992. (Illus.). 312p. pap. 70.00 (*0-86793-169-8*) Blackwell Sci.

Jones Strain-Counterstrain. Lawrence H. Jones et al. 1995. (Illus.). text 54.95 (*0-9645135-2-8*); pap. text, spiral bd. 39.95 (*0-9645135-4-4*) Jones Strain.

Jones's Animal Nursing. Bruce V. Jones & British Small Animal Veterinary Association Staff. Ed. by R. S. Pinniger. 2nd ed. 1976. LC 75-43703. (Pergamon International Library of Science, Technology, Engineering, & Social Studies). xviii, 496 p. (*0-08-020596-8*) Elsevier.

Jones's Animal Nursing. Bruce V. Jones. Ed. by D. R. Lane. (Illus.). 3rd ed. 1980. text 74.00 (*0-08-024945-0*); 3rd ed. 1980. pap. text 40.00 (*0-08-024944-2*); 4th ed. 1985. 620p. text 100.00 (*0-08-031982-3*); 4th ed. 1985. 620p. pap. text 51.00 (*0-08-031983-1*); 5th ed. 1989. 800p. pap. text 50.00 (*0-08-036157-9*, 0901; 0902; 0904) Elsevier (Pergamon Pr).

Jong's Community Dental Health. Morganstein Gluck. 4th ed. 1997. LC 97-9706. (Illus.). 400p. (C). (gr. 13). pap. text 41.00 (*0-8151-3488-6*, 27880) Mosby Inc.

Jordi - Lisa & David. Theodore I. Rubin. 18.95 (*0-89190-588-X*) Amereon Ltd.

Joseph Warren: Physician, Politician, Patriot. John Cary. 1986. (Illus.). 260p. lib. bdg. 69.50 (*0-313-25271-8*, CAJO, Greenwood Pr) Greenwood.

Joslin Diabetes Manual. Leo P. Krall & Richard Beaser. 12th ed. 1989. LC 88-6852. (Illus.). 437p. pap. text 19.95 (*0-8121-1120-6*) Lppncott W & W.

Joslin Guide to Diabetes: A Program for Managing Your Treatment. Richard S. Beaser et al. 1995. LC 95-12169. 352p. per. 15.00 (*0-684-80208-2*) S&S Trade Pap.

Joslin Guide to Diabetes Care. Joslin Diabetes Center Staff. 1994. pap. 14.00 (*0-671-79862-6*, Fireside) S&S Trade Pap.

Joslin's Diabetes Mellitus. C. Ronald Kahn & Gordon C. Weir. 13th ed. 1994. (Illus.). 1,068p. text 179.00 (*0-8121-1531-7*) Lppncott W & W.

Journal for the Psychoanalysis of Culture & Society Vol. 1-2: JPCS. Ed. by Mark Bracher. 1996. 170p. (C). pap. 14.00 (*1-883831-05-9*) Critical Pr.

Journal of Ambulatory Care Management Series, Set. Seth B. Goldsmith. 1994. pap. 166.00 (*0-8342-0669-2*) Aspen Pub.

Journal of Behavioral Economics: Winter 1985-Spring 1986 Symposium, Vol. XIV. Ed. by Richard E. Hattwick & Roger S. Frantz. 1986. 220p. pap. 8.00 (*0-931497-26-4*) WIU CBER.

Journal of Consulting & Clinical Psychology. Special Issue: Behavioral Medicine. Ed. by Edward B. Blanchard. 1992. 156p. pap. 16.00 (*1-55798-179-5*) Am Psychol.

Journal of Growth: A Workbook. Dee Frances. Ed. by Harry Koster. 1993. 258p. (Orig.). pap., wbk. ed. 9.95 (*0-9635341-5-7*) DDDD Pubns.

***Journal of Healthcare Information Management**, Vol. 15, No. 1. Julie Foreman. 2001. pap. 28.00 (*0-7879-5751-8*) Jossey-Bass.

***Journal of Healthcare Information Management, 2000**, Vol. 14, No. 4. Healthcare Information Management Staff. pap. 26.00 (*0-7879-5454-3*) Jossey-Bass.

Journal of Holistic Health, Vol. VI. Anastas Harris. 1981. (Illus.). 144p. pap. 12.00 (*0-939410-07-9*) Mandala Holistic.

Journal of Holistic Health, Vol. VII. Ed. by Alice DeBolt & Shelby Shapiro. 1982. (Illus.). 120p. pap. 12.00 (*0-939410-10-9*) Mandala Holistic.

Journal of Holistic Health, Vol. VIII. Ed. by Alice DeBolt & Shalby Shapiro. 1983. (*0-939410-12-5*) Mandala Holistic.

Journal of Holistic Health, Vol. IX. Shelby Shapiro. Ed. by Alice De Bolt. 1984. LC 78-59776. (Illus.). 144p. pap. 12.00 (*0-939410-13-3*) Mandala Holistic.

Journal of William Tully: Medical Student at Dartmouth, 1808-1809. Ed. by Oliver S. Hayward & Elizabeth Thomson. 1977. (Illus.). 17.50 (*0-88202-175-3*) Watson Pub Intl.

Journals of William A. Lindsay: An Ordinary Nineteenth-Century Physician's Surgical Cases. William A. Lindsay. Ed. by Katherine M. McDonell. 1989. LC 88-32003. (Illus.). xlix, 216p. 27.50 (*0-87195-029-4*) Ind Hist Soc.

Journey. Joseph B. Strauss. 1992. 236p. (Orig.). pap. 5.95 (*1-890419-04-4*) Fnd Chiropractic Educ.

Journey: A Breast Cancer Survival Guide. Allie F. Sawyer & Norma S. Jones. Ed. by Kathryn Hall. 1992. LC 92-62274. (Illus.). 192p. (Orig.). pap. 16.95 (*1-56664-012-1*) WorldComm.

Journey: Signposts from the Healing Road. Peter Reese. 1995. pap. 12.00 (*0-9629302-4-5*) Ramsey Found.

Journey Across the Life Span: Human Development & Health Promotion. Elaine Polan et al. 1997. LC 97-39790. (Illus.). 287p. (C). pap. text 21.95 (*0-8036-0196-4*) Davis Co.

Journey Across the Lifespan: Human Development & Health Promotion. Elaine Polan & Daphne C. Taylor. 1998. 287p. tchr. ed. 21.95 (*0-8036-0212-X*) Davis Co.

Journey Beyond Breast Cancer: From the Personal to the Political Taking an Active Role in Prevention, Diagnosis, & Your Own Healing. Virginia M. Soffa. 1994. (Illus.). 272p. pap. 14.95 (*0-89281-448-9*, Heal Arts VT) Inner Tradit.

Journey Beyond Trauma. John Petellat. Ed. by Joseph Jaeger. 1995. LC 95-61474. 133p. pap. 12.95 (*1-880254-24-7*) Vista.

Journey from Cognition to Brain to Gene: Perspectives from Williams Syndrome. Ed. by Ursula Bellugi & Marie E. St. George. 2001. LC 00-54892. (Illus.). 150p. pap. 25.00 (*0-262-52312-4*) MIT Pr.

Journey into Awareness: A Parent's Perspective on Children's Mental Health in Today's Society. Fred G. Beardsley, III. 1998. (Illus.). viii, 203p. pap. 12.50 (*0-9664485-0-2*) Bridgtte Rose.

Journey into Day: Meditations for New Cancer Patients. Rusty Freeman. 2000. LC 99-47478. 176p. pap. 13.00 (*0-8170-1350-4*) Judson.

Journey of Native American People with Serious Mental Illness: First National Conference. Ed. by A. Marie Sanchez & Frank D. McGuirk. 1996. (Illus.). 137p. (Orig.). (C). pap. text 35.00 (*0-7881-2826-4*) DIANE Pub.

Journey Through a Bypass: The Story of an Open Heart. David L. McKenna. 1998. 93p. pap. 5.99 (*0-89367-230-0*) Light & Life Comm.

Journey Through Brain Trauma: A Mother's Story of Her Daughter's Recovery. Louise R. Morningstar. 1998. LC 98-11005. 208p. pap. text 12.95 (*0-87833-988-4*) Taylor Pub.

***Journey Through Cancer: An Oncologist's Seven-Level Program for Healing & Transforming the Whole Person.** Jeremy Geffen. 2001. 304p. pap. 14.00 (*0-609-80704-8*, Three Riv Pr) Harmony Bks.

Journey Through Grief. Elizabeth B. Farnsworth. 1988. LC 88-818. 96p. (Orig.). pap. 8.95 (*0-932419-18-6*) Cherokee.

Journey Through Illness & Beyond. Brenda S. Lukeman & Noah T. Lukeman. 1995. LC 94-66317. 160p. (C). pap. 9.95 (*0-9641416-0-4*); 14.95 (*0-9641416-1-2*) Steppstone Pr.

Journey Through Suffering: How to Find Your Oasis in the Desert of Stress, Pain & Illness. Jim Hughes. 1995. (Illus.). pap. 14.95 (*0-9644616-7-6*) Whole Hlth Bks.

Journey to Brotherhood: Awakening, Healing & Connecting Men's Hearts. Frank Cardelle. 1991. 308p. 21.95 (*0-89876-153-0*) Gardner Pr.

Journey to Justice: A Woman's True Story of Breast Cancer & Medical Malpractice. Diane C. Chechik. Ed. by Eleanor S. Anderson. 2nd ed. 2000. LC 88-71206. (Illus.). 168p. (C). pap. 12.95 (*0-9620549-0-9*) Catalyst FL.

Journey to Recovery: A Complete Guide to Cancer Chemotherapy. Margot Fromer. 2000. 252p. pap. 12.95 (*1-58062-446-4*) Adams Media.

Journey to Well: Learning to Live after Spinal Cord Injury. Margie Williams. 1997. LC 96-95332. (Illus.). 252p. (Orig.). pap. 15.95 (*0-9655558-2-8*) Altarfire Pub.

Journey to Wholeness: And the Day Came When the Risk to Remain Tight in a Bud Was More Painful Than the Risk It Took to Bloom. Barbara M. Brewster. 1992. 256p. pap. text 14.95 (*0-9628608-1-6*) Four Winds OR.

Journey Toward Complete Recovery: Reclaiming Our Emotional, Spiritual & Sexual Wholeness. Michael Picucci. 1998. LC 98-7069. 244p. pap. 16.95 (*1-55643-286-0*) North Atlantic.

Journey with Grandpa: Our Family's Struggle with Alzheimer's Disease. Frwd. by Rosalie W. Honel & Peter V. Rabins. 1988. LC 88-45415. 224p. 22.95 (*0-8018-3721-9*) Johns Hopkins.

Journey Within: A Spiritual Path to Recovery. Ruth Fishel. 1987. LC 87-180. 180p. pap. 8.95 (*0-932194-41-9*) Health Comm.

Journeys Home I: Coming to Home Birth. Regina Adams & Blair Adams. 1989. LC 89-50807. 299p. (Orig.). pap. 9.95 (*0-916387-17-8*) Truth Forum.

Journeys into Cross-Cultural Psychology. Ed. by A. Bouvy et al. 1994. LC 95-119989. vi, 406p. pap. (*90-265-1403-4*) Swets.

Journeys Through Hell: Stories of Burn Survivors' Reconstruction of Self & Identity. Dennis J. Stouffer. 1994. 280p. (C). 86.50 (*0-8476-7891-1*); LC 93-8826. pap. 28.95 (*0-8476-7892-X*) Rowman.

Journeys with the Cancer Conqueror: Mobilizing Mind & Spirit. Greg Anderson. 1999. LC 99-22165. 240p. 14.95 (*0-7407-0020-0*) Andrews McMeel.

Joy-Full Holistic Remedies: How to Experience Your Natural Ability to Heal. 1999. LC 98-94200. (Illus.). 120p. pap. 12.95 (*0-9668742-0-X*) Joy-Full Pubng.

Joy, Inspiration, & Hope. Verena Kast. Tr. by Douglas Whitcher from GER. 1991. LC 90-47362. (Carolyn & Ernest Fay Series in Analytical Psychology: No. 1). 192p. 18.95 (*0-89096-470-X*) Tex A&M Univ Pr.

Joy of Breastfeeding. Linda McDonald. 1978. LC 77-18536. (Illus.). pap. 8.95 (*0-916198-07-3*) Oaklawn Pr.

Joy of Health: A Doctor's Guide to Nutrition & Alternative Medicine. Zoltan P. Rona. 2nd ed. 1999. LC 92-34054. (Illus.). 280p. pap. 12.95 (*0-87542-684-0*) Llewellyn Pubns.

Joy of Health: A Spiritual Concept of Integration & the Practicalities of Living. Kathy Oddenino. 1989. 300p. (Orig.). pap. 14.95 (*0-923081-00-3*) Joy Pubns MD.

Joy of Health & Fitness: A Scientific & Common Sense Approach to Healthy Life Style. Harbans S. Sraon. 1998. (Health & Fitness Ser.: Vol. 1). 95p. (YA). (gr. 10-12). pap. 14.99 (*0-9666861-0-1*) Mandil Pub Co.

Joy of Healthy Skin: A Lifetime Guide to Beautiful, Problem-Free Skin. Lynn Parentini. 1995. LC 95-37691. 38468p. text 24.95 (*0-13-127267-5*) P-H.

Joy of Natural Childbirth: Fifth Edition of Natural Childbirth & the Christian Family. Helen Wessel. 5th exp. rev. ed. 1994. LC 91-73769. Orig. Title: Natural Childbirth & the Christian Family. (Illus.). 363p. pap. 15.95 (*0-933082-20-7*) Bookmates Intl.

Joy of Solo Sex. Harold Litten. 3rd ed. 1993. Orig. Title: Solo Sex: Advanced Techniques. 193p. reprint ed. pap. 12.95 (*0-9626531-4-4*) Factor Pr.

Joy of Stress. Peter Hanson. 1987. (Illus.). 304p. pap. 10.95 (*0-8362-2412-4*) Andrews McMeel.

Joy of Suffering: The Psychoanalytic Theory & Therapy of Masochism. Shirley Panken. 1973. LC 73-96532. 256p. 35.00 (*0-87668-065-1*) Aronson.

Joy of Uncircumcising! Jim Bigelow. 2nd ed. 1998. (Illus.). 240p. (Orig.). pap. 19.95 (*0-934061-22-X*) Marketscope Bks.

Joy of Walking. Jack Scagnetti. 1979. 3.00 (*0-87980-370-3*) Wilshire.

Joy of Weight Loss: A Spiritual Guide to Easy Fitness. Norris J. Chumley. 2001. LC 00-66320. 192p. pap. 15.00 (*1-930051-19-0*) Lantern Books.

JST Caring: Nurses, Women, & Ethics. Helga Kuhse. 1997. LC 96-30173. 288p. pap. text 25.95 (*0-631-20211-0*); (C). text 60.95 (*0-631-20210-2*) Blackwell Pubs.

Jubilee Issue. Ed. by Richard F. Thompson. 1986. (Special Issue, Behavioral Neuroscience Ser.: Vol. 100, No. 6). 107p. pap. 16.00 (*0-912704-96-9*) Am Psychol.

Judaism & Psychoanalysis. M. Ostow. 1997. 320p. pap. (*1-85575-180-1*) Karnac Bks GBR. *Dist:* Other Pr LLC.

Judaism, Medicine & Healing. Ronald H. Isaacs. 1998. LC 97-33198. 208p. 30.00 (*0-7657-9997-9*) Aronson.

Judaism Without Christianity: An Introduction to the System of the Mishnah. Jacob Neusner. 1990. pap. 19.95 (*0-88125-333-2*) Ktav.

Jude's Herbal Home Remedies: Natural Health, Beauty & Home-Care Secrets. Jude C. Williams. 1999. LC 92-58. (Living with Nature Ser.). (Illus.). 320p. pap. 12.95 (*0-87542-869-X*) Llewellyn Pubns.

Judgement & Choice. Robin M. Hogarth. 2nd ed. 1987. LC 86-32481. 324p. 330.00 (*0-471-91479-7*) Wiley.

Judging Medicine. George J. Annas. 1988. LC 88-9024. (Contemporary Issues in Biomedicine, Ethics & Society Ser.). 456p. 59.50 (*0-89603-132-2*); pap. 39.50 (*0-89603-193-4*) Humana.

Judith's Pavilion: The Haunting Memories of a Neurosurgeon. Marc Flitter. 1997. LC 96-53575. 221p. 24.00 (*1-883642-31-0*) Steerforth Pr.

Judith's Pavilion: The Haunting Memories of a Neurosurgeon. Marc Flitter. 1998. LC 97-42587. 221p. pap. (*0-446-67472-9*) Warner.

Jugend in Ihrer Freizeit. Ed. by R. Schmitz-Scherzer. 1978. (Psychologische Praxis Ser.: Vol. 52). (GER., Illus.). 16.75 (*3-8055-2859-0*) S Karger.

Jukes: A Study in Crime, Pauperism, Disease, & Heredity. Richard L. Dugdale. 1973. LC 74-112542. (Rise of Urban America Ser.). (Illus.). reprint ed. 19.95 (*0-405-02451-7*) Ayer.

Julia's Mother: Life Lessons in the Pediatric ER. William Bonadio. 2001. 192p. reprint ed. pap. 11.95 (*0-312-27735-0*, St Martin Griffin) St Martin.

Jumbo Human Body Yearbook: Grade 5. Diana Van Camp. (Jumbo Human Body Ser.). 96p. (gr. 5). 15.95 (*0-8209-0070-2*, B JHBY 5) ESP.

Jumbo Human Body Yearbook: Grade 6. Diana Van Camp. (Jumbo Human Body Ser.). 96p. (gr. 6). 15.95 (*0-8209-0071-0*, B JHBY 6) ESP.

Jumbo Human Body Yearbook: Grade 7. Diana Van Camp. (Jumbo Human Body Ser.). 96p. (gr. 7). 15.95 (*0-8209-0072-9*, B JHBY 7) ESP.

Jumbo Nutrition Yearbook: Grade 3. Marilyn VanCamp. (Jumbo Nutrition Ser.). 96p. (gr. 3). 15.95 (*0-8209-0042-7*, B JNY 3) ESP.

Jumbo Nutrition Yearbook: Grade 4. Marilyn Hayes. (Jumbo Nutrition Ser.). 96p. (gr. 4). 15.95 (*0-8209-0043-5*, B JNY 4) ESP.

Jumbo Nutrition Yearbook: Grade 5. Marilyn Hayes. (Jumbo Nutrition Ser.). 96p. (gr. 5). 15.95 (*0-8209-0044-3*, B JNY 5) ESP.

Jung & Reich: The Body As Shadow. John P. Conger. 1988. (Orig.). 222p. 25.00 (*1-55643-038-8*); 224p. pap. 12.95 (*1-55643-037-X*) North Atlantic.

Jung & Searles: A Comparative Study. David Sedgwick. 1993. LC 93-3266. 192p. (C). 78.95 (*0-415-09698-7*, B0861) Routledge.

Jung & Tarot: An Archetypal Journey. Sallie Nichols. 1984. LC 80-53118. (Illus.). 416p. reprint ed. pap. 16.95 (*0-87728-515-2*) Red Wheel ME.

Jung & the East: A Dialogue with the Orient. John J. Clarke. 1994. LC 93-8078. 224p. (C). 78.95 (*0-415-07640-4*); (gr. 13). pap. 27.95 (*0-415-10419-X*) Routledge.

Jung & the Jungians on Myth: An Introduction. Steven F. Walker. 1994. LC 94-15753. (Theorists of Myth Ser.: Vol. 4). 216p. text 39.00 (*0-8240-3443-0*, H1163) Garland.

Jung & the Monotheisms: Judaism, Christianity, & Islam. Ed. by Joel Ryce-Menuhin. 1994. LC 93-8077. 288p. (C). pap. 31.95 (*0-415-10414-9*) Routledge.

Jung Cult. Richard Noll. 1997. LC 97-9823. 384p. per. 14.00 (*0-684-83423-5*) S&S Trade.

Jung Cult: Origins of a Charismatic Movement. Richard Noll. 1994. LC 94-4831. 408p. 49.50 (*0-691-03724-8*) Princeton U Pr.

Jung in Context: Modernity & the Making of a Psychology. Peter Homans. 2nd ed. 1995. 288p. pap. text 16.00 (*0-226-35112-2*) U Ch Pr.

Jungian Analysis. Ed. by Murray Stein. 2nd ed. 1995. LC 94-46180. (Reality of the Psyche Ser.). (Illus.). 474p. pap. 23.95 (*0-8126-9291-8*) Open Court.

Jungian Birth Charts. Arthur Dione. 1987. (Illus.). 256p. (Orig.). pap. (*0-85030-642-6*) Aqrn Pr GBR. *Dist:* HarperCollins Pubs.

Jungian Child Psychotherapy: Individuation in Childhood. Ed. by M. Davies & Mara Sidoli. 1988. 304p. pap. (*0-946439-47-8*) Karnac Bks GBR. *Dist:* Other Pr LLC.

Jungian Dreambook. Glenda G. Thomson-Daniel & Gabriel Thomson. Ed. by Yvonne McCall. 1997. LC 97-66528. (Illus.). 185p. (Orig.). (C). 20.00 (*1-887003-59-2*) Dancng Jester.

Jungian Literary Criticism, 1920-1980. Jos Van Meurs. 1991. LC 90-38018. pap. 18.95 (*0-938434-84-5*) Sigo Pr.

Jungian Perspectives on Clinical Supervision. Ed. by Paul Kugler. 1996. LC 82-14076. 208p. (Orig.). (C). pap. 25.00 (3-85630-552-1) Continuum.

Jungian Psychiatry. Heinz K. Fierz. 1995. 450p. pap. 19.95 (3-85630-521-1) Continuum.

Jungian Psychology after Jung. Mary-Ann Mattoon. 1994. LC 93-45880. 64p. (Orig.). pap. 7.95 (1-882275-03-9) Rnd Table Pr.

Jungian Psychology in Perspective. Mary-Ann Mattoon. 1985. 352p. pap. 18.95 (0-02-920650-2) Free Pr.

Jungian Thought in the Modern World. Ed. by Elphis Christopher & Hester Solomon. 1999. LC 00-269521. (Illus.). xxvi, 277p. (1-85343-466-3); pap. (1-85343-467-1) Free Assoc Bks GBR. *Dist:* Intl Spec Bk.

Jungians: A Comparative & Historical Perspective. Thomas B. Kirsch. 2000. 304p. 49.95 (0-415-15860-5) Routledge.

Jungle of the Mind. Edgar J. Swift. 1977. LC 70-134140. (Essay Index Reprint Ser.). reprint ed. 25.95 (0-8369-2334-0) Ayer.

Jung's Advice to the Players: A Jungian Reading of Shakespeare's Problem Plays, Vol. 57. Sally F. Porterfield. 1994. LC 94-5150. (Contributions in Drama & Theatre Studies Ser.: No. 57). 136p. 52.50 (0-313-29305-8, Greenwood Pr) Greenwood.

Jung's Map of the Soul: An Introduction. Murray Stein. 1998. LC 97-51485. 192p. pap. 18.95 (0-8126-9376-0) Open Court.

Jung's Quest for Wholeness: A Religious & Historical Perspective. Curtis D. Smith. 1990. LC 89-11313. 169p. (C). pap. text 22.95 (0-7914-0238-X) State U NY Pr.

Jung's Seminar on Nietzsche's Zarathustra, Vol. 99. Carl Gustav Jung. Ed. & Abr. by James L. Jarrett. abr. ed. 1997. LC 97-23727. (Bollingen XLV Ser.: Vol. 99). xxviii, 393p. pap. 21.95 (0-691-01738-7) Princeton U Pr.

Jung's Struggle with Freud. George Hogenson. rev. ed. 1994. LC 93-39285. 192p. pap. 5.95 (0-933029-81-0) Chiron Pubns.

Junior Bacteriologist. Jack Rudman. 1994. (Career Examination Ser.: C-392). pap. 27.95 (0-8373-0392-3) Nat Learn.

Junior Hospital Administrator. Jack Rudman. 1994. (Career Examination Ser.: C-400). pap. 29.95 (0-8373-0400-8) Nat Learn.

Junk Food Diet. Judith Wills. 1990. mass mkt. 3.95 (0-312-92182-9) St Martin.

Juran Prescription: Clinical Quality Management. Kathleen J. Goonan. 1995. LC 94-46126. (Jossey-Bass Health Ser.). 229p. 45.00 (0-7879-0096-6) Jossey-Bass.

Jurisdiction Competition Between Obstetricians & Nurse Midwives in Washington, Vol. O7. Phyllis A. Langton. 1991. 4.00 (1-888028-20-3) GWU Ctr WAS.

Jurisprudence, AIDS, HIV & Truth Disclosures: Index of New Information with Authors & Subjects. Science and Life Consultants Association Staff. 1992. LC 92-54225. 180p. 47.50 (1-55914-600-1); pap. 44.50 (1-55914-601-X) ABBE Pubs Assn.

Jurisprudence & Child Abuse Prevention: Index of New Information with Authors & Subjects. Science and Life Consultants Association Staff. 1992. LC 92-54227. 180p. 47.50 (1-55914-602-8); pap. 44.50 (1-55914-603-6) ABBE Pubs Assn.

Jurisprudence & Clinical Competence in the Health Sciences: Index of New Information with Authors & Subjects. Roy R. Zimmerman. rev. ed. 1998. 180p. 57.50 (0-7883-2072-6) ABBE Pubs Assn.

Jurisprudence & Consumer Product Safety: Index of New Information with Authors & Subjects. Science and Life Consultants Association Staff. 1992. LC 92-54244. 180p. 47.50 (1-55914-636-2); pap. 44.50 (1-55914-637-0) ABBE Pubs Assn.

Jurisprudence & Diagnostic Errors: Index of New Information with Authors & Subjects. Science and Life Consultants Association Staff. 1992. LC 92-54192. 180p. 47.50 (1-55914-534-X); pap. 44.50 (1-55914-535-8) ABBE Pubs Assn.

Jurisprudence & Doctor-Caused Diseases, Problems & Incidents: Index of New Information with Authors & Subjects. Science and Life Consultants Association Staff. 1992. LC 92-54193. 180p. 47.50 (1-55914-536-6); pap. 44.50 (1-55914-537-4) ABBE Pubs Assn.

Jurisprudence & Forensics: Index of Modern Information. Konrad S. Gunther. 1994. LC 94-35178. 57.50 (0-7883-0474-7); pap. 47.50 (0-7883-0475-5) ABBE Pubs Assn.

Jurisprudence & Medical Malpractice: Index of New Information with Authors & Subjects. Science and Life Consultants Association Staff. 1992. LC 92-54190. 180p. 47.50 (1-55914-530-7); 1992. LC 92-54190. 180p. pap. 44.50 (1-55914-531-5); 1998. 149p. reprint ed. 57.50 (0-7883-1988-4) ABBE Pubs Assn.

Jurisprudence & Medication Errors: Index of New Information with Authors & Subjects. Science and Life Consultants Association Staff. 1992. LC 92-54194. 180p. 47.50 (1-55914-538-2); pap. 44.50 (1-55914-539-0) ABBE Pubs Assn.

Jurisprudence & Organ Procurements: Index of Authors & Subjects. Leander L. O'hara. 1993. 180p. 47.50 (1-55914-938-8); pap. 44.50 (1-55914-939-6) ABBE Pubs Assn.

Jurisprudence in Health Affairs: Index of New Information with Authors & Subjects. Science and Life Consultants Association Staff. 1992. 180p. 47.50 (1-55914-714-8); pap. 44.50 (1-55914-715-6) ABBE Pubs Assn.

Jurisprudence in Health Biology: Index of Modern Information. Hanna U. Tyler. 1989. LC 88-48008. 150p. 47.50 (1-55914-096-8); pap. 44.50 (1-55914-097-6) ABBE Pubs Assn.

Jurisprudence in Medicine in Relation to the Law. John Ordronaux. 1973. LC 73-5158. (Mental Illness & Social Policy; the American Experience Ser.). reprint ed. 26.95 (0-405-05239-1) Ayer.

Jurisprudence, Medical Records & Systems: Index of New Information with Authors & Subjects. Science and Life Consultants Association Staff. 1992. LC 92-54191. 180p. 47.50 (1-55914-532-3); pap. 47.50 (1-55914-533-1) ABBE Pubs Assn.

Jurisprudence, Rights to Treatment in Prisons: Index of New Information with Authors, Subjects & Bibliography. Roy R. Zimmerman. 1995. LC 95-14592. 57.50 (0-7883-0750-9); pap. 47.50 (0-7883-0751-7) ABBE Pubs Assn.

Jurisprudent Physician: A Physician's Guide to Legal Process & Malpractice Litigation. Margaret M. Dean. 1999. LC 99-71509. 416p. pap. 69.99 (0-9670004-0-8) Legis.

Jury Instruction on Medical Issues, 1999 Cumulative Supplement: Pocketpart. Ronald W. Eades. 5th ed. 1999. 90p. (0-327-01594-2, 6141915) LEXIS Pub.

Jury Instructions on Medical Issues. Graham Douthwaite. 4th ed. 1992. 850p. 90.00 (0-87473-967-5, MICHIE) LEXIS Pub.

Jury of My Peers: A Surgeon's Encounter with the Malpractice Crisis. Howard C. Snider, Jr. 1988. 292p. reprint ed. 19.95 (0-9622607-0-3) Fountain AL.

Just as I Am... Toby Hall & Living & Dying & Grace. Ed. by Candace C. Hall. 1992. 106p. pap. 9.95 (0-916897-18-4) Andrew Mtn Pr.

Just Ask: A Handbook for Instructors of Students Being Treated for Mental Disorders. Howard Davidson. 1993. 174p. pap., tchr. ed. 12.95 (1-55059-058-8) Temeron Bks.

Just Beneath the Surface. Nicole Boand. Ed. by Joseph Jaeger. 1994. LC 93-61854. 200p. pap. 12.95 (1-880254-14-X) Vista.

Just Checking: Scenes from the Life of an Obsessive-Compulsive. Emily Colas. 1998. LC 98-15001. 176p. 22.00 (0-671-02437-X, PB Hardcover) PB.

***Just Coding Yearbook 2001.** Ed. by Ruthann Russo. 2001. 239p. pap. 119.95 (0-9713305-0-6) H P Three.

Just Doctoring: Medical Ethics in the Liberal State. Troyen A. Brennan. 1991. LC 91-10146. 301p. text 55.00 (0-520-07333-9) U CA Pr.

Just Get Me Through This! The Practical Guide to Breast Cancer. Deborah A. Cohen & Robert M. Gelfand. 2000. LC 00-709179. 272p. pap. 13.00 (1-57566-551-4, Knsington) Kensgtn Pub Corp.

Just Here Trying to Save a Few Lives: Tales of Life & Death from the ER. Pamela Grim. 2000. LC 00-103208. 320p. 23.95 (0-446-52423-9) Warner Bks.

Just How Smart Is Prozac? Makram K. Girgis. 1995. LC 95-196193. 152p. pap. 22.50 (0-87527-517-6) Green.

Just Say Everything: A Festschrift in Honor of Hyman Spotnitz. Intro. by Sara Sheftel. 1991. (Illus.). 304p. text 65.00 (0-9624534-0-4) Assn Modern Psy.

Just Take It Out! The Ethics & Economics of Cesarean Section & Hysterectomy. David C. Walters. 1999. LC 98-87849. 271p. pap. 16.95 (0-9667162-0-5) Topiary Pubg.

Just Talk to Me. Andre Bustanoby & Fay Bustanoby. 1981. 192p. (Orig.). pap. text 7.95 (0-310-22181-1, 9211P) Zondervan.

Just the Facts: A Pocket Guide to Basic Nursing. Veronica Peterson. 2nd ed. 1998. LC 98-23493. 368p. pap. text 19.95 (0-323-00152-1) Mosby Inc.

Just the Facts in Emergency Medicine. Cline. 2000. 344p. stu. ed., ring bd. 44.95 (0-07-134549-3) McGraw-Hill Prof.

Just the Working Life: Opposition & Accommodation in Daily Industrial Life. Marc Lendler. 1990. LC 89-70267. 224p. (gr. 13). text 74.95 (0-87332-608-3) M E Sharpe.

Just What Is the Word of Wisdom? John R. Christopher. 1991. pap. 2.00 (1-879436-05-1, 99105) Christopher Pubns.

Just What the Doctor Ordered. Walter Wilson. 1988. LC 87-37167. (Illus.). 168p. (Orig.). pap. 9.95 (0-89084-439-9) Bob Jones Univ.

Just What the Doctor Ordered: A Complete Guide to Drugs & Medications for Your Dog. Race Foster & Marty Smith. 2000. (Illus.). 248p. (C). reprint ed. pap. text 20.00 (0-7881-6907-6) DIANE Pub.

Just What the Doctor Ordered: Health & Grooming in the Classic Age of Advertising. Ad Nauseum. 2000. (Illus.). 32p. pap. 9.95 (1-58062-376-X) Adams Media.

Justice & Health Care. Ed. by Earl E. Shelp. 1981. (Philosophy & Medicine Ser.: No. 8). 252p. pap. text 51.50 (90-277-1251-4) Kluwer Academic.

Justice & Health Care: Comparative Perspectives. Ed. by Andrew Grubb & Maxwell J. Mehlman. 1996. LC 95-17812. 360p. 190.00 (0-471-95526-4) Wiley.

Justice & Justification: Reflective Equilibrium in Theory & Practice. Norman Daniels. 1996. (Cambridge Studies in Philosophy & Public Policy). 381p. (C). text 74.95 (0-521-46152-9) Cambridge U Pr.

Juvenile Delinquency in an English Middletown. Hermann Mannheim. 1970. LC 73-108226. (Criminology, Law Enforcement, & Social Problems Ser.: No. 109). (Illus.). 144p. reprint ed. 22.00 (0-87585-109-6) Patterson Smith.

Juvenile Delinquents, Their Condition & Treatment. Mary Carpenter. 1970. LC 76-108224. (Criminology, Law Enforcement, & Social Problems Ser.: No. 107). reprint ed. lib. bdg. 15.00 (0-87585-107-X) Patterson Smith.

Juvenile Homicide. Ed. by Elissa P. Benedek & Dewey G. Cornell. 1989. LC 88-7682. (Clinical Practice Ser.: No. 7). 247p. text 12.95 (0-88048-145-5, 8145) Am Psychiatric.

Juvenile Psychiatry & the Law. Richard Rosner & H. I. Schwartz. 1989. LC 88-657025. (Critical Issues in American Psychiatry & the Law Ser.: Vol. 4). (Illus.). 452p. (C). 90.00 (0-306-42958-6, Plenum Trade) Perseus Pubng.

Juvenile Rheumatoid Arthritis. Ed. by John J. Miller, III. 1979. LC 78-55290. (Illus.). 280p. 35.00 (0-88416-189-7) Mosby Inc.

***Juvenile Sexual Homicide.** Wade C. Myers. 2001. 185p. 79.95 (0-12-512303-5) Acad Pr.

K

K Plus Channels in Cardio-Vascular Medicine: From Basic Science to Clinical Practice. D. Escande & N. B. Standen. 1993. (Illus.). 370p. (0-387-59598-8) Spr-Verlag.

Kabalistic Healing. Shirley Chambers. 2000. LC 00-43571. (Healing Wisdom Ser.). (Illus.). xxiii, 216p. pap. 12.95 (0-658-00644-4) NTC Contemp Pub Co.

Kahuna Healing: Holistic Health & Healing Practices of Polynesia. Serge K. King. 1983. LC 82-42704. 212p. pap. 11.95 (0-8356-0572-8, Quest) Theos Pub Hse.

Kahuna La'au Lapa'au: The Practice of Hawaiian Herbal Medicine. June Gutmanis. Tr. by Theodore Kelsey. 1976. LC 76-1510. (Illus.). 144p. pap. 9.95 (0-89610-078-2) Island Heritage.

Kaiser Wilhelms - Akademie: Fur Das Militerarztliche Bildungswesen Von 1895 Bis 1910. Hermann Schmidt. 1995. (GER.). reprint ed. (3-487-10012-6) G Olms Pubs.

Kaleidoscope of Play Therapy Stories. Ed. by Emily Oe & Sherrie Mullen. 1996. LC 95-50408. 136p. 30.00 (1-56821-786-2) Aronson.

Kallawaya - Guerisseurs Itinerants des Andes (Kallawaya - Itinerant Healers in the Andes) Recherches sur les Pratiques Medicinales et Magiques (Research of Medicinal & Magical Practices) L. Girault. 1984.Tr. of Kallawaya. Itinerant Healers in the Andes - Research of Medicinal & Magical Practices. (FRE.). 668p. pap. (2-7099-0732-1) LInstitut Francais FRA. *Dist:* Balogh.

Kallawaya. Itinerant Healers in the Andes - Research of Medicinal & Magical Practices see Kallawaya - Guerisseurs Itinerants des Andes (Kallawaya - Itinerant Healers in the Andes): Recherches sur les Pratiques Medicinales et Magiques (Research of Medicinal & Magical Practices)

Kallikak Family: A Study in the Heredity of Feeble-Mindedness. Henry H. Goddard. 1976. LC 73-2966. (Classics in Psychology Ser.). reprint ed. 26.95 (0-405-05139-5) Ayer.

Kalman Jacob Mann - Reflections on a Life in Health Care. Kalman Jacob Mann. 1994. 334p. (965-09-0126-4, 66800) R Mass Ltd ISR. *Dist:* Lambda Pubs.

Kammerer & Gross' Medical Consultation: The Internist on Surgical, Obstetric, & Psychiatric Services. William S. Kammerer. Ed. by Richard J. Gross & Gregory M. Caputo. 3rd ed. 1998. LC 97-23571. 704p. text 89.00 (0-683-03639-4) Lppncott W & W.

Kampala Women Getting By: Wellbeing in the Time of AIDS. Sandra Wallman. 1996. LC 96-18181. (Eastern African Studies). (Illus.). 256p. (C). text 39.95 (0-8214-1158-6) Ohio U Pr.

Kampo: How the Japanese Updated Traditional Herbal Medicine. Akira Tsumura. 1991. (Illus.). 283p. 29.95 (0-87040-792-9) Japan Pubns USA.

Kampo Treatment: For Climacteric Disorders. Yoshiharu Shibata & Jean Wu. LC 97-4784. (Illus.). 272p. (Orig.). (C). pap. 29.95 (0-912111-51-8) Paradigm Publns.

Kansas Health Care in Perspective 2000. Ed. by Kathleen O'Leary Morgan & Scott E. Morgan. 2000. 21p. spiral bd. 19.00 (0-7401-0215-X) Morgan Quitno Corp.

Kansas Health Care Perspective, 1998. Ed. by Kathleen O'Leary Morgan & Scott E. Morgan. 1998. 20p. pap. 19.00 (1-56692-815-X) Morgan Quitno Corp.

Kansas Long-Term Care Handbook. Ed. by Molly M. Wood. 1999. 600p. ring bd. (1-890452-08-4) KS Bar.

Kansas University: Studies in Psychology, No. 1. Ed. by Raymond H. Wheeler. 1969. (Psychology Monographs General & Applied: Vol. 44). reprint ed. pap. 35.00 (0-8115-6433-9) Periodicals Srv.

Kant's Dove: The History of Transference in Psychoanalysis. Aldo Carotenuto. Tr. by Joan Tambureno from ITA. 1990. 184p. (Orig.). pap. 8.95 (0-933029-50-0) Chiron Pubns.

Kanzi: The Ape at the Brink of the Human Mind. E. Sue Savage-Rumbaugh et al. LC 94-9038. 299p. 1996. pap. 15.95 (0-471-15959-X); 1994. (Illus.). 24.95 (0-471-58591-2) Wiley.

Kaplan & Sadock's Comprehensive Textbook of Psychiatry. Benjamin J. Sadock & Virginia A. Sadock. 7th ed. 1999. 3,500p. 379.00 (0-7817-2388-4) Lppncott W & W.

Kaplan & Sadock's Synopsis of Psychiatry: Behavioral Sciences - Clinical Psychiatry. Harold I. Kaplan & Benjamin J. Sadock. 8th ed. 1998. LC 97-9138. (Illus.). 1,280p. pap. 75.00 (0-683-30330-9) Lppncott W & W.

Kaplan & Sadock's Synopsis of Psychiatry: Behavioral Sciences, Clinical Psychiatry. Harold I. Kaplan & Benjamin J. Sadock. 7th ed. 1994. (Illus.). 1280p. 55.00 (0-683-04530-X) Lppncott W & W.

Kaplan Careers in Nursing. Annette Vallano. 1999. LC 98-39430. (Kaplan Ser.). (Illus.). 256p. pap. 16.00 (0-684-85236-5) Kaplan.

Kaplan Success with Medical Words. Kaplan Staff. 1998. LC 98-29977. (Illus.). 144p. pap. 6.95 (0-684-85400-7) Kaplan.

Kaplan the Book of Medical School Lists. Adele Scheele. 1997. 180p. pap. 12.00 (0-684-84178-9) S&S Trade.

Kaposi's Sarcoma. Decio Cerimele. 1985. LC 84-13423. (Illus.). 168p. text 35.00 (0-88331-155-0) R B Luce.

Kaposi's Sarcoma. Ed. by Ch. L. Olweny et al. 1981. (Antibiotics & Chemotherapy Ser.: Vol. 29). (Illus.). xii, 104p. 77.50 (3-8055-2076-X) S Karger.

Kara Mia: The Story of Sudden Loss & Slow Recovery in a Teenager with Long QT Syndrome. Maryann Anglim & Walter Allan. 1997. (Illus.). 250p. (Orig.). pap. 12.95 (0-9656501-0-3) Seahorse Press.

***Karch's Pathology of Drug Abuse.** Steven B. Karch. 3rd ed. 2001. 568p. 89.95 (0-8493-0343-5, 0343) CRC Pr.

Karen Horney: A Psychoanalyst's Search for Self-Understanding. Bernard J. Paris. 1994. LC 94-14935. (Illus.). 288p. 45.00 (0-300-05956-6) Yale U Pr.

Karl Kraus & the Soul Doctors see Anti-Freud: Karl Kraus's Criticism of Psychoanalysis & Psychiatry

Karl Mannheim & the Crisis of Liberalism: The Secret of These New Times. David Kettler & Volker Meja. 1998. 372p. (C). text 44.95 (1-56000-188-7) Transaction Pubs.

Kaspar Hauser Syndrome of Psychosocial Dwarfism: Deficient Statural, Intellectual, & Social Growth Induced by Child Abuse. John Money. 1992. LC 92-11008. 290p. (C). 38.00 (0-87975-754-X) Prometheus Bks.

***Kathy Smith's Moving Through Menopause: The Complete Program for Exercise, Nutrition & Total Wellness.** Kathy Smith. 2002. LC 2001-53640. (Illus.). 272p. pap. (0-446-67871-6) Warner.

Kathy Smith's Walkfit for a Better Body. Kathy Smith & Susanna Levin. 1994. LC 93-48765. 176p. (Orig.). pap. (0-446-67048-0) Warner.

Katzenstein & Askin's Surgical Pathology of Non-Neoplastic Lung Disease. Anna-Luise A. Katzenstein et al. Ed. by Lesley Day. 3rd ed. 1997. LC 96-21235. (Major Problems in Pathology Ser.). (Illus.). 512p. text 84.00 (0-7216-5755-9) Saunders.

Katzung's Pharmacology: Examination & Board Review. Bertram G. Katzung & Anthony J. Trevor. 6th ed. 2001. 640p. (C). pap. 39.95 (0-8385-8147-1) McGraw-Hill Prof.

Kaufman Speech Praxis Test for Children. Nancy R. Kaufman. 1995. pap. text, stu. ed. 15.95 (0-8143-2468-1); (gr. 1-7). text, stu. ed. 125.00 (0-8143-2467-3) Wayne St U Pr.

Kava: The Pacific Elixir: The Definitive Guide to Its Ethnobotany, History, & Chemistry. Vincent Lebot et al. 1997. LC 97-1057. (Illus.). 272p. pap. 19.95 (0-89281-726-7) Inner Tradit.

Kava Kava. Ronald G. Reichert. 1997. LC 97-27617. (Keats Good Herb Guides). 96p. pap. 4.95 (0-87983-870-1, 38701K, Keats Pubng) McGraw-Hill Trade.

Kawasaki Disease: Proceedings of the 5th International Kawasaki Disease Symposium, Fukuoka, Japan, 22-25 May 1995. Ed. by Hiroshisa Kato. 1995. LC 95-25124. (International Congress Ser.: No. 1093). 666p. 248.50 (0-444-82200-3, Excerpta Medica) Elsevier.

Keane's Essentials of Medical-Surgical Nursing. Susan C. DeWit. 3rd ed. 1992. (Illus.). tchr. ed. (0-7216-4508-9) Saunders.

Keep Abortion Safe & Legal: The Postcard Activist. PGW Staff. 1991. pap. 4.95 (1-879096-00-5) Postcard Activist.

Keep Moving, Keep Young: Gentle Yoga Exercises. Margaret Graham. 1996. (Illus.). 166p. pap. (0-340-62117-6) Hodder & Stought Ltd GBR. *Dist:* Lubrecht & Cramer, Trafalgar.

Keep off the Grass. Gabriel G. Nahas. 5th rev. ed. 1990. LC 90-3658. (Illus.). 400p. reprint ed. pap. 12.95 (0-8397-4384-X) Eriksson.

Keep Quit! A Motivational Guide to Life Without Smoking. Terry A. Rustin. 1996. LC 95-52662. 300p. pap. 12.95 (1-56838-104-2) Hazelden.

Keep Your Breasts: Preventing Breast Cancer the Natural Way. Susan Moss. LC 94-92245. 1994. (Illus.). 306p. reprint ed. pap. 19.95 (0-9642329-0-1); 5th rev. ed. 1998. 316p. pap. text 19.95 (0-9642329-1-X) Res Pubns CA.

J K L

Keep Your Smile Beautiful! A Guide to Quality Dentistry. Paul R. Chalifoux. Ed. by Richard Leslie. 1990. (Illus.). (Orig.). pap. text 30.00 (*0-9625549-0-1*) Chalifoux Pub.

Keepers of the Central Fire: Issues in Ecology for Indigenous Peoples. Lorelei Lambert-Colombda. 1998. LC 97-51179. (Illus.). 320p. pap. 23.95 (*0-88737-742-4*, 14-7424) Natl League Nurse.

Keeping America Sane: Psychiatry & Eugenics in the United States & Canada, 1880-1940. Ian R. Dowbiggin. 1997. LC 97-3425. (Cornell Studies in the History of Psychiatry). xvi, 245p. pap. (*0-8014-8398-0*); (Illus.). 288p. 39.95 (*0-8014-3356-8*) Cornell U Pr.

Keeping Buildings Healthy: How to Monitor & Prevent Indoor Environmental Problems. James T. O'Reilly et al. 1998. LC 98-3365. 384p. 97.50 (*0-471-29228-1*, VNR) Wiley.

Keeping Children from Harm's Way: How National Policy Affects Psychological Development. Annette U. Rickel & Evvie Becker. 1997. LC 97-20445. 334p. pap. 24.95 (*1-55798-443-3*) Am Psychol.

Keeping Control: Understanding & Overcoming Fecal Incontinence. Marvin M. Schuster & Jacqueline Wehmueller. 1994. LC 94-8431. 176p. pap. 14.95 (*0-8018-4916-0*) Johns Hopkins.

Keeping Face: A Plastic Surgeon's Guide to Preserving & Improving Nature's Gifts. Robert L. Cucin. 1985. (Illus.). 183p. 22.50 (*0-9608304-2-1*) Rocin.

Keeping Fit with Asta O'Donnell: An Exercise Program for Problem Backs. Asta O'Donnell & June Lipton. 1983. (Illus.). 103p. (Orig.). pap. 12.50 (*0-9610564-0-1*) J L Prods.

Keeping Livestock Healthy: A Veterinary Guide. N. Bruce Haynes. 1986. LC 85-22182. 336p. pap. 14.95 (*0-88266-409-3*) Storey Bks.

Keeping Livestock Healthy: A Veterinary Guide to Horses, Cattle, Pigs, Goats & Sheep. N. Bruce Haynes. 3rd rev. ed. 1994. LC 94-26886. (Illus.). 352p. pap. 19.95 (*0-88266-884-6*) Storey Bks.

Keeping Patients in the Dark: Should Prescription Medicines Be Advertised Direct to Consumers. Peter Cardy et al. 1999. (Choice in Welfare Ser.: No. 51). 45p. pap. (*0-255-36454-7*) Inst Economic Affairs GBR. *Dist:* Coronet Bks.

Keeping Track: A Personal Medical Record System. Eleanor Laumark & Victoria Christianson. 1981. LC 80-22042. (Illus.). (Orig.). pap. 7.95 (*0-912800-79-8*) Woodbridge Pr.

Keeping up the Good Work: A Practitioner's Guide to Mental Health Ethics. Leonard J. Haas & John L. Malouf. 2nd ed. 1995. LC 94-47583. 296p. 37.95 (*1-56887-012-4*, KUGWBBP, Prof Resc Pr) Pro Resource.

Keeping Your Child Healthy with Chinese Medicine: A Parent's Guide to the Care & Prevention of Common Childhood Diseases. Bob Flaws & Honora L. Wolfe. 1996. LC 96-84842. (Illus.). 185p. pap. 15.95 (*0-936185-71-6*) Blue Poppy Pr.

Kelevan. 1986. (Environmental Health Criteria Ser.: No. 66). 32p. pap. text 11.00 (*92-4-154266-7*, 1160066) World Health.

Kelley Textbook of Rheumatology Edward D. Harris, Jr. et al. 6th ed. 2000. LC 00-20042. (Illus.). 2060p. text 249.00 (*0-7216-8008-9*) Saunders.

Kelley's Essentials of Internal Medicine. H. David Humes. 2nd ed. 2001. LC 00-45338. (Illus.). xxiii, 920p. pap. text 49.95 (*0-7817-1937-2*) Lppncott W & W.

Kelley's Textbook of Internal Medicine. H. David Humes et al. 4th ed. 2000. 3,408p. text 115.00 (*0-7817-1787-6*) Lppncott W & W.

Kelp, Dulse & Other Supplements from the Sea. William R. Lee. 1983. (Good Health Guides). 30p. pap. 2.95 (*0-87983-313-0*, 33130K, Keats Pubng) McGraw-Hill Trade.

Kelp, the Health Giver. Eric F. Powell. 1982. pap. 2.95 (*0-87904-041-6*) Lust.

Kelp the Health Giver. Eric F. Powell. 1980. 35.00 (*0-85032-195-6*) St Mut.

KELS: The Kohlman Evaluation of Living Skills. Linda K. Thomson. 3rd ed. 1992. (Orig.). pap. text 35.00 (*0-910317-90-9*) Am Occup Therapy.

Kelvin Problem: Foam Structures of Minimal Surface Area. Denis Weaire. 1997. LC 97-223521. 320p. (*0-7484-0632-8*) Tay Francis Ltd GBR. *Dist:* Taylor & Francis.

Kempe's Operative Neurosurgery. Ed. by M. Salcman et al. 2nd ed. 2001. (Illus.). 269p. 179.00 (*0-387-98537-9*) Spr-Verlag.

Ken Wilber in Dialogue: Conversations with Leading Transpersonal Thinkers. Ed. by Donald J. Rothberg & Sean M. Kelly. 1998. LC 97-35286. (Illus.). 304p. pap. 16.95 (*0-8356-0766-6*, Quest) Theos Pub Hse.

Kendig's Disorders of the Respiratory Tract in Children. Victor Chernick & Thomas F. Boat. Ed. by Judy Fletcher. 6th ed. 1997. LC 96-42343. (Illus.). 1104p. text 205.00 (*0-7216-6541-1*) Saunders.

Kent's Minor Writings on Homeopathy. Klaus-Henning Gypser. 1987. 766p. (*3-7760-0946-2*) K F Haug Pubs DEU. *Dist:* Medicina Bio.

Kentucky Health Care in Perspective 2000. Ed. by Kathleen O'Leary Morgan & Scott E. Morgan. 2000. 21p. spiral bd. 19.00 (*0-7401-0216-8*) Morgan Quitno Corp.

Kentucky Health Care Perspective, 1998. Ed. by Kathleen O'Leary Morgan & Scott E. Morgan. 1998. 20p. pap. 19.00 (*1-56692-816-8*) Morgan Quitno Corp.

Kentucky Medicaid Eligibility Guide for Nursing Home Care. Joseph S. Whitehouse & Brian Borellis. 2000. xix, 116p. pap. 24.95 (*0-9704431-0-2*) Guiding Light.

Keratinization & Growth Regulation. Ed. by J. W. Mali. 1976. (Current Problems in Dermatology Ser.: Vol. 6). (Illus.). 250p. 85.25 (*3-8055-2294-0*) S Karger.

Keratinocyte: Methods. Ed. by Irene M. Leigh & Fiona M. Watt. 1996. LC 93-42614. 310p. text 85.00 (*0-521-45103-5*) Cambridge U Pr.

Keratinocyte Methods. Ed. by Irene M. Leigh. 1995. (Illus.). 223p. (C). pap. text 74.95 (*0-521-45013-6*) Cambridge U Pr.

Kernel of Truth in Freud. Philip Lawton. 1991. 154p. (C). pap. text 23.00 (*0-8191-8035-1*); lib. bdg. 46.00 (*0-8191-8034-3*) U Pr of Amer.

Kestenberg Movement Profile: Its Past, Present Applications & Future Directions. Penny Lewis & Susan Loman. 1990. LC 90-81441. 176p. (C). pap. text 12.00 (*1-881245-01-2*) Antioch New Eng.

Ketogenic Diet: A Treatment for Epilepsy. John M. Freeman et al. 3rd rev. ed. 2000. LC 00-35856. Orig. Title: The Epilepsy Diet Treatment: An Introduction to the Ketogenic Diet. (Illus.). 224p. pap. 24.95 (*1-888799-39-0*) Demos Medical.

Ketotifen in the Prophylactic Treatment of Bronchial Asthma. Ed. by H. Herzog. 1980. (Journal: Vol. 39). (Illus.). 54p. pap. 35.00 (*3-8055-1171-X*) S Karger.

Kevin & Me: Tourette Syndrome & the Magic Power of Music Therapy: A Mothers Story. Patricia Heenan. 2000. LC 00-57243. (Illus.). viii, 135p. 19.95 (*1-878267-02-7*) Hope Pr CA.

***Key Advances in Rheumatoid Arthritis.** I. Haslock et al. 2001. 100p. pap. (*1-85315-493-8*) Royal Soc of Medicine Pr Ltd GBR. *Dist:* Balogh.

***Key Advances in the Effective Management of Benign Prostatic Disease.** C. E. Clarke. 2001. 80p. pap. (*1-85315-490-3*) Royal Soc of Medicine Pr Ltd GBR. *Dist:* Balogh.

Key Aspects of Caring for the Acutely Ill: Technological Aspects, Patient Education, & Quality of Life. Ed. by Sandra G. Funk et al. 1995. 360p. 42.95 (*0-8261-8580-0*) Springer Pub.

Key Aspects of Caring for the Chronically Ill: Hospital & Home. Ed. by Sandra Funk et al. 1993. LC 94-2735. 368p. 44.95 (*0-8261-8080-9*) Springer Pub.

Key Aspects of Comfort: Management of Pain, Fatigue, & Nausea. Ed. by Sandra G. Funk et al. 1989. 352p. 44.95 (*0-8261-6760-8*) Springer Pub.

Key Aspects of Elder Care: Managing Falls, Incontinence, & Cognitive Impairment. Ed. by Sandra G. Funk et al. 1992. LC 92-7827. 368p. 44.95 (*0-8261-7720-4*) Springer Pub.

Key Aspects of Recovery: Improving Nutrition, Rest & Mobility. Ruth A. Wiese & Elizabeth M. Tornquist. 1990. LC 90-9630. 368p. 44.95 (*0-8261-7290-3*) Springer Pub.

Key Concepts in Psychotherapy Integration. Jerold Gold. 1996. LC 96-304. (Applied Clinical Psychology Ser.). (Illus.). 242p. (C). 42.50 (*0-306-45175-1*, Plenum Trade) Perseus Pubng.

Key Facts in Cardiology. A. A. Grace et al. 1991. 40p. (Orig.). pap. text (*0-443-04596-8*) Church.

Key Facts in Clinical Nutrition. Payne-Jame. 1995. pap. text 14.95 (*0-443-05182-8*) Saunders.

Key Facts in Diabetes. Moriarty. 1994. pap. text 12.95 (*0-443-04828-2*) Saunders.

Key Facts in Gastroenterology. Jonathan Halevy. 1986. LC 86-22670. (Topics in Gastroenterology Ser.). (Illus.). 214p. (C). spiral bd. 57.00 (*0-306-42309-X*, Kluwer Plenum) Kluwer Academic.

Key Facts in Immunology. David W. Scott & Jeffrey R. Dawson. 1984. (Illus.). 264p. (Orig.). pap. text (*0-443-08247-2*) Church.

Key Facts in Infection. M. R. Miller & E. Davies. 1993. 38p. spiral bd. (*0-443-04993-9*) Church.

Key Ideas in Personality Theories. James R. Scroggs. 1984. (Illus.). 341p. text 53.25 (*0-314-85296-4*) West Pub.

Key Issues for Counselling in Action. Windy Dryden. 1989. (Counselling in Action Ser.: Vol. 7). 118p. (C). 57.95 (*0-8039-8051-5*, 7326); pap. 22.95 (*0-8039-8052-3*, 7327) Sage.

Key Issues in Business Ethics. John Donaldson. 1989. 224p. (C). text 49.95 (*0-12-220541-3*) Dryden Pr.

Key Issues in Cross-Cultural Psychology: Selected Papers from the Twelfth International Congress of the International Association for Cross-Cultural Psychology Held in Pamplona-Iruna, Navarra, Spain, July 24-27, 1994. Ed. by Hector Grad et al. 1996. LC 96-12891. vi, 390p. (*90-265-1441-7*) Swets.

Key Issues in Mental Retardation Research. Ed. by William I. Fraser. 1990. 516p. (C). 125.00 (*0-415-01363-1*) Routledge.

Key Issues in Plastic & Cosmetic Surgery. Ed. by M. B. Habal et al. (Illus.). 1999. (Key Issues in Plastic & Cosmetic Surgery Ser.: Vol. 16). x, 170p. 198.25 (*3-8055-6970-X*); Vol. 17. 2001. vi, 166p. 198.25 (*3-8055-7167-4*) S Karger.

Key Legal & Ethical Issues in Living Donor Organ Transplantation. Austen Garwood-Gowers. 1999. LC 99-45175. (Medico-Legal Ser.). 246p. text (*0-7546-2029-8*) Ashgate Pub GBR. *Dist:* Ashgate Pub Co.

Key Medical Membrane Devices in the Late 1990s. Leos J. Zeman. 1997. LC 98-120878. (Report Ser.: No. C-208). 182p. 3250.00 (*1-56965-381-X*) BCC.

***Key Points in Hospital Medicine.** Robert M. Wachter et al. 2002. (*0-7817-3603-X*) Lppncott W & W.

Key Questions in Obstetrics & Gynaecology. R. J. Slade et al. 1994. 128p. (Orig.). pap. (*1-872748-73-2*) Bios Sci GBR. *Dist:* Coronet Bks.

Key Questions in Pediatrics. A. Billson et al. 1997. (Key Topics - Questions Ser.). (Illus.). 128p. pap. (*1-85996-116-9*) Bios Sci GBR. *Dist:* Bks Intl VA.

Key Questions in Radiology. P. Hulse et al. 1996. 128p. (Orig.). pap. (*1-85996-245-9*) Bios Sci GBR. *Dist:* Coronet Bks.

Key Techniques in Orthopaedic Surgery. Steven H. Stern. 2000. (Illus.). 320p. 119.00 (*0-86577-922-8*) Thieme Med Pubs.

Key to Genius: Manic-Depression & the Creative Life. D. Jablow Hershman & Julian Lieb. 1988. LC 87-32900. (Psychology Ser.). (Illus.). 220p. 30.00 (*0-87975-437-0*) Prometheus Bks.

Key to Health. Mahatma Gandhi. Tr. by Sushila Nayar from GUJ. 1982. 83p. (Orig.). pap. 2.00 (*0-934676-58-5*) Greenlf Bks.

Key to Medical Literacy. Shulman. 1995. (C). pap. 40.95 (*0-15-503620-3*) Harcourt Coll Pubs.

Key to Medical Terminology. Jane Rice. 1986. (Illus.). 384p. pap. text 21.95 (*0-13-515032-9*) P-H.

Key to Nature Cure. J. M. Jussawalla. 1992. (C). reprint ed. (*81-7154-692-7*) Popular Prakashan IND. *Dist:* S Asia.

Key Topics in Accident & Emergency. P. Howarth & R. Evans. 1994. 300p. (Orig.). pap. (*1-872748-67-8*) Bios Sci GBR. *Dist:* Coronet Bks.

Key Topics in Cardiovascular Medicine. P. Hambly. 1997. 184p. (*1-85996-211-4*) Bios Sci GBR. *Dist:* Coronet Bks.

Key Topics in General Surgery. C. Lattimer et al. 1996. (Key Topics Ser.). 304p. (Orig.). pap. (*1-872748-02-3*) Bios Sci GBR. *Dist:* Bks Intl VA.

Key Topics in Obstetrics & Gynocology. R. J. Slade et al. 1993. 296p. (Orig.). pap. (*1-872748-07-4*) Bios Sci GBR. *Dist:* Coronet Bks.

Key Topics in Oncology. G. D. Hall et al. 1998. (Key Topics Ser.). (Illus.). 304p. (Orig.). pap. text (*1-85996-105-3*) Bios Sci GBR. *Dist:* Bks Intl VA.

Key Topics in Oral Surgery. P. Wilson & K. Riden. 1998. (Key Topics Ser.). (Illus.). 304p. (Orig.). pap. text (*1-85996-030-8*) Bios Sci GBR. *Dist:* Bks Intl VA.

Key Topics in Orthopedic Surgery. I. Nugent et al. 1994. 300p. pap. (*1-872748-33-3*) Bios Sci GBR. *Dist:* Coronet Bks.

Key Topics in Otolaryngology. R. McRae et al. 1995. 368p. (Orig.). pap. (*1-872748-68-6*) Bios Sci GBR. *Dist:* Coronet Bks.

Key Topics in Pediatrics. A. E. Davies & A. L. Billson. 1994. 300p. (Orig.). pap. (*1-872748-58-9*) Bios Sci GBR. *Dist:* Coronet Bks.

Key Topics in Psychiatry. P. Sudbury et al. 1996. (Key Topics). 300p. pap. (*1-872748-17-1*) Bios Sci GBR. *Dist:* Coronet Bks.

Key Topics in Renal Medicine. C. R. Tomson & W. D. Plant. 1996. (Key Topics Ser.). 208p. (Orig.). pap. text (*1-85996-170-3*) Bios Sci GBR. *Dist:* Bks Intl VA.

Key Topics in Trauma. I. Greaves et al. 1997. (Key Topics Ser.). (Illus.). 352p. (Orig.). pap. (*1-85996-175-4*) Bios Sci GBR. *Dist:* Bks Intl VA.

Key Words in Physical Rehabilitation: A Guide to Contemporary Usage. Ed. by Shirley Cammack & Myron G. Eisenberg. 1995. LC 94-23159. 152p. 25.95 (*0-8261-8740-4*) Springer Pub.

Key Words in Psychosocial Rehabilitation: A Guide to Contemporary Usage. Ed. by Myron G. Eisenberg. 1994. LC 93-23647. 136p. 24.95 (*0-8261-8320-4*) Springer Pub.

Keyboard, Graphic & Handwriting Skills: Helping People with Motor Disabilities. Dorothy E. Penso. Ed. by Jo Campling. 1990. (Therapy in Practice Ser.: No. 15). 160p. pap. 23.00 (*0-412-32210-2*, A4415) Chapman & Hall.

Keyguide to Information Sources in Dentistry. M. Clennett. 1985. 300p. text 90.00 (*0-7201-1747-X*) Continuum.

Keyguide to Information Sources in Paramedical Sciences. Ed. by John Hewlett. 1990. 282p. 130.00 (*0-7201-2057-8*) Continuum.

Keyguide to Information Sources in Pharmacy. Barry Strickland-Hodge et al. 1989. 188p. 110.00 (*0-7201-1966-9*) Continuum.

Keyguide to Information Sources in Veterinary Medicine. Mike Gibb. 1990. 459p. 120.00 (*0-7201-2018-7*) Continuum.

Keyhole Concept in Neurosurgery: With Endoscope-Assisted Microsurgery & Case Studies. Alex Perneczky. 1999. (Illus.). 264p. 199.00 (*0-86577-709-8*) Thieme Med Pubs.

Keys for Regeneration. Ed. by C. H. Taban & B. Boilly. 1992. (Monographs in Developmental Biology: Vol. 23). (Illus.). x, 252p. 213.25 (*3-8055-5510-5*) S Karger.

Keys, Species & Host List, & Bibliography for Nasal Mites of North American Birds: Acarina: Rhinonyssinae, Turbinoptinae, Speleognathinae, & Cytoditidae. Danny B. Pence. 1975. (Special Publications: No. 8). (Illus.). 148p. (Orig.). pap. 6.00 (*0-89672-033-0*) Tex Tech Univ Pr.

Keys to Breast Feeding. William M. Sears. 1991. (Parenting Keys Ser.). 160p. pap. 6.95 (*0-8120-4540-8*) Barron.

Keys to Caring & Preparing for Your Newborn. William M. Sears. 1991. 160p. pap. 6.95 (*0-8120-4539-4*) Barron.

Keys to Child Safety & Care of Minor Childhood Injuries. Robert J. Vinci. 1992. (Parenting Keys Ser.). 160p. pap. 5.95 (*0-8120-4825-3*) Barron.

Keys to Childhood Illness. Norman B. Schell. 1992. pap. 5.95 (*0-8120-4852-0*) Barron.

Keys to Clinical Practice. Gorrie. 1994. pap. text 8.50 (*0-7216-5194-1*) Saunders.

Keys to Dealing with Childhood Allergies. Judy L. Bachman. 1992. (Parenting Keys Ser.). 160p. pap. 5.95 (*0-8120-4836-9*) Barron.

Keys to Dealing with Stuttering. Patricia M. Treiber. 1993. (Parenting Keys Ser.). pap. 5.95 (*0-8120-4666-8*) Barron.

Keys to Health. Eric A. Mein. 1995. 232p. mass mkt. 4.99 (*0-312-95616-9*, Tor Books) T Doherty Assocs.

Keys to Nursing Success. 2000. (C). (*0-13-031542-7*) P-H.

Keys to Nursing Success. Carol Carter & Katz. 2000. 348p. pap. 32.00 (*0-13-019575-8*) P-H.

Keys to Parenting the Asthmatic Child. Gerald L. Klein. 1994. (Barron's Parenting Keys Ser.). pap. 5.95 (*0-8120-1677-7*) Barron.

Keys to Parenting the Child with Autism. Marlene Targ Brill. 1994. (Parenting Keys Ser.). 208p. pap. 6.95 (*0-8120-1679-3*) Barron.

Keys to Parenting Twins. Karen Kerkhoff. 1992. pap. 6.95 (*0-8120-4851-2*) Barron.

Keys to the Asylum: A Dean, a Medical School, & Academic Politics. Daniel K. Bloomfield. 2000. 488p. pap. 24.95 (*0-9701022-0-8*) New Med.

Keys to Understanding Alzheimer's Disease. Gisele Wolf-Klein. 1992. pap. 6.95 (*0-8120-4758-3*) Barron.

Keywords Defined, 1991. Gregory A. Smith. 1993. 200p. pap. text (*0-9635538-0-1*) MEDTEXT Med.

Kick the Drug Habit: The Basic Guide. Clifton J. Alexander & Sandy Alexander. rev. ed. 1989. 134p. reprint ed. pap. 8.95 (*0-929658-00-0*) Antler Pub.

Kicking Addictive Habits Once & for All: A Relapse Prevention Guide. Dennis C. Daley. 1998. LC 97-43205. 224p. pap. 20.00 (*0-7879-4068-2*) Jossey-Bass.

Kicking the Depression Habit: Bouncing Back Chasing the Blues Away. Lorenzo Arbett. 1986. (Orig.). pap. 10.95 (*0-941122-01-8*) Lorenzo Prema.

Kicking Your Stress Habits: A Do-It-Yourself Guide for Coping with Stress. Donald A. Tubesing. 1981. LC 80-54046. 192p. (Orig.). (C). pap. 15.95 (*0-938586-00-9*) Whole Person.

Kid-Friendly Parenting with Deaf & Hard of Hearing Children: A Treasury of Fun Activities Toward Better Behavior. Denise C. Weston & Daria Medwid. 1995. LC 95-25434. (Illus.). 382p. pap. 24.95 (*1-56368-031-9*, Clerc Bks) Gallaudet Univ Pr.

Kidney. H. E. De Wardner. 5th ed. 1985. (Illus.). 604p. text (*0-443-02841-9*) Church.

Kidney Barry M. Brenner & Floyd C. Rector, Jr. 4th ed. 1990. (Illus.). 1. text (*0-7216-2616-5*); 2. text (*0-7216-2617-3*) Saunders.

***Kidney**, Set. Barry M. Brenner. 2000. (Illus.). 2652p. text 550.00 incl. cd-rom (*0-7216-9310-5*) Saunders.

Kidney, Set. Barry M. Brenner. 6th ed. 2000. LC 99-11888. (Illus.). 2652p. (C). text 395.00 (*0-7216-7998-6*) Saunders.

Kidney: Physiology & Pathophysiology. Donald W. Seldin. 3rd ed. 1999. 3,168p. text 425.00 (*0-397-58784-8*); text (*0-397-58786-4*) Lppncott W & W.

Kidney: Structure & Functions in Health & Disease. Homer W. Smith. 1951. (Illus.). 1072p. text 65.00 (*0-19-501140-6*) OUP.

Kidney & Body Fluids in Health & Disease. Ed. by Saulo Klahr. 1982. LC 84-1983. 616p. (C). 95.00 (*0-306-41062-1*); pap. 39.50 (*0-306-41660-3*) Kluwer Academic (Kluwer Plenum).

Kidney & Hypertension in Diabetes Mellitus. Ed. by Carl E. Mogensen. 1988. (Topics in Renal Medicine Ser.). (C). text 235.00 (*0-89838-958-5*) Kluwer Academic.

Kidney & Hypertension in Diabetes Mellitus. Ed. by Carl Erik Mogensen. 2000. 760p. 170.00 (*0-7923-7901-2*) Kluwer Academic.

Kidney & Hypertension in Diabetes Mellitus. Ed. by Carl E. Mogensen. 2nd ed. 1994. LC 94-14065. 576p. text 233.00 (*0-7923-2829-9*); 3rd ed. 1996. LC 96-48296. 608p. (C). text 157.50 (*0-7923-4353-0*) Kluwer Academic.

Kidney & Hypertension in Pregnancy. Priscilla S. Kincaid-Smith & Kenneth F. Fairley. 1993. LC 92-49139. 416p. text (*0-443-04536-4*) Church.

Kidney & Pancreas Transplantation: Detailed Surgical Procedures & Management Protocols. Ed. by Ingemar J. A. Davidson. 2nd ed. 1999. (Vademecum Ser.). 228p. spiral bd. 45.00 (*1-57059-646-8*) Landes Bioscience.

J
K
L

Kidney & Pregnancy. Ed. by G. M. Eisenbach & J. Brod. 1981. (Contributions to Nephrology Ser.: Vol. 25). (Illus.). vi, 170p. pap. 29.75 (*3-8055-1798-X*) S Karger.

Kidney & Proteins in Health & Disease. Ed. by C. P. Bianchi et al. 1988. (Contributions to Nephrology Ser.: Vol. 68). (Illus.). xi, 274p. 29.75 (*3-8055-4821-4*) S Karger.

Kidney & Urinary Tract. Ed. by W. S. Symmers et al. 3rd rev. ed. 1992. (Systemic Pathology Ser.: No. 8). (Illus.). 785p. text (*0-443-03171-1*) Church.

Kidney & Urinary Tract Diseases & Disorders Sourcebook: Basic Information about Kidney Stones, Urinary Incontinence, Bladder Disease, Endstage Renal Disease, Dialysis & More. Ed. by Linda M. Ross. 1997. LC 97-16533. (Health Reference Ser.: Vol. 21). xiii, 602p. lib. bdg. 78.00 (*0-7808-0079-6*) Omnigraphics Inc.

Kidney at a Glance. Christopher A. O'Callaghan & Barry Brenner. 2000. LC 00-28907. (At a Glance Ser.). (Illus.). 120p. (C). pap. 26.95 (*0-632-05206-6*) Blackwell Sci.

Kidney Disease in Primary Care. Ed. by Anil K. Mandal & N. Stanley Nahman. 1997. LC 97-37957. 400p. 49.95 (*0-683-30057-1*) Lppncott W & W.

Kidney Failure: Coping & Feeling Your Best. Anna Hollingsworth. 1994. LC 94-16751. (Illus.). 48p. (Orig.). pap. text 9.95 (*0-939838-37-0*) Pritchett & Hull.

Kidney Failure: Our Success Story. Anne Benjamin. 1984. 150p. 7.50 (*0-86516-050-3*) Bolchazy-Carducci.

Kidney Failure: The Facts. J. Stewart Cameron. 2nd ed. 1996. LC 96-8019. (Facts Ser.). (Illus.). 248p. pap. 19.95 (*0-19-262643-4*) OUP.

Kidney Failure & the Federal Government. Institute of Medicine Staff. Ed. by Richard A. Rettig & Norman G. Levinsky. 1991. 440p. text 49.95 (*0-309-04432-4*) Natl Acad Pr.

Kidney in Essential Hypertension. Ed. by Franz H. Messerli. 1983. (Developments in Cardiovascular Medicine Ser.). text 113.00 (*0-89838-616-0*) Kluwer Academic.

Kidney in Hypertension. Ed. by V. M. Campese & W. A. Hsueh. 1983. (American Journal of Nephrology: Vol. 3, No. 2-3). (Illus.). vi, 140p. pap. 88.75 (*3-8055-3648-8*) S Karger.

Kidney in Liver Disease. Ed. by Murray Epstein. 4th rev. ed. 1996. LC 95-46921. (Illus.). 561p. 99.00 (*1-56053-166-5*) Hanley & Belfus.

Kidney in Plasma Cell Dyscrasias. Ed. by Luigi Minetti. 1988. (Developments in Nephrology Ser.). (C). text 226.50 (*0-89838-385-4*) Kluwer Academic.

Kidney in Pregnancy. Vittorio E. Andreucci. 1985. LC 85-11437. (Topics in Renal Medicine Ser.). text 160.50 (*0-89838-741-8*) Kluwer Academic.

Kidney in Systemic Diseases. Ed. by Shaul G. Massry. 1977. (Contributions to Nephrology Ser.: Vol. 7). (Illus.). 29.75 (*3-8055-2445-5*) S Karger.

Kidney Metabolism & Function. Ed. by R. Dzurik et al. 1986. (Developments in Nephrology Ser.). text 209.50 (*0-89838-749-3*) Kluwer Academic.

Kidney, Proteins & Drugs. Ed. by C. P. Bianchi et al. 1991. (Contributions to Nephrology Ser.: Vol. 83). (Illus.). xii, 276p. 29.75 (*3-8055-5190-8*) S Karger.

Kidney, Proteins & Drugs: An Update. Ed. by C. P. Bianchi et al. 1993. (Contributions to Nephrology Ser.: Vol. 101). (Illus.). x, 270p. 49.75 (*3-8055-5668-3*) S Karger.

Kidney, Small Proteins & Drugs. Ed. by C. P. Bianchi. 1985. (Contributions to Nephrology Ser.: Vol. 42). (Illus.). x, 262p. 29.75 (*3-8055-3913-4*) S Karger.

Kidney Stones: Medical & Surgical Management. Ed. by Frederic L. Coe et al. 1995. LC 95-416. (Illus.). 1,136p. text 320.00 (*0-7817-0263-1*) Lppncott W & W.

Kidney Stones & Renal Calculi: Index of New Information. Edward R. Swienten. 1998. 160p. 57.50 (*0-7883-1704-0*); pap. 47.50 (*0-7883-1705-9*) ABBE Pubs Assn.

Kidney Stones Handbook. Gail Golomb. pap. (*0-09-637060-2*) Arrow Bks.

Kidney Stones Handbook: A Patient's Guide to Hope, Cure & Prevention. Gail Golomb. 1994. LC 95-119584. 192p. pap. 12.95 (*0-9637068-0-2*) Four Geez.

Kidney Today: Selected Topics in Renal Science. Ed. by Geoffrey Merton Berlyne. 1992. (Contributions to Nephrology Ser.: Vol. 100). (Illus.). viii, 296p. 49.75 (*3-8055-5555-5*) S Karger.

Kidney Transplant Rejection: Diagnosis & Treatment. Ed. by Kim Solez. 3rd ed. 1998. LC 98-15516. (Illus.). 680p. text 225.00 (*0-8247-0139-9*) Dekker.

Kidney Transplantation. Peter J. Morris. 4th ed. 1994. (Illus.). 576p. text 175.00 (*0-7216-4557-7*) Saunders.

Kids & Alcohol. Jamie Rattray et al. 1983. 200p. pap. 5.95 (*0-932194-13-3*, 22H93) Health Comm.

Kids & Drugs. Jamie Rattray et al. 1983. 208p. pap. text 5.95 (*0-932194-19-2*, 22H98) Health Comm.

Kids & Smoking. Jamie Rattray et al. 1983. 199p. pap. text 5.95 (*0-932194-14-1*, 22H49) Health Comm.

Kids Breathe Free: A Parent's Guide for Treating Children with Asthma. 1997. LC 97-49990. (Illus.). 32p. pap. 4.40 (*0-939838-46-X*) Pritchett & Hull.

Kid's Guide to E-Mail. Cara J. Stevens et al. 2000. LC 99-76522. (Illus.). 80p. (J). (gr. 3-7). pap. 6.95 (*0-7373-0352-2*, 03522W, Roxbury Pk Juvenile) Lowell Hse Juvenile.

Kids, Herbs, & Health: A Parent's Guide to Natural Remedies. Linda B. White & Sunny Mavor. 1999. LC 98-53519. (Illus.). 256p. pap. 21.95 (*1-883010-53-5*) Interweave.

Kids' Symptoms: From Birth to Teens. William Proctor & Ralph E. Minear. 1992. 352p. (Orig.). pap. 12.50 (*0-380-76228-5*, Avon Bks) Morrow Avon.

Kids Who Care. Robert Vlahakis. 1978. LC 78-60623. pap. 3.95 (*0-917428-06-4*, Dowling College) Global Pubns.

Kids with Celiac Disease: A Family Guide to Raising Happy, Healthy, Gluten-Free Children. Danna Korn. 2001. LC 00-65022. (Illus.). xx, 256p. pap. 17.95 (*1-890627-21-6*) Woodbine House.

Kiefergelenk im Zahnaerztlich-Prothetischen Fall: Eine Anatomisch-Radiographische Untersuchung. A. H. Geering. 1977. (GER., Illus.). 21.00 (*3-8055-2804-3*) S Karger.

Kill As Few Patients As Possible & Fifty-Six Other Essays on How to Be the World's Best Doctor. Arlan Cohn. 10th anniv. ed. 1987. 102p. pap. 9.95 (*0-89815-197-X*) Ten Speed Pr.

Killer Germs. Barry E. Zimmerman & David J. Zimmerman. 1996. LC 95-48235. (Illus.). 256p. pap. 15.95 (*0-8092-3390-8*, 339080, Contemporary) McGraw-Hill Trade.

Killer Germs: Rogue Diseases of the Twenty-First Century. Pete Moore. 2001. (Illus.). 240p. (*1-84222-150-7*) Carlton Bks Ltd GBR. *Dist:* Natl Bk Netwk.

Killers in the Brain: Essays in Science & Technology from the Royal Institution. Ed. by Peter Day. 1999. (Illus.). 184p. text 24.95 (*0-19-850540-X*) OUP.

Killing & Letting Die. Ed. by Bonnie Steinbock & Alastair Norcross. 2nd ed. 1994. LC 94-16793. ix, 431p. 35.00 (*0-8232-1562-8*) Fordham.

Killing & Letting Die. Ed. by Bonnie Steinbock. 2nd ed. 1994. LC 94-16793. ix, 431p. reprint ed. pap. 20.00 (*0-8232-1563-6*) Fordham.

Killing Cancer. Jason Winters. 3rd rev. ed. 1993. 100p. pap. 9.95 (*1-885026-11-0*) Vinton Pubng.

Killing Profession. Louise C. Gitzen. 1992. 177p. 10.00 (*0-9632708-0-X*) L C Gitzen.

Kilovoltage X-Ray Dosimetry for Radiotherapy. Chang-Ming Charlie Ma & Jan P. Seuntjens. 1998. LC 98-89979. (AAPM Proceedings Ser.: No. 11). 309p. text 90.00 (*1-888340-16-9*) AAPM.

Kin Selection in the Japanese Monkey. J. A. Kurland. Ed. by F. S. Szalay. 1977. (Contributions to Primatology Ser.: Vol. 11). (Illus.). 55.75 (*3-8055-2633-4*) S Karger.

Kinanthropometry. No. IV. Ed. by William Duquet & James A. Day. 1993. LC 93-34093. 320p. (C). 125.00 (*0-419-16770-6*, Spon) Routledge.

Kind Relations: A Novel. Robert Liddell et al. 1994. LC 95-122831. 288p. (*0-7206-0947-X*) P Owen Ltd GBR. *Dist:* Dufour.

Kinder-Dips Ed Unnewehr. 1995. 37.95 (*0-387-57018-7*) Spr-Verlag.

Kinderchirurgische Probleme in der paediatrische Praxis. Ed. by M. Bettex & A. Koch. 1980. (Paediatrische Fortbildungskurse fuer die Praxis Ser.: Vol. 49). (Illus.). pap. 35.75 (*3-8055-0232-X*) S Karger.

Kindergarten Is Too Late! Masaru Ibuka. 1980. 6.95 (*0-671-25363-8*, 25363, Fireside) S&S Trade Pap.

Kindergartner with AIDS & the Classroom. Monte L. Betz. 1992. LC 92-101. 261p. pap. 24.95 (*0-934753-61-X*) LRP Pubns.

Kindling, Vol. 4. Ed. by J. A. Wada. 1990. LC 96-2061. (Illus.). 490p. (C). text 156.00 (*0-306-43605-1*, Kluwer Plenum) Kluwer Academic.

Kindling & Synaptic Plasticity: The Legacy of Graham Goddard. Ed. by F. Morrell. 1991. xvi, 304p. 140.50 (*0-8176-3466-5*) Birkhauser.

Kindly Interest: The Men & Women of Concord Hospital & Its School of Nursing. Jill C. Wilson. 1989. LC 89-30560. (Illus.). 160p. 20.00 (*0-914659-41-3*) Phoenix Pub.

Kindly Medicine: Physio-Medicalism in America, 1836-1911. John S. Haller. 1997. LC 97-11030. (Illus.). 232p. 35.00 (*0-87338-577-2*) Kent St U Pr.

Kindred of the Wild: A Book of Animal Life. Charles G. Roberts. 1977. 28.95 (*0-8369-4253-1*, 6062) Ayer.

Kinematics & Dynamics of Machinery. Ed. by Vladimir Stajskal & Michael Valasek. 1996. LC 96-13969. (Mechanical Engineering Ser.: Vol. 106). (Illus.). 512p. text 175.00 (*0-8247-9731-0*) Dekker.

Kinesiology. David Paul Greene & Susan L. Roberts. 1999. LC 98-45273. pap. text 32.95 (*1-55664-416-7*) Mosby Inc.

Kinesiology: Application to Pathological Motion. Gary L. Soderberg. (Illus.). 1986. 378p. text 42.00 (*0-683-07857-7*); 2nd ed. 1997. LC 96-21426. 504p. 49.95 (*0-683-07851-8*) Lppncott W & W.

Kinesiology: Movement in the Context of Activity. David P. Greene & Susan L. Roberts. 1999. (Illus.). 256p. tchr. ed. (*1-55664-477-9*) Mosby Inc.

Kinesiology: Of the Human Body under Normal & Pathological Conditions. Arthur Steindler. fac. ed. 1977. (Illus.). 736p. 133.95 (*0-398-01846-4*) C C Thomas.

Kinesiology: Scientific Basis of Human Motion. Kathryn Luttgens et al. 8th ed. 1992. 704p. (C). text 50.50 net. (*0-697-11632-8*) Brown & Benchmark.

Kinesiology: Scientific Basis of Human Motion. Kathryn Luttgens & Nancy Hamilton. 9th ed. 1996. LC 95-83190. 696p. (C). text, lab manual ed. 76.88 (*0-697-24655-8*) McGrw-H Hghr Educ.

Kinesiology & Its Applications. 1991. lib. bdg. 79.95 (*0-8490-4972-0*) Gordon Pr.

Kinesiology Laboratory Manual for Physical Therapy Assistants. Mary A. Minor et al. 1997. (Illus.). 302p. (C). pap. text 28.95 (*0-8036-0203-0*) Davis Co.

Kinesiology Workbook. Jan F. Perry et al. 2nd ed. 1995. (Illus.). 206p. pap. 25.95 (*0-8036-0046-1*) Davis Co.

Kinesthetic Legacy: The Life & Works of Barbara Clark. Pamela Matt. 1993. (Illus.). 340p. (C). pap. 29.50 (*1-881914-25-9*) C Manuals Trust.

Kinetic Data Analysis: Design & Analysis of Enzyme & Pharmacokinetic Experiments. Ed. by Laszlo Endrenyi. 1981. LC 81-120. 438p. 89.50 (*0-306-40724-8*, Plenum Trade) Perseus Pubng.

Kinetic Drawing System for Family & School: A Handbook. Howard M. Knoff & H. Thompson Prout. 1985. 65p. pap. text 39.95 (*0-87424-208-8*, W-208A) Western Psych.

Kinetic-House-Tree-Person Drawings (K-H-T-P) An Interpretative Manual. Robert C. Burns. 1987. LC 86-26876. 232p. text 33.95 (*0-87630-448-X*) Brunner-Routledge.

Kinetic Models of Trace Element & Mineral Metabolism During Development. Ed. by K. N. Siva Subramanian & Meryl E. Wastney. 1995. LC 95-21093. 419p. 159.95 (*0-8493-4736-X*, 4736) CRC Pr.

Kinetics & Dynamics of Intravenous Anesthetics. Gerald M. Woerlee. 1992. (Developments in Critical Care, Medicine, & Anesthesiology Ser.). 268p. (C). text 171.00 (*0-7923-1506-5*) Kluwer Academic.

Kinetics & Patterns of Necrosis. Ed. by G. Jasmin. 1988. (Methods & Achievements in Experimental Pathology Ser.: Vol. 13). (Illus.). viii, 264p. 207.00 (*3-8055-4668-8*) S Karger.

Kingdom of Dreams. Josephine Schuyler & Phlippa D. Schuyler. 1966. 12.00 (*0-8315-0043-3*) Speller.

Kingdom of Evils: Psychiatric Social Work Presented in One Hundred Case Histories. Elmer E. Southard & Mary C. Jarrett. 1973. LC 73-2417. (Mental Illness & Social Policy; the American Experience Ser.). reprint ed. 47.95 (*0-405-05227-8*) Ayer.

King's American Dispensatory. John King, III. Ed. by Harvey Felter & John U. Lloyd. 1997. 2072p. reprint ed. 285.00 (*1-888483-02-4*) Eclectic Med.

King's Midwife. Nina R. Gelbart. 1998. LC 97-8421. (Illus.). 358p. text 48.00 (*0-520-21036-0*) U CA Pr.

Kinin System. Ed. by Stephen G. Farmer. 1997. LC 97-8628. (Handbook for Immunopharmacology Ser.). (Illus.). 349p. text 99.00 (*0-12-249340-0*) Morgan Kaufmann.

Kinins VA. Ed. by K. Abe et al. 1989. (Advances in Experimental Medicine & Biology Ser.: Vol. 247A). (Illus.). 688p. 130.00 (*0-306-43207-2*, Plenum Trade) Perseus Pubng.

Kinins VB. Ed. by K. Abe et al. 1989. (Advances in Experimental Medicine & Biology Ser.: Vol. 247B). (Illus.). 718p. 130.00 (*0-306-43208-0*, Plenum Trade) Perseus Pubng.

Kirk & Bistner's Handbook of Veterinary Procedures & Emergency Treatment. Stephen I. Bistner & Richard B. Ford. 6th ed. 1994. (Illus.). 912p. pap. text 63.00 (*0-7216-4972-6*) Saunders.

Kirk's Current Veterinary Therapy XII: Small Animal Practice. John D. Bonagura. Ed. by Ray Kersey. 1999. (Illus.). 1435p. text 85.00 (*0-7216-5523-8*) Saunders.

Kiss of Death: Chagas Disease in the Americas. Joseph Bastien. 1998. LC 98-18279. (Illus.). xxiv, 301p. 39.95 (*0-87480-559-7*) U of Utah Pr.

Kistner's Gynecology & Women's Health. Kenneth J. Ryan et al. 7th ed. 1999. LC 99-24042. (Illus.). 760p. (C). text (*0-323-00201-3*) Mosby Inc.

Kitchen of the Family Doctor see Cocina de Medico de Familia

Kitchen Table Wisdom: Stories That Heal. Rachel Naomi Remen. 1997. LC 96-5175. 368p. 14.00 (*1-57322-610-6*, Riverhead Books) Putnam Pub Group.

Klaus Thurau Festschrift. Ed. by M. F. Horster & T. Morgan. 1989. (Journal: Vol. 15, No. 2, 1989). (Illus.). iv, 88p. pap. 43.50 (*3-8055-4897-4*) S Karger.

Klein. Hanna Segal. 1989. 189p. reprint ed. pap. text (*0-946439-69-9*) Karnac Bks GBR. *Dist:* Other Pr LLC.

Kleines Diabetes-Lexikon. K. Bergis. 1988. (GER.). 225p. 49.95 (*0-7859-8271-X*, 3110116200) Fr & Eur.

Kleines Psychologisches Woerterbuch. Christian Michel. (GER.). 39.95 (*0-7859-8368-6*, 3451040549) Fr & Eur.

Kleines Woerterbuch Medizin: English-German. Urban Staff. 1989. 185p. 19.95 (*0-7859-8422-4*, 3541130903) Fr & Eur.

Kleines Worterbuch Medizin. 1989. (ENG & GER.). 185p. lib. bdg. 19.95 (*0-8288-3589-6*, F83080) Fr & Eur.

Kleptomania: The Compulsion to Steal - What Can Be Done? Marcus J. Goldman. 1997. LC 97-66565. 260p. pap. 14.95 (*0-88282-158-X*) New Horizon NJ.

Klinefelter Syndrome: Personal & Professional Guide. Probasco Gibbs. 1999. 100p. pap. 9.95 (*0-932970-97-4*) Prinit Pr.

Klinisch-Pharmakologische Modelle zur Pruefung von Corticoidexterna. H. Wendt & P. J. Frosch. 1982. (Illus.). 64p. pap. 28.75 (*3-8055-3537-6*) S Karger.

Klinische Aspekte des Faktor-XIII-Mangels. 1999. 248p. 56.50 (*3-8055-6864-9*) S Karger.

Klinische Chemie - Theorie, Praxis, Interpretation, 4: Vollstaendig neu Bearbeitete Auflage. Ed. by Jean-Pierre Colombo & Roland Richterich. 1978. (Illus.). 71.50 (*3-8055-2796-9*) S Karger.

***Klinische Liquordiagnostik.** Ed. by Uwe K. Zettl et al. 2001. (GER., Illus.). 352p. 84.00 (*3-11-016846-4*) De Gruyter.

Klinische Oekologie in der Paediatrie: Pediatrics & Ecology. Ed. by A. H. Einhorn & R. P. Zurbruegg. 1974. (Paediatrische Fortbildungskurse fuer die Praxis Ser.: Vol. 38). (Illus.). 201p. 35.75 (*3-8055-1653-3*) S Karger.

Knaurs Lexikon der Modernen Medizin: Knaurs Modern Lexicon of Medicine. Kurt Pollak. 1972. (GER.). 19.95 (*0-8288-6404-7*, M-7519) Fr & Eur.

Knaurs Woerterbuch der Medizin. Georg Narciss. 2nd ed. 1988. (GER.). 574p. 59.95 (*0-7859-8358-9*, 3426263610) Fr & Eur.

Knee: Basic Techniques. Sweeney. 1993. (Illus.). 220p. text 52.00 (*0-397-51181-7*) Lppncott W & W.

Knee: Clinical Applications. A. L. Logan. 1994. LC 93-39114. 192p. pap. 68.00 (*0-8342-0522-X*, 20522) Aspen Pub.

Knee: Form, Function, & Ligament Reconstruction. W. Mueller. 1985. (Illus.). 314p. 268.00 (*0-387-11716-4*) Spr-Verlag.

Knee: Form, Function, Pathology & Treatment. Robert L. Larson & William A. Grana. 1992. (Illus.). 715p. text 155.00 (*0-7216-3495-8*) Saunders.

Knee: Problems & Prevention - A Self-Help Guide. Vivian Grisogono. 1998. (Illus.). 224p. pap. (*0-7195-5538-8*) John Murray GBR. *Dist:* Trafalgar.

Knee & Its Related Structures 1972. (Courtroom Medicine Ser.). ring bd. 535.00 (*0-8205-1252-4*) Bender.

Knee & the Cruciate Ligaments: Anatomy, Biomechanics, Clinical Aspects, Reconstruction, Complications, Rehabilitation. Ed. by R. P. Jakob & H. U. Staubli. Tr. by Terry C. Telger from GER. 1992. LC 92-49767. (Illus.). 640p. 198.00 (*3-540-53818-6*); 637p. 240.00 (*0-387-53818-6*) Spr-Verlag.

Knee Arthroplasty. Ed. by Paul A. Lotke. 1994. LC 93-42856. (Master Techniques in Orthopaedic Surgery Ser.). (Illus.). 400p. text 199.00 (*0-7817-0032-9*) Lppncott W & W.

Knee-High Nutrition. Charles A. Salter & Carlotta S. De Lerma. Ed. by Sheila S. Darst. Date not set. LC 86-83400. (*0-89896-094-0*); pap. 14.95 (*0-89896-096-7*) Larksdale.

Knee Injuries—Index of New Information & Medical Research Bible. Forest P. Wymore. 1994. 150p. 57.50 (*0-7883-0100-4*); pap. 47.50 (*0-7883-0101-2*) ABBE Pubs Assn.

Knee Ligament Rehabilitation. Todd S. Ellenbecker. 2000. LC 99-89460. (Illus.). xvi, 465p. (C). text (*0-443-07534-4*) Church.

Knee Ligaments: Clinical Examination. G. Liorzou. Tr. by D. Finlayson from FRE. 1991. (Illus.). 108p. 158.00 (*0-387-53761-9*) Spr-Verlag.

Knee Ligaments: Structure, Function, Injury, & Repair. Wayne H. Akeson. 2nd ed. 2002. text 139.00 (*0-7817-1817-1*) Lppncott W & W.

Knee Pain: The Self-Help Guide. John Garrett & Rob Reznik. 2000. (Illus.). 268p. pap. 14.95 (*1-57224-194-2*) New Harbinger.

Knee Pain & Disability. Rene Cailliet. 3rd ed. 1991. LC 91-28232. (Pain Ser.). (Illus.). 287p. (C). pap. 23.95 (*0-8036-1622-8*) Davis Co.

Knee Sourcebook. Marc Darrow & Laura O'Hare. 2001. LC 2001-37282. (Illus.). 288p. pap. 14.95 (*0-7373-0544-4*, Contemporary) McGraw-Hill Prof.

Knee Surgery Ed. by Freddie H. Fu et al. 1995. LC 93-28416. (Illus.). 2975p. text 359.00 (*0-683-03389-1*) Lppncott W & W.

Knee Surgery: Complications, Pitfalls & Salvage. M. Mike Malek. 2000. LC 99-40673. (Illus.). 496p. 225.00 (*0-387-98294-9*) Spr-Verlag.

Knidische Medizin Pt. 1: Die Testimonien zur Aeltesten Knidischen Lehre und Analysen Knidischer Schriften im Corpus Hippocraticum. Hermann Grensemann. 1974. (Ars Medica, Sect. 2, Griechisch-Lateinische Medizin Ser.: Vol. 4). 173.10 (*3-11-004141-3*) De Gruyter.

Knife & Gun Club: Scenes from an Emergency Room. Eugene Richards. 1995. LC 88-39302. (Illus.). 240p. pap. 21.00 (*0-87113-624-4*, Atlntc Mnthly) Grove-Atltc.

Knife That Saves: Memoirs of a Lahey Clinic Surgeon. Herbert D. Adams. 1991. (Illus.). xi, 369p. 28.95 (*0-88135-072-9*, Countway Lib Med) Watson Pub Intl.

Knights Hospitallers in England: Being the Report of Prior Phillip De Thame to the Grand Master Elyan De Villanova for A. D. 1338. Philippus De Thame. Ed. by Lambert B. Larking. (Camden Society, London. Publications, First Ser.: No. 65). reprint ed. 75.00 (*0-404-50165-6*) AMS Pr.

Knochenmarkbiopsie. R. Bartl et al. 1984. (Illus.). xvi, 140p. 50.50 (*3-8055-3875-8*) S Karger.

Knock ou le Triomphe de la Medecine. Jules Romains, pseud. 1972. (FRE.). pap. 10.95 (*0-7859-2857-X*, 2070360601) Fr & Eur.

Knocking At the Gate of Life: Healing Exercises from the Official Manual of the People's Republic of China. Tr. by Edward C. Chang from CHI. 2000. LC 00-33574. (Illus.). 256p. pap. 24.95 (*1-57145-662-7*, Laurel Glen Pub) Advantage Pubs.

Knot at the End of Your Rope: Ten Ways to Hold on When You Are Stressed Out. Teresa B. Kindred. 2000. LC 99-13080. 160p. pap. 10.99 (*0-87788-457-9*, H Shaw Pubs) Waterbrook Pr.

Knotted Subject: Hysteria & Its Discontents. Elisabeth Bronfen. 1998. LC 97-45157. (Illus.). 466p. 65.00 (*0-691-01231-8*); pap. 19.95 (*0-691-01230-X*) Princeton U Pr.

Knotted Tongues: Stuttering in History & the Quest for a Cure. Benson Bobrick. Ed. by Deborah Baker. 1996. LC 95-25881. (Kodansha Globe Ser.). (Illus.). 240p. pap. 14.00 (*1-56836-121-1*, Kodansha Globe) Kodansha.

Know the Codes. Patricia D. Salvato & Carol E. Thompson. 1998. (Illus.). pap. 149.95 (*0-9665067-0-7*) Prefer Pub Co.

Know Your Medicines. Pat Blair. 1991. 144p. (C). (*0-86242-100-4*) Age Concern Eng GBR. *Dist:* St Mut.

Know Your Nutrition. Linda Clark. 1984. LC 80-84437. 276p. reprint ed. pap. 4.95 (*0-87983-401-3*, 34013K, Keats Pubng) McGraw-Hill Trade.

Know Your Poisonous Plants, Vol. 1. Wilma R. James. 1973. LC 73-13884. (Know Your Poisonous Plants Ser.: Vol. 1). (Illus.). 99p. pap. 8.95 (*0-87961-012-3*) Naturegraph.

Knowing about Diabetes for Non-Insulin Dependent (Maturity Onset) Diabetics. 2. P. H. Wise. 1983. 320p. pap. (*0-572-02021-X*) W Foulsham GBR. *Dist:* Trans-Atl Phila.

Knowing Feeling. Ed. by Donald L. Nathanson. 1996. LC 95-49392. 448p. 45.00 (*0-393-70214-6*) Norton.

Knowing Feeling: Affect, Script, & Psychotherapy. Ed. by Donald L. Nathanson. 2000. 425p. reprint ed. text 45.00 (*0-7881-9558-1*) DIANE Pub.

Knowing Human Movement. Steven G. Estes & Robert A. Mechikoff. 1999. LC 98-55944. 239p. (C). 50.00 (*0-205-15841-2*, Macmillan Coll) P-H.

Knowing Levels & Developmental Stages. Mark H. Bickhard & R. L. Campbell. 1986. (Contributions to Human Development Ser.: Vol. 16). 148p. 38.50 (*3-8055-4262-3*) S Karger.

Knowing Practice: The Clinical Encounter of Chinese Medicine. Judith Farquhar. 1996. (Studies in Ethnographic Imagination). 260p. (C). pap. text 30.00 (*0-8133-3016-5*) Westview.

Knowing What the Problem Is & Getting It Solved: State Reform in Long-Term Care. Harry Nelson. 1994. 28p. (Orig.). pap. text (*0-9629870-3-4*) Milbank Memorial.

Knowing Woman: A Feminine Psychology. Irene Claremont de Castillejo. 1973. LC 72-80470. 12.00 (*0-913430-01-3*) C G Jung Foun.

Knowing Woman: A Feminine Psychology. Irene C. De Castillejo. 1997. 192p. reprint ed. pap. 14.95 (*1-57062-204-3*) Shambhala Pubns.

Knowledge about Care & Caring: State of the Art & Future Developments. Patricia Benner et al. Ed. by Joanne S. Stevenson & Toni Tripp-Reimer. 1990. 165p. (Orig.). (C). pap. 14.50 (*1-55810-052-0*, G-177, Am Acad Nursing) Am Nurses Pub.

Knowledge & Authority in the Psychoanalytic Relationship. Ed. by Owen Renik. 1998. LC 97-29287. (Currents in the Quarterly Ser.: Vol. 2). 280p. pap. 40.00 (*0-7657-0139-1*) Aronson.

Knowledge & Decisions in Health Telematics: The Next Decade. Ed. by Pedro Barahona & J. P. Christensen. 1994. LC 93-8115. (Studies in Health Technology & Informatics: Vol. 12). 237p. 95.00 (*90-5199-152-5*) IOS Press.

Knowledge & Memory: The Real Story. Ed. by Robert S. Wyer, Jr. 1995. (Advances in Social Cognition Ser.: Vol. 8). 248p. text 49.95 (*0-8058-1445-0*) L Erlbaum Assocs.

Knowledge & the Scholarly Medical Traditions. Ed. by Don Bates. 1995. (Illus.). 383p. (C). LC 96-7762. text 74.95 (*0-521-48071-X*); pap. text 27.95 (*0-521-49975-5*) Cambridge U Pr.

Knowledge-Based Medical Records for Patients with HIV Infection. 1995. lib. bdg. 260.75 (*0-8490-8352-4*) Gordon Pr.

Knowledge Based Systems in Medicine: Methods, Applications & Evaluation: Proceedings of the Workshop "System Engineering in Medicine" Maastricht, March 16-18, 1989. Ed. by J. L. Talmon et al. 1991. (Lecture Notes in Medical Informatics: Vol. 47). 330p. 67.00 (*0-387-55011-9*) Spr-Verlag.

Knowledge, Concepts & Categories. Ed. by Koen Lamberts & David R. Shanks. 1997. LC 96-52838. (Studies in Cognition). (Illus.). 384p. pap. 37.95 (*0-262-62118-5*) MIT Pr.

Knowledge Coupling: New Premises & New Tools for Medical Care & Education. L. L. Weed. Ed. by M. H. Ball & Kathryn J. Hannah. 1995. (Computers in Health Care Ser.). (Illus.). 362p. 74.95 (*0-387-97537-3*) Spr-Verlag.

Knowledge, Difference & Power: Essays Inspired by Women's Ways of Knowing. Nancy Goldberger et al. 1998. 496p. pap. 17.00 (*0-465-03733-X*) Basic.

Knowledge Engineering in Health Informatics. Homer R. Warner et al. 1997. LC 96-44233. (Computers & Medicine Ser.). 262p. 71.95 (*0-387-94901-1*) Spr-Verlag.

Knowledge for Health Care Practice: A Guide to Using Research Evidence. Sarah J. Brown. Ed. by Thomas Eoyang. 1999. LC 98-27551. xiv, 256p. pap. text 25.00 (*0-7216-7803-3*) Saunders.

Knowledge for Nursing Practice. Barbara Vaughan & Kate Robinson. 1992. 256p. pap. text 42.00 (*0-7506-0414-X*) Buttrwrth-Heinemann.

Knowledge Gap: What Medicaid Beneficiaries Understand - & What They Don't - about Managed Care. Christine Molnar et al. 1996. 98p. (Orig.). mass mkt. 10.00 (*0-88156-200-9*) Comm Serv Soc NY.

Knowledge into Action: A Guide to Research Utilization. George P. Cernada. 1982. (Community Health Education Monographs: Vol. 1). 168p. pap. text 23.95 (*0-89503-031-4*) Baywood Pub.

Knowledge of Illness in a Sepik Society: A Study of the Gnau, New Guinea. Gilbert Lewis. 1975. (London School of Economics Monographs on Social Anthropology: No. 52). (Illus.). 379p. (C). text (*0-485-19552-6*) Athlone Pr GBR. *Dist:* Transaction Pubs, Humanities.

Knowledge, Power, & Practice: The Anthropology of Medicine & Everyday Life. Ed. by Shirley Lindenbaum & Margaret M. Lock. 1993. LC 92-28208. (Comparative Studies of Health Systems & Medical Care: Vol. 36). text 58.00 (*0-520-07784-9*); pap. text 22.50 (*0-520-07785-7*) U CA Pr.

Knowledge Representation in Medicine & Clinical Behavioural Science. L. J. Kohout & W. Bandler. 1986. LC 86-14032. (Abacus Bks.). (Illus.). xii, 212p. text 171.00 (*0-85626-442-3*) Gordon & Breach.

Knowledge Structures. Ed. by James A. Galambos et al. 1986. 296p. text 59.95 (*0-89859-816-8*) L Erlbaum Assocs.

Knowledge to Care: A Handbook for Care Assistants. Ed. by Christine A. McMahon & Joan Harding. 1993. LC 93-2082. 384p. pap. 32.95 (*0-632-03585-4*) Blackwell Sci.

Knowledge Utilization in Residential Child & Youth Care Practice. Ed. by Jerome Beker & Zvi C. Eisikovits. 1991. pap. 14.50 (*0-87868-427-1*) Child Welfare.

Koch Centennial Memorial. Ed. by Gareth M. Green et al. 1982. 136p. text 12.50 (*0-915116-17-0*) Am Lung Assn.

Kochar's Concise Textbook of Medicine. Ed. by Kesavan Kutty et al. 3rd ed. 1998. LC 97-42621. (Illus.). 800p. pap. 45.00 (*0-683-04798-1*) Lppncott W & W.

Kohabitations-und Fertilitaets-Stoerungen: Ein Leitfaden fuer die aerztliche Praxis. W. Nikolowski et al. 1977. (Illus.). 17.50 (*3-8055-2682-2*) S Karger.

Kohlberg Legacy for the Helping Professions. Lisa Kuhmerker. 2nd ed. 1994. LC 90-25862. 234p. (Orig.). pap. 21.95 (*0-9637034-1-2*) Religious Educ.

Kohut, Loewald & the Postmoderns: A Comparative Study of Self & Relationship. Judith Guss Teicholz. 1999. LC 98-47700. (Psychoanalytic Inquiry Book Ser.: No. 18). 320p. 47.50 (*0-88163-260-0*) Analytic Pr.

Kohut Seminars: On Self Psychology & Psychotherapy with Adolescents & Young Adults. Ed. by Miriam Elson. 1987. (Professional Bks.). 318p. 32.95 (*0-393-70041-0*) Norton.

Kohut's Legacy: Contributions to Self Psychology. Ed. by Paul E. Stepansky & Arnold Goldberg. 1992. 280p. reprint ed. pap. text 27.50 (*0-88163-162-0*) Analytic Pr.

Kolff, Willem J. Festschrift, Journal: Nephron, Vol. 36, No. 3, 1984. Ed. by R. L. Stephen. 1984. (Illus.). 52p. pap. 45.25 (*3-8055-3845-6*) S Karger.

Kollision von Gefuehl und Verstand. Gabriele Jilg. 1983. (European University Studies: Ser. 1, Vol. 648). (GER.). 204p. 36.00 (*3-261-05095-0*) P Lang Pubng.

Kombinationtherapie Insulin-Sulfonylharnstoff. Ed. by W. Bachmann & H. Mehnert. 1984. (Illus.). viii, 208p. 56.75 (*3-8055-3850-2*) S Karger.

Kombucha: Healthy Beverage & Natural Remedy from the Far East. Gunther W. Frank. 10th ed. 1995. (Illus.). 150p. pap. (*3-85068-337-0*) Ennsthaler.

Kombucha: How to & What It's All About. Alana Pascal & Lynne VanderKar. Ed. by Anina Maurier. 1995. LC 95-90065. (Illus.). 128p. (Orig.). pap. text 12.95 (*0-9645352-0-3*) Van der Kar Pr.

Kombucha Rediscovered! A Guide to the Medicinal Benefits of an Ancient Healing Tea. Klaus Kaufmann. 1995. LC 95-910814. (Illus.). 96p. pap. 10.95 (*0-920470-64-5*) Alive Bks.

Kompendium der Anaesthesiologie. P. Hoffmann & B. Schockenhoff. 1997. (GER., Illus.). 200p. (Orig.). pap. text 42.95 (*3-11-014158-2*) De Gruyter.

Kompendium der Inneren Medizin. U. Sprandel & F. Stark. 2nd rev. ed. 1990. xvi, 430p. pap. 25.25 (*3-8055-5018-9*) S Karger.

Kompendium der Medizinischen Psychologie. H. Feldmann. 1983. (Illus.). viii, 264p. pap. 17.50 (*3-8055-3673-9*) S Karger.

Kompendium der Psychiatrie und Psychotherapie: Bergruendet Von Th. Spoerri Lo. Auflage. Ed. by Harald J. Freyberger & Rolf-Dieter Stieglitz. 10th rev. ed. 1995. (Illus.). xvi, 578p. pap. 35.00 (*3-8055-6173-3*) S Karger.

Kompendium der Schutzimpfungen. M. Schaer. 4th rev. ed. 1991. (Illus.). x, 116p. pap. 25.25 (*3-8055-5257-2*) S Karger.

Kontaktlinsenvademekum. Ed. by H. Streitenberg. 2nd ed. 1988. (Illus.). x, 208p. pap. 28.75 (*3-8055-4753-6*) S Karger.

Kontinuitat und Innovation - 21 Jahre Universitare Chirurgie in Bochum. Ed. by R. Smektala. 2000. (Chirurgische Gastroenterologie Ser.: Band 15, suppl. 1). (GER.). 64p. pap. 36.50 (*3-8055-7036-8*) S Karger.

Kontrastmittel in der Kinderradiologie. Ed. by H. J. Kaufman. 1986. 118p. 52.25 (*3-8055-4439-1*) S Karger.

Konzeptualisierung Eines Schulpsychologischen Dienstes: Strukturelle, Methodische und Inhaltliche Aspekte der Psychologischen Intervention. Peter Gutzwiller. 1998. (Illus.). 202p. pap. 35.95 (*3-906759-46-6*) P Lang Pubng.

Korakenes: Medical Home Remedies & Beauty Hints of Greece. Joan A. Saetes. 1990. (Illus.). 75p. (Orig.). pap. 10.00 (*0-9646038-0-2*) Saetes & Saetes.

Korean Elderly Women in America: Everyday Life, Health & Illness. Keum-Young C. Pang. 1991. (Immigrant Communities & Ethnic Minorities in the U. S. & Canada Ser.: No. 69). 59.50 (*0-404-19479-6*) AMS Pr.

Koss' Diagnostic Cytology & Its Histopathologic, In Two Volumes. Leopold G. Koss. 4th ed. 1992. (Illus.). 1,824p. text 299.00 (*1-397-51049-7*) Lppncott W & W.

***Kozier & Erb's Techniques in Clinical Nursing.** Audrey Berman. 5th ed. 2001. LC 2001-34047. 700p. pap. 62.67 (*0-13-028157-3*, Prentice Hall) P-H.

Krankheiten des Hoheren Alters und Ihre Heilung Carl Canstatt. Ed. by Robert J. Kastenbaum. 1979. LC 78-22187. (Aging & Old Age Ser.). (GER., Illus.). reprint ed. lib. bdg. 53.95 (*0-405-11805-8*) Ayer.

Krause's Food, Nutrition, & Diet Therapy. Ed. by L. Kathleen Mahan & Sylvia Escott-Stump. 9th ed. 1996. (Illus.). tchr. ed. (*0-7216-5836-9*) Saunders.

Kreislauf des Jugendlichen bei Arbeit und Sport. H. Mellerowicz. 2nd ed. 1980. (Illus.). viii, 60p. pap. 14.00 (*3-8055-1140-X*) S Karger.

Kremers & Urdang's History of Pharmacy. Glenn Sonnedecker. 4th ed. 1986. 571p. (C). reprint ed. pap. text 25.00 (*0-931292-17-4*) Am Inst Hist Pharm.

Kristeva Reader. Julia Kristeva. Ed. by Toril Moi. 1986. LC 86-11706. 327p. pap. text 22.00 (*0-231-06325-3*) Col U Pr.

Kritische Bewertung aktueller Therapiemassnahmen in der Intensivmedizin. Ed. by J. Eckart. 1984. (Beitraege zur Intensiv und Notfallmedizin Ser.: Vol. 2). (Illus.). viii, 300p. pap. 87.00 (*3-8055-3763-8*) S Karger.

Krusen's Handbook of Physical Medicine & Rehabilitation. Frederic J. Kottke & Justus F. Lehmann. 4th ed. 1990. 1168p. text 158.00 (*0-7216-2985-7*) Saunders.

Kuby Immunology. Goldsby et al. 5th ed. 2003. text (*0-7167-4335-3*) W H Freeman.

Kuenstlerische Therapie see Fundamentals of Artistic Therapy: The Nature & Tasks of Painting Therapy

Kuenstliche Ernaehrung - Indikationen, Monitoring, Komplikationen, Therapie: Indirekte Kalorimetrie, Stabile Isotope. Ed. by G. Wolfram et al. 1990. (Beitraege zur Infusionstherapie und Klinische Ernaehrung Ser.: Vol. 25). (Illus.). 456p. 108.75 (*3-8055-5097-9*) S Karger.

Kuenstliche Ernaehrung zu Hause. Ed. by S. Kolb & D. Sailer. 1986. (Beitraege zur Infusionstherapie und Klinische Ernaehrung Ser.: Vol. 14). (Illus.). 264p. 68.75 (*3-8055-4281-X*) S Karger.

Kuhlman-Binet Test for Children of Pre-School Age, Vol. 2. Florence L. Goodenough. 1973. LC 73-9226. 146p. reprint ed. lib. bdg. 48.00 (*0-8371-6990-9*, CWGT, Greenwood Pr) Greenwood.

Kunst Spirituellen Heilens see Art of Spiritual Healing: Chakra & Energy Workbook

Kunst und Sehen: Eine Psychologie des Schopeferischen Auges. Rudolf Arnheim. 2nd ed. 1978. (Illus.). (C). 55.40 (*3-11-006682-3*) De Gruyter.

Kunst und Wissenschaft der Goettlichen Ganzheit. Herbert L. Beierle. 1981. pap. 20.00 (*0-940480-13-1*) UNIPress.

Kurdi I. V. Antibiotic Handbook. William J. Kurdi. Ed. by Kevin J. Kurdi. 1995. pap. 19.95 (*0-937142-01-8*) Med Nurs Educ.

Kurt Goldstein Reader: The Shaping of Neuropsychology. Kurt Goldstein. Ed. by R. W. Rieber. 1986. LC 78-22720. 32.50 (*0-404-60868-X*) AMS Pr.

Kurzes Lehrbuch der Organischen Chemie. Bernhard Schrader. 1985. (GER.). xii, 368p. pap. 36.95 (*3-11-010238-2*) De Gruyter.

Kynurenine & Serotonin Pathways: Progress in Tryptophan Research. Ed. by Robert Schwarcz et al. 1991. (Advances in Experimental Medicine & Biology Ser.: Vol. 294). (Illus.). 736p. (C). text 198.00 (*0-306-43929-8*, Kluwer Plenum) Kluwer Academic.

L

L-Arginine: Biological Aspects & Clinical Application. Oleg Eremin. 1997. LC 96-16764. (Medical Intelligence Unit Ser.). 161p. 99.00 (*1-57059-348-5*) Landes Bioscience.

L-Carnitine. Brian Leibovitz. 1999. (Good Health Guides). 48p. pap. 3.95 (*0-87983-962-7*, 39627K, Keats Pubng) McGraw-Hill Trade.

L-Carnitine & Its Role in Medicine: From Function to Therapy. Ed. by R. Ferrari et al. 1992. (Illus.). 433p. text 136.00 (*0-12-253940-0*) Acad Pr.

L-Glutamine & Its Uses. 1996. lib. bdg. 250.75 (*0-8490-5893-7*) Gordon Pr.

L-Tryptophan: Current Prospects in Medicine & Drug Safety. Ed. by Walter Kochen & Hans Steinhart. 1994. LC 94-16828. x, 458p. (C). lib. bdg. 306.15 (*3-11-013673-2*) De Gruyter.

La Mettrie: Medicine, Philosophy, & Enlightenment. Kathleen Wellman. 1992. LC 91-23992. 358p. text 42.95 (*0-8223-1204-2*) Duke.

Laaketieteen Sanakirja. Niilo Pesonen & E. Ponteva. 8th ed. 1987. (ENG, FIN, FRE & SWE.). 525p. 250.00 (*0-8288-1886-X*, M9984) Fr & Eur.

Laam in the Treatment of Opiate Addiction: A Treatment Improvement Protocal. Ed. by Sandra Clunies. 1999. 66p. (C). pap. text 20.00 (*0-7881-7592-0*) DIANE Pub.

Lab Assessment of Nutritional Status. Mary Litchford. 1998. 119p. spiral bd. 110.00 (*1-879575-82-5*) Acad Med Sys.

Lab Manual for Bailey & Scott's Diagnostic Microbiology. Beverly P. Gobat & Scott. 9th ed. 1998. (Illus.). 224p. (C). (gr. 13). pap. text, wbk. ed., lab manual ed. 22.00 (*0-8151-5034-2*, 23837) Mosby Inc.

Lab Packet for 100-Level A&P: Dual Semester Version. Duane P. Hill. 1999. (Illus.). 154p. (C). pap. 45.00 (*0-9674988-0-5*) Archipelago Pubg.

Lab Packet for 100-Level A&P: Semester 1 Version. Duane P. Hill. 1999. (Illus.). 73p. (C). pap. 25.00 (*0-9674988-1-3*) Archipelago Pubg.

Lab Packet for 100-Level A&P: Semester 2 Version. Duane P. Hill. 1999. (Illus.). 79p. (C). pap. 25.00 (*0-9674988-2-1*) Archipelago Pubg.

Lab Science Basics. Linne. 4th ed. 1999. text 26.00 (*0-323-00759-7*) Mosby Inc.

Lab Tests & Diagnose Procedure. Jane Vincent Corbett. 5th ed. 1999. LC 99-52568. (Illus.). 832p. pap. 34.96 (*0-8385-5588-8*) P-H.

Lab Volt Lab Manual. Steve Herman. 2nd ed. 1998. 416p. pap., lab manual ed. 21.95 (*0-8273-8552-8*) Delmar.

Labat's Regional Anesthesia: Techniques & Clinical Applications. John Adriani. 4th ed. 1985. (Modern Concepts of Medicine Ser.). (Illus.). 748p. 75.00 (*0-87527-187-1*) Green.

Label Reader's Pocket Dictionary of Food Additives. Mike Lapchick. 1992. 72p. (Orig.). pap. 2.95 (*0-9632015-3-0*) Timberline Pr.

Label Reader's Pocket Dictionary of Food Additives. Mike Lapchick & Cindy Appleseth. 1993. 128p. (Orig.). pap. 4.95 (*1-56561-027-X*) Wiley.

Labeling of Home-Use in Vitro Testing Products: Approved Guideline (1996) Contrib. by Rosanne M. Savol. 1996. 75.00 (*1-56238-299-3*, GP14-A) NCCLS.

Labor among Primitive Peoples, Showing the Development of the Obstetric Science of Today. George J. Engelmann. LC 75-23705. (Illus.). reprint ed. 47.50 (*0-404-13257-X*) AMS Pr.

Labor & Birth: A Guide for You. Linda Todd. 1998. (Illus.). 52p. 3.00 (*0-934024-03-0*) Intl Childbirth.

Labor & Delivery: The Proceedings of the 2nd World Congress on Labor & Delivery, May 1997, Rome, Italy. Ed. by Ermelando V. Cosmi. 1998. (Illus.). 586p. lib. bdg. 88.95 (*1-85070-973-4*, Parthenon Pbng) CRC Pr.

Labor & Women's Nutrition: A Study of Energy Expenditure, Fertility & Nutritional Status in Ghana. CFNPP Staff et al. 1993. (Working Papers). (C). pap. 7.00 (*1-56401-137-2*) Cornell Food.

Labor of Love: Mothers Share the Joy of Childbirth. Judith Zimmer. 1997. LC 96-35910. 242p. pap. 14.95 (*0-471-15703-1*) Wiley.

Labor of Love: The Perfect Pregnancy Planner. Janet Bartlett & Barbara McHale. 1993. 65p. spiral bd. 7.95 (*0-9629092-0-3*) Heart-Bound Bks.

Labor Progress Handbook: Early Interventions to Prevent & Treat Dystocia. Penny Simkin et al. 2000. LC 99-25452. (Illus.). pap. 29.95 (*0-632-05281-3*) Blackwell Sci.

Labor Support Forms: A Guide to Doula Charting. Cheri B. Grant. Ed. by Dana Blue. 1994. 45p. (C). stu. ed. 29.95 (*0-9640082-0-3*) M & W Prods.

Laboratories. 1992. (*0-86022-385-X*) Build Servs Info Assn GBR. *Dist:* St Mut.

Laboratoriumsdiagnostik: Normalbereich der Ergebnisse und Interpretation Abnormer Befunde. Ed. by E. Deutsch et al. 3rd ed. 1991. (Illus.). x, 1168p. 71.50 (*3-8055-5487-7*) S Karger.

Laboratory-Acquired Infections. Christopher Herbert Collins & D. A. Kennedy. 4th ed. 1999. LC 98-32458. 336p. (*0-7506-4023-5*) E A GBR. *Dist:* OUP.

Laboratory-Acquired Infections: History, Incidence, Causes, & Prevention. C. H. Collins. 3rd ed. 1993. LC 92-45169. (Illus.). 274p. text 75.00 (*0-7506-0642-8*) Buttrwrth-Heinemann.

Laboratory Activities for Therapeutic Modalities. Sara D. Brown & Chad Starkey. 2nd ed. 1998. (Illus.). 170p. pap. 23.95 (*0-8036-0353-3*) Davis Co.

Laboratory Anatomy of the Cat. Robert B. Chiasson & William J. Radke. 1995. LC 94-79883. 208p. (C). spiral bd. 39.06 (*0-697-24926-3*, WCB McGr Hill) McGrw-H Hghr Educ.

Laboratory Anatomy of the Cat. Robert B. Chiasson & Ernest Booth. 8th ed. 1988. 160p. (C). text 23.50 net. (0-697-04934-5, WCB McGr Hill) McGrw-H Hghr Educ.

Laboratory Anatomy of the Fetal Pig. Theron O. Odlaug & Robert B. Chiasson. 10th ed. 1994. 160p. (C). (gr. 11-12). spiral bd. 17.50 (0-697-15984-1, WCB McGr Hill) McGrw-H Hghr Educ.

Laboratory Anatomy of the Fetal Pig. Theron O. Odlaug et al. 11th ed. 1996. LC 96-61077. 176p. (C). spiral bd. 39.06 (0-697-33324-8, WCB McGr Hill) McGrw-H Hghr Educ.

Laboratory Anatomy of the Mink. David Klingener. 2nd ed. 1979. (Laboratory Anatomy Ser.). 64p. (C). spiral bd. (0-697-04629-X, WCB McGr Hill) McGrw-H Hghr Educ.

Laboratory Anatomy of the Pigeon. Robert B. Chiasson. 3rd ed. 1984. (Laboratory Anatomy Ser.). 84p. (C). spiral bd. 39.06 (0-697-04927-2) McGrw-H Hghr Educ.

Laboratory Anatomy of the Rabbit. Charles A. McLaughlin & Robert B. Chiasson. 3rd ed. 1990. (Laboratory Anatomy Ser.). 124p. (C). spiral bd. 39.06 (0-697-04931-0) McGrw-H Hghr Educ.

Laboratory & Clinical Dental Materials. Karl F. Leinfelder & Duane F. Taylor. Ed. by Douglas V. Moor. 3rd ed. 1982. (Dental Laboratory Technology Manuals Ser.). xiii, 202p. (C). pap. 34.95 (0-8078-7906-1) U of NC Pr.

Laboratory & Diagnostic Procedures with Nursing Diagnoses. Jane Vincent Corbett. 4th ed. 1996. LC 95-36448. 832p. (C). pap. text 43.00 (0-8385-5595-0, A5595-2) Appleton & Lange.

Laboratory & Diagnostic Test Handbook. M.K. Gaedeke. 1995. LC 95-19475. 864p. (C). pap. text 33.75 (0-8053-1359-1) Benjamin-Cummings.

Laboratory & Diagnostic Tests. Joyce L. Kee. 5th ed. 1998. LC 98-20408. 816p. (C). pap. 35.15 (0-8385-5596-9) P-H.

Laboratory & Diagnostic Tests: A Pocket Guide. Mary E. McMorrow & Louise Malarkey. Ed. by Thomas Eoyang. 1997. LC 97-41310. (Illus.). 480p. pap. 19.95 (0-7216-7303-1) Saunders.

Laboratory & Radiologic Tests for Primary Eye Care. Gail Burden & Steven A. Bryant. 1996. LC 96-18185. 252p. pap. text 44.99 (0-7506-9755-5) Buttrwrth-Heinemann.

Laboratory Animal Endocrinology: Hormonal Action, Control Mechanisms & Interactions with Drugs. David D. Woodman. 1997. LC 97-11248. 576p. 240.00 (0-471-97262-2) Wiley.

Laboratory Animal Houses. 1991. (0-86022-292-6) Build Servs Info Assn GBR. *Dist:* St Mut.

Laboratory Animal Science: Handbook on the Humane Use & Care of Animals in Research. Ed. by L. F. Van Zutphen et al. 1993. LC 93-7467. 404p. pap. 92.00 (0-444-81487-6) Elsevier.

Laboratory Assistant. Jack Rudman. 1994. (Career Examination Ser.: C-1879). reprint ed. pap. 27.95 (0-8373-1879-3) Nat Learn.

Laboratory Assistant (Bacteriology) Jack Rudman. 1994. (Career Examination Ser.: C-431). pap. 27.95 (0-8373-0431-8) Nat Learn.

Laboratory Basis for Anesthesiology. G. Dal Santo. 1993. 764p. text (1-57235-009-1) Piccin Nuova ITA. *Dist:* Scholium Intl.

Laboratory Biosafety Manual. 2nd ed. 1993. (CHI, ENG, FRE & SPA.). xi, 133p. pap. text 26.00 (92-4-154450-3, 1152213) World Health.

Laboratory Data & Patient Care. Ed. by P. L. Kerkhof & M. P. Van Dieijen-Visser. 1988. LC 87-35820. (Illus.). 190p. 55.00 (0-306-42800-8, Plenum Trade) Perseus Pubng.

Laboratory Decontamination & Destruction of Carcinogens in Laboratory Wastes: Some Aromatic Amines & 4-Nitrobiphenyl. Ed. by M. Castegnaro et al. 1985. (IARC Scientific Publications Ser.: No. 64). 100p. pap. 12.95 (0-19-723064-4) OUP.

Laboratory Decontamination & Destruction of Carcinogens in Laboratory Wastes: Some Polycyclic Heterocyclic Hydrocarbons. Ed. by M. Castegnaro et al. 1992. (IARC Scientific Publications Ser.: No. 114). (Illus.). 58p. pap. text 20.00 (92-832-2114-1) OUP.

Laboratory Design: Proposed Guideline (1994) Contrib. by Pennell C. Painter. 1994. 85.00 (1-56238-246-2, GP18-P) NCCLS.

Laboratory Diagnosis in Chiropractic Care. David J. Wickes. 1994. 400p. (0-683-09041-0) Lppncott W & W.

Laboratory Diagnosis in Neonatal Calf & Pig Diarrhea: Current Topics in Veterinary Medicine & Animal Science, No. 13. Ed. by P. W. De Leeuw & P. A. Guinee. 1981. 210p. text 101.50 (90-247-2527-5) Kluwer Academic.

Laboratory Diagnosis of Diseases Caused by Toxic Agents. F. William Sunderman. 1970. LC 77-96992. (Illus.). 610p. 32.50 (0-87527-079-4) Green.

Laboratory Diagnosis of Endocrine Diseases. F. William Sunderman. 1971. LC 72-171949. (Illus.). 712p. 37.50 (0-87527-080-8) Green.

Laboratory Diagnosis of Group A Streptococcal Infections. Dwight R. Johnson et al. 1997. (Illus.). 111p. (Orig.). pap. 28.80 (92-4-154495-3, 1150441) Am Soc Clinical.

Laboratory Diagnosis of Infectious Diseases. Ed. by A. Balows et al. 1988. (Illus.). 1101p. 425.00 (0-387-96755-9) Spr-Verlag.

Laboratory Diagnosis of Infectious Diseases: Principles & Practice, Vol. 2. Ed. by Edwin H. Lennette et al. 1988. (Illus.). 961p. 360.00 (0-387-96756-7) Spr-Verlag.

Laboratory Diagnosis of Kidney Diseases. F. William Sunderman. 1970. LC 73-76164. (Illus.). 604p. 29.50 (0-87527-077-8) Green.

Laboratory Diagnosis of Livestock Abortion. Clyde A. Kirkbride. 3rd ed. 1990. LC 90-9676. (Illus.). 274p. (C). pap. text 49.95 (0-8138-1593-2) Iowa U Pr.

Laboratory Diagnosis of Selected Inborn Errors of Metabolism, 4. Vicky A. LeGrys. 1984. LC 83-22941. (Methods in Laboratory Medicine Ser.: Vol. 4). 154p. 58.00 (0-275-91441-0, C1441, Praeger Pubs) Greenwood.

Laboratory Diagnosis of Viral Infections. Ed. by Edwin H. Lennette. 2nd exp. rev. ed. 1991. (Illus.). 800p. text 215.00 (0-8247-8585-1) Dekker.

Laboratory Diagnosis of Viral Infections Edwin H. Lennette & Thomas F. Smith. 3rd exp. rev. ed. 1999. LC 99-22924. (Illus.). 880p. text 195.00 (0-8247-1952-2) Dekker.

Laboratory Diagnostic Procedures in the Rheumatic Diseases. Ed. by Alan S. Cohen. 3rd rev. ed. 1985. (Illus.). 416p. text 99.00 (0-8089-1737-4, 790879, Grune & Strat) Harcrt Hlth Sci Grp.

Laboratory Equipment Markets: A Detailed Database on a 25 Billion Dollar Market. Market Intelligence Staff. 1992. 270p. 995.00 (1-56753-082-6) Frost & Sullivan.

Laboratory Exercises for Competency in Respiratory Care. Thomas J. Butler et al. 1998. LC 97-41975. (Illus.). 577p. pap. 51.95 (0-8036-0248-0) Davis Co.

Laboratory Exercises for Psychology 132. Ronald Growney. 1993. 53p. (C). text, stu. ed. 10.56 (1-56870-050-4) RonJon Pub.

Laboratory Exercises in Auditory Evoked Potentials. John A. Ferraro. 1997. LC 96-52550. 192p. pap., lab manual ed. 39.95 (1-56593-698-1, 1356) Thomson Learn.

Laboratory Exercises in Human Anatomy with Cat Dissections. Gerard J. Tortora. 3rd ed. 1993. (Illus.). 432p. (C). pap. text, lab manual ed. 54.00 (0-02-421021-8, Macmillan Coll) P-H.

Laboratory Exercises in Medical Microbiology. Robert Pollack et al. 1992. (Illus.). 172p. (C). pap. text, stu. ed. 18.25 (1-878045-15-6) Whittier Pubns.

Laboratory Exercises in Respiratory Care. Cynthia Shoup & Terrance Gilmore. 3rd ed. 1988. (Illus.). 622p. (C). (gr. 13). pap. text 37.95 (0-8016-4328-7, 04328) Mosby Inc.

***Laboratory Guide to Human Anatomy.** Radke. 2001. LC 2001-44409. (Illus.). 416p. pap. 41.95 (0-471-41413-1) Wiley.

Laboratory Guide to In Vitro Transcription. Felipe Sierra. 1990. (Biomethods Ser.: Vol. 2). 165p. 96.50 (0-8176-2357-4) Birkhauser.

Laboratory Haematology. Ed. by Israel Chanarin. 1989. (Illus.). 464p. text (0-443-03343-9) Church.

Laboratory Hamsters. Ed. by G. L. Van Hoosier, Jr. & Charles W. McPherson. 1987. (American College of Laboratory Animal Medicine Ser.). 456p. text 146.00 (0-12-714165-0) Acad Pr.

Laboratory Handbook of Dermatophytes: A Clinical Guide & Laboratory Manual of Dermatophytes & Other Filamentous Fungi from Skin, Hair & Nails. Julius Kane et al. 1997. LC 97-23344. (Illus.). 400p. text, lab manual ed. 129.95 (0-89863-157-2) Star Pub CA.

Laboratory Handbook of Medical Mycology. Michael R. McGinnis. 1980. text 104.00 (0-12-482850-7) Acad Pr.

Laboratory Helper (Men) Jack Rudman. 1994. (Career Examination Ser.: C-446). pap. 23.95 (0-8373-0446-6) Nat Learn.

Laboratory Helper (Women) Jack Rudman. 1994. (Career Examination Ser.: C-447). pap. 23.95 (0-8373-0447-4) Nat Learn.

Laboratory Histopathology. Woods. 1994. text 210.00 (0-443-04912-2) Saunders.

Laboratory Immunology & Serology. Zane. 1999. (Illus.). 416p. pap. text 34.95 (0-7216-5002-3) Saunders.

Laboratory Immunology & Serology. Neville J. Bryant. 3rd ed. 1992. pap. text 47.00 (0-7216-4212-8) Saunders.

Laboratory in Clinical Medicine. Charles H. Halsted & James A. Halsted. 2nd ed. 1981. (Illus.). 1083p. text 165.00 (0-7216-4479-1) Saunders.

Laboratory Instrumention. Ed. by Mary C. Haven et al. 4th ed. 1994. 512p. pap. 54.95 (0-442-01520-8, VNR) Wiley.

Laboratory Instruments & Data Management Systems: Design of Software User Interfaces & End-User Software Systems Validation, Operation, & Monitoring; Approved Guideline (1994) Contrib. by Emery J. Stephans. 1995. 75.00 (1-56238-284-5, GP19-A) NCCLS.

Laboratory Investigation of Liver Disease. Johnson & I. G. MacFarlane. 1989. (Illus.). 320p. pap. text (0-7020-1376-5) Bailliere Tindall.

Laboratory Investigations in Cell & Molecular Biology. Allyn Bregman. 3rd rev. ed. 1996. LC 95-54168. 336p. pap. 53.95 (0-471-14809-1) Wiley.

Laboratory Manual - Kinesiology & Neurophysiology. Barbara E. Gench & M. Hinson. 1993. (C). stu. ed. 20.04 (1-56870-081-4) RonJon Pub.

Laboratory Manual for Animal Technicians. Victoria B. Solberg. 1985. (Illus.). 174p. (Orig.). pap. text 32.95 (0-8138-1066-3) Iowa U Pr.

Laboratory Manual for General & Oral Pathology. Shigeo Eda et al. 1991. (Illus.). 257p. text 96.00 (4-87417-262-8) Quint Pub Co.

Laboratory Manual for Human Nutrition. T. Dashman. 1991. xv, 237p. pap. text 46.00 (3-7186-0513-9, Harwood Acad Pubs) Gordon & Breach.

Laboratory Manual for Human Nutrition. Theodore Dashman & Deborah E. Blocker. 2nd ed. 1996. 288p. pap. text 34.95 (3-7186-0608-9, Harwood Acad Pubs) Gordon & Breach.

Laboratory Manual for Introduction to Psychology, Custom Pub. Norman. 1993. (C). pap. text 7.25 net. (0-07-047216-5) McGraw.

Laboratory Manual in Medical Microbiology. Robert Pollack. 1992. (Illus.). 200p. (C). pap. text 18.25 (1-878045-13-X) Whittier Pubns.

Laboratory Manual of Human Anatomy & Physiology, Vol. 2. Donald R. Ferruzzi. 4th ed. 1990. (Illus.). 254p. pap. text 32.95 (0-9609098-4-2) Biomat Pub Co.

Laboratory Manual of Neuroanatomy. D. T. Yew & M. I. Chuah. 1986. 104p. text 30.00 (9971-5-0102-3) World Scientific Pub.

Laboratory Manual of Tests, Procedures & Data for Exercise Physiology. R. G. Eston & T. Reilly. 1995. (Illus.). 360p. (C). 80.00 (0-419-17880-5, Spon) Routledge.

Laboratory Manual T-A Therapeutic Modalities. Quillen. 3rd ed. 1994. 192p. (C). text, lab manual ed. 19.95 (0-8016-7921-4) Mosby Inc.

Laboratory Manual to Accompany Anatomy & Physiology. Gary A. Thibodeau. 1987. 304p. pap. text 17.95 (0-8016-4982-X) Mosby Inc.

Laboratory Manual to Accompany Anatomy & Physiology. Kevin T. Patton. 4th ed. 1998. (Illus.). 528p. tchr. ed. (0-323-00196-3) Mosby Inc.

Laboratory Manual to Accompany Human Anatomy & Physiology. John W. Hole, Jr. 6th ed. 1992. 472p. (C). text 38.50 net. (0-697-12276-X, WCB McGr Hill) McGrw-H Hghr Educ.

Laboratory Mathematics: Medical & Biological Applications. Joe B. Campbell & June M. Campbell. 5th ed. 1996. (Illus.). 496p. (C). (gr. 13). pap. text 33.00 (0-8151-1397-8, 25633) Mosby Inc.

Laboratory Medicine: Essentials of Anatomic & Clinical Pathology. John H. Dirckx. 2nd ed. 1995. 396p. pap. text 31.00 (0-934385-61-0) Hlth Prof Inst.

Laboratory Medicine: Test Selection & Interpretation. Ed. by Joan H. Howanitz & Peter J. Howanitz. 1991. (Illus.). 966p. text (0-443-08576-5) Church.

Laboratory Medicine: The Selection & Interpretation of Clinical Laboratory Studies. Ed. by Dennis A. Noe et al. 1993. LC 93-27740. (0-683-65483-7) Lppncott W & W.

Laboratory Medicine: The Selection & Interpretation of Clinical Laboratory Studies. Dennis A. Noe & Robert C. Rock. 1993. (Illus.). 1012p. 135.00 (0-683-06548-3) Lppncott W & W.

Laboratory Medicine & the Aging Process. Joseph A. Knight. 1996. 45.00 (0-89189-397-0) Am Soc Clinical.

Laboratory Medicine Casebook: Introduction to Clinical Reasoning. Jana Raskova et al. 1996. 334p. (C). pap. text 42.95 (0-8385-5574-8, A5574-7, Apple Lange Med) McGraw.

Laboratory Medicine in Obstetrics & Gynecology. Gerald D. Willett. 1994. (Illus.). 328p. pap. 39.95 (0-86542-290-7) Blackwell Sci.

Laboratory Methods for the Diagnosis of Sexually Transmitted Diseases. Ed. by Berttina B. Wentworth et al. 2nd ed. 1991. LC 84-20394. 272p. 40.00 (0-87553-128-8) Am Pub Health.

Laboratory Methods Immunology Ed. by Heddy Zola. 1990. Vol. 1. 280p. 225.00 (0-8493-4481-6, QR183); Vol. 2. 252p. 225.00 (0-8493-4482-4, QR183) CRC Pr.

Laboratory Policy & Procedure Guideline Manual. Billy J. Vanderpool. 1997. 281p. spiral bd. 135.00 (1-879575-81-7) Acad Med Sys.

Laboratory Practice of Clinical Toxicology. Eleanor Davidson Berman. 1996. LC 95-48096. (Illus.). 220p. pap. 40.95 (0-398-06582-9); text 59.95 (0-398-06581-0) C C Thomas.

Laboratory Procedure in Clinical Microbiology. Ed. by J. A. Washington, II. 2nd ed. 1985. (Illus.). 885p. 159.00 (0-387-96087-2) Spr-Verlag.

Laboratory Procedures for Medical Assistants. Craig A. Stepp & MaryAnn Woods. Ed. by Margaret Biblis. 1997. LC 97-6736. (Illus.). 400p. pap. text 31.95 (0-7216-5275-1) Saunders.

Laboratory Procedures for Vet Technology. Driskill. pap. text (0-7216-4548-8) Saunders.

Laboratory Procedures for Veterinary Technicians. Paul W. Pratt. 3rd ed. 1996. LC 96-43451. (Illus.). 672p. (C). (gr. 13). pap. text 35.00 (0-8151-7326-1, 27768) Mosby Inc.

Laboratory Processes. 1984. (Medical Ser.). (Illus.). 216p. pap. text 14.95 (0-935920-15-3, Ntl Pubs Blck) P-H.

Laboratory Profiles of Equine Diseases. Susan C. Eades & Denise I. Bounous. 1996. (Illus.). 304p. (C). (gr. 13). pap. text 72.00 (0-8151-1731-0, 26575) Mosby Inc.

Laboratory Profiles of Small Animal Diseases. Charles Sodikoff. 2nd ed. 1995. LC 96-121883. xiii, 435p. 77.95 (0-939674-37-8) Am Vet Pubns.

Laboratory Profiles of Small Animal Diseases. Charles H. Sodikoff. 2nd ed. 1995. (Illus.). 464p. (84-8174-198-1) Mosby-Doyma Libros ESP. *Dist:* Mosby Inc.

Laboratory Profiles of Small Animal Diseases: A Guide to Laboratory Diagnosis. Charles H. Sodikoff. 3rd ed. 2000. LC 2001-272261. (Illus.). 540p. pap. 79.95 (0-323-00956-5) Mosby Inc.

Laboratory Quality Management: QC & QA. George S. Cembrowski & R. Neill Carey. 1989. LC 89-6729. (Illus.). 264p. text 45.00 (0-89189-277-X) Am Soc Clinical.

Laboratory Reference for Clinical Neurophysiology. Jay A. Liveson & Dong M. Ma. 1992. (Illus.). 528p. text 69.50 (0-19-512924-5) OUP.

Laboratory-Related Measures of Patient Outcomes: An Introduction. Ed. by Michael G. Bissell. 2000. 819p. pap. text 49.00 (1-890883-26-3, AACC Pr) Am Assn Clinical Chem.

Laboratory Safety. ring bd. 160.00 (1-56238-235-7, SC10-L) NCCLS.

Laboratory Safety & Infection Control. Peggy P. Luebbert. 1990. (NLM Ser.: No. WA485). 50.00 incl. VHS (0-89189-303-2) Am Soc Clinical.

Laboratory Studies in Animal Diversity. Cleveland P. Hickman, Jr. 1994. (C). pap., lab manual ed. 14.69 (0-697-25985-4, WCB McGr Hill) McGrw-H Hghr Educ.

Laboratory Studies in Integrated Zoology. Frances M. Hickman. 8th ed. 1992. 420p. spiral bd. 23.95 (0-8016-6377-6) Mosby Inc.

Laboratory Technician. Jack Rudman. 1994. (Career Examination Ser.: C-1734). pap. 27.95 (0-8373-1734-7) Nat Learn.

Laboratory Technician Trainee. Jack Rudman. 1994. (Career Examination Ser.: C-2909). pap. 23.95 (0-8373-2909-4) Nat Learn.

Laboratory Techniques for the Branemark System. Ross L. Taylor & Gary F. Bergman. 1990. (Illus.). 79p. ring bd. 52.00 (0-86715-173-0) Quint Pub Co.

Laboratory Techniques in Brucellosis. G. G. Alton & Lois M. Jones. 2nd ed. 1975. (Monographs: No. 55). (ENG, FRE, RUS & SPA., Illus.). 92p. pap. text 35.00 (92-4-140055-2, 1140055) World Health.

Laboratory Techniques in Rabies. Ed. by F. Meslin et al. 2nd ed. 1996. LC 96-212237. (FRE.). 476p. (Orig.). (C). pap. text 115.00 (92-4-154479-1, 1150423) World Health.

Laboratory Techniques in Renal Cell & Molecular Biology. Ed. by Y. Tomino. 2000. (Illus.). viii, 210p. spiral bd. 128.00 (3-8055-6998-X) S Karger.

Laboratory Techniques in Thrombosis: A Manual. Jergen Jespersen et al. 2nd ed. 1998. LC 98-31123. 336p. 154.00 (0-7923-5317-X) Kluwer Academic.

***Laboratory Techniques in Thrombosis, a Manual.** Roger M. Bertina & F. Haverkate. Ed. by J. Jespersen. 2nd rev. ed. 2000. 336p. 89.00 (0-7923-6472-4, Kluwer Acad) Kluwer Academic.

Laboratory Test Handbook. David S. Jacobs et al. 4th ed. 1996. (Clinical Reference Library). 1600p. 54.75 (0-916589-36-6) Lexi-Comp.

Laboratory Test Handbook. David S. Jacobs et al. 3rd ed. 1994. 1500p. 46.50 (0-683-58912-1) Lppncott W & W.

Laboratory Test Handbook: Concise Edition. David S. Jacobs et al. 1996. (Clinical Reference Library). 1142p. pap. 31.75 (0-916589-29-3) Lexi-Comp.

Laboratory Testing for Cancer: Proceedings of Laboratory for Testing Cancer Conference, Feb. 14-15, 1977. Ed. by H. Schoenfeld et al. 1978. (Antibiotics & Chemotherapy Ser.: Vol. 22). (Illus.). 66.25 (3-8055-2765-9) S Karger.

Laboratory Tests: Implications for Nursing Care. Claire J. Byrne et al. 1981. (0-201-00088-1); 2nd ed. 1986. 756p. (C). pap. text 34.69 (0-201-12670-2) Addison-Wesley (Health Sci).

Laboratory Tests & Diagnostic Procedures. Cynthia C. Chernecky & Barbara J. Berger. Ed. by Barbara N. Cullen. 2nd ed. 1996. LC 96-43069. (Illus.). 1180p. pap. text 28.00 (0-7216-6793-7) Saunders.

Laboratory Tests & Diagnostic Procedures. Cynthia C. Chernecky & Barbara J. Berger. 3rd ed. 2001. LC 00-49228. (Illus.). xix, 1114p. 32.95 (0-7216-8609-5) Saunders.

Laboratory/Pathology Words & Phrases. Ed. by Sally C. Pitman. 2nd rev. ed. 1996. 648p. (Orig.). pap. 37.00 (0-934385-66-1) Hlth Prof Inst.

Labour Ward Manual. David T. Y. Liu. 2001. 320p. pap. 50.00 (0-7506-4337-4) Buttrwrth-Heinemann.

***Labour Ward Rules.** Fay. 2001. 152p. pap. text (0-7279-1635-1) BMJ Pub GBR. *Dist:* AIDC.

Labworks Exp. MSU 121 Intro. Joseph Crook. 1995. (Illus.). 136p. (C). pap. text 18.75 (0-86720-514-8) Jones & Bartlett.

Lacan. Malcolm Bowie. 1991. 224p. 26.95 (0-674-50852-1, BOWLAC) HUP.

Lacan. Alain Vanier. 2000. LC 00-51639. (Lacanian Clinical Field Ser.). xxiv, 104p. pap. 18.00 (1-892746-50-6) Other Pr LLC.

Lacan & the Human Sciences. Ed. by Alexandre Leupin. 1991. LC 90-39325. 191p. text 45.00 (0-8032-2894-5) U of Nebr Pr.

Lacan & the New Wave in American Psychoanalysis: The Subject & the Self. Ed. by Judith Feher Gurewich & Michel Tort. 1999. LC 99-26605. (Lacanian Clinical Field Ser.). 280p. pap. 22.00 (1-892746-03-4) Other Pr LLC.

Lacanian Psychotherapy with Children: The Broken Piano. Catherine Mathelin. 1998. LC 98-36956.

(Lacanian Clinical Field Ser.). 220p. pap. 17.95 (*1-892746-01-8*, 46018) Other Pr LLC.

Lacanian Subject: Between Language & Jouissnace. Bruce Fink. 1996. LC 94-49033. 236p. pap. 18.95 (*0-691-01589-9*) Princeton U Pr.

Lacan's Seminar on "Anxiety" An Introduction. Robert Harari. 2001. LC 00-66911. (Lacanian Clinical Field Ser.). (Illus.). 368p. pap. 27.00 (*1-892746-36-0*) Other Pr LLC.

Lachman's Case Studies in Anatomy. Rev. by Donald R. Cahill. 4th ed. 1996. (Illus.). 432p. pap. text 22.95 (*0-19-510297-5*) OUP.

Lack & Transcendence: The Problem of Death & Life in Psychotherapy, Existentialism, & Buddhism. David Loy. 1996. LC 95-255. 224p. (C). text 49.95 (*0-391-03860-5*) Brill Academic Pubs.

Lacrimal Gland, Tear Film & Dry Eye Syndromes: Basic Science & Clinical Relevance. Vol. 1. D. A. Sullivan. 1994. (Advances in Experimental Medicine & Biology Ser.: Vol. 350). (Illus.). 752p. (C). text 155.00 (*0-306-44676-6*, Kluwer Plenum) Kluwer Academic.

Lacrimal Gland, Tear Film & Dry Eye Syndromes 2: Basic Science & Clinical Relevance. Ed. by David A. Sullivan et al. 1998. LC 98-17987. (Advances in Experimental Medicine & Biology Ser.: No. 438). (Illus.). 1076p. (C). text 195.00 (*0-306-45812-8*, Kluwer Plenum) Kluwer Academic.

Lacrimal Surgery. Ed. by John V. Linberg. 1988. (Contemporary Issues in Ophthalmology Ser.: Vol. 5). (Illus.). 348p. text (*0-443-08582-X*) Church.

Lacrimal System. Ed. by O. P. Van Bijsterveld et al. 1991. LC 91-7055. (Illus.). 113p. pap. text (*90-6299-073-8*) Kugler NLD. *Dist:* Lib Res.

Lacrimal System, 1994. Ed. by J. Hurwitz et al. 1996. LC 95-31274. (*90-6299-131-9*) Kugler NLD. *Dist:* Lib Res.

Lactancia Materna. Lawrence. 4th ed. 1996. (C). text 73.88 (*84-8174-176-0*) Mosby Inc.

Lactate: Physiologic, Methodologic & Pathologic Approach. Ed. by P. R. Moret et al. 1980. (Illus.). 257p. 42.95 (*0-387-09829-1*) Spr-Verlag.

Lactate in Acute Conditions: Proceedings of the International Symposium, Basel, March, 1978. Ed. by H. Bossart & C. Perret. 1979. (Illus.). 77.50 (*3-8055-2968-6*) S Karger.

Lactation. Ed. by Bruce L. Larson. 1985. (Illus.). 276p. (C). 42.95 (*0-8138-1063-9*) Iowa U Pr.

Lactation: Physiology, Nutrition & Breast Feeding. Ed. by Margaret C. Neville & Marianne R. Neifert. 1983. LC 83-17652. 482p. 95.00 (*0-306-41311-6*, Plenum Trade) Perseus Pubng.

Lactation: The Breast-Feeding Manual for Health Professionals. Ed. by Gary M. Chan. 1996. LC 96-38181. 192p. pap. 40.00 (*0-944496-48-2*) Precept Pr.

Lactation Consultant's Topical Review & Bibliography of the Literature on Breastfeeding. Ed. by Mary-Margaret Coates. 1990. LC 90-61943. 188p. (Orig.). pap. 12.00 (*0-912500-39-5*) La Leche.

***Lactation Guide for Primary Care Providers.** Maureen H. Dann. 2001. (Illus.). (C). pap. text 24.95 (*0-7637-1818-1*, 1818-1) Jones & Bartlett.

Lactation Specialist Self-Study Series. Rebecca F. Black et al. 1998. 900p. pap. 125.00 (*0-7637-0664-7*) Jones & Bartlett.

Lactic Dehydrogenase Virus. Brian W. Mahy & K. E. Rowson. 1975. LC 74-34231. (Virology Monographs: Vol. 13). (Illus.). iv, 121p. 47.00 (*0-387-81270-9*) Spr-Verlag.

Lactoferrin: Structure & Function. Ed. by T. W. Hutchens et al. 1995. (Advances in Experimental Medicine & Biology Ser.: Vol. 357). (Illus.). 310p. (C). text 95.00 (*0-306-44734-7*, Kluwer Plenum) Kluwer Academic.

Lactoferrin: Structure, Function & Applications: Proceedings of the 4th International Conference on Lactoferrin: Structure, Function & Applications, Hokkaido, Japan, 18-22 May 1999. Ed. by Kei-ichi Shimazaki et al. 2000. LC 00-28811. (International Congress Ser.: Vol. 1195). 478p. 155.50 (*0-444-50317-X*, Excerpta Medica) Elsevier.

Lactoperoxidase System: Chemistry & Biological Significance. Kenneth Pruitt & Tenovuov. 1985. (Immunology Ser.: Vol. 27). (Illus.). 272p. text 165.00 (*0-8247-7298-9*) Dekker.

Lactose Intolerance. Merri L. Dobler. 1991. pap. 5.50 (*0-88091-097-6*, 0881) Am Dietetic Assn.

Lacunar & Subcortical Infarctions. Ed. by Geoffrey Donnan et al. 1995. (Illus.). 294p. text 98.00 (*0-19-262341-9*) OUP.

Lady Boys, Tom Boys, Rent Boys: Male & Female Homosexualities in Contemporary Thailand. Ed. by Peter A. Jackson & Gerard Sullivan. 1999. LC 98-55912. xviii, 237p. pap. 19.95 (*1-56023-119-X*, Harrington Park) Haworth Pr.

Lady Killer: Heart Disease: Women at Risk. Suzanne Cambre. Ed. by Anna Hollingsworth. 1995. LC 35-3309. (Illus.). 24p. pap. text 5.95 (*0-939838-38-9*) Pritchett & Hull.

Laetrile Control for Cancer. Glenn D. Kittler. 1963. 14.00 (*0-8392-1059-0*) Astor-Honor.

L'/Agenda de Mere see Mother's Agenda

Lakeside Master's Study of the Pulse: (Pin-hu Mo Hsueh) Shi-zhen Li. Tr. by Bob Flaws from CHI. 1998. LC 98-71824. 130p. pap. 15.95 (*1-891845-01-2*) Blue Poppy Pr.

Lam & Other Diseases Characterized by Smooth Muscle Proliferation. Ed. by Joel Moss. 1999. LC 99-11317. (Lung Biology in Health & Disease Ser.). (Illus.). 640p. text 225.00 (*0-8247-0214-X*) Dekker.

Lamarck & Modern Genetics. H. Graham Cannon. 1975. LC 75-10211. 152p. reprint ed. lib. bdg. 60.00 (*0-8371-8173-9*, CALA, Greenwood Pr) Greenwood.

Lamarck to Darwin: Contributions to Evolutionary Biology, 1809-1859. Ed. by H. Lewis McKinney. 1971. 124p. 10.00 (*0-87291-019-9*) Coronado Pr.

Lamaze Ready Reference Guide for Labor & Birth. Harriet R. Shapiro et al. 2nd rev. ed. 1997. (Illus.). 59p. spiral bd. 9.95 (*0-9624335-0-0*) Shapiro Kuba.

Lamb Problems: Detecting, Diagnosing, Treating. Laura Lawson. rev. ed. 1996. LC 92-7300. (Illus.). 264p. (Orig.). pap. 29.95 (*0-9633923-0-1*) LDF Pubns.

Lame Horse. James Rooney. 1984. (Illus.). 237p. reprint ed. text 19.95 (*0-914327-04-6*) Breakthrgh NY.

Lame Horse - Causes, Symptoms & Treatment. James R. Rooney. 1975. pap. 15.00 (*0-87980-308-8*) Wilshire.

Lameness in Cattle. P. R. Greenough et al. 2nd ed. 1991. (Illus.). 496p. (*0-85608-030-6*) Blackwell Sci.

Lameness of the Equine Foot. Turner. 1994. (C). text (*0-7216-3730-2*) Saunders.

Laminectomia Lumbar. Oliver D. Grin & Dorothy L. Bouwman. 1992. (Patient Education Ser.). (SPA., Illus.). 18p. (Orig.). pap. text 4.00 (*0-929689-54-2*) Ludann Co.

Lamisil: The Evidence. K. Casano & R. J. Hay. 2001. LC 2001-21756. (Illus.). 96p. lib. bdg. 77.95 (*1-84214-047-7*, Parthenon Pbng) CRC Pr.

Lanahan Cases in Developmental Psychopathology. Kayla F. Bernheim et al. 1999. LC 2001-274293. xi, 195p. (Orig.). (C). pap. text 20.50 (*0-9652687-5-6*) Lanahan Pubs.

Landmarks in Gene Regulation. Ed. by David S. Latchman. 1997. (Landmarks in Science & Medicine Ser.: Vol. 1). (Illus.). 320p. (C). pap. text (*1-85578-109-3*) Portland Pr Ltd GBR. *Dist:* Ashgate Pub Co.

Landmarks in Medicine. New York Academy of Medicine Staff. 1977. LC 74-142676. (Essay Index Reprint Ser.). 25.95 (*0-8369-2114-3*) Ayer.

Langman's Medical Embryology. Thomas W. Sadler & Jan Langman. 2000. LC 00-23226. 528p. pap. text 41.95 (*0-683-30650-2*) Lppncott W & W.

Langman's Medical Embryology. Thomas W. Sadler. 6th ed. 1990. (Illus.). 432p. pap. 33.00 (*0-683-07493-8*) Lppncott W & W.

Langman's Medical Embryology. Thomas W. Sadler & Sang-Ho Baik. 7th ed. 1997. (KOR., Illus.). 480p. (*962-356-022-2*) Lppncott W & W.

Langman's Medical Embryology. Thomas W. Sadler & Ming-Jia Jou. 7th ed. 1996. (CHI., Illus.). 480p. (*962-356-019-2*) Lppncott W & W.

Langstaff: A Nineteenth-Century Medical Life. Dacalyn Duffin. 1993. (Illus.). 400p. text 60.00 (*0-8020-2908-6*) U of Toronto Pr.

Language: Structure, Processing & Disorders. David N. Caplan. 1992. (Illus.). 400p. 55.00 (*0-262-03189-2*) MIT Pr.

Language Acquisition. Jill G. De Villiers & Peter A. De Villiers. 1990. 384p. 45.95 (*0-674-50931-5*) HUP.

Language Acquisition: Core Readings. Ed. by Paul Bloom. 1993. LC 93-27417. 624p. pap. 35.00 (*0-262-52187-3*) MIT Pr.

Language Acquisition Problems & Reading Disorders: Aspects of Diagnosis & Intervention. Ed. by Hannelore Grimm & Helmut Skowronek. 1993. LC 93-27052. (Prevention & Intervention in Childhood & Adolescence Ser.: No. 14). xii, 360p. (C). lib. bdg. 82.95 (*3-11-014120-5*) De Gruyter.

Language & Communication Disorders in Children. Deena K. Bernstein & Ellenmorris Tiegerman. 4th ed. 1997. LC 96-48262. 544p. 83.00 (*0-205-19894-5*) Allyn.

Language & Communication in Mental Retardation: Development, Processes, & Intervention. Sheldon Rosenberg & Leonard Abbeduto. 1993. (Topics in Applied Psycholinguistics Ser.). 272p. text 59.95 (*0-8058-0302-5*) L Erlbaum Assocs.

Language & Communication in Mentally Handicapped People. Michael Beveridge et al. 1989. 200p. 67.50 (*0-412-32390-7*) Chapman & Hall.

Language & Communication in Old Age: Multidisciplinary Perspectives. Ed. by Heidi E. Hamilton & Diana K. Harris. 1998. LC 98-38853. (Issues in Aging Ser.: Vol. 9). (Illus.). 350p. 60.00 (*0-8153-2356-5*, SS1104) Garland.

Language & Conceptualization. Ed. by Jan Nuyts & Eric Pederson. 1997. LC 96-8776. (Language, Culture & Cognition Ser.: No. 1). (Illus.). 289p. (C). text 69.95 (*0-521-55303-2*) Cambridge U Pr.

Language & Deafness. Peter V. Paul & Stephen P. Quigley. 2nd ed. 1994. 252p. (C). pap. text, stu. ed. 29.95 (*1-56593-363-X*, 0700) Thomson Learn.

Language & Hemispheric Specialization in Man: Cerebral Event-Related Potentials. Ed. by J. E. Desmedt. 1977. (Progress in Clinical Neurophysiology Ser.: Vol. 3). (Illus.). 85.25 (*3-8055-2629-6*) S Karger.

Language & Interpretation in Psychoanalysis. Marshall Edelson. 1984. LC 84-2547. xvi, 260p. pap. text 11.00 (*0-226-18433-1*) U Ch Pr.

Language & Language Disturbances. Kurt Goldstein. 1953. LC 48-11852. (Illus.). 386p. text 68.00 (*0-8089-0156-7*, 791650, Grune & Strat) Harcrt Hlth Sci Grp.

Language & Learning: An Interactional Perspective. Ed. by Gordon Wells & John Nicholls. 1985. LC 85-6728. (Contemporary Analysis in Education Ser.). 170p. pap. 29.95 (*1-85000-028-X*, Falmer Pr) Taylor & Francis.

Language & Learning: The Debate Between Jean Piaget & Noam Chomsky. Ed. by Massimo Piattelli-Palmarini. 1984. 445p. pap. 18.50 (*0-674-50941-2*) HUP.

Language & Learning: The Importance of Speech in Children's Development. James N. Britton. 2nd ed. 1993. LC 93-22156. 330p. pap. text 29.00 (*0-86709-335-8*, 0335) Boynton Cook Pubs.

Language & Mind. Steven Pinker. 2000. (Science Masters Ser.). 176p. pap. (*0-465-07270-4*) Basic.

Language & Motor Speech Disorders in Adults. Harvey Halpern. 1986. LC 86-569. (PRO-ED Studies in Communicative Disorders). (Illus.). 88p. (Orig.). pap. text 9.00 (*0-89079-089-2*, 1379) PRO-ED.

Language & Perception. George A. Miller & Philip N. Johnson-Laird. 1987. 773p. pap. 17.95 (*0-674-50948-X*, Belknap) HUP.

Language & Psychiatry. Harley C. Shands & James D. Meltzer. 1973. LC 73-77388. (Janua Linguarum, Ser. Minor: No. 165). 85p. pap. text (*90-279-2483-X*) Mouton.

Language & Psychology: Historical Aspects of Psycholinguistics. Arthur L. Blumenthal. 1980. LC 80-12611. 262p. reprint ed. 69.50 (*0-89874-167-X*) Elliots Bks.

Language & Schizophrenia. Janusz Wrobel. 1989. LC 89-38326. (Linguistic & Literary Studies in Eastern Europe: Vol. No. 33). viii, 132p. 42.00 (*90-272-1539-1*) J Benjamins Pubng Co.

Language & Space. Ed. by Paul Bloom et al. 1996. LC 95-36427. (Language, Speech, & Communication Ser.). (Illus.). 672p. 85.00 (*0-262-02403-9*, Bradford Bks) MIT Pr.

Language & Speech: Proceedings of the Fifth Convention of the Academia Eurasiana Neurochirurgica, Budapest, September 19-12, 1990. Ed. by E. Pasztor et al. 1993. (Acta Neurochirurgica Ser.: No. 56). (Illus.). 120p. 119.95 (*0-387-82386-7*) Spr-Verlag.

Language & the Elderly: A Clinical Perspective. Jane Maxim & Karen Bryan. 1994. LC 94-185437. (Illus.). 298p. (Orig.). (C). pap. text 59.95 (*1-56593-254-4*, 0048) Thomson Learn.

Language & Thought in Humans & Computers: Theory & Research in Psychology, Artificial Intelligence & Neural Science. Morton Wagman. 1998. LC 97-32997. 192p. 62.50 (*0-275-96179-6*, Praeger Pubs) Greenwood.

Language Communication & the Brain: A Neuropsychological Study. Mariusz Maruszewski. Tr. by Grace W. Shugar from POL. 1975. (Janua Linguarum, Series Major: No. 80). (Illus.). 217p. text (*90-279-3067-8*) Mouton.

Language Comprehension as Structure Building. Ed. by Morton A. Gernsbacher. 1990. 304p. (C). text 79.95 (*0-8058-0676-8*) L Erlbaum Assocs.

Language Comprehension in Ape & Child. E. Sue Savage-Rumbaugh et al. 1993. (Monographs of the Society for Research in Child Development: No. 233, Vol. 58, Nos. 3-4). 510p. (C). pap. text 19.50 (*0-226-73542-7*) U Ch Pr.

Language Delays & Disorders: From Research to Practice. Lydia R. Smiley & Peggy A. Goldstein. 1997. LC 97-28437. (Illus.). 352p. (Orig.). pap. text 39.95 (*1-56593-694-9*, 1384) Thomson Learn.

Language Development & Language Disorders: A Compendium of Lectures. Nancy E. Wood. 1960. (SRCD M Ser.: Vol. 25, No. 3). pap. 25.00 (*0-527-01585-7*) Periodicals Srv.

Language Development & the Disadvantaged Child. Galen Downes. 1978. 91p. (*0-7157-1631-X*) St Mut.

Language Development from Birth to 3. Moshe Anisfeld. 1984. LC 83-82493. 306p. (C). pap. text 37.50 (*0-89859-625-4*) L Erlbaum Assocs.

Language Development from 2 to 3. Lois Bloom. 1993. (Illus.). 524p. (C). pap. text 32.95 (*0-521-43583-8*) Cambridge U Pr.

Language Development in Exceptional Circumstances. Ed. by Dorothy Bishop & Kay Mogford-Bevan. 1988. (Illus.). 324p. text (*0-443-03800-7*) Church.

Language Disorders: A Functional Approach to Assessment & Intervention. Robert E. Owens. 3rd ed. 1998. LC 98-34366. 596p. 78.67 (*0-205-28703-4*) P-H.

Language Disorders Across the Lifespan. Betsy P. Vinson. 1998. LC 98-34416. 333p. pap. text 59.95 (*1-56593-977-8*) Thomson Learn.

Language Disorders from Infancy Through Adolescence: Assessment & Intervention. Rhea Paul. 2nd ed. 2000. (Illus.). 672p. text 63.00 (*0-323-00660-4*) Mosby Inc.

Language Disorders in Children. Frank R. Kleffner. 1973. LC 73-3116. (Studies in Communicative Disorders). 60p. (C). pap. text (*0-672-61292-5*, Bobbs) Macmillan.

Language Disorders in Children: An Introductory Clinical Perspective. Barbara A. Johnson. 1995. LC 94-36579. (Health & Life Science Ser.). (Illus.). 381p. (C). pap. text 59.95 (*0-8273-5533-5*) Delmar.

Language Disorders in Children & Adolescents. Rhea Paul. 1995. (Illus.). 624p. (gr. 13). text 58.00 (*0-8016-7927-3*, 07927) Mosby Inc.

Language Disorders in Children & Adults: Psycholinguistic Approaches to Therapy. Ed. by Shula Chiat et al. 1997. 280p. 65.00 (*1-56593-878-X*, 1720) Singular Publishing.

Language Disorders in Older Students: Preadolescents & Adolescents. Vicki L. Larson & Nancy L. McKinley. 1995. LC 94-34928. pap. 42.00 (*0-930599-29-2*) Thinking Pubns.

Language Disturbance & Intellectual Functioning: A Comparison of the Performance of Hemiplegic Patients with Aphasia & Hemiplegic Patients Without Aphasia in Non-Verbal Tasks of Intellectual Functioning. Carl K. Lubin. 1969. LC 68-17904. (Janua Linguarum, Series Minor: No. 48). (Orig.). pap. text (*3-10-800093-4*) Mouton.

Language Diversity & Education. David Corson. 2000. LC 00-20306. xi, 253p. pap. 29.95 (*0-8058-3449-4*) L Erlbaum Assocs.

Language for the Preschool Deaf Child. Grace M. Harris. 3rd ed. 1971. LC 77-167976. 360p. text 45.00 (*0-8089-0733-6*, 791913, Grune & Strat) Harcrt Hlth Sci Grp.

Language for Those Who Have Nothing: Mikhail Bakhtin & the Lanscape of Psychiatry. Peter Good. 2000. LC 00-52740. (Cognition & Language Ser.). 258p. 65.00 (*0-306-46502-7*, Kluwer Plenum) Kluwer Academic.

Language, Gender & Childhood. Ed. by Valerie Walkerdine et al. 1986. (History Workshop Ser.). 256p. (Orig.). pap. 18.95 (*0-7100-9977-0*, Routledge Thoemms) Routledge.

Language Habits in Human Affairs: An Introduction to General Semantics. Irving J. Lee. Ed. by Sanford I. Berman. 2nd ed. 1994. LC 94-36138. pap. 21.95 (*0-918970-41-5*) Intl Gen Semantics.

Language in Behavior. Richard W. Howell & Harold J. Vetter. 2nd ed. 1985. 299p. 50.95 (*0-89885-215-3*, Kluwer Acad Hman Sci) Kluwer Academic.

Language in Cognitive Development: The Emergence of the Mediated Mind. Katherine Nelson. 1998. (Illus.). 448p. (C). reprint ed. pap. text 22.95 (*0-521-62987-X*) Cambridge U Pr.

Language in Mental Retardation. Jean A. Rondal. 1996. 322p. (Orig.). pap. 45.00 (*1-56593-812-7*, 1590) Singular Publishing.

Language in Psychotherapy: Strategies of Discovery. R. L. Russell. 1987. LC 87-2511. (Emotions, Personality, & Psychotherapy Ser.). (Illus.). 368p. (C). text 80.00 (*0-306-42422-3*, Kluwer Plenum) Kluwer Academic.

Language, Learning & Deafness: Theory, Application & Classroom Management. Alice Streng et al. 1978. (Illus.). 240p. text 42.00 (*0-8089-1060-4*, 794412, Grune & Strat) Harcrt Hlth Sci Grp.

Language Learning Disabilities in School-Age Children & Adolescents: Some Principles & Applications. Ed. by Geraldine P. Wallach & Katherine G. Butler. 1994. LC 93-29233. (Illus.). 544p. (C). 93.00 (*0-675-22153-6*, Merrill Coll) P-H.

Language, Logic & Concepts. Ed. by Ray Jackendoff et al. 1999. LC 98-47084. (Illus.). 470p. 55.00 (*0-262-10078-9*, Bradford Bks) MIT Pr.

Language, Memory, & Aging. Ed. by Leah L. Light & Deborah M. Burke. 1988. (Illus.). 296p. (C). text 80.00 (*0-521-32942-6*) Cambridge U Pr.

Language, Memory, & Thought. John R. Anderson. 1976. LC 76-21791. 546p. (C). text 99.95 (*0-89859-107-4*) L Erlbaum Assocs.

Language, Mind, & Brain. Ed. by Thomas W. Simon & Robert J. Scholes. 1982. (Illus.). 288p. text 59.95 (*0-89859-153-8*) L Erlbaum Assocs.

Language of Biotechnology: A Dictionary of Terms. Ed. by Michael Cox et al. 2nd ed. 1995. LC 94-23812. (Professional Reference Book). (Illus.). 300p. 35.00 (*0-8412-2982-1*) Am Chemical.

Language of Change: Elements of Therapeutic Communication. Paul Watzlawick. 1993. 184p. pap. 13.95 (*0-393-31020-5*) Norton.

Language of Directions: A Programmed Workbook. Mary L. Rush. 1977. LC 77-87703. pap. text 14.95 (*0-88200-113-2*, C1321) Alexander Graham.

Language of Dreams. Patricia Telesco. 1997. LC 97-11608. (Illus.). 272p. pap. 16.95 (*0-89594-836-2*) Crossing Pr.

Language of Family Therapy: A Systemic Vocabulary & Sourcebook. Fritz B. Simon et al. 1985.Tr. of Sprache den Familientherapie-Ein Vokabular. (C). 30.00 (*0-9615519-1-7*); pap. 18.00 (*0-9615519-0-9*) Family Process.

Language of Fractures. Robert J. Schultz. 1976. LC 75-43698. 408p. reprint ed. 42.50 (*0-88275-369-X*) Krieger.

Language of Fractures. Robert J. Schultz. 2nd ed. 1990. (Illus.). 336p. 58.00 (*0-683-07612-4*) Lppncott W & W.

Language of Medicine. Davi-Ellen Chabner. 5th ed. 1996. (Illus.). pap., tchr. ed. (*0-7216-6027-4*) Saunders.

***Language of Medicine.** Davi-Ellen Chabner. 6th ed. 2000. pap., tchr. ed. 250.00 (*0-7216-8570-6*) Saunders.

Language of Medicine: A General Guide to Medical Care. Byron K. Cole. 1997. 365p. (Orig.). pap. 19.95 (*0-9656764-0-4*) Medical Info Assocs.

Language of Medicine: A Write-In Text Explaining Medical Terms. Davi-Ellen Chabner. 6th ed. 2000. LC 99-89410. (Illus.). xx, 947p. pap. text 42.95 (*0-7216-8569-2*) Saunders.

***Language of Medicine: And Miller-Keane Encyclopedia & Dictionary of Medicine, Nursing & Allied Health.** Davi-Ellen Chabner. 6th ed. 2000. pap. 64.95 (*0-7216-9312-1*) Saunders.

***Language of Medicine: And Mosby Medical, Nursing & Allied Health Dictionary.** Davi-Ellen Chabner. 6th ed. 2000. pap. 65.95 (*0-7216-9311-3*) Saunders.

J K L

***Language of Medicine: Examaster.** Davi-Ellen Chabner. 6th ed. 2000. pap. 750.00 (*0-7216-8571-4*) Saunders.

Language of Medicine: Exam/Testbank. Bruce A. Chabner. 5th ed. 1996. pap., suppl. ed. 200.00 (*0-7216-3339-0*) Saunders.

Language of Medicine: Its Evolution, Structure, Dynamics. John H. Dirckx. 2nd ed. 1983. LC 83-8863. 206p. 65.00 (*0-275-91388-0*, C1388, Praeger Pubs) Greenwood.

Language Of Medicine In English: Revised Edition. Ethel Tiersky. rev. ed. 1992. LC 91-39488. 132p. (C). pap. text 27.60 (*0-13-521444-0*) P-H.

Language of Motivation & Language of Actions. Maria Nowakowska. 1973. LC 72-94491. (Janua Linguarum, Ser. Major: No. 67). (Illus.). 272p. text (*90-279-2385-X*) Mouton.

Language of Psycho-Analysis. Jean Laplanche & Jean-Baptiste Pontalis. Tr. by Donald Micholson-Smith from FRE. 1974. LC 73-18418. 510p. (C). 36.00 (*0-393-01105-4*) Norton.

Language of Tears. Jeffrey A. Kottler. 1996. LC 96-11136. 242p. 22.00 (*0-7879-0265-9*) Jossey-Bass.

Language of the Self: The Function of Language in Psychoanalysis. Jacques Lacan. Tr. & Comment by Anthony Wilden. 1998. LC 98-137660. 368p. pap. text 18.95 (*0-8018-5817-8*) Johns Hopkins.

Language of Winnicott: A Dictionary & Guide to Understanding His Work. Jan Abram & Harry Karnac. 1997. LC 96-50065. 400p. 50.00 (*1-56821-700-5*) Aronson.

***Language Processing.** Simon Garrod. 2001. 448p. pap. (*0-86377-837-2*) Psychol Pr GBR. *Dist:* Taylor & Francis.

Language Processing & Language Acquisition. Ed. by Lyn Frazier. 1990. (C). lib. bdg. 159.00 (*0-7923-0659-7*) Kluwer Academic.

Language Processing in Social Context. Ed. by R. Dietrich & Carl F. Graumann. 1989. (Linguistics Ser.: No. 54). (Illus.). x,302p. 195.50 (*0-444-87144-6*, North Holland) Elsevier.

Language Processing in Spanish. Ed. by Manuel Carreiras et al. 1996. 384p. text 79.95 (*0-8058-1721-2*) L Erlbaum Assocs.

Language, Structure & Change: Frameworks of Meaning in Psychotherapy. Jay S. Efran et al. 1990. 224p. (C). text 29.95 (*0-393-70103-4*) Norton.

Language, Thought & Consciousness: An Essay in Philosophical Psychology. Peter Carruthers. 1998. 307p. (C). reprint ed. pap. text 29.95 (*0-521-63999-9*) Cambridge U Pr.

Language Transfer in Language Learning. Ed. by Susan M. Gass & Larry Selinker. rev. ed. 1992. LC 92-23741. (Language Acquisition & Language Disorders Ser.: Vol. No. 5). x, 236p. 62.00 (*1-55619-240-1*) J Benjamins Pubng Co.

Languages of the Brain: Experimental Paradoxes & Principles in Neuropsychology. Karl H. Pribram. 5th ed. 1982. 432p. reprint ed. text 35.00 (*0-913412-22-8*) Brandon Hse.

Languages of the Mind. Ray S. Jackendoff. 1992. LC 91-45159. 200p. 30.00 (*0-262-10047-9*) MIT Pr.

Languages of the Mind: Essays on Mental Representation. Ray S. Jackendoff. 1995. (Illus.). 216p. reprint ed. pap. text 15.00 (*0-262-60024-2*, Bradford Bks) MIT Pr.

Langurs of Abu: Female & Male Strategies of Reproduction. Sarah Blaffer Hrdy. (Illus.). 381p. 1980. pap. 17.50 (*0-674-51058-5*); 1977. 37.00 (*0-674-51057-7*) HUP.

Lantibiotics & Related Peptides. Ralph W. Jack & Hans-Georg Sahl. Date not set. LC 97-31727. (Biotechnology Intelligence Unit Ser.). 263p. 129.00 (*1-57059-515-1*) Landes Bioscience.

Lao Handbook of Maternal & Child Health. Aletha Robinson. 1980. pap. 1.95 (*0-9602790-1-6*) Hlth Frontiers.

Laparo-Endoscopic Surgery. Iris Brune. 2nd ed. 1996. (Illus.). 400p. 185.00 (*0-86542-900-6*) Blackwell Sci.

Laparoscopic Appearance of Endometriosis, Vol. I. D. C. Martin et al. Ed. by Dan C. Martin. 2nd ed. 1990. LC 90-60383. (Illus.). 57p. pap. text 14.00 (*0-9616747-3-3*) Resurge Pr.

Laparoscopic Appearance of Endometriosis: Color Atlas, Vol. III. D. C. Martin et al. Ed. by Dan C. Martin. 2nd ed. 1990. LC 90-60393. (Illus.). 69p. pap. text 38.00 (*0-9616747-6-8*) Resurge Pr.

***Laparoscopic Approach in Gastro-Oesophageal Surgery: Experimental & Epidemiological Studies.** Rune Sandbu. 2001. (Comprehensive Summaries of Uppsala Dissertations from the Faculty of Medicine Ser.: No. 1094). (Illus.). 87p. pap. (*91-554-5155-1*) Acta Univ SWE. *Dist:* Coronet Bks.

Laparoscopic Cholecystectomy. M. Chellappa. 1994. text 38.00 (*981-02-1094-9*) World Scientific Pub.

Laparoscopic Cholecystectomy: Difficult Cases & Creative Solutions. Avram M. Cooperman. 1992. (Illus.). 192p. 100.00 (*0-942219-28-7*) Quality Med Pub.

Laparoscopic Cholecystectomy: Problems & Solutions. David C. Dunn & Christopher J. Watson. 1992. (Illus.). 160p. 70.00 (*0-632-03444-0*) Blackwell Sci.

Laparoscopic Cholecystectomy: State of the Art - Journal: Digestive Surgery, Vol. 8, No. 2, 1991. Ed. by J. J. Jakimowicz & T. J. Ruers. 1991. (Illus.). 72p. pap. 45.25 (*3-8055-5439-7*) S Karger.

Laparoscopic Colorectal Surgery. Ed. by M. W. Buchler & L. Krahenbuhl. 1996. (Journal: Vol. 12, No. 5, 1995). (Illus.). 42p. pap. 50.50 (*3-8055-6282-9*) S Karger.

Laparoscopic Colorectal Surgery. Jager. 1996. text 180.00 (*0-443-07785-1*) Saunders.

Laparoscopic Colorectal Surgery. Ed. by Rama M. Jager & Steven D. Wexner. 1995. LC 95-35115. 333p. text (*0-443-08998-1*) Church.

Laparoscopic Colorectal Surgery. Jeffrey W. Milsom et al. 1995. LC 95-16248. (Illus.). 270p. 154.00 (*0-387-94470-2*) Spr-Verlag.

Laparoscopic Colorectal Surgery. Steven D. Wexner. 1999. LC 98-27804. (Protocols in General Surgery Ser.). (Illus.). 563p. 142.00 (*0-471-24030-3*) Wiley.

Laparoscopic Digestive Surgery. Ed. by Pierre Testas & Bernard J. Delaitre. 1994. LC 94-5562. (Clinical Surgery International Ser.: Vol. 19). (Illus.). text (*0-443-04823-1*) Church.

Laparoscopic Hernia Repair. Michael S. Kavic. 1997. (Illus.). 160p. text 75.00 (*90-5702-538-8*, Harwood Acad Pubs) Gordon & Breach.

Laparoscopic Hernia Repair: A New Standard? Ed. by M. W. Buechler et al. 1995. LC 95-1526. (Progress in Surgery Ser.: Vol. 21). (Illus.). viii, 194p. 139.25 (*3-8055-6047-8*) S Karger.

Laparoscopic Hernia Repair: Problems & Solutions. David C. Dunn & Donald Menzies. 1995. 160p. 136.95 (*0-86542-908-1*) Blackwell Sci.

Laparoscopic Hysterectomy & Oopherectomy: A Practical Manual & Colour Atlas. Jeffrey H. Phipps. 1993. LC 93-7324. (Illus.). 120p. text (*0-443-04929-7*) Church.

Laparoscopic Hysterectomy & Pelvic Floor Reconstruction. R. Garry & Harry Reich. 1993. (Illus.). 208p. 110.00 (*0-632-03465-3*) Blackwell Sci.

Laparoscopic Hysterectomy & Pelvic Floor Reconstruction. Ed. by C. Y. Liu. 1995. LC 95-40310. (Minimally Invasive Gynecology Ser.). (Illus.). 240p. 125.00 (*0-86542-383-0*) Blackwell Sci.

Laparoscopic Surgery. Garth H. Ballantyne et al. 1994. (Illus.). 736p. text 230.00 (*0-7216-6648-5*) Saunders.

Laparoscopic Surgery: A Colloquium. Ed. by Ronald C. Merrell & R. M. Olson. 1998. LC 98-15837. (Illus.). 343p. 141.00 (*0-387-98396-1*) Spr-Verlag.

Laparoscopic Surgery: Principles & Practice. Ed. by Daniel B. Jones et al. 1997. LC 96-49577. (Illus.). 489p. text 82.00 (*1-57626-007-0*) Quality Med Pub.

Laparoscopic Surgery: Recent Developments in Basic Research & Clinical Update. Ed. by L. Krahenbuhl & M. W. Buchler. 1998. (Digestive Surgery Ser.: Vol. 15, No. 2, 1998). (Illus.). 104p. pap. 70.50 (*3-8055-6677-8*) S Karger.

Laparoscopic Surgery: The Implications of Changing Practice, Vol. 8. Ed. by Michael Hobsley et al. 1997. (An Arnold Publication). 348p. (*0-340-60760-2*) E A GBR. *Dist:* OUP.

Laparoscopic Surgery in Gynecological Oncology. Dennis Querleu et al. 1999. LC 98-36147. (Illus.). 240p. 136.95 (*0-86542-692-9*) Blackwell Sci.

Laparoscopic Urology. Ed. by Ralph V. Clayman et al. 1992. LC 92-48957. (Illus.). 450p. pap. 90.00 (*0-942219-41-4*) Quality Med Pub.

Laparoscopic Urology. Ed. by Sakti Das & E. David Crawford. 1994. LC 93-47167. text 105.00 (*0-7216-3766-3*) Saunders.

Laparoscopic Urology. Ed. by Ralph V. Clayman & Elspeth M. McDougall. 2nd ed. 1997. 90.00 (*1-57626-025-9*, C2358) Quality Med Pub.

Laparoscopy: A Clinical Companion. Jean N. Saleh. 1988. (Illus.). 288p. text 115.00 (*0-7216-2126-0*) Saunders.

Laparoscopy & Imaging Techniques. G. Dagnini. Tr. by S. Pearcey from ITA. 1990. (Illus.). 206p. 217.00 (*0-387-50999-2*) Spr-Verlag.

Laparoscopy in Urology, Pt. 1. M. J. Coptcoat & M. R. Joyce. 1994. LC 93-11903. (Illus.). 192p. 99.95 (*0-632-03664-8*) Blackwell Sci.

Laparoscopy in Women's Health: A Guide for Women. Andrew Friedman. Ed. by Edward E. Wallach. 1996. (Women's Health Ser.). (Illus.). 32p. pap. 2.95 (*1-885274-16-5*) Health InfoNet Inc.

L'Aphasie see Living with Aphasia: Psychosocial Issues

Laproscopic Panhysterectomy with Reconstructive Posterior Culdeplasty & Vaginal Vault Suspension. Adam Ostrzenski. 1993. (Illus.). 126p. (C). lib. bdg. 78.00 (*0-9638210-0-8*) Med Sci Pub.

Large Amplitude Motion in Molecules II. Ed. by F. L. Boschke. 1979. (Topics in Current Chemistry Ser.: Vol. 82). (Illus.). 184p. 74.95 (*0-387-09311-7*) Spr-Verlag.

Large Animal Anesthesia: Principles & Techniques. Thomas W. Riebold et al. 2nd ed. 1995. LC 94-24471. (Illus.). 312p. text 54.95 (*0-8138-0774-3*) Iowa U Pr.

Large Animal Diseases. James A. Kennedy. 2000. 198p. (*1-58692-053-7*) Courier Custom.

Large Animal Internal Medicine. Timothy H. Ogilvie. 1997. LC 97-33109. (National Veterinary Medical Series for Independent Study). 600p. 35.95 (*0-683-18033-9*) Lppncott W & W.

Large Animal Internal Medicine. Bradford P. Smith. 3rd ed. (Illus.). 2112p. (*0-323-00946-8*) Mosby Inc.

Large Animal Internal Medicine: Diseases of Horses, Cattle, Sheep, & Goats. Ed. by Bradford P. Smith. 2nd ed. 1996. LC 95-47494. (Illus.). 2112p. (C). (gr. 13). text 160.00 (*0-8151-7724-0*, 23783) Mosby Inc.

Large Animal Urogenital Surgery. Dwight F. Wolfe & H. David Moll. 2nd ed. 1998. LC 98-26257. 600p. 99.00 (*0-683-09230-8*) Lppncott W & W.

Large Bowel Cancer: Clinical & Basic Science Research. 3. Ed. by Anthony J. Mastromarino & Michael G. Brattain. 1985. LC 85-515. (Cancer Research Monographs: Vol. 3). 204p. 62.50 (*0-275-91319-8*, C1319, Praeger Pubs) Greenwood.

Large Bowel Cancer: Policy, Prevention, Research & Treatment. Ed. by P. Rozen et al. 1991. (Frontiers of Gastrointestinal Research Ser.: Vol. 18). (Illus.). viii, 302p. 242.75 (*3-8055-5269-6*) S Karger.

Large Deviations. Frank den Hollander. 2000. LC 99-58913. (FIM Ser.: Vol. 14). 143p. text 49.00 (*0-8218-1989-5*) Am Math.

Large Fire Scene Operations. 1998. (Training in a Box Ser.). 50p. ring bd. 49.00 (*1-57927-038-7*) APCO Inst.

Large Group: Dynamics & Therapy. Ed. by Lionel Kreeger. 1994. 344p. pap. text (*0-946439-02-8*) Karnac Bks GBR. *Dist:* Other Pr LLC.

Large Loop Excision of the Transformation Zone: A Practical Guide to LLETZ. Ed. by Walter Prendiville. LC 92-49021. 1993. 180p. (gr. 13). 200.95 (*0-412-46240-0*); 1992. (*0-442-31708-5*) Chapman & Hall.

Large Macaws: Their Care, Breeding & Conservation. Joanne Abramson et al. Ed. by Joanne Abramson & Jorgen B. Thomsen. 1996. (Illus.). 552p. lib. bdg. 170.00 (*0-9635964-0-3*) Raintree Pubns.

Large-Scale Neuronal Theories of the Brain. Ed. by Christof Koch & Joel L. Davis. 1994. LC 93-29736. (Computational Neuroscience Ser.). (Illus.). 355p. 63.00 (*0-262-11183-7*, Bradford Bks) MIT Pr.

Larnyx. Marvin P. Fried. 1988. 700p. 120.00 (*0-316-29360-1*, Little Brwn Med Div) Lppncott W & W.

Larousse de la Medecine Andre Domart & Jacques Bourneuf. 1982. 480p. pap. 34.95 (*0-7859-4820-1*) Fr & Eur.

Larousse des Plantes Qui Guerissent: Dictionary of Healing Plants. Gerard Debuigne. 1974. (FRE.). 256p. 95.00 (*0-8288-6059-9*, M-6104) Fr & Eur.

Larousse Dictionnaire de la Medecine. Ed. by Andre Domart. 1991. (FRE.). 690p. pap. 16.95 (*0-7859-3944-X*, 2035010063) Fr & Eur.

Larousse Dictionnaire de la Psychologie. Norbert Sillamy. 1971. (FRE.). 250p. pap. 16.95 (*0-7859-7635-3*, 2030754099) Fr & Eur.

Larousse Dictionnaire de Psychiatrie et de Psychopathologie Clinique. Jacques Postel. 1993. (FRE.). 630p. pap. 29.95 (*0-7859-7685-X*, 2037202210) Fr & Eur.

Larousse Dictionnaire de Psychologie. Larousse Staff. 1991. (FRE.). 273p. pap. 28.95 (*0-7859-7684-1*, 2037202164) Fr & Eur.

Larousse Dictionnaire des Examens Medicaux. Didier Sicard. 1991. (FRE.). 328p. 79.95 (*0-7859-7669-8*, 2035101271) Fr & Eur.

Larousse Medical. Ed. by Larousse Staff. 1995. 1142p. 195.00 (*0-7859-9843-8*) Fr & Eur.

Larue D. Carter Memorial Hospital Case-Study: A Behaviorial Approach to Environmental Normalization in Mental Health Settings. Alfredo R. Missair & Bruce F. Meyer. 1983. (Illus.). 16p. pap. 8.00 (*0-912431-03-2*) Ctr Env Des Res.

Laryngeal Biomechanics. B. Raymond Fink & Robert J. Demarest. 1978. LC 77-26937. (Commonwealth Fund Publications). (Illus.). 176p. 42.50 (*0-674-51085-2*) HUP.

Laryngeal Cancer: Proceedings World Congress on Laryngeal Cancer (2nd: 1994 Sydney, N. S. W.) Ed. by Robert Smee & G. Patrick Bridger. 1995. LC 94-42694. (International Congress Ser.: No. 1063). 780p. 300.00 (*0-444-81810-3*) Elsevier.

Laryngeal Electromyography. Sataloff. 2002. pap. 40.00 net. (*0-7693-0168-1*) Singular Publishing.

Laryngeal Function in Phonation & Respiration. Ed. by Katherine Harris et al. 1991. (Illus.). 598p. (Orig.). (C). reprint ed. pap. text 75.00 (*1-879105-22-5*, A004) Singular Publishing.

Laryngectomee Rehabilitation. Ed. by Robert L. Keith & Frederic L. Darley. 3rd ed. 1994. LC 93-39466. (Illus.). (C). text 44.00 (*0-89079-590-8*, 6688) PRO-ED.

Laryngology & Head & Neck Surgery, Vol. 5. Hibbert. 6th ed. 1996. (Scott Brown's Otolaryngology Ser.: Vol. 4). 608p. (*0-7506-0599-5*) E A GBR. *Dist:* OUP.

Larynx. Ed. by Harvey M. Tucker. 2nd ed. 1993. (Illus.). 336p. text 99.00 (*0-86577-437-4*) Thieme Med Pubs.

Larynx: A Multidisciplinary Approach. Marvin P. Fried. 2nd ed. 1995. (Illus.). 672p. (C). (gr. 13). text 149.00 (*0-8016-8046-8*, 08046) Mosby Inc.

Laser: Its Clinical Uses in Eye Diseases. Ian J. Constable & Arthur S. Lim. 2nd ed. 1990. (Illus.). 207p. text (*0-443-04450-3*) Church.

Laser Ablation, Mechanisms & Applications: Proceedings of a Workshop Held in Oak Ridge, Tennessee, U. S. A., 8-10 April 1991. Ed. by J. C. Miller & R. F. Haglund, Jr. 1991. (Lecture Notes in Physics: Vol. 389). 362p. 59.95 (*0-387-97731-7*) Spr-Verlag.

Laser Acupuncture, an Introductory Textbook for Treatment of Pain, Paralysis, Spasticity & Other Disorders: Clinical & Research Uses of Laser Acupuncture from Around the World. Margaret A. Naeser & Xiu-Bing Wei. 1994. (Illus.). 218p. spiral bd. 44.95 (*0-9625651-2-1*) Boston Chinese Med.

Laser & Conventional Refractive Surgery. Ed. by Charles Claove. 1996. 416p. text (*0-7279-0918-5*) BMJ Pub GBR. *Dist:* AIDC.

Laser & Noncoherent Ocular Effects Vol. 2974: Epidemiology, Prevention & Treatment. Ed. by Bruce E. Stuck & Michael Belkin. 1997. LC 97-175320. 240p. 69.00 (*0-8194-2385-8*) SPIE.

Laser Applications in Medicine & Biology. M. L. Wolbarsht. (Illus.). (C). Vol. 4. 1989. 310p. text 110.00 (*0-306-43074-6*); Vol. 5. 1991. 392p. text 120.00 (*0-306-43753-8*) Kluwer Academic (Kluwer Plenum).

Laser Applications in Medicine & Dentistry. Ed. by Gregory B. Altshuler et al. 1996. (Europto Ser.: Vol. 2922). 472p. 110.00 (*0-8194-2324-6*) SPIE.

Laser Applications in Oral & Maxillofacial Surgery. Ed. by Guy A. Catone & Charles C. Alling, 3rd. 1997. LC 95-45035. 307p. text 99.00 (*0-7216-5020-1*) Saunders.

Laser-Assisted Transurethral Resection of the Prostate. Stacy J. Childs. 1993. LC 93-25355. (Illus.). 96p. 25.00 (*0-683-01540-0*) Lppncott W & W.

Laser-Doppler Blood Flowmetry. Ed. by A. P. Shepherd & P. A. Oberg. 1990. 416p. text 215.50 (*0-7923-0508-6*) Kluwer Academic.

Laser Eye Surgery. 1992. lib. bdg. 350.95 (*0-8490-5598-9*) Gordon Pr.

Laser Eye Surgery: A Bibliography, Set. 1995. lib. bdg. 625.95 (*0-8490-8359-1*) Gordon Pr.

Laser in der Medizin - Laser in Medicine: Proceedings of the 11th International Congress. W. Waudelich & R. Waidelich. 1994. (Illus.). 525p. 118.00 (*0-387-57441-7*) Spr-Verlag.

Laser in Urology: International Symposium, Luebeck, November 1985. Ed. by A. Hofstetter. 1986. (Journal: Vol. 12, Suppl. 1, 1986). vi, 58p. pap. 24.50 (*3-8055-4362-X*) S Karger.

Laser-Induced Interstitial Thermotherapy. Ed. by Gerhard J. Muller & Andre Roggan. 1995. LC 95-12212. (Institute Ser.: Vol. PM25). 566p. 95.00 (*0-8194-1859-5*) SPIE.

Laser Lithotripsy. Ed. by R. Steiner. 1988. (Illus.). 201p. 79.95 (*0-387-19480-0*) Spr-Verlag.

Laser Methods for Biomedical Applications Vol. 2965: ALT '96 International Symposium. Ed. by Alexander M. Prokhorov & Costas Fotakis. 1996. 212p. 59.00 (*0-8194-2369-6*) SPIE.

Laser-Optoelectronics in Medicine, 1989. Ed. by W. Waidelich. 1990.Tr. of Laser-Optoelektronik in der Medizin 1989. (Illus.). 440p. 97.00 (*0-387-51434-1*) Spr-Verlag.

Laser-Optoelektronik in der Medizin 1989 see Laser-Optoelectronics in Medicine, 1989

Laser Plastic Surgery: Resurfacing & Cutting. G. H. Sasaki. 1999. (Illus.). 328p. 165.00 (*0-387-98394-5*) Spr-Verlag.

Laser Skin Rejuvenation. Paul J. Carniol. 1998. LC 98-21400. 336p. text 110.00 (*0-7817-1561-X*) Lppncott W & W.

Laser Spectroscopy VII. T. W. Hansch & Y. R. Shen. 1985. (Series in Optical Sciences: Vol. 49). (Illus.). 419p. 71.95 (*0-387-15894-4*) Spr-Verlag.

Laser Surgery: Advanced Characterization, Therapeutics, & Systems III. 1992. 102.00 (*0-8194-0789-5*, 1643) SPIE.

Laser Surgery in Children. H. P. Berlien & P. P. Schmittenbecher. 1997. LC 97-18416. (Illus.). 206p. 135.00 (*3-540-62633-6*) Spr-Verlag.

Laser Surgery in Gynecology: A Clinical Guide. V. Cecil Wright & John C. Fisher. 1993. LC 92-15350. (Illus.). 352p. text 70.00 (*0-7216-4007-9*) Saunders.

Laser Surgery in Ophthalmology. Thomas A. Weingeist & Scott R. Sneed. 1992. (Illus.). 206p. (C). pap. text 135.00 (*0-8385-7903-5*, A7903-6, Apple Lange Med) McGraw.

Laser Surgery of the Posterior Segment. Steven M. Bloom & Alexander J. Brucker. 2nd ed. 1996. LC 96-47103. 432p. text 115.00 (*0-397-58423-7*) Lppncott W & W.

Laser Systems for Photobiology & Photomedicine. Ed. by Arthur N. Chester et al. 1991. (NATO Advanced Science Institutes Ser.: Vol. 252). (Illus.). 320p. (C). text 132.00 (*0-306-43886-0*, Kluwer Plenum) Kluwer Academic.

Laser Technology V Vol. 3188: Applications in Medicine & Ecology. Ed. by Wieslaw Wolinski & Alfreda Graczyk. 1997. LC 98-196854. 208p. 59.00 (*0-8194-2618-0*) SPIE.

Laser-Tissue Interaction & Tissue Optics II. Ed. by Hans J. Albrecht et al. 1996. (Europto Ser.: Vol. 2923). 212p. 66.00 (*0-8194-2325-4*) SPIE.

Laser-Tissue Interaction IX, Vol. 3254. Ed. by Steven L. Jacques. 1998. 526p. 107.00 (*0-8194-2693-8*) SPIE.

Laser-Tissue Interaction III. Ed. by S. L. Jacques. 1992. 20.00 (*0-8194-0792-5*, 1646) SPIE.

Laser-Tissue Interaction, Tissue Optics & Laser Welding III. Ed. by Guy P. Delacretaz et al. 1998. LC 98-145663. (Europto Ser.: Vol. 3195). 358p. 80.00 (*0-8194-2627-X*) SPIE.

Laser-Tissue Interaction VIII, Vol. 2975. Ed. by Steven L. Jacques. 1997. 472p. 107.00 (*0-8194-2386-6*) SPIE.

Laser-Tissue Interactions: Fundamentals & Applications. Markolf H. Niemz. 1996. LC 96-118. (Illus.). 297p. stu. ed. 125.00 (*3-540-60363-8*) Spr-Verlag.

J
K
L

Laser Treatment & Photocoagulation of the Eye. Ed. by Reginald Birngruber & V. P. Gabel. 1984. (Documenta Ophthalmologica Proceedings Ser.). text 225.00 (*90-6193-732-9*) Kluwer Academic.

Laser Treatment for Naevi. Toshio Ohshiro. 1995. LC 95-171066. 292p. 315.00 (*0-471-95243-5*) Wiley.

Laser Vision Breakthrough: Everything You Need to Consider Before Making the Decision. Stephen F. Brint et al. 4th ed. 2000. LC 99-89458. (Illus.). 352p. 24.95 (*0-7615-2087-2*) Prima Pub.

Laser Vision Correction: A New Age in Vision. Harold A. Stein et al. 1998. (Illus.). 96p. pap. 24.95 (*0-9666621-0-5*) Ethis Commns.

Lasers: The Perioperative Challenge. Kay Ball. 2nd ed. 1995. LC 94-47036. (Illus.). 448p. (C). (gr. 13). pap. text 35.95 (*0-8151-0524-X*, 24568) Mosby Inc.

Lasers & Optical Fibers in Medicine. Abraham Katzir. 1993. LC 93-12744. (Physical Techniques in Biology & Medicine Ser.). (Illus.). 317p. text 100.00 (*0-12-401940-4*) Acad Pr.

Lasers in Aesthetic Surgery. Ed. by Gregory Keller et al. 2000. (Illus.). 408p. 169.00 (*0-86577-850-7*) Thieme Med Pubs.

Lasers in Cardiovascular Medicine & Surgery: Fundamentals & Techniques. Ed. by George S. Abela. 1990. (Developments in Cardiovascular Medicine Ser.). (C). text 259.50 (*0-7923-0440-3*) Kluwer Academic.

Lasers in Chemical Analysis. Ed. by Gary M. Hieftje et al. 1981. LC 80-84082. (Contemporary Instrumentation & Analysis Ser.). (Illus.). 330p. 140.00 (*0-89603-027-X*) Humana.

Lasers in Cutaneous & Cosmetic Surgery. Gary P. Lask & Nicholas J. Lowe. Ed. by Judy Fletcher. 1999. LC 98-7037. (Illus.). xi, 167p. text (*0-443-07639-1*) Saunders.

Lasers in Dentistry. Ed. by Leo J. Miserendino & Robert M. Pick. 1995. LC 94-41152. (Illus.). 341p. text 98.00 (*0-86715-282-6*) Quint Pub Co.

Lasers in Dentistry III, Vol. 2973. Ed. by Harvey A. Wigdor et al. 1997. LC 97-193065. 252p. 69.00 (*0-8194-2384-X*) SPIE.

Lasers in Dentistry IV, Vol. 3248. Ed. by John D. Featherstone et al. 1998. LC 98-233178. 240p. 69.00 (*0-8194-2687-3*) SPIE.

Lasers in Dermatology: Bio-Optics & Treatment of Human Skin. Compiled by Optical Society of America Staff. 1997. LC 97-68772. (Technical Digest Series, 1997: Vol. 15). (Illus.). 72p. pap. 75.00 (*1-55752-513-7*) Optical Soc.

Lasers in Dermatology: Proceedings of the International Symposium, Ulm, September 26, 1989. Ed. by R. Steiner et al. 1991. (Illus.). 176p. 118.00 (*0-387-51863-0*) Spr-Verlag.

Lasers in Facial Aesthetic & Reconstructive Surgery. Brian S. Biesman. 1998. LC 98-21399. 124p. text 129.00 (*0-683-30414-3*) Lppncott W & W.

Lasers in General Surgery. Hira. 1997. 500p. (C). (gr. 13). pap. 121.00 (*0-412-49340-3*) Chapman & Hall.

Lasers in General Surgery. Stephen N. Joffe. 1989. (Illus.). 336p. 70.00 (*0-683-04460-5*) Lppncott W & W.

Lasers in Gynecology: Possibilities & Limitations. Ed. by G. Bastert & D. Wallwiener. 1992. (Illus.). 453p. 250.00 (*0-387-53409-1*) Spr-Verlag.

Lasers in Maxillofacial Surgery & Dentisty. Lewis Clayman & Paul Kuo. 1997. LC 96-36512. (Illus.). 252p. text 99.00 (*0-86577-566-4*) Thieme Med Pubs.

Lasers in Medicine. Leon Goldman & James R. Rockwell, Jr. 1971. LC 77-163181. (Illus.). x, 386p. text 453.00 (*0-677-02430-4*) Gordon & Breach.

Lasers in Medicine. R. W. Waynant & G. H. Pettit. 1997. (Lasers, Photonics, & Electro-Optics Ser.). (Illus.). 468p. (C). (*0-306-45549-8*, Plenum Trade) Perseus Pubng.

Lasers in Medicine & Dentistry: Diagnostics & Treatment. Ed. by Brij M. Khorana et al. 1996. (Europto Ser.: Vol. 2887). 246p. 85.00 (*0-8194-2288-6*) SPIE.

Lasers in Neurosurgery. Ed. by E. F. Downing et al. 1989. (Illus.). 130p. 71.95 (*0-387-82067-1*) Spr-Verlag.

Lasers in Neurosurgery. Ed. by Jon H. Robertson & W. Craig Clark. 1988. (Foundations of Neurological Surgery Ser.). (C). text 150.00 (*0-89838-966-6*) Kluwer Academic.

Lasers in Ophthalmic Surgery. David B. Karlin. 1994. (Illus.). 352p. 125.00 (*0-86542-260-5*) Blackwell Sci.

Lasers in Ophthalmology IV, Vol. 2930. Ed. by Reginald Birngruber et al. 1996. (Europto Ser.). 238p. 66.00 (*0-8194-2332-7*) SPIE.

Lasers in Otolaryngology. Davis. 1990. (Illus.). 224p. text 135.00 (*0-7216-3124-X*) Saunders.

Lasers in Otorhinolaryngology, & in Head & Neck Surgery. Ed. by H. Rudert & J. A. Werner. 1995. (Advances in OtoRhinoLaryngology Ser.: Vol. 49). (Illus.). xii, 264p. 215.75 (*3-8055-6087-7*) S Karger.

Lasers in Plastic Surgery. Michael I. Kulick. 1997. LC 96-53897. (Illus.). 211p. 207.00 (*0-387-94891-0*) Spr-Verlag.

Lasers in Skin Disease. Ronald G. Wheeland. Ed. by James Smith. 1988. (American Academy of Facial Plastic & Reconstructive Surgery Monograph Ser.: Vol. 5). (Illus.). 128p. text 95.00 (*0-86577-271-1*) Thieme Med Pubs.

Lasers in Surgery: Advanced Characterization, Therapeutics & Systems VIII. Ed. by R. Rox Anderson et al. 1998. LC 99-192207. (Proceedings of SPIE Ser.: Vol. 3245). 474p. 116.00 (*0-8194-2684-9*) SPIE.

***Lasers in Surgery: Advanced Characterization, Therapeutics, & Systems X: 22-23, 25 January 2000, San Jose, California.** Ed. by Rox Anderson. 2000. LC 00-711703. (Progress in Biomedical Optics & Imaging Ser.: No. 1). (Illus.). xvi, 638p. (*0-8194-3523-6*) SPIE.

Lasers in Surgery Vol. 2970: Advanced Characterization, Therapeutics & Systems VII. Ed. by R. Rox Anderson et al. 1997. 632p. 132.00 (*0-8194-2381-5*) SPIE.

Lasers in Surgery & Medicine: Principles & Practice. Ed. by Carmen A. Puliafito. 1996. LC 95-36635. 484p. 145.00 (*0-471-12070-7*, Wiley-Liss) Wiley.

***Lasers in the Musculoskeletal System.** Ed. by B. E. Gerber et al. 2001. 450p. 179.00 (*3-540-63761-3*) Spr-Verlag.

Lasers in Urological Surgery. Ed. by Alfons G. Hofstetter. 1997. LC 97-20861. (Illus.). 168p. 70.00 (*3-540-62452-X*) Spr-Verlag.

Lasers in Urology: Principles & Practice. Ed. by Jack Tinker & T. A. McNicholas. 1990. (Bloomsbury Series in Clinical Science). (Illus.). 168p. 143.00 (*0-387-19615-3*) Spr-Verlag.

Lasik. Ioannis Pallikaris & Dimitrios Siganos. 1997. LC 97-37263. (Illus.). 384p. text 149.00 (*1-55642-323-3*, 63233) SLACK Inc.

***LASIK: A Guide to Laser Vision Correction.** Ernest Kornmehl et al. 2001. LC 2001-3385. (Illus.). 130p. pap. 12.95 (*1-886039-54-2*) Addicus Bks.

LASIK: Clinical Co-Management. Milton M. Hom & Loretta B. Szczotka. 2000. LC 00-29752. (Illus.). 176p. pap. text 44.99 (*0-7506-7214-5*) Buttrwrth-Heinemann.

LASIK: Surgical Techniques & Complications. Lucio Buratto & Stephen Brint. 2nd ed. 624p. 2000. (SPA., Illus.). 215.00 (*1-55642-446-9*); 1999. LC 99-46441. 215.00 (*1-55642-432-9*) SLACK Inc.

LASIK Complications: Prevention & Management. Howard Gimbel & Ellen E. Anderson Penno. 1998. LC 98-34613. (Illus.). xvi, 223p. 80.00 (*1-55642-392-6*, 63926) SLACK Inc.

***Lasik Eye Surgery (Laser in Situ) (Kerato-Mileusis) Index of New Information & Guide-Book for Consumers, Reference & Research.** Harvey K. Melbone. 2002. 180p. 57.50 (*0-7883-2500-0*); pap. 47.50 (*0-7883-2501-9*) ABBE Pubs Assn.

Last Choice: Preemptive Suicide in Advanced Age. C. G. Prado. 2nd ed. 1998. LC 98-11103. 208p. pap. 20.95 (*0-275-96150-8*, Praeger Pubs) Greenwood.

Last Dance: Encountering Death & Dying. Lynne Ann DeSpelder & Albert L. Strickland. 5th ed. 1998. LC 98-3326. 672p. (C). text 51.95 (*0-7674-0217-0*, 0217-0) Mayfield Pub.

Last Diaries. Leo Tolstoy. Ed. by Robert J. Kastenbaum. Tr. by Lydia W. Kesich. 1979. LC 78-22222. (Aging & Old Age Ser.). reprint ed. lib. bdg. 27.95 (*0-405-11835-X*) Ayer.

Last Five Pounds: How to Lose Them & Leave Them Forever. Jamie Pope. Ed. by Julie Rubenstein. 1995. 384p. 23.00 (*0-671-88453-0*) PB.

Last Good Freudian. Brenda S. Webster. 2000. LC 00-20442. 193p. 24.95 (*0-8419-1395-1*) Holmes & Meier.

Last (Lose & Stay Trim) Program: A Holistic Approach to Weight Loss. Melissa Caron. 1997. 87p. ring bd. 29.00 (*0-9657924-0-4*, 1001) Write Prodns.

Last Mile to Huesca. Judith Keene. 1988. (Illus.). 178p. pap. (*0-86840-338-5*) New South Wales Univ Pr AUS. *Dist:* Intl Spec Bk.

Last Minute Optics: A Concise Review of Optics, Refraction & Contact Lenses. David G. Hunter & Constance E. West. 1996. LC 96-6823. (Illus.). 144p. pap. 35.00 (*1-55642-317-9*, 63179) SLACK Inc.

Last of the Lunatics. John Cawte. 1998. LC 00-303787. 272p. pap. (*0-522-84804-4*) Melbourne Univ Pr AUS. *Dist:* Paul & Co Pubs.

Last Physician: Walker Percy & the Moral Life of Medicine. Ed. by Carl Elliott & John D. Lantos. 1999. LC 99-14158. 208p. 45.95 (*0-8223-2336-2*); pap. 15.95 (*0-8223-2369-9*) Duke.

Last Resort: Psychosurgery & the Limits of Medicine. Jack D. Pressman. 1998. LC 97-14074. (Cambridge Studies in the History of Medicine). (Illus.). 574p. (C). text 49.95 (*0-521-35371-8*) Cambridge U Pr.

Last Secret: Daughters Sexually Abused by Mothers. Bobbie Rosencrans. Ed. by Euan Bear. 1997. LC 98-234806. 261p. pap. 20.00 (*1-884444-36-9*) Safer Soc.

Last Served? Gendering the HIV Pandemic. Cindy Patton. 1994. LC 94-11502. (Social Aspects of AIDS Ser.). pap. 19.95 (*0-7484-0190-3*) Taylor & Francis.

Last Valentine. James Michael Pratt. l.t. ed. 1998. LC 98-10748. 24.95 (*1-57490-133-8*, Beeler LP Bks) T T Beeler.

Last Wish. Betty Rollin. 1998. LC 98-19185. 272p. pap. text 12.00 (*1-891620-01-0*) PublicAffairs NY.

Last Witness: The Child Survivor of the Holocaust. Judith S. Kestenberg & Ira Brenner. 1996. LC 95-26268. 272p. text 38.50 (*0-88048-662-7*, 8662) Am Psychiatric.

Last Words on Evolution. 3. Ernst Haeckel. Tr. by Joseph McCabe from GER. 1977. LC 77-72191. (Contributions to the History of Psychology Ser.: Vol. 3, Pt. D). 285p. reprint ed. lib. bdg. 69.50 (*0-313-26947-5*, U6947, Greenwood Pr) Greenwood.

Last Writings on the Philosophy of Psychology Vol. 1: Preliminary Studies for Part II of Philosophical Investigations. Ludwig Josef Johann Wittgenstein. Ed. by Heikki Nyman & George H. Von Wright. Tr. by C. J. Luckhardt & M. A. Aue. 1996. 268p. (C). reprint ed. pap. text 17.95 (*0-226-90425-3*) U Ch Pr.

Last's Anatomy: Regional & Applied. Ed. by R. M. H. McMinn. 9th ed. 1994. LC 94-5560. (Illus.). text (*0-443-04662-X*) Church.

Late Adolescence: Psychoanalytic Studies. Ed. by David D. Brockman. 1985. LC 84-25181. xxxvi, 367p. 60.00 (*0-8236-2948-1*, 02948) Intl Univs Pr.

Late Effects of Treatment for Childhood Cancer. Daniel M. Green. 1991. (Current Clinical Oncology Ser.). 200p. pap. 99.95 (*0-471-56166-5*, Wiley-Liss) Wiley.

Late Graft Loss: Proceedings of the 28th Conference on Transplantation & Clinical Immunology, 3-5 June 1996. Ed. by J. L. Toutaine et al. 1997. LC 96-48786. (Transplantation & Clinical Immunology Ser.). 256p. (C). text 100.50 (*0-7923-4315-8*) Kluwer Academic.

Late Onset Neurometabolic Genetic Disorders: From Clinical to Molecular Aspects of Lysosomal & Peroxisomal Disease - Journal: Developmental Neuroscience, Vol. 13, Nos. 4-5. Ed. by N. Baumann et al. 1991. (Illus.). 196p. pap. 106.25 (*3-8055-5524-5*) S Karger.

Late Phase Allergic Reactions. Ed. by Walter Dorsch. 1990. 464p. lib. bdg. 129.00 (*0-8493-6743-3*, QR188) CRC Pr.

Late Potentials of the Auditory System. David L. McPherson. 1995. LC 95-34210. (Evoked Potentials Ser.). 170p. 39.95 (*1-56593-163-7*, 0473) Thomson Learn.

Late Sequelae in Oncology. Ed. by J. Dunst & R. Sauer. 1995. LC 94-45370. (Medical Radiology Ser.). (*3-540-56936-7*) Spr-Verlag.

Late-Stage Dementia Care: A Basic Guide. C. R. Kovach. 1996. LC 96-35127. 220p. 69.95 (*1-56032-514-3*); pap. 29.95 (*1-56032-515-1*) Taylor & Francis.

Late-Talking Children. Thomas Sowell. 1998. 224p. pap. 14.00 (*0-465-03835-2*) Basic.

Lateinisch-Griechisch Wortschatz in der Medizin. Ilse Becher. 3rd ed. 1991. (GER, GRE & LAT.). 255p. 59.95 (*0-7859-6874-1*, 3333006278) Fr & Eur.

Latency. Charles A. Sarnoff. 1981. LC 75-34707. 416p. reprint ed. 60.00 (*0-87668-233-6*) Aronson.

Latency by Herpes Simplex Viruses: Journal: Intervirology, 1991, Vol. 32, No. 2. Ed. by Kenneth I. Berns & R. W. Whitley. 1991. (Illus.). 52p. pap. 37.50 (*3-8055-5362-5*) S Karger.

Latent Herpes Virus Infections in Veterinary Medicine. Ed. by G. Wittmann et al. 1984. (Current Topics in Veterinary Medicine & Animal Science Ser.). 528p. text 252.50 (*0-89838-622-5*) Kluwer Academic.

Latent Inhibition & Conditioned Attention Theory. R. E. Lubow. 1989. (Problems in the Behavioral Sciences Ser.). (Illus.). 336p. (C). text 90.00 (*0-521-36307-1*) Cambridge U Pr.

***Latent Prostatic Carcinoma: Epidemiology - Biology - Clinical Significance - Detection & Prevention.** Ed. by H. Huland. 2001. (European Urology Ser.: Vol. 39). (Illus.). iv, 54p. pap., suppl. ed. 25.25 (*3-8055-7242-5*) S Karger.

Latente Adipositas: Ein Vergleich Latent und Manifest Ausgepragter Ebsucht. Regina Pencik. 1997. (Psychologie Ser.: Bd. 599). (Illus.). 157p. 31.95 (*3-631-32117-1*) P Lang Pubng.

Lateral Preferences & Human Behavior. C. Porac & S. Coren. 1981. (Illus.). 283p. 97.00 (*0-387-90596-0*) Spr-Verlag.

Lateralisation of Language in the Child. Ed. by Y. Lebrun & O. L. Zangwill. 1982. (Neurolinguistics Ser.: Vol. 10). 175p. (*90-265-0337-7*) Swets.

Laterality & Psychopathology. Ed. by P. Flor-Henry & J. H. Gruzelier. 1983. (Developments in Psychiatry Ser.: Vol. 6). 648p. 108.00 (*0-444-80481-1*, I-360-83) Elsevier.

Latest Achievements of Diabetes Research. F. Belfiore & Agata M. Rabuazzo. 1986. (Frontiers in Diabetes Ser.: Vol. 7). x, 298p. 216.75 (*3-8055-4261-5*) S Karger.

Latest Findings on the Aetiology & Therapy of Depression. Ed. by P. Kielholz & W. Poeldinger. 1987. (Journal: Vol. 19, Suppl. 2, 1986). (Illus.). vi, 270p. pap. 83.50 (*3-8055-4542-8*) S Karger.

Latest Studies on VDTs, 1993. Robin Y. Woo. 3rd ed. 1993. 176p. (C). pap. 10.00 (*1-879887-00-2*) Ctr Office Tech.

Latex Allergies & the Health Care Industry: Do OSHA's Actions Confuse or Clarify? : Hearing Before the Subcommittee on Oversight & Investigations of the Committee on Education & the Workforce, House of Representatives, One Hundred Sixth Congress, First Session, Hearing Held in Washington, DC, March 25, 1999. Ed. by U. S. Congress, House Committee on Education and the Workforce, Subcommittee on Oversight and Investigations. 1999. LC 99-490421. (*0-16-058701-8*) USGPO.

Latex Allergies & the Health Care Industry Congressional Hearing: Do OSHA's Actions Confuse or Clarify? Ed. by Charlie Norwood. 2000. 205p. pap. text 35.00 (*0-7567-0141-4*) DIANE Pub.

Latin American Psychology: A Guide to Research & Training. Gerardo Marin et al. 1987. LC 87-17409. 220p. pap. 29.95 (*0-912704-84-5*) Am Psychol.

Latin-English-Chinese Dictionary of Medical Terms. Commercial Press Staff. 1979. (CHI, ENG & LAT.). 761p. 95.00 (*0-8288-4815-7*, M9564) Fr & Eur.

Latin-Estonian-Russian Medical Dictionary. A. Valdes & J. V. Veski. (C). Vol. 1. 1982. 640p. (*0-7855-6446-2*); Vol. 2. 1983. 768p. (*0-7855-5058-5*) Collets GBR. *Dist:* St Mut.

Latin-Estonian-Russian Medical Dictionary, Vol. A-N. A. Vales & J. V. Veski. 1982. (EST, LAT & RUS.). 640p. (*0-7855-1759-6*) Collets GBR. *Dist:* St Mut.

Latin-Estonian-Russian Medical Dictionary, Vol. O-Z. A. Valdes & J. V. Veski. 1983. (EST, LAT & RUS.). 768p. (*0-7855-1758-8*) Collets GBR. *Dist:* St Mut.

Latin Readings in the History of Medicine. Robert J. Smutny. 1994. (ENG & LAT.). 456p. (Orig.). (C). pap. 45.50 (*0-8191-9766-1*) U Pr of Amer.

Latino Families in Therapy: A Guide to Multicultural Practice. Celia J. Falicov. 1998. LC 98-2636. (Guilford Family Therapy Ser.). (Illus.). 303p. text 36.00 (*1-57230-364-6*) Guilford Pubns.

Latino Folk Illness. L. M. Pachter. 1993. 110p. pap. text 82.00 (*2-88124-636-2*) Gordon & Breach.

Latino Folk Medicine: Healing Herbal Remedies from an Ancient Tradition. Anthony DeStefano. 2001. LC 00-110327. 208p. pap. 12.95 (*0-345-43836-1*, Ballantine) Ballantine Pub Grp.

Latino Health in the U. S. A Growing Challenge. Ed. by Carlos W. Molina & Marilyn Aguirre-Molina. 1994. LC 96-147979. 513p. pap. 42.50 (*0-87553-215-2*) Am Pub Health.

Latino Psychiatric Patient: Assessment & Treatment. Ernestina Carrillo & Alberto Lopez. 2001. LC 00-67625. 240p. pap. 28.95 (*0-88048-773-9*, 8773) Am Psychiatric.

Latino Task Force Report on the Year 2000: Health Promotion Objectives & Recommendations for California. 1993. 72p. (Orig.). (C). pap. text 25.00 (*0-7881-0088-2*) DIANE Pub.

Laugh a Day Keeps the Doctor Away. Irvin Shrewsbury Cobb. 1998. (Collected Works of Irvin S. Cobb). 246p. reprint ed. lib. bdg. 88.00 (*1-58201-595-3*) Classic Bks.

Laugh at Your Muscles: A Light Look at Fibromyalgia. Mark J. Pellegrino. 1995. (Illus.). 92p. (Orig.). pap. 5.95 (*0-9646891-4-6*) Anadem Pubng.

Laughing & Loving with Autism: A Collection of "Real Life" Warm & Humorous Stories. R. Wayne Gilpin. 1993. 127p. pap. 9.95 (*1-885477-04-X*) Fut Horizons.

Laughing Death: The Untold Story of Kuru. Vincent Zigas. 1990. LC 89-24706. (Illus.). 315p. 29.50 (*0-89603-111-X*) Humana.

Laughing Your Way to Good Health. Susan Vass. 1990. (Illus.). 72p. (Orig.). pap. 4.95 (*0-9627545-0-1*) HMR Pubns Grp.

Laughing Your Way to Passing the Pediatric Boards: The Seriously Funny Study Guide. 2000. (Illus.). 400p. pap. 99.95 (*0-9700287-0-9*) Medhumor.

Laughter & Tears: The Emotional Life of New Mothers. Elizabeth Bing. 1997. LC 96-46089. (Illus.). 304p. pap. 16.95 (*0-8050-4157-5*, Owl) H Holt & Co.

Launching the Antibiotic Era: Personal Accounts of the Discovery & Use of the First Antibiotics. Edward P. Abraham et al. Ed. by Zanvil A. Cohn & Carol L. Moberg. 1990. 112p. 25.00 (*0-87470-047-7*) Rockefeller.

Laura: A Case Study for the Modularity of Language. Jeni Yamada. 1990. LC 90-39106. (Issues in the Biology of Language & Cognition Ser.). (Illus.). 135p. 35.00 (*0-262-24030-0*) MIT Pr.

***Lavendar Couch: A Guide to Psychtherapy for Lesbians & Gay Men.** Michael Bettinger. 2001. LC 2001-22574. xv, 325p. pap. 15.95 (*1-55583-534-1*) Alyson Pubns.

Law & Ethics: A Guide for the Health Professional. Ed. by Nathan T. Sidley. 1984. LC 83-26565. 368p. 53.95 (*0-89885-155-6*, Kluwer Acad Hman Sci) Kluwer Academic.

Law & Ethics for Health Occupations. Karen Judson & Sharon Blesie. 1993. LC 93-18325. 20.00 (*0-02-800668-2*) Glencoe.

Law & Ethics for Medical Careers. Karen Judson & Sharon Hicks. 2nd ed. 1999. LC 98-29423. (YA). (gr. 6-12). stu. ed. 28.00 (*0-02-804755-9*) Glencoe.

Law & Ethics in Clinical Laboratory Science. Griffith. 1996. (C). pap. text (*0-7216-5319-7*) Saunders.

Law & Ethics in Diagnostic Imaging & Therapeutic Radiology: With Risk Management & Safety Applications. Ed. by Ann M. Obergfell. 1995. LC 95-10278. (Illus.). 208p. text 27.00 (*0-7216-5062-7*) Saunders.

Law & Ethics of the Veterinary Profession. James F. Wilson et al. Ed. by Suzanne Neilson. 1988. (Illus.). 550p. (C). 59.95 (*0-9621007-0-6*) Priority Press.

Law & Medical Men. R. Vashon Rogers, Jr. 1981. 214p. reprint ed. 40.00 (*0-8377-1032-4*, Rothman) W S Hein.

Law & Medical Practice: Rights, Duties, Claims, & Defences. Loane Skene. 1998. LC 99-488091. (*0-409-31178-2*) Buttrwrth-Heinemann.

Law & Medicine. Belinda Bennett. 1997. LC 97-157544. 191p. pap. (*0-455-21456-5*) LawBk Co AUS. *Dist:* Gaunt.

Law & Medicine: A Special Issue of Law in Context. Ed. by Kerry Petersen. 1994. pap. (*1-86324-025-X*) LaTrobe Univ AUS. *Dist:* Intl Spec Bk.

Law & Medicine: Cases & Materials. Walter J. Wadlington et al. 1991. LC 80-23725. (University Casebook Ser.). 1039p. reprint ed. text 38.95 (*0-88277-015-2*) Foundation Pr.

Law & Medicine in Canada. Gilbert Sharpe. 2nd ed. 1987. 680p. text 123.00 (*0-409-86590-7*, MICHIE) LEXIS Pub.

Law & Mental Health: Harmonizing Objectives: A Comparative Survey of Existing Legislation Together with Guidelines for Its Assessment & Alternative Approaches to Improvement. William J. Curran & T. Harding. 1977. (International Digest of Health Legislation Offprints: Vol. 28, No. 4). 159p. 25.00 (*92-4-169284-7*) World Health.

Law & Mental Health: International Perspectives, Vol. 2. Ed. by David N. Weisstub. 1986. (Law & Mental Health Ser.). 304p. 96.00 (*0-08-032781-8*, K130, J110, Pergamon Pr) Elsevier.

Law & Mental Health: Research & Policy. Ed. by Saleem A. Shah. 1986. LC 85-63002. (Annals of the American Academy of Political & Social Science Ser.: Vol. 484). (Orig.). text 26.00 (*0-8039-2694-4*); pap. text 17.00 (*0-8039-2695-2*) Sage.

Law & Mental Health Professionals: Arizona. Michael O. Miller & Bruce D. Sales. 1986. LC 86-10780. 357p. 59.95 (*0-912704-50-0*) Am Psychol.

Law & Mental Health Professionals: California. O. Brant Caudill & Kenneth S. Pope. 1995. LC 94-40248. 630p. text 59.95 (*1-55798-276-7*, 431-5100) Am Psychol.

Law & Mental Health Professionals: Delaware. Ann H. Britton & Timothy H. Rohs. 2000. LC 99-86786. (Law & Mental Health Professionals Ser.). xix, 349p. 59.95 (*1-55798-686-X*) Am Psychol.

Law & Mental Health Professionals: Florida. Randy K. Otto & John Petrila. 1996. LC 95-40356. 373p. (C). text 59.95 (*1-55798-322-4*, 431-5120) Am Psychol.

Law & Mental Health Professionals: Massachusetts. Jonathan Brant. Ed. by Bruce D. Sales & Michael O. Miller. 2nd ed. 1997. LC 97-19091. (Illus.). 285p. 59.95 (*1-55798-446-8*) Am Psychol.

Law & Mental Health Professionals: Michigan. Beth K. Clark & Charles R. Clark. 2000. LC 00-38096. (Law & Mental Health Professionals Ser.). xxi, 324p. 59.95 (*1-55798-715-7*) Am Psychol.

Law & Mental Health Professionals: Minnesota. Eric S. Janus et al. 1994. 442p. text 59.95 (*1-55798-230-9*) Am Psychol.

Law & Mental Health Professionals: Nevada. Krista Johns & Ronald Dillehay. 1998. LC 98-6248. (Law & Mental Health Professionals Ser.). 328p. 59.95 (*1-55798-507-3*) Am Psychol.

Law & Mental Health Professionals: New Jersey. James S. Wulach. 2nd ed. 1997. LC 97-30496. (Law & Mental Health Professionals Ser.). 455p. text 59.95 (*1-55798-371-2*, 431-5041) Am Psychol.

Law & Mental Health Professionals: New York. James S. Wulach. 1993. 383p. text 59.95 (*1-55798-195-7*) Am Psychol.

Law & Mental Health Professionals: Pennsylvania. Donald N. Bersoff et al. 1998. LC 98-25722. (Law & Mental Health Professionals Ser.). 392p. 59.95 (*1-55798-555-3*) Am Psychol.

Law & Mental Health Professionals: Texas. Daniel W. Shuman. 2nd ed. 1997. LC 97-1390. (Law & Mental Health Professionals Ser.). 347p. 59.95 (*1-55798-405-0*, 431-5025) Am Psychol.

Law & Mental Health Professionals: Washington. Ed. by Thomas D. Overcast et al. 1995. LC 95-5363. (Law & Mental Health Professionals Ser.). 492p. text 59.95 (*1-55798-278-3*, 431-5110) Am Psychol.

Law & Mental Health Professionals: Wisconsin. Leonard V. Kaplan & Robert D. Miller. 1995. LC 95-40357. 383p. 59.95 (*1-55798-313-5*, 431-5060) Am Psychol.

Law & Mental Health Professionals: Wyoming. George Blau. 1997. LC 97-32112. 541p. 59.95 (*1-55798-447-6*) Am Psychol.

***Law & Mental Health Professionals: Wyoming Supplement.** George Blau. 2001. (*1-55798-552-9*) Am Psychol.

Law & Mercury-Free Dentistry. Pamela D. Ousley. 1994. 260p. (Orig.). pap. 19.65 (*0-941011-11-9*) Bio-Probe.

Law & Nursing. Jean McHale et al. 2nd ed. 2001. (Illus.). 304p. pap. 35.00 (*0-7506-4806-6*) Buttrwrth-Heinemann.

Law & Occupational Injury, Disease, & Death. Warren Freedman. 1990. LC 89-10746. 199p. 65.00 (*0-89930-410-9*, FOP/, Greenwood Pr) Greenwood.

Law & Psychiatry III: Selected Papers Presented at the Fourth International Congress on Law & Psychiatry, Pembroke College, Oxford England, 19-22 July 1979. Ed. by David N. Weisstub. 1981. 100p. pap. 18.25 (*0-08-026113-2*, Pergamon Pr) Elsevier.

Law & Psychiatry in the Canadian Context. Ed. by David N. Weisstub. 1981. 150.00 (*0-08-023134-9*, Pergamon Pr) Elsevier.

Law & the American Health Care System. Rand E. Rosenblatt et al. 1997. LC 97-200705. (University Casebook Ser.). 1346p. text 62.50 net. (*1-56662-481-9*) Foundation Pr.

Law & the American Health Care System. Rand E. Rosenblatt. 2nd ed. 2001. (University Casebook Ser.). (*1-58778-076-3*) Foundation Pr.

Law & the Ecological Challenge: Amintaphil, Vol. 2. Ed. by Eugene E. Dais. 1979. LC 78-61842. 265p. lib. bdg. 42.00 (*0-930342-66-6*, 300220) W S Hein.

Law & the Mental Health Professions: Friction at the Interface. Ed. by Walter E. Barton & Charlotte J. Sanborn. 1978. LC 77-90226. xviii, 330p. (Orig.). 50.00 (*0-8236-2950-3*) Intl Univs Pr.

Law & the Mental Health System: Civil & Criminal Aspects. Ralph Reisner & Christopher Slobogin. 2nd ed. 1990. (American Casebook Ser.). 1117p. (C). text 54.50 (*0-314-73302-7*) West Pub.

Law & the Midwife. Rosemary Jenkins. 1995. LC 94-23377. (Illus.). 224p. pap. 37.95 (*0-632-03629-X*) Blackwell Sci.

Law & the Physician. Edward P. Richards & Katharine C. Rathbun. 2nd ed. 1999. 560p. 99.00 (*0-8342-1380-X*) Aspen Pub.

Law & the Postmodern Mind: Essays on Psychoanalysis & Jurisprudence. Ed. by David F. Carlson & Peter Goodrich. 1998. LC 97-33739. (Law, Meaning, & Violence Ser.). 328p. (C). text 55.00 (*0-472-10841-7*, 10841) U of Mich Pr.

Law & the Public's Health. Kenneth R. Wing. 5th ed. 1999. LC 99-24641. 56.00 (*1-56793-098-0*); LC 99-11046. xv, 343p. (*1-56793-103-0*) Health Admin Pr.

Law & the Public's Health: Supplemental Cases. Kenneth R. Wing. 5th ed. 1999. LC 99-11046. xv, 343p. pap. 56.00 (*1-56793-105-7*) Health Admin Pr.

Law & the Team Physician. Elizabeth M. Gallup. 1994. LC 93-47607. (Illus.). 192p. text 32.00 (*0-87322-662-3*, BGAL0662) Human Kinetics.

Law & the Treatment of Drug & Alcohol-Dependent Persons: A Comparative Study of Existing Legislation. L. Porter et al. 1986. 216p. pap. text 34.00 (*92-4-156093-2*, 1150243) World Health.

Law, Behavior, & Mental Health: Policy & Practice. Steven R. Smith & Robert G. Meyer. 772p. (C). 1988. pap. text 27.50 (*0-8147-7887-9*); 1987. text 75.00 (*0-8147-7857-7*) NYU Pr.

Law Enforcement & AIDS: Questions of Justice & Care. Ed. by Gad J. Bensinger & Cyprian Rowe. 1988. 58p. pap. text 7.00 (*0-942854-13-6*) Loyola U Crim.

Law Enforcement Officer & AIDS. 1991. lib. bdg. 75.95 (*0-8490-4947-4*) Gordon Pr.

Law, Ethics & Pathology. Denis Baron. 1999. 160p. pap. (*0-7506-0846-3*) E A GBR. *Dist:* OUP.

Law Every Nurse Should Know. Helen Creighton. 5th ed. 1986. (Illus.). 335p. pap. text 39.50 (*0-7216-1832-4*) Saunders.

Law for Doctors. Wai-Ching Leung. 2000. LC 00-20659. (Illus.). 208p. pap. 52.95 (*0-632-05243-0*) Blackwell Sci.

***Law for Doctors: Principles & Practicalities.** M. Branthwaite. 2000. 96p. pap. (*1-85315-465-2*) Royal Soc of Medicine Pr Ltd GBR. *Dist:* Balogh.

Law for Nurses. Gill Korgaonka & Diana Tribe. 1995. 205p. pap. (*1-85941-132-0*) Cavendish Pubng GBR. *Dist:* Gaunt.

Law for the Medical Office. 1984. (Illus.). xviii, 312p. (Orig.). pap. text 20.00 (*0-942732-00-6*); stu. ed. 20.00 (*0-942732-01-4*) Am Med Assts.

Law for the Medical Profession. Andrew Dix et al. 1988. 336p. 70.00 (*0-409-49318-X*) Buttrwrth-Heinemann.

Law for the Medical Profession. Kevin Nicholson & Rob Dixon. 2nd ed. 1996. LC 96-228827. 350p. pap. text 69.99 (*0-7506-8929-3*) Buttrwrth-Heinemann.

Law, Health & Medical Regulation. Shaun McVeigh & Sally Wheeler. 1993. (Contemporary Legal Issues Ser.). 250p. (*1-85521-283-8*) Dartmth Pub GBR. *Dist:* Ashgate Pub Co.

Law in a Therapeutic Key: Developments in Therapeutic Jurisprudence. Ed. by David B. Wexler & Bruce J. Winick. 2001. LC 96-85934. 1032p. reprint ed. pap. 65.00 (*0-89089-988-6*) Carolina Acad Pr.

Law in Optometric Practice. Stephen P. Taylor. 2002. (Illus.). 192p. pap. 44.99 (*0-7506-4578-4*) Buttrwrth-Heinemann.

Law (in Plain English) for Health Care Professionals. Leonard D. DuBoff. 1993. LC 92-39745. 206p. 50.00 (*0-471-58001-5*); pap. 14.95 (*0-471-58002-3*) Wiley.

Law in the Health & Human Services: A Guide for Social Workers, Psychologists, Psychiatrists & Related Professionals. annuals Donald T. Dickson. 1995. LC 94-23670. 640p. 35.00 (*0-02-907435-5*) Free Pr.

Law in the Practice of Psychiatry: A Handbook for Clinicians. Seymour L. Halleck. 1980. (Critical Issues in Psychiatry Ser.). 306p. 55.00 (*0-306-40373-0*, Plenum Trade) Perseus Pubng.

Law, Liability & Ethics for Medical Office Personnel. Myrtle Flight. 2nd ed. 1993. LC 92-48661. 258p. pap. 27.95 (*0-8273-3973-9*) Delmar.

Law, Liability, & Ethics for Medical Office Personnel: Instructor's Guide. Myrtle Flight. 2nd ed. 1994. 58p. pap. 14.00 (*0-8273-3974-7*) Delmar.

Law, Liability And Ethics for Medical Office Professionals. Myrtle Flight. 3rd ed. 1997. LC 97-9100. 272p. (C). pap. text 47.95 (*0-8273-8183-2*) Delmar.

Law, Liberty, & Psychiatry: An Inquiry into the Social Uses of Mental Health Practices. Thomas Szasz. 1989. LC 63-14187. 296p. reprint ed. pap. 19.95 (*0-8156-0242-1*) Syracuse U Pr.

Law, Medicine & Forensic Science. William J. Curran & E. Donald Shapiro. 3rd ed. 1982. LC 81-81207. 1181p. (C). 41.00 (*0-316-16510-7*) Aspen Law.

Law Medicine Notes: Progress in Medicolegal Relations. William J. Curran. Ed. by Arnold S. Relman. 1989. 450p. 38.50 (*0-910133-26-3*) Mass Med Pub Div.

Law-Medicine Relation - A Philosophical Exploration: Proceedings of the Eighth Trans-Disciplinary Symposium on Philosophy & Medicine Held at Farmington, Connecticut, November 9-11, 1978. Ed. by Stuart F. Spicker et al. 1981. (Philosophy & Medicine Ser.: No. 9). 322p. text 106.00 (*90-277-1217-4*) Kluwer Academic.

Law of Chemical & Pharmaceutical Invention: Patent & Nonpatent Protection. Jerome Rosenstock. 1995. LC 98-31958. 2082p. spiral bd. 175.00 (*0-7355-0264-1*) Panel Pubs.

Law of Disability Discrimination. Ruth Colker & Bonnie Poitras Tucker. 2nd ed. 1998. 734p. (C). 51.95 (*0-87084-240-4*) Anderson Pub Co.

Law of Evidence Irving Younger. 1979. 795.00 incl. VHS (*1-55917-389-0*, 840); VHS 795.00 (*1-55917-388-2*) Natl Prac Inst.

Law of Evidence & the Medical Record: A Trial Lawyer's Guide. Elliott B. Oppenheim. 5th ed. 1997. 120p. 125.00 (*1-930263-01-5*) Terra Firma NM.

Law of Health Care Organization & Finance: 1995 Supplement. Barry R. Furrow et al. 2nd ed. 1995. (American Casebook Ser.). 550p. (C). pap. text 14.00 (*0-314-06863-5*) West Pub.

Law of Health Records in North Carolina. Anne M. Dellinger & Joan G. Brannon. 1987. 86p. (Orig.). (C). pap. text 12.00 (*1-56011-093-7*, 87.04) Institute Government.

Law of Life & Human Health. G. R. Clements. 1998. 313p. reprint ed. pap. 26.00 (*0-7873-0177-9*) Hlth Research.

Law of Medical Liability in a Nutshell. Marcia M. Boumil & Clifford E. Elias. 1995. LC 95-35002. (Nutshell Ser.). 266p. (C). pap. 22.50 (*0-314-06660-8*) West Pub.

Law of Medical Malpractice. Margaret C. Jasper. 1996. LC 96-188008. (Legal Almanac Ser.). text 25.50 (*0-379-11233-7*) Oceana.

Law of Natural Healing: Developing the Body, Mind & Spirit Through Forces Within. Charles L. Gilson. 1991. lib. bdg. 79.95 (*0-8490-4497-9*) Gordon Pr.

Law of Natural Healing (1905) Charles L. Gilson. 1996. 154p. reprint ed. pap. 15.95 (*1-56459-882-9*) Kessinger Pub.

Law of Texas Medical Malpractice. Jim M. Perdue. LC 85-8205. 660p. 39.50 (*0-913797-08-1*) Houston Law Review.

Law on Medicines, Set. I. H. Harrison. 1987. text 745.50 (*0-85200-820-1*) Kluwer Academic.

Law on Medicines: A Comprehensive Guide. I. H. Harrison. 1986. text 339.00 (*0-85200-897-X*) Kluwer Academic.

Law on Medicines: Distribution & Selling. I. H. Harrison. 1986. lib. bdg. 281.00 (*0-85200-912-7*) Kluwer Academic.

Law on Medicines: Licensing & Manufacture. I. H. Harrison. 1986. text 339.00 (*0-85200-913-5*) Kluwer Academic.

Law, Psychiatry & Morality: Essays & Analysis. Alan A. Stone. 1984. LC 84-3000. 277p. pap. text 6.50 (*0-88048-209-5*, 8209) Am Psychiatric.

Law, Psychiatry & the Mental Health System. Alexander D. Brooks. 1974. 54.00 (*0-316-10970-3*) Aspen Law.

Law Reform & Human Reproduction. Ed. by Sheila A. McLean. 1992. (Medico-Legal Issues Ser.). 200p. (*1-85521-026-6*) Dartmth Pub GBR. *Dist:* Ashgate Pub Co.

Law Science & Medicine. Judith C. Areen et al. 1996. (University Casebook Ser.). 276p. pap. text (*1-56662-447-9*) Foundation Pr.

Law, Science & Medicine. Judith C. Areen et al. 1990. LC 84-8181. (University Casebook Ser.). 1494p. (C). reprint ed. text 44.50 (*0-88277-179-5*) Foundation Pr.

Law, Science & Medicine. Judith C. Areen et al. Ed. by Lawrence Gostin. 2nd ed. 1996. LC 96-13106. (University Casebook Ser.). 1445p. text 64.50 (*1-56662-338-3*) Foundation Pr.

Law, Science & Medicine: 1988 Supplement. Judith C. Areen et al. 1990. (University Casebook Ser.). 395p. reprint ed. pap. text 14.50 (*0-88277-702-5*) Foundation Pr.

Law Without Enforcement: Integrating Mental Health & Justice. Ed. by Nigel Eastman & Jill Peay. 1998. LC 00-266037. xviii, 238p. pap. (*1-901362-75-2*) Hart Pub GBR. *Dist:* Intl Spec Bk.

Lawful Exit: The Limits of Freedom for Help in Dying. Derek Humphry. 1993. 168p. (Orig.). pap. 9.95 (*0-9637280-0-8*) Norris Ln Pr.

Laws & Policies Affecting Adolescent Health. J. M. Paxman & R. J. Zuckerman. 1987. 310p. pap. text 49.00 (*92-4-156095-9*, 1150263) World Health.

Laws of Life: With Special Reference to the Physical Education of Girls. Elizabeth Blackwell. Ed. by Elizabeth M. Whatley. rev. ed. (Illus.). 133p. reprint ed. pap. text 8.95 (*0-940151-10-3*) Statesman-Exam.

Laws, Theories & Values: Biological Approaches to Understanding. Jorge A. Quintero. 2nd ed. 1980. LC 79-50190. (Illus.). 144p. 10.50 (*0-87527-147-2*) Green.

Lawson Tait: The Rebellious Surgeon, 1845 to 1899. John S. Shepherd. 1980. (Illus.). 250p. 25.00 (*0-87291-131-4*) Coronado Pr.

Lawson's Guide to Health Care Business Development & Marketing. Gary W. Lawson. 1994. LC 93-43473. (*0-939644-94-0*, Midgrd Press) Media Pub.

Lawsuit Prevention Techniques for Mental Health Professionals, Chemical Dependency Specialists & Clergy. Barbara E. Calfee. 1992. 135p. (Orig.). pap. 19.95 (*0-9633540-1-9*) ARC Pub.

Lawyers' Guide to Medical Proof Marshall Houts. 1967. ring bd. 1081.00 (*0-8205-1353-9*) Bender.

Lawyers' Medical Encyclopedia of Personal Injuries & Allied Specialties, Vols. 3, 4 & 5. Richard Patterson. 4th ed. 1996. 0.00 (*1-55834-638-4*) LEXIS Pub.

Lawyers on Psychology & Psychologists on Law. P. J. Van Koppen & D. J. Hessing. 1989. viii, 189p. (*90-265-0977-4*) Swets.

Lay Analysis: Life Inside the Controversy. Robert S. Wallerstein. 1998. LC 98-46417. 528p. 69.95 (*0-88163-285-6*) Analytic Pr.

Lay Man: About Mind see Idiota de Mente

***Lay My Burden Down: Suicide & the Mental Health Crisis among African Americans.** Alvin F. Poussaint & Amy Alexander. 2001. LC 2001-37472. 208p. pap. 14.00 (*0-8070-0959-8*) Beacon Pr.

Lay My Burden Down: Suicide & the Mental Health Crisis among African Americans. Alvin F. Poussaint & Amy Alexander. 2000. LC 00-8859. 194p. 23.00 (*0-8070-0960-1*) Beacon Pr.

Laying on of Hands. Kenneth E. Hagin. 1980. pap. 1.00 (*0-89276-250-0*) Faith Lib Pubns.

Layman's Guide to Acupuncture. Yoshio Manaka et al. 1972. LC 72-78590. (Illus.). 144p. 12.50 (*0-8348-0072-1*); pap. 10.95 (*0-8348-0107-8*) Weatherhill.

Layperson's Glossary on Functional Electrical Stimulation (FES) Jeanne O. Teeter. 1992. 9p. pap. text 5.00 (*1-888470-01-1*) FES Info Ctr.

Laywoman's Primer of Breast Cancer. Carl Livingston. 1980. (Illus.). 24p. (Orig.). pap. 2.50 (*0-937816-03-5*) Tech Data.

LD Child & the ADHD Child: Ways Parents & Professionals Can Help. Suzanne H. Stevens. rev. ed. 1996. LC 95-26401. Orig. Title: The Learning-Disabled Child. pap. 12.95 (*0-89587-142-4*) Blair.

Lead & Public Health: Dangers for Children. Erik Millstone. 1997. LC 97-22574. 240p. 75.00 (*1-56032-723-5*); pap. 24.95 (*1-56032-724-3*) Hemisp Pub.

Lead & Public Health Integrated Risk Assessment. Paul Mushak. 1999. (Pharmacology & Toxicology Ser.). 99.95 (*0-8493-8557-1*, 8557) CRC Pr.

Lead-Based Paint Poisoning: Children Not Fully Protected When Federal Agencies Sell Homes to Public. 1993. (Illus.). 48p. (Orig.). (C). pap. text 30.00 (*0-7881-0079-3*) DIANE Pub.

Lead Detection & Abatement Directory, 1993. Intro. by Larry Siegelman. 1992. 333p. pap. 100.00 (*0-9633003-2-6*) IAQ Pubns.

Lead Disclosure & Training: A Strategic & Regulatory Marketplace Review. Ed. by Larry Siegelman. 1997. 30p. (Orig.). pap. 100.00 (*0-9633003-6-9*) IAQ Pubns.

Lead Exposure & Child Development: An International Assessment. Ed. by M. Smith et al. 1989. (C). text 229.00 (*0-7462-0069-2*) Kluwer Academic.

Lead in Paint, Soil, & Dust: Health Risks, Exposure Studies, Control Measures, Measurement Methods, & Quality Assurance. Ed. by Michael E. Beard & S. D. Iske. 1995. LC 95-17787. 435p. 74.00 (*0-8031-1884-8*, STP1226) ASTM.

Lead Is a Silent Hazard. Richard M. Stapleton. 1995. LC 94-5320. 160p. pap. 11.95 (*0-8027-7449-0*) Walker & Co.

Lead Paint Primer: Questions & Answers on Lead Paint Poisoning. John Pesce & Amadeo J. Pesce. 1991. (Illus.). 150p. (Orig.). pap. 9.95 (*0-9628220-1-9*) Star Industries.

Lead Poisoning: Federal Health Care Programs Are Not Effectively Reaching At-Risk Children. Ed. by Bernice Steinhardt. 2000. (Illus.). 105p. (C). pap. text 25.00 (*0-7567-0016-7*) DIANE Pub.

Lead Poisoning in Childhood. Ed. by Siegfried M. Pueschel et al. 1996. LC 95-41441. 256p. 31.95 (*1-55766-232-0*) P H Brookes.

Lead Poisoning of America's School Children: An Action Plan. Dick Amann. 1991. 150p. (Orig.). text 99.50 (*0-917194-21-7*) Prog Studies.

Lead Poisoning Prevention: Directory of State Contacts, 1995-1996. National Conference of State Legislatures Staff. 1996. 193p. 20.00 (*1-55516-430-7*, 4648) Natl Conf State Legis.

Lead Tech '92 Proceedings: Solutions for a Nation at Risk, 1992-1993. Ed. by Robert Morrow. 1992. (Illus.). 650p. pap. 50.00 (*0-9633003-3-4*) IAQ Pubns.

***Lead Toxicity: Case Studies in Environmental Medicine.** Ed. by Pamela S. Wigington. rev. ed. 2001. 55p. pap. text 20.00 (*0-7567-1748-5*) DIANE Pub.

Leader: Psychohistorical Essays. Ed. by Charles B. Strozier & Daniel Offer. 1985. 340p. 70.00 (*0-306-41784-7*, Plenum Trade) Perseus Pubng.

Leaders & Followers Vol. 4: Challenges for the Future. Ed. by Trudy Heller et al. 1988. LC 86-15369. (Contemporary Studies in Applied Behavioral Science: Vol. 4). 279p. 73.25 (*0-89232-495-3*) Jai Pr.

Leaders in the Study of Animal Behavior. Ed. by Donald A. Dewsbury. 1985. LC 83-46153. (Illus.). 512p. 65.00 (*0-8387-5052-4*) Bucknell U Pr.

Leadership: A Compliance Guide to the JACHO Standards. Richard O. Schmidt & Mary Becker. 1997. (Illus.). 136p. (Orig.). pap. text 67.00 (*1-57839-003-6*) Opus Communs.

Leadership: The Key to Professionalization of Nursing. Bernhard & Michelle Walsh. 3rd ed. 1994. LC

JKL

94-241837. (Illus.). 223p. (C). (gr. 13). pap. text 35.00 (*0-8151-0526-6*, 24347) Mosby Inc.

***Leadership & Management.** Dennis P. L'Heureux. 2001. (HIMSS Guidebook Ser.). (Illus.). 104p. pap. 35.00 (*0-9704287-6-6*) Healthcare Info.

Leadership & Management According to Florence Nightingale. Beth T. Ulrich. 1992. (Illus.). 144p. (C). pap. 24.20 (*0-8385-5642-6*, A5642-2) Appleton & Lange.

Leadership & Management in Nursing: A New Legacy. 2001. (Professional Reference - Nursing Ser.). (C). pap. 34.95 (*0-8273-7957-9*) Delmar.

Leadership & Mangement in Nursing. Mary Ellen Grohar-Murray & Helen R. Dicroce. 2nd ed. 1996. LC 96-31743. 312p. (C). pap. 45.00 (*0-8385-5646-9*, A5646-3) P-H.

Leadership & Nursing Care Management. Ed. by Diane Huber. 1996. (Illus.). 683p. pap., tchr. ed. (*0-7216-6514-4*) Saunders.

Leadership & Nursing Care Management. Diane G. Huber. Ed. by Thomas Eoyang. 1995. (Illus.). 688p. pap. text 35.00 (*0-7216-4428-7*) Saunders.

Leadership & Nursing Care Management. Diane Huber. 2nd ed. 2000. LC 99-54402. (Illus.). 670p. pap. text (*0-7216-7699-5*) Saunders.

***Leadership & Nursing Care Management.** Diane Huber. 2nd ed. 2000. (Illus.). 708p. pap., stu. ed. 19.95 (*0-7216-9200-1*) Saunders.

Leadership & Nursing Care Management. Diane G. Huber. 2nd ed. 1996. pap. text, stu. ed. 14.95 (*0-7216-6819-4*) Saunders.

Leadership for Change: An Action Guide for Nurses. Dorothy A. Brooten et al. 2nd ed. 1988. LC 64-5153. 192p. text 19.95 (*0-397-54597-5*, Lippnctt) Lppncott W & W.

Leadership for Primary Health Care: Levels, Functions & Requirements Based on Twelve Case Studies. D. M. Flahault & M. I. Roemer. 1986. (Public Health Papers: No. 82). 79p. pap. text 8.00 (*92-4-130082-5*, 1110082) World Health.

Leadership Guide for Board Presidents & Committee Chairpersons. Darla Struck. 1993. ring bd. 103.00 (*0-8342-0404-5*, 04045) Aspen Pub.

Leadership in Dietetics: Achieving a Vision for the Future. Anne M. Barker et al. 1994. LC 94-31016. pap. 28.00 (*0-88091-137-9*) Am Dietetic Assn.

Leadership in Healthcare: Values at the Top. Carson F. Dye. 2000. LC 99-47342. (Ache Management Ser.). 145p. pap. 42.00 (*1-56793-114-6*, LHC-1090) Health Admin Pr.

Leadership in Nursing Practice. Boyle. 1999. pap. text (*0-7216-4915-7*) Harcourt.

Leadership Report: Key Issues Shaping the Future of Health Care. Alden T. Solovy. 1999. LC 99-199466. (Hospitals & Health Networks Ser.). 277 p. pap. text 149.00 (*1-55648-241-8*) AHPI.

Leadership Roles & Management Functions in Nursing: Theory & Application. Bessie L. Marquis & Carol J. Huston. 3rd ed. 2000. LC 99-14493. 608p. pap. text 35.95 (*0-7817-1923-2*) Lppncott W & W.

Leadership Skills for the Nurse Manager: Restructuring the Role of Management in Today's... Kathleen O. Mott. 1996. LC 96-7876. 240p. pap. 32.50 (*0-7863-0860-5*, Irwn Prfssnl) McGraw-Hill Educ Grp.

Leading & Managing in Nursing. Patricia S. Yoder Wise. 1998. (Illus.). 784p. tchr. ed., suppl. ed. (*0-8151-9849-3*) Mosby Inc.

Leading & Managing in Nursing. Patricia S. Yoder-Wise. 2nd ed. 1998. (Illus.). 768p. tchr. ed. (*1-55664-402-7*); LC 98-11710. (C). text (*1-55664-401-9*) Mosby Inc.

Leading Antenatal Classes. Judy Priest & Judith Schott. 1991. (Illus.). 256p. pap. text 37.50 (*0-7506-0050-0*) Buttrwrth-Heinemann.

Leading Causes of Death by Age, Sex, Race, & Hispanic Origins: United States, 1992. Paula Gardner et al. 1997. (Illus.). 94p. (C). pap. text 25.00 (*0-7881-4535-5*) DIANE Pub.

Leading the Cooperative School. David W. Johnson & Roger T. Johnson. 2nd rev. ed. 1994. LC 95-215266. (Illus.). 296p. pap. text, tchr. ed. 25.00 (*0-939603-20-9*) Interaction Bk Co.

Leading the Revolution in Health Care: Advancing Systems, Igniting Performance. Cathleen Krueger Wilson & Tim Porter-O'Grady. 2nd ed. 1999. LC 99-23936. (Illus.). xv, 484p. 59.00 (*0-8342-1367-2*, 13672) Aspen Pub.

Leading the Way: Practical Management Skills for the Long-Term Care Nurse. Karl Pillemer & Philip T. Johnson. Ed. by Martin Schumacher. 1997. 50p. 10.95 (*0-9653629-1-4*) Frontline Pub.

Leaf Protein & Its Biproducts in Human & Animal Nutrition. N. W. Pirie. 1987. 224p. text 64.95 (*0-521-33030-0*) Cambridge U Pr.

Lean Advantage 2: The Second Four Years. Clarence Bass. 1989. LC 84-71083. (Illus.). 231p. (Orig.). pap. 15.95 (*0-9609714-4-0*) Clarence Bass.

Lean Body Promise: An Owner's Manual. Vince Quas. 1990. LC 89-4162. (Illus.). 288p. (Orig.). pap. 15.95 (*0-925572-36-5*) Synesis Pr.

Leaping upon the Mountains: Men Proclaiming Victory over Sexual Child Abuse. Mike Lew. 2000. LC 99-85759. xlvii, 266p. pap. 19.95 (*1-55643-345-X*) North Atlantic.

Leaps: Facing Risks in Offering a Constructive Therapeutic Response When Unusual Measures Are Necessary. Roy M. Mendelsohn. 1992. LC 90-22584. 320p. 55.00 (*0-87668-566-1*) Aronson.

Leaps & Boundaries: Psychoanalysis Revisited. Doris Treisman. Ed. by Susan A. Gordon. 1989. (Illus.). 110p. (Orig.). (C). pap. 8.95 (*0-9624424-0-2*) Oceanides Pr.

Learn-a-Term: A Course in Medical Terminology. A. Brent Garber & Leroy Sparks. 1977. LC 77-82026. 168p. (C). pap. 61.00 (*0-912862-48-3*) Aspen Pub.

Learn about Alcohol. 1983. 16p. pap. 1.25 (*0-89486-205-7*, 1343B) Hazelden.

Learn about Alcohol & Pregnancy. 1983. 16p. pap. 1.25 (*0-89486-210-3*, 1348B) Hazelden.

Learn about Alcoholism. 1983. 16p. pap. 1.25 (*0-89486-206-5*, 1344B) Hazelden.

Learn about Anorexia & Bulimia. 1985. (Learn about Ser.). pap. 1.25 (*0-89486-270-7*) Hazelden.

Learn about Cocaine & Crack. 1983. 16p. pap. 1.25 (*0-89486-207-3*, 1345B) Hazelden.

Learn about Drinking & Driving. 1983. 16p. pap. 1.25 (*0-89486-209-X*, 1347B) Hazelden.

Learn about Families & Chemical Dependency. 1985. (Learn about Ser.). 16p. (Orig.). pap. 1.25 (*0-89486-269-3*, 1354B) Hazelden.

Learn about Marijuana. 1983. 16p. pap. 1.25 (*0-89486-208-1*, 1346B) Hazelden.

Learn about Prescription Drugs. 1984. 16p. (Orig.). (C). pap. 1.25 (*0-89486-240-5*, 1349B) Hazelden.

Learn about Youth & Drug Addiction. 1985. (Learn about Ser.). 15p. (Orig.). pap. 1.25 (*0-89486-252-9*, 1353B) Hazelden.

Learn to Read Chinese. Paul U. Unschuld. 450p. (C). Vol. 1. 1995. LC 94-16448. pap. text 30.00 (*0-912111-46-1*); Vol. 2. 1994. pap. text 30.00 (*0-912111-47-X*) Paradigm Publns.

Learning. Richard F. Luduena. 1995. LC 94-43218. 344p. pap. 64.95 (*0-471-01887-2*) Wiley.

Learning: Behavior & Cognition. David A. Lieberman. 2nd ed. 1992. (C). pap. 49.75 (*0-534-17400-0*); 3rd ed. 1999. LC 99-36080. 614p. spiral bd. 87.95 (*0-534-33925-5*) Brooks-Cole.

Learning Ability Test (LAT) Jack Rudman. 1994. (Career Examination Ser.: C-1062). pap. 23.95 (*0-8373-1062-8*) Nat Learn.

Learning about AIDS. Peter Aggleton et al. 1989. pap. text (*0-443-04181-4*) Church.

Learning about AIDS: Scientific Social Issues. Ed. by Peter Aggleton et al. 2nd ed. 1995. LC 94-16625. pap. text (*0-443-05178-X*) Church.

Learning about Learning Disabilities. Ed. by Bernice Y. Wong. 1991. (Illus.). 643p. (C). text 54.95 (*0-12-762530-5*) Acad Pr.

Learning about Lupus: A User Friendly Guide. Ed. by Mary E. Moore et al. rev. ed. 1997. LC 97-73837. (Illus.). 224p. pap. text 7.00 (*0-9659530-0-9*) LFDV Inc.

Learning about Lyme Disease. Jo A. Heltzel. 1992. (Illus.). 32p. (Orig.). pap. text 3.75 (*0-9633041-0-0*) Jo Ann Heltzel.

Learning about Sexuality: A Practical Beginning. Ed. by Sondra Zeidenstein & Kirsten Moore. 1996. 404p. pap. 20.00 (*0-87834-085-8*) Population Coun.

Learning about Your Oral Health (ps). (J). 11.20 (*0-934510-20-2*, W021);Level I. 11.20 (*0-934510-16-4*, W017);Level II. 11.20 (*0-934510-17-2*, W018);Level III. 11.20 (*0-934510-18-0*, W019);Level IV. 11.20 (*0-934510-19-9*, W020) Am Dental.

Learning & Behavior. Paul Chance. 3rd ed. 1993. LC 93-2435. pap. 46.50 (*0-534-17394-2*) Brooks-Cole.

Learning & Change in the Adult Years: A Developmental Perspective. Mark Tennant & Philip Pogson. 1995. LC 94-42160. (Jossey-Bass Higher & Adult Education Ser.). 240p. 37.00 (*0-7879-0082-6*) Jossey-Bass.

Learning & Cognition in the Mentally Retarded. Ed. by Penelope Brooks et al. 1984. LC 84-10289. 576p. text 115.00 (*0-89859-374-3*) L Erlbaum Assocs.

Learning & Education: Psychoanalytic Perspectives. Ed. by Kay H. Field et al. 1990. LC 89-35513. (Emotions & Behavior Monographs: No. 6). 1030p. 90.00 (*0-8236-2954-6*) Intl Univs Pr.

Learning & Individual Differences. Phillip L. Ackerman. 1989. LC 88-16317. (Psychology Ser.). 343p. (C). pap. text 27.95 (*0-7167-1985-1*) W H Freeman.

Learning & Instruction Vol. 3: European Research in an International Context: Selected Proceedings of the 1989 European Conference for Research on Learning & Instruction. Ed. by Mario Carretero et al. 1992. 614p. 112.00 (*0-08-041039-1*, Pergamon Pr) Elsevier.

Learning & Intelligence: Conversations with Skinner & Wheeler. Maureen Lapan & Raymond Houghton. 1995. 142p. (*0-7165-2584-4*) Irish Acad Pr IRL. *Dist:* Intl Spec Bk.

Learning & Memory. Gordon Staff. 2nd ed. 2000. LC 00-34043. (Psychology Ser.). (Illus.). 512p. 75.95 (*0-534-16914-7*) Brooks-Cole.

Learning & Memory: A Biological View. Ed. by Joe L. Martinez, Jr. & Raymond P. Kesner. 2nd ed. 1991. (Illus.). 563p. text 104.00 (*0-12-474992-5*); LC 90-29995. pap. text 53.00 (*0-12-474993-3*) Acad Pr.

Learning & Memory: Mechanisms of Information Storage in the Nervous System. Ed. by H. Matthies. 1986. 427p. 100.50 (*0-08-034186-1*, H222, H223, Pergamon Pr) Elsevier.

Learning & Physiological Regulation. Barry R. Dworkin. 1993. LC 92-564. (John D. & Catherine T. MacArthur Foundation Series on Mental Health & Development). (Illus.). 232p. (C). 26.50 (*0-226-17600-2*) U Ch Pr.

Learning & Psychosomatic Approach to the Nature & Treatment of Illness: 18th Annual Conference of the Society for Psychosomatic Research. Ed. by Peter G. Mellett. 1977. pap. 53.00 (*0-08-020881-9*, Pergamon Pr) Elsevier.

Learning & Teaching Therapy. Jay Haley. 1996. LC 95-50953. (Guilford Family Therapy Ser.). 235p. text 34.00 (*1-57230-035-3*, 0035) Guilford Pubns.

Learning As a Behavioral Adaptation. Frieman. 2001. LC 2001-43343. (Psychology Ser.). 580p. 67.95 (*0-534-34226-4*) Brooks-Cole.

Learning by Heart: AIDS & Schoolchildren in America's Communities. David L. Kirp. 1990. 305p. (Orig.). pap. 14.95 (*0-8135-1609-9*) Rutgers U Pr.

Learning Clinical Reasoning. Jerome P. Kassirer & Richard Kopelman. 1991. (Illus.). 350p. 35.00 (*0-683-04537-7*) Lppncott W & W.

Learning Connection: Effective Answers to Reading & Learning Difficulties. Steven R. Shapiro. 1989. (Illus.). 238p. (Orig.). (C). pap. text 14.95 (*0-9624688-0-0*) Lrning Cnnect.

Learning Counseling & Problem-Solving Skills. Leslie E. Borck & Stephen B. Fawcett. 1982. LC 82-2916. 160p. (Orig.). (C). text 44.95 (*0-917724-30-5*); pap. text 19.95 (*0-917724-35-6*) Haworth Pr.

Learning Diabilities Vol. 1: Neuropsychological Correlates & Treatment. Ed. by Dirk J. Bakker. 1989. x, 202p. (*90-265-0983-9*) Swets.

Learning Difficulties & Emotional Problems. Ed. by Roy I. Brown & Maurice Chazan. 1989. 239p. (C). pap. text 18.95 (*0-920490-89-1*) Temeron Bks.

Learning Disabilities. Lawrence J. O'Shea et al. 1997. LC 97-28717. 444p. 84.00 (*0-02-389321-4*) P-H.

Learning Disabilities. Betty B. Osman. 1988. mass mkt. 4.95 (*0-446-35554-2*) Warner Bks.

Learning Disabilities. Bob Gates. 3rd ed. 1997. LC 96-49999. pap. text (*0-443-05539-4*) Church.

Learning Disabilities: A Neuropsychological Perspective. Byron P. Rourke & Jerel E. Del Dotto. 1994. LC 94-65. (Developmental Clinical Psychology & Psychiatry Ser.: Vol. 30). 160p. (C). 74.95 (*0-8039-5353-4*, 5693); pap. 34.95 (*0-8039-5354-2*, 4594) Sage.

Learning Disabilities: Basic Concepts, Assessment Practices & Instructional Strategies. Patricia I. Myers & Donald D. Hammill. 4th ed. 1990. LC 89-29044. (Illus.). 593p. text 43.00 (*0-89079-225-9*, 1499) PRO-ED.

Learning Disabilities: Best Practices for Professionals. Ed. by William N. Bender. 1993. LC 92-31024. 334p. 38.00 (*1-56372-058-2*, 6930) PRO-ED.

Learning Disabilities: Educational Principles & Practices. Doris J. Johnson & Helmer R. Myklebust. 1967. LC 66-28287. 336p. (C). text 36.00 (*0-8089-0219-9*, 1804) PRO-ED.

Learning Disabilities: How to Recognize & Manage Learning & Behavioral Problems in Children. Trudy Carlson. 1997. LC 95-94110. 144p. (Orig.). pap. 14.95 (*0-9642443-2-2*) Benline Pr.

Learning Disabilities: Implications for Psychiatric Treatment. Ed. by Laurence L. Greenhill. 2000. LC 00-23123. (Review of Psychiatry Ser.: Vol. 19, No. 5). 196p. pap. 28.50 (*0-88048-383-0*, 8383) Am Psychiatric.

Learning Disabilities: New Directions for Assessment & Intervention. Ed. by Nancy C. Jordan & Josephine Goldsmith-Phillips. 1993. LC 93-22965. 432p. (C). 78.00 (*0-205-14124-2*, Longwood Div) Allyn.

Learning Disabilities: The Struggle from Adolescence Toward Adulthood. William M. Cruickshank et al. 1980. (Illus.). 304p. (C). pap. 19.95 (*0-8156-2221-X*) Syracuse U Pr.

Learning Disabilities: Theoretical & Research Issues. Ed. by H. L. Swanson & Barbara Keogh. 1990. 384p. (C). text 79.95 (*0-8058-0392-0*) L Erlbaum Assocs.

Learning Disabilities Vol. 2: Cognitive, Social, & Remedial Aspects. Ed. by J. J. Dumont. 1989. xii, 208p. (*90-265-0984-7*) Swets.

Learning Disabilities & Brain Function: A Neuropsychological Approach. William H. Gaddes & Dorothy Edgell. 3rd ed. 1996. LC 93-28185. (Illus.). 594p. 69.95 (*0-387-94041-3*) Spr-Verlag.

Learning Disabilities & Psychosocial Functioning: A Neuropsychological Perspective. Byron P. Rourke & Darren R. Fuerst. 1991. LC 91-16388. 198p. 32.00 (*0-89862-767-2*, 2767) Guilford Pubns.

Learning Disabilities & Social Activity. Ed. by Gerald S. Coles. 1985. 49.95 (*0-915340-15-1*) PJD Pubns.

Learning Disabilities in Children. Peter Burke & Katy Cigno. 2000. LC 99-87589. (Special Publication Number 8 of the British Ecological Socie Ser.). pap. 41.95 (*0-632-05104-3*) Blackwell Sci.

Learning Disabilities in the Primary Classroom. Leonora Harding. 1986. 208p. (C). (*0-7099-3785-7*); pap. (*0-7099-4764-X*) C Helm GBR. *Dist:* Routldge.

Learning Disabilities Spectrum: ADD, ADHD, & LD. Ed. by Arnold J. Capute et al. 1994. LC 93-39701. 265p. pap. text 32.50 (*0-912752-33-5*) York Pr.

Learning Disability & the Social Context of Caring. Open Learning Foundation Staff. 1997. 142p. pap. (*0-443-05735-4*) Church.

Learning Disability Intervention Manual. Stephen B. McCarney & Angela M. Bauer. rev. ed. 1989. 217p. reprint ed. pap. 25.00 (*1-878372-07-6*) Hawthorne Educ Servs.

Learning Disability Rating Procedure. Gerald J. Spadafore & Sharon J. Spadafore. 1981. 32p. (Orig.). 20.00 (*0-87879-266-X*) Acad Therapy.

Learning Disability Rating Procedure (LDRP) Gerald J. Spadafore & Sharon J. Spadafore. 1981. 32p. (gr. 1-12). pap. text 25.00 (*0-87879-265-1*) Acad Therapy.

Learning-Disabled Child see LD Child & the ADHD Child: Ways Parents & Professionals Can Help

Learning-Disabled Child. Ed. by Marvin I. Gottlieb et al. 1979. (Current Issues in Developmental Pediatrics Ser.). 448p. text 53.00 (*0-8089-1179-1*, 791692, Grune & Strat) Harcrt Hlth Sci Grp.

Learning Disorders: An Integration of Neuropsychological & Psychoanalytic Considerations. Arden Rothstein et al. 1988. 398p. 55.00 (*0-8236-2956-2*) Intl Univs Pr.

***Learning Disorders & Disorders of the Self in Children & Adolescents.** Joseph Palombo. 2001. LC 2001-24007. 384p. 32.00 (*0-393-70377-0*) Norton.

Learning ECGS. Mosby Staff. 1993. pap. text, wbk. ed. 10.00 (*0-8151-0043-4*) Mosby Inc.

Learning Experience Guide, Nursing. Anne K. Roe. 1989. (Nursing Education Ser.). 15.95 (*0-8273-4348-5*) Delmar.

Learning Experience Guides for Nursing Students: Instructor's Guide. Anne K. Roe et al. 5th ed. 1994. 65p. 15.95 (*0-8273-6172-6*) Delmar.

Learning for Leadership: Interpersonal & Intergroup. A. K. Rice. 1999. 212p. pap. (*1-85575-233-6*) Karnac Bks GBR. *Dist:* Other Pr LLC.

***Learning from Bristol: The Report of the Public Inquiry into Children's Heart Surgery at the Bristol Royal Infirmary 1984-1995.** Ian Kennedy. 2001. (*0-10-152072-7*) Statnry Office GBR. *Dist:* Balogh.

Learning from Our Mistakes: Difficulties & Failures in Feminist Therapy. Ed. by Marcia Hill & Esther D. Rothblum. 1998. LC 98-35594. 126p. pap. 14.95 (*0-7890-0670-7*); 29.95 (*0-7890-0653-7*) Haworth Pr.

Learning from the Patient. Patrick J. Casement. LC 90-14120. (Psychoanalysis Ser.). 384p. 1990. 45.00 (*0-89862-559-9*); 1992. reprint ed. pap. 25.00 (*0-89862-157-7*, 2157) Guilford Pubns.

Learning Human Anatomy: A Laboratory Text & Workbook. Julia F. Guy. 2nd ed. 1997. 360p. (C). spiral bd. 46.00 (*0-8385-5657-4*, A-5657-0) P-H.

Learning Human Skills: An Experiential & Reflective Guide for Nurses. Philip Burnard. 3rd ed. 1995. LC 95-30494. (Illus.). 288p. pap. text 37.50 (*0-7506-2441-8*) Buttrwrth-Heinemann.

Learning in Children: Progress in Cognitive Development Research. Ed. by J. Bisanz et al. 1983. (Cognitive Development Ser.). (Illus.). 201p. 84.95 (*0-387-90802-1*) Spr-Verlag.

Learning in Infants & Young Children. Michael Howe. 1976. LC 75-44902. 216p. reprint ed. pap. 10.95 (*0-8047-0973-4*) Stanford U Pr.

Learning Incorporated Dictionary of Learning Handicaps. Edward R. Welles. 3rd ed. 1970. 1.00 (*0-913692-01-8*) Learning Inc.

Learning Language Addiction Counseling. Miller. 1998. LC 98-29190. 243p. pap. text 53.00 (*0-205-26318-6*) P-H.

Learning Medical Terminology. Miriam G. Austrin & Harvey R. Austrin. 9th ed. 1998. tchr. ed. (*0-323-00282-X*) Mosby Inc.

***Learning Medical Terminology.** Miriam G. Austrin & Harvey R. Austrin. 9th ed. 1998. (Illus.). 464p. 38.00 incl. audio (*0-323-00281-1*) Mosby Inc.

Learning Medical Terminology: A Work Text. Miriam G. Austrin & Harvey R. Austrin. 1998. text incl. audio (*0-8151-0340-9*); 8th ed. tchr. ed. (*0-8151-7898-0*) Mosby Inc.

Learning Medical Terminology: A Worktext. Miriam G. Austrin & Harvey R. Austrin. 9th ed. 1999. LC 99-180737. (Illus.). 464p. 33.00 (*0-323-00279-X*) Mosby Inc.

***Learning Medical Terminology: Computerized Testbank.** Miriam G. Austrin & Harvey R. Austrin. 9th ed. 1998. (*0-323-00283-8*) Mosby Inc.

***Learning Medical Terminology: Text/Audiotape/Dictionary Package.** Miriam G. Austrin & Harvey R. Austrin. 9th ed. 1998. 61.00 incl. audio (*0-323-00641-8*) Mosby Inc.

***Learning Medical Terminology: Text/Dictionary Package.** Miriam G. Austrin & Harvey R. Austrin. 9th ed. 1998. (Illus.). 56.00 (*0-323-00640-X*) Mosby Inc.

Learning Medicine. Ed. by Peter Richards & Simon Stockill. 15th ed. 2000. 141p. (*0-7279-1462-6*) BMJ Pub GBR. *Dist:* AIDC.

Learning Medicine, 1994. Peter Richards. 12th ed. 1995. 120p. pap. text (*0-7279-0999-1*) BMJ Pub GBR. *Dist:* AIDC.

Learning Medicine, 1993. Peter Richards. 1992. (Illus.). 108p. pap. text (*0-7279-0820-0*) BMJ Pub GBR. *Dist:* AIDC.

Learning More Biochemistry: 100 Case-Oriented Problems. Richard F. Luduena. 1997. LC 96-46129. 303p. pap. 59.95 (*0-471-17054-2*) Wiley.

J
K
L

Learning, Motivation, & Cognition: The Functional Behaviorism of Robert C. Bolles. Ed. by Mark E. Bouton & Michael S. Fanselow. 1997. LC 97-25299. (Illus.). 451p. text 49.95 (*1-55798-436-0*, 431-6910) Am Psychol.

Learning Patterns among Women Professionals: Theory Grounded in the Lives of Nurses. Ed. by Edwin L. Simpson. 1991. LC 91-12429. 72p. (Orig.). lib. bdg. 10.95 (*1-879528-01-0*) Ed Studies Pr.

Learning Patterns & Temperament Styles: A Systematic Guide to Maximizing Student Achievement. Keith J. Golay. 1982. LC 82-62144. 109p. (Orig.). pap. text 12.00 (*0-9610076-0-5*) Manas-Sys.

Learning Performance of Retarded & Normal Children, No. 5—5. G. Orville Johnson & Kathryn A. Blake. 1977. LC 77-22852. (Syracuse University Special Education & Rehabilitation Monographs: No. 5). (Illus.). 216p. reprint ed. lib. bdg. 67.00 (*0-8371-9725-2*, JOLE) Greenwood.

Learning Pharmacology Through MCQ. B. J. Large & I. E. Hughes. 2nd ed. 1990. LC 89-21548. 258p. pap. 78.50 (*0-471-92708-2*) Wiley.

Learning Problems in the Classroom. Marianne Frostig & Phyllis Maslow. 1973. LC 73-1578. 368p. text 36.50 (*0-8089-0783-2*, 791452, Grune & Strat) Harcrt Hlth Sci Grp.

Learning Process in Psychoanalytic Supervision. Paul A. Dewald. 1987. 72.50 (*0-8236-2965-1*, BN#02965) Intl Univs Pr.

Learning Psychotherapy: Rationale & Ground Rules. Hilde Bruch. 1980. LC 74-83848. 166p. pap. 16.50 (*0-674-52026-2*) HUP.

Learning, Speech, & the Complex Effects of Punishment: Essays Honoring George J. Wischner. Ed. by Donald K. Routh. 1982. LC 82-18075. 248p. 49.50 (*0-306-40960-7*, Plenum Trade) Perseus Pubng.

Learning Strategies for Allied Health Students. Marilyn Melzer. 1995. LC 95-901. (Illus.). 368p. pap. text 26.95 (*0-7216-5603-X*) Saunders.

Learning Strategies in Nursing: Reading, Study, & Test-Taking. Marilyn Meltzer & Susan M. Palau. Ed. by Thomas Eoyang. 2nd ed. 1997. LC 96-20650. (Illus.). 400p. pap. text 26.00 (*0-7216-6342-7*) Saunders.

Learning Stress Management Skills: Companion Workbook to Teaching Stress Management Skills. Frances K. Wiggins & Suni Petersen. 1986. (Illus.). 59p. (Orig.). (C). stu. ed. 5.95 (*0-942937-02-3*) Rivijon Pr.

Learning Styles & the Nursing Profession. Ed. by Rita S. Dunn & Shirley A. Griggs. 1998. LC 97-49117. 116p. pap. 23.95 (*0-88737-771-8*) Natl League Nurse.

Learning Theory, Instructional Theory & Psychoeducational Design. Glenn E. Snelbecker. 1985. 544p. reprint ed. pap. text 40.00 (*0-8191-4836-9*) U Pr of Amer.

Learning Through Supervision & Mentorship to Support the Development of Infants, Toddlers & Their Families: A Sourcebook. Ed. by Emily Fenichel. 1992. 175p. (Orig.). pap. 18.95 (*0-943657-19-9*) ZERO TO THREE.

Learning to Care: Effective Goal Setting. (*0-340-43009-5*) E A GBR. *Dist:* Routldge.

Learning to Care for the Aged. Charlotte Epstein. 1977. pap. 10.95 (*0-87909-441-9*); text 12.95 (*0-87909-442-7*) P-H.

Learning to Care in Community Psychiatric Nursing. (*0-340-39918-X*) E A GBR. *Dist:* Routldge.

Learning to Care in Midwifery. (*0-340-41176-7*) E A GBR. *Dist:* Routldge.

Learning to Care in the Operating Department. Kate Nightingale et al. 2nd ed. 1995. 78p. pap. (*0-340-59492-6*) E A GBR. *Dist:* Routldge.

Learning to Care on the Genito-Urinary Ward. (*0-340-41308-5*) E A GBR. *Dist:* Routldge.

Learning to Care on the Medical Ward. (*0-340-37062-9*) E A GBR. *Dist:* Routldge.

Learning to Care on the Orthopaedic Ward. (*0-340-37061-0*) E A GBR. *Dist:* Routldge.

Learning to Care on the Paediatric Ward. (*0-340-41175-9*) E A GBR. *Dist:* Routldge.

Learning to Care on the Psychiatric Ward. (*0-340-38498-0*) E A GBR. *Dist:* Routldge.

Learning to Heal: The Development of American Medical Education. Kenneth M. Ludmerer. 1996. LC 95-31818. 359p. reprint ed. pap. text 18.95 (*0-8018-5258-7*) Johns Hopkins.

Learning to Heal: The Medical Profession in Colonial Mexico, 1767-1831. Luz M. Hernandez Saenz. 1997. LC 96-7585. (Ameican University Studies XXI: No. 17). X, 301p. (C). text 48.95 (*0-8204-3328-4*) P Lang Pubng.

Learning to Learn from Experience. Edward Cell. 1984. LC 83-9283. 245p. (C). text 50.50 (*0-87395-832-2*); pap. text 17.95 (*0-87395-833-0*) State U NY Pr.

Learning to Live Drug Free: A Curriculum Model for Prevention. Kathleen A. McCormick & Charles H. Flatter. 1994. (Illus.). 182p. (Orig.). (C). pap. text 30.00 (*0-7881-0450-0*) DIANE Pub.

Learning to Master Your Chronic Pain. Robert N. Jamison. 1996. LC 96-15431. (Illus.). 240p. pap. 27.45 (*1-56887-019-1*, MCPWBP, Prof Resc Pr) Pro Resource.

Learning to Play God. Robert Marion. 1993. mass mkt. 6.99 (*0-449-22192-X*) Fawcett.

Learning to Say Good-Bye: When a Child's Parent Dies. Eda LeShan. 1978. 128p. pap. 8.00 (*0-380-40105-3*, Avon Bks) Morrow Avon.

Learning to Say Goodbye: Dealing with Death & Dying. Rosalie Peck & Charlotte Stefanics. 1987. LC 87-70820. xx, 164p. 17.95 (*0-915202-71-9*) Accel Devel.

Learning Together: One School Reports. Betty M. Young. 1969. 107p. pap. 2.75 (*0-85225-537-3*) Ed Solutions.

Learning Together to Work Together for Health: Report on a WHO Study Group. WHO Staff. 1998. (Technical Report Ser.: No. 769). 72p. 9.00 (*92-4-120769-8*) World Health.

Learning Veterinary Terminology. Douglas F. McBride. 1996. LC 95-48284. (Illus.). 560p. (C). (gr. 13). pap. text 30.00 (*0-8151-5960-9*, 25550) Mosby Inc.

Least of These My Brethren. Daniel J. Baxter. 1998. LC 98-4555. 272p. (C). pap. 13.00 (*0-15-600588-3*) Harcourt.

Least Restrictive Alternative: Principles & Practices. D. Biklin et al. Ed. by H. Rutherford Turnbull, III. 1981. 80p. (Orig.). pap. 6.00 (*0-940898-06-3*) Am Assn Mental.

Least Worst Death: Essays in Bioethics on the End of Life. Margaret Pabst Battin. 1994. LC 93-8276. (Illus.). 320p. (C). pap. text 26.95 (*0-19-508265-6*) OUP.

Leavell & Thorup's Fundamentals of Clinical Hematology. Oscar A. Thorup, Jr. 5th ed. 1987. (Illus.). 1040p. text 135.00 (*0-7216-5679-X*) Saunders.

Leaving Abusive Partners: From the Scars of Survival to the Wisdom for Change. Cathy Kirkwood. 1993. 224p. (C). 69.95 (*0-8039-8685-8*, 9843); pap. 25.95 (*0-8039-8686-6*, 9844) Sage.

Leaving Home: The Therapy of Disturbed Young People. Jay Haley. 2nd rev. ed. 1997. LC 96-50983. 336p. (YA). 39.95 (*0-87630-845-0*) Brunner-Routledge.

Leaving the Bedside: Search for the Nonclinical Medical Career. American Medical Association Staff. 2nd ed. 1992. LC 94-143692. (Career Development Ser.). ix, 118p. 32.95 (*0-89970-464-6*) AMA.

***Leben bis Zuletzt - Finalversorgung von Tumorkranken.** Ed. by Hartmut Reiners. 2001. (GER.). 140p. pap. 20.00 (*3-11-017183-X*) De Gruyter.

Leber des Menschen, the Human Liver: Rasterelektonenmikroskopischer Atlas: A Scanning Electron Microscopic Atlas. F. J. Vonnahme. 1993. (Illus.). x, 100p. 71.50 (*3-8055-5585-7*) S Karger.

Lebererkrankungen: Praevention, Progressionshemmung, Rehabilitation. Ed. by R. Nilius & K. J. Paquet. 1995. (Illus.). viii, 232p. 143.50 (*3-8055-6171-7*) S Karger.

LEC Rat: A New Model for Hepatitis & Liver Cancer. Ed. by M. Mori et al. 1992. (Illus.). 360p. 212.00 (*0-387-70079-X*) Spr-Verlag.

Lecideicole Ascomyceten - Eine Revision der Obligat Lichenicolen Ascomyceten Auf Lecideoiden Flechten. Dagmar Triebel. Ed. by Volkmar Wirth et al. 1989. (Bibliotheca Lichenologica: Vol. 35). (GER., Illus.). 278p. (*3-443-58014-9*) Gebruder Borntraeger DEU. *Dist:* Balogh.

Lecithin Book. Carlson Wade. 1980. LC 80-82319. (Pivot Original Health Bks.). 128p. pap. 3.95 (*0-87983-226-6*, 32266K, Keats Pubng) McGraw-Hill Trade.

Lecithins. Ed. by B. F. Szuhaj & Gary R. List. 1985. 394p. 40.00 (*0-935315-09-8*) Am Oil Chemists.

Lecithins: Sources, Manufacture, Uses. Ed. by B. F. Szuhaj. 1989. 294p. 80.00 (*0-935315-27-6*) Am Oil Chemists.

Lectins: Biomedical Perspectives. Ed. by Arpad Pusztai & Susan Bardocz. 1994. LC 95-167849. 368p. (*0-7484-0177-6*) Tay Francis Ltd GBR. *Dist:* Taylor & Francis.

Lectins & Cancer. Ed. by H. J. Gabius & S. Gabius. 1991. (Illus.). 329p. 112.00 (*0-387-54224-8*) Spr-Verlag.

Lecture Notes in Emergency Medicine. David W. Yates et al. 2nd ed. 1999. LC 98-36149. (Lecture Notes). (Illus.). 416p. pap. 39.95 (*0-632-02766-5*) Blackwell Sci.

Lecture Notes in Medical Microbiology. Ed. by T. S. Elliott et al. 3rd ed. 1997. LC 96-2259. (Lecture Notes). (Illus.). 352p. pap. 36.95 (*0-632-02446-1*) Blackwell Sci.

Lecture Notes in Obstetrics. Geoffrey V.P Chamberlain. 7th ed. 1996. LC 96-11891. (Illus.). 296p. (Orig.). pap. text 29.95 (*0-86542-681-3*) Blackwell Sci.

Lecture Notes in Ophthalmology. Anthony J. Bron et al. 8th ed. 1997. LC 96-20972. (Illus.). 224p. pap. 38.95 (*0-86542-723-2*) Blackwell Sci.

Lecture Notes on Anatomy. D. B. Moffat. 2nd ed. 1993. LC 93-9734. (Lecture Notes Ser.). (Illus.). 424p. pap. 36.95 (*0-632-03696-6*) Blackwell Sci.

Lecture Notes on Cardiology. Keith D. Dawkins et al. 4th ed. 2001. (Lecture Notes). (Illus.). 288p. pap. 29.95 (*0-86542-864-6*) Blackwell Sci.

Lecture Notes on Clinical Anaesthesia. Carol L. Gwinnutt. 1997. LC 96-39563. (Illus.). 360p. pap. 38.95 (*0-86542-656-2*) Blackwell Sci.

Lecture Notes on Clinical Biochemistry. Lionel Whitby & A. F. Smith. 5th ed. 1993. LC 92-48270. (Illus.). 452p. pap. 29.95 (*0-632-03687-7*) Blackwell Sci.

Lecture Notes on Clinical Biochemistry. A. F. Smith et al. 6th ed. 1998. LC 97-43308. (Lecture Notes). (Illus.). 317p. pap. 38.95 (*0-632-04834-4*) Blackwell Sci.

Lecture Notes on Clinical Medicine. David Rubenstein et al. 5th ed. 1997. LC 97-10914. (Lecture Notes). (Illus.). 320p. (C). pap. 36.95 (*0-86542-925-1*) Blackwell Sci.

Lecture Notes on Clinical Pharmacology. John L. Reid et al. 5th ed. 1996. LC 96-859. pap. 29.95 (*0-08-654665-1*) Blackwell Sci.

Lecture Notes on Clinical Skills. Robert C. Turner & Roger A. Blackwood. 3rd ed. 1997. LC 96-13667. (Lecture Notes). (Illus.). 288p. pap. 38.95 (*0-86542-971-5*) Blackwell Sci.

Lecture Notes on Dermatology. Bobin A. Graham-Brown et al. 7th ed. 1996. LC 95-51162. (Illus.). 288p. pap. 36.95 (*0-86542-635-X*) Blackwell Sci.

Lecture Notes on Diseases of the Ear, Nose & Throat. Peter D. Bull. 8th ed. 1996. LC 95-39680. (Illus.). 113p. pap. 38.95 (*0-86542-634-1*) Blackwell Sci.

Lecture Notes on Epidemiology & Public Health. Richard Farmer et al. 4th ed. 1996. LC 95-26229. (Illus.). 288p. pap. 36.95 (*0-86542-611-2*) Blackwell Sci.

Lecture Notes on General Surgery. H. Ellis et al. 9th ed. 1998. LC 97-42474. (Lecture Notes). (Illus.). 386p. pap. 38.95 (*0-86542-768-2*) Blackwell Sci.

Lecture Notes on Geriatrics. Nicholas Coni & Stephen Webster. 5th ed. 1998. LC 97-22533. (Lecture Notes). (Illus.). 208p. pap. 38.95 (*0-86542-750-X*) Blackwell Sci.

Lecture Notes on Gynaecology. Geoffrey V.P. Chamberlain et al. 7th rev. ed. 1996. LC 95-21884. (Lecture Notes). (Illus.). 275p. pap. 29.95 (*0-632-03111-5*) Blackwell Sci.

Lecture Notes on Hematology. Nevin C. Hughes-Jones et al. 6th ed. 1996. LC 95-9604. (Illus.). 288p. pap. 38.95 (*0-632-04039-4*) Blackwell Sci.

Lecture Notes on History Taking & Examination. Robert C. Turner & R. Blackwood. 2nd ed. 1991. (Lecture Notes). (Illus.). 208p. pap. 21.50 (*0-632-02885-8*) Blackwell Sci.

Lecture Notes on Human Physiology. John J. Bray. 4th ed. 1999. LC 98-28849. (*0-86542-776-3*) Blackwell Sci.

Lecture Notes on Human Physiology. John J. Bray et al. 4th ed. 1999. LC 98-28849. (Lecture Notes). (Illus.). 400p. pap. 38.95 (*0-86542-775-5*) Blackwell Sci.

Lecture Notes on Immunology. Gordon Reeves et al. 3rd ed. 1996. LC 95-39681. (Lecture Notes). (Illus.). 226p. pap. 28.95 (*0-632-03812-8*) Blackwell Sci.

Lecture Notes on Immunology. Gordon Reeves & Ian Todd. 4th ed. 2000. LC 99-462342. (Lecture Notes). (Illus.). 280p. (C). pap. 31.95 (*0-632-05636-3*) Blackwell Sci.

***Lecture Notes on Molecular Medicine.** John R. Bradley et al. 2nd ed. 2001. (Lecture Notes). 152p. pap. 34.95 (*0-632-05839-0*) Blackwell Sci.

Lecture Notes on Neurology. Lionel Ginsberg & Ivan T. Draper. 7th ed. 1999. LC 98-48820. (Lecture Notes). (Illus.). viii, 199p. pap. 28.95 (*0-632-04827-1*) Blackwell Sci.

Lecture Notes on Obstetrics & Gynaecology. Geoffrey Chamberlain & Diana Hamilton-Fairly. 1999. LC 98-39642. (Illus.). vii, 295p. pap. 36.95 (*0-632-04957-X*) Blackwell Sci.

Lecture Notes on Obstetrics & Gynaecology. Ajoy K. Ghosh. 1985. (*0-7855-0741-8*) Current Dist IND. *Dist:* St Mut.

Lecture Notes on Ophthalmology. Patrick Trevor-Roper. 7th ed. 1986. (Lecture Notes). (Illus.). 138p. pap. 32.95 (*0-632-01585-3*) Blackwell Sci.

Lecture Notes on Orthopaedics. T. Duckworth. 3rd ed. 1992. LC 94-23689. (Lecture Notes). (Illus.). 400p. pap. 38.95 (*0-632-02781-9*) Blackwell Sci.

Lecture Notes on Paediatrics. Meadow. 5th ed. 1986. 17.95 (*0-8016-3372-9*) Mosby Inc.

***Lecture Notes on Paediatrics.** S. R. Meadow & Simon J. Newell. 7th ed. 2001. LC 2001-35386. (Lecture Notes). 256p. pap. 29.95 (*0-632-05065-9*) Blackwell Sci.

Lecture Notes on Pathology. R. E. Cotton. 4th ed. 1992. (Lecture Notes). (Illus.). 448p. pap. 34.95 (*0-632-03355-X*) Blackwell Sci.

Lecture Notes on Psychiatry. M. Sharpe et al. 8th ed. 1998. LC 97-42431. (Lecture Notes). (Illus.). 224p. pap. 38.95 (*0-632-03677-X*) Blackwell Sci.

Lecture Notes on Radiology. P. R. Patel. 1997. LC 97-10069. (Lecture Notes). (Illus.). 256p. pap. 38.95 (*0-632-04758-5*) Blackwell Sci.

Lecture Notes on Respiratory Disease. S. J. Bourke & R. A. L. Brewis. 5th ed. 1998. LC 98-3473. (Lecture Notes). (Illus.). 350p. pap. 38.95 (*0-632-04968-5*) Blackwell Sci.

Lecture Notes on Tropical Medicine. D. Bell et al. 4th ed. 1995. LC 94-33311. (Lecture Notes). 320p. pap. 36.95 (*0-632-03839-X*) Blackwell Sci.

Lecture Notes on Urology. John P. Blandy. 5th ed. 1998. LC 97-23639. (Lecture Notes). (Illus.). 288p. pap. 38.95 (*0-632-04202-8*) Blackwell Sci.

Lectureactive Nutrition. Saundersco. 1994. (C). 303.00 (*0-03-013414-5*) Harcourt Coll Pubs.

Lectures & Symposia of the 14th International Cancer Congress Vol. 1: Cancer Research & Treatment Today: Results, Trends & Frontiers. K. Lapis & S. Eckhardt. 1987. 266p. (C). (*963-05-4523-3*) Akade Kiado HUN. *Dist:* St Mut.

Lectures & Symposia of the 14th International Cancer Congress Vol. 2: Molecular Biology & Differentiation of Cancer Cells, Oncogenes, Growth Factors, Receptors. K. Lapis & S. Eckhardt. 1987. 361p. (C). (*963-05-4524-1*) Akade Kiado HUN. *Dist:* St Mut.

Lectures & Symposia of the 14th International Cancer Congress Vol. 3: Cytology, Pathology & Cancer Prognosis. K. Lapis & S. Eckhardt. 1987. 219p. (C). (*963-05-4525-X*) Akade Kiado HUN. *Dist:* St Mut.

Lectures & Symposia of the 14th International Cancer Congress Vol. 4: Carcinogenesis & Tumour Progression. Ed. by K. Lapis & S. Eckhardt. 1987. 334p. (C). (*963-05-4526-8*) Akade Kiado HUN. *Dist:* St Mut.

Lectures & Symposia of the 14th International Cancer Congress Vol. 5: Novel Approaches in Cancer Therapy. K. Lapis & S. Eckhardt. 1987. 387p. (C). (*963-05-4527-6*) Akade Kiado HUN. *Dist:* St Mut.

Lectures & Symposia of the 14th International Cancer Congress Vol. 6: Epidemiology, Prevention, Diagnosis. K. Lapis & S. Eckhardt. 1987. 365p. (C). (*963-05-4528-4*) Akade Kiado HUN. *Dist:* St Mut.

Lectures & Symposia of the 14th International Cancer Congress Vol. 7: Oncological Surgery. K. Lapis & S. Eckhardt. 1987. 223p. (C). (*963-05-4529-2*) Akade Kiado HUN. *Dist:* St Mut.

Lectures & Symposia of the 14th International Cancer Congress Vol. 8: Radiotherapy, Paediatric Oncology, Neurooncology. K. Lapis & S. Eckhardt. 1987. 352p. (C). (*963-05-4530-6*) Akade Kiado HUN. *Dist:* St Mut.

Lectures & Symposia of the 14th International Cancer Congress Vol. 10: Biological Response Modifiers, Leukaemias & Lymphomas. K. Lapis & S. Eckhardt. 1987. 133p. (C). (*963-05-4532-2*) Akade Kiado HUN. *Dist:* St Mut.

Lectures & Symposia of the 14th International Cancer Congress Vol. 11: Medical Oncology. K. Lapis & S. Eckhardt. 1987. 339p. (C). (*963-05-4533-0*) Akade Kiado HUN. *Dist:* St Mut.

Lectures & Symposia of the 14th International Cancer Congress Vol. 13: Education, Nursing, Organization. K. Lapis & S. Eckhardt. 1987. 336p. (C). (*963-05-4535-7*) Akade Kiado HUN. *Dist:* St Mut.

Lectures in Hair Structure & Chemistry for Cosmetology Teachers. A. H. Powitt. 1991. (Illus.). pap. 28.95 (*0-87350-354-6*) Milady Pub.

Lectures in Medical Psychology: An Introduction to the Care of Patients. Grete L. Bibring & Ralph J. Kahana. 1969. LC 68-57279. 289p. 42.50 (*0-8236-2970-8*) Intl Univs Pr.

Lectures in Psychiatry: The Functional Psychoses, Vol. 1. Ken Reed. 1985. (Illus.). 304p. 37.50 (*0-87527-339-4*) Green.

Lectures on Homeopathic Philosophy. James T. Kent. 1979. 244p. reprint ed. pap. 14.95 (*0-913028-61-4*) North Atlantic.

Lectures on Human & Animal Psychology, 1. Wilhelm M. Wundt. Tr. by J. Creighton from GER. 1977. LC 77-72191. (Contributions to the History of Psychology Ser.: Pt. D, Vol. I, Comparative Psychology). 454p. reprint ed. lib. bdg. 79.50 (*0-313-26945-9*, U6945) Greenwood.

Lectures on Human & Animal Psychology. Wilhelm M. Wundt. 470p. 120.00 (*1-85506-680-7*) Thoemmes Pr.

Lectures on Jung's Typology. Marie-Louise Von Franz & James Hillman. 1971. LC 86-17912. (Seminar Ser.: No. 4). 302p. (Orig.). (C). pap. 17.00 (*0-88214-104-X*) Spring Pubns.

Lectures on Language Performance. C. E. Osgood. 1980. (Language & Communication Ser.: Vol. 7). (Illus.). 276p. 91.00 (*0-387-09901-8*) Spr-Verlag.

Lectures on Psychology Women. Joan C. Chrisler et al. 2nd ed. 1999. LC 99-29468. 408p. pap. 39.38 (*0-07-234860-7*, McGrw-H College) McGrw-H Hghr Educ.

Lectures on the Elementary Psychology of Feeling & Attention. Edward B. Titchener. 1978. LC 73-2994. (Classics in Psychology Ser.). reprint ed. 25.95 (*0-405-05166-2*) Ayer.

Lectures on the Experimental Psychology of the Thought-Processes. Edward B. Titchener. 1978. LC 73-2995. (Classics in Psychology Ser.). reprint ed. 25.95 (*0-405-05167-0*) Ayer.

Lee McGregor's Synopsis of Surgical Anatomy. G. A. Decker & D. J. Du Plessis. 12th ed. 1986. (Illus.). 626p. pap. text (*0-7236-0801-6*) E A GBR. *Dist:* OUP.

Leflunomide: Proceedings of the Vienna Symposium, 12 October 1993. Ed. by R. R. Bartlett. 1994. LC 94-43800. (*3-7643-5150-0*); (*0-8176-5150-0*) Birkhauser.

Lefrancois: Psychologie Lernes. 1994. 39.95 (*0-387-57807-2*) Spr-Verlag.

Left Brain, Right Brain. Sally P. Springer & Georg Deutsh. 5th ed. 1997. LC 97-27803. (Series of Books in Psychology). 368p. pap. text 21.95 (*0-7167-3111-8*) W H Freeman.

Left for Dead. Dick Quinn et al. 1992. (Illus.). 200p. (Orig.). pap. 12.95 (*0-9632839-0-1*) R F Quinn.

Left-Handedness: Behavioral Implications & Anomalies. Ed. by Stanley Coren. 1990. (Advances in Psychology Ser.: No. 67). xviii,574p. 201.50 (*0-444-88438-6*, North Holland) Elsevier.

Left-Hander Syndrome: The Causes & Consequences of Left-Handedness. Stanley Coren. 1991. LC 91-26505. (Illus.). 375p. 27.95 (*0-02-906682-4*) Free Pr.

***Left Heart in Congenital Heart Disease.** Robert H. Anderson. 2002. (Illus.). 280p. pap. (*1-84110-056-0*) Greenwich Med GBR. *Dist:* JAMCO Dist.

Left Ventricular Dysfunction. Ed. by J. J. Kellermann & David H. Spodick. 1986. (Advances in Cardiology Ser.: Vol. 34). (Illus.). viii, 212p. 152.25 (*3-8055-4349-2*) S Karger.

Left Ventricular Hypertrophy. Sheridan. 1999. (C). text 89.00 (*0-443-06361-3*) Harcrt Hlth Sci Grp.

***Left Ventricular Hypertrophy & the Insulin Resistance Syndrome.** Johan Sundstrom. 2001. (Comprehensive Summaries of Uppsala Dissertations from the Faculty of Medicine Ser.: No. 992). (Illus.). 68p. pap. (*91-554-4919-0*) Uppsala Universitet SWE. *Dist:* Coronet Bks.

Leg Ulcers. Christine J. Moffatt & Peter Harper. 1997. LC 97-22896. (Access to Clinical Education Ser.). 197p. pap. text (*0-443-05533-5*) Church.

Leg Ulcers: A Practical Approach to Management. David Negus. 2nd ed. 1995. (Illus.). 232p. text (*0-7506-1697-0*) E A GBR. *Dist:* OUP.

Leg Ulcers: Diagnosis & Treatment. Ed. by Wiete Westerhof. 1993. LC 93-28116. 422p. 321.00 (*0-444-81427-2*) Elsevier.

Legacy: A History of the Tuskegee University School of Veterinary Medicine. Eugene W. Adams. 1995. LC 94-74577. (Illus.). 312p. 32.50 (*0-9645067-1-8*) Media Ctr.

Legacy & History of Roswell Park Cancer Institute, 1898-1998. Edwin A. Mirand. 1998. LC 98-18365. 216p. 35.00 (*1-57864-036-9*) Donning Co.

Legacy of B. F. Skinner: Concepts & Perspectives, Controversies & Misunderstandings. Robert D. Nye. 1991. LC 91-21644. (Psychology Ser.). 145p. (C). pap. 18.25 (*0-534-16944-9*) Brooks-Cole.

Legacy of Caring: The Society of Memorial Sloan-Kettering Cancer Center. Joan S. Straus. 1996. (Illus.). xiv, 298p. 44.95 (*0-9653303-0-3*); pap. 24.95 (*0-9653303-1-1*) Soc Mem Sloan-Kettering.

***Legacy of Dr. Lamaze: The Story of the Man Who Changed Childbirth: A Biography.** Caroline Gutmann. Tr. by Bruce Benderson from FRE. 2001. LC 2001-19274. (Illus.). 240p. 24.95 (*0-312-26190-X*) St Martin.

Legacy of Erich Fromm. Daniel Burston. 1991. LC 90-5348. (Illus.). 288p. 45.50 (*0-674-52168-4*, BURLEG) HUP.

Legacy of Leadership: Presidential Addresses from the Superintendents' Society & the National League for Nursing 1894-1952. Ed. by Nettie Birnbach & Sandra B. Lewenson. 1993. 416p. (C). pap. text 29.95 (*0-88737-575-8*, 14-2514) Natl League Nurse.

Legacy of Longevity: Health & Health Care in Later Life. Sidney M. Stahl. 342p. (C). 1991. 67.95 (*0-8039-4001-7*, 3267); 1990. pap. 34.95 (*0-8039-4002-5*, 3268) Sage.

Legacy of Narcissus: Moral Dilemmas in Modern Aesthetic Surgery. Jeffrey S. Isenberg. 2000. 110p. pap. text 28.00 (*1-55605-313-4*) Wyndham Hall.

Legacy of Sandor Ferenczi. Ed. by Lewis Aron & Adrienne Harris. 1996. LC 93-6594. 320p. reprint ed. 49.95 (*0-88163-149-3*) Analytic Pr.

Legacy of Sigmund Freud. Jacob A. Arlow. 1956. LC 56-9746. 35.00 (*0-8236-2980-5*) Intl Univs Pr.

Legacy of Solomon Asch: Essays in Cognition & Social Psychology. Ed. by Irvin Rock. 1990. 320p. text 69.95 (*0-8058-0440-4*) L Erlbaum Assocs.

***Legacy of War: Poetry, Prose, Painting & Physic.** Dianna Berry & Campbell Mackenzie. 1995. (History of Medicine Ser.). 52p. pap. (*1-85315-262-5*) Royal Soc of Medicine Pr Ltd GBR. *Dist:* Balogh.

Legacy of William Schwartz: Group Practice As Shared Interaction. Ed. by Alex Gitterman & Lawrence Shulman. 1986. LC 85-17586. (Social Work with Groups Ser.: Vol. 8, No. 4). 120p. text 39.95 (*0-86656-520-5*) Haworth Pr.

Legal & Ethical Aspects of Fetal Tissue Transplantation. Arthur R. Bauer. 1993. LC 93-42908. (Medical Intelligence Unit Ser.). 128p. 99.00 (*1-57059-021-4*) Landes Bioscience.

Legal & Ethical Aspects of HIV-Related Research. Sana Loue. 1995. LC 95-34011. (Illus.). 214p. 47.00 (*0-306-45055-0*, Plenum Trade) Perseus Pubng.

Legal & Ethical Aspects of Organ Transplantation. David Price. 2001. LC 00-24475. 512p. (C). text 74.95 (*0-521-65164-6*) Cambridge U Pr.

***Legal & Ethical Aspects of Telemedicine.** Ben Stanberry. 1998. 172p. pap. (*1-85315-354-0*) Royal Soc of Medicine Pr Ltd GBR. *Dist:* Balogh.

Legal & Ethical Considerations for Dental Hygienists & Assistants. Judith A. Davison. 1999. LC 00-699155. (Illus.). xxii, 378p. text (*1-55664-422-1*) Mosby Inc.

Legal & Ethical Dimensions for Mental Health Professionals. Patrick B. Malley. 1999. LC 98-31545. 367p. pap. 29.95 (*1-56032-687-5*) Hemisp Pub.

Legal & Ethical Issues. Killion & Dempsi. 2000. (Quick Look Nursing Ser.). 18.95 (*1-889325-48-1*) Fence Crk Pubng.

Legal & Ethical Issues in Health. Joan Aiken. 1999. LC 2001-49406. pap. text (*0-7216-6525-X*) Saunders.

Legal & Ethical Issues in Nursing. Ginny Wacker Guido. 3rd ed. 2000. LC 00-22586. xi, 484p. (C). pap. 37.60 (*0-8385-5659-0*) P-H.

Legal & Ethical Issues in Physical Therapy. Dolly Swisher & Carol Krueger-Brophy. 1998. LC 97-23859. 272p. text 39.99 (*0-7506-9788-1*) Buttrwrth-Heinemann.

Legal & Ethical Issues in the Management of the Dementing Elderly. Vol. 3. Mary Gilhooley. 1994. (Medico-Legal Issues Ser.). text (*1-85521-027-4*) Dartmth Pub GBR. *Dist:* Ashgate Pub Co.

Legal & Ethical Perspectives In Healthcare: An Integrated Approach. Raymond S. Edge. 1997. LC 97-6627. (Allied Health Ser.). 320p. (C). pap. text 37.95 (*0-8273-7684-7*) Delmar.

Legal & Healthcare Ethics for the Elderly. George P. Smith. 2nd. 1996. 207p. 69.95 (*1-56032-452-X*); 225p. pap. 29.95 (*1-56032-453-8*) Hemisp Pub.

Legal & Medical Liability in Health Sciences: Index of New Information & Research Bible. Roy R. Zimmerman. 1994. 180p. 57.50 (*0-7883-0098-9*); pap. 47.50 (*0-7883-0099-7*) ABBE Pubs Assn.

Legal Answer Book for Managed Care. Aspen Health Law Center Staff. 1995. 368p. 91.00 (*0-8342-0700-1*) Aspen Pub.

Legal Aspects of Anaesthesia. Ed. by J. F. Crul. 1989. (Developments in Critical Care, Medicine, & Anesthesiology Ser.). 146p. (C). lib. bdg. 80.00 (*0-7923-0393-8*) Kluwer Academic.

Legal Aspects of Child Abuse. Elizabeth Butler-Sloss & A. E. Levy. 1991. (Waterlow Practitioner's Library). 256p. 40.01 (*0-08-036906-5*) Macmillan.

Legal Aspects of Child Health Care. J. Hendrick. 1996. LC 96-85901. (Illus.). 224p. (Orig.). pap. 47.75 (*1-56593-340-0*, 0670) Singular Publishing.

Legal Aspects of Complementary Therapy Practice: A Guide for Health Care Professionals. Bridgit C. Dimond. 1998. LC 98-20834. xx, 462p. (C). text (*0-443-05615-3*) Church.

Legal Aspects of Documenting Patient Care. Ronald W. Scott. 2nd ed. 1999. LC 99-55592. 221p. 54.00 (*0-8342-1630-2*) Aspen Pub.

Legal Aspects of Health Care Administration. George D. Pozgar. 7th ed. tchr. ed. (*0-8342-1648-5*, 16485) Aspen Pub.

Legal Aspects of Health Care for the Elderly: An Annotated Bibliography, 7. Compiled by Marshall B. Kapp. 1988. LC 88-15428. (Bibliographies & Indexes in Gerontology Ser.: No. 7). 174p. lib. bdg. 62.95 (*0-313-26159-8*, KLG/, Greenwood Pr) Greenwood.

Legal Aspects of Health Information Management. Dana C. McWay. 1996. LC 96-8394. (Nursing Education Ser.). 302p. (C). 53.95 (*0-8273-5576-9*) Delmar.

Legal Aspects of Health Policy: Issues & Trends. Ed. by Ruth Roemer & George McKray. 1980. LC 79-8583. (Illus.). 473p. lib. bdg. 75.00 (*0-313-21430-1*, RIH/, Greenwood Pr) Greenwood.

Legal Aspects of Home Health Care. William D. Cabin & James C. Pyles. 1987. LC 87-28974. (*0-87189-897-7*) Aspen Pub.

Legal Aspects of International Drug Control. S. K. Chatterjee. 1981. 612p. 117.00 (*90-286-2091-5*) Kluwer Academic.

Legal Aspects of Medical Practice. Bernard Knight. 5th ed. 1992. (Illus.). 386p. pap. text (*0-443-04568-2*) Church.

Legal Aspects of Medicare & Medicaid Reimbursement: Payment for Hospital & Physician Services. Ed. by Terry S. Coleman. 1990. 199p. 35.00 (*0-918945-05-4*) Am Hlth Lawyers.

Legal Aspects of Medicare & Medicaid Reimbursement: Payment for Hospital & Physician Services. Terry S. Coleman. Ed. by Susan K. Chambers. 1990. LC 90-61619. (NHLA Focus Ser.). 216p. pap. 45.00 (*0-918945-06-2*) Am Hlth Lawyers.

Legal Aspects of Medicare & Medicaid Reimbursement: Payment for Hospital & Physician Services; Supplement RBRVS & the New Medicare Physician Fee Schedule. Ed. by Terry S. Coleman. 1990. 44p. 35.00 (*0-918945-13-5*) Am Hlth Lawyers.

Legal Aspects of Medicine. Ed. by J. R. Vevaina et al. 1989. 340p. 148.00 (*0-387-96831-8*) Spr-Verlag.

Legal Aspects of Midwifery Workbook. Dimond & Walters. 1997. LC 97-181671. 80p. pap. text, wbk. ed. 34.99 (*1-898507-43-0*) Buttrwrth-Heinemann.

Legal Aspects of Occupational Therapy. Bridgit C. Dimond. 1997. LC 96-9284. (Illus.). 400p. (Orig.). pap. 46.95 (*0-632-04074-2*) Blackwell Sci.

Legal Aspects of Optometry. John G. Classe. (Illus.). 764p. 1989. text 95.00 (*0-409-95043-2*); 2nd ed. 2001. 95.00 (*0-7506-7265-X*) Buttrwrth-Heinemann.

Legal Aspects of Physiotherapy. Bridgit C. Dimond. 2000. LC 99-89275. pap. 65.95 (*0-632-05108-6*) Blackwell Sci.

Legal Aspects of Sports Medicine. David L. Herbert & William G. Herbert. 2nd ed. 1995. LC 94-92196. 280p. pap. 39.95 (*0-944183-18-2*) PRC Pub.

Legal Boundaries of California Nursing Practice. Robert Anderson. 5th ed. 1997. 300p. pap. 20.00 (*0-942028-50-3*) Andrsn Cont Educ.

Legal Competence in Environmental Health. T. Moran. 1997. 208p. text (*0-412-71580-5*, Chap & Hall NY) Chapman & Hall.

Legal Competence in Environmental Health. Terence Moran. 1998. LC 98-171432. (Illus.). 352p. (C). 80.00 (*0-419-23000-9*, D5809, Spon) Routledge.

Legal Concepts & Issues in Emergency Care. N. Genell Lee. 2000. LC 00-41267. (Illus.). xix, 298p. pap. 39.25 (*0-7216-8324-X*) Saunders.

Legal Considerations in Healthcare Delivery. M. Cronin. 1993. 210p. (C). spiral bd. (*0-933195-26-5*) CA College Health Sci.

Legal Constraints on Public Hospitals: Purchasing Requirements, Property Disposal, & Conflicts of Interest; Open Meetings & Public Records. Warren J. Wicker & David M. Lawrence. 1986. (Hospital Law in North Carolina Ser.: Chap. 7). 52p. (C). ring bd. 10.50 (*1-56011-079-1*, 85.03G) Institute Government.

Legal Defense of Pathological Intoxication with Related Issues of Temporary & Self-Inflicted Insanity. Lawrence P. Tiffany & Mary Tiffany. 1990. LC 89-49429. 560p. 99.50 (*0-89930-548-2*, TPA/, Greenwood Pr) Greenwood.

Legal Documents for HR Professionals. Steven Mitchell Sack. 1997. 1p. (C). pap. text 69.95 incl. disk (*0-13-889056-0*) P-H.

Legal, Ethical & Political Issues in Nursing. Tonia D. Aiken. 1994. LC 93-46312. 297p. pap. 31.95 (*0-8036-0081-X*) Davis Co.

Legal-Ethical Considerations, Restrictions, & Obligations for Clinicians Who Treat Communicative Disorders. Franklin H. Silverman. 2nd ed. 1992. (Illus.). 258p. text 54.95 (*0-398-05783-4*) C C Thomas.

Legal Ethics for Management & Their Counsel, 1998 Edition. Len Biernat & R. Hunter Manson. 1998. LC 99-461912. 410p. (*0-327-00715-X*, 6056113) LEXIS Pub.

Legal Framework for Bioethics. Cosimo M. Mazzoni. 1998. LC 97-32491. (Nijhoff Law Specials Ser.). 256p. pap. text 81.00 (*90-411-0523-9*) Kluwer Law Intl.

Legal Guide for Long-Term Care Administrators. Peter J. Buttaro. 1999. LC 99-32771. (Long Term Care Administration Ser.). 245p. pap. 68.00 (*0-8342-1370-2*) Aspen Pub.

Legal Guide for Physicians. Joseph M. Taraska. 1987. 1300p. text 140.00 (*1-887515-01-1*) AHAB Press.

Legal Guide for Practicing Psychotherapy in Colorado. Louie V. Larimer, Jr. 1992. pap. 34.95 (*0-9633550-0-7*) Ctr Prof Develop.

Legal Handbook of Texas Nurses. Susan S. Murphy. 1995. LC 94-27848. 256p. pap. 17.95 (*0-292-75176-1*); text 35.00 (*0-292-75161-3*) U of Tex Pr.

Legal Issues & Ethical Dilemmas in Respiratory Care. Charles Carroll. 1996. LC 95-44083. (Illus.). 163p. (C). pap. text 19.95 (*0-8036-0126-3*) Davis Co.

Legal Issues & the Integrated Delivery System: An Executive Guide. American Academy of Health Care Attorneys Staff. Ed. by Deborah A. Randall. 1996. LC 96-8090. 104p. pap. 40.00 (*1-55648-159-4*, 118119) AHPI.

***Legal Issues Associated with Development & Implementation of Provider-Sponsored Managed Care Organizations.** Anne M. Murphy & Heather L. Fields. 2001. 65p. (C). reprint ed. pap. text 25.00 (*0-7567-0624-6*) DIANE Pub.

Legal Issues in Biotechnology & Human Reproduction. Warren Freedman. 1991. LC 90-20709. 240p. 67.95 (*0-89930-635-7*, FLI/, Quorum Bks) Greenwood.

Legal Issues in Clinical Supervision. M. Janelle Disney & Anthony M. Stephens. 1994. LC 93-36194. (ACA Legal Ser.: Vol. 10). 90p. pap. text 18.95 (*1-55620-128-1*, 72310) Am Coun Assn.

Legal Issues in Health Care Fraud & Abuse: Navigating the Uncertainties. Ed. by Carrie S. Valiant. 1994. 288p. 50.00 (*0-918945-16-X*) Am Hlth Lawyers.

Legal Issues in Healthcare Fraud & Abuse: Navigating the Uncertainties. David E. Matyas. 2nd ed. 1997. LC 96-70114. (NHLA Focus Ser.). 403p. 75.00 (*0-918945-19-4*) Am Hlth Lawyers.

Legal Issues in Marriage & Family Counseling. Patricia Stevens-Smith & Marcia M. Hughes. 1993. LC 92-31486. (ACA Legal Ser.: Vol. 7). 61p. pap. text 18.95 (*1-55620-104-4*, 72307) Am Coun Assn.

Legal Issues in Medicine. Ed. by Sheila A. McLean. 1981. 234p. text 76.95 (*0-566-00428-3*) Ashgate Pub Co.

Legal Issues in Mental Health Care. R. Wettstein & Barbara A. Weiner. 1993. (Illus.). 432p. (C). 60.00 (*0-306-43867-4*, Plenum Trade) Perseus Pubng.

Legal Issues in Nursing Management. Davidson. 1996. (C). text 40.95 (*0-8273-6606-X*) Delmar.

Legal Issues in Obstetrics. Vivienne Harpwood. 1996. LC 95-39633. (Medico-Legal Issues Ser.). (Illus.). 320p. text (*1-85521-313-3*) Dartmth Pub GBR. *Dist:* Ashgate Pub Co.

Legal Issues in Pediatrics & Adolescent Medicine. Angela R. Holder. 2nd enl. rev. ed. 1985. LC 85-2410. 512p. 65.00 (*0-300-03384-2*) Yale U Pr.

Legal Issues in Social Work, Counseling, & Mental Health. Robert G. Madden. 1998. LC 97-45285. (Sourcebooks for the Human Services). pap. 39.95 (*0-7619-1233-9*, 82056) Sage.

Legal Issues in Social Work, Counseling, Mental Health. Robert G. Madden. 1998. LC 97-45285. (Sourcebooks for the Human Services). 89.95 (*0-7619-1232-0*, 82055) Sage.

Legal Liability & Malpractice in Health Sciences: Index of New Information with References. Brian H. Armstrong. 1996. 150p. 57.50 (*0-7883-0814-9*); pap. 47.50 (*0-7883-0815-7*) ABBE Pubs Assn.

Legal Medical Quarterly, 1977-1980 1995. 525.00 (*0-8377-9106-5*, Rothman) W S Hein.

Legal Medicine. American College of Legal Medicine Staff. 4th ed. 1998. LC 97-43320. (Illus.). 688p. (C). (gr. 13). text 145.00 (*0-8151-3669-2*, 31390) Mosby Inc.

Legal Medicine in History. Ed. by Michael Clark & Catherine Crawford. 1994. LC 93-11582. (Cambridge History of Medicine Ser.). 378p. (C). text 74.95 (*0-521-39514-3*) Cambridge U Pr.

Legal Medicine, 1985. Ed. by Cyril H. Wecht. 1985. 416p. 110.00 (*0-275-90182-3*, C0182, Praeger Pubs) Greenwood.

Legal Medicine, 1987. Ed. by Cyril H. Wecht. 1988. LC 80-647751. 226p. 82.50 (*0-275-92595-1*, C2595, Praeger Pubs) Greenwood.

Legal Medicine, 1986. Ed. by Cyril H. Wecht. 1986. LC 86-47751. 267p. 78.75 (*0-275-92551-X*, C2551, Praeger Pubs) Greenwood.

Legal Medicine, 1994. Ed. by Cyril H. Wecht. 1994. 85.00 (*0-250-47780-7*, MICHIE) LEXIS Pub.

Legal Neurology & Malingering: Cases & Techniques. Warren F. Gorman. 1993. 420p. pap. 40.00 (*0-87527-507-9*) Green.

Legal Nurse Consulting: Principles & Practice. Ed. by American Association of Legal Nurses Staff. 1997. LC 97-50089. 800p. 75.00 (*1-57444-123-X*, SL123X) St Lucie Pr.

Legal Order & Mental Disorder. Amita Dhanda. 1999. LC 99-17486. 354p. 49.95 (*0-7619-9324-X*) Sage.

Legal Pitfalls for Health Care Managers. J. Fiesta. 1996. (Professional Reference Ser.). 31.50 (*0-8273-7479-8*, VNR) Wiley.

Legal Problems in Emergency Medicine. Alan P. Montague & Andrew Hopper. 1996. LC 96-10999. (Illus.). 176p. pap. text 49.95 (*0-19-262496-2*) OUP.

Legal Problems in Nursing Practice. Ann P. Young. 2nd ed. 1989. (Illus.). 264p. (Orig.). (C). (gr. 13). pap. text 34.95 (*0-412-44550-6*, Chap & Hall NY) Chapman & Hall.

Legal Rights of Persons with Epilepsy. Epilepsy Foundation of America Staff. 1992. 124p. pap. 14.95 (*0-916570-02-9*) Epilepsy Foundation of America.

Legal Rights of the Elderly: Everything You & Your Family Need to Know about Government Benefits, Health Care, Social Security, Veteran's Benefits, Medicare & Medicaid, & Guardianship. Sia Arnason et al. 1995. 319p. pap. 15.95 (*0-87224-079-7*, K1-1500) PLI.

Legal Risk Management: A Guide for Volunteers & Staff of the American Psychological Association. APA Staff. 1993. LC 93-34365. (*1-55798-221-X*) Am Psychol.

Legal Risks in the Long-Term Care Facility. Charlotte K. Eliopoulos. 2nd ed. 2001. 52p. pap. text 25.95 (*1-882515-04-8*) Hlth Educ Netwk.

Legal Speller with Useful Medical Terms. Sheila B. Sloane & John L. Dusseau. 2nd ed. 1982. 366p. pap. text 23.25 (*0-314-69679-2*) West Pub.

Legally Safe Mental Health Practice: Psycholegal Questions & Answers. Robert H. Woody. 1996. LC 96-3083. 121p. pap. 24.95 (*1-887841-04-0*, Psychosocial) Intl Univs Pr.

***Legend of Nietzsche's Syphilis**, 46. Richard Schain. 2001. LC 2001-23341. (Contributions in Medical Studies Ser.: Vol. 46). (Illus.). 152p. 62.95 (*0-313-31940-5*, GM1940, Greenwood Pr) Greenwood.

Legendary Abs II. Health for Life Staff. 1989. (Illus.). 48p. pap. 14.95 (*0-944831-20-6*) Health Life.

Legends & Legacies: A Look Inside: Four Decades of Surgery at the University of North Carolina at Chapel Hill, 1952-1993. Colin G. Thomas, Jr. & Mary J. Kagarise. 1997. LC 96-30175. (Illus.). lib. bdg. 65.00 (*0-9653036-0-8*) U NC School Med.

LeGette's Cholesterol Encyclopedia. Bernard LeGette. 1989. 256p. (Orig.). mass mkt. 3.95 (*0-446-35092-3*) Warner Bks.

Legg Calve-Perthes Disease. Ed. by John A. Herring. 1996. (Illus.). 72p. pap. 35.00 (*0-89203-122-0*) Amer Acad Ortho Surg.

Legg-Calve-Perthes Disease. Jacob F. Katz. 1984. LC 83-24780. 252p. 55.00 (*0-275-91437-2*, C1437, Praeger Pubs) Greenwood.

Legionella Environmental Sampling Guide. Matthew R. Freije. 1998. LC 98-96025. 32p. pap. 24.00 (*0-9649926-6-3*, 306) HC Info Res.

Legionellae Control in Health Care Facilities: A Guide for Minimizing Risk. Matthew R. Freije. Ed. by James M. Barbaree & Rex N. Olsen. 1996. LC 95-82252. 144p. pap. 79.00 (*0-9649926-4-7*, 104) HC Info Res.

Legionellosis. Ed. by Sheila M. Katz. 1985. Vol. I. LC 85-416. 232p. 132.00 (*0-8493-5233-9*, RC152); Vol. II. 224p. 127.00 (*0-8493-5234-7*) Franklin (CRC Reprint).

Legionnaires' Disease. 1983. (Euro Reports & Studies Ser.: No. 72). 100p. pap. text 4.00 (*92-890-1238-2*) World Health.

Legionnaires' Disease: Facts, Legal Issues, Risk. Matthew R. Freije. 1998. LC 98-96023. 20p. pap. 14.00 (*0-9649926-0-4*, 301) HC Info Res.

Legionnaires' Disease: Prevention & Control. Frank Rosa. 1993. LC 92-45807. 29.95 (*0-912524-79-0*) Busn News.

Legislating Death: Socio-Legal Studies on the Brain Death Controversy in Sweden. Dimitris Michailakis. 1995. (Studia Sociologica Upsaliensia: No. 40). 254p. pap. (*91-554-3500-9*) Uppsala Universitet SWE. *Dist:* Coronet Bks.

Legislating Medical Ethics: A Study of the New York State Do-Not-Resuscitate Law. Ed. by Robert Baker. 1995. LC 94-19575. (Philosophy & Medicine Ser.: 48). 476p. (C). lib. bdg. (*0-7923-2995-3*) Kluwer Academic NLD. *Dist:* Kluwer Academic.

Legislation on the Rehabilitation of People with Disabilities in Sixteen Member States of the Council of Europe. 5th ed. 1993. (*92-871-2316-0*) Council of Europe FRA. *Dist:* Manhattan Pub Co.

J
K
L

Legislation on Vacccination in the Member States of the European Economic Community. R. Senault & M. Manciaux. 1965. (International Digest of Health Legislation Offprints: Vol. 16, No. 2). 32p. 3.00 (*92-4-169162-X*) World Health.

Legislative & Regulatory Initiatives for the 106th Congress. 1999. 96p. pap. 19.95 (*1-55810-145-4*, 9904LR) Am Nurses Pub.

Legislative Base: Maternal & Child Health Services Block Grant. National Center for Education in Maternal and Child Health Staff. 1996. 608p. pap. (*1-57285-036-1*) Nat Ctr Educ.

Legislative Handbook for the Practice of Acupuncture & Oriental Medicine. Barbara B. Mitchell. 1995. 62p. 18.00 (*0-9670262-4-5*) Natl Acup Fndt.

Legislative Power & Healthy People. Vigdor Schreibman. 1987. LC 87-6206. (Essays on the Impact of the Constitution & Legal System on American Life & Government Ser.: No. 5). (Illus.). 81p. (Orig.). pap. 19.00 (*0-942539-10-9*) Amicas Pubns.

Legislative Responses to AIDS. Ed. by World Health Organization Staff. 1989. (C). lib. bdg. 113.50 (*0-7923-0128-5*) Kluwer Academic.

Legislative Responses to Organ Transplantation. Ed. by World Health Organization Staff. 1994. LC 92-48521. 534p. (C). lib. bdg. 187.50 (*0-7923-2147-2*) Kluwer Academic.

Legwork: An Inspiring Journey Through a Chronic Illness. Ellen B. MacFarlane & Patricia Burstein. 1994. LC 94-11726. (*0-02-578001-8*) Macmillan.

Lehratlanten der Radiologischen Diagnostik see Teaching Atlas of Urologic Radiology

Lehrbuch der Anorganischen Chemie. A.F. Holleman & Egon Wiberg. 1984. (GER., Illus.). xxx, 1451p. 92.35 (*3-11-007511-3*) De Gruyter.

Lehrbuch der Geschichte der Medizin und der Epidemischen Krankheiten Heinrich Haeser. 1971. lvii, 2992p. reprint ed. (*3-487-04016-6*) G Olms Pubs.

Lehrbuch der Phytotherapie see Herbal Medicine

Leishmaniases I: Biology & Epidemiology, Vol. 1. Ed. by W. Peters & R. Killick-Kendrick. 1987. 550p. text 104.00 (*0-12-552101-4*) Acad Pr.

Leishmaniasis: The Current States & New Strategies for Control. Ed. by D. T. Hart. 1989. (NATO ASI Series A, Life Sciences: Vol. 163). (Illus.). 1056p. 185.00 (*0-306-43146-7*, Plenum Trade) Perseus Pubng.

Leisure & Human Behavior. Gene Bammel & Lei L. Bammel. 3rd ed. 1995. LC 95-75475. 528p. (C). pap. 65.63 (*0-697-23330-8*) McGrw-H Hghr Educ.

Leisure & Play in Therapy. McCree. 1998. 140p. pap. text 36.00 (*0-12-784562-3*) Acad Pr.

Leisure & the American Dream. Compton & Ellis. 2000. (Illus.). 425p. (C). (gr. 13). 22.95 (*0-8016-1028-1*, 01028) Mosby Inc.

Leisure Education: Program Materials for Persons with Developmental Disabilities. Kenneth F. Joswiak. 1989. LC 89-51383. 141p. (C). 15.95 (*0-910251-33-9*) Venture Pub PA.

Leisure in Later Life: A Sourcebook for the Provision of Recreation Services for Elders. Michael J. Leitner & Sara F. Leitner. 1986. LC 85-17635. (Activities, Adaptation & Aging Ser.: Vol. 7, Nos. 3-4). 341p. text 49.95 (*0-86656-452-7*); pap. text 24.95 (*0-86656-476-4*) Haworth Pr.

Leisure, Social Integration & Volunteers. British Institute of Mental Handicap Staff. 1985. 28p. 30.00 (*0-906054-53-2*) St Mut.

Leisure Time Activities for Deaf-Blind Children. California State Department of Health Staff. LC 75-70066. 24.95 (*0-917002-06-7*) Joyce Media.

Leitfaden der Kardiotokographie. F. Jaisle. 1982. (Illus.). viii, 112p. pap. 28.75 (*3-8055-3444-2*) S Karger.

Leitfaden fur das Studium der Christlichen Wissenschaft, Gemut see Compendium for the Study of Christian Science, No. 4, Mind

Leitmotifs in Natural Morphology. Wolfgang U. Dressler et al. 1988. LC 87-21791. (Studies in Language Companion: No. 10). ix, 168p. (*90-272-3009-9*) J Benjamins Pubng NLD. *Dist:* J Benjamins Pubng Co.

Leksel Gamma Knife Society: Proceedings. Ed. by J. C. Ganz et al. 1995. (Journal: Vol. 64, Suppl. 1, 1995). (Illus.). vi, 274p. pap. 68.00 (*3-8055-6266-7*) S Karger.

Leksell Gamma Knife?? Society: Proceedings of the 9th International Meeting, Hong Kong, November, 1998. Ed. by J. C. Ganz et al. 1999. (Stereotactic & Functional Neurosurgery Ser.: Vol. 72, Suppl. 1). (Illus.). vi, 188p. pap. 45.25 (*3-8055-6982-3*) S Karger.

Leksell Gamma Knife Society: 8th International Meeting, Marseille, June 1997 - Proceedings. Ed. by J. C. Ganz et al. 1998. (Stereotactic & Functional Neurosurgery Ser.: Vol. 70, Suppl. 1). (Illus.). vi, 252p. pap. 78.25 (*3-8055-6793-6*) S Karger.

Leksell Gamma Knife Society: Proceedings, 7th International Meeting, Island of Lana'i, Hawaii, November 1995. Ed. by Jeremy C. Ganz et al. 1997. (Journal: Vol. 66, Supplement 1, 1996). (Illus.). vi, 374p. pap. 115.75 (*3-8055-6446-5*) S Karger.

Lemon Twist: No Salt Added Cookbook. Ree. 1989. LC 87-92238. 204p. pap. text 14.95 (*0-929622-00-6*) Nutrit Unltd Pubns.

Length of Stay by Diagnosis & Procedure, 1997: Geriatric. 1997. pap. 295.00 (*1-57372-074-7*) Solucient.

Length of Stay by Diagnosis & Procedure, 1997: Pediatric. 1997. pap. 295.00 (*1-57372-073-9*) Solucient.

Length of Stay by Diagnosis & Procedure, 1997: Southern. 1997. pap. 295.00 (*1-57372-071-2*) Solucient.

Length of Stay by Diagnosis & Procedure, 1997: United States. 1997. pap. 295.00 (*1-57372-068-2*) Solucient.

Length of Stay by Diagnosis & Procedure, 1997: Western. 1997. pap. 295.00 (*1-57372-072-0*) Solucient.

Length of Stay by Diagnosis, 1998: Geriatric. 1998. pap. 295.00 (*1-57372-110-7*) Solucient.

Length of Stay by Diagnosis, 1998: United States. 1998. pap. 295.00 (*1-57372-105-0*) Solucient.

Length of Stay by DRG & Payment Source, 1997: North Central. 1997. pap. 195.00 (*1-57372-082-8*) Solucient.

Length of Stay by DRG & Payment Source, 1997: Northeastern. 1997. pap. 195.00 (*1-57372-081-X*) Solucient.

Length of Stay by DRG & Payment Source, 1997: Southern. 1997. pap. 195.00 (*1-57372-083-6*) Solucient.

Length of Stay by DRG & Payment Source, 1997: United States. 1997. pap. 195.00 (*1-57372-080-1*) Solucient.

Length of Stay by DRG & Payment Source, 1997: Western. 1997. pap. 195.00 (*1-57372-084-4*) Solucient.

Lens: Proceedings of the Workshop on Aging of the Lens, Bonn, July 1977. Aging of the Lens Workshop Staff. Ed. by Otto Hockwin. 1978. (Interdisciplinary Topics in Gerontology Ser.: Vol. 12). (Illus.). 121.00 (*3-8055-2876-0*) S Karger.

Lens Design. Milton Laikin. 2nd exp. rev. ed. 1995. LC 94-44816. (Optical Engineering Ser.: Vol. 48). (Illus.). 464p. text 65.00 (*0-8247-9602-0*) Dekker.

Lens Disorders: A Clinical Manual of Cataract Diagnosis. Nicholas P. Brown & Anthony J. Bron. 1996. LC 94-32580. (Illus.). 256p. text 125.00 (*0-7506-1482-X*) Buttrwrth-Heinemann.

Lens Surfacing Handbook. Clifford W. Brooks. 1992. LC 91-10957. (Illus.). 138p. spiral bd. 44.99 (*0-7506-9186-7*) Buttrwrth-Heinemann.

***Lentiviral Vector Systems for Gene Transfer.** Ed. by Gary L. Buchschacher. 2001. LC 2001-4703. (Medical Intelligence Unit Ser.: Vol. 31). 140p. 119.00 (*1-58706-094-9*); pap. 69.00 (*1-58706-095-7*) Eurekah.

Leonardo Da Vinci: Psychoanalytic Notes on the Enigma. K. R. Eissler. 1961. LC 61-11610. (Illus.). 379p. 55.00 (*0-8236-3000-5*) Intl Univs Pr.

Leonhard Classification of Endogenous Psychoses: Cycloid Psychoses, Differentiated Nosology, Differentiated Therapy & Historical Aspects - Journal: Psychopathology, 1990, Vol. 23, Nos. 4-6. Ed. by H. Beckmann & M. Lanczik. 1991. (Illus.). 164p. pap. 106.25 (*3-8055-5373-0*) S Karger.

***Leonhart Fuchs: Das Kreuterbuch von 1543.** Klaus Dobat & W. Dressendorfer. 2001. (GER.). 960p. 39.99 (*3-8228-1297-8*) Taschen Amer.

***Leonhart Fuchs: Le Nouvel Herbier de 1543.** Klaus Dobat & W. Dressendorfer. 2001. (FRE., Illus.). 960p. 39.99 (*3-8228-1299-4*) Taschen Amer.

***Leonhart Fuchs: The New Herbal of 1543.** Klaus Dobat & W. Dressendorfer. 2001. (Illus.). 960p. 39.99 (*3-8228-1298-6*) Taschen Amer.

Leper Hospitals in Medieval Ireland. Gerard Lee. 1996. 72p. (*1-85182-271-2*) Four Cts Pr IRL. *Dist:* Intl Spec Bk.

Leprosy. Ed. by Robert C. Hastings & Diltor V. Opromolla. 2nd ed. 1994. LC 93-16295. (Medicine in the Tropics Ser.). 488p. text (*0-443-04405-8*) Church.

Leprosy in Children. F. M. Noussitou et al. 1976. pap. text 8.10 (*92-4-154053-2*, 1150095) World Health.

Leprosy in Rural India. K. Venkateswara Rao. 1992. (Illus.). xii, 500p. (*81-85445-43-5*) Manak Pubns Pvt Ltd IND. *Dist:* Nataraj Bks.

Leptospira & Leptospirosis. Solomon Faine. 1993. 368p. lib. bdg. 189.00 (*0-8493-6994-0*, QR729) CRC Pr.

Lesbian & Gay Psychology: Theory, Research & Clinical Applications. Ed. by Beverly Greene & Gregory M. Herek. 1994. LC 94-155258. (Contemporary Prespectives on Lesbian & Gay Issues Ser.: Vol. 1). xii, 243p. (C). 91.95 (*0-8039-5311-9*, 4853); pap. 41.95 (*0-8039-5312-7*, 4854) Sage.

Lesbian & Gay Youth: Care & Counseling. Caitlin Ryan & Donna Futterman. 1998. 256p. 47.50 (*0-231-11190-8*); LC 97-52339. pap. 22.50 (*0-231-11191-6*) Col U Pr.

Lesbian, Gay, & Bisexual Identities in Families: Psychological Perspectives. Ed. by Charlotte J. Patterson & Anthony R. D'Augelli. 1998. LC 97-44736. 320p. pap. 29.95 (*0-19-511050-1*); text 60.00 (*0-19-511049-8*) OUP.

Lesbian Health. Institute of Medicine Staff. Ed. by Andrea L. Solarz. 1999. LC 99-6101. 200p. pap. 19.95 (*0-309-06567-4*) Natl Acad Pr.

Lesbian Health: What Are the Issues? Ed. by Phyllis N. Stern. 1993. LC 93-3686. 20.95 (*1-56032-299-3*) Hemisp Pub.

***Lesbian Health Guide.** Ed. by Regan McClure & Anne Vespry. 1994. 266p. pap. (*1-895564-02-6*) Q Pr CAN. *Dist:* Stackpole.

Lesbian Lives: Psychoanalytic Narratives Old & New. Maggie Magee & Diana C. Miller. 1997. LC 97-35034. 448p. 55.00 (*0-88163-269-4*) Analytic Pr.

Lesbian Therapists & Their Therapy: From Both Sides of the Couch. Ed. by Nancy D. Davis et al. 1996. LC 96-13471. (Women & Therapy Ser.: Vol. 18, No. 2). 80p. 39.95 (*1-56024-800-9*, Haworth Pastrl); pap. 9.95 (*1-56023-082-7*, Harrington Park) Haworth Pr.

Lesbians & Gay Men: Chemical Dependency Treatment Issues. Intro. by Dava L. Weinstein. 2nd ed. 1993. LC 92-31975. (Journal of Chemical Dependency Treatment Ser.: Vol. 5, No. 1). (Illus.). 175p. pap. 14.95 (*1-56023-036-3*); lib. bdg. 54.95 (*1-56024-393-7*) Haworth Pr (Harrington Park).

Lesbians & Lesbian Families: Reflections on Theory & Practice. Joan Laird. 1999. LC 98-36503. 363p. 49.50 (*0-231-10252-6*); 384p. 21.50 (*0-231-10253-4*) Col U Pr.

Lesbians & Lesbianisms: A Post-Jungian Perspective. Claudetta Kulkarni. 1997. LC 96-52975. 256p. (C). 78.95 (*0-415-15510-X*) Routledge.

Lesbians & Lesbianisms: A Post-Jungian Perspective. Claudette Kulkarni. 1997. LC 96-52975. 256p. (C). pap. 26.95 (*0-415-15511-8*) Routledge.

Lesbians & Psychoanalysis: Revolutions in Theory & Practice. Ed. by Judith M. Glassgold & Suzanne Iasenza. 1995. LC 95-13612. 416p. 35.00 (*0-02-874006-8*) Free Pr.

Lesions in the Upper Respiratory Tract in Blood Dyscrasias. I. V. Skurkovich. 1974. 156p. 3.5 hd 45.50 (*0-7065-1429-7*) Coronet Bks.

Lesions of the Cerebral Midline. Ed. by Wolfgang T. Koos & G. Pendl. 1986. (Acta Neurochirurgica Ser.: Supplementum 35). (Illus.). 125p. 92.00 (*0-387-81883-9*) Spr-Verlag.

Lesions of the Jawbone: Radiographic Features. Vivian J. Harris. 1983. (Illus.). 192p. 32.50 (*0-87527-212-6*) Green.

Less Time to Do More: Psychotherapy on the Short-Term Inpatient Unit. Ed. by Ellen Leibenluft et al. 1993. LC 93-20081. 321p. text 19.95 (*0-88048-512-4*, 8512) Am Psychiatric.

L'Essai Therapeutiques Chez L'Homme see Clinical Trials

Lessons & the Legacy of the Pew Health Policy Program. Institute of Medicine Staff. Ed. by Jon A. Chilingerian & Corrine M. Kay. 1997. LC 97-210200. 360p. (C). pap. text 59.50 (*0-309-05825-2*) Natl Acad Pr.

Lessons for Science from the Seven Countries Study. Ed. by A. Keys. 1995. 236p. 70.00 (*0-387-70140-0*) Spr-Verlag.

Lessons for Science from the Seven Countries Study: A 35-Year Collaborative Experience. H. Blackburn et al. 1995. 240p. (C). 77.95 (*4-431-70140-0*) Spr-Verlag.

Lessons for the Right Brain: Complete Kit Kathleen Anderson & Pamela C. Miller. 1984. 64p. pap. text 44.00 (*0-88120-212-6*, 2700) PRO-ED.

Lessons for the Right Brain: Memory Workbook. Kathleen Anderson & Pamela C. Miller. 1984. 64p. pap. text 44.00 (*0-88120-213-4*, 2701) PRO-ED.

Lessons for the Right Brain: Thought Organization Workbook. Kathleen Anderson & Pamela C. Miller. 1984. 64p. pap. text 44.00 (*0-88120-216-9*, 2704) PRO-ED.

Lessons from Animal Diabetes: 75th Anniversary of the Insulin Industry. Ed. by Eleazar Shafrir. 1996. LC 96-216799. (Hormones in Health & Disease Ser.: Vol. 6). (Illus.). 440p. 135.00 (*0-8176-3876-8*) Birkhauser.

Lessons from Laron Syndrome (LS), 1966-1992: A Model of GH & IGF-I Action & Interaction. Ed. by Z. Laron & J. S. Parks. 1993. LC 93-14660. (Pediatric & Adolescent Endocrinology Ser.: Vol. 24). (Illus.). x, 368p. 321.75 (*3-8055-5671-3*) S Karger.

Lessons from the First 20 Years of Medicare: Research Implications for Public & Private Sector Policy. Ed. by Mark V. Pauly et al. 1989. LC 88-17368. (Health Economics, Health Management, & Health Policy Ser.). 412p. (C). text 45.00 (*0-8122-8118-7*) U of Pa Pr.

Lessons from the Intersexed. Suzanne J. Kessler. 1998. LC 97-39342. (C). 193p. text 48.00 (*0-8135-2529-2*); 224p. pap. text 18.00 (*0-8135-2530-6*) Rutgers U Pr.

Lessons in EKG Interpretation: A Basic Self-Instructional Guide. Charles P. Summerall, III. 2nd ed. 1991. (Illus.). 214p. pap. text (*0-443-08778-4*) Church.

Lessons Learned: Provision of Technical Assistance to States. P. Pizzo et al. Ed. by Noelle Beatty. 1993. 90p. (Orig.). pap. 9.00 (*0-943657-29-6*) ZERO TO THREE.

Lest We Forget: Orthopaedics at the Massachusetts General Hospital, 1900-1995. Carter R. Rowe. 1996. LC 96-5704. 30.00 (*0-87233-119-9*) Bauhan.

Let Go of Fear: Tackling Our Worst Emotion. Carlos G. Valles. 1993. LC 90-46506. 224p. pap. text 9.95 (*0-89243-554-2*, Liguori Triumph) Liguori Pubns.

Let Me Decide: The Health Care Directive That Speaks for You When You Can't. William Molloy & Virginia Mepham. 1994. LC 94-61128. 72p. 4.95 (*0-934104-09-3*) Woodland.

Let My Heart Attack Save Your Life: A Simple, Sound, Workable Weight Management Plan. Joseph Mason. 1998. 240p. pap. 14.95 (*0-471-34745-0*) Wiley.

Let the Art of Medicine Flourish: The Centennial History of the Rochester Academy of Medicine. Teresa K. Lehr. 2000. LC 00-27483. (Illus.). 111p. (*0-9665228-4-2*) Q Pubng VA.

Let There Be Light see Es Werde Licht: Praktischer Leitfaden fur Dinshahs 12-Farben Chromotherapie

Let Us All Sleep, Nature's Way. NaiKang Chang. 1989. (Illus.). (Orig.). pap. 12.95 (*0-9622374-0-X*) Jupiter Pub.

Let Your Alcoholic Suffer! A Battle Plan for Families of Alcoholics. Donald M. Lazo. Ed. by Erik Fair. 1999. (Illus.). 128p. (Orig.). pap. 11.95 (*0-913581-12-7*) Publitec.

Lethal Arrhythmias Resulting from Myocardial Ischemia & Infarction: Proceedings of Second Rappaport Symposium Haifa, Israel, March 13-16, 1988. Ed. by Michael R. Rosen & Yoram Palti. 1988. (Developments in Cardiovascular Medicine Ser.). (C). text 170.00 (*0-89838-401-X*) Kluwer Academic.

Lethal Harvest. William Cutrer & Sandra Glahn. 2000. LC 00-30951. 407p. pap. 10.99 (*0-8254-2371-6*) Kregel.

Lethal Medicine: The Story of America's Worst Drug Disaster. Moore. 1995. 23.00 (*0-671-87016-5*) S&S Trade.

Lethal Secrets. Annette Baran & Reuben Pannor. rev. ed. 1999. LC 93-20015. (Illus.). 187p. reprint ed. pap. 11.95 (*1-56743-020-1*, Amistad) HarperTrade.

Lethal Violence, 2000: A Sourcebook on Fatal Domestic, Acquaintance & Stranger Aggression. Ed. by Harold V. Hall. 1997. (Illus.). 800p. text 125.00 (*0-9649535-0-1*) Pac Inst Conflict.

***Let's All Get Well Soon: An Exploration of Health Perspectives.** Contrib. by Rene Gaudette & Maggie McGuffin-Gaudette. 2001. 312p. per. (*1-894802-01-2*) WPI3.

***Let's Go on Bypass.** David Hayes. 2001. (Illus.). 96p. pap. 10.00 (*0-9714865-0-6*) Citilites Pr.

Let's Really Make Love: Sex, the Family, & Education in the Twenty-First Century. Robert H. Rimmer. 1995. LC 95-2877. 296p. pap. 25.00 (*0-87975-964-X*) Prometheus Bks.

Let's Talk about Alcoholism. Robert A. Liebelt & Edward B. Truitt, Jr. 1989. (Illus.). 248p. (Orig.). pap. 15.95 (*0-926719-00-9*) Platte River Pr.

Let's Talk about When Someone You Love Has Alzheimer's Disease. Elizabeth Weitzman. 1998. (PowerKids Ser.). 24p. (J). (gr. k-3). reprint ed. pap. 6.95 (*1-56838-224-3*) Hazelden.

Letters for Tomorrow: A Journal for Expectant Moms & Dads. Robin F. Bernstein & Cathy Moore. 1995. LC 94-9466. 160p. 20.00 (*0-385-47515-2*) Doubleday.

Letters from Jenny. Ed. by Gordon W. Allport. 1965. LC 65-18327. (Illus.). 238p. (Orig.). (C). pap. 7.95 (*0-15-650700-5*, Harvest Bks) Harcourt.

Letters from Simon. I. H. Paul. 1996. LC 96-444465. 270p. (Orig.). pap. 29.95 (*0-8236-8130-0*, 23011) Intl Univs Pr.

Letters of Milton H. Erickson. Ed. by Jeffrey K. Zeig & Brent Geary. 2000. LC 00-33361. xix, 393p. 50.00 (*1-891944-11-8*) Zeig Tucker Theisen.

Letters of Owen Wangensteen to a Surgical Fellow - With a Memoir. Stacey B. Day. 1996. LC 96-78241. (Illus.). 240p. 59.50 (*0-934314-25-X*, B10-10) Intl Found Biosocial Dev.

Letters of Sigmund Freud to Eduard Silberstein, 1871-1881. Ed. by Walter Boehlich. Tr. by Arnold J. Pomerans. 1990. LC 90-39119. (Illus.). 204p. text 39.00 (*0-674-52827-1*) HUP.

Letters of Stephen Gardiner. Stephen Gardiner. Ed. by James A. Muller. 1990. reprint ed. lib. bdg. 90.00 (*0-8371-4223-7*, GALE, Greenwood Pr) Greenwood.

Letters to His Excellency Governor Manning on the Lunatic Asylum. Daniel H. Trezevant. 1973. LC 73-2423. (Mental Illness & Social Policy; the American Experience Ser.). reprint ed. 17.95 (*0-405-05232-4*) Ayer.

Letters to His Parents, 1839-1864. Rudolph Virchow. Ed. by L. Rather. 1990. (Resources in Medical History Ser.). 200p. 20.00 (*0-88135-090-7*, Sci Hist) Watson Pub Intl.

Letters to My Patients: A Guide to Healthy & Happy Living. Harlan O. Wright. 1995. 256p. 18.95 (*0-9648404-0-5*) Shallowater.

Letters to the People on Health & Happiness. Catherine Esther Beecher. 1972. LC 70-180554. (Medicine & Society in America Ser.). (Illus.). 228p. reprint ed. 19.95 (*0-405-03934-4*) Ayer.

Letting Go: Death, Dying, & the Law. Melvin I. Urofsky. 1994. LC 93-31027. 224p. reprint ed. pap. 14.95 (*0-8061-2635-3*) U of Okla Pr.

Letting Go of Anger: The Ten Most Common Anger Styles & What to Do about Them. Ronald T. Potter-Efron & Patricia S. Potter-Efron. 1995. LC 94-73923. 168p. pap. 13.95 (*1-57224-001-6*) New Harbinger.

Letting Go of Suffering. Karuna Poole. 1994. (Orig.). pap. 12.95 (*0-9643629-0-2*) K Poole.

Leucocyte Antigen Factsbook. Ed. by A. Neil Barclay et al. 2nd ed. 1997. LC 97-15939. (Factsbook Ser.). (Illus.). 640p. pap. text 49.95 (*0-12-078185-9*) Morgan Kaufmann.

Leucocyte Depletion & Its Clinical Usefulness: Proceedings of the 33rd Hokkaido Symposium on Transfusion Medicine. Thirty-third Hokkaido Symposium on Transfusion Med. Ed. by Sadayoshi Sekiguchi. 1993. LC 92-48510. (Illus.). 256p. 85.00 (*0-632-03716-4*) Blackwell Sci.

Leucocyte Typing. Ed. by A. J. Bernard et al. 1984. (Illus.). 814p. 139.00 (*0-387-12056-4*) Spr-Verlag.

Leucocyte Typing V: White Cell Differentiation Antigens. Set. Stuart F. Schlossman. 1995. (Illus.). text 325.00 (*0-19-262376-1*) OUP.

Leukaemia. J. A. Whittaker. 2nd ed. 1992. (Illus.). 704p. 235.00 (*0-632-02945-5*) Blackwell Sci.

Leukaemia & Related Disorders. J. A. Whittaker. 3rd ed. 1998. LC 97-31481. (Illus.). 840p. 314.95 (*0-86542-607-4*) Blackwell Sci.

Leukaemia Diagnosis. Barbara J. Bain. 2nd ed. 1999. LC 98-28846. (Illus.). 119.00 (*0-632-05165-5*) Blackwell Sci.

Leukaemia Diagnosis: A Guide to FAB Classification. Barbara J. Bain. 1990. (Illus.). 128p. (gr. 13). (*0-397-44608-X*, GM0006) Gower-Mosby.

Leukemia. Edward S. Henderson et al. 6th rev. ed. 1996. LC 95-11494. (Illus.). 608p. text 215.00 (*0-7216-5381-2*) Saunders.

Leukemia. Edward S. Henderson. 7th ed. 2001. text (*0-7216-9060-2*) Harcrt Hlth Sci Grp.

Leukemia: A Research Report. Ed. by Barry Leonard. 2nd ed. 1998. 63p. (C). pap. text 15.00 (*0-7881-7189-5*) DIANE Pub.

Leukemia: Advances in Research & Treatment. Ed. by Emil J. Freireich & Hagop Kantarjian. 1993. LC 92-49282. (Cancer Treatment & Research Ser.: No. 64). 432p. (C). text 280.50 (*0-7923-1967-2*) Kluwer Academic.

Leukemia: Just a Shadow. Mary A. Croskey. 1996. LC 97-221872. 80p. (Orig.). pap. 14.95 (*0-9654678-0-5*) Life Shadows.

Leukemia & Lymphoma Reviews. Ed. by Aaron Polliack. No. 1. 1992. 372p. text 176.00 (*3-7186-5251-X*); No. 3. 1994. 296p. text 116.00 (*3-7186-5490-3*); No. 4. 1995. 304p. text 105.00 (*3-7186-5760-0*) Gordon & Breach (Harwood Acad Pubs).

Leukemia & Lymphoma Reviews, No. 2. Ed. by Aaron Polliack. 1993. 294p. 78.00 (*3-7186-5374-5*) Kluwer Academic.

Leukemia Cell. Arnold Rubin & Samuel Waxman. 1979. (Uniscience Ser.). 192p. 112.00 (*0-8493-5009-3*, RC643, CRC Reprint) Franklin.

Leukemia-Lymphoma Cell Line Factsbook. Hans G. Drexler. 2000. LC 00-104886. (Factsbook Ser.). 608p. pap. 54.95 (*0-12-221970-8*) Acad Pr.

Leukemias. Ed. by J. Fleischer. 1993. LC 92-48828. (Illus.). 334p. 129.00 (*0-387-54782-7*) Spr-Verlag.

Leukemic Cell. Ed. by D. Catovsky. 2nd ed. 1991. (Methods in Hematology Ser.). (Illus.). 428p. text (*0-443-03867-8*) Church.

Leukocyte Adhesion Molecules. Ed. by Timothy A. Springer et al. 1991. (Illus.). 287p. 165.00 (*0-387-96983-7*) Spr-Verlag.

Leukocyte-Depleted Blood Products. Ed. by T. A. Lane & G. Myllylae. 1994. LC 94-9283. (Current Studies in Hematology & Blood Transfusion: No. 60). (Illus.). viii, 150p. 149.75 (*3-8055-5862-7*) S Karger.

***Leukocyte Depletion in Cardiac Surgery & Cardiology.** Ed. by G. Matheis et al. 2001. LC 2001-50195. (Illus.). 158p. 128.75 (*3-8055-7281-6*) S Karger.

Leukocyte Emigration & Its Sequelae. Ed. by H. Z. Movat. 1987. (Illus.). vi, 186p. 121.00 (*3-8055-4489-8*) S Karger.

Leukocyte Typing II: Human B Lymphocytes, Vol. 2. Ed. by E. L. Reinherz et al. 1985. (Illus.). 560p. 220.00 (*0-387-96176-3*) Spr-Verlag.

Leukocyte Typing II: Human Myeloid & Hematopoietic Cells, Vol. 3. Ed. by E. L. Reinherz et al. 1985. (Illus.). 366p. 174.00 (*0-387-96177-1*) Spr-Verlag.

Leukocyte Typing II: Human T Lymphocytes, Vol. 1. Ed. by E. L. Reinherz et al. 1985. (Illus.). 549p. 220.00 (*0-387-96175-5*) Spr-Verlag.

Leukolysins & Cancer. Ed. by Janet H. Ransom & John R. Ortaldo. 1988. LC 87-17221. (Contemporary Biomedicine Ser.: Vol. 8). (Illus.). 344p. 145.00 (*0-89603-125-X*) Humana.

Leukotrienes: New Concepts & Targets for Therapy. Ed. by Ian Rodger et al. 1998. 160p. 85.00 (*0-7923-8738-4*) Kluwer Academic.

Leukozytenseparation und Transfusion. V. Kretschmer. 1981. (Beitraege zur Infusionstherapie und Klinische Ernaehrung Ser.: Vol. 6). (Illus.). viii, 188p. 43.50 (*3-8055-1946-X*) S Karger.

Lev Vygotsky Vol. 1: Critical Assessments. Peter Lloyd & Charles Fernyhough. 1998. LC 98-9488. (*0-415-11152-8*) Routledge.

Lev Vygotsky Vol. 2: Critical Assessments. Peter Lloyd & Charles Fernyhough. 1998. LC 98-9488. (*0-415-11153-6*) Routledge.

Lev Vygotsky Vol. 3: Critical Assessments. Peter Lloyd & Charles Fernyhough. 1998. LC 98-9488. (*0-415-11154-4*) Routledge.

Lev Vygotsky Vol. 4: Critical Assessments. Peter Lloyd & Charles Fernyhough. 1998. LC 98-9488. (*0-415-11155-2*) Routledge.

Levels & Trends of Contraceptive Use as Assessed in 1987. 1989. (Population Studies). 137p. pap. 15.00 (*92-1-151176-3*, E.89.XIII.4) UN.

Levels & Trends of Contraceptive Use As Assessed in 1994. Department for Economic and Social Information and Pol. LC 97-114933. (Population Studies: No. 146). 171p. pap. 17.50 (*92-1-151310-3*, RG133) UN.

Levels of Cognitive Complexity: An Approach to the Measurement of Thinking. E. McDaniel & C. Lawrence. 1990. (Recent Research in Psychology Ser.). (Illus.). 97p. 58.95 (*0-387-97301-X*) Spr-Verlag.

Levels of Cognitive Development. Tracy S. Kendler. 1995. 208p. 45.00 (*0-8058-0680-6*) L Erlbaum Assocs.

Levene's Color Atlas of Dermatology. Gary White. 2nd ed. 1997. 29.95 (*0-7234-2552-3*) Mosby Inc.

Levene's Color Atlas of Dermatology. Gary White. 2nd ed. 1997. (Illus.). 384p. pap. (*84-8174-263-5*) Mosby-Doyma Libros ESP. *Dist:* Mosby Inc.

Lever's Histopathology of the Skin. Walter F. Lever & David E. Elder. 8th ed. 1997. LC 96-30912. 1,104p. text 225.00 (*0-397-51500-6*) Lppncott W & W.

Levin & O'Neal's the Diabetic Foot. John H. Bowker & Michael A. Pfeifer. 6th ed. 2001. LC 00-41142. (Illus.). xxv, 790p. (C). text (*1-55664-471-X*) Mosby Inc.

Levinas & Lacan: The Missed Encounter. Ed. by Sarah Harasym. 1998. LC 97-48472. (Series in Psychoanalysis & Culture). 256p. (C). text 65.50 (*0-7914-3959-3*); pap. text 22.95 (*0-7914-3960-7*) State U NY Pr.

Levine's Conservation Model: A Framework for Nursing Practice. Ed. by Karen M. Schaefer & Jane B. Pond. 1991. LC 91-9488. 282p. text 36.95 (*0-8036-7747-2*) Davis Co.

Levitt & Tapley's Technological Basis of Radiation Therapy. S. H. Levitt et al. 2nd ed. 1992. (Illus.). 414p. text 82.00 (*0-8121-1466-3*) Lppncott W & W.

Levitt & Tapley's Technological Basis of Radiation Therapy: Clinical Applications. Ed. by Seymour H. Levitt et al. 3rd ed. 1998. LC 98-3836. 500p. 99.00 (*0-683-30123-3*) Lppncott W & W.

Lewin Legacy. Ed. by E. H. Stivers & S. A. Wheelan. 1989. (Recent Research in Psychology Ser.). 281p. 71.95 (*0-387-96352-9*) Spr-Verlag.

Lewis-Gale Medical Center. Amy Phillips. Ed. by Phyllis Harholdt & Rodney Nelson. 1993. (Illus.). 250p. (C). 50.00 (*0-929690-21-4*) Herit Pubs AZ.

Lexical Ambiguity Resolution: Perspectives from Psycholinguistics, Neuropsychology & Artificial Intelligence. Ed. by Steven Small et al. 1988. LC 87-33939. 518p. (C). 46.00 (*0-934613-50-8*) Morgan Kaufmann.

Lexical Borrowing in American Sign Language. Robbin M. Battison. 1978. LC 78-59164. (Illus.). 240p. pap. text 18.95 (*0-932130-02-X*) Linstok Pr.

Lexicon Medicum: Or, Medical Dictionary. Robert Hooper. 2000. cd-rom 24.95 (*1-58211-221-5*) Quintin Pub RI.

Lexicon of Alcohol & Drug Terms. 1994. 65p. pap. text 17.00 (*92-4-154468-6*, 1150413) World Health.

Lexicon of Cross-Cultural Terms in Mental Health. WHO Staff. 1997. (*92-4-154505-4*) World Health.

Lexicon of Lunacy: Metaphoric Malady, Moral Responsibility, & Psychiatry. Thomas Szasz. 1993. 192p. (C). text 34.95 (*1-56000-065-1*) Transaction Pubs.

Lexicon of Medical Radiological Engineering: Lexikon der Radiologischen Technik der Medizin. Wilfried Angerstein. 4th ed. 1987. (GER.). 576p. 95.00 (*0-8288-1834-7*, M15430) Fr & Eur.

Lexicon of Medical Terminology: Medicinsk Terminologi Lexikon. B. I. Lindskog & B. L. Zetterberg. 1981. 620p. 250.00 (*0-8288-1884-3*, F22400) Fr & Eur.

Lexicon of Medicine: Medicinski Leksikon. Aleksandar Kostic. deluxe ed. 1981. (CRO & SER.). 917p. 150.00 (*0-8288-4668-5*, M9706) Fr & Eur.

Lexicon of Psychiatric & Mental Health Terms, Vol. 1. WHO Staff. 1989. 79p. 16.00 (*92-4-154242-X*); 2nd ed. 1994. 108p. pap. text 25.00 (*92-4-154466-X*, 1152309) World Health.

Lexicon of Psychiatry, Neurology, & Neurosciences. Frank J. Ayd, Jr. 2nd ed. 2000. LC 99-53906. 1,120p. pap. text 79.95 (*0-7817-2468-6*) Lppncott W & W.

Lexicon of Psychology, Psychiatry & Psychoanalysis. Ed. by Jessica Kuper. 1988. (Social Science Lexicons Ser.). 384p. pap. text 19.95 (*0-415-00233-8*) Routledge.

Lexicon of Usual Terms in Psychiatry, Neuropsychiatry & Psychopathology. Lise Moor. 3rd ed. 1980. (ENG, FRE & GER.). 236p. 49.95 (*0-8288-0584-9*, M 15383) Fr & Eur.

Lexikon Angiologie, Kardiologie. Ulrich Busch. 1992. (GER.). 312p. 75.00 (*0-7859-8423-2*, 3541171413) Fr & Eur.

Lexikon Chemischer Kurzbezeichnungen Von Arzneistoffen. 1970. (GER.). pap. 24.95 (*0-8288-6544-2*, M-7283) Fr & Eur.

Lexikon der Dentalen Technologie. Erich Korber. 1986. (GER.). 405p. 135.00 (*0-7859-8528-X*, 3876520967) Fr & Eur.

Lexikon der Gesundheit: Medizinisches Fachwoerterbuch. Wolfhart Draeger. (GER.). 19.95 (*0-7859-8329-5*, 3404621190) Fr & Eur.

Lexikon der Medizinischen Fachsprache, Set. Dagobert Tutsch. 1970. (GER.). 388p. pap. 19.95 (*0-7859-0840-4*, M-7249) Fr & Eur.

Lexikon der Medizinischen Psychologie: Lexicon of Medical Psychology. U. Tewes. 1977. (GER.). 24.95 (*0-8288-5488-2*, M7248) Fr & Eur.

Lexikon der Mikrobiologie und Infektologie. Promod M. Shah. 2nd ed. 1993. (GER.). 352p. 125.00 (*0-7859-8475-5*, 3794514386) Fr & Eur.

Lexikon der Musiktherapie. Hans-Helmut Decker-Voight. 1992. (GER.). 400p. 150.00 (*0-7859-8481-X*, 3801706362) Fr & Eur.

Lexikon der Praktischen Psychologie. Knoll Ludwig. 1993. (GER.). 488p. 29.95 (*0-7859-8543-3*, 3893501657) Fr & Eur.

Lexikon der Rechtsmedizin. Horst Hunger. 1993. (GER.). 309p. 225.00 (*0-7859-8315-5*, 3335002539) Fr & Eur.

Lexikon der Reproduktionstechnik. Franz Bauer. 2nd ed. 1986. (GER.). 634p. 75.00 (*0-7859-8533-6*, 3880133387) Fr & Eur.

Lexikon Medicum. B. Zlotnicki. 1973. (ENG, FRE, GER, LAT & POL.). 95.00 (*0-8288-6309-1*, M-6576) Fr & Eur.

Lexikon Medizinisch-Wissenschaftlicher Abkurzungen. Rolf Heister. 3rd ed. 1993. (GER.). 424p. 69.95 (*0-7859-8509-3*, 3825215490) Fr & Eur.

Lexique de Nutrition: Les Mots pour Comprendre. Jean-Pierre Ruasse. 1993. (FRE.). 45p. pap. 15.95 (*0-7859-5668-9*, 2908502100) Fr & Eur.

Lexique des Terme de Prothese Dentaire (Lexicon of Dental Prothetics Terminology) Evelyn Batarec. 2nd ed. 1980. (FRE.). 90p. pap. 29.95 (*0-7859-4805-8*, M6024) Fr & Eur.

Lexique des Termes de Parodontologie de Microbiologie Parodontale et Buccale et de Sciences Fondamentales. Robert Sinsoilliez. 1973. (FRE.). 112p. pap. 29.95 (*0-8288-6315-6*, M-6518) Fr & Eur.

Lexique des Termes Medicaux Avec Lexique Etymologique a L'Usage des Infirmiers. J. P. Harley. 1984. 116p. 35.00 (*0-8288-1810-X*) Fr & Eur.

Lexique des Termes Usuels de Psychiatrie. Jean Carrere & Jacques Dessaigne. 1976. (FRE.). 114p. pap. 39.95 (*0-8288-5738-5*, M6061) Fr & Eur.

LH-RH Agonists in Oncology. Ed. by K. Hoffken. 1988. (Illus.). 208p. 111.00 (*0-387-19070-8*) Spr-Verlag.

LH-RH & Its Analogues: Fertility & Anti-Fertility Aspects. Ed. by Manfred Schmidt-Gollwitzer & Rosemarie Schley. 1985. (New Developments in Biosciences Ser.). (Illus.). x, 357p. 89.25 (*3-11-010055-X*) De Gruyter.

LHRH & Its Analogs: Contraceptive & Therapeutic Applications, Pt. 1. Ed. by B. H. Vickery et al. 1984. 450p. text 244.50 (*0-85200-732-9*) Kluwer Academic.

LHRH & Its Analogs: Contraceptive & Therapeutic Applications, Pt. 2. Ed. by B. H. Vickery & J. J. Nestor, Jr. 1987. (C). text 255.50 (*0-85200-987-9*) Kluwer Academic.

LIA Guide for the Selection for Laser Eye Protection, Vol. 104. 5th ed. 2000. per. 20.00 (*0-912035-08-0*) Laser Inst.

LIA Guide to Medical Laser Safety. Ed. by Steven L. Trogel. 1997. (Illus.). 40p. pap. text 25.00 (*0-912035-07-2*) Laser Inst.

Liability & Risk Management in Home Health Care. Fay Rozovsky. 1998. LC 97-44706. 2352p. 155.00 (*0-8342-1067-3*) Aspen Pub.

Liability & Risk Management in Managed Care. Charles G. Benda & Fay Rozovsky. 1998. LC 98-131242. ring bd. 209.00 (*0-8342-1035-5*, S512) Aspen Pub.

Liability for Employee Grievances: Mental Stress & Wrongful Termination. Ed. by Richard B. Victor. 1988. LC 88-27895. 35.00 (*0-935149-17-1*, WC-88-6) Workers Comp Res Inst.

Liability in Medical Practice: A Reference for Physicians. N. S. Blackman & C. P. Bailey. 1990. x, 476p. text 77.00 (*3-7186-0506-6*); 476p. pap. text 38.00 (*3-7186-0512-0*) Gordon & Breach.

Liability Issues in Perinatal Nursing. Donna Miller-Slade. 1998. LC 98-27994. 368p. pap. text 42.95 (*0-397-55276-9*) Lppncott W & W.

***Liaison Mental Health Nursing.** Stephen Regel et al. 2001. (Illus.). 347p. pap. (*0-7020-2525-9*) W B Saunders GBR. *Dist:* Saunders.

Liaison Psychiatry & Teamwork. Lynch et al. 2000. 256p. pap. text (*0-7506-4298-X*) E A GBR. *Dist:* OUP.

Liber Amicorum for Emil Alfred Loeliger. Ed. by E. Briet. 1985. (Journal: Vol. 15, No. 4, 1985). (Illus.). 72p. pap. 51.50 (*3-8055-4146-5*) S Karger.

Liber Amicorum Presented to Prof. Dr. J. R. Blickman. L. Penning & C. J. Thijn. 1984. (Journal: Vol. 53, No. 4). (Illus.). 56p. 38.50 (*3-8055-3934-7*) S Karger.

Liberalization of Abortion Laws: Implications. Ed. by Abdel R. Omran. 1976. LC 75-42005. 305p. pap. 5.00 (*0-89055-115-4*) Carolina Pop Ctr.

Liberating Medicine. David Seedhouse. 1991. LC 90-12515. 198p. pap. 80.00 (*0-471-92844-5*) Wiley.

Liberating Solutions to Alcohol Problems: Treating Problem Drinkers Without Saying No. Doug Cameron. 1995. LC 94-47466. 296p. reprint ed. 50.00 (*1-56821-462-6*) Aronson.

Liberating Young Children from Sex Roles: Experiences in Day Care Centers, Play Groups, & Free Schools. Phyllis T. Greenleaf. 1986. (Illus.). 22p. (YA). (gr. 11-12). reprint ed. pap. text 5.95 (*0-940139-01-4*) Consortium RI.

Libido Sexualis: Studies in the Psychosexual Laws of Love Verified by Clinical Sexual Case Histories. Albert Moll. Tr. by David Berger from GER. LC 72-11288. reprint ed. 36.00 (*0-404-57481-5*) AMS Pr.

Libraries Without Limits: Changing Needs—changing Roles : Proceedings of the 6th European Conference of Medical & Health LibrariesUtrecht, 22-27 June 1998 / Ed. by Suzanne Bakker. 1999. LC 99-10144. 25p. (*0-7923-5626-8*) Kluwer Academic.

Library of Congress Classification: Class R: Medicine: Cumulative Schedule & Index. Larry D. Dershem et al. 1999th ed. 2000. LC 00-62721. (AALL Publications Ser.: No. 50). pap. (*0-8377-9342-4*, Rothman) W S Hein.

Library of Congress Classification: R: Medicine. Library of Congress Staff. 2000. LC 99-86967. (*0-8444-1004-7*) Lib Congress.

Library of Lesson Plans: How Administrators & Victims Can Handle a Hostage Situation. Bud Allen & Diana Bosta. 1982. 100p. ring bd. 49.95 (*0-939438-21-6*) Rae John.

Library of Lesson Plans: Stress Management. Bud Allen & Diana Bosta. 1981. 64p. vinyl bd. 49.95 (*0-939438-17-8*) Rae John.

Library of Lesson Plans Vol. 3, No. 2: Counseling & Interviewing. Bud Allen & Diana Bosta. 1981. 78p. vinyl bd. 29.95 (*0-939438-06-2*) Rae John.

Library Research Guide to Nursing: Illustrated Search Strategy & Sources. Katina Strauch et al. 2nd ed. 1992. (Library Research Guides Ser.: No. 8). 86p. pap. 18.00 (*0-87650-253-2*) Pierian.

Library Research Guide to Psychology. Nancy E. Douglas & Nathan Baum. 1984. LC 84-60640. (Library Research Guides Ser.: No. 7). pap. 15.00 (*0-87650-175-7*) Pierian.

Library Service to People with Disabilities: Ten Case Studies. Eunice G. Lovejoy. 1989. (Professional Librarian Ser.). 176p. 35.00 (*0-8161-1922-8*); 25.00 (*0-8161-1923-6*) Macmillan (Hall Reference).

Library Services in Mental Health Settings. Mary E. Johnson & Medical Library Association Staff. 1997. LC 97-5801. 45.00 (*0-8108-3306-9*) Scarecrow.

Library Use: A Handbook for Psychology. Jeffrey G. Reed & Pam M. Baxter. 2nd ed. 1992. 177p. (Orig.). (C). pap. text 19.95 (*1-55798-144-2*) Am Psychol.

Libre de Addiciones. Maria E. De Castillo et al. 1999.Tr. of Free from Addictions. (SPA.). 248p. pap. 15.00 (*968-39-0507-2*) Hazelden.

Libro Universal de Ilustraciones del Parto. Fran P. Hosken. 1982. (Childbirth Picture Bks.).Tr. of Universal Childbirth Picture Book. (SPA., Illus.). 76p. (Orig.). 7.00 (*0-942096-03-7*) WINNEWS.

Lice-Buster Book: What to Do When Your Child Comes Home with Head Lice. Lennie Copeland. 1996. LC 96-3183. (Illus.). 128p. (Orig.). pap. (*0-446-67249-1*) Warner.

Licensed Practical Nurse. Jack Rudman. 1994. (Career Examination Ser.: C-440). pap. 29.95 (*0-8373-0440-7*) Nat Learn.

Licensed to Practice. Sykes. 1985. text 18.95 (*0-7216-9894-8*) Saunders.

Licensing Exam Review Guide in Nursing Home Administration: 1000 Test Questions in the Nation Examination Format on the 1996 Domains of Practice. James E. Allen. 3rd ed. 1997. LC 96-47701. 208p. 34.95 (*0-8261-5922-2*) Springer Pub.

Licensure in Professional Psychology: Preparatory Techniques. Tony D. Crespi. 1994. LC 94-14145. 39.95 (*1-56032-310-8*) Taylor & Francis.

Lichtenstein Hernia Repairs, & How to Do Them . . . Right! Alex G. Shulman. 1996. (Illus.). 162p. spiral bd. 30.00 (*0-9653526-0-9*) Wagner Design.

Lids & Nasolacrimal System: Optometric Procedures. Eric E. Schmidt. 1997. LC 96-50471. (Illus.). 119p. pap. text 44.99 (*0-7506-9621-4*) Buttrwrth-Heinemann.

Liebman's Neuroanatomy Made Easy & Understandable. S. David Gertz & Rina Tadmor. 6th ed. 1996. LC 99-29749. 236p. pap. 31.00 (*0-8342-1632-9*) PRO-ED.

Life: The Human Being Between Life & Death; A Dialogue Between Medicine & Philosophy, Recurrent Issues & New Approaches. Anna-Teresa Tymieniecka & Zigniew Zalewski. 2000. LC 99-40299. (Analecta Husserliana Ser.: Vol. 64). xi, 319p. 154.00 (*0-7923-5962-3*) Kluwer Academic.

Life after a Death: A Study of the Elderly Widowed. Ann Bowling & Ann Cartwright. 1982. 239p. (*0-422-78230-0*, NO. 3712) Tavistock GBR. *Dist:* Routldge.

Life after a Heart Attack: Social & Psychological Factors Eight Years Later. Sydney Croog & Sol Levine. 1982. LC 81-6702. 328p. 45.95 (*0-89885-071-1*, Kluwer Acad Hman Sci) Kluwer Academic.

Life after Birth: Every Woman's Guide to the First Year of Motherhood. Wendy Blumfield. 1993. LC 92-32961. 144p. pap. 12.95 (*1-85230-351-4*) Element MA.

Life after Doomsday. Bruce D. Clayton. 1992. (Illus.). 202p. pap. 29.95 (*0-87364-175-2*) Paladin Pr.

Life after Grief: A Soul Journey after Suicide. Jack Clarke. 1989. LC 88-90968. 192p. (Orig.). pap. 9.95 (*0-929841-02-6*) Prsnl Pathways.

Life after Head Injury: The Experiences of Twenty Young People & Their Families. Jane Hubert. 1995. 128p. text (*1-85972-148-6*) Avebry GBR. *Dist:* Ashgate Pub Co.

Life after Medical School: Thirty-Two Doctors Describe How They Shaped Their Medical Careers. Leonard Laster. 1996. LC 95-5551. 320p. (C). 29.95 (*0-393-71030-0*) Norton.

Life after Stress. M. Shaffer. 1982. LC 81-17785. (Illus.). 288p. (C). 15.95 (*0-306-40869-4*, Plenum Trade) Perseus Pubng.

Life after Survival: A Therapeutic Approach for Adult Children of Alcoholics. Patricia A. Mansmann & Patricia A. Neuhausel. 2nd rev. ed. 1989. (Illus.). 88p. pap. text 6.95 (*0-940967-01-4*) Genesis Pub PA.

Life & Adventures of an Arkansas Doctor. David Rattlehead. Ed. by W. K. McNeil. 1989. LC 89-4692. 200p. 22.00 (*1-55728-086-X*) U of Ark Pr.

Life & Adventures of an Arkansaw Doctor. David Rattlehead. Ed. by W. K. McNeil. 1989. LC 89-4692. (Arkansas Classics Ser.). 200p. pap. 16.00 (*1-55728-079-7*) U of Ark Pr.

J K L

Life & Confessions of a Psychologist. G. Stanley Hall. Ed. by Walter P. Metzger. 1977. (Academic Profession Ser.). lib. bdg. 53.95 (0-405-10008-6) Ayer.

Life & Death: Philosophical Essays in Biomedical Ethics. Dan W. Brock. 1993. LC 92-20921. (Studies in Philosophy & Public Policy). 449p. (C). text 85.00 (0-521-41785-6) Cambridge U Pr.

Life & Death Debate: Moral Issues of Our Time. J. P. Moreland & Norman L. Geisler. 1990. LC 90-37862. 192p. pap. 19.95 (0-275-93702-X, B3702, Praeger Pubs) Greenwood.

Life & Death in Health Care Ethics. Helen Watt. 2000. LC 00-34483. vii, 97p. pap. 12.99 (0-415-21574-9) Routledge.

Life & Death in Psychoanalysis. Jean Laplanche. Tr. by Jeffrey Mehlman from FRE. 1976. LC 75-36928. 160p. reprint ed. pap. text 15.95 (0-8018-2730-2) Johns Hopkins.

Life & Death in the Nervous System: Role of Neurothropic Factors & Their Receptors. Ed. by C. F. Ibanez et al. 1995. LC 95-22623. (Wenner-Gren International Ser.). 498p. 186.00 (0-08-042527-5, Pergamon Pr) Elsevier.

Life & Death in the United States: Statistics on Life Expectancies, Diseases & Death Rates for the Twentieth Century. Russell O. Wright. 1997. LC 97-20045. (Illus.). 151p. per. 30.00 (0-7864-0320-9) McFarland & Co.

Life & Health: Targeting Wellness. Mark Dignan et al. 1991. (C). text 44.54 net. (0-07-037494-5); pap. text, stu. ed. 19.00 (0-07-037523-2) McGraw.

Life & Loss: A Guide to Help Grieving Children. Linda Goldman. 1994. LC 93-29333. (Illus.). 68p. (Orig.). pap. text 19.95 (1-55959-052-1) Accel Devel.

Life & Scientific & Medical Career of Benjamin Waterhouse: With Some Account of the Introduction of Vaccination in America. I. Bernard Cohen. 1980. Vol. 1. 37.95 (0-405-12522-4); Vol. 2. 37.95 (0-405-12523-2) Ayer.

Life & the Scientific & Medical Career of Benjamin Waterhouse: With Some Account of the Introduction of Vaccination in America, An Original Anthology. Set. Ed. by I. Bernard Cohen. 1980. LC 79-8004. (Three Centuries of Science in America Ser.). (Illus.). lib. bdg. 75.95 (0-405-12591-7) Ayer.

Life & Time of Ambroise Pare, 1510-1590. Ambroise Pare. Ed. by Francis R. Packard. 1972. LC 79-160607. (Illus.). reprint ed. (0-405-08834-5) Blom Pubns GBR. *Dist:* Ayer.

Life & Times of a Country Doctor. James E. Albrecht. 1993. (Illus.). 280p. pap. 18.00 (0-9639102-0-5) Jjea enter.

Life & Times of G. V. Black. Charles N. Pappas. 1983. (Illus.). 128p. (Orig.). pap. text 38.00 (0-931386-55-1) Quint Pub Co.

Life & Work of an Eminent Psychologist: Autobiography of Richard S. Lazarus. Richard S. Lazarus. 1998. LC 98-10419. 39.95 (0-8261-1179-3) Springer Pub.

Life & Worklife Expectancies. Hugh Richards & Jon R. Abele. 2000. LC 99-48922. (Illus.). 272p. kivar 65.00 (0-913875-36-8, 5368-R) Lawyers & Judges.

Life & Works of John Arbuthnot, M. D., Fellow of the Royal College of Physicians. George Atherton Aitken. 1992. (BCL1-PR English Literature Ser.). 516p. reprint ed. lib. bdg. 99.00 (0-7812-7318-8) Rprt Serv.

Life & Writings of Henry Pickering Bowditch: An Original Anthology. Set. Henry P. Bowditch. Ed. by I. Bernard Cohen. 1980. LC 79-7950. (Three Centuries of Science in America Ser.). (Illus.). lib. bdg. 88.95 (0-405-12531-3) Ayer.

Life As Theater: A Dramaturgical Sourcebook. Ed. by Dennis Brissett & Charles Edgley. 2nd ed. 1990. (Communication & Social Order Ser.). 477p. (C). lib. bdg. 56.95 (0-202-30362-4) Aldine de Gruyter.

Life Assurance Medicine Congress, 9th, Tel Aviv, March 1967: Proceedings. Ed. by M. Leffkowitz & H. Steinitz. 1968. vi, 368p. pap. 99.25 (3-8055-0910-3) S Karger.

Life at the Border. Leland M. Heller. 1987. (Illus.). 244p. pap. 20.00 (1-928947-01-8) Dyslimbia Pr.

Life Before Birth. Marjorie A. England. 2nd ed. 1997. 64.00 (0-7234-2474-8); (Illus.). 240p. pap. text 37.00 (0-7234-2475-6) Mosby Inc.

Life Before Birth: The Moral & Legal Status of Embryos & Fetuses. Bonnie Steinbock. 1996. 272p. (C). pap. 22.50 (0-19-510872-8) OUP.

Life Before Birth & a Time to Be Born. Peter W. Nathanielsz. 1992. LC 92-26052. (Illus.). 250p. 25.00 (0-916859-55-X) Promethean Pr.

Life Beyond Headaches. Jeffry Finnigan. 2nd ed. 1999. (Illus.). 160p. pap. 14.95 (0-9662786-0-7) Finnigan Clinic.

Life Care: The Inside Story. Elwood N. Chapman. Ed. by Follin Armfield. 1994. LC 94-70615. 136p. pap. 12.95 (1-56052-290-9) Crisp Pubns.

Life Care Planning for the Amputee: A Step-by-Step Guide. Roger O. Weed & Anne Sluis-Powers. 1990. (Life Care Planning Monographs). 162p. per. 26.95 (1-878205-09-9) St Lucie Pr.

Life Care Planning for the Brain Damaged Baby: A Step-by-Step Guide. Julie A. Kitchen et al. 1989. (Life Care Planning Monographs). 140p. (C). per. 26.95 (1-878205-00-5) St Lucie Pr.

Life Care Planning for the Spinal Cord Injured: A Step-by-Step Guide. Paul M. Deutsch. 1989. 88p. per. 26.95 (0-945019-08-4) St Lucie Pr.

Life Care Planning for the Ventilator Dependent Patient: A Step-by-Step Guide. Julie A. Kitchen et al. 1990. (Life Care Planning Monographs). 224p. per. 31.95 (1-878205-05-6) St Lucie Pr.

Life Challenge Inventory: A Self-Administered Life Stress Questionnaire & Handbook for Managing Life's Challenges in Personal, Family & Work Life. Ruth Schelkun. rev. ed. 1995. 84p. (Orig.). pap. 13.50 (0-933933-00-2) Human Netwrks.

Life Change Events Research, 1966-1978: An Annotated Bibliography of the Periodical Literature. Thomas E. Holmes & Ella M. David. 1984. LC 83-19287. 331p. 70.00 (0-275-91192-6, C1192, Praeger Pubs) Greenwood.

Life Change, Life Events, & Illness: Selected Papers. Ed. by Thomas H. Holmes & Ella M. David. 1989. LC 88-28610. 361p. 77.00 (0-275-92480-7, C2480, Praeger Pubs) Greenwood.

Life Chemistry Reports, Vol. 12. Ed. by J. V. Bannister. 1994. (Life Chemistry Reports: Vol. 12, No. 2). 102p. pap. text 211.00 (3-7186-5640-X) Gordon & Breach.

Life Chemistry Reports: Proceedings of the International Meeting on Antioxidants, Inflammation, Cardiovascular & Ophthalmic Diseases. Francisco Romero. 1994. (Life Chemistry Reports: Vol. 12). 104p. pap. text 215.00 (3-7186-5639-6) Gordon & Breach.

Life Chemistry Reports Vol. 11, No. 1: Aluminum in Chemistry, Biology & Medicine, Vol. 11. Paolo F. Zatta. 1994. (Life Chemistry Reports). 270p. pap. text 189.00 (3-7186-5567-5) Gordon & Breach.

Life Choices: Health Concepts & Strategies. Lori Turner et al. Ed. by Marshall. 2nd ed. 1992. 621p. (C). pap. text 46.50 (0-314-93383-2) West Pub.

Life Choices, Life Changes: Develop Your Personal Vision Through Imagework. Dina Glouberman. 1999. 336p. pap. (1-85538-499-X) Thorsons GBR. *Dist:* Natl Bk Netwk.

Life Course Approach to Chronic Disease Epidemiology: Tracing the Origins of Ill-Health from Early to Adult Life. Ed. by Diana Kuh & Yoav Ben-Shlomo. 1997. LC 97-9893. (Illus.). 336p. text 65.00 (0-19-262782-1) OUP.

Life-Cycle Assessment: Inventory Guideline & Principles. Battelle Memorial Institute Staff. 1994. 144p. lib. bdg. 54.95 (1-56670-015-9) Lewis Pubs.

Life Cycle Completed: Extended Version. Erik H. Erikson & Joan M. Erikson. 1998. LC 96-34622. 144p. pap. 11.00 (0-393-31772-2) Norton.

Life Cycle Group Work in Nursing. E. H. Janosik & L. B. Phipps. 1983. reprint ed. 38.75 (0-86720-388-9, 80-71075) Jones & Bartlett.

Life, Death & Decisions: Doctors & Nurses Reflect. McHaffie. 1997. LC 97-142928. 304p. pap. text 39.99 (1-898507-55-4) Buttrwrth-Heinemann.

Life, Death & Public Policy. Robert H. Blank. 1988. 187p. pap. 15.00 (0-87580-540-X) N Ill U Pr.

Life, Death, & the Law: A Sourcebook on Autonomy & Responsibility in Medical Ethics, Set. W. Noel Keyes. 1995. LC 95-18793. (Illus.). 1076p. 195.95 (0-398-06533-0); pap. 143.95 (0-398-06534-9) C C Thomas.

Life-Death Decisions in Health Care. Ed. by Lesley F. Degner & Janet I. Beaton. 1987. (Death Education, Aging & Health Care Ser.). 159p. 63.95 (0-89116-399-9) Hemisp Pub.

Life Extension: Adding Years to Your Life & Life to Your Years: A Practical Scientific Approach. Durk Pearson & Sandy Shaw. 1983. LC 80-27589. (Illus.). 600p. (Orig.). mass mkt. 10.95 (0-446-87990-8) Warner Bks.

Life-Extension, Purposeful Relaxation, Differential (Multiple) "Feeling" (Psychophysiological) Awareness & Communication. Russell E. Mason. 1975. 70.00 incl. audio (0-89533-018-0) F I Comm.

Life Flow One: The Solution for Heart Disease. Karl Loren. 1994. (Illus.). 300p. (1-882537-02-5) Bigelow Charter.

Life from Death: The Organ & Tissue Donation & Transplantation Source Book, with Forms. Phillip Williams. 1989. LC 88-24461. (Current Issues in Medicine & Law Ser.: Vol. 2). 252p. pap. 19.95 (0-936284-44-7) P Gaines Co.

Life Histories & Psychobiography: Explorations in Theory & Method. William M. Runyan. 1984. (Illus.). 302p. pap. text 21.95 (0-19-503486-4) OUP.

Life Histories of North American Gallinaceous Birds. Arthur C. Bent. 1963. (Illus.). pap. 10.95 (0-486-21028-6) Dover.

Life-Histories of Northern Animals: An Account of the Mammals of Manitoba, Set. Ernest Thompson Seton. 1974. LC 73-17845. (Natural Sciences in America Ser.). (Illus.). 1514p. reprint ed. 113.95 (0-405-05767-9) Ayer.

Life-Histories of the Northern Animals: An Account of the Mammals of Manitoba Ernest Thompson Seton. 1974. LC 73-17845. (Natural Sciences in America Ser.). (Illus.). 1514p. reprint ed. 1. 57.95 (0-405-05768-7); Vol. 2. 57.95 (0-405-05769-5) Ayer.

Life in a Mental Hospital. William J. Kurdi. Ed. by Kort Kurdi. 1978. LC 77-92103. pap. 8.95 (957-616-491-5) Med Nurs Educ.

Life in the Labyrinth. E. J. Gold. 2001. LC 86-82759. 278p. reprint ed. pap. 19.95 (0-89556-048-8) Gateways Bks & Tapes.

Life in the Womb: The Origin of Health & Disease. Peter W. Nathanielsz. 1999. LC 98-51356. (Illus.). 363p. 27.50 (0-916859-56-8) Promethean Pr.

Life Is a Shared Creation. Paul Brenner. 1981. 176p. (Orig.). pap. 6.95 (0-87516-454-4) DeVorss.

Life Isn't Just a Panic: Stories of Hope by Recovering Agoraphobics. Anita L. Pace et al. 1996. (Illus.). 256p. (Orig.). pap. 13.95 (0-9631666-3-8) Baby Steps Pr.

Life Itself: "Messiness Is Next to Goddessness" & Other Essays. John Boe. 1994. LC 94-19711. 184p. (Orig.). pap. 14.95 (0-933029-86-1) Chiron Pubns.

Life Log: Promoting a Lifetime of Good Health. Hillary M. Hulce et al. 1996. (Illus.). 80p. (Orig.). 12.95 (0-9652193-0-5) Help Yourself.

Life Management Skills: Taking Charge of Your Future. Driggers. 1998. LC 98-20900. 320p. (C). pap. text 36.95 (0-7668-0506-9) Delmar.

Life of a Bipolar Child: What Every Parent & Professional Needs to Know. Trudy Carlson. 2000. 288p. pap. 18.95 (0-9642443-7-3) Benline Pr.

Life of a Midwife: A Celebration of Midwifery. Midwifery Today Magazine Staff. 1997. LC 98-198139. (Illus.). 92p. pap. 25.00 (1-890446-05-X) Midwifery Today.

Life of a Science: The Development of a New Medicine. Kari Cantell. 1997. LC 98-198486. 239p. text 15.00 (981-02-3148-2) World Scientific Pub.

Life of Clara Barton William E. Barton. LC 71-86171. reprint ed. 78.50 (0-404-00730-9) AMS Pr.

Life of Dorothea Lynde Dix. Francis Tiffany. 1992. 392p. reprint ed. lib. bdg. 42.00 (0-8328-2271-X) Higginson Bk Co.

Life of Illness: One Woman's Journey. Carol T. Olson. 1992. LC 91-33457. (SUNY Series, The Body in Culture, History, & Religion). 203p. (C). text 18.50 (0-7914-1199-0) State U NY Pr.

Life of Paracelsus, & the Substance of His Teachings. Franz Hartman. Ed. by R. I. Robb & Helena P. Blavatsky. 2nd ed. 1997. LC 81-52063. (Secret Doctrine Reference Ser.). 240p. reprint ed. 16.00 (0-913510-71-8) Wizards.

Life of Sir Robert Jones. Frederick Watson. Ed. by William R. Phillips & Janet Rosenberg. 1980. LC 79-6928. (Physically Handicapped in Society Ser.). (Illus.). reprint ed. lib. bdg. 31.95 (0-405-13135-6) Ayer.

Life of the Mind. Hannah Arendt. 1981. LC 80-25403. (Harvest Book Ser.). 300p. pap. 16.00 (0-15-651992-5, Harvest Bks) Harcourt.

Life of the Mind. Jason W. Brown. 1988. (Comparative Cognition & Neuroscience Ser.). 440p. 99.95 (0-8058-0236-3); pap. text 45.00 (0-8058-0422-6) L Erlbaum Assocs.

Life of the Mind. Ornstein. 2001. (0-15-100423-4) Harcourt.

Life on Earth: Its Origin & Succession. John Phillips. Ed. by Stephen Jay Gould. 1980. LC 79-8343. (History of Paleontology Ser.). reprint ed. lib. bdg. 23.95 (0-405-12733-2) Ayer.

Life Reframing in Hypnosis: The Seminars, Workshops & Lectures of Milton H. Erickson, Vol. 2. Milton H. Erickson. Ed. by Ernest L. Rossi & Margaret O. Ryan. 1985. (Illus.). 330p. 19.95 (0-8290-3155-3); 39.50 (0-8290-1581-7); pap. 20.00 (0-8290-3160-X) Irvington.

Life Science. William L. Smallwood. 1972. (Challenges to Science Ser.). text 33.52 (0-07-058415-X) McGraw.

Life Sciences & Health Challenges. Susan Raymond. 1999. (Annals of the New York Academy of Sciences Ser.). 160p. pap. text 19.95 (0-8018-6300-7) Johns Hopkins.

Life Sciences & Health Challenges. Susan Raymond. 1998. 160p. pap. 30.00 (1-57331-148-0) NY Acad Sci.

Life Sciences on File. Diagram Group Staff. 1986. (Illus.). 304p. ring bd. 165.00 (0-8160-1284-9) Facts on File.

Life, Sex & Death: Selected Writings of William Gillespie. William H. Gillespie. Ed. & Intro. by Michael D. Sinason. 1995. LC 94-42274. (New Library of Psychoanalysis : Vol. 23). (Illus.). 224p. (C). pap. 27.95 (0-415-12805-6); (gr. 13). 84.95 (0-415-12804-8) Routledge.

Life Skills Training Level 3: Promoting Health & Personal Development/Teacher Manual. Gilbert J. Botvin. 1998. (Illus.). 112p. tchr. ed., ring bd. 55.00 (0-933665-04-0) Princeton Hlth.

Life Space Intervention: Talking with Children & Youth in Crisis. Mary M. Wood & Nicholas J. Long. 1991. LC 90-32277. 342p. pap. text 34.00 (0-89079-245-3, 1437) PRO-ED.

Life-Span Communication: Normative Processes. Ed. by J. F. Nussbaum. 1989. (Communication Textbook Ser.). 392p. 79.95 (0-8058-0195-2) L Erlbaum Assocs.

Life-Span Development. John W. Santrock. 5th ed. 1994. 736p. (C). text 53.50 net. (0-697-14503-4) Brown & Benchmark.

Life Span Development. John W. Santrock. 6th ed. 1996. LC 95-80202. 720p. (C). text 49.50 net. (0-697-23583-1) Brown & Benchmark.

Life-Span Development. John W. Santrock et al. 6th ed. 1996. 272p. (C). text, stu. ed. 20.62 (0-697-23585-8, WCB McGr Hill) McGrw-H Hghr Educ.

Life-Span Development. John W. Santrock. 7th ed. 1998. LC 98-12814. 652p. 43.00 net. (0-697-36439-9, Dshkn McG-Hill) McGrw-H Hghr Educ.

Life-Span Development: An Introduction. John W. Santrock. 5th ed. 1994. LC 93-73056. 736p. (C). text 48.50 net. (0-697-14504-2) Brown & Benchmark.

Life-Span Development & Behavior. David L. Featherman et al. Ed. by Paul B. Baltes et al. 1994. (Life-Span Development & Psychology Ser.: Vol. 12). 296p. 69.95 (0-8058-1507-4) L Erlbaum Assocs.

Life-Span Development & Behavior, Vol. 7. Ed. by Paul B. Baltes et al. 1986. 352p. (C). text 99.95 (0-89859-692-0) L Erlbaum Assocs.

Life-Span Development & Behavior. Paul B. Baltes et al. Ed. by David L. Featherman et al. Vol. 9. 1988. 400p. 99.95 (0-8058-0272-X); Vol. 10. 1990. 384p. 105.00 (0-8058-0609-1) L Erlbaum Assocs.

Life-Span Developmental Psychology: A European Perspective. Andreas Demetriou et al. 1998. LC 97-23240. 536p. pap. 59.95 (0-471-97078-6) Wiley.

Life-Span Developmental Psychology: Introduction to Research Methods. Paul B. Baltes et al. 1988. 280p. reprint ed. pap. text 34.50 (0-8058-0235-5) L Erlbaum Assocs.

Life-Span Human Development. Dale Goldhaber. 1986. 635p. (C). text 57.50 (0-15-550740-0, GOLD) Harcourt Coll Pubs.

Life-Span Human Development. Carol K. Sigelman & David R. Shaffer. 1990. LC 89-29685. 720p. (C). pap., stu. ed. 17.95 (0-534-12284-1); mass mkt. 52.25 (0-534-12282-5) Brooks-Cole.

Life-Span Human Development: Study Guide. Carol K. Sigelman. 2nd ed. 1994. (Psychology Ser.). pap., stu. ed. 18.25 (0-534-19579-2) Brooks-Cole.

Life-Span Human Development (International Version) Sigelman. 3rd ed. 1998. (Psychology Ser.). 704p. spiral bd. 83.95 (0-534-36362-8) Brooks-Cole.

Life Span Nutrition: Conception Through Life. Sharon Rady Rolfes & Linda DeBruyne. 2nd ed. 1997. LC 97-36769. (Health Sciences Ser.). 540p. spiral bd. 83.95 (0-534-53834-7) Brooks-Cole.

Life-Span Perspectives & Social Psychology. Ed. by Ronald P. Abeles. 1987. 200p. text 39.95 (0-89859-953-9) L Erlbaum Assocs.

Life Span Perspectives of Suicide: Time-Lines in the Suicide Process. Ed. by Antoon A. Leenaars. 1991. LC 96-2679. (Illus.). 342p. (C). text 59.50 (0-306-43620-5, Kluwer Plenum) Kluwer Academic.

Life-Span Plus. Prevention Magazine Editors. 1993. 422p. 8.98 (1-56731-025-7, MJF Bks) Fine Comms.

Life-Span Radiation Effects Studies in Animals: What Can They Tell Us? Ed. by R.C. Thompson & J. A. Mahaffey. 1986. 732p. pap. 57.50 (0-935470-70-0) Battelle.

Life Span Research on the Prediction of Psychopathology. Ed. by L. Erlenmeyer-Kimling et al. 1986. 328p. (C). text 65.00 (0-89859-587-8) L Erlbaum Assocs.

Life Strategies, Human Evolution, Environmental Design: Toward a Biological Theory of Health, Vol. I. Valerius Geist. 1979. LC 78-10807. (Illus.). 495p. 140.00 (0-387-90363-1) Spr-Verlag.

Life Stress & Coronary Heart Disease. Ulf De Faire & Torres Theorell. 1984. 130p. 18.50 (0-87527-201-0) Green.

***Life Stress, Distress, Anxiety & Depression in the Psychological Garden of Mental Illlness & the Complex Variations in Human Activities: Index of New Information for Consumers, Reference & Research.** Chester O. Donovan. 2002. 180p. 57.50 (0-7883-2424-1) ABBE Pubs Assn.

Life Style & Mortality: A Large-Scale Census-Based Cohort Study in Japan - Contributions to Epidemiology & Biostatistics, Vol. 6. T. Hirayama. 1990. (Illus.). viii, 138p. 169.75 (3-8055-5201-7) S Karger.

Life Support: A Family Clinical Guide. Michael P. Hahn. 1996. LC 96-13337. (Illus.). 317p. lib. bdg. 35.00 (0-7864-0153-2) McFarland & Co.

Life Support & Habitability Vol. II: Space Biology & Medicine. Ed. by Frank M. Sulzman & A. M. Genin. 1994. (Space Biology & Medicine Ser.). (Illus.). 423p. 99.95 (1-56347-082-9, 82-9(890)) AIAA.

Life-Sustaining Technologies & the Elderly. 1991. lib. bdg. 76.95 (0-8490-4974-1) Gordon Pr.

Life-Sustaining Technologies & the Elderly. Ed. by Office of Technology Assessment Task Force Staff. 1988. LC 65-20241. 450p. text 39.95 (0-397-53024-2) Lppncott W & W.

Life Table & Its Applications. Chin Long Chiang. 1983. LC 82-20331. 336p. (C). 46.50 (0-89874-570-5) Krieger.

Life Tastes Better Than Steak Eating Plan: A Diet for a Clogged Artery. Gerry Krag. 1997. 104p. pap. 12.95 (0-932212-96-4) Avery Color.

Life, the Lab, & Everything. Ian Wilkinson. 1996. 178p. pap. 20.00 (0-915274-85-X, 202676, AACC Pr) Am Assn Clinical Chem.

Life-Threatening Allergic Reactions: Understanding & Coping with Anaphylaxis. Deryk Williams et al. 1998. 112p. pap. (0-7499-1700-8) Piatkus Bks GBR. *Dist:* London Brdge.

Life-Threatening Coagulation Disorders in Critical Care Medicine. V. Hach-Wunderle & P. P. Nawroth. Tr. by T. C. Telger from GER. 1996. LC 96-29356. (Illus.). 90p. pap. 58.95 (3-540-61475-3) Spr-Verlag.

Life Threatening Emergencies in Dentistry. V. Chilo et al. 1988. 188p. text (1-57235-015-6) Piccin Nuova.

Life to the Fullest: Stories of People Coping with Diabetes. Dan Brannan. 1996. Orig. Title: Diabetes Doesn't Have to Be a Death Sentence. (Illus.). 221p. (Orig.). pap. 15.95 (0-9650228-1-1) D Brannan.

Life Transitions in the Older Adult: Issues for Nurses & Other Health Professionals. Ed. by Elizabeth A. Swanson & Toni Tripp-Reimer. 1999. LC 00-266439. (Advances in Gerontological Nursing Ser.). (Illus.). 208p. text 35.95 (*0-8261-9112-6*) Springer Pub.

Life under Extreme Conditions: Biochemical Adaptation. Ed. by G. Di Prisco. 1991. (Illus.). 144p. 78.95 (*0-387-53108-4*) Spr-Verlag.

Life Values & Adolescent Mental Health. Patricia Cohen & Jacob Cohen. 1995. (Research Monographs in Adolescence). 192p. text 45.00 (*0-8058-1774-3*) L Erlbaum Assocs.

Life with AIDS. Rose Weitz. 1991. LC 90-36219. 224p. (C). text 35.00 (*0-8135-1629-3*); pap. text 16.00 (*0-8135-1630-7*) Rutgers U Pr.

Life with Charlie: How to Cope with an Alzheimer's Spouse or Other Dementia Patient & Still Keep Your Sanity. Carol Heckman-Owen. 1992. LC 91-38235. (Illus.). 144p. pap. 9.95 (*0-934793-41-7*) Pathfinder CA.

Life with Chronic Illness: Social & Psychological Dimensions. Ariela Royer. 1998. LC 98-11133. 232p. 62.50 (*0-275-96123-0*, Praeger Pubs) Greenwood.

Life with Diabetes: A Series of Teaching Outlines. Ed. by American Diabetes Association. 1997. LC 97-22986. (Illus.). 683p. 75.00 (*0-945448-80-5*, 5507-01) Am Diabetes.

Life with the Pneumococcus: Notes from the Bedside, Laboratory & Library. Robert Austrian. 1985. LC 85-1001. (Illus.). 160p. 49.95 (*0-8122-7977-8*) U of Pa Pr.

Life Within: Celebration of a Pregnancy. Jean Hegland. 1991. LC 90-46690. 114p. 17.95 (*0-89603-196-9*) Humana.

Life Within Hidden Worlds: Psychotherapy in Prisons. Ed. by Jessica Williams Saunders. 2001. 144p. pap. (*1-85575-219-0*) Karnac Bks GBR. *Dist:* Other Pr LLC.

Life without Disease: The Pursuit of Medical Utopia. William B. Schwartz. 1998. LC 97-41639. (Illus.). 190p. text 22.00 (*0-520-21467-6*) U CA Pr.

Life Without End: The Transplant Story. P. J. Houlihan. 1987. 192p. (Orig.). pap. (*1-55021-017-3*) NC Ltd CAN. *Dist:* U of Toronto Pr.

Life Without Fear Vol. V: Chiropractice Major Philosophical Tenet. Frederick H. Barge. deluxe ed. 1995. LC 94-73474. 147p. pap. 24.95 (*1-885048-10-6*) Barge Chiropract.

Life Without Problems? The Achievements of a Therapeutic Community. Michael Little. 1995. 240p. (*1-85742-317-8*); pap. (*1-85742-316-X*) Arena GBR. *Dist:* Ashgate Pub Co.

Life Without Stress: A Survival Guide. George H. Green. 2nd ed. 1997. 198p. (Orig.). pap. 11.95 (*1-890669-00-8*, LWS-1) Biofeedback Ctr.

Life Work of Dr. Elisabeth Kubler-Ross & Its Impact on the Death Awareness Movement. Michele Chaban. 1998. LC 98-8630. (Symposium Ser.: Vol. 49). x, 365p. text 109.95 (*0-7734-8302-0*) E Mellen.

Life Worth Living: Practical Strategies for Reducing Depression in Older Adults. Pearl M. Mosher-Ashley & Phyllis W. Barnett. 2nd ed. 1997. LC 97-1679. 384p. (Orig.). pap. 31.95 (*1-878812-03-3*) Hlth Prof Pr.

LifeCare Guide to Alzheimer's Disease & Related Dementia. DCC Inc. Staff. 1999. 100p. pap. 14.95 (*1-58559-036-3*) LifeCare Inc.

LifeCare Guide to Care Options. DCC Inc., Staff. 1999. pap. 14.95 (*1-58559-004-5*) LifeCare Inc.

LifeFacts: AIDS. Jane Stangle. 1991. (Illus.). pap., tchr. ed. 199.00 (*1-56304-026-3*) J Stanfield.

LifeFacts: Managing Emotions. James Stanfield & Garilynn Stanfield. 1992. (Illus.). pap. text 199.00 incl. sl. (*1-56304-029-8*) J Stanfield.

Lifeline to Care with Dignity: Caring for the Memory Impaired. Kathie T. Erwin. 1997. 192p. pap. 14.95 (*1-887454-01-2*) Caremore Pubns.

Lifelines: Clinical Perspectives on Suicide. Ed. by Ellen L. Bassuk et al. 1982. LC 82-9105. 250p. 45.00 (*0-306-40971-2*, Plenum Trade) Perseus Pubng.

Lifelines: Living Longer, Growing Frail, Taking Heart. Muriel R. Gillick. 2000. LC 00-33941. 256p. 25.95 (*0-393-05002-5*) Norton.

Lifelong Management of Hypertension. H. Mitchell Perry. 1983. (Developments in Cardiovascular Medicine Ser.). text 176.50 (*0-89838-582-2*) Kluwer Academic.

Lifelong Motor Development. Carl P. Gabbard. 2nd ed. 1995. 480p. (C). text 40.00 net. (*0-697-23333-2*) Brown & Benchmark.

Lifeplan: Your Own Master Plan for Maintaining Health & Preventing Illness. Donald M. Vickery. rev. ed. 1990. LC 89-52083. 347p. pap. 8.75 (*0-9625327-0-3*, M14531) Vicktor.

Life's Beginnings: Our Life Before Birth Helps Us Trace Our Roots. W. J. Howard. 1991. LC 90-83709. (Illus.). 128p. (Orig.). pap. 9.95 (*0-9627341-7-9*) Coast Pub OR.

Life's Career - Aging: Cultural Variations on Growing Old. Ed. by Barbara G. Myerhoff & Andrei Simic. 1979. (Cross-Cultural Research & Methodology Ser.: Vol. 4). 252p. pap. 36.95 (*0-8039-6000-X*, 8654) Sage.

Life's Little Health Book. C. Buckley, Jr. 1993. 160p. pap. 5.95 (*0-9635231-4-7*) CTA Resrch Corp.

Life's Living Toward Dying: A Theological & Medical-Ethical Study. Vigen Guroian. 1996. LC 96-10808. 135p. pap. 12.00 (*0-8028-4190-2*) Eerdmans.

Lifes Preservative Against Self Killing (1637) John Sym. Ed. by Michael McDonald. 1989. (Tavistock Classic Reprints in the History of Psychiatry Ser.). 384p. 54.00 (*0-415-00639-2*) Routledge.

Life's Second Half. Jerome Ellison. 1978. 10.95 (*0-8159-6116-2*) Devin.

Lifesaving First Aid for Children: A Quick-Reference Guide. American Red Cross Staff. Ed. by Dan Preniszni. 2nd rev. ed. 1998. (Illus.). (*0-9665371-1-4*) Laerdal Med Corp.

Lifespan. Guy R. Lefrancois. (C). 2nd ed. 1987. 664p. pap. 31.00 net. (*0-534-07470-7*); 3rd ed. 1990. 714p. pap. 37.50 net. (*0-534-11754-6*) Wadsworth Pub.

Lifespan: Developmental Psychology. Jack Rudman. 1994. (Dantes Subject Standardized Tests Ser.: DANTES-64). pap. 27.95 (*0-8373-6664-X*) Nat Learn.

Lifespan: New Perspectives on Extending Human Longevity. Thomas J. Moore. 1994. 320p. pap. 12.00 (*0-671-88622-3*, Touchstone) S&S Trade Pap.

Lifespan: What Really Affects Human Longevity. Thomas J. Moore. 1993. LC 92-40669. (Illus.). 352p. 23.00 (*0-671-72966-7*) S&S Trade.

Lifespan & Factors Affecting It: Aging Theories in Gerontology. Daniel Hershey. 1998. (Illus.). 157p. reprint ed. pap. text 25.00 (*0-916961-04-4*) Basal Books.

Lifespan Developement. Jeffrey S. Turner. 5th ed. 1994. (C). pap. text, tchr. ed. 33.75 (*0-15-502422-1*) Harcourt Coll Pubs.

Lifespan Development. Janina M. Jolley & Mitchell. 1995. tchr. ed. 26.87 (*0-697-14498-4*) McGraw.

Lifespan Development. Leonie Sugarman. 1986. (New Essential Psychology Ser.). 198p. pap. 14.95 (*0-416-34390-2*, 1018) Routledge.

Lifespan Development. Ed. by Helen L. Bee. 2nd ed. 1997. LC 97-5362. 640p. (C). text 76.00 (*0-321-01121-X*) Allyn.

Lifespan Development. Jeffrey S. Turner. 5th ed. 1994. (C). pap. text, stu. ed. 32.50 (*0-15-502789-1*) Harcourt Coll Pubs.

Lifespan Development. Jeffrey S. Turner & Donald B. Helms. 5th ed. 1994. LC 93-80877. 640p. (C). text 86.00 (*0-15-500996-6*) Harcourt.

Lifespan Development: Test Bank. Jeffrey S. Turner. 5th ed. 1994. (C). pap. text, tchr. ed., suppl. ed. 44.50 (*0-15-502682-8*) Harcourt Coll Pubs.

Lifespan Development in a Mixed Economy of Care. Open Learning Foundation Staff. 1996. 112p. pap. (*0-443-05736-2*) Church.

Lifespan Developmental Psychology. Donald B. Irwin & Janet A. Simons. 1993. 592p. (C). pap. 74.69 (*0-697-06430-1*) McGrw-H Hghr Educ.

Lifespan Developmental Psychology. Irwin & Simons. 1994. 22.50 (*0-697-22457-0*) McGraw.

Lifespan Health Psychology: Nursing Problems & Interventions. C. R. Paton. 1992. 288p. pap. 43.25 (*1-56593-008-8*, 0249) Thomson Learn.

Lifespan Nutrition: Conception Through Aging. Sharon R. Rolfes et al. Ed. by Marshall. 1990. 528p. (C). mass mkt. 43.50 (*0-314-66811-X*) West Pub.

Lifespan of Human Development. Goldhab. 1986. (C). text (*0-15-540380-X*) Harcourt Coll Pubs.

Lifespan of Human Development. Anne V. Gormly. 6th ed. 1996. (C). pap. text, stu. ed. 34.50 (*0-15-504016-2*); pap. text, tchr. ed. 28.00 (*0-15-503922-9*) Harcourt Coll Pubs.

Lifespan Perspectives on the Family & Disability. Judy V. Berry & Michael L. Hardman. 1997. LC 97-16309. 288p. pap. text 64.00 (*0-205-19395-1*) Allyn.

***Lifespan Processes.** Towler. 1993. 184p. 32.60 (*0-536-58383-8*) Pearson Custom.

Lifespan Prolongation. Vladimir V. Frolkis & Khachik K. Muradian. 1991. (Illus.). 432p. lib. bdg. 250.00 (*0-8493-6741-7*, QP85) CRC Pr.

Lifestyle & Cancer Prevention. Ernest H. Rosenbaum et al. Ed. by Sheila Mahoney & Nancy Wiltsek. 1985. (Illus.). 49p. pap. 2.50 (*0-933161-05-0*) Better H Prog.

Lifestyle Capsules see Dynamic Living Workbook

Lifestyle for Longevity: How to Extend Your Life with Moderation, Joy & Ease. Norman D. Ford. Ed. by Emily McKeigue & Marah Ren. 1984. LC 82-62228. 176p. pap. 9.95 (*0-914918-63-X*, Whitford) Schiffer.

Lifestyle Management for Patients with Coronary Heart Disease. Nancy Houston Miller & Craig B. Taylor. 1995. LC 95-177. (Current Issues in Cardiac Rehabilitation Ser.: Vol. 2). 144p. (Orig.). pap. text 26.00 (*0-87322-441-8*, BHOU0441) Human Kinetics.

Lifestyle Medicine. James M. Rippe. 1999. LC 99-13000. (Illus.). xxv, 1363p. 131.95 (*0-86542-294-X*) Blackwell Sci.

Lifestyle Nutrition. Johanna Dwyer et al. 2000. LC 00-44413. (Lifestyle Medicine Ser.). (Illus.). xxiii, 232p. pap. 31.95 (*0-632-04548-5*) Blackwell Sci.

Lifestyle Redesign: Implementing the Well Elderly Program. Deborah Mandel et al. 1999. LC 99-219954. (Illus.). pap. 32.00 (*1-56900-120-0*) Am Occup Therapy.

Lifestyles of the Elderly: Diversity in Relationships, Health, & Caregiving. Ed. by L. Ade-Ridder & C. B. Hennon. 1989. (Illus.). 256p. 37.00 (*0-89885-447-4*, Kluwer Acad Hman Sci) Kluwer Academic.

Lifetime Body Grafs: Men's Edition. Bruce C. Vandre. 1990. (Illus.). 24p. (Orig.). pap. 4.95 (*0-942223-08-X*) VanPress.

Lifetime Body Grafs: Women's Edition. Bruce C. Vandre. 1990. (Illus.). 24p. (Orig.). pap. 4.95 (*0-942223-07-1*) VanPress.

Lifetime Fitness & Wellness: A Personal Choice. Melvin H. Williams. 3rd ed. 1992. 384p. (C). text 25.00 net. (*0-697-12670-6*) Brown & Benchmark.

Lifetime Weight Control: Seven Steps to Achieving & Maintaining a Healthy Weight. Patrick Fanning. 1994. 208p. pap. 13.95 (*0-934986-83-5*) New Harbinger.

***Lift: Wanting, Fearing & Having a Face-Lift.** Joan Kron. 2001. 264p. reprint ed. 24.00 (*0-7881-9921-8*) DIANE Pub.

Lift: Wanting, Fearing, & Having a Facelift. Joan Kron. 2000. 272p. pap. 13.95 (*0-14-027803-6*) Penguin Putnam.

Lifting the Bull: Overcoming Chronic Back Pain, Fibromyalgia & Environmental Illness. Diane Dawber. 1999. (Illus.). 176p. pap. (*1-55082-199-7*) Quarry Pr.

Lifting the Curse of Menstruation: A Feminine Appraisal of the Influence of Menstruation on Women's Lives. Ed. by Sharon Golub. 1985. LC 84-19804. 156p. pap. text 14.95 (*0-918393-06-X*, Harrington Park) Haworth Pr.

Lifting the Curse of Menstruation: A Feminist Appraisal of the Influence of Menstruation on Women's Lives. Ed. by Sharon Golub. 1983. LC 83-12723. (Women & Health Ser.: Vol. 8, Nos. 2-3). 156p. text 39.95 (*0-86656-242-7*); pap. text 2.95 (*0-86656-422-5*) Haworth Pr.

Ligament & Tendon Relaxation (Skeletal Disability) Treated by Prolotherapy (Fibro-Osseous Proliferation) George S. Hackett. 3rd ed. 1958. (Illus.). 160p. 32.95 (*0-398-05066-X*) C C Thomas.

Ligamentous Articular Strain: Osteopathic Manipulative Techniques for the Body. William T. Crow & Conrad Speece. 2001. (Illus.). 184p. (C). pap. 35.00 (*0-939616-31-9*) Eastland.

Ligaments & Ligamentoplasties. Ed. by L. H. Yahia. 1996. LC 96-17116. (Illus.). 416p. 198.00 (*3-540-61171-1*) Spr-Verlag.

Ligaments of the Knee. Ed. by Alfred J. Tria, Jr. 1995. LC 95-8982. (Illus.). text (*0-443-08954-X*) Church.

Light: Medicine of the Future: How We Can Use It to Heal Ourselves Now. Jacob Liberman. 1993. LC 90-748. (Illus.). 288p. pap. 16.95 (*1-879181-01-0*) Bear & Co.

Light & Biological Rhythms in Man. Ed. by L. Wetterberg. 1994. LC 93-21167. (Wenner-Gren International Ser.). 462p. 185.25 (*0-08-042279-9*, Pergamon Pr) Elsevier.

Light & Electronmicroscopic Neuropathology - Slow Virus Diseases. Ed. by Pawel P. Liberski. 1992. 448p. 239.00 (*0-8493-6725-5*, QR201) CRC Pr.

Light Around the Dark. Elizabeth D. Gee. 1992. (Center for Human Caring Ser.). 168p. pap. text 24.95 (*0-88737-554-5*, 14-2476) Natl League Nurse.

Light at the End of the Carpal Tunnel Vol. 1: A Guide to Understanding & Relief from the Pain of Nerve Problems. Scott M. Fried. 1998. LC 97-94105. (Illus.). xvi, 205p. (Orig.). 14.95 (*0-9659267-5-3*) Healing Bks.

Light Eating for Survival. Marcia Acciardo. 1978. (Illus.). 106p. (Orig.). pap. text 14.00 (*0-933278-05-5*) Twen Fir Cent.

Light Foods: An Assessment of Their Psychological, Sociocultural, Physiological, Nutritional, & Safety Aspects. J. Leathwood. 1995. LC 95-75553. (Illus.). 98p. pap. 22.50 (*0-944398-44-8*) ILSI.

Light in Biology & Medicine, Vol. 2. Ed. by R. H. Douglas et al. 1991. (Illus.). 582p. (C). text 186.00 (*0-306-44025-3*, Kluwer Plenum) Kluwer Academic.

Light in Biology & Medicine, Vol. 1. Ed. by R. H. Douglas et al. 1988. (Illus.). 474p. 110.00 (*0-306-42918-7*, Plenum Trade) Perseus Pubng.

***Light in the Darkness: A Physician Talks Openly about His Own Addiction to Sex.** St. George Lee. 2000. 200p. pap. 21.95 (*0-9679881-0-1*) Dragon Pr VA.

Light in the Heart of Darkness. Steven Silver. 2001. LC 2001-45249. 240p. 32.00 (*0-393-70366-5*) Norton.

Light in the Skull: An Odyssey of Medical Discovery. Ronald Glasser. 1997. LC 96-51607. 210p. 24.95 (*0-571-19916-X*) Faber & Faber.

Light, Lasers, & Synchrotron Radiation: A Health Risk Assessment. M. Grandolfo et al. 1991. LC 90-23013. (NATO Advanced Science Institutes Ser.: Vol. 242). (Illus.). 436p. (C). text 156.00 (*0-306-43733-3*, Kluwer Plenum) Kluwer Academic.

Light, Lean, & Low-Fat Recipes from the Rice Council. 1993. (Favorite All Time Recipes Ser.). (Illus.). 96p. 7.98 (*1-56173-966-9*, 2013102) Pubns Intl Ltd.

Light Microscopic Techniques in Biology & Medicine. J. James. 1976. text 155.50 (*90-247-1900-3*) Kluwer Academic.

Light, Radiation & You: How to Stay Healthy. John N. Ott. 1990. LC 81-69951. (Illus.). 175p. pap. 11.95 (*0-8159-6121-9*) Devin.

Light Scattering Imaging of Neural Tissue Function. Ed. by David M. Rector & John S. George. 2001. (Contemporary Clinical Neuroscience Ser.). 400p. 125.00 (*0-89603-844-0*) Humana.

Light Search: A Healing Journal. Linda H. Keiser. 1988. 80p. (Orig.). pap. 5.00 (*0-944135-05-6*) Archedigm Pubns.

Light Years Ahead: The Illustrated Guide to Full Spectrum & Colored Light in Mindbody Healing. Jacob Lieberman. 1999. (Illus.). 424p. reprint ed. pap. text 20.00 (*0-7881-6777-4*) DIANE Pub.

Light Years Ahead: The Illustrated Guide to Full Spectrum & Colored Light Mind Body Healing. Light Years Ahead Productions Staff. Ed. by Brian Breiling & Bethany Argisle. 1995. LC 95-20046. (Illus.). 256p. text 19.95 (*0-89087-762-9*) Celestial Arts.

Lighten up Your Body - Lighten up Your Life: Beyond Diet & Exercise - The Inner Path to Lasting Change. Lucia Capacchione et al. 1990. 92p. pap. 12.95 (*0-87877-150-6*, 643, New Page Bks) Career Pr Inc.

Lighting Candles: Hospital Memories of Vietnam's Montagnards. Hilary Smith. 1988. (Illus.). 120p. (Orig.). pap. 7.95 (*0-9621110-0-7*) H Smith.

Lightning Injuries: Electrical, Medical, Legal Aspects. Christopher J. Andrews. 1991. 208p. lib. bdg. 139.00 (*0-8493-5458-7*, RD96) CRC Pr.

Lightning Stick: Arrows, Wounds & Indian Legends. H. Henrietta Stockel. 1995. LC 94-43926. (Illus.). 176p. 24.95 (*0-87417-266-7*) U of Nev Pr.

Lights & Siren: Code 3. Glenn Asaeda. 1994. LC 93-93773. 216p. (Orig.). pap. text 7.99 (*1-56002-308-2*) Aegina Pr.

Lights & Sirens: A Writer's Guide to Emergency Rescue Professions. James Cowan & Lois Cowan. 1998. LC 97-48735. (Behind the Scenes Ser.). (Illus.). 272p. pap. 16.99 (*0-89879-806-X*, Wrtrs Digest Bks) F & W Pubns Inc.

Lights in the Darkness: For Survivors & Healers of Sexual Abuse. Ave Clark. 1993. LC 92-82000. 150p. pap. 8.95 (*1-878718-12-6*, Resurrection Pr) Catholic Bk Pub.

Light's Manual: Intertidal Invertebrates of the Central California Coast: S. F. Lights Laboratory & Field Text in Invertebrate Zoology. Ed. by Ralph Smith & James T. Carlton. 3rd rev. ed. 1974. LC 70-170726. (Illus.). 716p. text 65.00 (*0-520-02113-4*) U CA Pr.

Lights Out: Sleep, Sugar & Survival. T. S. Wiley & Bent Formby. 2001. 368p. reprint ed. pap. 14.95 (*0-671-03868-0*, PB Trade Paper) PB.

Lights, Sirens & Donuts. Chuck Swanson. 1997. LC 98-210111. 64 p. (*0-912981-26-1*) Hse BonGiovanni.

Lignes de Conduite pour l'Erradication de la Deficience en Vitamine A Et De la Xerophtalmie. G. Arroyave et al. Tr. by Marc Vincent. 1984. (FRE., Illus.). 83p. (Orig.). pap. text 3.50 (*0-935368-38-8*) ILSI.

Like a Natural Woman: The Black Woman's Guide to Alternative Healing. Ziba Kashef. 2001. LC 00-103526. 304p. 23.00 (*1-57566-630-8*, Dafina) Kensgtn Pub Corp.

Like Fathers, Like Sons: Portraits of Intimacy & Strain. Thomas J. Cottle. 1981. LC 81-2171. (Modern Sociology Ser.). 140p. pap. 39.50 (*0-89391-087-2*, Ablex) Greenwood.

Liking, Loving & Relating. Clyde Hendrick & Susan Hendrick. 1983. LC 82-14561. (Psychology Ser.). 306p. (C). pap. 18.00 (*0-534-01263-9*) Brooks-Cole.

Lilio de Medicina. Bernardo De Gordonio. Ed. by Cynthia M. Wasick. 1989. (Medieval Spanish Medical Texts Ser.: No. 25). (SPA.). 14p. 10.00 incl. fiche (*0-942260-93-7*) Hispanic Seminary.

Lilio de Medicina. Bernardo Gordonio. Ed. by John Cull & Brian Dutton. 1991. (Spanish Ser.: No. 31). (SPA.). xxii, 418p. 35.00 (*0-940639-64-5*) Hispanic Seminary.

Limb Amputation. Rosalind Ham & Leonard Cotton. Ed. by Jo Campling. 1990. (Therapy in Practice Ser.). 140p. pap. 23.00 (*0-412-34610-9*, A4413) Chapman & Hall.

Limb Deficient Child. Yoshio Setoguchi & Ruth Rosenfelder. fac. ed. 1982. (Illus.). 344p. (C). 59.95 (*0-398-04656-5*) C C Thomas.

Limb Development & Regeneration Ed. by John F. Fallon et al. 1993. (Progress in Clinical & Biological Research Ser.: Vol. 383A-B). Pt. A. 484p. 1.25 (*0-471-59793-7*); Pt. B. 468p. 1.25 (*0-471-59794-5*) Wiley (Wiley-Liss).

***Limb Loss Prevention & Prosthetic Engineering.** Ed. by Mindy L. Aisen. 2001. (Illus.). 64p. pap. text 20.00 (*0-7567-1672-1*) DIANE Pub.

Limb Prosthetics. A. Bennett Wilson, Jr. 6th ed. 1989. (Illus.). 136p. pap. 24.95 (*0-939957-22-1*) Demos Medical.

Limb Salvage: Major Reconstruction in Oncologic & Nontumoral Conditions, 5th International Symposium - St. Malo. ISOLS-GETO. Ed. by F. Langlais & B. Tomeno. 1991. (Illus.). 826p. 214.00 (*0-387-52861-X*) Spr-Verlag.

Limb Salvage in Musculoskeletal Oncology, 1987. Ed. by T. Yamamuro. 1989. (Illus.). 720p. 174.00 (*0-387-70030-7*) Spr-Verlag.

Limbic Motor Circuits & Neuropsychiatry. Ed. by Peter W. Kalivas & Charles D. Barnes. 1993. 416p. 136.95 (*0-8493-4441-7*, QP383) CRC Pr.

Limbic Seizures in Children. G. Avanzini et al. 2001. 256p. (*0-86196-595-7*) J Libbey Med GBR. *Dist:* Buttrwrth-Heinemann.

Limbic System. Robert L. Isaacson. 2nd ed. 1982. LC 82-9077. (Illus.). 342p. 45.00 (*0-306-40874-0*, Plenum Trade) Perseus Pubng.

Limita Primitiva a Experientei. Thomas H. Ogden. Ed. & Tr. by F. V. Vladescu. Tr. by D. Bucerzan. 1995.Tr. of Primitive Edge of Experience. (RUM.). 168p. pap. text 19.95 (*1-883881-11-0*, 770) S Freud RT&PF.

Limitation of Exposure to Ionizing Radiation. Intro. by Charles B. Meinhold. 1993. LC 93-7142. (Report Ser.: No. 116). 70p. (Orig.). pap. text 35.00 (*0-929600-30-4*) NCRP Pubns.

Limitation of Infarct Size. Ed. by H. Schmutzler et al. 1988. (Illus.). 270p. 79.95 (*0-387-19148-8*) Spr-Verlag.

Limitations & Prospects for Retinal Surgery: Proceedings of the Club Jules Gonin Meeting, 8th, Miami, 1972. Club Jules Gonin Meeting Staff et al. 1974. (Modern Problems in Ophthalmology Ser.: Vol. 12). (Illus.). 152.25 (*3-8055-1629-0*) S Karger.

Limited Radiography. Campeau. 2nd ed. 1998. LC 98-27596. (Allied Health Ser.). 352p. pap. text 49.95 (*0-7668-0205-1*) Delmar.

Limited Radiography: Instructor's Guide. Frances E. Campeau & M. Jeana Phelps. 1993. 50p. 14.00 (*0-8273-3336-6*) Delmar.

Limiting Donor Exposure in Hemotherapy. Ed. by James P. Aubuchon & Linda A. Issitt. 1994. LC 94-32345. (Illus.). 99p. (C). 40.00 (*1-56395-030-8*) Am Assn Blood.

Limits: The Role of the Law in Bioethical Decision Making. Roger B. Dworkin. 1996. LC 95-50697. (Medical Ethics Ser.). 224p. text 35.00 (*0-253-33075-0*) Ind U Pr.

Limits & Lies of Human Genetic Research: Dangers for Social Policy. Jonathan Michael Kaplan. 2000. LC 99-44899. (Reflective Bioethics Ser.). (Illus.). xi, 224p. (C). text 85.00 (*0-415-92637-8*) Routledge.

Limits for Intakes of Radionuclides by Workers International Commission on Radiological Protection. Ed. by F. D. Sowby. 1982. (International Commission on Radiological Protection Ser.: No. 30). 2500p. 445.00 (*0-08-028863-4*, Pergamon Pr) Elsevier.

Limits for Intakes of Radionuclides by Workers. Ed. by F. D. Sowby. 1982. (ICRP Publication Ser.: No. 30, Pt. 3). 128p. pap. 35.50 (*0-08-026834-X*, Pergamon Pr) Elsevier.

Limits for Intakes of Radionuclides by Workers: Index. International Commission of Radiological Protection Staff. 1982. (International Commission on Radiological Protection Ser.). 73p. pap. 13.50 (*0-08-028884-7*, Pergamon Pr) Elsevier.

Limits for Intakes of Radionuclides by Workers: Report Commission 2 ICRP ADPTD 7-78, Supercedes ICRP 2. ICRP Staff. 1980. (Radiation Protection Ser.: Vol. 30: PT1S). (*0-08-024941-8*) Pergamon Repr GBR. *Dist:* Franklin.

Limits for Intakes of Radionuclides by Workers Pt. 4: An Addendum. ICRP Staff. 1989. (ICRP Publication Ser.: No. 30). 172p. pap. 37.50 (*0-08-036886-7*, Pergamon Pr) Elsevier.

Limits of Biological Treatments for Psychological Distress: Comparisons with Psychotherapy & Placebo. Ed. by Seymour Fisher & Roger P. Greenberg. 1989. 376p. (C). text 79.95 (*0-8058-0138-3*) L Erlbaum Assocs.

Limits of Litigation: The Dalkon Shield Controversy. Ronald J. Bacigal. 1990. LC 90-81011. 160p. 14.00 (*0-89089-391-8*) Carolina Acad Pr.

Limits of Medicine: How Science Shapes Our Hope for the Cure. Edward S. Golub. 1997. LC 96-45668. 262p. pap. 14.95 (*0-226-30207-5*) U Ch Pr.

Limits of Principle: Deciding Who Lives & What Dies. Tom Koch. 1998. LC 98-23553. 192p. 40.00 (*0-275-96407-8*, Praeger Pubs) Greenwood.

Limits of Professional Power: National Health Care in the Federal Republic of Germany. Deborah A. Stone. 1995. LC 80-16864. (Illus.). 244p. 25.50 (*0-226-77553-4*) U Ch Pr.

Limits of Scientific Psychiatry: The Role of Uncertainty in Mental Health. John O. Beahrs. 1986. LC 86-11692. 250p. text 39.95 (*0-87630-420-X*) Brunner-Routledge.

Limits to Medicine: Medical Nemenis: The Expropriation of Health. Ivan Illich et al. 1999. 312p. reprint ed. pap. 17.95 (*0-7145-2993-1*) M Boyars Pubs.

Limpieza Interna: Como Librarse de la Contaminacion en los Musculos, las Arterias, y las Articul. Carlson Wade. 2000. (SPA.). 345p. pap. 14.00 (*0-7352-0191-9*) PH Pr.

Linac Radiosurgery: A Practical Guide. William A. Friedman et al. 1997. LC 97-7619. (Illus.). 176p. 97.00 (*0-387-94698-5*) Spr-Verlag.

Linda Miles Practice Dynamics. Linda Miles. 1986. 160p. 29.95 (*0-87814-301-7*) PennWell Corp.

Lindane. 1991. (Environmental Health Criteria Ser.: No. 124). (ENG, FRE & SPA.). 208p. pap. text 37.00 (*92-4-157124-1*, 1160124) World Health.

Linear Accelerators for Radiation Therapy. D. Greene & P. C. Williams. 2nd ed. 1997. LC 97-28042. (Medical Science Ser.). pap. 50.00 (*0-7503-0476-6*); 156.00 (*0-7503-0402-2*) Inst of Physics Pubng.

Linear Alkylbenzene Sulfonates & Related Compounds. 1996. (Environmental Health Criteria Ser.: Vol. 169). 328p. (C). pap. 62.00 (*92-4-157169-1*, 1160169) World Health.

Lingual & Gastric Lipases: Their Role in Fat Digestion. Ed. by Margit Hamosh. 1990. 248p. 143.00 (*0-8493-6863-4*, QP609, CRC Reprint) Franklin.

Lingual Orthodontics. Ed. by Rafi Romano. 1998. 211p. incl. cd-rom (*1-55009-040-2*) DEKR.

Linguistic Basis of Communication Disorders. Schwartz. 1998. 36.00 net. (*1-56593-137-8*) Singular Publishing.

Linguistic Levels in Aphasiology. Ed. by Evy Visch-Brink & Roelien Bastiaanse. 1998. LC 97-52722. (Neurogenic Communication Disorders Ser.). (Illus.). 250p. pap. 79.95 (*1-56593-860-7*, 1680) Thomson Learn.

Linguistics & Psychoanalysis: Freud, Saussure, Hjelmslev, Lacan & Others. Michel Arrive. 1992. LC 92-8213. (Semiotic Crossroads Ser.: Vol. No. 4). xvi, 180p. 62.00 (*1-55619-338-6*) J Benjamins Pubng Co.

Linguistics in Clinical Practice. Ed. by Kim Grundy. 2nd ed. 1995. (Illus.). 410p. (C). 59.95 (*1-56593-514-4*, 1186) Thomson Learn.

Link Between ADD & Addiction: Getting the Help You Deserve. Wendy Richardson. 1997. LC 97-5122. 320p. pap. 16.00 (*1-57683-004-7*) Pinon Press.

Link Between Language & Consciousness: A Practical Philosophy. Marlene Carpenter. 1991. 120p. (C). pap. text 21.50 (*0-8191-8090-4*); lib. bdg. 46.00 (*0-8191-8089-0*) U Pr of Amer.

Linkage of Psychological Components with Vocational Loss/Access - An Assessment/Forensic Tool: Appendix Listing DOT Titles & Temperaments. Michelle A. Rowe. Ed. by Norman Iden. 1998. 367p. pap. 49.95 (*0-9666080-0-3*) Rowe Rehab.

Linking Alcoholism Treatment Research with Clinical Practice. 1992. (Illus.). 56p. (Orig.). (C). pap. text 25.00 (*1-56806-071-8*) DIANE Pub.

Linking Housing & Health Services for Older Persons. Frwd. by Daniel M. Fox & Sheldon L. Goldberg. 1997. LC 97-160855. 48p. (Orig.). pap. (*1-887748-09-1*) Milbank Memorial.

Linking Links: Persons Who Prepare Others for Caregiving: Instructor's Lesson Plans. Whorl et al. Ed. by Wingborne. 1992. (Illus.). 50p. (Orig.). pap. text, stu. ed. 12.95 (*0-9629755-1-6*) Wingborne-Diaconal.

Linking Objects & Linking Phenomena. Vamik D. Volkan & Harold F. Searles. 1981. LC 81-14278. 330p. 60.00 (*0-8236-3030-7*) Intl Univs Pr.

Linscott's Directory of Immunological & Biological Reagents. William D. Linscott. 10th rev. ed. 1998. 377p. pap. 85.00 (*0-9604920-9-7*) Linscotts Direct.

Lip Balm. Prentice-Hall Staff. text 6.47 (*0-13-800376-9*) PH School.

Lip Reading Made Easy. Edward B. Nitchie. 1985. LC 84-52486. (Illus.). 130p. pap. 10.00 (*0-915179-22-9*) Loompanics.

Lipid Chromatographic Analysis. Ed. by Takayuki Shibamoto. 1993. (Chromatographic Science Ser.: Vol. 65). (Illus.). 424p. text 175.00 (*0-8247-8941-5*) Dekker.

Lipid Handbook. J. L. Harwood & Frank D. Gunstone. 2nd ed. 1997. LC 94-70866. (Illus.). 1312p. (C). (gr. 13). ring bd. 519.95 (*0-412-43320-6*, Chap & Hall CRC) CRC Pr.

Lipid Homeostasis & the Kidney. Ed. by W. F. Keane & B. L. Kasiske. 1993. (Journal: Vol. 19, No. 3, 1993). (Illus.). 96p. pap. 41.00 (*3-8055-5832-5*) S Karger.

Lipid Hormone-Based Drug Therapies. Lynn Gray. 1997. LC 98-120893. (Report Ser.: No. B-116). (Illus.). 191p. 3150.00 (*1-56965-379-8*, B-116) BCC.

Lipid Lowering Therapy & Progression of Coronary Atherosclerosis. Ed. by A. V. Bruschke. 1996. (Developments in Cardiovascular Medicine Ser.). 240p. (C). text 129.00 (*0-7923-3807-3*) Kluwer Academic.

Lipid Mediators in Allergic Diseases of the Respiratory Tract. Clive Robinson. 1994. 268p. lib. bdg. 225.00 (*0-8493-5416-1*, RC859) CRC Pr.

Lipid Mediators in Eye Inflammation. Ed. by Nicolas G. Bazan. 1990. (New Trends in Lipid Mediators Research Ser.: Vol. 5). (Illus.). x, 192p. 155.00 (*3-8055-5067-7*) S Karger.

Lipid Mediators in Ischemic Brain Damage & Experimental Epilepsy. Ed. by Nicolas G. Bazan. 1990. (New Trends in Lipid Mediators Research Ser.: Vol. 4). (Illus.). viii, 262p. 207.00 (*3-8055-5068-5*) S Karger.

Lipid Mediators in the Immunology of Shock. Ed. by M. Paubert-Braquet et al. 1988. LC 87-29239. (NATO ASI Series A, Life Sciences: Vol. 139). (Illus.). 540p. 135.00 (*0-306-42694-3*, Plenum Trade) Perseus Pubng.

Lipid Metabolism in Normoxic & Ischemic Heart. Ed. by Ger J. Van der Vusse. 1989. (Developments in Molecular & Cellular Biochemistry Ser.). Orig. Title: Molecular & Cellular Biochemistry. (C). reprint ed. text 199.50 (*0-7923-0479-9*) Kluwer Academic.

Lipid Metabolism in the Healthy & Diseased Heart: Proceedings of the 3rd International Symposium on Lipid Metabolism in the Normoxic & Ischemic Heart, September 9-10, 1991, Rotterdam, The Netherlands. Ed. by Ger J. Van der Vusse & Hans Stam. 1992. LC 92-23631. 208p. (C). text 210.50 (*0-7923-1850-1*) Kluwer Academic.

Lipid Peroxidation in Vivo: Evaluation & Application of Methods for Measurement. Eva Sodergren. 2000. (Comprehensive Summaries of Uppsala Dissertations from the Faculty of Medicine Ser.: No. 949). (Illus.). 78p. (Orig.). pap. (*91-554-4791-0*) Uppsala Universitet SWE. *Dist:* Coronet Bks.

Lipid Storage Disorders: Biological & Medical Aspects. Ed. by R. Salvayre et al. 1988. (NATO ASI Series A, Life Sciences: Vol. 150). (Illus.). 856p. 165.00 (*0-306-42928-4*, Plenum Trade) Perseus Pubng.

Lipids. J. M. Lowenstein. Ed. by Sidney P. Colowick & Nathan O. Kaplan. 1969. (Methods in Enzymology Ser.: Vol. 14). text 209.00 (*0-12-181871-3*) Acad Pr.

Lipids. Ed. by Sidney P. Colowick et al. 1981. (Methods in Enzymology Ser.: Vol. 71). Pt. C. text 188.00 (*0-12-181971-X*); Pt. D. text 188.00 (*0-12-181972-8*) Acad Pr.

Lipids, Pt. B. Ed. by John M. Lowenstein. 1975. (Methods in Enzymology Ser.: Vol. 35). text 199.00 (*0-12-181935-3*) Acad Pr.

Lipids: Current Perspectives. Ed. by D. John Betteridge. 1996. 312p. (C). text (*1-85317-231-6*) Mosby Inc.

Lipids & Cardiovascular Disease. Ed. by D. J. Galton & G. R. Thompson. 1990. (Illus.). 264p. text (*0-443-04327-2*) Church.

Lipids & Heart Diseases: A Guide for the Primary Care Team. Madaleine Ball & Jim Mann. 2nd ed. 1995. (Illus.). 184p. pap. text 39.50 (*0-19-262495-4*) OUP.

Lipids & Lipid Disorders. Feher. 2nd ed. 1997. text (*0-7234-2830-1*) Wolfe Publishing.

Lipids & Lipid Disorders: An Essential Slide Collection. Michael Feher & William Richmond. 100p. sl. (*0-397-46496-7*, GM0089) Gower-Mosby.

Lipids & Lipoproteins. Ed. by M. Fondu. 1980. (Journal: Vol. 24, Suppl. 1). (Illus.). iv, 212p. 42.75 (*3-8055-1266-X*) S Karger.

Lipids & Lipoproteins in Clinical Practice. Neil & McIntyre. 1990. 160p. (C). (gr. 13). text 59.00 (*0-7234-0946-3*) Mosby Inc.

Lipids & Related Compounds. Ed. by Alan A. Boulton et al. 1989. LC 88-8909. (Neuromethods Ser.: Vol. 7). (Illus.). 360p. 119.50 (*0-89603-124-1*) Humana.

Lipids & Renal Disease. Ed. by William F. Keane. 1991. (Contemporary Issues in Nephrology Ser.: Vol. 24). (Illus.). 216p. text (*0-443-08779-2*) Church.

Lipids & Syndromes of Insulin Resistance: From Molecular Biology to Clinical Medicine. Ed. by Steven M. Haffner et al. 1997. LC 97-18285. (Annals of the New York Academy of Sciences Ser.: No. 827). 582p. 160.00 (*1-57331-070-0*) NY Acad Sci.

Lipids & Syndromes of Insulin Resistance: From Molecular Biology to Clinical Medicine. Ed. by Iwar Klimes et al. 1997. LC 97-18285. (Annals of the New York Academy of Sciences Ser.: No. 827). 582p. pap. 160.00 (*1-57331-071-9*) NY Acad Sci.

Lipids & the Kidney. Ed. by William F. Keane & Bertram L. Kasiske. 1997. LC 97-2775. (Contributions to Nephrology Ser.: Vol. 120, 1997). (Illus.). x, 234p. 199.25 (*3-8055-6389-2*) S Karger.

Lipids & Tumors. Ed. by K. K. Carroll. 1975. (Progress in Biochemical Pharmacology Ser.: Vol. 10). (Illus.). 300p. 128.75 (*3-8055-1708-4*) S Karger.

Lipids & Women's Health. Ed. by Geoffrey P. Redmond. 1990. (Illus.). 260p. 108.00 (*0-387-97318-4*) Spr-Verlag.

Lipids in Infant Nutrition. Ed. by Yung-Sheng Huang & Andrew J. Sinclair. 1998. LC 98-14490. (Illus.). 304p. lib. bdg. 99.00 (*0-935315-92-6*, PC121) Am Oil Chemists.

Lipids of Human Milk. Robert G. Jensen. 1988. 224p. 129.00 (*0-8493-6559-7*, QP246, CRC Reprint) Franklin.

Lipmann Symposium: Energy, Regulation & Biosynthesis in Molecular Biology. Ed. by Dietmar Richter. 1974. 698p. (C). 138.50 (*3-11-004976-7*) De Gruyter.

Lipo-Corticotropic Hormones & Cushing's Disease. Ed. by G. Copinschi & P. Jaquet. 1981. (Journal: Vol. 13, No. 4-5). (Illus.). 152p. pap. 57.50 (*3-8055-3410-8*) S Karger.

Lipofuscin & Ceroid Pigments. Ed. by Ernesto Porta. 1989. (Advances in Experimental Medicine & Biology Ser.: Vol. 266). (Illus.). 393p. 110.00 (*0-306-43519-5*, Plenum Trade) Perseus Pubng.

Lipofuscin & Ceroid Pigments: State of the Art, 1995. Ed. by K. Kitani et al. 1996. (Journal: Vol. 41, No. 2, 1995). (Illus.). x, 330p. pap., suppl. ed. 50.50 (*3-8055-6259-4*) S Karger.

Lipoic Acid: The Metabolic Antioxidant. Richard A. Passwater. 1996. (Good Health Guides). 48p. pap. 3.95 (*0-87983-720-9*, 37209K, Keats Pubng) McGraw-Hill Trade.

Lipoic Acid in Health & Disease. Ed. by Fuchs et al. 1997. LC 97-22478. (Antioxidants in Health & Disease Ser.: Vol. 7). (Illus.). 504p. text 185.00 (*0-8247-0093-7*) Dekker.

Lipolysis: The Theory & Practice of Suction Lipectomy. Gregory P. Hetter. 1984. 448p. 125.00 (*0-316-35920-3*, Little Brwn Med Div) Lppncott W & W.

Lipomatous Tumors: Diagnosis & Primary Treatment. Ed. by I. De Wever & M. Stas. 1997. (Illus.). 161p. (Orig.). pap. (*90-6186-798-3*) Leuven Univ BEL. *Dist:* Coronet Bks.

Lipophilicity in Drug Action & Toxicology. Ed. by Bernard Testa et al. 1996. (Methods & Principles in Medicinal Chemistry Ser.: Vol. 4). (Illus.). 439p. 205.00 (*3-527-29383-3*, Wiley-VCH) Wiley.

Lipoplasty: The Theory & Practice of Blunt Suction Lipectomy. Gregory P. Hetter. 2nd ed. 1990. 360p. text 250.00 (*0-316-35918-1*, Little Brwn Med Div) Lppncott W & W.

Lipoprotein Metabolism. Ed. by S. Eisenberg. 1979. (Progress in Biochemical Pharmacology Ser.: Vol. 15). (Illus.). 112.25 (*3-8055-2985-6*) S Karger.

Lipoprotein Precipitation. M. Burstein & P. Legmann. 1982. (Monographs on Atherosclerosis: Vol. 11). (Illus.). viii, 132p. 84.50 (*3-8055-3512-0*) S Karger.

Lipoproteins. Ed. by Edward G. Perkins. 1993. 176p. pap. 35.00 (*0-935315-48-9*) Am Oil Chemists.

Lipoproteins & Atherosclerosis. Ed. by C. L. Malmendier & P. Alaupovic. 1987. LC 87-2345. (Advances in Experimental Medicine & Biology Ser.: Vol. 210). 266p. 69.50 (*0-306-42487-8*, Plenum Trade) Perseus Pubng.

Lipoproteins in Health & Disease. Ed. by John Betteridge & James Shepherd. 1998. LC 98-3650. (An Arnold Publication). 1332p. (*0-340-55269-7*) E A GBR. *Dist:* OUP, Routldge.

Liposome Drug Delivery Systems. Guru Betageri et al. 1993. LC 93-60519. 152p. 84.95 (*1-56676-030-5*) CRC Pr.

Liposome Methods & Protocols. Ed. by Subhash C. Basu & Manju Basu. 2002. (Methods in Molecular Biology Ser.). 250p. 89.50 (*0-89603-845-9*) Humana.

Liposome Technology. Gregory Gregoriadis. Vol. I. 1984. 288p. lib. bdg. 179.00 (*0-8493-5316-5*, RS201); Vol. 1. 2nd ed. 1992. 656p. 179.00 (*0-8493-6707-7*, RS201); Vol. II. 1984. 256p. lib. bdg. 179.00 (*0-8493-5317-3*) CRC Pr.

Liposome Technology, Vol. 2. Ed. by Gregory Gregoriadis. 2nd ed. 1992. 368p. 179.00 (*0-8493-6708-5*, RS201) CRC Pr.

Liposome Technology. Gregory Gregoriadis. Vol. III. 1984. 312p. lib. bdg. 179.00 (*0-8493-5318-1*, RS201); Vol. 3. 2nd ed. 1992. 432p. 179.00 (*0-8493-6709-3*, RS201) CRC Pr.

Liposomes: Rational Design. Ed. by Andrew S. Janoff. 1998. LC 98-46309. (Illus.). 488p. text 195.00 (*0-8247-0225-5*) Dekker.

Liposomes in Biomedical Applications. Ed. by Pang N. Shek. 1995. (Drug Testing & Delivery Ser). 304p. text 132.00 (*3-7186-5701-5*, Harwood Acad Pubs) Gordon & Breach.

Liposomes in Drug Delivery. Ed. by G. Gregoriadis et al. 1993. (Drug Targeting & Delivery Ser.). 256p. text 128.00 (*3-7186-5265-X*) Gordon & Breach.

Liposomes in Drug Delivery. Ed. by Gregory Gregoriadis et al. 1992. LC 92-49658. (Drug Targeting & Delivery Ser.: Vol. 2). (*3-7186-5248-X*) Gordon & Breach.

Liposomes in Gene Delivery. Danilo D. Lasic. 1997. LC 96-35300. (Illus.). 320p. spiral bd. 74.95 (*0-8493-3109-9*) CRC Pr.

Liposuction: New Hope for a New Figure Through the Art of Body Contouring. Leon Tcheupdjian. 1989. (Illus.). 244p. (Orig.). text 29.95 (*0-9621284-0-6*); pap. text 24.95 (*0-9621284-1-4*) Liposuction Inst Am.

Liposuction & Aesthetic Surgery. Gerald H. Pitman. 1992. (Illus.). 478p. LC 92-532. 200.00 (*0-942219-18-X*); 245.00 incl. VHS (*1-57626-041-0*, QMP) Quality Med Pub.

Lippincott Manual of Nursing Practice. Sandra M. Nettina. 7th ed. 2000. LC 00-34902. (Illus.). 1,776p. text 59.95 (*0-7817-2296-9*) Lppncott W & W.

Lippincott's Computed Tomography Review. Phlipt-Scroggins. 1995. 288p. pap. text 29.95 (*0-397-55157-6*) Lppncott W & W.

Lippincott's Critical Care Drug Guide. Contrib. by Marla J. De Jong & Amy Morrison Karch. 2000. LC 99-52557. 704p. spiral bd. 29.95 (*0-7817-2196-2*) Lppncott W & W.

Lippincott's Guide to Behavior Management in Home Care. Nina A. Klebanoff & Nina M. Smith. 1997. LC 96-53511. 448p. pap. text 27.95 (*0-397-55432-X*) Lppncott W & W.

Lippincott's Handbook of Medical Assisting Procedures. Julie B. Hosley & Elizabeth Molle-Matthews. 1998. LC 98-21796. 479p. spiral bd. 23.95 (*0-7817-1458-3*) Lppncott W & W.

Lippincott's Home Care Manual Package. Mary Ann Chestnut. 1997. pap. text 127.00 (*0-7817-1622-5*) Lppncott W & W.

Lippincott's Illustrated Review: Physiology. Harvey. 1993. text (*0-397-51141-8*) Lppncott W & W.

Lippincott's Illustrated Reviews: Biochemistry. Pamela C. Champe & Richard A. Harvey. 1987. LC 65-9665. 441p. text 25.95 (*0-397-50801-8*, Lippnctt); 2nd ed. 1994. (Illus.). 420p. pap. text 35.00 (*0-397-51091-8*) Lppncott W & W.

Lippincott's Magnetic Resonance Imaging Review. Shappell. 1996. LC 96-157742. 256p. pap. text 29.95 (*0-397-55156-8*) Lppncott W & W.

Lippincott's Manual of Psychiatric Nursing Care Plans. Judith M. Schultz & Sheila L. Dark Videbeck. 5th ed. 1997. LC 97-26210. 448p. pap. text 39.95 (*0-397-55417-6*) Lppncott W & W.

Lippincott's Need-to-Know: Research Survival Guide. Ann M. Doordan. 1997. LC 97-13229. 208p. pap. text 17.95 (*0-7817-1040-5*) Lppncott W & W.

Lippincott's Need-to-Know ECG Facts. Mary J. Boyer. 1997. 288p. pap. text 18.95 (*0-397-55461-3*) Lppncott W & W.

Lippincott's Need-to-Know Psychotropic Drug Facts. Katharine Bailey & Amy M. Karch. 1997. LC 97-42713. (Need-to-Know Ser.). 240p. pap. text 17.95 (*0-7817-1039-1*) Lppncott W & W.

Lippincott's Nursing Drug Guide 2001. Amy Morrison Karch. 2000. (Lippincott's Nursing Drug Guide Ser.). 1,456p. pap. text 32.95 (*0-7817-2556-9*) Lppncott W & W.

Lippincott's Pocket Manual of Nursing Practice. Sandra Nettina. 1996. LC 96-15107. 1,040p. pap. text 28.95 (*0-397-55355-2*) Lppncott W & W.

Lippincott's Review for NCLEX-PN. Barbara Kuhn Timby & Bennita Vaughans. 5th ed. 1998. LC 97-36376. 576p. pap. text 32.00 (*0-397-55471-0*) Lppncott W & W.

Lippincott's Review for NCLEX-RN. D. McGovern Billings. 6th ed. 1997. LC 97-3490. 736p. pap. text 29.95 (*0-397-55452-4*) Lppncott W & W.

Lippincott's Review Series: Maternal-Newborn Nursing. Barbara R. Stright. 3rd ed. 2000. LC 00-37250. (Lippincott's Review Ser.). (Illus.). xvi, 328p. pap. text 25.95 (*0-7817-2238-1*) Lppncott W & W.

Lippincott's Review Series: Medical-Surgical Nursing. Ray A. Hargrove-Huttel. 3rd ed. 2000. LC 00-39093. (Lippincott's Review Ser.). (Illus.). 688p. pap. text 25.95 (*0-7817-1964-X*) Lppncott W & W.

Lippincott's Review Series: Mental Health & Psychiatric Nursing. Ann Isaacs. 3rd ed. 2000. LC 00-27375. (Lippincott's Review Ser.). 336p. pap. text 25.95 (*0-7817-2188-1*) Lppncott W & W.

Lippincott's Review Series: Pediatric Nursing. Mary Muscari. 3rd ed. 2001. LC 00-30162. (Lippincott's Review Ser.). 432p. pap. text 25.95 (*0-7817-2187-3*) Lppncott W & W.

Lippincott's State Board Review for NCLEX-RN. Edwina A. McConnell & LuVerne W. Lewis. 4th ed. 1989. text 24.50 (*0-397-54722-6*, Lippnctt) Lppncott W & W.

Lippincott's Textbook for Clinical Medical Assisting. Julie B. Hosley & Elizabeth Molle-Matthews. 800p. 54.00 (*0-7817-2339-6*) Lppncott W & W.

Lippincott's Textbook of Clinical Medical Assisting. Julie B. Hosley. 1999. LC 98-45295. 800p. text 39.95 (*0-7817-1457-5*) Lppncott W & W.

Liquid Chromatography - Mass Spectrometry: Applications in Agricultural, Pharmaceutical & Environmental Chemistry, 42. Ed. by Mark A. Brown. 1989. LC 89-18611. (ACS Symposium Ser.: No. 420). (Illus.). 312p. 75.00 (*0-8412-1740-8*) Am Chemical.

Liquid Chromatography Detectors. Ed. by Thomas M. Vickrey. 1983. LC 83-7428. (Chromatographic Science Ser.: Vol. 23). (Illus.). 448p. text 210.00 (*0-8247-1916-6*) Dekker.

Liquid Chromatography in Clinical Analysis. Ed. by Pokar M. Kabra & Laurence J. Marton. 1981. LC 80-84083. (Biological Methods Ser.). 466p. 145.00 (*0-89603-026-1*) Humana.

Liquor Problem: A Summary of Investigations Conducted by the Committee of Fifty, 1893-1903. Fifty Committee. 1978. LC 70-112533. (Rise of Urban America Ser.). reprint ed. 19.95 (*0-405-02444-4*) Ayer.

Liquor Problem in All Ages. Daniel Dorchester. Ed. by Gerald N. Grob. 1981. LC 80-1268. (Addiction in America Ser.). (Illus.). reprint ed. lib. bdg. 71.95 (*0-405-13582-3*) Ayer.

Lisa: The Story of an Irish Drug Addict. 1988. 205p. pap. (*1-85371-011-3*) Poolbeg Pr IRL. *Dist:* Dufour.

List of Battles & Roster of Regimental Surgeons & Assistant Surgeons During the War of the Rebellion (with a New Index to Names) U. S. Pension Bureau Staff. 1990. LC 88-60668. (American Civil War Surgery Ser.: No. 11). 386p. reprint ed. 65.00 (*0-930405-10-2*) Norman SF.

List of Fellows, 1913. American College of Surgeons Staff. ix, 187p. reprint ed. 39.00 (*0-932051-29-4*) Rprt Serv.

Listen to Me: Communicating the Needs of People with Profound & Multiple Disabilities. Pat Fitton. 1994. LC 93-33895. 200p. pap. 24.95 (*1-85302-244-6*) Taylor & Francis.

Listen to Me Good: The Life Story of an Alabama Midwife. Margaret C. Smith & Linda J. Holmes. 1996. LC 96-15037. (Women & Health Ser.). (Illus.). 178p. pap. 18.00 (*0-8142-0701-4*) Ohio St U Pr.

Listen to the Children: A Study of the Impact on the Mental Health of Children of a Parent's Catastrophic Illness. Cancer Care, Inc. Staff & National Cancer Foundation, Inc. Staff. 1977. LC 77-94376. 2.50 (*0-9606494-1-7*) Cancer Care.

Listen to Us, We're Not That Stupid: The People's Prescription for What Really Ails America's Health Care System. John E. Skvarla, III & Frank Elliott. 1994. LC 93-38373. 197p. 16.95 (*0-930095-28-6*); pap. 12.00 (*0-930095-29-4*) Signal Bks.

Listen to Your Body: And Add 10-15 Happy Healthy Years to Your Life. Lyle M. Becker. Ed. by Nancy Marriott. 2000. LC 99-98131. 126p. pap. 9.95 (*0-9661143-1-0*) Caliana Pub.

***Listen to Your Body: The Wisdom of the Dao.** Bisong Guo & Andrew Powell. 2001. LC 2001-27358. (Illus.). 208p. pap. 19.95 (*0-8248-2466-0*); text 39.00 (*0-8248-2381-8*) UH Pr.

Listen to Your Pain: The Active Person's Guide to Understanding. Ben E. Benjamin & Gale Borden. 1984. LC 82-20066. (Illus.). pap. 18.95 (*0-14-006687-X*, Penguin Bks) Penguin Putnam.

Listen with Mother: Consulting Users of Maternity Services. Rosemary Dodds. 1996. LC 96-131133. 84p. pap. text 34.99 (*1-898507-48-1*) Buttrwrth-Heinemann.

Listening: An Introduction to the Perception of Auditory Events. Stephen Handel. 1989. LC 88-22502. 611p. 75.00 (*0-262-08179-2*, Bradford Bks) MIT Pr.

Listening & Interpreting: The Challenge of the Work of Robert Langs. Ed. by James O. Raney. 1984. LC 83-8816. 544p. 50.00 (*0-87668-624-2*) Aronson.

Listening & Talking: A Guide to Promoting Spoken Language in Hearing-Impaired Children. Elizabeth B. Cole. 1992. 201p. (Orig.). (C). pap. text 25.95 (*0-88200-172-8*) Alexander Graham.

Listening Process. Robert J. Langs. 1978. LC 78-68010. 688p. 40.00 (*0-87668-341-3*) Aronson.

Listening Subjects: Music, Psychoanalysis, Culture. David Schwarz. 1997. LC 96-39870. (Illus.). 248p. lib. bdg. 49.95 (*0-8223-1929-2*) Duke.

Listening to Children. Carol R. Lewis. 1992. LC 84-11154. 208p. pap. 35.00 (*0-87668-285-9*) Aronson.

Listening to Gynaecological Patients' Problems. D. Jenkins. 2nd ed. 1998. LC 98-33389. (Illus.). 112p. pap. 39.00 (*1-85233-109-7*) Spr-Verlag.

Listening to Learn: A Handbook for Parents of a Hearing-Impaired Child. Arlie J. Adam et al. 1990. (Centennial Celebration Ser.). 110p. (Orig.). pap. text 19.95 (*0-88200-166-3*) Alexander Graham.

Listening to Life Stories: A New Approach to Stress Intervention in Health Care. Bruce Rybarczyk & Albert Bellg. 1997. 168p. 36.95 (*0-8261-9570-9*) Springer Pub.

Listening to Prozac: A Psychiatrist Explores Antidepressant Drugs & the Remaking of the Self. Peter D. Kramer. rev. ed. 1997. LC 92-50733. 448p. pap. 13.95 (*0-14-026671-2*) Penguin Putnam.

Listening to Women Talk about Their Health: Issues & Evidence from India. Ed. by Pertti J. Pelto et al. 1994. (C). text (*81-241-0274-0*) Har-Anand Pubns IND. *Dist:* S Asia.

Listening to Your Hormones. Gillian Ford. 1997. LC 95-23405. 496p. pap. 19.95 (*0-7615-1002-8*) Prima Pub.

Listening to Your Inner Voice: Discover the Truth Within You & Let It Guide Your Way. Douglas Bloch. 1991. 232p. pap. 9.95 (*1-56838-079-8*) Hazelden.

***Lister's the Hand.** Paul Smith. 2001. (Illus.). 615p. (*0-443-06416-4*) Church GBR. *Dist:* Saunders.

Lite Delight. 1993. (Favorite All Time Recipes Ser.). (Illus.). 96p. 7.98 (*0-7853-0064-3*, 2014903) Pubns Intl Ltd.

Lite Sweet Delites: Sweetened with Sugar Substitutes. Lee M. Cirillo. 1989. LC 89-91755. (Illus.). 226p. (Orig.). pap. 13.50 (*0-9623225-0-4*) SCP Rochester.

Literacy & Language Analysis. Ed. by Robert J. Scholes. 1993. 232p. text 49.95 (*0-8058-0920-1*) L Erlbaum Assocs.

Literatur der Medizin. Johann S. Ersch. 1965. (Handbuch der Deutschen Literatur Seit der Mitte des 18. Jahrhunderts Bis Auf die Neueste Zeit Ser.: Vol. V). 750p. reprint ed. (*3-487-07250-5*) G Olms Pubs.

Literature & Aging: An Anthology. Ed. by Martin Kohn et al. 1992. LC 92-7855. (Literature & Medicine Ser.: No. 1). (Illus.). 456p. (Orig.). pap. 29.00 (*0-87338-466-0*) Kent St U Pr.

Literature & the Relational Self. Barbara A. Schapiro. (Literature & Psychoanalysis Ser.). 201p. (C). 1995. pap. text 19.50 (*0-8147-8022-9*); 1993. LC 93-12879. text 50.00 (*0-8147-7969-7*) NYU Pr.

Literature Guide to the GLC of Body Fluids. Austin V. Signeur. 1982. LC 82-490. (IFI Data Base Library). 396p. 110.00 (*0-306-65203-X*, Kluwer Plenum) Kluwer Academic.

Literature of Animal Science & Health. Ed. by Wallace C. Olsen. 1993. 400p. 89.50 (*0-8014-2886-6*) Cornell U Pr.

Literature of 1950-1973. Gail G. Milgram. 1975. 20.00 (*0-911290-44-3*) Rutgers Ctr Alcohol.

Literature of 1978-1979. Penny B. Page & Gail G. Milgram. 1979. 10.00 (*0-911290-10-9*) Rutgers Ctr Alcohol.

Literature of 1973-1978. Gail G. Milgram & Mark Keller. 1980. 20.00 (*0-911290-06-0*) Rutgers Ctr Alcohol.

Literature of the Life Sciences. David A. Kronick. 1985. (Medical Library Association). 219p. 27.50 (*0-8108-2432-9*) Scarecrow.

***Literature Review on Electroconvulsive Therapy (ECT), 1980-1995.** Ed. by Barry Leonard. 2001. 68p. (C). reprint ed. pap. text 25.00 (*0-7567-0671-8*) DIANE Pub.

Lithium: Actions & Mechanisms. Rif S. El-Mallakh. 1996. (Progress in Psychiatry Ser.: No. 50). 208p. text 32.00 (*0-88048-481-0*, 8481) Am Psychiatric.

Lithium: Clinical & Biological Aspects. Ed. by F. A. Freyhan. 1972. (International Pharmacopsychiatry Ser.: Vol. 5, No. 2-4). (Illus.). 192p. pap. 51.50 (*3-8055-1277-5*) S Karger.

Lithium: Current Applications in Science, Medicine & Technology. Ed. by Ricardo Bach. 1985. LC 84-22210. 442p. text 100.00 (*0-471-80073-2*) Krieger.

Lithium & Manic Depression: A Guide. John T. Bohn & James W. Jefferson. rev. ed. 1999. 31p. pap. 4.95 (*1-890802-18-2*) Madison Inst of Med.

Lithium & the Blood. Ed. by V. S. Gallicchio. 1991. (Lithium Therapy Monographs: Vol. 4). (Illus.). x, 150p. 137.50 (*3-8055-5279-3*) S Karger.

Lithium & the Cell: Pharmacology & Biochemistry. Ed. by Nicholas J. Birch. 1991. (Illus.). 351p. text 104.00 (*0-12-099300-7*) Acad Pr.

Lithium & the Endocrine System. Ed. by F. N. Johnson. 1987. (Lithium Therapy Monographs: Vol. 2). (Illus.). xiv, 226p. 172.25 (*3-8055-4606-8*) S Karger.

Lithium & the Kidney. Ed. by S. Christensen. 1990. (Lithium Therapy Monographs: Vol. 3). (Illus.). xii, 188p. 164.50 (*3-8055-5042-1*) S Karger.

Lithium Combination Treatment. Ed. by F. N. Johnson. 1987. (Lithium Therapy Monographs: Vol. 1). (Illus.). xiv, 274p. 172.25 (*3-8055-4475-8*) S Karger.

Lithium in Biology & Medicine. Ed. by G. N. Schrauzer & K. F. Klippel. 1991. 209p. 75.00 (*3-527-28203-3*, Wiley-VCH) Wiley.

Lithium Treatment of Manic-Depressive Illness: A Practical Guide. M. Schou. 5th rev. ed. 1993. (Illus.). viii, 56p. pap. 15.75 (*3-8055-5667-5*) S Karger.

Litigation Assistant: A Guide for the Defendant Physician. American College of Obstetricians and Gynecologists Staff. 2nd ed. 1998. LC 98-14138. 19.00 (*0-915473-45-3*) Am Coll Obstetric.

Little Black Book of Dermatology. Stanford I. Lamberg. 2000. LC 00-36086. (Little Black Book Ser.). (Illus.). 432p. pap. 38.95 (*0-632-04519-1*) Blackwell Sci.

Little Black Book of Geriatrics. Karen Gershman et al. 1997. LC 97-37996. (Illus.). 288p. 38.95 (*0-632-04328-8*) Blackwell Sci.

Little Black Book of Home Care Cues. Ed. by Minnie B. Rose. 1996. LC 96-31652. (Illus.). 144p. (Orig.). ring bd. 21.95 (*0-87434-880-3*) Springhouse Corp.

Little Black Book of Neurology: A Manual for Neurological House Officers. Ed. by Alan J. Lerner. 3rd ed. 1994. LC 94-22738. (Illus.). 456p. (C). (gr. 13). pap. text 37.95 (*0-8151-5440-2*, 24022) Mosby Inc.

Little Black Book of Primary Care: Pearls & References. Daniel K. Onion. 3rd ed. LC 98-17781. (Little Black Book Ser.). 1998. (Illus.). 923p. pap. 39.95 (*0-632-04345-8*); 1996. 700p. spiral bd. 34.95 (*0-86542-489-6*) Blackwell Sci.

Little Black Book of Primary Care: Pearls & References. Daniel K. Onion. 2nd ed. 1995. 600p. (C). pap. (*0-393-71024-6*) Norton.

Little Black Book of Psychiatry. David P. Moore. 1999. LC 99-24497. (Little Black Book Ser.). xix, 337p. pap. 34.95 (*0-86542-562-0*) Blackwell Sci.

***Little Black Book of Sports Medicine.** Thomas Howard. 2001. (Little Black Book Ser.). (Illus.). 288p. pap. 38.95 (*0-86542-581-7*) Blackwell Sci.

Little Black Book of Urology. Pamela Ellsworth & Stephen N. Rous. 2001. LC 00-67463. (Blackwell's Primary Care Essentials Ser.). (Illus.). xxviii, 206p. pap. 38.95 (*0-86542-585-X*) Blackwell Sci.

Little Book about Baby. Compiled by Gladys Pucillo. 1981. 6.95 (*0-8378-1932-6*) Gibson.

Little Book of Doctors' Rule No. II: A Compilation. Clifton K. Meador. 2nd ed. 1999. LC 99-63780. 128p. (C). pap. 9.95 (*1-56053-365-X*) Hanley & Belfus.

Little Book of Doctors' Rules. Clifton K. Meador. 1992. (Orig.). pap. 9.95 (*1-56053-061-8*) Hanley & Belfus.

Little Book of Nurses' Rules. Ed. by Rosalie Hammerschmidt & Clifton K. Meador. 1993. LC 92-75322. 128p. (Orig.). pap. 10.95 (*1-56053-065-0*) Hanley & Belfus.

Little, Brown's NCLEX-RN Examination Review. Irene M. Bobak et al. Ed. by Sally L. Lagerquist. rev. ed. 1996. LC 95-49688. (Illus.). 680p. pap. text 36.95 (*0-316-51279-6*, Little Brwn Med Div) Lppncott W & W.

Little, Brown's Nursing Q&A: Critical-Thinking Exercises. Sally L. Lagerquist. 1996. LC 96-10793. (RN NCLEX Review Ser.). 412p. pap. text 32.95 (*0-316-51298-2*) Lppncott W & W.

***Little Child.** Diane-Lynn Broda. deluxe ed. 2000. (Illus.). xi, 240p. spiral bd. 50.00 (*0-9705699-7-1*) D Lynns Wrld.

Little Green Book: Questions for Radiology Conference & Examination Preparation. Eric P. Tamm. 2000. LC 99-89610. 416p. pap. text 49.95 (*0-683-30635-9*) Lppncott W & W.

Little Herb Encyclopedia. Jack Ritchason. 126p. 1984. spiral bd. 16.95 (*0-913923-18-4*); 2nd ed. 1994. pap. 9.95 (*0-913923-89-3*) Woodland UT.

Little Locksmith: A Memoir. Katharine Butler Hathaway. Ed. by William R. Phillips & Janet Rosenberg. 1980. LC 79-6904. (Physically Handicapped in Society Ser.). reprint ed. lib. bdg. 25.95 (*0-405-13113-5*) Ayer.

Little Pearls of Wisdom Book: For the Successful Dental Team. Henry Robinson. 1995. LC 95-1025. 19.95 (*0-87814-442-0*) PennWell Corp.

Little Red Book. Hazelden Foundation Staff. rev. ed. 1988. LC 87-45705. (Hazelden Book Ser.). 176p. 10.00 (*0-06-255470-0*) Harper SF.

Little Red Book. James Jennings. rev. ed. 1996. 153p. 10.00 (*0-89486-004-6*, 1030A) Hazelden.

Little Words That Grew: A Guide to Using Proverbs in the Therapeutic Process. Gary Beaulieu. 1998. LC 98-17909. 177p. pap. 18.00 (*1-882883-37-3*) Idyll Arbor.

Live & Be Well. Harry R. Litchfield. 1972. LC 72-76583. 300p. 12.95 (*0-87212-022-8*) Libra.

Live & Learn: An Introduction to the Psychology of Growth & Change in Everyday Life. Guy Claxton. 1984. 288p. pap. (*0-335-09809-6*) OpUniv Pr.

Live Better - Live Longer Resourcebook: Make the Second Half of Your Life the Better Half. Richard A. Herman. 1994. LC 93-73514. 180p. (Orig.). Vol. 2. pap. 12.95 (*1-884258-07-7*); Vol. 3. pap. 12.95 (*1-884258-08-5*) AltaMira Pr.

Live Better - Live Longer Resourcebook Vol. 1: Make the Second Half of Your Life the Better Half. Richard A. Herman. 1994. LC 93-73514. 180p. pap. 12.95 (*1-884258-06-9*) AltaMira Pr.

Live Company: Psychoanalytic Therapy with Autistic, Abused & Borderline Psychotic Children. Anne Alvarez. 1992. LC 91-40447. 264p. (C). pap. 27.95 (*0-415-06097-4*) Routledge.

Live in the Balance: The Ground-Breaking East-West Nutrition Program. Linda Prout. 2000. LC 00-56051. (Illus.). xv, 302p. pap. 16.95 (*1-56924-615-7*) Marlowe & Co.

Live Longer & Love It. Gordon R. Heath. 1980. LC 80-81595. (Illus.). 78p. (Orig.). pap. 5.95 (*0-937092-00-2*) Methuselah Bks.

Live Longer Better: Dr. Anderson's Complete Antiaging Health Program. James W. Anderson & Maury M. Breecher. 1997. LC 97-31746. 288p. pap. 12.95 (*0-7867-0472-1*) Carroll & Graf.

Live Now, Age Later: Proven Ways to Slow down the Clock. Isadore Rosenfeld. 2000. 480p. mass mkt. (*0-446-60910-2*, Warner Vision) Warner.

Live Right for Your Type: The Individualized Prescription for Maximizing Health, Well-Being & Vitality in Every Stage of Your Life. Peter J. D'Adamo & Catherine Whitney. 2000. LC 00-56500. 416p. 24.95 (*0-399-14673-3*) Penguin Putnam.

Live to Ninety & Stay Young. Andrew Stewart. 1968. 184p. pap. 17.95 (*0-8464-1029-X*) Beekman Pubs.

Live to Ninety & Stay Young. Andrew Stewart. 1980. 35.00 (*0-85032-030-5*) St Mut.

Live Well, Sleep Well: The Holistic Way to a Good Night's Sleep. Dan Campbell. 2000. LC 00-58300. xiv, 187p. pap. 12.95 (*0-87604-426-7*) ARE Pr.

Live Your Health: The Art & Practice of Holistic Healing. Reuben Halpern & Joshua Halpern. 1980. (Healing Arts Ser.). 220p. 12.95 (*0-89496-028-8*); 196p. pap. 9.95 (*0-89496-020-2*) Ross Bks.

Liver. Ed. by Mark Feldman & Willis C. Maddrey. 1995. LC 95-22343. (Gastroenterology & Hepatology Ser.: Vol. 1). (Illus.). 290p. text 85.00 (*1-878132-78-4*) Current Med.

Liver: Biology & Pathobiology. Ed. by Irwin M. Arias et al. 3rd ed. 1994. LC 93-23602. 1,664p. text 325.00 (*0-7817-0133-3*) Lppncott W & W.

***Liver: Biology & Pathobiology.** Irwin M. Arias & J. L. Boyer. 4th ed. 2001. LC 00-69996. (Illus.). 1,088p. text 249.00 (*0-7817-2390-6*) Lppncott W & W.

Liver & Biliary Diseases. Neil Kaplowitz. 1992. (Illus.). 752p. 115.00 (*0-683-04528-8*) Lppncott W & W.

Liver & Its Complaints. Herbert M. Shelton et al. 1996. 39p. reprint ed. spiral bd. 11.00 (*0-7873-1018-2*) Hlth Research.

Liver & Nervous Systems. Ed. by D. Haussinger & K. Jungermann. 1998. LC 98-196326. (Falk Symposium Ser.). 416p. 210.00 (*0-7923-8742-2*) Kluwer Academic.

Liver & Pancreas: Guides to Clinical Aspiration Biopsy. Denise Frias-Hidvegi. 1988. LC 87-4177. (Illus.). 352p. 95.00 (*0-89640-146-4*) Igaku-Shoin.

Liver & Systemic Disease. Norman Gitlin. 1997. LC 97-3036. text (*0-443-05546-7*) Church.

Liver, Biliary Tract & Exocrine Pancreas. Ed. by W. S. Symmers & D. G. Wight. 3rd ed. 1993. LC 93-13798. (Systemic Pathology Ser.: No. 11). (Illus.). 450p. text (*0-443-03098-7*) Church.

Liver Biopsy Diagnoses & Reports. J. Ludwig. 1984. (Illus.). x, 158p. 50.50 (*3-8055-3841-3*) S Karger.

Liver Biopsy Evaluation: Histologic Diagnoses with Clinical Correlations. Gary C. Kanel & Jacob Korula. Date not set. LC 99-59400. (Illus.). 220p. text (*0-7216-7692-8*) Saunders.

Liver Biopsy Interpretation. Paul J. Scheuer. 5th ed. 1994. text 86.00 (*0-7020-1594-6*) Saunders.

Liver Book: A Comprehensive Guide to Diagnosis, Treatment & Recovery. Sanjiv Chopra. 2001. LC 00-49135. (Illus.). 304p. 27.95 (*0-7434-0584-6*, PB Hardcover) PB.

***Liver Book: A Comprehensive Guide to Diagnosis, Treatment & Recovery.** Sanjiv Chopra. 2002. 304p. pap. 13.00 (*0-7434-0585-4*, PB Trade Paper) PB.

Liver Cancer. Ed. by Joseph C. Bottino et al. 1985. (Developments in Oncology Ser.). text 219.00 (*0-89838-713-2*) Kluwer Academic.

Liver Cancer. Okuda. 1997. text 150.00 (*0-443-05481-9*) Saunders.

Liver Carcinogenesis: The Molecular Pathays. Ed. by George G. Skouteris. 1994. LC 94-31130. (NATO ASI Ser.: 88). 483p. 263.00 (*3-540-58371-8*) Spr-Verlag.

Liver Carcinogenesis: The Molecular Pathways. Ed. by George G. SKouteris. 1994. (NATO ASI Ser.: Vol. 88). 512p. 214.00 (*0-387-58371-8*) Spr-Verlag.

Liver Causes Heart Attacks. W. P. Neufeld. 1991. 159p. (Orig.). pap. 14.95 (*0-88925-816-3*) Gordon Soules Bk.

Liver Cell Carcinoma. Ed. by P. Bannasch et al. 1989. (Falk Symposium Ser.). (C). lib. bdg. 242.00 (*0-7462-0111-7*) Kluwer Academic.

Liver Cirrhosis. Ed. by J. L. Boyer & L. Bianchi. 1987. (Falk Symposium Ser.: No. 44). text 206.50 (*0-85200-993-3*) Kluwer Academic.

Liver Cirrhosis. Ed. by Paolo Gentilini & M. U. Dianzani. 1984. (Frontiers of Gastrointestinal Research Ser.: Vol. 8). (Illus.). vii, 280p. 129.75 (*3-8055-3724-7*) S Karger.

Liver Disease in Children: An Atlas of Angiography & Cholangiography. Francis Brunelle et al. 1994. (Illus.). 290p. 165.00 (*3-540-19674-9*); LC 93-33451. 145p. 195.00 (*0-387-19674-9*) Spr-Verlag.

Liver Diseases: Targeted Diagnosis & Therapy Using Specific Receptors & Ligands. Ed. by George Y. Wu & Catherine H. Wu. 1991. (Targeted Diagnosis & Therapy Ser.: Vol. 4). (Illus.). 376p. text 175.00 (*0-8247-8486-3*) Dekker.

Liver Diseases in Children. Frederick J. Suchy. 2nd ed. 2000. LC 00-56914. 1,008p. text 169.00 (*0-7817-2098-2*) Lppncott W & W.

Liver Disorders in Childhood. Mowat. 1998. 496p. pap. 115.00 (*0-7506-4200-9*) Buttrwrth-Heinemann.

J
K
L

Liver Disorders in Childhood. Alex P. Mowat. 3rd ed. 1994. LC 93-31532. (Illus.). 496p. 160.00 (*0-7506-1039-5*) Buttrwrth-Heinemann.

Liver Disorders Sourcebook. Howard Worman. 1999. LC 99-24103. 352p. pap. 17.95 (*0-7373-0090-6*) Lowell Hse.

Liver Drugs: From Experimental Pharmacology to Therapeutic Application. Ed. by D. Perrissoud & B. Testa. 1988. 288p. 218.00 (*0-8493-6734-4*, RC846) CRC Pr.

Liver Function Vol. 3: Measurement in Medicine. Ed. by Derek Cramp & Ewart R. Carson. 1990. 300p. 74.95 (*0-412-33950-1*, A4470) Chapman & Hall.

Liver Growth & Repair. Ed. by A. J. Strain & A. M. Diehl. 1998. (Illus.). 688p. pap. (*0-412-71260-1*) Kluwer Academic.

Liver Imaging: Current Trends & New Techniques. Joseph T. Ferrucci & David D. Stark. 1990. (Illus.). 576p. text (*0-9626521-0-5*) E A GBR. *Dist:* OUP.

Liver Innervation & the Neural Control of Hepatic Function. Shimazu. 1996. 484p. (*0-86196-535-3*) J Libbey Med GBR. *Dist:* Buttrwrth-Heinemann.

Liver Malignancies: Diagnostic & Interventional Radiology. Ed. by C. Bartolozzi & R. Lencioni. 1999. LC 99-23562. (Medical Radiology Ser.). (Illus.). 300p. 299.00 (*3-540-64756-2*) Spr-Verlag.

Liver Metastasis. Ed. by J. H. Van de Velde et al. 1984. (Developments in Oncology Ser.). text 211.50 (*0-89838-684-5*) Kluwer Academic.

Liver Metastasis: Biology, Diagnosis & Treatment. Ed. by O. J. Garden et al. 1998. LC 97-52056. (Illus.). 224p. 79.00 (*3-540-76075-X*) Spr-Verlag.

Liver Microcirculation & Hepatobiliary Function. Ed. by K. Messmer & Michael D. Menger. 1993. LC 93-23883. (Progress in Applied Microcirculation Ser.: Vol. 19). (Illus.). viii, 172p. 161.75 (*3-8055-5701-9*) S Karger.

Liver, Nutrition, & Bile Acids. Ed. by G. Galli & E. Bosisio. 1985. (NATO ASI Series A, Life Sciences: Vol. 90). 270p. 69.50 (*0-306-42011-2*, Plenum Trade) Perseus Pubng.

Liver Pathology & Alcohol: Drug & Alcohol Abuse Reviews. Ed. by Ronald R. Watson. 1991. LC 91-20879. (Drug & Alcohol Abuse Reviews Ser.: No. 2). (Illus.). 620p. 135.00 (*0-89603-206-X*) Humana.

Liver Pathophysiology: Proceedings of the Annual Meeting of the Italian National Programme on Liver Cirrhosis & Viral Hepatitis, Held at San Miniato, Italy, 13-14 January, 1994. Italian National Programme on Liver Cirrhosis and Vi. Ed. by Mario U. Dianzani & Paolo Gentilini. 1994. LC 94-6966. (International Congress Ser.: No. 1060). 306p. 212.50 (*0-444-81637-2*, Excerpta Medica) Elsevier.

Liver Stem Cells: Normal Development, Carcinogenesis, Response to Injury & Role in Gene Therapy. Stewart Sell. 1997. (Medical Intelligence Unit Ser.). 250p. pap. 89.95 (*0-412-13491-8*) Chapman & Hall.

Liver Stem Cells: Special Edition. Stewart Sell & Zoran Illic. 1997. LC 96-29706. 335p. 99.00 (*1-57059-426-0*) Landes Bioscience.

Liver Surgery Approached Through the Mitochondria. K. Ozawa. 1993. (Illus.). 222p. 132.25 (*3-8055-5716-7*) S Karger.

Liver Transplantation. Ed. by Roy Y. Calne. 2nd ed. 1987. 576p. text 115.00 (*0-8089-1858-3*, 790768, Grune & Strat) Harcrt Hlth Sci Grp.

Liver Transplantation: Practice & Management. Ed. by James Neuberger & Michael Lucey. 1994. 420p. pap. text (*0-7279-0787-5*) BMJ Pub GBR. *Dist:* AIDC.

Liver Transplantation & the Alcoholic Patient. Ed. by M. R. Lucey et al. 1994. (Illus.). 144p. (C). text 52.95 (*0-521-43332-0*) Cambridge U Pr.

Liver Tumors: Multidisciplinary Management. W. John Hodgson. 1988. (Illus.). 340p. 47.50 (*0-87527-351-3*) Green.

Liver Update, 1981: Proceedings of an International Symposium on Recent Advances in Liver Physiology & Disease. Ed. by Ralph Kirsch et al. 1981. 150p. (C). pap. text (*0-86961-138-0*) A A Balkema NLD. *Dist:* Ashgate Pub Co.

Lives at Risk. Hilary Ryglewicz & Bert Pepper. 1996. LC 96-366. (Illus.). 288p. 29.95 (*0-684-82807-3*) Free Pr.

Lives at Risk: Public Health in Nineteenth-Century Egypt. LaVerne Kuhnke. 1990. LC 89-33122. (Comparative Studies of Health Systems & Medical Care: Vol. 24). text 50.00 (*0-520-06364-3*) U CA Pr.

Lives, Events & Other Players: Studies in Psychobiology. Ed. by Joseph T. Coltrera. 1979. LC 79-51911. (Downstate Psychoanalytic Institute Twenty-Fifth Anniversary Ser.: Vol. IV). 40.00 (*0-87668-369-3*) Aronson.

Lives in Distress: The Paths of the Elderly to the Psychiatric Ward. Marjorie F. Lowenthal. Ed. by Leon Stein. 1980. LC 79-8675. (Growing Old Ser.). reprint ed. lib. bdg. 28.95 (*0-405-12791-X*) Ayer.

Lives in Process: Mildly Retarded Adults in a Large City. Ed. by Robert B. Edgerton. 1984. LC 84-2869. (Monographs of the American Association on Mental Retardation: No. 6). 192p. text 8.00 (*0-940898-13-6*) Am Assn Mental.

Lives of a Cell: Notes of a Biology Watcher. Lewis Thomas. 1978. LC 77-23762. 160p. pap. 13.00 (*0-14-004743-3*, Penguin Bks) Penguin Putnam.

Lives of Lesions: Chronology in Dermatopathology. A. Bernard Ackerman & Raqaz. 1984. (Illus.). 266p. text 94.50 (*0-8121-1215-6*) Lppncott W & W.

Lives of University Hospitals of Cleveland: The 125-Year Evolution of an Academic Medical Center. Mark Gottlieb. 1991. LC 91-66654. (Illus.). 352p. 21.95 (*0-940601-06-0*, Wilson St Press) Octavia Ohio.

Lives Written in Sand: Addiction Awareness & Recovery Strategies. Thomas Byrd. 1997. (Illus.). 354p. (Orig.). pap. text, per. 33.00 (*0-9653658-0-8*) Hallum Pub.

Livestock & Poultry Production see Modern Livestock & Poultry Production

Livestock Environment IV. 1993. LC 93-71585. 1274p. 76.75 (*0-929355-41-5*, P0393) Am Soc Ag Eng.

Livestock Nutrition. Leslie D. Kamstra. 1982. (Illus.). 223p. (C). pap. text 13.95 (*0-89641-081-1*) American Pr.

Livestock Nutrition. Richard Warner. 1999. 29.95 (*0-8493-8763-9*) CRC Pr.

Living a Caring-Based Program. Ed. by Anne Boykin. 1993. LC 94-171951. 188p. 20.95 (*0-88737-591-X*, 14-2536, NLN Pr) Natl League Nurse.

Living Allergy Free: How to Create & Maintain an Allergen & Irritant-Free Environment. M. Eric Gershwin & Edwin L. Klingelhofer. 1992. LC 91-45417. (Illus.). 294p. 39.50 (*0-89603-225-6*) Humana.

Living Anatomy. Metcalf & Metcald. 1991. (*0-8151-5894-7*) Mosby Inc.

Living Anatomy: A Workbook Using Computed Tomography, Magnetic Resonance, & Angiography. Squire & Robert A. Novelline. 1986. 35.00 (*0-8016-4746-0*) Mosby Inc.

Living Anatomy: A Working Atlas Using Computed Tomography, Magnetic Resonance & Angiography Images. Robert A. Novelline & Lucy F. Squire. 1986. LC 86-80893. (Illus.). 117p. (Orig.). pap. 39.95 (*0-932883-03-6*) Hanley & Belfus.

Living & Dying Well. Lewis Petrinovich. 1996. LC 96-6465. (Critical Issues in Social Justice Ser.). (Illus.). 374p. 54.50 (*0-306-45171-9*, Kluwer Plenum) Kluwer Academic.

Living & Dying Well. Lewis Petrinovich. 1998. LC 98-24299. (Illus.). 374p. pap. 24.95 (*0-262-66142-X*, Bradford Bks) MIT Pr.

Living & Dying with AIDS. P. I. Ahmed. 1991. (Illus.). 296p. (C). 47.50 (*0-306-43851-8*, Plenum Trade) Perseus Pubng.

Living & Relating: An Introduction to Phenomenology. Carol S. Becker. 1992. (Illus.). 224p. 63.95 (*0-8039-3902-7*, 3281); pap. 32.95 (*0-8039-3903-5*, 3282) Sage.

Living & Working in the Community. Ed. by Steven J. Friedman & Kenneth G. Terkelsen. 1990. (Issues in Community Mental Health Ser.). (C). pap. text 6.95 (*0-88135-055-9*, Prodist) Watson Pub Intl.

Living & Working with New Biomedical Technologies: Intersections of Inquiry. Ed. by Margaret Lock et al. 2000. LC 99-24537. (Cambridge Studies in Medical Anthropology: No. 8). (Illus.). 306p. (C). text 59.95 (*0-521-65210-3*) Cambridge U Pr.

Living & Working with Schizophrenia. J. J. Jeffries et al. 1990. 227p. pap. text 13.95 (*0-8020-6781-6*) U of Toronto Pr.

Living at the Boundary: The Collected Works of Laura Perls. Laura P. Perls. 1991. 240p. text 35.00 (*0-939266-15-6*) Gestalt Journal.

Living Better: Every Patient's Guide to Living with Illness. Carol J. Langenfeld & Douglas E. Langenfeld. 2001. LC 00-192583. 250p. pap. 14.95 (*0-9701545-1-8*) Patient Pr.

Living Beyond Breast Cancer: A Survivor's Guide for When Treatment Ends & the Rest of Your Life Begins. Marisa Weiss. 1998. LC 99-228910. 528p. pap. 16.00 (*0-8129-3066-5*, Crown) Crown Pub Group.

Living Beyond Breast Cancer: A Survivor's Guide for When Treatment Ends & the Rest of Your Life Begins. Marisa C. Weiss & Ellen Weiss. 2000. 506p. reprint ed. text 27.00 (*0-7881-9069-5*) DIANE Pub.

Living Beyond Food. Gregory L. Jantz. 1991. (Orig.). pap. 12.95 (*0-9628408-0-7*) Ctr Counsel Hlth Resc.

Living Can Be Hazardous to Your Health. Florian Raymond. 1996. 10.95 (*0-943873-43-6*) Elder Bks.

Living Control Systems II. William T. Powers. 1992. (Selected Papers of William T. Powers). (Illus.). 277p. (Orig.). (C). pap. text 22.00 (*0-9624154-2-1*) New View Pubns.

Living Creatively with Chronic Illness: Transcending the Loss, Pain & Frustration. Eugenie G. Wheeler & Joyce Dace-Lombard. Ed. by Eugene D. Wheeler. 1989. LC 89-9250. 240p. pap. 11.95 (*0-934793-17-4*) Pathfinder CA.

Living Downstream: A Scientist's Personal Investigation of Cancer & the Environment. Sandra Steingraber. 1998. LC 98-21955. 384p. pap. 14.00 (*0-375-70099-4*) Vin Bks.

Living Eye. Jean Starobinski. Tr. by Arthur Goldhammer from FRE. 1989. LC 88-29398. (Studies in Comparative Literature: No. 40). (Illus.). 264p. 45.50 (*0-674-53664-9*) HUP.

Living Fear Free: Overcoming Agoraphobia - The Anxiety & Panic Syndrome. Melvin D. Green. 1985. LC 85-80401. 173p. text 16.95 (*0-939637-00-6*) Fear Free.

Living Fit. Francis J. Nagle et al. 1988. 300p. (C). pap. text 23.75 (*0-8053-8180-5*) Benjamin-Cummings.

Living for Tomorrow: A Positive Approach to the Treatment of Cervical Cancer. Margaret Wilson. 1994. 272p. (Orig.). pap. (*0-85572-227-4*) Hill Content Pubng AUS. *Dist:* Seven Hills Bk.

Living Free. Neva Coyle. 1981. LC 81-3811. 128p. pap. 6.99 (*0-87123-346-0*) Bethany Hse.

Living from Your Soul. Karen Katafiasz. 1997. LC 97-72947. (Elf-Help Bks.). (Illus.). 88p. pap. 4.95 (*0-87029-303-6*, 20146) Abbey.

Living Function of Sleep, Life & Aging. Betty Yulin Ho. 1967. LC 79-13810. (System of Government in the Living Body Ser.). (Illus.). 56p. pap. 12.00 (*0-9600148-0-2*) Juvenescent.

Living Healthy in a Toxic World: Simple Steps to Protect You & Your Family from Everyday Chemicals, Poisons & Pollution. David Steinman & Michael Wisner. 1996. LC 95-43241. 208p. (Orig.). pap. 12.95 (*0-399-52206-9*, Perigee Bks) Berkley Pub.

Living Heart Cookbook. Antonio M. Gotto, Jr. 1994. 352p. pap. 14.00 (*0-671-88388-7*, Fireside) S&S Trade Pap.

Living High: Daily Marijuana Use among Adults. Herbert Hendin et al. 1987. LC 86-27634. 183p. 34.95 (*0-89885-329-X*, Kluwer Acad Hman Sci) Kluwer Academic.

Living in the Labyrinth: A Personal Journey Through the Maze of Alzheimer's Disease. Diane F. McGowin. 1993. 133p. pap. 10.95 (*0-943873-18-5*) Elder Bks.

Living in the Post-Mastectomy Body: Learning to Live in & Love Your Body Again. Rebecca Zuckweiler. 1998. LC 98-18466. (Illus.). 282p. pap. 19.95 (*0-88179-152-0*) Hartley & Marks.

Living in the Question: An Exploration of Formlessness, Change, & Healing. Michael J. Maley. 1995. (Illus.). (Orig.). pap. 13.95 (*0-9649741-0-X*) Bodysmart Pubns.

Living in the Real World Vol. III: Participants Manual - From the "A Path to Responsibility" Treatment Program. G. Richard Kishur. 1994. 189p. stu. ed., spiral bd. 19.95 (*1-885473-03-6*) Wood N Barnes.

Living in the Shadow of Death: Tuberculosis & the Social Experience of Illness in American History. Sheila M. Rothman. 1995. LC 95-19372. 332p. reprint ed. pap. text 17.95 (*0-8018-5186-6*) Johns Hopkins.

Living Inside Prison Walls: Adjustment Behavior. Victoria R. Derosia. 1998. LC 98-15659. 224p. 60.00 (*0-275-95895-7*, Praeger Pubs) Greenwood.

Living Laboratories: Women & Reproductive Technology. Robyn Rowland. 1992. LC 92-13199. 384p. 37.95 (*0-253-34999-0*); pap. 6.95 (*0-253-20760-6*, MB-760) Ind U Pr.

Living Lean by Choosing More. Cheryl Jennings-Sauer. 1989. LC 88-24823. (Illus.). 200p. (Orig.). pap. 14.95 (*0-87833-604-4*) Taylor Pub.

Living Life Free from Pain: Treating Arthritis, Joint Pain, Muscle Pain & Fibromyalgia with Maharishi Vedic Medicine. Kumuda Reddy & Cynthia Lane. 2000. (Illus.). 300p. pap. 18.95 (*1-929297-17-3*) Samhita Prodns.

Living Life Well: New Strategies for Hard Times. Patricia Robinson. 1996. (Illus.). 109p. (Orig.). pap., wbk. ed. 19.95 (*1-878978-27-6*) Context Pr.

Living Life's Emergencies: Text for Total Emergency Preparedness. Patrick LaValla & Robert C. Stoffel. rev. ed. 1992. (Illus.). (C). pap. 35.00 (*0-913724-40-8*) Emerg Response Inst.

Living Longer & Better. Harold Elrick. 1978. pap. 5.95 (*0-02-499950-4*, Macmillan Coll) P-H.

Living Longer & Livelier: Guidelines for Older Adults. James H. Humphrey. 1999. LC 99-52429. (Illus.). xvii, 187p. (*1-56072-745-4*, Nova Kroshka Bks) Nova Sci Pubs.

Living Longer & Stronger: The Six-Week Plan to Enhance & Extend Your Years Over Forty. Ellington Darden. 1995. LC 94-26838. 224p. pap. 14.95 (*0-399-51900-9*, Perigee Bks) Berkley Pub.

Living Longer, Growing Stronger: The Vital Role of Geriatric Medicine: Congressional Hearing. Ed. by Charles E. Grassley. 2000. 125p. (C). reprint ed. pap. text 25.00 (*0-7881-8694-9*) DIANE Pub.

Living Longer in the Boomer Age: Combining Alternative & Conventional Medicine for Maximum Health & Vitality. John L. Zenk. 1998. LC 98-73258. 160p. per. 9.95 (*1-889462-03-9*) Advanced Research Pr.

Living Longer, Living Better, Slowing Aging with the Longevity Factor see Longevity Factor: Chromium Picolinate

Living Longer, Living Stronger. Normal Wall. 1997. 200p. pap. 14.95 (*0-9639683-1-9*) Vitality Corp.

Living Longer with Heart Disease: The Noninvasive Approach That Will Save Your Life. Howard H. Wayne. 1998. LC 98-14179. 260p. 22.95 (*1-885987-12-9*, Health Info Pr) Practice Mgmt Info.

Living, Loving, & Laughing with Pain. Jacqueline J. Pliskin. 1995. 272p. pap. 19.95 (*0-9647480-0-2*) Words & Pict.

Living, Loving & Learning. Leo F. Buscaglia. 1982. LC 81-824284. 264p. 13.50 (*0-913590-88-6*) SLACK Inc.

Living Morphogenesis of the Heart. Maria Victoria De la Cruz & Roger R. Markwald. 1998. LC 99-158844. (Cardiovascular Molecular Morphogenesis Ser.). (Illus.). 232p. 95.00 (*0-8176-4037-1*) Birkhauser.

Living New World Monkeys (Platyrrhini) With an Introduction to Primates. Vol. 1. Philip Hershkovitz. 1978. LC 75-9059. (Living New World Monkeys Ser.: Vol. 1). (Illus.). 1132p. lib. bdg. 132.00 (*0-226-32788-4*) U Ch Pr.

***Living on Medicine: A Cultural Study of End-Stage Renal Disease.** Jeannie Devitt. 1998. pap. (*1-86465-002-8*) IAD Pr AUS. *Dist:* Intl Spec Bk.

***Living on the Margin: Women Writers on Breast Cancer.** Ed. by Hilda Raz. 2001. 304p. reprint ed. pap. 15.95 (*0-89255-270-0*) Persea Bks.

***Living on the Razor's Edge.** Matthew Selekman. 2002. LC 2001-44674. 320p. 32.00 (*0-393-70335-5*) Norton.

Living Outside the Nursing Home: A Care Giver's Guide to Giving Nursing Home Care at Home. Linda Faber-Czingula. 1996. (Illus.). 183p. ring bd. 12.95 (*1-890118-05-2*, QualityCare Pub) Convalescnt Cnslts.

Living Positively: A Guide for Parents & Careers of Children Affected by HIV. Christine Hogg. 1997. 41p. pap. (*1-874579-97-0*) Natl Childrens Bur GBR. *Dist:* Paul & Co Pubs.

Living Positively in a World with HIV-AIDS. Mark De Solla Price. 1995. LC 94-16832. (Orig.). pap. 10.00 (*0-380-77623-5*, Avon Bks) Morrow Avon.

Living Psychology Instructor's Manual. James Lugo. 1990. 118p. (C). pap. text (*1-56226-025-1*) CAT Pub.

Living Related Donor Liver Transplantation: Assessment of Graft Viability Based on the Redox Theory. K. Ozawa. 1994. (Illus.). xii, 212p. 195.00 (*3-8055-5800-7*) S Karger.

Living Skills for the Brain Injured Child & Adolescent: A Rehabilitation Workbook. Julie M. Buxton & Kelly B. Godfrey. 1999. 400p. (ps-12). wbk. ed. 39.95 (*0-937857-80-7*, 1350) Speech Bin.

Living Sober see Viviendo Sobrio

Living Sober. 1990. (RUS.). pap. 1.35 (*0-916856-27-5*) AAWS.

Living State II. Ed. by R. K. Mishra. 1985. 712p. 121.00 (*9971-978-26-1*) World Scientific Pub.

Living Stones of the Himalayas: Adventures of an American Couple in Nepal. Thomas Hale. 1993. LC 93-18398. 256p. pap. 19.99 (*0-310-38511-3*) Zondervan.

Living Through Loss: A Manual for Those Working with Issues of Terminal Illness & Bereavement. Fay W. Jacobsen et al. 1996. 200p. pap. (*1-85302-395-7*) Jessica Kingsley GBR. *Dist:* Taylor & Francis.

Living Through Mourning: Finding Comfort & Hope When a Loved One Has Died. Harriet S. Schiff. 1987. LC 86-30676. 320p. pap. 13.95 (*0-14-010309-0*, Penguin Bks) Penguin Putnam.

Living Through the Older Years. Ed. by Clark Tibbitts & Robert J. Kastenbaum. 1979. LC 78-22221. (Aging & Old Age Ser.). reprint ed. lib. bdg. 19.95 (*0-405-11834-1*) Ayer.

Living Tree: The Roots & Growth of Jewish Law. Elliot N. Dorff & Arthur Rossett. 1987. LC 86-14581. 680p. (C). pap. text 24.95 (*0-88706-460-4*) State U NY Pr.

Living Well. Cu Byer & Shainberg. 1991. (C). pap. text 48.00 (*0-673-39885-4*) Addson-Wesley Educ.

Living Well. 3. Fries. 3rd ed. 1999. 320p. pap. text 18.00 (*0-7382-0059-X*) Perseus Bks Grp.

Living Well: Health in Your Hands. Curtis O. Byer & Louis W. Shainberg. 2nd ed. 1997. LC 94-3413. (Health Science Ser.). (Illus.). 796p. (C). pap. text 48.95 (*0-673-52337-3*, 52337-3) Jones & Bartlett.

Living Well: Taking Care of Your Health in the Middle & Later Years. James F. Fries. 2nd ed. 1993. LC 93-23756. (Illus.). 352p. pap. 17.95 (*0-201-62615-2*) Addison-Wesley.

Living Well: The Gay Man's Essential Health Guide. Peter Shalit. 1998. LC 98-39946. 336p. pap. 17.95 (*1-55583-444-2*, Alyson Bks) Alyson Pubns.

***Living Well Past 60.** George H. Hess. 1993. 191p. pap. 9.95 (*0-943685-17-6*) Essential Science.

Living Well-Walter Reed. Fries. 2nd ed. 1994. pap. (*0-201-62614-4*) Addison-Wesley.

Living Well with Asthma. Michael R. Freedman et al. 1998. LC 97-48747. 213p. 34.95 (*1-57230-318-2*, C0318); pap. 15.95 (*1-57230-051-5*, C0051) Guilford Pubns.

Living Well with Chronic Illness. Gayle Heiss. 1992. 16p. pap. 2.00 (*0-936609-10-9*) QED Ft Bragg.

Living Well with Epilepsy. Robert J. Gumnit. 2nd ed. 1997. LC 97-31340. 176p. pap. 19.95 (*1-888799-11-0*) Demos Medical.

Living Well with Hearing Loss: A Guide for the Hearing Impaired & Their Families. Debbie Huning. 1992. LC 91-39471. 192p. pap. 12.95 (*0-471-54522-8*) Wiley.

Living Well with HIV & AIDS. Allen Gifford. 1996. 296p. pap. text 18.95 (*0-923521-35-6*) Bull Pub.

Living Well with Macular Degeneration: Practical Tips & Essential Information. Bruce P. Rosenthal & Kate Kelly. 2001. LC 00-66843. (Illus.). vi, 272p. pap. 12.95 (*0-451-20264-3*) NAL.

Living Well with Multiple Sclerosis: A Guide for Patient, Caregiver, & Family. David L. Carroll & Jon Dorman. 1993. LC 92-53396. 272p. (Orig.). pap. 13.00 (*0-06-096980-6*, Perennial) HarperTrade.

Living Well with Parkinsons. Glenna W. Atwood. 1991. LC 90-42200. 208p. pap. 16.95 (*0-471-52539-1*) Wiley.

Living Wellness: Directory & Journal of Holistic Practices & Providers Los Angeles 1998-1999 Living Wellness Staff. 1998. (Illus.). 127p. pap. 4.95 (*0-9666402-0-9*) Liv Wellness.

Living Wild Flower Remedies: The Stananovs Method. Ingrid Hobart & Harald W. Tietze. 2000. (Illus.). 107p. pap. 12.95 (*0-8464-5198-0*) Beekman Pubs.

Living with a Broken String. Mary C. Greene. 1988. LC 87-92172. 221p. 12.95 (*0-9619979-0-7*) M C Greene.

Living with a Chronic Condition: A Practitioner's Guide. Alison Crumbie et al. 2002. (Illus.). 240p. pap. 40.50 (*0-7506-4808-2*) Buttrwrth-Heinemann.

Living with a Deaf Dog. Susan C. Becker. 1997. (Illus.). viii, 84p. pap. 15.95 (*0-9660058-0-5*) S C Becker.

Living With a Hearing Problem: Coping Strategies & Devices for the Hearing Impaired. Fred M. Roberts. 1990. (Illus.). 184p. pap. 16.95 (*0-912746-10-6*) F M Roberts.

Living with a Learning Disability. Barbara Cordoni. rev. ed. 1991. 174p. pap. 17.95 (*0-8093-1668-4*) S Ill U Pr.

Living with a Sick Child in Hospital. Philip Darbyshire. 1994. 225p. pap. 36.95 (*0-412-61050-7*) Chapman & Hall.

Living with a Stranger. Valerie Stillwell. LC 98-133674. (Illus.). 14.50 (*0-88048-582-5*) Am Psychiatric.

Living with a Stranger: A Discourse on the Human Body. John S. Collis. 1999. LC 78-21307. reprint ed. pap. 4.95 (*0-8076-0912-9*) Braziller.

Living with ADD: A Workbook for Adults with Attention Deficit Disorder. M. Susan Roberts & Gerard J. Jansen. 1997. LC 96-71152. 176p. (Orig.). pap., wbk. ed. 17.95 (*1-57224-063-6*) New Harbinger.

Living with ADHD: A Practical Guide to Coping with Attention Deficit Hyperactivity Disorder. Rebecca Kajander. 1995. (Illus.). 72p. (Orig.). pap. text 9.95 (*1-884153-08-9*) Prk Nicollet.

Living with AIDS. Ed. by Stephen R. Graubard. 1990. LC 89-13951. 462p. pap. text 23.00 (*0-262-57079-3*) MIT Pr.

Living with AIDS: A Photographic Journal. Sal Lopes. 1997. (Illus.). 133p. reprint ed. text 15.00 (*0-7881-5077-4*) DIANE Pub.

Living with AIDS: A Survival Guide. Christina Dye. rev. ed. 1999. pap. 0.50 (*0-89230-235-6*) Do It Now.

Living with AIDS: Experiencing Ethical Problems. Miriam Cameron. 1993. (Illus.). 256p. (C). 68.95 (*0-8039-4778-X*, 4253); pap. 31.95 (*0-8039-4779-8*, 4254) Sage.

Living with Alzheimer's. Tom Smith. 2000. pap. (*0-85969-832-7*) Sheldon Pr GBR. *Dist:* Intl Pubs Mktg.

Living with Alzheimer's: Ruth's Story. Art Danforth. 1986. LC 86-21052. Orig. Title: The Book of Ruth. 224p. (Orig.). 15.95 (*0-939533-02-2*); pap. 9.95 (*0-939533-01-4*) Howarth Pr.

Living with Alzheimer's Disease: One Couple's Journey. Frances Siegel. 2000. LC 99-45213. (Illus.). xv, 65p. pap. 9.95 (*1-889059-81-1*) Regent Pr.

Living with an Empty Chair: A Guide Through Grief. Roberta Temes. 2nd ed. LC 83-12894. 110p. 1984. (Illus.). 12.95 (*0-8290-1473-X*); 1992. reprint ed. pap. 9.95 (*0-8290-1773-9*) Irvington.

Living with Angina. Tom Smith. 1997. LC 96-71156. 128p. pap. 12.95 (*1-57224-067-9*) New Harbinger.

Living with Anorexia & Bulimia. James Moorey. 1993. (Living with Ser.). 176p. (C). text (*0-7190-3369-1*) Manchester Univ Pr GBR. *Dist:* St Martin.

Living with Anxiety: A Practical Research-Based Plan for Managing Anxiety Problems. Bob Montgomery & Laurel Morris. 1995. (Orig.). 232p. pap. (*0-85091-425-6*); audio (*0-85091-539-2*) Lothian Pub AUS. *Dist:* Seven Hills Bk.

Living with Aphasia: Psychosocial Issues. D. Lafond et al. 1992. LC 92-49888.Tr. of L'Aphasie. (Illus.). 308p. (Orig.). (C). pap. text 49.95 (*1-56593-067-3*, 0372) Thomson Learn.

***Living with Arthritis: Everything You Need to Know.** John Marcus Thompson. 2001. (Your Personal Health Ser.). (Illus.). 320p. pap. 16.95 (*1-55209-611-4*) Firefly Bks Limited.

Living with Ataxia: An Information & Resource Guide. Martha A. Nance. 1997. LC 96-72598. pap. text 10.00 (*0-943218-09-8*) Natl Ataxia Found.

Living with Brain Injury: A Guide for Families. Richard C. Senelick & Cathy E. Ryan. 2nd rev. ed. 1998. LC 97-77008. (Illus.). 126p. pap. 8.95 (*1-891525-00-X*, HealthSouth Pr) HealthSouth.

Living with Brain Injury: A Guide for Families & Caregivers. Ed. by Sonia Acorn & Penny Offer. 1998. LC 99-181017. (Illus.). 416p. text 40.00 (*0-8020-4265-1*); 296p. pap. text 18.95 (*0-8020-8103-7*) U of Toronto Pr.

Living with Breast Cancer: 39 Women & One Man Speak Candidly about Surviving Breast Cancer. Perry Colmore. 1997. (Illus.). 84p. (Orig.). pap. 24.95 (*0-9655817-0-5*) Andover Townsman.

Living with Change & Choice in Health: Proceedings of the 1st Sigma Theta Tau, Alpha Rho Chapter, National Research Conference. Ed. by Janet F. Wang et al. 1986. (Illus.). 374p. (*0-930284-25-9*) Morgantown Print & Bind.

Living with Chronic Fatigue: New Strategies for Coping with & Conquering CFS. Susan Conant. 1990. LC 89-77048. 148p. pap. 9.95 (*0-87833-709-1*) Taylor Pub.

Living with Chronic Fatigue Syndrome: A Personal Story of the Struggle for Recovery. Timothy Kenny. 1994. LC 93-46715. 226p. pap. 12.95 (*1-56025-075-5*, Thunders Mouth) Avalon NY.

***Living With Chronic Heartburn: A Guide for Patients.** Paulo Pacheco. 2002. 200p. pap. 15.95 (*1-57826-102-3*) Hatherleigh.

Living with Chronic Illness. Pamela L. Robison. 1988. pap. 1.00 (*0-8309-0507-3*) Herald Pub Hse.

Living with Chronic Pain: One Day at a Time - Daily Meditations. Mark A. Zabawa. 1993. (Illus.). 380p. 8.95 (*0-9637353-0-6*) FE Chronic Pain.

Living with Diabetes. Heather MacLean & Barbara Oram. 1988. 227p. pap. 11.95 (*0-8020-6693-3*) U of Toronto Pr.

Living with Diabetes I: The British Diabetic Association Guide for those Treated with Insulin. John Day. 1998. LC 98-23733. 240p. pap. 38.50 (*0-471-97274-6*) Wiley.

Living with Disfigurement: Psychological Implications of Being Born with a Cleft Palate. Poppy Nash. 1995. LC 95-80355. (CEDR Ser.). 304p. (*1-85628-967-2*) Avebry GBR. *Dist:* Ashgate Pub Co.

Living with Down Syndrome. Jenny Bryan. 1999. LC 98-29145. 32 p. lib. bdg. 27.12 (*0-8172-5569-9*) Raintree Steck-V.

Living with Drugs. Michael Gossop. 4th ed. 1996. 239p. pap. (*1-85742-216-3*) Arena GBR. *Dist:* Ashgate Pub Co.

Living with Dying: A Guide to Palliative Care. Cicely M. Saunders et al. 3rd ed. 1995. (Illus.). 76p. pap. text 23.95 (*0-19-262514-4*) OUP.

Living with Epilepsy. Mark A. Mentzer & David C. Ziegler. 1981. LC 81-71463. (Illus.). 144p. (Orig.). pap. 7.95 (*0-9607240-0-1*) Bubba Pr.

Living with Epilepsy. Patsy Westcott. 1999. LC 98-29144. 32 p. lib. bdg. 27.12 (*0-8172-5570-2*) Raintree Steck-V.

Living with Genetic Disorder: The Impact of Neurofibromatosis 1. Joan Ablon. 1999. LC 99-11894. 216p. 62.50 (*0-86569-287-4*, T287, Auburn Hse) Greenwood.

Living with Grief When Illness Is Prolonged. Kenneth J. Doka. 1997. LC 97-6211. (*1-56032-703-0*) Hemisp Pub.

Living with Heart Disease. Marie R. Squillace & Kathy Delaney. rev. ed. 1999. (Illus.). 304p. pap. 16.95 (*0-7373-0082-5*) NTC Contemp Pub Co.

Living with Hepatitis B: A Survivor's Guide. Gregory T. Everson & Hedy Weinberg. 2001. LC 2001-59358. (Illus.). 240p. pap. 15.95 (*1-57826-084-1*) Hatherleigh.

***Living with Hepatitis C: Everything You Need to Know.** Jenny Heathcote et al. 2001. (Your Personal Health Ser.). 192p. pap. 14.95 (*1-55209-612-2*) Firefly Bks Limited.

Living with Heroin: The Impact of a Drugs 'Epidemic" on an English Community. Howard Parker et al. 1988. 192p. (*0-335-15565-0*); pap. (*0-335-15564-2*) OpUniv Pr.

Living with High Blood Pressure. Creative Street, Inc. Staff. 1988. 34.95 incl. VHS (*0-929079-01-9*) Creative Street.

Living with High Blood Pressure. Smith. pap. (*0-85969-633-2*) Society Prom Christ Know GBR. *Dist:* Intl Pubs Mktg.

Living with HIV: Experiment in Courage. Mary E. O'Brien. 1992. LC 91-44130. 248p. 67.00 (*0-86569-040-5*, T040); pap. 22.95 (*0-86569-203-3*, R203) Greenwood (Auburn Hse).

Living with Infertility. Concordia Publishing Staff. 1994. (Master's Touch Bible Study Ser.). pap. 4.50 (*0-570-09520-4*, 20-2461) Concordia.

Living with John: Caring for a Loved One with Alzheimer's Disease. Nellie Kidd-Madison. 2000. 112p. pap. 14.95 (*1-58741-061-3*) Wellness Inst.

Living with Juvenile Diabetes: A Practical Guide for Parents & Caregivers. Victoria Peurrung. rev. ed. 2000. LC 00-63374. (Illus.). 202p. pap. 14.95 (*1-57826-057-4*) Hatherleigh.

Living with Life-Threatening Illness: A Guide for Patients, Their Families & Caregivers. Kenneth J. Doka. 1998. LC 97-35541. 294p. pap. 28.00 (*0-7879-4048-8*) Jossey-Bass.

Living with Low Vision: Independence, Driving, & Low Vision Solutions. Daniel Gottlieb et al. 1996. (Illus.). 260p. (Orig.). pap., wbk. ed. 45.00 (*1-887617-52-3*) St Bart Pr Ltd.

Living with Lung Cancer. Ann G. Fettner. Date not set. pap. 15.00 (*0-465-04152-3*) Basic.

Living with Lung Cancer: A Guide for Patients & Their Families. Barbara G. Cox et al. 4th rev. ed. 1998. LC 97-50581. 144p. pap. 14.95 (*0-937404-53-5*) Triad Pub FL.

Living with Lupus: A Comprehensive Guide to Understanding & Controlling Lupus While Enjoying Your Life. Mark Horowitz & Marietta Abrams-Brill. 1994. LC 93-21066. (Illus.). 192p. pap. 12.95 (*0-452-27056-1*, Plume) Dutton Plume.

Living with Lupus: All the Knowledge You Need to Help Yourself. Sheldon P. Blau. 2000. LC 93-8896. (Illus.). 224p. pap. 15.00 (*0-201-60809-X*) Perseus Bks Grp.

Living with Medicine: A Family Guide. Mary E. Smith. 1987. 262p. pap. 9.95 (*0-89042-504-3*, 2504) Am Psychiatric.

Living with Multiple Sclerosis: A Handbook for Families. Robert Shuman & Janice Schwartz. rev. ed. 1994. LC 93-47116. 256p. reprint ed. pap. 12.95 (*0-02-082026-7*) Hungry Minds.

Living with Multiple Sclerosis: A Wellness Approach. George H. Kraft & Marci Catanzaro. 2nd rev. ed. 2000. LC 00-20502. 128p. pap. 18.95 (*1-888799-26-9*) Demos Medical.

Living with Multiple Sclerosis: Personal Accounts of Coping & Adaptation. Sarah Perry. 1994. (Developments in Nursing & Health Care Ser.). 272p. (*1-85628-893-5*) Avebry GBR. *Dist:* Ashgate Pub Co.

***Living with Muscular Dystrophy: Illness Experience, Activities of Daily Living, Coping, Quality of Life & Rehabilitation.** Birgitta Natterlund. 2001. (Comprehensive Summaries of Uppsala Dissertations from the Faculty of Medicine Ser.: No. 1025). 84p. (*91-554-4997-2*) Uppsala Universitet SWE. *Dist:* Coronet Bks.

Living with Pain. Kathleen M. Dillon. 2001. LC 00-68440. x, 175p. (*1-887905-47-2*) Pkway Pubs.

Living with Paradox: An Introduction to Jungian Psychology. Anne S. Harris. 1995. LC 95-22936. (Counseling Ser.). 247p. pap. text 38.95 (*0-534-21643-9*) Brooks-Cole.

Living with Parkinson's: A Guide for the Patient & Caregiver. Brookdale Center on Aging Staff & David Carroll. 1993. LC 91-50475. (Illus.). 256p. reprint ed. pap. 12.00 (*0-06-092367-9*, Perennial) HarperTrade.

Living with Parkinson's Disease. Kathleen E. Biziere & Matthias C. Kurth. 1996. LC 96-46633. 160p. pap. 24.95 (*1-888799-10-2*) Demos Medical.

Living with Parkinson's Disease: Don't Rush Me! I'm Coping As Fast As I Can. Jon R. Pierce. 1989. LC 89-63189. 176p. (Orig.). pap. text (*0-9630559-0-9*) J R Pierce.

Living with PCOS: Polycystic Ovary Syndrome. Angela Boss et al. 2000. LC 00-10670. (Illus.). xi, 156p. pap. 14.95 (*1-886039-49-6*) Addicus Bks.

Living with Rheumatoid Arthritis. Tammi L. Sholtzhauer & James L. McGuire. 1995. (Health Bks.). (Illus.). 240p. reprint ed. pap. 16.95 (*0-8018-5185-8*) Johns Hopkins.

Living with Schizophrenia. Stuart Emmons et al. 1997. LC 97-19055. (Psychological Disorders Ser.: Vol. 2). 200p. pap. 24.95 (*1-56032-556-9*) Hemisp Pub.

Living with Shingles: The Chronic Condition of the Reactivated Herpes Zoster Virus. Mary-Ellen Siegel & William Gray, Jr. 1998. LC 98-8031. 224p. 19.95 (*0-87131-828-8*) M Evans.

Living with Spina Bifida: A Guide for Families & Professionals. Adrian Sandler. 1997. LC 96-47697. 296p. (gr. 13). 49.95 (*0-8078-2352-X*); pap. 19.95 (*0-8078-4657-0*) U of NC Pr.

Living with Tourette's Syndrome. Elaine F. Shimberg. 1995. LC 95-20038. 256p. per. 13.00 (*0-684-81160-X*) S&S Trade Pap.

Living with Uncertainty: My Bout with Inoperable Cancer. John Wimber. 1996. 48p. (Orig.). pap. 4.99 (*0-9651509-0-9*) Vineyard Minist.

Living with Your Selves: A Survival Manual for People with Multiple Personalities. Sandra J. Hocking et al. 1992. LC 92-16514. 90p. (Orig.). pap. 9.95 (*1-877872-06-7*) Launch Pr.

Living Without Dieting. John P. Foreyt & G. Ken Goodrick. 1994. 224p. pap. 10.99 (*0-446-38269-8*) Warner Bks.

Living Without Fatigue. Richard Ribner. 160p. (Orig.). pap. 9.95 (*0-8159-6117-0*) Devin.

Living Without Oxygen: Closed & Open Systems in Hypoxia Tolerance. Peter W. Hochachka. 1980. LC 79-20221. (Illus.). 192p. 35.50 (*0-674-53670-3*) HUP.

Living Younger: A Physicians Formula. Murdock Head. 1989. LC 88-7513. 248p. (C). 19.95 (*0-910155-12-7*) Bartleby Pr.

Living Your Life with Lung Cancer. Frank V. Fossella, MD & Elizabeth Waxman, RN, MSN. 2001. (Illus.). 16p. pap. 7.95 (*1-891483-11-0*) PRR.

Livingstone. Reginald J. Campbell. 1972. LC 77-138212. (Illus.). 295p. (C). reprint ed. lib. bdg. 55.00 (*0-8371-5567-3*, CALI, Greenwood Pr) Greenwood.

Livre d'Images Universel de la Naissance. Fran P. Hosken. 1982. (Childbirth Picture Bks.).Tr. of Universal Childbirth Picture Book. (FRE., Illus.). 76p. (Orig.). pap. 7.00 (*0-942096-04-5*) WINNEWS.

Lo Esencial en Anatomia. Phillip Ameerally. 1998. (C). text 14.09 (*84-8174-363-1*) Mosby Inc.

Lo Esencial en Aparato Digesti. Cheshire. 1998. (C). text 14.09 (*84-8174-365-8*) Mosby Inc.

Lo Esencial en Sistema Nervios. Daniel Lasserson. 1998. (C). text 14.09 (*84-8174-367-4*) Mosby Inc.

Lo Que los Jovenes Deben Saber Acerca de las Drogas: What Youth Should Know about Drugs. Guillermo H. Perez. 1977. 80p. reprint ed. pap. 3.99 (*0-311-46070-4*) Casa Bautista.

Loc Clinical Neurology, No. 2. Paul W. Brazis. 2nd ed. 1990. 84.95 (*0-316-10743-3*, Little Brwn Med Div) Lppncott W & W.

Local Anaesthesia in Dentistry. Fraser McDonald et al. 2000. LC 00-40400. (Illus.). 96p. pap. text 32.00 (*0-7236-1063-0*) Buttrwrth-Heinemann.

Local & Regional Anaesthesia. Ed. by Per Rosenberg. 2001. (Fundamentals of Anaesthesia & Acute Medicine Ser.). (Illus.). 176p. pap. text (*0-7279-1480-4*) BMJ Pub GBR. *Dist:* AIDC.

Local & Regional Anesthesia from Birth to Adulthood. Bernard J. Dalens. 1995. LC 95-3775.Tr. of Anesthesie Locoregionale de la Naissance a L'age Adulte. (Illus.). 480p. text 129.00 (*0-683-09653-2*) Lppncott W & W.

Local Anesthesia. Markus D. Lipp et al. Tr. by Mark Coldwell et al from GER. 1993. LC 93-12264. (Illus.). 166p. text 60.00 (*0-86715-263-X*) Quint Pub Co.

Local Anesthesia for Dermatologic Surgery. Michael J. Auletta & Roy C. Grekin. 1990. (Practical Manuals in Dermatologic Surgery Ser.). (Illus.). 99p. pap. text (*0-443-08704-0*) Church.

Local Anesthesia of the Oral Cavity. J. Theodore Jastak et al. 1994. LC 94-8370. (Illus.). 296p. pap. text 35.00 (*0-7216-2357-3*) Saunders.

Local Anesthetics. 1986. (Medical Ser.). lib. bdg. 79.95 (*0-8490-3802-2*) Gordon Pr.

Local Anesthetics, Vol. 81. Ed. by Gary R. Strichartz. 1986. (Handbook of Experimental Pharmacology Ser.). (Illus.). 292p. 243.00 (*0-387-16361-1*) Spr-Verlag.

Local Cortical Circuits: An Electrophysiological Study. M. Abeles. 1982. (Studies of Brain Function: Vol. 6). (Illus.). 102p. 38.95 (*0-387-11034-8*) Spr-Verlag.

Local Drug Delivery/Molecular. Ed. by Elazer R. Edelman. 1995. text 63.00 (*0-7020-1910-0*) Saunders.

Local Flaps in Facial Reconstruction. Ed. by Shan R. Baker & Neil A. Swanson. 1994. (Illus.). 656p. (C). (gr. 13). text 196.00 (*0-8016-6925-1*, 06925) Mosby Inc.

Local Government in the German Federal System. Arthur B. Gunlicks. 1986. LC 86-6350. (Duke Press Policy Studies). (Illus.). xii, 247p. text 53.00 (*0-8223-0674-3*) Duke.

Local Government Responsibilities in Health Care. 1994. (Illus.). 24p. (Orig.). (C). pap. text 20.00 (*0-7881-1515-4*) DIANE Pub.

Local Health Departments: Fifteen Case Studies. Ed. by C. Arden Miller & Merry K. Moos. 1981. LC 81-68703. 528p. 12.00 (*0-87553-094-X*, 061) Am Pub Health.

Local Health Policy in Action: The Municipal Health Services Program. Eli Ginzberg et al. 1985. (Conservation of Human Resources Ser.: Vol. 24). 152p. 52.50 (*0-8476-7425-8*) Rowman.

Local Health Units for the Nation. Haven Emerson & Martha Luginbuhl. Ed. by Barbara G. Rosenkrantz. 1977. LC 76-25661. (Public Health in America Ser.). (Illus.). reprint ed. lib. bdg. 31.95 (*0-405-09816-2*) Ayer.

Local Hospitals in Ancient Rigime France: Rationalization, Resistance, Renewal, 1530-1789. Daniel Hickey. 1997. LC 98-123958. (McGill-Queen's Hannah Institute Studies in the History of Medicine, Health, & Society Ser.). (Illus.). 296p. (*0-7735-1540-2*) McG-Queens Univ Pr CAN. *Dist:* CUP Services.

Local Immune Responses of the GUT. Ed. by T. J. Newby & C. R. Stokes. 1984. LC 83-26321. 264p. 129.00 (*0-8493-5534-6*, QR186, CRC Reprint) Franklin.

Local Immunosuppression of Organ Transplants. Scott A. Gruber. 1996. LC 96-17732. 217p. pap. 89.95 (*0-412-11091-1*, QR188) Chapman & Hall.

Local Immunosuppression of Organ Transplants. Scott A. Gruber. 1996. (Medical Intelligence Unit Ser.). 258p. 99.00 (*1-57059-352-3*) Landes Bioscience.

Local Invasion & Spread of Cancer. Ed. by Kenneth W. Brunson. 1989. (Cancer Growth & Progression Ser.). (C). text 207.50 (*0-89838-996-8*) Kluwer Academic.

Local Organizations for Rural Health in Panama: Community Participation, Bureaucratic Reorientation, & Political Will. Gerard M. LaForgia. 1985. (Special Series on Rural Local Organization: No. 8). 153p. 7.50 (*0-86731-035-9*) Cornell CIS RDC.

Local Prostatic Carcinoma. Ed. by J. J. Rambeaud & F. Vincent. 1995. (Contributions to Oncology Ser.: Vol. 47). (Illus.). viii, 146p. 121.75 (*3-8055-5973-9*) S Karger.

Local Regulation of Ovarian Function. Ed. by N. O. Sjoberg et al. 1992. (Illus.). 331p. (C). lib. bdg. 85.95 (*1-85070-394-9*, Parthenon Pbng) CRC Pr.

Local Regulators in the Ovary - Paracrine & Autocrine Control. Ed. by H. Mori & Y. Yoshimura. 1994. (Journal: Vol. 41, Suppl. 1, 1994). (Illus.). iv, 68p. pap. 31.50 (*3-8055-5994-1*) S Karger.

Local Services for Mentally Handicapped People: The Community Team, the Community Unit, & the Role & Function of the Community Nurse, Social Worker & Some Other Members of the CMHT. G. B. Simon. 1985. 88p. 40.00 (*0-906054-31-1*); pap. 29.00 (*0-906054-30-3*) St Mut.

Localised Prostate Cancer: Recent Advances in Diagnosis & Treatment. Fernand Labrie et al. 1997. 319p. (Orig.). 68.95 (*1-898099-11-1*) Blackwell Sci.

Localization. Vol. 51, No. 3. Ed. by C. R. Catlow & Mackrodt. 1985. 42.00 (*0-85066-973-1*) Taylor & Francis.

Localization & Neuroimaging in Neuropsychology. Ed. by Andrew Kertesz. 1994. LC 93-37924. (Foundations of Neuropsychology Ser.). (Illus.). 662p. text 99.95 (*0-12-405045-X*) Acad Pr.

Localization in Clinical Neurology. Paul W. Brazis et al. 1985. 429p. 45.00 (*0-316-10721-2*, Little Brwn Med Div); 3rd ed. 1996. 638p. text 120.00 (*0-316-09992-9*) Lppncott W & W.

Localization of Brain Lesions & Developmental Functions. Daria Riva & Arthur Benton. 168p. (*0-86196-599-X*) John Libby GBR. *Dist:* Buttrwrth-Heinemann.

Localization of Putative Steroid Receptors, Vol. 1: Experimental Systems. Ed. by Louis P. Pertschuk & Sin H. Lee. 1985. 200p. 116.00 (*0-8493-6048-X*, RC268, CRC Reprint) Franklin.

J
K
L

Localization of Putative Steroid Receptors, Vol. II: Clinically Oriented Studies. Ed. by Louis P. Perschuk & Sin H. Lee. 1985. 184p. 106.00 (*0-8493-6049-8*, CRC Reprint) Franklin.

Localized Prostatic Cancer: Heinrich Warner Stiftung. Ed. by H. Huland. 1995. (Journal: Vol. 27, Suppl. 2, 1995). (Illus.). 48p. pap. 21.75 (*3-8055-6126-1*) S Karger.

Localized RNAs. Howard D. Lipshitz. 1995. LC 95-16554. (Molecular Biology Intelligence Unit Ser.). 318p. 99.00 (*1-57059-276-4*) Landes Bioscience.

Locally Interacting Systems & Their Application in Biology: Proceedings of the School - Seminar on Markov Interaction Processes in Biology, Held in Pushchino, Moscow Region, March, 1976. Ed. by R. L. Dobryshin et al. 1978. (Lecture Notes in Mathematics: Vol. 653). (Illus.). 202p. 27.95 (*0-387-08450-9*) Spr-Verlag.

***Locatelli & Singh's Handbook of Neurology.** Eduardo Raul Locatelli & Sanjay Pratap Singh. 2001. 208p. pap. 19.95 (*1-58808-104-4*) Intl Med Pub.

Locating Ambulance Dispatch Centers in an Urban Region: A Man-Computer Interactive Problem-Solving Approach. Jerry B. Schneider & John B. Symons, Jr. 1971. (Discussion Papers: No. 49). pap. 10.00 (*1-55869-070-0*) Regional Sci Res Inst.

Locating Health: Sociological & Historical Explorations. Ed. by Sue Scott et al. 1993. 288p. (*1-85628-367-4*) Avebry GBR. *Dist:* Ashgate Pub Co.

Locating Resources for Healthy People. 1995. lib. bdg. 250.95 (*0-8490-7578-5*) Gordon Pr.

Location of Acupoints. Compiled by China Academy of Traditional Chinese Medicine, Institute of Acupuncture and Moxibustion Staff. 1990. LC 93-242403. 276p. (*7-119-01368-8*) Beijing Foreign Lang.

Location of Acupoints. Delta Staff. 1995. (Illus.). 184p. (*983-9808-32-X*) Delta Edits MYS. *Dist:* Weatherhill.

Locking Out & Tagging Out Accidents: A Compliance Program for OSHA Standard 29 CFR 1910.147. Ennis, Lumsden, Boylston and Associates Staff. 1992. 150p. lib. bdg., ring bd. 385.00 (*0-87371-934-4*, L934) Lewis Pubs.

Locomotor Morphology of the Vampire Bat, Desmodus Rotundus. J. Scott Altenbach. 1979. (ASM Special Publications: No. 6). (Illus.). vi, 137p. 12.00 (*0-943612-05-5*) Am Soc Mammalogists.

Locomotor System of the Domestic Mammals. Ed. by R. Nickel et al. 1985. (Anatomy of the Domestic Animals Ser.: Vol. 1). (Illus.). 520p. 145.00 (*0-387-91259-2*) Spr-Verlag.

Log Blood Glucose Levels. Charles E. Hugenberger. 1992. 12p. pap. 3.95 (*1-885057-08-3*) C E Hugenberger.

Logan Turner's Diseases of the Nose, Throat & Ear. Arnold G. Maran. 10th ed. 1995. 456p. pap. text (*0-7506-1643-1*) E A GBR. *Dist:* OUP.

Logic of Biochemical Sequencing. David Blackman. 1993. LC 93-12778. 192p. lib. bdg. 54.95 (*0-8493-4497-2*, QP551) CRC Pr.

Logic of Life: A History of Heredity. Francois Jacob. Tr. by Betty E. Spillman. 1993. LC 92-35369. (Princeton Science Library). (Illus.). 358p. reprint ed. pap. 19.95 (*0-691-00042-5*) Princeton U Pr.

Logic of Medicine, Vol. 2. Edmond A. Murphy. 2nd ed. 1997. LC 96-20279. (Logic of Medicine Ser.: Vol. 2). 416p. pap. text 30.00 (*0-8018-5538-1*) Johns Hopkins.

Logic of Science in Psychoanalysis. Benjamin B. Wolman. 1984. LC 84-1891. 332p. text 69.50 (*0-231-05744-X*) Col U Pr.

Logical Learning Theory: A Human Teleology & Its Empirical Support. Joseph F. Rychlak. 1994. LC 93-49664. 387p. text 45.00 (*0-8032-3904-1*) U of Nebr Pr.

Logical Nursing Mathematics. Bruce L. Wilson. 1987. 128p. (C). (gr. 12). pap. 23.00 (*0-8273-2934-2*) Delmar.

Logistic Regression: A Self-Learning Text. David G. Kleinbaum. 1997. LC 93-27484. (Series in Statistics in the Health Sciences). (Illus.). 282p. 71.95 (*0-387-94142-8*) Spr-Verlag.

Logotherapy: New Help for Problem Drinkers. James C. Crumbaugh et al. 1981. LC 79-18635. 176p. text 27.95 (*0-88229-421-0*) Burnham Inc.

Logotherapy for the Helping Professional: Meaningful Social Work. David L. Guttmann. 1996. LC 95-36966. 264p. 44.95 (*0-8261-9020-0*) Springer Pub.

Loimographia: An Account of the Great Plague of London in 1665. William Boghurst. Ed. by J. F. Payne. LC 75-23686. reprint ed. 44.50 (*0-404-13239-1*) AMS Pr.

Loimologia: Or, An Historical Account of the Plague in London in 1665. Nathaniel Hodges. LC 75-23722. reprint ed. 49.50 (*0-404-13280-4*) AMS Pr.

Lois Remembers. Lois W. 1979. LC 79-6975. (Illus.). pap. 9.50 (*0-910034-23-0*) Al-Anon.

***London Lock: A Charitable Hospital for Venereal Disease, 1746-1952.** David Innes Williams. 1988. (History of Medicine Ser.). 166p. pap. (*1-85315-263-3*) Royal Soc of Medicine Pr Ltd GBR. *Dist:* Balogh.

London Specialist Postgraduate Hospitals. Frank Wellman & Paul Palmer. 1975. (King Edward's Hospital Fund Ser.). pap. 19.00 (*0-8464-0577-6*) Beekman Pubs.

Lonely Pain of Cancer: Home Care for the Terminally Ill. Kathleen L. Peabody & Margaret L. Mooney. Ed. by Bettye Ellison. 1991. LC 91-90114. (Illus.). 160p. (Orig.). (C). pap. 15.95 (*0-9629350-1-8*) Sharp Pub.

Long Acting Cephalosporins in Surgery. Ed. by K. Hell. 1989. (Journal: Vol. 21, Suppl. 1, 1989). 58p. pap. 20.00 (*3-8055-4971-7*) S Karger.

Long-Acting Nifedipine: End-Organ Protection & Prevention of Cardiovascular Disease: 3rd International Symposium, Berlin, September 1996: Proceedings. Ed. by Shimon Braun. 1997. (Cardiology Ser.: Vol. 88, Suppl. 3, 1997). (Illus.). iv, 74p. pap. 34.00 (*3-8055-6620-4*) S Karger.

Long Circulating Liposomes: Old Drugs, New Therapeutics. Ed. by Martin C. Woodle. 1997. LC 97-30426. (Biotechnology Intelligence Unit Ser.). 301p. 159.00 (*3-540-63082-1*) Spr-Verlag.

Long Darkness: Psychological & Moral Perspectives on Nuclear Winter. Ed. & Intro. by Lester Grinspoon. 1986. LC 85-40986. 217p. pap. 14.00 (*0-300-03664-7*, YF-31) Yale U Pr.

Long Dying of Baby Andrew. Peggy Stinson & Robert Stinson. 1983. 384p. 17.95 (*0-316-81635-3*, Little Brwn Med Div) Lppncott W & W.

Long Goodbye & Beyond: Coping with Alzheimers. Linda M. Combs. 1998. LC 97-77070. 160p. pap. 12.95 (*1-885221-83-5*) BookPartners.

Long Journey: Personal Stories of Living with Arthritis. William E. Byrd. 1991. LC 90-71986. (Illus.). 153p. (Orig.). pap. 13.95 (*1-56002-046-6*, Univ Edtns) Aegina Pr.

Long Life & How to Reach It. Joseph G. Richardson. Ed. by Barbara G. Rosenkrantz. 1977. LC 76-40640. (Public Health in America Ser.). reprint ed. lib. bdg. 19.95 (*0-405-09828-6*) Ayer.

Long Life Now: Strategies for Staying Alive. Lee R. Hitchcox. 1996. LC 95-19693. (Illus.). 388p. (Orig.). text 15.95 (*0-89087-763-7*) Celestial Arts.

Long QT Syndrome. Ed. by Peter J. Schwartz. 1997. LC 97-16499. (Clinical Approaches to Tachyarrhythmias Ser.: No. 7). (Illus.). 120p. 24.00 (*0-87993-680-0*) Futura Pub.

Long-Range Effects of Early Childhood Sexual Experiences. Allie Kilpatrick. 1992. 224p. LC 91-28233. pap. 27.50 (*0-8058-0914-7*); text 49.95 (*0-8058-0913-9*) L Erlbaum Assocs.

Long Road Called Goodbye. Charlotte A. Akin. 2000. LC 00-25772. (Illus.). xi, 244p. 25.00 (*1-881871-33-9*); pap. 17.00 (*1-881871-34-7*) Creighton U Pr.

Long Term. Frazier. 1995. 160p. pap. text 21.95 (*0-316-29419-5*, Little Brwn Med Div) Lppncott W & W.

Long-Term Ambulatory Electrocardiography. Jos R. Roelandt & P. G. Hugenholtz. 1982. text 126.50 (*90-247-2664-6*) Kluwer Academic.

Long-Term & Short-Term Assays for Carcinogens: A Critical Appraisal. Ed. by R. Montesano et al. 1987. (IARC Scientific Publications Ser.: No. 83). (Illus.). 580p. pap. 70.00 (*92-832-1183-9*) OUP.

Long-Term Animal Studies: Their Predictive Value for Man. Ed. by S. R. Walker & A. D. Dayan. 1986. text 124.00 (*0-85200-931-3*) Kluwer Academic.

Long-Term Care: A Dollar & Sense Guide. 1999. LC 97-190253. pap. 18.00 (*0-944847-22-6*) United Sr Hlth Co-op.

Long Term Care: An Annotated Bibliography, 25. Theodore H. Koff. 1995. LC 94-39768. (Bibliographies & Indexes in Gerontology Ser.: Vol. 25). 152p. lib. bdg. 59.95 (*0-313-28583-7*, Greenwood Pr) Greenwood.

Long-Term Care: Economic Impacts & Financing Dilemmas. 1990. 104p. 20.00 (*0-929852-02-8*) Natl Health Coun.

Long-Term Care: Federal, State & Private Options for the Future. Raymond C. O'Brien & Michael T. Flannery. 1997. LC 97-1573. (Haworth Health & Social Policy Ser.). 290p. (C). 49.95 (*0-7890-0173-X*); pap. 24.95 (*0-7890-0261-2*) Haworth Pr.

Long Term Care: For Activity Professionals, Recreational Therapists & Social Service Professionals. Elizabeth Best Martini et al. 3rd ed. 2000. 402p. (C). pap. text 35.00 (*1-882883-44-6*, B380) Idyll Arbor.

Long-Term Care: Knowing the Risk, Paying the Price. Ed. by Bruce Boyd. 1997. LC 97-176580. 248p. pap. text 30.00 (*1-879143-34-8*) Health Ins Assn Am.

Long-Term Care: Management, Scope & Practical Issues. Ed. by John A. Toner et al. 1993. LC 92-49112. 240p. (Orig.). (C). pap. text 19.95 (*0-914783-66-1*) Charles.

Long-Term Care: Managing Across the Continuum. John R. Pratt. 1999. LC 98-44807. 640p. 70.00 (*0-8342-1032-0*, 10320) Aspen Pub.

Long-Term Care: Principles, Programs & Policies. Rosalie A. Kane & Robert L. Kane. 1987. 462p. (C). 52.95 (*0-8261-6010-7*) Springer Pub.

Long-Term Care: Private Sector Elder Care Could Yield Multiple Benefits. 1995. (Illus.). 45p. (Orig.). (C). pap. text 25.00 (*0-7881-1755-6*) DIANE Pub.

Long Term Care: Test-Taking Review for Nurses Aide. Barbara A. Vitale & Patricia M. Nugent. 1990. (Illus.). 224p. (C). (gr. 13). pap. text 17.95 (*0-8016-5221-9*, 05221) Mosby Inc.

Long Term Care Administration: Teamwork & Effective Management. Ruby H. Neuhaus. 1990. 200p. (C). 59.00 (*0-8191-7860-8*); pap. 27.50 (*0-8191-7861-6*) U Pr of Amer.

Long-Term Care Administration: The Management of Institutional & Non-Institutional Components of the Continuum of Care. Ben Abramovice. 1987. LC 87-11949. (Series in Marketing & Health Services Administration: No. 1). 256p. (C). text 39.95 (*0-86656-399-7*) Haworth Pr.

Long-Term Care Administration Handbook. Ed. by Seth B. Goldsmith. 1993. LC 92-48287. 592p. 114.00 (*0-8342-0374-X*, 20374) Aspen Pub.

Long-Term Care Advocacy. Eric M. Carlson. 1999. LC 99-43080. 1050p. 144.00 (*0-8205-4153-2*) Bender.

Long-Term Care & Its Alternatives. Charles B. Inlander et al. 1996. LC 95-52968. (Illus.). 256p. pap. 16.95 (*1-882606-56-6*) Peoples Med Soc.

Long-Term Care & the Law: A Legal Guide for Health Care Professionals. George D. Pozgar et al. 1992. 510p. 96.00 (*0-8342-0289-1*, 20289) Aspen Pub.

Long-Term Care Case Management: Design & Evaluation. Robert Applebaum & Carol Austin. 1990. LC 90-9483. 192p. 29.95 (*0-8261-6430-7*) Springer Pub.

Long-Term Care Case Management: State Experiences & Implications for Federal Policy. 1995. (Illus.). 45p. (Orig.). (C). pap. text 25.00 (*0-7881-2377-7*) DIANE Pub.

Long-Term Care Clinical Assessment: A Guide for the Social Worker. David Liebert. 1999. (Illus.). 100p. (C). pap. 29.50 (*0-929442-55-5*) Prof Prnting & Pub.

***Long Term Care Competency Evaluation Preparation Manual: Nurse Aide Certification Study Guide.** Fred Reneau et al. 2nd ed. 2001. 192p. pap. 15.63 (*0-07-254974-2*) McGrw-H Hghr Educ.

Long-Term Care Compliance Manual. D. Scott Jones. Ed. by Claudia Hoffacker. 2000. 210p. pap. text 249.00 (*1-57839-079-6*) Opus Communs.

Long Term Care Compliance Resource Manual. L. E. Zimmerman et al. Ed. by Aspen Health Law and Compliance Center Staff & Charles County Nursing and Rehabilitation Center Staff. 2000. LC 00-22787. (Illus.). 480p. ring bd. 189.00 (*0-8342-1730-9*) Aspen Pub.

Long-Term Care Crisis: Elders Trapped in the No-Care Zone. Carroll L. Estes & James H. Swan. 1993. LC 92-30579. (Illus.). 352p. (C). 76.95 (*0-8039-3992-2*, 7743); pap. 37.95 (*0-8039-3993-0*, 7744) Sage.

Long-Term Care Documentation. Marilyn Stoner. 1999. 250p. (C). ring bd. 97.95 (*1-56930-079-8*) Delmar.

Long-Term Care Experience Report for 1997. Ed. by Jim Bugenhagen. 6th rev. ed. 1999. 70p. (C). pap. (*0-89382-594-8*, LTC-LR97) Nat Assn Insurance.

Long-Term Care Experience Report for 1998. Ed. by Jim Bugenhagen. 6th rev. ed. 2000. 70p. pap. 45.00 (*0-89382-663-4*) Nat Assn Insurance.

Long Term Care Facility Resident Assessment Instrument: User's Manual. James E. Allen. 1997. LC 97-3056. 496p. 42.95 (*0-8261-9900-3*) Springer Pub.

Long-Term Care for Older Persons: A Policy Perspective. Nancy Eustis et al. 1984. LC 83-7080. (Social Gerontology Ser.). 224p. (C). mass mkt. 20.00 (*0-534-02910-8*) Brooks-Cole.

Long-Term Care for the Elderly: A Factbook. David Rabin. 1986. (Illus.). 269p. pap. text 19.95 (*0-19-504106-2*) OUP.

Long-Term Care for the Elderly with Disabilities: Current Policy, Emerging Trends & Implications for the Twenty-First Century. Robyn J. Stone. 2000. LC 00-708685. (Illus.). viii, 87p. pap. (*1-887748-38-5*) Milbank Memorial.

Long Term Care for the Rural Elderly: New Directions in Services, Research, & Policy. Ed. by Graham D. Rowles et al. 1996. LC 96-28439. (Illus.). 216p. 39.95 (*0-8261-9380-3*) Springer Pub.

Long-Term Care for the 21st Century: A Common Sense Proposal to Support Family Caregiver - Congressional Hearing. Ed. by Charles E. Grassley. 2000. 74p. pap. text 20.00 (*0-7567-0152-X*) DIANE Pub.

Long Term Care Handbook: Legal, Operational & Financial Guideposts. Ed. by Thomas C. Fox et al. 1991. 377p. 35.00 (*0-918945-11-9*) Am Hlth Lawyers.

Long-Term Care Handbook: Resources for the Health Information Manager. Ed. by Teresa Ganser. 1999. 198p. pap. text 62.00 (*1-58426-027-0*, AB102499) Am Hlth Info.

Long-Term Care Investment Strategies: A Guide to Start-Ups, Facility Conversions & Strategic Alliances. Ronald E. Mills. 1995. LC 95-34923. 200p. (C). text 55.00 (*1-55738-622-6*, Irwn Prfssnl) McGraw-Hill Educ Grp.

Long-Term Care Nursing Assistant. Peggy A. Grubbs & Barbara A. Blasband. 1994. LC 94-18668. (C). 30.20 (*0-13-146747-6*) P-H.

Long-Term Care Nursing Assistant. Perspective Press Inc. Staff. 1995. (Illus.). 320p. (gr. 13). pap. text 24.95 (*0-8151-4550-0*, 25772) Mosby Inc.

Long Term Care Nursing Assistant. 2nd ed. (C). 2000. pap. 50.00 (*0-13-016390-2*); 2000. pap. 50.00 (*0-13-016401-1*); 2000. pap. 50.00 (*0-13-016402-X*); 1999. pap. 22.00 (*0-13-016399-6*) P-H.

Long-Term Care Nursing Assistant Training Manual. Ed. by Mary Ann Anderson et al. 2nd ed. 1996. LC 95-46849. (Illus.). 352p. (Orig.). pap. 29.95 (*1-878812-28-9*) Hlth Prof Pr.

Long Term Care Nursing Standards Manual, Policies, & Procedures, Suppl. 6. Ed. by O. Alice Leshem & Dorothy M. Varholak. 1995. ring bd. 189.00 (*0-8342-0331-6*, S5406) Aspen Pub.

Long-Term Care of Older People: A Practical Guide. Elaine Brody. 1977. LC 77-5944. 402p. 52.00 (*0-87705-274-3*, Kluwer Acad Hman Sci) Kluwer Academic.

Long-Term Care Planning Guide. Phyllis R. Shelton. 8th ed. 1998. Orig. Title: Health Benefits Guide for Seniors. (Illus.). vii, 151p. pap. 19.95 (*0-9633516-4-8*) Shelton Mktg.

***Long Term Care Survival Handbook.** Barbara Hegner & Joan Fritsch Needham. 2002. pap. 39.95 (*0-7668-3222-8*) Delmar.

Long Term Central Venous Catheters. Springhouse Publishing Company Staff. 1992. (Procedures Video Ser.). 36.95 incl. VHS (*0-87434-429-8*) Springhouse Corp.

Long Term Clinical Care of Parkinson's Disease: 3rd Symposium, Tokyo, April 1988. Ed. by T. Nakanishi. 1989. (Journal: Vol. 29, Suppl. 1, 1988). 38p. pap. 19.25 (*3-8055-4969-5*) S Karger.

Long Term Clinical Care of Parkinson's Disease: Journal: European Neurology, Vol. 30, Suppl. 1, 1990. Ed. by T. Nakanishi. 1990. vi, 42p. pap. text 21.00 (*3-8055-5161-4*) S Karger.

Long Term Clinical Care of Parkinson's Disease, 5th Symposium, Tokyo, April 1990. Ed. by T. Nakanishi. 1991. (Journal: Vol. 31, Suppl. 1, 1991). (Illus.). iv, 60p. pap. 28.00 (*3-8055-5401-X*) S Karger.

Long Term Clinical Care of Parkinson's Disease, Tokyo, April 1987: Second Symposium. Ed. by T. Nakanishi. 1988. (Journal: Vol. 28, Suppl. 1, 1988). vi, 42p. pap. 15.00 (*3-8055-4833-8*) S Karger.

Long-Term Consequences of Early Environment: Growth, Development & the Lifespan Developmental Perspective. Ed. by C. J. Henry & Stanley J. Ulijaszek. 1996. (Society for the Study of Human Biology Symposium Ser.: No. 37). (Illus.). 265p. (C). text 74.95 (*0-521-47108-7*) Cambridge U Pr.

Long-Term Hemodialysis. Nguyen-Khoa Man et al. 1995. LC 95-14248. 148p. (C). text 81.00 (*0-7923-3477-9*) Kluwer Academic.

Long-Term Intragastric pH Measurement in Man: Basic & Methodological Aspects - Journal: Digestive Diseases, Vol. 8, Suppl. 1, 1990. Ed. by W. Londong et al. 1990. (Illus.). vi, 98p. pap. 29.75 (*3-8055-5274-2*) S Karger.

Long-Term Intravenous Immunoglobulin Treatment in Patients with AIDS-Related Complex: Journal: Vox Sanguinis, Vol. 59, Suppl. 1, 1990. Ed. by B. A. Perret et al. 1990. (Illus.). iv, 60p. pap. 19.25 (*3-8055-5256-4*) S Karger.

Long-Term Management of Patients after Myocardial Infarction. Ed. by C. Tissa Kappagoda & P. V. Greenwood. 1987. (Developments in Cardiovascular Medicine Ser.). (C). text 104.50 (*0-89838-352-8*) Kluwer Academic.

Long Term Monitoring for Epilepsy. American Journal of EEG Technology Staff & American END Society Committee. 1995. (Illus.). iv, 178p. per. 25.00 (*1-57797-004-7*) ASET.

Long Term Oxygen Therapy: Scientific Basis & Clinical Application. Ed. by Walter J. O'Donohue, Jr. 1995. LC 94-48767. (Lung Biology in Health & Disease Ser.: Vol. 81). (Illus.). 416p. text 195.00 (*0-8247-9499-0*) Dekker.

Long-Term Potentiation: A Debate of Current Issues. Ed. by Michel Baudry & Joel L. Davis. 1991. (Bradford Series in Complex Adaptive Systems). 464p. 79.95 (*0-262-02330-X*, Bradford Bks) MIT Pr.

Long-Term Prognosis Following Valve Replacement: Proceedings. Conference on Cardiovascular Disease, 2nd, Snowmas. Ed. by J. H. Vogel. 1972. (Advances in Cardiology Ser.: Vol. 7). 86.25 (*3-8055-1299-6*) S Karger.

Long-Term Psychiatric Patients: A Study in Community Care. Susan Lonsdale et al. 1980. (*0-7855-0572-5*) Natl Inst Soc Work GBR. *Dist:* St Mut.

Long-Term Results & Indications in Otology & Otoneurosurgery. Ed. by R. Charachon & E. Garcia-Ibanez. 1991. LC 91-30815. (Illus.). 596p. lib. bdg. (*90-6299-070-3*) Kugler NLD. *Dist:* Lib Res.

Long-Term Results in Plastic & Reconstruction Surgery. Robert M. Goldwyn. 1980. 110.00 (*0-316-31972-4*); 110.00 (*0-316-31973-2*) Lppncott W & W (Little Brwn Med Div).

Long-Term Results in Vascular Surgery. James S. Yao & William H. Pearce. 1993. (Illus.). 494p. (C). pap. text 169.00 (*0-8385-9385-2*, A9385-4, Apple Lange Med) McGraw.

Long-Term Results of Arterial Interventions. Ed. by Alain Branchereau & Michael Jacobs. 1997. LC 97-3245. (Illus.). 354p. 95.00 (*0-87993-679-7*) Futura Pub.

Long-Term Retention of Knowledge & Skills. M. J. Farr. 1989. (Recent Research in Psychology Ser.). 151p. 79.95 (*0-387-96531-9*) Spr-Verlag.

Long-term Treatment of Depression, Vol. 3. S. A. Montgomery & F. Rouillon. 1992. LC 91-40088. (Perspectives in Psychiatry Ser.: No. 1951). 286p. 235.95 (*0-471-92892-5*, Wiley-Liss) Wiley.

Long-Term Treatments of Anxiety Disorders. Ed. by Robert F. Prien & Matig R. Mavissakalian. 1996. LC 95-46599. 464p. 58.00 (*0-88048-656-2*, 8656) Am Psychiatric.

J
K
L

Long-Time Clinical Care of Parkinson's Disease, Symposium, Tokyo, April 1986: Journal: European Neurology, Vol. 26, Suppl. 1, 1987. Ed. by T. Nakanishi. 1987. (Illus.). iv, 56p. pap. 18.50 (*3-8055-4590-8*) S Karger.

Long Way from Home: The Tuberculosis Epidemic among the Inuit. Pat S. Grygier. (McGill-Queen's Hannah Institute Studies in the History of Medicine, Health, & Society Ser.). (Illus.). 272p. 1997. pap. (*0-7735-1637-9*); 1994. LC 95-170470. (*0-7735-1216-0*) McG-Queens Univ Pr CAN. *Dist:* CUP Services.

Long Weekend 1897-1919: Part of a Life. Wilfred R. Bion. 1991. 288p. pap. (*1-85575-000-7*); 1990. 299p. reprint ed. pap. text (*0-9507895-0-X*) Karnac Bks GBR. *Dist:* Other Pr LLC, Brunner-Routledge.

Longer Life for Your Pet: How to Increase the Lifespan of Your Dog or Cat. Robert Gilmore. 1994. LC 94-96037. (Orig.). pap. 4.95 (*0-9640710-0-2*) Dr Goodhlth.

Longevity. 1999. (Fitness, Health & Nutrition Ser.). (Illus.). 144p. (YA). (gr. 7). 17.95 (*0-8094-6142-0*) Time-Life.

Longevity: An Alternative Medicine Definitive Guide. Russ DiCarlo et al. 2000. LC 00-44175. (Illus.). 441p. pap. 14.95 (*1-887299-28-9*) AlternMed Bks.

Longevity & Quality of Life. Claude Jasmin. Ed. by Robert Butler. 2000. 334p. text 149.00 (*0-306-46315-6*, Kluwer Plenum) Kluwer Academic.

Longevity Code: Your Personal Prescription for a Longer, Sweeter Life. Zorba Paster & Susan Meltsner. 2001. LC 00-27864. xvii, 448p. 25.00 (*0-609-60360-4*, Clarkson Potter) Crown Pub Group.

Longevity Equation: How to Eat As Much As You Like & Still Live over 100 Years to Tell about It! Richard G. Deeb. 1992. 246p. pap. text 11.95 (*0-9634020-0-5*) Long Life Pr.

Longevity Factor: Chromium Picolinate. Richard A. Passwater. 1993. LC 93-5147. Orig. Title: Living Longer, Living Better, Slowing Aging with the Longevity Factor. 88p. (Orig.). pap. 4.95 (*0-87983-619-9*, 36199K, Keats Pubng) McGraw-Hill Trade.

Longevity, Senescence, & the Genome. Caleb E. Finch. (John D. & Catherine T. MacArthur Foundation Series on Mental Health & Development). (Illus.). 1995. 858p. 65.00 (*0-226-24888-7*); 1994. xvi, 938p. pap. text 45.00 (*0-226-24889-5*) U Ch Pr.

Longevity Therapy: An Innovative Approach to Nursing Home Care of the Elderly. Bobbie R. Graubarth-Szyller & Julianna D. Padgett. 1989. LC 89-821. 176p. (Orig.). pap. 20.95 (*0-914783-30-0*) Charles.

Longitudinal Muscle in Esophageal Disease. O. Arthur Stiennon. 1995. LC 94-61983. (Illus.). 300p. (C). 150.00 (*0-9644594-0-X*) Radiology Pub.

Longitudinal Research in Alcoholism. Ed. by Donald W. Goodwin & Sarnoff A. Mednick. 1984. lib. bdg. 97.00 (*0-89838-133-9*) Kluwer Academic.

Longitudinal Research on Individual Development: Present Status & Future Prospectives. Ed. by David Magnusson & Paul Casaer. 1993. LC 93-18120. (European Network on Longitudinal Studies on Individual Development: Vol. 7). (Illus.). 267p. (C). text 74.95 (*0-521-43478-5*) Cambridge U Pr.

Longitudinal Studies of HIV Infection in Intravenous Drug Users. 1993. lib. bdg. 250.00 (*0-8490-8921-2*) Gordon Pr.

Longitudinal Study of Dyslexia. H. J. Gjessing & B. Karlsen. 1989. (Illus.). 349p. 181.00 (*0-387-96948-9*) Spr-Verlag.

Longliving of Soviet Georgia. G. Z. Pitskhelauri. Tr. by Gari Lesnoff-Caravaglia from RUS. 1982. LC 81-4176. (Illus.). 158p. 30.95 (*0-89885-073-8*, Kluwer Acad Hman Sci) Kluwer Academic.

Longterm Care of the Coronary Patient. Risteard Mulcahy. 1992. (Illus.). 124p. (Orig.). pap. text (*0-443-04673-5*) Church.

Lonidamine. Ed. by B. Silvestrini et al. 1984. (Journal: Vol. 41, Suppl. 1). (Illus.). iv, 124p. pap. 76.75 (*3-8055-3867-7*) S Karger.

Lonidamine: A New Pharmacological Approach to the Study & Control of Spermatogenesis & Tumors. Ed. by B. Silvestrini & A. Caputo. 1981. (Journal: Vol. 27, Suppl.). (Illus.). 120p. pap. 31.50 (*3-8055-3438-8*) S Karger.

Look after Yourself: The Health Handbook for Older People. Alan Stewart. 1991. (Illus.). 156p. (Orig.). pap. (*0-04-442259-8*) Allen & Unwin Pty AUS. *Dist:* Paul & Co Pubs.

Look at Relapse. Jacqueline Kennedy Onassis. 1974. 10p. pap. 1.65 (*0-89486-007-0*, 1380B) Hazelden.

Look Mom . . . No Cavities: How to Raise a Cavity Free Child. Gregory F. George & Jordana H. Geist. 1997. (Illus.). 68p. pap. 16.95 (*0-9662475-0-7*) PDC Pr.

Look, Now Hear This: Combined Auditory Training & Speechreading Instruction. Janet Jeffers & Margaret Barley. 1979. (Illus.). 230p. 32.95 (*0-398-03830-9*) C C Thomas.

Look You Like: Medical Answers to 400 Questions on Skin & Hair Care. Linda Allen Schoen & Paul Lazar. 1989. (Illus.). 336p. text 39.75 (*0-8247-8146-5*) Dekker.

Looking at Children. Bjorklund. 1992. (Psychology Ser.). pap., stu. ed. 20.95 (*0-534-13705-9*) Brooks-Cole.

Looking at Children: Field Experiences in Child Study. Richard Goldman et al. 1976. LC 76-15127. (Illus.). 174p. (ps-k). pap. 16.95 (*0-89334-001-4*) Humanics Pub Grp.

Looking at Type. Earle C. Page. 3rd ed. 1997. LC 83-2028. (Illus.). 40p. pap. 5.75 (*0-935652-09-4*) Ctr Applications Psych.

Looking Back: A Reader on the Histories of Deaf Communities & Their Sign Languages. Ed. by Renate Fischer & Harlan Lane. 1993. LC 93-245607. (International Studies on Sign Language & Communication of the Deaf: Vol. 20). (Illus.). 540p. (C). text (*3-927731-32-3*) Signum-Verlag DEU. *Dist:* Gallaudet Univ Pr.

Looking Back: Reminiscent Party Fun for Senior Citizens. Marge Knoth. 1996. (Illus.). 110p. (Orig.). per. 11.99 (*0-927935-01-5*) Valley Pr IN.

Looking for Love in All the Wrong Places: Overcoming Romantic & Sexual Addictions. Jed Diamond. 1989. 256p. reprint ed. mass mkt. 4.99 (*0-380-70774-8*, Avon Bks) Morrow Avon.

Looking Forward: A Guidebook for the Laryngectomee. Robert L. Keith. 3rd ed. 1995. LC 95-905. pap. 9.95 (*0-86577-567-2*) Thieme Med Pubs.

Looking Forward: The Next 40 Years. Ed. by John M. Templeton. 1997. 228p. pap. 14.95 (*1-890151-05-X*) Templeton Fnd.

Looking Good: Teenagers & Eating Disorders. Marion Crook. 1992. 128p. (Orig.). pap. (*1-55021-077-7*) NC Ltd CAN. *Dist:* U of Toronto Pr.

Looking Good, Living Long, Feeling Great: A Breakthrough 9-Step Program to Help You Look Your Best, Live a Long, Healthy Life & Feel Great in the Process. Edna W. Burt. 1992. LC 92-90004. 100p. (Orig.). pap. 14.95 (*0-9631972-0-7*) Edna FourCZNS.

Looking Inside: Life Lessons from a Multiple Personality in Pictures & Words. Judy Castelli. 2000. LC 00-106370. (Illus.). 112p. pap. 19.95 (*0-9702806-0-2*) Castelli Studios.

Looking into Mind: How to Recognize Who You Are & How You Know. Anthony Damiani. Ed. by Widsom's Goldenrod Staff. 1990. 298p. (Orig.). pap. 14.95 (*0-943914-50-7*) Larson Pubns.

Looking Out/Looking In. Ronald B. Adler. 8th ed. 1995. LC 95-75226. 388p. (C). text 50.00 (*0-15-501728-4*) Harcourt Coll Pubs.

Looking Within: How X-Ray, CT, MRI, Ultrasound, & Other Medical Images Are Created & How They Help Physicians Save Lives. Anthony B. Wolbarst. 1999. LC 98-3892. (Illus.). xiii, 206p. pap. 19.95 (*0-520-21182-0*); 219p. text 50.00 (*0-520-21181-2*) U CA Pr.

Loony-Bin Trip. Kate Millett. 2000. LC 00-36488. 316p. reprint ed. pap. 16.95 (*0-252-06888-2*) U of Ill Pr.

Lord God Made Them All. James Herriot. 1998. 384p. reprint ed. mass mkt. 7.99 (*0-312-96620-2*, Tor Books) T Doherty Assocs.

Lose to Win: A Cardiologist's Guide to Weight Loss & Nutritional Healing. Stephen T. Sinatra. 1992. (Illus.). 228p. 19.95 (*1-879111-26-8*) Lincoln-Bradley.

Lose Ugly Fat Fast. Sylvan R. Lewis. 1980. (Illus.). 128p. pap. 2.00 (*0-936320-04-4*) Compact Books.

Lose Weight Naturally. Mark Bricklin. 1993. LC 93-7731. 374p. 9.98 (*1-56731-027-3*, MJF Bks) Fine Comms.

Lose Weight Without Going Hungry. Sylvan R. Lewis. 1981. (Illus.). 128p. pap. 2.00 (*0-936320-10-9*) Compact Books.

Losing It - Naturally: A Complete Holistic Weight Loss Program. Loretta Washburn. 1999. LC 98-73917. 296p. pap. 12.95 (*1-57174-122-4*) Hampton Roads Pub Co.

Losing Weight Permanently: Secrets of the 2% Who Succeed. Gregory L. Jantz. 2000. LC 96-3837. 204p. pap. 11.99 (*0-87788-480-3*, H Shaw Pubs) Waterbrook Pr.

Losing Weight Thru Past Lives: Or, How I Lost 90 Pounds & Realized Ancient Monks Didn't Always Eat Well. Joe Vitale. 1986. 32p. (Orig.). pap. text 3.00 (*0-9617549-0-7*) Awareness Pubns.

Losing Your Pounds of Pain: Breaking the Link Between Abuse, Stress, & Overeating. Doreen L. Virtue. 1994. LC 94-15864. 256p. (Orig.). pap. 12.95 (*1-56170-095-9*, 158) Hay House.

Loss: Sadness & Depression. John Bowlby. 2000. LC 79-2759. (Basic Books Classics). 492p. pap. text 26.00 (*0-465-04238-4*) Basic.

Loss & Bereavement: Managing Change. Ros Weston et al. 1998. LC 98-20838. pap. 43.95 (*0-632-04787-9*) Blackwell Sci.

Loss & Bereavement in Childbearing. Rosemary Mander. 1994. LC 94-13658. (Illus.). 240p. pap. (*0-632-03826-8*) Blckwell Science.

Loss & Grief. Bob Wright. 1992. LC 92-30086. (Skills for Caring Ser.). (Illus.). 48p. pap. text (*0-443-04619-0*) Church.

Loss & Grief Recovery: Help Caring for Children with Disabilities, Chronic, or Terminal Illness. Joyce M. Ashton & Dennis Ashton. 1996. LC 95-40492. 203p. 31.95 (*0-89503-138-8*) Baywood Pub.

Loss & Restoration of Regenerative Capacity in Tissues & Organs of Animals. L. V. Polezhaev. Tr. by Bruce M. Carlson. 1972. LC 71-160029. 395p. 34.00 (*0-674-53920-6*) HUP.

Loss During Pregnancy or in the Newborn Period: Principles of Care with Clinical Cases & Analysis. Ed. by James R. Woods, Jr. & Jenifer L. Woods. 1997. LC 97-70847. (Illus.). 450p. text 34.95 (*0-9655310-0-7*) Jannetti Pubns.

Loss for Words: The Story of Deafness in a Family. Lou Ann Walker. 1987. LC 85-42597. 224p. reprint ed. pap. 13.00 (*0-06-091425-4*, PL/1425, Perennial) HarperTrade.

Loss, Grief, & Bereavement: A Guide for Counseling, 4. Ed. by Otto S. Margolis et al. 1985. LC 85-12260. 176p. 49.95 (*0-275-90144-0*, C0144, Praeger Pubs) Greenwood.

Loss of Loved Ones: The Effects of a Death in the Family on Personality Development. David M. Moriarty. 2nd ed. 1983. LC 79-50189. 312p. 27.50 (*0-87527-161-8*) Green.

Loss of Self. Donna Cohen. 2nd ed. 2001. LC 00-46077. 461p. 27.95 (*0-393-05016-5*) Norton.

Loss of Self: A Resource for the Care of Alzheimer's Disease & Related Disorders. Donna Cohen & Carl Eisdorfer. l.t. ed. 1987. (Illus.). 574p. reprint ed. lib. bdg. 20.95 (*1-55736-005-7*) BDD LT Grp.

Lost Boys: Reflections on Psychoanalysis & Countertransference. Frederick Berenstein. 1995. LC 94-45955. 120p. (C). 20.00 (*0-393-70188-3*) Norton.

Lost Chord: Reaching the Person with Dementia Through the Power of Music. Melanie Chavin. 1991. 95p. (Orig.). pap. text 17.95 (*1-879633-08-6*) Eldersong.

Lost Daughters: Recovered Memory Therapy & the People It Hurts. Reinder Van Til. 1997. LC 97-21298. 301p. pap. 18.00 (*0-8028-4272-0*) Eerdmans.

***Lost for Words: Psychoanalysis of Anorexia & Bulmia.** Em Farrell. 1995. pap. (*1-899209-02-6*) Process Pr GBR. *Dist:* Intl Spec Bk.

Lost in the Mirror: An Inside Look at Borderline Personality Disorder. Richard A. Moskovitz. 1996. 208p. pap. 12.95 (*0-87833-936-1*) Taylor Pub.

Lost in the Shuffle: The Co-Dependent Reality. Robert Subby. 1987. 160p. pap. text 8.95 (*0-932194-45-1*, 22H123) Health Comm.

Lost Reform: The Campaign for Compulsory Health Insurance in the United States from 1932 to 1943. Daniel S. Hirshfield. 1970. LC 71-115187. (Commonwealth Fund Publications). 235p. 26.50 (*0-674-53917-6*) HUP.

Lost Secrets of Ayurvedic Acupuncture: An Ayurvedic Guide to Acupuncture. Frank Ros. 1994. LC 93-80314. 206p. (Orig.). pap. 15.95 (*0-914955-12-8*) Lotus Pr.

Lost Souls. Ed. by Charles Boer. 2000. (Spring Journal Ser.: Vol. 65). pap. 17.50 (*1-882670-17-5*) Spring Jrnl.

Lost Steps of Reiki: The Channeled Messages of Wei Chi. Thomas A. Hensel & Kevin R. Emery. 1997. (Orig.). pap. 9.95 (*1-890405-02-7*) LightLines.

Lost Voices: Women, Chronic Pain, & Abuse. Nellie A. Radomsky. 1995. LC 94-29611. pap. 14.95 (*1-56023-864-X*) Haworth Pr.

Lost Voices: Women, Chronic Pain & Abuse. Nellie A. Radomsky. 1995. LC 94-29611. 172p. lib. bdg. 54.95 (*1-56024-921-8*, Harrington Park) Haworth Pr.

Lotus Seeds & Lucky Stars: Asian Myths & Traditions on Pregnancy & Birthing. Shu Shu Costa. 1998. LC 97-53269. (Illus.). 144p. 17.95 (*0-684-84397-8*) S&S Trade.

Louis Guttman on Theory & Methodology: Selected Writings. Ed. by Shlomit Levy. 1994. (Benchmark Ser.). 448p. (*1-85521-389-3*) Dartmth Pub GBR. *Dist:* Ashgate Pub Co.

Lourdes of Arizona. Carlos Amantea. 1989. 150p. pap. 10.95 (*0-917320-11-5*) Mho & Mho.

Love Against Hate. Karl Augustus Menninger. 1959. LC 42-50183. 320p. pap. 10.95 (*0-15-653892-X*, Harvest Bks) Harcourt.

Love & Addiction. Stanton Peele & Archie Brodsky. 1975. LC 74-5818. 284p. 16.95 (*0-8008-5041-6*) Taplinger.

Love & Anger: Essays on AIDS, Activism, & Politics. Peter F. Cohen. 1998. LC 97-51814. (Haworth Gay & Lesbian Studies). 194p. 39.95 (*0-7890-0455-0*); pap. 16.95 (*1-56023-930-1*) Haworth Pr (Harrington Park).

Love & Attachment: Contemporary Issues & Treatment Considerations. Carol Tosone & Theresa G. Aiello. 1999. LC 98-36489. 256p. 40.00 (*0-7657-0185-5*) Aronson.

Love & Fertility: How to Avoid or Achieve Pregnancy . . . Naturally! (Includes 6-month Record Keeping Chart) Mercedes A. Wilson. 2nd ed. 1992. (Illus.). 65p. pap. text 17.90 (*0-9633125-0-2*) Family Amer Fnd.

Love & Hate: The Natural History of Behavior Patterns. Irenaus Eibl-Eibesfeldt. Tr. by Geoffrey Strachan from GER. 1996. LC 95-37462. (Evolutionary Foundations of Human Behavior Ser.). (Illus.). 289p. pap. text 24.95 (*0-202-02038-X*) Aldine de Gruyter.

Love & Hope: Fromm & Education, Vol. 10. Adir Cohen. Ed. by Roy Evans. 1990. (Special Aspects of Education Ser.). xiv, 114p. pap. text 69.00 (*2-88124-294-4*) Gordon & Breach.

Love & Love Sickness: The Science of Sex; Gender. Difference & Pair Bonding. John Money. 1980. LC 79-3679. (Illus.). 256p. pap. text 17.95 (*0-8018-2318-8*) Johns Hopkins.

Love & Narcissism in Psychoanalytic Practice. Ed. by Herbert S. Strean. 1985. LC 85-7644. (Current Issues in Psychoanalytic Practice Ser.: Vol. 2, No. 1). 107p. text 3.95 (*0-86656-386-5*) Haworth Pr.

Love & Orgasm: A Revolutionary Guide to Sexual Fulfillment. Alexander Lowen. 1975. (Illus.). 319p. pap. 7.00 (*0-02-077320-X*) Macmillan.

Love & Sex after Forty: A Guide for Men & Women for Their Mid & Later Years. Robert N. Butler & Myrna I. Lewis. l.t. ed. 1987. (Illus.). 322p. reprint ed. lib. bdg. 19.95 (*1-55736-008-1*) BDD LT Grp.

Love As Passion: The Codification of Intimacy. Niklas Luhmann. Tr. by Jeremy Gaines & Doris L. Jones from ENG. 1998. LC 98-17103. (Cultural Memory in the Present Ser.). 248p. pap. 19.95 (*0-8047-3253-1*) Stanford U Pr.

Love Drug: Marching to the Beat of Ecstasy. Richard S. Cohen. 1998. LC 97-39231. 166p. 39.95 (*0-7890-0453-4*); pap. 19.95 (*0-7890-0454-2*) Haworth Pr (Hawrth Medical).

Love, Guilt & Reparation & Other Works, 1921-1945. Melanie Klein. 1984. LC 84-13766. (Writings of Melanie Klein: Vol. 1). 480p. (C). 45.00 (*0-02-918420-7*) Free Pr.

Love in America: Gender & Self-Development. Francesca M. Cancian. 1987. (Illus.). 224p. text 64.95 (*0-521-34202-3*) Cambridge U Pr.

Love Is a Journey: Couples Facing Cancer. Jan Latona & Gary J. Stricklin. 1999. LC 99-66209. (Illus.). xv, 127p. pap. 14.95 (*0-9673715-0-3*) Greyrock.

Love Is Ageless: Stories about Alzheimer's Disease. Ed. by Jessica Bryan. 1988. 200p. pap. 9.95 (*0-9619311-0-8*) Lompico Cr Pr.

***Love Is Ageless: Stories about Alzheimer's Disease.** Jessica Bryan et al. 2nd rev. ed. 2002. LC 87-91232. (Illus.). 300p. pap. 16.95 (*0-9619311-1-6*) Lompico Cr Pr.

Love Is Never Enough: How Couples Can Overcome Misunderstandings, Resolve Conflicts, & Solve Relationship Problems Through Cognitive Therapy. Aaron T. Beck. 1989. LC 88-45010. 432p. reprint ed. pap. 14.00 (*0-06-091604-4*, Perennial) HarperTrade.

Love Knot: Ties That Bind Cancer Partners. Robert Ross. 2000. LC 00-55822. (Illus.). 232p. (C). pap. text 15.95 (*0-7637-1412-7*, 1412-7) Jones & Bartlett.

Love Madness: Medicine, the Novel, & the Female Insanity, 1800-1865. Helen Small. 1998. (Illus.). 274p. reprint ed. pap. text 24.95 (*0-19-818491-3*) OUP.

Love, Medicine & Miracles: Lessons Learned about Self-Healing from a Surgeon's Experience with Exceptional Patients. Bernie S. Siegel. 60th ed. 1998. LC 89-46437. (Illus.). 256p. reprint ed. pap. 14.00 (*0-06-091983-3*, Perennial) HarperTrade.

Love, Miracles & Animal Healing: A Veterinarian's Journey from Physical Medicine to Spiritual Understanding. Allen M. Schoen & Pam Procter. 1995. LC 95-1389. 240p. 21.50 (*0-684-80207-4*) S&S Trade.

Love, Miracles & Animal Healing: A Veterinarian's Journey from Physical Medicine to Spiritual Understanding. Allen M. Schoen & Pam Proctor. 1996. 240p. per. 12.00 (*0-684-82273-3*, Fireside) S&S Trade Pap.

Love Relations: Normality & Pathology. Otto F. Kernberg. 1995. LC 94-38369. 224p. 50.00 (*0-300-06031-9*) Yale U Pr.

Love, Sex, Feminism. John Wilson. 1980. LC 79-24902. 125p. 52.50 (*0-275-91695-2*, C1695, Praeger Pubs) Greenwood.

Love Thine Enemas & Heal Thyself. Jerry G. Knox. 1997. (Illus.). 425p. pap. text 29.95 (*0-9625908-1-9*) Lifeknox Pub.

Love Your Body. Viktoras Kulvinskas. 1972. (Illus.). 94p. (Orig.). pap. text 9.95 (*0-933278-01-2*) Twen Fir Cent.

Love Your Heart Italian (Low-Cholesterol) Cookbook. Carole Kruppa. 1994. LC 93-44576. 280p. (Orig.). pap. 12.95 (*0-940625-81-4*) Surrey Bks.

Lovell & Winter's Pediatric Orthopaedics. Raymond T. Morrissy & Stuart L. Weinstein. 5th ed. 1552p. text (*0-7817-2580-1*); 1552p. text (*0-7817-2581-X*); 2000. 1,600p. text 325.00 (*0-7817-2582-8*) Lppncott W & W.

Lovell & Winter's Pediatric Orthopaedics. Ed. by Raymond T. Morrissy & Stuart L. Weinstein. 1995. LC 95-31125. Vol. 1. (*0-397-51598-7*); Vol. 2. (*0-397-51599-5*) Lppncott W & W.

Lovemaps: Clinical Concepts of Sexual-Erotic Health & Pathology, Paraphilia & Gender Transposition in Childhood, Adolescence & Maturity. John Money. LC 85-24153. (Illus.). 350p. (C). 1986. 34.50 (*0-8290-1589-2*); 1989. reprint ed. pap. 18.95 (*0-8290-1892-1*) Irvington.

Lovenotes: Music for the Unborn Child. Lorna Zemke. 1989. tchr. ed. 89.95 incl. audio, VHS (*0-9625034-1-X*) Silver Lake Col Pr.

Lover Within: Opening to Energy in Sexual Practice. Julie Henderson. Ed. by George Quasha. 1987. LC 86-30066. (Illus.). 118p. 18.95 (*0-88268-023-4*) Station Hill Pr.

Lovers, Killers, Husbands, Wives. Martin Blinder. 1985. 192p. mass mkt. 4.50 (*0-312-90219-0*) St Martin.

Love's Body. Norman O. Brown. 1990. 285p. pap. 17.95 (*0-520-07106-9*); LC 90-34738. text 50.00 (*0-520-07105-0*) U CA Pr.

Love's Executioner: And Other Tales of Psychotherapy. Irvin D. Yalom. 2000. (Perennial Classics Ser.). 304p. reprint ed. pap. 14.00 (*0-06-095834-0*) HarperCollins Pubs.

Love's Executioner: And Other Tales of Psychotherapy. Irvin D. Yalom. 1990. LC 89-46494. 288p. reprint ed. pap. 13.50 (*0-06-097334-X*, Perennial) HarperTrade.

Love's Hidden Symmetry: What Makes Love Work in Relationships. Bert Hellinger et al. 1998. LC 98-13152. 330p. 38.00 (*1-891944-00-2*) Zeig Tucker Theisen.

Lovesickness in the Middle Ages: The Viaticum & Its Commentaries. Mary F. Wack. 1990. LC 89-22450. (Middle Ages Ser.). (Illus.). 372p. (C). text 44.95 (*0-8122-8142-X*) U of Pa Pr.

LoveStart: Pre-Birth Bonding. Eve Marnie. (SPA.). 142p. (Orig.). pap. 10.00 (*84-86344-88-3*, 139) Hay House.

Loving an Alcoholic: Help & Hope for Significant Others. Jack Mumey. 1985. 192p. 13.95 (*0-8092-5182-5*) NTC Contemp Pub Co.

Loving & Letting Go: Parents Who Decide Against Medical Intervention. Deborah Davis. 1992. (Illus.). 64p. (Orig.). pap. 5.95 (*1-56123-060-X*, LLGC) Centering Corp.

Loving Hands: The/Traditional Art of Baby Massage. Frederick Leboyer. 1997. LC 97-25335. (Illus.). 144p. pap. 16.95 (*1-55704-314-0*) Newmarket.

Loving, Hating & Survival: A Handbook for All Who Work with Troubled Children & Young People. Ed. by Andrew Hardwick & Judith Woodhead. 1999. LC 98-40536. xxviii, 427p. text (*1-85742-424-7*, RJ499.3.L68) Arena GBR. *Dist:* Ashgate Pub Co.

Loving Tough, Loving Smart, Loving You: You & the Alcoholic. Arnie Wallace & Adryan Russ. 1990. LC 89-82160. 98p. (Orig.). per. 9.95 (*0-9625341-0-2*) Challenger CA.

Low Back & Leg Pain. James M. Cox. 5th ed. 1988. (Illus.). 20p. (*0-9616488-3-X*) Alef Bet Comns.

Low Back & Leg Pain from Herniated Cervical Disk. Herman Kabat. 1980. 154p. pap. 17.50 (*0-87527-246-0*) Green.

Low Back & Neck Pain: Causes & Conservative Treatment. P. C. Williams. 1982. (Illus.). 96p. spiral bd. 19.95 (*0-398-03193-2*) C C Thomas.

Low Back & Pelvis: Clinical Applications. Chris J. Hutcheson. 1996. 200p. pap. 64.00 (*0-8342-0689-7*, 20689) Aspen Pub.

Low Back Pain. William Hunter. 1985. 56p. 5.00 (*0-8187-0058-0*) Harlo Press.

Low Back Pain. Sam W. Wiesel et al. 2nd ed. 1989. (Illus.). 931p. 65.00 (*0-87473-449-5*, 62021-10, MICHIE) LEXIS Pub.

Low Back Pain. James Cox et al. 5th ed. 1990. (Illus.). 645p. 100.00 (*0-683-02152-4*) Lppncott W & W.

Low Back Pain: A Scientific & Clinical Overview. Ed. by James Weinstein & Steve Gordon. 1996. LC 96-44528. 480p. 105.00 (*0-89203-160-3*) Amer Acad Ortho Surg.

Low Back Pain: A Symptom-Based Approach to Diagnosis & Treatment. Karen S. Rucker et al. 2000. LC 00-36007. (Illus.). 400p. pap. text 59.99 (*0-7506-9485-8*) Buttrwrth-Heinemann.

***Low Back Pain: An Evidence-Based, Biopsychosocial Model for Clinical Management.** Ed. by Jane Derebery & John R. Anderson. 2001. LC 2001-6158. (*1-883595-34-7*, OEM Pr) OEM Health.

Low Back Pain: Clinical Diagnosis & Management. Leonard P. Seimon. 2nd ed. 1995. (Illus.). 352p. 99.00 (*0-939957-40-X*) Demos Medical.

Low Back Pain: Health Care Needs Asessment: The Epidemiologically Based Needs Assessment Reviews, Second Series. Wessex Institute for Health Research and Development. 1997. LC 97-13355. (*1-85775-201-5*) Radcliffe Med Pr GBR. *Dist:* Balogh.

Low Back Pain: Mechanisms, Diagnosis & Treatment. James M. Cox. 6th ed. 1998. LC 98-17984. 800p. 89.00 (*0-683-30358-9*) Lppncott W & W.

Low Back Pain: Medical Diagnosis & Comprehensive Management. David G. Borenstein et al. 2nd ed. 1994. LC 93-41601. text 79.00 (*0-7216-5411-8*) Saunders.

Low Back Pain Handbook: A Practical Guide for the Primary Care Clinician. Ed. by Andrew J. Cole & Stanley Herring. 1996. LC 96-20355. 475p. pap. 49.95 (*1-56053-152-5*) Hanley & Belfus.

Low Back Pain Handbook: Evaluation & Management. Brian D'Orazio. 1998. LC 98-40679. 336p. text 44.99 (*0-7506-9618-4*) Buttrwrth-Heinemann.

Low Back Pain Syndrome. Renee Cailliet. 5th ed. 1994. LC 94-22969. (Pain Ser.). (Illus.). 381p. pap. text 25.95 (*0-8036-1607-4*) Davis Co.

Low-Back Patient: Treatment by Physical Therapy. Joan G. Lafreniere. 1979. (C). (gr. 13). 31.50 (*0-89352-033-0*) Mosby Inc.

Low Birthweight in Minority & High-Risk Women: Patient Outcome Research Team (Port)-Final Report. Ed. by Robert L. Goldenberg. 1999. (Illus.). 100p. (C). reprint ed. pap. text 20.00 (*0-7881-8415-6*) DIANE Pub.

Low Blood Sugar. Clement G. Martin. 1985. LC 74-112735. 192p. pap. 5.00 (*0-671-76410-1*, Fireside) S&S Trade Pap.

Low Blood Sugar (Hypoglysemia) The Twentieth Century Epidemic? Martin L. Budd. 1983. LC 83-5053. 128 sp. (Orig.). pap. 9.95 (*0-8069-7792-2*) Sterling.

Low Calorie & Special Dietary Foods. Ed. by Basant K. Dwivedi. 1978. (Uniscience Ser.). 144p. 89.00 (*0-8493-5249-5*, RM258, CRC Reprint) Franklin.

Low-Calorie Foods & Food Ingredients. Ed. by Riaz Khan. 1993. LC 93-3183. 183p. (*0-7514-0004-1*) B Acad & Prof GBR. *Dist:* Aspen Pub.

Low-Calorie Foods Handbook. Aaron M. Altschul. 1993. (Food Science & Technology Ser.: Vol. 56). (Illus.). 608p. text 250.00 (*0-8247-8812-5*) Dekker.

Low-Calorie Sweeteners: Present & Future: ISA-IUFoST World Conference on Low-Calorie Sweeteners, Barcelona, April 1999. Ed. by A. Corti. 1999. LC 99-48944. (World Review of Nutrition & Dietetics Ser.: Vol. 85). (Illus.). xiv, 244p. 198.25 (*3-8055-6938-6*) S Karger.

Low Cholesterol Life: The Diet & Lifestyle Way to the New, Healthier You. Sylvan Lewis. 1992. mass mkt. 4.50 (*1-56171-075-X*) SPI.

Low-Dose Extrapolation of Cancer Risks: Issues & Persepectives. Ed. by W. Farland et al. 1995. LC 95-77850. (Illus.). 355p. pap. 50.00 (*0-944398-33-2*) ILSI.

Low-Dose Methotrexate-Therapy in Rheumatic Diseases. Ed. by R. Rau. 1986. (Rheumatology Ser.: Vol. 9). (Illus.). xii, 268p. 155.75 (*3-8055-4236-4*) S Karger.

Low-Fat for Life: An Integrated Program for Making the Change to a Healthier, Low-fat Lifestyle. Mike Heus et al. rev. ed. 1998. LC 93-91552. (Illus.). 494p. pap. 16.95 (*0-937373-05-2*) Micamar Pub.

Low-Fat Good Food Cookbook: Combo Prepack. Martin Katahn & Terri Katahn. 1994. LC 94-6548. pap. 209.10 (*0-393-31186-4*) Norton.

Low-Fat Living: Turn off the Fat Makers, Turn on the Fat Burners for Longevity, Energy, Weight Loss, Freedom from Disease. Robert K. Cooper & Leslie L. Cooper. 1996. LC 95-38190. (Illus.). 496p. 27.95 (*0-87596-295-5*) Rodale Pr Inc.

Low Flow Anaesthesia. Jan A. Baum. 2nd ed. 2001. LC 00-48639. (Illus.). 300p. text 85.00 (*0-7506-4672-1*) Buttrwrth-Heinemann.

Low-Flow Anaesthesia: The Theory & Practice of Low Flow, Minimum Flow & Closed System Anaesthesia. Jan A. Baum & Geoffrey Nunn. 1996. LC 96-167207. 192p. text 80.00 (*0-7506-2127-3*) Buttrwrth-Heinemann.

Low Friction Arthroplasty of the Hip: Theory & Practice. J. Charnley. 1978. (Illus.). 376p. 176.00 (*0-387-08893-8*) Spr-Verlag.

Low Level Radiation & Immune System Damage: An Atomic Era Legacy. Joseph J. Mangano. 1998. LC 98-18138. 240p. lib. bdg. 49.95 (*1-56670-334-4*, L1334) Lewis Pubs.

Low Molecular Weight Heparin & Its Clinical Use: Journal: Haemostasis, Vol. 16, No. 1, 1985. 1986. 124p. pap. 68.00 (*3-8055-4230-5*) S Karger.

Low Molecular Weight Heparin Therapy: An Evaluation of Clinical Trials Evidence. Monique Sarret et al. 1999. LC 99-39512. (Illus.). 488p. text 175.00 (*0-8247-8213-5*) Dekker.

Low-Molecular-Weight Heparins: A New Therapeutic Approach to Thrombosis Proceedings. Ed. by J. Monasterio & M. M. Samama. 1996. (Journal: Vol. 26, No. 2, 1996). (Illus.). iv, 66p. pap., suppl. ed. 21.75 (*3-8055-6277-2*) S Karger.

Low Molecular Weight Heparins: Pharmacology, In-Vivo & Ex-Vivo Effects & Clinical Results - Journal: Haemostasis, Vol. 18, Suppl. 2, 1988. Ed. by H. K. Breddin et al. 1988. (Illus.). iv, 88p. pap. 28.00 (*3-8055-4787-0*) S Karger.

Low Molecular Weight Heparins in Clinical Practice. Ed. by Doutremepuich. 1992. (Illus.). 264p. text 160.00 (*0-8247-8640-8*) Dekker.

Low Protein Cookery for Phenylketonuria. Virginia E. Schuett. 3rd ed. 1997. LC 97-5931. (Illus.). 572p. pap. 24.95 (*0-299-15384-3*) U of Wis Pr.

Low Protein Diet & Progression of Chronic Renal Failure. Ed. by M. Strauch & Sergio Giovannetti. 1986. (Contributions to Nephrology Ser.: Vol. 53). (Illus.). viii, 146p. 29.75 (*3-8055-4364-6*) S Karger.

Low-Protein Diets in Renal Patients: Composition & Absorption. Ed. by N. Gretz. 1989. (Contributions to Nephrology Ser.: Vol. 72). (Illus.). x, 106p. 29.75 (*3-8055-4963-6*) S Karger.

Low Risk Neonatal Nursing. Jack Rudman. (Certified Nurse Examination Ser.: CN-22). pap. 27.95 (*0-8373-6122-2*) Nat Learn.

Low Temperature Preservation of Foods & Living Matter. Ed. by Owen R. Fennema et al. 1973. (Food Science & Technology Ser.: Vol. 3). (Illus.). 616p. text 59.75 (*0-8247-1185-8*) Dekker.

Low Vision. Ed. by G. C. Woo. 1987. (Illus.). 577p. 98.00 (*0-387-96538-6*) Spr-Verlag.

Low Vision: Reflections of the Past, Issues for the Future. Ed. by Virginia E. Bishop et al. 1993. 181p. pap. 29.95 (*0-89128-218-1*) Am Foun Blind.

Low Vision: Research & New Developments in Rehabilitation: Proceedings of Vision 1993, the International Conference on Low Vision, 5-9 July 1993, Groningen, Netherlands. Ed. by A. C. Kooijman et al. 1994. LC 93-8028. (Studies in Health Technology & Informatics: Vol. 11). 596p. 130.00 (*90-5199-144-4*) IOS Press.

Low Vision & Blindness: Research & Development. Ed. by Tamara T. Sowell. 2000. (Illus.). 103p. (C). pap. text 25.00 (*0-7567-0202-X*) DIANE Pub.

Low Vision Handbook. Barbara Brown. 1997. LC 97-10169. (Basic Bookshelf for Eyecare Professionals Ser.). (Illus.). 160p. pap. text 30.00 (*1-55642-329-2*, 63292) SLACK Inc.

Low Vision in Optometric Practice: Principles & Practice. Christine Dickinson. 1998. LC 98-28062. (Illus.). 320p. pap. text 70.00 (*0-7506-2262-8*) Buttrwrth-Heinemann.

Low Vision Rehabilitation. Donald C. Fletcher. 1999. LC 98-41362. (Ophthalmology Monographs Ser.). xiv, 162 p. (*1-56055-170-4*) American Academic Assn for Peace in the Middle East.

Lowenfeld Lectures: Viktor Lowenfeld on Art Education & Therapy. Ed. by John A. Michael. 1982. LC 80-29265. (Illus.). 420p. (C). text 44.00 (*0-271-00283-2*) Pa St U Pr.

Lowenfeld Mosaic Test. Margaret Lowenfeld. 2nd ed. 1994. 560p. reprint ed. pap. (*0-9521788-1-8*) M Lowenfeld GBR. *Dist:* Intl Spec Bk.

Lower Brainstem & Bodily Homeostasis. William W. Blessing. 1997. (Illus.). 592p. text 89.50 (*0-19-507511-0*) OUP.

Lower Extremity Amputation. Wesley S. Moore & Malone. 1989. 352p. text 105.00 (*0-7216-6485-7*) Saunders.

Lower Extremity Amputation: A Guide to Functional Outcomes in Physical Therapy Management. Linda A. Karacoloff et al. 2nd ed. 1995. LC 92-7054. 288p. spiral bd. 75.00 (*0-8342-0291-3*) PRO-ED.

Lower Extremity & Spine in Sports Medicine. Ed. by James A. Nicholas. 2nd ed. 1994. LC 94-26126. (Illus.). 1808p. (C). (gr. 13). text 280.00 (*0-8151-6391-6*, 23615) Mosby Inc.

Lower Extremity Vascular Disease. Ed. by Kenneth Ouriel. 1995. LC 95-6842. text 152.00 (*0-7216-4749-9*) Saunders.

Lower Genital Tract Precancer. Albert Singer & John M. Monaghan. 2nd ed. 2000. LC 99-16649. (Illus.). 323p. 208.95 (*0-632-04769-0*) Blackwell Sci.

Lower Limb, Vol. 2. Matthew J. Kandel et al. 5th ed. 1988. LC 80-42183. (Lower Limb Ser.: Vol. 2). (Illus.). 242p. (C). pap. text (*0-443-03618-7*) Church.

Lower Limb, Vol. 7. 1972. (*0-443-00721-7*) Church.

Lower Urinary Tract Diseases of Dogs & Cats. Gerald V. Ling. 1995. LC 94-41538. (Illus.). 256p. (C). (gr. 13). text 90.00 (*0-8151-5446-1*, 23970) Mosby Inc.

Lower Your Blood Pressure with Food & Herbs. Date not set. pap. 6.95 (*1-930329-01-6*) R M Khalilullah.

Lowering Cholesterol in High-Risk Individuals & Populations. Ed. by Basil M. Rifkind. 1995. LC 94-45081. (Fundamental & Clinical Cardiology Ser.: No. 24). (Illus.). 392p. text 150.00 (*0-8247-9412-5*) Dekker.

Lowering the Risk: A Self-Care Plan for Relapse Prevention. Merlene Miller & Terence Gorski. 1991. 31p. pap. 4.00 (*0-8309-0609-6*) Herald Pub Hse.

Lowfat American Favorites. Goldie Silverman & Jacqueline B. Williams. 1990. (Nitty Gritty Cookbooks Ser.). (Illus.). 160p. pap. 8.95 (*0-911954-95-3*, Nitty Gritty Ckbks) Bristol Pub Ent CA.

LPN Nursing Pearls of Wisdom. Hunter S. Thompson. 1999. (Pearls of Wisdom Ser.). pap. 26.00 (*1-58409-002-2*) Boston Medical.

LPN to RN Transitions. Nicki Harrington et al. 1995. LC 95-40073. 416p. pap. text 28.95 (*0-397-55065-0*) Lppncott W & W.

LPN/LVN Review: Medical/Surgical Tutor. Gary W. Stogsdill. 1995. (LPN/LVN Nursing Ser.). (C). 20.95 (*0-8273-6545-4*) Delmar.

LSD: A Total Study. D. Siva Sankar et al. 1975. LC 72-95447. 69.95 (*0-9600290-3-6*) PJD Pubns.

LSD Psychotherapy: Exploring the Frontiers of the Hidden Mind. Stanislav Grof. 2nd ed. 1994. LC 92-1429. (Illus.). 352p. 34.95 (*0-89793-166-1*); pap. 22.95 (*0-89793-158-0*) Hunter Hse.

Luchevaia Diagnostika Endofitnogo Raka Zheludka see Radiodiagnosis of Endophytic Gastric Cancer

Lucid Dreaming: The Paradox of Consciousness During Sleep. Celia Green & Charles McCreery. 1994. LC 93-50637. 224p. (C). (gr. 13). pap. 19.95 (*0-415-11239-7*, B4223) Routledge.

Lucid Dreams. Celia Green. 1989. (C). 70.00 (*0-900076-00-3*) St Mut.

Luckmann & Sorensen's Medical-Surgical Nursing: A Psychophysiologic Approach. Ed. by Joyce M. Black & Esther Matassarin-Jacobs. 4th ed. 1993. (Illus.). tchr. ed. (*0-7216-3786-8*);Manual of Test Questions. (*0-7216-3891-0*) Saunders.

Luckmann's Core Princ Prac. Polaski. 1996. 100.00 (*0-7216-5998-5*) Harcourt.

Luckmann's Core Principles & Practice of Medical-Surgical Nursing. Arlene L. Polaski. 1996. LC 97-115800. 1776p. pap. text, stu. ed. 17.95 (*0-7216-6771-6*) Saunders.

Luckmann's Core Principles & Practice of Medical-Surgical Nursing. Arlene L. Polaski & Suzanne E. Tatro. 1996. 1776p. (*0-7216-5996-9*); 1776p. tchr. ed. (*0-7216-5995-0*); LC 96-166595. pap. text 19.95 (*0-7216-6817-8*) Saunders.

Luckmann's Core Principles & Practice of Medical-Surgical Nursing. Arlene L. Polaski & Suzanne E. Tatro. Ed. by Thomas Eoyang. 1996. (Illus.). 1840p. text 68.00 (*0-7216-5994-2*) Saunders.

***Luckmann's Core Principles & Practice of Medical-Surgical Nursing.** Arlene L. Polaski & Suzanne E. Tatro. 1996. (*0-7216-5997-7*) Saunders.

Ludwig Wittgenstein: Eine Existenzielle Deutung. L. Adler. 1976. 35.00 (*3-8055-2390-4*) S Karger.

Lumb & Jones' Veterinary Anesthesia. Ed. by John C. Thurmon et al. 3rd ed. 1996. LC 95-46509. (Illus.). 928p. 89.00 (*0-683-08238-8*) Lppncott W & W.

Lumbale Discectomie. Oliver D. Grin & Dorothy L. Bouwman. Tr. by John Vriend et al. 1992. (Patient Education Ser.). (DUT., Illus.). 18p. (Orig.). pap. text 4.00 (*0-929689-55-0*) Ludann Co.

Lumbar Disc Herniation. Franco Postacchini. 1999. LC 98-54151. (Illus.). 700p. 299.00 (*3-211-83118-5*) Spr-Verlag.

Lumbar Fusion & Stabilization. Ed. by K. Ono et al. 1993. LC 92-46674. (Illus.). 416p. 174.00 (*0-387-70116-8*) Spr-Verlag.

Lumbar Microdiskectomy. Oliver D. Grin & Dorothy L. Bouwman. 1993. (Patient Education Ser.). (Illus.). 24p. (Orig.). pap. text 4.00 (*0-929689-57-7*) Ludann Co.

Lumbar Spinal Stenosis. F. Postacchini. 1989. (Illus.). 230p. 120.00 (*0-387-82111-2*) Spr-Verlag.

Lumbar Spinal Stenosis. Marek Szpalski & Robert Gunzburg. 1999. LC 99-44476. 432p. text 129.00 (*0-7817-2380-9*) Lppncott W & W.

Lumbar Spine & Back Pain. Ed. by Malcolm I. Jayson. 4th ed. 1992. (Illus.). 637p. text (*0-443-04189-X*) Church.

Lumbar Spine Disorders: Current Concepts. Ed. by R. M. Aspden & R. W. Porter. 1995. LC 95-2988. 260p. text 74.00 (*981-02-2175-4*) World Scientific Pub.

Lumbar Spine Disorders Current Concepts, 2. 1996. 250p. lib. bdg. 41.00 (*981-02-2792-2*) World Scientific Pub.

Lumbar Spine Syndromes. Gunnar B. Andersson & T. W. McNeill. 1989. (Illus.). 250p. 118.00 (*0-387-82070-1*) Spr-Verlag.

Lumber Spine. International Society for the Study of the Lumber Spine. Ed. by Wiesel, Weinstein, Herkowitz, Dvorak, & Bell Staff et al. 2nd ed. 1996. LC 95-10052. (Illus.). 1056p. text 260.00 (*0-7216-4953-X*) Saunders.

Lumboischialgie. Ed. by W. Miller et al. 1982. (Fortbildungskurse fuer Rheumatologie Ser.: Vol. 6). (Illus.). xii, 264p. pap. 62.75 (*3-8055-2207-X*) S Karger.

Lumbosacral & Spinopelvic Fixation. Joseph Margulies. 1996. LC 93-34226. (Illus.). 960p. text 239.00 (*0-397-51388-7*) Lppncott W & W.

Luminous Essence: New Light on the Healing Body an Alternative Healer's Story. Daniel Santos. 1997. LC 97-4460. 288p. pap. 14.00 (*0-8356-0755-0*, Quest) Theos Pub Hse.

Lumps & Bumps: A Children's Book for Parents & a Parent's Book for Children. Denton L. Roberts. 1997. (Illus.). 22p. pap. 7.50 (*0-9613559-2-1*) Human Esteem Pub.

Luna Yoga: Vital Fertility & Sexuality. Adelheid Ohlig. Tr. by Meret Liebenstein from GER. 1995. LC 94-71324. (Best of Europe Ser.). (Illus.). 192p. (Orig.). pap. 11.95 (*0-9614620-6-X*) Ash Tree.

Lung: Molecular Basis of Disease. Jerome S. Brody. Ed. by Judy Fletcher. 1998. LC 97-27841. (Illus.). 240p. (C). text 50.00 (*0-7216-6814-3*) Saunders.

Lung: Scientific Foundations Ed. by Ronald G. Crystal et al. 2nd ed. 1996. LC 96-14140. 3,056p. text 389.00 (*0-397-51632-0*) Lppncott W & W.

Lung & Heart-Lung Transplantation. V. Gallucci et al. 1991. 166p. text (*1-57235-040-7*) Piccin Nuova.

Lung at Depth. Ed. by Claes Lundgren & John M. Miller. 1999. LC 99-22838. (Lung Biology in Health & Disease Ser.). (Illus.). 712p. text 250.00 (*0-8247-0158-5*) Dekker.

Lung Cancer. Ed. by Desmond N. Carney. 1995. (An Arnold Publication). 280p. (*0-340-56759-7*) E A GBR. *Dist:* OUP.

Lung Cancer. Robert J. Ginsberg. 2000. (ACS Atlas of Clinical Oncology Ser.). 352p. incl. cd-rom (*1-55009-099-2*) DEKR.

Lung Cancer. Ed. by Heine H. Hansen. 1986. (Cancer Treatment & Research Ser.). text 152.50 (*0-89838-763-9*) Kluwer Academic.

Lung Cancer. Ed. by Bruce E. Johnson & David H. Johnson. 1994. (Current Clinical Oncology Ser.). 368p. 160.00 (*0-471-01285-8*) Wiley.

Lung Cancer. Ed. by Robert B. Livingston. 1981. (Cancer Treatment & Research Ser.: No. 1). (Illus.). 320p. text 175.50 (*90-247-2394-9*) Kluwer Academic.

Lung Cancer. Jack A. Roth et al. 2nd ed. 1998. LC 97-37264. (Illus.). 400p. 115.95 (*0-86542-573-6*) Blackwell Sci.

Lung Cancer. Chris Williams. 2nd ed. 1995. (Facts Ser.). (Illus.). 152p. (C). reprint ed. pap. 19.95 (*0-19-262250-1*) OUP.

Lung Cancer, Vol. 2. John G. Gruhn. 1989. 75.00 (*0-938607-17-0*); 65.00 (*0-938607-10-3*) Field & Wood Inc Medical.

Lung Cancer: A Comprehensive Guide for Patients & Families. Lorraine Johnston. 2001. LC 00-65256. (Patient-Centered Guides Ser.). (Illus.). 500p. 27.95 (*0-596-50002-5*) OReilly & Assocs.

Lung Cancer: A Guide to Diagnosis & Treatment. Walter Scott. 2000. LC 00-8028. (Illus.). x, 156p. pap. 14.95 (*1-886039-43-7*) Addicus Bks.

Lung Cancer: A Practical Guide to Management. Fergus R. Macbeth. 1996. 148p. pap. text 23.00 (*3-7186-5860-7*, Harwood Acad Pubs) Gordon & Breach.

Lung Cancer: A Practical Guide to Management. Fergus R. Macbeth et al. 1996. 148p. text 60.00 (*3-7186-5859-3*, Harwood Acad Pubs) Gordon & Breach.

J
K
L

Lung Cancer: Advances in Basic & Clinical Research. Ed. by Heine H. Hansen. 1994. LC 94-10350. (Cancer Treatment & Research Ser.: Vol. 72). 416p. (C). text 318.00 (*0-7923-2835-3*) Kluwer Academic.

Lung Cancer: Principles & Practice. Harvey I. Pass. 2000. LC 99-51908. (Illus.). 1,408p. text 189.00 (*0-7817-1791-4*) Lppncott W & W.

Lung Cancer: Textbook for General Practitioners. Ed. by Europe Against Cancer Staff & H. H. Hansen. 1990. (EC Series for General Practitioners). (Illus.). 58p. 39.00 (*0-387-53075-4*) Spr-Verlag.

Lung Cancer: The Art of Detection by Conventional Radiography. Alfred Szamosi. Ed. by Swedish Heart and Lung Foundation Staff. 1995. (Illus.). 117p. 74.50 (*91-630-2980-4*) Coronet Bks.

Lung Cancer Chronicles. John A. Meyer. 1990. LC 89-11000. (Illus.). 250p. (Orig.). 35.00 (*0-8135-1492-4*); pap. 12.95 (*0-8135-1493-2*) Rutgers U Pr.

Lung Cancer Differentiation: Implications for Diagnosis & Treatment. Ed. by Samuel D. Bernal & Paul J. Hesketh. 1992. (Lung Biology in Health & Disease Ser.: Vol. 58). (Illus.). 496p. text 230.00 (*0-8247-8638-6*) Dekker.

Lung Cancer Handbook: Evaluation & Management. Christine M. Dela Cruz & Harubumi Kato. 1993. LC 92-1694. 189p. pap. text 35.00 (*3-7186-5294-3*) Gordon & Breach.

Lung Cancer, 1980: Post-Graduate Course II. Ed. by Heine H. Hansen & M. Roth. 1981. (International Congress Ser.: Vol. 525). pap. 47.25 (*0-444-90160-4*) Elsevier.

Lung Carcinomas. Ed. by Elizabeth M. McDowell. 1987. LC 86-33361. (Current Problems in Tumor Pathology Ser.). (Illus.). 410p. text (*0-443-03165-7*) Church.

Lung Circulation. Set, Vols. 1 & 2. D. M. Aviado. 1965. LC 64-24302. (*0-08-010988-8*) Pergamon Repr GBR. *Dist:* Franklin.

Lung Connective Tissue: Location, Metabolism, & Response to Injury. Ed. by John A. Pickrell. 1981. 224p. 98.95 (*0-8493-5749-7*, RC756) CRC Pr.

Lung Disease: State-of-the-Art, 1984-1986. Ed. by Reuben M. Cherniack. 1987. (Lung Disease: State-of-the-Art Ser.). (Illus.). 224p. 20.50 (*0-915116-05-7*, 9807) Am Lung Assn.

Lung Disease: State of the Art, 1986-1987. Ed. by Reuben M. Cherniack. 1988. (State of the Art Ser.). (Illus.). 202p. (*0-915116-06-5*, 9801) Am Lung Assn.

Lung Disease: State of the Art, 1987-1988. Ed. by Reuben M. Cherniack. 1989. (Illus.). 224p. 35.00 (*0-915116-07-3*, 9622) Am Lung Assn.

Lung Disease: State of the Art, 1988-1989. Ed. by Reuben M. Cherniack. 1990. (State of the Art Ser.). (Illus.). 230p. 50.00 (*0-915116-08-1*, 9620) Am Lung Assn.

Lung Disease: State of the Art, 1989-90. Ed. by Robert A. Klocke. 1991. (State of the Art Ser.). (Illus.). 226p. 60.00 (*0-915116-09-X*, 9611) Am Lung Assn.

Lung Disease: State of the Art, 1990-92. Ed. by Robert A. Klocke. (State of the Art Ser.). (Illus.). 348p. 65.00 (*0-915116-10-3*, 9775) Am Lung Assn.

Lung Disease: State of the Art, 1993-94. Ed. by Robert A. Klocke. (State of the Art Ser.). 256p. 50.00 (*0-915116-11-1*, 9776) Am Lung Assn.

Lung Disease: State of the Art, 1995-1996. ATS Staff. 1997. 356p. per. 65.00 (*0-7872-3709-4*) Kendall-Hunt.

Lung Disease in the Tropics. Ed. by Om P. Sharma. 1990. (Lung Biology in Health & Disease Ser.: Vol. 51). (Illus.). 624p. text 255.00 (*0-8247-8398-0*) Dekker.

Lung Disorders Sourcebook: Basic Consumer Health Information about Emphysema, Pneumonia & Other Lung Disorders. Ed. by Dawn D. Matthews. 2001. (Health Reference Ser.). 650p. lib. bdg. 78.00 (*0-7808-0339-6*) Omnigraphics Inc.

Lung Dosimetry Models for Inhaled Radon Progeny. Martonen Hofmann. 1994. (*0-8493-5830-2*) CRC Pr.

Lung Function: Assessment & Application in Medicine. J. E. Cotes & G. L. Leathart. 5th ed. 1993. LC 92-49426. 784p. 199.95 (*0-632-03526-9*) Blackwell Sci.

Lung Function in Children & Adolescents. Ed. by A. Zapletal et al. 1987. (Progress in Respiratory Research Ser.: Vol. 22). (Illus.). viii, 220p. 152.25 (*3-8055-4495-2*) S Karger.

Lung Function Tests: A Guide to Their Interpretation. William J. M. Kinnear. 1999. 162p. pap. (*1-897676-80-8*) Nottingham Univ Pr GBR. *Dist:* St Mut.

Lung Growth & Development. Ed. by John A. McDonald. 1997. LC 96-52512. (Lung Biology in Health & Disease Ser.: Vol. 100). (Illus.). 768p. text 235.00 (*0-8247-9772-8*) Dekker.

***Lung Hyaluronan & Lung Water in the Perinatal Period.** Hans Johnson. 2001. (Comprehensive Summaries of Uppsala Dissertations from the Faculty of Medicine Ser.: No. 1020). (Illus.). 59p. (*91-554-4989-1*) Uppsala Universitet SWE. *Dist:* Coronet Bks.

Lung in Rheumatic Diseases. Grant W. Cannon & Zimmerman. 1990. (Lung Biology in Health & Disease Ser.: Vol. 45). (Illus.). 576p. text 225.00 (*0-8247-8211-9*) Dekker.

Lung in Transition Between Health & Disease. Ed. by Peter T. Macklem & S. Permutt. 1979. (Lung Biology in Health & Disease Ser.: Vol. 12). (Illus.). 464p. text 190.00 (*0-8247-7750-6*) Dekker.

Lung Macrophages & Dendritic Cells. Ed. by Mary F. Lipscomb & Stephen W. Russell. 1997. LC 96-53510. (Lung Biology in Health & Disease Ser.: Vol. 102). (Illus.). 864p. text 235.00 (*0-8247-9817-1*) Dekker.

Lung Sounds: A Practical Guide. Robert H. Wilkins et al. 2nd ed. 1996. (Illus.). 114p. (C). (gr. 13). pap. text 43.00 incl. audio (*0-8151-9287-8*, 25632) Mosby Inc.

Lung Surfactant: Basic Research in the Pathogenesis of Lung Disorders. Ed. by B. Mueller & P. Von Wichert. 1994. (Progress in Respiratory Research Ser.: Vol. 27). (Illus.). x, 266p. 208.75 (*3-8055-5837-6*) S Karger.

Lung Surfactant: Cellular & Molecular Processing. Seamus A. Rooney. 1998. LC 98-9173. (Molecular Biology Intelligence Unit Ser.). 227p. pap. 99.00 (*1-57059-479-1*) Landes Bioscience.

Lung Transplantation. R. Hetzer. 1999. 80p. (*3-7985-1062-8*) D Steinkopff DEU. *Dist:* Spr-Verlag.

Lung Transplantation, No. 3. Ed. by Alec Patterson & Louis Couraud. 1995. LC 94-43203. (Current Topics in General Thoracic Surgery Ser.: Vol. 3). 612p. 256.50 (*0-444-81567-8*) Elsevier.

Lung Tumors. Ed. by B. Hoogstraten. 1988. (Illus.). 272p. 85.95 (*0-387-16920-2*) Spr-Verlag.

Lung Vascular Injury: Molecular & Cellular Response. Ed. by Arnold Johnson & Thomas J. Ferro. 1992. LC 92-18425. (Lung Biology in Health & Disease Ser.: Vol. 60). (Illus.). 368p. text 180.00 (*0-8247-8718-8*) Dekker.

Lung Viability after Circulatory Arrest: An Experimental Study in Rabbits. Dirk Van Raemdonck. 1998. (Acta Biomedica Lovaniensia Ser.). (Illus.). 166p. pap. (*90-6186-879-3*) Leuven Univ BEL. *Dist:* Coronet Bks.

Lung Volume Reduction Surgery. Ed. by Michael Argenziano & Mark E. Ginsburg. 2001. LC 2001-24308. (Illus.). 273p. 145.00 (*0-89603-848-3*) Humana.

***Lung Volume Reduction Surgery for Emphysema.** Ed. by Henry Fessler et al. 2002. 385p. text 110.00 (*0-521-65050-X*) Cambridge U Pr.

Lungs. Ed. by B. Corrin. 3rd ed. 1990. (Systemic Pathology Ser.: Vol. 5). (Illus.). 467p. text (*0-443-03094-4*) Church.

Lungscapes. Ed. by Pier C. Braga & Luigi Allegra. 1992. LC 92-9560. (Illus.). 112p. 115.00 (*0-387-55249-9*) Spr-Verlag.

Lupus: A Patient Care Guide for Nurses & Other Health Professionals. Terri Nass. Ed. by Julia Freeman & Anne Brown Rodgers. 2000. 130p. (C). reprint ed. pap. text 30.00 (*0-7567-0062-0*) DIANE Pub.

Lupus: Alternative Therapies That Work. Sharon Moore. 2000. LC 00-40843. 256p. pap. 14.95 (*0-89281-889-1*, Heal Arts VT) Inner Tradit.

Lupus: Molecular & Cellular Pathogenesis. Gary M. Kammer & George C. Tsokos. 1999. LC 99-13238. (Contemporary Immunology Ser.: Vol. 7). (Illus.). 728p. 195.00 (*0-89603-556-5*) Humana.

Lupus: My Search for a Diagnosis. Eileen Radziunas. 1989. LC 89-24683. 144p. pap. 9.95 (*0-89793-065-7*) Hunter Hse.

Lupus - What's It All About? Claudia Pagano & Mary M. Goulding. 1997. xi, 210p. pap. 14.95 (*0-9661036-3-7*) Abiding Health.

Lupus Erythematoles. Schneider. 1996. text 19.95 (*3-540-00962-0*) Spr-Verlag.

Lupus Handbook for Women: Up-to-Date Information on Understanding & Managing the Disease Which Affects One in Five Hundred Women. Robin Dibner & Carol Colman. 1994. LC 94-17984. 176p. per. 11.00 (*0-671-79031-5*) S&S Trade.

Lupus Nephritis. Ed. by Edmund J. Lewis et al. 1999. LC 98-39265. (Oxford Clinical Nephrology Ser.). (Illus.). 336p. text 125.00 (*0-19-262755-4*) OUP.

Lupus Novice: Toward Self-Healing. Laura Chester. 2nd exp. rev. ed. 1999. LC 99-11490. 224p. pap. 13.95 (*1-58177-020-0*, P2083) Barrytown Ltd.

Lupus Novice: Towards Self Healing. Laura Chester. Ed. by George Quasha. 1987. LC 87-9758. 192p. (C). 16.95 (*0-88268-037-4*) Station Hill Pr.

Lurleen B. Wallace Foundation: A Legacy of Love. Bruce L. Patterson. 1996. (Illus.). 128p. (Orig.). pap. 9.95 (*0-9652910-0-6*) Comprehen Cancer.

Lutte Contre L'Hypertension, Lucha Contra la Hypertension see Hypertension Control: Report of a WHO Expert Committee

Luyties Homeopathic Practice. Edward L. Perry. 1974. 165p. pap. 1.95 (*0-89378-052-9*) Formur Intl.

Lying & Its Detection: A Study of Deception & Deception Tests. John A. Larson et al. 1969. LC 69-16241. (Criminology, Law Enforcement, & Social Problems Ser.: No. 78). reprint ed. 30.00 (*0-87585-078-2*) Patterson Smith.

Lying-In: A History of Childbirth in America. Richard W. Wertz & Dorothy C. Wertz. exp. ed. 1989. LC 89-50512. 344p. (C). pap. 20.00 (*0-300-04087-3*) Yale U Pr.

Lyme Borreliosis. J. S. Axford & D. H. Rees. 1994. (NATO Advanced Science Institutes Ser.: Vol. 260). (Illus.). 344p. (C). text 115.00 (*0-306-44664-2*, Kluwer Plenum) Kluwer Academic.

Lyme Borreliosis II: Zentralblatt fuer Bakteriologie, Suppl. #18. Ed. by G. Stanek. 1994. (Illus.). 365p. (*3-437-11283-X*) Gustav Fischer DEU. *Dist:* Lubrecht & Cramer.

Lyme Disease. Globe Net Staff. 1995. 184p. 22.99 (*0-7872-1508-2*) Kendall-Hunt.

Lyme Disease. Ronald L. Hoffman. 1994. (Good Health Guides). pap. 3.95 (*0-87983-617-2*, 36172K, Keats Pubng) McGraw-Hill Trade.

Lyme Disease. Alvin Silverstein et al. 2000. LC 99-42674. (Library Ser.). (Illus.). 64p. (J). (gr. 5-7). lib. bdg. 24.00 (*0-531-11751-0*) F Watts.

Lyme Disease. Elaine Landau. 2000. (Illus.). 63p. (J). (gr. 5-7). reprint ed. text 17.00 (*0-7881-9055-5*) DIANE Pub.

Lyme Disease. Ed. by Daniel Rahn & Janine Evans. 5th ed. 1998. LC 97-3304. (Key Diseases Ser.). 254p. (Orig.). (C). pap. text 35.00 (*0-943126-58-4*) Amer Coll Phys.

Lyme Disease: A Mother's Perspective. Karen Angotti. 1993. 112p. (Orig.). pap. 6.95 (*0-9633902-3-6*) Anarek Pubns.

Lyme Disease: Molecular & Immunologic Approaches. Ed. by Steven E. Schutzer. 1992. LC 92-20115. (Current Communications in Cell & Molecular Biology Ser.: Vol. 6). 327p. 25.00 (*0-87969-377-0*) Cold Spring Harbor.

Lyme Disease: My Search for a Diagnosis. Linda Hanner. Ed. by Carol J. Frick. 1991. 215p. pap. 8.95 (*0-9622669-1-4*) Kashan Pub.

Lyme Disease: The Cause, the Cure, the Controversy. Alan G. Barbour. 1996. LC 95-40308. (Johns Hopkins Press Health Bks.). (Illus.). 272p. (C). 42.95 (*0-8018-5224-2*); pap. 16.95 (*0-8018-5245-5*) Johns Hopkins.

Lymph Node Biopsy see Lymph Node Pathology

Lymph Node Biopsy Interpretation. Ed. by Alfred G. Stansfeld & A. J. D'Ardenne. 2nd ed. 1992. (Illus.). 512p. text (*0-443-04072-9*) Church.

Lymph Node Pathology. Harry L. Ioachim. 2nd ed. 1993. LC 93-10712. Orig. Title: Lymph Node Biopsy. 736p. (C). reprint ed. text 225.00 (*0-397-50807-7*) Lppncott W & W.

Lymph Stasis: Pathophysiology, Diagnosis, & Treatment. Waldemar L. Olszewski. 1991. (Illus.). 592p. lib. bdg. 259.00 (*0-8493-6499-X*, RC646) CRC Pr.

Lymphatic & Non-Lymphatic Fluid Loss from the Peritoneal Cavity. Ed. by N. J. Ofsthun et al. 1993. (Journal: Vol. 10, Nos. 3-4, 1992). (Illus.). 132p. pap. 88.75 (*3-8055-5769-8*) S Karger.

Lymphatic Filariasis. 1984. (Technical Report Ser.: No. 702). 112p. pap. text 9.00 (*92-4-120702-7*) World Health.

Lymphatic Filariasis: The Disease & Its Control: Fifth Report of the WHO Expert Committee on Filariasis. 1992. (Technical Reports: No. 821). (ENG, FRE & SPA.). vi, 71p. pap. text 10.00 (*92-4-120821-X*, 1100821) World Health.

***Lymphatic Mapping & Probe Applications in Oncology.** Ed. by Omgo E. Nieweg. 2000. LC 00-711331. (Illus.). 416p. text 175.00 (*0-8247-0267-0*) Dekker.

Lymphatic Metastasis & Sentinel Lymphonodectomy: Future Perspectives. Ed. by P. M. Schlag & Umberto Veronesi. 2000. LC 99-55310. (Recent Results in Cancer Research Ser.: Vol. 157). (Illus.). 304p. 175.00 (*3-540-66642-7*) Spr-Verlag.

Lymphatic System. Thomas Braem. 1994. (Organs of the Human Anatomy: Vol. 10). 24p. (C). spiral bd. 12.95 (*1-878576-26-7*) Flash Anatomy Inc.

Lymphatic System & Cancer: Mechanisms & Clinical Management. Ed. by J. L. Meyer & J. M. Vaeth. 1994. LC 94-19604. (Frontiers of Radiation Therapy & Oncology Ser.: Vol. 28). (Illus.). x, 240p. 205.25 (*3-8055-5889-9*) S Karger.

Lymphatic Transport of Drugs. William N. Charman. 1992. 352p. lib. bdg. 159.00 (*0-8493-6394-2*, RM301) CRC Pr.

Lymphatics. 2nd ed. 432p. text (*0-7131-4410-6*) E A GBR. *Dist:* Routldge.

Lymphatics: Surgery, Lymphography & Diseases of the Chyle & Lymph Systems. J. B. Kinmonth. 2nd ed. 1988. 440p. text (*0-683-13052-8*) E A GBR. *Dist:* Williams & Wilkins.

Lymphocyte: Structure & Function. John J. Marchalonis. 2nd ed. 1987. (Immunology Ser.: Vol. 37). (Illus.). 440p. text 199.00 (*0-8247-7797-2*) Dekker.

Lymphocyte Activation. Ed. by L. E. Samelson. 1994. (Chemical Immunology Ser.: Vol. 59). (Illus.). xii, 220p. 182.75 (*3-8055-5976-3*) S Karger.

Lymphocyte Hybridomas: Second Workshop. Ed. by F. Melchers et al. 1979. (Illus.). 246p. 34.95 (*0-387-09670-1*) Spr-Verlag.

Lymphocyte Signalling: Mechanisms, Subversion, & Manipulation. Maggie Harnett & Kevin Rigley. 1997. LC 96-19084. 470p. 285.00 (*0-471-95903-0*) Wiley.

Lymphocytes in Comparative Immunology. Pilet. 1981. (Comparative Immunology & Microbiology Ser.). pap. 24.00 (*0-08-026841-2*, Pergamon Pr) Elsevier.

Lymphocytes in Immunotherapy of Cancer. Ed. by P. Koldovsky et al. 1989. (Illus.). 100p. 71.95 (*0-387-50457-5*) Spr-Verlag.

Lymphocytes in the Liver: Immunobiology, Pathology, & Host Defense. Ed. by I. Nicholas Crispe. 1999. LC 98-7962. (Illus.). 256p. 115.00 (*0-471-19218-X*, Wiley-Liss) Wiley.

Lymphocytes, Macrophages, & Cancer. Ed. by G. Mathe et al. 1976. LC 76-26538. (Recent Results in Cancer Research Ser.: Vol. 56). 35.00 (*3-540-07902-5*) Spr-Verlag.

Lymphocytic Choriomeningitis. Ed. by F. Lehmann-Grube. 1972. LC 70-167276. (Virology Monographs: Vol. 10). 47.00 (*0-387-81017-X*) Spr-Verlag.

Lymphoedema: Methods of Treatment & Control. Michael Foldi & Ethel Foldi. unabr. ed. 1993. 136p. pap. text (*0-646-22342-9*) Lymphoedema AUS. *Dist:* Medicina Bio.

Lymphohaematopoietic Growth Factors in Cancer Therapy. Ed. by R. Mertelsmann & U. Veronesi. 1990. (EOS Monographs). (Illus.). 90p. 62.95 (*0-387-53086-X*) Spr-Verlag.

Lymphohaematopoietic Growth Factors in Cancer Therapy II. Ed. by R. Mertelsmann. 1993. LC 92-49430. (Illus.). 132p. 123.00 (*0-387-55953-1*) Spr-Verlag.

Lymphoid Malignancy. Masao Hanaoka. 1989. 95.00 (*0-938607-24-3*) Field & Wood Inc Medical.

Lymphokines & the Immune Response. Ed. by Stanley Cohen. 1989. 304p. lib. bdg. 230.00 (*0-8493-6427-2*, QR185) CRC Pr.

Lymphoma. Ed. by A. C. Wotherspoon. 1997. LC 98-224243. (Cancer Surveys Ser.: No. 30). (Illus.). 360p. text 90.00 (*0-87969-519-6*) Cold Spring Harbor.

Lymphoma Project Report: Current Issues in Research & Treatment of AIDS-Associated Lymphoma. Michael Marco. 1995. (Illus.). 64p. (Orig.). (C). pap. text 20.00 (*0-7881-1841-2*) DIANE Pub.

Lymphomas. George P. Canellos et al. Ed. by Richard Lampert. 1997. LC 97-22034. (Illus.). 544p. text 175.00 (*0-7216-5030-9*) Saunders.

Lymphomas, Vol. I. Ed. by J. M. Bennett. 1981. text 226.00 (*90-247-2479-1*) Kluwer Academic.

Lymphomes Epidermotropes: Proceedings of the International Symposium, Bruxelles, March, 1977. Ed. by R. Schuppli. 1978. (Dermatologica Ser.: Vol. 157, No. 6). (Illus.). pap. 22.75 (*3-8055-2982-1*) S Karger.

Lymphoproliferative Diseases. Ed. by D. B. Jones & D. H. Wright. 1990. (Immunology & Medicine Ser.). (C). text 146.00 (*0-85200-965-8*) Kluwer Academic.

Lymphoproliferative Diseases: Pathogenesis, Diagnosis, Therapy. Ed. by P. K. Pattengale et al. 1985. (Developments in Oncology Ser.). text 147.00 (*0-89838-725-6*) Kluwer Academic.

Lymphoproliferative Disorders: Handbook of Investigation, Diagnosis & Management. J. A. Child. 1999. LC 97-77658. (Illus.). 420p. text (*0-412-58030-6*) E A GBR. *Dist:* OUP.

Lymphoproliferative Disorders of the Skin. Ed. by George F. Murphy & Martin C. Mihm. 1986. (Illus.). 316p. text (*0-409-95181-1*) E A GBR. *Dist:* OUP.

Lynch's Medical Laboratory Technology. Stanley S. Raphael. 4th ed. 1983. (Illus.). 864p. text 93.00 (*0-7216-7465-8*) Saunders.

Lynda Madaras Talks to Teens about AIDS: An Essential Guide for Parents, Teachers & Young People. Lynda Madaras. 1991. LC 87-31567. (Illus.). 128p. (YA). (gr. 7 up). 14.95 (*1-55704-010-9*) Newmarket.

Lyrical Analysis: The Unconscious Through Jane Eyre. Angelyn Spignesi. 1990. 368p. (Orig.). pap. 3.95 (*0-933029-54-3*) Chiron Pubns.

Lysenkoism in China: Proceeding of the 1956 Qingdao Genetics Conference. Ed. by Laurence Schneider. 1986. 120p. pap. text 38.95 (*0-87332-410-2*) M E Sharpe.

Lysine & Its Uses. 1996. lib. bdg. 250.75 (*0-8490-5879-1*) Gordon Pr.

Lysine, Tryptophan & Other Amino Acids. Robert Garrison, Jr. Ed. by Richard A. Passwater & Earl R. Mindell. 1982. (Good Health Guides). 32p. (Orig.). pap. 2.95 (*0-87983-268-1*, 32681K, Keats Pubng) McGraw-Hill Trade.

Lysophospholipids & Eicosanoids in Biology & Pathophysiology. Vol. 905. Ed. by Edward J. Goetzl & Kevin R. Lynch. 2000. 400p. 140.00 (*1-57331-213-4*) NY Acad Sci.

Lysosomal Storage Disease: Aspartylglycosaminuria. Ilkka Mononen & Nathan N. Aronson. 1997. 197p. pap. 89.95 (*0-412-11551-4*) Landes Bioscience.

Lysosomes: A Survey. E. Holtzman. 1976. (Cell Biology Monographs: Vol. 3). (Illus.). 300p. 98.00 (*0-387-81316-0*) Spr-Verlag.

M

M. C. Q. & Self Assessment Manual in Medicine. A. C. Tripathy. 1990. 224p. (C). (*81-85017-47-6*) Interprint IND. *Dist:* St Mut.

M. C. Q. in Clinical Subjects. L. C. Gupta. 1991. 324p. (C). (*0-7855-6742-9*) Interprint IND. *Dist:* St Mut.

M. C. Q. in Obstetrics & Gynecology. Ed. by A. C. Tripathy. 1990. 154p. (C). (*0-7855-6743-7*) Interprint IND. *Dist:* St Mut.

M. C. Q. in Ophthalmology. M. L. Agarwal. 1991. 185p. (C). (*81-85017-54-9*) Interprint IND. *Dist:* St Mut.

M. C. Q. in Pathology. V. H. Talib. 1991. 170p. (C). (*81-85017-55-7*) Interprint IND. *Dist:* St Mut.

M. C. Q. in Radiology. Ed. by L. C. Gupta. 1990. 172p. (C). (*81-85017-45-X*) Interprint IND. *Dist:* St Mut.

M. D. Anderson Solid. Steven A. Curley. Ed. by Raphael E. Pollock. 1998. LC 97-41042. (M. D. Anderson Solid Tumor Oncology Ser.). (Illus.). 266p. 95.00 (*0-387-98370-8*) Spr-Verlag.

M. D. Anderson Surgical Oncology Handbook. M. D. Anderson Hospital and Tumor Institute at the University of Texas Staff & Barry W. Feig. 2nd ed. 1998. LC 98-37038. 576p. pap. text 39.95 (*0-7817-1581-4*) Lppncott W & W.

M1 - Selective Muscarinic Antagonists in Peptic Ulcer Therapy: Journal: Pharmacology. Vol. 37, Suppl. 1, 1988. Ed. by W. Kromer et al. 1988. (Illus.). vi, 66p. pap. 21.75 (3-8055-4925-3) S Karger.

Ma Vie. Carl Gustav Jung. 1991. (FRE.). 528p. pap. 13.95 (0-7859-2618-6, 2070384071) Fr & Eur.

Ma Vie et la Psychoanlyse. Sigmund Freud. 1971. (FRE.). pap. 10.95 (0-7859-2834-0) Fr & Eur.

MAC-AE: Human Development 96/97. Freiberg. 24th ed. 1996. (0-697-31668-8, WCB McGr Hill) McGrw-H Hghr Educ.

MacArthur Communicative Development Inventories: User's Guide & Technical Manual & Forms. Larry Fenson et al. 1993. (Illus.). 100p. (Orig.). (C). pap. text 100.00 net. (1-56593-154-8, 0489) Thomson Learn.

MacArthur Competence Assessment Tool for Treatment (MacCAT-T) Thomas Grisso & Paul S. Appelbaum. 1998. LC 98-19161. 54p. pap. 24.45 (1-56887-041-8, Prof Resc Pr) Pro Resource.

Machine at the Bedside: Strategies for Using Technology in Patient Care. Ed. by Stanley J. Reiser & Michael Anbar. 1984. (Illus.). 384p. pap. text 27.95 (0-521-31832-7) Cambridge U Pr.

Machine in the Nursery: Incubator Technology & the Origins of Newborn Intensive Care. Jeffrey P. Baker. 1996. LC 95-40320. (Illus.). 256p. (C). 50.95 (0-8018-5173-4) Johns Hopkins.

Machine Takeover: The Growing Threat to Human Freedom in a Computer-Controlled Society. F. H. George. 1977. LC 76-27722. 208p. (0-08-021229-8) Pergamon Repr GBR. Dist: Franklin.

Macho Medicine: A History of the Anabolic Steroid Epidemic. William N. Taylor. 1991. LC 91-52506. 208p. (gr. 10-12). lib. bdg. 32.50 (0-89950-613-5) McFarland & Co.

Macht Als Gefahr Beim Helfer. Adolf Guggenbuehl-Craig. 5th ed. 1987. (Psychologische Praxis Ser.: No. 45). vi, 106p. pap. 16.75 (3-8055-4562-2) S Karger.

Mackie & McCartney's Medical Microbiology, Vol. 2. Collee et al. 13th ed. 1989. (Illus.). 928p. text (0-443-02332-8) Church.

MacLeod's Clinical Examination. Christopher R. Edwards. 8th ed. 1990. (Illus.). 432p. pap. text (0-443-04079-6) Church.

MacLeod's Clinical Examination. Munro. 9th ed. 1995. pap. text 31.50 (0-443-04856-8) Saunders.

Macmillan Biology. Creager. 1985. (gr. 9-12). lab manual ed. (0-02-277380-0) Macmillan.

Macmillan Health Encyclopedia, Set. Macmillan Library Reference Staff. 2nd ed. 1999. LC 99-23432. (Illus.). 864p. 395.00 (0-02-865036-0, Macmillan Ref) Gale.

Macmillan Health Encyclopedia, Vol. 9. 1993. 45.00 (0-02-897453-0, Macmillan Ref) Gale.

Macnab's Backache. John A. Mcculloch et al. 3rd ed. 1997. LC 96-21766. (Illus.). 795p. 99.00 (0-683-05797-9) Lppncott W & W.

Macrobiotic Home Remedies. Michio Kushi & Marc Van Cauwenberghe. 1985. LC 84-80643. (Illus.). 224p. (Orig.). pap. 19.95 (0-87040-554-3) Japan Pubns USA.

Macrobiotic Miracle: A Woman Cures Herself of Cancer. Virginia Brown & Susan Stayman. 1985. (Illus.). 240p. pap. 15.00 (0-87040-573-X) Japan Pubns USA.

Macrobiotic Resource Guide: A Directory to the Most Healthful, Affordable & Enviromentally Safe Foods, Products & Service. Alex Jack. 1997. 160p. pap. 10.95 (1-882984-26-9) One Peaceful World.

Macrobiotic Seminars of Michio Kushi: Classic Lectures on Health & Diet, Oriental Medicine, & Self-Healing. Michio Kushi. Ed. by Edward Esko. 1998. 96p. pap. 10.95 (1-882984-29-3) One Peaceful World.

Macrobiotics: An Invitation to Health & Happiness. George Ohsawa. 1984. 77p. reprint ed. pap. 5.95 (0-918860-02-4) G Ohsawa.

Macrobiotics & Oriental Medicine: An Introduction to Holistic Health. Michio Kushi & Phillip Janetta. 2000. (Illus.). 272p. reprint ed. pap. 22.00 (0-7881-9415-1) DIANE Pub.

Macrobiotics & Oriental Medicine: An Introduction to Holistic Health. Michio Kushi & Phillip Janetta. 1991. LC 85-81366. 288p. pap. 22.00 (0-87040-659-0) Japan Pubns USA.

Macrobiotics Beyond Food: A Guide to Health & Well-Being. Roanld E. Kotzsch. 1987. LC 86-81324. 242p. 27.00 (0-87040-674-4) Japan Pubns USA.

Macroelements, Water & Electrolytes in Sports Nutrition. Judy A. Driskell & Ira Wolinsky. 1999. LC 99-234359. (Nutrition in Exercise & Sport Ser.). 272p. 89.95 (0-8493-8196-7) CRC Pr.

Macrolides, Chemistry, Pharmacology & Clinical Uses. A. Bryskier. 1993. (Illus.). 714p. 235.00 (2-7184-0589-9) Blackwell Sci.

Macromolecular Aspects of Medical Biochemistry. J. P. Luzio & R. J. Thompson. 1990. (Illus.). 278p. (C). text 80.00 (0-521-26083-3); pap. text 28.95 (0-521-27828-7) Cambridge U Pr.

Macromolecular Biomaterials. Ed. by Garth W. Hastings & Paul Ducheyne. 1984. LC 83-7094. (Structure Property Relationship Biomaterials Ser.). 320p. 157.00 (0-8493-6263-6, R857, CRC Reprint) Franklin.

Macromolecular Biorecognition: Principles & Methods. Ed. by Irwin M. Chaiken et al. 1988. LC 87-29304. (Experimental Biology & Medicine Ser.: Vol. 19). (Illus.). 850p. (C). 145.00 (0-89603-141-1) Humana.

Macromolecular Concept & Strategy for Humanity in Science, Technology & Industry. Ed. by B. Ranby et al. 1996. (Illus.). 160p. 125.00 (3-540-60315-8) Spr-Verlag.

Macromolecular Interplay in Brain Associative Mechanisms. Ed. by A. Neugebauer. 1997. LC 98-214620. 350p. text 78.00 (981-02-3212-8) World Scientific Pub.

Macromolecular Reactions: Peculiarities, Theory & Experimental Approaches. Nicolai A. Plate et al. 1995. LC 94-30634. 450p. 345.00 (0-471-94392-4) Wiley.

Macromolecules. John G. Kirkwood. Ed. by P. L. Auer. 1967. (Documents on Modern Physics Ser.). xii, 192p. text 216.00 (0-677-00340-4) Gordon & Breach.

Macrophage, 1990. Ed. by R. Andreesen. 1991. (Journal: Vol. 59, No. 3, 1991). (Illus.). Pt. 1. 92p. pap. 51.50 (3-8055-5407-9); Pt. 2. 100p. pap. 51.50 (3-8055-5408-7) S Karger.

Macrophage, 1992: Abstracts, European Conference on Basic & Clinical Aspects of Macrophage Biology, Regensburg, FRG, September 1992. Ed. by R. Andreesen. 1992. (Journal: Vol. 60, Suppl. 1, 1992). (Illus.). x, 42p. pap. 24.50 (3-8055-5689-6) S Karger.

Macrophage-Pathogen Interactions. Ed. by Bruce S. Zwilling & Eisenstein. 1993. (Immunology Ser.: Vol. 60). (Illus.). 664p. text 245.00 (0-8247-9124-X) Dekker.

Macrophages & Cancer. Ed. by Gloria H. Heppner & Amy M. Fulton. 1988. 240p. 132.00 (0-8493-4998-2, QR188, CRC Reprint) Franklin.

Macrophages & the Nervous System. V. Hugh Perry. 1994. (Molecular Biology Intelligence Unit Ser.). 118p. 99.00 (1-57059-044-3, LN9044); 99.00 (1-57059-173-3) Landes Bioscience.

Macrophages in Anti-Inflammation: Molecular Mechanisms, Apoptosis & Tolerance Induction 2nd Teupitzer Colloquium, Teupitz, September 1999. Ed. by S. Goerdt et al. 2000. (Illus.). 128p. pap. 39.25 (3-8055-7061-9) S Karger.

Macroscopic Ocular Pathology. F. H. Stefani & G. Hasenfratz. 1987. (Illus.). 178p. 192.00 (0-387-17404-4) Spr-Verlag.

Macrosomy, Obesity & Cancer. Lev M. Berstein. 1996. (Illus.). 207p. (C). lib. bdg. 135.00 (1-56072-202-9) Nova Sci Pubs.

Macular & Retinal Diseases: New Approaches in the Diagnosis & Therapy of Macular & Retinal Diseases, Leipzig, November 1996. Ed. by Peter Wiedemann & Leon Kohen. 1997. LC 97-34801. (Developments in Ophthalmology Ser.: No. 29). (Illus.). viii, 100p. 119.25 (3-8055-6553-4) S Karger.

Macular Degeneration: A Comprehensive Guide to Treatment, Breakthroughs & Coping Strategies. Robert D'Amato & Joan Snyder. 2000. LC 00-28991. (Illus.). xix, 192p. pap. 14.95 (0-8027-1359-9) Walker & Co.

Macular Degeneration: Living Positively with Vision Loss. Betty Wason & James J. McMillan. 1998. LC 98-42145. (Illus.). 256p. pap. 14.95 (0-89793-239-0); 24.95 (0-89793-240-4) Hunter Hse.

Macular Degeneration: The Latest Scientific Discoveries & Treatments for Preserving Your Sight. Robert D'Amato & Joan Snyder. 2000. (Illus.). 192p. (gr. 8-12). pap. 14.95 (0-8027-7603-5) Walker & Co.

Macular Degeneration Handbook: Natural Ways to Prevent & Reverse It. Chet Cunningham. 1998. LC 98-61570. (Illus.). 278p. pap. 14.95 (1-887053-11-5) United Res CA.

Macular Disease. Lim Sternberg. 1995. 39.00 (0-316-06079-8, Little Brwn Med Div) Lppncott W & W.

Macular Disorders: An Illustrated Diagnostic Guide. Anthony A. Cavallerano & Rodney K. Gutner. 1997. LC 96-39906. (Illus.). 304p. text 105.00 (0-7506-9224-3) Buttrwrth-Heinemann.

Macular Hole: Pathogenesis, Diagnosis & Treatment. Steven A. Madreperla et al. 1998. LC 98-20598. (Illus.). 192p. pap. text 69.99 (0-7506-9960-4) Buttrwrth-Heinemann.

Macular Surgery. Jerald A. Bovino. 1994. (Illus.). 184p. (C). pap. text 139.00 (0-8385-6082-2, A6082-0, Apple Lange Med) McGraw.

Mad Among Us: A History of the Care of America's Mentally Ill. Gerald N. Grob. 1994. LC 93-40806. 400p. 24.95 (0-02-912695-9) Free Pr.

Mad Among Us: A History of the Care of America's Mentally Ill. Gerald N. Grob. 1995. (Illus.). 416p. (C). pap. 16.95 (0-674-54112-X) HUP.

Mad Cow Crisis: Health & the Public Good. Scott C. Ratzan. 1998. LC 97-38913. 272p. text 55.00 (0-8147-7510-1); pap. text 18.50 (0-8147-7511-X) NYU Pr.

Mad Cow Crisis: Health & the Public Good. Scott C. Ratzan. 1997. 256p. pap. text (1-85728-812-2) UCL Pr Ltd GBR. Dist: Taylor & Francis.

Mad Cow Crisis: Health & the Public Good. Ed. by Scott C. Ratzan. 1997. 256p. (1-85728-828-9) UCL Pr Ltd GBR. Dist: Taylor & Francis.

***Mad Cow Disease (Bovine Spongiform Encephalopathy, B. S. E.) Index of New Information & Guide for Reference & Research.** Ed. by Research and Development Division Staff & John C. Bartone. 2001. 180p. 44.50 (0-7883-2343-1); pap. 44.50 (0-7883-2344-X) ABBE Pubs Assn.

***Mad Cow Disease in America, Something Special & Other Plays.** Lance Tait. 2001. 300p. pap. 17.00 (1-893598-03-9) Enfield Pubs NH.

Mad Cows & Mother's Milk: The Perils of Poor Risk Communication. Douglas Powell & William Leiss. LC 99-203404. 1998. 320p. pap. (0-7735-1619-0); 1997. 308p. text (0-7735-1618-2) McG-Queens Univ Pr CAN. Dist: CUP Services.

Mad Dogs: The New Rabies Plague. Don Finley. 1998. LC 97-34672. (Louise Lindsey Merrick Natural Environment Ser.). (Illus.). 232p. pap. 14.95 (0-89096-822-5) Tex A&M Univ Pr.

Mad Parts of Sane People in Analysis. Ed. by Murray Stein. 1993. LC 92-39057. (Chiron Clinical Ser.). (Illus.). 240p. (Orig.). pap. 24.95 (0-933029-67-5) Chiron Pubns.

Mad, the Bad & the Innocent: The Criminal Mind on Trial. Barbara R. Kirwin. 1997. LC 97-7833. 320p. (gr. 8). 23.95 (0-316-49499-2) Little.

Mad to Be Normal: Conversations with R. D. Laing. Bob Mullan. 1995. LC 97-187487. 406p. (C). pap. (1-85343-395-0) Free Assoc Bks GBR. Dist: Intl Spec Bk, NYU Pr.

Mad Travelers: Reflections on the Reality of Transient Mental Illness. Ian Hacking. 1998. LC 98-20894. (Page-Barbour Lectures). 174p. 27.95 (0-8139-1823-5) U Pr of Va.

Made to Order: The Myth of Reproductive & Genetic Progress. Ed. by Patricia Spallone & Deborah L. Steinberg. 1987. (Athene Ser.). 256p. text 50.00 (0-08-034954-4); pap. text 19.95 (0-08-034953-6) Elsevier (Pergamon Pr).

Made-to-Person Therapy for Ulcer Disease. F. Di Mario et al. 1993. (Advances in Gastroenterology Ser.: No. 6). 216p. text (1-57235-022-9) Piccin Nuova.

Madeleine Leininger: Cultural Care Diversity & Universality Theory. Cheryl L. Reynolds & Madeleine Leininger. 1993. LC 93-5728. (Notes on Nursing Theories Ser.: Vol. 8). (Illus.). 64p. (C). pap. 14.95 (0-8039-5098-5, 3330) Sage.

Madkour's Brucellosis. M. Monir Madkour. 2nd enl. rev. ed. 2000. LC 00-28461. (Illus.). 300p. 139.00 (3-540-67272-9) Spr-Verlag.

Madness & Cure. Robert J. Langs. 1995. 296p. (C). text 38.95 (0-89876-218-9) Gardner Pr.

Madness & Democracy. Marcel Gauchet & Gladys Swain. Tr. by Catherine Porter from FRE. 1999. LC 98-45014. (New French Thought Ser.). xxvi, 323p. 35.00 (0-691-03372-2) Princeton U Pr.

Madness & Reason. Jennifer Radden. 1985. (Studies in Applied Philosophy). 176p. text 55.00 (0-04-170034-1); pap. text 16.95 (0-04-170035-X) Routledge.

Madness & Social Representations: Living with the Mad in One French Community. Denise Jodelet. Ed. by Gerard Duveen. Tr. by Tim Pownall. 1992. (Medicine & Society Ser.: No. 5). 316p. text 60.00 (0-520-07865-9) U CA Pr.

Madness & the Criminal Law. Norval Morris. LC 82-13435. (Studies in Crime & Justice). (C). 1998. 237p. lib. bdg. 24.00 (0-226-53907-5); 1995. 168p. pap. text 8.95 (0-226-53908-3) U Ch Pr.

Madness, Chaos, & Violence: Therapy with Families at the Brink. John Brendler et al. 1998. 220p. (C). text 20.00 (0-7881-5667-5) DIANE Pub.

Madness, Heresy, & the Rumor of Angels: The Revolt Against the Mental Health System. Seth Farber. 1993. LC 93-1276. 286p. 49.95 (0-8126-9199-7); pap. 18.95 (0-8126-9200-4) Open Court.

Madness in America: Cultural & Medical Perceptions of Mental Illness Before 1914. Lynn Gamwell & Nancy Tomes. 1995. LC 94-46520. (Cornell Studies in the History of Psychiatry). (Illus.). 192p. 47.50 (0-8014-3161-1) Cornell U Pr.

Madness in Its Place: Narratives of Severalls Hospital, 1913-1997. Diana Gittins. 1998. LC 97-39489. (Illus.). 256p. (C). pap. 27.95 (0-415-18388-X) Routledge.

Madness in Late Imperial China: From Illness to Deviance. Vivien W. Ng. 1990. LC 90-50237. 208p. 35.00 (0-8061-2297-8) U of Okla Pr.

Madness in Society: Chapters in the Historical Sociology of Mental Illness. George Rosen. 1968. LC 68-13112. 348p. pap. text 14.95 (0-226-72642-8, P913) U Ch Pr.

Madness of Ushers: Coping with Vision & Hearing Loss (Usher Syndrome Type II) Dorothy H. Stiefel. 1991. 92p. 10.00 (1-879518-06-6) Busn Living Pubns.

***Madness on the Couch: Blaming the Victim in the Heyday of Psychoanalysis.** Edward Dolnick. 2001. (Illus.). 368p. reprint ed. 25.00 (0-7567-5117-9) DIANE Pub.

Madness on the Couch: Blaming the Victim in the Heyday of Psychoanalysis. Edward Dolnick. 1998. LC 98-23737. (Illus.). 368p. 25.00 (0-684-82497-3) Simon & Schuster.

Madopar HBS. Ed. by C. David Marsden et al. 1987. (Journal: Vol. 27, Suppl. 1). (Illus.). vi, 142p. pap. 45.25 (3-8055-4692-0) S Karger.

Maduracion Osea. M. Sempe & C. Pavia. 1994. (SPA.). 147p. pap. (84-7978-154-8) Ediciones Diaz ESP. Dist: IBD Ltd.

Madwives: Schizophrenic Women in the 1950s. Carol A. Warren. 1991. LC 86-14620. 283p. (C). pap. text 17.00 (0-8135-1689-7) Rutgers U Pr.

Maedi-Visna & Related Diseases. Ed. by G. Petursson. 1989. (Developments in Veterinary Virology Ser.). (C). text 191.50 (0-7923-0481-0) Kluwer Academic.

Maelzel's Chess Player: Sigmund Freud & the Rhetoric of Deceit. Robert Wilcocks. 1993. 360p. (Orig.). (C). pap. text 28.95 (0-8476-7810-5); lib. bdg. 86.50 (0-8476-7809-1) Rowman.

***Maestro, Medical Detective.** Robert A. Norman. 2001. 160p. pap. 14.95 (1-891576-06-2) North Shore Pr.

Magazine Photo Collage: A Multicultural Assessment & Treatment Technique. Helen Landgarten. 1993. LC 93-16792. (Illus.). 224p. text 31.95 (0-87630-706-3) Brunner-Routledge.

Magic & Medicine of Plants. Reader's Digest Editorial Staff. 1986. LC 85-30101. (Illus.). 464p. 28.00 (0-89577-221-3) RD Assn.

***Magic Cancer Bullet: How a Tiny Orange Pill May Rewrite Medical History.** Dan Vasella. 2002. 288p. 24.95 (0-06-001030-4) HarperCollins Pubs.

Magic Chest: Where You Are, Where You've Been, Where You're Going. Cornelia H. Eulert. 1998. LC 97-43841. 160p. pap. 25.95 (1-56032-738-3) Hemisp Pub.

Magic, Faith & Healing: Studies in Primitive Psychiatry. Ed. by Ari Kiev. 1996. 496p. pap. 60.00 (1-56821-809-5) Aronson.

Magic Herbs for Arthritis, Rheumatism & Related Ailments. Richard M. Lucas. 1981. LC 80-22346. 248p. 14.95 (0-13-543900-0, Parker Publishing Co) P-H.

Magic Kits: Meaningful Activities for the Gifted in the Classroom Through Knowledge, Interests, Training & Stimulation. Janet Heuer et al. 1980. (Illus.). 56p. (gr. k-8). pap. 14.95 (0-936386-11-8, 640) Creative Learning.

Magic Menus. American Diabetes Association. 1996. LC 96-42081. 256p. pap. 14.95 (0-945448-72-4, 4707-01) Am Diabetes.

Magic Mind Power: Make It Work for You! Leslie M. LeCron. 2nd ed. 1982. 176p. reprint ed. pap. 8.95 (0-87516-496-X) DeVorss.

Magic, Myth & Medicine. Donald T. Atkinson. 1977. LC 72-8510. (Essay Index Reprint Ser.). reprint ed. 21.95 (0-8369-7316-X) Ayer.

Magic, Myths & Medicine. Richard Hunderfund. 1987. (Illus.). 22.95 (0-89863-115-7) Star Pub CA.

Magic of Humor in Caregiving. James R. Sherman. 1995. (Illus.). 80p. pap. 9.95 (0-935538-19-4) Pathway Bks.

Magic of Past Life Therapy. Richard A. Greene. 1992. ("Magic Of" Ser.: Vol. 2). 165p. (Orig.). pap. 14.95 (0-942783-03-4) Next Step Pubns.

Magic of Psychic Healing. Richard A. Greene. 1992. ("Magic Of" Ser.: Vol. 1). 189p. (Orig.). pap. 14.95 (0-942783-02-6) Next Step Pubns.

Magic of the Minimum Dose. Dorothy Shepherd. 1964. 15.95 (0-85032-112-3) Formur Intl.

Magic of the Minimum Dose. Dorothy Shepherd. 1980. 40.00 (0-85032-183-2) St Mut.

Magic or Medicine? An Investigation of Healing & Healers. Robert Buckman & Karl Sabbagh. 1995. LC 94-42853. 261p. 32.00 (0-87975-948-8) Prometheus Bks.

Magic, Science, & Health. Robert Thomas Anderson. 1995. LC 95-77909. 454p. (C). pap. text 58.95 (0-15-500828-5) Wadsworth Pub.

Magic Years. Selma Fraiberg. 1996. 320p. per. 13.00 (0-684-82550-3) S&S Trade.

Magic Years: Understanding & Handling the Problems of Early Childhood. Selma Fraiberg. 1966. LC 59-6073. 320p. pap. 11.00 (0-684-71768-9, Macmillan Ref) Gale.

Magical Child: Rediscovering Nature's Plan for Our Children. Joseph C. Pearce. 1992. 276p. pap. 15.00 (0-452-26789-7, Plume) Dutton Plume.

Magical Staff: The Vitalist Tradition in Western Medicine. Matthew Wood. 1992. (Illus.). 223p. (Orig.). pap. 14.95 (1-55643-127-9) North Atlantic.

Magicians, Theologicans & Doctors: Studies in Folk Medicine & Folklore As Reflected in the Rabbinical Responsa. H. J. Zimmels. 1997. LC 96-41934. 304p. pap. 40.00 (0-7657-5971-3) Aronson.

Magill's Medical Guide, 1998. Salem Press Staff. rev. ed. 1998. LC 98-27251. (Illus.). 2077p. (YA). (gr. 9-12). lib. bdg. 310.00 (0-89356-937-2) Salem Pr.

***Magill's Medical Guide 2001,** Set. 3rd rev. ed. 2001. (Illus.). 2766p. 325.00 (1-58765-003-7) Salem Pr.

Magnesium: Its Biologic Significance. Jerry K. Aikawa. 1981. 144p. 99.00 (0-8493-5871-X, QP535) CRC Pr.

Magnesium & Man. Warren E. Wacker. 1980. LC 80-14189. (Commonwealth Fund Publications). (Illus.). 171p. 35.50 (0-674-54225-8) HUP.

Magnesium & the Cardiovascular System Journal Vol. 4, Nos. 5-6: Magnesium. Ed. by J. Durlach & B. M. Altura. 1986. (Illus.). vi, 134p. pap. 62.75 (3-8055-4282-8) S Karger.

***Magnesium & the Insulin Resistance Syndrome.** Arvo Hanni. 2001. (Comprehensive Summaries of Uppsala Dissertations from the Faculty of Medicine Ser.: No. 1088). (Illus.). 69p. pap. (91-554-5142-X) Uppsala Universitet SWE. Dist: Coronet Bks.

Magnesium Deficiency. Ed. by M. J. Halpern & J. Durlach. 1985. (Illus.). viii, 248p. 162.75 (3-8055-3979-7) S Karger.

Magnesium, Diabetes & Carbohydrate Metabolism Journal: Magnesium, Vol. 2, Nos. 4-6. Ed. by J. Durlach & B. M. Altura. 1984. (Illus.). iv, 172p. pap. 85.25 (*3-8055-3865-0*) S Karger.

Magnesium Homeostasis. Ed. by G. A. Quamme. 1993. (Journal: Vol. 19, Nos. 4-5, 1993). (Illus.). 132p. pap. 81.00 (*3-8055-5881-3*) S Karger.

Magnesium in Biological Systems Environmental & Biological Aspects: Environmental & Biomedical Aspects. Bela Fazekastamas-Selmeczi & Pal Stefanovits. Ed. by T. Fazekas et al. 1994. LC 95-149500. 350p. pap. (*963-05-6681-8*) Akade Kiado HUN. *Dist:* Intl Spec Bk, St Mut.

Magnesium in Cellular Processes & Medicine. Ed. by B. M. Altura et al. 1987. iv, 244p. 172.25 (*3-8055-4369-7*) S Karger.

Magnesium in Clinical Medicine & Therapeutics Journal: Magnesium & Trace Elements, Vol. 10, Nos. 2-4, 1991-92. Ed. by M. Burton. 1993. (Illus.). 252p. pap. 35.75 (*3-8055-5696-9*) S Karger.

Magnesium, Stress & the Cardiovascular System. Ed. by B. M. Altura. 1986. (Journal: Vol. 5, No. 3-4, 1986). (Illus.). 120p. pap. 55.00 (*3-8055-4355-7*) S Karger.

Magnet Hospitals: Attraction & Retention of Professional Nurses. Margaret L. McClure et al. 1983. 150p. (Orig.). (C). pap. 16.25 (*1-55810-070-9*, G-160, Am Acad Nursing) Am Nurses Pub.

Magnet Therapy: An Alternatie Medicine Definitive Guide. Burton Goldberg et al. 2000. LC 00-44176. (Illus.). 256p. pap. 14.95 (*1-887299-21-1*) AlternMed Bks.

Magnetic & Other Properties of Oxides & Related Compounds: Spinels, Fe Oxides & Fe- Me-O-Compounds, Pt. B. 1980. (Illus.). 758p. 1215.00 (*0-387-09421-0*) Spr-Verlag.

Magnetic Field Therapy Handbook: Balancing Your Energy Field. R. Allen Walls. 1995. (Illus.). 107p. pap. 9.95 (*0-9621790-3-5*) Inner Search Found.

Magnetic Fields & Cancer in People Residing Near Swedish High Voltage Power Lines. Maria Feychting & Anders Ahlbom. 1994. (Illus.). 100p. (Orig.). (C). pap. text 35.00 (*0-7881-0772-0*) DIANE Pub.

Magnetic Healer's Guide: or Personal Experiences in Magnetic & Suggestive Healing (1903) J. O. Crone. 1996. 127p. reprint ed. pap. 13.50 (*1-56459-766-0*) Kessinger Pub.

Magnetic Miracles: Your Guide to the Use of Magnetics for Radiant Health. Catherine J. Norris. 2000. LC 00-708411. (Illus.). xx, 169p. pap. 14.99 (*0-9678931-0-0*) Energy Essentials.

Magnetic Resonance: Bioeffects, Safety & Patient Management. Frank G. Shellock & Emanuel Kanal. 2nd ed. 1996. LC 96-46644. 360p. pap. text 59.95 (*0-397-58437-7*) Lppncott W & W.

Magnetic Resonance: Symposium, Utrech, April 1985. Ed. by William Penn. 1986. (Journal: Vol. 55, No. 1-2, 1986). (Illus.). 108p. (Orig.). pap. 76.75 (*3-8055-4259-3*) S Karger.

Magnetic Resonance Angiography. Ed. by Ingolf P. Arlart et al. 1995. (Medical Radiology Ser.). (Illus.). 350p. 265.00 (*0-387-56896-4*); LC 95-31126. (*3-540-56896-4*) Spr-Verlag.

***Magnetic Resonance Angiography.** Ed. by L. P. Arlart et al. 2nd rev. ed. 2001. (Medical Radiology Diagnostic Imaging Ser.). (Illus.). 450p. 225.00 (*3-540-65091-1*) Spr-Verlag.

Magnetic Resonance Image Techniques. Ajay M. Parikh. 1991. (Illus.). 349p. (C). pap. text 69.95 (*0-8385-6084-9*, A6084-6, Apple Lange Med) McGraw.

Magnetic Resonance Imaging. David D. Stark & Walter G. Bradley. 3rd ed. 1998. LC 98-36686. (Illus.). 2800p. (C). (gr. 13). text 399.00 (*0-8151-8518-9*, 28607) Mosby Inc.

Magnetic Resonance Imaging. David D. Stark & William G. Bradley, Jr. 3rd ed. 1999. (Illus.). 2800p. (*84-8174-451-4*) Mosby-Doyma Libros ESP. *Dist:* Mosby Inc.

Magnetic Resonance Imaging: Mathematical Foundations, & Applications. Walter Schempp. 1998. LC 97-48760. 288p. 110.00 (*0-471-16736-3*) Wiley.

Magnetic Resonance Imaging: Physical & Biological Principles. Stewart C. Bushong. 2nd ed. 1995. LC 95-3071. (Illus.). 512p. (C). (gr. 13). text 56.00 (*0-8151-1342-0*, 24166) Mosby Inc.

Magnetic Resonance Imaging: Physical Principles & Sequence Design. E. Mark Haacke et al. 1999. LC 99-22880. (Illus.). 936p. 157.00 (*0-471-35128-8*) Wiley.

Magnetic Resonance Imaging: Principles, Methods & Techniques. Perry Sprawls. 2000. LC 00-34862. (Illus.). xvii, 173p. (*0-944838-97-9*) Med Physics Pub.

Magnetic Resonance Imaging & Computed Tomography: Clinical Neuro-Orbital Anatomy. Jonathan D. Wirtschafter et al. 1992. LC 92-49178. (*1-56055-010-4*) Am Acad Ophthal.

Magnetic Resonance Imaging & Computed Tomography of the Head & Neck. J. E. Gillespie & A. Gholkar. 1994. (Illus.). 248p. 169.95 (*0-412-45200-6*) Chapman & Hall.

Magnetic Resonance Imaging & Computed Tomography of the Head & Spine. C. Barrie Grossman. 2nd ed. (Illus.). 1996. 810p. text 115.00 (*0-683-03769-2*); 1989. 488p. 125.00 (*0-683-03768-4*) Lppncott W & W.

Magnetic Resonance Imaging & Spectroscopy in Sports Medicine. Ed. by M. Osteaux & K. Meirleir. 1991. (Illus.). 199p. 123.00 (*0-387-52548-3*) Spr-Verlag.

Magnetic Resonance Imaging & the Kidney: Metabolic Studies/Clinical Research. Z. H. Endre. Date not set. (*0-8247-9488-5*) Dekker.

Magnetic Resonance Imaging Atlas of the Extremities. Kang & Donald Resnick. 1990. 400p. text 205.00 (*0-7216-3071-5*) Saunders.

***Magnetic Resonance Imaging in a Flash!** Judy Wells. 2002. 32.95 (*0-7668-4339-4*) Delmar.

Magnetic Resonance Imaging in Coronary Artery Disease. Ed. by Ernst E. Van der Wall & Albert De Roos. 1991. (C). text 233.50 (*0-7923-0940-5*) Kluwer Academic.

Magnetic Resonance Imaging in Orthopaedics & Rheumatology. David W. Stoller et al. 1988. (Illus.). 404p. text 125.00 (*0-397-50958-8*) Lppncott W & W.

Magnetic Resonance Imaging in Orthopaedics & Sports Medicine. David W. Stoller. 2nd ed. 1996. 1,408p. text 499.00 (*0-397-58475-X*) Lppncott W & W.

Magnetic Resonance Imaging in Orthopaedics & Sports Medicine. David W. Stoller et al. 2nd ed. 1996. 1,408p. text 325.00 (*0-397-51542-1*) Lppncott W & W.

Magnetic Resonance Imaging of Bone & Soft Tissue Tumors & Their Mimics. A. M. De Schepper. 1989. (Series in Radiology). (C). text 160.00 (*0-7923-0343-1*) Kluwer Academic.

Magnetic Resonance Imaging of Carcinoma of the Urinary Bladder. Jelle O. Barentsz. 1990. (Series in Radiology). (C). text 206.50 (*0-7923-0838-7*) Kluwer Academic.

Magnetic Resonance Imaging of Central Nervous System Diseases. W. J. Huk et al. 1991. (Illus.). 450p. 415.00 (*0-387-17641-1*) Spr-Verlag.

Magnetic Resonance Imaging of CNS Disease: A Teaching File. Douglas H. Yock. 1994. LC 95-154083. (Illus.). 752p. (C). (gr. 13). text 143.00 (*0-8016-8098-0*, 08098) Mosby Inc.

Magnetic Resonance Imaging of Orthopedic Trauma. Stephen J. Eustace et al. 1999. LC 98-27271. 288p. 115.00 (*0-412-15211-8*) Chapman & Hall.

Magnetic Resonance Imaging of the Body. Jeffrey C. Weinreb & Helen C. Redman. 1987. (Advanced Exercises in Diagnostic Radiology Ser.). (Illus.). 272p. pap. text 45.00 (*0-7216-2059-0*) Saunders.

Magnetic Resonance Imaging of the Body. Charles B. Higgins et al. 3rd ed. 1996. LC 96-36164. 1,616p. text 325.00 (*0-397-51711-4*) Lppncott W & W.

Magnetic Resonance Imaging of the Brain & Spine. Ed. by Scott W. Atlas. 2nd ed. 1995. LC 95-6253. (Illus.). 1,696p. text 299.00 (*0-7817-0282-8*) Lppncott W & W.

Magnetic Resonance Imaging of the Elbow. Ed. by Russell C. Fritz. 1999. (Illus.). text 95.00 (*0-7817-0286-0*) Lppncott W & W.

Magnetic Resonance Imaging of the Thorax. Miriam Sperber & Marc C. Kaiser. 1987. (Illus.). 264p. (C). 65.00 (*0-87527-375-0*) Green.

Magnetic Resonance Imaging Technologist (MRI) Jack Rudman. (Admission Test Ser.: ATS-115). pap. 49.95 (*0-8373-5815-9*) Nat Learn.

Magnetic Resonance Imaging Text/CD-Rom Package. David D. Stark. 3rd ed. 1999. 570.00 incl. cd-rom (*0-323-00510-1*) Mosby Inc.

***Magnetic Resonance in Dementia.** J. Valk et al. 2001. LC 2001-32219. (Illus.). 400p. 199.00 (*3-540-41731-1*) Springer Pub.

Magnetic Resonance in Experimental & Clinical Oncology. Ed. by Jeffrey L. Evelhoch et al. 1990. (Developments in Oncology Ser.). (C). text 157.00 (*0-7923-0935-9*) Kluwer Academic.

Magnetic Resonance in Medicine. Peter A. Rinck. 3rd ed. 1993. 256p. 95.00 (*0-632-03781-4*) Blackwell Sci.

Magnetic Resonance in Medicine & Biology. M. A. Hopf & F. W. Smith. 1984. (Progress in Nuclear Medicine Ser.: Vol. 8). (Illus.). viii, 180p. 142.75 (*3-8055-3868-5*) S Karger.

Magnetic Resonance in Multiple Sclerosis. David H. Miller et al. 1997. LC 96-21044. (Illus.). 210p. (C). text 95.00 (*0-521-47325-X*) Cambridge U Pr.

Magnetic Resonance in Nephrourology: Clinical & Experimental Applications. Ed. by S. Pomer & W. E. Hull. 1993. LC 93-9946. (Illus.). 158p. 132.00 (*0-387-56450-0*) Spr-Verlag.

Magnetic Resonance Neuroimaging. Walter Kucharczyk. 1993. 496p. lib. bdg. 135.00 (*0-8493-4719-X*, RC349) CRC Pr.

Magnetic Resonance Neuroimaging. John Kucharczyk & Michael Moseley. 2nd ed. 1998. 130.00 (*0-8493-7607-6*) CRC Pr.

Magnetic Resonance (NMR) Imaging C. Leon Partain et al. 2nd ed. 1988. (Illus.). 1. 1808p. 250.00 (*0-7216-2516-9*); 2. 1808p. 315.00 (*0-7216-2517-7*); Set. text 555.00 (*0-7216-1340-3*) Saunders.

Magnetic Resonance of Myelin, Myelination, & Myelin Disorders, Vol. XII. M. S. Van der Knaap & J. Valk. 2nd rev. ed. 1996. (Illus.). 558p. 334.00 (*3-540-59277-6*) Spr-Verlag.

Magnetic Resonance of the Heart & Great Vessels: Clinical Applications. Ed. by J. Bogaert et al. (Medical Radiology Ser.). (Illus.). 2000. 286p. 75.00 (*3-540-67217-6*); 1998. LC 98-24570. 296p. 189.00 (*3-540-63448-7*) Spr-Verlag.

Magnetic Resonance of the Reproductive System. Shirley McCarthy & Florence P. Haseltine. 1986. 180p. 68.95 (*0-316-55374-3*, Little Brwn Med Div) Lppncott W & W.

Magnetic Resonance Scanning & Epilepsy. Ed. by Frederick Andermann et al. 1994. (NATO Advanced Science Institutes Ser.: Vol. 264). (Illus.). 334p. (C). text 105.00 (*0-306-44735-5*, Kluwer Plenum) Kluwer Academic.

Magnetic Resonance Spectroscopy & Imaging in Neurochemistry. Ed. by Herman Bachelard. 1997. LC 97-15443. (Advances in Neurochemistry Ser.: Vol. 8). (Illus.). 436p. (C). text 115.00 (*0-306-45520-X*, Kluwer Plenum) Kluwer Academic.

Magnetic Resonance Techniques in Clinical Trials in Multiple Sclerosis. M. Filippi et al. 1999. LC 98-51407. (Topics in Neuroscience Ser.). x, 192p. (*88-470-0041-6*) Spr-Verlag ITA. *Dist:* Spr-Verlag.

Magnetic Resonance Test & Syllabus, Vol. 31. William G. Bradley, Jr. et al. 1991. (Professional Self-Evaluation & Continuing Education Program Ser.). (Illus.). 800p. 190.00 (*1-55903-031-3*) Am Coll Radiology.

Magnetic Stimulation in Clinical Neurophysiology. Sudhansu Chokroverty. 1989. 308p. text 75.00 (*0-409-90151-2*) Buttrwrth-Heinemann.

Magnetic Therapy: Healing in Your Hands. Abbot George Burke. 1987. LC 80-22941. 83p. reprint ed. pap. 8.95 (*0-87516-588-5*) DeVorss.

Magnetic Therapy in Eastern Europe: A Review of 30 Years of Research. Jiri Jerabek & William Pawluk. 1998. (Illus.). 161p. pap. 39.95 (*0-9664227-0-8*) W Pawluk.

Magnetism in Medicine. Wilfried Andra. 1998. 512p. 205.00 (*3-527-40221-7*, Wiley-VCH) Wiley.

Magnetresonanztomographie Von Tumoren des HNO-Gebiets: Hypopharynx und Larynx. P. Held & H. Pickrahn. 1995. (Illus.). viii, 56p. pap. 28.00 (*3-8055-6023-0*) S Karger.

Magnetresonanztomographie von Tumoren des HNO-Gebiets: Nasopharynx, Oropharynx, Mundhohle und-Boden. P. Held et al. 1997. (Illus.). viii, 64p. pap. 28.00 (*3-8055-6495-3*) S Karger.

Magnets for Health: A Practical Guide. Jose Luis Hinojosa. 2000. LC 00-39108. (Illus.). x, 54p. pap. 19.95 (*1-56072-808-6*, Nova Kroshka Bks) Nova Sci Pubs.

Maharishi Ayur-Veda Global Campaign to Create a Disease-Free Society in Every Country. 1991. LC 91-71302. (Illus.). (*0-89186-054-1*) Age Enlight Pr.

Mai Jing *see* **Pulse Classic: A Translation of the Mai Jing**

Maillard Reactions in Food: Proceedings of the International Symposium, Uddevalla, Sweden, September 1979. C. Ericksson. 1982. (Progress in Food & Nutrition Science Ser.: Vol. 5). (Illus.). 500p. 170.00 (*0-08-025496-9*, Pergamon Pr) Elsevier.

Maillard Reactions in Foods & Medicine. Ed. by J. O'Brien et al. 1998. (Special Publications: Vol. 223). 480p. 145.00 (*0-85404-733-6*) Spr-Verlag.

Main Currents of Critical Psychology. M. H. Van Ijzendoorn et al. Tr. by M. Schoen. 1984. 250p. text 32.50 (*0-8290-1517-5*); pap. text 16.95 (*0-8290-1518-3*) Irvington.

Main Issues in Mental Health & Race. Ed. by David Ndegwa & D. Olajide. 2001. 278p. text 74.95 (*1-84014-812-8*) Ashgate Pub Co.

Main Lectures: Proceedings of the International Congress of Logopedics & Phoniatrics, 17th, Copenhagen, August, 1977 International Congress of Logopedics and Phoniatrics. Ed. by E. Loebell et al. 1977. (Folia Phoniatrics Ser.: Vol. 29, No. 1). (Illus.). 28.75 (*3-8055-2780-2*) S Karger.

Main Report: Proceedings of the International Association of Logopedics & Phoniatrics 18th Congress, Washington, D. C., August 1980. International Association of Logopedics and Phoniatr. Ed. by B. Fritzell et al. 1980. (Journal: Vol. 32, No. 2). (Illus.). 72p. pap. 28.75 (*3-8055-1235-X*) S Karger.

Maine Health Care in Perspective 2000. Ed. by Kathleen O'Leary Morgan & Scott E. Morgan. 2000. 21p. spiral bd. 19.00 (*0-7401-0218-4*) Morgan Quitno Corp.

Maine Health Care Perspective, 1998. Ed. by Kathleen O'Leary Morgan & Scott E. Morgan. 1998. 20p. pap. 19.00 (*1-56692-818-4*) Morgan Quitno Corp.

Maingot's Abdominal Operations Rodney Maingot & Michael J. Zinner. 10th ed. 1996. LC 96-28893. 2150p. (C). text 350.00 (*0-8385-6106-3*, A6106-7) McGraw-Hill Prof.

Maingot's Abdominal Operations Michael J. Zinner. 10th ed. 1997. text 115.00 (*0-8385-6118-7*) Appleton & Lange.

Maingot's Abdominal Operations. Rodney Maingot & Michael J. Zinner. 10th ed. 1998. LC 96-28893. (C). Vol. I. pap. text 175.00 (*0-8385-6104-7*, A-6104-2); Vol. II. pap. text 175.00 (*0-8385-6105-5*, A6105-9) McGraw (Apple Lange Med).

Mainstream Education for Hearing Impaired Children & Youth. Ed. by Gary W. Nix. 1976. LC 75-40319. 288p. text 50.00 (*0-8089-0925-8*, 793115, Grune & Strat) Harcrt Hlth Sci Grp.

Mainstreaming: A Practical Guide. James L. Paul et al. 1977. (C). 29.95 (*0-8156-0136-0*) Syracuse U Pr.

Mainstreaming Emotionally Disturbed Children. Ed. by A. J. Pappanikou & James L. Paul. 1981. (Special Education & Rehabilitation Monograph Ser.: No. 10). (C). pap. 18.95 (*0-8156-2246-5*) Syracuse U Pr.

Maintaining a Healthy State Within the Individual: Proceedings of the IFIP-IMIA Working Conf., Kobe, Japan, 8-11 April 1986. Ed. by E. K. Harris & T. Yasaka. 1987. 326p. 100.00 (*0-444-70270-9*, North Holland) Elsevier.

Maintaining Communication with Persons with Dementia: An Educational Program for Nursing Home Staff & Family Members. Ronald W. Toseland & Phillip McCallion. 1998. LC 97-43904. 125.00 (*0-8261-1207-2*); 29.95 (*0-8261-1229-3*) Springer Pub.

Maintaining Function in Older Adults. Linda A. Newman. 1995. LC 95-13936. (Illus.). 141p. pap. text 34.99 (*0-7506-9568-4*) Buttrwrth-Heinemann.

Maintaining the Miracle Vol. 1: An Owner's Manual for the Human Body. Ted D. Adams et al. (Illus.). 246p. reprint ed. pap. 17.95 (*0-9638937-7-7*) Capp Pubng.

Maintaining the Profession: A Fieldbook for Clinical Supervisors. William R. Olcott. 1996. 238p. 19.95 (*1-889346-00-4*) Rainmaker Pr.

Maintaining Your Gains: Cope Program for Depression. John H. Greist et al. 1999. (Illus.). 9p. pap. (*0-9702974-7-5*) Healthcare Sys.

Maintenance & Repair of Laboratory, Diagnostic Imaging, & Hospital Equipment. 1994. LC 96-127663. (CHI, ENG, FRE & SPA.). vi, 158p. pap. text 39.00 (*92-4-154463-5*, 1150423) World Health.

Maintenance Management. Harold Roffman. 1997. 187p. ring bd. 44.50 (*0-929442-05-9*, 2210pp) Prof Prnting & Pub.

Maintenance Pharmacotherapies for Neuropsychiatric Disorders. Stephanie Richards et al. 1999. LC 98-45218. 390p. text 59.95 (*0-87630-894-9*) Brunner-Routledge.

Major Accident Reporting System: Lessons Learned from Accidents Notified. G. Drogaris. 1993. LC 93-29726. 254p. 193.00 (*0-444-81665-8*) Elsevier.

Major Depression: Prevention & Treatment. Michael R. Lowry. 1984. 136p. 15.00 (*0-87527-186-3*) Green.

Major Fractures of the Pilon, the Talus, & the Calcaneus: Current Concepts of Treatment. Ed. by Joseph Schatzker & H. Tscherne. 1994. LC 92-49465. (Illus.). 259p. 155.00 (*0-387-55837-3*) Spr-Verlag.

Major Histocompatibility Complex Region of Domestic Animal Species. Ed. by Lawrence B. Schook & Susan J. Lamont. 1996. 336p. 104.95 (*0-8493-8032-4*, 8032) CRC Pr.

Major Incident Medical Management & Support: The Practical Approach. Advanced Life Support Group. 1995. 205p. pap. text (*0-7279-0928-2*) BMJ Pub GBR. *Dist:* AIDC.

Major Issues in Gereontological Nursing. Ed. by John Lantz. 4th rev. ed. 1999. (Illus.). 143p. pap. (*1-57801-037-3*) Western Schls.

Major Issues in Gerontological Nursing. John Lantz. Ed. by Barbara Halliburton. 3rd rev. ed. 1996. 127p. pap. 29.95 (*1-57801-009-8*) Western Schls.

Major Issues in the Life & Work of C. G. Jung. Ed. by William Schoenl. 1996. LC 96-32905. 104p. (Orig.). pap. text 21.50 (*0-7618-0470-6*); lib. bdg. 38.50 (*0-7618-0469-2*) U Pr of Amer.

Major Medicinal Plants: Botany, Culture & Uses. Julia F. Morton. fac. ed. 1977. (Illus.). 448p. 103.95 (*0-398-03673-X*) C C Thomas.

Major Psychological Assessment Instruments. Ed. by Charles S. Newmark. 2nd ed. 1996. LC 95-40858. 480p. (C). 78.00 (*0-205-16869-8*) Allyn.

Major Psychological Assessment Instruments, Vol. I. Charles S. Newmark. 1985. LC 85-753. (Major Psychological Assessment Instruments Ser.: Vol. I). 430p. text 97.00 (*0-205-08457-5*, H84577, Longwood Div) Allyn.

Major State Health Care Policies: Fifty State Profiles, 1997. Health Policy Tracking Service Staff. 6th ed. 1998. LC 98-228420. vi, 294 p. (*1-55516-819-1*) Natl Conf State Legis.

Major Theories of Personality Disorder. Ed. by John F. Clarkin & Mark F. Lenzenweger. 1996. LC 95-53935. 402p. 50.00 (*1-57230-082-5*, 0082) Guilford Pubns.

Majoring in Nursing: From Prerequisites to Postgraduate Study & Beyond. Janet R. Katz. Ed. by Carol Carter. 1999. LC 98-15168. 144p. pap. 11.00 (*0-374-52567-6*, Noonday) FS&G.

Make a Difference. Henry W. Foster. 1997. LC 96-48006. 256p. 23.00 (*0-684-82685-2*) S&S Trade.

Make Every Session Counts: Getting the Most Out of Your Brief Therapy. John D. Preston et al. 2nd ed. 2000. (Illus.). 140p. pap. 12.95 (*1-57224-190-X*) New Harbinger.

Make Room for Sentiment: A Physician's Story. Theodore E. Woodward et al. 1998. LC 98-15858. (Illus.). 278p. 23.80 (*0-9619119-1-3*) Medical Alumni Association of Univ.

Make Your Mark in Health Services. Rosemary Grebel & Phyllis Pogrund. (Make Your Mark Ser.). pap. text, tchr. ed. 5.31 (*0-8092-0831-8*, PO831-8) NTC Contemp Pub Co.

Make Your Medicine Safe: How to Prevent Side Effects from the Drugs You Take. Jay S. Cohen. 1998. LC 98-92458. pap. 7.50 (*0-380-79075-0*, Avon Bks) Morrow Avon.

Makepeace Experiment. Abram Tertz, pseud & Abram Tertz. 1989. 191p. reprint ed. pap. 17.00 (*0-8101-0838-0*) Northwestern U Pr.

Makers of Modern Medicine. James J. Walsh. 1977. LC 70-107741. (Essay Index Reprint Ser.). 24.95 (*0-8369-1538-0*) Ayer.

Makers of Psychology: The Personal Factor. Harvey Mindess. 1988. 182p. 35.95 (*0-89885-371-0*); pap. 20.95 (*0-89885-380-X*) Kluwer Academic (Kluwer Acad Hman Sci).

Making a Baby: Everything You Need to Know to Get Pregnant. Debra Fulghum Bruce & Samuel Thatcher. 2000. LC 00-190529. (Illus.). xix, 379p. pap. 14.00 (*0-345-43543-5*) Ballantine Pub Grp.

Making a Friend in Youth: Developmental Theory & Pair Therapy. Robert L. Selman & Lynn H. Schultz. 1996. LC 89-20362. (Illus.). 374p. 35.95 (*0-226-74790-5*) U Ch Pr.

Making a Friend in Youth: Developmental Theory & Pair Therapy. Robert S. Selman & Lynn Schultz. 1998. LC 97-43304. 373p. reprint ed. pap. text 25.95 (*0-202-30605-4*); lib. bdg. 49.95 (*0-202-30606-2*) Aldine de Gruyter.

Making a Healthy World: Agencies Actors & Policies in International Health. Meri Koivusalo. 1998. LC 97-36972. (C). (*1-85649-493-4*); pap. (*1-85649-494-2*) Zed Books GBR. *Dist:* St Martin.

Making a Medical Living: Doctors & Patients in the English Market for Medicine, 1720-1911. Anne Digby. 1994. (Cambridge Studies in Population, Economy & Society in Past Time: No. 24). (Illus.). 369p. (C). text 69.95 (*0-521-34526-X*) Cambridge U Pr.

Making & Meaning of Hospital Policy in the United States & Canada. Terry Boychuk. 1999. LC 98-58120. 200p. (C). text 50.00 (*0-472-10928-6*, 10928) U of Mich Pr.

***Making Babies: The Science of Pregnancy.** David Bainbridge. 2001. LC 2001-24166. (Illus.). 230p. 26.00 (*0-674-00653-4*) HUP.

Making Capitation Work: Clinical Operations in an Integrated Delivery System. Ed. by Gloria G. Mayer et al. 1995. ring bd. 189.00 (*0-8342-0677-3*, S178) Aspen Pub.

Making Change: Even Still More Observations of a Chiropractic Advocate. William D. Esteb. 1995. 240p. (Orig.). pap. text 24.95 (*0-9631711-4-3*) Back Talk Systs.

Making Change Work for You in Health Care. Richard S. Deems & K. C. Warner. Ed. by Karen M. Miller. 1998. LC 98-70378. (How to Bks.). 93p. pap. 14.95 (*1-884926-85-1*, CHANH) Amer Media.

Making Changes for Good: A Cognitive Behavioral Approach for Sex Offender Relapse Prevention. Gregory L. Little & Kenneth D. Robinson. 1998. 58p. pap. 18.00 (*0-940829-22-3*) Eagle Wing Bks.

Making Chaplaincy Work: Practical Approaches. Ed. by Laurel A. Burton. 1988. LC 88-541. (Journal of Health Care Chaplaincy Ser.: Vol. 1, No. 2). (Illus.). 98p. text 29.95 (*0-86656-743-7*) Haworth Pr.

Making Children Mind Without Losing Yours. Kevin Leman. 2nd ed. 2000. LC 00-37280. 272p. pap., stu. ed. 12.99 (*0-8007-5731-9*) Revell.

Making Collaborative Connections with Medical Providers: A Guide for Mental Health Professionals. L. Kevin Hamberger et al. 1999. LC 99-10456. 160p. pap. 32.95 (*0-8261-1258-7*) Springer Pub.

Making Connections: Adult Day Health Care for People with AIDS. Leah Mason. 1993. LC 92-44741. (Practical Guide Ser.). 10.00 (*1-881277-14-3*) United Hosp Fund.

Making Connections with Others: A Handbook on Interpersonal Practice. Deborah Davidson & Suzanne Peloquin. 1998. 168p. pap. text 35.00 (*1-56900-100-6*, 1142) Am Occup Therapy.

Making Contact. Virginia M. Satir. 1995. LC 75-28768. (Illus.). 96p. text 7.95 (*0-89087-119-1*) Celestial Arts.

Making Contact: Uses of Language in Psychotherapy. Leston L. Havens. 1986. 215p. reprint ed. pap. text 14.00 (*0-674-54316-5*) HUP.

Making Decisions about Children: Psychological Questions & Answers. H. Rudolph Schaffer. 2nd ed. 1998. LC 97-37882. 256p. pap. 32.95 (*0-631-20259-5*) Blackwell Pubs.

Making Disability: Exploring the Social Transformation of Human Variation. Paul C. Higgins. 1992. 302p. (C). text 57.95 (*0-398-05769-9*) C C Thomas.

Making Effective Referrals. Sharon Cheston. 1991. text 29.95 (*0-89876-170-0*) Gardner Pr.

Making Gray Gold: Narratives of Nursing Home Care. Timothy Diamond. 1998. LC 91-45755. (Women in Culture & Society Ser.). 296p. 24.95 (*0-226-14473-9*) U Ch Pr.

Making Health Care Equipment: Ideas for Local Design & Production. Adam Platt & Nicola Carter. 1990. (Illus.). 96p. pap. (*1-85339-067-4*) Intermed Tech GBR. *Dist:* Stylus Pub VA.

Making Health Care Reform Work: How the New Law Affects You & Your Employer. Peter M. Berkery, Jr. pap. 9.95 (*0-7863-0344-1*, Irwn Prfssnl) McGraw-Hill Educ Grp.

Making Health Certain (1921) R. Swinburne Clymer. 1998. 190p. reprint ed. pap. 14.95 (*0-7661-0503-2*) Kessinger Pub.

Making Health Communication Programs Work: A Planner's Guide. 1993. (Illus.). 131p. (Orig.). (C). pap. text 40.00 (*0-7881-0080-7*) DIANE Pub.

Making Health Reform Work: The View from the States. Ed. by John J. DiIulio, Jr. & Richard P. Nathan. 1994. LC 94-3690. 179p. (C). text 34.95 (*0-8157-1852-7*); pap. text 14.95 (*0-8157-1851-9*) Brookings.

Making Health Work: Human Growth in Modern Japan. Carl Mosk. 1996. LC 96-26629. (Studies in Demography: Vol. 8). (Illus.). 174p. (C). text 50.00 (*0-520-08315-6*) U CA Pr.

Making Healthy Tomorrows: Cardiac Fitness & a Healthier Lifestyle. Barry Franklin. 1993. 208p. pap. 12.95 (*1-881139-07-7*) Glovebox Guidebks.

Making Informed Medical Decisions: Where to Look & How to Use What You Find. Nancy Oster et al. Ed. by Linda Lamb. 2000. LC 00-36705. (Patient-Centered Guides Ser.). (Illus.). xvii, 364p. pap. 17.95 (*1-56592-459-2*, Patient-Centered) OReilly & Assocs.

Making Integrated Health Care Work: The Analysis Dean C. Coddington et al. 1996. (Health Ser.). 300p. (C). pap. 51.00 (*1-56829-010-1*, 4828) M G M A.

Making Integrated Health Care Work & Making Integrated Health Care Work: Case Studies, Vol. 1 & 2. Dean C. Coddington et al. 1996. text 75.00 (*1-56829-014-4*) M G M A.

Making Joint Decisions: Preventing & Relieving Arthritis Pain. Anne E. Hunt. Ed. by Eric A. Mein. 1991. (Natural Remedies for Common Ailments & Conditions Ser.). 83p. (Orig.). pap. 4.95 (*0-87604-279-5*, 364) ARE Pr.

Making Life Choices: Health Skills & Concepts. Frances S. Sizer & Eleanor N. Whitney. 1993. LC 92-39251. mass mkt., stu. ed. 61.50 (*0-314-01686-4*); mass mkt. 61.50 (*0-314-01158-7*) West Pub.

***Making Long-Term Care Affordable: Congressional Hearing.** Ed. by Evan Bayh. 2001. 130p. (C). reprint ed. pap. 30.00 (*0-7567-0982-2*) DIANE Pub.

Making Love: How to Be Your Own Sex Therapist. Patricia E. Raley. 1980. 288p. pap. 12.95 (*0-380-48819-1*, Avon Bks) Morrow Avon.

Making Love Again: Regaining Sexual Potency Through the New Injection Treatment. J. Francois Eid & Carol A. Pearce. 1993. LC 93-5918. (Illus.). 144p. pap. 15.95 (*0-87630-722-5*) Brunner-Routledge.

Making Managed Care Work for You: Strategies for Local Market Dominance. Genie James. 1996. LC 96-20990. 336p. text 45.00 (*0-7863-1012-X*, Irwn Prfssnl) McGraw-Hill Educ Grp.

Making Managed Health Care Work for Kids in Foster Care: A Guide to Purchasing Services. Ellen S. Battistelli. 1996. 80p. pap. 7.95 (*0-87868-683-5*) Child Welfare.

Making Managed Healthcare Work: A Practical Guide to Strategies & Solutions. Peter Boland. 1992. 620p. 127.00 (*0-8342-0391-X*) Aspen Pub.

Making Manufacturing Cells Work. Lee R. Nyman. 1993. 387p. text 60.00 (*0-07-047977-1*) McGraw-Hill Prof.

Making Medical Decisions: An Approach to Clinical Decision Making for the Practicing Physician. Richard A. Gross. 1999. LC 98-29289. 120p. (C). pap. text 18.00 (*0-943126-75-4*) Amer Coll Phys.

Making Medical History: The Life & Times of Henry E. Sigerist. Ed. by Elizabeth Fee & Theodore M. Brown. 1997. LC 96-8862. (Illus.). 408p. 42.95 (*0-8018-5355-9*) Johns Hopkins.

Making Medical Spending Decisions: The Law, Ethics & Economics of Rationing Mechanisms. Mark A. Hall. 1996. LC 96-24738. 312p. text 35.00 (*0-19-509219-8*) OUP.

Making Midwives Legal: Childbirth, Medicine, & the Law. Raymond G. DeVries. 1996. LC 96-6312. (Women & Health Ser.). Orig. Title: Regulating Birth. 232p. reprint ed. pap. text 19.95 (*0-8142-0703-0*) Ohio St U Pr.

Making Miracles: Exploration into the Dynamics of Self-Healing. Paul C. Roud. 1990. pap. 9.95 (*0-446-39118-2*) Warner Bks.

Making Miracles: Finding Meaning in Life's Chaos. Paul P. Pearsall. 1993. 320p. reprint ed. pap. 10.00 (*0-380-71948-7*, Avon Bks) Morrow Avon.

Making Monsters: False Memories, Psychotherapy, & Sexual Hysteria. Richard Ofshe & Ethan Watters. 1998. 340p. text 23.00 (*0-7881-5931-3*) DIANE Pub.

Making Monsters: False Memories, Psychotherapy, & Sexual Hysteria. Richard Ofshe & Ethan Watters. 1994. LC 94-15642. 340p. 23.00 (*0-684-19698-0*) S&S Trade.

Making Monsters: False Memories, Psychotherapy, & Sexual Hysteria. Richard Ofshe & Ethan Watters. 1996. LC 95-49014. 352p. (C). pap. 18.95 (*0-520-20583-9*) U CA Pr.

Making of a Fly: The Genetics of Animal Design. Peter A. Lawrence. 1992. LC 91-27871. (Illus.). 242p. pap. 49.95 (*0-632-03048-8*) Blackwell Sci.

Making of a Psychotherapist. N. Symington. 1997. 240p. pap. (*1-85575-139-9*) Karnac Bks GBR. *Dist:* Other Pr LLC.

Making of a Psychotherapist. Neville Symington. 1997. LC 96-43136. 240p. 37.50 (*0-8236-3083-8*, BN03083) Intl Univs Pr.

Making of a Social Disease: Tuberculosis in Nineteenth-Century France. David S. Barnes. 1995. LC 94-15230. 305p. text 55.00 (*0-520-08772-0*) U CA Pr.

Making of an Efficient Physician. Sherry A. Delio & George Hein. 1987. 110p. 7.00 (*0-89970-042-X*, OP653895WE) AMA.

Making of an Efficient Physician. Sherry A. Delio & George Hein. 1995. 100p. 52.50 (*1-56829-042-X*, 4694) M G M A.

Making of Blind Men. Robert A. Scott. 1981. LC 80-20558. 145p. (C). pap. text 24.95 (*0-87855-687-7*) Transaction Pubs.

Making of Cognitive Science: Essays in Honor of George A. Miller. Ed. by William Hirst. 1988. (Illus.). 296p. text 80.00 (*0-521-34255-4*) Cambridge U Pr.

Making of Man-Midwifery: Childbirth in England, 1660-1770. Adrian Wilson. 1995. LC 94-38976. (Illus.). 256p. (C). 39.50 (*0-674-54323-8*) HUP.

Making of Masculinities: The New Men's Studies. Ed. by Harry Brod. 1987. LC 86-28796. 304p. text 44.95 (*0-04-497035-8*); pap. text 22.95 (*0-04-497036-6*) Routledge.

Making of Mind: A Personal Account of Soviet Psychology. Aleksandr R. Luria. Ed. by Michael Cole & Sheila Cole. 1979. (Illus.). 234p. pap. 18.00 (*0-674-54327-0*) HUP.

Making of the Dentiste, 1650-1760. Roger King. 1998. LC 98-27420. (History of Medicine in Context Ser.). 288p. 84.95 (*1-84014-653-2*) Ashgate Pub Co.

Making of the Unborn Patient: A Social Anatomy of Fetal Surgery. Monica J. Casper. 1998. LC 97-39331. (Illus.). (C). 267p. text 50.00 (*0-8135-2515-2*); 304p. pap. text 20.00 (*0-8135-2516-0*) Rutgers U Pr.

Making Peace with Chronic Pain: A Whole-Life Strategy. Marlene Hunter. 1996. LC 96-29183. 192p. pap. 18.95 (*0-87630-821-3*) Brunner-Routledge.

Making Peace with Your Adult Children. S. L. Smith. 1991. LC 91-7157. (Illus.). 398p. (C). 23.95 (*0-306-43767-8*) Da Capo.

Making Phonology Functional: What Do I Do First? Shelley L. Velleman. 1998. LC 97-52015. 215p. text 49.99 (*0-7506-9525-0*) Buttrwrth-Heinemann.

Making Plant Medicine. Richard A. Cech. 2000. (Illus.). 296p. pap. 14.98 (*0-9700312-0-3*) Horizon Herbs.

Making Safety Work: Getting Management Commitment to Occupational Health & Safety. Andrew Hopkins. 1996. LC 96-146376. 224p. pap. (*1-86373-869-X*) Allen & Unwin Pty AUS. *Dist:* Paul & Co Pubs.

Making Sense. Ed. by Jerome S. Bruner & Helen Haste. 1988. 260p. 65.00 (*0-416-38240-1*); pap. 15.95 (*0-416-92490-5*, A1369) Routledge.

Making Sense of a Primary Care Led Health Service. Peter Littlejohns & Christina R. Victor. 1996. LC 96-25406. (*1-85775-048-9*) Radcliffe Med Pr GBR. *Dist:* Balogh.

Making Sense of Advance Directives. Nancy M. King. rev. ed. 1996. LC 95-42746. (Clinical Medical Ethics Ser.). 286p. pap. 19.95 (*0-87840-605-0*) Georgetown U Pr.

Making Sense of Advance Directives. Nancy M. King. 1991. 240p. (C). lib. bdg. (*0-7923-1163-9*) Kluwer Academic NLD. *Dist:* Kluwer Academic.

Making Sense of Audit. Donald Irvine & Sally Irvine. 2nd ed. 1997. LC 97-5656. (Business Side of General Practice Ser.). (*1-85775-119-1*) Radcliffe Med Pr GBR. *Dist:* Balogh.

***Making Sense of Clinical Governance: A Workbook for NHS Doctors, Nurses & Managers.** Roy Lilley. 1999. 160p. reprint ed. pap., wbk. ed. (*1-85775-425-5*) Radcliffe Med Pr GBR. *Dist:* Balogh.

***Making Sense of Dental Practice Finance.** Mervyn Bright & Sau-Kee Li. 1996. 150p. pap. (*1-85775-065-9*) Radcliffe Med Pr GBR. *Dist:* Balogh.

Making Sense of Dental Practice Management: The Business Side of General Dental Practice. Raj Rattan. 1996. LC 95-52760. 256p. pap. (*1-85775-017-9*) Radcliffe Med Pr GBR. *Dist:* Balogh.

Making Sense of Illness: Studies in Twentieth Century Medical Thought. Robert A. Aronowitz. 1998. LC 97-9805. (Cambridge Studies in the History of Medicine). 283p. (C). text 52.95 (*0-521-55234-6*) Cambridge U Pr.

Making Sense of Illness: The Social Psychology of Health & Disease. Alan Radley. 1994. 256p. 74.50 (*0-8039-8908-3*, 2797); pap. 25.95 (*0-8039-8909-1*, 2796) Sage.

Making Sense of Managed Care Vol. I: Building Blocks & Fundamentals. Ed. by Kimball Miller & Elaine Miller. 1997. LC 97-70473. 148p. 32.00 (*0-924674-51-2*) Am Coll Phys Execs.

Making Sense of Managed Care Vol. II: Strategic Positioning, Vol. 2. Ed. by Kimball Miller & Elaine Miller. 1997. LC 97-70473. 192p. 32.00 (*0-924674-52-0*) Am Coll Phys Execs.

Making Sense of Managed Care Vol. III: Operational Issues & Practical Answers, Vol. 3. Ed. by Kimball Miller & Elaine Miller. 1997. LC 97-70473. 206p. 32.00 (*0-924674-53-9*) Am Coll Phys Execs.

Making Sense of Menopause: Over One Hundred Fifty Women & Experts Share Their Wisdom, Experience & Common Sense Advice. Faye K. Cone. 1993. LC 93-2526. 384p. pap. 14.00 (*0-671-78638-5*, Fireside) S&S Trade Pap.

Making Sense of NHS Complaints & Disciplinary Procedures. David Pickersgill & Tony Stanton. 1997. LC 97-1119. (*1-85775-163-9*) Radcliffe Med Pr GBR. *Dist:* Balogh.

Making Sense of Personnel Management. Sally Irvine & Hilary Haman. 2nd ed. 1997. LC 97-5360. (Business Side of General Practice Ser.). (*1-85775-124-8*) Radcliffe Med Pr GBR. *Dist:* Balogh.

***Making Sense of Public Health Medicine.** Jim Connelly & Chris Worth. 1997. 160p. pap. (*1-85775-186-8*) Radcliffe Med Pr GBR. *Dist:* Balogh.

Making Sense of Research: An Introduction for Nurses. Gill Hek et al. 1996. (Illus.). 160p. pap. (*0-304-33338-7*) Cassell GBR. *Dist:* Cassell.

Making Sense of Research & Development. Ed. by Mark R. Baker & Simon Kirk. 1995. (*1-85775-094-2*) Radcliffe Med Pr GBR. *Dist:* Balogh.

Making Sense of Social Development. Ed. by Karen Littleton et al. 1999. LC 98-25642. (Illus.). vi, 278p. (C). (gr. 13). pap. 24.95 (*0-415-17374-4*, D6390) Routledge.

***Making Sense of Spirituality in Nursing Practice: An Interactive Approach.** Wilfred McSherry. 2001. (Illus.). 205p. pap. (*0-443-06356-7*) Church GBR. *Dist:* Saunders.

Making Sense of the ECG. Andrew Houghton & David Gray. 1997. (Illus.). 288p. pap. text (*0-340-67657-4*) E A GBR. *Dist:* OUP.

Making Sense of the Red Book. Norman Ellis & John Chisholm. 3rd ed. 1997. LC 97-22326. (Business Side of General Practice Ser.). (*1-85775-291-0*) Radcliffe Med Pr GBR. *Dist:* Balogh.

Making-Sense-Out-of-Suffering Therapy. Jack Wintz. 1996. LC 96-85000. (Illus.). 88p. pap. 4.95 (*0-87029-296-X*, 20156) Abbey.

Making Sense Together: The Intersubjective Approach to Psychotherapy. Peter Buirski & Pamela Haglund. 2001. LC 00-52204. 40.00 (*0-7657-0314-9*) Aronson.

Making Sense With Offenders: Personal Construct, Therapy & Change. Julia C. Houston. 1998. LC 97-33472. (Offender Rehabilitation Ser.). 292p. 130.00 (*0-471-95415-2*) Wiley.

Making Sense with Offenders: Personal Constructs, Therapy & Change. Julia Houston. 1998. LC 97-33472. (Offender Rehabilitation Ser.). 292p. pap. 75.00 (*0-471-96627-4*) Wiley.

Making the Best Medical Records & Documentation. 7th ed. 1995. 200p. pap. text 45.00 (*1-58383-159-2*, RECORD1) Robert D Keene.

Making the Connection: Keys to Quality Customer Service in Health Care. Pennie Myers & Don W. Nance. 1997. 60p. spiral bd., wbk. ed. 29.00 (*0-9620723-7-0*) MAS.

***Making the Decision: The Cancer Patient's Guide to Clinical Trials.** Marilyn Mulay. 2001. LC 2001-41285. (Illus.). (C). pap. text 24.95 (*0-7637-1690-1*, 1690-1, N L N Bart) Jones & Bartlett.

Making the Estrogen Decision. Susan M. Lark. Ed. by Phyllis Herman. 1996. (Good Health Guides). 48p. pap. 3.95 (*0-87983-696-2*, 36962K, Keats Pubng) McGraw-Hill Trade.

Making the Moments Count: Leisure Activities for Caregiving Relationships. Joanne A. Decker. 1997. LC 97-12488. 208p. 39.95 (*0-8018-5699-X*); pap. 15.95 (*0-8018-5700-7*) Johns Hopkins.

***Making the Most of Your Training Dollars.** Spath. 2002. LC 2001-38440. (J-B AHA Press Ser.: Vol. 11). 250p. 50.00 (*0-7879-5874-3*) Wiley.

Making the Patient Your Partner: Communication Skills for Doctors & Other Caregivers. Thomas S. Gordon & W. Edwards. 1997. LC 94-42698. 240p. pap. 21.95 (*0-86569-273-4*, Auburn Hse) Greenwood.

Making the Physician Network Work: Leadership, Design & Incentives. Lisa K. Rolfe & Paul Wehner. 1995. LC 95-11325. 116p. pap. 56.50 (*1-55648-142-X*, 164101) AHPI.

Making the Prostate Therapy Decision. Jeff Baggish. 1996. (Illus.). 208p. pap. 16.00 (*1-56565-433-1*); 1995. 208p. 22.95 (*1-56565-207-X*); 2nd rev. ed. 1998. 240p. pap. 16.00 (*1-56565-869-8*, 08698W) Lowell Hse.

Making the Prozac Decision. Carol Turkington & Eliot F. Kaplan. 3rd rev. ed. 1997. LC 98-231517. 272p. pap. 15.00 (*1-56565-803-5*, 08035W, Anodyne) Lowell Hse.

Making the Radiation Therapy Decision. David J. Brenner & Eric J. Hall. 1996. (Illus.). 216p. 27.00 (*1-56565-333-5*) Lowell Hse.

Making the Right Choice - Treatment Options in Cancer Surgery see Cancer Breakthrough You've Never Heard Of: Your Guide to Limited Surgery in the Treatment of Cancer

Making the Transition to Home Health Nursing: A Practical Guide. Denise Lovejoy. 1997. LC 97-16428. 200p. 32.95 (*0-8261-9740-X*) Springer Pub.

Making the Transition to Managed Behavioral Health Care: A Guide for Agencies & Practitioners. Anna Scheyett. 1997. LC 97-36711. 165p. pap. 21.95 (*0-87304-300-6*) Manticore Pubs.

Making Us Crazy: DSM: The Psychiatric Bible & the Creation of Mental Disorders. Herb Kutchins & Stuart A. Kirk. 1997. LC 97-22228. 320p. 28.95 (*0-684-82280-6*) Free Pr.

Making Use of Clinical Audit: A Guide to Practice in the Health Professions. Maurice Kogan & Sally J. Redfern. 1995. LC 95-10765. 192p. (*0-335-19543-1*) OpUniv Pr.

Making Use of Clinical Audit: A Guide to Practice in the Health Professions. Maurice Kogan & Sally J. Redfern. 1995. LC 95-10765. 192p. pap. 33.95 (*0-335-19542-3*) Taylor & Francis.

***Making Use of Guidelines in Clinical Practice.** Ed. by Allen Hutchinson & Richard Baker. 1999. 224p. pap. (*1-85775-088-8*) Radcliffe Med Pr GBR. *Dist:* Balogh.

Making Wise Medical Decisions: How to Get the Information You Need. Resources for Rehabilitation Staff. 1998. LC 98-23960. 219p. pap. 39.95 (*0-929718-21-6*) Resc Rehab.

Making Your Patient Your Partner: Communication Skills for Doctors & Other Caregivers. Thomas Gordon & W. Sterling Edwards. 1995. LC 94-42698. 240p. 58.00 (*0-86569-255-6*, Auburn Hse) Greenwood.

Malabsorption in Coeliac Sprue. O. J. Cluysenaer & J. H. Van Tongeren. 1977. pap. text 141.50 (*90-247-2000-1*) Kluwer Academic.

Malade Age en Pratique Medicale. Ed. by W. Meier-Ruge. 1990. (Geriatrie en Pratique Quotidienne Ser.: Vol. 1). viii, 256p. pap. 31.50 (*3-8055-5292-0*) S Karger.

Maladies Systemiques. M. F. Kahn & A. P. Peltier. 2nd ed. 1985. (FRE., Illus.). 950p. 125.00 (*2-257-12299-2*) S M P F Inc.

Malaria: A Survey of Existing Legislation. WHO Staff. 1956. (International Digest of Health Legislation Offprints: Vol. 7, No. 4). 32p. 3.00 (*92-4-169074-7*) World Health.

Malaria: Host Responses to Infection. Ed. by Mary M. Stevenson. 1989. 184p. 159.00 (*0-8493-4745-9*, RC159) CRC Pr.

Malaria: Molecular & Clinical Aspects. Ed. by Mats Wahlgren & Peter Perlmann. 1999. 578p. text 120.00 (*90-5702-446-2*, Harwood Acad Pubs) Gordon & Breach.

Malaria: Obstacles & Opportunities. Institute of Medicine Staff. Ed. by Stanley C. Oaks, Jr. et al. 1991. 328p. text 39.95 (*0-309-04527-4*) Natl Acad Pr.

Malaria: Parasite Biology, Pathogenesis, & Protection. Ed. by Irwin W. Sherman. 1998. LC 98-8261. (Illus.). 500p. 119.95 (*1-55581-131-0*) ASM Pr.

Malaria: Waiting for the Vaccine. G. Targett. 1992. LC 91-40008. 236p. 314.50 (*0-471-93100-4*, Wiley-Liss) Wiley.

Malaria - That Remains a Killer. N. L. Pal. 1994. pap. (*0-7855-2755-9*) Scientific Pubs IND. *Dist:* St Mut.

Malaria & Barbesiosis. Ed. by Miodrag Ristic et al. 1984. (New Perspectives in Clinical Microbiology Ser.). text 225.00 (*0-89838-675-6*) Kluwer Academic.

Malaria & Greek History. William H. Jones. LC 75-23729. reprint ed. 35.00 (*0-404-13287-1*) AMS Pr.

Malaria Capers: Tales of Parasites & People. Robert S. Desowitz. 1993. 288p. pap. 13.95 (*0-393-31008-6*) Norton.

Malaria Control & National Health Goals. 1982. (Technical Report Ser.: No. 680). 68p. pap. text 6.00 (*92-4-120680-2*) World Health.

Malaria Control As Part of Primary Health Care: Report of a WHO Study Group, 1984. WHO Staff. 1984. (Technical Report Ser.: No. 712). 73p. 8.00 (*92-4-120712-4*) World Health.

Malaria Immunology. Ed. by P. Pearlmann & Hans Wigzell. 1988. (Progress in Allergy Ser.: Vol. 41). (Illus.). x, 374p. 228.00 (*3-8055-4672-6*) S Karger.

Malaria-Immunology & Immunopathology. Ed. by Dan T. Spira & Charles L. Greenblatt. 1978. pap. 51.50 (*3-8055-2940-6*) S Karger.

Malaria in Panama. James S. Simmons. 1979. 30.95 (*0-405-10628-9*) Ayer.

Malaria in the Upper Mississippi Valley, 1760-1900. Erwin H. Ackerknecht. Ed. by Barbara G. Rosenkrantz. 1977. LC 76-25650. (Public Health in America Ser.). (Illus.). reprint ed. lib. bdg. 19.95 (*0-405-09805-7*) Ayer.

Malaria Methods & Protocols. Ed. by Denise L. Doolan. 2001. LC 2001-51656. (Methods in Molecular Medicine Ser.: Vol. 72). 650p. 135.00 (*0-89603-823-8*) Humana.

Malaria Vaccine Development: A Multi-Immune Response Approach. Ed. by Stephen L. Hoffman. 1996. LC 96-4661. 325p. 99.95 (*1-55581-111-6*) ASM Pr.

Malaria Vaccine Development: Pre-Erythrocytic Stages Proceedings of a Conference Held in Bethesda, Maryland, U. S. A. Ed. by S. L. Hoffmann & L. J. Martinez. 1990. (Bulletin of WHO Ser.: Suppl. to Vol. 68, 1990). 196p. pap. text 35.00 (*92-4-068680-0*, 1036801) World Health.

Malay Poisons & Charm Cures. John D. Gimlette. 2nd ed. LC 77-87027. reprint ed. 37.50 (*0-404-16821-3*) AMS Pr.

Maldescensus Testis. Ed. by A. Kelami & J. P. Pryor. 1984. (Progress in Reproductive Biology & Medicine Ser.: Vol. 10). (Illus.). viii, 176p. 144.50 (*3-8055-3791-3*) S Karger.

Male Aesthetic Surgery. Ed. by Daniel Marchac et al. 1996. (Illus.). 418p. text (*0-7506-9277-4*) E A GBR. *Dist:* OUP.

Male & Female Homosexuality: Psychological Approaches. Louis Diamant. 1987. (Clinical & Community Psychology Ser.). 292p. 63.95 (*0-89116-449-9*) Hemisp Pub.

Male Batterer: A Treatment Approach. Daniel J. Sonkin et al. 1985. 272p. 32.95 (*0-8261-5090-X*) Springer Pub.

Male Birth Control Pill. 1979. (Landmark Ser.). 25.50 (*0-8422-4110-8*) Irvington.

Male Body: A Physician's Guide to What Every Man Should Know About His Sexual Health. Abraham Morgentaler. 1993. LC 93-18035. 208p. pap. 10.00 (*0-671-86426-2*) S&S Trade.

Male Body: An Owner's Manual: The Ultimate Guide to Staying Healthy & Fit for Life. K. Winston Caine & Perry Garfinkel. Ed. by Men's Health Books Staff. 1996. LC 96-18195. (Illus.). 432p. pap. 19.95 (*0-87596-401-X*) Rodale Pr Inc.

Male Continence. John H. Noyes. 1975. 250.00 (*0-87968-231-0*) Gordon Pr.

Male Depression & Alcoholism: Pocketbook Edition. Ihsan M. Salloum et al. 2000. 97p. (*1-85317-894-2*) Martin Dunitz GBR. *Dist:* Blackwell Sci.

***Male Dermatology: Care & Disease.** N. Talanin. 2001. LC 2001-55372. (Illus.). 79.95 (*1-84214-107-4*, Parthenon Pbng) CRC Pr.

Male Factor in Human Infertility. Ed. by W. M. Thompson et al. 1984. (Studies in Fertility & Sterility). lib. bdg. 174.50 (*0-85200-810-4*) Kluwer Academic.

Male, Female: The Evolution of Human Sex Differences. David C. Geary. 1998. LC 98-26961. 410p. 49.95 (*1-55798-527-8*) Am Psychol.

Male, Female, Email: The Struggle for Relatedness in a Paranoid Society. Michael Civin. 2000. LC 99-43547. 260p. 25.95 (*1-892746-30-1*) Other Pr LLC.

Male Fertility & Infertility. Ed. by T. D. Glover & C. L. Barratt. 1999. LC 98-55696. (Illus.). 286p. (C). text 74.95 (*0-521-62375-8*) Cambridge U Pr.

Male Fertility & It's Regulation. T. J. Lobl & E. S. Hafez. 1985. (Advances in Reproductive Health Care Ser.). text 322.00 (*0-85200-805-8*) Kluwer Academic.

Male Genital System. Ed. by Ulrich Mohr. 1997. (Illus.). 64p. pap. text 29.95 (*92-832-0128-0*) OUP.

Male Homosexual Behavior & the Effects of AIDS Education: A Study of Behavior & Safer Sex in New Zealand & South Australia. B. R. Rosser. 1991. LC 91-4626. 264p. 77.00 (*0-275-93809-3*, C3809, Praeger Pubs) Greenwood.

Male Homosexuality: A Contemporary Psychoanalytic Perspective. Richard C. Friedman. 1990. pap. 19.00 (*0-300-04745-2*) Yale U Pr.

Male Impersonators: Men Performing Masculinity. Mark Simpson. 1993. LC 93-36054. (*0-304-32806-5*); pap. (*0-304-32808-1*) Cassell GBR. *Dist:* Sterling.

Male in Crisis. Karl Bednarik. Tr. by Helen Sebba from GER. 1981. LC 81-7122. 194p. reprint ed. lib. bdg. 45.50 (*0-313-22713-6*, BEMS, Greenwood Pr) Greenwood.

Male in Farm Animal Reproduction. Ed. by M. Courot. 1984. (Current Topics in Veterinary Medicine & Animal Science Ser.). text 247.50 (*0-89838-682-9*) Kluwer Academic.

Male Infertility. Ed. by T. B. Hargreave. (Clinical Practice in Urology Ser.). 1983. (Illus.). 326p. 94.00 (*0-387-12055-6*); 2nd ed. 1997. LC 97-39625. (Illus.). 466p. pap. 76.00 (*3-540-76216-7*); 2nd ed. 1994. LC 94-10499. (Illus.). 466p. 197.00 (*0-387-19840-7*); 2nd ed. 1994. LC 94-10499. (*3-540-19840-7*) Spr-Verlag.

Male Infertility: A Guide for the Clinician. Anne M. Jequier. 2000. LC 99-16293. (Illus.). viii, 375p. 177.95 (*0-632-05129-9*) Blackwell Sci.

Male Infertility: Clinical Investigation, Cause Evaluation & Treatment. Comhaire. 1996. (Illus.). 408p. 188.95 (*0-412-57250-8*, Chap & Hall NY) Chapman & Hall.

Male Infertility: Men Talking. Mary-Claire Mason. 1993. LC 93-11986. 224p. (C). text 69.95 (*0-415-07289-1*, B2423) Routledge.

Male Infertility & Sexual Dysfunction. Ed. by Wayne J. Hellstrom. 1997. LC 96-3247. (Illus.). 624p. 175.00 (*0-387-94859-7*) Spr-Verlag.

Male Infertility from A to Z: A Concise Encyclopedia. J. M. Hollanders et al. 1996. LC 96-23150. (Studies in Profertility: Vol. 4). 198p. lib. bdg. 71.95 (*1-85070-758-8*, M2922, Parthenon Pbng) CRC Pr.

Male Matters: Masculinity, Anxiety & the Male Body on the Line. Calvin Thomas. 1996. LC 95-17447. 264p. 17.95 (*0-252-06500-X*) U of Ill Pr.

Male-Mediated Developmental Toxicity. Ed. by D. R. Mattison & A. F. Olshan. 1994. (Reproductive Biology Ser.). (Illus.). 418p. (C). text 125.00 (*0-306-44815-7*, Kluwer Plenum) Kluwer Academic.

Male Menopause. Jed Diamond. 1997. LC 97-26509. 384p. text 22.95 (*1-57071-143-7*) Sourcebks.

Male-Midwife & the Female Doctor. Charles E. Rosenberg & Carroll-Smith Rosenberg. 1979. LC 73-20642. (Sex, Marriage & Society Ser.). (Illus.). 224p. reprint ed. 28.95 (*0-405-05810-1*) Ayer.

Male Ordered Health Care: The Inequities of Women. Shirlee Pasau-Buck & Edward M. Jones. 1994. LC 94-65426. 184p. pap. 9.95 (*0-9627246-2-9*) Power NY.

Male Rape: A Casebook of Sexual Aggressions. Ed. by Anthony M. Scacco, Jr. 1982. LC 81-667777. (Studies in Modern Society: Political & Social Issues: No. 15). (Illus.). 352p. 32.50 (*0-404-61621-6*); pap. 12.95 (*0-404-61622-4*) AMS Pr.

Male Reproductive Function. Christina Wang. 1999. LC 99-24999. (Endocrine Updates Ser.). (*0-7923-8520-9*) Kluwer Academic.

Male Reproductive Function & Semen. T. Mann & C. Lutwak-Mann. 1981. (Illus.). 498p. 142.00 (*0-387-10383-X*) Spr-Verlag.

Male Sexual Disorders. Justine Vale & Anthony V. Hirsh. 2001. (Illus.). 208p. pap. 59.95 (*0-632-05347-X*) Blackwell Sci.

Male Sexual Dysfunction. Ed. by Robert J. Krane et al. 1998. (Illus.). 352p. (*0-443-07848-3*) Church.

Male Sexual Dysfunction. Robert J. Krane & Michael B. Siroky. 1983. 86.95 (*0-316-50331-2*) Little.

Male Sexual Function: A Guide to Clinical Management. Ed. by John J. Mulcahy. 2001. LC 00-67292. (Current Clinical Urology Ser.). 397p. 125.00 (*0-89603-917-X*) Humana.

Male Sterility & Motility Disorders: Etiological Factors & Treatment. Ed. by Samir Hamamah et al. 1999. (Serono Symposia Ser.). (Illus.). 338p. 140.00 (*0-387-98673-1*) Spr-Verlag.

Male Stress Syndrome: How to Survive Stress in the '90s. Georgia Witkin. 2nd ed. 1994. LC 94-27468. 240p. 23.00 (*1-55704-206-3*) Newmarket.

Male Survivor: The Impact of Sexual Abuse. Matthew P. Mendel. 1994. 264p. 64.95 (*0-8039-5441-7*, 3683); pap. 32.95 (*0-8039-5442-5*, 3684) Sage.

Males with Eating Disorders. Ed. by Arnold E. Andersen. 1990. LC 89-23909. (Eating Disorders Monographs: No. 4). (Illus.). 274p. text 39.95 (*0-87630-556-7*) Brunner-Routledge.

Malformations. Ed. by Harold L. Klawans et al. rev. ed. 1987. 670p. 323.00 (*0-444-90461-1*) Elsevier.

Malformations of the External Genitalia. Ed. by M. Westenfelder. 1981. (Monographs in Pediatrics: Vol. 12). (Illus.). xiii, 112p. pap. 55.75 (*3-8055-1509-X*) S Karger.

Malformed Fetus & Stillbirth: A Diagnostic Approach. Robin M. Winter et al. 1988. 324p. 720.00 (*0-471-90946-7*) Wiley.

Malformed Infant & Child: An Illustrated Guide. Richard M. Goodman & Robert J. Gorlin. 1983. (Illus.). 464p. (C). pap. text 52.50 (*0-19-503255-1*) OUP.

Malic Acid & Magnesium for Fibromyalgia & Chronic Pain Syndrome. Billie Jay Sahley & Katherine M. Birkner. 7th rev. ed. 1999. (Illus.). 36p. pap. (*1-889391-15-8*) Pain & Stress.

Malignancies of the Genitourinary Tract. Ed. by A. Ackermann & V. Diehl. 1993. LC 92-49944. (*3-540-54433-X*) Spr-Verlag.

Malignancy & Chronic Inflammation in the Gastrointestinal Tract: New Concepts: Proceedings of the 81st Falk Symposium, Held in Berlin, Germany, November 3-5, 1994. Ed. by E. O. Riecken et al. 1995. LC 95-35759. text 73.50 (*0-7923-8889-5*) Kluwer Academic.

Malignant Bone Tumors. Allan W. Yasko. 2000. (ACS Atlas of Clinical Oncology Ser.). 448p. incl. cd-rom (*1-55009-136-0*) DEKR.

Malignant Brain Tumors. Ed. by David G. Thomas & David I. Graham. 1995. (Illus.). 377p. 180.00 (*3-540-19689-7*); 1994. 175.00 (*0-387-19689-7*) Spr-Verlag.

Malignant Catarrhal Fever in Asian Livestock. Ed. by P. W. Daniels & Purnomo Ronohardjo. 1988. 127p. (Orig.). pap. 100.50 (*0-949511-71-4*) St Mut.

Malignant Diseases of Infancy, Childhood & Adolescence. Arnold Altman & Allen D. Schwartz. 2nd ed. 1983. (Major Problems in Clinical Pediatrics Ser.: Vol. 18). text 160.00 (*0-7216-1211-3*) Saunders.

Malignant Hyperthermia. Ed. by Beverly A. Britt. 1987. (C). text 147.50 (*0-89838-960-7*) Kluwer Academic.

Malignant Hyperthermia: Current Concepts. Ed. by Nalda Felipe et al. 1989. (Illus.). 220p. (C). 32.00 (*0-926592-00-9*) Normed Verlag.

Malignant Hyperthermia: Proceedings of the 3rd International Symposium on Malignant Hyperthermia, 1994. Ed. by M. Morio et al. 1996. (Illus.). 272p. 175.00 (*4-431-70171-0*) Spr-Verlag.

Malignant Hyperthermia Membrane-Linked Diseases, Vol. III. S. Tsuyoshi Ohnishi. 1993. 352p. 170.00 (*0-8493-8093-6*, RD82) CRC Pr.

Malignant Liver Tumors: Current & Emerging Therapies. Pierre-Alain Clavien & Kim Lyerly. 1999. LC 98-49184. (Illus.). 168.95 (*0-632-04406-3*) Blackwell Sci.

***Malignant Liver Tumors: Current & Emerging Therapies.** Pierre Clavien et al. 2nd ed. 2002. (Illus.). (C). text 160.00 (*0-7637-1857-2*, 1857-2) Jones & Bartlett.

Malignant Lymphoma. Hancock. 2nd ed. 1999. (Illus.). 352p. pap. 128.95 (*0-412-61070-1*, Chap & Hall NY) Chapman & Hall.

Malignant Lymphoma: Biology, Natural History & Treatments. Alan C. Aisenberg. 1991. LC 90-13686. (Illus.). 395p. text 54.50 (*0-8121-1382-9*) Lppncott W & W.

Malignant Lymphoma: Diagnosis, Biology & Treatment. Wendy N. Erber. 1991. text 117.00 (*3-7186-5058-4*, Harwood Acad Pubs) Gordon & Breach.

Malignant Lymphomas: Biology & Treatment, Vol. VIII. Ed. by Gerassimos A. Pangalis. 1995. LC 95-33049. (ESO Monographs). (Illus.). 189p. 147.00 (*3-540-60122-8*) Spr-Verlag.

Malignant Lymphomas & Hodgkin's Disease: Experimental & Therapeutic Advances. Ed. by F. Cavalli et al. 1986. (Developments in Oncology Ser.). text 253.50 (*0-89838-727-2*) Kluwer Academic.

Malignant Lymphomas, Including Hodgkin's Disease: Diagnosis, Management, & Special Problems, No. 66. Ed. by Bruce W. Dana. 1993. LC 93-127. (Cancer Treatment & Research Ser.). 192p. (C). text 175.50 (*0-7923-2171-5*) Kluwer Academic.

Malignant Lymphoproliferative Diseases. Ed. by J. G. Van der Tweel et al. 1980. (Boerhaave Series for Postgraduate Medical Education: No. 17). (Illus.). 520p. text 226.00 (*90-6021-451-X*) Kluwer Academic.

Malignant Melanoma. Ed. by Rona M. MacKie. 1983. (Pigment Cell Ser.: Vol. 6). (Illus.). viii, 204p. 121.00 (*3-8055-3690-9*) S Karger.

Malignant Melanoma: Biology, Diagnosis, & Therapy. Ed. by Larry Nathanson. 1988. (Cancer Treatment & Research Ser.). (C). text 150.00 (*0-89838-384-6*) Kluwer Academic.

Malignant Mesothelioma. Ed. by Douglas W. Henderson. 1991. 390p. 120.00 (*0-89116-977-6*) Hemisp Pub.

Malignant Neoplasms in Childhood & Adolescence. Ed. by H. Riehm. 1986. (Monographs in Pediatrics: Vol. 18). (Illus.). viii, 396p. 130.50 (*3-8055-4206-2*) S Karger.

Malignant Sadness: The Anatomy of Depression. Lewis Wolpert. 2000. LC 99-45815. 208p. 24.00 (*0-684-87058-4*) Free Pr.

Malignant Skin Tumours. Anthony J. Emmett. Ed. by Michael G. O'Rourke. 2nd ed. 1991. (Illus.). 425p. text (*0-443-04089-3*) Church.

Malignant Tumors of the Ear, Nose, & Throat. V. S. Pogosov & V. F. Antoniv. 1984. (Illus.). 600p. 70.00 (*0-8236-3082-X*) Intl Univs Pr.

Malignant Tumors of the Skin. Ed. by A. C. Chu & R. L. Edelson. 1999. LC 00-500748. (Illus.). 464p. 175.00 (*0-340-74086-8*) OUP.

Malignant Tumors of the Thyroid: Clinical Concepts & Controversies. Ed. by R. H. Cobin & D. K. Sirota. 1992. (Illus.). 218p. 185.00 (*0-387-97570-5*) Spr-Verlag.

Malignant Tumours of the Mouth, Jaw & Salivary Glands. Ed. by J. D. Langdon & J. M. Henk. 2nd ed. 1995. 288p. (*0-340-55794-X*) E A GBR. *Dist:* OUP.

Malingering & Deception in Adolescents: Assessing Credibility in Clinical & Forensic Settings. Joseph T. McCann. 1997. LC 97-37671. 243p. 34.95 (*1-55798-460-3*, 431-7990) Am Psychol.

Malin's Clinical Diabetes. Malcolm Nattrass. 2nd ed. 1996. (Illus.). 430p. (*0-412-30860-6*) E A GBR. *Dist:* OUP.

Malnutrition in the Elderly. Ed. by O. Seiler & H. B. Staehelin. 1999. 140p. (C). (*3-7985-1166-7*) D Steinkopff DEU. *Dist:* Spr-Verlag.

Malnutrition in the Elderly: A National Crisis: A Focus on the Problems, Causes, Consequences, & Solutions. Kathy Cope. 1998. (Illus.). 77p. pap. text 20.00 (*0-7881-4814-1*) DIANE Pub.

Malpractice: A Guide for Mental Health Professionals. Ronald J. Cohen. 1979. LC 78-72147. 22.95 (*0-02-905790-6*) Free Pr.

Malpractice: A Trial Lawyer's Advice for Physicians. Walter G. Alton, Jr. 1977. 21.50 (*0-316-03500-9*, Little Brwn Med Div) Lppncott W & W.

Malpractice: What They Don't Teach You in Dental School. Jeffrey J. Tonner. 1995. LC 95-39879. 69.95 (*0-87814-460-9*) PennWell Corp.

Malpractice & Contact Lenses. Harvey M. Rosenwasser. 2nd ed. 1991. (Illus.). 136p. text 49.99 (*0-7506-9192-1*) Buttrwrth-Heinemann.

Malpractice & Contact Lenses: A Guide to Limiting Liability in Contact Lens Practice. Harvey M. Rosenwasser. 1988. 96p. (Orig.). (C). pap. 15.00 (*0-9620349-0-8*) Gillman-Marcuse.

Malpractice Epidemic: A Layman's Guide to Medical Malpractice. Bernard L. Remakus. Ed. by Cara O'Donnell. 1990. LC 89-17582. 22.95 (*0-87949-295-3*) Ashley Bks.

Malpractice in Health Occupations: Index of New Information. Gerald D. MacFarland. 1994. 150p. 57.50 (*0-7883-0050-4*); pap. 47.50 (*0-7883-0051-2*) ABBE Pubs Assn.

Malpractice Issues in Radiology. Leonard Berlin et al. 1998. LC 98-6639. (Illus.). 154p. (*1-890705-00-4*) Am Roentgen.

Malpractice Liability in the Helping & Healing Professions: A Survey Guide for Attorneys & Clients. Warren Freedman. 1995. LC 94-40461. 280p. 72.95 (*0-89930-908-9*, Quorum Bks) Greenwood.

Malpractice Prevention & Liability Control for Hospitals. James E. Orlikoff & William R. Fifer. 1981. LC 85-4063. vii, 146p. 24.75 (*0-939450-62-3*) AHPI.

Malpractice Suit: A Survival Guide for Physicians & their Families. Ed. by Graham Chedd et al. 1989. 123p. 295.00 incl. VHS (*0-9624044-0-3*) Eidetics.

Malthey, Robert Dedication. Ed. by Martine Jotterand-Bellomo & H. P. Klinger. 1982. (Cytogenetics & Cell Genetics Ser.: Vol. 34, Nos. 1-2). (Illus.). vi, 192p. pap. 139.25 (*3-8055-3650-X*) S Karger.

Maltreated Child: The Maltreatment Syndrome in Children; a Medical, Legal & Social Guide. Vincent J. Fontana & Douglas J. Besharov. 5th ed. 1995. LC 95-30664. (Illus.). 174p. pap. 33.95 (*0-398-06548-9*); text 42.95 (*0-398-06547-0*) C C Thomas.

Maltreatment & the School-Age Child: Developmental Outcomes & System Issues. Phyllis T. Howing et al. 1993. 177p. pap. 8.95 (*1-56024-292-2*) Haworth Pr.

Maltreatment in Early Childhood: Tools for Research-Based Intervention. Ed. by Kathleen Coulborn Faller. 2000. LC 99-87450. (Illus.). xii, 258p. 49.95 (*0-7890-0784-3*, Maltreatment & Trauma Pr); pap. text 24.95 (*0-7890-0819-X*) Haworth Pr.

Mama Can't Remember Anymore: Care Management of Aging Parents & Loved Ones. Nancy Wexler. 2nd rev. ed. 1997. pap. text 14.95 (*0-9629358-2-4*) Wein & Wein.

Mama Might Be Better off Dead: The Failure of Health Care in Urban America. Laurie K. Abraham. 1994. xii, 302p. pap. 13.00 (*0-226-00139-3*); 1993. LC 93-15514. 304p. 25.00 (*0-226-00138-5*) U Ch Pr.

Mama Sana, Bebe Sano: Una Guia en Espanol e ingles Sobre el Embarazo la Atencion Prenatal, el Nacimiento y el Cuidado. Aliza A. Lifshitz. 1999. LC 99-94862. (ENG & SPA., Illus.). pap. 15.00 (*0-380-79245-1*, Avon Bks) Morrow Avon.

Mammalian Behavior: The Theory & the Science. John P. Smith. 1990. LC 90-80105. 420p. pap. text 29.50 (*0-9627194-0-4*) Bench Mark Bks.

Mammalian Cell As a Microorganism: Genetic & Biochemical Studies in Vitro. Theodore T. Puck. 1972. LC 73-188127. 219p. (C). 28.95 (*0-8162-6980-7*); pap. text 26.95 (*0-8162-6970-X*) Holden-Day.

Mammalian Cell-Derived Recombinant Human Growth Hormone: Pharmacology, Metabolism & Clinical Results. Ed. by N. Stahnke & M. Zachmann. 1992. (Journal: Vol. 37, Suppl. 2, 1992). (Illus.). iv, 56p. pap. 26.25 (*3-8055-5743-4*) S Karger.

Mammalian Cell Transformation by Chemical Carcinogens. Nawin C. Mishra & Myron A. Mehlman. 1981. LC 82-51185. (Advances in Modern Environmental Toxicology Ser.: Vol. 1). (Illus.). 504p. pap. text 58.00 (*0-911131-01-9*) Specialist Journals.

Mammalian Cells: Probes & Problems, Proceedings. Ed. by C. R. Richmond et al. 1975. LC 75-600009. (ERDA Symposium Ser.). 324p. fiche 6.50 (*0-87079-267-9*, CONF-731007) DOE.

Mammalian Cytochromes P-450, Vol. 1. F. Peter Guengerich. 1987. LC 86-17640. 126.00 (*0-8493-6674-7*, CRC Reprint) Franklin.

Mammalian Neuroendocrinology. Paul V. Malven. 1993. 272p. (C). 89.95 (*0-8493-8757-4*, QP356) CRC Pr.

Mammalian Radiations: An Analysis of Trends in Evolution, Adaption & Behavior. John F. Eisenberg. LC 80-27940. (Illus.). 1983. 610p. pap. text 25.00 (*0-226-19538-4*); 1982. 620p. lib. bdg. 72.00 (*0-226-19537-6*) U Ch Pr.

Mammalian Sex Chromosomes & Sex-Determining Genes. Ed. by Ken C. Reed & Jennifer A. Graves. 1993. LC 92-1483. xviii, 410p. text 131.00 (*3-7186-5276-5*) Gordon & Breach.

Mammalian Tumor Cell Heterogeneity. Ed. by John T. Leith & Daniel L. Dexter. 1986. 160p. 94.00 (*0-8493-6162-1*, RC267, CRC Reprint) Franklin.

Mammalogy. Terry A. Vaughan. 3rd ed. 1986. LC 77-2111. 576p. (C). text 91.00 (*0-03-058474-4*) SCP.

Mammals of Kentucky. Roger W. Barbour & Wayne H. Davis. 1974. LC 74-7870. (Kentucky Nature Studies: Vol. 5). (Illus.). 368p. 29.00 (*0-8131-1314-8*) U Pr of KY.

Mammals of the Canyon Country. David M. Armstrong. 1982. (Illus.). 263p. (Orig.). (C). pap. 3.95 (*0-937407-01-1*) Canyonlands.

Mammary Development & Cancer. Ed. by S. Rudland et al. 1997. LC 98-110810. (Biochemical Society Symposium Ser.: Vol. 63). (Illus.). 319p. (C). text (*1-85578-087-9*) Portland Pr Ltd GBR. *Dist:* Ashgate Pub Co.

Mammary Gland: Development, Regulation & Function. M. C. Neville & C. W. Daniel. 1987. LC 87-18606. (Illus.). 648p. (C). text 135.00 (*0-306-42641-2*, Kluwer Plenum) Kluwer Academic.

Mammary Tumor Cell Cycle, Differentiation, & Metastasis: Advances in Cellular & Molecular Biology of Breast Cancer. Ed. by Robert B. Dickson & Marc E. Lippman. 1996. LC 96-4654. 448p. text 345.00 (*0-7923-3905-3*) Kluwer Academic.

Mammary Tumorigenesis & Malignant Progression: Advances in Cellular & Molecular Biology of Breast Cancer. Ed. by Robert B. Dickson & Marc E. Lippman. 1994. LC 93-40375. (Cancer Treatment & Research Ser.: Vol. 71). 384p. (C). text 290.00 (*0-7923-2647-4*) Kluwer Academic.

Mammographic Appearances. A. Willemin. 1973. (Illus.). 126.25 (*3-8055-1584-7*) S Karger.

Mammographic Imaging: A Practical Guide. Valerie F. Andolina et al. 2nd ed. 2001. LC 00-51463. (Illus.). xvii, 498p. text 63.00 (*0-7817-1696-9*) Lppncott W & W.

Mammographic Interpretation: A Practical Approach. Marc J. Homer. 2nd ed. 1996. LC 96-43895. (Illus.). 376p. text 99.00 (*0-07-029720-7*) McGraw-Hill Prof.

Mammography. P. Haehnel & C. Kleitz. 1988. (Illus.). 121p. 38.95 (*0-387-15328-4*) Spr-Verlag.

Mammography. Heinlein. 2000. text 59.00 (*0-323-00407-5*) Mosby Inc.

Mammography. Luz A. Venta. 1999. 400p. pap. text 80.00 (*0-7817-1663-2*) Lppncott W & W.

Mammography: Self-Assessment & Review. Linda Lefave. 1993. LC 93-3913. (Pretest Specialty Level Ser.). (Illus.). 100p. pap. 25.00 (*0-07-052017-8*) McGraw-Hill Prof.

Mammography: The Requisites. Rubin. 2000. (Illus.). 384p. (C). (gr. 13). text 79.00 (*0-8151-7481-0*, 27477) Mosby Inc.

Mammography Exam Review. Philipot. 1992. 224p. pap. text 29.95 (*0-397-55019-7*) Lppncott W & W.

Mammography for Radiologic Technologists. Gini Wentz & Ward C. Parsons. 2nd ed. 1996. (Illus.). 192p. pap. 49.95 (*0-07-105845-1*) McGraw-Hill Prof.

Mammography of the Breast: Index of New Information. Lizabeth L. Holtzer. 1995. LC 95-16306. 57.50 (*0-7883-0703-7*); pap. 47.50 (*0-7883-0704-5*) ABBE Pubs Assn.

Mammography Quality Control: The Why & How Book. Calvin P. Myers. 1997. (Illus.). 41p. pap. text 19.95 (*0-944838-83-9*) Med Physics Pub.

Man Against Aging. Robert S. Ropp. Ed. by Robert J. Kastenbaum. 1979. LC 78-22216. (Aging & Old Age Ser.). reprint ed. lib. bdg. 30.95 (*0-405-11829-5*) Ayer.

Man & Biologically Active Substances: Introduction to the Pharmacology of Health. I. I. Brekhman. 2nd ed. 1980. 90p. (*0-08-023169-1*) Pergamon Repr GBR. *Dist:* Franklin.

Man & Mu: The Cradle of Becoming & Unbecoming: Desiderata for Human Science. Stacey B. Day. 1998. LC 97-72905. (Illus.). 200p. (Orig.). (C). lib. bdg. 39.50 (*0-934314-00-4*) Intl Found Biosocial Dev.

Man & Nature in the Renaissance. Allen G. Debus. 1978. LC 77-91085. (Cambridge History of Science Ser.). (Illus.). 180p. pap. text 18.95 (*0-521-29328-6*) Cambridge U Pr.

Man & Wolf. Ed. by H. Frank. 1987. (Perspectives in Vertebrate Science Ser.). lib. bdg. 333.00 (*90-6193-614-4*) Kluwer Academic.

Man & Woman, War & Peace: The Strategist's Companion. Anthony Wilden. 1987. 328p. 27.50 (*0-7100-9867-7*, 98677, Routledge Thoemms) Routledge.

Man As the Measure: The Crossroads. Ed. by Daniel Adelson. 1972. LC 77-184153. (Community Psychology Ser.: Vol. 1). 146p. 35.95 (*0-87705-058-9*, Kluwer Acad Hman Sci) Kluwer Academic.

Man Behind the Syndrome. Peter H. Beighton & G. J. Beighton. 1991. (Illus.). 259p. reprint ed. 64.95 (*0-387-16218-6*) Spr-Verlag.

Man de Diagnos. Friedman. 1995. (SPA.). (*84-458-0091-4*) Ediciones Cientificas ESP. *Dist:* P H Brookes.

Man Enough: Fathers, Sons & the Search for Masculinity. Frank S. Pittman, III. 1994. LC 94-11093. 336p. (Orig.). pap. 14.95 (*0-399-51883-5*, Perigee Bks) Berkley Pub.

Man in the Yellow Hat: Theology & Psychoanalysis in Child Therapy. Dorothy Martyn. 1992. (American Academy of Religion Academy Ser.). (C). 197p. 24.95 (*1-55540-630-0*, 010176); 187p. pap. text 15.95 (*1-55540-631-9*) OUP.

Man in Transition . . . His Role As Father, Son, Friend & Lover. Kenneth Byers. 1990. 216p. (gr. 9 up). pap. 9.95 (*0-9619040-3-8*) Journeys Together.

Man-Made Medicine: Women's Health, Public Policy & Reform. Ed. by Kary L. Moss. 1996. LC 96-21855. 304p. text 49.95 (*0-8223-1811-3*); pap. text 15.95 (*0-8223-1816-4*) Duke.

Man, Medicine & Microbe: The Science of AIDS & Long-Term Survival. Neal A. Dickerson. 1993. LC 93-23191. (Politics of AIDS Ser.: Vol. 6). (Illus.). xii, 179p. pap. 15.00 (*0-930383-39-7*) Monument Pr.

Man Meets Microbes. Jamison. 2nd ed. 1984. (*0-409-10721-2*) Buttrwrth-Heinemann.

Man Program: Self-Help Counseling for Child Molesters. Jerry M. Goffman. 1986. LC 86-73818. 60p. pap. text 12.95 (*0-9612754-2-1*) Batterers Anon.

Man to Man: Surviving Prostate Cancer. Michael Korda. 1997. 272p. pap. 13.00 (*0-679-78123-4*) Vin Bks.

Man under Stress. Ed. by A.T. Welford. 1974. LC 74-5440. (Illus.). 144p. 36.00 (*0-85066-073-4*) Taylor & Francis.

Man Who Cures Cancer. William K. Eidem. 1996. 304p. 26.95 (*0-9651968-0-1*) Am Educ Systs.

Man Who Got Lost in Duty Free & Other Video-Illustrated Case Studies for Examinations. Andrew Levy. 1999. LC 99-24400. (Video Casebook Ser.: Vol. II). (Illus.). ix, 158p. pap. 38.95 incl. cd-rom (*0-632-05382-8*) Blackwell Sci.

***Man Who Lost Himself: The Terry Evanshen Story.** June Callwood. 2001. 320p. pap. 19.95 (*0-7710-1864-9*) McCland & Stewart.

Man Who Mistook His Wife for a Hat: And Other Clinical Tales. Oliver W. Sacks. 1998. LC 98-4723. (Illus.). 256p. pap. 14.00 (*0-684-85394-9*, Touchstone) S&S Trade Pap.

Man with a Shattered World: The History of a Brain Wound. Aleksandr R. Luria. 1987. LC 86-31866. 168p. pap. 14.95 (*0-674-54625-3*) HUP.

Man with the Miraculous Hands. Joseph Kessel. Tr. by Helen Weaver & Leo Raditsa. 1977. LC 70-160922. (Biography Index Reprint Ser.). reprint ed. 19.95 (*0-8369-8085-9*) Ayer.

Man Woman Book: How We Are. J. Bruce Evans. 1988. LC 89-42867. (Illus.). 112p. 9.95 (*0-937552-26-7*, QRP Bks) Quail Ridge.

Manage Your Fears, Manage Your Anger: A Psychiatrist Speaks. Abraham A. Low. 1995. LC 95-60989. 472p. 20.00 (*0-915005-05-0*) Willett Pub Co.

Managed Behavioral Health Care: An Industry Perspective. Sharon A. Shueman et al. 1994. LC 93-34578. (Illus.). 290p. (C). text 63.95 (*0-398-05897-0*) C C Thomas.

Managed Behavioral Health Market Share in the United States, 1998-1999. Monica E. Oss & John H. Clary. 5th rev. ed. 1998. (Illus.). 50p. spiral bd. 65.00 (*1-878586-15-7*, DR-1) Open Minds PA.

Managed Behavioral Health Services: An Annotated Bibliography: 1989-1994. Ed. by Jane Kramer & Saul Feldman. 1999. 76p. reprint ed. pap. text 20.00 (*0-7881-7651-X*) DIANE Pub.

Managed Behavioral Healthcare: History, Models, Strategic Challenges, & Future Course. Tom Trabin & Michael Freeman. 1995. (Managed Behavioral Healthcare Library). 35p. pap. 35.00 (*1-887452-01-X*) CentraLink.

Managed Behavioral Healthcare: Provider Training & Development. American Board of Certified Managed Care Providers. Ed. by Alex D'Alessandro. 1992. LC 92-48824. pap. 95.00 (*0-935255-77-X*) Of Course Pubns.

Managed Behavioral Healthcare Handbook. Ed. by E. Clarke Ross. 2001. LC 2001-21808. (Illus.). 350p. 76.00 (*0-8342-1727-9*) Aspen Pub.

Managed Behavioral Healthcare Manual. Margaret D. Bischel. 1997. 275p. ring bd. 225.00 (*1-893826-02-3*) Apollo Managed.

Managed Care. Ed. by Mark A. Hall & William S. Brewbaker, III. 1995. LC 96-75044. (Health Care Corporate Law Ser.: Vol. 4). 741p. ring bd. 209.00 (*0-316-34038-3*, 40383) Aspen Law.

Managed Care: A Nursing Perspective. Anita W. Finkelman. 2000. LC 00-34020. 528p. pap. 47.00 (*0-8053-8152-X*) P-H.

Managed Care: A Sourcebook for Occupational Therapy. Ed. by AOTA Staff. 1996. LC 96-227563. 160p. (Orig.). pap. text 35.00 (*1-56900-046-8*, 1161) Am Occup Therapy.

Managed Care: An Agency Guide to Surviving & Thriving. David Emenhiser et al. 1995. pap. text 9.95 (*0-87868-597-9*) Child Welfare.

Managed Care: Anatomy of a Mass Medical Movement. Richard D. Smith. 2000. (Illus.). 425p. pap. text 40.00 (*1-55605-294-4*) Wyndham Hall.

Managed Care: Financial, Legal & Ethical Issues. Ed. by David A. Bennahum. 1999. LC 98-50328. (Pilgrim Library of Ethics). xii, 247p. pap. 23.95 (*0-8298-1274-1*) Pilgrim OH.

Managed Care: Good But Not Perfect. 2000. (*0-8013-3032-7*) Addison-Wesley.

Managed Care: Integrating the Delivery & Financing of Health Care, Pt. A. Ed. by HIAA Staff. 1995. LC 97-125731. 251p. pap. 30.00 (*1-879143-26-7*) Health Ins Assn Am.

Managed Care: Integrating the Delivery & Financing of Health Care, Pt. B. Ed. by Jane Stein. 1996. 226p. pap. text 30.00 (*1-879143-29-1*) Health Ins Assn Am.

Managed Care: Integrating the Delivery & Financing of Health Care Study Manual. HIAA Staff. 64p. Pt. A. 1995. pap. 10.00 (*1-879143-27-5*); Pt. B. 1996. pap. 10.00 (*1-879143-30-5*) Health Ins Assn Am.

Managed Care: Made in America. Arnold Birenbaum. 1997. LC 97-5578. 208p. 45.00 (*0-275-95916-3*, Praeger Pubs) Greenwood.

Managed Care: Practice & Progress. Robert Royce. 1997. LC 96-29999. 248p. pap. (*1-85775-280-5*) Radcliffe Med Pr GBR. *Dist:* Balogh.

Managed Care: Practice Strategies for Nursing. Margaret M. Conger. 1999. LC 98-40281. 290p. 72.95 (*0-7619-0964-8*, 81171) Sage.

Managed Care: Practice Strategies for Nursing. Margret M. Conger. 1999. LC 98-40281. pap. 34.95 (*0-7619-0965-6*, 81172) Sage.

Managed Care: State Regulation. Aspen Health Law and Compliance Center Staff. 1998. LC 98-11538. (Current Issue Ser.). 160p. pap. 46.00 (*0-8342-1120-3*, 11203) Aspen Pub.

Managed Care: Strategies, Networks & Management. Montague Brown. 1993. (HCMR Ser.). 272p. pap. 55.00 (*0-8342-0504-1*, 20504) Aspen Pub.

Managed Care: What It Is & How It Works. Wendy Knight. 1998. LC 98-35906. 160p. pap. 39.00 (*0-8342-1089-4*, 10894) Aspen Pub.

Managed Care Pt. C: Integrating the Delivery & Financing of Health Care. Andrew Alcorn et al. Ed. by Julie Hopkins. 1998. (HIAA Insurance Education Ser.). (Illus.). 233p. pap. text 30.00 (*1-879143-46-1*) Health Ins Assn Am.

Managed Care Pt. C: Integrating the Delivery & Financing of Health Care Study Manual. Health Insurance Association of America Staff. 1998. (HIAA Insurance Education Ser.). 76p. pap., stu. ed. 10.00 (*1-879143-47-X*) Health Ins Assn Am.

Managed Care Acquisition Report, 1999. Irving Levin Associates, Inc. Staff. 1999. (Illus.). v, 180p. per. 495.00 (*1-930625-07-3*) I Levin.

Managed Care & Capitation: Issues in Nursing. Teri Britt et al. 1998. LC 98-3607. 30p. pap. 15.95 (*1-55810-141-1*) Am Nurses Pub.

Managed Care & Capitation Contracting for Home Health Agencies. Ino. 1996. LC 96-7927. ring bd. 129.00 (*0-8342-0614-5*) Aspen Pub.

Managed Care & Changing Health Care Markets. Michael Morrisey. 1998. LC 97-43998. 39.95 (*0-8447-4038-1*); 250p. pap. 16.95 (*0-8447-4039-X*) Am Enterprise.

Managed Care & Children with Special Health Care Needs. American Academy of Pediatrics Staff. 1997. 197p. pap. 29.95 (*0-910761-80-9*) Am Acad Pediat.

Managed Care & Chronic Illness: Challenges & Opportunities. Peter D. Fox & Teresa Fama. 1996. 368p. 75.00 (*0-8342-0844-X*, 20844) Aspen Pub.

Managed Care & Developmental Disabilities: Reconciling the Realities of Managed Care with the Individual Needs of Persons with Disabilities. Dale Mitchell. 2000. LC 99-62954. 200p. pap. 19.95 (*1-892696-07-X*) High Tide Pr.

Managed Care & Medical Cost Containment in Workers' Compensation: A National Inventory, 1995-1996. Stacey M. Eccleston. 1995. LC 95-39458. 320p. (Orig.). pap. 250.00 (*0-935149-54-6*, WC-95-4) Workers Comp Res Inst.

Managed Care & Public Health. Paul K. Halverson et al. 1995. LC 97-26357. 496p. 68.00 (*0-8342-0897-0*, 20897) Aspen Pub.

Managed Care & the Cardiac Patient. Ed. by Richard Ott et al. 1995. LC 94-40714. (Illus.). 334p. 54.00 (*1-56053-122-3*) Hanley & Belfus.

Managed Care & the Evaluation & Adoption of Emerging Medical Technologies. Steven Garber et al. 2000. (C). pap. 8.00 (*0-8330-2849-9*, MR-1195/1) Rand Corp.

Managed Care & the Evaluation & Adoption of Emerging Medical Technologies. Steven Garber et al. 2000. LC 00-267383. xviii, 70p. pap. 12.00 (*0-8330-2831-6*, MR-1195-NIMA) Rand Corp.

Managed Care & the Law: Liability & Risk Management. Charles G. Benda & Fay Rozovsky. 506p. ring bd. 145.00 (*0-316-17408-4*, 74084) Aspen Law.

Managed Care & You: The Consumer Guide to Managing Your Health Care. Michael E. Cafferky. 2nd ed. 1995. (Illus.). 224p. (Orig.). pap. 14.95 (*0-07-600759-6*, ME104) Practice Mgmt Info.

Managed Care & You: The Consumer Guide to Managing Your Healthcare. Michael E. Cafferky. 3rd rev. ed. 1997. LC 98-113154. 234p. pap. 12.95 (*1-885987-04-8*, ME083, Health Info Pr) Practice Mgmt Info.

Managed Care Answer Book: Forms & Checklists. annuals Sheryl T. Dacso & Clifford C. Dacso. Date not set. 400p. pap. 96.00 incl. disk (*1-56706-407-8*, 64078) Panel Pubs.

Managed Care Blues & How to Cure Them. Walter A. Zelman & Robert A. Berenson. 1998. LC 98-16018. 192p. 45.00 (*0-87840-679-4*); (Illus.). pap. 17.95 (*0-87840-680-8*) Georgetown U Pr.

Managed Care Challenge for Nurse Executives. American Organization of Nurse Executives Staff. 1996. LC 96-24117. (AONE Leadership Ser.). (Illus.). 110p. pap. 43.00 (*1-55648-164-0*, 154154) AHPI.

Managed Care Concepts. D. Cole & F. Vogenberg. 1996. (Orig.). pap. text 49.46 (*1-56870-226-4*) RonJon Pub.

Managed Care Contracting: A Guide for Health Care Professionals. Wendy Knight. 1997. LC 97-12838. 288p. 75.00 (*0-8342-0883-0*, 20883) Aspen Pub.

Managed Care Contracting: A Practical Guide for Health Care Executives. Thomas M. Reardon. 1998. LC 98-43360. 115p. 46.95 (*0-7879-4581-1*) Jossey-Bass.

Managed Care Contracting: Advising the Managed Care Organization. Maureen E. Corcoran. 1996. (Health Law & Business Ser.: No. 1700). 125.00 (*1-55871-332-8*) BNA.

Managed Care Contracting: Advising the Provider. Gary S. Davis. 1996. (Health Law & Business Ser.: No. 1800). 125.00 (*1-55871-333-6*) BNA.

Managed Care Contracting: Concepts & Applications for the Health Care Executive. Douglas Conrad et al. 1996. LC 96-3242. (Management Ser.). 146p. 20.00 (*1-56793-042-5*, 0979) Health Admin Pr.

Managed Care Contracting Handbook: Planning & Negotiating the Managed Care Relationship. Maria Todd. 1996. LC 96-23786. 240p. per. 65.00 (*0-7863-0999-7*, Irwn McGrw-H) McGrw-H Hghr Educ.

Managed Care Contracting Manual. 1997. 335.00 (*0-937925-68-3*, MCC) Capitol VA.

Managed Care Contracts Manual. Robert W. McAdams, Jr. et al. 1996. LC 95-47265. 492p. ring bd. 299.00 (*0-8342-0813-X*) Aspen Pub.

Managed Care Coordinator. Jack Rudman. (Career Examination Ser.: C-3686). pap. 34.95 (*0-8373-3686-4*) Nat Learn.

Managed Care Course: The Easy Way to Learn What You Can't Afford Not to Know. Alice Jane Lippner. 1997. (Illus.). 304p. pap. 65.00 (*0-9662096-0-5*) Infobriefings.

Managed Care Desk Reference, 1996-1997. Sarah E. Hutchinson & Glen Coulthard. 2nd ed. 1996. text 79.00 (*0-07-413105-2*, Irwn McGrw-H) McGrw-H Hghr Educ.

Managed Care Desk Reference, 1994: The Complete Guide to Terminology & Resources. Marianne F. Fazen. 1994. LC 94-172104. 352p. (Orig.). pap. 65.00 (*0-9639835-0-4*) HCS Pubns.

Managed Care Desk Reference, 1996-1997: The Complete Guide to Terminology & Resources. Marianne F. Fazen. Ed. by Jay Lechtman. 2nd rev. ed. Date not set. 200p. (C). 79.00 (*1-56329-322-6*) Ingenix Inc.

Managed Care Essentials: A Book of Readings. Health Administration Press Staff. 1999. LC 99-43249. ix, 319p. pap. 42.00 (*1-56793-112-X*) Health Admin Pr.

Managed Care Ethics: Essays on the Impact of Managed Care on Traditional Medical Ethics. John LaPuma. 1998. LC 97-41350. (Hatherleigh Guides to Mental Health Ser.). 224p. pap. 39.95 (*1-57826-012-4*) Hatherleigh.

Managed Care Facts, Trends & Data, 1999-2000. Ed. by Phoebe Eliopoulos. 4th rev. ed. 1999. 305p. pap. 275.00 (*0-929156-65-X*) Atlantic Info Services Inc.

MNO

Managed Care 1500, 1996-97 Edition: A Complete Guide to the Most Influential Managed Care Leaders & Organizations. Ed. by Richard Sorian. 1996. 200p. (Orig.). pap. 195.00 (*1-881393-65-8*) Faulkner & Gray.

Managed Care Handbook: How to Prepare Your Medical Practice for the Managed Care Revolution. James R. Lyle & Hoyt W. Torras. Ed. by Kathryn Swanson & Maureen Lynch. 2nd ed. 1996. LC 96-21217. 428p. (Orig.). pap. 49.95 (*1-57066-055-7*, ME074) Practice Mgmt Info.

Managed Care in a Time of Transition Proceedings. 1998. pap. 35.00 (*0-938959-56-5*) Soc Actuaries.

Managed Care in Dentistry. Bryan Quattlebaum. 1994. LC 94-23729. 44.95 (*0-87814-432-3*) PennWell Corp.

Managed Care in Medicaid: Lessons for Policy & Program Design. Robert E. Hurley et al. 1993. LC 92-48437. 215p. pap. text 20.00 (*0-910701-95-4*, 0930) Health Admin Pr.

Managed Care in the Inner City: The Uncertain Promise for Providers, Plans & Communities. Dennis P. Andrulis. 1999. LC 98-56051. (Illus.). 191p. 45.00 (*0-7879-4623-0*) Jossey-Bass.

Managed Care Law Manual. Aspen Health Law Center Staff. Ed. by Cynthia Conner. 1996. LC 93-44768. ring bd. 279.00 (*0-8342-0523-8*) Aspen Pub.

Managed Care Law Manual. Aspen Health Law Center Staff et al. 1994. ring bd. 345.00 (*0-8342-0541-6*) Aspen Pub.

Managed Care Legal Issues: A Practical Guide for Health Care Decision-Makers. Bruce A. Johnson & Gerald A. Niederman. 1996. LC 97-185721. 260p. (Orig.). pap. 25.00 (*1-56829-076-4*, 4906) M G M A.

Managed Care Liability: Examining Risks & Responsibilities in a Changing Health Care System. Ed. by David L. Leitner. 1997. LC 96-80429. 488p. pap. 74.95 (*1-57073-393-7*) Amer Bar Assn.

Managed Care Made Easy: Survival in the HMO Era. Vikram Khanna. 1997. LC 97-28567. 256p. pap. text 14.95 (*1-882606-26-4*) Peoples Med Soc.

Managed Care Made Simple. Robert A. Baldor. 1995. LC 95-9515. pap. 21.95 (*0-86542-474-8*); 2nd ed. 1998. LC 97-43321. (Illus.). 148p. pap. 26.95 (*0-632-04378-4*) Blackwell Sci.

Managed Care Manual. Scott Becker. 1998. LC 99-182082. 416p. pap. text 39.95 (*0-323-00077-0*) Mosby Inc.

Managed Care Manual. Evelyn Eskin et al. Ed. by David B. Wash. 1996. (Illus.). xii, 252p. (Orig.). spiral bd. 54.95 (*1-890045-00-4*) T L C Med Pub.

Managed Care Manual: Medicaid & State Health Reform. Larry S. Gage & William H. Von Oehsen. 1995. LC 95-214970. (Health Law Ser.). (*0-87632-294-1*) West Group.

Managed Care Manual: Medicaid, Medicare & State Health Reform. Larry S. Gage & William H. Von Oehsen. 1996. LC 97-169042. (Health Law Ser.). (*0-8366-1071-7*) West Group.

Managed Care Monograph. National Hospice Organization, Commercial Reimburs. 1993. 37p. 10.50 (*0-931207-21-5*) Natl Hospice.

Managed Care Operational Strategies: A Medical Office Survival Guide. Thomas Prince & Edward Mayberry. 1997. LC 97-204049. 500p. (C). 169.00 (*1-56329-404-4*) Ingenix Inc.

Managed Care, Outcomes, & Quality: A Practical Guide. Steven Isenberg. 1997. LC 97-17252. (Illus.). 352p. pap. 59.00 (*0-86577-687-3*) Thieme Med Pubs.

Managed Care Pharmacy: Principles & Practice. Ed. by Albert I. Wertheimer & Robert Navarro. 1999. LC 98-33388. (Illus.). 412p. pap. text 49.95 (*0-7890-0639-1*) Haworth Pr.

Managed Care Pharmacy Practice. Ed. by Robert P. Navarro. 1999. LC 99-29131. 656p. 55.00 (*0-8342-1205-6*) Aspen Pub.

Managed Care Plan for Medical Assistance, General Assistance Medical Care & Minnesota Care: A Report to the Minnesota Legislature. 1994. (Illus.). 95p. (Orig.). (C). pap. text 35.00 (*0-7881-0621-X*) DIANE Pub.

Managed Care Primer, Monograph 1. 1993. (Cardiovascular Specialist's Guide to Managed Care Ser.). (Illus.). 78p. (Orig.). pap. text (*1-882764-02-1*) Am Coll Cardiology.

Managed Care Provider's Toolbox. Margaret D. Bischel. 1998. (Illus.). 415p. ring bd. (*1-893826-04-X*) Apollo Managed.

Managed Care Quality: A Practical Guide. Al Assaf et al. 1997. LC 97-35083. 296p. 59.95 (*1-57444-073-X*) St Lucie Pr.

Managed Care Referral: Development & Management Strategies - How to Develop a Systematic Plan for Building Your Referral Business in Today's Healthcare Environment. John F. O'Malley. 1996. LC 96-3675. 288p. text 45.00 (*0-7863-0878-8*, Irwn Prfssnl) McGraw-Hill Educ Grp.

Managed Care Register. Contrib. by Russell Perkins. 1999. 700p. pap. 45.00 (*1-880874-56-3*) Dorland Hlthcare.

Managed Care Strategies: A Physician Practice Desk Reference. George B. Moseley, III. 1999. LC 98-32278. 609p. 87.00 (*0-8342-0735-4*, 07354) Aspen Pub.

Managed Care Strategies: A Strategy Guide for Healthcare Organizations. Jeff Rogers. 1996. (Illus.). 186p. wbk. ed. 49.00 (*0-923680-08-X*, 4203) Amer ComVision Inc.

Managed Care Success: Reducing Risk While Increasing Patient Satisfaction. James W. Saxton & Thomas L. Leaman. 1998. LC 98-9985. 320p. 62.00 (*0-8342-1023-1*, 10231) Aspen Pub.

Managed Care Survival Manual: The Rehabilitation Therapist's Guide to Capitation & Per-Case Payment. Brian Rasmussen. 1996. 122p. pap. 84.00 (*1-887759-02-6*, P-118) Am Phys Therapy Assn.

Managed Care Systems & Emerging Infections: Challenges & Opportunities for Strengthening Surveillance. Institute of Medicine Staff. 2000. LC 99-69869. (Illus.). 128p. pap. 25.00 (*0-309-06828-2*) Natl Acad Pr.

Managed Community Long-Term Care in Texas: Planning for the 21st Century. Jacqueline L. Angel. 1997. LC 97-73906. (Policy Research Project Report Ser.: Vol. 122). 163p. pap. 16.00 (*0-89940-732-3*) LBJ Sch Pub Aff.

Managed Competition: A Health Care System for Pennsylvania. 1993. 120p. (Orig.). (C). pap. text 35.00 (*0-7881-0026-2*) DIANE Pub.

Managed Competition & Its Potential to Reduce Health Spending. 1993. (Illus.). 43p. (C). pap. text 25.00 (*1-56806-421-7*) DIANE Pub.

Managed Competition & Its Potential to Reduce Health Spending. 1995. lib. bdg. 250.95 (*0-8490-7588-2*) Gordon Pr.

Managed Competition & Pharmaceutical Care: A Challenge for the Profession. Ed. by Dev S. Pathak & Alan Escovitz. LC 96-10194. (Journal of Research in Pharmaceutical Economics: Vol. 7, Nos. 1/2). 169p. (C). 1997. pap. 19.95 (*0-7890-0211-6*); 1996. 49.95 (*1-56024-821-1*) Haworth Pr (Pharmctl Prods).

Managed Dental Care: A Guide to Dental HMOs. Donald S. Mayes. Ed. by Mary Brennan. 1993. LC 93-78068. 248p. pap. 15.00 (*0-89154-464-X*) Intl Found Employ.

Managed Health Care: A Teaching Syllabus. Compiled by SFTM Task Force on Managed Health Care Staff. 1990. 112p. 12.00 (*0-942295-19-6*, 57) Soc Tchrs Fam Med.

Managed Health Care: Effect on Employers' Costs Difficult to Measure. 1994. (Illus.). 43p. (Orig.). (C). pap. text 25.00 (*0-7881-0706-2*) DIANE Pub.

Managed Health Care - Problems & Promises: Summary from 21st NCSL's Annual Meeting, July 1995. 1995. 12p. 15.00 (*1-55516-398-X*, 7302-2012) Natl Conf State Legis.

Managed Health Care Dictionary. Richard Rognehaugh. 2nd ed. 1998. LC 98-3103. 288p. pap. 22.00 (*0-8342-1144-0*, 11440) Aspen Pub.

Managed Health Care Guide for Caseworkers & Foster Parents. Ellen S. Battistelli. 1997. LC 97-19976. pap. 9.95 (*0-87868-682-7*, CWLA Pr) Child Welfare.

Managed Health Care Handbook. Peter R. Kongstvedt. 3rd ed. 2000. LC 96-13500. 1752p. 110.00 (*0-8342-0733-8*, 20733) Aspen Pub.

Managed Health Care Handbook. Peter R. Kongstvedt. 3rd ed. 1997. 115.50 (*0-7616-1753-1*) Morgan Kaufmann.

Managed Health Care Handbook. Peter R. Kongstvedt. 4th ed. 2000. LC 00-35580. xxxi, 1408p. 135.00 (*0-8342-1726-0*, 17260) Aspen Pub.

Managed Health Care in the Lab: Reengineering, Leadership & Best Value. Paul Bozzo. 1998. LC 98-21036. 224p. text 75.00 (*0-397-58773-2*) Lppncott W & W.

Managed Health Care Simplified: A Glossary of Terms. Austrin. 1999. 212p. (C). pap. text 17.95 (*0-7668-2050-5*) Delmar.

Managed Health Care Simplified: A Glossary of Terms. Michael S. Austrin. 1999. LC 99-56122. (Illus.). v, 212p. (*0-7668-2078-5*) Delmar.

Managed Healthcare Fellowship Leading Integration Forward: What Is Pharmacy's Role? 1996. 24p. (Orig.). pap. (*1-884033-13-X*) Bimark.

Managed Healthcare U. S. Evidence: U. S. Evidence & Lessons for the National Health Service. Robinson. 1997. LC 97-13906. (State of Health Ser.). 206p. (*0-335-19949-6*); pap. (*0-335-19948-8*) OpUniv Pr.

Managed Heart: Commercialization of Human Feeling. Arlie Russell Hochschild. 1983. LC 83-1399. 307p. (C). pap. text 18.95 (*0-520-05454-7*) U CA Pr.

Managed Home Healthcare: A Guide to Integrating Home Care Services into Managed Care. Carol Schaffer. 1999. 140p. pap. 93.00 (*0-929156-61-7*) Atlantic Info Services Inc.

Managed Medicare & Medicaid Factbook 2001. 5th rev. ed. 2001. 380p. spiral bd. 319.00 (*1-931467-01-3*) Atlantic Info Services Inc.

Managed Mental Health Care: A Guide for Practitioners, Employers, & Hospital Administrators. Thomas R. Giles. 1993. LC 92-49082. (Practitioner Guidebook Ser.). 192p. (C). 55.00 (*0-205-14838-7*, Longwood Div) Allyn.

Managed Mental Health Care: Major Diagnostic & Treatment Approaches Handbook for Providers. Ed. by S. Richard Sauber. 1997. LC 97-1084. (Mental Health Practice under Managed Care Ser.: No. 8). 352p. pap. 37.95 (*0-87630-812-4*) Brunner-Routledge.

Managed Mental Health Care: The Bradman Approach. Leo H. Bradman. 1992. 177p. pap. (*1-883945-01-1*) UniPsych Pr.

Managed Mental Health Care in the Public Sector: A Survival Manual, Vol. 4. Ed. by Kenneth Minkoff & David Pollack. 1997. LC 98-168725. 410p. pap. text 35.00 (*90-5702-537-X*, Harwood Acad Pubs) Gordon & Breach.

Managed Mental Health Services. Saul Feldman. 1992. (Illus.). 326p. (C). text 57.95 (*0-398-05759-1*) C C Thomas.

Managed Mental Healthcare Video Resource Manual. 1991. 86p. stu. ed. 30.00 (*1-883066-03-4*); VHS 195.00 (*1-883066-02-6*) Natl Comm Mental.

Managed Physical/Occupational Therapy & Rehabilitation Care Manual. Margaret D. Bischel. 1996. (Illus.). 275p. ring bd. 225.00 (*1-893826-01-5*) Apollo Managed.

Managed Service Restructuring in Health Care: A Strategic Approach in a Competitive Environment. Robert L. Goldman & Sanjib K. Mukherjee. 1995. LC 93-43876. 105p. lib. bdg. 39.95 (*1-56024-896-3*) Haworth Pr.

Managed Vision Benefits. Jesse Rosenthal & Mort Soroka. Ed. by Mary Jo Brzezinski. 2nd ed. 1998. LC 98-70020. 198p. pap. 40.00 (*0-89154-524-7*) Intl Found Employ.

Management Accounting for Healthcare Organizations. Bruce R. Neumann & Keith E. Boles. 5th rev. ed. 1998. LC 97-75989. 745p. 65.00 (*0-944496-60-1*) Teach-em.

Management & Administration of Radiation Safety Programs: 1998 Health Physics Society Summer School. Ed. by Charles E. Roessler. 1998. LC 98-66489. (Illus.). 603p. pap. text 40.95 (*0-944838-01-4*) Med Physics Pub.

Management & Biology of Carcinoma in Situ & Cancer of the Testis. Ed. by N. E. Skakkebaek et al. 1993. (Journal: Vol. 23, No. 1, 1993). (Illus.). iv, 256p. reprint ed. 78.50 (*3-8055-5768-X*) S Karger.

Management & Health of Farmed Deer. Ed. by H. W. Reid. 1988. (Current Topics in Veterinary Medicine & Animal Science Ser.). (C). text 137.50 (*0-89838-408-7*) Kluwer Academic.

Management & Leadership for Nurse Managers. Russell C. Swansburg. 1990. 576p. pap. 41.25 (*0-86720-439-7*) Jones & Bartlett.

Management & Leadership for Nurse Managers. Russell C. Swansburg. 2nd ed. 1996. LC 95-46565. (Nursing Ser.). (Illus.). 704p. (C). pap. text 50.95 (*0-86720-734-5*, 734-5) Jones & Bartlett.

Management & Leadership in Nursing. Warren F. Stevens. 1978. (Illus.). text 27.00 (*0-07-061260-9*) McGraw.

Management & Practice of Low Visual Acuity. Albert Dowie. 1989. (C). (*0-900099-24-0*) Assn Brit Dispen Opticians GBR. *Dist:* St Mut.

Management & Practices for the Health Professional. M. Cronin. 1994. 176p. (C). spiral bd. (*0-933195-64-8*) CA College Health Sci.

Management & Prevention of Diarrhea: Practical Guidelines. Ed. by World Health Organization Staff. 3rd ed. 1993. (CHI, ENG, FRE & SPA.). v, 50p. pap. text 12.00 (*92-4-154454-6*, 1153230) World Health.

Management & Prognosis of Severe Traumatic Brain Injury. Brain Trauma Foundation Staff. Ed. by Brain Trauma Foundation Staff. 2000. (Illus.). 286p. 175.00 (*0-9703144-0-X*) Brain Trauma.

Management & Supervision of Jail Inmates with Mental Disorders. Martin Drapkin & William C. Collins. 1999. 300p. ring bd. 133.50 (*1-887554-08-4*) Civic Res Inst.

Management & Therapy of Sickle Cell Disease. 1990. lib. bdg. 250.00 (*0-87700-885-X*) Revisionist Pr.

Management & Therapy of Sickle Cell Disease. Ed. by Clarice D. Reid et al. 3rd rev. ed. 1997. (Illus.). 114p. pap. text 40.00 (*0-7881-3853-7*) DIANE Pub.

Management & Treatment of Benign Cutaneous Vascular Lesions. Oon T. Tan. 1992. (Illus.). 225p. text 98.50 (*0-8121-1489-2*) Lppncott W & W.

Management by Objectives in Mental Health Services. Vernon R. Wiehe. 1974. 8.95 (*0-912164-10-7*) Masterco Pr.

Management Decision Making for Nurses: 101 Case Studies. Bessie L. Marquis & Carol J. Huston. 1987. (Illus.). 393p. text 26.95 (*0-397-54663-7*, Lippncott) Lppncott W & W.

Management Development in Maternal & Child Health & Family Planning Programme: Proceedings of an Intercountry Workshop. 1988. (SEARO Technical Publications Ser.: No. 11). 124p. pap. text 6.00 (*92-9022-150-X*) World Health.

Management for Clinicians. White. 1993. 160p. pap. (*0-340-57321-X*) E A GBR. *Dist:* Routldge.

Management for Community Health Practice. Marie L. Friedmann. 1983. LC 82-20188. (Illus.). 288p. (C). pap. text 42.95 (*0-534-01240-X*, 240-X) Jones & Bartlett.

Management for Doctors. Ed. by Jenny Simpson & Richard Smith. 1995. 200p. (Orig.). (C). pap. text (*0-7279-0858-8*) BMJ Pub GBR. *Dist:* AIDC.

Management for Health Professionals. N. Wheeler. 2000. (Illus.). 224p. pap. (*0-7487-4038-4*) Nelson Thornes GBR. *Dist:* Intl Spec Bk, Trans-Atl Phila.

Management for Hospital Doctors. Maurice Burrows et al. 1994. LC 93-37792. 336p. text 85.00 (*0-7506-0880-3*) Buttrwrth-Heinemann.

Management for Nurses & Health Care Professionals. Ed. by J. E. Clark & L. Copcutt. 1996. (Illus.). 242p. pap. (*0-443-05091-0*) Church.

Management for Opticians. Ray Dennis et al. 2nd ed. 1998. LC 98-27915. 295p. pap. text 49.99 (*0-7506-9756-3*) Buttrwrth-Heinemann.

Management for Results: A "How to" Workbook for Improving the Management of Your Veterinary Practice. Michael H. Riegger. 1992. 200p. pap. 59.95 (*0-929870-06-9*) Advanstar Commns.

Management for the Eyecare Practitioner. Irving Bennett. 1992. LC 92-49731. (Illus.). 220p. text 89.99 (*0-7506-9319-3*) Buttrwrth-Heinemann.

Management Guidelines for Adult Nurse Practitioners. Lynne M. Hektor Dunphy. 1998. LC 98-11268. (Illus.). 568p. pap. 38.95 (*0-8036-0229-4*) Davis Co.

Management Guidelines for Family Nurse Practitioners Working in Family Practice. Alice F. Running & Amy Berndt. 2002. (Illus.). 640p. pap. 38.95 (*0-8036-0810-1*) Davis Co.

Management Guidelines for Gerontologic Nurse Practitioners. Laurie Kennedy-Malone et al. 1999. LC 99-15302. (Illus.). 601p. (C). pap. text 38.95 (*0-8036-0297-9*) Davis Co.

Management Guidelines for Pediatric Nurse Practitioners. Nancy L. Hill & Linda Sullivan. 1999. LC 98-5907. (Illus.). 536p. pap. 38.95 (*0-8036-0230-8*) Davis Co.

Management Guidelines for the Treatment of Renal Anemia: Journal: American Journal of Nephrology, Vol. 10, Supplement 2, 1990. Ed. by Marsha Wolfson & W. M. Bennett. 1990. (Illus.). iv, 54p. pap. 18.50 (*3-8055-5276-9*) S Karger.

Management Guidelines for Women's Health Nurse Practitioners. Kathleen Brown. 1999. LC 99-26449. (Illus.). 437p. (C). pap. text 38.95 (*0-8036-0292-8*) Davis Co.

Management in Geratal Practice: Health Care for Older People. Ed. by Steve Gliffe et al. 1998. 177p. pap. text (*0-7279-1192-9*) BMJ Pub GBR. *Dist:* AIDC.

Management in Health Care Systems. J. H. Brown. 1984. 152p. 91.00 (*0-8493-5572-9*, RA393, CRC Reprint) Franklin.

Management in Neuro-Oncology. Ed. by J. G. Hildebrand. 1993. LC 92-49588. (*3-540-56095-5*); (Illus.). 116p. 111.00 (*0-387-56095-5*) Spr-Verlag.

Management in Nursing. Ed. by Marjorie Cuthbert et al. 1992. (Illus.). 327p. text (*0-7295-0380-1*) Bailliere Tindall.

Management in Nursing: An Experiential Approach That Makes Theory Work for You. Elaine L. La Monica. 1990. LC 90-9455. 464p. 51.95 (*0-8261-6580-X*) Springer Pub.

Management in Physical Therapy: An Integrated Science. Frank J. M. Walter. 1993. (Illus.). 304p. (C). (gr. 13). text 53.00 (*0-8016-6416-0*, 06416) Mosby Inc.

Management in Rehabilitation: A Case Study Approach. Charles P. Schuch & Darlene K. Sekerak. 1995. (Illus.). 143p. (C). pap. text 18.95 (*0-8036-7758-8*) Davis Co.

Management of Abdominal Hernias. Keith J. Devlin. 2nd ed. 1999. 344p. (*0-412-73820-1*) E A GBR. *Dist:* OUP.

Management of Acute & Chronic Pain. Ed. by Narinder Rawal et al. 1998. 231p. pap. text (*0-7279-1193-7*) BMJ Pub GBR. *Dist:* AIDC.

Management of Acute Coronary Syndromes. Christopher P. Cannon. 1998. LC 98-31266. (Contemporary Cardiology Ser.: Vol. 1). (Illus.). 680p. 135.00 (*0-89603-552-2*) Humana.

Management of Acute Myocardial Infarction. Ed. by Desmond Julian & Eugene Braunwald. 1994. (Frontiers in Cardiology Ser.). (Illus.). 433p. text 61.00 (*0-7020-1884-8*) Saunders.

Management of Acute Pain. Gilbert Park et al. 2nd ed. 2000. LC 00-32694. (Illus.). 208p. pap. text 44.95 (*0-19-262467-9*) OUP.

Management of Acute Respiratory Infections in Children: Practical Guidelines for Outpatient Care. 1995. (FRE.). 77p. (C). pap. 15.00 (*92-4-154477-5*, 1150430) World Health.

Management of Adnexal Cysts: Proceedings of the First European Congress of the Raoul Palmer Club of Gynecologic Endoscopy, Clermont-Ferrand, 10-11 September, 1992. Ed. by Maurice A. Bruhat. 1994. LC 93-26992. (Illus.). 264p. 125.00 (*0-632-03794-6*) Blackwell Sci.

Management of Adult Neurogenic Dysphagia. Maggie L. Huckabee et al. 1998. LC 98-27474. (Dysphagia Ser.). (Illus.). 350p. pap. 59.95 (*1-56593-731-7*, 1422) Thomson Learn.

Management of Advanced Prostate Cancer. Malcolm J. Coptcoat. 1996. 64p. pap. 54.95 (*0-86542-929-4*) Blackwell Sci.

Management of Aging: The University of Geneva Experience. Ed. by J. P. Michel & P. R. Hof. 1999. LC 99-32982. (Interdisciplinary Topics in Gerontology Ser.: Vol. 30). (Illus.). x, 267p. 172.25 (*3-8055-6860-6*) S Karger.

Management of Allergy in the 1990s. Ed. by M. A. Kaliner. 1989. LC 88-35245. (Illus.). 90p. (C). text 16.00 (*0-920887-53-8*) Hogrefe & Huber Pubs.

Management of Alzheimer's Disease. Ed. by Gordon K. Wilcock. 1993. LC 93-3404. 256p. (*1-871816-20-3*) Wrightson Biomed GBR. *Dist:* Taylor & Francis.

Management of Aneurysmal Subarachnoid Haemorrhage. Ed. by Iver A. Langmoen et al. 1999. LC 99-19266. (Acta Neurochirurgica Ser.: Vol. 72). (Illus.). 100p. 89.00 (*3-211-83256-4*) Spr-Verlag.

M N O

Management of Aneurysmal Subarachnoid Hemorrhage. Damirez Fossett. 1993. (Illus.). 276p. (Orig.). (C). pap. 12.95 (*0-929240-59-6*) EMIS.

Management of Antimicrobials in Infectious Diseases: Impact of Antibiotic Resistance. Ed. by Arch G. Mainous, III & Claire Pomeroy. 2000. LC 00-22071. (Infectious Disease Ser.). (Illus.). xiv, 350p. 99.50 (*0-89603-821-1*) Humana.

Management of Anxiety. Diana Keable. 2nd ed. 1997. LC 97-9852. pap. text (*0-443-06001-0*); 228p. (*0-443-05527-0*) Church.

Management of Aphasia. Ed. by Y. Lebrun & R. Hoops. 1978. (Neurolinguistics Ser.: Vol. 8). 124p. (*90-265-0280-X*) Swets.

Management of Arterial Hypertension: A Practical Guide for the Physician & Allied Health Workers. Alberto Zanchetti et al. 1985. v, 72p. pap. text 9.90 (*92-4-154197-0*, 1150235) World Health.

Management of Asthma During Pregnancy. Ed. by Allan T. Luskin. 1999. (Illus.). 74p. (C). reprint ed. pap. text 20.00 (*0-7881-7683-8*) DIANE Pub.

Management of Autistic Behavior. Richard L. Simpson & Madelyn Regan. l.t. ed. 1986. LC 88-30480. 450p. spiral bd. 41.00 (*0-89079-196-1*, 1481) PRO-ED.

Management of Back Pain. Richard W. Porter. 2nd ed. 1993. (Illus.). 368p. text (*0-443-04630-1*) Church.

Management of Bleeding after Open Heart Surgery. Rephael Mohr & Daniel A. Goor. 1997. LC 97-13740. (Medical Intelligence Unit Ser.). 219p. text 99.00 (*1-57059-056-7*) Landes Bioscience.

Management of Bleeding Disorders in Surgical Practice. C. D. Forbes & Alfred Cuschieri. 1992. (Illus.). 400p. 131.95 (*0-632-03368-1*) Blackwell Sci.

Management of Blood Transfusion Services. Ed. by S. F. Hollan et al. 1990. (CHI, ENG, FRE & SPA.). xii, 229p. pap. text 41.00 (*92-4-154406-6*, 1150345) World Health.

Management of Bloodborne Infections in Sports: A Practical Guide for Sports Health Care Providers & Coaches. Terry A. Zeigler. 1996. LC 96-44257. (Illus.). 96p. pap. text 18.00 (*0-88011-682-X*, BZEI0682) Human Kinetics.

Management of Brain-injured Children. Ed. by Richard E. Appleton & Tony Baldwin. 1998. (Illus.). 270p. pap. text 39.95 (*0-19-262793-7*) OUP.

Management of Breastfeeding, Module 4. Rebecca F. Black et al. 1998. LC 97-25569. (Lactation Specialist Self Study Ser.). (Illus.). 336p. (C). spiral bd. 43.95 (*0-7637-0193-9*, 0193-9) Jones & Bartlett.

Management of Cancer Pain. 1995. lib. bdg. 251.95 (*0-8490-6780-4*) Gordon Pr.

Management of Cancer Pain: Clinical Practice Guidelines. 1995. (Illus.). 257p. (Orig.). (C). pap. text 50.00 (*0-7881-2061-1*) DIANE Pub.

Management of Cancer Pain: Clinical Practice Guidelines. 1997. (Orig.). lib. bdg. 253.99 (*0-8490-8140-8*) Gordon Pr.

Management of Cardiac Arrhythmias. Ed. by Leonard I. Ganz. 2001. (Contemporary Cardiology Ser.). 500p. 125.00 (*0-89603-846-7*) Humana.

Management of Cardiac Arrhythmias - Update, 1990: Journal: Cardiology, Vol. 77, No. 3, 1990. Ed. by L. S. Dreifus. 1990. (Illus.). 124p. pap. 77.50 (*3-8055-5308-0*) S Karger.

Management of Cataract in Primary Health Care Services. 1990. (ENG, FRE & SPA.). vi, 43p. pap. text 13.50 (*92-4-154408-2*, 1150344) World Health.

*__Management of Cervical Metastases.__ Ed. by Jonas T. Johnson & Jack L. Gluckman. 2001. (Illus.). 200p. (*1-901865-85-1*) Isis Med.

Management of Child Health Services. Ed. by Michael Rigby et al. 1997. LC 97-68391. (Illus.). 208p. pap. text (*0-412-59660-1*) E A GBR. *Dist:* OUP.

Management of Childhood Brain Tumors. Ed. by Melvin Deutsch. 1990. (Foundations of Neurological Surgery Ser.). (C). text 303.50 (*0-7923-0669-4*) Kluwer Academic.

Management of Children with Emotional & Behavioural Difficulties. Ed. by Ved P. Varma. 1989. 176p. 49.95 (*0-415-02245-2*, A3876); pap. 16.95 (*0-415-02246-0*, A3880) Routledge.

Management of Chronic Headaches. Edward Blanchard & F. Andraisk. 1992. 216p. (C). pap. text 60.95 (*0-205-14285-0*, H4285) Allyn.

Management of Chronic Headaches: A Psychological Approach. Edward B. Blanchard & Frank Andrasik. 1985. (Psychology Practitioner Guidebooks). 200p. text 32.50 (*0-08-030963-1*); pap. text 16.95 (*0-08-030962-3*) Elsevier (Pergamon Pr).

Management of Chronic Lower Limb Ischemia. Ed. by Joseph Mills. 2000. (An Arnold Publication). 192p. (*0-340-75956-9*) E A GBR. *Dist:* OUP.

Management of Chronic Pain. Andrew Diamond & Stephen Coniam. 2nd ed. 1997. LC 96-30136. (Illus.). 190p. (C). text 59.50 (*0-19-262695-7*) OUP.

*__Management of Chronic Viral Hepatitis.__ Gordon. 2001. (Gastroenterology Ser.). 380p. 150.00 (*0-8247-0582-3*) Dekker.

Management of Clinical Allergy. Russell I. Williams. rev. ed. 1984. LC 83-90909. (Illus.). 198p. pap. text 22.00 (*0-9613013-0-9*) R I Williams.

Management of Common Metabolic Bone Disorders. G. A. Campbell et al. 1994. (Illus.). 180p. (C). text 80.00 (*0-521-43037-2*); pap. text 21.95 (*0-521-43623-0*) Cambridge U Pr.

Management of Common Musculoskeletal Disorders: Physical Therapy Principles & Methods. Darlene Hertling & Randolph M. Kessler. 3rd ed. 1995. LC 95-4483. (Illus.). 816p. spiral bd. 58.00 (*0-397-55150-9*) Lppncott W & W.

Management of Common Problems in Obstetrics & Gynecology. Ed. by Daniel R. Mishell, Jr. & Paul F. Brenner. 3rd ed. 1994. LC 93-28312. (Illus.). 912p. 99.95 (*0-86542-269-9*) Blackwell Sci.

Management of Communication & Language Deficits. Ed. by William H. Burke. 1996. (Professional Series on Traumatic Brain Injury: Vol. 20). 56p. (Orig.). pap. 9.50 (*1-882855-27-2*) HDI Pubs.

Management of Communication Disorders in Multicultural. Cheng et al. 1994. 448p. pap. 39.95 (*0-8016-6818-2*) Mosby Inc.

Management of Complex Cardiovascular Problems: The Consultant's Approach. Ed. by Thach N. Nguyen et al. 1999. LC 99-36190. (Illus.). 272p. pap. 45.00 (*0-87993-441-7*) Futura Pub.

*__Management of Complex Cardiovascular Problems: The Consultant's Approach.__ Ed. by Thach N. Nguyen et al. 2nd ed. 2001. LC 2001-40337. (Illus.). 424p. 54.00 (*0-87993-493-X*) Futura Pub.

Management of Countertransference with Borderline Patients. Glen O. Gabbard & Sallye M. Wilkinson. 1994. LC 93-47462. 254p. text 42.00 (*0-88048-563-9*, 8563) Am Psychiatric.

Management of Cumulative Trauma Disorders. Ed. by Martha J. Sanders. 1997. LC 96-50459. 378p. text 59.99 (*0-7506-9561-7*) Buttrwrth-Heinemann.

Management of Data in Clinical Trials. Eleanor McFadden. 1997. LC 97-1251. (Probability & Statistics Ser.). 232p. 89.95 (*0-471-30316-X*) Wiley.

Management of Depression. Stuart Checkley. 1998. LC 97-6410. (Illus.). 512p. 180.00 (*0-86542-987-1*) Blackwell Sci.

Management of Depressions with Monoamine Precursors. Ed. by Julien Mendlewicz & Herman M. Van Praag. 1983. (Advances in Biological Psychiatry Ser.: Vol. 10). (Illus.). vi, 202p. pap. 108.75 (*3-8055-3645-3*) S Karger.

Management of Diabetes Mellitus. Joia Schwartz & Sherwyn L. Schwartz. 3rd ed. 1993. 318p. pap. 12.95 (*0-929240-60-X*) EMIS.

Management of Diabetes Mellitus: Perspectives of Care Across the Life Span. Debra Haire-Joshu. 2nd ed. 1996. LC 95-26440. (Illus.). 912p. (C). (gr. 13). text 54.95 (*0-8151-4223-4*, 26652) Mosby Inc.

Management of Diabetic Foot Problems. George P. Kozak et al. 2nd ed. 1994. LC 93-37401. (Illus.). 336p. text 79.00 (*0-7216-3284-X*) Saunders.

Management of Diabetic Retinopathy. A. M. Hamilton et al. 1996. 220p. pap. text (*0-7279-0919-3*) BMJ Pub GBR. *Dist:* AIDC.

Management of Diarrhoea & Use of Oral Rehydration Therapy: A Joint WHO-UNICEF Statement. 2nd ed. 1985. 25p. pap. text 2.70 (*92-4-156086-X*, 1150237) World Health.

Management of Difficult Glaucoma. Ed. by Eve J. Higginbotham et al. 1993. LC 93-6951. 472p. 165.00 (*0-86542-257-5*) Blackwell Sci.

Management of Digestive & Liver Disorders in Infants & Children. Ed. by Jean-Paul Buts & Etienne M. Sokal. 1993. LC 92-48383. 688p. 300.00 (*0-444-81456-6*) Elsevier.

Management of Ear, Nose & Throat Disorders in Primary Care Practice. Clarence T. Sasaki et al. 1999. (Current Clinical Practice Ser.). 300p. 74.50 (*0-89603-705-3*) Humana.

Management of Eating Disorders & Obesity. Ed. by David J. Goldstein. 1999. LC 98-53443. (Nutrition & Health Ser.). (Illus.). xvi, 367p. 115.00 (*0-89603-407-0*) Humana.

Management of Ectopic Pregnancy. Richard E. Leach & Steven J. Ory. 1999. LC 99-16453. (Illus.). 202p. 70.95 (*0-632-04469-1*) Blackwell Sci.

Management of Emergencies for the Primary Health Care Physician. Ed. by World Health Organization, Eastern Mediterranean R. 1994. (Illus.). 344p. (gr. 13). pap. 47.95 (*0-412-54800-3*) Chapman & Hall.

Management of End-Stage Heart Disease. Eric Rose. 1998. LC 98-15838. 288p. text 135.00 (*0-316-75697-0*) Lppncott W & W.

Management of Epilepsy. Sudhansu Chokroverty. 1996. LC 96-16864. 414p. pap. text 49.99 (*0-7506-9754-7*) Buttrwrth-Heinemann.

Management of Epilepsy. Rosalind Troupin. (*0-444-00851-9*) Elsevier.

Management of Esophageal Disease. David B. Skinner & Ronald H. Belsey. 1988. (Illus.). 864p. text 225.00 (*0-7216-8337-1*) Saunders.

Management of Esophageal Varices: Journal: Digestive Diseases, Vol. 10, Suppl. 1, 1992. Ed. by C. Scarpignato & Irvin M. Modlin. 1992. (Illus.). iv, 104p. pap. 33.25 (*3-8055-5686-1*) S Karger.

Management of Facial, Head, & Neck Pain. Cooper. 1989. 352p. text 115.00 (*0-7216-2841-9*) Saunders.

Management of Facial Lines & Wrinkles. Andrew Blitzer et al. 1999. LC 99-35334. (Illus.). 360p. text 149.00 (*0-7817-1551-2*) Lppncott W & W.

Management of Gastric Cancer. Ed. by Paul H. Sugarbaker. 1991. (Cancer Treatment & Research Ser.). (C). text 260.50 (*0-7923-1102-7*) Kluwer Academic.

Management of Gastrointestinal Cancer. Ed. by Peter McCulloch & Andrew Kingsnorth. 1996. 416p. (*0-7279-1071-X*) BMJ Pub GBR. *Dist:* AIDC.

Management of Hazardous Waste Policy Guidelines & Code of Practice. M. Suess & J. Huismans. 1983. (WHO Regional Publications, European Ser.: No. 14). 100p. pap. text 16.00 (*92-890-1105-X*) World Health.

Management of Head & Neck Cancer: A Multidisciplinary Approach. Ed. by Rodney R. Million et al. 2nd ed. 1993. LC 93-18326. 944p. (C). text 199.00 (*0-397-51208-2*) Lppncott W & W.

Management of Health Care. Ed. by Rosemary Stewart. 1998. LC 98-12104. (International Library of Management). 368p. text (*1-85521-934-4*) Dartmth Pub GBR. *Dist:* Ashgate Pub Co.

Management of Health Information: Functions & Applications. John Mattingly. 1996. 64p. (C). pap. text, tchr. ed. 15.95 (*0-8273-7892-0*) Delmar.

Management of Health Information: Functions & Applications. Rozella Mattingly. 1996. LC 95-47449. (Allied Health Ser.). (Illus.). 429p. (C). 59.95 (*0-8273-6057-6*) Delmar.

Management of Heart Failure. Jay Cohn & Spencer Kubo. 1990. pap. 12.95 (*0-929240-17-0*) EMIS.

Management of High Quadriplegia. Ed. by Gale Whiteneck et al. 1988. LC 88-71753. (Illus.). 384p. text 99.95 (*0-939957-19-1*) Demos Medical.

Management of High-Risk Pregnancy. John T. Queenan. (Illus.). 3rd ed. 1993. 632p. 89.95 (*0-86542-187-0*); 4th ed. 1999. LC 99-24041. 14p. 104.95 (*0-632-04332-6*) Blackwell Sci.

Management of HIV Infection in Infants & Children. Yogev & Connor. 1991. 639p. 59.00 (*0-8016-5653-2*) Mosby Inc.

Management of HIV Infection in the Hospital. American Hospital Association Staff. 3rd rev. ed. 1988. LC 89-34355. Orig. Title: A Hospitalwide Approach to AIDS. 58p. pap. 15.00 (*0-87258-501-8*, 094642) Am Hospital.

Management of Home Care Services. Stephen Crystal et al. 1987. 192p. 24.95 (*0-8261-5660-6*) Springer Pub.

Management of Human Resources for Health: Report of a WHO Expert Committee, 1987. 1989. (Technical Report Ser.: No. 783). 61p. pap. text 8.00 (*92-4-120783-3*, 1100783) World Health.

Management of Impotence & Infertility. Ed. by E. Douglas Whitehead & Harris M. Nagler. 1994. (Illus.). 432p. text 119.00 (*0-397-51153-1*, Lippnctt) Lppncott W & W.

Management of Infected Arterial Grafts. Ed. by Keith D. Calligaro & Frank J. Veith. 1994. LC 94-7228. (Illus.). 243p. 75.00 (*0-942219-57-0*) Quality Med Pub.

Management of Infectious Complications in Cancer Patients. Ed. by Gary A. Noskin. 1998. LC 98-16254. (Cancer Treatment & Research Ser.). 312p. 295.00 (*0-7923-8150-5*) Kluwer Academic.

Management of Infertility: A Clinician's Manual. Brian M. Cohen. 2nd ed. 1991. 172p. pap. 12.95 (*0-929240-33-2*) EMIS.

Management of Intensive Care. Ed. by D. Reis Miranda et al. 1990. (Developments in Critical Care, Medicine, & Anesthesiology Ser.). (C). text 171.00 (*0-7923-0754-2*) Kluwer Academic.

Management of Intercurrent Illness & Complicated Advanced Disease: Advanced Cancer & Stroke As a Model. Ed. by James E. Cimino & Austin H. Kutscher. 1999. LC 98-71723. 120p. pap. 18.95 (*0-930194-34-9*) Ctr Thanatology.

Management of Intermediate & High Grade Lymphomas. 1995. lib. bdg. 251.99 (*0-8490-7584-X*); 1994. lib. bdg. 250.95 (*0-8490-8528-4*) Gordon Pr.

Management of Labor & Delivery. Robert K. Creasey et al. 1997. LC 96-39912. (Illus.). 593p. 104.95 (*0-86542-416-0*) Blackwell Sci.

Management of Limb Inequality. Ed. by Malcolm B. Menelaus. 1991. (Current Problems in Orthopaedics Ser.). (Illus.). 236p. text (*0-443-04298-5*) Church.

Management of Lipid Disorders: A Basis & Guide for Therapy. Sander J. Robins. 1997. (Illus.). 112p. (Orig.). pap. text (*0-89640-337-8*) Igaku-Shoin.

Management of Lithiasis: The Rational Deploy of Technology. Ed. by J. Talati. 1997. LC 96-32629. (Developments in Nephrology Ser.). 368p. (C). text 180.50 (*0-7923-4198-8*) Kluwer Academic.

Management of Low Back Pain in Primary Care. Richard Bartley & Paul Coffey. 2001. LC 00-60887. (Illus.). 198p. pap. text 34.99 (*0-7506-4787-6*) Buttrwrth-Heinemann.

Management of Low Vision. Silver. Date not set. 256p. pap. text (*0-7506-1468-4*) Buttrwrth-Heinemann.

Management of Lower Extremity Fractures. Verdell Williamson et al. 1998. LC 99-188174. (Illus.). iv, 126p. pap. 65.00 (*1-892665-00-X*) Natl Assn Ortho Nurse.

Management of Major Trauma. Colin E. Robertson & Anthony D. Redmond. 2nd ed. 1994. (Hardbooks in Emergency Medicine Ser.: Vol. 9). (Illus.). 208p. 59.95 (*0-19-262448-2*); 202p. pap. text 27.50 (*0-19-262447-4*) OUP.

Management of Mass Burn Casualties & Fire Disasters. Ed. by M Masellis. 1993. 352p. (C). text 178.50 (*0-7923-8804-6*) Kluwer Academic.

Management of Medical Technology: A Primer for Clinical Engineers. Joseph D. Bronzino & Vernon Roosa. Ed. by Robert J. Austin-LaFrance. 1992. LC 92-21070. (Biomedical Engineering Ser.). 451p. 69.99 (*0-7506-9252-9*) Buttrwrth-Heinemann.

Management of Medical Technology: Theory, Practice & Cases. Eliezer Geisler & Ori Heller. 1998. LC 97-41934. (Management of Medical Technology Ser.). 518p. lib. bdg. 154.00 (*0-7923-8054-1*) Kluwer Academic.

Management of Memory Disorders. Ed. by William H. Burke. 2nd ed. 1995. (Professional Series on Traumatic Brain Injury: Vol. 8). 44p. (Orig.). pap. 9.50 (*1-882855-39-6*) HDI Pubs.

Management of Migraine. Egilius L. Spierings. 1995. 150p. text 49.99 (*0-7506-9623-0*) Buttrwrth-Heinemann.

Management of Motor Disorders of Children with Cerebral Palsy. Ed. by David Scrutton. 1991. (Clinics in Developmental Medicine Ser.: No. 90). (Illus.). 101p. (C). text (*0-521-41210-2*) Mc Keith Pr GBR. *Dist:* Cambridge U Pr.

Management of Motor Speech Disorders in Children & Adults. Kathryn M. Yorkston. 2nd ed. 1999. LC 98-16735. (Illus.). xiii, 618p. 43.00 (*0-89079-784-6*) PRO-ED.

*__Management of Movement Disorders: The Challenge of 24-Hour Symptom Control: EFNS, Copenhagen, October 2000.__ Ed. by K. R. Chaudhuri. 2001. (Illus.). 26p. pap. 25.25 (*3-8055-7339-1*) S Karger.

Management of Multiple Sclerosis: An Interdisiplinary Approach. William Stuart et al. Date not set. 448p. 59.00 (*0-8342-0758-3*) Aspen Pub.

Management of Musculoskeletal Problems in the Haemophilias. Robert B. Duthie et al. 2nd ed. 1994. (Illus.). 298p. text 110.00 (*0-19-262317-6*) OUP.

Management of Neurological Disorders. Ed. by C. M. Wiles. 1995. 180p. pap. text (*0-7279-0903-7*) BMJ Pub GBR. *Dist:* AIDC.

Management of Non-Hodgkin's Lymphomas in Europe. Ed. by S. Monfardini & U. Veronesi. 1990. (ESO Intercity Reports). (Illus.). 92p. 68.95 (*0-387-52297-2*) Spr-Verlag.

Management of Normality: Critical Essays in Health & Welfare. Abram De Swaan. 1990. LC 89-10352. 228p. (C). pap. text 16.95 (*0-415-03200-8*, A4157) Routledge.

Management of Occupational Therapy. Zielfa Maslin. Ed. by Jo Campling. 1990. (Therapy in Practice Ser.). 144p. pap. 23.00 (*0-412-33380-5*, A4814) Chapman & Hall.

Management of Ocular Traumas & Other Emergencies. Mathew MacCumber. 4th ed. 1997. LC 97-26482. 512p. pap. text 75.00 (*0-397-51496-4*) Lppncott W & W.

Management of Office Emergencies. Chris Barton. 1998. LC 98-35485. (Illus.). 398p. pap. 35.00 (*0-07-006303-6*) McGraw-Hill Prof.

Management of Open Fractures. Charles M. Court-Brown et al. 9th ed. 1996. 360p. (*1-85317-114-X*) Martin Dunitz GBR. *Dist:* Mosby Inc.

Management of Oral Cancer. Nicholas D. Stafford & John Waldron. 1990. (Illus.). 224p. text 65.00 (*0-19-261609-9*) OUP.

Management of Orbital & Ocular Tumors. Joseph Mauriello. 1990. 145.00 (*0-938607-19-7*) Field & Wood Inc Medical.

Management of Pain. Michael A. Ashburn & Linda J. Rice. 1997. LC 97-36319. (Illus.). 729p. text (*0-443-07679-0*) Church.

Management of Pain Ed. by John J. Bonica. 2nd ed. 1990. LC 88-8983. (Illus.). 2195p. 295.00 (*0-8121-1122-2*) Lppncott W & W.

Management of Pain & Anxiety in Dental Practice. Raymond A. Dionne & J. C. Phero. 1991. 420p. pap. 94.50 (*0-444-81749-2*) Elsevier.

Management of Pain in the Hand & Wrist. Ed. by Parry C. Wynn. 1991. (Hand & Upper Limb Ser.). (Illus.). 173p. text (*0-443-04109-1*) Church.

Management of Patient Care: Putting Leadership Skills to Work. Thora Kron & Anne Gray. 6th ed. 1987. (Illus.). tchr. ed. (*0-7216-2842-7*); 320p. pap. text 34.00 (*0-7216-2064-7*) Saunders.

Management of Patients at High-Risk for Breast Cancer. Victor G. Vogel. 2000. LC 00-30391. (Illus.). 328p. 101.95 (*0-632-04323-7*) Blackwell Sci.

Management of Patients with Sexually Transmitted Diseases: Report of a WHO Study Group. 1991. (Technical Reports: No. 810). (CHI, ENG, FRE & SPA.). vii, 103p. pap. text 14.00 (*92-4-120810-4*, 1100810) World Health.

Management of Pediatric Fractures. Ed. by Robert M. Letts. 1993. (Illus.). 1296p. text (*0-443-08860-8*) Church.

Management of Pediatric Trauma. Ed. by William L. Buntain. 1995. LC 93-47168. (Illus.). 788p. text 185.00 (*0-7216-4547-X*) Saunders.

Management of Perioperative Complications in Gynecology. Vicki V. Baker & Gunter Deppe. Ed. by Bill Schmitt. 1996. LC 96-15894. (Illus.). 288p. text 78.95 (*0-7216-5881-4*) Saunders.

Management of Personnel in Health Sciences: Index of New Information with Authors & Subjects. Denise J. Randall. 1993. 180p. 47.50 (*1-55914-858-6*); pap. 44.50 (*1-55914-859-4*) ABBE Pubs Assn.

Management of Personnel in Long Term Care. Ed. by Mildred O. Hogstel. 1982. LC 82-20579. (Illus.). 336p. text 29.95 (*0-89303-231-X*) P-H.

Management of Persons Accidentally Contaminated with Radionuclides. 1980. LC 79-91648. (Report Ser.: No. 65). 213p. 50.00 (*0-913392-49-9*) NCRP Pubns.

Management of Persons with Chronic Neurologic Illness. Mark N. Ozer. 2000. LC 99-53895. (Illus.). 400p. pap. text 64.99 (*0-7506-7005-3*) Buttrwrth-Heinemann.

Management of Persons with Spinal Cord Injury. Mark N. Ozer. 1988. LC 88-70004. 128p. (Orig.). pap. 29.95 (*0-939957-10-8*) Demos Medical.

Management of Physical Education & Sport. Charles Augustus Bucher & March L. Krotee. 1992. 466p. 39.95 (*0-8016-7442-5*) Mosby Inc.

Management of Poisonous Snakebite. Thomas G. Glass, Jr. 1989. (Illus.). 210p. pap. text 39.95 (*0-9614759-1-9*) Glass Pub Co.

Management of Postoperative Pain. Margaret E. Dodson. 1988. (Current Topics in Anaesthesia Ser.). 284p. (*0-683-13018-8*) E A GBR. *Dist:* Williams & Wilkins.

Management of Prader-Willi Syndrome. Ed. by Louise R. Greenswag & Randall C. Alexander. 2nd ed. 1995. LC 94-29757. (Illus.). 393p. 88.00 (*0-387-94373-0*) Spr-Verlag.

Management of Prader-Willi Syndrome. Louise R. Greenswag & Randall C. Alexander. 2nd ed. 1995. LC 94-29757. xxi, 393p. (*3-540-94373-0*) Spr-Verlag.

Management of Primary Bone Tumors. 1995. lib. bdg. 259.95 (*0-8490-7583-1*) Gordon Pr.

Management of Prostate Cancer. Ed. by Eric A. Klein. 2000. LC 99-34212. (Current Clinical Urology Ser.). (Illus.). 384p. 125.00 (*0-89603-797-5*) Humana.

Management of Prostate Cancer: A European-American Encounter, International Symposium, Munich, November 1996. Ed. by Claude C. Schulman & E. David Crawford. 1997. (European Urology Ser.: Vol. 32, Suppl. 3, 1997). (Illus.). iv, 90p. pap. 41.00 (*3-8055-6559-3*) S Karger.

Management of Prostate Diseases see Atencion de las Enfermedades Prostaticas

Management of Prostate Diseases. Robert E. Weiss & William R. Fair. 2nd rev. ed. 1997. 141p. per. 21.95 (*1-884735-24-X*) Prof Comms.

Management of Prostatic Cancer. Ed. by D. N. Kirk & J. Edson Pontes. 1994. (Illus.). 350p. pap. 120.00 (*0-412-28310-7*) Chapman & Hall.

Management of Respiratory Tract Infections. John C. Bartlett. 1997. LC 97-13539. 120p. pap. 15.00 (*0-683-30236-1*) Lppncott W & W.

Management of Schistosomiasis. Patricia L. Rosenfield. 1979. (Resources for the Future Ser.). 148p. pap. text 11.00 (*0-8018-2328-5*) Johns Hopkins.

Management of Severe & Complicated Malaria: A Practical Handbook. Herbert M. Gilles. 1991. (ENG, FRE & SPA.). vi, 56p. pap. text 11.00 (*92-4-154436-8*, 1150368) World Health.

Management of Severe & Complicated Malaria: An Interactive Computer Program. 1995. pap. text 78.00 incl. disk (*92-4-156174-2*, 1990004) World Health.

Management of Spinal Cord Injury: Toward a Caring Curriculum: A New Pedagogy for Nursing. Cynthia M. Zejdlik. 2nd ed. 1992. LC 82-23904. (Nursing-Health Science Ser.). (Illus.). 700p. (C). text 127.95 (*0-86720-438-9*, 438-9) Jones & Bartlett.

Management of Spinal Disorders. Ed. by Dishan Singh & Aresh Hashemi-Nejad. 1998. (Stanmore Orthopedic Updates Ser.). 224p. text 68.00 (*90-5702-214-1*, Harwood Acad Pubs) Gordon & Breach.

Management of Strabismus & Amblyopia. John A. Pratt-Johnson & Geraldine Tillson. 1994. LC 93-28854. 69.00 (*0-86577-499-4*) Thieme Med Pubs.

Management of Surgical Emergencies. Shaw Somers & William E. Thomas. 1998. (Illus.). 415p. (C). pap. text (*0-7020-1976-3*) Saunders.

Management of Temporomandibular Disorders. 1997. lib. bdg. 252.99 (*0-8490-8151-3*); lib. bdg. 251.99 (*0-8490-8117-3*) Gordon Pr.

Management of Temporomandibular Disorders: Current Bibliographies in Medicine: January 1990 Through December 1995. Martha H. Glock & James A. Lipton. 1996. 42p. pap. text 25.00 (*0-7881-3344-6*) DIANE Pub.

Management of Temporomandibular Disorders & Occlusion. Jeffrey P. Okeson. 4th ed. 1998. LC 97-35663. (Illus.). 656p. (C). (gr. 13). text 69.00 (*0-8151-6939-6*, 27162) Mosby Inc.

Management of Temporomandibular Disorders & Occlusion. Jeffrey P. Okeson. 4th ed. 1998. (Illus.). 656p. (*84-8174-371-2*) Mosby-Doyma Libros ESP. *Dist:* Mosby Inc.

Management of Temporomandibular Joint Degenerative Diseases: Biologic Basis & Treatment Outcome. B. Stegenga & L. G. De Bont. 1996. LC 96-10280. (Illus.). 248p. 131.00 (*3-7643-5286-8*); 119.00 (*0-8176-5286-8*) Birkhauser.

Management of Terminal Malignant Disease. Ed. by Cicely M. Saunders & Nigel Sykes. 3rd ed. 1993. 320p. pap. (*0-340-56354-0*) E A GBR. *Dist:* OUP.

Management of the Acute Coronary Attack: The J. Frank Pantridge Festschrift. Ed. by John S. Geddes. 1986. 124p. text 66.00 (*0-12-278755-2*) Acad Pr.

Management of the Acutely Ill Neurological Patient. Ed. by James Grotta. 1993. (Illus.). 208p. text (*0-443-08870-5*) Church.

***Management of the Cleft Lip Palate.** A. Watson et al. 2001. 330p. (Orig.). (C). pap. (*1-86156-158-X*) Whurr Pub GBR. *Dist:* Taylor & Francis.

Management of the Frail Elderly by the Health Care Team. John R. Walsh. 1989. 216p. pap. 32.50 (*0-87527-349-1*) Green.

***Management of the HIV-Infected Patient.** Suzanne Crowe et al. 2nd ed. 2001. (Illus.). 512p. (*1-901865-28-2*) Isis Med GBR. *Dist:* Bks Intl VA.

Management of the HIV Patient-LCM. Wofsy. 1999. text 22.95 (*0-8385-6119-5*) Appleton & Lange.

Management of the Hypertensive Patient. Lawrence R. Krakoff. 1994. (Illus.). 325p. text (*0-443-08769-5*) Church.

Management of the Infertile Woman. Helen A. Carcio. 1998. LC 97-42828. (Illus.). 352p. pap. text 42.50 (*0-7817-1044-8*) Lppncott W & W.

Management of the Menopause: The Millennium Review 2000. Ed. by J. Studd. 1999. (Illus.). 344p. lib. bdg. 60.95 (*1-85070-079-6*, Parthenon Pbng) CRC Pr.

Management of the Mentally Disordered Offender in Prisons. Geoffrey N. Conacher. 1996. LC 97-156212. 144p. (*0-7735-1419-8*) McG-Queens Univ Pr CAN. *Dist:* CUP Services.

Management of the Patient with Cancer. Thomas F. Nealon. 3rd ed. 1986. (Illus.). 784p. text 170.00 (*0-7216-1075-7*) Saunders.

Management of the Perimenopausal & Postmenopausal Woman: A Total Wellness Program. Barbara Kass-Annese. 1998. LC 98-26136. 368p. pap. text 42.50 (*0-7817-1654-3*) Lppncott W & W.

Management of the Severely Disturbed Adolescent. William M. Easson. 1996. LC 96-23716. xiii, 353p. 55.00 (*0-8236-3091-9*) Intl Univs Pr.

Management of Trauma. Bessey. Date not set. text (*0-7216-5140-2*) Saunders.

Management of Trauma: Pitfalls & Practices. Ed. by Robert F. Wilson & Alexander J. Walt. 2nd ed. 1996. LC 96-28033. 1,120p. text 169.00 (*0-683-08722-3*) Lppncott W & W.

Management of Upper Limb Hypertonicity. Jodie Copley & Kathy Kuipers. 1999. LC 98-54875. 308p. 45.00 (*0-7616-1529-6*) Commun Skill.

Management of Upper Limb Hypertonicity. Jodie Coply & Kathy Kuipers. 1999. LC 98-54875. (Illus.). 308p. pap. 45.00 (*0-12-784596-8*) Acad Pr.

Management of Visual Impairment in Childhood. Ed. by Alistair Fielder et al. 1994. (Clinics in Developmental Medicine Ser.: No. 128). (Illus.). 213p. (C). text 64.95 (*0-521-45150-7*) Cambridge U Pr.

Management of Vitreo-Retinal Disease: A Surgical Approach. David Wong et al. 1998. LC 98-20113. (Illus.). 256p. pap. 99.00 (*3-540-76082-2*) Spr-Verlag.

Management of Voice Disorders. Members of the Department of Otolaryngology Staff et al. 1994. (Illus.). 256p. (C). pap. 55.00 (*1-56593-311-7*, 0464) Thomson Learn.

Management of Voice Disorders. Morrison. 1998. 288p. pap. 57.95 (*0-7693-0003-0*) Course Tech.

Management of Voice Disorders. Murray D. Morrison et al. 1993. LC 93-32952. (Illus.). 288p. (*0-412-35090-4*) E A GBR. *Dist:* OUP.

Management of Waste from Hospitals & Other Health Care Establishments. 1985. (EURO Reports & Studies: No. 97). 61p. pap. text 6.30 (*92-890-1263-3*, 1330097) World Health.

Management of Wounds & Burns. Jim Wardrope & June Edhouse. 2nd ed. 1999. LC 99-461795. (Oxford Handbooks in Emergency Medicine Ser.). (Illus.). 252p. pap. text 54.50 (*0-19-262999-9*) OUP.

Management on & off the Ward. Michael Walton. 1995. LC 95-1076. pap. 29.95 (*0-632-03447-5*) Blackwell Sci.

Management Options for Carotid Disease. Ed. by A. Ross Naylor & William C. Mackey. 2000. 415p. Price not set. (*0-7020-2432-5*) W B Saunders.

Management Practices for the Health Professional. Beaufort B. Longest, Jr. 1976. 13.95 (*0-87909-485-0*) P-H.

Management Principles for Physical Therapists. Larry Nosse & Deborah Friberg. 1991. (Illus.). 336p. 47.00 (*0-683-06576-9*) Lppncott W & W.

Management Problems in Health Care. Ed. by Gunter U. Fandel. 1988. (Illus.). 310p. 102.00 (*0-387-19243-3*) Spr-Verlag.

Management Procedures. Leslie Lee & Robert Comte. 1975. LC 74-18677. (Allied Health Ser.). pap. 6.35 (*0-672-61397-2*, Bobbs) Macmillan.

***Management Risk in Community Practice.** Andy Alaszewski. 2000. (Illus.). 208p. pap. (*0-7020-2603-4*) W B Saunders GBR. *Dist:* Saunders.

Management Services Organizations: Cases & Analysis. Thomas M. Gorey & American Medical Association Staff. 1997. LC 97-5171. 18.20 (*1-56793-057-3*) Health Admin Pr.

Management Simulations for Mental Health & Human Services Administration. Michael J. Austin. 1995. LC 78-12172. 436p. pap., stu. ed. 24.95 (*0-917724-07-0*) Haworth Pr.

Management Skills for Clinical Supervisor. Connelly. 1998. (Allied Health Ser.). pap. 31.50 (*0-8273-6154-8*) Delmar.

Management Skills for the New Health Care Supervisor. William Umiker. 3rd ed. 1998. LC 98-175781. xxiii, 423p. 58.00 (*0-8342-1091-6*, 10916) Aspen Pub.

Management Strategies for Family Planning Programs. John A. Ross et al. 1989. LC 89-6029. (Illus.). 71p. (Orig.). pap. 10.00 (*0-9620952-1-4*) CUCFP&FH.

Management Strategies for Improving Family Planning Services: The Family Planning Manager Compendium. Ed. by Janice Miller & James A. Wolff. 1996. (Illus.). 431p. spiral bd. 25.00 (*0-913723-37-1*) Mgmt Sci Health.

Management Systems for Safety. Jeremy Stranks. 1994. (Health & Safety in Practice Ser.). 192p. (Orig.). pap. (*0-273-60441-4*) Pitman Pub GBR. *Dist:* Trans-Atl Phila.

Managerial Innovation Change in the Metropolitan Hospital. Dalton E. McFarland. 1979. LC 79-14551. (Praeger Special Studies). 322p. 77.00 (*0-275-90390-7*, C0390, Praeger Pubs) Greenwood.

Managerial Process for National Health Development: Guiding Principles. 1981. text (*92-4-180005-4*) World Health.

Managerial Psychology. Harold J. Leavitt. 4th ed. 1997. LC 77-13852. lib. bdg. 19.00 (*0-226-46974-3*) U Ch Pr.

Managerial Psychology: Managing Behavior in Organizations. Harold J. Leavitt & Homa Bahrami. 5th ed. 1988. LC 87-16820. (Illus.). 364p. 29.95 (*0-226-46973-5*) U Ch Pr.

Managerialism & Nursing: Beyond Oppression & Profession. Michael Traynor. 1999. LC 98-42097. xiv, 192p. 95.00 (*0-415-17895-9*); pap. 31.95 (*0-415-17896-7*) Routledge.

Manager's Guide to Health & Safety at Work. Jeremy Stranks. 3rd ed. 1994. 206p. pap. 67.95 (*0-8464-1370-1*) Beekman Pubs.

Manager's Guide to Occupational Health Services. Robert J. McCunney. 1996. LC 98-179273. viii, 47 p. 27.00 (*1-883595-06-1*) OEM Health.

Managing a Veterinary Practice. Jevring. 1995. pap. text 39.00 (*0-7020-1987-9*) Saunders.

Managing a Veterinary Practice in Canada. Jack Douglas. 1994. 265p. pap. (*0-920513-11-5*) Sau1nders CAN. *Dist:* Saunders.

Managing Acute Symptoms. Town. 1995. (Nursing Education Ser.). pap. 20.95 (*0-8273-5683-8*) Delmar.

Managing Aging & Human Service Agencies. Edward E. Morgan, Jr. & John Hiltner. 1992. LC 91-5227. 168p. 27.95 (*0-8261-7810-3*) Springer Pub.

Managing AIDS: Organizational Responses in Seven European Countries. Ed. by Patrick Kenis & Bernd Marin. 1997. LC 98-149925. (Public Policy & Social Welfare Ser.: Vol. 18). (Illus.). 400p. pap. text (*1-85972-126-5*) Ashgate Pub GBR. *Dist:* Ashgate Pub Co.

Managing Alcoholism: Matching Clients to Treatment. Lars Lindstrom. 1992. (Illus.). 390p. text 69.50 (*0-19-261902-0*) OUP.

Managing & Being Managed: Preparation for Reintegrated Professional Nursing Practice. Teddy L. Langford. rev. ed. 1990. (Illus.). 352p. (C). pap. text 26.95 (*0-9626604-1-8*) Landover Pub.

Managing & Communicating: Your Questions & Answers. Lyn Longridge. 1998. LC 98-15830. (Practice Manager Library). (*1-85775-233-3*) Radcliffe Med Pr GBR. *Dist:* Balogh.

Managing & Coordinating Nursing Care. Janice Rider Ellis & Celia Love Hartley. 3rd ed. 1999. LC 99-41445. 384p. pap. text 31.95 (*0-7817-1757-4*) Lppncott W & W.

***Managing & Leading Innovation Health Care.** John Turnbull & Colin Beacock. 2001. (Illus.). 255p. pap. (*0-7020-2552-6*) W B Saunders GBR. *Dist:* Saunders.

Managing & Preventing Prostate Disorders: The Natural Alternatives. George L. Redmon. 2000. LC 99-45214. (Illus.). xviii, 179p. pap. 12.95 (*0-934252-97-1*) Hohm Pr.

Managing Anxiety: A Training Manual. Helen Kennerley. 2nd ed. 1995. LC 94-31575. (Illus.). 226p. pap. text 38.50 (*0-19-262442-3*) OUP.

Managing Asthma. M. Weinberger. 2nd ed. 2001. (Illus.). 350p. pap. 42.95 (*1-85070-972-6*, Parthenon Pbng) CRC Pr.

Managing Asthma in Primary Care. A. Crockett. 1993. LC 93-24248. (Illus.). 96p. pap. 34.95 (*0-632-03757-1*) Blackwell Sci.

Managing Attention & Learning Disorders in Late Adolescence & Adulthood: A Guide for Practitioners. Sam Goldstein. 1996. LC 96-6743. 512p. 105.00 (*0-471-07662-7*) Wiley.

Managing Attention Deficit Hyperactivity Disorder in Children: A Guide for Practitioners. Sam Goldstein & Michael Goldstein. 2nd ed. 1998. LC 97-36626. 896p. 105.00 (*0-471-12158-4*) Wiley.

Managing Attention Deficits. Ed. by William H. Burke. 2nd rev. ed. 1996. (Professional Series on Traumatic Brain Injury: Vol. 7). 52p. pap. 9.50 (*1-882855-49-3*) HDI Pubs.

Managing Attention Disorders in Children: A Guide for Practitioners. Sam Goldstein & Michael Goldstein. 1993. (Personality Processes Ser.). 464p. text 310.00 incl. VHS (*0-471-30317-8*) Wiley.

Managing Back Pain. Michael S. Melnick et al. 1989. (Orig.). pap. text 4.00 (*0-9616461-6-0*) Saunders Grp.

Managing Behavioural Treatment: Policy & Practice with Delinquent Adolescents. Clive R. Hollin et al. LC 94-16008. (International Library of Philosophy, Psychology, & Scientific Method). 256p. (C). 1995. pap. 29.95 (*0-415-05006-5*, A7778); 1994. text 62.95 (*0-415-05005-7*, A7774) Routledge.

Managing Biotechnology in Drug Development. Chi-Jen Lee. 1996. LC 96-1245. 192p. 119.95 (*0-8493-9466-X*) CRC Pr.

Managing Bloodborne Pathogens: Guidelines for Transit Managers. Erskine S. Walther. 7th ed. 1997. LC 94-77291. (Illus.). 102p. spiral bd. 50.00 (*1-885327-11-0*) Walther Cnslt.

Managing Cancer: The African American's Guide to Prevention, Diagnosis & Treatment. George Rawls et al. 2001. (Illus.). 360p. pap. 16.95 (*0-9675258-2-9*) Hilton Pubg.

Managing Cancer Pain. F. De Conno. 1996. LC 96-32806. pap. text 29.00 (*0-7923-4202-X*) Kluwer Academic.

Managing Care, Not Dollars: The Continuum of Mental Health Services. Ed. by Robert K. Schreter et al. 1997. 396p. text 57.00 (*0-88048-855-7*, 8855) Am Psychiatric.

Managing Change, Changing Medicine: Park Nicollet, Seventy-Five Years. James R. Hare, Jr. 1996. LC 96-37059. 300p. (Orig.). pap. 16.00 (*0-9655104-0-9*) Park Nicollet.

Managing Change in Health Care: Innovative Solutions for People-Based Organizations. M.K. Key. 1998. LC 98-50696. 35.00 (*0-07-134301-6*) McGraw.

Managing Child Nutrition Programs: Leadership for Excellence. Josephine M. Martin et al. 1999. LC 99-13065. 768p. 75.00 (*0-8342-0917-9*, 09179) Aspen Pub.

Managing Childhood Medical Emergencies: An Action Guide for Parents & Childcare Providers. Lori Thompson. 1994. (Illus.). (gr. 2 up). pap. text 25.00 (*0-201-49050-1*) Addison-Wesley.

Managing Children with Psychiatric Problems. Ed. by M. Elena Garralda. 1993. 228p. pap. text (*0-7279-0788-3*) BMJ Pub GBR. *Dist:* AIDC.

***Managing Children's Psychosocial Needs.** Rollins. 1993. tchr. ed. (*0-8342-1922-0*) PRO-ED.

Managing Chronic Behavioral Disorders: A Desktop Reference for Mental Health & Addiction Professionals. Ed. by Karienne Stovell. 1997. 350p. 149.00 (*1-884937-48-9*) Manisses Communs.

Managing Chronic Illness: A Biopsychosocial Perspective. Ed. by Perry M. Nicassio & Timothy W. Smith. 1995. LC 95-17909. (Application & Practice in Health Psychology Ser.). 425p. text 29.95 (*1-55798-300-3*) Am Psychol.

Managing Chronic Orofacial Pain with Transcutaneous Electroneural Stimulation. Errol Lader. 1986. LC 85-50702. (Illus.). 300p. pap. text 85.00 (*0-9610782-5-1*) Vadare.

Managing Client Care. Elizabeth F. Wywialowski. 2nd ed. (Illus.). 384p. 1997. tchr. ed. (*0-8151-4495-4*); 1996. (C). (gr. 13). pap. text 31.00 (*0-8151-9499-4*, 28208) Mosby Inc.

Managing Clinical Supervision. Mary A. Falvey. 2001. LC 00-66740. (Counseling Ser.). 224p. pap. text 41.95 (*0-534-53074-5*) Duxbury.

Managing Cocaine Craving. Hazelden Publishing Staff. 1996. pap. 3.00 (*0-89486-674-5*) Hazelden.

***Managing Communication in Healthcare.** Mark Darley. 2001. (Illus.). 255p. pap. (*0-7020-2413-9*) W B Saunders GBR. *Dist:* Saunders.

Managing Community Health Services. Ed. by Allan McNaught. 1990. 200p. pap. 27.50 (*0-412-31900-4*, A5043) Chapman & Hall.

Managing Conduct & Data Quality of Toxicology Studies. Ed. by B. K. Hoover et al. 1986. LC 85-63837. (Illus.). 352p. 50.00 (*0-911131-93-0*) Specialist Journals.

Managing Contraceptive Pill Patients. Richard P. Dickey. 9th ed. 1998. LC 98-194210. 351p. pap. (*0-929240-84-7*); 10th rev. ed. 2000. (Illus.). 245p. pap. 17.95 (*0-917634-05-5*) EMIS.

Managing Corporate Health Care Programs: A Primer for Executives. Paul R. Torrens & Gary S. Whitted. 1985. LC 85-6564. 426p. 65.00 (*0-275-90236-6*, C0236, Praeger Pubs) Greenwood.

Managing Costs in Clinical Laboratories: A Manager's Fiscal Guide to Laboratory Cost Effectiveness. Eleanor M. Travers. 1989. LC 88-32591. (Illus.). 300p. (Orig.). pap. text 39.95 (*0-07-065121-3*, ME106) Practice Mgmt Info.

Managing Crisis & Change in Health Care: The Organizational Response to HIV-AIDS. Chris Bennett & Ewan Ferlie. 1994. LC 93-50137. 160p. pap. (*0-335-15787-4*) OpUniv Pr.

Managing Crisis & Change in Health Care: The Organizational Response to HIV-AIDS. Chris Bennett & Ewan Ferlie. 1994. LC 93-50137. 160p. (*0-335-15788-2*) OpUniv Pr GBR. *Dist:* Taylor & Francis.

Managing Crisis & Risk in Mental Health Nursing. Ed. by Tony Ryan. 1999. LC 00-362785. (Illus.). xv, 200p. pap. (*0-7487-3336-1*) Nelson Thornes GBR. *Dist:* Intl Spec Bk.

Managing Danazol Patients. Richard P. Dickey. 2nd ed. 1992. 137p. pap. 12.95 (*0-929240-35-9*) EMIS.

Managing Diabetes on a Budget. Leslie Y. Dawson. 1996. LC 95-16705. 96p. pap. 7.95 (*0-945448-53-8*, 5002-01) Am Diabetes.

Managing Diversity in Health Care. Lee Gardenswartz. 1998. LC 98-14745. 304p. 45.00 (*0-7879-4041-0*) Jossey-Bass.

Managing Diversity in Health Care Manual: Proven Tools & Activities for Leaders & Trainers. Lee Gardenswartz. 1999. LC 99-6145. (Illus.). 224p. pap., wbk. ed. 120.00 incl. disk (*0-7879-4393-2*) Jossey-Bass.

Managing Doctors. Alan Bruce & Sandra Hill. 1996. LC 96-187337. 64p. pap. (*0-7486-0728-5*) Edinburgh U Pr GBR. *Dist:* Col U Pr.

Managing Emergency Services. Tye. 1997. (Career Education Ser.). tchr. ed. 14.00 (*0-8273-7373-2*) Delmar.

Managing Epilepsy: A Clinical Handbook. Malcolm P. Taylor. 2nd ed. 2000. LC 00-59904. (Illus.). ix, 204p. pap. 36.95 (*0-632-05882-X*) Blackwell Sci.

Managing Epilepsy in Primary Care. Malcolm P. Taylor. 1996. (Illus.). 192p. pap. 38.95 (*0-86542-972-3*) Blackwell Sci.

Managing Family Planning in General Practice. Sam Rowlands et al. 1997. LC 97-10270. 160p. pap. (*1-85775-205-8*) Radcliffe Med Pr GBR. *Dist:* Balogh.

Managing Fatigue in Transportation: Selected Papers from the 3rd Fatigue in Transportation Conference, Freemantle, Western Australia, 1998. Laurence R. Hartley. 1998. LC 98-36059. 474p. 113.00 (*0-08-043357-X*, Pergamon Pr) Elsevier.

Managing Field Operations: An Introduction to Incident Management. Stoffel et al. 1989. (Illus.). 80p. ring bd. 15.00 (*0-913724-42-4*) Emerg Response Inst.

Managing Fragmented Public Mental Health Services. Richard G. Frank & Laura L. Morlock. 1997. 52p. (Orig.). pap. (*1-887748-03-2*) Milbank Memorial.

Managing Genetic Information: Implications for Nursing Practice. American Nurses Association Staff. 1995. 60p. pap. text 14.95 (*1-55810-111-X*, NP-102) Am Nurses Pub.

Managing Hazardous Drugs: A Quick Reference for Safe Administration. Anne M. Zolaer. 1997. (Illus.). spiral bd. (*1-891814-01-X*) Found Care Mgmt.

Managing Hazardous Materials Incidents Vol. I: Emergency Medical Services: A Planning Guide for the Management of Contaminated Patients. 1996. (Illus.). 77p. (Orig.). (C). pap. text 40.00 (*0-7881-3710-7*) DIANE Pub.

Managing Hazardous Materials Incidents Vol. II: Hospital Emergency Departments: A Planning Guide for the Management of Contaminated Patients. Scott V. Wright. 1996. (Illus.). 72p. (Orig.). (C). pap. text 40.00 (*0-7881-3714-X*) DIANE Pub.

Managing Hazardous Materials Incidents Vol. III: Medical Management Guidelines for Acute Chemical Exposures. Jonathan Borak et al. 1996. 495p. reprint ed. pap. text 50.00 (*0-7881-3256-3*) DIANE Pub.

Managing Hazards in the Transfusion Service. Harold B. Anstall et al. 1993. 212p. 47.00 (*0-89189-324-5*) Am Soc Clinical.

Managing Headache in Primary Care. Peter J. Goadsby & Stephen D. Silberstein. rev. ed. 1997. 464p. pap. text 39.95 (*0-86542-672-4*) Blackwell Sci.

Managing Health Care. Ed. by John J. Glynn & David A. Perkins. 1995. pap. text 30.00 (*0-7020-1831-7*) Saunders.

Managing Health Care Construction Projects: A Practical Guide. Compiled by Michael Hemmes. 1993. LC 93-12888. 198p. pap. 48.00 (*1-55648-103-9*, 055100) AHPI.

Managing Health Care Demand. Robin E. Scott MacStravic et al. 1998. LC 97-47204. 576p. 79.00 (*0-8342-0927-6*, 09276) Aspen Pub.

Managing Health Care Resources. Price. 1998. LC 98-4643. (Illus.). 336p. (C). (gr. 13). pap. text 34.95 (*0-8151-2298-5*, 27516) Mosby Inc.

Managing Health Professionals. Michael J. Nelson. 1990. 216p. pap. 25.50 (*0-412-33350-3*, A4446) Chapman & Hall.

Managing Health Promotion: Developing Healthy Organizations & Communities. Ina Simnett. 1996. 248p. pap. 49.95 (*0-471-95814-X*) Wiley.

Managing Health Service Information. R. Sheaff. 1994. LC 94-27219. 217p. pap. (*0-335-15702-5*) OpUniv Pr.

Managing Health Services Organizations. Beaufort B. Longest, Jr. et al. 2nd ed. 1985. (Illus.). 550p. 42.50 (*0-7216-2045-0*) Saunders.

Managing Health Services Organizations. Jonathon S. Rakich et al. 3rd ed. 1992. LC 92-1466. 768p. 58.00 (*1-878812-09-2*) Hlth Prof Pr.

Managing Healthcare Compliance. Scott C. Withrow. 1999. LC 98-47637. 34p. 49.00 (*1-56793-096-4*) Health Admin Pr.

Managing Heart Failure in Primary Care. Henry J. Dargie et al. 1996. LC 96-27460. (Illus.). 256p. pap. 57.95 (*0-86542-966-9*) Blackwell Sci.

Managing Herpes: How to Live & Love with a Chronic STD. Charles Ebel. rev. ed. 1998. LC 97-78101. (Illus.). 238p. pap. 27.75 (*1-885833-03-2*) Am Social Health.

Managing Hospital-Based Patient Education. Ed. by Barbara E. Giloth. 1993. LC 92-48394. 458p. pap. 68.95 (*1-55648-097-0*, 070194) AHPI.

Managing Immunization in General Practice. Michael Ingram. 1995. LC 95-15758. 120p. pap. (*1-85775-155-8*) Radcliffe Med Pr GBR. *Dist:* Balogh.

Managing in Academics: A Health Center Model. Jill Ridky & George F. Sheldon. 1993. LC 93-23854. (Illus.). 359p. pap. 30.00 (*0-942219-11-2*) Quality Med Pub.

***Managing in Health & Social Care.** Vivienne Martin & Euan S. Henderson. 2001. LC 00-54871. pap. 27.95 (*0-415-25190-7*) Routledge.

Managing in the Emergency Medical Services: Principles & Practice. William Newkirk & William Linden. 1984. (C). 41.00 (*0-8359-4198-1*) P-H.

***Managing Inequality & Diversity in Health.** Carol Baxter. 2001. (Illus.). 255p. pap. (*0-7020-2520-8*) W B Saunders GBR. *Dist:* Saunders.

Managing Infectious Waste. Michael Garvin. 1995. LC 94-31278. 192p. lib. bdg. 65.00 (*0-87371-637-X*, L637) Lewis Pubs.

Managing Integrated Delivery Systems: A Framework for Action. David W. Young & Sheila M. McCarthy. 1999. LC 98-42820. 222p. 45.00 (*1-56793-093-X*) Health Admin Pr.

Managing Low Back Pain. Ed. by William H. Kirkaldy-Willis & Charles V. Burton. 3rd ed. 1992. (Illus.). 420p. text (*0-443-08789-X*) Church.

Managing Low Back Pain. William H. Kirkaldy-Willis & Thomas N. Bernard. Ed. by Marc Staruss. 4th ed. 1999. LC 99-19473. (Illus.). 475p. (C). text (*0-443-07948-X*) Church.

Managing Major Diseases: Pulmonary Disorders. Mosby Staff. 4th ed. 1999. LC 99-10468. text 29.95 (*0-323-00855-0*) Harcourt.

Managing Managed Care. Michael C. Roberts & Linda K. Hurley. 1997. LC 97-33280. (Clinical Child Psychology Library). 188p. pap. 21.50 (*0-306-45671-0*); (Illus.). 206p. (C). 45.00 (*0-306-45670-2*) Kluwer Academic (Kluwer Plenum).

Managing Managed Care: A Handbook for Mental Health Professionals. Michael Goodman et al. 2nd ed. 1996. (Managing Managed Care II Ser.: Vol. II). 272p. 37.00 (*0-88048-772-0*, 8772) Am Psychiatric.

Managing Managed Care: A Practical Guide for Audiologists & Speech-Language Pathologists. Dennis Arnst et al. 1994. 150p. pap. text 40.00 (*0-910329-82-6*, 0111906) Am Speech Lang Hearing.

Managing Managed Care: Quality Improvements in Behavioral Health. Institute of Medicine Staff. Ed. by Margaret Edmonds et al. 1997. LC 97-2004. 396p. text 49.95 (*0-309-05642-X*, Joseph Henry Pr) Natl Acad Pr.

Managing Managed Care in the Medical Practice: The Physician's Handbook for Success & Survival. American Medical Association Staff. 1996. (Practice Success Ser.). 116p. pap. 54.00 (*0-89970-757-2*, OP701095WE) AMA.

Managing Manic Depressive Disorders. Ed. by Ved Varma. 1997. LC 97-198770. 200p. text (*1-85302-347-7*) Jessica Kingsley GBR. *Dist:* Taylor & Francis.

Managing Medical Office Personnel: A Comprehensive Guide to Personnel Management in the Medical Office. Lynne R. Costain & Karen Moawad. Ed. by Gregg Rogers. rev. ed. 1994. 250p. reprint ed. stu. ed. 49.95 (*1-57066-006-9*, 5839M) Practice Mgmt Info.

Managing Medical Staff Change Through Bylaws & Other Strategies. Daniel A. Lang et al. 1995. 160p. pap. 56.50 (*1-55648-138-1*, 145104) AHPI.

Managing Medicine. Lawrence L. Weed. Ed. by Jay S. Wakefield. 3rd ed. 1983. (Illus.). 260p. pap. 20.00 (*0-917054-18-0*) Med Communications.

Managing Medicine: A Survival Guide. Di Sanderson & John Brown. 1997. 302p. pap. (*0-443-05655-2*) Royal Soc of Medicine Pr Ltd GBR. *Dist:* Balogh.

Managing Medicines: Public Policy & Therapeutic Drugs. P. Davis. 1997. LC 96-37264. 192p. pap. (*0-335-19292-0*) OpUniv Pr.

Managing Medicines: Public Policy & Therapeutic Drugs. Peter Davis. 1997. LC 96-37264. (State of Health Ser.). 192p. (*0-335-19293-9*) OpUniv Pr.

Managing Mental Health Care in the Community: Chaos & Containment. Angela Foster & Vega Z. Roberts. 1998. LC 98-15339. (Illus.). 240p. (C). 80.00 (*0-415-16796-5*); pap. 29.95 (*0-415-16797-3*) Routledge.

Managing Mental Health Problems: A Practical Guide for Primary Care. Nick Kates & Marilyn Craven. rev. ed. 1998. LC 94-17533. (Illus.). 390p. (C). 49.00 (*0-88937-124-5*) Hogrefe & Huber Pubs.

Managing Mental Health Service. A. Reynolds. 1999. LC 98-30735. (Health Services Management Ser.). (Illus.). 224p. pap. (*0-335-19833-3*); 170p. pap. (*0-335-19834-1*) OpUniv Pr.

Managing Migraine in Primary Care. Anne MacGregor. 1998. LC 98-46293. (Illus.). 239p. pap. 47.95 (*0-632-05083-7*) Blackwell Sci.

Managing Nutrition Care of the Coronary Patient in Different Health Care Settings. Penny M. Kris-Etherton et al. 2000. 250p. 55.00 (*0-8342-1093-2*, 10932) Aspen Pub.

Managing Obesity & Eating Disorders. Nancy Gustafson. Ed. by Becky Colgan. 1997. 210p. pap. 64.95 (*1-57801-007-1*) Western Schls.

Managing Operations. Bob Johnson. 1998. LC 98-229119. 256p. pap. text 29.95 (*0-7506-3809-5*) Buttrwrth-Heinemann.

***Managing Oral Anticoagulation Therapy**, Supplement #4. Ansell. 2001. 90p. spiral bd. 125.00 (*91-1-113753-3*) Aspen Pub.

Managing Oral Healthcare Delivery: A Resource for the Dental professional. Catherine L. Ganssle. 1994. LC 94-16965. (Health & Life Science Ser.). 304p. (C). pap. text 56.95 (*0-8273-5532-7*) Delmar.

Managing Osteoarthritis in Primary Care. Gillian Hosie & John Dickson. 2000. LC 99-44006. (Illus.). 144p. pap. 41.95 (*0-632-05353-4*) Blackwell Sci.

Managing Osteogenesis Imperfecta: A Medical Manual. Ed. by Pricisalla Wacaster. 1996. (Illus.). 250p. (Orig.). pap. text 24.95 (*0-9642189-3-3*) Osteogenesis Imper.

Managing Our Selves: Building a Community of Caring. Elizabeth Power. 1992. 115p. stu. ed. 17.95 (*1-883307-01-5*) EPower & Assocs.

Managing Our Selves: God in Our Midst. Elizabeth Power. 1993. 63p. reprint ed. stu. ed. 12.95 (*1-883307-02-3*) EPower & Assocs.

Managing Outcomes, Process & Cost in a Managed Care Environment. Roey Kirk. 1997. LC 96-48673. 272p. 75.00 (*0-8342-0912-8*) Aspen Pub.

Managing Outcomes Through Collaborative Care: The Application of Caremapping & Case Management. Ed. by Karen Zander. 1995. LC 94-47919. 207p. pap. text 59.95 (*1-55648-132-2*, 027103) AHPI.

Managing Pain. Reader's Digest Editorial Staff. 2001. LC 98-43587. (Health & Healing the Natural Way Ser.). (Illus.). 160p. 19.95 (*0-7621-0144-X*) RD Assn.

Managing Patient Expectations: The Art of Finding & Keeping Loyal Patients. Susan K. Baker. 1998. LC 98-15900. (Business & Management Ser.). 304p. 40.00 (*0-7879-4158-1*) Jossey-Bass.

Managing Pediatric Emergencies. Patricia A. Moloney-Harmon. 1984. (Cardiopulmonary Arrest Ser.). (Illus.). 104p. (Orig.). pap. text 9.50 (*0-932491-03-0*) Res Appl Inc.

Managing People During Stressful Times: The Psychologically Defensive Workplace. Seth Allcorn & Michael A. Diamond. 1997. LC 96-17925. 184p. 59.95 (*1-56720-082-6*, Quorum Bks) Greenwood.

Managing People in the Health Service. Jane Weightman. 2000. 176p. pap. 47.95 (*0-8464-5117-4*) Beekman Pubs.

Managing Post-Acute Care & Other Extented Care Services. Margaret D. Bischel. 1998. 405p. ring bd. 225.00 (*1-893826-09-0*) Apollo Managed.

Managing Post-Polio: A Guide to Living Well with Post-Polio Syndrome. Linda S. Halstead. Ed. by Linda S. Halstead. 1998. (Illus.). 256p. 25.00 (*1-886236-17-8*) ABI Prof Pubns.

Managing Primary Health Care: Implications of the Health Transition. Richard A. Heaver. 1995. LC 95-3247. (World Bank Discussion Papers: No. 276). 58p. pap. 22.00 (*0-8213-3175-2*, 13175) World Bank.

Managing Public Access Microcomputers in Health Sciences Libraries. Gale G. Hannigan & Janis F. Brown. 1990. 172p. 40.00 (*0-8108-2436-1*) Scarecrow.

Managing Quality: A Guide to System-Wide Performance Management in Health Care. Jacqueline M. Katz & Eleanor Green. 2nd ed. 1996. LC 96-15639. (Illus.). 326p. (C). (gr. 13). text 44.95 (*0-8151-4973-5*, 26254) Mosby Inc.

Managing Quality of Care in a Cost-Focused Environment. Ed. by Norbert Goldfield & David B. Nash. 1999. 227p. 55.00 incl. cd-rom (*0-924674-73-3*) Aspen Pub.

Managing Risk: Preventing Liability in Clinical Practice. Dan J. Tennenhouse. 1999. viii, 174p. pap. 64.00 (*1-930548-16-8*) Tennenhouse Prof Pubns.

Managing Risks of Organizational Accidents. James T. Reason. 1997. LC 97-24648. 200p. pap. (*1-84014-105-0*) Ashgate Pub GBR. *Dist:* Ashgate Pub Co.

Managing Safety & Health Programs. Raymond P. Boylston. 1990. 264p. text 60.95 (*0-442-31900-2*, VNR) Wiley.

Managing Scarcity: Priority Setting & Rationing in the National Health Service. P. Klein et al. 1996. (State of Health Ser.). 192p. pap. (*0-335-19446-X*) OpUniv Pr.

Managing Scarcity: Priority Setting & Rationing in the National Health Service. Rudolf Klein et al. 1996. LC 96-18743. (State of Health Ser.). 161p. (*0-335-19447-8*) OpUniv Pr.

Managing Schizophrenia. 84p. pap. text (*0-86471-059-3*) Adis Intl NZL. *Dist:* Lppncott W & W.

Managing Sensitive Projects: Lateral Approach. Olivier D'Herbemont & Bruno Cesar. 1998. LC 98-20625. 232p. (YA). (gr. 13). 29.95 (*0-415-92166-X*) Routledge.

Managing Sickle Cell Disease in Low-Income Families. Shirley A. Hill. 1994. LC 93-37361. (AK-Sg Ser.). x, 225p. text 69.95 (*1-56639-188-1*) Temple U Pr.

Managing Sinusitus. Edward A. Ullmann & Steve Miller. 1998. (Illus.). pap. 10.95 (*1-892039-02-8*) Bienestar.

Managing Skin Diseases. Philip C. Anderson & Kristin S. Malaker. 1998. LC 98-25827. 338p. pap. 39.95 (*0-683-30598-0*) Lppncott W & W.

***Managing Spinal Cord Injury: A Guide to Living Well with Spinal Cord Injury.** 2002. 27.00 (*1-886236-37-2*) ABI Prof Pubns.

Managing Stress. American Institute for Preventive Medicine Staff. 1993. LC 93-40575. (For Your Information Ser.). 9.50 (*1-56420-025-6*) New Readers.

Managing Stress. Ann Edworthy. 2000. LC 00-22496. (*0-335-20406-6*) Taylor & Francis.

Managing Stress. David Fontana. 1989. (Problems in Practice Ser.). 128p. (*0-901715-98-0*); pap. (*0-901715-97-2*) Brit Psychol Soc GBR. *Dist:* Routledge.

Managing Stress. Jenny Steinmetz et al. 1980. LC 80-66389. 220p. pap. 12.95 (*0-915950-44-8*) Bull Pub.

Managing Stress. Donald H. Weiss. 1987. LC 86-47825. (Successful Office Skills Ser.). 64p. pap. 4.00 (*0-8144-7673-2*) AMACOM.

Managing Stress. Brian L. Seaward. 2nd ed. 1997. (Health Science Ser.). (Illus.). 160p. (C). pap. text, tchr. ed. 13.95 (*0-7637-0474-1*, 0474-1) Jones & Bartlett.

Managing Stress: A Mindset for Health. Melody Madlem et al. 1996. LC 96-8732. (*1-56796-151-7*) WRS Group.

Managing Stress: Journal Workbook. Brian L. Seaward. 1994. LC 93-40223. 96p. pap. text 13.75 (*0-86720-841-4*) Jones & Bartlett.

Managing Stress: Principles & Strategies for Health & Well-Being. Brian L. Seaward. 2nd ed. 1996. LC 96-26129. (Health Science Ser.). (Illus.). 512p. pap. text 53.95 (*0-7637-0233-1*, 0233-1) Jones & Bartlett.

Managing Stress: Subjectivity & Power in the Workplace. Tim Newton. 1995. LC 94-69147. 176p. 74.50 (*0-8039-8643-2*, 2739); pap. 26.50 (*0-8039-8644-0*, 2738) Sage.

Managing Stress & Controlling Self-Defeating Behavior. Charles P. Giles. 1988. 150p. (Orig.). pap. text 7.95 (*0-935920-62-5*, Ntl Pubs Blck) P-H.

Managing Stress for Mental Fitness. Merill F. Raber & George Dyck. Ed. by Michael Crisp. 2nd rev. ed. 1993. LC 92-74205. (Fifty-Minute Ser.). 85p. pap. 12.95 (*1-56052-200-3*) Crisp Pubns.

Managing Stress in Families: Cognitive & Behavioural Strategies for Enhancing Coping Skills. Ian R. Falloon et al. 1993. LC 92-12221. (Strategies for Mental Health Ser.). (Illus.). 304p. (C). text 69.95 (*0-415-07192-5*, A7016) Routledge.

Managing Stroke. Stanley N. Cohen. 1999. LC 00-708872. (Illus.). xiii, 680p. 89.00 (*0-07-012045-5*) McGraw-Hill Med Pub.

Managing Technology in Healthcare. Ori Heller. Ed. by Eliezer Geisler. 1996. LC 96-24589. (Management of Medical Technology Ser.: Vol. 1). 256p. (C). lib. bdg. 145.00 (*0-7923-9750-9*) Kluwer Academic.

Managing Teenage Pregnancy: Access to Abortion, Contraception & Sex Education. James E. Allen & Deborah Bender. 1980. LC 79-89009. 300p. 77.00 (*0-275-90444-X*, C0444, Praeger Pubs) Greenwood.

Managing the Analytical Laboratory: Plain & Simple. Clifford L. Nilsen. 1996. 337p. ring bd. 179.00 (*1-57491-015-9*) IHS Health Grp.

Managing the Apprehensive Dental Patient: A Management Guide for the Dentist & Staff for Effective Practice Building & Internal Marketing. Robert F. Kroeger. 1987. LC 87-80789. (Illus.). 191p. (Orig.). (C). pap. 45.00 (*0-9618291-0-9*) Heritage Cinn.

Managing the Chemically Dependent Nurse: A Guide to Identification, Intervention & Retention. Anne M. Catanzarite. 1992. 203p. pap. 25.00 (*1-886624-09-7*) Creative Nursing.

Managing the Clinical Drug Development Process. David M. Cocchetto & R. V. Nardi. 1991. (Drugs & the Pharmaceutical Sciences Ser.: Vol. 51). (Illus.). 232p. text 150.00 (*0-8247-8595-9*) Dekker.

Managing the Continuum of Care. Connie J. Evashwick & Lawrence J. Weiss. 1987. 440p. 92.00 (*0-87189-640-0*) Aspen Pub.

Managing the Difficult Patient. Robert E. Hooberman & Barbara M. Hooberman. 1998. LC 97-19686. 382p. 59.95 (*1-887841-08-3*, Psychosocial) Intl Univs Pr.

***Managing the Dually Diagnosed Patient: Current Issues & Clinical Approaches.** Ed. by David F. O'Connell & Ellen P. Beyer. 2001. 271p. (C). pap. 27.95 (*0-7890-0877-7*) Haworth Pr.

***Managing the Dually Diagnosed Patient: Current Issues & Clinical Approaches.** Ed. by David F. O'Connell & Ellen P. Beyer. 2nd ed. 2002. 271p. (C). 49.95 (*0-7890-0876-9*) Haworth Pr.

Managing the Emergency Department: A Team Approach. American College of Emergency Physicians Staff. 1992. 120.00 (*0-07-000209-6*) McGraw.

Managing the Marginal & Unsatisfactory Performer. Lawrence L. Steinmetz. 2nd ed. 1985. LC 84-24284. (Business Ser.). 176p. 10.36 (*0-201-07837-6*) Addison-Wesley.

Managing the Medical Arms Race: Innovation & Public Policy in the Medical Device Industry. Susan B. Foote. 1992. (C). text 45.00 (*0-520-07591-9*) U CA Pr.

Managing the Medical Practice: The Physician's Handbook for Successful Practice Administration. Lauretta Mink. Ed. by Kay Stanley. 1996. (Practice Success Ser.). pap. 44.95 (*0-89970-755-6*, OP701295AFR) AMA.

***Managing the Message: A Tool Kit for Communicators.** Roy Lilley & Geoffrey Bowden. 2000. 168p. pap. (*1-85775-412-3*) Radcliffe Med Pr GBR. *Dist:* Balogh.

Managing the Outpatient Medical Practice: Strategies for a Changing Environment. Thomas Landholt & Coker Group Staff. 1998. LC 98-20745. (Illus.). 143p. 39.00 (*1-55648-242-6*) AHPI.

***Managing the Patient-Centered Pharmacy.** Ed. by Harry P. Hagel & John P. Rovers. 2002. 200p. per. 45.00 (*1-58212-010-2*) Am Pharm Assn.

Managing the Patient with Type II Diabetes. Andrew L. Wilson. 1997. LC 97-23911. 192p. pap. 39.00 (*0-8342-1018-5*) Aspen Pub.

Managing the Patient with Type II Diabetes. Andrew L. Wilson & Ila V. Mehra. 1997. LC 97-23911. (*0-8342-1004-5*) Aspen Pub.

Managing the Pharmacy Benefit Robert Navarro & Albert I. Wertheimer. 1996. LC 96-164710. xxii, 376 p. (*0-9651745-0-6*) Emron.

Managing the Physician's Office Laboratory: Responsive Management under Regulatory & Economic Restraints. Eleanor M. Travers. 1994. 250p. (Orig.). pap. text 59.95 (*0-07-600653-0*, ME107) Practice Mgmt Info.

Managing the Practice: Whose Business? June Huntington. 1995. LC 95-21406. (Primary Care Development Ser.). 140p. pap. (*1-85775-053-5*) Radcliffe Med Pr GBR. *Dist:* Balogh.

Managing the Quality of Health Care in Developing Countries. Willy L. De Geyndt. 1995. LC 94-36278. (Technical Papers: No. 258). 92p. pap. 22.00 (*0-8213-3092-6*, 13092) World Bank.

Managing the Residential Treatment Center in Troubled Times. Intro. by Gordon Northrup. 1994. LC 94-17286. (Residential Treatment for Children & Youth Ser.). 111p. 39.95 (*1-56024-676-6*) Haworth Pr.

Managing the Risks of Managed Care. Barbara J. Youngberg. 1995. 320p. ring bd. 190.00 (*0-8342-0732-X*) Aspen Pub.

Managing the Side Effects of Chemotherapy & Radiation Therapy: A Guide for Patients & Their Families. Marylin J. Dodd. 3rd ed. 1996. 198p. (Orig.). pap. 20.00 (*0-943671-12-4*) UCSF Schl Nursing.

Managing the Use of Fluoroscopy in Medical Institutions: Report of the Radiation Protection Committee Task Group #6. 1998. (Report Ser.: No. 58). 56p. pap. text 10.00 (*1-888340-13-4*) AAPM.

Managing the Veterinary Cancer Patient: A Practice Manual. Gregory K. Ogilvie & Antony S. Moore. 1995. LC 94-61975. 540p. pap. text 68.00 (*1-884254-20-9*) Vet Lrn Syst.

Managing the Violent Patient: A Clinician's Guide. Ed. by Patricia E. Blumenreich & Susan Lewis. 1993. LC 93-12563. 176p. text 24.95 (*0-87630-707-1*) Brunner-Routledge.

Managing to Be a Non-Smoker. Mike Dowd. 1991. 96p. pap. 9.95 (*0-9630260-9-7*) Dowd Hlthgrp.

Managing to Care: Case Management & Service System Reform. Ann E. P. Dill. 2000. LC 2001-22601. (Social Institutions & Social Change Ser.). 176p. pap. text 18.95 (*0-202-30612-7*); lib. bdg. 37.95 (*0-202-30611-9*) Aldine de Gruyter.

Managing Traumatic Stress Through Art: Drawing from the Center. Barry M. Cohen et al. 1995. LC 95-68155. xviii, 174p. (Orig.). pap. 22.95 (*0-9629164-7-1*) Sidran Pr.

Managing Type Two Diabetes: Your Invitation to a Healthier Lifestyle. Arlene Monk et al. 2nd rev. ed. 1996. LC 87-20218. 192p. 11.95 (*1-885115-26-1*) IDC Pubng.

Managing Urinary Incontinence in the Elderly. John Schnelle. 1991. LC 90-10430. 144p. 48.00 (*0-8261-7360-8*) Springer Pub.

***Managing Your Allergies: Natural Remedies for Better Living.** David Hazard. 2002. (Healthy Body, Healthy Soul Ser.). 112p. pap. 6.99 (*0-7369-0483-2*) Harvest Hse.

Managing Your Career in Nursing. Frances C. Henderson & Barbara O. McGettigan. 1986. 276p. (C). pap. text 17.25 (*0-201-12958-2*) Addison-Wesley.

Managing Your Career in Nursing. Barbara McGettigan & Frances Henderson. 2nd ed. 1994. LC 95-102019. 358p. pap. 34.95 (*0-88737-629-0*) Natl League Nurse.

Managing Your Child's Eating Problems During Cancer Treatments. 1995. (Illus.). 32p. (Orig.). (C). pap. text 15.00 (*0-7881-1964-8*) DIANE Pub.

Managing Your Computer Physique: How to Manage the Human Body in a Computer Environment. Maribeth C. Yarnell. 1994. (Illus.). 69p. (Orig.). pap. 12.95 (*1-885879-00-8*) Eaglecliff.

Managing Your Ewe: And Her Newborn Lambs. Laura Lawson. rev. ed. 1997. LC 93-79480. (Illus.). 352p. (Orig.). pap. 34.95 (*0-9633923-1-X*) LDF Pubns.

***Managing Your Headaches.** M. Green & Leah M. Green. 2001. LC 00-67909. (Illus.). xi, 116p. pap. 19.95 (*0-387-95238-1*) Spr-Verlag.

Managing Your Health Care: Making the Most of Your Medical Resources. Martin Gipson et al. 1996. LC 95-46188. 96p. pap. 9.95 (*0-934793-59-X*) Pathfinder CA.

Managing Your Healthcare: A Consumer Guide to Navigating Today's Health Care Systems. William F. McNally. 1997. 216p. pap. 19.95 (*1-886346-20-8*) Warde Pubs.

Managing Your Medical Practice. Charles Wold. 1988. 1278p. text 135.00 (*1-887515-00-3*) AHAB Press.

Managing Your Migraine: A Migraine-Sufferer's Practical Guide. Susan L. Burks. 1994. LC 94-4712. 264p. pap. 19.50 (*0-89603-324-4*) Humana.

Managing Your Stress: How to Relax & Enjoy. Jerry V. Teplitz & Shelly Kellman. rev. ed. 1985. LC 81-80175. (Illus.). 128p. pap. 15.00 (*0-87040-402-4*) Happiness Unltd.

Mandala: Path of Beauty. Joan Kellogg. 1992. 112p. pap. text 10.00 (*0-9631949-1-7*) Graphic Pub Williamsbrg.

Mandated Health Care: Issues & Strategies. Donald L. Westerfield. 1991. LC 90-14331. 224p. 60.00 (*0-275-93813-1*, C3813, Praeger Pubs) Greenwood.

Mandating Health Insurance. John C. Goodman et al. 1989. pap. 10.00 (*0-943802-40-7*, 136) Natl Ctr Pol.

***Mandatory Testing for Substance Abuse: Index of New Information & Guide-Book for Reference & Research.** Research and Development Division Staff. 2001. 180p. pap. 44.50 (*0-7883-2347-4*) ABBE Pubs Assn.

***Mandatory Testing for Substance Abuse: Index of New Information & Guide-Book for Reference & Research.** Ed. by Research and Development Division Staff & John C. Bartone. 2001. 180p. 47.50 (*0-7883-2346-6*) ABBE Pubs Assn.

Mandell, Douglas & Bennett's Principles & Practice of Infectious Diseases Gerald L. Mandell et al. 5th ed. 1999. LC 99-16736. (Illus.). text 295.00 (*0-443-07593-X*) Saunders.

Mandibular Growth Anomolies: Terminology, Aetiology, Diagnosis, Treatment. H. Obwegeser. 2000. LC 00-41903. (Illus.). 608p. 199.00 (*3-540-67214-1*) Spr-Verlag.

Mandibular Reconstruction. Arnold Komisar. 1997. LC 96-36513. (Illus.). 160p. text 89.00 (*0-86577-614-8*) Thieme Med Pubs.

***Maneater: And Other True Stories of a Life in Infectious Diseases.** Pamela Nagami. 2001. 288p. 24.95 (*1-58063-209-2*) Renaissance.

Maneuvering the Maze of Managed Care. Corooran. 1996. 28.00 (*0-02-874126-9*) Free Pr.

Maneuvering the Maze of Managed Care: A Survival Guide for Clinicians in Public & Private Settings. Kevin Corcoran. 1996. LC 95-47008. (Illus.). 352p. 35.00 (*0-684-82310-1*); 1995. 18.00 (*0-02-874062-9*) Free Pr.

Maneuvering the Maze of Managed Care: A Survival Guide for Clinicians in Public & Private Settings. Kevin Corcoran et al. 1996. LC 95-47008. 352p. 20.00 (*0-684-82309-8*) Free Pr.

Manganese. 1981. (Environmental Health Criteria Ser.: No. 17). 110p. pap. text 13.00 (*92-4-154077-X*, 1160017) World Health.

Manganese in Health & Disease. Dorothy Klimas-Tavantzis. 1993. 224p. 169.00 (*0-8493-7841-9*) CRC Pr.

Manhattan Health Pages: A Directory of Resources for Living Healthy in New York City. Lyn Skreczko & Virginia Bell. 1998. LC 98-66462. 300p. pap. 16.95 (*0-9641262-8-1*) Little Bkrm.

Manhood & Politics: A Feminist Reading in Political Thought. Wendy L. Brown. 1988. LC 87 12850. (New Feminist Perspectives Ser.). 248p. 82.00 (*0-8476-7576-9*) Rowman.

Manhood & Politics: A Feminist Reading in Political Thought. Wendy L. Brown. 2002. LC 87-12850. (New Feminist Perspectives Ser.). 248p. pap. 27.95 (*0-8476-7577-7*) Rowman.

Mania: Clinical & Research Perspectives. Ed. by Paul J. Goodnick. 1998. 478p. text 62.00 (*0-88048-728-3*, 8728) Am Psychiatric.

Manic-Depression: Illness or Awakening. Robert E. Kelly. Ed. by Jennifer Carey & Marjorie Pannell. 1995. (Illus.). 266p. 19.95 (*0-9639451-4-9*) Knowldge Unltd.

Manic Depression & Creativity. D. Jablow Hershman & Julian Lieb. 1998. LC 98-27043. 310p. reprint ed. pap. 22.00 (*1-57392-241-2*) Prometheus Bks.

Manic-Depressive Illness. Frederick K. Goodwin & Kay R. Jamison. 1990. (Illus.). 962p. text 78.50 (*0-19-503934-3*) OUP.

Manic-Depressive Illness: History of a Syndrome. Edward A. Wolpert. 1977. LC 76-46817. 604p. 90.00 (*0-8236-3095-1*) Intl Univs Pr.

Manic-Depressive Insanity & Paranoia. Emil Kraepelin. Tr. by R. Mary Barclay from GER. 1977. LC 75-16712. (Classics in Psychiatry Ser.). (Illus.). reprint ed. 40.95 (*0-405-07441-7*) Ayer.

Manifest Dream & Its Use in Therapy. Roy M. Mendelsohn. 1990. LC 93-30140. 300p. 50.00 (*0-87668-766-4*) Aronson.

Manifestations of Cancer & Treatment. Susan L. Groenwald. 1991. (Illus.). (C). pap. text 44.95 (*0-86720-304-8*, 304-8) Jones & Bartlett.

Manifesting Medicine: Bodies & Machines. Ed. by Robert Bud et al. 1999. 174p. text 46.00 (*90-5702-408-X*); pap. text 24.00 (*90-5702-430-6*) Gordon & Breach (Harwood Acad Pubs).

Manifesto for a New Medicine. James S. Gordon. 2000. 368p. pap. 15.00 (*0-201-89828-4*) Perseus Bks Grp.

Manifesto for a New Medicine: Your Guide to Healing Partnerships & the Wise Use of Alternative Therapies. James S. Gordon. 1999. 358p. text 25.00 (*0-7881-6182-2*) DIANE Pub.

Manifesto for the Nation. R. K. Allday. 1989. (C). text (*0-902662-00-7*) R K Pubns GBR. *Dist:* St Mut.

Manipulating Life: Debating the Genetic Revolution. Ed. by Gary E. McCuen. 1985. (Ideas in Conflict Ser.). (Illus.). 136p. (YA). (gr. 7-12). lib. bdg. 15.95 (*0-86596-054-2*) G E M.

Manipulation & Mobilization: Extremity & Spinal Techniques. Susan L. Edmond. 1992. LC 92-49998. 304p. (gr. 13). text 45.00 (*0-8016-6305-9*, 06305) Mosby Inc.

Manipulation of Mammalian Development, set. R. B. Gwatkin. 1986. LC 85-3406. (Developmental Biology Ser.). (Illus.). 402p. (C). text 95.00 (*0-306-42166-6*, Kluwer Plenum) Kluwer Academic.

Manipulation Therapy for the Naturopathic Physician. David J. Shipley. 1997. (Illus.). 172p. pap. text 42.00 (*0-9662564-0-9*) Ascelapias Pub.

Manipulations Viscerales see Visceral Manipulation

Manipulative Therapy in the Rehabilitation of the Motor System. Karel Lewit. 2nd ed. 1991. (Illus.). 320p. 70.00 (*0-7506-1123-5*) Buttrwrth-Heinemann.

Mannerisms of Speech & Gestures in Everyday Life. Sandor S. Feldman. 1969. LC 59-6713. 318p. reprint ed. pap. 24.95 (*0-8236-8144-0*, 023100) Intl Univs Pr.

Manpower Problem in Mental Hospitals: A Consultant Team Approach. Philip F. Seitz et al. 1977. LC 76-18935. xiii, 253p. (C). 37.50 (*0-8236-3110-9*) Intl Univs Pr.

Manpower Substitution in the Hospital Industry: A Study of New York City Voluntary & Municipal Hospital Systems. Myron D. Fottler. 1972. LC 73-173280. (Special Studies in U. S. Economic, Social & Political Issues). 52.50 (*0-275-06150-7*) Irvington.

Man's Anatomy Arnold Tobias & Allan Tobias. 4th ed. 1989. pap. (*1-86814-040-7*) Intl Spec Bk.

Man's Anatomy Vol. 1: Thorax & Abdomen. Arnold Tobias & Allan Tobias. 1989. pap. (*1-86814-037-7*) Intl Spec Bk.

Man's Anatomy Vol. 2: Head, Neck & Central Nervous System. Arnold Tobias & Allan Tobias. 1989. pap. (*1-86814-038-5*) Intl Spec Bk.

Man's Anatomy Vol. 3: Back & Limbs. Arnold Tobias & Allan Tobias. 1989. pap. (*1-86814-039-3*) Intl Spec Bk.

Man's Confidence. Jack W. Hayford. 1995. LC 96-103794. (Power-to-Become Ser.: No. 02). 89p. pap. 4.99 (*0-7852-7791-9*) Nelson.

Man's Greatest Fear: The Final Phase of Human Evolution. Tim Marshall. 1995. LC 96-104113. (Illus.). 180p. (Orig.). pap. 11.00 (*0-9645750-0-0*) Athena Bks.

Man's Health Sourcebook. Alfred M. Dashe. 2nd ed. 1999. LC 99-43149. (Illus.). 288p. pap. 17.95 (*0-7373-0109-0*, 01090W) NTC Contemp Pub Co.

Man's Health Sourcebook. Alfred M. Dashe. 2nd ed. 1997. (Illus.). 288p. reprint ed. pap. 15.00 (*1-56565-813-2*, Anodyne) Lowell Hse.

Man's Image & Identity. Jack W. Hayford. 1995. LC 96-103815. (Power-to-Become Ser.: No. 04). 92p. pap. 4.99 (*0-7852-7794-3*) Nelson.

Man's Image in Medicine & Anthropology. Ed. by Iago Galdston. 1963. LC 63-19871. (Institute of Social & Historical Medicine Monographs: No. 4). 525p. 67.50 (*0-8236-3120-6*) Intl Univs Pr.

Man's Search for Meaning: An Introduction to Logotherapy. Viktor E. Frankl. 4th ed. 1992. LC 92-21055. 192p. 20.00 (*0-8070-2918-1*) Beacon Pr.

Man's Search for Ultimate Meaning. Viktor E. Frankl. 2000. 208p. reprint ed. pap. text 13.50 (*0-7382-0354-8*) Perseus Bks Grp.

Manson's Tropical Disease. Cook. 20th ed. 1995. text 125.00 (*0-7020-1764-7*) Saunders.

Manter & Gatz's Essentials of Clinical Neuroanatomy & Neurophysiology. Sid Gilman & Sarah W. Newman. 9th ed. 1996. LC 95-49487. (Illus.). 309p. (C). pap. text 28.95 (*0-8036-0144-1*) Davis Co.

Manter & Gatz's Essentials of Clinical Neuroanatomy & Neurophysiology. Sid Gilman & Sarah Winans Newman. 10th ed. 2001. (Illus.). 305p. pap. 29.95 (*0-8036-0772-5*) Davis Co.

Manual & Atlas of Fine Needle Aspiration Cytology. Svente R. Orell et al. 2nd ed. 1992. (Illus.). 341p. text (*0-443-04239-X*) Church.

Manual Asymmetries in Motor Performance. Ed. by Digby Elliott & Eric A. Roy. 1996. LC 96-98. 272p. 104.95 (*0-8493-8999-2*) CRC Pr.

Manual Complete Urology Asia. Martin I. Resnick. 1989. 10.95 (*0-316-74052-7*, Little Brwn Med Div) Lppncott W & W.

Manual Complete Urology ISE. Martin I. Resnick. 1989. 15.95 (*0-316-74053-5*, Little Brwn Med Div) Lppncott W & W.

Manual de Diagnostico y Terapeutica Medica en Atencion Primaria. R. Ruiz de Adana. 2nd ed. 1996. (SPA.). 1221p. pap. (*84-7978-255-2*) Ediciones Diaz ESP. *Dist:* IBD Ltd.

Manual de Ejercicios Para Pacientes en el Post-Operatorio de Cabeza y Cuello. 1984. (SPA.). 5.00 (*0-940876-09-4*) City Hope.

Manual de Ejercicios Para Pacientes Mastecjomizada y con Remocion de Nodulas Axilares. 1984. (SPA.). 5.00 (*0-940876-08-6*) City Hope.

Manual de Ensenanza de Medicamentos En Espanol: A Guide to Patient Drug Information in Spanish. 1995.Tr. of Medication Teaching Manual. (SPA.). 760p. (Orig.). pap. text 70.00 (*1-879907-60-7*) Am Soc Hlth-Syst.

Manual de Neurofisiologia. D. P. Cardinali. 1992. (SPA.). 339p. pap. (*84-7978-005-3*) Ediciones Diaz ESP. *Dist:* IBD Ltd.

Manual de Odontologia Infantil. Ed. by Luis A. Marini. 1982. (SPA.). 463p. (Orig.). (C). 12.00 (*0-8477-2330-5*) U of PR Pr.

Manual de Pediatria Practica. M. Pombo Arias. 4th ed. 1992. (SPA.). 693p. (*84-7978-055-X*) Ediciones Diaz ESP. *Dist:* IBD Ltd.

Manual de Primeros Auxilios. Editorial America, S. A. Staff. Ed. by Maria E. Alvarez del Real. 1989. (SPA., Illus.). 224p. (Orig.). pap. 3.50 (*0-944499-06-6*) Editorial Amer.

***Manual de Radiologia para Tecnicos (Radiologic Science for Technologists)** 6th ed. 1997. (SPA., Illus.). 608p. (*84-8174-309-7*) Mosby-Doyma Libros ESP. *Dist:* Mosby Inc.

Manual de Tecnicas Quirurgicas. J. Sanchez Fernandez. 1992. (SPA.). 291p. pap. (*84-7978-058-4*) Ediciones Diaz ESP. *Dist:* IBD Ltd.

Manual Derm Asia, No. 4. Andreas Arndt. 1988. 10.95 (*0-316-05179-9*, Little Brwn Med Div) Lppncott W & W.

Manual DX Imaging ISE, No. 2. William H. Straub. 1989. 15.95 (*0-316-81888-7*, Little Brwn Med Div) Lppncott W & W.

Manual for Animal Health Auxiliary Personnel. 1984. 392p. (*92-5-101475-2*, F2582) FAO ITA. *Dist:* Bernan Associates.

***Manual for Assessing Ecological & Human Health Effects of Genetically Engineered Organisms: Introductory Materials & Supporting Text for Flowcharts.** Ed. by Mark Wheelis. 2001. 158p. (C). pap. 40.00 (*0-7567-0782-X*) DIANE Pub.

Manual for Assessing Health Practices & Designing Practice Policies: The Explicit Approach. Council of Medical Specialty Societies Task Force & David M. Eddy. 1992. 144p. pap. 34.00 (*0-943126-18-5*, MAH91) Amer Coll Phys.

Manual for Child Health Workers in Major Disasters. 1986. lib. bdg. 79.95 (*0-8490-3796-4*) Gordon Pr.

Manual for Clinical Psychology Trainees, No. 10. James P. Choca & Eric J. Van Denburg. 3rd ed. 1996. LC 96-8894. (Basic Principles into Practice Ser.: Vol. 10). 256p. pap. text 27.95 (*0-87630-814-0*) Brunner-Routledge.

Manual for Clinical Trials Nursing. Ed. by Angela Klimaszewski et al. 2000. (Illus.). 400p. pap. text 50.00 (*1-890504-12-2*) Oncology Nursing.

Manual for Eye Examination & Diagnosis. Mark W. Leitman. 4th ed. 1993. pap. 36.95 (*0-86542-339-3*); 5th ed. 2000. LC 00-31237. (Illus.). 98p. (C). pap. 41.95 (*0-632-04542-6*) Blackwell Sci.

Manual for Functional Training. Lynn M. Palmer et al. 3rd ed. 1992. LC 91-34541. (Illus.). 351p. pap. text 29.95 (*0-8036-6759-0*) Davis Co.

Manual for Health Officers. J. Scott MacNutt. Ed. by Barbara G. Rosenkrantz. 1977. LC 76-40634. (Public Health in America Ser.). (Illus.). reprint ed. lib. bdg. 54.95 (*0-405-09825-1*) Ayer.

Manual for Human Dissection: Photographs with Clinical Applications. Gerald Callas. 1994. (Illus.). 203p. (C). pap. 34.95 (*0-8385-6133-0*, A6133-1, Apple Lange Med) McGraw.

Manual for Intensive Brief & Emergency Psychotherapy Manual. Leopold Bellak. 1987. LC 87-23865. 50p. (Orig.). pap. text 9.50 (*0-918863-01-5*) CPS Inc.

Manual for IV Therapy Procedures. Shila Hayden. Ed. by Jill C. Brittenham. 3rd ed. 1992. LC 92-49992. (Illus.). 361p. (C). 25.00 (*1-878487-50-7*, ME221) Practice Mgmt Info.

Manual for Laboratory Work in Mammalian Physiology. Illus. by Fred E. D'Amour et al. 3rd ed. 1996. LC 65-17285. pap. text 23.00 (*0-226-13563-2*) U Ch Pr.

***Manual for Large Animal Internal Medicine.** Bradford P. Smith. 2001. (*0-323-00978-6*) Mosby Inc.

Manual for Management of Diabetes Mellitus. Juliana C. Chan et al. Date not set. pap. (*962-201-757-6*) Chinese Univ HKG. *Dist:* U of Mich Pr.

Manual for Midwives see Home Birth: Step-by-Step Instructions for Natural & Emergency Childbirth

Manual for Pharmacy Technician. Keresztes. 1997. pap. text (*0-7216-5007-4*) Saunders.

Manual for Pharmacy Technicians. 2nd rev. ed. 1998. LC 98-228601. 416p. 69.00 (*1-879907-79-8*); Pts. 1 & 2. 1993. 349p. ring bd. 50.00 (*1-879907-34-8*) Am Soc Hlth-Syst.

Manual for Professionals Who Work with the Substance Abusing Mentally Ill. Robert D. Thompson. 1989. (Illus.). 103p. (Orig.). pap. 15.00 (*0-9624700-0-7*) Arapahoe Mental Hlth Ctr.

Manual for Radiation Oncology Nursing Practice & Education. Ed. by Deborah Watkins-Broner et al. rev. ed. 1998. (Illus.). 80p. pap. text 30.00 (*1-890504-07-6*) Oncology Nursing.

Manual for Rapid Laboratory Viral Diagnosis. J. Almeida & P. Atanasiu. 1979. (WHO Offset Publications: No. 47). 48p. 4.00 (*92-4-170047-5*) World Health.

Manual for (Relatively) Painless Medical Spanish: A Self-Teaching Course. Ana Manilow Rajkovic. 1992. LC 91-47543. (ENG & SPA., Illus.). 249p. (C). pap. 16.95 (*0-292-75146-X*, UTP146X) U of Tex Pr.

Manual for Staging of Cancer. Irvin D. Fleming et al. 5th ed. 1997. LC 97-6756. (Illus.). 320p. pap. text 65.00 (*0-397-58414-8*) Lppncott W & W.

Manual for Targeted Intervention Research on Sexually Transmitted Illnesses with Community Members. Deborah L. Helitzer-Allen & Hubert A. Allen, Jr. 1994. (Illus.). vii, 122p. pap. text 25.00 (*0-9641694-0-1*) H Allen & Assocs.

Manual for the Child Behavior Checklist 4-18 & 1991 Profile. Thomas M. Achenbach. 1991. LC 90-72107. (Illus.). 478p. (Orig.). pap. 25.00 (*0-938565-08-7*) Res Ctr Child.

Manual for the Determination of the Clinical Role of Anaerobic Microbiology. Ed. by Lorraine S. Gall & Phyllis E. Riely. 1981. 96p. 58.00 (*0-8493-5935-X*, QR67, CRC Reprint) Franklin.

Manual for the Examination of Bone. Colin Anderson. 1982. 128p. 78.00 (*0-8493-0725-2*, RC930, CRC Reprint) Franklin.

Manual for the Laboratory Assistant. Seth A. Morgan. pap. 4.95 (*0-89741-007-6*) Gila River.

Manual for the Medical Officers of the United States Army. Charles Greenleaf. 1992. (American Civil War Medical Ser.: No. 9). 199p. reprint ed. 45.00 (*0-930405-39-0*) Norman SF.

Manual for the Primary Animal Health Care Worker. 1994. LC 96-127666. 326p. (*92-5-103258-0*, F32580) FAO ITA. *Dist:* Bernan Associates.

Manual for the Provision of Intrauterine Devices IUDS. R. Gray. 1980. (Nonserial Publication). 51p. pap. text 10.00 (*92-4-154143-1*, 1150121) World Health.

Manual for the Semistructured Clinical Interview for Children & Adolescents. Stephanie H. McConaughy & Thomas M. Achenbach. 1994. 385p. (Orig.). pap. 25.00 (*0-938565-32-X*) Res Ctr Child.

Manual for the Videofluorographic Study of Swallowing. Jerilyn A. Logemann. 2nd rev. ed. 1993. LC 92-41623. (C). spiral bd. 44.00 (*0-89079-584-3*, 6599) PRO-ED.

Manual for the Youth Self-Report & 1991 Profile. Thomas M. Achenbach. 1991. LC 90-72109. (Illus.). 385p. (Orig.). pap. 25.00 (*0-938565-09-5*) Res Ctr Child.

Manual for Theory & Practice of Counseling & Psychotherapy. Gerald Corey. 5th ed. 1995. LC 95-15144. (Counseling Ser.). 230p. pap., stu. ed. 16.50 (*0-534-33857-7*) Brooks-Cole.

Manual for Theory & Practice of Group Counseling. Gerald Corey. 2nd ed. 1984. (Psychology-Counseling Ser.). 160p. (C). pap. 12.00 (*0-534-03428-4*) Brooks-Cole.

Manual for Ultasonography in Medicine. Jeffrey I. Schwartz. Ed. by Laura Becker. 1996. 209p. (Orig.). text 55.00 (*0-9655671-0-9*) EMI Medical.

Manual Gastro ISE. Gregory L. Eastwood. 1988. 15.95 (*0-316-20399-8*, Little Brwn Med Div) Lppncott W & W.

Manual Gyn Asia. Carol S. Havens. 2nd ed. 1991. 10.95 (*0-316-35099-0*, Little Brwn Med Div) Lppncott W & W.

Manual Gyn-Onc ISE. M. Steven Piver. 1989. 15.95 (*0-316-70937-9*, Little Brwn Med Div) Lppncott W & W.

Manual ICU ISE. James M. Rippe. 2nd ed. 1989. 15.95 (*0-316-74713-0*, Little Brwn Med Div) Lppncott W & W.

Manual Joslin para la Diabetes: The Joslin Guide to Diabetes. Richard S. Beaser & Joan V. Hill. 1996. (SPA.). 352p. per. 15.00 (*0-684-82387-X*, Libros) S&S Trade Pap.

Manual Material Handling: Understanding & Preventing Back Trauma. Ed. by AIHA Ergonomics Committee. 1993. (Illus.). (C). reprint ed. pap. 40.00 (*0-932627-54-4*, 149-ER-89) Am Indus Hygiene.

Manual Medicine: Therapy. W. Schneider et al. 2001. (Illus.). 49.00 (*0-86577-926-0*) Thieme Med Pubs.

Manual Medicine - Diagnostics. Jiri Dvorak et al. 2nd ed. 1990. (Illus.). text 89.00 (*0-86577-306-8*) Thieme Med Pubs.

Manual Medicine - Therapy. Schneider. 1988. (Illus.). 160p. 69.00 (*0-86577-266-5*) Thieme Med Pubs.

Manual Merck de Diagnostico y Terapeutica. Merck and Co., Inc. Staff. Ed. by Robert Berkow. 9th ed. 1994. (SPA.). 3122p. 150.00 (*0-7859-9597-8*) Fr & Eur.

Manual Ocular, No. 3. Deborah Pavan-Langston. 1991. 10.95 (*0-316-69548-3*, Little Brwn Med Div) Lppncott W & W.

Manual of Acute Coronary Care: A Guide to Patient Management. M. J. Walsh. 1999. (Illus.). 118p. pap. text (*1-86036-011-4*) E A GBR. *Dist:* OUP.

Manual of Acute Hand Injuries. Ed. by David S. Martin & E. Dale Collins. 1997. LC 97-17955. (Illus.). 696p. (C). (gr. 13). pap. text 49.95 (*0-8151-5861-0*, 25196) Mosby Inc.

Manual of Acute Orthopaedic Therapeutics. Larry D. Iversen & Marc F. Swiontkowski. 4th ed. 1995. LC 94-22476. 368p. spiral bd. 39.95 (*0-316-43439-6*) Lppncott W & W.

Manual of Acute Orthopaedic Therapeutics: International. Larry D. Iversen. 3rd ed. 1986. 15.95 (*0-316-43433-7*, Little Brwn Med Div) Lppncott W & W.

Manual of Acute Pain Management in Children. Ian M. McKenzie. 1997. LC 97-3034. pap. text (*0-443-05321-9*) Church.

Manual of Admitting Orders & Therapeutics. Eric B. Larson & W. Conrad Lilies, Jr. 3rd ed. 1994. LC 93-26134. pap. text 31.95 (*0-7216-5268-9*) Saunders.

***Manual of Adolescent Substance Abuse Treatment.** Ed. by Todd Wilk Estroff. 2001. LC 2001-22179. 334p. pap. 42.95 (*0-88048-712-7*, 8712) Am Psychiatric.

Manual of Adult & Pediatric Medical Oncology. Ed. by S. Monfardini et al. 1987. (Illus.). 401p. 58.95 (*0-387-15347-0*) Spr-Verlag.

Manual of Advanced Prehospital Care. Gail Walraven. (Illus.). 1978. 430p. pap. text 15.95 (*0-87618-995-8*); 2nd ed. 1984. 416p. pap. text 28.00 (*0-89303-252-2*) P-H.

Manual of Advanced Veterinary Nursing. Alasdair Moore. 2000. (Manual of Veterinary Care Ser.). (Illus.). 250p. pap. text (*0-905214-51-X*) BSAVA GBR. *Dist:* Iowa U Pr.

Manual of Adverse Drug Interactions. J. P. Griffin & P. F. D'Arcy. 5th ed. 1997. LC 97-8345. 664p. 207.00 (*0-444-82406-5*) Elsevier.

Manual of Aesthetic Surgery. Ed. by J.C. Fisher et al. 1985. (Comprehensive Manuals of Surgical Specialties Ser.). (Illus.). 125p. 220.00 (*0-387-96045-7*) Spr-Verlag.

Manual of Aesthetic Surgery, Vol. 1. W. L. Mang. 2001. LC 00-61916. (Illus.). 250p. 215.00 incl. cd-rom (*3-540-66512-9*) Spr-Verlag.

Manual of Allergy & Immunology. Ed. by Glenn J. Lawlor, Jr. et al. 3rd ed. 1995. LC 94-26782. 608p. spiral bd. 39.95 (*0-316-51681-3*, Little Brwn Med Div) Lppncott W & W.

Manual of Ambulatory Care. Ed. by K. R. Epstein. 1995. LC 94-20423. (Illus.). 416p. pap. 44.95 (*0-86542-340-7*) Blackwell Sci.

Manual of Ambulatory General Surgery. Shukri K. Shami & Delilah A. Hassanally. 2000. LC 99-17030. (Illus.). xiii, 140p. (C). (*1-85233-131-3*) Spr-Verlag GBR. *Dist:* Spr-Verlag.

Manual of Ambulatory Pediatrics. Rose W. Boynton. 4th ed. 1998. LC 97-35923. 592p. spiral bd. 39.95 (*0-397-55472-9*) Lppncott W & W.

Manual of Ambulatory Surgery. Ed. by K. J. Kassity. 1982. (Comprehensive Manuals of Surgical Specialties Ser.). (Illus.). 266p. 155.00 (*0-387-90700-9*) Spr-Verlag.

Manual of Anesthesia. John C. Snow. 3rd ed. 1988. (Spiral Manual Ser.). spiral bd. 19.50 (*0-316-80223-9*, Little Brwn Med Div) Lppncott W & W.

Manual of Anesthesiology. John C. Snow. 2nd ed. 1982. 32.95 (*0-316-80222-0*, Little Brwn Med Div) Lppncott W & W.

Manual of Ankle & Foot Arthroscopy. Richard O. Lundeen. 1991. (Manuals in Podiatric Surgery Ser.). (Illus.). 121p. (Orig.). pap. text (*0-443-08694-X*) Church.

Manual of Antenatal Pathology & Hygiene: The Embryo. John W. Ballantyne. 1991. (Classics in Human Development Ser.: Issue 1). 697p. reprint ed. text 75.00 (*1-879554-00-3*) Greenwood-Gene.

Manual of Antibiotics & Infectious Diseases. John E. Conte, Jr. 9th ed. 2001. LC 2001-38998. pap. text 59.95 (*0-7817-2316-7*) Lppncott W & W.

Manual of Aphasia Therapy. Nancy Helm-Estabrooks & Martin L. Albert. 1991. LC 90-5630. (Illus.). 284p. pap. text 31.00 (*0-89079-404-9*, 1588) PRO-ED.

Manual of Arryth Asia. Stephen E. Vlay. 1988. 10.95 (*0-316-90478-3*, Little Brwn Med Div) Lppncott W & W.

Manual of Arryth ISE. Stephen E. Vlay. 1988. 15.95 (*0-316-90477-5*, Little Brwn Med Div) Lppncott W & W.

***Manual of Arthroscopic Surgery.** Michael L. Strobel. 2001. LC 00-69836. (Illus.). 1008p. 299.00 (*3-540-67346-6*) Spr-Verlag.

Manual of Articulation & Phonological Disorders: Infancy Through Adulthood. Ken M. Bleile. 1995. (Clinical Competence Ser.). (Illus.). 404p. (C). spiral bd. 53.95 (*1-56593-343-5*, 0641) Thomson Learn.

Manual of Asthma Management. O'Byrne. 1995. pap. text 52.50 (*0-7020-1781-7*) Saunders.

Manual of Asthma Management. Paul M. O'Byrne & Neil C. Thomson. 2nd ed. 2000. 681p. text, tchr. ed. (*0-7020-2529-1*) W B Saunders GBR. *Dist:* Saunders.

Manual of Athletic Taping: U. S. Version. Sports Medicine Council of British Columbia Staff. 1995. LC 95-180778. (Illus.). 117p. (C). pap. text 24.95 (*0-8036-0115-8*) Davis Co.

Manual of Avian Practice. Agnes E. Rupley. Ed. by Stephanie Donley. 1997. LC 96-34618. (Illus.). 576p. pap. text 49.00 (*0-7216-4083-4*) Saunders.

Manual of Basic Neuropathology. Jacques Poirier et al. 3rd ed. 1990. 292p. pap. text 40.00 (*0-7216-3464-8*) Saunders.

Manual of Bed Oncology. Dennis Albert Casciato. 1988. 10.95 (*0-316-13069-9*, Little Brwn Med Div) Lppncott W & W.

Manual of Biological Markers of Disease. R. N. Maini. Ed. by W. J. Van Venrooij. 1997. LC 96-31174. 744p. (C). lib. bdg. 330.00 (*0-7923-4242-9*) Kluwer Academic.

Manual of Biological Markers of Disease. Ed. by W. J. Van Venrooij. 1997. 744p. (C). pap. text 102.50 (*0-7923-4243-7*) Kluwer Academic.

Manual of Biological Markers of Disease: Basic Work. Ed. by W. J. Van Venrooij. 1996. LC 93-3227. 744p. (C). ring bd. 337.00 (*0-7923-2219-3*) Kluwer Academic.

Manual of Burns. W. S. McDougal et al. 1978. LC 78-18210. (Comprehensive Manuals of Surgical Specialties Ser.). (Illus.). 165p. 107.00 (*0-387-90319-4*) Spr-Verlag.

Manual of Canine & Feline Cardiology. Michael S. Miller & Larry P. Tiley. 2nd ed. 1994. (Illus.). 528p. pap. text 65.00 (*0-7216-5940-3*) Saunders.

Manual of Canine & Feline Cardiology. Larry Patrick Tilley & John-Karl Goodwin. 3rd ed. 1999. LC 00-30092. (Illus.). 575p. (C). text 64.00 (*0-7216-7721-5*) Saunders.

Manual of Canine & Feline Emergency & Critical Care. Ed. by Richard Hammond & Lesley King. 1999. LC 00-362435. (Illus.). viii, 366p. pap. (*0-905214-40-4*) BSAVA GBR. *Dist:* Iowa U Pr.

Manual of Canine & Feline Gastroenterology. Ed. by D. A. Thomas et al. 1996. (Illus.). 268p. pap. 82.95 (*0-8138-1597-5*) Iowa U Pr.

Manual of Canine & Feline Nephrology & Urology. Ed. by John Bainbridge & Jonathan Elliott. 1996. (BSAVA Ser.). (Illus.). 232p. pap. 82.95 (*0-8138-1879-6*) Iowa U Pr.

Manual of Canine & Feline Wound Management & Reconstruction. Ed. by John Williams & David A. Fowler. 1999. (Illus.). 200p. pap. (*0-905214-38-2*) BSAVA GBR. *Dist:* Iowa U Pr.

Manual of Cardiac Anesthesia. Ed. by Stephen J. Thomas & Jan L. Kramer. 2nd ed. 1993. (Illus.). 711p. pap. text (*0-443-08580-3*) Church GBR. *Dist:* Saunders.

Manual of Cardiac Anesthesia. Thomas. 3rd ed. 2000. text 69.00 (*0-443-07922-6*) Saunders.

Manual of Cardiac Surgery. Bradley J. Harland et al. 2nd ed. 1994. LC 93-47190. (Illus.). 378p. 258.00 (*0-387-94220-3*) Spr-Verlag.

Manual of Cardiac Surgery, Vol. I. B. J. Harlan et al. 1980. (Comprehensive Manuals of Surgical Specialties Ser.). (Illus.). 204p. 120.00 (*0-387-90393-3*) Spr-Verlag.

Manual of Cardiac Surgery, Vol. II. B. J. Harlan. 1981. (Comprehensive Manuals of Surgical Specialties Ser.). (Illus.). 143p. 187.00 (*0-387-90563-4*) Spr-Verlag.

Manual of Cardiac Surgical Intensive Care. 144p. pap. (*0-340-52855-9*) E A GBR. *Dist:* Routldge.

Manual of Cardiopulmonary Transplantation. A. Kirk et al. 1993. 80p. pap. text (*0-340-56756-2*) E A GBR. *Dist:* OUP.

Manual of Cardiovascular Anesthesiology. Charles Kingsley & Kane High. 1999. (Illus.). 656p. pap. text 39.95 (*0-07-034773-5*) McGraw-Hill Med Pub.

Manual of Cardiovascular Diagnosis & Therapy. Joseph S. Alpert & James M. Rippe. (Spiral Manual Ser.). 2nd ed. 1985. 426p. spiral bd. 21.00 (*0-316-03510-6*, Little Brwn Med Div); 4th ed. 1996. LC 95-24885. 416p. spiral bd. 39.95 (*0-316-03531-9*) Lppncott W & W.

Manual of Cardiovascular Diagnosis & Therapy, No. 3. Joseph S. Alpert. 1988. 10.95 (*0-316-03521-1*) Little.

Manual of Cardiovascular Medicine. Steven Marso et al. 1999. LC 99-42919. 896p. pap. text 39.95 (*0-683-30685-5*) Lppncott W & W.

Manual of Cataract & Intraocular Lens Surgery. Richard B. Packard & Fiona C. Kinear. 1991. (Illus.). 144p. (*0-443-04091-5*) Church.

Manual of Cataract Surgery. Robert M. Sinskey & Jay V. Patel. 1987. 99p. pap. text 50.00 (*0-7506-9958-2*) Buttrwrth-Heinemann.

Manual of Cataract Surgery. Robert M. Sinsky & Jay V. Patel. 1987. (Illus.). 99p. pap. text (*0-443-08395-9*) Church.

Manual of Chemical Peels: Superficial & Medium Depth. Mark G. Rubin. 1995. 200p. text 125.00 (*0-397-51506-5*) Lppncott W & W.

Manual of Child Development. Sundara Lingham & David R. Harvey. 1988. LC 87-15861. (Manual Ser.). (Illus.). 120p. pap. text (*0-443-03784-1*) Church.

Manual of Child Neurology. Owen B. Evans. 1986. (Illus.). 435p. (Orig.). text (*0-443-08435-1*) Church.

***Manual of Childhood Infections.** E. Graham Davies et al. 2001. (Illus.). 520p. pap. (*0-7020-2626-3*) W B Saunders GBR. *Dist:* Saunders.

Manual of Chiropractic Diagnosis & Therapeutics. National College of Chiropractic Staff. 1993. 500p. pap. 39.95 (*0-8016-6468-3*) Mosby Inc.

Manual of Clinical Child & Adolescent Psychiatry. Ed. by Kenneth S. Robson. 2nd rev. ed. 1994. LC 93-28362. Orig. Title: Manual of Clinical Child Psychiatry. 497p. spiral bd. 44.50 (*0-88048-528-0*, 8528) Am Psychiatric.

Manual of Clinical Child Psychiatry see Manual of Clinical Child & Adolescent Psychiatry

Manual of Clinical Dietetics. Chicago Dietetic Association Staff & South Surburban Dietetic Association Staff. 4th ed. 1992. LC 92-49557. ring bd. 62.00 (*0-88091-108-5*, 0127A) Am Dietetic Assn.

Manual of Clinical Dietetics. Chicago Dietetic Association Staff. 5th ed. 1996. LC 96-36492. 868p. 70.00 (*0-88091-153-0*) Am Dietetic Assn.

Manual of Clinical Evaluation. Mark D. Aronson & Thomas L. Delbanco. 1988. (Brown Spiral Manual Ser.). 350p. 31.95 (*0-316-05210-8*, Little Brwn Med Div) Lppncott W & W.

Manual of Clinical Exercise Testing, Prescription & Rehabilitation. Ziya Altug & Janet L. Hoffman. Ed. by Jerome L. Martin. 1992. LC 92-21898. (Illus.). 336p. (C). pap. text 40.48 (*0-8385-0241-5*, A0241-8) Appleton & Lange.

Manual of Clinical Hematology. Ed. by Joseph J. Mazza. 2nd ed. 1995. LC 94-26649. 496p. spiral bd. 39.95 (*0-316-55220-8*, Little Brwn Med Div) Lppncott W & W.

Manual of Clinical Hospital Psychiatry. Ed. by Ole J. Thienhaus. 2nd ed. 1995. 432p. spiral bd. 48.50 (*0-88048-550-7*, 8550) Am Psychiatric.

Manual of Clinical Hysteroscopy: Diagnostic & Therapeutic. R. F. Valle et al. 1998. LC 97-18022. (Illus.). 160p. 90.95 (*1-85070-641-7*, Parthenon Pbng) CRC Pr.

***Manual of Clinical Laboratory Immunology.** Noel R. Rose et al. 2001. 1,200p. 139.95 (*1-55581-215-5*) ASM Pr.

Manual of Clinical Laparoscopy. Michael P. Diamond et al. 1998. LC 97-18021. (Illus.). 120p. lib. bdg. 79.95 (*1-85070-640-9*, Parthenon Pbng) CRC Pr.

Manual of Clinical Microbiology. Ed. by Patrick R. Murray. 7th rev. ed. 1999. LC 98-46075. (Illus.). 1800p. 149.95 (*1-55581-126-4*) ASM Pr.

Manual of Clinical Nephrology. Jhoong S. Cheich et al. Ed. by Kurt H. Stenzel & Albert L. Rubin. 1981. 470p. text 180.50 (*90-247-2397-3*) Kluwer Academic.

Manual of Clinical Nutrition. Wiley Staff. 1994. 584p. 75.00 (*0-471-34916-X*) Wiley.

Manual of Clinical Oncology. Ed. by Dennis Albert Casciato & Barry B. Lowitz. 3rd ed. 1995. LC 95-9993. 720p. spiral bd. 39.95 (*0-316-13279-9*) Lppncott W & W.

Manual of Clinical Oncology. Dennis Albert Casciato & Barry B. Lowitz. 4th ed. 2000. LC 99-86180. (Illus.). 768p. spiral bd. 39.95 (*0-7817-2159-8*) Lppncott W & W.

Manual of Clinical Oncology. Ed. by Dennis Albert Casciato & Barry Bennett Lowitz. 4th ed. 2000. LC 99-86180. (Illus.). xviii, 750p. (*0-7817-2563-1*) Lppncott W & W.

Manual of Clinical Oncology: UICC International Union Against Cancer. Ed. by R. R. Love et al. 6th ed. 1994. LC 94-37384. (Illus.). 605p. 52.95 (*0-387-58193-6*) Spr-Verlag.

Manual of Clinical Problems in Adult Ambulatory Care: With Annotated Key References. Ed. by Laurie Dornbrand et al. 3rd ed. 1997. LC 97-1675. (Illus.). 800p. spiral bd. 39.95 (*0-316-19038-1*) Lppncott W & W.

Manual of Clinical Problems in Cardiology: With Annotated Key References. David Hillis et al. 5th ed. 1995. LC 94-34559. 592p. spiral bd. 39.95 (*0-316-36493-2*) Lppncott W & W.

Manual of Clinical Problems in Cardiology: With Annotated Key References, No. 3. L. David Hillis. 1987. 15.95 (*0-316-36403-7*) Little.

Manual of Clinical Problems in Infectious Disease. Nelson M. Gantz et al. 2nd ed. 1986. 420p. 28.50 (*0-316-30352-6*, Little Brwn Med Div) Lppncott W & W.

Manual of Clinical Problems in Infectious Disease. Ed. by Nelson M. Gantz. 4th ed. 1999. LC 98-46884. (Spiral Manual Ser.). (Illus.). 544p. spiral bd. 39.95 (*0-7817-1910-0*) Lppncott W & W.

Manual of Clinical Problems in Nephrology. Burton D. Rose & Robert Black. 1988. 375p. 31.95 (*0-316-75637-7*, Little Brwn Med Div) Lppncott W & W.

Manual of Clinical Problems in Neurology: With Annotated Key References. J. P. Mohr. 1984. (Spiral Manual Ser.). spiral bd. 21.00 (*0-316-57747-2*, Little Brwn Med Div) Lppncott W & W.

Manual of Clinical Problems in Obstetrics & Gynecology. Michel E. Rivlin et al. 5th ed. 1999. LC 99-25744. 528p. spiral bd. 39.95 (*0-7817-1723-X*) Lppncott W & W.

Manual of Clinical Problems in Obstetrics & Gynecology: With Annotated Key References. Michael E. Rivlin et al. 2nd ed. 1986. 448p. 22.50 (*0-316-74769-6*, Little Brwn Med Div) Lppncott W & W.

Manual of Clinical Problems in Oncology. Carol S. Portlock & Donald R. Goffinet. 2nd ed. 1986. 27.00 (*0-316-71425-9*, Little Brwn Med Div) Lppncott W & W.

Manual of Clinical Problems in Ophthalmology. John W. Gittinger. 1987. 10.95 (*0-316-31473-0*, Little Brwn Med Div) Lppncott W & W.

Manual of Clinical Problems in Pediatrics. Kenneth B. Roberts. 2nd ed. 1985. spiral bd. 22.50 (*0-316-74990-7*, Little Brwn Med Div) Lppncott W & W.

Manual of Clinical Problems in Pediatrics: With Annotated Key References. Kenneth B. Roberts. 5th ed. 2001. LC 00-42823. (Illus.). xviii, 540p. spiral bd. 39.95 (*0-7817-2893-2*) Lppncott W & W.

Manual of Clinical Problems in Psychiatry. Steven E. Hyman. 1990. 15.95 (*0-316-38725-8*) Little.

Manual of Clinical Problems in Psychiatry. Steven E. Hyman. 1990. 10.95 (*0-316-38723-1*, Little Brwn Med Div) Lppncott W & W.

Manual of Clinical Problems in Psychiatry: With Annotated Key References. Steven E. Hyman. 1990. 34.95 (*0-316-38722-3*, Little Brwn Med Div) Lppncott W & W.

Manual of Clinical Problems in Pulmonary Medicine. Richard A. Bordow. 1991. 10.95 (*0-316-10271-7*, Little Brwn Med Div) Lppncott W & W.

Manual of Clinical Problems in Pulmonary Medicine. Ed. by Richard A. Bordow et al. 2nd ed. 1985. (Spiral Manual Ser.). 24.50 (*0-316-10265-2*, Little Brwn Med Div) Lppncott W & W.

Manual of Clinical Procedures in the Dog & Cat. Stephen Crow. 2nd ed. 1997. 336p. pap. text 37.95 (*0-397-51588-X*) Lppncott W & W.

Manual of Clinical Psychopharmacology. Alan F. Schatzberg et al. 3rd ed. 1997. LC 96-24026. 499p. spiral bd. 52.95 (*0-88048-921-9*, 8921) Am Psychiatric.

M N O

Manual of Clinical Trauma Care: The First Hour. Susan B. Sheehy. 3rd ed. 1998. LC 98-26666. 464p. pap. text 37.95 (*0-323-00305-2*) Mosby Inc.

Manual of Combined Movements: Their Use in the Examination & Treatment of Mechanical VCDs. Brian C. Edwards. 1992. (Illus.). 131p. text (*0-443-04666-2*) Church.

Manual of Common Bedside Surgical Procedures. Herbert Chen et al. 2nd ed. 2000. LC 99-40830. (Illus.). 400p. spiral bd. 26.95 (*0-683-30792-4*) Lppncott W & W.

Manual of Complete Internal Medicine Asia, No. 4. Jerry L. Spivak. 1990. 10.95 (*0-316-80741-9*, Little Brwn Med Div) Lppncott W & W.

Manual of Complete Internal Medicine ISE, No. 4. Jerry L. Spivak. 1990. 15.95 (*0-316-80742-7*, Little Brwn Med Div) Lppncott W & W.

Manual of Complete Neph ISE. Burton D. Rose. 1988. 15.95 (*0-316-75635-0*, Little Brwn Med Div) Lppncott W & W.

Manual of Complete Pediatrics ISE, No. 3. Roberts. 1989. 15.95 (*0-316-74992-3*, Little Brwn Med Div) Lppncott W & W.

Manual of Contact Lens Prescribing & Fitting. Ed. by Milton M. Hom. 2nd ed. 2000. (Illus.). 496p. pap. 59.99 incl. cd-rom (*0-7506-7215-3*) Buttrwrth-Heinemann.

Manual of Cooperative Group Therapy for Aphasia. Jan R. Avent. 1997. LC 97-21508. (Illus.). 174p. pap. text 39.99 (*0-7506-9921-3*) Buttrwrth-Heinemann.

Manual of Cranial Computerized Tomography. K. Y. Chynn & N. Finby. 1982. (Illus.). vi, 106p. 172.25 (*3-8055-3432-9*) S Karger.

Manual of Critical Care Medicine. Ed. by M. H. Weil & P. L. DaLuz. 1978. LC 77-24959. (Illus.). 371p. 118.00 (*0-387-90270-8*) Spr-Verlag.

Manual of Critical Care Nursing. Swearingen. 4th ed. 2000. LC 2001-272268. (Illus.). xix, 796p. text 42.95 (*0-323-00998-0*) Mosby Inc.

***Manual of Critical Care X-Ray Interpretation.** Charles McAllister & Eamonn McAteer. 2001. (Illus.). 315p. pap. (*0-7020-2572-0*) W B Saunders GBR. *Dist:* Saunders.

Manual of Cutaneous Laser Techniques. Tina S. Alster. 2nd ed. 1999. LC 99-43217. (Illus.). 288p. text 149.00 (*0-7817-1960-7*, Lippnctt) Lppncott W & W.

Manual of Darkroom Technique: WHO Basic Radiological System. P. E. Palmer. 1985. (CHI, FRE & SPA.). 25p. pap. text 8.00 (*92-4-154178-4*, 1150238) World Health.

Manual of Dermatologic Therapeutics. Kenneth A. Arndt et al. 5th ed. 1995. LC 94-24451. 400p. spiral bd. 39.95 (*0-316-05175-6*) Lppncott W & W.

Manual of Dermatologic Therapeutics: With Essentials of Diagnosis. Kenneth A. Arndt. 6th ed. 2001. spiral bd. 39.95 (*0-7817-2170-9*) Lppncott W & W.

Manual of Dermatological Therapeutics. Kenneth A. Arndt. 3rd ed. 1983. 19.50 (*0-316-05181-0*, Little Brwn Med Div) Lppncott W & W.

Manual of Dermatology for Developing Countries. Orlando Canizares. 2nd ed. 1993. LC 92-49991. (Illus.). 392p. 85.00 (*0-19-262293-5*) OUP.

Manual of Dermatology in Chinese Medicine. Nissi Wang et al. 1996. LC 94-61962. (Illus.). 381p. (C). text 45.00 (*0-939616-20-3*) Eastland.

Manual of Developmental & Behavioral Problems in Children. Vidya Bhushan Gupta. 1998. LC 98-46421. (Pediatric Habilitation Ser.: Vol. 9). (Illus.). 336p. text 79.75 (*0-8247-1938-7*) Dekker.

Manual of Diagnosis & Professional Practice in Mental Retardation. Ed. by John W. Jacobson & James A. Mulick. 1996. 540p. 39.95 (*1-55798-341-0*) Am Psychol.

Manual of Diagnostic Imaging: A Clinician's Guide to Clinical Problem Solving. William H. Straub. 1984. (Spiral Manual Ser.). 320p. spiral bd. 21.00 (*0-316-81887-9*, Little Brwn Med Div) Lppncott W & W.

Manual of Diagnostic Ultrasound. Ed. by P. E. Palmer. 1995. (FRE & SPA., Illus.). 334p. (C). pap. 65.00 (*92-4-154461-9*, 1150393) World Health.

Manual of Dietetic Practice: Edited for the British Dietetic Association by Briony Thomas. Ed. by Briony Thomas. 2nd ed. 1994. LC 93-20867. (Illus.). 752p. pap. 89.95 (*0-632-03003-8*) Blackwell Sci.

Manual of District Health Management for Uganda. Gilbert Bukenya et al. 1997. LC 97-37032. 128p. pap. 20.00 (*1-56474-251-2*) Fithian Pr.

Manual of Dosimetry in Radiotherapy. John B. Massey. 1970. (Technical Reports: No. 110). (Illus.). (Orig.). pap. (*92-0-115370-8*, IDC110) IAEA AUT. *Dist:* Bernan Associates.

Manual of Drug & Alcohol Abuse: Guidelines for Teaching in Medical & Health Institutions. A. Arif & J. Westmeyer. 1988. LC 88-22414. (Illus.). 350p. (C). text 65.00 (*0-306-42890-3*, Kluwer Plenum) Kluwer Academic.

Manual of Drug Interactions for Anesthesiology. Robery A. Mueller & Dag B. Lundberg. 3rd ed. 1996. LC 96-29164. pap. text (*0-443-07764-9*) Church.

Manual of Electrocardiography. Gilbert H. Mudge, Jr. 1986. spiral bd. 32.95 (*0-316-58918-7*, Little Brwn Med Div) Lppncott W & W.

Manual of Emergency Airway Management. Ron M. Walls et al. 2000. LC 00-22742. 256p. pap. text 49.95 (*0-7817-2616-6*) Lppncott W & W.

Manual of Emergency Care. Susan B. Sheehy & Gail P. Lenehan. 5th ed. 1998. LC 98-8531. 672p. pap. text 42.95 (*0-323-00304-4*) Mosby Inc.

Manual of Emergency Drugs. Bryan E. Bledsoe. 1984. (Illus.). 217p. pap. text 26.00 (*0-89303-647-1*) P-H.

Manual of Emergency Medical Treatment for the Dental Team. Robert J. Braun & Bruce J. Cutilli. 2nd ed. 1998. LC 98-19198. 139p. pap. 30.95 (*0-683-30270-1*) Lppncott W & W.

Manual of Emergency Medicine. George L. Sternbach & Michael Jay Bresler. 6th ed. 1997. LC 97-27604. (Mosby Handbook Ser.). (Illus.). 640p. (C). (gr. 13). pap. text 35.95 (*0-8151-1142-8*, 27233) Mosby Inc.

Manual of Emergency Medicine: Diagnosis & Treatment. Jon L. Jenkins & Joseph Loscalzo. 1986. 493p. 24.50 (*0-316-46052-4*, Little Brwn Med Div) Lppncott W & W.

Manual of Emergency Medicine: Diagnosis & Treatment. Jon L. Jenkins & G. Richard Braen. 4th ed. 2000. LC 99-27742. (Illus.). xv, 672p. spiral bd. 39.95 (*0-7817-1726-4*) Lppncott W & W.

Manual of Emergency Nursing. Judy Selfridge-Thomas. 1995. LC 95-2409. (Illus.). 476p. pap. text 41.00 (*0-7216-5452-5*) Saunders.

Manual of Emergency Orthopaedics. Phillip M. Segelov. 1986. (Illus.). 234p. (Orig.). pap. text (*0-443-03341-2*) Church.

Manual of Emergency Orthopedics. William M. Green et al. 480p. (*0-683-03760-9*) Lppncott W & W.

Manual of Emergency Outpatient Technique, Vol. 1. Klippel. 2nd ed. 1996. (Illus.). 22.95 (*0-316-49869-6*, Little Brwn Med Div) Lppncott W & W.

Manual of Emergency Pediatrics. Ed. by Robert M. Reece. 4th ed. 1992. (Illus.). 586p. pap. text 69.00 (*0-7216-3289-0*) Saunders.

Manual of Endocrine Surgery. A. J. Edis et al. 2nd ed. 1984. (Comprehensive Manuals of Surgical Specialties Ser.). (Illus.). 325p. 187.00 (*0-387-90921-4*) Spr-Verlag.

Manual of Endocrinology & Metabolism. Norman Lavin. 1986. 770p. pap. text 21.00 (*0-316-51651-1*, Little Brwn Med Div) Lppncott W & W.

Manual of Endocrinology & Metabolism. Ed. by Norman Lavin. 2nd ed. 1993. LC 93-874. (Illus.). 736p. spiral bd. 39.95 (*0-316-51657-0*, Little Brwn Med Div) Lppncott W & W.

Manual of Endoscopic Aesthetic Surgery. Oscar M. Ramirez & Rollin K. Daniel. 1994. LC 94-30008. 61p. 291.00 (*0-387-92623-2*) Spr-Verlag.

Manual of English for the Overseas Doctor. Joy E. Parkinson. 4th ed. 1991. (Illus.). 286p. pap. text (*0-443-04188-1*); 5th ed. 1998. LC 98-31755. (*0-443-06136-X*) Church.

Manual of Epidemiology & Epidemiological Services in Malaria Programmes. R. H. Black. 1968. (Illus.). 223p. pap. text 8.00 (*92-4-154015-X*, 1150098) World Health.

Manual of Epidemiology for District Health Management. Ed. by J. P. Vaughan & R. H. Morrow. 1989. (ENG & FRE.). vii, 198p. pap. text 35.00 (*92-4-154404-X*, 1150335) World Health.

Manual of Equine Anaesthesia. K. W. Clarke & P. M. Taylor. 2nd ed. 1998. (Illus.). 194p. pap. text 37.00 (*0-7020-1806-6*) Saunders.

Manual of Equine Emergencies: Treatment & Procedures. James A. Orsini & Thomas J. Divers. Ed. by Stephanie Donley. 6th ed. 1998. LC 97-35784. (Illus.). 592p. (C). text 55.00 (*0-7216-2425-1*) Saunders.

Manual of Equine Neonatal Medicine. John E. Madigan. (Illus.). 2nd rev. ed. 1994. 363p. pap. text 29.95 (*0-9629517-0-6*); 3rd ed. 1997. 415p. pap. 42.00 (*0-9629517-1-4*) Live Oak CA.

Manual of Equine Practice. Reuben J. Rose & David R. Hodgson. 1992. LC 92-21745. (Illus.). 544p. pap. text 72.00 (*0-7216-3739-6*) Saunders.

Manual of Equine Practice. Reuben J. Rose & David R. Hodgson. Ed. by Stephanie Donley. 2nd ed. 1999. LC 98-28631. 750p. text 85.00 (*0-7216-8665-6*) Saunders.

Manual of ERCP. Martin. 1998. (C). text 169.00 (*0-443-05117-8*) Saunders.

Manual of Examination & Treatment of the Spine & Extremities. Carolyn Wadsworth et al. 1988. (Illus.). 229p. pap. 45.00 (*0-683-08600-6*) Lppncott W & W.

Manual of Examination of the Eyes. E. Landolt. 1979. LC 78-20773. (Classics in Ophthalmology Ser.). 328p. reprint ed. lib. bdg. 31.50 (*0-88275-843-8*) Krieger.

Manual of Exercise Testing. Victor F. Froelicher. 2nd ed. 1994. LC 93-38016. (Illus.). 304p. (C). (gr. 13). pap. text 59.00 (*0-8151-3346-4*, 23774) Mosby Inc.

Manual of Experimental Embryology. Viktor Hamburger. rev. ed. 1994. LC 60-14069. (Illus.). lib. bdg. 15.00 (*0-226-31471-5*) U Ch Pr.

Manual of Facial Growth: A Computer Analysis of Longitudinal Cephalometric Growth Data. S. N. Bhatia & B. C. Leighton. 1993. LC 93-2900. (Illus.). 554p. text 230.00 (*0-19-261770-2*) OUP.

Manual of Family Practice. Robert B. Taylor. 1996. LC 96-271. 592p. spiral bd. 36.95 (*0-316-83390-8*, Little Brwn Med Div) Lppncott W & W.

Manual of Feline Behaviour. Peter Neville & Valerie O'Farrell. Ed. by Christopher S. Ross. 1994. (Illus.). 84p. pap. text (*0-905214-24-2*) BSAVA GBR. *Dist:* Iowa U Pr.

Manual of First-Aid Practices for School Bus Drivers. William R. Nesbitt. 1998. (Illus.). 80p. pap. text 20.00 (*0-7881-7122-4*) DIANE Pub.

Manual of Free Flaps. Russell & Zamboni. 1999. (Illus.). 320p. (C). (gr. 13). text 195.00 (*0-8151-9013-1*, 29110) Mosby Inc.

Manual of Gastroenterologic Procedures. Ed. by Douglas A. Drossman. 3rd ed. 1992. LC 92-17142. (Illus.). 304p. spiral bd. 49.95 (*0-88167-944-5*, 2424) Lppncott W & W.

Manual of Gastroenterology: Diagnosis & Therapy. Gregory L. Eastwood & Canan Avunduk. 2nd ed. 1994. LC 93-47188. 512p. spiral bd. 45.00 (*0-316-19992-3*, Little Brwn Med Div) Lppncott W & W.

Manual of Gastrointestinal Fluoroscopy: Performance of Procedures. David J. Ott et al. 1996. (Illus.). 212p. (C). text 55.95 (*0-398-06555-1*) C C Thomas.

Manual of Gastrointestinal Procedures. Society of Gastroenterology Staff. Ed. by Kathleen G. Domkowski & Nancy S. Schlossberg. 4th rev. ed. 2000. (Illus.). x, 236p. spiral bd. 85.00 (*0-9702133-0-1*) Scty Gastro.

Manual of Gastrointestinal Procedures Pediatric Supplement: A Publication of the Society of Gastroenterology Nurses & Associates. Nancy Rayhorn. 2nd ed. 1995. 35p. pap. text 21.95 (*0-683-07182-3*) Lppncott W & W.

Manual of Gerontologic Nursing. Charlotte Eliopoulos. 2nd ed. 1998. LC 98-17792. 416p. 34.95 (*0-323-00177-7*) Mosby Inc.

Manual of GI Fluoroscopy. Bruce R. Javors. 1996. (Illus.). 232p. pap. 29.90 (*0-86577-607-5*) Thieme Med Pubs.

Manual of Gynecologic Surgery. B. J. Masterson. 2nd ed. 1986. (Comprehensive Manuals of Surgical Specialties Ser.). (Illus.). 379p. 357.00 (*0-387-96193-3*) Spr-Verlag.

Manual of Gynecology. Carol S. Havens. 3rd ed. 1995. 32.95 (*0-316-35014-1*) Little.

Manual of Gynecology, No. 3. Michael E. Rivlin. 1990. 15.95 (*0-316-74773-4*, Little Brwn Med Div) Lppncott W & W.

Manual of Haematology. Annabelle S. Baughan et al. 1986. LC 85-11286. (Illus.). 274p. pap. text (*0-443-02564-9*) Church.

Manual of High-Risk Pregnancy & Delivery. Elizabeth Stepp Gilbert & Judith S. Harmon. 2nd ed. 1998. LC 97-46588. (Illus.). 848p. (C). (gr. 13). pap. text 36.95 (*0-8151-4462-8*, 30688) Mosby Inc.

Manual of Histological Techniques. John D. Bancroft & Harry C. Cook. 1984. (Illus.). 274p. (Orig.). pap. text (*0-443-02870-2*) Church.

Manual of Histological Techniques & Their Diagnostic Applications. John D. Bancroft & Harry C. Cook. 2nd ed. 1994. LC 93-35533. text (*0-443-04534-8*) Church.

Manual of HIV - AIDS Therapy, 1997 Edition: Current Clinical Strategies. Douglas C. Princeton. 2nd ed. 1997. 102p. pap. 12.75 (*1-881528-05-7*) Current Clin Strat.

Manual of HIV Therapeutics. Ed. by William G. Powderly. 2000. LC 00-42824. (*0-7817-2551-8*) Lppncott W & W.

Manual of HIV Therapeutics. William G. Powderly. 2nd ed. 2001. LC 00-42824. (Illus.). 288p. spiral bd. 39.95 (*0-7817-3011-2*) Lppncott W & W.

Manual of HIV/AIDS Therapy for PDAs & Desktops: 2001. Douglas C. Princeton. rev. ed. 2000. (Current Clinical Strategies Ser.). 83p. pap. 28.95 incl. cd-rom (*1-881528-88-X*) Current Clin Strat.

Manual of Home Care for Arthritis. Judith K. Sands. 1989. pap. text 35.95 (*0-8273-4353-1*) Delmar.

Manual of Home Care Nursing Orientation. Carolyn J. Humphrey & Paula Milone-Nuzzo. 1995. LC 95-21179. 392p. ring bd. 159.00 (*0-8342-0512-2*, S147) Aspen Pub.

Manual of Home Health Nursing Procedures. Robyn Rice. 1994. (Illus.). 400p. (C). (gr. 13). text 115.00 (*0-8016-6945-6*, 06945) Mosby Inc.

Manual of Home Health Nursing Procedures: Update. Robyn Rice. 1998. (Illus.). 400p. (*1-55664-414-0*) Mosby Inc.

Manual of Hospital Administration. Howard S. Rowland & Beatrice L. Rowland. 1992. LC 92-10857. ring bd. 275.00 (*0-8342-0324-3*) Aspen Pub.

Manual of Hospital Paediatrics. Garry Hambleton. 1988. (Illus.). 360p. (Orig.). pap. text (*0-443-03512-1*) Church.

Manual of Human Resources & Labor Negotiations in Nursing. Flarey. 1997. (Professional Reference - Nursing Ser.). (C). text 74.95 (*0-8273-6690-6*) Delmar.

Manual of Hydrotherapy & Massage. Fred B. Moor et al. 1964. LC 64-23214. 169p. 12.99 (*0-8163-0023-2*, 13160-7) Pacific Pr Pub Assn.

Manual of Hypertension. J. D. Swales. 1995. LC 94-30757. (Illus.). 200p. pap. 52.95 (*0-86542-861-1*) Blackwell Sci.

Manual of I. V. Therapeutics. Lynn D. Phillips. 2nd ed. 1997. LC 96-40183. (Illus.). 644p. (C). pap. text 29.95 (*0-8036-0131-X*) Davis Co.

Manual of I. V. Therapeutics. Lynn Dianne Phillips. 3rd ed. 2001. (Illus.). 848p. (C). pap. 34.95 incl. cd-rom (*0-8036-0808-X*) Davis Co.

Manual of Immunocytochemical Techniques. K. J. Morrell et al. 1997. (Illus.). 208p. text (*0-443-04861-4*) Church.

Manual of Immunology Asia, No. 2. Glenn J. Lawlor, Jr. 1987. 10.95 (*0-316-51669-4*, Little Brwn Med Div) Lppncott W & W.

Manual of Immunology ISE, No. 2. Glenn J. Lawlor, Jr. 1987. 15.95 (*0-316-51667-8*, Little Brwn Med Div) Lppncott W & W.

Manual of Infection Control in Respiratory Care. Arthur J. McLaughlin. 1983. 179p. spiral bd. 27.50 (*0-316-56096-0*, Little Brwn Med Div) Lppncott W & W.

Manual of Instructions for Enlisting & Discharging Soldiers. Roberts S. Bartholow. 1991. (American Civil War Medical Ser.: No. 6). 276p. reprint ed. 45.00 (*0-930405-37-4*) Norman SF.

Manual of Intensive Care Medicine. James M. Rippe & Marie Csete. 1983. (Spiral Manual Ser.). 465p. spiral bd. 22.50 (*0-316-74708-4*, Little Brwn Med Div) Lppncott W & W.

Manual of Intensive Care Medicine: With Annotated Key References. Richard S. Irwin & James M. Rippe. 3rd ed. 2000. LC 99-87836. 960p. spiral bd. 39.95 (*0-7817-1986-0*) Lppncott W & W.

Manual of Internal Fixation. M. E. Mueller et al. 2nd rev. ed. 1979. LC 78-20743. (Illus.). 230.00 (*3-540-92113-3*) Spr-Verlag.

Manual of Internal Fixation. Ed. by M. E. Muller et al. 3rd rev. ed. 1995. (Illus.). 750p. 249.00 (*0-387-52523-8*) Spr-Verlag.

Manual of Internal Fixation in Small Animals. Ed. by H. P. Berlien & P. P. Schmittenbecher. 2nd enl. rev. ed. 1997. LC 97-20200. (Illus.). 286p. 250.00 (*3-540-63000-7*) Spr-Verlag.

Manual of Internal Fixation in the Cranio-Facial Skeleton: Techniques As Recommended by the AO/ASIF-Maxillofacial Group. Ed. by J. Prein. 1997. LC 97-35559. (Illus.). 227p. 185.00 (*3-540-61810-4*) Spr-Verlag.

Manual of Internal Fixation of the Spine. Ed. by John S. Thalgott & Max Aebi. 1995. (Principles & Techniques in Spine Surgery Ser.). 320p. text 169.00 (*0-397-51621-5*) Lppncott W & W.

Manual of Internal Medicine. Jerry L. Spivak. 4th ed. 1990. 32.95 (*0-316-80738-9*, Little Brwn Med Div) Lppncott W & W.

Manual of Introductory Clinical Medicine. Roger M. Macklis. 1984. 26.90 (*0-316-54248-2*) Little.

Manual of IV Medications. Lynn D. Phillips & Merrily A. Kuhn. 2nd ed. 1998. LC 98-2987. 784p. spiral bd. 31.95 (*0-7817-1546-6*) Lppncott W & W.

Manual of Lab & Diagnostic Tests for Nursing. Wilson. 1997. (Illus.). spiral bd. (*0-316-94410-6*) Lppncott W & W.

Manual of Laboratory & Diagnostic Tests. Frances T. Fischbach. 6th ed. 1999. LC 99-27740. (Illus.). 1,312p. pap. text 36.95 (*0-7817-1969-0*) Lppncott W & W.

Manual of Laparoscopic Surgery. Christian Klaiber & Joseph B. Petelin. 1993. LC 92-48741. (Illus.). 264p. 146.00 (*0-88937-091-5*) Hogrefe & Huber Pubs.

Manual of Liver Surgery. W. P. Longmire, Jr. & R. K. Tompkins. 1981. (Comprehensive Manuals of Surgical Specialties Ser.). (Illus.). 267p. 214.00 (*0-387-90212-0*) Spr-Verlag.

Manual of Lower Extremities Orthotics. Miles H. Anderson. 1978. (Illus.). 552p. 91.95 (*0-398-02217-8*) C C Thomas.

Manual of Lower Gastrointestinal Surgery. C. E. Welch et al. 1980. LC 79-9534. (Comprehensive Manuals of Surgical Specialties Ser.). (Illus.). 276p. 185.00 (*0-387-90205-8*) Spr-Verlag.

Manual of Mammalogy. Anthony F. DeBlase & Robert E. Martin. 2nd ed. 1980. 448p. (C). spiral bd. 40.63 (*0-697-04591-9*) McGrw-H Hghr Educ.

Manual of Materia Medica & Pharmacology. David M. Culbreth. 7th ed. 1996. 667p. reprint ed. pap. 35.00 (*0-7873-0229-5*) Hlth Research.

Manual of Maternal-Newborn Nursing. Patricia A. Dunn. 1996. LC 96-3206. 450p. spiral bd. 31.95 (*0-316-19659-2*) Lppncott W & W.

Manual of Medical Care. R. Timothy Coussons. 4th ed. 1990. 34.95 (*0-316-77493-6*, Little Brwn Med Div) Lppncott W & W.

Manual of Medical Care Asia, No. 4. R. Timothy Coussons. 1990. 10.95 (*0-316-77490-1*, Little Brwn Med Div) Lppncott W & W.

Manual of Medical Care of the Surgical Patient. Solomon Papper et al. 3rd ed. 1985. 304p. 24.50 (*0-316-69058-9*, Little Brwn Med Div) Lppncott W & W.

Manual of Medical Manipulation. Loic Burn. 1994. 128p. (C). pap. text 47.00 (*0-7923-8839-9*) Kluwer Academic.

Manual of Medical Mycology. John T. Crissey et al. 1995. LC 94-3339. (Illus.). 300p. 79.95 (*0-86542-363-6*) Blackwell Sci.

Manual of Medical Nutrition Therapy. Crozer-Chester Medical Center Clinical Nutrition S. 4th ed. 1998. 376p. ring bd. 100.00 (*0-9662274-0-9*) Crozer-Keystone.

Manual of Medical Procedures. Ed. by Michael J. Ford. 1987. (Illus.). 204p. pap. (*0-443-03598-9*) Church.

Manual of Medical Procedures. Paul M. Suratt & Robert S. Gibson. 1982. LC 82-3457. (Illus.). 400p. (C). (gr. 13). spiral bd. 27.95 (*0-8016-4850-5*, 04850) Mosby Inc.

Manual of Medical-Surgical Nursing. Debra Daly-Gawenda. 1996. LC 96-9848. (Nursing Fact Finder Ser.). 700p. spiral bd. 32.95 (*0-316-21792-1*) Lppncott W & W.

Manual of Medical Surgical Nursing Care: Interventions & Collaborative Management. Pamela L. Swearingen & Dennis G. Ross. 1999. (Illus.). 896p. 3rd ed. pap. (*84-8086-150-9*); 4th ed. pap. (*84-8174-465-4*) Mosby-Doyma Libros ESP. *Dist:* Mosby Inc.

Manual of Medical Surgical Nursing Care: Interventions & Collaborative Management. No. 4. Pamela L. Swearingen. 4th ed. 1998. LC 98-22562. (Illus.). 896p. (C). (gr. 13). pap. text 36.95 (*0-8151-2744-8*, 31305) Mosby Inc.

Manual of Medical Therapeutics. Washington University Department of Medicine et al. 25th ed. 1986. 500p. 22.50 (*0-316-92393-1*, Little Brwn Med Div) Lppncott W & W.

Manual of Medical Therapeutics. 28th ed. 1996. 99.95 (*1-56712-266-3*, F0300) Franklin Elect.

Manual of Medical Therapy. No. 26. Washington University Department of Medicine. 1989. 24.50 (*0-316-92400-8*, Little Brwn Med Div) Lppncott W & W.

Manual of Medical Therapy Asia. Washington University Department of Medicine. 26th ed. 1989. 10.95 (*0-316-92390-7*, Little Brwn Med Div) Lppncott W & W.

Manual of Medicinal Poisoning. V. Anantharaman & P. P. Tan. 1995. 280p. text 61.00 (*981-02-1093-0*) World Scientific Pub.

Manual of Medicine. Rodes. 1995. (SPA.). 73.00 (*84-458-0093-0*, Little Brwn Med Div) Lppncott W & W.

Manual of Mental & Physical Tests Guy M. Whipple. 1974. LC 73-2997. (Classics in Psychology Ser.). reprint ed. 47.95 (*0-405-05169-7*) Ayer.

Manual of Mental Subnormality. Roberto Moran. 1968. (SPA.). 482p. 7.00 (*0-8477-2900-1*) U of PR Pr.

Manual of Methods & Identification of Toxins in Seafood & Seafood Products. Mark L. Tamplin. 1999. 90.00 (*0-8493-8975-5*, 8975) CRC Pr.

Manual of Microcomputers Speech Language Pathology & Audiology. Katz. 1998. 27.00 net. (*1-56593-230-7*) Singular Publishing.

Manual of Microsurgery on the Laboratory Rat. Pt. 1. Ed. by J. J. Van Dongen et al. 1990. (Techniques in the Behavioral & Neural Sciences Ser.: No. 4). (Illus.). 294p. 210.00 (*0-444-81138-9*) Elsevier.

Manual of Microsurgery on the Laboratory Rat, Pt. 1. J. J. Van Dongen & R. Remie. 1990. (Techniques in the Behavioral & Neural Sciences Ser.: Vol. 4). 312p. pap. 66.50 (*0-444-81139-7*, TBN 4) Elsevier.

Manual of Middle Ear Surgery. Set. Mirkos Tos. 2000. 1480p. 427.00 (*0-86577-820-5*) Thieme Med Pubs.

Manual of Middle Ear Surgery Vol. 1: Approaches, Myringoplasty, Ossiculoplasty & Tympanoplasty. Vol. 1. M. Tos. 1993. (Illus.). 413p. 159.00 (*0-86577-498-6*) Thieme Med Pubs.

Manual of Middle Ear Surgery Vol. 2: Mastoid Surgery & Reconstructive Procedures. Vol. 2. M. Tos. 1995. (Illus.). 448p. 159.00 (*0-86577-589-3*) Thieme Med Pubs.

Manual of Middle Ear Surgery Vol. 3: External Auditory Canal. Vol. 3. Mirkos Tos. 1997. (Illus.). 384p. 149.00 (*0-86577-608-3*) Thieme Med Pubs.

Manual of Military Surgery. Samuel D. Gross. 1988. LC 88-60872. (American Civil War Surgery Ser.: No. 1). 186p. reprint ed. 45.00 (*0-930405-04-8*) Norman SF.

Manual of Military Surgery: Prepared for the Use of the Confederate States Army. Intro. by Samuel P. Moore & Ira M. Rutkow. 1989. LC 88-60874. (American Civil War Surgery Ser.: No. 2). (Illus.). 297p. reprint ed. 75.00 (*0-930405-14-5*) Norman SF.

Manual of Minor Surgery. John H. Packard. 1989. LC 88-60670. (American Civil War Surgery Ser.: No. 10). 288p. reprint ed. 45.00 (*0-930405-08-0*) Norman SF.

Manual of Monocular Subjective Refraction. Harry Freeman. 1989. (C). (*0-9507635-0-0*) Assn Brit Dispen Opticians GBR. *Dist:* St Mut.

Manual of Morphometry in Diagnostic Pathology. J. P. Baak & J. Oort. 1983. (Illus.). 230p. 78.95 (*0-387-11431-9*) Spr-Verlag.

Manual of Nail Disease & Surgery. Robert Baran et al. 2nd ed. 1997. LC 97-5904. (Illus.). 112p. pap. 83.95 (*0-86542-638-4*) Blackwell Sci.

Manual of Nail Disorders. P. Rich. 2001. 250p. 75.00 (*1-84214-035-3*, Parthenon Pbng) CRC Pr.

Manual of Natural Therapy: A Practical Guide to Alternative Medicine. Moshe Olshevsky et al. 1999. (Illus.). 386p. reprint ed. lib. bdg. 39.95 (*0-7351-0088-8*) Replica Bks.

Manual of Neonatal Care. John P. Cloherty & Ann R. Stark. 2nd ed. 1985. 688p. 25.50 (*0-316-14756-7*, Little Brwn Med Div) Lppncott W & W.

Manual of Neonatal Care. Ed. by John P. Cloherty & Ann R. Stark. 4th ed. 1997. LC 97-22777. (Illus.). 800p. spiral bd. 39.95 (*0-316-14765-6*) Lppncott W & W.

Manual of Neonatal Emergency X-Ray Interpretation. P. W. Meerstadt & Catherine Gyll. 1995. (Illus.). 301p. pap. text (*0-7020-1567-9*) W B Saunders GBR. *Dist:* Saunders.

Manual of Neonatal Intensive Care. N. R. Robertson. 3rd ed. 1993. 432p. pap. (*0-340-55572-6*) E A GBR. *Dist:* OUP.

*__Manual of Neonatal Intensive Care.__ N. R. C. Roberton & J. Rennie. 4th ed. 2001. (Arnold Publication). (Illus.). 496p. pap. text 29.95 (*0-340-72010-7*) OUP.

Manual of Neonatal Respiratory Care. Ed. by Sunil K. Sinha & Steven M. Donn. 2000. LC 99-39510. (Illus.). 600p. 89.00 (*0-87993-444-1*) Futura Pub.

Manual of Nephrology. Robert W. Schrier. 2nd ed. 1985. (Diagnosis & Therapy Ser.). 291p. 22.50 (*0-316-77478-2*, Little Brwn Med Div) Lppncott W & W.

Manual of Nephrology. Ed. by Robert W. Schrier. 5th ed. 1999. LC 99-33657. (Illus.). 320p. spiral bd. 39.95 (*0-7817-2172-5*) Lppncott W & W.

Manual of Nerve Conduction Studies. Ralph M. Buschbacher. 1999. (Illus.). 304p. pap. text 52.95 (*1-888799-36-6*) Demos Medical.

Manual of Nerve Conduction Velocity & Clinical Neurophysiology. Joel A. DeLisa et al. 3rd ed. 1994. LC 93-21370. 512p. spiral bd. 69.95 (*0-7817-0138-4*) Lppncott W & W.

Manual of Neural Therapy According to Huneke: Therapy with Local Anesthetics. Peter Dosch. 1985. (Illus.). 498p. (*3-7760-0702-8*) K F Haug Pubs DEU. *Dist:* Medicina Bio.

Manual of Neurologic Emergencies. Feske. 2001. 256p. pap. 35.00 (*0-7506-9838-1*) Buttrwrth-Heinemann.

Manual of Neurologic Therapeutics. Martin A. Samuels. 6th ed. 1998. LC 98-41269. 512p. spiral bd. 39.95 (*0-7817-1645-4*) Lppncott W & W.

Manual of Neurologic Therapeutics: With Essentials of Diagnosis. Martin A. Samuels. 3rd ed. 1986. (Spiral Manual Ser.). spiral bd. 22.50 (*0-316-76992-4*, Little Brwn Med Div) Lppncott W & W.

Manual of Neurology. J. P. Mohr. 2nd ed. 1989. 32.95 (*0-316-57748-0*, Little Brwn Med Div) Lppncott W & W.

Manual of Neurology Asia. No. 4. Martin A. Samuels. 1990. 10.95 (*0-316-76999-1*, Little Brwn Med Div) Lppncott W & W.

Manual of Neurology ISE. J. P. Mohr. 2nd ed. 1989. 15.95 (*0-316-57749-9*, Little Brwn Med Div) Lppncott W & W.

Manual of Neurology ISE. No. 4. Martin A. Samuels. 1990. 15.95 (*0-316-77001-9*, Little Brwn Med Div) Lppncott W & W.

Manual of Neurology NSG. Nancy Swift-Bandin & Ban. 2nd ed. 1982. 16.00 (*0-316-82541-7*) Little.

Manual of Newborn Care Plans. Mary L. Rang. 1981. (Spiral Manual Ser.). 14.00 (*0-316-73380-6*, Little Brwn Med Div) Lppncott W & W.

Manual of Normal Neonatal Care. N. R. Robertson. 2nd ed. 1996. (Arnold Publication). 368p. pap. 27.95 (*0-340-61375-0*) OUP.

Manual of Nuclear Medicine Imaging. Christopher C. Kuni & Rene P. Du Cret. 1996. LC 96-48078. (Illus.). 336p. pap. text 35.00 (*0-86577-568-0*) Thieme Med Pubs.

Manual of Nuclear Medicine Procedures. Ed. by James E. Carey et al. 4th ed. 1983. 248p. 139.00 (*0-8493-0708-2*, R78, CRC Reprint) Franklin.

*__Manual of Nursing.__ Vol. 1. (Illus.). pap. (*0-7021-2046-4*) Juta & Co ZAF. *Dist:* Intl Spec Bk.

Manual of Nursing Diagnosis, 1997-1998. Marjory Gordon. 1996. 512p. (C). (gr. 13). text 24.00 (*0-8151-3494-0*, 27933) Mosby Inc.

Manual of Nursing Staff Development. Brown & Stewart. 1995. (Illus.). 432p. (C). (gr. 13). text 98.00 (*0-8016-6609-0*, 06609) Mosby Inc.

Manual of Nursing Therapeutics: Applying Nursing Diagnoses to Medical Disorders. Pamela L. Swearingen. 1986. 556p. (C). pap. text 22.95 (*0-201-12940-X*, Health Sci) Addison-Wesley.

Manual of Nutritional Therapeutics. David H. Alpers. 3rd ed. 1995. (Spiral Manual Ser.). 624p. spiral bd. 39.95 (*0-316-03524-6*) Lppncott W & W.

Manual of Obstetric & Gynecologic Ultrasound. Richard Jaffe & Jacques S. Abramowicz. 1997. LC 96-53903. 336p. pap. text 49.95 (*0-397-51595-2*) Lppncott W & W.

Manual of Obstetrics. Arthur T. Evans & Kenneth R. Niswander. 6th ed. 2000. LC 99-48129. (Illus.). 560p. spiral bd. 39.95 (*0-7817-2404-X*) Lppncott W & W.

Manual of Obstetrics: Diagnosis & Therapy. Kenneth R. Niswander. 3rd ed. 1987. spiral bd. 22.50 (*0-316-61139-5*, Little Brwn Med Div) Lppncott W & W.

Manual of Obstetrics Asia. Kenneth R. Niswander. No. 3. 1987. 10.95 (*0-316-61135-2*); No. 4. 1991. 10.95 (*0-316-61171-9*) Lppncott W & W (Little Brwn Med Div).

Manual of Obstetrics ISE. No. 3. Kenneth R. Niswander. 1987. 15.95 (*0-316-61136-0*, Little Brwn Med Div) Lppncott W & W.

Manual of Ocular Diagnosis & Therapy. Deborah Pavan-Langston. 2nd ed. 1985. 494p. 24.50 (*0-316-69544-0*, Little Brwn Med Div) Lppncott W & W.

Manual of Ocular Diagnosis & Therapy. Ed. by Deborah Pavan-Langston. 4th ed. 1995. LC 95-31695. 506p. spiral bd. 39.95 (*0-316-69534-3*, Little Brwn Med Div) Lppncott W & W.

Manual of Ocular Diagnosis for Asia. Deborah Pavan-Langston. 1995. 32.95 (*0-316-69560-2*) Little.

Manual of Oculoplastic Surgery. Mark Levine. 2nd ed. 1996. LC 96-9211. (Illus.). 336p. text 79.99 (*0-7506-9634-6*, Focal) Buttrwrth-Heinemann.

Manual of Ophthalmology. John W. Gittinger. 1987. 15.95 (*0-316-31472-2*, Little Brwn Med Div) Lppncott W & W.

Manual of Oral & Maxillofacial Surgery. Massachusetts General Hospital Staff. Ed. by R. Bruce Donoff. 3rd ed. 1996. (Illus.). 448p. (C). (gr. 13). text 46.95 (*0-8151-2755-3*, 26586) Mosby Inc.

Manual of Orbital & Lacrimal Surgery. Alan A. McNab. 1994. LC 93-36802. (Illus.). 116p. text (*0-443-04791-X*) Church.

Manual of Orbital Lacrimal Surgery. McNab. 4th ed. 1998. 160p. pap. text 65.00 (*0-7506-3997-0*) Buttrwrth-Heinemann.

Manual of Organic Materia Medica: Drugs from Natural Sources. J. M. Maisch. 1992. (Alternative Medicine Ser.). lib. bdg. 275.95 (*0-8490-5441-9*) Gordon Pr.

Manual of Organizational Development: The Psychology of Change. Claire Huffington et al. 1997. 112p. pap. (*1-85575-128-3*) Karnac Bks GBR. *Dist:* Other Pr LLC.

Manual of Orthopaedic Terminology. No. 6. Carolyn T. Blauvelt & Fred Nelson. 6th ed. 1998. LC 98-10711. (Illus.). 475p. (C). (gr. 13). pap. text 36.95 (*0-8151-2787-1*, 31249) Mosby Inc.

Manual of Orthopedic Anesthesia & Related Pain Syndromes. Ralph L. Bernstein & Andrew D. Rosenberg. 1993. (Illus.). 496p. (Orig.). pap. text (*0-443-08843-8*) Church.

Manual of Otolaryngology: Diagnosis & Therapy. Strome Marshall. 1985. 212p. 25.50 (*0-316-81967-0*, Little Brwn Med Div) Lppncott W & W.

Manual of Outpatient Gynecology. Patti Tilton et al. 1986. 280p. 25.50 (*0-316-35097-4*, Little Brwn Med Div); 3rd ed. 1995. LC 95-16986. 320p. spiral bd. 39.95 (*0-316-35000-1*) Lppncott W & W.

Manual of Paediatric Dentistry. R. J. Andlaw & W. P. Rock. 4th ed. 1998. LC 96-39210. (C). pap. text (*0-443-05372-3*) Church.

Manual of Pain Management. Carol A. Warfield & Hilary Fausett. 2nd ed. 2001. pap. text 59.95 (*0-7817-2313-2*) Lppncott W & W.

Manual of Panic-Focused Psychodynamic Psychotherapy. Barbara Milrod et al. 1997. LC 96-41407. 128p. text 29.00 (*0-88048-871-9*, 8871) Am Psychiatric.

Manual of Patient Care in Neurosurgery. James R. Howe. 2nd ed. 1983. 22.50 (*0-316-37575-6*, Little Brwn Med Div) Lppncott W & W.

Manual of Patient Care Standards. Anne MacGuire. ring bd. 249.00 (*0-87189-765-2*, S15) Aspen Pub.

Manual of Pediatric Anesthesia. David J. Steward. 3rd ed. 1990. (Illus.). 446p. pap. text (*0-443-08573-0*); 4th ed. 1994. LC 94-34674. pap. text (*0-443-08942-6*) Church.

Manual of Pediatric Critical Care. Mary F. Hazinski. 1998. (Illus.). 700p. (C). (gr. 13). pap. text 39.95 (*0-8151-4230-7*, 24849) Mosby Inc.

Manual of Pediatric Critical Care. Narendra C. Singh. Ed. by Judy Fletcher. 1997. LC 96-7417. (Illus.). 448p. pap. text 42.00 (*0-7216-5949-7*) Saunders.

Manual of Pediatric Gastroenterology. Joseph F. Fitzgerald & Joseph H. Clark. 1988. (Illus.). 216p. pap. text (*0-443-08538-2*) Church.

Manual of Pediatric Gastroenterology & Nutrition. John H. Tripp & David C. Candy. 2nd ed. 1992. (Illus.). 192p. pap. text (*0-7506-1325-4*) E A GBR. *Dist:* OUP.

Manual of Pediatric Hematology & Oncology. Philip Lanzkowsky. 2nd ed. 1994. LC 94-32744. text (*0-443-08969-8*) Church.

Manual of Pediatric Intensive Care. Haresh M. Kirpalani et al. 1999. 300p. pap. (*1-55009-089-5*) DEKR.

Manual of Pediatric Nursing. Ed. by Janet M. Brucker & Kelly D. Wallin. 1996. LC 95-52479. (Peds Fact Finder Ser.). 450p. spiral bd. 29.95 (*0-316-11451-0*) Lppncott W & W.

Manual of Pediatric Nursing Practice. Massachusetts General Hospital Department of Nursi. Ed. by Barbara H. Pikl. 1981. pap. 16.00 (*0-316-54959-2*, Little Brwn Med Div) Lppncott W & W.

Manual of Pediatric Nutrition. Kristy M. P. Hendricks et al. 3rd ed. 1999. LC 2001-266340. (Illus.). xii, 596p. pap. (*1-55009-091-7*) DEKR.

Manual of Pediatric Nutrition. Wiley Staff. 3rd ed. 1997. 555p. pap. 59.95 (*1-56561-118-7*) Wiley.

Manual of Pediatric Therapeutics. Ed. by John W. Graef. 6th ed. 1997. LC 97-1436. (Illus.). 656p. spiral bd. 39.95 (*0-316-14171-2*) Lppncott W & W.

Manual of Pediatrics Emergency Nursing. Treesa E. Soud & Janice Steiner Rogers. 1997. LC 97-14312. (Illus.). 792p. (C). (gr. 13). pap. text 39.95 (*0-8016-7891-9*, 07891) Mosby Inc.

Manual of Pelvic Surgery. Ed. by M. J. Webb. 1994. (Illus.). 195p. 145.00 (*0-387-56865-4*) Spr-Verlag.

Manual of Perinatal Anesthesia & Critical Care. Diaz. 1991. (Illus.). 416p. pap. text 64.00 (*0-7216-1874-X*) Saunders.

Manual of Perioperative Care in Cardiac & Thoracic Surgery. Robert M. Bojar. 2nd ed. 1994. LC 93-31153. (Illus.). 512p. pap. 44.95 (*0-86542-347-4*) Blackwell Sci.

Manual of Perioperative Care in Cardiac Surgery. Robert M. Bojar & Kenneth G. Warner. 3rd ed. 1998. LC 98-33471. (Illus.). pap. 56.95 (*0-632-04365-2*) Blackwell Sci.

Manual of Peritoneal Dialysis. G. A. Coles. 1988. (C). pap. text 72.50 (*0-7462-0081-1*) Kluwer Academic.

Manual of Physical Medicine & Rehabilitation. Tan. 1997. LC 97-22255. (Illus.). 848p. (C). (gr. 13). text 36.95 (*0-8151-8708-4*, 25352) Mosby Inc.

Manual of Physical Status & Performance in Childhood Vol. 2: Physical Performance. Ed. by Alex F. Roche & Robert M. Malina. 1983. LC 82-16515. 814p. 145.00 (*0-306-41137-7*, Plenum Trade) Perseus Pubng.

Manual of Physical Therapy. Ed. by Otto D. Payton et al. 1989. (Illus.). 761p. text (*0-443-08499-8*) Church.

Manual of Pleural Procedures. Henri Colt & Praveen N. Mathur. 1998. 208p. pap. text 35.00 (*0-7817-1476-1*) Lppncott W & W.

Manual of Postoperative Management in Adult Cardiac Surgery. Carlos Moreno-Cabral et al. 1988. (Illus.). 112p. pap. 29.00 (*0-683-06146-1*) Lppncott W & W.

Manual of Practical Gynecological Oncology. Ed. by Basil Bloch et al. 1994. LC 94-72656. 216p. (gr. 13). pap. 43.95 (*0-412-56990-6*) Chapman & Hall.

Manual of Practical Neuropathology Techniques. Tim P. Dawson & J. S. Neal. 2000. (Illus.). 256p. pap. text 75.00 (*0-7506-9086-0*) Buttrwrth-Heinemann.

Manual of Primary Eye Care. Narciss Okhravi. 192p. 1997. LC 97-144804. (Illus.). text 45.00 (*0-7506-2221-0*); 1999. reprint ed. pap. text 37.50 (*0-7506-4467-2*) Buttrwrth-Heinemann.

Manual of Psychiatric Consultation & Emergency Care. Ed. by Frederick G. Guggenheim & Myron F. Weiner. 1984. LC 84-477. 400p. 60.00 (*0-87668-666-8*) Aronson.

Manual of Psychiatric Disorders. Ed. by George M. Simpson. 1995. (Illus.). 200p. (Orig.). pap. text (*0-9645991-0-4*) Impact Commun.

Manual of Psychiatric Emergencies. Ed. by Steven E. Hyman & George E. Tesar. 3rd ed. 1993. LC 93-1834. (Spiral Manual Ser.). (Illus.). 384p. spiral bd. 39.95 (*0-316-38728-2*) Lppncott W & W.

Manual of Psychiatric Quality Assurance: A Report of the APA Committee on Quality Assurance. Ed. by Marlon R. Mattson. 1992. LC 91-25954. 254p. pap. text 27.50 (*0-89042-232-X*, 2232) Am Psychiatric.

Manual of Psychiatric Therapeutics. Ed. by Richard I. Shader. 2nd ed. 1994. LC 93-25998. (Spiral Manual Ser.). (Illus.). 400p. spiral bd. 39.95 (*0-316-78223-8*, Little Brwn Med Div) Lppncott W & W.

Manual of Psychology. George F. Stout. 1977. LC 77-72191. (Contributions to the History of Psychology Ser.: Pt. A, Vol. IX, Orientations). 642p. reprint ed. lib. bdg. 99.75 (*0-313-26933-5*, U6933, Greenwood Pr) Greenwood.

Manual of Psychosocial Nursing Interventions: Promoting Mental Health in Medical-Surgical Settings. Lewis et al. 1989. 288p. text 44.00 (*0-7216-5763-X*) Saunders.

Manual of Pulmonary Function Testing. Gregg Ruppel. 7th ed. 1997. LC 97-26485. (Illus.). 384p. (C). (gr. 13). pap. text 36.00 (*0-8151-2299-3*, 27686) Mosby Inc.

Manual of Pulmonary Surgery. E. W. Humphrey. 1982. (Comprehensive Manuals of Surgical Specialties Ser.). (Illus.). 259p. 198.00 (*0-387-90732-7*) Spr-Verlag.

Manual of Quantitative Pathology in Cancer Diagnosis & Prognosis. J. P. Baak. 2nd ed. 1991. (Illus.). 616p. 250.00 (*0-387-51275-6*) Spr-Verlag.

Manual of Rabbit Medicine & Surgery. Paul Flecknell. 2000. (Illus.). 160p. pap. text (*0-905214-46-3*) BSAVA GBR. *Dist:* Iowa U Pr.

Manual of Radiographic Interpretation for General Practitioners: WHO Basic Radiological System. W. P. Cockshott et al. 1985. (CHI, FRE & SPA., Illus.). 216p. pap. text 34.00 (*92-4-154177-6*, 1150231) World Health.

Manual of Radiographic Technique: WHO Basic Radiological System. T. Holm et al. 1986. (CHI, FRE & SPA., Illus.). 256p. pap. text 30.00 (*92-4-154179-2*, 1150240) World Health.

Manual of Radiology. Charles E. Kahn. 1992. pap. text 25.00 (*0-07-033647-4*) McGraw.

Manual of Refraction. Albert E. Sloane & George E. Garcia. 3rd ed. 1979. 23.00 (*0-316-79844-4*, Little Brwn Med Div) Lppncott W & W.

Manual of Respiratory Care Procedures. Blodgett. 2nd ed. 1987. LC 65-8782. text 19.50 (*0-397-50714-3*, Lippnctt) Lppncott W & W.

Manual of Retinal Surgery. Andrew J. Packer. 2nd ed. 2001. LC 00-45465. (Illus.). 160p. pap. text 39.99 (*0-7506-7106-8*) Buttrwrth-Heinemann.

Manual of Retinal Surgery. Ed. by Andrew J. Packer. 1989. (Illus.). 126p. pap. text (*0-443-08605-2*) Church.

Manual of School Health. Helen Thomson & Keeta D. Lewis. 1986. (Illus.). 288p. (C). pap. text 45.94 (*0-201-15292-4*, Health Sci) Addison-Wesley.

Manual of Sclerotherapy. Neil S. Sadick. 1998. LC 99-16112. (Illus.). 288p. text 149.00 (*0-397-51742-4*) Lppncott W & W.

Manual of Sequential Art Activities for Classified Children & Adolescents. Rocco A. Fugaro. 1985. (Illus.). 246p. (C). pap. 43.95 (*0-398-05085-6*) C C Thomas.

Manual of Sexually Transmitted Diseases. H. Hunter Handsfield & Walter E. Stamm. 1983. 324p. (*0-07-060694-3*) McGraw.

Manual of Skin Surgery: A Practical Guide to Dermatologic Procedures. David J. Leffell & Marc D. Brown. 1997. LC 96-30884. 250p. pap. 79.95 (*0-471-13411-2*) Wiley.

Manual of Skull Base Dissection. Vol. 1. Ed. by Takanori Fukushima. 1996. LC 96-84288. (Illus.). 136p. (Orig.). ring bd. 180.00 (*0-9651986-0-X*) AF NeuroVid.

Manual of Small Animal Anesthesia. Robert R. Paddleford. Ed. by Ray Kersey. 2nd ed. 1998. LC 98-15368. (Illus.). 320p. (C). pap. text 39.95 (*0-7216-4060-5*) Saunders.

Manual of Small Animal Anesthesia & Analgesia. Ed. by Chris Seymour & Robin Gleed. 1999. LC 00-501296. (Illus.). 320p. pap. (*0-905214-48-X*) BSAVA GBR. *Dist:* Iowa U Pr.

Manual of Small Animal Arthrology. Ed. by John E. Houlton & Robert W. Collinson. 1994. (Illus.). 344p. pap. text 74.95 (*0-8138-2869-4*) Iowa U Pr.

***Manual of Small Animal Behavior.** Karen Overall. 2001. (*0-323-00890-9*) Mosby Inc.

Manual of Small Animal Cardiorespiratory Medicine & Surgery. Ed. by Virginia Fuentes & Simon Swift. 1998. (Illus.). 320p. pap. text (*0-905214-33-1*) BSAVA GBR. *Dist:* Iowa U Pr.

Manual of Small Animal Diagnostic Imaging. Ed. by Robin Lee. 1995. 200p. pap. (*0-905214-26-9*) BSAVA GBR. *Dist:* Iowa U Pr.

Manual of Small Animal Endocrinology. Ed. by Andrew Torrance & Carmel Mooney. 2nd ed. 1998. LC 98-166450. (British Small Animal Veterinary Association Manual Ser.). (Illus.). 250p. (C). pap. text (*0-905214-42-0*) BSAVA GBR. *Dist:* Iowa U Pr.

Manual of Small Animal Internal Medicine. Richard W. Nelson & C. Guillermo Couto. 1998. (Illus.). 944p. (C). (gr. 13). pap. text 39.95 (*0-8151-7297-4*, 27769) Mosby Inc.

***Manual of Small Animal Opthamology.** Ed. by Simon M. Petersen-Jones & Sheila Crispin. 2nd ed. 2001. (Illus.). 288p. pap. 134.95 (*0-905214-54-4*) Blackwell Sci.

Manual of Small Animal Postoperative Care. Robert A. Taylor & Robin A. McGehee. 1995. (Illus.). 220p. 35.00 (*0-683-08125-X*); 1994. LC 94-4929. (*0-8121-1765-4*) Lppncott W & W.

Manual of Small Animal Reproduction & Neonatology. Ed. by Gillian M. Simpson et al. 1998. (Illus.). 235p. pap. (*0-905214-36-6*) BSAVA GBR. *Dist:* Iowa U Pr.

Manual of Small Animal Surgical Therapeutics. Ed. by C. W. Betts & Stephen W. Crane. 1986. (Illus.). 424p. pap. text (*0-443-08327-4*) Church.

Manual of Small Animal Surgical Therapeutics. Ed. by C. W. Betts & Stephen W. Crane. 1986. (Illus.). 440p. text 49.00 (*0-7216-5924-1*) Saunders.

Manual of Soft-Tissue Tumor Surgery. J. P. Neifeld et al. 1983. (Comprehensive Manuals of Surgical Specialties Ser.). (Illus.). 214p. 217.00 (*0-387-90843-9*) Spr-Verlag.

Manual of Spectrofluorometric & Spectrophotometric Derivative Experiments. Allesia M. Gillespie, Jr. 1993. LC 93-26029. 224p. spiral bd. 69.95 (*0-8493-6390-X*) CRC Pr.

Manual of Sports Medicine. Safran. 1997. (Illus.). spiral bd. 32.95 (*0-316-77111-2*) Lppncott W & W.

Manual of Sports Surgery. Ed. by C. L. Shields. 1986. (Comprehensive Manuals of Surgical Specialties Ser.). (Illus.). 206p. 335.00 (*0-387-96415-0*) Spr-Verlag.

***Manual of Strabismus Surgery.** C. J. MacEwen & Richard Gregson. 2001. (Illus.). 256p. pap. 55.00 (*0-7506-5248-9*) Buttrwrth-Heinemann.

Manual of Stroke Rehabilitation. Karl J. Sandin & Kristin D. Mason. 1996. LC 95-44678. (Physical Medicine & Rehabilitation Clinical Practice Manuals Ser.). 194p. pap. text 49.99 (*0-7506-9489-0*) Buttrwrth-Heinemann.

Manual Of Structural Kinesiology. Clem W. Thompson & Ed D. Floyd. 14th ed. 2000. (Illus.). 288p. Price not set. (*0-07-232917-3*) McGraw.

Manual of Style: A Guide for Authors & Editors. American Medical Association Staff & Cheryl Iverson. 9th ed. 1997. LC 97-19246. 672p. 41.95 (*0-683-40206-4*) Lppncott W & W.

Manual of Surgery Asia, No. 7. Condon. 1988. 10.95 (*0-316-15260-9*, Little Brwn Med Div) Lppncott W & W.

Manual of Surgery ISE, No. 7. Condon. 1988. 15.95 (*0-316-15259-5*, Little Brwn Med Div) Lppncott W & W.

Manual of Surgery of the Gallbladder, Bile Ducts, & Exocrine Pancreas. R. E. Hermann. 1979. (Comprehensive Manuals of Surgical Specialties Ser.). (Illus.). 306p. 174.00 (*0-387-90351-8*) Spr-Verlag.

Manual of Surgical Pathology Gross Room Procedures. Juan Rosai. 1981. (Illus.). 132p. (C). pap. 29.95 (*0-8166-1027-4*) U of Minn Pr.

Manual of Surgical Therapeutics. Robert E. Condon & Lloyd M. Nyhus. 7th ed. 1988. 480p. 23.50 (*0-316-15261-7*, Little Brwn Med Div) Lppncott W & W.

Manual of Surgical Therapeutics. Ed. by Robert E. Condon & Lloyd M. Nyhus. 9th ed. 1996. LC 95-333. 34.95 (*0-316-15396-6*, Little Brwn Med Div) Lppncott W & W.

Manual of Surgical Therapeutics. Robert E. Condon & Lloyd M. Nyhus. 9th ed. 1995. LC 95-333. (Illus.). 439p. spiral bd. 39.95 (*0-316-15402-4*) Lppncott W & W.

Manual of Systematic Corneal Surgery. Arthur D. Steele & Colin M. Kirkness. 2nd ed. 1999. (Illus.). 164p. text 90.00 (*0-7506-3720-X*) Buttrwrth-Heinemann.

Manual of Systematic Corneal Surgery. Arthur D. Steele & Colin M. Kirkness. 1992. (Illus.). 104p. text (*0-443-04284-5*) Church.

Manual of Systematic Corneal Surgery 2Ed. Steele & Kirkness. 2nd ed. Date not set. 104p. pap. text (*0-7506-3722-6*) Buttrwrth-Heinemann.

Manual of Systematic Eyelid Surgery. J. R. O. Collin. 2nd ed. 1999. 184p. pap. text 85.00 (*0-7506-4572-5*); 3rd ed. 2001. (Illus.). 256p. pap. 65.00 (*0-7506-4550-4*) Buttrwrth-Heinemann.

Manual of Sytematic Eyelid Surgery. J. R. Collin. 2nd ed. 1989. (Illus.). 166p. text (*0-443-04009-5*) Church.

Manual of Tests for Syphilis. Ed. by Sandra A. Larsen et al. 8th ed. 1990. 208p. 30.00 (*0-87553-174-1*); 9th ed. 1998. LC 98-72440. 361p. pap. 48.00 (*0-87553-234-9*) Am Pub Health.

Manual of the Penicillia. K. B. Raper & Charlesthom. 1984. 172p. pap. (*0-7855-0380-3*) Intl Bks & Periodicals IND. *Dist:* St Mut.

Manual of Therapeutics for Addictions. Ed. by Norman S. Miller et al. 1997. LC 96-30946. 364p. pap. 72.50 (*0-471-56176-2*) Wiley.

Manual of Therapy for Skin Diseases. Timothy Berger et al. 1990. 349p. pap. text (*0-443-08477-7*) Church.

Manual of Thoracic Surgery. Arndt Von Hippel. 2nd ed. 1986. pap. 40.00 (*0-9615808-1-X*) Stone Age Pr.

Manual of Trauma & Emergency Surgery. Ed. by David V. Shatz. 2000. LC 99-22699. (*0-7216-6437-7*) Saunders.

Manual of Trauma Resuscitation, Anaesthesia & Intensive Care. Oakley. 1997. (Illus.). 320p. (C). text (*0-412-61850-8*, Chap & Hall NY) Chapman & Hall.

Manual of Travel Medicine: A Guide to Disease Prevention & Treatment. Seymour I. Schlager. 2002. spiral bd. (*0-7817-2032-X*) Lppncott W & W.

Manual of Travel Medicine & Health. Robert Steffen & Herbert L. DuPont. 1999. LC 00-701226. (Illus.). 515p. pap. (*1-55009-078-X*) DEKR.

Manual of Tropical Dermatology. J. H. Pettit et al. 1984. (Illus.). 260p. 171.00 (*0-387-90987-7*) Spr-Verlag.

Manual of Tropical Pediatrics. Ed. by M. D. Seear. 2000. LC 99-16936. (Illus.). 492p. (C). text 85.00 (*0-521-65835-7*) Cambridge U Pr.

Manual of Tumescent Liposculpture & Laser Cosmetic Surgery: Including the Weekend Alternative to the Facelift. William R. Cook. 1999. LC 98-50220. 240p. text 139.00 (*0-7817-1987-9*) Lppncott W & W.

Manual of Ultrasound. H. Lutz & R. Meudt. 1983. (Illus.). 140p. 73.95 (*0-387-12377-6*) Spr-Verlag.

Manual of Upper Gastrointestinal Surgery. William H. ReMine et al. 1985. (Comprehensive Manuals of Surgical Specialties Ser.). (Illus.). 124p. 162.00 (*0-387-96148-8*) Spr-Verlag.

Manual of Urologic Surgery. A. T. Cockett & Ken Koshiba. 1979. (Comprehensive Manuals of Surgical Specialties Ser.). (Illus.). 284p. 161.00 (*0-387-90423-9*) Spr-Verlag.

Manual of Urology. Michael B. Siroky. 1990. 32.95 (*0-316-79296-9*, Little Brwn Med Div) Lppncott W & W.

Manual of Urology Asia. Michael B. Siroky. 1990. 10.95 (*0-316-79298-5*, Little Brwn Med Div) Lppncott W & W.

Manual of Urology ISE. Michael B. Siroky. 1990. 15.95 (*0-316-79297-7*, Little Brwn Med Div) Lppncott W & W.

Manual of Vascular Access, Organ Donation, & Transplantation. John S. Najarian et al. 1984. (Comprehensive Manuals of Surgical Specialties Ser.). (Illus.). 340p. 240.00 (*0-387-90965-6*) Spr-Verlag.

Manual of Vascular Surgery, Pt. 1. E. J. Wylie et al. Ed. by R. H. Egdahl. 1980. LC 79-18226. (Comprehensive Manuals of Surgical Specialties Ser.). (Illus.). 320p. 99.00 (*3-540-90408-5*) Spr-Verlag.

Manual of Vascular Surgery, Vol. 2. E. J. Wylie et al. 1986. (Comprehensive Manuals of Surgical Specialties Ser.). (Illus.). 338p. 434.00 (*0-387-90409-3*) Spr-Verlag.

Manual of Veterinary Care. Sue Dallas. 2000. (Manual of Veterinary Care Ser.). (Illus.). 256p. pap. text (*0-905214-49-8*) BSAVA GBR. *Dist:* Iowa U Pr.

Manual of Veterinary Echocardiography. June A. Boon. 1998. LC 97-43333. 447p. 79.00 (*0-683-00938-9*) Lppncott W & W.

Manual of Veterinary Nursing. Margaret Moore. 2000. (Manual of Veterinary Care Ser.). (Illus.). 208p. pap. text (*0-905214-50-1*) BSAVA GBR. *Dist:* Iowa U Pr.

Manual of Visual Fields. Elliot B. Werner. 1990. (Manuals in Ophthalmology Ser.). (Illus.). 238p. text (*0-443-08689-3*) Church.

Manual of Voice Therapy. Rex J. Prater & Roger W. Swift. 1984. LC 90-50380. 288p. (C). spiral bd. 31.00 (*0-89079-279-8*, 1773) PRO-ED.

Manual of Voice Treatment. Moya L. Andrews. 2nd rev. ed. 1999. LC 98-37605. (Clinical Competence Ser.). (Illus.). 709p. spiral bd. 73.95 (*1-56593-998-0*, 1976) Thomson Learn.

Manual of Voice Treatment: Pediatrics to Geriatrics. Moya L. Andrews. 1994. LC 94-40347. (Clinical Competence Ser.). (Illus.). 632p. (C). pap. 59.95 (*1-56593-162-9*, 0472) Thomson Learn.

Manual on Assisted Reproduction. Ed. by T. Rabe et al. 2nd ed. 2000. LC 00-38608. (Illus.). 600p. 129.00 (*3-540-67299-0*) Spr-Verlag.

Manual on Community Pediatrics. Polnay. 2nd ed. 1996. pap. text 24.95 (*0-443-05352-9*) Saunders.

Manual on Drug Dependence. Ed. by J. F. Kramer & D. C. Cameron. 1975. pap. text 24.00 (*92-4-154045-1*, 1150113) World Health.

Manual on Drug Dependence. Gabriel G. Nahas. 1992. (Illus.). 268p. (Orig.). pap. 12.95 (*0-929240-46-4*) EMIS.

Manual on Radiation Sterilization of Medical & Biological Materials. 1973. (Technical Reports: No. 149). (Illus.). 327p. (Orig.). pap. (*92-0-115073-3*, IDC149) IAEA AUT. *Dist:* Bernan Associates.

Manual on Small Animal Surgery. Theresa Welch Fossum. 1999. LC 99-26587. 1024p. pap. text 52.00 (*0-323-00562-4*) Harcourt.

Manual on the Diagnosis of Rinderpest: Animal Health Manual. J. Anderson et al. 2nd ed. 1997. (Animal Health Ser.: No. 1). (Illus.). 143p. pap. (*92-5-103814-7*, F38147) FAO ITA. *Dist:* Bernan Associates.

Manual Oncology, No. 2. Carol S. Portlock. 1986. 15.95 (*0-316-71426-7*, Little Brwn Med Div) Lppncott W & W.

Manual para la Preparacion de Informes y Tesis. Irma G. Deserrano. 1992. LC 76-11003. (C). pap. 8.25 (*0-8477-2312-7*) U of PR Pr.

Manual Pediatra Practico. Beryl J. Rosenstein. 3rd ed. 1998. (C). text 24.49 (*84-8174-344-5*) Mosby Inc.

Manual Terapeutico para el Adulto Con Dificultades Del Habla y Lenguaje Tomo 1: Una Seleccion de Materiales de Estimulo. Kathryn Kilpatrick & Cynthia L. Jones. Tr. by Ingrid Bahler & Katherine G. Gatto. 1985. (SPA., Illus.). 433p. stu. ed. 37.00 (*1-880504-01-4*) Visit Nurse.

Manual Therapy. Ed. by Jensen & Farrell. 1993. 104p. pap. 30.00 (*0-912452-83-8*, P-87) Am Phys Therapy Assn.

Manual Therapy: Improve Muscle & Joint Functioning. L. A. Warmerdam. Ed. by Barbara Field. 1998. LC 00-500796. (Illus.). 329p. text (*0-9657910-0-9*) Pine NY.

Manual Therapy Case Studies. Spencer. 1998. 369p. pap. text 39.95 (*0-443-05696-X*) Saunders.

Manual Therapy of Peripheral Joints. Ed. by J. D. Boyling. 1998. (Illus.). 592p. text (*0-443-04349-3*) Church.

***Manual Therapy of the Spine: An Integrated Approach.** Mark Dutton. 2001. LC 2001-30679. 384p. pap. 59.95 (*0-07-137582-1*) McGraw-Hill Prof.

Manual Thermal Diagnosis. Jean-Pierre Barral. 1996. (Illus.). 130p. (C). text 35.00 (*0-939616-24-6*) Eastland.

***Manual to Accompany Conceptual Foundations: The Bridge to Professional Nursing Practice.** Joan L. Creasia & Barbara Parker. 3rd ed. 2001. LC 2001-30284. (Illus.). xv, 503p. pap. (*0-323-01227-2*) Mosby Inc.

Manual Urologic Surgery. H. Ramsey Fowler. 1990. 115.00 (*0-316-28951-5*, Little Brwn Med Div) Lppncott W & W.

Manual Vacuum Aspiration: A Summary of Clinical & Programmatic Experience Worldwide. Forrest C. Greenslade et al. 1993. LC 93-8963. pap. (*1-882220-03-X*) IPAS.

Manual Vacuum Aspiration Guide for Clinicians. Laura Yordy et al. 1993. LC 93-39549. pap. (*1-882220-04-8*) IPAS.

Manuel Alphabetique de Psychiatrie Clinique et Therapeutique. Ed. by Antoine Porot. 6th ed. 1984. (FRE.). 768p. 135.00 (*0-7859-4832-5*, M6391) Fr & Eur.

Manuel de Bacteriologie Clinique J. Freney et al. 1994. 1760p. pap. 149.50 (*2-906077-57-7*) Elsevier.

Manuel de Recherche Operationnele en Matiere de Planification Familiale. Andrew Fisher et al. 1991.Tr. of Handbook for Family Planning Operations Research Design. (FRE.). (*0-87834-055-6*) Population Coun.

Manuel Elementaire Pour Coconseillers see Fundamentals of Co-Counseling Manual

Manuel Merck de Diagnostic et Therapeutic. Robert Berkow. 1988. (FRE.). lib. bdg. 195.00 (*0-8288-3829-1*, F120190) Fr & Eur.

Manuel Pratique de Curietherapie see Practical Manual of Brachytherapy

Manufacture & Use of the Functional Foot Orthosis. R. J. Anthony. 1991. (Illus.). xiv, 220p. 172.25 (*3-8055-5298-X*) S Karger.

Manufacture of Madness: A Comparative Study of the Inquisition & the Mental Health Movement. Thomas Szasz. 1997. LC 96-48784. 426p. reprint ed. pap. 19.95 (*0-8156-0461-0*) Syracuse U Pr.

Manufacture of Medical & Health Products by Transgenic Plants. Esra Galun. 2000. 300p. (*1-86094-249-0*); pap. (*1-86094-254-7*) Imperial College GBR. *Dist:* World Scientific Pub.

Manufacturing Babies & Public Consent: Debating the New Reproductive Technologies. Jose Van Dyck. 1994. 224p. (C). pap. text 19.50 (*0-8147-8786-X*) NYU Pr.

***Manufacturing Victims: What the Psychology Industry Is Doing to People.** Tana Dineen. 3rd rev. ed. 2001. (Illus.). 320p. (*1-55207-032-8*) R Davies Pub.

Manuscript Sources of Medieval Medicine: A Book of Essays. Ed. by Margaret R. Schleissner. 1995. LC 94-15149. (Medieval Casebooks Ser.: Vol. 8). 224p. text 42.00 (*0-8153-0815-9*, H1576) Garland.

Many Colored Buffalo: Transformation Through the Council of Many Voices. William S. Taegel. Ed. by Edward Tick. 1990. LC 90-46541. (Frontiers in Psychotherapy Ser.). 192p. (C). 73.25 (*0-89391-739-7*); pap. 39.50 (*0-89391-740-0*) Greenwood (Ablex).

Many Dimensions of Family Practice. North American Symposium on Family Practice Staff. 1983. LC 80-14847. (Many Dimensions of Family Practic C Ser.). 340p. 45.00 (*0-87668-427-4*) Aronson.

Many Faces of Abuse: Treating the Emotional Abuse of High-Functioning Women. Joan Lachkar. 1998. LC 96-53035. 240p. 50.00 (*0-7657-0065-4*) Aronson.

Many Faces of Bereavement: The Nature & Treatment of Natural, Traumatic & Stigmatized Grief. Ginny Sprang & John McNeill. 1995. LC 95-16267. 216p. text 28.95 (*0-87630-756-X*) Brunner-Routledge.

Many Faces of Deceit: Omissions, Lies & Disguise in Psychotherapy. Helen K. Gediman & Janice S. Lieberman. 1996. LC 95-18353. 272p. 45.00 (*1-56821-592-4*) Aronson.

Many Faces of Homosexuality: Anthropological Approaches to Homosexual Behavior. Ed. by Evelyn Blackwood. 1986. LC 85-17757. (Journal of Homosexuality Ser.: Vol. 11, Nos. 3 & 4). 217p. pap. 19.95 (*0-918393-20-5*, Harrington Park) Haworth Pr.

Many Faces of Long-Term Care: Today's Bitter Pill or Tommorrow's Cure : Hearing Before the Special Committee on Aging, United States Senate, One Hundred Fifth Congress, First Session, Las Vegas, NV, January 12, 1998, Reno, NV, January 13, 1998. U. S. Staff. 1998. LC 98-175718. (Real Lives Ser.). iv, 426 p. (*0-16-056532-4*) USGPO.

Many Meanings of Play: A Psychoanalytic Perspective. Ed. by Albert J. Solnit et al. 1993. LC 92-48988. 358p. (C). 60.00 (*0-300-05438-6*) Yale U Pr.

Many Minds: Information for People Who Have Multiple Personalities. Lauren Lund & David Lund. 1993. (Illus.). 34p. (Orig.). pap. text 4.95 (*0-9637149-0-2*) Soft Words.

Many Sleepless Nights: The World of Organ Transplantation. Lee Gutkind. 1990. LC 89-40585. 368p. reprint ed. pap. 15.95 (*0-8229-5905-4*) U of Pittsburgh Pr.

Many Specialties, One Corps: A Pictorial History of the Medical Services [sic] Corps. David P. Gray. 1997. LC 97-3179. (Illus.). (*0-89865-994-9*) Donning Co.

Mao-B-Inhibitor Selegiline (R-(-)-Deprenyl) Ed. by P. Riederer & H. Przuntek. 1987. (Journals of Neural Transmission: Suppl. 25). (Illus.). 220p. 69.95 (*0-387-82009-4*) Spr-Verlag.

MAP: The Co-Creative White Brotherhood Medical Assistance Program. Machaelle S. Wright. 2nd ed. 1994. LC 94-65465. (Illus.). 318p. pap. 16.00 (*0-927978-19-9*, B-106) Perelandra Ltd.

Map, Compass, & Campfire: A Handbook for the Outdoorsman. Donald E. Ratliff. 1993. LC 64-8453. (Illus.). 64p. (gr. 10-12). reprint ed. pap. 7.95 (*0-8323-0129-9*) Binford Mort.

Map of the Mind: Toward a Science of Psychotherapy. Richard Brockman. 1998. LC 98-11890. (Illus.). 279p. 37.95 (*1-887841-14-8*, Psychosocial) Intl Univs Pr.

Mapping Fate: A Memoir of Family, Risk, & Genetic Research. Alice Wexler. 1996. LC 96-16801. (Illus.). 320p. (C). pap. 15.95 (*0-520-20741-6*) U CA Pr.

Mapping the Brain & Its Functions: Integrating Enabling Technologies into Neuroscience Research. Institute of Medicine Staff. Ed. by Constance M. Pecura & Joseph B. Martin. 1991. 180p. text 24.95 (*0-309-04497-9*) Natl Acad Pr.

Mapping the Human Genome: Reality, Morality, & Deity. Theodore C. Kent. 1995. 154p. (C). 50.00 (*0-8191-9784-X*); pap. 26.50 (*0-8191-9779-3*) U Pr of Amer.

Mapping the Mind. Rita Carter. 1999. LC 98-70490. (Illus.). 224p. 45.00 (*0-520-21937-6*) U CA Pr.

Mapping the Mind. Hunter B. Shirley. 1983. LC 82-24664. (Illus.). 376p. text 49.95 (*0-911012-19-2*) Burnham Inc.

Mapping the Mind: Domain Specificity in Cognition & Culture. Ed. by Lawrence A. Hirschfeld & Susan A. Gelman. 1994. (Illus.). 530p. (C). pap. text 32.95 (*0-521-42993-5*) Cambridge U Pr.

Mapping Your Future: A Lifework Planning Guide for Health Professionals. Leland R. Kaiser. Ed. by Alys Novak. 1990. 120p. 76.00 (*0-933948-26-3*) M G M A.

Mapping Your Risk Management Course in Ambulatory Care. American Hospital Association Staff. 1995. (Illus.). 52p. (Orig.). pap. 20.00 (*0-87258-694-4*) Am Hospital.

Mapping Your Risk Management Course in Home Health Care. American Hospital Association Staff. 1995. (Illus.). 32p. (Orig.). pap. 20.00 (*0-87258-701-0*) Am Hospital.

Mapping Your Risk Management Course in Integrated Delivery Networks. American Hospital Association Staff. 1995. (Illus.). 40p. (Orig.). pap. 20.00 (*0-87258-697-9*) Am Hospital.

Maps & Guide to Microdissection of the Rat Brain. Miklos Palkovits & Brownstein. 1987. (Illus.). 262p. (C). pap. text 70.00 (*0-8385-6159-4*, A6159-6, Apple Lange Med) McGraw.

Marathon of Faith. Rex E. Lee et al. 1996. LC 96-10450. xiii, 194p. 15.95 (*1-57345-163-0*) Deseret Bk.

Marburg & Ebola Virus Infections: A Guide for Their Diagnosis, Management & Control. D. Simpson. 1977. (WHO Offset Publications: No. 36). 28p. 4.00 (*92-4-170036-X*) World Health.

Marburg & Ebola Viruses. Ed. by Hans-Dieter Klenk et al. 1998. (Current Topics in Microbiology & Immunology Ser.: Vol. 235). (Illus.). 232p. 149.00 (*3-540-64729-5*) Spr-Verlag.

Marcello Malpighi & the Evolution of Embryology Howard B. Adelmann. 1966. (Publications in the History of Science). (Illus.). 2548p. 250.00 (0-8014-0004-X) Cornell U Pr.

March of Dimes Statbook: Statistics for Monitorins Maternal & Infant Health. March of Dimes Birth Defects Foundation Staff. 1997. LC 97-20539. (0-86525-078-2) March of Dimes.

March of Dimes Substance Abuse Curriculum for Obstetricians & Gynecologists. Cynthia Chazotte et al. Ed. by Rochelle K. Rosen et al. 1995. LC 95-36651. (0-86525-066-9) March of Dimes.

March of Medicine Laity Lectures. New York Academy of Medicine Staff. 1977. LC 78-142677. (Essay Index Reprint Ser.). No. 4. reprint ed. 19.95 (0-8369-2212-3); No. 5. 19.95 (0-8369-2115-1); No. 6. 19.95 (0-8369-2116-X); No. 7. 22.95 (0-8369-2117-8) Ayer.

March of Medicine Laity Lectures, 1943. New York Academy of Medicine Staff. 1977. LC 78-142677. (Essay Index Reprint Ser.). reprint ed. 19.95 (0-8369-2466-5) Ayer.

March of Medicine Laity Lectures, 1944. New York Academy of Medicine Staff. 1977. LC 78-142677. (Essay Index Reprint Ser.). reprint ed. 18.95 (0-8369-2467-3) Ayer.

Marcus Cardiac Imaging: A Companion to Braunwald's Heart Disease Eugene Braunwald et al. 2nd rev. ed. 1996. LC 95-19482. (Illus.). 1318p. text 215.00 (0-7216-4687-5) Saunders.

Marek's Disease I: Genetics & Virology. Gad Zeitlin et al. 1974. (Herpesvirus-Related Diseases Ser.). 27.50 (0-8422-7166-X) Irvington.

Marek's Disease II: Pathogenicity & Immunology. Ed. by H. Graham et al. 1974. (Herpesvirus-Related Diseases Ser.). 320p. text 31.50 (0-8422-7167-8) Irvington.

Mares, Foals & Foaling. Friedrich Andrist. 1990. pap. (0-85131-053-2) J A Allen GBR. *Dist:* St Mut.

Marfan Syndrome. Reed E. Pyeritz & Cheryll Gasner. (Illus.). 4th ed. 1994. 48p. pap. 4.00 (0-918335-09-4); 5th ed. Date not set. 44p. pap. text 5.00 (0-918335-10-8) Natl Marfan Foun.

Marfan Syndrome: A Booklet for Teachers. Barbara A. Bernhardt. 1992. pap. text 3.00 (0-918335-07-8) Natl Marfan Foun.

Marfan Syndrome: Physical Activity Guidelines for Physical Educators, Coaches & Physicians. Thomas J. Romeo. 77p. pap. 15.00 (0-918335-08-6); 1992. 78p. pap. 15.00 (0-918335-06-X) Natl Marfan Foun.

Margaret Newman: Health As Expanding Consciousness. Joanne Marchione. 1993. (Notes on Nursing Theories Ser.: Vol. 6). (Illus.). 60p. 29.95 (0-8039-4796-8, 4541); pap. 14.95 (0-8039-4797-6, 4542) Sage.

Margaret Sanger Story & the Fight for Birth Control. Lawrence Lader. 1975. LC 73-11855. (Illus.). 348p. reprint ed. lib. bdg. 69.50 (0-8371-7076-1, LAMS, Greenwood Pr) Greenwood.

Margin of Error: The Ethics of Mistakes in Clinical Medicine. Ed. by Susan B. Rubin & Laurie Zoloth. 2000. 384p. (C). lib. bdg. 65.00 (1-55572-078-1) Univ Pub Group.

Margin of Error: The Ethics of Mistakes in the Practice of Medicine. Ed. by Susan B. Rubin & Laurie Zoloth. 2000. 384p. pap. 29.95 (1-55572-053-6) Univ Pub Group.

Marguerite Maury's Guide to Aromatherapy. Daniele Ryman & Marguerite Maury. 1989. 108p. pap. (0-85207-163-9) C W Daniel GBR. *Dist:* Natl Bk Netwk.

Marguerite Maury's Guide to Aromatherapy. Ed. by Daniele Ryman. 3rd ed. 240p. pap. 26.95 (0-8464-4249-3) Beekman Pubs.

Maria Treben's Cures: Letters & Accounts of Cures Through the Herbal, "Health Through God's Pharmacy" Maria Treben. 4th ed. 1995. (Illus.). 100p. pap. text (3-85068-224-2) Ennsthaler AUT. *Dist:* Am Educ Systs.

Marihuana - Cannaboids: Neurobiology & Neurophysiology. Ed. by Andrei Bartke. 1992. 608p. 198.95 (0-8493-7931-8, QP801) CRC Pr.

Marihuana, America's New Drug Problem: A Sociologic Question with Its Basic Explanation Dependent on Biologic & Medical Principles. Robert P. Walton & E. M. Geiling. 1976. LC 75-17248. (Social Problems & Social Policy Ser.). 19.95 (0-405-07523-5) Ayer.

Marihuana & Medicine. Ed. by Gabriel G. Nahas et al. 1999. LC 99-13481. (Illus.). 848p. 145.00 (0-89603-593-X) Humana.

Marihuana-Biological Effects, Analysis, Metabolism, Cellular Responses, Reproduction & Brain: Proceedings of the Satellite Symposium to the International Congress of Pharmacology, 7th, Reims, 1978. International Congress of Pharmacology Staff. Ed. by Gabriel G. Nahas & William D. Paton. 1979. (Illus.). 777p. 85.50 (0-08-023759-2, Pergamon Pr) Elsevier.

Marihuana, the Forbidden Medicine. Lester Grinspoon & James B. Bakalar. rev. ed. 1997. LC 97-981. 312p. 45.00 (0-300-07085-3); pap. 17.95 (0-300-07086-1) Yale U Pr.

Marihuana, Tobacco, Alcohol, & Reproduction. Ernest L. Abel. 1983. 256p. 146.00 (0-8493-6480-9, RG580, CRC Reprint) Franklin.

Marijuana. M. S. Gold. 1989. LC 88-32427. (Drugs of Abuse: Vol. 1). (Illus.). 276p. (C). text 42.50 (0-306-43062-2, Kluwer Plenum) Kluwer Academic.

Marijuana. David L. Ohlms. Ed. & Intro. by GWC, Inc. Staff. rev. ed. 1993. 17p. 2.50 (1-56168-030-3, B106) GWC Inc.

Marijuana: Health Effects. Sara Macintosh. rev. ed. 2000. pap. 0.50 (0-89230-161-9) Do It Now.

Marijuana: Its Effects on Mind & Body. William J. Hermes et al. 1992. LC 91-17766. (Encyclopedia of Psychoactive Drugs Ser.: No. 1). (Illus.). 124p. (YA). (gr. 7-11). lib. bdg. 19.95 (0-87754-754-8) Chelsea Hse.

Marijuana: Medical Uses. Jim Parker. 1999. pap. 0.50 (0-89230-159-7) Do It Now.

Marijuana: Personality & Behavior. Sara Macintosh. rev. ed. 2000. pap. 0.50 (0-89230-160-0) Do It Now.

Marijuana & AIDS: Pot, Politics & PWAs in America. Robert C. Randall. 1991. LC 91-77140. 183p. (Orig.). pap. 12.95 (0-936485-07-8, Galen Pr DC) Lkng Glass Pubns.

Marijuana & Medicine: Assessment of the Science Base. Institute of Medicine Staff. Ed. by John A. Benson et al. 1999. LC 99-6484. 288p. 39.95 (0-309-07155-0) Natl Acad Pr.

Marijuana As Medicine: The Science Beyond the Controversy. Alison Mack & Janet Joy. 2000. LC 00-46058. (Illus.). xii, 199p. pap. 17.95 (0-309-06531-3) Natl Acad Pr.

Marijuana Chemistry. Michael Starks. 2nd ed. 1990. 199p. pap. 22.95 (0-914171-39-9) Ronin Pub.

Marijuana Effects on the Endocrine & Reproductive Systems. 1986. lib. bdg. 250.00 (0-8490-3518-X) Gordon Pr.

Marijuana Medical Handbook: A Guide to Therapeutic Use. Ed Rosenthal et al. 1996. 270p. pap. 16.95 (0-932551-16-5) Quick Am Pub.

Marijuana Medicine: A World Tour of the Healing & Visionary Powers of Cannabis. Christian Ratsch. 2001. LC 00-50572. (Illus.). 224p. pap. 24.95 (0-89281-933-2, Heal Arts VT) Inner Tradit.

Marijuana, Medicine & the Law: Direct Testimony of Witnesses on Marijuana's Medical Use. Ed. by Richard C. Randall. 1988. LC 88-80330. 502p. (Orig.). pap. 29.95 (0-936485-02-7, Galen Pr DC) Lkng Glass Pubns.

Marijuana, Medicine & the Law Vol. II: The Legal Argument. Ed. by Richard C. Randall. LC 88-80330. 484p. (Orig.). pap. 25.95 (0-936485-04-3, Galen Pr DC) Lkng Glass Pubns.

Marijuana Question? Ask Ed: The Encyclopedia of Marijuana. Ed Rosenthal. 1987. (Illus.). 284p. reprint ed. pap. 19.95 (0-932551-01-7) Quick Am Pub.

Marijuana Reappraised: Two Personal Accounts. Martin Croes & Andre McNicoll. 1977. LC 77-15695. 20p. pap. 1.00 (0-913098-08-6) Orion Society.

Marijuana Research Findings. 1992. lib. bdg. 88.95 (0-8490-8823-2) Gordon Pr.

Marijuana Research Findings: Marijuana Chemistry, Metabolism & Its Effect on Human Health. 1992. lib. bdg. 79.00 (0-8490-5463-X) Gordon Pr.

Marine Algae in Pharmaceutical Science. Ed. by Hoppe. 1979. (C). 180.80 (3-11-007375-7) De Gruyter.

Marine Biology. John Reseck, Jr. rev. ed. 1979. (Illus.). text 18.95 (0-8359-4276-7) P-H.

Marine Lipids. Rita Elkins. 1997. (Woodland Health Ser.). 32p. pap. text 3.95 (1-885670-50-8) Woodland UT.

Marine Mammal Sensory Systems. J. A. Thomas et al. 1993. LC 92-35373. (Illus.). 788p. (C). text 165.00 (0-306-44351-1, Kluwer Plenum) Kluwer Academic.

Marine Mammals of California. Robert T. Orr et al. rev. ed. 1972. LC 78-165233. (California Natural History Guides Ser.: No. 29). 92p. pap. 12.95 (0-520-06515-8) U CA Pr.

Marine Pollution & Sea Life. Ed. by Mario Ruivo. 1978. 100.00 (0-7855-6936-7) St Mut.

Marion Press: A Survey & a Checklist. Thomas A. Larremore & Amy Hopkins. 1981. LC 85-51272. 293p. reprint ed. 35.00 (0-938768-04-2) Oak Knoll.

Marital & Family Processes in Depression: A Scientific Foundation for Clinical Practice. Steven R. H. Beach. 2000. LC 00-29321. (Illus.). xx, 259p. 39.95 (1-55798-695-9) Am Psychol.

Marital & Family Therapy. Ira D. Glick et al. Ed. by John F. Clarkin & David R. Kessler. 3rd ed. 1987. LC 87-81507. 623p. text 19.95 (0-88048-525-6, 8525) Am Psychiatric.

Marital & Family Therapy. Ira D. Glick et al. 4th ed. 2000. LC 99-47724. (Illus.). xlviii, 739p. 44.00 (0-88048-548-5, 8548) Am Psychiatric.

Marital & Family Therapy. Ira D. Glick et al. 3rd ed. 1987. text 39.50 (0-8089-1878-8, Grune & Strat) Harcrt Hlth Sci Grp.

Marital Counseling: A Biblical Behavioral Cognitive Approach. Norman Wright. 1981. iii, 421p. 16.95 (0-938786-00-8) Chr Marriage.

Marital Instability & Divorce Outcomes: Issues for Therapists & Educators. Craig A. Everett. 1991. (Journal of Divorce & Remarriage Ser.: Vol. 15, Nos. 1-2). (Illus.). 209p. text 6.95 (1-56024-115-2) Haworth Pr.

Marital Pathology. British Medical Journal Editors Staff. 1980. 30.00 (0-7855-7317-8) St Mut.

Marital Relationship of Parents & the Emotionally Disturbed Child. Ezra F. Vogel. 1990. LC 90-13948. (Harvard Studies in Sociology: Vol. 18). 525p. text 35.00 (0-8240-2565-2) Garland.

Marital-Relationship Therapy Casebook: Theory & Application of the Intersystem Model. Ed. by Gerald R. Weeks & Larry Hof. 1994. LC 94-4079. 272p. text 39.95 (0-87630-733-0) Brunner-Routledge.

Marital Therapy: A Behavioral-Communications Approach. Philip H. Bornstein & Marcy T. Bornstein. 1986. (Psychology Practitioner Guidebooks). (Illus.). 160p. text 30.00 (0-08-031615-8); pap. text 15.95 (0-08-031614-X) Elsevier (Pergamon Pr).

Marital Therapy: A Combined Psychodynamic-Behavioral Approach. R. Taylor Segraves. 1982. LC 82-16653. (Critical Issues in Psychiatry Ser.). 314p. 45.00 (0-306-40936-4, Plenum Trade) Perseus Pubng.

Marital Therapy: A Hypnoanalytic Approach. John Scott, Sr. 1989. 250p. text 29.95 (0-8290-2411-5) Irvington.

Marital Therapy: Strategies Based on Social Learning & Behavior Exchange Principles. Neil S. Jacobson & Gayla Margolin. 1986. LC 79-728. 432p. text 47.95 (0-87630-199-5) Brunner-Routledge.

Marital Therapy in Britain Vol. 1: Context & Therapeutic Approaches. Wendy Dryden. 1985. 368p. pap. (0-335-09812-6) OpUniv Pr.

Marital Therapy in Britain Vol. 2: Special Areas. Wendy Dryden. 1985. 368p. pap. (0-335-09813-4) OpUniv Pr.

Marjorie Holmes' Secrets of Health, Energy, & Staying Young. Marjorie Holmes. rev. ed. 1989. 384p. mass mkt. 4.50 (0-380-70707-1, Avon Bks) Morrow Avon.

Marker Proteins in Inflammation: Proceedings of the Symposium; Lyon, France, April 22-25, 1981, Vol. 1. Robert M. Suskind. Ed. by Robert C. Allen et al. 1982. (Illus.). 608p. 180.80 (3-11-008625-5) De Gruyter.

Marker Proteins in Inflammation Vol. 3: Proceedings of the 3rd Symposium, Lyon, France, June 26-28, 1985. Ed. by Jacques Bienvenu et al. 1986. (Illus.). xv, 693p. lib. bdg. 296.15 (3-11-010639-6) De Gruyter.

Markers in Urology: Journal: European Urology, Vol. 21, Suppl. 1, 1992. Ed. by F. Di Silverio. 1992. (Illus.). iv, 116p. pap. 36.75 (3-8055-5612-8) S Karger.

Markers in Urology, Abstracts Vol. 19, Suppl. 2: Journal: European Urology. Vol. 19, Suppl. 1. Ed. by F. Di Silverio. 1991. xvi, 44p. pap. 18.50 (3-8055-5453-2) S Karger.

Markers of Human Neuroectodermal Tumors. Ed. by Gerard E. Staal & Cees W. van Veelen. 1986. 288p. 146.00 (0-8493-6414-0, RC280, CRC Reprint) Franklin.

Markers of Neuronal Injury & Degeneration. Ed. by Jan N. Johannessen. 1993. LC 93-13753. (Annals Ser.: Vol. 679). 432p. (0-89766-795-6); pap. 120.00 (0-89766-796-4) NY Acad Sci.

Market & Health. David Reisman. 1993. LC 93-17299. 254p. 45.00 (0-312-09981-9) St Martin.

Market-Driven Health Care: Who Wins, Who Loses in the Transformation of America's Largest Service Industry. Regina Herzlinger. 1996. LC 96-30199. 416p. 25.00 (0-201-48994-5) Perseus Pubng.

Market-Driven Nursing: Developing & Marketing Patient Care Services. American Organization of Nurse Executives Staff. 1999. LC 98-45912. (Aone Leadership Ser.). (Illus.). 172p. pap. 40.00 (1-55648-247-7) AHPI.

Market for Antifungals. Market Intelligence Staff. 1992. 310p. 3700.00 (1-56753-674-3, A2500) Frost & Sullivan.

Market for Decubitus Ulcer Treatment: Products, Drugs & Devices. 1986. 238p. 1950.00 (0-931634-50-4) FIND-SVP.

Market for Intravenous Therapy & Interal Nutrition (Europe) Market Intelligence Staff. 1992. 405p. 3800.00 (1-56753-784-7, E1584) Frost & Sullivan.

Market for Lasers in Medicine. Ed. by Peter Allen. 1989. 239p. pap. 1495.00 (0-941285-49-9) FIND-SVP.

Market Mechanisms & the Health Sector in Central & Eastern Europe. Alexander S. Preker & Richard G. Feachem. 1996. (Technical Papers: Vol. 293). 64p. pap. 22.00 (0-8213-3331-3, 13331) World Bank.

Market Profiles for Medicare Risk Contracting, 1997: North Central. 1997. pap. 310.00 (1-57372-086-0) Solucient.

Market Profiles for Medicare Risk Contracting, 1997: Northeastern. 1997. pap. 310.00 (1-57372-085-2) Solucient.

Market Profiles for Medicare Risk Contracting, 1997: Southern. 1997. pap. 310.00 (1-57372-087-9) Solucient.

Market Profiles for Medicare Risk Contracting, 1997: Western. 1997. pap. 310.00 (1-57372-088-7) Solucient.

Market Research in Health & Social Care. Mike Luckovich et al. 2000. LC 99-87923. (Illus.). xxi, 304p. 100.00 (0-415-20754-1); pap. 36.99 (0-415-20755-X) Routledge.

Marketing Allied Health Educational Programs: Eight Low Cost Steps You Need to Know. Patricia L. Hassel & David R. Palmer. 1992. LC 92-22068. 39.95 (1-881566-10-2) Eagle Pub & Comms.

Marketing Ambulatory Care Services. Ed. by William J. Winston. 1985. LC 84-27902. (Health Marketing Quarterly Ser.: Vol. 2, Nos. 2 & 3). 209p. text 6.95 (0-86656-387-3); pap. text 24.95 (0-86656-448-9) Haworth Pr.

Marketing an Orthopedic Practice. John B. Pinto. 1991. 160p. (Orig.). pap. 19.95 (1-879952-02-5) Inst Spine.

Marketing & Healthcare Organizations. Colin Gilligan & Robin Lowe. 1995. LC 95-24339. (1-85775-190-6) Radcliffe Med Pr GBR. *Dist:* Balogh.

Marketing & Retail Pharmacy. Colin Gilligan et al. 1997. LC 97-28563. (1-85775-202-3) Radcliffe Med Pr GBR. *Dist:* Balogh.

Marketing Approach to Physician Recruitment: Haworth Marketing Resources. James O. Hacker et al. 1995. LC 93-41669. (Illus.). 130p. lib. bdg. 39.95 (1-56024-898-X); pap. 14.95 (1-56024-899-8) Haworth Pr.

Marketing Dermatology. Cynthia Hough. 1997. (Illus.). 77p. pap. 26.00 (1-890018-13-9) Anadem Pubng.

Marketing for Health & Wellness Programs. Donald R. Self & James W. Busbin. 1990. LC 90-34020. (Health Marketing Quarterly Ser.: Vol. 7, Nos. 3 & 4). 248p. text 49.95 (1-56024-014-8) Haworth Pr.

Marketing for Mental Health Services. Ed. by William J. Winston. 1984. LC 83-27534. (Health Marketing Quarterly Ser.: Vol. 1, Nos. 2 & 3). 180p. text 39.95 (0-86656-278-8); pap. text 17.95 (0-86656-313-X) Haworth Pr.

Marketing for Therapists: A Handbook for Success in Managed Care. Ed. by Jeri Davis & Michael A. Freeman. 1996. LC 95-44177. (Psychology Ser.). 190p. pap. 35.00 (0-7879-0207-1) Jossey-Bass.

Marketing Health Behavior: Principles, Techniques, & Applications. L. W. Frederiksen et al. 1984. LC 84-3271. (Illus.). 216p. (C). 47.50 (0-306-41523-2, Plenum Trade) Perseus Pubng.

Marketing Health Care. Carole A. Letheren & Richard Mathieu. 1991. (Illus.). 127p. (C). text 29.95 (1-878487-32-9, ME043) Practice Mgmt Info.

Marketing Health Care into the Twenty-First Century: The Changing Dynamic. Alan K. Vitberg. 1996. LC 94-44795. (Haworth Marketing Resources Ser.). (Illus.). 210p. 39.95 (1-56024-979-X) Haworth Pr.

Marketing Healthcare to Women: Meeting New Demands for Products & Services. Patricia Braus. 1997. (Illus.). 200p. 42.50 (0-936889-40-3) Intertec Pub Bks.

Marketing in the NHS. W. R. Sheaff. 1990. (0-335-15428-X); pap. (0-335-15427-1) OpUniv Pr.

Marketing Long-Term & Senior Care Services. William J. Winston. 1984. LC 84-6716. (Health Marketing Quarterly Ser.: Vol. 1, No. 4). 113p. 39.95 (0-86656-289-3) Haworth Pr.

Marketing Management: Issues in Ambulatory Health Care. Robert/E. Sweeney. 1991. (Journal of Ambulatory Care Marketing: Vol. 4 No. 2). (Illus.). 192p. text 49.95 (1-56024-122-5) Haworth Pr.

Marketing Mental Health Services in a Managed Care Environment. Norman Winegar & John L. Bistline. 1994. LC 92-1697. (Illus.). 202p. pap. 14.95 (1-56024-362-7); lib. bdg. 49.95 (1-56024-361-9) Haworth Pr.

Marketing Pharmaceutical Services: Patron Loyalty, Satisfaction, & Preferences. Ed. by Harry A. Smith & Stephen J. Coons. 1992. 368p. pap. 24.95 (1-56024-209-4); LC 91-22251. (Illus.). 386p. lib. bdg. 59.95 (1-56024-208-6) Haworth Pr.

Marketing Pharmacy Services, 1990, Level 2. 1990. 182p. ring bd. 63.00 (1-879907-12-7, P322) Am Soc Hlth-Syst.

Marketing Planning for the Pharmaceutical Industry. John Lidstone. 1987. 250p. text (0-566-02630-9) Gower GBR. *Dist:* Ashgate Pub Co.

Marketing Planning for the Pharmaceutical Industry. John Lidstone & Janice MacLennan. 2nd ed. 1999. LC 98-41233. 146p. (0-566-08112-1) Ashgate Pub GBR. *Dist:* Ashgate Pub Co.

Marketing Public Health: Strategies to Promote Social Change. Michael Siegel & Lynn Doner. 1998. LC 98-24163. 208p. 58.00 (0-8342-1071-1, 10711) Aspen Pub.

Marketing Stragty for Home Health Care Agencies see Marketing Strategy for Home Health Care Agencies

Marketing Strategies: A Resource for Registered Dietitians. Marcia Ward. 1984. (Illus.). (Orig.). pap. 12.95 (0-9613444-0-7) M Ward.

Marketing Strategy for Home Health Care Agencies. Gwen N. Walker. 2000. Orig. Title: Marketing Stragty for Home Health Care Agencies. 180p. pap. 19.99 (0-9672052-1-2) Step Out On Faith.

Marketing Techniques for Physical Therapists. Kathryn Schaefer. 1993. LC 90-14570. 446p. 62.00 (0-8342-0208-5) PRO-ED.

Marketing the Continuum of Care: Hospital Marketing Strategies for Developing Community Service. Vicki Mason. 1997. LC 97-25979. (HFMA Healthcare Financial Management Ser.). 250p. 45.00 (0-7863-1154-1, Irwn Prfssnl) McGraw-Hill Educ Grp.

Marketing the Group Practice: Practical Methods for the Health Care Practitioner. Ed. by William J. Winston. 1983. LC 83-13039. (Health Marketing Quarterly Ser.: Vol. 1, No. 1). 107p. text 39.95 (0-86656-264-8) Haworth Pr.

Marketing to Managed Care Organizations. Kathleen S. Penkert. 1998. LC 97-42357. pap. 9.95 (0-87868-727-0, CWLA Pr) Child Welfare.

Marketing Your Clinical Practice: Ethically, Effectively, Economically. Neil Baum & Gretchen Henkel. 2nd ed. 2000. LC 99-59817. 502p. 82.00 (0-8342-1745-7) Aspen Pub.

Marketing Your Lactation Practice, Vol. 5. Rebecca Black & Linda J. Smith. 2002. (Illus.). 288p. (C). pap. text 43.95 (0-7637-1037-7, 1037-7) Jones & Bartlett.

Marketing Your Practice: Creating Opportunities for Success. American Psychological Association Staff. 1996. (APA Practitioner's Toolbox Ser.). 82p. pap. 29.95 (*1-55798-358-5*) Am Psychol.

Marketing Your Veterinary Practice. Shawn Messonnier. 1994. 168p. 29.95 (*0-939674-56-4*) Am Vet Pubns.

Marketing Your Veterinary Practice, Vol. II. Shawn Messonnier. 1997. LC 96-37947. (Illus.). 176p. (gr. 13). pap. text 28.95 (*0-8151-8583-9*, 28819) Mosby Inc.

Markets & Health Care: A Comparative Analysis. Wendy Ranade. 1998. LC 97-37202. 272p. (C). pap. 57.60 (*0-582-28985-8*) Longman.

Markets & Mortality: Economics, Dangerous Work & the Value of Human Life. Peter Dorman. 1996. 286p. (C). text 59.95 (*0-521-55306-7*) Cambridge U Pr.

Markets & Networks: Contracting in Community Health Services. R. Flynn et al. 1996. LC 96-22704. 192p. 108.95 (*0-335-19457-5*) Taylor & Francis.

Markets & Networks: Contracting in Community Health Services. Flynn et al. 1996. LC 96-22704. 192p. pap. (*0-335-19456-7*) OpUniv Pr.

Marking Residential Care Work: Structure & Culture in Children's Homes. Elizabeth Brown et al. 1998. LC 98-70907. (Dartington Social Research Ser.: Vol. 1). 176p. text (*1-84014-499-8*) Ashgate Pub GBR. *Dist:* Ashgate Pub Co.

Marmoset Periodontium in Health & Disease. Barnet M. Levy et al. Ed. by H. M. Myers. 1972. (Monographs in Oral Science: Vol. 1). 34.00 (*3-8055-1366-6*) S Karger.

Marmosets in Experimental Medicine: Proceedings. Conference on Marmosets in Experimental Medicine Staff. Ed. by J. Moor-Jankowski et al. 1978. (Primates in Medicine Ser.: Vol. 10). (Illus.). 133.25 (*3-8055-2750-0*) S Karger.

Marriage: Its Ethic & Religion. Peter T. Forsyth. 1996. 152p. pap. 17.00 (*1-57910-010-4*) Wipf & Stock.

Marriage: Its History, Character, & Results. Thomas L. Nichols. LC 78-22161. (Free Love in America Ser.). reprint ed. 36.50 (*0-404-60955-4*) AMS Pr.

Marriage-Analysis, Treatment & Results: Index of New Information with Authors & Subjects. Edith Marie Christos. 1992. (Illus.). 180p. 47.50 (*1-55914-696-6*); pap. 44.50 (*1-55914-697-4*) ABBE Pubs Assn.

Marriage & Family Enrichment. Wallace Denton. 1986. LC 86-308. (Journal of Psychotherapy & the Family Ser.: Vol. 2, No. 1). 125p. text 39.95 (*0-86656-495-0*) Haworth Pr.

Marriage & Family Therapy: A Sociocognitive Approach. Nathan Hurvitz & Roger A. Straus. 1991. LC 90-25788. (Marriage & the Family Ser.). 240p. (C). text 49.95 (*1-56024-060-1*); pap. text 19.95 (*1-56024-061-X*) Haworth Pr.

Marriage & Personal Development. Rubin Blanck & Gertrude Blanck. 1968. LC 68-9577. 191p. text 52.50 (*0-231-03150-5*) Col U Pr.

Marriage & the Family: New Directions, New Integrations. Ed. by John T. Chirban. (Series on Medicine, Psychology & Religion). (Illus.). 94p. (Orig.). pap. 4.95 (*0-916586-63-4*) Holy Cross Orthodox.

Marriage Dead or Alive. Adolf Guggenbuhl-Craig. Tr. by Murray Stein. 2000. 150p. pap. 15.00 (*0-88214-378-6*) Spring Pubns.

Marriage, Divorce & Children's Adjustment. Robert E. Emery. 2nd ed. 1999. LC 98-40280. (Developmental Clinical Psychology & Psychiatry Ser.). 160p. pap. 34.95 (*0-7619-0252-X*, 2166) Sage.

Marriage on the Rocks: Learning to Live with Yourself & An Alcoholic. Janet G. Woititz. 1986. 148p. pap. 6.95 (*0-932194-17-6*) Health Comm.

Married Lady's Companion: or Poor Man's Friend. Samuel K. Jennings. 2nd ed. 1978. LC 77-180580. (Medicine & Society in America Ser.). 308p. reprint ed. 23.95 (*0-405-03957-3*) Ayer.

Married to Medicine: An Intimate Portrait of Doctor's Wives. Carla Fine. 1981. LC 80-69372. 3.95 (*0-689-11128-2*) Atheneum Yung Read.

Married Widows: The Wives of Men in Long-Term Care. Maria C. Bartlett. 1993. LC 93-22707. (Studies on the Elderly in America). 136p. text 15.00 (*0-8153-1535-X*) Garland.

Married Woman's Private Medical Companion. A. M. Mauriceau. 1974. LC 73-20635. (Sex, Marriage & Society Ser.). 256p. reprint ed. 23.95 (*0-405-05811-X*) Ayer.

Marrow & Stem Cell Processing for Transplantation. Ed. by Larry C. Lasky & Phyllis Warkentin. 1995. (Illus.). (C). text 35.00 (*1-56395-042-1*) Am Assn Blood.

Marrow Protection: Transduction of Hematopoietic Cells with Drug Resistance Genes. Ed. by J. R. Bertino. 1999. LC 99-25603. (Progress in Experimental Tumor Research Ser.: Vol. 36). (Illus.). vii, 184p. 174.00 (*3-8055-6828-2*) S Karger.

Marrow Stromal Cell Culture. Ed. by Jon Beresford & Maureen Owen. 1998. LC 97-30196. (Handbooks in Practical Animal Cell Biology). (Illus.). (C). 165p. text 74.95 (*0-521-58021-8*); 168p. pap. text 27.95 (*0-521-58978-9*) Cambridge U Pr.

Marshall's Physiology of Reproduction Vol. 2: Reproduction Function in the Male. Ed. by G. E. Lamming. 4th ed. 1990. (Illus.). 704p. text (*0-443-01967-3*) Church.

Marshall's Physiology of Reproduction Vol. 3, Pt. 1 & 2: Pregnancy & Lactation. Ed. by D. Lamming. 4th ed. 1994. (Illus.). 1416p. (C). pap. text 239.95 (*0-412-56770-9*, Chap & Hall NY) Chapman & Hall.

Marsilio Ficino, Three Books on Life: A Critical Edition & Translation. Ed. by Carol V. Kaske & John R. Clark. 1998. (Medieval & Renaissance Texts & Studies: Vol. 57). 528p. reprint ed. 40.00 (*0-86698-041-5*, MR57) MRTS.

Martha E. Rogers: Her Life & Her Work. Ed. by Violet M. Malinski & Elizabeth A. Barrett. 1994. LC 94-6137. (Illus.). 366p. 50.00 (*0-8036-5807-9*) Davis Co.

Martha Rogers: The Science of Unitary Human Beings. Louette R. Lutjens. (Notes on Nursing Theories Ser.: Vol. 1). (Illus.). 40p. (C). 1992. 29.95 (*0-8039-4578-7*, 3029); 1991. pap. 14.95 (*0-8039-4229-X*, 3030) Sage.

Martin Buber-Carl Rogers Dialogue: A New Transcript with Commentary. Rob Anderson & Kenneth N. Cissna. 1997. LC 96-44106. (SUNY Series in Speech Communication). 138p. (C). text 16.50 (*0-7914-3437-0*); pap. text 14.95 (*0-7914-3438-9*) State U NY Pr.

Martindale Extra Pharmacopoeia. Ed. by James Reynolds. 31st ed. 1996. 2739p. text (*0-85369-342-0*) Pharmaceutical Pr GBR. *Dist:* Rittenhouse.

Martin's Quick-E - Critical Care: Clinical Nursing Reference. Martin Schiavenato. 1999. (Martin's Quick-E Clinical Reference Guide Ser.). (Illus.). 40p. spiral bd. 19.95 (*1-929693-02-8*) Bandido Bks.

Martin's Quick-E - E. R. Clinical Nursing Reference. Martin Schiavenato. 1999. (Martin's Quick-E Clinical Reference Guide Ser.). (Illus.). 40p. spiral bd. 19.95 (*1-929693-01-X*) Bandido Bks.

Martin's Quick-E - Med-Surg: Clinical Nursing Reference. Martin Schiavenato. 1999. (Martin's Quick-E Clinical Reference Guide Ser.). (Illus.). 46p. spiral bd. 19.95 (*1-929693-00-1*) Bandido Bks.

Martin's Quick-E - Peds: Clinical Nursing Reference. Martin Schiavenato. 1999. (Martin's Quick-E Clinical Reference Guide Ser.). (Illus.). 40p. spiral bd. 19.95 (*1-929693-03-6*) Bandido Bks.

Martin's Quick-E - Spanish Guide: Clinical Nursing Reference. Martin Schiavenato. 1999. LC 00-703266. (Martin's Quick-E Clinical Reference Guide Ser.). (ENG & SPA., Illus.). 34p. spiral bd. 19.95 (*1-929693-04-4*) Bandido Bks.

Martin's Quick-E Clinical Nursing Reference IV: Intravenous Nursing. Martin Schiavenato. 2000. (Martin's Quick-E Clinical Nursing Reference Ser.). 60p. pap. 19.95 (*1-929693-05-2*) Bandido Bks.

Martin's Quick-E Clinical Nursing Reference OB: Obstetric Nursing. Martin Schiavenato. 2000. (Martin's Quick-E Clinical Nursing Reference Ser.). (Illus.). 60p. pap. 19.95 (*1-929693-06-0*) Bandido Bks.

Marx & the Missing Link: Human Nature. W. Peter Archibald. 1992. LC 89-1978. 292p. (C). pap. 18.50 (*0-391-03754-4*) Brill Academic Pubs.

Mary, Ferrie & the Monkey Virus: The Story of an Underground Medical Laboratory. Edward T. Haslam. 3rd ed. 1997. (Illus.). 144p. (Orig.). 19.95 (*0-9643981-2-5*) Wrdswrth Communs.

Mary Fulstone: Recollections of a Country Doctor in Smith, Nevada. Intro. by Mary E. Glass. 1980. 110p. lib. bdg. 24.00 (*1-56475-183-X*); fiche (*1-56475-184-8*) U NV Oral Hist.

Mary Louise. Lyle Stuart. 128p. 6.00 (*0-8065-0282-7*) Barricade Bks.

Maryland Health Care in Perspective 2000. Ed. by Kathleen O'Leary Morgan & Scott E. Morgan. 2000. 21p. spiral bd. 19.00 (*0-7401-0219-2*) Morgan Quitno Corp.

Maryland Health Care Perspective, 1998. Ed. by Kathleen O'Leary Morgan & Scott E. Morgan. 1998. 20p. pap. 19.00 (*1-56692-819-2*) Morgan Quitno Corp.

Masaje, Tecnica de Beard (Beard's Massage) Giovanni De Domenico. 4th ed. 1997. (SPA., Illus.). 199p. (C). pap. (*84-8174-341-0*) Mosby-Doyma Libros ESP. *Dist:* Mosby Inc, Saunders.

Masculinities & Violence. Lee H. Bowker. 1998. LC 97-33904. (Research on Men & Masculinities Ser.). 91.95 (*0-7619-0451-4*, 800239); pap. 38.95 (*0-7619-0452-2*, 80024) Sage.

Masculinities in Organizations. Cliff Cheng. 1996. LC 96-10041. (Research on Men & Masculinities Ser.: Vol. 9). 288p. 91.95 (*0-7619-0223-6*, 2087); pap. 38.95 (*0-7619-0224-4*, 2088) Sage.

Masculinity & Femininity: Their Psychological Dimensions, Correlates, & Antecedents. Janet T. Spence & Robert L. Helmreich. 1978. LC 77-10693. 309p. pap. text 9.95 (*0-292-75052-8*) U of Tex Pr.

Masculinizing Hormonal Therapy for the Transgendered. Sheila Kirk. 1996. 64p. pap. 14.95 (*1-887796-02-9*) Together Lifeworks.

M*A*S*H: An Army Surgeon in Korea. Otto F. Apel & Pat Apel. 1998. LC 98-15170. (Illus.). 256p. 25.00 (*0-8131-2070-5*) U Pr of KY.

Mashkiki: Old Medicine Nourishing the New. Edwin W. Haller & Larry P. Aitken. 1992. 214p. (Orig.). 58.00 (*0-8191-8556-6*); pap. 28.50 (*0-8191-8557-4*) U Pr of Amer.

Mask of Sanity: An Attempt to Clarify Some Issues about the So-Called Psychopathic Personality. Hervey Cleckley. 5th ed. 1988. 471p. (C). reprint ed. text 25.00 (*0-9621519-0-4*) E S Cleckley.

Masked Depression. Ed. by Stanley Lesse. 1983. LC 73-17744. 394p. 60.00 (*0-87668-688-9*) Aronson.

***Masks of Madness: Orthomolecular Treatment of Mental Illness.** Abram Hoffer & Margot Kidder. 2001. (Illus.). 96p. pap. (*1-55082-260-8*) Quarry Pr CAN. *Dist:* SCB Distributors.

Maslow's Motivation & Personality. Robert Frager & James Fadiman. 3rd ed. 1997. 336p. (C). pap. 32.48 net. (*0-06-041987-3*) Addson-Wesley Educ.

Masochism: A Jungian View. Lyn Barrett Cowan. rev. ed. 1998. LC 82-16957. 138p. (C). pap. 15.00 (*0-88214-367-0*) Spring Pubns.

Masochism & the Emergent Ego. Esther Menaker. 1996. LC 96-10226. (Master Work Ser.). 384p. reprint ed. pap. 50.00 (*1-56821-837-0*) Aronson.

Mason's Basic Medical-Surgical Nursing. Ed. by Grace F. Bates. 6th ed. 1996. LC 96-9332. (Illus.). 835p. pap. 45.00 (*0-07-105428-6*) McGraw-Hill Prof.

Mass Action in the Nervous System: Examination of the Neurophysiological Basis of Adaptive Behavior Through the EEG. Walter J. Freeman. 1975. text 83.00 (*0-12-267150-3*) Acad Pr.

Mass Communication & Public Health. Charles K. Atkin & Lawrence Wallack. 1990. (Focus Editions Ser.: Vol. 121). (Illus.). 250p. (C). pap. 38.95 (*0-8039-3925-6*, 7976) Sage.

Mass Entertainment. Harold Mendelsohn. 1966. pap. 14.95 (*0-8084-0218-8*) NCUP.

Mass Health Examinations. 1971. (Public Health Papers: No. 45). pap. text 6.00 (*92-4-130045-0*, 1110045) World Health.

Mass Media Images & Impact on Health: A Sourcebook. Nancy Signorielli. 1993. LC 92-35546. 240p. lib. bdg. 65.00 (*0-313-27800-8*, SYY, Greenwood Pr) Greenwood.

Mass Psychogenic Illness: A Social Psychological Analysis. Ed. by Michael J. Colligan et al. 1982. 288p. 49.95 (*0-89859-160-0*) L Erlbaum Assocs.

Mass Spectral & GC Data of Drugs, Poisons, Pesticides, Pollutants & Their Metabolites, Pts. I, II & III. Karl Pfleger et al. 2nd enl. rev. ed. 1992. LC 92-49331. 3000p. lib. bdg. 825.00 (*0-89573-855-4*, Wiley-VCH) Wiley.

Mass Spectrometer. J. R. Majer. 1977. (Wykeham Science Ser.: No. 44). 160p. pap. 18.00 (*0-85109-550-X*) Taylor & Francis.

Mass Spectrometry Vol. 1: Clinical & Biomedical Applications, Vol. 1. Dominic M. Desiderio. 1993. (Illus.). 368p. (C). text 79.50 (*0-306-44261-2*, Kluwer Plenum) Kluwer Academic.

Mass Spectrometry in Cancer Research. Roboz. 1995. 225p. 159.95 (*0-8493-0167-X*) CRC Pr.

Mass Spectrometry in Environmental Sciences. Ed. by Francis W. Karasek et al. 1985. LC 84-13469. (Illus.). 598p. (C). 174.00 (*0-306-41552-6*, Plenum Trade) Perseus Pubng.

Mass Spectrometry of Peptides. Ed. by Dominic M. Desidereo. 1990. 440p. lib. bdg. 239.00 (*0-8493-6293-8*, QP551) CRC Pr.

Mass Spectrometry of Proteins & Peptides. Ed. by John R. Chapman. 2000. LC 99-41621. (Methods in Molecular Biology Ser.: Vol. 146). (Illus.). xiv, 538p. 125.00 (*0-89603-609-X*) Humana.

Mass Spectrometry of Steroids. Z. Zaretskii. 1975. 182p. 3.5 hd 58.00 (*0-7065-1453-X*) Coronet Bks.

Massachusetts Eye & Ear Infirmary Residents' Guide to Ocular Antimicrobial Therapy. Ed. by Thomas A. Ciulla & Ann Sullivan Baker. 1996. 88p. (C). pap. text 9.95 (*1-56881-062-8*) AK Peters.

Massachusetts Eye & Ear Infirmary Review Manual for Ophthalmology. Jeffrey C. Lamkin & Massachusetts Eye and Ear Infirmary Staff. 2nd ed. 1998. LC 98-27315. 320p. pap. text 75.00 (*0-7817-1763-9*) Lppncott W & W.

Massachusetts General Hospital Department of Nursing Teaching Guides for Patients with Neurologic Disorders. Massachusetts General Hospital Department of Nursi. 1984. (C). pap. text 27.95 (*0-8359-4342-9*) P-H.

Massachusetts General Hospital Guide to Menopause: What It Is, How to Treat It, How to Cope with It. Isaac Schiff et al. 1996. LC 95-15171. 336p. pap. 15.00 (*0-8129-2318-9*, Crown) Crown Pub Group.

Massachusetts General Hospital Guide to Psychiatry in Primary Care. Ed. by Theodore Stern et al. 1997. LC 97-48338. (Illus.). 720p. pap. 49.95 (*0-07-061498-9*) McGraw-Hill Prof.

Massachusetts General Hospital Handbook of General Hospital Psychiatry. Ned H. Cassem et al. 4th ed. 1998. (Illus.). 688p. pap. (*84-8174-338-0*) Mosby-Doyma Libros ESP. *Dist:* Mosby Inc.

Massachusetts General Hospital Handbook of Neurology. Alice W. Flaherty. 2000. (Illus.). 208p. pap. text 29.95 (*0-683-30576-X*) Lppncott W & W.

Massachusetts General Hospital Handbook of Pain Management. Ed. by David Borsook et al. 1996. LC 95-23369. 400p. pap. text 39.95 (*0-316-54946-0*, Little Brwn Med Div) Lppncott W & W.

Massachusetts General Hospital Psychiatry Update & Board Preparation. Theodore Stern. 1999. LC 00-702437. (Illus.). 679p. pap. 69.00 (*0-07-135435-2*) McGraw-Hill Prof.

Massachusetts Health Care in Perspective 2000. Ed. by Kathleen O'Leary Morgan & Scott E. Morgan. 2000. 21p. spiral bd. 19.00 (*0-7401-0220-6*) Morgan Quitno Corp.

Massachusetts Health Care Perspective, 1998. Ed. by Kathleen O'Leary Morgan & Scott E. Morgan. 1998. 20p. pap. 19.00 (*1-56692-820-6*) Morgan Quitno Corp.

Massachusetts Pharmaceutical Laws & Regulations for Law 351. Doug Pisano. 1999. (C). pap. text 24.80 (*1-56870-368-6*) RonJon Pub.

Massacre of the Innocents: Infanticide in Britain, 1800-1939. Lionel Rose. 1986. (Illus.). 215p. (C). 45.00 (*0-7102-0339-X*, Routledge Thoemms) Routledge.

Massage. Denise Brown. 1995. (Headway Lifeguides Ser.). (Illus.). 88p. pap. (*0-340-55949-7*) Hodder & Stought Ltd GBR. *Dist:* Lubrecht & Cramer, Trafalgar.

Massage: Index of Modern Information. Floyd J. Kazis. 1989. LC 88-47989. 150p. 47.50 (*1-55914-058-5*); pap. 44.50 (*1-55914-059-3*) ABBE Pubs Assn.

Massage Book. Hosler. 1982. (Runner's World Ser.). pap. 9.95 (*0-02-499560-6*, Macmillan Coll) P-H.

Massage Book. Barbara K. Koplan. 1982. (Runner's World Ser.). pap. 9.95 (*0-02-499550-9*, Macmillan Coll) P-H.

Massage During Pregnancy. Bette Waters. 2nd rev. ed. 1995. (Illus.). 177p. pap. 16.95 (*0-9665584-0-5*) Bluwaters Pr.

Massage for Common Ailments. Sara Thomas. 1989. pap. 9.95 (*0-671-67552-4*, Fireside) S&S Trade Pap.

Massage for Health & Healing: Ayurvedic & Spiritual Energy Approach. S. V. Govindan. 1996. (C). (*81-7017-330-2*) Abhinav IND. *Dist:* S Asia.

Massage for Nurses. Walker. 2001. pap. 15.95 net. (*0-7668-0692-8*) Delmar.

Massage for Pain Relief. Peijian Shen. 1996. LC 95-31371. pap. 15.95 (*0-679-76954-4*) Random.

Massage for Sports Health Care Professionals. Human Kinetics. 1999. 80p. pap. 69.00 incl. VHS (*0-7360-0208-1*) Human Kinetics.

Massage for Therapists. Margaret Hollis. 1987. 125p. pap. 23.50 (*0-632-01757-0*); 2nd ed. 1998. LC 98-15039. 208p. pap. 49.95 (*0-632-04788-7*) Blackwell Sci.

Massage National Exam Questions & Answers. Daphna R. Moore. 3rd rev. ed. 2000. (Illus.). 202p. pap. 39.95 (*1-892693-08-9*) Hughes Henshaw.

Massage Therapist's Guide to Pathology. Ed. by Ruth Werner & Ben E. Benjamin. 1998. LC 98-4257. 489p. 41.95 (*0-683-30210-8*) Lppncott W & W.

Massage Therapy: Principles & Practice. Susan G. Salvo. Ed. by Maureen Pfeiffer. 1999. LC 98-8139. (Illus.). 590p. (C). pap. text 52.00 (*0-7216-7419-4*) Saunders.

Massage Therapy: Theory & Practice. Jean Loving. 1998. LC 98-3419. 320p. pap. 48.00 (*0-8385-6161-6*) P-H.

Massage Therapy Career Guide. Capellini. 1998. LC 98-24161. (Massage Ser). (Illus.). 343p. (gr. 12). pap. text 26.95 (*1-56253-382-7*) Thomson Learn.

Massage Therapy Exam Questions. Daphna R. Moore & Gina Perrusquia. 2nd rev. ed. 1999. LC 99-12414. Orig. Title: How to Pass Your Massage Therapy Exams. 141p. pap. text 38.00 (*1-892693-02-X*) Hughes Henshaw.

Massage Therapy Healing Techniques Workbook. Julie Donnelly. rev. ed. 1996. (Illus.). 57p. pap., wbk. ed. 15.95 (*1-929632-00-2*) Julstro Pubns.

Massage Therapy in Ayurveda. Vaidya Bhagwan Dash. 1992. LC 91-908872. (Pancakarma Therapy of Ayurveda Ser.: No. 1). (C). (*81-7022-380-6*) Concept IND. *Dist:* S Asia.

Massive at Last! How to Build More Muscle Mass Than You Ever Thought Possible. Robert Kennedy & Dwayne Hines, II. 1997. LC 97-901067. (Illus.). 64p. pap. (*1-55210-007-3*) MuscleMag Intl CAN. *Dist:* BookWorld.

Massive Myths with Simple Solutions: Revolutionary Breakthrough in Drug Dependencies Derived from Psychopharmacology. Paul M. D'Amico. Ed. by Paul M. D'Amico. 1987. (Illus.). 290p. (YA). 10.00 (*0-89288-163-1*) Damico.

Massive Transfusion. Ed. by Leigh C. Jefferies & Mark E. Brecher. 1994. (Illus.). 166p. (C). text 45.00 (*1-56395-031-6*) Am Assn Blood.

Massry & Glassock's Textbook of Nephrology. Shaul G. Massry & Richard J. Glassock. 4th ed. 2000. 2,112p. text 375.00 (*0-683-30488-7*) Lppncott W & W.

Mast Cell Activation & Mediator Release. Ed. by K. Ishizaka. 1984. (Progress in Allergy Ser.: Vol. 34). (Illus.). xii, 336p. 172.25 (*3-8055-3713-1*) S Karger.

Mast Cell in Health & Disease. Ed. by Michael A. Kaliner & Dean D. Metcalfe. 1992. LC 92-49151. (Lung Biology in Health & Disease Ser.: Vol. 62). (Illus.). 858p. text 275.00 (*0-8247-8732-3*) Dekker.

Mast Cell Proteases in Immunology & Biology, No. 6. George H. Caughey. 1995. (Clinical Allergy & Immunology Ser.: Vol. 6). (Illus.). 352p. text 185.00 (*0-8247-9484-2*) Dekker.

Master Book of Herbalism. Paul Beyerl. 1984. (Illus.). 424p. pap. 14.95 (*0-919345-53-0*) Phoenix WA.

Master Builders of Modern Psychology: From Freud to Skinner. J. D. Keehn. 1996. LC 95-51968. 216p. (C). text 40.00 (*0-8147-4685-3*) NYU Pr.

Master Chohans of the Color Rays. John-Roger. 1979. LC 79-88974. pap. 8.00 (*0-914829-14-9*) Mandeville LA.

Master Clinicians on Treating the Regressed Patient. Ed. by L. Bryce Boyer & Peter L. Giovacchini. 1990. LC 89-6975. (Master Clinicians on Treating the Regressed Patient Ser.: Vol. 1). 408p. 60.00 (0-87668-834-2) Aronson.

Master Feeding Program. Bernard Jensen. 1988. pap. 12.99 (0-932615-12-0) B Jensen.

Master Guide for Passing the Respiratory Care Credentialing Exams. Rick Meyer. 4th ed. 1999. 566p. pap. text 53.33 (0-13-013832-0) P-H.

Master Guide for Passing the Respiratory Care Credentialing Exams. Rick Meyer et al. 4th ed. 1999. LC 99-43212. (Cancer Chemotherapy Annual Ser.). 632p. 182.50 (0-444-50074-X) Elsevier.

Master Guide for Passing the Respiratory Credentialing Exams. Terrance M. Krider et al. 2nd ed. 1989. 472p. pap. 29.95 (0-931263-01-8) Educ Res Consortium.

Master Hand: A Study of the Origin & Meaning of Right & Left Sidedness & Its Relation to Personality & Language. Abram Blau. LC 78-72790. (Brainedness, Handedness, & Mental Abilities Ser.). reprint ed. 49.50 (0-404-60854-X) AMS Pr.

Master Hua's Classic of the Central Viscera. Hua Tuo. Ed. by Bob Flaws. Tr. by Yang Shou-zhong from CHI. 1993. LC 93-71096. 250p. pap. 21.95 (0-936185-43-0) Blue Poppy Pr.

***Master Medicine: Microbiology & Infection.** T. J. J. Inglis. 2nd ed. 2001. (Illus.). 251p. pap. (0-443-07095-4) Church GBR. *Dist:* Saunders.

***Master Medicine: Psychiatry.** Shon Lewis & Elspeth Guthrie. 2001. (Illus.). 251p. pap. text (0-443-06276-5) Church GBR. *Dist:* Saunders.

***Master Medicine - Pathology: A Core Text of Basic Pathological Processes with Self Assessment.** Paul Bass & Claire du Boulay. 2nd ed. 2001. (Master Medicine Ser.). (Illus.). 160p. pap. (0-443-07094-6) Church GBR. *Dist:* Saunders.

***Master of Lucid Dreams.** Olga Kharitidi. 2001. pap. 14.95 (1-57174-329-4) Hampton Roads Pub Co.

Master Office Manual. Wayne Wood. 1992. (Office Manual Ser.). 172p. 89.00 (1-890018-01-5) Anadem Pubng.

Master Secrets of Hypnosis & Self-Hypnosis. Kurt Tepperwein. Ed. by Christian Godefroy. Tr. by R. Sullivan from FRE. 1991. LC 91-73801. 535p. 38.00 (0-941683-15-X) Instant Improve.

Master Stress. Malcolm Newell. 1995. pap. (0-949142-16-6) Stirling Pr AUS. *Dist:* Intl Spec Bk.

Master Techniques in Ophthalmalic Surgery. Roy. 1995. (Illus.). 1,277p. text 110.00 (0-683-07410-5) Lppncott W & W.

Master Techniques in Orthopaedic Surgery: Trauma. Ed. by Donald A. Wiss. 1998. LC 98-15918. 768p. text 199.00 (0-397-51703-3) Lppncott W & W.

Master the Techniques of Ophthalmic Surgery. Ed. by F. Hampton Roy & Renee Tindall. 1994. LC 94-7614. (Illus.). (0-8121-1679-8) Lppncott W & W.

Master Tong's Acupuncture: An Ancient Alternative Style in Modern Clinical Practice. Tr. & Comment by Miriam Lee. 1992. LC 92-73391. (Illus.). 240p. pap. 21.95 (0-936185-37-6) Blue Poppy Pr.

Master Your Panic . . . & Take Back Your Life! Twelve Treatment Sessions to Overcome High Anxiety. Denise F. Beckfield. 2nd ed. 1998. LC 97-51465. 304p. pap. 15.95 (1-886230-08-0) Impact Pubs CA.

MasterCases: Orthopaedic Trauma. Clayton R. Perry. 1999. (Illus.). 456p. 95.00 (0-86577-782-9) Thieme Med Pubs.

MasterCases in Neurosurgery: Peripheral Nerve Surgery. Seth M. Zeidman. 2001. (Illus.). 320p. pap. 59.00 (0-86577-860-4) Thieme Med Pubs.

MasterCases in Shoulder & Elbow Surgery. Felix H. Savoie. 2001. (Illus.). 480p. 95.00 (0-86577-873-6) Thieme Med Pubs.

MasterCases in Spine Surgery. Alexander R. Vaccaro. 2000. (Illus.). 430p. 149.00 (0-86577-924-4) Thieme Med Pubs.

Mastering Anxiety: The Nature & Treatment of Anxious Conditions. R. A. Kleinknecht. 1991. LC 91-2218. (Illus.). 292p. (C). 23.95 (0-306-43769-4) Da Capo.

Mastering APA Style: Student's Workbook & Training Guide. Harold Gelfand & Charles J. Walker. 1990. 238p. (Orig.). (C). pap. 19.95 (1-55798-085-3) Am Psychol.

Mastering Bach Flower Therapies: A Guide to Diagnosis & Treatment. Mechthild Scheffer. 1996. LC 96-5716. (Illus.). 144p. pap. 14.95 (0-89281-630-9, Heal Arts VT) Inner Tradit.

Mastering Chronic Pain: A Professional's Guide to Behavioral Treatment. Robert N. Jamison. 1996. LC 96-16713. 192p. otabind 34.45 (1-56887-018-3, MCPBP, Prof Resc Pr) Pro Resource.

***Mastering Coding: Tools, Techniques & Practical Applications.** Marsha Diamond. 2001. (Illus.). pap., tchr. ed. (0-7216-9040-8); pap., stu. ed., wbk. ed. (0-7216-9042-4) Saunders.

Mastering Documentation. Springhouse Publishing Company Staff et al. 1994. LC 94-29557. 416p. 39.95 (0-87434-749-1) Springhouse Corp.

Mastering Documentation. 2nd ed. 1999. LC 98-42247. 448p. spiral bd. 44.95 (0-87434-952-4) Springhouse Corp.

Mastering Dysrhythmias. Kevin R. Brown & Sheldon Jacobson. 1987. LC 87-15448. (Illus.). 295p. (C). pap. 20.00 net. (0-8036-1251-6) Delmar.

Mastering Expert Testimony: A Courtroom Handbook for Mental Health Professionals. William T. Tsushima & Robert M. Anderson, Jr. 1996. 224p. 45.00 (0-8058-1888-X); pap. 19.50 (0-8058-1889-8) L Erlbaum Assocs.

Mastering Family Therapy: Journeys of Growth & Transformation. Salvador Minuchin et al. 1996. LC 96-22887. 272p. 80.00 (0-471-15558-6) Wiley.

Mastering Geriatric Care. Ed. by Patricia Schull. 1996. LC 96-28895. (Illus.). 480p. (Orig.). spiral bd. 44.95 (0-87434-871-4) Springhouse Corp.

Mastering Medical-Surgical Nursing. SPC Staff. 1997. LC 97-22241. (Illus.). 736p. spiral bd. 44.95 (0-87434-909-5) Springhouse Corp.

Mastering Medical Terminology. Peggy Stanfield & Yh Hui. 3rd ed. 2002. (Illus.). 736p. (C). pap. text 49.95 (0-7637-1480-1, 1480-1) Jones & Bartlett.

Mastering Medicine: The Most Current, Concise & Comprehensive Guide to Medical Education. Zia Hashemi. 1995. LC 95-94427. (Illus.). 135p. (Orig.). pap. 12.95 (0-9645956-7-2) Z Hashemi.

Mastering NABPLEX. Kosegarten. 2000. (Essentials of Medical Imaging Ser.). 359p. pap. 34.95 (0-07-134538-8) McGraw-Hill Prof.

Mastering New Medical Terminology. Christine Stanfield & Pogorzala. 2nd ed. 1995. (Nursing Ser.). (Illus.). 192p. (C). pap. text, tchr. ed. 14.95 (0-86720-733-7, 733-7) Jones & Bartlett.

Mastering Path-Based Patient Care. Patrice L. Spath. 1995. (Illus.). 210p. 50.00 (1-929955-02-2) Brown Spath.

Mastering Psychology. Lester A. Lefton. 3rd ed. 1988. 680p. (C). pap. text 34.00 (0-205-10626-9, H0626-5) Allyn.

Mastering Records Completion: Successful Strategies from Medical Records Briefing. Rob Stuart. 1997. 140p. pap. text 87.00 (1-57839-019-2) Opus Communs.

Mastering Resistance: A Practical Guide to Family Therapy. Carol M. Anderson & Susan Stewart. 1983. LC 82-21033. (Guilford Family Therapy Ser.). 259p. text 35.00 (0-89862-044-9, 2044) Guilford Pubns.

Mastering Statistics: A Guide for Health Service Professionals & Researchers. Kelvin Jordan et al. 1998. pap. (0-7487-3325-6) Nelson Thornes GBR. *Dist:* Intl Spec Bk, Trans-Atl Phila.

Mastering the Marketplace: Taking Your Practice to the Top Ross Clark. Incl. Taking Your Practice to the Top. 358p. pap. Not sold separately (0-935078-57-6); The Workbook. (Illus.). 158p. pap. Not sold separately (0-935078-58-4); LC 96-60136. 1996. Set pap. 89.95 (0-935078-65-7) Veterinary Hlthcare.

***Mastering the Negotiation Process: A Practical Guide for the Healthcare Executive.** Christopher L. Laubach. 2002. LC 2001-51517. (1-56793-170-7) Health Admin Pr.

Mastering the New Medical Terminology Through Self-Instructional Modules: Principles & Practices. Peggy S. Stanfield & Yiu H. Hui. 2nd ed. 1995. LC 94-31116. (Illus.). 592p. (C). pap. text 49.95 (0-86720-686-1, 686-1) Jones & Bartlett.

Mastering the Nursing Process: A Case Method Approach. Jean D. Leuner et al. 1990. LC 89-71523. (Illus.). 494p. (Orig.). (C). pap. text 26.95 (0-8036-5588-6) Davis Co.

Mastering the Objective Structured Clinical Examination & Clinical Skills Assessment. Jo-Ann Reteguiz & Beverly Cornel-Avendano. 1999. LC 98-55698. (Illus.). 336p. pap. 39.95 (0-07-135012-8) McGraw-Hill Prof.

Mastering the Oral Boards: An Oral Board Review System. G. A. Smith. 1994. 250p. (Orig.). pap. text, per. 149.95 (0-9635538-4-4) MEDTEXT Med.

Mastering the Reimbursement Process. American Medical Association Staff. 2nd ed. 1999. 200p. pap. 49.95 (0-89970-762-9, OP080095WE) AMA.

Mastering the Zone: The Next Step in Achieving SuperHealth Permanent Fat Loss. Barry Sears & Mary Goodbody. 1997. LC 96-39111. (Illus.). 384p. 25.00 (0-06-039190-1, ReganBooks) HarperCollins Pubs.

Mastering Your Moods. Melvyn Kinder. 1994. LC 93-26169. 288p. 21.00 (0-671-78223-1) S&S Trade.

Masters of Bedlam: The Transformation of the Mad-Doctoring Trade. Andrew T. Scull et al. 1996. LC 96-12051. (Illus.). 408p. 75.00 (0-691-03411-7) Princeton U Pr.

Masters of Medicine: An Historical Sketch of the College of Medical Sciences of the University of Minnesota, 1888-1966. J. Arthur Myers. 1968. LC 68-8890. (Illus.). 942p. 22.50 (0-87527-058-1); pap. 17.50 (0-87527-140-5) Green.

Masters of Social Psychology: Freud, Mead, Lewin, & Skinner. James A. Schellenberg. 1979. 152p. pap. text 17.95 (0-19-502622-5) OUP.

Mastery Motivation Vol. 12: Origins, Conceptualizations & Applications. Ed. by Robert H. MacTurk & George A. Morgan. 1995. LC 96-136371. (Advances in Applied Developmental Psychology Ser.: Vol. 12). (Illus.). 336p. pap. 39.50 (1-56750-203-2, Ablex) Greenwood.

Mastery Motivation Vol. 12: Origins, Conceptualizations & Applications, 12. Robert H. MacTurk & George A. Morgan. Ed. by Gallaudet University Press Staff & Colorado State University Staff. 1995. LC 96-136371. (Advances in Applied Developmental Psychology Ser.: Vol. 12). (Illus.). 336p. 77.00 (1-56750-146-X, Ablex) Greenwood.

Mastery of Cardiothoracic Surgery. Ed. by Larry R. Kaiser & Irving Kron. 1997. LC 97-23282. (Illus.). 1,008p. text 225.00 (0-316-48210-2) Lppncott W & W.

Mastery of Cardiothoracic Surgery. Larry R. Kaiser & Irving L. Kron. 1997. LC 97-23282. 1053p. text (0-7817-1423-0) Lppncott W & W.

Mastery of Endoscopic & Laparoscopic Surgery. Steve Eubanks et al. 1998. LC 98-32156. (Illus.). xx, 619p. text 225.00 (0-316-26865-8) Lppncott W & W.

Mastery of Plastic & Reconstructive Surgery. Ed. by Mimis Cohen. 1994. LC 93-33838. 2,736p. text 399.00 (0-316-15003-7) Lppncott W & W.

Mastery of Submission: Inventions of Masochism. John K. Noyes. 1997. LC 96-51035. (Cornell Studies in the History of Psychiatry). (Illus.). 256p. 29.95 (0-8014-3345-2) Cornell U Pr.

Mastery of Surgery. Lloyd M. Nyhus et al. 3rd ed. 1996. LC 96-9115. (0-316-61751-2, Little Brwn Med Div) Lppncott W & W.

Mastery of Surgery, Set. Lloyd M. Nyhus & Robert Baker. 1984. 1540p. 240.00 (0-316-61742-3, Little Brwn Med Div) Lppncott W & W.

Mastery of Your Anxiety & Worry. Michelle G. Craske et al. 1992. 150p. stu. ed. 19.95 (1-880659-04-2) Graywind Pubns.

Mastology—Breast Diseases: Proceedings of the 8th International Congress on Senology, Breast Diseases, 8-12 May, 1994, Rio de Janeiro, Brazil. Antonio S. S. Figueira Fo. 1995. LC 95-45214. (International Congress Ser.: No. 1067). 422p. 218.50 (0-444-82102-3, Excerpta Medica) Elsevier.

Masturbation: From Infancy to Senescence. Ed. by Irwin M. Marcus & John J. Francis. 1975. LC 73-16855. 634p. 75.00 (0-8236-3150-8) Intl Univs Pr.

Matching Consultation, Assessment, & Intervention. Donald J. Dickinson. 1993. LC 93-79581. (Illus.). 310p. (C). pap. text 18.00 (0-9637951-4-7) Hart-Whitlow Pubs.

Matching Law: A Research Review. Michael Davison & Dianne McCarthy. 1987. 296p. 59.95 (0-89859-923-7) L Erlbaum Assocs.

Matching Law: Papers in Psychology & Economics. Richard J. Herrnstein et al. 1997. LC 96-31500. (Illus.). 368p. 33.95 (0-674-06459-3) HUP.

Matching Metaphors: Companion Teaching Tales to Teaching Stress Management Skills. Frances K. Wiggins. 1987. 45p. (Orig.). (C). pap. 6.50 (0-942937-03-1) Rivijon Pr.

Matching People with Services in Long-Term Care. Ed. by Zev Harel & Ruth Dunkle. 1995. LC 95-3183. (Illus.). 304p. 42.95 (0-8261-8950-4) Springer Pub.

Materia Medica of Ayureda. Bhagwan D. Vaidya. 1991. (C). text 18.50 (0-8364-2781-5) S Asia.

Materia Medica of Ayurveda. Bhagavan D. Dash & Lalitesh Kashyap. 1988. (C). (0-8364-2325-9) Concept IND. *Dist:* S Asia.

Materia Medica of Ayurveda. Bhagwan Dass. 1988. (C). (0-7855-2283-2) Scientific GBR. *Dist:* St Mut.

Materia Medica of Indo-Tibetan Medicine. Vaidya B. Dash. 1987. 647p. (C). (81-85132-00-3) Classics India Pubns IND. *Dist:* S Asia.

Materia Medica of the Hindus. U. C. Dutt. 1995. (C). reprint ed. (0-8364-2915-X) Mittal Pubs Dist IND. *Dist:* S Asia.

Materia Medica of Tibetan Medicine. Vaidya B. Dash. 1994. LC 93-908512. (C). (81-7030-387-7) Sri Satguru Pubns IND. *Dist:* S Asia.

Materia Medica of W. India. A. Dymock. 1986. (C). (0-7855-2264-6) Scientific GBR. *Dist:* St Mut.

Material Discourses of Health & Illness. Ed. by Lucy Yardley. 1997. 256p. (C). 78.95 (0-415-13823-X) Routledge.

Material Discourses of Health & Illness. Ed. by Lucy Yardley & Jane M. Ussher. 1997. 256p. (C). pap. 26.95 (0-415-13824-8) Routledge.

Materiales Dentales. Craig. 6th ed. 1996. (C). text 29.42 (84-8174-188-4) Mosby Inc.

Materials & Strategies for the Education of Trainable Mentally Retarded Learners. James P. White. 1990. LC 90-38465. (Source Books on Education: Vol. 24). 366p. text 50.00 (0-8240-6345-7, SS476) Garland.

Materials for the Physical Anthropology of the Eastern European Jews. Maurice Fishberg. 1905. (American Anthropological Association Memoirs Ser.). 25.00 (0-527-00500-2) Periodicals Srv.

Materials in Dentistry: Principles & Applications. Jack L. Ferracane. 1994. (Illus.). 384p. (C). pap. text 40.00 (0-397-54955-5, Lippncott) Lppncott W & W.

***Materials in Dentistry: Principles & Applications.** Jack L. Ferracane. 2nd ed. 2001. LC 00-69159. (Illus.). xiv, 354p. pap. text 40.00 (0-7817-2733-2) Lppncott W & W.

Materials Management in the Operating Room. Mary Starr. 1993. (Illus.). 122p. (Orig.). pap. 55.00 (0-87258-644-8, 142901) Am Hospital.

Materials Science & Implant Orthopedic Surgery. Ram Kossowsky & Nir Kossovsky. 1986. text 218.00 (90-247-3409-6) Kluwer Academic.

Materials Science & Technology: A Comprehensive Treatment, Medical & Dental Materials, Vol. 14. Ed. by D. F. Williams. 1992. (Illus.). 469p. 390.00 (3-527-26827-8, Wiley-VCH) Wiley.

Materials Science of Synthetic Membranes. Ed. by Douglas R. Lloyd. 1984. LC 84-21652. (ACS Symposium Ser.: No. 269). 494p. lib. bdg. 87.95 (0-8412-0887-5) Am Chemical.

Materials Testing & Biocompatibility: Index of New Information & Medical Research Bible. Steve K. Martinez. rev. ed. 1997. 183p. 57.50 (0-7883-1564-1); pap. 47.50 (0-7883-1565-X) ABBE Pubs Assn.

Materials Used in Pharmaceutical Formulation. A. T. Florence. LC 85-210857. (Critical Reports on Applied Chemistry Ser.). 35.00 (0-632-01257-9) Blackwell Sci.

Maternal - Newborn Nursing: Theory & Practice. Nichols. 1715p. Price not set. (0-7216-6252-8) Saunders.

Maternal & Child Health: Programs, Problems, & Policy in Public Health. Jonathan B. Kotch. 1997. LC 96-48785. (Illus.). 496p. 55.00 (0-8342-0771-0, 20771) Aspen Pub.

Maternal & Child Health Nurse. Jack Rudman. 1994. (Certified Nurse Examination Ser.: CN-9). pap. 27.95 (0-8373-6109-5) Nat Learn.

Maternal & Child Health Nursing. A. Joy Ingalls & M. Constance Salerno. 4th ed. 1987. pap. text 15.95 (0-8016-2412-6) Mosby Inc.

Maternal & Child Health Nursing: Care of the Childbearing & Childrearing Family. Adele Pillitteri. 3rd ed. 1998. LC 98-22348. 1,800p. text 83.95 (0-7817-1547-4) Lppncott W & W.

Maternal & Child Health Statistics: Russian Federation & United States, Selected Years 1985-1995. National Center for Health Statistics Staff. 1998. LC 98-15066. (International Vital & Health Statistics Ser.). 120p. (0-8406-0545-5) Natl Ctr Health Stats.

Maternal & Child Nursing. Betty L. Broom et al. 9th ed. 1999. LC 99-10442. text 45.95 (0-323-00322-2) Mosby Inc.

Maternal & Child Nursing - Associate. Jack Rudman. (Regents College Proficiency Examination Ser.: Vol. 22). 43.95 (0-8373-5472-2) Nat Learn.

Maternal & Child Nursing, Associate. Jack Rudman. 1994. (Regents College Proficiency Examination Ser.: CPEP-22). pap. 23.95 (0-8373-5422-6) Nat Learn.

Maternal & Child Nursing, Associate Degree. Jack Rudman. (ACT Proficiency Examination Program Ser.: Vol. 37). 43.95 (0-8373-5587-7); 1994. pap. 23.95 (0-8373-5537-0) Nat Learn.

Maternal & Child Nursing, Baccalaureate. Jack Rudman. 1994. (Regents College Proficiency Examination Ser.: CPEP-23). pap. 23.95 (0-8373-5423-4) Nat Learn.

Maternal & Child Nursing, Baccalaureate Degree. Jack Rudman. (ACT Proficiency Examination Program Ser.: Vol. 38). 43.95 (0-8373-5588-5); 1994. pap. 23.95 (0-8373-5538-9) Nat Learn.

Maternal & Child Oral Health Regional Workshops: Summary Report. Jane E. Steffensen. 1994. 52p. pap. text (1-57285-002-7) Nat Ctr Educ.

Maternal & Fetal Thyroid Function in Pregnancy. Ed. by J. G. Thorpe Beeston & K. H. Nicolaides. 1995. (Illus.). 128p. lib. bdg. 71.95 (1-85070-611-5, Parthenon Pbng) CRC Pr.

Maternal & Infant Health Care. Ed. by Mary J. Houston. 1984. LC 96-6398. (Illus.). 205p. pap. (0-443-02813-3) Church.

Maternal & Infant Nursing Care. Elizabeth J. Dickason. 3rd ed. 1997. (Illus.). (C). (gr. 13). 128p. pap. text, stu. ed. 14.95 (0-8151-2518-6, 29926); LC 97-10756. 928p. text 55.00 (0-8151-2517-8, 29925) Mosby Inc.

Maternal & Neonatal Nursing. Aileen MacLaren. 1993. LC 93-37753. (Concepts & Activities Ser.). (Illus.). 448p. pap. 23.95 (0-87434-576-6) Springhouse Corp.

Maternal Anthropometry & Pregnancy Outcomes: A WHO Collaborative Study. 1995. (WHO Bulletin Supplement Ser.: No. 73). 98p. pap. text 20.00 (92-4-068730-0) World Health.

Maternal Care for the Reduction of Perinatal & Neonatal Mortality: A Joint WHO-UNICEF Statement. 1986. 22p. pap. text 2.70 (92-4-156099-1, 1150248) World Health.

Maternal Child Health Nursing Research Digest. Ed. by Joyce J. Fitzpatrick & Kristen S. Montgomery. 1999. LC 99-23404. 244p. text 34.95 (0-8261-1294-3) Springer Pub.

Maternal-Child Home Health Aide Training Manual. Mary Ann Chestnut. 1997. LC 97-25842. 224p. pap. text 42.50 (0-7817-1204-1) Lppncott W & W.

Maternal-Child Nursing Care. Shannon E. Perry & Donna L. Wong. 1997. LC 97-8667. (Illus.). 1848p. (C). (gr. 13). text 79.00 (0-8151-2837-1, 29893) Mosby Inc.

Maternal-Child Nursing Care. Donna L. Wong. 1998. (Illus.). 448p. (C). (gr. 13). stu. ed. (0-8151-2473-2, 31054) Mosby Inc.

Maternal-Child Nursing Care: Includes Testbank. Donna L. Wong & Shannon E. Perry. 1998. (Illus.). tchr. ed. (0-8151-2537-2) Mosby Inc.

Maternal Deprivation. Michael Rutter. 1991. 288p. pap. (0-14-013526-X) Pnguin Bks Ltd GBR. *Dist:* Trafalgar.

Maternal Disease in Pregnancy. K. H. Nicolaides. 2001. (Diploma in Fetal Medicine Ser.). (Illus.). 150p. lib. bdg. 67.95 (1-84214-061-2, Parthenon Pbng) CRC Pr.

Maternal Drug Abuse & Drug Exposed Children: Understanding the Problem. 1994. (Illus.). 82p. (Orig.). (C). pap. text 25.00 (0-7881-1480-8) DIANE Pub.

Maternal Employment & Children's Development: Longitudinal Research. A. E. Gottfried & A. W.

Gottfried. 1988. LC 88-15167. (Studies in Work & Industry). (Illus.). 316p. (C). 52.50 (*0-306-42867-9*, Plenum Trade) Perseus Pubng.

Maternal, Fetal & Neonatal Physiology: A Clinical Perspective. Blackburn. 1991. (Illus.). 735p. text 95.00 (*0-7216-2936-9*) Saunders.

Maternal-Fetal Endocrinology. Ed. by Dan Tulchinsky & Brian A. Little. 2nd ed. 1994. LC 93-9931. (Illus.). 448p. text 79.00 (*0-7216-4232-2*) Saunders.

Maternal Fetal Interface. Ed. by Anthony Carter et al. 1998. LC 98-30167. (Trophoblast Research Ser.: Vol. 12). (Illus.). 448p. 120.00 (*1-58046-043-7*) Univ Rochester Pr.

Maternal-Fetal Medicine. Robert K. Creasy & Robert Resnick. Ed. by Lisette Bralow. 4th ed. 1998. LC 98-12044. (Illus.). 1152p. (C). text 139.00 (*0-7216-7605-7*) Saunders.

Maternal-Fetal Medicine: Principles & Practice. Ed. by Robert K. Creasy & Robert Resnik. 3rd ed. 1993. LC 92-48215. (Illus.). 1168p. (C). text 135.00 (*0-7216-6590-X*) Saunders.

Maternal-Fetal Toxicology: A Clinician's Guide. Ed. by Gideon Koren. 2nd exp. rev. ed. 1994. (Medical Toxicology Ser.: Vol. 2). (Illus.). 848p. text 215.00 (*0-8247-8841-9*) Dekker.

Maternal Genetic Disease. Nelson Isada & Evans Johnson. 1996. LC 95-4745. 272p. (C). pap. text 95.00 (*0-8385-6164-0*, A6164-6, Apple Lange Med) McGraw.

Maternal Health & Infant Survival. C. Arden Miller. 2nd ed. 1991. LC 91-62010. 52p. reprint ed. pap. text 7.50 (*0-943657-14-8*) ZERO TO THREE.

Maternal Health Services: Index of New Information with References. Maurice K. Hobden. 1997. 160p. 57.50 (*0-7883-1542-0*); pap. 47.50 (*0-7883-1543-9*) ABBE Pubs Assn.

Maternal-Infant Care Planning. Melson et al. 3rd ed. 1998. LC 98-36726. 384p. pap. 39.95 (*0-87434-951-6*) Springhouse Corp.

Maternal-Infant Nursing Care. Elizabeth J. Dickason & Martha O. Schultz. 3rd ed. 1998. (Illus.). tchr. ed. (*0-8151-2563-1*) Mosby Inc.

Maternal-Infant Nursing Care: Text, Student Learning Guide Package, Set. Elizabeth J. Dickason et al. 3rd ed. 1998. (Illus.). (C). text, stu. ed. (*0-8151-2521-6*) Mosby Inc.

Maternal-Infant Nursing Care Plans. Karla Luxner. unabr. ed. 1999. (Nursing Care Plans Ser.). 309p. pap. 39.95 (*1-56930-099-2*) Delmar.

Maternal-Infant Nursing Care Pocket Handbook. Elizabeth J. Dickason. 3rd ed. 1998. (Illus.). 400p. (C). (gr. 13). pap. text 14.95 (*0-8151-2519-4*, 29927) Mosby Inc.

Maternal Journal. Linda Schwartz et al. 1982. LC 82-4736. (Illus.). 80p. (Orig.). pap. 5.95 (*0-912800-99-2*) Woodbridge Pr.

Maternal Journal: Your Personal Pregnancy Guide. Matthew Bennett. 1999. (Illus.). 28p. per. 10.00 (*0-671-31798-9*) S&S Trade.

Maternal Mortality: A Global Factbook. Compiled by C. AbouZahr & E. Royston. 1991. 608p. pap. text 50.00 (*92-4-159001-7*, 1930024) World Health.

Maternal, Neonatal, & Women's Health Nursing. Lynna Littleton & Joan Engebretson. 2001. LC 2001-32460. (Illus.). 1256p. (C). text 68.95 (*0-7668-0121-7*) Delmar.

Maternal, Neonatal & Women's Health Nursing Student's Activity Book. MacLaren et al. 1991. 304p. pap., stu. ed. 17.95 (*0-87434-360-7*) Springhouse Corp.

Maternal-Neonatal Nursing. Lynne Conrad. 3rd ed. 1996. LC 96-29145. (Springhouse Notes Ser.). (Illus.). 192p. (Orig.). pap. 26.95 (*0-87434-860-9*) Springhouse Corp.

Maternal Neonatal Nursing: A Holistic Approach. Staley. 1996. (Professional Reference - Nursing Ser.). 60.95 (*0-8273-7785-1*); 18.95 (*0-8273-7786-X*); 10.50 (*0-8273-7787-8*); 10.50 (*0-8273-7788-6*) Delmar.

Maternal Newborn. Patricia A. Ladewig et al. Ed. by Debra Hunter. 2nd ed. 1990. 889p. (C). pap. text 9.95 (*0-201-53238-7*) Addison-Wesley.

Maternal-Newborn Home Care Manual. Mary A. Chestnut. 1997. LC 97-25845. 208p. pap. text 42.50 (*0-397-55474-5*) Lppncott W & W.

Maternal-Newborn Nursing. National Student Nurses' Association, Inc. Staff. 1994. LC 93-37630. (NSNA Review Ser.). 263p. (C). pap. 21.50 (*0-8273-5674-9*) Delmar.

Maternal-Newborn Nursing. Georgiana M. Stamps & Gasparis. 1991. LC 91-5208. (Nursetest: A Review Ser.). 272p. pap. 21.95 (*0-87434-304-6*) Springhouse Corp.

Maternal Newborn Nursing. Sally B. Olds. Ed. by Patti Cleary. 4th ed. 1992. 1328p. (C). pap. text 18.75 (*0-8053-5581-2*) Addison-Wesley.

Maternal-Newborn Nursing: Theories. Francine H. Nichols. 1997. pap. text, stu. ed. 17.95 (*0-7216-6258-7*) Saunders.

Maternal-Newborn Nursing: Theory & Practice. Francine H. Nichols & Elaine Zwelling. 1997. 1715p. tchr. ed. (*0-7216-6249-8*) Saunders.

Maternal-Newborn Nursing: Theory & Practice. Francine H. Nichols & Elaine Zwelling. Ed. by Ilze Rader. 1997. LC 96-15371. 1344p. text 66.95 (*0-7216-6777-5*) Saunders.

***Maternal-Newborn Nursing: Theory & Practice, ExaMaster.** Francine H. Nichols. 1997. (Illus.). text 250.00 (*0-7216-6251-X*) Saunders.

Maternal-Newborn Nursing Care: The Nurse, the Family & the Community. Patricia W. Ladewig. 4th ed. 1997. 288p. (C). pap. text, wbk. ed. 27.19 (*0-8053-5628-2*) Addison-Wesley.

Maternal-Newborn Nursing Care: The Nurse, the Family, & the Community, with Student Disk. Patricia Ladewig et al. 4th ed. 1997. LC 97-37686. (Illus.). 896p. (C). pap. text 71.24 (*0-8053-5622-3*) Addison-Wesley.

Maternal-Newborn Plans of Care: Guidelines for Planning & Documenting Client Care. Marilynn E. Doenges & Mary F. Moorhouse. 3rd ed. 1999. LC 98-31646. (Illus.). 580p. (C). pap. text 37.95 (*0-8036-0320-7*) Davis Co.

Maternal Nutrition & Child Health. Douglas R. Shanklin. 2000. LC 00-23479. (Illus.). 316p. pap. text 42.95 (*0-398-07075-X*); 2nd ed. text 59.95 (*0-398-07074-1*) C C Thomas.

Maternal Nutrition & Pregnancy Outcome. Ed. by Carl L. Keen et al. 1993. LC 93-21708. (Annals Ser.: Vol. 678). (*0-89766-753-0*); pap. 110.00 (*0-89766-754-9*) NY Acad Sci.

Maternal Nutrition & Pregnancy Outcomes: Anthropometric Assessment. Ed. by K. Krasovec et al. 1991. (PAHO Scientific Publications: No. 529). (ENG & SPA.). ix, 214p. pap. text 50.00 (*92-75-11529-X*, 1610529) World Health.

Maternal Overprotection. David M. Levy. 1966. (C). pap. 2.50 (*0-393-00349-3*) Norton.

Maternal Personality, Evolution, & the Sex Ratio: Do Mothers Control the Sex of the Infant? Valerie J. Grant. 1998. LC 97-14825. 240p. (C). 78.95 (*0-415-15879-6*) Routledge.

Maternal Physician: A Treatise on the Nurture & Management of Infants from the Birth until Two Years Old Being the Result of Sixteen Years' Experience in the Nursery. American Matron Staff. 2nd ed. 1972. LC 70-180581. (Medicine & Society in America Ser.). 294p. reprint ed. 20.95 (*0-405-03958-1*) Ayer.

Maternal Serum Screening for Fetal Genetic Disorders. Ed. by Sherman Elias & Joe L. Simpson. 1992. LC 92-16757. (Illus.). 139p. text (*0-443-08867-5*) Church.

Maternal Substance Abuse & the Developing Nervous System. Ed. by Ian S. Zagon & Theodore A. Slotkin. 1992. LC 92-7145. (Illus.). 377p. text 73.00 (*0-12-775225-0*) Acad Pr.

Maternal/Pediatric Nursing for Practical Nursing. Shapiro. 1994. (LPN/LVN Nursing Ser.). tchr. ed. 16.95 (*0-8273-4994-7*) Delmar.

Maternity: Letters from Working Women. Margaret L. Davies. 1990. 211p. pap. 13.95 (*0-86068-028-2*) Trafalgar.

Maternity - Women's Health Nursing. Paulette D. Rollant & Karen A. Piotrowski. 1995. LC 95-20708. (Mosby's Review Ser.). (Illus.). 560p. (C). (gr. 13). pap. text 24.95 incl. 3.5 hd (*0-8151-7246-X*, 24859) Mosby Inc.

Maternity & Gynecologic Care: The Nurse & the Family. Irene M. Bobak et al. 4th ed. 1988. (Illus.). 1408p. (C). trans. 75.00 (*0-8016-0470-2*) Mosby Inc.

Maternity & Pediatric Nursing. Paulette Rollant et al. 2nd ed. 2000. LC 00-45226. (Illus.). xxix, 639p. 27.95 incl. cd-rom (*0-323-01216-7*) Mosby Inc.

Maternity & Woman's Health. Deitra Leonard Lowdermilk. 7th ed. 2000. pap. text (*0-323-01180-2*) Mosby Inc.

Maternity & Women's Health Care. Deitra L. Lowdermilk & Irene M. Bobak. 6th ed. 1996. (Illus.). 328p. (C). (gr. 13). pap. text, stu. ed. 19.95 (*0-8151-5579-4*, 28012) Mosby Inc.

Maternity & Women's Health Care. Deitra L. Lowdermilk et al. 6th ed. 1997. (Illus.). tchr. ed. (*0-8151-5578-6*) Mosby Inc.

Maternity & Women's Health Care. Deitra Leonard Lowdermilk et al. 7th ed. 2000. (Illus.). 1215p. text 69.00 (*0-323-00961-1*) Mosby Inc.

***Maternity & Women's Health Care: Computer Test Bank.** Deitra Leonard Lowdermilk et al. 7th ed. 2000. 500.00 (*0-323-00963-8*) Mosby Inc.

***Maternity & Women's Health Care: Instructor's Resource Manual.** Deitra Leonard Lowdermilk et al. 7th ed. 2000. (Illus.). 250.00 (*0-323-00962-X*) Mosby Inc.

Maternity & Women's Healthcare. C. V. Mosby Company Staff. 6th ed. 1999. 66.00 (*0-323-01063-6*) Mosby Inc.

Maternity Care. Helen Farrer. 2nd ed. 1990. (Illus.). 224p. pap. text (*0-443-04209-8*) Church.

Maternity Care: Resources for Family-Centered Practice Beveryl H. Johnson et al. 1997. (Family-Centered Care Ser.). 140p. ring bd. 40.00 (*0-9642014-9-6*) Inst Fmly Ctr.

***Maternity Leave Breast Feeding Plan.** William G. Wilkoff. 2002. (Illus.). pap. 12.00 (*0-7432-1345-9*, Fireside) S&S Trade Pap.

Maternity Massage: A Healthy Indulgence a Welcome Relief. Connie Cox. 1994. LC 94-66358. 98p. pap. 12.95 (*1-885044-01-1*) Stress Less.

Maternity Nursing. Jack Rudman. 1994. (ACT Proficiency Examination Program Ser.: PEP-58). 43.95 (*0-8373-5933-3*, PEP-58); pap. 23.95 (*0-8373-5908-2*) Nat Learn.

Maternity Nursing. Janice Holmes. 2nd ed. 1995. (Nursing Education Ser.). text 57.50 (*0-8273-5531-9*) Delmar.

Maternity Nursing. Connolly-Lauder & Schwartz. 3rd ed. 1998. 222p. (C). per. 47.95 (*0-7872-4568-2*, 41456801) Kendall-Hunt.

Maternity Nursing. Van Hoozer. 3rd ed. 1999. (Illus.). 154p. (*0-8385-7087-9*, A7087-8) Appleton & Lange.

Maternity Nursing. Zimbler. 3rd ed. 1999. (Illus.). 320p. pap. text, stu. ed. 30.40 (*0-8385-7113-1*, Medical Exam) Appleton & Lange.

Maternity Nursing. Irene M. Bobak et al. 4th ed. (Illus.). tchr. ed. (*0-8151-0615-7*) Mosby Inc.

Maternity Nursing. Deitra Leonard Lowdermilk et al. 5th ed. 1998. LC 98-33732. xx, 932p. 54.00 (*0-323-00215-3*) Mosby Inc.

Maternity Nursing. Deitra L. Lowdermilk et al. 5th ed. 1998. (Illus.). tchr. ed. (*0-323-00217-X*) Mosby Inc.

Maternity Nursing. Deitra Leonard Lowdermilk et al. 5th ed. 1999. (Illus.). 952p. stu. ed. 72.95 (*0-323-00865-8*) Mosby Inc.

Maternity Nursing. Karen A. Piotrowski. 5th ed. 1998. (Illus.). 224p. stu. ed. (*0-323-00216-1*) Mosby Inc.

***Maternity Nursing: An Introductory Text.** Arlene Burroughs & Gloria Leifer. 2000. pap., tchr. ed. (*0-7216-9172-2*) Saunders.

Maternity Nursing: An Introductory Text. Arlene Burroughs. 6th ed. 1992. (Illus.). pap., tchr. ed. (*0-7216-4507-0*) Saunders.

Maternity Nursing: An Introductory Text. Burroughs. 7th ed. (C). text (*0-8089-2119-3*, Grune & Strat) Harcrt Hlth Sci Grp.

Maternity Nursing: An Introductory Text. Arlene Burroughs. Ed. by Ilze Rader. 7th ed. 1997. LC 97-7111. (Illus.). 608p. pap. text 31.50 (*0-7216-2473-1*) Saunders.

Maternity Nursing: An Introductory Text. Arlene Burroughs. 7th ed. 1997. (Illus.). pap., tchr. ed. (*0-7216-2496-0*) Saunders.

Maternity Nursing: Care of the Childbearing Family. Mary A. Scoloveno et al. 3rd rev. ed. 1999. LC 98-31091. (Illus.). 1232p. (C). 82.00 (*0-8385-7083-6*) Appleton & Lange.

Maternity Nursing: Family, Newborn & Women's Health Care. Sharon J. Reeder et al. 18th ed. 1996. LC 96-15970. 1,328p. text 64.95 (*0-397-55166-5*) Lppncott W & W.

Maternity Nursing IRK. Janice Holmes. 1997. (Nursing Education Ser.). tchr. ed. 51.50 (*0-8273-7216-7*); stu. ed. 20.95 (*0-8273-7217-5*) Delmar.

Math & Dosage Calculations for Health Occupations: Instructor's Guide. Dawe. 1999. tchr. ed. 12.21 (*0-02-800678-X*) Glencoe.

Math & Meds for the Nurse. Delores F. Saxton. 1998. LC 97-44437. (Student Material TV). (Illus.). 400p. (C). pap. text 48.95 (*0-8273-7331-7*) Thomson Learn.

Math Calculations in Respiratory Therapy. Ray Sibberson. 1994. 200p. (*0-683-07732-5*) Lppncott W & W.

Math Concepts for Food Engineering. Ed. by R. W. Hartel et al. 1997. LC 97-60545. 177p. 34.95 (*1-56676-564-1*) CRC Pr.

Math for Health Professionals. B. Louise Whisler. 3rd ed. 1992. 320p. (C). pap. text 37.50 (*0-86720-447-8*) Jones & Bartlett.

Math for Meds: Dosages & Solutions. Laurie D. Munday. 8th rev. ed. 2000. LC 00-266127. (Illus.). 306p. pap. text 34.95 (*0-918082-09-9*, 30,000) WI Pubns Inc.

Math for Nurses. Miller. 2nd ed. 1996. (Mathematics Ser.). pap. 46.95 (*0-534-20616-6*) Brooks-Cole.

Math for Nurses: A Pocket Guide to Dosage Calculation & Drug Administration. Mary Jo Boyer. 4th ed. 1998. LC 97-42716. 320p. spiral bd. 16.95 (*0-7817-1021-9*) Lppncott W & W.

Math for Nurses: A Problem Solving Approach. Sally I. Lipsey & Donna D. Ignatavicius. 1993. (Illus.). 256p. pap. text 28.00 (*0-7216-6481-4*); (C). pap. text, tchr. ed. (*0-7216-6496-2*) Saunders.

Math Modeling in Social & Biomedical Sciences. Edward Beltrami. 1992. (C). 50.00 (*0-86720-292-0*) Jones & Bartlett.

Math Principles & Practice: Preparing for Health Career Success. Michele Benjamin-Chung. 1998. LC 98-28717. 176p. pap. text 38.00 (*0-8359-5272-X*) P-H.

Math-Pro: Preparation for Real World Medical Administration. Cynthia R. Butters. 1992. pap. 19.95 (*0-397-54904-0*) Lppncott W & W.

Mathematical Analysis of Biomedical Images, 1996 Workshop On. 1996. LC 96-77115. 350p. pap. 70.00 (*0-8186-7367-2*, PRO7367) IEEE Comp Soc.

Mathematical Analysis of the Electrical Activity of the Brain. Ed. by M. N. Livanov et al. Tr. by John S. Barlow. 1968. LC 68-17621. (Illus.). 113p. 22.95 (*0-674-55400-0*) HUP.

Mathematical & Statistical Approaches to AIDS Epidemiology. C. Castillo-Chavez. 1990. (Lecture Notes in Biomathematics: Vol. 83). 405p. 69.95 (*0-387-52174-7*) Spr-Verlag.

Mathematical Approaches to Problems in Resource Management & Epidemiology. Ed. by C. Castillo-Chavez et al. 1989. (Lecture Notes in Biomathematics: Vol. 81). 327p. 61.95 (*0-387-51820-7*) Spr-Verlag.

Mathematical Aspects of Chemical & Biochemical Problems & Quantum Chemistry: Proceedings of the SIAM-AMS Seminar, New York, 1974. Ed. by Donald S. Cohen. 1974. LC 74-26990. (SIAM-AMS Proceedings Ser.: Vol. 8). 153p. text 47.00 (*0-8218-1328-5*, SIAMS-8) Am Math.

Mathematical Aspects of Physiology. Ed. by Frank C. Hoppensteadt. 1981. LC 81-1315. (Lectures in Applied Mathematics: No. 19). 394p. text 60.00 (*0-8218-1119-3*, LAM/19) Am Math.

Mathematical Concepts in Clinical Science. Steven Tiger et al. 1999. LC 99-49101. (Illus.). 302p. pap. 34.00 (*0-13-011549-5*) P-H.

Mathematical Concepts in Nursing: A Workbook. H. Readey & W. Readey. 1980. pap. text 17.56 (*0-201-06166-X*, Health Sci) Addison-Wesley.

Mathematical Epidemiology of Infectious Diseases: Model Building, Analysis & Interpretation. O. Diekmann. 2000. LC 99-52964. (Mathematical & Computational Biology Ser.). (Illus.). 320p. 150.00 (*0-471-98682-8*) Wiley.

Mathematical Methods for DNA Sequences. Ed. by Michael S. Waterman. 1988. 288p. lib. bdg. 215.95 (*0-8493-6664-X*, QP624) CRC Pr.

Mathematical Methods in Clinical Practice. Ed. by Gurii I. Marchuk & N. I. Nisevich. 1980. (Illus.). 150p. (*0-08-025493-4*) Pergamon Repr GBR. *Dist:* Franklin.

Mathematical Methods in Medicine. Richard Ernest Bellman. 1983. (Series in Modern Applied Mathematics: Vol. 1). 268p. text 52.00 (*9971-950-20-0*); pap. text 30.00 (*9971-950-21-9*) World Scientific Pub.

Mathematical Methods in Sample Surveys. Howard G. Tucker. 1998. LC 98-29452. 206p. 24.00 (*981-02-2617-9*) World Scientific Pub.

Mathematical Modeling: Applications in Emergency Health Services. Ralph B. D'Agostino et al. 1984. LC 84-12917. (Emergency Health Services Review Ser.: Vol. 2, Nos. 2-3). 118p. 29.95 (*0-86656-373-3*) Haworth Pr.

Mathematical Modeling in Epidemiology. J. C. Frauenthal. 1980. (Universitext Ser.). 118p. 59.95 (*0-387-10328-7*) Spr-Verlag.

Mathematical Modeling in Experimental Nutrition: Proceedings of a Conference Held in Davis, California, August 17-20, 1997. Ed. by Andrew J. Clifford. 1998. LC 98-8315. (Advances in Experimental Medicine & Biology Ser.: Vol. 445). (Illus.). 436p. (C). text 125.00 (*0-306-46020-3*, Kluwer Plenum) Kluwer Academic.

Mathematical Modeling in Tumor Growth & Progression. Ed. by Seth Michelson. 1997. (Invasion & Metastasis Ser.: Vol. 16, No. 4-5, 1997). (Illus.). 100p. pap. 48.75 (*3-8055-6548-8*) S Karger.

Mathematical Modeling of Pharmacokinetic Data. David W. Bourne. 1995. LC 94-61269. 139p. 104.95 (*1-56676-204-9*) CRC Pr.

Mathematical Modeling of the Immune Response. Daniela Prikrylova. 1992. 224p. 125.00 (*0-8493-6753-0*, QR186) CRC Pr.

Mathematical Modelling in Biomedicine. Y. Cherruault. 1986. text 144.00 (*90-277-2149-1*) Kluwer Academic.

Mathematical Modelling in Medicine. Ed. by J. T. Ottensen & M. Danielsen. 2000. LC 99-68339. (Studies in Health Technology & Informatics: Vol. 71). (Illus.). viii, 235p. 80.00 (*1-58603-026-4*) IOS Press.

Mathematical Modelling of Immune Response in Infectious Diseases, Vol. 395. G. I. Marchuk. 1997. LC 97-12156. (Mathematics & Its Applications Ser.). text 187.00 (*0-7923-4528-2*) Kluwer Academic.

Mathematical Models in Immunology. Gurii I. Marchuk. Ed. by A. V. Balakrishnan. 1983. LC 83-8269. (Translations Series in Mathematics & Engineering). (Illus.). 378p. pap. text 98.00 (*0-911575-01-4*) Optimization Soft.

Mathematical Models in Immunology. G. I. Mnarchuk. 1983. (Illus.). xxv, 351p. 89.95 (*0-387-90901-X*) Spr-Verlag.

Mathematical Models in Medical & Health Science. Ed. by Mary Ann Horn et al. 1998. LC 98-38746. (Innovations in Applied Mathematics Ser.). (Illus.). 496p. text 60.00 (*0-8265-1310-7*) Vanderbilt U Pr.

Mathematical Models in Medical Diagnosis. M. C. Miller, III et al. 1981. LC 81-5170. 187p. 62.95 (*0-275-91349-X*, C1349, Praeger Pubs) Greenwood.

Mathematical Models in Medicine, Vol. 2. M. Witten. 1988. (Computers & Mathematics with Applications Ser.: No. 301). 310p. 95.00 (*0-08-036377-6*, Pergamon Pr) Elsevier.

Mathematical Models in Medicine: Diseases & Epidemics, Vol. 7, Nos. 5-12. Ed. by M. Witten. 1987. 1100p. 182.50 (*0-08-034692-8*, Pergamon Pr) Elsevier.

Mathematical Models in Microbial Population Dynamics. Ed. by Richard B. Philp. 1981. 288p. 164.00 (*0-8493-6110-9*, RM340, CRC Reprint) Franklin.

Mathematical Models in the Social Management & Life Sciences. D. N. Burghes & A. D. Wood. 1980. LC 79-40989. (Mathematics & Its Applications Ser.). 287p. pap. 41.95 (*0-470-27073-X*) P-H.

Mathematical Physiology. J. Keener et al. 1998. LC 98-14499. (Interdisciplinary Applied Mathematics Ser.: Vol. 8). (Illus.). 785p. 69.95 (*0-387-98381-3*) Spr-Verlag.

Mathematical Problems in the Biological Sciences. Sol I. Rubinow. 1973. (CBMS-NSF Regional Conference Series in Applied Mathematics: No. 10). vii, 90p. pap. text 21.00 (*0-89871-008-1*) Soc Indus-Appl Math.

Mathematical Problems in the Biological Sciences: Proceedings. Ed. by R. Bellman. 1962. LC 50-1183. (Proceedings of Symposia in Applied Mathematics Ser.: Vol. 14). 250p. text 36.00 (*0-8218-1314-5*, PSAPM/14) Am Math.

Mathematical Psychology & Psychophysiology. Ed. by Stephen Grossberg. 1981. LC 81-3500. (SIAM-AMS Proceedings Ser.: 13). 318p. text 51.00 (*0-8218-1333-1*, SIAMS/13) Am Math.

Mathematical Psychology & Psychophysiology. Ed. by Stephen Grossberg. 1981. 330p. 59.95 (*0-89859-182-1*) L Erlbaum Assocs.

Mathematical Psychology in Progress. Ed. by E. E. Roskam. 1989. (Recent Research in Psychology Ser.). 385p. 79.95 (*0-387-51686-7*) Spr-Verlag.

Mathematical Structure of the Human Sleep-Wake Cycle. Steven H. Strogatz. 1986. (Lecture Notes in Biomathematics: Vol. 69). 247p. 46.95 (*0-387-17176-2*) Spr-Verlag.

Mathematical Structures of Epidemic Systems. Vincenzo Capasso. 1993. LC 93-10042. (Lecture Notes in Biomathematics: Vol. 97). 297p. 69.95 (*0-387-56526-4*) Spr-Verlag.

Mathematical Techniques for Biology & Medicine. William Simon. 1987. 320p. reprint ed. pap. 10.95 (*0-486-65247-5*) Dover.

Mathematical Theory of Infectious Diseases. 2nd ed. (*0-85264-231-8*) Lubrecht & Cramer.

Mathematics & Computer Science in Medical Imaging. Ed. by Max A. Viergever & Andrew E. Todd-Pokropek. 1988. (NATO ASI Ser.: Vol. 39). 546p. 153.00 (*0-387-18672-7*) Spr-Verlag.

Mathematics & Medicine: How Serious Is the Injury? William Sacco et al. 1987. (Contemporary Applied Mathematics Ser.). (Illus.). 61p. (Orig.). (YA). (gr. 9 up). pap. text 11.95 (*0-939765-06-3*, G103) Janson Pubns.

Mathematics & Physics of Emerging Biomedical Imaging. National Research Council Staff. 1996. LC 95-72622. 260p. (Orig.). pap. text 29.00 (*0-309-05387-0*) Natl Acad Pr.

Mathematics & Physics of Neutron Radiography. A. A. Harms & D. R. Wyman. 1986. text 107.50 (*90-277-2191-2*) Kluwer Academic.

***Mathematics & Simulation in Medicine & the Life Sciences.** Frank C. Hoppensteadt & Charles S. Peskin. Ed. by J. E. Marsden et al. 2nd ed. 2001. LC 2001-32010. (Texts in Applied Mathematics: Vol. 10). (Illus.). 350p. 49.95 (*0-387-95072-9*) Spr-Verlag.

Mathematics & Statistics in Anaesthesia. Steven Cruickshank. 1998. LC 97-53170. (Illus.). 268p. pap. text 49.50 (*0-19-262312-5*) OUP.

Mathematics for Health Careers. Carol Castellon et al. 1993. LC 93-15623. (C). pap. 26.50 (*0-8273-5569-6*) Delmar.

Mathematics for Health Careers: Instructor's Guide. Carol Castellon et al. 1994. 52p. tchr. ed. 12.95 (*0-8273-6357-5*) Delmar.

Mathematics for Health Occupations. Kathi Dunlap. 1991. 200p. (C). mass mkt. 28.50 (*0-8273-4173-3*) Delmar.

Mathematics for Health Occupations. Dennis Bila et al. 1986. 526p. reprint ed. stu. ed. (*0-935115-04-8*); pap. text 18.36 (*0-87626-570-0*) Instruct Tech.

Mathematics for Health Sciences. Keith Roberts & Leo Michels. 1996. LC 81-12234. (Mathematics Ser.). 423p. (C). mass mkt. 41.25 (*0-8185-0478-1*) Brooks-Cole.

Mathematics for the Biological Sciences. Jagdish C. Arya & Robin W. Lardner. 1979. LC 78-13424. (Illus.). 705p. 100.00 (*0-13-562439-8*) P-H.

Mathematics for the Health Sciences. Paul T. Olsen & Sandra Murrell. 1981. (Developmental & Precalculus Math Ser.). (Illus.). 432p. pap. text (*0-201-04647-4*) Addison-Wesley.

Mathematics for the Health Sciences. John B. Scott & E. L. Hutton. 1978. 205p. pap. text 19.95 (*0-89641-009-9*) American Pr.

Mathematics in Medicine & the Life Sciences. Frank C. Hoppensteadt & C. S. Peskin. Ed. by F. John et al. 1996. LC 91-4945. (Texts in Applied Mathematics: Vol. 10). (Illus.). 252p. 49.95 (*0-387-97639-6*) Spr-Verlag.

Mathematics of Cell Electrophysiology. Cronin. 1981. (Lecture Notes in Pure & Applied Mathematics Ser.: Vol. 63). (Illus.). 144p. pap. text 125.00 (*0-8247-1157-2*) Dekker.

Mathematics of Drugs & Solutions with Clinical Applications. Judith Knight Richardson & Lloyd I. Richardson. 5th ed. 1993. (Illus.). 188p. (C). (gr. 13). pap. text 27.00 (*0-8016-7895-1*) Mosby Inc.

Mathematics of Radiology & Nuclear Medicine. Herbert L. Jackson. rev. ed. 1991. LC 70-107201. (Illus.). 167p. reprint ed. 10.20 (*0-87527-019-0*) Green.

Mathematics Recovered for the Natural & Medical Sciences. Dennis Rosen. 1992. (Illus.). 224p. (C). (gr. 13). ring bd. 49.95 (*0-412-41040-0*, A6503, Chap & Hall CRC) CRC Pr.

Mathematics Review for Health Physics Technicians. K. Paul Steinmeyer et al. 1994. 412p. pap. text 35.00 (*0-9630191-1-2*) RSA Pubns.

Mathematics, the Gas Laws & the Respiratory Practitioner. C. Peters. 1988. 33p. (C). pap. 15.00 (*0-933195-37-0*) CA College Health Sci.

Mating. M. Ronald Minge et al. 1982. 352p. pap. 9.95 (*0-940162-01-6*) Red Lion.

Matkailualan Ammattisanasto. Honelin. 1987. (ENG & FIN.). 130p. pap. 95.00 (*0-8288-7813-7*) Fr & Eur.

Matrix & Matrix Regulation: Basis for a Holistic Theory in Medicine. Alfred Pischinger. Ed. by Hartmut Heine. Tr. by Norman Mac Lean from GER. 1991. (Illus.). 221p. (C). text (*2-8043-4000-7*) Edits Haug Intl BEL. *Dist:* Medicina Bio.

Matrix Metalloproteinase Inhibitors in Cancer Therapy. Ed. by Neil J. Clendeninn & Krysztof Appelt. 2000. LC 99-89543. (Cancer Drug Discovery & Development Ser.). (Illus.). xi, 262p. 135.00 (*0-89603-668-5*) Humana.

Matrix of the Mind: Object Relations & the Psychoanalytic Dialogue. Thomas H. Ogden. 1994. LC 85-13404. 288p. reprint ed. pap. 40.00 (*1-56821-051-5*) Aronson.

Matrons, Medics & Maladies: Edinburgh Royal Infirmary in the 1840's. Bill Yule. 2000. LC 00-303243. (Illus.). 236p. pap. (*1-86232-091-8*) Tuckwell Pr GBR. *Dist:* General Distrib Services.

Matter, Mind & Medicine: Transforming the Clinical Method. Jacques Kriel. 2000. (Value Inquiry Book Ser.: Vol. 93). XXXII, 157p. pap. 39.00 (*90-420-0799-0*) Rodopi.

Matter of Balance: Personal Strategies for Alcohol & Other Drugs. Holstein et al. 1995. (Illus.). 180p. (C). pap. text 23.00 (*0-926544-12-8*) CNS.

Matter of Life. W. Coda Martin. 1965. 6.95 (*0-8159-6202-9*) Devin.

Matter of Life & Death: Health, Illness & Medicine in McLean County. Lucinda M. Beier. 1996. (Illus.). 312p. (Orig.). 40.00 (*0-943788-09-9*); pap. 15.00 (*0-943788-08-0*) McLean County.

Matters of Life & Death: Jewish Bio-Ethics. Elliot N. Dorff. 1998. LC 97-36295. 474p. 34.95 (*0-8276-0647-8*) JPS Phila.

Matty's Heart: A Child's & Parents' Guide to Open Heart Surgery. Jean Clabough. Ed. by Debbie Polk & M. W. Cocalis. 1995. LC 94-71677. (Child's & Parent's Medical Storybooks Ser.: Vol. 1). (Illus.). 55p. (J). (gr. k-6). lib. bdg. 14.95 (*0-9638662-3-0*) Aletheia CA.

Maturation of Fetal Body Systems: Proceedings of the WHO Scientific Group, Geneva, 1973. WHO Staff. 1974. (Technical Reports: No. 540). pap. text 5.00 (*92-4-120540-7*, 1100540) World Health.

Maturation of Neurotransmission: Proceedings of the Satellite Symposium, Sainte-Vincent, August, 1977. Satellite Symposium on Maturational Aspects of Neu. Ed. by Antonia Vernadakis et al. 1978. (Illus.). 68.00 (*3-8055-2833-7*) S Karger.

Maturation of the Therapeutic Community: An Organic Approach to Health & Mental Health. Maxwell Jones. 1976. LC 75-11002. 169p. 32.95 (*0-87705-264-6*, Kluwer Acad Hman Sci) Kluwer Academic.

Maturation Phenomenon in Cerebral Ischemia: Proceedings of the Satelite Symposium of the International Congress on Neuropathology, 11th, Tokyo, September 11-12, 1990. Ed. by Umeo Ito et al. 1992. (Illus.). 208p. 82.95 (*0-387-54871-8*) Spr-Verlag.

Maturation Phenomenon in Cerebral Ischemia Vol. II: Neuronal Recovery & Plasticity, No. II. Ed. by Umeo Ito et al. 1997. LC 96-36379. (Illus.). 225p. 84.00 (*3-540-61673-X*) Spr-Verlag.

Maturational Processes & the Facilitating Environment: Studies in the Theory of Emotional Development. Donald Woods Winnicott. 1965. 296p. 45.00 (*0-8236-3200-8*, 03200) Intl Univs Pr.

Mature Gravida. Virginia A. Passero. Ed. by Karla Damus et al. 1995. LC 95-33586. (*0-86525-067-7*) March of Dimes.

Maudsley Handbook of Practical Psychiatry. Ed. by David P. Goldberg & Bethlem Royal Hospital and the Maudsley Hospital Staff. 3rd ed. 1997. LC 97-3039. (Oxford Medical Publications). (Illus.). 294p. pap. 27.50 (*0-19-262853-4*) OUP.

Mausner & Bahn Epidemiology: An Introductory Text. Judith S. Mausner & Shira Kramer. 2nd ed. 1985. (Illus.). 361p. pap. text 40.95 (*0-7216-6181-5*) Saunders.

Mawson's Diseases of the Ear. Harold Ludman. 5th ed. 688p. pap. (*0-7131-4580-3*) E A GBR. *Dist:* Routldge.

Mawsouat Al Toubiya. Hamad A. Saamak. Ed. by Yousseff Farhat. 1990.Tr. of Medical Encyclopedia. (ARA., Illus.). 2880p. 699.00 (*1-58311-002-X*) Eastern Corp.

Max Brodel: The Man Who Put Art into Medicine. R. W. Crosby & J. Cody. 1993. (Illus.). 352p. 81.95 (*0-387-97563-2*) Spr-Verlag.

Maxillary & Trimalar Fractures: Applied Pathophysiology & Repair: Self-Instructional Package. Arnold Komisar et al. 2nd ed. 1994. LC 94-31838. (Self-Instructional Package Ser.). (Illus.). 75p. pap. text 25.00 (*1-56772-015-3*) AAO-HNS.

Maxillofacial & Dental Emergencies. John Hawkesford & James G. Banks. 1994. (Oxford Handbooks in Emergency Medicine Ser.: Vol. 7). (Illus.). 196p. 65.00 (*0-19-262391-5*); 192p. pap. text 29.50 (*0-19-261997-7*) OUP.

Maxillofacial Injuries Ed. by N. L. Rowe & J. L. Williams. (Illus.). 2nd ed. 1994. 1067p. (C). text (*0-443-04591-7*); Set. 1985. 1080p. text (*0-443-01509-0*) Church.

***Maxillofacial Surgery**, Set. Peter Ward-Booth et al. 1999. (Illus.). 1500p. (*0-443-05853-9*) Church GBR. *Dist:* Saunders.

***Maxillofacial Trauma.** Yadranko Ducic et al. Ed. by Robert H. Maisel. 2001. LC 2001-22635. (Monograph). (Illus.). 148p. pap. text 75.00 (*1-56772-034-X*, 5206290) AAO-HNS.

Maxillofacial Trauma: An International Perspective. Ed. by John R. Jacobs. 1983. LC 82-18116. 303p. 79.50 (*0-275-91398-8*, C1398, Praeger Pubs) Greenwood.

Maximal Myocardial Perfusion As a Measure of the Functional Significance of Coronary Artery Disease: From a Pathoanatomic to a Pathophysiologic Interpretation of the Coronary Arteriogram. Nico H. Pijls. 1991. (Developments in Cardiovascular Medicine Ser.). 208p. text 137.50 (*0-7923-1430-1*) Kluwer Academic.

Maximizing Mobility after Stroke: Nursing the Acute Patient. George I. Turnbull & Patricia A. Bell. 1985. LC 85-71509. (Illus.). 84p. pap. text 16.95 (*0-914783-10-6*) Charles.

Maximizing Psychotherapeutic Gains & Preventing Relapse in Emotionally Distressed Clients. John W. Ludgate. 1995. LC 95-20029. (Practitioner's Resource Ser.). 81p. pap. 16.95 (*1-56887-014-0*, MPGBP, Prof Resc Pr) Pro Resource.

Maximizing the Arthritis Cure: A Step-by-Step Program to Faster, Stronger Healing During Any Stage of the Cure. Jason Theodosakis et al. 1998. LC 97-47099. (Illus.). 224p. 22.95 (*0-312-18134-5*) St Martin.

Maximizing the Role of Nutrition in Diabetes Management. American Diabetes Association. 1994. 64p. pap. 24.95 (*0-945448-42-2*, 5607-01) Am Diabetes.

Maxims of Madness. Michael A. Roybal. 1993. 137p. (Orig.). pap. 8.00 (*0-9639456-0-2*) Maximedia NM.

Maximum Metabolism: The Diet Breakthrough for Permanent Weight Loss. Robert M. Giller. 1990. pap. 13.95 (*0-425-12180-1*) Berkley Pub.

Maximum Permissible Body Burdens & Maximum Permissible Concentrations of Radionuclides in Air & in Water for Occupational Exposures. 1959. (Report Ser.: No. 22). pap. 20.00 (*0-913392-06-5*) NCRP Pubns.

Maxwell Quick Medical Reference. Robert W. Maxwell. (Illus.). 32p. (Orig.). (C). 1995. pap. text 7.95 (*0-9645191-0-0*); 3rd rev. ed. 1996. pap. text 7.95 (*0-9645191-1-9*) Mxwll Pub.

Maya-Spanish Crosses in Yucatan. George D. Williams. 1931. (HU PMP Ser.: Vol. 13, No. 1). 25.00 (*0-527-01228-9*) Periodicals Srv.

Maye's Midwifery. Betty R. Sweet. 12th ed. 1996. (Illus.). 915p. pap. text (*0-7020-1757-4*) W B Saunders GBR. *Dist:* Saunders.

Maynaud Features, Acrocyanosis, Cryoimmunoproteins. Ed. by E. Davis. 1982. (Advances in Microcirculation Ser.: Vol. 10). (Illus.). viii, 116p. 85.25 (*3-8055-2790-X*) S Karger.

Mayo Clinic Diet Manual: A Handbook of Nutrition Practices. Jennifer K. Nelson et al. 7th ed. 1994. LC 93-43747. (Illus.). 912p. (C). (gr. 13). pap. text 75.00 (*0-8151-6348-7*, 23782) Mosby Inc.

Mayo Clinic Examinations in Neurology. Mayo Clinic Staff. 7th ed. 1997. LC 97-26131. (Illus.). 528p. (C). (gr. 13). text 62.95 (*0-8151-9319-X*, 26881) Mosby Inc.

Mayo Clinic Family Health Book: The Ultimate Home Medical Reference. David E. Larson. 2nd rev. ed. 1996. LC 96-23661. (Illus.). 1456p. 45.00 (*0-688-14478-0*, Wm Morrow) Morrow Avon.

Mayo Clinic Guide to Self-Care see Clinica Mayo Guia de Autocuidados

Mayo Clinic Guide to Self Care see Clinica Mayo: Guia de Autocuidades

Mayo Clinic Guide to Self-Care: Answers for Everyday Health Problems. Ed. by Philip T. Hagen. 2nd ed. 1999. LC 98-68087. (Mayo Clinic on Health Ser.). 279p. pap. 19.95 (*0-9627865-7-8*) Mayo Fndtn Med Ed & Res.

Mayo Clinic Heart Book. Mayo Clinic Staff. 1993. LC 93-25353. 368p. 26.00 (*0-688-09972-6*, Wm Morrow) Morrow Avon.

Mayo Clinic Heart Book. Ed. by Bernard J. Gersh. 2nd rev. ed. 2000. LC 99-53785. (Illus.). viii, 406p. 30.00 (*0-688-17642-9*, Wm Morrow) Morrow Avon.

Mayo Clinic Manual of Nuclear Medicine. Ed. by Michael K. O'Connor. 1996. LC 96-11649. 592p. pap. text (*0-443-07765-7*) Church.

Mayo Clinic on Arthritis: Brings You the Answers You Need for Managing Arthritis from the World Renowned Mayo Clinic. Ed. by Gene G. Hunder. 1999. LC 98-67333. (Mayo Clinic on Health Ser.). (Illus.). 188p. pap. 14.95 (*1-893005-00-3*) Mayo Fndtn Med Ed & Res.

***Mayo Clinic on Chronic Pain.** David Swanson. l.t. ed. 2001. 292p. (*0-7089-4349-7*, Ulverscroft) F A Thorpe GBR. *Dist:* Ulverscroft US.

Mayo Clinic on Chronic Pain: Lead a More Active & Productive Life with Answers from the World Renowned Mayo Clinic. Ed. by David Swanson. 1999. LC 98-68086. (Mayo Clinic on Health Ser.). (Illus.). 178p. pap. 14.95 (*1-893005-02-X*) Mayo Fndtn Med Ed & Res.

***Mayo Clinic on Depression: Answers to Help You Understand, Recognize & Manage Depression.** Ed. by Keith G. Kramlinger. 2001. LC 00-136715. (Mayo Clinic on Health Ser.). (Illus.). 216p. pap. 14.95 (*1-893005-17-8*) Mayo Fndtn Med Ed & Res.

Mayo Clinic on Digestive Health: Enjoy Better Digestion with Answers to More Then 12 Common Conditions. John E. King. 2000. (Mayo Clinic on Health Ser.). (Illus.). 204p. pap. 14.95 (*1-893005-04-6*) Mayo Fndtn Med Ed & Res.

Mayo Clinic on Healthy Aging: Answers to Help You Make the Most of the Rest of Your Life. Ed. by Edward T. Creagan. 2001. LC 00-135980. (Illus.). 192p. pap. 14.95 (*1-893005-07-0*) Mayo Fndtn Med Ed & Res.

Mayo Clinic on Healthy Weight: How to Determine & Achieve the Weight That's Best for You. Ed. by Donald D. Hensrud. 2000. LC 00-130630. (Mayo Clinic on Health Ser.). (Illus.). 196p. pap. 14.95 (*1-893005-05-4*) Mayo Fndtn Med Ed & Res.

Mayo Clinic on High Blood Pressure. Ed. by Sheldon G. Sheps. l.t. ed. 2000. 344p. (*0-7089-4301-2*, Ulverscroft) F A Thorpe GBR. *Dist:* Ulverscroft US.

Mayo Clinic on High Blood Pressure: Brings You the Answers You Need for Treating & Preventing High Blood Pressure From the World Renowned Mayo Clinic. Ed. by Sheldon G. Sheps. 1999. LC 98-68088. (Mayo Clinic on Health Ser.). 192p. pap. 14.95 (*1-893005-01-1*) Mayo Fndtn Med Ed & Res.

Mayo Clinic on Managing Diabetes: Practical Answers to Help You Enjoy a Healthy & Active Life. Ed. by Maria Collazo-Clavell. 2001. (Illus.). 216p. pap. 14.95 (*1-893005-06-2*) Mayo Fndtn Med Ed & Res.

Mayo Clinic on Prostate Disease. Ed. by David M. Barrett. 2000. pap. 14.95 (*1-57566-541-7*, Knsington) Kensgtn Pub Corp.

Mayo Clinic on Prostate Health: Answers from the World Renowned Mayo Clinic on Prostate Inflammation, Enlargement, Cancer. Ed. by David M. Barrett. 2000. LC 99-85835. (Mayo Clinic on Health Ser.). (Illus.). ix, 178p. pap. 14.95 (*1-893005-03-8*) Mayo Fndtn Med Ed & Res.

Mayo Clinic's Complete Guide for Family Physicians & Residents in Training. Robert L. Bratton. 1999. LC 00-500863. (Illus.). 364p. pap. 60.00 (*0-07-134683-X*) McGraw-Hill Prof.

Mayo Internal Medicine Board Review, 2000-2001. Mayo Clinic Department of Internal Medicine Staff & Udaya B.S. Prakash. 2000. 1,006p. pap. text 99.00 (*0-7817-2393-0*) Lppncott W & W.

Mayo Internal Medicine Board Review, 1996-1997. Ed. by Udaya B. Prakash. 1996. 1000p. 89.95 (*0-9627865-2-7*) Mayo Fndtn Med Ed & Res.

Mayo Internal Medicine Board Review, 1994-1995. Ed. by Udaya B. Prakash. 1994. 1000p. text 89.95 (*0-9627865-1-9*) Mayo Fndtn Med Ed & Res.

May's Manual of the Diseases of the Eye. James H. Allen. 1974. LC 74-10746. 442p. reprint ed. 48.50 (*0-88275-190-5*) Krieger.

MBA in Five Days: A Handbook for Health-Care Professionals. J. S. Sanfilippo. 2001. LC 2001-50001. 200p. lib. bdg. 57.95 (*1-84214-074-4*, Parthenon Pbng) CRC Pr.

MBD: The Family Book about Minimal Brain Dysfunction. Richard A. Gardner. 1973. LC 72-96533. (Illus.). 192p. 40.00 (*0-87668-853-9*) Aronson.

McAlpine's Multiple Sclerosis. W. B. Matthews et al. 2nd ed. 1990. (Illus.). 401p. text (*0-443-04047-8*) Church.

McAlpine's Multiple Sclerosis. D. A. Compston et al. 3rd ed. 1998. (Illus.). 440p. text (*0-443-05008-2*) Church.

MCAT - Medical College Admission Test: Comprehensive Manual Self Study. David M. Tarlow. 2nd rev. ed. 1999. (Illus.). 135p. (C). pap. text 19.95 (*1-57732-089-1*) Datar Pub.

MCAT - Medical College Admission Test: For Comprehensive Review. David M. Tarlow. 7th rev. ed. 1996. (Illus.). 140p. (Orig.). (C). pap., stu. ed. 19.95 (*1-57732-000-X*) Datar Pub.

MCAT - Medical College Admission Test No. 1: Practice Exam Annotated Answers. David M. Tarlow. 2nd rev. ed. 1999. 20p. (C). pap. text 6.95 (*1-57732-091-3*) Datar Pub.

MCAT - Medical College Admission Test No. 1: Practice Examination. David M. Tarlow. 2nd rev. ed. 1999. 40p. (C). pap. text 18.95 (*1-57732-090-5*) Datar Pub.

MCAT - Medical College Admission Test No. 2: Practice Exam Annotated Answers. David M. Tarlow. 2nd rev. ed. 1999. 20p. (C). pap. text 6.95 (*1-57732-093-X*) Datar Pub.

MCAT - Medical College Admission Test No. 2: Practice Examination. David M. Tarlow. 2nd rev. ed. 1999. 40p. (C). pap. text 18.95 (*1-57732-092-1*) Datar Pub.

MCAT - Medical College Admission Test No. 3: Practice Exam Annotated Answers. David M. Tarlow. 2nd rev. ed. 1999. 20p. (C). pap. text 6.95 (*1-57732-095-6*) Datar Pub.

MCAT - Medical College Admission Test No. 3: Practice Examination. David M. Tarlow. 2nd rev. ed. 1999. 40p. (C). pap. text 18.95 (*1-57732-094-8*) Datar Pub.

MCAT - Medical College Admission Test No. 4: Practice Exam Annotated Answers. David M. Tarlow. 2nd rev. ed. 1999. (C). pap. text 6.95 (*1-57732-097-2*) Datar Pub.

MCAT - Medical College Admission Test No. 4: Practice Examination. David M. Tarlow. 2nd rev. ed. 1999. 40p. (C). pap. text 18.95 (*1-57732-096-4*) Datar Pub.

MCAT - Medical College Admission Test No. 5: Practice Exam Annotated Answers. David M. Tarlow. 2nd rev. ed. 1999. (C). pap. text 6.95 (*1-57732-099-9*) Datar Pub.

MCAT - Medical College Admission Test No. 5: Practice Examination. David M. Tarlow. 2nd rev. ed. 1999. 40p. (C). pap. text 18.95 (*1-57732-098-0*) Datar Pub.

MCAT - Medical College Admission Test - Core Content. David M. Tarlow. 2nd rev. ed. 1999. (Illus.). 400p. pap. text 49.95 (*1-57774-029-7*) Educ Tsting Cnslts.

MCAT Essentials. Daniel Roth. 1998. LC 97-16631. (Illus.). 200p. pap. 15.95 (*0-683-30105-5*) Lppncott W & W.

MCAT Exam No. 5 Annotated Answers (Medical College Admissions Test) David M. Tarlow. 7th ed. 1996. (Orig.). (C). pap. 5.95 (*1-57732-010-7*) Datar Pub.

MCAT Exam No. 4 Annotated Answers (Medical College Admissions Test) David M. Tarlow. 7th ed. 1996. (Orig.). pap. 5.95 (*1-57732-009-3*) Datar Pub.

M
N
O

MCAT Exam No. 4 (Medical College Admission Test) David M. Tarlow. 7th ed. 1996. 40p. (Orig.). (C). pap. 19.95 (*1-57732-004-2*) Datar Pub.

MCAT Exam No. 1 Annotated Answers (Medical College Admissions Test) David M. Tarlow. 1996. pap. 5.95 (*1-57732-006-9*) Datar Pub.

MCAT Exam No. 1 (Medical College Admission Test) David M. Tarlow. 7th ed. 1996. 40p. (Orig.). pap. 19.95 (*1-57732-001-8*) Datar Pub.

MCAT Exam No. 3 Annotated Answers (Medical College Admission Test) David M. Tarlow. 7th ed. 1996. (Orig.). pap. 5.95 (*1-57732-008-5*) Datar Pub.

MCAT Exam No. 3 (Medical College Admission Test) David M. Tarlow. 7th ed. 1996. (Illus.). pap. 19.95 (*1-57732-003-4*) Datar Pub.

MCAT Exam No. 2 Annotated Answers (Medical College Admissions Test) David M. Tarlow. 7th ed. 1996. (Orig.). pap. 5.95 (*1-57732-007-7*) Datar Pub.

MCAT Exam No. 2 (Medical College Admission Test) David M. Tarlow. 7th rev. ed. 1996. 40p. (Orig.). pap. 19.95 (*1-57732-002-6*) Datar Pub.

MCAT Exam No. 5 (Medical College Admission Test) David M. Tarlow. 7th ed. 1996. (Orig.). pap. 19.95 (*1-57732-005-0*) Datar Pub.

MCAT (Medical College Admission Test) David M. Tarlow. 1992. (Practice Examination Ser.: No. 4). 40p. pap. 16.95 (*0-931572-10-X*) Datar Pub.

MCAT (Medical College Admission Test) Practice Examination. David M. Tarlow. 1992. (Practice Examination Ser.). 40p. (Orig.). No. 1. pap. 16.95 (*0-931572-07-X*); No. 2. pap. 16.95 (*0-931572-08-8*); No. 3. pap. 16.95 (*0-931572-09-6*); No. 5. pap. 16.95 (*0-931572-11-8*) Datar Pub.

MCAT, 1998. Kaplan Staff. 1997. 20.00 (*0-684-83673-4*) S&S Trade.

MCAT, 1998: Complete Review. Kaplan Staff. 1997. 60.00 incl. cd-rom (*0-684-83672-6*) S&S Trade.

MCAT Practice Examination: Annotated Master Answer Guide. David M. Tarlow. 1992. No. 1. 4.95 (*0-931572-32-0*); No. 2. 4.95 (*0-931572-33-9*); No. 3. 4.95 (*0-931572-34-7*); No. 4. 4.95 (*0-931572-35-5*); No. 5. 4.95 (*0-931572-36-3*) Datar Pub.

MCAT Preparation Guide. Miriam S. Willey' & Barbara M. Jarecky. 1995. LC 94-44915. 144p. pap. text 17.50 (*0-8131-0847-0*) U Pr of KY.

MCAT Sample Exams. Stefan Bosworth et al. 2nd ed. 1996. LC 96-209878. 240p. pap. 13.95 (*0-02-861312-0*, Arc) Hungry Minds.

MCAT Sample Tests with CD. Stefan Bosworth et al. 1999. (Illus.). 256p. pap. 34.95 incl. cd-rom (*0-02-863253-2*, Arc) Hungry Minds.

MCAT Success. Peterson's Guides Staff. 4th ed. 1999. (Peterson's MCAT Success Ser.). 364p. pap. text 16.95 (*0-7689-0297-5*) Petersons.

MCAT Success 1999. Peterson's Guides Staff. 1998. (Peterson's MCAT Success Ser.). 356p. pap. text 16.95 (*0-7689-0149-9*) Petersons.

MCAT SuperCourse. Stefan Bosworth et al. 4th ed. 1997. 720p. 39.95 (*0-02-861711-8*, Arc) Hungry Minds.

MCAT Supercourse. Stefan Bosworth et al. 22nd ed. 1996. 720p. 35.00 (*0-02-861083-0*) Macmillan.

McCracken's Removable Partial Prosthodontics. Glen P. McGivney & Alan B. Carr. 10th ed. 1999. LC 99-37063. (Illus.). 576p. (C). text (*0-323-00678-7*) Mosby Inc.

McCracken's Removable Partial Prosthodontics, No. 9. Glenn P. McGivney & Castleberry. 9th ed. 1994. (Illus.). 544p. (C). (gr. 13). text 79.00 (*0-8016-7964-8*, 07964) Mosby Inc.

McDonald's Blood Flow in Arteries. 3rd ed. (*0-340-52944-X*) E A GBR. *Dist:* Routldge.

McDonald's Blood Flow in Arteries: Theoretical, Experimental & Clinical Principles. Wilmer W. Nichols & Michael F. O'Rourke. 4th ed. 1997. LC 97-21356. (Illus.). 576p. 150.00 (*0-340-64614-4*) OUP.

McDougall Program. John A. McDougall. 1998. 448p. pap. 15.95 (*0-452-27266-1*, Plume) Dutton Plume.

McDougall Program: Twelve Days to Dynamic Health. John A. McDougall. 1991. LC 91-19489. 448p. reprint ed. pap. 14.95 (*0-452-26639-4*, Plume) Dutton Plume.

McDougall Program for a Healthy Heart: A Life-Saving Approach to Preventing & Treating Heart Disease. John A. McDougall. 1998. (Illus.). 430p. text 25.00 (*0-7881-5356-0*) DIANE Pub.

McDougall Program for a Healthy Heart: A Life-Saving Approach to Preventing & Treating Heart Disease. John A. McDougall. l.t. ed. 1997. LC 96-46142. (Spec-Hall Ser.). lib. bdg. 25.95 (*0-7838-2013-5*, Macmillan Ref) Gale.

McDougall's Medicine: A Challenging Second Opinion. John A. McDougall. 1986. LC 85-21686. 298p. pap. 12.95 (*0-8329-0448-1*) New Win Pub.

***McElroy's Essential Emergency Medicine.** Stephen McElroy. 2001. 250p. pap. 19.95 (*1-58808-103-6*) Intl Med Pub.

McGill Medicine: The First Half Century, 1829-1885. Joseph Hanaway. 1996. LC 97-114151. (Illus.). 288p. (*0-7735-1324-8*) McG-Queens Univ Pr CAN. *Dist:* CUP Services.

McGlamry's Comprehensive Textbook of Foot Surgery. Alan S. Banks et al. 3rd ed. 2000. LC 00-42036. 2,304p. text 369.00 (*0-683-30471-2*) Lppncott W & W.

McGraw-Hill Pocket Guide to Managed Care. John La Puma & David L. Schiedermayer. 1996. 200p. reprint ed. pap. text 14.95 (*1-57066-105-7*, ME108) Practice Mgmt Info.

MCGs in Paediatrics. Jagdish M. Gupta & John Beveridge. 2nd ed. 1996. 280p. pap. (*0-412-73340-4*) E A GBR. *Dist:* OUP.

McIlwraith & Turner's Equine Surgery: Advanced Techniques. C. Wayne McIlwraith et al. 2nd ed. 1998. LC 98-15576. 430p. 99.00 (*0-683-05770-7*) Lppncott W & W.

McMinn's Color Atlas of Human Anatomy. Peter H. Abrahams et al. 4th ed. 1998. (Illus.). 368p. (*84-8174-151-5*) Mosby-Doyma Libros ESP. *Dist:* Mosby Inc.

McPherson's Respiratory Care Equipment. Cairo Pilbeam. 6th ed. 1999. LC 98-55692. (Illus.). 787p. (gr. 13). text 55.00 (*0-8151-2148-2*, 30759) Mosby Inc.

MCQ Companion to General & Systematic Pathology. Simon S. Cross. 1992. 208p. (Orig.). pap. text (*0-443-04367-1*) Church.

MCQ Companion to General & Systematic Pathology. S. S. Cross. 2nd ed. 1998. 216p. pap. (*0-443-05281-6*) Church.

MCQ Companion to Grainger & Allison's Diagnostic Radiology, Vol. 1. J. Cockburn & A. Mitchell. Ed. by R. G. Grainger & D. V. Allison. 1998. 320p. pap. (*0-443-05941-1*) Church.

MCQ Companion to the Textbook of Anaesthesia. D. Fell et al. 2nd ed. 1998. 300p. pap. (*0-443-05346-4*) Church.

MCQ Examinations in Psychiatry. John M. Eagles & David A. Alexander. 1986. 272p. pap. text (*0-08-032472-X*) Aberdeen U Pr GBR. *Dist:* Macmillan.

MCQ in Obstetrics Gynecology & Contraception. D. Dawn. 1985. (C). (*0-7855-4656-1*) Current Dist IND. *Dist:* St Mut.

MCQ Tutor: Basic Science in Obstetrics & Gynecology. Victor R. Tindall. 1987. 140p. pap. text (*0-7506-0784-X*) E A GBR. *Dist:* OUP.

MCQ Tutor for Principles & Practice of Surgery. Diamond. 1996. pap. text 21.00 (*0-443-05192-5*) Harcourt.

MCQ Tutor in Anaesthesia: Clinical Practice. Colin A. Pinnock & Robert M. Haden. 1993. 304p. (Orig.). pap. text (*0-443-04610-7*) Church.

MCQ Tutor in Anaesthesia Pt. 1: FRCA. Colin A. Pinnock & Robert P. Jones. 1993. LC 93-29089. (*0-443-04963-7*) Church.

MCQ Tutor in Basic Sciences for Anaesthesia. Colin A. Pinnock & Robert P. Jones. 1993. 240p. (Orig.). pap. text (*0-443-04611-5*) Church.

MCQs & OSCEs for the Primary FRCA. Edward Doyle & Paul Goggin. 1997. LC 96-39853. 168p. pap. text 35.00 (*0-7506-2338-1*) Buttrwrth-Heinemann.

MCQs & Revision Aid in Occupational Medicine. Ken Addley. 1995. LC 95-30546. (Illus.). 176p. pap. text (*0-7506-2394-2*) E A GBR. *Dist:* OUP.

MCQ's for MRCOG, Pt. II. Patrick Hogston. 1995. 96p. (C). pap. text 22.00 (*0-7923-8882-8*) Kluwer Academic.

MCQ's for MRCOG, Pt. 2. K. Khaled. 1998. 144p. pap. (*0-443-06122-X*) Church.

MCQs for MRCOPHTH for the Royal College of Ophthalmologists Examinations. Ivor S. Levy. 1994. 80p. (C). pap. text 21.50 (*0-7923-8848-8*) Kluwer Academic.

MCQs for MRCP Pt. 1: General Medicine. M. J. Ford & D. M. Matthews. 2nd ed. 1995. 225p. pap. (*0-443-05083-X*) Church.

MCQ's for MRCP Pt. 1: General Medicine. Michael J. Ford & David M. Matthews. 2nd rev. ed. 1995. LC 94-34014. (*0-663-05083-9*) Silver.

MCQs for MRCP part 1, Pt. 1. N. I. Johnson & A. Pozniak. 1992. 98p. 21.95 (*0-387-16215-1*) Spr-Verlag.

MCQs for Psychiatric Studies. Chris Freeman. 1988. 162p. (Orig.). pap. text (*0-443-03230-0*) Church.

MCQs for the DRCOG. Matthew Hoghton & Patrick Hogston. 1991. 160p. (Orig.). pap. text (*0-443-04469-4*) Church.

MCQs for the DRCOG. Matthew Hoghton. 2nd ed. 2000. 175p. (Orig.). Price not set. (*0-443-06247-1*) Harcrt Hlth Sci Grp.

MCQs for the Final FRCA. Henderson. 1998. (C). pap. text (*0-7020-2347-7*) Bailliere Tindall.

MCQs for the MRCP, Part 1. Alimuddin Zumla et al. 1993. LC 93-14889. (Illus.). 240p. (gr. 13). pap. text 29.95 (*0-412-49290-3*) Chapman & Hall.

MCQs for the MRCP: Clinical Chemistry, Haematology & Infectious Disease, Pt. 1. Contrib. by David W. Galvani. 1999. LC 99-12516. vii, 108p. (*0-7020-2306-X*) Saunders Ents.

MCQs for the MRCP: Paediatrics. N. G. S. Barakat & Maria O'Callaghan. 1994. 160p. pap. text (*0-7506-2029-3*) E A GBR. *Dist:* OUP.

MCQs for the MRCPsych Pt. I: Examination. Jane Marshall. 1995. LC 93-16822. 224p. pap. text, stu. ed., suppl. ed. (*0-7506-1871-X*) E A GBR. *Dist:* OUP.

MCQs for the MRCPsych Pt. II: Clinicl Topics. Roger Howells. 1995. LC 93-16822. 240p. pap. text, stu. ed., suppl. ed. (*0-7506-1869-8*) E A GBR. *Dist:* OUP.

MCQs for the Paediatric MRCP. A. P. Winrow & G. Supramaniam. 1996. LC 96-6477. 188p. pap. text (*0-443-05354-5*) Church.

MCQs for the PLAB Examination. Kavita Dutta. 1998. 288p. pap. text (*0-7506-4004-9*) E A GBR. *Dist:* OUP.

MCQS for the Primary FRCA. C. R. Bailey & A. Pearce. 1999. LC 98-45216. 260p. (C). pap. text (*0-7020-2160-1*) W B Saunders GBR. *Dist:* Saunders.

MCQ's in Anaesthesia. Ganado. 1998. pap. text (*0-443-05915-2*) Church.

MCQs in Anaesthesiology for the FRCA. Andrea Kelleher. 1994. LC 94-219051. 96p. (C). pap. text 22.00 (*0-7923-8854-2*) Kluwer Academic.

MCQ's in Anatomy. Lumley. 2nd ed. 1988. 272p. pap. (*0-443-03574-1*) Church.

MCQ's in Anatomy: A Self-Testing Supplement to Essential Anatomy. J. S. Lumley & J. L. Craven. 3rd ed. 1996. LC 95-40796. pap. text (*0-443-04977-7*) Church.

MCQ's in Applied Basic Science for Basic Surgical Training. S. Jacob & R. C. Samuel. 2000. LC 99-58757. 255p. Price not set. (*0-443-06349-4*) Harcrt Hlth Sci Grp.

MCQs in Applied Basic Sciences for the Primary FRCS. K. M. Mokbel. 1992. (C). pap. text 22.50 (*0-7923-8994-8*) Kluwer Academic.

MCQs in Basic & Clinical Physiology. Dom Colbert. 1996. 350p. pap. text 29.95 (*0-19-262736-8*) OUP.

MCQs in Cardiology for the MRCP, Pt. I. Ed. by D. Sandler. 1992. (C). pap. text 22.50 (*0-7923-8999-9*) Kluwer Academic.

MCQ's in Clinical Imaging. Asif Saifuddin. 1993. LC 92-49566. 400p. (gr. 13). pap. 45.50 (*0-412-47970-2*) Chapman & Hall.

MCQs in Clinical Medicine. R. R. Baliga. 2nd ed. 1999. LC 99-29016. pap. text 16.00 (*0-7020-2296-9*) Saunders.

MCQS in Clinical Nuclear Medicine. David Scullion et al. 1997. 230p. pap. text (*90-5702-109-9*) GBSP NLD. *Dist:* Gordon & Breach.

MCQS in Clinical Nuclear Medicine. David Scullion et al. 1997. 230p. text 65.00 (*90-5702-146-3*, Harwood Acad Pubs) Gordon & Breach.

MCQS in Clinical Pathology. Bint. 1995. pap. text 21.00 (*0-7020-1782-5*) Saunders.

MCQS in Clinical Pharmacology. Laurence. 2nd ed. 1988. pap. text 27.95 (*0-443-03416-8*) Saunders.

MCQs in General Medicine. Ed. by J. R. Lawrence & J. D. Hunter. 1989. 216p. (Orig.). pap. text (*0-443-03425-7*) Church.

MCQs in General Pathology. F. G. Smiddy & J. L. Turk. 2nd ed. 1996. LC 96-25829. pap. text (*0-443-05419-3*) Church.

MCQ's in Human Physiology. Oliver Wendell Holmes & Sheila Jennett. 1995. LC 95-69152. (Illus.). 472p. (Orig.). pap. 37.95 (*0-412-56210-3*, Chap & Hall NY) Chapman & Hall.

MCQs in Integrated Sciences. Wai-Ching Leung. 1999. LC 99-11697. (*0-443-06239-0*) Church.

MCQS in Medical Virology: A Study Guide. Steven H. Myint & William L. Irving. 1994. LC 93-74445. (Illus.). 200p. (Orig.). (C). (gr. 13). pap. text 35.95 (*0-412-47620-7*, Chap & Hall NY) Chapman & Hall.

MCQ's in Medicine for MRCP, Pt. 1. A. Provan. 1989. 208p. pap. (*0-443-04220-9*) Church.

MCQs in Obstetrics & Gynaecology. D. M. Gibb & John W. Studd. 1983. LC 82-14694. 310p. (C). pap. text (*0-443-02283-6*) Church.

MCQs in Optometry. Robert Fletcher & Katherine M. Oliver. 1996. LC 95-39175. (Illus.). 192p. pap. text 37.50 (*0-7506-2187-7*) Buttrwrth-Heinemann.

MCQ's in Otolaryngology. R. S. Dhillon et al. 2nd ed. 1999. LC 00-265014. 272p. pap. (*0-7506-2165-6*) E A GBR. *Dist:* OUP.

MCQs in Paediatrics. J. M. Gupta & J. Beveridge. 1993. 246p. (gr. 13). pap. 26.95 (*0-412-48310-6*) Chapman & Hall.

MCQS in Paediatrics. T. G. Marshall et al. 1999. LC 98-46987. 410p. pap. text (*0-7020-2249-7*) W B Saunders GBR. *Dist:* Saunders.

MCQS in Paediatrics. Speight. 1984. pap. text 27.95 (*0-443-03653-5*) Saunders.

MCQs in Pharmacology. Bryan V. Robinson. 1980. 286p. reprint ed. pap. text (*0-443-03873-2*) Church.

MCQs in Physiology. C. A. Browne & R. Luff. 1996. 176p. (*0-412-75640-4*) E A GBR. *Dist:* OUP.

MCQS in Physiology. Jennett. 1986. pap. text 21.00 (*0-443-03620-9*) Saunders.

MCQS in Sports Medicine. Conor O'Brien. 1999. 151p. pap. text 32.50 (*0-7506-2949-5*) Buttrwrth-Heinemann.

MCQS in Surgery. D. Das. 1987. (C). (*0-8110-0134-2*) Current Dist IND. *Dist:* St Mut.

MCQS in Surgery: Student Self-Assessment. C. P. Shearman & N. C. Hickey. 1994. 220p. pap. text (*0-7020-1761-2*) W B Saunders GBR. *Dist:* Saunders.

MCQs in the Physics of Diagnostic Imaging. D. J. Dowsett et al. 1999. (An Arnold Publication). 352p. pap. (*0-340-74088-4*) E A GBR. *Dist:* OUP.

MCQ's in Undergraduate Obstetrics & Gynaecology. Ian Johnson & Ken Dowell. 2nd ed. 1994. LC 94-4028. pap. text (*0-443-04959-9*) Church.

MCQS in Veterinary Nursing. Ed. by College of Animal Welfare Staff. 2nd ed. 2005. 128p. Pt. 1. pap. 18.00 (*0-7506-4699-3*); Pt. 2. pap. 18.00 (*0-7506-4700-0*) Buttrwrth-Heinemann.

MCRP Pt. 1: A System Based Tutorial. C. A, O'Callaghan. 1997. (Illus.). pap. 30.95 (*0-632-04781-X*) Blackwell Sci.

MCSE: The Electives in a Nutshell. Michael Moncur. Ed. by Tim O'Reilly. 1998. LC 00-699756. (In a Nutshell Ser.). (Illus.). 372p. pap. 24.95 (*1-56592-482-7*) OReilly & Assocs.

MD-MBA: Physicians on the New Frontier of Medical Management. Ed. by Arthur Lazarus. 1998. LC 97-78156. 240p. pap. 45.00 (*0-924674-61-X*) Am Coll Phys Execs.

MDI-R, Multiaxial Diagnostic Inventory (Revised Edition) Professional Manual. William F. Doverspike. rev. ed. 1999. LC 99-27193. 100p. pap. 44.95 (*1-56887-051-5*, Prof Resc Pr) Pro Resource.

MDR Domestic 2000, Set. Ed. by Medical Economics Staff. 20th rev. ed. 2000. (Medical Device Register, Domestic Edition Ser.). (Illus.). 3500p. 325.00 (*1-56363-348-5*) Med Econ.

MDR International, 2000. Ed. by Medical Economics Staff. rev. ed. 2000. (Illus.). 1100p. 275.00 (*1-56363-349-3*, PDR) Med Econ.

Mds+ Reference Manual (Lt Blue) Eliot Press Staff. 1993. (C). (gr. 13). 34.95 (*0-9628976-4-7*, 25281) Eliot Pr.

Me: Understanding Myself & Others. Audrey Riker. 1977. 11.96 (*0-02-665070-3*); 2nd ed. (Illus.). pap., tchr.'s training gde. ed. 15.67 (*0-02-665080-0*); 2nd ed. (Illus.). stu. ed. 7.78 (*0-02-665090-8*) Glencoe.

Me & My Marrow: A Kid's Guide to Bone Marrow Transplants. Karen Crowe. 2000. (Illus.). 48p. (J). (gr. 3-8). pap. 5.95 (*0-9702446-0-6*) Fujisawa Health.

Me I Know: A Study of Adult Identity. S. Krauss Whitbourne. 1986. (Illus.). 264p. 78.95 (*0-387-96261-1*) Spr-Verlag.

Meal Planning for Diabetes in Pregnancy: Practical Applications. Johanna C. Burani. 1990. 60p. spiral bd. 29.95 (*1-879339-13-7*) Infinity Impress.

Meal Service Study Course. Iowa Dietetic Association Staff et al. 2nd ed. 1991. LC 91-24467. (Illus.). 104p. pap. text, per. 24.95 (*0-8138-0866-9*) Iowa U Pr.

Meal System for the Elderly: Conventional Food in Novel Form. Jurgen Schmandt. 1977. (Policy Research Project Report Ser.: No. 16). 150p. pap. 3.00 (*0-89940-609-2*) LBJ Sch Pub Aff.

Meals for Good Health. Karen Graham & Canadian Diabetes Association Staff. 1999. (Illus.). 232p. (*1-55056-569-9*) Hushion Hse.

***Meals That Heal over 150 Simple Everyday Recipes That Help Prevent & Treat Disease.** Anne Egan & Regina Ragone. 2001. LC 2001-2168. (Illus.). 416p. 29.95 (*1-57954-419-3*) Rodale Pr Inc.

Meaning: An Odyssey in Medicine. Rudi Binder. 1998. 291p. (YA). per. 11.95 (*1-893309-01-0*, 2) Red Maple Pubg.

Meaning & Categorization. R. M. Frumkina & A. V. Mikhejev. 1996. 203p. 95.00 (*1-56072-143-X*) Nova Sci Pubs.

Meaning & Cognitive Structure: Issues in the Computational Theory of Mind. Ed. by Zenon W. Pylyshyn & William Demopoulos. 1986. LC 86-10801. (Theoretical Issues in Cognitive Science Ser.: Vol. 3). 264p. (C). 85.00 (*0-89391-372-3*, Ablex) Greenwood.

Meaning & Context: A Introduction to the Psychology of Language. Ed. by H. Hermann. (Cognition & Language Ser.). (Illus.). 308p. (C). 90.00 (*0-306-42197-6*, Kluwer Plenum) Kluwer Academic.

Meaning & Void: Inner Experience & the Incentives in People's Lives. Eric Klinger. 1978. LC 77-73546. (Illus.). 426p. pap. 19.95 (*0-8166-0856-3*) U of Minn Pr.

Meaning in Child Language. Laurence B. Leonard. 1986. LC 76-45665. 272p. text 52.50 (*0-8089-0977-0*, 792510, Grune & Strat) Harcrt Hlth Sci Grp.

Meaning in Therapy. James Yoder. 1988. 192p. (Orig.). pap. text (*0-932281-05-2*) Quill Pubns GA.

Meaning-Making: Therapeutic Processes in Adult Development. Mary B. Carlsen. 1988. (Professional Bks.). 264p. 25.95 (*0-393-70049-6*) Norton.

Meaning of a Disability: The Lived Experience of Paralysis. Albert B. Robillard. 1999. LC 98-36637. 208p. 59.50 (*1-56639-675-1*); pap. 19.95 (*1-56639-676-X*) Temple U Pr.

Meaning of Addiction: An Unconventional View. Stanton Peele. 1998. LC 98-19896. (Psychology Ser.). 224p. reprint ed. pap. 28.00 (*0-7879-4382-7*) Jossey-Bass.

Meaning of Addiction: Compulsive Experience & Its Interpretations. Stanton Peele. 1985. LC 79-4750. 203p. pap. 27.95 (*0-669-13835-5*) Jossey-Bass.

Meaning of AIDS: Implications for Medical Science, Clinical Practice, & Public Health Policy. Ed. by Eric T. Juengst & Barbara Koenig. 1989. LC 88-25464. 218p. 65.00 (*0-275-92646-X*, C2646, Praeger Pubs) Greenwood.

Meaning of Culture in Pediatric Rehabilitation & Health Care. Ed. by Suzann K. Campbell & Irma J. Wilhelm. 1992. LC 91-35397. (Physical & Occupational Therapy in Pediatrics Ser.). 72p. pap. text 19.95 (*1-56024-262-0*) Haworth Pr.

Meaning of Grief: A Dramaturgical Approach to Understanding Emotion, 8. Larry Cochran & Emily Claspell. 1987. LC 86-27156. (Contributions in Psychology Ser.: No. 8). 189p. 60.00 (*0-313-25607-1*, CMG/, Greenwood Pr) Greenwood.

M
N
O

Meaning of Health. Paul Tillich. Ed. by Perry D. LeFevre. 1984. LC 83-83035. 251p. text 25.00 (*0-913552-21-6*) Exploration Pr.

Meaning of Illness. Mark Kidel & Susan Rowe-Leete. 1988. 224p. pap. text 13.95 (*0-415-00192-7*) Routledge.

Meaning of Illness: A Phenomenological Account of the Different Perspectives of Physician & Patient. S. Kay Toombs. 1993. (Philosophy & Medicine Ser.). 184p. (C). pap. text (*0-7923-2443-9*) Kluwer Academic NLD. *Dist:* Kluwer Academic.

Meaning of Illness: Selected Psychoanalytic Writings. Georg Groddeck. 1977. LC 76-46813. 290p. 42.50 (*0-8236-3205-9*) Intl Univs Pr.

Meaning of Things: Symbols in the Development of the Self. Mihaly Csikszentmihalyi & Eugene Rochberg-Halton. 1981. LC 81-1443. 330p. pap. text 32.95 (*0-521-28774-X*) Cambridge U Pr.

Meanings for Manhood: Constructions of Masculinity in Victorian America. Ed. by Mark C. Carnes & Clyde Griffen. 1990. LC 90-32943. 288p. lib. bdg. 48.00 (*0-226-09364-6*); pap. text 17.95 (*0-226-09365-4*) U Ch Pr.

Meanings of Macho: Being a Man in Mexico City. Matthew Gutmann. 1996. LC 95-49535. (Men & Masculinity Ser.: Vol. 3). (Illus.). 318p. (C). pap. text 18.95 (*0-520-20236-8*) U CA Pr.

Meanings of Menopause: Historical, Medical, & Clinical Perspectives. Ed. by Ruth Formanek. 1990. 352p. text 59.95 (*0-88163-080-2*) Analytic Pr.

Measles: A History. Andrew Cliff et al. 1994. (Illus.). 500p. text 184.95 (*0-631-16235-6*) Blackwell Pubs.

Measles & Poliomyelitis: Vaccines, Immunization, & Control. Ed. by Eduard Kurstak. 1993. (Illus.). 422p. 169.00 (*0-387-82436-7*) Spr-Verlag.

Measure & Manage Stress. Herbert S. Kindler & Marilyn Ginsburg. Ed. by Chris Carrigan. 1994. LC 93-74715. 155p. (Orig.). pap. 16.95 (*1-56052-288-7*) Crisp Pubns.

Measure for Measure: Calorie & Carbohydrate Recipes. Ed. by Elizabeth O'Reilly. 1974. (Illus.). spiral bd. 11.95 (*0-433-24220-5*) Coronet Bks.

Measure It, Manage It: Laying the Foundation for Benchmarking Health Care Foodservice Operations. Lynne M. Richards. 1997. LC 97-33559. (*0-88091-157-3*) Am Dietetic Assn.

Measure of Malpractice: Medical Injury, Malpractice Litigation, & Patient Compensation. Paul C. Weiler et al. 1993. LC 92-1705. 200p. (C). 37.95 (*0-674-55880-4*) HUP.

Measure of My Days: The Journal of a Country Doctor. David Loxterkamp. 1997. LC 96-54704. 333p. lib. bdg. 40.00 (*0-87451-799-0*) U Pr of New Eng.

Measure of Our Days: New Beginnings at Life's End. Jerome Groopman. 1997. LC 97-11693. 320p. 23.95 (*0-670-87570-8*, Viking) Viking Penguin.

Measurement & Evaluation of Health Education. Mark B. Dignan. 3rd ed. 1995. LC 94-30631. (Illus.). 210p. (C). text 54.95 (*0-398-05935-7*) C C Thomas.

Measurement & Management of Clinical Outcomes in Mental Health. John S. Lyons et al. 1997. LC 96-42269. 304p. 105.00 (*0-471-15429-6*) Wiley.

Measurement in Elderly Chronic Care Populations. Ed. by M. Powell Lawton et al. 1997. LC 97-28766. (Illus.). 272p. 43.95 (*0-8261-9990-9*) Springer Pub.

Measurement in Health Promotion & Protection. T. Abelin & Z. Brzezinski. 1987. (WHO Regional Publications, European Ser.: No. 22). 682p. text 80.00 (*92-890-1113-0*) World Health.

Measurement in Hearing & Balance. Ed. by S. D. Stephens. 1988. (Advances in Audiology Ser.: Vol. 5). (Illus.). xx, 220p. 191.50 (*3-8055-4714-5*) S Karger.

Measurement in Laboratory Medicine: A Primer on Control & Interpretation. P. W. Strike. 1995. LC 95-36225. (Illus.). 360p. pap. text 75.00 (*0-7506-2259-8*) Buttrwrth-Heinemann.

Measurement in Neurological Rehabilitation. Derick T. Wade. 1992. 408p. pap. text 62.50 (*0-19-261954-3*) OUP.

Measurement in Nursing Research. Carolyn F. Waltz et al. 2nd ed. 1991. LC 90-14072. (Illus.). 533p. (C). 59.00 (*0-8036-9047-9*) Davis Co.

Measurement of Absorbed Dose in a Phantom Irradiated by a Single Beam of X or Gamma Rays, No. 23. International Commission on Radiation Units and Measurements Staff. 1973. LC 72-97332. 40.00 (*0-913394-16-5*) Intl Comm Rad Meas.

Measurement of Absorbed Dose of Neutrons & Mixtures of Neutrons & Gamma - Rays. 1961. (Report Ser.: No. 25). pap. 20.00 (*0-913392-08-1*) NCRP Pubns.

Measurement of Air Pollutants: Guide to the Selection of Methods. Morris Katz. 1969. 123p. pap. text 23.00 (*92-4-154006-0*, 1150099) World Health.

Measurement of Biological Shape & Shape Change. Fred L. Bookstein. 1978. LC 78-15923. (Lecture Notes in Biomathematics: Vol. 24). (Illus.). 28.00 (*0-387-08912-8*) Spr-Verlag.

Measurement of Cardiac Function. Ed. by John H. McNeill. 1996. LC 96-31525. (Methods in Pharmacology Ser.). 144p. spiral bd. 74.95 (*0-8493-3332-6*) CRC Pr.

Measurement of Cardiovascular Function. Ed. by John H. McNeill. 1996. LC 96-31524. (Methods in the Life Sciences - Methods in Pharmacology Ser.). (Illus.). 128p. spiral bd. 74.95 (*0-8493-3331-8*) CRC Pr.

***Measurement of Community Health: The Social Health Index.** Yoku Shaw-Taylor. 2002. 112p. pap. 24.50 (*0-7618-2126-0*) U Pr of Amer.

Measurement of Free Radicals in Human Disease Process. Dalal. 1992. (*0-8493-0173-4*, CRC Reprint) Franklin.

Measurement of Health: Concepts & Indicators, 31. James S. Larson. 1991. LC 90-44840. (Contributions in Medical Studies Ser.: No. 31). 192p. 52.95 (*0-313-27339-1*, LMH, Greenwood Pr) Greenwood.

Measurement of Intelligence. Lewis M. Terman. 1979. LC 74-21431. (Classics in Child Development Ser.). 376p. reprint ed. 43.95 (*0-405-06480-2*) Ayer.

Measurement of Intelligence. Edward Lee Thorndike et al. 1976. LC 73-2993. (Classics in Psychology Ser.). reprint ed. 38.95 (*0-405-05165-4*) Ayer.

Measurement of Intelligence by Drawings. Florence L. Goodenough. 1976. LC 74-21410. (Classics in Child Development Ser.). 196p. reprint ed. 28.95 (*0-405-06462-4*) Ayer.

Measurement of Joint Motion. Cynthia C. Norkin et al. 2nd ed. 1996. (CHI., Illus.). 272p. (*962-356-018-4*) Lppncott W & W.

Measurement of Joint Motion: A Guide to Goniometry. Cynthia C. Norkin et al. 2nd ed. 1994. (Illus.). 241p. text 26.95 (*0-8036-6579-2*) Davis Co.

Measurement of Levels of Health: Published under Joint Sponsorship of WHO & IEA. W. W. Holland et al. 1979. (WHO Regional Publications, European Ser.: No. 7). 456p. 50.00 (*92-9020-107-X*, 1310007) World Health.

Measurement of Levels of Health: Report of a Study Group. 1957. (Technical Report Ser.: No. 137). 29p. pap. text 3.00 (*92-4-120137-1*) World Health.

Measurement of Metabolic Bone Disease. Ed. by F. I. Tovey & T. C. Stamp. 1995. LC 95-3667. (Medical Measurement Ser.: Vol. 1). 160p. lib. bdg. 63.95 (*1-85070-465-1*, Parthenon Pbng) CRC Pr.

Measurement of Nervous Habits in Normal Children, Vol. 3. Willard C. Olson. 1970. LC 73-9228. 97p. reprint ed. lib. bdg. 48.00 (*0-8371-6991-7*, CWOH, Greenwood Pr) Greenwood.

***Measurement of Nursing Outcomes: Professional & Education Focus.** Ed. by Carolyn Feher Waltz & Louise Sherman Jenkins. 2001. LC 00-54928. 352p. (*0-8261-1417-2*) Springer Pub.

Measurement of Nursing Outcomes Vol. 1: Measuring Client Outcomes, Vol. 1. Carolyn F. Waltz & Ora L. Strickland. 1988. 592p. (C). 65.95 (*0-8261-5271-6*) Springer Pub.

Measurement of Nursing Outcomes Vol. 2: Measuring Nursing Performance, Practice, Education & Research. Ora L. Strickland & Carolyn F. Waltz. 1988. 512p. (C). 89.00 (*0-8261-5272-4*) Springer Pub.

Measurement of Nursing Outcomes Vol. 3: Measuring Clinical Skills & Professional Development in Education & Practice, Vol. 3. Ed. by Carolyn F. Waltz & Ora L. Strickland. 1990. 432p. (C). 62.95 (*0-8261-5273-2*) Springer Pub.

Measurement of Nursing Outcomes Vol. 4: Measuring Client Self-Care & Coping Skills, Vol. 4. Ed. by Ora L. Strickland & Carolyn F. Waltz. 1991. 368p. (C). 59.95 (*0-8261-5274-0*) Springer Pub.

Measurement of Pain in Infants & Children. Ed. by G. Allen Finley & Patrick J. McGrath. 1998. LC 98-44901. (Progress in Pain Research & Management Ser.: Vol. 10). (Illus.). 224p. 67.00 (*0-931092-20-5*) Intl Assn Study Pain.

Measurement of Population Growth, Methods & Result, Vol. 6. P. Kuczynski. 1969. (Demographic Monographs). viii, 256p. text 160.00 (*0-677-02220-4*) Gordon & Breach.

Measurement of Returns to Adult Health: Morbidity Effects on Wage Rates in Cote d'Ivoire & Ghana. T. Paul Schultz & Aysit Tansel. 1993. LC 93-9458. (Living Standards Measurement Study Working Papers: No. 95). 71p. 6.95 (*0-8213-2379-2*, 12379) World Bank.

Measurement of Short-Range Radiations. International Atomic Energy Agency Staff. 1973. (Technical Reports: No. 150). (Illus.). 114p. pap. (*92-0-125173-4*, IDC150) IAEA AUT. *Dist:* Bernan Associates.

Measurement of Stress, Trauma, & Adaptation. Ed. by B. Hudnall Stamm. 1996. LC 96-9819. x, 445p. (Orig.). pap. 55.00 (*1-886968-02-0*, STMS) Sidran Pr.

Measurement of the Intelligence of Young Children by an Object-Fitting Test, Vol. 5. Ruth E. Atkins. 1970. LC 75-12673. (University of Minnesota Institute of Child Welfare Monographs: No. 5). (Illus.). 89p. reprint ed. lib. bdg. 48.00 (*0-8371-8083-X*, CWAI) Greenwood.

Measurement of the Public Health Importance of Bilharziasis: Report of a WHO Scientific Group, 1967. 1967. (Technical Report Ser.). 93p. pap. text 5.00 (*92-4-120349-8*, 1100349) World Health.

Measurement Techniques in Space Plasmas: Particles. Robert F. Pfaff et al. Ed. by Joseph E. Borovsky & David T. Young. 1998. LC 98-18386. (Geophysical Monograph Ser.: Vol. 102). 90.00 (*0-87590-085-2*) Am Geophysical.

Measurements & Landmarks in Physical Anthropology. Frederick W. Jones. 1969. (BMB Ser.: No. 63). (Illus.). reprint ed. 25.00 (*0-527-02169-5*) Periodicals Srv.

Measurements for Long-Term Care. Sarah R. Beaton & Susan A. Voge. 1998. LC 97-33870. 61.95 (*0-8039-5388-7*, 3649) Sage.

Measurements in Cardiology. Ed. by P. M. Sutton. 1999. (Measurements in Medicine Ser.). (Illus.). 286p. lib. bdg. 74.95 (*1-85070-463-5*, Parthenon Pbng) CRC Pr.

Measurements in Pediatric Radiology. H. Pettersson & Hans Ringertz. 1991. (Illus.). 185p. 97.00 (*0-387-19665-X*) Spr-Verlag.

Measurements of Mechanical Ability. John L. Stenquist. LC 73-177744. (Columbia University. Teachers College. Contributions to Education Ser.: No. 130). reprint ed. 37.50 (*0-404-55130-0*) AMS Pr.

Measures for Clinical Practice: A Sourcebook. Kevin Corcoran & Joel Fischer. 1987. LC 86-25819. 576p. 45.00 (*0-02-906681-6*) Free Pr.

Measures for Clinical Practice Vol. 1: Couples, Families, & Children. Joel Fischer & Kevin Corcoran. 2nd ed. 1994. LC 93-32384. 39.95 (*0-02-906685-9*) Free Pr.

Measures for Clinical Practice Vol. 2: Adults. Joel Fischer & Kevin Corcoran. 2nd ed. 1994. LC 93-32384. (Measures for Clinical Practice Ser.: Vol. 2). 715p. 49.95 (*0-02-906686-7*) Free Pr.

Measures of Family Function for Research & Practice. Kathleen J. Sawin & Marcia Harrigan. Ed. by Pierre Woog. 1994. LC 94-38528. (Illus.). 144p. 27.95 (*0-8261-8900-8*) Springer Pub.

Measures of Man: Methodologies in Biological Anthropology. Ed. by Eugene Giles & Jonathan S. Friedlaender. 1976. LC 76-28638. (Museum Press Ser.). (Illus.). 696p. 42.00 (*0-87365-800-0*); pap. 27.00 (*0-87365-782-9*) Peabody Harvard.

Measures of Medicine: Benefits, Harms & Costs. S. Schoth & Richard K. Riegelman. 1994. 320p. pap. 39.95 incl. disk (*0-86542-280-X*) Blackwell Sci.

Measures of Personality & Social Psychological Attitudes, Vol. 1. Ed. by John P. Robinson et al. 1990. LC 90-91. (Measures of Personality & Social Psychological Attitudes Ser.). 753p. pap. text 69.95 (*0-12-590244-1*) Acad Pr.

***Measures of Physical Function in the Elderly: Complete Guide.** Todd Gitlin. 1994. 52.00 (*0-8342-1954-9*) PRO-ED.

Measuring & Evaluating the Radiography Student's Educational Achievement. Robert J. Parelli. 1997. 28p. (Orig.). pap., wbk. ed. 10.00 (*1-880359-10-3*) Par Rad.

Measuring & Improving Patient Satisfaction. Patrick J. Shelton. 2000. LC 00-20622. (Illus.). 300p. 68.00 (*0-8342-1074-6*, 10746) Aspen Pub.

Measuring & Managing Ambulatory Care Outcomes. Jean Carroll. 1996. ring bd. 225.00 (*0-8342-0776-1*, S194) Aspen Pub.

Measuring & Managing Healthcare Quality: Procedures, Techniques, & Protocols, Set. Norbert Goldfield et al. 1995. ring bd. 239.00 (*0-8342-0265-4*) Aspen Pub.

Measuring & Managing Patient Satisfaction. William J. Krowinski & Steven R. Steiber. 2nd rev. ed. 1996. LC 96-22064. (Illus.). 266p. pap. 60.00 (*1-55648-157-8*, 136108) AHPI.

Measuring & Recording of Joint Motion: Instrumentation & Techniques. Ed. by John J. Gerhardt et al. 2nd ed. 1990. LC 89-7515. 140p. 37.00 (*0-920887-33-3*) Hogrefe & Huber Pubs.

Measuring Avoidable Deaths & Diseases in New York State. Willine Carr et al. 1988. (Paper Ser.: No. 8). 56p. 5.00 (*0-934459-40-1*) United Hosp Fund.

Measuring Behavioral Health Outcomes. R. P. Hawkins et al. 1999. LC 98-47605. (Clinical Child Psychology Library). (Illus.). (C). 200p. 75.00 (*0-306-46080-7*); 180p. pap. 24.95 (*0-306-46081-5*) Perseus Pubng (Plenum Trade).

Measuring Cognitive Impairment. Folstein. 2000. (Illus.). 320p. (C). pap. text 34.95 (*0-8151-2931-9*, 31820) Mosby Inc.

Measuring Country Performance on Health: Selected Indicators for 115 Countries. Jian Wang. 1999. LC 98-50177. (Health, Nutrition, & Population Ser.). 368p. pap. 30.00 (*0-8213-4409-9*) World Bank.

Measuring Disease. Ann Bowling. 1994. LC 94-28081. 17.99p. pap. text (*0-335-19225-4*) OpUniv Pr.

Measuring Disease: A Review of Disease-Specific Quality of Life Measurement Scales. Ann Bowling. 2nd ed. 2001. LC 00-60647. (*0-335-20641-7*) OpUniv Pr GBR. *Dist:* Taylor & Francis.

Measuring Disease: A Review of Disease-Specific Quality of Life Measurement Scales. Ann Bowling. 2nd ed. 2001. LC 00-60647. 400p. (gr. 13). text 105.00 (*0-335-20642-5*) Routledge.

Measuring Emotions in Infants & Children. Ed. by Carroll E. Izard. 1982. LC 81-10032. (Cambridge Studies in Social & Emotional Development: No. 3). (Illus.). 352p. text 69.95 (*0-521-24171-5*) Cambridge U Pr.

Measuring Emotions in Infants & Children, Vol. 2. Ed. by Carroll E. Izard & Peter B. Read. 1986. (Cambridge Studies in Social & Emotional Development: No. 7). (Illus.). 288p. text 80.00 (*0-521-32367-3*) Cambridge U Pr.

Measuring Environment Across the Life Span: Emerging Methods & Concepts. Ed. by Sarah L. Friedman & Theodore D. Wachs. 1999. LC 98-49321. (Illus.). 419p. 49.95 (*1-55798-561-8*) Am Psychol.

Measuring Expenditures for Essential Public Health Services. Kay W. Eilbert et al. 1998. (Illus.). 98p. (C). reprint ed. pap. text 25.00 (*0-7881-4205-4*) DIANE Pub.

Measuring Forensic Psychiatric & Mental Health Nursing Interactions. David K. Robinson & Val Reed. 1996. LC 96-84008. (Developments in Nursing & Health Care Ser.). 252p. (*1-85972-221-0*) Avebry GBR. *Dist:* Ashgate Pub Co.

Measuring Functioning & Well-Being: The Medical Outcomes Study Approach. Ed. by Anita L. Stewart & John E. Ware, Jr. 1991. LC 91-34579. 479p. text 64.95 (*0-8223-1212-3*) Duke.

Measuring Health: A Guide to Rating Scales & Questionnaires. Ian McDowell & Claire Newell. 2nd ed. 1996. LC 95-20980. (Illus.). 544p. (C). text 62.50 (*0-19-510371-8*) OUP.

Measuring Health: A Review of Quality of Life Measurement Scales. Ann Bowling. 2nd ed. 1997. LC 96-50373. pap. (*0-335-19754-X*) OpUniv Pr.

Measuring Health & Medical Outcomes. Jenkinson. 1994. LC 94-12568. (Social Research Today Ser.: Vol. 3). 224p. (*1-85728-083-0*); pap. (*1-85728-084-9*) UCL Pr Ltd GBR. *Dist:* Taylor & Francis.

Measuring In Vivo Oxidative Damage: A Practical Approach. J. Lunec. 2000. LC 99-47679. (Illus.). 192p. 99.95 (*0-471-81848-8*) Wiley.

***Measuring Mental Health Needs.** Ed. by Graham Thornicroft. 2nd rev. ed. 2001. pap. (*1-901242-60-9*) Royal Coll Psych GBR. *Dist:* Balogh.

Measuring Minds: Henry Herbert Goddard & the Origins of American Intelligence Testing. Leila Zenderland. 1998. (Cambridge Studies in the History of Psychology). (Illus.). 478p. (C). text 64.95 (*0-521-44373-3*) Cambridge U Pr.

Measuring Movement & Locomotion. Klaus-Peter Ossenkopp. 1996. (Medicine Ser.). pap. 89.95 (*0-412-10321-4*, VNR) Wiley.

Measuring Occupational Performance: Supporting Best Practice in Occupational Therapy. Mary Law et al. 2000. LC 00-30067. (Illus.). viii, 302p. pap. 36.00 (*1-55642-298-9*, 32989) SLACK Inc.

Measuring Outcomes. Deborah K. Wall. 1997. LC 97-17398. (Illus.). 96p. pap. 40.00 (*0-944496-52-0*) Precept Pr.

Measuring Outcomes: Desktop Reference for Behavioral Healthcare Providers. Ed. by Anne M. Christner. 3rd rev. ed. 1998. 550p. 149.00 (*1-884937-51-9*) Manisses Communs.

Measuring Outcomes in Ambulatory Care. Dale S. Benson. 1992. LC 92-49961. 192p. (Orig.). pap. 49.95 (*1-55648-094-6*, 169106) AHPI.

Measuring Outcomes in Children's Services. John Mordock. 1998. 75.00 (*1-884937-47-0*) Manisses Communs.

Measuring Outcomes in Speech-Language Pathology. Carol M. Frattali. 1998. LC 97-26377. (Illus.). 500p. 59.00 (*0-86577-718-7*) Thieme Med Pubs.

Measuring Outcomes in Speech-Language Pathology. Carol Frattali. 1997. LC 97-26377. (*3-13-109731-0*) G Thieme DEU. *Dist:* Thieme Med Pubs.

Measuring Patient Changes in Mood, Anxiety, & Personality Disorders: Toward a Core Battery. Ed. by Hans H. Strupp et al. 1997. LC 97-7469. 544p. 49.95 (*1-55798-414-X*, 431-8590) Am Psychol.

Measuring Patient Reported Health Status in Advanced HIV Disease: HIV-PARSE Survey Instrument. Sandra H. Berry et al. 1994. LC 94-32313. pap. 9.00 (*0-8330-1584-2*, MR-342-NIAID) Rand Corp.

Measuring Personality Adjustment in Children 9 to 13 Years of Age. Carl Ransom Rogers. LC 76-177202. (Columbia University. Teachers College. Contributions to Education Ser.: No. 458). reprint ed. 37.50 (*0-404-55458-X*) AMS Pr.

Measuring Quality Improvement in Healthcare: A Guide to Statistical Process Control Applications. Raymond G. Carey & Robert C. Lloyd. 1995. LC 95-5101. 208p. pap. 26.95 (*0-527-76293-8*) Product Pr.

Measuring Self-Concept Across the Life Span: Issues & Instrumentation. Barbara M. Byrne. 1996. LC 95-45591. (Measurement & Instrumentation in Psychology Ser.). 297p. 39.95 (*1-55798-332-1*); pap. text 29.95 (*1-55798-346-1*) Am Psychol.

Measuring Sex Stereotypes: A Thirty-Nation Study. John E. Williams & Deborah L. Best. rev. ed. 1990. (Cross-Cultural Research & Methodology Ser.: Vol. 6). (Illus.). 376p. (C). pap. 36.95 (*0-8039-3814-4*, 7386); 96.95 (*0-8039-3815-2*, 7377) Sage.

Measuring Stress: A Guide for Health & Social Scientists. Ed. by Sheldon Cohen et al. 1997. (Illus.). 256p. reprint ed. pap. text 29.50 (*0-19-512120-1*) OUP.

Measuring the Burden of Disease & the Cost-Effectiveness of Health Interventions: A Case Study in Guinea. Prabhat Jha. 1996. LC 96-31866. (Technical Papers: No. 333). 48p. pap. 22.00 (*0-8213-3727-0*) World Bank.

Measuring the Health Behavior of Adolescents: The Youth Risk Behavior Surveillance System & Recent Reports on High Risk Adolescents. 1995. (Illus.). 96p. (Orig.). (C). pap. text 30.00 (*0-7881-2321-1*) DIANE Pub.

Measuring the Health of Persian Gulf Veterans: Workshop Summary. Institute of Medicine Staff. 1998. LC 99-175490. 42p. pap. text 10.00 (*0-309-06245-4*) Natl Acad Pr.

Measuring the Locational Efficiency of the Urban Hospital. Jerry B. Schneider. 1967. (Discussion Papers: No. 11). pap. 10.00 (*1-55869-074-3*) Regional Sci Res Inst.

Measuring the Mind: Psychological Theory & Educational Controversy in England, C. 1860-C. 1990. Adrian Wooldridge. 1995. LC 93-29889. 458p. (C). text 90.00 (*0-521-39515-1*) Cambridge U Pr.

Measuring the Quality of Health Care. 1999. 42p. 12.00 (*0-309-06387-6*) Natl Acad Pr.

Meat Inspector. Jack Rudman. 1994. (Career Examination Ser.: C-517). pap. 29.95 (*0-8373-0517-9*) Nat Learn.

Meat Inspector Trainee. Jack Rudman. 1994. (Career Examination Ser.: C-518). pap. 23.95 (*0-8373-0518-7*) Nat Learn.

Mechanical Ability of Deaf Children. Mildred B. Stanton. LC 74-177747. (Columbia University. Teachers College. Contributions to Education Ser.: No. 751). reprint ed. 37.50 (*0-404-55751-1*) AMS Pr.

Mechanical Circulatory Support. 1997. (Illus.). 226p. 64.00 (*3-7985-1046-6*) Spr-Verlag.

Mechanical Circulatory Support. Ed. by Terence Lewis et al. 1995. (An Arnold Publication). 400p. (*0-340-57602-2*) E A GBR. *Dist:* OUP.

Mechanical Devices for Cardiopulmonary Assistance: Proceedings of the Symposium, Boston, 1970. Symposium, Boston Staff. Ed. by R. H. Bartlett et al. 1971. (Advances in Cardiology Ser.: Vol. 6). 59.25 (*3-8055-1163-9*) S Karger.

Mechanical Factors of Digestion. Walter B. Cannon. 1987. LC 86-10161. 20.00 (*0-88135-082-6*) Watson Pub Intl.

Mechanical Loading of Bones & Joints. Hideaki Takahashi. 1999. LC 99-19475. (Illus.). 330p. 169.00 (*4-431-70242-3*) Spr-Verlag.

Mechanical Low Back Pain: Perspectives in Functional Anatomy. James A. Porterfield & Carl DeRosa. Ed. by Margaret Biblis. 2nd ed. 1998. LC 97-14398. (Illus.). 304p. text 45.00 (*0-7216-6837-2*) Saunders.

Mechanical Man: John B. Watson & the Beginnings of Behaviorism. Kerry W. Buckley. 1989. LC 88-24081. 233p. 30.00 (*0-89862-744-3*) Guilford Pubns.

Mechanical Neck Pain: Perspectives in Functional Anatomy. James A. Porterfield & Carl DeRosa. 1994. (Illus.). 272p. text 46.00 (*0-7216-6640-X*) Saunders.

***Mechanical Support for Cardiac & Respiratory Failure in Pediatric Patients.** Ed. by Brian W. Duncan. 2001. LC 2001-28064. (Illus.). xiv, 369p. text 165.00 (*0-8247-0275-1*) Dekker.

Mechanical Systems for Health Care Facilities. J. Robin Barrick. 1993. (Management & Compliance Ser.: Vol. 8). (Illus.). 308p. ring bd. 110.00 (*0-87258-654-5*, 055216) Am Hospital.

Mechanical Ventilation. Lonny J. Ashworth. 1998. (CPG Mentor - Patient Cases in Respiratory Care Ser.: Unit 6). (*0-8151-2290-X*) Mosby Inc.

Mechanical Ventilation. Ed. by F. Lemaire. 1991. (Illus.). 198p. 76.95 (*0-387-53322-2*) Spr-Verlag.

Mechanical Ventilation. Springhouse Publishing Company Staff. 1992. (Procedures Video Ser.). 36.95 incl. VHS (*0-87434-373-9*) Springhouse Corp.

Mechanical Ventilation. Payne. 3rd ed. 1999. pap. text, stu. ed. 18.95 (*0-8151-4376-1*) Mosby Inc.

Mechanical Ventilation: A Practice Approach. Ed. by Suhail A. Raoof & Faroque Khan. 1998. LC 97-3305. 186p. (Orig.). (C). pap. text 40.00 (*0-943126-57-6*) Amer Coll Phys.

Mechanical Ventilation: And Other Measures of Respiratory Support for Adult... Rashed A. Hasan & Michael D. Pappas. 2000. 90p. pap. 19.95 (*0-9704158-1-8*) R A Hasan.

Mechanical Ventilation: Physiological & Clinical Applications. Pilbeam. 3rd ed. 1998. LC 97-40495. (Illus.). 460p. (C). (gr. 13). pap. text 43.00 (*0-8151-2600-X*, 31083) Mosby Inc.

Mechanical Ventilation & Assisted Respiration: Past, Present & Future. Ake Grenvik et al. 1991. (Contemporary Management in Critical Care Ser.: Vol. 1, No. 1). (Illus.). 190p. text (*0-443-08828-4*) Church.

Mechanics & Biophysics of Hearing: Proceedings of a Conference Held at the University of Wisconsin, Madison, WI June 25-29, 1990. Ed. by C. D. Geisler. 1991. (Lecture Notes in Biomathematics: Vol. 87). 418p. 69.95 (*0-387-97473-3*) Spr-Verlag.

Mechanics, Heat, & the Human Body: An Introduction to Physics. Howard D. Goldick. 2000. LC 00-44586. (Illus.). 212p. pap. text 34.80 (*0-13-922816-0*) P-H.

Mechanics of Deformable Media. A. B. Bhatia & R. N. Singh. 1986. (Graduate Student Series in Physics). (Illus.). 204p. (C). pap. 49.00 (*0-85274-500-1*) Inst of Physics Pubng.

Mechanics of Disease. David O. Slauson et al. 2nd ed. 1990. LC 76-56215. (Illus.). 560p. text 59.95 (*0-683-07743-0*) Lppncott W & W.

Mechanics of Environmental Carcinogenesis, Vol. I. Barrett. 1987. 160p. 182.00 (*0-8493-4671-1*) CRC Pr.

Mechanics of Hearing. Ed. by E. De Boer & Max A. Viergever. 1983. text 126.50 (*90-247-2878-9*) Kluwer Academic.

Mechanics of Human Joints: Physiology, Pathophysiology, & Treatment. Verna Wright. Ed. by Eric L. Radin. 1993. (Illus.). 480p. text 225.00 (*0-8247-8763-3*) Dekker.

***Mechanics of Motor Proteins & the Cytoskeleton.** Jonathon Howard. 2001. LC 2001-17017. (Illus.). xvi, 367p. text 59.95 (*0-87893-334-4*) Sinauer Assocs.

Mechanics of Muscle. Daniel J. Schneck. 1991. (Monographs in Biomedical Engineering). (Illus.). 350p. (C). text 80.00 (*0-8147-7935-2*) NYU Pr.

Mechanics of Surgery. Charles Truax. 1988. LC 87-31483. (Illus.). 1024p. reprint ed. 155.00 (*0-930405-01-3*) Norman SF.

Mechanics of the Feeding of the Mallard (Anas Platryrhynchos L.) the Lingual Apparatus & the Suctio-Pressure Pump Mechanism of Straining. G. A. Zweers et al. 1977. (Contributions to Vertebrate Evolution Ser.: Vol. 3). (Illus.). 44.50 (*3-8055-2424-2*) S Karger.

Mechanics of the Spine. Robert Allen & Peter McCarthy. 2002. 256p. 55.00 (*0-7506-2455-8*) Buttrwrth-Heinemann.

Mechanism - Prevention - Treatment of Aspiration Pneumonia: Theodor Billroth's M.D. Thesis in 1852 on Cervical Vagotomy. Theodor Billroth. fac. ed. 1994. (LAT.). 50p. (C). pap. text 19.50 (*0-930329-67-8*) Kabel Pubs.

Mechanism - Treatment - Prevention of Aspiration Pneumonia (Theodor Billroth) Karel B. Absolon & J. Lee Sedwitz. 1999. (Illus.). 102p. (C). text 29.50 (*0-930329-70-8*) Kabel Pubs.

Mechanism & Management of Corneal Graft Rejection. John C. Hill. 1996. LC 96-1852. (*90-6299-127-0*) Kugler NLD. *Dist:* Lib Res.

Mechanism & Management of Headache. Peter J. Goadsby & James W. Lance. 6th ed. 1998. LC 98-15127. 336p. text 95.00 (*0-7506-3728-5*) Buttrwrth-Heinemann.

Mechanism & New Approach on Drug Resistance of Cancer Cells: Proceedings of the International Symposium on the Mechanism & New Approach on Drug Resistance of Cancer Cells, Sapporo, 15-17 October 1992. Ed. by Tamotsu Miyazaki et al. 1993. LC 93-15706. (International Congress Ser.: No. 1026). 348p. 166.75 (*0-444-81480-9*, Excerpta Medica) Elsevier.

Mechanism of Action, Safety & Efficacy of Intrauterine Devices. 1987. (Technical Reports: No. 753). 91p. pap. text 12.00 (*92-4-120753-1*, 1100753) World Health.

Mechanism of Denial: The Manifest Content of the Dream. Ed. by Bernard D. Fine et al. 1969. LC 79-75242. (Kris Study Group Monographs: No. 3). 113p. text 27.50 (*0-8236-3210-5*) Intl Univs Pr.

Mechanism of Evolution: A New Look at Old Ideas. M. I. Wolsky & A. Wolsky. 1976. (Contributions to Human Development Ser.: Vol. 4). (Illus.). 160p. 38.50 (*3-8055-2347-5*) S Karger.

Mechanism of Human Facial Expression. Duchenne De Boulogne. Tr. by R. Andrew Cuthbertson. 1990. (Studies in Emotion & Social Interaction). (Illus.). 304p. (C). text 59.95 (*0-521-36392-6*) Cambridge U Pr.

Mechanism of Myofilament Sliding in Muscle Contraction. H. Sugi & G. H. Pollack. 1993. (Advances in Experimental Medicine & Biology Ser.: Vol. 332). (Illus.). 882p. (C). text 175.00 (*0-306-44525-5*, Kluwer Plenum) Kluwer Academic.

Mechanism of Tumor Promotion: Cellular Responses to Tumor Promoters, Vol. IV. Ed. by Thomas J. Slaga. 1984. 168p. 98.00 (*0-8493-6524-4*, RC268, CRC Reprint) Franklin.

Mechanism of Tumor Promotion: Tumor Promotion in Internal Organs. Ed. by Thomas J. Slaga. 208p. I. 1983. 111.00 (*0-8493-6521-X*, RC268); II. 1984. 125.00 (*0-8493-6522-8*, RC268); III. 1984. 118.00 (*0-8493-6523-6*, RC268) Franklin (CRC Reprint).

Mechanisms & Concepts in Toxicology. Norman Aldrige. 1996. LC 96-137508. 288p. 99.95 (*0-7484-0413-9*); 254p. 44.95 (*0-7484-0414-7*) Taylor & Francis.

***Mechanisms & Management of Cardiac Arrhythmias.** Garratt & Clifford Statter. 2001. 176p. pap. text (*0-7279-1194-5*) BMJ Pub GBR. *Dist:* AIDC.

Mechanisms & Management of Headache. James W. Lance. 5th ed. 1993. 288p. text 85.00 (*0-7506-0575-8*) Buttrwrth-Heinemann.

Mechanisms & Models in Rheumatoid Arthritis. John A. Edwards. 1995. (Illus.). 548p. text 105.00 (*0-12-340440-1*) Acad Pr.

Mechanisms & Models in Toxicology. Ed. by P. L. Chambers et al. 1987. (Archives of Toxicology Ser.: Supp. 11). (Illus.). 347p. 134.00 (*0-387-17614-4*) Spr-Verlag.

Mechanisms & Recent Advances in Therapy of Hypertension. Ed. by H. Liebau. 1977. (Contributions to Nephrology Ser.: Vol. 8). (Illus.). 29.75 (*3-8055-2671-7*) S Karger.

Mechanisms & Reversal of Multidrug Resistance in Cancer: The Other Alternatives. Ed. by John A. Kellen. 1995. LC 95-1582. 278p. 99.00 (*0-8176-3775-3*) Birkhauser.

Mechanisms & Specificity of HIV Entry into Host Cells. Ed. by N. Duzgunes. 1991. (Advances in Experimental Medicine & Biology Ser.: Vol. 300). (Illus.). 222p. (C). text 102.00 (*0-306-44008-3*, Kluwer Plenum) Kluwer Academic.

Mechanisms in B-Cell Neoplasia. Ed. by F. Melchers & M. Potter. 1986. (Current Topics in Microbiology & Immunology Ser.: Vol. 132). (Illus.). 374p. 106.00 (*0-387-17048-0*) Spr-Verlag.

Mechanisms in B-Cell Neoplasia, 1988. Ed. by M. Potter & F. Melchers. 1988. (Current Topics in Microbiology & Immunology Ser.: Vol. 141). (Illus.). 336p. 123.00 (*0-387-50212-2*) Spr-Verlag.

Mechanisms in B-Cell Neoplasia, 1992: Workshop at the National Cancer Institute, National Institutes of Health, Bethesda, MD, U. S. A., April 21-23, 1992. Ed. by Michael B. Oldstone et al. 1992. (Current Topics in Microbiology & Immunology Ser.: Vol. 182). (Illus.). 528p. 189.00 (*0-387-55658-3*) Spr-Verlag.

Mechanisms in Blood Coagulation, Fibrinolysis & the Complement System. Torben Halkier. Tr. by Paul Woolley. 1992. (Illus.). 483p. (C). text 110.00 (*0-521-38187-8*) Cambridge U Pr.

Mechanisms in Pigmentation: Proceedings of the International Pigment Cell Conference, 8th, Sydney, March, 1972. International Pigment Cell Conference Staff. Ed. by V. J. McGovern & P. Russel. 1973. (Pigment Cell Ser.: Vol. 1). (Illus.). 115.00 (*3-8055-1480-8*) S Karger.

Mechanisms in Respiratory Toxicology Paul Nettesheim & Hanspeter R. Witschi. 1982. Vol. I. 288p. 168.00 (*0-8493-5689-X*, RC732); Vol. II. 240p. 138.00 (*0-8493-5690-3*) Franklin (CRC Reprint).

Mechanisms in Symptom Formation: Proceedings. Congress of International College of Psychosomatic. Ed. by H. Musaph. 1974. (Psychotherapy & Psychosomatics Ser.: Vol. 23, No. 1-6). 300p. 83.50 (*3-8055-1689-4*) S Karger.

Mechanisms in the Pathogenesis of Enteric Diseases: Proceedings of the First International Rushmore Conference Held in Rapid City, South Dakota, September 28-30, 1995. Ed. by Prem S. Paul et al. 1997. LC 97-5561. (Advances in Experimental Medicine & Biology Ser.: No. 412). (Illus.). 452p. 125.00 (*0-306-45519-6*, Kluwer Plenum) Kluwer Academic.

Mechanisms in Tobacco Carcinogenesis. Ed. by D. Hoffmann & C. C. Harris. 1986. LC 86-12956. (Banbury Reports: No. 23). 428p. 80.00 (*0-87969-223-5*) Cold Spring Harbor.

Mechanisms of Age Cognition Relations in Adulthood. Timothy A. Salthouse. 1992. (John M. Memorial Lecture). 152p. text 29.95 (*0-8058-1129-X*) L Erlbaum Assocs.

Mechanisms of Airways Obstruction in Human Respiratory Disease: Proceedings of the International Symposium, Tygerberg, South Africa, 1978. Ed. by Jay A. Nadel et al. 1979. 425p. 130.00 (*0-86961-107-0*) Ashgate Pub Co.

Mechanisms of Anesthetic Action in Skeletal, Cardiac & Smooth Muscle. Ed. by T. J. Blanck & D. M. Wheeler. 1991. (Advances in Experimental Medicine & Biology Ser.: Vol. 301). (Illus.). 320p. (C). text 132.00 (*0-306-44011-3*, Kluwer Plenum) Kluwer Academic.

Mechanisms of Apoptotic Cell Death. Ed. by Martin Kroenke. 1996. (Journal: Vol. 6, No. 6, 1996). (Illus.). iv, 78p. pap. 28.00 (*3-8055-6453-8*) S Karger.

Mechanisms of Arrhythmias. Michiel J. Janse. Ed. by A. John Camm. 1993. LC 93-11901. (Clinical Approaches to Tachyarrhythmias Ser.: Vol. 1). (Illus.). 72p. pap. 15.00 (*0-87993-569-3*) Futura Pub.

Mechanisms of B Cell Neoplasia 1998 15th Workshop: Proceedings of the Workshop Held at the Basel Institute for Immunology 4th - 6th October 1998, No. 246. Ed. by F. Melchers et al. 1999. (Current Topics in Microbiology & Immunology Ser.). (Illus.). 430p. 250.00 (*3-540-65759-2*) Spr-Verlag.

Mechanisms of Brain Laterilization. V. L. Bianki. 1993. (Monographs in Neuroscience: Vol. 4). 296p. text 94.00 (*2-88124-460-2*) Gordon & Breach.

Mechanisms of Cancer Metastasis: Potential Therapeutic Implications. Ed. by Kenneth V. Honn et al. 1985. (Developments in Oncology Ser.). text 160.50 (*0-89838-765-5*) Kluwer Academic.

Mechanisms of Carcinogenesis. Ed. by Elisabeth K. Weisburger. 1988. (Cancer Growth & Progression Ser.). (C). text 213.50 (*0-89838-991-7*) Kluwer Academic.

Mechanisms of Carcinogenesis by Dichloroacetate (DCA) & Trichloroacetate (TCA) Richard J. Bull & Anja J. Stauber. 1998. LC 98-8262. (Illus.). xx, 93p. (*0-89867-962-1*) Am Water Wks Assn.

Mechanisms of Carcinogenesis in Risk Identification. Ed. by Harri Vainio et al. 1992. (IARC Scientific Publications Ser.: No. 116). (Illus.). 630p. pap. text 145.00 (*92-832-2116-8*) OUP.

Mechanisms of Cell Injury & Cell Death. B. A. Fowler. 1990. 86p. text 96.00 (*2-88124-411-4*) Gordon & Breach.

Mechanisms of Cerebral Hypoxia & Stroke. Ed. by G. Somjen. 1988. LC 88-25293. (Advances in Behavioral Biology Ser.: Vol. 35). (Illus.). 486p. 110.00 (*0-306-43015-0*, Plenum Trade) Perseus Pubng.

Mechanisms of Cocaine Abuse & Toxicity. 1993. lib. bdg. 262.75 (*0-8490-8912-3*) Gordon Pr.

Mechanisms of Differentiation Ed. by Paul B. Fisher. 1990. Vol. 1. 176p. 153.00 (*0-8493-4947-8*, QH607); Vol. 2. 216p. 166.00 (*0-8493-4948-6*, QH607) CRC Pr.

Mechanisms of Disease: An Introduction to Clinical Science. Ed. by S. Tomlinson et al. 1997. LC 96-39361. (Illus.). 531p. (C). pap. text 34.95 (*0-521-46738-1*); text 95.00 (*0-521-46180-4*) Cambridge U Pr.

Mechanisms of DNA Damage & Repair: Implications for Carcinogenesis & Risk Assessment. Ed. by Michael G. Simic et al. 1986. LC 86-9363. (Basic Life Sciences Ser.: Vol. 38). 594p. 110.00 (*0-306-42288-3*, Plenum Trade) Perseus Pubng.

***Mechanisms of DNA Tumor Virus Transformation.** Ed. by L. Rosenthal. 2001. (Monographs in Virology: Vol. 22). (Illus.). x, 160p. 128.75 (*3-8055-7247-6*) S Karger.

Mechanisms of Drug Interactions. Ed. by P. F. D'Arcy et al. 1996. (Handbook of Experimental Pharmacology Ser.: Vol. 122). (Illus.). 400p. 349.00 (*3-540-60204-6*) Spr-Verlag.

***Mechanisms of Drug Resistance in Epilepsy: No. 243.** Novartis staff. 2002. 300p. 125.00 (*0-470-84146-X*) Wiley.

Mechanisms of Drugs in Anaesthesia. 2nd ed. 448p. (*0-340-55157-7*) E A GBR. *Dist:* Routldge.

Mechanisms of Epileptogenesis: The Transition to Seizure. Ed. by Marc A. Dichter. 1988. LC 88-25274. (Illus.). 298p. 79.50 (*0-306-43010-X*, Plenum Trade) Perseus Pubng.

Mechanisms of Everyday Cognition. Ed. by James M. Puckett & Hayne W. Reese. 1993. (West Virginia Series on Lifespan Developmental Psychology). 256p. text 59.95 (*0-8058-0976-7*) L Erlbaum Assocs.

Mechanisms of Fetal Allograft Survival. Gary W. Wood. 1997. (Medical Intelligence Unit Ser.). 250p. pap. 89.95 (*0-412-11601-4*) Chapman & Hall.

Mechanisms of Fibre Carcinogenesis. Ed. by A. B. Kane et al. 1997. LC 97-162025. (IARC Scientific Publications Ser.: No. 140). (Illus.). 170p. pap. text 89.50 (*92-832-2140-0*) OUP.

Mechanisms of Heart Failure. Ed. by Pawan K. Singal et al. 1996. LC 95-14335. (Developments in Cardiovascular Medicine Ser.: Vol. 167). 480p. (C). text 236.00 (*0-7923-3490-6*) Kluwer Academic.

Mechanisms of Host Resistance to Infectious Agents, Tumors, & Allografts. Ed. by Ralph Steinman & Robert J. North. 1986. LC 86-60123. (Illus.). 480p. pap. 25.00 (*0-87470-042-6*) Rockefeller.

Mechanisms of Immue Regulation. Ed. by R. D. Granstein. 1994. (Chemical Immunology Ser.: Vol. 58). (Illus.). xiv, 338p. 248.75 (*3-8055-5786-8*) S Karger.

Mechanisms of Injury in Renal Disease & Toxicity. Ed. by Robin S. Goldstein. 1994. 320p. lib. bdg. 259.00 (*0-8493-8873-2*, TP8873) CRC Pr.

Mechanisms of Inorganic & Organometallic Reactions, Vol. 1. Ed. by M. V. Twigg. 1983. LC 83-2140. 390p. 115.00 (*0-306-41142-3*, Plenum Trade) Perseus Pubng.

Mechanisms of Intelligence: Ashby's Writings on Cybernetics. W. Ross Ashby. Ed. by Roger Conant. 1981. (Systems Inquiry Ser.). 394p. (Orig.). (C). pap. text 17.95 (*0-914105-04-3*) Intersystems Pubns.

Mechanisms of Invasion & Metastasis. Marc M. Mareel et al. 1991. (Illus.). 584p. 251.00 (*0-8493-6254-7*, RC269) CRC Pr.

Mechanisms of Language Acquisition. Brian MacWhinney. 1987. (Carnegie-Mellon Symposium Ser.). 480p. (C). pap. 55.00 (*0-89859-973-3*) L Erlbaum Assocs.

Mechanisms of Learning & Motivation: A Memorial Volume to Jerzy Konorski. Ed. by A. Dickinson & R. A. Boakes. 1979. 460p. 79.95 (*0-89859-460-X*) L Erlbaum Assocs.

Mechanisms of Lung Injury. H. M. Mehendale. 1989. 90p. text 84.00 (*2-88124-410-6*) Gordon & Breach.

Mechanisms of Lymphocyte Activation & Immune Regulation. Ed. by Sudhir Gupta et al. 1987. LC 87-7005. (Illus.). 348p. 85.00 (*0-306-42568-8*, Plenum Trade) Perseus Pubng.

Mechanisms of Lymphocyte Activation & Immune Regulation Vol. 4: Cellular Communications. S. Gupta & T. A. Waldmann. 1992. LC 92-26881. (Advances in Experimental Medicine & Biology Ser.: Vol. 323). (Illus.). 214p. (C). text 85.00 (*0-306-44312-0*, Kluwer Plenum) Kluwer Academic.

Mechanisms of Lymphocyte Activation & Immune Regulation Vol. 5: Molecular Basis of Signal Transduction. S. Gupta et al. 1994. (Advances in Experimental Medicine & Biology Ser.: 365). (Illus.). 274p. (C). text 95.00 (*0-306-44897-1*, Kluwer Plenum) Kluwer Academic.

Mechanisms of Lymphocyte Activation & Immune Regulation 3. Ed. by S. Gupta et al. 1991. (Advances in Experimental Medicine & Biology Ser.). (Illus.). 268p. (C). text 114.00 (*0-306-43922-0*, Kluwer Plenum) Kluwer Academic.

Mechanisms of Lymphocyte Activation & Immune Regulation 7: Molecular Determinants of Microbial Immunity: Proceedings of the 7th International Conference Held in Newport Beach, California, February 6-8, 1998. Ed. by Sudhir Gupta et al. 1998. LC 98-40455. (Advances in Experimental Medicine & Biology Ser.: No. 452). 223p. (C). text 85.00 (*0-306-46033-5*, Kluwer Plenum) Kluwer Academic.

Mechanisms of Lymphocyte Activation & Immune Regulation II. Ed. by S. Gupta et al. 1989. (Illus.). 150p. 65.00 (*0-306-43250-1*, Plenum Trade) Perseus Pubng.

Mechanisms of Lymphocyte Activation & Immune Regulation VI: Cell Cycle & Programmed Cell Death in the Immune System. Ed. by Sudhir Gupta & John Cohen. 1996. LC 96-29392. (Advances in Experimental Medicine & Biology Ser.: Vol. 406). (Illus.). 279p. 102.00 (*0-306-45483-1*, Kluwer Plenum) Kluwer Academic.

Mechanisms of Lymphocyte Extravasation. Ed. by S. Ratner. 1992. (Journal: Vol. 12, No. 2, 1992). (Illus.). 92p. pap. 52.25 (*3-8055-5657-8*) S Karger.

Mechanisms of Microbial Disease. Moselio Schaechter et al. 2nd ed. 1993. (Illus.). 996p. pap. 42.00 (*0-683-07606-X*) Lppncott W & W.

Mechanisms of Microbial Disease. Moselio Schaechter. 3rd ed. 1998. LC 98-3835. 896p. pap. 45.00 (*0-683-07605-1*) Lppncott W & W.

Mechanisms of Motion-Induced Vomiting. Ed. by N. G. Daunton et al. 1983. (Journal: Vol. 23, No. 1-2). (Illus.). 80p. pap. 45.25 (*3-8055-3790-5*) S Karger.

Mechanisms of Peptic Ulcer Healing. Ed. by F. Halter et al. 1991. (C). text 225.50 (*0-7923-8955-7*) Kluwer Academic.

Mechanisms of Physical & Emotional Stress. Ed. by George P. Chrousos et al. 1988. LC 88-28384. (Illus.). 542p. 125.00 (*0-306-43017-7*, Plenum Trade) Perseus Pubng.

Mechanisms of Platelet Activation & Control. K. S. Authi et al. 1994. LC 93-32065. (Advances in Experimental Medicine & Biology Ser.: Vol. 334). (Illus.). 286p. (C). text 89.50 (*0-306-44631-6*, Kluwer Plenum) Kluwer Academic.

Mechanisms of Progression in Renal Disease. Ed. by J. Floege. 1999. (Kidney & Blood Pressure Research Ser.: Vol. 22, No. 1 (1999)). (Illus.). 90p. pap. 34.00 (*3-8055-6876-2*) S Karger.

Mechanisms of Psychological Influence on Physical Health: With Special Attention to the Elderly. Ed. by John M. Neale & L. L. Carstensen. 1989. (Illus.). 196p. 69.50 (*0-306-43116-5*, Plenum Trade) Perseus Pubng.

Mechanisms of Quality in Long-Term Care: Service & Clinical Outcomes. 1991. (NLN-Ross Laboratories Long-Term Care Conferences Ser.). (Illus.). 128p. (C). pap. text 5.95 (*0-88737-506-5*, 41-2382) Natl League Nurse.

Mechanisms of Receptor Regulation. Ed. by Stanley T. Crooke & George H. Poste. 1985. LC 85-28339. (New Horizons in Therapeutics Ser.). (Illus.). 458p. (C). text 150.00 (*0-306-42125-9*, Kluwer Plenum) Kluwer Academic.

Mechanisms of Renal Injury & Repair Vol. 21, No. 4-5: Mineral & Electrolyte Metabolism, 1995. Ed. by Manuel Martinez-Maldonado. 1995. (Journal: Vol. 21, No. 4-5, 1995). (Illus.). 122p. pap. 86.25 (*3-8055-6209-8*) S Karger.

Mechanisms of Secondary Brain Damage. Ed. by A. Baethmann et al. 1986. LC 86-22671. (NATO ASI Series A, Life Sciences: Vol. 115). 416p. 95.00 (*0-306-42397-9*, Plenum Trade) Perseus Pubng.

Mechanisms of Secondary Brain Damage: Current State. Ed. by A. Baethmann et al. 1993. LC 92-49078. (Acta Neurochirurgica Ser.: No. 57). (*3-211-82421-9*); 140.00 (*0-387-82421-9*) Spr-Verlag.

Mechanisms of Secondary Brain Damage in Cerebral Ischemia & Trauma, Vol. 66. Ed. by A. Baethmann et al. 1996. LC 96-3928. (Acta Neurochirurgica Ser.: No. 66). (Illus.). 150p. suppl. ed. 149.00 (*3-211-82817-6*) Spr-Verlag.

Mechanisms of Speech. N. I. Zinkin. 1968. LC 68-15534. (Janua Linguarum, Ser. Major: No. 13). (Illus.). (C). text (*90-279-0607-6*) Mouton.

Mechanisms of Stimulus-Response Coupling in Platelets. Ed. by J. Westwick et al. 1986. LC 85-12135. (Advances in Experimental Medicine & Biology Ser.: Vol. 192). 456p. 110.00 (*0-306-42073-2*, Plenum Trade) Perseus Pubng.

Mechanisms of Tinnitus. Ed. by Jack A. Vernon & Aage R. Moller. 1994. LC 94-27956. 272p. (C). 78.00 (*0-205-14083-1*, Longwood Div) Allyn.

Mechanisms of Transdermeal Drug Delivery. Ed. by Russell O. Potts & Richard A. Guy. 1997. LC 97-20470. (Drugs & the Pharmaceutical Sciences Ser.: Vol. 82). (Illus.). 376p. text 175.00 (*0-8247-9863-5*) Dekker.

***Mechanisms of Vasodilatation: 8th International Symposium on Mechanisms of Vasodilatation, Boston, Mass., May-June 2001: Abstracts.** 2001. 32p. pap. 25.25 (*3-8055-7269-7*) S Karger.

Mechanisms of Vasodilatation: Proceeding of the International Congress of Physiological Sciences, Official Satellite Symposium, 27th, Wilrijk, July 1977. International Congress of Physiological Sciences. Ed. by P. M. Vanhoutte & Isadore Leusen. 1978. (Illus.). 85.25 (*3-8055-2841-8*) S Karger.

Mechanisms of Vasodilatation Abstracts: Journal: Blood Vessels, Vol. 23, No. 2, 1986. Ed. by P. M. Vanhoutte. 1986. 60p. pap. 27.00 (*3-8055-4361-1*) S Karger.

Mechanisms of Vasodilation Symposium, Abstracts. Mechanisms of Vasodilatation Symposium Staff. Ed. by P. M. Vanhoutte. 1980. (Journal: Vol. 17, No. 3). 56p. pap. 32.25 (*3-8055-1252-X*) S Karger.

Mechanisms of Viral Carcinogenesis: From Hypercarcinogenic State to Normo- or Hypocarcinogenic States. Ed. by O. Hino. 1995. (Journal: Vol. 38, Nos. 3 & 4, 1995). (Illus.). 128p. pap. 80.00 (*3-8055-6275-6*) S Karger.

Mechanisms of Viral Toxicity in Animal Cells. Luis Carrasco. 1987. 208p. 120.00 (*0-8493-6742-5*, CRC Reprint) Franklin.

Mechanisms Regulating Lactation & Infant Nutrient Utilization. Mary F. Picciano & Bo Lonnerdal. 1992. (Contemporary Issues in Clinical Nutrition Ser.). 480p. 420.00 (*0-471-56134-7*) Wiley.

Mechanisms/Interferon Actions. Pfeffer. 1987. Vol. I. 152p. 89.00 (*0-8493-6146-X*); Vol. II. 200p. 113.00 (*0-8493-6147-8*) Franklin (CRC Reprint).

Mechanistic Basis & Relevance of Kidney Tumors in Male Rats for Use in Risk Assessment. 1994. (Illus.). 84p. pap. 54.00 (*0-89867-741-6*, 90655) Am Water Wks Assn.

Mechanistic Relationships Between Development & Learning: Report of the Dahlem Workshop on Mechanistic Relationships Between Development & Learning, Berlin, January 19-25, 1997. Thomas J. Carew et al. 1998. LC 98-17869. (Dahlem Workshop Reports). 336p. 165.00 (*0-471-97702-0*) Wiley.

Mechanobiology: Cartilage & Condrocyte. Ed. by J. F. Stoltz. 2000. LC 99-69689. (Biomedical & Health Research Ser.: Vol. 42). (Illus.). vii, 190p. 102.00 (*1-58603-051-5*) IOS Press.

***Mechanobiology: Osteoarthritis & Skeletal Regeneration & Osteoporosis & Bone Functional Adaptation.** Ed. by Tamara T. Sowell. 2001. 127p. (C). pap. text 25.00 (*0-7567-0590-8*) DIANE Pub.

MED Inc. How Consolidation Is Shaping Tomorrow's Health Care System. Sandy Lutz et al. 1998. LC 97-40890. 212p. 35.00 (*0-7879-4040-2*) Jossey-Bass.

Med-Math: Dosage Calculation, Preparation & Administration. Grace Henke. 3rd ed. 1998. LC 98-8269. 368p. pap. text 32.95 (*0-7817-1028-6*) Lppncott W & W.

Med School Mayhem. David J. Fletcher. 1980. LC 80-65389. (Illus.). 345p. pap. 10.95 (*0-935510-01-X*) F Fergeson.

Med School Survival Guide: How to Make the Challenges of Medical School Seem Like Small Stuff. Jennifer Danek. 2000. LC 00-20105. 192p. pap. 12.00 (*0-609-80595-9*, STU014000, Three Riv Pr) Crown Pub Group.

Med Study: The Internal Medicine Board Review Robert A. Hannaman. 7th rev. ed. 1997. 400p. ring bd. 395.00 (*0-9640788-3-X*) MedStudy.

Med Terminology: Student-Centered Appr/Flashcards. Elmer W. Moisio & Marie A. Moisio. 2001. (C). 8.00 net. (*0-7668-1527-7*) Thomson Learn.

Medcin: A New Nomenclature for Clinical Medicine. Ed. by Peter S. Goltra. 1997. LC 96-52993. 717p. 94.00 (*0-387-94953-4*) Spr-Verlag.

Meddive. Kathy Work & Jon Kushner. Ed. by Michael K. Bielmaier & Michael S. Klush. 1991. (Illus.). 123p. (C). pap. text 22.00 (*0-929905-05-9*) Dive Rescue.

Meddling with Mythology: AIDS & the Social Construction of Knowledge. Rosaline S. Barbour & Guro Huby. 1998. LC 97-49216. 304p. (C). 90.00 (*0-415-16389-7*); pap. 27.95 (*0-415-16390-0*) Routledge.

Medecine, Vol. 2. Pierre de Graciansky. 1979. (FRE.). lib. bdg. 155.00 (*0-7859-3843-5*) Fr & Eur.

Medecine: Histoire & Doctrines. Charles Daremberg. 2nd ed. 1976. LC 75-13257. (History of Ideas in Ancient Greece Ser.). (FRE.). reprint ed. 35.95 (*0-405-07300-3*) Ayer.

Medecine, Maladie et Societe: Recueli de Textes Presentes et Commentes. Claudine Herzlich. 1970. (Textes de Sciences Sociales Ser.: No. 4). pap. (*90-279-6757-1*) Mouton.

***MedEMT: A Learning System for Prehospital Care.** 2001. suppl. ed., wbk. ed. 81.93 (*0-13-073419-5*) P-H.

MedEMT: A Learning System for Prehospital Care. Victory Technologies, Inc. Staff et al. 2000. (Illus.). 896p. pap. 59.00 (*0-8385-6369-4*) P-H.

***MedEMT: A Learning System for Prehospital Care.** Mark G. Wills & Grant Goold. 2000. 896p. suppl. ed 61.67 (*0-13-019744-0*) P-H.

***MedEMT: A Learning System for Prehospital Care.** Wills & Goold. 2001. 400p. reprint ed. suppl. ed. 32.00 (*0-13-093986-2*) P-H.

MedEMT Learning System for Prehospital Care. 2000. 400p. tchr. ed. 63.00 (*0-8385-6384-8*) Allyn.

MedEMT Multiple User Insert. 1998. (C). (*0-8385-6381-3*, Medical Exam) Appleton & Lange.

Medi-Cal County Data Book. unabr. ed. 1999. (Illus.). 138p. spiral bd. (*1-929008-19-8*) CA HlthCare Fnd.

Medi-Cal Outstationing in California: Findings from a Statewide Survey. Jennifer Blackburn & Ingrid Aguirre-Happordt. unabr. ed. 1999. (Illus.). 38p. pap. (*1-929008-15-5*) CA HlthCare Fnd.

Medi-Record: Female. Ruben Trottman. 1996. (Illus.). 208p. per. 39.95 (*0-9632430-1-2*) Medi-Record.

Medi-Record: Male. Ruben Trottman. 1996. (Illus.). 208p. per. 39.95 (*0-9632430-0-4*) Medi-Record.

Media & Family Planning with Supplement. Richard J. Udry. 1974. LC 74-5075. 9.75 (*0-89055-123-5*) Carolina Pop Ctr.

Media & Mental Distress. Ed. by Greg Philo. 1997. LC 96-9069. (Illus.). 135p. (C). pap. 46.40 (*0-582-29219-0*) Longman.

Medical Imaging, 1997 Vol. 3037: Ultrasonic Transducer Engineering. Ed. by K. Kirk Shung. 1997. LC 97-175332. 220p. 59.00 (*0-8194-2448-X*) SPIE.

Median Longitudinal Cervical Somatotomy. A. Pansini & P. Conti. 1986. 158p. text (*1-57235-044-X*) Piccin Nuova.

Mediastinal Surgery. Thomas W. Shields. 1991. LC 90-13346. (Illus.). 400p. text 99.00 (*0-8121-1362-4*) Lppncott W & W.

Mediastinal Tumors. Ed. by D. E. Wood & C. R. Thomas, Jr. 1995. (Illus.). 144p. 110.00 (*3-540-58750-0*) Spr-Verlag.

Mediastinum. E. R. Heitzman. 2nd ed. 1988. (Illus.). 355p. 231.00 (*0-387-18727-8*) Spr-Verlag.

Mediators & Drugs in Gastrointestinal Motility II: Endogenous & Exogenous Agents. Ed. by G. Bertaccini. 1982. (Handbook of Experimental Pharmacology Ser.: Vol. 59, II). (Illus.). 386p. 272.00 (*0-387-11333-9*) Spr-Verlag.

Mediators in Airway Hyperreactivity. Ed. by E. P. Nijkamp et al. 1990. (Agents & Actions Supplements Ser.: Vol. 31). 296p. 87.50 (*0-8176-2513-5*) Birkhauser.

Mediators in the Cardiovascular System: Regional Ischemia. Ed. by K. Schror & Cecil R. Pace-Asciak. 1995. (Agents & Actions Supplements Ser.: Vol. 45). LC 94-43433. (*3-7643-5130-6*); (Illus.). 340p. 104.00 (*0-8176-5130-6*) Birkhauser.

Mediators of Pulmonary Inflammation. Ed. by Michael A. Bray & Wayne Anderson. 1991. (Lung Biology in Health & Disease Ser.: Vol. 54). (Illus.). 688p. text 255.00 (*0-8247-8442-1*) Dekker.

Mediators of Sepsis. Ed. by L. G. Thijs & M. Lamy. 1992. LC 92-32047. (Update in Intensive Care & Emergency Medicine Ser.: Vol. 16). (Illus.). 414p. 142.00 (*0-387-55841-1*) Spr-Verlag.

Mediators of the Immediate Type Inflammatory Reaction: Proceedings of the Collegium Internationale Allergologicum Symposium, 11th, Heidelberg, May 1976. Collegium Internationale Allergologicum Symposium. Ed. by K. O. Rother. 1977. (Monographs in Allergy: Vol. 12). (Illus.). 85.25 (*3-8055-2660-1*) S Karger.

Medic: The Mission of an American Military Doctor in Occupied Japan & Wartorn Korea. Crawford F. Sams. Ed. by Zabelle Zakarian. 1998. LC 97-35989. (Illus.). 344p. (C). (gr. 13). 35.95 (*0-7656-0030-7*, East Gate Bk) M E Sharpe.

Medic Life: Creating Success in EMS. John Becknell. 1995. LC 95-872. pap. text 9.95 (*0-8151-3046-5*) Jems Comm.

Medicaid: Oregon's Managed Care Program & Implications for Expansion. 1992. 71p. (Orig.). (C). pap. text 25.00 (*1-56806-008-4*) DIANE Pub.

Medicaid: Restructuring Approaches Leave Many Questions. 1995. (Illus.). 25p. (Orig.). (C). pap. text 25.00 (*0-7881-1805-6*) DIANE Pub.

Medicaid: States Turn to Managed Care to Improve Access & Control Costs. 1993. (Illus.). 102p. (Orig.). (C). pap. text 35.00 (*1-56806-588-4*) DIANE Pub.

Medicaid: Waiver Program for Developmentally Disabled Is Promising, but Poses Some Risks. 1996. (Illus.). 48p. (Orig.). (C). pap. text 25.00 (*0-7881-3460-4*) DIANE Pub.

Medicaid at the Crossroads: A Report of the Kaiser Commission on the Future of Medicaid. Diane Rowland et al. 1992. 90p. (Orig.). pap. 5.00 (*0-944525-10-5*) H J Kaiser.

Medicaid Claims Examiner. Jack Rudman. 1994. (Career Examination Ser.: C-2691). pap. 27.95 (*0-8373-2691-5*) Nat Learn.

Medicaid Cost Containment: Long-Term Care Reimbursment. Robert J. Buchanan. 1987. LC 85-45028. 200p. 36.50 (*0-8386-3271-8*) Fairleigh Dickinson.

Medicaid Cost Explosion: Causes & Consequences: Report of the Kaiser Commission on the Future of Medicaid. Judith Feder et al. 1993. (Orig.). pap. text 10.00 (*0-944525-12-1*) H J Kaiser.

Medicaid Distribution Formula: Hearing Before the Committee on Finance, United States Senate, One Hundred Fourth Congress, First Session, July 27, 1995. U. S. Congress, Senate Committee on Finance. 1997. LC 97-187239. (Illus.). (*0-16-054989-2*) USGPO.

Medicaid Drug Fraud: Drug Diversion Schemes & "Pill Mills" 1994. (Illus.). 53p. (Orig.). (C). pap. text 30.00 (*0-7881-0200-1*) DIANE Pub.

Medicaid Drug Fraud, Medical Malpractice, & Reliability of Claims Processing for Medicare, Pt. B. 1994. (Illus.). 98p. (Orig.). (C). pap. text 30.00 (*0-7881-1034-9*) DIANE Pub.

Medicaid Expansions for Prenatal Care: State & Local Implementation. 1994. 80p. (Orig.). (C). pap. text 25.00 (*0-7881-0628-7*) DIANE Pub.

Medicaid Financing Crisis: Balancing Responsibilities, Priorities & Dollars. Diane Rowland et al. 1994. 222p. (C). pap. 21.95 (*0-87168-514-0*, 93-04S) Transaction Pubs.

Medicaid Financing for Mental Health & Substance Abuse Services for Children & Adolescents. Harriette B. Fox et al. 1997. (Illus.). 69p. (C). reprint ed. pap. text 20.00 (*0-7881-4596-7*) DIANE Pub.

Medicaid for Long-Term Nursing Home Care. Richard Moran Enders. 2000. 13p. pap. 15.00 (*0-9627964-9-2*) SOS Clinton.

***Medicaid Fraud & Abuse: Assessing State & Federal Responses - Congressional Hearing.** Ed. by Fred Upton. 2001. 85p. reprint ed. pap. 25.00 (*0-7567-1160-6*) DIANE Pub.

Medicaid Fraud & Abuse: Assessing State & Federal Responses : Hearing Before the Subcommittee on Oversight & Investigations of the Committee on Commerce, House of Representatives, One Hundred Sixth Congress, First Session, November 9, 1999. Ed. by U. S. Congress, House Committee on Commerce, Subcommittee on Oversight and Investigations. 1999. LC 00-273836. (Illus.). iii, 85p. (*0-16-059890-7*) USGPO.

***Medicaid Funding for School - Based Services: Congressional Hearings.** Ed. by William V. Roth, Jr. 2001. 83p. (C). reprint ed. pap. text 25.00 (*0-7567-0959-8*) DIANE Pub.

Medicaid Home Care Options for Disabled Children. Linda A. Hall. Ed. by Karen Glass. 1990. 60p. (Orig.). pap. text 20.00 (*1-55877-062-3*) Natl Governor.

Medicaid in Schools: Improper Payments Demand Improvements in HCFA Oversight. Ed. by Carolyn Yocom & William Hamel. 2000. (Illus.). 57p. (C). pap. text 20.00 (*0-7567-0298-4*) DIANE Pub.

Medicaid Long-Term Care: Successful State Efforts to Expand Home Services While Limiting Costs. 1995. (Illus.). 68p. (Orig.). (C). pap. text 20.00 (*0-7881-1861-7*) DIANE Pub.

Medicaid, Managed Behavioral Health, & Implications for Public Policy: Report of the Hawaii Medicaid Project & Other Readings. N. A. Cummings et al. 1993. (Readings in Behavioral Health Ser.: No. 2). 60p. pap. text (*0-9637577-0-9*) Fnd Behav Hlth.

Medicaid Managed Care: Challenges in Implementing Safeguards for Children with Special Needs. Kathryn G. Allen. 2000. (Illus.). 65p. pap. 20.00 (*0-7567-0296-8*) DIANE Pub.

Medicaid Managed Care: Defining the Issues for Women with HIV/AIDS. Leslie R. Wolfe et al. 1996. 16p. (Orig.). pap. 5.00 (*1-877966-29-0*) Ctr Women Policy.

Medicaid Managed Care: Serving the Disabled Challenges State Programs. 1996. (Illus.). 66p. (Orig.). (C). pap. text 25.00 (*0-7881-3490-6*) DIANE Pub.

Medicaid Managed Care: Serving Women with HIV/AIDS. Belinda Rochelle et al. 1997. 74p. pap. 18.00 (*1-877966-40-1*) Ctr Women Policy.

***Medicaid Managed Care: State's Safeguards for Children with Special Needs Vary Significantly.** Walter Ochinko & Karen Doran. 2001. 63p. pap. text 20.00 (*0-7567-1758-2*) DIANE Pub.

Medicaid Manual: How to Qualify for Medicaid. Richard T. Taps. 1994. 120p. pap. 12.95 (*0-9640442-2-6*) Silver Press.

Medicaid Policy in California, 1980-1987, with Special Reference to Pregnant Women & Infants. Eve L. Schenker et al. 1993. LC 93-25929. pap. 13.00 (*0-8330-1421-8*, MR-146-AHCPR) Rand Corp.

Medicaid Prenatal Care: States Improve Access & Enhance Services, but Face New Challenges. 1995. (Illus.). 44p. (Orig.). (C). pap. text 20.00 (*0-7881-1859-5*) DIANE Pub.

***Medicaid Reform.** Ed. by Linda F. Wolf. 2001. (Illus.). 183p. (C). reprint ed. pap. text 30.00 (*0-7567-1208-4*) DIANE Pub.

Medicaid Reform: The Governors' View: Hearing Before the Committee on Commerce, U. S. House of Representatives. Ed. by Michael Bilirakis. 1998. 89p. (C). pap. text 20.00 (*0-7881-4970-9*) DIANE Pub.

Medicaid Reform: The Governors' View: Hearing Before the Subcommittee on Health & Environment of the Committee on Commerce, House of Representatives, One Hundred Fifth Congress, First Session, March 11, 1997. U. S. Congress, House Committee on Commerce, Subcommittee on Health and the Environment. 1997. LC 97-186917. (Illus.). (*0-16-054912-4*) USGPO.

Medicaid Reform & the American States: Case Studies on the Politics of Managed Care. Ed. by Mark R. Daniels. 1998. LC 97-23657. 320p. 72.50 (*0-86569-263-7*, Auburn Hse) Greenwood.

Medicaid since 1980: Cost, Coverage, & the Shifting Alliance Between the Federal Government & the States. Teresa A. Coughlin et al. 1994. 200p. pap. text 23.00 (*0-87766-618-0*); lib. bdg. 49.00 (*0-87766-617-2*) Urban Inst.

Medicaid Source Book: Background Data & Analysis. 1993. (Illus.). 510p. pap. 44.00 (*0-16-006301-9*, 052-070-06848-5) USGPO.

Medicaid Survival Kit. Martha P. King & Stephen M. Christian. 1996. LC 99-162571. 322p. 75.00 (*1-55516-655-5*, 6654) Natl Conf State Legis.

Medicaid Waivers: California's Use of a Federal Option. Valerie Lewis. 2000. (Illus.). 27p. pap. (*1-929008-28-7*) CA HlthCare Fnd.

Medical - Surgical Care Planning. Nancy M. Holloway. 2nd ed. 1992. LC 92-20351. 768p. 36.95 (*0-87434-489-1*) Springhouse Corp.

Medical - Surgical Market, '94. Market Intelligence Staff. 1994. 346p. 595.00 (*1-56753-934-3*) Frost & Sullivan.

Medical - Surgical Nursing: An Integrated Approach - Study Guide. Duncan White. 1997. (LPN/LVN Nursing Ser.). 272p. (C). mass mkt., stu. ed. 13.75 (*0-8273-7681-2*) Delmar.

Medical Abacus: Review of Clinical Formulas & How to Use Them. D. Rifkind. 2000. LC 98-44811. (Illus.). 72p. 24.95 (*1-85070-023-0*, Parthenon Pbng) CRC Pr.

Medical Abbreviations: 15,000 Conveniences at the Expense of Communications & Safety. Neil M. Davis. 10th rev. ed. 2001. 432p. pap. 22.95 (*0-931431-10-7*) N M Davis.

Medical Abbreviations: Abkurzungen in der Medizin. Albrecht Schertel. 3rd ed. 1984. (ENG, FRE & GER.). 200p. pap. 39.95 (*0-8288-0587-3*, M 7292) Fr & Eur.

Medical Abbreviations & Eponyms. Sheila B. Sloane. Ed. by Margaret Biblis. 2nd ed. 1997. LC 96-28595. 880p. pap. text 39.00 (*0-7216-7088-1*) Saunders.

Medical Accelerator Safety Considerations: Report of AAPM Radiation Therapy Committee Task Group, No. 35. J. Purdy et al. 1996. (AAPM Report Ser.: No. 56). 16p. reprint ed. (*1-888340-01-0*) AAPM.

Medical Accidents Handbook: A Practical Guide for Patients & Their Advisors. AVMA Staff. 1999. LC 00-266152. 448p. pap. 65.00 (*0-471-96642-8*) Wiley.

Medical Acronyms, Eponyms, & Abbreviations. Marilyn F. Delong. Ed. by Kathryn Swanson. 3rd ed. 1995. LC 94-40393. 400p. (C). pap. 15.95 (*1-57066-007-7*, ME063) Practice Mgmt Info.

Medical Acronyms, Eponyms, & Abbreviations. Marilyn F. DeLong. 3rd rev. ed. 1997. LC 96-78925. 332p. pap. 12.95 (*1-885987-05-6*, ME077, Health Info Pr) Practice Mgmt Info.

Medical Acronyms, Eponyms & Mnemonics. Ed. by Kimberly N. Jones. 1999. (Pocket Brain Ser.: No. 2). 70p. pap. text 9.95 (*0-9651162-5-5*) Wysteria Ltd.

Medical Administration: Management Techniques. A. Everette James. 1994. 158p. pap. 24.95 (*0-87527-511-7*) Green.

Medical ADP Systems: Defense's Tools & Methodology for Managing CHCs Performance Needs Strengthening. Helen Lew. 1998. (Illus.). 44p. pap. text 30.00 (*0-7881-4507-X*) DIANE Pub.

Medical Advances. Steve Parker. 1998. LC 97-17985. (20th Century Inventions Ser.). (Illus.). 48p. (gr. 4-9). lib. bdg. 18.98 (*0-8172-4896-X*) Raintree Steck-V.

Medical Advances: A User Friendly Guide to the Latest Technology. Dan Burrus & Patti Thomsen. 1991. 131p. (Orig.). pap. 12.95 (*1-880136-52-X*) Intl Mgmt Pubns.

Medical Advisor: The Complete Guide. Time-Life Books Editors. 1996. LC 95-45803. (Illus.). 1152p. 39.95 (*0-8094-6737-2*) Time-Life.

Medical Advisor: The Complete Guide to Alternative & Conventional Treaments. Ed. by Time-Life Books Editors. 2nd ed. 2000. LC 00-45576. (Illus.). 1152p. (*0-7370-1622-1*) Time-Life Bks GBR. *Dist:* AOL Time Warner.

Medical Advisor - Home Education. Time-Life Books Editors. 1999. 29.95 (*0-7835-5301-3*) Time-Life.

Medical Advisor Home Edition: The Complete Guide to Alternative & Conventional Treatments. Time-Life Books Editors. 1997. LC 97-10717. (Illus.). 960p. pap. 19.95 (*0-7835-5250-5*) Time-Life.

Medical Aide. Jack Rudman. 1994. (Career Examination Ser.: C-1364). pap. 23.95 (*0-8373-1364-3*) Nat Learn.

Medical Almanac. Ed. by Pasquale J. Accardo. 1992. LC 91-20882. (Illus.). 254p. 49.50 (*0-89603-181-0*) Humana.

Medical Anatomy & Clinical Research: Index of Modern Authors & Subjects with Guide for Rapid Research. John C. Bartone. 1991. LC 90-56294. 160p. 47.50 (*1-55914-372-X*); pap. 44.50 (*1-55914-373-8*) ABBE Pubs Assn.

Medical & Applied Virology. Ed. by Murray Sanders et al. 1968. LC 67-26005. (Illus.). 428p. 22.50 (*0-87527-069-7*) Green.

Medical & Biological Dictionary Italian-English - English-Italian. G. Delfino. 1996. (ENG & ITA.). 2144p. (*88-08-08854-5*) Zanichelli ITA. *Dist:* IBD Ltd.

Medical & Biological Engineering in the Future of Health Care. Ed. by Joseph D. Andrade. 1994. LC 94-8413. (Illus.). 176p. (Orig.). (C). pap. 24.95 (*0-87480-454-X*) U of Utah Pr.

Medical & Biological Terminologies: Classical Origins. John Scarborough. 1998. LC 92-54139. (Classical Culture Ser.: Vol. 13). 320p. (Orig.). pap. 19.95 (*0-8061-3029-6*) U of Okla Pr.

Medical & Dental Associates, P. C. Insurance Forms Preparation. Gense & Lucinda Joy. 2nd ed. 1990. (Medical Assisting Ser.). 352p. pap. 21.95 (*0-538-70056-4*) S-W Thomson.

Medical & Dental Associates, P. C. Insurance Forms Preparation. Chapman. 3rd ed. 1997. 336p. (C). pap. text 43.95 (*0-8273-7560-3*) Delmar.

Medical & Dental Associates, P. C. Insurance Forms Preparation. Gense. 3rd ed. 1997. (Medical Assisting Ser.). pap. 18.95 (*0-538-71191-4*) S-W Thomson.

Medical & Dental Space Planning for the 1990s. Jain Malkin. 2nd ed. 1989. (Illus.). 144p. text 92.95 (*0-442-26485-2*, VNR) Wiley.

Medical & Dental Suction & Irrigation Equipment Markets: Environment & Infection Control Issues Encourage Innovations. Market Intelligence Staff. 1993. 279p. 1695.00 (*1-56753-451-1*) Frost & Sullivan.

Medical & Economical Botany. John Lindley. 1988. (C). (*0-7855-2294-8*) Scientific GBR. *Dist:* St Mut.

Medical & Environmental Aspects of Anaerobes. Ed. by Brian I. Duerden et al. 1992. 280p. (*1-871816-13-0*) Wrightson Biomed GBR. *Dist:* Taylor & Francis.

Medical & Genetic Aspects of Purebred Dogs II. Ross D. Clark & Joan R. Stainer. 2nd ed. 1994. LC 94-1762. 687p. (C). 103.50 (*0-9641609-0-0*) Cortlandt Grp.

Medical & Health Business Including Economic Competition: Index of New Information. Mary R. Klingenhagen & Jay Klingenhagen. 1995. LC 95-15404. 57.50 (*0-7883-0736-3*); pap. 47.50 (*0-7883-0737-1*) ABBE Pubs Assn.

Medical & Health Care Books & Serials in Print 1998, Vols. 1 & 2. Bowker Staff. 1998. 249.95 (*0-8352-3992-6*) Bowker LLC.

Medical & Health Costs of Care, Illness & Disability: Index of New Information with References. Allen Z. Buckner. rev. ed. 1997. 182p. 57.50 (*0-7883-1582-X*) ABBE Pubs Assn.

Medical & Health Costs of Care, Illness & Disability: Index of New Information with References. Allen Z. Buckner & Vincent Z. De Leo. rev. ed. 1997. 182p. pap. 47.50 (*0-7883-1583-8*) ABBE Pubs Assn.

***Medical & Health Information Directory** 14th ed. 2002. 650.00 (*0-7876-5326-8*); 275.00 (*0-7876-5327-6*); 275.00 (*0-7876-5328-4*); 275.00 (*0-7876-5329-2*) Gale.

Medical & Health Information Directory, Set. 13th ed. 2001. 650.00 net. (*0-7876-3479-4*) Gale.

Medical & Health Information Directory Vol. 1: Organizations, Agencies & Institutions. Karen Backus. 13th ed. 2001. 275.00 net. (*0-7876-3482-4*) Gale.

Medical & Health Information Directory Vol. 3: Health Services. 13th ed. 2001. 275.00 net. (*0-7876-3488-3*) Gale.

Medical & Health Practices & Defensive Medicine: New Research Bible of Current Trends. Herbert H. Newson. 1994. 160p. 57.50 (*0-7883-0200-0*); pap. 47.50 (*0-7883-0201-9*) ABBE Pubs Assn.

Medical & Health Sciences Word Book. Ann Roe-Hafer. 3rd ed. 1992. 448p. 12.00 (*0-395-60664-0*) HM.

Medical & Healthcare Books & Serials in Print, 1999: An Index to Literature in the Health Sciences, Set. Ed. by Bowker Staff. 1999. 265.95 (*0-8352-4068-1*) Bowker LLC.

Medical & Healthcare Marketplace Guide. 7th ed. 1991. (*0-926700-04-9*) MLR Pub.

Medical & Healthcare Marketplace Guide. Ed. by Robert Smith. 15th ed. 2001. 1000p. pap. 690.00 (*1-880874-58-X*) Dorland Hlthcare.

Medical & International Cooperation of Local & World Health Problems: Index of New Information. Tom Y. Appler. 1998. 57.50 (*0-7883-1806-3*); pap. 47.50 (*0-7883-1807-1*) ABBE Pubs Assn.

Medical & Legal Liability in Health Sciences: Index of New Information. Roy R. Zimmerman. 1994. 150p. 57.50 (*0-7883-0078-4*); pap. 47.50 (*0-7883-0079-2*) ABBE Pubs Assn.

Medical & Life-Style Risk Factors Affecting Fetal Mortality, 1989-1990. Donna L. Hoyert. 1996. LC 96-30479. (Vital & Health Statistics Ser.: Series 20, No 31). (*0-8406-0517-X*) Natl Ctr Health Stats.

Medical & Nutritional Complications of Alcoholism: Mechanisms & Management. Charles S. Lieber. 1992. (Illus.). 598p. (C). 132.00 (*0-306-43558-6*, Kluwer Plenum) Kluwer Academic.

Medical & Orthopedic Issues of Active & Athletic Women. Ed. by Rosemary Agostini. 1994. LC 94-75825. (Illus.). 530p. (Orig.). pap. 50.95 (*1-56053-019-7*) Hanley & Belfus.

Medical & Paramedical Dictionary English-French. W. J. Gladstone. 1996. Orig. Title: Dictionnaire Anglais-Francais des Sciences Medicales & Paramedicales. 1282p. (*2-224-02446-0*) Maloine FRA. *Dist:* IBD Ltd.

Medical & Psychiatric Issues for Counselors. Brian Daines et al. 1996. (Professional Skills for Counselors Ser.). 160p. 57.95 (*0-8039-7506-6*, 1003); pap. 19.95 (*0-8039-7507-4*, 1004) Sage.

Medical & Psychological Hypnosis: How It Benefits Patients. Corydon Hammond. 1994. 23p. pap. text 5.00 (*1-886610-00-2*) Am Soc Clin Hyp Pr.

Medical & Psychosocial Aspects of Chronic Illness & Disability. Donna R. Falvo. 2nd ed. 1999. LC 99-46280. xxi, 464p. 55.00 (*0-8342-1198-X*) Aspen Pub.

Medical & Scientific Reports & Research on Efficiency & Performance in the Health Sciences. American Health Research Institute Staff. 1993. 180p. 47.50 (*1-55914-870-5*); pap. 44.50 (*1-55914-871-3*) ABBE Pubs Assn.

Medical & Service Delivery Guidelines for Family Planning: Russian Edition. AVSC International Staff. Ed. by Inna Sacci & Vera Grigorieva. 2nd ed. 1999. (RUS.). 250p. pap. (*1-885063-21-0*) EngenderHlth.

Medical & Social Aspects of Alcohol Abuse. Ed. by Boris Tabakoff et al. 1983. LC 83-4786. 420p. 80.00 (*0-306-41221-7*, Plenum Trade) Perseus Pubng.

Medical & Social Problems of the Disabled. V. Kallio. 1982. (Euro Reports & Studies Ser.: No. 73). 35p. pap. text 4.00 (*92-890-1239-0*) World Health.

Medical & Surgical Aspects of Renovascular Hypertension. Ed. by J. Rosenthal & H. E. Franz. 1976. (Contributions to Nephrology Ser.: Vol. 3). (Illus.). 200p. 29.75 (*3-8055-2341-6*) S Karger.

Medical & Surgical Care for Children with Down Syndrome: A Guide for Parents. Ed. by D. C. Van Dyke et al. 1995. LC 95-1177. (Topics in Down Syndrome Ser.). (Illus.). 395p. pap. 14.95 (*0-933149-54-9*) Woodbine House.

***Medical & Surgical Equipment Words.** Stedman's. 3rd ed. 2001. 600p. pap. text 38.95 (*0-7817-2703-0*) Lppncott W & W.

Medical & Surgical History of the Civil War, Set. Ed. by James I. Robertson, Jr. 1992. Orig. Title: The Medical & Surgical History of the War of the Rebellion. (Illus.). reprint ed. 1800.00 (*0-916107-86-8*) Broadfoot.

Medical & Surgical History of the Civil War Index, Set. Ed. by James I. Robertson, Jr. 1992. 1400p. 400.00 (*0-916107-95-7*) Broadfoot.

Medical & Surgical History of the War of the Rebellion see Medical & Surgical History of the Civil War

Medical & Surgical Management of Adrenal Disease. Joseph C. Cerny. 1999. LC 96-54024. 240p. text 120.00 (*0-683-30344-9*) Lppncott W & W.

Medical & Surgical Management of Adrenal Diseases. Joseph C. Cerny. 1997. LC 96-54024. (*4-260-14339-5*) Igaku-Shoin.

Medical & Surgical Management of Adrenal Diseases. Ed. by Joseph C. Cerny. 1997. LC 96-54024. (Illus.). 224p. text (*0-89640-339-4*) Igaku-Shoin.

Medical & Surgical Management of Prostate Cancer. Ed. by Richard G. Middleton, Jr. 1996. LC 95-52984. (Topics in Clinical Urology Ser.). (Illus.). 184p. 59.00 (*0-89640-293-2*) Igaku-Shoin.

Medical & Surgical Therapeutics of the Foot & Ankle. David E. Marcinko. 1992. (Illus.). 968p. 125.00 (*0-683-05549-6*) Lppncott W & W.

Medical & Veterinary Entomology. D. S. Kettle. 2nd ed. 1995. LC 96-182455. (CAB International Publication). (Illus.). 736p. pap. text 70.00 (*0-85198-969-1*) OUP.

Medical Annual, 1983. D. J. Gray. 1983. (Illus.). 320p. pap. text (*0-7236-0688-9*) Buttrwrth-Heinemann.

Medical Annual, 1982-83. Ronald B. Scott & James Fraser. 1982. (Illus.). 408p. pap. text (*0-7236-0655-2*) Buttrwrth-Heinemann.

Medical Anthropology: Contemporary Theory & Method. Ed. by Thomas R. Johnson. 1996. LC 95-40052. 584p. pap. 35.00 (*0-275-95265-7*, Greenwood Pr) Greenwood.

Medical Anthropology & African American Health. Eric J. Bailey. 2000. LC 99-21244. (Illus.). 272p. 68.00 (*0-89789-592-4*, Bergin & Garvey) Greenwood.

Medical Anthropology & the World System: A Critical Perspective. Hans A. Baer et al. 1997. LC 97-16134. 288p. 77.00 (*0-89789-424-3*); pap. 24.95 (*0-89789-539-8*) Greenwood (Bergin & Garvey).

Medical Anthropology in Ecological Perspective, 3. Ann McElroy & Patricia K. Townsend. 3rd ed. 1996. LC 96-30556. 464p. (C). pap. text 41.00 (*0-8133-8610-1*) Westview.

Medical Anthropology of the Jaunsaris. S. N. Rizvi. 1991. (C). text (*81-7211-012-X*) Northern Bk Centre IND. *Dist:* S Asia.

Medical Aphorisms, Bks. 1-5. Moses Maimonides. Ed. by Gerrit Bos. 2000. (Graeco-Arabic Sciences Ser.). (ARA & ENG.). 320p. 29.95 (*0-8425-2474-6*) Brigham.

Medical Application of Liposomes. Ed. by K. Yagi. 1986. (Illus.). viii, 204p. 124.50 (*3-8055-4404-9*) S Karger.

***Medical Applications of Computer Modelling** Ed. by T. B. Martonen. Incl. Medical Applications of Computer Modelling Vol. 1: Cardiovascular & Ocular Systems. LC 99-68728. 304p. 2000. text (*1-85312-613-6*); Medical Applications of Computer Modelling Vol. 2: The Respiratory System. LC 99-69346. (Illus.). 345p. 2001. text (*1-85312-808-2*); (Advances in Computational Bioengineering Ser.). 664p. text (*1-85312-809-0*) WIT Pr GBR. *Dist:* Computational Mech MA.

Medical Applications of Computer Modelling Vol. 1: Cardiovascular & Ocular Systems. Ed. by T. B. Martonen. 2000. LC 99-68728. (Advances in Computational Bioengineering Ser.: Vol. 3). 304p. text (*1-85312-613-6*) WIT Pr GBR. *Dist:* Computational Mech MA.

Medical Applications of Computer Modelling Vol. 2: The Respiratory System. Ed. by T. B. Martonen. 2001. LC 99-69346. (Advances in Computational Bioengineering Ser.: Vol. 4). (Illus.). 345p. text (*1-85312-808-2*) WIT Pr GBR. *Dist:* Computational Mech MA.

Medical Applications of Controlled Release Ed. by Robert S. Langer & Donald L. Wise. 1985. Vol. I: Classes of Systems. 272p. 155.00 (*0-8493-5405-6*, RS201); Vol. II: Applications & Evaluation. 248p. 137.00 (*0-8493-5406-4*, RS201) Franklin (CRC Reprint).

Medical Applications of Fluorescent Excitation Analysis. Leon Kaufman. 1979. 176p. 104.00 (*0-8493-5507-9*, QP519, CRC Reprint) Franklin.

Medical Applications of Lasers in Dermatology, Cardiology, Gynecology, Ophthalmology & Dentistry II, Ed. by Gregory B. Altshuler et al. 1997. LC 98-145664. (Europto Ser.: Vol. 3192). 306p. 99.00 (*0-8194-2624-5*) SPIE.

Medical Applications of Lasers in Dermatology, Cardiology, Gynecology, Ophthalmology & Dentistry II. Ed. by Peter Bjerring et al. 1999. (Europto Ser.: Vol. 3564). 89.00 (*0-8194-3026-9*) SPIE.

Medical Applications of Liposomes. D. D. Lasic & Demetrios Papahadjopoulos. 1998. LC 98-22644. 794p. 236.50 (*0-444-82917-2*) Elsevier.

Medical Applications of Natural Family Planning: A Contemporary Approach to Women's Health Care. Thomas W. Hilgers. 1991. (Illus.). 183p. (Orig.). pap. text 29.95 (*0-9626485-1-5*) Pope Paul Sixth.

***Medical Appraisal, Selection & Revalidation: A Professional's Guide to Good Practice.** J. Gatrell & T. White. 2000. 64p. (*1-85315-400-8*) Royal Soc of Medicine Pr Ltd GBR. *Dist:* Balogh.

Medical Armageddon. Michael L. Culbert. rev. ed. 1997. LC 97-69817. (Illus.). 830p. pap. 29.95 (*0-9636487-5-6*) C&C Communs.

Medical Aromatherapy: Healing with Essential Oils. Kurt Schnaubelt. 1999. LC 97-46512. (Illus.). 300p. pap. 16.95 (*1-883319-69-2*) Frog Ltd CA.

Medical Art & Science of Relaxation in Sickness & Health: Index of New Information with Authors & Subjects. Sally M. Frost. 1993. 180p. 47.50 (*1-55914-906-X*); pap. 44.50 (*1-55914-907-8*) ABBE Pubs Assn.

Medical Aspects of Balance of Diabetes in Juveniles: Part I: Medical Aspects. Proceedings of the 3rd Beilinson, Symposium, Tel Aviv, April-May 1975. International Beilinson Symposium Staff. Ed. by Z. Laron. 1977. (Pediatric & Adolescent Endocrinology Ser.: Vol. 2). (Illus.). 85.25 (*3-8055-2388-2*) S Karger.

Medical Aspects of Biochemistry. William E. Schreiber. 1984. 304p. 22.50 (*0-316-77473-1*, Little Brwn Med Div) Lppncott W & W.

Medical Aspects of Boxing. Jordan. 1992. 352p. lib. bdg. 119.00 (*0-8493-4281-3*, RC1220) CRC Pr.

Medical Aspects of Crime. William N. East. 1980. lib. bdg. 79.95 (*0-8490-3160-5*) Gordon Pr.

Medical Aspects of Developmental Disabilities in Children Birth to Three. Blackman. 3rd ed. 1995. LC 96-44579. 320p. pap. 48.00 (*0-8342-0759-1*) PRO-ED.

Medical Aspects of Disability: A Handbook for the Rehabilitation Professional. Ed. by Myron G. Eisenberg et al. 2nd ed. 1999. LC 98-50679. 744p. text 62.95 (*0-8261-7971-1*) Springer Pub.

Medical Aspects of Early Intervention. James A. Blackman. 1995. 240p. pap. 45.00 (*0-8342-0648-X*) Aspen Pub.

Medical Aspects of Mortality Statistics. Ed. by H. Bostrom & N. Ljungstedt. 1981. (Illus.). 388p. (Orig.). pap. text 64.00 (*91-22-00440-8*) Coronet Bks.

Medical Aspects of Nuclear - Biological - Chemical Defensive Operations. 1991. lib. bdg. 75.00 (*0-8490-4198-8*) Gordon Pr.

Medical Aspects of Personal Injury Litigation. Michael Barnes et al. 1997. LC 97-23811. 141.95 (*0-632-04176-5*) Blackwell Sci.

Medical Aspects of Radiation Accidents. Eugene L. Saenger & AEC Technical Information Center Staff. 1963. 369p. 44.50 (*0-87079-268-7*, TID-18867); fiche 9.00 (*0-87079-388-8*, TID-18867) DOE.

Medical Assessment of Fitness to Dive. David Elliott. 1994. (Illus.). 302p. 78.75 (*0-9525162-0-9*, D746) Best Pub Co.

Medical Assistant. Julie B. Hosley. 1997. LC 96-34495. 768p. text 52.95 (*0-397-55096-0*) Lppncott W & W.

Medical Assistant. Jack Rudman. 1994. (Career Examination Ser.: C-1365). pap. 27.95 (*0-8373-1365-1*) Nat Learn.

Medical Assistant. Marian G. Cooper et al. 6th ed. 1993. tchr. ed. (*0-8151-2663-8*); 1993. (Illus.). 624p. (C). (gr. 13). text 43.00 (*0-8016-7445-X*, 01012); 1992. LC 92-48690. text 36.95 (*0-8016-1012-5*) Mosby Inc.

Medical Assistant: Administrative & Clinical. Mary E. Kinn et al. 7th ed. 1993. (Illus.). tchr. ed. (*0-7216-6718-X*); LC 93-6719. 864p. text 39.95 (*0-7216-4691-3*); pap. text, stu. ed. 17.95 (*0-7216-6719-8*) Saunders.

Medical Assistant: Administrative & Clinical. Mary E. Kinn & MaryAnn Woods. 8th ed. 1999. LC 98-36106. (Illus.). xxxi, 1144p. (C). text 45.00 (*0-7216-7299-X*) Saunders.

***Medical Assistant: Administrative & Clinical, Including Student Manual.** Mary E. Kinn & MaryAnn Woods. 8th ed. 2000. (Illus.). (C). stu. ed. 72.00 (*0-7216-8778-4*) Saunders.

Medical Assistant: An Intermediate Level of Health Care Personnel. Ed. by D. M. Pitcairn & D. M. Flahault. 1974. (Public Health Papers: No. 60). pap. text 10.00 (*92-4-130060-4*, 1110060) World Health.

Medical Assistant: Clinical Calculations. Watts. 2nd ed. 1989. (Medical Assisting Ser.). pap., tchr. ed. 12.00 (*0-8273-3079-0*) Delmar.

Medical Assistant: Clinical Calculations. Edith A. Watts. 2nd ed. 1989. (Medical Assisting Ser.). (gr. 11-12). pap. 28.95 (*0-8273-3078-2*) Delmar.

Medical Assistant: Program Review & Exam Preparation. Patricia Hurlbut. rev. ed. 1997. LC 97-24421. 352p. pap. 35.15 (*0-8385-6266-3*, A-6266-9) P-H.

Medical Assistant Clinical Comp. Keir. 1989. (Medical Assisting Ser.). Section 1. 2nd ed. 10.95 (*0-8273-5257-3*); Section 3. 3rd ed. 10.95 (*0-8273-5260-3*); Section 4. 2nd ed. 10.95 (*0-8273-5261-1*) Delmar.

Medical Assistant Examination Review. Laverne Dreizen. 4th ed. 1989. LC 92-83815. 280p. (C). pap. text 14.00 (*0-8385-5772-4*, A5772-7) Appleton & Lange.

Medical Assisting. Keir. 1986. (Medical Assisting Ser.). tchr. ed. 22.00 (*0-8273-2388-3*) Delmar.

Medical Assisting. Jack Rudman. (Occupational Competency Examination Ser.: Vol. 26). 47.95 (*0-8373-5776-4*); 1994. pap. 27.95 (*0-8373-5726-8*) Nat Learn.

Medical Assisting. Keir. 4th ed. 1998. (Medical Assisting Ser.). (C). pap. text, suppl. ed. 49.95 (*0-8273-7716-9*) Delmar.

Medical Assisting. Keir et al. 4th ed. 1998. (Medical Assisting Ser.). 320p. (C). tchr. ed., spiral bd. 79.95 (*0-8273-7714-2*) Delmar.

***Medical Assisting: A Commitment to Service: Administrative Competencies.** Margaret Townsend Warren. 2002. LC 00-61742. (Illus.). xvi, 376p. pap. incl. cd-rom (*0-7638-1325-7*) EMC-Paradigm.

Medical Assisting: A Patient-Centered Approach to Administrative & Clinical Competencies. Barbara Prickett-Ramutkowski. 1999. (Illus.). (gr. 6-12). stu. ed., wbk. ed. 19.75 (*0-02-802429-X*) Glencoe.

Medical Assisting: Administration & Clinical Compensation. Keir et al. 4th ed. 1997. (Medical Assisting Ser.). (C). 480p. pap. text, tchr. ed. 24.00 (*0-8273-7715-0*); 464p. pap. text, wbk. ed. 24.00 (*0-8273-7713-4*) Delmar.

Medical Assisting: Administrative & Clinical Competencies. Lucille Keir et al. 3rd ed. 1993. LC 92-49820. 778p. pap. 62.95 (*0-8273-5919-5*); 3rd ed. 1993. pap., tchr. ed. 25.00 (*0-8273-5313-8*); 3rd ed. 1993. text, stu. ed. 22.95 (*0-8273-5314-6*); 3rd ed. 1992. LC 92-49820. 778p. text 46.95 (*0-8273-5311-1*); 4th ed. 1997. LC 97-16219. 848p. (C). 66.95 incl. disk (*0-8273-7712-6*) Delmar.

Medical Assisting: Administrative & Clinical Competencies: Teacher's Resource Kit. Lucille Keir et al. 3rd ed. 1993. 251p. 74.95 (*0-8273-5694-3*) Delmar.

Medical Assisting: Advanced Clinical Skills Manual. Shea. 1996. (Medical Assisting Ser.). 96p. pap., tchr. ed. 14.00 (*0-8273-5642-0*) Delmar.

Medical Assisting: Clinical & Administrative Competencies. Lucille Keir et al. 2nd ed. 1989. 495p. (gr. 12). pap., tchr. ed. 22.00 (*0-8273-3508-3*, 2388-3) Delmar.

Medical Assisting: Clinical Competencies. Connie Krebs & Barbara A. Wise. 1994. LC 93-43603. 612p. (C). pap. 36.00 (*0-8273-4986-6*) Delmar.

Medical Assisting: Clinical Competencies: Instructor's Guide. Connie Krebs & Barbara A. Wise. 1993. 137p. pap. 18.00 (*0-8273-4987-4*) Delmar.

Medical Assisting: Clinical Skills Manual. Donna Shea & Adrienne L. Carter-Ward. 1995. LC 94-30041. (Health & Life Science Ser.). 592p. (C). otabind 47.95 (*0-8273-5641-2*) Delmar.

***Medical Assisting - A Commitment to Service: Administrative Competencies.** Ed. by Margaret Townsend Warren et al. 2002. 992p. 71.43 incl. cd-rom (*0-7638-1324-9*) EMC-Paradigm.

Medical Assisting - Clinical Competencies: Workbook. Connie Krebs & Barbara A. Wise. 1994. 325p. (C). pap. 18.95 (*0-8273-4988-2*) Delmar.

Medical Assisting Exam Review: Preparation For The CMA & RMA Exams. J. P. Cody. 1997. LC 97-4806. (Medical Assisting Ser.). 416p. (C). pap. text 44.95 (*0-8273-7183-7*) Delmar.

Medical Assisting Examination Guide: A Comprehensive Review for Certification. Karen Lane. 2nd ed. 1995. (Illus.). 267p. (C). pap. text 31.95 (*0-8036-0039-9*) Davis Co.

Medical Assisting Program. Pat Moeck. 1999. pap. text 17.36 (*1-56870-366-X*) RonJon Pub.

Medical Audiology. Wynne. 2000. pap. 52.75 net. (*0-7693-0004-9*) Thomson Learn.

Medical Audit: Rationale & Practicalities. Ed. by Simon P. Frostick et al. 1993. (Illus.). 457p. pap. text 39.95 (*0-521-44604-X*) Cambridge U Pr.

Medical Audit & General Practice. Ed. by Marshall Marinker. 2nd ed. 1995. 250p. pap. text (*0-7279-0908-8*) BMJ Pub GBR. *Dist:* AIDC.

Medical Audit in Primary Health Care. Ed. by Martin S. Lawrence & Theo Schofield. 1993. LC 92-48416. (Oxford Medical Publications). (Illus.). 270p. pap. text 34.50 (*0-19-262267-6*) OUP.

Medical Bacteriology. J. Douglas Sleigh & Morag C. Timbury. 3rd ed. 1990. (Student Notes Ser.). (Illus.). 438p. pap. text (*0-443-04147-4*) Church.

Medical Bacteriology. Ed. by N. C. Dey. 14th ed. 1988. (C). (*0-7210-0123-8*) Current Dist IND. *Dist:* St Mut.

***Medical Basis for Nuclear Accident Preparedness: The Clinical Care of Victims.** R. C. Ricks & M. E. Berger. 2002. 323p. lib. bdg. 97.95 (*1-84214-090-6*, Parthenon Pbng) CRC Pr.

Medical Basis for Radiation Accident Preparedness. Ed. by Robert C. Ricks & S. A. Fry. 1991. 548p. 175.00 (*0-444-01585-X*) P-H.

Medical Basis of Psychiatry. Paula Clayton. Ed. by George Winokur. 2nd ed. 1994. LC 93-22601. (Illus.). 624p. text 72.00 (*0-7216-6484-9*) Saunders.

Medical Bibliography in an Age of Discontinuity. Scott Adams. 1981. 244p. 20.00 (*0-8108-2433-7*) Scarecrow.

Medical Bill Survival Guide: What You Need to Know Before You Pay a Dime. Pat Palmer et al. 2000. (Illus.). 208p. mass mkt. (*0-446-60862-9*) Warner.

Medical Billing: The Bottom Line: An Entrepreneur's Guide. Claudia A. Yalden. Date not set. (Orig.). pap. 24.95 (*1-880325-39-X*) Borderlnds NH.

Medical Biochemistry. John Baynes & Marek H. Dominiczak. 1999. (Illus.). 560p. pap. 39.95 (*0-7234-3012-8*) Mosby Inc.

Medical Biochemistry. Nadhipuram V. Bhagavan. 2nd ed. 2001. 1060p. 84.95 (*0-12-095440-0*) Acad Pr.

Medical Biochemistry at a Glance. Ben D. Greenstein et al. 1996. LC 95-36168. (Illus.). 112p. pap. 28.95 (*0-86542-980-4*) Blackwell Sci.

Medical Biochemistry for the Tropics. J. K. Candlish. 1977. text (*0-7020-0619-X*) Bailliere Tindall.

Medical Biology of Bees: Index of New Information for Reference & Research. James G. Jinno. 1997. 150p. pap. 47.50 (*0-7883-1333-9*) ABBE Pubs Assn.

Medical Biology of Grief-Reactions & Management: Index of New Information. Jennifer W. Quinn. 1997. 150p. 57.50 (*0-7883-1384-3*); pap. 47.50 (*0-7883-1385-1*) ABBE Pubs Assn.

Medical Biology of Yohimbine & Its Easy Use in Male Sex Erectile Dysfunction: Index of New Information with Authors, Subjects, Research Categories & References. Henry Z. Poche. 1997. 167p. 57.50 (*0-7883-1590-0*); pap. 47.50 (*0-7883-1591-9*) ABBE Pubs Assn.

Medical Biostatistics. Abhaya Indrayan & Sanjeev B. Sarmukaddam. 2000. LC 00-50448. (Biostatistics Ser.). (Illus.). text 195.00 (*0-8247-0426-6*) Dekker.

Medical Blemishes: Untrue Stories about Real Problems. Loren Humphrey. 1997. 133p. pap. 9.95 (*1-890622-24-9*) Leathers Pub.

Medical Blunders: Amazing True Stories of Mad, Bad & Dangerous Doctors. Robert M. Youngson & Ian Schott. 1999. 405p. pap. 17.95 (*0-8147-9689-3*) NYU Pr.

Medical Blunders: Amazing True Stories of Mad, Bad, & Dangerous Doctors. Robert M. Youngson et al. 1996. 416p. (C). text 55.00 (*0-8147-9678-8*) NYU Pr.

Medical Boards - Step 1 Made Ridiculously Simple. Andreas Carl. 2nd ed. 1999. (Illus.). 367p. (C). pap. text 24.95 (*0-940780-39-9*) MedMaster.

***Medical Boards - Step 1 Made Ridiculously Simple.** Andreas Carl. 3rd rev. ed. 2001. (Illus.). 367p. pap. 24.95 (*0-940780-52-6*) MedMaster.

***Medical Boards - Step 2 Made Ridiculously Simple.** Andreas Carl. 2001. (Illus.). 356p. pap. 24.95 (*0-940780-55-0*) MedMaster.

Medical Boards - Step 2 Made Ridiculously Simple. Andreas Carl. 1999. LC 97-122209. 356p. pap. text 24.95 (*0-940780-28-3*) MedMaster.

Medical Boards Step 3 Made Ridiculously Simple. Andreas Carl. 1999. (Illus.). 285p. pap. text 22.95 (*0-940780-37-2*) MedMaster.

***Medical Boards Step 3 Made Ridiculously Simple.** Andreas Carl. 2nd rev. ed. 2001. 286p. pap. 22.95 (*0-940780-54-2*) MedMaster.

Medical Book Illustration: A Short History. John L. Thornton & Carole Reeves. 1984. (Medical Bks.: Vol. 2). (Illus.). (*0-906672-07-4*) Oleander Pr.

Medical Book of Remedies: 50 Ways to Ease Back Pain. Billy Glisan. 1998. (Illus.). 80p. text 20.00 (*0-7881-5391-9*) DIANE Pub.

Medical Book of Remedies: 50 Ways to Manage Diabetes. Jean Betschart. 1999. LC 00-501826. (*0-7853-3557-9*) Pubns Intl Ltd.

Medical Book of Remedies for People over 40. Consumer Guide Editors. 1996. LC 97-141346. 640p. pap. 7.99 (*0-451-82319-2*) NAL.

Medical Botany: A Herbal Guide to Health. William J. Simmonite. 1992. lib. bdg. 88.00 (*0-8490-8705-8*) Gordon Pr.

Medical Botany: A Herbal Guide to Health. William J. Simmonite. 1996. 191p. reprint ed. spiral bd. 13.00 (*0-7873-0794-7*) Hlth Research.

Medical Botany: Plants Affecting Man's Health. Walter H. Lewis & Memory P. Elvin-Lewis. 1982. LC 76-44376. 544p. pap. 59.95 (*0-471-86134-0*) Wiley.

Medical Brain Teasers, Puzzles & Games. Deena Silverman. 1993. 117p. (C). pap. 24.50 (*0-8273-5635-8*) Delmar.

***Medical Breakthroughs 2001: The Latest Advances in Preventing, Treating & Curing Nearly 100 Common Diseases.** Reader's Digest Editorial Staff. 2002. (Illus.). 256p. pap. 19.95 (*0-7621-0305-1*) RD Assn.

Medical Briefs: A Dictionary of Realtime Briefs for Court Reporters Laurie Boucke. 1998. LC 98-8417. 1380p. pap. 75.00 (*1-888580-02-X*) White-Boucke.

Medical Care. 8.50 (*0-8224-4365-1*) Globe Fearon.

Medical Care & Risks of Dysfunctional Chronic Pain: Abstract, Executive Summary, Final Report & Appendices A-C. Michael Van Korff. 1998. (Illus.). 99p. (C). reprint ed. pap. text 25.00 (*0-7881-4505-3*) DIANE Pub.

Medical Care for the American People: Proceedings of the Committee on the Costs of Medical Care, October, 1932. Medical Care Costs Committee. 1977. LC 75-180569. (Medicine & Society in America Ser.). 242p. reprint ed. 19.95 (*0-405-03944-1*) Ayer.

Medical Care for the Elderly: Acute & Chronic Care. Ed. by I. M. Smith et al. 1982. LC 80-26495. 276p. text 35.00 (*0-88331-158-5*) R B Luce.

Medical Care for the Poor & Indigent: Index of Modern Information. Nellie M. Jacobs. 1989. LC 88-47987. 150p. 47.50 (*1-55914-062-3*); pap. 44.50 (*1-55914-063-1*) ABBE Pubs Assn.

Medical Care in Down Syndrome: A Preventive Medicine Approach, No. 8. Paul T. Rogers & Harry Coleman. 1992. (Pediatric Habilitation Ser.: Vol. 8). (Illus.). 360p. text 85.00 (*0-8247-8684-X*) Dekker.

Medical Care in the Nursing Home. Joseph G. Ouslander et al. 1991. 461p. text 58.00 (*0-07-047949-6*) McGraw-Hill Med Pub.

Medical Care in the Nursing Home. Joseph G. Ouslander et al. 2nd ed. 1996. LC 96-43576. (Illus.). 565p. text 62.00 (*0-07-048209-8*) McGraw-Hill Prof.

Medical Care in the United States: The Debate Before 1940 Ed. by Charles E. Rosenberg. 433.00 (*0-8153-0321-1*) Garland.

Medical Care Law. Edward P. Richards, III & Katharine C. Rathbun. 2nd ed. 1999. LC 99-22815. 109.00 (*0-8342-1603-5*) Aspen Pub.

Medical Care, Medical Costs: The Search for a Health Insurance Policy. Rashi Fein. 1999. 256p. lib. bdg. 26.95 (*0-7351-0186-8*) Replica Bks.

Medical Care of Refugees. Ed. by Richard H. Sandler & Thomas C. Jones. 1987. (Illus.). 432p. text 42.50 (*0-19-504181-X*) OUP.

***Medical Care of Terminally Ill Patients.** Robert E. Enck. 2nd ed. 2001. LC 00-13053. 256p. 68.00 (*0-8018-6765-7*); (Illus.). pap. text 31.50 (*0-8018-6766-5*) Johns Hopkins.

Medical Care of the Adolescent Athlete. Eugene F. Luckstead & Donald E. Greydanus. 1993. (Illus.). 325p. pap. 45.95 (*1-878487-18-3*, 5847M) Practice Mgmt Info.

Medical Care of the Dying Patient. Ed. by Robert DeBellis et al. 1982. 34.95 (*0-405-13947-0*) Ayer.

Medical Care of the Liver Transplant Patient. Paul G. Killenberg & Pierre A. Clavien. 1997. LC 96-6592. (Illus.). 200p. (Orig.). text 95.00 (*0-86542-524-8*) Blackwell Sci.

Medical Care of the Nursing Home Resident: What Physicians Need to Know. Ed. by Richard W. Besdine et al. 1996. LC 96-12363. 175p. pap. 29.00 (*0-943126-48-7*) Amer Coll Phys.

Medical Care of the Pregnant Patient. Richard S. Abrams & Paul Wexler. 1983. 404p. 49.95 (*0-316-00470-7*, Little Brwn Med Div) Lppncott W & W.

Medical Care of the Pregnant Patient. Richard V. Lee et al. 2000. LC 99-12514. (Women's Health Ser.). (Illus.). xxvii, 866p. pap. 55.00 (*0-943126-81-9*, 330301190) Amer Coll Phys.

Medical Care of the Soul: A Practical & Healing Guide to End-of-Life Issues for Families, Patients, & Healthcare Providers. Bruce G. Bartlow. 2000. LC 00-29644. x, 289p. pap. 18.00 (*1-55566-254-4*); (Illus.). 32.50 (*1-55566-253-6*) Johnson Bks.

***Medical Care of The Transplant Liver Patient.** Paul G. Killenberg. 2nd ed. 2001. LC 00-68003. (Illus.). 480p. pap. 99.95 (*0-632-04566-3*) Blackwell Sci.

Medical Care of Women. Phyllis L. Carr et al. 1995. LC 94-34774. (Illus.). 874p. text 105.00 (*0-7216-3779-5*) Saunders.

***Medical Care Output & Productivity.** David M. Cutler & Ernst R. Berndt. 2001. LC 00-67235. (Studies in Income & Wealth: Vol. 62). (Illus.). xii, 611p. 75.00 (*0-226-13226-9*) U Ch Pr.

Medical Care Reform: A Guide to Issues & Choices. Henry A. Shenkin. 1993. 168p. pap. 14.95 (*0-9638888-4-6*) Oakvale Pr.

Medical Care System: A Conceptual Model. Michael Long. 1994. LC 94-34492. (Illus.). 176p. pap. 17.50 (*1-56793-016-6*, 0946) Health Admin Pr.

Medical Case Management: Forms, Checklists, & Guidelines. annuals Aspen Reference Group Staff. Ed. by Rufus Howe. 1995. 506p. ring bd., suppl. ed. 225.00 (*0-8342-0624-2*, S173) Aspen Pub.

Medical Catheter Markets: New Applications, Technologies, & Safety Issues Overcome Cost Containment. Market Intelligence Staff. 1992. 245p. (Orig.). 1895.00 (*1-56753-057-5*) Frost & Sullivan.

Medical Catheters & Catheterizations - Harmful Reactions, Errors, Punctures, Migrations, Displacements & Complications: Index of New Information. Roy R. Zimmerman. rev. ed. 1997. 145p. 57.50 (*0-7883-1574-9*); pap. 47.50 (*0-7883-1575-7*) ABBE Pubs Assn.

Medical Causes. Tanya L. Stone. 1997. LC 97-25244. (Celebrity Activists Ser.). (Illus.). 64p. (YA). (gr. 5-9). 24.40 (*0-8050-5233-X*) TFC Bks NY.

Medical Causes of Deaths in Hospitals: Index of New Information & Medical Research Bible. Joel P. Travis. 1994. 150p. 47.50 (*0-7883-0128-4*); 1994. 150p. pap. 47.50 (*0-7883-0129-2*); 1998. 145p. 57.50 (*0-7883-2088-2*); 1998. 145p. pap. 47.50 (*0-7883-2089-0*) ABBE Pubs Assn.

Medical Cell Biology. Steven R. Goodman. 2nd ed. 1997. LC 97-26571. 352p. pap. text 32.95 (*0-397-58427-X*) Lppncott W & W.

Medical Center Occupational Health & Safety. Robert J. McCunney. 1999. LC 99-14496. 448p. text 59.95 (*0-7817-2198-9*) Lppncott W & W.

Medical Charities, Medical Politics: The Irish Dispensary System & the Poor Law, 1836-1872. Ronald D. Cassell. 1997. LC 97-3751. (Royal Historical Society Studies in History). 192p. 60.00 (*0-86193-228-5*, Royal Historical Soc) Boydell & Brewer.

Medical Choice in a Mexican Village. James C. Young & Linda C. Garro. 1994. (Illus.). 233p. (C). reprint ed. pap. text 14.50 (*0-88133-785-4*) Waveland Pr.

Medical Claim Game - & How to Win It. G. J. Watkins. 1995. LC 91-66284. (Illus.). 125p. pap. 14.95 (*0-9639152-1-5*) Shadow Pubns.

Medical, Clinical, Pharmacological & Therapeutic Dictionary: Dictionnaire Medical, Clinique, Pharmacologique et Therapeutique. Alain Blacque-Belair. 3rd ed. 1981. 1938p. 150.00 (*0-8288-1789-8*, M6036) Fr & Eur.

Medical College Admission Test (MCAT) Jack Rudman. 1994. (Admission Test Ser.: ATS-11). pap. 27.95 (*0-8373-5011-5*) Nat Learn.

Medical College Admission Test Student Guide. David M. Tarlow. rev. ed. 1993. LC 78-53092. (Illus.). pap. 15.95 (*0-931572-00-2*) Datar Pub.

Medical College Admissions Test (MCAT) - Core Content. David M. Tarlow. 1996. (Medical Examinations Ser.). (Illus.). 575p. (Orig.). (C). pap. 49.95 (*1-57774-000-9*) Educ Tsting Cnslts.

Medical Complications During Pregnancy. Ed. by Gerard N. Burrow & Thomas F. Ferris. 4th ed. 1994. LC 94-25450. (Illus.). 633p. text 87.00 (*0-7216-5150-X*) Saunders.

Medical Complications in Labor & Delivery. Bernard Gonick et al. 1995. LC 95-21120. 240p. pap. 29.95 (*0-86542-475-6*) Blackwell Sci.

Medical Computing & Applications. David Ellis. 1987. LC 86-21333. (Computers & Their Applications Ser.). 325p. 44.95 (*0-470-20766-3*) P-H.

Medical Concepts & Penal Policy. Gerry Johnstone. 1996. 204p. pap. (*1-85941-021-9*) Cavendish Pubng GBR. *Dist:* Gaunt.

Medical Conduct Investigator. Jack Rudman. 1994. (Career Examination Ser.: C-2287). reprint ed. pap. 27.95 (*0-8373-2287-1*) Nat Learn.

Medical Consequences of Natural Disasters. L. Beinin. 1985. (Illus.). 160p. pap. 78.00 (*0-387-15506-6*) Spr-Verlag.

Medical Consequences of the Chernobyl Nuclear Accident. Ed. by P. V. Ramzaev. 1994. 237p. lib. bdg. 145.00 (*1-56072-111-1*) Nova Sci Pubs.

Medical Consultation: The Internist on Surgical, Obstetric & Psychiatric Services. William S. Kammerer & Richard J. Gross. 2nd ed. 1990. (Illus.). 696p. 75.00 (*0-683-04506-7*) Lppncott W & W.

Medical Consultations - Practice, Methods, Preferences, Importance & Necessity: Index of New Information with Authors & Subjects. Eric S. Anderson. 1993. 180p. 47.50 (*1-55914-910-8*); pap. 44.50 (*1-55914-911-6*) ABBE Pubs Assn.

Medical Control of Populations: Index of New Information with Authors, Subjects & References. Webster K. Harmonsen. 1996. 150p. 57.50 (*0-7883-1340-1*); pap. 47.50 (*0-7883-1341-X*) ABBE Pubs Assn.

Medical Cornea: Corneal & Refractive Surgery. Ed. by Richard E. Selser, Jr. 1994. LC 94-2839. (Illus.). xii, 192p. text (*90-6299-106-8*) Kugler NLD. *Dist:* Lib Res.

Medical Cost Containment in Workers' Compensation: Innovative Approaches. Ed. by Richard B. Victor. 1987. LC 87-27900. 35.00 (*0-935149-06-6*, WC-87-1) Workers Comp Res Inst.

Medical Cost Crisis! A Common-Sense Solution. Don W. Larson. 1993. 240p. 24.00 (*0-9635576-0-2*) Bond Pub MN.

Medical Costs in Workers' Compensation: Interstate Comparisons, Minnesota, & Other Selected States. Greg Gifford. 1998. (Illus.). 127p. (C). reprint ed. pap. text 25.00 (*0-7881-7473-8*) DIANE Pub.

Medical Costs in Workers' Compensation: Trends & Interstate Comparisons. Leslie I. Boden & Charles A. Fleischman. 1989. LC 89-24975. 70p. 35.00 (*0-935149-22-8*, WC-89-5) Workers Comp Res Inst.

Medical Curiosities. Robert Youngson. 1997. LC 97-19502. 352p. pap. 10.95 (*0-7867-0432-2*) Carroll & Graf.

Medical Cyclotrons in Nuclear Medicine: Proceedings of the Medical Cyclotron Users Conference, 4th, Miami, 1976. Medical Cyclotron Users Conference Staff. Ed. by H. Roesler et al. 1977. (Progress in Nuclear Medicine Ser.: Vol. 4). 86.25 (*3-8055-2670-9*) S Karger.

Medical Dangers to Health & Energy in Our Drinking Water in the United States: Index of New Information. American Health Research Institute Staff. 1994. 150p. 57.50 (*0-7883-0070-9*); pap. 47.50 (*0-7883-0071-7*) ABBE Pubs Assn.

Medical Dark Ages Circa 1984: Cancer Alternative Therapies' Cure Rates. Ralph R. Hovnanian. 2nd ed. 1985. LC 81-90082. 288p. pap. 1.00 (*0-9607774-0-7*) Hovnanian.

***Medical Data Analysis: Second International Symposium, ISMDA 2001, Madrid, Spain, October 2001: Proceedings.** Jose Crespo et al. 2001. LC 2001-55105. (Lecture Notes in Computer Science Ser.: Vol. 2199). pap. (*3-540-42734-1*) Springer Pub.

Medical Data Mining & Knowledge Discovery. Ed. by K. J. Cios. 2001. LC 00-52451. (Studies in Fuzziness & Soft Computing: Vol. 60). (Illus.). 514p. 121.00 (*3-7908-1340-0*) Spr-Verlag.

Medical Data Portfolio. Burgus C. Garrison. 1992. LC 92-90468. 96p. pap., stu. ed. 12.00 (*0-9633245-0-0*, TXU438774) B C Garrison.

Medical Decision Making. Harold C. Sox et al. 1988. 406p. (C). pap. text 49.99 (*0-7506-9288-X*) Buttrwrth-Heinemann.

Medical Decision Making: Diagnostic Strategies & Expert Systems: Proceedings of the IFIP-IMIA International Working Conference on Computer-Aided Medical Decision Making, Prague, Czechoslovakia, 30 September to 4 October, 1985. Ed. by F. Gremey et al. 1985. 394p. 112.00 (*0-444-87840-8*, North Holland) Elsevier.

Medical Decisions & "Advance Directives" Index of New Information Including "Do-Not-Resuscitate" Orders, Accuracy of Judgments & Legal Aspects. American Health Research Institute Staff. rev. ed. 1997. (Illus.). 189p. 57.50 (*0-7883-0674-X*); pap. 47.50 (*0-7883-0673-1*) ABBE Pubs Assn.

M
N
O

Medical Defense Against Mustard Gas: Toxic Mechanisms & Pharmacological Implications. Bruno Papirmeister et al. 1991. (Illus.). 376p. 150.00 (*0-8493-4257-0*, RA1247) CRC Pr.

Medical, Dental & Pharmaceutical Auxiliaries: A Survey of Existing Legislation. 1968. (International Digest of Health Legislation Offprints: Vol. 19, No. 1). (ENG & FRE.). 143p. pap. text 9.00 (*92-4-169191-3*, 1956801) World Health.

Medical-Dental Terminology: Syllabus. LeGrand H. Woolley. 2nd ed. 1974. (gr. 11-12). pap. text 9.95 (*0-89420-003-8*, 217705) Natl Book.

Medical Department of the Army: Its History, Activities & Organization. James A. Tobey. LC 72-3061. (Brookings Institution. Institute for Government Research. Service Monographs of the U. S. Government: No. 45). reprint ed. 24.00 (*0-404-57145-X*) AMS Pr.

Medical Department of the United States Army from 1775 to 1873. U. S. Surgeon General's Office Staff. Ed. by Harvey E. Brown. LC 75-23763. reprint ed. 45.00 (*0-404-13369-X*) AMS Pr.

Medical Department of the United States Army in the World War. U. S. Surgeon General's Office Staff. Ed. by Gerald N. Grob. 1980. LC 78-22593. (Historical Issues in Mental Health Ser.). reprint ed. lib. bdg. 42.95 (*0-405-11943-7*) Ayer.

Medical Department of the United States in the Civil War. Louis C. Duncan. 1987. 400p. reprint ed. 28.50 (*0-942211-30-8*) Olde Soldier Bks.

Medical Detectives. Berton Roueche. rev. ed. 1991. 432p. pap. 14.95 (*0-452-26588-6*, Plume) Dutton Plume.

Medical Device Accidents: With Illustrative Cases. L. A. Geddes. 1998. LC 97-44271. (Illus.). 256p. 74.95 (*0-8493-9236-5*) CRC Pr.

Medical Device & Equipment Design: Usability Engineering & Ergonomics. Ed. by Michael E. Wiklund. 1995. 382p. 139.00 (*0-935184-69-4*) IHS Health Grp.

Medical Device Industry: Science Technology & Regulation in a Competitive Environment. Estrin. 1990. (Illus.). 976p. text 295.00 (*0-8247-8268-2*) Dekker.

Medical Device Industry Factbook. Ed. by Amy Allen. 3rd rev. ed. 1996. (Illus.). 190p. pap. 45.00 (*1-884551-02-5*) Canon Comns.

Medical Device Marketing Opportunities: Turkey. ECRI Staff. 85p. pap. text 17.95 (*0-941417-29-8*) ECRI.

Medical Device Markets: A Detailed Database on a 41 Billion Dollar Market. Market Intelligence Staff. 1992. 240p. 995.00 (*1-56753-085-0*) Frost & Sullivan.

Medical Device Packaging Handbook. Ed. by Max Sherman. 2nd ed. 1998. LC 98-36296. (Illus.). 416p. text 175.00 (*0-8247-0199-2*) Dekker.

Medical Device Quality Assurance & Regulatory Compliance. Richard C. Fries. 1998. LC 98-27991. (Illus.). 496p. text 185.00 (*0-8247-0177-1*) Dekker.

Medical Device Quality Systems Manual - For GMP & ISO 9001-9002 Compliance: (Includes PC-Word 7.0 Diskettes) Gunther Gumpp. Ed. by Brisitte Gumpp. 1998. (C). text, lab manual ed. 500.00 (*1-881006-55-7*) Qual Cont Systs Srvs.

Medical Device Register International, 2001: MDR International. Medical Economics Staff. rev. ed. 2001. (Illus.). 1,100p. 275.00 (*1-56363-384-1*, PDR) Med Econ.

Medical Device Register, 2001: MDR Medical Economics Staff. rev. ed. 2001. (Medical Device Register, Domestic Edition Ser.). (Illus.). 3500p. 325.00 (*1-56363-383-3*, PDR) Med Econ.

Medical Device Regulation: Assessment of European System's Value As a Model for the EDA. 1996. 48p. (Orig.). (C). pap. text 20.00 (*0-7881-2868-X*) DIANE Pub.

Medical Device Tracking System, 1993. Ed. by Ronni P. Solomon. 1993. 300p. ring bd. 295.00 (*0-941417-26-3*) ECRI.

Medical Device Vigilance/Monitoring: European Device Directives Compliance. Robin N. Stephens. 1997. LC 96-51891. 225p. 194.00 (*1-57491-030-2*) IHS Health Grp.

Medical Devices: FDA Review Time. 1996. (Illus.). 87p. (Orig.). (C). pap. text 30.00 (*0-7881-2766-7*) DIANE Pub.

Medical Devices: International Perspectives on Health & Safety. Ed. by C. W. Van Gruting. 1994. LC 94-24486. 678p. 366.00 (*0-444-89242-7*) Elsevier.

Medical Devices: Obtaining FDA Market Clearance. Jonathan S. Kahan. 1995. 289p. (Orig.). pap. 195.00 (*1-882615-24-7*) Parexel Intl.

Medical Devices: Validation & Routine Control. 1994. (Illus.). 20p. (Orig.). pap. text 86.00 (*1-57020-015-7*, ST1135-209) Assn Adv Med Instrn.

Medical Devices & Equipment - Design, Supplies, Failures, Control, Contaminations & Alarms: Index & Research Bible. American Health Research Institute Staff. 1995. 160p. 57.50 (*0-7883-0220-5*); pap. 47.50 (*0-7883-0221-3*) ABBE Pubs Assn.

Medical Devices & the Year 2000 Problem: ECRI's Step-by-Step Guide for Addressing the Year 2000 Problem in Healthcare Facilities. ECRI Staff. 1998. (Illus.). 12p. reprint ed. pap. 125.00 (*0-941417-65-4*) ECRI.

Medical Devices Used in Home Health Care. 1994. 48p. (Orig.). (C). pap. text 25.00 (*0-7881-0829-8*) DIANE Pub.

Medical Diagnosis & Treatment of Alcoholism. Ed. by Nancy K. Mello & Jack H. Mendelson. 1992. (Illus.). 656p. text 65.00 (*0-07-041491-2*) McGraw-Hill Med Pub.

Medical Diagnosis Asia. Friedman. No. 4. 1987. 9.95 (*0-316-29381-4*); No. 5. 1991. 10.95 (*0-316-29388-1*) Lppncott W & W (Little Brwn Med Div).

Medical Diagnosis Codes: A Consumer's Guide to the Classification of Diseases. Ed. by James Davis. 1999. LC 96-78923. 1375p. pap. 29.95 (*1-885987-06-4*, ME076, Health Info Pr) Practice Mgmt Info.

Medical Diagnosis of Child Maltreatment: A Guide for Medical Providers. Jean Smith et al. 1999. (Illus.). 288p. pap. text 35.00 (*0-07-069765-5*) McGraw-Hill Med Pub.

Medical Diagnostic Electronics Products: Market Share Analysis, 1991. Market Intelligence Staff. 1992. 246p. (Orig.). 1495.00 (*1-56753-064-8*) Frost & Sullivan.

Medical Diagnostic Kits & Products. 1992. 124p. 2450.00 (*0-89336-868-7*, C-045N) BCC.

Medical Diagnostic Kits & Products. Barbara Breindel. 1997. LC 98-100567. (Report Ser.: No. C-045U). 138p. 3150.00 (*1-56965-386-0*) BCC.

Medical Dictionary see Diccionario Medico

Medical Dictionary. Stedman. 1995. 20308p. 55.00 (*0-395-73855-5*) HM.

Medical Dictionary. D. W. Unseld. 1982. (ENG & GER.). 88.00 (*3-8047-0992-3*) Adlers Foreign Bks.

Medical Dictionary. S. Jedraszko. 2nd ed. 1980. (ENG & POL.). 431p. (*0-8288-0574-1*, M 7983) Fr & Eur.

Medical Dictionary. Glenn T. Rogers. 2nd ed. 1997. (ENG & SPA.). pap. text (*0-07-053580-9*); pap. text (*0-07-055680-6*) McGraw.

Medical Dictionary, Set. E. Veillon & Albert Nobel. 1983. (ENG, FRE, GER & ITA.). 1344p. 295.00 (*0-8288-1892-4*) Fr & Eur.

Medical Dictionary: Spanish/English/Spanish. Ruiz Torres. 9th ed. 1999. (ENG & SPA.). 956p. 295.00 (*0-320-00699-9*) Fr & Eur.

Medical Dictionary: English-German see Springer GroBworterbuch Medizin: Deutsch-Englisch

Medical Dictionary, English-German, German-English. C. Eichhorst. 1998. (ENG & GER.). 150.00 incl. cd-rom (*0-7859-9627-3*) Fr & Eur.

Medical Dictionary, English-Spanish/Spanish-English. Mosby Staff. 1996. (ENG & SPA.). 370p. 95.00 (*0-7859-9644-3*) Fr & Eur.

Medical Dictionary for Health Related Professionals. Hearl. 2000. (C). pap. 26.50 net. (*0-7668-0221-3*) Thomson Learn.

Medical Dictionary for Stenotypists. George P. Andrews. 1994. (Realtime Machine Shorthand Ser.). 526p. (C). pap. text 52.00 (*0-938643-32-0*, 555) Stenotype Educ.

Medical Dictionary for Tropical Regions: Dictionnaire Medical pour les Regions. Bernard Pierre & Genevieve Pierre. 2nd ed. 1988. (FRE.). 850p. pap. 75.00 (*0-8288-1823-1*) Fr & Eur.

Medical Dictionary in Six Languages. Bert Spilker. 1994. LC 94-30921. 688p. text 129.00 (*0-7817-0182-1*) Lppncott W & W.

Medical Dictionary of Symptoms & Syndromes: Dictionnaire Medical des Symptomes et Syndromes. Raymond Villey. 2nd ed. 1982. (FRE.). 312p. 95.00 (*0-8288-1831-2*, M15604) Fr & Eur.

Medical Dictionary of the English & German Languages. Dieter W. Unseld. 8th ed. 1982. (ENG & GER.). 593p. 125.00 (*0-8288-0573-3*, M8016) Fr & Eur.

Medical Dictionary of Women: Dictionnaire Medical de la Femme. Lucien Bouccara. 1981. 500p. 29.95 (*0-8288-1792-8*, M15419) Fr & Eur.

Medical Dictionary Student Value Pack. Contrib. by Stedman's Medical Dictionary Staff. 27th ed. 2000. LC 99-56094. (Illus.). 2098p. stu. ed. 59.95 incl. cd-rom (*0-7817-2727-8*) Lppncott W & W.

Medical Direction in Long-Term Care: A Guidebook for the Future. Ed. by Steven A. Levenson. 2nd ed. 1993. LC 93-72380. 694p. 65.00 (*0-89089-547-3*) Carolina Acad Pr.

Medical Direction in the Nursing Home: Principles & Concepts for Physician-Administrators. James J. Pattee & Orlo J. Otteson. 1991. 405p. 49.50 (*0-9629614-0-X*) North Ridge Pr.

Medical Directors: What, Why, How. George E. Linney, Jr. & Barbara J. Linney. 1993. LC 92-74400. 44p. (Orig.). (C). pap. text 20.00 (*0-924674-19-9*) Am Coll Phys Execs.

Medical Directory, 1990, Set. 90th ed. 1990. 4000p. 150.00 (*0-582-06163-6*, Saint James) Gale.

Medical Directory, 1994. Churchill Livingstone. 1994. (Illus.). 4672p. text (*0-582-23418-2*) Church.

Medical Disability Advisor: Workplace Guidelines for Disability Duration. Presley Reed. 1994. LC 91-14155. 275.00 (*0-934753-52-0*) LRP Pubns.

Medical Discourse & Systemic Frames of Comprehension, 42. Ronald Chenail. Ed. by Roy Freedle. 1991. LC 90-14418. (Advances in Discourse Processes Ser.: Vol. 42). 144p. 85.00 (*0-89391-707-9*, Ablex) Greenwood.

Medical Discoveries: Medical Breakthroughs & the People Who Developed Them. F. Freiman. 1996. LC 96-42696. (*0-7876-0892-0*, UXL) Gale.

Medical Discoveries: Medical Breakthroughs & the People Who Developed Them. Fran L. Freiman. 1996. LC 96-42696. (*0-7876-0891-2*, UXL) Gale.

Medical Discoveries: Medical Breakthroughs & the People Who Discover Them Fran L. Freiman. 1997. LC 96-42696. (Illus.). 442p. (gr. 4-7). text 105.00 (*0-7876-0890-4*, GML14099-110188, UXL) Gale.

Medical Discoveries of Edward Bach, Physician. Weeks. (*0-85207-001-2*) C W Daniel GBR. *Dist:* Natl Bk Netwk.

Medical Discoveries of Edward Bach, Physician. Nora Weeks. 16th ed. 144p. pap. 11.95 (*0-8464-4250-7*) Beekman Pubs.

Medical Disorders During Pregnancy. Ed. by William M. Barron et al. 3rd ed. 2000. 649p. 89.95 (*0-323-00772-4*) Mosby Inc.

Medical Disorders During Pregnancy, Vol. 2. John M. Barron & Marshall D. Lindheimer. 2nd ed. 1994. (Illus.). 576p. (C). (gr. 13). text 92.00 (*0-8016-8002-6*, 08002) Mosby Inc.

***Medical Disorders in Obstetric Practice.** Michael DeSwiet. 4th ed. 2001. LC 2001-52784. (Illus.). 680p. 139.95 (*0-632-05395-X*) Blackwell Sci.

Medical Disorders of Alcoholism: Pathogenesis & Treatment. Charles S. Lieber. 1982. (Major Problems in Internal Medicine Ser.: Vol. 22). (Illus.). 608p. text 120.00 (*0-7216-5774-5*) Saunders.

Medical Disposables Markets: A Detailed Database on a 45 Billion Dollar Market. Market Intelligence Staff. 1992. 340p. 995.00 (*1-56753-084-2*) Frost & Sullivan.

Medical Dissertations of Psychiatric Interest. Oskar Diethelm. 1971. 36.75 (*3-8055-1201-5*) S Karger.

Medical Divination. H. Tomlinson. 1980. 35.00 (*0-85032-133-6*) St Mut.

Medical Doctors of Maryland in the C. S. A. Daniel D. Hartzler. 1979. 98p. pap. 20.00 (*0-942211-72-3*) Olde Soldier Bks.

Medical Dosage Calculations. June L. Olsen. 5th ed. 1991. 246p. (C). pap. text 25.95 (*0-8053-5603-7*) Addison-Wesley.

Medical Drug Reference. Contrib. by Mosby Staff. 2000. (Mosby's Medical Drug Reference Ser.). (Illus.). 1152p. text 31.95 (*0-8151-3657-9*, 31228) Mosby Inc.

Medical Drugs on Trial: An Expose of the Disease Industrialists. 1992. lib. bdg. 79.95 (*0-8490-8795-3*) Gordon Pr.

Medical Economics & Health Finance. Steven R. Eastaugh. 1981. LC 81-3450. (C). 352p. 35.00 (*0-86569-065-0*); 340p. pap. 15.00 (*0-86569-066-9*) Greenwood (Auburn Hse).

Medical Education: Annotated Bibliography, 1946-1955. 1958. (ENG & FRE.). 391p. pap. text 12.00 (*92-4-152003-5*, 1150101) World Health.

Medical Education: Curriculum & Financing Strategies Needed to Encourage Primary Care Training. 1995. (Illus.). 50p. (Orig.). (C). pap. text 40.00 (*0-7881-1710-6*) DIANE Pub.

Medical Education, Accreditation, & the Nation's Health: Reflections of an Atypical Dean. Andrew D. Hunt. 1991. LC 90-50845. 200p. (C). text 22.00 (*0-87013-288-1*) Mich St U Pr.

Medical Education & Health Care: A Pluridimensional Paradigm. Jasbir S. Bajaj & Indian Institute of Advanced Study Staff. 1998. LC 98-903260. xiv, 218p. (*81-85952-51-5*) Indian Inst.

Medical Education in the U. S. Before the Civil War. William F. Norwood. 1975. LC 72-165726. (American Education, Ser, No. 2). reprint ed. 30.95 (*0-405-03714-7*) Ayer.

Medical Education in the United States & Canada. Abraham Flexner. 1979. LC 78-180575. (Medicine & Society in America Ser.). 368p. reprint ed. 24.95 (*0-405-03952-2*) Ayer.

Medical Education in Transition. Commission on Medical Education, Sciences of Medic. Ed. by Roseann M. Jones. 1992. LC 92-64117. 146p. (Orig.). pap. (*0-942054-05-9*) R W Johnson Found.

Medical Effectiveness & Outcomes Management: Issues, Methods & Case Studies. Ed. by Patrice L. Spath. 1996. LC 95-46552. 327p. pap. 80.00 (*1-55648-150-0*, 169110) AHPI.

Medical Effectiveness Directory, 1995. 1995. 45.00 (*1-56925-028-6*, MED2) Capitol Publns.

Medical Effects of Free Radicals: Index of New Information with Authors & Subjects. American Health Research Institute Staff. 1995. LC 95-16341. 57.50 (*0-7883-0775-4*); 1995. LC 95-16341. pap. 47.50 (*0-7883-0776-2*); 1994. LC 92-54213. 173p. 57.50 (*0-7883-0384-8*); 1994. 173p. pap. 47.50 (*0-7883-0385-6*) ABBE Pubs Assn.

Medical Effects of Ionizing Radiation. Fred A. Mettler & Arthur C. Upton. 2nd ed. 1995. 464p. text 140.00 (*0-7216-6646-9*) Saunders.

Medical Electrical Equipment, General Requirements for Safety UL 2601-1. Underwriters Laboratories, Inc. Staff. 2nd ed. 1997. (C). pap. text 175.00 (*0-7629-0227-2*) Underwrtrs Labs.

Medical Electron Accelerators. Clarence J. Karzmark et al. 1992. LC 92-49307. 336p. text 125.00 (*0-07-105410-3*) McGraw-Hill Educ Grp.

Medical Emergencies. Ed. by Robert G. Sherding. 1984. (Contemporary Issues in Small Animal Practice Ser.: Vol. 1). (Illus.). 389p. pap. text (*0-443-08333-9*) Church.

***Medical Emergencies in Dentistry.** Jeffrey Bennett. 2001. 510p. pap. (*0-7216-8481-5*) Saunders.

Medical Emergencies in the Dental Office. Stanley F. Malamed. 4th rev. ed. 1992. LC 92-49542. (Illus.). 480p. (C). (gr. 13). pap. text 52.00 (*0-8016-6386-5*, 06386); 5th ed. 1999. LC 99-40660. (*1-55664-420-5*) Mosby Inc.

Medical Emergency! The St. Luke's-Roosevelt Hospital Center Book of Emergency Medicine. Stephen G. Lynn & Pamela Weintraub. 1999. (Illus.). 385p. pap. text 20.00 (*0-7881-6067-2*) DIANE Pub.

Medical Emergency Dispatcher. Jack Rudman. 1994. (Career Examination Ser.: C-2331). pap. 27.95 (*0-8373-2331-2*) Nat Learn.

Medical Employer's Guide: A Handbook of Employment Laws & Regulations. Amy L. Greenspan. 7th rev. ed. 2000. 670p. spiral bd. 120.00 (*1-56759-042-X*) Summers Pr.

Medical Encyclopedia see Mawsouat Al Toubiya

Medical Encyclopedia: World Book Rush-Presbyterian-St. Luke's Medical Center. Ed. by World Book, Inc. Staff. 8th ed. 1999. (YA). (gr. 4 up). (*0-7166-4206-9*) World Bk.

Medical Encyclopedia of Moses Maimonides. Fred Rosner. 1998. LC 97-41034. 288p. 50.00 (*0-7657-5997-7*) Aronson.

Medical Engineering in Japan: Research & Development. Ed. by K. Atsumi & F. Kajiya. 1987. (C). pap. text 278.50 (*0-89838-973-9*) Kluwer Academic.

Medical English for German Doctors. H. Kleinsorge. 1990. (ENG & GER.). lib. bdg. 115.00 (*0-8288-3590-X*, F106950) Fr & Eur.

Medical English Usage & Abusage. Edith Schwager. 1990. LC 90-7644. 232p. lib. bdg. 19.95 (*0-89774-590-6*, Oryx) Greenwood.

Medical Enlightenment of the Eighteenth Century. Ed. by Andrew Cunningham & Roger French. 1990. (Illus.). 342p. (C). text 90.00 (*0-521-38235-1*) Cambridge U Pr.

Medical Entomology for Students. Michael W. Service. 1996. LC 95-71091. (*0-412-71230-X*) Kluwer Academic.

Medical Epidemiology. Raymond S. Greenberg et al. 3rd ed. 2000. (Lange Medical Bks.). (Illus.). 215p. pap. 39.95 (*0-8385-6295-7*) McGraw-Hill Prof.

Medical Eponyms from A to Z. Yvonne T. Sesi. 1997. LC 96-61223. 212p. pap. 18.95 (*0-9642134-0-0*) Univ Scripts.

Medical Equipment Technician. Jack Rudman. 1994. (Career Examination Ser.: C-2654). pap. 29.95 (*0-8373-2654-0*) Nat Learn.

***Medical Errors: A Look at the IOM Report: Congressional Hearing.** Ed. by James M. Jeffords. 2001. 179p. (C). pap. text 35.00 (*0-7567-1095-2*) DIANE Pub.

***Medical Errors: Improving Quality of Care & Consumer Information: Congressional Hearing.** Ed. by Michael Bilirakis. 2001. (Illus.). 180p. (C). pap. text 35.00 (*0-7567-1103-7*) DIANE Pub.

***Medical Errors: Understanding Adverse Drug Events: Congressional Hearing.** Ed. by James M. Jeffords. 2001. (Illus.). 218p. (C). pap. text 40.00 (*0-7567-1097-9*) DIANE Pub.

Medical Ethics. Ed. by Robert S. Downie. 1996. LC 96-608. (International Research Library of Philosophy). (Illus.). 520p. (*1-85521-631-0*) Dartmth Pub GBR. *Dist:* Ashgate Pub Co.

Medical Ethics. Bernard Haring. 1990. 254p. (C). (*0-85439-391-9*) St Paul Pubns GBR. *Dist:* St Mut.

Medical Ethics. Robert M. Veatch. (Illus.). (C). 1989. text 46.95 (*0-86720-074-X*, 074-X); 2nd ed. 1996. LC 96-24292. 480p. text 58.95 (*0-86720-974-7*, 974-7) Jones & Bartlett.

***Medical Ethics.** Alistair Campbell et al. 3rd ed. 2002. 252p. (Orig.). pap. text 45.95 (*0-19-558445-7*) OUP.

Medical Ethics: A Patient-Centered Approach. James E. Giles. 1983. 224p. 18.95 (*0-87073-314-1*); LC 82-10294. pap. 13.95 (*0-87073-315-X*) Schenkman Bks Inc.

Medical Ethics: A Primer for Students. Robert Orr & Fred Chay. 2001. 128p. pap. 9.95 (*0-9666809-6-0*) Christ Med & Dental Assns.

Medical Ethics: A Reference Handbook. Lawrence H. Berlow. 1997. (Contemporary Ethical Issues Ser.). (Illus.). 256p. 39.50 (*0-87436-930-4*, FN-1718) ABC-CLIO.

Medical Ethics: Applying Theories & Principles to the Patient Encounter. Ed. by Matt Weinberg. 2000. LC 00-40658. (Illus.). 576p. pap. 60.00 (*1-57392-652-3*) Prometheus Bks.

Medical Ethics: Codes, Opinions & Statements. Ed. by Mark A. Rothstein et al. 2000. LC 99-55490. (Illus.). xxxix, 1074p. pap. 255.00 (*1-57018-100-4*, 1100-PRYY) BNA Books.

Medical Ethics: Essays on Abortion & Euthanasia. Robert L. Barry. 1989. (American University Studies: Ser. VII, Vol. 45). XI, 308p. (C). text 41.95 (*0-8204-0925-1*) P Lang Pubng.

Medical Ethics: Evolution, Rights & the Physician. Henry A. Shenkin. 1990. (Episteme Ser.). 500p. (C). lib. bdg. (*0-7923-1031-4*) Kluwer Academic NLD. *Dist:* Kluwer Academic.

***Medical Ethics: For Undergraduate Medical Students.** Lisa Schwartz et al. 2001. (Illus.). 255p. (C). pap. (*0-7020-2543-7*) W B Saunders GBR. *Dist:* Saunders.

Medical Ethics: Policies, Protocols, Guidelines & Programs. Ed. by John F. Monagle & David C. Thomasma. 1995. LC 92-21893. ring bd. 279.00 (*0-8342-0349-9*) Aspen Pub.

Medical Ethics: Principles, Persons & Problems. John M. Frame. 1988. 160p. pap. 9.99 (*0-87552-261-0*) P & R Pubng.

Medical Ethics: Sources of Catholic Teaching. Ed. by Kevin D. O'Rourke & Philip Boyle. 2nd ed. 1993. LC 93-4895. 368p. (Orig.). pap. text 35.00 (*0-87840-540-2*) Georgetown U Pr.

Medical Ethics: Sources of Catholic Teaching. Kevin D. O'Rourke & Philip Boyle. 3rd rev. ed. 1999. LC 98-44647. 442p. (Orig.). pap. 37.50 (*0-87840-722-7*) Georgetown U Pr.

Medical Ethics & Human Life: Doctor, Patient & Family in the New Technology. John E. Thomas. 1983. 482p. pap. (*0-88866-625-X*); 595p. text (*0-88866-624-1*) Edgar Kent.

Medical Ethics & Medical Education: XIVth CIOMS Round Table Conference Bilingual English/Spanish. Z. Bankowski & J. Bernardelli. 1981. (CIOMS Round Table Proceedings Ser.: No. 14). pap. text 20.00 (*92-9036-006-2*) World Health.

Medical Ethics at the Dawn of the 21st Century. Raphael Cohen-Almagor. 2000. LC 00-40186. (Annals of the New York Academy of Sciences Ser.: Vol. 913). vii, 265p. pap. (*1-57331-300-9*) NY Acad Sci.

Medical Ethics at the Dawn of the 21st Century, Vol. 913. Ed. by Raphael Cohen-Almagor. 2000. LC 00-40186. (Annals of the New York Academy of Sciences Ser.: Vol. 913). vii, 265p. 125.00 (*1-57331-299-1*) NY Acad Sci.

Medical Ethics for Physicians & Health Providers. Jay E. Kantor. 1999. 224p. 75.00 (*1-57309-368-8*) Intl Scholars.

Medical Ethics for Physicians-in-Training. J. E. Kantor. 1989. (Illus.). 242p. (C). text 44.50 (*0-306-43194-7*, Kluwer Plenum) Kluwer Academic.

Medical Ethics, Human Choices: A Christian Perspective. Ed. by John Rogers. 1988. LC 87-29747. 176p. (Orig.). pap. 12.99 (*0-8361-3460-5*) Herald Press.

Medical Ethics in Antiquity: Philosophical Perspectives on Abortion & Euthanasia. Paul Carrick. 1985. (Philosophy & Medicine Ser.: No. 18). 264p. pap. text 64.50 (*90-277-1915-2*); lib. bdg. 112.00 (*90-277-1825-3*) Kluwer Academic.

Medical Ethics in Practice: The Ethics Advisory Group at Boston's Beth Israel Hospital: A Case Study. Terry R. Bard. 1990. (Death Education, Aging & Health Care Ser.). 128p. 53.95 (*1-56032-056-7*) Hemisp Pub.

Medical Ethics in the Ancient World. Paul Carrick. 2001. (Clinical Medical Ethics Ser.). (Illus.). 248p. pap. text 27.50 (*0-87840-849-5*) Georgetown U Pr.

Medical Ethics in the Renaissance. Winfried Schleiner. 1997. LC 95-7359. (Illus.). 256p. pap. 28.95 (*0-87840-601-8*) Georgetown U Pr.

Medical Ethnobiology of the Highland Maya of Chiapas, Mexico: The Gastrointestinal Diseases. Elois A. Berlin & Brent Berlin. 1996. 352p. 105.00 (*0-691-03741-8*) Princeton U Pr.

Medical Evaluation of Physically & Sexually Abused Children. Carole Jenny. 1996. LC 96-4507. (APSAC Study Guides Ser.: Vol. 3). 128p. pap. 129.95 (*0-7619-0397-6*, 2556) Sage.

Medical Evaluation of Psychiatric Patients. R. B. Schiffer et al. 1988. LC 88-25380. (Illus.). 268p. (C). text 49.50 (*0-306-42957-8*, Kluwer Plenum) Kluwer Academic.

Medical Evaluation of the Surgical Patient. Alan G. Adler et al. 1985. (Blue Bk.). (Illus.). 304p. pap. text 36.95 (*0-7216-1146-X*) Saunders.

*__Medical Evidence: A Handbook for Doctors.__ Roger Clements et al. 2001. 136p. pap. (*1-85315-387-7*) Royal Soc of Medicine Pr Ltd GBR. *Dist:* Balogh.

Medical Examination Review: Pediatrics. V. A. LaCerva. 7th ed. 1986. (Clinical Sciences Ser.: Vol. 11, No. 7). 250p. pap. 18.00 (*0-444-01036-X*) Elsevier.

Medical Examination Review Vol. 2: Medicine. M. A. Baker. 9th ed. 1987. pap. 18.00 (*0-444-01126-9*) Elsevier.

Medical Examinations: A Preparation Guide. V. Bhushan Bhardwaj. 1979. (Illus.). pap. 9.00 (*0-668-03944-2*, Arc) Hungry Minds.

Medical Examiner. Jack Rudman. 1994. (Career Examination Ser.: C-486). pap. 49.95 (*0-8373-0486-5*) Nat Learn.

Medical Executive Committee Handbook. Hugh P. Greeley et al. Ed. by Meaghan Dwyer. 1999. LC 00-268204. (Illus.). vi, 206p. pap. text 87.00 (*1-57839-033-8*) Opus Communs.

Medical Expenditures for People with Disabilities in the United States. 1997. lib. bdg. 250.95 (*0-8490-8214-5*) Gordon Pr.

Medical Expense Insurance. Ed. by Jane Stein. 1997. LC 98-206181. 309p. pap. text 30.00 (*1-879143-40-2*) Health Ins Assn Am.

Medical Expense Insurance Study Manual. HIAA Staff. 1997. 80p. pap., stu. ed. 10.00 (*1-879143-41-0*) Health Ins Assn Am.

Medical Experimentation & the Protection of Human Rights: Proceedings of the XIIth CIOMS Round Table Conference. N. Howard-Jones & Z. Bankowski. 1979. (CIOMS Round Table Proceedings Ser.: No. 12). pap. text 25.00 (*92-9036-002-X*) World Health.

Medical Facilities. Meisei Publications Editorial Staff. 1994. (New Concept in Architecture & Design Ser.). (Illus.). 224p. (*4-87246-294-7*) Tenpo Syst Study JPN. *Dist:* Bks Nippan.

Medical Facilities Auditor. Jack Rudman. 1994. (Career Examination Ser.: C-2058). reprint ed. pap. 39.95 (*0-8373-2058-5*) Nat Learn.

Medical Factors & Psychological Disorders: A Handbook for Psychologists. R. L. Morrison & A. S. Bellack. 1987. LC 87-7903. (Illus.). 392p. (C). 90.00 (*0-306-42425-8*, Plenum Trade) Perseus Pubng.

Medical Family Therapy: Psychosocial Treatment of Families with Health Problems. Susan H. McDaniel et al. 1992. LC 92-11151. 352p. 50.00 (*0-465-04437-9*) Basic.

*__Medical Family Tree.__ Frances Boulden. 2001. 72p. spiral bd. (*0-9713098-0-9*) F C B.

Medical Fees in the United States, 1999. Ed. by ADP Context Software Staff & James B. Davis. 1999. 380p. pap. 119.95 (*1-57066-129-4*, 9935) Practice Mgmt Info.

Medical Fees in the United States 2000. Ed. by ADP Context Software Staff & James B. Davis. 2000. pap. text 119.95 (*1-57066-167-7*, 20035) Practice Mgmt Info.

*__Medical Fees in the United States 2001.__ annuals ADP Context Staff. 2001. pap. text 119.95 (*1-57066-197-9*, 21035) Practice Mgmt Info.

Medical Fictionary. H. C. Wolford. 1998. 80p. pap. 7.95 (*0-9654563-4-X*, Big Tree Bks) Easy Money Pr.

Medical Filing. Claeys. 1993. (Medical Assisting Ser.). pap. 14.95 (*0-538-70675-9*) S-W Thomson.

Medical Filing. Terese Claeys. 2nd ed. 1996. 112p. LC 96-9526. (Illus.). pap. text 32.95 (*0-8273-8177-8*); pap., tchr. ed. (*0-8273-8178-6*) Delmar.

Medical First Aid Guide for Use in Accidents Involving Dangerous Goods (MFAG) International Maritime Organization Staff. 1991. text (*0-89771-875-5*) Intl Maritime Org GBR. *Dist:* St Mut.

Medical First Aid Guide for Use in Accidents Involving Dangerous Goods MFAG 1994. International Maritime Organization Staff. 1994. pap. (*0-7855-0500-8*) Intl Maritime Org GBR. *Dist:* St Mut.

Medical Flora: Or Manual of the Medical Botany of the United States of North America, Set. Constantine S. Rafinesque. LC 75-23755. (Illus.). reprint ed. 60.00 (*0-404-13191-3*) AMS Pr.

Medical Fringe & Medical Orthodoxy, 1750-1850: A Volume in the Wellcome Institute. William F. Bynum & R. S. Porter. 1986. (History of Medicine Ser.). 288p. (*0-7099-3959-0*) C Helm GBR. *Dist:* Routldge.

Medical Futility: And the Evaluation of Life-Sustaining Interventions. Ed. by Marjorie B. Zucker & Howard D. Zucker. 1997. 219p. (C). text 74.95 (*0-521-56020-9*); pap. text 27.95 (*0-521-56877-3*) Cambridge U Pr.

Medical Gas & Vacuum Systems. Gary D. Slack. 1993. (Management & Compliance Ser.: Vol. 3). (Illus.). 108p. ring bd. 110.00 (*0-87258-480-1*, 055215) Am Hospital.

Medical Genetic & Behavioral Aspects of Purebred Cats. Ross D. Clark. 1992. 253p. 64.95 (*0-9634124-0-X*) Cortlandt Grp.

Medical Genetics. George Sack. 1998. LC 99-175561. (Illus.). 512p. pap. 45.00 incl. audio compact disk (*0-07-057998-9*) McGraw-Hill Prof.

Medical Genetics. George H. Sack. 1998. LC 99-175561. 45.00 (*0-07-134203-6*) McGraw.

Medical Genetics. Lynn B. Jorde et al. 2nd ed. 1998. LC 98-7537. (Illus.). 384p. (C). (gr. 13). pap. text 41.95 (*0-8151-4608-6*, 31253) Mosby Inc.

*__Medical Genetics.__ Lynn B. Jorde et al. 2nd rev. ed. 2001. (Illus.). 388p. reprint ed. pap. 43.95 (*0-323-01253-1*) Mosby Inc.

Medical Genetics. Lynn B. Jorde et al. 2nd ed. 1999. (Illus.). 384p. pap. (*84-8174-423-9*); pap. (*84-8174-161-2*) Mosby-Doyma Libros ESP. *Dist:* Mosby Inc.

*__Medical Genetics: An Illustrated Color Text.__ Michael Connor & Douglas Wilcox. 2001. (Illus.). 142p. pap. (*0-443-05809-1*) Church GBR. *Dist:* Saunders.

Medical Genetics: An Illustrated Outline. Andrew P. Read. 1989. (Illus.). 160p. (gr. 13). text (*0-397-44571-7*, GM0043) Gower-Mosby.

Medical Genetics: Principles & Practice. James J. Nora et al. 4th ed. 1994. LC 93-19984. (Illus.). 420p. 42.50 (*0-8121-1663-1*) Lppncott W & W.

Medical Genetics & Society. Ed. by N. Fujiki et al. 1991. LC 91-7099. (Illus.). 106p. pap. text (*90-6299-077-0*) Kugler NLD. *Dist:* Lib Res.

Medical Gentleman: James J. Waring, M. D. Patricia Paton. 1993. LC 93-23589. (*0-942576-02-0*); pap. (*0-942576-33-0*) CO Hist Soc.

Medical Geographic Research in Latin America. Ed. by C. Weil. 1982. 100p. pap. 18.00 (*0-08-028895-2*, Pergamon Pr) Elsevier.

Medical Geography. Melinda S. Meade & Robert J. Earickson. 2nd ed. 2000. LC 00-37658. (Illus.). 501p. 50.00 (*1-57230-558-4*, C0558) Guilford Pubns.

Medical Geography South & Southeast Asia. Ed. by Ashok K. Dutt. 1981. (Illus.). 78p. pap. 24.00 (*0-08-026762-9*, Pergamon Pr) Elsevier.

Medical Graduates of Foreign Nations: Index of New Information Including Social & Professional Discrimination, Selection, Performance & Problems. Darrell R. Rhodes. 1997. 135p. 57.50 (*0-7883-1636-2*); pap. 47.50 (*0-7883-1637-0*) ABBE Pubs Assn.

Medical Greek & Latin Workbook. James A. McCulloch. 2nd ed. 1984. 212p. spiral bd. 35.95 (*0-398-04905-X*) C C Thomas.

Medical Group Practice Legal & Administrative Guide. Aspen Health Law and Compliance Center Staff. 1998. LC 98-12742. ring bd. 219.00 (*0-8342-1100-9*) Aspen Pub.

Medical Group Practice Legal & Administrative Guide. Aspen Reference Group Staff. 1998. 189.00 (*0-8342-1068-1*, S470) Aspen Pub.

Medical Group Practices Face the Uncertain Future: Challenges, Opportunities & Strategies. John D. Blair et al. 1995. 63p. (Orig.). pap. text 27.00 (*1-56829-009-8*) M G M A.

Medical Group Practices in the U. S., 1999 Edition. American Medical Association Staff. 1999. 99.95 (*0-89970-958-3*) AMA.

Medical Group Treatment in Turbulent Times: How Physicial Leadership Can Optimize Health Plan, Hospital, & Medical Group Performance. Paul A. Sommers. 1998. LC 97-50421. (Illus.). 484p. lib. bdg. 79.95 (*0-7890-0487-9*) Haworth Pr.

Medical Guide to Hazardous Marine Life. Paul S. Auerbach. 3rd rev. ed. 1997. LC 96-79063. (Illus.). 72p. pap. 19.95 (*0-941332-55-1*, D267) Best Pub Co.

Medical Guidelines & Outcomes at Work. 1993. 52.00 (*1-56925-012-X*, MGOW) Capitol Publns.

Medical Guidelines for Determining Prognosis in Selected Non-Cancer Diseases. National Hospice Organization Standards and Accredit & National Hospice Organization Medical Guidelines T. 2nd ed. 1996. 58p. (Orig.). pap. 11.85 (*0-931207-50-9*, 713008) Natl Hospice.

Medical Halacha for Everyone see Comprehensive Guide to Medical Halachah

Medical Handbook for Medical. K. Majumdar. 1989. (C). (*0-89771-355-9*) Current Dist IND. *Dist:* St Mut.

Medical Handbook for Mountaineers. Peter Steele. 1988. (Illus.). 248p. reprint ed. pap. 29.50 (*0-09-468570-3*) Trans-Atl Phila.

Medical Handbook for Pilots. 1997. (Illus.). 74p. reprint ed. pap. text 25.00 (*0-7881-4618-1*) DIANE Pub.

Medical Handbook for Senior Citizens & Their Families. Howard A. Thornton. 1989. LC 87-30821. 383p. 75.00 (*0-86569-171-1*, Auburn Hse) Greenwood.

Medical Handbook for the Medical Representative. M. Majumder. 7th ed. 1989. (C). (*0-7855-4666-9*) Current Dist IND. *Dist:* St Mut.

Medical Harm: Historical, Conceptual & Ethical Dimensions of Iatrogenic Illness. Virginia A. Sharpe & Alan I. Faden. 1998. LC 97-11814. (Illus.). 292p. (C). pap. text 29.95 (*0-521-63490-3*) Cambridge U Pr.

Medical Health Care Career Prep Path. Zephyr Tate-Mann. 2000. 24p. pap. 10.00 (*0-8059-4895-3*) Dorrance.

Medical Health of the World: Index of New Information with Authors & Subjects. Science and Life Consultants Association Staff. rev. ed. 1994. LC 94-34919. 157p. 57.50 (*0-7883-0356-2*); pap. 47.50 (*0-7883-0357-0*) ABBE Pubs Assn.

Medical Hieroglyphs. Avice H. Kerr. 1970. LC 75-131216. 14.75 (*0-918558-01-8*) Enterprise Calif.

Medical Histories of Confederate Generals. Jack D. Welsh. 1994. LC 94-8673. 297p. 35.00 (*0-87338-505-5*) Kent St U Pr.

Medical Histories of Union Generals. Jack D. Welsh. 1997. LC 96-13353. 442p. (C). (gr. 9-12). 35.00 (*0-87338-552-7*) Kent St U Pr.

Medical History: Index of Modern Authors & Subjects with Guide for Rapid Research. Arthur Schlefman. rev. ed. 1994. LC 94-34373. 129p. 57.50 (*0-7883-0372-4*); pap. 47.50 (*0-7883-0373-2*) ABBE Pubs Assn.

Medical History & Physical Examination in Companion Animals. Ed. by Adam Rijnberk & H. W. De Vries. Tr. by B. E. Belshaw from DUT. 1995. LC 94-29947.Tr. of Anamnese en Lichamelijk Onderzoek bij Gezelschapsdieren. x, 376p. lib. bdg. 169.00 (*0-7923-3037-4*) Kluwer Academic.

Medical History of Current & Old Wars: Index of New Information. Gregg V. Goldin. 1995. LC 95-19211. 57.50 (*0-7883-0660-X*); 1995. LC 95-19211. pap. 47.50 (*0-7883-0661-8*); 1994. 150p. 57.50 (*0-7883-0034-2*); 1994. 150p. pap. 47.50 (*0-7883-0035-0*) ABBE Pubs Assn.

Medical Hypnosis: An Introduction & Clinical Guide. Roberta Temes. Ed. by Marc Staruss. 1998. LC 98-25700. (Medical Guides to Complementary & Alternative Medicine). (Illus.). 140p. (C). text (*0-443-06010-X*) Church.

Medical I Ching: Oracle of the Healer Within. Miki Shima. Ed. by Robert Flaws. 1992. LC 92-73393. (Illus.). 265p. (Orig.). pap. 21.95 (*0-936185-38-4*) Blue Poppy Pr.

Medical Illustration Source Book. (Illus.). 7th ed. 1994. 192p. 50.00 (*1-883486-01-7*); 8th ed. 1996. 232p. 50.00 (*1-883486-04-1*); 10th ed. 1997. 230p. 50.00 (*1-883486-05-X*); 11th ed. 1998. 184p. 50.00 (*1-883486-06-8*) Assn Med Illus.

*__Medical Illustration Source Book.__ 14th ed. 2001. (Illus.). 170p. 50.00 (*1-883486-09-2*) Assn Med Illus.

Medical Image Computing & Computer-Assisted Intervention - MICCAI 2000: Third International Conference, Pittsburgh, PA, U. S. A., October 11-14, 2000, Proceedings. Ed. by Scott L. Delp et al. 2000. LC 00-48256. (Lecture Notes in Computer Science: Vol. 1935). 1275p. pap. 99.00 (*3-540-41189-5*) Spr-Verlag.

Medical Image Computing & Computer-Assisted Intervention - MICCAI'98: First International Conference, Cambridge, MA, U. S. A., October 11-13, 1998, Proceedings. Ed. by Scott L. Delp et al. 1998. LC 98-45053. (Lecture Notes in Computer Science: Vol. 1496). 1280p. pap. 129.00 (*3-540-65136-5*) Spr-Verlag.

Medical Image Computing & Computer-Assisted Intervention - MICCAI'99: Second International Conference, Cambridge, U. K., September 19-22, 1999, Proceedings. Ed. by Chris Taylor et al. 1999. LC 99-49729. (Lecture Notes in Computer Science: Vol. 1679). 1261p. pap. 116.00 (*3-540-66503-X*) Spr-Verlag.

Medical Image Databases. Stephen T. Wong. 1998. LC 98-33987. (International Series in Engineering & Computer Science). 398p. 140.00 (*0-7923-8289-7*) Kluwer Academic.

Medical Image Management Markets: Telemedicine Is Here: PACS & Teleradiology Lead the Way. Market Intelligence Staff. 1992. 215p. (Orig.). 1895.00 (*1-56753-079-6*) Frost & Sullivan.

Medical Image Processing: The Mathematics of Medical Imaging. James A. Green. 1999. LC 94-77688. Vol. 2. (Illus.). 232p. 49.20 (*1-890121-18-5*, 03/02/01) Grnwd Resch.

Medical Image Registration. J. V. Hajnal et al. 2001. LC 2001-28031. (Biomedical Engineering Ser.). (Illus.). 382p. 79.95 (*0-8493-0064-9*) CRC Pr.

Medical Images: Formation, Handling, & Evaluation. Ed. by Andrew E. Todd-Pokropek & Max A. Viergever. 1993. LC 92-48909. (NATO ASI Ser.: No. 98). (Illus.). 700p. 250.00 (*0-387-56131-5*) Spr-Verlag.

Medical Imaging. Peter Scally. 2000. LC 98-55265. (Oxford Core Texts). (Illus.). 304p. pap. text 39.95 (*0-19-263056-3*) OUP.

Medical Imaging, No. 1. Ed. by H. J. Kaufmann. 1980. (Medical Imaging Ser.). (Illus.). vi, 142p. pap. 13.25 (*3-8055-3056-0*) S Karger.

Medical Imaging: A Concise Textbook. Ed. by Eugene R. Jacobs. 1987. LC 87-2644. (Illus.). 570p. 49.50 (*0-89640-126-X*) Igaku-Shoin.

Medical Imaging: Analysis of Multimodiality 2-3D Images. Ed. by L. Beolchi & M. H. Kuhn. 1995. LC 94-7342. (Studies in Health Technology & Informatics: Vol. 19). 216p. 103.00 (*90-5199-210-6*) IOS Press.

Medical Imaging: Selected Reprints. Ed. by Stephen J. Riederer. 1995. (Reprint Bks.). (Illus.). 144p. per. 26.00 (*0-917853-57-1*, RB-65) Am Assn Physics.

*__Medical Imaging: Techniques & Technology.__ Martin Fox. 2001. (Biomedical Engineering Ser.). 312p. text 89.95 (*0-8493-9691-3*, 9691) CRC Pr.

Medical Imaging - The Assessment of Image Quality. ICRU Staff. Ed. by W. Roger Ney. 1995. (ICRU Report Ser.: No. 54). 100p. (Orig.). pap. text 60.00 (*0-913394-53-X*) Intl Comm Rad Meas.

Medical Imaging, 1998: Image Display. Ed. by Yongmin Kim & Seong K. Mun. 1998. LC 98-227269. (Proceedings of SPIE Ser.: Vol. 3335). 710p. 124.00 (*0-8194-2780-2*) SPIE.

Medical Imaging, 1998: Image Processing. Ed. by Kenneth M. Hanson. 1998. LC 99-182755. (Proceedings of SPIE Ser.: Vol. 3338). 1614p. 166.00 (*0-8194-2783-7*) SPIE.

Medical Imaging 1998: PACS Design & Evaluation: Engineering & Clinical Issues. Ed. by Steven C. Horii & G. James Blaine. 1998. LC 98-226770. (Proceedings of SPIE Ser.: Vol. 3339). 616p. 116.00 (*0-8194-2784-5*) SPIE.

Medical Imaging, 1998: Physics of Medical Imaging. Ed. by James T. Dobbins & John M. Boone. 1998. LC 98-227297. (Proceedings of SPIE Ser.: Vol. 3336). 856p. 132.00 (*0-8194-2781-0*) SPIE.

Medical Imaging, 1998: Physiology & Function from Multidimensional Images. Ed. by Eric A. Hoffman. 1998. LC 98-227288. (Proceedings of SPIE Ser.: Vol. 3337). 396p. 80.00 (*0-8194-2782-9*) SPIE.

Medical Imaging, 1998 Vol. 3340: Image Perception. Ed. by Harold L. Kundel. 1998. 148p. 48.00 (*0-8194-2785-3*) SPIE.

Medical Imaging, 1998 Vol. 3341: Ultrasonic Transducer Engineering. Ed. by K. Kirk Shung. 1998. 292p. 69.00 (*0-8194-2786-1*) SPIE.

Medical Imaging, 1997 Vol. 3031: Image Display. Ed. by Yongmin Kim. 1997. LC 97-200314. 876p. 132.00 (*0-8194-2442-0*) SPIE.

Medical Imaging, 1997 Vol. 3032: Physics of Medical Imaging. Ed. by Richard L. Van Metter & Jacob Beutel. 1997. LC 97-193057. 556p. 107.00 (*0-8194-2443-9*) SPIE.

Medical Imaging, 1997 Vol. 3033: Physiology & Function from Multidimensional Images. Ed. by Eric A. Hoffman. 1997. LC 97-193071. 472p. 80.00 (*0-8194-2444-7*) SPIE.

Medical Imaging, 1997 Vol. 3034: Image Processing. Ed. by Kenneth M. Hanson. 1997. LC 97-200957. 1182p. 158.00 (*0-8194-2445-5*) SPIE.

Medical Imaging, 1997 Vol. 3035: PACS Design & Evaluation: Engineering & Clinical Issues. Ed. by Steven C. Horii & G. James Blaine. 1997. LC 97-200313. 652p. 124.00 (*0-8194-2446-3*) SPIE.

Medical Imaging 1996: 11-13 February, 1996, Newport Beach, California. Eric A. Hoffman et al. 1996. LC 95-72069. xi, 526p. 85.00 (*0-8194-2084-0*) SPIE.

Medical Imaging of Focal Liver Lesions: Clinico-Radiologic Approach. Kohkan Shamsi & A. M. DeSchepper. 1994. LC 94-22473. 144p. 178.50 (*0-444-81919-3*) Elsevier.

Medical Imaging of the Spleen. Ed. by A. M. De Schepper & F. Vanhoenacker. 2000. LC 99-40699. (Medical Radiology Ser.). (Illus.). 192p. 119.00 (*3-540-65535-2*) Spr-Verlag.

Medical Imaging VI: Image Capture, Formatting, & Display. 1992. 76.00 (*0-8194-0805-0*, 1653) SPIE.

Medical Imaging VI: Image Processing. 1992. 110.00 (*0-8194-0804-2*, 1652) SPIE.

Medical Imaging VI: Instrumentation. 1992. 56.00 (*0-8194-0803-4*, 1651) SPIE.

Medical Imaging VI: PACS Design & Evaluation. 1992. 20.00 (*0-8194-0806-9*, 1654) SPIE.

Medical Imaging Systems Techniques & Applications: Brain & Skeletal Systems. Ed. by Cornelius T. Leondes. 1997. (International Series in Engineering, Technolog, & Applied Science: Vol. 2). 258p. text (*90-5699-541-3*) GBSP NLD. *Dist:* Gordon & Breach.

Medical Imaging Systems Techniques & Applications: Cardiovascular Systems. Ed. by Cornelius T. Leondes. 1997. (Gordon & Breach International Ser.). 226p. text (*90-5699-509-X*) GBSP NLD. *Dist:* Gordon & Breach.

Medical Imaging Systems Techniques & Applications: Computational Techniques. Ed. by Cornelius T. Leondes. 1998. (International Series in Engineering, Technolog, & Applied Science: Vol. 6). 264p. text (*90-5699-620-7*) GBSP NLD. *Dist:* Gordon & Breach.

Medical Imaging Systems Techniques & Applications: Diagnosis Optimization Techniques. Ed. by Cornelius T. Leondes. 1997. (International Series in Engineering, Technolog, & Applied Science: Vol. 3). 336p. text (*90-5699-595-2*) GBSP NLD. *Dist:* Gordon & Breach.

Medical Imaging Systems Techniques & Applications: General Anatomy, Vol. 4. Ed. by Cornelius T. Leondes. 1997. (International Series in Engineering, Technolog, & Applied Science). 334p. text (*90-5699-597-9*) GBSP NLD. *Dist:* Gordon & Breach.

Medical Imaging Systems Techniques & Applications: Modalities. Ed. by Cornelius T. Leondes. 1997. (Gordon & Breach International Ser.). 340p. text (*90-5699-610-X*) GBSP NLD. *Dist:* Gordon & Breach.

***Medical Imaging 2000: 13-15 February 2000, San Diego, California.** Ed. by Chin-Tu Chen & Anne V. Clough. 2000. LC 00-711276. (Progress in Biomedical Optics & Imaging Ser.: No. 1). (Illus.). ix, 550p. (*0-8194-3595-3*) SPIE.

Medical Imitations of Illness with Pretense & Shams Including Munchausen's Syndrome. Shirley L. Sinclair. rev. ed. 1997. 171p. 57.50 (*0-7883-1554-4*); pap. 47.50 (*0-7883-1555-2*) ABBE Pubs Assn.

***Medical Immunology.** Ed. by Gabriel Virella. 2001. 656p. 85.00 (*0-8247-0550-5*) Dekker.

Medical Immunology. Ed. by D. P. Stites. 10th ed. 2001. 814p. pap. 64.95 (*0-8385-6300-7*) McGraw-Hill Prof.

Medical Immunology for Students. Playfair. 1995. pap. text 26.95 (*0-443-05000-7*) Saunders.

***Medical Immunology for Students.** J. H. L. Playfair & P. M. Lydyard. 2001. (Illus.). 125p. pap. (*0-443-06420-2*) Church GBR. *Dist:* Saunders.

Medical Importance of the Normal Microflora. Contrib. by G. W. Tannock. 1999. LC 99-27093. (Illus.). 492p. (*0-412-79390-3*) Kluwer Academic.

Medical Index of Severity of Illness & Sick Roles: Judgemental Signs, Symptoms, Rules & Controversy. Science and Life Consultants Staff. 1997. 151p. 57.50 (*0-7883-1656-7*); pap. 47.50 (*0-7883-1657-5*) ABBE Pubs Assn.

Medical Infobahn for Europe: Proceedings of MIE2000 & GMD2000. Ed. by Arie Hasman. 2000. LC 00-106864. (Studies in Health Technology & Informatics: 77). (Illus.). xx, 1274p. 126.00 (*1-58603-063-9*) IOS Press.

Medical Informatics. Goble. 1996. (ITCP Computer Science Ser.). pap. 39.95 (*1-85032-238-4*) ITCP.

Medical Informatics: Computer Applications in Health Care. Edward H. Shortliffe. Ed. by K. J. Hannah et al. 2nd ed. 2000. LC 99-89476. (Health Informatics Ser.). (Illus.). 768p. 69.95 (*0-387-98472-0*) Spr-Verlag.

Medical Informatics: The Essentials. F. T. De Dombal. 1996. LC 96-205533. 144p. pap. text 37.50 (*0-7506-2162-1*, Focal) Buttrwrth-Heinemann.

Medical Informatics Europe, 1984: Proceedings. Ed. by F. H. Roger et al. 1984. (Lecture Notes in Medical Informatics: Vol. 24). 778p. 81.95 (*0-387-13374-7*) Spr-Verlag.

Medical Informatics Europe, 1988: Proceedings Oslo, Norway, August 17-20, 1988. Ed. by Bjarte G. Solheim et al. 1988. (Lecture Notes in Medical Informatics: Vol. 35). 764p. 135.00 (*0-387-50138-X*) Spr-Verlag.

Medical Informatics Europe, 1990 Vol. 40: Proceedings Glasgow, Scotland, August 20-23, 1990. R. R. O'Moore et al. Ed. by O. Rienhoff & D. A. Lindberg. 1990. (Lecture Notes). 820p. 146.00 (*0-387-52936-5*) Spr-Verlag.

Medical Informatics Europe '99. Ed. by Peter Kokol et al. 1999. LC 99-65239. (Studies in Health Technology & Informatics: Vol. 68). (Illus.). xvii, 1009p. 142.00 (*0-9673355-1-5*) IOS Press.

Medical Informatics '96. Ed. by J. Brender et al. 1996. LC 96-77454. (Studies in Health Technology & Informatics: Vol. 34). 1100p. 143.00 (*90-5199-278-5*, 278-5) IOS Press.

Medical Information: A Profile. Barry S. Hodge & Barbara C. Allan. 1986. LC 85-19726. (Professional Librarian Ser.). 145p. 40.00 (*0-86729-163-X*, Hall Reference) Macmillan.

Medical Information on the Internet. Robert Kiley. 1996. pap. (*0-443-05699-4*, K1162) Church.

Medical Information on the Internet: A Guide for Health Professionals. Robert Kiley. 2nd ed. 1999. LC 98-48320. xiv, 160p. (*0-443-06194-7*) Church.

Medical Injuries in the Martial Arts. Richard B. Birrer & Christina D. Birrer. 1981. LC 80-24773. (Illus.). 240p. pap. 31.95 (*0-398-04134-2*) C C Thomas.

Medical Inquiries & Observations Benjamin Rush. 4th ed. 1972. LC 76-180588. (Medicine & Society in America Ser.). 1070p. reprint ed. Set. 65.95 (*0-405-03968-9*); Vol. 1. 33.95 (*0-405-03969-7*); Vol. 2. 33.95 (*0-405-03970-0*) Ayer.

Medical Insects & Arachnids. Ed. by Richard P. Lane & Roger W. Crosske. 1993. LC 92-49000. (*0-04-124000-6*) Chapman & Hall.

Medical Inspector. Jack Rudman. 1994. (Career Examination Ser.: C-487). pap. 44.95 (*0-8373-0487-3*) Nat Learn.

Medical Instrument Nurses - Allied Health. Richard Aston & Katherine K. Brown. 2nd ed. 1994. (Nursing-Health Science Ser.). (Illus.). 336p. (C). pap. text 44.95 (*0-86720-688-8*, 688-8) Jones & Bartlett.

***Medical Instrumentation: A Guide for Patient Care Technology.** L. Street. 2002. LC 2001-55374. (Illus.). 200p. lib. bdg. 49.95 (*1-84214-127-9*, Parthenon Pbng) CRC Pr.

Medical Instrumentation: Application & Design. Ed. by John G. Webster. 3rd ed. 1997. LC 97-4385. 720p. text 98.95 (*0-471-15368-0*) Wiley.

Medical Insurance Made Easy. Jill L. Brown. 2001. LC 00-49271. (Illus.). ix, 415p. pap. text 52.00 (*0-7216-9187-0*) Harcrt Hlth Sci Grp.

Medical Insurance Manual for Dentists: Maximizing Reimbursements. Rose Nierman. 1995. LC 95-25462. (Pennwell Bks.). 89.95 (*0-87814-459-5*) PennWell Corp.

Medical Insurance Paperwork: Conquering the Chaos. Connie Clark. 1992. (Illus.). 192p. (Orig.). pap. 18.95 (*0-9643510-0-5*) Med Ins Servs.

***Medical Internet Directory.** Michale D. Gainey & Milton C. Heuston. 4th ed. 2001. 39.95 (*0-9675465-1-6*) Heuston Consult.

Medical Internet Toolkit, 1998. Ed. by Jennifer Wayne-Doppke. 1998. (Illus.). 210p. pap. 97.00 (*0-9645360-6-4*) Cor Hlthcare.

Medical Interview. Mack Lipkin, Jr. et al. LC 94-6511. 1996. 643p. 115.00 (*0-387-94257-2*); 1994. 138.00 (*3-540-94257-2*) Spr-Verlag.

Medical Interview: A Functional & Operational Approach. Steven A. Cohen & Cole. 1990. (Illus.). 224p. (C). (gr. 13). pap. text 32.95 (*0-8016-0345-5*, 00345) Mosby Inc.

Medical Interview: Gateway to the Doctor-Patient Relationship. C. Knight Aldrich. 1993. LC 93-18395. (Illus.). 126p. lib. bdg. 19.95 (*1-85070-487-2*, Parthenon Pbng) CRC Pr.

Medical Interview: Mastering Skills for Clinical Practice. John L. Coulehan & Marian R. Block. 3rd ed. 1997. LC 97-6737. (Illus.). 287p. (C). pap. text 29.95 (*0-8036-0267-7*) Davis Co.

Medical Interview: The Three-Function Approach. Steven A. Cole. 2nd ed. 2000. LC 2001-280605. (Illus.). 220p. (C). pap. text 32.00 (*0-8151-1992-5*, 30377) Mosby Inc.

Medical Intuition: How to Combine Inner Resources with Modern Medicine. Ruth Berger. 1995. LC 95-19107. (Illus.). 160p. (Orig.). pap. 9.95 (*0-87728-851-8*) Red Wheel ME.

Medical Issues & Health Care Reform in Russia. Vicki L. Hesli & Margaret H. Mills. 1999. LC 99-41404. (Studies in Health & Human Services: Vol. 35). (Illus.). xii, 322p. text 99.95 (*0-7734-7933-3*) E Mellen.

Medical Issues & the Eating Disorders: The Interface. Ed. by Allan S. Kaplan & Paul E. Garfinkel. 1993. LC 92-48961. (Eating Disorders Monographs: No. 7). (Illus.). 224p. text 35.95 (*0-87630-681-4*) Brunner-Routledge.

Medical Itch. Claude Benjamin. 1964. (Illus.). 14.95 (*0-8392-1067-1*) Astor-Honor.

Medical Job Interview. Colin Mumford. 2000. (Illus.). 56p. pap. 23.95 (*0-632-05527-8*) Blackwell Sci.

Medical Jurisprudence. J. Jhala & R. Raju. 1990. (C). text 135.00 (*0-89771-481-4*) St Mut.

Medical Justice: A Guide to Fair Provision. Sara E. Austin. 2001. LC 00-22977. (International Healthcare Ethics Ser.: Vol. 5). 144p. 46.95 (*0-8204-4935-0*) P Lang Pubng.

Medical Keyboarding, Typing & Transcribing: Techniques & Procedures. Marcy O. Diehl & Marilyn Takahashi Fordney. Ed. by Margaret Biblis. 4th ed. 1997. LC 96-41729. (Illus.). 544p. pap. text 43.00 (*0-7216-6858-5*) Saunders.

Medical Keyboarding, Typing & Transcribing: Techniques & Procedures. Mary O. Diehl & Marilyn Takahashi Fordney. 4th ed. 1997. (Illus.). pap., tchr. ed. (*0-7216-6859-3*) Saunders.

Medical Knowledge: Doubt & Certainty. Ed. by Clive Seale & Stephen Pattison. 1994. LC 93-23599. pap. (*0-335-19251-3*) OpUniv Pr.

***Medical Knowledge: Doubt & Certainty.** Ed. by Clive Swale et al. 2nd ed. 2001. (Health & Disease Ser.). 208p. pap. (*0-335-20834-7*) OpUniv Pr GBR. *Dist:* Taylor & Francis.

Medical Knowledge for Fun. Richard Worcester. 1995. LC 95-34795. 108p. lib. bdg. 19.95 (*1-85070-685-9*, Parthenon Pbng) CRC Pr.

Medical Laboratory Diagnostics. Ursala Spranger & Jurgen Grove. 1993. (ENG, FRE & GER.). 500p. (*3-86177-053-9*) A Hatier DEU. *Dist:* Paul & Co Pubs.

Medical Laboratory Management: Forms, Checklists & Guidelines. Ed. by Sara N. Di Lima & Suzanne Niemeyer. 1995. LC 94-34047. ring bd. 249.00 (*0-8342-0667-6*) Aspen Pub.

Medical Laboratory Management & Supervision: Operations, Review, & Study Guide. Lionel A. Varnadoe. 1996. LC 95-42716. (Illus.). 321p. (C). 33.95 (*0-8036-8861-X*) Davis Co.

Medical Laboratory Management Report 2000 Yearbook. Sherrye Henry. Ed. by Jan Christian Bernabe. 1999. (Illus.). 200p. pap. 199.00 (*1-58673-014-2*) IOMA.

Medical Laboratory Procedures. Mary E. Wedding. 2nd ed. 1997. LC 97-984. (Illus.). 427p. pap. 41.95 (*0-8036-0052-6*) Davis Co.

Medical Laboratory Technician. Jack Rudman. 1994. (Career Examination Ser.: C-2323). pap. 27.95 (*0-8373-2323-1*) Nat Learn.

Medical Landmarks, U. S. A. A Travel Guide to Historical Sites, Architectural Gems, Remarkable. Martin Lipp. 70th ed. 1990. LC 90-5507. 384p. pap. text 45.00 (*0-07-037974-2*) McGraw-Hill Med Pub.

Medical Language. Devi Ellen Chabner. 2000. LC 00-55720. 175p. pap. text 12.95 (*0-7216-8582-X*) Saunders.

Medical Language. Collins. Date not set. tchr. ed. (*0-314-06959-3*) West Pub.

Medical Language. Layman. 1994. audio 107.25 net. (*0-8273-6923-9*) Delmar.

Medical Language. Dale P. Layman. 1995. (Medical Terminology Ser.). 62.95 (*0-8273-6924-7*) Delmar.

Medical Language: A Programmed Body-System Approach. Peggy M. Krueger. 1995. 221p. tchr. ed. 20.00 (*0-8273-5639-0*) Delmar.

Medical Language: A Programmed Body-System Approach. Dale P. Layman. 544p. 1995. text 42.95 incl. audio (*0-8273-6925-5*); 1994. (C). text 46.00 incl. audio (*0-8273-6922-0*) Delmar.

Medical Language Processing: Computer Management of Narrative Data. Naomi Sager et al. 1987. 320p. (C). text 51.75 (*0-201-16810-3*) Addison-Wesley.

Medical Language Specialist. Lindsey. (Medical Assisting Ser.). 1997. pap. 21.95 (*0-8273-6052-5*); 1995. pap., tchr. ed. 12.00 (*0-8273-6053-3*) Delmar.

Medical Larousse. R. Valenti & M. G. Malesani. 1987. (ITA.). 1040p. 295.00 (*0-8288-7346-1*) Fr & Eur.

Medical Laser Endoscopy. Ed. by Dennis M. Jensen & Jean M. Brunetaud. 1990. (Developments in Gastroenterology Ser.). (C). text 299.50 (*0-7923-0579-5*) Kluwer Academic.

Medical Lasers: Science & Clinical Practice. J. A. Carruth & A. McKenzie. 1986. (Illus.). 280p. 116.00 (*0-85274-560-5*) Inst of Physics Pubng.

Medical Lasers & Their Safe Use. David H. Sliney & Stephen L. Trokel. LC 92-2299. (Illus.). 1994. 230p. 86.95 (*0-387-97856-9*); 1992. 264p. (*3-540-97856-9*) Spr-Verlag.

Medical Law. Michael Davies. 1996. 374p. pap. (*1-85431-504-8*) Blackstone Pr GBR. *Dist:* Gaunt.

Medical Law & Ethics. Bonnie F. Frengen. 2001. LC 2001-36202. (Illus.). 304p. (C). 30.67 (*0-8359-5138-3*) P-H.

Medical Law & Ethics. Michel Lipman. 1993. LC 93-1344. 139p. (C). pap. 19.60 (*0-13-064585-0*) P-H.

Medical Law, Ethics & Bioethics for Ambulatory Health Care. Marcia A. Lewis & Carol A. Tamparo. 4th ed. 1998. LC 97-50565. (Illus.). 295p. (C). pap. text 22.95 (*0-8036-0348-7*) Davis Co.

Medical Law for the Attending Physician: A Case-Oriented Analysis. Salvatore F. Fiscina. 1982. LC 82-5559. (Medical Humanities Ser.). 495p. 44.95 (*0-8093-1045-7*) S Ill U Pr.

Medical Law Reports. Ed. by Geoffrey M. Hall. (C). Vol. 1. 1992. (*0-9514449-2-1*); Vol. 2. 1990. (*0-9514449-7-2*); Vol. 3. 1990. (*0-9514449-3-X*) Busn & Med GBR. *Dist:* St Mut.

Medical Law Text, Cases & Materials. John Devereux. 1997. LC 98-111617. xxv, 440p. pap. (*1-876213-11-6*) Cavendish Pubng GBR. *Dist:* Gaunt.

Medical Legacy of Moses Maimonides. Fred Rosner. 1997. LC 97-16874. xii, 308p. 29.50 (*0-88125-573-4*) Ktav.

Medical Legal Advisor. Salvatore F. Fiscina & Janet B. Seifert. 1996. LC 96-10386. 320p. (C). (gr. 13). pap. text 37.95 (*0-8151-3302-2*, 26930) Mosby Inc.

Medical-Legal Correspondence Course. RiskCare Staff. 1980. 111p. reprint ed. pap. text 199.00 (*1-893929-02-7*) RiskCare.

Medical-Legal Evaluation of Hearing Loss. Robert A. Dobie. 2nd ed. 2001. LC 2001-16081. pap. 61.50 net. (*0-7693-0052-9*) Singular Publishing.

Medical-Legal Evaluation of Hearing Loss. Robert A. Dobie. 1998. (Illus.). 398p. reprint ed. pap. 69.95 (*0-7693-0023-5*, 2024) Thomson Learn.

Medical-Legal Evaluation of Hearing Loss. Robert A. Dobie. 1993. LC 93-5118. 400p. text 81.95 (*0-442-01266-7*, VNR) Wiley.

Medical Legal Issues in Long-Term Care: Regulations & Risk Management Safeguards Pennsylvania Physicians Need to Know. RiskCare Staff. 1999. 75p. pap. text 79.00 (*1-893929-03-5*) RiskCare.

Medical Letter Handbook of Adverse Drug Interactions, 1998. Martin A. Rizack. rev. ed. 1998. 377p. 18.00 (*0-9660510-1-7*) Med Letter.

Medical Letter Handbook of Adverse Drug Interactions (IC-162) 1995. 99.95 (*1-56712-263-9*, F0682) Franklin Elect.

Medical Letter Handbook of Adverse Interactions, 2000. rev. ed. 2000. 455p. 23.00 (*0-9660510-5-X*) Med Letter.

Medical Letter Handbook of Antimicrobial Therapy: 2000 Edition. Ed. by Mark Abramowicz. 2000. 214p. 12.00 (*0-9660510-6-8*) Med Letter.

Medical Lexicon: A Dictionary of Medical Science: Containing a Concise Explanation of the Various Subjects & Terms of Anatomy, Physiology, Pathology, Hygiene. Robley Dunglison. 2000. 1131p. cd-rom 19.95 (*1-58211-300-9*) Quintin Pub RI.

Medical Lexicon: Lexikon der Medizin. Dagobert Tutsch. 2nd ed. 1982. (GER.). 714p. 49.95 (*0-8288-1841-X*, M7250) Fr & Eur.

Medical Liability: Cases & Materials. Salvatore F. Fiscina et al. 1990. LC 90-37048. (American Casebook Ser.). 487p. (C). 55.00 (*0-314-75264-1*) West Pub.

Medical Liability: Teacher's Manual to Accompany. Salvatore F. Fiscina et al. 1990. (American Casebook Ser.). 146p. pap. text (*0-314-81774-3*) West Pub.

Medical Liability for Pediatricians. American Academy of Pediatrics Staff. 5th ed. 1995. 176p. pap. 49.95 (*0-910761-72-8*) Am Acad Pediat.

Medical Libraries - Roles, Services & Challenges: Index of Modern Authors & Subjects with Guide for Rapid Research. American Health Research Institute Staff. 1991. LC 90-56303. 160p. 47.50 (*1-55914-402-5*); pap. 44.50 (*1-55914-403-3*) ABBE Pubs Assn.

Medical Library Association Guide to Managing Health Care Libraries. Ed. by Ruth Holst & Sharon A. Phillips. 2000. LC 00-55399. (Illus.). xi, 371p. pap. 75.00 (*1-55570-397-6*) Neal-Schuman.

***Medical Library Association Guide to Providing Consumer Health Information.** Donald A. Barclay & Deborah Halsted. 2001. (Illus.). 200p. pap. 55.00 (*1-55570-418-2*) Neal-Schuman.

Medical Library Budget & Expenditure Report. Primary Research Staff. 1994. 110p. 82.50 (*0-9626749-6-6*) Primary Research.

Medical Licensure & Discipline in the United States. Robert C. Derbyshire. 1978. LC 78-17712. 183p. reprint ed. lib. bdg. 62.50 (*0-313-20528-0*, DEML, Greenwood Pr) Greenwood.

Medical Litigation Alert. Ed. by James B. Rosenblum & Ira Zarin. 1990. ring bd. 250.00 (*0-9626905-0-3*) Med Litigation.

Medical Lives & Scientific Medicine at Michigan, 1891-1969. Ed. by Joel D. Howell. 1993. LC 93-37106. 208p. (C). text 55.00 (*0-472-10465-9*, 10465) U of Mich Pr.

Medical Log Book. Ed. by Wysteria Staff. 2000. (Pocket Brain Ser.: No. 3). 175p. ring bd. 19.95 (*0-9651162-8-X*) Wysteria Ltd.

Medical Mafia. Lanctot. 1995. pap. (*0-9644126-0-8*) Heres The Key.

Medical Malpractice David W. Louisell & William Henry Louisell. 1960. ring bd. 963.00 (*0-8205-1370-9*) Bender.

Medical Malpractice. Ed. by Duncan Yaggy & Patricia Hodgson. 1987. LC 86-32981. x, 128p. (C). text 39.95 (*0-8223-0722-7*) Duke.

Medical Malpractice. David M. Harney. 3rd ed. 1993. 849p. 95.00 (*1-55834-108-0*, MICHIE) LEXIS Pub.

Medical Malpractice: A Comprehensive Analysis. Vasanthakumar N. Bhat. 2001. LC 00-52554. (Illus.). 288p. 64.00 (*0-86569-279-3*, Auburn Hse) Greenwood.

Medical Malpractice: A Preventive Approach. William O. Robertson. 1985. LC 84-40322. 212p. text 20.00 (*0-295-96162-7*) U of Wash Pr.

Medical Malpractice: A Primer for Orthopaedic Residents & Fellows. AAOS Committee on Professional Liability Staff. 1994. 73p. 40.00 (*0-89203-093-3*) Amer Acad Ortho Surg.

Medical Malpractice: Bases of Liability. Michael D. McCafferty & Steven M. Meyer. 1985. LC 84-23580. 494p. text 125.00 (*0-07-044837-X*) Shepards.

Medical Malpractice: Guide to Medical Issues Lee S. Goldsmith. 1986. ring bd. 1188.00 (*0-8205-1432-2*) Bender.

Medical Malpractice: Handling Obstetric & Neonatal Cases. Michael D. Volk & Melvin D. Morgan. 1986. LC 86-10230. (Medical Malpractice Ser.). 1212p. text 125.00 (*0-07-043122-1*) Shepards.

Medical Malpractice: Law, Tactics, & Ethics. Frank M. McClellan. 1993. 296p. (C). text 69.95 (*1-56639-065-6*) Temple U Pr.

Medical Malpractice: Maine's Use of Practice Guidelines to Reduce Costs. 1994. (Illus.). 100p. (Orig.). (C). pap. text 40.00 (*0-7881-0395-4*) DIANE Pub.

Medical Malpractice: Pharmacy Law. David B. Brushwood. 1986. text 125.00 (*0-07-008576-5*) Shepards.

Medical Malpractice: Psychiatric Care-1998. 1998. pap. text, suppl. ed. 75.00 (*0-7355-0189-0*) Aspen Pub.

Medical Malpractice: Theory, Evidence, & Public Policy. Patricia M. Danzon. 1985. (Illus.). 312p. 45.95 (*0-674-56115-5*) HUP.

Medical Malpractice & the American Jury. Neil Vidmar. 1997. 336p. (C). reprint ed. pap. text 22.95 (*0-472-08479-8*, 08479) U of Mich Pr.

Medical Malpractice Claims Investigation: A Step-by-Step Approach. Nancy Acerbo-Avalone & Katherine Kremer. 1995. LC 96-28261. 288p. 82.00 (*0-8342-0860-1*, 20860) Aspen Pub.

Medical Malpractice Handbook: The Plaintiff. Bruce Livingston & Stephen Morewitz. 1996. LC 93-42754. 113p. pap. 46.95 (*1-880921-65-0*) Austin & Winfield.

Medical Malpractice in New York. New York State Bar Association Staff. Ed. & Pref. by Robert Devine. 1993. LC 92-63000. 570p. 115.00 (*0-942954-54-8*) NYS Bar.

Medical Malpractice in Nineteenth Century America. Kenneth De Ville. (American Social Experience Ser.: No. 19). (C). 1992. pap. text 19.50 (*0-8147-1848-5*); 1990. text 50.00 (*0-8147-1832-9*) NYU Pr.

Medical Malpractice Lawsuit: A Case Study. George Parker. 2000. 198p. lib. bdg. 45.00 (*1-56072-470-6*); (Illus.). pap. 17.95 (*1-56072-340-8*, Nova Kroshka Bks) Nova Sci Pubs.

Medical Malpractice on Trial. Paul C. Weiler. 1991. LC 90-15600. 256p. 39.50 (*0-674-56120-1*, WEIMED) HUP.

Medical Management of AIDS. Merle A. Sande. 6th ed. 1999. LC 98-43930. (Illus.). xx, 636p. (C). text 60.00 (*0-7216-8102-6*) Saunders.

Medical Management of AIDS in Women. Ed. by Deborah Cotton & D. H. Watts. 1996. LC 95-48022. 488p. 132.00 (*0-471-07674-0*) Wiley.

Medical Management of Atherosclerosis. Ed. by John C. Larosa. 1998. LC 97-50182. (Illus.). 352p. text 145.00 (*0-8247-0149-6*) Dekker.

Medical Management of Cerebral Ischemia Vol. 17, Suppl. 1, 1978: Journal: European Neurology. Ed. by H. E. Kaeser. 1979. (Illus.). pap. 50.50 (*3-8055-3077-3*) S Karger.

Medical Management of Chronic Myelogenous Lukemia. Ed. by Hagop Kantarjian & Moshe Talpaz. 1998. LC 98-38123. (Illus.). 464p. text 185.00 (*0-8247-9901-1*) Dekker.

Medical Management of Heart Disease. Burton E. Sobel. 1996. LC 96-4747. (Illus.). 584p. text 115.00 (*0-8247-9315-3*) Dekker.

Medical Management of Hematological Malignant Diseases. Ed. by Hagop M. Kantarjian & Emily J. Freireich. 1998. LC 98-16879. (Illus.). 592p. text 195.00 (*0-8247-9886-4*) Dekker.

Medical Management of HIV & AIDS. Ed. by Ann Millar. 1995. LC 95-40049. (Illus.). 260p. 141.00 (*3-540-19958-6*) Spr-Verlag.

Medical Management of HIV Infection: 1995 Edition. John Bartlett. 1995. 260p. 17.95 (*0-924428-09-0*) Phys Sci Pub.

Medical Management of Liver Disease. Edward L. Krawitt. 1999. LC 99-32710. (Clinical Guides to Medical Management Ser.). (Illus.). 664p. text 185.00 (*0-8247-1968-9*) Dekker.

Medical Management of Long-Term Disability. Ed. by David Green. 2nd ed. 1996. LC 96-26646. (Rehabilitation Institute of Chicago Publication Ser.). (Illus.). 351p. text 74.99 (*0-7506-9604-4*) Buttrwrth-Heinemann.

Medical Management of Pregnancy Complicated by Diabetes. American Diabetes Association. 2nd ed. 1995. 136p. pap. 39.95 (*0-945448-44-9*, 5401-01) Am Diabetes.

Medical Management of Prostate Cancer, No. II. Ed. by I. Denis. 1991. (ESO Monographs). (Illus.). 100p. 64.95 (*0-387-53443-1*) Spr-Verlag.

Medical Management of Pulmonary Diseases. Gerald S. Davis & Elizabeth A. Seward. 1999. LC 99-37340. (Clinical Guides to Medical Management Ser.). (Illus.). xxvii, 795p. text 250.00 (*0-8247-6002-6*) Dekker.

Medical Management of Radiation Accidents. Ed. by Fred A. Mettler, Jr. et al. 1989. 416p. 208.95 (*0-8493-4865-X*, RA1231) CRC Pr.

Medical Management of Radiation Accidents. Igor Gusev et al. 2nd ed. 2001. LC 00-52909. (Illus.). 640p. 139.95 (*0-8493-7004-3*) CRC Pr.

Medical Management of Rheumatic Musculoskeletal & Connective Tissue Diseases. Grahame et al. 1997. LC 97-22374. (Illus.). 408p. text 150.00 (*0-8247-9847-3*) Dekker.

Medical Management of Stroke: A Guide for Rehabilitation Specialists. Scott Silliman. 1997. 325p. 49.00 (*0-8342-0890-3*, 20890) Aspen Pub.

Medical Management of the Surgical Patient. Geno J. Merli & Howard H. Weitz. Ed. by Ray Kersey. 2nd ed. 1998. LC 97-39759. (Illus.). 496p. (C). pap. text 39.95 (*0-7216-6976-X*) Saunders.

Medical Management of the Violent Patient. K. Tardiff. 1999. LC 99-26167. (Medical Psychiatry Ser.). (Illus.). 512p. text 195.00 (*0-8247-9906-2*) Dekker.

Medical Management of Type 1 Diabetes. Ed. by Jay S. Skyler. 3rd ed. 1998. LC 98-4108. (Clinical Education Ser.). (Illus.). 246p. pap. 39.95 (*0-945448-92-9*, 5403-01) Am Diabetes.

Medical Management of Type 2 Diabetes. Ed. by Bruce R. Zimmerman. 4th ed. 1998. LC 98-4107. (Clinical Education Ser.). (Illus.). 139p. pap. 39.95 (*0-945448-93-7*, 5404-01) Am Diabetes.

Medical Manager. Humphrey. 1995. (Medical Assisting Ser.). pap., stu. ed. 16.95 (*0-538-71308-9*); stu. ed. 24.00 (*0-538-71312-7*) S-W Thomson.

Medical Manager. Personalized Programming Staff. 1992. (Medical Terminology Ser.). pap., stu. ed. 16.95 (*0-538-70539-6*) S-W Thomson.

Medical Manager. Ed. by Anthony Young. 1999. (Illus.). 289p. pap. text (*0-7279-1376-X*) BMJ Pub GBR. *Dist:* AIDC.

Medical Manager: Managed Care System - Student Edition - IML. Gartee. 1998. 120p. tchr. ed. 14.95 (*0-8273-8407-6*) Delmar.

Medical Manager: Managed Care System, Version 8.10. Richard Gartee. 1998. LC 98-149905. 336p. (C). pap. text, stu. ed. 55.95 (*0-8273-8406-8*) Delmar.

Medical Manager (R), Student Edition: Version 9.20 for Windows (TM) Richard Gartee. 9th ed. 2000. LC 00-712785. (Illus.). 350p. stu. ed., spiral bd. 67.95 (*0-7668-2841-7*) Delmar.

Medical Manager, Student Edition, Computerized Practice Management Version 5.3. Richard Gartee & Doris Humphrey. 2nd ed. 1995. 288p. pap., stu. ed. incl. disk (*0-538-71311-9*); pap., stu. ed. (*0-8273-8073-9*) S-W Thomson.

Medical Manager, Version 8.10. Gartee. 3rd ed. 1997. 320p. (C). mass mkt., stu. ed. 61.95 (*0-8273-8592-7*) Delmar.

Medical Managment of Emesis. 1997. 85.00 (*1-85317-267-7*) Mosby Inc.

Medical Mandarins: The French Academy of Medicine in the Nineteenth & Early Twentieth Centuries. George Weisz. 1995. (Illus.). 328p. text 57.50 (*0-19-509037-3*) OUP.

Medical Manpower in the European Community. Ed. by H. Viefhues. 1988. (Illus.). 238p. 79.95 (*0-387-18733-2*) Spr-Verlag.

Medical Manual for Chinese Family. Ming Tat Wong. (CHI.). 200p. pap. 18.00 (*0-9635700-0-5*) J Wong.

Medical Marijuana Referenda Movement in America: Congressional Hearing. Ed. by Bill McCollum. 2001. (Illus.). 188p. (C). reprint ed. pap. text 35.00 (*0-7567-0654-8*) DIANE Pub.

Medical Marriage: The New Partnership Between Orthodox & Complementary Medicine. Ed. by Cornelia Featherstone & Lori Forsyth. 1997. (Illus.). 640p. (Orig.). (C). pap. (*1-899171-16-9*) Findhorn Pr GBR. *Dist:* Words Distrib.

Medical Marriages. Ed. by Glen O. Gabbard & Roy W. Menninger. 1988. LC 88-14653. 182p. 34.00 (*0-88048-260-5*, 8260) Am Psychiatric.

***Medical Mass Screening for Health & Disease: Research Survey Index with Reference Bibliography.** Colette O. Babbit. 2001. pap. 39.50 (*0-7883-2563-9*) ABBE Pubs Assn.

Medical Materials Industry Review. 1996. 317p. 1500.00 (*1-56965-415-8*, DMU95) BCC.

Medical Materials Industry Review. Ed. by Melvin Schlechter & Dori A. Horn. 1995. 251p. 1500.00 (*1-56965-340-2*) BCC.

Medical Mathematics. Thomas J. Taylor. 1975. LC 74-79839. (Allied Health Ser.). pap. 4.55 (*0-672-61393-X*, Bobbs) Macmillan.

Medical Matters: A Handbook for Medical Secretaries. Rozema. 3rd ed. 1997. pap. 0.00 (*0-582-80907-X*) Addison-Wesley.

Medical Mavericks. Hugh D. Riordan. LC 88-63321. (Orig.). Vol. 1. 1988. 102p. pap. 7.95 (*0-942333-07-1*); Vol. 2. 1989. 120p. pap. 7.95 (*0-942333-09-8*) Bio-Comns Pr.

Medical Meanings: A Glossary of Word Origins. Ed. by William S. Haubrich. 1997. LC 96-29494. 253p. (C). pap. text 29.95 (*0-943126-56-8*) Amer Coll Phys.

Medical Measurements of Pain by Research Scientists: Index of New Information with References. Marcella K. Javorekko. 1996. 150p. 57.50 (*0-7883-0796-7*); pap. 44.50 (*0-7883-0797-5*) ABBE Pubs Assn.

Medical, Mental & Emotional Factors in Human Personality Disorders: Index of New Information with Authors, Subjects & Bibliography. Roger M. Mocker. rev. ed. 1994. 155p. 57.50 (*0-7883-0406-2*); pap. 47.50 (*0-7883-0407-0*) ABBE Pubs Assn.

Medical Micro Lab: Learning Guide. Smith. 1989. (Medical Lab Technician Ser.). tchr. ed. 12.00 (*0-8273-4373-6*) Delmar.

Medical Microbiology. Robert F. Boyd & Joseph J. Marr. 1980. (Illus.). 760p. 35.00 (*0-316-10432-9*, Little Brwn Med Div) Lppncott W & W.

Medical Microbiology. Samuel Baron. 2nd ed. 1986. 1296p. (C). text 50.36 (*0-201-10146-7*, Health Sci) Addison-Wesley.

Medical Microbiology. Cedric Mims et al. 2nd ed. 1998. (Illus.). 592p. pap. 45.00 (*0-7234-2781-X*) Mosby Inc.

Medical Microbiology. Patrick R. Murray. 3rd ed. 1997. LC 97-18902. (Illus.). 736p. (C). (gr. 13). pap. text 49.00 (*0-8151-9035-2*, 29126) Mosby Inc.

Medical Microbiology. Patrick R. Murray et al. 3rd ed. 1998. (Illus.). 736p. pap. (*84-8174-162-0*) Mosby-Doyma Libros ESP. *Dist:* Mosby Inc.

Medical Microbiology. Ed. by Samuel Baron. 4th ed. 1996. LC 95-50499. (Illus.). (C). 55.00 (*0-9631172-1-1*) U TX MB Microb.

Medical Microbiology. Patrick R. Murray et al. 4th ed. 2001. 826p. pap. text (*0-323-01213-2*) Mosby Inc.

Medical Microbiology. C. G. Thomas. 6th ed. 1988. (Illus.). 416p. text (*0-7020-1270-X*) Bailliere Tindall.

Medical Microbiology: A Laboratory Study. William G. Wu. 3rd ed. 1995. (Illus.). 420p. (C). spiral bd. 32.95 (*0-89863-180-7*) Star Pub CA.

Medical Microbiology: A Short Course. Ellen Barron et al. 1994. LC 93-16481. (Illus.). 1072p. (Orig.). pap. 84.95 (*0-471-56728-0*, Wiley-Liss) Wiley.

Medical Microbiology: General Concepts. Ed. by Samuel Baron. 1996. LC 96-4860. (Illus.). pap. 12.00 (*0-9631172-2-X*) U TX MB Microb.

Medical Microbiology - A Guide to Microbial Infections: Pathogenesis, Immunity, Laboratory Diagnosis & Control. Ed. by D. Greenwood et al. 15th ed. 1997. (Illus.). 690p. pap. (*0-443-05454-1*) Church.

Medical Microbiology at a Glance. S. H. Gillespie & Kathleen Bamford. 2000. LC 99-26884. (At a Glance Ser.). (Illus.). 117p. pap. 24.95 (*0-632-05026-8*) Blackwell Sci.

Medical Microbiology Illustrated. Stephen H. Gillespie. 1999. (Arnold Publication). 296p. pap. 40.00 (*0-7506-4415-X*) OUP.

Medical Milestones in Cole County, Missouri: A History of the Cole County Medical Society. Joseph S. Summers, Jr. 1988. 200p. text 35.00 (*0-916109-06-2*) Summers Pub.

Medical Millennium. Ed. by H. Lee. 2000. LC 99-44527. (Illus.). 120p. lib. bdg. 49.95 (*1-85070-466-X*, Parthenon Pbng) CRC Pr.

Medical Millennium. William H. Hay. 1993. 133p. reprint ed. spiral bd. 14.00 (*0-7873-0386-0*) Hlth Research.

Medical Ministry. Ellen Gould Harmon White. 1963. reprint ed. 12.99 (*0-8163-0157-3*, 13371-0) Pacific Pr Pub Assn.

Medical Mischief, You Say! Degerminating the Germ Theory. Nell Rogers & Guy Rogers. 1996. reprint ed. spiral bd. 8.50 (*0-7873-0735-1*) Hlth Research.

Medical Mishaps: Pieces of the Puzzle. Ed. by Linda Mulcahy et al. 1998. LC 98-21881. (Illus.). xix, 265p. (*0-335-20258-6*) OpUniv Pr.

Medical Mishaps: Pieces of the Puzzle. Linda Mulcahy et al. 1998. LC 98-21881. (Illus.). xix, 265p. (*0-335-20259-4*) OpUniv Pr.

Medical Money Mess: A Survivor's Guide to Health Care Costs & Health Insurance in the 1980's. Hugh E. Wilson & Robert Valentine. rev. ed. 1986. LC 85-117532. 120p. pap. 9.95 (*0-933811-02-0*) MCS Pubns KY.

Medical Monitoring & Screening in the Workplace: Results of a Survey. 1992. 84p. (Orig.). (C). pap. text 30.00 (*0-941375-59-5*) DIANE Pub.

Medical Monitoring Markets: A Detailed Database on a 6 Billion Dollar Market. Market Intelligence Staff. 1992. 480p. 995.00 (*1-56753-087-7*) Frost & Sullivan.

Medical Monitoring of Hostile Environments: Index of New Information. Hugh G. Gartzky. 1998. 57.50 (*0-7883-1832-2*); pap. 47.50 (*0-7883-1833-0*) ABBE Pubs Assn.

Medical Monopoly Versus Your Right to Freedom of Choice in Health Care. 1992. lib. bdg. 75.00 (*0-8490-5261-0*) Gordon Pr.

Medical Motifs. Macagba. 1998. pap. 1.00 (*0-486-28256-2*) Dover.

***Medical Multimedia.** 1995. pap. (*1-871516-63-3*) Intellect GBR. *Dist:* Intl Spec Bk.

Medical Mycology. Dode Grigoriu et al. Tr. by D. Q. Stephenson. 1987. LC 87-3153.Tr. of Traite de Mycologie Medicale. (Illus.). 482p. text 149.00 (*0-920887-18-X*) Hogrefe & Huber Pubs.

Medical Mycology. S. Nolting & K. Fegler. 1987. 208p. 29.95 (*0-387-17606-3*) Spr-Verlag.

Medical Mycology: A Self-Instructional Text. Martha E. Kern. 2nd ed. 1997. LC 96-46605. (Illus.). 242p. pap. 37.95 (*0-8036-0036-4*) Davis Co.

Medical Mycology & Human Mycoses. Everette S. Beneke & Alvin L. Rogers. 1996. LC 95-47079. (Illus.). 239p. (C). 54.95 (*0-89863-175-0*) Star Pub CA.

Medical Mycology Protocols. Ken A. Haynes & David C. Coleman. 1999. (Methods in Molecular Medicine Ser.). (Illus.). 400p. 74.50 (*0-89603-533-6*) Humana.

Medical Negligence. Malcolm Khan & Michelle Robson. 1997. LC 97-127677. (Medico-Legal Ser.). 432p. pap. (*1-85941-022-7*) Cavendish Pubng GBR. *Dist:* Gaunt.

Medical Negligence: A Practical Guide. Charles J. Lewis. 1995. 600p. (*1-86012-073-3*); 1992. 567p. (*0-85459-643-7*) Tolley Pubng GBR. *Dist:* St Mut.

Medical Negligence: Cost-Effective Case Management. Iain S. Goldrein & Margaret R. De Hass. 1997. pap. (*0-406-99920-1*, MICHIE) LEXIS Pub.

Medical Negligence: Managing Medical Disputes, 1. Susan Rodway & Simon Levene. 2000. 260p. (*1-902558-05-7*) Palladian Law GBR. *Dist:* Gaunt.

Medical Negligence: The Cranium, Spine & Nervous System. John Garfield & Christopher Earl. 1999. LC 99-17519. 131.95 (*0-632-05183-3*) Blackwell Sci.

Medical Negligence Case Law. Rodney Nelson-Jones & Frank Burton. 1990. 432p. (C). text (*1-85190-087-X*) Tolley Pubng GBR. *Dist:* St Mut.

Medical Negligence Law: Seeking a Balance. Andrew F. Phillips. 1997. LC 96-32164. (Medico-Legal Issues Ser.). (Illus.). 248p. text (*1-85521-643-4*) Dartmth Pub GBR. *Dist:* Ashgate Pub Co.

Medical Neurology. David Chadwick et al. 1989. (Illus.). 506p. pap. text (*0-443-03051-0*) Church.

Medical Neuropsychology: The Impact of Disease on Behavior. R. E. Tarter et al. 1988. LC 87-36138. (Critical Issues in Neuropsychology Ser.). (Illus.). 366p. (C). 65.00 (*0-306-42741-9*, Plenum Trade) Perseus Pubng.

Medical Neuroscience. T. Pritchard & K. Alloway. 1998. (Integrated Medical Sciences Ser.). (C). pap. 29.95 (*1-889325-29-5*) Blackwell Sci.

Medical Neurosciences: An Approach to Anatomy, Pathology, & Physiology by Systems & Levels. Eduardo E. Benarroch. 4th ed. 1998. LC 98-24218. 640p. pap. text 39.95 (*0-7817-1426-5*) Lppncott W & W.

Medical Neurotoxicology: Occupational & Environmental Causes of Neurological Dysfunction. Ed. by Peter G. Blain & John B. Harris. 1999. LC 99-16934. (An Arnold Publication). (Illus.). 388p. text (*0-340-59665-1*) E A GBR. *Dist:* OUP.

Medical Nirds Quickie. Afshine Emrani. 1997. (Nirds Quickie Ser.). 180p. pap. 9.95 (*0-9654687-0-4*) Emrani Publns.

Medical Nursing of Small Animals. Joanne Masters. 2001. 300p. pap. 45.00 (*0-7506-5171-7*) Buttrwrth-Heinemann.

Medical Nutrition & Disease. Lisa Hark & Gail Morrison. 1996. LC 96-26674. 288p. pap. 32.95 (*0-86542-491-8*) Blackwell Sci.

Medical Nutrition & Disease. Gail Morrison & Lisa Hark. 2nd ed. 1999. LC 99-24988. (Illus.). 354p. pap. 39.95 (*0-632-04339-3*) Blackwell Sci.

Medical Nutrition from Marz. Russell B. Marz. 2nd ed. 1998. (Illus.). 587p. text 69.95 (*1-882550-28-5*, Omni Pr) Quiet Lion Pr.

Medical Nutrition Therapy: A Case Study Approach. Marcia Nahikian-Nelms & Anderson. 2001. 400p. pap. text 50.95 (*0-534-52410-9*) Thomson Learn.

Medical Nutrition Therapy: Case Studies for the Dietary Manager. Litchford. 1997. 166p. spiral bd. 21.00 (*0-7872-3605-5*) Kendall-Hunt.

Medical Nutrition Therapy Across the Continuum of Care. American Dietetic Association Staff. 1997. 200p. ring bd. 80.00 incl. VHS, disk (*0-88091-149-2*) Am Dietetic Assn.

Medical Odysseys: The Different & Sometimes Unexpected Pathways to Twentieth-Century Medical Discoveries. Allen B. Weisse. 1991. LC 90-8387. 237p. (C). pap. 15.95 (*0-8135-1617-X*) Rutgers U Pr.

Medical Office Administrative Procedures. Mary A. Frew & David R. Frew. 2nd ed. 1989. LC 88-31065. (Illus.). 439p. (C). pap. 29.95 (*0-8036-3862-0*) Davis Co.

Medical Office Applications Using Your Epson. Susan Dodson. 1985. pap. 16.95 (*0-8359-4492-1*) P-H.

Medical Office Design: Territory & Conflict. Henry F. Doble, Jr. 1982. 200p. (C). pap. 42.50 (*0-87527-243-6*) Green.

Medical Office Pharmacology. 2000. tchr. ed. 21.00 (*0-13-030721-1*) P-H.

Medical Office Pharmacology. Barb R. Struck. 2000. LC 00-29859. 224p. pap. 41.00 (*0-8359-5290-8*) P-H.

Medical Office Policy Manual. Medical Management Institute Staff. 1996. LC 95-39519. (Illus.). 199p. (Orig.). pap. text 44.95 (*0-07-600796-0*, ME109) Practice Mgmt Info.

Medical Office Practice. Martha Foster. 1975. LC 75-4051. (Allied Health Ser.). pap. 6.25 (*0-672-61381-6*, Bobbs) Macmillan.

Medical Office Practice. Atkinson. 6th ed. 1998. (Allied Health Ser.). 128p. (C). pap. text 57.95 (*0-7668-0605-7*) Delmar.

Medical Office Practice - IML. Atkinson. 6th ed. 1998. tchr. ed. 25.95 (*0-7668-0855-6*) Delmar.

Medical Office Practice Set. Phillip S. Atkinson & Deborah Begg. 4th ed. 1990. (C). pap. 29.95 (*0-538-70010-6*, RL40DC) S-W Thomson.

Medical Office Practice Set. Phillip S. Atkinson. 5th ed. 1994. (Medical Assisting Ser.). (C). 36.00 (*0-538-71204-X*) S-W Thomson.

Medical Office Procedures. Karonne Becklin & Edith Sunnarborg. 1999. tchr. ed. 14.00 (*0-02-804746-X*) Glencoe.

Medical Office Procedures. Karonne J. Becklin & Edith Sunnarborg. 4th ed. 1995. LC 95-35495. pap. 53.00 (*0-02-802531-8*) Glencoe.

Medical Office Procedures. Karonne Becklin & Edith Sunnarborg. 4th ed. 1999. wbk. ed. 35.00 incl. disk (*0-02-804881-4*) Glencoe.

***Medical Office Procedures.** Karonne J. Becklin. 5th ed. 2002. LC 2001-54797. pap. (*0-07-826261-5*) Glencoe.

Medical Office Procedures Manual. Ann Ehrlich. 3rd ed. 1993. (Illus.). 28.95 (*0-940012-35-9*) Colwell Syst.

Medical Office Procedures with Medical Pegboard-Complete Set. Contrib. by Eleanor K. Flores & Dorothy A. Taylor. 4th ed. 1999. LC 99-31969. 128p. pap. text 64.95 (*0-7668-1645-1*) Delmar.

Medical Office Projects. Mark E. Abell. 1999. (Illus.). 128p. pap. text 29.95 (*0-538-72127-8*) S-W Thomson.

Medical Office Transcription: An Introduction to Medical Transcription. Karonne Becklin & Edith Sunnarborg. 1998. tchr. ed. 9.60 incl. disk (*0-02-802242-4*); 128p. text, wbk. ed. 27.50 incl. disk (*0-02-802240-8*) Glencoe.

Medical Officer. Jack Rudman. 1994. (Career Examination Ser.: C-488). pap. 39.95 (*0-8373-0488-1*) Nat Learn.

Medical Officer (Departmental) Jack Rudman. 1994. (Career Examination Ser.: C-489). pap. 39.95 (*0-8373-0489-X*) Nat Learn.

Medical Offset Effect & Public Health Policy: Mental Health Industry in Transition. John L. Fiedler & Jonathan B. Wight. 1989. LC 88-28927. 216p. 75.00 (*0-275-92859-4*, C2859, Praeger Pubs) Greenwood.

Medical Oncology: A Comprehensive Review. Ed. by Richard Pazdur. 2nd ed. 1995. 520p. 49.95 (*0-9641823-1-9*) PRR.

Medical Orthodoxy & the Future of Psychoanalysis. K. R. Eissler. 1965. LC 65-18721. 592p. 87.50 (*0-8236-3240-7*) Intl Univs Pr.

Medical Parasitology. Ralph L. Muller & John Baker. 1989. (Illus.). 200p. (gr. 13). text (*0-397-44609-8*, GM0059) Gower-Mosby.

Medical Parasitology. N. C. Dey. rev. ed. 1984. (C). (*0-7855-4660-X*) Current Dist IND. *Dist:* St Mut.

Medical Parasitology. Edward K. Markell et al. Ed. by Adrianne Williams. 8th ed. 1998. LC 98-15802. (Illus.). viii, 501p. (C). text 49.95 (*0-7216-7634-0*) Saunders.

Medical Parasitology: A Practical Approach. Ed. by S. Gillespie & P. M. Hawkey. 1995. (Practical Approach Ser.: Vol. 152). (Illus.). 314p. pap. text 65.00 (*0-19-963300-2*) OUP.

Medical Parasitology: A Self-Instructional Text. Ruth Leventhal & Russell F. Cheadle. (Illus.). 4th ed. 1995. LC 95-4649. 178p. (C). pap. 39.95 (*0-8036-0041-0*); 5th ed. 2002. LC 2001-53881. 304p. per. 43.95 (*0-8036-0788-1*) Davis Co.

Medical Patents in the Health Sciences Including Legislative Actions: Index of New Information. Albert E. Goldring. 1996. 150p. 57.50 (*0-7883-0912-9*); 1996. 150p. pap. 47.50 (*0-7883-0913-7*); 1997. 135p. 57.50 (*0-7883-1592-7*); 1997. 135p. pap. 47.50 (*0-7883-1593-5*) ABBE Pubs Assn.

Medical Pegboard Procedure: Contents Only. Taylor. 2nd ed. 1992. (Medical Assisting Ser.). pap. 32.95 (*0-538-70438-1*) S-W Thomson.

Medical Pegboard Procedures. 2nd ed. 1992. (Medical Assisting Ser.). 39.95 (*0-538-70437-3*) Delmar.

Medical Pegboard Procedures. Dorothy A. Taylor et al. 3rd ed. 1995. 80p. (C). text, tchr. ed. 14.00 (*0-8273-7551-4*) Delmar.

Medical Pegboard Procedures, Pegboard Only. Taylor et al. 3rd ed. 1996. text, tchr. ed. 11.95 (*0-8273-7550-6*) Delmar.

Medical Pegboard Procedures, Set. Dorothy A. Taylor et al. 3rd ed. 1995. LC 95-42299. tchr. ed. 62.95 (*0-8273-7548-4*) Delmar.

Medical Periodicals: Index of Functions, History & Standards. Alphonse R. Abell. 1989. LC 88-48002. 150p. 47.50 (*1-55914-086-0*); pap. 44.50 (*1-55914-087-9*) ABBE Pubs Assn.

Medical Pharmacology at a Glance. M. J. Neal. 3rd ed. 1997. LC 97-2123. (At a Glance Ser.). (Illus.). 104p. pap. 29.95 (*0-86542-719-4*) Blackwell Sci.

***Medical Phrase Index: A Comprehensive Reference to the Terminology of Medicine.** Jean Lorenzini. 4th ed. 2001. 1800p. text 54.95 (*1-57066-185-5*, ME128) Practice Mgmt Info.

Medical Phrase Index: A One-Step Reference to the Terminology of Medicine. Jean A. Lorenzini & Laura Lorenzini-Ley. Ed. by Gregg Rogers & Kathryn Swanson. 3rd ed. 1994. LC 93-42123. 1300p. 49.95 (*1-878487-58-2*, ME052) Practice Mgmt Info.

Medical Physicists & Malpractice. Robert J. Shalek & David S. Gooden. 1996. LC 96-17117. 128p. text 27.00 (*0-944838-64-2*); pap. text 21.00 (*0-944838-65-0*) Med Physics Pub.

Medical Physics: 2nd Mexican Symposium. Ed. by Marla-Ester Brandan et al. 1998. LC 98-86572. (Conference Proceedings Ser.: Vol. 440). (Illus.). x, 232p. (C). 85.00 (*1-56396-807-X*) Am Inst Physics.

***Medical Physics: Fifth Mexican Symposium.** Ed. by F. A. Barrios et al. 2001. (AIP Conference Proceedings Ser.: Vol. 593). 213p. 135.00 (*0-7354-0036-9*) Am Inst Physics.

Medical Physics: Fourth Mexican Symposium: Merida, Yucatan, Mexico, 1-4 March 2000. Ed. by J. J. Alvarado-Gil et al. 2000. LC 00-108312. (Conference Proceedings Ser.: Vol. 538). (Illus.). vii, 262p. (C). 125.00 (*1-56396-963-7*) Am Inst Physics.

Medical Physics & Biomedical Engineering. B. H. Brown. 1999. LC 99-23505. (Medical Science Ser.). (Illus.). xxvi, 736p. 180.00 (*0-7503-0367-0*) Inst of Physics Pubng.

Medical Physics & Biomedical Engineering. B. H. Brown et al. 1999. LC 99-23505. (Medical Science Ser.). (Illus.). xxvi, 736p. pap. text 60.00 (*0-7503-0368-9*) Inst of Physics Pubng.

Medical Physics Handbook of Nuclear Medicine. Mark T. Madsen. 1992. (Illus.). 114p. (Orig.). (C). pap. text 16.95 (*0-944838-14-6*) Med Physics Pub.

Medical Physics Handbook of Radiation Therapy. Ed. by Ann E. Wright. 1992. (Illus.). 127p. (Orig.). (C). pap. text 16.95 (*0-944838-17-0*) Med Physics Pub.

Medical Physics Handbook of Units & Measures. John Freim, Jr. & Arnold Feldman. 1992. 47p. pap. text 7.95 (*0-944838-30-8*) Med Physics Pub.

Medical Physics of CT & Ultrasound: Tissue Imaging & Characterization. Ed. by Gary D. Fullerton & James A. Zagzebski. 1980. (Medical Physics Monograph Ser.: No. 6). 717p. text 50.00 (*1-888340-08-8*) AAPM.

Medical Physics of CT & Ultrasound: Tissue Imaging & Characterization: Proceedings of the AAPM 1980 Summer School Held at the University of Wisconsin - La Cross, Wisconsin, July 20-26, 1980. Ed. by Gary D. Fullerton & James A. Zagzebski. 1980. (American Association of Physicists in Medicine Symposium Ser.: No. 6). 725p. 50.00 (*0-88318-279-3*) Am Inst Physics.

Medical Physiology. Ernie Boulpaep & Walter Boron. 1995. 1000p. (C). text (*0-7216-3256-4*) Saunders.

Medical Physiology. Ed. by Rodney A. Rhoades & George A. Tanner. 1995. LC 94-24639. (Illus.). 864p. text 62.00 (*0-316-74228-7*, Little Brwn Med Div) Lppncott W & W.

Medical Physiology: Objectives & Multiple Choice Questions. Graham Mitchell. 2nd ed. 1986. 153p. (C). pap. text 35.00 (*0-409-10727-1*) Buttrwrth-Heinemann.

Medical Plastics: Degradation Resistance & Failure Analysis. 1998. LC 98-65533. (SPE/ PDL Ser.). 215p. text 160.00 (*1-884207-60-X*) William Andrew.

Medical Politics - Actions, Status & Reactions: Index of Modern Progress. Science and Life Consultants Association Staff. rev. ed. 1994. LC 94-32481. 151p. 57.50 (*0-7883-0240-X*); pap. 47.50 (*0-7883-0241-8*) ABBE Pubs Assn.

Medical Portraits, Supplement 10. 1983. suppl. ed. 420.00 (*0-8161-1391-2*, Macmillan Ref) Gale.

Medical Power & Social Knowledge. Bryan S. Turner. 2nd ed. 1995. LC 95-70832. 288p. 69.95 (*0-8039-7598-8*, 1561); pap. 24.95 (*0-8039-7599-6*, 1562) Sage.

Medical Power in Prisons: The Prison Medical Service in England, 1774-1988. Joe Sim. 1990. (Crime, Justice & Social Policy Ser.). 224p. (*0-335-15183-3*); pap. (*0-335-15182-5*) OpUniv Pr.

Medical Practice Accounting & Finance: A Practical Guide for Physicians, Dentists & Other Medical Practitioners. Rose Marie Bukics & Donald R. Chambers. 1995. LC 95-223119. 200p. (C). text 45.00 (*1-55738-617-X*, Irwn Prfssnl) McGraw-Hill Educ Grp.

Medical Practice Change Management: Strategies & Techniques for the Changing Business of Healthcare. Peter D. Lucash. 1996. LC 96-45342. 240p. text 45.00 (*0-7863-0998-9*, Irwn McGrw-H) McGrw-H Hghr Educ.

Medical Practice Consolidation: Structural & Legal Issues. Peter N. Grant et al. 1996. (Health Law & Business Ser.: No. 1200). 125.00 (*1-55871-339-5*) BNA.

Medical Practice, Defensive Medicine & Legal Issues: Index of New Information with Authors, Subjects, Research Categories & References. Darnella Devitto. 1995. 160p. 57.50 (*0-7883-0728-2*); 1995. pap. 47.50 (*0-7883-0729-0*); 1998. 160p. 57.50 (*0-7883-2086-6*); 1998. 160p. pap. 47.50 (*0-7883-2087-4*) ABBE Pubs Assn.

Medical Practice Forms: Every Form You Need to Succeed. Keith C. Borglum. 1998. 300p. (Orig.). pap. text 44.95 (*1-57066-083-2*) Practice Mgmt Info.

***Medical Practice Forms: Every Form You Need to Succeed.** Keith Borglum & Diane Cate. 2nd ed. 2001. (Illus.). 400p. pap. text 54.95 (*1-57066-212-6*, ME097) Practice Mgmt Info.

Medical Practice in Rural Communities. C. F. Mutel & K. J. Donham. 1983. (Illus.). 168p. 58.00 (*0-387-91224-X*) Spr-Verlag.

Medical Practice in the Current Health Care Environment: A Handbook for Residents & Medical Students. Ed. by Janine C. Edwards & Robert M. Donati. 1994. LC 94-19801. 169p. pap. text 17.95 (*0-8018-4966-7*) Johns Hopkins.

Medical Practice Management. Dean C. Kramer. 1982. 288p. 19.50 (*0-316-50322-3*, Little Brwn Med Div) Lppncott W & W.

Medical Practice Management Book. 8th ed. 1998. 225p. pap. text 65.00 (*1-58383-160-6*, PERMGT1) Robert D Keene.

Medical Practice Management Desk Book. Charles H. Walsh & Morton Walker. 1982. LC 81-19972. 208p. 49.95 (*0-13-572701-4*) P-H.

Medical Practice Management Handbook. Reed Tinsley. 2000. 900p. 119.00 incl. cd-rom (*0-15-607122-3*) Harcourt Prof.

Medical Practice Performance Management Manual: How to Evaluate Employees. Courtney Price & Alys Novak. 1993. (Employee Performance Management Ser.). 234p. (Orig.). pap. 85.00 (*1-56829-027-6*) M G M A.

Medical Practice Valuation Guidebook 1999/2000: Including the Influence of Managed Care. Mark O. Dietrich. 1998. (Pocket Primer Ser.). pap. 95.00 (*1-893190-00-5*) Windsor Profess.

Medical Practice Valuation Guidebook 2001/2002: Including Comprehensive Financial Analysis & the Influence of Managed Care. Mark O. Dietrich. 2nd ed. 2001. (Illus.). 480p. pap. 115.00 (*1-893190-09-9*) Windsor Profess.

Medical Practices in the Civil War. Susan Provost Beller. 1998. LC 92-14960. (Illus.). 96p. reprint ed. pap. 9.99 (*0-9663758-0-7*, 01) OurStory.

Medical Prescriptions—Abuse, Choices, Control, Evaluation, Habits, Generics & Computerization: Index of New Information with Authors, Subjects, & Bibliography. Darlee M. Bentley. 1996. LC 96-12514. 57.50 (*0-7883-0820-3*); pap. 47.50 (*0-7883-0821-1*) ABBE Pubs Assn.

Medical Primatology, 1970: Proceedings. Conference on Experimental Medicine and Surgery in P. Ed. by E. I. Goldsmith & J. Moor-Jankowski. 1971. 243.50 (*3-8055-1227-9*) S Karger.

Medical Privacy Legislation: Implications for Workers' Compensation. Romona P. Tanabe et al. 2000. LC 00-47309. 255p. pap. 50.00 (*0-935149-95-3*, WC-00-4) Workers Comp Res Inst.

Medical Problem Solving: An Analysis of Clinical Reasoning. Arthur S. Elstein et al. 1978. LC 77-21505. (Illus.). 352p. 51.95 (*0-674-56125-2*) HUP.

Medical Problems in Athletes. Karl B. Fields & Peter A. Fricker. 1997. LC 97-13110. (Illus.). 464p. pap. 104.95 (*0-86542-480-2*) Blackwell Sci.

Medical Problems in Dentistry. Crispian Scully et al. 4th ed. 1998. LC 97-51176. 592p. (*0-7236-1056-8*) John Wright GBR. *Dist:* Buttrwrth-Heinemann.

Medical Profession in 19th Century Florida: A Biographical Register. Ashby E. Hammond. 1996. LC 96-43502. (*0-929595-08-4*) Univ Florida Lib.

Medical Professional Liability & the Delivery of Obstetrical Care, Vol. I. Institute of Medicine Staff. 1989. 256p. text 29.95 (*0-309-03982-7*) Natl Acad Pr.

Medical Professional Liability & the Delivery of Obstetrical Care: An Interdisciplinary Review, Vol. II. Ed. by Victoria P. Rostow et al. 1989. 256p. text 35.00 (*0-309-03986-X*) Natl Acad Pr.

Medical Professions Admission Guide: Strategy for Success. Ed. by Brice W. Corder. 3rd ed. 1994. 142p. (C). pap. 15.95 (*0-911899-11-1*) NAAHP Inc.

Medical Professions & Drug Addiction: Six Studies, 1882 to 1932, An Original Anthology. Gerald N. Grob. 1981. LC 80-1206. (Addiction in America Ser.). lib. bdg. 37.95 (*0-405-13560-2*) Ayer.

***Medical Profile Journal.** 2001. (Illus.). 24p. mass mkt. (*0-9712221-1-8*, 76223-2); 24p. mass mkt. (*0-9712221-0-X*); 128p. ring bd. (*0-9712221-2-6*, 76223-3) Robbe Health Intl.

Medical Progress & Social Reality: A Reader in Nineteenth-Century Medicine & Literature. Ed. by Lilian R. Furst. 2000. LC 00-26534. (SUNY Series, The Margins of Literature). xiv, 314p. (C). text 66.50 (*0-7914-4803-7*) State U NY Pr.

Medical Proof of Social Securities Disability. David A. Morton, III. 1983. LC 83-16800. 585p. (C). reprint ed. text 58.50 net. (*0-314-72082-0*) West Pub.

Medical Proof of Social Securities Disability: 1995-1996 Supplement. David A. Morton, 3rd. 1995. (Miscellaneous Treatise Ser.). 400p. (C). pap. text, suppl. ed. (*0-314-08334-0*) West Pub.

Medical Prosthetic Devices & Artificial Organs. Ed. by Peter Allen. 1983. 279p. pap. 295.00 (*0-931634-35-0*) FIND-SVP.

Medical Protestants: The Eclectics in American Medicine, 1825-1939. John S. Haller, Jr. 1993. LC 93-7389. (Medical Humanities Ser.). (Illus.). 352p. (C). 51.95 (*0-8093-1894-6*) S Ill U Pr.

Medical-Psychiatric Practice. Ed. by Alan Stoudemire & Barry S. Fogel. Vol. 1. 1991. 645p. text 29.95 (*0-88048-425-X*, 8425); Vol. 2. 1993. (Medical-Psychiatric Practice Ser.: Vol. 2). 657p. text 29.95 (*0-88048-426-8*, 8426) Am Psychiatric.

Medical Psychiatry: Theory & Practice, Set. Ed. by Enrique S. Garza-Trevino. 1989. 1300p. (C). text 74.00 (*9971-5-0774-9*) World Scientific Pub.

Medical Psychology of Adolescents: Index of New Information. American Health Research Institute Staff. 1996. 150p. 57.50 (*0-7883-0924-2*); 1996. 150p. pap. 47.50 (*0-7883-0925-0*); 1998. 165p. 57.50 (*0-7883-1956-6*); 1998. 165p. pap. 47.50 (*0-7883-1957-4*) ABBE Pubs Assn.

Medical Psychology of Alcohol Drinking & Addiction: Index of New Information with References. Helen R. Haggert. rev. ed. 1997. 177p. 57.50 (*0-7883-1568-4*); pap. 47.50 (*0-7883-1569-2*) ABBE Pubs Assn.

Medical Psychology of Breast Cancer: Index of New Information. Ruth K. Leeson. 1997. 153p. 57.50 (*0-7883-1500-5*); 1997. 153p. pap. 47.50 (*0-7883-1501-3*); 1996. 150p. 57.50 (*0-7883-0908-0*); 1996. 150p. pap. 47.50 (*0-7883-0909-9*) ABBE Pubs Assn.

Medical Psychology of Crime - Including Patients. American Health Research Institute Staff. 1996. 150p. pap. 47.50 (*0-7883-0919-6*) ABBE Pubs Assn.

Medical Psychology of Crime - Including Patients: Index of New Information for Reference & Research. American Health Research Institute Staff. 1996. 150p. 57.50 (*0-7883-0918-8*) ABBE Pubs Assn.

Medical Psychology of Delusions in Normal & Abnormal Behaviors: Index of New Information & Bibliography. Gladys G. Petronno. 1996. 150p. 57.50 (*0-7883-0984-6*); pap. 47.50 (*0-7883-0985-4*) ABBE Pubs Assn.

Medical Psychology of Homosexuality Male & Female: Index of New Information with References. Charder R. Eksteen. 1996. 150p. 57.50 (*0-7883-0812-2*); 1996. 150p. pap. 47.50 (*0-7883-0813-0*); 1997. 169p. 57.50 (*0-7883-1598-6*); 1997. 169p. pap. 47.50 (*0-7883-1599-4*) ABBE Pubs Assn.

Medical Psychology of Parents & Parenting: Index & Reference Book of New Information. Francis M. Vizzier. 1996. 150p. 57.50 (*0-7883-0910-2*); 1997. 159p. 57.50 (*0-7883-1556-0*); 1997. 159p. pap. 47.50 (*0-7883-1557-9*) ABBE Pubs Assn.

Medical Psychology of Placebo Effects-Myths, Magic & Reality: Index of New Information for the Health Sciences. William W. Wheeler. 1997. 147p. 57.50 (*0-7883-1382-7*); pap. 47.50 (*0-7883-1383-5*) ABBE Pubs Assn.

Medical Psychology of Regression & Factorial Elements of Personality: Index of New Information with Authors & Subjects. Anita M. Wolman. 1993. 180p. 47.50 (*1-55914-904-3*); pap. 44.50 (*1-55914-905-1*) ABBE Pubs Assn.

Medical Psychology of Shame, Self-Blame & Guilt: Index of New Information. Joyce C. Kirkland. 1998. 160p. 57.50 (*0-7883-1662-1*); pap. 47.50 (*0-7883-1663-X*) ABBE Pubs Assn.

Medical Psychology of Spouse Abuse: Index of New Information with Authors & Subjects. Willard T. Brainard. rev. ed. 1994. LC 94-34611. 57.50 (*0-7883-0424-0*); 131p. pap. 47.50 (*0-7883-0425-9*) ABBE Pubs Assn.

Medical Psychology of the Id, Ego & Superego: Index of Modern Authors & Subjects with Guide for Rapid Research. Nita C. Galanakis. 1991. LC 90-56275. 160p. 47.50 (*1-55914-332-0*); pap. 44.50 (*1-55914-333-9*) ABBE Pubs Assn.

Medical Psychology of (Tobacco) Smoking: Index of New Information with Authors, Subjects & References. Roger S. Ingalsbe. 1997. 150p. 57.50 (*0-7883-1390-8*); pap. 47.50 (*0-7883-1391-6*) ABBE Pubs Assn.

Medical Psychosomatics: Index of Modern Authors & Subjects with Guide for Rapid Research. Tony A. Pellicano. 1991. LC 90-56289. 160p. 47.50 (*1-55914-382-7*); pap. 44.50 (*1-55914-383-5*) ABBE Pubs Assn.

Medical Psychotherapy, Vol. 8. ABMP Staff. 1995. 240p. pap. text 6.95 (*0-7872-0963-5*) Kendall-Hunt.

Medical Publishing in Nineteenth Century America: Lea of Philadelphia, William Wood & Company of New York City & F. E. Boericke of Philadelphia with a Checklist of Wood's Library of Standard Medical Authors & Specimen Catalogues. Francesco Cordasco. 1990. (Illus.). 225p. 47.50 (*0-940198-06-1*) St Aedans Pr & Bk.

Medical Purchasing Specialist. Jack Rudman. 1994. (Career Examination Ser.: C-2448). pap. 27.95 (*0-8373-2448-3*) Nat Learn.

Medical Q & A. Emanual Grodsky. Ed. by Ross McElroy. (Realtime Machine Shorthand Ser.). (C). 1993. 142p. pap. text, stu. ed. 34.75 (*0-938643-24-X*, 410); 1992. 175p. pap., tchr. ed. 37.25 (*0-938643-25-8*, 610) Stenotype Educ.

Medical Quality & the Law: Final Report of the 1989 Chief Justice Earl Warren Conference on Advocacy in the United States. Michael E. Carbine. 1989. 116p. (Orig.). pap. 25.00 (*0-941916-60-X*) Roscoe Pound Inst.

Medical Radiation Detectors: Fundamental & Applied Aspects. Ed. by N. F. Kember. 1994. (Medical Science Series). (Illus.). 236p. 110.00 (*0-7503-0319-0*) Inst of Physics Pubng.

Medical Radiation Exposure of Pregnant & Potentially Pregnant Women. 1977. LC 77-80439. (Report Ser.: No. 54). 39p. pap. text 20.00 (*0-913392-36-7*) NCRP Pubns.

Medical Radiation Physics: Report of a Joint IAEA/WHO Expert Committee, 1968. 1968. (Technical Report Ser.: No. 390). 19p. pap. text 3.00 (*92-4-120390-0*, 1100390) World Health.

Medical Radiesthesia & Radionics: An Introduction. Vernon D. Wethered. 1957. 196p. pap. 17.95 (*0-8464-1032-X*); 4th ed. (Illus.). 192p. 17.95 (*0-8464-4251-5*) Beekman Pubs.

Medical Radiographic Techniques. Robert Zimmerman. 1975. LC 74-18672. (Allied Health Ser.). pap. 8.35 (*0-672-61392-1*, Bobbs) Macmillan.

Medical Radiography: Self-Assessment & Review. Linda Lefave. 1995. LC 95-14113. (Specialty Level PreTest Ser.). (Illus.). 286p. pap. 28.00 (*0-07-052078-X*) McGraw-Hill Prof.

Medical Radioisotope Scintigraphy. International Atomic Energy Agency Staff. 1968. Vol. 1. pap. (*92-0-010069-4*, ISP193-1); Vol. 2. pap. (*92-0-010169-0*, ISP193-2) IAEA AUT. *Dist:* Bernan Associates.

Medical Radioisotope Scintigraphy 1972. International Atomic Energy Agency Staff. 1973. Vol. 1. pap. (*92-0-010173-9*, ISP315-1); Vol. 2. pap. (*92-0-010273-5*, ISP315-2) IAEA AUT. *Dist:* Bernan Associates.

Medical Radiology Technician. Jack Rudman. 1994. (Career Examination Ser.: C-1367). pap. 27.95 (*0-8373-1367-8*) Nat Learn.

Medical Radiology Technologist. Jack Rudman. 1994. (Career Examination Ser.: C-490). pap. 29.95 (*0-8373-0490-3*) Nat Learn.

Medical Radionuclides: Radiation Dose & Effects, Proceedings. Ed. by Roger J. Cloutier et al. 1970. LC 70-606556. (AEC Symposium Ser.). 528p. pap. 21.25 (*0-87079-269-5*, CONF-691212); fiche 9.00 (*0-87079-270-9*, CONF-691212) DOE.

Medical Record Abstraction & Guidelines for Assessing Quality of Care for Hospitalized Patients with AIDS-Related Pneumocystis Carinii Pneumonia. Charles Bennett. 1994. 172p. (Orig.). (C). pap. text 45.00 (*0-7881-1055-1*) DIANE Pub.

Medical Record Abstraction Form & Guidelines for Assessing the Appropriateness of Hysterectomy. 1995. (Illus.). 174p. (Orig.). (C). pap. text 45.00 (*0-7881-2298-3*) DIANE Pub.

Medical Record Abstraction Form & Guidelines for Assessing the Appropriateness of Hysterectomy. Elizabeth A. McGlynn et al. 1993. LC 93-4601. pap. 9.00 (*0-8330-1394-7*, MR-239-HF) Rand Corp.

Medical Record Abstraction Form & Guidelines for Assessing the Quality of Prenatal Care. Elizabeth A. McGlynn et al. 1993. LC 93-4622. pap. 9.00 (*0-8330-1393-9*, MR-238-HF) Rand Corp.

Medical Record Librarian. Jack Rudman. 1994. (Career Examination Ser.: C-491). pap. 27.95 (*0-8373-0491-1*) Nat Learn.

Medical Record Management see Health Information Management

Medical Record Management. Edna K. Huffman. 9th ed. 1990. 35.15 (*0-917036-16-6*) Physicians Rec.

Medical Record Technician. Jack Rudman. 1994. (Career Examination Ser.: C-2329). pap. 27.95 (*0-8373-2329-0*) Nat Learn.

Medical Records. Anne M. Dellinger. 1987. (Hospital Law in North Carolina Ser.: Chap. 8). 67p. (C). ring bd. 10.50 (*1-56011-080-5*, 85.03H) Institute Government.

Medical Records: Getting Yours. Sidney M. Wolfe & Diann Johnson. rev. ed. 1995. (Illus.). 72p. (C). pap. text 10.00 (*0-937188-56-5*) Pub Citizen.

Medical Records & How They Affect Legal Issues. Arleen N. Kaizer. 1994. 127p. pap. 32.80 (*0-89412-232-0*) Aegean Park Pr.

Medical Records & the Law. William Roach, Jr. 3rd ed. 1998. LC 98-25735. 368p. 67.00 (*0-8342-1104-1*, 11041) Aspen Pub.

Medical Records Assistant. Jack Rudman. 1994. (Career Examination Ser.: C-2952). pap. 27.95 (*0-8373-2952-3*) Nat Learn.

Medical Records Clerk. Jack Rudman. 1994. (Career Examination Ser.: C-2309). reprint ed. pap. 27.95 (*0-8373-2309-6*) Nat Learn.

Medical Records Confidentiality in a Changing Health Care Environment: Congressional Hearing. Ed. by James M. Jeffords. 2000. 118p. (C). pap. 25.00 (*0-7567-0291-7*) DIANE Pub.

Medical Records Confidentiality in the Modern Delivery of Health Care: Congressional Hearing. Ed. by Michael Bilirakis. 2000. 121p. pap. text 30.00 (*0-7567-0138-4*) DIANE Pub.

Medical Records Examination Review. Susan P. Bailey. 1989. 224p. pap. 25.75 (*0-444-01485-3*) Elsevier.

***Medical Records for Attorneys.** Laurence M. Deutsch. 2001. LC 2001-92170. (Illus.). 464p. text 99.00 (*0-8318-0817-9*, BK11) Am Law Inst.

Medical Records for Lawyers. Ali Malsher. 2000. (*1-85811-259-1*) EMIS GBR. *Dist:* Gaunt.

Medical Records Handbook for the Physician's Office. Barbara O. Wesley. Ed. by Kimberly Koschemann & Debra Farris. 1999. 84p. pap. (*1-893621-01-4*) TX Med Assn.

Medical Records in Health Information. Kathleen Waters. 2nd ed. 1996. 700p. 52.00 (*0-8342-0251-4*) Aspen Pub.

Medical Records Policy & Procedure Guideline Manual. Mary J. Zellner. 1991. stu. ed. 80.00 (*1-879575-11-6*) Acad Med Sys.

Medical Records Privacy: Congressional Hearing. Ed. by James M. Jeffords. 2000. 77p. pap. 25.00 (*0-7567-0289-5*) DIANE Pub.

Medical Records Review Kristyn S. Appleby & Joanne Tarver. 3rd ed. 1995. LC 98-49309. 656p. 100.00 (*0-7355-0337-0*) Panel Pubs.

Medical Records Review & Analysis. Charles C. Sharpe. 1999. LC 98-47758. 224p. 65.00 (*0-86569-283-1*, Auburn Hse) Greenwood.

Medical Records Review, 2000. Kristyn S. Appleby. 3rd ed. 1999. pap. text, suppl. ed. 56.00 (*0-7355-1284-1*) Aspen Pub.

Medical Records Technology. Alice Mosier & Frank J. Pace. 1975. LC 74-18676. (Allied Health Ser.). pap. 9.95 (*0-672-61396-4*, Bobbs) Macmillan.

Medical Reference, Set. Bantam Books Inc. Editors Staff. 1992. mass mkt. 20.95 (*0-553-62870-4*) Bantam.

Medical Reference Works, 1969-1972. Compiled by Joy S. Richmond. 1973. LC 67-30664. pap. 7.50 (*0-8108-2440-X*) Scarecrow.

Medical Referrals for Health Science Practices & Business: Index of New Information with Authors & Subjects. Gene J. Whittlesby. 1993. 180p. 47.50 (*1-55914-908-6*); pap. 44.50 (*1-55914-909-4*) ABBE Pubs Assn.

Medical Rehabilitation of Traumatic Brain Injury. Ed. by Lawrence J. Horn & Nathan D. Zasler. 1996. (Illus.). 642p. 110.00 (*1-56053-070-7*) Hanley & Belfus.

Medical Rehabilitation Outcomes Research. Marcus J. Fuhrer. 1997. LC 96-31051. 464p. 67.00 (*1-55766-274-6*) P H Brookes.

Medical Rehabilitation Services: Forms, Checklists & Guidelines. Aspen Reference Group Staff. Ed. by Sara N. Di Lima & Sandra J. Painter. 1995. LC 94-41112. ring bd. 209.00 (*0-8342-0668-4*, S175) Aspen Pub.

Medical Relations Officer. Jack Rudman. 1994. (Career Examination Ser.: C-3351). pap. 34.95 (*0-8373-3351-2*) Nat Learn.

Medical Reports of the U. S. Office of Research Integrity: Index of New Information & Bibliography. Brian L. Longnecker. 1996. 150p. 57.50 (*0-7883-0996-X*); pap. 47.50 (*0-7883-0997-8*) ABBE Pubs Assn.

Medical Research - Priorities & Responsibilities: Proceedings of the Round Table Conference of CIOM-WHO-UNESCO, Geneva, Oct., 1969. CIOM-WHO-UNESCO Conference Staff. 1970. 156p. pap. text 7.20 (*92-4-156031-2*, 1830004) World Health.

Medical Research & the Jungle of Science: A New System for Universal Organization of All Subjects with Permanent Listing of All Publications, Authors & Contributors. John C. Bartone. rev. ed. 1996. (Illus.). 170p. 65.50 (*0-7883-1022-4*); pap. 55.50 (*0-7883-1023-2*) ABBE Pubs Assn.

***Medical Research at the Office for National Statistics: A Review.** Ed. by Morris Greenberg & Michel P. Coleman. 2000. (Studies on Medical & Population Subjects: No. 65). 132p. pap. (*0-11-621390-6*, SMPS 65) Statnry Office GBR. *Dist:* Balogh.

Medical Research Centres. 1990. 1000p. text 470.00 (*0-582-06123-7*) Longman.

Medical Research in the Health Sciences: Index of New Information with Authors & Subjects. Science and Life Consultants Association Staff. 1992. LC 92-54206. 180p. 47.50 (*1-55914-564-1*); pap. 44.50 (*1-55914-565-X*) ABBE Pubs Assn.

Medical Research Novel in English & German, 1900-1950. Phillip A. Scott. 1992. LC 91-78363. (ENG & GER.). 144p. (C). 24.95 (*0-87972-551-6*); pap. 13.95 (*0-87972-552-4*) Bowling Grn St Univ.

Medical Research of Current & Past Wars: Index of New Information. Gregg V. Goldin. 1995. LC 95-19212. 57.50 (*0-7883-0658-8*); 1994. 150p. 57.50 (*0-7883-0032-6*); 1994. 150p. pap. 47.50 (*0-7883-0033-4*) ABBE Pubs Assn.

Medical Research of Deception in Health Sciences Vol. I: Directory of Authors & Index of New Information, Vol. 1. Brian Z. Yardela. 1997. 170p. 57.50 (*0-7883-0964-1*); pap. 47.50 (*0-7883-0965-X*) ABBE Pubs Assn.

Medical Research of Deception in Health Sciences Vol. 2: Directory of Authors & Index of New Information. Brian Z. Yardela. 1997. 59p. pap. 47.50 (*0-7883-0967-6*);Vol. 2. 159p. 57.50 (*0-7883-0966-8*) ABBE Pubs Assn.

Medical Research of Leisure Activities - Active, Passive or Dangerous: Index of New Information. Virginia C. Venezia. 1997. 167p. 57.50 (*0-7883-1606-0*); 1997. 167p. pap. 47.50 (*0-7883-1607-9*); 1996. 150p. 57.50 (*0-7883-0844-0*); 1996. 150p. pap. 47.50 (*0-7883-0845-9*) ABBE Pubs Assn.

Medical Research of Sexual Partners: Index of New Information. American Health Research Institute Staff. 1996. 150p. 57.50 (*0-7883-0914-5*); pap. 47.50 (*0-7883-0915-3*) ABBE Pubs Assn.

Medical Research of Women's Health: Index & Reference Book of New Information. Angel A. Decker. 1996. 150p. 57.50 (*0-7883-0900-5*); pap. 47.50 (*0-7883-0901-3*) ABBE Pubs Assn.

Medical Research on Arctic & Antarctic Expeditions. A. L. Matusov. 1972. 216p. 3.5 hd 56.00 (*0-7065-1282-0*) Coronet Bks.

Medical Research Support - What's Going on in the U. S. A. Index of New Information & Research Bible. Science and Life Consultants Association Staff. 1996. LC 96-12494. 57.50 (*0-7883-1066-6*); 1996. LC 96-12494. pap. 47.50 (*0-7883-1067-4*); 1995. 160p. 57.50 (*0-7883-0224-8*); 1995. 160p. pap. 44.50 (*0-7883-0225-6*) ABBE Pubs Assn.

Medical Research Technician. Jack Rudman. 1994. (Career Examination Ser.: C-3352). pap. 34.95 (*0-8373-3352-0*) Nat Learn.

Medical Responsibility: Paternalism, Informed Consent & Euthanasia. Ed. by Wade L. Robison & Michael S. Pritchard. 1979. LC 79-87656. (Contemporary Issues in Biomedicine, Ethics & Society Ser.). 230p. 59.50 (*0-89603-007-5*) Humana.

Medical Review Criteria Guidelines for Managed Care. Margaret D. Bischel. 1997. (Illus.). 605p. ring bd. 495.00 (*1-893826-00-7*) Apollo Managed.

Medical Review Officer Handbook. Theodore F. Shults. 7th ed. Date not set. pap. text 125.00 (*0-9637094-4-5*) Quadrangle Res.

Medical Review Officer Handbook. Theodore F. Shults. Ed. by Jennifer Harrington. 7th ed. 1999. pap. text 125.00 (*0-9637094-7-X*) Quadrangle Res.

Medical Review Officer Manual: A Guide to Evaluating Urine Drug Analysis for Implementation of the Mandatory Guidelines for Federal Workplace Drug Testing Programs. 1991. lib. bdg. 69.75 (*0-8490-4341-7*) Gordon Pr.

Medical Review Officer's Guide to Drug Testing. Ed. by Robert B. Swotinsky. 1992. 272p. pap. 89.50 (*0-471-28445-9*, VNR) Wiley.

Medical Review Officer's Manual: MROCC's Guide to Drug Testing. Robert B. Swotinsky & Donna R. Smith. 1999. LC 99-12452. 213p. pap. text 45.00 (*1-883595-24-X*, 23053, OEM Pr) OEM Health.

Medical Revolution in Minnesota: A History of the University of Minnesota Medical School. Leonard G. Wilson. 1989. LC 88-29563. (Illus.). 612p. 55.00 (*0-9620884-0-4*) Midewiwin.

Medical Risk & the Right to an Informed Consent in Clinical Care & Clinical Research. Dennis J. Mazur. 1998. LC 98-86506. 183p. pap. 48.00 (*0-924674-64-4*) Am Coll Phys Execs.

Medical Risks: 1991 Compendium of Mortality & Morbidity. Ed. by Richard B. Singer et al. 1994. LC 94-18560. (Illus.). 344p. 125.00 (*0-275-94553-7*, Praeger Pubs) Greenwood.

Medical Risks: Trends in Mortality by Age & Time Elapsed Ed. by Edward A. Lew & Jerzy Gajewski. 1990. LC 90-7707. Set. 1512p. 195.00 (*0-275-93786-0*, C37860); Vol. 1. 368p. 195.00 (*0-275-93787-9*, C37861); Vol. 2. 368p. 195.00 (*0-275-93788-7*, C37862) Greenwood (Praeger Pubs).

Medical Savings Accounts: The Singapore Experience. Thomas A. Massaro & Yu-Ning Wong. 1996. 22p. pap. 10.00 (*1-56808-071-9*, 203) Natl Ctr Pol.

Medical School: Getting in, Staying in, Staying Human. Keith Russell Ablow. 7th rev. ed. 1990. 144p. pap. 14.95 (*0-312-04349-X*) St Martin.

Medical School Admission Requirements, 1997-98, United States & Canada. Ed. by Cynthia T. Bennett. 47th ed. 1996. xiii, 407p. (Orig.). pap. 20.00 (*1-57754-000-X*) Assn Am Med Coll.

Medical School Admission Requirements, 1998-99, United States & Canada. Ed. by Cynthia T. Bennett. 48th rev. ed. 1997. 416p. (C). pap. 25.00 (*1-57754-003-4*) Assn Am Med Coll.

Medical School Admission Requirements, 1999-2000, United States & Canada: United States & Canada, 1998-1999. Ed. by Kimberly S. Varner. 49th ed. 1998. xvi, 416p. pap. 25.00 (*1-57754-007-7*) Assn Am Med Coll.

Medical School Admission Requirements, United States & Canada, 2000-2001. Ed. by Kimberly S. Varner. 50th ed. 1999. (C). pap. 25.00 (*1-57754-011-5*) Assn Am Med Coll.

Medical School Admission Success. Stanley Zaslau. Ed. by Paul L. McGrath. 1995. 182p. pap. text 25.00 (*1-886468-04-4*) FMSG.

Medical School Admissions: The Insider's Guide. John A. Zebala et al. 5th rev. ed. 1999. LC 99-23877. 192p. pap. 14.95 (*0-914457-94-2*) Mustang Pub.

Medical School Companion. Mary M. Ross-Dolen. 1996. LC 96-202427. (Princeton Review Ser.). 178p. pap. 15.00 (*0-679-76462-3*) Villard Books.

Medical School Dean: Reflections & Directions. D. Kay Clawson & Emery A. Wilson. 1999. LC 99-60111. (Illus.). 256p. 21.95 (*0-913383-63-5*) McClanahan Pub.

Medical School Interview. Randall Zielinski. 1984. 18p. pap. 2.00 (*0-911899-00-6*) NAAHP Inc.

Medical School Is Born: A History of the Conception, Gestation & Infancy of the University of Kentucky College of Medicine. Robert Strauss. 1996. LC 96-77768. (Illus.). 224p. (C). 18.95 (*0-913383-48-1*) McClanahan Pub.

Medical Schools - Activities, Trends & Progress: Index of New Information with Authors, Subjects & Bibliography. Norbert G. Alden. 1993. 180p. 47.50 (*1-55914-804-7*); pap. 44.50 (*1-55914-805-5*) ABBE Pubs Assn.

Medical School's Mission & the Population's Health: Medical Education in Canada, the United Kingdom, the United States, & Australia. Ed. by K. L. White & J. E. Connelly. 1992. LC 96-. (Illus.). 281p. 79.00 (*0-387-97733-3*) Spr-Verlag.

***Medical School's Mission & the Population's Health: Medical Education in Canada, the United Kingdom, the United States, & Australia.** Ed. by Kerr L. White & Julia E. Connelly. 1992. (Illus.). xi, 281p. (C). pap. 9.50 (*0-387-97772-4*) Spr-Verlag.

Medical Science & Democratic Truth: Doctors & Revolution in Nepal. Vincanne Adams. 1998. LC 97-18016. (Cambridge Studies in Medical Anthropology: No. 6). (Illus.). 263p. (C). text 69.95 (*0-521-58486-8*); pap. text 24.95 (*0-521-58548-1*) Cambridge U Pr.

Medical Science Applies to Crime Mystery: Index of New Information. Henry H. Hetterman. rev. ed. 1997. 163p. 57.50 (*0-7883-1158-1*); pap. 47.50 (*0-7883-1159-X*) ABBE Pubs Assn.

Medical Science under Dictatorship. Leo Alexander. 1996. 32p. (Orig.). pap. 4.00 (*0-930429-03-6*) Bibliographic Pr.

Medical Sciences Knowledge Profile Examination (MSKP) Jack Rudman. (Admission Test Ser.: Vol. 86). 89.95 (*0-8373-5186-3*); 1994. pap. 69.95 (*0-8373-5086-7*) Nat Learn.

Medical Sciences 1998. Ed. by James G. Anderson & Meyer Katzper. 1998. 201p. 80.00 (*1-56555-138-9*) Soc Computer Sim.

Medical Secretary & Receptionists. Michael Drury. 6th ed. 1998. pap. text 21.00 (*0-7020-1643-8*) Harcourt.

Medical Secretary's & Assistant's Encyclopedic Dictionary. Leonard Karlin & Muriel S. Karlin. 1983. 241p. 19.95 (*0-13-572909-2*) P-H.

Medical Secretary's Handbook. Green. 1998. (C). pap. text 25.00 (*0-7020-2103-2*) Saunders.

Medical Secrets: Questions You Will Be Asked on Rounds, in the Clinic, on Oral Exams. Ed. by Anthony J. Zollo, Jr. 2nd rev. ed. 1996. LC 96-47625. (Secrets Ser.). (Illus.). 600p. pap. 39.00 (*1-56053-172-X*) Hanley & Belfus.

Medical Secrets: Spanish Edition. Anthony J. Zollo, Jr. 1993. (SPA.). 78.75 (*0-8016-7212-0*) Mosby Inc.

Medical Semiotics. Eugen Baer. Ed. by John Deely & Brooke Williams. 1988. (Sources in Semiotics Ser.: Vol. VII). (Illus.). 434p. (C). 72.00 (*0-8191-6705-3*) U Pr of Amer.

Medical Series. C. Richard Harper & H. Stacy Vereen. Ed. by Becky Dean et al. 1998. 24p. reprint ed. pap. 7.95 (*1-891726-15-3*) Aviation Info.

Medical Services & the Hospital in Britain, 1860-1939. Steven Cherry. 1996. (New Studies in Economic & Social History: No. 28). 106p. (C). text 39.95 (*0-521-57126-X*); pap. text 11.95 (*0-521-57784-5*) Cambridge U Pr.

Medical Services Market: Increasing Cost Constraints Put 20 Billion Dollar Business Up for Grabs. Market Intelligence Staff. 1992. 379p. (Orig.). 1295.00 (*1-56753-036-2*) Frost & Sullivan.

Medical Services Specialist. Jack Rudman. 1994. (Career Examination Ser.: C-2746). pap. 34.95 (*0-8373-2746-6*) Nat Learn.

Medical Side of Benjamin Franklin. William Pepper. 1970. (Illus.). 137p. reprint ed. 15.00 (*0-87266-039-7*) Argosy.

Medical Sign Language: Easily Understood Definitions of Commonly Used Medical, Dental & First Aid Terms. W. Joseph Garcia. 1983. (Illus.). 726p. 107.95 (*0-398-04805-3*); pap. 82.95 (*0-398-04806-1*) C C Thomas.

Medical Simulation for Word Processing. 1988. text 15.40 (*0-13-573015-5*, Macmillan Coll) P-H.

Medical Skills of Ancient Egypt. J. Worth Estes. 1989. LC 89-6004. 16.95 (*0-88135-093-1*); 1989. LC 89-6004. pap. 10.95 (*0-88135-099-0*); 1993. LC 93-16127. (Illus.). xv, 198p. pap. 15.95 (*0-88135-178-4*, Sci Hist) Watson Pub Intl.

Medical Social Work: The Pre-Professional Paradox. Toba S. Kerson. 1981. LC 80-23646. 320p. text 32.50 (*0-8290-0237-5*) Irvington.

Medical Social Work Coordinator. Jack Rudman. 1994. (Career Examination Ser.: C-2578). pap. 34.95 (*0-8373-2578-1*) Nat Learn.

Medical Social Worker. Jack Rudman. 1994. (Career Examination Ser.: C-521). pap. 29.95 (*0-8373-0521-7*) Nat Learn.

Medical Society of Copenhagen, 1772-1972. J. Genner. 1972. (Acta Historica Scientarium Ser.: No. 27). 345p. (Orig.). pap. (*87-7492-066-9*) Odense Univ.

Medical Sociologists at Work. Ed. by Ray H. Elling & M. Sokolowska. 1977. LC 76-6204. 347p. text 39.95 (*0-87855-139-5*) Transaction Pubs.

Medical Sociology. William C. Cockerham. 8th ed. 2000. LC 00-62322. (Illus.). 432p. 58.00 (*0-13-016557-3*) P-H.

Medical Sociology: A Comparative Perspective. Duane A. Matcha. 1999. LC 99-13142. (Illus.). 420p. (C). 65.00 (*0-205-26309-7*) Allyn.

Medical Solution to the Health Care Crisis. Julian Lieb. 1993. 129p. pap. 19.50 (*0-87527-512-5*) Green.

Medical Spanish. 1997. (Made Easy Ser.). pap. 9.99 (*0-9657083-0-6*) A B Anup.

Medical Spanish. Gail L. Bongiovanni. 3rd ed. 1999. LC 99-54045. (SPA., Illus.). 176p. pap. 24.95 (*0-07-134550-7*) McGraw-Hill Prof.

Medical Spanish: A Conversational Approach. Maria A. Di Lorenzo-Kearon. 1982. 256p. (Orig.). pap. 195.00 incl. audio (*0-88432-079-0*, AFMS20) J Norton Audio-Forum.

***Medical Spanish: A Conversational Approach.** Maria Dilorenzo Kearon & Thomas P. Kearon. 2nd ed. 2000. (ENG & SPA.). pap., stu. ed. (*0-03-026659-9*) Harcourt Coll Pubs.

Medical Spanish: An Instant Translator. Isam Nasr et al. 1996. LC 95-39974. (SPA., Illus.). 394p. pap. text 20.95 (*0-7216-6052-5*) Saunders.

Medical Spanish: Conversational Approach. Maria A. Kearon & Thomas P. Kearon. 1981. 256p. (C). pap. text 38.00 (*0-15-557880-4*) Harcourt Coll Pubs.

Medical Spanish: Interviewing the Latino Patient: A Cross-Cultural Perspective. Teresa Gonzalez-Lee & Harold J. Simon. 1990. LC 89-70896. (ENG & SPA.). 256p. (C). pap. text 76.00 incl. audio (*0-13-572512-7*, PH5127) P-H.

Medical Spanish: The Instant Survival Guide. Cynthia J. Wilber & Susan Lister. 3rd ed. 1995. LC 95-13931. 403p. spiral bd. 44.99 (*0-7506-9597-8*, Focal) Buttrwrth-Heinemann.

Medical Spanish in Pediatrics: An Instant Translator. Isam Nasr & Marco Cordero. 2000. LC 00-26970. xvii, 379p. pap. text (*0-7216-8447-5*) Saunders.

Medical Spanish Made Incredibly Easy. Lisa A. Atchley. 2000. LC 00-33880. (Made Incredibly Easy Ser.). (ENG & SPA., Illus.). v, 310p. 32.95 (*1-58255-040-9*) Springhouse Corp.

Medical Spanish Made Ridiculously Simple. Trudy Espinoza-Abrams. rev. ed. 2000. 106p. pap. text 12.95 (*0-940780-45-3*) MedMaster.

Medical Specialist. Jack Rudman. 1994. (Career Examination Ser.: C-1965). reprint ed. pap. 39.95 (*0-8373-1965-X*) Nat Learn.

Medical Specialist, Set. 1995. lib. bdg. 5005.99 (*0-8490-6652-2*); 1992. lib. bdg. 2995.95 (*0-8490-8874-7*) Gordon Pr.

Medical Speciality Selector: A Medical Speciality Referral Guide. Presley Reed. 1996. 200p. (Orig.). pap. text 65.00 (*1-889010-00-6*) Reed Grp Ltd.

Medical Specialization in Relation to Health Needs. 1985. 67p. pap. 8.00 (*92-890-1035-5*, 1340023) World Health.

MNO

Medical Speech Language Pathology. Alex F. Johnson & Barbara Jacobson. 1997. LC 97-41324. (Illus.). 672p. 79.00 (*0-86577-688-1*) Thieme Med Pubs.

Medical Speech-Language Pathology: A Practitioner's Guide. Alex F. Johnson & Barbara H. Jacobson. 1997. LC 97-41324. 75.00 (*3-13-110531-3*) Thieme Med Pubs.

Medical Staff: Legal Issues. Ed. by Michael M. Biehl & Cathleen S. Biehl. 1990. 136p. 30.00 (*0-918945-07-0*) Am Hlth Lawyers.

Medical Staff Credentialing: A Practical Guide. Fay Rozovsky et al. 1993. LC 93-33354. (Illus.). 120p. pap. 49.00 (*1-55648-112-8*, 145102) AHPI.

Medical Staff Handbook: A Guide to Joint Commission Standards. Joint Commission on Accreditation of Healthcare Organizations. 1999. (Illus.). 211p. pap. 50.00 (*0-86688-536-6*, MS-500) Joint Comm Hlthcare.

Medical Staff Leaders Practical Guide. Richard E. Thompson. 3rd rev. ed. 1995. 200p. pap. text 97.00 (*1-885829-28-0*) Opus Communs.

Medical Staff Management Forms, Policies, & Procedures for Health Care Providers. Ed. by Christine Mobley & Sheryl Deutsch. 1995. LC 94-49233. ring bd. 239.00 (*0-8342-0539-4*) Aspen Pub.

Medical Staff Peer Review: A Strategy for Motivation & Performance. Daniel A. Lang. 1991. LC 90-14532. 146p. (Orig.). pap. 42.50 (*1-55648-065-2*, 145157) AHPI.

***Medical Staff Peer Review: Motivation & Performance in the Era of Managed Care.** rev. ed. 2000. 308p. pap. 37.00 (*0-7879-5600-7*) Jossey-Bass.

Medical Staff Privileges. Lewis M. Levin. Ed. by Melanie C. Karaffa. 1992. 220p. (C). text 49.95 (*1-878487-36-1*, ME046) Practice Mgmt Info.

Medical Staff Privileges & Peer Review: A Legal Guide for Healthcare Professionals. Jonathan P. Tomes. 1994. LC 94-170692. 304p. (C). text 60.00 (*1-55738-603-X*, Irwn Prfssnl) McGraw-Hill Educ Grp.

Medical Statistics: A Commonsense Approach. Michael J. Campbell & David Machin. 3rd ed. 1999. LC 99-13004. (Illus.). 218p. pap. 34.95 (*0-471-98721-2*) Wiley.

Medical Statistics at a Glance. Avid Petrie & Caroline Sabin. 2000. LC 99-45806. (At a Glance Ser.). (Illus.). xxxi, 448p. (C). pap. 24.95 (*0-632-05075-6*) Blackwell Sci.

Medical Statistics from Graunt to Farr: Proceedings of the Royal College of Physicians of London, February, 1943. Royal College of Physicians of London Staff & Major Greenwood. Ed. by Barbara G. Rosenkrantz. 1977. LC 76-25665. (Public Health in America Ser.). (Illus.). reprint ed. lib. bdg. 18.95 (*0-405-09820-0*) Ayer.

Medical Statistics on Microcomputers. R. A. Brown & J. Swanson Beck. 1990. 103p. pap. text (*0-7279-0290-3*) BMJ Pub GBR. *Dist:* AIDC.

Medical Statistics on Personal Computers. Ed. by R. A. Brown & J. Swanson Beck. 2nd ed. 1994. 160p. pap. text (*0-7279-0771-9*) BMJ Pub GBR. *Dist:* AIDC.

Medical Stenographer. Jack Rudman. 1994. (Career Examination Ser.: C-1368). pap. 23.95 (*0-8373-1368-6*) Nat Learn.

Medical Stewardship: Fulfilling the Hippocratic Legacy. Ed. by M. Oliver Kepler. 1981. LC 80-25457. 280p. 77.00 (*0-313-22489-7*, KMS/, Greenwood Pr) Greenwood.

Medical Student USMLE Pts. II & III: Pearls of Wisdom. Scott H. Plantz et al. 1998. pap. 32.00 (*1-890369-10-1*) Boston Medical.

Medical Student's Desk Reference: 1999 Edition. Ken Bookstein. l.t. ed. 1999. 226p. (C). pap. 18.95 (*0-9660645-1-8*) Bookstein Pub.

Medical Student's Guide to Successful Residency Matching, 1994-1995. Lee T. Miller. 1994. (Illus.). 112p. 9.95 (*0-683-05996-3*) Lppncott W & W.

Medical Student's Guide to Top Board Scores. P. Thomas Rogers. 1994. (Illus.). 236p. (Orig.). (C). pap. text 24.95 (*0-9632231-0-0*) Innovat Pub & Graph.

Medical Student's Pocket Reference. Ken Bookstein. 1996. vi, 259p. pap. text 10.95 (*0-9660645-0-X*) Bookstein Pub.

Medical Student's Pocket Reference: 1999 Edition. Ken Bookstein. rev. ed. 1999. 322p. pap. 12.50 (*0-9660645-2-6*) Bookstein Pub.

Medical Studies of Aggression: Index of New Information. American Health Research Institute Staff. 1996. 150p. 57.50 (*0-7883-0922-6*); pap. 47.50 (*0-7883-0923-4*) ABBE Pubs Assn.

Medical Studies of Gunshot Wounds: Index of New Information with Authors, Subjects & References. American Health Research Institute Staff. 1996. 150p. 57.50 (*0-7883-0926-9*); pap. 47.50 (*0-7883-0927-7*) ABBE Pubs Assn.

Medical Studies of Hallucinogens: Index of Modern Authors & Subjects with Guide for Rapid Research. Salvatore A. Velazo. rev. ed. 1994. LC 94-24710. 150p. 57.50 (*0-7883-0452-6*); 139p. pap. 47.50 (*0-7883-0453-4*) ABBE Pubs Assn.

Medical Studies of Human Cadavers - Normal & Diseased: Index of New Information. American Health Research Institute Staff. 1996. 150p. 57.50 (*0-7883-0978-1*); pap. 47.50 (*0-7883-0979-X*) ABBE Pubs Assn.

Medical Studies of Polygraphs & Other Lie Detectors: Index of Modern Authors & Subjects with Guide for Rapid Research. Science and Life Consultants Association Staff. rev. ed. 1997. 193p. 57.50 (*0-7883-0944-7*); pap. 47.50 (*0-7883-0945-5*) ABBE Pubs Assn.

Medical Studies of Saliva: Index of Modern Authors & Subjects with Guide for Rapid Research. Larsen K. Lozzi. 1991. LC 90-56295. 160p. 47.50 (*1-55914-366-5*); pap. 44.50 (*1-55914-367-3*) ABBE Pubs Assn.

Medical Studies of Violence: Index of New Information. American Health Research Institute Staff. 1996. 150p. 57.50 (*0-7883-0920-X*); pap. 47.50 (*0-7883-0921-8*) ABBE Pubs Assn.

Medical Subject Analysis of a Selected Bibliography Concerning General Counseling. American Health Research Institute Staff. Ed. by John C. Bartone. rev. ed. 1994. LC 94-34597. 161p. 57.50 (*0-7883-0238-8*); pap. 47.50 (*0-7883-0239-6*) ABBE Pubs Assn.

Medical Supervision in Radiation Work. 1960. (Technical Report Ser.). 31p. pap. text 3.00 (*92-4-120196-7*) World Health.

Medical Supply Management after Natural Disaster. 1983. (Technical Publications: Vol. 443). 8.00 (*92-75-11438-2*) PAHO.

Medical Supply Technician. Jack Rudman. 1994. (Career Examination Ser.: C-3353). pap. 27.95 (*0-8373-3353-9*) Nat Learn.

Medical Support: Army Air Forces in World War II. Mae M. Link & Hubert A. Coleman. 1992. 1027p. pap. text (*0-912799-69-2*) AFH & MP.

Medical Support in Divisions, Separate Brigades, & Armored Cavalry Regiment. 1995. lib. bdg. 258.99 (*0-8490-6651-4*) Gordon Pr.

Medical, Surgical & Anesthetic Nursing for Veterinary Technicians. Ed. by P. W. Pratt. 2nd ed. 1994. LC 94-70822. 621p. 32.00 (*0-939674-49-1*) Am Vet Pubns.

Medical-Surgical Care Planning. Ed. by Nancy M. Holloway. 3rd ed. 1998. LC 98-17557. 896p. pap. 42.95 (*0-87434-925-7*) Springhouse Corp.

Medical-Surgical Nurse. Jack Rudman. 1994. (Certified Nurse Examination Ser.: CN-11). pap. 27.95 (*0-8373-6111-7*) Nat Learn.

Medical Surgical Nursing. Keegan. 1998. (Nursing Education Ser.). tchr. ed. 51.50 (*0-8273-7204-3*); stu. ed. 16.00 (*0-8273-7205-1*); text 65.95 (*0-8273-7203-5*) Delmar.

Medical Surgical Nursing. Reeves. 1998. 37.00 (*0-07-134657-0*) McGraw.

Medical-Surgical Nursing. Charlene Reeves et al. 1998. LC 98-20549. (McGraw-Hill Nursing Core Ser.). (Illus.). 600p. pap. 39.95 (*0-07-105480-4*) McGraw-Hill Prof.

Medical-Surgical Nursing. Paulette D. Rollant & Deborah A. Ennis. 1995. LC 95-24828. (Mosby's Review Ser.). (Illus.). 544p. (C). (gr. 13). pap. text 24.95 incl. 3.5 hd (*0-8151-7249-4*, 24862) Mosby Inc.

Medical Surgical Nursing. Jack Rudman. 1994. (Regents College Proficiency Examination Ser.: CPEP-24). pap. 23.95 (*0-8373-5424-2*) Nat Learn.

Medical-Surgical Nursing. Jack Rudman. 1994. (College Level Examination Ser.: CLEP-37). pap. 27.95 (*0-8373-5337-8*) Nat Learn.

Medical-Surgical Nursing. Marilyn S. Sommers. 1991. LC 91-4836. (Nursetest: A Review Ser.). 320p. pap. 21.95 (*0-87434-303-8*) Springhouse Corp.

Medical Surgical Nursing. Wilson. 2002. (C). pap. 18.00 net. (*0-7668-1381-9*); pap. 20.25 net. (*0-7668-1382-7*) Delmar.

Medical-Surgical Nursing. Susan Wilson & Steward Brown. 2002. pap. 58.50 net. (*0-7668-1378-9*) Delmar.

Medical-Surgical Nursing. Ignatavici. 2nd ed. 1994. (C). pap. text, stu. ed. 17.95 (*0-7216-4865-7*) Harcourt.

Medical-Surgical Nursing. Donna D. Ignatavici. 2nd ed. 1994. 76.00 (*0-7216-5908-X*) Saunders.

Medical-Surgical Nursing. Springhouse Publishing Company Staff. 2nd ed. 1999. LC 99-23705. (Nursetest Ser.). 352p. pap. 27.95 (*1-58255-003-4*) Springhouse Corp.

Medical-Surgical Nursing. Audree Reynolds. 2nd rev. ed. 1998. (Outline Ser.). (Illus.). 275p. (C). per. 22.95 (*1-56930-068-2*) Delmar.

Medical-Surgical Nursing. Mildred Boyd & Barbara Tower. 3rd ed. 1996. LC 96-29017. (Springhouse Notes Ser.). (Illus.). 416p. pap. 26.95 (*0-87434-861-7*) Springhouse Corp.

Medical-Surgical Nursing. Barbara C. Long. 3rd ed. 1992. 78.00 (*0-8016-7416-6*) Mosby Inc.

***Medical-Surgical Nursing**, Set. Joyce M. Black et al. 6th ed. 2001. (Illus.). 2240p. 85.00 (*0-7216-8197-2*) Saunders.

Medical-Surgical Nursing: A Nursing Process Approach. Ed. by Donna D. Ignatavicius et al. 2nd ed. 1995. (Illus.). (*0-7216-4866-5*); tchr. ed. (*0-7216-4864-9*) Saunders.

Medical-Surgical Nursing: A Nursing Process Approach. Donna D. Ignatavicius et al. 2nd ed. 1994. LC 94-14942. (Illus.). 2490p. text 74.00 (*0-7216-4863-0*) Saunders.

Medical-Surgical Nursing: A Nursing Process Approach. Barbara C. Long et al. 3rd ed. (Illus.). 1993. 1728p. tchr. ed. (*0-8151-4282-X*); 1993. 193p. pap. text, stu. ed. (*0-8016-7417-4*); 1992. LC 92-49614. 1728p. (C). (gr. 13). text 72.00 (*0-8016-6672-4*, 06672) Mosby Inc.

Medical-Surgical Nursing: A Nursing Process Approach. Barbara C. Long et al. 3rd ed. 1993. (Illus.). 1728p. (*84-8174-270-8*) Mosby-Doyma Libros ESP. *Dist:* Mosby Inc.

Medical-Surgical Nursing: Assessment & Management of Clinical Problems. Ed. by Sharon M. Lewis et al. 4th ed. 1995. LC 95-30732. (Illus.). 2176p. (C). (gr. 13). text 75.00 (*0-8151-5301-5*, 24617) Mosby Inc.

Medical-Surgical Nursing: Assessment & Management of Clinical Problems. Sharon M. Lewis et al. 4th ed. stu. ed. (*0-8151-5299-X*); 1996. (Illus.). 2176p. (C). (gr. 13). text 81.00 (*0-8151-5373-2*, 28963) Mosby Inc.

Medical-Surgical Nursing: Assessment & Management of Clinical Problems. Sharon Lewis et al. 4th ed. 1996. 368p. stu. ed. (*0-8151-5524-7*) Mosby Inc.

Medical-Surgical Nursing: Assessment & Management of Clinical Problems. Sharon M. Lewis et al. 5th ed. 1999. (Illus.). stu. ed. (*0-323-00258-7*); LC 99-23884. 2176p. (C). text 80.00 (*1-55664-430-2*) Mosby Inc.

***Medical-Surgical Nursing: Assessment & Management of Clinical Problems**, Set. Sharon M. Lewis et al. 5th ed. 2000. (Illus.). 85.00 (*0-323-01048-2*) Mosby Inc.

Medical-Surgical Nursing: Assessment & Management of Clinical Problems: Skidmore Drug Guide Package Sharon Lewis et al. 4th ed. 1996. (*0-323-00496-2*) Mosby Inc.

Medical-Surgical Nursing: Assessment & Management of Clinical Problems: Text & Skidmore Drug Guide Package. Sharon Lewis et al. 4th ed. 1996. (Illus.). (*0-323-00495-4*) Mosby Inc.

Medical-Surgical Nursing: Clinical Management for Continuity of Care. Joyce M. Black & Esther Matassarin-Jacobs. 5th ed. 1997. (Illus.). 2772p. pap., stu. ed. 18.95 (*0-7216-6950-6*); tchr. ed. (*0-7216-6400-8*) Saunders.

Medical-Surgical Nursing: Clinical Management for Continuity of Care. Joyce M. Black & Esther Matassarin-Jacobs. Ed. by Thomas Eoyang. 5th ed. 1997. LC 96-7419. (Illus.). 2395p. 75.00 (*0-7216-6399-0*) Saunders.

Medical-Surgical Nursing: Clinical Management for Continuity of Care, Test Manual. Joyce M. Black & Esther Matassarin-Jacobs. 5th ed. 1997. (Illus.). 2399p. (*0-7216-7086-5*) Saunders.

***Medical-Surgical Nursing: Clinical Management for Continuity of Care, ExaMaster.** Joyce M. Black & Esther Matassarin-Jacobs. 5th ed. 1997. (*0-7216-7085-7*) Saunders.

***Medical-Surgical Nursing: Clinical Management for Continuity of Care, Including Study Guide.** Joyce M. Black & Esther Matassarin-Jacobs. 1997. (Illus.). 5th ed. 87.00 (*0-7216-7570-0*); Set stu. ed. 92.00 (*0-7216-7571-9*) Saunders.

***Medical-Surgical Nursing: Clinical Management for Positive Outcomes.** Joyce Black et al. 6th ed. 2001. (Illus.). 576p. pap., stu. ed. 19.95 (*0-7216-9341-5*) Saunders.

Medical-Surgical Nursing: Concepts & Clinical Practice. Wilma J. Phipps et al. 5th ed. (Illus.). stu. ed. (*0-8016-8131-6*); 6th ed. 1998. stu. ed. (*0-323-00311-7*); 6th ed. 1998. LC 98-30558. (Illus.). xxiv, 2388p. text 80.00 (*0-323-00310-9*); Includes Testbank. 6th ed. 1998. (Illus.). 2336p. tchr. ed. (*0-323-00527-6*) Mosby Inc.

Medical-Surgical Nursing: Concepts & Clinical Practice: Text-Skidmore Drug Guide Package. Wilma J. Phipps et al. 6th ed. 1998. (Illus.). 2336p. (*0-323-00740-6*) Mosby Inc.

Medical-Surgical Nursing: Critical Thinking in Medical-Surgical Settings Lewis & Winningham. 1996. text 99.00 (*0-8151-4496-2*, 30630); 1995. text 93.00 (*0-8151-9672-5*, 29185) Mosby Inc.

Medical-Surgical Nursing: Diagnoses & Interventions. Ed. by Pamela L. Swearingen. 2nd ed. 1995. LC 95-42113. (Pocket Guide Ser.). 544p. (C). (gr. 13). pap. text 22.95 (*0-8151-8692-4*, 26103) Mosby Inc.

Medical-Surgical Nursing: Foundations for Clinical Practice. Ed. by Frances D. Monahan & Marianne Neighbors. 2nd ed. 1998. (Illus.). 2175p. tchr. ed. (*0-7216-7007-5*); pap. (*0-7216-7553-0*) Saunders.

Medical-Surgical Nursing: Foundations for Clinical Practice. Frances D. Monahan & Marianne Neighbors. Ed. by Barbara N. Cullen. 2nd ed. 1998. LC 96-51069. (Illus.). 2000p. text 72.95 (*0-7216-7006-7*) Saunders.

***Medical-Surgical Nursing: Foundations for Clinical Practice - ExaMaster.** Frances Donovan Monahan & Marianne Neighbors. 1998. (*0-7216-7008-3*) Saunders.

***Medical-Surgical Nursing: Review & Rationales.** Mary A. Hogan & Tomas M. Madayag. 2001. 512p. pap. 24.95 (*0-13-030457-3*) P-H.

Medical-Surgical Nursing: Total Patient Care. Gail Harkness & Judith R. Dincher. 9th ed. (Illus.). 1997. tchr. ed. (*0-8151-4182-3*); 1997. stu. ed., wbk. ed. (*0-8151-4594-2*); 1995. pap. text, wbk. ed. 19.95 (*0-8151-4183-1*) Mosby Inc.

Medical Surgical Nursing: Total Patient Care. Gail A. Harkness & Judith R. Dincher. 10th ed. 1998. (Illus.). 1312p. tchr. ed. (*0-323-00245-5*); 391p. wbk. ed. (*0-323-00246-3*); LC 98-46228. xvi, 1477p. (C). text 49.00 (*0-323-00247-1*) Mosby Inc.

Medical-Surgical Nursing: View Studies. Sharon M. Lewis. 4th ed. 1997. (C). (gr. 13). pap. text 150.00 (*0-8151-9523-0*, 29394) Mosby Inc.

***Medical-Surgical Nursing Across the Health Care Continuum.** Donna D. Ignatavicius et al. 3rd ed. 1999. (Illus.). 2232p. 85.00 (*0-7216-6980-8*) Saunders.

Medical-Surgical Nursing Across the Health Care Continuum. Donna D. Ignatavicius et al. Ed. by Robin Carter. 3rd ed. 1998. LC 98-38329. (Illus.). 2205p. (C). text 76.00 (*0-7216-6981-6*) Saunders.

Medical-Surgical Nursing Care Planning Guides. Susan P. Ulrich et al. Ed. by Barbara N. Cullen. 4th ed. 1998. LC 97-7514. 880p. pap. text 39.95 (*0-7216-6031-2*) Saunders.

Medical-Surgical Nursing Care Plans. Barbara Engram. 1993. LC 92-49864. 814p. (C). mass mkt. 38.25 (*0-8273-3413-3*) Delmar.

Medical-Surgical Nursing Care Plans: Nursing Diagnoses & Interventions. Marie S. Jaffe. 3rd ed. 1996. LC 95-4744. (Illus.). 456p. (C). pap. 47.00 (*0-8385-6263-9*, A6263-6) P-H.

Medical Surgical Nursing Clinical Handbook: Critical Thinking in Client Care. Susan Gauthier. 1996. LC 96-4741. 624p. (C). pap. text 27.19 (*0-8053-3522-6*) Addison-Wesley.

Medical Surgical Nursing CTB. Keegan. 1998. (Nursing Education Ser.). 52.50 (*0-8273-7206-X*) Delmar.

Medical Surgical Nursing Lab Manual. Gloria Hankins. 3rd ed. 1993. 336p. (C). pap. text 60.00 (*0-536-58369-2*) Pearson Custom.

Medical-Surgical Nursing Study Guide. Mary S. Nichols & Barbara W. Engam. 1987. (Illus.). 350p. pap. text 16.95 (*0-8016-3856-9*) Mosby Inc.

Medical-Surgical Policy & Procedure Guideline Manual. Diane I. Howery. 1991. stu. ed. 90.00 (*1-879575-15-9*) Acad Med Sys.

Medical-Surgical Supplies Market in Freestanding Outpatient Healthcare Delivery Centers. Ed. by Nal-Dutton Staff. 1987. (Marketing Research Reports). 1975.00 (*0-86621-863-7*, A1684) NAL.

Medical Surveillance for Hazardous Waste. Shirley Conibear. 1990. text (*0-442-31901-0*, VNR) Wiley.

Medical Surveillance of Populations for Health & Disease with Global Watch for Transmission & Infections: Index of New Information. Lester B. Ramsey. rev. ed. 1997. 149p. 57.50 (*0-7883-1628-1*); pap. 47.50 (*0-7883-1629-X*) ABBE Pubs Assn.

Medical Surveillance of Populations for Health & Disease with Global Watch for Transmission of Infections: Index of New Information. Lester B. Ramsey. 1996. 150p. 47.50 (*0-7883-0830-0*); pap. 47.50 (*0-7883-0831-9*) ABBE Pubs Assn.

Medical Surveillance Program. Mark M. Moran. 1992. (OSHA Written Compliance Programs Ser.: No. 19). (Illus.). 24p. ring bd. 169.00 (*1-890966-12-6*) SafetyCertified.

Medical Synonyms: Synonyme der Medizin. Martin E. Westarp & Hans P. Ditz. 1983. (GER.). 280p. 39.95 (*0-8288-1843-6*) Fr & Eur.

Medical Talk & Medical Work: The Liturgy of the Clinic. Paul Atkinson. 1995. 192p. 69.95 (*0-8039-7730-1*, 1207); pap. 24.95 (*0-8039-7731-X*, 1208) Sage.

Medical Teaching in Ambulatory Care: A Practical Guide. Warren Rubenstein & Yves Talbot. 1992. LC 91-5183. (Medical Education Ser.: Vol. 15). 144p. 27.95 (*0-8261-7690-9*) Springer Pub.

Medical Technical Assistant. Jack Rudman. 1994. (Career Examination Ser.: C-492). pap. 27.95 (*0-8373-0492-X*) Nat Learn.

Medical Technician. Jack Rudman. 1994. (Career Examination Ser.: C-512). pap. 29.95 (*0-8373-0512-8*) Nat Learn.

Medical Technician Instructor. Jack Rudman. 1994. (Career Examination Ser.: C-1370). pap. 39.95 (*0-8373-1370-8*) Nat Learn.

Medical Technician Trainee. Jack Rudman. 1994. (Career Examination Ser.: C-1371). pap. 27.95 (*0-8373-1371-6*) Nat Learn.

Medical Technologies & the Science of Progress: Index of New Information with Authors, Subjects, Research Categories & References. Science and Life Consultants Association Staff. 1997. 170p. 57.50 (*0-7883-1446-7*); pap. 47.50 (*0-7883-1447-5*) ABBE Pubs Assn.

Medical Technologist. Jack Rudman. 1994. (Career Examination Ser.: C-493). pap. 29.95 (*0-8373-0493-8*) Nat Learn.

Medical Technology. Lisa Yount. annot. ed. 1998. LC 97-17679. (Milestones in Discovery & Invention Ser.). (Illus.). 160p. (gr. 6-12). 19.95 (*0-8160-3568-7*) Facts on File.

Medical Technology: A Nursing Perspective. D. W. Hill & R. Summers. 1993. LC 93-40111. 204p. pap. 44.75 (*1-56593-229-3*, 0562) Singular Publishing.

Medical Technology: Emerging Markets for the 21st Century. Ed. by BioWorld Today Staff & BBI Editorial Staff. 2001. pap. 349.00 (*1-931107-03-3*) Am Health Consults.

Medical Technology: For Some Cardiac Pacemaker Leads, the Public Health Risks Are Still High. 1993. 52p. (Orig.). (C). pap. text 25.00 (*1-56806-907-3*) DIANE Pub.

Medical Technology: Inventing the Instruments. Robert Mulcahy. 1997. LC 96-4939. (Innovators Ser.). (Illus.). 144p. (YA). (gr. 5-12). lib. bdg. 21.95 (*1-881508-34-X*) Oliver Pr MN.

Medical Technology: Quality Assurance Needs Stronger Management Emphasis & Higher Priority. 1993. (Illus.). 100p. (Orig.). (C). pap. text 30.00 (*1-56806-330-X*) DIANE Pub.

Medical Technology & Society: An Interdisciplinary Perspective. Joseph Bronzino & Vincent K. Smith. 1990. (Sloan NLA Ser.). (Illus.). 580p. 80.00 (*0-262-02300-8*) MIT Pr.

Medical Technology & the Cost of the Medicare Program. 1992. lib. bdg. 288.00 (*0-8490-5478-8*) Gordon Pr.

Medical Technology Assessment: A Model for Informed Decision Making. Kathleen R. Ciccone & Thomas J. Chesnut. rev. ed. 1992. 100p. stu. ed. 100.00 (*0-915963-09-4*) Bader Assoc Inc.

Medical Technology Assessment Directory. Institute of Medicine Staff. 1988. 712p. text 250.00 (*0-309-03829-4*) Natl Acad Pr.

Medical Technology, Ethics & Economics. Joseph Bronzino et al. 1990. (C). text 46.00 net. (*0-07-008002-X*) McGraw.

Medical Technology Examination Review. Ali A. Hossaini et al. 1978. LC 78-1743. (Arco Medical Review Ser.). pap. text 12.00 (*0-668-04365-2*, Arc) Hungry Minds.

Medical Technology Examination Review & Study Guide. Anna P. Ciulla & Georganne K. Buescher. 2nd rev. ed. 1992. (Illus.). 512p. (C). pap., stu. ed. 42.51 (*0-8385-6310-4*, A6310-5) P-H.

Medical Technology for the Neonate. 1984. (Illus.). 119p. pap. text 30.00 (*0-910275-39-4*, TAR9-209) Assn Adv Med Instrn.

Medical Technology, Health Care, & the Consumer. Ed. by Allen D. Spiegel et al. 1981. LC 79-25559. 352p. 45.95 (*0-87705-498-3*, Kluwer Acad Hman Sci) Kluwer Academic.

Medical Terminology. Robert C. Anderson. 1992. 52p. (C). 13.95 incl. audio (*0-9634298-3-3*) Cricket Sci.

Medical Terminology. Nancy Scanlon. 1988. (C). pap. 17.80 (*0-13-572785-5*) P-H.

Medical Terminology. Peggy S. Stanfield. 1990. 560p. (Orig.). pap. 36.25 (*0-86720-409-5*) Jones & Bartlett.

Medical Terminology. 3rd ed. 1998. (C). 54.00 (*0-8087-9627-5*) Pearson Custom.

Medical Terminology. J. Patrick Fisher. 4th ed. 1993. pap. 20.00 (*0-02-800875-8*); pap. (*0-02-800877-4*); tchr. ed. (*0-02-800876-6*) Macmillan.

Medical Terminology. Genevieve L. Smith et al. 6th ed. 1991. text 35.75 (*0-8273-4563-1*) Delmar.

Medical Terminology. Smith. 7th ed. 1995. (C). pap. text 29.95 (*0-8273-6550-0*) Delmar.

Medical Terminology: A Programmed Approach. Genevieve L. Smith et al. 7th ed. 1994. LC 80-17970. (Illus.). 512p. mass mkt. 36.75 (*0-8273-6304-4*) Delmar.

Medical Terminology: A Programmed Systems Approach. Genevieve L. Smith et al. 8th ed. 1998. LC 98-24810. 560p. (C). spiral bd. 57.95 (*0-7668-0063-6*) Delmar.

Medical Terminology: A Programmed Systems Approach - IML. Smith & Davis. 1998. 176p. tchr. ed. 24.95 (*0-7668-0065-2*) Delmar.

Medical Terminology: A Programmed Systems Approach Text/Tape Package. Genevieve Love Smith et al. 8th ed. 1998. 560p. spiral bd. 69.95 incl. 3.5 hd (*0-7668-0117-9*) Delmar.

Medical Terminology: A Programmed Text. Smith. 7th ed. 1995. (Medical Terminology Ser.). 64.95 incl. disk (*0-8273-6919-0*) Delmar.

Medical Terminology: A Programmed Text. Smith et al. 7th ed. (RT-Medical Terminolgy Ser.). (C). 1995. 256p. text, tchr. ed. 20.00 (*0-8273-6918-2*); 1994. 480p. text 44.75 incl. audio (*0-8273-6917-4*) Delmar.

Medical Terminology: A Programmed Text, Testbank. Genevieve L. Smith et al. 6th ed. 1991. 64.95 (*0-8273-4567-4*) Delmar.

Medical Terminology: A Self-Learning Text. Jacqueline J. Birmingham. 3rd ed. 1999. LC 98-42213. xv, 570p. pap. text 31.95 (*0-323-00406-7*); tchr. ed. (*0-323-00456-3*) Mosby Inc.

Medical Terminology: A Short Course. Bruce A. Chabner. 1990. (Illus.). 240p. text 17.95 (*0-7216-2939-3*) Saunders.

Medical Terminology: A Short Course. Davi-Ellen Chabner. 1991. (Illus.). 238p. (C). pap. text, tchr. ed. (*0-7216-3508-3*) Saunders.

***Medical Terminology: A Short Course.** Davi-Ellen Chabner. 2nd ed. 1999. (Illus.). 316p. pap., tchr. ed. (*0-7216-8125-5*) Saunders.

Medical Terminology: A Short Course. Davi-Ellen Chabner. Ed. by Andrew Allan. 2nd ed. 1999. LC 98-48477. (Illus.). 316p. (C). text 18.95 (*0-7216-8124-7*) Saunders.

***Medical Terminology: A Student-Centered Approach.** Marie A. Moisio. 2002. 39.95 (*0-7668-1522-6*); 49.95 incl. audio (*0-7668-1526-9*) Delmar.

Medical Terminology: A Systems Approach. Barbara A. Gylys & Mary E. Wedding. 4th ed. 1999. (Illus.). 398p. 41.95 incl. cd-rom (*0-8036-0395-9*); 34.95 incl. audio (*0-8036-0396-7*); LC 98-48638. 31.95 (*0-8036-0394-0*) Davis Co.

Medical Terminology: A Text/Workbook. Alice V. Prendergast et al. 4th ed. 1996. LC 96-35083. 416p. (C). pap., wbk. ed. 46.00 (*0-8053-9368-4*) Addison-Wesley.

Medical Terminology: Activities. Wistreich. 1993. tchr. ed. 51.25 (*0-697-14743-6*, WCB McGr Hill) McGrw-H Hghr Educ.

Medical Terminology: An Anatomy & Physiology Systems Approach. Fremgen. 1997. 463p. pap. 55.33 incl. cd-rom (*0-8359-5274-6*) P-H.

***Medical Terminology: An Anatomy & Physiology Systems Approach.** Bonnie F. Fremgen & Suzanne Frucht. 2nd ed. 2001. LC 2001-46154. 640p. pap. 53.33 (*0-13-031182-0*) P-H.

Medical Terminology: An Illustrated Guide. Barbara Janson Cohen. 3rd ed. 1997. LC 97-4344. 592p. spiral bd. 37.95 (*0-7817-1411-7*) Lppncott W & W.

Medical Terminology: Building a Vocabulary. Nancy N. Scanlan. 1988. (Medical Ser.). 123p. (C). pap. 12.95 (*0-935920-57-9*, Ntl Pubs Blck) P-H.

Medical Terminology: Building Blocks for Health Careers. Kinn. 1989. pap., tchr. ed. 14.00 (*0-8273-3339-0*) Delmar.

Medical Terminology: Exercises in Etymology. Charles W. Dunmore & Rita M. Fleischer. 2nd ed. 1985. LC 85-4350. (Illus.). 305p. (C). pap. 29.95 (*0-8036-2946-X*) Davis Co.

Medical Terminology: Hsie. Smith. 1986. 13.00 (*0-12-650364-8*) Acad Pr.

Medical Terminology: Instructor's Activity & Resource Kit. Ann Ehrlich. 2nd ed. 1993. 221p. text, tchr. ed. 32.95 (*0-8273-5563-7*) Delmar.

Medical Terminology: Instructor's Guide. Wistreich. 1993. tchr. ed. 51.25 (*0-697-14243-4*, WCB McGr Hill) McGrw-H Hghr Educ.

Medical Terminology: Self-Directed Approach. Dale P. Layman. 1998. pap. 29.95 (*0-8273-5611-0*) Delmar.

Medical Terminology: The Language of Health Care. Margorie C. Willis. 1996. 550p. pap. text 36.95 (*0-683-09055-0*) Lppncott W & W.

Medical Terminology App. Smith. 1986. bds. 41.00 (*0-12-650362-1*) Harcourt.

Medical Terminology Challenge. Gladys Pucillo. 1995. (Medical Terminology Ser.). 79.95 (*0-8273-7430-5*, VNR) Wiley.

Medical Terminology Coloring Workbook. Date not set. (Illus.). (C). pap. text (*0-13-013934-3*) P-H.

Medical Terminology Companion Dictionary: For Stenotypists. George P. Andrews & Beverly L. Ritter. 1992. (Realtime Machine Shorthand Ser.). 69p. (C). pap. text 8.75 (*0-938643-29-0*, 543) Stenotype Educ.

Medical Terminology Essentials. Alice G. Ettinger & Pamala F. Burch. 1999. 26.95 (*0-7638-0303-0*) EMC-Paradigm.

Medical Terminology Essentials: Instructor's Guide. Alice G. Ettinger & Pamala F. Burch. 1999. 14.00 (*0-7638-0315-4*) EMC-Paradigm.

Medical Terminology Flash Cards. Ann Ehrlich. 1993. text 18.95 (*0-8273-5562-9*) Delmar.

Medical Terminology for Health Careers. Alice G. Ettinger & Pamala F. Burch. 1998. LC 98-9864. (*0-7638-0093-7*) Paradigm MN.

Medical Terminology for Health Careers. Alice G. Etttinger & Pamala F. Burch. 1999. 59.95 incl. cd-rom (*0-7638-0201-8*) EMC-Paradigm.

Medical Terminology for Health Professional. Ann Ehrlich. 1988. (Medical Terminology Ser.). 64.95 incl. 3.5 ld (*0-8273-3023-5*) Delmar.

Medical Terminology for Health Professionals. Ann Ehrlich. (Medical Terminology Ser.). 1988. pap., tchr. ed. 24.00 (*0-8273-3037-5*); 1988. pap. 25.95 (*0-8273-3036-7*); 3rd ed. 1997. 62.95 (*0-8273-7841-6*); 3rd ed. 1997. 244p. tchr. ed. 39.95 (*0-8273-7843-2*); 3rd ed. 1996. 176p. pap., tchr. ed. 24.95 (*0-8273-7842-4*) Delmar.

Medical Terminology for Health Professions. Ann Ehrlich. 2nd ed. 1993. LC 92-9897. 427p. text, tchr. ed. 24.00 (*0-8273-4976-9*); 2nd ed. 1993. LC 92-9897. 427p. 124.95 incl. audio (*0-8273-4979-3*); 2nd ed. 1992. LC 92-9897. 427p. text 35.95 (*0-8273-4975-0*); 2nd ed. 1992. LC 92-9897. 427p. text 62.95 (*0-8273-4977-7*); 3rd ed. 1997. 99.95 incl. audio (*0-8273-7840-8*); 3rd ed. 1996. 512p. (C). pap. 44.75 incl. audio (*0-8273-8212-X*) Delmar.

Medical Terminology for Health Professions. Ann Erlich. 3rd ed. 1996. LC 96-4882. (Medical Terminology Ser.). (Illus.). 528p. (C). mass mkt. 57.95 incl. disk (*0-8273-7839-4*) Delmar.

Medical Terminology for Health Professions. Ann Ehrlich. 4th ed. 2000. 544p. pap. 57.95 (*0-7668-1297-9*) Delmar.

Medical Terminology for Medical Students. William B. Tyrrell. 2nd ed. 1989. (Illus.). 202p. (C). pap. text 42.95 (*0-398-05550-5*) C C Thomas.

Medical Terminology for Stenotypists. Beverly L. Ritter & George P. Andrews. 1992. (Realtime Machine Shorthand Ser.). 189p. (C). pap. text, tchr. ed. 30.75 (*0-938643-54-1*, 651) Stenotype Educ.

Medical Terminology for Stenotypists: Anatomy & Physiology. Beverly L. Ritter & George P. Andrews. 1994. (Realtime Machine Shorthand Ser.). (Illus.). 675p. (C). pap. text 61.25 (*0-938643-27-4*, 451) Stenotype Educ.

Medical Terminology for the Allied Health Professional: An A & P Systems Approach. Bonnie F. Fremgen. 1996. LC 96-21729. 624p. pap. 42.00 (*0-8359-4991-5*) P-H.

Medical Terminology from Greek & Latin. Sandra R. Patterson & Lawrence S. Thompson. 1978. LC 77-93780. (GRE & LAT.). xii, 275p. reprint ed. pap. 25.00 (*0-87875-484-9*) Whitston Pub.

Medical Terminology in Action. George A. Wistreich. 1993. 624p. (C). pap. 60.94 (*0-697-10896-1*) McGrw-H Hghr Educ.

Medical Terminology Instructor's Guide. Genevieve L. Smith. 6th ed. 1991. pap., tchr. ed. 18.00 (*0-8273-4565-8*) Delmar.

Medical Terminology Made Comprehensible: Medizinische Fachsprache Verstaendlich Gemacht. Eduard Strauss & E. Ruediger. 1981. 94p. 19.95 (*0-8288-1853-3*) Fr & Eur.

Medical Terminology Made Easy. Jean T. Dennerll. 1997. 64p. text, tchr. ed. 14.00 (*0-8273-8137-9*); 1993. LC 92-48740. 296p. text 24.95 (*0-8273-5278-6*); 2nd ed. 1997. (C). 28.00 incl. audio (*0-8273-8139-5*) Delmar.

Medical Terminology Made Easy. Jean T. Dennerll & Genevieve L. Smith. 2nd ed. 1997. LC 97-21616. 336p. (C). pap. text 41.95 (*0-8273-8136-0*) Delmar.

Medical Terminology Made Incredibly Easy. Contrib. by Springhouse Corporation Staff. 2001. LC 00-41974. (Made Incredibly Easy Ser.). (Illus.). vi, 354p. 32.95 (*1-58255-041-7*) Springhouse Corp.

Medical Terminology Review Challenge. Mary E. Kinn. 1987. LC 86-24019. 168p. (C). (gr. 12). pap. 25.95 (*0-8273-2688-2*, 2688-2) Delmar.

Medical Terminology Simplified: A Programmed Learning Approach by Body Systems. Barbara A. Gylys. 2nd ed. 1998. (Illus.). 500p. pap. text 44.95 incl. audio compact disk (*0-8036-0345-2*) Davis Co.

Medical Terminology Simplified: A Programmed Learning Approach by Body Systems. Barbara A. Gylys & Regina M. Masters. 2nd ed. 1998. LC 97-43006. 506p. pap. 36.95 (*0-8036-0344-4*) Davis Co.

Medical Terminology with Human Anatomy: Instructor's Guide. Jane Rice. 4th ed. 1999. 240p. pap., tchr. ed. 29.20 (*0-8385-6291-4*, Medical Exam) Appleton & Lange.

Medical Terminology with Human Anatomy & Student Disk. Jane Rice. 4th ed. 1998. LC 98-15836. 696p. pap. 50.67 (*0-8385-6274-4*) P-H.

Medical Terms: Their Roots & Origins. A. R. Tindall. 1997. LC 97-26853. 230p. pap. (*90-265-1498-0*) Swets.

Medical Terms & Abbreviations. SPC Staff. 1997. LC 97-27804. (Healthcare Professional Guides: Vol. 1). (Illus.). 336p. spiral bd. 26.95 (*0-87434-911-7*) Springhouse Corp.

Medical Terms Made Easy. Dennerll. 1993. 25.95 incl. audio (*0-8273-5907-1*); text 36.95 incl. audio (*0-8273-5918-7*) Delmar.

Medical Testimony on Victims of Torture: A Physician's Guide to Political Asylum Cases. Nancy Arnison et al. 1991. 46p. pap. text 7.00 (*1-879707-02-0*) Phy Human Rights.

Medical Testing & Health Insurance. 1991. (Orig.). lib. bdg. 79.95 (*0-8490-4340-9*) Gordon Pr.

Medical Tests Sourcebook: Basic Consumer Health Information about Medical Test. Ed. by Joyce Shannon. 1999. LC 99-35456. (Health Reference Ser.). (Illus.). xv, 691p. lib. bdg. 78.00 (*0-7808-0243-8*) Omnigraphics Inc.

Medical Textiles for Implantation: Proceedings of the 3rd International ITV Conference on Biomaterials, Stuttgart, June 14-16, 1989. H. I. Planck et al. 1991. (Illus.). 357p. 119.00 (*0-387-52741-9*) Spr-Verlag.

Medical Theories in Hippocrates: Early Texts & the "Epidemics" Volker Langholf. 1990. (Untersuchungen zur Antiken Literatur und Geschichte Ser.: No. 34). vi, 285p. (C). lib. bdg. 127.70 (*3-11-011956-0*) De Gruyter.

Medical Therapeutics: A Pocket Companion. Eric B. Larson & Paul G. Ramsey. Ed. by Ray Kersey. 3rd ed. 1997. (Illus.). 720p. pap. text 29.95 (*0-7216-5126-7*) Saunders.

Medical Thinking. S. C. Schwartz & T. Griffin. 1986. (Contributions to Psychology & Medicine Ser.). (Illus.). 277p. 104.00 (*0-387-96315-4*) Spr-Verlag.

Medical Topography of Upper Canada. John Douglas. 1986. LC 85-14626. 9.95 (*0-88135-078-8*) Watson Pub Intl.

Medical Training in the European Community. Ed. by Commission of the European Communities. 1987. 96p. 52.80 (*0-387-17761-2*) Spr-Verlag.

Medical Transciptionist's Handbook - IML. Blake. 2nd ed. 1998. 96p. tchr. ed. 12.95 (*0-8273-8324-X*) Delmar.

Medical Transcribing Machine Operator. Jack Rudman. 1994. (Career Examination Ser.: C-3203). pap. 23.95 (*0-8373-3203-6*) Nat Learn.

Medical Transcription. Blanche Ettinger & Alice Ettinger. Ed. by Sheri Coalson et al. 1996. LC 96-33434. 472p. (C). pap., stu. ed. 29.95 (*1-56118-654-6*) Paradigm MN.

Medical Transcription. Blanche Ettinger & Alice G. Ettinger. 1997. (C). 272p. pap. text, tchr. ed. 14.00 (*1-56118-655-4*); stu. ed., ring bd. 150.00 incl. audio (*1-56118-656-2*) Paradigm MN.

Medical Transcription: Fundamentals & Practice. 2nd ed. 1999. (C). cd-rom 500.00 (*0-13-017965-5*) P-H.

Medical Transcription: Fundamentals & Practice. Sally Pitman et al. 2nd ed. 1999. LC 99-36720. 494p. pap. 51.00 (*0-13-013833-9*) P-H.

Medical Transcription & Terminology: An Integrated Approach. Florence Maloney & Lois Burns. 1996. LC 96-662. (Medical Assisting Ser.). (Illus.). 336p. (C). text 47.95 incl. disk (*0-8273-6374-5*) Delmar.

Medical Transcription at the Lexington Medical Group. J. Patrick Fisher & Dianne K. Frantz. 1990. 400p. text 28.55 (*0-02-685570-4*) Glencoe.

Medical Transcription Curriculum: MDT 1 Course. S. Turley. 1993. 524p. (C). ring bd. (*0-933195-47-8*) CA College Health Sci.

Medical Transcription for Health Information Managers. 1994. 98p. pap. text 60.00 incl. audio (*0-934385-59-9*) Hlth Prof Inst.

Medical Transcription Guide: Do's & Dont's. Marilyn Takahashi Fordney & Marcy O. Diehl. Ed. by Maureen Pfeiffer. 2nd ed. 1999. LC 98-28552. (Illus.). 635p. pap. text 46.25 (*0-7216-7650-2*) Saunders.

Medical Transcription Power Building: Student Key & Guide. Bruce Tennant. 1983. 90p. (gr. 10-12). pap. text 9.95 (*0-89420-222-7*, 470020) Natl Book.

Medical Transcription Power Building: Student Key & Guide. Bruce Tennant. 1983. 90p. pap. 111.95 incl. audio (*0-89420-224-3*, 470000) Natl Book.

Medical Transcription Self-Assessment. No. 1. 1995. 31p. stu. ed. 35.00 incl. audio (*0-935229-28-0*); No. 2. 1996. 27p. stu. ed. 35.00 incl. audio (*0-935229-30-2*, MTSA-2) Am Assoc Med.

Medical Transcription with Advanced Terminology. Lois R. Tutherly. 1987. LC 86-23962. 384p. (C). tchr. ed. 16.00 (*0-8273-2588-6*); pap. 36.95 (*0-8273-2587-8*) Delmar.

***Medical Transcription Workbook.** Health Professions Institute Staff. 2001. pap. 53.33 (*0-13-094089-5*) P-H.

Medical Transcriptionist's Handbook. Rachelle S. Blake. 1993. 352p. pap., tchr. ed. (*0-538-70678-3*) S-W Thomson.

Medical Transcriptionist's Handbook. Blake. 2nd ed. 1997. 112p. (C). mass mkt., wbk. ed. 9.25 (*0-8273-8323-1*) Delmar.

Medical Treason: Nurses on Drugs. Joyce E. Strom-Paikin. 1988. LC 89-60104. 311p. 21.95 (*0-88282-043-5*) New Horizon NJ.

Medical Treatment of Epilepsy. Ed. by Stanley R. Resor, Jr. & Henn Kutt. 1991. (Neurological Disease & Therapy Ser.: Vol. 10). (Illus.). 760p. text 255.00 (*0-8247-8549-5*) Dekker.

Medical Treatment of Self & Hypochondria: Index of Modern Authors & Subjects with Guide for Rapid Research. Samuel M. Morris. 1991. LC 90-56315. 160p. 47.50 (*1-55914-414-9*); pap. 44.50 (*1-55914-415-7*) ABBE Pubs Assn.

Medical Treatments of Foreign Objects: Invasions, Penetrations & Migrations in the Human Body Including Drug Smuggling in Body Cavities. Science and Life Consultants Association Staff. 1996. 150p. pap. 47.50 (*0-7883-1301-0*) ABBE Pubs Assn.

Medical Treatments of Foreign Objects: Invasions, Penetrations & Migrations in the Human Body Including Drug Smuggling in Body Cavities. Science and Life Consultants Staff. 1996. 150p. 57.50 (*0-7883-1300-2*) ABBE Pubs Assn.

Medical Triangle: Physicians, Politicians, & the Public. Eli Ginzberg. 1992. 328p. (C). pap. 18.50 (*0-674-56326-3*); 1990. 360p. 34.50 (*0-674-56325-5*) HUP.

Medical Trivia. James M. Navratil. 1998. LC 86-82986. 200p. 12.50 (*0-937557-06-4*) Litarvan Lit.

Medical Typewriting. Patsy C. Smith. 2nd ed. 1983. (Illus.). 128p. text 17.12 (*0-07-058925-9*) McGraw.

Medical Typing & Transcribing: Techniques & Procedures. Marcy O. Diehl & Marilyn Takahashi Fordney. 2nd ed. 1984. (Illus.). 450p. tchr. ed. 7.50 (*0-7216-2009-4*) Saunders.

Medical Typing & Transcribing: Techniques & Procedures. Mary O. Diehl & Marilyn Takahashi Fordney. 3rd ed. 1991. (Illus.). pap., tchr. ed. (*0-7216-3736-1*) Saunders.

Medical Typing Practice. Kathleen B. Root & Edward E. Byers. 2nd ed. 1967. (gr. 9-12). text 37.74 net. (*0-07-053585-X*) McGraw.

Medical Use of Snake Venom Proteins. Ed. by Kurt F. Stocker. 1990. 280p. 210.00 (*0-8493-5846-9*, RM666) CRC Pr.

Medical Uses of Anti-Oxidants for Cancer Prevention: Index of New Information with Authors, Subjects & Bibliography. American Health Research Institute Staff. 1995. LC 95-16102. 57.50 (*0-7883-0470-4*); pap. 47.50 (*0-7883-0471-2*) ABBE Pubs Assn.

Medical Uses of Ionizing Radiation & Radioisotopes. Joint EAEA-WHO Expert Committee. 1972. (Technical Reports: No. 492). 56p. pap. text 4.00 (*92-4-120492-3*, 1100492) World Health.

Medical Uses of Statistics. Ed. by John C. Bailar, III & Frederick Mosteller. 2nd ed. 1992. (Illus.). 480p. text 65.00 (*0-910133-36-0*) Dekker.

Medical Uses of Television As a Media for Health, Dangers, News, Advertising & Brain-Washing: Index of New Information for World Review. John C. Bartone. 1997. (Illus.). 160p. 57.50 (*0-7883-1396-7*); pap. 47.50 (*0-7883-1397-5*) ABBE Pubs Assn.

Medical Value of Psychoanalysis. Franz Gabriel Alexander. Ed. by Chicago Institute for Psychoanalysis Staff. 1985. LC 84-22475. (Classics in Psychoanalysis Monographs: No. 2). vi, 278p. 42.50 (*0-8236-3285-7*, BN03285) Intl Univs Pr.

Medical Virology. David O. White & Frank Fenner. 4th ed. 1994. LC 93-48068. (Illus.). 603p. text 67.00 (*0-12-746642-8*) Acad Pr.

Medical Virology. Morag C. Timbury. 9th ed. 1991. (Illus.). 196p. pap. text (*0-443-04148-2*) Church.

M N O

Medical Virology, No. 8. Ed. by Luis M. De la Maza & E. M. Peterson. 1989. (Illus.). 342p. 85.00 (*0-306-43361-3*, Plenum Trade) Perseus Pubng.

Medical Virology, No. 9. Ed. by L. M. De la Meza & E. M. Peterson. 1990. LC 89-657524. (Illus.). 270p. 85.00 (*0-306-43700-7*, Plenum Trade) Perseus Pubng.

Medical Virology, Vol. 10. Ed. by Luis M. De la Maza & E. M. Peterson. 1991. (Illus.). 312p. (C). text 114.00 (*0-306-44010-5*, Kluwer Plenum) Kluwer Academic.

Medical Visits to Medicare Patients: Physician Coding Practice. Sally Trude. 1992. LC 92-9017. pap. 7.50 (*0-8330-1224-X*, R-4055-HCFA) Rand Corp.

Medical Warrior: Fighting Corporate Socialized Medicine. Miguel A. Faria, Jr. 1997. LC 97-72144. 207p. (Orig.). pap. 23.95 (*0-9641077-2-4*) Hacienda Pub.

Medical Waste Disposal. Calvin R. Brunner. 1996. LC 95-95256. (Illus.). 560p. (C). text 150.00 (*0-9621774-1-5*) Incinerat Consults.

Medical Waste Management & Disposable Markets: Regulations, Regulations & More Regulations Promote Rapid Technological Innovations. Market Intelligence Staff. 1992. 315p. 1895.00 (*1-56753-382-5*) Frost & Sullivan.

Medical Waste Management & Disposal. U. S. Environmental Protection Agency Staff et al. 1991. LC 90-23201. (Pollution Technology Review Ser.: No. 200). (Illus.). 541p. 125.00 (*0-8155-1264-3*) Noyes.

Medical Waste Management & Disposal Markets. Ed. by Frost and Sullivan Staff. 1997. 343p. spiral bd. 2450.00 (*0-7889-0694-1*, 5401-15) Frost & Sullivan.

Medical Waste Tracking Act of 1988: A Legislative History of Public Law 100-582, Set. Ed. by Bernard D. Reams. 1993. LC 93-78606. (Federal Health Law Ser.: Part 8). 4068p. 395.00 (*0-89941-848-1*, 307940) W S Hein.

Medical Wit & Humor: Index of Modern Writings. Mary R. Bartone. 1995. LC 95-16708. 57.50 (*0-7883-0480-1*) ABBE Pubs Assn.

Medical Wit & Wisdom: The Best Medical Quotations from Hippocrates to Groucho Marx. Ed. by Jess M. Brallier. 1993. LC 93-83465. (Illus.). 288p. 15.95 (*1-56138-289-2*) Running Pr.

Medical Word Book. Sheila Sloane-Dusseau. (Illus.). 3rd ed. 1990. 1168p. pap. text 41.00 (*0-7216-3243-2*); 4th ed. 1999. LC 2001-20706. xii, 1501p. pap. text 34.95 (*0-7216-7626-X*) Saunders.

Medical Word Building. Park-Davis and Company Staff. 1970. 125p. pap. 19.95 (*0-87489-043-8*) Practice Mgmt Info.

Medical Word Finder: A Reverse Medical Dictionary. Betty Hamilton & Barbara Guidos. 1987. LC 86-28462. 177p. text 49.95 (*1-55570-011-X*) Neal-Schuman.

Medical Word Processing Simulation. Linda F. Klafehn & Marilyn G. Fowler. 1985. (Word Processing Ser.). 117p. text 19.50 (*0-471-88528-2*) P-H.

Medical Work in America. Eliot Freidson. 1989. LC 89-5448. 304p. (C). pap. 25.00 (*0-300-04158-6*) Yale U Pr.

Medical Work, Medical Knowledge & Health Care: A Reader. Ed. by Ellen Annandale et al. 2000. 360p. pap. 29.95 (*0-631-22327-4*) Blackwell Pubs.

Medical Works of Richard Mead. Richard Mead. LC 75-23740. reprint ed. 94.50 (*0-404-13550-1*) AMS Pr.

Medical World of Early Modern France. Laurence Brockliss & Colin Jones. 1997. LC 96-33516. (Illus.). 982p. text 150.00 (*0-19-822750-7*) OUP.

Medical Writing: A Prescription for Clarity. Neville W. Goodman & Martin B. Edwards. 2nd ed. 1997. LC 95-51694. (Illus.). 239p. (C). pap. text 31.95 (*0-521-49876-7*) Cambridge U Pr.

Medical Writing & Communicating. John J. Gartland. 1992. 250p. 39.00 (*1-55572-018-8*) Univ Pub Group.

Medical Writing in Drug Development: A Practical Guide for Pharmaceutical Research. Robert J. Bonk. 1998. LC 97-18243. (Illus.). 139p. (C). 42.00 (*0-7890-0174-8*); pap. 19.95 (*0-7890-0449-6*) Haworth Pr (Pharmctl Prods).

Medical X-Ray Electron Beam & Gamma-Ray Protection for Energies up to 50 MeV: Equipment Design, Performance & Use. 1989. LC 89-2975. (Report Ser.: No. 102). 139p. (Orig.). pap. text 45.00 (*0-929600-03-7*) NCRP Pubns.

Medical X-Ray Techniques in Diagnostic Radiology. G. J. Van der Plaats. 1979. lib. bdg. 79.50 (*90-247-2155-5*) Kluwer Academic.

Medicalese: A Humorous Medical Dictionary. Peter K. Meyer. Ed. by Catherine Graves. 1994. LC 93-74044. (Illus.). 96p. (Orig.). pap. 9.95 (*0-9628186-1-5*) Avian Cetacean.

Medicalization of Obstetrics: Personnel, Practice, & Instruments. Ed. by Philip K. Wilson. 1996. LC 96-794. (Childbirth Ser.: Vol. 2). (Illus.). 424p. reprint ed. text 88.00 (*0-8153-2231-3*) Garland.

Medicalized Motherhood: Perspectives from the Lives of African American & Jewish Women. Jacquelyn S. Litt. 2000. LC 99-43560. xi, 189p. text 50.00 (*0-8135-2781-3*) Rutgers U Pr.

Medically Assisted Conception: An Agenda for Research. Institute of Medicine Staff. 1989. 370p. pap. text 29.00 (*0-309-04128-7*) Natl Acad Pr.

Medically Complex Child: The Transition to Home Care. N. J. Hochstadt & D. Yost. 1991. xix, 323p. text 69.00 (*3-7186-0520-1*, Harwood Acad Pubs) Gordon & Breach.

Medically Complex Child: The Transition to Home Care. N. Hochstadt & D. Yost. 1991. xix, 323p. pap. text 43.00 (*3-7186-0521-X*) Gordon & Breach.

Medically Important Fungi: A Guide to Identification. Ed. by Davise H. Larone. 3rd ed. 1995. LC 94-40202. (Illus.). 274p. 59.95 (*1-55581-091-8*) ASM Pr.

Medically Important Insects & Arachnids. Ed. by Richard P. Lane & Roger W. Crosskey. 1993. (Illus.). 576p. (C). (gr. 13). pap. text 239.95 (*0-412-40000-6*, A9482) Chapman & Hall.

Medically Refractory Rest Angina. Ed. by Douglass Andrew Morrison & Patrick W. Serruys. 1992. (Illus.). 480p. text 190.00 (*0-8247-8630-0*) Dekker.

Medical/Surgical Nursing: An Integrated Approach. Duncan White. 1997. (LPN/LVN Nursing Ser.). 128p. pap. text, tchr. ed. 16.95 (*0-8273-7680-4*) Delmar.

Medical/Surgical Nursing: An Integrated Approach. Lois White & Gena Duncan. 1997. LC 97-17371. (LPN/LVN Nursing Ser.). 1162p. (C). 71.95 (*0-8273-6371-0*) Delmar.

Medicamentos Indigenas. Ed. by Maria E. Alvarez del Real. 1988. (SPA., Illus.). 448p. pap. 4.00 (*0-944499-42-2*) Editorial Amer.

Medicaments et Aliments, Approche Ethnopharmacologique (Medicines & Foods, Ethnopharmacological Approach) E. Schroder et al. 1996. (ENG & FRE.). 418p. pap. (*2-7099-1320-8*) LInstitut Francais FRA. *Dist:* Balogh.

Medicare: 85 Commonly Asked Questions. rev. ed. 1996. 28p. (C). pap. text 15.00 (*0-7881-2691-1*) DIANE Pub.

Medicare: A Handbook in the History & Issues of Health Care Services for the Elderly. Ed. by William A. Pearman & Phillip Starr. 1988. LC 88-2423. 166p. text 10.00 (*0-8240-8391-1*) Garland.

Medicare: Advancing Towards the 21st Century, 1966-1996. Ed. by Linda F. Wolf. 1997. (Illus.). 237p. (Orig.). (C). pap. text 50.00 (*0-7881-4495-2*) DIANE Pub.

Medicare: Increased HMO Oversight Could Improve Quality & Access to Care. 1996. (Illus.). 44p. reprint ed. pap. text 20.00 (*0-7881-3211-3*) DIANE Pub.

***Medicare & Choice: An Examination of the Risk Adjuster: Congressional Hearing.** Ed. by Michael Bilirakis. 2001. 117p. (C). reprint ed. pap. text 25.00 (*0-7567-1633-0*) DIANE Pub.

***Medicare & Choice: Plan Withdrawals Indicate Difficulty of Providing Choice While Achieving Savings.** William J. Scanlon. 2001. (Illus.). 67p. (C). pap. text 25.00 (*0-7567-0893-1*) DIANE Pub.

Medicare & Choice Interim Final Rule: Regulations Effective July 27, 1998 Including CCH Executive Summary & Medicare & Choice Provisions from the Balanced Budget Act of 1997. CCH Editorial Staff. 1998. (Health Law Professional Ser.). 320p. pap. 49.95 (*0-8080-0283-X*) CCH INC.

Medicare & Coding for Ophthalmology. Robert D. Keene. 2000. 245p. pap. 145.00 (*1-58383-084-7*) Robert D Keene.

Medicare & Graduate Medical Education. James Baumgardner. 1995. (Illus.). 49p. (Orig.). (C). pap. text 25.00 (*0-7881-2559-1*) DIANE Pub.

***Medicare & Medicaid: Implementing State Demonstrations for Dual Eligibles Has Proven Challenging.** Ed. by Kathryn G. Allen & Walter Ochinko. 2001. 51p. (C). pap. 25.00 (*0-7567-0900-8*) DIANE Pub.

Medicare & Medicaid: The 1965 & 1967 Social Security Amendments. Margaret Greenfield. 1983. LC 82-25157. 143p. reprint ed. lib. bdg. 59.50 (*0-313-23841-3*, GRME, Greenwood Pr) Greenwood.

Medicare & Medicaid Claims & Procedures Harvey L. McCormick. 1986. LC 86-9150. 1440p. text (*0-314-97401-6*) West Pub.

Medicare & Medicaid Data Book. 1990. lib. bdg. 600.00 (*0-8490-4047-7*) Gordon Pr.

Medicare & Medicaid Laws & Regulations: Vol. 1: Medicare & Medicaid Laws; Vol. 2: Medicare & Medicaid Regulations, Vol. 2. 1997. 2700p. pap. 145.00 (*0-8080-0196-5*, 5472) CCH INC.

Medicare & Medicaid Laws & Regulations As of August 20, 1998, Set. CCH Inc. Staff. 1998. (Vol. 1: Laws Ser.). 2958p. pap. 150.00 (*0-8080-0289-9*) CCH INC.

Medicare & Medicaid Laws & Regulations As of January 1, 2000 CCH Editorial Staff. 2000. 2650p. pap. text 160.00 (*0-8080-0462-X*) CCH INC.

Medicare & Medicaid Managed Care: A Strategic Guide to Serving Dually Eligible Persons Throughout the Continuum. Catholic Health Association of the United States Staff. 1998. LC 98-221767. (Mission in Action Ser.). xv, 131 p. pap. 40.00 (*0-87125-244-9*) Cath Health.

Medicare & Medicaid Patient & Program Protection Act of 1987: A Legislative History of Pub. Law No. 98-507, Set. Ed. by Bernard D. Reams. 1990. LC 89-83920. (Federal Health Law Ser.: Part 5). 1932p. lib. bdg. 185.00 (*0-89941-695-0*, 305960) W S Hein.

***Medicare & Medicaid, Statistical Supplement (2000)** Earl Hoffman. Ed. by Linda F. Wolf. 2001. (Illus.). 348p. (C). pap. text 50.00 (*0-7567-1549-0*) DIANE Pub.

Medicare & Private Sector Health Care Quality Measurement, Assurance, & Improvement: Hearing Before the Subcommittee on Health of the Committee on Ways & Means, House of Representatives, One Hundred Fourth Congress, First Session, March 21, 1995. U. S. Congress, House Committee on Ways and Means, Subcommittee on Health. 1997. LC 97-153835. (Illus.). (*0-16-053976-5*) USGPO.

Medicare & the American Health Care System: Report to the Congress. Donald A. Young et al. 1997. (Illus.). 152p. pap. text 35.00 (*0-7881-4676-9*) DIANE Pub.

Medicare & You: 2000. Frwd. by Donna E. Shalala & Nancy-Ann M. DeParle. rev. ed. 2000. (Illus.). 51p. 15.00 (*0-7567-0082-5*) DIANE Pub.

***Medicare & You, 2001.** Frwd. by Donna E. Shalala & Nancy-Ann M. DeParle. 2001. 73p. (C). pap. text (*0-7567-1091-X*) DIANE Pub.

Medicare Answer Book. Connacht Cash. 304p. 2nd ed. 1998. LC 98-65682. pap. 19.95 (*0-9633145-4-8*); 3rd ed. 1999. LC 99-89280. pap. 19.95 (*0-9633145-5-6*) Race Pt Pr.

Medicare at Risk: Emerging Fraud in Medicare Programs: Congressional Hearing. Ed. by Susan M. Collins. 2000. 326p. (C). reprint ed. pap. text 40.00 (*0-7881-8773-2*) DIANE Pub.

Medicare Benefits for Recipients Living in Mexico: Proceedings of a Conference. Policy Research Project Staff. 1999. (U. S. - Mexican Occasional Paper Ser.: Vol. 8). 166p. pap. 20.00 (*0-89940-580-0*) LBJ Sch Pub Aff.

***Medicare Billing Guide 2001.** Ingenix, Inc. Staff. pap. 99.95 (*1-56337-319-X*) Ingenix Inc.

Medicare Billing Guide 2000. Medicode, Med-Index Division Staff. 2000. (C). 80.00 (*1-56337-328-9*) Thomson Learn.

Medicare Claims Management for Home Health Agencies. Andrea L. Dumat. 1999. LC 98-32279. ring bd. 179.00 (*0-8342-1220-X*, 1220X) Aspen Pub.

***Medicare Compliance Manual 2001.** annuals James Davis & Maxine Lewis. 2001. 1000p. ring bd. 129.95 (*1-57066-198-7*, 21047) Practice Mgmt Info.

Medicare Compliance Manual 2000. annuals James B. Davis & Maxine Lewis. Ed. by James B. Davis & Maxine Lewis. rev. ed. 2000. (Illus.). 956p. ring bd. 129.95 (*1-57066-168-5*, 20047) Practice Mgmt Info.

Medicare Computer Systems: Year 2000 Challenges Put Benefits & Services in Jeopardy. Ed. by Mark E. Heatwole. 1999. (Illus.). 49p. (C). pap. text 20.00 (*0-7881-7644-7*) DIANE Pub.

Medicare Contractors: Despite Its Efforts, H C F A Cannot Ensure Their Effectiveness or Integrity. Ed. by Richard L. Hembra. 1999. 80p. (C). pap. text 20.00 (*0-7881-8464-4*) DIANE Pub.

Medicare Fraud & Abuse: Congressional Hearing. Ed. by Bob Packwood. 1999. 108p. (C). reprint ed. pap. text 25.00 (*0-7881-8090-8*) DIANE Pub.

Medicare Fraud & Abuse: Understanding the Law. National Health Lawyers Association Staff et al. 1986. LC 86-61317. 300p. 36.00 (*0-918945-01-1*) Am Hlth Lawyers.

Medicare Fraud Prevention & Enforcement Efforts: Congressional Hearing. Ed. by Susan Collins. 2000. 51p. pap. text 20.00 (*0-7567-0277-1*); (C). pap. text 20.00 (*0-7567-0299-2*) DIANE Pub.

***Medicare Fraud Prevention, The Medicare Enrollment Process: Congressional Hearing.** Ed. by Susan M. Collins. 2001. (Illus.). 254p. (C). reprint ed. pap. 35.00 (*0-7567-0292-5*) DIANE Pub.

Medicare Handbook: 1994 Edition. 1994. lib. bdg. 255.95 (*0-8490-9037-7*) Gordon Pr.

Medicare Handbook: Complete Guide to Medicare Hospital & Medical Insurance Eligibility, Claims & Appeal. 1991. lib. bdg. 300.00 (*0-8490-5156-8*) Gordon Pr.

***Medicare Handbook 2001.** Judith Stein & Alfred J. Chipin. 2001. pap. 125.00 (*0-7355-2365-7*) Aspen Pub.

Medicare HMO Payment Policies: Hearing Before the Subcommittee on Health of the Committee on Ways & Means, House of Representatives, One Hundred Fifth Congress, First Session, February 25, 1997. Contrib. by U. S. Congress, House Committee on Ways and Means, Subcommittee on Health. 1997. LC 98-133431. (Illus.). (*0-16-055956-1*) USGPO.

Medicare HMO's: HCFA Can Promptly Eliminate Hundreds of Millions in Excess Payments. Jonathan Ratner. 1998. (Illus.). 58p. pap. text 20.00 (*0-7881-4762-5*) DIANE Pub.

Medicare HMOs: Making Them Work for the Chronically Ill. Richard Kronick & Joy De Beyer. 1998. LC 98-40045. 238p. 44.00 (*1-56793-091-3*) Health Admin Pr.

Medicare HMOs: Potential Effects of a Limited Enrollment Period Policy. 1997. (Illus.). 48p. pap. text 30.00 (*1-57979-225-1*) DIANE Pub.

Medicare HMOs: Rapid Enrollment Growth Concentrated in Selected States. 1996. (Illus.). 39p. (Orig.). pap. text 20.00 (*0-7881-3207-5*) DIANE Pub.

Medicare Home Health: Hearing Before the Subcommittee on Oversight & Investigations of the Committee on Commerce, House of Representatives, 105th Congress, 1st Session, October 29, 1997. USGPO Staff. 1998. LC 98-152312. iii, 130p. pap. (*0-16-056111-6*) USGPO.

Medicare Home Health Agencies: Certification Process Ineffective in Excluding Problem Agencies. Ed. by William J. Scanlon. 1999. 48p. pap. text 20.00 (*0-7881-7891-1*) DIANE Pub.

Medicare Home Health Agencies: Closures Continue, with Little Evidence Beneficiary Access Is Impaired. Ed. by William J. Scanlon. 2000. (Illus.). 54p. (C). pap. text 20.00 (*0-7881-8893-3*) DIANE Pub.

Medicare Home Health Care: Hearing Before the Subcommittee on Health & Environment of the Committee on Commerce, House of Representatives, One Hundred Fifth Congress, First Session, March 5, 1997. Contrib. by U. S. Congress, House Committee on Commerce, Subcommittee on Health and the Environment. 1997. LC 97-187350. (Illus.). (*0-16-055056-4*) USGPO.

Medicare Home Health Care: Prospective Payment System Will Need Refinement As Data Become Available. William J. Scanlon. 2000. 51p. (C). pap. text 20.00 (*0-7567-0297-6*) DIANE Pub.

***Medicare Improper Payments: While enhancements Hold Promise for Measuring Potential Fraud & Abuse, Challenges Remain.** Kay Daly & Jim Kernen. 2001. 51p. (C). pap. 25.00 (*0-7567-0896-6*) DIANE Pub.

Medicare Made Easy. Charles B. Inlander. 3rd ed. 1992. pap. 13.41 (*0-201-63219-5*) Addison-Wesley.

Medicare Made Easy: Everything You Need to Know to Make Medicare. Charles B. Inlander. 1989. pap. 10.53 (*0-201-17269-0*) Addison-Wesley.

Medicare Made Easy: Everything You Need to Know to Make Medicare Work for You. Charles B. Inlander. 1991. pap. 11.95 (*0-201-57089-0*) Addison-Wesley.

Medicare Made Simple: A Consumer's Guide to the Medicare Program. Denise L. Knaus. Ed. by Kathryn Swanson & Maureen Lynch. 1996. 450p. (Orig.). pap. 12.95 (*1-885987-00-5*, ME070, Health Info Pr) Practice Mgmt Info.

Medicare Managed Care: Securing Beneficiary Protections. Geraldine Dallek. 1998. (Illus.). 66p. pap. text 25.00 (*0-7881-7079-1*) DIANE Pub.

Medicare Managed Care Resource Information Directory. 1996. lib. bdg. 259.95 (*0-8490-6361-2*) Gordon Pr.

***Medicare, Medicaid & S-Chip Adjustment Act of 1999: Congressional Report.** Ed. by William V. Roth, Jr. 2001. 73p. reprint ed. pap. 20.00 (*0-7567-1177-0*) DIANE Pub.

Medicare-Medicaid Nursing Home Information for California, Set. 1991. lib. bdg. 600.95 (*0-8490-5076-6*) Gordon Pr.

Medicare-Medicaid Nursing Home Information for Florida, Set. 1991. lib. bdg. 199.75 (*0-8490-5083-9*) Gordon Pr.

Medicare-Medicaid Nursing Home Information for New Jersey, Set. 1991. lib. bdg. 175.99 (*0-8490-5074-X*) Gordon Pr.

Medicare-Medicaid Nursing Home Information for New York, Set. 1991. lib. bdg. 199.95 (*0-8490-5077-4*) Gordon Pr.

Medicare-Medicaid Nursing Home Information for Texas, Set. 1991. lib. bdg. 545.95 (*0-8490-5075-8*) Gordon Pr.

Medicare Now & in the Future. Marilyn Moon. 1996. 285p. 61.00 (*0-87766-652-0*) Urban Inst.

Medicare Physician Payments: Need to Refine Practice Expence Values During Transition & Long Term. Robert F. Dee. Ed. by William J. Scanlon. 2000. (Illus.). 55p. (C). reprint ed. pap. text 25.00 (*0-7567-0511-8*) DIANE Pub.

Medicare Policy & Procedure Manual. Diane P. Atchinson. 1996. (Illus.). 487p. 225.00 (*1-929162-00-6*) DPA Assocs.

Medicare Policy & Procedure Manual for Long Term Care Facilities. Diane P. Atchinson. Ed. by Diana Johnson. 2nd ed. 1998. 427p. ring bd. 225.00 (*1-929162-02-2*) DPA Assocs.

Medicare Practice Manual. Legal Counsel for the Elderly Staff. 1990. 314p. pap. 25.00 (*0-933945-05-1*) Legal Coun Elderly.

Medicare Prenatal Care. 1994. 48p. pap. text 30.00 (*1-57979-120-4*) DIANE Pub.

***Medicare Prescription Drug Benefit: Congressional Hearing.** Ed. by William V. Roth, Jr. l.t. ed. 2001. 172p. (C). reprint ed. pap. 25.00 (*0-7567-0961-X*) DIANE Pub.

Medicare Private Contracting: Paternalism Or Autonomy? John S. Hoff & American Enterprise Institute for Public Policy Research Staff. 1998. LC 99-163570. viii, 73p. (*0-8447-7123-6*) Am Enterprise.

Medicare Provider-Sponsored Organizations: A Practical Guide to Development & Certification. Peter N. Grant & William R. Hirsch. 1998. LC 98-27335. 66p. pap. 38.00 (*1-55648-243-4*) AHPI.

Medicare RBRVS: The Physicians' Guide, 1997 Edition. American Medical Association Staff. rev. ed. 1997. 496p. pap. 59.95 (*0-89970-860-9*, OP059697WE) AMA.

Medicare RBRVS: The Physicians' Guide 2000. 2000. 66.95 (*1-57947-028-9*) AMA.

Medicare Reform: The Private-Sector Impact. Employee Benefit Research Institute Staff. 1985. LC 85-25266. 156p. (Orig.). 39.95 (*0-86643-044-X*, 85-25266); pap. 19.95 (*0-86643-045-8*) Empl Benefit Res Inst.

Medicare Reform: The Private-Sector Impact; An EBRI-ERF Policy Forum. Employee Benefit Research Institute Staff. 1986. 168p. (C). reprint ed. text 31.00 (*0-8191-5537-3*) U Pr of Amer.

Medicare Reimbursement & the Quality of Hospital Care. Michael J. McGinty. 1994. 137p. (Orig.). (C). pap. text 40.00 (0-7881-1053-5) DIANE Pub.

Medicare Rules & Compliance Regulations. 11th ed. 2001. 300p. 75.00 (1-58383-132-0, MCCR1) Robert D Keene.

Medicare Rules & Regulations 1998: A Survival Guide to Policies, Procedures & Payment Reform. annuals Denise Knaus. rev. ed. 1998. (Illus.). 380p. pap. text 49.95 (1-57066-124-3, 9843) Practice Mgmt Info.

***Medicare Rules & Regulations 2001.** annuals Maxine Lewis. 2001. 250p. pap. text 59.95 (1-57066-199-5, 21043) Practice Mgmt Info.

Medicare Rules & Regulations 2000: A Survival Guide to Policies, Procedures & Payment Reform. annuals Maxine Lewis. Ed. by Maxine Lewis. rev. ed. 2000. (Illus.). 404p. pap. text Price not set. (1-57066-148-0, 20043) Practice Mgmt Info.

***Medicare Self-Referral Laws: Congressional Hearing.** Ed. by William Thomas. 2001. 150p. reprint ed. pap. text 30.00 (0-7567-1486-9) DIANE Pub.

Medicare Supplement Insurance Model Regulations Compliance Manual. 1993. 98p. (C). pap. 25.00 (0-89382-291-4) Nat Assn Insurance.

Medicare Supplement Loss Ratio Report in 1990. 1991. 136p. (C). per. 75.00 (0-89382-181-0) Nat Assn Insurance.

Medicare Supplement Loss Ratios in 1992. 1993. 176p. ring bd. 75.00 (0-89382-252-3) Nat Assn Insurance.

Medicare Supplement Loss Ratios in 1998. Ed. by Jim Bugenhagen. 7th rev. ed. 1998. 122p. reprint ed. pap. (0-89382-531-X, MED-BB97) Nat Assn Insurance.

Medicare Supplement Loss Ratios in 1991: Annual Edition. 1992. 142p. (C). per. 75.00 (0-89382-214-0) Nat Assn Insurance.

Medicare Supplement Loss Ratios Report. Ed. by Jim Bugenhagen. rev. ed. 1995. 140p. (C). ring bd. 100.00 (0-89382-364-3, MED-BB) Nat Assn Insurance.

Medicare Supplement Loss Ratios Report for 1995. 7th rev. ed. 1996. (C). ring bd. 100.00 (0-89382-426-7, MED-BB) Nat Assn Insurance.

Medicare System of Perspective Payment: Implications for Medical Education & Practice. Ed. by Mohan L. Garg & Barbara M. Barzansky. 1986. LC 85-30052. 238p. 70.00 (0-275-92009-7, C2009, Praeger Pubs) Greenwood.

Medicare Transaction System: Success Depends upon Correcting Critical Managerial & Technical Weaknesses. Mark E. Heatwole. 1998. (Illus.). 83p. (C). pap. text 25.00 (0-7881-4042-6) DIANE Pub.

Medicare Waste, Fraud & Abuse, a Regional Perspective: Hearing Before the Subcommittee on Oversight & Investigations of the Committee on Commerce, House of Representatives, 105th Congress, Second Session, March 2, 1998. 1998. LC 98-175808. iii, 63p. (0-16-056545-6) USGPO.

Medicare+Choice Final Rule: Regulations Effective 7/31/2000. CCH Inc. Staff. 2000. 450p. pap. text 69.00 (0-8080-0512-X) CCH INC.

Medicare's New Hospital Payment System: Is It Working? Louise B. Russell. 1989. 120p. text 32.95 (0-8157-7624-1); LC 89-22079. pap. text 12.95 (0-8157-7623-3) Brookings.

Medicare's Prospective Payment System: Strategies for Evaluating Cost, Quality & Medical Technology. 1992. lib. bdg. 275.00 (0-8490-5481-8) Gordon Pr.

Medicate Me Again. Judith G. Marshall. 1994. 132p. pap. text 10.00 (0-934385-62-9) Hlth Prof Inst.

Medicated Intrauterine Devices: Physiological & Clinical Aspects. Ed. by E. S. Hafez & W. A. Van Os. 1980. (Developments in Obstetrics & Gynecology Ser.: No. 5). (Illus.). 245p. text 199.50 (90-247-2371-X) Kluwer Academic.

Medicating Schizophrenia: A History. Sheldon Gelman. 1999. LC 98-47002. ix, 274p. (C). text 52.00 (0-8135-2642-6) Rutgers U Pr.

Medication Administration for Unlicensed Personnel. Division of Mental Retardation Staff. 1998. (Illus.). pap. 29.95 (1-928752-06-3) Mc Gowan Pubns.

Medication Administration for Unlicensed Personnel. Tennessee Department of Mental Health Staff. 1999. (Illus.). 352p. pap. 35.95 (1-928752-14-4) Mc Gowan Pubns.

Medication Administration for Unlicensed Personnel: Training Guide. Illus. by Bonnie Kline. 1999. 164p. pap. 249.95 (1-928752-21-7) Mc Gowan Pubns.

Medication Calculation & Administration. Welborn. 1995. pap. (0-7216-5001-5) Saunders.

Medication Cards for Clinical Use. Linda Skidmore-Roth. 7th ed. 1993. 728p. (C). pap. 29.81 (0-8385-6313-9, A6313-9) Appleton & Lange.

Medication Errors. Ed. by Michael R. Cohen. 1999. LC 99-31972. (Illus.). 380p. text 70.00 (0-917330-89-7) Am Pharm Assn.

Medication Errors: Risk Management Remedies. RiskCare Staff. 2000. 104p. pap. 150.00 (1-893929-16-7) RiskCare.

Medication Errors: The Nursing Experience. Zane R. Wolfe. 1993. LC 93-5886. (Real Nursing Ser.). 209p. pap. 23.75 (0-8273-6262-5) Delmar.

Medication Management & the Elderly: A Monograph. Carol O. Long. 2000. 10p. pap. 16.00 (1-930304-09-9) Home Care Univ.

Medication Teaching Aids. Springhouse Publishing Company Staff. 2nd rev. ed. 1998. LC 98-19030. (Illus.). 432p. pap. 36.95 (0-87434-942-7) Springhouse Corp.

Medication Teaching Manual see Manual de Ensenanza de Medicamentos En Espanol: A Guide to Patient Drug Information in Spanish

Medication Teaching Manual: The Guide to Patient Counseling. 6th rev. ed. 1994. LC 95-123096. 608p. pap. text 66.00 (1-879907-51-8) Am Soc Hlth-Syst.

Medication Teaching Manual: The Guide to Patient Drug Information. 7th rev. ed. 1998. LC 98-187236. 1253p. spiral bd. 81.00 (1-879907-81-X) Am Soc Hlth-Syst.

Medications: A Guide for the Health Professions. Karen Lane & Linda Reed. 2nd rev. ed. 1998. LC 98-27995. (Illus.). 350p. pap. 34.95 (0-8036-0378-9) Davis Co.

Medications & Math for Allied Health Professions. Rice. 2000. (Allied Health Ser.). (Illus.). 480p. (C). pap. 26.50 (0-7668-1090-9) Delmar.

Medications & Math for the Nurse. Jane Rice. (LPN/LVN Nursing Ser.). 6th ed. 1988. (gr. 11-12). pap. 33.95 (0-8273-2841-9); 8th ed. 1997. LC 97-13780. 652p. (C). pap. text 49.95 (0-8273-8328-2) Delmar.

Medications & Math for the Nurse - IML. Rice. 8th ed. 1998. 96p. tchr. ed. 15.95 (0-8273-8329-0) Delmar.

Medications & Mathematics for Nursing. Jane Rice & Esther G. Skelley. 7th ed. 1993. LC 92-18283. 620p. text 33.95 (0-8273-5119-4) Delmar.

Medications & Mathematics for the Nurse: Instructor's Guide. Jane Rice & Esther G. Skelley. 7th ed. 1993. 87p. pap. 12.95 (0-8273-5120-8) Delmar.

Medications Development: Drug Discovery, Databases, & Computer-Aided Drug Design. 1994. (Illus.). 288p. (C). pap. text 65.00 (0-7881-1137-X) DIANE Pub.

Medications Development: Drug Discovery, Databases, & Computer-Aided Drug Design. 1997. lib. bdg. 250.99 (0-8490-7734-6) Gordon Pr.

Medications Development: Drug Discovery, Databases & Computer-Aided Drug Design. 1994. lib. bdg. 295.00 (0-8490-8400-8) Gordon Pr.

Medications for Attention Disorders (ADHD/ADD) & Related Medical Problems. Edna D. Copeland & Stephen C. Copps. 2nd rev. ed. 1995. (Illus.). 420p. 37.00 (1-886941-00-9) Spec Pr FL.

Medications for School-Age Children: Effects on Learning & Behavior. Ronald T. Brown & Michael G. Sawyer. 1998. LC 97-50080. (Guilford School Practitioner Ser.). 228p. text 30.00 (1-57230-316-6, 0316) Guilford Pubns.

Medications Guide: Basic Guide to Physical & Pyschiatric Medications for Recreational Therapy. Thomas K. Skalko et al. 1994. 58p. (Orig.). pap. text 14.00 (1-889435-03-1) Am Therapeutic.

Medications Used in Oral Surgery: A Self-Instructional Guide, Bk. 3. James R. Hooley & Robert J. Whitacre. 3rd rev. ed. 1984. 112p. pap. 19.95 (0-89939-032-3) Stoma Pr.

Medications Without Prescriptions. Ephim Berkin. Ed. by Leonora Chernyakhovskaya. 2000. (RUS., Illus.). 224p. pap. 12.00 (1-893552-07-1) Mir Collection.

Medicina Antiqua: Vienna, Cod. Vind. 93. Intro. by Peter Murray Jones. 1999. (Manuscripts in Miniature Ser.). (Illus.). 380p. text 95.00 (1-872501-20-6) Gordon & Breach.

Medicina Cientifica en el Siglo XIX Mexico. Fernando M. Cortes. (Ciencia para Todos Ser.). (SPA.). pap. 6.99 (968-16-2709-1) Fondo CA.

Medicina Gerocomica. John Floyer. Ed. by Robert J. Kastenbaum. 1979. LC 78-22199. (Aging & Old Age Ser.). reprint ed. lib. bdg. 18.95 (0-405-11838-4) Ayer.

Medicina Natural: Retorno a Nuestra Esencia. Efraibn Rodriquez Malavbe. 1999. LC 98-50215. (0-8477-0365-7) U of PR Pr.

***Medicina Natural en el Hogar.** Keith Scott & Linda Scott. 1998.Tr. of Natural Home Pharmacy. (SPA., Illus.). 144p. (84-89960-25-9) Jaguar Ed ESP. *Dist:* Libros Fronteras.

Medicina Plinii - Concordantiae in Medicinam Plinii. Ed. by Anna R. Corsini & Maria P. Segoloni. 1989. (Alpha-Omega, Reihe A Ser.: Bd. CI). vi, 351p. 160.00 (3-487-09182-8) G Olms Pubs.

Medicina y Salud: Nueva Enciclopedia Completa. Richard J. Wagman. Tr. by Maria T. Sanz & Pedro Larios A. 1992. (SPA., Illus.). 1390p. 59.95 (0-915741-33-4) C D Stampley Ent.

Medicinal & Aromatic Plants XI. Ed. by Y. P. S. Bajaj. 1999. (Biotechnology in Agriculture & Forestry Ser.: Vol. 43). (Illus.). 439p. 275.00 (3-540-63911-X) Spr-Verlag.

Medicinal & Aromatic Plants V. Y. P. S. Bajaj. 1993. (Biotechnology in Agriculture & Forestry Ser.: Vol. 24). (Illus.). 350p. 344.00 (0-387-56008-4) Spr-Verlag.

Medicinal & Aromatic Plants IV. Ed. by Y. P. S. Bajaj. 1993. (Biotechnology in Agriculture & Forestry Ser.: Vol. 21). (Illus.). 464p. 402.00 (0-387-54644-8) Spr-Verlag.

Medicinal & Aromatic Plants IX, Vol. 37. Ed. by Y. P. S. Bajaj. 1996. (Illus.). 432p. 339.00 (3-540-60597-5) Spr-Verlag.

Medicinal & Aromatic Plants VI. Ed. by Y. P. S. Bajaj. 1994. (Biotechnology in Agriculture & Forestry Ser.: Vol. 26). (Illus.). 426p. 319.00 (0-387-56391-1) Spr-Verlag.

Medicinal & Aromatic Plants II. Ed. by Y. P. S. Bajaj. 1989. (Biotechnology in Agriculture & Forestry Ser.: Vol. 7). (Illus.). 545p. 329.00 (0-387-19196-8) Spr-Verlag.

Medicinal & Aromatic Plants X. Ed. by Y. P. S. Bajaj. 1997. (Biotechnology in Agriculture & Forestry Ser.: Vol. 41). (Illus.). 460p. 249.00 (3-540-62727-8) Spr-Verlag.

Medicinal & Other Uses of North American Plants. Charlotte Erichsen-Brown. 1989. pap. 12.95 (0-486-25951-X) Dover.

Medicinal & Pharmaceutical Chemistry. J. B. Stenlake. 1979. (Foundations of Molecular Pharmacology Ser.: Vol. 1). (Illus.). 936p. (C). text (0-485-11171-3) Athlone Pr GBR. *Dist:* Transaction Pubs, Humanities.

Medicinal & Poisonous Plants of India. Jean F. Caius. 1986. 528p. (C). (0-7855-2273-5) Scientific GBR. *Dist:* St Mut.

Medicinal Chemistry. Heras. 1981. 25.00 (0-08-026198-1, Pergamon Pr) Elsevier.

Medicinal Chemistry: A Biochemical Approach. Thomas Nogrady. 2nd ed. 1988. (Illus.). 542p. pap. text 49.95 (0-19-505369-9) OUP.

Medicinal Chemistry: An Introduction. Thomas. 2000. 568p. pap. 45.00 (0-471-48935-2); 99.95 (0-471-98807-3) Wiley.

Medicinal Chemistry: Principles & Practice. Ed. by Frank D. King. 1997. 340p. (C). (0-85186-494-5, R6494) Royal Soc Chem GBR. *Dist:* Spr-Verlag.

Medicinal Chemistry: The Role of Organic Chemistry in Drug Research. Ed. by C. R. Ganellin & S. M. Roberts. 2nd ed. 1993. (Illus.). 324p. text 76.00 (0-12-274120-X) Acad Pr.

Medicinal Chemistry: Today & Tomorrow: Proceedings of the AFMC International Medicinal Chemistry Symposium Held in Tokyo, Japan, 3-8 September 1995. M. Yamazaki et al. 1997. LC 96-38942. 292p. (Orig.). text 99.95 (0-632-04272-9) Blackwell Sci.

Medicinal Chemistry for the Twenty-First Century. 1992. 120.00 (0-632-03408-4) Blackwell Sci.

Medicinal Fatty Acids in Inflammation. J. M. Kremer. 1998. LC 98-35853. (Progress in Inflammation Research Ser.). 154p. 109.00 (3-7643-5854-8) Birkhauser.

Medicinal Fatty Acids in Inflammation. Joel Kremer. 1998. LC 98-35853. (PIR, Progress in Inflammation Research Ser.). 109.00 (0-8176-5854-8) Birkhauser.

Medicinal Floral Ecology in Central India: A Case Study of the Narmada Basin. Rajendra Kumar Deoll. 1994. 238p. pap. (81-7054-186-7) Print Hse IND. *Dist:* St Mut.

Medicinal Flowers: Puspayurveda Medicinal Flowers of India & Adjacent Regions. Gyanendra Pandey. 1992. (Indian Medical Science Ser.: No. 14). (C). 18.00 (81-7030-351-6) S Asia.

Medicinal Herbal Therapy: A Pharmacist's View Point. Steven G. Ottariano. 1999. LC 98-22339. (Illus.). 192p. pap. 14.95 (0-9637077-6-0) Nicolin Flds.

Medicinal Herbs & Essential Oils. Anthony Gardiner. 1997. (Illus.). 64p. 7.98 (0-7858-0713-6) Bk Sales Inc.

***Medicinal Mushrooms for Immune Enhancement: Argaricus Blazei Murill.** Beth M. Ley. 2nd ed. 2001. LC 00-12992. (Health Learning Handbook Ser.). (Illus.). 40p. pap. 4.95 (1-890766-15-1) B L Pubns.

Medicinal Natural Products: A Biosynthetic Approach. Paul M. Dewick. 1997. LC 97-12100. 476p. 235.00 (0-471-97477-3); pap. 72.95 (0-471-97478-1) Wiley.

***Medicinal Natural Products - A Biosynthetic Approach.** Paul M. Dewick. 2nd ed. 2001. LC 2001-26766. 500p. 115.00 (0-471-49640-5); pap. 55.00 (0-471-49641-3) Wiley.

Medicinal Plant Industry. R. O. Wijesekera. 1991. 280p. per. 314.95 (0-8493-6669-0, SB293) CRC Pr.

Medicinal Plants, Vol. 1. Vimala Ramalingam et al. Ed. by N. Singh & H. C. Mital. 1974. 161p. text 25.50 (0-8422-7240-2) Irvington.

Medicinal Plants, Vols. 1-4. R Bentley. 1999. reprint ed. pap. (81-7089-167-1) Intl Bk Distr IND. *Dist:* St Mut.

Medicinal Plants: A Source Guide. 1991. lib. bdg. 76.00 (0-8490-4907-5) Gordon Pr.

Medicinal Plants: An Expanding Role in Development. John Lambert et al. 1996. LC 96-13421. (World Bank Technical Papers: No. 320). 32p. pap. 22.00 (0-8213-3613-4, 13613) World Bank.

Medicinal Plants: An Illustrated & Descriptive Guide to Plants Indigenous to & Naturalized in the United States Which Are Used in Medicine, Set. Charles F. Millspaugh. 1980. 1132p. lib. bdg. 200.00 (0-8490-3103-6) Gordon Pr.

Medicinal Plants: Can Utilization & Conservation Coexist? Jennie W. Sheldon et al. 1997. LC 97-16472. (Advances in Economic Botany Ser.: Vol. 12). 104p. pap. 14.50 (0-89327-406-2) NY Botanical.

Medicinal Plants: Culture, Utilization & Phytopharmacology. Thomas S. C. Li. 2000. LC 00-104016. 517p. ring bd. 134.95 (1-56676-903-5) CRC Pr.

Medicinal Plants: New Vistas of Research. Ed. by J. N. Govil et al. 1992. (Glimpses in Plant Research Ser.: Vol. X). (Illus.). Pt. 1. 286p. (1-55528-272-5); Pt. 2. 300p. (1-55528-273-3) Today Tomorrow IND. *Dist:* Lubrecht & Cramer, Scholarly Pubns.

Medicinal Plants: Rescuing a Global Heritage. John Lambert et al. 1997. LC 96-52234. (Technical Paper Ser.: No. 355). 80p. pap. 22.00 (0-8213-3856-0, 13856) World Bank.

Medicinal Plants: Their Role in Health & Biodiversity. Timothy R. Tomlinson. 1998. LC 98-10113. (Illus.). 208p. (C). text 39.95 (0-8122-3431-6) U of Pa Pr.

Medicinal Plants & Folklores: A Strategy Towards Conquest of Human Ailments. V. K. Singh. 1989. 230p. (1-55528-212-1) Today Tomorrow IND. *Dist:* Lubrecht & Cramer, Scholarly Pubns.

Medicinal Plants & Their History. Edith G. Wheelwright. 1974. LC 74-78815. (Illus.). 288p. reprint ed. pap. 7.95 (0-486-23103-8) Dover.

Medicinal Plants for Forest Conservation & Health Care. 1998. (Non-Wood Forest Products Ser.: No. 11). 164p. pap. (92-5-104063-X, F4063X) FAO ITA. *Dist:* Bernan Associates.

Medicinal Plants in China. 1989. (WHO Regional Publications: No. 2). 327p. pap. text 50.00 (92-9061-102-2, 1510002) World Health.

Medicinal Plants in the Biblical World. Ed. by Walter Jacob & Irene Jacob. 1990. (Horticulture & Technology in the Biblical World Ser.: No. I). 160p. (Orig.). reprint ed. pap. 12.00 (0-929699-02-5) Rodef Shalom Pr.

Medicinal Plants in Viet Nam. 1992. (WHO Regional Publications: No. 3). 410p. pap. text 45.00 (92-9061-101-4, 1510003) World Health.

Medicinal Plants of Bombay Presidency. S. P. Agharkar. 1991. (C). text (81-7233-017-0) Scientific Pubs IND. *Dist:* St Mut.

Medicinal Plants of China, Set. James A. Duke & Edward S. Ayensu. 1985. LC 84-4867. (Medicinal Plants of the World Ser.: No. 4). (Illus.). 99.00 (0-917256-20-4) Ref Pubns.

Medicinal Plants of Himalaya. Gyanendra Pandey. 1995. (C). (81-7030-464-4) Sri Satguru Pubns IND. *Dist:* S Asia.

Medicinal Plants of India, Set. S. K. Jain & Robert A. DeFilipps. 1991. LC 90-8051. (Medicinal Plants of the World Ser.: No. 5). 99.00 (0-917256-39-5) Ref Pubns.

Medicinal Plants of India & Pakistan. J. F. Dastur. 1988. (C). (0-7855-2269-7) Scientific GBR. *Dist:* St Mut.

Medicinal Plants of North Africa. Loutfy Boulos. Ed. by Edward S. Ayensu. 1983. LC 82-20412. (Medicinal Plants of the World Ser.: No. 3). (Illus.). 300p. 45.00 (0-917256-16-6) Ref Pubns.

Medicinal Plants of the Arid Zones. L. C. Chopra & B. K. Abrol. 1983. 96p. (1-55528-035-8) Today Tomorrow IND. *Dist:* Lubrecht & Cramer, Scholarly Pubns.

Medicinal Plants of the Desert & Canyon West. Michael Moore. 1989. LC 87-21954. (Illus.). 200p. pap. 13.95 (0-89013-182-1) Museum NM Pr.

Medicinal Plants of the Guianas. Robert A. DeFilipps. Date not set. (Medicinal Plants of the World Ser.: No. 7). (Illus.). (0-917256-47-6) Ref Pubns.

Medicinal Plants of the Mountain West. Michael Moore. 1979. (Illus.). 216p. pap. 13.95 (0-89013-104-X) Museum NM Pr.

Medicinal Plants of the Pacific Northwest: A Digest of Anthropological Writings about Native American Uses. Illus. by Rachel Hallett & Julie Gomez. 1999. 210p. 35.00 (0-9624868-3-3) Longevity Herb Pr.

Medicinal Plants of the World: Chemical Constituents, Traditional & Modern Medicinal Uses. Ivan A. Ross. 1998. LC 98-34758. (Illus.). xi, 415p. 99.50 (0-89603-542-5) Humana.

Medicinal Plants of the World Vol. 2: Chemical Constituents, Traditional & Modern Medicinal Uses. Ivan A. Ross. 2001. LC 98-34758. (Illus.). 504p. 99.50 (0-89603-877-7) Humana.

Medicinal Plants of Vietnam, Cambodia & Laos. Nguyen Van Duong. 1993. LC 93-92625. 528p. (Orig.). (C). pap. 31.00 (0-9637303-1-2) N Van Duong.

Medicinal Plants of West Africa. Edward S. Ayensu. Ed. by Keith Irvine. 1978. LC 78-3110. (Medicinal Plants of the World Ser.: No. 1). (Illus.). 45.00 (0-917256-07-7) Ref Pubns.

Medicinal Resources of the Tropical Forest: Biodiversity & Its Importance to Human Health. Ed. by Michael J. Balick et al. 1996. LC 95-13809. (Biology & Resource Management in the Tropics Ser.). (Illus.). 464p. 79.00 (0-231-10170-8) Col U Pr.

Medicinal Resources of the Tropical Forest: Biodiversity & its Importance to Human Health. Ed. by Michael J. Balick et al. 1996. (Biology & Resource Management in the Tropics Ser.). (Illus.). 440p. pap. 37.00 (0-231-10171-6) Col U Pr.

Medicinal Wild Plants of the Prairie: An Ethnobotanical Guide. Kelly Kindscher. 1992. LC 91-38471. (Illus.). xii, 324p. 25.00 (0-7006-0526-6); pap. 14.95 (0-7006-0527-4) U Pr of KS.

Medicine. (How Things Work Ser.). (Illus.). 144p. 1999. (J). (gr. 3). 19.95 (0-8094-7870-6); 1991. lib. bdg. 25.93 (0-8094-7871-4) Time-Life.

Medicine. Nick Arnold. 1999. (Tomorrow's Technology Ser.). (Illus.). 32p. (J). lib. bdg. 16.95 (1-929298-39-0) Thameside Pr.

Medicine. Ed. by John S. Axford. 1996. LC 96-21661. (Essentials Ser.). (Illus.). 800p. pap. 80.95 (0-632-02707-X) Blackwell Sci.

Medicine. O'Neill. 1997. pap. text 24.95 (0-443-05078-3) Saunders.

M N O

Medicine. Steve Parker. 2000. LC 00-503619. (Eyewitness Books Ser.). (Illus.). 64p. (J). (gr. 4-7). 15.95 (*0-7894-5580-3*, D K Ink) DK Pub Inc.

Medicine. Mark C. Fishman et al. 4th ed. 1996. LC 96-6181. 672p. spiral bd. 36.00 (*0-397-51464-6*) Lppncott W & W.

Medicine: A Guide for Prospective Students. Patrick Mackerras. 1996. 137p. (*0-644-36056-9*) Aust Gov Pub AUS. *Dist:* Accents Pubns.

Medicine: A Guide for Study & Practice. Ellis H. Friedman & Roger E. Moshy. 2nd ed. 1992. LC 91-30652. 630p. pap. 176.95 (*0-471-93166-7*, Wiley-Interscience) Wiley.

Medicine: A Primary Care Approach. Richard H. Rubin et al. 1996. LC 95-21763. (STARS Ser.). (Illus.). 517p. pap. text 33.95 (*0-7216-5200-X*) Saunders.

Medicine: An Illustrated History. Albert S. Lyons & R. Joseph Petrucelli. 1978. (Illus.). text 42.95 (*0-8109-1054-3*) Abrams.

Medicine: Diagnosis & Treatment. Robert W. Schier. 1988. (Illus.). 600p. 39.95 (*0-316-77484-7*, Little Brwn Med Div) Lppncott W & W.

Medicine: Essentials of Clinical Practice. Richard Wilkins & Norman Levinsky. 3rd ed. 1983. 1013p. 38.00 (*0-316-94092-5*, Little Brwn Med Div) Lppncott W & W.

Medicine: Health & Illness. 2000. 34p. (C). 8.60 (*0-536-61930-1*) Pearson Custom.

Medicine: Preserving the Passion. Ed. by P. R. Manning & L. DeBakey. 1988. (Illus.). 297p. 74.95 (*0-387-96361-8*) Spr-Verlag.

Medicine: The Year in Review, 1992. Medical Tribune, Inc. Staff. 1992. 320p. 49.95 (*0-931861-81-0*) Med Tribune.

Medicine - Alternative & Complementary Systems, Methods & Treatments: Index of New Information. Louis D. Volente. 1997. 160p. 57.50 (*0-7883-1594-3*); pap. 47.50 (*0-7883-1595-1*) ABBE Pubs Assn.

Medicine - An Art or a Science. Arnold Galambos. 1984. reprint ed. 6.00 (*0-88078-001-0*) Univ Sci Publns.

Medicine: A History of Healing: Ancient Traditions to Modern Practices. Roy Porter. 1998. (Illus.). 224p. pap. text 24.95 (*1-56924-708-0*) Marlowe & Co.

Medicine among the American Indians. Eric P. Stone. LC 75-23657. (Clio Medica Ser.: 7). (Illus.). reprint ed. 32.50 (*0-404-58907-3*) AMS Pr.

Medicine & Anthropology. New York Academy of Medicine Staff. Ed. by Iago Galdston. 1977. LC 71-142678. (Essay Index Reprint Ser.). 19.95 (*0-8369-2118-6*) Ayer.

Medicine & Christian Morality. Thomas J. O'Donnell. 3rd rev. ed. 1996. LC 96-20352. 336p. (Orig.). pap. 19.95 (*0-8189-0765-7*) Alba.

Medicine & Culture. Lynn Payer. 1996. LC 96-27481. 208p. pap. 15.00 (*0-8050-4803-0*) H Holt & Co.

Medicine & Health Care. Ed. by Saul Jarcho. 1977. LC 76-29724. (Great Contemporary Issues Ser.). lib. bdg. 29.95 (*0-405-09850-2*) Ayer.

Medicine & Health Care in the U. S. S. R. Ed. by Sergei Burenkov. 1985. LC 85-14460. 315p. 47.50 (*0-8236-3310-1*, 03310) Intl Univs Pr.

Medicine & Health Care into the Twenty-First Century. Shyamal K. Majumdar & David B. Nash. 1995. LC 95-67144. (Illus.). xii, 613p. 50.00 (*0-945809-11-5*) Penn Science.

Medicine & Hygiene in the Works of Flavius Josephus. Samuel S. Kottek. 1994. LC 94-905. (Studies in Ancient Medicine: Vol. 9). xii, 217p. 84.50 (*90-04-09941-7*) Brill Academic Pubs.

Medicine & Its Technology: An Introduction to the History of Medical Instruments, 7. Audrey B. Davis. 1981. LC 80-25202. (Contributions in Medical History Ser.: No. 7). (Illus.). 285p. 69.50 (*0-313-22807-8*, DMT/, Greenwood Pr) Greenwood.

Medicine & Jewish Law. Fred Rosner. 1991. LC 89-49410. 216p. 35.00 (*0-87668-790-7*) Aronson.

Medicine & Jewish Law. Ed. by Fred Rosner. 1993. LC 89-49410. (Medicine & Jewish Law Ser.: Vol. I). Vol. I. 216p. pap. 25.00 (*1-56821-028-0*); Vol. II. 184p. pap. 25.00 (*0-87668-574-2*) Aronson.

Medicine & Labour: The Politics of a Profession. Watkins. 1987. (C). pap. (*0-85315-639-5*) Lawrence & Wishart GBR. *Dist:* NYU Pr.

***Medicine & Literature: The Doctors Companion to the Classics.** John Salinsky. 2001. 248p. pap. (*1-85775-535-9*) Radcliffe Med Pr GBR. *Dist:* Balogh.

Medicine & Mankind. Ed. by Iago Galdston. 1977. LC 70-142632. (Essay Index Reprint Ser.). 19.95 (*0-8369-2108-9*) Ayer.

Medicine & Mental Illness. Marvin E. Lickey & Barbara Gordon. 1991. Orig. Title: Drugs for Mental Illness. 459p. (C). pap. text 22.95 (*0-7167-2196-1*) W H Freeman.

Medicine & Modernity: Public Health & Medical Care in Nineteenth-& Twentieth-Century Germany. Ed. by Manfred Berg & Geoffrey Cocks. 1997. LC 96-15487. (Publications of the German Historical Institute, Washington, D.C.). 252p. text 74.95 (*0-521-56411-5*) Cambridge U Pr.

Medicine & Money: A Study of the Role of Beneficence in Health Care Cost Containment, 30. Frank H. Marsh & Mark Yarborough. 1990. LC 90-2718. (Contributions in Medical Studies Ser.: No. 30). 184p. 55.00 (*0-313-26357-4*, MMM/, Greenwood Pr) Greenwood.

Medicine & Moral Reasoning. Ed. by K. W. Fulford et al. 1994. 217p. (C). pap. text 21.95 (*0-521-45946-X*) Cambridge U Pr.

Medicine & Morality in Haiti: The Contest for Healing Power. Paul Brodwin. 1996. (Cambridge Studies in Medical Anthropology: No. 3). (Illus.). (C). 250p. text 69.95 (*0-521-57029-8*); 256p. pap. text 27.95 (*0-521-57543-5*) Cambridge U Pr.

Medicine & Nursing: Professions in a Changing Health Service. Sylvia Walby et al. 1994. 224p. 74.50 (*0-8039-8741-2*); pap. 25.95 (*0-8039-8742-0*, 9430) Sage.

Medicine & Pharmacy in American Political Prints, 1765-1870. William Helfand. 1978. (Illus.). 84p. 11.00 (*0-931292-07-7*) Am Inst Hist Pharm.

Medicine & Public Health: The Power of Collaboration. Roz D. Lasker. 1997. LC 97-42385. 176p. (C). pap. text (*0-924143-05-3*) NY Acad Med.

Medicine & Public Health: The Power of Collaboration. Roz D. Lasker et al. 1998. LC 98-51607. 178p. 26.00 (*1-56793-100-6*) Health Admin Pr.

Medicine & Public Health in the Arctic & Antarctic: Selected Papers from a Conference. K. Andersen et al. 1963. (Public Health Papers: No. 18). 169p. pap. text 6.00 (*92-4-130018-3*, 1110018) World Health.

Medicine & Religion c.1300: The Case of Arnau de Vailanova. Joseph Ziegler. 1998. LC 98-229102. (Oxford Historical Monographs). 352p. text 80.00 (*0-19-820726-3*) OUP.

Medicine & Science. New York Academy of Medicine Staff. Ed. by Iago Galdston. 1977. LC 75-142679. (Essay Index Reprint Ser.). 19.95 (*0-8369-2122-4*) Ayer.

Medicine & Science in Aquatic Sports. Ed. by Y. Mutoh et al. 1994. (Medicine & Sport Science Ser.: Vol. 39). (Illus.). xii, 236p. 215.75 incl. 5.25 hd (*3-8055-5981-X*) S Karger.

Medicine & Shakespeare in the English Renaissance. F. David Hoeniger. 1992. LC 90-50400. 408p. 60.00 (*0-87413-425-0*) U Delaware Pr.

Medicine & Society in America. Ed. by Jennifer Hanson. 1997. LC 97-77588. (Perspectives on History Ser.: Pt. III). (Illus.). 60p. pap. 6.95 (*1-57960-019-0*) Disc Enter Ltd.

Medicine & Society in America, Set. Ed. by Charles E. Rosenberg. 1972. 1073.00 (*0-405-03930-1*) Ayer.

Medicine & Society in America, 1660-1860. Richard H. Shryock. 1962. LC 60-6417. 190p. pap. 14.95 (*0-8014-9093-6*) Cornell U Pr.

Medicine & Society in Later Medieval England. Carole Rawcliffe. 1998. (History Paperbacks Ser.). (Illus.). 256p. pap. (*0-7509-1497-1*) Sutton Pub Ltd GBR. *Dist:* Intl Pubs Mktg.

Medicine & Surgery for Dentistry. Stephen R. Porter. 2nd ed. 1999. LC 99-10540. (Colour Guide Ser.). 142p. (*0-443-06169-6*) Harcrt Hlth Sci Grp.

Medicine & Surgery for Lawyers. A. J. Buzzard et al. 1986. xxi, 675p. (*0-455-20675-9*) LawBk Co AUS. *Dist:* Gaunt.

Medicine & Surgery of South American Camelids: Llama, Alpaca, Vicuna, Guanaco. Murray E. Fowler. 2nd ed. 1998. LC 97-53127. (Illus.). 558p. 99.95 (*0-8138-0397-7*) Iowa U Pr.

Medicine & the Allied Sciences: A Medical Course, Set. 1992. lib. bdg. 1500.95 (*0-8490-8703-1*) Gordon Pr.

Medicine & the American Revolution: How Diseases & Their Treatments Affected the Colonial Army. Oscar Reiss. 1998. LC 98-20088. 286p. lib. bdg. 48.50 (*0-7864-0338-1*) McFarland & Co.

Medicine & the Bible. Ed. by Bernard Palmer. 1992. 272p. reprint ed. pap. (*0-85364-423-3*) Paternoster Pr GBR. *Dist:* McClelland & Stewart, OM Literature.

Medicine & the Ethics of Care. Diana Fritz Cates & Paul Lauritzen. 2000. LC 00-61026. (Moral Traditions & Moral Arguements Ser.). xxxiv, 331p. text 55.00 (*0-87840-824-X*) Georgetown U Pr.

Medicine & the Family: A Feminist Perspective. Lucy M. Candib. 1995. LC 95-7114. xxiv, 360p. 38.00 (*0-465-02374-6*) Basic.

Medicine & the Five Senses. Ed. by William F. Bynum & Roy Porter. 1993. 349p. (C). text 74.95 (*0-521-36114-1*) Cambridge U Pr.

Medicine & the Information Age. Jeffrey S. Rose. 1998. LC 97-77013. (Illus.). xx, 278p. 50.00 (*0-924674-57-1*) Am Coll Phys Execs.

Medicine & the Internet: Introducing Online Resources & Terminology. Bruce McKenzie. 2nd ed. 1997. LC 97-219195. (Illus.). 372p. pap. text 29.50 (*0-19-262852-6*) OUP.

Medicine & the Law. Ed. by Bernard M. Dickens. 1993. LC 93-16964. (C). lib. bdg. 150.00 (*0-8147-1846-9*) NYU Pr.

Medicine & the Management of Living: Taming the Last Great Beast. William R. Arney & Bernard J. Bergen. 1984. LC 83-24380. (Illus.). x, 216p. 25.00 (*0-226-02792-9*) U Ch Pr.

Medicine & the Marketplace: The Moral Dimensions of Managed Care. Kenman L. Wong. 1999. LC 98-30622. 219p. 32.00 (*0-268-01440-X*) U of Notre Dame Pr.

Medicine & the Raj: British Medical Policy in India, 1835-1911. Anil Kumar. 1998. LC 97-43728. 248p. (C). 39.95 (*0-7619-9233-2*) Sage.

Medicine & the Reign of Technology. Stanley J. Reiser. 1981. LC 77-87389. (Illus.). 328p. (Orig.). pap. text 24.95 (*0-521-28223-3*) Cambridge U Pr.

Medicine & the War. Ed. by William H. Taliaferro. 1977. LC 70-37923. (Essay Index Reprint Ser.). reprint ed. 27.95 (*0-8369-2629-3*) Ayer.

Medicine & Western Civilization. Ed. by David J Rothman et al. (Illus.). 450p. (C). 1996. LC 95-7203. pap. text 22.95 (*0-8135-2190-4*); 1995. text 50.00 (*0-8135-2189-0*) Rutgers U Pr.

Medicine As a Human Experience. David H. Rosen & Stanley J. Reiser. 1985. 192p. pap. 79.00 (*0-8391-2037-0*, 12037) Aspen Pub.

Medicine As Ministry: Reflections on Ethics, Suffering & Hope. Margaret E. Mohrman. 1995. LC 95-18069. 120p. (Orig.). pap. 12.95 (*0-8298-1073-0*) Pilgrim OH.

Medicine at the Crossroads: A Global View from Agriculture to Complementary Medicine. Cordell E. Logan. 1993. (Illus.). 444p. (Orig.). (C). pap. 19.95 (*0-9636519-0-0*) C E Logan.

Medicine at the Threshold of a New Consciousness. Michaela Glocker. 1998. 128p. pap. text (*0-904693-92-9*) Temple Lodge GBR. *Dist:* Anthroposophic.

Medicine at War. Brendan O'Keefe. 1994. (Official History of Australia's Involvement in Southeast Asian Conflicts Ser.: Vol. III). (Illus.). 536p. (*1-86373-301-9*) Allen & Unwin Pty AUS. *Dist:* Paul & Co Pubs.

Medicine Avenue: The Story of Medical Advertising in America. William Castagnoli et al. 1998. (Illus.). 128p. 60.00 (*0-9667793-0-4*) Med Ad Hall Fame.

Medicine Betrayed: The Participation of Doctors in Human Rights Abuses. British Medical Association Staff. 1992. LC 92-28909. 288p. (C). pap. (*1-85649-104-8*); text (*1-85649-103-X*) Zed Books GBR. *Dist:* St Martin.

Medicine Cards. Jamie Sams et al. exp. rev. ed. 1999. (Illus.). 240p. 29.95 (*0-312-20491-4*) St Martin.

Medicine Civilization. David J. Rothman. 1992. (C). pap. text 12.95 (*0-691-02439-1*) Princeton U Pr.

Medicine et les Medecins en France a l'Epoque de la Renaissance. Charles A. Wickersheimer. LC 75-23770. (FRE.). reprint ed. 55.50 (*0-404-13396-7*) AMS Pr.

Medicine, Ethics & Law. Mark Ockelton. 1987. 111p. (Orig.). pap. 33.50 (*3-515-04935-5*) Coronet Bks.

Medicine, Ethics & the Third Reich: Historical & Contemporary Issues. Ed. by John J. Michalczyk. 1994. LC 94-25916. (Illus.). 240p. (Orig.). pap. 19.95 (*1-55612-752-9*, LL1752) Sheed & Ward WI.

Medicine Family Vision: Deep-Heart Sharing in the Wisdom & Guidance of the Earth. Jai J. Daemion. 1997. LC 96-76583. (Illus.). 400p. (Orig.). pap. 16.95 (*0-9651534-3-6*, 1010) Ajna Media.

Medicine for Anaesthetists. Michael D. Vickers & Ian Power. 4th ed. 1999. LC 98-34371. (Illus.). xi, 415p. 173.95 (*0-86542-637-6*) Blackwell Sci.

Medicine for Beginners. Richard Clark & Tony Pinchuck. 1984. 4.95 (*0-86316-006-9*); pap. 4.95 (*0-86316-007-7*) Writers & Readers.

Medicine for Disasters. Peter J. Baskett & R. O. Weller. 1988. (Illus.). 494p. text (*0-7236-0949-7*) John Wright GBR. *Dist:* Buttrwrth-Heinemann.

Medicine for Examinations. R. J. Epstein. 3rd ed. 1996. LC 96-6832. 192p. pap. text (*0-443-05377-4*) Church.

Medicine for Examinations: A Streamlined Approach to Revision. R. J. Epstein. 2nd ed. 1990. (Illus.). 384p. pap. text (*0-443-04149-0*) Church.

Medicine for Nurses. 13th ed. (*0-7131-4344-4*) E A GBR. *Dist:* Routldge.

Medicine for PDAs & Desktops: 2001 Edition. Paul D. Chan et al. rev. ed. 1999. (Current Clinical Strategies Ser.). 100p. cd-rom 28.95 (*1-881528-84-7*) Current Clin Strat.

Medicine for Student. G. Golwalla. 14th ed. 1989. (C). (*0-7855-4673-1*) Current Dist IND. *Dist:* St Mut.

Medicine for the Coming Age. Lisa Sand. 1999. (Illus.). pap. (*1-86163-068-9*) Capall Bann Pubng GBR. *Dist:* Holmes Pub.

Medicine for the Mind: Coping Skills for People Who Are Surviving Cancer. Jacqueline Grekin. Date not set. pap. (*0-9659685-2-9*) J Grekin.

Medicine for the Outdoors: A Guide to Emergency Medical Procedures & First Aid for Wilderness Travelers. Paul S. Auerbach. 1986. (Illus.). 24.95 (*0-316-05928-5*); pap. 12.95 (*0-316-05929-3*) Lppncott W & W (Little Brwn Med Div).

Medicine for the Practicing Physician. J. Willis Hurst. 2nd ed. 1988. (Illus.). 1857p. pap. text 110.00 (*0-409-95176-5*) Buttrwrth-Heinemann.

Medicine for the Practicing Physician. J. Willis Hurst. 4th ed. 1996. LC 96-1711. 2241p. (C). pap. text 155.00 (*0-8385-6317-1*, A6317-0, Apple Lange Med) McGraw.

Medicine for the Twenty-First Century. Keith Mason. 1993. 180p. pap. 14.95 (*1-85230-329-8*) Element MA.

Medicine for the Whole Person: A Critique of Scientific Medicine. Erich K. Ledermann. 1997. LC 97-16364. 192p. pap. 16.95 (*1-86204-056-7*) Element MA.

Medicine from Art to Science: The Role of Complexity & Evolution. Giovanni Felice Azzone. 1998. (Veneto Institute of Sciences, Letters & Arts Sciences Ser.: Vol. 1). 197p. (YA). (gr. 12 up). 60.00 (*90-5199-390-0*) IOS Press.

Medicine from the Black Death to the French Disease. Ed. by Roger K. French et al. 1998. LC 98-2502. (History of Medicine in Context Ser.). (Illus.). 280p. text (*1-85928-382-9*) Scolar Pr GBR. *Dist:* Ashgate Pub Co.

Medicine from the Mountains: Medicinal Plants of the Sierra Nevada. Kimball Chatfield. 1997. LC 97-92169. (Illus.). 219p. pap. 17.95 (*0-9658001-0-5*) Range Light.

Medicine Hands: Massage Therapy for People with Cancer. Gayle MacDonald. 1999. (Illus.). 192p. pap. (*1-899171-77-0*) Findhorn Pr GBR. *Dist:* Lantern Books.

Medicine, Health, & Risk: Sociological Approaches. Ed. by Jonathan Gabe. 1996. LC 95-14115. (Sociology of Health & Illness Monograph Ser.: Vol. 1). 176p. pap. 24.95 (*0-631-19484-3*) Blackwell Pubs.

Medicine in a Changing Society. New York Academy of Medicine Staff. Ed. by Iago Galdston. 1977. LC 70-142680. (Essay Index Reprint Ser.). 19.95 (*0-8369-2123-2*) Ayer.

Medicine in a Tropical Environment: Proceedings of the International Symposium, South Africa, 1976. Ed. by J. H. Gear. 1977. 832p. (*0-86961-097-X*) A A Balkema NLD. *Dist:* Ashgate Pub Co.

Medicine in America: A Short History. James H. Cassedy. 1991. LC 91-7058. (American Moment Ser.). 200p. pap. text 16.95 (*0-8018-4208-5*) Johns Hopkins.

Medicine in Canada. William B. Howell. LC 75-23659. (Clio Medica Ser.: 9). (Illus.). reprint ed. 34.50 (*0-404-58909-X*) AMS Pr.

Medicine in Canadian Society: Historical Perspectives. Ed. by Samuel E. Shortt. 1981. LC 80-90100. 506p. pap. (*0-7735-0369-2*) McGill-Queens Univ Pr CAN. *Dist:* CUP Services.

Medicine in Chicago: A Chapter in the Social & Scientific Development of a City, 1850- 1950. Thomas N. Bonner. 2nd ed. 1991. 352p. text 42.50 (*0-252-01760-9*) U of Ill Pr.

Medicine in China: A History of Ideas. Paul U. Unschuld. 1985. LC 84-2415. (Comparative Studies of Health Systems & Medical Care: Vol. 13). pap. 19.95 (*0-520-06216-7*) U CA Pr.

Medicine in China: A History of Pharmaceutics. Paul U. Unschuld. 1985. LC 83-4937. (Comparative Studies of Health Systems & Medical Care: Vol. 14). text 95.00 (*0-520-05025-8*) U CA Pr.

Medicine in Colonial Massachusetts, 1620-1820. Ed. by Philip Cash et al. 1980. LC 80-68589. (Illus.). xxiv, 425p. text 35.00 (*0-8139-0908-2*) U Pr of Va.

Medicine in England During the Reign of George III. Arnold Chaplin. LC 75-23695. reprint ed. 38.00 (*0-404-13244-8*) AMS Pr.

Medicine in Europe. Ed. by Tessa Richards. 1992. 164p. pap. text (*0-7279-0319-5*) BMJ Pub GBR. *Dist:* AIDC.

Medicine in Great Britain from the Restoration to the Nineteenth Century, 1660-1800: An Annotated Bibliography, 8. Compiled by Samuel J. Rogal. 1992. LC 91-39004. (Bibliographies & Indexes in Medical Studies: No. 8). 272p. lib. bdg. 78.75 (*0-313-28115-7*, RMH, Greenwood Pr) Greenwood.

Medicine in History: A World History Companion. Janet Ann Harbour. 2001. lib. bdg. 60.00 (*1-57607-088-3*) ABC-CLIO.

***Medicine in India.** O. P. Jaggi. Ed. by O. P. Jaggi. 2001. (History of Science, Philosophy, & Culture in Indian Civilization Ser.: Vol. IX: Part 1). 448p. text 55.00 (*0-19-565126-X*) OUP.

Medicine in Maryland: The Practice & the Profession, 1799-1999. Jane Eliot Sewell. 1999. LC 98-43609. (Illus.). 264p. 42.50 (*0-8018-6127-6*) Johns Hopkins.

Medicine in Old Age. S. C. Allen & J. C. Brocklehurst. 4th ed. 1998. LC 97-37958. (C). pap. text (*0-443-05778-8*) Church.

Medicine in Persia. Cyril Elgood. LC 75-23665. (Clio Medica Ser.: No. 14). (Illus.). reprint ed. 34.50 (*0-404-58914-6*) AMS Pr.

Medicine in Quotations: Views of Health & Disease Through the Ages. Ed. by Edward J. Huth & T. J. Murray. 2000. LC 99-57212. xvi, 524p. 49.00 (*0-943126-83-5*) Amer Coll Phys.

***Medicine in Society: Behavioural Sciences for Medical Students.** Ed. by Christopher Dowrick. 2001. (Arnold Publication). 216p. (Orig.). pap. text (*0-340-76027-3*) E A GBR. *Dist:* OUP.

Medicine in Society: Historical Essays. Ed. by Andrew Wear. 1992. 407p. (C). text 74.95 (*0-521-33351-2*); pap. text 27.95 (*0-521-33639-2*) Cambridge U Pr.

Medicine in Sports Training & Coaching. Ed. by J. Karvonen et al. 1992. (Medicine & Sport Science Ser.: Vol. 35). (Illus.). x, 244p. 214.00 (*3-8055-5517-2*) S Karger.

Medicine in the Athens of the West: The History & Influence of the Lexington-Fayette County Medical Society. Porter Mayo. 1999. LC 99-65231. (Illus.). 352p. 24.95 (*0-913383-64-3*) McClanahan Pub.

Medicine in the British Isles. D'Arcy Power. LC 75-23651. (Clio Medica Ser.: No. 2). reprint ed. 32.50 (*0-404-58902-2*) AMS Pr.

Medicine in the English Middle Ages. Faye M. Getz. 1998. LC 98-3534. (Illus.). 192p. 35.00 (*0-691-08522-6*) Princeton U Pr.

Medicine in the Life Sciences 1450 Through 1700. James Bono. 1999. 22.95 (*0-8057-9513-8*, Macmillan Ref) Gale.

Medicine in the Litigation Process. Giovanna Roccamo & John B. Haydon. 1999. LC 00-343546. xl, 886p. text (*0-459-23829-9*) Carswell CAN. *Dist:* Carswell.

Medicine in the Making of Modern Britain, 1700-1920. Christopher J. Lawrence. 1994. LC 93-33387. (Historical Connections Ser.). 112p. (Orig.). (C). pap. 17.95 (*0-415-09168-3*, B3713) Routledge.

Medicine in the Postwar World: The March of Medicine, 1947, Laity Lectures, No. 12. New York Academy of Medicine Staff. 1977. LC 78-167392. (Essay Index Reprint Ser.). reprint ed. 18.95 (*0-8369-2468-1*) Ayer.

Medicine in the 20th Century. Ed. by Roger Cooter & John Pickstone. 2000. 970p. 120.00 (*90-5702-479-9*, Harwood Acad Pubs) Gordon & Breach.

Medicine in the West. Ed. by James O. Breeden. 1982. (Illus.). 86p. (Orig.). pap. text 15.00 (*0-89745-025-6*) Sunflower U Pr.

Medicine in Virginia in the Eighteenth Century. Wyndham B. Blanton. LC 80-12669. reprint ed. 78.00 (*0-404-13238-3*) AMS Pr.

Medicine in Virginia in the Seventeenth Century. Wyndham B. Blanton. 1977. LC 77-180556. (Medicine & Society in America Ser.). (Illus.). 430p. reprint ed. 28.95 (*0-405-03936-0*) Ayer.

Medicine Is the Best Laughter. Ed. & Compiled by Gideon Bosker. 1994. LC 94-44178. (Illus.). 208p. (C). (gr. 13). text 35.95 (*0-8016-8113-8*, 08113) Mosby Inc.

Medicine Is the Best Laughter, Vol. II. Gideon Bosker. 1998. LC 99-182200. (Medicine is the Best Laughter Ser.: Vol. II). (Illus.). 208p. (C). (gr. 13). text 29.95 (*0-8151-9640-7*, 31797) Mosby Inc.

Medicine Journeys: Ten Stories. Carl Ginsburg. 1991. LC 91-90402. 72p. (Orig.). pap. 10.00 (*0-916185-00-1*) Ctr Pr NM.

Medicine, Law & Public Policy. Ed. by Nicholas N. Kittrie et al. LC 75-793. (Studies in Modern Society: Political & Social Issues: No. 8). 37.50 (*0-404-10426-6*) AMS Pr.

Medicine, Law & Social Change: How Bioethics, Feminism & Rights Movements Are Affecting Decision Making. Leanna Darvall. 1993. (Medico-Legal Issues Ser.). 153p. (*1-85521-077-0*) Dartmth Pub GBR. *Dist:* Ashgate Pub Co.

Medicine, Literature & Eponyms: Encyclopedia of Medical Eponymns Derived from Literary Characters. A. E. Rodin & Jack Key. 1989. LC 88-542. 370p. pap. 32.50 (*0-89464-960-4*); (C). lib. bdg. 44.50 (*0-89464-277-4*) Krieger.

Medicine Looks at the Humanities. Ed. by J. D. Newell & Ira W. Gabrielson. 1987. LC 87-17925. 206p. (C). 51.00 (*0-8191-6607-3*) U Pr of Amer.

Medicine Made Clear: House Calls from a Maine Country Doctor. Michael A. LaCombe. Ed. by Edward L. Francis. 1989. (Illus.). 400p. 21.95 (*0-9623199-0-2*) Dirigo Bks.

Medicine Made Memorable. McDermott. 1998. (C). pap. text (*0-443-05195-X*) Church.

Medicine, Magic & Religion. William H. Rivers. LC 76-44784. reprint ed. 32.50 (*0-404-15967-2*) AMS Pr.

Medicine Man. Owen T. Stratton. Ed. by Owen S. Stratton. 1989. LC 89-40224. (Western Frontier Library: Vol. 56). (Illus.). 272p. 24.95 (*0-8061-2241-2*) U of Okla Pr.

Medicine Man: A Sociological Study of the Character & Evolution of Shamanism. John L. Maddox. LC 75-23737. reprint ed. 45.00 (*0-404-13294-4*) AMS Pr.

Medicine-Man of the American Indian & His Cultural Background. William T. Corlett. LC 75-23699. reprint ed. 47.50 (*0-404-13249-9*) AMS Pr.

Medicine, Media & Morality: Pulitzer Prize Winning Articles on Health-Related Problems. Ed. by Heinz Dietrich Fischer. 1992. 264p. (C). lib. bdg. 31.50 (*0-89464-692-3*) Krieger.

Medicine Meets Virtual Reality: Art, Science, Technology. Ed. by J. Westwood & K. Morgan. 1998. LC 97-78103. (Studies in Health Technology & Informatics: Vol. 50). 500p. (YA). (gr. 12 up). 98.00 (*90-5199-386-2*) IOS Press.

Medicine Men of the Apache: A Paper from the Ninth Annual Report of the Bureau of American Ethnology 1887-1888. John G. Bourke. 1983. LC 77-135517. (Beautiful Rio Grande Classics Ser.). (Illus.). 187p. reprint ed. lib. bdg. 22.50 (*0-87380-050-8*) Popular E Commerce.

Medicine, Monopolies & Malice: How the Medical Establishment Tried to Destroy Chiropractic in the U. S. Chester A. Wilk. 2nd ed. 2000. 245p. reprint ed. pap. 12.95 (*0-9701625-0-2*) C Wilks.

Medicine, Morals, & the Law. Sheila A. McLean & Gerry Maher. 1983. 113p. text 87.95 (*0-566-00533-6*) Ashgate Pub Co.

Medicine, Mortality & the Book Trade. Ed. by Robin Myers & Michael Harris. 1998. LC 99-47430. (Publishing Pathways Ser.). 170p. 39.95 (*1-884718-81-7*, No. 53864RB) Oak Knoll.

Medicine News. Philip Gates. 2000. (History News Ser.). (Illus.). 32p. (YA). (gr. 4-9). pap. 6.99 (*0-7636-0986-2*) Candlewick Pr.

Medicine, Nutrition, Demography, & Slavery. Ed. by Paul Finkelman. 1990. LC 89-23625. (Articles on American Slavery Ser.: Vol. 15). 384p. reprint ed. text 20.00 (*0-8240-6795-9*) Garland.

Medicine of ER: Or, How We Almost Die. Alan D. Ross & Harlan Gibbs. 2000. 232p. reprint ed. 22.00 (*0-7881-9379-1*) DIANE Pub.

Medicine of the Cherokee: The Way of Right Relationship. J. T. Garrett & Michael T. Garrett. 1996. LC 96-16156. 352p. pap. 14.00 (*1-879181-37-1*) Bear & Co.

Medicine of the Fetus & Mother. E. Albert Reece & John C. Hobbins. 2nd ed. 1998. LC 98-29286. 1,840p. text 169.00 (*0-397-51862-5*) Lppncott W & W.

Medicine of the Prophet. Ibn Qayyim al-Jawziyya. Tr. by Penelope Johnstone from ARA. 1996. (ARA & ENG.). 350p. (*0-946621-19-5*); pap. (*0-946621-22-5*) Islamic Texts GBR. *Dist:* Intl Spec Bk.

Medicine, Patients & the Law. Margaret Brazier. pap. (*0-14-012749-6*) Pnguin Bks Ltd GBR. *Dist:* Trafalgar.

Medicine, Philosophy & Religion in Ancient China: Researches & Reflections. Nathan Sivin. 1995. LC 95-19571. 296p. (*0-86078-493-2*) Variorum GBR. *Dist:* Ashgate Pub Co.

Medicine Quest: In Search of Nature's Healing Secrets. Mark J. Plotkin. 2000. LC 99-42822. 304p. 22.95 (*0-670-86937-6*) Viking Penguin.

Medicine, Rationality, & Experience: An Anthropological Perspective. Byron J. Good. 1994. LC 92-45254. (Lewis Henry Morgan Lectures: No. 1990). 260p. (C). pap. text 21.95 (*0-521-42576-X*) Cambridge U Pr.

Medicine Recall. James D. Bergin. 1997. LC 97-11939. (Recall Ser.). 928p. pap. text 29.95 (*0-683-18098-3*) Lppncott W & W.

Medicine, Science & Art. Alfred E. Cohn. 1977. LC 72-86742. (Essay Index Reprint Ser.). 19.95 (*0-8369-1126-1*) Ayer.

Medicine, Science & Art. Alfred E. Cohn. 1982. (Essay Index Reprint Ser.). reprint ed. lib. bdg. 15.50 (*0-8290-0840-3*) Irvington.

Medicine Society. Paul Scriven. 1992. LC 92-53724. 230p. pap. 18.95 (*0-87013-315-2*) Mich St U Pr.

*__Medicine That Walks: Medicine, Disease & Canadian Plains Aboriginal People, 1880-1945.__ Maureen Lux. 2001. (Illus.). xii, 300p. text 50.00 (*0-8020-4728-9*); pap. text 22.95 (*0-8020-8295-5*) U of Toronto Pr.

Medicine Through the Ages. Peter Mantin & Richard Pulley. 2nd ed. 1996. (Key History for GCSE Ser.). (Illus.). 112p. pap. (*0-7487-3026-5*) Nelson Thornes GBR. *Dist:* Trans-Atl Phila.

Medicine Today: The March of Medicine, 1946 (Laity Lectures, No. 11) New York Academy of Medicine Staff. 1977. LC 71-167393. (Essay Index Reprint Ser.). reprint ed. 19.95 (*0-8369-2469-X*) Ayer.

Medicine, Tradition, & Development in Kenya & Tanzania, 1920-1970. Ann Beck. 1981. 114p. 12.00 (*0-918456-44-4*) African Studies Assn.

Medicine, 2001: Current Clinical Strategies. Paul D. Chan, MD. rev. ed. 1999. (Current Clinical Strategies Medical Book Ser.). 100p. pap. text 14.95 (*1-881528-83-9*) Current Clin Strat.

Medicine Unbound: The Human Body & the Limits of Medical Intervention. Ed. by Robert H. Blank & Andrea L. Bonnicksen. 1994. LC 94-41829. 287p. 57.50 (*0-231-08148-0*) Col U Pr.

Medicine Way: How to Live the Teachings of the Native American Medicine Wheel: A Shamanic Path to Self-Mastery. Kenneth Meadows. rev. ed. 1997. LC 92-194584. (Earth Quest Ser.). 256p. pap. 17.95 (*1-86204-022-2*) Element MA.

Medicine Ways: Disease, Health & Survival among Native Americans. Ed. by Clifford E. Trafzer & Diane Weiner. 2000. LC 00-55867. (Contemporary Native American Communities Ser.: Vol. 5). 324p. 69.00 (*0-7425-0254-6*); pap. 24.95 (*0-7425-0255-4*) Rowman.

Medicine Wheels: Native American Vehicles of Healing. Roy I. Wilson. 2001. LC 94-2388. 154p. pap. 16.95 (*0-8245-1416-5*) Crossroad NY.

Medicine Woman Inner Guidebook: A Woman's Guide to Her Unique Powers. Carol Bridges. rev. ed. 1987. (Illus.). 279p. (Orig.). pap., stu. ed. 21.00 (*0-945111-00-2*) Earth Nation.

Medicine Women, Curanderas & Women Doctors. Bobette Perrone et al. 1993. LC 89-4901. (Illus.). 272p. pap. 15.95 (*0-8061-2512-8*) U of Okla Pr.

Medicine Worth Paying For: Assessing Medical Innovations. Ed. by Howard S. Frazier & Frederick Mosteller. 1995. LC 94-48899. (Illus.). 336p. (C). text 46.50 (*0-674-56362-X*) HUP.

Medicine's Deadly Dust: A Surgeons Wake-Up Call to Society. Richard F. Edlich & Julia A. Woods. 1997. 224p. 24.95 (*0-918339-45-6*) Vandamere.

Medicine's Dilemmas: Infinite Needs vs. Finite Resources. William L. Kissick. 1994. LC 94-1137. (Yale FastBack Ser.). (Illus.). 240p. 15.00 (*0-300-05964-7*); pap. 14.00 (*0-300-05965-5*) Yale U Pr.

*__Medicines, Ethics & Practice__, No. 24. Royal Pharmaceutical Society of Great Britain Staff. 2000. (Pharmaceutical Medicines, Ethics, & Practice Ser.: Vol. 24). 136p. pap. (*0-85369-486-8*) Pharmaceutical Pr GBR. *Dist:* Rittenhouse.

*__Medicines, Ethics & Practice: A Guide for Pharmacists.__ 2001. 136p. (*0-85369-476-1*) Pharmaceutical Pr GBR. *Dist:* Rittenhouse.

Medicines for the Union Army: The United States Army Laboratories During the Civil War. George Winston Smith. 2000. LC 00-31924. (Pharmaceutical Heritage Ser.). (Illus.). x, 197p. (C). pap. 24.95 (*0-7890-0947-1*); lib. bdg. 69.95 (*0-7890-0946-3*) Haworth Pr (PPP).

Medicines from Nature. Peggy Thomas. 1997. LC 96-47686. (Health & Medicine Ser.). (Illus.). 128p. (YA). (gr. 7-12). 25.90 (*0-8050-4168-0*) TFC Bks NY.

Medicines from the Bible. M. DeWaal. 1994. pap. 8.95 (*0-942272-37-4*) Original Pubns.

*__Medicines in the Elderly.__ Armour & Cairns. 2001. 416p. pap. (*0-85369-446-X*) Pharmaceutical Pr GBR. *Dist:* Rittenhouse.

Medicine's Lighter Moments. Ted L. Grisell. 1994. LC 94-14863. 184p. pap. 19.95 (*1-877633-19-4*) Luthers.

Medicines Management for Clinical Nurses. Ed. by Karen A. Luker & David J. Wolfson. 1998. LC 98-35983. 348p. pap. 47.95 (*0-632-04247-8*) Blackwell Sci.

Medicines, Medical Devices & the Law. Ed. by John O'Grady. 1999. LC 00-361513. xiii, 412p. pap. text (*1-900151-07-3*) Greenwich Med GBR. *Dist:* JAMCO Dist.

Medicine's 10 Greatest Discoveries. Meyer Friedman & Gerald W. Friedland. LC 98-19921. (Illus.). 296p. 2000. pap. 14.95 (*0-300-08278-9*); 1998. 40.00 (*0-300-07598-7*) Yale U Pr.

Medicinisches Woerterbuch: English-German, German-English. C. Eichorst. 2nd ed. 1989. 703p. 95.00 (*0-7859-7093-2*) Fr & Eur.

Medicion del Estado de la Saluld: Genero, Carga de Morbilidad y Establecimiento de Prioridades... Kara Hanson. 2000. (Publicaciones Ocasionales Ser.: Vol. 5). (SPA.). pap. 14.00 (*92-75-32285-6*) PAHO.

Medico-Legal Aspects of Reproduction & Parenthood. J. K. Mason. 2nd ed. 1998. LC 97-38226. (Medico-Legal Ser.). 300p. pap. (*1-85521-816-X*); 413p. text (*1-84014-065-8*) Ashgate Pub GBR. *Dist:* Ashgate Pub Co.

Medico-Legal Decisions in Arkansas. Tracey Brown & Mimi Lowery. 1986. 200p. pap. 25.00 (*0-938339-04-4*) Nook Pubs.

Medico-Legal Decisions in Colorado. Tracey Brown & Mimi Lowery. 1986. 250p. (Orig.). pap. 25.00 (*0-938339-06-0*) Nook Pubs.

Medico-Legal Decisions in Florida. Tracey Brown & Mimi Lowery. 1986. 250p. pap. 25.00 (*0-938339-03-6*) Nook Pubs.

Medico-Legal Decisions in Louisiana. Tracey Brown & Mimi Lowery. 1986. 250p. (Orig.). pap. 25.00 (*0-938339-01-X*) Nook Pubs.

Medico-Legal Decisions in Missouri. Tracey Brown & Mimi Lowery. 1986. 200p. pap. 25.00 (*0-938339-02-8*) Nook Pubs.

Medico-Legal Decisions in Tennessee. Tracey Brown & Mimi Lowery. 1986. 225p. (Orig.). pap. 25.00 (*0-938339-05-2*) Nook Pubs.

Medico-Legal Directory. Ed. by Geoffrey M. Hall. 1992. (*0-9514449-1-3*) Busn & Med GBR. *Dist:* St Mut.

Medico-Legal Reporting in Orthopaedic Trauma. M. A. Foy & P. S. Fagg. 1995. (Illus.). 496p. ring bd. (*0-443-04834-7*) Church.

*__Medico-Legal Reporting Orthopaedic Trauma.__ Michael A. Foy & Phillip S. Fagg. 3rd ed. 2001. (Illus.). 510p. (*0-443-06374-5*) Church GBR. *Dist:* Saunders.

Medico-Legal Treatise on Malpractice & Medical Evidence: Comprising the Elements of Medical Jurisprudence. John J. Elwell. 1996. 588p. reprint ed. 85.00 (*0-8377-2107-5*, Rothman) W S Hein.

Medico Mnemonica: A Collection of Fun, Fibald, Irreverent & Quite Witty Mnemonics for Medical Students. Evan Marlowe. 1997. LC 96-49033. (Illus.). 186p. (Orig.). (C). pap. text 12.95 (*1-57066-056-5*, ME075) Practice Mgmt Info.

Medico-Social Aspects of Child Abuse (Recommendation & Explanatory Memorandum), No. R(93)2. 1995. (*92-871-2616-X*) Council of Europe FRA. *Dist:* Manhattan Pub Co.

Medicolegal Aspects of Moral Offences. L. Thoinot. Tr. by Arthur W. Weysse from FRE. 1997. xv, 487p. reprint ed. 152.00 (*1-56169-333-2*) Gaunt.

Medicolegal Consequences of Trauma. William H. Simon & George E. Ehrlich. 1992. (Illus.). 536p. text 115.00 (*0-8247-8745-5*) Dekker.

Medicolegal Essentials in Health. Payne. 1996. pap. text 32.00 (*0-443-05240-9*) Saunders.

Medicolegal Examination, Evaluation, & Report Bernard J. Ficarra. 1986. Set, Vols. I & II. 95.00 (*0-8493-6956-8*, RA1055); Vol. I. 304p. 129.00 (*0-8493-6957-6*, RA1055); Vol. II. 368p. 152.00 (*0-8493-6958-4*, RA1055) Franklin (CRC Reprint).

Medicolegal Fees in California: An Assessment. Leslie I. Boden. 1994. LC 93-50720. 50.00 (*0-935149-45-7*, WC-94-1) Workers Comp Res Inst.

Medicolegal Forms with Legal Analysis: Documenting Issues in the Patient-Physician Relationship. AMA Staff. 2nd ed. 1999. LC 00-265579. (Illus.). xiv, 223p. pap. text 44.95 (*0-89970-905-2*) AMA.

Medicolegal Issues for Radiographers. Robert J. Parelli. 1991. 115p. (C). pap. text 23.95 (*0-9628440-2-0*) Bellwether-Cross.

Medicolegal Issues for Radiographers. Robert J. Parelli. 4th ed. 1998. 184p. spiral bd. 80.00 (*1-880359-15-4*) Par Rad.

Medicolegal Issues for Radiographers. Robert J. Parelli. 3rd ed. 1996. 216p. 45.00 (*1-57444-081-0*) St Lucie Pr.

Medicolegal Reporting in Orthopaedic Trauma. Ed. by Michael A. Foy & Phillip S. Fagg. 1990. (Illus.). 528p. text (*0-443-03918-6*) Church.

Medicolegal Reporting in Surgery. B. J. Jones. 1996. (Illus.). 314p. (*0-443-05160-7*) Church.

Medicosocial Work & Nursing: The Changing Needs. 1983. (Euro Reports & Studies Ser.: No. 79). 70p. pap. text 7.00 (*92-890-1245-5*) World Health.

Medics: A Documentation of Paramedics Working in the Harlem Community. Richard Falco. 1986. (Illus.). 88p. 26.95 (*0-941062-21-X*) Begos & Rosenberg.

Medics & Nurses. William B. Sinclair. 1989. (Confusion Beyond Imagination Ser.: Bk. 5). (Illus.). 243p. 25.00 (*0-937577-08-1*); pap. 17.00 (*0-937577-09-X*) J F Whitley.

Medic's Pocket Reference. Ed. by William F. Minikiewicz. 1997. (Illus.). iv, 120p. (Orig.). pap. 12.95 (*0-9656879-0-2*) Medic Pub SC.

Medieval & Early Renaissance Medicine: An Introduction to Knowledge & Practice. Nancy G. Siraisi. 1990. LC 89-20368. (Illus.). 264p. pap. text 17.00 (*0-226-76130-4*); lib. bdg. 37.50 (*0-226-76129-0*) U Ch Pr.

Medieval Coroner. R. F. Hunisett. 1986. LC 85-48162. (Cambridge Studies in English Legal History). 230p. reprint ed. 60.00 (*0-912004-31-2*) Gaunt.

Medieval Health Handbook: Tacuinum Sanitatis. Luisa C. Arano. Tr. by Oscar Ratti & Adele Westbrook from ITA. 1992. LC 75-21725. (Illus.). 156p. reprint ed. pap. 20.00 (*0-8076-1277-4*) Braziller.

Medieval Iconography: A Research Guide. John B. Friedman et al. 1998. LC 97-42974. (Garland Medieval Bibliographies Ser.: Vol. 20). 464p. text 95.00 (*0-8153-1753-0*) Garland.

Medieval Medicine. James J. Walsh. LC 75-23766. reprint ed. 37.50 (*0-404-13393-2*) AMS Pr.

Medieval Medicine in Illuminated Manuscripts. Peter M. Jones. rev. ed. 1998. LC 98-169988. (Illus.). 900p. reprint ed. text 40.00 (*0-7123-0657-9*) U of Toronto Pr.

Medieval Psychology, 14. Simon Kemp. 1990. LC 89-29782. (Contributions in Psychology Ser.: No. 14). 192p. 60.00 (*0-313-26734-0*, KMP/, Greenwood Pr) Greenwood.

Medigap Insurance: A License to Steal. Frank W. Pandozzi. 1990. 61p. (Orig.). pap. 9.95 (*0-9628734-0-3*) Aa Zz Pub.

Medikamentoese Therapie des Genital- Und Mammakarzinoms. M. Kaufmann et al. 4th enl. rev. ed. 1989. (Illus.). 106p. pap. 28.00 (*3-8055-5069-3*) S Karger.

Medinfo '86: Proceedings of the World Conference on Medical Informatics, 12th, Washington, D.C., 26-30 October, 1986, Set. World Conference on Medical Informatics. Ed. by R. Salamon et al. 1986. (IFIP Transactions Ser.: No. 5). 1184p. 302.50 (*0-444-70110-9*, North Holland) Elsevier.

Medinfo, 1977: Proceedings of the World Conference, 2nd. Ed. by David B. Shires & H. K. Wolf. 1977. (IFIP Transactions Ser.). 1090p. 179.50 (*0-7204-0754-0*, North Holland) Elsevier.

MediQuik Cards. SPC Staff. 11th ed. 1997. 28.95 incl. disk (*0-87434-879-X*) Springhouse Corp.

Mediquiz, Vol. 2. Ed. by Alfred J. Bollet & Allan H. Bruckheim. (Illus.). 344p. 50.00 (*0-935466-04-5*) Pierson Pubs.

Mediscams: How to Spot & Avoid Healthcare Scams, Medical Frauds & Quackery, from the Local Physician to the Major Healthcare Providers & Drug Manufacturers. Chuck Whitlock. 2001. 304p. 24.95 (*1-58063-180-0*) Renaissance.

Meditation & Yoga Retreats: An International Directory. Compiled by Frieda Carrol. 1983. 200p. ring bd. 23.95 (*0-913597-06-6*) Prosperity & Profits.

Meditation Therapy: Short-Term Decision-Making for Couples & Families in Crisis. Janet M. Wiseman. 1990. 216p. 34.95 (*0-669-20421-8*) Lxngtn Bks.

Meditations for Healing. Larry Moen & Patty Smith. rev. ed. 1994. LC 93-34926. (Illus.). 264p. reprint ed. pap. 11.95 (*1-880698-69-2*) US Pub FL.

Meditations for the Terminally Ill & Their Families. Ed. by Judy Osgood. 1989. LC 88-36326. (Gilgal Meditations Ser.). 72p. pap. 5.95 (*0-916895-05-X*) Gilgal Pubns.

Meditations for Transformation. Larry Moen. 2nd rev. ed. 1994. LC 93-34925. 247p. pap. 11.95 (*1-880698-33-1*) US Pub FL.

Meditations on Diabetes: Strengthening Your Spirit for Every Season. Catherine Feste. 1999. 255p. pap. 13.95 (*1-58040-001-9*, 00019Q) Am Diabetes.

Meditations on the Gospel According to St. Matthew: A Devotional Commentary. Ed. by Leo Zanchettin. 1997. LC 98-104684. 320p. pap. 22.95 (*0-932085-12-1*) Word Among Us.

Meditative Therapy: Facilitating Inner-Directed Healing. Michael L. Emmons & Janet Emmons. 1999. LC 98-7501. (Practical Therapist Ser.: Vol. 3). 230p. pap. 27.95 (*1-886230-11-0*) Impact Pubs CA.

Meditators & Drugs in Gastrointestinal Motility I: Morphological Basis & Neurophysiological Control. Ed. by G. Bertaccini. 1982. (Handbook of Experimental Pharmacology Ser.: Vol. 59, I). (Illus.). 468p. 312.00 (*0-387-11296-0*) Spr-Verlag.

Mediterranean Diets. Ed. by Artemis P. Simopoulos & Francesco Visioli. 2000. LC 00-27361. (World Review of Nutrition & Dietetics Ser.: Vol. 87). (Illus.). xvi, 184p. 198.25 (*3-8055-7066-X*) S Karger.

Mediterranean Diets in Health & Disease. Ed. by Gene A. Spiller. 1995. LC 90-41112. (Illus.). 320p. (C). 121.00 (*0-442-00449-4*) Aspen Pub.

MediTrends, 1995-1996. American Hospital Association Staff. 3rd ed. 1995. 100p. pap. 75.00 (*0-87258-708-8*, 012010) Am Hospital.

M N O

Medium Secure Psychiatric Provision in the Private Sector. Katrina R. Moss. 1998. LC 98-73023. 168p. text (*1-84014-310-X*) Ashgate Pub GBR. *Dist:* Ashgate Pub Co.

Medizin. G. Alexander. 1983. 95.00 (*0-8288-1856-8*, M15409) Fr & Eur.

Medizin Von A Boz Z. 1973. (GER.). 464p. pap. 48.00 (*0-7859-0701-7*, M7553) Fr & Eur.

Medizingeschichte Japans. Erhard Rosner. 1989. LC 89-30046. (Handbuch der Orientalistik Ser.: Vol. 5/3/5). (GER.). vi, 135p. (Orig.). pap. 128.00 (*90-04-08815-6*) Brill Academic Pubs.

Medizinische Erklaerung der Maennlichen Homosexualitaet aus der Antike. P. H. Schrijvers. 1985. (Caelius Aurelianus de Morbis Chronicis Ser.: Vol. 9). (GER.). vi, 75p. (Orig.). pap. (*90-6032-266-5*) B R Gruner NLD. *Dist:* Humanities.

Medizinische Informatik, Biometrie und Epidemiologie. Ed. by Hans-Juergen Seelos. 1997. (GER.). xvi, 299p. (Orig.). (C). pap. text 42.95 (*3-11-014317-8*) De Gruyter.

Medizinische Universitaets Poliklinik Basel, 100 Jahre. Ed. by J. B. Obrecht & U. C. Dubach. 1975. (Illus.). 100p. 26.00 (*3-8055-2280-0*) S Karger.

Medizinisches Sachwoeterbuch: German-English-French-Latin. Albert Nobel. 1987. (ENG, FRE & GER.). 846p. 150.00 (*0-7859-6961-6*) Fr & Eur.

Medizinisches Woerterbuch. Urban Kaps. 17.95 (*0-8288-7823-4*, M7555) Fr & Eur.

Medizinisches Woerterbuch. Margaret Minker. 1992. (GER.). 320p. 29.95 (*0-7859-8496-8*, 3809400580) Fr & Eur.

Medizinisches Woerterbuch. Boss. 36th ed. 1994. (GER.). 864p. 49.95 (*0-7859-7443-1*, 3541159464) Fr & Eur.

Medizinisches Woerterbuch: Medical Dictionary. E. Veillon & Albert Nobel. 6th rev. ed. 1989. (ENG, FRE & GER.). 1329p. 350.00 (*0-8288-6606-6*, M4673) Fr & Eur.

MedLearn's CPT Coding Workbook. 1997. 485350p. pap. text 49.00 (*1-889115-20-7*) Med Learn.

MedLearn's CPT Coding Workbook: Instructor's Edition. 1997. 350p. 89.00 (*1-889115-21-5*) Med Learn.

MEDLINE: A Guide to Effective Searching. Brian S. Katcher. 1999. LC 99-64479. (Illus.). 160p. (C). pap. text 29.00 (*0-9673445-0-6*) Ashbury Pr.

MEDLINE for Health Professionals: How to Search PubMed on the Internet. David Hutchinson. 1998. (Illus.). 176p. pap. 29.95 (*0-9651412-6-8*) New Wind.

MedStudy: The Internal Medicine Board Review. Robert A. Hannaman. 9th ed. 2001. 450p. 395.00 (*0-9640788-5-6*) MedStudy.

MedStudy - A Condensed. Robert A. Hannaman. 8th ed. 1999. 450p. ring bd. 395.00 (*0-9640788-4-8*) MedStudy.

Med/Surg Policy & Procedure Guideline Manual. Diane Johnson. 1998. 195p. spiral bd. 125.00 (*1-879575-89-2*) Acad Med Sys.

Med'Toons. Stephen Goldberg. 1999. (Illus.). 145p. pap. text 8.95 (*0-940780-40-2*) MedMaster.

Medullary Thyroid Carcinoma. L. J. Deftos. 1983. (Beitraege Zur Onkologie, Contributions to Oncology Ser.: Vol. 17). (Illus.). x, 114p. pap. 72.25 (*3-8055-3703-4*) S Karger.

Medullary Thyroid Carcinoma. Ed. by F. Raue et al. 1992. LC 92-2297. (Recent Results in Cancer Research Ser.: Vol. 125). (Illus.). 216p. 104.00 (*0-387-55372-X*) Spr-Verlag.

Medulloblastomas in Children: New Concepts in Tumor Biology, Diagnosis & Treatment. Ed. by Paul M. Zeltzer & Carl Pochedly. 1986. LC 86-15105. 274p. 77.00 (*0-275-92164-6*, C2164, Praeger Pubs) Greenwood.

Meeting at the Crossroads: Women's Psychology & Girls' Development. Lyn M. Brown & Carol Gilligan. 1992. LC 92-14312. 240p. text 19.95 (*0-674-56464-2*) HUP.

Meeting Basic Competencies in Practical Science & Health: A Workstudy Book to Improve Daily Living Skills. Eileen L. Corcoran. 1985. (Illus.). 72p. 2.50 (*0-88323-210-3*, 237); tchr. ed. 0.50 (*0-88323-154-9*, 245) Pendergrass Pub.

Meeting Freud's Family. Paul Roazen. 1993. LC 93-22734. (Illus.). 256p. 30.00 (*0-87023-873-6*) U of Mass Pr.

Meeting GMP & ISO Expectations for Product Development. Carol DeSain & Charmaine V. Sutton. 1996. LC 98-148363. 183p. (Orig.). pap. 145.00 (*1-882615-31-X*) Parexel Intl.

Meeting JCAHO Restraint & Seclusion Standards. Eric D. Joseph. Ed. by Nancy Webster. 1997. 73p. pap. 25.00 (*0-916499-69-3*) Care Educ Grp.

Meeting Patient's Needs: Quality Care in a Changing Environment. Lynn Rogut & Avery Hudson. 1995. (Papers). pap. 12.00 (*1-881277-27-5*) United Hosp Fund.

Meeting Physical & Health Needs of Children with Disabilities: Teaching Student Participation & Management. Kathryn W. Heller. 2000. LC 00-22004. 480p. pap. text 91.95 (*0-534-34837-8*) Wadsworth Pub.

Meeting the Challenge: Living with Chronic Illness. Audrey Kron & Lawrence Kron. Ed. by Edith Brioda. 1998. (Illus.). 200p. (Orig.). pap. 14.00 (*0-9633877-1-5*) A Kron.

Meeting the Challenge of Community-Acquired Respiratory Tract Infections: The Role of Cephalosporins. Ed. by G. L. Petrikkos & W. Koenig. 1993. (Journal: Vol. 60, Suppl. 1, 1993). (Illus.). vi, 58p. pap. 28.00 (*3-8055-5754-X*) S Karger.

Meeting the Challenge of HIV Infection in Family Foster Care. Constance M. Ryan & L. Jean Emery. 1991. 96p. pap. 10.95 (*0-87868-440-9*) Child Welfare.

Meeting the Challenge of Progressive Multiple Sclerosis. Patricia K. Coyle & June Halper. 2001. LC 00-69370. (Illus.). ix, 128p. pap. 19.95 (*1-888799-46-3*) Demos Medical.

Meeting the Competency Challenge in Behavioral Health Care. Ed. by Cathy Cecere. 2000. 240p. 117.00 (*0-9679474-0-5*) C & R Pubns.

Meeting the Nation's Needs for Biomedical & Behavioral Scientists. National Research Council Staff. 1994. LC 94-66477. 174p. (Orig.). (C). pap. text 27.00 (*0-309-05086-3*) Natl Acad Pr.

Meeting the Need for Long-Term Care. Denise Iona. 1998. 126p. (Orig.). pap. (*1-893360-00-8*) Inkslingers Res.

Meeting the Needs of People with Vision Loss: A Multidisciplinary Perspective. Ed. by Susan L. Greenblatt. 1991. pap. 24.95 (*0-929718-07-0*) Resc Rehab.

Meeting the Patients' Needs in the Climacteric: The Proceedings of a Symposium Held at the 15th World Congress on Fertility & Sterility, Montpellier, France, September 1995. Ed. by J. C. Colau. 1996. LC 96-33684. (Illus.). 84p. ring bd. (*1-85070-761-8*, Parthenon Pbng) CRC Pr.

Meetings with Jung: Conversations Recorded During the Years 1946-1961. E. A. Bennet. 1995. LC 81-40459. 214p. pap. 12.95 (*3-85630-501-7*) Continuum.

Meganutrients: A Prescription for Total Health. H. L. Newbold. 1987. 422p. 19.95 (*0-89586-566-1*, Price Stern) Penguin Putnam.

Megargee's Guide to Obtaining a Psychological Internship. Edwin I. Megargee. 3rd ed. 1997. LC 97-27628. 255p. pap. 21.95 (*1-56032-750-2*) Hemisp Pub.

Meharry Medical College. Charles V. Roman. 1977. LC 71-38019. (Black Heritage Library Collection). reprint ed. 26.95 (*0-8369-8986-4*) Ayer.

Mejores Remedios Caseros (The Best Home Remedies) 220 Consejos Practicos para Vencer Problemas Comunes de la Salud (220 Practical Tips to Conquer Common Health Conditions) Ed. by Abel Delgado & Prevention Magazine Health Book Staff. 1998. LC 98-30434. (SPA.). 192p. pap. 12.95 (*1-57954-030-9*) Rodale Pr Inc.

Melancholia: A Disorder of Movement & Mood: A Phenomenological & Neurobiological Review. Ed. by Gordon Parker & Dusan Hadzi-Pavlovic. 1996. (Illus.). 352p. (C). text 90.00 (*0-521-47275-X*) Cambridge U Pr.

Melancholia & Depression: From Hippocratic Times to Modern Times. Stanley W. Jackson. 1990. 451p. (C). reprint ed. pap. 25.00 (*0-300-04614-6*) Yale U Pr.

Melancholy Muse: Chaucer, Shakespeare & Early Medicine. Carol F. Heffernan. 1995. LC 95-4368. (Language & Literature Ser.: Vol. 19). 200p. (C). text 48.00 (*0-8207-0262-5*) Duquesne.

Melancholy Scene of Devastation: The Public Response to the 1793 Yellow Fever Epidemic. J. Worth Estes & Billy G. Smith. 1997. LC 96-54741. 35.95 (*0-88135-192-X*) Watson Pub Intl.

Melanie Klein. Julia Segal. 1992. (Key Figures in Counselling & Psychotherapy Ser.). (Illus.). 160p. (C). 57.95 (*0-8039-8476-6*, 9279); pap. 25.95 (*0-8039-8477-4*, 9280) Sage.

Melanie Klein. J. M. Petot. Tr. by Christine Trollope from FRE. 1991. Vol. 1. 324p. 50.00 (*0-8236-3328-4*); Vol. 2. 300p. 50.00 (*0-8236-3329-2*) Intl Univs Pr.

Melanie Klein: Her World & Her Work. Phyllis Grosskurth. 1995. LC 94-42683. 544p. 50.00 (*1-56821-445-6*) Aronson.

Melanie Klein: Her World & Her Work. Phyllis Grosskurth. 1987. LC 86-26963. (Illus.). 544p. pap. text 19.50 (*0-674-56470-7*) HUP.

Melanie Klein Today Vol. 2: Developments in Theory & Practice: Mainly Practice. Ed. by Elizabeth B. Spillius. 1989. 272p. 49.95 (*0-415-01044-6*); 322p. (C). pap. 29.99 (*0-415-01045-4*) Routledge.

Melanin: Its Role in Human Photoprotection. Ed. by Lisa Zeise et al. 1995. LC 94-61229. (Illus.). 320p. 65.00 (*0-9632105-2-1*); pap. 50.00 (*0-9632105-3-X*) Valdenmar.

Melanins & Melanogenesis. Guiseppe Prota. 1992. LC 92-11108. (Illus.). 290p. text 69.00 (*0-12-565970-9*) Acad Pr.

Melanocyte Stimulating Hormone-Control, Chemistry & Effects: Proceedings of the International Symposium of MSH, Amsterdam, 1976. International Symposium of MSH Staff. Ed. by F. J. Tilders et al. 1977. (Frontiers of Hormone Research Ser.: Vol. 4). 86.25 (*3-8055-2635-0*) S Karger.

Melanocytic Tumors: A Guide to Diagnosis. Alastair J. Cochran et al. 1996. LC 96-4715. (Biopsy Interpretation Ser.). 448p. text 129.00 (*0-397-51633-9*) Lppncott W & W.

***Melanoma.** Thompson et al. 2001. (Illus.). 400p. (*1-901865-65-7*) Isis Med GBR. *Dist:* Bks Intl VA.

Melanoma: Prevention, Detection & Treatment. Catherine M. Poole & Dupont Guerry. 1998. LC 97-39658. (Illus.). 176p. 35.00 (*0-300-07361-5*); pap. 15.95 (*0-300-07362-3*) Yale U Pr.

Melanoma: The New Biotherapeutics for Solid Tumors. Ed. by Ernest C. Borden. 2002. LC 2001-39468. (Current Clinical Oncology Ser.). 400p. 135.00 (*0-89603-876-9*) Humana.

Melanoma & Naevi. Ed. by J. M. Elwood. 1988. (Pigment Cell Ser.: Vol. 9). (Illus.). viii, 156p. 100.00 (*3-8055-4639-4*) S Karger.

Melanoma Antigens & Antibodies. Ed. by Ralph A. Reisfeld & Soldano Ferrone. 1982. LC 82-5288. 462p. 95.00 (*0-306-40852-X*, Plenum Trade) Perseus Pubng.

Melanoma Research: Genetics, Growth Factors, Metastases & Antigens. Ed. by Larry Nathanson. 1991. (Cancer Treatment & Research Ser.). (C). text 172.50 (*0-7923-0895-6*) Kluwer Academic.

Melanoma Techniques & Protocols: Molecular Diagnosis, Treatment & Monitoring. Ed. by Brian J. Nickoloff. 2001. LC 00-63353. (Methods in Molecular Medicine Ser.: Vol. 61). (Illus.). xv, 366p. 119.50 (*0-89603-684-7*) Humana.

Melanomas: Basic Properties & Clinical Behavior: Proceedings of the International Pigment Cell Conference, 9th, Houston, Texas, Jan., 1975, Pt. 1. International Pigment Cell Conference Staff. Ed. by V. Riley. 1977. (Pigment Cell Ser.: Vol. 2). (Illus.). 476p. 133.25 (*3-8055-2369-6*) S Karger.

Melanotropins. Alex N. Eberle. 1988. (Illus.). xx, 556p. 277.50 (*3-8055-4678-5*) S Karger.

Melatonin. Woodland Publishing Staff. 1999. (Woodland Health Ser.). 32p. pap. 3.95 (*1-885670-22-2*) Woodland UT.

Melatonin: A Universal Photoperiodic Signal with Diverse Actions: International Symposium, Hong Kong, September 1995. Ed. by Russell J. Reiter et al. 1996. LC 96-44662. (Frontiers of Hormone Research Ser.: Vol. 21, 1996). (Illus.). viii, 208p. 198.25 (*3-8055-6344-2*) S Karger.

Melatonin: Binding Sites in Endocrine & Immune Systems. Ed. by G. M. Brown et al. 1994. (Journal: Vol. 3, No. 2, 1994). (Illus.). 60p. pap. 30.50 (*3-8055-6007-9*) S Karger.

Melatonin: Biosynthesis, Physical Effects & Clinical Applications. Hing-Sing Yu. 1992. 560p. lib. bdg. 249.00 (*0-8493-6900-2*, QP572) CRC Pr.

Melatonin: Clinical Perspectives. Ed. by Andrew Miles et al. 1988. (Illus.). 304p. 80.00 (*0-19-261652-8*) OUP.

Melatonin: From Contraception to Breast Cancer Prevention. Michael Cohen. 1995. (Illus.). 180p. (Orig.). (C). pap. 75.00 (*1-880613-10-7*) Sheba Pr.

Melatonin: The Anti-Aging Hormone. Suzanne LeVert. 1998. LC 95-94265. (Orig.). pap. 5.99 (*0-380-78304-5*, Avon Bks) Morrow Avon.

Melatonin: Your Body's Natural Wonder Drug. Russel J. Reiter & Jo Robinson. 1996. 416p. mass mkt. 6.99 (*0-553-57484-1*) Bantam.

Melatonin - Current Status & Perspectives: Proceedings of an International Symposium on Melatonin, Held in Bremen, F. R. Germany, September 18-30, 1980. Ed. by N. Birau & W. Schlott. 1981. (Advances in the Biosciences Ser.: Vol. 29). 420p. 66.00 (*0-08-026400-X*, Pergamon Pr) Elsevier.

Melatonin & the Biological Clock. Dallas Clouatre et al. 1996. (Good Health Guides). 48p. pap. 3.95 (*0-87983-734-9*, 37349K, Keats Pubng) McGraw-Hill Trade.

Melatonin & the Mammalian Pineal Gland. J. Arendt. 1994. (Illus.). 352p. (C). (gr. 13). pap. text 143.95 (*0-412-53600-5*, Chap & Hall NY) Chapman & Hall.

Melatonin & the Pineal: Symposium No. 117. CIBA Foundation Staff. 1985. 320p. 128.00 (*0-471-91086-4*) Wiley.

Melatonin & the Pineal Gland, from Basic Science to Clinical Application: Proceedings of the International Symposium on Melatonin & the Pineal Gland,from Basic Science to Clinical Application, Paris, 6-9 September 1992. Ed. by Yvan Touitou et al. 1993. LC 92-48538. (International Congress Ser.: Vol. 1017). 394p. 150.50 (*0-444-89583-3*, Excerpta Medica) Elsevier.

Melatonin Hypothesis: Breast Cancer & Use of Electric Power. Ed. by Richard G. Stevens et al. 1997. LC 96-27522. 776p. 87.50 (*1-57477-020-9*) Battelle.

Melatonin in Humans. Ed. by Richard J. Wurtman & F. Waldhauser. 1986. (Journals of Neural Transmission: Suppl. 2). (Illus.). 330p. 133.00 (*0-387-81927-4*) Spr-Verlag.

Melatonin in Psychiatric & Neoplastic Disorders. Ed. by Mohammad Shafii & Sharon L. Shafii. 1998. LC 97-3183. (Progress in Psychiatry Ser.: Vol. 55). 344p. text 44.00 (*0-88048-919-7*, 8919) Am Psychiatric.

Melatonin in the Promotion of Health. Ronald R. Watson. 1998. LC 98-45986. (Modern Nutrition Ser.). (Illus.). 240p. 94.95 (*0-8493-8564-4*) CRC Pr.

Melatonin, Panic Attacks, Anti-Aging & Insomnia. 1996. lib. bdg. 250.95 (*0-8490-5896-1*) Gordon Pr.

Melatonin Report. Billie Jay Sahley. 5th ed. 1996. (Illus.). 20p. pap. text 3.95 (*0-9625914-6-7*) Pain & Stress.

Melatonin Rhythm Generating System: Developmental Aspects. Ed. by D. C. Klein. 1983. (Illus.). 250p. 137.50 (*3-8055-3460-4*) S Karger.

Melbourne Medical School, 1862-1962. K.F. Russell. 1977. 39.95 (*0-522-84113-9*) Intl Spec Bk.

Melissa Extract: The Natural Remedy for Herpes. Jan De Vries. 1996. (Good Health Guides). 48p. pap. 3.95 (*0-87983-719-5*, 37195K, Keats Pubng) McGraw-Hill Trade.

Mellen History of Medicine Plinio Prioreschi. Incl. Vol. 1. Primitive & Ancient Medicine. LC 91-29934. 672p. 1991. lib. bdg. 129.95 (*0-7734-9661-0*); (*0-7734-9715-3*) E Mellen.

Melloni's Illustrated Dictionary of Medical Abbreviations. B. John Melloni & Ida G. Dox. 1998. LC 98-11886. (Illus.). 492p. 29.95 (*1-85070-708-1*, Parthenon Pbng) CRC Pr.

Melloni's Illustrated Dictionary of Obstetrics & Gynecology. I. G. Dox & J. L. Melloni. 2000. LC 99-56573. (Illus.). 402p. 43.95 (*1-85070-710-3*, Parthenon Pbng) CRC Pr.

Melloni's Illustrated Dictionary of the Musculoskeletal System. B. John Melloni et al. 1998. LC 98-2796. (Illus.). 314p. lib. bdg. 32.95 (*1-85070-667-0*, Parthenon Pbng) CRC Pr.

Melloni's Illustrated Medical Dictionary. Ida Dox et al. 3rd ed. 1994. LC 92-48306. (Illus.). 536p. 31.95 (*1-85070-479-1*, Parthenon Pbng) CRC Pr.

Melloni's Illustrated Medical Dictionary. Ida G. Dox & B. John Melloni. 4th ed. 2001. (Illus.). 800p. (C). lib. bdg. 39.95 (*1-85070-094-X*, Parthenon Pbng) CRC Pr.

Melloni's Pocket Illustrated Medical Dictionary. I. G. Dox. 2001. 400p. 29.00 (*1-84214-051-5*, Parthenon Pbng) CRC Pr.

Melmon & Morrelli's Clinical Pharmacology: Basic Principles in Therapeutics. Kenneth L. Melmon et al. 3rd ed. 1992. (Illus.). 1141p. pap. text 65.00 (*0-07-105385-9*) McGraw-Hill Med Pub.

Melting the Darkness: The Dyad & Principles of Clinical Practice. Warren S. Poland. 1996. LC 96-4643. 328p. 45.00 (*1-56821-816-8*) Aronson.

Meltzer's Intensive Coronary Care. Kathleen Dracup. 5th ed. 1995. LC 95-5351. 368p. (C). pap. text 51.00 (*0-8385-4276-X*, A4276-0) Appleton & Lange.

Membrane Abnormalities & Disease Ed. by Mariano Tao. 1982. Vol. 1. 160p. 94.00 (*0-8493-6160-5*, RB152); Vol. 2. 192p. 101.00 (*0-8493-6161-3*) Franklin (CRC Reprint).

Membrane Abnormalities in Hypertension, Vol. 1. C. Kwan. Ed. by Chiu-Yin Kwan. 1989. LC 88-26305. 208p. 116.00 (*0-8493-4527-8*, RC685, CRC Reprint) Franklin.

Membrane Abnormalities in Hypertension, Vol. 2. Ed. by Chiu-Yin Kwan. 1989. LC 88-23605. 224p. 123.00 (*0-8493-4528-6*, RC685, CRC Reprint) Franklin.

Membrane Alterations in Cancer. Ed. by Akira Makita et al. 1983. (Gann Monographs on Cancer Research: No. 29). 312p. 85.00 (*0-306-41565-8*, Plenum Trade) Perseus Pubng.

Membrane Anomalies of Tumor Cells. Ed. by F. Homburger & Donald F. Wallach. 1978. (Progress in Experimental Tumor Research Ser.: Vol. 22). (Illus.). 129.75 (*3-8055-2775-6*) S Karger.

Membrane Associated Abnormalities - Sickle Cell Diseases - Membrane Linked Diseases, Vol. II. S. Tsuyoshi Ohnishi. 1993. 304p. 125.00 (*0-8493-8092-8*, RC641) CRC Pr.

Membrane Biochemistry. Edith Sim. 1982. (Outline Studies in Biology). 80p. pap. 9.95 (*0-412-23810-1*, NO. 6691) Chapman & Hall.

Membrane Biogenesis & Protein Targeting. Ed. by Walter Neupert & Roland Lill. 1992. LC 92-24428. (New Comprehensive Biochemistry Ser.: Vol. 22). 344p. 197.75 (*0-444-89638-4*) Elsevier.

Membrane Digestion: Physiology & Pathology. Ed. by A. M. Ugolve. 1990. 68.00 (*0-8493-7126-0*, QP) CRC Pr.

Membrane Dynamics & Transport of Normal & Tumor Cells: International Symposium, Debrecen, Hungary, July 6-10, 1983. J. C. Somogyi. 1984. (Symposia Biologica Hungarica Ser.: No. 26). 388p. (C). (*963-05-3889-X*) Akade Kiado HUN. *Dist:* St Mut.

Membrane Fluidity: Biophysical Techniques & Cellular Regulation. Ed. by Morris Kates & Arnisa Kuksis. 1980. LC 79-93347. (Experimental Biology & Medicine Ser.: Vol. 1). (Illus.). 464p. 119.50 (*0-89603-020-2*) Humana.

Membrane Hypothesis of Aging. Roberta W. Imre. 1994. 220p. lib. bdg. 210.00 (*0-8493-6738-7*) CRC Pr.

Membrane Separation in Biotechnology. McGregor. 1986. (Bioprocess Technology Ser.: Vol. 1). (Illus.). 408p. text 195.00 (*0-8247-7465-5*) Dekker.

Membrane Spectroscopy. Ed. by E. Grell. 1981. (Molecular Biology, Biochemistry & Biophysics Ser.: Vol. 31). (Illus.). 498p. 155.00 (*0-387-10332-5*) Spr-Verlag.

Membrane Structure in Disease & Drug Therapy. G. Zimmer. 2000. LC 00-29049. (Illus.). xxi, 530p. text 195.00 (*0-8247-0361-8*) Dekker.

***Membrane Transport & the Human Small Intestine: Relation to Mucosal Protection, Intestinal Anaphylaxis & Nitric Oxide.** Tina W. Knutson. 2000. (Comprehensive Summaries of Uppsala Dissertations from the Faculty of Medicine Ser.: No. 910). (Illus.). 83p. (Orig.). pap. (*91-554-4662-0*) Uppsala Universitet SWE. *Dist:* Coronet Bks.

Membrane Transport of Antineoplastic Agents. Ed. by I. D. Goldman. 1986. (International Encyclopedia of Pharmacology & Therapeutics Ser.: Section 118). (Illus.). 421p. 198.00 (*0-08-032007-4*, Pergamon Pr) Elsevier.

Membrane Transporters. Michael Kavanaugh. 2000. (Handbooks of Receptors & Channels Ser.). 94.95 (0-8493-8323-4) CRC Pr.

Membrane Transporters as Drug Targets. Ed. by G. L. Amidon & W. Sadee. 1999. LC 99-37278. (Pharmaceutical Biotechnology Ser.: Vol. 12). (Illus.). xxv, 528p. (C). (0-306-46094-7, Plenum Trade) Perseus Pubng.

***Membranes & Filters for Hemodialysis Database, 2001.** C. Ronco et al. 2000. cd-rom 234.00 (3-8055-7062-7) S Karger.

Membranes & Sensory Transduction. Ed. by Giuliano Colombetti & Francesco Lenci. 1984. LC 84-3373. 396p. 95.00 (0-306-41439-2, Plenum Trade) Perseus Pubng.

Membranes & Transport. Ed. by Anthony N. Martonosi. 1982. LC 82-3690. Vol. 1. 722p. 110.00 (0-306-40853-8); Vol. 2. 712p. 110.00 (0-306-40854-6) Perseus Pubng (Plenum Trade).

Memento de l'Investigateur Promoteur. T. Dupin-Spriet & A. Spriet. 1999. 70p. 52.25 (3-8055-6844-4) S Karger.

Memmler's Structure & Function of the Human Body. Barbara Janson Cohen & Dena Lin Wood. 7th ed. 2000. 416p. pap. text 34.95 (0-7817-2438-4) Lppncott W & W.

Memmler's Structure of Function of the Human Body. Barbara Janson Cohen & Dena Lin Wood. 8th ed. 2000. LC 99-37062. 416p. text 36.95 (0-7817-2113-X) Lppncott W & W.

Memmler's Study Guide for Structure & Function of the Human Body. Barbara Janson Cohen & Dena Lin Wood. 7th ed. 2000. 336p. pap. text 18.95 (0-7817-2115-6) Lppncott W & W.

Memmler's Study Guide for the Human Body in Health & Disease. Barbara Janson Cohen & Dena Lin Wood. 9th ed. 1999. 376p. pap. text 19.95 (0-7817-2111-3) Lppncott W & W.

Memmler's the Human Body in Health & Disease. Barbara Janson Cohen & Dena Lin Wood. 9th ed. 1999. 519p. text 39.95 (0-7817-2439-2) Lppncott W & W.

Memoir of James Jackson, Jr., M. D., with Extracts from His Letters to His Father & Medical Cases Collected by Him. James Jackson. 1972. LC 72-180579. (Medicine & Society in America Ser.). 452p. reprint ed. 28.95 (0-405-03956-5) Ayer.

Memoirs of a Woman Doctor. Nawal Al-Sa'Dawi. Tr. by Catherine Cobham. 1989. 101p. pap. 8.95 (0-87286-223-2) City Lights.

Memoirs of Childhood & Youth. Albert Schweitzer et al. Ed. & Tr. by Kurt Bergel & Alice R. Bergel. 1997. LC 96-49619. 96p. 19.95 (0-8156-0446-7) Syracuse U Pr.

Memoirs of Eighty Years. Thomas G. Hake. LC 73-131509. reprint ed. 45.00 (0-404-03025-4) AMS Pr.

Memoirs of Pliny Earle, M. D. with Extracts from His Diary & Letters (1830-1892) & Selections from His Professional Writings (1839-1891) Pliny Earle. Ed. by F. B. Sanborn. 1973. LC 73-2396. (Mental Illness & Social Policy; the American Experience Ser.). reprint ed. 31.95 (0-405-05204-9) Ayer.

Memoirs of the Life & Services of Daniel Drake, M. D. Edward D. Mansfield. 1993. reprint ed. lib. bdg. 89.00 (0-7812-5386-1) Rprt Serv.

Memoirs of the Life & Services of Daniel Drake, M. D., Physician, Professor, & Author. Edward D. Mansfield. 1975. LC 75-108. (Mid-American Frontier Ser.). reprint ed. 34.95 (0-405-06875-1) Ayer.

Memoirs of William Williams Keen, M. D. William W. Keen. Ed. by W. W. James. 1990. LC 90-90402. 345p. (Orig.). pap. 18.00 (0-9628197-0-0) W W Keen James.

Memoirs on Paris Hospitals: Resource in Medical History. Jacques Tenon. 1997. LC 91-14970. 405p. 39.95 (0-88135-074-5) Watson Pub Intl.

Memorial Candles: Children of the Holocaust. Dina Wardi. 1992. LC 91-847. (International Library of Group Psychotherapy & Group Process). (C). 288p. pap. 27.95 (0-415-06099-0, A7026); 272p. text 59.95 (0-415-06098-2, A7022) Routledge.

Memories, Dreams, Reflections. Carl Gustav Jung. Ed. by Aniela Jaffe. Tr. by Richard Winston & Clara Winston. rev. ed. 1989. LC 88-37040. xiii, 430p. pap. 14.00 (0-679-72395-1) Vin Bks.

Memories of an Iowa Veterinarian. John W. Sutcliffe. 1990. (Illus.). pap. 7.50 (0-943164-15-X) Geronima.

Memories, Thoughts & Convictions. Bernhard Naunyn. 1994. LC 94-2999. (Resources in Medical History Ser.).Tr. of Erinnerungen, Gedanken und Meinungen. 30.00 (0-88135-059-1, Sci Hist) Watson Pub Intl.

Memorix Clinical Medicine. Conrad Droste & Martin Von Planta. 1999. 376p. pap. (0-412-56050-X) E A GBR. *Dist:* OUP.

Memorix Emergency Medicine. S. Muller. Tr. by Andersen Burrows. 1997. LC 95-67603. (Illus.). 324p. pap. (0-412-56040-2) E A GBR. *Dist:* OUP.

Memorix Gynecology. Thomas Rabe. 1996. (Memorix Ser.). 288p. (J). pap. (0-412-56060-7) E A GBR. *Dist:* OUP.

Memorix Medical & Biochemical Abbreviations. John Gibson & O. Potparic. 1998. LC 96-86060. 232p. pap. (0-412-78490-4) E A GBR. *Dist:* OUP.

Memorix Neurology. Peter Berlit. 1996. (Memorix Ser.). (Illus.). 304p. pap. (0-412-56070-4) E A GBR. *Dist:* OUP.

Memorix Obstetrics. Thomas Rabe. Tr. by A. Davis & R. Davis. 1996. LC 94-72653. (Memorix Ser.). (Illus.). 304p. pap. (0-412-56080-1) E A GBR. *Dist:* OUP.

Memorix Pediatrics. D. Harms & J. Scharf. 1999. (Memorix Ser.). (Illus.). 560p. pap. (0-412-73830-9) E A GBR. *Dist:* OUP.

Memorix Surgery. J. Hussman. Tr. by Albert Davis. 1997. LC 96-86266. 312p. pap. 27.95 (0-412-62910-0) Chapman & Hall.

Memory. Ed. by Patricia Fara et al. 1998. LC 98-17394. (Darwin College Lectures). (Illus.). 207p. (C). text 29.95 (0-521-57210-X) Cambridge U Pr.

Memory. Ed. by Edward C. Carterette et al. 2nd ed. 1998. (Handbook of Perception & Cognition Ser.). (Illus.). 586p. reprint ed. pap. text 39.95 (0-12-102571-3) Morgan Kaufmann.

Memory: A Cognitive Approach. Gillian Cohen et al. 2nd ed. 1993. LC 92-40621. (Open Guides to Psychology Ser.). pap. 25.00 (0-335-19079-0) OUP.

Memory: Interdisciplinary Approaches. Ed. by P. R. Solomon et al. 1990. (Illus.). 300p. 108.00 (0-387-96724-9) Spr-Verlag.

Memory: Phenomena, Experiment, & Theory. Alan J. Parkin. 1993. LC 92-35260. pap. 29.95 (0-631-15712-3) Blackwell Pubs.

Memory: Systems, Process, or Function? Ed. by Jonathan K. Foster & Marko Jelicic. 1999. LC 98-34162. (Debates in Psychology Ser.). (Illus.). 310p. pap. text 36.50 (0-19-852406-4) OUP.

Memory, Amnesia, & the Hippocampal System. Neal J. Cohen & Howard Eichenbaum. 1995. (Illus.). 344p. reprint ed. pap. 32.00 (0-262-53132-1, Bradford Bks) MIT Pr.

Memory & Affect in Development: The Minnesota Symposia on Child Psychology. Ed. by Charles A. Nelson. 1993. (Minnesota Symposium on Child Psychology Ser.: Vol. 26). 288p. text 59.95 (0-8058-1261-X) L Erlbaum Assocs.

Memory & Awareness in Anaesthesia. Benno Bonke et al. 1990. 396p. (90-265-1020-9) Swets.

Memory & Cognition. Walter Kintsch. 1982. LC 81-18648. 496p. reprint ed. 42.50 (0-89874-403-2) Krieger.

Memory & Hypnotic Age Regression: Developmental Aspects of Cognitive Function Explored Through Hypnosis. Robert Reiff & Martin Scheerer. 1970. LC 59-13120. 253p. 40.00 (0-8236-3340-3) Intl Univs Pr.

Memory & Language Impairment in Children & Adults: New Perspectives. Ronald B. Gillam. 1998. LC 98-27277. 228p. pap. 39.00 (0-8342-1213-7) PRO-ED.

Memory & Remembering: Everyday Memory in Context. John A. Groeger. 1997. LC 96-51084. 302p. (C). pap. 32.95 (0-582-29220-4) Longman.

Memory & Testimony in the Child Witness. Maria S. Zaragosa et al. 1995. (Applied Psychology: Individual, Social & Community Issues Ser.: Vol. 1). 320p. 79.95 (0-8039-5554-5, 3449) Sage.

Memory & Testimony in the Child Witness, No. 1. Ed. by Maria S. Zaragosa et al. 1995. LC 94-32593. (Applied Psychology Ser.: Vol. 1). 320p. pap. 42.95 (0-8039-5555-3, 3450) Sage.

Memory & the Brain. Magda B. Arnold. 1984. 544p. text 99.95 (0-89859-290-9) L Erlbaum Assocs.

Memory & the Brain. Larry R. Squire. 1987. (Illus.). 336p. pap. text 29.95 (0-19-504208-5) OUP.

Memory Bank for Chemotherapy. Fredrica A. Preston. 1987. (Illus.). 256p. (C). spiral bd. 19.95 (0-683-06972-1, 972-1) Jones & Bartlett.

Memory Bank for Chemotherapy. Fredrica A. Preston & Cecilia Wilfinger. 3rd ed. 1996. LC 96-21045. (Illus.). 288p. (C). spiral bd. 34.95 (0-86720-740-X, 740-X) Jones & Bartlett.

Memory Bank for Hemodynamic Monitoring. Gary W. Ervin & Sylvia Long. 1993. (Illus.). 240p. (C). spiral bd. 29.95 (0-86720-646-2, 646-2) Jones & Bartlett.

Memory Bank for HIV Medications. Gail M. Wilkes. 1994. (Nursing-Health Science Ser.). (Illus.). 368p. (C). spiral bd. 39.95 (0-86720-685-3, 685-3) Jones & Bartlett.

Memory Bank for Intravenous Therapy. Sharon M. Weinstein. 2nd ed. 1992. (Nursing-Health Science Ser.). (Illus.). 288p. (C). spiral bd. 31.95 (0-86720-326-9, 326-9) Jones & Bartlett.

Memory Bank for Medications. Kostin & Evans. 2nd ed. 1992. (Nursing-Health Science Ser.). (Illus.). 274p. (C). spiral bd. 29.95 (0-86720-329-3, 329-3) Jones & Bartlett.

Memory Change in the Aged. David F. Hultsch et al. 1998. LC 98-16538. (Illus.). 354p. (C). text 59.95 (0-521-47361-6) Cambridge U Pr.

Memory Consolidation: Psychobiology of Cognition. Ed. by Herbert Weingartner & Elizabeth S. Parker. 1984. 288p. (C). text 59.95 (0-89859-323-9) L Erlbaum Assocs.

Memory Defects in Organic Psychoses. Jonathan Liljencrants. 1974. (Psychology Monographs General & Applied: Vol. 32). reprint ed. 55.00 (0-8115-1431-5) Periodicals Srv.

Memory, Dementia, & Perception of Time, Music, & Faces, Section 11. Ed. by H. Spinnler & F. Boller. 1993. (Handbook of Neuropsychology Ser.: Vol. 8). 456p. 313.00 (0-444-89975-8) Elsevier.

Memory Development: Universal Changes & Individual Differences. Ed. by Franz E. Weinert & Marion Perlmutter. 1988. 432p. text 79.95 (0-8058-0148-0) L Erlbaum Assocs.

Memory Development Between 2 & 20. M. Pressley & Wolfgang Schneider. 1988. (Cognitive Development Ser.). (Illus.). 274p. 49.50 (0-387-96742-7) Spr-Verlag.

Memory Disorders: Research & Clinical Practice. Ed. by Takehiko Yanagihara & Ronald C. Petersen. 1991. (Neurological Disease & Therapy Ser.: Vol. 9). (Illus.). 536p. text 199.00 (0-8247-8489-8) Dekker.

Memory Dynamics: A Complete Memory System. William Fauver & Robert L. Birch. 1981. 59.95 (0-939036-01-0); spiral bd. 39.95 (0-939036-00-2) Knowledge Bank.

Memory Dynamics System for Memory & Learning Improvement: Summary of the Theory & Methods. William Fauver. 1982. 31p. pap. 6.95 (0-939036-02-9) Knowledge Bank.

Memory Enhancement Program for Older Adults. Prem S. Fry & May D. Caprio-Prevette. 1997. LC 95-32416. 310p. spiral bd. 99.00 (0-8342-0728-1) PRO-ED.

Memory for Everyday & Emotional Events. Ed. by Nancy L. Stein et al. 1996. LC 96-35580. 496p. text 99.95 (0-8058-1443-4) L Erlbaum Assocs.

Memory for Odors. Ed. by Frank R. Schab & Robert G. Crowder. 1995. 200p. text 39.95 (0-8058-0728-4) L Erlbaum Assocs.

Memory Function & Aging-Related Disorders. Ed. by John E. Morley et al. 1992. LC 91-5089. 352p. 48.95 (0-8261-7710-7) Springer Pub.

Memory Functioning in Dementia. Ed. by Lars B. Ackman. 1992. LC 92-11600. xii,300p. 157.00 (0-444-88920-5, North Holland) Elsevier.

Memory Improvement Programs for Older Adults: A Training Manual. Janet Fogler & Lynn Stern. 1987. 58p. (Orig.). pap. 10.00 (0-9627777-0-6) Memory Skills.

Memory in Everyday Life. Ed. by Graham M. Davies & Robert H. Logie. 1993. LC 93-14511. (Advances in Psychology Ser.: Vol. 100). 568p. 166.00 (0-444-88997-3, North Holland) Elsevier.

Memory in Historical Perspective. Ed. by D. J. Herrmann & R. Chaffin. 1988. (Recent Research in Psychology Ser.). (Illus.). 254p. 90.00 (0-387-96705-2) Spr-Verlag.

Memory in Neurodegenerative Disease: Biological, Cognitive, & Clinical Perspectives. Ed. by Alexander I. Troster. 1998. LC 97-46776. (Illus.). 432p. (C). text 95.00 (0-521-57192-8) Cambridge U Pr.

Memory in Oral Traditions: The Cognitive Psychology of Epic, Ballads & Counting-Out Rhymes. David C. Rubin. 1997. (Illus.). 400p. reprint ed. pap. text 26.00 (0-19-512032-9) OUP.

Memory in the Cerebral Cortex: An Empirical Approach to Neural Networks in the Human & NonHuman Primate. Joaquin M. Fuster. 1994. LC 94-8307. (Illus.). 372p. 55.00 (0-262-06171-6, Bradford Bks) MIT Pr.

Memory, Learning & Higher Function. Charles D. Woody. 1984. 483p. 115.00 (0-387-90994-X) Spr-Verlag.

Memory Loss - Changing Tracks - Growing Older: Don't Act Your Age. Hankins Parker. 1994. (Illus.). (Orig.). pap. 5.00 (0-85132-200-X) Park Hurst Pubs.

Memory Notebook of Nursing, Vol. I. JoAnn Zerwekh & Jo Carol Claborn. 1994. (Illus.). 134p. (C). pap. text, stu. ed. 19.95 (0-9628210-5-5) Nursing Ed Consultants.

Memory Notebook of Nursing Vol. II: A New & Different Collection of Visual Images. JoAnn Zerwekh & Jo C. Claborn. 1997. (Illus.). 158p. pap., stu. ed. 24.95 (0-9628210-8-X) Nursing Ed Consultants.

Memory of Childhood Trauma: A Clinician's Guide to the Literature. Susan L. Reviere. 1996. LC 96-10813. 178p. 38.95 (1-57230-109-0); pap. 21.00 (1-57230-110-4, 0110) Guilford Pubns.

Memory Problems & Alzheimers Disease. 1994. lib. bdg. 250.00 (0-8490-5672-1) Gordon Pr.

Memory Quest: Trauma & the Search for Personal History. Elizabeth A. Waites. 1996. LC 96-32288. 288p. 35.00 (0-393-70234-0) Norton.

Memory System of the Brain. John Z. Young. 1986. LC 85-30577. 136p. reprint ed. lib. bdg. 59.50 (0-313-25096-0, YOME, Greenwood Pr) Greenwood.

Memory Systems, 1994. Ed. by Daniel L. Schacter & Endel Tulving. 1994. LC 93-36582. 415p. (C). 70.00 (0-262-19350-7, Bradford Bks) MIT Pr.

Memory Trace: Its Formation & Its Fate. Pref. by Erich Goldmeier. 1982. (Illus.). 288p. text 59.95 (0-89859-172-4) L Erlbaum Assocs.

Memory Wars: Freud's Legacy in Dispute. Frederick C. Crews et al. 1995. LC 95-37847. 300p. 22.95 (0-940322-04-8) NY Rev Bks.

MemoryMinder: Personal Health Journal. Frances E. Wilkins. rev. ed. 2001. (Illus.). 224p. spiral bd. 14.95 (0-9637968-0-1) MemoryMinder.

Men & Books. Ed. by Earl F. Nation. 1987. (Illus.). x, 67p. reprint ed. 20.00 (0-937543-01-2) Sacrum Pr.

Men & Family Planning. Bruce Stokes. 1980. pap. (0-916468-40-2) Worldwatch Inst.

***Men & Heart Disease: An Atlas of Racial & Ethnic Disparities in Mortality.** Elizabeth Barnett. 2002. (Illus.). 231p. (C). pap. text 45.00 (0-7567-1893-7) DIANE Pub.

Men & Heart Disease: An Atlas of Racial & Ethnic Disparities in Mortality. Elizabeth Barnett et al. 2000. (Illus.). pap. text (0-9665085-2-1) Prevention Ctr.

Men & Sex: New Psychological Perspectives. Ronald F. Levant & Gary R. Brooks. 1997. LC 97-12813. 283p. 95.00 (0-471-16903-X) Wiley.

Men & Their Sex. Robert L. Rowan. 1982. LC 80-25539. (Illus.). 168p. pap. 12.95 (0-8290-0446-7) Irvington.

Men & Women in Biological Perspective: A Review of the Literature. Aman U. Khan. 1984. LC 84-6802. 240p. 32.95 (0-275-91438-0, C1438, Praeger Pubs) Greenwood.

Men at Work. Charles A. Oakley. Ed. by Leon Stein. 1977. LC 77-70522. (Illus.). reprint ed. lib. bdg. 33.95 (0-405-10190-2) Ayer.

Men Behind Bars: Sexual Exploitation in Prison. Wayne S. Wooden & Jay Parker. 1982. LC 82-12242. 264p. 19.95 (0-306-41074-5, Plenum Trade) Perseus Pubng.

Men Freeing Men: Exploding the Myth of the Traditional Male. Ed. by Francis Baumli. 1985. LC 85-21487. 352p. (Orig.). pap. 16.95 (0-9615480-0-2) New Atlantis.

Men Healing Shame: An Anthology. Ed. by Roy U. Shenk & John Everingham. 1995. (Focus on Men Ser.: Vol. 7). (Illus.). 352p. 44.95 (0-8261-8800-1) Springer Pub.

Men in Crisis see Mosaic of Despair: Human Breakdowns in Prison

Men in Groups: Insights, Interventions & Psychoeducational Work. Michael P. Andronico. 1995. LC 95-20968. (Measurement & Instrumentation in Psychology Ser.). 435p. pap. 29.95 (1-55798-618-5) Am Psychol.

Men in Therapy: The Challenge of Change. Jo Ann Allen et al. 1991. (Family Therapy Ser.). 284p. reprint ed. pap. 18.95 (0-89862-485-1) Guilford Pubns.

Men in Transition: Theory & Therapy. Ed. by Kenneth Solomon & Norman B. Levy. 1982. LC 82-15134. 518p. 79.50 (0-306-40976-3, Plenum Trade) Perseus Pubng.

Men Surviving Incest. T. Thomas. 1989. LC 89-13881. 100p. (Orig.). pap. 9.95 (0-9613205-8-3) Launch Pr.

Men under Stress. Roy R. Grinker, Sr. & John Speigel. 1985. reprint ed. (0-89197-645-0) Irvington.

Men Who Batter Women. Adam Jukes. 1999. LC 98-38319. xiv, 192p. pap. 18.99 (0-415-04099-X) Routledge.

Men Who Control Women's Health: The Miseducation of Obstetrician-Gynecologists. Diane H. Scully. 1994. LC 93-45686. (Athene Ser.: Vol. 40). 304p. (C). pap. 18.95 (0-8077-6273-3) Tchrs Coll.

***Men Who Rape: The Psychology of the Offender.** Groth. 2001. 248p. pap. text 20.00 (0-7382-0624-5) Perseus Bks Grp.

Men with Sexual Problems & What Women Can Do to Help Them. Eva Margolies. 2001. LC 00-67545. xii, 293p. 40.00 (0-7657-0317-3) Aronson.

Men, Women, & Infertility: Intervention & Treatment Strategies. Aline P. Zoldbrod. 1993. LC 92-49301. 256p. 39.95 (0-669-27270-1) Lxngtn Bks.

Men, Women & Madness. Joan Busfield. 1996. (C). pap. text 19.00 (0-8147-1281-9) NYU Pr.

Men, Women & Madness: Understanding Gender & Mental Disorder. Joan Busfield. Ed. by Jo Campling. 1996. LC 95-42253. 296p. (C). text 50.00 (0-8147-1278-9) NYU Pr.

Men, Women & Prostate Cancer: A Medical & Psychological Guide for Women & the Men They Love. Barbara Rubin Wainrib et al. 2nd rev. ed. 2000. LC 99-75278. (Illus.). 287p. pap. 15.95 (1-57224-182-9) New Harbinger.

Menace in the West: Colorado & the American Experience with Drugs, 1873-1963. Henry O. Whiteside. 1997. LC 97-9940. (Illus.). 136p. (Orig.). pap. 12.95 (0-942576-38-1) CO Hist Soc.

Mendelian Genetics: A Problem-Solving Approach. Ruth C. Von Blum et al. 1979. (gr. 11-12). pap. text 6.95 (0-933694-00-8, COM 4223A) COMPress.

Mendelian Inheritance in Man: A Catalog of Human Genes & Genetic Disorders Victor A. McKusick. 12th ed. LC 97-26291. 1998. 3,972p. 250.00 (0-8018-5742-2); 1997. (0-8018-5743-0) Johns Hopkins.

Mending Bodies, Saving Souls: A History of Hospitals. Guenter B. Risse. 1999. LC 98-40966. (Illus.). 752p. text 39.95 (0-19-505523-3) OUP.

Mending Minds: A Guide to Today's Psychiatry. Leonard L. Heston. 1991. LC 91-25061. (Series of Books in Psychology). (Illus.). 233p. (C). pap. text 16.95 (0-7167-2167-8) W H Freeman.

Mending Ourselves: Expressions of Healing & Self-Integration. Ed. by Lynn Wasnak. 1993. (Illus.). 272p. (Orig.). pap. 12.95 (0-9637277-0-2) Many Voices Pr.

Mengele: The Complete Story. Gerald Posner & John Ware. 2000. LC 00-43061. (Illus.). xxvii, 364p. reprint ed. pap. 18.95 (0-8154-1006-9) Cooper Sq.

Meniere's & Its Management. Tom Wilmot. 1984. (Illus.). 132p. (C). 31.95 (0-398-04965-3) C C Thomas.

Meniere's Disease. Jeffrey P. Harris. 1999. (Illus.). xiii, 419p. (90-6299-162-9) Kugler NLD. *Dist:* Lib Res.

Meniere's Disease. Ed. by M. Kitahara. 1990. (Illus.). 220p. 64.00 (0-387-70056-0) Spr-Verlag.

Meniere's Disease. Ed. by Joseph B. Nadol, Jr. 1989. LC 89-19868. (Illus.). 568p. lib. bdg. (90-6299-052-5) Kugler NLD. *Dist:* Lib Res.

Meniere's Disease: An Information Book for People with Meniere's Disease. V. K. Barton. 1991. 136p. pap. (0-646-05022-2) Menieres Aust AUS. *Dist:* St Mut.

Meniere's Disease: Perspectives in the 90's. Ed. by R. Filipo & Maurizio Barbara. 1994. LC 94-23038. (Illus.). 586p. lib. bdg. (90-6299-112-2) Kugler NLD. *Dist:* Lib Res.

M N O

Meniere's Disease: What You Need to Know. P. J. Haybach. Ed. by Jerry L. Underwood. 1998. LC 98-220287. (Illus.). 300p. pap. 24.95 (*0-9632611-1-8*) Vestibular.

Meniere's Disease: What You Need to Know. P. J. Heybach. Ed. by Jerry L. Underwood. 1998. LC 98-220287. (Illus.). 300p. 34.95 (*0-9632611-2-6*) Vestibular.

Meningiomas. Ed. by Ossama Al-Mefty. 1990. 656p. text 189.00 (*0-88167-713-2*, 2188) Lppncott W & W.

Meningiomas & Their Surgical Management. Henry M. Schmidek. 1991. (Illus.). 480p. text 255.00 (*0-7216-3114-2*) Saunders.

Meningitis. Karen Roos. 1996. (One Hundred Maxims in Neurology Ser.). (Illus.). 224p. pap. 35.00 (*0-340-60879-X*) OUP.

Meningococcal Disease. Ed. by Keith Cartwright. 1995. LC 94-32088. 324p. 245.00 (*0-471-95259-1*) Wiley.

Meningococcal Disease: Methods & Protocols. Ed. by Andrew J. Pollard & Martin C. J. Maiden. 2001. LC 2001-16676. (Methods in Molecular Medicine Ser.: Vol. 67). 728p. 145.00 (*0-89603-849-1*) Humana.

Meningococcal Vaccines: Methods & Protocols. Ed. by Andrew J. Pollard & Martin C. J. Maiden. 2001. LC 2001-16674. (Methods in Molecular Medicine Ser.: Vol. 66). (Illus.). 421p. 120.00 (*0-89603-801-7*) Humana.

Menninger: The Family & the Clinic. Lawrence J. Friedman. 1991. LC 91-30510. (Illus.). xx, 484p. reprint ed. pap. 15.95 (*0-7006-0513-4*) U Pr of KS.

Menopausal Memoir: Letters from Another Climate. Anne Herrmann. 1997. LC 97-31420. (Illus.). 111p. 39.95 (*0-7890-0296-5*); pap. 14.95 (*1-56023-919-0*) Haworth Pr (Harrington Park).

Menopausal Years: The Wise Womans Way: Alternative Approaches for Women 30-90. Susun S. Weed. 1992. LC 92-70069. (Wise Woman Healing Ser.: No. 3). (Illus.). 228p. (Orig.). (C). pap. 9.95 (*0-9614620-4-3*) Ash Tree.

Menopause. 1993. (Illus.). 36p. (C). pap. text 20.00 (*1-56806-398-9*) DIANE Pub.

Menopause. 1999. ring bd. 109.95 (*1-84214-015-9*, Parthenon Pbng) CRC Pr.

Menopause. Sarah Brewer. 1997. pap. (*0-7225-3389-6*) Thorsons GBR. *Dist:* Natl Bk Netwk.

Menopause. Ed. by Herbert J. Buchsbaum. 1983. (Clinical Perspectives in Obstetrics & Gynecology Ser.). (Illus.). 225p. 90.00 (*0-387-90825-0*) Spr-Verlag.

Menopause. Raymond G. Burnett. 1987. (Illus.). 144p. pap. 12.75 (*0-8092-4677-5*, 467750, Contemporary) McGraw-Hill Trade.

Menopause. Reginald B. Cherry. 1999. LC 00-500781. (God's Pathway to Healing Ser.: Vol. 1). 120p. pap. 5.99 (*1-57778-118-X*) Albury Pub.

***Menopause.** Health Canada Staff. 96p. pap. (*0-660-15911-2*) Can7 Govern Pub CAN. *Dist:* Intl Spec Bk.

***Menopause.** Jill Wright. 2002. 128p. pap. (*1-85703-724-3*) How To Bks GBR. *Dist:* Midpt Trade.

Menopause: A Guide to Health & Happiness. James E. Huston. 1998. LC 97-36897. (Illus.). 256p. 25.95 (*0-8160-3675-6*); pap. 15.95 (*0-8160-3693-4*) Facts on File.

Menopause: A Medical Guide for Women. Winnifred B. Cutler et al. 2nd rev. ed. 1993. LC 93-28386. 432p. pap. 14.95 (*0-393-30995-9*) Norton.

Menopause: A Midlife Passage. Ed. by Joan Callahan. 1993. LC 92-41565. 240p. 31.95 (*0-253-31312-0*); pap. 13.95 (*0-253-20817-3*) Ind U Pr.

Menopause: A Self-Care Manual. Judy Costlow et al. rev. ed. 1989. (Illus.). 72p. 5.00 (*0-9622933-1-8*) Santa Fe Health.

Menopause: A Woman Doctor's Guide: Essential Facts and up-to-the-Minute Information for a Woman. Lois Jovanovic & Suzanne LeVert. 2000. 256p. mass mkt. 6.99 (*1-57566-601-4*, Knsington) Kensgtn Pub Corp.

Menopause: Biological & Clinical Consequences of Ovarian Failure: Evaluation & Management. Ed. by Stanley G. Korenman. 1990. (Serono Symposia, U. S. A. Ser.). (Illus.). 270p. (C). text 55.00 (*1-878601-00-8*) Serono Symposia USA.

Menopause: Biology & Pathology. Ed. by Rogerio A. Lobo et al. 2000. LC 99-67667. (Illus.). xvii, 672p. 159.95 (*0-12-453790-1*) Acad Pr.

Menopause: Comprehensive Management. Bernard A. Eskin. 4th ed. 2000. LC 99-45757. (Illus.). 326p. 80.95 (*1-85070-090-7*, Parthenon Pbng) CRC Pr.

Menopause: Comprehensive Management. Ed. by Bernard A. Eskin. 3rd ed. 1993. (Illus.). text 65.00 (*0-07-019619-2*) McGraw-Hill Med Pub.

Menopause: Endocrinology & Management. Ed. by David B. Seifer & Elizabeth A. Kennard. 1999. LC 99-32278. (Contemporary Endocrinology Ser.: Vol. 18). (Illus.). 288p. 115.00 (*0-89603-677-4*) Humana.

Menopause: How to Combine the Best of Traditional & Alternative Therapies. Milton Hammerly. 2001. 352p. pap. 7.95 (*1-58062-480-4*) Adams Media.

Menopause: How You Can Benefit from Diet, Vitamins. Michael T. Murray. 1994. LC 93-41651. 192p. pap. 12.95 (*1-55958-427-0*) Prima Pub.

Menopause? Nothing to Be Afraid Of. Maria Kuman. pap. 20.00 (*1-893637-15-8*) Hlth & Hap.

Menopause: Questions You Have... Answers You Need. Lisa Bonnell Samalonis. 1999. LC 98-31192. (Illus.). 192p. pap. 12.95 (*1-882606-45-0*) Peoples Med Soc.

Menopause: Self Help Book. Susan M. Lark. 4th rev. ed. 1995. LC 89-25292. 224p. text 18.95 (*0-89087-592-8*) Celestial Arts.

Menopause & Beyond: A Fitness Plan for Life. Leora Myers. Ed. by Laura Kath. 1995. (Illus.). 208p. (Orig.). reprint ed. pap. 12.95 (*0-9647666-0-4*) Adelaide Pr.

Menopause & Estrogen: Natural Alternatives to Hormone Replacement Therapy. Ellen Hodgson Brown & Lynn Walker. 2nd ed. 1997. LC 96-53863. (Illus.). 197p. (Orig.). pap. 14.95 (*1-883319-53-6*) Frog Ltd CA.

Menopause & Homeopathy: A Guide for Women in Mid-Life. Ifeoma Ikenze. 1999. LC 98-19873. (Illus.). 250p. pap. 16.95 (*1-55643-291-7*) North Atlantic.

***Menopause & its Treatment: What You Need to Know.** M. Whitehead. 2002. 80p. 29.95 (*1-84214-130-9*, Parthenon Pbng) CRC Pr.

Menopause & the Heart. Ed. by M. Neves-E-Castro & M. Birkhauser. 1999. LC 98-32248. (Illus.). 138p. lib. bdg. 85.95 (*1-85070-071-0*, Parthenon Pbng) CRC Pr.

Menopause & the Mind: The Complete Guide to Coping with the Cognitive Effects of Perimenopause & Menopause - Including Memory Loss, Foggy Thinking & Verbal Slips. Simon and Schuster Staff & Claire Warga. 2000. 400p. pap. 14.00 (*0-684-85479-1*) S&S Trade.

Menopause & the Spirit Filled Woman: Something Every Man Needs to Know. Charles M. Washington. Date not set. 130p. (*0-9638436-3-X*) Indelble Ink.

Menopause at the Millennium: Proceedings of the 9th World Congress on the Menopause. Takeshi Aso & T. Yanaihara. 2000. (Illus.). 574p. lib. bdg. 126.95 (*1-85070-709-X*, Parthenon Pbng) CRC Pr.

Menopause Book: A Guide to Health & Well-Being for Women. Sheldon H. Cherry & Carolyn D. Runowicz. 1995. LC 95-2054. 272p. pap. 11.95 (*0-02-860416-4*) Mac Bks.

Menopause Book: A Guide to Health & Well-Being for Women. Sheldon H. Cherry & Carolyn D. Runowicz. 2000. (Illus.). 252p. reprint ed. pap. text 12.00 (*0-7881-9012-1*) DIANE Pub.

Menopause Book: A Guide to Health & Well-Being for Women After Forty. Sheldon H. Cherry & Carolyn Runowicz. 1994. (Illus.). 320p. 20.00 (*0-02-524758-1*) Macmillan.

Menopause Core Curriculum. 2000. stu. ed. 60.00 (*0-9701251-0-0*) N Amer Men.

Menopause, Hormone Therapy, & Women's Health. 1992. 126p. (Orig.). (C). pap. text 30.00 (*1-56806-042-4*) DIANE Pub.

Menopause, Hormones & Cancer. B. Wren. Ed. by M. Neves-E-Castro. 2001. LC 2001-55371. (Illus.). 250p. lib. bdg. 89.95 (*1-85070-628-X*, Parthenon Pbng) CRC Pr.

Menopause Madness. Pat Ross. 1998. LC 97-39014. 96p. per. 10.00 (*0-684-84227-0*, Fireside) S&S Trade Pap.

Menopause, Me & You: The Sound of Women Pausing. Ann M. Voda. 1997. LC 96-52108. (Haworth Innovations in Feminist Studies). 396p. (Illus.). (C). 59.95 (*1-56023-911-5*); pap. 24.95 (*1-56023-922-0*) Haworth Pr (Harrington Park).

Menopause Naturally. Carolyn Dean. Ed. by Phyllis Herman. 1995. (Good Health Guides). 48p. pap. 3.95 (*0-87983-681-4*, 36814K, Keats Pubng) McGraw-Hill Trade.

Menopause Self Help Book: A Woman's Guide to Feeling Wonderful for the Second Half of Her Life. Susan M. Lark. rev. ed. 1999. (Illus.). 239p. pap. text 17.00 (*0-7881-6074-5*) DIANE Pub.

Menopause, Stress & Amino Acid Therapy. 1996. lib. bdg. 252.75 (*0-8490-5898-8*) Gordon Pr.

Menopause the Natural Way: Six Step Natural Program to Health, Menopause with Nutrition, Herbal Medicine, Exercise & Mind Body Techniques. Deborah Gordon et al. 2001. LC 00-65439. (Women's Natural Health Ser.). (Illus.). 256p. pap. 14.95 (*0-471-37957-3*) Wiley.

Menopause Without Medicine. Linda Ojeda. 4th rev. ed. 2000. LC 00-38884. (Illus.). xii, 354p. pap. 15.95 (*0-89793-281-1*); 25.95 (*0-89793-282-X*) Hunter Hse.

Men's Health. Ed. by Tony Harrison & Karen Dignan. 1999. LC 98-54878. (Illus.). xii, 222p. (*0-443-05919-5*) Church.

Men's Health. Ed. by Tom O'Dowd & David Jewell. 1998. (Oxford General Practice Ser.: No. 41). (Illus.). 290p. pap. text 68.00 (*0-19-262581-0*) OUP.

Men's Health: Perspectives, Diversity & Paradox. Mike Luckovich et al. 1999. LC 99-32983. pap. 49.95 (*0-632-05288-0*) Blackwell Sci.

Men's Health & Illness: Gender, Power & the Body. Ed. by Donald J. Sabo & David Frederick Gordon. 1995. LC 95-17398. (Research on Men & Masculinities Ser.: Vol. 8). 320p. 91.95 (*0-8039-4814-X*, 4733); pap. 38.95 (*0-8039-5275-9*, 4734) Sage.

Men's Health & the Hormone Revolution. Siegfried Meryn et al. Tr. by Warner Patels. 2000. (Illus.). 350p. pap. (*1-55321-103-0*) NDE Pub CAN. *Dist:* IPG Chicago.

Men's Health Concerns Sourcebook: Basic Information about Health Issues That Affect Men. Ed. by Allan R. Cook. 1998. LC 98-33612. (Health Reference Ser.: Vol. 38). (Illus.). 600p. 78.00 (*0-7808-0212-8*) Omnigraphics Inc.

Men's Health Problems. Loretta H. Kurban. 1991. (Orig.). pap. 8.00 (*0-938863-22-3*) HCI Pr.

Men's Health Sourcebook: Everything You Need to Know. Alfred M. Dashe. 1996. 288p. 25.00 (*1-56565-465-X*) Lowell Hse.

Men's Reproductive Health. Janice Swanson & Katherine Forrest. 1984. (Focus on Men Ser.). (Illus.). 416p. 41.95 (*0-8261-4200-1*) Springer Pub.

Menstrual & Pre-Menstrual Tension. Jan De Vries. 1992. (Well Woman Ser.). 160p. pap. (*1-85158-417-X*) Mainstream Pubng GBR. *Dist:* Trafalgar.

Menstrual Cramps: Self Help Book. Susan M. Lark. 3rd rev. ed. 1995. LC 95-14861. 224p. text 16.95 (*0-89087-771-8*) Celestial Arts.

Menstrual Cycle: Physiology, Reproductive Disorders & Infertility. Michael Ferin et al. 1993. LC 92-1058. (Illus.). 264p. text 63.50 (*0-19-506193-4*) OUP.

Menstrual Disorders. Annette Scambler et al. 1992. LC 92-2319. (Experience of Illness Ser.). (Illus.). 128p. (C). (gr. 13). pap. 18.99 (*0-415-04646-7*, A9766) Routledge.

Menstrual Disorders & Menopause: Etiology, Maintenance & Treatment. Linda R. Gannon. 1985. LC 85-3629. 304p. 67.00 (*0-275-90103-3*, C0103, Praeger Pubs) Greenwood.

Menstrual Health in Women's Lives. Ed. by Alice J. Dan & Linda L. Lewis. LC 90-11178. (Illus.). 312p. 1992. text 37.50 (*0-252-01784-6*); 1991. pap. text 17.95 (*0-252-06209-4*) U of Ill Pr.

Menstruation & Psychoanalysis. Mary J. Lupton. 1993. LC 92-39667. 240p. text 34.95 (*0-252-02012-X*); pap. text 14.95 (*0-252-06315-5*) U of Ill Pr.

***Menstruation Disturbances: Index of New Information & Guide-Book for Consumers, Reference & Research.** Estelle S. Dornato. 2002. 180p. 57.50 (*0-7883-2528-0*); pap. 47.50 (*0-7883-2529-9*) ABBE Pubs Assn.

Menstruation, Health & Illness. Ed. by Diana L. Taylor & Nancy F. Woods. 1991. (Health Care for Women International Publication). 410p. 75.00 (*1-56032-132-6*) Hemisp Pub.

Mental Affections of Childhood & Youth. J. Langdon Down. 1991. (Classics in Developmental Medicine Ser.: No. 5). 185p. (C). text (*0-521-41330-3*) Mc Keith Pr GBR. *Dist:* Cambridge U Pr.

Mental & Interest Tests, Their Evaluation & Comparative Effectiveness As Factors of Prognosis in Secondary Education. Leo H. King. LC 77-176957. (Columbia University. Teachers College. Contributions to Education Ser.: No. 444). reprint ed. 37.50 (*0-404-55444-X*) AMS Pr.

Mental & Physical Measurements of Working Children. Henry T. Wooley. 1974. (Psychology Monographs General & Applied: Vol. 18). reprint ed. pap. 55.00 (*0-8115-1417-X*) Periodicals Srv.

Mental & Physical Traits of a Thousand Gifted Children. Lewis M. Terman et al. 2nd rev. ed. 1925. (Genetic Studies of Genius: Vol. I). xiii, 648p. 82.00 (*0-8047-0009-5*) Stanford U Pr.

Mental & Social Disorder in Sub-Saharan Africa: The Case of Sierra Leone, 1787-1990, 147. Leland V. Bell. 1991. LC 91-14922. (Contributions in Afro-American & African Studies Ser.: No. 147). 224p. 62.95 (*0-313-27942-X*, BLQ, Greenwood Pr) Greenwood.

Mental & Social Life of Babies: How Parents Create Persons. Kenneth Kaye. 1994. LC 82-6965. (Illus.). 288p. (C). pap. text 11.00 (*0-226-42848-6*) U Ch Pr.

Mental Birth Control. Mildred Jackson & Terri Teague. Ed. by Paul Ghelev. 1978. (Illus.). pap. 3.00 (*0-932516-00-9*) Lawton-Teague.

Mental Capacity: Medical & Legal Aspects of the Aging. J. Brooke Aker et al. 1977. (Trial Practice Ser.). 372p. text 95.00 (*0-07-000756-X*) Shepards.

Mental Competency: Index of New Information with Authors, Subjects & References. Larry J. Cantrell. 1996. 150p. 57.50 (*0-7883-1274-X*); pap. 47.50 (*0-7883-1275-8*) ABBE Pubs Assn.

Mental Conflicts & Misconduct. William Healy. 1969. LC 69-16237. (Criminology, Law Enforcement, & Social Problems Ser.: No. 88). reprint ed. 24.00 (*0-87585-088-X*) Patterson Smith.

Mental Defectives: Their History, Treatment & Training. Martin W. Barr. 1973. LC 73-2383. (Mental Illness & Social Policy; the American Experience Ser.). reprint ed. 31.95 (*0-405-05191-3*) Ayer.

Mental Des Cellules *see* **Mind of the Cells**

Mental Development in the Child. William Preyer. Tr. by H.W. Brown from GER. LC 78-72818. (Brainedness, Handedness, & Mental Abilities Ser.). reprint ed. 42.50 (*0-404-60887-6*) AMS Pr.

Mental Development of the Child: Summary of Modern Psychological Theory. Karl Buhler. Tr. by Oscar Oeser from GRE. 1978. LC 74-21403. (Classics in Child Development Ser.). 190p. reprint ed. 30.95 (*0-405-06456-X*) Ayer.

Mental Disability: 1990 Supplement. Michael L. Perlin. 3rd ed. 1990. (*0-87473-705-2*, 65814-10, MICHIE) LEXIS Pub.

Mental Disability Law: Civil & Criminal, Set. Michael L. Perlin. 1989. 240.00 (*0-87473-422-3*, 65810-10, MICHIE) LEXIS Pub.

Mental Disease & Social Welfare. Horatio M. Pollock. 1976. LC 75-17237. (Social Problems & Social Policy Ser.). (Illus.). reprint ed. 20.95 (*0-405-07506-5*) Ayer.

Mental Disease in History: A Selection of Translated Readings. Ed. by J. Thomas Dalby. 1997. LC 96-33891. (Reshaping of Psychoanalysis Ser.: No. 7). XIX, 264p. (C). text 51.95 (*0-8204-3056-0*) P Lang Pubng.

Mental Diseases: A Public Health Problem. James V. May. Ed. by Gerald N. Grob. 1980. LC 78-22574. (Historical Issues in Mental Health Ser.). reprint ed. lib. bdg. 40.95 (*0-405-11927-5*) Ayer.

Mental Disorder among Prisoners: Toward an Epidemiologic Inventory. Nathaniel J. Pallone. 1991. 186p. (C). text 49.95 (*0-88738-383-1*) Transaction Pubs.

Mental Disorder & the Criminal Law: A Study in Medico-Sociological Jurisprudence. S. Sheldon Glueck. 1993. LC 93-78309. 693p. reprint ed. 75.00 (*0-89941-843-0*, 307840) W S Hein.

Mental Disorder As a Criminal Defense. Henry Weihofen. 1954. LC 54-8478. 530p. lib. bdg. 42.00 (*0-89941-607-1*, 500580) W S Hein.

Mental Disorder in the Criminal Process: Stan Stress & the Vietnam-Sports Conspiracy, 72. Grant H. Morris & Allen C. Snyder. 1993. LC 92-21355. (Contributions in Legal Studies Ser.: No. 72). 324p. 72.50 (*0-313-28761-9*, GM8761, Greenwood Pr) Greenwood.

Mental Disorders. Ed. by Bruce A. Thyer & John S. Wodarski. 1998. LC 97-15312. (Handbook of Empirical Social Work Practice Ser.: Vol. 1). 528p. 99.95 (*0-471-15361-3*) Wiley.

Mental Disorders & Cognitive Deficits in MS. K. Jensen et al. 1988. (Current Problems in Neurology Ser.: Vol. 10). 224p. (*0-86196-180-3*) J Libbey Med GBR. *Dist:* Bks Intl VA.

Mental Disorders & Genetics. 1996. lib. bdg. 251.75 (*0-8490-6042-7*) Gordon Pr.

Mental Disorders & Genetics: Bridging the Gap Between Research & Society. 1995. (Illus.). 58p. (Orig.). (C). pap. text 30.00 (*0-7881-2508-7*) DIANE Pub.

Mental Disorders & the Law. Kok L. Peng et al. 1994. LC 94-943831. 360p. (Orig.). pap. (*9971-69-188-4*) Sngapore Univ Pr SGP. *Dist:* Coronet Bks.

Mental Disorders in HIV-1 Infection & AIDS. Norman Sartorius et al. 1993. (WHO Expert Series on Neuroscience: Vol. 5). (Illus.). 90p. text 24.00 (*0-88937-096-6*) Hogrefe & Huber Pubs.

Mental Disorders in Later Life. Ed. by Oscar J. Kaplan & Leon Stein. 1980. LC 79-8673. (Growing Old Ser.). (Illus.). reprint ed. lib. bdg. 53.95 (*0-405-12789-8*) Ayer.

Mental Disorders in Older Adults: Fundamentals of Assessment & Treatment. Steven H. Zarit & Judy M. Zarit. 1998. LC 98-22968. 418p. text 42.00 (*1-57230-368-9*, C0368) Guilford Pubns.

Mental Disorders in the Elderly: New Therapeutic Approaches - Rome, April, 1997. Ed. by Nicoletta Brunello et al. 1998. LC 97-52828. (International Academy for Biomedical & Drug Research Ser.: Vol. 13, 1997). (Illus.). vi, 192p. 189.75 (*3-8055-6536-4*) S Karger.

Mental Disorders, Suicide. Ed. by American Public Health Association Staff et al. 1972. LC 74-186673. (Vital & Health Statistics Monographs). (Illus.). 331p. 44.00 (*0-674-56735-8*) HUP.

Mental Effects of Heroin. Ann Holmes. Ed. by Carol C. Nadelson. 1998. LC 98-33640. (Encyclopedia of Psychological Disorders Ser.). (Illus.). 89p. 22.95 (*0-7910-4899-3*) Chelsea Hse.

Mental Evolution in Animals: With a Posthumous Essay on Instinct by Charles Darwin. George J. Romanes. LC 71-96472. reprint ed. 55.00 (*0-404-05389-0*) AMS Pr.

Mental Evolution in Man: Origin of Human Faculty. George J. Romanes. 1975. LC 74-21426. (Classics in Child Development Ser.). 466p. reprint ed. lib. bdg. 40.95 (*0-405-06475-6*) Ayer.

Mental Fatigue: Index of New Information for Reference & Research. Fritz O. Sanders. 1997. 150p. 57.50 (*0-7883-1328-2*); pap. 47.50 (*0-7883-1329-0*) ABBE Pubs Assn.

Mental Fatigue: Index of New Information with Authors, Subjects & References. Larry J. Cantrell. 1996. 150p. 57.50 (*0-7883-1272-3*); pap. 47.50 (*0-7883-1273-1*) ABBE Pubs Assn.

Mental Fatigue - Analysis, Procedures, Tests, Factors, Results & Advice: Index of New Information with Authors, Subjects, Research Categories & References. Carla Dodenhoff. 1995. 160p. 57.50 (*0-7883-0688-X*); pap. 47.50 (*0-7883-0689-8*) ABBE Pubs Assn.

Mental Growth & Personality Development: A Longitudinal Study. Lester W. Sontag et al. 1958. (SRCD M Ser.: Vol. 23, No. 2). 25.00 (*0-527-01574-1*) Periodicals Srv.

Mental Growth of Children from Two to Fourteen Years: Study of the Predictive Value of the Minnesota Pre-School Scales, Vol. 20. Florence L. Goodenough & Katharine Maurer. 1975. LC 70-141548. (University of Minnesota Institute of Child Welfare Monographs: No. 20). (Illus.). 130p. reprint ed. lib. bdg. 48.00 (*0-8371-5895-8*, CWGM) Greenwood.

Mental Growth of the Pre-School Child. Arnold L. Gesell. 1968. reprint ed. 59.00 (*0-403-00127-7*) Scholarly.

Mental Handicap. Aelred S. Shanley. 1986. pap. text 43.00 (*0-443-02793-5*) Saunders.

Mental Handicap: A Multi-Disciplinary Approach. Michael Craft et al. 1985. text (*0-7020-1085-5*) Bailliere Tindall.

Mental Healing & Personal Welfare: Index of New Information. Holly K. Young. 1998. 160p. 57.50 (*0-7883-1728-8*); pap. 47.50 (*0-7883-1729-6*) ABBE Pubs Assn.

Mental Health. Ed. by C. S. Aneshensel & J. C. Phelan. 1999. LC 99-38201. (Handbooks of Sociology & Social Research Ser.). (Illus.). 600p. (C). (*0-306-46069-6*, Plenum Trade) Perseus Pubng.

Mental Health. Dubray. 1993. mass mkt. 16.75 (*0-314-02889-7*) West Pub.

Mental Health. Ed. by Jennifer Hurley. 1998. LC 98-33944. (Current Controversies Ser.). 192p. (YA). (gr. 9-12). pap. 17.45 (*1-56510-952-X*); lib. bdg. 27.45 (*1-56510-953-8*) Gale (Greenhaven Pr).

Mental Health: A Report of the Surgeon General. Ed. by Howard H. Goldman et al. 2000. 487p. (C). pap. text 40.00 (*0-7881-8976-X*) DIANE Pub.

***Mental Health: A Report of the Surgeon General: Executive Summary, Directory of Mental Health Resources, Fact Sheets & Catalog of Materials.** Frwd. by Donna E. Shalala. 2001. 60p. reprint ed. pap. 25.00 (*0-7567-1301-3*) DIANE Pub.

Mental Health: Nursing Edition. Karen L. Fontaine. 4th ed. 1998. LC 98-23779. 612p. 61.00 (*0-8053-1644-2*, Prentice Hall) P-H.

Mental Health: Philosophical Perspectives. Ed. by H. Tristram Engelhardt & Stuart F. Spicker. 1977. LC 77-24974. (Philosophy & Medicine Ser.: No. 4). 324p. text 97.50 (*90-277-0828-2*) Kluwer Academic.

***Mental Health: Planning for One Billion People.** Tsung-yi Lin & Leon Eisenberg. 1985. 244p. pap. (*0-7748-0233-2*) UBC Pr.

Mental Health - Psychiatric Nursing: A Holistic Life-Cycle Approach. Ed. by Ruth P. Rawlins et al. 3rd ed. 1992. LC 92-49347. (Illus.). 960p. (C). (gr. 13). text 57.00 (*0-8016-6331-8*, 06331) Mosby Inc.

Mental Health Act 1983. Great Britain, Department of Health Staff & Great Britain Welsh Office. 1998. LC 98-205724. viii, 138 p. (*0-11-322112-6*) Gale.

Mental Health Administration: Principles & Practice Walter E. Barton & Gail M. Barton. 1982. LC 81-7064. 845p. I. 56.95 (*0-89885-061-4*); II. 56.95 (*0-89885-062-2*) Kluwer Academic (Kluwer Acad Hman Sci).

Mental Health Aide. Jack Rudman. 1994. (Career Examination Ser.: C-1372). pap. 27.95 (*0-8373-1372-4*) Nat Learn.

Mental Health & Aging. Ed. by Eugene Aronowitz & Eleanor M. Bromberg. 1986. LC 86-22684. pap. 6.95 (*0-88135-051-6*) Watson Pub Intl.

Mental Health & Aging: Progress & Prospects. Michael A. Smyer. 1993. LC 93-32953. 192p. 29.95 (*0-8261-8380-8*) Springer Pub.

Mental Health & Deafness. Peter Hindley. 1998. 250p. (Orig.). pap. text (*1-897635-39-7*) Whurr Pub GBR. *Dist:* Singular Publishing.

Mental Health & Deafness. Ed. by Peter Hindley & Nick Kitson. 1998. (Illus.). 256p. (Orig.). pap. 59.95 (*1-56593-748-1*, 1452) Singular Publishing.

Mental Health & Going to School: The Woodlawn Program of Assessment, Early Intervention, & Evaluation. Sheppard G. Kellam et al. 1979. LC 74-10341. pap. text 6.50 (*0-226-42969-5*) U Ch Pr.

Mental Health & Industry: Planning for the 1980's. Ed. by Sherman N. Kieffer et al. 1980. LC 80-18057. (Problems of Industrial Psychiatric Medicine Ser.: Vol. 6). 210p. 35.95 (*0-87705-085-6*, Kluwer Acad Hman Sci) Kluwer Academic.

Mental Health & Law. Leo Stone. 1995. pap. 30.00 (*1-56821-559-2*) Aronson.

Mental Health & Long-Term Physical Illness. Ed. by Eugene Aronowitz & Eleanor M. Bromberg. 1984. 96p. pap. 6.95 (*0-88135-001-X*, N Watson) Watson Pub Intl.

Mental Health & Mental Illness. Patricia D. Barry. 6th ed. 1997. LC 97-16220. 480p. pap. text 30.95 (*0-397-55473-7*) Lppncott W & W.

Mental Health & Mental Illness: Policies, Programs & Services. Phillip Fellin. 1996. LC 95-71917. 258p. (C). pap. text 37.00 (*0-87581-398-4*, MHMI) F E Peacock Pubs.

Mental Health & People of Color: Curriculum Development & Change. Ed. by Jay Chunn, II et al. 1982. LC 83-295. (Illus.). 688p. 34.95 (*0-88258-097-3*) Howard U Pr.

Mental Health & Politics: A History of the Mental Health Services in Northern Ireland. Pauline Prior. 1993. 208p. (*1-85628-540-5*) Avebry GBR. *Dist:* Ashgate Pub Co.

Mental Health & Psychiatric Nursing. O'Connell. 1999. pap. text (*0-7216-6853-4*) Saunders.

Mental Health & Psychiatric Nursing. Linda E. Reese & Gasparis. 1991. LC 91-5211. (Nursetest: A Review Ser.). 288p. pap. 21.95 (*0-87434-306-2*) Springhouse Corp.

Mental Health & Psychiatric Nursing. Margaret Benner. 3rd ed. 1996. LC 96-29146. (Springhouse Notes Ser.). (Illus.). 208p. pap. 26.95 (*0-87434-862-5*) Springhouse Corp.

Mental Health & Psychiatric Nursing: A Caring Approach. Janet L. Davies & Ellen H. Janosik. 1991. (Illus.). 768p. (C). text 68.95 (*0-86720-442-7*, 442-7) Jones & Bartlett.

Mental Health & Psychiatry in Africa: An Annotated Bibliography. David Westley. 1993. LC 93-20491. 224p. (*1-873836-90-2*) H Zell Pubs GBR. *Dist:* Seven Hills Bk.

Mental Health & Religion. Loewenthal. 1994. 256p. pap. 41.50 (*1-56593-356-7*, 0680) Singular Publishing.

Mental Health & Social Change: Fifty Years of Orthopsychiatry, No. 7. Ed. by Fortune V. Mannino. LC 74-26634. (Studies in Modern Society: Political & Social Issues). 34.50 (*0-404-11277-3*) AMS Pr.

Mental Health & the Economy. Ed. by Louis A. Ferman & Jeanne P. Gordus. 1979. LC 79-25809. 423p. pap. text 15.00 (*0-911558-68-3*) W E Upjohn.

Mental Health & the Elderly: Social Work Perspective. Ed. by Francis J. Turner. 1992. LC 92-14579. 539p. 39.95 (*0-02-932795-4*) Free Pr.

Mental Health & the Environment. Ed. by Hugh L. Freeman. 1985. LC 84-9421. (Illus.). 490p. pap. (*0-443-02780-3*) Church.

Mental Health & the Law. Sales. 1994. 39.00 (*0-02-927655-1*) S&S Trade.

Mental Health & the Planned Environment: More than Bricks & Mortar? David Halpern. 1995. LC 95-11983. 240p. 89.95 (*0-7484-0235-7*); pap. 29.95 (*0-7484-0236-5*) Taylor & Francis.

Mental Health & Violence. 1985. LC 85-19098. 129p. pap. 6.95 (*0-88135-050-8*) Watson Pub Intl.

Mental Health Assessment in Occupational Therapy: An Integrative Approach to the Evaluative Process. Barbara J. Hemphill. 1988. LC 86-42925. 281p. pap. 35.00 (*1-55642-004-8*) SLACK Inc.

Mental Health Assessments, 2. Gwen Howe. 1998. LC 99-161854. (Living with Serious Mental Illness Ser.). 152p. pap. 22.95 (*1-85302-458-9*) Taylor & Francis.

Mental Health Benefits: A Purchaser's Guide. William M. Glazer & Nancy N. Bell. Ed. by Mary Jo Brzezinski. 1993. LC 93-77214. 206p. (Orig.). pap. 40.00 (*0-89154-459-3*) Intl Found Employ.

Mental Health Care & National Health Insurance: A Philosophy of & an Approach to Mental Health Care for the Future. David Upton. 1983. LC 83-8049. 334p. 65.00 (*0-306-41235-7*, Plenum Trade) Perseus Pubng.

Mental Health Care & Social Policy. Ed. by Philip Brown. 1985. 428p. pap. 19.95 (*0-7102-0472-8*, Routledge Thoemms) Routledge.

Mental Health Care & Substance Abuse: A Review of Evidence on Insurance Coverage & Utilization. Jeffrey Robin. 1992. (Illus.). 69p. (Orig.). (C). pap. text 25.00 (*1-56806-131-5*) DIANE Pub.

Mental Health Care Delivery: Innovations, Impediments & Implementation. Ed. by Isaac M. Marks & Robert A. Scott. 1990. (Illus.). 280p. (C). text 80.00 (*0-521-38494-X*) Cambridge U Pr.

Mental Health Care for Allied Health & Nursing Professionals. H. Steven Moffic et al. 1989. 240p. pap. 27.50 (*0-87527-344-0*) Green.

Mental Health Care in Crisis. Anny Brackx & Catherine Grimshaw. 1988. 192p. (C). text 49.95 (*0-7453-0221-1*) Westview.

Mental Health Care in Prisons: Index of New Information with Authors, Subjects & Bibliography. Stuart L. Wymer. rev. ed. 1999. 155p. 57.50 (*0-7883-1980-9*); pap. 47.50 (*0-7883-1981-7*) ABBE Pubs Assn.

Mental Health Computing. Kenric W. Hammond & Mathew G. Hile. Ed. by Marvin J. Miller. 1996. LC 95-37689. (Computers & Medicine Ser.). (Illus.). 491p. 95.00 (*0-387-94580-6*) Spr-Verlag.

Mental Health Concepts. Waughfield. 4th ed. 1997. 96p. pap. text, tchr. ed. 12.00 (*0-8273-8219-7*); LC 97-9720. 448p. (C). pap. text 52.95 (*0-8273-8218-9*) Delmar.

***Mental Health Concepts.** Claire G. Waughfield. 5th ed. 2001. LC 2001-47700. 448'p. 48.95 (*0-7668-3830-7*) Delmar.

Mental Health Concepts: Instructor's Guide. Natalie Kalman et al. 3rd ed. 1993. 65p. pap. 15.00 (*0-8273-4981-5*) Delmar.

Mental Health Concepts & Techniques for the Occupational Therapy Assistant. Mary Beth Early. 3rd ed. 1999. 564p. text 45.95 (*0-7817-1975-5*) Lppncott W & W.

Mental Health Consultation Field. Ed. by Saul Cooper & William F. Hodges. 1983. (Community Psychology Ser.: Vol. XI). 247p. (C). 34.95 (*0-89885-130-0*); pap. 24.95 (*0-89885-286-2*) Kluwer Academic (Kluwer Acad Hman Sci).

Mental Health Consultation in Nursing Homes. Michael A. Smyer et al. Ed. by Steven H. Zarit. 1990. (Clinical Gerontology Ser.). 240p. (C). pap. text 18.50 (*0-8147-7911-5*) NYU Pr.

Mental Health Counseling: Theory & Practice. David B. Hershenson & Paul W. Power. 1987. (General Psychology Ser.: No. 144). 448p. 60.00 (*0-08-033147-5*, J115); pap. 22.50 (*0-08-033146-7*) Elsevier (Pergamon Pr).

Mental Health Counselors Clinical Practice Companion: A Continuing Education Program. PTI-AMHCA Staff & AMHCA Staff. 1999. pap. text 195.00 (*0-7872-6384-2*) Kendall-Hunt.

Mental Health Counselor's Handbook. Ed. by G. Seiler. 1989. (Illus.). 300p. 35.00 (*0-89885-476-8*, Kluwer Acad Hman Sci) Kluwer Academic.

Mental Health Diagnostic Desk Reference: Visual Guides & More for Learning to Use the Diagnostic & Statistical Manual (DSM-IV) Ed. by Carlton E. Munson. 2000. LC 99-20779. 396p. 59.95 (*0-7890-1075-5*, Hawrth Medical); LC 99-20779. 396p. pap. text 24.95 (*0-7890-1076-3*); 2nd ed. LC 00-47282. (Illus.). xxvii, 337p. (C). pap. text 24.95 (*0-7890-1465-3*) Haworth Pr.

Mental Health Diagnostic Desk Reference: Visual Guides & More for Learning to Use the Diagnostic & Statistical Manual (DSM-IV-TR) Ed. by Carlton E. Munson. 2nd ed. 2000. LC 00-47282. (Illus.). xxvii, 337p. (C). 59.95 (*0-7890-1464-5*) Haworth Pr.

Mental Health Disorders Sourcebook: Basic Consumer Health Information about Anxiety Disorders, Depression & Other Mood Disorders & More. Ed. by Karen Bellenir. 2nd ed. 2000. LC 99-49596. (Health Reference Ser.). (Illus.). xiii, 605p. lib. bdg. 78.00 (*0-7808-0240-3*) Omnigraphics Inc.

Mental Health Disorders Sourcebook: Basic Information about Schizophrenia, Depression, Bipolar-Disorder, Phobias & Other Disorders. Ed. by Karen Bellenir. 1995. LC 95-36873. (Health Reference Ser.: Vol. 9). viii, 548p. lib. bdg. 78.00 (*0-7808-0040-0*) Omnigraphics Inc.

Mental Health Financing & Programming a Legislator's Guide. Rebecca T. Craig & Barbara Wright. Ed. by Shirley Michaels. 1988. (Illus.). 135p. (Orig.). pap. 15.00 (*1-55516-679-2*, 6619) Natl Conf State Legis.

Mental Health Geriatric Consultant. Jack Rudman. 1994. (Career Examination Ser.: C-1582). pap. 39.95 (*0-8373-1582-4*) Nat Learn.

***Mental Health Handbook for Schools.** Mary Atkinson & Garry Hornby. 2002. LC 2001-40809. pap. (*0-415-20829-7*) Routledge.

***Mental Health in a Mad World.** James A. Magner. 2001. 303p. reprint ed. 23.90 (*1-929291-09-4*) Roman Cath Bks.

Mental Health in a Multi-Ethnic Society: A Multi-Disciplinary Handbook. Ed. by Suman Fernando. 1995. LC 95-8129. 256p. (C). pap. 27.95 (*0-415-10537-4*) Routledge.

Mental Health in Africa & the Americas Today. Samuel O. Okpaku. 1993. 507p. (C). pap. text 49.95 (*0-916085-01-5*) Chrisolith Bks.

Mental Health in Black America. Harold W. Neighbors & James S. Jackson. 1996. LC 95-50210. (C). 248p. 54.95 (*0-8039-3539-0*, 7291); pap. 26.95 (*0-8039-3540-4*, 7290) Sage.

Mental Health in Children. Ed. by D. Siva Sankar. LC 74-27252. Vol. 1. 1975. 49.95 (*0-9600290-7-9*); Vol. 2. 1976. 49.95 (*0-9600290-8-7*); Vol. 3. 1976. 49.95 (*0-9600290-9-5*) PJD Pubns.

Mental Health in Children, Vol. 5. D. Siva Sankar. (*0-915340-04-6*) PJD Pubns.

Mental Health in Europe: Ends, Beginnings, & Rediscoveries. Shulamit Ramon. 1996. LC 95-53929. 224p. text 59.95 (*0-312-16066-6*) St Martin.

Mental Health in Indian Schools. M. Kapur. 1997. LC 97-31052. 26.00 (*0-7619-9206-5*, 82433) Sage.

Mental Health in Late Life: The Adaptive Process. Marguerite D. Kermis. 1986. (Illus.). 392p. (C). pap. text 47.95 (*0-86720-353-6*, 353-6) Jones & Bartlett.

Mental Health in Our Future Cities. David Goldberg. 1998. LC 99-165888. xii, 290p. 59.95 (*0-86377-546-2*) Taylor & Francis.

Mental Health in Primary Care. Linda D. Oakley. 1996. LC 97-118473. 480p. (C). (gr. 13). pap. text 31.95 (*0-8151-7310-5*, 28195) Mosby Inc.

Mental Health in Remote Rural Developing Areas: Concepts & Cases. Committee on Therapeutic Care & Group for the Advancement of Psychiatry Staff. 1995. (GAP Reports: No. 139). 230p. text 12.95 (*0-87318-207-3*, 7207) Am Psychiatric.

Mental Health in the Nursing Home. T. L. Brink. 1990. LC 90-4667. (Clinical Gerontologist Ser.: Vol. 9, Nos. 3-4). 226p. text 39.95 (*1-56024-010-5*); pap. text 19.95 (*1-56024-011-3*) Haworth Pr.

Mental Health in the Nursing Home: An Educational Approach for Staff. Ed. by David M. Blau & Anne O. Freed. 1983. 138p. (Orig.). pap. 27.50 (*0-8236-3362-4*, 03362) Intl Univs Pr.

Mental Health in the Workplace: A Practical Psychiatric Guide. Ed. by Jeffrey P. Kahn. 1992. 462p. 120.00 (*0-471-28418-1*, VNR) Wiley.

Mental Health in the Workplace: An Employer's & Manager's Guide. Donna R. Kemp. 1994. LC 93-27708. 296p. 67.95 (*0-89930-703-5*, Quorum Bks) Greenwood.

Mental Health in Your School: A Guide for Teachers & Others Working in Schools. Young Minds Staff. 1996. LC 97-100824. 64p. pap. (*1-85302-407-4*) Jessica Kingsley GBR. *Dist:* Taylor & Francis.

Mental Health Information Systems: Problems & Prospects. Ed. by E. M. Bennett & Barry Trute. 1983. LC 83-23683. (Studies in Health & Human Services: Vol. 1). 318p. 99.95 (*0-88946-125-2*) E Mellen.

Mental Health Interventions for the Aging. Ed. by Arthur M. Horton, Jr. 1982. 208p. 60.00 (*0-275-90821-6*, C0821, Praeger Pubs) Greenwood.

Mental Health Issues & Aging: Building on the Strengths of Older Persons. Carolyn Tice. 1995. LC 95-43480. (Social Work Ser.). 300p. 23.87 (*0-534-20754-5*) Brooks-Cole.

Mental Health Issues & Aging: Building on the Strengths of Older Persons. Carolyn Tice. 1999. (Social Work Ser.). pap. 26.75 net. (*0-534-76778-8*) Wadsworth Pub.

Mental Health Issues of the Mexican Origin Population in Texas: Proceedings of the Fifth Robert L. Sutherland Seminar. Ed. by Reymundo Rodriguez & Marion T. Coleman. 1987. 240p. (Orig.). pap. 9.45 (*0-943463-00-9*) Hogg Found.

Mental Health Law: Major Issues. David B. Wexler. 1981. LC 80-20523. (Perspectives in Law & Psychology Ser.). 280p. 49.50 (*0-306-40538-5*, Plenum Trade) Perseus Pubng.

Mental Health Law in Context: Doctors Orders. Michael Cavadino. 1989. (Medico-Legal Issues Ser.). (Illus.). 192p. text (*1-85521-024-X*) Dartmth Pub GBR. *Dist:* Ashgate Pub Co.

Mental Health Matters in Primary Care. Elaine Millar & Mark Walsh. 2000. (Illus.). 160p. pap. (*0-7487-4528-9*) Nelson Thornes GBR. *Dist:* Intl Spec Bk, Trans-Atl Phila.

Mental Health, Mental Retardation & Substance Abuse Laws of Virginia Annotated 1998. Ed. by Gail D. Haskins. annot. ed. 1998. LC 99-180384. 442p. (*0-327-06098-0*, 35458-13) LEXIS Pub.

Mental Health Nurse: Views of Practice & Education. Stephen Tilley. 1997. LC 97-26992. 240p. pap. 38.95 (*0-632-03999-X*) Blackwell Sci.

Mental Health Nursing. David Arthur et al. 1992. (Illus.). 260p. (*0-7295-1209-6*) Bailliere Tindall.

Mental Health Nursing. Paulette D. Rollant. 1996. LC 95-33378. (Review Ser.). (Illus.). 416p. (C). 23.95 (*0-8151-7247-8*, 24860) Mosby Inc.

Mental Health Nursing: An Evidence-Based Approach. Robert Newell & Kevin Gournay. 2000. LC 99-34393. pap. text (*0-443-05873-3*) Church.

***Mental Health Nursing: An Introductory Text.** Barbara B. Bauer & Signe S. Hill. 2000. (Illus.). 382p. pap., tchr. ed. (*0-7216-7754-1*) Saunders.

Mental Health Nursing: An Introductory Text. Barbara B. Bauer & Signe S. Hill. 2nd ed. 2000. LC 99-29020. (Illus.). 430p. (C). pap. text (*0-7216-7753-3*) Saunders.

Mental Health Nursing: From First Principles to Professional Practice. Wright. 1992. 554p. pap. 63.75 (*1-56593-022-3*, 0265) Thomson Learn.

Mental Health Nursing: From First Principles to Professional Practice. Ed. by Harry Wright & Martin Giddey. 1992. LC 92-48991. (*0-412-41210-1*) Chapman & Hall.

***Mental Health Nursing: Review & Rationales.** Mary A. Hogan & George B. Smith. 2001. 384p. pap. 24.95 (*0-13-030458-1*) P-H.

Mental Health Nursing: The Art of Compassionate Care. Peter Watkins. 2000. LC 00-57172. (Illus.). 228p. pap. text 35.00 (*0-7506-4119-3*) Buttrwrth-Heinemann.

Mental Health Nursing: The Nurse-Patient Journey. Ed. by Verna B. Carson & Elizabeth N. Arnold. 1996. (Illus.). 1332p. tchr. ed. (*0-7216-6820-8*) Saunders.

Mental Health Nursing: The Nurse-Patient Journey: Robert Carson. 2nd ed. 2000. 205p. pap., tchr. ed. (*0-7216-8057-7*) Saunders.

***Mental Health Nursing: The Nurse-Patient Journey, ExaMaster.** Verna Benner Carson. 2000. 500.00 (*0-7216-8061-5*) Saunders.

Mental Health Nursing in the Community. Nancy Worley. 1996. (Illus.). 496p. (C). (gr. 13). pap. text 35.95 (*0-8151-9429-3*, 27462) Mosby Inc.

Mental Health of Adolescents & Young Persons. Proceedings of the WHO Technical Conference, Stockholm, 1969. A. R. May et al. 1971. (Public Health Papers: No. 41). 72p. pap. 5.00 (*92-4-130041-8*, 1110041) World Health.

Mental Health of Ethnic Minorities. Ed. by Felicisima C. Serafica et al. 1990. LC 89-26597. 360p. 69.50 (*0-275-93111-0*, C3111, Praeger Pubs) Greenwood.

Mental Health of Immigrants & Refugees. Ed. by Wayne H. Holtzman & Thomas H. Bornemann. 1990. 348p. (Orig.). pap. 9.00 (*0-943463-10-6*) Hogg Found.

Mental Health of Older Populations. Martin R. Prince & Sube Banerjee. 2001. (Illus.). 224p. pap. (*0-7506-4860-0*) E A GBR. *Dist:* OUP.

Mental Health of the Child: Program Reports. National Institute of Mental Health Staff. Ed. by Julius Segal. 1973. 19.95 (*0-405-03149-1*) Ayer.

Mental Health on the Community College Campus. Ed. by Gerald Amada. 2nd ed. 1985. 152p. (Orig.). (C). pap. text 23.50 (*0-8191-4915-2*); lib. bdg. 55.50 (*0-8191-4914-4*) U Pr of Amer.

Mental Health Outcome Evaluation. David C. Speer. 1998. LC 97-80314. (Illus.). 121p. text 34.95 (*0-12-656575-9*) Morgan Kaufmann.

Mental Health Outcome Measures. Graham Thornicroft & Michele Tansella. 1996. LC 96-15971. 208p. 106.00 (*3-540-61073-1*); (*0-387-61073-1*) Spr-Verlag.

Mental Health Parity: What Can It Accomplish in a Market Dominated by Managed Care? Alan L. Otten. 1998. (Illus.). 44p. pap. (*1-887748-21-0*) Milbank Memorial.

Mental Health Parity Act: Despite New Federal Standards; Mental Health Benefits Remain Limited. Ed. by John Dicken. 2000. 64p. pap. text 20.00 (*0-7567-0321-2*) DIANE Pub.

Mental Health Policy & Practice Today. Ted R. Watkins & James W. Callicutt. 1997. LC 96-51206. 400p. (C). 86.95 (*0-8039-7138-9*, 2679); pap. 44.95 (*0-8039-7139-7*, 2678) Sage.

Mental Health Practice in Geriatric Health Care Settings. Peter A. Lichtenberg. 1997. LC 97-21734. 212p. 49.95 (*0-7890-0117-9*); pap. 24.95 (*0-7890-0435-6*) Haworth Pr.

Mental Health Practitioner & the Law: A Comprehensive Handbook. Lawrence E. Lifson & Robert I. Simon. 1999. LC 97-41510. 416p. 52.95 (*0-674-69721-9*) HUP.

Mental Health Problems & Older Adults. Greg Hinrichsen. 1990. LC 90-40319. (Choices & Challenges Ser.). 300p. lib. bdg. 45.00 (*0-87436-240-7*) ABC-CLIO.

Mental Health Problems & the Nursing Home Resident. Marylou Hughes. 1988. 174p. (C). 19.50 (*1-877735-21-3*, 2136PP) Prof Prnting & Pub.

Mental Health Procedural Tables. Shaw and Sons Ltd. Staff. 1988. (C). pap. (*0-7219-0196-4*) Scientific GBR. *Dist:* St Mut.

Mental Health Professionals' Book Guide, 1990. Ed. by Aronson, Jason, Inc. Staff. 1990. LC 89-18515. 92p. pap. 1.00 (*0-87668-800-8*) Aronson.

Mental Health Professional's Guide to Managed Care. Ed. by Rodney L. Lowman & Robert J. Resnick. 1994. LC 93-47570. 191p. pap. text 24.95 (*1-55798-232-5*) Am Psychol.

Mental Health Professionals in Medical Settings. Jo Ellen Patterson et al. 2001. LC 00-50050. 272p. 40.00 (*0-393-70338-X*) Norton.

Mental Health Promotion: Paradigms & Practice. Keith Tudor. 1996. LC 95-4477. 336p. (C). pap. 29.95 (*0-415-10106-9*); (Illus.). 85.00 (*0-415-10105-0*) Routledge.

Mental Health Promotion: Policy, Practice & Partnerships. Gary F. McCulloch & Judy Boxer. 1997. (Illus.). 256p. pap. (*0-7020-1981-X*) W B Saunders.

Mental Health Protocols for Occupational Therapy. Catana Brown et al. 1993. 32p. (C). pap. text 6.50 (*0-935273-06-9*) Chess Pub.

Mental Health Psychiatric Nursing. Janosik. 1996. 34.95 (*0-316-45757-4*, Little Brwn Med Div) Lppncott W & W.

Mental Health Psychiatric Nursing: A Continuum of Care. Ed. by Joan Norris et al. 1989. pap. text, tchr. ed. 12.95 (*0-8273-4325-6*); 12.95 (*0-8273-4326-4*) Delmar.

Mental Health, Racism & Sexism. Ed. by Charles V. Willie et al. 1995. 512p. pap. (*0-7484-0392-2*) Tay Francis Ltd GBR. *Dist:* Taylor & Francis.

Mental Health, Racism & Sexism. Charles V. Willie et al. Ed. by Bertram S. Brown. rev. ed. 1995. 440p. (C). pap. 22.95 (*0-8229-5549-0*); text 49.95 (*0-8229-3869-3*) U of Pittsburgh Pr.

Mental Health Research in Texas: Retrospect & Prospect. Ed. by Charles M. Bonjean & Donald J. Foss. 1990. 400p. (Orig.). pap. 8.50 (*0-943463-09-2*) Hogg Found.

Mental Health Resource Guide. Contrib. by Resources for Rehabilitation Staff. 2000. LC 00-62632. 224p. pap. 39.95 (*0-929718-27-5*) Resc Rehab.

Mental Health Response to Mass Emergencies: Theory & Practice. Ed. by Mary Lystad. 1988. LC 88-5025. (Psychosocial Stress Ser.: No. 12). 454p. text 56.95 (*0-87630-514-1*) Brunner-Routledge.

Mental Health Service Delivery Guidelines. Ed. by AOTA Staff. 1996. 176p. (Orig.). pap. text 25.00 (*1-56900-037-9*, 1135) Am Occup Therapy.

Mental Health Service Evaluation. Ed. by Helle C. Knudsen & Graham Thornicroft. 1996. (Studies in Social & Community Psychiatry). (Illus.). 399p. (C). text 95.00 (*0-521-46088-3*) Cambridge U Pr.

Mental Health Services - Law & Practice. Larry Gostin. 1986. (C). ring bd. (*0-7219-0197-2*) Scientific GBR. *Dist:* St Mut.

Mental Health Services—Status, Trends & Practices: Index of New Information. American Health Research Institute Staff. 1998. 160p. 57.50 (*0-7883-1652-4*); pap. 47.50 (*0-7883-1653-2*) ABBE Pubs Assn.

Mental Health Services & Sectors of Care. Enola Knisley Proctor et al. 1999. LC 99-17012. 117p. 49.95 (*0-7890-0760-6*) Haworth Pr.

Mental Health Services for Older Adults: Implications for Training & Practice in Geropsychology. Ed. by Bob G. Knight et al. 1995. LC 95-23757. 158p. pap. text 19.95 (*1-55798-334-8*) Am Psychol.

Mental Health Services in Developing Countries: Proceedings of the WHO Seminar on the Organization of Mental Health Services, Addis Ababa, 1973. WHO Staff. Ed. by T. A. Baasher et al. 1975. (Offset Publications: No. 22). pap. text 18.00 (*92-4-170022-X*, 1120022) World Health.

Mental Health Services in Europe. A. R. May. 1976. (Offset Publications: No. 23). pap. text 12.00 (*92-4-170023-8*, 1120023) World Health.

Mental Health Services in Europe: Ten Years On. H. L. Freeman et al. 1985. (Public Health in Europe Ser.: No. 25). 112p. pap. text 11.00 (*92-890-1161-0*, 1320025) World Health.

Mental Health Services in Pilot Study Areas: Report on a European Study. 1987. text 70.00 (*92-890-1046-0*) World Health.

Mental Health Services in Southern Countries of the European Region. 1988. (Euro Reports & Studies Ser.: No. 107). 46p. pap. text 6.00 (*92-890-1273-0*) World Health.

Mental Health Services in the United States & England: Struggling for Change: Collected Papers Prepared for the Joint United States-England Conference on Mental Health Services Princeton, New Jersey, February 25-28, 1990. Ed. by Jeffrey C. Merrill. 1991. LC 91-61190. (Illus.). 160p. (Orig.). pap. (*0-942054-03-2*) R W Johnson Found.

Mental Health Social Work Observed. Mike Fisher et al. 1984. (*0-7855-0842-2*) Natl Inst Soc Work GBR. *Dist:* St Mut.

Mental Health Technology Bible. Larry D. Rosen & Michelle M. Weil. 1997. LC 96-42475. 256p. pap. 80.00 incl. cd-rom (*0-471-17618-4*) Wiley.

Mental Health Through Will-Training: A System of Self Help in Psychotherapy As Practiced by Recovery, Incorporated. Abraham A. Low. 3rd ed. 1997. LC 97-60039. 448p. (C). reprint ed. text 20.00 (*0-915005-06-9*) Willett Pub Co.

Mental Health, United States, 1996. Ed. by Ronald W. Manderscheid & Mary A. Sonnenschein. (Illus.). 1998. 249p. (C). pap. text 45.00 (*0-7881-4889-3*); 1996. 260p. pap. text 45.00 (*1-57979-154-9*) DIANE Pub.

Mental Health, United States, 1994. Ed. by Ronald W. Manderscheid & Mary A. Sonnenschein. 1995. (Illus.). 192p. (Orig.). (C). pap. text 45.00 (*0-7881-1833-1*) DIANE Pub.

Mental Health Work in the Community: Theory & Practice in Social Work & Community Psychiatric Nursing. Michael Sheppard. 1991. 224p. 65.00 (*1-85000-978-3*); pap. 34.95 (*1-85000-979-1*) Taylor & Francis (Falmer Pr).

Mental Health Worker: Psychiatric Aide. Beverly Marshburn. Ed. by Kay Cox-Stevens. 1999. LC 97-77991. (Clinical Allied Healthcare Ser.). (Illus.). 540p. pap. text 44.95 (*0-89262-437-X*) Career Pub.

Mental Health Worker: Psychiatric Aide: Instructor's Guide. Beverly Marshburn. Ed. by Kay Cox-Stevens. 1999. (Clinical Allied Healthcare Ser.). (Illus.). 464p. tchr. ed., ring bd. 99.95 (*0-89262-445-0*) Career Pub.

Mental Hygiene in Twentieth-Century America, Four Studies, 1921-1924: An Original Anthology. Ed. by Gerald N. Grob. 1980. LC 78-22586. (Historical Issues in Mental Health Ser.). (Illus.). lib. bdg. 40.95 (*0-405-11937-2*) Ayer.

Mental Hygiene Nursing Program Coordinator. Jack Rudman. 1994. (Career Examination Ser.: C-2665). pap. 34.95 (*0-8373-2665-6*) Nat Learn.

Mental Hygiene Therapy Assistant. Jack Rudman. 1994. (Career Examination Ser.: C-2188). pap. 27.95 (*0-8373-2188-3*) Nat Learn.

Mental Hygiene Treatment Team Leader. Jack Rudman. 1994. (Career Examination Ser.: C-1885). pap. 29.95 (*0-8373-1885-8*) Nat Learn.

Mental Illness. Tom Campbell. 1991. (Medico-Legal Issues Ser.: Vol. 5). text (*1-85521-028-2*) Dartmth Pub GBR. *Dist:* Ashgate Pub Co.

Mental Illness: A Homecare Guide. Aristide H. Esser & Sylvia Lacey. 1989. 274p. pap. 12.95 (*0-471-61157-3*) Wiley.

Mental Illness: Can It Be Cured? Prevented? Irving G. Walmann. 3rd annot. rev. ed. 2001. LC 00-191825. (Illus.). 164p. pap. 9.95 (*0-9663299-6-1*) ALMA Pub.

Mental Illness: Cracking The Code to Its Meaning. Melvin P. Firestone. 1993. 250p. 29.95 (*0-9635627-0-3*) Eileen Bks.

Mental Illness: Key Area Handbook. Department of Health Staff. 1994. 180p. pap. (*0-11-321829-X*, HM1829X) Statnry Office GBR. *Dist:* Bernan Associates.

Mental Illness: Law & Public Policy. Ed. by Baruch A. Brody & H. Tristram Engelhardt. 1980. (Philosophy & Medicine Ser.: No. 5). 272p. text 94.00 (*90-277-1057-0*) Kluwer Academic.

Mental Illness & Psychology. Michel Foucault. 1986. 90p. pap. 14.95 (*0-520-05919-0*) U CA Pr.

Mental Illness & Public Health Care. Ed. by James M. Humber & Robert F. Almeder. 2001. (Biomedical Ethics Reviews Ser.). 142p. 44.50 (*1-58829-021-2*) Humana.

Mental Illness & Social Policy: The American Experience. Set. Ed. by Gerald N. Grob et al. 1973. 1390.00 (*0-405-05190-5*) Ayer.

Mental Illness & the Economy. M. Harvey Brenner. 1973. LC 72-85144. 320p. 34.00 (*0-674-56875-3*) HUP.

Mental Illness for Caregivers. Irving G. Walmann. 1998. LC 98-70655. (Illus.). 118p. pap. 9.95 (*0-9663299-5-3*) ALMA Pub.

Mental Illness Heal Yourself. Mary M. Harris. unabr. ed. 1993. LC 93-73310. (Heal Your Self Ser.). (Illus.). 125p. (Orig.). pap. 14.95 (*0-9636781-9-1*, 560) BBCS.

Mental Illness in General Health Care: An International Study. Ed. by Norman Sartorius & T. B. Usturn. 1996. LC 94-43206. 410p. 200.00 (*0-471-95491-8*) Wiley.

Mental Illness in Perspective. Robert A. Clark. 1973. 101p. (Orig.). 3.75 (*0-910286-34-5*); pap. 2.95 (*0-910286-29-9*) Boxwood.

Mental Illness in the Family: Issues & Trends. Ed. by Beverley Abosh & April Collins. 1996. 410p. text 45.00 (*0-8020-2905-1*); LC 96-164563. 280p. pap. text 15.95 (*0-8020-7412-X*) U of Toronto Pr.

Mental Illness in the United States: Epidemiological Estimates. Bruce P. Dohrenwend. 1980. LC 79-18725. 161p. 45.00 (*0-275-90471-7*, C0471, Praeger Pubs) Greenwood.

Mental Illness, Stigma & Self-Help: The Founding of Recovery, Inc. Abraham A. Low. 1991. 174p. reprint ed. 20.00 (*0-915005-04-2*) Willett Pub Co.

Mental Imagery Abstracts: The Journal of Mental Imagery, 1977-1989. Ed. by Akhter Ahsen. 1989. LC 89-62538. 302p. pap. text 29.95 (*0-913412-42-2*) Brandon Hse.

Mental Imagery in Health Care: An Introduction to Contemporary Therapeutic Practice. H. Graham. 1995. 192p. pap. text 41.50 (*1-56593-333-8*, 0663) Singular Publishing.

Mental Imagery in Health Care: An Introduction to Therapeutic Practice. Helen Graham. 1995. 183p. pap. 34.95 (*0-412-56940-X*) Chapman & Hall.

Mental Immunity Phenomenon: Constructive Difficulties in the Child's World. Jonathan Shatil. Tr. by Sara Kitai from HEB. 1998. LC 98-16692. 256p. (C). 36.00 (*0-7618-1114-1*) U Pr of Amer.

Mental Incarceration: It's All in Your Mind. Michelle Caple Taylor. 2000. pap. 16.00 (*0-7388-3622-2*) Xlibris Corp.

Mental Life of Monkeys & Apes. Robert M. Yerkes. 1979. LC 79-22241. (History of Psychology Ser.). 180p. 50.00 (*0-8201-1341-7*) Schol Facsimiles.

Mental Load & Stress in Activity. Ed. by W. Bachmann et al. 1983. 136p. 76.00 (*0-444-86349-4*, I-107-82) Elsevier.

Mental Models. Dedre Gentner et al. 1983. 352p. (C). text 39.95 (*0-89859-242-9*) L Erlbaum Assocs.

Mental Models & the Interpretation of Anaphora. Alan Garnham. 2000. LC 00-59251. (Essays in Cognitive Psychology Ser.). 192p. (*1-84169-128-3*) Psychol Pr GBR. *Dist:* Taylor & Francis.

Mental Processes: Index of Modern Information. Willard W. Welkston. 1990. LC 88-47959. 150p. 47.50 (*1-55914-208-1*); pap. 44.50 (*1-55914-209-X*) ABBE Pubs Assn.

Mental Processes: Studies in Cognitive Science. H. Longuet-Higgins & H. Christopher. 1987. (Explorations in Cognitive Science Ser.). 508p. 55.00 (*0-262-12119-0*) MIT Pr.

Mental Representation: A Reader. Ed. by Stephen P. Stich & Ted A. Warfield. 1994. LC 93-31974. (Illus.). 448p. pap. 37.95 (*1-55786-477-2*) Blackwell Pubs.

Mental Representation in Health & Illness. Ed. by J. A. Skelton et al. 1991. (Contributions to Psychology & Medicine Ser.). (Illus.). 284p. 51.95 (*0-387-97401-6*) Spr-Verlag.

Mental Representation of Trait & Autobiographical Knowledge of the Self. Ed. by Robert S. Wyer, Jr. & Thomas K. Srull. 1993. (Advances in Social Cognition Ser.: Vol. 5). 200p. pap. 24.50 (*0-8058-1312-8*); text 45.00 (*0-8058-1310-1*) L Erlbaum Assocs.

Mental Retardation. Robert B. Edgerton. 1979. LC 78-27199. (Developing Child Ser.). (Illus.). 125p. 26.95 (*0-674-56885-0*) HUP.

Mental Retardation. Robert B. Edgerton et al. 1979. LC 78-27199. (Developing Child Ser.). (Illus.). 125p. pap. text 8.95 (*0-674-56886-9*) HUP.

Mental Retardation. Bernard Schlanger. 1973. LC 73-9613. (Studies in Communicative Disorders). (C). pap. (*0-672-61289-5*, Bobbs) Macmillan.

Mental Retardation: A Review of Research. Ed. by Harvey A. Stevens & Rick Heber. 1994. LC 64-15808. lib. bdg. 17.50 (*0-226-77388-4*) U Ch Pr.

Mental Retardation: A Source Guide. 1991. lib. bdg. 250.00 (*0-8490-4864-8*) Gordon Pr.

Mental Retardation: Definition, Classification & Systems of Support. Ruth A. Luckasson et al. 9th ed. 1992. 189p. 79.00 (*0-940898-30-6*); 54p. pap., stu. ed. 22.95 (*0-940898-35-7*) Am Assn Mental.

Mental Retardation: Developing Pharmacotherapies. Ed. by John J. Ratey. 1991. LC 90-14485. (Progress in Psychiatry Ser.: No. 32). 162p. text 12.95 (*0-88048-452-7*, 8452) Am Psychiatric.

Mental Retardation: Nature, Cause & Management. George S. Baroff. 2nd ed. 1986. (Illus.). 400p. (C). 66.95 (*0-89116-263-1*) Hemisp Pub.

Mental Retardation: The Developmental-Difference Controversy. D. Balla & Edward F. Zigler. 1982. (Illus.). 352p. (C). text 69.95 (*0-89859-170-8*) L Erlbaum Assocs.

Mental Retardation & Developmental Disabilities. Ed. by Phillip J. McLaughlin & Paul Wehman. 2nd ed. 1996. LC 95-38189. 411p. (C). text 41.00 (*0-89079-643-2*, 7639) PRO-ED.

Mental Retardation & Developmental Disabilities, Vol. 13. Ed. by Joseph Wortis. 1984. LC 73-647002. 226p. 65.00 (*0-306-41456-2*, Plenum Trade) Perseus Pubng.

Mental Retardation & Mental Health: Classification, Diagnosis, Treatment, Services. Ed. by Jack A. Stark et al. 1990. (Disorders of Human Learning, Behavior, & Communication Ser.). (Illus.). 464p. 44.00 (*0-387-96577-7*) Spr-Verlag.

Mental Retardation & Sterilization: A Problem of Competency & Paternalism. Ed. by Ruth Macklin & Willard Gaylin. 1981. LC 81-7393. (Hastings Center Series in Ethics). 274p. 39.50 (*0-306-40689-6*, Plenum Trade) Perseus Pubng.

Mental Retardation-Approaches to Institutional Change. Charles C. Cleland & Jon D. Swartz. 1969. LC 69-19945. 288p. text 68.00 (*0-8089-0100-1*, 790865, Grune & Strat) Harcrt Hlth Sci Grp.

Mental Retardation Handbook. Martin N. Levine. 1989. 147p. pap. text 39.50 (*0-87424-230-4*, W-230) Western Psych.

Mental Retardation in Social Context. Duane F. Stroman. 1989. LC 89-5455. 368p. (Orig.). (C). pap. 33.00 (*0-8191-7393-2*) U Pr of Amer.

Mental Retardation in the Year 2000. Ed. by L. Rowitz. 1992. (Disorders of Human Learning, Behavior, & Communication Ser.). (Illus.). 389p. 143.00 (*0-387-97474-1*) Spr-Verlag.

Mental Retardation, Its Nature & Incidence: A Population Survey of the State of Delaware. Joseph F. Jastak et al. LC 62-19658. 184p. 26.50 (*0-87413-103-0*) U Delaware Pr.

Mental Retardation Programs: How Does Massachusetts Compare? Edward Moscovitch. 1991. (Pioneer Paper Ser.: No. 4). 100p. (Orig.). pap. 10.00 (*0-929930-06-1*) Pioneer Inst.

Mental Retardation Sourcebook: Basic Consumer Health Information about Mental Retardation & Its Causes, Including down Syndrome, Fetal Alcohol Syndrome, Fragile X Syndrome, Genetic Conditions, Injury ... Ed. by Joyce Brennfleck Shannon. 2000. LC 00-21692. (Health Reference Ser.). xiii, 642p. 78.00 (*0-7808-0377-9*) Omnigraphics Inc.

Mental State of Hystericals. Pierre Janet. 557p. 120.00 (*1-85506-681-5*) Thoemmes Pr.

Mental State of Hystericals, 2. Pierre Janet. 1977. LC 77-72191. (Contributions to the History of Psychology Ser.: Pt. 2, Medical Psychology). 535p. reprint ed. lib. bdg. 75.00 (*0-313-26941-6*, U6941, Greenwood Pr) Greenwood.

Mental Status Examination in Neurology. Richard L. Strub & F. William Black. 4th ed. 1999. LC 99-24985. (Illus.). 208p. pap. text 28.95 (*0-8036-0427-0*) Davis Co.

Mental Status Schedules & Psychiatric Rating Scales: Index of New Information for Reference & Research. Larry W. Lingeman. 1997. 160p. 57.50 (*0-7883-1326-6*); pap. 47.50 (*0-7883-1327-4*) ABBE Pubs Assn.

Mental Symptoms, Vol. 1. H. Barthel. 1987. 734p. 156.00 (*3-7760-0559-9*) Medicina Bio.

Mentality of Apes. Wolfgang Kohler. 1976. (Illus.). 352p. reprint ed. pap. 3.95 (*0-87140-108-8*) Liveright.

Mentality of the Arriving Immigrant. E. H. Mullan. 1970. LC 77-129408. (American Immigration Collection. Series 2). (Illus.). reprint ed. 15.95 (*0-405-00562-8*) Ayer.

Mentally Disordered Offender. Seymour L. Halleck. 1987. 214p. pap. text 12.95 (*0-88048-270-2*, 8270) Am Psychiatric.

Mentally Disordered Offender in an Era of Community Care: New Directions in Provision. Ed. by William Watson & Adrian Grounds. 1993. LC 92-48693. (Illus.). 238p. (C). text 69.95 (*0-521-40342-1*) Cambridge U Pr.

Mentally Disordered Offenders: Managing People Nobody Owns. David Webb. 1999. LC 98-53740. (*0-415-18009-0*) Routledge.

Mentally Disordered Offenders: Managing People Nobody Owns David Webb & Robert Harris. 1999. LC 98-53740. 224p. pap. 27.95 (*0-415-18010-4*) Routledge.

Mentally Disordered Offenders: Perspectives from Law & Social Science. J. Monahan & H. J. Steadman. 1983. LC 83-2329. (Perspectives in Law & Psychology Ser.: Vol. 6). (Illus.). 318p. (C). 62.50 (*0-306-41151-2*, Plenum Trade) Perseus Pubng.

Mentally Ill Child Grows Up: Transitions to the World of Work. Bertram J. Black. 1993. LC 93-31218. 222p. text 31.95 (*0-87630-711-X*) Brunner-Routledge.

Mentally Ill in Jail: Planning for Essential Services. Henry J. Steadman et al. 1988. LC 88-24157. (Guilford Law & Behavior Ser.). 242p. 33.95 (*0-89862-279-4*) Guilford Pubns.

Mentally Ill in Urban America: An Original Anthology. Ed. by Gerald N. Grob. 1980. LC 78-22575. (Historical Issues in Mental Health Ser.). (Illus.). lib. bdg. 48.95 (*0-405-11928-3*) Ayer.

Mentally Ill Mothers & Their Children. Henry Grunebaum et al. 2nd ed. LC 82-10911. 1996. xvii, 414p. pap. text 12.00 (*0-226-31022-1*); 1993. xvii, 378p. lib. bdg. 30.00 (*0-226-31029-9*) U Ch Pr.

Mentally Ill Offenders & the Criminal Justice System: Issues in Forensic Services. Ed. by Nancy J. Beran & Beverly G. Toomey. 1979. LC 78-19782. 193p. 62.50 (*0-275-90330-3*, C0330, Praeger Pubs) Greenwood.

Mentally Impaired Elderly: Strategies & Interventions to Maintain Function. Ed. by Ellen D. Taira. 1991. LC 91-20816. (Physical & Occupational Therapy in Geriatrics Ser.). (Illus.). 169p. lib. bdg. 39.95 (*1-56024-168-3*) Haworth Pr.

Mentally Retarded & Normal Children: A Comparative Study of Their Family Conditions. Manju Biswas. 1980. 157p. (*0-940500-50-7*) Sterling IND. *Dist:* Asia Bk Corp.

Mentally Retarded Child. Abraham Levinson. enl. rev. ed. 1978. LC 77-25884. (Illus.). 187p. reprint ed. lib. bdg. 48.50 (*0-313-20123-4*, LEMR, Greenwood Pr) Greenwood.

Mentally Subnormal Child. Date not set. (Technical Report Ser.). 46p. pap. text 3.00 (*92-4-120075-8*) World Health.

Mentor Connection in Nursing. Ed. by Connie Vance & Roberta K. Olson. 1998. LC 97-41971. (Illus.). 220p. 39.95 (*0-8261-1174-2*) Springer Pub.

Mentor Manual: For Adults Who Work with Pregnant & Parenting Teens. Frederick H. Kanfer et al. 1995. LC 95-131150. (Orig.). pap. 18.95 (*0-87868-580-4*) Child Welfare.

Mentoring & Nurturing Communication in Health Contexts: A Special Issue of "Health Communication" Ed. by Jeffery Pittam & Cynthia Gallois. 1998. pap. (*0-8058-9821-2*) L Erlbaum Assocs.

Mentoring & Preceptorship: A Guide to Support Roles in Clinical Practice. Alison Morton-Cooper & Anne Palmer. 1993. LC 93-19829. 192p. pap. 24.95 (*0-632-03596-X*) Blackwell Sci.

Mentoring in General Practice. Rosslynne Freeman. 1998. LC 98-27560. 240p. pap. text 45.00 (*0-7506-3940-7*) Buttrwrth-Heinemann.

Mentoring Strategic Change in Healthcare: An Action Guide. Chip Caldwell. 1995. (Illus.). 262p. 32.00 (*0-87389-224-0*, H0787) ASQ Qual Pr.

Menu - Connections for Healthy... Mullen et al. 5th ed. 1999. 36.30 net. (*0-697-29420-X*) McGraw.

Menu Engineering: A Practical Guide to Menu Analysis. Michael L. Kasavana & Donald I. Smith. rev. ed. 1990. 167p. (Orig.). (C). pap. text 24.95 (*0-932235-06-9*) Hosp Pubns.

MEPC: Obstetrics & Gynecology. R. Douglas Ross. 1997. 411p. (C). pap. 21.95 (*0-8385-6328-7*) McGraw-Hill Prof.

MEPC: Optometry. Linda Casser et al. 4th ed. 1994. (Illus.). 416p. (C). pap. 39.95 (*0-8385-7449-1*, A7449-0, Apple Lange Med) McGraw.

MEPC: Pharmacology. Joseph Krzanowski, Jr. 8th ed. 1996. (Illus.). 267p. (C). pap. text 21.95 (*0-8385-6227-2*, A6227-1, Apple Lange Med) McGraw.

MEPC: Preventive Medicine & Public Health. Richard Hart. 10th ed. 1996. 265p. (Orig.). (C). pap. text 21.95 (*0-8385-6319-8*, A6319-6, Apple Lange Med) McGraw.

MEPC Review for USMLE Step 2 Step 2. Samuel L. Jacobs. 1996. 392p. (C). pap. 34.95 (*0-8385-6270-1*, A6270-1) McGraw-Hill Prof.

MEPC Review of Neurology. Paul S. Slosberg. 10th ed. 1995. LC 93-10813. (Illus.). 267p. (C). pap. text 24.95 (*0-8385-5778-3*, A5778-4, Apple Lange Med) McGraw.

MEPC Review of Pathology. Olusegun Fayemi. 10th ed. 1999. LC 94-121308. (Medical Examination Review Ser.). (Illus.). 319p. (C). pap. text 21.95 (*0-8385-8441-1*, A8441-6, Apple Lange Med) McGraw.

MEPC USMLE Step 1 Review. Olusegun Fayemi. 1996. LC 96-132039. (USMLE Step 1 Review Ser.). (Illus.). 455p. (C). pap. text 34.95 (*0-8385-6269-8*, A6269-3, Apple Lange Med) McGraw.

MEPC USMLE Step 3 Review. Carlyle H. Chan. 3rd ed. 1996. 280p. (C). pap. text 34.95 (*0-8385-6339-2*, A6339-4, Apple Lange Med) McGraw.

Mercado Atlas of Foot Anatomy. O. A. Mercado. 1995. Orig. Title: An Atlas of Podiatric Anatomy. (Illus.). spiral bd. 50.00 (*0-940542-05-6*) Carolando.

Merchant & the Parrot see Oriental Stories As Tools in Psychotherapy

Merchants of Life: An Account of the American Pharmaceutical Industry. Tom Mahoney. 1977. LC 77-167381. (Essay Index Reprint Ser.). reprint ed. 22.95 (*0-8369-2608-0*) Ayer.

Merck Manual: Arabic Language Edition. Ed. by Robert Berkow. Date not set. (ARA.). 150.00 (*0-7859-9677-X*) Fr & Eur.

Merck Manual: Centennial Edition. Ed. by Robert Berkow et al. 17th ed. 1999. (Manual of Diagnosis & Therapy Ser.). (Illus.). 35.00 (*0-911910-10-7*) Merck.

Merck Manual: Chinese Language Edition. Ed. by Robert Berkow. Date not set. (CHI.). 150.00 (*0-7859-9676-1*) Fr & Eur.

Merck Manual: Czech Language Edition. Ed. by Robert Berkow. Date not set. (CZE.). 150.00 (*0-7859-9680-X*) Fr & Eur.

Merck Manual: El Manual Merck. Sharp Merck & Dohme Merck. 7th ed. 1986. (SPA.). 75.00 (*0-8288-1869-X*, S37592) Fr & Eur.

Merck Manual: French Language Edition. Ed. by Robert Berkow. Date not set. (FRE.). 225.00 (*0-7859-9675-3*) Fr & Eur.

Merck Manual: German Language Edition. Ed. by Robert Berkow. Date not set. (GER.). 195.00 (*0-7859-9674-5*) Fr & Eur.

Merck Manual: Hungarian Language Edition. Ed. by Robert Berkow. Date not set. (HUN.). 150.00 (*0-7859-9669-9*) Fr & Eur.

Merck Manual: Italian Language Edition. Ed. by Robert Berkow. Date not set. (ITA.). 150.00 (*0-7859-9672-9*) Fr & Eur.

Merck Manual: Japanese Language Edition. Ed. by Robert Berkow. Date not set. (JPN.). 295.00 (*0-7859-9681-8*) Fr & Eur.

Merck Manual: Polish Language Edition. Ed. by Robert Berkow. Date not set. (POL.). 150.00 (*0-7859-9670-2*) Fr & Eur.

Merck Manual: Portuguese Language Edition. Ed. by Merck Editors. Date not set. (POR.). 150.00 (*0-7859-9662-1*) Fr & Eur.

Merck Manual: Russian Language Edition. Ed. by Merck Editors. Date not set. (RUS.). 195.00 (*0-7859-9663-X*) Fr & Eur.

Merck Manual: Turkish Language Edition. Ed. by Merck Editors. Date not set. (TUR.). 150.00 (*0-7859-9664-8*) Fr & Eur.

Merck Manual for Veterinarians: El Manual Merck de Veterinaria. Sharp Merck & Dohme. 2nd ed. 1981. (SPA.). 1386p. 75.00 (*0-8288-2389-8*, S39845) Fr & Eur.

Merck Manual of Geriatrics. Ed. by Robert Berkow et al. 2nd ed. 1995. LC 96-168522. 25.00 (*0-911910-66-2*) Merck.

Merck Manual of Medical Information: Home Edition. Ed. by Robert Berkow et al. 1997. LC 96-80494. (Illus.). 1509p. 29.95 (*0-911910-87-5*) Merck.

Merck Manual of Medical Information: Home Edition. Ed. by Robert Berkow. 2000. 1536p. pap. 19.95 (*0-671-02726-3*, Star Trek) PB.

Merck Veterinary Manual. Ed. by Merck Editors. 8th rev. ed. 1998. 32.00 (*0-911910-29-8*) Merck.

Mercury As a Global Pollutant: Human Health Issues. Brian Wheatley & R. E. Wyzga. 1997. LC 97-28626. text 95.00 (*0-7923-4679-3*) Kluwer Academic.

Mercury Bibliography Update Covering Research Published Between 1991-1993: 1404 Citations, 610 Abstracts. Mats Hanson. 117p. spiral bd. 19.95 (*0-941011-12-7*) Bio-Probe.

Mercury Contamination in Man & His Environment. 1972. (Technical Reports: No. 137). (Illus.). 181p. (Orig.). pap. (*92-0-115172-1*, IDC137) IAEA AUT. *Dist:* Bernan Associates.

Mercury Free: The Wisdom Behind the Global Consumer Movement to Ban "Silver" Dental Fillings. James E. Hardy. 1996. (Illus.). 270p. 24.95 (*0-9649301-1-0*); 264p. pap. 6.95 (*0-9649301-0-2*) Gabriel Rose.

Mercury in Your Mouth Vol. 1: The Truth about Silver Dental Fillings. Quicksilver Associates Staff. rev. ed. 1994. LC 95-67129. 208p. (Orig.). pap. 14.95 (*0-9643870-0-X*) Quicksilv Pr.

Mercury Poisoning, No. 1. Eusebio Mayz et al. 1972. LC 72-13563. (Illus.). 220p. (C). text 29.50 (*0-8422-7072-8*) Irvington.

Mercury Poisoning, No. 2. J.W. Daniel et al. 1972. LC 72-13563. (Illus.). 220p. (C). text 32.50 (*0-8422-7073-6*) Irvington.

Mercury Poisoning from Dental Amalgam - A Hazard to Human Brain. Patrick Stortebecker. 1986. 213p. reprint ed. 20.00 (*0-941011-01-1*) Bio-Probe.

Mergers & Acquisitions Healthcare Sourcebook. 1989. 495.00 (*0-926700-01-4*) MLR Pub.

Mergers & Acquisitions Healthcare Sourcebook. Ed. by Robert C. Smith, Jr. 2nd ed. 1990. 300p. pap. 495.00 (*0-926700-03-0*) MLR Pub.

Mergers in Health Care: The Performance of Multi-Institutional Organizations, Vol. 7. Ed. by Richard M. Scheffler et al. 1987. (Advances in Health Economics & Health Services Research Ser.). 300p. 73.25 (*0-89232-573-9*) Jai Pr.

Mergers of Teaching Hospitals in Boston, New York & Northern California. John A. Kastor. 2001. LC 2001-27374. (Illus.). 504p. (C). text 59.50 (*0-472-11196-5*, 11196) U of Mich Pr.

Merging Language Intervention with Classroom Practices: A Practical Guide for the Speech Language Pathologist. Eileen Eisner. 1998. LC 97-14964. spiral bd. 34.00 (*0-89079-751-X*, 8459) PRO-ED.

Merging Medical Practices. Keith M. Korenchuk. 1994. 147p. 45.00 (*1-56829-041-1*, 4619) M G M A.

Merging Medical Staffs. Albert L. Fritz et al. Ed. by David Beardsley. 1999. LC 00-501818. (Illus.). viii, 37p. pap. text 49.00 (*1-57839-058-3*) Opus Communs.

Meridia: The Weight-Loss Breakthrough. Othniel J. Seiden. 1998. LC 98-18596. 256p. pap. 14.00 (*0-7615-1654-9*, Prima Health) Prima Pub.

Merleau-Ponty: Language & the Act of Speech. Wayne J. Froman. 1982. LC 81-65292. 256p. 36.50 (*0-8387-5015-X*) Bucknell U Pr.

Merleau-Ponty & Psychology. Ed. by Keith Hoeller. 1985. 270p. (Orig.). pap. 20.00 (*0-914857-02-9*) Rev Exist Psych.

***Merriam Webster's Medical Desk Dictionary.** 2001. 894p. pap. text 19.95 (*0-7668-6175-9*) Delmar.

Merriam-Webster's Medical Desk Dictionary. Ed. by Merriam-Webster, Inc. Staff. 1998. (Illus.). 928p. 49.95 incl. cd-rom (*0-87779-027-2*) Merriam-Webster Inc.

Merriam Webster's Medical Desk Dictionary. Ed. by Merriam-Webster, Inc. Staff. rev. ed. 1993. LC 96-15564. 928p. 25.95 (*0-87779-125-2*) Merriam-Webster Inc.

Merriam Webster's Medical Dictionary see Webster's New Explorer Medical Dictionary

Merriam-Webster's Medical Dictionary. Merriam-Webster, Inc. Staff. 1995. 800p. mass mkt. 6.99 (*0-87779-914-8*) Merriam-Webster Inc.

Merriam-Webster's Medical Office Handbook. Merriam-Webster, Inc. Staff. 2nd rev. ed. 1996. 544p. 19.95 (*0-87779-235-6*) Merriam-Webster Inc.

***Merrill's Atlas of Radiographic Positions & Radiologic Procedures.** Philip W. Ballinger & Euhene D. Frank. 9th ed. 1999. (Illus.). tchr. ed. (*0-323-00789-9*) Mosby Inc.

Merrill's Atlas of Radiographic Positions & Radiologic Procedures, Set. Philip W. Ballinger. 9th ed. 1999. (Illus.). 1696p. text 169.00 (*0-8151-2650-6*, 31648) Mosby Inc.

Merrill's Atlas of Radiographic Positions & Radiologic Procedures. Philip W. Ballinger & Eugene D. Frank. 9th ed. 1999. (Illus.). 1692p. Vol. 1. LC 98-52916. text 67.00 (*0-8151-2651-4*, 31649); Vol. 2. LC 98-52916. text 67.00 (*0-8151-2652-2*, 31650); Vol. 3. text 67.00 (*0-8151-2653-0*, 31651) Mosby Inc.

Merrill's Atlas of Radiographic Positions & Radiologic Procedures: Atlas Posiciones Radiograficas. Philip W. Ballinger & Eugene D. Frank. 8th ed. 1999. (SPA., Illus.). 1696p. (*84-8174-174-4*) Mosby-Doyma Libros ESP. *Dist:* Mosby Inc.

***Merrill's Atlas of Radiographic Positions & Radiologic Procedures: Computerized Testbank.** Philip W. Ballinger & Euhene D. Frank. 9th ed. 1999. (Illus.). (*0-323-00672-8*) Mosby Inc.

Merrill's Atlas-Radiographic Positions & Radiologic Procedures. Philip W. Ballinger. 8th ed. 1995. tchr. ed. (*0-8151-6219-7*) Mosby Inc.

Merritt's Neurology. Lewis P. Rowland. 10th ed. 2000. 1,024p. text 110.00 (*0-683-30474-7*) Lppncott W & W.

Merritt's Neurology: Companion Handbook. Lewis P. Rowland. 10th ed. 2001. LC 2001-29419. (Illus.). pap. text 45.00 (*0-683-30496-8*) Lppncott W & W.

Mesencephalic Trigeminal Nucleus in the Cat. N. E. Lazarov. 2000. LC 99-49732. (Advances in Anatomy, Embryology & Cell Biology Ser.: Vol. 153). (Illus.). 96p. pap. 72.00 (*3-540-66524-2*) Spr-Verlag.

Mesmer & Animal Magnetism: A Chapter in the History of Medicine. Frank A. Pattie. 1994. LC 93-41168. (Illus.). 303p. 39.95 (*0-9622393-5-6*) Edmonston Publ.

Mesmerism: The Discovery of Animal Magnetism (1779); A New Translation. Franz A. Mesmer. Ed. & Tr. by Joseph Bouleur from FRE. 1997. (Orig.). pap. 7.95 (*1-55818-382-5*) Holmes Pub.

Mesmerism in India, 10. James Esdaile. 1977. LC 77-72191. (Contributions to the History of Psychology Ser.: Vol. X, Pt. A, Orientations). 654p. reprint ed. lib. bdg. 99.75 (*0-313-26934-3*, U6934, Greenwood Pr) Greenwood.

Mesmerism in India & Its Practical Application in Surgery & Medicine. James Esdaile. 1989. (C). (*81-206-0456-3*) Asian Educ Servs IND. *Dist:* S Asia.

Mesmerism in India & Its Practical Application in Surgery & Medicine. James Esdaile. 1976. LC 75-16702. (Classics in Psychiatry Ser.). reprint ed. 28.95 (*0-405-07429-8*) Ayer.

Mesolimbic Dopamine System: From Motivation to Action. Ed. by Paul Willner & Jrgen Scheel-Kruger. 1991. LC 90-12986. 674p. 575.00 (*0-471-92886-0*) Wiley.

Mesothelial Cell & Mesothelioma. Ed. by Marie-Claude Jaurand & Jean Bignon. 1994. LC 94-16595. (Lung Biology in Health & Disease Ser.: Vol. 78). (Illus.). 368p. text 185.00 (*0-8247-9232-7*) Dekker.

Mesothelioma: The Story of an Illness. Brenda McKessock. 1994. LC 95-233331. 240p. pap. (*1-874640-21-1*) Argyll Pubng GBR. *Dist:* St Mut.

Mesotheliomas of Animals: A Comprehensive, Tabular Compendium of the World's Literature. E. B. Ilgren. 1993. 384p. 179.00 (*0-8493-4308-9*, RC280) CRC Pr.

Messages Men Hear: Constructing Masculinities. Ian M. Harris. 1995. LC 94-37988. 224p. 85.00 (*0-7484-0229-2*) Taylor & Francis.

Messages of Despair, Messages of Hope: A Guide to the Recovery from Eating Disorders. Mary Orndorff. 1990. 70p. 8.95 (*0-9636536-0-1*) Garkakee.

***Meta-Study of Qualitative Health Research: A Practical Guide to Meta-Analysis & Meta-Synthesis.** Barbara L. Paterson. 2001. LC 00-12991. (Methods in Nursing Research Ser.: Vol. 3). (Illus.). xiii, 162p. pap. 24.95 (*0-7619-2415-9*) Sage.

Metabolic Activation & Toxicity of Chemical Agents to Lung Tissue & Cells. Ed. by Theodore E. Gram. 1993. LC 92-49048. (International Encyclopedia of Pharmacology & Therapeutics Ser.: Section 138). 324p. 176.00 (*0-08-041177-0*, Pergamon Pr) Elsevier.

Metabolic Activation of Drugs & Other Xenobiotics in Hapatocellular Carcinoma. Grace S. Lau. 1998. 320p. pap. text (*962-201-744-4*) Chinese Univ HKG. *Dist:* U of Mich Pr.

Metabolic & Degenerative Diseases of the Central Nervous System: Pathology, Biochemistry, & Genetics. Ed. by Jorge Cervos-Navarro & Henry Urich. 1995. LC 95-15211. (Illus.). 873p. text 129.95 (*0-12-165250-5*) Acad Pr.

Metabolic & Endocrine Disturbances in Renal Diseases. Ed. by Shaul G. Massry et al. 1986. (Contributions to Nephrology Ser.: Vol. 49). (Illus.). viii, 224p. 29.75 (*3-8055-4143-0*) S Karger.

Metabolic & Endocrine Problems in the Elderly. W. J. MacLennan & N. R. Peden. 1989. (Illus.). 205p. 80.00 (*0-387-19541-6*) Spr-Verlag.

Metabolic & Endocrine Problems of the Horse. Ed. by Tim Watson. 1998. (Illus.). 260p. (C). text (*0-7020-2241-1*) W B Saunders GBR. *Dist:* Saunders.

Metabolic & Molecular Bases of Disease Cohen. 1990. (Illus.). 2248p. text 375.00 (*0-7020-1493-1*) Saunders.

Metabolic & Molecular Bases of Inherited Disease. Ed. by Charles R. Scriver et al. 7th ed. 1997. cd-rom 345.00 (*0-07-864187-X*) McGraw-Hill Med Pub.

Metabolic & Molecular Bases of Inherited Disease Charles R. Scriver et al. 8th ed. 2000. (Illus.). 5568p. text 550.00 (*0-07-913035-6*) McGraw-Hill Prof.

Metabolic & Nutritional Abnormalities in Kidney Disease. Ed. by G. Guarnieri et al. 1992. (Contributions to Nephrology Ser.: Vol. 98). (Illus.). viii, 196p. 49.75 (*3-8055-5582-2*) S Karger.

Metabolic & Pediatric Eye Disease: Proceedings of the International Society on Metabolic Eye Disease Symposium, 3rd. International Society on Metabolic Eye Disease Sta. Ed. by Heskel M. Haddad. 1980. (Illus.). 240p. pap. 55.00 (*0-08-024950-7*, Pergamon Pr) Elsevier.

Metabolic Arrest & the Control of Biological Time. Peter W. Hochachka & Michael Guppy. 1987. LC 86-14860. (Illus.). 256p. 45.50 (*0-674-56976-8*) HUP.

***Metabolic Basis of Common Inherited Diseases.** Gordon H. Williams. 2001. (Illus.). 900p. (*0-7216-8678-8*) Saunders.

Metabolic Bone Disease. Ed. by Louis V. Avioli & Stephen M. Krane. 3rd ed. 1997. (Illus.). 811p. text 179.95 (*0-12-068700-3*) Morgan Kaufmann.

Metabolic Bone Disease: Cellular & Tissue Mechanisms. Ed. by Cherk S. Tam et al. 1988. 272p. 168.00 (*0-8493-6422-1*, RC931, CRC Reprint) Franklin.

Metabolic Bone Disease & Clinically Related Disorders. Louis V. Avioli & Stephen M. Krane. 2nd ed. 1990. (Illus.). 912p. text 270.00 (*0-7216-2766-8*) Saunders.

Metabolic Consequences of Changing Dietary Patterns. Ed. by A. P. Simopoulos. 1996. LC 96-15858. (World Review of Nutrition & Dietetics Ser.: Vol. 79, 1996). (Illus.). xv, 226p. 221.00 (*3-8055-6296-9*) S Karger.

Metabolic Control of Disease. Philip K. Bondy & Leon E. Rosenberg. 8th ed. 1980. LC 78-52722. (Illus.). text 225.00 (*0-7216-1844-8*) Saunders.

Metabolic Control of Eating, Energy Expenditure & the Bioenergetics of Obesity. Ed. by A. P. Simopoulos. 1992. (World Review of Nutrition & Dietetics Ser.: Vol. 70). (Illus.). xii, 176p. 204.50 (*3-8055-5595-4*) S Karger.

Metabolic Diseases: Foundations of Clinical Management, Genetics & Pathology. Enid Gilbert-Barness & Lewis Barness. 2000. (Illus.). 1014p. 279.00 (*1-881299-11-2*) Eaton Pub Co.

Metabolic Diseases in Farm Animals. Jack M. Payne. 1979. 38.95 (*0-433-24750-9*) Coronet Bks.

Metabolic Diseases in Pediatric Practice. Mary G. Ampola. 1982. text 39.00 (*0-316-03796-6*, Little Brwn Med Div) Lppncott W & W.

Metabolic Disorders & Nutrition Correlated with Skin. Ed. by B. J. Vermeer et al. 1991. (Current Problems in Dermatology Ser.: Vol. 20). (Illus.). x, 216p. 217.50 (*3-8055-5361-7*) S Karger.

Metabolic Disorders & Their Prevention in Farm Animals. Ed. by L. Vrzgula. 1991. (Developments in Animal & Veterinary Science Ser.: No. 24). 390p. 183.50 (*0-444-98734-7*) Elsevier.

Metabolic Disorders, Methods of Examination. Ed. by W. Straub. 1981. (Developments in Ophthalmology Ser.: Vol. 4). (Illus.). v, 218p. 144.50 (*3-8055-2014-X*) S Karger.

Metabolic Disturbances in the Predialytic Phase of Chronic Renal Failure. Ed. by R. Schmicker et al. 1988. (Contributions to Nephrology Ser.: Vol. 65). (Illus.). viii, 140p. 29.75 (*3-8055-4739-0*) S Karger.

Metabolic Effects of Dietary Carbohydrates. Ed. by I. MacDonald. 1986. (Progress in Biochemical Pharmacology Ser.: Vol. 21). (Illus.). x, 274p. 186.25 (*3-8055-4229-1*) S Karger.

Metabolic Effects of Dietary Fructose. Ed. by Sheldon Reiser & Judith Hallfrisch. 1987. LC 86-31687. 176p. 105.00 (*0-8493-6457-4*, QP702, CRC Reprint) Franklin.

Metabolic Encephalopathies, Therapy & Prognosis. Di Donato. 1995. 216p. (*0-86196-489-6*) J Libbey Med GBR. *Dist:* Buttrwrth-Heinemann.

Metabolic-Endocrine Responses to Food Intake in Infancy. Ed. by G. Zoppi. 1982. (Monographs in Pediatrics: Vol. 16). (Illus.). viii, 116p. pap. 56.75 (*3-8055-3477-9*) S Karger.

Metabolic Engineering: Principles & Methodologies. Gregory N. Stephanopoulos et al. 1998. LC 98-84372. (Illus.). 725p. (C). 99.95 (*0-12-666260-6*) Acad Pr.

Metabolic Feedback: Burn Calories Faster. D. M. Foster. 1987. 24p. (Orig.). pap. 3.00 (*0-938451-04-9*) Selena Pr.

Metabolic Homeostasis: A Syllabus for Those Concerned with the Care of Patients. Nathan B. Talbot et al. 1959. LC 59-14732. (Commonwealth Fund Publications). 144p. pap. 18.00 (*0-674-57000-6*) HUP.

Metabolic Modifiers: Effects on the Nutrient Requirements of Food-Producing Animals. National Research Council, Subcommittee on Metabolism Staff. 1994. LC 94-13922. 96p. (Orig.). (C). pap. text 27.95 (*0-309-04997-0*) Natl Acad Pr.

Metabolic Myopathies. Hilton. 1995. text 72.00 (*0-7020-1607-1*) Saunders.

Metabolic, Nutritional, & Endocrine Disorders: International Nomenclature of Diseases. 1991. xxiii, 464p. pap. text 25.00 (*92-4-154432-5*, 1820006) World Health.

Metabolic Problems of the Newborn: Journal: Biology of the Neonate, Vol. 58, Suppl. 1, 1990. Ed. by Firmino F. Rubaltelli. 1990. (Illus.). iv, 108p. pap. 35.00 (*3-8055-5304-8*) S Karger.

Metabolic Regulation: A Human Perspective. K. N. Frayn. Ed. by Keith Snell. 1996. (Frontiers in Metabolism Ser.: No. 1). (Illus.). 284p. (Orig.). (C). pap. text (*1-85578-048-8*) Portland Pr Ltd GBR. *Dist:* Ashgate Pub Co.

Metabolic Support for the Critically Ill Patient. Ed. by D. W. Wilmore & Y. A. Carpentier. 1993. LC 93-28459. (Update in Intensive Care & Emergency Medicine Ser.: Vol. 17). 455p. 130.00 (*0-387-57154-X*) Spr-Verlag.

Metabolic Support of the Stunned Myocardium: An Experimental Study on the Influence of Lipid Emulsions on Myocardial Performance. Marc Van De Velde. 2000. (Acta Biomedica Lovaniensia Ser.: Vol. 213). (Illus.). 134p. pap. (*90-5867-030-9*) Leuven Univ BEL. *Dist:* Coronet Bks.

Metabolism. Carole J Coffee. 1997. (Integrated Medical Sciences Ser.). (C). pap. 29.95 (*1-889325-26-0*) Blackwell Sci.

Metabolism & Artificial Nutrition in the Critically Ill. G. Guarnieri & F. Iscra. 1999. LC 99-34124. (Topics in Anaesthesia & Critical Care Ser.). 251p. (C). (*88-470-0042-4*) Spr-Verlag ITA. *Dist:* Spr-Verlag.

Metabolism & Nutrition in Liver Disease. Ed. by E. Holm & H. Kasper. 1985. (Falk Symposium Ser.). text 225.00 (*0-85200-907-0*) Kluwer Academic.

Metabolism & Reaction of Anti Cancer Drugs Garth Powis. 1994. 368.50 (*0-08-042355-8*, Pergamon Pr) Elsevier.

Metabolism & Toxicity of Fluoride. G. M. Whitford. (Monographs in Oral Science: Vol. 13). (Illus.). 1989. x, 160p. 128.00 (*3-8055-4942-3*); 2nd rev. ed. 1996. xiv, 156p. 172.25 (*3-8055-6247-0*) S Karger.

Metabolism at a Glance. J. D. Salway. 1994. LC 93-45782. (At a Glance Ser.). (Illus.). 96p. pap. 27.95 (*0-632-03258-8*) Blackwell Sci.

Metabolism at a Glance. Jack G. Salway. 2nd ed. 1999. LC 98-48798. (At a Glance Ser.). (Illus.). 111p. pap. 29.95 (*0-632-05274-0*) Blackwell Sci.

Metabolism-Dependent Activation of Food & Environmental Mutagens in Endothelial Cells. Anita Annas. 2000. (Comprehensive Summaries of Uppsala Dissertations from the Faculty of Pharmacy Ser.: No. 226). (Illus.). 46p. pap. (*91-554-4708-2*) Uppsala Universitet SWE. *Dist:* Coronet Bks.

Metabolism of Amino Acids & Amines. Ed. by H. Tabor & C. W. Tabor. 1971. (Methods in Enzymology Ser.: Vol. 17). (C). Pt. A. text 209.00 (*0-12-181874-8*); Pt. B. text 209.00 (*0-12-181877-2*) Acad Pr.

Metabolism of Anabolic-Androgenic Steroids. Victor A. Rogozkin. 1991. (Illus.). 168p. lib. bdg. 225.00 (*0-8493-6415-9*, QP) CRC Pr.

Metabolism of Trace Metals in Man. Ed. by Owen M. Rennert & Wayiee Chan. 1984. Vol. I. 192p. 110.00 (*0-8493-5798-5*, QP534); Vol. II. 168p. 99.00 (*0-8493-5799-3*, QP534) Franklin (CRC Reprint).

Metabolites 3: Lipids, Amino Acids & Related Compounds, Vol. 8, Metabolites 3: Lipids, Amino Acids and Rel. Hans U. Bergmeyer. 3rd ed. 1985. LC 84-105641. (Illus.). 629p. 320.00 (*3-527-26048-X*, Wiley-VCH) Wiley.

Metabolize: The Personalized Program for Weight Loss. Kenneth Baum & Richard Trubo. 2000. 304p. pap. 13.95 (*0-399-52638-2*, Perigee Bks) Berkley Pub.

Metabotropic Glutamate Receptors. Ed. by P. Jeffrey Conn & Jitendra Patel. 1994. LC 94-18190. (Receptors Ser.). (Illus.). 300p. text 140.00 (*0-89603-291-4*) Humana.

Metacognition & Cognitive Neuropsychology: Monitoring & Control Processes. Ed. by Giuliana Mazzoni & Thomas O. Nelson. 1998. LC 98-5819. 200p. (*0-8058-2662-9*) L Erlbaum Assocs.

Metal & Ceramic Biomaterials: Strength & Surface, Vol. II. Ed. by Paul Ducheyne & Garth W. Hastings. 1984. 184p. 108.00 (*0-8493-6262-8*, R857, CRC Reprint) Franklin.

Metal Carcinogenesis Testing: Principles & In Vitro Methods. Max Costa. 1980. LC 80-80444. (Biological Methods Ser.). (Illus.). 170p. 99.50 (*0-89603-017-2*) Humana.

Metal Complexes in Solution. E. A. Jenne et al. 1986. 318p. pap. text (*1-57235-053-9*) Piccin Nuova.

Metal Compounds in Cancer Therapy. Ed. by Simon P. Fricker. 1994. LC 94-72007. (Metals in Health & Disease Ser.: No. 1). 256p. (C). (gr. 13). pap. text 149.95 (*0-412-54280-3*) Chapman & Hall.

Metal Ions in Biological Systems Vol. 30: Metalloenzymes Involving Amino Acid-Residue & Related Radicals. Helmut Sigel. 1994. (Illus.). 536p. text 245.00 (*0-8247-9093-6*) Dekker.

Metal Metabolism & Disease. Max E. Rafelson. 1986. (Journal: Vol. 4, No. 1, 1986). (Illus.). 112p. pap. 36.75 (*3-8055-4264-X*) S Karger.

Metal Neurotoxicity. Ed. by Stephen C. Bondy. 1987. 198p. 117.00 (*0-8493-4941-9*, RC347, CRC Reprint) Franklin.

Metal Poisoning in Fish. Elsa M. Sorensen. 1991. (Illus.). 384p. 157.95 (*0-8493-4268-6*, SH177) CRC Pr.

Metalinguistic Awareness in Children. Ed. by William E. Tunmer et al. 1983. (Language & Communication Ser.: Vol. 15). (Illus.). 238p. 49.00 (*0-387-12432-2*) Spr-Verlag.

Metalinguistic Development. Jean E. Gombert. Tr. by Tim Pownall. 1992. LC 91-41761. 246p. pap. text 29.95 (*0-226-30209-1*); lib. bdg. 66.00 (*0-226-30208-3*) U Ch Pr.

Metalinguistic Functioning in Children. Judith A. Bowey. 1988. 81p. (C). (*0-7300-0551-8*) Deakin Univ AUS. *Dist:* St Mut.

Metalinguistic Performance & Interlinguistic Competence. David Birdsong. 1989. (Language & Communication Ser.: Vol. 25). 246p. 86.95 (*0-387-50351-X*) Spr-Verlag.

Metallopharmaceuticals I: DNA Interactions Ed. by Michael J. Clarke et al. 1999. LC 99-21036. (Topics in Biological Inorganic Chemistry Ser.: Vol. 1). (Illus.). 240p. 129.00 (*3-540-64889-5*) Spr-Verlag.

Metallothionein III: Biological Roles & Medical Implications. Ed. by K. T. Suzuki et al. 1994. LC 93-41417. 118.00 (*0-8176-2769-3*) Birkhauser.

Metallothionein in Biology & Medicine. Curtis D. Klaassen & K. T. Suzuki. 1991. (Illus.). 432p. lib. bdg. 189.00 (*0-8493-8832-5*) CRC Pr.

Metals & Micronutrients: Uptake & Utilization by Plants. D. A. Robb & S. Pierpoint. 1983. text 136.00 (*0-12-589580-1*) Acad Pr.

Metals & Oxidative Damage in Neurological Disorders. Ed. by James R. Connor. 1997. LC 97-30552. (Illus.). 396p. (C). text 114.00 (*0-306-45534-X*, Kluwer Plenum) Kluwer Academic.

Metals & the Immune System. S. Evans. 1999. (Metals in Health & Disease Ser.). (Illus.). 250p. pap. 99.95 (*0-412-62140-1*, Chap & Hall NY) Chapman & Hall.

Metals & the Skin: Topical Effects & Systemic Absorption. Richard H. Guy & Jurij J. Hostynek. 1999. LC 99-25576. (Illus.). 448p. text 195.00 (*0-8247-9385-4*) Dekker.

Metals in Bone. Ed. by Nicholas D. Priest. 1985. text 225.00 (*0-85200-909-7*) Kluwer Academic.

Metamedicine: Power & Medicine, the 21st Century Way. Vida C. Baron & Norman Baron. 1990. (Illus.). 203p. (Orig.). pap. 14.95 (*0-9624701-0-4*) Barez Pub.

Metamorphosis: Reflections on Recovery. Judith McDaniel. 1989. LC 89-80611. 80p. pap. 7.95 (*0-932379-61-3*); lib. bdg. 16.95 (*0-932379-62-1*) Firebrand Bks.

Metaphor in Psychotherapy: Clinical Applications of Stories & Allegories. Henry T. Close. 1998. LC 98-7500. (Practical Therapist Ser.: Vol. 4). 320p. 34.95 (*1-886230-10-2*) Impact Pubs CA.

Metaphor Therapy: Using Client-Generated Metaphors in Psychotherapy. Richard R. Kopp. 1995. LC 94-47346. 216p. text 25.95 (*0-87630-779-9*) Brunner-Routledge.

Metaphoric Body: Guide to Expressive Therapy Through Images & Archetypes. Nira Ne'eman & Lea Barthal. 1993. 200p. pap. 25.95 (*1-85302-152-0*) Taylor & Francis.

Metaphors in the History of Psychology. Ed. by David E. Leary. (Cambridge Studies in the History of Psychology). (Illus.). 397p. (C). 1994. pap. text 27.95 (*0-521-42152-7*); 1990. text 74.95 (*0-521-37166-X*) Cambridge U Pr.

Metaphors of Aging in Science & the Humanities. Ed. by James E. Birren et al. 1991. LC 91-12798. 272p. (C). text 33.95 (*0-8261-7440-X*) Springer Pub.

Metaphors of Consciousness. R. S. Valle & R. Von Eckartsberg. rev. ed. 1981. LC 80-24803. (Illus.). 544p. (C). pap. 37.50 (*0-306-43119-X*, Plenum Trade) Perseus Pubng.

Metaphors of Consciousness. Ed. by Ronald S. Valle & Rolf Von Eckartsberg. rev. ed. 1981. LC 80-24803. 544p. 45.00 (*0-306-40520-2*, Plenum Trade) Perseus Pubng.

Metaprograms. Wyatt Woodsmall. 1998. (Advanced Neuro Linguistic Programming Applications Ser.). 115p. spiral bd. 35.00 (*1-892876-03-5*) Next Step Pr.

Metaskills: The Spiritual Art of Therapy. Amy Mindell. 1995. LC 94-68554. 192p. (Orig.). pap. 12.95 (*1-56184-119-6*) New Falcon Pubns.

Metastasis. CIBA Foundation Staff. 1989. LC 88-8494. (CIBA Foundation Symposia Ser.: No. 141). 266p. 128.00 (*0-471-91513-0*) Wiley.

Metastasis: Basic Research & Its Clinical Application. Ed. by H. Rabes et al. 1992. (Beitraege Zur Onkologie, Contributions to Oncology Ser.: Vol. 44). x, 394p. 68.75 (*3-8055-5610-1*) S Karger.

Metastasis-Dissemination. Ed. by Elizier Gorelik. 1989. (Cancer Growth & Progression Ser.). (C). text 207.50 (*0-89838-997-6*) Kluwer Academic.

Metastasis Research Protocols Vol. 1: Analysis of Cells & Tissues. Ed. by Susan A. Brooks & Udo Schumacher. 2001. LC 2001-16931. (Methods in Molecular Medicine Ser.: Vol. 57). 336p. 99.50 (*0-89603-610-3*) Humana.

Metastasis Research Protocols Vol. 2: Cell Behavior in Vitro & in Vivo. Ed. by Susan A. Brooks & Udo Schumacher. 2001. LC 2001-16931. (Methods in Molecular Medicine Ser.: Vol. 58). 380p. 99.50 (*0-89603-615-4*) Humana.

Metastatic Bone Disease: Fundamental & Clinical Aspects. Ed. by I. J. Diel et al. 1993. LC 93-46632. (*3-540-57356-9*) Spr-Verlag.

Metastatic Disease of the Musculoskeletal System. Ed. by John Heinerman et al. 2000. (Illus.). 400p. text 125.00 (*1-57626-088-7*) Quality Med Pub.

Meteorology & Weather Factors: Index of New Information with Authors, Subjects & Bibliography. Gilbert J. Umanski. rev. ed. 1995. LC 95-16706. 137p. 57.50 (*0-7883-0354-6*); pap. 47.50 (*0-7883-0355-4*) ABBE Pubs Assn.

Metered Dose Inhaler Technology. Tol S. Purewal. Ed. by David J. Grant. 1998. LC 97-41982. (Illus.). 280p. 194.00 (*1-57491-065-5*) IHS Health Grp.

Methadone: Experiences & Issues. Ed. by Carl D. Chambers & Leon Brill. 1973. LC 72-6122. 411p. 52.00 (*0-87705-072-4*, Kluwer Acad Hman Sci) Kluwer Academic.

Methadone Maintenance in the Management of Opioid Dependence: An International Review. Ed. by Awni Arif & Joseph Westermeyer. 1990. LC 89-78368. 128p. 50.00 (*0-275-93392-X*, C3392, Praeger Pubs) Greenwood.

Methadone Maintenance Treatment & Other Opioid Replacement Therapies. Richard P. Mattick & Wayne Hall. Ed. by Jeff Ward. 1997. LC 99-459989. 480p. text 52.00 (*90-5702-238-9*, Harwood Acad Pubs) Gordon & Breach.

Methadone Treatment for Opioid Dependence. Eric C. Strain & Maxine L. Stitzer. 1999. LC 98-50962. (Johns Hopkins Paperback Ser.). (Illus.). 368p. pap. text 26.95 (*0-8018-6137-3*) Johns Hopkins.

Methamphetamine: A New Deadly Neighbor: Congressional Hearing. Ed. by Jon Kly. 1999. (Illus.). 71p. (C). reprint ed. pap. text 20.00 (*0-7881-8434-2*) DIANE Pub.

Method & Practice in Aristotle's Biology. Michael Boylan. 1983. LC 82-23708. (Illus.). 300p. lib. bdg. 62.00 (*0-8191-2952-6*) U Pr of Amer.

Method, Directions, & Examples: Baccalaureate Program, Pt. I. Ed. by Lucille Knopf. 1982. 66p. 35.00 (*0-88737-081-0*, 19-1909) Natl League Nurse.

Method, Directions, & Examples: Diploma Program, Pt. I. Ed. by Lucille Knopf. 1982. 59p. 35.00 (*0-88737-083-7*, 19-1911) Natl League Nurse.

Method for Constructing Complete Annual United States Life Tables. Robert N. Anderson. 2000. 32p. pap. 3.00 (*0-16-050256-X*) USGPO.

Method for Constructing Complete Annual United States Life Tables. Robert N. Anderson & National Center for Health Statistics Staff. 1999. LC 99-58350. (Vital & Health Statistics Ser.). pap. (*0-8406-0560-9*) Natl Ctr Health Stats.

Method in Madness: Case Studies in Cognitive Neuropsychiatry. Peter W. Halligan & John C. Marshall. 1996. 320p. 49.95 (*0-86377-441-5*); pap. 24.95 (*0-86377-442-3*) L Erlbaum Assocs.

Methode d'Evaluation Rapide pour la Nutrition et les Soins de Sante Primaires. Susan C. Scrimshaw & Elena Hurtado. 1991. (Reference Ser.). 74p. pap. 10.95 (*0-87903-114-X*) UCLA Lat Am Ctr.

Methoden der Klinischen Kapillarmikroskopie. Ed. by F. Mahler et al. 1986. (Illus.). 168p. pap. 68.75 (*3-8055-4409-X*) S Karger.

Methodenentwicklungen Zur Identitaetspruefung Pflanzlicher Drogen Mit Weiterfuehrenden Untersuchungen an Den Infloreszenzen Von Calendula Officinalis L. Mit Weiterfuehrenden Untersuchungen an den Infloreszenzen von Calendula L. Wolfgang Heisig. 1991. (Dissertationes Botanicae Ser.: Band 167). (GER., Illus.). vi, 162p. pap. (*3-443-64079-6*) Gebruder Borntraeger DEU. *Dist:* Balogh.

***Methodes d' Aveugle pour les Essais Cliniques.** 2000. (FRE.). 172p. 68.75 (*3-8055-7118-6*) S Karger.

Methodist Hospital of Houston. Marilyn M. Sibley. 1990. (Illus.). 256p. 19.95 (*0-87611-088-X*) Tex St Hist Assn.

Methodological & Biostatistical Foundations of Clinical Neuropsychology. Ed. by Byron P. Rourke et al. 1992. xii, 556p. (*90-265-1165-5*); pap. (*90-265-1245-7*) Swets.

Methodological & Statistical Advances in the Study of Individual Differences. Ed. by Cecil R. Reynolds & Victor L. Willson. 1985. LC 85-17042. (Perspectives on Individual Differences Ser.). (Illus.). 492p. (C). 114.00 (*0-306-41962-9*, Plenum Trade) Perseus Pubng.

Methodological Approaches in Pharmacoepidemiology: Application to Spontaneous Reporting. Ed. by B. Begaud. 1993. 180p. 149.50 (*0-444-81577-5*) Elsevier.

Methodological Issues & Strategies in Clinical Research. Ed. by Alan E. Kazdin. 2nd ed. 825p. 1998. LC 97-42491. text 59.95 (*1-55798-481-6*, 431-602A); 1998. LC 97-42491. pap. text 39.95 (*1-55798-482-4*, 431-603A); 1992. (Illus.). pap. text 39.95 (*1-55798-167-1*) Am Psychol.

Methodological Issues for Health Care Surveys. Brneda G. Cox & Steven Cohen. 1985. (Statistics: Textbooks & Monographs: Vol. 61). (Illus.). 480p. text 185.00 (*0-8247-7323-3*) Dekker.

Methodological Issues in Aging Research. Ed. by K. Warner Schaie et al. 1988. 272p. 36.95 (*0-8261-5400-X*) Springer Pub.

Methodological Issues in AIDS Behavioral Research. D. G. Ostrow & R. C. Kessler. 1993. (AIDS Prevention & Mental Health Ser.). (Illus.). 374p. (C). text 59.00 (*0-306-44439-9*, Kluwer Plenum) Kluwer Academic.

Methodological Problems in Migraine Trails. Ed. by F. Clifford Rose. 1987. (Journal: Vol. 6, No. 4). (Illus.). iv, 80p. pap. 48.00 (*3-8055-4677-7*) S Karger.

Methodological Problems of Clinical Trials in Dementia. Ed. by Clifford F. Rose. 1990. (Journal: Vol. 9, No. 4, 1990). (Illus.). 60p. pap. 39.25 (*3-8055-5239-4*) S Karger.

Methodologies for Monitoring & Evaluating Vitamin A Deficiency Intervention Programs. Ed. by Guillermo Arrogave et al. 1989. LC 89-83358. 66p. pap. text 3.50 (*0-944398-04-9*) ILSI.

Methodology for Analytical Toxicology, Vol. I. Ed. by Irving Sunshine. 1975. 478p. 270.00 (*0-8493-0716-3*, RA1221, CRC Reprint) Franklin.

Methodology for Analytical Toxicology, Vol. II. Irving Sunshine. 1982. 272p. 149.00 (*0-8493-0717-1*, RA1221, CRC Reprint) Franklin.

Methodology for Assessment of Medical IT Based Systems. Ed. by J. Brender. 1997. (Studies in Health Technology & Informatics: Vol. 42). 308p. 73.00 (*90-5199-337-4*) IOS Press.

Methodology for Family Studies of Genetic Factors: Proceedings of the WHO Scientific Group, Geneva, 1970. WHO Staff. 1971. (Technical Reports: No. 466). pap. text 5.00 (*92-4-120466-4*, 1100466) World Health.

Methodology for Student Drug-Use Surveys. R. Smart & P. Hughes. 1980. (WHO Offset Publications: No. 50). 55p. 7.00 (*92-4-170050-5*) World Health.

Methodology for the Human Sciences: Systems of Inquiry. Donald E. Polkinghorne. 1984. LC 82-5895. (Series in Transpersonal & Humanistic Psychology). 349p. (C). pap. text 19.95 (*0-87395-664-8*) State U NY Pr.

Methodology for the Serum Bactericidal Test: Tentative Guideline (1992), Vol. 7. 1992. 75.00 (*1-56238-142-3*, M21-T) NCCLS.

Methodology in Human Fatigue Assessment: Symposium on Methodology in Human Fatigue Assessment, Kyoto, Japan, 1969. 1971. LC 72-304858. 200p. 42.00 (*0-85066-049-1*) Taylor & Francis.

Methodology in Microcirculation: Proceedings of the European Conference on Microcirculation 7th, Aberdeen, Aug-Sept, 1972. European Conference on Microcirculation Staff. Ed. by D. H. Lewis & J. Ditzel. 1974. (Bibliotheca Anatomica Ser.: No. 11). 248.75 (*3-8055-1571-5*) S Karger.

Methodology of Clinical Drug Trials. A. Spriet et al. 2nd rev. ed. 1994. LC 94-136937. (Illus.). viii, 270p. 123.50 (*3-8055-5856-2*) S Karger.

Methodology of Measuring the Impact of Family Planning Programmes on Fertility: Addendum Manual IX. (Population Studies: No. 66). 38p. pap. 8.00 (*92-1-151160-7*, E.78.XIII.4) UN.

Methodology of Nutritional Surveillance: 27th Report of a Joint FAO/UNICEF/WHO Expert Committee. 1976. (Technical Report Ser.: No. 593). 66p. pap. text 7.00 (*92-4-120593-8*, 1100593) World Health.

Methodology of the Evaluation of Psychotropic Drugs. Ed. by D. Benkert et al. 1990. (Psychopharmacology Ser.: Vol. 8). (Illus.). 191p. 103.00 (*0-387-52094-5*) Spr-Verlag.

Methods & Applications in Mental Health Surveys. Ed. by Shosuke Suzuki & Robert Roberts. 1991. text (*0-86008-473-6*) U of Tokyo JPN. *Dist:* Col U Pr.

Methods & Data Analysis for Cross-Cultural Research. Fons Van De Vijver & Kwok Leung. 1997. LC 96-51274. (Cross-Cultural Psychology Ser.: Vol. 1). 200p. 86.95 (*0-7619-0106-X*, 1765) Sage.

Methods & Folklore. Ed. by Philip K. Wilson. 1996. LC 96-794. (Childbirth Ser.: Vol. 3). (Illus.). 464p. reprint ed. text 88.00 (*0-8153-2232-1*) Garland.

Methods & Materials of Dental Hygiene. Parker. pap. (*0-7216-6014-2*); pap. text, lab manual ed. (*0-7216-6015-0*) Saunders.

Methods & Models for Education in Parapsychology. D. Scott Rogo. 1973. LC 73-75209. (Parapsychological Monographs: No. 14). pap. 5.00 (*0-912328-22-3*) Parapsych Foun.

Methods & Models for Studying the Individual. Robert B. Cairns et al. 1998. LC 98-19777. 308p. 73.95 (*0-7619-1451-X*, 82527); pap. 39.95 (*0-7619-1452-8*, 82528) Sage.

Methods & Techniques in Virology. Ed. by Payment & Trudel. 1993. LC 93-1766. (Illus.). 336p. text 165.00 (*0-8247-9101-0*) Dekker.

***Methods & Tools for Object-Oriented Modelling & Knowledge-Based Simulation of Complex Biomedical Systems.** Mikael Hakman. 2000. (Comprehensive Summaries of Uppsala Dissertations from the Faculty of Medicine Ser.: No. 913). (Illus.). 54p. pap. (*91-554-4674-4*) Uppsala Universitet SWE. *Dist:* Coronet Bks.

Methods Cardiac Electrophysiology. Ed. by Michael J. Walker & Michael K. Pugsley. 1997. LC 97-25186. (CRC Press Methods in Pharmacology Ser.). 224p. per. 84.95 (*0-8493-3334-2*) CRC Pr.

Methods, Directions, & Examples: Associate Degree Program, Pt. I. Ed. by Lucille Knopf. 1982. 74p. 35.00 (*0-88737-082-9*, 19-1910) Natl League Nurse.

Methods for Biological Monitoring: A Manual for Assessing Human Exposure to Hazardous Substances. Ed. by Theodore J. Kneip & John V. Crable. 1988. 512p. 60.00 (*0-87553-148-2*) Am Pub Health.

Methods for Cohort Studies of Chronic Airflow Limitation. C. Florey & S. Leeder. 1982. (WHO Regional Publications, European Ser.: No. 12). 134p. pap. text 19.00 (*92-890-1103-3*) World Health.

Methods for Cutaneous Investigation. Robert L. Rietschel & Thomas S. Spencer. 1990. (Cosmetic Science & Technology Ser.: Vol. 9). (Illus.). 248p. text 150.00 (*0-8247-8264-X*) Dekker.

Methods for Detecting DNA Damaging Agents in Humans: Applications in Cancer Epidemiology & Prevention. Ed. by H. Bartsch et al. 1988. (IARC Scientific Publications Ser.: No. 89). (Illus.). 544p. pap. 115.00 (*92-832-1189-8*) OUP.

Methods for Determining Bactericidal Activity of Antimicrobial Agents: Tentative Guideline (1992), Vol. 7. 1992. 75.00 (*1-56238-144-X*, M26-T) NCCLS.

M N O

Methods for Dilution Antimicrobial Susceptibility Tests for Bacteria That Grow Aerobically: Approved Standard (1993) Contrib. by James H. Jorgensen. 3rd ed. 1993. 85.00 (1-56238-209-8, M7-A3) NCCLS.

Methods for Genetic Risk Assessment. Ed. by David J. Brunsick. 1994. LC 93-5520. 272p. lib. bdg. 120.00 (1-56670-039-6, L1039) Lewis Pubs.

***Methods for 'In Vivo' Optical Imaging of the Central Nervous System.** Ron Frostig. 2001. (Methods & New Frontiers in Neuroscience Ser.). 256p. text 89.95 (0-8493-2389-4) CRC Pr.

Methods for Investigating Localized Clustering of Disease. Ed. by F. E. Alexander & P. Boyle. 1997. LC 97-183624. (IARC Scientific Publications Ser.: No. 135). (Illus.). 264p. pap. text 89.50 (92-832-2135-4) OUP.

Methods for Quality Control in Diagnostic Microbiology. Ed. by J. Michael Miller & Berttina B. Wentworth. 1985. LC 85-3991. 368p. 45.00 (0-87553-121-0) Am Pub Health.

Methods for Specifying Acoustic Properties of Tissue Mimicking Phantoms & Objects: Stage I. 1995. (Illus.). 13p. pap. 24.00 (1-930047-21-5, TMP) Am Inst Ultrasound.

Methods for the Analysis of Human Chromosome Aberrations. K. E. Buckton & Harold J. Evans. 1973. pap. text 12.00 (92-4-154031-1, 1150105) World Health.

Methods for the Economic Evaluation of Health Care Programmes. Michael F. Drummond et al. 2nd ed. 1997. LC 97-10273. (Illus.). 316p. pap. text 42.50 (0-19-262773-2) OUP.

Methods for the Study of Personality in Young Children. Ed. by E. Lerner. 1941. (SRCD M Ser.: Vol. 6, No. 4). 25.00 (0-527-01520-2) Periodicals Srv.

Methods in Aging Research. Byang Pal Yu. 2nd ed. 1998. LC 98-14354. 720p. 139.95 (0-8493-3112-9) CRC Pr.

Methods in Analytical Psychology: An Introduction. Hans Dieckmann. Tr. by Boris Matthews from GER. 1991. 240p. (Orig.). pap. 24.95 (0-933029-48-9) Chiron Pubns.

Methods in Angiology: A Physical-Technical Introduction Written for Clinicians by Physicians. Ed. by Marc Verstraete. 1980. (Instrumentation & Techniques in Clinical Medicine Ser.: No. 2). (Illus.). 525p. text 296.00 (90-247-2376-0) Kluwer Academic.

Methods in Animal Physiology. Ed. by Zdenek Deyl & Joseph Zicha. 1988. 448p. lib. bdg. 295.00 (0-8493-6965-7, QP43) CRC Pr.

Methods in Astmology. Ed. by Luigi Allegra et al. 1993. LC 93-14963. (Illus.). 477p. 174.00 (0-387-56428-4) Spr-Verlag.

Methods in Behavioral Pharmacology. Ed. by Frans Van Haaren. 1993. LC 93-8396. (Techniques in the Behavioral & Neural Sciences Ser.: Vol. 10). 692p. 300.00 (0-444-81444-2) Elsevier.

Methods in Behavioral Research. Paul C. Cozby. 7th ed. 2000. LC 00-21365. (Illus.). xiii, 370p. (0-7674-1063-7) Mayfield Pub.

Methods in Biliary Research. Ed. by Maurizio Muraca. 1994. 336p. lib. bdg. 210.00 (0-8493-8701-9, 8701) CRC Pr.

Methods in Biomedical Magnetic Resonance Imaging & Spectroscopy Ian R. Young. 2000. LC 00-42265. (Encyclopedia of Nuclear Magnetic Resonance Ser.). (Illus.). 1480p. 900.00 (0-471-98804-9) Wiley.

Methods in Cartilage Research. Ed. by A. Maroudas & K. Kuettner. 1990. 392p. text 188.00 (0-12-473280-1) Acad Pr.

Methods in Cell Biology Vol. 55: Laser Tweezers in Cell Biology. Ed. by Leslie Wilson et al. 1997. LC 97-218856. (Methods in Cell Biology, Ser.: Vol. 55). (Illus.). 228p. pap. text 64.95 (0-12-639370-2) Morgan Kaufmann.

Methods in Chemical Neuroanatomy. Ed. by Anders T. Bjorklund & Tomas B. Hokfelt. 1983. (Handbooks of Chemical Neuroanatomy: No. 1). 548p. 336.00 (0-444-90281-3, Excerpta Medica) Elsevier.

Methods in Clinical Toxicology. Orsulak. 1999. 420p. 73.95 (0-8493-7883-4) CRC Pr.

Methods in Comparative Psychoacoustics. Ed. by G. M. Klump et al. 1995. LC 94-45873. (BioMethods Ser.: Vol. 6). x, 345p. 98.50 (0-8176-5079-2) Birkhauser.

Methods in Developmental Toxicology & Biology. Renate Thiel & Stephen Klug. 1997. (Illus.). 240p. 170.00 (0-632-04187-0) Blackwell Sci.

Methods in DNA Amplification. Ed. by Arndt Rolfs et al. 1994. LC 94-43082. (Illus.). 262p. (C). text 95.00 (0-306-44908-0, Kluwer Plenum) Kluwer Academic.

Methods in Enzymology. Sidney P. Colowick. 1998. (C). text 115.00 (0-12-182197-8); Vol. 305. 1999. (Methods in Enzymology Ser.: Vol. 305). 640p. 129.95 (0-12-182206-0); Vol. 310. 1999. (Methods in Enzymology Ser.: Vol. 310). (Illus.). 582p. 99.95 (0-12-182211-7); Vol. 312. 2000. (Methods in Enzymology Ser.: Vol. 312). 540p. 129.95 (0-12-182213-3); Vol. 313. 1999. (Methods in Enzymology Ser.: Vol. 313). (Illus.). 279p. 105.00 (0-12-182214-1); Vol. 314. 1999. (Methods in Enzymology Ser.: Vol. 314). (Illus.). 515p. 105.00 (0-12-182215-X); Vol. 315. 1997. (Methods in Enzymology Ser.: Vol. 315). 774p. 119.95 (0-12-182216-8); Vol. 316. 1997. (Methods in Enzymology Ser.: Vol. 316). 657p. 129.95 (0-12-182217-6); Vol. 317. 1997. (Methods in Enzymology Ser.: Vol. 317). 466p. 129.95 (0-12-182218-4) Acad Pr.

Methods in Enzymology, Vol. 318. Ed. by D. W. Celander. 1997. (Methods in Enzymology Ser.: Vol. 318). (Illus.). 431p. 129.95 (0-12-182219-2) Acad Pr.

Methods in Enzymology, Vol. 319. Sidney P. Colowick. 2000. (Methods in Enzymology Ser.: Vol. 319). (Illus.). 626p. 119.95 (0-12-182220-6) Acad Pr.

Methods in Enzymology: Caged Compounds, Vol. 291. Sidney P. Colowick. Ed. by Gerard Marriott. 1998. (Illus.). 529p. (C). text 99.95 (0-12-182192-7) Acad Pr.

***Methods in Enzymology: G Protein Pathways, Part B: G Proteins & Their Regulators**, 344. Ed. by Ravi Iyengar & John D. Hildebrandt. 2001. (Methods in Enzymology Ser.: Vol. 344). 813p. 129.95 (0-12-182245-1) Acad Pr.

Methods in Enzymology: Ion Channels, Vol. 293. Sidney P. Colowick. 1998. (Illus.). 805p. (C). text 110.00 (0-12-182194-3) Acad Pr.

Methods in Enzymology Vol. 289: Solid-Phase Peptide Synthesis. Ed. by John N. Abelson et al. 1997. (Illus.). 780p. text 110.00 (0-12-182190-0) Morgan Kaufmann.

Methods in Enzymology Vol. 290: Molecular Chaperones, Vol. 290. Ed. by George H. Larimer & Thomas O. Baldwin. 1998. (Illus.). 500p. text 99.95 (0-12-182191-9) Acad Pr.

Methods in Enzymology Vol. 294, Pt. C: Ion Channels. Ed. by Michael P. Conn et al. 1998. (Illus.). 788p. (C). 115.00 (0-12-182195-1) Acad Pr.

Methods in Enzymology Vol. 295: Energetics of Biological Macromolecules. Ed. by John N. Abelson et al. 1998. (Illus.). 548p. (C). 99.95 (0-12-182196-X) Acad Pr.

Methods in Enzymology Vol. 300: Oxidants & Antioxidants. Sidney P. Colowick. Ed. by John N. Abelson et al. 1998. (Illus.). 530p. (C). 99.95 (0-12-182201-X) Acad Pr.

Methods in Enzymology Vol. 301, Pt. C: Nitric Oxide. Sidney P. Colowick. Ed. by John N. Abelson et al. 1998. (Illus.). 589p. (C). 99.95 (0-12-182202-8) Acad Pr.

***Methods in Enzymology Vol. 336, Pt. A: Microbial Growth in Biofilms.** Ed. by John N. Abelson & Melvin I. Simon. 2001. (Biomedical Sciences Ser.). 600p. 129.95 (0-12-182237-0) Acad Pr.

***Methods in Enzymology Vol. 340: Drug-Nucleic Acid Interactions**, 340. Ed. by Jonathan B. Chaires & Michael J. Waring. 2001. 705p. 129.95 (0-12-182241-9) Acad Pr.

***Methods in Enzymology Vol. 343, Pt. A: Ribonucleases: G Protein Pathways.** Ed. by Ravi Iyengar & John D. Hildebrandt. 2001. 817p. 129.95 (0-12-182244-3) Acad Pr.

Methods in Genetic Epidemiology. N. E. Morton et al. 1983. (Contributions to Epidemiology & Biostatistics Ser.: Vol. 4). (Illus.). x, 262p. pap. 131.25 (3-8055-3668-2) S Karger.

Methods in Immunohematology. W. John Judd. 2nd ed. 1994. LC 93-81030. xxii, 476p. pap. text 30.00 (0-935643-04-4) Mont Sci Pubns.

Methods in Immunotoxicology, Vol. 1. Ed. by Gary B. Burleson et al. 1995. LC 95-979. 552p. 339.50 (0-471-56196-7, Wiley-Liss) Wiley.

Methods in Immunotoxicology, Vol. 2. Ed. by Gary R. Burleson et al. 1995. LC 95-979. 496p. 339.50 (0-471-56197-5, Wiley-Liss) Wiley.

***Methods in Medical Ethics.** Ed. by Jeremy Sugarman & Daniel P. Sulmasy. 2001. LC 2001-23268. (Illus.). xiv, 314p. pap. 39.95 (0-87840-873-8) Georgetown U Pr.

Methods in Medicine. J. Ridderikhoff. 1989. 240p. (C). lib. bdg. (1-55608-080-8) Kluwer Academic NLD. *Dist:* Kluwer Academic.

Methods in Microbiology, Vol. 11. Ed. by John R. Norris & T. Bergen. 1979. text 209.00 (0-12-521511-8) Acad Pr.

Methods in Microbiology, Vol. 12. Ed. by John R. Norris & D. W. Ribbons. 1979. text 209.00 (0-12-521512-6) Acad Pr.

Methods in Microbiology, Vol. 19. Ed. by R. R. Colwell & R. Grigorova. 1988. 518p. text 136.00 (0-12-521519-3) Acad Pr.

Methods in Molecular Genetics Vol. 4: Molecular Virology Techniques, Pt. A. Ed. by Kenneth W. Adolph. 1994. (Illus.). 410p. text 104.00 (0-12-044306-6) Acad Pr.

Methods in Molecular Genetics Vol. 5: Gene & Chromosome Analysis, Pt. C. Ed. by Kenneth W. Adolph. 1994. (Illus.). 402p. text 104.00 (0-12-044307-4) Acad Pr.

Methods in Molecular Genetics, Vol. 2: Gene & Chromosome Analysis, Pt. B. Kenneth W. Adolph. 1993. (Illus.). 369p. text 104.00 (0-12-044303-1) Acad Pr.

Methods in Neurobiology. Ed. by Robert Lahue. 1981. LC 80-15623. Vol. 1. 614p. 110.00 (0-306-40517-2); Vol. 2. 682p. 110.00 (0-306-40518-0) Perseus Pubng (Plenum Trade).

Methods in Neuroendocrinology. Louis D. Van de Kar. 1998. LC 98-3241. (Cellular & Molecular Neuropharmacology Ser.). 256p. otabind 94.95 (0-8493-3363-6, 3363) CRC Pr.

Methods in Neurology. A. K. Bagchi. 1989. (C). (0-89771-377-X) Current Dist IND. *Dist:* St Mut.

Methods in Neuronal Modeling: From Ions to Networks. Ed. by Christof Koch & Idan Segev. 2nd ed. 1998. LC 97-17166. (Computational Neuroscience Ser.). (Illus.). 687p. 70.00 (0-262-11231-0, Bradford Bks) MIT Pr.

Methods in Neurosciences: Neurobiology of Cytokines, Vol. 17. Ed. by Errol B. De Souza & P. Michael Conn. 1993. (Illus.). 327p. text 104.00 (0-12-185283-0) Acad Pr.

Methods in Neurosciences Vol. 2: Cell Culture. Ed. by P. Michael Conn. 1990. 424p. text 104.00 (0-12-185253-9) Acad Pr.

Methods in Neurosciences Vol. 4: Electrophysiology & Microinjection. Ed. by P. Michael Conn. 1991. (Illus.). 504p. pap. 73.00 (0-12-185258-X) Acad Pr.

Methods in Neurosciences Vol. 7: Lesions & Transplantation. Ed. by P. Michael Conn. 1991. (Illus.). 496p. spiral bd. 48.00 (0-12-185264-4) Acad Pr.

Methods in Neurosciences Vol. 9: Gene Expression in Neural Tissues. Ed. by P. Michael Conn. 1992. (Illus.). 492p. pap. 48.00 (0-12-185268-7) Acad Pr.

Methods in Neurosciences Vol. 18: Lipid Metabolism in Signaling Systems. Ed. by P. Michael Conn & John N. Fain. 1993. (Illus.). 357p. text 104.00 (0-12-185285-7) Acad Pr.

Methods in Neurosciences Vol. 19: Ion Channels of Excitable Cells. Ed. by Toshio Narahashi & P. Michael Conn. 1994. (Illus.). 387p. text 104.00 (0-12-185287-3) Acad Pr.

Methods in Neurosciences Vol. 20: Pulsatility in Neuroendocrine Systems. Ed. by Jon E. Levine & P. Michael Conn. 1994. (Illus.). 510p. text 104.00 (0-12-185289-X) Acad Pr.

Methods in Neurosciences Vol. 21: Providing Pharmacological Access to the Brain, Alternate Approaches. Ed. by Thomas R. Flanagan et al. 1994. (Illus.). 508p. text 104.00 (0-12-185291-1) Acad Pr.

Methods in Neurosciences Vol. 22: Neurobiology of Steroids. Ed. by E. Ron De Kloet et al. 1994. (Illus.). 552p. text 104.00 (0-12-185292-X) Acad Pr.

Methods in Neurosciences Vol. 23: Peptidases & Neuropeptide Processing. Ed. by A. Ian Smith & P. Michael Conn. 1995. (Illus.). 407p. text 90.00 (0-12-185293-8) Acad Pr.

Methods in Neurosciences Vol. 24: Neuroimmunology. Ed. by P. Michael Conn et al. 1995. (Illus.). 434p. (C). text 59.95 (0-12-185294-6) Acad Pr.

Methods in Neurosciences Vol. 26: PCR in Neuroscience. Ed. by Gobinda Sarkar & P. Michael Conn. 1995. (Illus.). 455p. pap. 58.00 (0-12-619255-3) Acad Pr.

Methods in Neurosciences Vol. 30: Paradigms of Neural Injury. Ed. by P. Michael Conn & Jose R. Perez-Polo. 1996. (Illus.). 335p. text 85.00 (0-12-185300-4) Acad Pr.

Methods in Neurosciences Vol. 31: Nitric Oxide Synthase: Characterization & Functional Analysis. Ed. by P. Michael Conn & Mahin D. Maines. 1996. LC 96-200801. (Methods in Neurosciences Ser.: Vol. 31). (Illus.). 354p. text 89.00 (0-12-185301-2) Acad Pr.

Methods in Neurotransmitter & Neuropeptide Research. Ed. by S. H. Parvez et al. 1994. LC 93-13620. Pt. 1. 432p. 228.50 (0-444-81369-1); Pt. 1. 432p. pap. 70.50 (0-444-81674-7); Pt. 2. 424p. 228.50 (0-444-81368-3); Pt. 2. 424p. pap. 70.50 (0-444-81675-5) Elsevier.

Methods in Nonradioactive Detection in Biological Systems. Gary C. Howard. 1994. LC 92-49351. (Illus.). 294p. (C). pap. text 65.00 (0-8385-6946-3, A6946-6, Apple Lange Med) McGraw.

Methods in Observational Epidemiology. Jennifer L. Kelsey et al. 2nd ed. 1996. LC 95-47816. (Monographs in Epidemiology & Biostatistics: 26). (Illus.). 448p. (C). text 52.50 (0-19-508377-6) OUP.

Methods in Pharmacology Vol. 5: Myocardial Biology. Ed. by Arnold Schwartz. 1984. LC 74-34441. 248p. 69.50 (0-306-41684-0, Plenum Trade) Perseus Pubng.

Methods in Pharmacology Vol. 6: Methods Used in Adenosine Research. Ed. by David M. Paton. 1985. LC 84-26638. 400p. 95.00 (0-306-41872-X, Plenum Trade) Perseus Pubng.

Methods in Pharmacology Vol. 7: Molecular & Cellular Biology of Pharmacological Targets. H. Glossmann & J. Striessnig. 1993. (Illus.). 288p. (C). text 89.50 (0-306-44424-0, Kluwer Plenum) Kluwer Academic.

Methods in Protein Sequence Analysis. Ed. by Marshall Elzinga. 1982. LC 82-80733. (Experimental Biology & Medicine Ser.: Vol. 3). 607p. 145.00 (0-89603-038-5) Humana.

Methods in Protein Sequence Analysis. K. Imahori & F. Sakiyama. 1993. LC 93-7788. (Illus.). 326p. (C). text 89.50 (0-306-44488-7, Kluwer Plenum) Kluwer Academic.

Methods in Pulmonary Research. S. Uhlig & Aubrey E. Taylor. 1998. LC 98-14358. xxiv, 541p. (0-8176-5427-5) Birkhauser.

Methods in Pulmonary Research. Ed. by S. Uhlig & Aubrey E. Taylor. 1998. LC 98-14358. 320p. 130.00 (3-7643-5427-5) Birkhauser.

Methods in Renal Toxicology. Ed. by Rudolfs K. Zalups & Lawrence H. Lash. 1996. (Methods in Toxicology Ser.). 448p. 139.95 (0-8493-3341-5) CRC Pr.

Methods in Studying Cardiac Membranes, Vol. I. Ed. by N. S. Ohalla. 1984. 320p. 181.00 (0-8493-5995-3, QP114, CRC Reprint) Franklin.

Methods in Studying Cardiac Membranes, Vol. II. Ed. by Naranjan S. Dhalla. 1984. 344p. 189.00 (0-8493-5996-1, QP114, CRC Reprint) Franklin.

Methods in Teaching Consultation-Liaison Psychiatry. Ed. by M. S. Hale. 1990. (Advances in Psychosomatic Medicine Ser.: Vol. 20). (Illus.). x, 144p. 85.25 (3-8055-5080-4) S Karger.

Methods in the Neurosciences: Intracellular Perfusions of Excitable Cells, Vol. 5, Intracellular Perfusion of Excitable Cells. Ed. by Platon G. Kostyuk & O. A. Krishtal. 99th ed. 1984. (IBRO Handbook Ser.: No. 1-569). 146p. 365.00 (0-471-90379-5, Wiley-Interscience) Wiley.

Methods in Toxicology: Male Reproductive Toxicology, Vol. 3, Pt. A. Ed. by Charles A. Tyson et al. 1993. (Illus.). 389p. 58.00 (0-12-461208-3) Acad Pr.

Methods in Toxicology, Vol. 1, Pt. B: In Vitro Toxicity Indicators. Ed. by Charles A. Tyson & John M. Frazier. 1994. (Illus.). 497p. 58.00 (0-12-461204-0); text 104.00 (0-12-461203-2) Acad Pr.

Methods in Toxicology, Vol. 2: Mitochondrial Dysfunction. Ed. by Charles A. Tyson et al. 1993. (Illus.). 502p. pap. 58.00 (0-12-461206-7) Acad Pr.

Methods in Toxicology, Vol. 3, Pt. B: Female Reproductive Toxicology. Ed. by Jerrold J. Heindel & Robert E. Chapin. 1993. (Illus.). 404p. 58.00 (0-12-461210-5) Acad Pr.

Methods of Analysis for Processed Fruits & Vegetables, Vol. 31. 1980. 14p. pap. 4.50 (92-5-100813-2, F1886) Bernan Associates.

Methods of Assessing the Reinforcing Properties of Abused Drugs. Ed. by M. A. Bozarth. 1987. (Illus.). 658p. 71.95 (0-387-96625-0) Spr-Verlag.

Methods of Assessment of Avoidable Blindness. WHO Staff. 1980. (WHO Offset Publications: No. 54). 42p. 4.00 (92-4-170054-8) World Health.

Methods of Cell Separation Ed. by Nicholas Catsimpoolas. LC 77-11018. (Biological Separations Ser.). (Illus.). 1980. 55.00 (0-306-40377-3); 1979. 59.50 (0-306-40094-4); 1977. 59.50 (0-306-34604-4) Perseus Pubng (Plenum Trade).

Methods of Electrophysiology Recordings. Jeffery D. Kocsis. 1999. 450p. 72.95 (0-8385-6324-4, Medical Exam) Appleton & Lange.

Methods of Enzymatic Analysis Metabolites Two: Tri- & Dicarboxylic Acids, Purines, Pyrimidines & Derivatives, Coenzymes, Inorganic Compounds, Vol. 7, Metabolites 2: Tri- and Dicarboxylic Acids. Ed. by Hans U. Bergmeyer. 3rd ed. 1985. 642p. 325.00 (3-527-26047-1, Wiley-VCH) Wiley.

Methods of Enzymatic Analysis. Metabolites 1: Carbohydrates, Vol. 6, Metabolites 1: Carbohydrates. Ed. by Hans U. Bergmeyer. 3rd ed. 1984. 701p. 320.00 (3-527-26046-3, Wiley-VCH) Wiley.

Methods of External Hyperthermic Heating. J. W. Hand et al. 1990. (Clinical Thermology Ser.: Vol. 2). (Illus.). 143p. 118.00 (0-387-50976-3) Spr-Verlag.

Methods of Family Research: Biographies of Research Projects, Vol. I. Ed. by Irving E. Sigel & Gene H. Brody. 1989. 352p. 69.95 (0-89859-826-5) L Erlbaum Assocs.

Methods of Fertility Regulation-Advances in Research & Clinical Experience: A Report. WHO Staff. 1971. (Technical Reports: No. 473). 48p. pap. text 5.00 (92-4-120473-7, 1100473) World Health.

Methods of Genome Analysis: A Gene Hunter's Guide. Alan J. Buckler & David E. Houseman. Date not set. (Illus.). 250p. pap. 39.95 (0-19-509341-0) OUP.

Methods of Hyperthermia Control. T. C. Cetas et al. 1990. (Clinical Thermology Ser.: Vol. 3). (Illus.). 130p. 125.00 (0-387-50978-X) Spr-Verlag.

Methods of Immunological Analysis, Vol. 1, Fundamentals, Vol. 1, Fundamentals. Ed. by Rene F. Masseyeff et al. 1992. LC 92-49344. 716p. 425.00 (3-527-27906-7, Wiley-VCH) Wiley.

Methods of Pesticide Exposure Assessment: Proceedings of a Workshop Held in Ottawa, Canada, October 5-8, 1993. Ed. by Patricia B. Curry et al. 1995. (NATO Challenges of Modern Society Ser.: Vol. 19). (Illus.). 236p. 89.50 (0-306-45130-1, Kluwer Plenum) Kluwer Academic.

Methods of Protein & Nucleic Acid Research: Immunoelectrophoresis - Application of Radioisotopes. L. A. Osterman. 1988. (Illus.). 220p. 159.00 (0-387-13094-2) Spr-Verlag.

Methods of Radiochemical Analysis. 1966. (ENG & FRE., Illus.). 163p. pap. text 16.00 (92-4-154019-2, 1150106); 1959. (Technical Report Ser.: No. 173). 116p. pap. text 5.00 (92-4-120173-8) World Health.

Methods of Research in Social Psychology. Elliot Aronson et al. 2nd ed. 1989. 376p. (C). text 81.88 (0-07-002466-9) McGrw-H Hghr Educ.

Methods of Sleep Research. Ed. by S. Kubicki & W. M. Herrmann. 1985. (Illus.). 222p. pap. (0-89574-201-2) Gustav Fischer DEU. *Dist:* Lubrecht & Cramer, Balogh.

Methods of Urine Drug Testing. Alphonse Poklis. Date not set. (Methods in Analytical Toxicology Ser.). 50.00 (0-8493-7882-6) CRC Pr.

Methods, Sex & Madness. Derek Layder & Julia O. Davidson. 1994. LC 94-5596. (Illus.). 240p. (C). pap. 26.95 (0-415-09764-9, B4626) Routledge.

Methods to Defend the Natural Cold & Flu. C. M. Hawkes. 1998. pap. text 7.95 (1-58054-016-3) Woodland UT.

Methods Toward a Science of Behavior & Experience. William J. Ray. (C). 4th ed. 1993. 480p. text 45.50 (0-534-17838-3); 5th ed. 1996. LC 96-12020. 496p. pap. 52.25 (0-534-20346-9) Brooks-Cole.

Methods Toward a Science of Behavior & Experience: Study Guide & Activities Workbook. William J. Ray. 5th ed. 1996. (Psychology Ser.). (C). mass mkt., stu. ed., wbk. ed. 20.00 (*0-534-34389-9*) Brooks-Cole.

Methods Toward Scientific Behavior & Explanation. Ray. 4th ed. 1992. (Psychology Ser.). pap., stu. ed., wbk. ed. 20.00 (*0-534-17840-5*) Brooks-Cole.

Methods Used in Establishing Permissible Levels in Occupational Exposure to Harmful Agents: Report of a WHO Expert Committee with the Participation of ILO, 1977. 1977. (Technical Report Ser.: No. 601). 68p. pap. text 8.00 (*92-4-120601-2*, 1100601) World Health.

Methods Used in the U. S. S. R. Proceedings of the WHO Expert Committee, Moscow, Dec. 12-19, 1972. WHO Staff. 1975. pap. text 30.00 (*92-4-156043-6*, 1150114) World Health.

Methomyl. 1995. (Health & Safety Guides Ser.: No. 96). 27p. (C). pap. text 4.50 (*92-4-151097-8*, 1860097) Am Soc Clinical.

Methomyl. rev. ed. 1996. (Environmental Health Criteria Ser.: Vol. 178). (FRE & SPA.). 150p. (C). pap. 30.00 (*92-4-157178-0*, 1160178) World Health.

Methotrexate. Ed. by B. N. Cronstein. 2000. LC 00-29751. (Milestones in Drug Therapy Ser.). 250p. 159.00 (*3-7643-5959-5*) Birkhauser.

Methyl Bromide. 1995. (Environmental Health Criteria Ser.: Vol. 166). (FRE & SPA.). 324p. (C). pap. 62.00 (*92-4-157166-7*, 1160166) World Health.

Methyl Ethyl Ketone. 1993. (Environmental Health Criteria Ser.: No. 143). (ENG, FRE & SPA.). 161p. pap. text 36.00 (*92-4-157143-8*, 1160143) World Health.

Methyl Isobutyl Ketone. 1990. (Environmental Health Criteria Ser.: No. 117). (ENG, FRE & SPA.). 79p. pap. text 19.00 (*92-4-157117-9*, 1160117) World Health.

Methyl Parathion. 1993. (Environmental Health Criteria Ser.: No. 145). (ENG, FRE & SPA.). 244p. pap. text 45.00 (*92-4-157145-4*, 1160145) World Health.

Methyldopa in Hypertension. Alberto Zanchetti. 1978. LC 78-68086. 3.00 (*0-911910-96-4*) Merck-Sharp-Dohme.

Methylene Chloride. 2nd ed. Date not set. (Environmental Health Criteria Ser.: No. 164). 242p. (C). pap. 41.40 (*92-4-157164-0*, 1160164) Am Soc Clinical.

Methylmercury. 1990. (Environmental Health Criteria Ser.: No. 101). 144p. pap. text 26.00 (*92-4-157101-2*, 1160101) World Health.

Methylotrophs: Microbiology, Biochemistry & Genetics. Ching T. Hou. 1984. 192p. 112.00 (*0-8493-5992-9*, QR92, CRC Reprint) Franklin.

Methylphenate HCL (Ritalin) Index of New Information with Authors, Subjects & References. Kevin B. Armstrong. 1997. 131p. 57.50 (*0-7883-1252-9*); pap. 47.50 (*0-7883-1253-7*) ABBE Pubs Assn.

Methylxanthines & Phosphodiesterase Inhibitors in the Treatment of Airways Disease: Proceedings of a Meeting Held by the Royal Society of Medicine's Section of Respiratory Medicine, RSM, London, November 1993. Ed. by John F. Costello & Priscilla J. Piper. 1994. LC 94-16137. (Illus.). 200p. (C). lib. bdg. 46.95 (*1-85070-597-6*, Parthenon Pbng) CRC Pr.

Metodologia de Investigacion en Epidemiologia. I. Rebagliato et al. 1996. (SPA.). 223p. pap. (*84-7978-265-X*) Ediciones Diaz ESP. *Dist:* IBD Ltd.

Mexican American Fertility Patterns. Frank D. Bean & Gray Swicegood. 1985. (Mexican American Monographs: No. 10). 192p. text 20.00 (*0-292-75087-0*) U of Tex Pr.

Mexican Macaws: Comparative Osteology. Lyndon L. Hargrave. 1970. LC 72-125168. (Anthropological Papers: No. 20). 67p. pap. 7.95 (*0-8165-0212-9*) U of Ariz Pr.

Mexican Remedies: Homegrown Wisdom. Annette Sandoval. 1998. 192p. pap. 6.99 (*0-425-16155-2*) Berkley Pub.

Meyler's Side Effects of Drugs: An Encyclopedia of Adverse Reactions & Interactions. Ed. by M. N. Dukes. 12th ed. 1992. (Side Effects of Drugs Ser.: Vol. 12). 1308p. 288.00 (*0-444-89524-8*) Elsevier.

Meyler's Side Effects of Drugs: An Encyclopedia of Adverse Reactions & Interactions. Ed. by M. N. G. Dukes. 13th ed. 1996. 1610p. 288.00 (*0-444-82405-7*) Elsevier.

MGH Board Review of Anesthesiology. Mark Dershwitz et al. 5th ed. 1998. LC 98-21937. (Illus.). 302p. (C). pap. 54.95 (*0-8385-6348-1*) McGraw-Hill Prof.

***MGH Guide to Risk Assessment in Breast Cancer.** Kevin Hughes & Constance Roche. 2002. (Illus.). (C). pap. text 34.95 (*0-7637-1860-2*, 1860-2) Jones & Bartlett.

MHC Ligands & Peptide Motifs. Hans-Georg Rammensee & Jutta Bachmann. 1997. LC 97-18997. (Molecular Biology Intelligence Unit Ser.). text 99.00 (*1-57059-460-0*) Landes Bioscience.

MHC Molecules & Antigen Processing. Clifford V. Harding. 1997. LC 97-578. (Molecular Biology Intelligence Unit Ser.). 162p. 99.00 (*1-57059-428-7*) Landes Bioscience.

MHC Plus X. Ed. by P. Ivanyi. 1989. (Illus.). 247p. 132.00 (*0-387-50247-5*) Spr-Verlag.

Mi Bebe y Yo: Una Guia Esencial para el Embarazo. Deborah D. Stewart. Tr. by Ricardo Perugorria & Ana C. Matiella. 3rd rev. ed. 1998.Tr. of Baby & Me: The Essential Guide to Pregnancy. (SPA., Illus.). 160p. pap. 10.95 (*1-884255-04-3*) Willapa Bay.

Mi Medula y Yo: Guia de Trasplantes de Medula para Ninos. Karen Crowe. Tr. by Dana Levy. 2000. (SPA., Illus.). 48p. (J). (gr. 3-8). pap. 5.95 (*0-9702446-1-4*) Fujisawa Health.

Miami Cochlear Implant, Auditory, & Tactile Skills Curriculum: CHATS. Kathleen C. Vergara & Lynn W. Miskiel. 1994. LC 94-74538. 327p. pap. text 75.00 (*1-886887-00-4*) Intell Hearing.

Miasmas & Disease: Public Health & Environment in the Pre-Industrial Age. Carlo M. Cipolla. Tr. by Elizabeth Potter from ITA. 1992. LC 91-30385. 144p. (C). 37.50 (*0-300-04806-8*) Yale U Pr.

Mice, Myths, & Men. R. J. Fry. 1994. LC 95-1235. (L.S. Taylor Lectures in Radiation Protection & Measurements: No. 18). 61p. pap. text 25.00 (*0-929600-41-X*) NCRP Pubns.

Michael Fordham: Innovations in Analytical Psychology. James Astor. 1995. LC 94-48784. (Makers of Modern Psychotherapy Ser.). (C). 288p. 78.95 (*0-415-09348-1*); 304p. pap. 27.95 (*0-415-09349-X*) Routledge.

Michael's Story: The Story of a Burn Victim. Joan Brunette. 1995. 105p. (Orig.). (YA). (gr. 7-12). pap. 6.95 (*1-57515-085-9*) PPI Pubng.

Michel Delacroix. Michel Delacroix. Ed. by Michelle L. Cassanetti. 1987. LC 86-83287. (Illus.). 200p. 150.00 (*0-941393-05-4*) Lublin Graph.

Michel Salmon Anatomic Studies, Set. G. Ian Taylor et al. 1993. LC 93-21903. Orig. Title: Les Arteres des Muscles des Membres et du Tronc, Les Vois Anastomotiques Arterielles des Membres. (Illus.). 307p. 90.00 (*0-942219-27-9*) Quality Med Pub.

Michels's Retinal Detachment. Charles P. Wilkinson & Thomas A. Rice. 2nd ed. 1996. LC 96-4878. Orig. Title: Retinal Detachment. (Illus.). 1184p. (C). (gr. 13). text 210.00 (*0-8151-9416-1*, 26954) Mosby Inc.

Michigan Health Care in Perspective 2000. Ed. by Kathleen O'Leary Morgan & Scott E. Morgan. 2000. 21p. spiral bd. 19.00 (*0-7401-0221-4*) Morgan Quitno Corp.

Michigan Health Care Perspective, 1998. Ed. by Kathleen O'Leary Morgan & Scott E. Morgan. 1998. 20p. pap. 19.00 (*1-56692-821-4*) Morgan Quitno Corp.

Michigan Manual: A Guide to Neonatal Intensive Care. Steven M. Donn. 2nd ed. 1997. LC 97-20394. (Illus.). 464p. 37.50 (*0-87993-676-2*) Futura Pub.

Michigan Manual of Clinical Diagnosis: The Basis of Cost-Effective Medical Practice. Richard D. Judge et al. 1997. LC 97-34667. 416p. spiral bd. 39.95 (*0-316-47581-5*, Little Brwn Med Div) Lppncott W & W.

Michigan Poor Law: Its Development & Administration with Special Reference to State Provision for Medical Care of the Indigent. Isabel Bruce & Edith Eickhoff. 1976. LC 75-17210. (Social Problems & Social Policy Ser.). reprint ed. 25.95 (*0-405-07482-4*) Ayer.

Micmac Medicines: Remedies & Recollections. Laurie Lacey. 1993. (Illus.). 128p. pap. (*1-55109-041-4*) Nimbus Publ.

Micro- & Nanofabricated Structures & Devices for Biomedical Environmental Applications, Vol. 3258. Ed. by Paul L. Gourley. 1998. LC 98-171717. 236p. 69.00 (*0-8194-2697-0*) SPIE.

***Micro- & Nanotechnology for Biomedical & Environmental Applications: 26-27 January 2000, San Jose, California, USA.** Ed. by Raymond P. Mariella. 2000. LC 00-709187. (Progress in Biomedical Optics Ser.: No. 1). (Illus.). x, 184p. (*0-8194-3528-7*) SPIE.

Micro-Acupuncture Comprehensive Manual & Prescription Index. Ralph Alan Dale. 2001. (Illus.). 400p. 125.00 (*1-877589-06-3*) Dialectic Pubng.

Micro-dialysis as a Tool in Pharmacokinetic-Pharmacodynamic Studies Investigating the Brain Distribution & Effect Delay of Morphine & Morphine-6-Glucuronide. Marcel Rene Bouw. 2000. (Comprehensive Summaries of Uppsala Dissertations from the Faculty of Pharmacy Ser.: 221). (Illus.). 58p. (Orig.). pap. (*91-554-4659-0*) Uppsala Universitet SWE. *Dist:* Coronet Bks.

Micro-Endoscopic Surgery of the Paranasal Sinuses & the Skull Base. Ed. by Aldo C. Stamm & Wolfgang Draf. 2000. LC 00-39481. (Illus.). 608p. 275.00 (*3-540-66629-X*) Spr-Verlag.

Micro Silver Bullet: A Preliminary Scientifically Documented Answer to the Three Largest Epidemics in the World. M. Paul Farber. 5th rev. ed. Date not set. 700p. pap. text 29.95 (*1-887742-01-8*) Prof Phys Pub.

Microalbuminuria: Biochemistry, Epidemiology & Clinical Practice. Peter H. Winocour et al. 1998. LC 98-25128. (Illus.). 260p. (C). pap. text 64.95 (*0-521-45703-3*) Cambridge U Pr.

Microanalysis & Quantification. Ed. by Jasmin Gaetan & L. Proschek. 1984. (Methods & Achievements in Experimental Pathology Ser.: Vol. 11). (Illus.). vi, 190p. 142.75 (*3-8055-3717-4*) S Karger.

Microanatomical Aspects for Neurosurgeons & Neuroradiologists. Wolfgang Seeger. 2000. (Illus.). 440p. 298.00 (*3-211-83376-5*) Spr-Verlag.

Microanatomy & Function of the Spleen. Birte Steiniger & Peter Barth. 1999. LC 99-32588. (Advances in Anatomy, Embryology & Cell Biology Ser.: Vol. 151). (Illus.). 96p. pap. 78.00 (*3-540-66161-1*) Spr-Verlag.

Microbe Hunters. Paul De Kruif. 1966. LC 67-34588. 337p. pap. 7.95 (*0-15-659413-7*, Harvest Bks) Harcourt.

Microbe Hunters - Then & Now. Ed. by Hilary Koprowski & Michael B. Oldstone. 1996. LC 96-28898. (Illus.). 456p. 45.00 (*0-936741-11-2*) Medi-Ed Pr.

Microbes & Malignancy: Infection as a Cause of Human Cancers. Ed. by Julie Parsonnet. 1999. LC 98-22168. (Illus.). 480p. text 79.95 (*0-19-510401-3*) OUP.

Microbes & Minie Balls: An Annotated Bibliography of Civil War Medicine. Frank R. Freemon. 1993. LC 92-23153. (Illus.). 256p. 39.50 (*0-8386-3484-2*) Fairleigh Dickinson.

Microbes in Action: A Laboratory Manual of Microbiology. Harry W. Seeley, Jr. 4th ed. 1990. LC 89-71383. (Illus.). 351p. (C). pap. text 44.95 (*0-7167-2100-7*) W H Freeman.

Microbes Versus Mankind: The Coming Plague. Laurie Garrett. Ed. by Karen Rohan & Nancy L. Hoepli-Phalon. 1996. LC 96-84227. (Headline Ser.: No. 309). (Illus.). 72p. (YA). pap. text 5.95 (*0-87124-169-2*) Foreign Policy.

Microbial Antigenodiagnosis: General Considerations, I. Ed. by Konrad Wicher. 1987. 274p. 156.00 (*0-8493-6345-4*, CRC Reprint) Franklin.

Microbial Antigenodiagnosis: Practical Application, Set. Ed. by Konrad Wicher. 1987. 274p. 349.00 (*0-8493-6344-6*, RC113) CRC Pr.

Microbial Antigenodiagnosis: Practical Application, II. Ed. by Konrad Wicher. 1987. 274p. 104.00 (*0-8493-6346-2*, CRC Reprint) Franklin.

Microbial Cell Cycle. Ed. by Paul Nurse & Eva Streiblova. 1984. 304p. 164.00 (*0-8493-5574-5*, QR73, CRC Reprint) Franklin.

Microbial Development. Ed. by Richard Losick & Lucy Shapiro. 1984. LC 84-9599. (Monographs: Vol. 16). 303p. 60.00 (*0-87969-172-7*); pap. 35.00 (*0-87969-173-5*) Cold Spring Harbor.

Microbial Disease. Ed. by Pierre J. Vinken et al. 1988. 662p. 309.50 (*0-444-90480-8*) Elsevier.

Microbial Diseases: A Veterinarian's Guide to Laboratory Diagnosis. G. R. Carter & M. M. Chengappa. 1993. LC 92-35999. 318p. (C). text 49.95 (*0-8138-0671-2*) Iowa U Pr.

Microbial Diseases of Occupations, Sports & Recreations. C. H. Collins et al. 1996. LC 96-38862. 184p. pap. (*0-7506-2183-4*) E A GBR. *Dist:* OUP.

Microbial Ecology & Infectious Disease. Ed. by Eugene Rosenberg. 1998. LC 98-30758. 340p. 89.95 (*1-55581-148-5*) ASM Pr.

Microbial Infections: Role of Biological Response Modifiers. H. Friedman et al. 1992. LC 92-21809. (Advances in Experimental Medicine & Biology Ser.: Vol. 319). (Illus.). 358p. (C). text 105.00 (*0-306-44237-X*, Kluwer Plenum) Kluwer Academic.

Microbial Limit & Bioburden Tests: Validation Approaches & Global Requirements. Lucia Clontz. 1998. LC 97-41282. (Illus.). 240p. 189.00 (*1-57491-062-0*) IHS Health Grp.

Microbial Metabolism in the Digestive Tract. Michael J. Hill. 1986. 264p. 150.00 (*0-8493-5936-8*, QR171, CRC Reprint) Franklin.

Microbial Pathogenesis: Current & Emerging Issues: Proceedings of the 2nd Annual Indiana Conference. Ed. by Donald J. LeBlanc et al. 1998. LC 98-73482. (Illus.). 179p. text (*0-9655149-1-9*) IN Univ Schl Dentstry.

Microbial Pathogenesis & Immune Response II: Proceedings of a New York Academy of Sciences Conference, October 25-28, 1995, Vol. 797. Ed. by Edwin W. Ades et al. 1996. 90.00 (*1-57331-016-6*) NY Acad Sci.

Microbial Physiology. Ian W. Dawes & Ian W. Sutherland. 2nd ed. 1991. (Basic Microbiology Ser.). (Illus.). 304p. 54.95 (*0-632-02463-1*) Blackwell Sci.

Microbial Quality Assurance in Pharmaceuticals: Cosmetics & Toiletries. Bloomfield et al. 1988. (Pharmaceutical Technology Ser.). 264p. 62.95 (*0-470-21122-9*) P-H.

Microbial Resistance to Drugs. Ed. by L. E. Bryan. 1989. (Handbook of Experimental Pharmacology Ser.: Vol. 91). (Illus.). 451p. 332.00 (*0-387-50318-8*) Spr-Verlag.

Microbial Surface Components & Toxins in Relation to Pathogenesis. Ed. by E. Z. Ron & S. Rottem. 1991. (FEMS Symposium Ser.: No. 51). (Illus.). 210p. (C). text 107.00 (*0-306-43908-5*, Kluwer Plenum) Kluwer Academic.

Microbial Toxins in Foods & Feeds: Cellular & Molecular Modes of Action. Ed. by A. E. Pohland et al. 1990. LC 90-14343. (Illus.). 634p. (C). text 198.00 (*0-306-43716-3*, Kluwer Plenum) Kluwer Academic.

Microbio Pat Care W/lm-wb&mm P. Morello. 6th ed. 1998. 89.50 net. (*0-07-228988-0*) McGraw.

Microbioglia: General. Garcia. 1999. (C). text 78.20 (*84-8174-170-1*) Mosby Inc.

Microbiol & Parasitic Infection. Brian I. Duerden et al. 7th ed. 1993. 448p. pap. (*0-340-56018-5*) E A GBR. *Dist:* OUP.

Microbiologia Clinica. Inglis. 1999. (C). text 13.62 (*84-8174-413-1*) Mosby Inc.

Microbiologia Medica. Mims. 2nd ed. 1999. (C). text 60.64 (*84-8174-396-8*) Mosby Inc.

Microbiological & Parasitic Diseases of the Dog & Cat. Ed. by P. J. Quinn et al. 1997. (Illus.). 500p. text (*0-7020-1985-2*) W B Saunders GBR. *Dist:* Saunders.

Microbiological Methods Pt. 1: Estimation of the Population of Microorganisms on Product. 1995. (Illus.). 16p. (Orig.). pap. 74.00 (*1-57020-049-1*, 11737-1-209) Assn Adv Med Instrn.

Microbiologist. Jack Rudman. 1994. (Career Examination Ser.: C-2477). pap. 29.95 (*0-8373-2477-7*) Nat Learn.

Microbiology. I. Edward Alcamo. 1994. (Blond's Medical Guides Ser.). (Illus.). 181p. (C). pap. text 19.99 (*0-945819-41-2*) Sulzburger & Graham Pub.

Microbiology. Cynthia F. Norton. 1981. LC 80-23350. (Life Sciences Ser.). (Illus.). 850p. (C). tchr. ed. (*0-201-05308-X*); text (*0-201-05304-7*); stu. ed. (*0-201-05307-1*) Addison-Wesley.

Microbiology. Jack Rudman. 1994. (College Level Examination Ser.: Vol. CLEP-35). pap. 27.95 (*0-8373-5335-1*) Nat Learn.

Microbiology. T. J. Inglis. 2nd ed. 1997. LC 96-51002. (Colour Guide Ser.). (*0-443-05772-9*) Harcrt Hlth Sci Grp.

Microbiology. B. Larsen. 2nd ed. 1997. LC 97-41309. pap. 45.00 (*0-915473-37-2*) Am Coll Obstetric.

Microbiology. Jacquelyn R. Marshall. 2nd ed. 1994. LC 93-38266. (Clinical Laboratory Manual Ser.). 160p. (C). mass mkt. 28.95 (*0-8273-5363-4*) Delmar.

Microbiology: 2000 Multiple-Choice Questions & Answers. 1999. 310p. spiral bd. 25.95 (*1-893720-03-9*) Biotest.

Microbiology: A Centenary Perspective. Ed. by Wolfgang K. Joklik et al. 1999. LC 99-20173. 99.95 (*1-55581-162-0*); pap. 59.95 (*1-55581-169-8*) ASM Pr.

***Microbiology: A Laboratory Manual.** James G. Cappuccino & Natalie Sherman. 6th ed. 2001. LC 2001-17096. (Illus.). 477p. 45.00 (*0-8053-7648-8*) Benjamin-Cummings.

Microbiology: A Photographic Atlas for the Laboratory. Steven K. Alexander & Dennis Strete. 2000. LC 00-34585. (Illus.). 193p. pap., suppl. ed. 27.60 (*0-8053-2732-0*) Benjamin-Cummings.

Microbiology: Diversity, Disease, & the Environment. Abigail A. Salyers & Dixie B. Whitt. 2000. LC 00-55129. (Illus.). 500p. pap. text 59.00 (*1-891786-01-6*) Fitzgerald Sci.

Microbiology: Medical Exam Review. KIM Staff. 10th ed. 1991. (Basic Sciences Ser.). 18.50 (*0-444-01627-9*, BAS) Elsevier.

***Microbiology: Principles & Health Science Applications.** Lois Bergquist & Barbara Pogosian. 2000. (Illus.). pap., tchr. ed. 75.00 (*0-7216-9178-1*) Saunders.

Microbiology: Review for New National Boards. Gerald V. Stokes. 1993. 194p. pap. 25.00 (*0-8036-0713-X*) Davis Co.

Microbiology: Review for New National Boards. Gerald V. Stokes. 1993. LC 93-77103. (Illus.). 193p. pap. 25.00 (*0-9632873-2-X*) J & S Pub VA.

***Microbiology: Self-Assessment & Review.** Richard C. Tilton. 10th ed. 2001. (Pretest Self-Assessment & Review Ser.). (Illus.). 220p. pap. 24.95 (*0-07-137495-7*) McGraw-Hill Prof.

Microbiology & Epidemiology of Infection for Health Science Students. J. Sedgwick & Peter Meers. 1995. (Illus.). 352p. pap. text 41.50 (*1-56593-350-8*, 0674) Singular Publishing.

***Microbiology & Immunlgy for Health-Related Professionals.** Hay Jensen. 2000. 492p. 47.00 (*0-536-62214-0*) Pearson Custom.

Microbiology & Immunology. Arthur G. Johnson et al. (Board Review Ser.). (Illus.). 2nd ed. 1992. LC 92-49680. 284p. 19.95 (*0-683-04465-6*); 3rd ed. 1996. LC 96-7007. 297p. pap. text 26.95 (*0-683-18005-3*) Lppncott W & W.

Microbiology & Immunology. Richard M. Hyde. 4th rev. ed. 1995. LC 95-2578. (Oklahoma Notes). (Illus.). 229p. 24.95 (*0-387-94392-7*) Spr-Verlag.

Microbiology & Immunology - An Encyclopedic Approach. M. K. Majundar. 1989. (C). (*0-89771-367-2*) Current Dist IND. *Dist:* St Mut.

Microbiology & Immunology for the Health Team. Peter R. Stewart et al. 1985. pap. 27.95 (*0-471-33385-9*) Wiley.

Microbiology & Infectious Disease. Gabriel T. Virella. 3rd ed. 1997. LC 96-5707. (National Medical Series for Independent Study). 575p. pap. text 29.00 (*0-683-06235-2*) Lppncott W & W.

Microbiology for Health Careers. Elizabeth Fong. 4th ed. LC 86-19720. 256p. (C). (gr. 11-12). 1987. pap., instr.'s gde. ed. 16.00 (*0-8273-2566-5*); 1986. pap. 27.95 (*0-8273-2565-7*) Delmar.

Microbiology for Health Careers. Elizabeth Fong et al. 5th ed. 1994. 101p. tchr. ed. 16.00 (*0-8273-6050-9*) Delmar.

Microbiology for Health Careers. Elizabeth Fong. 6th ed. 1998. LC 98-53502. (Allied Health Ser.). 456p. (C). pap. text 41.95 (*0-7668-0917-X*) Delmar.

Microbiology for Health Careers: Instructor's Manual. Lakomia. 6th ed. 1999. 96p. tchr. ed. 14.95 (*0-7668-0918-8*) Delmar.

Microbiology for Health Science. Marcus M. Jensen & Donald N. Wright. 4th ed. 1996. LC 96-28137. 530p. 101.33 (*0-13-251464-8*) P-H.

Microbiology for Public Health & Environmental Engineers. J. N. Lester & R. M. Sterritt. 1988. 284p. text 65.00 (*0-419-12760-7*); pap. text 29.50 (*0-419-12770-4*) Routledge (Spon).

Microbiology for the Health Sciences. Deborah Simon. 1996. 90p. (C). spiral bd., lab manual ed. 19.95 (*0-7872-2342-5*) Kendall-Hunt.

Microbiology for Veterinary Technicians. M. Ikram & E. Hill. 1994. LC 90-83303. (Illus.). 275p. pap. text 29.00 (*0-939674-30-0*) Am Vet Pubns.

Microbiology in Clinical Practice. Shanson. 3rd ed. 1998. 520p. pap. (*0-7506-3110-4*) E A GBR. *Dist:* OUP.

Microbiology in Patient Care. Josephine A. Morello et al. (C). 5th ed. 1993. 592p. text, stu. ed. 32.50 net. (*0-697-13784-8*); 6th ed. 1997. LC 97-14452. 576p. text 56.00 net. (*0-697-25763-0*) McGrw-H Hghr Educ (WCB McGr Hill).

Microbiology of Animals & Animal Products. Ed. by J. B. Woolcock. 1991. (World Animal Science Ser.: Vol. A6). 278p. 183.50 (*0-444-43010-5*) Elsevier.

Microbiology of Chlamydia, Vol. I. Ed. by Almen L. Barron. 1988. 256p. 149.00 (*0-8493-6877-4*, QR201, CRC Reprint) Franklin.

Microbiology of Landfill Sites. Eric Senior. 2nd ed. 1995. LC 94-27855. 224p. lib. bdg. 85.00 (*0-87371-968-9*, L968) Lewis Pubs.

***Microbiology with Health Care Applications.** Isaiah Amiel Benathen. 2nd ed. 2001. 568p. (C). per., lab manual ed. 39.95 (*0-89863-215-3*) Star Pub CA.

Microbiology with Health Care Applications: A Laboratory Manual. Isaiah Amiel Benathen. 1993. (Illus.). 416p. (C). pap. 32.95 (*0-89863-150-5*) Star Pub CA.

Microcapsules & Nanoparticles in Medicine & Pharmacy. M. Donbrow. 1991. 360p. lib. bdg. 249.00 (*0-8493-6986-X*, RS201) CRC Pr.

Microcirculation & Inflammation: Vessel Wall, Inflammatory Cells, Mediator Interaction. Ed. by K. Messmer & F. Hammersen. 1987. (Progress in Applied Microcirculation Ser.: Vol. 12). xvi, 330p. pap. 130.50 (*3-8055-4552-5*) S Karger.

Microcirculation in Cancer Metastasis. F. William Orr et al. 1991. LC 96-6236. (Illus.). 328p. 202.00 (*0-8493-6154-0*, RC269) CRC Pr.

Microcirculation in Chronic Venous Insufficiency: 15th Bodensee Symposium on Microcirculation, June 1998. Ed. by K. Messmer. 1999. LC 99-30254. (Progress in Applied Microcirculation Ser.: Vol. 23, 1999). (Illus.). x, 216p. 149.75 (*3-8055-6821-5*) S Karger.

Microcirculation in Diabetes. Ed. by E. Davis. 1979. (Advances in Microcirculation Ser.: Vol. 8). (Illus.). 100.00 (*3-8055-2916-3*) S Karger.

Microcirculation in Inflammation: Proceedings of the European Conference on Microcirculation, 10th, Cagliari, Oct. 24, 1978. European Conference on Microcirculation Staff. Ed. by J. W. Irwin & G. Hauck. 1979. (Bibliotheca Anatomica Ser.: No. 17). (Illus.). pap. 42.75 (*3-8055-3016-1*) S Karger.

Microcirculation in Organ Transplantation. Ed. by K. Messmer et al. 1994. LC 95-14205. (Progress in Applied Microcirculation Ser.: Vol. 21). (Illus.). x, 126p. 129.75 (*3-8055-5849-X*) S Karger.

Microcirculation in Venous Disease. P. D. Coleridge Smith. 2nd ed. 1998. LC 97-49120. (Medical Intelligence Unit Ser.). 99.00 (*1-57059-476-7*) Landes Bioscience.

Microcirculation of the Alimentary Tract: Physiology & Pathophysiology. Ed. by A. Koo et al. 1983. 400p. 75.00 (*9971-950-75-8*) World Scientific Pub.

Microcirculation of the Brain: A Synoptic View by World Experts. Ed. by M. Tomita et al. 1992. 283p. (C). text 195.00 (*1-56072-014-X*) Nova Sci Pubs.

Microcirculatory Approach to Asian Traditional Medicine: Strategy for the Scientific Evaluation: Selected Proceedings from the Satellite Symposium of the 2nd Asian Congress for Microcirculation, Beijing, China, 17 August 1995. Ed. by Hideyuji Niimi et al. 1996. LC 96-17518. (International Congress Ser.: No. 1117). 206p. 112.50 (*0-444-82343-3*, Excerpta Medica) Elsevier.

Microcirculatory Approaches to Current Therapeutic Problems: Lung in Shock, Organ Transplantation, Diabetic Microangiopathy. Proceedings. Conference on Microcirculation, 6th European, Aalb. Ed. by J. Ditzel & D. H. Lewis. 1971. (Illus.). 45.25 (*3-8055-1186-8*) S Karger.

Microcirculatory Disorders in the Heart & Brain. Ed. by Hideyuki Nimi. 1991. xv, 195p. text 223.00 (*3-7186-5090-8*, Harwood Acad Pubs) Gordon & Breach.

Microcompartmentation. Ed. by Dean P. Jones. 1988. 272p. 155.00 (*0-8493-4779-3*, QH604, CRC Reprint) Franklin.

Microcomputer Applications. California College for Health Sciences Staff. 1990. 96p. (C). spiral bd. (*0-933195-27-3*) CA College Health Sci.

Microcomputer Applications in Health Education. Robert S. Gold. 1990. 304p. (C). text 25.00 net. (*0-697-10628-4*) Brown & Benchmark.

Microcomputer Applications in Medicine & Bioengineering: Proceedings, ISMM Symposium, New York, U. S. A., October 22-24, 1984. Ed. by M.H. Hamza. 1984. 107p. 60.00 (*0-88986-067-X*, 073) ACTA Pr.

Microcomputer Programs in Medicine, Vol. I. Derek Enlander. 1983. (Illus.). 116p. 80.00 (*0-88672-000-1*) Med Software.

Microcomputer Resource Book for Special Education: How to Use the Microcomputer with Handicapped Children. Dolores Hagen. 1984. text 34.00 (*0-8359-4345-3*) P-H.

M
N
O

Microcomputers & Physiological Simulation. James E. Randall. 1980. pap. (*0-201-06128-7*) Addison-Wesley.

Microcosms in Ecological Research: Proceedings. Ed. by John P. Giesy. 1980. LC 80-23472. (DOE Symposium Ser.). 1139p. fiche 9.00 (*0-87079-454-X*, CONF-781101) DOE.

Microcounseling: Innovations in Interviewing, Counseling, Psychotherapy & Psychoeducation. Allen E. Ivey & Jerry Authier. 2nd ed. 1978. (Illus.). 624p. pap. 65.95 (*0-398-06175-0*); text 95.95 (*0-398-03712-4*) C C Thomas.

Microdialysis in the Neurosciences. T. E. Robinson & J. B. Justice, Jr. 1991. (Techniques in the Behavioral & Neural Sciences Ser.: Vol. 7). 450p. 180.50 (*0-444-81194-X*); pap. 71.50 (*0-444-89375-X*) Elsevier.

Microdosimetry & Its Applications. H. H. Rossi. 1995. (Illus.). 321p. 58.95 (*3-540-58541-9*) Spr-Verlag.

Microembolism Syndrome. Ed. by Tom Saldeen. 1979. (Illus.). 240p. (Orig.). pap. text 32.50 (*91-22-00295-2*) Coronet Bks.

Microencapsulation of Drugs. Ed. by Tony L. Whateley. 1992. LC 92-49642. (Drug Targeting & Delivery Ser.: Vol. 1). 309p. text 141.00 (*3-7186-5247-1*) Gordon & Breach.

Microenvironment & Vision. Ed. by J. B. Sheffield & S. R. Hilfer. 1987. (Cell & Developmental Biology of the Eye Ser.). (Illus.). 247p. 205.00 (*0-387-96540-8*) Spr-Verlag.

Microenvironment of the Human Thymus: Thymus Update, Vol. 1. Ed. by Marion D. Kendall & M. A. Ritter. 1988. xii, 306p. text 189.00 (*3-7186-4806-7*) Gordon & Breach.

Microinjection. Ed. by J. Feramisco et al. 1999. LC 98-43502. (Methods & Tools in Biosciences & Medicine Ser.). 350p. 128.00 (*3-7643-5973-0*) Birkhauser.

Microinjection. Ed. by Juan Carlos Lacal et al. 1999. LC 98-43502. (Methods & Tools in Biosciences & Medicine Ser.). (Illus.). 350p. spiral bd. 98.00 (*3-7643-6019-4*) Birkhauser.

Microinjection. Juan Carlos Lacal. 1999. LC 98-43502. (Methods & Tools in Biosciences & Medicine Ser.). 248p. pap. (*0-8176-6019-4*) Birkhauser.

Microlaryngoscopy & Endolaryngeal Microsurgery. Oskar Kleinsasser. Tr. by Philip M. Stell from GER. 3rd ed. 1992. (Illus.). 130p. 139.00 (*1-56053-006-5*) Hanley & Belfus.

Microlenses: Coupling Light to Optical Fibers. Ed. by Huey-Daw Wu & Frank S. Barnes. 1990. LC 90-4081. 512p. 89.95 (*0-87942-259-9*, PC02493) Inst Electrical.

Micromanipulation by Light in Biology & Medicine: Laser Microbeam & Optical Tweezers. K. O. Greulich. 1999. LC 97-29317. 300p. 129.00 (*3-7643-3873-3*) Birkhauser.

Micromanipulation by Light in Biology & Medicine: Laser Microbeam & Optical Tweezers. Karl O. Greulich. Ed. by D. L. Farkas. 1998. LC 97-29317. (Methods in Bioengineering Ser.). (Illus.). 450p. 79.95 (*0-8176-3873-3*) Spr-Verlag.

Micromotives & Macrobehavior. Thomas C. Schelling. 1978. (Fels Lectures on Public Policy Analysis). (Illus.). 252p. (C). pap. text 12.00 (*0-393-09009-4*) Norton.

Micromovement in Orthopaedics. Alan R. Smith. 1993. (Illus.). 342p. text 95.00 (*0-19-262306-0*) OUP.

Microneuro-Surgery. Yasargil. 1995. 1300.00 (*0-86577-658-X*) Thieme Med Pubs.

Microneurosurgery. M. Gazi Yasargil. (Illus.). Vol. 1. 1984. 386p. 219.00 (*0-86577-141-3*); Vol. 3A. 1987. 432p. text 219.00 (*0-86577-258-4*); Vol. 3B. 1988. 596p. text 219.00 (*0-86577-259-2*) Thieme Med Pubs.

Microneurosurgery, Vols. 3A & 3B. Yasargil. 1988. 399.00 (*0-86577-656-3*) Thieme Med Pubs.

Microneurosurgery, Vols. 4A & 4B. M. G. Yasargil. 1995. 489.00 (*0-86577-657-1*) Thieme Med Pubs.

Microneurosurgery Vol. IVB: Microsurgery of CNS Tumors, Vol. 4B. M. G. Yasargil. 1995. LC 97-202615. (Illus.). 552p. 269.00 (*0-86577-546-X*) Thieme Med Pubs.

Microneurosurgical Atlas. K. Sugita. 1985. (Illus.). 275p. 383.00 (*0-387-15110-9*) Spr-Verlag.

***Micronutrients & HIV Infection.** Ed. by Henrik Friis. 2001. LC 2001-25684. (Illus.). 272p. 99.95 (*0-8493-0085-1*) CRC Pr.

***Micronutrients in Health & Disease.** Ed. by Ian Bremner et al. 1999. (British Medical Bulletin Ser.: Vol. 55, No. 3). 215p. pap. (*1-85315-435-0*) Royal Soc of Medicine Pr Ltd GBR. *Dist:* Balogh.

Micronutrients in Health & in Disease Prevention. Ed. by Adrianne Bendich & C. E. Butterworth. 1991. (Illus.). 504p. text 175.00 (*0-8247-8539-8*) Dekker.

Microorganismos. 1968. (Serie de Biologia: No. 6). (SPA.). pap. 3.50 (*0-8270-6065-3*) OAS.

Microorganisms & Autoimmune Diseases. Ed. by H. Friedman et al. 1996. LC 96-25100. (Infectious Agents & Pathogenesis Ser.). (Illus.). 275p. (C). text 95.00 (*0-306-45236-7*, Kluwer Plenum) Kluwer Academic.

Microorganisms As Model Systems for Studying Evolution. Ed. by Robert P. Mortlock. 1984. LC 84-17938. (Monographs in Evolutionary Biology). 344p. 95.00 (*0-306-41788-X*, Plenum Trade) Perseus Pubng.

Microorganisms in Foods: Their Significance & Methods of Enumeration, Vol. 1. International Commission on Microbiological Specifcations Staff. 2nd ed. 1978. LC 77-17842. 907p. text 60.00 (*0-8020-2293-6*) U of Toronto Pr.

Microorganisms in Foods Bk. 2: Sampling for Microbiological Analysis; Principles & Specific Applications. Internal Commission on Microbiological Specificati. 1986. 448p. text 55.00 (*0-8020-5693-8*) U of Toronto Pr.

Microparticulate Systems for the Delivery of Proteins & Vaccines. Smadar Cohen & Howard Bernstein. 1996. LC 96-25983. (Drugs & the Pharmaceutical Sciences Ser.: Vol. 77). (Illus.). 552p. text 195.00 (*0-8247-9753-1*) Dekker.

Micropollutants in River Sediments: Report on a WHO Working Group. 1982. (Euro Reports & Studies Ser.: No. 61). 85p. pap. text 8.00 (*92-890-1227-7*) World Health.

Microscale Syntheses. Zanger-Mckee & McKee. 1999. pap. text 37.00 (*0-697-33008-7*) McGraw.

Microscope. Saville Bradbury. 1968. (*0-08-012848-3*) Pergamon Repr GBR. *Dist:* Franklin.

Microscope & How to Use It. George Stehli. 1970. (Illus.). 160p. reprint ed. pap. 4.95 (*0-486-22575-5*) Dover.

Microscopic & Spectroscopic Imaging of the Chemical State. Michael D. Morris. 1993. (Practical Spectroscopy Ser.: Vol. 16). (Illus.). 504p. text 225.00 (*0-8247-9104-5*) Dekker.

Microscopic Diagnosis in Forensic Pathology. Joshua A. Perper & Cyril H. Wecht. 1980. (Illus.). 488p. 91.95 (*0-398-03969-0*) C C Thomas.

Microscopic Haematology: A Practical Guide for the Laboratory. Gillian Rozenberg. 1997. 160p. pap. text 48.00 (*90-5702-247-8*, Harwood Acad Pubs) Gordon & Breach.

Microscopic Haematology: A Practical Guide to the Haematology Laboratory. Gillian Rozenberg. 1996. 160p. text (*90-5702-093-9*) GBSP NLD. *Dist:* Gordon & Breach.

Microscopic Procedures for Primary Care Providers. Shirley Lowe. 1998. LC 98-22966. 272p. spiral bd. 39.95 (*0-7817-1432-X*) Lppncott W & W.

JMSA Proceedings: Microscopy & Microanalysis, 1995. Ed. by G. W. Bailey et al. 1995. 1132p. 225.00 (*1-56700-032-0*) Begell Hse.

Microscopy & Microsurgery of Larynx & the Laryngopharynx. V. S. Pogosov & V. F. Antoniv. 1987. 37.50 (*0-8236-3363-2*, BN#03363) Intl Univs Pr.

***Microscopy Tutor.** 1997. cd-rom 195.00 (*0-7817-1217-3*) Lppncott W & W.

Microsociology: Discourse, Emotion & Social Structure. Thomas J. Scheff. 1997. (Illus.). 230p. 35.95 (*0-226-73666-0*) U Ch Pr.

Microsoft Excel 2000 QuickTorial. Patricia Murphy. 1999. LC 98-47588. (Computer Applications Ser.). 208p. pap. text 22.95 (*0-538-68853-X*) S-W Thomson.

Microspheres & Drug Therapy: Pharmaceutical, Immunological & Medical Aspects. Ed. by S. S. Davis et al. 1985. 448p. 168.25 (*0-444-80577-X*) Elsevier.

Microspheres & Regional Cancer Therapy. Neville Willmott. 1993. 256p. lib. bdg. 179.00 (*0-8493-6952-5*, RC271) CRC Pr.

Microspheres Medical & Biological Applications. Ed. by Alan Rembaum & Zoltan A. Tokes. 1988. LC 88-7343. 272p. 140.00 (*0-8493-6571-6*, RS201, CRC Reprint) Franklin.

Microstructure Analysis of the Execution of Complex Motor Actions: Methods & Results. N. D. Gordeeva et al. 1989. (*0-8364-2559-6*) Oxford IBH IND. *Dist:* S Asia.

Microsurgery: Transplantation-Replantation: An Atlas-Text. Harry J. Buncke. 1991. LC 90-6142. 832p. text 275.00 (*0-8121-0981-3*) Lppncott W & W.

Microsurgery Forum. 1997. 250p. 40.00 (*981-02-2616-0*) World Scientific Pub.

Microsurgery in Female Infertility. Victor Gomel. 1983. 132.95 (*0-316-31988-0*, Little Brwn Med Div) Lppncott W & W.

Microsurgery in Orthopaedic Practice. P. C. Leung & Y. D. Gu. 1995. LC 94-43237. 360p. text 61.00 (*9971-5-0860-5*) World Scientific Pub.

Microsurgery of Cataract, Vitreous & Astigmatism: Proceedings of the Ophthalmic Microsurgery Study Group Symposium, 5th, London, June 1974. Ophthalmic Microsurgery Study Group Symposium Staf. Ed. by J. Kersley & D. Pierse. 1976. (Advances in Ophthalmology Ser.: Vol.33). 400p. 155.75 (*3-8055-2323-8*) S Karger.

Microsurgery of Cerebral Aneurysms. Zentaro Ito. 1985. (Illus.). 350p. 520.75 (*90-219-3062-5*, Excerpta Medica) Elsevier.

Microsurgery of Cerebral Veins. Wolfgang Seeger. 1985. (Illus.). 418p. 214.00 (*0-387-81807-3*) Spr-Verlag.

Microsurgery of Intracranial Tumors Wolfgang Seeger. 1998. 664p. 350.00 (*0-387-91500-1*, S2307) Spr-Verlag.

Microsurgery of Intracranial Tumors Vol. 1: Supratentorial Tumors, Vol. 1. Wolfgang Seeger et al. 1995. LC 95-12163. 232.00 (*3-211-82677-7*) Spr-Verlag.

Microsurgery of Intracranial Tumors Vol. 2: Special Lesions of the Midline & Rhombenecephalon, Vol. 2. Wolfgang Seeger et al. 1995. LC 95-12163. (Illus.). 373p. 217.00 (*3-211-82678-5*) Spr-Verlag.

Microsurgery of Ocular Injuries. Ed. by R. C. Troutman. 1972. (Advances in Ophthalmology Ser.: Vol. 27). 85.25 (*3-8055-1355-0*) S Karger.

Microsurgery of the Anterior & Posterior Segments for the Eye. Ed. by Michael J. Roper-Hall. 1982. (Developments in Ophthalmology Ser.: Vol. 5). (Illus.). vi, 134p. pap. 78.50 (*3-8055-2711-X*) S Karger.

Microsurgery of the Brain, Set. Wolfgang Seeger. 1981. (Illus.). 727p. 260.00 (*0-387-81573-2*) Spr-Verlag.

Microsurgery of the Cornea: An Atlas & Textbook. Joaquin Barraquer. 1984. 400p. text 231.00 (*84-85835-03-4*) Gordon & Breach.

Microsurgery of the Cranial Base. Wolfgang Seeger. 416p. 1984. (Illus.). 207.00 (*0-387-81769-7*); 1983. 189.00 (*3-211-81769-7*) Spr-Verlag.

Microsurgery of the Eye: Main Aspects. Ed. by S. N. Fyodorov. 1987. (Illus.). 280p. (C). text 295.00 (*0-941743-65-9*) Nova Sci Pubs.

Microsurgery of the Spinal Cord & Surrounding Structure: Anatomical & Technical Principles. Wolfgang Seeger. 1982. 410p. 185.00 (*3-211-81648-8*) Spr-Verlag.

Microsurgery of the Spinal Cord & Surrounding Structures: Anatomical & Technical Principles. Wolfgang Seeger. 1982. (Illus.). 410p. 203.00 (*0-387-81648-8*) Spr-Verlag.

Microsurgery of the Spine. John A. McCulloch. 1998. 688p. text 199.00 (*0-397-51861-7*) Lppncott W & W.

Microsurgery of the Temporo-Medical Region. R. R. Renella. 1989. (Illus.). 203p. 126.00 (*0-387-82144-9*) Spr-Verlag.

Microsurgery Retinal Detachment. Mireille Bonnet. 2nd ed. 1989. 120.00 (*0-938607-12-X*) Field & Wood Inc Medical.

Microsurgery Update, 1982-1984. Ed. by F. Bigar. 1985. (Developments in Ophthalmology Ser.: Vol. 11). (Illus.). x, 206p. 110.50 (*3-8055-4004-3*) S Karger.

Microsurgical Anatomy. Zhong Shizhen et al. 1985. text 445.50 (*0-85200-904-6*) Kluwer Academic.

Microsurgical Anatomy of the Brain: A Stereo Atlas. Gary E. Kraus & Gregory J. Bailey. 1994. LC 93-5757. (Illus.). 272p. 249.00 (*0-683-04780-9*) Lppncott W & W.

Microsurgical Anatomy of the Skull Base & Approaches to the Cavernous Sinus. Kalmon D. Post et al. 1996. (Illus.). 450p. 189.00 incl. 5.25 hd (*0-86577-598-2*) Thieme Med Pubs.

Microsurgical Approach to Cerebro-Spinal Lesions. Ed. by H. Krayenbuehl et al. 1978. (Progress in Neurological Surgery Ser.: Vol. 9). (Illus.). 170.50 (*3-8055-2819-1*) S Karger.

Microsurgical Approaches to the Target Areas of the Brain. Wolfgang Seeger. 1993. (Illus.). 300p. 179.00 (*3-211-82406-5*) Spr-Verlag.

Microsurgical Approaches to the Target Areas of the Brain. Wolfgang Seeger et al. 1993. LC 92-49017. (Illus.). 300p. 220.00 (*0-387-82406-5*) Spr-Verlag.

Microsurgical Carotid Endarterectomy. Ed. by Julian E. Bailes & Robert F. Spetzler. 1995. (Illus.). 208p. text 159.00 (*0-7817-0149-X*) Lppncott W & W.

Microsurgical Dissection of the Cranial Base. J. Diaz Day et al. 1996. 176p. text (*0-443-07550-6*) Church.

Microsurgical Models in Rats for Transplantation Researh. Ed. by A. Thiede et al. 1985. (Illus.). 420p. 221.00 (*0-387-13221-X*) Spr-Verlag.

Microsurgical Procedures. Ed. by Viktor E. Meyer & Michael J. Black. 1991. (Illus.). 268p. text (*0-443-03463-X*) Church.

Microsurgical Reconstruction of the Cancer Patient. Mark Schusterman. 1997. LC 96-29739. 352p. text 199.00 (*0-397-51391-7*) Lppncott W & W.

Microsurgical Reconstruction of the Extremities. L. Gordon. 1988. (Illus.). 186p. 199.00 (*0-387-96632-3*) Spr-Verlag.

Microsurgical Reconstruction of the Head & Neck. Ed. by Shan R. Baker. 1989. (Illus.). 366p. text (*0-443-08587-0*) Church.

Microvascual Surgery & Free Tissue Transfer. 288p. (*0-340-54925-4*) E A GBR. *Dist:* Routldge.

Microvascular & Neurological Complication of Diabetes. Ed. by G. Crepaldi et al. 1988. (FIDIA Research Ser.: Vol. 10). 328p. 162.00 (*0-387-96619-6*) Spr-Verlag.

Microvascular Bone Reconstruction. Michael B. Wood & Alain Gilbert. 1998. 224p. text (*0-948269-71-5*) Martin Dunitz GBR. *Dist:* Mosby Inc.

Microvascular Corrosion Casting in Scanning Electron Microscopy: Techniques & Applications. S. H. Aharinejad & A. Lametschwandtner. 1993. LC 92-48882. 400p. 159.00 (*0-387-82377-8*) Spr-Verlag.

Microvascular Free Flaps in Head & Neck Reconstruction. Richard L. Arden & John M. Truelson. 1998. LC 97-36821. (Monograph Ser.). (Illus.). 130p. pap. text 60.00 (*1-56772-057-9*, 5206265) AAO-HNS.

Microvascular Motricity & Haemorheology Effects of Buflomedil: Journal: Blood Vessels, Vol. 28, Suppl. 1. Ed. by Marcos Intaglietta. 1991. (Illus.). iv, 48p. pap. 16.75 (*3-8055-5491-5*) S Karger.

Microvascular Networks: Experimental & Theoretical Studies. Ed. by A. S. Popel & P. C. Johnson. 1986. (Illus.). x, 226p. 172.25 (*3-8055-4323-9*) S Karger.

Microvascular Perfusion & Transport in Health & Disease. Ed. by P. F. McDonagh. 1986. (Illus.). x, 254p. 209.75 (*3-8055-4394-8*) S Karger.

Microvascular Reconstruction. R. T. Manktelow. 1986. (Illus.). 221p. 450.00 (*0-387-15271-7*) Spr-Verlag.

Microvascular Surgery. David S. Soutar. 1993. 145.00 (*0-316-80470-3*, Little Brwn Med Div) Lppncott W & W.

Microvascular Surgery of the Extremities. Zhongjia Yu. Tr. by Bingfang Zeng. 1993. LC 92-2302. 298.00 (*3-540-55273-1*); (Illus.). 528p. 350.00 (*0-387-55273-1*) Spr-Verlag.

Microvascular Therapeutic Advances in Venous Disorders Vol. 15, Suppl. 1: Journal: Int. J. Microcirc., 1995. Ed. by C. Allegra & A. Bollinger. 1995. (Journal: Vol. 15, Suppl. 1, 1995). (Illus.). iv, 56p. pap. 26.25 (*3-8055-6253-5*) S Karger.

Microwave Fixation of Labile Metabolites: Proceedings of an Official Satellite Symposium of the 8th International Congress of Pharmacology Held in Tokyo, Japan, 25 July 1981. Ed. by Yosh Maruyama et al. 1983. (Advances in the Biosciences Ser.: 45). (Illus.). 191p. 55.00 (*0-08-029829-X*, Pergamon Pr) Elsevier.

Micturition. Ed. by J. O. Drife et al. 1990. (Illus.). 356p. 125.00 (*0-387-19614-5*) Spr-Verlag.

Mid-Level Practitioners: Their Role in Providing Quality Health Care. Sara R. McGonagle. 1992. (Working Papers Ser.: No. 64). 42p. pap. 5.50 (*0-89940-546-0*) LBJ Sch Pub Aff.

Middle Age Is Not a Disease. James R. Sherman. 1985. LC 84-63051. pap. 3.95 (*0-935538-07-0*) Pathway Bks.

Middle Atlantic Projectile Point Typology & Nomenclature. W. Jack Hranicky. 3rd ed. 1994. LC 95-198211. (Special Publications: No. 33). 110p. pap. 19.00 (*1-884626-22-X*) Archeolog Soc.

Middle-Class Waifs: The Psychodynamic Treatment of Affectively Disturbed Children. Elaine V. Siegel. 1991. 280p. text 42.50 (*0-88163-098-5*) Analytic Pr.

Middle Ear: The Role of Ventilation in Disease & Surgery. H. Takahashi. 2000. LC 00-50987. (Illus.). 120p. 89.00 (*4-431-70306-3*) Spr-Verlag.

***Middle Ear - The Inflammatory Response in Children with Otitis Media with Effusion & the Impact of Atopy: Clinical & Histochemical Studies.** David S. Hurst. 2000. (Comprehensive Summaries of Uppsala Disertations from the Faculty of Medicine: No. 978). (Illus.). 60p. (Orig.). pap. (*91-554-4887-9*) Uppsala Universitet SWE. *Dist:* Coronet Bks.

Middle Ear Implant: Implantable Hearing Aids. Ed. by K. I. Suzuki. 1988. (Advances in Audiology Ser.: Vol. 4). (Illus.). x, 174p. 128.00 (*3-8055-4620-3*) S Karger.

Middle Ear Structures, Organogenesis & Congenital Defects. Ed. by B. Ars & P. Van Cauwenberge. 1991. LC 91-12019. (Illus.). 98p. pap. text (*90-6299-074-6*) Kugler NLD. *Dist:* Lib Res.

Middle Eastern Clinical Medicine. M. A. Kassimi & M. J. Farebrother. 1994. LC 94-68784. 608p. pap. 54.95 (*0-412-60040-4*) Chapman & Hall.

Middle Ground: Coping with Physical & Emotional Pain. John Guzman & Jean Dixen. unabr. ed. 1996. (Illus.). 84p. (Orig.). pap. 14.95 (*0-9655573-0-8*) Ivory Tower CA.

Middle Years: New Psychoanalytic Perspectives. John M. Oldham & Robert S. Liebert. 1990. 304p. (C). 37.50 (*0-300-04418-6*) Yale U Pr.

Midlife & Older Women in Latin America & the Caribbean. 1989. (ENG & SPA.). x, 424p. pap. text 50.00 (*92-75-12021-8*, 1630002) World Health.

Midlife Health: A Woman's Practical Guide to Feeling Good. Ada P. Kahn & Linda H. Holt. 1989. 384p. mass mkt. 5.99 (*0-380-70719-5*, Avon Bks) Morrow Avon.

Midlife, Madness, or Menopause: Does Anyone Know What's Normal? Patricia Richter & Roger Duvivier. 1995. 264p. pap. 12.95 (*1-56561-059-8*) Wiley.

Midlife, Madness, or Menopause: Does Anyone Know What's Normal? Patricia J. Richter. 1995. 264p. pap. 14.95 (*0-471-34685-3*) Wiley.

Midnight Meal & Other Essays about Doctors, Patients, & Medicine. Jerome Lowenstein. 1997. LC 96-26159. 144p. 19.00 (*0-300-06816-6*) Yale U Pr.

Midstream: An Intimate Journal of Loss & Discovery. Le Anne Schreiber. 1996. LC 96-17584. 320p. pap. 14.95 (*1-55821-493-3*, Lyons) Globe Pequot.

Midwife Challenge. Ed. by Sheila Kitzinger. 1991. 288p. pap. 12.95 (*0-04-440845-5*) NYU Pr.

Midwife Challenge. Ed. by Sheila Kitzinger. 1989. pap. (*0-86358-235-4*) Pandora GBR. *Dist:* Harper SF.

Midwife Through the Dying Process: Stories of Healing & Hard Choices at the End of Life. Timothy E. Quill. 1996. LC 96-26475. 208p. 29.00 (*0-8018-5516-0*) Johns Hopkins.

Midwifery. Linda V. Walsh. 2001. LC 2001-20138. (Illus.). xxi, 550p. text 69.95 (*0-7216-4716-2*) Harcrt Hlth Sci Grp.

Midwifery. Set. Pauline M. Sellers. 1995. pap. (*0-7021-2882-1*) Juta & Co ZAF. *Dist:* Intl Spec Bk, Gaunt.

Midwifery. P. McCall Sellars. 1992. Vol. 1. (*0-7021-2925-9*); Vol. 2. (*0-7021-2926-7*) Juta & Co ZAF. *Dist:* Gaunt.

Midwifery & Herbs. Willa Shaffer. 1987. pap. 3.95 (*0-913923-19-2*) Woodland UT.

Midwifery & Medicine in Early Modern France: Louise Bourgeois. Wendy Perkins. 1996. 240p. text (*0-85989-471-1*) Univ Exeter Pr GBR. *Dist:* David Brown.

Midwifery & the Law. 1990. pap. 5.95 (*0-914257-08-0*) Mothering Magazine.

Midwifery & the Medicalization of Childbirth: Comparative Perspectives. Ed. by Edwin Van Teijlingen et al. 1999. LC 99-14711. xii, 393p. lib. bdg. 59.00 (*1-56072-680-6*) Nova Sci Pubs.

Midwifery Handbook: A Practical Guide to Prenatal & Postpartum Care. Linda Wheeler. 1997. LC 96-49608. 288p. spiral bd. 44.00 (*0-397-55360-9*) Lppncott W & W.

Midwifery, Mind & Spirit: Emerging Issues of Care. Jennifer Hall. 2000. LC 00-29749. 134p. pap. text 32.00 (*0-7506-4297-1*) Buttrwrth-Heinemann.

Midwifery Research Database Miriad Supplement, No. 1. Ed. by Mary J. Renfrew & Felicia McCormick. 1997. LC 97-152752. 60p. pap. text, suppl. ed. 44.99 (*1-898507-46-5*) Buttrwrth-Heinemann.

Midwifery Theory & Practice. Ed. by Philip K. Wilson. 1996. LC 96-794. (Childbirth Ser.: Vol. 1). (Illus.). 488p. reprint ed. text 94.00 (*0-8153-2230-5*) Garland.

Midwife's Practical Directory: Woman's Confidential Friend. Thomas Hersey. 1974. LC 73-20627. (Sex, Marriage & Society Ser.). 362p. reprint ed. 33.95 (*0-405-05803-9*) Ayer.

Midwife's Tale: An Oral History from Handywoman to Professional Midwife. Nicky Leap & Billie Hunter. 1993. (Illus.). 238p. pap. (*1-85727-041-X*) Scarlet Pr GBR. *Dist:* LPC InBook.

Midwives & Management. Rosemary E. Cross. 1996. 216p. pap. text 29.99 (*1-898507-20-1*) Buttrwrth-Heinemann.

Midwives & Mothers: The Re-Emergence of Midwifery in Canada. Elizabeth Allemang et al. Date not set. 175p. pap. (*0-929005-58-9*) Sec Story Pr CAN. *Dist:* LPC InBook.

Midwives & Safer Motherhood. Murray. 1996. mass mkt. 24.00 (*0-7234-2122-6*) Mosby Inc.

Midwives in History & Society. Jean Towler & Joan Bramall. 1986. LC 85-26508. (Illus.). 288p. (Orig.). pap. (*0-7099-2453-4*) C Helm GBR. *Dist:* Routldge.

Midwives of Seventeenth-Century London. Doreen Evenden. 2000. LC 99-26518. (Cambridge Studies in the History of Medicine). (Illus.). 280p. (C). text 64.95 (*0-521-66107-2*) Cambridge U Pr.

Midwives, Research & Childbirth, Vol. II. Ed. by Sarah Robinson & Ann Thomson. 1990. 256p. pap. 34.95 (*0-412-31650-1*, A4455) Chapman & Hall.

***Midwives, Research & Childbirth**, Vol. IV. Robinson. 1995. pap. 34.95 (*0-412-45840-3*) Chapman & Hall.

Midwives, Society & Childbirth: Debates & Controversies in the Modern Period. Ed. by Hilary Marland & Anne M. Rafferty. 1997. LC 96-41125. (Studies in the Social History of Medicine). 292p. (C). 90.00 (*0 415 13328-9*) Routledge.

Midwives to the Dying. Miriam Schneider & Jan S. Bernard. 1992. (Illus.). 64p. (Orig.). pap. 12.95 (*0-9632553-0-4*) Angels Work.

Mielograma. Oliver D. Grin & Dorothy L. Bouwman. 1992. (Patient Education Ser.). (SPA., Illus.). 10p. (Orig.). pap. text 4.00 (*0-929689-53-4*) Ludann Co.

Mighty. Brian Porter. 1991. 645p. (C). text 34.95 (*1-881814-99-8*) Pace Pr MA.

Migraine. M. A. Budd. 1998. pap. (*0-7225-3326-8*, 902696Q) Thorsons GBR. *Dist:* Natl Bk Netwk.

***Migraine: A Neuroinflammatory Disease?** Ed. by Egiluis L. H. Spierings & Margarita Sanchez del Rio. 2002. LC 2001-52408. (*3-7643-6231-6*) Birkhauser.

Migraine: An Annotated Bibliography of Treatment Sources. Compiled by Gerald Wade. 1986. 41p. 12.00 (*0-937755-00-1*) Cypress Creek Pubns.

Migraine: Everything You Need to Know. Valerie South. 1996. (Illus.). 220p. pap. 14.95 (*1-55013-784-0*) Firefly Bks Limited.

Migraine: Manifestations, Pathogenesis & Management. Robert A. Davidoff. 1994. LC 94-16409. (Contemporary Neurology Ser.: No. 42). (Illus.). 400p. (C). 85.00 (*0-8036-2360-7*) OUP.

Migraine: Pharmacology & Genetics. Ed. by M. Sandler et al. 1996. (Illus.). 344p. (*1-86036-006-8*) E A GBR. *Dist:* OUP.

Migraine: Questions & Answers. Egilius L. Spierings. 1996. (Illus.). 120p. pap. 15.95 (*1-873413-60-2*) Merit Pub Intl.

Migraine: The Complete Guide. American Council for Headache Education Staff et al. 1994. LC 93-27843. 304p. pap. 12.95 (*0-440-50458-9*) Dell.

Migraine & Other Headaches. Marcia Wilkinson & Anne MacGregor. Ed. by David R. Goldmann. 2000. LC 98-43379. (ACP Home Medical Guides Ser.). (Illus.). 96p. pap. 6.95 (*0-7894-4164-0*, D K Ink) DK Pub Inc.

Migraine Headache: Prevention & Treatment by Phytotherapy, Herbal Medicine. Ela Ronen & Bernice Baefour. 1993. 68p. (Orig.). pap. 15.95 (*0-9638677-0-9*) E M D Ent.

Migraine Headache Prevention & Management. Seymour Diamond. 1990. (Illus.). 256p. text 135.00 (*0-8247-8212-7*) Dekker.

Migraine Headaches & the Food You Eat: 200 Recipes for Relief. Agnes Peg Hartnell. 1997. 272p. pap. 12.95 (*0-471-34686-1*) Wiley.

Migraine in Perspective. 1999. 96p. pap. text (*0-86471-053-4*) Adis Intl NZL. *Dist:* Lppncott W & W.

***Migraine in Women: Epidemiological, Clinical, Genetic & Experimental Aspects.** Peter Mattson. 2000. (Comprehensive Summaries of Uppsala Dissertations from the Faculty of Medicine Ser.: No. 924). 54p. pap. (*91-554-4706-6*) Uppsala Universitet SWE. *Dist:* Coronet Bks.

Migraine Killers That Zap Headaches Now. Douglas Hunt. 1998. 272p. pap. 19.95 (*0-9663040-0-4*) Rosebud Pubns.

Migraine Prevention. Victor A. Young. 1978. LC 78-61831. 156p. 3.95 (*0-9603694-0-6*) V Young.

Migraines: A Natural Approach. Sue Dyson. 1998. LC 98-84064. (Illus.). 240p. pap. 10.95 (*1-56975-140-4*) Ulysses Pr.

Migraines & More - Conquered. Louis M. Hale. 1987. 160p. 14.95 (*0-941219-75-5*) Phillips Pub MA.

Migration & Health: Towards an Understanding of the Health Care Needs of Ethnic Minorities. M. Colledge. 1987. 210p. pap. text 17.00 (*92-890-1045-2*, 1340032) World Health.

Migration & Homing of Lymphoid Cells. Ed. by Alan Husband. 1988. Vol. I. 240p. 121.00 (*0-8493-6508-2*, QR185); Vol. II: A Common Mucosal Immune System Revisited. 224p. 113.00 (*0-8493-6509-0*, QR185) Franklin (CRC Reprint).

MIK Medical Information Kit: Your Memory File for Faster, Safer Health Care. Carol H. Jones. 1998. 48p. ring bd. 17.95 (*0-9664061-0-9*) Hlth Care Excell.

Mikrofiltration und Andere Tranfusions-Probleme in der Intensivmedizin. Ed. by H. Busch. 1979. (Beitraege zur Infusionstherapie und Klinische Ernaehrung Ser.: Band 3). (Illus.). pap. 15.00 (*3-8055-3057-9*) S Karger.

Mikrozirkulation des Skelettmuskels. Ed. by K. Messmer & F. Hammersen. 1985. (Illus.). viii, 162p. pap. 64.50 (*3-8055-3919-3*) S Karger.

Mikrozirkulation in Malignen Tumoren. Ed. by P. W. Vaupel & F. Hammersen. 1983. (Mikrozirkulation in Forschung und Klinik Ser.: Vol. 2). (Illus.). vi, 126p. pap. 39.25 (*3-8055-3762-X*) S Karger.

Mikrozirkulation und arterielle Verschlusskrankheiten, Muenchen, November 1980. Ed. by K. Messmer & Bengt Fagrell. 1982. (Illus.). vi, 222p. pap. 42.75 (*3-8055-2417-X*) S Karger.

Mikrozirkulation und Entzuendung: Beziehungen Zwischen Gefaesswand Entzuendungszellen und Mediatoren. Ed. by K. Messmer & F. Hammersen. 1988. (Illus.). xvi, 358p. pap. 130.50 (*3-8055-4656-4*) S Karger.

Milady's Theory & Practice of Therapeutic Massage. Mark F. Beck. 2nd ed. 1994. LC 93-28234. 693p. pap. 48.95 (*1-56253-120-4*) Thomson Learn.

Milady's Theory & Practice of Therapeutic Massage: Curriculum Guide. Mark F. Beck. 2nd ed. 1993. 3p. 2.75 (*1-56253-121-2*) Milady Pub.

Milagrosas Hierbas Curativas. John Heinerman. 2000. (SPA.). 608p. pap. 14.00 (*0-7352-0212-5*) PH Pr.

Milagrosos Alimentos Curativos. Rex Adams. 2000. (SPA.). 316p. pap. 14.00 (*0-7352-0195-1*) PH Pr.

Milagrosos Alimentos Curativos de la Biblia. Reese P. Dubin. 2000. (SPA.). 480p. pap. 14.00 (*0-7352-0210-9*) PH Pr.

Milan Approach to Family Therapy. Guido L. Burbatti & Laura Formenti. 1988. LC 87-19595. 221p. 40.00 (*0-87668-972-1*) Aronson.

Milan Family Therapy: Variant & Invariant Methods. Esther Gelcer et al. 1990. LC 89-18346. 280p. 45.00 (*0-87668-807-5*) Aronson.

Milan Systemic Family Therapy: Conversations in Theory & Practice. Luigi Boscolo et al. 1987. LC 87-71985. 352p. 47.00 (*0-465-04596-0*) Basic.

Milani-Comparetti Motor Development Screening Test for Infants & Young Children: A Manual. Wayne Stuberg. 3rd ed. 1992. reprint ed. spiral bd. 20.00 (*1-889843-02-4*) Munroe-Meyer Inst.

Mild Brain Injury: A Special Issue of "Applied Neuropsychology" Ed. by Thomas L. Bennett & Michael J. Raymond. 1997. 83p. pap. (*0-8058-9868-9*) L Erlbaum Assocs.

Mild Head Injury. Ed. by Harvey S. Levin et al. 1989. (Illus.). 304p. text 49.50 (*0-19-505301-X*) OUP.

Mild Head Injury: A Guide to Management. Philip Wrightson & Dorothy Gronwall. 1999. LC 99-19511. (Illus.). 194p. text 34.50 (*0-19-262939-5*) OUP.

Mild Traumatic Brain Injury: A Therapy & Resource Manual. Elizabeth S. Green et al. 1997. LC 97-25314. (Neurogenic Communication Disorders Ser.). 282p. (Orig.). pap. 49.95 (*1-56593-827-5*, 1622) Thomson Learn.

Mildly Handicapped Conditions. Ed. by Margaret C. Wang et al. 1988. (Handbooks of Special Education: Vol. 2). 406p. 142.00 (*0-08-033384-2*, Pergamon Pr) Elsevier.

Mildly Handicapped Student. Ed. by Ted L. Miller & Earl Davis. 1982. (Illus.). 526p. text 52.00 (*0-8089-1441-3*, 792926, Grune & Strat) Harcrt Hlth Sci Grp.

Milestones in Health & Medicine. Anne S. Harding. 2000. LC 00-32660. (Illus.). 272p. (YA). (gr. 8 up). lib. bdg. 59.95 (*1-57356-140-1*, Oryx) Greenwood.

Milestones in Hypertension, Issue No. 2. Ed. by Claudia Stahl. 1999. (*1-57130-039-2*) Medicine Grp USA.

Milestones in Hypertension, Vol. 4. Ed. by Dave Varnum. 2000. (*1-57130-045-7*) Medicine Grp USA.

Milestones in Medicine. New York Academy of Medicine Staff. 1977. LC 73-142681. (Essay Index Reprint Ser.). 23.95 (*0-8369-2119-4*) Ayer.

Milestones in Midwifery & the Secret Instrument: The Birth of the Midwifery Forceps. Walter Radcliffe. 1989. (Illus.). 193p. reprint ed. 75.00 (*0-930405-20-X*) Norman SF.

Milieu Therapy: Significant Issues & Innovative Applications. Ed. by Jacquelyn Sanders. 1993. LC 93-15448. (Residential Treatment for Children & Youth Ser.: Vol. 10, No. 3). 121p. lib. bdg. 39.95 (*1-56024-409-7*) Haworth Pr.

Militararztlichen Bildungsanstalten Von Ihrer Grundung Bis Zur Gegenwart. Otto Schickert. 1985. (GER.). reprint ed. (*3-283-07697-9*) G Olms Pubs.

Military Orders: Fighting for the Faith & Caring for the Sick. Ed. by Malcolm C. Barber. 1994. LC 94-17896. (Illus.). 432p. text (*0-86078-438-X*) Variorum GBR. *Dist:* Ashgate Pub Co.

Military Physicians: Dod's Medical School & Scholarship Program. 1996. (Illus.). 93p. (Orig.). (C). pap. text 25.00 (*0-7881-2751-9*) DIANE Pub.

Military Physicians: DOD's Medical School & Scholarship Program. 1995. (Illus.). 94p. pap. text 35.00 (*1-57979-121-2*) DIANE Pub.

Military Psychiatry: A Comparative Perspective, 57. Ed. by Richard A. Gabriel. 1986. LC 86-12107. (Contributions in Military Studies Ser.: No. 57). 225p. 55.00 (*0-313-25491-5*, GML/, Greenwood Pr) Greenwood.

Military Psychology: An Introduction. Christopher Cronin. 1998. (Illus.). 324p. (C). text 66.00 (*0-536-00565-6*) Pearson Custom.

Military Retirement: Social, Economic & Mental Health Dilemmas. John S. McNeil et al. 1983. (Illus.). 156p. text 52.50 (*0-86598-078-0*) Rowman.

Military Strategies for Sustainment of Nutrition & Immune Function in the Field. Institute of Medicine Staff. 1999. LC 98-89702. (Illus.). xiii, 708p. pap. 80.00 (*0-309-06345-0*) Natl Acad Pr.

Military Telemedicine On-Line Today, 1995 National Forum. 1996. LC 94-75388. 192p. pap. 50.00 (*0-8186-5860-6*, PR05860) IEEE Comp Soc.

Milk: The Deadly Poison. Robert Cohen. unabr. ed. 1998. LC 97-94585. (Illus.). 317p. 24.95 (*0-9659196-0-9*) Argus Pub.

Milk & Lactation: Proceedings of the Symposium, Campione, Sept. 1973. Symposium, Campione Staff. Ed. by N. Kretchmer et al. 1975. (Modern Problems in Pediatrics Ser.: Vol. 15). (Illus.). 250p. 85.25 (*3-8055-2056-5*) S Karger.

Milk & Mortality: The Connection Between Milk Drinking & Coronary Heart Disease. David B. Gordon. 1999. LC 99-94557. (Illus.). vii, 207p. 35.00 (*0-9671605-0-2*) Gordon Bks.

Milk Hygiene: Report of the FAO-WHO Expert Committee on Milk Hygiene, 3rd, Geneva, 1969. FAO-WHO Expert Committee on Milk Hygiene. (Technical Reports: No. 453). 1970. 82p. pap. text 5.00 (*92-4-120453-2*, 1100453); 1957. (ENG & SPA.). 54p. pap. 3.00 (*92-4-120124-X*) World Health.

Milk Intolerances & Rejection. Ed. by J. Delmont. 1983. (Illus.). x, 170p. pap. 121.75 (*3-8055-3546-5*) S Karger.

Milk Proteins. Ed. by C. A. Barth & E. Schlimme. 1989. 240p. 54.00 (*0-387-91349-1*) Spr-Verlag.

***Milk Soy Protein Intolerance (MSPI) Guidebook/ Cookbook.** Tamara Field. 2001. pap. 14.94 (*0-533-13841-8*) Vantage.

Milk Thistle. Woodland Publishing Staff. 1999. (Woodland Health Ser.). 32p. pap. text 3.95 (*1-885670-24-9*) Woodland UT.

Milk Thistle: A Step-by-Step Guide. Jill Nice & Jill Rosemary Davies. 2000. (In a Nutshell Ser.). (Illus.). 64p. 7.95 (*1-86204-710-3*) Element MA.

Millennium Management: "Better, Faster, Cheaper" Strategies for Managing 21st Century Healthcare Organizations. Russell C. Coile, Jr. 1998. LC 98-19872. 215p. 49.00 (*1-56793-084-0*) Health Admin Pr.

Miller-Keane Encyclopedia & Dictionary of Medicine, Nursing & Allied Health. Marie O'Toole. Ed. by Thomas Eoyang. 6th ed. 1997. LC 97-151513. 2016p. text 35.95 (*0-7216-6278-1*) Saunders.

Miller's Anatomy of the Dog. Howard E. Evans. 3rd ed. 1993. LC 92-32950. (Illus.). 1056p. text 99.00 (*0-7216-3200-9*) Saunders.

Miller's Clinical Case Companion. Neal H. Cohen. 1994. pap. (*0-443-08961-2*) Church.

Miller's Guide to the Dissection of the Dog. Howard E. Evans & Alexander DeLahunta. 4th ed. 1995. 420p. text 39.00 (*0-7216-5748-6*) Saunders.

Million Clinical Multiaxial Inventory: A Clinical Research Information Synthesis. Ed. by Robert J. Craig. 1993. 312p. text 69.95 (*0-8058-1145-1*) L Erlbaum Assocs.

Milne's Dermatopathology. Ed. by Rona M. Mackie. 2nd ed. 1988. 368p. (C). text (*0-683-13060-9*) E A GBR. *Dist:* Williams & Wilkins.

Milwaukee Evaluation of Daily Living Skills: Evaluation in Long-Term Psychiatric Care (MEDLS) Carol A. Leonardelli. 1988. LC 88-42542. 136p. pap. 25.00 (*1-55642-039-0*) SLACK Inc.

Milwaukee Project: Preventing Mental Retardation in Children at Risk. Howard L. Garber. 1988. 464p. (C). 15.00 (*0-940898-16-0*) Am Assn Mental.

Mimesis & Alterity: A Particular History of the Senses. Michael Taussig. 1992. LC 92-35584. 288p. (C). (gr. 13). pap. 25.95 (*0-415-90687-3*, A7365) Routledge.

Miminal Access Coloproctology. Ed. by Maurice E. Arregui & Jonathan M. Sackier. 1995. LC 94-45687. (*1-870905-68-7*) Radcliffe Med Pr GBR. *Dist:* Balogh.

Miminally Invasive Techniques in Thoracic Medicine & Surgery. Ed. by Martin R. Hetzel. 1994. LC 94-68239. 336p. (gr. 13). 171.95 (*0-412-49530-9*) Chapman & Hall.

Mims' Pathogenesis of Infectious Disease. Cedric A. Mims et al. 5th ed. 2000. LC 00-105900. (Illus.). 450p. 64.95 (*0-12-498264-6*); pap. 44.95 (*0-12-498265-4*) Acad Pr.

Mind: Its Origin, Evolution, Structure & Functioning. Malcolm I. Hale. 1989. (Illus.). 300p. (Orig.). pap. 7.95 (*0-9623691-0-1*) Hale-Van Ruth.

Mind: Our Greatest Gift. Ed. by Margaret Leuverink. 1995. (Mananam Ser.). (Illus.). 111p. 7.00 (*1-880687-09-7*) Chinmaya Pubns.

Mind: Perception & Thought in Their Constructive Aspects. Paul Schilder. 1977. LC 72-165805. (Select Bibliographies Reprint Ser.). reprint ed. 31.95 (*0-8369-5962-0*) Ayer.

Mind & Brain: Or The Correlation of Consciousness Thomas Laycock. 1976. LC 75-16715. (Classics in Psychiatry Ser.). (Illus.). reprint ed. 75.95 (*0-405-07443-3*) Ayer.

Mind & Brain: Principles of Neuropsychology. Alberta S. Gilinsky. 1984. LC 83-24740. 550p. 75.00 (*0-275-91170-5*, C1170, Praeger Pubs) Greenwood.

Mind & Brain Sciences in the 21st Century. Ed. by Robert L. Solso. 1997. LC 96-43751. (Illus.). 374p. 38.50 (*0-262-19385-X*, Bradford Bks) MIT Pr.

Mind & Common Sense: Philosophical Essays on Common Sense Psychology. Ed. by Radu J. Bogdan. 1991. 218p. (C). text 64.95 (*0-521-40201-8*) Cambridge U Pr.

Mind & Destiny: A Social Approach to Psychoanalytic Theory. Robert Seidenberg & Hortence S. Cochrane. 1964. LC 64-16918. 39.95 (*0-8156-2061-6*) Syracuse U Pr.

Mind & Heart in Human Sexual Behavior: Owning & Sharing Our Personal Truths. Alan P. Bell. 1997. LC 97-33435. (Illus.). 408p. 40.00 (*0-7657-0135-9*) Aronson.

Mind & Immunity: Behavioral Immunology. Steven Locke & Mady Hornig-Rohan. 1983. LC 83-81107. 258p. 82.50 (*0-275-91400-3*, C1400, Praeger Pubs) Greenwood.

Mind & Its Depths. Richard Wollheim. 224p. 1994. pap. 18.50 (*0-674-57612-8*); 1993. LC 92-12738. 32.50 (*0-674-57611-X*) HUP.

Mind & Its Discontents: An Essay in Discursive Psychiatry. Grant Gillett. 1999. LC 00-265816. 462p. text 55.00 (*0-19-852313-0*) OUP.

Mind & Its Treatment: A Psychoanalytic Approach. Veikko Tahka. 1993. LC 92-49559. 509p. 72.50 (*0-8236-3367-5*) Intl Univs Pr.

Mind & Mood of Aging: Mental Health Problems of the Community Elderly in New York & London. Barry J. Gurland et al. 1983. LC 83-294. 192p. text 49.95 (*0-917724-28-3*) Haworth Pr.

Mind & Tissue: Russian Research Perspective on the Human Brain. Raymond Peat. 2001. LC 00-191607. 173p. pap. 10.00 (*0-9702913-4-5*, 500) R Peat.

Mind As Behavior & Studies in Empirical Idealism. Edgar A. Singer. LC 75-3386. (Philosophy in America Ser.). reprint ed. 45.00 (*0-404-59382-8*) AMS Pr.

Mind Body & Health: Toward an Integral Medicine. Ed. by James S. Gordon et al. 1984. 269p. 43.95 (*0-89885-150-5*); pap. 21.95 (*0-89885-188-2*) Kluwer Academic (Kluwer Acad Hman Sci).

Mind, Body & Immunity. Rachel Charles. 1996. pap. 9.99 (*0-7493-2416-3*) Buttrwrth-Heinemann.

Mind, Body & Soul: A Guide to Living with Cancer. Nancy Hassett Dahm. Ed. by Robert F. Schirmer. unabr. ed. 2001. LC 00-134425. 335p. 27.95 (*0-9702904-0-3*, 2050-1) Taylor Hill.

Mind Body in Action: MBA - Multi-Dimensional Health & Fitness. Steve Beard. 1995. (Illus.). 165p. (Orig.). pap. 15.95 (*0-9642982-9-5*) NuLife Pubg.

Mind-Body Maturity: Psychological Approaches to Sports, Exercise, & Fitness. Louis Diamant. 1991. 304p. 79.95 (*0-89116-892-3*) Hemisp Pub.

Mind-Body Medicine: A Clinician's Guide to Psychoneuroimmunology. Alan Watkins. 1997. 314p. (C). pap. text (*0-443-05526-2*) Church.

Mind Body Medicine Vol. 1: The Stages of Healing. Lewis E. Mehl & Gayle H. Peterson. (Frontiers of Consciousness Ser.). (Illus.). 250p. (*0-8290-2468-9*) Irvington.

Mind-Body Problem: A Psychobiological Approach. Mario Bunge. 1980. (Foundations & Philosophy of Science & Technology Ser.: Vol. 1). (Illus.). 245p. (*0-08-024720-2*) Pergamon Repr GBR. *Dist:* Franklin.

Mind-Body Problems: Psychotherapy with Psychosomatic Disorders. Janet S. Finell. 1997. LC 96-38977. 376p. 70.00 (*1-56821-654-8*) Aronson.

***Mind Body Spirit: A complete Guide to Holistic Therapies for Achieving & Maintaining Optimum Health.** Jane Alexander. 2001. (*1-84222-267-8*) Carlton Bks Ltd GBR. *Dist:* Natl Bk Netwk.

Mind-Body-Spirit: Connecting with Your Creative Self. Mary Braheny & Diane Halperin. 1989. 64p. 7.95 (*1-55874-039-2*) Health Comm.

Mind-Body Therapies: A Select Bibliography of Books in English. R. Monro et al. 1987. 176p. text 90.00 (*0-7201-1811-5*) Continuum.

Mind, Brain, & Adaptation in the 19th Century: Cerebral Localization & Its Biological Context from Gall to Ferrier. Robert M. Young. 1990. (History of Neuroscience Ser.: No. 3). 304p. text 39.95 (*0-19-506389-9*) OUP.

Mind, Brain & Function: Essays in the Philosophy of Mind. J. I. Biro & Robert W. Shahan. 1982. LC 81-40296. 208p. 29.95 (*0-8061-1783-4*) U of Okla Pr.

Mind Brain Behavior: Discussions of B. F. Skinner & J. R. Searle. Ilham Dilman. 1988. 128p. (C). lib. bdg. 49.95 (*0-415-00006-8*) Routledge.

Mind, Brain, Behavior: The Mind-Body Problem & the Philosophy of Psychology. Martin Carrier & Juergen Mittelstrass. 1995. x, 314p. (C). pap. text 29.95 (*3-11-014954-0*) De Gruyter.

Mind-Brain Continuum: Sensory Processes. Ed. by Rodolfo R. Llinas & Patricia S. Churchland. 1996. LC 95-46160. (Illus.). 329p. (C). 60.00 (*0-262-12198-0*, Bradford Bks) MIT Pr.

Mind Bugs: The Origins of Procedural Misconception. Kurt Vanlehn. 1990. LC 89-12493. (Learning, Development, & Conceptual Change Ser.). 368p. 42.00 (*0-262-22036-9*, Bradford Bks) MIT Pr.

Mind, Character, & Personality: Guidelines to Mental & Spiritual Health Ellen Gould Harmon White. 1978. 1. 12.99 (*0-8127-0148-8*); 2. 12.99 (*0-8127-0149-6*) Review & Herald.

Mind, Culture & Activity: Seminal Papers from the Laboratory of Comparative Human Cognition. Ed. by Michael Cole et al. 1997. (Illus.). 517p. (C). text 69.95 (*0-521-55238-9*); pap. text 24.95 (*0-521-55823-9*) Cambridge U Pr.

Mind Food & Smart Pills: A Sourcebook for the Vitamins, Herbs & Drugs That Can Increase Intelligence, Improve Memory & Prevent Brain Aging. Ross Pelton & Taffy C. Pelton. 1989. 336p. pap. 13.95 (*0-385-26138-1*) Doubleday.

Mind Game see Witchdoctors & Psychiatrists: The Common Roots of Psychotherapy & Its Future

Mind Game: Witchdoctors & Psychiatrists. E. Fuller Torrey. 1994. LC 87-70297. 236p. 50.00 (*0-87668-689-7*) Aronson.

Mind Games: American Culture & the Birth of Psychotherapy. Eric Caplan. 1998. LC 98-16999. (Medicine & Society Ser.: Vol. 9). 246p. text 45.00 (*0-520-21169-3*) U CA Pr.

Mind Games: Are We Obsessed with Therapy? Robert A. Baker. 1996. LC 96-3035. (Illus.). 476p. 36.00 (*1-57392-071-1*) Prometheus Bks.

Mind in Conflict. Charles Brenner. 1982. LC 82-21391. v, 266p. (Orig.). 40.00 (*0-8236-3365-9*) Intl Univs Pr.

Mind in Context: Interactionist Perspectives on Human Intelligence. Ed. by Robert J. Sternberg & Richard K. Wagner. 1994. LC 93-221756. (Illus.). 259p. (C). text 74.95 (*0-521-41114-9*); pap. text 27.95 (*0-521-42287-6*) Cambridge U Pr.

Mind in Disorder: Psychoanalytic Models of Pathology. John E. Gedo. 1987. 264p. text 39.95 (*0-88163-068-3*) Analytic Pr.

Mind in Sleep: Psychology & Psychophysiology. Ed. by Steven J. Ellman & John Antrobus. 2nd ed. 1991. LC 90-39136. (Personality Processes Ser.). 588p. 240.00 (*0-471-52556-1*) Wiley.

Mind in Society: The Development of Higher Psychological Processes. L. S. Vygotsky. Ed. by Michael Cole et al. 1978. LC 77-26023. (Illus.). 173p. pap. 16.50 (*0-674-57629-2*) HUP.

Mind Is Not the Heart: Recollections of a Woman Physician. Eva J. Salber. 1993. LC 88-33557. (Illus.). 304p. pap. 16.95 (*0-8223-1365-0*); xvi, 284p. text 49.95 (*0-8223-0910-6*) Duke.

Mind-Made Disease: A Clinician's Guide to Recent Research. Ed. by R. Rosser. 1982. (Journal of Psychosomatic Research: No. 25). (Illus.). 144p. pap. 30.00 (*0-08-027957-0*, Pergamon Pr) Elsevier.

***Mind M.A.P. (Multimedia for Abnormal Psychology.** Lauren B. Alloy. 1999. stu. ed. 22.50 incl. cd-rom (*0-07-236233-2*) McGrw-H Hghr Educ.

***Mind Maps in Pathology.** Peter Dervan & Michele Harrison. 2001. LC 2001-37990. 12op. (*0-443-07054-7*) Church GBR. *Dist:* Saunders.

Mind, Matter, & Gravitation. Haakon Forwald. 1969. LC 72-97212. (Parapsychological Monographs: No. 11). pap. 5.00 (*0-912328-15-0*) Parapsych Foun.

Mind, Matter, Motion: Prescription Running, Your Animal Therapy in the 21st Century. Eugene R. Smith & Elaine N. Smith. Ed. by Elaine N. Smith. 2nd l.t. ed. 1983. LC 82-99857. (Philosophy & Lifestyle Ser.). (Illus.). 264p. (Orig.). reprint ed. pap. 10.00 (*0-9608910-0-5*) Mind-Matter-Motion.

Mind Matters. Marguerite Iwersen. 1981. LC 80-67158. 123p. (Orig.). pap. 5.50 (*0-87516-421-8*) DeVorss.

Mind Matters: Psychological Medicine in Holistic Practice. J. R. Millenson. 1995. LC 94-61963. (Illus.). 337p. (Orig.). (C). pap. text 29.95 (*0-939616-21-1*) Eastland.

Mind Mending Medicine: "Insights from God's Word" John J. Feeney. 2000. LC 00-50700. (Illus.). 224p. pap. 12.00 (*1-877633-58-5*) Luthers.

Mind Mood Pill Book: A Concise Guide to the Most Widely Used Psychiatric Drugs. Robert E. Hales et al. 2000. LC 00-33664. (Illus.). 400p. pap. 19.95 (*0-553-38004-4*) Bantam.

Mind Myths: Exploring Popular Assumptions about the Mind & Brain. Sergio Della Sala. 1999. LC 98-38574. 310p. pap. 49.95 (*0-471-98303-9*) Wiley.

Mind Object: Precocity & Pathology of Self Sufficiency. Ed. by Edward G. Corrigan & Pearl-Ellen Gordon. 1995. LC 95-9997. 264p. 50.00 (*1-56821-480-4*) Aronson.

Mind of a Savant: Language Learning & Modularity. Neil Smith & Ianthi Tsimpli. 1995. (Illus.). 256p. (C). pap. 30.95 (*0-631-19017-1*) Blackwell Pubs.

Mind of Its Own: Tourette's Syndrome, a Story & a Guide. Ruth D. Bruun & Bertel Bruun. 1994. LC 93-14081. (Illus.). 192p. (C). 32.50 (*0-19-506587-5*) OUP.

Mind of Man: Being a Natural System of Mental Philosophy. Alfred Smee. LC 78-72825. (Brainedness, Handedness, & Mental Abilities Ser.). (Illus.). reprint ed. 39.50 (*0-404-60893-0*) AMS Pr.

Mind of One's Own: A Kleinian View of Self & Object. Robert A. Caper. 1998. LC 98-25734. (New Library of Psychoanalysis). 208p. (C). 85.00 (*0-415-19911-5*, D6620); pap. 31.95 (*0-415-19912-3*, D6624) Routledge.

Mind of the Cells. SATPREM Staff. Tr. by Luc Venet from FRE. 1982. LC 82-15659.Tr. of Mental Des Cellules. 215p. pap. 8.95 (*0-938710-06-0*) Inst Evolutionary.

Mind of the Child William Preyer. 1977. LC 73-2985. (Classics in Psychology Ser.). reprint ed. 47.95 (*0-405-05156-5*) Ayer.

Mind of Your Newborn Baby. David Chamberlain. 3rd ed. 1998. LC 97-46583. Orig. Title: Babies Remember Birth. 225p. reprint ed. pap. 14.95 (*1-55643-264-X*) North Atlantic.

Mind Out of Matter: Topics in the Physical Foundations of Consciousness & Cognition. Gregory R. Mulhauser. 1998. LC 98-22509. (Studies in Cognitive Systems). 120.00 (*0-7923-5103-7*) Kluwer Academic.

Mind over Back Pain. John E. Sarno. 1986. pap. 4.50 (*0-425-12700-1*); (Illus.). 128p. pap. 6.50 (*0-425-08741-7*) Berkley Pub.

Mind over Labor. Carl Jones. 1988. LC 87-7126. (Handbooks Ser.). 208p. pap. 12.95 (*0-14-046762-9*, Penguin Bks) Penguin Putnam.

Mind over Malignancy: Living with Cancer. Wayne D. Gersh et al. 1997. LC 97-66076. 168p. pap. 12.95 (*1-57224-082-2*) New Harbinger.

Mind over Mood: Change How You Feel by Changing the Way You Think. Dennis Greenberger & Christine A. Padesky. 1995. LC 95-8223. (Illus.). 243p. pap. 21.00 (*0-89862-128-3*, 2128) Guilford Pubns.

Mind, Self, & Society: From the Standpoint of a Social Behaviorist. George Herbert Mead. Ed. by Charles W. Morris. 1967. 448p. pap. text 15.95 (*0-226-51668-7*) U Ch Pr.

Mind Styles Model: Theory, Principles & Practice. Anthony F. Gregorc. 1998. 28p. pap. 5.00 (*0-934481-06-7*) Gregorc Assocs.

Mind That Found Itself. Clifford W. Beers. 5th ed. 1981. LC 80-5256. (Contemporary Community Health Ser.). 228p. (C). (gr. 11-12). reprint ed. pap. 15.95 (*0-8229-5324-2*) U of Pittsburgh Pr.

Mind Unfolded: Essays on Psychology's Historic Texts. Daniel N. Robinson. 1978. 539p. LC 78-58510. pap. 19.95 (*0-313-27077-5*, P7077); LC 78-53510. lib. bdg. 92.50 (*0-313-27076-7*, U7076) Greenwood.

Mind Wars. Ron Dalrymple. 1981. 175p. text 12.95 (*0-935882-02-2*) Celestial Gifts.

Mind Within the Net: Models of Learning, Thinking & Acting. Manfred Spitzer. (Bradford Book Ser.). (Illus.). 1999. LC 98-10911. 320p. 27.50 (*0-262-19406-6*, Bradford Bks); 2000. 376p. reprint ed. pap. 17.95 (*0-262-69236-8*) MIT Pr.

Mindblindness: An Essay on Autism & Theory of Mind. Simon Baron-Cohen. 1995. LC 94-36470. (Learning, Development, & Conceptual Change Ser.). 300p. 50.00 (*0-262-02384-9*, Bradford Bks) MIT Pr.

Mind/Body Health: The Effects of Attitudes, Emotions & Relationships. Brent Q. Hafen et al. 1995. LC 95-13437. 656p. pap. text 60.00 (*0-205-17211-3*) Allyn.

Mind/Body Integration: Essential Readings in Biofeedback. E. Peper et al. 1979. LC 78-27224. (Illus.). 606p. (C). 90.00 (*0-306-40102-9*, Plenum Trade) Perseus Pubng.

***Minding the Body: Psychotherapy in Cases of Chronic & Life-Threatening Illness.** Ellyn Kaschak. 2001. LC 00-54706. (Women & Therapy Monograph Ser.: Vol. 23, No. 1). 148p. pap. text 19.95 (*0-7890-1368-1*) Haworth Pr.

***Minding the Body: Psychotherapy in Cases of Chronic & Life-Threatening Illness.** Ed. by Ellyn Kaschak. 2001. LC 00-54706. (Women & Therapy Monograph Ser.: Vol. 23, No. 1). 148p. 49.95 (*0-7890-1367-3*) Haworth Pr.

Minding the Whole Person: Cultivating a Healthy Lifestyle from Youth Through the Senior Years. William F. Haynes. 1994. LC 94-12238. (Campion Book Ser.). 178p. pap. 14.95 (*0-8294-0778-2*) Loyola Pr.

***Mind/Mood Pill Book.** Robert E. Hales. 2001. 496p. mass mkt. 6.99 (*0-553-58035-3*) Bantam.

Minds & Money: The Mental Health Business in America. Leo H. Bradman & David T. Volz. Ed. by Ronald C. Harshman. 1994. LC 93-60952. 350p. 38.00 (*1-883945-04-6*); pap. 24.00 (*1-883945-00-3*) UniPsych Pr.

***Minds, Brains, & Learning: Understanding the Psychological & Education Relevance of Neuroscientific Research.** James P. Byrnes. 2001. LC 00-67750. (Illus.). x, 214p. 42.00 (*1-57230-651-3*); pap. 25.00 (*1-57230-652-1*) Guilford Pubns.

Mind's Extensive View: Samuel Johnson as a Critic of Poetic Language. N. Jain. 1991. 183p. (*0-902965-25-5*) Clunie Pr GBR. *Dist:* Other Pr LLC.

Mind's New Science: A History of Cognitive Revolution. Howard Gardner. 1987. LC 87-47555. 448p. pap. 25.00 (*0-465-04635-5*) Basic.

Mind's Past. Michael S. Gazzaniga. 1998. LC 97-32505. (Illus.). 216p. text 22.50 (*0-520-21320-3*) U CA Pr.

Mind's Staircase: Stages in the Development of Human Intelligence. Ed. by Robbie Case. 1992. 424p. pap. 45.00 (*0-8058-1190-7*); text 79.95 (*0-8058-0324-6*) L Erlbaum Assocs.

Mind's We: Contextualism in Cognitive Psychology. Dianne F. Gillespie. 1992. LC 91-39988. 232p. (C). 26.95 (*0-8093-1675-7*) S Ill U Pr.

Minefields in Their Hearts: The Mental Health of Children in War & Communal Violence. Ed. by Roberta J. Apfel & Bennett Simon. 1996. LC 96-10976. 256p. 40.00 (*0-300-06570-1*) Yale U Pr.

Minerais para Ruminantes Em Pastejo Em Regioes Tropicais. Joseph H. Conrad et al. Tr. by Valeria P. Euclides from ENG. 1984. LC 84-72136.Tr. of Minerals for Grazing Ruminants in Tropical Regions. (POR., Illus.). (Orig.). (*0-916287-03-3*) Univ Fla Food.

Mineral Absorption in the Monogastric GI Tract: Chemical, Nutritional, & Physiological Aspects. Ed. by F. R. Dintzis & J. A. Laszlo. 1989. (Advances in Experimental Medicine & Biology Ser.). (Illus.). 208p. 69.50 (*0-306-43200-5*, Plenum Trade) Perseus Pubng.

Mineral & Metal Neurotoxicology. Ed. by Masayuki Yasui et al. 1996. LC 96-5735. 480p. 169.95 (*0-8493-7664-5*) CRC Pr.

Mineral Aspects of Dentistry. F. C. Driessens. 1982. (Monographs in Oral Science: Vol. 10). (Illus.). xvi, 216p. 128.75 (*3-8055-3469-8*) S Karger.

Mineral Fibers & Health. F. D. Liddell & Klara Miller. 1991. (Illus.). 376p. lib. bdg. 229.00 (*0-8493-6646-1*, RC1231) CRC Pr.

Mineral Nutrition of Fruit Crops. T. K. Bose & S. K. Mitra. 1986. 850p. (C). (*81-85109-44-3*) Naya Prokash IND. *Dist:* S Asia.

Minerales para Rumiantes en Pastoreo en Regiones Tropicales. Ed. by Lee R. McDowell et al. 1984. LC 84-71582.Tr. of Minerals for Grazing Ruminants in Tropical Regions. (SPA., Illus.). 106p. (Orig.). (*0-916287-01-7*) Univ Fla Food.

Mineralocorticoids & Hypertension. K. A. Meurer. Ed. by W. Kaufman et al. 1983. (International Boehringer Mannheim Symposia Ser.). (Illus.). 237p. 56.95 (*0-387-12391-1*) Spr-Verlag.

Minerals for Grazing Ruminants in Tropical Regions see Minerales para Rumiantes en Pastoreo en Regiones Tropicales

Minerals for Grazing Ruminants in Tropical Regions. L. R. McDowell. 3rd ed. 1997. LC 97-20222. (Bulletin Ser.). (*0-916287-23-8*) Univ Fla Food.

Mineraux pour les Ruminants de Paturage des Regions Tropicales. Joseph H. Conrad et al. 1984. LC 84-72137.Tr. of Minerals for Grazing Ruminants in Tropical Regions. (FRE., Illus.). (Orig.). (*0-916287-02-5*) Univ Fla Food.

Mini-Consults in Dermatology Vol. III: Gross & Microscopic Symposium, American Academy of Dermatology Staff & Antoinette F. Hood. 2nd ed. 1996. (Illus.). 1500p. (C). text 179.00 (*0-8151-1552-0*) Mosby Inc.

Mini Medical Encyclopedia: Mini-Encyclopedie Medicale. P. Letonturier. 8th ed. 1984. (FRE.). 416p. 25.00 (*0-8288-1816-9*, M8935) Fr & Eur.

Mini-Module, No. MS3: Skillbuilding in Medicine-Surgery. Ed. by American Association for Medical Transcription Staff. 1995. (Exploring Transcription Practices Ser.). 16p. (C). text, stu. ed. 30.00 incl. audio (*0-935229-26-4*) Am Assoc Med.

Mini-Module, No. R1: Skillbuilding in Radiology. Ed. by American Association for Medical Transcription Staff. 1993. (Exploring Transcription Practices Ser.). 16p. (C). stu. ed. 30.00 incl. audio (*0-935229-19-1*) Am Assoc Med.

Mini-Module, No. R2: Skillbuilding in Radiology. Ed. by American Association for Medical Transcription Staff. 1994. (Exploring Transcription Practices Ser.). 16p. (C). text, stu. ed. 30.00 incl. audio (*0-935229-24-8*) Am Assoc Med.

Mini Nutritional Assessment (MNA) Research & Practice in the Elderly: 1st Nestle Clinical & Performance Nutrition Workshop, Mini Nutritional Assessment (MNA) - MNA in the Elderly, Lausanne, October 1997. Ed. by B. J. Vellas et al. 1999. LC 99-18247. (Nestle Nutrition Workshop Ser.). (Illus.). 196p. 137.50 (*3-8055-6803-7*) S Karger.

Minilaparotomy under Local Anaesthesia: A Curriculum for Doctors & Nurses, Participant's Handbook. AVSC International Staff. Ed. by Ruth Mullen. 1995. (Illus.). 72p. stu. ed. 8.00 (*1-885063-08-3*) EngenderHlth.

Minilaparotomy under Local Anaesthesia: A Curriculum for Doctors & Nurses, Trainer's Package. AVSC International Staff. Ed. by Ruth Mullen. 1993. (Illus.). 140p. pap. text 75.00 (*1-885063-07-5*) EngenderHlth.

MNO

Minimal Access Cardiothoracic Surgery. Anthony P. Yim et al. Ed. by Richard Lampert. 1999. LC 99-36532. (Illus.). xxv, 693p. (C). text 295.00 (*0-7216-7723-1*) Saunders.

Minimal Access General Surgery. David Rosin. 1994. LC 93-41152. (*1-870905-72-5*) Radcliffe Med Pr GBR. *Dist:* Balogh.

Minimal Access Gynaecology. Ed. by Stephen Grochmal. 1994. LC 94-37495. (*1-870905-73-3*) Radcliffe Med Pr GBR. *Dist:* Balogh.

Minimal Access Orthopedics. David Hunt. 1996. LC 95-1976. (*1-870905-58-X*) Radcliffe Med Pr GBR. *Dist:* Balogh.

Minimal Access Surgery for Nurses & Technicians. Ed. by Fiona A. Hall. 1994. LC 94-8610. (*1-870905-63-6*) Radcliffe Med Pr GBR. *Dist:* Balogh.

Minimal Access Surgical Oncology. Ed. by Frederick Greene & David Rosin. 1995. LC 95-5161. (*1-85775-080-2*) Radcliffe Med Pr GBR. *Dist:* Balogh.

***Minimal Access Therapy for Vascular Disease.** Bell et al. 2001. (Illus.). 256p. (*1-901865-27-4*) Isis Med GBR. *Dist:* Bks Intl VA.

Minimal Access Thoracic Surgery. K. Manncke. 1999. LC 97-78061. (Illus.). 296p. text (*0-412-81600-8*) E A GBR. *Dist:* OUP.

Minimal Brain Dysfunction: A Prospective Study. Paul L. Nichols & Ta-Chuan Chen. 1981. LC 80-18739. 352p. text 69.95 (*0-89859-074-4*) L Erlbaum Assocs.

Minimal Brain Dysfunction: Facts or Fiction. Ed. by Alex F. Kalverboer et al. 1978. (Advances in Biological Psychiatry Ser.: Vol. 1). (Illus.). 34.00 (*3-8055-2864-7*) S Karger.

Minimal Model Approach & Determinants of Glucose Tolerance. Ed. by Richard N. Bergman & Jennifer C. Lovejoy. 1997. LC 97-18553. (Pennington Center Nutrition Ser.: Vol. 7). 424p. text 110.00 (*0-8071-2238-6*) La State U Pr.

Minimal Neopasia. Ed. by Ekkehard Grundmann & L. Beck. 1988. (Recent Results in Cancer Research Ser.: Vol. 106). (Illus.). 194p. 106.00 (*0-387-18455-4*) Spr-Verlag.

Minimal Rationality. Christopher Cherniak. 1990. 176p. reprint ed. pap. 15.95 (*0-262-53087-2*, Bradford Bks) MIT Pr.

Minimal Residual Disease in Acute Leukemia. Ed. by B. Lowenberg & A. Hagenbeek. 1984. (Developments in Oncology Ser.). 382p. text 211.50 (*0-89838-630-6*) Kluwer Academic.

Minimal Residual Disease in Acute Leukemia, 1986. Ed. by A. Hagenbeek & B. Lowenberg Hagenbeek. 1986. (Developments in Oncology Ser.). lib. bdg. 170.50 (*0-89838-799-X*) Kluwer Academic.

Minimal Residual Disease in Melanoma: Biology, Detection & Clinical Relevance. Ed. by Uwe Reinhold et al. 2000. (Recent Results in Cancer Research Ser.: Vol. 158). (Illus.). 264p. 125.00 (*3-540-67349-0*) Spr-Verlag.

Minimally Invasive Abdominal Surgery. Ed. by K. Kremer et al. 2001. (Illus.). 396p. 199.00 (*0-86577-639-3*) Thieme Med Pubs.

Minimally Invasive Cancer Management. Ed. by F. L. Greene & B. T. Heniford. 2000. LC 00-41902. (Illus.). 408p. 129.00 (*0-387-98710-X*) Spr-Verlag.

Minimally Invasive Cardiac Surgery, Vol. II. Mehmet C. Oz & Daniel Goldstein. 1998. LC 98-30788. (Contemporary Cardiology Ser.: Vol. 2). 256p. 135.00 (*0-89603-635-9*) Humana.

Minimally Invasive Endonasal Sinus Surgery: Principles, Techniques, Results, Complications, Revision Surgery. Contrib. by Werner G. Hosemann. 2000. LC 99-52609. viii, 134p. (*3-13-124611-1*) G Thieme.

Minimally Invasive Endonasal Sinus Surgery: Principles, Techniques, Results, Complications, Revision Surgery. Werner G. Hosemann. 2000. LC 99-52609. (Illus.). viii, 134p. 99.00 (*0-86577-907-4*) Thieme Med Pubs.

Minimally Invasive Neurosurgery I. Ed. by B. L. Bauer & D. Hellwig. 1992. (Acta Neurochirurgica Ser.: Vol. 54). 200p. 108.00 (*0-387-82321-2*) Spr-Verlag.

Minimally Invasive Neurosurgery II. Ed. by B. L. Bauer & D. Hellwig. 1995. (Acta Neurochirurgica Ser.: Vol. 61). 115p. 88.00 (*0-387-82593-2*) Spr-Verlag.

Minimally Invasive Restorations with Bonding. Michel Degrange & Jean-Francois Roulet. 1997. LC 96-37504. (Illus.). 280p. 98.00 (*0-86715-327-X*) Quint Pub Co.

Minimally Invasive Surgery: Principles & Outcomes. Ed. by Charles Andrus et al. 1998. 416p. text 128.00 (*90-5702-261-3*, ECU107, Harwood Acad Pubs) Gordon & Breach.

Minimally Invasive Surgery & New Technology. Ed. by Felicien M. Steichen & Roger Welter. 1993. LC 93-38895. (Illus.). 763p. 130.00 (*0-942219-51-1*) Quality Med Pub.

Minimally Invasive Surgery in Gastrointestinal Cancer. Ed. by Miguel A. Cuesta & Alexander G. Nagy. 1993. LC 93-29876. (Illus.). text (*0-443-04987-4*) Church.

***Minimally Invasive Surgical Techniques,** Vol. 1. 1997. text 133.95 (*1-56593-900-X*) Singular Publishing.

Minimally Invasive Therapy of the Brain. Antonio A. De Salles & Robert B. Lufkin. 1996. LC 96-44702. 189.00 (*0-86577-641-5*) Thieme Med Pubs.

Minimizing Medical Mistakes. Richard K. Riegelman. 1991. 32.95 (*0-316-74523-5*, Little Brwn Med Div) Lppncott W & W.

Minimizing the Risk of Legionella in Cooling Towers & Other HVAC Equipment. Matthew R. Freije. 1998. LC 98-92505. 18p. pap. 19.00 (*0-9649926-3-9*, 304) HC Info Res.

Mining the Silver Lining: Taking Triumph from Tragedy. Billy J. Branson. 1988. 224p. (Orig.). pap. 9.95 (*0-925048-00-3*) Sun-Coyote Pr.

Minireviews of the Neurosciences from Life Sciences, Vols. 13-15. Ed. by Bernard B. Brodie & R. Bressler. 1975. LC 75-8733. 493p. (*0-08-019724-8*) Pergamon Repr GBR. *Dist:* Franklin.

Ministering to Abortion's Aftermath. Bill Banks & Sue Banks. 1982. 144p. (Orig.). pap. 5.95 (*0-89228-057-3*) Impact Christian.

Minister's Handbook of Mental Disorders. Joseph W. Ciarrocchi. 1993. LC 93-11092. (Integration Bks.). 224p. pap. 16.95 (*0-8091-3403-9*) Paulist Pr.

Ministry & Meaning: A Religious History of Catholic Health Care in the United States. Christopher J. Kauffman. 1995. LC 95-1123. 384p. 29.95 (*0-8245-1459-9*) Crossroad NY.

Ministry & Medicine in Human Relations. New York Academy of Medicine Staff. Ed. by Iago Galdston. 1977. LC 77-142682. (Essay Index Reprint Ser.). 19.95 (*0-8369-2120-8*) Ayer.

Ministry to the Sick & Dying. Jude J. McGeehan. 1981. (Synthesis Ser.). pap. 1.00 (*0-8199-0836-3*, Frncscn Herld) Franciscan Pr.

Minnesota Health Care in Perspective 2000. Ed. by Kathleen O'Leary Morgan & Scott E. Morgan. 2000. 21p. spiral bd. 19.00 (*0-7401-0222-2*) Morgan Quitno Corp.

Minnesota Health Care Perspective, 1998. Ed. by Kathleen O'Leary Morgan & Scott E. Morgan. 1998. 20p. pap. 19.00 (*1-56692-822-2*) Morgan Quitno Corp.

Minnesota Multiphasic Personality Inventory (MMPI) Index of Modern Authors & Subjects with Guide for Rapid Research. Remley L. Rannigan. 1991. 200p. 47.50 (*1-55914-280-4*); pap. 44.50 (*1-55914-281-2*) ABBE Pubs Assn.

Minnesota Public Health Goals, 1995. Ed. by Barry Leonard. 1998. (Illus.). 185p. pap. text 35.00 (*0-7881-7186-0*) DIANE Pub.

Minnesota Symposia on Child Psychology, Vol. 11. Ed. by W. Andrew Collins. 1978. 286p. 59.95 (*0-89859-113-9*) L Erlbaum Assocs.

MinnesotaCare: A Progress Report on the Coordination of Medical Assistance & the MinnesotaCare Plan. 1994. (Illus.). 94p. (Orig.). (C). pap. text 35.00 (*0-7881-0380-6*) DIANE Pub.

Minor & Trace Elements in Breast Milk: Report of a Joint WHO/IAEA Collaborative Study. WHO Staff. 1989. 171p. 30.00 (*92-4-156121-1*) World Health.

Minor Emergencies. Philip M. Buttaravoli & Thomas O. Stair. 1999. LC 99-40670. (Illus.). xvii, 526p. pap. text 34.95 (*0-323-00756-2*) Mosby Inc.

Minor Head Trauma. Ed. by Steven Mandel et al. 1993. LC 92-49619. (Illus.). 347p. 163.00 (*0-387-97943-3*) Spr-Verlag.

Minor Illness Manual. Gina Johnson et al. 1997. LC 97-3787. (*1-85775-285-6*) Radcliffe Med Pr GBR. *Dist:* Balogh.

***Minor Illness Manual.** Ed. by Gina Johnson et al. 2nd exp. rev. ed. 2000. 142p. (*1-85775-482-4*) Radcliffe Med Pr GBR. *Dist:* Balogh.

***Minor Illness or Major Disease? Responding to Symptoms in the Pharmacy.** Edwards & Stillman. 3rd ed. 2000. 224p. pap. (*0-85369-447-8*) Pharmaceutical Pr GBR. *Dist:* Rittenhouse.

Minor Injuries & Repairs. John A. Grossman. 1992. LC 92-1565. (Illus.). (gr. 13). (*1-56375-080-5*) Gower-Mosby.

Minor Injuries Unit Handbook: A Guide for A & E Senior House Officers Emergency Nurse Practitioners & General Practitioners. Matthew Cooke et al. 1998. LC 98-26929. 190p. (*0-7506-3451-0*) E A GBR. *Dist:* OUP.

***Minor Surgery.** Price & Sinclair. 2001. (Fast Facts Ser.). (Illus.). 100p. pap. (*1-903734-01-0*) Health Pr GBR. *Dist:* JAMCO Dist.

Minor Surgery: A Text & Atlas. John S. Brown. 2nd ed. 1992. (Illus.). 344p. (C). (gr. 13). mass mkt. 99.95 (*0-412-44910-2*, Chap & Hall NY) Chapman & Hall.

Minor Surgery: A Text & Atlas. John S. Brown & John Alexander-Williams. 2nd ed. 1992. LC 92-49983. (*0-442-31713-1*) Chapman & Hall.

Minor Surgery: A Text & Atlas. John Stuart Brown. 4th ed. 2001. (An Arnold Publication). 469p. text (*0-340-76113-X*) E A GBR. *Dist:* OUP.

Minor Surgery in Orthodontics. Ed. by Jean-Paul Schatz & Jean-Pierre Joho. 1992. LC 92-21763. (Illus.). 188p. text 98.00 (*0-86715-248-6*) Quint Pub Co.

Minor Surgery in Practice. Vija K. Sodera. 1995. LC 93-31378. (Illus.). 378p. (C). text 74.95 (*0-521-44466-7*) Cambridge U Pr.

Minor Traumatic Brain Injury Handbook: Diagnosis & Treatment. Gary W. Jay. 2000. LC 00-37818. 376p. 79.95 (*0-8493-1955-2*) CRC Pr.

Minorities & Cancer. Ed. by L. A. Jones. 1989. (Illus.). 334p. 126.00 (*0-387-96950-0*) Spr-Verlag.

Minorities & Family Therapy. Ed. by George W. Saba et al. LC 89-26981. (Journal of Psychotherapy & the Family Ser.: Vol. 6, Nos. 1 & 2). 237p. reprint ed. 1995. pap. 19.95 (*1-56024-565-4*); 1990. (C). 49.95 (*0-86656-777-1*) Haworth Pr.

Minority Alzheimer's Caregivers: Removing Barriers to Community Services. J. Neil Henderson et al. 1989. LC 89-64011. 100p. stu. ed., ring bd. 20.00 (*0-9622070-1-2*) USF SGC.

Minority Children in Therapy. Man Keung Ho. 1992. 224p. (C). 68.95 (*0-8039-3912-4*, 3643); LC 91-41972. (Illus.). pap. 34.95 (*0-8039-3913-2*, 3644) Sage.

Minority Health Issues for an Emerging Majority: The 4th National Forum on Cardiovascular Health, Pulmonary Disorders, & Health Resources. Ed. by Shiriki Kumanyika & John Karefa-Smart. 1998. (Illus.). 129p. (C). pap. text 25.00 (*0-7881-7292-1*) DIANE Pub.

Minority Mental Health. Jones Staff. 1982. (C). text (*0-03-047056-0*) Harcourt Coll Pubs.

Minority Student's Guide to Success in Health Careers. Edward James & Karen E. Hamilton. 1997. LC 96-107079. (Planning Guide Ser.). 198p. (Orig.). pap. 12.50 (*0-941406-51-2*) Lppncott W & W.

Minoxidil (Rogaine) Index of New Information with Authors & Subjects. Science and Life Consultants Association Staff. rev. ed. 1994. 105p. LC 31-242. 57.50 (*0-7883-0342-2*); pap. 47.50 (*0-7883-0343-0*) ABBE Pubs Assn.

***MIR: A Novel ERM-Like Protein in the Nervous System.** Per-Andres Olsson. 2001. (Comprehensive Summaries of Uppsala Dissertatons from the Faculty of Medicine: No. 1052). (Illus.). 45p. pap. (*91-554-5061-X*) Uppsala Universitet SWE. *Dist:* Coronet Bks.

Miracle & a Privilege: Recounting a Half-Century of Surgical Advance. Francis D. Moore. 1995. LC 95-1645. (Illus.). 488p. (C). 29.95 (*0-309-05188-6*, Joseph Henry Pr) Natl Acad Pr.

Miracle Cures: Dramatic New Scientific Discoveries Revealing the Healing Powers of Herbs, Vitamins, & Other Natural Remedies. Jean Carper. 1998. 308p. text 25.00 (*0-7881-5907-0*) DIANE Pub.

Miracle Cures: Dramatic New Scientific Discoveries Revealing the Healing Powers of Herbs, Vitamins, & Other Natural Remedies. Jean Carper. 1998. LC 97-13747. 320p. pap. 14.00 (*0-06-098436-8*, Perennial) HarperTrade.

Miracle Exercises That Can Save Your Life! Edwin Flatto. 11th rev. ed. 1998. Orig. Title: Encyclopedia of Therapeutic Exercises. (Illus.). 394p. pap. 19.95 (*0-935540-05-9*) Plymouth Pr.

Miracle Eye Cure: Microcurrent Stimulation. Edward Kondrot. 2001. LC 00-127491. (Illus.). 300p. pap. 24.95 (*1-55643-401-4*) North Atlantic.

Miracle Healing Power of Chelation Therapy. Intro. by Morton Walker. 1984. (Illus.). 257p. 18.95 (*0-915421-00-3*) Fischer Pub.

Miracle Healing Power Through Nature's Pharmacy. William L. Fischer. Ed. by Juilene McKnight-Osborne. 1986. LC 85-81689. (Illus.). 202p. (Orig.). pap. 17.95 (*0-915421-04-6*) Fischer Pub.

Miracle Hormones . . . Naturally. Paul Yanick. 1998. 256p. pap. 13.00 (*1-57566-197-7*, Knsington) Kensgtn Pub Corp.

Miracle Medicine Herbs. Richard M. Lucas. 1991. LC 90-22314. (Reward Bks.). 224p. (C). text 24.95 (*0-13-585142-4*, Busn) P-H.

Miracle Medicines of the Rainforest: A Doctor's Revolutionary Work with Cancer & AIDS Patients. Thomas David. Tr. by J. Michal Beasley from GER. 1997. LC 97-22873. (Illus.). 144p. pap. 19.95 (*0-89281-746-1*, Heal Arts VT) Inner Tradit.

Miracle Nutrient: Coenzyme Q10. Emile G. Bliznakov & Gerry Hunt. 1986. 256p. mass mkt. 6.99 (*0-553-26233-5*) Bantam.

Miracle of Garlic. Paavo O. Airola. 1984. 48p. pap. 3.95 (*0-932090-08-7*) Health Plus.

Miracle of Mind Power. Dan Custer. 1985. 263p. (C). reprint ed. pap. 9.95 (*0-930298-20-9*) Westwood Pub Co.

Miracle of Natural Hormones. David Brownstein. 2nd rev. ed. 1999. (Illus.). 204p. pap. 14.95 (*0-9660882-0-4*) Med Alternat.

Miracle Protein: Secret of Natural Cell-Tissue Rejuvenation. Carlson Wade. 1976. 12.95 (*0-13-585653-1*); pap. 4.95 (*0-13-585588-8*) P-H (Reward).

Miracles & the Modern Religious Imagination. Robert B. Mullin. 1996. LC 96-13505. 336p. 45.00 (*0-300-06696-1*) Yale U Pr.

Miracles Do Happen: A Physician's Experiences with Alternative Medicine. C. Norman Shealy. 1995. LC 95-51001. 288p. pap. 15.95 (*1-85230-688-2*) Element MA.

Miracles of Military Medicine. Albert Q. Maisel. 1977. LC 70-167382. (Essay Index Reprint Ser.). reprint ed. 25.95 (*0-8369-2561-0*) Ayer.

Miracles of Minerals: The Human Need for 90 Plus Elements from a Cell's Point of View. Albert E. Carter. 1995. 224p. (Orig.). pap. text 14.95 (*1-887995-00-5*) Amer Institute Res.

Miracles of Urine Therapy. C. P. Mithal. 1990. 82p. pap. 4.95 (*0-8464-4821-1*) Beekman Pubs.

Miraculous Breakthroughs for Prostate & Impotency Problems. William L. Fischer. Ed. by Rebekah Schreffler. rev. ed. 1994. (Illus.). 222p. 24.95 (*0-915421-19-4*) Fischer Pub.

Miraculous World of Your Unborn Baby. Nikki Bradford. 1998. LC 97-46417. (Illus.). 160p. pap. 14.95 (*0-8092-2928-5*, 292850, Contemporary) McGraw-Hill Trade.

Mirage of Health: Utopias, Progress, & Biological Change. Rene Jules Dubos. 1987. 236p. LC 87-9566. pap. 16.00 (*0-8135-1260-3*); text 35.00 (*0-8135-1259-X*) Rutgers U Pr.

MIRD Cellular S Values: Self-Absorbed Dose per Unit Cumulated Activity for Selected Radionuclides & Monoenergetic Electron & Alpha Particle Emitters Incorporated into Different Cell Compartments. SNM MIRD Committee. 1997. LC 96-51086. pap. text 70.00 (*0-932004-46-6*) Soc Nuclear Med.

MIRD Head & Brain Dosimetry: Absorbed Fractions of Energy & Absorbed Dose Per Unit Cumulated Activity Within Pediatric & Adult Head & Brain Models for Use in Nuclear Medicine Internal Dosimetry. Lionel G. Bouchet et al. 1999. (Illus.). 206p. pap. 70.00 (*0-932004-70-9*) Soc Nuclear Med.

MIRD Primer for Absorbed Dose Calculations. Ed. by Robert Loevinger et al. rev. ed. 1991. LC 91-4858. (Illus.). 128p. text 49.00 (*0-932004-38-5*) Soc Nuclear Med.

Mirena - The Levonorgestrel Intrauterine System: The New Contraceptive Option for Parous Women. Ed. by E. D. Johansson. 1998. LC 97-46788. (Illus.). 86p. lib. bdg. 38.95 (*1-85070-037-0*, Parthenon Pbng) CRC Pr.

Miriam Adahan Handbook: Nobody's Perfect - Maintaining Emotional Health, Vol. 1. Miriam Adahan. 1994. 263p. 12.95 (*1-56871-047-X*) Targum Pr.

Mirror of Coitus: An Edition with English Translation & Edition of the Fifteenth-Century Speculum al Foderi. Ed. & Tr. by Michael Solomon. 1990. (Medieval Spanish Medical Texts Ser.: No. 29). (SPA.). xxviii, 142p. 12.50 (*0-940639-48-3*) Hispanic Seminary.

Mirror of the Body. Anna Kaye & Don C. Matchan. 1978. LC 77-8717. (Illus.). 160p. (Orig.). pap. 6.95 (*0-89407-010-X*) Strawberry Hill.

Mirrored Lives: Aging Children & Elderly Parents. Tom Koch. 1990. LC 90-7457. 240p. 67.00 (*0-275-93671-6*, C3671, Praeger Pubs) Greenwood.

Mirrors of Madness: Patroling the Psychic Border. Bruce Luske. 1990. (Social Problems & Social Issues Ser.). 143p. pap. text 25.95 (*0-202-30423-X*); lib. bdg. 47.95 (*0-202-30422-1*) Aldine de Gruyter.

MIS Spanish-English Clinical Medical Translator. Contrib. by Medical Information Systems Staff. 2nd ed. 1998. LC 00-266238. (ENG & SPA.). 132p. (*1-891953-00-1*) Medical Info.

Misadministration of Radioactive Material in Medicine - Scientific Background. Intro. by Charles B. Meinhold. 1991. LC 91-35005. (Commentary Ser.: No. 7). 49p. pap. text 25.00 (*0-929600-22-3*) NCRP Pubns.

Miscarriage: A Man's Book. Rick Wheat. Ed. by Joy Johnson. 1995. 24p. pap. 3.50 (*1-56123-082-0*, MMBC) Centering Corp.

***Miscarriage: A Woman Doctor's Guide: The Support & Facts You Need to Get Through Pregnancy Loss.** Lynn Friedman & Irene Daria. 2001. 208p. mass mkt. 6.99 (*1-57566-649-9*, Knsington) Kensgtn Pub Corp.

Miscarriage: For Parents Experiencing Fetal Death. Joy Johnson & S. M. Johnson. rev. ed. 1980. LC 98-45174. (Illus.). 24p. pap. 3.50 (*1-56123-007-3*, MISC) Centering Corp.

Miscarriage: Sharing the Grief, Facing the Pain, Healing the Wounds. Walter Williamson. 1987. 14.95 (*0-8027-0947-8*) Walker & Co.

Miscarriage: The Facts. Gillian C. Lachelin. 2nd ed. 1996. LC 95-39063. (Facts Ser.). (Illus.). 96p. (C). pap. 19.95 (*0-19-262613-2*) OUP.

Miscarriage: Women Sharing from the Heart. Marie Allen & Shelly Marks. 1993. LC 92-22852. 272p. pap. 17.95 (*0-471-54834-0*) Wiley.

Miscarriage - A Shattered Dream. Sherokee Ilse & Linda H. Burns. rev. ed. 1995. 64p. pap. 9.95 (*0-9609456-3-6*) Wntergrn.

Miscellaneous Tracts Relating to Natural History, Husbandry, & Physick: Calender of Flora Is Added. Carl Linnaeus. Ed. by Frank N. Egerton, 3rd. 1978. LC 77-74237. (History of Ecology Ser.). reprint ed. lib. bdg. 31.95 (*0-405-10406-5*) Ayer.

Miscellaneous Writings of J. H. Tilden, M. D. J. H. Tilden. 1996. 232p. reprint ed. spiral bd. 21.00 (*0-7873-1083-2*) Hlth Research.

Misdiagnosis: Woman As a Disease. Karen M. Hicks. 1994. LC 93-48592. 256p. pap. 19.95 (*1-882606-10-8*) Peoples Med Soc.

Mishell's Textbook of Infertility, Contraception & Reproductive Endocrinology. Rogerio A. Lobo et al. 4th ed. 1997. LC 96-52003. (Illus.). 896p. 209.95 (*0-86542-385-7*) Blackwell Sci.

***Misinformed Consent: Experiences of Hysterectomized Women.** Lise Cloutier-Steele. 2001. 208p. LC 2001-41324. 42.95 (*1-882360-05-2*); pap. 23.95 (*1-882360-06-0*) ATL Pr Sci.

Mismanaged Care: How Corporate Medicine Jeopardizes Your Health. Michael E. Makover. 1998. LC 98-38860. 296p. 28.00 (*1-57392-248-X*) Prometheus Bks.

Mismatch Negativity. Ed. by R. Naatanen. 2000. (Audiology & Neuro-Otology Ser.: 5). (Illus.). 150p. pap. 39.25 (*3-8055-7100-3*) S Karger.

Misplaced Loyalties. Esther Menaker. 1995. LC 94-24042. xxi, 205p. pap. text 24.95 (*1-56000-816-4*) Transaction Pubs.

Missed Connections: Hard of Hearing in a Hearing World. Barbara Stenross. 1999. LC 98-30716. (Illus.). 128p. 39.50 (*1-56639-681-6*); pap. 16.95 (*1-56639-682-4*) Temple U Pr.

Missiles to Learning: Beyond the Left/Right Brain. Beverly B. Casebeer. Ed. by Betty Lou Kratoville. 1996. LC 96-208557. (Illus.). 206p. (Orig.). pap. 18.00 (*1-57128-018-9*, 018-9) Acad Therapy.

Missing Diagnosis. C. Orian Truss. 2nd ed. 1986. 175p. (Orig.). 25.00 (*0-9615758-2-4*) Missing Diag.

Missing Link? A Persuasive New Look at Heart Disease As It Relates to Mercury. Michael F. Ziff & Sam Ziff. 1991. (Illus.). 184p. (Orig.). pap. 12.00 (*0-941011-08-9*) Bio-Probe.

Missing Medical Text: Humane Patient Care. Anthony R. Moore. 1978. 29.95 (*0-522-84139-2*) Intl Spec Bk.

Missing Patient. J. L. Lu. 1978. pap. 2.75 (*0-9601768-0-2*) J L Lu.

Mission & Method: The Early Nineteenth-Century French Public Health Movement. Ann F. La Berge. 1992. (Cambridge History of Medicine Ser.). (Illus.). 396p. (C). text 95.00 (*0-521-40406-1*) Cambridge U Pr.

Mission Management Vol. 2: A New Synthesis. Ed. by Elaine R. Rubin. 1998. LC 98-19149. pap. 30.00 (*1-879694-12-3*) AAH Ctrs.

Mission Matters: A Report on the Future of Voluntary Health Care Institutions. J. David Seay & Bruce C. Vladeck. 1987. 47p. 5.00 (*0-934459-36-3*) United Hosp Fund.

Mission to Korea: Thirty-Eight Years Below the Thirty-Eighth. Joe B. Hopper. 1999. LC 98-68425. (Illus.). 288p. pap. 18.95 (*1-57736-127-X*) Providence Hse.

Missionaries of Science: The Rockefeller Foundation & Latin America. Ed. by Marcos Cueto. 1994. LC 93-24416. (Philanthropic Studies). 196p. (C). 24.95 (*0-253-31583-2*) Ind U Pr.

Missionary Leadership: By Motivation & Communication. Roland Muller. 2000. pap. 16.00 (*0-7388-3990-6*) Xlibris Corp.

Missionary Medicine in China: A Study of Two Canadian Protestant Missions in China Before 1937. Yuet-Wah Cheung. 1988. LC 88-173. (Illus.). 192p. (C). lib. bdg. 44.50 (*0-8191-6901-3*) U Pr of Amer.

Mississippi Health Care in Perspective 2000. Ed. by Kathleen O'Leary Morgan & Scott E. Morgan. 2000. 21p. spiral bd. 19.00 (*0-7401-0223-0*) Morgan Quitno Corp.

Mississippi Health Care Perspective, 1998. Ed. by Kathleen O'Leary Morgan & Scott E. Morgan. 1998. 20p. pap. 19.00 (*1-56692-823-0*) Morgan Quitno Corp.

Mississippi Valley's Great Yellow Fever Epidemic of 1878. Khaled J. Bloom. 1993. LC 93-2965. x, 296p. (C). text 42.50 (*0-8071-1824-9*) La State U Pr.

Missouri Cancer Control Resource Directory. 1993. 131p. (Orig.). (C). pap. text 35.00 (*1-56806-307-5*) DIANE Pub.

Missouri Health Care in Perspective 2000. Ed. by Kathleen O'Leary Morgan & Scott E. Morgan. 2000. 21p. spiral bd. 19.00 (*0-7401-0224-9*) Morgan Quitno Corp.

Missouri Health Care Perspective, 1998. Ed. by Kathleen O'Leary Morgan & Scott E. Morgan. 1998. 20p. pap. 19.00 (*1-56692-824-9*) Morgan Quitno Corp.

Missouri's Early Home Remedies. Betty Hams et al. 1992. (Illus.). 181p. (Orig.). pap. text 9.95 (*1-878488-53-8*) Quixote Pr IA.

Mistake Making: With Sections on Stuttering & Psychotherapy. Kenneth L. Artiss. 1996. 298p. pap. text 38.50 (*0-7618-0309-2*) U Pr of Amer.

Mistaken Beliefs about Relapse. Terence T. Gorski & Merlene Miller. 1988. 32p. pap. text 4.00 (*0-8309-0511-1*) Herald Pub Hse.

Mistaken Seven: Eyewitness Identification of the "Gentlemen Bandit" R. Buckhout. 1985. (Monographs: No. CR-48). 4.00 (*1-55524-049-6*) Ctr Respon Psych.

Misteltherapie & Immunologische Forschung: Arbeitstagung, Hercecke, Mai, 1996. Ed. by Arndt Buessing et al. 1996. (Journal: Vol. 3, Supplement 1, 1996). (GER., Illus.). iv, 20p. pap. 40.00 (*3-8055-6445-7*) S Karger.

Mr. Dooley in Peace & War. Finley P. Dunne. 1972. 250.00 (*0-87968-249-3*) Gordon Pr.

Mr. Dooley in the Hearts of His Countrymen. Finley P. Dunne. 1972. 250.00 (*0-87968-248-5*) Gordon Pr.

Mr. Dooley's Opinions. Finley P. Dunne. 1973. 250.00 (*0-87968-161-6*) Gordon Pr.

Mr. Spectroscopy: Clinical Applications & Techniques. Ian R. Young & H. Cecil Charles. 1997. 264p. (*1-85317-068-2*) Martin Dunitz GBR. *Dist:* Mosby Inc.

Mistletoe. Ed. by H. Franz. 1986. (Journal: Vol. 1, Suppl. 1). (Illus.). vi, 70p. pap. 24.50 (*3-8055-4465-0*) S Karger.

Mistletoe: The Genus Viscum. A. Bussing. 2000. (Medicinal & Aromatic Plants - Industrial Profiles Ser.: Vol. 16). 216p. 105.00 (*90-5823-092-9*, Harwood Acad Pubs) Gordon & Breach.

Mistress of Her Own Thoughts: Ella Freeman Sharpe & the Practice of Psychoanalysis. Ed. by Maurice J. Whelan. 2000. 260p. pap. (*1-900877-26-0*) Rebus Pr Ltd GBR. *Dist:* Intl Spec Bk, Other Pr LLC.

Misuse of Drugs. Ed. by British Medical Association Staff. 1997. 160p. text 37.00 (*90-5702-259-1*); pap. text 20.00 (*90-5702-260-5*) Gordon & Breach (Harwood Acad Pubs).

Misuse of Drugs. Don Mathias. 1988. 251p. pap. 54.00 (*0-409-78816-3*, NZ, MICHIE) LEXIS Pub.

Misuse of Drugs. P. Bucknell & H. Ghodse. (Criminal Law Library). Suppl. 1. 1986. 128p. pap. 8.25 (*0-08-033081-9*); Supplement No. 3. 1989. 192p. pap. 30.00 (*0-08-036914-6*) Macmillan.

Misuse of Persons: Analyzing Pathological Dependency. Stanley J. Coen. 1992. LC 91-47096. 344p. text 49.95 (*0-88163-139-6*) Analytic Pr.

Mit Hippokrates zur Organgewinnung? Medizinische Ethik und Sprache. Ed. by Horst D. Scholosser. 1998. (Frankfurter Forschungen zur Kultur und Sprachwissenschaft Ser.: Band 1). (GER.). 278p. pap. 48.95 (*3-631-33006-5*) P Lang Pubng.

Mit Quinoa Sich eine Neue Welt Erschliessen: Ueber 100 Kockrezepte Sowie Texte Rund. C. Ibisch. 1995. (Illus.). 191p. pap. (*3-931251-02-0*) Martina Galunder DEU. *Dist:* Balogh.

Mitochondria: Structure, Biogenesis & Transducing Functions. Henry Tedeschi. 1976. (Cell Biology Monographs: Vol. 4). (Illus.). 180p. 87.95 (*0-387-81317-9*) Spr-Verlag.

Mitochondria 1977: Genetics & Biogenesis of Mitochondria. Ed. by W. Bandlow et al. 1977. (C). 215.40 (*3-11-007321-8*) De Gruyter.

Mitochondrial Diseases: Models & Methods. Ed. by Patrick Lestienne. 1999. LC 99-25405. (Illus.). 350p. 156.00 (*3-540-64177-7*) Spr-Verlag.

Mitochondrial Disorders in Neurology. A. H. Schapira & Dimauro. 2001. LC 2001-52902. (Blue Books of Practical Neurology: Vol. 26). 288p. 99.00 (*0-7506-7288-9*) Buttrwrth-Heinemann.

Mitochondrial Disorders in Neurology. Ed. by A. H. Schapira & Salvatore DiMauro. 1993. LC 93-41988. (International Medical Reviews Ser.: Vol. 14). 254p. text 85.00 (*0-7506-0585-5*) Buttrwrth-Heinemann.

Mitochondrial Free Radical Theory of Aging. Aubrey D. N. J. de Grey. 1999. LC 99-27037. (Molecular Biology Intelligence Unit Ser.: Vol. 9). (Illus.). 212p. 99.00 (*1-57059-564-X*) Landes Bioscience.

Mitosenes & Related Antitumor Drugs: Rational Design & Cytostatic Agents. Marc Maliepaard. 1996. LC 96-960. (Molecular Biology Intelligence Unit Ser.). 126p. pap. 89.95 (*0-412-10511-X*, RC271) Chapman & Hall.

Mitosenes & Related Antitumor Drugs: Rational Drug Design of Cytostatic Agents. Marc Maliepaard. 1995. (Medical Intelligence Unit Ser.). 139p. 99.00 (*1-57059-335-3*) Landes Bioscience.

Mitosis. Abramoff. Date not set. 1.20 (*0-7167-9015-7*) W H Freeman.

Mitosis & Apoptosis. I. D. Bowen et al. 1997. (Illus.). 240p. pap. 44.95 (*0-412-71070-6*, Chap & Hall NY) Chapman & Hall.

Mitoxantrone for Injection Concentrate: Clinical Use in Bladder Cancer. Ed. by Chris Fellner. 1996. 7p. (Orig.). (*1-57130-020-1*) Medicine Grp USA.

Mitoxantrone for Injection Concentrate: Clinical Use in Hormone-Resistant Prostate Cancer. Ed. by Chris Fellner. 1996. 7p. (Orig.). (*1-57130-019-8*) Medicine Grp USA.

Mitoxantrone for Injection Concentrate: Clinical Use in Leukemia. Ed. by Chris Fellner. 1995. (Orig.). pap. (*1-57130-015-5*) Medicine Grp USA.

Mitoxantrone for Injection Concentrate: Clinical Use in Ovarian Cancer. Ed. by Chris Fellner. 1996. (Orig.). (*1-57130-017-1*) Medicine Grp USA.

Mitral Valve: Floppy Mitral Valve, Mitral Valve Prolapse, Mitral Valvular Regurgitation. Ed. by Harisios Boudoulas & Charles F. Wooley. 2nd ed. 2000. (Illus.). 780p. 145.00 (*0-87993-448-4*) Futura Pub.

Mitral Valve Prolapse. 1979. (Landmark Ser.). 25.50 (*0-8422-4123-X*) Irvington.

Mitral Valve Prolapse: The Heart with a Different Beat. Nancy Tkaczuk. Ed. & Illus. by Nancy R. Hull. rev. ed. 1992. LC 86-22549. 16p. pap. text 6.50 (*0-939838-20-6*) Pritchett & Hull.

Mixed Blessings: Intensive Care for Newborns. Jeanne H. Guillemin & Lynda L. Holmstrom. 1990. 336p. reprint ed. pap. text 19.95 (*0-19-506659-6*) OUP.

MMPI: A Comprehensive, Annotated Bibliography, 1940-1964 (Minnesota Multiphasic Personality Inventory) Earl S. Taulbee et al. 1977. LC 72-87108. viii, 603p. 50.00 (*0-87875-037-1*) Whitston Pub.

MMPI: A Contemporary Normative Study of Adolescents. Robert C. Colligan & Kenneth P. Offord. Ed. by Glenn R. Caddy. 1992. (Developments in Clinical Psychology Ser.). 640p. (C). 130.00 (*0-89391-872-5*); pap. 49.50 (*0-89391-985-3*) Greenwood (Ablex).

MMPI: An Interpretive Manual. Roger L. Greene. 1980. (Illus.). 306p. text 34.95 (*0-8089-1279-8*, 791720, Grune & Strat) Harcrt Hlth Sci Grp.

MMPI: Clinical & Research Trends. Ed. by Charles S. Newmark. 1979. LC 79-17777. (Praeger Special Studies). 464p. 49.95 (*0-03-048926-1*, Praeger Pubs) Greenwood.

MMPI-A: Assessing Adolescent Psychopathology. Robert P. Archer. (C). 1992. 472p. text 39.95 (*0-8058-1113-3*); 2nd ed. 1996. 512p. 39.95 (*0-8058-2343-3*) L Erlbaum Assocs.

MMPI-A Casebook. Robert P. Archer et al. 1994. LC 94-5851. 223p. pap. 38.00 (*0-911907-14-9*) Psych Assess.

MMPI-A Content Scales: Assessing Psychopathology in Adolescents. Carolyn L. Williams et al. 1992. (MMPI-A Monograph Ser.). 192p. (C). text 29.95 (*0-8166-2144-6*) U of Minn Pr.

MMPI & MMPI-2: Interpretation Manual for Counselors & Clinicians. Jane C. Duckworth & Wayne P. Anderson. 4th ed. 1994. LC 94-19528. 552p. 49.95 (*1-56032-377-9*) Accel Devel.

MMPI Handbook: Clinical Interpretation, Vol. 1. W. Grant Dahlstrom et al. rev. ed. 1972. LC 74-172933. (MMPI Handbook Ser.: Vol. 1). (Illus.). 2p. text 49.95 (*0-8166-0589-0*) U of Minn Pr.

MMPI (Minnesota Multiphasic Personality Inventory) in Testing, Medicine & Psycology: Guidebook for Reference & Research. Remley L. Rannigan. rev. ed. 1998. 150p. 57.50 (*0-7883-1070-4*); pap. 47.50 (*0-7883-1071-2*) ABBE Pubs Assn.

MMPI Patterns of American Minorities. W. Grant Dahlstrom et al. 1986. 440p. text 44.95 (*0-8166-1530-6*) U of Minn Pr.

MMPI-2 Correlates for Outpatient Community Mental Health Settings. John R. Graham et al. 1999. LC 99-20293. (Illus.). xx, 598p. 60.00 (*0-8166-2564-6*) U of Minn Pr.

MMPI-2 in Psychological Treatment. James Neal Butcher. 1990. (Illus.). 208p. (C). text 32.95 (*0-19-506344-9*) OUP.

MMPI-2 Tutorial Workbook. Robert R. Reilly & Barbara A. Reilly. 1991. 212p. pap. text 22.00 (*0-89079-267-4*, 1510) PRO-ED.

Mnemonics for Anatomy Students: A Guide to Memory Aids for the Students of Anatomy. David J. Gerrick. 1975. pap. 4.00 (*0-916750-38-8*) Dayton Labs.

Mnemonics Rhetoric & Poetics for Medics, Vol. II. Carolyn F. Pedley et al. 1984. (Illus.). 175p. (Orig.). pap. 10.95 (*0-9612242-3-1*) Harbinger Med Pr NC.

Mnemonics Rhetoric & Poetics for Medics, Vol. III. Robert L. Bloomfield & Carolyn F. Pedley. 1990. (Illus.). 165p. pap. 9.75 (*0-9612242-6-6*) Harbinger Med Pr NC.

Mobbing: Emotional Abuse in the American Workplace. Noa Davenport et al. 1999. LC 00-699536. (Illus.). 213p. pap. 14.95 (*0-9671803-0-9*) Civil Society.

Mobile Receptor Hypothesis: Membrane Receptor Lateral Movement in Signal Transduction. David A. Jans. 1997. LC 97-5905. (Molecular Biology Intelligence Unit Ser.). 99.00 (*1-57059-437-6*) Landes Bioscience.

Mobilisation of the Nervous System. David S. Butler. 1991. (Illus.). 265p. text (*0-443-04400-7*) Church.

Mobilisation of the Spine: A Primary Handbook of Clinical Methods. Gregory P. Grieve. 5th ed. 1991. (Illus.). 426p. (Orig.). pap. text (*0-443-04236-5*) Church.

Mobility: Theory & Practice. Werner Schneider et al. 1992. LC 92-403. (Flexibook Ser.). 9.90 (*0-86577-435-8*) Thieme Med Pubs.

Mobility & Transport for Elderly & Handicapped Persons. Ed. by Norman Ashford et al. 1982. (Transportation Studies: Vol. 2). xi, 383p. text 228.00 (*0-677-16380-0*) Gordon & Breach.

Mobilization for the Neurologically Involved Child: Assessment & Application Strategies for Pe. Sandra Brooks-Scott. 1997. (Illus.). 151p. pap. text 55.00 (*0-12-785061-9*) Acad Pr.

Mobilizing Against AIDS. Eve K. Nichols. enl. rev. ed. 1989. LC 88-30100. (Illus.). 387p. 42.00 (*0-674-57763-9*); pap. text 12.95 (*0-674-57762-0*) HUP.

Mocrocirculation in Circulatory Disorders. Ed. by K. Messmer et al. 1988. (Illus.). 551p. 160.00 (*0-387-70034-X*) Spr-Verlag.

Mode of Action. Ed. by H. Schoenfeld & Alain L. De Weck. 1971. (Antibiotics & Chemotherapy Ser.: Vol. 17). 45.25 (*3-8055-1225-2*) S Karger.

Mode of Action of Autonomic Drugs. Budh D. Bhagat. 1979. LC 78-58696. (Illus.). 170p. text 32.95 (*0-932126-00-6*); pap. text 29.50 (*0-932126-01-4*) Graceway.

Model Compliant Standard Operating Procedures for Biological Vaccines Current Good Manufacturing Practices. Date not set. (*1-893091-74-0*) F R Parker.

Model Compliant Standard Operating Procedures for Biological Vaccines in Good Clinical Practices. Date not set. (*1-893091-73-2*) F R Parker.

Model Compliant Standard Operating Procedures for Medical Device Current Good Manufacturing Practices. Date not set. (*1-893091-77-5*) F R Parker.

Model Compliant Standard Operating Procedures for Medical Device Manufacturers Current Good Clinical Practices. Date not set. (*1-893091-76-7*) F R Parker.

Model Compliant Standard Operating Procedures for Pharmaceutical Drugs, Current Good Manufacturing Practices. Date not set. (*1-893091-75-9*) F R Parker.

Model of Human Occupation: Theory & Application. Ed. by Gary Kielhofner. 2nd ed. 1995. LC 95-7615. (Illus.). 416p. pap. 52.95 (*0-683-04601-2*) Lppncott W & W.

Model Patient: My Life as an Incurable Wise-Ass. Karen Duffy. 2000. LC 00-60264. (Illus.). 272p. 24.00 (*0-06-019725-0*, Cliff Street) HarperTrade.

Model-Perinatal Autopsy Protocol. MacPherson. 1995. (Illus.). 60p. pap. text 10.00 (*1-881041-16-6*) Am Registry Path.

Model Practices in Service Delivery in Child & Family Mental Health. Ed. by Michael C. Roberts. 1996. LC 95-47987. 456p. text 79.95 (*0-8058-1651-8*); pap. text 45.00 (*0-8058-1652-6*) L Erlbaum Assocs.

Model Systems of Development & Aging of the Nervous System. Ed. by Antonia Vernadakis. 1987. (C). text 210.50 (*0-89838-838-4*) Kluwer Academic.

Model Tuberculosis Exposure Control Plan. Terry J. Gile. 1996. 36p. wbk. ed. 69.00 (*0-9625414-4-3*) Clinical Lab Mgmnt Assn.

Model Tuberculosis Exposure Control Plan (Workbook & Training Kit) Terry J. Gile. 1996. 85p. ring bd., wbk. ed. 125.00 (*0-9625414-6-X*) Clinical Lab Mgmnt Assn.

Modeles Clinico-Pharmacologiques pour l'Experimentation de Corticoides a Usage Externe. H. Wendt & P. J. Frosch. 1982. (Illus.). 64p. pap. 28.75 (*3-8055-3548-1*) S Karger.

Modeling & Analysis in Biomedicine: Proceedings of the 4th Course of the International School of Pure & Applied Biostructure, Erice, Italy, Oct. 18-27,1982. Ed. by C. Nicolini. 1984. 552p. 108.00 (*9971-950-81-2*) World Scientific Pub.

Modeling & Control in Biomedical Systems: Proceedings of the International Federation of Automatic Control Symposium, Gavelston, Texas, U. S. A., 27-30 March 1994. Ed. by B. W. Patterson & International Federation of Automatic Control, Tri. 1994. LC 94-3756. 598p. pap. 40.00 (*0-08-042224-1*, Pergamon Pr) Elsevier.

Modeling & Data Treatment in the Pharmaceutical Sciences. Jens T. Carstensen. 1996. LC 96-60624. 270p. 169.95 (*1-56676-440-8*) CRC Pr.

Modeling & Parameter Estimation in Respiratory Control. Ed. by Michael C. Khoo. 1990. LC 90-7301. (Illus.). 220p. (C). text 95.00 (*0-306-43530-6*, Kluwer Plenum) Kluwer Academic.

Modeling Disease Transmission & Its Prevention by Disinfection. Ed. by Christon J. Hurst. 1996. (Illus.). 424p. (C). text 100.00 (*0-521-48131-7*) Cambridge U Pr.

Modeling Growth & Individual Differences in Spatial Tasks. Hoben Thomas & Arnold Lohaus. 1993. (Monographs of the Society for Research on Child Development). 200p. pap. text 15.00 (*0-226-79602-7*) U Ch Pr.

Modeling HIV Transmission & AIDS in the United States. Herbert W. Hethcote & James W. Van Ark. 1992. LC 92-27862. (Lecture Notes in Biomathematics: Vol. 95). 234p. 58.95 (*0-387-55904-3*) Spr-Verlag.

***Modeling in Medical Decision Making: A Bayesian Approach.** Parmigiani. 2002. (Statistics in Practice Ser.). 278p. 69.95 (*0-471-98608-9*) Wiley.

Modeling Methodology for Physiology & Medicine. Richard E. Carson & Claudio Cobelli. 2000. LC 00-104369. (Biomedical Engineering Ser.). (Illus.). xiv, 421p. 79.95 (*0-12-160245-1*) Acad Pr.

Modeling Ruminant Digestion & Metabolism. Baldwin. 1995. LC 95-68053. (Illus.). 592p. (C). pap. text 299.95 (*0-412-59160-X*, Chap & Hall NY) Chapman & Hall.

Modeling Sensorineural Hearing Loss. Ed. by Walter Jesteadt. 1997. LC 96-49676. 432p. 99.95 (*0-8058-2230-5*) L Erlbaum Assocs.

Modeling the Demand for Cocaine. S. M. Everingham & C. Peter Rydell. 1994. 79p. pap. 15.00 (*0-8330-1553-2*, MR-332) Rand Corp.

Modelling & Control in Biomedical Systems. Ed. by E. Carson & Derek A. Linkens. 1997. LC 97-42725. (IFAC Ser.). 378p. pap. 74.50 (*0-08-042601-8*, Pergamon Pr) Elsevier.

Modelling & Control in Biomedical Systems: Proceedings of the IFAC Symposium, Venice, Italy, April 6-8, 1988. Ed. by C. Cobelli & L. Mariani. (IFAC Ser.: 8901). (Illus.). 1989. 686p. 36.00 (*0-08-035732-6*); 1988. 683p. pap. 30.00 (*0-08-036609-0*) Elsevier (Pergamon Pr).

Modelling & Simulation of Neurons & Neural Networks with Temporal-Pattern Learning Capability. C. Torras. 1985. (Lecture Notes in Biomathematics: Vol. 63). 227p. 39.95 (*0-387-16046-9*) Spr-Verlag.

Modelling Brain Function: The World of Attractor Neural Networks. Daniel J. Amit. (Illus.). (C). 1992. 522p. pap. text 32.95 (*0-521-42124-1*); 1989. 528p. text 95.00 (*0-521-36100-1*) Cambridge U Pr.

***Modelling Hospital Resource Use: A Different Approach to the Planning & Control of Health Care Systems.** Ed. by P. H. Millard & S. I. McClean. 1994. 125p. pap. (*1-85315-218-8*) Royal Soc of Medicine Pr Ltd GBR. *Dist:* Balogh.

Modelling of Livestock Production Systems. Ed. by S. Korver & J. A. Van Arendonk. 1988. (Current Topics in Veterinary Medicine & Animal Science Ser.). (C). text 130.50 (*0-89838-373-0*) Kluwer Academic.

Modelling the Stress-Strain Relationship in Work Settings. Meni Koslowsky. 1998. LC 97-45074. (Progress in Psychology Ser.). (Illus.). 232p. (C). 78.95 (*0-415-15320-4*) Routledge.

Modell's Drugs in Current Use & New Drugs, 2000. Ed. by Elizabeth A. Duthie. 46th ed. 2000. (Modell's Drugs in Current Use & New Drugs Ser.). 328p. pap. 29.95 (*0-8261-1326-5*) Springer Pub.

***Modell's Drugs in Current Use & New Drugs, 2001.** Ed. by Movses Hovsepian. 47th ed. 2001. 360p. pap. 29.95 (*0-8261-1396-6*) Springer Pub.

Models & Integrations Vol. 3: Rochester Symposium on Developmental Psychopathology. Ed. by Dante Cicchetti & Sheree L. Toth. 1991. (Illus.). 352p. 85.00 (*1-878822-04-7*) Univ Rochester Pr.

Models & Techniques in Medical Imaging Research. Eric N. Milne et al. 1983. LC 82-13141. 596p. 120.00 (*0-275-91404-6*, C1404, Praeger Pubs) Greenwood.

Models for Assessing Drug Absorption & Metabolism. Ed. by Ronald T. Borchardt et al. 1996. (Pharmaceutical Biotechnology Ser.: Vol. 8). (Illus.). 436p. (C). text 95.00 (*0-306-45243-X*, Kluwer Plenum) Kluwer Academic.

Models for Change in Social Group Work. Marian F. Fatout. 1992. LC 91-29645. (Modern Applications of Social Work Ser.). 231p. pap. text 27.95 (*0-202-36078-4*); lib. bdg. 48.95 (*0-202-36077-6*) Aldine de Gruyter.

Models for Genetics. Wolfgang Balzer & Chris M. Dawe. 1997. LC 97-19725. (Illus.). 183p. pap. 42.95 (*0-8204-3283-0*) P Lang Pubng.

Models for Infectious Human Diseases: Their Structure & Relation to Data. Ed. by V. Isham & G. Medley. 1996. LC 95-23452. (Publications of the Newton Institute: No. 6). (Illus.). 514p. (C). text 110.00 (*0-521-45339-9*) Cambridge U Pr.

Models for Measuring Quality in Managed Care: Analysis & Impact. Ed. by Jonathan Seltzer & David Nash. 1997. (Medical Outcomes & Guidelines Practice Library II). (Illus.). 384p. (Orig.). pap. 145.00 (*1-57987-001-5*) Faulkner & Gray.

Models for Mental Disorder: Conceptual Models in Psychiatry. Peter J. Tyrer & Derek Steinberg. 3rd ed. 1998. LC 97-41382. 158p. pap. 49.95 (*0-471-97433-1*) Wiley.

Models for Multidisciplinary Arrangements: A State-by-State Review of Options. American Psychological Association Staff & McDermott, Will and Emery Staff. 1996. LC 96-27361. (APA Practitioner's Toolbox Ser.). 135p. 29.95 (*1-55798-363-1*) Am Psychol.

Models for Psychotherapy: A Primer. Ed. by J. D. Haldane et al. 1983. 96p. pap. text 10.00 (*0-08-028446-9*, Pergamon Pr) Elsevier.

Models in Dermatology, Vol. 4. Ed. by Howard I. Maibach & N. J. Lowe. 1989. x, 298p. 321.75 (*3-8055-4761-7*) S Karger.

Models in Dermatology, 1987, Vol. 3. Ed. by Howard I. Maibach & N. J. Lowe. 1987. xvi, 204p. 217.50 (*3-8055-4239-9*) S Karger.

Models of Addiction. Ed. by Don C. Fowles. 1988. (Special Issue, Journal of Abnormal Psychology Ser.: Vol. 97, No. 2). 131p. pap. 16.00 (*1-55798-026-8*) Am Psychol.

Models of Anaerobic Infection. Ed. by M. J. Hill. 1984. (New Perspectives in Clinical Microbiology Ser.). text 160.50 (*0-89838-688-8*) Kluwer Academic.

Models of Brain Function. Ed. by Rodney M. Cotterill. 1990. (Illus.). 590p. (C). text 130.00 (*0-521-38503-2*) Cambridge U Pr.

Models of Brief Psychodynamic Therapy: A Comparative Approach. Stanley B. Messer & C. Seth Warren. LC 95-23628. 374p. 1998. pap. 25.00 (*1-57230-340-9*, C0340); 1995. text 39.95 (*1-57230-024-8*, 0024) Guilford Pubns.

Models of Causality in Psychopathology: Toward Dynamic, Synthetic & Nonlinear Causal Models of Behavior Disorders. Stephen N. Haynes. 1991. (General Psychology Ser.). 328p. text (*0-08-040624-6*) PPI GBR. *Dist:* Elsevier.

Models of Cognition: A Review of Cognitive Science. Ed. by Noel E. Sharkey. 1989. LC 88-7473. 320p. (C). 78.50 (*0-89391-528-9*, Ablex) Greenwood.

Models of Collaboration. Mary Susan E. Fishbaugh. 1997. LC 96-41881. 208p. pap. text 40.00 (*0-205-18441-3*) Allyn.

Models of Collaboration: A Guide for Mental Health Professionals Working with Physicians & Health Care Practitioners. David B. Seaburn et al. 1996. LC 96-15804. 304p. 35.00 (*0-465-09580-1*) Basic.

Models of Depressive Disorders: Psychological, Biological & Genetic Perspectives. J. J. Mann. 1989. (Depressive Illness Ser.: Vol. 2). (Illus.). 198p. (C). text 49.50 (*0-306-43277-3*, Kluwer Plenum) Kluwer Academic.

Models of Family Therapy. Williams A. Griffan. 1998. LC 98-31347. pap. text 32.95 (*0-87630-886-8*) Brunner-Routledge.

Models of Information Processing in the Basal Ganglia. Ed. by James C. Houk et al. 1994. LC 94-14822. (Computational Neuroscience Ser.). 394p. 60.00 (*0-262-08234-9*, Bradford Bks) MIT Pr.

Models of Inpatient Group Psychotherapy. Virginia Brabender & April Fallon. 1993. (Illus.). 716p. text 59.95 (*1-55798-174-4*) Am Psychol.

Models of Learning, Memory & Choice: Selected Papers. Ed. by William K. Estes. 1982. LC 82-9823. 395p. 72.00 (*0-275-90786-4*, C0786, Praeger Pubs) Greenwood.

Models of Lung Disease: Microscopy & Structural Methods. Joan Gil. 1990. (Lung Biology in Health & Disease Ser.: Vol. 47). (Illus.). 1032p. text 275.00 (*0-8247-8096-5*) Dekker.

Models of Mental Disorders: A New Comparative Psychiatry. W. T. McKinney. 1988. LC 88-2335. (Illus.). 212p. (C). text 55.00 (*0-306-42746-X*, Kluwer Plenum) Kluwer Academic.

Models of Noncommunicable Diseases: Health Status & Health Service Requirements. Ed. by F. Gotthard Schettler et al. 1993. LC 92-2326. (Supplement zu den Sitzungsberichten der Mathematisch-Naturwissenschaftlichen Klasse Ser.: Vol. 1992). (Illus.). 196p. 22.00 (*3-540-55217-0*); 21.95 (*0-387-55217-0*) Spr-Verlag.

Models of Nursing in Practice: A Pattern for Practical Care. Paul McGee. 1998. (Illus.). 152p. pap. (*0-7487-3343-4*) Nelson Thornes GBR. *Dist:* Intl Spec Bk, Trans-Atl Phila.

Models of Oculomotor Behavior & Control. Ed. by B. L. Zuber. 1981. 304p. 170.00 (*0-8493-5679-2*, QP477, CRC Reprint) Franklin.

Models of Psychological Space. J. Eliot. 1987. LC 87-9770. (Illus.). 203p. 151.00 (*0-387-96549-1*) Spr-Verlag.

Models of the Mind: A Psychoanalytic Theory. John E. Gedo & Arnold I. Goldberg. 1976. LC 73-77132. 236p. pap. text 16.95 (*0-226-28487-5*, P695) U Ch Pr.

Models of the Mind: Their Relationship to Clinical Work. Ed. by Arnold Rothstein. 1985. LC 85-10844. (Monograph 1 of the American Psychanalytic Association Ser.). x, 160p. 27.50 (*0-8236-3410-8*) Intl Univs Pr.

Models, Theories, & Concepts. James P. Smith. 1994. LC 93-49560. (Advanced Nursing Ser.). (Illus.). 192p. pap. (*0-632-03865-9*) Blckwell Science.

Moderation As a Goal or Outcome of Treatment for Alcohol Problems: A Dialogue. Ed. by Mark B. Sobell & Linda C. Sobell. 1987. LC 87-7443. (Drugs & Society Ser.: Vol. 1, Nos. 2-3). 127p. text 39.95 (*0-86656-669-4*) Haworth Pr.

Moderators of Competence. Ed. by Edith D. Neimark et al. 1985. (Jean Piaget Symposia Ser.). 240p. (C). text 49.95 (*0-89859-531-2*) L Erlbaum Assocs.

Modern Aesthetic Surgeon: Confronting a Medical Paradox in an Aging World. Jeffrey Scott Isenberg. 2000. 96p. pap. text 28.00 (*1-55605-315-0*) Wyndham Hall.

Modern Ailments, Ancient Remedies. Gillian Kerr & Yvonne Bloomfield. 1999. LC 99-17080. 160p. 12.98 (*0-7651-1681-2*) Smithmark.

Modern Analysis of Antibiotics. Adorjan Aszalos. 1986. (Drugs & the Pharmaceutical Sciences Ser.: Vol. 27). (Illus.). 568p. text 250.00 (*0-8247-7358-6*) Dekker.

Modern Analytical Chemistry. Harvey. 2000. (Illus.). 800p. (C). (gr. 13). text 61.95 (*0-8151-4208-0*, 26564) Mosby Inc.

Modern & Healthy Body Care: Recipes for Professional, Natural Skin & Hair Care Products. Karin Bombeli. Ed. by Peter Ansdell. unabr. ed. 1997. LC 97-92195. (Illus.). ix, 105p. (Orig.). pap. 19.90 (*0-9658528-0-6*, B01-97) Somerset Bks.

Modern Applied Biostatistical Methods: Using S-Plus. Steve Selvin. 1998. LC 97-19777. (Illus.). 480p. text 49.95 (*0-19-512025-6*) OUP.

Modern Applied Psychology. Arnold P. Goldstein & Leonard Krasner. 1987. 300p. text 45.00 (*0-08-034501-8*); pap. text 19.95 (*0-08-034500-X*) Elsevier (Pergamon Pr).

Modern Approach to Benign Esophageal Disease: Diagnosis & Surgical Therapy. Ed. by Cedric G. Bremner et al. 1995. LC 98-114000. (Illus.). 243p. text 65.00 (*0-942219-96-1*) Quality Med Pub.

Modern Approaches to Endometriosis. Ed. by Eric J. Thomas & John A. Rock. 1991. 304p. text 140.50 (*0-7923-8901-8*) Kluwer Academic.

Modern Approaches to the Dementias Pt. I: Etiology & Pathophysiology. Ed. by Clifford F. Rose. 1985. (Interdisciplinary Topics in Gerontology Ser.: Vol. 19). (Illus.). x, 230p. 155.00 (*3-8055-3980-0*) S Karger.

Modern Approaches to the Dementias Pt. II: Clinical & Therapeutic Aspects. Ed. by F. Clifford Rose. 1985. (Interdisciplinary Topics in Gerontology Ser.: Vol. 20). (Illus.). x, 202p. 137.50 (*3-8055-3981-9*) S Karger.

Modern Approaches to the Treatment of Hypertension. Ed. by Edward A. Babayan et al. 1976. 21.75 (*3-8055-2400-5*) S Karger.

Modern Approaches to the Treatment of Initial Stages of Breast Cancer. V. P. Letyagin et al. 1989. (Soviet Medical Reviews Ser.: Vol. 3). iv, 84p. pap. text 87.00 (*3-7186-4912-8*) Gordon & Breach.

Modern ART in the 2000's: Andrology in the Nineties. Ed. by W. Ombelet et al. 1998. LC 98-10330. (Studies in Profertility: Vol. 8). (Illus.). 238p. lib. bdg. 63.95 (*1-85070-043-5*) CRC Pr.

Modern Aspects of Ancient Acupuncture. Maria Kuman. 1997. (Illus.). 196p. pap. 20.00 (*1-893637-05-0*) Hlth & Hap.

Modern Aspects of Gold Therapy. Ed. by M. Schattenkirchner & W. Mueller. 1983. (Rheumatology Ser.: Vol. 8). (Illus.). viii, 232p. 113.25 (*3-8055-3630-5*) S Karger.

Modern Aspects of Medicine, Vol. 3, No. 5. H. Baum & I. Roman. 1980. (Illus.). 133p. pap. 14.50 (*0-08-027378-5*, Pergamon Pr) Elsevier.

Modern Attitudes in Psychiatry. New York Academy of Medicine Staff. 1977. LC 70-142683. (Essay Index Reprint Ser.). 19.95 (*0-8369-2121-6*) Ayer.

Modern Biology & Its Human Implications. J. A. Butler. 1976. LC 76-27619. 119p. pap. 12.00 (*0-8448-1007-X*, Crane Russak) Taylor & Francis.

Modern Blood Banking & Transfusion Practices. Denise M. Harmening. 4th ed. 1999. LC 98-54477. (Illus.). 592p. 55.95 (*0-8036-0419-X*) Davis Co.

Modern Breast & Pelvic Examinations: A Handbook for Health Professionals. Lila A. Wallis. 4th rev. ed. 1980. viii, 104p. pap. 15.95 (*0-9678633-0-9*) Nat Council on Womens Health.

Modern Cardiovascular Physiology. Carl R. Honig. 2nd ed. 1988. (Illus.). 336p. 40.00 (*0-316-37213-7*, Little Brwn Med Div) Lppncott W & W.

Modern Cellular Automata: Theory & Applications. K. Preston, Jr. & M. J. Duff. 1984. LC 84-11672. (Advanced Applications in Pattern Recognition Ser.). (Illus.). 368p. (C). 95.00 (*0-306-41737-5*, Plenum Trade) Perseus Pubng.

Modern Chromatographic Analysis of Vitamins. Ed. by Deleenheer et al. 2nd ed. 1992. (Chromatographic Science Ser.: Vol. 60). (Illus.). 592p. text 225.00 (*0-8247-8626-2*) Dekker.

Modern Coloproctology: Surgical Grand Rounds from St. Mark's Hospital. John M. Northover. 1993. 208p. (*0-340-55258-1*) E A GBR. *Dist:* OUP.

Modern Colposcopy: A Practical Approach. Michael Campion et al. 1991. (Illus.). 280p. (Orig.). (C). pap. text (*0-9629655-0-2*) Educ Systems.

Modern Concepts in Gastroenterology, Vol. 1. Ed. by Alan B. Thomson et al. 1986. (Topics in Gastroenterology Ser.). (Illus.). 392p. (C). text 126.00 (*0-306-42303-0*, Kluwer Plenum) Kluwer Academic.

Modern Concepts in Gastroenterology, Vol. 2. E. Shaffer & A. B. Thomson. 1989. (Topics in Gastroenterology Ser.). (Illus.). 310p. (C). text 105.00 (*0-306-43125-4*, Kluwer Plenum) Kluwer Academic.

Modern Concepts in Gastroenterology, Vol. 3. A. B. Thomson & E. Shaffer. 1992. (Topics in Gastroenterology Ser.). (Illus.). 378p. (C). text 105.00 (*0-306-43980-8*, Kluwer Plenum) Kluwer Academic.

Modern Concepts in Penicillium & Aspergillus Classification. R. A. Samson. 1990. LC 90-7008. (NATO Advanced Science Institutes Ser.: Vol. 185). (Illus.). 488p. (C). text 135.00 (*0-306-43516-0*, Kluwer Plenum) Kluwer Academic.

Modern Concepts in the Management of Fissure Caries. R. C. Paterson et al. 1991. (Illus.). 80p. pap. text 42.00 (*1-85097-013-0*) Quint Pub Co.

Modern Concepts of Acute & Chronic Hepatitis. G. Gitnick. 1989. LC 88-22557. (Illus.). 358p. (C). text 75.00 (*0-306-42895-4*, Kluwer Plenum) Kluwer Academic.

Modern Contraception: Updates from the Contraception Report. David A. Grimes et al. 1997. LC 97-60969. vi, 265 p. (*0-9651745-1-4*) Emron.

Modern Dental Assisting. Hazel O. Torres. 5th ed. 1995. text 67.00 (*0-7216-6161-0*) Saunders.

Modern Dental Assisting. Hazel O. Torres et al. 5th ed. 1995. (Illus.). 775p. tchr. ed. (*0-7216-5054-6*); 976p. text 52.50 (*0-7216-5053-8*) Saunders.

Modern Dermatologic Radiation Therapy. H. L. Goldschmidt & R. G. Panizzon. 1990. (Illus.). 165p. 143.00 (*0-387-97328-1*) Spr-Verlag.

Modern Developments in Cholinergie (Muscarinic) Receptors & Drugs. Ed. by Pieter A. Van Zwieten & Eduard Schonbaum. 1989. LC 88-30087. (Progress in Pharmacology Ser.: Vol. 7, No. 1). 122p. pap. (*0-89574-277-2*) Gustav Fischer DEU. *Dist:* Lubrecht & Cramer, Balogh.

Modern Diagnostic & Surgical Arthroscopy of the Temporomandibular Joint. Glenn T. Clark et al. 1992. LC 92-11625. (Illus.). 192p. text 165.00 (*0-7216-6591-8*) Saunders.

Modern Drug Use. Ronald D. Mann. 1984. text 242.50 (*0-85200-717-5*) Kluwer Academic.

Modern Eclectic Therapy: A Functional Orientation to Counseling & Psychotherapy. Joseph Hart. 1983. LC 83-11088. 408p. 75.00 (*0-306-41213-6*, Plenum Trade) Perseus Pubng.

Modern Electrochemistry: An Introduction to an Interdisciplinary Area, Vol. 2. J. O. Bockris & A. K. Reddy. 1970. LC 68-19518. (Illus.). 810p. (C). text 47.00 (*0-306-25002-0*, Kluwer Plenum) Kluwer Academic.

Modern Epidemic: A History of Tuberculosis in Japan. William Johnston. 1995. LC 95-5509. (Harvard East Asian Monographs: No. 162). 450p. (C). text 45.00 (*0-674-57912-7*) HUP.

Modern Epidemiology. Kenneth J. Rothman & Sander Greenland. 2nd ed. LC 97-23369. 1998. (Illus.). 752p. text 79.95 (*0-316-75780-2*); 1997. (*0-7817-1049-9*) Lppncott W & W.

Modern Era of Coronary Thrombolysis, 160. Ed. by Richard C. Becker. 1994. LC 94-30680. (Developments in Cardiovascular Medicine Ser.). 320p. (C). text 180.00 (*0-7923-3063-3*) Kluwer Academic.

Modern Freudians: Contemporary Psychoanalytic Technique. Ed. by Carolyn Ellman et al. 1998. LC 98-12097. (Library of Clinical Psychoanalysis). 336p. 40.00 (*0-7657-0158-8*) Aronson.

Modern Head & Neck Imaging. A. L. Baert et al. Ed. by S. K. Mukherji et al. 1998. LC 98-17985. (Medical Radiology Ser.). (Illus.). 261p. 189.00 (*3-540-62549-6*) Spr-Verlag.

Modern Head & Neck Imaging. Ed. by S. K. Mukherji & J. A. Castelijns. 2000. (Medical Radiology Ser.). (Illus.). 272p. pap. 75.00 (*3-540-66344-4*) Spr-Verlag.

Modern Health Care Administration. Richard M. Hodgetts & Dorothy M. Cascio. 1982. 496p. (C). tchr. ed. (*0-15-561401-0*) SCP.

Modern Herbal. M. Grieve. Ed. by C. F. Leyel. 1971. LC 72-169784. (Illus.). reprint ed. Vol. 1. pap. 9.95 (*0-486-22798-7*); Vol. 2. pap. 9.95 (*0-486-22799-5*) Dover.

Modern Hernia Repair: The Embryological & Anatomical Basis of Surgery. Lee J. Skandalakis et al. 2nd rev. ed. 1995. (Illus.). 560p. lib. bdg. 140.95 (*1-85070-585-2*, Parthenon Pbng) CRC Pr.

Modern Higher Education: A Wholistic View. Richard Crews. 1993. 89p. (Orig.). (C). pap. text 11.95 (*0-945864-48-5*) Columbia Pacific U Pr.

Modern Horse Herbal. Hilary P. Self. 1996. (Illus.). 176p. (*1-872082-85-8*) Kenilworth Pr GBR. *Dist:* Half Halt Pr.

Modern Ideas of Evolution. J. William Dawson. 1977. pap. 8.95 (*0-88202-167-2*, Sci Hist) Watson Pub Intl.

Modern Imaging of the Alimentary Tube. M. Ando. Ed. by Alexander R. Margulis. 1997. LC 97-13066. (Medical Radiology Ser.). (Illus.). 363p. 169.00 (*3-540-61441-9*) Spr-Verlag.

Modern Imaging of the Alimentary Tube. Ed. by Alexander R. Margulis. 1999. (Medical Radiology Ser.). (Illus.). 384p. pap. 75.00 (*3-540-66345-2*) Spr-Verlag.

Modern Infectious Disease Epidemiology. Johan Giesecke. 1994. 264p. pap. (*0-340-59237-0*) E A GBR. *Dist:* OUP.

Modern Inhalation Anesthetics. Ed. by Maynard B. Chenoweth. 1972. LC 76-156998. (Handbook of Experimental Pharmacology Ser.: Vol. 30). (Illus.). 175.00 (*0-387-05135-X*) Spr-Verlag.

Modern Instrumental Delivery. John P. O'Grady. 1988. (Illus.). 288p. 40.00 (*0-683-06632-3*) Lppncott W & W.

Modern Intravenous Therapy Procedures. William J. Kurdi. Ed. by James K. Kurdi. 1995. pap. text 34.95 (*0-937142-00-X*) Med Nurs Educ.

Modern Lifestyles, Lower Energy Intake & Micronutrient Status. Ed. by K. Pietrzik & I. G. Macdonald. 1991. (ILSI Human Nutrition Reviews Ser.). (Illus.). 212p. 110.00 (*0-387-19629-3*) Spr-Verlag.

Modern Livestock & Poultry Production. James R. Gillespie. Orig. Title: Livestock & Poultry Production. 4th ed. 1991. text 52.95 (*0-8273-4087-7*); 4th ed. 1990. pap., tchr. ed. 12.00 (*0-8273-4088-5*); 5th ed. 1996. 128p. tchr. ed. 16.00 (*0-8273-6734-1*); 5th ed. 1995. LC 95-15278. 1040p. (C). 82.95 (*0-8273-6733-3*) Delmar.

Modern Livestock & Poultry Production CTB. James R. Gillespie. 5th ed. 1996. (Agriculture Ser.). 100.00 (*0-8273-7493-3*) Delmar.

Modern Management Methods & the Organization of Health Services. 1974. (Public Health Papers: No. 55). pap. text 10.00 (*92-4-130055-8*, 1110055) World Health.

Modern Management of Cervical Spine Syndromes. Donald R. Murphy. 1999. LC 99-35198. (Illus.). 747p. pap. 95.00 (*0-8385-6386-4*) McGraw-Hill Prof.

Modern Management of Myelomeningocele. Wilton H. Bunch et al. 1972. LC 75-161035. (Illus.). 320p. 22.50 (*0-87527-097-2*) Green.

Modern Management of Spinal Injury. S. Mahmoud Rezaian. 1996. (Illus.). 152p. pap. 50.00 (*0-8059-3966-0*) Dorrance.

Modern Management of the Menopause. Ed. by Goran Berg & Mats Hammar. 1994. LC 94-1746. (International Congress, Symposium, & Seminar Ser.: Vol. 8). 626p. lib. bdg. 82.95 (*1-85070-544-5*, Parthenon Pbng) CRC Pr.

Modern Manual Therapy of the Vertebral Column. Ed. by Gregory P. Grieve. 1986. (Illus.). 898p. text (*0-443-03009-X*) Church.

Modern Medical Assisting. Gail A. Chester. Ed. by Adrianne Williams. 1998. LC 97-30097. (Illus.). 768p. (C). pap. text 52.00 (*0-7216-4997-1*) Saunders.

***Modern Medical Assisting: Curriculum Guide.** Gail A. Chester. 1998. (Illus.). 831p. tchr. ed. (*0-7216-8465-3*) Saunders.

Modern Medical Chemistry. John Taylor. 1994. 500p. (C). pap. text 72.00 (*0-13-590399-8*) P-H.

Modern Medical Language. C. Edward Collins & Juanita J. Davies. 1996. LC 96-135119. 750p. (C). pap. text 69.95 (*0-314-06702-7*) West Pub.

Modern Medical Language Act Cards. Collins & Davies. 1996. (Medical Terminology). (C). 21.75 net. (*0-314-08925-X*) Brooks-Cole.

Modern Medical Office: A Reference. Doris D. Humphrey & Kathie Sigler. 2nd ed. 1990. text, stu. ed. 21.95 (*0-538-70101-3*) S-W Thomson.

Modern Medicine: Lay Perspectives & Experiences. Williams. 1996. 288p. (*1-85728-317-1*); pap. (*1-85728-318-X*) UCL Pr Ltd GBR. *Dist:* Taylor & Francis.

Modern Medicine & Jewish Ethics. Fred Rosner. 1986. LC 86-2910. (C). text 29.50 (*0-88125-407-X*) Ktav.

Modern Medicine for the MRCP. Kevin Davies et al. 1996. 135p. pap. text (*0-7020-2112-1*) W B Saunders GBR. *Dist:* Saunders.

Modern Methods of Clinical Investigation. Institute of Medicine Staff. Ed. by Annetine C. Gelijns. 1990. (Medical Innovation at the Crossroads Ser.: Vol. 1). 244p. text 24.95 (*0-309-04286-0*) Natl Acad Pr.

Modern Methods of Inducing Abortion. Ed. by David T. Baird et al. 1995. LC 95-14056. (Illus.). 220p. 99.95 (*0-86542-819-0*) Blackwell Sci.

M N O

Modern Methods of Pharmaceutical Analysis, Vol. I. Roger E. Schirmer. 1981. 304p. 119.95 (*0-8493-5244-4*, RS189, CRC Reprint) Franklin.

Modern Methods of Pharmaceutical Analysis, Vol. 1. 2nd ed. 1990. 416p. 159.00 (*0-8493-5266-5*, RS189) CRC Pr.

Modern Methods of Pharmaceutical Analysis, Vol. II. Roger E. Schirmer. 1982. 288p. 150.00 (*0-8493-5245-2*, RS189, CRC Reprint) Franklin.

Modern Methods of Pharmaceutical Analysis, Vol. 2. 2nd ed. 1990. 464p. 159.00 (*0-8493-5267-3*, RS189) CRC Pr.

Modern Methods of Pharmaceutical Analysis, Vol. III. Roger E. Schirmer. 1982. 256p. 81.50 (*0-8493-5246-0*, CRC Reprint) Franklin.

Modern Methods of Pharmaceutical Analysis: A Textbook for Pharmacy Students & Pharmaceutical Chemists. David G. Watson. 1999. LC 98-32446. (Illus.). xi, 337p. (*0-443-05986-1*) Saunders.

Modern Methods of Radiology in Otorhinolaryngology: Proceedings of the International Congress, 5th, Copenhagen, June, 1976. International Congress of Radiology in Otorhinolaryngology. Ed. by C. R. Pfaltz et al. 1978. (Advances in OtoRhinoLaryngology Ser.: Vol. 24). (Illus.). 115.75 (*3-8055-2707-1*) S Karger.

Modern Microbiology: Principles & Applications. Edward A. Birge. 1991. 496p. (C). text 56.00 net. (*0-697-07628-8*, WCB McGr Hill) McGrw-H Hghr Educ.

Modern Microscopies: Techniques & Applications. P. J. Duke & A. G. Michette. 1989. (Illus.). 266p. (C). text 102.00 (*0-306-43288-9*, Kluwer Plenum) Kluwer Academic.

Modern Miracle Men. John D. Ratcliff. 1977. LC 79-37770. (Essay Index Reprint Ser.). reprint ed. 28.95 (*0-8369-2619-6*) Ayer.

Modern Modalities for the Diagnosis of Hematologic Neoplasms. Tsieh Sun et al. 2nd ed. 1993. LC 93-33311. (*0-89189-366-0*) Am Soc Clinical.

Modern Modalities for the Diagnosis of Hematologic Neoplasms: Color Atlas-Text. Chin-Yang Li et al. 1996. LC 95-36945. (Illus.). 272p. 158.50 (*0-89640-292-4*) Igaku-Shoin.

Modern Multidimensional Scaling Theory & Applications. Ingwer Borg & Patrick J. Groenen. 1996. LC 96-30269. (Statistics Ser.). (Illus.). 471p. 82.95 (*0-387-94845-7*) Spr-Verlag.

Modern Neuromuscular Technique. L. Chaitow. 1996. text 45.00 (*0-443-05298-0*) Saunders.

Modern Neuromuscular Techniques. L. Chaitow. 1997. 24p. pap. (*0-443-05977-2*) Church.

Modern Neurosurgery, Vol. I. Ed. by M. Brock. 1982. (Illus.). 400p. 79.95 (*0-387-10972-2*) Spr-Verlag.

Modern Neurosurgery of Meningiomas & Pituitary Adenomas. Ed. by R. Fahlbusch et al. 1996. (Acta Neurochirurgica Ser.: Vol. 65). (Illus.). 150p. suppl. ed. 149.00 (*3-211-82779-X*) Spr-Verlag.

Modern NMR-Spectroscopy. H. Duddeck & W. Dietrich. 1989. 230p. 39.95 (*0-387-91348-3*) Spr-Verlag.

Modern Nutrition in Health & Disease. Ed. by Maurice E. Shils et al. 9th ed. 1998. LC 98-38505. 2,100p. text 110.00 (*0-683-30769-X*) Lppncott W & W.

Modern Nutrition in Health & Disease James A. Olson et al. 8th ed. 1993. (Illus.). 1. 2200p. lib. bdg. 67.50 (*0-8121-1751-4*); 2. 3036p. lib. bdg. 67.50 (*0-8121-1752-2*); Set. 2200p. lib. bdg. 99.50 (*0-8121-1485-X*) Lppncott W & W.

Modern Operative Techniques in Liver Surgery. Bernard Launois & Glyn G. Jamieson. 1993. LC 92-49203. 160p. text (*0-443-04616-6*) Church.

Modern Parasitology: A Textbook of Parasitology. Ed. by F. E. Cox. 2nd ed. 1993. LC 93-7085. (Illus.). 276p. pap. 58.95 (*0-632-02585-9*) Blackwell Sci.

Modern Pathology of AIDS & Other Retroviral Infections. Ed. by A. T. Haase et al. 1990. (Illus.). viii, 230p. 167.00 (*3-8055-5079-0*) S Karger.

Modern Persecution: Or Insane Asylums Unveiled, As Demonstrated by the Report of the Investigating Committee of the Legislature of Illinois Elizabeth P. Packard. 1973. LC 73-2410. (Mental Illness & Social Policy; the American Experience Ser.). reprint ed. 57.95 (*0-405-05220-0*) Ayer.

Modern Perspectives in Otology. Ed. by B. H. Colman & C. R. Pfaltz. 1983. (Advances in OtoRhinoLaryngology Ser.: Vol. 31). (Illus.). xii, 252p. 172.25 (*3-8055-3641-0*) S Karger.

Modern Perspectives in World Psychiatry. Ed. by John G. Howells. 1971. (Illus.). (C). Set. 787p. text 32.00 (*0-8464-1155-5*); Vol. 2. 787p. 32.00 (*0-8464-1332-9*); Vol. 3. 32.00 (*0-8464-1333-7*) Beekman Pubs.

Modern Pharmaceutics, No. 72. Ed. by Gilbert S. Banker & Christopher T. Rhodes. 3rd ed. 1995. LC 95-33238. (Drugs & the Pharmaceutical Sciences Ser.: Vol. 72). (Illus.). 960p. text 195.00 (*0-8247-9371-4*) Dekker.

Modern Pharmacology. Ed. by Charles R. Craig & Robert E. Stitzel. 2nd ed. 1986. 1115p. (C). 44.50 (*0-316-15925-5*); 4th ed. 1994. LC 93-35535. 49.95 (*0-316-15932-8*) Lppncott W & W (Little Brwn Med Div).

Modern Pharmacology: International. Craig. 3rd ed. 1990. 30.00 (*0-316-15929-8*, Little Brwn Med Div) Lppncott W & W.

Modern Pharmacology with Clinical Applications. Craig. 5th ed. 1997. LC 96-23366. 848p. pap. text 52.95 (*0-316-15934-4*) Lppncott W & W.

Modern Practical Prescriptions of Acupuncture & Moxibustion. Xiaoping Ji. Tr. by Maoxin Chen & Shuting Li. 1996. (Illus.). 297p. pap. 29.50 (*1-880132-22-2*) Sci Pr NY.

Modern Psychoanalysis: New Directions & Perspectives. Ed. by Judd Marmor. 1995. LC 95-16725. 752p. pap. text 39.95 (*1-56000-825-3*) Transaction Pubs.

Modern Psychoanalysis of the Schizophrenic Patient. Hyman Spotnitz. 1969. LC 68-29401. 240p. pap. text 55.00 (*0-8089-0469-8*, 794285, Grune & Strat) Harcrt Hlth Sci Grp.

Modern Psychoanalytic Concepts in a General Psychology Pts. 1 & 2: Including General Concepts & Principles & Motivation. Allan Rosenblatt & James Thickstrun. 1978. LC 77-14712. (Psychological Issues Monographs: Nos. 42 & 43). 348p. text 52.50 (*0-8236-3430-2*) Intl Univs Pr.

Modern Psychology. Philip L. Harriman. 1975. (Quality Paperback Ser.: No. 20). 316p. (Orig.). reprint ed. pap. 14.00 (*0-8226-0020-X*) Littlefield.

Modern Psychometrics: The Science of Psychological Assessment. John Rust & Susan Golombok. (International Library of Philosophy, Psychology, & Scientific Method). 1989. 192p. 49.95 (*0-415-03058-7*); 2nd ed. 1999. LC 98-47962. (Illus.). 240p. pap. 31.95 (*0-415-20341-4*) Routledge.

Modern Sex. Cloyd J. Julian. 1985. pap. text 26.00 (*0-03-071899-6*) Holt R&W.

Modern Society & Mental Disease. Carney Landis & James D. Page. Ed. by Gerald N. Grob. 1980. LC 78-22571. (Historical Issues in Mental Health Ser.). (Illus.). reprint ed. lib. bdg. 19.95 (*0-405-11924-0*) Ayer.

Modern South Africa in Search of a Soul: Perspectives on the Wilderness Within. Ed. by Graham Saayman. 1990. (Illus.). 247p. 27.50 (*0-938434-56-X*) Sigo Pr.

Modern Spectrochemical Analysis of Metals: An Introduction for Users of Arc/Spark Instrumentation. V. B. Thomsen. 1996. LC 96-86487. 220p. 156.00 (*0-87170-578-8*, 6540) ASM.

Modern Statistical Methods in Chronic Disease Epidemiology: Proceedings of a Conference Sponsored by SIAM Institute for Mathematics & Society & Supported by the Department of Energy. Ed. by Suresh H. Moolgavkar & Ross L. Prentice. 1986. LC 86-1597. 282p. 155.00 (*0-471-83904-3*, Wiley-Interscience) Wiley.

Modern Stereotactic Neurosurgery. Ed. by L. Dade Lunsford. 1988. (C). text 309.50 (*0-89838-950-X*) Kluwer Academic.

Modern Strategy for Preclinical Pharmaceutical R & D: Towards the Virtual Research Company. David Cavalla et al. 1997. LC 96-37234. 228p. 155.00 (*0-471-97117-0*) Wiley.

Modern Surgical Care: Physiologic Foundations & Clinical Applications. Thomas A. Miller. 2nd ed. 1998. LC 97-50113. 1454p. 145.00 (*1-57626-060-7*) Quality Med Pub.

Modern Surgical Management of Endometriosis. Camran Nezhat et al. 1995. LC 94-19130. (Illus.). 317p. 158.00 (*0-387-94243-2*) Spr-Verlag.

Modern Surgical Pathology Weidner. 1999. (C). text (*0-7216-7253-1*) Saunders.

Modern Technology of Radiation Oncology: A Compendium for Medical Physicists & Radiation Oncologists. Ed. by Jacob Van Dyk. 1999. LC 99-31932. (Illus.). 1072p. pap. 145.95 (*0-944838-22-7*); text 175.95 (*0-944838-38-3*) Med Physics Pub.

Modern Theory & Method in Group Training. William G. Dyer. 1981. LC 80-24641. 268p. (C). reprint ed. text 23.00 (*0-89874-280-3*) Krieger.

Modern Therapeutics in Rheumatic Diseases. Ed. by George C. Tsokos et al. 2001. LC 00-53529. 700p. 145.00 (*0-89603-916-1*) Humana.

Modern Transfusion Medicine: A Practical Approach. Ed. by Derwood H. Pamphilon. 1995. LC 94-5411. 288p. 144.95 (*0-8493-8922-4*) CRC Pr.

Modern Transfusion Therapy Ed. by Janice P. Dutcher. 1989. Vol. 1. 304p. 225.00 (*0-8493-6247-4*, RM171); Vol. 2. 352p. 216.00 (*0-8493-6248-2*, RM171) CRC Pr.

Modern Treatment of Alzheimer's Disease: 4th EFNS Congress, Lisbon, September 1999. Ed. by J. M. Orgogozo. 2000. (Dementia & Geriatric Cognitive Disorders Ser.: Vol 11). (Illus.). iv, 34p. pap. 25.25 (*3-8055-7151-8*) S Karger.

Modern Treatment of Severe Burns. Z. Y. Fang et al. Ed. by N. Li & S. D. Ge. 1992. (Illus.). 334p. 247.00 (*0-387-54028-8*) Spr-Verlag.

Modern Trends in Aging Research. Y. Courtois et al. 1987. (Colloque de L'INSERM Ser.). (ENG & FRE.). 620p. lib. bdg. 85.00 (*2-85598-309-6*) S M P F Inc.

Modern Trends in Biothermokinetics. S. Schuster et al. 1994. (Illus.). 512p. (C). text 135.00 (*0-306-44579-4*, Kluwer Plenum) Kluwer Academic.

Modern Trends in Huin Leukemia. 1976. (Illus.). 576p. 87.95 (*0-387-79785-8*) Spr-Verlag.

Modern Trends in Human Leukemia, No. VIII. Ed. by Rolf Neth et al. 1990. (Haematology & Blood Transfusion Ser.: Vol. 32). (Illus.). 532p. 224.00 (*0-387-50967-4*) Spr-Verlag.

Modern Trends in Human Leukemia IX: New Results in Clinical & Biological Research Including Pediatric Oncology; Organized on Behalf of the Deutsche Gesellschaft fur Hamatologie und Onkologie, Wilsede, June 17-21, 1990. Ed. by Rolf Neth et al. 1992. LC 92-2334. (Haematology & Blood Transfusion Ser.: Vol. 35). (Illus.). 480p. 239.00 (*0-387-54360-0*); pap. 198.00 (*3-540-54360-0*) Spr-Verlag.

Modern Trends in Human Leukemia Three. Ed. by Rolf Neth et al. 1979. (Illus.). 599p. 100.00 (*0-387-08999-3*) Spr-Verlag.

Modern Vaccinology. Ed. by Edward Kurstak. 1994. (Illus.). 408p. (C). text 85.00 (*0-306-44820-3*, Kluwer Plenum) Kluwer Academic.

Modern Vascular Surgery. Ed. by John B. Chang. Vol. 5. 1992. LC 92-2307. 519p. 217.00 (*0-387-97864-X*); Vol. 5. 1992. LC 92-2307. 520p. (*3-540-97864-X*); Vol. 6. 1994. (Illus.). 607p. 214.00 (*0-387-94187-8*) Spr-Verlag.

Modern Witchcraft & Psychoanalysis. M. D. Faber. 1993. LC 91-58949. 192p. 32.50 (*0-8386-3488-5*) Fairleigh Dickinson.

Modern Woman in Search of Soul: A Jungian Guide to the Visible & Invisible Worlds. June Singer. rev. ed. 1998. LC 97-48983. (Jung on the Hudson Bks.). Orig. Title: Seeing Through the Visible World: Jung Gnosis & Chaos. 256p. pap. 18.95 (*0-89254-041-9*) Nicolas-Hays.

Modern X-Ray Analysis on Single Crystals. Peter Luger. 1980. 312p. 77.70 (*3-11-006830-3*) De Gruyter.

Moderne Endoskoskopie im Kindesalter: Proceedings of Kinderchirurgisches Symposium, Obergurgl, January 1977. Kinderchirurgisches Symposium Staff. Ed. by E. Bern Rossi & P. Wurnig. 1978. (Paediatrische Fortbildungskurse fuer die Praxis Ser.: Bd. 46). (Illus.). 35.75 (*3-8055-2799-3*) S Karger.

Modernity, Medicine & Health: Medical Sociology Towards 2000. Graham Scambler & Paul Higgs. 1998. LC 97-34889. 264p. (C). 85.00 (*0-415-14938-X*); pap. 26.95 (*0-415-14939-8*) Routledge.

Modes & Morals of Psychotherapy. Perry London. 2nd ed. 1986. LC 84-29769. (Clinical & Community Psychology Ser.). 350p. (C). 79.95 (*0-89116-290-9*); pap. 27.95 (*0-89116-350-6*) Hemisp Pub.

Modes of Action of GnRH & GnRH Analogs. Ed. by W. F. Crowley, Jr. & P. Michael Conn. 1992. (Serono Symposia Ser.). (Illus.). 378p. 209.00 (*0-387-97802-X*) Spr-Verlag.

Modes of Medical Instruction: A Semiotic Comparison of Textbooks of Medicine & Popular Home Medical Books. Joan Y. Kahn. 1983. LC 83-2379. (Approaches to Semiotics Ser.: No. 65). xx, 342p. (*90-279-3070-8*) Mouton.

Modest Livestock & Poultry Product. Gillespie. 3rd ed. 1989. (Agriculture Ser.). text, tchr. ed. 12.00 (*0-8273-3278-5*) Delmar.

Modifiability of Response to Taste Stimuli in the Preschool Child. Marguerite E. Gauger. LC 77-176799. (Columbia University. Teachers College. Contributions to Education Ser.: No. 348). reprint ed. 37.50 (*0-404-55348-6*) AMS Pr.

Modification of Tumor Development in Rodents. Ed. by N. Ito & H. Sugano. 1991. (Progress in Experimental Tumor Research Ser.: Vol. 33). (Illus.). viii, 236p. 200.00 (*3-8055-5242-4*) S Karger.

Modified Essay Questions for the MRCGP Examination. Ed. by T. S. Murray. 1995. LC 95-34949. 204p. pap. 39.95 (*0-86542-646-5*) Blackwell Sci.

Modified Lipoproteins in the Pathogenesis of Atherosclerosis. Sampath Pathasarathy. 1994. (Medical Intelligence Unit Ser.). 115p. 99.00 (*1-57059-080-X*, LN9080) Landes Bioscience.

Modified Nucleosides & Cancer: Workshop, Freiburg, FRG, 1981. Ed. by G. Nass. 1983. (Recent Results in Cancer Research Ser.: Vol. 84). (Illus.). 432p. 99.00 (*0-387-12024-6*) Spr-Verlag.

Modifiers Made Easy. Ed. by Kathy Brouch. 1999. 200p. (C). pap. 99.95 (*1-56329-536-9*) Thomson Learn.

Modifiers Made Easy 2000. Medicode, Med-Index Division Staff. 1999. (C). 75.95 (*1-56337-346-7*) Thomson Learn.

***Modifiers Made Easy 2001.** Ingenix, Inc. Staff. pap. 79.95 (*1-56337-320-3*) Ingenix Inc.

Modular Approaches to the Study of the Mind. Noam Chomsky. 1984. LC 82-62962. (Distinguished Graduate Research Lectures). 118p. 15.00 (*0-916304-56-6*) SDSU Press.

Modular Brain. Richard M. Restak. 1994. LC 93-42298. 256p. 22.00 (*0-684-19544-5*, Macmillan Ref) Gale.

Modular Deficits in Alzheimer-Type Dementia. Ed. by Myrna F. Schwartz. 1991. 456p. 60.00 (*0-262-19298-5*, Bradford Bks) MIT Pr.

Modular Psychology. Myers. 6th ed. 2000. pap. text, stu. ed. 17.00 (*0-7167-5180-1*) Worth.

Modularity of Mind. Jerry A. Fodor. 1983. LC 82-24892. (Bradford Monograph Ser.). 216p. (C). pap. 15.95 (*0-262-56025-9*) MIT Pr.

Modularity of Orthopedic Implants. Ed. by Donald C. Marlowe et al. 1997. LC 97-7308. (STP Ser.: No. 1301). (Illus.). 236p. pap. 63.00 (*0-8031-2415-5*, STP1301) ASTM.

Modulation & Mediation of Cancer by Vitamins. Ed. by K. N. Prasad & Frank L. Meyskens. 1983. (Illus.). x, 350p. 143.50 (*3-8055-3526-0*) S Karger.

Modulation of Aging Process by Dietary Restriction. Ed. by Byung P. Yu. 1994. 304p. lib. bdg. 190.95 (*0-8493-4994-X*) CRC Pr.

Modulation of Cellular Responses in Toxicity. Ed. by Corrado L. Galli et al. 1995. (NATO ASI Ser.: Vol. 93). 371p. 204.00 (*3-540-60010-8*) Spr-Verlag.

Modulation of Dopaminergic Neurotransmission by Other Neurotransmitters. Ed. by Charles R. Ashby, Jr. 1995. LC 95-43990. 240p. 159.95 (*0-8493-4780-7*) CRC Pr.

Modulation of Liver Cell Expression. Ed. by Werner Reutter et al. 1987. (Falk Symposium Ser.: No. 43). text 268.50 (*0-85200-677-2*) Kluwer Academic.

Modulation of MHC Antigen Expression & Disease. Ed. by G. Eric Blair et al. 1995. (Illus.). (C). 458p. text 110.00 (*0-521-49578-4*); 480p. pap. (*0-521-49921-6*) Cambridge U Pr.

***Modulation of Nitric Oxide/Cyclic GMP Signal Transduction in the Injured Vascular Wall.** Peter Sinnaeve. 2001. (Acta Biomedica Lovaniensia Ser.: No. 239). (Illus.). 111p. pap. (*90-5867-143-7*) Leuven Univ BEL. *Dist:* Coronet Bks.

Modulation von Zelloberflaechenstrukturen. A. Raedler & Elisabeth Raedler. 1984. (Bibliotheca Anatomica Ser.: No. 25). (Illus.). vi, 82p. 41.75 (*3-8055-3755-7*) S Karger.

Modulators of Immune Responses: The Evolutionary Trail. Ed. by J. S. Stolen et al. 1996. LC 95-67853. (Illus.). 600p. (C). pap. text 85.00 (*1-887052-00-3*) SOS Pubns NJ.

Module 5, Monitoring the Pharmacist's Care Plan: Advancing Pharmaceutical Care. Carla Frye. 1994. (Clinical Skills Program Ser.). 100p. (C). text 65.00 (*1-879907-49-6*) Am Soc Hlth-Syst.

Modules for Basic Nursing Skills, Volumes I and II. Janice R. Ellis et al. 6th ed. 1996. LC 95-37176. 720p. pap. text 36.95 (*0-397-55170-3*); 816p. pap. text 36.95 (*0-397-55171-1*) Lppncott W & W.

Modules for Medication Administration. Barbarito & D'Amico. 1998. 190p. (C). spiral bd. 49.95 (*0-7872-4691-3*, 41469102) Kendall-Hunt.

Moe's Textbook of Scoliosis & Other Spinal Deformities. Ed. by David S. Bradford et al. 3rd ed. 1994. LC 94-11860. (Illus.). 672p. text 155.00 (*0-7216-5533-5*) Saunders.

Mohave Ethnopsychiatry & Suicide: Psychiatric Knowledge & the Psychic Disturbances of an Indian Tribe. George Devereux. 1995. (Bureau of American Ethnology Ser.). 586p. lib. bdg. 119.00 (*0-7812-4175-8*) Rprt Serv.

Mohave Ethnopsychiatry & Suicide: The Psychiatric Knowledge & the Psychic Disturbances of an Indian Tribe. George Devereux. reprint ed. 95.00 (*0-403-03650-X*) Scholarly.

MOHR's Guide see Healthcare Safety Sourcebook

MOHs. Terence M. Davidson. 1999. LC 99-47753. (Self-Instructional Package Ser.). (Illus.). 121p. pap. text 25.00 (*1-56772-028-5*, 5506360) AAO-HNS.

Moh's Micrographic Surgery. Mikail. 1991. (Illus.). 432p. text 170.00 (*0-7216-3415-X*) Saunders.

MOHS Surgery: Fundamentals & Techniques. Kenneth G. Gross et al. 1998. LC 98-13759. 331p. text 139.00 (*0-323-00012-6*) Mosby Inc.

Molecular - Cellular Mechanisms of Immunomodulatory Drugs. Etienne C. Dupont & Cathy Walker. 1993. (*0-8493-4809-9*, 4809, CRC Reprint) Franklin.

Molecular Analysis of Cancer. Ed. by Jacqueline Boultwood & Carrie Fidler. 2001. LC 2001-24306. (Methods in Molecular Medicine Ser.: Vol. 68). (Illus.). 328p. 99.50 (*0-89603-622-7*) Humana.

Molecular & Biochemical Aspects of Progesterone Function. Judith Ramaley et al. 1972. 173p. text 29.75 (*0-8290-2380-1*) Irvington.

Molecular & Biomolecular Electronics: Developed from a Symposium Sponsored by the Division of Biochemical Technology of the American Chemical Society at the 4th Annual Chemical Congress of North America (202nd National Meeting of the American Chemical Society), New York, NY, 8/25-8/30, 1991, Vol. 24. Chemical Congress of North America Staff. Ed. by Robert R. Birge. 1994. LC 94-28455. (Advances in Chemistry Ser.: No. 240). (Illus.). 608p. 150.00 (*0-8412-2698-9*) Am Chemical.

Molecular & Cell Biological Aspects of Gastoenteropancreatic Neuroendocrine Tumor Disease. Ed. by Bertram Wiedenmann. 1994. LC 94-27923. 145.00 (*0-89766-897-9*) NY Acad Sci.

Molecular & Cell Biological Aspects of Gastoenteropancreatic Neuroendocrine Tumor Disease. Ed. by Bertram Wiedenmann et al. 1994. LC 94-27923. (Annals Ser.: Vol. 733). (Illus.). 535p. pap. 145.00 (*0-89766-898-7*) NY Acad Sci.

Molecular & Cell Biology of Human Gene Therapeutics. Ed. by George Dickson. 1995. LC 95-67601. (Molecular & Cell Biology of Human Diseases Ser.). (Illus.). 424p. (C). pap. text 167.95 (*0-412-62550-4*, Chap & Hall NY) Chapman & Hall.

Molecular & Cell Biology of Liver Fibrogenesis: Proceedings of the International Falk Symposium Held in Marburg, Germany, 22-23 January 1992. Ed. by A. M. Gressner & G. Ramadori. 1992. LC 92-23629. 576p. text 268.50 (*0-7923-8980-8*) Kluwer Academic.

Molecular & Cell Biology of Muscular Dystrophy. Ed. by Terence Partridge. 1993. LC 92-48393. (Molecular & Cell Biology of Human Diseases Ser.). (Illus.). 320p. (C). (gr. 13). pap. text 143.95 (*0-412-43440-7*, A9501) Chapman & Hall.

Molecular & Cell Biology of Sexually Transmitted Diseases. Ed. by David Wright & Len Archard. 1992. LC 92-17402. (Molecular & Cell Biology of Human Diseases Ser.). (Illus.). 304p. (C). (gr. 13). pap. text 155.95 (*0-412-36510-3*, A7028) Chapman & Hall.

Molecular & Cell Biology of the Liver. Ed. by Albert V. LeBouton. 1993. 560p. lib. bdg. 229.00 (*0-8493-8891-0*, QP185) CRC Pr.

Molecular & Cell Biology of Type 2 Diabetes & Its Complications: 5th International Diabetes Conference, Turin, April 10 - 12, 1997. Ed. by Francesco Belfiore et al. 1998. LC 98-10210. (Frontiers in Diabetes Ser.: Vol. 14). (Illus.). x, 260p. 97.50 (*3-8055-6644-1*) S Karger.

Molecular & Cellular Aspects of Allergy: Proceedings of the Collegium Internationale Allergologicum Symposium, 10th, Copenhagen, 1974. Collegium Internationale Allergologicum Symposium. Ed. by B. Diamant et al. 1975. (International Archives of Allergy & Immunology Ser.: Vol. 49, No. 1-2). (Illus.). 250p. pap. 88.75 (*3-8055-2166-9*) S Karger.

Molecular & Cellular Aspects of Carcinogen Screening Tests. Ed. by R. Montesano et al. 1986. (IARC Scientific Publications Ser.: No. 27). (Illus.). 372p. 43.00 (*0-19-723027-X*) OUP.

Molecular & Cellular Aspects of Periimplanation Processes. S. K. Dey. 1995. LC 95-21136. (Serono Symposia Ser.). (Illus.). 361p. 163.00 (*0-387-94569-5*) Spr-Verlag.

Molecular & Cellular Aspects of Reproduction. Ed. by Dharam S. Dhindsa & Om P. Bahl. 1986. LC 86-20533. (Advances in Experimental Medicine & Biology Ser.: Vol. 205). 392p. 85.00 (*0-306-42403-7*, Plenum Trade) Perseus Pubng.

Molecular & Cellular Aspects of the Drug Addiction. Ed. by A. Goldstein. 1989. (Illus.). 238p. 88.00 (*0-387-96827-X*) Spr-Verlag.

Molecular & Cellular Aspects of Vascular Smooth Muscle in Health & Disease: Proceedings - Journal: Blood Vessels, Vol. 15, Nos. 1-3. U. S. Japan Cooperative Symposium Staff. Ed. by D. F. Bohr & F. Takenha. 1978. (Illus.). 75.75 (*3-8055-2857-4*) S Karger.

Molecular & Cellular Basis of Inflammation. Charles N. Serhan & Peter A. Ward. 1998. LC 98-47837. (Current Inflammation Research Ser.). 352p. 135.00 (*0-89603-595-6*) Humana.

Molecular & Cellular Basis of Visual Acuity. Ed. by S. R. Hilfer & J. B. Sheffield. 1984. (Cell & Developmental Biology of the Eye Ser.). (Illus.). 184p. 92.00 (*0-387-90964-8*) Spr-Verlag.

Molecular & Cellular Biochemistry see Lipid Metabolism in Normoxic & Ischemic Heart

Molecular & Cellular Biology of Multidrug Resistance in Tumor Cells. I. B. Roninson. 1990. (Illus.). 424p. (C). text 120.00 (*0-306-43547-0*, Kluwer Plenum) Kluwer Academic.

Molecular & Cellular Biology of Prostate Cancer. Ed. by James P. Karr et al. 1991. (Advances in Experimental Medicine & Biology Ser.). (Illus.). 396p. (C). text 144.00 (*0-306-43884-4*, 305, Kluwer Plenum) Kluwer Academic.

Molecular & Cellular Biology of the Allergic Response. Ed. by Arnold I. Levinson & Yvonne Paterson. 1994. LC 94-4449. (Clinical Allergy & Immunology Ser.: Vol. 3). (Illus.). 473p. text 185.00 (*0-8247-8876-1*) Dekker.

Molecular & Cellular Biology of Wound Repair. Ed. by R. A. Clark & P. M. Henson. 1988. LC 87-37683. (Illus.). 620p. 125.00 (*0-306-42716-8*, Plenum Trade) Perseus Pubng.

Molecular & Cellular Biology of Wound Repair. Ed. by Richard A. Clark. 2nd ed. 1996. (Illus.). 600p. (C). text 135.00 (*0-306-45159-X*, Kluwer Plenum) Kluwer Academic.

Molecular & Cellular Effects of Nutrition on Disease Process. Grant M. Pierce. 1998. LC 98-3954. (Developments in Molecular & Cellular Biochemistry Ser.). 237p. (*0-7923-8171-8*) Kluwer Academic.

Molecular & Cellular Endocrine Pathology. Lucia Stefaneanu et al. 1998. LC 97-42372. pap. 159.95 (*0-412-11271-X*) Chapman & Hall.

Molecular & Cellular Endocrinology of the Testis. G. Verhoeven & U. F. Habenicht. 1994. LC 94-35138. (Ernst Schering Research Foundation Ser.: Supp. 1). (Illus.). xiv, 298p. text 56.00 (*0-387-58337-8*) Spr-Verlag.

Molecular & Cellular Gerontology. Olivier Toussaint. 2000. LC 00-34861. (Annals of the New York Academy of Sciences Ser.: Vol. 908). (Illus.). ix, 350p. (*1-57331-272-X*) NY Acad Sci.

Molecular & Cellular Gerontology, Vol. 908. Ed. by Olivier Toussaint et al. 2000. LC 00-34861. (Annals of the New York Academy of Sciences Ser.: Vol. 908). (Illus.). ix, 350p. 90.00 (*1-57331-271-1*) NY Acad Sci.

Molecular & Cellular Mechanisms of Anesthetics. Sheldon H. Roth & Keith W. Miller. 1986. LC 85-28274. (Illus.). 502p. (C). text 150.00 (*0-306-42128-3*, Kluwer Plenum) Kluwer Academic.

Molecular & Cellular Mechanisms of Cardiovascular Regulation. Ed. by M. Endoh et al. 1996. 464p. 250.00 (*4-431-70180-X*) Spr-Verlag.

Molecular & Cellular Mechanisms of Neuronal Plasticity: Basic & Clinical Implications. Ed. by Y. H. Ehrlich. 1999. LC 98-31763. (Advances in Experimental Medicine & Biology Ser.: 466). (Illus.). 235p. (C). text 125.00 (*0-306-46040-8*, Kluwer Plenum) Kluwer Academic.

Molecular & Cellular Mechanisms of Toxicity. Ed. by Francesco De Matteis & Lewis L. Smith. 1995. LC 95-16810. 240p. 199.95 (*0-8493-9229-2*, 9229) CRC Pr.

Molecular & Cellular Pediatric Endocrinology. Stuart Handwerger. 1999. LC 98-50918. (Contemporary Endocrinology Ser.: Vol. 10). (Illus.). 328p. 135.00 (*0-89603-406-2*) Humana.

Molecular & Cellular Targets for Anti Epileptic Drugs. Avanzini. 1997. 272p. (*0-86196-554-X*) J Libbey Med GBR. *Dist:* Buttrwrth-Heinemann.

Molecular & Clinical Advances in Anticancer Drug Resistance. Ed. by Robert F. Ozols. 1991. (Cancer Treatment & Research Ser.). 320p. (C). text 204.50 (*0-7923-1212-0*) Kluwer Academic.

Molecular & Clinical Advances in Pituitary Disorders - 11993: Proceedings of the 3rd International Pituitary Congress. Ed. by Shlomo Melmed. 1993. 400p. pap. 30.00 (*0-9637943-0-2*) Endocrine Res.

Molecular & Clinical Aspects of Bacterial Vaccine Development. Ed. by Dlawer A. Ala'Aldeen & Carlos E. Hormaeche. 1995. LC 94-43839. 376p. 285.00 (*0-471-95564-7*) Wiley.

Molecular & Clinical Implications for Allergy in the 21st Century. Ed. by A. L. Sheffer & S. J. Galli. 1995. (Journal: Vol. 107, No. 1-3, 1995). (Illus.). 474p. pap. 213.25 (*3-8055-6206-3*) S Karger.

Molecular & Developmental Biology of Cartilage. Benoit De Crombrugghe & New York Academy of Medicine Staff. 1996. LC 96-1721. (Annals of the New York Academy of Sciences Ser.). 367p. pap. 110.00 (*1-57331-011-5*) NY Acad Sci.

Molecular & Functional Aspects of Blood Group Antigens. Ed. by Leslie E. Silberstein. 1995. (Illus.). 245p. (C). text 50.00 (*1-56395-048-0*) Am Assn Blood.

Molecular & Genetic Analysis of Human Traits. Gustavo Maroni. 2000. LC 00-23792. (Illus.). xii, 274p. pap. 60.95 (*0-632-04369-5*) Blackwell Sci.

Molecular & Genetic Aspects of Obesity. Ed. by George A. Bray & Donna H. Ryan. 1996. LC 95-35680. (Pennington Center Nutrition Ser.: Vol. 5). (Illus.). 712p. (C). text 110.00 (*0 8071-2025-1*) La State U Pr.

Molecular & Genetic Basis of Neurological Disease. Roger N. Rosenberg et al. 2nd ed. 1996. LC 96-47652. 1430p. text 380.00 (*0-7506-9668-0*) Buttrwrth-Heinemann.

Molecular & Immune Mechanisms of Pathogenesis of Cutaneous Leishmaniasis. Felix J. Tapia et al. 1996. LC 96-9384. (Medical Intelligence Unit Ser.). 219p. 99.00 (*1-57059-353-1*) Landes Bioscience.

Molecular & Quantum Pharmacology. Ed. by Ernst Bergmann & Bernard Pullman. 1975. LC 74-83002. (Jerusalem Symposia on Quantum Chemistry & Biochemistry Ser.: No. 7). 522p. text 261.50 (*90-277-0525-9*) Kluwer Academic.

Molecular & Subcellular Cardiology: Effects of Structure & Function: Proceedings of the Ninth Goldberg Workshop Held in Haifa, Israel, December 4-8, 1994. Ed. by Samuel Sideman & Rafael Beyar. 1995. LC 95-25128. (Advances in Experimental Medicine & Biology Ser.: Vol. 382). (Illus.). 372p. 110.00 (*0-306-45123-9*, Kluwer Plenum) Kluwer Academic.

Molecular Approaches to Human Polygenic Diseases. CIBA Foundation Staff. 1987. LC 87-13374. (CIBA Foundation Symposia Ser.: No. 130). 284p. 128.00 (*0-471-91096-1*) Wiley.

Molecular Approaches to Parasitology. Ed. by John C. Boothroyd & Richard Komuniecki. 1995. (MBL Lectures in Biology: Vol. 12). 560p. 257.00 (*0-471-10342-X*); LC 94-41923. pap. 120.00 (*0-471-10341-1*) Wiley.

Molecular Approaches to the Study of Allergens. Ed. by B. A. Baldo. 1990. (Monographs in Allergy: Vol. 28). (Illus.). viii, 166p. 185.25 (*3-8055-5213-0*) S Karger.

Molecular Approaches to Tumor Immunotherapy. Ed. by Yang Liu. 1997. LC 97-41654. 300p. lib. bdg. 55.00 (*981-02-2793-0*) World Scientific Pub.

Molecular Aspects of Ammoniagenesis. Ed. by H. Endou et al. 1991. (Contributions to Nephrology Ser.: Vol. 92). (Illus.). x, 228p. 49.75 (*3-8055-5368-4*) S Karger.

Molecular Aspects of Anticancer Drug-DNA Interactions, Vol. II. Ed. by Michael J. Waring & Stephen Neidle. 1994. (Topics in Molecular & Structural Biology Ser.). 336p. 110.00 (*0-8493-7773-0*, Z7773) CRC Pr.

Molecular Aspects of Asian Medicines Vol. 1: The Orient. Ed. by A. Mori & T. Satoh. 1996. 69.95 (*0-915340-20-8*) PJD Pubns.

Molecular Aspects of Cancer & Its Therapy. Andrzej Mackiewicz & Pravinkumar B. Sehgal. 1998. LC 97-32691. (Molecular & Cell Biology Updates Ser.). (*0-8176-5724-X*) Birkhauser.

Molecular Aspects of Cancer & Its Therapy. Ed. by Andrzej Mackiewicz & Pravinkumar B. Sehgal. 1997. LC 97-32691. (Molecular & Cell Biology Updates Ser.). (Illus.). 300p. text 125.00 (*3-7643-5724-X*) Birkhauser.

Molecular Aspects of Chemotherapy. Edward Borowski & David Shugar. 1990. (Illus.). 272p. 78.00 (*0-08-036848-4*, Pergamon Pr) Elsevier.

Molecular Aspects of Chemotherapy: Proceedings of the 3rd International Symposium, Gdansk, Poland, June 19-21, 1991. Ed. by David Shugar et al. 1993. (Illus.). 400p. 163.00 (*0-387-54874-2*) Spr-Verlag.

Molecular Aspects of Development & Aging of the Nervous System. Ed. by Jean M. Lauder et al. 1989. LC 89-70995. (Advances in Experimental Medicine & Biology Ser.: Vol. 265). (Illus.). 335p. 89.50 (*0-306-43408-3*, Plenum Trade) Perseus Pubng.

Molecular Aspects of Human Cytomegalovirus Diseases. Ed. by Yechiel Becker et al. 1993. LC 92-49467. (Frontiers of Virology Ser.: Vol. 2). (*3-540-55948-5*); (Illus.). 486p. 150.00 (*0-387-55948-5*) Spr-Verlag.

Molecular Aspects of Human Disease. Ed. by John W. Gorrod et al. 1989. 279p. 74.95 (*0-470-21298-5*); Vol. 2. 284p. 74.95 (*0-470-21303-5*) P-H.

Molecular Aspects of Idiopathic Urolithiasis. R. Nath et al. 1984. (Illus.). 176p. pap. 59.00 (*0-08-031697-2*, Pergamon Pr) Elsevier.

Molecular Aspects of Immunoglobulin Subclasses. Farouk Shakib. 1990. (Illus.). 328p. 177.00 (*0-08-037504-9*, Pergamon Pr) Elsevier.

Molecular Aspects of Inflammation: 42 Colloquium, 11-13, April 1991. Ed. by Helmut Sies et al. 1992. (Colloquium der Gesellschaft fur Biologische Chemie in Mosbach Baden Ser.: Vol. 42). (Illus.). 288p. 173.00 (*0-387-53654-X*) Spr-Verlag.

Molecular Aspects of Medicine, ser. vol. 2. H. Baum. 1979. (Molecular Aspects of Medicine Ser.). pap. 18.25 (*0-08-025888-3*, no. 6, Pergamon Pr) Elsevier.

Molecular Aspects of Medicine, Vol. 2. Ed. by H. Baum & J. Gergely. 1980. LC 80-40473. (Illus.). 453p. 85.00 (*0-08-026355-0*, Pergamon Pr) Elsevier.

Molecular Aspects of Medicine, Vol. 3, No. 6. 1981. pap. 14.50 (*0-08-027978-3*, Pergamon Pr) Elsevier.

Molecular Aspects of Medicine. Ed. by H. Baum et al. (Illus.). Vol. 4. 1982. 452p. 180.00 (*0-08-030007-3*); Vol. 5. 1983. 470p. 180.00 (*0-08-030429-X*); Vol. 6. 1984. 584p. 180.00 (*0-08-031724-3*) Elsevier (Pergamon Pr).

Molecular Aspects of Medicine, Vol. 7. Ed. by H. Baum et al. 1985. (Illus.). 554p. (*0-08-033239-0*, H210, H125) PPL GBR. *Dist:* Elsevier.

Molecular Aspects of Medicine Vol. 1: Complete. Ed. by H. Baum & J. Gergely. 1978. 600p. 85.00 (*0-08-020277-2*, Pergamon Pr) Elsevier.

Molecular Aspects of Monooxygenases & Bioactivation of Toxic Compounds. Ed. by Emel Arinc et al. 1991. (NATO Advanced Science Institutes Ser.: Vol. 202). (Illus.). 508p. (C). text 180.00 (*0-306-43823-2*, Kluwer Plenum) Kluwer Academic.

Molecular Aspects of Myeloid Stem Cell Development, No. 211. Ed. by L. Wolff & A. S. Perkins. 1995. (Current Topics in Microbiology & Immunology Ser.: Vol. 211). (Illus.). 298p. 152.00 (*3-540-60414-6*) Spr-Verlag.

Molecular Aspects of Oxidative Drug Metabolizing Enzymes: Their Signigicance in Environmental Toxicology, Chemical Carcinogenesis & Health. Ed. by Emel Arinc et al. 1995. LC 94-47314. (NATO ASI Ser.: Vol. 90). 614p. 312.00 (*3-540-58856-6*) Spr-Verlag.

Molecular Aspects of Picornavirus Infection & Detection. Ed. by Bert L. Semler & Ellie Ehrenfeld. 1989. (Illus.). 335p. text 79.95 (*1-55581-009-8*) ASM Pr.

Molecular Aspects of Placental & Fetal Autacoids. Ed. by Gregory E. Rice & Shaun P. Brennecke. 1993. LC 92-48814. 480p. 232.00 (*0-8493-6239-3*, QP281) CRC Pr.

Molecular Aspects of the Rheumatic Diseases. W. V. Williams. 1995. (Journal: Vol. 13, No. 2 - 3, 1994). (Illus.). 136p. pap. 36.75 (*3-8055-6136-9*) S Karger.

Molecular Bacteriology: Experimental & Diagnostic Applications. Ed. by Neil Woodford & Alan Johnson. 1998. (Methods in Molecular Medicine Ser.: Vol. 15). (Illus.). 675p. 79.50 (*0-89603-463-1*) Humana.

Molecular Bacteriology: Protocols & Clinical Applications. Ed. by Neil Woodford & Alan Johnson. 1998. LC 98-14185. (Methods in Molecular Medicine Ser.: Vol. 15). (Illus.). 692p. 135.00 (*0-89603-498-4*) Humana.

Molecular Bases of Anesthesia. Eric Moody & Phil Skolnick. 2000. LC 00-64136. (Pharmacology & Toxicology Ser.). (Illus.). 352p. 139.95 (*0-8493-8555-5*) CRC Pr.

Molecular Bases of Axonal Growth & Pathfinding. Ed. by U. Drescher et al. 1997. LC 97-40498. (Illus.). 296p. pap. 69.00 (*3-540-63522-X*) Spr-Verlag.

Molecular Basis of Aging. Ed. by Alvaro Macieira-Coelho. 1995. LC 95-15170. 576p. 199.95 (*0-8493-4786-6*, 4786) CRC Pr.

Molecular Basis of Autoimmune Hepatitis. Ian G. McFarlane. 1996. (Molecular Biology Intelligence Unit Ser.). 197p. 99.00 (*1-57059-339-6*) Landes Bioscience.

Molecular Basis of Axon Growth & Nerve Pattern Formation. Ed. by Hajime Fujisawa. 1997. LC 97-226309. (Taniguchi Symposia on Brain Sciences Ser.: Vol. 20, 1997). (Illus.). x, 280p. 259.25 (*3-8055-6587-9*) S Karger.

Molecular Basis of Bacterial Pathogenesis. Ed. by Barbara H. Iglewski & Virginia L. Clark. 1991. (Illus.). 473p. (C). pap. text 56.00 (*0-12-370390-5*) Acad Pr.

Molecular Basis of Blood Diseases. George Stamatoyannopoulos et al. 2nd ed. 1993. LC 92-48879. (Illus.). 752p. text 210.00 (*0-7216-4735-9*) Saunders.

Molecular Basis of Blood Diseases. George Stamatoyannopoulos. 3rd ed. 1999. LC 00-29714. 1028p. (C). text 336.25 (*0-7216-7671-5*) Saunders.

Molecular Basis of Cancer. Peter B. Farmer & John M. Walker. 1989. 358p. (Orig.). pap. 39.95 (*0-471-82755-X*) Krieger.

Molecular Basis of Cancer. Berk Mendelsohn et al. 2nd ed. 1999. LC 2001-20592. (Illus.). xvi, 691p. text 185.00 (*0-7216-7291-4*) Saunders.

Molecular Basis of Cardiology. Ed. by R. Roberts. 1992. (Molecular Basis of Clinical Medicine Ser.). (Illus.). 544p. pap. 49.95 (*0-86542-196-X*) Blackwell Sci.

Molecular Basis of Cardiovascular Disease: A Companion to Braunwald's Heart Disease. Kenneth R. Chien. Ed. by Richard Zorab. 1998. LC 98-34730. (Illus.). 592p. (C). text 135.00 (*0-7216-6401-6*) Saunders.

Molecular Basis of Cellular Defence Mechanisms. Gregory R. Bock & Jamie Goode. 1997. LC 96-43728. (CIBA Foundation Symposia Ser.: Vol. 204). 260p. 128.00 (*0-471-96567-7*) Wiley.

Molecular Basis of Dementia. Ed. by John Growdon et al. 2000. LC 00-48683. (Annals of the New York Academy of Sciences Ser.: Vol. 920). (Illus.). xii, 339p. 140.00 (*1-57331-283-5*) NY Acad Sci.

Molecular Basis of Dementia. John H. Growdon. 2000. LC 00-48683. (Annals of the New York Academy of Sciences Ser.: Vol. 920). (Illus.). xii, 339p. (*1-57331-284-3*) NY Acad Sci.

Molecular Basis of Human Cancer. Ed. by Claudio Nicolini. 1991. (NATO Advanced Science Institutes Ser.: Vol. 209). (Illus.). 224p. (C). text 114.00 (*0-306-44018-0*, Kluwer Plenum) Kluwer Academic.

Molecular Basis of Human Cancer: Genomic Instability & Molecular Mutation in Neoplastic Transformation. Ed. by William B. Coleman & Gregory J. Tsongalis. 2001. LC 2001-16560. (Illus.). 590p. 145.00 (*0-89603-634-0*) Humana.

Molecular Basis of Human Disease: And Approaches to Its Treatment. Wallace Snipes & Neena Agarwala. 1992. LC 92-38825. (Illus.). 310p. (C). pap. text 19.95 (*0-9612798-5-0*) Woodburn Pr.

Molecular Basis of Human Nutrition. Tom Sanders & Peter Emery. 2000. (Lifelines Ser.). (Illus.). 200p. pap. (*0-7484-0753-7*) Tay Francis Ltd GBR. *Dist:* Taylor & Francis.

Molecular Basis of Lymphokine Action. Ed. by David R. Webb et al. 1987. LC 87-26151. (Experimental Biology & Medicine Ser.: Vol. 18). 512p. 145.00 (*0-89603-139-X*) Humana.

Molecular Basis of Medical Cell Biology. Gerald M. Fuller et al. 1997. LC 98-125598. (Lange Medical Bks.). (Illus.). 231p. (C). pap. text 34.95 (*0-8385-1384-0*, A-1384-5, Apple Lange Med) McGraw.

Molecular Basis of Medicine. Arthur M. Feldman & Daug. 1993. 700p. 49.00 (*1-55664-169-9*) Mosby Inc.

Molecular Basis of Neurological Disorders & Their Treatment. Ed. by A. Albano et al. 1991. (Illus.). 264p. (C). (gr. 13). pap. text 197.95 (*0-412-40410-9*, A6117) Chapman & Hall.

Molecular Basis of Neuropharmacology: A Foundation for Clinical Neuroscience. Steven E. Hyman et al. 2001. LC 00-51549. (Illus.). 539p. pap. 49.95 (*0-8385-6379-1*) McGraw-Hill Prof.

Molecular Basis of Oncology. Ed. by Emil J. Freireich & Sanford A. Stass. 1995. LC 94-43841. (Molecular Basis of Clinical Medicine Ser.). 300p. pap. 59.95 (*0-86542-254-0*) Blackwell Sci.

Molecular Basis of Oxidation Damage by Leukocytes. Algirdas J. Jesaitis. 1992. 368p. 129.00 (*0-8493-6363-2*, OR185) CRC Pr.

Molecular Basis of Reproductive Endocrinology. Ed. by Peter C. Leung et al. 1992. LC 92-2304. (Serono Symposia Ser.). (Illus.). 311p. 130.00 (*0-387-97861-5*); 312p. (*3-540-97861-5*) Spr-Verlag.

Molecular Basis of Sex & Differentiation: A Comparative Study of Evolution, Mechanism & Control in Microorganisms. Milton H. Saier, Jr. & G. R. Jacobson. 1984. (Illus.). 216p. 105.00 (*0-387-96007-4*) Spr-Verlag.

Molecular Basis of Sex Hormone Receptor Function: New Targets for Intervention. H. Gronemeyer et al. 1998. LC 98-26256. (Ernst Schering Research Foundation Ser.). (Illus.). 250p. 79.00 (*3-540-64702-3*) Spr-Verlag.

Molecular Basis of Smell & Taste Transduction - Symposium No. 179. Ed. by Derek J. Chadwick et al. 1993. LC 93-28783. (CIBA Foundation Symposia Ser.: No. 179). 298p. 128.00 (*0-471-93946-3*) Wiley.

Molecular Basis of Thrombosis & Hemostasis. Ed. by Katherine A. High & Harold R. Roberts. 1995. LC 94-43114. (Illus.). 688p. text 225.00 (*0-8247-9501-6*) Dekker.

Molecular Basis of Viral & Microbial Pathogenesis. R. Rott & W. Goebel. 1988. (Colloquium der Gesellschaft fur Biologische Chemie in Mosbach Baden Ser.: Vol. 38). (Illus.). 185p. 69.00 (*0-387-18606-9*) Spr-Verlag.

Molecular Basis of Viral Replication. Ed. by R. Perez Bercoff. 1987. LC 87-15226. (NATO ASI Series A, Life Sciences: Vol. 136). (Illus.). 594p. 135.00 (*0-306-42619-6*, Plenum Trade) Perseus Pubng.

Molecular Biochemistry of Human Diseases, Vol. 1. Felix A. De La Iglesia. Ed. by George Feuer. 1985. LC 84-7156. 240p. 133.00 (*0-8493-6205-9*, RC627, CRC Reprint) Franklin.

Molecular Biochemistry of Human Diseases. George Feuer & Felix De La Iglesia. LC 84-7156. Vol. II. 1986. 272p. 145.00 (*0-8493-6206-7*, RB112, CRC Reprint); Vol. 3. 1990. 384p. 231.00 (*0-8493-6207-5*, RB112) Franklin.

Molecular Biological Clinical Medicine. Ralph C. Williams. 1992. (C). pap. text 79.95 (*0-8385-6213-2*, A6213-1, Apple Lange Med) McGraw.

***Molecular Biological Techniques as a Tool in Diagnostic Pathology: Applications in B-Cell Lymphoproliferative Disease, Medullary Thyroid Carcinoma & Cervical Carcinoma.** Mansour Alemi. 2000. (Comprehensive Summaries of Uppsala Dissertations from the Faculty of Medicine Ser.: No. 909). (Illus.). 61p. pap. (*91-554-4658-2*) Uppsala Universitet SWE. *Dist:* Coronet Bks.

Molecular Biology & Biotechnology: A Comprehensive Desk Reference. Ed. by R. A. Meyers. 1995. 1072p. pap. 150.00 (*0-471-18634-1*) Wiley.

Molecular Biology & Cell Regulation of the Placenta. Ed. by Richard K. Miller & Henry A. Thiede. 1991. (Trophoblast Research Ser.: Vol. 5). (Illus.). 488p. (C). 85.00 (*0-9630864-0-5*) Verav Med.

Molecular Biology & Its Application to Medical Mycology. Ed. by Bruno Maresca et al. 1993. LC 92-49124. (NATO ASI Ser.: Vol. 69). (*3-540-54609-X*); 257p. 212.00 (*0-387-54609-X*) Spr-Verlag.

Molecular Biology & Physiology of Insulin & Insulin-Like Growth Factors. Ed. by Mohan K. Raizada & D. LeRoith. 1991. (Advances in Experimental Medicine & Biology Ser.: Vol. 293). (Illus.). 498p. (C). text 186.00 (*0-306-43928-X*, Kluwer Plenum) Kluwer Academic.

Molecular Biology Approach to the Neurosciences. Ed. by Hermona Soreq. 1984. LC 84-7341. (IBRO Handbook Ser.: No. 1-569). 270p. pap. 315.00 (*0-471-90437-6*) Wiley.

Molecular Biology for Obstetricians & Gynecologists. P. R. Bennett & G. E. Moore. 1991. (Illus.). 192p. 75.00 (*0-632-02744-4*) Blackwell Sci.

Molecular Biology for Oncologists. John Yarnold. 2nd ed. 1996. LC 96-84903. pap. 44.95 (*0-412-71270-9*, Y0202) Chapman & Hall.

Molecular Biology in Blood Transfusion. C. Th. Smit Sibinga & Harvey G. Klein. 2000. (Developments in Hematology & Immunology Ser.). 296p. 125.00 (*0-7923-6534-8*) Kluwer Academic.

Molecular Biology in Cancer Medicine. Ed. by Razelle Kurzrock & Moshe Talpaz. 2nd ed. 1999. 679p. (*1-85317-676-1*) Martin Dunitz.

Molecular Biology in Cancer Medicine. Razelle Kurzrock & Moshe Talpaz. 1995. (Illus.). 456p. text 89.50 (*0-19-521173-1*) OUP.

Molecular Biology in Critical Medicine. Reed E. Pyeritz. 1995. pap. text 30.00 (*0-07-051102-0*) McGraw.

***Molecular Biology in Health Sciences: Index of New Information with Authors & Subjects.** Ed. by Research and Development Division Staff & John C. Bartone. 2001. 185p. 47.50 (*0-7883-2318-0*); pap. 44.50 (*0-7883-2319-9*) ABBE Pubs Assn.

Molecular Biology in Histopathology. Ed. by John Croaker. 1994. LC 93-50921. (Molecular Medical Science Ser.). 190p. 190.00 (*0-471-94093-3*) Wiley.

Molecular Biology in Medicine. Timothy M. Cox & John Sinclair. 1997. LC 96-21997. (Illus.). 384p. pap. 77.95 (*0-632-02785-1*) Blackwell Sci.

Molecular Biology in Medicine: A Practical Guide for the Health Care Physician. Timothy L. Reudelhuber & Christian Deschepper. Date not set. (*0-8247-9411-7*) Dekker.

Molecular Biology in Toxicology. Ed. by Alvaro Puga & Kendall Wallace. 1998. LC 98-17547. 582p. text 135.00 (*1-56032-592-5*) Hemisp Pub.

Molecular Biology of Adenoviruses. L. Philipson et al. 1975. LC 75-6658. (Virology Monographs: Vol. 14). (Illus.). iv, 115p. 47.00 (*0-387-81284-9*) Spr-Verlag.

Molecular Biology of Alzheimer's Disease. Ed. by Caleb E. Finch & Peter Davies. 1988. (Current Communications in Molecular Biology Ser.). (Illus.). 197p. (C). pap. text 25.00 (*0-87969-319-3*) Cold Spring Harbor.

Molecular Biology of Alzheimer's Disease: Genes & Mechanisms Involved in Amyloid Generation. Christian Haass. 1998. (Illus.). 330p. text 120.00 (*90-5702-381-4*) Gordon & Breach.

Molecular Biology of Autoimmune Disease. Ed. by A. G. Demaine et al. 1990. (NATO ASI Ser.: Vol. 38). (Illus.). 404p. 159.00 (*0-387-51771-5*) Spr-Verlag.

Molecular Biology of B-Cell & T-Cell Development. John G. Moore & Ellen Rothenberg. 1998. LC 98-12613. (Contemporary Immunology Ser.). (Illus.). 608p. 185.00 (*0-89603-536-0*) Humana.

Molecular Biology of Cancer. Finlay J. MacDonald & C. Ford. 1996. (Medical Perspectives Ser.). (Illus.). 160p. (Orig.). pap. text (*1-85996-225-4*) Bios Sci GBR. *Dist:* Bks Intl VA.

Molecular Biology of Cardiac Development & Growth. Paul Barton et al. 1995. LC 95-31277. (Molecular Biology Intelligence Unit Ser.). 268p. 99.00 (*1-57059-302-7*) Landes Bioscience.

Molecular Biology of Cell Determination & Cell Differentiation. L. W. Browder. 1988. LC 85-3406. (Developmental Biology Ser.). (Illus.). 460p. (C). text 105.00 (*0-306-42735-4*, Kluwer Plenum) Kluwer Academic.

Molecular Biology of Diabetes Pt. I: Autoimmunity & Genetics; Insulin Synthesis & Secretion. Ed. by Boris Draznin & Derek LeRoith. 1994. LC 94-27263. (Illus.). 424p. text 145.00 (*0-89603-286-8*) Humana.

Molecular Biology of Diabetes Pt. II: Insulin Action, Effects on Gene Expression & Regulation & Glucose Transport. Ed. by Boris Draznin & Derek Le Roith. 1994. LC 94-27263. (Illus.). 568p. 145.00 (*0-89603-287-6*) Humana.

Molecular Biology of Digestive Diseases. Ed. by Philip Quirke. 1994. 128p. pap. text (*0-7279-0827-8*) BMJ Pub GBR. *Dist:* AIDC.

Molecular Biology of DNA Methylation. R. L. Adams & R. H. Burdon. 1985. (Molecular Biology, Biochemistry & Biophysics Ser.). (Illus.). 257p. 96.00 (*0-387-96161-5*) Spr-Verlag.

***Molecular Biology of Down Syndrome.** Ed. by G. Lubec. 1999. (Journals of Neural Transmission: Suppl. 57). (Illus.). 350p. pap. 102.00 (*3-211-83377-3*) Spr-Verlag.

Molecular Biology of Erythropoiesis. Ed. by J. L. Ascensao et al. 1989. (Advances in Experimental Medicine & Biology Ser.: Vol. 271). (Illus.). 240p. 79.50 (*0-306-43532-2*, Plenum Trade) Perseus Pubng.

Molecular Biology of Hematopoiesis. Ed. by L. Sachs et al. 1992. 650p. (C). lib. bdg. (*0-946707-30-8*) Intercept UK GBR. *Dist:* Spr-Verlag.

***Molecular Biology of Hematopoiesis & Treatment of Leukemia & Cancer: 13th Symposium, New York, N. Y., July 2000 - Proceedings.** Ed. by N. G. Abraham et al. 2001. (Acta Haematologica Ser.: Vol. 105, No. 3). (Illus.). 78p. pap. 25.25 (*3-8055-7273-5*) S Karger.

Molecular Biology of Hematopoiesis & Treatment of Leukemia & Cancer: 13th Symposium, New York, N.Y., July 2000: Abstracts. Ed. by N. G. Abraham et al. 2000. (Acta Haematologica Ser.: Vol. 103). vi, 116p. pap. 39.25 (*3-8055-7113-5*) S Karger.

Molecular Biology of Hematopoiesis & Treatment of Leukemias & Lymphomas: 10th Symposium, Hamburg, July 1997 - Proceedings. Ed. by N. G. Abraham et al. 1998. (Acta Haematologica Ser.: Vol. 90, No. 3, 1998). (Illus.). 76p. pap. 43.50 (*3-8055-6681-6*) S Karger.

Molecular Biology of Hematopoiesis & Treatment of Leukemias & Lymphomas: 10th Symposium, Hamburg, July 1997: Abstracts. Ed. by N. G. Abraham et al. 1997. (Acta Haematologica Ser.: Vol. 98, Suppl. 1, 1997). vi, 128p. pap. 48.75 (*3-8055-6550-X*) S Karger.

Molecular Biology of Hematopoiesis & Treatment of Myeloproliferative Diseases: 11th Symposium, Bornio, June 1998 - Abstracts. Ed. by N. G. Abraham et al. 1998. (Acta Haematologica Ser.: Vol. 100, Suppl. 1). iv, 72p. pap. 33.25 (*3-8055-6729-4*) S Karger.

Molecular Biology of Hematopoiesis 5. Ed. by Nader G. Abraham et al. 1996. (Illus.). 737p. (C). text 179.00 (*0-306-45318-5*, Kluwer Plenum) Kluwer Academic.

Molecular Biology of Hematopoiesis Proceedings: Proceedings. Ed. by Nader G. Abraham et al. 1996. (Acta Haematologica Ser.: Vol. 95, No. 3-4, 1996). (Illus.). iv, 128p. pap. 44.00 (*3-8055-6319-1*) S Karger.

Molecular Biology of Hemopoesis. Ed. by M. Tavassaoli et al. 1988. LC 88-28836. (Advances in Experimental Medicine & Biology Ser.: Vol. 241). (Illus.). 350p. 89.50 (*0-306-43022-3*, Plenum Trade) Perseus Pubng.

Molecular Biology of HIV & AIDS. Ed. by A. M. Lever. 1996. LC 95-19768. (Molecular Medical Science Ser.). 232p. 137.95 (*0-471-96094-2*) Wiley.

Molecular Biology of Human Hepatitis Viruses. J. Monjardino. 1997. LC 98-214266. 150p. text 24.00 (*1-86094-048-X*) World Scientific Pub.

Molecular Biology of Insect Disease Vectors: A Methods Manual. Ed. by Julian M. Crampton et al. 1996. LC 96-70874. (Illus.). 416p. pap. (*0-412-73660-8*) Kluwer Academic.

Molecular Biology of Iridoviruses. Ed. by Gholamreza Daria. 1989. (Developments in Molecular Virology Ser.). text 210.50 (*0-7923-0506-X*) Kluwer Academic.

Molecular Biology of Lung Disease. Ed. by Peter J. Barnes & Robert A. Stockley. 1994. LC 93-28488. (Illus.). 384p. 125.00 (*0-632-03344-4*) Blackwell Sci.

Molecular Biology of Multiple Sclerosis. W. C. Russell. 1997. LC 96-9436. 320p. 235.00 (*0-471-96966-4*) Wiley.

Molecular Biology of Neuropsychiatric Disease. Ed. by F. Owen. 1993. LC 93-31644. (Molecular & Cell Biology of Human Diseases Ser.). (Illus.). 220p. (C). (gr. 13). pap. text 143.95 (*0-412-47800-5*) Chapman & Hall.

Molecular Biology of Neuroreceptors & Ion Channels. Ed. by A. Maelicke. 1989. (NATO ASI Ser.: Vol. 32). (Illus.). 675p. 252.00 (*0-387-50380-3*) Spr-Verlag.

Molecular Biology of Opportunistic Infections in AIDS. Ed. by S. Myint & Alan Cann. 1992. (Molecular & Cell Biology of Human Diseases Ser.). (Illus.). 320p. (C). (gr. 13). pap. text 155.95 (*0-412-45330-4*, A7991) Chapman & Hall.

Molecular Biology of Paget's Disease. P. Sharpe. 1996. (Medical Intelligence Unit Ser.). 200p. (C). pap. 89.95 (*0-412-10731-7*) Chapman & Hall.

Molecular Biology of Paget's Disease. Paul T. Sharpe. 1996. LC 96-3238. (Medical Intelligence Unit Ser.). 214p. 99.00 (*1-57059-388-4*) Landes Bioscience.

Molecular Biology of Steroid & Nuclear Hormone Receptors. Leonard P. Freedman. Ed. by M. Karin. 1997. LC 97-21837. (Progress in Gene Expression Ser.). (Illus.). 272p. 109.00 (*0-8176-3952-7*) Birkhauser.

Molecular Biology of the Cell. Bruce Alberts et al. 3rd rev. ed. 1994. LC 93-45907. (Illus.). 1408p. text 73.95 (*0-8153-1619-4*); pap. text 63.00 (*0-8153-1620-8*) Garland.

Molecular Biology of the Cytoskeleton. Ed. by Gary G. Borisy et al. 1984. LC 84-17566. 512p. 62.00 (*0-87969-174-3*) Cold Spring Harbor.

Molecular Biology of the Female Reproduction System. Ed. by J. K. Findlay. 1994. LC 93-30113. (Illus.). 457p. text 99.00 (*0-12-256365-4*) Acad Pr.

Molecular Biology of the Gene, Vol. II. James Dewey Watson et al. 4th rev. ed. 1987. (Molecular Biology of the Gene Ser.: Vol. II). (Illus.). 419p. (C). text 67.00 (*0-8053-9613-6*) Benjamin-Cummings.

Molecular Biology of the Hepatitis B Virus. Alan McLachlan. 1991. (Illus.). 312p. lib. bdg. 229.00 (*0-8493-5516-8*, QR749) CRC Pr.

Molecular Biology of the Human Brain. Ed. by Edward G. Jones. 1988. 212p. (C). lib. bdg. 48.00 (*0-8451-2671-7*) Krieger.

Molecular Biology of the Islets of Langerhans. Ed. by Hiroshi Okamoto. 1990. (Illus.). 362p. (C). text 90.00 (*0-521-36204-0*) Cambridge U Pr.

Molecular Biology of the Lung R. A. Stockley. 1998. LC 98-36983. (Respiratory Pharmacology & Pharmacotherapy Ser.). 650p. (C). (*3-7643-5969-2*) Birkhauser CHE. *Dist:* Spr-Verlag.

Molecular Biology of the Lung. Robert Stockley. 1998. LC 98-36983. (Respiratory Pharmacology & Pharmacotherapy Ser.). 195.00 (*0-8176-5968-4*) Birkhauser.

Molecular Biology of the Lung Vol. 1: Emphysema & Infection. R. A. Stockley. 1999. (Respiratory Pharmacology & Pharmacotherapy Ser.). 224p. 195.00 (*3-7643-5857-2*) Birkhauser.

Molecular Biology of the Lung Vol. II: Asthma & Cancer. R. A. Stockley. 1998. LC 98-36983. (Respiratory Pharmacology & Pharmacotherapy Ser.). 216p. (C). (*3-7643-5968-4*) Birkhauser CHE. *Dist:* Spr-Verlag.

Molecular Biology of the Male Reproductive System. Ed. by D. M. De Kretser. 1993. LC 93-17236. (Illus.). 483p. text 99.00 (*0-12-209030-6*) Acad Pr.

Molecular Biology of the Neuron. Ed. by R. Wayne Davies & Brian J. Morris. 1998. (Molecular & Cellular Neurobiology Ser.). (Illus.). 416p. text 95.00 (*1-85996-240-8*) OUP.

Molecular Biology of the Skin: The Keratinocyte. Ed. by Michel Darmon & M. Blumenberg. 1993. LC 92-48406. (Illus.). 291p. text 99.00 (*0-12-203455-4*) Acad Pr.

Molecular Biotechnology: Therapeutic Applications & Strategies. Sunil Maulik & Salil Patel. 1996. LC 96-2733. 223p. pap. 74.95 (*0-471-11681-5*, Wiley-Liss) Wiley.

Molecular Cardiology for the Cardiologist. Bernard Swynghedauw. (Developments in Cardiovascular Medicine Ser.). 2nd ed. 1998. LC 98-40587. 301p. (*0-7923-8323-0*); No. 172. 1995. LC 95-21870. 272p. (C). text 109.00 (*0-7923-3622-4*) Kluwer Academic.

Molecular Cell Biology. H. Lodish & J. E. Darnell. 3rd ed. 1995. (C). pap. text, stu. ed. 27.95 (*0-7167-2672-6*); pap. text, tchr. ed., suppl. ed. 11.95 (*0-7167-2703-X*) W H Freeman.

Molecular, Cellular & Clinical Aspects of Angiogenesis: Proceedings of a NATO ASI Held in Porto Carras, Halkidiki, Greece, June 16-27, 1995, Vol. A285. Ed. by Michael Maragoudakis. 1996. LC 96-21623. (NATO ASI Series A: Vol. 285). (Illus.). 302p. 126.00 (*0-306-45315-0*) Plenum.

Molecular Components of Hepatitis B Virus. Mark A. Feitelson. 1985. (Developments in Molecular Virology Ser.). text 91.00 (*0-89838-696-9*) Kluwer Academic.

Molecular Control of Haemopoiesis - Symposium No. 148. CIBA Foundation Staff. 1990. LC 89-24869. (CIBA Foundation Symposia Ser.: No. 148). 242p. 128.00 (*0-471-92561-6*) Wiley.

Molecular Design & Modeling - Concepts & Applications Pt. B: Antibodies & Antigens, Nucleic Acids, Polysaccharides, & Drugs. Ed. by John N. Abelson et al. 1991. (Methods in Enzymology Ser.: Vol. 203). (Illus.). 764p. text 136.00 (*0-12-182104-8*) Acad Pr.

Molecular Diagnosis. S. Jeffery et al. 1999. (Medical Perspectives Ser.). (Illus.). 134p. pap. 36.95 (*0-387-91511-7*) Spr-Verlag.

Molecular Diagnosis & Treatment of Melanoma. John M. Kirkwood. 1998. LC 97-52827. (Illus.). 330p. text 150.00 (*0-8247-0102-X*) Dekker.

Molecular Diagnosis of Cancer. Ed. by Finbarr Cotter. 1996. (Methods in Molecular Medicine Ser.: Vol. 6). (Illus.). 236p. 99.50 (*0-89603-341-4*) Humana.

Molecular Diagnosis of Genetic Diseases. Ed. by Rob Elles. 1996. (Methods in Molecular Medicine Ser.: Vol. 5). (Illus.). 372p. 99.50 (*0-89603-346-5*) Humana.

Molecular Diagnosis of Genetic Diseases. Ed. by Rob Elles & Roger Mountford. 2nd ed. 2001. (Methods in Molecular Medicine Ser.). 700p. 125.00 (*0-89603-932-3*) Humana.

Molecular Diagnostic Methods for Infectious Diseases: Approved Guideline, (1995) Contrib. by Russel K. Enns. 1995. 75.00 (*1-56238-288-8*, MM3-A) NCCLS.

Molecular Diagnostics: For the Clinical Laboratorian. Ed. by William B. Coleman & Gregory J. Tsongalis. 1996. LC 96-37505. (Pathology & Laboratory Medicine Ser.: Vol. 1). (Illus.). 400p. 99.50 (*0-89603-373-2*) Humana.

Molecular Diagnostics: Research Towards Application. Ed. by Ralph Rapley & Matthew R. Walker. 1993. LC 92-43669. (Illus.). 480p. 125.00 (*0-632-03528-5*) Blackwell Sci.

Molecular Diagnostics of Human Cancer. Ed. by Mark Furth & Melvyn Greaves. 1989. (Cancer Cells Ser.: No. 7). (Illus.). 414p. 95.00 (*0-87969-324-X*) Cold Spring Harbor.

Molecular Diagnostics of Infectious Diseases. Ed. by Udo Reischl. 1997. (Methods in Molecular Medicine Ser.: Vol. 13). (Illus.). 648p. spiral bd. 109.50 (*0-89603-398-8*) Humana.

Molecular Diversity & Combinatorial Chemistry: Libraries & Drug Discovery. Ed. by Irwin M. Chaiken & Kim D. Janda. 1996. (ACS Conference Proceedings Ser.). (Illus.). 336p. text 115.00 (*0-8412-3450-7*) Am Chemical.

Molecular Diversity in Drug Design. Ed. by Philip M. Dean & Richard A. Lewis. 253p. text 150.00 (*0-7923-5980-1*) Kluwer Academic.

Molecular Dosimetry & Human Cancer: Analytical, Epidemiological, & Social Considerations. John D. Groopman & Paul L. Skipper. 1991. 488p. 119.00 (*0-8493-8800-7*, RC268) CRC Pr.

Molecular Dynamics in Biological Membranes. Milton H. Saier, Jr. & C. D. Stiles. 1975. LC 75-12923. (Heidelberg Science Library: Vol. 22). (Illus.). 129p. (Orig.). 54.95 (*0-387-90142-6*) Spr-Verlag.

Molecular Dynamics in the Developing Drosophila Eye. Daisuke Yamamoto. 1996. (Molecular Biology Intelligence Unit Ser.). (Illus.). 197p. (C). pap. 89.95 (*0-412-11321-X*) Chapman & Hall.

Molecular Endocrinology: Genetic Analysis of Hormones & Their Receptors. Ed. by G. Rumsby & S. Farrow. 1997. (Human Molecular Genetics Ser.). (Illus.). 300p. (*1-85996-235-1*) Bios Sci GBR. *Dist:* Bks Intl VA.

Molecular Endocrinology of Cancer. Ed. by Jonathan Waxman. 1996. (Cancer Ser.). (Illus.). 440p. (C). text 100.00 (*0-521-46067-0*) Cambridge U Pr.

Molecular Epidemiology: Principles & Practices. Ed. by Paul A. Schulte & Frederica Perera. 1998. (Illus.). 588p. pap. text 49.95 (*0-12-632346-1*) Morgan Kaufmann.

Molecular Epidemiology of Tropical Diseases: Hemoparasites & Their Vectors. Ed. by Frans Jongejan et al. 1998. LC 98-13136. (Annals of the New York Academy of Sciences Ser.: Vol. 849). 503p. 140.00 (*1-57331-141-3*); 550p. pap. 140.00 (*1-57331-142-1*) NY Acad Sci.

Molecular Evolution of Chromosomes. Michele Calos. 2000. (Illus.). 300p. 50.00 (*0-19-509957-5*) OUP.

Molecular Evolution of Physiological Processes: Proceedings: Symposium on Molecular Evolution of Physiological Process (47th: 1993: Woods Hole, Mass.) Ed. by Douglas M. Fambrough. 1995. LC 94-65642. (Society of General Physiologists Ser.: Vol. 49). 297p. pap. 50.00 (*0-87470-055-8*) Rockefeller.

Molecular Evolutionary Genetics. R. J. MacIntyre. 1985. LC 85-19312. (Monographs in Evolutionary Biology). (Illus.). 632p. (C). text 135.00 (*0-306-42042-2*, Kluwer Plenum) Kluwer Academic.

Molecular Foundations of Psychiatry. Steven E. Hyman & Eric J. Nestler. 1992. LC 92-7017. 239p. text 41.95 (*0-88048-353-9*, 8353) Am Psychiatric.

Molecular Genetic Medicine, Vol. 4. Ed. by Theodore Friedmann. 1994. (Illus.). 188p. text 67.00 (*0-12-462004-3*) Acad Pr.

Molecular Genetic Studies of Three Autosomal Recessive Disorders: Sjogren-Larsson Syndrome, Glutathione Synthetase Deficiency & Congenital Ichthyosis. Maritta Pigg. 2000. (Comprehensive Summaries of Uppsala Dissertations from the Faculty of Medicine Ser.: No. 928). (Illus.). 56p. pap. (*91-554-4718-X*) Uppsala Universitet SWE. *Dist:* Coronet Bks.

Molecular Genetics. J. T. Hancock. 1999. LC 99-15300. (Biomedical Sciences Explained Ser.). (Illus.). 200p. pap. (*0-7506-3253-4*) E A GBR. *Dist:* OUP.

Molecular Genetics & Colorectal Neoplasia: A Primer for the Clinician. James M. Church et al. 1996. LC 96-13339. (Illus.). 128p. pap. 39.95 (*0-89640-299-1*) Igaku-Shoin.

Molecular Genetics & Gene Therapy of Cardiovascular Diseases. Ed. by Stephen C. Mockrin. 1996. LC 95-25992. (Fundamental & Clinical Cardiology Ser.: Vol. 26). (Illus.). 616p. text 235.00 (*0-8247-9408-7*) Dekker.

Molecular Genetics & Therapy of Leukemia. Ed. by Emil J. Freireich & Hagop Kantarjian. 1996. LC 96-4656. (Cancer Treatment & Research Ser.: Vol. 84). 352p. (C). text 278.50 (*0-7923-3912-6*) Kluwer Academic.

Molecular Genetics, Biochemistry & Clinical Aspects of Inherited Disorders of Purine & Pyrimidine Metabolism. Ed. by U. Gresser. 1993. (Illus.). 210p. (*3-540-56774-7*) Spr-Verlag.

Molecular Genetics for the Clinician. D. J. Brock. 1993. LC 92-9574. (Illus.). 301p. (C). text 85.00 (*0-521-41179-3*); pap. text 31.95 (*0-521-42325-2*) Cambridge U Pr.

Molecular Genetics in Diagnosis & Research. Ed. by Robert W. Allen & James P. AuBuchon. 1995. LC 95-35428. (Illus.). 161p. (C). 45.00 (*1-56395-044-8*) Am Assn Blood.

Molecular Genetics in Hearing Research. Ed. by Matthew C. Holley & Marcelo N. Rivolta. 1997. (Journal: Vol. 2, Nos. 1 & 2, 1997). (Illus.). iv, 112p. pap. 61.00 (*3-8055-6475-9*) S Karger.

Molecular Genetics in Hypertension. Florent Soubrier. 1997. (Medical Intelligence Unit Ser.). 250p. 89.95 (*0-412-13081-5*) Chapman & Hall.

Molecular Genetics in Surgical Oncology. J. F. Moley. 1994. (Medical Intelligence Unit Ser.). 115p. 99.00 (*1-879702-18-5*) Landes Bioscience.

Molecular Genetics of Biological Rhythms. Ed. by Michael W. Young. 1992. LC 92-29091. (Cellular Clocks Ser.: Vol. 4). (Illus.). 336p. text 165.00 (*0-8247-8774-9*) Dekker.

***Molecular Genetics of Cancer.** Ed. by John K. Cowell. 2nd ed. 2001. 550p. 120.00 (*0-12-150100-0*) Acad Pr.

Molecular Genetics of Coronary Artery Disease: Candidate Genes & Processes in Atherosclerosis. Ed. by Robert S. Sparkes et al. 1992. (Monographs in Human Genetics: Vol. 14). (Illus.). xviii, 454p. 278.50 (*3-8055-5558-X*) S Karger.

Molecular Genetics of Endocrine Disorders. Ed. by R. V. Thakker. 1997. LC 97-66898. (Illus.). 508p. (*0-412-58970-2*) E A GBR. *Dist:* OUP.

Molecular Genetics of Haemostasis & Its Inherited Disorders. Edward G. Tuddenham & David N. Cooper. 1994. (Oxford Monographs on Medical Genetics: No. 25). (Illus.). 604p. text 145.00 (*0-19-261661-7*) OUP.

Molecular Genetics of Human Inherited Disease. Ed. by Duncan J. Shaw. 1995. LC 95-10485. (Molecular Medical Science Ser.). 260p. 147.50 (*0-471-93459-3*) Wiley.

Molecular Genetics of Inherited Eye Disorders. Ed. by Alan F. Wright & Barrie Jay. 1994. (Modern Genetics Ser.: Vol. 2). (Illus.). xiv, 528p. text 116.00 (*3-7186-5493-8*) Gordon & Breach.

Molecular Genetics of Muscle Disease: Duchenne & Other Dystrophies. Ed. by A. J. Buller et al. 1989. (Illus.). 222p. text (*0-443-04199-7*) Church.

Molecular Genetics of Pediatric Solid Tumors: Basic Concepts & Recent Advances. Ed. by Gian P. Tonini et al. 1992. LC 91-35383. xiv, 382p. text 132.00 (*3-7186-5080-0*) Gordon & Breach.

Molecular Genetics of Sex Determination. Ed. by Stephen S. Wachtel. 1993. LC 93-8302. (Illus.). 518p. text 99.00 (*0-12-728960-7*) Acad Pr.

Molecular Genetics of X-Linked Alport Syndrome. Caiying Guo. 1995. (Acta Biomedica Lovaniensia Ser.: Vol. 109). (Illus.). v, 85p. (Orig.). pap. (*90-6186-681-2*) Leuven Univ BEL. *Dist:* Coronet Bks.

Molecular Gerontology: Research Status & Strategies. Ed. by Suresh I. Rattan & Olivier Toussaint. 1997. LC 96-37284. 224p. (C). text 69.50 (*0-306-45491-2*, Kluwer Plenum) Kluwer Academic.

Molecular Haematology. Ed. by Andrew Provan & John Gribbin. 2000. LC 99-16528. (Illus.). xv, 240p. 208.95 (*0-632-05037-3*) Blackwell Sci.

Molecular Immunological Considerations in Malaria Vaccine Development. Michael F. Good. 1993. 288p. 179.00 (*0-8493-5258-4*, QR189) CRC Pr.

Molecular Immunology. Ed. by B. David Hames & David M. Glover. 2nd ed. 1996. (Frontiers in Molecular Biology Ser.). (Illus.). 404p. (C). text 115.00 (*0-19-963379-7*) OUP.

Molecular Immunology: A Textbook. Ed. by M. Zouhair Atassi et al. 1984. (Immunology Ser.: 22). (Illus.). 744p. text 95.00 (*0-8247-7045-5*, 7045-5) Dekker.

Molecular Immunology of Complex Carbohydrates. Ed. by A. M. Wu. 1988. LC 88-2532. (Advances in Experimental Medicine & Biology Ser.: Vol. 228). (Illus.). 882p. 165.00 (*0-306-42818-0*, Plenum Trade) Perseus Pubng.

Molecular Investigation of Mucopolysaccharidosis Type II (Hunter Syndrome) in Man. Stanislav L. Karsten. 2000. (Comprehensive Summaries of Uppsala Dissertations from the Faculty of Medicine Ser.: No. 938). (Illus.). 55p. pap. (*91-554-4746-5*) Uppsala Universitet SWE. *Dist:* Coronet Bks.

Molecular Mechanics & Conformational Analysis in Drug Design. Gyorgy M. Keseru & Istvan Kolossvary. 1999. LC 98-42144. (Illus.). 136.95 (*0-632-05289-9*) Blackwell Sci.

Molecular Mechanisms in Astroglia. Elisabeth Hansson. 1997. (Neuroscience Intelligence Unit Ser.). 250p. pap. 89.95 (*0-412-13471-3*) Chapman & Hall.

***Molecular Mechanisms in Cervical Carcinogenesis: Studies of Clonality, Somatic Genetic Alterations & Human Papillomavirus Variants in Cervical Pre-Invasive & Invasive Cancer.** Zhonhmin Guo. 2000. (Comprehensive Summaries of Uppsala Dissertations from the Faculty of Medicine Ser.: No. 920). (Illus.). 60p. pap. (*91-554-4698-1*) Uppsala Universitet SWE. *Dist:* Coronet Bks.

Molecular Mechanisms in Secretions. Ed. by Niels A. Thorn et al. 1988. (Alfred Benzon Symposium Ser.: No. 25). (Illus.). 668p. 175.00 (*87-16-06953-6*) Coronet Bks.

Molecular Mechanisms in Striated Muscle. S. V. Perry. 1996. (Lezioni Lincee Lectures). (Illus.). 178p. (C). pap. text 21.95 (*0-521-57916-3*) Cambridge U Pr.

Molecular Mechanisms of Adrenal Steroidogenesis & Aspects of Regulation & Application. Ed. by Klaus Ruckpaul & Horst Rein. 1991. (Frontiers in Biotransformation Ser.: Vol. 3). 251p. (*0-7484-0025-7*) Tay Francis Ltd GBR. *Dist:* Taylor & Francis.

Molecular Mechanisms of Aging. Ed. by F. Gotthard Schettler & K. Beyreuther. 1990. (Sitzungsberichte der Heidelberger Akademie der Wissenschaften Ser., Mathematisch-Naturwissenschaftliche Klasse, Jahrgang 1991: Suppl. 2). (Illus.). 206p. 36.00 (*0-387-52732-X*) Spr-Verlag.

Molecular Mechanisms of Alcohol: Neurobiology & Metabolism. Ed. by Grace Y. Sun et al. 1989. LC 89-19848. (Experimental Biology & Medicine Ser.: Vol. 21). 411p. 119.50 (*0-89603-170-5*) Humana.

Molecular Mechanisms of Cancer Predisposition. Neil F. Sullivan & Anne E. Willis. 1994. LC 94-38487. (Molecular Biology Intelligence Unit Ser.). 150p. 99.00 (*1-57059-193-8*) Landes Bioscience.

Molecular Mechanisms of Dementia. Ed. by Wilma Wasco & Rudolph Tanzi. 1996. LC 96-38858. (Contemporary Neuroscience Ser.). (Illus.). 328p. 145.00 (*0-89603-371-6*) Humana.

Molecular Mechanisms of Drug Action. Christopher J. Coulson. 2nd ed. 1993. LC 93-32329. 300p. (*0-7484-0068-0*); pap. (*0-7484-0078-8*) Tay Francis Ltd GBR. *Dist:* Taylor & Francis.

Molecular Mechanisms of Epithelial Cell Junctions: From Development to Disease. Ed. by Sandra Citi. 1994. (Molecular Biology Intelligence Unit Ser.). 118p. 99.00 (*1-57059-091-5*, LN9091) Landes Bioscience.

Molecular Mechanisms of Fever. Matthew J. Kluger. 1999. (Annals of the New York Academy of Sciences Ser.). 320p. pap. text 22.50 (*0-8018-6301-5*) Johns Hopkins.

Molecular Mechanisms of Fever. Ed. by Matthew J. Kluger et al. 1998. LC 98-31202. (Annals of the New York Academy of Sciences Ser.: Vol. 856). 308p. 100.00 (*1-57331-133-2*); xii, 308 p. pap. 100.00 (*1-57331-134-0*) NY Acad Sci.

Molecular Mechanisms of Hormone Action. U. Gehring et al. 1990. (Colloquium der Gesellschaft fur Biologische Chemie in Mosbach Baden Ser.: Vol. 40). (Illus.). 204p. 97.00 (*0-387-51607-7*) Spr-Verlag.

Molecular Mechanisms of Hypercoagulable States. Andrew I. Schafer. 1997. LC 97-14453. (Medical Intelligence Unit Ser.). 250p. pap. 89.95 (*0-412-13071-8*) Chapman & Hall.

Molecular Mechanisms of Hypercoagulable States. Andrew I. Schafer. 1997. (Medical Intelligence Unit Ser.). 203p. 99.00 (*1-57059-453-8*) Landes Bioscience.

Molecular Mechanisms of Immune Regulation. Ed. by Rakesh Srivastava et al. 1991. 286p. 125.00 (*1-56081-092-0*, Wiley-VCH) Wiley.

Molecular Mechanisms of Immune Responses in Insects. Ed. by Paul T. Brey & Dan E. Hultmark. 1997. (Illus.). 256p. (*0-412-71280-6*) Kluwer Academic.

Molecular Mechanisms of Neurodegenerative Diseases. Ed. by Marie-Francoise Chesselet. 2000. LC 00-32041. (Contemporary Clinical Neuroscience Ser.). (Illus.). xiii, 410p. 125.00 (*0-89603-804-1*) Humana.

Molecular Mechanisms of Pre-Eclampsia - MIU. Bradley W. Arbogast. 1996. (Medical Intelligence Unit Ser.). 250p. pap. 89.95 (*0-412-11471-2*) Chapman & Hall.

Molecular Mechanisms of the Immune Response. Ed. by W. F. Bodmer & M. J. Owen. 1994. (Cancer Surveys Ser.: Vol. 22). (Illus.). 190p. (C). 56.25 (*0-87969-442-4*) Cold Spring Harbor.

Molecular Mechanisms of Water Transport. Thomas Zeuthen. 1996. (Medicine Ser.). pap. 89.95 (*0-412-10311-7*, VNR) Wiley.

Molecular Medical Bacteriology, Vol. 2. Sussman. 1998. 750p. (*0-12-677532-X*) Acad Pr.

Molecular Medicine. John Bradley et al. 1995. LC 95-8412. (Lecture Notes). viii, 151p. 29.95 (*0-632-03851-9*) Blackwell Sci.

Molecular Medicine: An Introductory Text. R. J. Trent. 2nd ed. 1997. LC 96-26054. pap. text (*0-443-05366-9*) Church.

Molecular Medicine: Clinical Implications. Benz. 1993. 55.00 (*0-397-44610-1*) Lppncott W & W.

Molecular Medicine of Viral Hepatitis. Tim J. Harrison & Arie J. Zuckerman. 1997. LC 96-28960. (Molecular Medical Science Ser.). 282p. 129.95 (*0-471-96996-6*) Wiley.

Molecular Methods for Virus Detection. Ed. by Danny L. Wiedbrauk & Daniel H. Farkas. 1995. LC 94-28603. (Illus.). 386p. pap. 63.00 (*0-12-748920-7*) Acad Pr.

Molecular Modelling & Drug Design. Ed. by Andrew Vinter & Mark Gardner. 1994. LC 93-42952. (Topics in Molecular & Structural Biology Ser.). 110.00 (*0-8493-7772-2*) CRC Pr.

Molecular Modulation of Chemical Presynaptic Neurotransmission. Nathan Moskowitz. 1985. 258p. 72.50 (*0-275-91320-1*, C1320, Praeger Pubs) Greenwood.

Molecular Nephrology: Kidney Function in Health & Disease. Ed. by Detlef Schlondorff & Joseph V. Bonventre. 1995. LC 95-23371. (Illus.). 960p. text 250.00 (*0-8247-9508-3*) Dekker.

Molecular Neuro-Oncology & Its Impact on the Clinical Management of Brain Tumours. Ed. by O. D. Wiestler et al. 1994. (Recent Results in Cancer Research Ser.). (Illus.). 200p. 105.00 (*0-387-57351-8*) Spr-Verlag.

Molecular Neurobiological Techniques. Ed. by Alan A. Boulton et al. 1989. LC 89-2053. (Neuromethods Ser.: Vol. 16). (Illus.). 310p. 104.50 (*0-89603-140-3*) Humana.

Molecular Neurobiology: Frontiers in Molecular Biology. Ed. by David M. Glover & B. David Hames. 1990. (Frontiers in Molecular Biology Ser.). (Illus.). 216p. 58.00 (*0-19-963042-9*) OUP.

Molecular Neurobiology: Recombinant DNA Approaches. S. Heinemann & J. Patrick. 1987. LC 87-2512. (Current Topics in Neurobiology Ser.). (Illus.). 316p. (C). text 89.50 (*0-306-42440-1*, Kluwer Plenum) Kluwer Academic.

Molecular Neurobiology & Brain Ischemia. K. Oki Shimoji. 1996. LC 96-26702. (Illus.). 166p. 74.95 (*4-431-70184-2*) Spr-Verlag.

Molecular Neurobiology of Epilepsy. E. A. Cavalheiro et al. Ed. by J. Engel, Jr. et al. 1992. LC 92-18550. (Epilepsy Research Ser.: No. 9). xvi,412p. 289.50 (*0-444-89711-9*) Elsevier.

Molecular Neurobiology of Pain. Ed. by David Borsook. 1997. LC 97-36742. (Progress in Pain Research & Management Ser.: Vol. 9). (Illus.). 384p. 76.00 (*0-931092-19-1*) Intl Assn Study Pain.

Molecular Neurobiology of the Mammalian Brain. P. L. McGeer et al. 2nd ed. 1987. LC 86-25333. (Illus.). 800p. (C). pap. text 49.50 (*0-306-42511-4*, Kluwer Plenum) Kluwer Academic.

Molecular Neurobiology of the Mammalian Brain. P. L. McGeer et al. 2nd ed. 1987. LC 86-25333. (Illus.). 800p. (C). 95.00 (*0-306-42329-4*, Plenum Trade) Perseus Pubng.

Molecular Neuropathology. Ed. by Gareth W. Roberts & Julia M. Polak. 1995. (Postgraduate Medical Science Ser.: No. 4). (Illus.). 199p. (C). pap. text 21.95 (*0-521-42558-1*) Cambridge U Pr.

Molecular Neuropathology of Aging. Ed. by Peter Davies & Caleb E. Finch. 1988. LC 87-15673. (Banbury Reports: No. 27). (Illus.). 484p. text 80.00 (*0-87969-227-8*) Cold Spring Harbor.

Molecular Neurovirology: Pathogenesis of Viral CNS Infections. Ed. by Raymond P. Roos. 1992. LC 91-20851. (Illus.). 625p. 155.00 (*0-89603-222-1*) Humana.

Molecular Oncology & Clinical Applications. Ed. by A. Cittadini et al. 1993. LC 93-2395. (Molecular & Cell Biology Updates Ser.). (Illus.). 448p. 131.00 (*0-8176-2915-7*) Birkhauser.

***Molecular Pathogenesis of Cervical Carcinoma: Analysis of Clonality, HPV 16 Sequence Variations & Loss of Heterozygosity.** Xinrong Hu. 2001. (Comprehensive Summaries of Uppsala Dissertations from the Faculty of Medicine Ser.: No. 1080). (Illus.). 76p. (C). pap. (*91-554-5127-6*) Acta Univ SWE. *Dist:* Coronet Bks.

Molecular Pathogenesis of Diabetes Mellitus. Ed. by Richard D. Leslie. 1997. LC 96-24159. (Frontiers of Hormone Research Ser.: Vol. 22, 1997). (Illus.). viii, 228p. 198.25 (*3-8055-6373-6*) S Karger.

Molecular Pathogenesis of Gastrointestinal Infections. T. Wadstrom et al. 1991. (FEMS Symposium Ser.: No. 58). (Illus.). 352p. (C). text 110.00 (*0-306-44020-2*, Kluwer Plenum) Kluwer Academic.

Molecular Pathogenesis of HTLV-1: A Current Perspective. Ed. by O. John Semmes & Marie-Louise Hammarskjold. 1998. LC 00-501882. (Illus.). 256p. 50.00 (*1-886236-19-4*) ABI Prof Pubns.

Molecular Pathogenesis of MODYs. Ed. by F. M. Matschinsky & M. A. Magnuson. 2000. LC 99-49965. (Frontiers in Diabetes Ser.: Vol. 15). (Illus.). x, 271p. 168.00 (*3-8055-6950-5*) S Karger.

Molecular Pathology. Antoni Horst. 1991. (Illus.). 440p. lib. bdg. 239.00 (*0-8493-6088-9*, RB113) CRC Pr.

Molecular Pathology. Ed. by Jonathan R. Salisbury. 1997. LC 97-201783. 168p. pap. (*0-7484-0571-2*) Tay Francis Ltd GBR. *Dist:* Taylor & Francis.

Molecular Pathology. Wolfe. 1997. text (*0-7216-4871-1*) Saunders.

Molecular Pathology: Approaches to Diagnosing Human Disease in the Clinical Laboratory. Ed. by Ruth A. Heim & Lawrence M. Silverman. 1994. LC 93-74307. 274p. 69.00 (*0-89089-544-9*) Carolina Acad Pr.

Molecular Pathology of Autoimmune Disease. Ed. by Constantin A. Bona et al. 1993. LC 92-49272. 795p. text 234.00 (*3-7186-0555-4*) Gordon & Breach.

Molecular Pathology of Early Cancer. Ed. by Sudhir Srivastava et al. 1997. LC 97-75194. (Illus.). 481p. 99.00 (*90-5199-373-0*) IOS Press.

Molecular Pathology of Gastroenterological Cancer: Application to Clinical Practice. Ed. by E. Tahara. 1997. LC 97-4383. (Illus.). 250p. 180.00 (*4-431-70195-8*) Spr-Verlag.

***Molecular Pathology of Insulin-Dependent Diabetes Mellitus.** Ed. by M. G. Von Herrath. 2001. (Current Directions in Autoimmunity Ser.: Vol. 4). (Illus.). viii, 340p. 250.50 (*3-8055-7240-9*) S Karger.

Molecular Pathology of Nerve & Muscle: Noxious Agents & Genetic Lesions. Ed. by Antony D. Kidman et al. 1984. (Experimental & Clinical Neuroscience Ser.). 416p. 129.50 (*0-89603-057-1*) Humana.

Molecular Pathology of the Prions. Ed. by Harry F. Baker. 2001. (Methods in Molecular Medicine Ser.: Vol. 59). 250p. 99.00 (*0-89603-924-2*) Humana.

Molecular Pharmacology. Terrence P. Kenakin. 1996. LC 96-39098. (Illus.). 300p. (Orig.). pap. 65.95 (*0-86542-540-X*) Blackwell Sci.

Molecular Physiology & Pharmacology of Cardiac Ion Channels & Transporters. Ed. by M. Morad et al. 1996. LC 95-51375. (Developments in Cardiovascular Medicine Ser.: Vol. 182). 624p. (C). text 331.50 (*0-7923-3913-4*) Kluwer Academic.

Molecular Probe Markets: Hoffman-La Roche Bids for Dominance. Market Intelligence Staff. 1992. 230p. (Orig.). 1895.00 (*1-56753-379-5*) Frost & Sullivan.

Molecular Probes of the Nervous System Vol. 1: Selected Methods for Antibody & Nucleic Acid Probes. Susan Hockfield et al. 1993. (Illus.). 336p. text 21.25 (*0-87969-351-7*) Cold Spring Harbor.

Molecular Protocols in Transfusion Medicine. Greg Denomme et al. 2000. LC 99-68336. (Illus.). 200p. 99.95 (*0-12-209370-4*) Acad Pr.

Molecular Radiobiology. N. B. Strazhevskaya. 1975. 224p. 3.5 hd 67.00 (*0-7065-1432-7*) Coronet Bks.

Molecular Regulation of Arousal States. Ed. by Ralph Lydic. 1997. LC 97-21353. (Cellular & Molecular Neuropharmacology Ser.). 256p. per. 94.95 (*0-8493-3361-X*) CRC Pr.

***Molecular Regulators in Cartilage & Bone Formation.** Thomas Engstrand. 2001. (Comprehensive Summaries of Uppsala Dissertations from the Faculty of Medicine Ser.: No. 1024). 62p. (*91-554-4996-4*) Uppsala Universitet SWE. *Dist:* Coronet Bks.

Molecular Signaling & Regulation in Glial Cells: A Key to Remyelination & Functional Repair. Ed. by G. Jeserich et al. 1997. LC 96-49970. (Illus.). 390p. 157.00 (*3-540-62076-1*) Spr-Verlag.

Molecular Similarity in Drug Design. Ed. by P. M. Dean. 1994. (Illus.). 360p. pap. (*0-7514-0221-4*) B Acad & Prof GBR. *Dist:* Routldge.

Molecular Specialization & Symmetry in Membrane Function. Ed. by Arthur K. Solomon & Manfred L. Karnovsky. 1978. LC 77-134. (Harvard Books in Biophysics: Vol. 2). 406p. 51.95 (*0-674-58179-2*) HUP.

Molecular Theory of Radiation Biology. K. H. Chadwick & H. P. Leenhouts. 1981. (Monographs in Theoretical & Applied Genetics: Vol. 5). (Illus.). 377p. 120.00 (*0-387-10297-3*) Spr-Verlag.

Molecular Virology. D. R. Harper & C. Grose. 1994. (Medical Perspectives Ser.). 160p. pap. (*1-872748-57-0*) Bios Sci GBR. *Dist:* Coronet Bks.

Molecular Volumes in Chemistry & Biology: Applications Including Partitioning Toxicity. John C. McGowan & Alan Mellors. 1986. LC 86-10520. 259p. 65.95 (*0-470-20353-6*) P-H.

Molecularising Biology & Medicine: New Practices & Alliances, 1930s to 1970s. Soraya De Chadarevain & Harmke Kamminga. 1998. (Studies in the History of Science, Technology & Medicine Ser.: Vol. 6). 350p. text 70.00 (*3-7186-5908-5*, Harwood Acad Pubs) Gordon & Breach.

Molecularizing Biology & Medicine: New Practices & Alliances, 1930s to 1970s. Chadarevain. 1998. 292p. text 59.00 (*90-5702-293-1*) Gordon & Breach.

Molecule & Mental Illness. Samuel H. Barondes. 1992. LC 92-35150. vi, 215p. text 32.95 (*0-7167-5041-4*) W H Freeman.

Molecules, Cells & Disease. J. L. Van Lancker. 1977. LC 77-893. (Springer Study Edition Ser.). (Illus.). 311p. 99.00 (*0-387-90242-2*) Spr-Verlag.

Molecules, Miracles & Medicine. Andrew Lasslo. 2000. 89p. pap. 12.99 (*0-87527-533-8*) Green.

Molecules of Emotion: Why You Feel the Way You Feel. Candace B. Pert. 1997. LC 97-17463. 304p. 25.00 (*0-684-83187-2*) S&S Trade.

Molecules Within Us: Our Body in Health & Disease. Charles A. Pasternak. 1998. LC 98-26173. (Illus.). 350p. (C). 26.95 (*0-306-45987-6*) Da Capo.

Molekularbiologie In der Viszeralchirurgie. 1999. (Chirurgische Gastroenterologie Ser.). 100p. 44.50 (*3-8055-6830-4*) S Karger.

Molluscan Neuro-Endocrinology. Ed. by J. L. Lever & H. H. Boer. 1983. (Illus.). 268p. 32.00 (*0-444-85572-6*, North Holland) Elsevier.

Mollusken. Ihre Bedeutung fuer Wissenschaft, Medizin, Handel und Kultur (Mollusks. Their Importance for Research, Medicine, Commerce & Culture) Dora Godan. 1996. (Illus.). 203p. (*3-8263-3131-1*) Blckwell Wissenschafts DEU. *Dist:* Balogh.

Molybdenim Enzymes. Ed. by Thomas G. Spiro. 1985. LC 85-6343. (Metal Ions in Biology Ser.). 624p. (C). text 150.00 (*0-471-88542-8*) Krieger.

Mom & Dad Are Divorced, but I'm Not: Parenting after Divorce. Hal W. Anderson & Gail S. Anderson. 1981. LC 80-27602. 284p. text 28.95 (*0-88229-522-5*) Burnham Inc.

Moment of Transition: Two Neuroscientific Articles by Sigmund Freud. Sigmund Freud. Ed. by Mark Solms & Michael Saling. 1990. 192p. reprint ed. pap. text (*0-946439-92-3*) Karnac Bks GBR. *Dist:* Other Pr LLC.

Momentous Events, Vivid Memories. David H. Pillemer. 1998. LC 97-47043. (Illus.). 256p. 36.50 (*0-674-58205-5*) HUP.

Moments of Engagement: Intimate Psychotherapy in a Technological Age. Peter D. Kramer. 2000. 260p. reprint ed. text 25.00 (*0-7881-6450-3*) DIANE Pub.

Moments of Engagement: Intimate Psychotherapy in a Technological Age. Peter D. Kramer. 1989. 260p. (C). 24.95 (*0-393-70075-5*) Norton.

M
N
O

Moments of Engagement: Intimate Psychotherapy in a Technological Age. Peter D. Kramer. 1994. 272p. pap. 11.95 (*0-14-023790-9*, Penguin Bks) Penguin Putnam.

Moments of Unreason: The Practice of Canadian Psychiatry & the Homewood Retreat, 1883-1923. Cheryl K. Warsh. 1989. (Illus.). 304p. (C). text (*0-7735-0701-9*) McG-Queens Univ Pr CAN. *Dist:* CUP Services.

Moments on Maple Avenue: The Reality of Abortion. Louise K. Howe. 1986. 224p. mass mkt. 3.95 (*0-446-34015-4*) Warner Bks.

Mommy, I Can't Sit Still: Coping with Hyperactive & Aggressive Children. K. Daniel O'Leary. Ed. by Joan S. Dunphy. 132p. 1989. LC 84-2104. pap. 10.95 (*0-88282-055-9*); 1984. 13.95 (*0-88282-000-1*) New Horizon NJ.

Mommy I'm Hungry: How to Feed Your Child Nutritiously. Patricia McEntire. 1982. LC 81-68292. 168p. pap. 3.00 (*0-917982-11-8*, Cougar Books) Capitol Enquiry.

Moms Don't Get Sick. Pat Brack. 1990. LC 90-60228. (Illus.). 124p. (Orig.). pap. 10.95 (*0-937603-07-4*) Melius Pub.

Mom's Marijuana: Insights about Living. Dan Shapiro. 2000. LC 00-38275. (Illus.). 256p. 20.00 (*0-609-60569-0*) Harmony Bks.

*__Mom's Medicine: How to Protect Your Kids, Husband, & Parents Against 100 Health Conditions & Medical Emergencies.__ Contrib. by Prevention Health Books for Women Staff. 2001. LC 2001-19873. 560p. pap. 17.95 (*1-57954-490-8*) Rodale Pr Inc.

*__Mom's Medicine: How to Protect Your Kids, Husband, & Parents Against 100 Health Conditions & Medical Emergencies.__ Contrib. by Prevention Health Books for Women Staff. 2001. LC 2001-19873. xvi, 544p. (*1-57954-469-X*) Rodale Pr Inc.

*__Mom's Medicine: How to Protect Your Kids, Husband & Parents Against More Than 100 Health Conditions & Medical Emergencies.__ Prevention Health Books for Women Staff. 2001. (Illus.). 560p. pap. 17.95 (*1-57954-509-2*) Rodale Pr Inc.

Moms with ADD: A Self-Help Manual. Christine A. Adamec. 2000. LC 00-44684. xv, 224p. pap. 14.95 (*0-87833-175-1*) Taylor Pub.

Monclonal Antibodies in Diagnostic Immunohistochemistry. Ed. by Mark R. Wick & Gene P. Siegal. 1988. (Clinical & Biochemical Analysis Ser.: Vol. 24). (Illus.). 664p. text 250.00 (*0-8247-7838-3*) Dekker.

Money: Rx for Physicians: Secrets for Building Wealth. Steven C. Camp. 2000. LC 00-45137. pap. 14.95 (*1-887620-02-8*) Trunkey Pub.

Money Matters: The Fee in Psychotherapy & Psychoanalysis. William G. Herron & Shelia R. Welt. 1994. LC 92-1564. 203p. pap. 19.95 (*0-89862-305-7*, 2305) Guilford Pubns.

Money, Medicine, & Malpractice in American Society. Iain Hay. 1992. LC 91-25188. 280p. 72.50 (*0-275-93952-9*, C3952, Praeger Pubs) Greenwood.

Monitoring & Assessment of Adverse Drug Effects. 1987. 35p. pap. text 10.00 (*92-9036-027-5*, 1840007) World Health.

Monitoring & Compliance Vol. 4: The Political Economy of Inspection. David Hemenway. Ed. by William Breit & Kenneth G. Elzinga. 1985. LC 84-29980. (Political Economy & Public Policy Ser.: Vol. 4). 137p. 78.50 (*0-89232-477-5*) Jai Pr.

Monitoring & Evaluating Programmes Module 5: Facilitator's Guide. Martine Hilton. 1993. (Primary Health Care Management Advancement Programme Modules Ser.). 67p. pap. text (*1-882839-11-0*) Aga Khan Fnd.

Monitoring & Evaluating Programmes Module 5: User's Guide. Lynne M. Franco et al. 1993. (Primary Health Care Management Advancement Programme Modules Ser.). 111p. pap. text (*1-882839-03-X*) Aga Khan Fnd.

Monitoring & Evaluation: Anesthesia Services. Ed. by Robert Fromberg. 1987. LC 90-60439. 38p. pap. 25.00 (*0-86688-124-7*) Joint Comm Hlthcare.

Monitoring & Evaluation of Oral Health: Report of a WHO Expert Committee, 1987. 1989. (Technical Report Ser.: No. 782). 69p. pap. text 9.00 (*92-4-120782-5*, 1100782) World Health.

Monitoring Child Health in the United States: Selected Issues & Policies. Ed. by Deborah K. Walker & Julius B. Richmond. 1984. (Illus.). 256p. 20.00 (*0-674-58551-8*) HUP.

Monitoring Children's Health: Key Indicators. C. Arden Miller et al. 2nd ed. 1989. 176p. 17.50 (*0-87553-162-8*) Am Pub Health.

Monitoring Elder Compliance & Response: A Self Learning Programme for Community Nurses. S. D. Moir. 1996. 125p. spiral bd. (*0-443-05525-4*) Church.

Monitoring for Adverse Drug Reactions. Ed. by Stuart Walker. 1985. text 147.50 (*0-85200-876-7*) Kluwer Academic.

Monitoring for Drug Safety. Ed. by W. H. Inman. 2nd ed. 1986. text 350.00 (*0-85200-721-3*) Kluwer Academic.

Monitoring for Health Hazards at Work. Indira Ashton & F. S. Gill. 3rd ed. 1999. LC 99-32635. (Illus.). xxi, 304p. pap. 64.95 (*0-632-05041-1*) Blackwell Sci.

Monitoring in Anaesthesia & Intensive Care. Ed. by P. Hutton & C. Prys-Roberts. 1994. (Illus.). 463p. text (*0-7020-1407-9*) W B Saunders GBR. *Dist:* Saunders.

Monitoring in Anesthesia. Casey D. Blitt. 3rd ed. 1994. text (*0-443-08912-4*) Church.

Monitoring in Anesthesia. Lawrence J. Saidman & N. Ty Smith. 3rd enl. ed. 1993. (Illus.). 576p. text 165.00 (*0-7506-9067-4*) Buttrwrth-Heinemann.

Monitoring in Patients with Optical Tissue Sensors. 1993. 139.95 (*0-8493-4581-2*) CRC Pr.

Monitoring Medicaid Managed Care: Developing & Assessment & Evaluation Program. Melvin I. Krasner. 1995. LC 95-37658. (Special Reports). 52p. pap. 25.00 (*1-881277-25-9*) United Hosp Fund.

Monitoring of Cerebral Blood Flow & Metabolism in Intensive Care: Proceedings of an International Symposium, Berlin, October 1992. Ed. by A. W. Unterberg et al. 1994. LC 93-23371. (Illus.). 133p. 101.00 (*0-387-82484-7*) Spr-Verlag.

Monitoring of Industrial Sickness. Banarsi Misra. 1990. (C). text (*81-7100-266-8*) Deep & Deep Pubns IND. *Dist:* S Asia.

Monitoring of National AIDS Prevention & Control Programmes: Guiding Principles. 1988. (WHO AIDS Ser.: No. 4). (ENG, FRE, RUS & SPA.). iii, 27p. pap. text 8.00 (*92-4-121004-4*, 1870004) World Health.

Monitoring of Radioactive Effluents from Nuclear Facilities. International Atomic Energy Agency Staff. 1978. (Proceedings Ser.). (Illus.). 610p. pap. (*92-0-020078-8*, ISP466) IAEA AUT. *Dist:* Bernan Associates.

Monitoring of Vital Parameters During Extracorporal Circulation. H. P. Kimmich. 1981. (Illus.). x, 334p. pap. 164.50 (*3-8055-2059-X*) S Karger.

Monitoring Patient Care: Are Your Patients Safe? Meridith B. Cox. 1999. (Risk Management Ser.). (Orig.). (C). pap. text 30.00 (*0-912665-23-8*) BusinessWatch.

Monitoring the Central Nervous System. Ed. by Peter S. Sebel & William Fitch. 1994. LC 93-42920. (Illus.). 496p. 136.95 (*0-632-03648-6*) Blackwell Sci.

Monitoring the Changes in Use of Medicare Posthospital Services. Andrea Steiner & C. R. Neu. 1993. LC 93-3542. pap. 9.00 (*0-8330-1361-0*, MR-153-HCFA) Rand Corp.

Monitoring the Worker for Exposure & Disease: Scientific Legal & Ethical Considerations in the Use of Biomarkers. Nicholas A. Ashford et al. 1990. LC 89-43479. (Johns Hopkins Series in Environmental Toxicology Ser.). 240p. pap. text 20.95 (*0-8018-3989-0*) Johns Hopkins.

Monitoring Toxic Substances. Ed. by Dennis Schuetzle. 1979. LC 78-27490. (ACS Symposium Ser.: No. 94). 49.95 (*0-8412-0480-2*); pap. 27.95 (*0-8412-0656-2*) Am Chemical.

*__Monitoring Universal Salt Iodization Programs: Key Resources in Its Prevention & Elimination.__ Ed. by Kevin M. Sullivan et al. 1995. (Micronutrient Initiative Ser.). 108p. pap. (*0-660-16000-5*) IDRC-CRDI CAN. *Dist:* Stylus Pub VA.

*__Monitoring Vitamin A Programs.__ Jenny Cervinskas et al. 1998. 112p. pap. (*1-894217-00-4*) IDRC-CRDI CAN. *Dist:* Stylus Pub VA.

Monoamine Oxidase: Basic & Clinical Aspects. Ed. by H. Yasuhara et al. 1993. 256p. 135.00 (*90-6764-146-4*) Coronet Bks.

Monoamine Oxidase & Its Selective Inhibitors. Ed. by H. Beckmann & P. Riederer. 1983. (Modern Problems of Pharmacopsychiatry Ser.: Vol. 19). (Illus.). x, 354p. 172.25 (*3-8055-3595-3*) S Karger.

Monoamine Oxidase Inhibitors in Neurological Diseases. Ed. by Lieberman et al. 1994. (Neurological Disease & Therapy Ser.: Vol. 21). (Illus.). 400p. text 175.00 (*0-8247-9082-0*) Dekker.

Monoclonal Antibodies. Ed. by Peter Allen. 1988. 300p. pap. 1795.00 (*0-941285-26-X*) FIND-SVP.

Monoclonal Antibodies. Ed. by Peter C. Beverley. 1986. LC 85-19512. (Illus.). 352p. (*0-443-02990-3*) Church.

Monoclonal Antibodies: A Manual of Techniques. Heddy Zola. 1987. 232p. 239.00 (*0-8493-6476-0*) CRC Pr.

Monoclonal Antibodies: A Practical Guide. Ed. by J. H. Peters & H. Baumgarten. 1992. LC 92-30163. (Laboratory Ser.). (Illus.). 488p. 74.95 (*0-387-50843-0*) Spr-Verlag.

Monoclonal Antibodies: Applications in Clinical Oncology. Agamemnon A. Epenetos. 1991. (Illus.). 352p. (gr. 13). pap. 209.95 (*0-412-41090-7*) Chapman & Hall.

Monoclonal Antibodies: Principles & Applications. Ed. by J. R. Birch & E. S. Lennox. 1995. LC 94-39791. 344p. 120.00 (*0-471-05147-0*) Wiley.

Monoclonal Antibodies: Principles & Practice. James W. Goding. 3rd ed. 1996. (Illus.). 512p. text 49.95 (*0-12-287023-9*) Acad Pr.

Monoclonal Antibodies: Production, Engineering & Clinical Application. Ed. by Mary A. Ritter & Heather M. Ladyman. 1995. (Postgraduate Medical Science Ser.: No. 2). (Illus.). 496p. (C). pap. text 41.95 (*0-521-42503-4*) Cambridge U Pr.

Monoclonal Antibodies No. 2: Applications in Clinical Oncology. Ed. by Agamemnon A. Epenetos. 1993. LC 92-49123. 560p. (gr. 13). pap. 295.95 (*0-412-48100-6*) Chapman & Hall.

Monoclonal Antibodies & Breast Cancer. Ed. by Roberto L. Ceriani. 1985. (Developments in Oncology Ser.). text 127.00 (*0-89838-739-6*) Kluwer Academic.

Monoclonal Antibodies & Functional Cell Lines: Progress & Applications. Ed. by Roger H. Kennett et al. 1984. LC 84-4877. 444p. 95.00 (*0-306-41567-4*, Plenum Trade) Perseus Pubng.

Monoclonal Antibodies & T Cell Products. David H. Katz. 1982. LC 81-21604. 184p. 110.00 (*0-8493-6580-5*, QR186) Franklin.

Monoclonal Antibodies, Cytokines & Arthritis: Mediators of Inflammation & Therapy. Ed. by Thomas Kresina. 1991. (Infectious Disease & Therapy Ser.: Vol. 7). (Illus.). 512p. text 225.00 (*0-8247-8116-3*) Dekker.

Monoclonal Antibodies for Therapy, Prevention & in Vivo Diagnosis of Human Disease. Ed. by H. Van de Donk & W. Hennessen. 1990. (Developments in Biological Standardization Ser.: Vol. 71). (Illus.). xiv, 248p. pap. 61.00 (*3-8055-5115-0*) S Karger.

Monoclonal Antibodies in Cancer. Ed. by Stewart Sell & Ralph A. Reisfeld. 1985. LC 85-4735. (Contemporary Biomedicine Ser.: Vol. 6). 428p. 119.50 (*0-89603-068-7*) Humana.

Monoclonal Antibodies in Cardiovascular Diseases. Ban A. Khaw et al. 1993. LC 93-8769. (Illus.). 325p. text 115.00 (*0-8121-1611-9*) Lppncott W & W.

Monoclonal Antibodies in Clinical Medicine. Ed. by A. McMichael & J. Fabre. 1982. text 157.00 (*0-12-485580-6*) Acad Pr.

Monoclonal Antibodies in Drug Development. Ed. by J. Thomas August. 1982. (Illus.). 237p. (Orig.). 24.00 (*0-9609094-0-0*) Am Phar & Ex.

Monoclonal Antibodies in Immunoscintigraphy. Jean-Francois Chantal. 1989. (Illus.). 440p. 259.00 (*0-8493-4716-5*, RC78) CRC Pr.

Monoclonal Antibodies in Transplantation. Lucienne Chatenoud. 1995. LC 95-24139. (Medical Intelligence Unit Ser.). 181p. 89.00 (*1-57059-269-1*) Landes Bioscience.

Monoclonal Antibodies in Tumor Therapy: Present Stage, Chances & Limitations. Ed. by Louis A. Kuhlmann et al. 1988. (Contributions to Oncology Ser.: Vol. 32). (Illus.). x, 178p. 51.50 (*3-8055-4763-3*) S Karger.

Monoclonal Antibodies Therapy. Ed. by H. Waldmann. 1988. (Progress in Allergy Ser.: Vol. 45). (Illus.). x, 174p. 120.00 (*3-8055-4803-6*) S Karger.

Monoclonal Antibodies to Receptors: Probes for Receptor Structure & Function. Ed. by M. Greaves. 1984. (Receptors & Recognition Series B: Vol. 17). 250p. (C). text 75.00 (*0-412-25330-5*, 9015) Chapman & Hall.

Monoclonal Antibody-Based Therapy of Cancer. Ed. by Michael L. Grossbard. 1998. LC 98-29118. (Illus.). 472p. text 195.00 (*0-8247-0196-8*) Dekker.

Monoclonal Antibody Markets. Market Intelligence Staff. 1994. 320p. 2295.00 (*0-7889-0057-9*) Frost & Sullivan.

Monoclonal Antibody Markets: Enormous Potential in Diagnostic & Therapeutic Products, Cancer Leads the Way. Market Intelligence Staff. 1992. 267p. (Orig.). 1995.00 (*1-56753-048-6*) Frost & Sullivan.

Monoclonal Antibody Production. Ed. by Shelley Minden. 1996. (Biomedical Library). 225p. pap. 795.00 (*1-57936-007-6*) Drug & Market Dev.

Monoclonal Antibody Production. National Research Council Staff. 1999. LC 00-502202. (Illus.). xiv, 59p. pap. 18.00 (*0-309-06447-3*) Natl Acad Pr.

Monoclonal Antibody Purification. Ed. by Shelley Minden. 1996. (Biomedical Library). pap. 795.00 (*1-57936-020-3*) Drug & Market Dev.

Monoclonal Antibody Therapy of Human Cancer. Ed. by Kenneth F. Foon & Alton C. Morgan, Jr. 1985. (Developments in Oncology Ser.). text 97.50 (*0-89838-754-X*) Kluwer Academic.

Monoclonal Hybridoma Antibodies: Techniques & Applications. Ed. by John G. Hurrell. 1982. 240p. 139.00 (*0-8493-6511-2*, QR186, CRC Reprint) Franklin.

Monograph of the Stipitate Steroid Fungi. Derek A. Reid. 1965. (Illus.). pap. 96.00 (*3-7682-5418-6*) Lubrecht & Cramer.

Monograph on Dengue-Dengue Haemorrhagic Fever. Compiled by P. Thongcharoen. 1994. (WHO Regional Publications: No. 22). ix, 163p. pap. text 15.00 (*92-9022-124-0*, 1560022) World Health.

Monograph on the Complications of Unsafe Abortion in Africa. Stephen N. Kinoti et al. 1995. LC 97-950106. (Orig.). pap. text (*0-929817-38-9*) JHPIEGO.

Monograph on the Epidemic of Poliomyelitis (Infantile Paralysis) in New York City in 1946. Haven Emerson. Ed. by Barbara G. Rosenkrantz. 1977. LC 76-25662. (Public Health in America Ser.). (Illus.). reprint ed. lib. bdg. 41.95 (*0-405-09817-0*) Ayer.

Monographic Dictionary of Medicine & Health see Diccionario Monografico de Medicina y Salud

Monographs on Infancy: An Original Anthology. Judith K. Gardner & Howard Gardner. 1975. LC 74-21702. 316p. reprint ed. 27.95 (*0-405-06472-1*) Ayer.

Mononitrates: International Symposium, Held at the Royal Society of Medicine, London , June 1986. Ed. by M. Weiss et al. 1987. (Journal: Vol. 74, Suppl. 1, 1987). (Illus.). viii, 80p. pap. 28.00 (*3-8055-4626-2*) S Karger.

Mononuclear Phagocytes. Ed. by Ralph Van Furth. 1985. text 642.00 (*0-89838-732-9*) Kluwer Academic.

Mononuclear Phagocytes in Cell Biology. Ed. by Gabriel Lopez-Berestein & Jim Klostergaard. 1992. 256p. lib. bdg. 189.00 (*0-8493-4706-8*, QR185) CRC Pr.

Monophasic Action Potentials: Basics & Clinical Application. Ed. by M. R. Franz et al. 1997. LC 97-4382. (Illus.). 241p. 120.00 (*3-540-63152-6*) Spr-Verlag.

Monopoly, M. D. James Gettins. 1997. 227p. (Orig.). pap. 11.95 (*1-57901-014-8*) Intl Promotions.

Monsoon Season. William Q. Wu. 1996. LC 96-60262. 10.00 (*1-885854-01-3*) UniStar Pubng.

Mont Reid Surgical Handbook. Scott Berry. 4th ed. 1997. LC 97-4039. (Illus.). 920p. (C). (gr. 13). pap. text 35.95 (*0-8151-1007-3*, 29155) Mosby Inc.

Montana Health Care in Perspective, 2000. Ed. by Kathleen O'Leary Morgan & Scott E. Morgan. 2000. 21p. spiral bd. 19.00 (*0-7401-0225-7*) Morgan Quitno Corp.

Montana Health Care Perspective, 1998. Ed. by Kathleen O'Leary Morgan & Scott E. Morgan. 1998. 20p. pap. 19.00 (*1-56692-825-7*) Morgan Quitno Corp.

Monte Carlo Calculations in Nuclear Medicine: Applications in Diagnostic Imaging. Ed. by M. Ljungberg & M. A. King. 1998. LC 98-11380. (Medical Science Ser.). (Illus.). 256p. 99.00 (*0-7503-0479-0*) Inst of Physics Pubng.

Montessori Based Activities for Persons with Dementia, Vol. 1. Illus. by Cameron J. Camp. 1999. 76p. pap. 46.50 (*0-9676343-1-8*) Myers Resear Inst.

Month of Birth, Creativity, & the "Two Classes of Men" Vol. 1: A Prenatal Influence of the Sum's Radiation on the Left-Right "Configuration" of the Brain. Giovanni Marzullo. 1996. LC 96-92663. 304p. 24.95 (*0-9652322-9-8*, 223) Per Aspera.

Monthly Nutrition Companion: Up-to-Date Tips from the World's Foremost Nutrition Experts. American Dietetic Association Staff & Roberta Larson Duyff. 1997. LC 98-231231. 224p. pap. 6.95 (*1-56561-099-7*) Wiley.

Monuments of Mars: A City on the Edge of Forever. Richard C. Hoagland. 4th rev. ed. 1996. LC 96-39041. (Illus.). 526p. (C). pap. 25.00 (*1-883319-30-7*) Frog Ltd CA.

Mood. W. N. Morris. 1989. (Social Psychology Ser.). (Illus.). 261p. 107.00 (*0-387-96978-0*) Spr-Verlag.

Mood & Anxiety Disorders. Ed. by A. John Rush. 1997. 379p. pap. 69.95 (*0-683-30516-6*) Lppncott W & W.

Mood Apart: Depression, Mania & Other Afflictions of the Self. Peter C. Whybrow. 1998. 288p. pap. 13.00 (*0-465-04726-2*) Basic.

Mood Disorders: Systematic Medication Management. Ed. by A. John Rush. 1997. LC 97-21357. (Modern Problems of Pharmacopsychiatry Ser.: Vol. 25, 1996). (Illus.). viii, 262p. 224.50 (*3-8055-6223-3*) S Karger.

Mood Disorders: Toward a New Psychobiology. P. C. Whybrow et al. 1984. LC 84-3339. (Critical Issues in Psychiatry Ser.). (Illus.). 244p. (C). text 42.50 (*0-306-41568-2*, Kluwer Plenum) Kluwer Academic.

Mood Disorders Throughout the Lifespan. Ed. by Kenneth I. Shulman et al. 1996. LC 96-15350. 464p. 105.00 (*0-471-10477-9*, Wiley-Liss) Wiley.

Mood Genes: Hunting for Origins of Mania & Depression. Samuel H. Barondes. 1998. LC 98-4678. 237p. text 24.95 (*0-7167-2943-1*) W H Freeman.

Mood Medicine: Consciousness & the Healing of Mind & Body by the Brain, Set. 1992. (Alternative Medicine Ser.). lib. bdg. 555.95 (*0-8490-5340-4*) Gordon Pr.

Moonlight, Magnolias, & Madness: Insanity in South Carolina from the Colonial to the Progressive Eras. Peter McCandless. 1996. LC 95-16641. (Illus.). 432p. (C). lib. bdg. 55.00 (*0-8078-2251-5*) U of NC Pr.

Morag - Myself or Mother Hen? Ed. by Moira Walker. 1995. LC 95-9568. (In Search of a Therapist Ser.). 160p. pap. 30.95 (*0-335-19224-6*) Taylor & Francis.

Moral Agoraphobia Vol. 25: The Challenge of Egoism, Vol. 25. Kim Chong Chong. 1996. LC 95-16202. (Revisioning Philosophy Ser.). 104p. (C). text 34.95 (*0-8204-2839-6*) P Lang Pubng.

Moral Challenge of Alzheimer Disease. Stephen G. Post. 1995. LC 95-13505. 160p. 32.50 (*0-8018-5174-2*) Johns Hopkins.

Moral Challenge of Alzheimer Disease: Ethical Issues from Diagnosis to Dying. Stephen Garrard Post. 2nd ed. 2000. LC 99-50625. 192p. 39.95 (*0-8018-6409-7*) Johns Hopkins.

Moral Challenges of Health Care Management. John R. Griffith. 1992. LC 92-48699. 153p. text 40.00 (*0-910701-93-8*, 0928) Health Admin Pr.

Moral Dimensions of Marriage & Family Therapy. August G. Lageman. 1993. LC 92-33573. 138p. (C). pap. 25.50 (*0-8191-8966-9*) U Pr of Amer.

Moral Domain: Essays in the Ongoing Discussion Between Philosophy & the Social Science. Ed. by Thomas E. Wren. 1990. (Studies in Contemporary German Social Thought). 440p. 52.95 (*0-262-23147-6*) MIT Pr.

Moral Evaluation of Contraception & Sterilization: A Dialogical Study. Gary M. Atkinson & Albert S. Moraczewski. 1979. LC 79-90971. viii, 115p. (Orig.). pap. 4.95 (*0-935372-05-9*) NCBC.

Moral Issues in Health Care. Terrence McConnell. 2nd ed. 1996. LC 96-19413. (Philosophy Ser.). 288p. (C). pap. text 33.95 (*0-534-24744-X*) Wadsworth Pub.

Moral Issues in Mental Retardation. Ed. by Ronald S. Laura & Adrian F. Ashman. 1985. LC 84-29329. 224p. (*0-7099-1692-2*) C Helm GBR. *Dist:* Routldge.

M N O

Moral Issues in Psychology: Personalist Contributions to Selected Problems. Ed. by James M. DuBois. 1996. LC 96-36306. 182p. pap. text 32.00 (*0-7618-0543-5*); lib. bdg. 50.50 (*0-7618-0542-7*) U Pr of Amer.

Moral Judgment of the Child. Jean Piaget. Tr. by Marjorie Gabain. 1965. 416p. pap. 17.95 (*0-02-925240-7*) Free Pr.

Moral Military. Sidney Axinn. 1990. 264p. pap. 22.95 (*0-87722-780-2*) Temple U Pr.

Moral Panics. Kenneth Thompson. 1998. LC 97-28401. 176p. (C). 70.00 (*0-415-11976-6*); pap. 18.95 (*0-415-11977-4*) Routledge.

Moral Problems & Mental Health. Richard Egenter & Paul Matussek. 1967. 190p. (Orig.). pap. 4.95 (*0-8189-0095-4*) Alba.

Moral Psychology. Daniel K. Lapsley. 1996. LC 96-6852. (Developmental Psychology Ser.). 304p. (C). pap. text 29.00 (*0-8133-3033-5*) Westview.

Moral Theory & Medical Practice. K. W. Fulford. 1990. (Illus.). 333p. (C). pap. text 22.95 (*0-521-38869-4*) Cambridge U Pr.

Morality & Health. Ed. by Paul Rozin. 1997. LC 96-52813. 432p. (C). 90.00 (*0-415-91581-3*); pap. 27.95 (*0-415-91582-1*) Routledge.

***Morality & the Machine.** Stacey L. Edgar. rev. ed. 2002. (Illus.). (C). pap. text 47.95 (*0-7637-1767-3*, 1767-3) Jones & Bartlett.

Morality, Mortality: Death & Whom to Save from It, Vol. 1. F. M. Kamm. 1998. (Oxford Ethics Ser.). (Illus.). 352p. reprint ed. pap. 19.95 (*0-19-511911-8*) OUP.

Morality, Philosophy & Practice: Historical & Contemporary Readings & Studies. Abraham Edel et al. 1988. 656p. (C). text 50.74 net. (*0-07-554364-8*) McGraw.

Morals & Politics of Psychology: Psychological Discourse & the Status Quo. Isaac Prilleltensky. 1994. LC 93-37494. (SUNY Series, Alternatives in Psychology). 283p. (C). pap. text 22.95 (*0-7914-2038-8*) State U NY Pr.

Morbid Craving for Morphia: Die Morphiumsucht. Edward Levinstein. Ed. by Gerald N. Grob. Tr. by Charles Harrer. 1981. LC 80-1259. (Addiction in America Ser.). reprint ed. lib. bdg. 16.95 (*0-405-13602-1*) Ayer.

Morbidity & Mortality of Dialysis. 1994. lib. bdg. 250.00 (*0-8490-8404-0*) Gordon Pr.

Morbidity Statistics: Twelfth Report of the WHO Expert Committee on Health Statistics. 1968. (Technical Report Ser.). 29p. pap. text 3.00 (*92-4-120389-7*, 1100389) World Health.

Morbus Hodgkin und Non-Hodgkin-Lymphome: Fortschritte der Diagnostik und Aktuelle Therapiekonzepte, 2, Uberarbeitete Auflage. Ed. by V. Diehl et al. 1998. (GER.). 170p. pap. 56.50 (*3-8055-6744-8*) S Karger.

***Morcelised Impacted Cortico-Cancellous Bone Allografts in Revision Surgery for Endoprosthetic Loosening with Osteolysis: Experimental & Clinical Studies.** Gosta Ullmark. 2001. (Comprehensive Summaries of Uppsala Dissertations from the Faculty of Medicine Ser.: No. 1075). (Illus.). 73p. pap. (*91-554-5118-7*) Uppsala Universitet SWE. *Dist:* Coronet Bks.

Mord & Mordmotiv: Ein Gerichtsmedizinischer Pitaval Zusammengestellt aus Fachzeitschriften des 19. Jahrhunderts. Ed. by W. Duerwald. 1987. (Gerichtliche Medizin im 19. Jahrhundert Ser.: Vol. 1). xx, 290p. 71.50 (*3-8055-4777-3*) S Karger.

More Advice from the Back Doctor. Hamilton Hall. 1992. (Illus.). 256p. mass mkt. 5.95 (*0-7710-3769-4*) McCland & Stewart.

More Alike Than Different: Treating Severely Dissociative Trauma Survivors. Margo Rivera. 1996. 520p. text 50.00 (*0-8020-0450-4*); LC 97-129923. 400p. pap. text 24.95 (*0-8020-7238-0*) U of Toronto Pr.

More Annie Stories: Therapeutic Storytelling Techniques. Doris Brett. 1992. LC 91-46084. 224p. 16.95 (*0-945354-47-9*) Am Psychol.

***More Aromatherapy Recipes from Around the World.** 2001. pap. incl. audio compact disk (*0-7322-7135-5*) Colns AUS. *Dist:* Consort Bk Sales.

More Case Presentations in Paediatric & Intensive Care. N. S. Morton et al. 2nd ed. 2000. LC 00-62114. (Illus.). 160p. pap. text 28.50 (*0-7506-4215-7*) Buttrwrth-Heinemann.

More Chicken Soup & Other Folk Remedies. Joan Wilen & Lydia Wilen. 2000. LC 00-702857. (Illus.). 352p. pap. 14.00 (*0-345-44062-5*, Ballantine) Ballantine Pub Grp.

More Excellent Way: A Teaching on the Spiritual Roots of Disease. Henry W. Wright. 2000. xvi,296p. pap. text 24.95 (*0-9678059-0-2*) Pleasant Vally GA.

More Exercises in Fetal Monitoring. Barry S. Schifrin. 1993. (Illus.). 208p. (C). (gr. 13). pap. text 43.00 (*0-8151-7566-3*, 22102) Mosby Inc.

More Harm Than Help: The Ramifications for Rape Survivors of Mandatory HIV Testing of Rapists. Lisa Bowleg & Kathleen D. Stoll. 1991. (Violence Against Women Ser.). (Orig.). (C). pap. 10.00 (*1-877966-08-8*) Ctr Women Policy.

More Instant Teaching Tools for Health Care Educators. Michele L. Deck. 1998. LC 99-178835. 272p. pap. text 36.95 (*0-323-00085-1*) Mosby Inc.

***More Joy As He Leads: Dora M. Taylor Nurse in British Honduras/Belize.** 2001. (Illus.). 224p. pap. 12.00 (*0-9672285-5-7*) MecPublishing.

More Laughing & Loving with Autism. R. Wayne Gilpin. 1994. 108p. pap. 9.95 (*1-885477-12-0*) Fut Horizons.

More Magic of the Minimum Dose. Dorothy Shepherd. 1974. 17.95 (*0-85032-056-9*) Formur Intl.

More Management for Results: A "How to" Workbook for Improving the Management of Your Veterinary Practice. Michael H. Riegger. 1995. 300p. pap. 59.95 (*0-929870-32-8*) Advanstar Commns.

More MRCP, Pt. 1. N. I. Johnson & C. Bunker. 1988. 100p. 16.00 (*0-387-19507-6*) Spr-Verlag.

More Natural Remedies. Agatha M. Thrash et al. 1984. (Illus.). pap. 6.95 (*0-942658-06-X*) NLB.

More Oral Sadism & the Vegetarian Personality. Glenn C. Ellenbogen. 1996. LC 96-783. 192p. pap. 13.95 (*0-87630-795-0*, 7950) Brunner-Routledge.

More Pages off the Doctor's Pad. Harold C. Klein. Ed. by Miriam S. Klein. 1999. 104p. pap. 9.95 (*1-879653-20-6*) Lakeside Pr.

More Than Just a Meal: The Art of Eating Disorders. Susan R. Makin. 1999. LC 99-43182. (Illus.). 208p. pap. text (*1-85302-805-3*) Jessica Kingsley GBR. *Dist:* Taylor & Francis.

Morfologia del Ojo: Histologia y Estructura Microscopica, Cornea, y Esclera. G. K. Smelser et al. Tr. by Norma Boschetti. 1980. LC 78-15614. (Illus.). 380p. 18.00 (*0-8477-2322-4*) U of PR Pr.

Moringa: Nature's Medicine Cabinet. Sanford Holst. 2000. LC 00-133478. (Illus.). 122p. pap. 9.95 (*1-887263-16-0*) Sierra Sunrise Pub.

Morita Therapy & the True Nature of Anxiety-Based Disorders (Shinkeishitsu) Shoma Morita. Ed. by Peg LeVine. Tr. by Akihisa Kondo. 1998. LC 97-35187. (Illus.). 160p. (C). text 19.50 (*0-7914-3765-5*) State U NY Pr.

Moritz Schlick. Ed. by Brian F. McGuinness. 1985. 156p. text 88.00 (*90-277-2096-7*) Kluwer Academic.

Morning Report: Internal Medicine. Thomas P. Archer et al. 1999. LC 99-33659. (Illus.). 373p. pap. 39.95 (*0-07-006692-2*) McGraw-Hill Prof.

Morning Star of the Reformation. Andy Thomson. 1988. LC 90-155223. 134p. (J). (gr. 7-12). pap. 6.49 (*0-89084-453-4*, 034637) Bob Jones Univ.

Moroney's Surgery for Nurses. Ed. by Malcolm R. Colmer. 16th ed. 1987. LC 85-26938. (Illus.). 624p. text (*0-443-03355-2*) Church.

Morphinism & Narcomanias from Other Drugs: Their Etiology, Treatment, & Medicolegal Relations. T. D. Crothers. Ed. by Gerald N. Grob. 1981. LC 80-1220. (Addiction in America Ser.). reprint ed. lib. bdg. 33.95 (*0-405-13577-7*) Ayer.

Morphogene des Humanpathogenen Pilzes Candida Albicans: Isolierung und Charakterisierung der Gene EFG1 und RFG1. Volker R. Stoldt. 1995. (Bibliotheca Mycologica: Vol. 162). (GER., Illus.). iii, 86p. (*3-443-59064-0*) Gebruder Borntraeger DEU. *Dist:* Balogh.

Morphogenesis: The Cellular & Molecular Processes of Developmental Anatomy. Jonathan B.L. Bard. 1992. (Developmental & Cell Biology Monographs: No. 23). (Illus.). 325p. (C). pap. text 29.95 (*0-521-43612-5*) Cambridge U Pr.

Morphogenesis of Endothelium. Ed. by Werner Risau & Gabor M. Rubanyi. 2000. 312p. 120.00 (*90-5823-061-9*, Harwood Acad Pubs) Gordon & Breach.

Morphogenesis of Lung Cancer. Ed. by Yukio Shimosato et al. Vol. I. 1982. 184p. 108.00 (*0-8493-6526-0*, RC280); Vol. II. 1983. 224p. 129.00 (*0-8493-6527-9*, RC280) Franklin (CRC Reprint).

Morphogenesis of T-Even Bacteriophages. B. F. Poglazov. 1973. (Monographs in Developmental Biology: Vol. 7). 47.00 (*3-8055-1645-2*) S Karger.

Morphogenesis of the Arteries of the Pelvic Extremity. C. Funke & H. J. Kuhn. Ed. by F. Beck et al. 1998. LC 98-29669. (Advances in Anatomy, Embryology & Cell Biology Ser.: Vol. 144). (Illus.). 132p. pap. 95.00 (*3-540-64706-6*) Spr-Verlag.

Morpholine. (C). 1995. (Health & Safety Guides Ser.: No. 92). 28p. pap. text 5.00 (*92-4-151092-7*, 1860092); 1996. (Environmental Health Criteria Ser.: Vol. 179). (FRE & SPA.). 163p. pap. 36.00 (*92-4-157179-9*, 1160179) World Health.

Morphologic & Functional MR of the Kidneys & Adrenal Glands. Gabriel Krestin. 1990. 115.00 (*0-938607-40-5*) Field & Wood Inc Medical.

Morphological & Functional Aspects of Placental Dysfunction. Ed. by Hiroaki Soma. 1982. (Contributions to Gynecology & Obstetrics Ser.: Vol. 9). (Illus.). viii, 180p. pap. 111.50 (*3-8055-3510-4*) S Karger.

Morphological Basis of Human Reproductive Function. G. Spera & D. M. DeKretser. 1987. LC 87-42790. (Illus.). 264p. (C). text 89.50 (*0-306-42738-9*, Kluwer Plenum) Kluwer Academic.

Morphological Diagnosis of Skin Disease: A Study of the Living Gross Pathology of the Skin. Robert Jackson. 1998. (Illus.). 496p. 79.00 (*1-896918-02-6*) Manticore Pubs.

Morphological Investigations of Single Neurons in Vitro. Ed. by Gloria E. Meredith & Gordon W. Arbuthnott. 1993. LC 93-10269. (IBRO Handbook Ser.: No. 16). 210p. pap. 295.00 (*0-471-93928-5*) Wiley.

Morphological Tumor Markets. Ed. by G. Seifert. 1987. (Current Topics in Pathology Ser.: Vol. 77). (Illus.). 398p. 214.00 (*0-387-16733-1*) Spr-Verlag.

Morphology & Function in MRI of the Cardiovascular & Renal Systems. G. K. Von Schulthess. 1988. (Illus.). 144p. 158.00 (*0-387-19061-9*) Spr-Verlag.

Morphology in Lung Transplantation: Proceedings of the Congress of Experimental Surgery Symposium, 7th, Amsterdam, April 1972. Congress of Experimental Surgery Symposium Staff. Ed. by R. H. Wildevuur. 1973. (Illus.). 85.25 (*3-8055-1441-7*) S Karger.

***Morphology Methods: Cell & Molecular Biology Techniques.** Ed. by Ricardo V. Lloyd. 2001. LC 2001-16959. (Illus.). xvi, 422p. 125.00 (*0-89603-955-2*) Humana.

Morphology of Experimental Respiratory Carcinogenesis: Proceedings. Ed. by Paul Nettesheim et al. 1970. LC 73-609398. (AEC Symposium Ser.). 500p. pap. 20.50 (*0-87079-277-6*, CONF-700501); fiche 9.00 (*0-87079-278-4*, CONF-700501) DOE.

Morphology of the Blood. Giuseppe D'Onofrio & Gina Zini. Tr. by Barbara J. Bain. 1998. LC 97-51175. 400p. (*0-7506-4055-3*) E A GBR. *Dist:* OUP.

Morphology of the Rat Brain Ventricles, Ependyma & Periventricular Structures. A. Mitro & M. Palkovits. 1981. (Bibliotheca Anatomica Ser.: No. 21). (Illus.). x, 110p. pap. 85.25 (*3-8055-2546-X*) S Karger.

Morphology, Phonology & Aphasia. Ed. by J. L. Nespoulous & P. Villiard. 1990. (Neuropsychology Ser.). (Illus.). 286p. 107.00 (*0-387-97183-1*) Spr-Verlag.

Morphometric Tools for Landmark Data: Geometry & Biology. Fred L. Bookstein. 1992. 455p. (C). text 110.00 (*0-521-38385-4*) Cambridge U Pr.

Morphometry. Ed. by Piero Tosi & G. Mariuzzi. 1987. (Journal: Vol. 4, No. 1-2, 1986). (Illus.). 112p. pap. 62.75 (*3-8055-4563-0*) S Karger.

Mort Safety Assurance Systems. W. Johnson. 1980. (Occupational Safety & Health Ser.: Vol. 4). (Illus.). 544p. text 140.00 (*0-8247-6897-3*) Dekker.

Mortal Men: Living with Asymptomatic HIV. Richard MacIntyre. 1999. LC 98-8501. 256p. (C). 26.00 (*0-8135-2596-9*) Rutgers U Pr.

Mortal Peril: Our Inalienable Right to Health Care? Richard A. Epstein. 2000. LC 96-46024. 528p. 27.50 (*0-201-13647-3*) Perseus Bks Grp.

Mortality & Health Policy. 1984. 30.00 (*92-1-151098-8*, E 84.XIII.4) UN.

Mortality from Malignant Neoplasms, 1955-1965 1970. (World Health Statistics Ser.). (ENG & FRE.). 1147p. pap. text 110.00 (*92-4-056008-4*, 1151107) World Health.

Mortality of Children under Age 5: World Estimates & Projections, 1950-2025. 1988. (Population Studies: No. 105). 50p. 9.50 (*92-1-151169-0*, E.88.XIII.4) UN.

Mortality Statistics - Child, Infant & Perinatal. 1998. (OPCS Series, 1996: No. 29). 81p. pap. (*0-11-621048-6*, HM10486) Statnry Office GBR. *Dist:* Bernan Associates.

Mortality Surveillance System: Models from the First Year. 1992. LC 92-48958. (Vital & Health Statistics Ser.: Series 20, No. 21). (*0-8406-0468-8*) Natl Ctr Health Stats.

Mortality Trends for Alzheimer's Disease, 1979-91. Donna L. Hoyert. 1995. LC 95-50806. (Vital & Health Statistics Ser.: Series 20, No. 28). (*0-8406-0511-0*) Natl Ctr Health Stats.

Morton's Medical Bibliography. Ed. by Jeremy M. Norman. 5th ed. 1991. 1046p. text (*0-85967-897-0*) Scolar Pr GBR. *Dist:* Ashgate Pub Co.

Mosaic of Care: Frail Elderly & Their Families in the Real World. Jaber F. Gubrium. 1990. 192p. 31.95 (*0-8261-7570-8*) Springer Pub.

Mosaic of Contemporary Psychiatry Perspectives. Ed. by A. Kales & M. Greenblatt. 1992. (Illus.). 448p. 99.00 (*0-387-97760-0*) Spr-Verlag.

Mosaic of Despair: Human Breakdowns in Prison. Hans Toch. rev. ed. 1992. LC 92-17878. Orig. Title: Men in Crisis. 452p. text 19.95 (*1-55798-177-9*) Am Psychol.

Mosby Buyer's Guide to Ten Essential Herbs. Mosby Staff. 1997. 96p. pap. text 10.00 (*1-57857-004-2*) Mosby Consmer Hlth.

***Mosby Drug Cards, 2001 Edition.** Joseph A. Albanese & Patricia A. Nutz. 11th ed. 2001. 445p. pap. 31.95 (*0-323-00794-5*) Mosby Inc.

Mosby Medical Encyclopedia. Walter D. Glanze. rev. ed. 1992. (Illus.). 1024p. (Orig.). pap. 19.95 (*0-452-26672-6*, Plume) Dutton Plume.

Mosby Patient Teaching Guides for Health Promotion. Mosby Staff. 1997. 32p. (C). (gr. 13). pap. text 24.95 (*0-8151-2574-7*, 31313) Mosby Inc.

Mosby Soundbytes - Education. Mosby Staff. 1996. 36.00 (*0-8151-4440-7*) Mosby Inc.

***Mosby Soundbytes - Health Care Managers.** Mosby Inc. Staff. 1996. 36.00 (*0-8151-4442-3*) Mosby Inc.

***Mosby Soundbytes - Psychiatry.** Mosby Inc. Staff. 1996. 36.00 (*0-8151-3712-5*) Mosby Inc.

Mosby's ABCs of Test Taking for Nurses: Anchor Your Anxiety, Build Your Basic. Paulette D. Rollant. 1999. LC 99-10465. (Illus.). 240p. (C). (gr. 13). pap. text 21.95 (*0-8151-3858-X*, 31669) Mosby Inc.

Mosby's Ace the Boards: General Clinical Sciences. Anthony J. Alario. 1999. LC 98-51164. 336p. (C). (gr. 13). pap. text 28.95 (*0-8151-3715-X*, 31410) Mosby Inc.

Mosby's Ace the Boards: USMLE Step 1 Review, Physiology, Windows. Uwe Ackermann. 1996. LC 96-8434. (Ace the Boards Win Ser.). (Illus.). 304p. pap. text 31.95 (*0-8151-0054-X*, 27044) Mosby Inc.

Mosby's Anatomy & Physiology Lab Manual. Kathleen B. Sloan. 1990. (Illus.). 312p. (C). (gr. 13). pap. text 18.95 (*0-8016-5986-8*, 05986) Mosby Inc.

Mosby's Assesstest: 1999 Secured Version. Dolores F. Saxton et al. 1998. 86p. (*0-323-00290-0*) Mosby Inc.

Mosby's Assesstest: 1999 Unsecured Version. Dolores F. Saxton et al. 1998. 72p. (*0-323-00291-9*) Mosby Inc.

Mosby's Assesstest Unsecured. Dolores F. Saxlon. 2000. 32.00 (*0-323-01272-8*) Mosby Inc.

Mosby's Assisting with Patient Care. Bernardine Gorek. 1999. (Illus.). 336p. stu. ed. (*0-323-00753-8*) Mosby Inc.

Mosby's Assisting with Patient Care. Sheila A. Sorrentino. 1998. (Illus.). 912p. (C). (gr. 13). pap. text 35.00 (*0-8151-2033-8*, 31707) Mosby Inc.

Mosby's Assisting with Patient Care: Includes Testbank. Sheila A. Sorrentino. 1999. (Illus.). tchr. ed. (*0-8151-2034-6*) Mosby Inc.

Mosby's Atlas & Text of Clinical Imaging. Jamie Weir & Alison D. Murray. 1998. (Illus.). 256p. pap. (*84-8174-402-6*) Mosby-Doyma Libros ESP. *Dist:* Mosby Inc.

Mosby's Basic Science for Soft Tissue & Movement Therapies. Sandy Fritz et al. 1999. (Illus.). 644p. pap., tchr. ed. (*0-323-00463-6*); 1998. LC 98-14479. pap. text 36.00 (*0-323-00284-6*); 2nd ed. 1999. (Illus.). 644p. pap. 71.95 (*0-323-00933-6*) Mosby Inc.

Mosby's Biomedical Science Series: Understanding Immunology. Roth Coe-Clough. 1997. LC 97-9892. (Illus.). 240p. (gr. 13). pap. text 23.00 (*0-8151-8582-0*, 28791) Mosby Inc.

***Mosby's Clinical Medical Assisting.** 1994. wbk. ed. 13.95 (*0-8151-0518-5*) Mosby Inc.

Mosby's Clinical Nursing. June Thompson. 4th ed. 1997. 1848p. text 49.95 (*0-8151-2573-9*, 31312) Mosby Inc.

Mosby's Clinical Nursing. June Thompson. 5th ed. 2001. 1652p. text (*0-323-01195-0*) Mosby Inc.

Mosby's Clinical Skills for Medical Assistants. Sharron M. Zakus. 4th ed. 1999. LC 00-66999. (Illus.). 752p. text 52.00 (*0-323-00766-X*) Mosby Inc.

Mosby's Color Atlas & Text of Diabetes & Endocrinology. Peter E. Belchetz & Peter Hammond. 6th ed. 1999. (Illus.). 304p. 39.95 (*0-7234-3104-3*) Mosby Inc.

Mosby's Color Atlas & Text of Gastroenterology. Richard J. Aspinall & Simon D. Taylor-Robinson. 1999. (Illus.). 304p. 39.95 (*0-7234-3103-5*) Mosby Inc.

Mosby's Complementary & Alternative Therapies. Lyn Freeman. 2000. (Illus.). 608p. 49.00 (*0-323-00697-3*) Mosby Inc.

Mosby's Comprehensive Review of Dental Hygiene. Michele L. Darby. 4th ed. 1997. LC 97-34800. (Illus.). 912p. (C). (gr. 13). pap. text 45.95 (*0-8151-2267-5*, 29189) Mosby Inc.

Mosby's Comprehensive Review of Nursing. Dolores F. Saxton et al. 1999. 912p. pap. (*84-8174-212-0*) Mosby-Doyma Libros ESP. *Dist:* Mosby Inc.

Mosby's Comprehensive Review of Nursing. Ed. by Patricia Mary Nugent et al. 16th ed. 1998. LC 99-184202. (Illus.). 928p. pap. text 29.95 (*0-323-00286-2*) Mosby Inc.

Mosby's Comprehensive Review of Practical Nursing. Mary O. Eyles. 1999. 39.95 (*0-323-00313-3*) Mosby Inc.

Mosby's Comprehensive Review of Practical Nursing for NCLEX-PN. Ed. by Mary O. Eyles. 12th ed. 1997. LC 97-17859. (Illus.). 648p. (C). (gr. 13). pap. text 27.95 incl. disk (*0-8151-2388-4*, 31041) Mosby Inc.

Mosby's Comprehensive Review of Practical Nursing for NCLEX-PN. Mary O. Eyles. 13th ed. 2000. (Illus.). 735p. 29.95 (*0-323-01166-7*) Mosby Inc.

Mosby's Comprehensive Review of Radiography. William J. Callaway. 2nd ed. 1998. LC 97-41998. (Illus.). 336p. (C). (gr. 13). pap. text 32.95 (*0-8151-2900-9*, 31811) Mosby Inc.

Mosby's Conventional Medicine, Alternative Medicine. Green. 1998. (Illus.). 112p. pap. text 12.95 (*0-916363-17-1*) Beechwood Hlthbks.

Mosby's CPG Mentor - Patient Cases in Respiratory Care Series Lonny J. Ashworth. 1998. (*0-8151-2276-4*) Mosby Inc.

***Mosby's Crash Course: Cells & Genetics.** Emma Jones & Anna Morris. 1998. (Illus.). 216p. 26.95 (*0-7234-3135-3*) Mosby Inc.

***Mosby's Crash Course: History & Physical Examination.** James Marsh. 1998. (Illus.). 252p. 26.95 (*0-7234-3146-9*) Mosby Inc.

***Mosby's Crash Course: Immune System, Blood & Lymphatics.** Saimah Arif & Arjmand Mufti. 1998. (Illus.). 240p. text 26.95 (*0-7234-2993-6*) Mosby Inc.

Mosby's Crash Course: Internal Medicine. Ed. by Daniel A. Horton-Szar. 1998. (*0-7234-3114-0*) Mosby Inc.

***Mosby's Crash Course: Musculoskeletal System.** Sona Biswas & Rehana Iqbal. 1998. (Illus.). 288p. 26.95 (*0-7234-3127-2*) Mosby Inc.

***Mosby's Crash Course: Obstetrics & Gynaecology.** Mark Broadbent et al. 1999. (Illus.). 288p. (*0-7234-3151-5*) Mosby Inc.

***Mosby's Crash Course: Paediatrics.** Mark Gardiner & Christine Budd. 1999. (Illus.). 288p. 26.95 (*0-7234-3139-6*) Mosby Inc.

***Mosby's Crash Course: Pathology.** Bethan Goodman Jones. 1998. (Illus.). 288p. 26.95 (*0-7234-3142-6*) Mosby Inc.

***Mosby's Crash Course: Pharmacology.** Magali Taylor & Peter Reide. 1998. pap. 26.95 (*0-7234-3125-6*) Mosby Inc.

***Mosby's Crash Course: Renal & Urinary Systems.** Nisha Nirpuri & Pratiksha Patel. 1998. (Illus.). 240p. 26.95 (*0-7234-3126-4*) Mosby Inc.

Mosby's Critical Care Nursing Consultant. Janet Hicks Keen. Ed. by Pamela L. Swearingen. 1997. LC 97-6318. (Illus.). 544p. (C). (gr. 13). text 49.95 (*0-8151-3178-X*, 29561) Mosby Inc.

Mosby's Critical Care Nursing Consultant. Pamela L. Swearingen & Janet H. Keen. 1997. LC 97-6318. (*0-08-151378-X*) Elsevier.

Mosby's Critical Care Nursing Reference. Susan B. Stillwell. 2nd ed. 1996. LC 95-51676. (Illus.). 816p. (C). (gr. 13). text 34.95 (*0-8151-8241-4*, 26898) Mosby Inc.

Mosby's Dental Dictionary. Thomas J. Zwemer. 1998. LC 97-41342. (Illus.). 704p. (YA). (gr. 13). text 39.95 (*0-8151-9888-4*, 29172) Mosby Inc.

Mosby's Dental Drug Reference. Mosby-Year Book Staff. 4th ed. 1998. pap. 33.95 (*0-323-00501-2*) Mosby Inc.

Mosby's Dental Drug Reference. Tommy W. Gage & Frieda Atherton Pickett. 5th ed. 2000. 830p. 34.95 (*0-323-01196-9*) Mosby Inc.

Mosby's Desktop Primary Care Consultant: Rapid Access to Current Diagnosis Treatments. Fred F. Ferri. 1998. LC 98-3837. (Illus.). xxiv, 1124p. (C). (gr. 13). text 54.95 (*0-8151-0317-4*, 30998) Mosby Inc.

Mosbys Diagnostic & Laboratory Test, 1900-2000. Kathleen D. Pagana. 4th ed. 1998. LC 98-27246. (Illus.). xxiii, 967p. 27.95 (*0-323-00288-9*) Mosby Inc.

Mosby's Diagnostic & Laboratory Test Reference. Kathleen Deska Pagana & Timothy James Pagana. 4th ed. 1999. (Illus.). 990p. spiral bd. (*84-8174-142-6*) Mosby-Doyma Libros ESP. *Dist:* Mosby Inc.

Mosby's Diagnostic & Laboratory Test Reference. Kathleen Pagana & Timothy Pagana. 5th ed. 2000. LC 00-56248. (Illus.). 1005p. 29.95 (*0-323-01178-0*) Mosby Inc.

Mosby's Drug Guide for Nurses. Linda Skidmore. 3rd ed. 1999. (C). text (*0-323-01130-6*) Mosby Inc.

Mosby's Drug Guide for Nurses. Linda Skidmore-Roth. 3rd ed. 1998. (*0-323-00500-4*); LC 98-23778. (Illus.). 1568p. 29.95 (*0-323-00308-7*) Mosby Inc.

Mosby's Drug Guide for Nurses. Linda Skidmore. 4th ed. 2000. 1430p. pap. text 34.95 (*0-323-01174-8*) Mosby Inc.

Mosby's Drug Reference: British Edition. Linda Skidmore-Roth. 1991. (*0-8016-4586-7*) Mosby Inc.

Mosby's Emergency Department Patient Teaching Guides. Jean A. Proehl & Linell M. Jones. (Illus.). 1998. 168p. (*1-55664-564-3*); 1997. LC 97-15759. 128p. (C). text 72.00 (*0-8151-3829-6*, 30305) Mosby Inc.

***Mosby's Emergency Department Patient Teaching Guides.** Jean A. Proehl & Linell M. Jones. 1998. (Illus.). 128p. 185.00 incl. cd-rom (*0-323-00125-4*) Mosby Inc.

Mosby's Emergency Dictionary: Quick Reference. William Garcia. 2nd ed. 1997. LC 97-34822. (Illus.). 512p. (C). (gr. 13). pap. text 33.95 (*0-8016-7941-9*, 07941) Mosby Inc.

Mosby's Emergency Nursing Reference. Pamela Stinson Kidd & Patricia Sturt. 1996. (Illus.). 896p. pap. (*84-8174-319-4*) Mosby-Doyma Libros ESP. *Dist:* Mosby Inc.

Mosby's Emergency Nursing Reference. Pamela S. Kidd. 2nd ed. 2000. LC 2001-272298. (Illus.). xv, 959p. pap. text 37.95 (*0-323-01108-X*) Mosby Inc.

Mosby's EMT: Intermediate Test Generator. Richard Campbell. 1999. 60.00 (*0-323-01067-9*) Mosby Inc.

Mosby's EMT - Basic Textbook. Walt A. Stoy & Center for Emergency Medicine Staff. 1995. LC 95-24140. (Illus.). 704p. (C). (gr. 13). text 37.95 (*0-8151-7958-8*, 25207) Mosby Inc.

Mosby's EMT Basic Computerized Test Generator, DOS. Barbara Aehlert. 1996. ring bd. 61.00 (*0-8151-1473-7*) Mosby Inc.

***Mosby's EMT Basic Computerized Test Generator, DOS: Windows.** Barbara Aehlert. 1996. ring bd. 61.00 incl. disk (*0-8151-1472-9*) Mosby Inc.

Mosby's EMT-Basic Hardcover. Walt A. Stoy. 1996. pap., wbk. ed. (*0-8151-9653-9*); text, wbk. ed. (*0-8151-9654-7*) Mosby Inc.

Mosby's EMT-Basic Textbook. Walt A. Stoy. 1996. tchr. ed. (*0-8151-7960-X*); 1996. wbk. ed. (*0-8151-7959-6*); 1995. (Illus.). (C). pap. (*0-8151-8055-1*, 27238) Mosby Inc.

Mosby's Essentials for Nursing Assistants. Sheila Sorrentino. 1997. (Illus.). tchr. ed. (*0-8151-5258-2*) Mosby Inc.

***Mosby's Essentials for Nursing Assistants.** Sheila A. Sorrentino & Bernie Gorek. 2nd ed. 2001. (Illus.). 400p. pap. (*0-323-01324-4*) Mosby Inc.

***Mosby's Essentials for Nursing Assistants: Instructor's Guide.** Sheila A. Sorrentino & Bernie Gorek. 2001. pap., tchr. ed. (*0-323-01326-0*) Mosby Inc.

Mosby's Expert Rapid Response. Mosby Staff. 1998. 448p. pap. text 36.95 (*0-323-00548-9*) Mosby Inc.

Mosby's Family Practice Sourcebook, 1999: Current Literature & Medical Evidence in Patient Care. Kenneth G. Marshall. 1999. LC 98-15925. (Illus.). 405p. (C). pap. text 54.95 (*0-8151-2785-5*, 31801) Mosby Inc.

Mosby's Family Practice Sourcebook, 2000. Kenneth G. Marshall. 1999. (Illus.). 512p. (C). text 59.00 (*1-55664-468-X*) Mosby Inc.

Mosby's First Responder Textbook. Walt A. Stoy. 1997. LC 96-79893. (Illus.). 352p. (C). (gr. 13). pap. text 29.95 (*0-8151-8279-1*, 28070) Mosby Inc.

Mosby's Fundamentals of Medical Assistants. Eggars & Sharron M. Zakus. 2nd ed. 1990. (Illus.). (gr. 13). 736p. text 39.95 (*0-8016-4280-9*, 04280); 208p. pap. text, stu. ed. 16.95 (*0-8016-5293-6*, 05293) Mosby Inc.

Mosby's Fundamentals of Medical Assisting. Sharron M. Zakus et al. 2nd ed. 1990. tchr. ed. (*0-8151-2702-2*) Mosby Inc.

Mosby's Fundamentals of Therapeutic Massage. Sandra Fritz. 1995. tchr. ed. (*0-8151-3253-0*); wbk. ed. (*0-8151-3301-4*);Set. (C). text, wbk. ed. (*0-8151-3323-5*) Mosby Inc.

Mosby's Fundamentals of Therapeutic Message. Sandy Fritz. 2nd ed. 1999. LC 99-14180. (Illus.). 681p. text 49.00 (*0-323-00677-9*) Harcourt.

Mosby's GenRx: 1999 Edition. Genrx. 1998. (Mosby's Physicians GenRx Ser.). 72.95 (*0-323-00625-6*) Mosby Inc.

Mosby's GenRx: A Comprehensive Reference for Generic & Brand Prescription Drugs. Mosby's GenRx Staff. 11th ed. 2000. (Mosby's Physicians GenRx Ser.). (Illus.). 2750p. 49.95 (*0-323-00629-9*) Mosby Inc.

Mosby's Genrx Retail Direct Mail 1998. Mosby-Year Book Staff. 1997. (C). text 69.95 (*0-8151-4418-0*, 30812) Mosby Inc.

Mosby's Guide to Physical Examination. Henry M. Seidel. 1991. 816p. (gr. 13). text 175.00 (*0-8016-6520-5*) Mosby Inc.

Mosby's Guide to Physical Examination. Henry M. Seidel et al. 3rd ed. 1995. (Illus.). tchr. ed. (*0-8151-6136-0*) Mosby Inc.

Mosby's Guide to Physical Examination. Jean Giddens. 4th ed. 1998. (Illus.). 256p. stu. ed., wbk. ed. (*0-323-00309-5*) Mosby Inc.

Mosby's Guide to Physical Examination. Henry M. Seidel. 4th ed. 1998. LC 98-27245. 1008p. text 58.00 (*0-323-00178-5*); (Illus.). tchr. ed. (*0-323-00451-2*) Mosby Inc.

Mosby's Guide to Physical Examination. Henry M. Seidel et al. 4th ed. 1999. (Illus.). 992p. (*84-8174-165-5*) Mosby-Doyma Libros ESP. *Dist:* Mosby Inc.

Mosby's Handbook of Diseases. Rae Langford & June M. Thompson. 1996. LC 95-52142. 624p. (C). (gr. 13). text 26.95 (*0-8151-8771-8*, 25183) Mosby Inc.

Mosby's Handbook of Diseases. Rae W. Langford & June D. Thompson. 2nd ed. 2000. LC 00-267725. xv, 591p. pap. text 26.95 (*0-323-00895-X*) Mosby Inc.

Mosby's Handbook of Herbs & Natural Supplement. Paul Skidmore. 2001. text (*0-323-01208-6*) Mosby Inc.

Mosby's Home Care & Hospice Drug Handbook. Tina M. Marrelli et al. 1999. LC 00-698994. (Illus.). xx, 759p. (C). (gr. 13). text 26.95 (*0-8151-1226-2*, 31777) Mosby Inc.

Mosby's Home Health Client. Karen Martin. 2000. (Illus.). 96p. text, tchr. ed. 24.95 (*0-8151-8589-8*, 28841) Mosby Inc.

Mosby's Home Health Client Teaching. Karen Martin. 1997. (Illus.). 416p. (C). (gr. 13). text 114.00 (*0-8151-2296-9*, 29975) Mosby Inc.

Mosby's Home Health Client Teaching Guides: RX for Teaching. 3rd rev. ed. 1999. (Illus.). 96p. text 24.95 (*0-8151-8590-1*, 28842) Mosby Inc.

Mosby's Home Health Nursing Pocket Consultant. C. V. Mosby. 1994. LC 95-136742. (Illus.). 352p. (C). (gr. 13). spiral bd. 29.95 (*0-8151-6125-5*, 25341) Mosby Inc.

Mosby's Manual of Diagnostic & Laboratory Tests. Kathleen D. Pagana & Timothy Pagana. 1998. LC 97-40589. (Illus.). 960p. (C). (gr. 13). pap. text 29.95 (*0-8151-5586-7*, 29626) Mosby Inc.

Mosby's Maternal-Newborn Patient Teaching Guides. Carol Schlef. 2000. LC 99-12448. (Illus.). 252p. pap. 72.00 (*0-323-00465-2*) Mosby Inc.

***Mosby's Maternal-Newborn Patient Teaching Guides.** Carol Schlef. 2000. (Illus.). 252p. 185.00 incl. cd-rom (*0-323-00957-3*) Mosby Inc.

Mosby's Medical Assisting Examination Review. Joanna Bligh. 1999. LC 2001-34267. (Illus.). 320p. (C). text 38.95 (*0-323-00349-4*) Mosby Inc.

Mosby's Medical Drug Reference, 2003-2004. Ellsworth et al. 2002. 1184p. pap. text 32.95 (*0-8151-3658-7*, 31229) Mosby Inc.

Mosby's Medical, Nursing & Allied Health Dictionary. Kenneth N. Anderson & C. V. Mosby. 4th ed. 1993. (Illus.). 2208p. (C). (gr. 13). text 32.95 (*0-8016-7225-2*, 07225) Mosby Inc.

Mosby's Medical, Nursing & Allied Health Dictionary. Kenneth N. Anderson et al. 5th ed. 1998. (Illus.). 2112p. (*84-8174-380-1*) Mosby-Doyma Libros ESP. *Dist:* Mosby Inc.

Mosby's Medical, Nursing & Allied Health Dictionary. Kenneth Anderson et al. 5th ed. LC 97-33687. 1998. 34.95 (*1-55664-566-X*); 1997. (Illus.). 2112p. (C). (gr. 13). text 32.95 (*0-8151-4800-3*, 29948) Mosby Inc.

Mosby's Medical Surfari: Guide to Exploring Internet & Discover. Gibbs. 2nd ed. 2000. 24.95 incl. cd-rom (*1-55664-558-9*) Mosby Inc.

Mosby's 1999 Nursing Drug Reference & Review Cards. Joseph A. Albanese & Patricia A. Nutz. 9th ed. 1998. 300p. (C). (gr. 13). text 29.95 (*0-8151-2056-7*, 27777) Mosby Inc.

Mosby's Nursing Drug Database, 1999. Mosby Staff. 1998. pap. 39.95 (*0-323-00659-0*) Mosby Inc.

Mosby's Nursing Drug Reference. Linda Skidmore-Roth. 1998. (Mosby's Nursing Drug Reference Ser.). 1185p. pap. 29.95 (*0-323-00307-9*) Harcrt Hlth Sci Grp.

Mosby's Nursing Drug Reference 2001. Linda Skidmore-Roth. 2000. (Mosby's Nursing Drug Reference Ser.). (Illus.). 1280p. pap. text 31.95 (*0-323-00981-6*) Mosby Inc.

Mosby's Oncology Nursing Certification Review. Cynthia C. Chernecky & Sue Schlesselman. 2000. LC 99-38245. x, 328p. (*0-323-00960-3*) Mosby Inc.

***Mosby's Online Computer Adaptive Test (CAT) for NCLEX-RN.** Dolores F. Saxton. 2000. (*0-323-00817-8*) Mosby Inc.

Mosby's OTC Drugs: A Resource for Health Professionals. Richard P. Donjon & Bryon J. Goeckner. 1998. LC 98-39429. (Illus.). 464p. (C). (gr. 13). text 29.95 (*0-8151-8395-X*, 31695) Mosby Inc.

Mosby's Outdoor Emergency Medical Guide. David H. Manhoff. 1996. LC 96-164036. (Illus.). 66p. spiral bd. 12.95 (*0-916363-14-7*) Mosby Inc.

Mosby's Paramedic Text. Mick J. Sanders & Kim McKenna. 1996. (C). (gr. 13). reprint ed. text, wbk. ed. 59.95 (*0-8151-2470-8*, 31259) Mosby Inc.

Mosby's Paramedic Textbook. Mick J. Sanders. 1995. 1008p. (gr. 13). text 51.95 (*0-8016-4315-5*, 28181); 2nd ed. 2000. LC 00-702859. (Illus.). xxiv, 1606p. 64.95 (*0-323-00652-3*) Mosby Inc.

***Mosby's Paramedic Textbook.** Mick J. Sanders & Kim McKenna. 2nd ed. 2000. (Illus.). tchr. ed. 40.00 (*0-323-01264-7*) Mosby Inc.

Mosby's Paramedic Workbook. Mick J. Sanders. 2nd ed. 2000. 26.95 (*0-323-00951-4*) Mosby Inc.

Mosby's Patient Carelink. Mosby Staff. 1998. 160p. (*0-8151-4457-1*) Mosby Inc.

Mosby's Patient Teaching Guides. 1996. (Illus.). 226p. 72.95 (*0-8151-3315-4*) Mosby Inc.

Mosby's Patient Teaching Guides. Mosby Staff. 1994. (C). (gr. 13). spiral bd. 52.95 (*0-8151-5862-9*, 25114) Mosby Inc.

Mosby's Patient Teaching Guides: Update 3, Update 3. Mosby Staff. 1998. (Illus.). 40p. (*0-323-00073-8*) Mosby Inc.

Mosby's Patient Teaching Guides with Updates 2 & 3. Mosby Staff. 1998. (*0-323-00227-7*) Mosby Inc.

Mosby's Patient Teaching Guides with Updates 2 & 3: Tips. Mosby Staff. 1998. (*0-8151-6196-4*) Mosby Inc.

Mosby's Pediatric Nursing Reference. Ed. by Cecily L. Betz & Linda A. Sowden. 3rd ed. 1996. LC 95-26736. (Illus.). 672p. (C). (gr. 13). pap. text 33.95 (*0-8151-0599-1*, 26571) Mosby Inc.

Mosby's Pediatric Nursing Reference. Betz. 4th ed. 1999. 743p. text 34.95 (*0-323-00935-2*) Mosby Inc.

Mosby's Pediatric Patient Teaching Guides. Jane W. Ball. 1998. LC 97-37998. (Illus.). 224p. (C). (gr. 13). text 74.95 (*0-8151-1558-X*, 29994) Mosby Inc.

Mosby's Pediatric Patient Teaching Guides. Jane W. Ball. 1998. LC 97-37607. (Illus.). 225p. (C). text 129.00 (*0-8151-2577-1*) Mosby Inc.

Mosby's Perfect Pregnancy. Thompson. 1998. (Illus.). 112p. pap. text 12.95 (*0-916363-15-5*) Beechwood Hlthbks.

Mosby's Pharmacology in Nursing. Contrib. by McKenry Staff. 20th ed. 1998. 58.00 (*0-323-01275-2*) Mosby Inc.

Mosby's Pharmacology in Nursing. Leda M. McKenry & Evelyn Salerno. 20th ed. 1998. 96p. (C). pap. text, stu. ed. (*0-8151-4516-0*, 30650); 21st ed. 2001. LC 00-56838. (Illus.). 1344p. text 59.00 (*0-323-01005-9*); Vol. 20. 20th ed. 1997. LC 98-220129. (Illus.). 1200p. (C). (gr. 13). text 56.00 (*0-8151-4515-2*, 30649) Mosby Inc.

Mosby's Pharmacology in Nursing: Includes Testbank. Contrib. by Leda M. McKenry & Evelyn Salerno. 20th ed. 1998. tchr. ed. (*0-8151-2132-6*) Mosby Inc.

***Mosby's Pharmacology in Nursing: Instructor's Electronic Resource.** Leda M. McKenry. 21st ed. 2001. (Illus.). 750.00 (*0-323-01008-3*) Mosby Inc.

Mosby's Pharmacology in Nursing: Quick Medication Administration Reference. Leda M. McKenry & Evelyn Salerno. 1998. LC 99-174426. (Illus.). (*1-55664-481-7*) Mosby Inc.

Mosby's Pharmacology in Nursing Package. Leda M. McKenry. 20th ed. 1998. 1392p. (C). (gr. 13). text 63.00 (*0-8151-4517-9*, 30651) Mosby Inc.

Mosby's Pharmacology Patient Teaching Guide. Leda M. McKenry. 1999. (Illus.). ring bd. 139.00 incl. cd-rom (*0-8151-2934-3*); LC 98-45346. 400p. (C). text 59.95 (*0-8151-2933-5*, 31829) Mosby Inc.

Mosbys Physical Examination Handbook. Seidel. 2nd ed. 1998. LC 98-27273. (Illus.). 320p. pap. text 25.95 (*0-323-00179-3*) Mosby Inc.

Mosby's PN Assesstest. Mary O. Eyles. 3rd ed. 1995. 48p. (C). (gr. 13). pap. text 29.95 (*0-8151-9775-6*, 25329) Mosby Inc.

Mosby's Pocket Dictionary of Medicine, Nursing & Allied Health. Kenneth N. Anderson & Lois E. Anderson. 3rd ed. 1998. 1312p. (*84-8174-301-1*) Mosby-Doyma Libros ESP. *Dist:* Mosby Inc.

Mosby's Pocket Dictionary of Medicine, Nursing & Allied Health, Vol. 3. Kenneth N. Anderson et al. 3rd ed. 1998. LC 98-3311. (Mosby's Pocket Dictionary of Medicine, Nursing & Allied Heal Ser.). 1312p. (YA). (gr. 13). text 25.95 (*0-8151-3166-6*, 28931) Mosby Inc.

Mosby's Primary Care Patient Teaching Guides. Mosby Staff. 2nd rev. ed. Date not set. ring bd. 39.95 (*0-8151-8399-2*) Mosby Inc.

Mosby's Psychiatric Nursing Study Guide: Instructor's Resource Manual. Mosby Staff. 1997. (C). (gr. 13). text (*0-8151-2131-8*, 30751) Mosby Inc.

Mosby's Questions & Answers for NCLEX-PN. Mary O. Eyles. 2nd ed. 1998. LC 99-181156. 320p. (C). text 26.95 (*0-323-00151-3*) Mosby Inc.

Mosby's Quick Review: Neuroscience. Mosby Staff. 1999. 350p. text 29.95 incl. cd-rom (*0-323-00836-4*) Mosby Inc.

Mosby's Rapid Review Series: Medical-Surgical Nursing. Paulette D. Rollant & Deborah E. Ennis. 2nd ed. 2000. LC 00-45243. (Illus.). xxvii, 468p. 24.95 (*0-323-01177-2*) Mosby Inc.

Mosby's Resource Guide to Children with Disabilities & Chronic Illness. Ed. by Helen M. Wallace et al. 1996. LC 96-10609. (Illus.). 528p. (C). (gr. 13). text 59.00 (*0-8151-9051-4*, 28151) Mosby Inc.

Mosby's Review Cards: Marternity Women Health Nursing. Multi-Resources Incorporation et al. 1997. (Mosby's Review Cards Ser.). 273p. text 22.95 (*0-8151-7382-2*, 28138) Mosby Inc.

***Mosby's Review Cards: Medical-Surgical Nursing.** Paulette D. Rollant & Karen A. Piotrowski. 1997. (Rollant Nursing Review Ser.). 270p. 24.95 (*0-8151-7375-X*) Mosby Inc.

Mosby's Review Cards: Mental Health Nursing. Multi-Resources Incorporation et al. 1997. (Mosby's Review Cards Ser.). 232p. text 22.95 (*0-8151-7378-4*, 28137) Mosby Inc.

***Mosby's Review Cards: Nursing Pharmacology.** Paulette D. Rollant & Karen Hill. 1997. (Rollant Nursing Review Ser.). 236p. 24.95 (*0-8151-7380-6*) Mosby Inc.

Mosby's Review Cards: Pediatric Nursing. Multi-Resources Incorporation Staff et al. 1997. (Mosby's Review Cards Ser.). 190p. text 22.95 (*0-8151-7377-6*, 28136) Mosby Inc.

Mosby's Review for Long-Term Care Certification for Practical & Vocational Nurses. Mary O. Eyles. 1996. LC 96-138897. 224p. (C). (gr. 13). pap. text 25.95 (*0-8151-3170-4*, 29307) Mosby Inc.

Mosby's Review for the Clinical Competency Test: Large Animal Medicine & Surgery. Corrine R. Sweeney. 1997. 264p. (C). (gr. 13). pap. text 39.95 (*0-8151-4443-1*, 30740) Mosby Inc.

Mosby's Review for the Clinical Competency Test: Small Animal Medicine & Surgery. Ellen Miller. 1997. LC 98-231811. 264p. (C). (gr. 13). pap. text 39.95 (*0-8151-4379-6*, 31125) Mosby Inc.

Mosby's Review Questions for NCLEX-RN. Delores F. Saxton. 3rd ed. 1997. LC 97-1041. 736p. (C). (gr. 13). pap. text 28.95 (*0-8151-2836-3*, 30965) Mosby Inc.

Mosby's Rounds: Interactive Case Studies in Internal Medicine, Windows. Timothy Rice. 1995. 32p. incl. disk (*0-8151-6478-5*) Mosby Inc.

Mosby's Spanish/English-English/Spanish Medical Dictionary. Ed. by Mosby Staff. 1996. (ENG & SPA.). 275.00 (*0-7859-9704-0*) Fr & Eur.

Mosby's Sports Therapy: Taping Guide. Robert Kennedy. 1995. LC 95-165980. 144p. spiral bd. 16.95 (*0-8151-5198-5*, 26955) Mosby Inc.

Mosby's Success in Medicine: Anatomy (Ibm) Mosby Staff. 1996. (Illus.). 480p. (C). (gr. 13). pap. text 29.95 incl. 3.5 hd (*0-8151-8974-5*, 29056) Mosby Inc.

Mosby's Success in Medicine: Biochemistry (Ibm) Mosby Staff. 1996. 400p. (C). (gr. 13). pap. text 29.95 (*0-8151-8985-0*, 29062) Mosby Inc.

Mosby's Success in Medicine: Physiology (IBM) Mosby Staff. 1996. (Illus.). 304p. (C). (gr. 13). pap. text 29.95 (*0-8151-8914-1*, 29046) Mosby Inc.

Mosby's Survival Guide to Medical Abbreviations, Acronyms, Symbols, Prefixes & Suffixes. June M. Campbell. 1994. LC 95-119665. 608p. (C). (gr. 13). text 24.95 (*0-8151-1398-6*, 25635) Mosby Inc.

Mosby's Textbook & Workbook for Nursing Assistants. Sheila A. Sorrentino. 4th ed. 1995. 1p. (gr. 13). pap. text 40.00 (*0-8151-8028-4*, 25742) Mosby Inc.

Mosby's Textbook for Long-Term Care & Workbook Package. Sheila Sorrentino & Bernardine Gorek. 3rd ed. 1999. (Illus.). 912p. pap., wbk. ed. 42.00 (*0-323-00707-4*) Mosby Inc.

Mosby's Textbook for Long Term Care Assistants. Sheila Sorrentino & Jean Hogan. 2nd ed. 1994. (Illus.). tchr. ed. (*0-8151-7945-6*); tchr. ed. (*0-8151-7946-4*) Mosby Inc.

Mosby's Textbook for Long Term Care Assistants. Sheila Sorrentino. 3rd ed. 1999. tchr. ed. (*0-323-00711-2*) Mosby Inc.

Mosby's Textbook for Long-Term Care Assistants. Sheila Sorrentino. 3rd ed. 1999. LC 99-461782. 724p. text 34.00 (*0-323-00709-0*) Mosby Inc.

Mosby's Textbook for Long Term Care Assistants: LTC Textbook & Workbook Package. Sheila A. Sorrentino & Jean Hogan. 2nd ed. 1994. (Illus.). wbk. ed. (*0-8151-7887-5*) Mosby Inc.

Mosby's Textbook for Nursing Assistants. Sheila A. Sorrentino. 3rd ed. 1991. (Illus.). 528p. (gr. 13). text 28.95 (*0-8016-6589-2*, 06589); 4th ed. 1996. (Illus.). tchr. ed. (*0-8016-6273-7*); 4th ed. 1996. tchr. ed. (*0-8151-8027-6*); 4th ed. 1996. 268p. pap. text, wbk. ed. 17.95 (*0-8151-5057-1*) Mosby Inc.

Mosbys Textbook for Nursing Assistants. Shelia A. Sorentino. 5th ed. 1999. 884p. pap. text 34.95 (*0-323-00924-7*) Mosby Inc.

Mosby's Textbook for Nursing Assistants. Sheila A. Sorrentino. 5th ed. 2000. 884p. (*0-323-00926-3*) Mosby Inc.

Mosby's Textbook for Nursing Assistants. Relda Kelly & Sheila A. Sorrentino. 1996. wbk. ed. 41.00 (*0-8151-8599-5*, 28309) Mosby Inc.

Mosby's Textbook for Nursing Assistants. Gilbert Sorrentino. 5th ed. 1999. LC 00-266132. xxiv, 884p. text 39.00 (*0-323-00923-9*) Harcourt.

***Mosby's Textbook for Nursing Assistants: Computerized Testbank.** Bernie Gorek. 5th ed. 2000. 500.00 (*0-323-00925-5*) Mosby Inc.

Mosby's Textbook for Nursing Assistants: Text & Seed Package. Sheila A. Sorrentino. 4th ed. 1996. (Illus.). (*0-8151-8239-2*) Mosby Inc.

Mosby's Textbook for the Home Care Aide. Joan M. Birchenall & Mary E. Streight. tchr. ed. (*0-8151-0728-5*); 1997. pap. text, wbk. ed. 16.00 (*0-8151-0727-7*) Mosby Inc.

Mosby's Textbook for the Home Care Aide: Instructor's Resource Kit. Joan M. Birchenall. 1997. (Illus.). tchr. ed. (*0-8151-0730-7*) Mosby Inc.

Mosby's Tour Guide to Alternative Medicine. Marilyn Freedman. 1997. (C). (gr. 13). pap. text 10.00 (*0-8151-2198-9*, 30952) Mosby Inc.

Mosby's Tour Guide to Alternative Medicine. Mosby Staff. 1997. 160p. pap. text 10.00 (*1-57857-003-4*) Mosby Consmer Hlth.

Mosby's Tour Guide to Nursing School: A Student's Road Survival Guide. Melodie Chenevert. 3rd ed. 1994. LC 94-32030. (Illus.). 216p. (C). (gr. 13). pap. text 21.95 (*0-8151-1539-3*, 24868) Mosby Inc.

Mosby's 2000 Assess Test: A Practice Exam for RN Licensure (Secured) Dolores F. Saxton et al. 2000. 35.00 (*0-323-00563-2*) Mosby Inc.

***Mosby's 2000 Nursing Drug Database CD-ROM.** Linda Skidmore-Roth. 1999. pap. 39.95 incl. cd-rom (*0-323-00692-2*) Mosby Inc.

Mosby's 2000 Nursing Drug Reference & Review Cards. Joseph A. Albanese & Patricia A. Nutz. 10th ed. 1999. 448p. (C). text (*0-323-00795-3*) Mosby Inc.

***Mosby's 2001 Assess Test: A Practice Exam.** Dolores F. Saxton et al. 2001. 72p. 35.00 (*0-323-01215-9*) Mosby Inc.

Mosby's USMLE Step 1 Reviews: Pathology. John Wurzel et al. 1997. LC 96-44703. (Ace the Boards Ser.). (Illus.). 624p. (C). (gr. 13). pap. text 29.95 incl. disk (*0-8151-9276-2*, 28895) Mosby Inc.

Mosby's USMLE Step 1 Reviews: Anatomy. N. Anthony Moore. 1996. LC 96-2738. (Ace the Boards Ser.). (Illus.). 480p. (C). (gr. 13). pap. text 29.95 incl. 3.5 hd (*0-8151-6905-1*, 27051) Mosby Inc.

Mosby's USMLE Step 1 Reviews: Histology & Cell Biology. E. Robert Burns & M. Donald Cave. 1996. LC 95-52478. (Ace the Boards Ser.). (Illus.). 272p. (C). (gr. 13). pap. text 30.00 incl. audio compact disk (*0-8151-1338-2*, 27045) Mosby Inc.

Mosby's USMLE Step 1 Reviews: Microbiology & Immunology. Ken S. Rosenthal & James S. Tan. 1996. LC 95-52095. (Ace the Boards Ser.). (Illus.). 344p. (C). (gr. 13). pap. text 30.00 incl. 3.5 hd (*0-8151-7349-0*, 27042) Mosby Inc.

Mosby's USMLE Step 1 Reviews: Neuroscience. Anthony J. Castro. 1996. LC 96-22065. (Ace the Boards Ser.). (Illus.). 496p. (C). (gr. 13). pap. text 30.00 (*0-8151-1479-6*, 27046); pap. text 30.00 (*0-8151-1480-X*, 28956) Mosby Inc.

Mosby's USMLE Step 1 Reviews: Pharmacology. Sam J. Enna et al. 1996. (Illus.). 416p. (C). (gr. 13). pap. text 30.00 incl. 3.5 hd (*0-8151-3112-7*, 27049) Mosby Inc.

Mosby's USMLE Step 3 Reviews: Specialty Clinical Sciences. Joseph L. Donnelly & Randolph B. Lipscher. 1996. (Ace the Boards Ser.). (Illus.). 504p. (C). (gr. 13). pap. text 38.00 incl. disk (*0-8151-2734-0*, 27047) Mosby Inc.

Mosby's USMLE Step 2 Reviews: General Clinical Sciences. Alfred J. Bollet. 1996. LC 96-4742. (Ace the Boards Ser.). (Illus.). 552p. (C). (gr. 13). pap. text 37.00 (*0-8151-0723-4*, 27048) Mosby Inc.

Mosby's USMLE Step 2 Reviews: Surgery. Koutlas. 1999. (Ace the Boards Ser.). (Illus.). 480p. (C). (gr. 13). text 29.95 (*0-8151-3703-6*, 31407) Mosby Inc.

Mosby's Visual Guide to Massage Essentials. Sandra Fritz. 1997. 128p. pap. text 16.00 (*1-57857-002-6*) Mosby Consmer Hlth.

Mosby's Visual Guide to Massage Essentials. Sandra Fritz. 1997. LC 96-29696. (C). (gr. 13). 15.00 (*0-8151-3968-3*) Mosby Inc.

Mosby's Workbook for Long-Term Care Assistants. Relda Kelly. 3rd ed. 1999. (Illus.). 332p. pap., wbk. ed. 16.95 (*0-323-00708-2*) Mosby Inc.

Mosby's Workbook for Nursing Assistants. Sheila A. Sorrentino. 5th ed. 2000. pap. 42.95 (*0-323-01047-4*) Mosby Inc.

Moscow Lectures on Psychoanalysis. Ed. by Arnold Rothstein. 1991. LC 91-30974. 186p. (C). 30.00 (*0-8236-3435-3*) Intl Univs Pr.

Mosher Survey. Clelia D. Mosher. Ed. by James MaHood & Kristine Wanburg. 1980. LC 79-48014. 490p. lib. bdg. 30.95 (*0-405-13090-2*) Ayer.

Moss & Adams' Heart Disease in Infants, Children & Adolescents: Including the Fetus & Young Adult Hugh D. Allen et al. 6th ed. 2001. Orig. Title: Adams' Heart Disease in Infants, Children, & Adolescents. 1,632p. text 299.00 (*0-683-30742-8*) Lppncott W & W.

Moss' Heart Disease in Infants, Children & Adolescents, Set. Ed. by Forrest Adams. 4th ed. 1989. 1085p. text 172.00 (*0-683-00052-7*) Lppncott W & W.

***Moss' Radiation Oncology: Rationale, Technique.** James D. Cox & Kie Kian Ang. 8th ed. 2001. (Illus.). 1020p. (*0-323-01258-2*) Mosby Inc.

Moss' Radiation Oncology: Rationale, Technique & Results. James D. Cox. 7th ed. 1993. LC 93-34732. (Illus.). 1040p. (C). (gr. 13). text 155.00 (*0-8016-6940-5*, 06940) Mosby Inc.

Moss' Radiation Oncology: Rationale, Technique & Results. Ed. by James D. Cox. 7th rev. ed. 1992. LC 93-34732. 40.00 (*0-8016-6906-5*) Mosby Inc.

Most Common Manual for Medical Students. Steven M. Grosso. 2nd ed. 1997. (Orig.). pap. 14.95 (*1-883205-29-8*) Intl Med Pub.

Most Commons in Medicine. Edward F. Goljan. Date not set. LC 99-48221. 635p. text (*0-7216-8759-8*) Saunders.

Most Commons in Pathology & Laboratory Medicine. Edward F. Goljan. Ed. by William Schmitt. 1999. LC 98-38024. 516p. (C). pap. text 19.95 (*0-7216-7992-7*) Saunders.

Most Commons in Surgery. Edward F. Goljan & Paul P. Koro. 2001. LC 2001-20285. 658p. (*0-7216-9291-5*) Saunders.

Most Excellent Homish Apothecarye, No. 43. Von Brunveig Hieronymus. 1968. LC 68-54620. reprint ed. 30.00 (*90-221-0043-X*) Walter J Johnson.

Most Excellent Works of Chirurgerye Made M. T. Vignon. Johannes De Vigo. Tr. by B. Traheron. 1968. LC 68-54639. (English Experience Ser.: No. 67). 540p. reprint ed. 83.00 (*90-221-0067-7*) Walter J Johnson.

Most Frequent Diagnoses & Procedures for DRGs, by Insurance Status. Ed. by Cassandra Swartz. 1998. (Illus.). 132p. reprint ed. pap. text 30.00 (*0-7881-4246-1*) DIANE Pub.

Most Satisfactory Man: The Story of Theodore Brevard Hayne, Last Martyr of Yellow Fever. Charles S. Bryan. 1996. LC 95-50693. (Illus.). 220p. text 19.95 (*1-57003-123-1*) U of SC Pr.

Mostly Macro: A Guide to Healthy Cuisine for the Discriminating Palate. Lisa Turner. 1995. LC 94-48512. (Illus.). 192p. pap. 16.95 (*0-89281-534-5*, Heal Arts VT) Inner Tradit.

Mot d'Esprit et Sa Relation a L'Inconscient. Sigmund Freud. 1992. (FRE.). pap. 14.95 (*0-7859-2830-8*) Fr & Eur.

Mother & Child Health: Delivering the Services. Cicely D. Williams et al. 3rd ed. 1994. LC 93-16378. (Illus.). 416p. text 59.95 (*0-19-508148-X*); pap. text 35.00 (*0-19-508149-8*) OUP.

Mother & Fetus: Changing Notions of Maternal Responsibility, 36. Robert H. Blank. 1992. LC 91-38029. (Contributions in Medical Studies Ser.: No. 36). 224p. 60.00 (*0-313-27639-0*, BOF/, Greenwood Pr) Greenwood.

Mother Is Born: Preparing for Motherhood During Pregnancy. Merete Leonhardt-Lupa. 1995. LC 94-29716. 176p. 17.75 (*0-89789-353-0*, Bergin & Garvey) Greenwood.

Mother Knows Best: How to Live Through & Love Your Child's First Four Years! Karen Javitch & Amy Friedman. 1982. (Illus.). 208p. pap. 6.95 (*0-89709-032-2*) Liberty Pub.

Mother Nature, Father Time: Tales of Medicine. Robert A. Norman. 1998. 190p. pap. 14.95 (*1-891576-05-4*) North Shore Pr.

Mother Nature's Herbal. Judy Griffin. 2000. LC 00-37144. (Illus.). 384p. 10.99 (*0-517-16228-8*) Random Hse Value.

Mother Nature's Herbal: Herbs for Healthy Living. Judy Griffin. 1997. LC 96-43893. (Whole Life Ser.). (Illus.). 400p. pap. 19.95 (*1-56718-340-9*, K-340-9) Llewellyn Pubns.

Mother to Be: A Guide to Pregnancy & Birth for Women with Disabilities. Judith Rogers & Molleen Matsumura. 1991. 424p. pap. 39.95 (*0-939957-30-2*) Demos Medical.

Mother-to-Mother Baby Care Book. Barbara Wilcox Sills & Jeannie Henry. 1980. LC 79-15708. 14.95 (*0-913290-18-1*) Camaro Pub.

Mother with Child: Transformation Through Children. Kathryn A. Rabuzzi. 1994. LC 92-45765. 192p. 31.95 (*0-253-34769-6*) Ind U Pr.

Mothercare New Guide to Pregnancy & Child Care: An Illustrated Guide to Caring for Your Child from Pregnancy Through Age Five. Ed. by Penny Stanway. rev. ed. 2000. LC 99-87127. (Mothercare Ser.). (Illus.). 320p. per. 22.00 (*0-7432-0103-5*) S&S Trade.

Mothercare's New Guide to Pregnancy & Childcare: An Illustrated Guide to Caring for Your Child from Pregnancy Through Age Five. Ed. by Penny Stanway. 1994. LC 94-1161. (Illus.). 304p. per. 20.00 (*0-671-50095-3*) S&S Trade Pap.

Motherhood after Miscarriage. Kathleen Diamond. 1991. 252p. pap. 10.95 (*1-55850-043-X*) Adams Media.

Motherhood & Mental Health. Ian F. Brockington. 1996. (Illus.). 630p. text 102.50 (*0-19-262126-2*) OUP.

Motherhood & Mourning: Perinatal Death. Larry G. Peppers & Ronald J. Knapp. 1980. LC 80-286. 165p. 58.00 (*0-275-91760-6*, C1760, Praeger Pubs) Greenwood.

Motherhood by Choice: Pioneers in Women's Health & Family Planning. Perdita Huston. 1992. LC 91-44239. (Illus.). 192p. (gr. 9-12). pap. 14.95 (*1-55861-069-3*) Feminist Pr.

Motherhood Constellation: A Unified View of Parent Infant Psychotherapy. Daniel N. Stern. 1995. LC 94-24388. 288p. pap. 45.00 (*0-465-02602-8*) Basic.

Motherhood Optional: A Psychological Journey. Phyllis Z. Tobin & Barbara Aria. 1998. LC 97-29367. 376p. 23.95 (*0-7657-0127-8*) Aronson.

Mothering. Rudolph Schaffer. 1977. (Developing Child Ser.). (Illus.). 128p. 23.50 (*0-674-58745-6*); pap. text 9.50 (*0-674-58746-4*) HUP.

Mothering: Toward a New Psychoanalytic Construction. Silvia Vegetti-Finzi. Tr. by Kathrine Jason. 1995. LC 95-38876. (Feminism & Psychoanalysis Ser.). 196p. 30.00 (*0-89862-334-0*, C2334) Guilford Pubns.

Mothering & Ambivalence. Ed. by Wendy Hollway & Brid Featherstone. 1997. LC 97-224465. 216p. (C). 80.00 (*0-415-13910-4*); pap. 25.99 (*0-415-13911-2*) Routledge.

Mothering the Mother: How a Doula Can Help You Have a Shorter, Easier, Healthier Birth. Marshall H. Klaus et al. 2000. LC 92-35509. 168p. pap. 18.00 (*0-201-63272-1*) Perseus Bks Grp.

Mother's Agenda. Satprem Staff & Mother. LC 80-472990.Tr. of L'Agenda de Mere. (Orig.). Vol. 2, 1961. 1981. 500p. pap. 12.50 (*0-938710-01-X*); Vol. 3, 1962. 1982. 540p. pap. text 12.50 (*0-938710-02-8*) Inst Evolutionary.

Mothers & Medicine: A Social History of Infant Feeding, 1890-1950. Rima D. Apple. 1987. LC 87-40137. (Wisconsin Publications in the History of Science & Medicine: Vol. 7). (Illus.). 280p. pap. text 18.95 (*0-299-11484-8*) U of Wis Pr.

Mothers, Babies, & Cocaine: The Role of Toxins in Development. Ed. by Michael Lewis et al. 1995. 408p. pap. 37.50 (*0-8058-1584-8*); text 79.95 (*0-8058-1583-X*) L Erlbaum Assocs.

Mothers, Babies & Health in Later Life. D. J. Barker. 2nd ed. 1998. LC 98-14947. ix, 217p. (*0-443-06165-3*) Church.

Mothers Bereaved by Stillbirth, Neonatal Death or Sudden Infant Death Syndrome: Patterns of Distress & Recovery. Frances M. Boyle. 1997. LC 97-70894. (Illus.). 160p. text (*1-85972-149-4*) Ashgate Pub GBR. *Dist:* Ashgate Pub Co.

Mother's Book of Home Medical Tests for Infants & Children. Herbert Haessler & Raymond Harris. 1998. LC 98-10365. (Illus.). 240p. pap. 14.95 (*0-8092-3037-2*, 303720, Contemporary) McGraw-Hill Trade.

Mother's Guide to a Healthier Pregnancy & Easier Birth. Jeanine L. LaBaw & Mary M. Lepley. 1991. (Illus.). 24.95 incl. audio (*0-9627583-0-2*) Lifesounds.

Mother's Herbal: Caring for Yourself & Your Family with Natural Remedies. Anne McIntyre. 2000. (Illus.). 224p. pap. 24.95 (*1-86204-744-8*) Element MA.

Mothers of Psychoanalysis: Helene Deutsch, Karen Horney, Anna Freud, & Melanie Klein. Janet Sayers. 1993. 336p. pap. 12.95 (*0-393-30942-8*) Norton.

Mother's Tears: Understanding the Mood Swings That Follow Childbirth. Arlene Huysman. 1998. LC 97-52079. 192p. 23.95 (*1-888363-70-3*) Seven Stories.

MotherWit: A Guide to Healing & Psychic Development. Diane Mariechild. rev. ed. 1989. (Illus.). 192p. pap. 14.95 (*0-89594-358-1*) Crossing Pr.

Motif Reference Manual, Vol. 6B. Antony Fountain & Paula Ferguson. 2nd ed. 2000. LC 00-709434. (Definitive Guides to the X Window System Ser.: Vol. 6). (Illus.). xiii, 1154p. pap. 49.95 (*1-56592-654-4*) OReilly & Assocs.

Motility of Vertebrate Cells in Culture & in the Organism. G. Haemmerli & P. Strauli. 1985. (Experimental Biology & Medicine Ser.: Vol. 10). (Illus.). x, 266p. 121.00 (*3-8055-4135-X*) S Karger.

Motion & Space Sickness. Ed. by George H. Crampton. 1990. 496p. lib. bdg. 219.00 (*0-8493-4703-3*, RC103) CRC Pr.

Motion Palpation & Chiropractic Technic: Principles Dynamic Chiropractic. R. C. Schafer & Leonard J. Faye. 1989. LC 88-93050. (Illus.). 500p. (C). text 59.00 (*0-924889-00-4*) Motion Palpat Inst.

Motion Picture Prescription: 200 Movies to Help You Heal Life's Problems. Gary Solomon. 1995. LC 95-237. 242p. pap. 12.95 (*0-944031-27-7*) Aslan Pub.

Motion Sickness. Terry O'Neal. Ed. by Andrea Burrise. 2000. 112p. pap. 11.95 (*0-9679446-0-0*) Motion Pubns.

Motivated Brain: A Neurophysiological Analysis of Human Behavior. P. V. Simonov. 1991. (Monographs in Psychobiology). vii, 280p. text 160.00 (*2-88124-444-0*) Gordon & Breach.

Motivating Blood Donors in Today's World: Recruitment & Retention. Ed. by Merlyn H. Sayers. 1998. pap. text (*1-56395-095-2*) Am Assn Blood.

Motivating Donors in Today's World: Recruitment & Retention. Lorraine Kohr & Marilyn Sayers. 1998. LC 98-173369. xviii, 318 p. (*1-56395-075-8*, AABB Pr) Am Assn Blood.

Motivating Health Behavior. John P. Elder et al. 1993. LC 93-12430. 388p. (C). mass mkt. 44.25 (*0-8273-4963-7*) Delmar.

Motivating the Unmotivated. Dick Hartman. 1987. LC 87-50744. (Illus.). (Orig.). pap. 8.95 (*0-9619238-0-6*) Valley Hill Pub.

Motivation: The Organization of Action. Douglas G. Mook. 2nd ed. 1995. LC 95-32839. (C). text 56.00 (*0-393-96717-4*) Norton.

Motivation: Theory & Research. Ed. by Michael Drillings & Harold F. O'Neil. 1994. 328p. pap. 29.95 (*0-8058-1287-3*); text 69.95 (*0-8058-1286-5*) L Erlbaum Assocs.

Motivation: Theory & Research. Herbert L. Petri. 2nd ed. 1985. 432p. (C). mass mkt. 40.50 (*0-534-05382-3*) Brooks-Cole.

Motivation: Theory, Research & Applications. Herbert L. Petri. 3rd ed. 1991. 434p. (C). text 46.20 (*0-534-14364-4*) Brooks-Cole.

Motivation & Action. Heinz Heckhausen. 1991. (Illus.). 504p. 86.95 (*0-387-54204-3*) Spr-Verlag.

Motivation & Culture. Donald Munro et al. 1997. LC 96-51882. 256p. (C). 85.00 (*0-415-91509-0*) Routledge.

Motivation & Economic Mobility. Martha S. Hill et al. 1985. LC 85-18017. 192p. (Orig.). pap. text 20.00 (*0-87944-304-9*) Inst Soc Res.

Motivation & Emotion. Decatanzaro. 1998. LC 98-7523. 352p. 76.00 (*0-13-849159-3*) P-H.

Motivation & Emotion. Phil Evans. 1989. 160p. 39.50 (*0-415-01475-1*); pap. 13.95 (*0-415-01476-X*) Routledge.

Motivation & Emotion: Evolutionary, Physiological, Cognitive & Social Influences. David C. Edwards. 1998. LC 98-19717. (Advanced Psychology Texts Ser.). 467p. 74.95 (*0-7619-0832-3*, 80727) Sage.

Motivation & Explanation: An Essay on Freud's Philosophy of Science. Nigel Mackay. 1989. (Psychological Issues Monographs: No. 56). 260p. 37.50 (*0-8236-3474-4*) Intl Univs Pr.

Motivation & Learning: Applying Contingency Management Techniques. Ed. by Mark L. Berman. 1972. LC 70-160894. 222p. pap. 24.95 (*0-87778-023-4*) Educ Tech Pubns.

Motivation & Personality: Handbook of Thematic Content Analysis. Ed. by Charles P. Smith. 1992. (Illus.). 726p. (C). text 130.00 (*0-521-40052-X*) Cambridge U Pr.

Motivation & Self-Regulation Across the Life-Span. Ed. by Jutta Heckhausen & Carol S. Dweck. 1998. LC 97-32110. (Illus.). 472p. (C). text 64.95 (*0-521-59176-7*) Cambridge U Pr.

Motivation & the Neural & Neurohumoral Factors in Regulation of Behaviour: Recent Development of Neurobiology in Hungary, Vol. 10. Ed. by K. Lissak & P. Molnar. 1982. (Recent Developments of Neurobiology in Hungary Ser.: No. 10). 331p. (C). (*963-05-2993-9*) Akade Kiado HUN. *Dist:* St Mut.

Motivation Assessment Scale (MAS) Administration Guide. V. Mark Durand & Daniel B. Crimmins. 1992. 64p. (Orig.). (C). pap. text 49.00 (*1-882322-00-2*) Monaco & Assocs.

Motivation, Behavior & Emotional Health: An Everyman's Interpretation. Donald M. Wonderly. 1991. 576p. (C). pap. text 51.00 (*0-8191-8384-9*) U Pr of Amer.

Motivation, Emotion, & Goal Direction in Neural Networks. Ed. by Daniel S. Levine & Samuel J. Leven. 1992. 472p. (C). text 99.95 (*0-8058-0447-1*) L Erlbaum Assocs.

Motivation in Functional Systems. Ed. by K. V. Sudakov et al. 1987. (Systems Research in Physiology Ser.: Vol. 1). xvi, 364p. text 376.00 (*2-88124-193-X*) Gordon & Breach.

Motivation, Intention, & Volition. Ed. by F. Halisch & Julius Kuhl. 1987. (Illus.). 436p. 123.00 (*0-387-16191-0*) Spr-Verlag.

Motivation, Motor & Sensory Processes of the Brain: Electrical Potentials, Behavior & Clinical Use. Ed. by H. H. Kornhuber & L. Deecke. 1981. (Progress in Brain Research Ser.: Vol. 54). 812p. 322.00 (*0-444-80196-0*) Elsevier.

Motivation, Planning & Action: A Relational Theory of Behavior Dynamics. J. M. Nuttin. 1984. 259p. (Orig.). pap. (*90-6186-154-3*) Leuven Univ BEL. *Dist:* Coronet Bks.

Motivation Profile. Gregory Engel & Lowell J. Arthur. 1998. 24p. pap., stu. ed. 5.95 (*1-884180-00-0*) LifeStar.

Motivational Enhancement Therapy Manual: A Clinical Research Guide for Therapists Treating Individuals with Alcohol Abuse & Dependence. William R. Miller et al. 1994. 121p. (Orig.). (C). pap. text 35.00 (*0-7881-1476-X*) DIANE Pub.

Motivational Interviewing: Preparing People to Change Addictive Behavior. William R. Miller & Stephen Rollnick. LC 91-16597. 348p. 1991. 39.95 (*0-89862-566-1*); 1992. reprint ed. pap. 23.00 (*0-89862-469-X*, 2469) Guilford Pubns.

Motives & Mechanisms: An Introduction to the Psychology of Action. Rom Harre et al. 1985. 192p. 35.00 (*0-416-36230-3*, 9467); pap. 12.95 (*0-416-36240-0*, 9468) Routledge.

Motives & Thoughts: Psychoanalytic Essays in Honor of David Rapaport. Ed. by Robert R. Holt. 1967. LC 67-20615. (Psychological Issues Monographs: No. 18-19, Vol. 5, Nos. 2-3). 214p. (Orig.). 60.00 (*0-8236-3480-9*); pap. 42.50 (*0-8236-3460-4*) Intl Univs Pr.

Motives, Personality & Society. David C. McClelland. 1984. LC 84-2033. (Centennial Psychology Ser.). 502p. 65.00 (*0-275-91224-8*, C1224, Praeger Pubs) Greenwood.

Motor Activity & Movement Disorders: Research Issues & Applications. Ed. by Klaus-Peter Ossenkopp et al. 1995. LC 95-40459. (Contemporary Neuroscience Ser.). (Illus.). 392p. 145.00 (*0-89603-327-9*, RC376) Humana.

Motor & Cognitive Functions of the Prefrontal Cortex. Ed. by A. M. Thierry et al. 1994. LC 93-37169. (Research & Perspectives in Neurosciences Ser.). (Illus.). 182p. 63.95 (*0-387-57128-0*) Spr-Verlag.

Motor Assessment of the Developing Infant. Martha C. Piper & Johanna Darrah. 1994. LC 93-24914. (Illus.). 224p. text 46.00 (*0-7216-4307-8*) Saunders.

Motor Control. Ed. by G. N. Gantchev et al. 1987. LC 87-2326. 232p. 65.00 (*0-306-42560-2*, Plenum Trade) Perseus Pubng.

Motor Control: Concepts & Issues. Ed. by D. R. Humphrey & H. J. Freund. 1991. LC 90-13046. (Dahlem Workshop Reports). 518p. 343.95 (*0-471-92919-0*) Wiley.

Motor Control & Learning: A Behavioral Emphasis. Richard A. Schmidt & Timothy D. Lee. 3rd ed. 1998. LC 98-15263. (Illus.). 512p. 65.00 (*0-88011-484-3*, BSCH0484) Human Kinetics.

Motor Control & Motor Learning in Rehabilitation. Carolyn Crutchfield & Marylou R. Barnes. 1993. (Illus.). 520p. (C). text 50.00 (*0-936030-06-2*) Stokesville Pub.

Motor Control & Physical Therapy: Theoretical Framework & Practical Applications. Ed. by Patricia C. Montgomery & Barbara Connolly. 1991. (Illus.). 240p. (Orig.). (C). pap. text 34.95 (*1-879971-00-3*) Chattanga Grp.

Motor Control & Sensory Motor Integration: Issues & Directions. Ed. by Denis J. Glencross & Jan P. Piek. 1995. LC 95-41895. (Advances in Psychology Ser.: Vol. 111). 462p. 126.00 (*0-444-81921-5*, QP454) Elsevier.

Motor Coordination Disorders in Children. David Sugden & Helen Wright. 1998. LC 98-19704. (Developmental Clinical Psychology & Psychiatry Ser.). 136p. 49.95 (*0-7619-0999-0*, 81333) Sage.

Motor Development in Children: Aspects of Coordination & Control. Ed. by M. G. Wade & H. T. Whiting. 1986. lib. bdg. 278.50 (*90-247-3389-8*) Kluwer Academic.

Motor Development in Early & Later Childhood: Longitudinal Approaches. Ed. by Alex F. Kalverboer et al. 1993. (Illus.). 403p. (C). text 100.00 (*0-521-40101-1*) Cambridge U Pr.

Motor Development of Children with Down Syndrome: Birth to Six Years. Ron French & Jack Share. rev. ed. 1993. (Illus.). 125p. reprint ed. tchr. ed. 35.00 (*1-878276-46-8*) Educ Systs Assocs Inc.

Motor Disorders. David S. Younger. 1999. LC 98-32461. 576p. text 159.00 (*0-316-97600-8*) Lppncott W & W.

Motor Learning & Control. Charles H. Shea et al. 1993. LC 92-2485. 368p. (C). 88.00 (*0-13-605684-9*) P-H.

Motor Learning & Synaptic Plasticity in the Cerebellum. Ed. by Paul J. Cordo et al. 1997. LC 97-1229. (Illus.). 208p. (C). text 100.00 (*0-521-59286-0*); pap. text 37.95 (*0-521-59705-6*) Cambridge U Pr.

***Motor Neurobiology of the Spinal Cord.** Ed. by Timothy C. Cope. 2001. LC 2001-25610. (Methods & New Frontiers in Neuroscience Ser.). (Illus.). 337p. 119.95 (*0-8493-0006-1*) CRC Pr.

Motor Neuron Disease. 1995. (Illus.). 468p. 155.00 (*3-540-19685-4*) Spr-Verlag.

Motor Neuron Disease. Ed. by P. N. Leigh & Michael Swash. 1995. LC 94-14875. (Illus.). 486p. 135.00 (*0-387-19685-4*) Spr-Verlag.

Motor Neuron Disease. Ed. by A. C. Williams. 1994. LC 93-32613. 776p. 207.95 (*0-412-54780-5*, Chap & Hall NY) Chapman & Hall.

***Motor Neurone Disease.** Beresford. 1995. pap. 28.95 (*0-412-55640-5*) Chapman & Hall.

Motor Neurone Disease. Ed. by Gourie Devi. 1987. (C). (*81-204-0195-6*) Oxford IBH IND. *Dist:* S Asia.

Motor Neurone Disease. Oliver. pap. (*0-85969-705-3*) Society Prom Christ Know GBR. *Dist:* Intl Pubs Mktg.

Motor Neurone Disease. Ian Robinson & Margaret Hunter. 1998. LC 97-32221. (Experience of Illness Ser.). 160p. (C). pap. 24.95 (*0-415-09711-8*) Routledge.

Motor Neurone Disease (Amyotrophic Lateral Sclerosis) S. Beresford. 1995. 196p. pap. 41.50 (*1-56593-318-4*, 0648) Singular Publishing.

Motor Performance in Adolescence. Anna Espenschade. 1940. (SRCD Ser.: Vol. 5, No. 1). 25.00 (*0-527-01513-X*) Periodicals Srv.

Motor Relearning Programme for Stroke. Janet H. Carr & Roberta B. Shepherd. 2nd ed. 1987. 198p. (C). 79.00 (*0-87189-312-6*) Aspen Pub.

Motor Speech Disorders. Frederick L. Darley et al. 1975. LC 74-25475. (Illus.). 304p. text 68.00 (*0-7216-2878-8*) Saunders.

Motor Speech Disorders. James Paul Dworkin. 1991. 351p. (C). (gr. 13). text 49.95 (*1-55664-223-7*) Mosby Inc.

Motor Speech Disorders: Substrates & Differential. Joseph R. Duffy. 1995. (Illus.). 480p. (gr. 13). text 54.00 (*0-8016-6944-8*, 06944) Mosby Inc.

Motor Speech Disorders in Children. Ed. by Anthony J. Caruso & Edythe A. Strand. 1999. LC 99-17630. (Illus.). 384p. 45.00 (*0-86577-762-4*) Thieme Med Pubs.

Motor Thalamus. Ed. by P. L. Gildenberg et al. 1993. (Journal: Vol. 60, Nos. 1-3, 1993). (Illus.). 156p. pap. 109.75 (*3-8055-5756-6*) S Karger.

Motor Unit Types, Recruitment & Plasticity in Health & Disease. Ed. by J. E. Desmedt. 1981. (Progress in Clinical Neurophysiology Ser.: Vol. 9). (Illus.). x, 418p. 128.75 (*3-8055-1929-X*) S Karger.

Motor Vehicle Collision Injuries: Mechanisms, Diagnosis & Management. Lawrence Nordhoff. 1995. 391p. 91.00 (*0-8342-0727-3*) Aspen Pub.

Motorcycle Sex: Or Freud Would Never Understand the Relationship Between Me & My Motorcycle. Gregory W. Frazier. 2nd ed. 1999. LC 94-202752. (Illus.). 150p. (Orig.). (C). pap. 22.95 (*0-935151-19-2*) Arrowstar Pub.

Motorspeech & Related Oropharyngeal Disorders in Children. Sheppard. 2001. 44.00 net. (*1-56593-699-X*) Thomson Learn.

Motorsports Medicine: Race Faster! Longer! Safer! Harlen C. Hunter & Rick Stoff. 1992. LC 92-39754. (Illus.). 250p. pap. 19.95 (*0-9634819-0-8*) Lake Hill Pr.

Mots Pour le Dire see Words to Say It

Mould's Medical Anecdotes: Omnibus Edition. Richard F. Mould. 1996. LC 96-9553. (Illus.). 496p. pap. 35.00 (*0-7503-0390-5*) Inst of Physics Pubng.

Mt. Sinai Clinical Handbook of Surgery: A Case-Oriented Approach. Mount Sinai Hospital, New York, N. Y. Staff. Ed. by Joel J. Bauer. 1998. LC 98-6114. 800p. spiral bd. 34.95 (*0-683-18001-0*) Lppncott W & W.

Mount Sinai School of Medicine Complete Book of Nutrition. Victor Herbert. 1990. 35.00 (*0-312-05129-8*) St Martin.

Mountain Medicine. A. B. Guthrie. 1991. 5.95 (*0-89174-057-0*) Comstock Edns.

Mountain Sickness: Prevention Recognition & Treatment. Peter Hackett. 2nd ed. 1997. (Climber's Guides). (Illus.). 80p. reprint ed. pap. 8.50 (*0-930410-10-6*) Amer Alpine Club.

Mountaineering First Aid: A Guide to Accident Response & First Aid Care. Jan D. Carline et al. 4th ed. 1996. LC 96-15825. (Illus.). 144p. pap. 10.95 (*0-89886-478-X*) Mountaineers.

Mountaineering Medicine. Fred Darvill, Jr. 14th rev. ed. 1998. LC 98-9968. (Illus.). 116p. pap. 7.95 (*0-89997-207-1*) Wilderness Pr.

Mounting a Prenatal Care Campaign in Your Community. Dana Hughes. Ed. by Children's Defense Fund Staff. 1986. 44p. (Orig.). pap. 3.00 (*0-938008-56-0*) Childrens Defense.

Mourning the Living: Families Coping with the Losses of Substance Abuse. Ed. by Florence Selder et al. rev. ed. 2000. reprint ed. pap. (*0-930194-85-3*) Ctr Thanatology.

Mouse Brain in Stereotaxic Coordinates. George Paxinos & Keith B. J. Franklin. 2nd deluxe ed. 2001. LC 00-107124. 296p. spiral bd. 189.95 incl. cd-rom (*0-12-547637-X*) Acad Pr.

Mouse Ear Inflammation Models & Their Pharmacological Applications. Miklos Gabor. 2000. 336p. (*963-05-7704-6*) Akade Kiado HUN. *Dist:* Intl Spec Bk, St Mut.

Mouse Histopathology. Ed. by J. M. Faccini et al. 1990. 226p. 173.00 (*0-444-81345-4*) Elsevier.

Mouse in Biomedical Research Vol. 4: Experimental Biology & Oncology. Ed. by Henry L. Foster et al. 1982. 545p. text 188.00 (*0-12-262504-8*) Acad Pr.

Mouse Models in the Study of Genetic Neurological Disorders. Ed. by Brian Popko. 1999. LC 98-55684. (Advances in Neurochemistry Ser.: Vol. 9). (Illus.). 366p. (C). text 149.00 (*0-306-45965-5*, Kluwer Plenum) Kluwer Academic.

Mousetraps & the Moon: The Strange Ride of Sigmund Freud & the Early Years of Psychoanalysis. Robert Wilcocks. 2000. LC 00-30153. xix, 290p. 75.00 (*0-7391-0158-7*) Lxngtn Bks.

Mouthsounds. Frederick R. Newman. 1980. LC 80-51513. (Illus.). 128p. pap. 6.95 (*0-89480-128-7*, 427) Workman Pub.

Movement & Allied Disorders in Childhood. Ed. by Mary M. Robertson & Valsamma Eapen. 1996. LC 95-9400. 342p. 215.00 (*0-471-95324-5*) Wiley.

Movement & Drama in Therapy. Audrey G. Wethered. 2nd ed. 1993. 128p. pap. 27.00 (*1-85302-199-7*) Taylor & Francis.

Movement & Mental Imagery: Outlines of a Motor Theory of the Complexer Mental Processes. Margaret F. Washburn. 1978. LC 73-2996. (Classics in Psychology Ser.). reprint ed. 20.95 (*0-405-05168-9*) Ayer.

Movement & Rhythmic Activities for the Mentally Retarded. Cynthia D. Crain. 1981. (Illus.). 136p. 28.95 (*0-398-04174-1*) C C Thomas.

Movement Control. Ed. by Paul Cordo & Stevan R. Harnad. 1994. (Illus.). 288p. (C). text 74.95 (*0-521-45241-4*); pap. text 28.95 (*0-521-45607-X*) Cambridge U Pr.

Movement Control: An Interdisciplinary Forum. Ed. by R. Jacobs & W. E. Rikkert. 1992. 108p. (Orig.). pap. text (*90-5383-035-9*) VU Univ Pr NLD. *Dist:* Paul & Co Pubs.

***Movement Discomfort & Disorders (Dyskinesias) Index of New Information & Guide-Book for Consumers, Reference & Research.** Jonathan L. Blakiston. 2002. 180p. 57.50 (*0-7883-2408-X*); pap. 47.50 (*0-7883-2409-8*) ABBE Pubs Assn.

Movement Disorder Surgery: Progress & Challenges. Ed. by A. M. Lozano. 2000. LC 00-37076. (Progress in Neurological Surgery Ser.: Vol. 15). (Illus.). x, 404p. 243.50 (*3-8055-6990-4*) S Karger.

Movement Disorders. Ed. by Nandkumar S. Shah & Alexander G. Donald. 1986. LC 86-4884. (Illus.). 424p. (C). text 120.00 (*0-306-42135-6*, Kluwer Plenum) Kluwer Academic.

Movement Disorders, No. 3. Ed. by C. David Marsden & Stanley Fahn. 3rd ed. 1994. (BIMR Ser.: Vol. 12). (Illus.). 529p. text 105.00 (*0-7506-1412-9*) Buttrwrth-Heinemann.

Movement Disorders: A Contemporary Model for Stroke Rehabilitation. Susan Ryerson & Kathryn Levit. 1996. LC 96-48529. text (*0-443-08913-2*) Church.

Movement Disorders: Neurologic Principles & Practice. Ed. by Raymond L. Watts & William C. Koller. 1997. LC 96-35518. (Illus.). 779p. text 155.00 (*0-07-035203-8*) McGraw-Hill Prof.

Movement Disorders in Childhood. Harvey S. Singer & Joseph Jankovic. 2001. (Illus.). 304p. 125.00 (*0-7506-9852-7*) Buttrwrth-Heinemann.

Movement Disorders in Children. Ed. by H. Forssberg & H. Hirschfeld. 1992. (Medicine & Sport Science Ser.: Vol. 36). (Illus.). viii, 302p. 61.00 (*3-8055-5556-3*) S Karger.

Movement Disorders in Neurology & Neuropsychiatry. Anthony B. Joseph & Robert R. Young. 2nd ed. 1998. LC 98-8767. (Illus.). xxi, 726p. 173.95 (*0-86542-523-X*) Blackwell Sci.

Movement Is Fun: A Preschool Movement Program. Susan Young & Liz Keplinger. 1988. LC 88-60761. 150p. (Orig.). pap. 14.00 (*1-882068-01-7*) Sensory Integration.

Movement Science. Ed. by Carolee Winstein & H. Knecht. 1991. 256p. pap. 30.00 (*0-912452-78-1*, P-81) Am Phys Therapy Assn.

Movement Skill Assessment. Allen W. Burton & Daryl E. Miller. 1997. LC 97-21938. (Illus.). 416p. text 37.00 (*0-87322-975-4*, BBUR0975) Human Kinetics.

Movement, Stability & Low Back Pain: The Essential Role of the Pelvis. Andry Vleeming. 1997. LC 97-20042. pap. text (*0-443-05574-2*) Church.

Movies & Mental Illness. M. Boyd & Danny Wedding. 1998. LC 98-38002. 272p. pap. 25.00 (*0-07-068990-3*) McGrw-H Hghr Educ.

Moving & Learning: Test & Lessons Plan Manual, No. 2. Nichols. 1990. 46.95 (*0-8016-3687-6*) Mosby Inc.

Moving & Shaking American Medicine: The Structure of a Socioeconomic Transformation, 57. Betty Leyerle. 1984. LC 83-22646. (Contributions in Economics & Economic History Ser.: No. 57). 218p. 65.00 (*0-313-24020-5*, LIP/, Greenwood Pr) Greenwood.

Moving Experience: A Practical Guide to Psychological Survival. Gail Meltzer & Elaine Grandjean. 1989. (*1-85359-058-4*); pap. (*1-85359-057-6*) Multilingual Matters GBR. *Dist:* Taylor & Francis, U of Toronto Pr.

Moving Forward: A Book for Ileostomy Patients. Kay Marshall. 1990. (Illus.). 32p. pap. text 3.95 (*0-916999-07-6*) HERC Pubng.

Moving Free: A Total Program of Post-Mastectomy Exercises. Carol Walter & Lenore H. Miller. 1981. LC 80-2735. (Illus.). pap. (*0-672-52686-7*) Macmillan.

Moving from Parameters to Pathways: A Guide for Developing & Implementing Critical Pathways. Deborah K. Wall & Mitchell M. Proyect. 1997. LC 97-24163. 154p. pap. 40.00 (*0-944496-55-5*) Precept Pr.

Moving Frontiers in Invertebrate Virology. T. W. Tinsley & K. A. Harrap. Ed. by Joseph L. Melnick. 1972. (Monographs in Virology: Vol. 6). (Illus.). 34.00 (*3-8055-1464-6*) S Karger.

Moving Frontiers in Veterinary Immunology. Ed. by R. Pandey. 1987. (Progress in Veterinary Microbiology & Immunology Ser.: Vol. 4). (Illus.). xii, 252p. 182.75 (*3-8055-4632-7*) S Karger.

Moving in on Occupational Injury. David Worth. 2000. LC 00-22816. (Illus.). 370p. pap. text 55.00 (*0-7506-4198-3*) Buttrwrth-Heinemann.

Moving in on Pain: Conference Proceedings. Ed. by Michael D. Shacklock. 1995. LC 96-122656. 224p. pap. text 49.99 (*0-7506-8926-9*) Buttrwrth-Heinemann.

Moving Medicine: The Life Work of Milton Trager, M. D. Jack Liskin. 1996. LC 96-31343. 176p. 24.95 (*0-88268-196-6*) Station Hill Pr.

Moving Points in Nephrology: Festschrift in Honor of Professor Geoffrey M. Berlyne. Ed. by E. Bourke et al. 1992. (Contributions to Nephrology Ser.: Vol. 102). (Illus.). xvi, 254p. 49.75 (*3-8055-5642-X*) S Karger.

Moving Psychotherapy: Theory & Application of Pesso System- Psychomotor Therapy. John S. Crandell. Ed. by Albert Pesso. 1990. LC 90-1623. 306p. text 39.95 (*0-914797-72-7*) Brookline Bks.

Moving Right along after Heart Surgery. Susan G. Burrows & Carole A. Gassert. Ed. by Karen Hubbard. l.t. rev. ed. 1999. (Illus.). 56p. pap. 6.50 (*0-939838-49-4*) Pritchett & Hull.

***Moving Temporomandibular Joint Research into the 21st Century.** Ed. by A. W. English & C. S. Stohler. 2001. (Cells Tissues Organs 2001 Ser.: Vol. 169, No. 3). (Illus.). 146p. pap. 39.25 (*3-8055-7229-8*) S Karger.

Moving the Mountain with the Never-Give-Up Diaries Kitty M. Jones. (Illus.). 222p. reprint ed. Level 1. rev. ed. 15.00 (*1-878502-01-8*); Level 2. rev. ed. 15.00 (*1-878502-02-6*); Level 3. rev. ed. 15.00 (*1-878502-03-4*); Level 4. rev. ed. 15.00 (*1-878502-04-2*); Set. 2nd rev. ed. (*1-878502-00-X*) Never-Give-Up Weight.

Moving Through Pregnancy. Elisabeth D. Bing. 1975. LC 74-17673. 144p. pap. (*0-672-52095-8*) Macmillan.

***Moyamoya Disease.** Ed. by Kiyonobu Ikezaki & Christopher M. Loftus. 2001. LC 2001-22993. (*1-879284-80-4*) Am Assn Neuro.

Mozart Effect. Don Campbell. 2000. pap. 14.00 (*0-380-79013-0*, Quil) HarperTrade.

Mozart Effect: Tapping the Power of Music to Heal the Body, Strengthen the Mind & Unlock the Creative Spirit. Don Campbell. 1997. LC 97-27570. 352p. 24.00 (*0-380-97418-5*, Avon Bks) Morrow Avon.

MR Angiography Applications in Pediatric Intracranial Vascular Lesions. R. Nuri Sener. 1997. pap. 32.50 (*0-87527-526-5*) Green.

MR-Atlas des Muskuloskelettalen Systems see MRI Atlas of the Musculoskeletal System

MR Cholangiopancreatography: Techniques, Results & Clinical Indications. P. Pavone & R. Passariello. 1996. LC 96-30464. (Illus.). 160p. 129.00 (*3-540-61349-8*) Spr-Verlag.

***MR Imaging & Spectroscopy of Central Nervous System Infection.** Ed. by Rakesh K. Gupta & Robert B. Lufkin. 2001. LC 2001-23697. 95.00 (*0-306-46551-5*, Kluwer Plenum) Kluwer Academic.

MR Imaging of Laryngeal Cancer. Gordon B. Snow et al. 1991. (Series in Radiology). (C). text 175.00 (*0-7923-1101-9*) Kluwer Academic.

MR Imaging of the Skull & Brain: A Correlative Text-Atlas. K. Sartor. Ed. by W. Loeffler et al. 1995. (Illus.). 820p. 298.00 (*0-387-52293-X*) Spr-Verlag.

MR in Pediatric Neuroradiology. Samuel M. Wolpert et al. Ed. by H. Verdain Barnes. 1991. (Illus.). 491p. (C). (gr. 13). text 125.00 (*0-8016-5370-3*, 05370) Mosby Inc.

MR Mammography (MRM) Werner A. Kaiser. 1993. LC 92-49786. 350p. (*3-540-55083-6*); (Illus.). 225.00 (*0-387-55083-6*) Spr-Verlag.

***MRCGP: Preparation & Passing.** John J. Ferguson. 2000. 194p. pap. (*1-85315-468-7*) Royal Soc of Medicine Pr Ltd GBR. *Dist:* Balogh.

MRCGP Workbook. Maskrey. 1994. LC 94-234055. (C). pap. text, wbk. ed. 34.00 (*0-443-04985-8*) Harcourt.

MRCOG: MCQS Clinical Obstetrics & Gynecology. K. W. Sharif & J. Jordan. 1997. pap. text (*0-7020-2120-2*) W B Saunders GBR. *Dist:* Saunders.

MRCOG Pt. 1: MCP's: Basic Science for Obstetrics & Gynaecology. Khaldoun W. Sharif et al. 1995. 226p. pap. text (*0-7020-1970-4*) W B Saunders GBR. *Dist:* Saunders.

MRCOG Survival Guide. Khaldoun W. Sharif & Judith B. Weaver. 2nd ed. 2000. LC 99-28975. xi, 226p. (*0-7020-2545-3*) W B Saunders.

MRCOG Survival Guide: Postgraduate Self-Assessment. Khaldoun W. Sharif & Judith B. Weaver. 1994. (Illus.). 258p. pap. text (*0-7020-1828-7*) W B Saunders GBR. *Dist:* Saunders.

Mrcogo, Pt. 1. Tim Chard & Richard J. Lilford. 1987. 122p. 29.50 (*0-387-19501-7*); 2nd ed. 1992. LC 92-13661. 127p. 29.95 (*0-387-19767-2*) Spr-Verlag.

MRCP: 500 MCQ's for MRCP, Pt. 1. Baliga. 1997. pap. text 28.00 (*0-7020-2243-8*) Harcourt.

***MRCP Masterclass.** Royal College of Physicians Staff. 2001. (Medical Masterclass Ser.). (Illus.). 1200.00 (*0-632-05567-7*) Blackwell Sci.

MRCP (Paediatrics) Pt. 1: MCQ's. Simon Hannam et al. 1997. 255p. pap. text (*0-7020-1875-9*) W B Saunders GBR. *Dist:* Saunders.

MRCP Pediactrics. Maconochie. 1999. (C). pap. text 40.00 (*0-7020-2381-7*) Harcourt.

MRCPsych Tutor Pt. 1: MCQs. Kam Bhui et al. 1992. 72p. pap. text (*0-7020-1642-X*) W B Saunders GBR. *Dist:* Saunders.

MRCS: MCQs for the Surgical Membership. P. A. Sylvester et al. 1997. 240p. pap. text (*0-7506-2606-2*) E A GBR. *Dist:* OUP.

MRCS Examination: MCQS & EMQS. Paul Chatrath & Omar Rahim. 1999. LC 99-35373. 34.95 (*0-632-05402-6*) Blackwell Sci.

MRI: A Conceptual Overview. Sunder S. Rajan. 1997. LC 96-37408. (Illus.). 167p. pap. 39.95 (*0-387-94911-9*) Spr-Verlag.

MRI: Central Nervous System. Walter Kucharczyk. 1990. (Illus.). 279p. (gr. 13). (*0-397-44670-5*, GM0080) Gower-Mosby.

MRI: The Basics. Ray H. Hashemi & William G. Bradley, Jr. 1997. LC 96-9064. 360p. text 59.95 (*0-683-18240-4*) Lppncott W & W.

MRI & CT Atlas of Correlative Imaging in Otolaryngology. Vijay M. Rao et al. 1993. 383p. (C). pap. text 169.00 (*0-8385-6526-3*, A6526-6, Apple Lange Med) McGraw.

MRI & CT of the Brain. Gillespie. 1999. (Illus.). 256p. pap. 96.95 (*0-412-73080-4*, Chap & Hal NY) Chapman & Hall.

MRI & CT of the Dog. J. Assheuer & M. Sager. 1996. (Illus.). 482p. 199.95 (*0-86542-825-5*) Blackwell Sci.

MRI & CT of the Musculoskeletal System. John L. Bloem & David J. Satoris. 1991. (Illus.). 672p. 150.00 (*0-683-00875-7*) Lppncott W & W.

MRI, Arthroscopy & Surgical Anatomy of the Joints. David W. Stoller. 1998. 704p. 450.00 (*0-7817-1836-8*); LC 98-22297. text 279.00 (*0-7817-1666-7*) Lppncott W & W.

MRI-Arthroscopy Correlative Atlas. Mark D. Miller et al. Ed. by Richard Lampert. 1997. LC 96-44085. (Illus.). 264p. text 152.00 (*0-7216-6054-1*) Saunders.

***MRI at a Glance.** Catherine Westbrook. 2001. (At a Glance Ser.). (Illus.). 96p. pap. 19.95 (*0-632-05619-3*) Blackwell Sci.

MRI Atlas for Technologists. Carolyn Kaut. 1999. (Radiographic Technology Ser.). (C). 595.00 (*0-8273-7262-0*) Delmar.

MRI Atlas for Technologists: Clinical Application. Carolyn Kaut. (Radiographic Technology Ser.). 1999. text, tchr. ed. 14.00 (*0-8273-7265-5*); 1996. text 79.95 (*0-8273-7264-7*) Delmar.

MRI Atlas for Technologists: Clinical Application CTB. Carolyn Kaut. 1996. (Radiographic Technology Ser.). 64.95 (*0-8273-7266-3*) Delmar.

MRI Atlas for Technologists: Clinical Applications. Carolyn Kaut. 1999. (Radiographic Technology Ser.). (C). 595.00 (*0-8273-7267-1*) Delmar.

MRI Atlas for Technologists: Physical Principles. Carolyn Kaut. 1999. (Radiographic Technology Ser.). text, tchr. ed. 14.00 (*0-8273-7261-2*) Delmar.

MRI Atlas of Central Nervous System Tumors. L. Cecconi et al. Ed. & Contrib. by E. Tettamanti. 1992. (Illus.). 291p. 274.00 (*0-387-82304-2*) Spr-Verlag.

MRI Atlas of Sectional Anatomy of the Head & Neck. William C. Yuh et al. 1993. (Illus.). 384p. text (*0-443-08892-6*) Church.

MRI Atlas of Soft Tissue Tumours. Moskovic. 2001. (Illus.). 224p. pap. 109.95 (*0-412-60030-7*, Chap & Hall NY) Chapman & Hall.

MRI Atlas of the Abdomen. Ed. by John A. Markisz & Elias Kazam. 1997. (Illus.). 256p. 125.00 (*0-86542-398-9*) Blackwell Sci.

MRI Atlas of the Abdomen. H. Weissleder. Ed. by David D. Stark. 1988. 66.00 (*0-8493-2750-4*) CRC Pr.

MRI Atlas of the Chest & Neck: Normal Anatomy & Pathology. John A. Markisz et al. 1997. LC 97-4962. (Illus.). 306p. 135.00 (*0-86542-391-1*) Blackwell Sci.

MRI Atlas of the Head & Neck. Anton N. Hasso. 1993. LC 93-16858. (Illus.). 216p. text 133.95 (*0-412-04381-5*) OUP.

MRI Atlas of the Human Cerebellum. Ed. by Jeremy D. Schmahmann. 2000. LC 00-100269. (Illus.). xiv, 167p. (C). 149.95 (*0-12-625665-9*) Acad Pr.

MRI Atlas of the Musculoskeletal System. Lawrence Bassett et al. 1988. 153.00 (*0-8493-2751-2*) CRC Pr.

MRI Atlas of the Musculoskeletal System. Torsten B. Moller & Emil Reif. 1993. LC 93-2493.Tr. of MR-Atlas des Muskuloskelettalen Systems. 308p. 278.95 (*0-86542-291-5*) Blackwell Sci.

MRI Atlas of the Pelvis: Normal Anatomy & Pathology. John A. Markisz et al. 1993. LC 92-14015. (Illus.). 248p. 135.00 (*0-683-05557-7*) Lppncott W & W.

MRI, Cardiovascular System. Ed. by Gerald G. Blackwell et al. 1992. LC 92-1484. (gr. 13). text (*1-56375-000-7*) Gower-Mosby.

MRI-CT & Pathology in Head & Neck Tumors: A Correlative Study. Roland Chisin et al. 1989. (Series in Radiology). (C). text 213.50 (*0-7923-0227-3*) Kluwer Academic.

MRI for Radiographers. P. T. English & C. Moore. 1995. (Illus.). 187p. 114.00 (*3-540-19750-8*) Spr-Verlag.

MRI for Radiographers. Philip T. English & Christine Moore. 1995. LC 94-41660. (Illus.). 195p. 98.00 (*0-387-19750-8*) Spr-Verlag.

MRI for Technologists. Peggy Woodward. 2nd ed. 2000. LC 00-32110. (Illus.). 408p. pap. 55.00 (*0-07-135318-6*) McGraw-Hill Prof.

MRI in Medicine: The Nottingham Conference. Ed. by Peter Mansfield. 1995. LC 95-31244. 333p. pap. 109.95 (*0-412-07391-9*, Chap & Hall NY) Chapman & Hall.

MRI in Practice. Catherine Westbrook & Carolyn Kaut. 1993. LC 93-9653. 296p. pap. 39.95 (*0-632-03587-0*); 2nd ed. 1999. LC 97-45782. (Illus.). 320p. pap. 52.95 (*0-632-04205-2*) Blackwell Sci.

MRI Manual. Robert B. Lufkin. 2nd ed. 1997. LC 97-20148. (Illus.). 480p. (C). (gr. 13). pap. text 64.95 (*0-8151-5665-0*, 27077) Mosby Inc.

MRI of Musculoskeletal Masses. Alan Laorr & Clyde A. Helms. 1996. LC 96-24302. (Illus.). 384p. text 139.50 (*0-89640-320-3*) Igaku-Shoin.

MRI of Musculoskeletal System. William E. Palmer. 1994. 700.00 (*1-56815-021-0*) Mosby Inc.

MRI of the Abdomen & Pelvis: A Text-Atlas. Richard C. Semelka et al. 1997. LC 96-46195. 744p. 247.00 (*0-471-16164-0*) Wiley.

MRI of the Brain: Normal Anatomy & Normal Variants. Vimal H. Patel & Lawrence Friedman. Ed. by Sandra Valkoff. 1996. LC 96-41701. 325p. text 89.00 (*0-7216-6945-X*) Saunders.

***MRI of the Brain & Spine.** Scott W. Atlas. 3rd ed. 2002. cd-rom (*0-7817-3623-4*) Lppncott W & W.

MRI of the Brain I. William G. Bradley & Michael Brant-Zawadzki. 2nd ed. 2000. 240p. text 99.00 (*0-7817-2568-2*) Lppncott W & W.

MRI of the Brain II. Michael Brant-Zawadzki & William G. Bradley. 2nd ed. 2000. 240p. text 99.00 (*0-7817-2569-0*) Lppncott W & W.

MRI of the Central Nervous System: A Pathology Atlas. Ed. by K. Mori. 1991. (Illus.). 241p. 176.00 (*0-387-70069-2*) Spr-Verlag.

MRI of the Extremities. Kang. 2nd ed. 1999. LC 2001-49842. text (*0-7216-5264-6*) Saunders.

MRI of the Female Pelvis. Kaori Togashi. 1993. LC 93-38533. (Illus.). 336p. 125.00 (*0-89640-253-3*) Igaku-Shoin.

MRI of the Foot & Ankle. Ed. by Andrew L. Deutsch et al. 1992. 400p. text 165.00 (*0-88167-899-6*) Lppncott W & W.

MRI of the Head & Neck. J. Vignand. 1999. 660p. (gr. 13). pap. 215.50 (*0-412-56030-5*) Chapman & Hall.

MRI of the Head & Neck. Robert B. Lufkin. 2nd ed. 2001. LC 00-55879. (LWW MRI Teaching File Ser.). (Illus.). vii, 244p. text 99.00 (*0-7817-2572-0*) Lppncott W & W.

MRI of the Head & Neck: Functional Anatomy - Clinical Findings - Pathology - Imaging. T. J. Vogl. enl. rev. ed. 1992. (Illus.). 269p. 198.00 (*0-387-54306-6*) Spr-Verlag.

MRI of the Knee. Marc Fenstermacher. 1997. (Body MRI Ser.). cd-rom (*0-412-14351-8*) E A GBR. *Dist:* OUP.

MRI of the Knee. Jerrold H. Mink et al. 2nd ed. 1992. LC 92-17023. 502p. text 165.00 (*0-88167-936-4*, 2417) Lppncott W & W.

MRI of the Knee. Ed. by Peter L. Munk & Clyde A. Helms. 2nd ed. 1996. LC 96-12935. 384p. text 159.00 (*0-397-51642-8*) Lppncott W & W.

MRI of the Musculoskeletal System. Harry K. Genant et al. 1993. (Illus.). 688p. text 225.00 (*0-7216-4295-0*) Saunders.

MRI of the Musculoskeletal System. Phoebe Kaplan et al. 2001. LC 00-58854. (Illus.). 605p. 95.00 (*0-7216-9027-0*) Saunders.

MRI of the Musculoskeletal System. Martin Vahlensieck et al. Tr. by Peter Winter from GER. 2000. LC 99-52542. (Illus.). xii, 394p. 149.00 incl. trans. (*0-86577-875-2*) Thieme Med Pubs.

MRI of the Musculoskeletal System. Mini Nutan Pathria & Karence K. Chan. 2nd ed. 2001. LC 00-59370. (LWW MRI Teaching File Ser.). (Illus.). x, 212p. text 99.00 (*0-7817-2571-2*) Lppncott W & W.

MRI of the Musculoskeletal System. Thomas H. Berquist. 4th ed. 2000. LC 00-42431. 1,136p. text 199.00 (*0-7817-2574-7*) Lppncott W & W.

MRI of the Musculoskeletal System: A Teaching File. Andrew Deutsch. 2nd ed. 1996. 768p. text 175.00 (*0-397-51672-X*) Lppncott W & W.

MRI of the Pelvis. Hedvig Hricak. 1992. (Illus.). 562p. (C). pap. text 199.00 (*0-8385-6527-1*, A6527-4, Apple Lange Med) McGraw.

MRI of the Shoulder. Lynn Steinbach. 1998. LC 97-49684. 288p. text 199.00 (*0-397-51468-9*) Lppncott W & W.

MRI of the Shoulder. Michael B. Zlatkin. 1991. 188p. text 125.00 (*0-88167-800-7*); 2nd ed. 2002. text 149.00 (*0-7817-1590-3*) Lppncott W & W.

MRI of the Spine. Thomas E. St. Amour et al. 1993. LC 93-7902. 864p. text 250.00 (*0-7817-0027-2*) Lppncott W & W.

MRI of the Spine. Jeffrey S. Ross. 2nd ed. 2000. LC 99-48216. 240p. text 99.00 (*0-7817-2528-3*) Lppncott W & W.

MRI Optimization: A Hands on Approach. Peggy Woodward & Gary Schwartz. 1996. LC 96-30379. (Illus.). 219p. pap. 48.00 (*0-07-071801-6*) McGraw-Hill Prof.

MRI Physics for Physicians. A. L. Horowitz. 1990. (Illus.). 113p. 25.00 (*0-387-96904-7*) Spr-Verlag.

MRI Physics for Radiologists: A Visual Approach. Alfred L. Horowitz. 3rd ed. 1997. LC 94-33017. (Illus.). 180p. 46.95 (*0-387-94372-2*) Spr-Verlag.

MRI Principles: A Guide for the Mathematically Illiterate. Donald G. Mitchell. Ed. by Lisette Brawlow. 1998. LC 98-12902. (Illus.). 288p. (C). text 59.00 (*0-7216-6759-7*) Saunders.

MRI Study Guide & Exam Review. Rundle. 1997. (C). pap. text, stu. ed. (*0-7216-6880-1*) Saunders.

MRI Study Guide for Technologists. Kenneth S. Meacham. 1995. LC 95-10164. (Illus.). 171p. 44.95 (*0-387-94489-3*) Spr-Verlag.

MRI Survival Guide. Jim D. Cardoza & Robert J. Herfkens. 1994. LC 93-41765. 240p. text 69.95 (*0-7817-0180-5*) Lppncott W & W.

Mrna Formation & Function. Ed. by Joel D. Richter. 1997. LC 97-33343. (Illus.). 395p. text 85.00 (*0-12-587545-2*) Morgan Kaufmann.

MS: Immunological, Diagnostic & Therapeutic Aspects. F. Clifford Rose & Jones Staff. 1987. (Current Problems in Neurology Ser.: Vol. 3). 272p. (*0-86196-109-9*) J Libbey Med GBR. *Dist:* Bks Intl VA.

MS, Lupus & Me (And That's Not All!) Bess K. Harvey. 2nd ed. 1992. 70p. pap. 7.95 (*0-9640635-0-6*) Golden Lght.

MSM. Woodland Publishing Staff. 1999. (Woodland Health Ser.). pap. 3.95 (*1-58054-026-0*) Woodland UT.

Mucosal Biopsy of the Gastrointestinal Tract. Richard Whitehead. Ed. by Lesley Day. 5th ed. 1997. LC 96-20545. (Illus.). 487p. text 110.00 (*0-7216-6192-0*) Saunders.

Mucosal Immunity in HIV Infection: Proceedings of the International Symposium, Berlin, June 6-7, 1997. Ernst-Otto Riecken. Ed. by Reiner Ullrich et al. 1998. (Pathobiology Ser.: Vol. 66, Nos. 3 & 4, 1998). (Illus.). 82p. pap. 55.75 (*3-8055-6739-1*) S Karger.

Mucosal Immunobiology. Ed. by L. A. Hanson. 1988. (Monographs in Allergy: Vol. 24). (Illus.). x, 330p. 221.75 (*3-8055-4680-7*) S Karger.

Mucosal Immunology. Ed. by Pearay Ogra et al. 2nd ed. 1998. LC 98-36839. (Illus.). 1628p. (C). 199.95 (*0-12-524725-7*) Acad Pr.

Mucosal Immunology & Ocular Disease. Ed. by Manfred Zierhut & John V. Forrester. 2000. LC 99-48103. (Illus.). 264p. text (*90-70430-37-1*) Aeolus Press NLD. *Dist:* Swets & Zeitlinger.

Mucosal Vaccines. Ed. by Hiroshi Kiyono et al. 1996. LC 96-19774. (Illus.). 479p. (C). text 89.95 (*0-12-410580-7*) Acad Pr.

Mucus Secretions & Cystic Fibrosis. Ed. by G. G. Forstner. 1977. (Modern Problems in Pediatrics Ser.: Vol. 19). (Illus.). 96.75 (*3-8055-2678-4*) S Karger.

Muir's Textbook of Pathology. J. R. Anderson. 12th ed. 1988. 1284p. pap. text (*0-683-13001-3*) E A GBR. *Dist:* Williams & Wilkins.

Muir's Textbook of Pathology. 13th ed. 1040p. (*0-340-66233-6*) E A GBR. *Dist:* Routldge.

Mujer, el SIDA y el Activismo: The Spanish Language Edition of Women, AIDS, & Activism - The ACT UP-NY Women & AIDS Book Group. Ed. by Cynthia Chris & Monica Pearl. 1992. 340p. 25.00 (*0-89608-455-8*); pap. 10.00 (*0-89608-454-X*) South End Pr.

Mujeres e Iglesia: Sexualidad y Aborto en America Latina. Ed. by Ana M. Portugal. 1989. (SPA., Illus.). 146p. (Orig.). pap. 10.00 (*0-915365-15-4*) Cath Free Choice.

Muller & Kirk's Small Animal Dermatology. Danny W. Scott et al. (Illus.). 5th ed. 1995. LC 94-4949. 1232p. text 135.00 (*0-7216-4850-9*); 6th ed. 2000. LC 00-30093. xi, 1528p. text 145.00 (*0-7216-7618-9*) Saunders.

Multi-Axial Classification of Child Psychiatric Disorders. D. Shaffer et al. 1975. pap. text 16.20 (*92-4-154050-8*, 1150115) World Health.

Multi-Company - Multi-Country Clinical Trials: Implementation, Monitoring, & Regulations. Ed. by Rhona Simmons. 1993. (Illus.). 303p. 159.00 (*0-935184-49-X*) IHS Health Grp.

Multi-Disciplinary Teamwork: Community Mental Handicap Teams. Morag McGrath. 1991. (Care in the Community Studies). 217p. text (*1-85628-152-3*) Avebry GBR. *Dist:* Ashgate Pub Co.

Multi-Facility Systems: The VA Experience. Ed. by R. M. Kolodner. 1997. LC 96-25988. (Computers in Health Care Ser.). (Illus.). 515p. pap. text 71.95 (*0-387-94837-6*) Spr-Verlag.

***Multi-Lead ST-Monitoring in the Early Assessment of Patients with Suspected or Confirmed Unstable Coronary Artery Disease.** Tomas Jernberg. 2000. (Comprehensive Summaries of Uppsala Dissertations from the Faculty of Medicine Ser.: No. 966). (Illus.). 89p. (Orig.). pap. (*91-554-4837-2*) Uppsala Universitet SWE. *Dist:* Coronet Bks.

Multi-Modal Approach to Creative Art Therapy. Arthur Robbins. 1994. LC 94-236986. 250p. text 23.00 (*1-85302-262-4*) Taylor & Francis.

Multi-Organ Donor: Selection & Management. Robert S. Higgins et al. 1997. LC 97-10438. (Illus.). 400p. 105.00 (*0-86542-395-4*) Blackwell Sci.

Multi-State Information System: Proceedings of the Fifth Annual National Users Group Conference. Ed. by Jeffrey Johnsen. 1981. 133p. pap. 10.00 (*0-936934-01-8*) N S Kline Inst.

Multi-Systemic Auto-Immune Diseases: An Integrated Approach: Dermatological & Internal Aspects. Ed. by Louis Kater & Harold B. De La Faille. 1995. LC 95-6498. 372p. 310.00 (*0-444-81896-0*) Elsevier.

Multi-Systemic Structural-Strategic Interventions for Child & Adolescent Behavior Problems. Ed. by Patrick H. Tolan. 1990. LC 89-26684. (Journal of Psychotherapy & the Family Ser.: Vol. 6, Nos. 3-4). (Illus.). 168p. text 4.95 (*0-86656-974-X*) Haworth Pr.

Multiaxial Classification of Child & Adolescent Psychiatric Disorder: The ICD-10 Classification of Mental & Behavioural Disorders in Children & Adolescents. World Health Organization Staff. 1997. 310p. (C). text 80.00 (*0-521-58133-8*) Cambridge U Pr.

Multiaxial Presentation of the ICD-10 for Use in Adult Psychiatry. World Health Organization Staff. 1997. LC 96-51767. (Illus.). 166p. (C). text 64.95 (*0-521-58502-3*) Cambridge U Pr.

Multicentre Study on Low Birth Weight & Infant Mortality in India, Nepal, & Sri Lanka. 1994. (SEARO Regional Health Papers: No. 25). x, 78p. pap. text 10.00 (*92-9022-194-1*, 1580025) World Health.

Multicentre Trials. Ed. by H. Helmchen & Norman Sartorius. 1981. (Modern Problems of Pharmacopsychiatry Ser.: Vol. 16). (Illus.). xii, 116p. 68.75 (*3-8055-2806-X*) S Karger.

Multicultural Challenge in Health Education. Ana C. Matiella. 1994. LC 93-44540. 34.95 (*1-56071-355-0*) ETR Assocs.

Multicultural Clients: Professional Handbook for Health Care Providers & Social Workers. Sybil M. Lassiter. 1995. LC 94-30927. 224p. lib. bdg. 69.50 (*0-313-29140-3*, Greenwood Pr) Greenwood.

Multicultural Counseling & Psychotherapy: A Lifespan Perspective. Leroy G. Baruth et al. 2nd ed. 1998. LC 98-7606. 426p. pap. text 76.00 (*0-13-271925-8*, Merrill Coll) P-H.

Multicultural Counseling Competencies: Individual & Organizational Development. Derald W. Sue et al. 1998. LC 97-45323. (Multicultural Aspects of Counseling Ser.). 89.95 (*0-8039-7130-3*, 2697) Sage.

Multicultural Counseling Competencies: Individual & Organizational Development. Derald Wing Sue et al. 1998. LC 97-45323. (Multicultural Aspects of Counseling Ser.). pap. 34.95 (*0-8039-7131-1*, 2696) Sage.

Multicultural Counseling in a Divided & Traumatized Society: The Meaning of Childhood & Adolescence in South Africa, 32. Joyce Hickson & Susan Kriegler. 1996. LC 95-41697. (Contributions in Psychology Ser.: Vol. 32). 200p. 62.50 (*0-313-28554-3*, Greenwood Pr) Greenwood.

Multicultural Healthcare & Rehabilitation of Older People. Ed. by Amanda J. Squires. 1991. 192p. (C). (*0-340-54362-0*) Age Concern Eng GBR. *Dist:* St Mut.

Multicultural Human Services for AIDS Treatment & Prevention: Policy, Perspectives, & Planning. Ed. by Marcia Bok. 1993. LC 92-48833. (Journal of Multicultural Social Work Ser.: Vol. 2, No. 3). (Illus.). 134p. 39.95 (*1-56024-414-3*); pap. 12.95 (*1-56023-038-X*, Harrington Park) Haworth Pr.

Multicultural Imagination: Race, Color & the Unconscious. Michael V. Adams. 1996. LC 96-7561. 296p. (C). pap. 29.95 (*0-415-13838-8*); (Illus.). 89.95 (*0-415-13837-X*) Routledge.

Multicultural Multimodal Multisystems Approach to Working with Culturally Different Families. Sharon-Ann Gopaul-McNicol. 1997. LC 96-33195. 160p. 60.00 (*0-275-95560-5*, Praeger Pubs) Greenwood.

Multicultural Pharmaceutical Education. Ed. by Barry Bleidt. LC 92-49896. (Journal of Pharmacy Teaching Ser.: Vol. 3, No. 2). 151p. 1996. pap. 14.95 (*0-7890-0071-7*, Pharmctl Prods); 1992. (Illus.). 39.95 (*1-56024-356-2*) Haworth Pr.

Multiculturalism & Learning Style: Teaching & Counseling Adolescents. Rita Dunn & Shirley A. Griggs. 1995. LC 94-36775. 296p. 72.50 (*0-275-94762-9*, Praeger Pubs) Greenwood.

Multicultural/Multiracial Psychology: Mestizo Perspectives in Personality & Mental Health. Manual Ramirez, III. 1998. LC 97-5664. 296p. 50.00 (*0-7657-0073-5*) Aronson.

***Multidimensional Assessment of People with Chronic Pain: An Occupational Therapy Perspective.** Marie-Louise Schult. 2001. (Comprehensive Summaries of Uppsala Dissertations from the Faculty of Medicine Ser.: No. 993). (Illus.). 71p. pap. (*91-554-4921-2*) Uppsala Universitet SWE. *Dist:* Coronet Bks.

Multidimensional Chromatography: Techniques & Applications. Ed. by Hernan J. Cortes. 1989. (Chromatographic Science Ser.: Vol. 50). (Illus.). 424p. text 170.00 (*0-8247-8136-8*) Dekker.

Multidimensional Description of Child Personality: A Manual for the Personality Inventory for Children, 1990 Edition. Robert D. Wirt et al. 1990. LC 79-57301. 192p. pap. 58.50 (*0-87424-152-9*, W-152B) Western Psych.

Multidimensional Scaling. Mark L. Davison. 1992. LC 91-30195. 256p. (C). reprint ed. lib. bdg. 44.95 (*0-89464-662-1*) Krieger.

Multidimensional Solid-State NMR & Polymers. K. Schmidt-Rohr & H. W. Spiess. 1994. (Illus.). 512p. text 111.00 (*0-12-626630-1*) Acad Pr.

Multidisciplinary Analysis of Controversies in the Management of Prostate Cancer. Ed. by D. S. Coffey et al. 1988. LC 88-18004. (Illus.). 350p. 89.50 (*0-306-42927-6*, Plenum Trade) Perseus Pubng.

Multidisciplinary Approach to Health Care Ethics. Drew E. Hinderer & Sara R. Hinderer. 2000. LC 00-24568. xi, 192p. (*0-7674-1302-4*) Mayfield Pub.

Multidisciplinary Approach to Myelin Diseases. Ed. by G. Serlupi Crescenzi. 1987. LC 87-29227. (NATO ASI Series A, Life Sciences: Vol. 142). (Illus.). 416p. 110.00 (*0-306-42776-1*, Plenum Trade) Perseus Pubng.

Multidisciplinary Approach to Myelin Diseases 2. S. Salvati. 1994. (NATO Advanced Science Institutes Ser.: Vol. 258). (Illus.). 274p. (C). text 95.00 (*0-306-44634-0*, Kluwer Plenum) Kluwer Academic.

Multidisciplinary Approach to Rehabilitation. Shrawan Kumar. 2000. LC 99-56946. (Illus.). 400p. text 49.99 (*0-7506-7067-3*) Buttrwrth-Heinemann.

Multidisciplinary Approaches to Cholinesterase Functions. A. Shafferman & B. Velan. 1993. (Illus.). 310p. (C). text 95.00 (*0-306-44315-5*, Kluwer Plenum) Kluwer Academic.

M N O

Multidisciplinary Atlas of Breast Surgery. David W. Kinne. 1997. LC 97-4343. 208p. text 175.00 (*0-397-51467-0*) Lppncott W & W.

Multidisciplinary Care of Cancer Patients. Council of Europe Staff. 1992. (*92-871-2043-9*) Council of Europe FRA. *Dist:* Manhattan Pub Co.

Multidisciplinary Gerontology: A Structure for Research in Gerontology in a Developed Country. Ed. by I. R. Mackay. 1977. (Interdisciplinary Topics in Gerontology Ser.: Vol. 11). (Illus.). 53.25 (*3-8055-2679-2*) S Karger.

***Multidisciplinary Handbook of Child & Adolescent Mental Health for Front Line Professionals.** Nisha Dogra. 2001. LC 2001-50398. 176p. pap. (*1-85302-929-7*) Jessica Kingsley.

Multidisciplinary Pain Center: Organization & Personnel Functions for Pain Management. Ed. by Jawahar N. Ghia. 1988. (Current Management of Pain Ser.). (C). text 134.00 (*0-89838-359-5*) Kluwer Academic.

Multidisciplinary Treatment of Soft Tissue Sarcomas. Ed. by Jaap Verweij et al. 1993. LC 93-9299. (Cancer Treatment & Research Ser.: Vol. 67). 208p. (C). text 198.50 (*0-7923-2183-9*) Kluwer Academic.

Multidrug Resistance: Cancer Cells & Multiple Chemotherapeutic Drugs. 1995. lib. bdg. 255.95 (*0-8490-7564-5*) Gordon Pr.

Multidrug Resistance in Cancer Cells: Molecular, Biochemical, Physiological, & Biological Aspects. Ed. by Sudhir Gupta & Takashi Tsuruo. 1996. LC 96-13797. 522p. 265.00 (*0-471-96712-2*) Wiley.

Multigenerational Family Therapy. David S. Freeman. LC 91-7953. (Illus.). 420p. 1992. lib. bdg. 59.95 (*1-56024-125-X*); 1991. pap. 24.95 (*1-56024-126-8*) Haworth Pr.

Multihandicapped: Serving the Severely Disabled. Jack M. Gootzeit. 1981. 300p. text 32.50 (*0-8290-0556-0*); pap. text 16.95 (*0-8290-0269-3*) Irvington.

Multilevel Approach to the Study of Motor Control & Learning. Debra J. Rose. 1996. LC 96-24476. 331p. 67.00 (*0-02-403621-8*) Allyn.

Multilevel Health Effects Research: From Molecules to Man. Ed. by J. F. Park & R. A. Pelroy. 1990. LC 89-18083. (Proceedings of the 27th Hanford Symposium on Health & the Environment Ser.). 492p. pap. text 57.50 (*0-935470-55-7*) Battelle.

Multilingual Dictionary of Disaster Medicine & International Relief: English, Francais, Espanole, (Arabic) S. W. Gunn. 1989. (C). lib. bdg. 158.50 (*0-89838-409-5*) Kluwer Academic.

Multilingual Dictionary of Narcotic Drugs & Psychotropic Substances under International Control. 508p. 42.00 (*92-1-048056-2*, M.93.XI.2) UN.

Multilingual Dictionary of Narcotics Drug & Psychotropic Substances under International Control. 37.00 (*92-1-048005-8*, E/F/R/S.83.XI.5) UN.

Multilingual Health Education Resource Guide. Pref. by Margot Pfleger & Mizzette Fuenzalida. 2nd ed. 1996. 151p. pap. text 25.00 (*0-7881-8939-5*) DIANE Pub.

Multilingual Manual for Medical History-Taking. Louis Del Guercio. 1972. (FRE.). 178p. pap. 39.95 (*0-7859-9618-4*) Fr & Eur.

Multimedia Edition of Educational Psychology: Developing Learners. Jeanne Ellis Ormrod. 3rd ed. 2000. 773p. pap. 69.00 (*0-13-032298-9*) P-H.

Multimethod Assessment of Chronic. Paul Karoly & Mark P. Jensen. 1987. (C). 54.95 (*0-205-14386-5*, H4386) Allyn.

Multimethod Assessment of Chronic Pain. Paul Karoly & Mark P. Jensen. 1987. (Psychology Practitioner Guidebooks). 192p. text 30.00 (*0-08-032377-4*); pap. text 15.95 (*0-08-032376-6*) Elsevier (Pergamon Pr).

Multimodal Psychiatric Music Therapy for Adults, Adolescents, & Children: A Clinical Manual. Michael D. Cassity & Julia E. Cassity. 1993. 250p. pap. text 30.00 (*0-9643602-0-9*); 3rd exp. ed. 1998. LC 95-45524. 256p. 24.95 (*0-918812-85-2*) MMB Music.

Multimodal Therapy in Oncology Nursing. Ed. by Marcia C. Liebman & Dawn Camp-Sorrell. 1996. LC 96-10353. (Illus.). 528p. (C). (gr. 13). pap. text 37.95 (*0-8151-5422-4*, 25466) Mosby Inc.

Multimodality Therapy in Gynecologic Oncology. Ed. by B. U. Sevin et al. 1996. LC 96-14486. 89.00 (*0-86577-588-5*) Thieme Med Pubs.

Multimodality Treatment of Lung Cancer. Ed. by Arthur T. Skarin. 2000. LC 00-267825. (Lung Biology in Health & Disease Ser.: Vol. 140). (Illus.). 496p. text 195.00 (*0-8247-0236-0*) Dekker.

Multinational Pharmaceutical Companies: Principles & Practice. Bert Spilker. 2nd ed. 1993. 848p. text 159.00 (*0-7817-0100-7*) Lppncott W & W.

Multiparticulate Oral Drug Delivery. Ghebre-Sellassie. 1994. (Drugs & the Pharmaceutical Sciences Ser.: Vol. 65). (Illus.). 496p. text 225.00 (*0-8247-9191-6*) Dekker.

Multiperspective Case Formulation: A Step Towards Treatment Integration. Priyanthy Weerasekera. 348p. (Orig.). 1996. pap. 29.50 (*0-89464-976-0*); 1995. (C). 38.50 (*0-89464-814-4*) Krieger.

Multiphase Biomedical Materials. Ed. by T. Tsuruta & A. Nakajima. 1989. 202p. (*90-6764-109-X*) VSP NLD. *Dist:* Coronet Bks.

Multiplane Transesophageal Echocardiography. Ed. by Jos R. Roelandt & Natesa G. Pandian. 1995. 257p. text (*0-443-07950-1*) Church.

Multiple AIDS-Related Loss: A Handbook for Understanding & Surviving a Perpetual Fall. David Nord. 1997. LC 96-53419. (Series in Death, Dying & Bereavement). xxi, 308p. 64.95 (*1-56032-581-X*); pap. 29.95 (*1-56032-582-8*) Taylor & Francis.

Multiple Auditory Areas. Ed. by Clinton N. Woolsey. 1982. LC 81-81433. (Cortical Sensory Organization Ser.: Vol. 3). (Illus.). 276p. 119.50 (*0-89603-032-6*) Humana.

Multiple Chemical Interactions. Edward J. Calabrese. 1990. (Illus.). 736p. lib. bdg. 139.00 (*0-87371-146-7*, L146) Lewis Pubs.

Multiple Chemical Sensitivity: A Scientific Overview. Ed. by Frank L. Mitchell. 1995. LC 94-74818. (Illus.). 669p. text 135.00 (*0-911131-53-1*) Specialist Journals.

Multiple Choice Questions. H. L. Beynon et al. 1991. (Complete MRCP Ser.). (Illus.). 265p. (Orig.). pap. text (*0-443-04308-6*) Church.

Multiple Choice Questions Pt. 1: MRCP. Ed. by H. L. Beynon et al. 2nd ed. 1998. 328p. pap. (*0-443-05691-9*) Church.

Multiple Choice Questions Clinical Examination. Nicholas J. Talley & Simon O'Connor. 1996. (Illus.). 144p. (Orig.). pap. 31.95 (*0-632-04153-6*) Blackwell Sci.

Multiple Choice Questions for MRCP. P. Joshi. 2nd ed. 1995. 320p. pap. text, stu. ed., suppl. ed. (*0-7506-2048-X*) E A GBR. *Dist:* OUP.

Multiple Choice Questions for the MRCPsych Pt. II: Basic Sciences Examination. Gin S. Malhi. 2000. LC 99-58726. 181p. pap. text (*0-7506-4089-8*) E A GBR. *Dist:* OUP.

Multiple Choice Questions in Anatomy. 96p. pap. (*0-340-50785-3*) E A GBR. *Dist:* Routldge.

Multiple Choice Questions in Anatomy for the FRCS. McDiarmid. 1995. 80p. pap. 14.95 (*0-340-59433-0*) Trafalgar.

Multiple Choice Questions in Clinical Pharmacology. James M. Ritter et al. 1995. 168p. pap. text (*0-340-55932-2*) E A GBR. *Dist:* OUP.

Multiple Choice Questions in Clinical Pharmacology for the Higher Level Examination. McCarthy. 1992. 192p. pap. 14.95 (*0-340-55792-3*) Trafalgar.

Multiple Choice Questions in Dermatology. S. K. Goolamali. 1992. 144p. (C). (gr. 13). pap. text 16.00 (*0-8151-3539-4*, 21909) Mosby Inc.

Multiple Choice Questions in Gynaecology & Obstetrics. Richard J. Lilford & Marcus E. Setchell. 3rd ed. 88p. pap. (*0-340-58896-9*) E A GBR. *Dist:* OUP, Routldge.

Multiple Choice Questions in Haematology. Baglin. 2nd ed. 1992. 112p. pap. text 9.95 (*0-340-55303-0*) Trafalgar.

Multiple Choice Questions in Medicine. Debra King & Susan J. Benbow. 1993. LC 93-34658. 248p. (gr. 13). pap. 29.95 (*0-412-45710-5*, Chap & Hall NY) Chapman & Hall.

Multiple Choice Questions in Orthopaedics. M. Farooque & L. C. Gupta. 1991. 182p. (C). (*81-85017-58-1*) Interprint IND. *Dist:* St Mut.

Multiple Choice Questions in Paraclinical Subjects. L. C. Gupta. 1991. 292p. (C). (*81-85017-59-X*) Interprint IND. *Dist:* St Mut.

Multiple Choice Questions in Pathology. Brown. 3rd ed. 80p. pap. text (*0-340-55164-X*) E A GBR. *Dist:* Routldge.

Multiple Choice Questions in Pathology for the FRCS. McDiarmid. 1995. 80p. pap. 14.95 (*0-340-59434-9*) Trafalgar.

Multiple Choice Questions in Pharmacology: With Answers & Explanatory Comments. D'Mello. 2nd ed. 80p. pap. text (*0-340-54321-3*) E A GBR. *Dist:* Routldge.

Multiple Choice Questions in Veterinary Nursing. Barbara Cooper. 1997. LC 97-185352. 132p. Vol. 1. pap. text 25.00 (*0-7506-3611-4*); Vol. 2. pap. text 25.00 (*0-7506-3612-2*) Buttrwrth-Heinemann.

Multiple Choice Questions on Surgical Diagnosis. R. Visvanathan & J. S. P. Lumley. 2000. (Illus.). 144p. pap. (*0-7506-4730-2*) E A GBR. *Dist:* OUP.

Multiple Cholecystokinin Receptors in the CNS. Ed. by Colin T. Dourish et al. 1992. (Illus.). 580p. text 130.00 (*0-19-857756-7*) OUP.

Multiple Congenital Anomalies: A Catalogue of Recognizable Syndromes. Robin M. Winter & Michael Baraitser. 1991. 1300p. 279.95 (*0-442-31316-0*) Chapman & Hall.

Multiple Congenital Anomalies: A Diagnostic Compendium. Ed. by Michael Baraitser & Winter. 1992. (Illus.). 352p. (C). 467.95 (*0-412-49190-7*, Chap & Hall NY) Chapman & Hall.

Multiple Congenital Anomalies: A Diagnostic Compendium. Ed. by Michael Baraitser & R. Winter. 1990. (Illus.). 1448p. (C). (gr. 13). text 907.95 (*0-412-29130-4*) Chapman & Hall.

Multiple Crises of Marital Separation & Divorce. Gerald Jacobson. 1982. (Seminars in Psychiatry Ser.). 357p. text 54.00 (*0-8089-1483-9*, 792159, Grune & Strat) Harcrt Hlth Sci Grp.

Multiple Drug Resistance in Cancer: Cellular, Molecular, & Clinical Approaches. Ed. by M. Clynes. 1994. LC 93-44250. 400p. (C). text 204.50 (*0-7923-2669-5*) Kluwer Academic.

Multiple Exposures: Chronicles of the Radiation Age. Catherine Caufield. 1990. LC 89-20637. (Illus.). 312p. pap. 16.95 (*0-226-09785-4*) U Ch Pr.

Multiple Facets of Therapeutic Transactions. Chaya Roth & Steven D. Kulb. 1997. LC 96-43562. 308p. 45.00 (*0-8236-3487-6*, BN03487) Intl Univs Pr.

Multiple Forms of Enzymes. Ed. by R. J. Haschen et al. 1982. (Advances in Clinical Enzymology Ser.: Vol. 2). 250p. 121.00 (*3-8055-2921-X*) S Karger.

Multiple Intelligences: The Theory in Practice. Howard Gardner. 1993. LC 92-53241. 272p. 23.00 (*0-456-01821-2*) Basic.

Multiple Medical Impairment Study. MIB, Inc. Staff & SOA/ AAIM/ HOLUA-IHOU Mortality and Morbidity Liaison Committee. 1998. LC 98-39856. 95.00 (*0-9665356-0-X*) CMAS Bks.

Multiple Monitores Electro-Convulsive Therapy. Barry M. Maletzky. 1981. LC 80-23111. 256p. 143.00 (*0-8493-5940-6*, RC485, CRC Reprint) Franklin.

Multiple Muscle Systems: Biomechanics & Movements Organization. Ed. by J. Winters & S. L. Woo. 1990. (Illus.). 801p. 76.00 (*0-387-97307-9*) Spr-Verlag.

Multiple Myeloma. Gosta Gahrton & Brian G. Durie. 1996. (Arnold Publication). (Illus.). 232p. (C). 89.50 (*0-340-57603-0*) OUP.

Multiple Myeloma & Other Paraproteinaemias. I.W. Delamore. 1987. LC 86-9666. (Illus.). 377p. text (*0-443-03134-7*) Church.

Multiple Neurology & the Law: Private Litigation & the Public Policy. H. Richard Beresford. 1998. LC 97-34794. (Contemporary Neurology Ser.: No. 51). (Illus.). 208p. (C). 89.00 (*0-8036-0168-9*) OUP.

Multiple Organ Dysfunction & Failure: Pathophysiology & Clinical Implications. Ed. by Virginia H. Secor. 2nd ed. 1996. (Illus.). 480p. (C). (gr. 13). text 59.95 (*0-8151-4325-7*, 29188) Mosby Inc.

Multiple Organ Dysfunction Syndrome: Examining the Role of Eicosanoids & Procoagulants. John G. Williams. 1996. (Medical Intelligence Unit Ser.). 158p. 99.00 (*1-57059-325-6*) Landes Bioscience.

Multiple Organ Dysfunction Syndrome: Examining the Role of Eicosanoids & Procoagulants. Ed. by John G. Williams. 1996. LC 95-50752. (Medicine Ser.). 153p. pap. 89.95 (*0-412-10301-X*, VNR) Wiley.

Multiple Personalites, Multiple Disorders: Psychiatric Classification & Media Influence. Carol S. North et al. 1993. LC 92-49904. (Oxford Psychiatry Ser.: No. 1). (Illus.). 296p. (C). text 45.00 (*0-19-508095-5*) OUP.

Multiple Personality, Allied Disorders & Hypnosis. Eugene L. Bliss. 1986. 282p. text 45.00 (*0-19-503658-1*) OUP.

Multiple Personality & Dissociation, 1791-1992: A Complete Bibliography. Ed. by Carole Goettman et al. 2nd ed. 1994. LC 94-7179. xii, 156p. pap. 9.95 (*0-9629164-5-5*) Sidran Pr.

Multiple Personality Disorder: Diagnosis, Clinical Features & Treatment. Colin A. Ross. 1989. LC 89-14608. 400p. 120.00 (*0-471-61515-3*) Wiley.

Multiple Personality Disorder from the Inside Out. Ed. by Barry M. Cohen et al. 1991. LC 91-60530. (Illus.). xxii, 245p. (Orig.). pap. 18.95 (*0-9629164-0-4*) Sidran Pr.

Multiple Personality Disorders in the Netherlands: A Study on Reliability & Validity of the Diagnosis. Suzette Boon & Nel Draijer. 1993. 262p. pap. (*90-265-1361-5*) Swets.

Multiple Pregnancy: Epidemiology, Gestation & Perinatal Outcome. Louis G. Keith et al. 1995. (Illus.). 722p. lib. bdg. 107.95 (*1-85070-666-2*, Parthenon Pbng) CRC Pr.

Multiple Pregnancy & Delivery. Ed. by Stanley A. Gall. 1996. LC 96-3728. (Illus.). 368p. (C). (gr. 13). text 69.00 (*0-8151-3406-1*, 24729) Mosby Inc.

Multiple Psychotherapy. Rudolf Dreikurs et al. 1984. LC 84-71164. 146p. (Orig.). pap. 10.00 (*0-918560-31-4*) Adler Sch Prof Psy.

Multiple Realities in Clinical Practice. John S. Kafka. 1989. LC 88-38238. 208p. (C). 35.00 (*0-300-04350-3*) Yale U Pr.

Multiple Risk Factors in Cardiovascular Disease: Strategies of Prevention of Coronary Heart Disease, Cardiac Failure, & Stroke. Ed. by Antonio M. Gotto, Jr. et al. 1998. LC 98-15831. (Medical Science Symposia Ser.). 388p. 119.00 (*0-7923-5023-5*) Kluwer Academic.

Multiple Risk Factors in Cardiovascular Diseases. Ed. by Antonio M. Gotto, Jr. et al. 1992. LC 92-49870. (Medical Science Symposia Ser.: Vol. 1). 284p. text 166.50 (*0-7923-1938-9*) Kluwer Academic.

Multiple Risk Factors in Cardiovascular Diseases: Vascular & Organ Protection. Ed. by A. M. Gotto, Jr. et al. 1995. LC 95-22833. (Medical Science Symposia Ser.: Vol. 8). 456p. text 170.00 (*0-7923-3503-1*) Kluwer Academic.

Multiple Sclerosis. David Barne. 2000. (Questions & Answers Ser.). (Illus.). 120p. pap. 26.95 (*1-873413-86-6*) Merit Pub Intl.

Multiple Sclerosis. Jan De Vries. 1985. (By Appointment Only Ser.). 125p. pap. (*0-906391-98-9*) Mainstream Pubng GBR. *Dist:* Trafalgar.

Multiple Sclerosis. Louis J. Rosner & Shelley Ross. 1992. 256p. 13.00 (*0-671-77809-9*, Fireside) S&S Trade Pap.

Multiple Sclerosis. Ed. by Jorg Kesselring. 2nd ed. 1996. (Illus.). 230p. (C). text 74.95 (*0-521-48018-3*) Cambridge U Pr.

Multiple Sclerosis, Vol. 51. Donald W. Paty & George C. Ebers. 1997. LC 97-3052. (Contemporary Neurology Ser.: No. 50). (Illus.). 612p. (C). 150.00 (*0-8036-6784-1*) OUP.

Multiple Sclerosis: A Dragon with a Hundred Heads. Peter P. Michael. 1981. LC 79-10954. 22.95 (*0-87949-170-1*) Ashley Bks.

Multiple Sclerosis: A Guide for Families. Rosalind C. Kalb. 1998. LC 97-49252. 207p. pap. 24.95 (*1-888799-14-5*) Demos Medical.

Multiple Sclerosis: A Guide for Patients & Their Families. Ed. by Labe C. Scheinberg & Nancy J. Holland. 2nd ed. 1987. 288p. text 27.50 (*0-88167-254-8*); pap. text 35.00 (*0-88167-255-6*) Lppncott W & W.

***Multiple Sclerosis: A Guide for Rehabilitation & Health Care Professionals.** Ed. by Phillip D. Rumrill, Jr. & Mary Hennessey. 2001. (Illus.). 230p. text 47.95 (*0-398-07227-2*) C C Thomas.

Multiple Sclerosis: A Guide for the Newly Diagnosed. Nancy J. Holland et al. 1996. LC 96-35928. 128p. pap. 21.95 (*1-888799-06-4*) Demos Medical.

***Multiple Sclerosis: A Guide for the Newly Diagnosed.** Nancy J. Holland et al. 2nd ed. 2001. 120p. pap. 21.95 (*1-888799-60-9*) Demos Medical.

Multiple Sclerosis: A Neuropsychiatric Disorder. Ed. by Uriel Halbreich. 1993. LC 92-22041. (Progress in Psychiatry Ser.: No. 37). 192p. text 32.00 (*0-88048-463-2*, 8463) Am Psychiatric.

Multiple Sclerosis: A Personal Exploration. Alexander Burnfield. 1997. (Human Horizons Ser.). (Illus.). 192p. (Orig.). pap. (*0-285-65018-1*) Souvenir Pr Ltd GBR. *Dist:* IPG Chicago.

Multiple Sclerosis: A Self-Care Guide to Wellness. Nancy J. Holland et al. 1998. LC 98-7854. (Illus.). 164p. spiral bd. 9.00 (*0-929819-09-8*) Paralyzed Vets.

Multiple Sclerosis: A Self-Help Guide to Its Management. Judy Graham. rev. ed. 1990. 160p. pap. 12.95 (*0-89281-242-7*, Heal Arts VT) Inner Tradit.

Multiple Sclerosis: Advances in Trial Design, Treatment, & Future Perspectives. Ed. by D. E. Goodkin & R. A. Rudick. 1997. LC 96-12736. (Illus.). 364p. 139.00 (*3-540-76018-0*) Spr-Verlag.

Multiple Sclerosis: Approaches to Management. Ed. by Lorraine De Souza & Jo Campling. 1990. (Therapy in Practice Ser.). 140p. pap. 23.00 (*0-412-32230-7*, A4411) Chapman & Hall.

Multiple Sclerosis: Clinical & Pathogenetic Basis. Cedric S. Raine. 1996. (Illus.). 448p. (*0-412-30890-8*) E A GBR. *Dist:* OUP.

Multiple Sclerosis: Control of the Disease. W. R. Russell. 1976. 84p. pap. text 18.25 (*0-08-021002-3*, Pergamon Pr) Elsevier.

Multiple Sclerosis: Diagnosis, Medical Management & Rehabilitation. Jack S. Burks & Kenneth P. Johnson. 2000. LC 00-35858. (Illus.). 616p. 210.00 (*1-888799-35-8*) Demos Medical.

Multiple Sclerosis: How I Won the Battle. Yvonne A. Fischer. 1999. 70p. pap. (*0-7392-0134-4*, PO3055) Morris Pubng.

***Multiple Sclerosis: Psychosocial & Vocational Interventions.** Robert Fraser et al. 2002. 200p. pap. 39.95 (*1-888799-59-5*) Demos Medical.

***Multiple Sclerosis: The Facts.** W. B. Matthews & Margaret Rice-Oxley. 4th ed. 2001. LC 2001-45165. (Oxford Medical Publications). 140p. pap. (*0-19-850898-0*) OUP.

Multiple Sclerosis: The Facts You Need. Paul O'Connor. 1999. (Your Personal Health Ser.). 156p. pap. 14.95 (*1-55209-367-0*) Firefly Bks Limited.

Multiple Sclerosis: The Questions You Have - The Answers You Need. Rosalind C. Kalb. 2nd rev. ed. 2000. LC 00-35857. 592p. pap. 39.95 (*1-888799-43-9*) Demos Medical.

Multiple Sclerosis & Having a Baby: Everything You Need to Know about Conception, Pregnancy & Parenthood. Judy Graham. 1999. LC 99-18416. 192p. pap. 12.95 (*0-89281-788-7*, Heal Arts VT) Inner Tradit.

Multiple Sclerosis & Other Demyelinating Diseases. Ed. by Pierre J. Vinken & George W. Bruyn. 1971. 277.50 (*0-444-10019-9*) Elsevier.

Multiple Sclerosis Diet Book: A Low-Fat Diet for the Treatment of MS, Heart Disease & Stroke. Roy L. Swank & Barbara Dugan. 1987. LC 86-16819. (Illus.). 416p. 29.95 (*0-385-23279-9*) Doubleday.

Multiple Sclerosis East & West. Ed. by Y. Kuroiwa & L. T. Kurland. 1983. (Illus.). vi, 398p. 172.25 (*3-8055-3674-7*) S Karger.

Multiple Sclerosis Fact Book. Richard Lechtenberg. 2nd ed. 1995. LC 94-25306. (Illus.). 235p. (C). pap. text 23.95 (*0-8036-0074-7*) Davis Co.

Multiple Sclerosis Research in Europe. Ed. by O. R. Hommes. 1986. text 248.00 (*0-85200-917-8*) Kluwer Academic.

Multiple Selves, Multiple Voices: Working with Trauma, Violation, & Dissociation. Phil Mollon. 1999. LC 96-1476. (Clinical Psychology & Personality Ser.). 228p. pap. 49.95 (*0-471-96330-5*) Wiley.

Multiple Somatic Areas. Ed. by Clinton N. Woolsey. 1981. LC 81-81433. (Cortical Sensory Organization Ser.: Vol. 1). (Illus.). 268p. 119.50 (*0-89603-030-X*) Humana.

Multiple System Atrophy. N. Quinn & Gregor Wenning. 1913. 264p. 85.00 (*0-7506-2359-4*) Buttrwrth-Heinemann.

Multiple Systems Organ Failure: Hepatic Regulation of Systemic Host Defense. George M. Matuschak. 1993. (Illus.). 408p. text 199.00 (*0-8247-9059-6*) Dekker.

Multiple Trauma. R. Wilder. 1984. (Progress in Critical Care Medicine Ser.: Vol. 1). (Illus.). xii, 288p. 82.75 (*3-8055-3823-5*) S Karger.

Multiple Unit - Agency Response for Fire. 1998. (Training in a Box Ser.). 36p. ring bd. 49.00 (1-57927-037-9) APCO Inst.

Multiple Victimization of Children: Conceptual, Developmental, Research & Treatment Issues. Ed. by B. B. Rossman & Mindy S. Rosenberg. 1998. LC 98-10643. 341p. 49.95 (0-7890-0361-9); pap. 24.95 (0-7890-0382-1) Haworth Pr (Maltreatment & Trauma Pr).

Multiple Visual Areas. Ed. by Clinton N. Woolsey. 1982. LC 81-81433. (Cortical Sensory Organization Ser.: Vol. 2). (Illus.). 242p. 119.50 (0-89603-031-8) Humana.

Multiple Voices: Narrative in Systemic Family Psychotherapy. Renos K. Papadoupoulos & John Byng-Hall. 1998. LC 97-44057. 304p. (C). 85.00 (0-415-92084-1); pap. 25.95 (0-415-92085-X) Routledge.

Multiple's Guide to Harmonized Family Living: A Healthy Alternative, or Prelude, to Integration. Tammy C. Whitman & Susan C. Shore. 1994. LC 94-70635. (Illus.). 128p. (Orig.). pap. 16.95 (1-884390-03-X) Art Endeavors.

Multiplicity of Dreams: Memory, Imagination & Consciousness. Harry T. Hunt. 1989. LC 88-27908. (Illus.). 288p. (C). 42.50 (0-300-04330-9) Yale U Pr.

Multiplicity of Dreams: Memory, Imagination, & Consciousness. Harry T. Hunt. 1991. 288p. (C). reprint ed. pap. 18.00 (0-300-04985-4) Yale U Pr.

Multiply Handicapped Hearing Impaired Child. Ed. by Sanford E. Gerber & George T. Mencher. 1983. 448p. text 41.00 (0-8089-1618-1, 792878, Grune & Strat) Harcrt Hlth Sci Grp.

Multipotential Stem Cells in the Brain. Jack Price. 1997. (Neuroscience Intelligence Unit Ser.). 250p. 89.95 (0-412-13461-6) Chapman & Hall.

Multiprofessional Education of Health Personnel. 1995. (92-871-2653-4) Council of Europe FRA. *Dist:* Manhattan Pub Co.

Multiprofessional Handbook of Child Sexual Abuse: Integrated Management, Therapy, & Legal Intervention. Tilman Furniss. 1991. 384p. (C). pap. 47.95 (0-415-05563-6, A5265) Routledge.

Multipurpose Serological Serveys & WHO Serum Reference Banks: Proceedings of the WHO Scientific Group, Geneva, 1969. WHO Staff. 1970. (Technical Reports: No. 454). 95p. pap. text 7.00 (92-4-120454-0, 1160454) World Health.

Multisensory Control of Posture: Proceedings of an International Symposium on Sensory Interaction in Posture & Movement Control Held in Smolenice, Slovakia, September 9-11, 1994, As a Satellite Symposium to the European Neuroscience Association Meeting of 1994. Ed. by T. Mergner & F. Hlavacka. 1995. LC 95-30547. (Illus.). 370p. 95.00 (0-306-45101-8, Kluwer Plenum) Kluwer Academic.

Multiskilled Health Care Workers: Issues & Approaches to Cross-Training. Sherry Makely. Ed. by Lana Christian. 1997. 288p. pap. 34.95 (0-9652954-3-5) Pine Ridge Publns.

Multiskilled Radiologic Technologist: A Competency-Based Approach. Belinda Escamilla et al. 2001. (Illus.). 250p. pap. 29.00 (0-8036-0547-1) Davis Co.

Multiskilled Respiratory Therapist: A Competency-Based Program. David W. Chang et al. 3rd ed. 2000. (Illus.). 252p. (C). pap. text 29.95 (0-8036-0380-0) Davis Co.

Multiskilling: Advanced Patient Care Skills For The Health Care Provider. Denise York. 1997. LC 97-34658. (Delmar's Multiskilling Ser.). 138p. (C). pap. text, tchr. ed. 22.95 (0-8273-8523-4) Delmar.

Multiskilling: Dietary Practice for the Health Care Provider. Jo Ann R. Airaghi & Rebecca S. Galvin. 2nd abr. rev. ed. 1999. LC 98-51789. (Allied Health Ser.). 30p. (C). pap. text 22.95 (0-7668-0514-X) Delmar.

Multiskilling: Electrocardiography for the Health Care Provider. Kovanda & Karen Brisindine. 1997. LC 97-37683. 64p. (C). pap. text 22.95 (0-8273-8522-6) Delmar.

Multiskilling: Electrocardiography for the Health Care Provider - IML. Kovanda & Brisendine. 1998. 24p. tchr. ed. 16.00 (0-7668-0487-9) Delmar.

Multiskilling: Health Unit Coordination for the Health Care Provider. Emerick & Graham. 1998. (Home Care Aide Ser.). 64p. (C). pap. text 18.95 (0-7668-0213-2) Delmar.

Multiskilling: Phlebotomy Collection Procedures for the Health Care Provider. Beverly M. Kovanda. 1997. LC 97-28487. 126p. (C). pap. text 22.95 (0-8273-8452-1) Delmar.

Multiskilling: Phlebotomy for the Health Care Provider - IML. Kovanda. 1998. 80p. tchr. ed. (0-7668-0737-1) Delmar.

Multiskilling: Point Of Care Testing for the Health Care Provider. Beverly M. Kovanda. 1997. LC 97-26293. 85p. (C). pap. text 22.95 (0-8273-8453-X) Delmar.

Multiskilling: Point of Care Testing for the Health Care Provider - IML. Kovanda. 1998. 56p. tchr. ed. (0-7668-0738-X) Delmar.

Multiskilling: Respiratory Care for the Health Care Provider. Sills. 1997. LC 97-42387. 128p. (C). pap. text 22.95 (0-7668-0075-X) Delmar.

Multiskilling: Team Building for the Health Care Provider. Makeley Kovanda. 1998. (Home Care Aide Ser.). 48p. (C). pap. text 18.95 (0-8273-8524-2) Delmar.

Multiskilling & Aural Rehabilitation. Carole E. Johnson & Jeffrey L. Danhauer. 1999. LC 99-10767. (Illus.). xvi, 365p. 57.50 net. (1-56593-905-0) Thomson Learn.

Multisystem Diseases. Ed. by Graeme R. Catto. 1989. (New Clinical Applications in Nephrology Ser.). (C). text 91.00 (0-7462-0060-9) Kluwer Academic.

Multitesting Database Acquisition: Current Approaches; Proceedings of the Washington-Alaska Regional Medical Program Conference, Everett, Wash., 1973. Washington-Alaska Regional Medical Program Confere. 1973. LC 73-16454. 197p. 6.00 (0-917054-06-7) Med Communications.

Multivariable Analysis: A Practical Guide for Clinicians. Mitchell H. Katz. 1999. LC 98-39350. (Illus.). 208p. (C). text 85.00 (0-521-59301-8) Cambridge U Pr.

Multivariate Analysis in Behavioral Research: For Medical & Social Science Students. A. E. Maxwell. 2nd ed. 1977. 164p. (gr. 13). pap. 54.95 (0-412-14300-3, NO. 6193) CRC Pr.

Multivariate Applications in Substance Use Research. Ed. by Jennifer S. Rose et al. 1999. LC 99-28611. (Multivariate Applications Ser.). 450p. (0-8058-2942-3) L Erlbaum Assocs.

Multivariate Applications in the Social Sciences. Nancy Hirschberg & Lloyd G. Humphreys. 1982. 304p. (C). text 59.95 (0-89859-152-X) L Erlbaum Assocs.

Multivariate Approaches for the Behavioral Sciences: A Brief Text. G. Frank Lawlis & Douglas Chatfield. 1974. (Illus.). 153p. (Orig.). pap. text 5.00 (0-89672-051-9) Tex Tech Univ Pr.

Multivariate Design & Statistics. Steve Miller. 1986. (New Essential Psychology Ser.). 224p. pap. 7.95 (0-416-34930-7, 1019) Routledge.

Multivariate Personality Research. Ed. by Ralph Dreger. 1972. 17.50 (0-87511-029-0) Claitors.

Multivariate Statistical Methods in Behavioral Research. R. Darrell Bock. 2nd ed. 1985. pap. 40.00 (0-89498-014-9) Sci Ware.

Mummies, Disease & Ancient Cultures. Ed. by Aidan Cockburn et al. 2nd ed. 1998. LC 97-26894. (Illus.). 424p. (C). text 90.00 (0-521-58060-9); pap. text 34.95 (0-521-58954-1) Cambridge U Pr.

Mummies Old & New - Their Health, Disease & Research Investigations: Index of New Information. Andris G. Chien. 1998. 150p. 57.50 (0-7883-2038-6); pap. 47.50 (0-7883-2039-4) ABBE Pubs Assn.

Munchausen Syndrome by Proxy: Issues in Diagnosis & Treatment. Alex V. Levin & Mary S. Sheridan. 1996. LC 95-3324. 480p. 49.95 (0-02-918606-4) Jossey-Bass.

Munchausen Syndrome by Proxy Abuse: A Practical Approach. Ed. by D. Mary Eminson & R. J. Postlethwaite. 2000. LC 99-46238. 336p. pap. (0-7506-4072-3) E A GBR. *Dist:* OUP.

Mundo Visto a los Ochenta Anos: Impresiones de un Arteriosclerotico. Santiago R. Cajal. Ed. by Robert J. Kastenbaum. 1979. LC 78-22214. (Aging & Old Age Ser.). (SPA.). reprint ed. lib. bdg. 23.95 (0-405-11827-9) Ayer.

Municipal Health Department Practice for the Year 1923: In America's 100 Largest Cities. 1974. LC 73-11911. (Metropolitan America Ser.). 810p. reprint ed. 56.95 (0-405-05429-7) Ayer.

Municipal Waste Combustion Study: Assessment of Health Risks Associated with Municipal Waste Combustion Emissions. Radian Corp. Staff. 1989. 248p. 78.95 (0-89116-071-X) Hemisp Pub.

Mur Contre la Malaria: Du Nouveau dans la Prevention des Deces Dus au Paludisme (Net Gain, a New Method for Preventing Malaria Deaths) Christian Lengeler et al. 1997. (FRE.). 300p. pap. (0-88936-831-7) IDRC-CRDI CAN. *Dist:* Stylus Pub VA.

Murals of the Mind: Images of a Psychiatric Community. Jay Harris & Cliff Joseph. 1973. LC 72-8793. (Illus.). 274p. 40.00 (0-8236-3490-6) Intl Univs Pr.

Murderous Science: Elimination by Scientific Selection of Jews, Gypsies, & Others in Germany, 1933-1945. Benno Mueller-Hill. Tr. by George R. Fraser from GER. 1997. LC 97-40085. (Illus.). 200p. (C). pap. 29.00 (0-87969-531-5) Cold Spring Harbor.

Murdoch vs. Freud: A Freudian Look at an Anti-Freudian. Jack Turner. 1993. LC 92-2925. (American University Studies: Ser. IV, Vol. 146). 148p. (C). text 35.95 (0-8204-1857-9) P Lang Pubng.

Murphy's Law: Doctors. Arthur Bloch. 2000. LC 00-28281. (Illus.). 240p. (YA). 7.99 (0-8431-7581-8, Price Stern) Penguin Putnam.

Muscarinic Agonists & the Treatment of Alzheimer's Disease. Ed. by Abraham Fisher. 1996. (Neuroscience Intelligence Unit Ser.). 197p. pap. 89.95 (0-412-10331-1, RC523) Chapman & Hall.

Muscarinic Agonists & the Treatment of Alzheimer's Disease. Abraham Fisher. 1996. LC 95-48062. (Neuroscience Intelligence Unit Ser.). 197 p. 99.00 (1-57059-326-4) Landes Bioscience.

Muscarinic & Nicotinic Stimulant Actions Autonomic Ganglia, Vol. 1. D. Bovet & A. Vurgen. 1966. LC 66-22361. (International Encyclopedia of Pharmacology & Therapeutics Ser.: Sec. 12). (0-08-012062-8) Pergamon Repr GBR. *Dist:* Franklin.

Muscarinic Receptor Subtypes in Smooth Muscle. Eglan. 1997. LC 96-26614. (Pharmacology & Toxicology Ser.). 208p. 149.95 (0-8493-8549-0) CRC Pr.

Muscarinic Receptors. Ed. by Joan Heller Brown. 1989. LC 89-15539. (Receptors Ser.). 496p. 145.00 (0-89603-156-X) Humana.

Muscarinic Receptors in Airways Diseases. J. Zaagsma et al. 2001. LC 00-51949. (Progress in Inflammation Research Ser.). (Illus.). xi, 266p. 149.00 (3-7643-5988-9) Birkhauser.

Muscle Adaptation in the Craniofacial Region. Ed. by D. S. Carlson & J. A. McNamara. 1978. (Craniofacial Growth Ser.: Vol. 8). (Illus.). 252p. 45.00 (0-929921-05-4) UM CHGD.

Muscle Afferents & Spinal Control of Movement. IBRO Symposium Staff. Ed. by L. Jami et al. 1992. LC 92-48946. 484p. 207.00 (0-08-041979-8, Pergamon Pr) Elsevier.

Muscle & Bone. Paul-Victor Winters. 1995. 32p. (Orig.). pap. 8.00 (0-9624178-5-8) Slapering Hol.

Muscle Biopsy: Techniques. Mike A. Loughlin. 1993. (Illus.). 242p. text 97.50 (0-7506-1406-4) Buttrwrth-Heinemann.

Muscle Building 101: The Fundamentals of Shaping Your Physique. Robert Kennedy & Dwayne Hines, II. 1997. LC 97-901205. (Illus.). 112p. pap. (1-55210-008-1) MuscleMag Intl CAN. *Dist:* BookWorld.

Muscle Contraction: Its Regulatory Mechanism. Ed. by Setsuro Ebashi et al. 1980. (Illus.). 549p. 94.00 (0-387-10411-9) Spr-Verlag.

Muscle Damage. Ed. by Stanley Salmons. 1997. (Illus.). 260p. text 65.00 (0-19-262753-8) OUP.

Muscle Diseases. Anthony H. V. Schapira & Robert C. Griggs. 1999. LC 99-20297. 432p. text 99.00 (0-7506-7085-1) Buttrwrth-Heinemann.

Muscle Disorders in Childhood. Victor Dubowitz. 2nd ed. 1995. 549p. text 125.00 (0-7020-1437-0) Saunders.

***Muscle Disorders in Childhood.** Victor Dubowitz. 2001. (Illus.). 605p. (0-7020-2580-1) W B Saunders GBR. *Dist:* Saunders.

Muscle Energy Manual Vol. 1: Concepts & Mechanisms the Musculoskeletal Screen Cervical Region Evaluation & Treatment. Fred L. Mitchell, Jr. & P. Kai-Galen Mitchell. 1995. LC 95-77816. (Illus.). 228p. pap. text 59.00 (0-9647250-1-0) MET Pr.

Muscle Energy Manual Vol. 2: Evaluation & Treatment of the Thoracic Spine, Lumbar Spine & Rib Cage Fred L. Mitchell, Jr. & P. Kai-Galen Mitchell. 1998. LC 95-77816. (Illus.). 240p. (Orig.). pap. text 68.00 (0-9647250-2-9) MET Pr.

Muscle Fatigue Mechanisms in Exercise & Training. Ed. by P. Marconnet et al. 1992. (Medicine & Sport Science Ser.: Vol. 34). (Illus.). viii, 244p. 215.75 (3-8055-5483-4) S Karger.

Muscle Foods. D. Kinsman. 1992. text (0-442-00610-1) Chapman & Hall.

Muscle Imaging. Ed. by James Fleckenstein et al. 1996. LC 95-36652. (Illus.). 461p. 184.00 (0-387-94231-9) Spr-Verlag.

Muscle, Matrix & Bladder Function: Proceedings of a Symposium Held in Philadelphia, Pennsylvania, March 18-19, 1994, Vol. 385. Ed. by Stephen A. Zderic. 1995. LC 95-45640. (Advances in Experimental Medicine & Biology Ser.: Vol. 385). (Illus.). 282p. 95.00 (0-306-45193-X, RC919, Kluwer Plenum) Kluwer Academic.

Muscle Membranes in Diseases of Muscle. Ed. by Robert E. Mrak. 1985. 168p. 99.00 (0-8493-5622-9, RC925, CRC Reprint) Franklin.

***Muscle Morphology & the Insulin Resistance Syndrome: A Population-Based Study of 70 Year-Old Men in Uppsala.** Anu Hedman. 2001. (Comprehensive Summaries of Uppsala Dissertations from the Faculty of Medicine Ser.: No. 1063). (Illus.). 58p. pap. (91-554-5083-0) Acta Univ SWE. *Dist:* Coronet Bks.

Muscle Pain: Understanding Its Nature, Diagnosis & Treatment. Siegfried Mense & David Simons. 2000. LC 00-41262. (Illus.). 400p. text 54.95 (0-683-05928-9) Lppncott W & W.

Muscle Pain, Myofascial Pain & Fibromyalgia: Recent Advances. Ed. by Leonardo Vecchiet & Maria Adele Giamberardino. 1999. LC 99-39599. (Journal of Musculoskeletal Pain Ser.: Vol. 7, Nos. 1/2). 360p. 89.95 (0-7890-0795-9); pap. text 49.95 (0-7890-0828-9) Haworth Pr.

Muscle Pain Relief in 90 Seconds: The Fold & Hold Method. Dale L. Anderson. 1994. 160p. pap. 12.95 (0-471-34689-6) Wiley.

Muscle Pain Relief in Ninety Seconds: The Fold & Hold Method. Dale Anderson. 1995. LC 98-234774. (Illus.). 176p. pap. 10.95 (1-56561-058-X) Wiley.

Muscle Pain Syndromes & Fibromyalgia: Pressure Algometry for Quantification of Diagnosis & Treatment Outcome. Ed. by Andrew A. Fischer. 1998. LC 98-12625. 158p. 39.95 (0-7890-0510-7, Hawrth Medical) Haworth Pr.

Muscle Physiology & Cardiac Function. Lincoln E. Ford. 2000. (Illus.). 413p. (C). text 60.00 (1-884125-72-7) Cooper Pubng.

Muscle Relaxants. 1995. 158.00 (0-387-70168-0) Spr-Verlag.

Muscle Relaxants in Anaesthesia. Ed. by Nigel J. N. Harper & M. J. Pollard. 1995. (Illus.). 280p. text (0-340-55155-0) E A GBR. *Dist:* OUP.

Muscle Scanning: Interpreting EMG Scans Barbara J. Headley. 1990. (Illus.). 95p. (Orig.). pap. 14.00 (0-929538-05-6) Innovat Systems.

Muscle Spasm, Pain & Marijuana Therapy: Testimony from Federal & State Court Proceedings on Marijuana's Medical Use. Ed. by Robert C. Randall. 1991. LC 91-71175. (Marijuana, Medicine & the Law Ser.). 237p. pap. 14.95 (0-936485-06-X, Galen Pr DC) Lkng Glass Pubns.

Muscle Strength. Ed. by Karin Harms-Ringdahl. 1995. LC 92-48964. (International Perspectives in Physical Therapy Ser.: No. 8). (Illus.). 288p. pap. text (0-443-04336-1) Church.

Muscle Testing Handbook. Virginia Pact et al. 1984. 194p. 36.95 (0-316-68768-5, Little Brwn Med Div) Lppncott W & W.

Muscle Transplantation. Ed. by G. Freilinger et al. 1981. (Illus.). 320p. 123.00 (0-387-81636-4) Spr-Verlag.

Muscles: A Study Aid for Students of the Allied Health Professions. Delia Barreto. 1974. (Illus.). 48p. (C). pap. 3.00 (0-87936-005-4) Scholium Intl.

Muscles: Testing & Function. Florence P. Kendall et al. 4th rev. ed. 1993. LC 92-49150. (Illus.). 448p. 60.95 (0-683-04576-8) Lppncott W & W.

Muscles Alive: Their Functions Revealed by Electromyography. John V. Basmajian & Carlo J. DeLuca. 5th ed. 1985. (Illus.). 562p. 65.00 (0-683-00414-X) Lppncott W & W.

Muscles & Molecules: Uncovering the Principles of Biological Motion. Gerald H. Pollack. 1990. 300p. (C). 55.00 (0-9626895-0-5) Ebner & Sons.

Muscles & Movements: A Basis for Human Kinesiology. John V. Basmajian & M. A. MacConaill. rev. ed. 1977. LC 76-6883. 412p. 42.50 (0-88275-398-3) Krieger.

Muscles as Molecular & Metabolic Machines. Peter W. Hochachka. 1994. LC 94-6564. 176p. 104.95 (0-8493-2468-8, 2468) CRC Pr.

Muscles in Action: An Approach to Manual Muscle Testing. Joan H. Cole et al. 1988. (Illus.). 184p. pap. (0-443-03613-6) Church.

Muscles in Motion: Surface EMG Analysis of the Human Body Range of Motion. Gabriel E. Sella. 3rd ed. 1997. LC 93-93665. (C). 120.00 (1-884325-00-9) G E Sella.

Muscles, Masses & Motion: The Physiology of Normality, Hypotonicity, Spasticity & Rigidity. E. Geoffrey Walsh. 1993. (Clinics in Developmental Medicine Ser.: No. 125). (Illus.). 220p. (C). text 64.95 (0-521-43229-4) Cambridge U Pr.

Muscles, Nerves, & Movement: Kinesiology in Daily Living. Barbara Tyldesley & June I. Grieve. 2nd ed. 1996. LC 96-13775. (Illus.). 360p. pap. 54.95 (0-632-04096-3) Blackwell Sci.

Muscular Analysis of Everyday Activities. Elaine Bukowski. 2000. 80p. pap. text (1-55642-507-4) SLACK Inc.

Muscular Dynamics: Electromyographic Assessment of Energy & Motion. Gabriel E. Sella. 2000. LC 00-92685. (Illus.). 350p. text 120.00 (1-884325-14-9) G E Sella.

Muscular Dystrophy. Alan Emery. 2nd ed. 2000. LC 00-268816. (Oxford Medical Publications). (Illus.). xii, 166p. pap. text 19.95 (0-19-263217-5) OUP.

Muscular Dystrophy: Biomedical Aspects. Ed. by Setsuro Ebashi & E. Ozawa. 1983. (Illus.). 302p. 73.95 (0-387-12342-3) Spr-Verlag.

Muscular Dystrophy: Methods & Protocols. Ed. by Katherine M. D. Bushby & Louise V. B. Anderson. 2000. (Methods in Molecular Medicine Ser.: Vol. 43). (Illus.). 436p. 99.50 (0-89603-695-2) Humana.

Muscular Dystrophy: The Facts. Alan E. Emery. 1994. (Facts Ser.). (Illus.). 148p. pap. text 19.95 (0-19-262449-0) OUP.

Muscular Dystrophy & Allied Diseases: Impact on Patients, Family & Staff. Ed. by Leon I. Charash et al. 1988. LC 86-82709. (Current Thanatology Ser.). 90p. pap. 15.95 (0-930194-38-1) Ctr Thanatology.

Muscular Dystrophy & Other Neuromuscular Diseases: Psychosocial Issues. Leon I. Charash et al. 1991. (Loss, Grief & Care Ser.: Vol. 4 Nos. 3 & 4). (Illus.). 270p. text 49.95 (1-56024-077-6) Haworth Pr.

Muscular Dystrophy, 1976: Proceedings of the Symposium, Jerusalem, 1976. Muscular Dystrophy Symposium Staff. Ed. by Gordon C. Robin & George Falewski de Leon. 1977. (Illus.). 42.75 (3-8055-2680-6) S Karger.

Muscule Hypertrophy of Genetic Origin & Its Use to Improve Beef Production. J. W. King & F. Menissier. 1982. text 249.00 (90-247-2637-9) Kluwer Academic.

Musculo Skeletal Diseases & Homeopathy. Luc De Schepper. 1994. 200p. (Orig.). (C). pap. 39.95 (0-942501-02-0) Full of Life.

Musculo Skeletal MRI & Ultrasound: A Correlative Atlas & Teaching File. 2000. (Illus.). 576p. text 145.00 (0-8151-1200-9, 31718) Mosby Inc.

Musculo-Skeletal Problems in Emergency Medicine. Jim Wardrope & Bryan English. 1998. (Oxford Handbooks in Emergency Medicine Ser.). (Illus.). 348p. pap. text 47.50 (0-19-262862-3) OUP.

Musculoskeletal Aspects of Haemophilia. E. C. Rodriguez-Merchan et al. 2000. LC 00-23044. (Illus.). 256p. 159.00 (0-632-05671-1) Blackwell Sci.

Musculoskeletal Assessment: An Integrated Approach. Barbara M. Edwardson. 1992. LC 92-13349. (Illus.). 224p. (Orig.). (C). pap. text 34.95 (1-879105-69-1, 0332) Thomson Learn.

Musculoskeletal Assessment: Joint Range of Motion & Manual Muscle Strength. Hazel Clarkson. 1989. (Illus.). 384p. (C). pap. text 42.00 (*0-683-01711-X*) Lppncott W & W.

Musculoskeletal Assessment: Joint Range of Motion & Manual Muscle Strength. Hazel M. Clarkson. 2nd ed. 2000. LC 99-33414. 448p. spiral bd. 49.95 (*0-683-30384-8*) Lppncott W & W.

Musculoskeletal Clinical Metrology. Nicholas Bellamy. 1993. 384p. (C). text 254.00 (*0-7923-8828-3*) Kluwer Academic.

Musculoskeletal Disease Test & Syllabus. William A. Murphy, Jr. et al. 1994. (Professional Self-Evaluation & Continuing Education Program Ser.: Vol. 37). (Illus.). 900p. 220.00 (*1-55903-036-4*) Am Coll Radiology.

Musculoskeletal Disorders: Common Problems. Barbara M. Edwardson. 1995. (Illus.). 318p. (Orig.). (C). pap. text 42.95 (*1-56593-170-X*, 0469) Thomson Learn.

Musculoskeletal Disorders: Healing Methods from Chinese Medicine & Orthopaedic Medicine. Alon Marcus. 1999. LC 98-34889. 650p. 85.00 (*1-55643-282-8*) North Atlantic.

Musculoskeletal Disorders & Congenital Deformities. Arnold J. Rudolph. 1997. (Atlas of the Newborn Ser.: Vol. 2). (Illus.). incl. cd-rom (*1-55009-032-1*) DEKR.

***Musculoskeletal Disorders & the Workplace: Low Back & Upper Extremities.** Institute of Medicine Staff. 2001. LC 2001-906. (Illus.). xv, 492p. 59.95 (*0-309-07284-0*) Natl Acad Pr.

Musculoskeletal Disorders of the Lower Extremities. Ed. by Lawrence M. Oloff. 1994. LC 93-7250. text 142.00 (*0-7216-3716-7*) Saunders.

***Musculoskeletal Disorders Related to Pregnancy: Physical Therapy Assessment & Treatment.** Downie. 2001. (Illus.). 180p. pap. (*0-443-06282-X*) Church GBR. *Dist:* Saunders.

Musculoskeletal Drug Therapy for Geriatric Patients. Ed. by Marie A. Chisholm & James W. Cooper. 2000. LC 99-55307. (Journal of Geriatric Drug Therapy Ser.). (Illus.). 89p. pap. text 19.95 (*0-7890-0824-6*, Pharmctl Prods) Haworth Pr.

Musculoskeletal Drug Therapy for Geriatric Patients. Ed. by Marie A. Chisolm & James W. Cooper. 2000. LC 99-55307. (Journal of Geriatric Drug Therapy Ser.). 89p. 29.95 (*0-7890-0789-4*, Pharmctl Prods) Haworth Pr.

Musculoskeletal Examination. Jeffery Gross et al. 1995. LC 95-25651. (Illus.). 300p. pap. 49.95 (*0-86542-410-1*) Blackwell Sci.

Musculoskeletal Function: An Anatomy & Kinesiology Laboratory Manual. Dortha Esch & Marvin Lepley. 1974. LC 73-93577. (Illus.). 134p. pap. 9.95 (*0-8166-0716-8*) U of Minn Pr.

Musculoskeletal Imaging. John A. Markisz. 1991. 159.95 (*0-316-54613-5*, Little Brwn Med Div) Lppncott W & W.

Musculoskeletal Imaging: A Teaching File. Felix S. Chew. 1998. LC 99-15483. (Illus.). xxvi, 644p. text 159.00 (*0-683-30175-6*) Lppncott W & W.

Musculoskeletal Imaging: Diagnostic & Therapeutic Procedures. Ed. by Jacqueline C. Hodge. 1997. LC 96-45275. (Vademecum Ser.). (Illus.). xii, 250p. 98.00 (*3-8055-6496-1*) S Karger.

Musculoskeletal Imaging: The Requisites. David J. Sartoris. 1995. LC 95-25625. (Requisites Ser.). (Illus.). 432p. (C). (gr. 13). text 85.00 (*0-8151-8002-0*, 26257) Mosby Inc.

Musculoskeletal Infection. Ed. by John L. Esterhai, Jr. et al. 1991. 459p. 85.00 (*0-89203-053-4*) Amer Acad Ortho Surg.

Musculoskeletal Injection Skills: Principles & Practice. Monica Kesson & Elaine Atkins. 2001. (Illus.). 208p. pap. 50.00 (*0-7506-4372-2*) Buttrwrth-Heinemann.

Musculoskeletal Injuries. William D. Arnold & John P. Lyden. 1987. (Illus.). 800p. text (*0-07-044994-5*) McGraw.

Musculoskeletal Magnetic Resonance. Edward J. Easton, Jr. & John A. Powers. 1985. 178p. 41.50 (*0-316-20402-1*, Little Brwn Med Div) Lppncott W & W.

Musculoskeletal Manifestations of AIDS. Jamshid Tehranzadeh. 1994. 181p. (Orig.). (C). pap. text 37.50 (*0-87527-509-5*) Green.

***Musculoskeletal Matters in Primary Care.** Gill Wakley et al. 2001. 120p. pap. (*1-85775-434-4*) Radcliffe Med Pr GBR. *Dist:* Balogh.

Musculoskeletal Medicine: The Spine. Loic Burn. 1990. (C). text 173.50 (*0-7923-8913-1*) Kluwer Academic.

Musculoskeletal Pain: Principles of Physical Diagnosis & Physical Treatment. David A. Zohn & John M. Mennell. 2nd ed. 1987. 261p. 65.00 (*0-316-98897-9*, Little Brwn Med Div) Lppncott W & W.

Musculoskeletal Pain Emanating from the Head & Neck: Current Concepts in Diagnosis, Management, & Cost Containment. Ed. by Murray E. Allen. 1996. LC 96-31753. (Journal of Musculoskeletal Pain: Vol. 4, No. 4). 202p. (C). 34.95 (*0-7890-0005-9*) Haworth Pr.

Musculoskeletal Pain, Myofascial Pain Syndrome, & the Fibromyalgia Syndrome: Proceedings from the Second World Congress on Myofascial Pain & Fibromyalgia. Ed. by Bente Danneskiold-Samsoe & Birger Lund. 1993. LC 93-30041. (Journal of Musculoskeletal Pain: Vol. 1, Nos. 3-4). (Illus.). 334p. pap. text 49.95 (*1-56024-508-5*); lib. bdg. 89.95 (*1-56024-485-2*) Haworth Pr.

Musculoskeletal Primary Care. Sharon J. Gates & Pekka A. Mooar. 1998. LC 98-38544. 368p. pap. text 39.95 (*0-7817-1430-3*) Lppncott W & W.

Musculoskeletal Radiology. Sergio Fernandez-Tapia. 1999. 472p. pap. text 80.00 (*0-7817-1662-4*) Lppncott W & W.

***Musculoskeletal Shockwave Therapy.** Coombs et al. 2000. (Greenwich Medical Media Ser.). (Illus.). 336p. (*1-84110-058-7*) Greenwich Med GBR. *Dist:* JAMCO Dist.

Musculoskeletal Soft-Tissue Aging: Impact on Mobility. Ed. by Joseph A. Buckwalter et al. 1994. LC 93-41652. 423p. 105.00 (*0-89203-086-0*) Amer Acad Ortho Surg.

Musculoskeletal System. John M. Mennell. 1991. LC 91-4866. 208p. 102.00 (*0-8342-0255-7*) Aspen Pub.

***Musculoskeletal System.** Philip Sambrook et al. 2001. (Illus.). 175p. (*0-443-07015-6*) Church GBR. *Dist:* Saunders.

Musculoskeletal System: An Integrated Textbook of Diagnosis & Medical Surgical Management of Musculoskeletal Disorders. D. I. Rowley & John A. Dent. 1997. LC 96-85637. (Illus.). 360p. pap. (*0-412-62700-0*) E A GBR. *Dist:* OUP.

Musculoskeletal System Course. Competence Assurance Systems Staff. 1981. (Illus.). pap. text 45.00 (*0-89147-066-2*) CAS.

Musculoskeletal Ultrasound. Ed. by Bruno D. Fornage. 1995. LC 94-44679. (Clinics in Diagnostic Ultrasound Ser.: Vol. 30). text (*0-443-08909-4*) Church.

Musculoskeletal Ultrasound. Marnix Van Holsbeek. 1990. (Illus.). 344p. (C). (gr. 13). text 110.00 (*0-8151-8975-3*, 22127) Mosby Inc.

Musculoskeletal Ultrasound. Marnix Van Holsbeeck. 2nd ed. 1999. LC 00-58417. (Illus.). 448p. (C). text 149.00 incl. cd-rom (*0-323-00018-5*) Mosby Inc.

Musculoskeletl Imaging: The Requisite. Manaster. 2nd ed. 2001. 554p. text (*0-323-01189-6*) Mosby Inc.

Mushroom Hunters Guide & Common Poisonous Plants. W. G. Farlow. 1982. LC 82-72605. (Illus.). 60p. (Orig.). pap. 4.95 (*0-89708-084-X*) And Bks.

Music - Motion & Emotion: The Developmental-Integrative Model in Music Therapy. Chava Sekeles. 1996. (Illus.). 192p. per. 29.95 (*0-918812-88-7*) MMB Music.

Music & Medicine. Dorothy M. Schullian & Max Schoen. 1977. LC 78-142693. (Essay Index Reprint Ser.). 29.95 (*0-8369-2132-1*) Ayer.

Music & Memory: An Introduction. Bob Snyder. 2000. LC 99-86731. (Illus.). xxii, 291p. (C). 75.00 (*0-262-19441-4*) MIT Pr.

Music & Psychology: A Mutual Regard, Vol. 2, No. 1. Stephen McAdams. 1987. (Contemporary Music Review Ser.). viii, 320p. pap. text 74.00 (*3-7186-0382-9*) Gordon & Breach.

Music & Self-Management Methods: A Physicological Model. Joseph P. Scartelli. 1989. (Horizon Ser.: Vol. 7). 41p. (Orig.). pap. text 11.50 (*0-918812-53-4*, ST 150) MMB Music.

Music & Sound in the Healing Arts: An Energy Approach. John Beaulieu. Ed. by George Quasha. 1987. LC 87-10076. 150p. (C). 19.95 (*0-88268-057-9*); pap. 14.95 (*0-88268-056-0*) Station Hill Pr.

Music & the Cognitive Sciences: Proceedings from the "Symposium on Music & the Cognitive Sciences," 14-18 March 1988 Paris, France. Ed. by Stephen McAdams & I. Deilege. 1989. (Contemporary Music Review Ser.: Vol. 4). x, 468p. pap. text 96.00 (*3-7186-4953-5*) Gordon & Breach.

Music & Your Mind: Listening with a New Consciousness. Helen L. Bonny. 1990. pap. 10.95 (*0-88268-094-3*) Station Hill Pr.

Music As Cognition: The Development of Thought & Sound. Mary L. Serafine. 1988. (Illus.). 288p. text 57.50 (*0-231-05742-3*) Col U Pr.

Music at the Edge: Music Therapy Experiences of a Musician with AIDS. Colin Lee. 1996. LC 95-25782. 192p. (C). pap. 34.95 incl. audio compact disk (*0-415-12464-6*); (Illus.). text 89.95 incl. audio compact disk (*0-415-12463-8*) Routledge.

Music, Cognition, & Computerized Sound: An Introduction to Psychoacoustics. Ed. by Perry R. Cook. 2001. (Illus.). 384p. pap. 34.95 (*0-262-53190-9*) MIT Pr.

Music Curriculum Guidelines for Moderately Retarded Adolescents. Mary R. Beal & Janet P. Gilbert. 1982. 122p. (C). pap. 29.95 (*0-398-04757-X*) C C Thomas.

Music Education for the Deaf. Eleanor M. Edwards. 1974. LC 74-76260. 248p. (Orig.). (C). pap. 6.00 (*0-914562-00-2*) Merriam-Eddy.

Music for Developing Speech & Language Skills in Children: A Guide for Parents & Therapists. Donald E. Michel & Janet L. Jones. 1991. (MMB Horizon Ser.: Vol. 9). 49p. (Orig.). pap. text 9.95 (*0-918812-69-0*, ST 233) MMB Music.

Music for Life: Aspects of Creative Music Therapy with Adult Clients. Gary Ansdell. 1995. LC 95-14419. 237p. pap. (*1-85302-299-3*) Jessica Kingsley GBR. *Dist:* Taylor & Francis.

Music for Living: Enriching the Lives of Profoundly Mentally Handicapped People. M. Wood. 1984. 78p. 35.00 (*0-906054-47-8*) St Mut.

Music, Mind & Brain: The Neuropsychology of Music. Ed. by Manfred Clynes. 1982. LC 82-546. (Illus.). 444p. (C). text 107.00 incl. lp (*0-306-40908-9*, Kluwer Plenum) Kluwer Academic.

Music, Musicians & Health Influences: Index of Modern Authors & Subjects with Guide for Rapid Research. Melvin M. Galloway. 1996. 160p. 57.50 (*0-7883-0942-0*) ABBE Pubs Assn.

Music Techniques in Therapy, Counseling & Special Education. Jayne Standley. 1991. LC 91-30003. 225p. (Orig.). pap. text 19.95 (*0-918812-64-X*, ST230) MMB Music.

Music Therapy: An Introduction. Jacqueline S. Peters. 1987. 186p. (C). text 37.95 (*0-398-05284-0*); 2nd ed. 2000. LC 99-88599. 486p. 79.95 (*0-398-07042-3*) C C Thomas.

Music Therapy: Art Beyond Words. Leslie Bundt. 1994. 224p. (C). pap. 29.95 (*0-415-08703-1*) Routledge.

Music Therapy & Its Relationship to Current Treatment Theories. Even Ruud. rev. ed. 1980. 85p. reprint ed. per. 9.95 (*0-918812-14-3*) MMB Music.

Music Therapy & Medicine: Theoretical & Clinical Approaches. Ed. by Cheryl Dileo. 1999. (*1-884914-00-4*) Amer Music Therapy.

Music Therapy & Music in Special Education Vol. 1: The International State of the Art Ed. by Rosalie R. Pratt & Barbara Hesser. 1989. (ISME Edition Ser.: Vol. No. 3). 180p. per. 11.95 (*0-918812-61-5*, ST 189) MMB Music.

Music Therapy & Music in Special Education Vol. 2: The International State of the Art Pref. by Rosalie R. Pratt. 1989. (ISME Edition Ser.: Vol. 4). 163p. per. 11.95 (*0-918812-62-3*, ST 191) MMB Music.

Music Therapy Clinical Training Manual. Robert Ellis Krout & Mary Elinor Boyle. 1988. 84p. (Orig.). (C). pap. text, training bk. ed. 11.95 (*0-918812-52-6*, ST 003) MMB Music.

Music Therapy for Living: The Principle of Normalization Embodied in Music Therapy. Edith H. Boxill. 1989. (Horizon Ser.: Vol. 6). 39p. (Orig.). pap. text 10.50 (*0-918812-54-2*, ST 179) MMB Music.

Music Therapy for the Autistic Child. Juliette Alvin & Auriel Warwick. 2nd ed. 1992. (Illus.). 164p. pap. text 22.00 (*0-19-816276-6*) OUP.

Music Therapy for the Developmentally Disabled. Edith H. Boxill. 1985. LC 84-15752. (Illus.). 270p. text 36.00 (*0-89079-190-2*, 2054) PRO-ED.

Music Therapy in Child Psychosis. Rolando O. Benenzon. 1982. (Illus.). 112p. (C). text 29.95 (*0-398-04646-8*) C C Thomas.

Music Therapy in Health & Education. Ed. by Margaret Heal & Tony Wigram. 1993. 304p. pap. (*1-85302-175-X*) Jessica Kingsley GBR. *Dist:* Taylor & Francis.

Music Therapy in the Treatment of Adults with Mental Disorders. Ed. by Robert F. Unkefer. 1990. 225p. 45.00 (*0-02-873032-1*, Macmillan Ref) Gale.

Music Therapy Research: Quantitative & Qualitative Perspectives. Ed. by Barbara L. Wheeler. 1995. 616p. (C). pap. text 45.00 (*0-9624080-3-4*) Barcelona Pubs.

Music Therapy Research & Practice in Medicine: From Out of the Silence. David Aldridge. 1996. 352p. text (*1-85302-296-9*) Jessica Kingsley GBR. *Dist:* Taylor & Francis.

Music Therapy Sourcebook: A Collection of Activities Categorized & Analyzed. Cecilia Schulberg. 1981. LC 80-12945. 296p. pap. 22.95 (*0-89885-281-1*, Kluwer Acad Hman Sci) Kluwer Academic.

Music Therapy, Theory & Manual: Contributions to the Knowledge of Nonverbal Contexts. Rolando O. Benenzon. 2nd ed. LC 96-6334. (Illus.). 296p. 1997. pap. text 46.95 (*0-398-06612-4*); 1996. text 62.95 (*0-398-06611-6*) C C Thomas.

Musical Savants: Exceptional Skill in Mentally Retarded. Leon K. Miller. 1989. 272p. (C). text 49.95 (*0-8058-0034-4*) L Erlbaum Assocs.

Musical Structure & Cognition. Ed. by Peter Howell et al. 1985. text 145.00 (*0-12-357170-7*) Acad Pr.

Musicians & the Prevention of Hearing Loss. Marshall Chasin. 1996. (Illus.). 204p. (Orig.). pap. 45.00 (*1-56593-626-4*, 1298) Thomson Learn.

MusicMedicine Vol. 1: International Society for Music in Medicine, Fourth International MusicMedicine Symposium Ed. by Ralph Spintge & Roland Droh. 1992. 424p. per. 29.95 (*0-918812-72-0*, ST 249) MMB Music.

Muslim Tradition in Psychotherapy & Modern Trends. Syed A. Rizvi. 1995. 25.50 (*1-56744-160-2*) Kazi Pubns.

Mutable Brain: Dynamic & Plastic Features of the Developing & Mature Brain. Ed. by Jon H. Kaas. 2000. (Brain Plasticity & Reorganization Ser.: Vol. 1). 376p. 65.00 (*90-5823-081-3*, Harwood Acad Pubs) Gordon & Breach.

Mutagen-Induced Chromosome Damage in Man. Harold J. Evans & D. Lloyd. 1979. LC 78-60354. 355p. 55.00 (*0-300-02315-4*) Yale U Pr.

Mutagenicity, Carcinogenicity, & Teratogenicity of Industrial Pollutants. Ed. by Micheline Kirsch-Volders. 1984. LC 83-11126. 350p. 85.00 (*0-306-41148-2*, Plenum Trade) Perseus Pubng.

Mutant Oncogenes: Targets for Therapy. Ed. by Nicholas R. Lemoine & Agamemnon A. Epenetos. 1993. LC 92-48907. 224p. (gr. 13). text 132.95 (*0-412-48110-3*) Chapman & Hall.

Mutative Metaphors in Psychotherapy. Murray Cox & Alice Theilgaard. 1987. 280p. (C). pap. (*0-422-61810-1*); lib. bdg. (*0-422-61800-4*) Tavistock GBR. *Dist:* Routldge.

Muted Consent: A Casebook in Modern Medical Ethics. Jan Wojcik. 1978. LC 77-89472. (Science & Society: Series in Science, Technology, & Human Values: Vol. 1). 169p. pap. 7.95 (*0-931682-02-9*) Purdue U Pubns.

Mutual Goal Setting in Patient Care. Jo Anne Horsley. 1982. (Using Research to Improve Nursing Practice Ser.). pap. text 44.00 (*0-8089-1510-X*, 792061, Grune & Strat) Harcrt Hlth Sci Grp.

Muy Macho: Latino Men Confront Their Manhood. Ed. & Intro. by Ray Gonzalez. 1996. LC 95-49859. (Illus.). 256p. pap. 14.00 (*0-385-47861-5*) Doubleday.

MVA in the Treatment of Incomplete Abortion see Ameu en el Tratamiento del Aborto Incompleto: Experiencia Clinica y Programatica

MVA in the Treatment of Incomplete Abortion. Traci L. Baird et al. 1995. LC 95-4492. pap. (*1-882220-08-0*) IPAS.

My Adventure with Lupus: Living with a Chronic Illness. Robert L. Yocum. 1995. 180p. (Orig.). pap. text 12.95 (*1-888824-02-6*) Bridgeport Bks.

My Analysis with Freud. Joseph Wortis. 1994. LC 94-34614. (Master Work Ser.). 234p. pap. text 45.00 (*1-56821-394-8*) Aronson.

My Body . . . Handle with Care: Your Personal Life History . . . of Medical & Health Care. Edward P. Swertz. unabr. ed. 1997. 144p. pap. 12.95 (*0-9661764-0-5*) Exten Inc.

My Child's Care. Laura Nieboer. 1992. 50p. 25.00 (*1-881782-00-X*) State Art.

My Cook Book: Tutor's Notes. R. M. Marshall. 1985. 9p. 40.00 (*0-906054-44-3*) St Mut.

My Detour on Life's Highway: A Survivor's Story of Stem Cell Transplant. Rosemary Champagne. 1999. (Illus.). 80p. pap. 7.95 (*0-9650315-7-8*) Glacier Publng.

My Divided Brain. W. R. Baker. 1999. LC 98-41210. 80p. pap. 11.00 (*1-56474-298-9*) Fithian Pr.

My Experience with Clinical Depression. Gerald F. Mundfrom. rev. ed. 1990. Orig. Title: Purged. (Illus.). 191p. reprint ed. pap. 7.50 (*0-9615494-1-6*) Mercy & Truth.

My Experience with Depression: And How I Overcame It. 150p. 16.00 (*0-9624825-3-6*) Achivmnt USA.

My Fading Full Moon: A Husband's Journal. Boen Hallum. 1984. LC 84-61706. 200p. 14.00 (*0-9608854-3-9*) B Hallum.

My Father Forgets. Lynn McAndrews. 1991. LC 90-91658. 110p. (Orig.). pap. 8.95 (*0-9626683-0-3*) Nrthrn Expressions.

My Fifty-Five Years in Medicine. Constance Friess. 1995. 12.95 (*0-533-11165-X*) Vantage.

My Fifty Years of Nursing: Give Us to Go Blithely. Doris Schwartz. 2nd ed. 1995. LC 94-24237. 216p. 28.95 (*0-8261-8920-2*) Springer Pub.

My First Year As a Doctor: Real World Stories from America's M. D.s. Ed. by Melissa S. Ramsdell. 1994. LC 94-4990. (First Year Career Ser.). 144p. 19.95 (*0-8027-1290-8*); pap. 9.95 (*0-8027-7418-0*) Walker & Co.

My Healing from Breast Cancer. Barbara Joseph. Ed. by Phyllis Herman. 1996. 392p. pap. 14.95 (*0-87983-711-X*, 3711XK, Keats Pubng) McGraw-Hill Trade.

My Healing Secrets. Boris R. Chaitow. 1980. 35.00 (*0-85032-163-8*) St Mut.

My Heart's Health: A New Revolutionary View. D. Sodi-Pallares. 1989. 198p. pap. text (*1-57235-064-4*) Piccin Nuova.

My Herbal Water Cure: An Encyclopedia of Herbology. Sebastian Kneipp. 1991. lib. bdg. 79.95 (*0-8490-4255-0*) Gordon Pr.

My Ivory Cellar: Photo-Synthesis & Plants. John N. Ott. (Illus.). 12.95 (*0-8159-6217-7*) Devin.

My Life As a Male Anorexic. Michael Krasnow. 1996. LC 95-43399. (Illus.). 152p. 29.95 (*0-7890-6029-9*); pap. 12.95 (*1-56023-883-6*, Harrington Park) Haworth Pr.

My Life in My Hands: Living on with Cystic Fibrosis. Doug Lab & Olivia K. Lab. Ed. by Robyn Witkin. 1990. 163p. pap. 7.50 (*0-9629216-0-2*) LabPro Pr.

My Lifetime Tidbits of Preventive Medicine. Frank Smith. 1997. (Illus.). 110p. (Orig.). pap. 12.95 (*1-57502-345-8*, PO1140) Morris Pubng.

My Love, My Care, My Spouse: A Chronicle of Parkinson's Disease. Eva B. Popper. 1988. LC 88-90551. 75p. (Orig.). pap. text 6.95 (*0-945520-09-3*) PSGA.

***My Medical Journal.** Eleanor Welling. l.t. rev. ed. 2001. 153p. spiral bd. 9.95 (*0-9602118-0-2*, MMJ-1) CnE Varieties.

My Mind Is Out to Get Me: Humor & Wisdom in Recovery. Compiled by Ron B. 1994. 180p. pap. 6.95 (*1-56838-010-0*) Hazelden.

My Mother Made Me Do It see Overcoming the Legacy of Overeating: How Your Mother Influenced Your Eating Patterns & How You Can Change Them

My Patients with Tales: The Experiences of a Wisconsin Veterinarian. Robert W. Pope. 1999. (Illus.). 120p. pap. 11.25 (*0-9669829-0-8*, 0101) Pause Pub Co.

My Personal Health History. William E. Pitts. 1999. 95p. 19.95 (*0-9671388-0-9*) Bea Pubg.

My Pregnancy Record Book. Dorling Kindersley Publishing Staff. 1998. (Illus.). 64p. 9.95 (*0-7894-4122-5*) DK Pub Inc.

M N O

My Psychosis, My Bicycle, & I: The Self-Organization of Madness. Fritz B. Simon. 1996. LC 95-21424. 304p. 45.00 (*1-56821-647-5*) Aronson.

My Pulse Is Not What It Used to Be: The Leadership Challenges in Health Care. Irwin M. Rubin & C. Raymond Fernandez. 1991. LC 91-65593. 104p. (Orig.). pap. 40.00 (*0-9629561-0-4*) Temenos Found.

My Report of Findings: More Observations of a Chiropractic Advocate. William D. Esteb. 1993. 240p. (Orig.). pap. text 24.95 (*0-9631711-1-9*) Back Talk Systs.

My Shaping-Up Years: The Early Life of Labor's Great Reporter. Art Shields. 1983. LC 82-21176. (Illus.). 292p. (Orig.). 14.00 (*0-7178-0597-2*); pap. 4.95 (*0-7178-0571-9*) Intl Pubs Co.

My Sister's Keeper: Learning to Cope with a Sibling's Mental Illness. Margaret Moorman. 1993. 320p. pap. 17.00 (*0-14-023121-8*, Penguin Bks) Penguin Putnam.

My Son, My Sorrow: The Tragic Tale of Dr. Kevorkian's Youngest Patient. Carol Loving. 1998. LC 97-66563. (Illus.). 300p. 22.95 (*0-88282-161-X*) New Horizon NJ.

My Special Brother. Lena Schiff. 1991. 250p. (C). 17.95 (*1-56062-102-8*, CFR116H); pap. 14.95 (*1-56062-101-X*, CFR116S) CIS Comm.

My Story of the War: A Woman's Narrative of Four Year's Personal Experience As Nurse in the Union Army. Mary A. Livermore. 1975. LC 72-2612. (American Women Ser.: Images & Realities). (Illus.). 704p. reprint ed. 46.95 (*0-405-04466-6*) Ayer.

My Three Mothers & Other Passions. Sophie Freud. 1991. 351p. (C). pap. text 17.50 (*0-8147-2600-3*) NYU Pr.

My Work with Borderline Patients. Harold F. Searles. 1986. LC 86-20639. 432p. 60.00 (*0-87668-930-6*) Aronson.

***My Year Off: Rediscovering Life after a Stroke.** Robert McCrum. 2001. 231p. reprint ed. 25.00 (*0-7881-9891-2*) DIANE Pub.

My Years with Ayn Rand: The Truth Behind the Myths. Nathaniel Branden. 1999. LC 98-25440. 480p. pap. 19.00 (*0-7879-4513-7*) Jossey-Bass.

***Myalgic Encephalomyelitis/Chronic Fatigue Syndrome & Enteroviral-Mediated Organ Pathology.** John Richardson. 2001. LC 00-54146. (Illus.). 284p. 59.95 (*0-7890-1127-1*, Haworth Pastrl) Haworth Pr.

Myalgic Encephalomyelitis/Chronic Fatigue Syndrome & Enteroviral-Mediated Organ Pathology. John Richardson. 2001. LC 00-54146. (Illus.). 284p. (C). pap. text 24.95 (*0-7890-1128-X*, Hawrth Medical) Haworth Pr.

Myasthenia Gravis. Ed. by Marc H. De Baets & Hans J. Oosterhuis. 1993. LC 92-49515. 288p. lib. bdg. 198.00 (*0-8493-6343-8*, RC935) CRC Pr.

Myasthenia Gravis. Christian Hermann, Jr. et al. 1973. (Illus.). 220p. (C). text 32.50 (*0-8422-7074-4*) Irvington.

Myasthenia Gravis. A. Szobor. 1989. (Illus.). 229p. (*963-05-5312-0*) Akade Kiado HUN. *Dist:* Intl Spec Bk, St Mut.

Myasthenia Gravis: Disease Mechanism & Immunointervention. Premkumar Christadoss. 2000. 208p. 78.00 (*0-7923-6278-0*) Kluwer Academic.

Myasthenia Gravis: European Conference on Myasthenia Gravis, Maastricht, 1st, June 1987. Ed. by M. De Baets et al. 1988. (Monographs in Allergy: Vol. 25). (Illus.). viii, 160p. 109.75 (*3-8055-4736-6*) S Karger.

Myasthenia Gravis: The Immunobiology of an Autiommune Disease. Bianca M. Conti-Fine et al. 1997. (Molecular Intelligence Unit Ser.). 230p. pap. 89.95 (*0-412-11791-6*) Chapman & Hall.

Myasthenia Gravis: The Immunobiology of an Autoimmune Disease. Bianca M. Conti-Fine et al. 1996. LC 96-41316. (Neuroscience Intelligence Unit Ser.). 212p. 99.00 (*1-57059-406-6*) Landes Bioscience.

Myasthenia Gravis & Related Diseases: Disorders of the Neuromuscular Junction. Ed. by David P. Richman. 1998. LC 97-52826. (Annals of the New York Academy of Sciences Ser.: No. 841). 838p. 160.00 (*1-57331-119-7*); pap. 160.00 (*1-57331-120-0*) NY Acad Sci.

Myasthenia Gravis & Related Disorders: Experimental & Clinical Aspects. Ed. by Audrey S. Penn et al. 1993. LC 93-8239. (Annals Ser.: Vol. 681). (*0-89766-755-7*); pap. 165.00 (*0-89766-756-5*) NY Acad Sci.

Mycobacteria: Molecular Biology & Virulence. Colin Ratledge & Jeremy Dale. 1999. LC 99-24452. (Illus.). x, 406p. 209.95 (*0-632-05304-6*) Blackwell Sci.

Mycobacteria & Human Disease. John M. Grange. 2nd ed. 1996. (Arnold Publication). (Illus.). 240p. (C). 75.00 (*0-340-64563-6*) OUP.

Mycobacteria Protocols. Ed. by Tanya Parish & Neil G. Stoker. 1998. LC 98-22177. (Methods in Molecular Biology Ser.: Vol. 101). (Illus.). 488p. 99.50 (*0-89603-471-2*) Humana.

Mycobacterial Infections of Zoo Animals. Ed. by Richard J. Montali. 1979. LC 77-60860. (Research Symposia of the National Zoological Park Ser.: No. 1). (Illus.). 276p. text 30.00 (*0-87474-644-2*, MOMI); pap. text 18.95 (*0-87474-645-0*, MOMIP) Smithsonian.

Mycobacterial Skin Disease. Ed. by Marwali Harahap. 1989. (New Clinical Applications in Dermatology Ser.). (C). text 121.50 (*0-7462-0119-2*) Kluwer Academic.

Mycobacterium Avium—Complete Infection: Progress in Research & Treatment. Ed. by Joyce A. Korvick & Constance A. Benson. 1995. LC 95-31147. (Lung Biology in Health & Disease Ser.: Vol. 87). (Illus.). 344p. text 150.00 (*0-8247-9403-6*) Dekker.

Mycobacterium Tuberculosis: Interactions with the Immune System. M. Bendinelli & H. Friedman. 1988. LC 88-4128. (Infectious Agents & Pathogenesis Ser.). (Illus.). 448p. (C). text 115.00 (*0-306-42724-9*, Kluwer Plenum) Kluwer Academic.

Mycobacterium Tuberculosis Protocols. Tanya Parish & Neil G. Stoker. 2001. LC 00-40977. (Methods in Molecular Medicine Ser.: Vol. 54). (Illus.). xiv, 403p. 135.00 (*0-89603-776-2*) Humana.

Mycological Contributions Celebrating the 70th Birthday of Clark T. Rogerson. Frwd. by Gary J. Samuels. 1989. LC 88-29648. (Memoirs Ser.: No. 49). (Illus.). 374p. pap. text 37.00 (*0-89327-336-8*) NY Botanical.

Mycological Dictionary. Karl Berger. 2nd ed. 1980. (CZE, ENG, FRE, GER & LAT.). 432p. 125.00 (*0-8288-0068-5*, M15339) Fr & Eur.

Mycological Papers No. 161: Aspergillus Species on Stored Products. Z. Kozakiewicz. 1989. 188p. 63.00 (*0-85198-632-3*) C A B I Pub.

Mycoplasma Protocols. Ed. by Roger J. Miles & Robin A. J. Nicholas. 1998. LC 98-4288. (Methods in Molecular Biology Ser.: Vol. 104). (Illus.). 336p. 99.50 (*0-89603-525-5*) Humana.

Mycoplasmosis in Animals: Laboratory Diagnosis. Ed. by Howard W. Whitford et al. 1994. LC 93-24447. (Illus.). 186p. (C). text 69.95 (*0-8138-2491-5*) Iowa U Pr.

Mycoses—Index of New Information & Medical Research Bible. Martha R. Stein. 1995. LC 95-16710. 150p. 57.50 (*0-7883-0102-0*); pap. 47.50 (*0-7883-0103-9*) ABBE Pubs Assn.

Mycoses in AIDS Patients. Ed. by H. Vanden Bossche et al. 1990. (Illus.). 348p. (C). text 114.00 (*0-306-43704-X*, Kluwer Plenum) Kluwer Academic.

Mycoses International Nomenclature of Diseases Vol. II: Infectious Diseases, 2. Date not set. (International Nomenclature of Diseases Ser.: No. 2). pap. text 15.00 (*92-9036-007-0*) World Health.

Mycosis of the Eye & Its Adnexa. W. Behrens-Baumann. 1999. LC 99-35330. (Developments in Ophthalmology Ser.: Vol. 32). (Illus.). xii, 202p. 195.00 (*3-8055-6915-7*) S Karger.

Mycotaxon Cumulative Index for Volumes XLI-LX (1991-1996) Karen D. Gettelman et al. 1998. 296p. pap. 35.00 (*0-930845-07-2*) Mycotaxon Ltd.

Mycotic Diseases in Europe. 1987. (Euro Reports & Studies Ser.: No. 105). 84p. pap. text 9.00 (*92-890-1271-4*) World Health.

Mycotoxins. 1979. (Environmental Health Criteria Ser.: No. 11). 127p. pap. text 19.00 (*92-4-154071-0*, 1160011) World Health.

Mycotoxins & Animal Foods. John E. Smith & Rachel S. Henderson. 1991. (Illus.). 864p. lib. bdg. 395.00 (*0-8493-4904-4*, SF757) CRC Pr.

Mycotoxins & Phytoalexins. Raghubir P. Sharma et al. 1991. (Telford Press Ser.). 800p. 195.00 (*0-8493-8833-3*) CRC Pr.

Mycotoxins, Cancer & Health. Donna H. Ryan. Ed. by George A. Bray. 1991. LC 90-13706. (Pennington Center Nutrition Ser.: Vol. 1). (Illus.). 352p. text 65.00 (*0-8071-1679-3*) La State U Pr.

Mycotoxins, Nephropathy & Urinary Tract Tumors. M. Castegnaro et al. 1992. (IARC Scientific Publications Ser.: No. 115). (Illus.). 358p. pap. text 98.00 (*92-832-2115-X*) OUP.

Myelin. Ed. by Pierre Morell. 2nd ed. 1984. LC 84-9975. (Illus.). 566p. (C). text 132.00 (*0-306-41540-2*, Kluwer Plenum) Kluwer Academic.

Myelination & Demyelination: Implications for Multiple Sclerosis. Ed. by S. U. Kim. 1989. (Illus.). 284p. 75.00 (*0-306-43118-1*, Plenum Trade) Perseus Pubng.

Myelodysplastic Syndromes. Ed. by G. J. Mufti & D. A. Galton. 1992. (Illus.). 256p. text (*0-443-04083-4*) Church.

Myelodysplastic Syndromes. Ed. by F. Schmalzi & G. J. Mufti. 1992. (Illus.). 336p. 181.00 (*0-387-52966-7*) Spr-Verlag.

Myelodysplastic Syndromes: Approach to Diagnosis & Treatment. Harold R. Schumacher & Sucha Nand. 1995. LC 94-13053. (Illus.). 264p. 98.50 (*0-89640-266-5*) Igaku-Shoin.

Myelodysplastic Syndromes - Advances in Research & Treatment: Proceedings of the International Sympopsium on Myelodsyplastic Syndrdomes, National Cancer Center, Tokyo, Japan, 13-14 October 1994. International Symposium on Myelodyspastic Syndromes Staff. Ed. by Takeo Nomura. 1995. LC 95-4214. (International Congress Ser.: No. 1080). 428p. 233.00 (*0-444-82050-7*) Elsevier.

***Myelodysplastic Syndromes & Secondary Acute Myelogenous Leukemia: Directions for the New Millennium.** Azra Raza & Suneel D. Mundle. 2001. (Cancer Treatment & Research Ser.: Vol. 108). 296p. 180.00 (*0-7923-7396-0*) Kluwer Academic.

Myeloma: Biology & Management. Ed. by James Malpas et al. 2nd ed. 1998. LC 97-18025. (Illus.). 686p. text 175.00 (*0-19-262882-8*) OUP.

Myeloma Poetry. Muriel R. Kulwin. 1996. 60p. 15.00 (*1-889080-11-X*) Doublem Bks.

***Myelopathy, Radiculopathy & Peripheral Entrapment Syndromes.** Ed. by David H. Durrant & Jerome Martin True. 2001. (Illus.). 450p. 129.95 (*0-8493-0926-3*) CRC Pr.

Myers-Briggs Type Indicator: A Critical Review & Practical Guide. R. Bayne. 1996. 186p. pap. text 55.00 (*1-56593-353-2*, 0677) Singular Publishing.

Myles Textbook for Midwives. Ed. by V. Ruth Bennett & Linda K. Brown. 12th ed. 1993. LC 93-3748. 876p. pap. text (*0-443-04581-X*) Church.

Myoblast Transfer Therapy. Ed. by R. C. Griggs & G. Karpati. 1990. (Advances in Experimental Medicine & Biology Ser.: Vol. 280). (Illus.). 330p. (C). text 132.00 (*0-306-43714-7*, Kluwer Plenum) Kluwer Academic.

Myocardial & Skeletal Muscle Bioenergetics. Ed. by Nachman Brautbar. 1986. LC 86-4883. (Advances in Experimental Medicine & Biology Ser.: Vol. 194). 692p. 130.00 (*0-306-42237-9*, Plenum Trade) Perseus Pubng.

Myocardial Biopsy: Diagnostic Significance. H. D. Bolte. 1980. (Illus.). 146p. 43.00 (*0-387-10063-6*) Spr-Verlag.

Myocardial Contrast Two Dimensional Echocardiography. Ed. by Samuel Meerbaum & Richard Melzer. 1989. (Developments in Cardiovascular Medicine Ser.). (C). text 182.50 (*0-7923-0205-2*) Kluwer Academic.

Myocardial Damage: Early Detection by Novel Biochemical Markers, Vol. 205. Juan C. Kaski & David W. Holt. 1998. LC 98-8191. (Developments in Cardiovascular Medicine Ser.). 212p. 82.00 (*0-7923-5140-1*) Kluwer Academic.

Myocardial Energy Metabolism. Ed. by J. W. De Jong. 1988. (Developments in Cardiovascular Medicine Ser.). (C). text 195.50 (*0-89838-394-3*) Kluwer Academic.

Myocardial Hypertrophy. Franklin & Harold Sandler. 1990. 60.00 (*0-88258-023-X*) Howard U Pr.

Myocardial Infarction: From Trials to Practice. Ed. by Stephen G. Ball. 1995. 224p. (*1-871816-26-2*) Wrightson Biomed GBR. *Dist:* Taylor & Francis.

Myocardial Infarction: Measurement & Intervention, Developments in Cardiovascular Medicine, No. 14. Ed. by Galen S. Wagner. 1982. 500p. text 249.00 (*90-247-2513-5*) Kluwer Academic.

Myocardial Infarction: Proceedings of the Cardiovascular Disease Conference, 3rd, Snowmass at Aspen, CO, Jan. 1972. Cardiovascular Disease Conference Staff. Ed. by J. H. Vogel. 1973. (Advances in Cardiology Ser.: Vol. 9). 85.25 (*3-8055-1373-9*) S Karger.

Myocardial Infarction at Young Age: Proceedings. Ed. by H. Roskamm. 1982. (Illus.). 228p. 39.95 (*0-387-11090-9*) Spr-Verlag.

Myocardial Infarction Community Registers. 1976. (Public Health in Europe Ser.: No. 5). 232p. 22.00 (*92-9020-124-X*, 1320005) World Health.

Myocardial Infarction in the Spectrum of Ischemic Heart Disease: Proceedings of the Symposium, March 1977. Symposium, Palm Springs, Calif. Staff. Ed. by J. R. See et al. 1978. (Advances in Cardiology Ser.: Vol. 23). (Illus.). 76.75 (*3-8055-2753-5*) S Karger.

Myocardial Injury: Laboratory Diagnosis. Johannes Mair & Bernd Puschendorf. 1996. LC 96-27642. (Medical Intelligence Unit Ser.). 204p. 89.95 (*1-57059-303-5*) Landes Bioscience.

Myocardial Ischemia. Ed. by Naranjan S. Dhalla et al. 1987. (Developments in Cardiovascular Medicine Ser.). text 161.50 (*0-89838-866-X*) Kluwer Academic.

Myocardial Ischemia: Mechanisms, Reperfusion, Protection. Ed. by M. Karmazyn. 1996. LC 96-4758. xii, 515p. 189.95 (*0-8176-5269-8*);Vol. 76. 528p. 209.00 (*3-7643-5269-8*) Birkhauser.

Myocardial Ischemia & Arrhythmia. Ed. by M. Zehender et al. 1995. 276p. 67.00 (*0-387-91455-2*) Spr-Verlag.

Myocardial Ischemia & Reperfusion. Michael V. Cohen. 1998. LC 98-7849. (Developments in Molecular & Cellular Biochemistry Ser.). 207p. (*0-7923-8173-4*) Kluwer Academic.

Myocardial Ischemia Arrhytmia. 1995. (Illus.). 301p. 73.95 (*3-7985-0956-5*) Spr-Verlag.

Myocardial Metabolism, 2. V. N. Smirnov & A. Katz. 1987. (Cardiology of the Soviet Medical Reviews Supplement, Section A.: Vol 2). xii, 674p. text 436.00 (*3-7186-0311-X*) Gordon & Breach.

Myocardial Perfusion, Reperfusion, Coronary Venous Retroperfusion. Ed. by Samuel Meerbaum. 1990. 160p. 102.00 (*0-387-91362-9*) Spr-Verlag.

Myocardial Preconditioning. Cherry L. Wainwright. 1996. (Medicine Ser.). pap. 89.95 (*0-412-10401-6*, VNR) Wiley.

Myocardial Preconditioning. Cherry L. Wainwright & James R. Parratt. 1995. (Medical Intelligence Unit Ser.). 266p. 99.00 (*1-57059-333-7*) Landes Bioscience.

Myocardial Preservation, Preconditioning & Adaptation. Dipak K. Das et al. 1996. LC 96-21067. (Annals of the New York Academy of Sciences Ser.: Vol. 793). 150.00 (*1-57331-024-7*) NY Acad Sci.

Myocardial Preservation, Preconditioning, & Adaptation. Dipak K. Das et al. 1996. LC 96-21067. (Annals of the New York Academy of Sciences Ser.). pap. 150.00 (*1-57331-025-5*) NY Acad Sci.

Myocardial Protection & the KATP Channel, No. 179. Ed. by Derek M. Yellon & Garrett J. Gross. 1996. LC 95-41178. (DICM Ser.: Vol. 179). 232p. (C). text 151.50 (*0-7923-3791-3*) Kluwer Academic.

Myocardial Protection in Cardiac Surgery. Ed. by Arthur J. Roberts. 1987. (Cardiothoracic Surgery Ser.: Vol. 3). (Illus.). 640p. text 250.00 (*0-8247-7638-0*) Dekker.

***Myocardial Repolarization: From Gene to Bedside.** Ed. by Ali Oto & Gunter Breithardt. 2001. LC 2001-33460. (Illus.). 416p. 105.00 (*0-87993-477-8*) Futura Pub.

Myocardial Revascularization: A Surgical Atlas. Quentin R. Stiles et al. 1976. LC 75-30304. 49.00 (*0-316-81500-4*, Little Brwn Med Div) Lppncott W & W.

Myocardial Revascularization Bibliography. Ed. by Joe R. Utley. 1989. LC 89-81062. (Cardiothoracic Surgery Monographs). 600p. pap. text 50.00 (*0-9623617-7-1*) Cardiothoracic Rsch.

Myocardial Revascularization in Acute Conditions. Ed. by S. G. Degre. 1986. (Bibliotheca Cardiologica Ser.: No. 39). (Illus.). vi, 146p. 100.00 (*3-8055-4142-2*) S Karger.

Myocardial Viability. Ed. by Ami E. Iskandrian & E. Van der Wall. 2nd ed. 2000. LC 99-89525. (Illus.). 240p. 118.00 (*0-7923-6161-X*) Kluwer Academic.

Myocardial Viability: A Clinical & Scientific Treatise. Ed. by Vasken Dilsizian. 1999. LC 99-39509. (Illus.). 550p. 125.00 (*0-87993-437-9*) Futura Pub.

Myocardial Viability: Detection & Clinical Relevance. Ed. by Abdulmassih S. Iskandrian & Ernst E. Van der Wall. 1994. LC 94-13373. (Developments in Cardiovascular Medicine Ser.: Vol. 154). 212p. (C). text 148.50 (*0-7923-2813-2*) Kluwer Academic.

Myocardium. Ed. by Glenn A. Langer. 2nd ed. 1997. LC 97-15596. (Illus.). 405p. text 69.95 (*0-12-436570-1*) Morgan Kaufmann.

Myocardium: Proceedings. Conference on Canberra, 1973. Ed. by Ralph Reader. 1974. (Advances in Cardiology Ser.: Vol. 12). 300p. 117.50 (*3-8055-1690-8*) S Karger.

Myocardium at Risk & Viable Myocardium: Evaluation by SPET. Jaume Candell-Riera et al. 2000. LC 00-51441. (Developments in Cardiovascular Medicine Ser.: Vol. 234). (Illus.). 256p. 93.00 (*0-7923-6724-3*) Kluwer Academic.

Myofascial & Fascial-Ligamentous Approaches in Osteopathic Manipulative Medicine. Harry Friedman et al. 2000. LC 00-131503. (Illus.). 120p. pap. 39.95 (*0-9701841-1-5*) S F I M M S Pr.

Myofascial Exams & Biofeedback: Can EMG Validate Trigger Points? Barbara J. Headley & Barbara A. North. 1990. (Illus.). 101p. (Orig.). pap. 14.00 (*0-929538-08-0*) Innovat Systems.

Myofascial Manipulation: Theory & Clinical Applications. Robert I. Cantu & Alan J. Grodin. 2nd ed. 2000. LC 00-61843. 261p. 79.00 (*0-8342-1779-1*, 17791) PRO-ED.

***Myofascial Pain: An Introduction & Guide to Treatment.** P. E. Baldry. 2001. (Illus.). 476p. (*0-443-07003-2*) Church GBR. *Dist:* Saunders.

Myofascial Pain & Dysfunction: The Trigger Point Manual, Volume 2: The Lower Extremities. Janet G. Travell & David G. Simons. 1992. (Illus.). 628p. 102.00 (*0-683-08367-8*) Lppncott W & W.

Myofascial Release: The Search for Excellence. John F. Barnes & Art Marzano. 1990. 254p. 64.95 (*1-929894-00-7*) M F R Treatment Ctrs.

Myofascial Release & It's Application to Neuro-Developmental Treatment. Regi Boehme. 1991. (Illus.). 87p. (Orig.). (C). pap. text 20.00 (*1-879801-00-0*) Boehme Wkshps.

***Myofibrillogenesis.** Dipak K. Dube. 2001. LC 00-69765. (Cardiovascular Molecular Morphogenesis Ser.: Vol. 6). (Illus.). 272p. 149.00 (*0-8176-4226-9*) Birkhauser.

Myologik Vol. 3: Atlas of Human Pectoral Musculature in Clay. Jon Zahourek. 1995. (Myologic Anatomy Ser.). (Illus.). 122p. pap. text 19.95 (*1-887087-03-6*) Zahourek Systs.

Myologik Vol. 4: Atlas of Human Pelvic Musculature in Clay. Jon Zahourek. 1995. (Myologic Anatomy Ser.). (Illus.). 126p. pap. text 19.95 (*1-887087-04-4*) Zahourek Systs.

Myology. Andrew G. Engel. 2nd ed. 1. (*0-07-019558-7*); 2. (*0-07-019559-5*) McGraw.

Myology, Set. Ed. by Andrew G. Engel & Clara Franzini-Armstrong. 2nd ed. 1994. (Illus.). 2500p. text 395.00 (*0-07-911134-3*) McGraw-Hill Prof.

Myomectomy. Eric J. Bieber & Victoria M. Maclin. 1998. LC 98-21524. (Minimally Invasive Gynecology Ser.: Vol. 3). (Illus.). 310p. 105.00 (*0-86542-381-4*) Blackwell Sci.

Myopain '98: Abstracts from the 4th World Congress on Myofascial Pain & Fibromyalgia, Silvi Marina, Italy, August 24-27, 1998. Leonardo Vecchiet & Maria A. Giamberardino. 1998. LC 98-22001. (Journal of Musculoskeletal Pain Ser.). 40.00 (*0-7890-0549-2*, Hawrth Medical) Haworth Pr.

Myopain '95: Abstracts from the 3rd World Congress of Myofacial Pain & Fibromyalgia, San Antonio, Texas, U. S. A. July 30-August 3, 1995. Ed. by I. Jon Russell. 1995. LC 95-23108. 35.00 (*0-7890-0000-8*, Hawrth Medical) Haworth Pr.

Myopathies. Ed. by Pierre J. Vinken et al. 1992. LC 92-48375. 686p. 272.50 (*0-444-81281-4*) Elsevier.

Myopia: Prevalence & Progression. National Research Council Staff. 1989. 126p. pap. text 15.00 (*0-309-04081-7*) Natl Acad Pr.

Myopia & Nearwork. Mark Rosenfield & Bernard Gilmartin. 1998. LC 98-10422. 232p. text 65.00 (*0-7506-3784-6*) Buttrwrth-Heinemann.

Myopia & the Control of Eye Growth - Symposium No. 155. CIBA Foundation Staff. 1991. LC 90-13012. (CIBA Foundation Symposia Ser.: No. 155). 266p. 128.00 (*0-471-92692-2*) Wiley.

Myopia Control Vol. 39-3: Behavioral Aspects of Vision Care. 1998. (Illus.). 162p. pap. 20.00 (*0-943599-25-3*) OEPF.

Myopia Myth: The Truth about Nearsightedness & How to Prevent It. Donald S. Rehm. 1983. LC 83-80453. (Illus.). 165p. reprint ed. pap. 15.00 (*0-9608476-0-X*) Intl Myopia.

Myopia Updates: Proceedings of the 6th International Conference on Myopia. Ed. by Takashi Tokoro. 1997. LC 97-30100. (Illus.). 400p. 159.00 (*4-431-70199-0*) Spr-Verlag.

Myopia Updates II. International Conference on Myopia Staff. Ed. by L. L. Lin et al. 1999. LC 99-51551. (Illus.). 200p. pap. 90.00 (*4-431-70275-X*) Spr-Verlag.

Mysteria, Jung & the Ancient Mysteries: Extracts from the Collected Works of C. G. Jung. Richard Nool. 1994. LC 94-34815. (C). pap. 14.95 (*0-691-03647-0*) Princeton U Pr.

Mysteries of Attention. James S. Hans. 1993. LC 92-9021. 292p. (C). text 64.50 (*0-7914-1391-8*); pap. text 21.95 (*0-7914-1392-6*) State U NY Pr.

Mysteries of Human Reproduction. Raymond W. Bernard. 1994. 126p. reprint ed. spiral bd. 14.50 (*0-7873-1157-X*) Hlth Research.

Mysteries of the Mind. Richard M. Restak. 2000. LC 00-27688. (*0-7922-7640-X*); LC 00-27668. (Illus.). 256p. 35.00 (*0-7922-7941-7*) Natl Geog.

Mysteries of the Rainforest: 20th Century Medicine Man. Elaine Pascoe. 1997. LC 96-47736. (New Explorers Ser.). (Illus.). 48p. (YA). (gr. 5 up). lib. bdg. 18.95 (*1-56711-229-3*, Blackbirch Pr) Gale.

Mystery in Western Medicine. David Greaves. 1996. (Avebury Series in Philosophy). 176p. text (*1-85972-441-8*) Avebury GBR. *Dist:* Ashgate Pub Co.

Mystery of Alzheimer's: A Guide for Carers. Elizabeth Forsythe. 1997. (Illus.). 202p. pap. (*1-85626-220-0*) Cathie Kyle GBR. *Dist:* Trafalgar.

Mystery of Alzheimer's: Sunrise to Sunset & Beyond. Harold E. Wagner. Ed. by Fern Wagner & Laura Aymond. abr. ed. 1998. LC 98-93223. (Illus.). 160p. pap. 19.50 (*0-9665600-0-0*) H E W.

Mystery of Goodness & the Positive Moral Consequences of Psychotherapy. Mary Nicholas. 1994. LC 93-27992. 288p. (C). 30.00 (*0-393-70166-2*) Norton.

Mystery of Healing: Journeys Through Alternative Medicine. Stephen A. Appelbaum. 1998. LC 98-38700. 288p. pap. 16.95 (*1-57129-062-1*) Brookline Bks.

Mystery of Human Relationship: Alchemy & the Transformation of Self. Nathan Schwartz-Salant. 1998. LC 97-21851. (Illus.). 264p. pap. 26.95 (*0-415-15389-1*); (C). 94.95 (*0-415-08971-9*) Routledge.

Mystery of Sex: Race Regeneration. R. Swinburne Clymer. 1950. 273p. 9.95 (*0-932785-32-8*) Philos Pub.

Mystery of Things. Christopher Bollis. 1999. LC 98-53607. 256p. pap. 29.99 (*0-415-21232-4*); xi, 203p. text 90.00 (*0-415-21231-6*) Routledge.

Mystery Patient's Guide to Gaining & Retaining Patients. Suzanne Boswell. 1997. LC 96-50954. 49.95 (*0-87814-654-7*) PennWell Corp.

Mystic Healers & Medicine Shows: Blazing Trails to Wellness in the Old West & Beyond. Gene Fowler, Jr. 1997. LC 96-34432. (Illus.). 208p. pap. 14.95 (*0-941270-95-5*) Ancient City Pr.

Mystical Chorus: Jung & the Religious Dimension. Donald Broadribb. 1996. LC 95-193988. 276p. (Orig.). pap. (*1-86429-019-6*) Millennium Bks AUS. *Dist:* Morehouse Pub.

Mystical Christianity: A Psychological Commentary on the Gospel of John. John A. Sanford. 1994. 352p. reprint ed. pap. 24.95 (*0-8245-1412-2*) Crossroad NY.

Mystical Diets: Paranormal, Spiritual, & Occult Nutrition & Practices. Jack Raso & Stephen Barrett. 1993. LC 92-40828. (Consumer Health Library). 299p. 31.00 (*0-87975-761-2*) Prometheus Bks.

Mystical Magical Marvelous World of Dreams. Wilda B. Tanner. 1996. (Illus.). 400p. pap. 17.75 (*0-945027-02-8*) Sparrow Hawk Pr.

Mystical Medicine. Warren Peters. 1995. LC 95-61242. 96p. per. 7.95 (*1-57258-044-5*) TEACH Servs.

Mysticism & Mental Healing. Manly P. Hall. pap. 4.95 (*0-89314-336-7*) Philos Res.

Mysticism, Freudianism & Scientific Psychology. Knight Dunlap. 1977. (Select Bibliographies Reprint Ser.). reprint ed. 19.95 (*0-8369-5838-1*) Ayer.

Mystics & Medics: A Comparison of Mystical & Psychotherapeutic Encounters. Ed. by Reuven P. Bulka. 1979. LC 79-87593. 120p. pap. 16.95 (*0-87705-377-4*, Kluwer Acad Hman Sci) Kluwer Academic.

Mystics, Magicians & Medicine People: Tales of a Wanderer. Doug Boyd. 1995. 173p. (C). pap. 11.95 (*1-56924-880-X*) Marlowe & Co.

Mystified Fortune-Teller & Other Tales from Psychotherapy. Gerald Amada. 1998. LC 97-34255. 216p. 24.95 (*1-56833-099-5*) Madison Bks UPA.

Mystique of Dreams: A Search for Utopia Through Senoi Dream Theory. G. William Domhoff. 1985. 156p. pap. text 16.95 (*0-520-06021-0*) U CA Pr.

Myth of Addiction: An Application of the Psychological Theory of Attribution to Illicit Drug Use. John B. Davies. 1992. xii, 180p. text 71.00 (*3-7186-5197-1*, Harwood Acad Pubs) Gordon & Breach.

Myth of ADHD & Other Learning Disabilities: Parenting Without Ritalin. Jan Strydom. 2000. 304p. pap. 14.99 (*1-56384-180-0*, Vital Issue Pr) Huntington Hse.

Myth of Analysis: Three Essays in Archetypal Psychology. James Hillman. 1998. LC 97-32837. 320p. pap. 17.95 (*0-8101-1651-0*) Northwestern U Pr.

Myth of Atlas: Families & the Therapeutic Story. Maurizio Andolfi et al. 1989. LC 89-32190. 256p. text 35.95 (*0-87630-549-4*) Brunner-Routledge.

Myth of Heterosexual AIDS: How a Tragedy Has Been Distorted by the Media & Partisan Politics. Michael Fumento. 1993. LC 93-26358. 496p. pap. 14.95 (*0-89526-729-2*) Regnery Pub.

Myth of Meaning: In the Work of C. G. Jung. Aniela Jaffe. 1995. 214p. pap. 14.00 (*3-85630-500-9*) Continuum.

Myth of Mental Illness, Revised Edition. Thomas S. Szasz. rev. ed. 1984. LC 84-47742. 320p. pap. 14.00 (*0-06-091151-4*, CN 1151, Perennial) HarperTrade.

Myth of Psychology. Fred Newman. 1991. LC 91-76608. 229p. pap. 12.95 (*0-9628621-2-6*) All Stars Project.

Myth of Psychotherapy: Mental Healing As Religion, Rhetoric, & Repression. Thomas Szasz. 1988. LC 87-30150. (Illus.). 238p. (C). reprint ed. pap. 17.95 (*0-8156-0223-5*) Syracuse U Pr.

Myth of the A. D. D. Child: 50 Ways to Improve Your Child's Behavior & Attention Span Without Drugs, Labels or Coercion. Thomas Armstrong. 1997. 320p. pap. 13.95 (*0-452-27547-4*, Plume) Dutton Plume.

Myth of the First Three Years: A New Understanding of Early Brain Development & Lifelong Learning. John T. Bruer. 1999. LC 99-34934. 256p. pap. 25.00 (*0-684-85184-9*) Free Pr.

Mythic Artery: The Magic of Music Therapy. Carolyn B. Kenny. 1982. xiv, 154p. (Orig.). (C). pap. text 12.00 (*0-917930-60-6*); lib. bdg. 27.00 (*0-917930-74-6*) Ridgeview.

Mythic Tarot. Juliet Sharman-Burke et al. 1986. 224p. pap. 24.95 (*0-671-61863-6*, Fireside) S&S Trade Pap.

Mythos & Logos in the Thought of Carl Jung: The Theory of the Collective Unconscious in Scientific Perspective. Walter A. Shelburne. 1988. LC 87-10210. 180p. (C). text 64.50 (*0-88706-693-3*); pap. text 21.95 (*0-88706-695-X*) State U NY Pr.

***Myths & Facts about Colorectal Cancer: What You Need to Know.** Richard Pazdur, MD & Melanie Royce, MD. 2nd ed. 2001. (Myths & Facts Series). (Illus.). 48p. pap. 9.95 (*1-891483-12-9*) PRR.

***Myths & Facts about Lung Cancer: What You Need to Know.** John C. Ruckdeschel. 2nd rev. ed. 2002. (Illus.). 80p. pap. 9.95 (*1-891483-15-3*) PRR.

Myths & Facts about Ovarian Cancer: What You Need to Know. M. Steven Piver, MD & Gamal Eltabbakh, MD. 2nd ed. 2000. LC 00-132234. (Illus.). 64p. pap. 9.95 (*1-891483-07-2*) PRR.

***Myths & Facts about Ovarian Cancer: What You Need to Know.** M. Steven Piver & Gamal Eltabbakh. 3rd rev. ed. 2002. (Illus.). 60p. pap. 9.95 (*1-891483-14-5*) PRR.

Myths & Realities about the Decentralization of Health Systems. Ed. by Riitta-Liisa Kolehmainen-Aitken. 1999. LC 99-25251. 192p. lib. bdg. 39.95 (*0-913723-56-8*) Mgmt Sci Health.

Myths in Medical Care: Causes & Effects. Henry A. Shenkin. 2000. 220p. pap. 15.95 (*1-58244-081-6*) Rutledge Bks.

Myths, Misconceptions & Heroics: The Story of the Treatment of Hypertension from the 1930's. Marvin Moser. 1997. 68p. pap. 22.00 (*0-9626020-4-3*) Le Jacq Commns.

Myths of Gender: Biological Theories about Women & Men. Anne Fausto-Sterling. 2nd rev. ed. 1992. LC 85-47561. 272p. 20.00 (*0-465-04792-0*) Basic.

N

N-Acetyl-L-Cysteine & Its Uses. 1996. lib. bdg. 250.75 (*0-8490-5912-7*) Gordon Pr.

N-Hexane. 1991. (Environmental Health Criteria Ser.: No. 122). (ENG, FRE & SPA.). 164p. pap. text 32.00 (*92-4-157122-5*, 1160122) World Health.

N-Nitroso Compounds in Carcinogenesis: Occurrence & Biological Effects. H. Bartsch. 1986. (IARC Scientific Publications Ser.: No. 41). (Illus.). 672p. 75.00 (*0-19-723041-5*) OUP.

N-Oxidation of Drugs: Biochemistry, Pharmacology & Toxicology. Peter Hlavica & L. A. Damani. 1991. (Illus.). 416p. (C). (gr. 13). pap. text 309.95 (*0-412-36030-6*, A5561) Chapman & Hall.

N-3 Fatty Acids: Prevention & Treatment in Vascular Disease. Ed. by S. D. Kristensen et al. 1996. LC 95-49885. (Current Topics in Cardiovascular Diseases Ser.). (Illus.). 244p. 110.00 (*3-540-76001-6*) Spr-Verlag.

N-3 Fatty Acids & Vascular Disease: Backgound & Pathophysiology - Hyperlipidaemia - Renal Diseases- Ischaemic Heart Disease. Ed. by R. DeCaterina et al. 1995. 166p. 49.00 (*0-387-19837-7*) Spr-Verlag.

NAB Study Guide: How to Prepare for the Nursing Home Administrator's Examination. Sorenson and Rock Staff et al. Ed. by James E. Allen. 3rd rev. ed. Date not set. (C). pap. 65.00 (*0-9635064-3-9*) Nat Assn Bds Exam.

NaCl Transport in Epithelia. Ed. by R. Greger. 1988. (Advances in Comparative & Environmental Physiology Ser.: Vol. 1). (Illus.). 321p. 142.00 (*0-387-18700-6*) Spr-Verlag.

Nadas' Pediatric Cardiology. Ed. by Donald C. Fyler. 1991. (Illus.). 784p. 99.00 (*0-932883-94-X*) Hanley & Belfus.

NAFTA & Trade in Medical Services Between the U. S. & Mexico. David C. Warner. 1997. LC 96-78430. (U. S. - Mexican Policy Report Ser.: Vol. 7). 384p. pap. 21.00 (*0-89940-326-3*) LBJ Sch Pub Aff.

NAGNA's CNA Code of Ethics & Federal Regulation Handbook. Lori Porter & Lisa Cantrell. 1996. 31p. wbk. ed. 4.99 (*0-9662101-1-5*) NAGNA.

Na+/H+ Exchanger. Larry Fliegel. 1996. (Molecular Biology Intelligence Unit Ser.). (Illus.). 297p. pap. 89.95 (*0-412-10471-7*) Landes Bioscience.

Naikan Psychotherapy: Meditation for Self-Development. David K. Reynolds. 1983. LC 82-21862. 184p. 17.50 (*0-226-71029-7*) U Ch Pr.

Nail Disorders: Common Presenting Signs, Differential Diagnosis & Treatment. Robert Baran et al. 1991. (Illus.). 188p. text (*0-443-08800-4*) Church.

Nail in Health & Disease. Nardo Zaias. 2nd ed. 1992. (Illus.). 255p. (C). pap. text 165.00 (*0-8385-6645-6*, A6645-4, Apple Lange Med) McGraw.

Nail Surgery: Text & Atlas. Edward A. Krull et al. 1997. 432p. text 159.00 (*0-7817-0154-6*) Lppncott W & W.

Nails: Therapy, Diagnosis, Surgery. Richard K. Scher. 2nd ed. 1997. LC 96-36756. (C). text 160.00 (*0-7216-7026-1*) Harcourt.

Naked Empress: Or The Great Medical Fraud. Hans Ruesch. 3rd rev. ed. 1982. (Illus.). 202p. pap. text (*3-905280-02-7*) Civis CHE. *Dist:* U of Mich Pr.

Naked to the Bone: Medical Imaging in the Twentieth Century. Bettyann H. Kevles. 2000. LC 97-46598. (Illus.). 378p. pap. 18.00 (*0-201-32833-X*) Perseus Bks Grp.

Naked to the Bone: Medical Imaging in the Twentieth Century. Bettyann H. Kevles. 1997. LC 96-2844. (Illus.). 400p. (C). 35.95 (*0-8135-2358-3*) Rutgers U Pr.

Naloxone, Flumazenil & Dantrolene As Antidotes. T. J. Meredith et al. 1994. LC 93-32098. (IPCS-CES Evaluation of Antidotes Ser.: No. 1). 114p. (C). text 49.95 (*0-521-45459-X*) Cambridge U Pr.

***Naltrexone & Alcoholism Treatment: Treatment Improvement Protocol.** Ed. by Stephanie S. O'Malley. 2001. 94p. (C). reprint ed. pap. text 30.00 (*0-7567-0605-X*) DIANE Pub.

Nameless Diseases. Terra Ziporyn. 1992. LC 91-36660. 288p. 24.95 (*0-8135-1800-8*) Rutgers U Pr.

Naming the Shadows: A New Approach to Individual & Group Psychotherapy for Adult Survivors of Childhood Incest. Susan Roth & Ronald Batson. 1997. LC 97-1617. 224p. 29.95 (*0-684-83704-8*) Free Pr.

Nan-Ching - The Classic of Difficult Ideas. Paul U. Unschuld. 1986. LC 84-28049. (Comparative Studies of Health Systems & Medical Care: Vol. 18). 700p. 95.00 (*0-520-05372-9*) U CA Pr.

NANDA Nursing Diagnoses: Definitions & Classifications, 1995-1996. North American Nursing Diagnosis Association Staff. Ed. by North American Nursing Diagnosis Association Staff. rev. ed. 1995. 124p. (C). pap. 11.00 (*0-9637042-1-4*) Nursecom Inc.

NANDA Nursing Diagnoses: Definitions & Classifications 1997-1998. NANDA Staff. 1996. 120p. (C). pap. 11.00 (*0-9637042-3-0*) Nursecom Inc.

Nanise: A Navajo Herbal. Vernon O. Mayes & Barbara Bayless Lacy. 1990. pap. 27.00 (*0-912586-62-1*) Dine College Pr.

Nanomedicine Vol. 1: Basic Capabilities. Robert A. Freitas, Jr. 1999. LC 99-48974. (Illus.). 600p. 99.00 (*1-57059-645-X*) Landes Bioscience.

Nanotechnology in Medicine & the Biosciences. Richard Coombs & Dennis Robinson. 1996. (Developments in Nanotechnology Ser.). 320p. text 90.00 (*2-88449-080-9*) Gordon & Breach.

Narcissism: A New Theory. Neville Symington. 1993. LC 93-238309. 160p. pap. text (*1-85575-047-3*) Karnac Bks GBR. *Dist:* Other Pr LLC.

Narcissism: Psychoanalytic Essays. Bela Grunberger. 1990. 332p. reprint ed. pap. 24.95 (*0-8236-8155-6*, BN 23491) Intl Univs Pr.

Narcissism: The Self & Society. Reuben Fine. 1986. 384p. text 64.50 (*0-231-05732-6*) Col U Pr.

Narcissism & Intimacy: Love & Marriage in an Age of Confusion. Marion F. Solomon. 1992. LC 88-21981. pap. 13.95 (*0-393-30916-9*) Norton.

Narcissism & the Interpersonal Self. Ed. by John Fiscalini & Alan L. Grey. 1993. LC 92-35506. (Personality, Psychopathology & Psychotherapy: Theoretical & Clinical Perspectives Ser.). (Illus.). 384p. (C). text 61.50 (*0-231-07010-1*) Col U Pr.

Narcissism & the Psychotherapist. Sheila R. Welt & William G. Herron. 1990. LC 89-27520. 356p. 42.00 (*0-89862-398-7*) Guilford Pubns.

Narcissistic - Borderline Couple: A Psychoanalytic Perspective on Marital Treatment. Joan Lachkar. 1992. LC 91-28228. 224p. text 41.95 (*0-87630-634-2*) Brunner-Routledge.

Narcissistic & Borderline Disorders: An Integrated Developmental Approach. James F. Masterson. 18th ed. 1989. LC 81-38540. 260p. text 38.95 (*0-87630-292-4*) Brunner-Routledge.

Narcissistic Condition: A Fact of Our Lives & Times. Ed. by Marie C. Nelson. 1977. LC 76-20724. (Self-in-Process Ser.: Vol. 1). 300p. 43.95 (*0-87705-250-6*, Kluwer Acad Hman Sci) Kluwer Academic.

Narcissistic Family: Diagnosis & Treatment. Stephanie Donaldson-Pressman & Robert H. Pressman. 1994. LC 93-40133. (*0-02-925434-5*) Free Pr.

Narcissistic Family: Diagnosis & Treatment. Stephanie Donaldson-Pressman & Robert H. Pressman. 1997. LC 97-16678. 192p. pap. 30.00 (*0-7879-0870-3*) Jossey-Bass.

Narcissistic Pursuit of Perfection. Arnold Rothstein. 2nd rev. ed. 1985. LC 84-25159. 327p. 50.00 (*0-8236-3494-9*, 03493) Intl Univs Pr.

Narcissistic States & the Therapeutic Process. Sheldon Bach. LC 85-1440. 1993. 280p. pap. 40.00 (*0-87668-304-9*); 1985. 250p. 45.00 (*0-87668-893-8*) Aronson.

Narcissistic Wounds: Clinical Perspectives. Judy Cooper & Nilda Maxwell. 1995. LC 95-35828. 280p. pap. 25.00 (*1-56821-747-1*) Aronson.

Narcissus & Oedipus: The Children of Psychoanalysis. Vicoria Hamilton. 1982. 304p. 37.50 (*0-7100-0869-4*, Routledge Thoemms) Routledge.

Narcolepsy: A Funny Disorder That's No Laughing Matter. Marguerite J. Utley. 1995. LC 95-90011. (Illus.). 166p. 18.00 (*0-9643328-1-7*); pap. 12.00 (*0-9643328-0-9*) M J Utley.

Narcolepsy Primer, 1991: A Guide for Physicians, Patients, & Their Families. Meeta Goswami. 1991. 18p. pap. 6.00 (*0-9667122-0-X*) Meeta Goswami.

Narcotic Drug Diseases & Allied Ailments: Pathology, Pathogenesis, & Treatment. George E. Pettey. Ed. by Gerald N. Grob. 1981. LC 80-1246. (Addiction in America Ser.). (Illus.). reprint ed. lib. bdg. 49.95 (*0-405-13616-1*) Ayer.

Narcotic Drug Problem. Ernest S. Bishop. 1976. LC 75-17204. (Social Problems & Social Policy Ser.). reprint ed. 18.95 (*0-405-07476-X*) Ayer.

Narcotic Drugs: Estimated World Requirements for 1990, Statistics for 1988. 184p. 35.00 (*92-1-048045-7*, EFS.89.XI.3) UN.

Narcotic Drugs: Estimated World Requirements for 1991; Statistics for 1989. 1990. 35.00 (*92-1-048047-3*, MU90.XI.4) UN.

Narcotic Drugs: Estimated World Requirements for 1992 - Statistics for 1990. 1991. 184p. 36.00 (*92-1-048050-3*, 91.XI.2) UN.

Narcotic Drugs & Psychotropic Substances Laws of India. B. V. Kumar & R. K. Tewari. 1989. xx, 617p. text (*81-220-0151-3*) Konark Pubs Pvt Ltd IND. *Dist:* Advent Bks Div.

Narcotic Plants of the Old World, Used in Rituals & Everyday Life: An Anthology of Texts from Ancient Times to the Present. Hedwig Schleiffer. 1979. (Illus.). (Orig.). pap. text 10.00 (*0-934454-00-0*); lib. bdg. 17.50 (*0-934454-01-9*) Lubrecht & Cramer.

Narcotics: Dangerous Painkillers. George Glass. 1998. LC 97-44384. (Drug Abuse Prevention Library). (Illus.). 64p. (YA). (gr. 7-12). lib. bdg. 17.95 (*0-8239-2719-9*, DRNARC) Rosen Group.

Narcotics & Drug Abuse - A to Z. 1990. LC 78-173860. Vol. 1. (*0-87514-004-1*); Vol. 2. (*0-87514-005-X*); Vol. 3. (*0-87514-006-8*) Croner.

Narcotics & Reproduction: A Bibliography. Compiled by Ernest L. Abel. 1983. LC 83-13252. 215p. lib. bdg. 75.00 (*0-313-24052-3*, ABN/, Greenwood Pr) Greenwood.

Narcotics & the Law. William B. Eldridge. 2nd ed. 1967. LC 67-25528. lib. bdg. 17.50 (*0-226-20315-8*) U Ch Pr.

Narcotics Education Assistant. Jack Rudman. 1994. (Career Examination Ser.: C-2503). pap. 29.95 (*0-8373-2503-X*) Nat Learn.

Narcotics Menace. St. Charles. 1952. 5.95 (*0-87505-229-0*) Borden.

Narcotics Security Assistant. Jack Rudman. 1994. (Career Examination Ser.: C-1378). pap. 27.95 (*0-8373-1378-3*) Nat Learn.

Narrating Psychology: How Psychology Gets Made. Mary Vander Goot. 1987. LC 87-50856. 280p. (C). text 32.00 (*1-55605-015-1*); pap. text 20.00 (*1-55605-014-3*) Wyndham Hall.

Narrative & the Cultural Construction of Illness & Healing. Ed. by Cheryl Mattingly & Linda C. Garro. 2000. LC 00-31629. ix, 279p. text 45.00 (*0-520-21824-8*); pap. text 17.95 (*0-520-21825-6*) U CA Pr.

Narrative Based Medicine. Ed. by Trisha Greenhalgh & Brian Hurwitz. 1998. 286p. pap. (*0-7279-1223-2*) BMJ Pub GBR. *Dist:* AIDC.

Narrative Discourse in Normal Aging & Neurologically-Impaired Adults. Ed. by Hiram H. Brownell & Yves Joanette. 1993. LC 93-15128. (Illus.). 354p. (Orig.). (C). pap. text 65.00 (*1-56593-083-5*, 0388) Thomson Learn.

Narrative Enlarging. Verle Waters. 1995. pap. 24.95 (*0-88737-641-X*) Natl League Nurse.

Narrative Gerontology: Theory, Research & Practice. Gary M. Kenyon et al. 2001. LC 00-53811. (Illus.). xviii, 358p. (*0-8261-1389-3*) Springer Pub.

Narrative Means to Therapeutic Ends. Michael James Denham White & David Epston. 1990. LC 89-48776. 230p. (C). 27.00 (*0-393-70098-4*) Norton.

Narrative of the Life & Medical Discoveries of Samuel Thomson, Containing an Account of His System of Practice & the Manner of Curing. Samuel Thomson. 1972. LC 79-180594. (Medicine & Society in America Ser.). 186p. reprint ed. 19.95 (*0-405-03976-X*) Ayer.

Narrative Psychology: The Storied Nature of Human Conduct. Ed. by Theodore R. Sarbin. 1986. LC 86-8130. 321p. 68.50 (*0-275-92103-4*, C2103, Praeger Pubs) Greenwood.

Narrative Solutions in Brief Therapy. Joseph B. Eron & Thomas W. Lund. LC 96-2355. (Guilford Family Therapy Ser.). 288p. 1998. pap. 22.00 (*1-57230-420-0*, C0420); 1996. 42.00 (*1-57230-126-0*) Guilford Pubns.

Narrative Study of Lives. Ruthellen Josselson & Amia Lieblich. 1993. LC 93-6581. (Narrative Study of Lives Ser.: Vol. 1). (Illus.). 232p. (C). pap. 38.95 (*0-8039-4813-1*, 4452) Sage.

Narrative Study of Lives, Vol. 5. Amia Lieblich & Ruthellen Josselson. 1997. 244p. 86.95 (*0-7619-0324-0*, 2481); pap. 38.95 (*0-7619-0325-9*, 2482) Sage.

Narrative Therapies with Children & Adolescents. Ed. by Craig Smith & David Nylund. 1997. LC 97-35905. 469p. text 45.00 (*1-57230-253-4*, C0253) Guilford Pubns.

Narrative Therapy: The Social Construction of Preferred Realities. Jill Freedman & Gene Combs. 1996. LC 95-53127. 320p. 39.00 (*0-393-70207-3*, RC489) Norton.

Nasal & Sinus Surgery. Steven C. Marks. 2000. LC 00-38803. (Illus.). xvi, 489p. text 214.00 (*0-7216-7804-1*) Saunders.

Nasal Manifestations of Systemic Diseases. Michael Schatz & Robert S. Zeiger. 1991. (Illus.). 116p. text 48.00 (*0-936587-03-2*) OceanSide Pubns.

Nasal Neoplasia. Dennis H. Kraus & Howard Levine. 1996. LC 96-41026. (Rhinology & Sinusology Ser.). 79.00 (*0-86577-655-5*) Thieme Med Pubs.

Nasal Plastic Surgery. E. Gaylon McCollough. 1994. LC 93-26436. (Illus.). 400p. text 152.00 (*0-7216-4067-2*) Saunders.

Nasal Polyps: Epidemiology, Pathogenesis & Treatment. Guy A. Settipane et al. 1997. LC 96-70568. (Illus.). 200p. 98.00 (*0-936587-09-1*) OceanSide Pubns.

Nasal Systemic Drug Delivery. Yie W. Chien et al. 1989. (Drugs & the Pharmaceutical Sciences Ser.: Vol. 39). (Illus.). 320p. text 175.00 (*0-8247-8093-0*) Dekker.

Nasal Toxicity & Dosimetry of Inhaled Xenibiotics: Implications for Human Health. Ed. by Chemical Industry Institute of Toxicology Staff et al. 1995. LC 94-29943. 450p. 125.00 (*1-56032-366-3*) Taylor & Francis.

Nasal Tumors in Animals & Man Ed. by Sherman F. Stinson & Gerd K. Reznik. 1983. Vol. I. 296p. 162.00 (*0-8493-5577-X*, RC271); Vol. II. LC 82-1277. 288p. 157.00 (*0-8493-5578-8*, RC280); Vol. III. LC 82-1277. 280p. 156.00 (*0-8493-5579-6*, RC271) Franklin (CRC Reprint).

Nasalcrom in Clinical Practice. Robert N. Ross. 1983. LC 83-81193. (Illus.). 40p. (*0-914132-04-0*) Fisons Corp.

Nasenplastik und Sonstige Gesichtsplastik nebst Mammaplastik see Jacques Joseph's Rhinoplasty & Facial Plastic Surgery with a Supplement on Mammaplasty

Nashville Medicine: A History. James Summerville. 1998. (Illus.). 175p. 29.95 (*0-9668380-0-9*) Assoc Publ.

Nasopharyngeal Carcinoma. Ed. by C. Andrew Van Hasselt & Alan G. Gibb. 1991. (Illus.). 286p. 99.50 (*962-201-542-5*) Coronet Bks.

Nasorespiratory Function & Craniofacial Growth. Ed. by J. A. McNamara. 1985. (Craniofacial Growth Ser.: Vol. 9). (Illus.). 332p. reprint ed. 59.00 (*0-929921-06-2*) UM CHGD.

NASPE/CAP Educational Guidelines: Pacing & Electrophysiology. Ed. by Lois Schurig et al. 2nd ed. 1997. LC 97-2755. (Illus.). 640p. 45.00 (*0-87993-672-X*) Futura Pub.

Natal Charting: How to Master the Techniques of Birth Chart Construction. John Filbey. 1988. LC 84-670142. (Illus.). 192p. (Orig.). pap. (*0-85030-246-3*) Aqrn Pr GBR. *Dist:* Harper SF.

Nathan & Oski's Hematology of Infancy & Childhood. David G. Nathan & Stuart H. Orkin. Ed. by Richard Lampert. 5th ed. 1997. LC 96-41120. (Illus.). 2096p. text 295.00 (*0-7216-5951-9*) Saunders.

National Admissions to Substance Abuse Treatment Services: The Treatment Episode Data Set, 1992-1995. Barbara Ray et al. 1998. (Illus.). 91p. (C). pap. text 25.00 (*0-7881-4907-5*) DIANE Pub.

National & International Standardization of Radiation Dosimetry International Atomic Energy Agency Staff. 1979. (Proceedings Ser.). pap. (*92-0-010478-9*, ISP471-1);Vol. 2. pap. (*92-0-010578-5*, ISP471-2) IAEA AUT. *Dist:* Bernan Associates.

National Arthritis Action Plan: A Public Health Strategy. Susan B. Toal. Ed. by Phyllis L. Moir. 2000. (Illus.). 58p. pap. text 20.00 (*0-7567-0042-6*) DIANE Pub.

National Association for the Protection of the Insane & the Prevention of Insanity Ed. by Gerald N. Grob. 1980. LC 78-22578. (Historical Issues in Mental Health Ser.). reprint ed. lib. bdg. 18.95 (*0-405-11930-5*) Ayer.

National Black Health Leadership Directory: 1992 Edition. Nathaniel Wesley. 1991. 200p. 65.00 (*0-9631990-0-5*) NRW Assocs.

National Black Health Leadership Directory: 1993 Edition. Ed. by Nathaniel Wesley, Jr. 1993. (*0-9631990-1-3*) NRW Assocs.

National Black Health Leadership Directory, 1996-97. Ed. by Nathaniel Wesley, Jr. 1996. 200p. pap. 75.00 (*0-9631990-3-X*) NRW Assocs.

National Cancer Control Programmes: Policies & Managerial Guidelines. 1995. LC 96-117924. (FRE & SPA.). 134p. (C). pap. 32.00 (*92-4-154474-0*, 1150422) World Health.

National Certifying Examination for Physician's Assistants (PA) Jack Rudman. 1994. (Admission Test Ser.: ATS-91). pap. 29.95 (*0-8373-5091-3*) Nat Learn.

National Childhood Encephalopathy Study: A 10-Year Follow-Up. Nicola Madge et al. 1993. (Illus.). 128p. (C). pap. text 19.95 (*0-521-45883-8*) Cambridge U Pr.

National Commission on Nursing Implementation Project: Models for the Future of Nursing. 1988. 80p. pap. 14.95 (*0-88737-427-1*, 15-2251) Natl League Nurse.

National Conference on Drug Abuse Prevention Research, 1996: Presentations, Papers & Recommendations. Ed. by Susan L. David. 2000. (Illus.). 182p. reprint ed. pap. text 35.00 (*0-7567-0050-7*) DIANE Pub.

National Dental Assistant Boards (NDAB) Jack Rudman. (Admission Test Ser.: Vol. 87). 59.95 (*0-8373-5187-1*); 1994. pap. 39.95 (*0-8373-5087-5*) Nat Learn.

National Dental Boards (NDB) Jack Rudman. (Admission Test Ser.: Vol. 36). 89.95 (*0-8373-5136-7*); 1996. pap. 69.95 (*0-8373-5036-0*);Pt. I. 1996. pap. 49.95 (*0-8373-6955-X*);Pt. II. 69.95 (*0-8373-6981-9*);Pt. II. 1994. pap. 49.95 (*0-8373-6956-8*) Nat Learn.

National Dental Hygiene Boards (NDHB) Jack Rudman. (Admission Test Ser.: Vol. 51). 59.95 (*0-8373-5151-0*); 1994. pap. 39.95 (*0-8373-5051-4*) Nat Learn.

National Diet & Nutrition Survey: Children Aged 1 & 1/2 to 4 & 1/2 Years. HMSO Staff. 1995. 412p. pap. (*0-11-691611-7*, HM16117) Statnry Office GBR. *Dist:* Bernan Associates.

National Directory of AIDS Care. Nancy Shenker & Shawn D. Phillps. 6th ed. 1996. 500p. pap. 54.90 (*0-925133-46-9*) Volt Directory.

National Directory of Drug Abuse & Alcoholism Treatment & Prevention Programs. 1986. lib. bdg. 200.00 (*0-8490-3508-2*) Gordon Pr.

National Directory of Drug Abuse & Alcoholism Treatment Programs (1998) Ed. by Rick Albright & Deborah Trunzo. 2000. 550p. (C). pap. text 60.00 (*0-7567-0165-1*) DIANE Pub.

National Directory of Four Year Colleges, Two Year Colleges, & Post High School Training Programs for Young People with Learning Disabilities. Ed. by P. M. Fielding & John R. Moss. 7th ed. 1994. pap. 29.95 (*0-937660-10-8*) PIP.

National Directory of Health Care Critical Pathways: Fall 1996 Edition. Ed. by Marilyn Lang. 2nd ed. 1996. 135p. pap. text 98.00 (*0-9645360-2-1*) Cor Hlthcare.

National Directory of Integrated Healthcare Delivery Systems. Gwen, B. Lareau. Ed. by Phyllis Harris. 2nd ed. 1999. 557p. pap. text 395.00 (*1-882364-31-7*, Amer Busn Pub) Hlth Res Pub.

National Directory of Psychotherapy Training Institutes. Ed. by Laurie A. Baum & Bette G. Pounds. 1993. LC 93-574. 224p. pap. 21.95 (*0-87630-720-9*) Brunner-Routledge.

***National Disaster Medical System (NDMS) Annual Conference (1992) Conference.** Ed. by Connie Boatright & Pete Brewster. 2001. (Illus.). 600p. (C). reprint ed. pap. text 65.00 (*0-7567-1450-8*) DIANE Pub.

National Drug Policies. 1979. (Public Health in Europe Ser.: No. 12). 99p. 10.00 (*92-9020-131-2*, 1320012) World Health.

National Environmental Health Programmes: Proceedings of the WHO Expert Committee on National Environmental Health Programmes & Their Planning, Organization & Administration, Geneva, 1969. WHO Staff. 1970. (Technical Reports: No. 439). 56p. pap. text 5.00 (*92-4-120439-7*, 1100439) World Health.

***National Evaluation of the Housing Opportunities for Persons with Aids Program (HOPWA)** Dave Pollack. 2001. (Illus.). 250p. (C). pap. text 40.00 (*0-7567-1334-X*) DIANE Pub.

National Exposure Registry: Policies & Procedures Manual. rev. ed. 1995. 44p. (C). pap. text 25.00 (*0-7881-1981-8*) DIANE Pub.

***National Fee Analyzer 2001.** Ingenix, Inc. Staff. pap. 149.95 (*1-56337-366-1*) Ingenix Inc.

National Government & Public Health. J. A. Tobey. 1978. LC 77-74961. (American Federalism-the Urban Dimension Ser.). (Illus.). lib. bdg. 38.95 (*0-405-10503-7*) Ayer.

National Guide to Funding in Aids. Ed. by Gina-Marie Cantarella. 1999. LC 00-500751. xlvi, 216p. 75.00 (*0-87954-882-7*) Foundation Ctr.

***National Guide to Funding in AIDS.** Foundation Center Staff. 2nd ed. 2001. 268p. 115.00 (*0-87954-950-5*, GFA2) Foundation Ctr.

National Guide to Funding in Health. Foundation Center Staff. 5th ed. 1997. LC 91-38072. 1195p. pap. text 150.00 (*0-87954-710-3*) Foundation Ctr.

National Guide to Funding in Health. 6th ed. 1999. 1195p. 150.00 (*0-87954-876-2*) Foundation Ctr.

***National Guide to Funding in Health.** Foundation Center Staff. 7th ed. 2001. 2032p. 155.00 (*0-87954-951-3*, HLTH7) Foundation Ctr.

National Health Care: An Annotated Guide to the Current Literature. Ed. by N. G. Arashvili. annot. ed. 1994. 204p. pap. text 95.00 (*1-56072-113-8*) Nova Sci Pubs.

National Health Care: Issues & Background. Ed. by C. J. Spreding. 1993. 290p. (C). lib. bdg. 135.00 (*1-56072-109-X*) Nova Sci Pubs.

National Health Care: Law, Policy, Strategy. Donald L. Westerfield. 1993. LC 92-40184. 224p. 62.50 (*0-275-94474-3*, C4474, Praeger Pubs) Greenwood.

National Health Development Networks in Support of Primary Health Care. 1986. (WHO Offset Publications: No. 94). 53p. pap. text 10.00 (*92-4-170094-7*, 1120094) World Health.

National Health Education Standards: Achieving Health Literacy. AAHE Staff et al. 1995. 79p. (Orig.). pap. 3.00 (*0-88314-611-8*, 301-10035) AAHPERD.

National Health Insurance: Benefits, Costs, & Consequences. Karen Davis. 1975. LC 77-91832. (Studies in Social Economics). 182p. 29.95 (*0-8157-1760-1*); pap. text 10.95 (*0-8157-1759-8*) Brookings.

National Health Insurance & Health Resources: The European Experience. Jan Blanpain et al. 1978. LC 77-25818. 320p. 29.95 (*0-674-26955-1*) HUP.

National Health Interview Survey: Research for the 1995-2004 Redesign. David Judkins. 1999. 127p. pap. 13.00 (*0-16-050096-6*) USGPO.

National Health Interview Survey: Research for the 1995-2004 Redesign. Ed. by Monroe Sirken. 2000. (Illus.). 119p. reprint ed. pap. text 25.00 (*0-7567-0200-3*) DIANE Pub.

National Health Planning in Developing Countries: Report of a WHO Expert Committee, 1967. 1967. (Technical Report Ser.). 40p. pap. text 6.00 (*92-4-120350-1*, 1100350) World Health.

National Health Program Book: A Source Guide for Advocates. David Himmelstein & Steffie Woolhandler. 1994. pap. 11.95 (*1-56751-018-3*); lib. bdg. 29.95 (*1-56751-019-1*) Common Courage.

National Health Service? The Restructuring of Health Care in Britain since 1979. John Mohan. 1995. LC 94-22962. 286p. text 59.95 (*0-312-12410-4*) St Martin.

National Health Service & the Labour Market. J. A. Stilwell & R. A. Wilson. 1992. 322p. (*1-85628-390-9*) Avebry GBR. *Dist:* Ashgate Pub Co.

National Health Service Corps: Opportunities to Stretch Scarce Dollars & Improve Provider Placement. 1996. (Illus.). 59p. (Orig.). (C). pap. text 20.00 (*0-7881-3106-0*) DIANE Pub.

National Health Systems & Their Reorientation Towards Health for All Guidance for Policy-Making. B. Kleczkowski et al. 1984. (Public Health Papers: No. 77). 120p. pap. text 11.00 (*92-4-130077-9*, 1110077) World Health.

National Health Systems of the World, Vols. I & II. Milton I. Roemer. 1993. (Illus.). 1056p. 140.00 (*0-19-508623-6*) OUP.

National Health Systems of the World: The Issues, Vol. 2. Milton I. Roemer. 1993. 368p. text 59.50 (*0-19-507845-4*) OUP.

National Health Systems of the World Vol. 1: Countries, Vol. 1. Milton I. Roemer. 1991. (Illus.). 688p. text 89.50 (*0-19-505320-6*) OUP.

National Healthlines Directory (TM), 1994: Toll-Free 800 Numbers. Herner and Company Staff. rev. ed. 1994. LC 92-71167. viii, 194p. pap. 30.00 (*0-87815-065-X*) Info Resources.

***National Hospital Discharge Survey 1999: Annual Summary with Detailed Diagnosis & Procedure Data.** Jennifer R. Popovic. 2001. 212p. per. 27.00 (*0-16-050921-1*) USGPO.

National Household Survey on Drug Abuse. 1992. (Illus.). 121p. (Orig.). (C). pap. text 30.00 (*1-56806-135-8*) DIANE Pub.

National Household Survey on Drug Abuse: Main Findings, 1996. Angela Brittingham et al. 1998. (Illus.). 328p. (C). pap. text 45.00 (*0-7881-7419-3*) DIANE Pub.

National Household Survey on Drug Abuse: Population Estimates, 1992. 1994. (Illus.). 125p. (Orig.). (C). pap. text 30.00 (*0-7881-0818-2*) DIANE Pub.

National Human Exposure Assessment Survey (NHEXAS) Ed. by Edo Pellizzari. 1995. (Journal of Exposure Analysis & Environmental Epidemiology Ser.: Vol. 5, No. 3). (Illus.). pap. text (*0-911131-72-8*) Specialist Journals.

National Inpatient Profile 1997: Diagnoses. 1998. ring bd. (*1-880678-63-2*) Solucient.

National Inpatient Profile 1997: Diagnoses & Procedures. 1998. ring bd. (*1-880678-78-0*) Solucient.

National Inpatient Profile 1997: Procedures. 1998. ring bd. (*1-880678-74-8*) Solucient.

National Institues of Health (NIH) Consensus Conference on Cervical Cancer. Ed. by Barnett S. Kramer. 2000. (Illus.). 148p. reprint ed. pap. text 30.00 (*0-7567-0245-3*) DIANE Pub.

National Institutes of Health 1994. lib. bdg. 395.00 (*0-8490-8433-4*) Gordon Pr.

National Link Study, 1997. 1998. ring bd. (*1-880678-38-1*) Solucient.

National Listing of Medicare Providers Furnishing Kidney Dialysis & Transplant Services. (Orig.). 1996. lib. bdg. 253.95 (*0-8490-6929-7*); 1994. lib. bdg. 250.00 (*0-8490-9053-9*) Gordon Pr.

***National Listing of Medicare Providers Furnishing Kidney Dialysis & Transplant Services 2001.** 2001. 284p. per. 35.00 (*0-16-050946-7*) USGPO.

National Listing of Medicare Providers Furnishing Kidney Dialysis & Transplant Services, January 1997. 1997. 224p. per. 16.00 (*0-16-049080-4*) USGPO.

National Listing of Medicare Providers Furnishing Kidney Dialysis & Transplant Services, January 1999. 1999. 262p. per. 26.00 (*0-16-050134-2*) USGPO.

National Managed Care Leadership Directory: Key Contacts in Today's Leading Managed Care Organization. Brad Bangerter. Ed. by Laura Bangerter & Mirid Weidner. 11th rev. ed. 1999. 426p. pap. 185.00 (*0-9639238-3-8*) HlthQuest Pubs.

National Medical Boards (NMB) Jack Rudman. (Admission Test Ser.: Vol. 23). 89.95 (*0-8373-5123-5*); 1994. pap. 69.95 (*0-8373-5023-9*);Pt. I. 69.95 (*0-8373-6975-4*);Pt. I. 1994. pap. 49.95 (*0-8373-6950-9*);Pt. II. 69.95 (*0-8373-6976-2*);Pt. II. 1994. pap. 49.95 (*0-8373-6951-7*) Nat Learn.

National Medical Directory. Jean Carper. 1985. (Orig.). pap. 11.95 (*0-671-49974-2*) PB.

National Mental Health Association: Eighty Years of Prevention. Ed. by Robert E. Hess & Jean DeLeon. 1989. LC 89-19799. (Prevention in Human Services Ser.: Vol. 6, No. 2). (Illus.). 306p. text 9.95 (*0-86656-943-X*) Haworth Pr.

National Newborn Screening Report (1991) Final Report. 1996. (Illus.). 110p. (Orig.). (C). pap. text 25.00 (*0-7881-2680-6*) DIANE Pub.

National Nursing Home License Exam Study Guide: A Comprehensive Preparation Guide for Administrators & Directors of Nursing. Melissa Tracey & Kenneth M. Bowman. 1996. LC 96-22260. 216p. text 80.00 (*0-7863-0973-3*, Irwn Prfssnl) McGraw-Hill Educ Grp.

National Organ Transplant Act of 1984: A Legislative History of Pub. Law No. 98-507, Set. Ed. by Bernard D. Reams. 1990. LC 89-83919. (Federal Health Law Ser.: Part 1). 2466p. lib. bdg. 225.00 (*0-89941-691-8*, 305920) W S Hein.

National Pharmacy Boards (NPB) Jack Rudman. (Admission Test Ser.: Vol. 47). 69.95 (*0-8373-5147-2*); 1994. pap. 49.95 (*0-8373-5047-6*) Nat Learn.

National Plan for Research on Child & Adolescent Mental Disorders. 1990. (Illus.). 80p. pap. 6.00 (*0-16-021851-9*, S/N 017-024-01395-1) USGPO.

National Plan for Research on Child & Adolescent Mental Disorders. Ed. by Lewis L. Judd. 2000. 64p. (C). pap. text 20.00 (*0-7881-8941-7*) DIANE Pub.

National Pool & Waterpark Lifeguard CPR Training. Jeff Ellis & NSC Staff. 2nd ed. 1998. (Illus.). 104p. (C). pap. text, tchr. ed. 30.00 (*0-7637-0983-2*, 0983-2) Jones & Bartlett.

National Pool & Waterpark Lifeguard CPR Training. Jeff Ellis et al. 2nd ed. 1999. LC 98-21019. (Illus.). 224p. (C). pap. text 45.00 (*0-7637-0793-7*, 0793-7) Jones & Bartlett.

National Psychology Boards (NPsyB) Jack Rudman. (Admission Test Ser.: Vol. 89). 69.95 (*0-8373-5189-8*); 1994. pap. 49.95 (*0-8373-5089-1*) Nat Learn.

National Psychology in International Relations. Franz E. Winkler. 1976. 35p. reprint ed. pap. 1.50 (*0-913098-10-8*) Orion Society.

National Registry of Community Mental Health Services. 3rd ed. 1991. 158p. pap. 29.50 (*1-883066-04-2*) Natl Comm Mental.

National Renal Diet: Renal Dietitians Dietetic Practice Group of the American Dietetic. 1993. LC 93-27161. (*0-88091-116-6*) Am Dietetic Assn.

National Safety Council - First Aid - CPR I-III: Instructor's Manual. National Safety Council Staff. 2nd ed. 1993. 216p. pap. text 15.00 (*0-86720-795-7*) Jones & Bartlett.

National Strategy for Prevention of Drug Abuse & Drug Trafficking. 1986. lib. bdg. 200.00 (*0-8490-3505-8*) Gordon Pr.

National Study of Health & Growth. Roberto J. Rona & Susan Chinn. 1999. LC 99-14303. (Illus.). 144p. text 98.50 (*0-19-262919-0*) OUP.

National Summary State Medicaid Manage Care Programs, 1999: Program Descriptions as of June 30, 1999. 2000. 419p. per. 38.00 (*0-16-050396-5*) USGPO.

National Survey of Family Growth, Cycle IV: Evaluation of Linked Design. 1993. LC 93-24687. (Vital & Health Statistics Ser.: Series 2, No. 117). (*0-8406-0482-3*) Natl Ctr Health Stats.

National Survey of Problems & Competencies among Four- to Sixteen-Year Olds. Thomas M. Achenbach et al. 1992. (Child Development Monographs: No. 225, Vol. 56, No. 3). (Illus.). 136p. pap. text 15.00 (*0-226-00221-7*) U Ch Pr.

National Survey of State Medicaid Managed Care Programs. 1997. lib. bdg. 250.95 (*0-8490-8246-3*) Gordon Pr.

National Survey Results on Drug Use: Secondary School Students, College Students & Young Adults 1997. lib. bdg. 600.95 (*0-8490-8242-0*) Gordon Pr.

M N O

National Symposium on Medical & Public Health: Response to Bioterrorism. Ed. by Joseph E. McDade. 2000. (Illus.). 76p. pap. text 25.00 (0-7881-8531-4) DIANE Pub.

National Therapeutics for Infants & Children: Workshop Summary. Sumner J. Yaffe. 2000. 136p. pap. 30.75 (0-309-06937-8) Natl Acad Pr.

National Toxicology Chemical Data Compendium, Vol. 3. Keith. 1991. 832p. 204.95 (0-87371-717-1) CRC Pr.

National Toxicology Program Chemical Data Compendium. Keith. 1991. Vol. 1. 992p. 204.95 (0-87371-715-5); Vol. 2. 1664p. 278.95 (0-87371-716-3); Vol. 4. 896p. 278.95 (0-87371-718-X) CRC Pr.

National Toxicology Program Chemical Data Compendium, Vol. 5. Lawrence H. Keith. 1992. 1216p. 278.95 (0-87371-719-8) CRC Pr.

National Toxicology Program Chemical Data Compendium. Keith. 1991. Vol. 6. 1472p. 278.95 (0-87371-720-1); Vol. 7. 1440p. 278.95 (0-87371-721-X); Vol. 8. 880p. 194.95 (0-87371-722-8) CRC Pr.

National Toxicology Program's Chemical Database, Set. Lawrence H. Keith & Douglas B. Walters. 1991. 1995.00 incl. 5.25 hd (0-87371-695-7) Lewis Pubs.

National Toxicology Program's Chemical Database, Vol. 1: Chemical Names & Synonyms. Lawrence H. Keith & Douglas B. Walters. 1993. 288p. lib. bdg. 65.00 (0-87371-703-1); Vol. 1. 1991. ring bd. 235.00 (0-87371-687-6, L687) Lewis Pubs.

National Toxicology Program's Chemical Database, Vol. 2: Chemical & Physical Properties, Vol. 2. Lawrence H. Keith & Douglas B. Walters. 1991. 235.00 (0-87371-688-4, L688) Lewis Pubs.

National Toxicology Program's Chemical Database, Vol. 3: Standards & Regulations, Vol. 3. Lawrence H. Keith & Douglas B. Walters. 1991. 199.00 (0-87371-689-2, L689) Lewis Pubs.

National Toxicology Program's Chemical Database, Vol. 4: Medical Hazards & Symptoms of Exposure, Vol. 4. Lawrence H. Keith & Douglas B. Walters. 1991. ring bd. 220.00 (0-87371-690-6, L690) Lewis Pubs.

National Toxicology Program's Chemical Database, Vol. 5: Medical First Aid. Lawrence H. Keith & Douglas B. Walters. 1992. 94p. lib. bdg. 335.00 incl. 3.5 hd (0-87371-707-4); Vol. 5. 1991. 199.00 (0-87371-691-4, L691) Lewis Pubs.

National Toxicology Program's Chemical Database, Vol. 6: Personal Protective Equipment, Vol. 6. Lawrence H. Keith & Douglas B. Walters. 1991. ring bd. 220.00 (0-87371-692-2, L692) Lewis Pubs.

National Toxicology Program's Chemical Database, Vol. 7: Hazardous Properties & Uses. Lawrence H. Keith & Douglas B. Walters. 1992. 84p. lib. bdg. 359.00 (0-87371-709-0); Vol. 7. 1991. ring bd. 220.00 (0-87371-693-0, L693) Lewis Pubs.

National Toxicology Program's Chemical Database, Vol. 8: Shipping Classifications & Regulations, Vol. 8. Lawrence H. Keith & Douglas B. Walters. 1991. ring bd. 220.00 (0-87371-694-9, L694) Lewis Pubs.

National Toxicology Program's Chemical Solubility Compendium. Lawrence H. Keith & Douglas B. Walters. 1991. 448p. lib. bdg. 185.00 (0-87371-653-1, L653) Lewis Pubs.

National Toxicology Program's Chemical Solubility Database. Lawrence H. Keith & Douglas B. Walters. 1991. 32p. lib. bdg. 260.00 incl. 3.5 hd, 5.25 hd (0-87371-652-3, L652) Lewis Pubs.

National Tuberculosis Association, 1904-1954: A Study of the Voluntary Health Movement in the United States. Richard H. Shryock. Ed. by Barbara G. Rosenkrantz. 1977. LC 76-40645. (Public Health in America Ser.). (Illus.). reprint ed. lib. bdg. 35.95 (0-405-09831-6) Ayer.

National Veterinary Boards (NBE) (NVB) Jack Rudman. (Admission Test Ser.: ATS-50). pap. 69.95 (0-8373-5050-6) Nat Learn.

National Veterinary Boards (NBE) (NVB) Anatomy, Physiology, Pathology, Pt. 1. Jack Rudman. (Admission Test Ser.: ATS-50A). pap. 39.95 (0-8373-6960-6) Nat Learn.

National Veterinary Boards (NBE) (NVB) Pt. II: Pharmacology, Therapeutics, Parasitology, Hygiene. Jack Rudman. (Admission Test Ser.: Vol. 50B). 59.95 (0-8373-6986-X);Pt. 2. 1994. pap. 39.95 (0-8373-6961-4) Nat Learn.

National Veterinary Boards (NBE) (NVB) Pt. III: Physical Diagnosis, Medicine, Surgery, Pt. 3. Jack Rudman. 1994. (Admission Test Ser.: ATS-50C). pap. 39.95 (0-8373-6962-2) Nat Learn.

National Veterinary Boards (NBE) (NVE) Pt. III: Physical Diagnosis, Medicine, Surgery. Jack Rudman. (Admission Test Ser.: Vol. 50C). 59.95 (0-8373-6987-8) Nat Learn.

Nation's Health. Lee & Estes. 2nd ed. 1989. (Illus.). (C). pap. text 25.00 (0-86720-423-0, 423-0) Jones & Bartlett.

Nation's Health. Philip R. Lee & Carroll L. Estes. 3rd ed. 1990. (Illus.). 576p. pap. text 37.50 (0-86720-428-1, 428-1) Jones & Bartlett.

Nation's Health. Ed. by Philip R. Lee & Carroll L. Estes. 4th ed. 1994. LC 93-41200. 432p. pap. 46.25 (0-86720-840-6) Jones & Bartlett.

Nation's Health. Philip R. Lee et al. 5th ed. 1997. LC 97-5162. (Health Science Ser.). (Illus.). 448p. pap. text 52.95 (0-7637-0405-9, 0405-9) Jones & Bartlett.

Nation's Physician Workforce: Options for Balancing Supply & Requirements. Institute of Medicine Staff. Ed. by Kathleen N. Lohr et al. 1996. LC 95-72889. 124p. pap. text 22.00 (0-309-05431-1) Natl Acad Pr.

Nationwide Medical Transcription Service Directory 2000. Compiled by Denise M. Schultheis. 2000. 304p. pap. 39.95 (1-877810-88-6) Rayve Prodns.

Native American Healing. Howard Badhand. 2001. LC 2001-35777. 160p. pap. 11.95 (0-658-00727-0, Keats Pubng) McGraw-Hill Trade.

Native American Medicine: Indians of North America. Nancy Bonvillain. 1997. LC 97-11427. (Indians of North America Ser.). (Illus.). 120p. (YA). (gr. 8 up). lib. bdg. 19.95 (0-7910-4041-0) Chelsea Hse.

Native American Voices: Native American Health Educators Speak Out. Ed. by Audrey M. Koertvelyessy. 1997. 29.95 (0-88737-677-0, 14-6770, NLN Pr) Natl League Nurse.

Native Aquatic Bacteria: Enumeration, Activity & Ecology - STP 695. Ed. by J. W. Costerton & R. R. Colwell. 1979. 219p. 25.00 (0-8031-0526-6, STP695) ASTM.

Native Healer: Initiation into an Ancient Art. Lake Medicine Grizzly Bear. 1991. pap. 13.00 (0-8356-0667-8, Quest) Theos Pub Hse.

Native North American Shamanism: An Annotated Bibliography, 38. Compiled by Shelley Anne Osterreich. 1998. LC 98-28015. (Bibliographies & Indexes in American History Ser.: Vol. 38). 128p. lib. bdg. 65.00 (0-313-30168-9, Greenwood Pr) Greenwood.

Native Plants, Native Healing. Tis Mal Crow. 2000. LC 00-46573. (Illus.). 143p. pap. 12.95 (1-57067-105-2) Book Pub Co.

Native Society & Disease in Colonial Ecuador. Suzanne A. Alchon. 1992. (Cambridge Latin American Studies: No. 71). (Illus.). 165p. (C). text 54.95 (0-521-40186-0) Cambridge U Pr.

Natnl Fund Nrsg/ CC+ Comm. A. Kozier. 1995. text 61.88 (0-201-30253-5) Addison-Wesley.

Natriuretic Peptides & Congestive Heart Failure. C. Wei. 1998. (Medical Intelligence Unit Ser.). 200p. (C). 89.95 (0-412-11401-1) Chapman & Hall.

Natural Alternatives (O. T. C.) to Over-the-Counter & Prescription Drugs. Michael T. Murray. 1998. 384p. reprint ed. pap. 15.00 (0-688-16627-X, Quil) HarperTrade.

Natural Alternatives (O. T. C.) to Over-the-Counter & Prescription Drugs. Michael T. Murray. 1994. LC 93-14152. 383p. 25.00 (0-688-12358-9, Wm Morrow) Morrow Avon.

Natural Alternatives (p Rozac) to Prozac. Michael T. Murray. 1996. LC 95-47489. 192p. 20.00 (0-688-14684-8, Wm Morrow) Morrow Avon.

Natural Alternatives to Antibiotics. Ray C. Wunderlich, Jr. 1995. (Good Health Guides). 47p. pap. 3.95 (0-87983-684-9, 36849K, Keats Pubng) McGraw-Hill Trade.

Natural Alternatives to HRT Cookbook: Understanding Estrogen & Foods That Benefit Your Health. Marilyn Glenville. 2001. (Illus.). 192p. pap. 17.95 (1-58761-025-6) Celestial Arts.

Natural Alternatives to Prozac. Michael T. Murray. 1998. 240p. pap. 10.00 (0-688-16628-8, Quil) HarperTrade.

Natural & Artificial Control of Hearing & Balance. Ed. by J. H. Allum et al. 1993. LC 93-11042. (Progress in Brain Research Ser.: Vol. 97). 452p. 273.50 (0-444-81252-0) Elsevier.

Natural & Artificial Minds. Ed. by Robert G. Burton. 1993. LC 92-35020. (SUNY Series, Scientific Studies in Natural & Artificial Intelligence). 245p. (C). text 64.50 (0-7914-1507-4); pap. text 22.95 (0-7914-1508-2) State U NY Pr.

Natural & Healthy Childhood. Jessie R. Thomson. (Orig.). pap. 12.95 (0-8464-4257-4) Beekman Pubs.

Natural & Herbal Family Remedies. Cynthia Black. 1997. LC 96-53552. (Storey Publishing Bulletin Ser.: Vol. A-168). pap. 2.95 (0-88266-716-5) Storey Bks.

Natural & Living Biomaterials. Ed. by Garth W. Hastings & Paul Ducheyne. 1984. 192p. 105.00 (0-8493-6264-4, QP88, CRC Reprint) Franklin.

Natural & Mesmeric Clairvoyance: With the Practical Application of Mesmerism in Surgery & Medicine. James Esdaile. 1975. LC 75-7378. (Perspectives in Psychical Research Ser.). reprint ed. 26.95 (0-405-07028-4) Ayer.

Natural & Synthetic Neurotoxins. Ed. by Alan L. Harvey. 1993. (Neuroscience Perspectives Ser.). (Illus.). 386p. text 83.00 (0-12-329870-9) Acad Pr.

Natural Answers for Women's Health Questions: A Comprehensive A-Z Guide to Drug-Free Mind-Body Remedies. D. Lindsey Berkson. 2002. LC 2001-57563. 496p. pap. 15.00 (0-684-86514-9, Fireside) S&S Trade Pap.

Natural Antidepressants. Syd Baumel. 1998. (Good Health Guides). 48p. pap. 3.95 (0-87983-900-7, 39007K, Keats Pubng) McGraw-Hill Trade.

Natural Antioxidants: Chemistry, Health. Ed. by Feridoon Shahibi. 1997. (Illus.). 432p. lib. bdg. 105.00 (0-935315-77-2, PC111) Am Oil Chemists.

Natural Antioxidants in Human Health & Disease. Ed. by Balz Frei. 1994. LC 94-7646. (Illus.). 588p. text 104.00 (0-12-266975-4) Acad Pr.

Natural Asthma & Allergy Management. Celeste White. 1997. LC 96-95414. iv, 114p. (Orig.). pap. 8.95 (0-9653024-1-5) Keswick Hse.

Natural Auto Antibodies: Their Physiologocal Role & Regulatory Significance. Yehuda Shoenfeld. 1992. 368p. lib. bdg. 219.00 (0-8493-5501-X, QR186) CRC Pr.

Natural Behavior in Humans & Animals. American Psychological Association Staff. 1981. (Human Behavior Curriculum Project Ser.). 55p. (Orig.). tchr. ed. 9.95 (0-8077-2614-1); pap. text 3.95 (0-8077-2613-3) Tchrs Coll.

Natural Cat Care. Bruce Fogel. 1997. LC 98-31107. (Illus.). 160p. 24.95 (0-7894-4123-3) DK Pub Inc.

Natural Childbirth after Cesarean: A Practical Guide. Karis Crawford & Johanne Walters. 1996. (Illus.). 218p. (Orig.). pap. 14.95 (0-86542-490-X) Blackwell Sci.

Natural Childbirth & the Christian Family see Joy of Natural Childbirth: Fifth Edition of Natural Childbirth & the Christian Family

Natural Childbirth Self-Taught. Chan Thomas. 1993. 111p. (Orig.). otabind 7.95 (1-884600-00-X) Bengal Tiger.

Natural Childbirth the Bradley Way. Susan McCutcheon & Peter Rosegg. rev. ed. 256p. 1999. pap. 16.95 (0-452-27658-6); 1996. LC 96-333. (Illus.). pap. 17.95 (0-452-27659-4) Dutton Plume (Plume).

Natural Choices for Menopause. Marilyn Glenville. 1999. 256p. mass mkt. 5.99 (0-312-97013-7) St Martin.

Natural Cold/Flu Defense. Woodland Publishing Staff. 1997. (Woodland Health Ser.). 32p. pap. 3.95 (1-885670-90-7) Woodland UT.

Natural Compounds in Cancer Therapy. John C. Boik. 2001. (Illus.). 521p. pap. 32.00 (0-9648280-1-4) OR Med Pr.

Natural Conception Through Personal Hormone Monitoring. Ed. by J. Bonnar. 1996. (Illus.). 68p. 27.95 (1-85070-718-9, Parthenon Pbng) CRC Pr.

Natural Cures & Gentle Medicines: That Work Better Than Dangerous Drugs or Risky Surgery. FC and A Publishing Staff. 2000. 368p. 27.96 (1-890957-35-6); pap. 9.99 (1-890957-36-4) FC&A Pub.

Natural Cures for the Common Cold: Powerful, Drug-Free Remedies Proven to Work. Carol Turkington. 1999. LC 98-35534. (Health Ser.). (Illus.). 216p. pap. 11.95 (0-936197-38-2) Harbor Pr.

Natural Death with Dignity: Protecting Your Right to Refuse Medical Treatment. Lee R. Kerr & Delnetta J. Kerr. 1991. 170p. (Orig.). 29.95 (0-9628237-1-6); pap. 19.95 (0-9628237-0-8) Kerr Pubns.

Natural Dental Wellness. Soaring Bear. 1980. (Illus.). 90p. (Orig.). pap. 9.95 (0-9607518-0-7) Dental-Info.

Natural Dog Care: A Complete Guide to Holistic Health Care for Dogs. Celeste Yarnall. 1998. LC 98-8453. (Illus.). 320p. pap. 16.95 (1-885203-47-0) Jrny Editions.

Natural Estrogen Diet: Healthy Recipes for Perimenopause & Menopause. Lana Liew et al. 1999. LC 98-52737. (Illus.). x, 212p. reprint ed. pap. 13.95 (0-89793-246-3) Hunter Hse.

Natural Eye Care: An Encyclopedia: Complementary Treatments for Improving & Saving Your Eyes. Marc Grossman & Glen Swartwout. 1999. LC 98-55416. (Illus.). x, 196p. pap. 16.95 (0-87983-704-7, 37047K, Keats Pubng) McGraw-Hill Trade.

Natural Foods: The Safe Way to Health. Otto Carque. 1998. (Illus.). 350p. reprint ed. pap. text 35.00 (0-87556-858-0) Saifer.

Natural Foods & Nutrition: A Report. Center for Self-Sufficiency, Research Division Staff. 1983. 50p. ring bd. 39.95 (0-910811-67-9) Ctr Self Suff.

Natural Garden Book: A Holistic Approach to Gardening. Peter Harper & Jeremy Light. 1994. LC 93-19439. 288p. pap. 25.00 (0-671-74323-6, Fireside) S&S Trade Pap.

Natural Goodness of Man: The Study of Behavior Without a Goal. Norman R. Maier. 1982. LC 81-20092. (Illus.). 264p. reprint ed. lib. bdg. 72.50 (0-313-23340-3, MAFRU, Greenwood Pr) Greenwood.

Natural Guide to Colon Health. Louise Tenney. 1997. 224p. pap. text 12.95 (1-885670-45-1) Woodland UT.

Natural Guide to Good Health: Nutritional Balance for a Life Time. Mark Curley & Sandra Curley. 1990. LC 90-70943. 185p. (Orig.). pap. 14.95 (0-9626875-9-6) Supreme Pub.

Natural Guide to Treating High Blood Pressure. S. Streicher-Lankin. 1998. pap. 9.99 (0-7615-1554-2) Prima Pub.

Natural Guide to Women's Health. Lynda Wharton. 1996. LC 95-81600. 270p. 6.98 (1-56731-095-8, MJF Bks) Fine Comms.

Natural Healing: Alternative/Complementary Resources for Total Health. S. Jeanne Gunn. 1999. LC 98-72445. (Illus.). 288p. pap. 19.95 (1-58151-013-6) BookPartners.

Natural Healing & Herbs: A Reference Guide in the Proper Dosage of Herbal Preparations. 1991. lib. bdg. 250.00 (0-8490-5105-3) Gordon Pr.

Natural Healing & Prevention Secrets. James Robinson & Nancy Nielson. pap. 19.95 (0-9638596-1-7) Amer Pubng.

Natural Healing for Babies & Children. Aviva J. Romm. 1996. (Illus.). 256p. (Orig.). pap. text 16.95 (0-89594-786-2) Crossing Pr.

Natural Healing for Dogs. Susanne Bonisch. 1996. LC 96-19222. (Illus.). 96p. pap. 10.95 (0-8069-8120-2) Sterling.

Natural Healing for Dogs A-Z. Cheryl Schwartz. 2001. (Illus.). 156p. pap. 11.95 (1-56170-793-7, L478) Hay House.

Natural Healing for Dogs & Cats. Diane Stein. 1993. (Illus.). 190p. pap. 16.95 (0-89594-614-9) Crossing Pr.

Natural Healing for Parasites. Anne L. Gittleman. 1995. 16p. pap. 2.95 (0-9647080-0-0) Healing Wisdom.

Natural Healing for Schizophrenia: A Compendium of Nutritional Methods. Eva Edelman. 1996. LC 96-83505. (Illus.). 208p. (Orig.). (C). pap. 24.95 (0-9650976-2-5) Borage Bks.

Natural Healing for Schizophrenia: A Compendium of Nutritional Methods see Natural Healing for Schizophrenia & Other Common Mental Disorders

Natural Healing for Schizophrenia & Other Common Mental Disorders. Eva Edelman. 2nd rev. ed. 1998. LC 98-92417. Orig. Title: Natural Healing for Schizophrenia: A Compendium of Nutritional Methods. (Illus.). 256p. pap. 24.95 (0-9650976-6-8) Borage Bks.

***Natural Healing for Schizophrenia & Other Common Mental Disorders.** Eva Edelman. 3rd rev. ed. 2001. Orig. Title: Natural Healing for Schizophrenia: A Compendium of Nutritional Methods. (Illus.). 256p. pap. 26.95 (0-9650976-7-6) Borage Bks.

Natural Healing for Women: Caring for Yourself with Herbs, Homeopathy & Essential Oils. Susan Curtis & Romy Fraser. 1992. 422p. pap. (0-04-440645-2) Pandora GBR. *Dist:* Routldge.

Natural Healing Handbook: Get Back to Health . . . Naturally. Beth M. Ley. 2nd ed. 1995. 328p. pap. 14.95 (0-9642703-1-5) B L Pubns.

Natural Healing in Gynecology: A Manual for Women. Rina Nissim. 1986. 220p. pap. (0-86358-069-6) Pandora GBR. *Dist:* Harper SF.

Natural Healing Remedies 1999: The Smartest, Quickest Ways to Guard Your Health. Prevention Magazine Health Book Staff. 1999. LC 99-206905. (Illus.). (1-57954-054-6) Rodale Pr Inc.

Natural Healing Secrets: An A to Z Guide to the Best Home Remedies. Random House Value Publishing Staff. 1998. 176p. 8.99 (0-517-16046-3) Random Hse Value.

Natural Healing Through Ayurveda. Subhash Ranade. 1993. 238p. pap. 14.95 (1-878423-13-4) Morson Pub.

Natural Healing Through Cell Salts. Skye Weintraub. 1996. pap. text 12.95 (1-885670-29-X) Woodland UT.

Natural Healing with Aromatherapy. PH Editorial Staff. 1996. (C). pap. text 5.95 (0-13-258963-X) P-H.

Natural Healing with Chinese Herbs. Hong-yen Hsu. 1993. 30.00 (0-941942-05-8) Orient Heal Arts.

Natural Healing with Herbs: The Complete Reference Book for the Use of Herbs. Humbart Santillo. Ed. by Subhuti Dharmananda. 1993. LC 84-553. (Illus.). 408p. reprint ed. pap. 16.95 (0-934252-08-4) Hohm Pr.

Natural Healing with Tibb Medicine: Medicine of the Prophet. Ibn A. Al-Jawziyya. Tr. by Muhammad M. Al-Akili. 1994. LC 92-85137. 384p. (Orig.). (C). pap. 16.95 (1-879405-07-5) Pearl Pub Hse.

Natural Health at 50+ The Vital Guide to Living Longer & Looking Good. Christina Scott-Moncrieff. 2001. LC 00-42540. (Illus.). 192p. 24.95 (0-7621-0294-2) RD Assn.

Natural Health First-Aid Guide: The Definitive Handbook of Natural Remedies for Treating Minor Emergencies. Natural Health Magazine Editors & Mark Mayeell. 1994. LC 93-11906. 560p. pap. 14.00 (0-671-79273-3) PB.

Natural Health First-Aid Guide: The Definitive Handbook of Natural Remedies for Treating Minor Emergencies. Ed. by Mark Mayell. 2000. 544p. reprint ed. text 24.00 (0-7881-6986-6) DIANE Pub.

Natural Health for African Americans: The Physician's Guide. Marcellus A. Walker & Kenneth B. Singleton. 1999. LC 98-24371. (Physicians' Guide to Healing Ser.). 320p. pap. (0-446-67369-2) Warner.

Natural Health Guide to Beating Supergerms: Use Vitamins & Nutrients to Turn Your Body into the Ultimate Germ Killer. Richard P. Huemer et al. 1997. LC 96-29498. 368p. per. 14.00 (0-671-53764-4) PB.

Natural Health Guide to Headache Relief. Ed. by Peter Maas. 1997. LC 97-144755. 304p. per. 14.00 (0-671-51899-2, PB Trade Paper) PB.

***Natural Health Magazine Complete Guide to Safe Herbs: What Every Consumer Should Know about Interactions & Side Effects for Hundreds of Herbs, Drugs, Supplements, & Foods.** Chris D. Meletis & Rachel Streit. 2001. LC 2001-42263. (Illus.). 256p. 29.95 (0-7894-8073-5) DK Pub Inc.

Natural Health, Natural Medicine. Houghton Mifflin Company Staff. rev. ed. 1998. LC 94-42040. 370p. pap. 13.00 (0-395-91155-9) HM.

Natural Healthcare for Your Child: Trustworthy Information on the Prevention, Causes & Treatment of the Diseases & Ailments Which are Common from Birth Through the Teenage Years. Phylis A. Austin et al. 1990. (Illus.). 268p. (Orig.). pap. 9.95 (1-878726-01-3) Fam Hlth Pubns.

Natural History of a Delinquent Career. Clifford R. Shaw. 1969. LC 68-56042. (Illus.). 280p. reprint ed. lib. bdg. 68.00 (0-8371-0654-0, SHDC, Greenwood Pr) Greenwood.

Natural History of Alcoholism. George E. Vaillant. 1983. LC 82-11696. (Illus.). 384p. 32.00 (0-674-60375-3) HUP.

Natural History of Alcoholism: Causes, Patterns, & Paths to Recovery. George E. Vaillant. 1985. 384p. pap. text 14.95 (*0-674-60376-1*) HUP.

Natural History of Alcoholism Revisited. George E. Vaillant. 1995. LC 94-41749. (Illus.). 384p. text 46.50 (*0-674-60377-X*, VAINAR); pap. text 18.00 (*0-674-60378-8*, VAINAY) HUP.

Natural History of Cerebral Palsy. Bronson Crothers & Richmond S. Paine. 1991. (Classics in Developmental Medicine Ser.: No. 2). (Illus.). 300p. (C). text (*0-521-41327-3*) Mc Keith Pr GBR. *Dist:* Cambridge U Pr.

Natural History of Coronary Atherosclerosis. Constantin Velican & Doina Velican. 1989. LC 88-8128. 416p. 242.00 (*0-8493-6935-5*, RC685, CRC Reprint) Franklin.

Natural History of Homosexuality. Francis M. Mondimore. 1996. LC 96-16191. (Illus.). 252p. pap. 17.95 (*0-8018-5440-7*) Johns Hopkins.

Natural History of Mania, Depression, & Schizophrenia. George Winokur & Ming T. Tsuang. 1996. 336p. text 44.50 (*0-88048-726-7*, 8726) Am Psychiatric.

Natural History of Orthopaedic Disease: A Gatekeeper's Guide. Ed. by Lewis Cozen. 1993. (Illus.). 600p. (Orig.). 20.00 (*0-9637929-0-3*) Dr L Cozen Pub.

Natural History of Rabies. Ed. by George M. Baer. 2nd ed. 1991. 640p. 375.00 (*0-8493-6760-3*, QR201) CRC Pr.

Natural History of the Mammalia. George R. Waterhouse. Ed. by Keir B. Sterling. 1978. LC 77-83843. (Biologists & Their World Ser.). (Illus.). reprint ed. lib. bdg. 93.95 (*0-405-10739-0*) Ayer.

Natural History of Viruses. Christopher Andrewes. 1967. (World Naturalist Ser.). (Illus.). (C). 8.00 (*0-393-06277-5*) Norton.

Natural History of Vision. Nicholas J. Wade. 1998. LC 97-22697. (Bradford Book Ser.). (Illus.). 486p. 65.00 (*0-262-23194-8*, Bradford Bks) MIT Pr.

Natural Home Pharmacy see Medicina Natural en el Hogar

Natural Home Physician. Powell. 1975. 164p. (*0-85032-092-5*) C W Daniel GBR. *Dist:* Natl Bk Netwk.

Natural Home Physician. Eric F. Powell. 288p. pap. 17.95 (*0-8464-4316-3*) Beekman Pubs.

Natural Home Physician. Eric F. Powell. 1980. (*0-85032-189-1*) C W Daniel GBR. *Dist:* Natl Bk Netwk.

Natural Home Remedies: A Step-by-Step Guide. Karen Hurrell. 1997. LC 97-18373. (In a Nutshell Ser.). (Illus.). 64p. 7.95 (*1-86204-108-3*) Element MA.

***Natural Hormone Balance: Look Younger Feel Stronger & Live Life with Exuberance.** Suzannah Olivier. 2001. 192p. pap. 10.00 (*0-7432-1869-8*) S&S Trade.

Natural Hormone Balance for Women: Look Younger, Feel Stronger, & Live Life with Exuberance. Uzzi Reiss & Martin Zucker. 2001. LC 00-49139. (Illus.). xxiii, 294p. 26.95 (*0-7434-0665-6*, PB Hardcover) PB.

Natural Hormone Replacement: For Women over 45. Jonathan V. Wright & John Morgenthaler. 1997. LC 97-65916. (Illus.). 128p. pap. 9.95 (*0-9627418-0-9*) Smart Pubns CA.

Natural Immunity. David Nelson. 1990. 844p. text 132.00 (*0-12-514555-1*) Acad Pr.

Natural Immunity & Biological Response International Symposium, Honolulu, Nov. 1985. Ed. by Eva Lotzova. 1985. (Journal: Vol. 4, No. 5, 1985). 64p. pap. 28.00 (*3-8055-4243-7*) S Karger.

Natural Immunity, Cancer & Biological Response Modification. Ed. by Eva Lotzova. 1986. (Illus.). xii, 324p. 191.50 (*3-8055-4412-X*) S Karger.

Natural Immunity to Normal Hemopoietic Cells. Bent Rolstad. 1993. 256p. 189.00 (*0-8493-4837-4*, QR185) CRC Pr.

Natural Inheritance. Francis Galton. 1989. LC 72-1633. reprint ed. 40.00 (*0-404-08129-0*) AMS Pr.

Natural Killer Cell & Its Interaction with Immune & Non-Immune Cell: Second Meeting of the Society for Natural Immunity, Taormina, May 1994. Ed. by A. Santoni & C. Riccardi. 1994. (Journal: Vol. 13, No. 4, 1994). (Illus.). 70p. pap. 38.50 (*3-8055-5999-2*) S Karger.

Natural Killer Cells: Biology & Clinical Application, Sixth International Natural Killer Cell Workshop, Goslar, July 1989. Ed. by R. E. Schmidt. 1990. (Illus.). xii, 318p. 257.50 (*3-8055-5200-9*) S Karger.

Natural Killer Cells: Their Definition, Functions, Lineage & Regulation. Ed. by Eva Lotzova. 1993. (Journal: Vol. 12, Nos. 4-5, 1993). (Illus.). 128p. pap. 40.00 (*3-8055-5875-9*) S Karger.

Natural Killer Cells & Host Defense. Ed. by Edwin W. Ades & C. Lopez. 1989. (Illus.). xiv, 302p. 256.75 (*3-8055-4791-9*) S Karger.

***Natural Language Processing in Medicine: Design, Implementation & Evaluation of an Analyser for Dutch.** Peter Spyns. 2000. (Illus.). 355p. pap. (*90-5867-069-4*) Leuven Univ BEL. *Dist:* Coronet Bks.

Natural Limitations of Youth: The Predispositions That Shape the Adolescent Character. John J. Mitchell. 1998. LC 97-40928. (Developments in Clinical Psychology Ser.). 77.00 (*1-56750-372-1*); pap. 39.50 (*1-56750-373-X*) Greenwood (Ablex).

Natural Medicine. Shaykh Nazim Al-Naqshbandi. 2000. 64p. (C). pap. (*1-898863-10-5*) Zero Prods GBR. *Dist:* Kazi Pubns.

Natural Medicine & Medicare: How to Solve the Medicare Crisis & Improve Our Health Care. Joseph E. Pizzorno. 1997. pap. text 16.00 (*1-880831-18-X*) Aletheia Pr.

Natural Medicine Chest & Home Remedies Handbook. Ed. by Denise Domb. 1994. LC 94-220557. 72p. pap. 4.95 (*0-9636334-8-1*) AlternMed Bks.

Natural Medicine Childre. Julian Scott. 1990. LC 89-63649. 192p. pap. 15.00 (*0-380-75876-8*, Avon Bks) Morrow Avon.

***Natural Medicine First Aid Remedies: Self-Care Treatments for 100 Common Conditions.** Stephanie Marohn. 2001. (Illus.). 446p. pap. 22.95 (*1-57174-218-2*) Hampton Roads Pub Co.

Natural Medicine for Allergies: The Best Alternative Methods for Quick Relief. Glenn S. Rothfeld & Suzanne LeVert. 1996. LC 96-2738. 288p. pap. 13.95 (*0-87596-286-6*) Rodale Pr Inc.

Natural Medicine for Arthritis: The Best Alternative Methods for Relieving Pain & Stiffness: from Food & Herbs to Acupuncture & Homeopathy. Glenn S. Rothfeld & Suzanne LeVert. 1996. LC 96-13305. 288p. pap. 13.95 (*0-87596-287-4*) Rodale Pr Inc.

Natural Medicine for Back Pain. Glenn S. Rothfeld & Suzanne LeVert. l.t. ed. 1997. LC 96-39213. (Spec-Hall Ser.). 328p. lib. bdg. 23.95 (*0-7838-2026-7*, Macmillan Ref) Gale.

Natural Medicine for Back Pain: The Best Alternative Methods for Banishing Backache from Acupressure & Chiropractic to Nutrition & Yoga. Glenn Rothfeld et al. 1996. LC 95-31025. (Illus.). 224p. (Orig.). pap. 11.95 (*0-87596-288-2*) Rodale Pr Inc.

Natural Medicine for Heart Disease: The Best Alternative Methods to Prevent & Treat High Cholesterol, High Blood Pressure, Stroke, Chest Pain, & Other Circulatory Problems. Glenn Rothfeld et al. 1996. LC 95-24445. 233p. (Orig.). pap. 11.95 (*0-87596-289-0*) Rodale Pr Inc.

Natural Medicine vs. Orthodox Medicine. Karen Bradstreet. 1997. (Woodland Health Ser.). 32p. pap. 3.95 (*1-58054-014-7*) Woodland UT.

Natural Medicines & Cures Your Doctor Never Tells You About. FC and A Publishing Staff. 1999. 366p. pap. 9.99 (*0-915099-76-4*); 1998. 370p. 27.96 (*0-915099-81-0*) FC&A Pub.

Natural Medicines Comprehensive Database. Therapeutic Research Faculty Staff. 1999. 164p. pap. 92.00 (*0-9676136-0-4*); 2nd rev. ed. pap. 92.00 (*0-9676136 2 0*) Theraptc Res.

Natural Medicines Comprehensive Database. Therapeutic Research Faculty Staff. Ed. by Jeff M. Jellin. 3rd rev. ed. 1999. 1530p. pap. 92.00 (*0-9676136-4-7*) Theraptc Res.

Natural Menopause. Miriam Stoppard. 1998. LC 97-48453. (DK Healthcare Ser.). (Illus.). 96p. pap. 7.95 (*0-7894-3090-8*) DK Pub Inc.

Natural Menopause: The Complete Guide. Susan Perry et al. Ed. by James Broll. 2nd rev. ed. 2000. LC 96-27094. 272p. pap. 16.00 (*0-201-47987-7*) Perseus Bks Grp.

Natural Menopause: The Complete Guide to a Woman's Most Misunderstood Passage. Susan Perry & Katherine A. O'Hanlan. 1993. (Illus.). 224p. pap. 10.95 (*0-201-62477-X*) Addison-Wesley.

Natural Mind: An Investigation of Drugs & Higher Consciousness. Andrew Weil. 1998. LC 98-28464. 240p. pap. 14.00 (*0-395-91156-7*) HM.

Natural Mothering: A Guide to Holistic Therapies for Pregnancy, Birth, & Early Childhood. Nicky Wesson. 1997. LC 97-10399. (Illus.). 240p. pap. 14.95 (*0-89281-733-X*, Heal Arts VT) Inner Tradit.

Natural Options: A Natural Healthcare Guide. Barbara H. Sharp. 1995. (Illus.). 112p. (Orig.). pap. 12.95 (*0-9649166-4-9*, 1) Nat Hlth Res.

***Natural Pain Relief: A Practical Handbook for Self-Help.** Jan Sadler. 2001. pap. (*0-85207-350-X*) C W Daniel.

Natural Pain Relief: A Practical Handbook for Self-Help. Jan Sadler. 1997. LC 96-43238. 160p. pap. 10.95 (*1-85230-924-5*) Element MA.

Natural Pain Relief: Techniques for Miraculous Healing. Scott Lux. 1997. ix, 112p. pap. 10.95 (*0-9609324-1-0*) Wisdom of Pain.

Natural Painkillers. Nikki Bradford. 1998. pap. (*0-7528-1603-9*) Orion GBR. *Dist:* Trafalgar.

Natural Path for Horses - A Guide to Homeopathy & Other Alternative Therapies. Cheyanne West. 1999. LC 99-93105. 257p. pap. (*0-9619435-2-1*) A Natural Path.

Natural Pet Cures: The Definitive Guide to Natural Remedies for Dogs & Cats. John Heinerman. 1998. LC 98-18803. (Illus.). 352p. 26.95 (*0-13-258484-0*) P-H.

Natural Pharmacist. Prima Publishing Staff. 1999. text 491.32 (*0-7615-9016-1*) Prima Pub.

Natural Pharmacist: Complementary Treatments for Diabetes. Kathi Head. 2000. LC 98-49613. (Natural Pharmacist Ser.). 208p. pap. 6.99 (*0-7615-1755-3*, Prima Health) Prima Pub.

Natural Pharmacist: Natural Treatment for Colds & Flus. Anna M. Barton. 2000. LC 99-57540. (Natural Pharmacist Ser.). 176p. pap. 9.99 (*0-7615-2469-X*, Prima Health) Prima Pub.

Natural Pharmacist: Natural Treatment for Diabetes. Prima Publishing Staff. 2000. (Natural Pharmacist Ser.). 176p. pap. 9.99 (*0-7615-2463-0*, Prima Health) Prima Pub.

Natural Pharmacist: Natural Treatments for Menopause. Prima Publishing Staff. 2000. (Natural Pharmacist Ser.). 176p. pap. 9.99 (*0-7615-2471-1*, Prima Health) Prima Pub.

Natural Pharmacist: Natural Treatments to Improve Memory. Prima Publishing Staff. 2000. (Natural Pharmacist Ser.). 144p. pap. 9.99 (*0-7615-2465-7*, Prima Health) Prima Pub.

Natural Pharmacist: Reducing Cancer Risk. Richard Harkness. 2000. LC 98-48205. (Illus.). 208p. pap. 6.99 (*0-7615-1557-7*, TNP) Prima Pub.

Natural Pharmacist: Treating Osteoporosis. Sheila Dunn-Merritt et al. 2000. LC 00-105937. (Natural Pharmacist Ser.). (Illus.). 208p. pap. 6.99 (*0-7615-1618-2*, Prima Health) Prima Pub.

Natural Pharmacist: Treating Varicose Veins & Improving Circulation. Richard Conant. 2000. LC 2001-133025. (Natural Pharmacist Ser.). 192p. pap. 6.99 (*0-7615-1617-4*, Prima Health) Prima Pub.

Natural Pharmacist: Your Complete. Prima Publishing Staff. 1999. pap. 9.99 (*0-7615-2476-2*, Prima Health) Prima Pub.

Natural Pharmacist: Your Complete Guide. S. Fulder & B. Tabachnik. 1999. pap. 6.99 (*0-7615-1757-X*) Prima Pub.

Natural Pharmacist: Your Complete Guide to Ginko & Memory. Stephen Dentali. 2000. LC 98-50708. (Illus.). 176p. pap. 6.99 (*0-7615-1552-6*) Prima Pub.

Natural Pharmacist: Your Complete Guide to Herbs. Steven Bratman. 2000. LC 98-22156. (Natural Pharmacist Ser.). 274p. pap. 7.99 (*0-7615-1671-9*) Prima Pub.

Natural Pharmacist: Your Complete Guide to Memopause. Joanne Snow. 2000. LC 98-38774. (Natural Pharmacist Ser.). (Illus.). 208p. pap. 6.99 (*0-7615-1560-7*) Prima Pub.

Natural Pharmacist: Your Complete Guide to PMS. Helen Batchelder. 2000. LC 98-49608. (Natural Pharmacist Ser.). (Illus.). 192p. pap. 6.99 (*0-7615-1615-8*) Prima Pub.

Natural Pharmacist: Your Complete Guide to Reducing Cancer Risk. Anna M. Barton. 2000. LC 98-49607. (Natural Pharmacist Ser.). (Illus.). 192p. pap. 6.99 (*0-7615-1559-3*) Prima Pub.

Natural Pharmacist: Your Complete Guide to St John's Wort & Depression. Steven Bratman. 2000. LC 98-17492. (Natural Pharmacist Ser.). (Illus.). 176p. pap. 6.99 (*0-7615-1553-4*) Prima Pub.

Natural Pharmacist: Your Natural Health Guide to Arthritis. Gloria Bucco & Ron Hobbs. 2000. LC 98-50705. (Natural Pharmacist Ser.). (Illus.). 208p. pap. 6.99 (*0-7615-1556-9*) Prima Pub.

Natural Pharmacist - Natural Health Bible: From the Most Trusted Alternative Health Site in the World—Your A-Z Guide to Over 300 Conditions, Herbs, Vitamins & Supplements. David Kroll. Ed. by Steven Bratman. 2nd rev. ed. 2000. LC 00-53744. (Natural Pharmacist Ser.). (Illus.). 528p. pap. 19.99 (*0-7615-2448-7*, Prima Health) Prima Pub.

Natural Pharmacist: Drug-Herb-Vitamin Interactions Bible: From A-Z, Know the Dangers & Benefits of Combining Drugs, Herbs & Vitamins. Steven Bratman. Ed. by Richard Harkness & Steven Bratman. 2001. LC 00-66908. (Natural Pharmacist Ser.). 448p. pap. 19.99 (*0-7615-3013-4*, Prima Health) Prima Pub.

Natural Pharmacist Guide to Antioxidants. Lisa Chavis. 1999. pap. 9.99 (*0-7615-1561-5*) Prima Pub.

Natural Pharmacy: An Illustrated Guide to Natural Medicine. Miriam Polunin & Christopher Robbins. 1992. (Illus.). 144p. pap. 18.95 (*0-02-036041-X*) Mac Bks.

Natural Pharmacy: From the Top Experts in the Field, Your Essential Guide to Vitamins, Herbs, Minerals & Homeopathic Remedies. Schuyler W. Lininger, Jr. et al. rev. ed. 1999. LC 99-56624. 640p. pap. 24.95 (*0-7615-1967-X*) Prima Pub.

Natural Pharmacy Products: A Guide. 1991. lib. bdg. 77.95 (*0-8490-5118-5*) Gordon Pr.

Natural Pharmacy Products Guide. 1994. (Alternative Medicine Ser.). lib. bdg. 255.95 (*0-8490-9020-2*) Gordon Pr.

Natural Physician: Your Health Guide for Common Ailments. Mark Stengler. 2nd ed. 1997. 230p. pap. 12.95 (*0-920470-46-7*) Alive Bks.

Natural Pregnancy A-Z. Carolle Jean-Murat. 2001. (Illus.). 156p. pap. 11.95 (*1-56170-794-5*, L479) Hay House.

Natural Pregnancy A-Z. Carolle Jean Murat. 2000. LC 99-45797. (Illus.). 159p. 19.95 (*1-56170-709-0*, L461) Hay House.

Natural Pregnancy Book: Herbs, Nutrition, & Other Holistic Choices. Aviva J. Romm. 1997. LC 97-11514. (Illus.). 304p. pap. 19.95 (*0-89594-819-2*) Crossing Pr.

Natural Prescriptions for Women: What to Do - & When to Do It - to Solve Dozens of Female Health Problems - Without Drugs. For Women Editors & Susan Berg. 1998. LC 98-10112. (Illus.). 512p. 29.95 (*0-87596-433-8*) Rodale Pr Inc.

Natural Prescriptions for Women: What to Do - & When to Do It - to Solve More Than 100 Female Problems. Ed. by Prevention Magazine Health Book Staff & Susan Berg. 2000. LC 98-10112. (Illus.). 576p. pap. 17.95 (*0-87596-434-6*) Rodale Pr Inc.

Natural Procreation Alternatives: For Men with Low Sperm Counts in Childbearing Efforts. Howard W. Gabriel, III. 1987. 16p. 14.95 incl. audio (*0-936997-14-1*, T87-12) M & H Enter.

Natural Products: Rapid Utilization of Sources for Drug Discovery & Development. Ed. by Nancy Mulford. 1995. (Biomedical Library). 352p. pap. 795.00 (*1-57936-009-2*) Drug & Market Dev.

Natural Products As Antiviral Agents. C. K. Chu & H. G. Cutler. 1993. LC 92-27287. (Illus.). 288p. (C). text 95.00 (*0-306-44346-5*, Kluwer Plenum) Kluwer Academic.

Natural Products Drug Discovery: New Technologies to Increase Efficiency & Speed. Ed. by Wendy Mori. 1997. (Illus.). (Orig.). pap. (*1-57936-044-0*) Drug & Market Dev.

Natural Progesterone: The Multiple Roles of a Remarkable Hormone. John R. Lee. 4th rev. ed. 2000. (Illus.). VIII, 156p. pap. 12.00 (*0-9643737-3-4*) BLL Pubng.

Natural Progesterone: The Natural Way to Alleviate Symptoms of Menopause, PMS & Other Hormone-Related Problems. Anna Rushton & Shirley Bond. 1999. pap. (*0-7225-3766-2*) Thorsons GBR. *Dist:* Natl Bk Netwk.

Natural Progesterone: Wild Yam. Woodland Publishing Staff. 1999. pap. text 3.95 (*1-885670-25-7*) Woodland UT.

Natural Progesterone Cream. C. Norman Shealy. 1998. (Good Health Guides). 48p. pap. 3.95 (*0-87983-889-2*, 38892K, Keats Pubng) McGraw-Hill Trade.

Natural Prostate Cure: A Practical Guide to Using Diet & Supplements in a Healthy Prostate. Roger Mason. 2000. LC 00-134970. 72p. pap. 6.95 (*1-884820-61-1*) SAFE GOODS.

Natural Prozac: Leaning to Release Your Body's Own Anti-Depressants. Joel C. Robertson & Tom Monte. 1998. LC 96-33513. 240p. pap. 14.00 (*0-06-251354-0*) Harper SF.

Natural Psychology & Human Transformation. Na'im Akbar. rev. ed. 1995. 54p. pap. 8.00 (*0-935257-04-7*) Mind Prods Assocs.

Natural Radiation Environment III: Proceedings Ed. by Thomas F. Gesell et al. 1980. LC 80-607130. (DOE Symposium Ser.). 1789p. fiche 5.00 (*0-87079-458-2*, CONF-780422);Set. pap. 52.75 (*0-87079-129-X*, CONF-780422) DOE.

Natural Relief for Your Child's Asthma: A Guide to Controlling Asthma & Reducing Your Child's. Steven J. Bock et al. 1999. LC 98-43771. (Illus.). 304p. pap. 13.95 (*0-06-095289-X*) HarperCollins Pubs.

Natural Relief from Headaches, Insomnia & Stress. David Hoffmann. 1999. LC 99-25559. 240p. pap. 14.95 (*0-87983-982-1*, 39821K, Keats Pubng) McGraw-Hill Trade.

Natural Remedies. 1998. 208p. pap. (*0-14-019543-2*) Pnguin Bks Ltd GBR. *Dist:* Trafalgar.

Natural Remedies. Day. 1996. (Threshold Picture Guide Ser.: No. 35). (Illus.). 24p. pap. 12.00 (*1-872082-79-3*) Half Halt Pr.

Natural Remedies. Norman D. Ford. 1995. 352p. 8.98 (*0-88365-901-8*) Galahad Bks.

Natural Remedies: A Manual. Agatha M. Thrash et al. 1983. 172p. (Orig.). pap. 6.95 (*0-942658-05-1*) NLB.

Natural Remedies for Allergies: Safe Self-Help Measures for Treating a Wide Range of Modern Allergies. Paul Morgan. 1999. 128p. reprint ed. text 25.00 (*0-7881-6783-9*) DIANE Pub.

Natural Remedies for Better Health. Ingrid Sherman. 2nd rev. ed. 1994. LC 90-39261. (Illus.). 224p. pap. 8.95 (*0-87961-213-4*) Naturegraph.

Natural Remedies for Common Ailments. Constance Mellor. 1980. 134p. 17.95 (*0-8464-1073-7*) Beekman Pubs.

Natural Remedies for Common Ailments Handbook. Celeste White. 1996. LC 96-94470. ii, 63p. (Orig.). pap. 7.95 (*0-9653024-0-7*) Keswick Hse.

Natural Remedies for Dogs & Cats. C. J. Puotinen. 1998. LC 99-22191. (Keats Good Herb Guides). xii, 244p. pap. 14.95 (*0-87983-827-2*, 38272K, Keats Pubng) McGraw-Hill Trade.

Natural Remedies for Hayfever: Self-Help Measures for Treating the Symptoms of Hayfever Naturally. Paul Morgan. 2000. (Illus.). 128p. text 27.00 (*0-7881-6983-1*) DIANE Pub.

Natural Remedies for Pet Ailments. John Heinerman. 1998. (C). pap. 12.95 (*0-13-258476-X*, Macmillan Coll) P-H.

Natural Remedies for Stress. Judith Sachs. 1996. LC 96-38495. 528p. (C). text 22.95 (*0-13-243338-9*) P-H.

Natural Remedies for Women. Ed. by Prevention Magazine Health Book Staff. 2000. LC 2001-265041. viii, 279p. mass mkt. 5.99 (*0-312-97503-1*, St Martins Paperbacks) St Martin.

Natural Remedies from the Chinese Cupboard: Healing Foods & Herbs. Fang Jing Pei. 1998. LC 98-34671. 128p. pap. 10.95 (*0-8348-0459-X*) Weatherhill.

Natural Remedy Bible: Everyone's Guide to the Natural of Healing. John B. Lust & Michael Tierra. Ed. by Paul McCarthy. 1990. 384p. reprint ed. mass mkt. 6.99 (*0-671-66127-2*) PB.

Natural Remedy Book for Dogs & Cats. Diane Stein. 1994. LC 94-22084. (Illus.). 341p. pap. 16.95 (*0-89594-686-6*) Crossing Pr.

Natural Remedy Book for Women. Diane Stein. 1992. (Illus.). 348p. (Orig.). pap. 16.95 (*0-89594-525-8*) Crossing Pr.

Natural Resistance to Tumors & Viruses. Ed. by O. Haller. 1981. (Current Topics in Microbiology & Immunology Ser.: Vol. 92). (Illus.). 128p. 59.00 (*0-387-10732-0*) Spr-Verlag.

Natural Supports in School, at Work, & in the Community for People with Severe Disabilities. Ed. by Jan Nisbet. 1992. LC 92-9855. 368p. text 30.00 (*1-55766-101-4*) P H Brookes.

Natural Therapeutics. Henry Lindlahr. 108p. Vol. II. 1981. (*0-85207-148-5*); Vol. III. 1983. (*0-85207-155-8*); Vol. IV. 1985. pap. (*0-85207-171-X*) C W Daniel GBR. *Dist:* Natl Bk Netwk.

Natural Therapeutics Vol. 6: Iridiagnosis & Other Diagnostic Methods. Henry Lindlahr. 5th ed. 1996. 327p. reprint ed. spiral bd. 22.00 (*0-7873-0563-4*) Hlth Research.

Natural Therapies for Mitral Valve Prolapse. Ronald L. Hoffman. 1997. (Good Health Guides). 48p. pap. 3.95 (*0-87983-765-9*, 37659K, Keats Pubng) McGraw-Hill Trade.

Natural Therapy for Your Arthritic Cat. Shawn Messonnier. 1998. (Pet Care Naturally Ser.). 64p. pap. 4.95 (*0-87983-880-9*, Keats Pubng) McGraw-Hill Trade.

Natural Therapy for Your Arthritic Dog. Shawn Messonnier. 1998. (Pet Care Naturally Ser.). 64p. pap. 4.95 (*0-87983-879-5*, Keats Pubng) McGraw-Hill Trade.

Natural Toxicants in Feeds, Forages, & Poisonous Plants. Peter R. Cheeke. 1997. LC 97-937. 496p. pap. 58.75 (*0-8134-3128-X*) Interstate.

Natural Toxins: Proceedings of the 6th International Symposium on Animal, Plant & Microbial Toxins, Uppsala, August, 1979. D. Eaker. Ed. by Torkel Wadstrom. 1980. LC 80-40898. (Illus.). 704p. (*0-08-024952-3*) Pergamon Repr GBR. *Dist:* Franklin.

Natural Toxins: Toxicology, Chemistry, & Safety. N. Bhushan Mandava et al. 1992. 370p. (C). pap. text 79.15 (*1-880293-01-3*) Alaken.

Natural Treatment of Carpal Tunnel Syndrome. Ray C. Wunderlich, Jr. 1993. (Good Health Guides). (Illus.). 48p. (Orig.). pap. 3.95 (*0-87983-609-1*, 36091K, Keats Pubng) McGraw-Hill Trade.

Natural Treatment of Fibroid Tumors & Endometriosis. Susan M. Lark. 1995. (Good Health Guides). 48p. pap. 3.95 (*0-87983-690-3*, 36903K, Keats Pubng) McGraw-Hill Trade.

Natural Treatments & Remedies: For Over 400 of the World's Most Common Ailments. Global Health Research, Staff. 1995. (Illus.). 192p. pap. (*0-921202-11-3*) Gloh CAN. *Dist:* BookWorld.

Natural Treatments for Hyperactivity. Skye Weintraub. 1996. 318p. pap. text 12.95 (*1-885670-36-2*) Woodland UT.

Natural Treatments for Infertility. Karen Bradstreet. 1997. (Woodland Health Ser.). 32p. pap. text 3.95 (*1-58054-002-3*) Woodland UT.

Natural Treatments for Insomnia. Marian Broida. 2000. (Natural Pharmacist Ser.). pap. 9.99 (*0-7615-3011-8*) Prima Pub.

Natural Treatments for Osteoporosis. Sheila Dunn-Merritt. 2000. (Natural Pharmacist Ser.). 176p. pap. 9.99 (*0-7615-3010-X*) Prima Pub.

Natural Treatments for Varicose Veins. Richard Conant. 2000. (Natural Pharmacist Ser.). 176p. pap. 9.99 (*0-7615-3012-6*) Prima Pub.

Natural Way: Arthritis & Rheumatism. Pat Young. 1995. (Natural Way Ser.). (Illus.). 128p. pap. 5.95 (*1-85230-629-7*) Element MA.

Natural Way: Asthma; A Comprehensive Guide to Gentle, Safe & Effective Treatment. Roy Ridgeway. 1994. LC 94-25493. (Natural Way Ser.). (Illus.). 128p. pap. 5.95 (*1-85230-492-8*) Element MA.

Natural Way: Back Pain. Helena Bridge. 1995. LC 94-47047. (Natural Way Ser.). (Illus.). 128p. pap. 5.95 (*1-85230-581-9*) Element MA.

Natural Way: Cancer. Pat Young. 1996. LC 96-12362. (Natural Way Ser.). (Illus.). 128p. pap. 5.95 (*1-85230-799-4*) Element MA.

Natural Way: Colds & Flu. Penny Davenport. 1995. LC 94-47032. (Natural Way Ser.). (Illus.). 128p. pap. 5.95 (*1-85230-630-0*) Element MA.

Natural Way: Diabetes: A Comprehensive Guide to Effective Treatment. Catherine Steven. 1995. LC 95-30817. (Natural Way Ser.). (Illus.). 128p. pap. 5.95 (*1-85230-705-6*) Element MA.

Natural Way: Eczema: A Comprehensive Guide to Gentle, Safe & Effective Treatment. Sheena Meredith. 1994. LC 94-25492. (Natural Way Ser.). (Illus.). 128p. pap. 5.95 (*1-85230-493-6*) Element MA.

Natural Way: Heart Disease: A Comprehensive Guide to Effective Treatment. Richard Thomas. 1994. LC 94-13149. (Natural Way Ser.). (Illus.). 128p. pap. 5.95 (*1-85230-494-4*) Element MA.

Natural Way: Irritable Bowel Syndrome: A Comprehensive Guide to Gentle, Safe & Effective Treatment. Nigel Howard. 1995. LC 94-42101. (Natural Way Ser.). (Illus.). 128p. pap. 5.95 (*1-85230-583-5*) Element MA.

Natural Way: Migraine: A Comprehensive Guide to Gentle, Safe & Effective Treatment. Eileen Herzberg. 1994. LC 94-25918. (Natural Way Ser.). (Illus.). 128p. pap. 9.95 (*1-85230-495-2*) Element MA.

Natural Way: Multiple Sclerosis - A Comprehensive Guide to Effective Treatment. Richard Thomas. 1995. LC 95-30334. (Natural Way Ser.). (Illus.). 128p. pap. 5.95 (*1-85230-715-3*) Element MA.

Natural Way: Premenstrual Syndrome. Jane Sullivan. 1996. LC 95-44032. (Natural Way Ser.). (Illus.). 128p. pap. 5.95 (*1-85230-805-2*) Element MA.

Natural Way: Psoriasis. Hilary Bower. 1996. LC 96-2737. (Natural Way Ser.). (Illus.). 128p. pap. 5.95 (*1-85230-832-X*) Element MA.

Natural Way - Cystitis: A Comprehensive Guide to Effective Treatment. Jacqueline C. Young. 1997. LC 97-3508. (Natural Way Ser.). (Illus.). 128p. pap. 5.95 (*1-85230-889-3*) Element MA.

Natural Way for Dogs & Cats: Natural Treatments & Remedies for Your Pet. Midi Fairgrieve. 1999. (Illus.). pap. (*1-85158-973-2*) Mainstream Pubng.

Natural Way for Dogs & Cats: Natural Treatments, Remedies & Diet for Your Pet. Midi Fairgrieve. 2001. (Illus.). 240p. pap. (*0-85207-344-5*) C W Daniel GBR. *Dist:* Natl Bk Netwk.

Natural Way Infertility: A Comprehensive Guide to Effective Treatment. Belinda Whitworth. 1997. LC 96-42371. (Natural Way Ser.). (Illus.). 128p. pap. 5.95 (*1-85230-925-3*) Element MA.

Natural Way to a Healthy Prostate. Michael B. Schachter. 1995. (Good Health Guides). 48p. pap. 3.95 (*0-87983-650-4*, 36504K, Keats Pubng) McGraw-Hill Trade.

Natural Way to Better Babies see Healthy Parents, Better Babies: A Couple's Guide to Pre-Conception Health Care

Natural Way to Sexual Health. Henry G. Bieler & Sarah Nichols. Ed. by Jerome Fried. 1972. LC 72-83312. 231p. text 12.95 (*0-912880-03-1*) Charles Pub.

Natural Way to Vibrant Health. N. W. Walker. rev. ed. 1995. 132p. pap. 7.95 (*0-89019-035-6*) Norwalk Pr.

Natural Ways to Relieve the Common Discomforts of Pregnancy. Carl Jones. Ed. by Phyllis Herman. 1996. (Good Health Guides). 48p. pap. 3.95 (*0-87983-699-7*, 36997K, Keats Pubng) McGraw-Hill Trade.

Natural Well Woman: A Complete Guide to Health & Well-Being for Life. Penny Stanway. 2000. (Illus.). 224p. pap. 24.95 (*1-86204-791-X*) Element MA.

Natural Women's Health: A Guide to Healthy Living for Women of Any Age. Lynda Wharton. 1995. LC 94-73921. 274p. pap. 13.95 (*1-57224-007-5*) New Harbinger.

Naturalistic Articulation Carryover Experiences. Nanette C. Dahlke. 1990. (Illus.). stu. ed. 13.95 (*0-9626939-2-8*) Janelle Pubns.

Naturalists Guide to Self-Hypnosis. Garry De Young. 1988. pap. 3.00 (*0-936128-10-0*) De Young Pr.

Naturally Healthy Babies & Children: A Commonsense Guide to Herbal Remedies, Nutrition & Health. Aviva Romm. 2000. LC 00-34453. (Illus.). ix, 437p. pap. 16.95 (*1-58017-285-7*) Storey Bks.

Naturally Healthy Pregnancy: The Essential Guide to Nutritional & Botanical Medicine for the Child Bearing Years. Shonda Parker. 3rd ed. 2000. LC 2001-276840. (Illus.). 323p. pap. 14.99 (*1-929125-12-7*) Loyal Pubng.

Naturally Occurring Antioxidants. Richard A. Larson. 1997. LC 97-8169. 224p. lib. bdg. 89.95 (*0-87371-957-3*) Lewis Pubs.

Naturally Occurring Biological Immunosuppressive Factors & Their Relationship to Disease. Russell H. Neubauer. 1979. 304p. 170.00 (*0-8493-5243-6*, RC268, CRC Reprint) Franklin.

Naturally Occurring Phorbol Esters. Fred J. Evans. 1986. 366p. 182.00 (*0-8493-5117-0*, RS341, CRC Reprint) Franklin.

Naturally Processed Peptides. Ed. by A. Sette. 1993. (Chemical Immunology Ser.: Vol. 57). (Illus.). xii, 240p. 215.75 (*3-8055-5755-8*) S Karger.

Nature & Causes of Homosexuality. Ed. by Noretta Koertge. 1982. LC 81-6960. (Journal of Homosexuality Ser.: Vol. 6, No. 4). 100p. text 39.95 (*0-86656-148-X*) Haworth Pr.

Nature & Extent of Lead Poisoning in Children in the U. S. A Report to Congress. Paul Mushak & Annemarie F. Crocetti. 1999. (Illus.). 700p. (Orig.). (C). reprint ed. pap. text 60.00 (*0-7881-3383-7*) DIANE Pub.

Nature & Nurture in Psychiatry: A Predisposition-Stress Model of Mental Disorders. Joel Paris. 1999. LC 98-26811. 368p. 49.50 (*0-88048-781-X*, 8781) Am Psychiatric.

Nature & Organization of Retroviral Genes in Animal Cells. D. R. Strayer & D. H. Gillespie. 1980. (Virology Monographs: Vol. 17). (Illus.). 117p. 58.00 (*0-387-81563-5*) Spr-Verlag.

Nature & Origin of Amyloid Fibrils: Symposium, No. 199. CIBA Foundation Staff. 1996. LC 96-2872. (CIBA Foundation Symposia Ser.). 266p. 128.00 (*0-471-96361-5*) Wiley.

Nature & Origin of the Biological World. E. J. Ambrose. 1982. 190p. 78.95 (*0-470-27513-8*); pap. 38.95 (*0-470-27514-6*) P-H.

Nature & Treatment of Anxiety Disorders. C. Barr Taylor & Bruce A. Arnow. 1988. 368p. 45.00 (*0-02-932981-7*) Free Pr.

Nature & Treatment of Stuttering: New Directions. Richard F. Curlee & Gerald M. Siegel. 2nd ed. 1996. LC 96-22777. 452p. 80.00 (*0-205-16336-X*) Allyn.

Nature & Treatment of the Stress Response: A Practical Guide for Clinicians. G. S. Everly, Jr. & R. Rosenfeld. 1981. (Illus.). 232p. (C). 42.50 (*0-306-40677-2*, Plenum Trade) Perseus Pubng.

Nature Doctor: A Manual of Traditional & Complementary Medicine. H. C. Vogel. (GER., Illus.). 704p. reprint ed. 29.98 (*0-941683-27-3*) Instant Improve.

Nature Doctor: A Manual of Traditional & Complementary Medicine. H. C. Vogel. 1991. 29.95 (*0-87983-618-0*, Keats Pubng) McGraw-Hill Trade.

Nature Doctors: Pioneers in Naturopathic Medicine. Friedhelm Kirchfeld & Wade Boyle. 1993. (Illus.). 360p. (Orig.). pap. text 29.95 (*1-962351-85-8*) Univ OK Archeol.

Nature-Guided Therapy: Brief Integrative Strategies for Health & Wellbeing. George Burns. 1998. LC 97-44772. 250p. 35.95 (*0-87630-850-7*) Taylor & Francis.

Nature Has a Remedy. Bernard Jensen. 1979. 246p. reprint ed. pap. 12.99 (*0-932615-05-8*) B Jensen.

Nature Heals: The Psychological Essays of Paul Goodman. Paul Goodman. Ed. by Taylor Stoehr. rev. ed. 1991. 300p. pap. 24.95 (*0-939266-11-3*) Gestalt Journal.

Nature of Alcohol & Drug-Related Problems. Ed. by Malcolm H. Lader et al. 1992. (Society for the Study of Addiction Monograph Ser.: No. 2). (Illus.). 228p. text 69.95 (*0-19-262138-6*) OUP.

Nature of Animal Healing: The Definitive Holistic Medicine Guide to Caring for Your Dog & Cat. Martin Goldstein. 2000. 368p. pap. 16.00 (*0-345-43919-8*) Ballantine Pub Grp.

Nature of Cognition. Ed. by Robert J. Sternberg. LC 97-47622. (Bradford Book Ser.). (Illus.). 688p. 1999. pap. 39.95 (*0-262-69212-0*); 1998. 100.00 (*0-262-19405-8*) MIT Pr (Bradford Bks).

Nature of Communication Disorders. Orlando L. Taylor. 1986. 310p. text 44.99 (*0-7506-9857-8*) Buttrwrth-Heinemann.

Nature of Concepts: Evolution, Structure & Representation. Ed. by Philip Van Loocke. 1999. LC 99-185358. (Frontiers of Cognitive Science Ser.: No. 2). (Illus.). viii, 254 p. (C). 99.99 (*0-415-17963-7*, D6238) Routledge.

Nature of Consciousness: Philosophical Debates. Ed. by Ned J. Block et al. 1997. LC 96-17500. (Illus.). 608p. pap. 37.95 (*0-262-52210-1*); 95.00 (*0-262-02399-7*) MIT Pr (Bradford Bks).

Nature of Grief: The Evolution & Psychology of Reactions to Loss. John Archer. 1999. LC 98-20134. (Illus.). 336p. (C). 90.00 (*0-415-17857-6*); pap. 32.95 (*0-415-17858-4*) Routledge.

Nature of Human Feelings: With Exercises in Intimacy. Laurence C. Smith, Jr. 1990. 164p. (Orig.). pap. text 10.95 (*0-9625114-0-4*) BSA Pub.

Nature of Human Nature. Ellsworth Faris. abr. ed. 1977. (Midway Reprint Ser.). pap. text 10.00 (*0-226-23815-6*) U Ch Pr.

Nature of Human Nature & Other Essays in Social Psychology. Ellsworth Faris. 1977. LC 69-17575. (Essay Index Reprint Ser.). 23.95 (*0-8369-0073-1*) Ayer.

Nature of Hypnosis. Paul Schilder. 1956. LC 56-5485. 204p. pap. 24.95 (*0-8236-8156-4*, 23500); 30.00 (*0-8236-3500-7*) Intl Univs Pr.

Nature of Hypnosis & Suggestion. Milton H. Erickson. Ed. by Ernest L. Rossi. 1980. (Collected Papers of Milton H. Erickson on Hypnosis: Vol. I). 570p. (C). pap. 39.95 (*0-8290-1206-0*); text 59.95 (*0-8290-0542-0*) Ardent Media.

Nature of Hysteria. Niel Micklem. 1995. LC 95-18320. 144p. (C). 47.95 (*0-415-12186-8*) Routledge.

Nature of Intelligence. Ed. by Lauren B. Resnick. 1976. 364p. text 69.95 (*0-89859-137-6*) L Erlbaum Assocs.

Nature of "Intelligence" & the Principles of Cognition. Charles E. Spearman. 1977. LC 73-2990. (Classics in Psychology Ser.). reprint ed. 26.95 (*0-405-05163-8*) Ayer.

Nature of Learning Disabilities: Critical Elements of Diagnosis & Classification. Kenneth A. Kavale & Steven R. Forness. 1995. 448p. pap. 39.95 (*0-8058-1607-0*); text 89.95 (*0-8058-1606-2*) L Erlbaum Assocs.

Nature of Man: Studies in Optimistic Philosophy. Elie Metchnikoff. Ed. by Robert J. Kastenbaum. Tr. by P. Chalmers Mitchell. 1977. LC 76-19582. (Death & Dying Ser.). (Illus.). reprint ed. lib. bdg. 31.95 (*0-405-09578-3*) Ayer.

Nature of Man. Regimen in Health. Humours. Amorphisms. Regimen 1-3. Dreams., Vol. 4. Tr. by W. H. Jones. 1931. (Nature of Man. Regimen in Health. Humours. Amorphisms. Regim Ser.: No. 150). 582p. 19.95 (*0-674-99166-4*) HUP.

Nature of Nursing: Reflections after 25 Years. Virginia A. Henderson. 2nd ed. 1991. (Illus.). 128p. (C). reprint ed. pap. text 19.95 (*0-88737-494-8*) Natl League Nurse.

Nature of Nursing Work. Alan Pearson. 1996. pap. (*0-949823-69-4*) Deakin Univ AUS. *Dist:* St Mut.

Nature of Qualitative Evidence. Janice M. Morse et al. 2001. LC 00-11774. (Illus.). xv, 321p. pap. 31.95 (*0-7619-2285-7*) Sage.

Nature of Stuttering. Charles G. Van Riper. 2nd ed. 1982. (Illus.). 496p. text 43.95 (*0-13-610709-5*) P-H.

Nature of the Learning Process. Harvey Jackins. 1966. pap. 2.00 (*0-911214-14-3*) Rational Isl.

Nature of Their Bodies: Women & Their Doctors in Victorian Canada. Wendy Mitchinson. 1991. 765p. text 60.00 (*0-8020-5901-5*); 750p. pap. text 22.95 (*0-8020-6840-5*) U of Toronto Pr.

Nature of Theoretical Thinking in Nursing. Hesook S. Kim. 2nd ed. 2000. LC 99-54403. (Illus.). 272p. 39.95 (*0-8261-1306-0*) Springer Pub.

Nature of Thought: Essays in Honor of D. O. Hebb. Ed. by Peter W. Jusczyk & Raymond M. Klein. 1990. LC 80-18697. (Illus.). 256p. text 49.95 (*0-89859-034-5*) L Erlbaum Assocs.

Nature, Pregnancy, Sexuality. R. Perkins. 1985. 33.00 (*0-275-91321-X*, C1321, Praeger Pubs) Greenwood.

Nature, the Healer. John T. Richter & Vera M. Richter. 1996. reprint ed. spiral bd. 23.50 (*0-7873-0719-X*) Hlth Research.

Nature's Alternatives to Phen-Fen. Rita Elkias. 1996. 96p. pap. text 7.95 (*1-58054-015-5*) Woodland UT.

Nature's Aphrodisiacs. Nancy L. Nickell. 1999. LC 98-47924. 186p. pap. 14.95 (*0-89594-890-7*) Crossing Pr.

Nature's Cures: From Acupressure & Aromatherapy to Walking & Yoga—The Ultimate Guide to the Best, Scientifically Proven, Drug-Free Healing Methods. Michael Castleman. 1995. LC 95-22150. 528p. 27.95 (*0-87596-301-3*) Rodale Pr Inc.

Nature's Free Herbal Pharmacy - Herbal Healing Using Nature's Wild Foods & Wild Herbs. Ken Larson. 1997. (Illus.). 160p. pap. 10.95 (*0-9642497-3-1*) Rhema Pubng.

Nature's Healing Agents: The Medicines of Nature. R. S. Clymer. 1963. xx, 256p. lthr. 20.00 (*0-916285-54-5*) Humanitarian.

Nature's Healing Agents: The Medicines of Nature. R. Swinburne Clymer. 4th enl. rev. ed. 1996. (Illus.). 230p. pap. 10.95 (*0-916638-51-0*) Meyerbooks.

Nature's Miracle Medicines: Amazing Remedies from Mother Earth. Consumer Guide Editors. 2000. pap. 5.99 (*0-7853-4048-3*) NAL.

Nature's Path to Supreme Health: A Self-Reliant Guide to Living Supremely Healthy, Full of Energy. 1999. (Illus.). 330p. pap. (*0-7392-0495-5*, PO3861) Morris Pubng.

Nature's Prozac. Judith Sachs. 1998. LC 96-38495. (Illus.). 528p. (C). pap. 14.95 (*0-13-887654-1*) PH Pr.

Nature's 7 Doctors: Let Nature Make You Well. H. E. Kirschner. 1982. (Illus.). 128p. pap. 3.95 (*0-88007-153-2*) Woodbridge Pr.

Nature's Sports Pharmacy: A Natural Approach to Peak Athletic Performance. Frederick C. Hatfield & Frederick C. Hatfield, II. 1999. LC 96-1350. (Illus.). ix, 230p. pap. 14.95 (*0-8092-3221-9*, 322190, Contemporary) McGraw-Hill Trade.

Nature's Thumbprint: The New Genetics of Personality. Peter S. Neubauer & Alexander Neubauer. 1996. LC 95-37858. 224p. (C). pap. 18.50 (*0-231-10441-3*) Col U Pr.

Nature's Thumbprint: The Role of Genetics in Human Development. Peter B. Neubauer. 1990. 17.26 (*0-201-09254-9*) Addison-Wesley.

Nature's Way to Nutrition & Vibrant Health. Robert Scrutton. 1977. reprint ed. pap. 3.00 (*0-87980-344-4*) Wilshire.

Naturgemasse Hausapotheke see Home Remedies: Herbal & Homeopathic Treatments for Use at Home

Naturheilkunde In der Dermatologie. 1999. iv, 36p. 26.25 (*3-8055-6883-5*) S Karger.

Naturopathic Treatment of Colds & Infectious Diseases. Erich Rauch. Tr. by David M. Fogg from GER. 1993. (Illus.). 83p. (Orig.). pap. (*2-8043-4003-1*) K F Haug Pubs DEU. *Dist:* Medicina Bio.

Naturopathy: Understanding the Healing Power of Nature. Stewart Mitchell. 236th ed. 1998. LC 98-21514. (Health Essentials Ser.). (Illus.). 128p. 9.95 (*1-86204-303-5*) Element MA.

Naturopathy for Horses. Gerd Emich. 1994. 320p. (*0-85131-600-X*) J A Allen GBR. *Dist:* Trafalgar.

Nausea & Vomiting. HPNA Staff. 1999. 68p. pap. text 15.00 (*0-7872-6009-6*) Kendall-Hunt.

Nausea & Vomiting: Recent Research & Clinical Advances. Walter Kucharczyk. 1991. 272p. lib. bdg. 123.00 (*0-8493-6781-6*, RB150) CRC Pr.

Navaho Symbols of Healing: A Jungian Exploration of Ritual, Image, & Medicine. Donald Sandner. 1991. (Illus.). 304p. reprint ed. pap. 14.95 (*0-89281-434-9*, Heal Arts VT) Inner Tradit.

Navajo: Basic Medical. Alan Wilson. 1992. 141p. pap. text 18.95 (*0-88432-535-0*, AFNV94) J Norton Audio-Forum.

Navajo Aging: The Transition from Family to Institutional Support. Stephen J. Kunitz & Jerrold E. Levy. 1991. LC 91-3178. (Illus.). 191p. 39.00 (*0-8165-1260-4*) U of Ariz Pr.

Navajo Dictionary of Diagnostic Terminology: Navajo Medical Terminology. 1991. pap. 10.00 (*0-912586-68-0*) Dine College Pr.

Navajo Food Practices, Customs, & Holidays. Suzanne Pelican & Karen Bachman-Carter. 1992. (Ethnic & Regional Food Practices Ser.). pap. 10.00 (*0-88091-083-6*, 0867) Am Dietetic Assn.

Navajo Indian Medical Ethnobotany. Leland C. Wyman & Stuart K. Harris. LC 76-43902. (Univ. of New Mexico Bulletin Anthropological Ser.: Vol. 3, No. 5). reprint ed. 34.50 (*0-404-15761-0*) AMS Pr.

Navajo Infancy: An Ethological Study of Child Development. James S. Chisholm. 1983. LC 83-12258. (Evolutionary Foundations of Human Behavior Ser.). 279p. (C). lib. bdg. 49.95 (*0-202-01169-0*) Aldine de Gruyter.

Navajo Medicine Man Sand Paintings. Gladys A. Reichard. 1977. LC 77-73298. (Illus.). 132p. reprint ed. pap. 12.95 (*0-486-23329-4*) Dover.

***Navajo Nation Health Care System.** H. Bishara. 2001. pap. (*0-9711097-0-2*) Bistai Pr.

Naval Surgeon: Life & Death at Sea in the Age of Sail. J. Worth Estes. 1998. LC 97-31845. 39.95 (*0-88135-194-6*) Watson Pub Intl.

Navigating Midlife: Using Typology As a Guide. Eleanor Corlett & Nancy Millner. 1993. LC 93-4374. 420p. pap. 17.95 (*0-89106-061-8*, 7394, Davies-Black Pub) Consulting Psychol.

Navigating Research. Langford. 2001. text (*0-323-01012-1*); text, tchr. ed. (*0-323-01015-6*) Mosby Inc.

Navigating Research. Rae W. Langford. 2000. (Illus.). 448p. 35.00 (*0-323-00947-6*) Mosby Inc.

Navigating the NHS: Core Issues for Clinicians. Ed. by Peter Lees. 1996. (*1-85775-106-X*) Radcliffe Med Pr GBR. *Dist:* Balogh.

Navigating the Yellow Stream: A Voyage into the Cesspool of Urine Collection for Drug Testing. Paul Crumrine. 1991. LC 91-66421. 192p. pap. 9.95 (*0-9631221-0-X*) Nest Egg Pr.

Navigating Through a Strange Land: A Book for Brain Tumor Patients & Their Families. Tricia A. Roloff. 1995. LC 94-25863. (Illus.). 248p. pap. 16.95 (*0-9641214-1-7*) Indigo Pr AR.

***Navigating Through a Strange Land: A Book for Brain Tumor Patients & Their Families.** Tricia Ann Roloff. 2nd ed. 2001. LC 2001-40728. 256p. pap. 19.95 (*1-57749-108-4*) Fairview Press.

Nazi War on Cancer. Robert Proctor. 2000. LC 98-49405. (Illus.). 365p. pap. 16.95 (*0-691-07051-2*) Princeton U Pr.

NCA Review for the Clinical Laboratory Sciences. James L. Bender. 1985. 315p. pap. text 19.50 (*0-316-08889-7*, Little Brwn Med Div) Lppncott W & W.

NCA Review for the Clinical Laboratory Sciences. NCA Staff. 2nd ed. 1989. 32.95 (*0-316-59925-5*, Little Brwn Med Div) Lppncott W & W.

NCA Review for the Clinical Laboratory Sciences. Beck. 3rd ed. 1996. LC 96-16315. 264p. pap. text 36.00 (*0-316-59942-5*, Little Brwn Med Div) Lppncott W & W.

NCCLS Collection of ASTM Computerized System Standards. ring bd. 250.00 (*1-56238-252-7*, SC14-L) NCCLS.

NCG to Wound Care. Cathy T. Hess. 2nd ed. 1997. LC 97-26211. (Illus.). 400p. 28.95 (*0-87434-906-0*) Springhouse Corp.

NCLEX: PMIC's Comprehensive Review for the Registered Nurse Licensing Exam. Gisela Nily et al. Ed. by Maureen Lynch & Adrienne DiDonata. 1998. LC 98-21936. 600p. (Orig.). pap. text 34.95 (*1-57066-045-X*, ME073) Practice Mgmt Info.

NCLEX, 1998. Kaplan Staff. 1997. 34.95 incl. cd-rom (*0-684-83684-X*) S&S Trade.

NCLEX-PN: A Comprehensive Study Guide. Joann Zerwekh & Jo Carol Claborn. 3rd ed. 1997. (C). stu. ed. 29.95 (*0-9628210-7-1*) Nursing Ed Consultants.

NCLEX Q & A. L.L.C. Lishing. 1999. (Princeton Review Ser.). pap. (*0-375-75188-2*) Random.

NCLEX Review. S. Fields & R. N. Yurchuck. pap. (*0-444-01242-7*) Elsevier.

NCLEX-RN. Research and Education Association Staff. 2000. 600p. pap. text 24.95 (*0-87891-865-5*) Res & Educ.

NCLEX-RN: A Comprehensive Study Guide. JoAnn Zerwekh & Jo Carol Claborn. 3rd ed. 1997. 700p. pap., stu. ed. 29.95 incl. disk (*0-9628210-3-9*) Nursing Ed Consultants.

NCLEX-RN: A Study for Practical Nursing. JoAnn Zerwekh & Jo Carol Claborn. 2nd ed. 1997. LC 96-93049. (Illus.). 550p. (C). pap., stu. ed. 24.95 incl. disk (*0-9628210-6-3*) Nursing Ed Consultants.

NCLEX RN, 1998-99. Kaplan Staff. 1998. 336p. 34.95 incl. cd-rom (*0-684-84763-9*) S&S Trade.

NCLEX-RN, 1999-2000 ed. Kaplan Staff. 1999. (Kaplan NCLEX-RN Ser.). 368p. pap. text 34.95 (*0-684-85671-9*) S&S Trade.

NCLEX-RN Practice: Questions & Answers Made Incredibly Easy. Springhouse Publishing Company Staff. 1999. LC 99-37059. (Made Incredibly Easy Ser.). 800p. pap. 34.95 (*1-58255-017-4*) Springhouse Corp.

NCLEX-RN Questions & Answers: More Than 2,000 Questions & Answers for NCLEX-RN Success. Princeton Review Publishing Staff. 1999. (Princeton Review Ser.). 892p. pap. 27.95 (*0-375-75291-9*) Random.

NCLEX-RN Review. Springhouse Publishing Company Staff. 1999. LC 99-40804. (Made Incredibly Easy Ser.). (Illus.). 800p. pap. 34.95 (*1-58255-016-6*) Springhouse Corp.

NCLEX-RN (TM)-RN 101: How to Pass. Sylvia Rayfield & Loretta Manning. 2nd ed. 1996. 264p. (C). pap. 24.95 incl. disk (*0-9643622-1-X*) ICAN LA.

ND-YAG Laser in Ophthalmology: Principles & Clinical Applications of Photodistribution. Roger F. Steinert & Carmen A. Puliafito. 1985. (Illus.). 154p. text 98.00 (*0-7216-1320-9*) Saunders.

NDA Book Ed. by FOI Services, Inc. Staff. 1996. Set. pap. 289.00 (*1-880626-09-8*); Vol. I. pap. (*1-880626-07-1*); Vol. II. pap. (*1-880626-08-X*) FOI Services.

NDH Pocket Guide to Drug Dosages. Springhouse Publishing Company Staff. 2nd ed. 2000. LC 00-699760. vi, 362p. pap. 19.95 (*1-58255-045-X*) Springhouse Corp.

NDR, '96. George R. Spratto. 1996. (Professional Reference - Nursing Ser.). 1392p. pap. 26.95 (*0-8273-6644-2*) Delmar.

Neal's Common Foot Disorders: Diagnosis & Management. Donald L. Lorimer et al. 6th ed. 1997. LC 96-37052. pap. text (*0-443-05258-1*) Church.

Near-Death Experience: An Annotated Bibliography. Terry K. Basford. 1990. LC 89-78521. 192p. text 10.00 (*0-8240-6349-X*, SS481) Garland.

Near Misses in Anesthesia. John M. Lewis & Tionette H. Fontrier. 1988. 112p. pap. text 36.50 (*0-409-90111-3*) Buttrwrth-Heinemann.

Near Misses in Cardiac Surgery: Great Saves. Miles E. Lee. 1992. 112p. pap. text (*0-7506-9391-6*) E A GBR. *Dist:* OUP.

Near Misses in Neuroanesthesia. Terri W. Blackburn & Garfield B. Russell. 2001. (Illus.). 208p. pap. 34.99 (*0-7506-7065-7*) Buttrwrth-Heinemann.

Near Misses in Pediatric Anesthesia. Brock-Utne. 1998. LC 98-39866. 128p. pap. text 34.99 (*0-7506-7018-5*) Buttrwrth-Heinemann.

Near Misses in Pulmonary & Cardiothoracic Critical Care. Joseph Varon et al. 1999. LC 98-54232. 136p. pap. text 34.99 (*0-7506-7117-3*) Buttrwrth-Heinemann.

Near Visual Acuity Tests. Matthias Sachsenweger. 1987. (C). text 73.50 (*0-85200-664-0*) Kluwer Academic.

Nebraska Health Care in Perspective, 2000. Ed. by Kathleen O'Leary Morgan & Scott E. Morgan. 2000. 21p. spiral bd. 19.00 (*0-7401-0226-5*) Morgan Quitno Corp.

Nebraska Health Care Perspective, 1998. Ed. by Kathleen O'Leary Morgan & Scott E. Morgan. 1998. 20p. pap. 19.00 (*1-56692-826-5*) Morgan Quitno Corp.

Nebraska Symposium on Motivation, 1984: Psychology & Gender. Ed. by Theo B. Sonderegger & Richard A. Dienstbier. 1985. LC 53-11655. (Nebraska Symposium on Motivation Ser.: Vol. 32). 326p. text 45.00 (*0-8032-4152-6*); pap. text 25.00 (*0-8032-9150-7*) U of Nebr Pr.

Nebraska Symposium on Motivation, 1988: Socioemotional Development. Ed. by Ross A. Thompson. 1990. LC 53-11655. (Nebraska Symposium on Motivation Ser.: Vol. 36). 492p. text 45.00 (*0-8032-4421-5*); pap. text 25.00 (*0-8032-9415-8*) U of Nebr Pr.

Nebraska Symposium on Motivation, 1991: Psychology & Aging. Ed. by Theo B. Sonderegger. 1991. LC 53-11655. (Nebraska Symposium on Motivation Ser.: Vol. 39). 276p. text 45.00 (*0-8032-4222-0*); pap. text 25.00 (*0-8032-9210-4*, Bison Books) U of Nebr Pr.

Nebraska Symposium on Motivation, 1992: Developmental Perspectives on Motivation. Ed. by Janis E. Jacobs. 1993. LC 53-11655. (Nebraska Symposium on Motivation Ser.: Vol. 40). 299p. text 45.00 (*0-8032-2575-X*); pap. text 25.00 (*0-8032-7576-5*) U of Nebr Pr.

Nebraska Symposium on Motivation, 1996: Alcohol & Addictive Behavior. Ed. by P. Clayton Rivers & Richard A. Dienshier. 1987. LC 53-11655. (Nebraska Symposium on Motivation Ser.: No. 34). 346p. text 45.00 (*0-8032-3880-0*); pap. text 25.00 (*0-8032-8925-1*) U of Nebr Pr.

Nebraska Symposium on Motivation, 1993: Integrative View of Motivation, Cognitive, & Emotion. William D. Spaulding. 1994. LC 53-11655. 265p. text 45.00 (*0-8032-4233-6*) U of Nebr Pr.

Necessary Illusion - Art As "Witness" Resonance & Attunement to Forms & Feelings. Gilbert J. Rose. 1996. LC 95-8950. 148p. 27.50 (*0-8236-3510-4*) Intl Univs Pr.

Necessary Toughness: Facing Defenses & Diabetes. Jonathan Hayes & Robert L. Briggs. 1993. LC 93-11172. 7.95 (*0-945448-30-9*, 4807-01) Am Diabetes.

Necessity among Us: The Owen Sound General & Marine Hospital, 1891-1985. David Gagan. 1990. 180p. text 30.00 (*0-8020-3462-4*) U of Toronto Pr.

Neck, Vol. 3. Ed. by Hahns H. Naumann. 2nd ed. 1997. (Illus.). 450p. 199.00 (*0-86577-624-5*) Thieme Med Pubs.

Neck & Arm Pain. Rene Cailliet. 3rd ed. 1990. LC 90-13849. (Pain Ser.). (Illus.). 226p. pap. 21.95 (*0-8036-1610-4*) Davis Co.

Neck & Back Pain: The Scientific Evidence of Causes, Diagnosis, & Treatment. Alf L. Nachemson & Egon Jonsson. 2000. LC 00-23914. 512p. text 110.00 (*0-7817-2760-X*) Lppncott W & W.

Neck Care. Andrew Cole. 1999. (Illus.). 24p. pap. 1.42 (*0-934230-47-1*) Medic Pub.

Neck Injuries. Syed M. Babar. 1999. LC 99-33583. 160p. pap. 89.00 (*1-85233-637-4*) Spr-Verlag.

Neck Pain. Henry L. Feffer et al. 2nd ed. 1992. (Illus.). 456p. 85.00 (*0-87473-823-7*, 62016-10, MICHIE) LEXIS Pub.

Neck Pain: Medical Diagnosis & Comprehensive Management. David G. Borenstein et al. Ed. by Richard Lampert. 1996. 512p. text 89.00 (*0-7216-5412-6*) Saunders.

Neck, Upper Back, Shoulder & Arm Pain. James M. Cox. 1992. (Illus.). 11p. (Orig.). (C). pap. text 2.00 (*0-9616488-9-9*) Alef Bet Comns.

Necropsy: Procedures & Basic Diagnostic Methods for Practicing Veterinarians. Albert C. Strafuss. 1988. (Illus.). 262p. (C). text 61.95 (*0-398-05375-8*) C C Thomas.

Necropsy Guide: Rodents & the Rabbit. Ed. by Donald B. Feldman & John C. Seely. 1988. 176p. 208.95 (*0-8493-4934-6*, SF997) CRC Pr.

Need a Doctor? Janus. 1981. 64p. pap. text 8.95 (*0-8224-5057-7*) Globe Fearon.

Need for Better Focus in the Rural Health Care Clinic Program- Part II: Hearing Before the Subcommittee on Human Resources of the Committee on Government Reform & Oversight, House of Representatives, One Hundred Fifth Congress, First Session, September 11, 1997. USGPO Staff. 1998. LC 98-167877. iii, 126 p. (*0-16-056433-6*) USGPO.

Need for Food Supplements. 1996. lib. bdg. 250.75 (*0-8490-5885-6*) Gordon Pr.

Need for Healthcare. Rod Sheaff. 1996. LC 95-25911. (Social Ethics & Policy Ser.). 240p. (C). 90.00 (*0-415-10111-5*); pap. 27.95 (*0-415-10112-3*) Routledge.

Need to Have Enemies & Allies: From Clinical Practice to International Relationships. Vamik D. Volkan. 1988. LC 87-32763. 298p. (C). 35.00 (*0-87668-999-3*) Aronson.

Needful, New & Necessarie Treatise of Chyrugerie. John Banister. 1971. LC 73-171732. (English Experience Ser.: No. 300). 276p. reprint ed. 22.00 (*90-221-0300-5*) Walter J Johnson.

Needle Biopsy of the Thyroid: Current Concepts. J. Martin Miller et al. 1983. LC 82-16667. 289p. 93.95 (*0-275-91403-8*, C1403, Praeger Pubs) Greenwood.

Needle Exchange & AIDS Prevention: Advances & Controversies in Public Health & Social Policy. Merrill Singer. 1997. 134p. pap. text (*90-5699-598-7*) GBSP NLD. *Dist:* Gordon & Breach.

Needle Exchange Evaluation Report. 1992. (Illus.). 57p. (Orig.). (C). pap. text 25.00 (*1-56806-087-4*) DIANE Pub.

Needle Sharing among Intravenous Drug Abusers: National & International Perspectives. 1992. lib. bdg. 79.95 (*0-8490-8824-0*) Gordon Pr.

***Needs Assessment in Occupational Therapy: Studies of Persons with Long-Term/Recurrent Pain.** Maria Mullersdort. 2001. (Comprehensive Summaries of Uppsala Dissertations from the Faculty of Medicine Ser.: No. 1065). 82p. pap. (*91-554-5086-5*) Acta Univ SWE. *Dist:* Coronet Bks.

Needs Assessment of Human Problems. Steve Baldwin et al. 1998. LC 97-41334. (Illus.). 256p. pap. text 37.50 (*0-7506-2435-3*) Buttrwrth-Heinemann.

Negative Schizophrenic Symptoms: Pathophysiology & Clinical Implications. Ed. by John F. Greden & Rajiv Tandon. 1991. LC 90-535. (Progress in Psychiatry Ser.: No. 28). 290p. text 12.95 (*0-88048-192-7*, 8192) Am Psychiatric.

Negative Staining & Cryoelectron Microscopy: The Thin Film Techniques. J. R. Harris. 1998. (Microscopy Handbook Ser.: No. 35). 224p. (C). pap. (*1-85996-120-7*) Bios Sci GBR. *Dist:* Bks Intl VA.

Negative Symptom & Cognitive Deficit Treatment Response in Schizophrenia. Ed. by Richard S. E. Keefe & Joseph P. McEvoy. 2000. LC 00-23099. (Illus.). xiv, 201p. 87.00 (*0-88048-785-2*, 8785) Am Psychiatric.

Negative vs. Positive Schizophrenia. Ed. by Andreas Marneros et al. 1991. (Illus.). 466p. 134.00 (*0-387-54388-0*) Spr-Verlag.

Neglected & Abused: A Physician's Year in Haiti. Joseph F. Bentivegna. 1990. (Illus.). 180p. (Orig.). (C). pap. 12.95 (*0-9626001-0-5*) Michelle Pub.

Neglected Cause of Stroke: Occlusion of the Smaller Intracranial Arteries & Their Diagnosis by Cerebral Angiography. B. Albert Ring. 1969. LC 68-55659. (Illus.). 220p. 12.00 (*0-87527-066-2*) Green.

Neglected Children: Research, Practice, & Policy. Howard Dubowitz. 1999. LC 98-40296. 320p. pap. 31.95 (*0-7619-1842-6*, 81210) Sage.

Neglected Factors in Pharmacology & Neuroscience Research. Volkert Claassen. 1994. LC 94-16419. (Techniques in the Behavioral & Neural Sciences Ser.: Vol. 12). 496p. 260.50 (*0-444-81871-5*) Elsevier.

Negotiating at an Uneven Table: A Practical Approach to Working with Difference & Diversity. Phyllis B. Kritek. 1994. LC 94-27889. 354p. (C). pap. text 34.95 (*1-55542-670-0*, 670-0) Jones & Bartlett.

Negotiating at an Uneven Table: A Practical Approach to Working with Difference & Diversity. Phyllis B. Kritek. 1996. (Conflict Resolution Ser.). 368p. reprint ed. pap. 30.00 (*0-7879-0254-3*) Jossey-Bass.

Negotiating Consent in Psychotherapy. Patrick O'Neill. 1998. LC 98-25349. (Qualitative Studies in Psychology). 200p. pap. text 18.50 (*0-8147-6195-X*) NYU Pr.

Negotiating Health Care: The Social Context of Chronic Illness. Sally E. Thorne. 1993. (Illus.). 280p. (C). pap. 32.95 (*0-8039-4918-9*, 47863) Sage.

Negotiating Health Insurance in the Workplace: A Basic Guide. Suzanne S. Taylor. 1992. LC 92-11190. 346p. trans. 48.00 (*0-87179-731-3*) BNA Books.

Negotiating Parent-Adolescent Conflict: A Behavioral-Family Systems Approach. Arthur L. Robin & Sharon L. Foster. 1989. LC 87-31502. (Guilford Family Therapy Ser.). 338p. 39.95 (*0-89862-072-4*) Guilford Pubns.

Negotiating Positive Identity in a Group Care Community: Reclaiming Uprooted Youth. Intro. by Zvi Levy. 1993. LC 93-34917. (Child & Youth Services Ser.: Vol. 16, No. 2). (Illus.). 141p. lib. bdg. 39.95 (*1-56024-514-X*) Haworth Pr.

Negotiating Realities: Making Sense of Interaction Between Patients Diagnosed As Neurotic & Nurses. Stephen Tilley. 1995. 448p. (C). text (*1-85628-939-7*) Avebry GBR. *Dist:* Ashgate Pub Co.

Negotiation for Health & Social Service Professionals. Keith Fletcher. 1997. LC 98-150929. 160p. text (*1-85302-549-6*) Jessica Kingsley GBR. *Dist:* Taylor & Francis.

Negotiations for Health Care Materials Manager: A Systematic Approach. Thomas F. Guernsey & Kathe Klare. 1993. (Illus.). 106p. (Orig.). pap. 60.00 (*0-87258-645-6*, 142902) Am Hospital.

Negro Child Welfare in North Carolina. Wiley B. Sanders. 1968. LC 68-55782. (Criminology, Law Enforcement, & Social Problems Ser.: No. 18). (Illus.). reprint ed. 24.00 (*0-87585-018-9*) Patterson Smith.

Neighborhood Network Conversations on Nutrition. Ruth L. Cohen. 1992. 150p. (Orig.). pap. 11.50 (*0-9633720-0-9*) Environ Comms.

Neighborhood Networks for Humane Mental Health Care. Arthur J. Naparstek et al. 1982. 238p. 42.50 (*0-306-41051-6*, Plenum Trade) Perseus Pubng.

Neisseriae, 1990: Proceedings of the 7th International Neisseria Conference Berlin, Federal Republic of Germany, Sept. 9-14, 1990. Ed. by Mark Achtman et al. 1991. (Illus.). xx, 752p. (C). lib. bdg. 261.55 (*3-11-012712-1*) De Gruyter.

Nelson Essentials of Pediatrics. Behrman. 3rd ed. 1998. pap. text 32.50 (*0-8089-2052-9*, Grune & Strat) Harcrt Hlth Sci Grp.

Nelson Essentials of Pediatrics. Richard E. Behrman & Robert M. Kliegman. 3rd ed. 1998. LC 97-15484. (Illus.). 736p. pap. text 42.50 (*0-7216-7229-9*) Saunders.

Nelson Handbook on Pediatric Therapeutics. Richard E. Behrman. 1995. (C). pap. text (*0-7216-5018-X*) Saunders.

Nelson-Jones & Burton: Medical Negligence Case Law. Rodney Nelson-Jones & Frank Burton. 2nd ed. 1995. (*0-406-03601-2*, NJBM2, MICHIE) LEXIS Pub.

Nelson Review of Pediatrics. Richard E. Behrman et al. Ed. by Lisette Bralow. 1996. LC 95-52571. 208p. pap. text 29.00 (*0-7216-5579-3*) Saunders.

Nelson Textbook of Pediatrics. Richard E. Behrman et al. Ed. by Waldo E. Nelson. 15th ed. 1995. LC 95-17879. (Illus.). 2245p. text 105.00 (*0-7216-5578-5*) Saunders.

Nelson Textbook of Pediatrics. Richard E. Behrman et al. 16th ed. 2000. LC 98-50604. (Illus.). xlvii, 2414p. text 110.00 (*0-7216-7767-3*) Saunders.

***Nelson Textbook of Pediatrics.** Richard E. Behrman et al. 16th ed. 2000. (Illus.). 2414p. 175.00 incl. cd-rom (*0-7216-9273-7*) Saunders.

Nelson Textbook of Pediatrics: Pocket Companion. Richard E. Behrman et al. 16th ed. 2000. (Illus.). 510p. text (*0-7216-7770-3*) Saunders.

Nelson Textbook of Pediatrics Pocket Companion. Ed. by Richard E. Behrman. 1993. LC 93-9371. (Illus.). 546p. pap. text 25.00 (*0-7216-3968-2*) Saunders.

***Nelson's Pocket Book of Pediatric Antimicrobial Therapy PDA 2002-2003.** John S. Bradley & John D. Nelson. 15th ed. 2002. 29.95 (*0-7817-3703-6*) Lppncott W & W.

Nelson's Textbook of Pediatrics. Behrman. 15th ed. (C). text (*0-8089-2154-1*, Grune & Strat) Harcrt Hlth Sci Grp.

Nelson's 2000-2001 Pocket Book of Pediatric Antimicrobial Therapy. John D. Nelson & John S. Bradley. 14th ed. 2000. 120p. pap. text 19.95 (*0-7817-2570-4*) Lppncott W & W.

Neo-Tech Cures Alcoholism, Drug Abuse, Neurosis. Gary Twitchell. 1990. 160p. pap. 29.95 (*0-911752-63-3*) Neo-Tech Pub.

Neoantology: Management, Procedures, On-Call Problems, Diseases & Drugs. Tricia L. Gomella. 4th rev. ed. 1999. (Illus.). 620p. (C). spiral bd. 39.95 (*0-8385-6687-1*, A-6687-6, Apple Lange Med) McGraw.

Neocarzinostatin: The Past, Present, & Future of an Anticancer Drug. H. Maeda et al. 1997. LC 96-47101. (Illus.). 304p. 211.00 (*4-431-70187-7*) Spr-Verlag.

Neocortex: Ontogeny & Phylogeny. Ed. by B. L. Finlay et al. 1991. LC 91-21500. (NATO Advanced Science Institutes Ser.: Vol. 200). (Illus.). 272p. (C). text 114.00 (*0-306-43808-9*, Kluwer Plenum) Kluwer Academic.

Neocortical Development. Shirley A. Bayer & Joseph Altman. 1991. 272p. text 169.00 (*0-88167-778-7*) Lppncott W & W.

Neocortical Dynamics & Human EEG Rhythms. Paul L. Nunez. 1995. LC 94-5465. (Illus.). 728p. text 98.50 (*0-19-505728-7*) OUP.

Neocortical Epilepsies, Vol. 84. Ed. by Peter D. Williamson et al. 2000. LC 00-30739. (Advances in Neurology Ser.: Vol. 84). (Illus.). 688p. text 169.00 (*0-7817-1872-4*) Lppncott W & W.

NeoFax. Thomas Young & O. Barry Magnum. 13th ed. 2000. (Clinicofax Ser.). 264p. spiral bd. 28.00 (*1-888703-13-X*) Neofax.

Neonatal & Pediatric Pulmonary Graphics: Principle & Clinical Applications. Ed. by Steven M. Donn. 1997. LC 97-39522. (Illus.). 443p. 85.00 (*0-87993-645-2*) Futura Pub.

Neonatal & Pediatric Respiratory Care. Whitaker. 1993. (C). pap. text, tchr. ed. 10.00 (*0-8273-3851-1*) Delmar.

Neonatal & Pediatric Respiratory Care. Barbara G. Wilson et al. 3rd ed. 1999. (Illus.). 576p. (C). text (*0-323-00164-5*) Mosby Inc.

Neonatal & Pediatric Ultrasonography. Ed. by Diane S. Babcock. 1992. (Clinics in Diagnostic Ultrasound Ser.: Vol. 24). (Illus.). 251p. text (*0-443-08606-0*) Church.

Neonatal & Perinatal Screening: The Asian Pacific Perspective. Ed. by Stephen T. Lam & Calvin C. Pang. 1997. LC 98-139431. xii, 199p. (*962-201-765-7*) Chinese Univ HKG. *Dist:* U of Mich Pr.

Neonatal Anesthesia. Ed. by D. Ryan Cook & Joseph H. Marcy. 1988. LC 87-27309. 300p. text 52.50 (*0-941022-10-2*) Davies Pubng.

***Neonatal Cardiology.** Michael Artman et al. 2001. LC 2001-44906. (Illus.). 768p. text 125.00 (*0-07-007098-9*) McGraw-Hill Prof.

Neonatal Care Policy & Procedure Guideline Manual. Mel Pepper and Janet Adams. 1997. 260p. spiral bd. 110.00 (*1-879575-85-X*) Acad Med Sys.

Neonatal Cerebral Ultrasound. Janet M. Rennie. 1997. LC 96-13980. (Illus.). 252p. (C). text 95.00 (*0-521-45079-9*) Cambridge U Pr.

Neonatal Critical Care Nursing: Outline Core Content. AACN Staff. 1997. pap. (*0-7216-5898-9*) Saunders.

Neonatal Decision Making. Sheldon B. Korones. 1992. LC 92-49370. (Clinical Decision Making Ser.). 286p. (C). (gr. 13). text 74.95 (*1-55664-148-6*) Mosby Inc.

Neonatal Dermatology. Eichenfiel. 1997. LC 00-50070. (Illus.). 512p. text 145.00 (*0-7216-7810-6*) Saunders.

Neonatal Disease & Congenital Disorders: RCP 308 Course. Wojciechowski et al. 1994. 270p. (C). ring bd. 39.95 (*0-933195-75-3*) CA College Health Sci.

Neonatal EEG. American Journal of END Technology Staff. 1998. (Illus.). per. 28.00 (*1-57797-008-X*) ASET.

Neonatal Emergency. Diane Charsha. 1997. No. 1. text, wbk. ed. (*0-8151-2377-9*); No. 2. text, wbk. ed. (*0-8151-2378-7*); No. 3. text, wbk. ed. (*0-8151-2380-9*) Mosby Inc.

Neonatal Formulary. Compiled by Northern Neonatal Network Staff. 1996. 199p. pap. text (*0-7279-1030-2*) BMJ Pub GBR. *Dist:* AIDC.

***Neonatal Formulary.** Northern Neonatal Network Staff. 3rd ed. 2001. 288p. pap. (*0-7279-1547-9*) BMJ Pub GBR. *Dist:* AIDC.

Neonatal Group B Streptococcal Infections. Ed. by K. K. Christensen et al. 1985. (Antibiotics & Chemotherapy Ser.: Vol. 35). (Illus.). x, 350p. 215.00 (*3-8055-3953-3*) S Karger.

Neonatal Haematology & Immunology II: Proceedings of the International Symposium, Gottingen, Germany, 13-15 May 1993. Ed. by Marietta Xanthou et al. 1993. LC 93-38871. (International Congress Ser.: Vol. 1038). 220p. 177.25 (*0-444-81656-9*, Excerpta Medica) Elsevier.

Neonatal Heart Disease. R. M. Freedom et al. 1991. 912p. (Illus.). 385.00 (*0-387-19639-0*); 225.00 (*3-540-19639-0*) Spr-Verlag.

Neonatal Hematology & Immunology III: Proceedings of the Third Neonatal Hematology & Immunology Symposium, Held in Washington, D. C., U. S. A. on 29 September - 1 October 1996, Vol. 113. Ed. by J. A. Bellanti et al. 1997. LC 97-5558. (International Congress Ser.: Vol. 1131). 262p. 137.50 (*0-444-82573-8*, Excerpta Medica) Elsevier.

Neonatal Immune Thrombocytopenia. Bussell. 1991. (*0-8493-6469-8*, CRC Reprint) Franklin.

Neonatal Infectious Diseases. Diane Charsha. 1997. No. 1. pap., wbk. ed. (*0-8151-2367-1*); No. 2. text, wbk. ed. (*0-8151-2368-X*); No. 3. wbk. ed. (*0-8151-2369-8*) Mosby Inc.

Neonatal Intensive Care Handbook. Boyd W. Goetzman & Richard P. Wennberg. 3rd ed. 1999. LC 98-54475. (*0-323-00814-3*) Mosby Inc.

Neonatal Intensive Care Handbook. Boyd W. Goetzman & Richard P. Wennberg. 3rd ed. 1999. (Illus.). 768p. (*84-8174-472-7*) Mosby-Doyma Libros ESP. *Dist:* Mosby Inc.

Neonatal Intensive Care Nursing. Glenys Boxwell. 2000. LC 99-55486. (Illus.). xxix, 455p. (*0-415-20339-2*) Routledge.

Neonatal Intensive Care Nursing. Jack Rudman. (Certified Nurse Examination Ser.: CN-25). pap. 27.95 (*0-8373-6125-7*) Nat Learn.

Neonatal Jaundice. Ed. by M. Jeffrey Maisels & Jon F. Watchko. 2000. (Monographs in Clinical Pediatrics: Vol. 11). 228p. 70.00 (*90-5702-626-0*, Harwood Acad Pubs) Gordon & Breach.

Neonatal Kidney & Fluid-Electrolytes. Ed. by Jose Strauss. 1983. text 125.00 (*0-89838-575-X*) Kluwer Academic.

Neonatal Medications & Nutrition: A Comprehensive Guide. Karin E. Zenk et al. 1999. LC 99-25645. (Illus.). 600p. pap. 39.95 (*1-887571-03-5*); 2nd ed. 2000. LC 99-59774. pap. 39.95 (*1-887571-07-8*) NICU Ink.

Neonatal Medicine. Ed. by Leo Stern. 1987. 1250p. (gr. 13). 224.50 (*0-89352-229-5*, MA229) Mosby Inc.

Neonatal Meningitis. Pamela A. Davies & P. T. Rudd. 1995. (Clinics in Developmental Medicine Ser.: No. 132). (Illus.). 185p. text 59.95 (*0-901260-96-7*) Cambridge U Pr.

Neonatal Neurology. Gerald M. Fenichel. 3rd ed. 1989. (Illus.). 250p. pap. text (*0-443-08700-8*) Church.

Neonatal Nurse Practitioner. Jack Rudman. (Certified Nurse Examination Ser.: CN-21). pap. 27.95 (*0-8373-6121-4*) Nat Learn.

***Neonatal Nursing.** 1994. (Illus.). pap. (*0-7487-5792-9*) Nelson Thornes GBR. *Dist:* Intl Spec Bk.

Neonatal Nursing. Ed. by Doreen Crawford & Maryke Morris. 1994. 400p. pap. 37.50 (*0-412-48730-6*) Chapman & Hall.

Neonatal-Pediatric Respiratory Care. Koff. 2nd ed. 1993. (Illus.). 525p. (gr. 13). text 54.00 (*0-8016-6518-3*, 06518) Mosby Inc.

Neonatal-Perinatal Medicine: Diseases of the Fetus & Infant. Avary A. Fanaroff & Richard J. Martin. 6th ed. 1996. LC 96-47141. (Illus.). 1904p. (C). (gr. 13). text 180.00 (*0-8151-3205-0*, 24740) Mosby Inc.

Neonatal-Perinatal Medicine: Diseases of the Fetus & Infant. Avroy A. Fararoff & Richard J. Martin. 7th ed. 1920p. (*0-323-00929-8*) Mosby Inc.

Neonatal Physical Assessment: Gestational Age & Size Evaluation, No. 1. Diane Charsha. 1997. wbk. ed. (*0-8151-2354-X*) Mosby Inc.

Neonatal Physical Assessment: Musculoskeletal & Skin Assessment. Diane Charsha. 1997. (*0-8151-2356-6*) Mosby Inc.

Neonatal Physical Assessment: Respiratory & Cardiovascular Assessment, No. 2. Diane Charsha. 1997. wbk. ed. (*0-8151-2355-8*) Mosby Inc.

Neonatal Repiratory Disorders. Anthony Milner et al. 1996. (Illus.). 528p. (*0-340-55242-5*) E A GBR. *Dist:* OUP.

Neonatal Skin: Structure & Function. Howard I. Maibach & Edward K. Boisits. 1982. (Dermatology Ser.: Vol. 1). (Illus.). 296p. text 145.00 (*0-8247-1860-7*) Dekker.

Neonatal Surgery of the Cleft Lip & Palate. 1997. 400p. text 44.00 (*981-02-3116-4*) World Scientific Pub.

Neonatal Tumours. Ed. by Prem Puri & Rajendra Surana. 1996. LC 96-13126. (Illus.). 160p. 140.00 (*3-540-19938-1*) Spr-Verlag.

Neonatal Vade-Mecum. Peter J. Fleming. 2nd ed. 448p. (Orig.). pap. text (*0-340-53869-4*) E A GBR. *Dist:* Routldge.

Neonatal/Pediatric Respiratory Care: A Critical Care Pocket Guide. Dana Oakes. 3rd ed. 1996. (Illus.). 320p. ring bd. 19.95 (*0-932887-08-2*) Health Ed Pubns.

Neonatology. Thomas. 2nd ed. 1998. (C). pap. text 16.95 (*0-443-05885-7*) Saunders.

Neonatology. Roslyn Thomas & David R. Harvey. 2nd ed. 1997. LC 96-39722. (Colour Guide Ser.). (*0-443-05774-5*) Harcrt Hlth Sci Grp.

Neonatology: A Practical Guide. Alistair G. Philip. Ed. by Judy Fletcher. 4th ed. 1996. LC 95-9516. (Illus.). 400p. pap. text 50.00 (*0-7216-4776-6*) Saunders.

Neonatology Word Book. Hazel Tank & Catherine Gilliam. 1991. 102p. (Orig.). (C). pap. text 30.00 (*0-935229-10-8*) Am Assoc Med.

Neoplasia & Cell Differentiation. Ed. by G. V. Sherbet. 1973. (Illus.). 121.75 (*3-8055-1581-2*) S Karger.

Neoplasia in Infancy & Childhood. Ed. by H. S. Rosenberg & J. Bernstein. 1986. (Perspectives in Pediatric Pathology Ser.: Vol. 9). viii, 248p. 191.50 (*3-8055-4373-5*) S Karger.

Neoplasma & Related Lesions of the Head & Neck: Based on the Proceedings of the 59th Annual Anatomic Pathology Slide Seminar of the American Society of Clinical Pathologists. Stacey E. Mills et al. 1994. LC 94-21116. 126p. 35.00 (*0-89189-385-7*) Am Soc Clinical.

Neoplasms - Prevention & Control: Index of New Information with Authors, Subjects & Bibliography. Mumford C. Yeatman. 1993. 180p. 47.50 (*1-55914-816-0*); pap. 44.50 (*1-55914-817-9*) ABBE Pubs Assn.

Neoplasms—Prevention, Control & Results: Index of New Information for Reference & Research. John C. Bartone. 1997. 160p. 57.50 (*0-7883-1666-4*); pap. 47.50 (*0-7883-1667-2*) ABBE Pubs Assn.

Neoplasms of the Colon, Rectum, & Anus. Philip H. Gordon & Santhat Nivatvongs. 2000. (Illus.). 368p. text 110.00 (*1-57626-124-7*) Quality Med Pub.

Neoplasms of the Liver. Kunio Okuda & Kamal G. Ishak. 1987. (Illus.). 420p. 391.00 (*0-387-70020-X*) Spr-Verlag.

Neoplasms of the Lung: Based on the Proceedings of the 57th Annual Anatomic Pathology Slide Seminar of the American Society of Clinical Pathologists, September 26-27, 1991, New Orleans, Louisiana. 1994. LC 93-5551. 35.00 (*0-89189-348-2*) Am Soc Clinical.

Neoplasms with Follicular Differentiation. A. Bernard Ackerman. 1992. LC 91-34968. (Illus.). 650p. text 150.00 (*0-8121-1542-2*) Lppncott W & W.

Neoplasms with Follicular Differentiation. A. Bernard Ackerman et al. 2nd rev. ed. 2001. LC 99-98185. (Histologic Diagnosis of Neoplastic Skin Diseases Ser.). 1,109p. 225.00 (*1-893357-11-2*) Ardor Scrib.

Neoplastic Diseases. Ed. by C. Julian Rosenthal. 1991. LC 91-62100. 891p. 129.00 (*0-944496-24-5*) Precept Pr.

Neoplastic Diseases in Childhood, Set. Ed. by Carl Pochedly et al. 1995. LC 93-12664. 1600p. text 473.00 (*3-7186-5340-0*) Gordon & Breach.

Neoplastic Diseases of the Blood. Peter H. Wiernik et al. 3rd ed. 1995. LC 95-31180. 1240p. text (*0-443-07600-6*) Church.

Neoplastic Hematopathology. Daniel M. Knowles. (Illus.). 1992. 1640p. 229.00 (*0-683-04735-3*); 2nd ed. 1998. LC 00-41238. xxiv, 1957p. text 299.00 (*0-683-30246-9*) Lppncott W & W.

Neoplastic Process & the Nervous System. Ed. by R. E. Kavetskii. 1960. 248p. text 66.00 (*0-7065-0124-1*) Coronet Bks.

Neoplastic Transformation in Human Cell Culture: Mechanisms of Carcinogenesis. Ed. by Johng S. Rhim & Anatoly Dritschilo. 1991. LC 91-35328. (Experimental Biology & Medicine Ser.: Vol. 25). (Illus.). 408p. 145.00 (*0-89603-227-2*) Humana.

Nephrogenesis. Ed. by A. S. Woolf. 1996. (Journal: Vol. 4, No. 2, 1996). (Illus.). 70p. pap. 45.25 (*3-8055-6294-2*) S Karger.

Nephrologic Problems of the Newborn. Ed. by J. F. Pascual & P. L. Calcagno. 1979. (Contributions to Nephrology Ser.: Vol. 15). (Illus.). pap. 29.75 (*3-8055-2947-3*) S Karger.

Nephrologie im Kindesalter III. Ed. by O. Oetliker & E. Bern Rossi. 1978. (Paediatrische Fortbildungskurse fuer die Praxis Ser.: Bd. 45). (GER., Illus.). 46.25 (*3-8055-2825-6*) S Karger.

Nephrologie Pediatrique. P. Royer et al. 3rd ed. 1983. (Collection Pediatrie Ser.). (FRE., Illus.). 652p. lib. bdg. 75.00 (*2-257-12397-2*) S M P F Inc.

Nephrology. Ed. by Jamison & R. Wilkinson. 1997. (Illus.). 1172p. (*0-412-60930-4*) E A GBR. *Dist:* OUP.

Nephrology. M. Legrain. 1987. 400p. (gr. 13). 17.00 (*0-89352-230-9*) Mosby Inc.

Nephrology. Ed. by Rachael Robinson. 1984. (Illus.). 884p. 367.00 (*0-387-96072-4*) Spr-Verlag.

Nephrology. Ed. by Francesco Paolo Schena. 2000. (Clinical Medicine Ser.). (Illus.). 520p. Price not set. (*0-07-709525-1*) McGraw-Hill Med Pub.

Nephrology: Diuretics: Basic, Pharmacological, & Clinical Aspects. Ed. by Vittorio E. Andreucci & Antonio Dal Canton. 1987. (Developments in Nephrology Ser.). 640p. (C). text 208.00 (*0-89838-885-6*) Kluwer Academic.

Nephrology: Proceedings of the XIth International Congress of Nephrology, Set. Ed. by M. Hatano. 1991. (Illus.). 1800p. 290.00 (*0-387-70074-9*) Spr-Verlag.

Nephrology & Dialysis Updated. Ed. by G. D'Amico & G. Colasanti. 1988. (Contributions to Nephrology Ser.: Vol. 61). (Illus.). vi, 298p. 29.75 (*3-8055-4673-4*) S Karger.

Nephrology & Transplantation, 1986. Jon C. Ransom. 1986. pap. text 24.95 (*0-914899-04-X*) Current Lit Pubns.

Nephrology & Transplantation, 1987. Jon C. Ransom. 1987. 340p. pap. text 24.95 (*0-914899-05-8*) Current Lit Pubns.

Nephrology & Transplantation, 1988. Jon C. Ransom. 1988. 436p. pap. text 29.95 (*0-914899-06-6*) Current Lit Pubns.

Nephrology & Urology for the Pediatrician. Bernard Gauthier et al. 1982. 54.95 (*0-316-30524-3*, Little Brwn Med Div) Lppncott W & W.

Nephrology & Urology in the Aged Patient. Ed. by Dimitrious G. Oreopoulos et al. 1993. LC 92-48668. text 392.50 (*0-7923-2019-0*) Kluwer Academic.

Nephrology for the House Officer. C. Craig Tisher. 2nd ed. 1992. LC 92-49487. (Illus.). 336p. pap. 21.95 (*0-683-08276-0*) Lppncott W & W.

Nephrology Forum. Ed. by J. J. Cohen et al. 1982. (Illus.). 383p. 117.00 (*0-387-90764-5*) Spr-Verlag.

Nephrology Grand Rounds: Clinical Issues in Nephrology. Ed. by Martin Zeier & Eberhard Ritz. 1998. LC 98-22539. (Contributions to Nephrology Ser.: Vol. 123). (Illus.). viii, 202p. 198.25 (*3-8055-6718-9*) S Karger.

Nephrology, 1985. Jon C. Ransom. 1985. 337p. pap. text 24.95 (*0-914899-03-1*) Current Lit Pubns.

Nephrology, 1984. Jon C. Ransom. 1984. 338p. (Orig.). pap. text 24.95 (*0-914899-01-5*) Current Lit Pubns.

Nephrology Nursing. Francine Hekelman & Carol Ostendarp. 1979. (Illus.). text 33.95 (*0-07-027948-9*) McGraw.

Nephrotic Syndrome. J. Stewart Cameron & Richard J. Glassock. 1987. (Kidney Disease Ser.: Vol. 8). (Illus.). 1080p. text 299.00 (*0-8247-7361-6*) Dekker.

Nephrotoxicity. J. B. Hook. 1986. 86p. text 70.00 (*2-88124-420-3*) Gordon & Breach.

Nephrotoxicity: In Vitro & in Vivo, Animals to Man. Ed. by Peter H. Bach & E. A. Lock. 1989. (Illus.). 788p. 145.00 (*0-306-43153-X*, Plenum Trade) Perseus Pubng.

Nephrotoxicity in the Experimental & Clinical Situation. Ed. by Peter H. Bach & E. A. Lock. 1987. (Developments in Nephrology Ser.). (C). Pt. 1. lib. bdg. 179.50 (*0-89838-977-1*); Pt. 2. text 195.50 (*0-89838-980-1*) Kluwer Academic.

Nephrotoxicity of Clinically Relevant Drugs. Ed. by William M. Bennett. 1994. (Journal: Vol. 2, No. 4, 1994). (Illus.). 76p. pap. 41.75 (*3-8055-6091-5*) S Karger.

Nernstach - Neurophysiology. Gunther. 1994. 81.25 net. (*0-697-22926-2*) McGraw.

Nerve - Muscle Interaction. Gerta Vrbova et al. 2nd ed. 1994. 256p. (C). (gr. 13). pap. text 131.95 (*0-412-40490-7*) Chapman & Hall.

Nerve & Muscle. R. D. Keynes & David J. Aidley. 2nd ed. 1992. (Illus.). 191p. (C). pap. text 20.95 (*0-521-42255-8*) Cambridge U Pr.

Nerve & Muscle: Membranes, Cells & Systems. R. B. Stein. 1980. LC 80-15028. (Illus.). 274p. 35.00 (*0-306-40512-1*, Plenum Trade) Perseus Pubng.

Nerve Block for Common Pain. Richard E. Cytowic. 1991. (Illus.). 96p. 37.95 (*0-387-97147-5*) Spr-Verlag.

Nerve Cells & Animal Behaviour. David G. Young. 1989. (Illus.). 248p. text 69.95 (*0-521-30705-8*); pap. text 24.95 (*0-521-31443-7*) Cambridge U Pr.

Nerve Cells & Nervous Systems: An Introduction to Neuroscience. A. Brown. 1994. (Illus.). 265p. 59.95 (*0-387-19637-4*) Spr-Verlag.

Nerve Conduction Studies. Kathryne Hammer. 1982. (Illus.). 166p. spiral bd. 38.95 (*0-398-04519-4*) C C Thomas.

Nerve Conduction Studies for the Technologist. American Journal of END Technology Staff. 2nd ed. 1999. spiral bd. 25.00 (*1-57797-007-1*) ASET.

Nerve Growth & Guidance. Ed. by C. D. McCaig. 1996. (Frontiers in Neurobiology Ser.: No. 2). 188p. (C). text (*1-85578-085-2*) Portland Pr Ltd GBR. *Dist:* Ashgate Pub Co.

Nerve Injuries. David G. Kline & Alan R. Hudson. 1995. LC 94-12233. (Illus.). 624p. text 150.00 (*0-7216-3264-5*) Saunders.

Nerve Injuries & Their Repair: A Critical Appraisal. Sydney Sunderland. 1990. (Illus.). 538p. text (*0-443-04161-X*) Church.

Nerve Injury & Repair. Goran Lundborg. 1988. (Illus.). 256p. text (*0-443-03528-8*) Church.

Nerve, Muscle & Synapse. Bernard Katz. 1966. (New Biology Ser.). text (*0-07-033374-2*) McGraw.

Nerve-Muscle Cell Trophic Communication. Ed. by Hugo L. Fernandez & J. Alejandro Donoso. 1988. 224p. 146.00 (*0-8493-6660-7*, QP364, CRC Reprint) Franklin.

Nerves & the Gastrointestinal Tract. Ed. by M. V. Singer & H. Goebell. 1989. (Falk Symposium Ser.). (C). lib. bdg. 324.50 (*0-7462-0114-1*) Kluwer Academic.

Nervine Herbs. Rita Elkins. 1997. (Woodland Health Ser.). 32p. pap. 3.95 (*1-885670-32-X*) Woodland UT.

Nervous Disorders & Religion: A Study of Souls in the Making. John G. McKenzie. 1981. LC 79-8719. 183p. reprint ed. lib. bdg. 35.00 (*0-313-22192-8*, MCND, Greenwood Pr) Greenwood.

Nervous System. Thomas Braem. 1994. (Organs of the Human Anatomy: Vol. 3). 88p. (C). spiral bd. 15.95 (*1-878576-28-3*) Flash Anatomy Inc.

Nervous System. Helen Frost. Ed. by Gail Saunders-Smith. 2000. LC 00-24558. (Human Body Systems Ser.). (Illus.). 24p. (J). (ps-2). lib. bdg. 14.60 (*0-7368-0651-2*, Pebble Bks) Capstone Pr.

Nervous System: Its Function & Its Interaction with the World. Lloyd D. Partridge & L. Donald Partridge. 1992. (Illus.). 593p. 75.00 (*0-262-16134-6*, Bradford Bks) MIT Pr.

Nervous System Pt. 2: Anatomy & Physiology. Illus. by Frank H. Netter. 2000. (*0-914168-24-X*) Icon Lrning Systs.

Nervous System & the Heart. Ed. by Gert J. Ter Horst. 2000. LC 99-25404. (Illus.). 584p. 145.00 (*0-89603-693-6*) Humana.

Nervous System Course. Competence Assurance Systems Staff. 1983. (Illus.). pap. text 60.00 (*0-89147-069-7*) CAS.

Nervous System, Muscle & Eyes. Ed. by R. O. Weller. 3rd ed. 1990. (Systemic Pathology Ser.: Vol. 4). (Illus.). 776p. text (*0-443-03312-9*) Church.

Nervous System of Invertebrates: An Evolutionary & Comparative Approach. Ed. by O. Breidbach et al. 1995. LC 94-35125. (Exs Ser.: Vol. 72). 448p. 145.50 (*0-8176-5076-8*) Birkhauser.

Nervous Systems Regeneration in the Invertebrates: Invertebrate Neural Regeneration. S. B. Moffett. 1996. (Zoophysiology & Ecology Ser.: Vol. 34). (Illus.). 208p. 158.00 (*3-540-59454-X*) Spr-Verlag.

Net Gain: A New Method for Preventing Malaria Deaths. Ed. by Christian Lengeler et al. 1996. 260p. pap. (*0-88936-792-2*) IDRC-CRDI CAN. *Dist:* Stylus Pub VA.

NetHealer: Your Guide to Choosing Alternative Health Care. Michael Wolff. 1997. 200p. pap. 12.95 (*1-889670-24-3*) Wolff New Media.

Netherlands Ophthalmological Society, 168th Meeting, Rotterdam, December 1973: Proceedings. 1976. (Journal: Vol. 173, No. 3-4). 52.25 (*3-8055-2218-5*) S Karger.

Netter Atlas of Human Anatomy. Rittenhouse Book Distributors Staff. 2nd ed. 1998. LC 97-75710. (The Novartis Medical Education Program Ser.). 596p. lib. bdg. 84.95 (*0-914168-80-0*) Icon Lrning Systs.

Netter Collection of Medical Illustrations. Frank H. Netter & Ernst Oppenheimer. 1997. LC 97-76569. (Illus.). (*0-914168-75-4*); (*0-914168-76-2*); (*0-914168-78-9*) Icon Lrning Systs.

M N O

***Netter's Altlas of Physiology.** John T. Hansen & Bruce M. Koeppen. 2001. (Illus.). 250p. (C). pap. 45.00 (*1-929007-01-9*) Icon Lrning Systs.

***Netter's Atlas of Embryology.** Larry Cochard. 2001. (Illus.). 250p. (C). pap. 45.00 (*0-914168-99-1*) Icon Lrning Systs.

***Netter's Orthopedic Primer.** Walter Greene. 2002. (Illus.). 600p. (C). pap. 50.00 (*1-929007-02-7*) Icon Lrning Systs.

***Netter's Pocket Atlas of Orthopedic Anatomy.** John Thompson. 2001. LC 00-130477. (Illus.). 350p. pap. 37.95 (*0-914168-94-0*) Icon Lrning Systs.

***Netter's Textbook of Internal Medicine.** Marschall Runge. 2002. (Illus.). 600p. (C). pap. 50.00 (*1-929007-00-0*) Icon Lrning Systs.

Netvet: Mosby's Veterinary Guide to the Internet, Vol. 1. Kenneth R. Boschert & Henry James. 1997. LC 98-151846. (Illus.). 275p. (gr. 13). pap. text 24.95 incl. 3.5 hd (*0-8151-2935-1*, 31825) Mosby Inc.

Network Models in Population Biology. E. R. Lewis. 1977. LC 77-5873. (Biomathematics Ser.: Vol 7). 59.95 (*0-387-08214-X*) Spr-Verlag.

Network Therapy for Alcohol & Drug Abuse. Marc Galanter. enl. ed. 1999. LC 98-52868. 264p. pap. 22.00 (*1-57230-441-3*, C0441) Guilford Pubns.

Networking Families in Crisis: Intervention Strategies with Families & Social Networks. Uri Rueveni. 1979. LC 78-8024. 162p. 32.95 (*0-87705-374-X*, Kluwer Acad Hman Sci) Kluwer Academic.

Networking in Brucellosis Research: Report of the United Nations University Brucellosis Research Network. 236p. 35.00 (*92-808-0756-0*, E. 91.III. A. 8) UN.

Networks: Aging of Cell Membranes & Molecules. Ed. by Marguerite M. Kay. 1991. (Journal: Vol. 37, Nos. 1-3, 1991). (Illus.). 180p. pap. 117.50 (*3-8055-5391-9*) S Karger.

Networks of Innovation: Vaccine Development at Merck, Sharp & Dohme, & Mulford, 1895-1995. Louis Galambos & Jane E. Sewell. 1997. (Illus.). 288p. (C). reprint ed. pap. text 17.95 (*0-521-62620-X*) Cambridge U Pr.

Networks of Meaning: A Bridge Between Mind & Matter. Christine Hardy. 1998. LC 98-14932. 232p. 60.00 (*0-275-96035-8*, Praeger Pubs) Greenwood.

Networks That Work: A Guide to Dental Networking. Cheryl Maesaka. 1999. 100p. pap. 15.95 (*0-88100-105-8*) Natl Writ Pr.

Neue Akquisitionen in der Neonatologie: Nouvelles Acquisitions en Neonatologie. Ed. by E. Bern Rossi. 1988. (Paediatrische Fortbildungskurse fuer die Praxis Ser.: Vol. 62). (Illus.). x, 660p. pap. 34.00 (*3-8055-4742-0*) S Karger.

Neue Aspekte in der Behandlung der Herzinsuffizienz: Oberrheinisches Kardiologen - Symposium. Ed. by F. Burkhart. 1980. (Journal: Vol. 65, Suppl. 1, 1980). (Illus.). pap. 16.75 (*3-8055-0652-X*) S Karger.

Neue Erfahrungen Mit Oxazaphosphorinen unter Besonderer Beruecksichtigung des Uroprotektors Uromitexan. Ed. by H. Burkert & G. A. Nagel. 1980. (Beitraege Zur Onkologie, Contributions to Oncology Ser.: Band 5). (Illus.). 126p. pap. 25.25 (*3-8055-1381-X*) S Karger.

Neue Therapeutische Strategien in der Haematologischen Onkologie. Ed. by H. Loeffler. 1989. (Beitraege Zur Onkologie, Contributions to Oncology Ser.: Vol. 36). (Illus.). vi, 115p. 47.00 (*3-8055-5046-4*) S Karger.

Neuere Aspekte der Kinderkardiiology, Set. Ed. by E. Bern Rossi & F. Wyler. 1978. (Paediatrische Fortbildungskurse fuer die Praxis Ser.: Vol. 47). (FRE & GER., Illus.). pap. 32.25 (*3-8055-2865-5*) S Karger.

Neuere Aspekte der Kinderkardiology. Ed. by F. Stocker et al. 1980. (Paediatrische Fortbildungskurse fuer die Praxis Ser.: Vol. 51). (Illus.). vi, 130p. pap. 50.50 (*3-8055-0926-X*) S Karger.

Neuman Systems Model. Ed. by Betty M. Neuman. 3rd ed. 1994. LC 94-30479. 608p. (C). pap. 59.00 (*0-8385-6701-0*, A6701-5) P-H.

Neural & Neurohumoral Organization of Motivated Behaviour: The 4th Conference in Interbrain Held in Pecs, Hungary, May 19-23, 1975. K. Lissak. 1978. 267p. (C). (*963-05-1316-1*) Akade Kiado HUN. *Dist:* St Mut.

Neural Aspects of Human Movement: Implications for Control & Coordination. C. M. Bakker et al. 1993. LC 93-211584. viii, 96p. pap. (*90-265-1322-4*) Swets.

Neural Bases of Motor Behaviour: Proceedings of the NATO Advanced Study Institute on Multi-Sensory Control of Movement, Trieste, Italy, 3-12 July 1994. Ed. by Francesco Lacquinniti & Paolo Viviani. 1996. (NATO Advanced Study Institutes Ser.: Series D, Vol. 85). 356p. (C). text 180.50 (*0-7923-4009-4*) Kluwer Academic.

Neural Bases of Speech, Hearing, & Language. Ed. by David Kuehn et al. 1989. LC 87-2825. (Illus.). 315p. text 38.00 (*0-316-50491-2*, 1722) PRO-ED.

Neural Bases of Violence & Aggression. William S. Fields & W. H. Sweet. 1975. LC 72-13847. (Illus.). 640p. 37.50 (*0-87527-102-2*) Green.

Neural Basis of Behavior. Ed. by A. L. Beckman. 1982. (Illus.). 350p. text 53.95 (*0-88331-162-3*) R B Luce.

Neural Basis of Behavioral Adaptations: Proceedings of an International Symposium in Honour of Professor Dr. Franz Huber Held in the Evangelische Akademie Tutzing, FRC. Ed. by Klaus Schildberger & Nobert Elsner. 1994. LC 93-38296. (Fortschritte der Zoologie Ser.: No. 39). xii, 284p. (*3-437-30680-4*) Gustav Fischer DEU. *Dist:* Lubrecht & Cramer, Balogh.

Neural Basis of Feeding & Reward. Ed. by B. G. Hoebel & D. Novin. 1982. (Illus.). 575p. (Orig.). pap. text 39.95 (*0-940090-02-3*) Haer Inst.

Neural Basis of Motor Control. Vernon B. Brooks. 1986. (Illus.). 344p. pap. text 49.50 (*0-19-503684-0*) OUP.

Neural Basis/Visual Function. J. Cronly-Dillon. 1991. 137.00 (*0-8493-7504-5*) CRC Pr.

Neural Blockage in Clinical Anesthesia & Management of Pain. Ed. by Michael J. Cousins. 3rd ed. 1997. LC 97-26333. 1,200p. text 199.00 (*0-397-51159-0*) Lppncott W & W.

Neural Cartography: How Does the CNS Use Sensory Maps? Ed. by Thomas E. Finger. 1987. (Journal: Vol. 31, No. 1, 1988). 56p. pap. 85.25 (*3-8055-4724-2*) S Karger.

Neural Cell Culture: A Practical Approach. Ed. by James Cohen & Graham Wilkin. 1996. (Practical Approach Ser.: Vol. 165). (Illus.). 268p. (C). pap. text 55.00 (*0-19-963484-X*) OUP.

Neural Cell Specification: Molecular Mechanisms & Neurotherapeutic Implications: Proceedings of the Third Altschul Symposium Held in Saskatoon, Canada, May 12-14, 1994. Ed. by Bernard H. Juurlink et al. 1995. (Altschul Symposia Ser.: Vol. 3). (Illus.). 324p. 110.00 (*0-306-45185-9*, Kluwer Plenum) Kluwer Academic.

Neural Codes & Distributed Representations: Foundations of Neural Computation. Ed. by Laurence Abbott & Terrence J. Sejnowski. 1998. LC 98-14783. (Computational Neuroscience Ser.). (Illus.). xxiii, 345p. pap. 32.00 (*0-262-51100-2*, Bradford Bks) MIT Pr.

Neural Computation of Pattern Motion: Modeling Stages of Motion Analysis in the Primate Visual Cortex. Margaret E. Sereno. 1993. LC 92-19630. (Neural Network Modeling & Connectionism Ser.). (Illus.). 190p. 35.00 (*0-262-19329-9*, Bradford Bks) MIT Pr.

Neural Connections, Mental Computation. Ed. by Lynn Nadel & Lynn A. Cooper. 1992. (Illus.). 368p. reprint ed. pap. text 27.50 (*0-262-64029-5*, Bradford Bks) MIT Pr.

Neural Control of Macronutrient Selection: Neural & Metabolic Control of Macronujtrient Intake. Hans-Rudolf Berthoud & Randy J. Seeley. 1999. LC 99-29233. (Illus.). 528p. 89.95 (*0-8493-2752-0*, 2752) CRC Pr.

Neural Control of Movement: Proceedings of the 32nd Congress of the International Union of Physiological Sciences (IUPS), Held in Glasgow, Scotland, August 1-6, 1992. Ed. by William R. Ferrell & Uwe Proske. 1995. LC 95-8372. (Illus.). 326p. 95.00 (*0-306-45016-X*, Kluwer Plenum) Kluwer Academic.

Neural Control of Skilled Human Movements. Ed. by F. W. Cody. 1995. (Studies in Physiology: Vol. 3). (Illus.). 120p. (Orig.). (C). pap. text (*1-85578-081-X*) Portland Pr Ltd GBR. *Dist:* Ashgate Pub Co.

Neural Control of the Cardiovascular System & Orthostatic Regulation: Proceedings Basel, 1975. Ed. by H. Denolin et al. 1976. (Cardiology Ser.: Vol. 61, Suppl. 1). (Illus.). 250p. 61.00 (*3-8055-2260-6*) S Karger.

Neural Development & Plasticity. R. Ranney Mize & Reha S. Erzurumlu. 1996. LC 96-41471. (Progress in Brain Research Ser.). 434p. 207.00 (*0-444-82433-2*) Elsevier.

Neural Development & Schizophrenia: Theory & Research, No. 275. Ed. by Sarnoff A. Mednick & J. Meggin Hollister. 1995. LC 95-3584. (NATO ASI Ser.: Ser. A, Vol. 275). (Illus.). 272p. (C). text 89.50 (*0-306-44996-X*) Plenum.

Neural Dynamics of Adaptive Sensory-Motor Control. Stephen Grossberg & M. Kuperstein. enl. ed. 1989. (Neural Networks Research & Applications Ser.: Vol. 1). (Illus.). 450p. pap. text 35.00 (*0-08-036827-1*, Pergamon Pr) Elsevier.

Neural Function. Michael Wang & Alan Freeman. 1986. 208p. 21.00 (*0-316-92148-3*, Little Brwn Med Div) Lppncott W & W.

Neural Hormones & Reproduction: Proceedings of the International Symposium on Brain-Endocrine Interaction, 3rd, Wurzberg, July, 1977. International Symposium on Brain-Endocrine Interac. Ed. by D. E. Scott et al. 1978. (Brain-Endocrine Interaction Ser.: Vol. III). (Illus.). 172.25 (*3-8055-2798-5*) S Karger.

Neural Mechanisms & Cardiovascular Disease: Proceedings of the International Symposium Held in S. Margherita Ligure, Italy, in May 1985. Ed. by A. Malliani et al. 1987. (FIDIA Research Ser.). 642p. 196.00 (*0-387-96454-1*) Spr-Verlag.

Neural Mechanisms in Animal Behavior. Ed. by A. M. Granda & W. N. Hayes. 1972. (Illus.). 39.25 (*3-8055-1558-8*) S Karger.

Neural Mechanisms in Behavior: A Texas Symposium. Ed. by D. McFadden. 1980. (Illus.). 308p. 102.00 (*0-387-90468-9*) Spr-Verlag.

Neural Mechanisms in Disorders of Movement. A. R. Crossman & M. A. Sambrook. 1988. (Current Problems in Neurology Ser.: Vol. 9). 224p. (*0-86196-164-1*) J Libbey Med GBR. *Dist:* Bks Intl VA.

Neural Mechanisms in Taste. Ed. by Robert H. Cagan. 1989. 240p. 159.00 (*0-8493-5834-5*, QP456) CRC Pr.

***Neural Mechanisms of Anesthesia.** Ed. by Joseph F. Antognini et al. 2002. (Contemporary Clinical Neuroscience Ser.). 600p. 165.00 (*0-89603-997-8*) Humana.

Neural Mechanisms of Salivary Gland Secretion. Ed. by J. R. Garrett et al. 1999. (Frontiers of Oral Biology Ser.: Vol. 11). (Illus.). viii, 200p. 174.00 (*3-8055-6880-0*) S Karger.

Neural Mechanisms of Salivary Gland Secretion/ Glandular Mechanisms of Salivary Gland Secretion. Ed. by J. R. Garrett et al. 2000. (Frontiers of Oral Biology Ser.: Vols. 10 & 11). (Illus.). xx, 464p. 283.50 (*3-8055-6964-5*) S Karger.

Neural Membranes. Ed. by Grace Y. Sun et al. 1983. LC 83-6106. (Experimental & Clinical Neuroscience Ser.). (Illus.). 584p. 140.00 (*0-89603-052-0*) Humana.

Neural Modeling & Neural Networks. Ed. by F. Ventriglia. 1994. LC 93-34085. (Studies in Neurosciences). 360p. 173.00 (*0-08-042277-2*, Pergamon Pr) Elsevier.

Neural Modeling of Brain & Cognitive Disorders. 1996. LC 96-35593. 425p. lib. bdg. 60.00 (*981-02-2879-1*) World Scientific Pub.

Neural Monitoring: The Prevention of Intraoperative Injury. Ed. by Steven K. Salzman. 1990. LC 90-4625. (Neurotrauma Ser.). (Illus.). 336p. 145.00 (*0-89603-189-6*) Humana.

Neural Networks & Brain Function. Edmund T. Rolls & Alessandro Treves. 1997. LC 97-41669. (Illus.). 428p. text 115.00 (*0-19-852433-1*); pap. text 52.50 (*0-19-852432-3*) OUP.

Neural Networks & Psychopathology: Connectionist Models in Practice & Research. Ed. by Dan J. Stein & Jacques Ludik. 1999. LC 98-5826. (Illus.). 385p. (C). text 95.00 (*0-521-57163-4*) Cambridge U Pr.

Neural Networks in Biomedicine: Proceedings of the Course. F. Masulli & P. G. Morasso. 1994. 300p. text 91.00 (*981-02-1744-7*) World Scientific Pub.

Neural Organization: Structure, Function & Dynamics. Michael A. Arbib et al. 1997. LC 96-44543. 328p. 75.00 (*0-262-01159-X*, Bradford Bks) MIT Pr.

Neural Plasticity & Regeneration, Vol. 128. Ed. by F. R. Seiler. 2000. LC 00-50396. (Progress in Brain Research Ser.: Vol. 128). (Illus.). 392p. 152.00 (*0-444-50209-2*, Excerpta Medica) Elsevier.

Neural Prostheses: Materials, Physiology & Histopathology of Electrical Stimulation of the Nervous System. J. J. Bernstein. 1977. (Journal: Vol. 14, No. 1 2). (Illus.). 61.50 (*3-8055-2640-7*) S Karger.

Neural Prostheses: Replacing Motor Function after Disease or Disability. Richard B. Stein et al. 1992. (Illus.). 360p. text 68.00 (*0-19-507216-2*) OUP.

Neural Prosthesis & Neurostimulation. Ed. by Philip L. Gildenberg et al. 1981. (Applied Neurophysiology Ser.: Vol. 45, No. 1-2). (Illus.). iv, 208p. pap. 68.00 (*3-8055-3500-7*) S Karger.

Neural Protheses: Reversing the Vector of Surgery. Ed. by Robert J. Maciunas. 2000. 372p. 95.00 (*1-879284-73-1*) Am Assn Neuro.

Neural Regulation in the Vertebrate Endocrine System: Neuroendocrine Regulation. Ed. by P. D. Prasada Rao & Richard E. Peter. 1999. LC 99-30042. (Illus.). (*0-306-46127-7*) Plenum.

Neural Regulation of Brain Circulation. Ed. by Christer Owman & J. E. Hardebo. 1987. (Fernstrom Foundation Ser.: No. 8). 632p. 357.00 (*0-444-80777-2*) Elsevier.

***Neural Repair, Transplantation & Rehabilitation.** Roger A. Barker & Stephen B. Dunnett. 2001. 336p. pap. (*0-86377-629-9*) Psychol Pr GBR. *Dist:* Taylor & Francis.

Neural Representation of Temporal Patterns: Proceedings of a Symposium Held in Durham, North Carolina, April 29-May 2, 1993. Ed. by Ellen Covey et al. 1996. 274p. (C). text 95.00 (*0-306-45199-9*, Kluwer Plenum) Kluwer Academic.

Neural Stimulation Ed. by Joel B. Myklebust et al. 1985. Vol. I. 168p. 100.00 (*0-8493-5253-3*, RC350); Vol. II. 176p. 101.00 (*0-8493-5254-1*, RC350) Franklin (CRC Reprint).

Neural Substrates of Limbic Epilepsy. Makram K. Girgis. 1981. (Illus.). 206p. (C). 42.50 (*0-87527-238-X*) Green.

Neural Tissue Transplantation Research: Proceedings in Life Sciences. Ed. by R. B. Wallace & G. D. Das. 1983. (Illus.). 243p. 152.00 (*0-387-90833-1*) Spr-Verlag.

Neural Transplantation, CNS Neuronal Injury & Regeneration. Joe Marwak. 1994. 304p. 141.95 (*0-8493-8683-7*, RD124) CRC Pr.

Neural Transplantation in Cerebellar Ataxia. Lazaros C. Triarhou. 1996. LC 96-34818. (Neuroscience Intelligence Unit Ser.). 160p. 99.00 (*1-57059-395-7*) Landes Bioscience.

Neural Transplantation in Neurodegenerative Disease - Novartis Foundation Symposium 231: Current Status & New Directions, Vol. 231. Novartis Foundation Symposium Staff. 2000. LC 00-43390. (CIBA Foundation Symposia Ser.: Vol. 231). 334p. 125.00 (*0-471-49246-9*) Wiley.

Neural Transplants: Development & Function. Ed. by John R. Sladek, Jr. & Don M. Gash. 1984. 444p. 95.00 (*0-306-41587-9*, Plenum Trade) Perseus Pubng.

Neural Tube Defects, No. 181. CIBA Foundation Staff. 1994. (CIBA Foundation Symposia Ser.: Vol. 181). 310p. 128.00 (*0-471-94172-7*) Wiley.

Neurally Mediated Syncope: Pathophysiology, Investigations & Treatment. Jean-Jacques Blanc et al. 1996. (Bakken Research Center Ser.: No. 10). (Illus.). 188p. 55.00 (*0-87993-644-4*) Futura Pub.

Neuro-Anaesthetic Practice. Ed. by Hugo Van Aken. 1995. 320p. (Orig.). (C). pap. text (*0-7279-0909-6*) BMJ Pub GBR. *Dist:* AIDC.

Neuro-Immune Interactions in Neurologic & Psychiatric Disorders. Ed. by Paul H. Patterson et al. 1999. LC 99-36334. (Research & Perspectives in Neurosciences Ser.). (Illus.). 180p. 104.00 (*3-540-66013-5*) Spr-Verlag.

Neuro-Immunology for the Clinician. Loren A. Rolek & Yadollah Harati. 1997. LC 96-50466. 440p. text 99.00 (*0-7506-9616-8*) Buttrwrth-Heinemann.

Neuro-Immunology of Fever. Ed. by Tamas Bartfai & David Ottoson. 1992. LC 92-48954. (Wenner-Gren International Ser.). 300p. 188.00 (*0-08-042001-X*, Pergamon Pr) Elsevier.

Neuro-Linguistic Programming, Vol. 1. Robert Dilts et al. 1980. LC 80-50147. 26.95 (*0-916990-07-9*) META Pubns.

Neuro-Linguistic Programming in Alcoholism Treatment. Ed. by Chelly M. Sterman. LC 90-34784. 186p. 1996. pap. 19.95 (*0-7890-0081-4*); 1990. (Addiction Treatment Ser.: Vol. 3). (Illus.). 39.95 (*1-56024-002-4*) Haworth Pr.

Neuro-Muscular Testing with Surface EMG. Gabriel E. Sella. 1995. 410p. (C). pap. text 120.00 (*1-884325-08-4*) G E Sella.

Neuro-Oncology. Ed. by P. Paoletti et al. 1991. (Developments in Oncology Ser.). (C). text 243.00 (*0-7923-1215-5*) Kluwer Academic.

Neuro Oncology. Ed. by Clifford F. Rose & William S. Fields. 1985. (Progress in Experimental Tumor Research Ser.: Vol. 29). (Illus.). xiv, 274p. 200.00 (*3-8055-4054-X*) S Karger.

Neuro-Oncology, Pt. 1. P. J. Vinken et al. 1997. LC 97-50465. (Handbooks of Clinical Neurology). 448p. 209.00 (*0-444-81286-5*) Elsevier.

Neuro-Oncology: Gliomas & Other Primary Tumors of the Brain & Spinal Cord. Ed. by P. J. Vinken et al. Pt. II. 1998. 614p. 224.00 (*0-444-81287-3*); Pt. III. 1997. 548p. 225.00 (*0-444-81288-1*) Elsevier.

***Neuro-Oncology: Scientific Basis & Clinical Practice.** William R. Shapiro. 2001. (Illus.). 635p. (*0-443-06580-2*) Church GBR. *Dist:* Saunders.

Neuro-Oncology: The Essentials. Mark Bernstein. 1999. (Illus.). 736p. 149.00 (*0-86577-880-9*) Thieme Med Pubs.

Neuro-Oncology for Nurses. Douglas Guerrero. 1998. xiv, 330p. pap. text (*1-86156-087-7*) Whurr Pub.

Neuro-Ophthalmic System: Clinical Procedures. Patricia A. Modica. 1999. LC 98-46226. (Optometric Series). 163p. spiral bd. 44.99 (*0-7506-9620-6*) Buttrwrth-Heinemann.

Neuro-Ophthalmological Disorders: Diagnostic Work-Up & Management. Ed. by Ronald J. Tusa & Steven A. Newman. 1994. (Neurological Disease & Therapy Ser.: Vol. 31). (Illus.). 664p. text 225.00 (*0-8247-8839-7*) Dekker.

Neuro-Ophthalmology. Joel S. Glaser. 3rd ed. 1999. LC 99-24157. 688p. text 149.00 (*0-7817-1729-9*) Lppncott W & W.

Neuro-Ophthalmology, Vol. 2. Ed. by Simmons Lessell & J. T. Van Dalen. 1982. 404p. 184.00 (*0-444-90210-4*, Excerpta Medica) Elsevier.

Neuro-Ophthalmology: A Practical Text. Nancy M. Newman. 1992. (Illus.). 484p. (C). pap. text 125.00 (*0-8385-6698-7*, A6698-3, Apple Lange Med) McGraw.

Neuro-Ophthalmology: Clinical Signs & Symptoms. Thomas J. Walsh. 3rd ed. 1991. LC 91-14153. (Illus.). 642p. text 98.50 (*0-8121-1462-0*) Lppncott W & W.

Neuro-Ophthalmology: Diagnosis. Nicholas J. Volpe et al. 2000. LC 00-38805. (Illus.). xi, 756p. text 100.00 (*0-7216-6533-0*) Saunders.

Neuro-Ophthalmology Now! 1988. 107.00 (*0-387-17270-X*) Spr-Verlag.

Neuro-Ophthalmology Review Manual. Lanning B. Kline & Frank J. Bajandas. 5th ed. 2000. LC 00-57413. 288p. pap. text 45.00 (*1-55642-470-1*) SLACK Inc.

Neuro-Ophthamology. Newman. 2nd ed. 1999. text 97.00 (*0-8385-6697-9*) Appleton & Lange.

Neuro-Optometric Rehabilitation. William V. Padula. Ed. by Sally M. Corngold. 3rd rev. ed. 2000. 212p. reprint ed. lib. bdg. 29.50 (*0-943599-65-2*) OEPF.

Neuro-Otology & Skull Base Surgery. Paulus Willem Van den Broek et al. 1984. (Advances in OtoRhinoLaryngology Ser.: Vol. 34). (Illus.). viii, 280p. 142.75 (*3-8055-3887-1*) S Karger.

***Neuro-Protective Agents & Therapeutic Uses: Index of New Information & Guide-Book for Consumers, Reference & Research.** Carole E. Spandola. 2002. 180p. pap. 47.50 (*0-7883-2567-1*) ABBE Pubs Assn.

Neuro Rehabilitation. Darcy P. Umphred. 3rd ed. 1995. 176p. (gr. 13). pap. text, stu. ed. 19.95 (*0-8151-9109-X*, 28572) Mosby Inc.

***Neuro-Triage Telephone Advice.** Linda M. Selwa. 2002. LC 2001-52451. (*0-7506-7419-9*) Buttrwrth-Heinemann.

***Neuroanaesthesia.** George Hall & Judith Dinsmore. 2001. (Anaesthesia in a Nutshell Ser.). (Illus.). 128p. pap. 26.50 (*0-7506-5009-5*) Buttrwrth-Heinemann.

Neuroanatomica Clinica Hecha Ridiculamente Simple. Stephen Goldberg. 1985. (SPA.). 89p. (Orig.). pap. text 12.95 (*0-940780-03-8*) MedMaster.

M N O

Neuroanatomical Basis of Clinical Neurology. Orhan Arslan. 2001. LC 00-48301. (Illus.). 432p. (C). pap. 49.95 (1-85070-578-X, Parthenon Pbng) CRC Pr.

Neuroanatomical Pathways. Raphael Poritsky. 1984. (Illus.). 152p. pap. text 23.00 (0-7216-1276-8) Saunders.

Neuroanatomical Tract-Tracing Methods 2: Recent Progress. L. Heimer & L. Zaborszky. 1989. (Illus.). 424p. (C). text 95.00 (0-306-43165-3, Kluwer Plenum) Kluwer Academic.

Neuroanatomy. James D. Fix. 1991. (Board Review Ser.). 337p. 19.95 (0-683-03250-X) Lppncott W & W.

Neuroanatomy. P. A. Roberts. (Oklahoma Notes). (Illus.). 1991. xi, 100p. pap. 13.95 (0-387-97477-6); 1989. 84p. (C). 11.95 (0-387-96335-9) Spr-Verlag.

Neuroanatomy. William DeMyer. 2nd ed. 1997. LC 97-18904. (National Medical Series for Independent Study). (Illus.). 480p. pap. text 29.00 (0-683-30075-X) Lppncott W & W.

Neuroanatomy. James D. Fix. 2nd ed. 1995. (Board Review Ser.). (Illus.). 428p. pap. text 26.95 (0-683-03249-6) Lppncott W & W.

Neuroanatomy. P. A. Roberts. 3rd ed. 1992. (Oklahoma Notes). (Illus.). 128p. 13.95 (0-387-97777-5) Spr-Verlag.

Neuroanatomy: 3D-Stereoscopic Atlas of the Human Brain. Martin C. Hirsch & Thomas Kramer. 1999. LC 99-52139. (Illus.). 360p. 49.00 incl. cd-rom (3-540-65998-6) Spr-Verlag.

Neuroanatomy: A Functional Atlas of Parts & Pathways. Ray Poritsky. 1992. (Illus.). 300p. pap., stu. ed. 34.00 (1-56053-008-1) Hanley & Belfus.

Neuroanatomy: A Programmed Text, Vol. 1. Richard L. Sidman & Murray Sidman. 1965. 645p. spiral bd. 45.95 (0-316-78985-2, Little Brwn Med Div) Lppncott W & W.

Neuroanatomy: An Atlas of Structures, Sections & Systems. Duane E. Haines. 3rd ed. 1991. (Illus.). 252p. spiral bd. 27.00 (0-683-03815-X); 5th ed. 2000. LC 99-24992. 272p. spiral bd. 37.95 (0-683-30649-9) Lppncott W & W.

Neuroanatomy: An Illustrated Colour Text. A. R. Crossman & D. Neary. 1995. LC 95-6580. (Illus.). pap. text (0-443-04479-1) Church.

Neuroanatomy: An Illustrated Colour Text. A. R. Crossman & D. Neary. 2nd ed. 2000. LC 00-46276. 190p. pap. text 39.95 (0-443-06216-1) Saunders.

Neuroanatomy: Basic & Applied. M. J. Fitzgerald. 3rd ed. 1996. (C). text 41.00 (0-7020-1994-1) Harcourt.

***Neuroanatomy: Basic & Clinical.** M. J. T. FitzGerald & Jean Folan-Curran. 4th ed. 2001. (Illus.). 300p. pap. (0-7020-2558-5) W B Saunders GBR. *Dist:* Saunders.

Neuroanatomy: Dissection of the Sheep Brain. Bruce Oakley & Rollie Schafer. 1980. (Illus.). 32p. (C). pap. text 7.95 (0-472-08691-X, 08691) U of Mich Pr.

Neuroanatomy: Selected Papers of Walle J. H. Nauta. Walle J. Nauta. 1993. LC 93-10358. (Contemporary Neuroscientists Ser.). (Illus.). 614p. 120.00 (0-8176-3539-4) Birkhauser.

Neuroanatomy & Neuropathology: A Clinical Guide for Neuropsychologists. Ralph M. Reitan & Deborah Wolfson. 1985. LC 85-61660. (Illus.). 353p. tchr. ed. (0-934515-05-0); text 39.95 (0-934515-03-4) Neuropsych Pr.

Neuroanatomy & Physiology of Abdominal Vagal Afferents. Sue Ritter. 1992. 336p. 127.95 (0-8493-8881-3, QM471) CRC Pr.

Neuroanatomy & the Neurologic Exam: A Thesaurus of Synonyms, Similar-Sounding Non-Synonyms, & Terms of Variable Meaning. Terence R. Anthoney. 1993. LC 93-13864. 656p. 131.95 (0-8493-8631-4, QM541) CRC Pr.

Neuroanatomy Atlas. John H. Martin. 2nd ed. 1996. 578p. (C). pap. text 69.95 (0-8385-6694-4, A6694-2, Apple Lange Med) McGraw.

Neuroanatomy for Medical Students. J. S. Wilkinson. 2nd ed. 1992. (Illus.). 272p. pap. text (0-7506-1447-1) John Wright GBR. *Dist:* Buttrwrth-Heinemann.

Neuroanatomy for Medical Students. J. L. Wilkinson. 3rd ed. 1998. LC 98-9508. 256p. pap. text 55.00 (0-7506-3469-3) Buttrwrth-Heinemann.

Neuroanatomy Laboratory Guide. Jose G. Frontera. 1970. 220p. pap. 5.00 (0-8477-2310-0) U of PR Pr.

Neuroanatomy Primer: Color to Learn. M. Evelyn McNeill. 1997. LC 96-46125. (Illus.). 230p. 27.95 (0-683-30067-9) Lppncott W & W.

Neuroanesthesia. Ed. by J. O. Johnson et al. 1997. LC 96-6583. (Developments in Critical Care, Medicine, & Anesthesiology Ser.: Vol. 32). 444p. text 207.50 (0-7923-4426-X) Kluwer Academic.

Neuroanesthesia Handbook. David J. Stone et al. rev. ed. 1996. LC 95-34090. (Illus.). 496p. (C). text 44.00 (0-8151-8145-0, 25770) Mosby Inc.

Neuroaudiology: Case Studies. Frank E. Musiek et al. 1993. LC 93-9066. (Illus.). 320p. (Orig.). (C). pap. text 65.00 (1-56593-217-X, 0577) Thomson Learn.

Neurobehavioral Aspects of Cerebrovascular Disease. Ed. by Robert A. Bornstein & Gregory G. Brown. 1991. (Illus.). 384p. text 68.00 (0-19-505431-8) OUP.

Neurobehavioral Aspects of Multiple Sclerosis. Ed. by Stephen M. Rao. 1990. (Illus.). 288p. text 42.50 (0-19-505400-8) OUP.

Neurobehavioral Assessment. Robert M. Stowe. 1999. (Illus.). 288p. pap. (0-07-061825-9) McGraw-Hill Med Pub.

Neurobehavioral Assessment Format (NAF) A Manual for the Clinical Assessment of Patients with Neurologically Related Disorders. Andrew W. Siegal et al. 1996. 400p. lib. bdg. 89.95 (1-57444-038-1, SL0381) St Lucie Pr.

Neurobehavioral Consequences of Closed Head Injury. Harvey S. Levin et al. 1982. (Illus.). 280p. (C). text 47.50 (0-19-503008-7) OUP.

Neurobehavioral Plasticity: Learning, Development & Response to Brain Insults. Ed. by Norman E. Spear et al. 1995. 488p. text 99.95 (0-8058-1425-6) L Erlbaum Assocs.

Neurobehavioral Recovery from Head Injury. Ed. by Harvey S. Levin et al. 1987. (Illus.). 446p. text 49.95 (0-19-504287-5) OUP.

Neurobehavioral Toxicology. 464p. (0-7131-4518-8) E A GBR. *Dist:* Routldge.

Neurobehavioral Treatment of Epilepsy. Ed. by David I. Mostofsky & Yngve Loyning. 1993. 352p. text 69.95 (0-8058-1106-0) L Erlbaum Assocs.

Neurobehavioural Disorders. Pierre J. Vinken et al. 1985. (Handbooks of Clinical Neurology: Vol. 46(2)). 700p. 356.50 (0-444-90357-7) Elsevier.

Neurobiologic Mechanisms in Manipulative Therapy. Ed. by I. M. Korr. 1978. LC 78-4667. (Illus.). 488p. (C). text 125.00 (0-306-31150-X, Kluwer Plenum) Kluwer Academic.

Neurobiologic View of Speech Production & the Dysarthrias. Ronald Netsell. 1991. (Illus.). 164p. (C). reprint ed. pap. text 37.95 (1-879105-25-X, 0080) Thomson Learn.

Neurobiological & Clinical Consequences of Stress: From Normal Adaptation to Post-Traumatic Stress Disorder. Ed. by Matthew J. Friedman et al. 1995. (Illus.). 576p. text 159.00 (0-7817-0177-5) Lppncott W & W.

Neurobiological & Developmental Basis for Psychotherapeutic Intervention. Ed. by Michael Moskowitz et al. 1997. LC 97-23572. (Illus.). 288p. text 50.00 (0-7657-0097-2) Aronson.

Neurobiological Approaches to Human Disease. Ed. by Dirk Hellhammer et al. 1988. LC 87-16813. (Neuronal Control of Bodily Function Ser.: Vol. 2). 451p. (C). text 69.00 (0-920887-27-9) Hogrefe & Huber Pubs.

Neurobiological Basis of Human Locomotion. Ed. by Muneo Shimamura et al. 1991. text (4-7622-4646-8) Busn Ctr Acad JPN. *Dist:* Intl Spec Bk.

Neurobiological Basis of Memory & Behavior. H. Rahmann & M. Rahmann. 1992. (Illus.). 292p. 148.00 (0-387-97545-4) Spr-Verlag.

Neurobiological Issues in Autism. E. Schopler & G. B. Mesibov. 1987. (Current Issues in Autism Ser.). (Illus.). 440p. (C). text 71.00 (0-306-42451-7, Kluwer Plenum) Kluwer Academic.

Neurobiological Mechanisms of Drugs of Abuse. Ed. by Syed F. Ali. 2000. LC 00-61300. (Annals of the New York Academy of Sciences Ser.: Vol. 914). (Illus.). xi, 440p. 140.00 (1-57331-279-7) NY Acad Sci.

Neurobiological Mechanisms of Drugs of Abuse: Cocaine, Ibogaine & Substituted Amphetamines. Syed F. Ali. 2000. LC 00-61300. (Annals Ser.: Vol. 914). (Illus.). xi, 440p. (1-57331-280-0) NY Acad Sci.

Neurobiological Mechanisms of Opiate Withdrawal. G. F. Koob et al. 1996. (Neuroscience Intelligence Unit Ser.). 200p. (C). pap. 89.95 (0-412-11061-X) Chapman & Hall.

Neurobiological Mechanisms of Opiate Withdrawal. Rafael Maldonado & Luis Stinus. 1996. LC 96-8139. (Neuroscience Intelligence Unit Ser.). 196p. 99.00 (1-57059-347-7) Landes Bioscience.

Neurobiologische Forschung und Psychiatrische Therapie. Ed. by Wolfgang P. Kaschka. 1996. (Illus.). viii, 232p. pap. 121.75 (3-8055-6310-8) S Karger.

Neurobiology. Ed. by David Robinson. 1998. LC 97-37177. (Illus.). 371p. (C). pap. 39.95 (3-540-63546-7) Spr-Verlag.

Neurobiology. David Robinson. 1997. LC 97-37177. (0-7492-8151-0) Spr-Verlag.

Neurobiology. Gordon M. Shepherd. 3rd ed. 1994. (Illus.). 784p. (C). text 85.00 (0-19-508842-5); pap. text 57.95 (0-19-508843-3) OUP.

Neurobiology: Ionic Channels, Neurons & the Brain. North Atlantic Treaty Organization Staff et al. Ed. by Vincent Torre & Franco Conti. 1997. LC 96-29397. (NATO ASI Series A: Vol. 289). (Illus.). 404p. (C). text 150.00 (0-306-45480-7) Plenum.

Neurobiology: Molecules, Cells & Systems. Gary Matthews. 2nd ed. 2000. LC 00-63014. (Illus.). 563p. 79.95 (0-632-04496-9) Blackwell Sci.

Neurobiology & Cell Physiology of Chemoreception. P. G. Data et al. 1993. (Advances in Experimental Medicine & Biology Ser.: Vol. 337). (Illus.). 466p. (C). text 135.00 (0-306-44575-1, Kluwer Plenum) Kluwer Academic.

Neurobiology & Clinical Aspects of the Outer Retina. M. B. A Djamgoz et al. 1995. LC 95-67595. (Illus.). 520p. (C). pap. text 239.95 (0-412-60080-3, Chap & Hall NY) Chapman & Hall.

Neurobiology in the Treatment of Eating Disorders. Hans Hoek et al. 1998. LC 97-48993. (Clinical & Neurobiological Advances in Psychiatry Ser.). 546p. 185.00 (0-471-98102-8) Wiley.

Neurobiology of Aggression & Impulsivity. Michael Maes & Emil F. Coccaro. 1998. LC 98-19062. (Clinical & Neurobiological Advances in Psychiatry Ser.). 228p. 150.00 (0-471-98101-X) Wiley.

Neurobiology of Alzheimer's Disease. Ed. by David Dawbarn & Shelley J. Allen. 2nd ed. 2000. LC 00-45314. (Molecular & Cellular Neurobiology Ser.). (Illus.). 426p. pap. text 59.50 (0-19-852459-5) OUP.

Neurobiology of Alzheimer's Disease, Vol. 777. Ed. by Richard J. Wurtman et al. 1996. LC 95-48168. 439p. pap. 115.00 (0-89766-974-6); text 115.00 (0-89766-973-8) NY Acad Sci.

Neurobiology of Amino Acids, Peptides & Trophic Factors. Ed. by James A. Ferrendelli et al. 1988. (Topics in Neurosciences Ser.). (C). text 150.00 (0-89838-360-9) Kluwer Academic.

Neurobiology of Autism. Margaret L. Bauman. Ed. by Thomas L. Kemper. 1997. LC 93-5358. (Johns Hopkins Series in Psychiatry & Neuroscience Ser.). (Illus.). 272p. pap. text 39.95 (0-8018-5680-9) Johns Hopkins.

Neurobiology of Central D1-Dopamine Receptors. Ed. by George R. Breese & Ian Creese. 1986. (Advances in Experimental Medicine & Biology Ser.: Vol. 204). 228p. 69.50 (0-306-42383-9, Plenum Trade) Perseus Pubng.

Neurobiology of Central Nervous System Trauma. Steven K. Salzman & Alan I. Faden. 1994. (Illus.). 368p. text 98.00 (0-19-507230-8) OUP.

Neurobiology of Cerebrospinal Fluid 2. Ed. by James H. Wood. 1983. LC 79-21731. 1002p. 145.00 (0-306-40969-0, Plenum Trade) Perseus Pubng.

Neurobiology of Cholinergic & Adrenergic Transmitters. Ed. by E. Heldman et al. 1981. (Monographs in Neural Sciences: Vol. 7). (Illus.). xvi, 200p. pap. 77.50 (3-8055-0828-X) S Karger.

Neurobiology of Cingulate Cortex & Limbic Thalamus: A Comprehensive Handbook. Ed. by Brent A. Vogt & Michael Gabriel. 1993. LC 93-18429. (Illus.). 650p. 219.00 (0-8176-3568-8) Birkhauser.

Neurobiology of Cocaine: Cellular & Molecular Mechanisms. Ed. by Ronald P. Hammer, Jr. 1995. LC 95-7021. 272p. 139.95 (0-8493-8311-0, 8311) CRC Pr.

Neurobiology of Cocaine Addiction: From Bench to Bedside. Ed. by Joseph Herman & Barry Stimmel. 1997. LC 96-39364. (Journal of Addictive Diseases Ser.: Vol. 15, No. 4). 129p. (C). 49.95 (0-7890-0031-8); pap. text 19.95 (0-7890-0300-7) Haworth Pr.

Neurobiology of Cognition. Ed. by Peter D. Eimas. 1990. LC 90-5517. (Cognitive Special Issues Ser.). 256p. pap. 27.95 (0-262-55019-9) MIT Pr.

Neurobiology of Comparative Cognition. Ed. by David S. Olton & R. Kesner. 1990. (Roitblat Bever Olton Ser.). 488p. (C). text 99.95 (0-8058-0133-2) L Erlbaum Assocs.

Neurobiology of Computation: Proceedings of the 3rd Annual Computation & Neural Systems Conference. Conference on Computation & Neural Systems Staff. Ed. by James M. Bower. 1995. LC 94-41228. 464p. (C). text 218.00 (0-7923-9543-3) Kluwer Academic.

Neurobiology of Decision-Making. Ed. by A. R. Damasio et al. 1995. (Research & Perspectives in Neurosciences Ser.). (Illus.). 192p. 108.00 (3-540-60143-0) Spr-Verlag.

Neurobiology of Disease. Ed. by Alan L. Pearlman & Robert C. Collins. 1989. (Illus.). 504p. text 55.00 (0-19-505318-4); pap. text 45.00 (0-19-505319-2) OUP.

Neurobiology of Disease: Contributions from Neuroscience to Clinical Neurology. Ed. by H. Bostock et al. 1996. LC 95-33564. (Illus.). 463p. (C). text 110.00 (0-521-45132-9) Cambridge U Pr.

Neurobiology of Drug Abuse: Learning & Memory. 1992. lib. bdg. 88.75 (0-8490-8822-4) Gordon Pr.

Neurobiology of Drug Use. Ed. by Joe Marwah. 1987. (Monographs in Neural Sciences: Vol. 13). (Illus.). viii, 164p. 128.00 (3-8055-4561-4) S Karger.

Neurobiology of Food & Fluid Intake. E. M. Stricker. 1990. (Handbook of Behavioral Neurobiology Ser.: Vol. 10). (Illus.). 576p. (C). text 125.00 (0-306-43458-X, Kluwer Plenum) Kluwer Academic.

Neurobiology of Incontinence - Symposium No. 151. CIBA Foundation Staff. 1990. LC 90-12321. (CIBA Foundation Symposia Ser.: No. 151). 346p. 128.00 (0-471-92687-6) Wiley.

Neurobiology of Ischemic Brain Damage. Ed. by Bo K. Siesjo et al. 1993. LC 93-201359. (Progress in Brain Research Ser.: Vol. 96). 398p. 231.50 (0-444-89603-1) Elsevier.

Neurobiology of Learning & Memory. Grau. 2001. (Psychology Ser.). pap. 28.00 net. (0-534-36767-4) Brooks-Cole.

Neurobiology of Learning & Memory. Ed. by Joe L. Martinez, Jr. & Raymond P. Desner. 1998. LC 98-84370. (Illus.). 456p. 69.96 (0-12-475655-7) Acad Pr.

Neurobiology of Learning & Memory. G. Shaw et al. 1990. (Advanced Series in Neuroscience: Vol. 2). 868p. (C). reprint ed. text 109.00 (9971-5-0865-6); pap. text 55.00 (9971-5-0868-0) World Scientific Pub.

Neurobiology of Memory: Concepts, Findings, Trends. Yadin Dudai. 1989. (Illus.). 352p. pap. text 41.95 (0-19-854229-1) OUP.

Neurobiology of Mental Illness. Ed. by Dennis S Charney et al. 1999. LC 98-27421. (Illus.). 984p. text 150.00 (0-19-511265-2) OUP.

Neurobiology of Motivation & Reward. J. R. Stellar & Eliot Stellar. 1985. (Illus.). 255p. 85.95 (0-387-96092-9) Spr-Verlag.

Neurobiology of Motor Programme Selection. Jenny Kien et al. 1992. (SINS Ser.: Vol. 4). 290p. 188.00 (0-08-041986-0, Pergamon Pr) Elsevier.

Neurobiology of Neural Networks. Ed. by Daniel Gardner. 1993. LC 93-9125. (Computational Neuroscience Ser.). (Illus.). 241p. 45.00 (0-262-07150-9, Bradford Bks) MIT Pr.

Neurobiology of Opiates. Ed. by Ronald P. Hammer, Jr. Ph.d. 1992. 432p. 131.95 (0-8493-7932-6, RM328) CRC Pr.

Neurobiology of Primary Dementia. Marshal F. Folstein & Association for Research in Nervous and Mental Disease Staff. 1998. LC 97-27523. 440p. 63.50 (0-88048-915-4, 8915) Am Psychiatric.

Neurobiology of Puberty. Ed. by T. M. Plant & P. A. Lee. 1995. 368p. 79.95 (1-898099-06-5) Blackwell Sci.

Neurobiology of Reproduction in the Female Rat. J. W. Everett. 1989. (Monographs in Endocrinology: Vol. 32). (Illus.). 133p. 119.00 (0-387-51157-1) Spr-Verlag.

Neurobiology of Reproductive Behavior. Ed. by L. E. Muske. 1993. (Journal: Vol. 42, No. 4-5, 1993). (Illus.). 84p. pap. 42.75 (3-8055-5852-X) S Karger.

Neurobiology of Saccadic Eye Movements. Ed. by R. H. Wurts et al. 1989. (Reviews of Oculomotor Research Ser.: Vol. 3). 472p. 298.25 (0-444-81017-X) Elsevier.

Neurobiology of Sensory Systems. Ed. by R. N. Singh & N. J. Strausfeld. 1989. LC 89-22960. (Illus.). 632p. 140.00 (0-306-43377-X, Plenum Trade) Perseus Pubng.

Neurobiology of Spinal Cord Injury. Ed. by Robert G. Kalb & Stephen M. Strittmatter. 2000. LC 99-23563. (Contemporary Neuroscience Ser.). 304p. 125.00 (0-89603-672-3) Humana.

Neurobiology of Stereotyped Behavior. Ed. by Steven J. Cooper & Colin T. Dourish. 1990. (Illus.). 308p. text 75.00 (0-19-852160-X) OUP.

Neurobiology of Taste & Smell. Ed. by Thomas E. Finger & Wayne L. Silver. 1991. 462p. (C). reprint ed. lib. bdg. 89.50 (0-89464-616-8) Krieger.

Neurobiology of the Inner Retina. Ed. by R. Weiler & Neville N. Osborne. 1989. (NATO ASI Ser.: Vol. 31). (Illus.). 529p. 200.00 (0-387-50378-1) Spr-Verlag.

Neurobiology of the Locus Coeruleus Vol. 88: Progress in Brain Research. Ed. by C. D. Barnes & O. Pompeiano. 1991. 642p. 323.50 (0-444-81394-2) Elsevier.

Neurobiology of the Nucleus Accumbens. Ed. by R. B. Chronister & J. F. De France. 1981. (Illus.). 380p. (Orig.). pap. 39.95 (0-940090-00-7) Haer Inst.

Neurobiology of the Trace Amines: Analytical, Physiological, Pharmacological, Behavioral & Clinical Aspects. Ed. by Alan A. Boulton et al. 1984. LC 84-626. (Illus.). 597p. 139.00 (0-89603-063-6) Humana.

Neurobiology of the Trace Elements Vol. 2: Neurotoxicology & Neuropharmacology. Ed. by Ivor E. Dreosti & Richard M. Smith. 1983. LC 83-8413. (Contemporary Neuroscience Ser.). 323p. 119.50 (0-89603-047-4) Humana.

Neurobiology of Violence. Jan Volavka. 1995. LC 94-40145. 448p. text 56.00 (0-88048-543-4, 8543) Am Psychiatric.

Neurobiology Progression. G. A. Kerkut. (Progress in Neurobiology Ser.: Vol. 14). 1980. pap. 63.00 (0-08-026048-9, no. 2); ser. vol. 4. 1980. pap. 28.00 (0-08-026042-X, 1); ser. vol. 13. 1979. pap. 21.00 (0-08-024898-5, no. 3); ser. vol. 13. 1979. pap. 18.50 (0-08-024899-3, no. 4); ser. vol. 14. 1980. pap. 29.00 (0-08-026019-5, no. 1) Elsevier (Pergamon Pr).

Neuroblastoma. Ed. by G. M. Brodeur et al. 2000. 610p. 182.50 (0-444-50222-X) Elsevier.

Neuroblastoma: Molecular Genetics in Diagnosis & Therapy. Ed. by M. Sluyser & A. Voue. 1988. 168p. 49.95 (0-470-21237-3) P-H.

Neuroblastoma: Tumor Biology & Therapy. Ed. by Carl Pochedly. 1990. 424p. 169.00 (0-8493-0157-2, RC280) CRC Pr.

Neurocardiology. Ed. by John A. Armour & Jeffrey L. Ardell. 1994. LC 93-41500. (Illus.). 456p. (C). text 75.00 (0-19-507304-5) OUP.

Neurocardiology. Richard A. Johnson et al. 1985. (Major Problems in Neurology Ser.). (Illus.). 416p. text 98.00 (0-7216-1375-6) Saunders.

Neurochemical Correlates of Cerebral Ischemia Vol. 7: Advances in Neurochemistry. N. G. Bazan et al. 1992. (Illus.). 392p. (C). text 110.00 (0-306-43944-1, 441, Kluwer Plenum) Kluwer Academic.

Neurochemical Studies on Monoaminergic Neutotransmitters in the Central Nervous System. 001. Patrick Herregodts. 1994. (Illus.). 174p. pap. (90-70289-93-8) VUB Univ Pr BEL. *Dist:* Paul & Co Pubs.

Neurochemistry: Cellular, Molecular & Clinical Aspects: Proceedings of the 11th European Society for Neurochemistry Meeting Held in Groningen, The Netherlands, June 15-20, 1996. Ed. by Albert Teelken et al. 1998. LC 97-36254. (Illus.). 1190p. (C). text 294.00 (0-306-45705-9, Kluwer Plenum) Kluwer Academic.

Neurochemistry & Clinical Disorders Circuitry of Some Psychiatric & Psychosomatic Syndromes. Ed. by Fuad Lechin & Bertha Van der Dijs. 1989. LC 88-19263. 208p. 139.00 (0-8493-6595-3, RC483, CRC Reprint) Franklin.

Neurochemistry in Clinical Application: Proceedings of the International Neuropharmacology Held in Guangzhou, China, November 9-11, 1992, Vol. 363.

Ed. by Lily C. Tang & Steven J. Tang. 1995. (Advances in Experimental Medicine & Biology Ser.: Vol. 363). (Illus.). 226p. (C). text 79.50 (*0-306-44836-X*, Kluwer Plenum) Kluwer Academic.

Neurochemistry of Drug Dependence: From Molecular Targets to Behavioral Consequences. Ed. by S. Wonnacott & S. S. Lunt. 1994. (Biochemical Society Symposium Ser.: Vol. 59). (Illus.). 223p. (C). text (*1-85578-034-8*) Portland Pr Ltd GBR. *Dist:* Ashgate Pub Co.

Neurochemistry of Drugs of Abuse: Cocaine, Ibogaine, & Substituted Amphetamines. Ed. by Syed F. Ali. 1998. LC 98-3824. (Annals of the New York Academy of Sciences Ser.: Vol. 844). 300p. 140.00 (*1-57331-145-6*); 362p. pap. 140.00 (*1-57331-146-4*) NY Acad Sci.

Neurochemistry of Hepatic Coma. Ed. by E. E. Polli. 1971. (Experimental Biology & Medicine Ser.: Vol. 4). 30.50 (*3-8055-1187-6*) S Karger.

Neurochemistry of the Vestibular System. Alvin J. Beitz & John H. Anderson. 1999. LC 99-38971. (Illus.). 432p. 129.95 (*0-8493-7679-3*) CRC Pr.

Neurocritical Care. Ed. by Thomas P. Bleck. Date not set. 352p. text 65.00 (*0-07-005925-X*) McGraw-Hill Med Pub.

Neurocritical Care. Ed. by Werner Hacke et al. 1994. LC 93-48232. (Illus.). 1076p. 125.00 (*0-387-56443-8*) Spr-Verlag.

Neurocysticercosis: A Clinical Handbook. Oscar H. Brutto et al. 1998. LC 98-11617. (*90-265-1513-8*) Swets.

Neurocytochemical Methods. Ed. by A. Calas & D. Eugene. 1991. (NATO ASI Ser.: Vol. 58). (Illus.). 335p. 217.00 (*0-387-53148-3*) Spr-Verlag.

Neurocytology: Fine Structure of Neurons, Nerve Processes, & Neuroglial Cells. Ennio Pannese. 1994. LC 93-18191. 99.00 (*0-86577-456-0*) Thieme Med Pubs.

Neurocytopathology. John M. Andrews & G. Berry Schumann. 1992. (Illus.). 352p. 125.00 (*0-683-00227-9*) Lppncott W & W.

Neurodegeneration & Neuroprotection in Parkinson's Disease. Charles W. Olanow & M. B. Youdim. 1996. (Neuroscience Perspectives Ser.). (Illus.). 224p. text 65.00 (*0-12-525445-8*) Acad Pr.

Neurodegeneration Methods & Protocols. Jean Harry & Hugh A. Tilson. 1999. LC 98-46592. (Methods in Molecular Medicine Ser.: Vol. 22). 328p. 99.50 (*0-89603-612-X*) Humana.

Neurodegenerative Dementias. Ed. by John Q. Trojanowski & Christopher Clark. 1999. (Illus.). 491p. text 125.00 (*0-07-065093-4*) McGraw-Hill Prof.

Neurodegenerative Diseases. Donald B. Caine. 1994. LC 93-13286. (Illus.). 992p. text 220.00 (*0-7216-4349-3*) Saunders.

Neurodegenerative Diseases. Ed. by G. Jolles & J. M. Stutzman. 1994. (Rhone-Poulenc Rorer Round Table Conferences Ser.). (Illus.). 320p. text 79.00 (*0-12-388185-4*) Acad Pr.

Neurodegenerative Diseases: Molecular & Cellular Mechanisms & Therapeutic Advances. Ed. by Gary Fiskum. 1996. LC 96-5688. (GWUMC Department of Biochemistry & Molecular Biology Annual Spring Symposium Ser.). (Illus.). 467p. (C). text 162.00 (*0-306-45298-7*, Kluwer Plenum) Kluwer Academic.

***Neurodegenerative Disorders: Loss of Function Through Gain of Function.** K. Beyreuther et al. 2001. LC 00-69232. (Research & Perspectives in Alzheimer's Disease Ser.). (Illus.). xiv, 189p. 69.95 (*3-540-41218-2*) Spr-Verlag.

Neurodevelopment, Aging, & Cognition. Ed. by Henryk M. Wisniewski et al. 1992. LC 92-396. (Illus.). xiv, 396p. 140.50 (*0-8176-3599-8*) Birkhauser.

Neurodevelopment & Adult Psychopathology. Ed. by Matcheri S. Keshavan & Robin M. Murray. 1997. (Illus.). 298p. (C). text 150.00 (*0-521-48104-X*); pap. text 54.95 (*0-521-48565-7*) Cambridge U Pr.

Neurodevelopmental Approach to Specific Learning Disorders. Ed. by Kingsley Whitmore & Guy Willems. 1999. LC 99-231944. (Clinics in Developmental Medicine Ser.: Vol. 145). (Illus.). ix, 304p. (C). text (*1-898683-11-5*) Mc Keith Pr GBR. *Dist:* Cambridge U Pr.

Neurodevelopmental Basis of Schizophrenia. John L. Waddington. 1996. (Medicine Ser.). pap. 89.95 (*0-412-10081-9*, VNR) Wiley.

Neurodevelopmental Basis of Schizophrenia. John L. Waddington & Peter F. Buckley. 1996. LC 95-37078. 177p. 89.95 (*1-57059-306-X*) Landes Bioscience.

Neurodevelopmental Disorders. Ed. by Helen Tager-Flusberg. 1999. LC 98-26850. (Development Cognitive Neuroscince Ser.). (Illus.). 614p. 75.00 (*0-262-20116-X*, Bradford Bks) MIT Pr.

Neurodevelopmental Disorders: Diagnosis & Treatment. Randi Jenssen Hagerman. 1999. LC 98-54687. (Developmental Perspectives in Psychiatry Ser.). (Illus.). 224p. text 65.00 (*0-19-512314-X*) OUP.

Neurodevelopmental Problems in Early Childhood: Assessment & Management. Drillien & Drummond. 1978. (Illus.). 512p. (gr. 13). 89.95 (*0-632-00409-6*, B-1475-9) Mosby Inc.

Neurodevelopmental Strategies for Managing Communication Disorders in Children with Severe Motor Dysfunction. Ed. by M. Beth Langley & Linda J. Lombardino. 1991. LC 90-9166. 342p. text 39.00 (*0-89079-422-7*, 1942) PRO-ED.

Neurodynamics & Psychology. Ed. by Michael Oaksford & Gordon Brown. 1994. (Illus.). 400p. text 79.95 (*0-12-523515-1*) Acad Pr.

NeuroDynamix: Computer Models for Neurophysiology. W. Otto Friesen & Jonathan A. Friesen. 1994. (Computational Neuroscience Ser.). (Illus.). 224p. (C). pap. text 38.95 (*0-19-508282-6*) OUP.

Neurodystrophies & Neurolipidoses. George W. Bruyn & Hugo W. Moser. 1996. LC 96-51995. (Handbooks of Clinical Neurology). 790p. 256.50 (*0-444-81285-7*) Elsevier.

Neuroembryology: The Selected Papers of Viktor Hamburger. Viktor Hamburger. 1990. 384p. 96.50 (*0-8176-3459-2*) Birkhauser.

Neuroendocrine - Immune Network. Ed. by Serem Freier. 1989. 272p. lib. bdg. 217.00 (*0-8493-4625-8*, QP356) CRC Pr.

Neuroendocrine Immune Basis of the Rheumatic Disease: The First International Conference. Ed. by H. L. Bradlow. 1999. LC 99-26842. 520p. lib. bdg. 140.00 (*1-57331-215-0*) NY Acad Sci.

Neuroendocrine Immune Basis of the Rheumatic Diseases. M. Cutolo. 1999. LC 99-26842. (Annals Ser.). pap. (*1-57331-216-9*) NY Acad Sci.

***Neuroendocrine-Immune Interactions.** Ed. by R. C. Gaillard. 2001. (Illus.). 134p. 170.50 (*3-8055-7282-4*) S Karger.

Neuroendocrine Neoplasms of the Larynx: Journal: Oto-Rhino-Laryngology, Vol. 53, No. 4, 1991. Ed. by A. Ferlito. 1991. (Illus.). 84p. pap. 55.00 (*3-8055-5445-1*) S Karger.

Neuroendocrine Perspectives, Vol. 6. Ed. by J. A. Wass & M. F. Scanlon. 1988. (Illus.). 353p. 159.00 (*0-387-96636-6*) Spr-Verlag.

Neuroendocrine Perspectives, Vol. 7. 1989. (Illus.). 178p. 93.00 (*0-387-96828-8*) Spr-Verlag.

Neuroendocrine Perspectives, Vol. 8. Ed. by E. E. Muller & R. M. MacLeod. 1990. (Illus.). 182p. 117.00 (*0-387-97365-6*) Spr-Verlag.

Neuroendocrine Regulation & Altered Behavior. Ed. by Pavel D. Hrdina & R. L. Singhal. 1981. LC 81-81689. 416p. (C). 85.00 (*0-306-40840-6*, Kluwer Plenum) Kluwer Academic.

Neuroendocrine Regulation of Behavior. Jay Schulkin. 1998. LC 97-41739. (Illus.). 334p. (C). text 110.00 (*0-521-45385-2*); pap. text 39.95 (*0-521-45985-0*) Cambridge U Pr.

Neuroendocrine Regulation of Fertility: Proceedings. International Symposium on Neuroendocrine Regulation Staff. Ed. by T. C. Anand Kumar. 1976. (Illus.). 133.25 (*3-8055-2199-5*) S Karger.

Neuroendocrine Research Methods, Vol. 1 & 2. B. Greenstein. 1991. xxxxix, 1,040p. text 515.00 (*3-7186-5101-7*, Harwood Acad Pubs) Gordon & Breach.

Neuroendocrinological Aspects of Neurosurgery. Ed. by J. D. Pickard et al. 1990. (Acta Neurochirurgica Ser.: Supplement 47). (Illus.). 135p. 126.00 (*0-387-82160-0*) Spr-Verlag.

Neuroendocrinology. Charles B. Nemeroff. 1992. LC 91-46098. 640p. lib. bdg. 110.00 (*0-8493-8844-9*, QP356) CRC Pr.

Neuroendocrinology, Vol. V. Warren R. Selman. 1992. LC 92-5836. (Concepts in Neurosurgery Ser.). (Illus.). 418p. 90.00 (*0-683-07665-5*) Lppncott W & W.

Neuroendocrinology: A Clinical Text. Mary L. Forsling & Ashley Grossman. 1986. LC 86-7122. 206p. text 27.95 (*0-914783-14-9*) Charles.

Neuroendocrinology: Retrospect & Perspectives. Ed. by H. W. Korf & K. H. Usadel. 1997. LC 97-42699. (Illus.). 444p. 129.00 (*3-540-63629-3*) Spr-Verlag.

Neuroendocrinology & Pituitary Disease. Ed. by Stanley G. Korenman & Mark E. Molitch. 1999. LC 99-34471. (Atlas of Clinical Endocrinology Ser.: Vol. 4). (Illus.). 240p. 131.95 (*0-632-04405-5*) Blackwell Sci.

Neuroendocrinology in Physiology & Medicine. Ed. by P. Michael Conn & Marc E. Freeman. 2000. LC 99-10139. (Contemporary Endocrinology Ser.). 592p. 125.00 (*0-89603-725-8*) Humana.

Neuroendocrinology, 1988: 31st International Henri-Pierre Klotz Days of Clinical Endocrinology, Paris, May 1988. Ed. by A. Enjalbert & J. J. Legros. 1989. (Journal: Vol. 31, Nos. 1-2, 1989). (Illus.). 104p. pap. 75.75 (*3-8055-5037-5*) S Karger.

Neuroendocrinology of Aging. Ed. by Joseph Meites. 1983. LC 83-10937. 400p. 85.00 (*0-306-41310-8*, Plenum Trade) Perseus Pubng.

Neuroendocrinology of Female Reproductive Function: Proceedings of the 2nd International Capri Conference on Neuroendocrine & Peripheral Disorders of Female Reproductive System—Pathophysiology & Therapies, Capri, May 1992. Ed. by U. Montemagno et al. 1993. LC 93-5174. (International Congress, Symposium, & Seminar Ser.: No. 4). (Illus.). 450p. ring bd. (*1-85070-509-7*, Parthenon Pbng) CRC Pr.

Neuroendocrinology of Gastrointestinal Ulceration: Hans Selye Symposia on Neuroendocrinology & Stress; Vol. 2, Vol. 2. Ed. by Sandor Szabo et al. 1995. LC 95-14350. (Hans Selve Symposia on Neuroendocrinology & Stress Ser.: Vol. 2). (Illus.). 246p. (C). text 95.00 (*0-306-44988-9*, Kluwer Plenum) Kluwer Academic.

Neuroendocrinology of Leptin. Ed. by U. R. Ehud. 1999. LC 99-40628. (Frontiers of Hormone Research Ser.: Vol. 26). (Illus.). x, 130p. pap. 147.00 (*3-8055-6921-1*) S Karger.

Neuroendocrinology of Reproduction: Physiology & Behavior. Ed. by Norman T. Adler. 1981. LC 80-28245. 576p. 75.00 (*0-306-40600-4*); pap. 37.50 (*0-306-40611-X*) Perseus Pubng (Plenum Trade).

Neuroendocrinology of Sex Steroids: Basic Knowledge & Clinical Implications. Ed. by W. G. Rossmanith & W. A. Scherbaum. 1993. (New Developments in Biosciences Ser.: No. 6). viii, 222p. (Orig.). (C). pap. text 98.50 (*3-11-013616-3*) De Gruyter.

Neuroendoscopy. Cohen. Date not set. text (*0-7216-7442-9*) Saunders.

Neuroendoscopy. Kim H. Manwaring & Kerry R. Crone. 1991. 121p. 40.00 (*0-913113-57-3*) M Liebert.

Neuroepidemiology. Ed. by Devera G. Schoenberg. 1990. 384p. 195.00 (*0-8493-5237-1*, RC346) CRC Pr.

Neuroepidemiology: Theory & Method. Ed. by Craig Molgaard. 1993. (Illus.). 381p. text 27.00 (*0-12-504220-5*) Acad Pr.

Neuroethology. Jorg-Peter Ewert. 1980. (Illus.). 342p. 58.95 (*0-387-09790-2*) Spr-Verlag.

Neuroethology of the Mauthner System, 1991 Vol. 37, No. 5: Journal: Brain, Behavior & Evolution. Ed. by R. C. Eaton. 1991. (Illus.). 88p. pap. 69.75 (*3-8055-5449-4*) S Karger.

Neurofibromatoses. Ed. by R. A. Hughes & S.M. Huson. 1994. (Illus.). 512p. (C). (gr. 13). 188.95 (*0-412-38920-7*) Chapman & Hall.

Neurofibromatosis: Phenotype, Natural History & Pathogenesis. J. M. Friedman. 3rd ed. 1999. LC 99-27988. (Illus.). 400p. 110.00 (*0-8018-6285-X*) Johns Hopkins.

Neurofibromatosis Type 1 in Childhood. Kathryn North. 1997. LC 97-181243. (International Review of Child Neurology Ser.). (Illus.). 142p. (C). (*1-898683-13-1*) Mc Keith Pr GBR. *Dist:* Cambridge U Pr.

Neurofilament. 1994. (*0-8493-8880-5*) CRC Pr.

Neurofunctional Systems: 3D Reconstructions in Correlated Neuroimaging. H. J. Kretschmann & Wolfgang Weinrich. 1998. LC 97-31484. (Illus.). 160p. 99.00 (*0-86577-708-X*) Thieme Med Pubs.

Neurogastroenterology. Ed. by Enrico Corazziari. 1996. (Illus.). xix, 410p. (Orig.). (C). pap. text 91.45 (*3-11-015343-2*) De Gruyter.

Neurogenesis of Central Respiratory Rhythm: Electrophysiological, Pharmacological & Pathological Aspects. Ed. by A. L. Bianchi & M. Denavit Saubie. 1985. text 322.00 (*0-85200-903-8*) Kluwer Academic.

Neurogenetic Directory, Pt. 2. Ed. by Pierre J. Vinken & George W. Bruyn. 1982. 280.50 (*0-7204-7200-8*) Elsevier.

Neurogenetics & Neuro-Ophthalmology. Ed. by A. F. Deutman & J. R. Cruysberg. 1979. (Documenta Ophthalmologica Proceedings Ser.: No. 17). text 255.50 (*90-6193-159-2*) Kluwer Academic.

Neurogenic Communication Disorders: A Functional Approach. Linda Worrall. 1999. LC 99-48698. (Illus.). 384p. 59.00 (*0-86577-868-X*) Thieme Med Pubs.

Neurogenic Disorders of Language. Robin. 2001. 40.00 net. (*1-56593-703-1*) Thomson Learn.

Neurogenic Hypertension: A Synthesis & Review. C. J. Dickinson. 1991. 94.95 (*0-442-31414-0*) Chapman & Hall.

Neurogenic Inflammation. Ed. by Pierangelo Geppetti & Peter Holzer. 1996. LC 95-38900. 338p. 224.95 (*0-8493-7646-7*) CRC Pr.

Neuroglia. Helmut Kettenmann & Bruce R. Ransom. 1995. (Illus.). 1104p. text 195.00 (*0-19-507847-0*) OUP.

Neuroglia in the Aging Brain. Ed. by Jean S. de Vellis. 2001. (Contemporary Neuroscience Ser.). 536p. 165.00 (*0-89603-594-8*) Humana.

Neurohumoral Control of Blood Vessel Tone: Springfield Blood Vessel Symposium. Ed. by T. J. Lee. 1987. (Journal: Vol. 24, No. 3). (Illus.). 80p. pap. 42.75 (*3-8055-4604-1*) S Karger.

Neurohumoral Maintenance of Immune Homeostasis. Viktor M. Klimenko & Elenor K. Shkhinek. Ed. by Samuel A. Corson & Elizabeth O. Corson. 1995. LC 84-8771. (Illus.). 184p. lib. bdg. 38.50 (*0-226-45042-2*) U Ch Pr.

Neurohumoral Mechanisms of Aging. Ed. by V. V. Frolkis. 1988. (Journal: Vol. 34, No. 1-2, 1988). 96p. pap. 76.75 (*3-8055-4797-8*) S Karger.

Neurohumoral Regulation of Coronary Flow. Ed. by W. H. Van Gilst. 1993. LC 94-119974. (Developments in Cardiovascular Medicine Ser.). 160p. (C). text 85.50 (*0-7923-2588-5*) Kluwer Academic.

Neurohypophysial Hormones & Similar Polypeptides. Ed. by E. Berde et al. 1968. (Handbook of Experimental Pharmacology Ser.: Vol. 23). (Illus.). 184.00 (*0-387-04149-4*) Spr-Verlag.

Neurohypophysis: Psychological & Clinical Aspects. Ed. by Seymour Reichlin. 1984. LC 84-4861. 240p. 65.00 (*0-306-41642-5*, Kluwer Plenum) Kluwer Academic.

Neurohypophysis: Recent Progress of Vasopressin & Oxytocin Ressearch: Proceedings of the 1st Joint World Congress of Neurohypophysis & Vasopressin, Nasu, Tochigi, Japan, 16-21 July 1995. Ed. by Toshikazu Saito et al. 1995. LC 95-44867. (International Congress Ser.: No. 1098). 702p. 292.00 (*0-444-82231-3*, Excerpta Medica) Elsevier.

Neuroimaging William W. Orrison. 1999. LC 97-39761. (Illus.). xvii, 1776p. text (*0-7216-6799-6*) Saunders.

Neuroimaging: A Companion to Adams & Victor's Principles of Neurology. Ed. by Jack O. Greenberg. 1994. LC 93-41639. 614p. text 125.00 (*0-07-024308-5*) McGraw-Hill Med Pub.

Neuroimaging: A Window to the Neurological Foundations of Learning & Behavior in Children. Ed. by G. Reid Lyon & Judith M. Rumsey. 1996. (Illus.). 288p. (Orig.). text 49.95 (*1-55766-256-8*, 2568) P H Brookes.

Neuroimaging: Basic Science. Ed. by Erin D. Bigler. 1996. LC 96-29400. (Human Brain Function Ser.: Vol. 1). (Illus.). 334p. (C). text 75.00 (*0-306-45228-6*, Kluwer Plenum) Kluwer Academic.

Neuroimaging: Clinical & Physical Principles. Ed. by Robert A. Zimmerman et al. 1999. LC 97-28144. (Illus.). 1656p. 195.00 (*0-387-94963-1*) Spr-Verlag.

Neuroimaging: Clinical Applications. Ed. by Erin D. Bigler. 1996. (Human Brain Function Ser.: Vol. 2). (Illus.). 382p. (C). text 75.00 (*0-306-45229-4*, Kluwer Plenum) Kluwer Academic.

Neuroimaging & Developmental Neurophysiology in Child Psychiatric Disorders. Bernard Garreau & J. L. Beaulieu. 1997. LC 97-42376. x, 289p. (*2-287-63634-X*) Spl France Editions FRA. *Dist:* Spr-Verlag.

Neuroimaging & the Psychiatry of Late Life. Ed. by David Ames & Edmond Chiu. 1998. LC 96-52958. (Illus.). 251p. (C). text 110.00 (*0-521-49505-9*) Cambridge U Pr.

Neuroimaging in Child Neuropsychiatric Disorders. Ed. by B. Garreau. 1998. (Illus.). 289p. 149.00 (*3-540-63634-X*) Spr-Verlag.

Neuroimaging in Epilepsy: Principles & Practice. Gregory Cascino & Clifford R. Jack. 1996. LC 96-32628. 289p. text 165.00 (*0-7506-9716-4*) Buttrwrth-Heinemann.

***Neuroimmune Circuits, Drugs of Abuse & Infectious Diseases.** Ed. by Herman Friedman et al. 2001. LC 00-52729. (Advances in Experimental Medicine & Biology Ser.: Vol. 492). (Illus.). 310p. 110.00 (*0-306-46466-7*, Kluwer Plenum) Kluwer Academic.

Neuroimmunodegeneration. Paul K. Wong & William S. Lynn. 1998. LC 98-23047. (Biotechnology Intelligence Unit Ser.). (*1-57059-484-8*) Landes Bioscience.

Neuroimmunoendocrinology. Ed. by J. Edwin Blalock. 3rd enl. rev. ed. 1997. (Chemical Immunology Ser.: Vol. 69, 1997). (Illus.). xiv, 228p. 194.00 (*3-8055-6524-0*) S Karger.

Neuroimmunology. Ed. by Jeremy Brockes. 1982. LC 82-3679. (Current Topics in Neurobiology Ser.). 272p. 65.00 (*0-306-40955-0*, Plenum Trade) Perseus Pubng.

Neuroimmunomodulation: Molecular Aspects, Integrative Systems, & Clinical Advances. Ed. by Samuel M. McCann et al. 1998. LC 98-15845. (Annals of the New York Academy of Sciences Ser.: No. 840). 866p. 160.00 (*1-57331-072-7*); pap. 160.00 (*1-57331-073-5*) NY Acad Sci.

Neuroimmunomodulation: Proceedings of the 1st International Workshop. Novera H. Spector. 1988. xxii, 306p. pap. text 208.00 (*0-677-21960-1*) Gordon & Breach.

Neuroimmunomodulation - the State of the Art: Proceedings of the 2nd International Congress ISNIM (International Society for Neuroimmunomodulation), Held in Paestum, Salerno, Italy, Sept. 12-17, 1993. Ed. by Nicola Fabris et al. 1994. LC 94-39175. (Annals Ser.: Vol. 741). (*0-89766-909-6*) NY Acad Sci.

Neuroinflammation: Mechanisms & Management. Ed. by Paul L. Wood. 1997. LC 99-207058. (Contemporary Neuroscience Ser.). (Illus.). 392p. 155.00 (*0-89603-416-X*) Humana.

***Neuroinflammatory Mechanisms in Alzheimer's Disease: Basic & Clinical Research.** J. Rogers. 2001. (Illus.). 250p. 149.00 (*3-7643-6074-7*) Birkhauser.

Neuroinformatics: An Overview of the Human Brain Project. Ed. by Stephen H. Koslow & Michael F. Huerta. 1997. (Progress in Neurinformatics Research Ser.). 384p. (C). text 79.95 (*0-8058-2099-X*) L Erlbaum Assocs.

Neurolaryngology. Ed. by Minoru Hirano et al. 1991. (Illus.). 304p. (Orig.). (C). reprint ed. pap. text 65.00 (*1-879105-19-5*, A031) Singular Publishing.

Neuroleptic-Induced Movement Disorders: A Comprehensive Survey. Ed. by Ramzy Yassa et al. 1996. (Illus.). 512p. (C). text 120.00 (*0-521-43364-9*) Cambridge U Pr.

Neuroleptics. Ed. by D. P. Bobon et al. 1970. (Modern Problems of Pharmacopsychiatry Ser.: Vol. 5). 41.00 (*3-8055-0530-2*) S Karger.

Neurolinguistic Approaches to Stuttering: Proceedings of the International Symposium on Stuttering, Brussels, 1972. International Symposium on Stuttering Staff. Ed. by Y. Lebrun & Richard Hoops. 1973. (Janua Linguarum, Series Major: No. 70). (Illus.). (*90-279-2417-1*) Mouton.

Neurolinguistic Aspects of the Japanese Writing System. Michel Paradis & Nancy Hildebrandt. 1985. (Perspectives in Neurolinguistics, Neuropsychology & Psycholinguistics Ser.). text 89.95 (*0-12-544965-8*) Acad Pr.

M N O

Neurolinguistics: Historical & Theoretical Perspectives. C. P. Bouton. 1990. LC 90-7853. (Applied Psycholinguistics & Communication Disorders Ser.). (Illus.). 286p. (C). 65.00 (*0-306-43691-4*, Plenum Trade) Perseus Pubng.

Neurolinguistics & Linguistic Aphasiology: An Introduction. David N. Caplan. 1987. (Cambridge Studies in Speech Science & Communication). (Illus.). 512p. text 95.00 (*0-521-32420-3*); pap. text 34.95 (*0-521-31195-0*) Cambridge U Pr.

Neurologia Pediatrica-Princ y. Kenneth F. Swaiman. 1996. (C). text 196.15 (*84-8086-191-6*) Mosby Inc.

Neurologic & Neurosurgical Emergencies. Julio Cruz. Ed. by Richard Zorab. 1998. LC 98-7038. (Illus.). 624p. (C). text 145.00 (*0-7216-6105-X*) Saunders.

Neurologic Aspects of Substance Abuse. John C. Brust. 2002. 475p. 95.00 (*0-7506-7313-3*) Buttrwrth-Heinemann.

Neurologic Athletic Head & Spinal Injuries. Robert Cantu. 2000. LC 99-57426. (Illus.). 430p. text 84.50 (*0-7216-8339-8*) Saunders.

Neurologic Complications in Organ Transplant Recipients. Eelco F. M. Wijdicks. 1999. LC 98-49668. 272p. text 99.00 (*0-7506-7066-5*) Buttrwrth-Heinemann.

Neurologic Complications of Cancer. Jerome B. Posner. 1995. (Contemporary Neurology Ser.: No. 45). (Illus.). 496p. (C). 99.00 (*0-8036-0006-2*) OUP.

Neurologic Differential Diagnosis. Mark Mumenthaler. Tr. by Otto Appenzeller. 2nd ed. 1992. (GER., Illus.). 192p. (C). pap. text 49.00 (*0-86577-432-3*) Thieme Med Pubs.

Neurologic Disease in Women. Ed. by Peter W. Kaplan. 1998. LC 98-4136. (Illus.). 472p. 150.00 (*1-888799-15-3*) Demos Medical.

Neurologic Disorders, No. 1. Esther Chipps. 1992. (Illus.). 336p. (C). (gr. 13). text 36.00 (*0-8016-1372-8*, 01372) Mosby Inc.

Neurologic Disorders in Women. Ed. by Merit E. Cudkowicz & Michael C. Irizarry. 1997. LC 96-50469. 184p. text 64.99 (*0-7506-9745-8*) Buttrwrth-Heinemann.

Neurologic Emergencies in Infancy & Childhood. John M. Pellock & Edwin C. Myer. 2nd ed. 1993. (Illus.). 425p. text 95.00 (*0-7506-9419-X*) Buttrwrth-Heinemann.

Neurologic Injury During Cardiac Surgery IV Abstract Booklet: Emerging Consensus. Ed. by Silent Partners, Inc. Staff. 1999. 36p. pap. (*1-878353-48-9*) Silent Partners.

Neurologic Localization & Diagnosis. Karl E. Misulis. 1996. LC 95-50501. 217p. pap. text 34.99 (*0-7506-9636-2*) Buttrwrth-Heinemann.

Neurologic Pearls. Orrin Devinsky et al. 2000. LC 99-46439. (Illus.). 320p. (C). pap. text 19.95 (*0-8036-0433-5*) Davis Co.

Neurologic Rehabilitation. Bruce H. Dobkin. 1996. LC 95-46567. (Contemporary Neurology Ser.: No. 47). (Illus.). 360p. (C). 99.00 (*0-8036-0169-7*) OUP.

Neurologic Skills: Examination, History, & Localization for Students & House Officers. Thomas H. Glick. 1993. LC 92-49587. (Illus.). 472p. pap. 46.95 (*0-86542-292-3*) Blackwell Sci.

Neurological Adverse Reactions to Anticancer Drugs. Ed. by J. G. Hildebrand & U. Veronesi. 1990. (ESO Monographs). (Illus.). 112p. 59.00 (*0-387-53263-3*) Spr-Verlag.

Neurological Anatomy in Relation to Clinical Medicine. Alf Brodal. 3rd ed. 1981. (Illus.). 1053p. text 89.00 (*0-19-502694-2*) OUP.

Neurological & Neurosurgical. Nikas. Date not set. text (*0-7216-6001-0*) Saunders.

Neurological & Neurosurgical Nursing. (*0-7131-4521-8*) E A GBR. *Dist:* Routldge.

Neurological & Psychiatric Disorders, Neurogenomics No. 1: Drug Discovery, Development & Market Analysis. Stan M. Goldin & Timothy Tankosic. Ed. by Susan C. DiClemente & Laura Carter. 1997. (Illus.). 1792p. spiral bd. (*1-57936-094-7*, 936) Drug & Market Dev.

Neurological & Psychiatric Disorders, Neurogenomics No. 2: Drug Discovery, Development & Market Analysis - Neurogene Compendium, Market Analysis, Blueprints for Drug Discovery. Stan M. Goldin. Ed. by Susan C. DiClemente & Laura Carter. 1997. (Illus.). 700p. spiral bd. (*1-57936-092-0*, 936) Drug & Market Dev.

Neurological & Psychiatric Disorders, Neurogenomics No. 3: Drug Discovery, Development & Market Analysis - Company Profiles. Stan M. Goldin & Timothy Tankosic. Ed. by Susan C. DiClemente & Laura Carter. 1997. 488p. spiral bd. (*1-57936-093-9*, 936) Drug & Market Dev.

Neurological Aspects of Substance Abuse. John C. Brust. 1993. (Illus.). 289p. text 99.95 (*0-7506-9005-4*) Buttrwrth-Heinemann.

Neurological Assessment of the Pre-Term & Full-Term Newborn Infant. Libby Dubowitz & Victor Dubowitz. 1991. LC 65-80377. (Clinics in Developmental Medicine Ser.: No. 79). (Illus.). 104p. (C). text (*0-521-41204-8*) Mc Keith Pr GBR. *Dist:* Cambridge U Pr.

Neurological Assessment of the Preterm & Full-Term Newborn Infant. Lilly M. Dubowitz et al. 2nd ed. 2000. (Clinics in Developmental Medicine Ser.: No. 148). (Illus.). 150p. (C). text (*1-898683-15-8*) Mc Keith Pr GBR. *Dist:* Cambridge U Pr.

Neurological Complications of Cancer. Ed. by Ronald G. Wiley. 1995. LC 94-41748. (Neurological Disease & Therapy Ser.: Vol. 37). (Illus.). 568p. text 210.00 (*0-8247-8840-0*) Dekker.

Neurological Complications of HIV-AIDS. Said. 1998. (Illus.). 202p. text (*0-7020-1836-8*) Bailliere Tindall.

Neurological Differential Diagnosis. John Patten. 2nd ed. 1996. LC 95-14336. 350p. 75.00 (*3-540-19937-3*) Spr-Verlag.

Neurological Disabilities: Assessment & Treatment. Susan Bennett. 1998. LC 97-52018. 272p. text 41.95 (*0-397-55151-7*) Lppncott W & W.

Neurological Disorders. Connie Goldsmith. 2001. LC 00-11949. (Amazing Brain Ser.). (Illus.). 64p. (YA). (gr. 6-10). 21.95 (*1-56711-422-9*, Blackbirch Pr) Gale.

Neurological Disorders. Ed. by J. D. Parkes et al. 1987. (Treatment in Clinical Medicine Ser.). 227p. 59.30 (*0-387-17013-8*) Spr-Verlag.

Neurological Disorders: Course & Treatment. Ed. by Thomas Brandt et al. 1996. LC 95-15214. (Illus.). 1150p. text 159.95 (*0-12-125830-0*) Acad Pr.

Neurological Dysfunction & Nursing Interventions. Joyce Taylor & Sally Ballenger. 1979. (Illus.). text 35.95 (*0-07-063170-0*) McGraw.

Neurological Emergencies. Ed. by R. A. Hughes. 1994. 350p. (C). pap. text (*0-7279-0756-5*) BMJ Pub GBR. *Dist:* AIDC.

Neurological Evaluation of the Psychogenic Patient. Ed. by W. L. Smith et al. 1982. 160p. (C). text 20.00 (*0-88331-163-1*) R B Luce.

Neurological Examination Made Easy. Geraint Fuller. 1993. LC 92-48187. (Illus.). 232p. pap. text (*0-443-04294-2*) Church.

Neurological Examination of the Full-Term Newborn Infant. Heinz F. Prechtl & David Beintema. 2nd ed. 1991. (Clinics in Developmental Medicine Ser.: No. 63). (Illus.). 76p. (C). reprint ed. text (*0-521-41199-8*) Mc Keith Pr GBR. *Dist:* Cambridge U Pr.

Neurological Examination of the Newborn. N. O'Doherty. 1986. text 124.00 (*0-85200-877-5*) Kluwer Academic.

Neurological Investigations. Ed. by Rac Hughes. 1997. 511p. (*0-7279-1080-9*) BMJ Pub GBR. *Dist:* AIDC.

Neurological Organization of Ocular Movement. Ed. by R. Daroff & A. Neetens. 1989. LC 90-5225. (Illus.). 562p. lib. bdg. (*90-6299-067-3*) Kugler NLD. *Dist:* Lib Res.

***Neurological Physiotherapy.** Susan Edwards. 2nd ed. 2001. (Illus.). 285p. pap. (*0-443-06440-7*) Church GBR. *Dist:* Saunders.

Neurological Physiotherapy: A Problem-Solving Approach. Ed. by Susan Edwards. 1996. LC 96-1650. 212p. pap. text (*0-443-04887-8*) Church.

***Neurological Physiotherapy: Basis Evidence for Practice.** Ed. by Cecily J. Partridge. 2001. 200p. (Orig.). (C). pap. (*1-86156-225-X*) Whurr Pub GBR. *Dist:* Taylor & Francis.

Neurological Rehabilitation. Richard Greenwood. 1997. LC 97-204472. (Illus.). xiii, 640p. (*0-86377-484-9*) Psychol Pr GBR. *Dist:* Taylor & Francis.

Neurological Rehabilitation. Ed. by L. S. Illis. 2nd ed. 1994. LC 93-41918. (Illus.). 592p. 149.00 (*0-632-03282-0*) Blackwell Sci.

Neurological Rehabilitation. Vol. 3. Darcy A. Umphred. 3rd ed. 1995. (Illus.). 1056p. (C). (gr. 13). text 81.00 (*0-8016-7925-7*, 07925) Mosby Inc.

Neurological Side of Neuropsychology. Richard E. Cytowic. 1996. LC 95-1528. (Illus.). 529p. 70.00 (*0-262-03231-7*, Bradford Bks) MIT Pr.

Neurological Sports Medicine: A Guide for Physicians & Athletic Trainers. Ed. by Julian E. Bailes & Arthur L. Day. 2000. 310p. pap. 65.00 (*1-879284-75-8*) Am Assn Neuro.

Neurological Surgery: A Comprehensive Reference Guide to the Diagnosis & Management of Neurosurgical Problems. Julian R. Youmans. Ed. by Richard Zorab. 4th ed. 1995. LC 94-33455. (Illus.). 3648p. text 835.00 (*0-7216-5141-0*) Saunders.

Neurological Surgery: A Comprehensive Reference Guide to the Diagnosis & Management of Neurosurgical Problems Julian R. Youmans. 2nd ed. 1989. 2600p. 1. (*0-7216-9652-X*); 2. (*0-7216-9653-8*); 3. (*0-7216-9654-6*) Saunders.

Neurological Surgery: A Comprehensive Reference Guide to the Diagnosis & Management of Neurosurgical Problems, 4th Edition. Ed. by Julian R. Youmans. 4th ed. 1996. (Illus.). 4242p. incl. cd-rom (*0-7216-6845-3*) Saunders.

Neurological Therapeutics. D. L. Davidson & J. A. Lenman. 1981. 350p. pap. 64.95 (*0-8464-1216-0*) Beekman Pubs.

Neurologically-Impaired Child: Doman-Delacato Techniques Reappraised. Robert A. Cummins. 1988. 272p. lib. bdg. (*0-7099-4859-X*) C Helm GBR. *Dist:* Routldge.

Neurology. Robert C. Collins. Ed. by William Schmitt. 1997. LC 96-48724. 224p. pap. text 36.95 (*0-7216-5992-6*) Saunders.

Neurology. Michael Donaghy. 1997. LC 97-11745. (Oxford Core Texts). (Illus.). 228p. pap. text 29.50 (*0-19-262795-3*) OUP.

Neurology. Alex Habel & Rod Scott. 1998. LC 98-23208. (Illus.). 104p. pap. (*0-7506-2445-0*) E A GBR. *Dist:* OUP.

Neurology. Christopher N. Martyn. 1990. (Student Notes Ser.). (Illus.). 296p. pap. text (*0-443-03307-2*) Church.

Neurology. 2nd ed. 1984. (Medical Ser.). (Illus.). 64p. (C). 12.95 (*0-935920-23-4*, Ntl Pubs Blck) P-H.

Neurology. Trend. 2nd ed. 1998. (C). pap. text (*0-443-05884-9*) Church.

Neurology. Patrick Trend et al. 2nd ed. 1997. LC 97-17396. (Colour Guide Ser.). (*0-443-05807-5*) Harcrt Hlth Sci Grp.

Neurology. Mark Mumenthaler. 3rd ed. 1990. (Flexibook Ser.). (Illus.). 551p. text 32.00 (*0-86577-317-3*) Thieme Med Pubs.

Neurology. Elizabeth K. White. 3rd ed. 1993. LC 92-48848. (Regents - Prentice-Hall Medical Assistant Kit Ser.). pap. 16.40 (*0-13-036823-7*) P-H.

Neurology: A Concise Clinical Text. Michael Swash. 1989. (Illus.). 250p. text (*0-7020-1382-X*) Bailliere Tindall.

Neurology: An Illustrated Collection. Geraint Fuller & Mark R. Manford. 1999. (Illus.). 129p. text 31.00 (*0-443-05374-X*) Mosby Inc.

***Neurology: Diagnosis in Colour.** Malcolm Parsons & Michael Johnson. 2001. (Illus.). 365p. pap. (*0-7234-3179-5*) Mosby Inc.

Neurology: Problems in Primary Care. James L. Bernat & Frederick M. Vincent. Ed. by Melanie C. Karaffa. 2nd ed. 1993. LC 93-6786. (Problems in Primary Care Ser.). (Illus.). 900p. pap. text 49.95 (*1-878487-85-X*, 5855M) Practice Mgmt Info.

Neurology: What Shall I Do? Dayfydd Thomas & Bev Daily. 2nd ed. 1996. LC 97-178844. 128p. pap. text 35.00 (*0-7506-3195-3*) Buttrwrth-Heinemann.

Neurology & Clinical Neuroscience. Roger A. Brumback. Ed. by Rita R. Claudet. 2nd ed. 1996. LC 96-13784. (Oklahoma Notes). 186p. pap. 24.95 (*0-387-94635-7*) Spr-Verlag.

Neurology & General Medicine. Michael J. Aminoff. 2nd ed. 1995. text (*0-443-08933-7*) Church.

Neurology & Neuroscience 2000: An Internet Resource Guide. 2000. 500p. pap. 24.95 (*0-9676811-9-7*) eMedguides.

Neurology & Neurosurgery Illustrated. Kenneth W. Lindsay & Ian Bone. 3rd ed. 1997. LC 97-16820. pap. text (*0-443-05061-9*) Church.

Neurology & Psychiatry: A Meeting of Minds. Ed. by J. Mueller. 1989. (Illus.). xiv, 290p. 195.00 (*3-8055-4712-9*) S Karger.

Neurology & Trauma. Randolph W. Evans. Ed. by Bill Schmidt. 1996. LC 95-42805. (Illus.). 544p. text 104.00 (*0-7216-4352-3*) Saunders.

Neurology Examination Made Easy. Geraint Fuller. 2nd ed. 1998. LC 98-40972. (C). pap. text (*0-443-06166-1*) Church.

Neurology for General Practitioners. Roy Beran. 1996. (Illus.). 224p. text 50.00 (*0-07-470205-X*) McGraw-Hill Med Pub.

Neurology for Non-Neurologists. Wiederholt. 3rd ed. 1995. 368p. pap. text 43.00 (*0-7216-4191-1*) Saunders.

Neurology for Psychiatrists. Gin S. Malhi et al. 2000. 120p. pap. (*1-85317-922-1*) Martin Dunitz GBR. *Dist:* Blackwell Sci.

Neurology for the Boards. James D. Geyer & Janice M. Keating. 1998. LC 98-4651. 320p. pap. text 55.00 (*0-7817-1722-1*) Lppncott W & W.

Neurology for the Non-Neurologist. William J. Weiner & Christopher G. Goetz. 4th ed. 1999. LC 99-11318. (Illus.). xvii, 504p. pap. text 59.95 (*0-7817-1707-8*) Lppncott W & W.

Neurology for the Psychiatry Specialty Board Review. Leon A. Weisberg. 1992. LC 92-16164. (Continuing Education in Psychiatry Ser.: Vol. 2). 160p. pap. 21.95 (*0-87630-684-9*); 2nd ed. 1998. LC 97-36014. (Brunner/Mazel Continuing Education in Psychiatry & Psychol Ser.: Vol. 7). 162p. pap. 24.95 (*0-87630-868-X*) Brunner-Routledge.

Neurology for the Speech-Language Pathologist. Russell Love & Rhonda G. Webb. 4th ed. 2000. (Illus.). 344p. pap. text 39.99 (*0-7506-7252-8*) Buttrwrth-Heinemann.

Neurology in Clinical Practice Walter G. Bradley et al. 3rd ed. 1999. LC 99-31264. (Illus.). xxiii, 2296p. text 460.00 (*0-7506-9973-6*) Buttrwrth-Heinemann.

Neurology in Practice. Y. L. Yu et al. 2nd ed. 1997. 168p. pap. (*962-209-445-7*) HK Univ Pr HKG. *Dist:* Intl Spec Bk, Coronet Bks.

Neurology in Primary Care. Andrea C. Adams. 2000. LC 00-31824. (Illus.). 304p. per. 34.95 (*0-8036-0538-2*) Davis Co.

Neurology in Primary Care. Joseph H. Friedman. 1998. 232p. pap. text 24.99 (*0-7506-7036-3*) Buttrwrth-Heinemann.

Neurology in Science, Medicine & Disease: Index of New Information with Authors & Subjects. Julia M. Knouse. 1993. 180p. 47.50 (*1-55914-884-5*); pap. 44.50 (*1-55914-885-3*) ABBE Pubs Assn.

Neurology of AIDS. Howard E. Gendelman et al. 1997. LC 97-9987. 672p. (*0-412-08631-X*) E A GBR. *Dist:* OUP.

Neurology of Aphasia. Ed. by H. S. Kirshner & F. R. Freemon. 1982. (Neurolinguistics Ser.: Vol. 12). 224p. (*90-265-0409-8*) Swets.

Neurology of Critical Illness. Eelco F. M. Wijdicks. 1995. LC 94-16409. (Contemporary Neurology Ser.: No. 43). (Illus.). 384p. 90.00 (*0-8036-9316-8*) OUP.

Neurology of Eye Movements. R. John Leigh & David S. Zee. 3rd ed. 1999. (Contemporary Neurology Ser.: No. 55). (Illus.). 656p. text 195.00 incl. cd-rom (*0-19-512973-3*) OUP.

Neurology of Hereditary Metabolic Diseases of Children. Gilles Lyon et al. 2nd ed. 1996. LC 95-23487. (Illus.). 379p. text 79.00 (*0-07-000389-0*) McGraw-Hill Prof.

Neurology of the Elderly. Richard Godwin-Austin & M. J. Bendall. 1990. (Illus.). 148p. 69.00 (*0-387-19593-9*) Spr-Verlag.

Neurology of the Newborn. Joseph J. Volpe. (Illus.). 3rd ed. 1994. 876p. text 97.00 (*0-7216-3690-X*); 4th ed. 2000. LC 00-58851. 995p. text 105.00 (*0-7216-8448-3*) Saunders.

Neurology of Thinking. D. Frank Benson. 1994. LC 93-6521. (Illus.). 328p. (C). text 59.50 (*0-19-505882-8*) OUP.

Neurology of Vision. Jonathan D. Trobe. 2000. LC 00-55052. (Contemporary Neurology Ser.: 60). (Illus.). 472p. text 120.00 (*0-19-512978-4*) OUP.

Neurology Pearls of Wisdom: Over 2500 Questions. Labanowski. 1998. (Pearls of Wisdom Ser.). (Illus.). pap. 88.00 (*1-890369-12-8*) Boston Medical.

Neurology Practical Guidelines. Ed. by Lechtenberg & Schutta. 1997. LC 97-36796. (Neurological Disease & Therapy Ser.). (Illus.). 544p. text 165.00 (*0-8247-0104-6*) Dekker.

Neurology Recall. James Q. Miller & Nathan B. Fountain. 1997. LC 97-2668. (Recall Ser.). 360p. pap. text 29.95 (*0-683-18216-1*) Lppncott W & W.

Neurology Resident's Training Program. Epilepsy Foundation of America Staff. 66.95 incl. VHS (*0-916570-16-9*) Epilepsy Foundation of America.

Neurology Secrets: Questions You Will be Asked on Rounds, in the Clinic & on Oral Exams. Loren A. Rolak. 2nd ed. 1998. LC 98-21152. 425p. pap. 39.95 (*1-56053-251-3*) Hanley & Belfus.

Neurology Short Case. John G. L. Morris. 1992. 96p. pap. (*0-340-54923-8*) E A GBR. *Dist:* OUP.

Neuromodules & Brain Function. Giovanni Biggio et al. 1984. (Advances in the Biosciences Ser.). 460p. 73.00 (*0-08-030782-5*, Pergamon Pr) Elsevier.

Neuromonitoring in Brain Injury. Ed. by Ross Bullock et al. 2000. LC 99-46769. (Acta Neurochirurgica Ser.: Vol. 75). (Illus.). 79p. 54.00 (*3-211-83379-X*) Spr-Verlag.

Neuromorphological Plasticity: Proceedings of the Symposium, Dallas, Texas, April 1972. American Association of Anatomists, Cajal Club Mee. Ed. by J. Bernstein & D. C. Goodman. 1973. (Brain, Behavior & Evolution Ser.: Vol. 8, Nos. 1-2). (Illus.). 164p. reprint ed. 42.50 (*3-8055-1703-3*) S Karger.

Neuromorphometry. Weis. 1998. 600p. (*0-12-742730-9*) Acad Pr.

Neuromotor Mechanisms in Human Communication. Doreen Kimura. 1993. LC 92-49194. (Oxford Psychology Ser.: No. 20). (Illus.). 208p. text 55.00 (*0-19-505492-X*) OUP.

Neuromuscular Block. Stanley Feldman. 1996. LC 95-45603. 208p. text 85.00 (*0-7506-1764-0*) Buttrwrth-Heinemann.

Neuromuscular Diagnostics & Association. Karen Scotti. 1999. pap. text 45.00 (*0-8385-6709-6*, Medical Exam) Appleton & Lange.

Neuromuscular Disease: From Basic Mechanisms to Clinical Management. Ed. by F. S. Deymeer. 2000. LC 00-30965. (Monographs in Clinical Neuroscience: Vol. 18). (Illus.). viii, 196p. 164.50 (*3-8055-7056-2*) S Karger.

Neuromuscular Diseases: A Practical Approach to Diagnosis & Management. Michael Swash & Martin S. Schwartz. 3rd ed. 1997. LC 96-39564. (Illus.). 504p. 198.00 (*3-540-76025-3*) Spr-Verlag.

Neuromuscular Diseases: Expert Clinicians' Views. Rahman Pourmand. 2001. LC 00-65179. (Illus.). 520p. text 125.00 (*0-7506-7019-3*) Buttrwrth-Heinemann.

Neuromuscular Diseases During Development. Fernando Cornelio. 1997. 168p. (*0-86196-541-8*) J Libbey Med GBR. *Dist:* Buttrwrth-Heinemann.

Neuromuscular Disorders in Clinical Practice. Bashar Katirji & Henry J. Kaminski. 2001. (Illus.). 1416p. 295.00 (*0-7506-7169-6*) Buttrwrth-Heinemann.

Neuromuscular Disorders of Infancy & Childhood: A Clinician's Approach. Basil T. Darras. 2001. 1000p. 285.00 (*0-7506-7190-4*) Buttrwrth-Heinemann.

Neuromuscular Fatigue: Proceedings of the Symposium, Amsterdam, the Netherlands, 9-11 April 1992. Ed. by A. J. Sargeant & D. Kernell. 1993. 210p. pap. (*0-444-85763-X*) Royal Netherlands Acad NLD. *Dist:* Elsevier.

Neuromuscular Maturation of the Human Infant. Myrtle B. McGraw. 1991. (Classics in Developmental Medicine Ser.: No. 4). (Illus.). 117p. (C). text (*0-521-41329-X*) Mc Keith Pr GBR. *Dist:* Cambridge U Pr.

Neuromuscular Physiology. Bill Garoutte. 1997. (Illus.). 500p. (Orig.). pap. 24.00 (*0-9643644-1-7*) Mill Valley Med.

Neuromuscular Transmission: Basic & Applied Aspects. Ed. by Angela Vincent & Dennis Wary. 1992. LC 92-23209. 304p. 188.00 (*0-08-041983-6*, Pergamon Pr) Elsevier.

Neuromuscular Transmission: Basic & Applied Aspects. Ed. by Angela Vincent & D. Wray. 1991. (Studies in Neuroscience). (*0-7190-2598-2*) Manchester Univ Pr GBR. *Dist:* St Martin.

Neuromusculoskeletal Examination & Assessment: A Handbook for Therapists. Nicola J. Petty & Ann P. Moore. 1998. LC 97-33318. pap. text (*0-443-05980-2*) Church.

***Neuromusculoskeletal Examination & Assessment: A Handbook for Therapists.** Nicola J. Petty & Ann P. Moore. 2001. (Illus.). 395p. pap. *(0-443-07061-X)* Church GBR. *Dist:* Saunders.

Neuron, Brain & Behaviour: Proceedings of the Annual Meeting of the European Brain & Behaviour Society, Novi Sad, Yugoslavia, 19th, 23-25 August, 1987. Ed. by M. Bajic. 1988. (Advances in the Biosciences Ser.: Vol. 70). 236p. 94.00 *(0-08-035597-8,* Pergamon Pr) Elsevier.

Neuron in Tissue Culture. L. W. Haynes. 1999. LC 98-22011. (IBRO Handbook Ser.: Vol. 18). (Illus.). 752p. 395.00 *(0-471-97505-2)* Wiley.

Neuronal Aging & Its Implications in Human Neurological Pathology. 1981. (Technical Report Ser.: No. 665). 88p. pap. text 6.00 *(92-4-120665-9)* World Health.

Neuronal Cooperativity. Ed. by James E. Kruger. 1991. (Synergetics Ser.: Vol. 49). (Illus.). 324p. 124.00 *(0-387-53155-6)* Spr-Verlag.

Neuronal Cytoskeleton. Ed. by Nobutaka Hirokawa. 1994. LC 93-29823. (Taniguchi Symposia on Brain Sciences Ser.: No. 16). 84.95 *(0-8493-7741-2)* CRC Pr.

Neuronal Degeneration & Regeneration: From Basic Mechanisms to Prospects for Therapy. F. W. Van Leeuwen. 1998. LC 98-36940. (Progress in Brain Research Ser.). 550p. 229.00 *(0-444-82817-6)* Elsevier.

Neuronal Development. Ed. by Nicholas C. Spitzer. 1982. LC 82-3693. (Current Topics in Neurobiology Ser.). (Illus.). 478p. 89.50 *(0-306-40956-9,* Plenum Trade) Perseus Pubng.

Neuronal Ensembles: Strategies for Recording & Decoding. Howard B. Eichenbaum & Joel L. Davis. 1998. LC 97-28317. 267p. 126.00 *(0-471-17940-X)* Wiley.

Neuronal-Glial Cell Interrelationships. Ed. by T. A. Sears. 1982. (Dahlem Workshop Reports Ser.: Vol. 20). (Illus.). 375p. 42.95 *(0-387-11329-0)* Spr-Verlag.

Neuronal Grafting & Alzheimer's Disease. Ed. by F. Gage et al. 1989. (Research & Perspectives in Alzheimer's Disease Ser.). (Illus.). 201p. 86.95 *(0-387-51197-0)* Spr-Verlag.

Neuronal Man: The Biology of the Mind. Jean-Pierre Changeux. Tr. by Laurence Garey. 1997. LC 97-209028. (Princeton Science Library). 368p. pap. 19.95 *(0-691-02666-1)* Princeton U Pr.

Neuronal Morphology of Avian Telencaephalon. Tombol. 1995. (SINS Ser.). *(0-08-041990-9,* Pergamon Pr) Elsevier.

Neuronal Networks of the Hippocampus. Roger D. Traub & Richard Miles. 1991. (Illus.). 301p. (C). text 59.95 *(0-521-36481-7)* Cambridge U Pr.

Neuronal Nicotinic Receptors: Pharmacology & Therapeutic Opportunities. Ed. by Stephen P. Arneric & Jorge D. Brioni. 1998. LC 98-17280. (Illus.). 421p. 199.00 *(0-471-24743-X)* Wiley.

Neuronal Operations in the Visual Cortex. Guy A. Orban. 1984. (Studies of Brain Function: Vol. 11). (Illus.). 367p. 102.00 *(0-387-11919-1)* Spr-Verlag.

Neuronal Plasticity: Building a Bridge from the Laboratory to the Clinic. Ed. by Jordan Grafman & Yves Christen. 1998. LC 98-38384. (Research & Perspectives in Neurosciences Ser.). (Illus.). 201p. 119.00 *(3-540-64357-5)* Spr-Verlag.

Neuronal Receptors, Endogenous Ligands & Biotechnical Approaches. Ed. by M. E. Vartanian. 1989. LC 88-13259. 149p. 35.00 *(0-8236-3558-9)* Intl Univs Pr.

Neurones Without Impulses. Ed. by Alan Roberts & B. M. Bush. 1981. LC 79-42572. (Society for Experimental Biology Seminar Ser.: No. 6). (Illus.). 304p. pap. text 29.95 *(0-521-29935-7)* Cambridge U Pr.

Neurons: Directory of Authors of New Medical & Scientific Reviews with Subject Index. Science and Life Consultants Association Staff. 1995. 160p. 57.50 *(0-7883-0598-0)*; pap. 47.50 *(0-7883-0599-9)* ABBE Pubs Assn.

Neurons & Networks: An Introduction to Neuroscience. John E. Dowling. 1992. (Illus.). 447p. (C). 58.50 *(0-674-60820-8)* HUP.

Neurons, Networks, & Motor Behavior. Ed. by Paul S. Stein et al. 1997. LC 97-1551. (Computational Neuroscience: A Bradford Book Ser.). (Illus.). 262p. 60.00 *(0-262-19390-6,* Bradford Bks) MIT Pr.

Neuronuclear Medicine. Ed. by O. Juge & A. Donath. 1981. (Progress in Nuclear Medicine Ser.: Vol. 7). (Illus.). viii, 176p. 135.00 *(3-8055-2319-X)* S Karger.

Neuroophthalmology. Roy W. Beck & Craig H. Smith. 1987. (Illus.). 256p. 64.95 *(0-316-08651-7,* Little Brwn Med Div) Lppncott W & W.

Neuropaediatrie III, III. Ed. by J. Luetschg. 1986. (Paediatrische Fortbildungskurse fuer die Praxis Ser.: Vol. 60). (Illus.). xii, 92p. pap. 47.00 *(3-8055-4232-1)* S Karger.

Neuropaediatrie II. Ed. by F. Vassella. 1982. (Paediatrische Fortbildungskurse fuer die Praxis Ser.: Vol. 55). (Illus.). xiv, 190p. pap. 71.50 *(3-8055-3434-5)* S Karger.

Neuropathic Bladder in Childhood. M. Borzyskowski & A. R. Mundy. 1991. (Clinics in Developmental Medicine Ser.: No. 111). (Illus.). 120p. (C). text *(0-521-41194-7)* Mc Keith Pr GBR. *Dist:* Cambridge U Pr.

Neuropathies. Ed. by Pierre J. Vinken et al. 1987. 668p. 320.50 *(0-444-90478-6)* Elsevier.

Neuropathogenic Viruses & Immunity. S. Specter et al. 1992. (Infectious Agents & Pathogenesis Ser.). (Illus.). 376p. (C). text 95.00 *(0-306-43785-6,* Kluwer Plenum) Kluwer Academic.

Neuropathological Diagnostic Criteria for Brain Banking. Ed. by F. F. Cruz-Sanchez et al. 1995. LC 94-7342. (Biomedical & Health Research Ser.: Vol. 10). 166p. 77.00 *(90-5199-208-4)* IOS Press.

Neuropathological Surgery. Spoor. 1992. 105.00 *(0-316-80814-8,* Little Brwn Med Div) Lppncott W & W.

Neuropathology. David Ellison. 1998. 2484p. pap. 425.00 incl. cd-rom *(0-7234-3136-1)*; 1997. text 299.00 *(0-7234-2550-7)* Mosby Inc.

Neuropathology: Based on the 1989 IAP Annual Long Course. P. A. Cancilla & F. Stephen Vogel. 1990. (Illus.). 160p. 69.00 *(0-683-01430-7)* Lppncott W & W.

Neuropathology & Basic Neuroscience. Ed. by Roger A. Brumback & Richard W. Leech. 1995. LC 94-42193. (Oklahoma Notes). 289p. 24.95 *(0-387-94389-7)* Spr-Verlag.

Neuropathology & Genetics of Dementia. Ed. by Markus Tolnay & Alphonse Probst. 2001. LC 00-67413. (Advances in Experimental Medicine & Biology Ser.: Vol. 487). (Illus.). xiii, 255p. 90.00 *(0-306-46558-2,* Kluwer Plenum) Kluwer Academic.

Neuropathology & Ophthalmologic Pathology in AIDS: A Color Atlas. Umberto De Girolami et al. 1991. (Illus.). 165p. text *(0-7506-9239-1)* E A GBR. *Dist:* OUP.

Neuropathology Manual. Fredrich Klutzow. 1996. (Illus.). 264p. 30.00 *(0-89189-358-X)* Am Soc Clinical.

Neuropathology of AIDS. Ed. by Harry V. Vinters & Karl H. Anders. 1989. 240p. 210.00 *(0-8493-5074-3,* RC607) CRC Pr.

Neuropathology of Dementia. Ed. by Margaret M. Esiri & James H. Morris. 1997. LC 96-27783. (Illus.). 454p. (C). text 150.00 *(0-521-43311-8)* Cambridge U Pr.

Neuropathology of Dementing Disorders. Ed. by William R. Markesbery. 1998. LC 97-9715. (Arnold Publication). (Illus.). 416p. text 195.00 *(0-340-59037-8)* OUP.

Neuropathology of Epilepsy. Ed. by F. Scaravilli. 1997. LC 97-29351. 300p. 58.00 *(981-02-3170-9)* World Scientific Pub.

Neuropeptide Y & Drug Development. Ed. by Lars Grundemar & Stephen R. Bloom. 1996. (Illus.). 224p. text 75.00 *(0-12-304990-3)* Morgan Kaufmann.

Neuropeptide y Protocols. Ambikaipakan Balasubramaniam. 2000. LC 00-20392. (Methods in Molecular Biology Ser.: Vol. 153). (Illus.). 256p. 99.50 *(0-89603-662-6)* Humana.

Neuropeptides: Basic & Clinical Advances. Ed. by Jacqueline N. Crawley & Stafford McLean. 1996. LC 96-6767. (Annals of the New York Academy of Sciences Ser.: No. 780). 255p. 100.00 *(0-89766-989-4)* NY Acad Sci.

Neuropeptides Vol. 897: Structure & Function in Biology & Behavior. Ed. by Curt A. Sandman et al. 1999. 443p. 120.00 *(1-57331-225-8)* NY Acad Sci.

Neuropeptides & Immunoregulation. Ed. by B. Scharrer et al. 1994. LC 93-32233. (Illus.). 174p. 131.00 *(0-387-57188-4)* Spr-Verlag.

Neuropeptides & Stress. Ed. by T. Tache et al. 1988. (Hans Selve Symposia on Neuroendocrinology & Stress Ser.). (Illus.). 345p. 116.00 *(0-387-96748-6)* Spr-Verlag.

Neuropeptides in Development & Aging. Bill E. Beckwith. 1997. LC 97-5944. (Annals of the New York Academy of Sciences Ser.). pap. 120.00 *(1-57331-067-0)* NY Acad Sci.

Neuropeptides in Respiratory Medicine. Ed. by Michael A. Kaliner et al. 1994. LC 94-5869. (Clinical Allergy & Immunology Ser.: Vol. 4). (Illus.). 720p. text 245.00 *(0-8247-9199-1)* Dekker.

Neuropeptides in the Spinal Cord. Ed. by F. Nyberg et al. 1995. LC 93-11042. (Progress in Brain Research Ser.: Vol. 104). (Illus.). 438p. 200.00 *(0-444-81719-0)* Elsevier.

Neuropharmacological Basis of Reward. Jeffrey M. Liebman & Steven J. Cooper. 1989. (Illus.). 444p. text 75.00 *(0-19-852176-6)* OUP.

Neuropharmacology. Trevor W. Stone. 1997. LC 95-4264. (Biochemical & Medicinal Chemistry Ser.). (Illus.). 160p. (C). pap. text 27.50 *(0-7167-4510-0)* OUP.

Neuropharmacology: Clinical Applications. Ed. by Walter B. Essman & L. Valzelli. 1982. (Illus.). 500p. text 60.00 *(0-88331-164-X)* R B Luce.

Neuropharmacology Methods in Epilepsy Research. Steven L. Peterson & Timothy E. Albertson. 1998. LC 98-9863. (CRC Press Methods in the Life Sciences Ser.). 304p. per. 129.95 *(0-8493-3362-8)* CRC Pr.

Neuropharmacology of Epilepsy: Pathophysiology & Drug Mechanisms. Robert A. Gross & Timothy J. Greenamyre. 1999. (Illus.). 125.00 *(0-89603-522-0)* Humana.

Neuropharmacology of Polyamines. Ed. by Chris J. Carter. 1994. (Neuroscience Perspectives Ser.). (Illus.). 336p. text 83.00 *(0-12-161640-1)* Acad Pr.

Neuropharmacology Reviews, Vol. 1. A. V. Valdman. 1990. (Soviet Medical Reviews Ser.: Sect. G, Vol 1). xii, 228p. pap. text 506.00 *(3-7186-4884-9)* Gordon & Breach.

Neuropharmacology Reviews Vol. 2, Pt. 1.2: Investigation of the Mechanisms of Action of Non-Benzodiazepine Anxiolytics, Vol. 2. I. V. Komissarov. 1992. (Soviet Medical Reviews Ser.: Section G). 230p. pap. text 94.00 *(3-7186-5249-8,* Harwood Acad Pubs) Gordon & Breach.

Neuropharmacology Reviews Vol. 2, Pt. 2.2: Present-Day Problems in Experimental Psychopharmacology of Nootropic Drugs, Vol. 2. T. A. Voronina. 1992. (Soviet Medical Reviews Ser.: Section G). 212p. pap. text 110.00 *(3-7186-5282-X,* Harwood Acad Pubs) Gordon & Breach.

Neuropharmacology Reviews Vol. 2, Pt. 3: Blood-Brain Barrier, Vol. 2. S. Borisenko. 1992. 78p. pap. text 80.00 *(3-7186-5285-4,* Harwood Acad Pubs) Gordon & Breach.

Neurophilosophy: Toward a Unified Science of the Mind-Brain. Patricia S. Churchland. (Illus.). 384p. 1989. pap. 29.95 *(0-262-53085-6)*; 1986. LC 85-23706. 60.00 *(0-262-03116-7)* MIT Pr (Bradford Bks).

Neurophilosophy & Alzheimer's Disease. Ed. by Yves Christen & Patricia S. Churchland. 1992. (Research & Perspectives in Alzheimer's Disease Ser.). (Illus.). 153p. 100.00 *(0-387-54779-7)* Spr-Verlag.

Neurophsiological Correlates of Relaxation & Psychopathology. Ed. by B. Taneli et al. 1987. (Advances in Biological Psychiatry Ser.: Vol. 16). (Illus.). vi, 214p. 143.50 *(3-8055-4449-9)* S Karger.

Neurophysics of Human Behavior: Explorations at the Interface of the Brain, Mind & Information. Mark E. Furman & Fred Gallo. 2000. LC 00-23640. 376p. 79.95 *(0-8493-1308-2)* CRC Pr.

Neurophysiological & Behavioural Research in Psychiatry: Report of a WHO Scientific Group, 1968. 1968. (Technical Report Ser.: No. 381). 33p. pap. text 5.00 *(92-4-120381-1,* 1100381) World Health.

Neurophysiological & Clinical Aspects of Vestibular Disorders. Ed. by C. R. Pfaltz. 1983. (Advances in OtoRhinoLaryngology Ser.: Vol. 30). (Illus.). xii, 372p. 171.50 *(3-8055-3607-0)* S Karger.

Neurophysiological Basis for the Treatment of Cerebral Palsy. Karel Bobath. 2nd ed. 1991. (Clinics in Developmental Medicine Ser.: No. 75). (Illus.). 98p. (C). text *(0-521-41202-1)* Mc Keith Pr GBR. *Dist:* Cambridge U Pr.

Neurophysiological Basis of Cerebral Blood Flow. Mraovtich. 1995. 424p. *(0-86196-272-9)* J Libbey Med GBR. *Dist:* Buttrwrth-Heinemann.

Neurophysiological Basis of Mind: The Principles of Neurophysiology. John C. Eccles. 1988. LC 88-16029. (Genes Cells, & Organisms Ser.). 332p. text 10.00 *(0-8240-1377-8)* Garland.

Neurophysiological Basis of Patient Treatment: Peripheral Components of Motor Control, Vol. III. Carolyn A. Crutchfield & Marylou R. Barnes. 1984. (Illus.). pap. 35.00 *(0-936030-03-8)* Stokesville Pub.

Neurophysiological Basis of Patient Treatment: Reflexes in Motor Development, Vol. II. Marylou R. Barnes et al. 1978. LC 72-87895. (Illus.). pap. 35.00 *(0-936030-01-1)* Stokesville Pub.

Neurophysiological Correlates of Mental Disorders. Ed. by B. Saletu et al. 1985. (Advances in Biological Psychiatry Ser.: Vol. 15). (Illus.). vi, 114p. 74.00 *(3-8055-3969-X)* S Karger.

Neurophysiological Correlates of Normal Cognition & Psychopathology. Ed. by C. Perris et al. 1984. (Advances in Biological Psychiatry Ser.: Vol. 13). (Illus.). viii, 232p. pap. 85.25 *(3-8055-3737-9)* S Karger.

Neurophysiological Examination of the Newborn Infant. Ed. by J. A. Eyre. 1992. (Clinics in Developmental Medicine Ser.: No. 120). (Illus.). 207p. (C). text 64.95 *(0-521-41276-5)* Cambridge U Pr.

Neurophysiological Insights into Teaching. Marion F. Stuart. 1963. LC 62-21040. (Illus.). xvi, 125p. (Orig.). pap. text 14.95 *(0-87015-114-2)* Pacific Bks.

Neurophysiological Techniques I: Basic Methods & Concepts. Ed. by Alan A. Boulton et al. 1990. LC 89-26855. (Neuromethods Ser.: Vol. 14). (Illus.). 408p. 109.50 *(0-89603-160-8)* Humana.

Neurophysiological Techniques II: Applications to Neural Systems. Ed. by Alan A. Boulton et al. 1990. LC 90-44264. (Neuromethods Ser.: Vol. 15). (Illus.). 391p. 109.50 *(0-89603-185-3)* Humana.

Neurophysiologische Grundlagen der Hirnleistungsstorungen: Erkennen, Verstehen, Rehabilitieren. Gino Gschwend. 2000. (GER.). 148p. pap. 35.00 *(3-8055-6999-8)* S Karger.

Neurophysiology. P. P. Newman. 1980. (Illus.). 455p. text 35.00 *(0-88331-165-8)* R B Luce.

Neurophysiology. Roger Carpenter. 3rd ed. 1996. (Illus.). 322p. pap. *(0-340-60880-3)* E A GBR. *Dist:* OUP.

Neurophysiology. Roger Carpenter. 2nd ed. 1990. 24.00 *(0-340-50634-2)* Trafalgar.

Neurophysiology: Applications in the Behavioural & Biomedical Sciences. K. A. Clarke. 1989. (Ellis Horwood Series in Eurosciences). 150p. 59.95 *(0-470-21554-2)* P-H.

Neurophysiology & Emotion. Ed. by David C. Glass. 1967. LC 67-31389. (Illus.). 256p. 13.00 *(0-87470-006-X)* Rockefeller.

Neurophysiology & Neuropsychology of Motor Development. Ed. by Kevin J. Connolly & Hans Forssberg. 1997. LC 98-107760. (Clinics in Developmental Medicine Ser.: No. 143). (Illus.). 350p. (C). *(1-898683-10-7)* Mc Keith Pr GBR. *Dist:* Cambridge U Pr.

Neurophysiology & Psychophysiology: Experimental & Clinical Applications. Ed. by G. C. Galbraith et al. 1988. 416p. 79.95 *(0-89859-946-6)* L Erlbaum Assocs.

Neurophysiology & Standards of Spinal Cord Monitoring. Ed. by T. B. Ducker & R. H. Brown. 1988. (Illus.). 388p. 127.00 *(0-387-96634-X)* Spr-Verlag.

Neurophysiology of Consciousness: Selected Papers of Benjamin Libet. Benjamin Libet. 1993. LC 93-16896. (Contemporary Neuroscientists Ser.). (Illus.). 424p. 120.00 *(0-8176-3538-6)* Birkhauser.

Neurophysiology of Ingestion. Ed. by D. A. Booth. 1993. LC 93-34148. (Studies in Neurosciences). 186p. 180.00 *(0-08-041988-7,* Pergamon Pr) Elsevier.

Neurophysiology of the Jaws & Teeth. Anthony Taylor. 1990. text 90.00 *(0-333-42362-3)* Intl Spec Bk.

Neurophysiology of the Vestibular System. Ed. by E. Pirodda. 1988. (Advances in OtoRhinoLaryngology Ser.: Vol. 41). (Illus.). xii, 244p. 148.75 *(3-8055-4766-8)* S Karger.

Neuroplasticity: A New Therapeutic Tool in the CNS Pathology. Ed. by R. Masland et al. 1988. (FIDIA Research Ser.: Vol. 12). 245p. 112.00 *(0-387-96620-X)* Spr-Verlag.

Neuroplasticity & Repair in the Central Nervous System: Implications for Health Care. WHO Staff. 1983. (WHO Offset Publications: No. 73). 56p. 5.00 *(92-4-170073-4)* World Health.

Neuroprosthetics: From Basic Research to Clinical Applications:Biomedical & Health Research Program (Biomed) of the European Union, Concerted Action:Restoration of Muscle Activity Through Fes & Associated Technology (Raft) J. Quintern & R. Riener. 1996. LC 96-20390. (Illus.). 654p. 141.00 *(3-540-61084-7)* Spr-Verlag.

Neuroprotection. Ed. by Peter Rudolf Bar & M. Flint Beal. 1997. LC 97-12545. (Illus.). 584p. text 225.00 *(0-8247-9876-7)* Dekker.

Neuroprotection in Neurodegeneration. Ed. by M. B. Youdim et al. 1995. 73.00 *(0-387-82542-8)* Spr-Verlag.

Neuroprotective Agents: 3rd International Conference. Ed. by William Slikker & Bruce Trembly. 1997. LC 97-26504. (Annals of the New York Academy of Sciences Ser.). 438p. pap. 120.00 *(1-57331-093-X)* NY Acad Sci.

Neuroprotective Agents: Clinical & Experimental Aspects. Ed. by Bruce Trembly & William Slikker, Jr. 1995. LC 95-21866. (Annals of the New York Academy of Sciences Ser.: Vol. 765). *(0-89766-945-2)*; pap. *(0-89766-946-0)* NY Acad Sci.

Neuroprotective Agents: Clinical & Experimental Aspects, 3rd International Conference, Vol. 825. William Slikker, Jr. & Bruce Trembly. 1997. LC 97-26504. 120.00 *(1-57331-092-1)* NY Acad Sci.

Neuroprotective Agents: Fourth International Conference. Contrib. by Bruce Trembly et al. 1999. LC 99-47061. (Annals of the New York Academy of Sciences Ser.: Vol. 890). (Illus.). xi, 537p. *(1-57331-222-3)* NY Acad Sci.

Neuroprotective Agents: Fourth International Conference. Bruce Trembly & William Slikker. 1999. LC 99-47061. (Annals of the New York Academy of Sciences Ser.: Vol. 890). (Illus.). xi, 537p. *(1-57331-223-1)* NY Acad Sci.

***Neuroprotective Agents Vol. 939: Fifth International Conference.** Ed. by William J. Slikker, Jr. & Bruce Trembly. 2001. 500p. 150.00 *(1-57331-352-1)* NY Acad Sci.

Neuroprotective Strategies for Early Intervention in Acute Ischaemic Stroke: Janssen-Cilag Satellite Meeting to the 3rd World Stroke Congress & the 5th European Stroke Conference, Munich, September 1996. Ed. by Werner Hacke. 1997. (Journal: Vol. 7, Supplement 2, 1997). (Illus.). iv, 40p. pap. 21.75 *(3-8055-6463-5)* S Karger.

Neuropsychiatric Disorders. Gareth W. Roberts. 1993. 228p. (C). (gr. 13). *(1-56375-510-6)* Gower-Mosby.

Neuropsychiatric Features of Medical Disorders. James W. Jefferson & John R. Marshall. 1981. LC 81-2550. (Critical Issues in Psychiatry Ser.). 404p. 80.00 *(0-306-40674-8,* Kluwer Plenum) Kluwer Academic.

Neuropsychiatric Guide to Modern Everyday Psychiatry. Michael A. Taylor. 1993. LC 92-49025. xi, 530p. 55.00 *(0-02-932455-6)* Free Pr.

Neuropsychiatric Manifestations of Systemic Lupus Erythemafosus, Vol. 823. Ed. by Patricia M. Moore & Robert G. Lahita. 1997. LC 97-28522. (Annals of the New York Academy of Sciences Ser.: No. 823). 336p. 110.00 *(1-57331-080-8)* NY Acad Sci.

Neuropsychiatric Manifestations of Systemic Lupus Erythematosus. P. M. Moore & Robert G. Lahita. 1997. LC 97-28522. (Annals of the New York Academy of Sciences Ser.: No. 823). 336p. pap. 110.00 *(1-57331-081-6)* NY Acad Sci.

Neuropsychiatric Study in Children. Michael Rutter et al. 1991. (Clinics in Developmental Medicine Ser.: Vols. 35 & 36). (Illus.). 272p. (C). text *(0-521-41198-X)* Mc Keith Pr GBR. *Dist:* Cambridge U Pr.

Neuropsychiatry: A Comprehensive Textbook. Barry S. Fogel et al. 1996. (Illus.). 1,064p. text 189.00 (*0-683-03305-0*) Lppncott W & W.

Neuropsychiatry & Mental Health Services. Ed. by Fred Ovsiew. 1999. LC 98-39584. 448p. 61.95 (*0-88048-730-5*, 8730) Am Psychiatric.

Neuropsychiatry & the War: A Bibliography with Abstracts & Supplement I, October, 1918 Ed. by Frankwood E. Williams. 1976. LC 75-16690. reprint ed. 36.95 (*0-405-07420-4*) Ayer.

Neuropsychiatry in Old Age: An Update. Franz Muller-Spahn. 1996. (Psychiatry in Progress Ser.: Vol. 3). 32.00 (*0-88937-137-7*) Hogrefe & Huber Pubs.

Neuropsychiatry, Neuropsychology, & Clinical Neuroscience. R. Joseph. 2nd rev. ed. 1996. LC 95-38650. (Illus.). 864p. 139.00 (*0-683-04485-0*) Lppncott W & W.

Neuropsychiatry of Limbic & Subcortical Disorders. Stephen Salloway et al. 1998. LC 97-34481. (Journal of Neuropsychiatry & Clinical Neurosciences). 232p. 49.50 (*0-88048-942-1*, 8942) Am Psychiatric.

Neuropsychiatry of Multiple Sclerosis. Anthony Feinstein. 1999. LC 98-46888. (Illus.). 214p. (C). text 69.95 (*0-521-57274-6*) Cambridge U Pr.

Neuropsychiatry of Personality Disorders. John J. Ratey. 1994. LC 94-32669. (Neuropsychiatry Ser.). (Illus.). 352p. 69.95 (*0-86542-293-1*) Blackwell Sci.

Neuropsychiatry of Traumatic Brain Injury. Ed. by Jonathan M. Silver et al. 1994. LC 93-11646. 832p. text 82.95 (*0-88048-538-8*, 8538) Am Psychiatric.

Neuropsychological Aging Inventory (NAI) W. D. Oswald & U. M. Fleischmann. 2001. 300p. 79.00 (*0-88937-215-2*) Hogrefe & Huber Pubs.

Neuropsychological Analysis of Problem Solving. A. R. Luria & L. S. Tsvetkova. Tr. by Tichinas Staff from RUS. 1990. LC 90-83131. (Classics in Soviet Psychology Ser.). 256p. 57.95 (*1-878205-10-2*) St Lucie Pr.

Neuropsychological & Behavioral Aspects of Diabetes: Contributions to Psychology & Medicine. Ed. by C. S. Holmes. 1989. (Illus.). 283p. 141.00 (*0-387-97075-4*) Spr-Verlag.

Neuropsychological Aspects of Lyme Disease: A Special Issue of "Applied Neuropsychology" Ed. by Richard F. Kaplan. 1999. 48p. pap. 20.00 (*0-8058-9817-4*) L Erlbaum Assocs.

Neuropsychological Assessment. Muriel D. Lezak. 3rd ed. 1995. LC 94-38337. (Illus.). 1056p. text 72.50 (*0-19-509031-4*) OUP.

Neuropsychological Assessment & Intervention. Charles J. Golden et al. 1992. (Illus.). 314p. (C). 59.95 (*0-398-05754-0*) C C Thomas.

Neuropsychological Assessment & the School-Age Child: Issues & Procedures. Ed. by John E. Obrzut & George W. Hynd. 1981. (Illus.). 448p. (C). text 40.95 (*0-8089-1381-6*, 792109, Grune & Strat) Harcrt Hlth Sci Grp.

Neuropsychological Assessment in Clinical Practice: A Guide to Test Interpretation & Integration. Gary Groth-Marnat. 2000. LC 99-19227. 672p. 89.95 (*0-471-19325-9*) Wiley.

Neuropsychological Assessment of Dementia & Depression in Older Adults: A Clinician's Guide. Ed. by Martha Storandt & Gary R. VandenBos. 1994. (Illus.). 219p. pap. 29.95 (*1-55798-437-9*) Am Psychol.

Neuropsychological Assessment of Neuropsychiatric Disorders. Ed. by Igor Grant & Kenneth M. Adams. 2nd ed. 1996. LC 95-49329. (Illus.). 672p. text 76.50 (*0-19-509073-X*) OUP.

Neuropsychological Case Histories: A Comparative Analysis. Ivan G. Ainyette. unabr. ed. 1998. LC 96-93042. (Illus.). 304p. text 50.00 (*0-9655600-0-7*) NY Neurosci Pr.

Neuropsychological Differentiation of Dementia Syndrome. M. M. Derix. 1994. LC 94-9130. 184p. (*90-265-1312-7*) Swets.

Neuropsychological Disorders Associated with Subcortical Lesions. Ed. by Guiseppe Vallar et al. 1992. (Illus.). 522p. text 115.00 (*0-19-854677-7*) OUP.

Neuropsychological Evaluation in Vocational Planning. Jay Uomoto. Ed. by Robert Fraser & David Clemmons. 1991. LC 91-73657. (Traumatic Brain Injury Rehabilitation Training Ser.). (Illus.). 120p. per. 29.95 (*1-878205-06-4*) St Lucie Pr.

Neuropsychological Evaluation of Head Injury. Lawrence C. Hartlage. Ed. by Harold H. Smith, Jr. 1990. LC 89-43626. (Practitioner's Resource Ser.). 68p. pap. 15.95 (*0-943158-47-8*, NEHIBP, Prof Resc Pr) Pro Resource.

Neuropsychological Evaluation of the Older Adult: A Clinician's Guidebook. Joanne Green. 2000. LC 99-68194. (Illus.). xiv, 311p. 59.95 (*0-12-298190-1*) Morgan Kaufmann.

Neuropsychological Evaluation of the Spanish Speaker. A. Ardila et al. 1994. (Critical Issues in Neuropsychology Ser.). (Illus.). 216p. (C). text 37.50 (*0-306-44149-7*, Kluwer Plenum) Kluwer Academic.

Neuropsychological Explorations of Memory & Cognition: Essays in Honor of Nelson Butters. Ed. by Laird S. Cermak. 1995. LC 94-41856. (Critical Issues in Neuropsychology Ser.). 352p. 54.50 (*0-306-44983-8*, Kluwer Plenum) Kluwer Academic.

Neuropsychological Foundations of Learning Disabilities: A Handbook of Issues, Methods & Practice. John E. Obrzut. 1996. 848p. pap. text 99.00 (*0-12-524039-2*) Acad Pr.

Neuropsychological Function & Brain Imaging. Erin D. Bigler et al. 1989. (Critical Issues in Neuropsychology Ser.). (Illus.). 370p. (C). text 75.00 (*0-306-43045-2*, Kluwer Plenum) Kluwer Academic.

Neuropsychological Impairments of Short-Term Memory. Ed. by Guiseppe Vallar & Tim Shallice. 1990. (Illus.). 538p. (C). text 120.00 (*0-521-37088-4*) Cambridge U Pr.

***Neuropsychological Interventions: Clinical Research & Practice.** Maureen Downey-Lamb et al. Ed. by Paul Eslinger. 2002. 360p. 50.00 (*1-57230-744-7*) Guilford Pubns.

Neuropsychological Outcomes Research. Ed. by Rodney D. Vanderloeg. 1999. 56p. pap. (*0-8058-9810-7*) L Erlbaum Assocs.

Neuropsychological Rehabilitation. Ed. by Anne-Lise Christensen & Barbara P. Uzzell. 1988. (C). text 85.50 (*0-89838-374-9*) Kluwer Academic.

Neuropsychological Rehabilitation. Ed. by Manfred Meier et al. 1987. LC 87-154. 468p. text 57.95 (*0-89862-702-8*) Guilford Pubns.

Neuropsychological Studies in Aphasia. Aleksandr R. Luria. 1977. (Neurolinguistics Ser.: Vol. 6). 184p. (*90-265-0244-3*) Swets.

Neuropsychological Studies of Non-Focal Brain Damage. Ed. by H. A. Whitaker. 1988. (Neuropsychology Ser.). (Illus.). 308p. 189.00 (*0-387-96605-6*) Spr-Verlag.

***Neuropsychological Tests: Index of New Information & Guide-Book for Reference & Research.** Ed. by Research and Development Division Staff & John C. Bartone. 2001. 180p. 47.50 (*0-7883-2600-7*); pap. 44.50 (*0-7883-2601-5*) ABBE Pubs Assn.

Neuropsychological Theories of Lashley & Hebb. Jack Orbach. 1998. 412p. (C). 77.00 (*0-7618-1165-6*) U Pr of Amer.

Neuropsychological Toxicology: Identification & Assessment of Human Neurotoxic Syndromes. D. E. Hartman. 1988. (Illus.). 320p. 49.50 (*0-08-034944-7*, Pergamon Pr) Elsevier.

Neuropsychological Toxicology: Identification & Assessment of Human Neurotoxic Syndromes. David E. Hartman. 2nd ed. 1995. LC 87-14795. (Critical Issues in Neuropsychology Ser.). (Illus.). 548p. (C). text 71.00 (*0-306-44922-6*, Kluwer Plenum) Kluwer Academic.

Neuropsychological Treatment after Brain Injury. Anne-Lise Christensen. Ed. by David W. Ellis. 1989. (Foundations of Neuropsychology Ser.). (C). text 227.50 (*0-7923-0014-9*) Kluwer Academic.

Neuropsychological Treatments of Dyslexia. Dirk J. Bakker. 1990. (Illus.). 112p. pap. text 19.95 (*0-19-506132-2*) OUP.

Neuropsychological Validation of Learning Disability Subtypes. Ed. by Byron P. Rourke. 1990. LC 90-3912. 398p. 45.00 (*0-89862-446-0*) Guilford Pubns.

Neuropsychology. Ed. by Alan A. Boulton et al. 1990. LC 89-26859. (Neuromethods Ser.: Vol. 17). (Illus.). 381p. 139.50 (*0-89603-133-0*) Humana.

Neuropsychology. Michael S. Gazzaniga. 1979. LC 78-21459. (Handbook of Behavioral Neurobiology Ser.: Vol. 2). (Illus.). 586p. (C). text 125.00 (*0-306-35192-7*, Kluwer Plenum) Kluwer Academic.

Neuropsychology. Ed. by Gerald Goldstein et al. 1998. LC 97-42120. (Human Brain Function Ser.). (Illus.). 516p. (C). text 115.00 (*0-306-45646-X*, Kluwer Plenum) Kluwer Academic.

Neuropsychology. Kevin W. Walsh. 2nd ed. 1987. (Illus.). 429p. (*0-443-03858-9*) Church.

Neuropsychology. Ed. by Dahlia W. Zaidel. 2nd ed. 1994. LC 94-14627. (Handbook of Perception & Cognition Ser.). (Illus.). 342p. text 64.95 (*0-12-775290-0*) Acad Pr.

***Neuropsychology: From Theory to Practice.** David G. Andrewes. 2001. LC 2001-19340. (*1-84169-103-8*) Psychol Pr GBR. *Dist:* Taylor & Francis.

Neuropsychology & Cognition. Rattihalli N. Malatesha. 1987. lib. bdg. 375.00 (*90-247-2752-9*) Kluwer Academic.

Neuropsychology & Neurolinguistics. Egon Weigl. 1980. (Janua Linguarum, Series Major: No. 78). text (*90-279-7956-1*) Mouton.

Neuropsychology Casebook. D. L. Orsini et al. 1988. (Illus.). 270p. 93.00 (*0-387-96681-1*) Spr-Verlag.

Neuropsychology for Clinical Practice: Etiology, Assessment, & Treatment of Common Neurological Disorders. Ed. by Russell L. Adams et al. 1996. LC 95-49944. (APA Clinical Psychology Bks.). 546p. 69.95 (*1-55798-298-8*, 431-7540) Am Psychol.

Neuropsychology for Lawyers & Health Science Professionals. Robert J. Sbordone & Ronald E. Saul. 2nd ed. 2000. LC 00-23929. (Illus.). 489p. 99.95 (*0-8493-0204-8*) CRC Pr.

Neuropsychology for Occupational Therapists: Assessment of Perception & Cognition. June Grieve. 1993. LC 93-19447. 176p. pap. 29.95 (*0-632-03303-7*) Blackwell Sci.

Neuropsychology for the Attorney. Robert J. Sbordone. 2nd ed. 1996. 350p. lib. bdg. 89.95 (*1-57444-131-0*); 1995. LC 91-70189. (Illus.). 392p. lib. bdg. 95.00 (*1-878205-26-9*) St Lucie Pr.

Neuropsychology, Neuropsychiatry & Behavioral Neurology. R. Joseph. 1990. LC 89-16319. (Critical Issues in Neuropsychology Ser.). (Illus.). 412p. (C). text 54.50 (*0-306-43136-X*, Kluwer Plenum) Kluwer Academic.

Neuropsychology of Aggression. Ed. by Joel S. Milner. 1991. 208p. (C). text 147.50 (*0-7923-1245-7*) Kluwer Academic.

Neuropsychology of Aging. Diana S. Woodruff-Pak. 1997. (Understanding Aging Ser.). (Illus.). 352p. (C). 86.95 (*1-55786-454-3*); LC 96-37330. pap. 40.95 (*1-55786-455-1*) Blackwell Pubs.

Neuropsychology of Alcoholism: Implications for Diagnosis & Treatment. Ed. by Oscar A. Parsons et al. 1987. LC 86-29583. 414p. 55.00 (*0-89862-696-X*) Guilford Pubns.

Neuropsychology of Alzheimer's Disease & Other Dementias. Ed. by Randolph W. Parks et al. 1993. LC 92-49274. (Illus.). 698p. text 79.00 (*0-19-506612-X*) OUP.

Neuropsychology of Anxiety: An Inquiry into the Functions of the Septo-Hippocampal System. Jeffrey A. Gray & Neil McNaughton. 2nd ed. 2000. LC 2001-280232. (Oxford Psychology Ser.: No. 33). (Illus.). 560p. text 95.00 (*0-19-852270-3*) OUP.

Neuropsychology of Attention. R. A. Cohen. 1993. (Critical Issues in Neuropsychology Ser.). (Illus.). 566p. (C). text 85.00 (*0-306-43953-0*, Kluwer Plenum) Kluwer Academic.

Neuropsychology of Cardiovascular Disease. Ed. by Shari R. Waldstein & Merrill F. Elias. 2000. LC 00-42246. 304p. 55.00 (*0-8058-3103-7*) L Erlbaum Assocs.

***Neuropsychology of Childhood Epilepsy.** Ed. by Isabelle Jambaque et al. 2001. LC 2001-23703. (Advances in Behavioral Biology Ser.: Vol. 50). (Illus.). 286p. 95.00 (*0-306-46522-1*, Kluwer Plenum) Kluwer Academic.

Neuropsychology of Degenerative Brain Diseases. Robert G. Knight. 1992. 360p. text 69.95 (*0-8058-0927-9*) L Erlbaum Assocs.

Neuropsychology of Developmental Stuttering. Bernard-Thomas Hartman & Stephen F. Austin. 1994. LC 94-143. 158p. (C). pap. text 34.95 (*1-56593-384-2*, 0763) Thomson Learn.

Neuropsychology of Dreams. Mark Solms. 1996. LC 96-21693. (Institute for Research in Behavioral Neuroscience Ser.). 304p. 69.95 (*0-8058-1585-6*) L Erlbaum Assocs.

Neuropsychology of Emotion. Joan C. Borod. 2000. LC 99-45300. (Series in Affective Science). (Illus.). 536p. text 69.50 (*0-19-511464-7*) OUP.

Neuropsychology of Epilepsy. T. L. Bennett. 1992. (Critical Issues in Neuropsychology Ser.). (Illus.). 336p. (C). text 54.50 (*0-306-43948-4*, Kluwer Plenum) Kluwer Academic.

Neuropsychology of Everyday Life: Assessment & Basic Competencies. Ed. by David E. Tupper & Keith D. Cicerone. 1990. (C). lib. bdg. 132.50 (*0-7923-0671-6*) Kluwer Academic.

Neuropsychology of Everyday Life: Issues in Development & Rehabilitation. Ed. by David E. Tupper & Keith D. Cicerone. 1990. (C). lib. bdg. 132.50 (*0-7923-0847-6*) Kluwer Academic.

Neuropsychology of Eye Movement. Ed. by C. W. Johnston & F. Priozzolo. 1988. (Harry Whitaker's Neuropsychology & Neurolinguistics Ser.). 296p. (C). text 59.95 (*0-89859-796-X*) L Erlbaum Assocs.

Neuropsychology of Face Perception & Facial Expression. Raymond Bruyer. 1986. 344p. (C). text 89.95 (*0-89859-602-5*) L Erlbaum Assocs.

Neuropsychology of HIV Infection. Igor Grant & Alex Martin. 1994. LC 93-26567. (Illus.). 402p. (C). text 65.00 (*0-19-507225-1*) OUP.

Neuropsychology of Individual Differences. Ed. by Philip A. Vernon. 1994. LC 94-7647. (Illus.). 272p. text 59.95 (*0-12-718670-0*) Acad Pr.

Neuropsychology of Individual Differences: A Developmental Perspective. Ed. by Lawrence C. Hartlage & Cathy F. Telzrow. 1985. (Perspectives on Individual Differences Ser.). (Illus.). 346p. (C). 84.00 (*0-306-41986-6*, Plenum Trade) Perseus Pubng.

Neuropsychology of Learning Disabilities: Essentials of Subtype Analysis. Ed. by Byron P. Rourke. 1985. LC 84-10860. 351p. 45.00 (*0-89862-644-7*, 2644) Guilford Pubns.

Neuropsychology of Memory. Ed. by Larry R. Squire & Nelson Butters. 2nd ed. 620p. reprint ed. 1993. pap. 42.00 (*0-89862-158-5*, 2158); 1992. 69.95 (*0-89862-881-4*) Guilford Pubns.

Neuropsychology of Mental Disorders: A Practical Guide. Leonard F. Koziol & Chris E. Stout. 1994. LC 94-2876. (Illus.). 338p. (C). text 73.95 (*0-398-05905-5*) C C Thomas.

Neuropsychology of Mental Imagery. Ed. by M. Behrmann et al. 1995. 258p. pap. 63.00 (*0-08-042733-2*, Pergamon Pr) Elsevier.

Neuropsychology of Perinatal Complications. Ed. by Jeffrey W. Gray & Raymond S. Dean. 1990. 256p. 39.95 (*0-8261-5890-0*) Springer Pub.

Neuropsychology of Visual Perception. Ed. by Jason W. Brown. 1989. (Institute for Research in Behavioral Neuroscience Ser.). 280p. 59.95 (*0-8058-0284-3*) L Erlbaum Assocs.

Neuropsychopharmacology: Proceedings of the XVIth C. I. N. P. Congress, Munich, August, 15-19 1988. Set. Ed. by William E. Bunney, Jr. et al. 1990. (Illus.). 845p. 368.00 (*0-387-50252-1*) Spr-Verlag.

Neuropsychopharmacology of the Trace Amines: Experimental & Clinical Aspects. Ed. by Alan A. Boulton et al. 1986. LC 85-24904. 510p. 145.00 (*0-89603-099-7*) Humana.

Neuropsychotherapy Community Integration: Brain Illness, Emotions & Behavior. Tedd Judd. 1999. LC 99-33665. (Critical Issues in Neuropsychology Ser.). 372p. 79.95 (*0-306-46170-6*, Kluwer Plenum) Kluwer Academic.

Neuropsychotic Manifestations of Systematic Lupus Erythematosus. Patricia M. Moore. 1999. (Annals of the New York Academy of Sciences Ser.). 350p. pap. text 22.50 (*0-8018-6216-7*) Johns Hopkins.

Neuroradiology. Ruth G. Ramsey. 3rd ed. 1994. LC 93-26474. (Illus.). 1056p. text 175.00 (*0-7216-3657-8*) Saunders.

Neuroradiology: A Pattern Approach. J. Randy Jinkins. 1997. LC 97-6721. 1,200p. text 249.00 (*0-397-51494-8*) Lppncott W & W.

Neuroradiology: Applications in Neurology & Neurosurgery. Ed. by Stanley Van den Noort & Elliot M. Frohman. 1988. LC 82-642121. 204p. pap. 24.00 (*0-930195-03-5*) Inst Mind Behavior.

Neuroradiology—The Requisites. Robert I. Gorssman & David M. Yousem. 1994. LC 94-229702. (Illus.). 562p. (C). (gr. 13). text 89.00 (*0-8016-6492-6*, 06492) Mosby Inc.

Neuroradiology & Head & Neck Imaging. Ed. by Jesus Rodriguez-Carbajal. 1998. LC 99-19267. (Illus.). xvi, 583p. pap. text 80.00 (*0-7817-1447-8*) Lppncott W & W.

Neuroradiology Companion: Methods, Guidelines & Imaging Fundamentals. Mauricio Castillo. 2nd ed. 1998. LC 98-26851. 384p. pap. text 65.00 (*0-7817-1695-0*) Lppncott W & W.

Neuroradiology Test & Syllabus, Vol. 28. Peter E. Weinberg et al. 1990. (Professional Self-Evaluation & Continuing Education Program Ser.). (Illus.). 1050p. 330.00 (*1-55903-028-3*) Am Coll Radiology.

Neuroradiology Test & Syllabus Second Series: Test & Syllabus, Vol. 42, Series 2. Eric J. Russell et al. 1998. LC 98-3648. (Professional Self-Evaluation Program Ser.: Vol. 42). (Illus.). 600p. 220.00 (*1-55903-042-9*) Am Coll Radiology.

Neuroreceptor Mechanisms in the Brain. Ed. by S. Kito et al. 1991. (Advances in Experimental Medicine & Biology Ser.: Vol. 287). (Illus.). 510p. (C). text 174.00 (*0-306-43821-6*, Kluwer Plenum) Kluwer Academic.

Neuroreceptors. Ed. by Ferdinand Hucho. 1982. (Illus.). 367p. 123.10 (*3-11-008855-X*) De Gruyter.

Neuroreceptors in Health & Disease. Ed. by J. Marwaha & W. J. Anderson. 1984. (Monographs in Neural Sciences: Vol. 10). (Illus.). viii, 256p. 129.75 (*3-8055-3715-8*) S Karger.

Neuroregulation of Autonomic, Endocrine & Immune Systems. Ed. by R. Frederickson et al. 1986. (Topics in the Neurosciences Ser.). text 208.00 (*0-89838-800-7*) Kluwer Academic.

Neuroregulatory Mechanisms in Aging. Ed. by Maynard H. Makman & George B. Stefano. 1993. LC 93-21169. (Studies in Neurosciences). 212p. 180.00 (*0-08-041989-5*, Pergamon Pr) Elsevier.

Neurorehabilitation. Namerow. Date not set. text (*0-7216-5646-3*) Saunders.

Neurorehabilitation: A Multisensory Approach. Shereen D. Farber. 1982. (Illus.). 282p. pap. text 47.00 (*0-7216-3571-7*) Saunders.

Neuroscience. Ed. by Philip H. Abelson et al. 1986. LC 84-24524. (Illus.). 516p. (C). 54.50 (*0-87168-309-1*, 84-13S) AAAS.

Neuroscience. Lundy. 1998. LC 97-50316. (C). text 49.95 (*0-7216-4717-0*) Saunders.

Neuroscience. Dale Purves et al. 2nd ed. 2000. LC 00-59496. (Illus.). xviii, 681p. (*0-87893-742-0*) Sinauer Assocs.

Neuroscience: Exploring the Brain. Mark F. Bear et al. 2nd ed. 2001. LC 00-46513. (Illus.). 888p. text 62.95 (*0-683-30596-4*) Lppncott W & W.

***Neuroscience: Focus on Acute & Chronic Pain.** Ed. by Mario Tiengo. 2001. LC 00-54932. (Topics in Anaesthesia & Critical Care Ser.). (Illus.). xii, 120p. (C). pap. (*88-470-0134-X*) Spr-Verlag ITA. *Dist:* Spr-Verlag.

Neuroscience: From Neural Networks to Artificial Intelligence - Proceedings of a U. S.-Mexico Seminar Held in the City of Xalapa in the State of Veracruz in December 9-11, 1991. Ed. by Pablo Rudomin et al. 1993. LC 93-18575. (Research Notes in Neural Computing Ser.: Vol. 4). 579p. 79.95 (*0-387-56501-9*) Spr-Verlag.

Neuroscience: From the Molecular to the Cognitive. Ed. by Floyd E. Bloom. 1994. LC 94-12298. (Progress in Brain Research Ser.: Vol. 100). 300p. 242.00 (*0-444-81678-X*) Elsevier.

***Neuroscience: Self-Assessment & Review.** Allan Siegel. 4th ed. 2001. (Pretest Self-Assessment & Review Ser.). (Illus.). 300p. pap. 24.95 (*0-07-137350-0*) McGraw-Hill Prof.

Neuroscience & Behavior: An Introduction. Ed. by D. M. Atrens & J. S. Curthoys. 2nd ed. 1982. 214p. text 55.00 (*0-12-066850-5*) Acad Pr.

M
N
O

Neuroscience & Connectionist Theory. Ed. by Mark A. Gluck & David E. Rumelhart. 1990. (Developments in Connectionist Theory Ser.). 424p. 125.00 (*0-8058-0504-4*); pap. 65.00 (*0-8058-0619-9*) L Erlbaum Assocs.

Neuroscience Approached Through Cell Culture. Steven E. Pfeiffer. Vol. I. 1982. 256p. 140.00 (*0-8493-6340-3*, QP356); Vol. II. 1983. 192p. 114.00 (*0-8493-6341-1*, QP356) Franklin (CRC Reprint).

Neuroscience at a Glance. Roger A. Barker & Stephen Barasi. 1999. LC 98-22073. (At a Glance Ser.). (Illus.). 128p. pap. 22.95 (*0-86542-869-7*); (*0-86542-872-7*) Blackwell Sci.

Neuroscience Critical Care: Pathophysiology & Patient Management. Marshall et al. 1990. (Illus.). 464p. text 89.00 (*0-7216-2790-0*) Saunders.

Neuroscience for Rehabilitation. Helen Cohen. 2nd ed. 1998. LC 98-24809. (Illus.). 544p. text 46.95 (*0-397-55465-6*) Lppncott W & W.

Neuroscience for the Study of Communicative Disorders. Subhash C. Bhatnagar & Orlando J. Andy. 1995. LC 94-19356. (Illus.). 521p. pap. text 47.95 (*0-683-00740-8*) Lppncott W & W.

Neuroscience in Medicine. P. Michael Conn. 1994. (Illus.). 688p. text 42.50 (*0-397-51279-1*) Lppncott W & W.

Neuroscience Labfax. Ed. by Marina A. Lynch & Shane M. O'Mara. 1997. LC 96-47962. (Labfax Ser.). (Illus.). 288p. text 59.95 (*0-12-460490-0*) Morgan Kaufmann.

Neuroscience, Memory, & Language: Papers Presented at a Symposium Series Cosponsored by the National Institute of Mental Health & the Library of Congress. Ed. by Richard D. Broadwell. 1995. LC 94-37346. (Decade of the Brain Ser.: Vol. 1). 1p. pap. (*0-8444-0847-6*); (Illus.). 160p. 33.00 (*0-8444-0815-8*) Lib Congress.

Neuroscience Nursing. Ellen Barker. 1994. (Illus.). 848p. (C). (gr. 13). text 61.95 (*0-8016-6470-5*, 06470) Mosby Inc.

Neuroscience of Animal Intelligence: From the Seahare to the Seahorse. E. M. Macphail. Ed. by Herbert S. Terrace. 1993. LC 92-31167. (Animal Intelligence Ser.). (Illus.). 506p. (C). text 75.50 (*0-231-06144-7*) Col U Pr.

Neuroscience of Communication. Donald B. Webster. 1995. (Singular Textbook Ser.). (Illus.). 326p. (Orig.). (C). pap. 38.95 (*1-56593-114-9*, 0417) Thomson Learn.

Neuroscience of Communication. Douglas B. Webster. 2nd rev. ed. 1998. LC 98-24475. 379p. pap. text 60.95 (*1-56593-985-9*, 1950) Thomson Learn.

Neuroscience of Human Movement: A Primer. Charles T. Leonard. 1997. LC 98-221239. (Illus.). 272p. (gr. 13). pap. text 25.00 (*0-8151-5371-6*, 26560) Mosby Inc.

Neuroscience of Mental Health: A Report on Neuroscience Research. Ed. by Stephen H. Koslow. 1997. (Illus.). 182p. (C). reprint ed. pap. text 45.00 (*0-7881-4694-7*) DIANE Pub.

Neuroscience of the Mind on the Centennial of Freud's "Project for a Scientific Psychology" On the Centennial of Freud's Project for a Scientific Psychology. Ed. by Robert M. Bilder & F. Frank LeFever. 1998. LC 98-13652. (Annals of the New York Academy of Sciences Ser.: Vol. 843). 80.00 (*1-57331-062-X*) NY Acad Sci.

Neuroscience Protocols. Ed. by Floris G. Wouterlood. 1993. LC 93-29391. 314p. ring bd. 342.50 (*0-444-89539-6*) Elsevier.

Neuroscience Protocols, Module 6. Floris G. Wouterlood. 1995. 122p. ring bd. 130.00 (*0-444-82342-5*) Elsevier.

Neuroscience Protocols. Ed. by Floris G. Wouterlood. 1996. Module 7. 250p. ring bd. 133.00 (*0-444-82466-9*); Module 8. 156p. ring bd. 118.00 (*0-444-82512-6*) Elsevier.

Neuroscience Year: Encyclopedia of Neuroscience, Supplement 2. Ed. by Barry Smith & George Adelman. 1991. (Illus.). xiii, 158p. 87.50 (*0-8176-3507-6*) Birkhauser.

Neuroscience Year: Supplement 1 to the Encyclopedia of Neuroscience. George Adelman. 1989. 200p. 87.50 (*0-8176-3383-9*) Birkhauser.

Neurosciences: 2nd Study Program. Ed. by F. O. Schmit. 1970. (Illus.). 1069p. 60.00 (*0-87470-014-0*) Rockefeller.

Neurosciences: 4th Study Program. Ed. by Francis O. Schmitt & Frederic G. Worden. 1979. 1201p. 105.00 (*0-262-19162-8*) MIT Pr.

Neurosciences: Paths of Discovery II. Ed. by F. E. Samson. 1992. (Illus.). xvi, 352p. 97.00 (*0-8176-3503-3*) Birkhauser.

Neurosciences: The Basics. Brian A. Curtis. 1990. LC 90-5577. 172p. text 26.00 (*0-8121-1309-8*) Lppncott W & W.

Neuroscientific Principles of Swallowing & Dysphagia. Arthur J. Miller. 1998. LC 98-8532. (Illus.). 300p. pap. 69.95 (*1-56593-859-3*, 1678) Thomson Learn.

***Neuroscientist's Guide to Classical Conditioning.** Ed. by J. W. Moore. 2001. (Illus.). 304p. 110.00 (*0-387-98787-8*) Spr-Verlag.

Neurosen - Mythen, Modelle, Fakten: Ein Beitrag zur Genese Neurotischer Stoerungen. H. G. Zapotoczky. Ed. by P. Berner. 1976. (Bibliotheca Psychiatrica Ser.: No. 153). (Illus.). 180p. 38.50 (*3-8055-2310-6*) S Karger.

Neuroses & Character Types: Clinical Psychoanalytic Studies. Helene Deutsch. 1965. LC 65-15288. xii, 388p. (Orig.). 57.50 (*0-8236-3560-0*) Intl Univs Pr.

Neurosis & Human Growth: The Struggle Toward Self-Realization. Karen Horney. 1991. 391p. pap. 16.95 (*0-393-30775-1*) Norton.

Neurosonography of the Pre-Term Neonate. Ed. by E. G. Grant. 1986. (Illus.). 116p. 104.00 (*0-387-96219-0*) Spr-Verlag.

Neurosonology. Ed. by Charles H. Tegeler et al. 1995. LC 95-32584. (Illus.). 528p. (C). (gr. 13). text 169.00 (*0-8151-8792-0*, 24076) Mosby Inc.

Neurospeak: Transforms Your Body While You Read. Robert Masters. 1994. 124p. pap. 14.00 (*0-8356-0707-0*, Quest) Theos Pub Hse.

Neurospsychological Assessment & Intervention with Children & Adolescents. Lawrence C. Hartlage & Cathy F. Telzrow. 1986. LC 86-70324. 192p. (C). pap. 26.45 (*0-943158-15-X*, NABP, Prof Resc Pr) Pro Resource.

Neurosteroids: A New Regulatory Function in the Nervous System. Ed. by Etienne-Emile Baulieu et al. 1999. LC 99-10461. (Contemporary Endocrinology Ser.: Vol. 16). (Illus.). 396p. 145.00 (*0-89603-545-X*) Humana.

Neurosurgeon's Notebook. Chris Adams. 1998. (Illus.). 19p. pap. 48.95 (*0-632-05154-X*) Blackwell Sci.

Neurosurgery. Alan Crockard et al. 3rd rev. ed. 2000. LC 99-28832. (Illus.). 1301p. 619.95 (*0-632-04838-7*) Blackwell Sci.

Neurosurgery, Set. 2nd ed. Ed. by Robert H. Wilkins & Setti S. Rengachary. Incl. text (*0-07-070313-2*); text (*0-07-070314-0*); text (*0-07-070315-9*); (C). LC 95-35870. (Illus.). 4272p. 1995. Set text 595.00 (*0-07-079991-1*) McGraw-Hill Prof.

Neurosurgery: An Introductory Text. Peter M. Black & Eugene Rossitch. 1995. (Illus.). 248p. text 49.95 (*0-19-504448-7*); pap. text 24.95 (*0-19-504449-5*) OUP.

Neurosurgery & Medical Ethics. Ed. by H. August van Alphen. 1999. LC 99-33462. (Acta Neurochirurgica Ser.: Vol. 74). (Illus.). 120p. 75.00 (*3-211-83348-X*) Spr-Verlag.

Neurosurgery Board Review: Questions & Answers for Self-Assessment. Cargill H. Alleyne, Jr. & Daniel L. Barrow. 2nd ed. 1997. LC 96-29700. (Illus.). 254p. pap. 39.95 (*0-86577-706-3*) Thieme Med Pubs.

Neurosurgery for Spasticity: A Multidisciplinary Approach. Ed. by M. P. Sindou et al. 1991. (Illus.). 219p. 174.00 (*0-387-82225-9*) Spr-Verlag.

Neurosurgery of Complex Tumors & Vascular Lesions. Ed. by S. Kobayashi et al. 1996. (Illus.). 480p. (*0-443-07870-X*) Church.

Neurosurgery, Ophthalmic Surgery, ENT. Ed. by Gunther O. Schlag et al. 1994. LC 94-27186. (Fibrin Sealing in Surgical & Nonsurgical Fields Ser.: Vol. 5). 231p. 74.95 (*0-387-58014-X*) Spr-Verlag.

Neurosurgical & Medical Management of Pain: Trigeminal Neuralgia, Chronic Pain & Cancer Pain. Ed. by Ronald Brisman. 1989. (C). text 145.00 (*0-89838-405-2*) Kluwer Academic.

Neurosurgical Applications of Transcranial Doppler Sonography. A. Harders. 1986. (Illus.). 10p. 47.95 (*0-387-81938-X*) Spr-Verlag.

Neurosurgical Aspects of Epilepsy: Proceedings of the 4th Advanced Seminar in Neurosurgical Research of the European Association of Neurosurgical Societies, May 17-18, 1989, Bressco die Teolo, Padova, Italy. Ed. by J. D. Pickard et al. 1990. (Acta Neurochirurgica Ser.: No. 50). (Illus.). viii, 144p. 128.00 (*0-387-82227-5*) Spr-Verlag.

Neurosurgical Classics II. Ed. by Robert H. Wilkins & Gloria K. Wilkins. 2000. 592p. 85.00 (*1-879284-74-X*) Am Assn Neuro.

Neurosurgical Intensive Care. Ed. by Brian T. Andrews. 1993. LC 92-49880. (Illus.). 450p. text 79.00 (*0-07-001849-9*) McGraw-Hill Educ Grp.

Neurosurgical Issues in Otolaryngology: Principles & Practice of Collaboration. Contrib. by Moises A. Arriaga & J. Diaz Day. 1999. LC 99-23052. 416p. text 149.00 (*0-7817-1579-2*) Lppncott W & W.

Neurosurgical Management of Pain. Ed. by Robert M. Levy & Richard B. North. 1996. LC 95-23662. (Illus.). 379p. 192.00 (*0-387-94256-4*) Spr-Verlag.

Neurosurgical Operative Atlas. Ed. by Setti S. Rengachary & Robert H. Wilkins. Vol. 4. 1995. (Illus.). 257p. ring bd. 165.00 (*1-879284-39-1*); Vol. 5. 1996. (Illus.). 250p. ring bd. 165.00 (*1-879284-41-3*); Vol. 6. 1997. 277p. 165.00 (*1-879284-50-2*) Am Assn Neuro.

Neurosurgical Operative Atlas, Vols. 1-9. American Association of Neurological Surgeons Staff. 1500p. 1237.50 (*0-683-07234-X*) Am Assn Neuro.

***Neurosurgical Pain Management.** Kenneth A. Follett. 2001. (Illus.). 500p. (*0-7216-9241-9*) Saunders.

Neurosurgical Review. Christopher D. Sturm & Thomas R. Forget. 1998. LC 98-46841. 323p. 30.00 (*1-57626-115-8*) Quality Med Pub.

Neurosurgical Review Vol. 12, Supplement 1: Advances in Neurotraumatology. Ed. by R. A. Frowein et al. 1989. 619p. (C). pap. text 152.35 (*3-11-011240-X*) De Gruyter.

Neurosurgical Standards, Cerebral Aneurysms, Malignant Gliomas. Ed. by K. Piscol et al. 1992. (Advances in Neurosurgery Ser.: Vol. 20). (Illus.). 401p. pap. 79.00 (*0-387-54838-6*) Spr-Verlag.

Neurosurgical Treatment of Chronic Pain: Physiologica & Pathologic Mechanisms of Human Pain. J. M. Gybels & W. H. Sweet. 1989. (Pain & Headache Ser.: Vol. 11). (Illus.). xvi, 444p. 168.75 (*3-8055-4885-0*) S Karger.

Neurosyphilis: Modern Systematic Diagnosis & Treatment Preserved in One Hundred & Thirty-Seven Case Histories. Elmer E. Southard & Harry C. Solomon. 1973. LC 73-2418. (Mental Illness & Social Policy; the American Experience Ser.). reprint ed. 37.95 (*0-405-05228-6*) Ayer.

Neurotherapeutics: Emerging Strategies. Ed. by Linda M. Pullan & Jitendra Patel. 1995. LC 95-381027. (Contemporary Neuroscience Ser.). (Illus.). 444p. 145.00 (*0-89603-306-6*) Humana.

Neurotic & Psychotic Language Behavior. Ed. by Ruth Wodak & Pete Van de Craen. 1987. 525p. pap. (*0-905028-76-7*); 630p. text (*0-905028-77-5*) Multilingual Matters GBR. *Dist:* Taylor & Francis.

Neurotic Child & Adolescent. Ed. by M. Hossein Etezady. 1990. LC 89-18246. 440p. 65.00 (*0-87668-808-3*) Aronson.

Neurotic Constitution. Alfred Adler. 1980. LC 74-39684. (Select Bibliographies Reprint Ser.). reprint ed. 34.95 (*0-8369-9925-8*) Ayer.

Neurotic Disorders in the Elderly. Ed. by James Lindesay. 1995. (Illus.). 260p. (C). text 79.50 (*0-19-262396-6*) OUP.

Neurotic Personality of Our Time. Karen Horney. 1994. 256p. pap. 12.95 (*0-393-31097-3*) Norton.

Neurotic Styles. David Shapiro. 1999. pap. 22.00 (*0-465-09502-X*, TB5003) Basic.

Neurotic's Handbook. Robert L. McKinley. 1977. 131p. (C). pap. 10.00 (*0-9609644-0-1*) Candle Bks.

Neurotoxic Factors in Parkinson's Disease & Related Disorders. Ed. by Michael Storch & Michael A. Collins. 2001. LC 00-52731. (Illus.). 280p. 120.00 (*0-306-46529-9*, Kluwer Plenum) Kluwer Academic.

Neurotoxic Side Effects of Prescription Drugs. John C. Brust. 1996. LC 96-23662. 435p. pap. text 49.99 (*0-7506-9663-X*) Buttrwrth-Heinemann.

Neurotoxicity: Identifying & Controlling Poisons of the Nervous System. 1992. lib. bdg. 186.96 (*0-8490-8790-2*) Gordon Pr.

Neurotoxicity: Identifying & Controlling Poisons of the Nervous System. U. S. Congress, Office of Technology Assessment Staff. 1992. (Illus.). 384p. (C). (gr. 13). text 64.95 (*0-442-01047-8*) Chapman & Hall.

Neurotoxicology. M. B. Abou-Donia. 1989. 444p. text 107.00 (*2-88124-406-8*) Gordon & Breach.

Neurotoxicology. Mohammed B. Abou-Donia. 1992. 640p. lib. bdg. 149.00 (*0-8493-8895-3*, RC347) CRC Pr.

Neurotoxicology. Blum & Manzo. 1985. (Drug & Chemical Toxicology Ser.: Vol. 3). (Illus.). 704p. text 255.00 (*0-8247-7283-0*) Dekker.

Neurotoxicology. Hugh A. Tilson. 2nd ed. 1999. LC 98-48639. (Target Organ Toxicology Ser.). (Illus.). xiv, 386p. 140.00 (*1-56032-720-0*) Taylor & Francis.

Neurotoxicology: A Clinical Source Book. Peter G. Bernad. 1998. LC 98-85162. text 105.00 (*0-327-00132-1*, 66067-10) LEXIS Pub.

Neurotoxicology: A Clinical Sourcebook, 1999 Supplement. Peter G. Bernad. 1999. 72p. (*0-327-01487-3*, 6606610) LEXIS Pub.

Neurotoxicology: Approaches & Methods. Ed. by Louis W. Chang & William Slikker. 1995. LC 94-40509. (Illus.). 851p. text 149.95 (*0-12-168055-X*) Acad Pr.

Neurotoxicology Handbook. Ed. by Edward J. Massaro. 2001. LC 2001-39605. 672p. 175.00 (*0-89603-795-9*) Humana.

***Neurotoxins: Index of New Information & Research Reference Bible.** Ed. by Research and Development Division Staff & John C. Bartone. 2001. 180p. 47.50 (*0-7883-2452-7*); pap. 44.50 (*0-7883-2453-5*) ABBE Pubs Assn.

Neurotransmission & Hearing Loss: Basic Science, Diagnosis & Management. Charles I. Berlin. 1997. LC 97-937. (Illus.). 184p. (Orig.). 55.00 (*1-56593-834-8*, 1630) Thomson Learn.

Neurotransmitter Actions & Interactions: Proceedings of a Satellite Symposium of the 12th International Society for Neurochemistry Meeting, Algarve, Portugal, April 29-30, 1989. Ed. by M. B. Youdim & Keith F. Tipton. 1990. (Journals of Neural Transmission: Suppl. 29). (Illus.). 292p. 192.00 (*0-387-82142-2*) Spr-Verlag.

Neurotransmitter Actions in the Vertebrate Nervous System. Ed. by Michael A. Rogawski & Jeffrey L. Barker. 1985. 536p. 125.00 (*0-306-41991-2*, Plenum Trade) Perseus Pubng.

Neurotransmitter & Dementia. Ed. by C. G. Gottfries & Joyce Nakamura. 1990. (Journals of Neural Transmission: Suppl. 30). 120p. 56.95 (*0-387-82190-2*) Spr-Verlag.

Neurotransmitter Balances Regulating Behavior. Ed. by E. F. Domino & J. M. Davis. 1975. LC 75-21131. (Illus.). 240p. 30.00 (*0-916182-00-2*) NPP Bks.

Neurotransmitter Interactions & Cognitive Function. Ed. by Edward D. Levin et al. 1992. LC 92-17848. xiv, 362p. 132.00 (*0-8176-3617-X*) Birkhauser.

Neurotransmitter Receptors Ed. by Sam J. Enna & H. D. Yamamura. 1980. (Receptors & Recognition Series B: Vols. 9 & 10). Pt. 1: Amino Acids, Peptides & Benzodiazepines. 49.95 (*0-412-16250-4*, NO. 6399); Set. 105.00 (*0-412-23130-1*, NO. 2178) Chapman & Hall.

Neurotransmitter Receptors in Actions of Antipsychotic Medications. Michael S. Lidow. 2000. LC 00-25387. (Pharmacology & Toxicology Ser.). (Illus.). 272p. 99.95 (*0-8493-0744-9*) CRC Pr.

Neurotransmitter Release & Its Modulation: Biochemical Mechanisms, Physiological Function & Clinical Relevance. Ed. by David A. Powis & Stephen J. Bunn. 1995. (Illus.). 374p. (C). text 90.00 (*0-521-44068-8*); pap. text 32.95 (*0-521-44616-3*) Cambridge U Pr.

Neurotransmitter Release & Uptake. Sakire Pogun. 1997. LC 97-4076. (NATO ASI Ser.). (Illus.). 344p. 157.00 (*3-540-62479-1*) Spr-Verlag.

Neurotransmitter Revolution: Serotonin, Social Behavior, & the Law. Michael T. McGuire. Ed. by Roger D. Masters. 1993. LC 92-49968. 272p. (C). 41.95 (*0-8093-1792-3*); pap. 21.95 (*0-8093-1801-6*) S Ill U Pr.

Neurotransmitters & Drugs. Z. L. Kruk & C. J. Pycock. 3rd ed. 1991. (Illus.). 208p. (gr. 13). pap. 148.95 (*0-412-36100-0*, A5559); (C). pap. text 52.95 (*0-412-36110-8*, A5563) Chapman & Hall.

Neurotransmitters & Pain Control. Ed. by H. Akil & J. W. Lewis. 1987. (Pain & Headache Ser.: Vol. 9). (Illus.). x, 306p. 128.00 (*3-8055-4579-7*) S Karger.

Neurotransmitters in Embryogenesis. G. A. Buznikov. 1990. (Soviet Scientific Reviews Supplement Ser., Physicochemical Biology). 424p. pap. text 462.00 (*3-7186-4877-6*) Gordon & Breach.

Neurotransmitters in Epilepsy. R. Fariello & G. Avanzini. Ed. by Jerome Engel, Jr. et al. 1992. LC 92-18549. (Epilepsy Research Ser.: No. 8). xvi,408p. 216.50 (*0-444-89710-0*) Elsevier.

Neurotransmitters in Neuronal Plasticity & Psychiatric Disorders: Proceedings of the 10th Workshop on Neurotransmitters & Diseases, Tokyo, Japan, 5 June, 1993. Ed. by M. Toru. 1994. (International Congress Ser.: Vol. 1061). 112p. 136.50 (*0-444-81806-5*, Excerpta Medica) Elsevier.

Neurotransmitters in the Human Brain: Proceedings of a Conference in Honor of Istyan Tork Held in New South Wales, Sydney, February 5, 1994. Ed. by George T. Paxinos et al. 1995. (Advances in Behavioral Biology Ser.: Vol. 43). (Illus.). 254p. (C). text 85.00 (*0-306-44915-3*, Kluwer Plenum) Kluwer Academic.

Neurotransmitters, Receptors, & Drug Action. Ed. by Walter B. Essman. 1980. LC 79-23862. (Illus.). 220p. text 39.50 (*0-88331-166-6*) R B Luce.

Neurotrauma. Ed. by Raj K. Narayan et al. 1996. LC 95-40277. (Illus.). 1600p. text 275.00 (*0-07-045662-3*) McGraw-Hill Prof.

Neurotrophic Factors. Ed. by Alan A. Boulton et al. 1993. (Neuromethods Ser.: Vol. 25). (Illus.). 440p. 140.00 (*0-89603-249-3*) Humana.

Neurotrophic Factors. Ed. by Sandra E. Loughlin & James H. Fallon. 1992. LC 92-11683. (Illus.). 607p. text 104.00 (*0-12-455830-5*) Acad Pr.

Neurotrophic Factors. Ed. by Yasuzo Tsukada & Eric Shooter. 1993. (Taniguchi Symposia on Brain Sciences Ser.: No. 15). 99.95 (*0-8493-7755-2*, QP552) CRC Pr.

***Neurotrophic Factors & Their Receptors in the Developing Avian Retina & Its Tectal Target.** Miriam Karlsson. 2001. (Illus.). 79p. pap. (*91-554-5062-8*) Uppsala Universitet SWE. *Dist:* Coronet Bks.

Neurovasc Immun: Vasoactive Neurotrans & Modul-Cell Immun. Thomas C. Moore. 1992. 480p. 199.00 (*0-8493-6894-4*, QP356) CRC Pr.

Neurovascular Compression of the Cranial Nerves in Neurological & Systemic Disease. Ed. by Peter J. Hamlyn. 1999. LC 98-47916. 292p. 177.50 (*0-444-82977-6*) Elsevier.

Neurovascular Neuro-Ophthalmology. M. J. Kupersmith & A. Berenstein. 1992. LC 92-49714. (Illus.). 554p. 330.00 (*0-387-55636-2*) Spr-Verlag.

Neurovascular Surgery: Specialized Neurosurgical Techniques. Ed. by F. Marguth et al. 1979. (Advances in Neurosurgery Ser.: Vol. 7). (Illus.). 394p. 63.95 (*0-387-09675-2*) Spr-Verlag.

Neurypnology. James Braid. 1976. LC 75-16688. (Classics in Psychiatry Ser.). reprint ed. 25.95 (*0-405-07418-2*) Ayer.

Neutral Proteases of Mast Cells. Ed. by L. B. Schwartz. 1990. (Monographs in Allergy: Vol. 27). viii, 166p. 148.00 (*3-8055-5162-2*) S Karger.

Neutral Transplantation & Regeneration. Ed. by R. B. Wallace & G. D. Das. 1985. (Proceedings in Life Sciences Ser.). (Illus.). 330p. 312.00 (*0-387-96160-7*) Spr-Verlag.

Neutron Capture Gamma-Ray Spectroscopy. 1969. (Proceedings Ser.). (Illus.). 708p. (Orig.). pap. (*92-0-130369-6*, ISP235) IAEA AUT. *Dist:* Bernan Associates.

Neutron Contamination from Medical Electron Accelerators. Intro. by Warren K. Sinclair. 1984. LC 84-19848. (Report Ser.: No. 79). 132p. pap. text 35.00 (*0-913392-70-7*) NCRP Pubns.

Neutron Monitoring for Radiation Protection Purposes. International Atomic Energy Agency Staff. 1974. (Proceedings Ser.). (Illus.). Vol. 1. pap. (*92-0-020173-3*, ISP318-1); Vol. 2. pap. (*92-0-020273-X*, ISP318-2) IAEA AUT. *Dist:* Bernan Associates.

Neutron Radiography. John P. Barton & Peter Von der Hardt. 1983. text 411.50 (*90-277-1528-9*) Kluwer Academic.

Neutrophil: Cellular Biochemistry & Physiology. Ed. by Maurice B. Hallett. 1989. 288p. lib. bdg. 239.00 (*0-8493-4808-0*, QR185) CRC Pr.

Neutrotraumatology: Progress & Perspectives - Proceedings of the International Conference on Recent Advances in Neurotraumatology Porto,

Portugal, November 1990. Ed. by A. Martins Da Silva et al. 1992. (Acta Neurochirurgica Ser.: No. 55). (Illus.). 90p. 96.95 (*0-387-82378-6*) Spr-Verlag.

Nevada Health Care in Perspective, 2000. Ed. by Kathleen O'Leary Morgan & Scott E. Morgan. 2000. 21p. spiral bd. 19.00 (*0-7401-0227-3*) Morgan Quitno Corp.

Nevada Health Care Perspective, 1998. Ed. by Kathleen O'Leary Morgan & Scott E. Morgan. 1998. 20p. pap. 19.00 (*1-56692-827-3*) Morgan Quitno Corp.

Never Be Tired Again! David C. Gardner & Grace J. Beatty. 1990. LC 89-45791. (Illus.). 384p. reprint ed. pap. 13.00 (*0-06-097298-X*, Perennial) HarperTrade.

Never Die Young: Or How to Survive ACLS! David P. Doernbach & Jane Huff. 2nd ed. 1993. (Illus.). 195p. pap. text 24.00 (*0-9638043-0-8*) Vital Signs.

Never Get Naked on Your First Visit: A Patient's Survival Guide. David H. Ellig. 1992. LC 90-92333. (Illus.). 310p. (Orig.). pap. 19.95 (*0-9628311-0-7*) Med Ed Az.

Never Old - The Ultimate Success Story: Secrets of Perpetual Youth, Health & CE Mindpower Revealed. Jesse A. Dawn. 1995. (Illus.). 264p. (Orig.). pap. 9.95 (*0-9636589-0-5*) Wrld Changing.

Never Question the Miracle: A Surgeon's Story. Rose-Marie Toussaint & Anthony E. Santaniello. 1998. LC 97-37566. 336p. 24.95 (*0-345-40723-7*) Ballantine Pub Grp.

New Actions of Parathyroid Hormone. Ed. by Shaul G. Massry & T. Fujita. 1989. (Illus.). 494p. 110.00 (*0-306-43418-0*, Plenum Trade) Perseus Pubng.

New Actions of Parathyroid Hormone. Y. Nishizawa & M. Smogorzewski. 1995. (Journal: Vol. 21, Nos. 1-3, 1995). (Illus.). 244p. pap. 129.75 (*3-8055-6195-4*) S Karger.

New Advances in Diuretic Treatment. Ed. by St. H. Taylor. 1994. (Journal: Vol. 84, Suppl. 2, 1994). (Illus.). iv, 172p. pap. 52.25 (*3-8055-6001-X*) S Karger.

New Advances in Histamine Research. Kenji Tasaka. 1995. LC 94-39978. 110.00 (*0-387-70137-0*) Spr-Verlag.

New Advances in Renal Ammonia Metabolism. Ed. by A. C. Schoolwerth et al. 1985. (Contributions to Nephrology Ser.: Vol. 47). (Illus.). x, 238p. 29.75 (*3-8055-4009-4*) S Karger.

New Age: Problems & Potential. Kenneth R. Pelletier. 1985. (Broadside Editions Ser.). 44p. (Orig.). (C). pap. 4.95 (*0-931191-02-5*) Rob Briggs.

New Age of Healing: Anthology. 1979. 96p. pap. 5.95 (*0-911336-78-8*) Sci of Mind.

New Agenda for Medical Missions. Ed. by D. Merrill Ewert. 1993. (MAP International Monograph). 136p. (Orig.). reprint ed. pap. text 6.95 (*1-879148-05-6*) MAP Intl.

New Agenda for Women's Health & Nutrition. Contrib. by International Bank for Reconstruction and Development Staff. 1994. LC 94-29586. (Development in Practice Ser.). 116p. pap. 22.00 (*0-8213-3009-8*, 13009) World Bank.

New Aird's Companion in Surgical Studies. K. C. Burnand & A. E. Young. 1993. (Illus.). 1440p. text (*0-443-03831-7*) Church.

New Aird's Companion in Surgical Studies. Ed. by K. G. Burnand & A. E. Young. 2nd ed. 1998. (Illus.). 1248p. text (*0-443-05326-X*) Church.

New American Acupuncture: Acupuncture Osteopathy: The Myofascial Release of the Bodymind's Holding Patterns. Mark Seem. Ed. by Bob Flaws. 1993. LC 93-71097. (Illus.). 175p. pap. 22.95 (*0-936185-44-9*) Blue Poppy Pr.

New American Diet System. Sonja L. Connor & William E. Connor. 1992. LC 90-20518. (Illus.). 576p. pap. 26.00 (*0-671-75503-X*, Fireside) S&S Trade Pap.

New American Pocket Medical Dictionary. Ed. by Nancy Roper. 2nd ed. 1988. (Illus.). 368p. pap. text (*0-443-08581-1*) Church.

New American Pocket Medical Dictionary. Nancy Roper. 2nd ed. 1988. 372p. pap. 17.00 (*0-684-19031-1*, Macmillan Ref) Gale.

New & Exploratory Therapeutic Agents for Asthma. Ed. by Michael Yeadon & Zuzana Diamant. 1999. LC 00-269886. (Lung Biology in Health & Disease Ser.: Vol. 139). (Illus.). 528p. text 185.00 (*0-8247-7861-8*) Dekker.

New & Re-Emerging Market for Human Vaccines. Contrib. by Sandra Graham. 1995. 187p. 2750.00 (*1-56965-045-4*, C-171) BCC.

New & Resurgent Infections: Prediction, Detection, & Management of Tomorrow's Epidemics. B. M. Greenwood & Kevin De Cock. 1998. LC 97-46506. 236p. 99.95 (*0-471-98174-5*) Wiley.

New & Untried Course: Woman's Medical College & Medical College of Pennsylvania, 1850-1998. Steven J. Peitzman. 2000. LC 99-45850. (Illus.). xiii, 322p. text 60.00 (*0-8135-2815-1*); pap. text 22.00 (*0-8135-2816-X*) Rutgers U Pr.

New Anesthetic Agents, Devices & Monitoring Techniques. Theodore H. Stanley & W. Clayton Petty. 1983. text 112.50 (*90-247-2796-0*) Kluwer Academic.

New Angiotherapy. Ed. by Tai-Ping Fan & Elise C. Kohn. 2001. LC 00-50029. (Illus.). 640p. 150.00 (*0-89603-464-X*) Humana.

New Animal Doctor's Answer Book. Michael W. Fox. rev. ed. 1991. LC 84-6973. Orig. Title: The Animal Doctor's Answer Book. (Illus.). 320p. pap. 14.95 (*1-55704-035-4*) Newmarket.

New Anthology of Orthopaedics. Mercer Rang. 2000. LC 99-88684. 587p. text 79.00 (*0-7216-7141-1*) Harcrt Hlth Sci Grp.

New Antibacterial Strategies. Ed. by Harold C. Neu. 1991. (Illus.). 340p. (Orig.). pap. text (*0-443-04448-1*) Church.

New Anticancer Drugs. Ed. by S. K. Carter. 1980. (Recent Results in Cancer Research Ser.: Vol. 70). (Illus.). 229p. 66.00 (*0-387-09682-5*) Spr-Verlag.

New Anticoagulants for the Cardiovascular Patient. E. Roque Pifarre. 1997. LC 96-51845. 65.00 (*1-56053-220-3*) Hanley & Belfus.

New Anticonvulsant Drugs. Brian S. Meldrum & Roger J. Porter. 1986. (Current Problems in Epilepsy Ser.: Vol. 4). (Illus.). 350p. (*0-86196-063-7*) J Libbey Med GBR. *Dist:* Bks Intl VA.

New Antiepileptic Drug Development: Preclinical & Clinical Aspects. Ed. by Jacqueline A. French et al. 1993. LC 93-8273. (Epilepsy Research Ser.: Vol. 10). 272p. 230.50 (*0-444-89987-1*) Elsevier.

New Antiepileptic Drugs in Psychiatry: Symposium, Schloss Elmau, March 1998, No.38. Ed. by J. Walden & H. Grunze. 1998. (Neuropsychobiology Ser.: No.3). (Illus.). 94p. pap. 29.00 (*3-8055-6761-8*) S Karger.

New Antiviral Strategies. Ed. by S. R. Norrby. 1989. (Frontiers of Infectious Diseases Ser.). (Illus.). 288p. pap. text (*0-443-04166-0*) Church.

New Applications of Accelerators & Nuclear Detectors to Medical Diagnosis, Vol. 3, No. 2. Ed. by P. Min & Robert Klapisch. 1988. (Nuclear Science Applications Ser.: Sec. A, Vol. 3, No. 2). 92p. text 173.00 (*3-7186-4825-3*) Gordon & Breach.

New Applications of Interpersonal Psychotherapy. Ed. by Gerald L. Klerman & Myrna M. Weissman. 1993. LC 92-48959. 408p. text 56.00 (*0-88048-511-6*, 8511) Am Psychiatric.

New Approach in the Treatment of Climacteric Disorders. Ed. by H. P. Schneider & Andrea R. Genazzani. 1993. (New Developments in Biosciences Ser.: No. 7). (Illus.). viii, 53p. (Orig.). (C). pap. text 44.65 (*3-11-013471-3*) De Gruyter.

New Approach to Women & Therapy. Miriam Greenspan. 2nd ed. 1993. LC 92-34036. (*0-8306-4167-X*); pap. 12.95 (*0-8306-4168-8*) McGraw-Hill Educ Grp.

New Approaches for Antifungal Drugs. Ed. by Prabhavathi B. Fernandes. 1992. LC 92-11106. x, 201p. 105.00 (*0-8176-3602-1*); (*3-7643-3602-1*) Birkhauser.

New Approaches in Cancer Pharmacology: Drug Design & Development. Ed. by Paul Workman. 1993. LC 92-49597. (*3-540-56089-0*); (Illus.). 116p. 95.00 (*0-387-56089-0*) Spr-Verlag.

New Approaches in Cancer Pharmacology: Drug Design & Development. Ed. by P. Workman. 2nd ed. 1994. LC 94-27065. (Series in Surface Sciences: Vol. 20). 280p. 53.95 (*0-387-58415-3*) Spr-Verlag.

New Approaches in Cancer Pharmacology: Drug Design & Development II. Ed. by P. Workman. 1994. LC 94-27065. (Monographs of the European School of Oncology). (Illus.). 104p. 86.95 (*0-387-58153-7*) Spr-Verlag.

New Approaches in Cardiac Mechanics. Ed. by Kazuo Kitamura et al. 1986. x, 330p. text 189.00 (*2-88124-126-3*) Gordon & Breach.

New Approaches in the Diagnosis & Management of Cardiovascular Disease: Proceedings of the Conference on Cardiovascular Disease, 9th, Snowmass-at-Aspen, Aspen, Colorado, January, 1978. Conference on Cardiovascular Disease Staff. Ed. by John H. Vogel. 1979. (Advances in Cardiology Ser.: Vol. 26). 71.50 (*3-8055-2914-7*) S Karger.

New Approaches to Breeding for Improved Plant Protein. International Atomic Energy Agency Staff. 1969. (Panel Proceedings Ser.). (Illus.). 193p. pap. (*92-0-111069-3*, ISP212) IAEA AUT. *Dist:* Bernan Associates.

New Approaches to Counseling & Communication: How to Improve Your Skills in Patient Care: Proceedings of the Advances in Patient Care Conference, 4th, 1977. Advances in Patient Care Conference Staff. Ed. by Spring Zoog & Stephen R. Yarnall. 1977. 20.00 (*0-917054-14-8*) Med Communications.

New Approaches to Health Education in Primary Health Care: Report of a WHO Expert Committee, 1983. 1983. (Technical Report Ser.: No. 690). 44p. pap. text 5.00 (*92-4-120690-X*, 1100690) World Health.

New Approaches to Stabilisation of Vaccines Potency: WHO Headquarters, May 1995. Ed. by F. Brown. 1996. (Developments in Biological Standardization Ser.: Vol. 87). xii, 364p. pap. 278.25 (*3-8055-6309-4*) S Karger.

New Approaches to the Management of Allergic Diseases: Proceedings of the Collegium Internationale Allergologicum, 12th, New Orleans, LA, Sept. 1978. Collegium Internationale Allergologicum Staff. Ed. by Lawrence M. Lichtenstein & G. J. Gleich. 1979. (Monographs in Allergy: Vol. 14). (Illus.). pap. 126.25 (*3-8055-3039-0*) S Karger.

New Approaches to the Treatment of Leukaemia. Ed. by Emil J. Freireich & U. Veronesi. 1990. (ESO Monographs). (Illus.). 193p. 118.00 (*0-387-52261-1*) Spr-Verlag.

New Art of Keeping Fit: Modern Methods for Men. Joseph Edmundson. rev. ed. 1978. LC 63-13393. (Illus.). 10.95 (*0-87523-144-6*) Emerson.

New Arthritis Breakthrough: The Only Medical Therapy Clinically Proven to Produce Long-Term Improvement & Remission: RA, Lupus, Juvenile RA, Fibromyalgia, Scleroderma, Spondyloarthropathy, & Other Inflammatory Forms of Arthritis. Henry Scammell. 1998. LC 97-61592. 256p. pap. 22.95 (*0-87131-843-1*) M Evans.

New Arthritis Cures: All the Treatments That Work for Your Arthritis Pain. Brenda Adderly & Amal Das. 1999. 208p. 24.95 (*0-89526-332-7*, LifeLine Press) Regnery Pub.

New Arthritis Relief Diet: Proven Steps to Stop Inflammation, Prevent Joint Damage, Decrease Medication & Improve the Quality of Your Life. James Scala. 1998. LC 97-34927. 272p. pap. 13.95 (*0-452-27951-8*) Dutton Plume.

New Aspects in Diabetes: Treatment Strategies with Alphaglucosidase Inhibitors. Ed. by P. J. Lefebvre & E. Standl. 1993. (Illus.). xii, 306p. (C). lib. bdg. 98.50 (*3-11-013469-1*) De Gruyter.

New Aspects in Physiological Antitumor Substances. Ed. by G. Gillissen & K. E. Theurer. 1985. (Illus.). x, 228p. pap. 35.00 (*3-8055-4002-7*) S Karger.

New Aspects in the Diagnosis & Treatment of Hodgkin's Disease. Ed. by V. Diehl et al. 1989. (Recent Results in Cancer Research Ser.: Vol. 17). (Illus.). 283p. 137.00 (*0-387-51124-5*) Spr-Verlag.

New Aspects in the Regulation of Prostatic Function. Ed. by G. Aumuller et al. 1989. (Clinical & Experimental Urology Ser.). (Illus.). 186p. text (*3-88603-318-X*) W Zuckschwerdt DEU. *Dist:* Scholium Intl.

New Aspects in the Treatment of Failing Heart. Ed. by H. Yasuda & H. Kawaguchi. 1992. LC 92-49576. (Illus.). 256p. 139.00 (*0-387-70110-9*) Spr-Verlag.

New Aspects in the Treatment of Pulmonary & Upper Airways Diseases. Ed. by G. Allegra & J. A. Nahkosteen. 1987. (Journal: Vol. 51, Suppl. 1, 1987). iv, 68p. pap. 22.75 (*3-8055-4592-4*) S Karger.

New Aspects of Allergic Diseases, Immuno-Regulation & Immunodeficiencies. Ed. by L. A. Hanson et al. 1987. (Journal: Vol. 82, No. 3-4, 1987). (Illus.). viii, 332p. pap. 120.00 (*3-8055-4568-1*) S Karger.

New Aspects of Cochlear Mechanics & Inner Ear Pathophysiology. Ed. by C. R. Pfaltz. 1990. (Advances in OtoRhinoLaryngology Ser.: Vol. 44). (Illus.). x, 170p. 146.25 (*3-8055-5020-0*) S Karger.

New Aspects of Complement Structure & Function. Anna Erdei. 1994. 120p. 99.00 (*1-57059-158-X*, LN9158) Landes Bioscience.

New Aspects of Fundamental Problems of Larynology & Otology. Ed. by C. R. Pfaltz. 1984. (Advances in OtoRhinoLaryngology Ser.: Vol. 32). (Illus.). viii, 200p. 138.50 (*3-8055-3701-8*) S Karger.

New Aspects of Haemophilia Treatment. Ed. by Harold R. Roberts. 1996. (Journal: Vol. 26, No. 1, 1996). (Illus.). vi, 166p. pap., suppl. ed. 53.25 (*3-8055-6279-9*) S Karger.

New Aspects of Human Ethology: Proceedings of the 13th Conference of the International Society for Human Ethology Held in Vienna, Austria, August 5-10, 1996. Ed. by Alain Schmitt et al. 1997. LC 97-30572. (Illus.). 252p. 107.00 (*0-306-45695-8*, Kluwer Plenum) Kluwer Academic.

New Aspects of Human Polymorphonuclear Leukocytes. Ed. by Walter H. Horl & P. J. Schollmeyer. 1991. (Advances in Experimental Medicine & Biology Ser.). (Illus.). 236p. (C). text 107.00 (*0-306-43906-9*, Kluwer Plenum) Kluwer Academic.

New Aspects of Pathophysiology & Treatment of Polycycstic Ovary Syndrome: Journal: Hormone Research, Vol. 33. Ed. by Y. Nakamura & Y. Taketani. 1990. (Illus.). vi, 50p. 24.50 (*3-8055-5262-9*) S Karger.

New Aspects of Physiology & Pathology of Luteal Phase: Journal: Hormone Research, Vol. 37, Suppl. 1, 1992. Ed. by H. Mori & A. Miyake. 1992. (Illus.). iv, 80p. pap. 36.75 (*3-8055-5625-X*) S Karger.

New Aspects of Thrombolytic Therapy for Acute Myocardial Infarction. Sorin V. Pislaru. 1998. (Acta Biomedica Lovaniensia Ser.). (Illus.). 126p. pap. (*90-6186-888-2*) Leuven Univ BEL. *Dist:* Coronet Bks.

New Aspects of Vitreoretinopathology. Ed. by C. Gailloud et al. 1979. (Modern Problems in Ophthalmology Ser.: Vol. 20). (Illus.). 226.25 (*3-8055-3038-2*) S Karger.

New Aspects on Hirudin: Journal: Haemostasis, Vol. 21, Suppl. 1, 1991. Ed. by J. Fareed et al. 1991. (Illus.). vi, 174p. pap. 55.00 (*3-8055-5389-7*) S Karger.

New Aspects on Respiratory Failure. Ed. by E. Rugheimer. 1991. (Illus.). 341p. 107.00 (*0-387-51445-7*) Spr-Verlag.

New Aspects on Thromboembolism. Ed. by U. Hedner. 1993. (Journal: Vol. 23, Suppl. 1, 1993). (Illus.). iv, 228p. pap. 70.50 (*3-8055-5745-0*) S Karger.

New Avenues & Perspectives in the Management of Advanced Prostate Cancer: Paris, September 1996. Ed. by Laurent Boccon-Gibod. 1997. (European Urology Ser.: Vol. 31, Suppl. 1997). (Illus.). iv, 40p. pap. 21.75 (*3-8055-6487-2*) S Karger.

New Baby Therapy. Lisa Engelhardt. 1998. LC 97-77583. (Elf-Help Bks.). (Illus.). 88p. pap. 4.95 (*0-87029-307-9*, 20140) Abbey.

New Bach Flower Body Maps: Treatment by Topical Application. Dietmar Kramer. 1995. LC 95-48845. (Illus.). 237p. pap. 19.95 (*0-89281-531-0*, Heal Arts VT) Inner Tradit.

New Bach Flower Therapies: Healing the Emotional & Spiritual Causes of Illness. Dietmar Kramer. 1995. LC 94-49148. 168p. pap. 12.95 (*0-89281-529-9*, Heal Arts VT) Inner Tradit.

New Back Doctor: The Program or Lifetime Relief from Back Pain. Hamilton Hall. 1995. (Illus.). 272p. mass mkt. 7.99 (*0-7704-2619-0*) Bantam.

New Beginning: A Book for Urostomy Patients. Kay Marshall. 1988. (Illus.). pap. text (*0-916999-05-X*) HERC Pubng.

New Beginnings: Healing Through Communication. Russ Bedord. 1995. LC 94-93982. 272p. (Orig.). pap. 24.95 (*0-9644918-6-9*) Regenics Pr.

New Beyond Peek-a-Boo & Pat-a-Cake: Activities for Baby's First 24 Months. Evelyn M. Munger & Susan J. Bowdon. 3rd ed. 1993. LC 93-1421. 256p. spiral bd. 15.95 (*0-8329-0504-6*) New Win Pub.

New Biomedical Materials: Basic & Applied Studies. Ed. by D. Chapman & P. I. Haris. 1998. LC 97-77017. (Biomedical & Health Research Ser.: Vol. 16). 197p. 86.00 (*90-5199-365-X*, 365-X) IOS Press.

New Biotechnology in Oral Research. Ed. by H. M. Myers. 1989. (Illus.). x, 170p. 128.00 (*3-8055-4916-4*) S Karger.

New Bodytalk: Self-Help for All Your Health Problems. Michael Van Straten. 1994. (Illus.). 302p. pap. (*0-7472-4156-2*) Headline Bk Pub GBR. *Dist:* Trafalgar.

New Book of Health. Frank Osborne & Judy Goldstein. 1996. 402p. (Orig.). pap. 19.95 (*0-9638596-7-6*) Amer Pubng.

New Book on Healing. Hanna Kroeger. 1996. LC 98-102067. (Illus.). 155p. pap. 7.50 (*1-883713-17-X*) Hanna Kroeger.

New Brain Imaging Techniques in Cerebrovascular Disease. Cahn & Lassen. 1985. (Current Problems in Neurology Ser.: Vol. 2). 136p. (*0-86196-060-2*) J Libbey Med GBR. *Dist:* Bks Intl VA.

New Cancer Sourcebook: Basic Information about Major Forms & Stages of Cancer. Ed. by Allan R. Cook. 1996. LC 95-33730. (Health Reference Ser.: Vol. 12). xi, 1313p. lib. bdg. 78.00 (*0-7808-0041-9*) Omnigraphics Inc.

New Cancer Survivors: Living with Grace, Fighting with Spirit. Natalie Davis Spingarn. 1999. LC 99-25087. 256p. pap. 16.95 (*0-8018-6267-1*); 47.00 (*0-8018-6266-3*) Johns Hopkins.

New Cancer Therapies: The Patient's Dilemma. Penny Williams. 2000. (Illus.). 224p. pap. 16.95 (*1-55209-485-5*) Firefly Bks Limited.

New Careers in Nursing. Florence Downs & Dorothy A. Brooten. 1985. LC 82-18449. (Illus.). 192p. pap. 12.95 (*0-668-05255-4*, Arc) Hungry Minds.

New Certificate Practical Chemistry. Samuel O. Acquaah. 1983. LC 83-82066. 112p. (*0-8187-0054-8*) Harlo Press.

New Challenges in Surfactant Research: Proceedings of the 15th International Workshop on Surfactant Replacement, Kos, June 2000. Ed. by C. Papagaroufalis et al. 2000. (Biology of the Neonate Ser.: Vol. 77, Suppl. 1 (2000)). (Illus.). iv, 30p. pap. 25.25 (*3-8055-7094-5*) S Karger.

New Child Protection Team Handbook. Donald C. Bross et al. 1988. LC 88-2542. 658p. text 30.00 (*0-8240-8519-1*) Garland.

New Choices in Natural Healing. Prevention Magazine Editors. 1997. 800p. mass mkt. 6.99 (*0-553-57690-9*) Bantam.

New Choices in Natural Healing: Over 1,000 of the Best Self-Help Remedies from the World of Alternative Medicine. Ed. by Bill Gottlieb. 1997. LC 95-15907. (Illus.). 687p. pap. 18.95 (*0-87596-364-1*) Rodale Pr Inc.

New Choices in Natural Healing: Over 1,800 of the Best Self-Help Remedies from the World of Alternative Medicine. Ed. by Bill Gottlieb. 1995. LC 95-15907. (Illus.). 704p. 27.95 (*0-87596-257-2*) Rodale Pr Inc.

New Choices in Natural Healing for Dogs & Cats. Amy D. Shojai & Prevention for Pets Editors. 2001. (Illus.). 480p. pap. 16.95 (*1-57954-461-4*) Rodale Pr Inc.

New Choices in Natural Healing for Women: Drug-Free Remedies from the World of Alternative Medicine. Sara A. O'Donnell et al. 1997. LC 97-2481. (Illus.). 544p. 29.95 (*0-87596-387-0*) Rodale Pr Inc.

New Choices in Natural Healing for Women: Drug-Free Remedies from the World of Alternative Medicine. Prevention Magazine Health Book Staff. 1998. 640p. mass mkt. 6.99 (*0-553-57980-0*) Bantam.

New Civil War: The Psychology, Culture & Politics of Abortion. Ed. by Linda J. Beckman & S. Marie Harvey. 1998. LC 98-3553. (Psychology of Women Bks.: Div. 35). (Illus.). 432p. text 49.95 (*1-55798-517-0*) Am Psychol.

New Class of Renally Active Compounds with Antihypertensive, Diuretic, Uricosuric Properties: Proceedings of the Symposium, Montreal, June 17, 1978. Symposium, Montreal Staff. Ed. by G. Lemieux & T. H. Steele. 1979. (Nephron Ser.: Vol. 23 Suppl. 1). (Illus.). pap. 32.25 (*3-8055-3002-1*) S Karger.

New Clinical & Epidemiological Data on Dipyrone: Yokohama, July 28, 1992. World Conference on Clinical Pharmacology and Therap. Ed. by Kay Brune. 1993. LC 93-25354. 26.00 (*0-8176-2916-5*) Birkhauser.

New Cognitive Neurosciences. Michael S. Gazzaniga. 2nd ed. 1999. LC 98-52869. (Illus.). xiv, 1419p. 129.95 (*0-262-07195-9*) MIT Pr.

New Compendium of Materials Medica (Pharmaceutical Botany & China Medicinal Plants) Ling Yeouruenn. 1996. 292p. (*7-03-003789-8*) Sci Pr CHN. *Dist:* Lubrecht & Cramer.

New Concepts for Topical Use of Natural Retinoids: Retinaldehyde in Perspective, Satellite Symposium Held at the 7th EADV Meeting, Nice, October 1998: Proceedings. Ed. by J. H. Saurat & A. Vahlquist. 1999. (Dermatology Ser.: Vol. 199, Suppl. 1). (Illus.). iv, 64p. pap. 25.25 (*3-8055-6914-9*) S Karger.

New Concepts in AIDS Pathogenesis. Luc Montagnier & Marie-Lise Gougeon. 1993. LC 93-4765. (Illus.). 344p. text 155.00 (*0-8247-9127-4*) Dekker.

New Concepts in Anxiety. Ed. by Mike Briley & Sandra E. File. 1991. text (*0-333-53414-X*) Intl Spec Bk.

New Concepts in Blood Formation Cell Generation in Malignant & Benign Tissues: Adult & Embryonic Tissues from Humans & Animals in Chronic Ischemic Conditions, Acute Rhuematic Fever & Coronary Occlusion with Myocardial Infarction. Hemprova G. McDonald. 1995. LC 89-90849. (Cardiac Muscle Ser.: Vol. II). (Illus.). 117p. (C). 90.00 (*0-9627824-1-6*) Diagnostic & Cell.

***New Concepts in Cerebral Ischemia.** Ed. by Rick C. S. Lin. 2001. (Methods & New Frontiers in Neuroscience Ser.). 328p. 119.95 (*0-8493-0119-X*) CRC Pr.

New Concepts in Diabetes & Its Treatment. Ed. by F. Belfiore & C. E. Mogensen. 2000. LC 99-57726. (Illus.). viii, 218p. 172.25 (*3-8055-6907-6*) S Karger.

New Concepts in Immunopathology of CNS Infections. Phillip K. Peterson & Jack S. Remington. 2000. LC 00-23231. (Illus.). 368p. 104.95 (*0-632-04528-0*) Blackwell Sci.

New Concepts in Lipid Research in Honor of Stina & Einar Stenhagen, Vol. 16. Ed. by Ralph T. Holman. 1978. (Progress in the Chemistry of Fats & Other Lipids Ser.). 86.00 (*0-08-022663-9*, Pergamon Pr) Elsevier.

New Concepts in Stroke Pathophysiology & Prevention. Ed. by N. M. Bornstein & A. G. Turpie. 1994. (Journal: Vol. 4, Suppl. 1, 1994). (Illus.). iv, 48p. pap. 22.75 (*3-8055-5966-6*) S Karger.

New Concepts in Surgical Correction of Dentofacial Deformities, Vol. 3. William H. Bell. 1985. (Illus.). 850p. text 235.00 (*0-7216-1739-5*) Saunders.

New Concepts in the Pathogenesis of NIDDM. C. G. Ostenson et al. 1993. LC 93-29031. (Advances in Experimental Medicine & Biology Ser.: Vol. 334). (Illus.). 326p. (C). text 89.50 (*0-306-44563-8*, Kluwer Plenum) Kluwer Academic.

New Concepts of a Blood-Brain Barrier: Proceedings of a Symposium in Honor of Michael Bradbury Held in London, England, July 4-6, 1994. Ed. by John Greenwood et al. 1996. (Illus.). 344p. 95.00 (*0-306-45204-9*, Kluwer Plenum) Kluwer Academic.

New Conceptual Aspects of Negative Symptoms: Journal: Psychopathology, 1995, Vol. 28, No. 1. Ed. by H. Gerbaldo & C. Mundt. 1994. (Illus.). 64p. pap. 46.25 (*3-8055-6105-9*) S Karger.

New Concise Guide to Homeopathy: An Introduction to the Understanding & Use of Homeopathy. Nigel Garion-Hutchings. 1995. LC 94-49125. 160p. pap. 10.95 (*1-85230-634-3*) Element MA.

New Concordance of Cranial Chronic Pain. Gelb. 1994. text (*0-7234-2041-6*) Wolfe Publishing GBR. *Dist:* Mosby Inc.

New Connection: A Problem Solving Approach to Chemical Dependency. John Frykman. rev. ed. 1992. LC 74-156775. 151p. pap. 11.95 (*0-916147-04-5*) Regent Pr.

New Deal Medicine: The Rural Health Programs of the Farm Security Administration. Michael R. Grey. 1999. LC 98-18240. (Illus.). 260p. 44.50 (*0-8018-5939-5*) Johns Hopkins.

New Developments in Anti-Rheumatic Drugs Ed. by Kim D. Rainsford & G. P. Velo. 1989. (Inflammation & Drug Therapy Ser.). 272p. (C). text 154.00 (*0-7462-0080-3*) Kluwer Academic.

New Developments in Behavior Therapy: From Research to Clinical Application. Ed. by Cyril M. Franks. 1984. LC 83-26402. (Supplement to Child & Family Behavior Therapy Ser.: No. 1). 589p. text 89.95 (*0-86656-241-9*); pap. text 39.95 (*0-86656-178-1*) Haworth Pr.

New Developments in Behavioral Research: Theory, Method, & Application: In Honor of Sidney W. Bijou. Ed. by B. C. Etzel et al. 1977. 656p. 59.95 (*0-89859-459-6*) L Erlbaum Assocs.

New Developments in Biosciences: Their Implication for Laboratory Animal Science. Ed. by Anton C. Beynen & H. A. Solleveid. 1987. 480p. (C). text 306.50 (*0-89838-354-4*) Kluwer Academic.

New Developments in Cardiac Assist Devices, Vol. 6. Ed. by Safuh Attar. 1985. LC 85-6585. (Surgical Science Ser.: No. 6). 222p. 77.00 (*0-275-91330-9*, C13306, Praeger Pubs) Greenwood.

New Developments in Cardiac Nuclear Imaging. Ed. by Ami E. Iskandrian & Mario S. Verani. 1998. LC 97-29167. (Illus.). 288p. 85.00 (*0-87993-670-3*) Futura Pub.

New Developments in Cervical Cancer Screening & Prevention. Joseph Monsonego & Eduard Franco. 1997. LC 96-37506. (Illus.). 464p. 168.95 (*0-632-04765-8*) Blackwell Sci.

New Developments in Clinical Instrumentation. Ed. by Leroy Hersh. 1981. 160p. 96.00 (*0-8493-5305-X*, RB38, CRC Reprint) Franklin.

New Developments in Dietary Fiber: Physiological, Physicochemical & Analytical Aspects. Ed. by Ivan Furda & Charles J. Brine. (Advances in Experimental Medicine & Biology Ser.: Vol. 270). (Illus.). 338p. (C). text 114.00 (*0-306-43583-7*, Kluwer Plenum) Kluwer Academic.

New Developments in Home Care Services for the Elderly: Innovations in Policy, Program, & Practice. Ed. by Lenard W. Kaye. 1995. LC 95-48902. 290p. 45.00 (*1-56024-794-0*) Haworth Pr.

New Developments in Medical Research: Nih & Patient Groups : Hearing Before the Subcommittee on Health & Environment of the Committee on Commerce, House of Representatives, One Hundred Fifth Congress, Second Session March 26, 1998. USGPO Staff. 1998. LC 98-176158. iii, 150p. (*0-16-056546-4*) USGPO.

New Developments in Quantitative Coronary Arteriography. Ed. by Johan H. Reiber & Patrick W. Serruys. 1988. (Developments in Cardiovascular Medicine Ser.). (C). text 226.50 (*0-89838-377-3*) Kluwer Academic.

New Developments in Research on Adult Cognition. Chris Brotherton. 1991. (C). (*1-85041-036-4*) Univ Nottingham GBR. *Dist:* St Mut.

New Developments in Statistics for Psychology & the Social Sciences. Ed. by A. D. Lovie & Frederick Mosteller. 1986. 200p. (*0-901715-46-8*, 1020) Brit Psychol Soc GBR. *Dist:* Routledge.

New Developments in Statistics for Psychology & the Social Sciences. A. D. Lovie et al. 2nd ed. 1992. 200p. (C). lib. bdg. (*1-85433-017-9*, A5028) Brit Psychol Soc GBR. *Dist:* Routledge.

New Developments in Telemedicine. Feedback Research Services Staff. 1997. (Illus.). 200p. spiral bd. 100.00 (*1-889713-10-4*) Feedback Rsch.

New Developments in the Management of Urolithiasis. Ed. by James E. Lingeman & Glenn M. Preminger. 1996. LC 95-32960. (Topics in Clinical Urology Ser.). (Illus.). 216p. 69.50 (*0-89640-287-8*) Igaku-Shoin.

New Developments in the Therapy of Allergic Disorders & Asthma. Ed. by S. Z. Langer & Martin K. Church. 1994. LC 93-40209. (International Academy for Biomedical & Drug Research Ser.: Vol. 6). (Illus.). vi, 136p. 139.25 (*3-8055-5748-5*) S Karger.

New Developments in Therapeutic Enzyme Inhibitors & Receptor Blockers. 1996. 207p. 3400.00 (*1-56965-353-4*, C-202) BCC.

New Developments of the Aetiogenesis of Chronic Pancreatitis - Implications for Treatment & Disease Prophylaxis: Symposium Held During the World Congresses of Gastroenterology, Vienna, September 1998, Vol.59. Ed. by Joan M. Braganza. 1998. (Digestion Ser.: Vol. 59, Suppl. 4). (Illus.). iv, 60p. pap. 48.00 (*3-8055-6804-5*) S Karger.

New Diabetes Without Fear: Take Control of Your Life. Joseph I. Goodman & W. Watts Biggers. rev. ed. 1995. LC 94-96769. 176p. mass mkt. 5.99 (*0-380-77761-4*, Avon Bks) Morrow Avon.

New Diabetic Cookbook. Mabel Cavaiani. 4th rev. ed. 1996. 432p. pap. 14.95 (*0-8092-3164-6*, 316460, Contemporary) McGraw-Hill Trade.

New Diabetic Cookbook. Mabel Cavaiani. rev. ed. 1989. 384p. reprint ed. pap. 14.95 (*0-8092-4251-6*) NTC Contemp Pub Co.

New Diagnostic Methods in Oncology & Hematology. Ed. by D. Huhn. 1998. LC 98-22181. (Illus.). 258p. pap. 65.00 (*3-540-63578-5*) Spr-Verlag.

New Dictionary of Medical Ethics. Ed. by Kenneth Boyd. 1997. 285p. pap. (*0-7279-1001-9*) BMJ Pub GBR. *Dist:* AIDC.

New Dictionary of Sign Language: Employing the Eshkol-Wachmann Movement Notation System. Enya Cohen et al. 1977. (Approaches to Semiotics Ser.: No. 50). text (*90-279-3334-0*) Mouton.

New Dimensions in Healing: Healing & the Future. Torkom Saraydarian. 1992. LC 91-75267. 916p. 50.00 (*0-929874-20-X*); pap. 40.00 (*0-929874-21-8*) TSG Pub Found.

New Dimensions in Mental Health-Psychiatric Nursing. Markian E. Kalkman & Anne B. Davis. 5th ed. 1980. text 31.95 (*0-07-033253-3*) McGraw.

New Dimensions in Women's Health. Linda Lewis Alexander & Judith H. LaRosa. 2nd ed. 1994. (Illus.). 440p. (C). pap. text 56.95 (*0-7637-1083-0*, 1083-0) Jones & Bartlett.

New Dimensions in Women's Health. Linda Alexander et al. 2nd ed. 2000. LC 00-63927. (Nursing Ser.). (Illus.). 532p. (C). text 56.95 (*0-7637-0552-7*, 0552-7) Jones & Bartlett.

New Dimensions of Warfarin Prophylaxis. Ed. by Stanford Wessler et al. 1987. (Illus.). 320p. 75.00 (*0-306-42588-2*, Plenum Trade) Perseus Pubng.

New Dimensions of Women's Health. Linda Lewis Alexander & Judith H. LaRosa. 1994. LC 93-50822. (Health Science Ser.). (Illus.). 464p. (C). text 56.95 (*0-86720-777-9*, 777-9) Jones & Bartlett.

New Directions for Medical Education. Ed. by H. G. Schmidt et al. 1989. (Frontiers of Primary Care Ser.). (Illus.). 300p. 71.95 (*0-387-96390-1*) Spr-Verlag.

New Directions for Mental Health Services. Carl A. Taube et al. 1990. 325p. 51.95 (*1-56032-140-7*) Hemisp Pub.

New Directions in Affective Disorders. Ed. by Bernard Lerer & Samuel Gershon. 1989. (Illus.). 732p. 244.00 (*0-387-96769-9*) Spr-Verlag.

New Directions in Anti-Cancer Chemotherapy. Ed. by Michel E. Marty. 1994. (Journal: Vol. 51, Suppl. 1, 1994). (Illus.). iv, 40p. pap. 19.25 (*3-8055-6080-X*) S Karger.

New Directions in Attitude Measurement. Ed. by Dagmar Krebs & Peter Schmidt. 1993. LC 93-24296. xiv, 378p. (C). lib. bdg. 121.55 (*3-11-013871-9*) De Gruyter.

New Directions in Attribution Research, Vol. 3. Ed. by John H. Harvey et al. 1981. 560p. text 89.95 (*0-89859-098-1*) L Erlbaum Assocs.

New Directions in Behavioral Development. Ed. by Sidney W. Bijou & Emilio Ribes. 1996. (Illus.). 189p. (C). text 29.95 (*1-878978-24-1*) Context Pr.

New Directions in Cancer Treatment. Ed. by Ian T. Magrath. 1989. (Illus.). 631p. 107.00 (*0-387-19063-5*) Spr-Verlag.

New Directions in Childhood Psychopathology: Developmental Considerations, Vol. 1. Ed. by Saul I. Harrison & John F. McDermott, Jr. 1979. LC 78-70232. (Illus.). xviii, 609p. (C). 90.00 (*0-8236-3570-8*) Intl Univs Pr.

New Directions in Childhood Psychopathology Vol. 2: Deviations in Development. Ed. by Saul I. Harrison & John F. McDermott, Jr. 1982. LC 78-70232. xix, 566p. 85.00 (*0-8236-3571-6*) Intl Univs Pr.

New Directions in Children's Mental Health. Ed. by Jalal Shamsie. 1979. LC 79-17844. text 25.00 (*0-88331-167-4*) R B Luce.

New Directions in Dream Interpretation. Ed. by Gayle Delaney. 1993. LC 92-33941. (SUNY Series in Dream Studies). 308p. (C). pap. text 25.95 (*0-7914-1606-2*) State U NY Pr.

New Directions in Health Care: Consequences for the Elderly. Emily Goodman. 1986. (Papers: No. 5). 36p. 5.00 (*0-934459-30-4*) United Hosp Fund.

New Directions in Health Care Policies: Improving Cost Control & Effectiveness. OECD Staff. 1995. LC 96-147497. (Health Care Policy Studies: No. 7). 15p. (Orig.). pap. (*92-64-14545-1*) Org for Econ FRA. *Dist:* OECD.

New Directions in Health Psychology. Harold E. Schroeder. 1990. 53.95 (*0-89116-925-3*) Hemisp Pub.

New Directions in Invertebrate Immunology. Ed. by K. Soderhall et al. 1995. LC 95-67854. (Illus.). 494p. (C). text 95.00 (*0-9625505-9-0*) SOS Pubns NJ.

New Directions in Medicine: A Directory of Learning Opportunities. Raymond F. Rosenthal & James S. Gordon. 1984. pap. 15.95 (*0-931211-00-X*) Aurora Assocs.

New Directions in Memory & Aging: Proceedings of the George A. Talland Memorial Conference. Leonard W. Poon. Ed. by James L. Fozard et al. 1980. LC 79-27548. (Illus.). 572p. text 115.00 (*0-89859-035-3*) L Erlbaum Assocs.

New Directions in Parapsychological Research. Joseph H. Rush. 1964. LC 64-22612. (Parapsychological Monographs: No. 4). pap. 5.00 (*0-912328-07-X*) Parapsych Foun.

New Directions in Pediatric Hemotherapy. Ed. by Stephen M. Capon & Linda A. Chambers. 1996. (Illus.). 144p. pap. text 65.00 (*1-56395-064-2*, PC97-960014) Am Assn Blood.

New Directions in Pharmaceutical Tablet Manufacture, No. C-135. Business Communications Co., Inc. Staff. 1991. 156p. 2250.00 (*0-89336-816-4*) BCC.

New Directions in Public Health Care: A Prescription for the 1980's. Cotton M. Lindsay. 3rd ed. 1980. 308p. text 39.95 (*0-87855-394-0*); pap. text 24.95 (*0-917616-37-5*) Transaction Pubs.

New Directions in Sex Therapy: Innovations & Alternatives. Peggy J. Kleinplatz. 2001. LC 00-66741. (Illus.). xxxiii, 375p. 44.95 (*0-87630-967-8*) Brunner-Routledge.

New Directions in Tardive Dyskinesia Research. Ed. by R. H. Belmaker & J. Bannet. 1983. (Modern Problems of Pharmacopsychiatry Ser.: Vol. 21). (Illus.). vi, 222p. 109.75 (*3-8055-3735-2*) S Karger.

New Directions in the Psychological Treatment of Serious Mental Illness. Ed. by Diane T. Marsh. 1993. LC 93-23930. 224p. 75.00 (*0-275-94428-X*, C4428, Praeger Pubs) Greenwood.

New Directions in the Psychophysiology of Individual Differences: A Symposium of Papers from the 22nd Annual Meeting of the Society for Psychophysiological Research, Minneapolis, 21-24 October 1982. Ed. by R. M. Stelmack. 1983. 76p. pap. 15.25 (*0-08-030844-9*, Pergamon Pr) Elsevier.

New Directions in Understanding Dementia & Alzheimer's Disease. Ed. by T. Zandi & R. J. Ham. 1990. LC 90-14297. (Advances in Experimental Medicine & Biology Ser.: Vol. 282). (Illus.). 174p. (C). text 95.00 (*0-306-43728-7*, Kluwer Plenum) Kluwer Academic.

New Disability History: American Perspectives. Ed. by Paul K. Longmore & Lauri Umansky. 2000. LC 00-11661. (History of Disability Ser.). (Illus.). vi, 416p. 65.00 (*0-8147-8563-8*); pap. 23.95 (*0-8147-8564-6*) NYU Pr.

New Discoveries in Medicine: Their Effect on the Public Health. Paul R. Hawley. 1977. LC 76-37922. (Essay Index Reprint Ser.). reprint ed. 22.95 (*0-8369-2594-7*) Ayer.

New Drug Approval in Brazil. Ivo Ferreira. 1995. LC 98-148823. (Worldwide Pharmaceutical Regulation Ser.). 62p. (Orig.). pap. 100.00 (*1-882615-21-2*) Parexel Intl.

New Drug Approval in Canada. Eileen McMahon. 1995. (Worldwide Pharmaceutical Regulation Ser.). (Orig.). pap. 100.00 (*1-882615-20-4*) Parexel Intl.

New Drug Approval in France. Gillian Ivers-Read & Colin Scott. 1996. (Worldwide Pharmaceutical Regulation Ser.). 104p. (Orig.). pap. 100.00 (*1-882615-16-6*) Parexel Intl.

New Drug Approval in Germany. Christian Hinze & Barbara Sickmuller. 1995. (Worldwide Pharmaceutical Regulation Ser.). 55p. (Orig.). pap. 100.00 (*1-882615-15-8*) Parexel Intl.

New Drug Approval in Italy. Guiliana Tabusso & Nadia Peviani. 1995. (Worldwide Pharmaceutical Regulation Ser.). 94p. (Orig.). pap. 100.00 (*1-882615-17-4*) Parexel Intl.

New Drug Approval in Japan. William J. Currie. 1995. (Worldwide Pharmaceutical Regulation Ser.). 64p. (Orig.). pap. 125.00 (*1-882615-14-X*) Parexel Intl.

New Drug Approval in South Korea. Suk C. Lee. 1995. (Worldwide Pharmaceutical Regulation Ser.). 92p. (Orig.). pap. 100.00 (*1-882615-22-0*) Parexel Intl.

New Drug Approval in the European Union. Paul T. Evers. 1995. (Worldwide Pharmaceutical Regulation Ser.). 97p. (Orig.). pap. 150.00 (*1-882615-12-3*) Parexel Intl.

New Drug Approval in the United Kingdom. Paul T. Evers. 1995. (Worldwide Pharmaceutical Regulation Ser.). 111p. (Orig.). pap. 100.00 (*1-882615-18-2*) Parexel Intl.

New Drug Approval in the United States. Mark Mathieu. 1995. (Worldwide Pharmaceutical Regulation Ser.). (Orig.). pap. 100.00 (*1-882615-13-1*) Parexel Intl.

New Drug Approval Process. Ed. by Richard Guarino. 2nd exp. rev. ed. 1992. LC 92-23366. (Drugs & the Pharmaceutical Sciences Ser.: Vol. 56). (Illus.). 500p. text 180.00 (*0-8247-8801-X*) Dekker.

New Drugs. Thomas W. Feeley. 1995. 39.00 (*0-316-27684-7*, Little Brwn Med Div) Lppncott W & W.

New Drugs. Ed. by John Feely. 2nd ed. pap. text (*0-7279-0297-0*); 3rd ed. 1994. 464p. pap. text (*0-7279-0821-9*) BMJ Pub GBR. *Dist:* AIDC.

New Drugs: Discovery & Development. Alan A. Rubin. 1978. (Drugs & the Pharmaceutical Sciences Ser.: Vol. 5). (Illus.). 328p. text 175.00 (*0-8247-6634-2*) Dekker.

New Drugs, Concepts & Results in Cancer Chemotherapy. Ed. by Franco M. Muggia. 1991. (Cancer Treatment & Research Ser.). 176p. (C). text 147.50 (*0-7923-1253-8*) Kluwer Academic.

New Drugs for Asthma Therapy Vol. 34: Agents & Actions Supplement. Ed. by I. D. Chapman et al. 1991. ix, 548p. 164.00 (*0-8176-2505-4*) Birkhauser.

New Drugs in Allergy & Asthma. Ed. by Trevor T. Hansel & John Morley. 1993. (Agents & Actions Supplements Ser.: Vol. 43). 307p. 99.50 (*0-8176-2870-3*) Spr-Verlag.

New Drugs in Oncology. Ed. by W. Queisser & H. H. Fiebig. 1989. (Beitraege Zur Onkologie, Contributions to Oncology Ser.: Vol. 37). (Illus.). 302p. 68.75 (*3-8055-5047-2*) S Karger.

New Economic Health Care: Drugs Case Mix & Patients' Length of Stay. Raymond A. Arons. 1984. LC 84-6831. 256p. 60.00 (*0-275-91421-6*, C1421, Praeger Pubs) Greenwood.

New Endocrinology of Cancer. Charles Coombes & Jonathan Waxman. 1988. 176p. (*0-683-13011-0*) E A GBR. *Dist:* Williams & Wilkins.

New England Journal of Medicine, Vol. 1, No. 1. deluxe ed. 1987. 112p. 35.00 (*0-910133-20-4*) Mass Med Pub Div.

New English-Italian Dictionary of the Medical Sciences: Nuovo Dizionario Inglese-Italiano delle Scienze Mediche. L. Bussi & M. T. Cognazzo. 1987. 864p. 150.00 (*0-8288-1846-0*, M14387) Fr & Eur.

New Epidemics: Proceedings of the International Seminar on Nuclear War & Planetary Emergencies - 21st Session Erice, Italy 19-24 August, 1996. Ed. by K. Goebel. 1997. (Science & Culture Ser.). 260p. 68.00 (*981-02-3232-2*) World Scientific Pub.

New Era in Bioenergetics. Ed. by Yasuo Mukohata. 1992. (Illus.). 308p. text 73.00 (*0-12-509854-5*) Acad Pr.

New Era of Lipid-Lowering Drug Alternative: Journal: Cardiology, Vol. 76, Suppl. 1, 1989. Ed. by R. I. Levy. 1989. (Illus.). iv, 102p. pap. 23.25 (*3-8055-5023-5*) S Karger.

New Ethics for the Public's Health. Ed. by Dan E. Beauchamp & Bonnie Steinbock. 1999. LC 99-23617. (Illus.). 400p. text 67.50 (*0-19-512438-3*); pap. text 39.95 (*0-19-512439-1*) OUP.

New Events & Facts in Diabetes. F. Belfiore. 1982. (Frontiers in Diabetes Ser.: Vol. 2). (Illus.). x, 190p. 99.25 (*3-8055-3541-4*) S Karger.

New Experimental Modalities in the Control of Neoplasia. Ed. by Prakash Chandra. 1986. LC 86-22709. (NATO ASI Series A, Life Sciences: Vol. 102). 414p. 95.00 (*0-306-42464-9*, Plenum Trade) Perseus Pubng.

New Face of the NHS. Ed. by Peter Spurgeon. 2nd ed. 1998. 306p. pap. (*0-443-05969-1*) Royal Soc of Medicine Pr Ltd GBR. *Dist:* Balogh.

New Facts about Fiber Health Builder, Disease Fighter, Vital Nutrient: How Fiber Supplements Can Enhance

Your Health. Betty Kamen. 6th rev. ed. 1997. (Illus.). 139p. pap. 9.95 (*0-944501-05-2*) Nutrition Encounter.

New Facts on Mental Disorders. Neil A. Dayton. Ed. by Gerald N. Grob. 1980. LC 78-22558. (Historical Issues in Mental Health Ser.). (Illus.). reprint ed. lib. bdg. 37.95 (*0-405-11912-7*) Ayer.

New Findings on Aclarubicin in the Treatment of Acute Myeloid Leukemia. Ed. by W. Hiddemann & R. Mertelsmann. 1990. (Illus.). 88p. 18.95 (*0-387-52613-7*) Spr-Verlag.

New Findings on HSV-Induced Retinitis in the Von Szily Model. H. J. Thiel. 1994. LC 95-104225. 100p. pap. text 63.00 (*0-7506-9588-9*) Buttrwrth-Heinemann.

New Findings with Anxiolytic Drugs: Journal: Psychopathology, Vol. 22, Suppl. 1. Ed. by Samuel Gershon & J. Bruinvels. 1989. vi, 78p. pap. 26.25 (*3-8055-5016-2*) S Karger.

New Foundations in Health: Six Stories. Frwd. by Daniel M. Fox et al. 1999. 168p. pap. (*1-887748-27-X*) Milbank Memorial.

New Frontiers in Cancer Causation: Proceedings of the 2nd International Conference on Theories of Carcinogenesis. Ed. by Olav H. Iversen. 1993. 432p. (*1-56032-251-9*) Tay Francis Ltd GBR. *Dist:* Taylor & Francis.

New Frontiers in Cytology. Ed. by K. Goeritler et al. 1988. (Illus.). 450p. 256.00 (*0-387-19168-2*) Spr-Verlag.

New Frontiers in Mammary Pathology, 1986. Ed. by K. H. Hollman & J. M. Verley. 1986. (Developments in Oncology Ser.). text 278.50 (*0-89838-852-X*) Kluwer Academic.

New Frontiers in Medical Device Technology. Ed. by Arye Rosen & Harel D. Rosen. 1995. LC 94-26892. (Microwave & Optical Components Ser.). 364p. 120.00 (*0-471-59189-0*) Wiley.

New Frontiers in Medical Sciences: Redefining Hyaluronan: Proceedings of the Symposium on New Frontiers in Medical Sciences, Held in Padua, Italy, 17-19 June 1999. Symposium on New Frontiers in Medical Sciences Staff et al. 2000. LC 00-42983. (International Congress Ser.: No. 1196). (Illus.). 382p. 144.00 (*0-444-50357-9*, Excerpta Medica) Elsevier.

New Frontiers in Psychosocial Occupational Therapy. Ed. by Anne Hiller-Scott. 1998. LC 98-36240. 176p. 29.95 (*0-7890-0652-9*) Haworth Pr.

New Frontiers in Renal Stone Disease: International ASTIF Meeting, Fiuggi, July 1998. Ed. by Vittorio E. Andreucci. 1998. (Nephron Ser.: Vol. 81, Supplement 1 (1999)). (Illus.). iv, 104p. pap. 34.00 (*3-8055-6818-5*) S Karger.

New Frontiers in Stress Research: Modulation of Brain Function. Ed. by Aharon Levy et al. 1998. (Illus.). 320p. text 125.00 (*90-5702-266-4*, Harwood Acad Pubs) Gordon & Breach.

New Frontiers in the Study of Gene Functions. G. Poste & S. T. Crooke. 1987. LC 86-30313. (New Horizons in Therapeutics Ser.). (Illus.). 218p. (C). text 75.00 (*0-306-42502-5*, Kluwer Plenum) Kluwer Academic.

New Frontiers of the Mind: The Story of the Duke Experiments. Joseph B. Rhine. 1972. LC 71-178080. (Illus.). 275p. reprint ed. lib. bdg. 49.75 (*0-8371-6279-3*, RHNF, Greenwood Pr) Greenwood.

New Generation of Antipsychotic Drugs: Novel Mechanisms of Action. N. Brunello et al. Ed. by N. Brunello et al. 1993. (International Academy for Biomedical & Drug Research Ser.: Vol. 4). (Illus.). vi, 150p. 146.25 (*3-8055-5654-3*) S Karger.

New Generation of Quinolones. C. Siporin et al. 1990. (Infectious Disease & Therapy Ser.: Vol. 5). (Illus.). 368p. text 155.00 (*0-8247-8224-0*) Dekker.

New Generation Vaccines. Myron M. Levine. 2nd ed. 1997. LC 97-12541. (Illus.). 1240p. text 225.00 (*0-8247-0061-9*) Dekker.

New Generation Vaccines: The Role of Basic Immunology. G. Poste et al. 1994. (NATO Advanced Science Institutes Ser.: Vol. 261). (Illus.). 232p. (C). text 85.00 (*0-306-44666-9*, Kluwer Plenum) Kluwer Academic.

New Genetics & Clinical Practice. D. J. Weatherall. 3rd ed. 1991. (Illus.). 392p. pap. 35.00 (*0-19-261905-5*) OUP.

New God-Image: A Study of Jung's Key Letters Concerning the Evolution of the Western God-Image. Edward F. Edinger. 1996. LC 95-51642. (Illus.). 206p. (Orig.). pap. 24.95 (*0-933029-98-5*, 985) Chiron Pubns.

New Governance: Strategies for an Era of Health Reform. Russell C. Coile, Jr. 1994. LC 93-44914. 241p. text 22.00 (*1-56793-007-7*, 0940) Health Admin Pr.

New Guidelines for Surviving Prostate Cancer. James Lewis, Jr. & E. Roy Berger. 1997. LC 95-50596. (Illus.). 460p. pap. 22.95 (*1-883257-13-1*) Hlth Edu Lit.

New Guidelines for Surviving Prostrate Cancer. James Lewis, Jr. & Roy Berger. 1996. pap. 18.95 (*0-915253-47-X*) Wilkerson Pub Co.

New Hampshire Health Care in Perspective 2000. Ed. by Kathleen O'Leary Morgan & Scott E. Morgan. 2000. 21p. spiral bd. 19.00 (*0-7401-0228-1*) Morgan Quitno Corp.

New Hampshire Health Care Perspective, 1998. Ed. by Kathleen O'Leary Morgan & Scott E. Morgan. 1998. 20p. pap. 19.00 (*1-56692-828-1*) Morgan Quitno Corp.

New Hampshire Personal Injury: Tort & Insurance Practice, 1988-1993, Vols. 8 & 9. Richard B. McNamara. 1988. (New Hampshire Practice Ser.). 950p. 140.00 (*0-88063-489-8*, MICHIE) LEXIS Pub.

New Handbook of Health & Preventive Medicine. Kurt Butler & Lynn Rayner. rev. ed. 1990. LC 90-32513. (Illus.). 450p. reprint ed. pap. 25.00 (*0-87975-581-4*) Prometheus Bks.

New Handbook Of Multicultural Assessment: Clinical, Psychological, & Educational Applications. Ed. by Lisa A. Suzuki et al. 2nd rev. ed. 2000. LC 00-59008. (Illus.). 640p. 65.00 (*0-7879-5177-3*, G873-E2F) Jossey-Bass.

New Handbook of Psychotherapy & Counseling with Men: A Comprehensive Guide to Settings, Problems & Treatment Approaches Ed. by Gary R. Brooks & Glenn E. Good. 2001. LC 00-10041. Set. 544p. 112.50 (*0-7879-5606-6*, J038-Y2t); Vol. 2. 384p. 112.50 (*0-7879-5604-X*, J035-Y2T) Jossey-Bass.

New Harvard Guide to Psychiatry. Armand M. Nicholi. 1988. LC 87-24115. (Illus.). 864p. 58.00 (*0-674-61540-9*, Belknap) HUP.

New Healing Herbs. Michael Castleman. 2001. LC 00-11434. (Illus.). xiv, 465p. pap. 17.95 (*1-57954-304-9*) Rodale Pr Inc.

New Herball, Pts. 2-3. William Turner. Ed. by George T. Chapman et al. 1996. 850p. (C). text 225.00 (*0-521-44549-3*) Cambridge U Pr.

New Holistic Herbal. David Hoffmann. 3rd ed. 1991. 284p. pap. 16.95 (*1-85230-193-7*, NEHOLP) Element MA.

New Hope!!! There Is New Hope for the Drug & Alcohol Abuser - You Too Can Be Healed! Ruth E. Norman. 1984. (Illus.). 48p. (Orig.). (C). pap. 4.00 (*0-932642-96-9*) Unarius Acad Sci.

New Hope for People with Bipolar Disorder. Jan Fawcett et al. 2000. LC 00-44127. (New Hope Ser.). (Illus.). 352p. pap. 18.95 (*0-7615-3008-8*, Prima Health) Prima Pub.

New Hope for People with Borderline Personality Disorder: Your Friendly, Authoritative Guide to the Latest in Traditional & Complementary Solutions. Neil R. Bockian & Nora Elizabeth Villagran. 2002. LC 2001-36979. (New Hope Ser.). 304p. pap. 18.95 (*0-7615-2572-6*, Prima Health) Prima Pub.

New Hope for People with Diabetes: Your Friendly, Authoritative Guide to the Latest in Traditional & Complementary Solutions. Porter Shimer. 2001. LC 2001-21482. (New Hope Ser.). 320p. pap. 18.95 (*0-7615-2571-8*, Prima Health) Prima Pub.

New Hope for People with Fibromyalgia: Your Friendly, Authoritative Guide to the Latest in Traditional & Complementary. Theresa Foy DiGeronimo. 2001. LC 2001-21490. (New Hope Ser.). 320p. pap. 18.95 (*0-7615-2098-8*, Prima Health) Prima Pub.

New Hope for People with Lupus: Your Friendly, Authoritative Guide to the Latest in Traditional & Complementary Solutions. Sara J. Henry. 2002. LC 2001-55456. (New Hope Ser.). 304p. pap. 18.95 (*0-7615-2097-X*) Prima Pub.

New Hope for People with Weight Problems: Your Friendly, Authoritative Guide to the Latest in Traditional & Complementary Solutions. Lawrence J. Cheskin & Ron Sauder. 2002. 304p. pap. 22.00 (*0-7615-1160-1*, Prima Lifesty) Prima Pub.

New Horizon for Psychotherapy: Autonomy As a Profession. Ed. by Robert R. Holt. 1971. LC 77-143391. 418p. 62.50 (*0-8236-3580-5*) Intl Univs Pr.

New Horizons: A Guide to Sexuality after Spinal Cord Injury. Pam Bieluniss. Ed. by Betty Garee. 1995. LC 95-67324. 100p. (Orig.). pap. 7.95 (*0-915708-42-6*) Cheever Pub.

New Horizons No. 3: Multiple Organ Failure. Ed. by David Bihari & Frank B. Cerra. 1989. (*0-936145-52-8*) SCCM Fullerton.

New Horizons & the Future of Heart Valve Bioprotheses: Is Glutaraldehyde a Villain? Ed. by Shlomo Gabbay & Robert W. Frater. 1995. (Illus.). 310p. (*1-878353-37-3*) Silent Partners.

New Horizons for Failing Heart Syndrome. Ed. by S. Sasayama. 1996. LC 95-44936. (*3-540-70151-6*); 125.00 (*4-431-70151-6*); (Illus.). x, 238p. 117.00 (*0-387-70151-6*) Spr-Verlag.

New Horizons in Allergy Immunotherapy: Proceedings of the Second International Conference on the Molecular Biology of Allergens & the Atopic Immune Research Held in Quebec City, Canada, February 18-22, 1995. Ed. by Alec Sehon et al. 1997. LC 96-50090. (Advances in Experimental Medicine & Biology Ser.: No. 409). (Illus.). 494p. (C). text 129.50 (*0-306-45498-X*, Kluwer Plenum) Kluwer Academic.

New Horizons in Health: An Integrative Approach. National Research Council Staff et al. Ed. by Burton H. Singer & Carol D. Ryff. 2001. LC 00-12474. 224p. pap. 39.00 (*0-309-07296-4*) Natl Acad Pr.

New Horizons in Neonatal Screening: Proceedings of the Nineth International Neonatal Screening Symposium, & the 2nd Meeting of the International Society for Neonatal Screening, Lille, France, 13-17 September 1993. Ed. by Jean-Pierre Farriaux & Jean-Louis Dhondt. 1994. LC 93-46349. (International Congress Ser.: Vol. 1041). 406p. 216.00 (*0-444-81602-X*) Elsevier.

New Horizons in Neuropsychology: Proceedings of the 9th Tokyo Metropolitan Institute of Neuroscience (TMIN) Symposium 'New Horizons in Neuropsychology', Tokyo, 24-25 November 1993. Tokyo Metropolitan Institute of Neuroscience Sympo. Ed. by Morihiro Sugishita. 1994. LC 94-37535. 242p. 184.75 (*0-444-81757-3*) Elsevier.

New Horizons in Pediatric Exercise Science. Ed. by Cameron J. Blimkie & Oded Bar-Or. 1995. LC 95-7588. 264p. text 42.00 (*0-87322-528-7*, BBLI0528) Human Kinetics.

New Horizons in Reproductive Medicine. Cristos Coutifaris & Luigi Mastroianni. 1997. LC 96-37080. (International Congress, Symposium, & Seminar Ser.: Vol. 12). (Illus.). 620p. lib. bdg. 107.95 (*1-85070-793-6*, M3604, Parthenon Pbng) CRC Pr.

New Horizons in the Pharmaceutical Industry. Business Communications Co., Inc. Staff. 1990. 245p. 2450.00 (*0-89336-566-1*, C-072) BCC.

New Horizons with Biological Response Modifiers in Haematological Malignancies. Ed. by J. M. Goldman. 1993. (Acta Haematologica Ser.: Vol. 89, Suppl. 1, 1993). (Illus.). vi, 34p. pap. 17.50 (*3-8055-5801-5*) S Karger.

New Hospital Supervisor. Nancy L. Diekelmann & Martin M. Broadwell. 1977. (Illus.). pap. text (*0-201-00773-8*) Addison-Wesley.

New Hypnosis in Family Therapy. Daniel L. Araoz & Esther Negley-Parker. 1988. LC 87-25960. 304p. text 35.95 (*0-87630-491-9*) Brunner-Routledge.

New Hypnosis in Sex Therapy: Cognitive-Behavioral Methods for Clinicians. Daniel L. Araoz. 1998. LC 97-34484. 208p. pap. 40.00 (*0-7657-0137-5*) Aronson.

New Ideas in Psychoanalysis: The Process of Change in a Humanistic Science. Ed. by Calvin F. Settlage & Reed Brockbank. 1985. 364p. text 49.95 (*0-88163-040-3*) Analytic Pr.

New Ideas in Therapy: Introduction to an Interdisciplinary Approach, 10. Ed. by Douglas H. Ruben & Dennis J. Delprato. 1987. LC 86-31922. (Contributions in Psychology Ser.: No. 10). (Illus.). 235p. 68.00 (*0-313-24845-1*, RNI/, Greenwood Pr) Greenwood.

New Ideas on the Structure of the Nervous System in Man & Vertebrates. Santiago Ramon Y Cajal. Tr. by Larry W. Swanson & Neely Swanson from FRE. 1990. 200p. 37.95 (*0-262-18141-X*) MIT Pr.

New Illustrated Family Medical & Health Guide. Consumer Guide Editors. rev. ed. 1993. (Illus.). 448p. 14.98 (*1-56173-600-7*, 3210102) Pubns Intl Ltd.

New Illustrated Medical Encyclopedia. Robert E. Rothenberg. 1990. 19.98 (*0-88365-762-7*) Galahad Bks.

New Immunology: Molecules to Medicine. S. Umlauf. 1998. (Illus.). 250p. text 45.00 (*0-8176-3968-3*) Birkhauser.

New Immunosuppressive Modalities & Antirejection Approaches in Organ Transplantation. Ed. by Jerzy W. Weglinski. 1994. LC 94-25392. (Medical Intelligence Unit Ser.). 130p. 99.00 (*1-57059-136-9*) Landes Bioscience.

New Informants: The Betrayal of Confidentiality in Psychoanalysis & Psychotherapy. Christopher Bollas & David Sundelson. 1995. LC 95-14299. 232p. 35.00 (*1-56821-595-9*) Aronson.

New Initiatives & Approaches in Health Care Quality. 1995. (Illus.). 242p. (C). pap. text 45.00 (*0-7881-2280-0*) DIANE Pub.

New Injection Treatment for Impotence: Medical & Psychological Aspects. Gorm Wagner & Helen S. Kaplan. 1993. LC 92-49232. (Illus.). 248p. text 32.95 (*0-87630-689-X*) Brunner-Routledge.

New Insights in Gynecology & Obstetrics: Research & Practice. Ed. by B. Ottesen & A. Tabor. 1998. LC 98-15899. (Illus.). 336p. lib. bdg. 137.95 (*1-85070-966-1*, Parthenon Pbng) CRC Pr.

New Insights in Vertebrate Kidney Function. Ed. by J. Anne Brown et al. 1993. (Society for Experimental Biology Seminar Ser.: No. 52). (Illus.). 403p. (C). text 100.00 (*0-521-38324-2*) Cambridge U Pr.

***New Insights into Retinal Degenerative Diseases.** Ed. by Robert E. Anderson et al. 2001. LC 2001-38936. (*0-306-46679-1*, Kluwer Plenum) Kluwer Academic.

New Insights into the Clinical Profile of Norfloxacin: Journal: European Urology, Vol. 17, Suppl. 1. Ed. by S. R. Norrby. 1990. (Illus.). iv, 52p. pap. 17.50 (*3-8055-5198-3*) S Karger.

New Insights on Renin-Angiotensin System in the Kidney. Ed. by N. Yanagawa & C. E. Palant. 1991. (Journal: Vol. 14, No. 4-5, 1991). (Illus.). 76p. pap. 72.25 (*3-8055-5378-1*) S Karger.

New International Directions in HIV Prevention for Gay & Bisexual Men. Ed. by Michael T. Wright et al. 1998. LC 98-27620. 212p. pap. 22.95 (*1-56023-116-5*); 167p. 49.95 (*0-7890-0538-7*) Haworth Pr (Harrington Park).

New International Health Order. Charles O. Pannenborg. 1980. 476p. lib. bdg. 72.00 (*90-286-0239-9*) Kluwer Academic.

New Interpretation of Dreams: Maps for Psychotherapy & the General Reader. 1997. (Illus.). 302p. pap. 30.00 (*0-9662185-0-7*) J P Gustafson.

New Invitation Bridges . . . A Curriculum for Persons with Disabilities Vol. 1: Fall. Ed. by Hilda R. Davis. 1995. 72p. pap. text 14.95 (*0-687-71978-X*) Abingdon.

New Invitation Bridges . . . A Curriculum for Persons with Disabilities Vol. 1: Winter. Ed. by Hilda R. Davis. 1995. 72p. pap. text 14.95 (*0-687-71979-8*) Abingdon.

New Invitation Bridges . . . A Curriculum for Persons with Disabilities Vol. 3: Summer. Ed. by Hilda R. Davis. 1998. 72p. pap. text 14.95 (*0-687-71989-5*) Abingdon.

New Ischemic Syndromes: Beyond Angina & Infarction. Derek M. Yellon & Shahbudin H. Rahimtoola. 1997. 254p. pap. text 59.95 (*1-881063-06-2*) Lppncott W & W.

New Jersey: Environment & Cancer. Eustace A. Dixon. Ed. by V. Eugene Vivian. 1982. (Illus.). 410p. (C). pap. 19.95 (*0-942848-01-2*) Eureka Pubns.

New Jersey Guide to Nursing Homes: And Other Care Facilities for the Elderly. Ed. by Roby McClellan. 1997. LC 97-77548. 252p. pap. 19.95 (*0-9661654-0-3*) Guide Inc.

New Jersey Health Care in Perspective 2000. Ed. by Kathleen O'Leary Morgan & Scott E. Morgan. 2000. 21p. spiral bd. 19.00 (*0-7401-0229-X*) Morgan Quitno Corp.

New Jersey Health Care Perspective, 1998. Ed. by Kathleen O'Leary Morgan & Scott E. Morgan. 1998. 20p. pap. 19.00 (*1-56692-829-X*) Morgan Quitno Corp.

New Kind of Doctor: The General Practitioner's Part in the Health of the Community. Julian T. Hart. 1988. (C). pap. (*0-85036-300-4*) MRLN GBR. *Dist:* Paul & Co Pubs.

New Knowledge in the Biomedical Sciences. Ed. by William B. Bondeson et al. 1982. 242p. text 106.00 (*90-277-1319-7*) Kluwer Academic.

New Language for Psychoanalysis. Roy Schafer. 1981. LC 75-18185. 432p. pap. 20.00 (*0-300-02761-3*) Yale U Pr.

New Language of Change: Constructive Collaboration in Psychotherapy. Steven Friedman. 1997. LC 92-49093. 464p. pap. 25.00 (*1-57230-282-8*, C0282) Guilford Pubns.

New Language of Change: Constructive Collaboration in Psychotherapy. Ed. by Steven Friedman. 1993. LC 92-49093. 464p. 46.95 (*0-89862-145-3*) Guilford Pubns.

New Leadership in Health Care Management: The Physician Executive. Ed. by Wesley Curry. 2nd ed. 1994. LC 94-72291. 329p. 45.00 (*0-924674-30-X*) Am Coll Phys Execs.

New Leafing: A Journey from Grief. Doreen Gandy. 1985. LC 85-70002. (Illus.). (Orig.). pap. 5.95 (*0-9614529-0-0*) Celilo Pubns.

New Learning Medicine. Contrib. by Peter Richards & Simon Stockill. 14th ed. 1997. 148p. pap. (*0-7279-1155-4*) BMJ Pub GBR. *Dist:* AIDC.

New Life in the Neighborhood: How Persons with Retardation & Other Disabilities Can Help Make a Good Community Better. Robert Perske. 1980. LC 80-15517. (Illus.). 80p. (Orig.). pap. text 14.00 (*0-687-27800-7*) Abingdon.

New Light on Delinquency & Its Treatment: Results of a Research Conducted for the Institute of Human Relations, Yale University. William Healy & Augusta F. Bronner. 1969. LC 79-90525. 226p. reprint ed. lib. bdg. 65.00 (*0-8371-2253-8*, HENL) Greenwood.

New Light on William Harvey. W. Pagel. 1975. (Illus.). 200p. 78.50 (*3-8055-2209-6*) S Karger.

New Literature on Fetal Alcohol Exposure & Effects: A Bibliography, 1983-1988, 4. Compiled by Ernest L. Abel. 1990. LC 89-28641. (Bibliographies & Indexes in Medical Studies: No. 4). 245p. lib. bdg. 68.50 (*0-313-27329-4*, ANL/, Greenwood Pr) Greenwood.

New Living Heart: Learn How the Heart Works, the Latest Medical Treatments & Procedures & How to Protect Yourself from All Types of Cardiovascular Diseases. Michael E. DeBakey. 1997. LC 97-365. (Illus.). xvi, 495p. pap. text 18.95 (*1-55850-722-1*) Adams Media.

New Living Heart Diet. Michael E. DeBakey et al. rev. ed. 1996. LC 95-40787. (Illus.). 416p. per. 16.00 (*0-684-81188-X*, Fireside) S&S Trade Pap.

New Look at Some Old Mechanisms in Human Newborns: Taste & Tactile Determinants of State, Affect, & Action. Elliott M. Blass & Vivian Ciaramitaro. 1994. (Monographs of the Society for Research in Child Development: No. 239). 112p. pap. text 15.00 (*0-226-05699-6*) U Ch Pr.

New Look at Tumour Immunology. Ed. by A. J. McMichael & W. F. Bodmer. 1992. (Cancer Surveys Ser.: Vol. 13). (Illus.). 208p. (C). text 66.00 (*0-87969-370-3*) Cold Spring Harbor.

New Macrolides, Azalides & Streptogramin in Clinical Practice. Acar et al. Ed. by Harold C. Neu et al. 1995. (Infectious Disease & Therapy Ser.: Vol. 18). (Illus.). 552p. text 199.00 (*0-8247-9311-0*) Dekker.

New Macrolides, Azalides, & Streptogramins: Pharmacology & Clinical Applications. Lowell S. Young et al. Ed. by Harold C. Neu & Stephen H. Zinner. 1993. (Infectious Disease & Therapy Ser.: Vol. 8). (Illus.). 256p. text 155.00 (*0-8247-9038-3*) Dekker.

New Manual for Managing Dental Office Personnel: A Management Tool for Structuring & Administering Personnel Policies in the Dental Practice. Karen Moawad & Lynne R. Costain. 1992. 368p. 79.95 (*0-87814-372-6*, D4293) PennWell Corp.

New Manual of Interventional Cardiology. Mark Freed et al. unabr. ed. 1997. 821p. text 84.95 (*1-890114-25-1*) Physicians Pr.

New Manual of Interventional Cardiology. Freed. 2nd ed. 1996. 84.95 (*0-9633886-5-7*, F0567) Physicians Pr.

New Medicaid: Issues & Prospects. Ed. by Frank J. Thompson & John J. Dilulio, Jr. 1997. LC 97-45316. 310p. text 42.95 (*0-8157-8450-3*) Brookings.

New Medical Devices: Invention, Development & Use. National Academy of Engineering Staff. 1988. 204p. 34.50 (*0-309-03847-2*); pap. 24.50 (*0-309-03846-4*) Natl Acad Pr.

New Medical Dictionary. Igakushoin. 2nd ed. 1984. (ENG & JPN.). 1045p. 150.00 (*0-8288-1849-5*, F18860) Fr & Eur.

New Medical Encyclopedia: Nueva Enciclopedia Medica G. Venzmer. 1980. (SPA.). 820p. 150.00 (*0-8288-1880-0*, S34777) Fr & Eur.

New Medical Follies. Morris Fishbein. LC 75-23711. reprint ed. 37.50 (*0-404-13262-6*) AMS Pr.

New Medical Marketplace: A Physician's Guide to Health Care Economics in the 1990s. Anne M. Stoline et al. 2nd rev. ed. 1993. LC 92-48457. 352p. pap. text 19.95 (*0-8018-4583-1*) Johns Hopkins.

New Medical Model: A Challenge for Biomedicine? H. Balner. 1989. 96p. pap. (*90-265-1067-5*) Swets.

New Medical-Pharmaceutical Dictionary. A. M. Oweida. 1970. (ARA & ENG.). 2404p. 150.00 (*0-8288-6550-7*, M-9766) Fr & Eur.

New Medical Therapies - Addictions. Ed. by Lisa Henderson. 2000. (New Medical Therapies Ser.). 14p. pap. 7.99 (*1-930624-05-0*) CenterWatch.

New Medical Therapies - Colorectal Cancer. Ed. by Lisa Henderson. 2000. (New Medical Therapies Ser.). 14p. pap. 7.99 (*1-930624-06-9*) CenterWatch.

New Medical Therapies - Hypertension/Heart Disease. Ed. by Lisa Henderson. 2000. (New Medical Therapies Ser.). 14p. pap. 7.99 (*1-930624-04-2*) CenterWatch.

***New Medical Therapies - Leukemia.** Ed. by Lisa Henderson. 2001. (New Medical Therapies Ser.). 14p. pap. 7.99 (*1-930624-16-6*) CenterWatch.

***New Medical Therapies - Melanoma.** Ed. by Lisa Henderson. 2001. (New Medical Therapies Ser.). 14p. pap. 7.99 (*1-930624-19-0*) CenterWatch.

***New Medical Therapies - Migraine.** 1999. (New Medical Therapies Ser.). 7.99 (*0-9673029-9-4*) CenterWatch.

***New Medical Therapies - Osteoporosis.** 2000. (New Medical Therapies Ser.). 7.99 (*0-9673029-4-3*) CenterWatch.

***New Medical Therapies - Prostate Cancer.** 2000. (New Medical Therapies Ser.). 7.99 (*0-9673029-8-6*) CenterWatch.

***New Medical Therapies - Schizophrenia.** Ed. by Lisa Henderson. 2001. (New Medical Therapies Ser.). 14p. pap. 7.99 (*1-930624-17-4*) CenterWatch.

***New Medications for Drug Abuse.** Ed. by Stanley D. Glick & Isabelle Maisonneuve. 2001. 220p. pap. 26.00 (*0-8018-6697-9*) NY Acad Sci.

New Medications for Drug Abuse, Vol. 909. Ed. by Stanley D. Glick & Isabelle Maisonneuve. 2000. LC 00-30527. (Annals of the New York Academy of Sciences Ser.: Vol. 909). (Illus.). x, 282p. 65.00 (*1-57331-275-4*) NY Acad Sci.

New Medications for Drugs of Abuse. Stanley D. Glick et al. 2000. LC 00-30527. (Annals of the New York Academy of Sciences Ser.: Vol. 909). (Illus.). x, 282p. pap. (*1-57331-276-2*) NY Acad Sci.

New Medicine & the Old Ethics. Albert R. Jonsen. 1992. (Illus.). 192p. (C). pap. 15.50 (*0-674-61726-6*); 1990. LC 90-33157. 176p. 23.50 (*0-674-61725-8*) HUP.

New Medicine Man: A Different Kind of Health Care for the Elderly. Hugh A. Scott. 1992. LC 91-24245. 192p. (Orig.). pap. 9.95 (*1-56474-004-8*) Fithian Pr.

New Medicines: The Practice of Medicine & Public Policy. Rock Carling Fellowship Staff & Richard Sykes. 2000. 220p. pap. (*0-11-702676-X*) Statnry Office GBR. *Dist:* Balogh.

New Methods & Technologies for Functional Genomics: Drug Discovery from Gene to Screen. Ed. by Susan Gilbert. 1997. (Biomedical Library). pap. (*1-57936-030-0*) Drug & Market Dev.

New Methods for Old-Age Research. Christine L. Fry et al. 1986. LC 85-26792. 325p. (Orig.). 62.95 (*0-89789-063-9*); pap. 24.95 (*0-89789-034-5*) Greenwood (Bergin & Garvey).

New Methods of Sensory Visual Testing. Ed. by M. Wall & A. A. Sadun. 1989. (Illus.). 137p. 68.00 (*0-387-96865-2*) Spr-Verlag.

New Mexico Health Care in Perspective 2000. Ed. by Kathleen O'Leary Morgan & Scott E. Morgan. 2000. 21p. spiral bd. 19.00 (*0-7401-0230-3*) Morgan Quitno Corp.

New Mexico Health Care Perspective, 1998. Ed. by Kathleen O'Leary Morgan & Scott E. Morgan. 1998. 20p. pap. 19.00 (*1-56692-830-3*) Morgan Quitno Corp.

New Microbiotests for Routine Toxicity Screening & Biomonitoring. Ed. by Guido Persoone et al. 2000. LC 00-38631. (Illus.). xvii, 550p. 99.50 (*0-306-46406-3*, Kluwer Plenum) Kluwer Academic.

New Microsurgical Concepts (Posterior & Anterior Segments) Ed. by J. Draeger & R. Winter. 1987. (Developments in Ophthalmology Ser.: Vol. 14). (Illus.). xii, 208p. 156.75 (*3-8055-4545-2*) S Karger.

New Midwifery: Reflections on Renaissance & Regulation. Ed. by Farah M. Shroff. 1997. 368p. pap. (*0-88961-224-2*) Womens Pr CAN. *Dist:* U of Toronto Pr.

New Model of Health & Disease. George Vithoulkas. 1991. LC 92-161429. 216p. (Orig.). pap. 14.95 (*1-55643-087-6*) North Atlantic.

New Mother's Body Book. Jacqueline Shannon. 1994. LC 93-46066. 288p. pap. 9.75 (*0-8092-3795-4*, 379540, Contemporary) McGraw-Hill Trade.

New Neuroethology on the Move: Proceedings of the 26th Goettingen Neurobiology 1998. Norbert Elsner. 1998. pap. 79.00 (*0-86577-806-X*) Thieme Med Pubs.

New No-Pill, No-Risk Birth Control: The Latest Findings on Natural Family Planning, the Method for Postponing Pregnancy Without Using Drugs, Chemicals, IUDs or Barrier Devices. Nona Aguilar. 1985. LC 85-42927. (Illus.). 240p. pap. 12.95 (*0-89256-300-1*, Rawson Assocs) Macmillan.

New Nurse. E. Michael Hanton. 1974. LC 74-79614. 122p. 10.00 (*0-914698-01-X*); pap. 6.95 (*0-914698-02-8*) New Nurse.

New Nutrients Against Cancer. Judi Quilici-Timmcke. 1998. LC 99-185182. 48p. pap. 3.95 (*0-87983-890-6*, Keats Pubng) McGraw-Hill Trade.

New Nutrition: Medicine for the Millennium. Michael Colgan. 1995. (Your Personal Guide to Health Ser.). (Illus.). 261p. 24.95 (*0-9624840-6-7*); pap. 14.95 (*0-9624840-7-5*) Colgan Inst.

New Older Woman: A Dialogue for the Coming Century. Peggy Downs et al. 1995. LC 95-42795. 196p. text 12.95 (*0-89087-769-6*) Celestial Arts.

New Option in Low-Dose Oral Contraception: Expanding the Gestadene Choice. Ed. by P. Lopes & S. R. Killick. 1996. LC 96-33683. (Illus.). 70p. lib. bdg. 27.95 (*1-85070-739-1*, Parthenon Pbng) CRC Pr.

New Orleans' Charity Hospital: A Story of Physicians, Politics, & Poverty. John E. Salvaggio. 1992. LC 91-44719. (Illus.). 264p. (C). text 45.00 (*0-8071-1613-0*) La State U Pr.

New Ourselves, Growing Older. Paula B. Doress-Worters & Diana L. Siegal. 1996. 31.00 (*0-8446-6844-3*) Peter Smith.

New Ourselves, Growing Older: Revised & Updated. Paula B. Doress-Worters & Diana L. Siegal. 1994. LC 93-48494. (Illus.). 560p. per. 20.00 (*0-671-87297-4*, Touchstone) S&S Trade Pap.

New Outline of Social Psychology. Martin Gold. 1997. LC 96-54814. 287p. 29.95 (*1-55798-408-5*, 431-6840) Am Psychol.

New Paradigm for Informed Consent. Irene S. Switankowsky. 1998. LC 97-50149. (Illus.). 160p. 34.50 (*0-7618-1016-1*) U Pr of Amer.

New Pathways in Medical Education: Learning to Learn at Harvard Medical School. Ed. by Daniel C. Tosteson et al. 1994. (Illus.). 192p. pap. text 22.50 (*0-674-61739-8*, TOSNEX) HUP.

New Pathways to Medical Education: Learning to Learn to at Harvard Medical School. Ed. by Daniel C. Tosteson et al. 1994. LC 94-11196. (Illus.). 192p. text 39.00 (*0-674-61738-X*, TOSNEW) HUP.

New Pediatrics: A Profession in Transition. Dorothy Pawluch. 1996. LC 96-1029. (Social Problems & Social Issues Ser.). 187p. lib. bdg. 43.95 (*0-202-30534-1*) Aldine de Gruyter.

New Personality Self-Portrait: Why You Think, Work, Love & Act the Way You Do. John M. Oldham & Lois B. Morris. rev. ed. 1995. LC 95-12233. Orig. Title: The Personality Self-Portrait. 464p. pap. 14.95 (*0-553-37393-5*) Bantam.

New Perspectives in Diagnosis & Treatment of Kidney Disease. Ed. by G. Colasanti & G. D'Amico. 1987. (Contributions to Nephrology Ser.: Vol. 55). (Illus.). vi, 258p. 29.75 (*3-8055-4393-X*) S Karger.

New Perspectives in Early Emotional Development. Ed. by John G. Warhol. unabr. ed. 1998. (Pediatric Round Table Ser.). (Illus.). 300p. pap. text 10.00 (*0-931562-19-8*) J & J Consumer Prods.

New Perspectives in Hemodialysis, Peritoneal Dialysis, Arteriovenous Hemofiltration, & Plasmapheresis. Ed. by Walter H. Horl & P. J. Schollmeyer. 1989. LC 89-22951. (Advances in Experimental Medicine & Biology Ser.). (Illus.). 226p. 69.50 (*0-306-43376-1*, Plenum Trade) Perseus Pubng.

New Perspectives in Histamine Research. Ed. by H. Timmerman & H. Van der Goot. 1991. (Agents & Actions Supplements Ser.: Vol. 33). 448p. 136.50 (*0-8176-2507-0*) Birkhauser.

New Perspectives in Lung Cancer. Ed. by N. Thatcher & S. Spiro. 1994. 203p. pap. text (*0-7279-0786-7*) BMJ Pub GBR. *Dist:* AIDC.

New Perspectives in Molecular & Clinical Management of Gastrointestinaltumors. Ed. by E. D. Kreuser & P. M. Schlag. 1996. LC 95-39447. (Recent Results in Cancer Research Ser.: Vol. 142). (Illus.). 480p. 157.00 (*3-540-60498-7*) Spr-Verlag.

New Perspectives in Nuclear Medicine. Ed. by Peter H. Cox & E. Touja. 1986. (Monographs in Nuclear Medicine: Vol. 2). xxviii, 414p. text 489.00 (*2-88124-131-X*) Gordon & Breach.

New Perspectives in Nuclear Medicine Vol. 1: Clinical in Vitro Studies. P. H. Cox & E. Touja. 1986. xxx, 394p. (*2-88124-129-8*) Gordon & Breach.

New Perspectives in Nuclear Medicine Vol. 2: Instrumentation, Laboratory Investigations & in Vitro Studies. P. H. Cox & E. Touja. 1986. (*2-88124-130-1*) Gordon & Breach.

New Perspectives in Psychoanalysis. Ed. by Harold Kelman. 1965. 5.00 (*0-393-01028-7*) Norton.

New Perspectives on Adolescent Risk Behavior. Ed. by Richard Jesor. 1998. LC 97-49944. (Illus.). 576p. (C). text 59.95 (*0-521-58432-9*); pap. text 21.95 (*0-521-58607-0*) Cambridge U Pr.

New Perspectives on Benign Prostatic Hypertrophy (BPH) Paul D. Miller. 2001. (New Perspectives Ser.). (Illus.). 124p. pap. text 26.95 (*1-873413-62-9*) Merit Pub Intl.

New Perspectives on Dermatological Infections (Handbook) J. Bikowski. 1995. 9.95 (*1-873413-16-5*) Merit Pub Intl.

New Perspectives on Genetic Markers & Diseases among Jewish People. Batsheva Bonne-Tamir. 1992. (Illus.). 488p. text 69.50 (*0-19-506817-3*) OUP.

New Perspectives on Human Abortion. Ed. by Thomas W. Hilgers et al. 1981. LC 81-51983. 504p. lib. bdg. 55.00 (*0-313-27079-1*, U7079) Greenwood.

New Perspectives on Hypertension. Adrian Brady. 2001. (New Perspectives Ser.). 128p. pap. text 29.95 (*1-873413-67-X*) Merit Pub Intl.

New Perspectives on Psychotherapy & Homosexualities. Ed. by Christopher Shelley. 1998. 275p. (*1-85343-403-5*); pap. (*1-85343-404-3*) Free Assoc Bks GBR. *Dist:* Intl Spec Bk, NYU Pr.

New Perspectives on the Treatment of Obesity & Redux: A Comprehensive Overview. Ed. by Stylianos Nicolaidis. 1996. LC 96-36686. (Illus.). 150p. pap. text 36.00 (*0-12-518170-1*) Acad Pr.

New Perspectives on Therapeutics in the Elderly. Mark T. Kinirons. 2001. (New Perspectives Ser.). (Illus.). 128p. pap. text 26.95 (*1-873413-08-4*) Merit Pub Intl.

New Pesticide User's Guide. Bert L. Bohmont. 1983. (C). (*0-8359-4891-9*); text 45.00 (*0-8359-4890-0*) P-H.

New Pharmacological & Epidemiological Data in Analgesics Research. Kay Brune. 1990. 60p. 25.00 (*0-8176-2452-X*) Birkhauser.

New Pharmacological Approaches to the Therapy of Depressive Disorders. Ed. by G. Racagni et al. 1993. (International Academy for Biomedical & Drug Research Ser.: Vol. 5). (Illus.). vi, 196p. 194.00 (*3-8055-5746-9*) S Karger.

New Pharmacotherapy of Schizophrenia. Ed. by Alan Breier. 1996. (Clinical Practice Ser.: No. 36). 272p. text 33.50 (*0-88048-491-8*, 8491) Am Psychiatric.

New Phrenology: The Limits of Localizing Cognitive Processes in the Brain. William R. Uttal. 2001. LC 00-52534. (Life & Mind Ser.). (Illus.). 317p. 42.00 (*0-262-21017-7*) MIT Pr.

New Physician's Guide to Legal Medicine. RiskCare Staff & Chad D. Kollas. 1997. 59p. pap. text 19.00 (*1-893929-06-X*) RiskCare.

New Plant Sources for Drugs & Foods from the New York Botanical Garden Herbarium. Siri V. Von Reis & Frank J. Lipp. 1982. LC 81-6280. (Illus.). 376p. 47.95 (*0-674-61765-7*) HUP.

New Possibilities for Weight Reduction. Ed. by J. C. Somogyi. 1986. (Bibliotheca Nutritio et Dieta Ser.: No. 39). (Illus.). xx, 68p. 68.75 (*3-8055-4416-2*) S Karger.

New Practice Handbook: A Guide to Establishing a Successful Medical Practice. Maryann Szostak-Ricardo. 1994. 115p. stu. ed. 49.95 (*1-57066-029-8*) Practice Mgmt Info.

New Prescription: Marijuana As Medicine. Martin Martinez. Ed. by Francis Podrebarac. 2nd ed. 2000. 142p. pap. text 14.95 (*0-932551-35-1*) Quick Am Pub.

New Prescription Drug Reference Guide. Consumer Guide Editors. 1993. (Illus.). 448p. 14.98 (*1-56173-601-5*, 3210801) Pubns Intl Ltd.

New Primal Scream: Primal Therapy 20 Years On. Arthur Janov. 2000. 432p. pap. (*0-349-10203-1*) Little Brown GBR. *Dist:* Trafalgar.

New Pritikin Program. Robert C. Pritikin. Ed. by Julie Rubenstein. 1991. 464p. reprint ed. mass mkt. 6.99 (*0-671-73194-7*) PB.

New Procedures in Nuclear Medicine. Ed. by Richard P. Spencer. 1989. LC 88-26260. 224p. 134.00 (*0-8493-4592-8*, R895, CRC Reprint) Franklin.

New Protein Foods in Human Health: Nutrition, Prevention & Therapy. F. H. Steinke et al. 1991. (Illus.). 232p. 129.00 (*0-8493-6904-5*, TX558) CRC Pr.

New Psychiatry. Jack M. Gorman. 1996. LC 96-2878. (Illus.). 416p. 27.50 (*0-312-14690-6*) St Martin.

New Psychiatry. Wilbur. 1994. 23.99 (*0-02-933220-6*) S&S Trade.

New Psychiatry: The Essential Guide to State-of-the-Art Therapy, Medication, & Emotional Health. Jack M. Gorman. 1998. (Illus.). 389p. text 27.00 (*0-7881-5563-6*) DIANE Pub.

New Psychology of Women: Gender, Culture & Ethnicity. Hilary M. Lips. 1999. LC 98-19271. xviii, 413p. (C). pap. text 40.00 (*1-55934-334-6*, 334-6) Mayfield Pub.

New Psychometrics: Science, Psychology, & Measurement. Paul Kline. 1998. LC 98-13276. 208p. (C). 89.95 (*0-415-18751-6*) Routledge.

New Psychotherapy for Traditional Men. Gary R. Brooks. 1998. LC 97-45455. 272p. 43.00 (*0-7879-4123-9*) Jossey-Bass.

New Public Health. John Ashton & Howard Seymour. 1988. 160p. (*0-335-15555-3*); pap. (*0-335-15550-2*) OpUniv Pr.

New Public Health. Theodore H. Tulchinsky & Elena V. Varavikova. 1999. LC 99-66055. (Illus.). xxi, 882p. (C). pap. 69.95 (*0-12-703350-5*) Acad Pr.

New Public Health. Hibbert W. Hill. Ed. by Barbara G. Rosenkrantz. 1977. LC 76-40630. (Public Health in America Ser.). (Illus.). reprint ed. lib. bdg. 20.95 (*0-405-09823-5*) Ayer.

New Radiance Metaphysical & Holistic Florida Directory. Barbara Casey. 1997. pap. 7.95 (*1-889131-35-0*) CasAnanda.

New Radiotracers in Cardiac Imaging: Principles & Approach. Raymond Taillefer. 1998. LC 98-38333. 224p. text 159.00 (*0-8385-6749-5*) McGraw-Hill Prof.

New Reproductive Techniques: A Legal Perspective. Douglas J. Cusine. (Medico-Legal Issues Ser.). 1990. pap. (*1-85521-007-X*); 1988. 280p. text (*0-566-05410-8*) Dartmth Pub GBR. *Dist:* Ashgate Pub Co.

***New Reproductive Technologies & the Health Care System: The Case for Evidence-Based Medicine.** 809p. pap. (*0-662-21385-8*) Can7 Govern Pub CAN. *Dist:* Intl Spec Bk.

***New Reproductive Technologies & the Science, Industry, Education & Social Welfare Systems in Canada.** 493p. pap. (*0-662-21379-3*) Can7 Govern Pub CAN. *Dist:* Intl Spec Bk.

New Research & Child Witnesses Pt. I: A Special Issue of Applied Developmental Science. Ed. by Michael Lamb. 1999. 72p. pap. 20.00 (*0-8058-9800-X*) L Erlbaum Assocs.

New Research in Psychiatry. Ed. by H. Hafner & E. M. Wolpert. rev. ed. 1996. LC 96-931354. (Illus.). 190p. text 38.00 (*0-88937-174-1*) Hogrefe & Huber Pubs.

New Research on Child Witnesses Pt. II: A Special Issue in Applied Developmental Science. Ed. by Michael E. Lamb. 1999. 80p. pap. 20.00 (*0-8058-9795-X*) L Erlbaum Assocs.

New Research on the Aetiology & Surgery of Retinal Detachment: Proceedings of the Jules Gorin Club, 9th Meeting, La Baule, May 1974. Gorin, Jules, Club Staff. Ed. by E. B. Streiff. 1975. (Modern Problems in Ophthalmology Ser.: Vol. 15). (Illus.). xiv, 338p. 132.75 (*3-8055-2141-3*) S Karger.

New Roles for Psychiatrists in Organized Systems of Care. Ed. by Jeremy A. Lazarus & Steven S. Sharfstein. 1998. LC 97-50111. (Issues in Psychiatry Ser.). 271p. pap. text 36.00 (*0-88048-758-5*, 8758) Am Psychiatric.

New Rules: Regulation, Markets & the Quality of American Health Care. Troyen A. Brennan & Donald M. Berwick. 1995. LC 95-30487. (Health Ser.). 404p. 50.00 (*0-7879-0149-0*) Jossey-Bass.

New Rules of Healthcare Marketing: 23 Strategies for Success. Arthur C. Sturm. 1998. LC 97-42425. xvii, 117p. pap. 33.00 (*1-56793-074-3*) Health Admin Pr.

New Rules of Measurement: What Every Psychologist & Educator Should Know. Ed. by Susan E. Embretson & Scott L. Hershberger. 1999. LC 98-24513. 272p. 69.95 (*0-8058-2860-5*) L Erlbaum Assocs.

New School Health Handbook: A Ready Reference for School Nurses & Educators. Jerry Newton et al. 1997. LC 97-7189. 388p. text 34.95 (*0-13-614652-X*) P-H.

New Science: Self-Esteem Psychology. Robert N. Campbell. 1984. LC 84-5085. 354p. (Orig.). lib. bdg. 61.00 (*0-8191-3892-4*) U Pr of Amer.

New Science of Technical Analysis: Using the Statistical Techniques of Neuroscience. Clifford Sherry. 1994. 300p. text 60.00 (*1-55738-502-5*, Irwn Prfssnl) McGraw-Hill Educ Grp.

New Self: Self Therapy with Transactional Analysis. Muriel James & Louis M. Savary. 1977. LC 76-55632. (Illus.). pap. 8.61 (*0-201-03463-8*) Addison-Wesley.

New Sex Therapy: Active Treatment of Sexual Dysfunctions. Helen S. Kaplan. 1974. LC 73-7729. 554p. text 52.95 (*0-87630-083-2*) Brunner-Routledge.

New Short Textbook of Chemical Pathology. 288p. pap. text (*0-340-37686-4*) E A GBR. *Dist:* Routldge.

New Short Textbook of Psychiatry. 280p. pap. (*0-340-40543-0*) E A GBR. *Dist:* Routldge.

New Siwalik Primates: Their Bearing on the Question of Evolution of Man & the Anthropoidea. G. E. Pilgrim. LC 77-86436. (India Geological Survey: Records of the Geological Survey of India Ser.: Vol. 45). reprint ed. 15.00 (*0-404-16675-X*) AMS Pr.

New Sjogren's Syndrome Handbook. Sjogren's Syndrome Foundation Staff. Ed. by Steven Carsons & Elaine K. Harris. 1998. LC 97-44421. (Illus.). 256p. 25.00 (*0-19-511724-7*) OUP.

New Statistical Procedures for the Social Sciences: Modern Solutions to Basic Problems. Randy Wilcox. 1987. 442p. 89.95 (*0-89859-936-9*) L Erlbaum Assocs.

New Strategies for Treating Children's Articulation & Phonological Disorders. Ken Bleile. 1998. 110.00 incl. VHS (*1-58041-017-0*, 0112092) Am Speech Lang Hearing.

New Strategies in Clinical Nutrition. Ed. by P. Furst. 1993. (Clinical Nutrition Ser.: Vol. 33). (Illus.). 88p. text (*3-88603-462-3*) W Zuckschwerdt DEU. *Dist:* Scholium Intl.

New Strategies in Fungal Disease. Ed. by John E. Bennett et al. 1992. (Frontiers of Infectious Diseases Ser.). (Illus.). 312p. (Orig.). pap. text (*0-443-04684-0*) Church.

New Super Antioxidant Plus. Richard A. Passwater. 1992. 46p. pap. 3.95 (*0-87983-589-3*, 35893K, Keats Pubng) McGraw-Hill Trade.

New Supernutrition. Richard A. Passwater. 1991. 337p. mass mkt. 6.99 (*0-671-70071-5*) PB.

M
N
O

New Syntheses with Carbon Monoxide. Ed. by Jurgen Falbe. 1980. (Reactivity & Structure Ser.: Vol. 11). (Illus.). 465p. 229.00 (*0-387-09674-4*) Spr-Verlag.

New Systemic Ideas from the Italian Mental Health Movement. Laura Fruggeri et al. 1992. 112p. pap. text (*1-85575-016-3*) Karnac Bks GBR. *Dist:* Other Pr LLC.

New Targets in Cancer Chemotherapy. David J. Kerr. 1994. 236p. 189.00 (*0-8493-4905-2*, RC268) CRC Pr.

New Techniques in Reconstructive Urology. Jack W. McAninch. 1996. (Illus.). 160p. (*0-89640-281-9*) Igaku-Shoin.

New Techniques of Osteosynthesis of the Hand. F. Schuind. 1990. (Reconstruction Surgery & Traumatology Ser.: Vol. 21). (Illus.). x, 156p. 137.50 (*3-8055-5194-0*) S Karger.

New Technologies & Concepts for Reducing Drug Toxicities. Harry Salem & Steven I. Baskin. 1992. 176p. lib. bdg. 95.00 (*0-8493-8896-1*, RA1238) CRC Pr.

New Technologies & the Future of Food & Nutrition. Ed. by Gerald E. Gaull & Ray A. Goldberg. 1991. LC 91-18915. 192p. 120.00 (*0-471-55408-1*) Wiley.

New Technologies for Liver Resections. Ed. by R. Dionigi & Juan Madariaga. 1997. LC 97-6443. (Medical Intelligence Unit Ser.). (Illus.). xiv, 268p. 98.00 (*3-8055-6564-X*) S Karger.

New Technologies in Clinical Laboratory Science. Ed. by K. Shinton. 1985. text 147.50 (*0-85200-927-5*) Kluwer Academic.

New Technologies in Hospital Information Systems. Ed. by J. Dudeck et al. 1997. LC 97-75049. (Studies in Health Technology & Informatics: Vol. 45). 250p. 86.00 (*90-5199-363-3*, 363-3) IOS Press.

New Technologies in Reproductive Medicine, Neonatology & Gynecology: The Proceedings of the 1st International Symposium, Folgaria, Italy. Ermelando V. Cosmi. 1999. LC 99-21828. (Illus.). 368p. lib. bdg. 96.95 (*1-85070-065-6*, Parthenon Pbng) CRC Pr.

New Technologies in the Fight Against Transboundary Animal Diseases. Prod. by Food and Agriculture Organization of the United Nations Staff. 2000. (Animal Production & Health Papers: No. 145). 130p. pap. (*92-5-104358-2*, F43582) FAO ITA. *Dist:* Bernan Associates.

New Technology in Medical Plastics. Ed. by M. Weiselberg & R. H. Bauman. 1990. 177p. reprint ed. pap. 42.00 (*0-938648-20-9*) T-C Pr CA.

New Themes in Palliative Care. David Clark et al. 1997. LC 97-12123. 336p. pap. (*0-335-19605-5*) OpUniv Pr.

New Themes in Palliative Care. Clark et al. 1997. LC 97-12123. 306p. (*0-335-19606-3*) OpUniv Pr.

New Theory of Arthritis Based on the Edgar Cayce Readings. Carol Baraff. 1981. 43p. 2.00 (*1-882545-01-X*) Herit Pubns.

New Therapeutic Agents in Thrombosis & Thrombolysis. Ed. by Loscalzo & Arthur A. Sasahara. 1997. LC 97-12542. (Illus.). 700p. text 225.00 (*0-8247-9866-X*) Dekker.

New Therapeutic Indications of Antidepressants: Workshop, Bruges, March 1996. Ed. by Julien Mendlewicz et al. 1997. LC 97-4322. (International Academy for Biomedical & Drug Research Ser.: Vol. 12, 1997). (Illus.). vi, 138p. 139.25 (*3-8055-6436-8*) S Karger.

New Therapeutic Strategies in Nephrology: Proceedings of the 3rd International Meeting on Current Therapy in Nephrology. Ed. by Vittorio E. Andreucci & Antonio D. Canton. 1991. (Developments in Nephrology Ser.). 576p. text 197.00 (*0-7923-1199-X*) Kluwer Academic.

New Therapeutic Uses of Calcium Channel Blockers. Ed. by H. Glossmann. 1990. (Journals of Neural Transmission: Suppl. 31). (Illus.). 65p. 52.95 (*0-387-82200-3*) Spr-Verlag.

New Therapeutic Visions. Ed. by Arnold Goldberg. 1992. (Progress in Self Psychology Ser.: Vol. 8). 288p. text 45.00 (*0-88163-150-7*) Analytic Pr.

New Therapies for Neonatal Respiratory Failure: A Physiological Approach. Ed. by Bruce R. Boynton et al. 1994. (Illus.). 377p. (C). text 95.00 (*0-521-43161-1*) Cambridge U Pr.

New "Thin" You: The Simple Safe Secret to Lose Weight Once & Forever Naturally. A. Tony Martin. 1999. LC 99-75513. 180p. reprint ed. pap. 9.95 (*1-884820-56-5*) SAFE GOODS.

New Thinking on Financing & Regulating Long-Term Care. Wendy Fox-Grage. 1998. 20.00 incl. audio (*1-55516-821-3*) Natl Conf State Legis.

New Treatment of Alcohol & Substance Abuse in Akhter Absen's Eidetic Image Therapy. Toni Nixon. 1997. 308p. pap. 25.00 (*0-913412-39-2*) Brandon Hse.

New Treatment of Diseases: Therapeutics Founded upon Histology & Cellular Pathology. W. H. Schussler. 1991. lib. bdg. 79.95 (*0-8490-4106-6*) Gordon Pr.

New Treatments for Chemical Addictions. Ed. by Elinore F. McCance-Katz & Thomas R. Kosten. 1998. LC 98-6546. (Review of Psychiatry Series, Ser.). 211p. pap. text 39.00 (*0-88048-838-7*, 8838) Am Psychiatric.

New Treatments for Opiate Dependence. Ed. by Susan M. Stine & Thomas R. Kosten. 1997. LC 97-3244. (Substance Abuse Ser.). 286p. text 40.00 (*1-57230-190-2*, 0190) Guilford Pubns.

New Trends & Developments in Carotid Artery Disease. Ed. by Alain Branchereau & Michael Jacobs. 1998. LC 98-6275. (Illus.). 284p. 110.00 (*0-87993-403-4*) Futura Pub.

New Trends in Aging Research. Ed. by Giancarlo Pepeu et al. 1989. (FIDIA Research Ser.: Vol. 15). 237p. 79.00 (*0-387-96911-X*) Spr-Verlag.

New Trends in Allergy. Ed. by G. Burg & Johannes Ring. 1981. (Illus.). 333p. 79.95 (*0-387-10346-5*) Spr-Verlag.

New Trends in Allergy, No. III. Ed. by B. Przybilla & Johannes Ring. 1991. (Illus.). 575p. 249.00 (*0-387-52993-4*) Spr-Verlag.

New Trends in Allergy IV, Together with Environmental Allergy & Allergotoxicology III: Joint International Symposium, Hamburg, April 29-May 1, 1995. Johannes Ring et al. 1996. LC 96-42937. (Illus.). 376p. 199.00 (*3-540-61120-7*) Spr-Verlag.

New Trends in Antivirals: Highlighting Antisense Oligonucleotides. BCC Staff. 1990. 156p. 2450.00 (*0-89336-619-6*, C109) BCC.

New Trends in Cerebral Hemodynamics & Neurosonology: Proceedings of the 10th International Symposium on Cerebral Hemodynamics, Munich, Germany, 29 August-1 September, 1996. Jurgen Klingelhofer et al. 1997. LC 97-41501. 864p. 261.50 (*0-444-82631-9*) Elsevier.

New Trends in Clinical Pharmacology. D. Bartko et al. 1988. (Current Problems in Neurology Ser.: Vol. 7). 320p. (*0-86196-146-3*) J Libbey Med GBR. *Dist:* Bks Intl VA.

New Trends in Conceptual Representation: Challenges to Piaget's Theory. Ellin K. Scholnick. 1983. (Jean Piaget Symposia Ser.). 304p. (C). text 59.95 (*0-89859-260-7*) L Erlbaum Assocs.

New Trends in Diagnosis & Management of Stroke. Ed. by Klaus Poeck et al. 1987. (Illus.). 147p. 33.10 (*0-387-18369-8*) Spr-Verlag.

New Trends in Ganglioside Research: Neurochemical & Neuroregenerative Aspects. Ed. by Robert W. Ledeen et al. 1988. (FIDIA Research Ser.: Vol. 14). 660p. 189.00 (*0-387-96797-4*) Spr-Verlag.

New Trends in Gastric Cancer. Ed. by P. I. Reed et al. 1990. (Developments in Oncology Ser.). (C). text 123.00 (*0-7923-8917-4*) Kluwer Academic.

New Trends in Haemostasis: Coagulation Proteins, Endothelium, & Tissue Factors. Ed. by F. Gotthard Schettler et al. 1990. (Sitzungsberichte der Heidelberger Akademie der Wissenschaften Ser., Mathematisch-Naturwissenschaftliche Klasse, Jahrgang 1991: Suppl. 3). (Illus.). 280p. 45.00 (*0-387-53275-7*) Spr-Verlag.

New Trends in Heart Transplantation. Ed. by M. Havel. 1989. (Bibliotheca Cardiologica Ser.: No. 43). viii, 168p. 127.00 (*3-8055-4792-7*) S Karger.

New Trends in Hepatology, Vol. 15. Ed. by Paolo Gentilini. 1996. 352p. (C). text 129.00 (*0-7923-8703-1*) Kluwer Academic.

New Trends in Hepatology, 1996: Proceedings of the Falk Symposium No. 92, St. Petersburg. Ed. by W. Gerok et al. 1997. (Falk Symposium Ser.: No. 92). 256p. text 120.50 (*0-7923-8723-6*) Kluwer Academic.

New Trends in Management of Cerebro-Vascular Malformation: Proceedings of the International Conference, Verona, Italy, June 8-12, 1992. Ed. by A. Pasqualin & R. Da Pian. 1994. LC 94-7680. 600p. 280.00 (*0-387-82528-2*) Spr-Verlag.

New Trends in Management of Cerebro-Vascular Malformation: Proceedings of the International Conference, Verona, Italy, June 8-12, 1992. Ed. by A. Pasqualin & R. DaPian. 1994. LC 94-7680. (*3-211-82528-2*) Spr-Verlag.

New Trends in Medical Technologies & Hospital Management: French Experiences. Asian Productivity Organization Staff. 1991. 126p. pap. text 15.00 (*92-833-2099-9*, 320999) Product Pr.

New Trends in Nuclear Neurology & Psychiatry. Costa. 1993. 192p. (*0-86196-401-2*) J Libbey Med GBR. *Dist:* Buttrwrth-Heinemann.

New Trends in Osteoarthritis. Ed. by E. C. Huskisson & G. Katona. 1982. (Rheumatology Ser.: Vol. 7). (Illus.). vi, 198p. 69.75 (*3-8055-3487-6*) S Karger.

New Trends in Patient Education: A Trans-Cultural & Inter-Disease Approach: Proceedings of the Patient Education 2000 Congress, Geneva, 1-4 June 1994. Ed. by Jean-Philippe Assal et al. 1995. (International Congress Ser.: Vol. 1076). 400p. 185.00 (*0-444-82234-8*) Elsevier.

New Trends in Pharmacokinetics. Ed. by A. Rescigno & A. K. Thakur. 1992. (NATO Advanced Science Institutes Ser.: Vol. 221). (Illus.). 456p. (C). text 168.00 (*0-306-44089-X*, Kluwer Plenum) Kluwer Academic.

New Trends in Radiopharmaceutical Synthesis, Quality Assurance & Regulatory Control. Ed. by A. M. Emran. 1991. (Illus.). 536p. (C). text 174.00 (*0-306-44035-0*, Kluwer Plenum) Kluwer Academic.

New Trends in Referred Pain & Hyperalgesia. Ed. by L. Vecchiet et al. 1993. LC 93-10736. (Pain Research & Clinical Management Ser.). 468p. 251.50 (*0-444-89631-7*) Elsevier.

New Trends in Reproductive Medicine. Ed. by K. H. Broer & I. Turanli. 1996. LC 95-44731. (Illus.). 448p. 147.00 (*3-540-58981-3*) Spr-Verlag.

New Trends in Suicide Prevention. Julien Mendlewicz. Ed. by J. Wilmotte. 1982. (Bibliotheca Psychiatrica Ser.: No. 162). (Illus.). vi, 106p. pap. 41.75 (*3-8055-3430-2*) S Karger.

New Trends in the Diagnosis & Therapy of Non-Alzheimer's Dementia. Ed. by K. A. Jellinger & M. Windisch. 1996. (Journals of Neural Transmission: Vol. 47). 290p. 131.00 (*3-211-82823-0*) Spr-Verlag.

New Trends in the Therapy of Liver Disease: Proceedings of the International Symposium on Tirrenia, June, 1974. Ed. by A. Bertelli. 1975. 300p. 54.50 (*3-8055-2118-9*) S Karger.

New Trends in Ulcer Disease. F. Di Mario et al. 1988. 314p. text (*1-57235-018-0*) Piccin Nuova.

New Trends in Urinary Tract Infections. Ed. by H. C. Neu & J. D. Williams. 1988. (Illus.). x, 358p. 214.00 (*3-8055-4637-8*) S Karger.

New Types of Cardiovascular Diseases: Topics in Clinical Cardiology. Ed. by J. Willis Hurst. 1994. LC 93-11899. (Illus.). 312p. 69.50 (*0-89640-245-2*) Igaku-Shoin.

New Vaccine Development - Establishing Priorities Vol. 2: Diseases of Importance in Developing Countries. Institute of Medicine Staff. 1986. 432p. pap. text 43.50 (*0-309-03679-8*) Natl Acad Pr.

New Vaccine for Child Safety. Murl Harmon. 1976. LC 76-8726. (Illus.). pap. 7.50 (*0-917066-00-6*) Safety Now.

New View of Insanity: The Duality of the Mind Proved by the Structure, Functions, & Diseases of the Brain, & by the Phenomena of Mental Derangement. Arthur L. Wigan. LC 78-72829. (Brainedness, Handedness, & Mental Abilities Ser.). reprint ed. 37.50 (*0-404-60897-3*) AMS Pr.

New Vistas in Depression. Ed. by S. Z. Langer et al. 1982. (Illus.). 339p. 69.50 (*0-08-027388-2*, Pergamon Pr) Elsevier.

New Vistas in Parkinson's Disease. Ed. by T. Caraceni et al. 1986. (Journals of Neural Transmission: Suppl. 22). (Illus.). 280p. pap. 68.00 (*0-387-81929-0*) Spr-Verlag.

New Vistas in Psychology: An Anthroposophical Contribution. Stewart C. Easton. 1986. 146p. pap. (*0-85440-454-6*) R Steiner Pr GBR. *Dist:* Anthroposophic.

New Vocabulary of Medical Terms (Uj Magyar Orvosi Szotar) J. Brencsan. 1993. 544p. (*963-05-6497-1*) Akade Kiado HUN. *Dist:* St Mut.

New Way to Fly: An Alternative Way to Achieve Freedom from Alcohol & Drugs. Ken Mills. 1987. LC 87-60845. 184p. (Orig.). pap. text 6.95 (*0-942267-00-1*) Profile Press.

New Way to Take Charge of Your Medical Treatment: A Patient's Guide. Barbara Hardt & Katharine R. Halkin. 1994. LC 94-38467. 144p. (Orig.). pap. 10.95 (*1-56833-034-0*) Madison Bks UPA.

New Ways to Care for Older People: Building Systems Based on Evidence in Managed Care. Ed. by Evan Calkins et al. 1998. LC 98-38606. (Illus.). 280p. 42.95 (*0-8261-1220-X*) Springer Pub.

New Well Pregnancy Book. Mike Samuels & Nancy H. Samuels. rev. ed. 1996. LC 96-7186. 496p. per. 20.00 (*0-684-81057-3*, Fireside) S&S Trade Pap.

New Woman, New Earth: Sexist Ideologies & Human Liberation. Rosemary Radford Ruether. 1995. LC 95-16969. 256p. (C). pap. 14.00 (*0-8070-6503-X*) Beacon Pr.

New World Plants & Their Uses: A Guide to Selected Literature & Genetic Resources 1980-1993. Joanne Meil. 1995. (Illus.). 39p. (Orig.). (C). pap. text 20.00 (*0-7881-1613-4*) DIANE Pub.

New York Academy of Medicine, 1947-1997: Enhancing the Health of the Public. Marvin Lieberman & Leon J. Warshaw. 1998. LC 97-29698. 428p. 69.50 (*0-89464-984-1*) Krieger.

New York City Community Health Atlas. Compiled by Division of Research, Analysis, and Planning Staff. 1985. LC 85-675630. 40.00 (*0-934459-15-0*) United Hosp Fund.

New York City Community Health Atlas, 1988. Melvin I. Krasner. 1988. LC 85-645644. 216p. 40.00 (*0-934459-51-7*) United Hosp Fund.

New York City Community Health Atlas, 1994. Melvin I. Krasner. 1994. LC 94-6675. 192p. 50.00 (*1-881277-00-3*) United Hosp Fund.

New York City Health Facts: A Profile from the National Health Interview Survey. United Hospital Fund Staff. 1989. 56p. 20.00 (*0-934459-54-1*) United Hosp Fund.

New York City Health Trends, 1979-1989. 1993. 56p. pap. 20.00 (*0-934459-99-1*) United Hosp Fund.

New York City's Hospital Occupancy Crisis: Caring for a Changing Patient Population. Bigel Institute for Health Policy Staff & United Hospital Fund Staff. 1988. 36p. 25.00 (*0-934459-50-9*) United Hosp Fund.

New York End-of-Life Issues: Health Care Proxies, Living Wills, & Do-Not-Resuscitate Orders. James R. Sahlem & Mary E. Roche. 1996. (*1-57588-340-6*, 308630) W S Hein.

New York Health Care in Perspective 2000. Ed. by Kathleen O'Leary Morgan & Scott E. Morgan. 2000. 21p. spiral bd. 19.00 (*0-7401-0231-1*) Morgan Quitno Corp.

New York Health Care Perspective, 1998. Ed. by Kathleen O'Leary Morgan & Scott E. Morgan. 1998. 20p. pap. 19.00 (*1-56692-831-1*) Morgan Quitno Corp.

New York Hospital: A History of the Psychiatric Service, 1771-1936. William L. Russell. 1973. LC 73-2414. (Mental Illness & Social Policy; the American Experience Ser.). reprint ed. 40.95 (*0-405-05224-3*) Ayer.

New York State Office of Mental Health Psychotherapeutic Drug Manual. Ed. by Julie M. Zito. 3rd rev. ed. 1994. LC 93-17909. (General & Clinical Psychiatry Ser.). 334p. 105.00 (*0-471-30530-8*) Wiley.

New York Times Guide to Alternative Health: A Consumer Reference. Jane E. Brody & Denise Grady. 2001. LC 2001-17160. (Illus.). xvii, 394p. pap. 16.00 (*0-8050-6743-4*, Times Bks) H Holt & Co.

New York Times Natural Foods Dieting Book. Yvonne Y. Tarr. 1972. LC 75-190484. (*0-8129-0277-7*, Crown) Crown Pub Group.

New York University Medical Center Family Guide to Staying Healthy in a Risky Environment. Ed. by Arthur C. Upton & Eden Graber. 1993. LC 93-2634. (Illus.). 960p. 32.50 (*0-671-76815-8*) S&S Trade.

New Yorker Book of Doctor & Psychiatrist Cartoons. New Yorker Magazine Editors. 1996. (Illus.). 96p. pap. 10.00 (*0-679-76573-5*) Knopf.

New York's Health Care System: Making the Transition to Managed Care & Competition. Ed. by Martin A. Strosberg. 1997. LC 97-77569. (Dialogues on Public Policy Ser.). pap. 25.95 (*0-9658339-3-3*) Educ Intl Pr.

New York's Role As a Center for Health Care: An Analysis of Nonresident Patients Served by New York City Hospitals. Steven Finkler et al. 1986. (Papers: No. 4). 40p. 5.00 (*0-934459-29-0*) United Hosp Fund.

Newark Experiment: A New Direction for Urban Health Care. John Kolesar. 1975. 3.00 (*0-943136-14-8*) Ctr Analysis Public Issues.

***Newborn at High Risk of Brain Damage: EURAIBI International Workshop, Siena, April 2001, Europe Against Infant Brain Injury.** Ed. by G. Buonocore. 2001. (Biology of the Neonate Ser.: Vol. 79, No. 3-4). (Illus.). iv, 142p. pap. 39.25 (*3-8055-7212-3*) S Karger.

Newborn Baby. V. C. Harrison et al. 5th ed. 1994. (Illus.). 464p. (C). reprint ed. pap. text (*0-7021-1848-6*) Juta & Co ZAF. *Dist:* Intl Spec Bk.

***Newborn Brain: Neuroscience & Clinical Applications.** Ed. by Philippe Evrard et al. 2001. (Illus.). 336p. text 130.00 (*0-521-79338-6*) Cambridge U Pr.

Newborn Child. David G. Vulliamy & Peter G. Johnston. 6th ed. 1987. LC 87-10324. (Illus.). 273p. pap. text (*0-443-03668-3*) Church.

Newborn Child. Peter G. B. Johnston & David G. Vulliamy. 8th ed. 1998. LC 97-15115. (Illus.). pap. (*0-443-05510-6*) Church.

Newborn Death: For Parents Experiencing the Death of an Infant. Joy Johnson et al. 1997. (SPA.). 3.50 (*1-56123-113-4*) Centering Corp.

Newborn Feeding & Care Kit for Cleft Lip and/or Palate Infants. Renee L. Howard. (Illus.). 24p. (Orig.). (C). pap. 5.00 (*0-935801-00-6*) Howard & Assocs.

Newborn in the Intensive Care Unit: A Neuropsychoanalytic Prevention Model. Romana Negri. 1994. 288p. pap. text (*1-85575-073-2*) Karnac Bks GBR. *Dist:* Other Pr LLC.

Newborn Intensive Care: Resources for Family-Centered Practice. Janice L. Hanson et al. 1997. (Family-Centered Care Ser.). 142p. ring bd. 45.00 (*0-9642014-7-X*) Inst Fmly Ctr.

Newborn Intensive Care: What Every Parent Needs to Know. Ed. by Jeanette G. Zaichkin. 1996. LC 96-21773. (Illus.). 463p. (Orig.). pap. 24.95 (*0-9622975-8-5*) NICU Ink.

Newborn Intensive Care: What Every Parent Needs to Know. Ed. by Jeanette Goodnow Zaichkin. 2nd ed. 2000. LC 00-45230. (Illus.). xii, 460p. pap. 24.95 (*1-887571-05-1*) NICU Ink.

Newborn Medicine & Society: European Background & American Practice (1750-1975) Murdina M. Desmond. 1998. LC 97-43737. 26.95 (*1-57168-219-8*) Eakin Press.

Newborns at Risk: Medical Care & Psychoeducational Intervention. Gail L. Ensher & David A. Clark. 2nd ed. 1994. 400p. 69.00 (*0-8342-0555-6*) PRO-ED.

Newcastle Disease. Ed. by David J. Alexander. 1988. (Developments in Veterinary Virology Ser.). (C). text 240.00 (*0-89838-392-7*) Kluwer Academic.

Newe Iewell of Health. Conrad Gesner. 1971. LC 73-171759. (English Experience Ser.: No. 381). 540p. reprint ed. 75.00 (*90-221-0381-1*) Walter J Johnson.

Newer Dimensions of Patient Care, Set. Esther L. Brown. Incl. Pt. 1. Use of the Physical & Social Environment of the General Hospital for Therapeutic Purposes. 160p. 1961. pap. 16.50 (*0-87154-183-1*); Pt. 2. Improving Staff Motivation & Competence in the General Hospital. 194p. 1962. pap. 19.95 (*0-87154-184-X*); Pt. 3. Patients As People. 164p. 1965. pap. 14.95 (*0-87154-185-8*); 160p. (*0-87154-182-3*) Russell Sage.

Newer Tests & Procedures in Pediatric Gastroenterology. Ed. by G. Dinari et al. 1989. (Frontiers of Gastrointestinal Research Ser.: Vol. 15). (Illus.). vii, 332p. 258.50 (*3-8055-4646-7*) S Karger.

Newer Tests & Procedures in Pediatric Gastroenterology: Function & Laboratory Tests; Nutrition, 2. Ed. by G. Dinari et al. 1989. (Frontiers of Gastrointestinal Research Ser.: Vol. 16). (Illus.). viii, 296p. 233.25 (*3-8055-4900-8*) S Karger.

NewGAP. John McLeod & Rita McLeod. 1990. 40p. (Orig.). pap. text 24.00 (*0-87879-892-7*); 22.00 (*0-87879-893-5*); 6.00 (*0-87879-894-3*) Acad Therapy.

Newly Independent States (NIS) Industrial Directories Vol. 16: Medical Equipment Industry. Russian Information and Business Center, Inc. Staff. 1997. 200p. pap. 99.00 (*1-57751-216-2*) Intl Business Pubns.

M N O

Newspaper: A Subscription for Success. Lisa C. O'Connor. Ed. by Cindy Drolet & C. Gilles-Brown. rev. ed. 1999. (Language for Living Ser.). 143p. spiral bd. 38.00 (*0-9609464-8-9*, 8004) Imaginart Intl.

Newsweek Medical School Admissions Adviser. Lofftus & Kaplan Staff. 4th ed. 2002. 272p. 20.00 (*0-7432-1399-8*) Kaplan.

Newton Messagepad Version of Practical Guide to the Care of the Medical Patient. Fred F. Ferri. 3rd ed. 1996. 2p. (C). (*0-8151-3168-2*) Mosby Inc.

Next: The Coming Era in Medicine, Vol. 1. Holcomb B. Noble. 1988. pap. 9.95 (*0-316-61134-4*, Little Brwn Med Div) Lppncott W & W.

***Next Generation: Third Wave Feminist Psychotherapy.** Ed. by Ellyn Kaschak. 2001. LC 2001-24982. 162p. (C). (Women & Therapy Monograph: Vol. 23, No. 2). 29.95 (*0-7890-1409-2*); pap. 19.95 (*0-7890-1410-6*) Haworth Pr (Haworth Pastrl).

Next-Generation Nursing Information Systems: Essential Characteristics for Professional Practice. Rita Zielstorff et al. 1993. (Illus.). 59p. (C). pap. text 14.95 (*1-55810-083-0*, NP-83) Am Nurses Pub.

***Next Generation of AIDS Patients: Service Needs & Vulnerabilities.** Ed. by George J. Huba et al. 2001. LC 2001-24048. (Home Health Care Services Quarterly Ser.). (Illus.). xxi, 130p. (C). pap. text 34.95 (*0-7890-1362-2*); 170p. 59.95 (*0-7890-1361-4*) Haworth Pr.

***Next Nine Months: A Guide to Your Body after Giving Birth.** Paula M. Siegel. 2001. (Illus.). 278p. pap. 11.00 (*0-7881-9809-2*) DIANE Pub.

Next Step: Etiology & Treatment of Addiction. Joseph Rosenfeld. 1995. LC 95-16788. 15.95 (*0-938475-06-1*) Lighthouse Inst.

Next Step Forward: Music Therapy with the Terminally Ill. Ed. by Jenny A. Martin. 1989. 95p. spiral bd. 17.95 (*0-930194-46-2*) Ctr Thanatology.

Next Step on the Ladder: Assessment & Management of the Multi-Handicapped Child. G. B. Simon. 1985. 144p. 70.00 (*0-906054-27-3*); pap. 65.00 (*0-906054-26-5*) St Mut.

NFNA Flight Nursing Review Manual. Ed. by Angela Golden et al. Date not set. 128p. pap. text 33.00 (*0-935890-21-1*) Emerg Nurses IL.

NGNA Care Curriculum for Gerontological Nurses & Associates. National Gerontological Nursing Association Staff. 1995. LC 96-119375. (Illus.). 768p. (C). (gr. 13). pap. text 46.95 (*0-8151-6424-6*, 24848) Mosby Inc.

NGNA Core Curriculum for Gerontological Advance Practice Nurses. Ann S. Luggen et al. 1998. LC 98-9043. 717p. 122.95 (*0-7619-1300-9*, 82309); pap. 79.95 (*0-7619-1301-7*, 82310) Sage.

Ngoma: Discourses of Healing in Central & Southern Africa. John M. Janzen. 1992. (Comparative Studies of Health Systems & Medical Care: Vol. 34). (C). text 50.00 (*0-520-07265-0*) U CA Pr.

NHA Practice Examination C. Robert Haacker. 1998. 10.00 (*0-929442-46-6*, 2213PP) Prof Prnting & Pub.

NHA Practice Examination D. Robert Haacker. 1998. 10.00 (*0-929442-45-8*, 2212PP) Prof Prnting & Pub.

NHA Practice Examination E. Robert Haacker. rev. ed. 1999. 10.00 (*0-929442-47-4*, 2219PP) Prof Prnting & Pub.

NHS & Ideological Conflict. Paul Higgs. 1993. 233p. (*1-85628-346-1*) Avebury Technical GBR. *Dist:* Ashgate Pub Co.

***NHS Budget Holder's Survival Guide.** David Bailey. 1994. 85p. pap. (*0-582-24467-6*) Royal Soc of Medicine Pr Ltd GBR. *Dist:* Balogh.

NHS Complaints: Litigation & Professional Discipline. Vivienne Harpwood. 1996. 250p. pap. (*1-85941-012-X*) Cavendish Pubng GBR. *Dist:* Gaunt.

NHS Data Book. John Fry et al. 1984. text 90.50 (*0-85200-735-3*) Kluwer Academic.

NHS Wales: Putting Patients First, Command Paper 3841. 1998. LC 98-147247. (Command Papers: 81011068). (*0-10-138412-2*, HM84122) Statnry Office GBR. *Dist:* Bernan Associates.

Nicaraguan Revolution in Health: From Somoza to the Sandinistas. John M. Donahue. 1986. LC 85-31562. 188p. 57.75 (*0-89789-101-5*); 173p. pap. 18.95 (*0-89789-170-8*) Greenwood (Bergin & Garvey).

Nicht-Seminomatoese Hodentumoren. Ed. by H. J. Illiger et al. 1982. (Beitraege Zur Onkologie, Contributions to Oncology Ser.: Vol. 8). (Illus.). x, 298p. pap. 43.50 (*3-8055-3065-X*) S Karger.

Nickel. 1991. (Environmental Health Criteria Ser.: No. 108). (ENG, FRE & SPA.). 383p. pap. text 60.00 (*92-4-157108-X*, 1160108) World Health.

Nickel & the Skin. Ed. by Howard I. Maibach. 1989. 232p. 166.95 (*0-8493-6976-2*, RL803) CRC Pr.

Nickel Toxicology. Ed. by Stanley S. Brown & F. William Sunderman, Jr. 1981. text 104.00 (*0-12-137680-X*) Acad Pr.

Nicotine: An Old-Fashioned Addiction. Jack E. Henningfield. 1985. LC 84-14956. (Encyclopedia of Psychoactive Drugs Ser.: No. 1). (Illus.). 124p. (YA). (gr. 8-12). lib. bdg. 19.95 (*0-87754-751-3*) Chelsea Hse.

Nicotine & Related Alkaloids: Absorption, Distribution, Metabolism & Excretion. Ed. by John W. Gorrod & John Wahren. 1993. LC 93-25262. 320p. (C). (gr. 13). pap. text 226.95 (*0-412-55740-1*) Chapman & Hall.

Nicotine, Caffeine & Social Drinking: Behaviour & Brain Function. Ed. by Jan Snel & Monicque Lorist. 1997. 488p. text 68.00 (*90-5702-218-4*, Harwood Acad Pubs) Gordon & Breach.

Nicotine Psychopharmacology: Molecular, Cellular, & Behavioural Aspects. S. Wonnacott et al. 1990. (Illus.). 448p. 80.00 (*0-19-261614-5*) OUP.

Nicotine Replacement: A Critical Evaluation. Ed. by Ovide F. Pomerleau & Cynthia S. Pomerleau. 1992. 325p. pap. 29.95 (*1-56024-250-7*) Haworth Pr.

Nicotine Safety & Toxicity. Ed. by Neal L. Benowitz. 1998. LC 97-46155. (Illus.). 224p. text 59.50 (*0-19-511496-5*) OUP.

Nicotine, Smoking, & the Low Tar Program. Ed. by Nicholas J. Wald & P. Froggatt. 1989. (Illus.). 256p. 75.00 (*0-19-261729-X*) OUP.

Niehs Report on Health Effects from Exposure to Power-Line Frequency Electric & Magnetic Fields. Ed. by Kenneth Olden. 1999. 67p. (C). pap. text 20.00 (*0-7881-8373-7*) DIANE Pub.

Nietzsche & Jung: Quest for Wholeness. Patricia E. Dixon. 1999. LC 89-13134. (Contemporary Existentialism Ser.). XVI, 459p. (C). text 68.00 (*0-8204-1161-2*) P Lang Pubng.

Nietzsche & Psychoanalysis. Daniel Chapelle. 1993. LC 92-35535. 258p. (C). text 22.50 (*0-7914-1527-9*) State U NY Pr.

Nietzsche und Freud. Reinhard Gasser. 1997. (Monographien und Texte Zur Nietzsche-Forschung Ser.: Vol. 38). (GER.). 800p. (C). lib. bdg. 289.00 (*3-11-014960-5*) De Gruyter.

Nietzsche's Presence in Freud's Life & Thought: On the Origins of a Psychology of Dynamic Unconscious Mental Functioning. Ronald Lehrer. 1994. LC 94-571. 370p. (C). text 69.50 (*0-7914-2145-7*); pap. text 24.95 (*0-7914-2146-5*) State U NY Pr.

Night & Shift Work - Biological & Social Aspects: Proceedings of the 5th International Symposium on Night & Shift Work-Scientific Committee on Shift Work of the Permanent Commission & International Association on Occupational Health (PCIAIH, Rouen, 12-16 May 1980. Ed. by Alain Reinberg et al. 1981. (Illus.). 509p. 85.50 (*0-08-025516-7*, Pergamon Pr) Elsevier.

Night Chant: A Navaho Ceremony. Washington Matthews. 1995. LC 95-32398. (Illus.). 376p. reprint ed. pap. 19.95 (*0-87480-491-4*); text 25.00 (*0-87480-490-6*) U of Utah Pr.

Night Thoughts: Reflections of a Sex Therapist. Avodah K. Offit. rev. ed. 1995. LC 94-45758. (Master Work Ser.). 256p. pap. 25.00 (*1-56821-458-8*) Aronson.

Night Vision: Basic, Clinical & Applied Aspects. Ed. by R. F. Hess et al. 1990. (Illus.). 562p. (C). text 120.00 (*0-521-32736-9*) Cambridge U Pr.

Nightmare in the Greenhouse: The True Story of a Woman's Fight for Survival. Neva Kent. 1995. vi, 118p. (Orig.). pap. 9.95 (*0-9650712-1-9*) Teller Press.

Nightmare of Success: The Fallacy of the Super-Success Dream. William J. Ruzicka. 1973. LC 73-90028. 155p. 6.95 (*0-914372-01-7*) Peninsula Pubns.

Nightmares & Human Conflict. John Mack. 1989. 288p. text 64.50 (*0-231-07102-7*); pap. text 22.50 (*0-231-07103-5*) Col U Pr.

Nils Alwall Festschrift. Ed. by C. M. Kjellstrand. 1984. (Journal: Vol. 39, No. 2). (Illus.). 88p. pap. 48.00 (*3-8055-4001-9*) S Karger.

Nimodipine: Pharmacological & Clinical Results in Cerebral Ischemia. Ed. by A. Scriabine et al. 1991. (Illus.). 277p. 86.95 (*0-387-53405-9*) Spr-Verlag.

Nine Lives: The Emotional Experience in General Practice. K. Sanderson. 1991. 156p. pap. (*0-902965-28-X*) Clunie Pr GBR. *Dist:* Other Pr LLC.

1989 Forensic Services Directory. 1989. 1300p. 87.50 (*0-9602962-5-5*) Natl Forensic.

1989-2000 Portfolio of Award-Winning Floor Plans. Ed. by Veterinary Healthcare Communications Staff. 2000. 74.95 (*0-935078-80-0*) Veterinary Hlthcare.

1983 Travis Papers in the Integration of Psychology & Theology. Ed. by Christopher H. Rosik & H. Newton Malony. 1986. pap. 10.00 (*0-9609928-5-5*) Integ Pr.

1900-1970. Joseph I. Waring. reprint ed. 10.00 Reprint.

1980 Annual Handbook for Group Facilitators. Ed. by J. William Pfeiffer & John E. Jones. 9th ed. 1986. LC 73-92841. (Human Resource Development Ser.). (Illus.). 296p. pap. 99.00 (*0-88390-096-3*); pap. 49.00 (*0-88390-097-1*) Jossey-Bass (Pffr & Co).

1998-99 AAHSA Continuing Care Retirement Community Salary & Benefits Report. 1998. 281p. pap. 250.00 (*0-939326-38-8*) Hosp & Hlthcare.

1998-99 AAHSA Nursing Home Salary & Benefits Report. 1998. 370p. pap. 250.00 (*0-939326-39-6*) Hosp & Hlthcare.

1998-99 Home Care Salary & Benefits Report. 1998. 424p. pap. 250.00 (*0-939326-40-X*) Hosp & Hlthcare.

1998-99 Hospital Salary & Benefits Report. 1998. 336p. pap. 295.00 (*0-939326-42-6*) Hosp & Hlthcare.

1998-99 Hospice Salary & Benefits Report. 1998. 260p. pap. 195.00 (*0-939326-41-8*) Hosp & Hlthcare.

1998-99 Nursing Department Report. 1998. pap. 195.00 (*0-939326-44-2*) Hosp & Hlthcare.

1998 Annual Survey Report. Susan L. MacLean. 1999. 500.00 (*0-935890-33-5*) Emerg Nurses IL.

1998 Behavioral Outcomer & Guideliner Sourcebook: A Practical Guide to Measuring, Managing & Standardizing Mental Health & Substance Abuse Treatment. Ed. by Kenneth M. Coughlin. 1997. 672p. pap. 295.00 (*1-57987-030-9*) Faulkner & Gray.

1998 Year Book of Oncology. Robert F. Ozols. 2nd ed. 1998. (Illus.). 408p. (C). (gr. 13). text 86.00 (*0-8151-9710-1*, 24997) Mosby Inc.

1998 Year Book of Psychiatry & Applied Mental Health. Talbott. 1998. (Illus.). 528p. text 73.00 (*0-8151-9733-0*, 25020) Mosby Inc.

1998 CLC Integrative Medicine: A Balanced Account of the Data. Steven Wirth & May Farkas. Ed. by Sandra Wirth & Larry Reed. rev. ed. 1998. (Illus.). 80p. pap. text 7.95 (*0-9661161-3-5*, 161-35) Creat Logic.

1998 Clinician's Therapeutic Quickie. Afshine A. Emrani. 1998. pap. 9.95 (*0-9654687-3-9*) Emrani Publns.

1998 Comparative Performance Data Sourcebook. Ed. by Gwen Segre. 1997. 496p. pap. 245.00 (*1-57987-033-3*) Faulkner & Gray.

1998 Computers in Cardiology Conference. IEEE, Engineering in Medicine and Biology Staff. Ed. by IEEE, Institute of Electrical and Electronics Engineers, Inc. Staff. 1998. LC 80-641097. 850p. pap. 182.00 (*0-7803-5200-9*, 98CH36292) Inst Electrical.

1998 Directory to Medical Product Manufacturing Consultants. 1998. 164p. pap. 10.00 (*1-884551-04-1*) Canon Comns.

1998 Ed Database Summary. Susan L. MacLean. 1999. 30.00 (*0-935890-32-7*) Emerg Nurses IL.

1998 Fee Schedule & Payment Policies for Physicians' Medicare Services. CCH Editorial Staff. 1997. (Health Law Professional Ser.). 300p. pap. 45.00 (*0-8080-0200-7*) CCH INC.

1998 Guide to Healthcare Resources on the Internet. Ed. by John W. Hoben. 1997. 638p. pap. 245.00 (*1-57987-034-1*) Faulkner & Gray.

1998 Guide to Intranets in Healthcare: A Comprehensive Guide to New Developments in Networks, Extranets & Electronic Commerce. Jeffery Muscarella. Ed. by Luci Koizumi. 1997. (Illus.). pap. 245.00 (*1-57987-032-5*) Faulkner & Gray.

1998 Guidelines for Treatment of Sexually Transmitted Diseases. Centers for Disease Control and Prevention Staff & U. S. Department of Health & Human Services Staff. 1998. 116p. (C). pap. 7.95 (*1-883205-45-X*) Intl Med Pub.

1998 Health Care Almanac & Yearbook: The Single Volume Desk Reference for Facts, Figures & Resources. Ed. by Luci Koizumi & Daniel Moskowitz. 1997. (Illus.). 576p. pap. 195.00 (*1-57987-043-0*) Faulkner & Gray.

1998 Health Network & Alliance Sourcebook. Ed. by Daniel Moskowitz. 1997. (Illus.). 642p. pap. 250.00 (*1-57987-042-2*) Faulkner & Gray.

1998 International Conference on Information Technology Applications in Biomedicine. IEEE, Engineering in Medicine and Biology Staff. 1998. LC 98-179886. 166p. pap. 114.00 (*0-7803-4973-3*, 98EX188) IEEE Standards.

1998 Medicaid Managed Care Sourcebook. Ed. by Kenneth M. Coughlin & Lois Wingerson. 1997. 558p. pap. 245.00 (*1-57987-041-4*) Faulkner & Gray.

1998 Medicaid Managed Behavioral Care Sourcebook. Ed. by Ken Coughlin. 1997. (Illus.). 495p. pap. text 195.00 (*1-57987-008-2*) Faulkner & Gray.

1998 Medicare Explained. CCH Editorial Staff. 1998. (Health Law Professional Ser.). 200p. pap. 25.00 (*0-8080-0215-5*) CCH INC.

1998 Medicare & Medicaid Benefits. Ed. by CCH Editorial Staff. rev. ed. 1998. (Health Law Professional Ser.). 340p. pap. text 10.00 (*0-8080-0214-7*) CCH INC.

1998 Nursing Licensure Guidelines: State Information Manual for Nursing in U. S. Doctor's Licensure Group, Inc. Staff. 1998. 290p. 65.00 (*1-887617-57-4*) St Bart Pr Ltd.

1998 OR Product Directory. Ed. by Deb Reno. 1998. 458p. pap. 25.00 (*1-888460-01-6*) AORN.

1998 Physician. 1998. 368p. pap. 250.00 (*0-939326-37-X*) Hosp & Hlthcare.

1998 Reference Guide to the Occupational Therapy Code of Ethics. AOTA Staff. rev. ed. 1999. LC 00-501889. 58p. pap. 20.00 (*1-56900-113-8*, 1139) Am Occup Therapy.

1998 Rehabilitation Services Administration Consumer Satisfaction Survey. M. Davis & F. J. Meaney. 1998. (*1-888557-90-7*) No Ariz Univ.

1998 Residency Directory. Accreditation Services Division Staff. rev. ed. 1997. Vol. 2. 176p. pap. text 19.00 (*1-879907-74-7*, P509); Vols. 1 & 2. 324p. pap. text 31.00 (*1-879907-73-9*, P508) Am Soc Hlth-Syst.

1998 Risk Management for Health Care Provider Groups. Ed. by Lois Wingerson. 1997. 496p. pap. 235.00 (*1-57987-006-6*) Faulkner & Gray.

1998 State Medical Licensure Guidelines: Information Manual for Physicians in the U. S. Worldwide Medical Services Staff. 1998. 136p. 89.00 (*1-887617-59-0*) St Bart Pr Ltd.

1998 Year Book Neonatal & Perinatal Medicine. Avary A. Fanaroff. 2nd ed. 1998. (Illus.). 480p. (C). (gr. 13). text 80.00 (*0-8151-9644-X*, 24981) Mosby Inc.

1998 Year Book Neurology & Neurosurgery. Walter G. Bradley. 1998. (Illus.). 440p. (C). (gr. 13). text 78.00 (*0-8151-9648-2*, 24985) Mosby Inc.

1998 Year Book Obstetrics & Gynecology. Daniel R. Mishell. 2nd ed. 1998. (Illus.). 600p. (C). (gr. 13). text 79.00 (*0-8151-9704-7*, 24991) Mosby Inc.

1998 Year Book of Medicine. Cline. 1998. (Illus.). 752p. (C). (gr. 13). text 75.00 (*0-8151-3156-9*, 26975) Mosby Inc.

1998 Year Book of Anesthesia & Pain Management. John H. Tinker. 2nd ed. 1998. (Illus.). 504p. (C). (gr. 13). text 79.00 (*0-8151-8781-5*, 24436) Mosby Inc.

1998 Year Book of Cardiology. Robert C. Schlant. 2nd ed. 1998. (Illus.). 576p. (C). (gr. 13). text 79.00 (*0-8151-7539-6*, 24312) Mosby Inc.

1998 Year Book of Chiropractic. Lawrence Phillips. 1997. (Illus.). 448p. (C). (gr. 13). text 73.00 (*0-8151-6737-7*, 21967) Mosby Inc.

1998 Year Book of Critical Care Medicine. Parrillo. 1998. (Illus.). 432p. (C). (gr. 13). text 78.00 (*0-8151-9605-9*, 24944) Mosby Inc.

1998 Year Book of Dentistry. Meskin. 1998. (Illus.). 528p. (C). (gr. 13). text 73.00 (*0-8151-7084-X*, 27509) Mosby Inc.

1998 Year Book of Dermatologic Surgery. Hubert T. Greenway. 1998. (Illus.). 368p. (C). (gr. 13). text 88.00 (*0-8151-9608-3*, 24947) Mosby Inc.

1998 Year Book of Dermatology. Sober. 1998. (Illus.). 512p. (C). (gr. 13). text 81.00 (*0-8151-9613-X*, 24950) Mosby Inc.

1998 Year Book Of Diagnostic Radiology. Anne G. Osborn. 1998. (Illus.). 640p. (C). (gr. 13). text 79.00 (*0-8151-9616-4*, 24953) Mosby Inc.

1998 Year Book of Digestive Diseases. Norton J. Greenberger. 1998. (Illus.). 264p. (C). (gr. 13). text 77.95 (*0-8151-9619-9*, 24956) Mosby Inc.

1998 Year Book of Drug Therapy. Louis Lasagna. 1998. (Illus.). 408p. (C). (gr. 13). text 79.95 (*0-8151-5296-5*, 24747) Mosby Inc.

1998 Year Book of Emergency Medicine. David K. Wagner. 2nd ed. 1998. (Illus.). 456p. (C). (gr. 13). text 83.00 (*0-8151-9623-7*, 24960) Mosby Inc.

1998 Year Book of Endocrinology. John D. Bagdade. 2nd ed. 1998. (Illus.). 432p. (C). (gr. 13). text 79.00 (*0-8151-9626-1*, 24963) Mosby Inc.

1998 Year Book of Geriatrics & Gerontology. Burton. 1998. (Illus.). 424p. (C). (gr. 13). text 69.95 (*0-8151-9631-8*, 24968) Mosby Inc.

1998 Year Book of Hand Surgery. Peter C. Amadio et al. 1998. (Illus.). 444p. (C). text 80.00 (*0-8151-0163-5*, 25764) Mosby Inc.

1998 Year Book of Infectious Diseases. Gerald T. Keusch. 1998. (Illus.). 400p. (C). (gr. 13). text 80.00 (*0-8151-9387-4*, 24592) Mosby Inc.

1998 Year Book of Nuclear Medicine. Ed. by Alexander Gottschalk. 1998. (Illus.). 504p. (C). (gr. 13). text 86.00 (*0-8151-3821-0*, 25463) Mosby Inc.

1998 Year Book of Occupational & Environmental Health. Edward A. Emmett. 2nd ed. 1998. (Illus.). 360p. (C). (gr. 13). text 74.95 (*0-8151-9707-1*, 24994) Mosby Inc.

1998 Year Book of Ophthalmology. Wilson. 2nd ed. 1998. (Illus.). 408p. (C). (gr. 13). text 82.00 (*0-8151-9713-6*, 25000) Mosby Inc.

1998 Year Book of Orthopaedics. Clement B. Sledge. 2nd ed. 1998. (Illus.). 488p. (C). (gr. 13). text 83.00 (*0-8151-9716-0*, 25003) Mosby Inc.

1998 Year Book of Pathology & Laboratory Medicine. Steve Raab. 2nd ed. 1998. (Illus.). 568p. (C). (gr. 13). text 83.00 (*0-8151-9722-5*, 25009) Mosby Inc.

1998 Year Book of Pediatrics. James A. Stockman. 2nd ed. 1998. (Illus.). 680p. (C). (gr. 13). text 67.95 (*0-8151-9725-X*, 25012) Mosby Inc.

1998 Year Book of Plastic & Reconstructive Surgery. Ronald D. Miller. 2nd ed. 1998. (Illus.). 352p. (C). (gr. 13). text 82.00 (*0-8151-9728-4*, 25015) Mosby Inc.

1998 Year Book of Pulmonary Disease. Jett James Jett. 2nd ed. 1998. (Illus.). 472p. (C). (gr. 13). text 79.00 (*0-8151-9736-5*, 25023) Mosby Inc.

1998 Year Book of Sports Medicine. Roy J. Shephard. 2nd ed. 1998. (Illus.). 472p. (C). (gr. 13). text 74.95 (*0-8151-9740-3*, 25027) Mosby Inc.

1998 Year Book of Surgery. Edward M. Copeland, III. 2nd ed. 1998. (Illus.). 576p. (C). (gr. 13). text 74.00 (*0-8151-9743-8*, 25030) Mosby Inc.

1998 Year Book of Urology. Vincent T. Andriole. 2nd ed. 1998. (Illus.). 384p. (C). (gr. 13). text 82.00 (*0-8151-2548-8*, 24061) Mosby Inc.

1998 Year Book of Vascular Surgery. Porter. 1998. (Illus.). 544p. (C). (gr. 13). text 86.00 (*0-8151-9800-0*, 25037) Mosby Inc.

1998 Year Book of Podiatry. Ed. by Stephen J. Kominsky. 2nd ed. 1998. 348p. (C). (gr. 13). text 69.95 (*0-8151-9731-4*) Mosby Inc.

1995 Almanac of Hospital Financial & Operating Indicators. William O. Cleverley. 1995. 516p. pap. 350.00 (*1-882733-04-5*) Ctr Hlthcare IPS.

1995 Almanac of Hospital Financial & Operating Indicators. Timothy Carse & Jeffrey Cleverley. 2nd ed. 1996. text 350.00 (*0-07-413128-1*, Irwn McGrw-H) McGrw-H Hghr Educ.

1995 China Medical Market Report Vol. 1: An Indepth Market Study on China's Pharmaceutical, Biotechnology & Medical Device Markets. Deborah Miller & Shannon Shi. 1995. 100p. (Orig.). pap. 79.95 (*0-9657889-0-3*) Golden Tri Org.

1995 Computers in Cardiology. IEEE, Engineering in Medicine and Biology Staff. Ed. by IEEE, Institute of Electrical and Electronics Engineers, Inc. Staff. 1995. LC 80-641097. 900p. pap. text 150.00 (*0-7803-3053-6*, 95CH35874); 900p. lib. bdg. 150.00 (*0-7803-3054-4*, 95CB35874); fiche 150.00 (*0-7803-3055-2*, 95CM35874) Inst Electrical.

1995 First Regional Conference of the IEEE Engineering in Medicine & Biology Society Proceedings. IEEE, Engineering in Medicine and Biology Staff. Ed. by IEEE, Institute of Electrical and Electronics Engineers, Inc. Staff. 1995. 450p. pap. (*0-7803-2711-X*, 95TH8089); mic. film (*0-7803-2712-8*, 95TH8089) Inst Electrical.

1995 Fourteenth Southern Biomedical Engineering Conference. IEEE, Engineering in Medicine and Biology Staff. Ed. by IEEE, Society Staff. 1995. LC 94-77907. 350p. pap. (*0-7803-2083-2*, 95TH0703-9); fiche (*0-7803-2084-0*, 95TH0703-9) Inst Electrical.

1995 IEEE Engineering in Medicine & Biology 17th Annual Conference: Basic & Applied Biomedical Engineering - Building Block for Health Care. IEEE, Engineering in Medicine and Biology Staff. Ed. by IEEE, Institute of Electrical and Electronics Engineers, Inc. Staff. 1995. LC 94-73760. 2000p. pap. text 222.00 (*0-7803-2475-7*, 95CH35746); 2000p. lib. bdg. 222.00 (*0-7803-2476-5*, 95CB35746); fiche 222.00 (*0-7803-2477-3*, 95CM35746); cd-rom 222.00 (*0-7803-2478-1*, 95CH35746) Inst Electrical.

1995 Physician Salary Survey Report. annuals 19th ed. 1995. pap. 250.00 (*0-939326-88-4*) Hosp & Hlthcare.

1995-1996 AAO Yearbook: Osteopathic Vision. Ed. by Myron C. Beal. 1996. (Illus.). 205p. (Orig.). (C). pap. 40.00 (*0-940668-04-1*) Am Acad Osteopathy.

1995-96 Home Care Salary & Benefits Report. annuals 5th ed. 1995. (Orig.). pap. 250.00 (*0-939326-91-4*) Hosp & Hlthcare.

1995-96 Hospice Salary & Benefits Report. annuals 4th ed. 1995. (Orig.). pap. 195.00 (*0-939326-92-2*) Hosp & Hlthcare.

1995-96 Hospital Salary & Benefits Report. annuals 25th ed. 1995. 304p. (Orig.). pap. 250.00 (*0-939326-90-6*) Hosp & Hlthcare.

1995-96 Management Company Report. 13th ed. 1995. pap. 495.00 (*0-939326-94-9*) Hosp & Hlthcare.

1995-96 Nursing Department Report. annuals 4th ed. 1995. pap. 195.00 (*0-939326-93-0*) Hosp & Hlthcare.

1995-96 Nursing Home Salary & Benefits Report. annuals 17th ed. 1995. pap. 250.00 (*0-939326-89-2*) Hosp & Hlthcare.

1994 Almanac of Hospital Financial & Operating Indicators. William O. Cleverley. 1994. 516p. pap. 350.00 (*1-882733-02-9*) Ctr Hlthcare IPS.

1994 Dallas, Fort Worth Medical Directory. American Medical Sales School, Inc. Staff. Ed. & Intro. by Diane Huggins. rev. ed. 1994. (Illus.). 737p. 42.50 (*1-882328-02-7*) Am Med Sales.

1994 Physician Salary Survey Report. annuals 18th ed. 1994. 247p. pap. 250.00 (*0-939326-81-7*) Hosp & Hlthcare.

1994-95 Nursing Department Report. annuals 3rd ed. 1994. 152p. (Orig.). pap. 195.00 (*0-939326-86-8*) Hosp & Hlthcare.

1994-95 Nursing Home Salary & Benefits Report. annuals 16th ed. 1994. pap. 250.00 (*0-939326-82-5*) Hosp & Hlthcare.

1999 Behavioral Outcomes & Guidelines Sourcebook. Ed. by Kenneth M. Coughlin. 1998. 736p. pap. 295.00 (*1-57987-091-0*) Faulkner & Gray.

1999 Year Book of Endocrinology. 3rd ed. 1999. (Illus.). 460p. text 82.00 (*0-8151-9627-X*, 24964) Mosby Inc.

1999 CLC Integrative Medicine: A Balanced Account of the Data. Steven Wirth & Sandra Wirth. Ed. by Mary Farkas & Larry Reed. 1998. (Illus.). 88p. 7.95 (*0-9661161-1-9*, 161-1-9, Boitumelo Pub) Creat Logic.

1999 Coding Workbook: Physician's Office. Covell. 6th ed. 1999. (C). pap., wbk. ed. 25.95 (*0-7668-0853-X*) Thomson Learn.

1999 Consultants Directory: A Comprehensive Directory to Medical Device Industry Consultants. Susan Wallace. 1999. 164p. pap. 10.00 (*1-884551-05-X*) Canon Comns.

1999 Disease Management Sourcebook. Ed. by Lois Wingerson. 1998. 570p. pap. 250.00 (*1-57987-085-6*) Faulkner & Gray.

1999 Environmental Assessment: Rising to the Challenge of a New Century. Ed. by Daniel P. Bourque et al. 1999. (Illus.). 114p. pap. 9.00 (*0-9667828-1-X*) VHA Inc.

1999 Guide to Healthy Restaurant Eating: What to Eat in America's Most Popular Family & Chain Restaurants. Hope Warshaw. 1998. LC 98-35395. 192p. pap. 13.95 (*1-58040-004-3*, 00043Q) Am Diabetes.

1999 Guide to Intranets in Health Care. Ed. by Jeffrey W. Muscarella & Luci Koizumi. 1998. (Illus.). 352p. pap. 275.00 (*1-57987-106-2*) Faulkner & Gray.

1999 HCPCS: Level II Codes. 1999. 240p. pap. 65.00 (*1-58383-010-3*, HCPCS9) Robert D Keene.

1999 Health Network & Alliance Sourcebook: Purchasing & Selling Strategies for Payers & Providers, Including Blue Book Network, Coalition & Alliance Directories. Ed. by Daniel B. Moskowitz. 1998. (Illus.). 544p. pap. 265.00 (*1-57987-099-6*) Faulkner & Gray.

1999 IEEE 25th Annual Northeast Bioengineering Conf. IEEE, Engineering in Medicine and Biology Staff. 1999. LC 88-646567. 144p. pap. (*0-7803-5486-9*, 99CH36355) Inst Electrical.

1999 Medicaid Managed Behavioral Care Sourcebook: Strategies & Opportunities for Providers & Purchasers. Ed. by Ken Coughlin. 1998. LC 99-192066. (Illus.). 560p. pap. 225.00 (*1-57987-047-3*) Faulkner & Gray.

1999 Medicaid Managed Care Sourcebook. Ed. by Kenneth M. Coughlin. 1998. 560p. pap. 265.00 (*1-57987-105-4*) Faulkner & Gray.

1999 Medical Outcomes & Guidelines Sourcebook: A Progress Report & Resource Guide on Medical Outcomes Research & Practice Guidelines: Developments Data, & Implementation. Laura Newman. 1998. (Illus.). pap. 295.00 (*1-57987-084-8*) Faulkner & Gray.

1999 Medical Quality Management Sourcebook: A Comprehensive Guide to Measuring Quality & Applying the Results. Ed. by Ken Coughlin. rev. ed. 1998. 608p. pap. 250.00 (*1-57987-087-2*) Faulkner & Gray.

1999 Medicare & Medicaid Benefits. CCH Editorial Staff. rev. ed. 1999. 48p. pap. 10.00 (*0-8080-0308-9*) CCH INC.

1999 Medicare Explained. CCH Editorial Staff. 1999. 224p. pap. 25.00 (*0-8080-0307-0*) CCH INC.

1999 Medicare Managed Care Sourcebook. Ed. by Melissa Glim. 1998. 546p. pap. 275.00 (*1-57987-104-6*) Faulkner & Gray.

1999 Mosby's Genrx: Internet Version. Mosby Staff. 2nd ed. 1998. 195.00 (*0-323-00588-8*) Mosby Inc.

1999 National Correct Coding Manual. 5th ed. 1999. 250p. pap. 250.00 (*1-58383-052-9*) Robert D Keene.

1999 Oncology Nursing Drug Handbook - Hoechst. Gail Wilkes et al. 3rd ed. 1998. (Illus.). (C). pap. text 50.00 (*0-7637-0987-5*) Jones & Bartlett.

1999 Patient Resources on the Internet. Ed. by Eric Levy. 1998. 512p. pap. 195.00 (*1-57987-044-9*) Faulkner & Gray.

1999 Physician ICD-9-CM: International Classification of Diseases, Clinical Modification. Medicode Staff. 9th ed. 1998. iii, 774p. (C). pap. 51.95 (*1-56337-285-1*) Thomson Learn.

1999 Physician Salary Survey Report, Vol. 23. 1999. 390p. pap. 250.00 (*0-939326-46-9*) Hosp & Hlthcare.

1999 Post Acute Outcomes Sourcebook: A Guide to Methods, Measures, & Strategies in Post-Acute Care. Ed. by Lois Wingerson. 1998. (Illus.). 496p. pap. 245.00 (*1-57987-049-X*) Faulkner & Gray.

1999 RBRVS: Resource Based Relative Value Scale. 1999. 250p. pap. 65.00 (*1-58383-008-1*, RBRVS9) Robert D Keene.

1999 Residency Directory Contrib. by Accreditation Services Division Staff. rev. ed. 1998. 448p. pap. text 31.00 (*1-879907-83-6*);Vol. 2. 256p. pap. text 31.00 (*1-879907-84-4*) Am Soc Hlth-Syst.

1999 Social Security Benefits Including Medicare. CCH Editorial Staff. rev. ed. 1999. 64p. pap. 10.00 (*0-8080-0309-7*) CCH INC.

1999 Telemedicine Sourcebook. Ed. by Eric Levy & Kenneth Coughlin. 1998. 512p. pap. 275.00 (*1-57987-046-5*) Faulkner & Gray.

1999-2000 Home Care Salary & Benefits Report, Vol. 9. 1999. 420p. pap. 250.00 (*1-893772-01-2*) Hosp & Hlthcare.

1999-2000 Hospice Salary & Benefits Report. 1999. 260p. pap. 195.00 (*1-893772-03-9*) Hosp & Hlthcare.

1999-2000 Hospital Salary & Benefit Report, Vol. 29. 1999. 320p. pap. 295.00 (*1-893772-00-4*) Hosp & Hlthcare.

1999-2000 AAHSA Nursing Home Salary & Benefits Report. 1999. 370p. pap. 250.00 (*0-939326-49-3*) Hosp & Hlthcare.

1999-2000 AAHSA Continuing Care Retirement Community Salary & Benefits Report, Vol. 2. 1999. 300p. pap. 250.00 (*0-939326-48-5*) Hosp & Hlthcare.

1999 Veterinary Drug Guide. Delmar Publishing Staff. 1999. (C). mass mkt. 22.50 (*0-7668-0754-1*) Delmar.

1999 Wellness & Prevention Sourcebook. Ed. by Eric Levy. 1998. 496p. pap. 235.00 (*1-57987-081-3*) Faulkner & Gray.

1999 Year Book Allergy & Clinical Immunology. Lanny J. Rosenwasser. 1999. 79.00 (*0-8151-9600-8*, 24939) Mosby Inc.

1999 Year Book Neurology & Neurosurgery. Bradley. 2nd ed. 1999. (Illus.). 448p. text 81.00 (*0-8151-9649-0*, 24986) Mosby Inc.

1999 Year Book Obstetrics & Gynecology. 1999. (Illus.). 608p. text 82.00 (*0-8151-9705-5*, 24992) Mosby Inc.

1999 Year Book of Anesthesia & Pain Management. Date not set. 75.95 (*0-8151-9601-6*) Mosby Inc.

1999 Year Book of Anesthesiology & Pain Management. John H. Tinker et al. 1999. 82.00 (*0-323-00645-0*) Mosby Inc.

1999 Year Book of Cardiology. Schlant. 1999. (Illus.). 475p. text 82.00 (*0-8151-9602-4*, 24941) Mosby Inc.

1999 Year Book of Chiropractic. Lawrence. 1998. (Illus.). 416p. text 78.00 (*0-8151-9603-2*, 24942) Mosby Inc.

1999 Year Book of Critical Care Medicine. 1999. (Illus.). 350p. text 81.00 (*0-8151-9606-7*, 24945) Mosby Inc.

1999 Year Book of Dentistry. 1999. (Illus.). 520p. text 74.95 (*0-8151-7085-8*, 27510) Mosby Inc.

1999 Year Book of Dermatologic Surgery. 1999. 350p. text 84.95 (*0-8151-9610-5*) Mosby Inc.

1999 Year Book of Dermatology & Dermatologic Surgery. Bruce H. Thiers. 1999. 500p. text 84.00 (*0-8151-9614-8*, 24951) Mosby Inc.

1999 Year Book of Diagnostic Radiology. 1999. 83.00 (*0-8151-9617-2*, 24954) Mosby Inc.

1999 Year Book of Drug Therapy. 1999. 79.95 (*0-8151-9621-0*) Mosby Inc.

1999 Year Book of Emergency Medicine. 3rd ed. 1999. (Illus.). 408p. text 85.00 (*0-8151-9624-5*, 24961) Mosby Inc.

1999 Year Book of Family Practice. 3rd ed. 1999. (Illus.). 488p. text 69.00 (*0-8151-9630-X*, 24967) Mosby Inc.

1999 Year Book of Gastroenterology. 1999. (Illus.). 315p. text 79.00 (*0-8151-9620-2*, 24957) Mosby Inc.

1999 Year Book of Geriatrics & Gerontology. Date not set. 69.95 (*0-8151-9632-6*) Mosby Inc.

1999 Year Book of Hand Surgery. 1999. (Illus.). 360p. text 83.00 (*0-8151-0164-3*, 25765) Mosby Inc.

1999 Year Book of Hematology. Spivak. 3rd ed. 1998. 594p. (C). (gr. 13). text 82.95 (*0-8151-9635-0*) Mosby Inc.

1999 Year Book of Medicine. 1999. (Illus.). 670p. text 78.00 (*0-8151-2902-5*, 31813) Mosby Inc.

1999 Year Book of Neonatal & Perinatal Medicine. 3rd ed. 1999. (Illus.). 400p. text 83.00 (*0-8151-9645-8*, 24982) Mosby Inc.

1999 Year Book of Nephrology, Hypertension & Mineral Metabolism. 2nd ed. 1999. (Illus.). 283p. text 86.00 (*0-8151-9647-4*, 24984) Mosby Inc.

1999 Year Book Of Nuclear Medicine. 1999. (Illus.). 448p. text 88.00 (*0-8151-3822-9*, 25464) Mosby Inc.

1999 Year Book of Oncology. Simone. 3rd ed. 1999. (Illus.). 500p. text 86.00 (*0-8151-9711-X*, 24998) Mosby Inc.

1999 Year Book of Ophthalmology. 3rd ed. 1999. (Illus.). 500p. text 84.00 (*0-8151-9714-4*, 25001) Mosby Inc.

1999 Year Book of Orthopaedics. Sledge. 3rd ed. 1999. (Illus.). 450p. text 86.00 (*0-8151-9717-9*, 25004) Mosby Inc.

1999 Year Book of Pathology. 3rd ed. 1999. (Illus.). 536p. text, lab manual ed. 85.00 (*0-8151-9723-3*, 25010) Mosby Inc.

1999 Year Book of Pediatrics. 3rd ed. 1999. (Illus.). 632p. text 71.00 (*0-8151-9726-8*, 25013) Mosby Inc.

1999 Year Book of Plastic & Reconstructive Surgery. 3rd ed. 1999. 400p. text 85.00 (*0-8151-9729-2*, 25016) Mosby Inc.

1999 Year Book of Podiatry. Date not set. 73.00 (*0-8151-9732-2*) Mosby Inc.

1999 Year Book of Psychiatry. 2nd ed. 1999. (Illus.). 456p. text 76.00 (*0-8151-9734-9*, 25021) Mosby Inc.

1999 Year Book of Pulmonary Disease. 3rd ed. 1999. (Illus.). 539p. text 79.00 (*0-8151-9737-3*, 25024) Mosby Inc.

1999 Year Book of Rheumatology, Arthritis & Musculoskeletal Disease. 1999. (Illus.). 376p. text 86.00 (*0-8151-9738-1*, 25025) Mosby Inc.

1999 Year Book of Sports Medicine. 3rd ed. 1999. (Illus.). 450p. text 77.95 (*0-8151-9741-1*, 25028) Mosby Inc.

1999 Year Book of Surgery. 3rd ed. 1999. (Illus.). 552p. text 76.95 (*0-8151-9744-6*, 25031) Mosby Inc.

1999 Year Book of Thoracic & Cardiac Surgery. 1999. 79.95 (*0-8151-9745-4*, 25032) Mosby Inc.

1999 Year Book of Urology. 3rd ed. 1999. (Illus.). 550p. text 84.00 (*0-8151-2549-6*, 24062) Mosby Inc.

1999 Year Book of Vascular Surgery. 2nd ed. 1999. (Illus.). 560p. text 87.95 (*0-8151-9801-9*, 25038) Mosby Inc.

1997-98 Compensation Report on Management Employees in Hospital, Nursing Home, & Home Care Management Companies. 1998. 200p. pap. 495.00 (*0-939326-36-1*) Hosp & Hlthcare.

1997 Annual Statement Instructions - Limited Health Services Organizations (LHSO) Ed. by Patti Carli. 6th rev. ed. 1997. 108p. (C). ring bd. 75.00 (*0-89382-471-2*, ASI-SM) Nat Assn Insurance.

1997 Annual Statement Instructions - Hospital, Medical, Dental Service & Indemnity Corporation (HMDI) Ed. by Patti Carli. 6th rev. ed. 1997. 252p. (C). ring bd. 75.00 (*0-89382-469-0*, ASI-MM) Nat Assn Insurance.

1997 Annual Statement Instructions - Health Maintenance Organization. Ed. by Patti Carli. 7th rev. ed. 1997. 137p. (C). ring bd. 175.00 (*0-89382-468-2*, ASI-HM) Nat Assn Insurance.

1997 Annual Survey Report. Susan L. MacLean. 1999. (Illus.). 500.00 (*0-935890-31-9*) Emerg Nurses IL.

1997 AVMA Convention Notes. 1997. pap. (*1-882691-11-3*) Am Veterinary Med Assn.

1997 Behavioral Outcomes & Guidelines Sourcebook. Ed. by Ken Coughlin. 1996. (Illus.). 575p. pap. text 295.00 (*1-881393-93-3*) Faulkner & Gray.

1997 Book of Vascular Surgery. Ed. by John M. Porter. 1997. (Illus.). 560p. (C). (gr. 13). text 86.00 (*0-8151-6800-4*, 22715) Mosby Inc.

1997 Computers in Cardiology. IEEE, Engineering in Medicine and Biology Staff. Ed. by Institute of Electrical and Electronics Engineers, Inc. Staff. 1997. LC 80-641097. 776p. pap. text (*0-7803-4445-6*, 97CH36184); lib. bdg. (*0-7803-4446-4*, 97CH36184) Inst Electrical.

1997 Directory of Community Blood Centers. 1997. pap. text 70.00 (*1-56395-089-8*) Am Assn Blood.

1997 Directory of Key Health Legislators & Legislative Staff. Compiled by NCSL Health Care Program Staff. 1997. 79p. 20.00 (*1-55516-651-2*, 6661) Natl Conf State Legis.

1997 Directory to Medical Product Manufacturing Consultants. 1997. 164p. (Orig.). pap. 10.00 (*1-884551-03-3*) Canon Comns.

1997 Ed Database Summary. Susan L. MacLean. 1999. (Illus.). 30.00 (*0-935890-30-0*) Emerg Nurses IL.

1997 Guide to Behavioral Resources on the Internet: A Review of Mental Health & Substance Abuse Web Sites, Mailing Lists & Support Forms. Ed. by Kenneth M. Coughlin. 1997. (Illus.). 519p. (Orig.). pap. text 245.00 (*1-881393-99-2*) Faulkner & Gray.

1997 Health Care Almanac & Yearbook. Ed. by Luci S. Koizumi & Daniel B. Moskowitz. 1996. 480p. (Orig.). pap. text 195.00 (*1-881393-94-1*) Faulkner & Gray.

1997 Healthcare Alliance & Network Sourcebook. Ed. by John Reichard. 1996. 700p. pap. 265.00 (*1-881393-22-4*) Faulkner & Gray.

1997 Healthcare Guide to the Internet: An Annotated Listing of Internet Resources for the Healthcare Professional. Jennifer Wayne-Doppke. 2nd ed. 1997. (Illus.). 140p. (Orig.). pap. 68.00 (*0-9645360-4-8*) Cor Hlthcare.

1997 IEEE 23rd Northeast Bioengineering Conference. IEEE, Engineering in Medicine and Biology Staff. Ed. by Institute of Electrical and Electronics Engineers, Inc. Staff. 1997. LC 88-646567. 250p. pap. text (*0-7803-3848-0*, 97CH36045); lib. bdg. (*0-7803-3849-9*, 97CH36045); fiche (*0-7803-3850-2*, 97CH36045) Inst Electrical.

1997 IEEE Engineering in Medicine & Biology Annual Conference. IEEE, Engineering in Medicine and Biology Staff. 1997. LC 99-226406. 2400p. pap. text 384.00 (*0-7803-4262-3*, 97CH36136); lib. bdg. (*0-7803-4263-1*, 97CH36136) Inst Electrical.

1997 Indian Medical Market Report Vol. 1: An Indepth Market Study on India's Pharmaceutical, Biotechnology & Medical Device Industries. Amiya Nayak et al. 1997. 167p. (Orig.). pap. 299.95 (*0-9657889-1-1*) Golden Tri Org.

1997 International Conference on Information Technology Applications in Biomedicine Proceedings. Ed. by V. Eck & Ivan Krekule. 1997. LC 97-80277. 80p. pap. (*0-7803-4318-2*, 97TH8342) Inst Electrical.

1997 Life Safety Code Field Guide for Health Care Facilities. David M. Birk & James K. Lathrop. 1998. (Illus.). 176p. pap. text 145.00 (*1-57839-045-1*) Opus Communs.

1997 Managed Home Care Sourcebook. Ed. by David Bech. 1997. LC 98-233104. (Illus.). 575p. pap. text 195.00 (*1-881393-97-6*) Faulkner & Gray.

1997 Medicaid Managed Care Sourcebook. Ed. by Lois Wingerson. 1996. 560p. (Orig.). pap. text (*1-881393-95-X*) Faulkner & Gray.

1997 Medical Outcomes & Guidelines Sourcebook: A Progress Report & Resource Guide on Medical Outcomes Research & Practice Guidelines: Developments, Data, & Documentation. 1996. 800p. (Orig.). (C). pap. 295.00 (*1-881393-66-6*) Faulkner & Gray.

1997 National Directory of Fire Chiefs & Emergency Departments. Tr. by Laura J. Gross. 6th ed. 1997. 1080p. 70.00 (*1-880245-14-0*) SPAN Pub.

1997-1998 Absite Combat Manual. Hratch L. Karamanoukian et al. Ed. by John Pryor. unabr. ed. 1997. 295p. spiral bd. 59.00 (*0-9663292-0-1*) Magalhaes Sci Pr.

1997-1998 Oncology Nursing Drug Handbook. Gail M. Wilkes et al. 2nd ed. 1997. LC 97-3045. (Nursing Ser.). (Illus.). 752p. pap. text 42.50 (*0-7637-0369-9*, 0369-9) Jones & Bartlett.

1997-98 Hospital Salary & Benefits Report. 1997. 227p. pap. 295.00 (*0-939326-30-2*) Hosp & Hlthcare.

1997-98 Home Care Salary & Benefits Report. 1997. 420p. pap. 250.00 (*0-939326-32-9*) Hosp & Hlthcare.

1997-98 Hospice Salary & Benefits Report. 1997. 260p. pap. 195.00 (*0-939326-33-7*) Hosp & Hlthcare.

1997-98 Nursing Department Report. 1997. 168p. pap. 195.00 (*0-939326-35-3*) Hosp & Hlthcare.

1997-98 AAHSA Nursing Home Salary & Benefits Report. 1997. 280p. pap. 250.00 (*0-939326-34-5*) Hosp & Hlthcare.

1997-98 Nursing Home Salary & Benefits Report. 19th ed. 1997. 300p. pap. 250.00 (*0-939326-29-9*) Hosp & Hlthcare.

1997-98 Workers' Compensation Managed Care Sourcebook. Ed. by Gwen C. Segre. 1997. LC 98-183719. (Illus.). 480p. pap. text 235.00 (*1-57987-005-8*) Faulkner & Gray.

1997-99 Handbook of Emergency Cardiovascular Care for Healthcare Providers. 1997. (Illus.). 58p. pap. 7.95 (*0-87493-629-2*) Am Heart.

1997 Nursing Licensure Guidelines: Information Manual for Nurses in the United States of America. Jason F. Janoulis & Brenda H. Janoulis. 1997. 224p. pap. 89.00 (*1-887617-54-X*) St Bart Pr Ltd.

1997 Nursing Licensure Guidelines: State, Provincial, Territorial Information Manual for Nurses in the United States of America & Canada. Jason F. Janoulis & Brenda H. Janoulis. 1997. 150.00 incl. audio compact disk (*1-887617-55-8*) St Bart Pr Ltd.

1997 Physician Salary Survey Report. 21st ed. 1997. 392p. pap. 250.00 (*0-939326-28-0*) Hosp & Hlthcare.

1997 Physicians' GenRx. Ed. by David R. Avery & Ralph E. McDonald. 7th rev. ed. 1999. LC 99-33332. (Illus.). 880p. (C). (gr. 13). text 64.95 (*0-8151-9017-4*, 31745) Mosby Inc.

1997 Report of the Committee on Infectious Diseases. American Academy of Pediatrics Staff. 24th ed. 1997. 764p. pap. 84.95 (*0-910761-85-X*) Am Acad Pediat.

1997 Shanghai International Conference on Laser Medicine & Surgery, Vol. 3344. Ed. by Jing Zhu. 1998. LC 00-500824. 80.00 (*0-8194-2791-8*) SPIE.

1997 State Health Care Expenditure Report. Frwd. by Daniel M. Fox et al. 1999. (Illus.). 192p. pap. (*1-887748-25-3*) Milbank Memorial.

1997 State Medical Licensure Guidelines: Information Manual for MD & DO Physicians in the United States of America. Jason F. Janoulis & Brenda H. Janoulis. 1997. pap. 125.00 incl. audio compact disk (*1-887617-56-6*) St Bart Pr Ltd.

1997 Supplement to Coping with Psychiatric & Psychological Testimony. Jay Ziskin. Ed. by John T. Dunn. 1997. 192p. pap. 75.00 (*1-879689-08-1*) Law & Psych.

1997 Symposium on Cannabinoids, Vol. 1. Ed. by Patricia Reggio. 1997. (*0-9658053-0-1*) Intl Cannabinoid.

1997-98 Physician Practice Acquisition Resource Book. William O. Cleverley & Patrick J. Knott. 1997. 280p. pap. 295.00 (*1-882733-09-6*) Ctr Hlthcare IPS.

1997 Year Book of Sports Medicine. annuals Roy J. Shephard. 1998. (Illus.). 560p. (C). (gr. 13). text 74.95 (*0-8151-9739-X*, 25026) Mosby Inc.

1997 Year Book of Allergy & Clinical Immunology. Lanny J. Rosenwasser. 4th ed. 1997. (Illus.). 520p. (C). (gr. 13). text 74.95 (*0-8151-7278-8*, 23107) Mosby Inc.

1997 Year Book of Anesthesia & Pain Management. John H. Tinker. 1997. (Illus.). 568p. (C). (gr. 13). text 79.00 (*0-8151-8780-7*, 24435) Mosby Inc.

1997 Year Book of Dentistry. Lawrence Meskin. 1997. (Illus.). 552p. (C). (gr. 13). text 73.00 (*0-8151-7083-1*, 27508) Mosby Inc.

1997 Year Book of Dermatology. Arthur J. Sober. 1997. (Illus.). 696p. (C). (gr. 13). text 81.00 (*0-8151-9611-3*, 24949) Mosby Inc.

1997 Year Book of Digestive Diseases. Norton J. Greenberger. 1997. (Illus.). 544p. (C). (gr. 13). text 81.00 (*0-8151-9618-0*, 24955) Mosby Inc.

1997 Year Book of Drug Therapy. Louis Lasagna. 1997. (Illus.). 488p. (C). (gr. 13). text 79.95 (*0-8151-5295-7*, 24746) Mosby Inc.

1997 Year Book of Endocrinology. John D. Bagdade. 1997. (Illus.). 512p. (C). (gr. 13). text 79.00 (*0-8151-9625-3*, 24962) Mosby Inc.

1997 Year Book of Family Practice. Alfred O. Berg. 1997. (Illus.). 592p. (C). (gr. 13). text 66.95 (*0-8151-9628-8*, 24965) Mosby Inc.

1997 Year Book of Medicine. Ed. by Martin J. Cline et al. 1997. (Illus.). 1024p. (C). (gr. 13). text 75.00 (*0-8151-3155-0*, 26974) Mosby Inc.

1997 Year Book of Neurology & Neurosurgery. Walter G. Bradley. 1997. (Illus.). 608p. (C). (gr. 13). text 78.00 (*0-8151-1209-2*, 23003) Mosby Inc.

1997 Year Book of Obstetrics & Gynecology & Women's Health. Morrow et al. 1997. (Illus.). 728p. (C). (gr. 13). text 79.00 (*0-8151-6019-4*, 22714) Mosby Inc.

1997 Year Book of Occupational & Environmental Health. Edward A. Emmett. 1997. (Illus.). 392p. (C). (gr. 13). text 74.95 (*0-8151-9706-3*, 24993) Mosby Inc.

1997 Year Book of Ophthalmology. Wilson. 1997. (Illus.). 608p. (C). (gr. 13). text 82.00 (*0-8151-9712-8*, 24999) Mosby Inc.

1997 Year Book of Pathology & Laboratory Medicine. Ed. by Mark Stoler. 1997. (Illus.). 472p. (C). (gr. 13). text 83.00 (*0-8151-9721-7*, 25008) Mosby Inc.

1997 Year Book of Pediatrics. James A. Stockman. 1997. (Illus.). 744p. (C). (gr. 13). text 67.95 (*0-8151-9724-1*, 25011) Mosby Inc.

1997 Year Book of Plastic & Reconstructive Surgery. Ronald D. Miller. 1997. (Illus.). 480p. (C). (gr. 13). text 82.00 (*0-8151-9727-6*, 25014) Mosby Inc.

1997 Year Book of Podiatry. Ed. by Stephen J. Kominsky. 1997. (Illus.). 392p. (C). (gr. 13). text 73.00 (*0-8151-9730-6*, 25017) Mosby Inc.

1997 Year Book of Psychiatric & Applied Mental Health. John A. Talbott. 1997. (Illus.). 616p. (C). (gr. 13). text 73.00 (*0-8151-8945-1*, 24105) Mosby Inc.

1997 Year Book of Pulmonary Diseases. Petty. 1997. (Illus.). 560p. (C). (gr. 13). text 79.00 (*0-8151-9735-7*, 25022) Mosby Inc.

1997 Year Book of Rheumatology. Ed. by John S. Sergent. 4th ed. 1997. (Illus.). 480p. (C). (gr. 13). text 86.00 (*0-8151-7863-8*, 23010) Mosby Inc.

1997 Year Book of Surgery. Edward M. Copeland, III. 1997. (Illus.). 672p. (C). (gr. 13). text 74.00 (*0-8151-9742-X*, 25029) Mosby Inc.

1996 Mercer Guide to Social Security & Medicare. Dale Detlefs & Robert J. Myers. 24th ed. 1995. 200p. pap. 9.95 (*1-880754-96-7*) W M Mercer.

1996 Annual Statement Instructions - Health Maintenance Organizations. Ed. by Todd Sells. 7th rev. ed. 1996. 82p. (C). ring bd. 175.00 (*0-89382-408-9*, ASI-HM) Nat Assn Insurance.

1996 Blue Book of Optometrists. 1995. 447p. pap. 95.00 incl. disk (*0-7506-9682-6*) Buttrwrth-Heinemann.

1996 Computers in Cardiology. IEEE, Engineering in Medicine and Biology Staff. 1996. LC 80-641097. 850p. pap. text (*0-7803-3710-7*, 96CH36012); lib. bdg. (*0-7803-3711-5*, 96CH36012); fiche (*0-7803-3712-3*, 96CH36012) Inst Electrical.

1996 Consumer RX Drug Price Guide Vol. 1: Spring Issues. 1996. (Consumer RX Drug Price Guide Ser.). 128p. (Orig.). pap. 19.95 (*0-9652203-0-3*) Greystone Pubng.

1996 15th Southern Biomedical Engineering Conference. IEEE, Engineering in Medicine and Biology Staff. Ed. by IEEE, Institute of Electrical and Electronics Engineers, Inc. Staff. 1996. LC 96-212640. 350p. pap. 128.00 (*0-7803-3131-1*, 96TH8154); fiche 128.00 (*0-7803-3132-X*, 96TM8154) Inst Electrical.

1996 Healthcare Guide to the Internet. Ed. by Jennifer Wayne-Doppke. 1996.Tr. of Nineteen Ninety-Six Healthcare Guide to the Inter. (Illus.). 123p. (Orig.). pap. text 68.00 (*0-9645360-1-3*) Cor Hlthcare.

Nineteen Ninety-Six Healthcare Guide to the Inter see 1996 Healthcare Guide to the Internet

1996 Home Health Care Law, Vol. 1. Fay Rozovsky. 1996. 65.00 (*0-316-76103-6*, Little Brwn Med Div) Lppncott W & W.

1996 National Emergency Department Annual Survey Report Summary. Contrib. by Susan L. MacLean et al. unabr. ed. 1997. 78p. pap. 30.00 (*0-935890-16-5*) Emerg Nurses IL.

1996 National Emergency Department Database Survey. Contrib. by Susan L. MacLean et al. unabr. ed. 1997. 311p. pap. 500.00 (*0-935890-17-3*) Emerg Nurses IL.

1996-97 Almanac of Hospital Financial & Operating Indicators. William O. Cleverley. 1996. (Illus.). 520p. pap. 350.00 (*1-882733-07-X*) Ctr Hlthcare IPS.

1996-97 Supplement to Health Law, Cases, Materials & Problems. Barry R. Furrow et al. 1996. (American Casebook Ser.). 350p. pap. text, suppl. ed. (*0-314-20598-5*) West Pub.

1996 Physician Salary Survey Report. 1996. 384p. (Orig.). pap. 250.00 (*0-939326-95-7*) Hosp & Hlthcare.

1996 Physicians Fee & Coding Guide. James R. Lyle & Hoyt W. Torras. 1996. pap. 109.95 (*1-879249-14-6*) HlthCare Consult.

1996 Resident Year Book of Surgery. Edward Copeland. 5th ed. 1998. LC 98-4103. (Illus.). 528p. (C). (gr. 13). text 67.00 (*0-8151-2952-1*, 31833) Mosby Inc.

1996-97 Hospital Salary & Benefits Report. 1996. 300p. pap. 250.00 (*0-939326-97-3*) Hosp & Hlthcare.

1996-97 Nursing Home Salary & Benefits Report. 1996. 288p. (Orig.). pap. 250.00 (*0-939326-96-5*) Hosp & Hlthcare.

1996-97 Nursing Department Report. 5th ed. 1996. 152p. pap. 195.00 (*0-939326-26-4*) Hosp & Hlthcare.

1993 Bioengineering Conference. Ed. by N. A. Langrana et al. 1993. LC 93-71951. (BED Ser.: Vol. 24). 677p. 70.00 (*0-7918-0682-0*) ASME.

1993-1994 Debate on Health Care: Did the Polls Mislead the Policy Makers? Bowman. 1995. 50p. (Orig.). pap. 9.95 (*0-8447-7031-0*) Am Enterprise.

1992 Columbus & Franklin County Cancer Incidence: Assessment & Mapping 5 Leading Cancer Sites. Columbus Health Department Staff. 1998. (Columbus Community Health Assessment Ser.: Vol. 8). (Illus.). iii, 93p. pap. (*1-888492-54-6*) Columbus Hlth.

1992 Directory of Toxicology Laboratories Offering Contract Services (DOTLOCS) Ed. by Ralph I. Freudenthal. 1992. LC 90-81989. 272p. (Orig.). 99.95 (*0-9623813-4-9*) Aribet Bks.

1992 National Directory of Fire Chiefs, Rescue & Emergency Departments, Vol. I. Ed. by Steve Cywinski. 1992. 30.00 (*1-880245-02-7*) SPAN Pub.

1992-93 Dallas-Fort Worth Medical Director. Ed. by Diane E. Huggins. 1992. (Illus.). 826p. pap. 42.50 (*1-882328-01-9*) Am Med Sales.

1992-93 Home Care Salary & Benefits Report. 2nd ed. 1992. pap. 250.00 (*0-939326-71-X*) Hosp & Hlthcare.

1978. pap. 5.00 (*0-89970-132-9*, OP-051) AMA.

1978 Annual Handbook for Group Facilitators. Ed. by J. William Pfeiffer & John E. Jones. 7th ed. 1978. LC 73-92841. (Human Resource Development Ser.). (Illus.). 295p. pap. 99.00 (*0-88390-098-X*); pap. 49.00 (*0-88390-099-8*) Jossey-Bass (Pffr & Co).

1979 Annual Handbook for Group Facilitators. Ed. by John E. Jones & J. William Pfeiffer. 8th ed. 1979. LC 73-92841. (Human Resource Development Ser.). (Illus.). 295p. pap. 99.00 (*0-88390-093-9*); 205p. pap. 49.00 (*0-88390-095-5*) Jossey-Bass (Pffr & Co).

1939-1989: Fifty Years Progress in Allergy. A Tribute to Paul Kallos. Ed. by B. H. Waksman. 1990. (Chemical Immunology Ser.: Vol. 49). (Illus.). xii, 284p. 219.25 (*3-8055-5076-6*) S Karger.

Nineteenth Century Medical Attitudes Toward Alcoholic Addiction: Six Studies, 1814 to 1867, an Original Anthology. Ed. by Gerald N. Grob. 1981. LC 80-1204. (Addiction in America Ser.). lib. bdg. 40.95 (*0-405-13562-9*) Ayer.

Nineteenth-Century Origins of Neuroscientific Concepts. Edwin Clarke & L. S. Jacyna. 1998. 593p. (C). pap. text 17.00 (*0-7881-5669-1*) DIANE Pub.

XIXes Journees Nationales de Neonatologie, 1989. Ed. by J. P. Relier. 1989. (Progres en Neonatologie Ser.: Vol. 9). (Illus.). 268p. pap. 115.75 (*3-8055-5060-X*) S Karger.

1997 Orlando Conference Abstracts & Resources: The American Occupational Therapy Association's 1997 Annual Conference & Exposition, Friday, April 11—Tuesday, April 15, 1997, Orange County Convention Center Orlando, Florida. AOTA Staff. 1997. LC 98-182954. (*1-56900-072-7*) Am Occup Therapy.

Ninety-Nine Days & Get Up: A Pre- & Post-Release Survival Manual for Inmates & Their Loved Ones. Ned Rollo. 2nd ed. 1988. (Information Ser.). 29p. (Orig.). pap. 3.95 (*1-878436-04-X*) OPEN TX.

Ninety-Three Health Benefits Planning Guide for Seniors. Phyllis Shelton. Ed. by Michael Goforth. 1993. 50p. (Orig.). pap. 10.00 (*0-9633516-0-5*) Shelton Mktg.

Nino Campesino Deshabilitado: Una Guia Para Promotores de Salud, Trabajadores de Rehabilitation y Familias. David B. Werner. Ed. by Elizabeth De Avila & Martin Lamarque. 1990. LC 86-81738. (SPA., Illus.). 672p. (Orig.). pap. 22.00 (*0-942364-07-4*) Hesperian Found.

Nino de Dos a Cinco Anos. Editorial America, S. A. Staff. Ed. by Maria E. Del Real. 1990. (SPA., Illus.). 264p. (Orig.). pap. (*0-944499-69-4*) Editorial Amer.

Nino de Seis a Trece Anos. Editorial America, S. A. Staff. Ed. by Maria E. Del Real. 1990. (SPA., Illus.). 304p. (Orig.). pap. (*0-944499-88-0*) Editorial Amer.

Nino Insoportable. Doris J. Rapp. Tr. by Lydia J. Zaragoza. 1988. Orig. Title: The Impossible Child. (SPA., Illus.). 170p. pap. 12.95 (*1-880509-01-6*); VHS 16.95 (*1-880509-02-4*) Practical Allergy.

1998 Year Book of Family Practice. Berg. 1998. (Illus.). 472p. text 66.95 (*0-8151-9629-6*, 24966) Mosby Inc.

1999 Yearbook of Otolaryngology-Head & Neck Surgery. Paparella. 2nd ed. 1999. (Illus.). 350p. text 79.00 (*0-8151-9719-5*, 25006) Mosby Inc.

1998 Year Book of Nephrology, Hypertension & Mineral Metabolism. Steve Schwab. 1998. (Illus.). 312p. text 83.00 (*0-8151-9646-6*, 24983) Mosby Inc.

1998 Year Book of Otolaryngology - Head & Neck Surgery. Paparella. 1998. (Illus.). 368p. text 76.00 (*0-8151-9718-7*, 25005) Mosby Inc.

Ninth Street Notebook: Voice of a Nurse in the City. Veneta Masson. 2001. LC 00-90481. 208p. pap. 18.00 (*0-9673688-1-2*) Sage Femme Pr.

NIOSH Manual of Analytical Methods: Sampling & Analytical Methods for Monitoring Occupational Exposures to Toxic Substances in Air & Biological Samples. Ed. by Peter M. Eller & Mary E. Cassinelli. 1994. (Illus.). 625p. (C). pap. text 95.00 (*0-7881-1500-6*) DIANE Pub.

Nishkamakarma. John G. Finch. 1982. LC 82-83498. (Orig.). (C). pap. 10.00 (*0-9609928-0-4*) Integ Pr.

Nisoldipine CC Investigators' Meeting, Wiesbaden, Germany, May 1996: Proceedings - Sessions I & II. Ed. by G. Heusch & J. L. Palma-Gamiz. 1996. (Journal: Vol. 88, Supplement 1, 1997). (Illus.). iv, 72p. pap. 33.25 (*3-8055-6464-3*) S Karger.

Nisoldipine Coat-Core. Ed. by M. F. Rousseau. 1999. LC 99-33461. (Illus.). x, 62p. pap. 41.00 (*3-540-66049-6*) Spr-Verlag.

Nitrate Therapy & Nitrate Tolerance: Current Concepts & Controversies. Ed. by D. Rezakovic & J. S. Alpert. 1993. LC 92-49386. (Illus.). x, 548p. 252.25 (*3-8055-5669-1*) S Karger.

Nitrates III - Cardiovascular Effects: Proceedings. Ed. by H. J. Engel & P. R. Lichtlen. 1981. (Illus.). 597p. 61.95 (*0-387-10761-4*) Spr-Verlag.

Nitrates Updated: Current Use in Angina, Ischemia, Infarction & Failure. Ed. by Udho Thadani. 1997. LC 95-14210. 236p. (C). text 174.00 (*0-7923-3466-3*) Kluwer Academic.

Nitric Oxide: Roles in Neuronal Communication & Neurotoxicity. Ed. by Hiroshi Takagi et al. 1994. LC 94-15352. (Taniguchi Symposia on Brain Sciences Ser.: No. 17). 89.95 (*0-8493-7776-5*) CRC Pr.

Nitric Oxide & Infection. Ferric C. Fang. 1999. LC 99-30078. (C). text (*0-306-46147-1*, Kluwer Plenum) Kluwer Academic.

Nitric Oxide & Radicals in the Pulmonary Vasculature. E. Kenneth Weir et al. 1996. LC 95-36634. (Illus.). 528p. 85.00 (*0-87993-631-2*) Futura Pub.

Nitric Oxide & the Cardiovascular System. Ed. by Joseph Loscalzo & Joseph A. Vita. 2000. LC 99-54493. (Contemporary Cardiology Ser.: Vol. 4). 616p. 175.00 (*0-89603-620-0*) Humana.

Nitric Oxide & the Kidney: Physiology & Pathophysiology. Michael S. Goligorsky & Steven S. Gross. 1997. LC 96-48721. 488p. 89.95 (*0-412-08061-3*) Kluwer Academic.

Nitric Oxide & the Lung. Ed. by Warren M. Zapol & Kenneth D. Bloch. 1996. LC 96-35124. (Lung Biology in Health & Disease Ser.: Vol. 98). (Illus.). 497p. text 195.00 (*0-8247-9725-6*) Dekker.

Nitric Oxide, Cytochromes P450, & Sexual Steroid Hormones. Ed. by Jack R. Lancaster & J. F. Parkinson. 1997. LC 97-25453. (Ernst Schering Research Foundation Ser.: Vol. 21). (Illus.). 307p. 53.95 (*3-540-63050-3*) Spr-Verlag.

Nitric Oxide in Bone & Joint Disease. Ed. by M. V. Hukkanen et al. 1998. LC 98-14672. (Postgraduate Medical Science Ser.: No. 7). (Illus.). 206p. (C). text 90.00 (*0-521-59220-8*) Cambridge U Pr.

Nitric Oxide in Health & Disease. Jill Lincoln et al. 1997. (Biomedical Research Topics Ser.). (Illus.). 377p. (C). text 120.00 (*0-521-55038-6*); pap. text 45.95 (*0-521-55977-4*) Cambridge U Pr.

Nitrogen & Energy Nutrition of Ruminants. Raymond L. Shirley. 1986. (Animal Feeding & Nutrition Ser.). text 94.00 (*0-12-640260-4*) Acad Pr.

Nitrogen Cycling in Ecosystems of Latin America & the Caribbean. C. P. Robertson et al. 1982. text 211.50 (*90-247-2719-7*) Kluwer Academic.

Nitrogen, Electrolytes Water & Metabolism. Ed. by Miloslav Rechcigl, Jr. 1979. (Comparative Animal Nutrition Ser.: Vol. 3). (Illus.). 113.25 (*3-8055-2829-9*) S Karger.

Nitroglycerin 5. Ed. by Bodo E. Strauer. 1987. 125p. (C). pap. text 63.10 (*3-11-010879-8*) De Gruyter.

Nitroglycerin 7: Progress in Therapy. 1990. LC 91-28638. 103p. pap. 63.10 (*3-11-013396-2*) De Gruyter.

Nitrosamines & Human Cancer. Ed. by Peter N. Magee. 1982. LC 82-12952. (Banbury Reports: Vol. 12). 599p. 67.00 (*0-87969-211-1*) Cold Spring Harbor.

NK Cell Medicated Cytotoxicology: Receptors, Signaling & Mechanics. Eva Lotzova. 1992. 512p. lib. bdg. 239.00 (*0-8493-6267-9*, QR188) CRC Pr.

NK Cells & Natural Immunity. Ed. by B. Bonavida & S. Golup. 1995. (Journal: Vol. 14, 2, 1995). (Illus.). 60p. pap. 47.00 (*3-8055-6263-2*) S Karger.

NK Cells in the Liver. Ed. by Luc Bouwens. 1995. LC 95-1069. (Medical Intelligence Unit Ser.). 136p. text 79.00 (*1-57059-249-7*) Landes Bioscience.

NLN Criteria for Appraisal of Baccalaureate Programs: A Critical Hermeneutic Analysis. Nancy Diekelmann et al. Ed. by Linda Moody & Moira Shannon. 1989. 80p. 17.95 (*0-88737-429-8*) Natl League Nurse.

Nlp: The New Technology. Steve Andreas. 1996. 352p. pap. 14.95 (*0-688-14619-8*, Quil) HarperTrade.

***NMDA Antagonists As Potential Analgesic Drugs.** Ed. by D. J. S. Sirinathsinghji & R. G. Hill. 2002. LC 2001-43881. (*3-7643-6011-9*) Birkhauser.

NMDA Receptor. Ed. by Graham L. Collingridge & Jeffrey C. Watkins. 2nd ed. 1995. LC 94-10163. (Illus.). 516p. pap. text 54.50 (*0-19-262502-0*) OUP.

NMDA Receptor Related Agents: Biochemistry, Pharmacology & Behavior. Ed. by T. Kameyama et al. 1991. LC 90-64353. (Illus.). 414p. text 75.00 (*0-916182-08-8*) NPP Bks.

NMR: A Primer for Medical Imaging. Gerald L. Wolfe & Carol Popp. 1983. 96p. 30.95 (*0-316-95099-8*, Little Brwn Med Div) Lppncott W & W.

NMR: Principles & Applications to Biomedical Research. Ed. by J. W. Pettegrew. 1989. (Illus.). 618p. 133.00 (*0-387-97094-0*) Spr-Verlag.

NMR - Basic Principles & Progress Vol. 22: Solid-State NMR; Inorganic Matter, Vol. 31; Vol II. Ed. by P. Diehl et al. 1994. (Illus.). 215p. 220.00 (*0-387-57190-6*) Spr-Verlag.

NMR - Basic Principles & Progress Vol. 22: Solid-State NMR; Methods, Vol. 30; Vol. I. Ed. by B. Blumich et al. 1994. (Illus.). 281p. 186.00 (*0-387-57189-2*) Spr-Verlag.

NMR Data Processing. Jeffrey C. Hoch & Alan S. Stern. 1996. LC 96-4981. 196p. 87.50 (*0-471-03900-4*) Wiley.

NMR Imaging: Recent Developments & Future Prospects. Ed. by P. Mansfield & H. L. Hahn. 1990. (Philosophical Transactions of the Royal Society, Series B: Vol. 334, 1990). (Illus.). 175p. text 95.00 (*0-85403-426-9*) Scholium Intl.

NMR in Biomedicine: The Physical Basis. Ed. by Eiichi Fukushima. (Key Papers in Physics). (Illus.). 170p. 1997. 69.95 (*0-88318-603-9*); 1989. pap. 43.95 (*0-88318-609-8*) Spr-Verlag.

NMR in Drug Design. Ed. by David J. Craik. 1995. LC 95-34213. (Analytical Biotechnology Ser.). 496p. 209.95 (*0-8493-7824-9*, 7824) CRC Pr.

NMR in Medicine: The Instrumentation & Clinical Applications: Proceedings of the AAPM 1985 Summer School Held at the University of Portland, Portland, Oregon, August 4-9, 1985. Ed. by Stephen R. Thomas & Robert L. Dixon. 1986. (American Association of Physicists in Medicine Symposium Ser.: No. 14). 608p. 70.00 (*0-88318-497-4*) Am Inst Physics.

NMR in Medicine & Biology: Structure Determination, Tomography, In-Vivo Spectroscopy. K. H. Hausser & H. R. Kalbitzer. 1991. (Illus.). 240p. 95.00 (*0-387-53195-5*) Spr-Verlag.

NMR in Physiology & Biomedicine. Ed. by Robert J. Gillies. 1994. LC 94-930. (Illus.). 471p. text 104.00 (*0-12-283980-3*) Acad Pr.

NMR of Biological Macromolecules, 87. Ed. by Chariklia I. Stassinopoulou. 1994. 357p. 206.00 (*0-387-58269-X*) Spr-Verlag.

NMR of Proteins & Nucleic Acids. Kurt Wuthrich. 1986. LC 86-7834. (Baker Lectures). 320p. 105.00 (*0-471-82893-9*) Wiley.

NMR Spectra of Simple Heterocycles. T. J. Batterham. 1982. LC 80-11724. 560p. reprint ed. lib. bdg. 69.50 (*0-89874-140-8*) Krieger.

NMR Spectroscopy & Its Application to Biomedical Research. Sustana K. Sarkar. 1996. LC 96-45701. 406p. 209.00 (*0-444-89410-1*) Elsevier.

NMR Spectroscopy & Stereoregularity of Polymers. K. Matsuzaki et al. 1996. (Illus.). xviii, 278p. 287.00 (*3-8055-6298-5*) S Karger.

NMR Spectroscopy in Drug Research. Ed. by Jerzy W. Jaroszewski et al. 1988. (Alfred Benzon Symposium Ser.: No. 26). (Illus.). 606p. 162.50 (*87-16-06955-2*) Coronet Bks.

NMR Spectroscopy in Psychiatric Brain Disorders. Ed. by Henry A. Nasrallah & Jay W. Pettegrew. 1995. LC 94-34269. (Progress in Psychiatry Ser.: No. 47). 272p. text 16.95 (*0-88048-483-7*, 8483) Am Psychiatric.

NMR Techniques in Catalysis. Ed. by Alexis T. Bell & Alexander Pines. 1994. LC 93-43400. (Chemical Industries Ser.: Vol. 55). (Illus.). 448p. text 215.00 (*0-8247-9173-8*) Dekker.

NMS Anatomy. Ernest W. April. 2nd ed. 1990. (National Medical Ser.). 610p. 26.00 (*0-683-06200-X*) Lppncott W & W.

NMS Genetics. J. Friedman et al. 1992. (National Medical Ser.). 250p. 26.00 (*0-683-06218-2*) Lppncott W & W.

NMS Neuroanatomy. William DeMyer. 1990. (National Medical Ser.). 380p. 26.00 (*0-683-06236-0*) Lppncott W & W.

NMS Pediatrics. Paul H. Dworkin. 2nd ed. 1991. (National Medical Ser.). 460p. 27.00 (*0-683-06246-8*) Lppncott W & W.

NMS Pharmacology. L. Jacobs. 3rd ed. 1991. (National Medical Ser.). 336p. 26.00 (*0-683-06250-6*) Lppncott W & W.

NMS Surgery. Bruce E. Jarrell & R. Anthony Carabasi, III. 4th ed. 2000. LC 00-20850. 720p. pap. text 32.00 (*0-683-30615-4*) Lppncott W & W.

No: The Positive Response to Alcohol. Jerry D. Hull. 1989. LC 93-212959. (Christian Response to Contemporary Social Issues Ser.). 104p. pap. 9.99 (*0-8341-1301-5*) Beacon Hill.

NO & Nervous System Plasticity: Journal. Ed. by Sean Murphy. 1997. (Journal: Vol. 19, No. 3, 1997). (Illus.). 74p. pap. 40.00 (*3-8055-6525-9*) S Karger.

***No Apologies for Ritalin.** Vidya Bhushan Gupta. 2000. 176p. pap. (*0-930958-09-8*, EP8012AD) Excptnl Parent.

No Appointment Necessary: The Hospital Emergency Department in the Medical Services World. Julius A. Roth & Dorothy Douglas. 1983. 324p. pap. text 27.50 (*0-8290-1255-9*) Irvington.

No Beggars Just Balloons: A Practical Approach to Self-Transformation. Ted L. Orcutt. 1989. 248p. 19.95 (*0-9623434-2-0*) Global Village.

No Bull Diet: A Lifetime Beyond Dieting. Howard A. Rose. 1992. pap. 10.00 (*0-9631828-0-3*) Hart Mktg.

No Butts about It: How to Want to Stop Smoking. John R. Parker. 3rd ed. 1989. (Illus.). 88p. (Orig.). pap. 6.95 (*0-912095-00-8*) Johmax Bks Inc.

No Cellulite Cookbook: The First Cookbook-Menu Planner to Help You Fight Those Lumps, Bumps & Bulges. Penelope Perryman & Kirsten West. 1983. 256p. 14.38 (*0-02-595900-X*) Macmillan.

No Drugs Allowed: An Elementary Drug Education Curriculum. Berneta K. Sherck. Ed. by Erla K. Williams. 1989. (Illus.). 120p. 75.00 (*0-935589-19-8*) Elite Pub IN.

No-Drugs Guide to Better Health. Eleanore B. Busch & Bernd W. Busch. 1983. 223p. 19.95 (*0-13-623090-3*); pap. 5.95 (*0-13-623082-2*) P-H (Parker Publishing Co).

No-Hysterectomy Option: Your Body—Your Choice. Herbert A. Goldfarb. 2nd rev. ed. 1997. LC 96-29848. 288p. pap. 16.95 (*0-471-16557-3*) Wiley.

No Less a Woman: Femininity, Sexuality & Breast Cancer. Deborah H. Kahane. 2nd ed. 1995. LC 95-37552. (Illus.). 320p. pap. 14.95 (*0-89793-187-4*) Hunter Hse.

No Longer a Victim. Carol J. Cole. 1996. (Illus.). 196p. (Orig.). pap. 19.95 (*1-890961-02-7*) C Communs.

No Longer Patient: Feminist Ethics & Health Care. Susan Sherwin. 1992. 304p. pap. 22.95 (*1-56639-061-3*) Temple U Pr.

No Milk: A Revolutionary Solution to Back Pain & Headaches. Daniel A. Twogood. 1992. (Illus.). (Orig.). (C). pap. text (*0-9631125-0-3*) Wilhelmina.

No More Allergies: Identifying & Eliminating Allergies & Sensitivity Reactions to Everything in Your Environment. Gary Null. 1992. LC 92-50149. (Gary Null's Natural Health Library). 421p. pap. 14.95 (*0-679-74310-3*) Villard Books.

No More Amoxicillin. Mary Ann Block. 1998. LC 99-188647. 144p. pap. 12.00 (*1-57566-316-3*, Knsington) Kensgtn Pub Corp.

No More Antibiotics: Preventing & Treating Ear & Respiratory Infections the Natural Way. Mary A. Block. 2000. 128p. mass mkt. 5.99 (*1-57566-500-X*) Kensgtn Pub Corp.

No More Black Days: Complete Freedom from Depression, Eating Disorders & Other Compulsive Behaviors. Lauri A. Mallord. 1992. 128p. pap. 5.95 (*0-9630069-0-8*, 1000) Whi Stone.

No More Dying: The Conquest of Aging & the Extension of Human Life. Joel Kurtzman & Phillip Gordon. 1976. LC 75-32856. 19.95 (*0-87477-055-6*) ETC Pubns.

No More Heroes: Madness & Psychiatry in War. Richard A. Gabriel. 1988. pap. 7.95 (*0-8090-1539-0*) Hill & Wang.

No More Hot Flashes & Other Good News. Penny W. Budoff. 1989. 376p. mass mkt. 5.99 (*0-446-35879-7*) Warner Bks.

No More Kidney Stones. John S. Rodman et al. 1996. LC 95-52786. 240p. pap. 16.95 (*0-471-12587-3*) Wiley.

No More Morning Sickness: A Survival Guide for Pregnant Women. Miriam Erick. 1993. LC 92-43578. 192p. pap. 12.95 (*0-452-26983-0*, Plume) Dutton Plume.

No More Ritalin. Mary Ann Block. 1997. 160p. mass mkt. 5.99 (*1-57566-239-6*) Kensgtn Pub Corp.

No More Sleepless Nights. Peter J. Hauri & Shirley Linde. 2nd rev. ed. 1996. LC 96-7758. (Illus.). 304p. pap. 16.95 (*0-471-14904-7*) Wiley.

No More Snoring: A Proven Program to Conquer Snoring & Sleep Apnea. Victor Hoffstein & Shirley Linde. 1998. LC 98-16096. 192p. pap. 12.95 (*0-471-24375-2*) Wiley.

No Mountain Too High. Andrea Gabbard. 1998. LC 98-7824. (Illus.). 240p. pap. text 16.00 (*1-58005-008-5*) Seal Pr WA.

No New Baby: For Siblings Whose Brother or Sister Dies. Marilyn Gryte. 1988. (SPA.). 4.95 (*1-56123-114-2*) Centering Corp.

No One Prepared Me for This. Kathleen V. Nielson. 1991. (Orig.). pap. 9.95 (*0-9622967-0-8*) IHC Home Health.

No Place for Borders: The HIV/AIDS Epidemic & Development in Asia & the Pacific. Ed. by Godfrey Linge & Doug Porter. 1998. LC 98-176591. 191p. pap. (*1-86448-307-5*) Allen & Unwin Pty AUS. *Dist:* Paul & Co Pubs.

No Place for Borders: The HIV/AIDS Epidemic & Development in Asia & the Pacific. Doug Porter & Godfrey J. Linge. 1997. LC 96-52306. 224p. text 49.95 (*0-312-17354-7*) St Martin.

No Place Like Home: As Nursing Homes Profit from Pain, Communities Fight to Reform Them. Ed. & Pref. by Eric R. Bates. 1992. (Southern Exposure Ser.). (Illus.). 64p. (Orig.). (C). pap. 5.00 (*0-943819-54-7*) Inst Southern Studies.

No Red Meat: Over 300 Delicious Lowfat, Low-Cholestrol Recipes. Brenda J. Shriver & Ann Tinsley. 1989. LC 89-11632. (Illus.). 320p. pap. 18.00 (*1-55561-021-8*) Fisher Bks.

No Safe Place: Toxic Waste, Leukemia & Community Action. Phil Brown & Edwin J. Mikkelsen. 1997. 284p. pap. text 18.95 (*0-520-21248-7*) U CA Pr.

No-Scalpel Vasectomy: An Illustrated Guide for Surgeons. Betty Gonzales. 2nd ed. 1997. LC 96-36490. (Illus.). 59p. 20.00 (*0-9604536-6-0*) EngenderHlth.

No Small Part: A History of Regional Organizations in American Psychology. Ed. by James L. Pate et al. 1993. LC 93-37085. 227p. text 29.95 (*1-55798-215-5*) Am Psychol.

No Sugar Added: Or Redesigning Our Children's Future. Nicholas Krilanovich. 1982. (Illus.). 300p. 14.00 (*0-941098-00-1*) November Bks.

No-Talk Therapy for Children & Adolescents. Martha B. Straus. 1999. LC 98-44978. 288p. 27.00 (*0-393-70286-3*) Norton.

No Time for Fear. Diane Fessler. 1997. 255p. reprint ed. pap. 22.95 (*0-87013-440-X*) Mich St U Pr.

No Time for Tears. Lora W. Hughes. 1985. LC 85-8644. (Illus.). 305p. reprint ed. pap. 7.95 (*0-8032-7229-4*, Bison Books); text 40.00 (*0-8032-2336-6*) U of Nebr Pr.

No Time to Lose: Getting More from HIV Prevention. Monica S. Ruiz & Institute of Medicine Staff. 2001. LC 00-65369. (Illus.). xxiii, 225p. 39.95 (*0-309-07137-2*) Natl Acad Pr.

No Time to Teach? A Nurse's Guide to Patient & Family Education. Contrib. by Fran London. 1999. LC 99-14488. (Illus.). 448p. pap. text 32.95 (*0-7817-1644-6*) Lppncott W & W.

No Voice Is Ever Wholly Lost. Louise J. Kaplan. 1995. LC 94-47923. 288p. 24.00 (*0-671-79868-5*) S&S Trade.

No Water in My Cup. Ratibor-Ray M. Jurjevich. 1968. LC 68-9415. 12.95 (*0-87212-010-4*) Libra.

No Water in My Cup: Experiences & a Controlled Study of Psychotherapy of Delinquent Girls. Ratibor-Ray M. Jurjevich. 1968. 194p. 8.95 (*0-930711-03-3*) Ichthys Bks.

Noah Smernoff: A Life in Medicine. Robert T. King. 1990. (Great Basin History of Medicine Ser.: No. 1). (Illus.). 144p. lib. bdg. 26.00 (*1-56475-001-9*); fiche (*1-56475-352-2*) U NV Oral Hist.

Nobel Lectures in Physiology or Medicine 1971-1980. J. Lindsten. 1992. 690p. text 122.00 (*981-02-0790-5*); pap. text 61.00 (*981-02-0791-3*) World Scientific Pub.

Nobel Lectures in Physiology or Medicine 1981-1990. J. Lindsten. 1993. 640p. text 118.00 (*981-02-0792-1*); pap. text 55.00 (*981-02-0793-X*) World Scientific Pub.

Nobel Lectures in Physiology or Medicine, 1991-1995. 1997. 300p. text 33.00 (*981-02-3061-3*) World Scientific Pub.

Nobel Lectures in Physiology or Medicine, 1991-1995. Nils Ringertz. 1997. 300p. pap. text 19.00 (*981-02-3062-1*) World Scientific Pub.

Nobody Likes a Smartass: Expert Testimony by Psychologists. R. Buckhout. 1976. (Monographs: No. CR-44). 5.00 (*1-55524-045-3*) Ctr Respon Psych.

Nobody's Child: The Marie Balter Story. Marie Balter. 1991. 17.95 (*0-201-57073-4*) Addison-Wesley.

Nobody's Children: Orphans of the HIV Epidemic. Steven F. Dansky. 1997. LC 96-48940. (Haworth Social Ser.). 178p. pap. 14.95 (*1-56023-923-9*, Harrington Park) Haworth Pr.

Nobody's Fault. Slightly Off Center Writers Group Staff. 1995. (Orig.). pap. 8.95 (*1-56721-114-3*) Twnty-Fifth Cent Pr.

Nociception & Pain in Animals: Measurement Techniques & Procedures. Martin Kavaliers. 1997. (Neuroscience Intelligence Unit Ser.). 250p. 89.95 (*0-412-13441-1*) Chapman & Hall.

Nocturnal Enuresis: The Child's Experience. Richard J. Butler. 1995. LC 94-32797. (Illus.). 192p. pap. text 39.00 (*0-7506-2132-X*) Buttrwrth-Heinemann.

NOD Mice & Related Strains: Research Applications in Diabetes, AIDS, Cancer & Other Diseases. Edward Leiter & Mark Atkinson. 1999. LC 97-31480. (Molecular Biology Intelligence Unit Ser.). 182p. 99.00 (*1-57059-466-X*) Landes Bioscience.

Noise & Health. Ed. by Thomas H. Fay. 1991. (Illus.). 110p. text 35.00 (*0-924143-01-0*) NY Acad Med.

Noise & Your Health. Billy R. Boyd. 1996. 32p. pap. 3.50 (*0-9616792-6-3*) Taterhill.

***Noise Induced Hearing Loss.** Linda M. Luxon et al. 2001. 300p. (C). text (*1-86156-154-7*) Whurr Pub GBR. *Dist:* Taylor & Francis.

***Nolen-Hoeksema Abnormal Psychology: With Taking Sides, MindMap & Making the Grade.** Susan Nolen-Hoeksema. 2nd ed. 2000. 779p. (C). 82.50 incl. cd-rom (*0-07-241380-8*) McGrw-H Hghr Educ.

NOLS Wilderness First Aid. Tod Schimelpfenig et al. 2nd ed. 1992. LC 92-19090. (NOLS Library). (Illus.). 368p. pap. 14.95 (*0-8117-3084-0*) Stackpole.

Nomenclature Anatomique Illustree. Guntz. 1975. (FRE.). 512p. pap. 69.95 (*0-8288-5941-8*, M6307) Fr & Eur.

Nomenclature of Organic Compounds: Principles & Practice. Ed. by J. H. Fletcher et al. 1974. LC 73-92675. (Advances in Chemistry Ser.: No. 126). 337p. 54.95 (*0-8412-0191-9*); pap. 34.95 (*0-8412-0234-6*) Am Chemical.

Nomenclature of Organic Compounds: Principles & Practice. Robert B. Fox & Warren H. Powell. 2nd ed. 2001. LC 99-43801. (American Chemical Society Publication). (Illus.). xvii, 437p. text 215.00 (*0-8412-3648-8*) Am Chemical.

Nomina Anatomica Veterinaria & Nomina Histologica. 1983. 267p. 15.00 (*0-9600444-5-0*) Wld Assn Vet.

Nomina Simplicium Medicinarum ex Synonymariis Medii Aevi Collecta: Semantische Untersuchungen zum Fachwortschatz Hoch- & Spaetmittelalterlicher Drogenkunde. Willem F. Daems. 1993. LC 92-42058. (Studies in Ancient Medicine: Vol. 6). (GER.). 563p. 186.00 (*90-04-09672-8*) Brill Academic Pubs.

Non-Anticoagulant Actions of Glycosaminoglycans. Ed. by Job Harenberg et al. 1996. LC 96-10228. (Protein Binding Studies). (Illus.). 288p. (C). text 107.00 (*0-306-45299-5*, Kluwer Plenum) Kluwer Academic.

Non-Authentic Nature of Freud's Observations, Set, Vols. 1-2. Max Scharnberg. 1993. (Uppsala Studies in Education: Nos. 47-48). (Orig.). pap. 82.50 (*91-554-3122-4*) Coronet Bks.

Non-Automated Sphygmomanometers. 1994. 15p. pap. 73.00 (*1-57020-020-3*, SP9-209) Assn Adv Med Instrn.

Non-Cardiac Thoracic Interventions. 1997. LC 96-52547. (Radiologic Interventions Ser.). (*4-260-14288-7*) Igaku-Shoin.

Non-Cardiac Thoracic Interventions. Alan Matsumoto. 1997. LC 96-52547. (Radiologic Interventions Ser.). (Illus.). 384p. (*0-89640-288-6*) Igaku-Shoin.

Non-Coronary Angioplasty & Interventional Radiological Treatment of Vascular Malformations. Laszlo Szlavy & Juan M. Taveras. 1994. (Illus.). 700p. text 179.00 (*0-683-08066-0*) Lppncott W & W.

Non-Disabling Surgical Rehabilitation of the Forefoot. Milton D. Roven. 1976. LC 76-176177. (Illus.). 416p. 32.50 (*0-87527-123-5*) Green.

Non-Disseminated Breast Cancer: Controversial Issues in Management. G. H. Fletcher et al. 1993. LC 93-20548. (Medical Radiology Ser.). (Illus.). 168p. 166.00 (*0-387-54514-X*) Spr-Verlag.

Non-Drug European Secret. Michael Loes. 1999. pap. 5.95 (*1-893910-03-2*) Freedom Pr Inc.

Non-Drug Treatments for Essential Hypertension. Edward B. Blanchard et al. 1988. (Psychology Practitioner Guidebooks). 224p. text 35.00 (*0-08-032809-1*); pap. text 17.95 (*0-08-032808-3*) Elsevier (Pergamon Pr).

Non-Epileptic Seizures. Ed. by John R. Gates & A. James Rowan. 2nd ed. 1999. LC 99-55305. 344p. text 99.00 (*0-7506-7026-6*) Buttrwrth-Heinemann.

Non-Fluent Aphasia in a Multilingual World. Lise Menn et al. 1995. LC 95-14639. (Studies in Speech Pathology & Clinical Linguistics: Vol. 5). xvii, 212p. 72.00 (*1-55619-391-2*); pap. 27.95 (*1-55619-392-0*) J Benjamins Pubng Co.

Non-Governmental Organizations & Health in Developing Countries. Andrew Green & Ann Matthias. 1997. LC 96-27850. (Illus.). 240p. text 59.95 (*0-312-16428-9*) St Martin.

Non-Heart-Beating Organ Transplantation: Medical & Ethical Issues in Procurement. Institute of Medicine Staff. 1997. LC 98-114047. 104p. (C). pap. text 22.00 (*0-309-06424-4*) Natl Acad Pr.

Non-Heart-Beating Organ Transplantation: Practice & Protocols. Institute of Medicine Staff. 2000. 174p. pap. 42.00 (*0-309-06641-7*) Natl Acad Pr.

Non-Hodgkin's Lymphomas. Ed. by Ian T. Magrath. 2nd ed. 1997. 1174p. (*0-340-55793-1*) E A GBR. *Dist:* OUP.

Non-Hodgkin's Lymphomas: Making Sense of Diagnosis, Treatment & Options. Lorraine Johnston. Ed. by Linda Lamb. 1999. LC 98-55468. (Patient-Centered Guides Ser.). (Illus.). xx, 556p. pap. 24.95 (*1-56592-444-4*) OReilly & Assocs.

Non-Hodgkin's Lymphomas: New Techniques & Treatments. Ed. by J. J. Sotto et al. 1985. (Illus.). viii, 232p. 141.00 (*3-8055-4064-7*) S Karger.

Non-Human Primates As Models for Study of Human Reproduction: Proceedings of the International Primatological Society 7th Congress, Bangalore, January, 1979. International Primatological Society Staff. Ed. by T. C. Anand Kumar. 1980. (Illus.). 252p. pap. 77.50 (*3-8055-0540-X*) S Karger.

Non-Invasive Cardiac Imaging. Gibson. 1990. text 105.00 (*0-443-04200-4*) Saunders.

Non Invasive Cardiovascular Monitoring. Bernard Hayes. Ed. by C. E. Hahn & A. P. Adams. 1997. (Illus.). 229p. pap. (*0-7279-1038-8*) BMJ Pub GBR. *Dist:* AIDC.

Non-Invasive Diagnostics of the Left Heart: Biochemical Disturbances. B. Y. Kantor et al. 1998. 214p. (C). lib. bdg. 125.00 (*1-56072-243-6*) Nova Sci Pubs.

Non-Invasive Imaging of Atherosclerosis. Ed. by Michele Mercuri et al. 1997. LC 97-37849. (Developments in Cardiovascular Medicine Ser.: No. 199). 245p. text 159.50 (*0-7923-8036-3*) Kluwer Academic.

Non-Invasive Measurements of Bone Mass & Their Clinical Application. Ed. by S. H. Cohn. 1981. 240p. 138.00 (*0-8493-5789-6*, RC930, CRC Reprint) Franklin.

Non-Invasive Mechanical Methods in Cardiology & Cardivascular Dynamics: Proceedings of the World Congress, 4th, Amsterdam, April 14-16, 1975. World Congress on Ballistocardiography and Cardiovas. Ed. by W. J. Goedhard. 1976. (Bibliotheca Cardiologica Ser.: No. 35). 275p. 123.50 (*3-8055-2295-9*) S Karger.

Non-Invasive Respiratory Support. A. K. Simonds. 1995. (Illus.). 192p. pap. (*0-412-56840-3*) E A GBR. *Dist:* OUP.

Non-Invasive, Semi-Invasive Surgical Procedures, No. C-140. Business Communications Co., Inc. Staff. 1991. 189p. 2250.00 (*0-89336-831-8*) BCC.

Non-Invasive Techniques in Cardiology Journal: Cardiology, Vol. 71, No. 2-3, 1984. Ed. by J. S. Borer. 1984. (Illus.). 112p. pap. 69.75 (*3-8055-3886-3*) S Karger.

Non-Invasive Thermometry of the Human Body. Ed. by Michio Miyakawa et al. 1995. LC 95-20156. 272p. 169.95 (*0-8493-4738-6*, 4738) CRC Pr.

Non-Isotopic In Situ Hybridization: Applications to Clinical Diagnosis & Molecular Gene. Matteo Adinolfi & Angela F. Davies. 1994. (Medical Intelligence Unit Ser.). 114p. 99.00 (*1-879702-85-1*, LN0285) Landes Bioscience.

Non-Lymphoid Leukemias in Children. Ed. by Carl Pochedly. 1985. 256p. 45.00 (*0-275-90009-6*, C0009, Praeger Pubs) Greenwood.

Non-Mammalian Models for Research on Ageing. Ed. by F. A. Lints. 1985. (Interdisciplinary Topics in Gerontology Ser.: Vol. 21). (Illus.). viii, 288p. 172.25 (*3-8055-4019-1*) S Karger.

Non-Mathematical Approach to Basic MRI. Hans J. Smith & Frank Ranallo. 1989. LC 87-28170. (Illus.). 200p. (C). pap. text 23.95 (*0-944838-02-2*) Med Physics Pub.

Non-Mendelian Genetics in Humans: Medelian & Non-Mendelian. Harry Ostrer. 1998. LC 97-20620. (Oxford Monographs on Medical Genetics: No. 35). (Illus.). 216p. text 42.50 (*0-19-506877-7*) OUP.

***Non-neoplastic Diseases of the Anorectum: An Interdisciplinary Approach.** P. Fruhmorgen & H. P. Bruch. 2001. (Falk Symposium Ser.: Vol. 118). 272p. 133.00 (*0-7923-8766-X*) Kluwer Academic.

Non-Neoplastic Diseases of the Anorectum: Proceedings of the 64th Falk Symposium, Held in Titisee - Black Forest, Germany, October 11-13, 1991. Ed. by L. Demling & P. Fruhmorgen. 1992. LC 92-15602. 400p. (C). text 191.50 (*0-7923-8979-4*) Kluwer Academic.

Non-Neuronal Cells in Alzheimer's Disease. M. Nicolini & Paolo F. Zatta. 1995. 200p. text 61.00 (*981-02-2092-8*) World Scientific Pub.

Non-Occupational Exposure to Mineral Fibres. Ed. by J. Bignon et al. 1989. (IARC Scientific Publications Ser.: No. 90). (Illus.). 550p. pap. text 115.00 (*92-832-1190-1*) OUP.

Non-Operative Aspects of Pediatric Surgery. Richard Owings. 1973. LC 72-176176. 160p. 10.00 (*0-87527-118-9*) Green.

Non-Opioid Analgesics in the Treatment of Acute Pain: Johannesbergs Slott, Sweden, March 14th, 1996. Michael J. Parnham. 1997. LC 97-513. (*0-8176-5680-4*); (*3-7643-5680-4*) Birkhauser.

Non-Opioids in Pain Management: Vancouver, August 19, 1996. Michael J. Parnham. 1997. LC 97-10915. (*0-8176-5700-2*); 19.00 (*3-7643-5700-2*) Birkhauser.

Non Palpable Breast Lesions. Ed. by M. R. Christiaens & I. De Wever. 1996. (Surgical Oncology Ser.: No. 3). (Illus.). 126p. (Orig.). pap. (*90-6186-734-7*) Leuven Univ BEL. *Dist:* Coronet Bks.

Non-Pharmacologic Therapy of Hypertension. Ed. by M. Donald Blaufox & H. G. Langford. 1987. (Bibliotheca Cardiologica Ser.: No. 41). (Illus.). vi, 150p. 121.75 (*3-8055-4459-6*) S Karger.

***Non-Prescription Medicines.** Nathan. 2nd ed. 2002. (*0-85369-506-7*) Pharmaceutical Pr GBR. *Dist:* Rittenhouse.

M N O

Non-Profit Hospitals: Their Structure, Human Resources, & Economic Importance. Thomas A. Barocci. 1980. LC 80-22075. 251p. 67.00 (*0-86569-054-5*, Auburn Hse) Greenwood.

Non-Reproductive Actions of Sex Steroids: Symposium No. 191. CIBA Foundation Staff. 1995. LC 95-6957. (CIBA Foundation Symposia Ser.: Vol. 191). 307p. 128.00 (*0-471-95513-2*) Wiley.

Non-Specific Aspects of Treatment. Ed. by Norman Sartorius & M. Shepherd. 1989. LC 88-13504. 160p. 39.00 (*0-920887-32-5*) Hogrefe & Huber Pubs.

Non-Specific Factors Influencing Host Resistance: A Reexamination. Ed. by W. Braun & J. Ungar. 1973. (Illus.). 116.75 (*3-8055-1598-7*) S Karger.

Non-Specific Mesenteric Lymphadenitis. V. Tuchel. 1972. 55.75 (*3-8055-1251-1*) S Karger.

Non-Standard Medical Electives in the U. S. A. & Canada, 1998-1999. Kenneth V. Iserson. 1998. LC 98-22346. pap. 31.95 (*1-883620-00-7*) Galen AZ.

Non-Steroidal Regulations in Reproductive Biology & Medicine: Proceedings of a Satellite Symposium to the 8th International Congress of Pharmacology, Tokyo, 26-27 July 1981. Vol. 34. T. Fujii & C. P. Channing. 1982. (Illus.). 266p. 87.50 (*0-08-027976-7*, H130, Pergamon Pr) Elsevier.

Non-Surgical Relief for Chronic Pain: Reconstructive Therapy. 1996. lib. bdg. 251.75 (*0-8490-5883-X*) Gordon Pr.

Non-Trycyclic & Non-Monamine Oxydase Inhibitors. Ed. by H. E. Lehmann. 1982. (Modern Problems of Pharmacopsychiatry Ser.: Vol. 18). (Illus.). viii, 212p. 100.00 (*3-8055-3428-0*) S Karger.

Non-Ulcer Dyspepsia. F. Di Mario et al. 1991. (Advances in Gastroenterology Ser.: No. 3). 130p. text (*1-57235-019-9*) Piccin Nuova.

Non-Vasoactive Renal Hormones. Ed. by G. M. Eisenbach & Jan Brod. 1978. (Contributions to Nephrology Ser.: Vol. 13). (Illus.). pap. 29375.00 (*3-8055-2895-7*) S Karger.

Non-Verbal Intelligence Tests for Use in China. Herman C. Liu. LC 76-177001. (Columbia University. Teachers College. Contributions to Education Ser.: No. 126). reprint ed. 37.50 (*0-404-55126-2*) AMS Pr.

Non-Verbal Intimacy & Exchange: A Special Issue of Journal of Nonverbal Behavior. Ed. by Miles L. Patterson. 1985. (Illus.). 169p. (Orig.). pap. 14.95 (*0-89885-224-2*, Kluwer Acad Hman Sci) Kluwer Academic.

Non-Viral Genetic Therapeutics: Advances, Challenges & Applications for Self-Assembling Systems. Ed. by Bari Walsh. 1996. (Biomedical Library). pap. 795.00 (*1-57936-019-X*) Drug & Market Dev.

Nonadrenergic Innervation of Blood Vessels G. Burnstock & S. G. Griffith. 1988. LC 87-24283. Vol. I: Putative Neurotransmitters. 176p. 95.00 (*0-8493-6681-X*, QP109); Vol. II: Regional Innervation. 256p. 140.00 (*0-8493-6682-8*, QP109) Franklin (CRC Reprint).

Noncondensed Aromatic Derivatives. V. St. Georgiev. 1983. (Survey of Drug Research in Immunologic Disease Ser.: Vol. 3). Part II. x, 582p. 426.75 (*3-8055-3687-9*); Pt. I. xii, 656p. 426.25 (*3-8055-3566-X*) S Karger.

Noncondensed Aromatic Derivatives. Pt. III. Vassil St. Georgiev. 1984. (Survey of Drug Research in Immunologic Disease Ser.: Vol. 4). x, 334p. 252.25 (*3-8055-3799-9*) S Karger.

Noncondensed Aromatic Derivatives. V. St. Georgiev. (Survey of Drug Research in Immunologic Disease Ser.: Vol. 5). Pt. IV. 1984. x, 606p. 426.25 (*3-8055-3856-1*); Pt. V. 1985. x, 586p. 426.25 (*3-8055-3962-2*); Pt. VII. 1987. xiv, 794p. 687.00 (*3-8055-4240-2*) S Karger.

Nondescription Drug. Consumer Guide Editors. 1997. pap. 7.99 (*0-451-19063-7*, Sig) NAL.

Nondiscriminatory Multifactored Assessment: A Sourcebook. David W. Barnett. 1983. (Illus.). 214p. pap. 20.95 (*0-89885-082-7*, Kluwer Acad Hman Sci) Kluwer Academic.

None Can Be Called Deformed. Vernon Mallinson. Ed. by William R. Phillips & Janet Rosenberg. 1980. LC 79-6917. (Physically Handicapped in Society Ser.). reprint ed. lib. bdg. 24.95 (*0-405-13124-0*) Ayer.

None of These Diseases: A Famous Doctor's Biblical Prescription for Healthier & Happier Living. S. I. McMillen. 2nd ed. 1993. LC 63-13359. (Illus.). 160p. (YA). (gr. 10). reprint ed. mass mkt. 5.99 (*0-8007-8030-2*, Spire) Revell.

Nongenotoxic Carcinogenesis. Ed. by A. Cockburn & L. Smith. 1994. (Ernst Schering Research Foundation Ser.: Vol. 10). (Illus.). 252p. 69.95 (*0-387-58342-4*) Spr-Verlag.

Nongonococcal Urethritis & Other Selected Sexually Transmitted Diseases of Public Health Importance. 1981. (Technical Report Ser.: No. 660). 142p. pap. text 9.00 (*92-4-120660-8*) World Health.

Nonhuman Environment in Normal Development & in Schizophrenia. Harold F. Searles. 1960. LC 60-9579. (Monograph Series on Schizophrenia: No. 5). 464p. 70.00 (*0-8236-3660-7*) Intl Univs Pr.

Nonhuman Primate Models for Human Diseases. Ed. by W. Richard Dukelow. 1983. LC 82-4519. 208p. 123.00 (*0-8493-6466-3*, RB125, CRC Reprint) Franklin.

Nonhuman Primates in Biomedical Research: Diseases. Ed. by B. Taylor Bennett et al. 1998. LC 94-49352. (American College of Laboratory Animal Medicine Ser.). (Illus.). 512p. 132.00 (*0-12-088665-0*) Acad Pr.

***Noni: Aspirin of the Ancients.** Diana Fairechild. 3rd l.t. rev. ed. 2001. (Illus.). 192p. pap. 9.95 (*1-892997-81-9*) Flyana.

Noninfectious Diseases of Wildlife. Ed. by Anne Fairbrother et al. 2nd ed. 1996. LC 96-33967. (Illus.). 246p. text 52.95 (*0-8138-0451-5*) Iowa U Pr.

Noninstitutional Senior Market for Healthcare Products & Services. Ed. by Peter Allen. 2nd ed. 1984. 250p. pap. 295.00 (*0-931634-46-6*) FIND-SVP.

Noninsulin-Dependent Diabetes: A Management Guide for Patients. 1994. (Illus.). 90p. (Orig.). (C). pap. text 20.00 (*0-7881-1033-0*) DIANE Pub.

Noninvasive Access to Cardiovascular Dynamics: Experimental & Applied. Ed. by G. Juznic et al. 1979. (Bibliotheca Cardiologica Ser.: No. 37). (Illus.). pap. 122.75 (*3-8055-2970-8*) S Karger.

Noninvasive Approaches to Pain Management in the Terminally Ill. Ed. by Caryn S. Feldman. 1992. LC 92-1485. (Hospice Journal: Vol. 8, Nos. 1-2). (Illus.). 232p. lib. bdg. 49.95 (*1-56024-300-7*); pap. text 19.95 (*1-56024-301-5*) Haworth Pr.

Noninvasive Assessment of the Visual System. Ed. by Dean Yager. 1997. LC 96-72423. (Trends in Optics & Photonics Ser.: Vol. 11). (Illus.). 209p. pap. 55.00 (*1-55752-471-8*) Optical Soc.

Noninvasive Cardiac Assessment Technology. Ed. by Dhanjoo N. Ghista. 1989. (Advances in Cardiovascular Physics Ser.: Vol. 6). (Illus.). x, 190p. 165.25 (*3-8055-4839-7*) S Karger.

Noninvasive Diagnosis of Kidney Disease. G. Lubec. 1983. (Continuing Education Ser.: Vol. 3). (Illus.). xii, 368p. 85.25 (*3-8055-3051-X*) S Karger.

Noninvasive Diagnosis of Vascular Disease. Ed. by Falls B. Hershey et al. 1984. LC 83-22310. (Illus.). 371p. text 52.50 (*0-941022-01-3*) Davies Pubng.

Noninvasive Diagnostic Techniques in Ophthalmology. Ed. by Barry R. Masters. 1990. (Illus.). 649p. 236.00 (*0-387-96992-6*) Spr-Verlag.

Noninvasive Electrocardiology. Moss. 1995. text 65.00 (*0-7020-1925-9*) Saunders.

Noninvasive Electrocardiology in Clinical Practice. Wojciech Zareba et al. 2001. LC 00-49487. (Illus.). xiv, 489p. 98.00 (*0-87993-467-0*) Futura Pub.

Noninvasive Evaluation of Hemodynamcis in Congenital Heart Disease: Doppler Ultrasound Applications in the Adult & Pediatric Patient with Congenital Heart Disease. Ed. by James V. Chapman & George R. Sutherland. 1990. (Developments in Cardiovascular Medicine Ser.). (C). text 268.50 (*0-7923-0836-0*) Kluwer Academic.

Noninvasive Imaging of Cardiac Metabolism. Ed. by Ernst E. Van der Wall. 1987. (Developments in Cardiovascular Medicine Ser.). text 272.50 (*0-89838-812-0*) Kluwer Academic.

Noninvasive Imaging of Congenital Heart Disease: Before & after Surgical Reconstruction. Alvin J. Chin. 1994. LC 93-39613. (Illus.). 400p. 128.00 (*0-87993-574-X*) Futura Pub.

Noninvasive Respiratory Monitoring. Ed. by Michael L. Nochomovitz & Neil S. Cherniak. 1986. (Contemporary Issues in Pulmonary Disease Ser.: Vol. 3). (Illus.). 229p. text (*0-443-08342-8*) Church.

Noninvasive Vascular Diagnosis. Ed. by Ali F. AbuRahma & John J. Bergan. 1999. LC 98-50138. 504p. (C). (*1-85233-128-3*) Spr-Verlag GBR. *Dist:* Spr-Verlag.

Noninvasive Vascular Laboratory: Current Issues & Clinical Developments. Ed. by Marsha M. Neumyer & Arthur I. Auer. Date not set. text (*0-941022-28-5*) Davies Pubng.

Nonionizing Radiation Protection. Ed. by Michael J. Seuss & D. A. Benwell-Morison. 2nd ed. 1989. (WHO Regional Publications, European Ser.: No. 25). xiv, 346p. pap. text 34.40 (*92-890-1101-7*, 1310025) World Health.

Nonionizing Radiation Protection. Suess & Benwell-Morison. 2nd ed. 1989. (WHO Regional Publications, European Ser.: No. 25). 350p. text 43.00 (*92-890-1116-5*) World Health.

Nonisotropic Probing, Blotting, & Sequencing. Ed. by Larry J. Kricka. 2nd ed. 1995. LC 94-24916. (Illus.). 518p. 42.00 (*0-12-426292-9*) Acad Pr.

Nonlinear Analysis of Physiological Data. Ed. by H. Kantz et al. 1998. LC 98-5675. (Illus.). 352p. 59.95 (*3-540-63481-9*) Spr-Verlag.

Nonlinear Biomedical Signal Processing Vol. II: Dynamic Analysis & Modeling, Vol. 2. Metin Akay. 2000. LC 00-27777. (Biomedical Engineering Ser.). (Illus.). 364p. 110.00 (*0-7803-6012-5*, PC5862, Wiley-IEEE) Wiley.

Nonlinear Dynamical Analysis of the EEG: Proceedings of the 2nd Annual Conference. B. H. Jansen & M. E. Brandt. 1993. 384p. text 95.00 (*981-02-1204-6*) World Scientific Pub.

Nonlinear Dynamics & Structures in Biology & Medicine: Optical & Laser Technologies. Ed. by Valery V. Tuchin. 1997. LC 96-72140. 206p. 59.00 (*0-8194-2468-4*) SPIE.

Nonlinear Psychophysical Dynamics. Robert A. Gregson. 1988. 232p. 49.95 (*0-8058-0015-8*) L Erlbaum Assocs.

Nonmammalian Animal Models for Biomedical Research. Ed. by Avril D. Woodhead & Katherine Vivirito. 1989. 408p. 298.00 (*0-8493-4763-7*, QL55) CRC Pr.

Nononcogenic Avian Viruses. Ed. by R. Pandey. 1989. (Progress in Veterinary Microbiology & Immunology Ser.: Vol. 5). (Illus.). viii, 136p. 100.00 (*3-8055-4827-3*) S Karger.

Nonparametric Statistics in Health Care Research: Statistics for Small Samples & Unusual Distributions. Marjorie A. Pett. 1997. LC 96-35711. 400p. (C). 81.95 (*0-8039-7038-2*, 2825); pap. 39.95 (*0-8039-7039-0*, 2824) Sage.

Nonparametrics: Statistical Methods Based on Ranks. Lehmann. rev. ed. 2000. 480p. 86.00 (*0-13-997735-X*) P-H.

Nonpharmacological Management of Atrial Fibrillation. Ed. by Francis D. Murgatroyd & John Camm. 1997. LC 97-4340. (Illus.). 560p. 120.00 (*0-87993-665-7*) Futura Pub.

Nonpharmacological Therapy of Arrhythmias for the 21st Century: The State of the Art. Ed. by Igor Singer et al. 1998. LC 98-4105. (Illus.). 992p. 125.00 (*0-87993-690-8*) Futura Pub.

Nonphysician & Family Health in Sub-Sahara Africa. Ed. by Ronald S. Waife & Marianne C. Burkhart. 1981. (FRE.). 141p. 7.00 (*0-933853-11-4*) Pathfinder Fund.

Nonprescription Drugs: Value of a Pharmacist-Controlled Class Has Yet to Be Determined. 1996. 136p. (Orig.). (C). pap. text 20.00 (*0-7881-2934-1*) DIANE Pub.

Nonprescription Product Therapeutics. W. Steven Pray. 1999. LC 98-22505. 850p. pap. text 85.00 (*0-683-30126-8*) Lppncott W & W.

Nonprescription Products: Patient Assessment Handbook. Ed. by Lynn Limon et al. 1996. LC 96-79456. (Illus.). 456p. (Orig.). pap. 42.00 (*0-917330-82-X*, T270) Am Pharm Assn.

Nonprofit & For-Profit HMOs: Converging Practices but Different Goals? Harry Nelson. 1997. 36p. (Orig.). pap. (*1-887748-13-X*) Milbank Memorial.

Nonprofit Personnel Polices, Suppl. No. 4. Ed. by John Gillis. 1995. LC 96-51519. 178.00 (*0-8342-0410-X*, S130) Aspen Pub.

Nonsmoker Solution. Lynn H. Christensen. 1994. LC 94-94331. 192p. pap. 10.95 (*0-9641059-1-8*) Crystal VA.

Nonsteroidal Anti-Inflammatory Drugs. Ed. by N. J. Lowe & C. Hensby. 1989. (Pharmacology & the Skin Ser.: Vol. 2). (Illus.). x, 158p. 129.75 (*3-8055-4898-2*) S Karger.

Nonsteroidal Anti-Inflammatory Drugs: Mechanisms & Clinical Uses. Ed. by Alan J. Lewis & Daniel E. Furst. 2nd ed. 1993. LC 93-34984. (Illus.). 480p. text 240.00 (*0-8247-8856-7*) Dekker.

Nonsurgical Management of Acute Low Back Pain: Cutting Through the AHCPR Guidelines. Ed. by Erwin G. Gonzalez & Richard S. Materson. 1997. LC 97-45695. (Illus.). 272p. 125.00 (*1-888799-13-7*) Demos Medical.

Nonsynaptic Diffusion Neurotransmission & Late Brain Reorganization. Paul Bach-y-Rita. 1995. LC 95-2187. 232p. pap. 69.95 (*0-939957-77-9*) Demos Medical.

Nontraditional Families: Parenting & Child Development. Ed. by Michael E. Lamb. 1982. (Illus.). 372p. text 79.95 (*0-89859-178-3*) L Erlbaum Assocs.

***Nontraditional Methods of Sensing Stress, Strain & Damage in Materials,** Vol. 2. Ed. by George F. Lucas et al. 2001. LC 2001-280091. (STP Ser.: Vol. 1323). (Illus.). 213p. pap. text 75.00 (*0-8031-2882-7*, STP1323) ASTM.

Nontraditional Methods of Sensing Stress, Strain & Damage in Materials & Structure. George T. Lucas & David A. Stubbs. 1997. LC 97-18165. (Illus.). 231p. pap. 52.00 (*0-8031-2403-1*, STP1318) ASTM.

Nonverbal Aspects of Psychotherapy. Peter H. Waxer. 1978. LC 78-71280. 105p. 50.00 (*0-275-90321-4*, C0321, Praeger Pubs) Greenwood.

Nonverbal Behavior: Perspectives, Applications & Intercultural Insights. Ed. by Aaron W. Wolfgang. 1997. LC 84-10899. 500p. (C). pap. text 38.00 (*0-88937-008-7*) Hogrefe & Huber Pubs.

Nonverbal Behavior & Social Psychology. Richard Heslin & Miles Patterson. 1982. (Perspectives in Social Psychology Ser.). 196p. 54.50 (*0-306-40952-6*, Plenum Trade) Perseus Pubng.

Nonverbal Communication: The Unspoken Dialogue. Judee K. Burgoon et al. 2nd ed. 1995. 535p. (C). pap. 46.88 (*0-07-008995-7*) McGrw-H Hghr Educ.

Nonverbal Communication & Marital Interaction. Patricia Noller. 1984. (International Series in Experimental Social Psychology: Vol. 9). (Illus.). 250p. text 104.00 (*0-08-027927-9*, CRC Reprint) Franklin.

Nonverbal Learning Disabilities: The Syndrome & the Model. Byron P. Rourke. 1989. LC 89-1958. 253p. 35.00 (*0-89862-378-2*, 2378) Guilford Pubns.

Nonverbal Vocal Communication: Comparative & Developmental Approaches. Ed. by H. Papousek et al. 1992. (Studies in Emotion & Social Interaction). (Illus.). 319p. (C). text 59.95 (*0-521-41265-X*) Cambridge U Pr.

Nonviolent Crisis Intervention: Learning to Defuse Explosive Behavior. Algene Caraulia & Linda Steiger. Ed. by Eugene T. Wyka & Sandra Christensen. 1997. LC 97-156982. 139p. text 59.00 (*0-9651733-2-1*) Crisis Prevent.

Nonviral Vectors for Gene Therapy. Leaf Huang et al. 1999. LC 99-63092. (Illus.). xxv, 442p. 99.95 (*0-12-358465-5*) Acad Pr.

Nonviral Vectors for Gene Therapy: Methods & Protocols. Ed. by Mark A. Findeis. 2001. (Methods in Molecular Medicine Ser.: Vol. 65). 450p. 99.00 (*0-89603-712-6*) Humana.

***Nordic Lights: New Initiatives in Health Care Systems.** 1995. (Illus.). pap. (*87-7838-144-4*) Odense Univ DNK. *Dist:* Intl Spec Bk.

Nordic Radioecology: The Transfer of Radionuclides Through Nordic Ecosystems to Man. Ed. by H. Dahlgaard. 1994. LC 95-188023. (Studies in Environmental Science: Vol. 62). 498p. 222.00 (*0-444-81617-8*) Elsevier.

Norfolk & Western: A History. E. F. Striplin. rev. ed. 1997. LC 96-71382. (Illus.). 250p. reprint ed. pap. text 21.95 (*0-9633254-6-9*) Norfolk & Wstrn HS.

Normal Aging 1: Reports from the Duke Longitudinal Study, 1955-1969. Ed. by Erdman B. Palmore. 1970. LC 74-132028. xxiv, 431p. text 49.95 (*0-8223-0238-1*) Duke.

Normal Aging 3: Reports from the Duke Longitudinal Studies, 1975-84. Ed. by George L. Maddox et al. 1985. LC 85-1598. (Illus.). xx, 468p. (C). text 49.95 (*0-8223-0624-7*) Duke.

Normal Aging 2: Reports from the Duke Longitudinal Study, 1970-1973. Erdman B. Palmore. 1974. LC 74-132028. xix, 316p. text 49.95 (*0-8223-0311-6*) Duke.

Normal Alcoholic. William F. Kraft. 1999. LC 99-13593. 159p. pap. 9.95 (*0-8189-0853-X*) Alba.

Normal & Abnormal Breath Sounds. Springhouse Publishing Company Staff. 1989. 112p. audio 34.95 (*0-87434-201-5*) Springhouse Corp.

Normal & Abnormal Development: The Influence of Primitive Reflexes on Motor Development. Mary R. Fiorentino. 1980. (Illus.). 80p. 22.95 (*0-398-02278-X*) C C Thomas.

Normal & Abnormal Development of Cortex. Ed. by Albert M. Galaburda & Yves Christen. 1997. LC 97-22615. (Research & Perspectives in Neurosciences Ser.). (Illus.). 199p. 102.00 (*3-540-63208-5*) Spr-Verlag.

Normal & Abnormal Epidermal Keratinization. Ed. by M. S. Seigi & I. A. Bernstein. 1983. (Current Problems in Dermatology Ser.: Vol. 11). (Illus.). x, 344p. pap. 144.50 (*3-8055-3752-2*) S Karger.

Normal & Abnormal Heart Sounds. SPC Staff. 1989. 144p. audio 34.95 (*0-87434-202-3*) Springhouse Corp.

Normal & Abnormal Processes in the Basic Sciences. National Medical School Review Staff. 1996. LC 96-22910. (Board Simulator Ser.). 253p. pap. 24.95 (*0-683-06331-6*) Lppncott W & W.

Normal & Abnormal Processes in the Basic Sciences: A Body Systems-Based Review for USMLE Step 1. National Medical School Review Staff & Gerald D. Barry. 2nd ed. 1997. LC 97-6602. (Board Simulator Ser.). 375p. pap. text 25.95 (*0-683-30297-3*) Lppncott W & W.

Normal & Abnormal Swallowing: Imaging in Diagnosis & Therapy. Ed. by B. Jones & Martin W. Donner. 1990. (Illus.). 235p. 169.00 (*0-387-97347-8*) Spr-Verlag.

Normal & Disordered Phonology in Children. Carol Stoel-Gammon & Carla Dunn. 1985. LC 84-15309. (Illus.). 238p. (Orig.). text 36.00 (*0-89079-150-3*, 1328) PRO-ED.

Normal & Disturbed Motility of the Gastrointestinal Tract. Andre J. Smout & Louis M. Akkermans. 1992. 320p. (*1-871816-15-7*) Wrightson Biomed GBR. *Dist:* Taylor & Francis.

Normal & Malignant Liver Cell Growth: Proceedings: International Falk Workshop (1998: Halle, Germany) Ed. by W. E. Fleig. 1999. LC 99-188037. 247p. 180.00 (*0-7923-8748-1*) Kluwer Academic.

Normal & Pathlogic Development of the Human Brain & Spinal Cord. Maria Dambska & Krystyna E. Wisniewski. 1999. 208p. pap. text 79.00 (*0-86196-591-4*) Buttrwrth-Heinemann.

Normal & the Pathological. Georges Canguilhem. Tr. by Carolyn R. Fawcett & Robert S. Cohen from FRE. 1989. LC 88-20626. 327p. reprint ed. 28.95 (*0-942299-58-2*) Zone Bks.

Normal & the Pathological. Georges Canguilhem. Tr. by Carolyn R. Fawcett from FRE. 1989. LC 88-20626. 327p. reprint ed. pap. 16.95 (*0-942299-59-0*) Zone Bks.

Normal Baby: The Sensorimotor Processes of the First Year. Cheryl Colangelo et al. 2nd rev. ed. 1986. (Illus.). (C). pap. text (*0-911681-03-5*) Valhalla Rehab.

Normal Child: Some Problems of the Early Years & Their Treatment. Ronald S. Illingworth. 10th ed. 1991. (Illus.). 450p. (Orig.). pap. text (*0-443-04455-4*) Church.

Normal Child & Adolescent. Tamhne. 11th ed. 1999. (C). pap. text (*0-443-05707-9*) Church.

Normal Child & Adolescent Development. Ralph Gemelli. 1996. 596p. text 75.50 (*0-88048-258-3*, 8258) Am Psychiatric.

Normal Child Development: An Annotated Bibliography of Articles & Books Published 1950-1969. Janice B. Schulman & Robert C. Prall. 1971. LC 71-178971. 336p. text 53.00 (*0-8089-0742-5*, 793923, Grune & Strat) Harcrt Hlth Sci Grp.

Normal Family Processes. Ed. by Froma Walsh. LC 81-7197. (Guilford Family Therapy Ser.). 1982. 486p. text 43.95 (*0-89862-051-1*); 2nd ed. 1993. 511p. 52.00 (*0-89862-090-2*, 2090) Guilford Pubns.

Normal Findings in CT & MRI. Torsten B. Moeller. 2000. LC 99-33663. (Illus.). 250p. pap. 32.00 (*0-86577-864-7*) Thieme Med Pubs.

Normal Findings in Radiography. Torsten B. Moeller. 2000. LC 99-40799. (Illus.). 280p. pap. 32.00 (*0-86577-871-X*) Thieme Med Pubs.

Normal Human Anatomy. Arnold J. Smolen. 1994. text 700.00 (*1-56815-022-9*) Mosby Inc.

Normal Life: A Study of War & Industrially Injured Pensioners. Sally Sainsbury. 1993. 230p. (*1-85628-482-4*) Avebury Technical GBR. *Dist:* Ashgate Pub Co.

Normal Lung. John R. Murray. 2nd ed. 1986. (Illus.). 377p. text 47.00 (*0-7216-6613-2*) Saunders.

Normal Lymph Node Topography: A CT-Atlas. E. Richter & T. Feyerabend. 1990. (Illus.). 153p. 175.00 (*0-387-52549-1*) Spr-Verlag.

Normal, Malignant Hematopoiesis & New Advances: Proceedings of the Sixth Pezcoller Symposium Held in Rovereto, Italy, June 29-July 1, 1994, Vol. 6. Ed. by Enrico Mihich et al. 1995. LC 95-37107. (Pezcoller Foundation Symposia Ser.: Vol. 6). (Illus.). 260p. 95.00 (*0-306-45136-0*, Kluwer Plenum) Kluwer Academic.

Normal Microflora: An Introduction to Microbes Inhabiting the Human Body. G. W. Tannock. 1994. 115p. (C). (gr. 13). pap. text 53.95 (*0-412-55040-7*) Chapman & Hall.

Normal Psychology of the Aging Process. Ed. by Norman E. Zinberg & Irving Kaufman. enl. rev. ed. 1978. LC 77-92178. 285p. 45.00 (*0-8236-3641-0*) Intl Univs Pr.

Normal Radiographic Anatomy. B. K. Omar. 1983. (*0-7855-0795-7*) Current Dist IND. *Dist:* St Mut.

Normal Testicular Descent & the Aetiology of Cryptorchidism. John M. Hutson et al. 1995. LC 95-24947. (Advances in Anatomy, Embryology & Cell Biology Ser.: Vol. 132). (Illus.). 75p. 93.00 (*3-540-60283-6*) Spr-Verlag.

***Normal Tissue Reactions in Radiotherapy & Oncology Vol. 37: International Symposium, Marburg, April 2000.** Ed. by W. Dorr et al. 2001. (Frontiers of Radiation Therapy & Oncology Ser.). (Illus.). 200p. 171.50 (*3-8055-7284-0*) S Karger.

Normal Values in Pregnancy. M. M. Ramsay. 2nd ed. 2000. 160p. pap. text (*0-7020-2527-5*) W B Saunders GBR. *Dist:* Saunders.

Normal Variant & Pitfalls. Volger. 1986. text 172.00 (*0-7216-1457-4*) Saunders.

Normalities & Abnormalities in Human Movement. Ed. by B. Kirkcaldy. 1989. (Medicine & Sport Science Ser.: Vol. 29). (Illus.). xiv, 214p. 148.75 (*3-8055-4823-0*) S Karger.

Normality & Pathology in Childhood: Assessments of Development. Anna Freud. 1966. LC 65-17007. (Writings of Anna Freud: Vol. 6). 273p. (Orig.). 45.00 (*0-8236-6875-4*); pap. 25.95 (*0-8236-8165-3*, 26875) Intl Univs Pr.

Normality & Pathology in Cognitive Functions. Ed. by A. Ellis. 1982. text 135.00 (*0-12-237480-0*) Acad Pr.

Norman Geschwind: Selected Publications. Norman Geschwind et al. 1997. LC 96-37401. 592p. text 59.99 (*0-7506-9753-9*) Buttrwrth-Heinemann.

Normas para la Realizacion del Estudio Pelvico Femenino Por Medio de Ultrasonido. 1995.Tr. of Standards for the Performance of the Ultrasound Examination of the Female. (SPA.). 8p. pap. 10.00 (*1-930047-03-7*, GFPS) Am Inst Ultrasound.

Normas para la Realizacion del Estudio Vascular/Doppler Por Ultrasonido. 1992.Tr. of Standards for Performance of the Vascular/Doppler Ultrasound Examination. (SPA.). 16p. pap. 10.00 (*1-930047-04-5*, GVDS) Am Inst Ultrasound.

Normas para Llevar A Cabo el Examen Obstetrico Prenatal Con Ultrasonido. 1994.Tr. of Standards for Performance of the Antepartum Obstetrical Ultrasound. (SPA.). 8p. pap. 10.00 (*1-930047-05-3*, GAOBS) Am Inst Ultrasound.

Normative Health Care Measures. 1996. (*1-57372-032-1*); 1995. (*1-57372-001-1*) Solucient.

Normative Model of Physical Therapist Assistant Education: Version 99. 1999. 232p. pap. 67.00 (*1-887759-64-6*) Am Phys Therapy Assn.

Norplant Implants Guidelines for Family Planning Service Programs. Ed. by Noel McIntosh et al. 2nd rev. ed. 1996. (RUS., Illus.). (Orig.). pap. 15.00 (*0-929817-02-8*) JHPIEGO.

Norplant Implants Guidlines for Family Planning Service Programs: A Problem-Solving Reference Manual. Ed. by Noel McIntosh et al. 2nd ed. 1995. (Illus.). pap. text 15.00 (*0-929817-09-5*) JHPIEGO.

Norris & Campbell's Anaesthetics, Resuscitation & Intensive Care. Donald Campbell & Alistair A. Spence. 7th ed. 1990. (Illus.). 254p. pap. text (*0-443-04067-2*) Church.

Norris & Campbell's Anaesthetics, Resuscitation & Intensive Care. David Campbell & Alastair A. Spence. 8th ed. 1998. LC 96-26056. pap. text (*0-443-04886-X*) Church.

North American Indians & Alaska Natives: Abstracts of the Psychological & Behavioral Literature, 1967-1994. Ed. by Joseph E. Trimble & Weldon M. Bagwell. 1995. LC 95-17645. (Bibliographies in Psychology Ser.: No. 15). 272p. pap. 19.95 (*1-55798-311-9*) Am Psychol.

North Carolina Area Health Education Centers: A Brief History. Henry S. Uhl. Ed. by Karen Klein. 1993. (Illus.). 88p. (C). pap. text (*0-9621194-6-6*) Stratford NC.

North Carolina Eldercare Sourcebook: A Resource Guide for Older Adults & Caregivers. Carla S. Rogg & Oskar H. Rogg. 1995. (Orig.). spiral bd. 24.95 (*0-9631939-4-5*) Care Solutions.

North Carolina Health Care in Perspective 2000. Ed. by Kathleen O'Leary Morgan & Scott E. Morgan. 2000. 21p. spiral bd. 19.00 (*0-7401-0232-X*) Morgan Quitno Corp.

North Carolina Health Care Perspective, 1998. Ed. by Kathleen O'Leary Morgan & Scott E. Morgan. 1998. 20p. pap. 19.00 (*1-56692-832-X*) Morgan Quitno Corp.

North Carolina Senior Resource Guide: A Resource Guide for Older Adults, Caregivers & Eldercare Professional. Carla S. Rogg & Oskar H. Rogg. 1995. 277p. (Orig.). pap. 19.95 (*0-9631939-7-X*) Care Solutions.

North Dakota Health Care in Perspective 2000. Ed. by Kathleen O'Leary Morgan & Scott E. Morgan. 2000. 21p. spiral bd. 19.00 (*0-7401-0233-8*) Morgan Quitno Corp.

North Dakota Health Care Perspective, 1998. Ed. by Kathleen O'Leary Morgan & Scott E. Morgan. 1998. 20p. pap. 19.00 (*1-56692-833-8*) Morgan Quitno Corp.

North Enough: AIDS & Other Clear-Cuts. Jan Zita Grover. 1997. LC 96-75891. 150p. (Orig.). pap. 12.95 (*1-55597-235-7*) Graywolf.

North Texas Eldercare Sourcebook: A Resource Guide for Older Adults, Caregivers & Eldercare Professionals. Carla S. Rogg & Oskar H. Rogg. 1995. 186p. (Orig.). pap. 14.95 (*0-9631939-3-7*) Care Solutions.

Northeast Asia. Ed. by Takeatsu Kimura et al. 1996. LC 96-4659. (International Collation of Traditional & Folk Medicine Ser.: Vol. 1). 240p. (*981-02-2589-X*) World Scientific Pub.

Northern Nurse. Elliot Merrick. 1994. LC 94-29285. (Illus.). 336p. reprint ed. pap. 14.00 (*0-88150-299-5*) Countryman.

Norwegian-English, English-Norwegian Medical Dictionary. Kass. 1993. (ENG & NOR.). 104p. 49.95 (*0-7859-7505-5*, 8257305588) Fr & Eur.

Nose. Ed. by P. Van Cauwenberge et al. 1998. (Illus.). xii, 356p. (*90-6299-147-5*) Kugler NLD. *Dist:* Lib Res.

Nosography. Knud H. Faber. 2nd rev. ed. 1976. LC 75-23706. (Illus.). reprint ed. 45.00 (*0-404-13258-8*) AMS Pr.

Nosology & Research Methods in Psychiatry: Festschrift in Honor of Professor Jules Angst. Ed. by C. Scharfetter. 1995. (Journal: Vol. 28, No. 1, 1995). (Illus.). iv, 98p. pap. 31.50 (*3-8055-6265-9*) S Karger.

Nostradamus's Dream Interpretations. Dita Arzt-Wegman. 1999. Orig. Title: Umfangreiches Agyptisches Traum-Deutungs Buch by Nostradamus. (Illus.). 175p. pap. (*0-9686022-0-7*) VPI1 CAN. *Dist:* Allnce Hse.

Not a Total Waste: The True Story of a Mother, a Son & AIDS. B. M. Lloyd. 1994. LC 93-93482. (Illus.). 270p. pap. 16.95 (*0-88962-540-9*) Mosaic.

Not All of Us Are Saints: A Doctor's Journey with the Poor. David Hilfiker. 1994. LC 94-4717. 288p. 20.95 (*0-8090-3921-4*) Hill & Wang.

Not by Faith Alone: A Biblical Study of the Catholic Doctrine of Justification. Robert A. Sungenis. 1997. 774p. (Orig.). pap. 24.95 (*1-57918-009-4*, 3671) Queenship Pub.

Not by the Color of Their Skin: The Impact of Racial Differences on the Child's Development. Marjorie McDonald. 1971. LC 73-134334. Orig. Title: Integration & Skin Color. 242p. 37.50 (*0-8236-3690-9*); pap. 24.95 (*0-8236-8166-1*, 23690) Intl Univs Pr.

Not Entirely Benign Procedure: Four Years As a Medical Student. Perri Klass. 1994. LC 94-50781. 288p. reprint ed. pap. 14.00 (*0-452-27258-0*, Plume) Dutton Plume.

Not from the Apes: A History of Man's Origin & Evolution. Bjorn Kurten. 1984. LC 84-1842. pap. text 19.50 (*0-231-05815-2*) Col U Pr.

Not-God: A History of Alcoholics Anonymous. Ernest Kurtz. 1998. LC 79-88264. 436p. pap. 14.50 (*0-89486-065-8*, 1036A, Hazelden-Pittman) Hazelden.

Not Just Another Namebook: How & Why the Numerical Patterns Hidden Within Your Name Influence Your Daily Life, Love Life & Bank Account. Maryanna Korwitts & Jim Gash. 1995. pap. 19.95 (*1-887270-02-7*) Spiritpoint Pr.

Not Just the Cleaning Lady: A Hygienist's Guide to Survival. Catherine A. Schmidt. 1998. LC 97-47790. 29.95 (*0-87814-672-5*) PennWell Corp.

Not My Child: A Mother Confronts Her Child's Sexual Abuse. Patricia Crowley. 1991. 320p. mass mkt. 4.95 (*0-380-71276-8*, Avon Bks) Morrow Avon.

Not Now . . . I'm Having a No Hair Day: Humor & Healing for People with Cancer. Christine Clifford. 1996. LC 96-10027. (Illus.). 110p. (Orig.). pap. 9.95 (*1-57025-120-7*) Pfeifer-Hamilton.

Not Our Baby, Vol. 1. Sharon Clark. 1984. (Illus.). 149p. 17.95 (*0-920490-43-3*) Temeron Bks.

Not What the Doctor Ordered: How to End the Medical Monopoly in Pursuit of Managed Care. Jeffrey C. Bauer. 2nd rev. ed. 1997. LC 97-43100. (HFMA Healthcare Financial Management Ser.). (Illus.). 240p. 24.95 (*0-07-006721-X*) McGraw.

Not Yet Pregnant: Infertile Couples in Contemporary America. Larry L. Greil. 1991. LC 90-21142. 250p. (C). pap. 14.95 (*0-8135-1683-8*); text 40.00 (*0-8135-1682-X*) Rutgers U Pr.

Notable Advances in the Understanding & Treatment of Mentally Handicapped Children. J. E. Wallace. 1957. LC 58-1578. (Augustana College Library Occasional Papers, Wallin Lecture: No. 1). 20p. pap. 1.00 (*0-910182-22-1*) Augustana Coll.

Note of an Anatomist. Frank Gonzalez-Crussi. 1986. 144p. pap. 4.95 (*0-15-667430-0*, Harvest Bks) Harcourt.

Notes & Abstracts: International Neutron Therapy Workshop. Yosh Maruyama. 1991. (Nuclear Science Applications Ser.). 56p. pap. text 101.00 (*3-7186-5122-X*, Harwood Acad Pubs) Gordon & Breach.

Notes for the DRCOG. J. Anthony & P. Kaye. 3rd ed. 1995. (Illus.). 215p. pap. (*0-443-04713-8*) Church.

***Notes for the DRCOG.** Jo Anthony & Peter Kaye. 4th ed. 2001. (Illus.). 255p. pap. (*0-443-06418-0*) Church GBR. *Dist:* Saunders.

Notes for the MRCGP. K. T. Palmer. 3rd ed. 1998. LC 97-46538. 336p. pap. 49.95 (*0-86542-777-1*) Blackwell Sci.

Notes from the Field in Commmunication for Child Survival. Ed. by Renata E. Seidel. 1993. LC 93-17710. 15.00 (*0-89492-102-9*) Acad Educ Dev.

***Notes in Neuroanaesthesia & Critical Care.** Arun K. Gupta & Andrew C. Summors. 2001. (Illus.). 302p. pap. (*1-84110-035-8*) Greenwich Med GBR. *Dist:* JAMCO Dist.

Notes on Asylums for the Insane in America. John C. Bucknill. 1973. LC 73-2391. (Mental Illness & Social Policy; the American Experience Ser.). reprint ed. 15.95 (*0-405-05199-9*) Ayer.

Notes on Child Study. Edward Lee Thorndike. 1979. LC 74-21432. (Classics in Child Development Ser.). 162p. reprint ed. 23.95 (*0-405-06481-0*) Ayer.

Notes on Feline Internal Medicine. Willoughby & Gaskell. 1996. pap. (*0-632-03399-1*) Blackwell Sci.

Notes on Hospitals. Florence Nightingale. 1976. lib. bdg. 150.00 (*0-8490-2357-2*) Gordon Pr.

Notes on Human Physiology: By an Experienced Teacher. 3rd ed. 1977. 539p. (*0-7855-0820-1*) Current Dist IND. *Dist:* St Mut.

Notes on Medical Bacteriology. Sleigh. 5th ed. 1998. (C). pap. text (*0-443-05847-4*) Church.

Notes on Medical Bacteriology. J. Douglas Sleigh & Morag C. Timbury. 5th ed. 1998. LC 97-39910. (*0-443-05848-2*) Church.

Notes on Medical Virology. Morag C. Timbury. 11th ed. 1998. LC 97-8837. pap. text (*0-443-05845-8*) Church.

Notes on Nursing: What It Is, & What It Is Not. Florence Nightingale. 1969. LC 79-79233. 140p. pap. 4.95 (*0-486-22340-X*) Dover.

Notes on Nursing: What It Is, & What It Is Not. Florence Nightingale et al. 1992. LC 92-15476. 168p. text 30.95 (*0-397-55007-3*) Lppncott W & W.

Notes on Nursing: What It Is, & What It Is Not. Florence Nightingale. 1987. 140p. reprint ed. lib. bdg. 21.95 (*0-89966-604-3*) Buccaneer Bks.

Notes on Nursing Notes. Fay Yocum. 1999. 200p. pap. (*0-9637649-5-0*) Awareness Prods.

Notes on Nursing, Replica Edition: What It Is & What It Is Not. Florence Nightingale. 1946. 79p. text 21.95 (*0-397-54000-0*, 64-01046, Lippnctt) Lppncott W & W.

Notes on Paediatrics: Neonatology. Alex Habel & Rod Scott. 1998. LC 98-23206. (Illus.). 144p. pap. (*0-7506-2446-9*) E A GBR. *Dist:* OUP.

Notes on Pathology, Part II. Ed. by Current Dist Staff. 1976. 260p. (*0-7855-0799-X*) Current Dist IND. *Dist:* St Mut.

Notes on Pathology Pt. 1: By an Experienced Teacher. 1976. 298p. (*0-7855-0744-2*) Current Dist IND. *Dist:* St Mut.

Notes on Pharmaco-Therapeutics: By an Experienced Teacher. 3rd ed. 1974. 284p. (*0-7855-0821-X*) Current Dist IND. *Dist:* St Mut.

Notes on Radiological Diagnosis. Laurence S. Lau & John F. DeCampo. 1985. 216p. pap. text 46.00 (*0-7216-1936-3*) Saunders.

Notes on Surgery: By an Experienced Teacher. 2nd ed. 1987. 379p. reprint ed. (*0-7855-0822-8*) Current Dist IND. *Dist:* St Mut.

Notes on Symptom Control in Hospice & Palliative Care: U. S. A. Version. Peter Kaye. rev. ed. 1995. (Illus.). 427p. pap. text 28.95 (*0-9623438-1-1*) Hospice Education.

Notes on the Human Ecology of Glen Canyon. Angus M. Woodbury. (Glen Canyon Ser.: No. 26). reprint ed. 20.00 (*0-404-60674-1*) AMS Pr.

Notes on the Mental Health Act, 1983. Ralph L. Kilby. 1983. (C). (*0-7219-0204-9*) Scientific GBR. *Dist:* St Mut.

Notes on the Plague Years: AIDS in Marseilles. Bernard Paillard. Tr. by Berkeley Frank from FRE. 1998. LC 98-28154. (Social Problems & Social Issues Ser.). 313p. pap. text 24.95 (*0-202-30555-4*) Aldine de Gruyter.

Notes Surgical Nursing. Fream. 3rd ed. 1986. pap. text 27.00 (*0-443-03380-3*) Saunders.

Noteworthy Publications by African-American Surgeons: In Commemoration of the 100th Anniversary of the National Medical Association. Vernon J. Henderson & Claude H. Organ, Jr. ltd. ed. 1995. (Illus.). 414p. 75.00 (*0-9617380-2-2*) C H Organ.

Notification of Communicable Diseases: A Survey of Existing Legislation. WHO Staff. 1958. (International Digest of Health Legislation Offprints: Vol. 9, No. 4). 51p. 3.00 (*92-4-169094-1*) World Health.

Notions of the Deaf & Dumb Before Instruction. Harvey P. Peet. 1973. 59.95 (*0-8490-0740-2*) Gordon Pr.

Notter's Essentials of Nursing Research. Jacqueline R. Hott & Wendy C. Budin. 6th ed. 1999. LC 98-39259. xii, 212p. 29.95 (*0-8261-1599-3*) Springer Pub.

Nourishing a Happy Affair: Nutrition Alternatives for Individual & Family Needs. Leslie Cohen. 1983. LC 82-16226. (Illus.). 150p. (Orig.). pap. 5.95 (*0-943914-02-7*) Larson Pubns.

***Nourishing Your Daughter: How to Keep Your Daughter from Emotional & Physical Battles with Her Weight.** Carol Beck. 2001. LC 00-68476. (Illus.). 224p. pap. 13.95 (*0-399-52707-9*, Perigee Bks) Berkley Pub.

Nouveau Dictionary Medicaments. G. Huchon. 1998. (FRE.). 27.95 (*0-320-00361-2*) Fr & Eur.

Nouveau Dictionnaire Medical. Edmond Schuller. 1987. (FRE.). 349p. 39.95 (*0-7859-8011-3*, 2737300495) Fr & Eur.

Nouveau Larousse de la Medecine, No. 2. Andre Domart & Jacques Bourneuf. 1988. 1152p. 155.00 (*0-7859-4827-9*) Fr & Eur.

Nouveau Larousse Medical. Maurice Fontaine. deluxe ed. 1969. (FRE.). 1956p. 135.00 (*0-7859-4550-4*) Fr & Eur.

Nouvelles Conferences d'Introduction a la Psychanalyse. Sigmund Freud. 1989. (FRE.). pap. 12.95 (*0-7859-2818-9*) Fr & Eur.

Nova Scotia Conference on Early Identification of Hearing Loss, Halifax, Nova Scotia, September 9-11, 1974. Nova Scotia Conference on Early Identification of Hearing Loss. Ed. by Georges T. Mencher. 1976. 42.75 (*3-8055-2296-7*) S Karger.

Novak's Gynecology. Jonathan S. Berek et al. 12th ed. 1996. LC 96-16316. (Illus.). 1,359p. text 125.00 (*0-683-00593-6*) Lppncott W & W.

Novak's Gynecology Self-Assessment & Review: Study Guide for Novak's Gynecology. David L. Olive et al. 1997. LC 97-50305. 380p. 39.95 (*0-683-00589-8*) Lppncott W & W.

Novak's Textbook of Gynecology. Howard W. Jones. Ed. by Jones, 3rd & Anne C. Wentz. 11th ed. 1988. (Illus.). 919p. 82.00 (*0-683-04469-9*) Lppncott W & W.

Novantrone Mitoxantrone for Injection Concentrate: Initial Therapy of Acute Nonlymphocytic Leukemia. Ed. by Chris Fellner. 1995. (Orig.). pap. (*1-57130-014-7*) Medicine Grp USA.

Novarits Foundation Symposium 215: Immumnological Tolerance, Vol. 215. Gregory Bock & Jamie Goode. 1998. LC 98-14471. (Novartis Foundation Symposium Ser.). 248p. 125.00 (*0-471-97843-4*) Wiley.

Novartis Foundation Symposium. Novartis staff. 2000. LC 00-33015. (Novartis Foundation Symposium Ser.: Vol. 230). (Illus.). 292p. 125.00 (*0-471-49203-5*) Wiley.

Novartis Foundation Symposium 217 Genetics & Tuberculosis, Vol. 217. Derek Chadwick & Gail Cardew. 1998. LC 98-23836. (Novartis Foundation Symposium Ser.). 280p. 125.00 (*0-471-98261-X*) Wiley.

Novel Approach to Sexuality & Disability. Georgie Maxfield. Ed. by Fanny Toner. 1996. (Illus.). 195p. (Orig.). pap. 7.95 (*0-9654069-0-3*) Nrthrn NV Amputee.

Novel Approaches in Anticancer Drug Design: Molecular Modelling - New Treatment Strategies. Ed. by W. J. Zeller et al. 1995. (Beitraege Zur Onkologie, Contributions to Oncology Ser.: Vol. 49). (Illus.). viii, 196p. 143.50 (*3-8055-6043-5*) S Karger.

Novel Approaches to Selective Treatments of Human Solid Tumors: Laboratory & Clinical Correlation. Y. M. Rustum. 1994. (Advances in Experimental Medicine & Biology Ser.: Vol. 339). (Illus.). 332p. (C). text 95.00 (*0-306-44592-1*, Kluwer Plenum) Kluwer Academic.

Novel Approaches to the Treatment of Alzheimer's Disease. Ed. by E. M. Meyer et al. 1989. LC 89-26615. (Advances in Behavioral Biology Ser.: No. 36). (Illus.). 400p. 110.00 (*0-306-43402-4*, Plenum Trade) Perseus Pubng.

Novel Calcium-Binding Proteins: Fundamentals & Clinical Implications. Ed. by C. W. Heizmann. 1991. (Illus.). 624p. 184.00 (*0-387-53277-3*) Spr-Verlag.

Novel Chemotherapeutic Agents: Preactivation in the Treatment of Cancer & AIDS. K. S. Gulliya. 1996. (Medical Intelligence Unit Ser.). (Illus.). 200p. (C). pap. 89.95 (*0-412-11301-5*) Chapman & Hall.

Novel Chemotherapeutic Agents: Preactivation in the Treatment of Cancer & AIDS. K. S. Gulliya. 1996. LC 96-17729. (Medical Intelligence Unit Ser.). 233p. 99.00 (*1-57059-350-7*) Landes Bioscience.

Novel Cytokine Inhibitors. Ed. by G. A. Higgs & B. Henderson. 2000. (Progress in Inflammation Research Ser.). (Illus.). 400p. 155.00 (*3-7643-5942-0*) Birkhauser.

Novel Delivery Systems for Oral Vaccines. Ed. by Derek T. O'Hagan. 1994. LC 93-40167. 288p. lib. bdg. 189.00 (*0-8493-4866-8*, 4866) CRC Pr.

Novel Diarrhea Viruses: Symposium. CIBA Foundation Staff. 1987. LC 86-32597. (CIBA Foundation Symposia Ser.: No. 128). 280p. 128.00 (*0-471-91094-5*) Wiley.

Novel Drug Delivery Systems. Yie W. Chien. 2nd enl. rev. ed. 1991. (Drugs & the Pharmaceutical Sciences Ser.: Vol. 50). (Illus.). 816p. text 250.00 (*0-8247-8520-7*) Dekker.

Novel Infectious Agents & the Central Nervous System. CIBA Foundation Staff. 1988. LC 87-31740. (CIBA Foundation Symposia Ser.: No. 135). 288p. 128.00 (*0-471-91512-2*) Wiley.

Novel Methods in Molecular & Cellular Biochemistry of Muscle. William C. Claycomb. Ed. by Grant N. Pierce. 1997. LC 96-39968. (Developments in Molecular & Cellular Biochemistry Ser.). 304p. (C). text 289.50 (*0-7923-4387-5*) Kluwer Academic.

Novel Molecular Approaches to Anti-Inflammatory Therapy. Ed. by W. Pruzanski & P. Vadas. 1995. LC 95-1382. (Agents & Actions Supplements Ser.: Vol. 46). 69.50 (*0-8176-5096-2*) Birkhauser.

***Novel Non-Surgical Porcine Model of Chronic Left Ventricular Dysfunction: Identification of Myocardial Viability Using Different Diagnostic Techniques.** Monika Szilard. 2001. (Illus.). 121p. pap. (*90-5867-146-1*) Leuven Univ BEL. *Dist:* Coronet Bks.

Novel Peripheral Neurotransmitters. Ed. by Christopher Bell. 1991. (International Encyclopedia of Pharmacology & Therapeutics Ser.: No. 135). (Illus.). 388p. 142.50 (*0-08-040691-2*, Pergamon Pr) Elsevier.

Novel Pharmacological Interventions for Alcoholism. Ed. by C. A. Naranjo & Edward M. Sellers. 1991. (Illus.). 378p. 98.00 (*0-387-97741-4*) Spr-Verlag.

Novel Strategies in the Design & Production of Vaccines: Proceedings of the 39th OHOLO Conference Held in Eilat, Israel, May 7-11, 1995. Ed. by Sara Cohen & Avigdor Shafferman. 1996. (Illus.). 214p. 85.00 (*0-306-45211-1*, Kluwer Plenum) Kluwer Academic.

Novel Synergy of Auriculotherapy. Kinesiology & Temporomandibular Dysfunction (TMD) Treatment Protocols for the Quantitative Characterization & Treatment Of: Hyperacusis - a Pain-Causing Ultra-Sensitivity to Normal Sounds. Meyer R. Rosen. 1994. LC 94-77159. 112p. pap. 60.00 (*0-9641617-0-2*) Interact Cnslting.

Novel Systems for the Study of Human Disease. OECD Staff. 1998. LC 98-146020. 400p. pap. (*92-64-16011-6*, 93-98-02-1-P) Org for Econ FRA. *Dist:* OECD.

Novel Therapeutic Agents for the Treatment of Autoimmune Diseases. Ed. by Vibeke Strand & David L. Scott. 1996. LC 96-18671. (Illus.). 332p. text 150.00 (*0-8247-9748-5*) Dekker.

Novel Therapeutics from Modern Biotechnology: From Laboratory to Human Testing. Ed. by Dale L. Oxender & Leonard E. Post. 1999. LC 99-16259. (Illus.). 250p. pap. 106.00 (*3-540-65927-7*) Spr-Verlag.

Novel Therapies for CNS Injuries: Rationales & Results. Ed. by Patti L. Peterson & John W. Phillis. 1995. LC 95-645. 416p. 264.95 (*0-8493-7652-1*, 7652) CRC Pr.

Now Breathe: A Very Personal Journal of Breast Cancer. Claudia Sternbach. 1999. LC 98-83286. 156p. pap. 13.95 (*0-9653800-4-1*) Whiteaker Pr.

Now Dare Everything: Tales of HIV-Related Psychotherapy. Steven Dansky. 1994. LC 92-48376. pap. 17.95 (*1-56023-037-1*, Harrington Park) Haworth Pr.

Now Dare Everything: Tales of HIV-Related Psychotherapy. Steven F. Dansky. 1994. LC 92-48376. (Illus.). 332p. lib. bdg. 49.95 (*1-56024-398-8*) Haworth Pr.

Now I Lay Me Down: Suicide & the Elderly. Ed. by David Lester & Margot Tallmer. 1994. LC 93-25814. 252p. (Orig.). pap. 22.95 (*0-914783-65-3*) Charles.

Now That Baby Can Crawl, Walk & Run, Bk. 1. 2000. 100p. pap. 14.95 (*0-9654700-1-6*) F R Parker.

Now That You Know: What Every Parent Should Know about Homosexuality. Betty Fairchild & Nancy Hayward. 1981. LC 78-22251. 240p. pap. 6.95 (*0-15-667702-4*, Harvest Bks) Harcourt.

Now That You're Pregnant. Louise Edeiken & Johanna Antar. 1992. LC 91-34634. 192p. pap. 12.00 (*0-02-079031-7*) Hungry Minds.

Now They Lay Me down to Sleep: What You Don't Know about Anesthesia & Surgery May Harm You. William G. Pace & Frederick W. Ernst. 1996. LC 96-19515. 180p. pap. 12.00 (*0-9651454-0-9*) F W Ernst.

Noxious Weeds of Victoria. W. T. Parsons. 1981. reprint ed. 45.00 (*0-909605-00-9*) Intl Spec Bk.

NSAID-Induced Gastroduodenal Damage Vol. 12, Supplement 1, 1994: Prevention & Treatment. Ed. by C. Scarpignato. 1995. (Journal: Vol. 13, Supplement 1, 1994). (Illus.). iv, 106p. pap. 34.00 (*3-8055-6068-0*) S Karger.

NSAIDs: A Profile of Adverse Effects. Ed. by Ivan Borda & Raymond Koff. 1992. (Illus.). 240p. 39.00 (*1-56053-018-9*) Hanley & Belfus.

NSC- First Aid & CPR Standard Web Enhanced. National Safety Council Staff. 2nd ed. 1998. (Illus.). 160p. (C). pap. text 5.70 (*0-7637-0897-6*) Jones & Bartlett.

NSNA Review Series: Critical Care Nursing. VEC Staff. 1996. LC 96-26301. (NSNA Review Ser.). (Illus.). 224p. (C). pap. 31.95 (*0-8273-7642-1*) Delmar.

NSNA Review Series: Health Assessment/Physical Examination. Ed. by Teresa W. Julian et al. 1995. LC 94-33067. (NSNA Review Ser.). 224p. (C). pap. 31.95 (*0-8273-6483-0*) Delmar.

NSNA's NCLEX - RN Review 1992. Alice M. Stein. 1992. text 29.95 (*0-8273-4836-3*) Delmar.

NSUCO Oculomotor Test. W. C. Maples. Ed. by Willard Bleything. 1994. (Illus.). 60p. (Orig.). (C). lib. bdg. 18.00 (*0-943599-74-1*) OEPF.

Nuances of Technique in Dynamic Psychotherapy. Mardi J. Horowitz. 1989. LC 89-30865. 288p. 50.00 (*0-87668-859-8*) Aronson.

Nuclear Accident Dosimetry Systems. International Atomic Energy Agency Staff. 1970. (Panel Proceedings Ser.). (Illus.). 200p. pap. (*92-0-021070-8*, ISP241) IAEA AUT. *Dist:* Bernan Associates.

Nuclear Accidents: Harmonization of the Public Health Response. 1989. (Euro Reports & Studies Ser.: No. 110). 111p. pap. text 10.00 (*92-890-1276-5*) World Health.

Nuclear Analytical Methods in the Life Sciences. Ed. by Rolf Zeisler & Vincent P. Guinn. 1991. (Illus.). 792p. 170.00 (*0-89603-202-7*) Humana.

Nuclear, Biological & Chemical Warfare. L. W. McNaught. 1984. (Brassey's Battlefield Weapons Systems & Technology Ser.: Vol. 4). 60p. text 35.95 (*0-08-028328-4*); pap. text 19.95 (*0-08-028329-2*) Elsevier (Pergamon Pr).

Nuclear Cardiac Imaging: Equilibrium & Gated First Pass Radionuclide Angiocardiography. Frans J. Wackers et al. 1992. (C). text 500.00 incl. disk (*1-56815-013-X*) Mosby Inc.

Nuclear Cardiac Imaging: Principles & Applications. Ami S. Iskandrian & Mario S. Verani. 2nd ed. 1996. LC 95-31109. (Illus.). 464p. (C). 180.00 (*0-8036-0071-2*) OUP.

Nuclear Cardiology. Ed. by Manuel D. Cerqueira. 1993. LC 93-31087. (Practical Cardiac Diagnosis Ser.). (Illus.). 280p. pap. 44.95 (*0-86542-248-6*) Blackwell Sci.

Nuclear Cardiology: State of the Art & Future Directions. Zaret Beller. 2nd ed. 1998. LC 98-33551. (Illus.). 668p. (C). (gr. 13). text 129.00 (*0-8151-1740-X*, 30422) Mosby Inc.

Nuclear Cardiology & Cardiac Magnetic Resonance. Ernst E. Van der Wall. 1992. LC 92-15313. 285p. (C). text 185.00 (*0-7923-1780-7*) Kluwer Academic.

Nuclear Cardiology in Everyday Practice. Ed. by J. Candell-Riera & D. Ortega-Alcalde. 1994. LC 93-24826. (Developments in Cardiovascular Medicine Ser.: Vol. 146). 396p. (C). text 243.00 (*0-7923-2374-2*) Kluwer Academic.

Nuclear Cardiovascular Imaging: Current Clinical Practice. Ed. by Milton J. Guiberteau. 1989. (Illus.). 248p. text (*0-443-08577-3*) Church.

Nuclear Chemistry: Theory & Applications. Ed. by Gregory R. Choppin & J. Ryberg. 1980. (Illus.). pap. 275.00 (*0-08-023823-8*); 294.00 (*0-08-023826-2*) Elsevier (Pergamon Pr).

Nuclear Contamination of Water Resources. Institution of Civil Engineers Staff. 1990. 268p. text (*0-7277-1527-5*) T Telford GBR. *Dist:* RCH.

Nuclear Emergency - How to Protect Your Family from Nuclear Radiation, Fallout & Terrorism. Ken Larson. 1997. 144p. pap. 10.95 (*0-9642497-2-3*) Rhema Pubng.

Nuclear Energy Simplified: An Overview of the Nuclear Technology of Reactors, Space & Medicine. Frank L. Bouquet. 1992. (Illus.). 130p. (Orig.). pap. 40.00 (*1-56216-074-5*); text 70.00 (*1-56216-073-7*) Systems Co.

Nuclear Handbook for Medical Service Personnel. 1995. lib. bdg. 255.75 (*0-8490-6554-2*); 1995. lib. bdg. 256.75 (*0-8490-6629-8*); 1991. lib. bdg. 79.95 (*0-8490-4125-2*) Gordon Pr.

Nuclear Hepatology: A Textbook of Hepatobiliary Diseases. Gerbail T. Krishnamurthy & Shakuntala Krishnamurthy. 2000. LC 00-21831. (Illus.). 330p. 169.00 (*3-540-65917-X*) Spr-Verlag.

Nuclear Imaging in Clinical Cardiology. M. L. Simmons & Johan H. Reiber. 1984. (Developments in Cardiovascular Medicine Ser.). 254p. text 174.50 (*0-89838-599-7*) Kluwer Academic.

Nuclear Imaging in Drug Discovery, Development, & Approval. Ed. by H. Donald Burns et al. 1992. LC 92-48930. x, 339p. 70.00 (*0-8176-3601-3*) Birkhauser.

Nuclear Imaging of the Chest. Yong W. Bahk et al. 1997. LC 97-29699. (Illus.). 336p. 175.00 (*3-540-62766-9*) Spr-Verlag.

Nuclear Localization of Growth Factors & of Monoclonal Antibodies. Ed. by Ewa M. Rakowicz-Szulczynska. 1993. LC 93-12471. 224p. lib. bdg. 179.00 (*0-8493-4713-0*, QP552) CRC Pr.

Nuclear Magnetic Resonance, Pt. C. Ed. by John N. Abelson et al. 1994. (Methods in Enzymology Ser.: Vol. 239). (Illus.). 813p. text 125.00 (*0-12-182140-4*) Acad Pr.

Nuclear Magnetic Resonance in Biology & Medicine: A Special Issue of the Journal Life Chemistry Reports, Vol. 1, Part 4. Jack Cohen et al. 1983. (Life Chemistry Reports: Vol. 1, No. 4). ii, 176p. pap. text 171.00 (*3-7186-0170-2*) Gordon & Breach.

Nuclear Medical Physics, Set. Ed. by Lawrence E. Williams. 1987. 357.00 (*0-8493-4677-0*, R895, CRC Reprint) Franklin.

Nuclear Medical Physics. L. Williams. 1987. LC 87-10262. reprint ed. Vol. 1. 256p. 130.00 (*0-8493-4678-9*); Vol. 3. 192p. 112.00 (*0-8493-4680-0*) Franklin (CRC Reprint).

Nuclear Medicine see Handbook of Nuclear Medicine

***Nuclear Medicine.** David Greenberg & William D. Leslie. 2001. (Vademecum Ser.). 254p. spiral bd. 45.00 (*1-57059-644-1*) Eurekah.

Nuclear Medicine: Diagnosis & Therapy. Ed. by John C. Harbert et al. 1996. LC 95-20599. (Illus.). 1200p. text 225.00 (*0-86577-570-2*) Thieme Med Pubs.

Nuclear Medicine: Factors Influencing the Choice & Use of Radionuclides in Diagnosis & Therapy. 1982. LC 81-84121. (Report Ser.: No. 70). 175p. 45.00 (*0-913392-57-X*) NCRP Pubns.

Nuclear Medicine: Principles & Practice Mark A. Boles et al. Ed. by Robert E. Henkin. 1995. (Illus.). 1852p. (C). (gr. 13). text 309.00 (*0-8016-7701-7*, 07701) Mosby Inc.

Nuclear Medicine: Quantitative Procedures. Heinz W. Wahner. 1983. 49.50 (*0-316-91748-6*, Little Brwn Med Div) Lppncott W & W.

Nuclear Medicine: Self-Study Program 1 Ed. by Barry A. Siegel & Peter T. Kirchner. 1988. LC 88-6549. (Illus.). 105.00 (*0-932004-30-X*) Soc Nuclear Med.

Nuclear Medicine: Self-Study Program 2: Instrumentation. Peter T. Kirchner & Barry A. Siegel. 1996. LC 95-48204. 70p. (Orig.). pap. 63.00 (*0-932004-44-X*) Soc Nuclear Med.

Nuclear Medicine: Teaching File. M. Reza Habibian. 1999. LC 98-45018. 944p. text 150.00 (*0-683-30122-5*) Lppncott W & W.

Nuclear Medicine: Technology & Techniques. Donald R. Bernier et al. 4th ed. 1997. LC 97-6999. (Illus.). 544p. (C). (gr. 13). text 91.00 (*0-8151-1991-7*, 30346) Mosby Inc.

Nuclear Medicine: The Requisites. James H. Thrall. 2nd ed. 2000. LC 2001-271703. (Radiology Requisites Ser.). (Illus.). x, 419p. text 89.00 (*0-323-00537-3*) Mosby Inc.

Nuclear Medicine Vol. IV, Unit 1: Self-Study Program 4: Oncology Overview. Thomas P. Haynie et al. 1997. LC 97-153510. (Illus.). 50p. pap. 20.00 (*0-932004-51-2*) Soc Nuclear Med.

Nuclear Medicine—The Requisites. James H. Thrall & Harvey A. Ziessman. 1994. (Illus.). 384p. (C). (gr. 13). text 79.00 (*0-8016-6674-0*, 06674) Mosby Inc.

Nuclear Medicine & Biology Advances: Proceedings of the Third World Congress on Nuclear Medicine & Biology, August 29 - September 2, 1982, Paris, France Ed. by C. Raynaud. 1983. 3685p. (*0-08-026405-0*) Pergamon Repr GBR. *Dist:* Franklin.

Nuclear Medicine & Lung Disease. J. L. Baulieu et al. 1993. (Illus.). 136p. 167.00 (*0-387-59605-4*) Spr-Verlag.

Nuclear Medicine Annual, 2000. Ed. by Leonard M. Freeman. 2000. 288p. text 129.00 (*0-7817-2573-9*) Lppncott W & W.

***Nuclear Medicine Annual, 2001.** Ed. by Leonard M. Freeman. 2001. (Nuclear Medicine Annual Ser.). (Illus.). 300p. text 129.00 (*0-7817-3102-X*) Lppncott W & W.

Nuclear Medicine Board Review: Questions & Answers for Self-Assessment. Richard Goldfarb et al. 1997. LC 97-41323. 176p. pap. 24.00 (*0-86577-703-9*) Thieme Med Pubs.

Nuclear Medicine Handbook for Achieving Compliance with NRC Regulations. Katherine M. Elliott et al. 1997. LC 97-9525. 159p. pap. text 35.00 (*0-932004-50-4*) Soc Nuclear Med.

Nuclear Medicine Imaging. Owens. 1999. text (*0-7216-6089-4*) Saunders.

Nuclear Medicine in Clinical Diagnosis & Treatment Ed. by I. P. Murray & P. J. Ell. 1995. LC 94-34613. (Illus.). 1388p. text (*0-443-04710-3*) Church.

Nuclear Medicine in Clinical Diagnosis & Treatment. I. P. Murray & P. J. Ell. 2nd ed. 1999. (*0-443-05861-X*) Church.

Nuclear Medicine in Clinical Practice: 100 Self-Assessment Case Studies. Ignac Fogelman et al. 1997. LC 97-67752. (Illus.). 212p. pap. (*0-412-45830-6*) E A GBR. *Dist:* OUP.

Nuclear Medicine in Clinical Urology & Nephrology. W. Newlon Tauxe & Eva V. Dobovsky. 1992. (Illus.). 358p. (C). pap. text 110.00 (*0-8385-6983-8*, A6983-9, Apple Lange Med) McGraw.

Nuclear Medicine in Gastroenterology. Ed. by Hans J. Biersack & Peter H. Cox. 1991. (Developments in Nuclear Medicine Ser.). 264p. text 180.50 (*0-7923-1074-8*) Kluwer Academic.

Nuclear Medicine in Pharmaceutical Research. A. C. Perkins. 1999. 178p. 99.00 (*0-7484-0688-3*) Taylor & Francis.

Nuclear Medicine Physics: The Basics. Ramesh Chandra. 5th ed. 1998. LC 97-15681. (Illus.). 198p. pap. 49.95 (*0-683-30092-X*) Lppncott W & W.

Nuclear Medicine Science & Safety. Perkins. 200p. (*0-86196-470-5*) J Libbey Med GBR. *Dist:* Bks Intl VA.

Nuclear Medicine Science & Safety. Alan C. Perkins. 2001. 192p. (*0-86196-605-8*) J Libbey Med GBR. *Dist:* Buttrwrth-Heinemann.

Nuclear Medicine Self-Study Program Vol. IV, Unit 4: Nuclear Medicine Oncology: PET Tumor Imaging. Sudha Challa & Carl K. Hoh. Ed. by Thomas P. Haynie. 1999. LC 99-34619. 28.00 (*0-932004-62-8*) Soc Nuclear Med.

Nuclear Medicine Self-Study Program, Cardiology Vol. II, Unit 4: Radionclide Assessment of Congenital Heart Disease & Cardiac PET. Michale W. Dae. 1998. LC 98-27502. 127p. pap. text 49.00 (*0-932004-54-7*) Soc Nuclear Med.

Nuclear Medicine Self-Study Program, Cardiology Vol. III, Unit 1: Physical & Technical Aspects of Nuclear Cardiology. Elias H. Botvinick et al. 1997. LC 97-25005. (Nuclear Medicine Self-Study Program III). (Illus.). 96p. pap. 35.00 (*0-932004-52-0*) Soc Nuclear Med.

Nuclear Medicine Self-Study Program, Cardiology Vol. III, Unit 2: Pharmacological Stress Self-Study Program 3. Elias H. Botvinick. 1998. LC 98-26415. 195p. pap. text 63.00 (*0-932004-60-1*) Soc Nuclear Med.

Nuclear Medicine: Self-Study Program IV Vol. IV Unit 2: Conventional Tumor Imaging. Patrice K. Rehm. 1997. LC 97-41360. (Conventional Tumor Imaging Ser.: No. 2). (Illus.). pap. text 35.00 (*0-932004-53-9*) Soc Nuclear Med.

Nuclear Medicine Self-Study Program Oncology Vol. IV, Unit 3: Self-Study Program 4 Antibody Tumor Imaging. Nabi H. Abdel. 1999. LC 98-49229. 49p. pap. 20.00 (*0-932004-61-X*) Soc Nuclear Med.

Nuclear Medicine Therapy. Alan C. Perkins & D. M. Lewis. 2001. 200p. (*0-86196-570-1*) John Libby GBR. *Dist:* Buttrwrth-Heinemann.

Nuclear Mentality: A Psychosocial Analysis of the Arms Race. Lynn Barnett. Ed. by Ian Lee. 1989. 192p. (C). pap. (*0-7453-0393-5*) Pluto GBR GBR. *Dist:* Stylus Pub VA.

Nuclear Mentality: A Psychosocial Analysis of the Arms Race. Ed. by Lynn Barnett & Ian Lee. 1989. 192p. (C). text 42.00 (*0-7453-0392-7*) Westview.

Nuclear Oncogenes. Ed. by Frederick W. Alt et al. 1987. (Illus.). 194p. (Orig.). pap. text 30.00 (*0-87969-305-3*) Cold Spring Harbor.

Nuclear Oncology. Ed. by Cumali Aktolun & W. Newlon Tauxe. 1999. LC 99-10449. (Illus.). 472p. 189.00 (*3-540-64760-0*) Spr-Verlag.

Nuclear Oncology: Diagnosis & Therapy. Iraj Khalkhali et al. 2000. LC 00-48746. (Illus.). 608p. text 149.00 (*0-7817-1990-9*) Lppncott W & W.

***Nuclear Organization of Gene Expression in Adenovirus Infected Cells.** Anders Aspegren. 2001. (Comprehensive Summaries of Uppsala Dissertations from the Faculty of Medicine Ser.: No. 1067). (Illus.). 48p. pap. (*91-554-5095-4*) Acta Univ SWE. *Dist:* Coronet Bks.

Nuclear Particles in Cancer Treatment. John F. Fowler. 1981. (Medical Physics Handbook Ser.: No. 8). (Illus.). 190p. 19.00 (*0-85274-521-4*) Inst of Physics Pubng.

Nuclear Pharmacy: An Introduction to the Clinical Application of Radiopharmaceuticals. Henry M. Chilton & Richard L. Witcofski. 1986. LC 85-23910. (Illus.). 190p. text 35.00 (*0-8121-1021-8*) Lppncott W & W.

Nuclear Power - Accidental Releases - Principles of Public Health Action: Report on a WHO Meeting. 1984. (Who Regional Publications, European Ser.: No. 16). 62p. pap. text 12.00 (*92-890-1107-6*) World Health.

Nuclear Power - Health Implications of Transuranium Elements: Report on a Working Group. 1982. (WHO Regional Publications, European Ser.: No. 11). 88p. pap. text 14.00 (*92-890-1102-5*) World Health.

Nuclear Power & Health: The Implications for Health of Nuclear Power Production. 1994. (WHO Regional Publications: No. 51). xviii, 145p. pap. text 26.00 (*92-890-1315-X*, 1310051) World Health.

Nuclear Radiation: What It Is, How to Detect It, How to Protect Yourself from It. Gregory H. Piesinger. 1980. LC 80-24001. (Illus.). 127p. (Orig.). (C). pap. 9.95 (*0-937224-00-6*) Dyco Inc.

Nuclear Radiology (Fourth Series) Test & Syllabus. James H. Thrall et al. 1990. (Professional Self-Evaluation & Continuing Education Program Ser.: Vol. 30). (Illus.). 750p. 190.00 (*1-55903-030-5*) Am Coll Radiology.

Nuclear Submicroscopy. G. Jasmin & R. Simard. 1986. (Methods & Achievements in Experimental Pathology Ser.: Vol. 12). (Illus.). viii, 300p. 249.75 (*3-8055-4137-6*) S Karger.

Nuclear Techniques in Diagnostic Medicine. Ed. by P. P. van Rijk. 1986. text 401.00 (*0-89838-744-2*) Kluwer Academic.

Nuclear Tests: Long-Term Consequences in the Semipalatinsk/Altai Region. NATO Staff. Ed. by Charles S. Shapiro et al. 1998. LC 97-39008. (NATO ASI Ser.: Vol. 36). (Illus.). 204p. 110.00 (*3-540-63805-9*) Spr-Verlag.

Nuclear War & Radioactive Fallout: Index of New Information with Authors, Subjects & References. Henry A. Reddy. 1997. 150p. 57.50 (*0-7883-1320-7*); pap. 47.50 (*0-7883-1321-5*) ABBE Pubs Assn.

Nuclear Wastelands: A Global Guide to Nuclear Weapons Production & Its Health & Environmental Effects. Ed. by Arjun Makhijani et al. 1995. LC 95-945. 666p. 65.00 (*0-262-13307-5*) MIT Pr.

Nucleic Acid Amplification Techniques for Virus Detection in Transfusion Medicine. Ed. by Gregor Caspari. 1998. (Infusionstherapie und Transfusionsmedizin Ser.: Vol. 25, No. 2-3). (Illus.). 140p. pap. 58.25 (*3-8055-6717-0*) S Karger.

Nucleic Acid-Based Diagnosis. S. Jeffery et al. 1997. (Medical Perspective Ser.). 176p. pap. (*1-85996-190-8*) Bios Sci GBR. *Dist:* Coronet Bks.

Nucleic Acid Sequences Handbook. Christian Gautier et al. 1982. LC 81-19904. 320p. Vol. 1. 78.75 (*0-275-90798-8*, C07981); Vol. 2. 85.00 (*0-275-90799-6*, C07992) Greenwood (Praeger Pubs).

Nucleic Acid Targeted Drug Design. Ed. by C. Propst & Thomas Perun. 1992. LC 92-17585. (Illus.). 644p. text 225.00 (*0-8247-8662-9*) Dekker.

Nucleic Acids, Pt. D. Ed. by Lawrence Grossman & Kivie Moldave. 1971. (Methods in Enzymology Ser.: Vol. 21). text 209.00 (*0-12-181884-5*) Acad Pr.

Nucleic Acids, Pts. A-B. Ed. by Lawrence Grossman et al. (Methods in Enzymology Ser.: Vol. 12). (C). 1968. text 209.00 (*0-12-181856-X*); 1967. text 209.00 (*0-12-181854-3*) Acad Pr.

Nucleic Acids & Protein Synthesis, Pt. C. Ed. by Kivie Moldave & Lawrence Grossman. 1971. (Methods in Enzymology Ser.: Vol. 20). text 209.00 (*0-12-181883-7*) Acad Pr.

Nucleic Acids & Protein Synthesis, Pt. E. Ed. by Lawrence Grossman & Kivie Moldave. 1974. (Methods in Enzymology Ser.: Vol. 29). text 199.00 (*0-12-181892-6*) Acad Pr.

Nucleic Acids & Protein Synthesis, Pt. F. Ed. by Lawrence Grossman & Kwie Molve. 1974. (Methods in Enzymology Ser.: Vol. 30). text 199.00 (*0-12-181893-4*) Acad Pr.

Nucleic Acids & Protein Synthesis, Pt. H. Ed. by Kivic Moldave & Lawrence Grossman. 1979. (Methods in Enzymology Ser.: Vol. 60). 896p. text 121.00 (*0-12-181960-4*) Acad Pr.

Nucleic Acids & Proteins in Plants II: Structure, Biochemistry & Physiology of Nucleic Acids. Ed. by B. Parthier & D. Boulter. 1982. (Encyclopedia of Plant Physiology Ser.: Vol. 14 B). (Illus.). 774p. 337.00 (*0-387-11140-9*) Spr-Verlag.

Nucleic Acids & Proteins Synthesis, Pt. G. Ed. by Kivic Moldave & Lawrence Grossman. 1979. (Methods in Enzymology Ser.: Vol. 59). 939p. text 121.00 (*0-12-181959-0*) Acad Pr.

Nucleolus Ribosome Biogenesis. A. A. Hadjiolov. 1985. (Cell Biology Monographs: Vol. 12). (Illus.). 290p. 123.95 (*0-387-81790-5*) Spr-Verlag.

Nucleoside Analogs in Cancer Therapy. Bruce D. Cheson et al. 1997. LC 97-11276. (Basic & Clinical Oncology Ser.). (Illus.). 488p. text 199.00 (*0-8247-9850-3*) Dekker.

Nucleosides & Nucleotides As Antitumor & Antiviral Agents. C. K. Chu & D. C. Baker. 1993. LC 93-13432. (Illus.). 346p. (C). text 95.00 (*0-306-44520-4*, Kluwer Plenum) Kluwer Academic.

Nucleotide Analogues As Antiviral Agents. Ed. by John C. Martin. 1989. LC 89-15114. (ACS Symposium Ser.: No. 401). (Illus.). 175p. text 50.00 (*0-8412-1659-2*) Am Chemical.

Nucleotide Antagonists As Anticancer Drugs. Richard I. Christopherson & Stephen D. Lyons. 2000. 95.00 (*0-8493-4309-7*) CRC Pr.

Nude Mouse in Oncology Research. Epie Boven & Benjamin Winograd. 1991. (Illus.). 352p. lib. bdg. 229.00 (*0-8493-6531-7*, RC267) CRC Pr.

Nuestros Cuerpos, Nuestras Vidas. Boston Women's Health Collective Staff. 2000. LC 99-461970.Tr. of Our Bodies, Ourselves. (SPA., Illus.). 604p. pap. 24.95 (*1-58322-024-0*, SC0240) Seven Stories.

Nueva Enciclopedia de Medicina y Salud: Para el Hogar Moderno. Richard J. Wagman. Tr. by Maria T. Sanz & Pedro Larios A. 1992. (SPA., Illus.). 1390p. 59.95 (*0-915741-35-0*) C D Stampley Ent.

Nueva Guia De Ginecologia. Garcia Del Real Eduardo. 1999. (SPA.). pap. text 18.95 (*84-7880-977-5*) Planeta.

Nuevas Perspectivas en Atencion Primaria de Salud. J. M. Aranda Regules. 1994. (SPA.). 399p. pap. (*84-7978-114-9*) Ediciones Diaz ESP. *Dist:* IBD Ltd.

Numb Toes & Aching Soles: Coping with Peripheral Neuropathy. John A. Senneff. 2000. LC 99-62350. xxix, 300p. 29.95 (*0-9671107-2-6*); pap. 22.95 (*0-9671107-1-8*) MedPress.

Number & Time: Reflections Leading Toward a Unification of Depth, Psychology & Physics. Marie-Louise Von Franz. Tr. by Andrea Dykes from GER. 1986. LC 73-86467. (Studies in Jungian Thought). 332p. pap. 28.00 (*0-8101-0532-2*) Northwestern U Pr.

Numbers for Blood Bankers. Ed. by Joy L. Fridey et al. 1995. LC 95-44611. (Illus.). 107p. (C). 40.00 (*1-56395-045-6*) Am Assn Blood.

Numerical Computer Methods. Ed. by John N. Abelson et al. 1992. (Methods in Enzymology Ser.: Vol. 210). (Illus.). 718p. text 125.00 (*0-12-182111-0*) Acad Pr.

Numerical Computer Methods, Pt. B. Ed. by Michael L. Johnson et al. 1994. (Methods in Enzymology Ser.: Vol. 240). (Illus.). 857p. text 125.00 (*0-12-182141-2*) Acad Pr.

Numerical Methods in the Biomedical Sciences. E. H. Twizell. 1988. (Mathematics & Its Applications Ser.). 300p. 73.95 (*0-470-21002-8*) P-H.

Numerical Proportions of the Sexes at Birth. John B. Nichols. 1906. (American Anthropological Association Memoirs Ser.: No. 4). 25.00 (*0-527-00503-7*) Periodicals Srv.

Nunn's Applied Respiratory Physiology. J. F. Nunn. 4th ed. 1999. (Illus.). 608p. text 100.00 (*0-7506-1336-X*) Buttrwrth-Heinemann.

Nunn's Applied Respiratory Physiology. Andrew Lumb et al. 5th ed. 1999. LC 99-40687. 687p. text 120.00 (*0-7506-3107-4*) Buttrwrth-Heinemann.

Nuova Encyclopedia Medica Garzanti. 1993. (ITA.). 1328p. pap. text 82.00 (*0-913298-94-8*) S F Vanni.

Nurse. Jack Rudman. 1994. (Career Examination Ser.: C-532). pap. 27.95 (*0-8373-0532-2*) Nat Learn.

Nurse Abuse: Impact & Resolution. Ed. by Laura G. Vonfrolio et al. 2nd rev. ed. 1996. 300p. pap. 15.00 (*1-888315-02-4*) Power NY.

Nurse Administrator. Jack Rudman. 1994. (Career Examination Ser.: C-2913). pap. 34.95 (*0-8373-2913-2*) Nat Learn.

Nurse Aide in Long Term Care. Betty J. Walston & Keith E. Walston. 1995. 352p. 38.60 net. (*0-8273-8787-3*) Delmar.

Nurse Aide in Long-Term Care: Instructor's Guide. Betty J. Walston & Keith E. Walston. 3rd ed. 1994. 298p. tchr. ed. 19.00 (*0-8273-5471-1*) Delmar.

Nurse Allocation. Iain M. Banks. 1972. (Illus.). spiral bd. 16.95 (*0-433-01165-3*) Coronet Bks.

Nurse Anesthesia: Clinical Textbook. John J. Nagelhout & Karen L. Zaglaniczny. Ed. by Maura Connor. 1996. (Illus.). 1375p. pap. text 130.00 (*0-7216-6479-2*) Saunders.

Nurse Anesthesia: Pretest Self-Assessment & Review. Ed. by Francis R. Gerbasi. 1997. LC 97-21700. (Pretest Specialty Level Ser.). (Illus.). 155p. pap. 39.95 (*0-07-052080-1*) McGraw-Hill Prof.

Nurse Anesthesia Handbook. John J. Nagelhout & Karen L. Zaglaniczny. Ed. by Maura Connor. 1997. LC 96-20547. (Illus.). 1397p. pap. text 42.95 (*0-7216-6694-9*) Saunders.

Nurse Apprentice, 1860-1977. Ann Bradshaw. 2000. LC 00-42042. 286p. 79.95 (*0-7546-0172-2*) Ashgate Pub Co.

Nurse As Caregiver for the Dying Patient & His Family. Ed. by Ann M. Earle & Nina Arson-Dizzo. 1976. LC 76-14441. 252p. 12.50 (*0-930194-31-4*) Ctr Thanatology.

Nurse As Counselor. Virgil Parsons & Beverly Meyer. 1985. (C). pap. 18.95 (*0-8359-5011-5*) P-H.

Nurse as Educator: Principle of Teaching & Learning. Susan B. Bastable. 1997. LC 97-7066. (Nursing Ser.). (Illus.). 432p. (C). pap. text 47.95 (*0-7637-0310-9*, 0310-9) Jones & Bartlett.

Nurse as Educator: Principles of Teaching & Learning. Susan B. Bastable. 2nd ed. 2001. (Illus.). 416p. (C). pap. text 46.95 (*0-7637-1441-0*, 1441-0, N L N Bart) Jones & Bartlett.

Nurse As Executive. Barbara Stevens-Barnum & Darlene M. Kerfoot. 4th ed. 1995. 369p. pap. 72.00 (*0-8342-0571-8*, 20571) Aspen Pub.

Nurse As Group Leader. Carolyn C. Clark. 3rd ed. 1994. LC 94-3104. (Teaching of Nursing Ser.: Vol. 3). 304p. (C). text 32.95 (*0-8261-2333-3*) Springer Pub.

Nurse As Healer. Lynn Keegan. 1993. LC 93-26361. (Nurse as Healer Ser.). 228p. (C). mass mkt. 21.50 (*0-8273-6156-4*) Delmar.

Nurse As Manager. Joyce L. Schweiger. 1989. LC 80-17456. 194p. pap. text 32.20 (*0-8273-4360-4*) Delmar.

Nurse As Manager Handbook. Joyce L. Schweiger. 1989. LC 86-9126. (Red Bks.). 600p. pap. text 33.95 (*0-8273-4361-2*) Delmar.

Nurse as the Wounded Healer: From Trauma to Transformation. Marion Conti-O'Hare. 2001. (Illus.). 192p. (C). pap. text 24.95 (*0-7637-1568-9*, 1568-9) Jones & Bartlett.

Nurse As Therapist: A Behavioural Model. Ed. by Philip J. Barker & Douglas Fraser. 1985. LC 85-10935. 250p. (Orig.). pap. (*0-7099-3253-7*) C Helm GBR. *Dist:* Routldge.

Nurse Assistant in Long-Term Care: A Rehabilitative Approach. Hazel M. Castillo. 1992. (Illus.). 528p. (gr. 13). pap. text 27.00 (*0-8016-0945-3*, 00945) Mosby Inc.

Nurse Assistant Test Preparation. Wanda Smith. 1994. LC 94-35572. (Test Prep Ser.). 192p. pap. 31.80 (*0-8359-4925-7*) P-H.

Nurse Case Management in the 21st Century. Ed. by Elaine L. Cohen. 1995. LC 95-41096. (Illus.). 288p. (C). text 43.95 (*0-8151-1518-0*, 25106) Mosby Inc.

Nurse-Client Interaction: Implementing the Nursing Process. Sandra J. Sundeen. 6th ed. 1997. LC 97-42735. (Illus.). 376p. (C). (gr. 13). pap. text 29.00 (*0-8151-2605-0*, 31075) Mosby Inc.

Nurse Communicates. April Sieh & Louise Brentin. Ed. by Maura Connor. 1997. LC 96-30276. (Illus.). 352p. pap. text 26.00 (*0-7216-4173-3*) Saunders.

Nurse Consultant's Handbook. Belinda Puetz & Linda J. Shinn. 1997. LC 96-47041. 248p. 39.95 (*0-8261-9520-2*) Springer Pub.

Nurse Education. 224p. pap. (*0-340-55786-9*) E A GBR. *Dist:* Routldge.

Nurse Educator in Academia: Strategies for Success. Theresa M. Valiga & Helen J. Streubert. 1991. LC 90-10437. (Teaching of Nursing Ser.: Vol. 13). 240p. 34.95 (*0-8261-7150-8*) Springer Pub.

Nurse Educators 1999. National League for Nursing Staff. 2nd ed. 2001. 128p. (C). pap. text 32.95 (*0-7637-1439-9*, 1439-9, N L N Bart) Jones & Bartlett.

Nurse Educators 1997: Findings from the RN & LPN Faculty Census. NLN Staff. 1999. (Illus.). 72p. (C). pap. text 33.95 (*0-7637-1011-3*, 1011-3, N L N Bart) Jones & Bartlett.

Nurse Entrepreneur: Building the Bridge of Opportunity. Carolyn S. Zagury et al. Ed. by Maryann Liotta. 3rd rev. ed. 1995. LC 94-61762. 227p. pap., wbk. ed. 24.95 (*1-880254-28-X*) Vista.

***Nurse Executive Resource Manual.** Julian Cicatiello. 2001. LC 2001-22077. (Illus.). ring bd. 249.00 (*0-8342-1931-X*) Aspen Pub.

Nurse GS4-GS7. Jack Rudman. 1994. (Career Examination Ser.: C-533). pap. 27.95 (*0-8373-0533-0*) Nat Learn.

Nurse Instructor. Jack Rudman. 1994. (Career Examination Ser.: C-2108). reprint ed. pap. 34.95 (*0-8373-2108-5*) Nat Learn.

Nurse Leadership Development: A Training Program for Developing Nurse Intrapreneurs. Laura J. McCarthy & Carolyn S. Zagury. Ed. by Mary L. Diecker et al. 1997. LC 91-75022. (Illus.). 346p. pap. 79.00 (*1-880254-00-X*) Vista.

Nurse Manager: A Practical Guide to Better Employee Relations. June B. Pugh & Mary A. Woodard-Smith. Ed. by Thomas Eoyang. 2nd ed. 1996. LC 96-28574. (Illus.). 125p. pap. text 14.95 (*0-7216-6445-8*) Saunders.

Nurse Manager's Answer Book. Ruth I. Hansten & Marilynn J. Washburn. 1993. LC 93-4978. 256p. pap. 32.00 (*0-8342-0501-7*, 20501) Aspen Pub.

Nurse Manager's Problem Solver. Tim Porter-O'Grady. 1994. LC 94-2184. (Illus.). 322p. (C). (gr. 13). pap. text 33.95 (*0-8016-7945-1*, 07945) Mosby Inc.

Nurse Manager's Survival Guide: Practical Answers to Everyday Problems. Tina M. Marrelli. 2nd ed. 1997. LC 96-37670. (Illus.). 400p. (C). (gr. 13). pap. text 29.95 (*0-8151-5672-3*, 28206) Mosby Inc.

Nurse-Midwife Discusses Pregnancy & Childbirth. Barbara Graves. 1994. 6.00 (*0-910304-14-9*) Budlong.

Nurse, Pharmacology & Drug Therapy. Marshal Shlafer. Ed. by Debra Hunter. 1989. 1432p. (C). text 55.95 (*0-201-12796-2*); trans. 175.00 (*0-201-57837-9*) Addison-Wesley.

Nurse, Pharmacology & Drug Therapy. Marshall Shlafer. 3rd ed. 2001. (C). text (*0-8053-7247-4*) Addison-Wesley.

Nurse-Physician Collaboration: Care of Adults & the Elderly. Eugenia L. Siegler & Fay W. Whitney. 1994. LC 94-19260. (Advanced Practice Nursing & Geriatric Nursing Ser.). (Illus.). 264p. 35.95 (*0-8261-8500-2*) Springer Pub.

***Nurse Practitioner Manual.** Sue Cross & Myfamwy Rimmer. 2001. (Illus.). 400p. pap. (*0-7020-2518-6*) W B Saunders GBR. *Dist:* Saunders.

Nurse Practitioner Protocols. Matthew M. Cohen & Anni Lanigan. 264p. rev. ed. 1991. disk (*0-924381-14-0*); 2nd rev. ed. 1995. pap. 55.00 (*0-924381-24-8*); 2nd rev. ed. 1995. ring bd. 85.00 (*0-924381-23-X*) Sunbelt Med Pubs.

Nurse Practitioners: Clinical Skills & Professional Issues. Mike Walsh et al. 1999. LC 99-15486. 320p. pap. text 45.00 (*0-7506-3990-3*) Buttrwrth-Heinemann.

Nurse Practitioner's Business Practice & Legal Guide. Carolyn Buppert. 1998. LC 98-39952. 496p. 89.00 (*0-8342-1185-8*, 11858) Aspen Pub.

Nurse Practitioner's Clinical Companion. Springhouse Publishing Company Staff. 2000. LC 99-52581. (Illus.). 480p. pap. 42.95 (*1-58255-006-9*) Springhouse Corp.

Nurse Practitioner's Drug Handbook. Ed. by Springhouse Publishing Company Staff. 3rd ed. 2000. (Illus.). spiral bd. 42.95 (*0-87434-997-4*) Springhouse Corp.

Nurse Practitioners in Primary Care. Naomi Chambers. 1998. LC 98-198331. 144p. pap. (*1-85775-298-8*) Radcliffe Med Pr GBR. *Dist:* Balogh.

***Nurse Prescribers' Formulary, 2001-2003.** Mehta. 2002. 320p. (*0-85369-496-6*) Pharmaceutical Pr GBR. *Dist:* Rittenhouse.

Nurse Remembers. Eula A. Sforza. 1991. (Illus.). 233p. pap. 22.50 (*0-9636567-0-8*) E A Sforza.

Nurse Saver: An Organizational Too! Kevan J. Burns & Caroline E. Burns. 1998. (Illus.). 24p. wbk. ed. 25.00 (*0-9663913-0-6*) Nurse Saver.

Nurse-Social Worker Collaboration in Managed Care: A Model of Community Case Management. Joellen W. Hawkins et al. 1997. LC 97-22490. (Illus.). 240p. 37.95 (*0-8261-9830-9*) Springer Pub.

Nurse Staffing & Patient Outcomes in the Inpatient Hospital Setting. Contrib. by American Nurses' Association Staff. 2000. LC 00-42363. ix, 53p. pap. 24.95 (*1-55810-151-9*) Am Nurses Pub.

Nurse Teachers as Researchers: Research in Practice. 280p. pap. (*0-340-66193-3*) E A GBR. *Dist:* Routldge.

NurseNotes: Maternal-Newborn Nursing. Irene M. Bobak. 1997. LC 96-9117. 288p. pap. text 28.95 (*0-7817-1128-2*) Lppncott W & W.

NurseNotes: Medical-Surgical Nursing. Nelson. 1997. LC 96-23717. 448p. pap. text 26.95 (*0-7817-1130-4*) Lppncott W & W.

NurseNotes: Pediatric Nursing. Geraldine C. Colombrari & Diane M. Billings. 1997. LC 96-20788. (Nursenotes Ser.). 288p. pap. text 28.95 (*0-7817-1129-0*) Lppncott W & W.

NurseNotes: Psychiatric-Mental Health Nursing. Diane M. Billings. 1997. LC 96-9116. (Nursenotes Ser.). 272p. pap. text 28.95 (*0-7817-1127-4*) Lppncott W & W.

Nurse's Aide. Jack Rudman. 1994. (Career Examination Ser.: C-535). pap. 23.95 (*0-8373-0535-7*) Nat Learn.

Nurses & Doctors at Work: Rethinking Professional Boundaries. Deidre Wicks. 1998. LC 99-178837. xvii, 202p. 95.00 (*0-335-20274-8*); pap. text 29.95 (*0-335-20273-X*) Taylor & Francis.

Nurses & Families: A Guide to Family Assessment & Intervention. Lorraine M. Wright & Maureen Leahey. 3rd ed. 1999. LC 99-42916. (Illus.). 358p. (C). pap. text 25.95 (*0-8036-0371-1*) Davis Co.

Nurses & Family Health Promotion: Concepts, Assessment & Interventions. Ed. by Perri J. Bomar. 2nd ed. 1995. LC 95-19486. (Illus.). 429p. pap. text 38.95 (*0-7216-3795-7*) Saunders.

Nurses & Health Care. Ed. by Elizabeth Lucas. 1976. pap. 24.95 (*0-8464-0679-9*) Beekman Pubs.

***Nurses & Nursing: Influencing Policy.** Ed. by Pippa Gough & Nicola Walsh. 2000. 128p. pap. (*1-85775-353-4*) Radcliffe Med Pr GBR. *Dist:* Balogh.

Nurses & the Law: A Guide to Principles & Applications. Nancy J. Brent. 2nd ed. 2001. LC 00-49269. (Illus.). xiv, 529p. 38.00 (*0-7216-9195-1*) Saunders.

Nurses & Work Satisfaction: An Index for Measurement. Paula L. Stamps. 2nd ed. 1997. LC 97-18700. 42.00 (*1-56793-061-1*) Health Admin Pr.

Nurses As Consultants: ESS Concepts & Processes. Susan Norwood. 1997. LC 97-22981. 336p. pap. text 41.00 (*0-8053-5427-1*, Prentice Hall) P-H.

Nurse's Atlas of Dermatology. Theodore Rosen et al. 1983. 203p. 25.50 (*0-316-75705-5*, Little Brwn Med Div) Lppncott W & W.

Nurse's Book of Courage. Helene K. Nawrocki. 1993. 61p. pap. 14.95 (*0-9636792-0-1*) Ctr Nursing Excell.

Nurse's Clinical Guide to Dosage Calculations. Belle Erickson & Catherine M. Todd. 2nd rev. ed. 1994. LC 94-3506. 224p. spiral bd. 32.95 (*0-87434-703-3*) Springhouse Corp.

Nurse's Clinical Guide to Maternity Care. Springhouse Publishing Company Staff. 2nd ed. 1998. LC 97-42636. (Nurse's Clinical Guide Ser.). (Illus.). 512p. spiral bd. 34.95 (*0-87434-883-8*) Springhouse Corp.

Nurse's Clinical Guide to Neonatal Care. Springhouse Publishing Company Staff. 2nd ed. 1998. LC 97-42704. (Nurse's Clinical Guide Ser.). 400p. spiral bd. 32.95 (*0-87434-884-6*) Springhouse Corp.

Nurse's Clinical Guide to Psychiatric & Mental Health Care. Linda C. Copel. 1995. LC 95-32425. (Illus.). 384p. pap. 27.95 (*0-87434-720-3*) Springhouse Corp.

Nurse's Clinical Guide to Psychiatric & Mental Health Care. Linda C. Copel. 2nd ed. 1999. LC 99-35195. (Nurse's Clinical Guide Ser.). 416p. spiral bd. 32.95 (*0-87434-986-9*) Springhouse Corp.

Nurse's Clinical Pocket Manual: Nursing Diagnoses, Care Planning & Documentation. Mary F. Moorhouse & Marilynn E. Doenges. 1990. 477p. (C). spiral bd. 18.95 (*0-8036-6314-5*) Davis Co.

Nurses, Computers & Information Technology. Procter. 1992. 118p. pap. 34.95 (*1-56593-019-3*, 0262) Thomson Learn.

Nurses Counselling: The View from the Practitioners. Ed. by Philip Burnard & Ian Hulatt. 1996. LC 96-14626. 192p. pap. text 40.00 (*0-7506-2004-8*) Buttrwrth-Heinemann.

Nurse's Directory of Capitol Connections. 4th rev. ed. 1997. 90p. ring bd. 25.00 (*0-9659713-0-9*) Sharp Legis.

Nurse's Dosage Calculator. Springhouse Publishing Company Staff. 1998. (Illus.). 24p. 24.95 incl. disk (*0-87434-974-5*) Springhouse Corp.

Nurse's Drug Handbook. Suzanne Loebl & George R. Spratto. 6th ed. 1991. pap. 33.95 (*0-8273-4527-5*) Delmar.

Nurse's Drug Reference, 1990. George R. Spratto. 2nd ed. 1990. (Professional Reference - Nursing Ser.). pap. 25.95 (*0-8273-4277-2*) Delmar.

Nurse's Guide for Teaching Patients Undergoing Cancer Chemotherapy. 1984. lib. bdg. 250.00 (*0-87700-543-5*) Revisionist Pr.

Nurse's Guide to Cancer Care. Constance S. Kirkpatrick. 1986. LC 86-17666. 304p. 68.50 (*0-8476-7500-9*); pap. 29.50 (*0-8476-7501-7*) Rowman.

Nurse's Guide to Cardiac Rhythm Interpretation: Implications for Patient Care. Sara Paul & Jennifer D. Hebra. Ed. by Barbara N. Cullen. 1998. LC 97-36629. (Illus.). 405p. (C). pap. text 27.95 (*0-7216-5906-3*) Saunders.

Nurse's Guide to Caring for Elders. Mary Carroll & L. Jane Brue. 1987. 240p. (C). pap. 29.95 (*0-8261-5520-0*) Springer Pub.

Nurses' Guide to Clinical Procedures. Jean Smith-Temple & Joyce Young Johnson. 3rd ed. 1997. LC 97-15075. (Illus.). 768p. spiral bd. 30.95 (*0-397-55464-8*) Lppncott W & W.

***Nurses' Guide to Consumer Health Websites.** Ed. by Joyce J. Fitzpatrick. 2001. 280p. pap. 33.95 (*0-8261-1435-0*) Springer Pub.

Nurse's Guide to Diet Therapy. Lois H. Bodinski. 2nd ed. 1989. pap. text 33.50 (*0-8273-4209-8*) Delmar.

Nurse's Guide to Home Care of the Elderly. Sheryl Zang. 1998. LC 98-22344. 560p. spiral bd. 27.50 (*0-7817-1542-3*) Lppncott W & W.

Nurses' Guide to Home Care Procedures. Ed. by Joyce Young Johnson et al. 1997. LC 97-19139. (Illus.). 704p. spiral bd. 31.00 (*0-397-55468-0*) Lppncott W & W.

Nurse's Guide to Home Health Care. Tina M. Marrelli. 1997. LC 97-18701. (Illus.). 448p. (C). (gr. 13). spiral bd. 26.95 (*0-8151-5558-1*, 29633) Mosby Inc.

Nurse's Guide to Marketing. Ruth R. Alward. 1990. (Home Care Aide Ser.). pap. 43.45 (*0-8273-4203-9*) Delmar.

Nurse's Guide to Successful Management. Jo A. McGuffin. 1999. LC 98-43530. xvii, 332p. spiral bd. 29.95 (*0-323-00388-5*) Mosby Inc.

Nurses' Guide to Understanding Laboratory & Diagnostic Tests. Denise D. Wilson. 1998. LC 98-3764. 576p. pap. text 27.95 (*0-7817-1834-1*) Lppncott W & W.

Nurse's Handbook for High-Dose Chemotherapy. Sakurai. 1997. pap. text (*0-7216-6958-1*) Saunders.

Nurses Handbook for Home Care Procedures. Marie S. Jaffe. 1992. (Nursing Education Ser.). pap. 31.50 (*0-8273-4508-9*) Delmar.

Nurse's Handbook of Complementary & Alternative Therapies. Springhouse Publishing Company Staff. 1998. LC 98-21445. (Illus.). 416p. spiral bd. 34.95 (*0-87434-898-6*) Springhouse Corp.

Nurses' Handbook of Complementary Therapies. Ed. by Denise F. Rankin-Box. 1995. LC 94-41151. pap. text (*0-443-05180-1*) Church.

Nurse's Handbook of Complementary Therapies: U. S. A. Edition. Ed. by D. Rankin-Box & V. Slater. 1996. (Illus.). 190p. pap. (*0-443-07791-6*) Church.

Nurses' Handbook of Health Assessment. Janet Weber. 4th ed. 2000. LC 00-34814. (Illus.). 576p. spiral bd. 26.95 (*0-7817-2331-0*) Lppncott W & W.

Nurse's Handbook of Home Infusion Therapy. SPC Staff. Ed. by Patricia Schull. 1997. LC 97-65077. (Springhouse Home Care Ser.). (Illus.). 224p. pap. 26.95 (*0-87434-908-7*) Springhouse Corp.

Nurse's Handbook of Patient Education. Shirin F. Pestonjee. 1999. LC 99-36721. 274p. 36.95 (*1-58255-018-2*) Springhouse Corp.

Nurse's Homecare Companion. Springhouse Publishing Company Staff. 1998. LC 97-50211. 512p. spiral bd. 32.95 (*0-87434-894-3*) Springhouse Corp.

Nurses' Illustrated Physiology. Ann B. McNaught & Robin Callander. 4th rev. ed. 1989. (Illus.). 158p. pap. text (*0-443-02703-X*) Church.

Nurses in Family Planning: Counseling, Patient Advocacy & Clinical Care. Mickey Gillmor-Kahn et al. 1982. LC 82-84278. (Illus.). 300p. pap. text 19.95 (*0-8290-0927-2*) Irvington.

Nurses in Managed Care. Stutz. 1999. (C). pap. text (*0-7216-8147-6*) Saunders.

Nurses in Texas: Nurse Aides to Advanced Nurse Practitioners, 1971-1991. Olive Roen. 1992. (Working Papers Ser.: No. 62). 84p. pap. 5.50 (*0-89940-544-4*) LBJ Sch Pub Aff.

Nurses in the Courtroom: Cases & Commentary for Concerned Professionals. Barbara E. Calfee. 1992. 250p. (Orig.). pap. text 25.00 (*0-9633540-2-7*) ARC Pub.

Nurses in the Workplace. Marie E. Cowart & William J. Serow. 1992. (Illus.). 304p. 49.95 (*0-8039-4313-X*, 3147) Sage.

***Nurses Know! What Happened to Health Care? What Can We Do about It?** Edward M. Pallette. 2001. x, 320p. pap. 15.95 (*0-9710104-3-9*) Empathy Pubng.

Nurse's Legal Handbook. Springhouse Publishing Company Staff. 4th ed. 2000. LC 99-51494. 432p. pap. 36.95 (*0-87434-991-5*) Springhouse Corp.

Nurse's Liability for Malpractice: A Programmed Course. Eli P. Bernzweig. 6th ed. 1995. LC 95-30160. (Illus.). 496p. (C). (gr. 13). pap. text 37.00 (*0-8151-0702-1*, 26104) Mosby Inc.

Nurses Manage: Issues of Nurses & Management in the General Hospital. Carol Hawley et al. 1995. 368p. (*1-85972-107-9*) Avebry GBR. *Dist:* Ashgate Pub Co.

Nurse's Managed Care Manual. Ed. by David B. Nash & Patricia Carroll. 1997. (Illus.). 260p. (Orig.). spiral bd. 54.95 (*1-890045-01-2*) T L C Med Pub.

Nurse's Manual of Laboratory & Diagnostic Tests. Bonita M. Cavanaugh. 3rd rev. ed. 1999. LC 98-50920. (Illus.). 1033p. pap. 35.95 (*0-8036-0363-0*) Davis Co.

Nurse's Manual of Laboratory Test & Diagnostic Procedures. Louise M. Malarkey & Mary E. McMorrow. Ed. by Thomas Eoyang. 2nd ed. 1999. LC 99-11885. (Illus.). 895p. pap. text (*0-7216-7812-2*) Saunders.

Nurse's Manual of Laboratory Tests & Diagnostic Procedures. Louise M. Malarkey & Mary E. McMorrow. Ed. by Ton Eoyang. 1996. LC 95-17715. (Illus.). 1005p. pap. text 31.50 (*0-7216-3774-4*) Saunders.

Nurse's Med Deck. Judith Hopfer Deglin. 7th ed. 2000. (Illus.). 34.95 (*0-8036-0587-0*) Davis Co.

Nurse's Med Deck: Ring Version. Judith Hopfer Deglin. 7th ed. 2000. (Illus.). pap. 29.95 (*0-8036-0588-9*) Davis Co.

Nurses' Medication Errors: An Interpretative Study of Experiences. Marianne Arndt. 1994. LC 95-167614. (Illus.). XVIII, 408p. pap. 59.95 (*3-631-47209-9*) P Lang Pubng.

Nurses, Nurse Practitioners: Evolution to Advanced Practice. Ed. by Mathy D. Mezey & Diane O. McGivern. 1993. LC 93-13719. 400p. 32.95 (*0-8261-7770-0*) Springer Pub.

Nurses, Nurse Practitioners: Evolution to Advanced Practice. Mathy D. Mezey & Diane O'Neill-McGivern. 2nd ed. 1998. LC 98-26293. (Series on Advanced Practice Nursing). 39.95 (*0-8261-7771-9*) Springer Pub.

Nurses of a Different Stripe: A History of the Columbia University School of Nursing, 1892-1992. Gary Goldenberg. 1992. LC 91-77490. (Illus.). 288p. 20.00 (*0-9631670-0-6*) Col U Sch Nursing.

Nurses of All Nations: A History of the International Council of Nurses, 1899-1999. Barbara L. Brush. 1999. LC 98-37564. 240p. pap. text 37.95 (*0-7817-1904-6*) Lppncott W & W.

Nurse's Photolibrary, Vol. 1. Springhouse Publishing Company Staff. 1993. LC 92-48480. 23.95 (*0-87434-511-1*) Springhouse Corp.

Nurse's Pocket Companion. Springhouse Publishing Company Staff. Ed. by Patricia Schull. 2nd ed. 1996. LC 96-6927. (Illus.). 672p. spiral bd. 39.95 (*0-87434-859-5*) Springhouse Corp.

Nurse's Pocket Guide: Nursing Diagnosis, Interventions, & Rationales. Marilynn E. Doenges & Mary F. Moorhouse. 7th ed. 2000. LC 99-58309. xii, 697p. (C). spiral bd. 24.95 (*0-8036-0525-0*) Davis Co.

Nurse's Quest for a Professional Identity. Helen A. Cohen. 1981. pap. (*0-201-01157-3*) Addison-Wesley.

Nurse's Questions/Women's Questions: The Impact of the Demographic Revolution & Feminism on United States Working Women, 1946-1986. Susan Leighow. 1996. LC 94-44165. (American University Studies: Vol. 5). VIII, 209p. (C). text 39.95 (*0-8204-2755-1*) P Lang Pubng.

Nurse's Quick Reference to Common Laboratory & Diagnostic Tests. Frances T. Fischbach. 2nd ed. 1997. LC 97-8629. 560p. spiral bd. 21.95 (*0-7817-1031-6*) Lppncott W & W.

Nurse's Shift Work Handbook. Ruth R. Alward & Timothy H. Monk. 1993. (Illus.). 147p. (Orig.). (C). pap. text 21.95 (*1-55810-087-3*, NP-82) Am Nurses Pub.

Nurses Story. Carol Gino. rev. ed. 1997. LC 96-95308. 336p. pap. 14.95 (*1-889853-03-8*) Aah-ha Bks.

***Nurse's Survival Guide to the Ward.** Ann Richards. 2001. (Illus.). 335p. pap. (*0-443-05395-2*) Church GBR. *Dist:* Saunders.

Nurse's Survival Handbook. Barbara Acello. Ed. by Molly Sullivan. 3rd ed. 1999. 350p. (Orig.). (C). per. 38.95 (*1-56930-040-2*) Delmar.

Nurses Taking the Lead: Personal Qualities of Effective Leadership. Fay L. Bower. 2000. LC 99-31083. (Illus.). 315p. (C). pap. text (*0-7216-8169-7*) Saunders.

Nurses Work: An Analysis of the U. K. Nursing Labour Market. Ed. by James Buchan et al. 1998. LC 98-771462. (Developments in Nursing & Health Care Ser.). 160p. text (*1-84014-386-X*) Ashgate Pub GBR. *Dist:* Ashgate Pub Co.

Nurses' Work, the Sacred & the Profane. Zane R. Wolf. 1988. LC 87-35770. (Studies in Health, Illness & Caregiving). (Illus.). 324p. (C). pap. text 21.50 (*0-8122-1266-5*) U of Pa Pr.

Nurses's Clinical Guide: Medication Administration. Springhouse Publishing Company Staff. 2000. LC 99-57636. (Illus.). vi, 506p. pap. 32.95 (*1-58255-024-7*) Springhouse Corp.

Nurses's Illustrated Handbook of Home Health Procedures. Springhouse Publishing Company Staff. 1998. LC 98-11706. (Springhouse Home Care Ser.). (ENG & SPA., Illus.). xii, 528p. spiral bd. 36.95 (*0-87434-960-5*) Springhouse Corp.

Nursing. (Quick Study Academic Ser.). 4p. pap. 3.95 (*1-57222-174-7*) Barcharts.

***Nursing.** pap. 38.50 (*0-412-60500-7*) Chapman & Hall.

Nursing. 2nd ed. 360p. pap. (*0-340-63188-0*) E A GBR. *Dist:* Routldge.

Nursing: A Knowledge Base for Practice. (*0-340-51492-2*) E A GBR. *Dist:* Routldge.

Nursing: A Knowledge Base for Practice. Abigayl Perry. 2nd ed. 1997. (Illus.). 400p. pap. 34.95 (*1-56593-819-4*, 1610) Singular Publishing.

Nursing: Art & Science. Ed. by Alison L. Kitson. 1992. LC 92-32252. 156p. pap. 47.75 (*1-56593-063-0*, 0369) Singular Publishing.

Nursing: Concepts of Practice. Dorothea E. Orem. 5th ed. 1995. LC 94-47916. (Illus.). 448p. (C). (gr. 13). pap. text 39.00 (*0-8151-6552-8*, 24728) Mosby Inc.

Nursing: Concepts of Practice. Dorothea E. Orem et al. 6th ed. 2001. LC 00-49614. (Illus.). xviii, 542p. 45.00 (*0-323-00864-X*) Mosby Inc.

Nursing: From Education to Practice, Rx for Success. Helen Hodges et al. 1988. 368p. (C). pap. 36.21 (*0-8385-7019-4*, A7019-1) P-H.

Nursing: Human Science & Human Care. Jean Watson. 1988. 128p. pap. 32.95 (*0-88737-417-4*, 15-2236) Natl League Nurse.

Nursing: Human Science & Human Care. Jean Watson & NLN Staff. 1999. (Illus.). 128p. (C). pap. text 34.95 (*0-7637-1111-X*, 1111-X, N L N Bart) Jones & Bartlett.

Nursing: Its Hidden Agendas. 192p. pap. (*0-340-55726-5*) E A GBR. *Dist:* Routldge.

Nursing: Reflecting on an Evolving Practice. Judy Lumby. 1991. (C). pap. (*0-7300-1263-8*, NPR300) Deakin Univ AUS. *Dist:* St Mut.

Nursing: The Career of a Lifetime. Shirley H. Fondiller & Barbara J. Nerone. 2001. 200p. pap. 27.95 (*0-88737-655-X*) Natl League Nurse.

Nursing: The Fine Art: An Illustrated History. M. Patricia Donahue. 2nd ed. 1995. LC 95-26093. (Illus.). 560p. (C). (gr. 13). text 56.95 (*0-8151-2727-8*, 26817) Mosby Inc.

Nursing: The Philosophy & Science of Caring. Jean Watson. 1985. LC 78-71220. pap. 27.50 (*0-87081-154-1*) Univ Pr Colo.

***Nursing: The Reflective Approach to Adult Nursing Practice.** 2nd ed. 1996. (Illus.). pap. (*0-7487-5834-8*) Nelson Thornes GBR. *Dist:* Intl Spec Bk.

Nursing: The Reflective Approach to Adult Nursing Practice. A. Faulkner. 2nd ed. 1996. (Illus.). 576p. (C). pap. text 47.99 (*1-56593-432-6*, 1101) Singular Publishing.

Nursing a Problem. Lesley MacKay. 1989. (*0-335-09902-5*); pap. (*0-335-09901-7*) OpUniv Pr.

Nursing Administration. Jack Rudman. 1994. (Certified Nurse Examination Ser.: CN-16). pap. 27.95 (*0-8373-6116-8*) Nat Learn.

Nursing Administration: From Concepts to Practice. Laura C. Young & Arlene N. Hayne. 1988. (Illus.). 400p. text 52.00 (*0-7216-1810-3*) Saunders.

Nursing Administration: Managing Patient Care. Ed. by Jaqueline A. Dienemann. 2nd ed. 1997. LC 97-14107. 544p. (C). 68.00 (*0-8385-6986-2*, A-6986-2) P-H.

Nursing Administration (Advanced) Jack Rudman. 1994. (Certified Nurse Examination Ser.: CN-17). pap. 27.95 (*0-8373-6117-6*) Nat Learn.

Nursing Administration Handbook. Howard S. Rowland & Beatrice L. Rowland. 4th ed. 1997. LC 96-39566. 768p. 108.00 (*0-8342-0926-8*, 20926) Aspen Pub.

Nursing Administration in the 21st Century. Sarah E. Allison & Katherine E. Renpenning. 1999. LC 98-25382. xxi, 298p. 66.95 (*0-7619-1455-2*, 82489) Sage.

Nursing Administration in the 21st Century: A Self-Care Theory Approach. Sarah E. Allison & Katherine McLaughlin-Renpenning. 1998. LC 98-25382. xxi, 298p. pap. 32.95 (*0-7619-1456-0*, 82490) Sage.

Nursing Administration Manual for Long-Term Care Facilities. Charlotte Eliopoulos. 3rd ed. 2001. 435p. 95.00 (*1-882515-00-5*) Hlth Educ Netwk.

Nursing Adolescents: Psychology, Research & Practice. Jayne Taylor & Dave Muller. 1994. LC 94-38761. (Illus.). 224p. pap. 38.95 (*0-632-03625-7*) Blackwell Sci.

Nursing & Allied Health School Entrance Examinations. Marion F. Gooding. 13th ed. 1995. LC 95-36421. 496p. 15.95 (*0-02-860578-0*, Arc) Hungry Minds.

Nursing & Care Home Care Plans. Linda Faber-Czingula. 1996. 150p. ring bd. (*1-890118-07-9*, QualityCare Pub) Convalescnt Cnslts.

Nursing & Computers: An Anthology. Ed. by K. A. Rieder et al. 1989. (Computers & Medicine Ser.). (Illus.). 441p. 74.95 (*0-387-96937-3*) Spr-Verlag.

Nursing & Computers: An Anthology, 1987-1996. Ed. by Virginia K. Saba et al. 1997. LC 97-12462. (Computers & Medicine Ser.). (Illus.). 675p. 92.00 (*0-387-94955-0*) Spr-Verlag.

Nursing & Health Care for the Homeless. Ed. by Juanita K. Hunter. 1993. LC 92-2172. 235p. (C). text 64.50 (*0-7914-1349-7*); pap. text 21.95 (*0-7914-1350-0*) State U NY Pr.

Nursing & Malpractice Risks: Understanding the Law. Becky Colgan & Barbara J. Youngberg. 3rd ed. 1996. 160p. (C). pap. text 49.95 (*1-878025-91-0*) Western Schls.

Nursing & Nursing Education: Public Policies & Private Actions. Institute of Medicine Staff. 1983. 336p. pap. text 24.95 (*0-309-03346-2*) Natl Acad Pr.

Nursing & Politics Power Thru Practice. Abigail Masterson. 1999. LC 98-31647. (*0-443-05991-8*) Church.

Nursing & Thanatolgy. 1982. 18.95 (*0-405-13095-3*) Ayer.

Nursing & the American Health Care Delivery System. Joellen B. Hawkins & Loretta P. Higgins. 4th ed. 1993. (Illus.). 224p. (Orig.). pap. text 16.00 (*0-913292-46-X*) Tiresias Pr.

Nursing & the Continuum of Care. M. Patricia Donahue & American Organization of Nurse Executives Staff. 1998. LC 98-9874. (AONE Leadership Ser.). 138p. pap. 40.00 (*1-55648-235-3*) AHPI.

Nursing & the Continuum of Care. M. Patricia Donahue & American Organization of Nurse Executives Staff. 1998. LC 98-9874. (AONE Leadership Ser.). (*1-55664-823-5*) Mosby Inc.

Nursing & the Disabled: Across the Lifespan. Ardella M. Fraley. 1992. (Nursing-Health Science Ser.). (Illus.). (C). text 54.95 (*0-86720-314-5*, 314-5) Jones & Bartlett.

Nursing & the Experience of Illness: Phenomenology in Practice. Irena Madjar. 1999. LC 98-33321. xvi, 198p. 90.00 (*0-415-20782-7*); pap. 27.95 (*0-415-20783-5*) Routledge.

Nursing & the Injustices of the Law. Megan-Jane Johnstone. 1994. (Illus.). 349p. pap. text (*0-7295-1418-8*) Bailliere Tindall.

Nursing & the Law. T. Verschoor et al. 1997. LC 97-162542. 120p. (*0-7021-3542-9*) Juta & Co ZAF. *Dist:* Intl Spec Bk, Gaunt.

Nursing & the Law. Darlene M. Trandel-Korenchuk & Keith M. Trandel-Korenchuk. 5th ed. 1997. LC 97-36619. 400p. 57.00 (*0-8342-0570-X*, 20570) Aspen Pub.

Nursing & the Older Patient. Lynne Swiatczak & Steve Wright. 3rd ed. 1998. (Illus.). 224p. pap. (*0-7487-3353-1*) Nelson Thornes GBR. *Dist:* Intl Spec Bk, Trans-Atl Phila.

Nursing Approach to the Evaluation of Child Maltreatment. Angelo P. Giardino & Eileen R. Giardino. 2001. (Illus.). 250p. 42.95 (*1-878060-51-1*) GW Medical.

Nursing as a Spiritual Practice: Contemporary Applicaton of Florence Nightingale's Views. Janet Macrae. 2001. LC 00-64096. xi, 130p. (*0-8261-1387-7*) Springer Pub.

Nursing As a Therapeutic Activity: An Ethnography. Steven J. Ersser. 1997. LC 97-70634. (Developments in Nursing & Health Care Ser.). 392p. (C). text (*1-85972-658-5*) Ashgate Pub GBR. *Dist:* Ashgate Pub Co.

Nursing As Caring: A Model for Transforming Practice. Anne Boykin & Savina Schoenhofer. 1993. LC 93-23021. 26.95 (*0-88737-601-0*) Natl League Nurse.

Nursing as Caring: A Model for Transforming Practice. Anne Boykin & Savina O'Bryan-Schoenhofer. 2nd ed. 2000. LC 00-48369. (Illus.). 96p. pap. text 24.95 (*0-7637-1643-X*, 1643-X) Jones & Bartlett.

Nursing As Therapy. McMahon. 1991. 234p. pap. 43.25 (*1-56593-012-6*, 0253) Singular Publishing.

Nursing As Therapy. Richard McMahon & Alan Pearson. 2nd ed. 1998. (Illus.). 336p. pap. (*0-7487-3326-4*) Nelson Thornes GBR. *Dist:* Aspen Pub.

Nursing Assessment - Bloodborne Valuepack. National Safety Council Staff et al. 1993. (Nursing-Health Science Ser.). (C). text 57.50 (*0-86720-690-X*) Jones & Bartlett.

Nursing Assessment & Diagnosis. Janis P. Bellack & Barbara J. Edlind. 2nd ed. 1992. (Nursing-Health Science Ser.). (Illus.). 864p. (C). text 65.95 (*0-86720-436-2*, 436-2) Jones & Bartlett.

Nursing Assistant. Joan F. Needham. 1999. (Home Care Aide Ser.). tchr. ed. 18.00 (*0-8273-6488-1*); wbk. ed. 12.95 (*0-8273-6487-3*); pap. 27.95 (*0-8273-6486-5*) Delmar.

Nursing Assistant. Perspective Press Staff. 1995. (Illus.). 304p. (gr. 13). (*0-8151-4747-3*, 24904) Mosby Inc.

Nursing Assistant. Jack Rudman. 1994. (Career Examination Ser.: C-534). pap. 23.95 (*0-8373-0534-9*) Nat Learn.

Nursing Assistant. Pulliam. 2nd ed. 1997. pap., tchr. ed. 23.20 (*0-8359-5161-8*); 144p. pap., wbk. ed. 17.27 (*0-8359-5162-6*) P-H.

Nursing Assistant. Barbara R. Hegner & Esther Caldwell. 6th ed. 1992. pap., stu. ed. 19.95 (*0-8273-4802-9*); 1992. pap. 31.00 (*0-8273-4800-2*); 1991. tchr. ed. 25.50 (*0-8273-4799-5*) Delmar.

Nursing Assistant. Barbara R. Hegner. 8th ed. 1998. (Home Care Aide Ser.). (C). pap., wbk. ed. 18.50 (*0-8273-9062-9*) Delmar.

Nursing Assistant: A Nursing Process Approach. Barbara R. Hegner. 7th ed. 1995. (Home Care Aide Ser.). 786p. (C). text 35.50 (*0-8273-6286-2*) Delmar.

Nursing Assistant: A Nursing Process Approach. Barbara R. Hegner & Ester Caldwell. 7th rev. ed. 1996. (Home Care Aide Ser.). 768p. mass mkt. 34.50 (*0-8273-8414-9*) Delmar.

Nursing Assistant: A Nursing Process Approach. Barbara R. Hegner & Esther Caldwell. 7th rev. ed. 1997. 168p. tchr. ed. (*0-8273-8499-8*); 1996. LC 94-13479. 768p. mass mkt. 32.00 (*0-8273-8394-0*) Delmar.

Nursing Assistant: A Nursing Process Approach (HC) Barbara R. Hegner. 8th ed. 1998. LC 98-9510. (Home Care Aide Ser.). 700p. (C). 54.95 (*0-8273-9063-7*) Delmar.

Nursing Assistant: A Nursing Process Approach (SC) Barbara R. Hegner et al. 8th abr. rev. ed. 1998. (Home Care Aide Ser.). 700p. (C). pap. text 48.95 (*0-8273-9058-0*) Delmar.

Nursing Assistant: Acute & Long-Term Care. Jolynn Pulliam. 2nd ed. 1997. LC 97-12604. 336p. pap. text 33.40 (*0-8359-5141-3*) P-H.

***Nursing Assistant: Acute, Subacute & Long-Term Care.** Jolynn Pulliam. 3rd ed. 2001. 412p. pap. 32.00 (*0-13-093950-1*) P-H.

Nursing Assistant: CTB IBM 3.5/5.25. Barbara R. Hegner. 1995. (Home Care Aide Ser.). 68.25 (*0-8273-6289-7*) Delmar.

Nursing Assistant: Laser Disc User Manual. Barbara R. Hegner. 7th ed. 1994. (Home Care Aide Ser.). pap. 12.95 (*0-8273-7045-8*, VNR) Wiley.

Nursing Assistant: Nursing Procedures & Application. Barbara R. Hegner. 7th ed. 1995. (Home Care Aide Ser.). 164p. (C). tchr. ed. 25.50 (*0-8273-6288-9*) Delmar.

Nursing Assistant: Nursing Procedures Approach. Doyle. 5th ed. 1989. (Home Care Aide Ser.). pap. 25.95 (*0-8273-3370-6*); wbk. ed. 18.95 (*0-8273-3369-2*) Delmar.

Nursing Assistant: Spanish Edition Instructor's Guide. Barbara R. Hegner & Esther Caldwell. 6th ed. 1993. 106p. pap., tchr. ed. 21.00 (*0-8273-5800-8*) Delmar.

Nursing Assistant: Spanish Edition Workbook. Barbara R. Hegner. 6th ed. 1993. 297p. pap. 18.00 (*0-8273-5801-6*) Delmar.

Nursing Assistant Level 5 Workbook. Kelly. 5th ed. 1999. 453p. pap. text, wbk. ed. 17.95 (*0-323-01046-6*) Mosby Inc.

Nursing Assistant Complete Test Bank (IBM) Barbara R. Hegner. 6th ed. 1992. (Home Care Aide Ser.). 64.95 (*0-8273-4842-8*) Delmar.

Nursing Assistant Fundamentals: A Patient-Centered Approach. June Eastmond et al. (gr. 6-12). 704p. stu. ed. 15.00 (*0-02-802425-7*); 1998. text, stu. ed. 39.75 (*0-02-802441-9*) Glencoe.

Nursing Assistant Fundamentals: A Patient-Centered Approach Instructor's Annotated. June Eastmond et al. annot. ed. 704p. tchr. ed. 38.15 (*0-02-802426-5*) Glencoe.

Nursing Assistant Instructors Resource Kit. Barbara R. Hegner. 6th ed. 1992. pap. 74.95 (*0-8273-4875-4*) Delmar.

Nursing Assistant IRK. Barbara R. Hegner. 7th ed. 1995. 528p. tchr. ed. 78.95 (*0-8273-7046-6*) Delmar.

Nursing Assistant Procedures Viewer's Manual. Barbara Kast. 1993. 241p. 16.75 (*0-8273-5557-2*) Delmar.

Nursing Assistant Review for Competency Evaluation. SheilaA. Sorrentino. 2nd ed. 1996. (Illus.). 176p. (C). (gr. 13). pap. text 15.00 (*0-8151-8625-8*, 28734) Mosby Inc.

Nursing Assistant Review for Competency Evaluation: Textbook for Nursing Assistants & Reviews. Sheila A. Sorrentino. 4th ed. 1996. (Illus.). 160p. (0-8151-8626-6) Mosby Inc.

***Nursing Assistant Review Self-Assessment Disk.** Sheila A. Sorrentino. 1996. pap. 17.95 incl. disk (0-8151-8627-4) Mosby Inc.

Nursing Assistant Workbook. Barbara R. Hegner. 7th ed. 1995. 560p. stu. ed. 19.45 (0-8273-6287-0) Delmar.

Nursing Assistants: A Basic Study Guide. Beverly Robertson. 5th rev. ed. 1998. (Illus.). 184p. pap. text 13.95 (1-880246-09-0) First Class Bks.

Nursing Assistant's Casebook of Elder Care. George H. Weber & George J. McCall. 1987. LC 87-12434. 238p. pap. 21.95 (0-86569-166-5, Auburn Hse) Greenwood.

Nursing Assisting: A Nursing Process Approach. Barbara R. Hegner. 7th rev. ed. 1996. 560p. wbk. ed. 20.00 (0-8273-8426-2) Delmar.

Nursing Assisting: Essentials for Long-Term Care - IML. Barbara Acello. 1998. 224p. tchr. ed. 13.95 (0-8273-8451-3) Delmar.

Nursing Assisting: Essentials of Long-Term Care. Barbara Acello. 1998. LC 98-17776. 384p. (C). pap. text 33.95 (0-8273-8450-5) Delmar.

Nursing Assisting: In Service Training Manual. Joan Fox-Rose. 1999. LC 99-24986. 416p. 177.95 (0-7668-0516-6) Delmar.

Nursing Assisting in Long-Term Care. Barbara R. Hegner. 1988. (Home Care Aide Ser.). pap. 29.95 (0-8273-2959-8); pap., tchr. ed. 17.00 (0-8273-2960-1) Delmar.

Nursing Attendants: Your Role Working in Psychiatry. Gloria Elliott. 1994. (Illus.). 60p. (Orig.). pap. text 8.00 (0-9640929-5-6) Good Sign NY.

Nursing Beyond the Year 2000: Report of a WHO Study Group. 1994. LC 95-103037. (Technical Reports: No. 842). (ENG, FRE & SPA.). iv, 21p. pap. text 6.00 (92-4-120842-2, 1100842) World Health.

Nursing Boards Review: American Journal of Nursing. American Journal of Nursing Staff et al. 10th ed. 1996. LC 92-28146. (Illus.). 624p. (C). (gr. 13). pap. text 30.95 (0-8151-0080-9, 27082) Mosby Inc.

Nursing Book. College. 1984. 6.95 (0-316-15182-3, Little Brwn Med Div) Lppncott W & W.

Nursing Calculations. John D. Gatford. (Orig.). 2nd ed. 1987. LC 86-17145. 106p. pap. text (0-443-03533-4); 3rd ed. 1990. 128p. pap. text (0-443-04347-7) Church.

Nursing Calculations. Gatford. 4th ed. 1994. pap. text 7.95 (0-443-04920-3) Saunders.

Nursing Care. Ed. by Moya Jolley & Brykczynska Gosia. 1992. 224p. pap. 56.00 net. (0-340-53920-8) Thomson Learn.

Nursing Care: Summary of a European Study. 1987. pap. text 13.00 (92-890-1040-1) World Health.

Nursing Care During the Labor Process. Janet S. Malinowski et al. 3rd ed. 1989. LC 88-30981. (Illus.). 433p. (C). pap. text 26.95 (0-8036-5803-6) Davis Co.

Nursing Care for Alcohol & Substance Abuse. Sisneg. 1997. (C). pap. text 19.95 (0-8273-5529-7) Delmar.

Nursing Care for Children. Sandra R. Mott. Ed. by Debra Hunter. 2nd ed. 1990. 1907p. (C). pap. text 9.95 (0-201-52924-6) Addison-Wesley.

Nursing Care for Myocardial Infarction: Physiological Basis of Cardiovascular Nursing. Marilyn B. Rubin. 1977. LC 76-6218. (Illus.). 200p. 14.50 (0-87527-151-0) Green.

Nursing Care in an Aging Society. Ed. by Donna M. Corr & Charles A. Corr. 1990. LC 90-9601. 368p. 38.95 (0-8261-6630-X) Springer Pub.

Nursing Care in Radiation Oncology. Karen Hassey Dow et al. Ed. by Barnara N. Cullen. 2nd ed. 1997. (Illus.). 400p. text 72.50 (0-7216-2347-6) Saunders.

Nursing Care of Adolescents. Jeanne Howe. 1979. (Illus.). text 31.95 (0-07-030585-4) McGraw.

Nursing Care of Adults. Ed. by Frances D. Monahan et al. 1994. (Illus.). tchr. ed. (0-7216-4926-2) Saunders.

Nursing Care of Adults. Ed. by James P. Smith. 1995. (Advanced Nursing Ser.). pap. 38.95 (0-632-03994-9) Blackwell Sci.

Nursing Care of Adults, Test Manual. Ed. by Frances D. Monahan et al. 1994. (Illus.). (0-7216-3504-0) Saunders.

Nursing Care of Adults with Orthopaedic Conditions. Mourad. 2nd ed. 1989. LC 87-279. 576p. text 41.95 (0-8273-4315-9) Delmar.

Nursing Care of Children. Jean W. Ashwill. 1997. 1479p. pap., stu. ed. 16.50 (0-7216-7285-X) Saunders.

Nursing Care of Children. Ed. by James P. Smith. 1995. LC 95-20874. (Advanced Nursing Ser.). pap. 39.95 (0-632-03995-7) Blackwell Sci.

Nursing Care of Children: Principles & Practice. Jean W. Ashwill & Susan C. Droske. Ed. by Ilze Rader. 1997. LC 96-16728. (Illus.). 1264p. pap. text 61.95 (0-7216-6488-1) Saunders.

Nursing Care of Children: Principles & Practice. Jean Weiler Ashwill & Susan Colvert Droske. 1997. (Illus.). tchr. ed. (0-7216-6502-0) Saunders.

***Nursing Care of Children: Principles & Practice - Ashwill/Gorrie Package.** Jean Weiler Ashwill & Gorrie. 1997. 101.00 (0-7216-7994-3) Saunders.

***Nursing Care of Children: Principles & Practice - ExaMaster.** Jean Weiler Ashwill. 1997. (0-7216-6500-4) Saunders.

***Nursing Care of Children: Principles & Practice - Text & Study Guide.** Jean Weiler Ashwill & Susan Colvert Droske. 1997. (Illus.). 81.00 (0-7216-7565-4) Saunders.

Nursing Care of Children & Families. Sandra R. Mott. Ed. by Debra Hunter. 2nd ed. 1990. 1907p. (C). text 78.75 (0-201-12923-X); stu. ed. (0-201-12924-8) Addison-Wesley.

Nursing Care of Geriatric Emergencies. Christine W. Bradway. 1996. (Series on Geriatric Nursing). (Illus.). 304p. 44.95 (0-8261-9010-3) Springer Pub.

Nursing Care of Infants & Children. Lucille F. Whaley. 2nd ed. 1987. text 25.00 (0-8016-5461-0); 4th ed. 1991. 2096p. (0-8016-5387-8); 4th ed. 1991. 2096p. (0-8016-5381-9); 4th ed. 1991. 2096p. (0-8016-5403-3) Mosby Inc.

Nursing Care of Older Adults: Diagnoses, Outcomes & Interventions. Meridean Maas. 2000. LC 00-45203. (Illus.). xxvii, 834p. 57.00 (0-323-01259-0) Mosby Inc.

Nursing Care of Older Adults: Theory & Practice. Carol A. Miller. 3rd ed. 1998. LC 98-45982. (Illus.). 752p. pap. text 41.00 (0-7817-1623-3) Lppncott W & W.

Nursing Care of Survivors of Family Violence. Jacquelyn Campbell. 2nd ed. 1993. LC 92-48726. (Illus.). 416p. (C). (gr. 13). pap. text 35.00 (0-8016-6378-4, 06378) Mosby Inc.

Nursing Care of the Addicted Client. Karen Allen et al. 1996. LC 95-50020. 384p. pap. text 41.95 (0-397-55204-1) Lppncott W & W.

Nursing Care of the AIDS/HIV Patient. Carol R. Kneisl. 1997. (Nursing Education Ser.). text 41.95 (0-8273-6737-6) Delmar.

Nursing Care of the Burn-Injured Patient. Rita B. Trofino. 1991. LC 90-15722. (Illus.). 466p. 49.95 (0-8036-8658-7) Davis Co.

Nursing Care of the Child with Cancer. Association of Pediatric Oncology Nurses. Ed. by Genevieve V. Foley et al. 2nd ed. 1993. (Illus.). 548p. text 70.00 (0-7216-4006-0) Saunders.

Nursing Care of the Clients with Substance Abuse. Eleanor J. Sullivan. 1995. LC 94-30146. (Illus.). 528p. (C). (gr. 13). pap. text 37.95 (0-8016-7881-1, 07881) Mosby Inc.

Nursing Care of the Critically Ill Child. Mary F. Hazinski. 2nd ed. 1991. (Illus.). 1152p. (C). (gr. 13). text 64.95 (0-8016-5312-6, 05312) Mosby Inc.

Nursing Care of the Elderly. Joan Cagley-Knight. Ed. by John Lantz. 4th rev. ed. 1998. (Illus.). 277p. pap. 39.95 (1-57801-031-4) Western Schls.

Nursing Care of the General Pediatric Surgical Patient. Chris J. McKenna et al. 2000. LC 00-23254. 544p. 91.00 (0-8342-1170-X) Aspen Pub.

Nursing Care of the HIV Positive Patient. Lori A. DeLorenzo. 3rd ed. 1999. (Illus.). 238p. pap. (1-57801-043-8) Western Schls.

Nursing Care of the Immunocompromised Patient. M. Linda Workman et al. 1992. (Illus.). 320p. pap. text 33.00 (0-7216-3213-0) Saunders.

Nursing Care of the Organ-Tissue Transplant Recipient. Sigardson-Poor & Haggerty. 1990. (Illus.). 384p. text 70.00 (0-7216-2882-6) Saunders.

Nursing Care of the Person Who Smokes. Patricia G. Rienzo. 1992. 216p. 33.95 (0-8261-7620-8) Springer Pub.

Nursing Care of the Skin. Penzer. 2002. (Illus.). 196p. pap. 34.99 (0-7506-2834-0) Buttrwrth-Heinemann.

Nursing Care Plans: Nursing Diagnosis & Intervention. Meg Gulanick. 4th ed. 1997. LC 97-41319. 1248p. (C). (gr. 13). pap. text 37.95 (0-8151-2471-6, 31214) Mosby Inc.

Nursing Care Plans & Documentation: Nursing Diagnoses & Collaborative Problems. Lynda J. Carpenito. 3rd ed. 1998. LC 98-46595. 848p. pap. text 39.95 (0-7817-1742-6) Lppncott W & W.

Nursing Care Report Card for Acute Care. American Nurses Association Staff. 1995. pap. text 34.95 (1-55810-112-8, NP-101) Am Nurses Pub.

Nursing Care Studies. Riddle. 1993. pap. text 58.95 (0-443-04995-5); 1989. pap. text 11.00 (0-443-03939-9); Vol. 3. 1988. pap. text 11.00 (0-443-03936-4); Vol. 4. 1989. pap. text 11.00 (0-443-03937-2); Vol. 5. 1989. pap. text 11.00 (0-443-03938-0) Saunders.

Nursing Case Management. Olga Cotera. 1998. 131p. spiral bd. 125.00 (1-879575-94-9) Acad Med Sys.

Nursing Case Management: From Concept to Evaluation. Elaine L. Cohen & Toni G. Cesta. 2nd ed. 1996. (Illus.). 368p. (C). (gr. 13). text 41.95 (0-8151-1906-2, 28201) Mosby Inc.

Nursing Case Management: From Essentials to Advanced Practice. Elaine L. Cohen & Toni G. Cesta. 3rd ed. 2000. LC 00-711206. (Illus.). xix, 614p. 49.95 (0-323-01135-7) Mosby Inc.

Nursing Centers: The Time Is Now. Ed. by Barbara Murphy. 1995. 279p. pap. 33.95 (0-88737-623-1, 41-2629, NLN Pr) Natl League Nurse.

Nursing Children: Psychology, Research, & Practice. Dave J. Muller et al. 2nd ed. 1992. LC 92-20109. 41.50 (1-56593-023-1, 0266) Thomson Learn.

Nursing Children: Psychology, Research & Practice. Jayne Taylor et al. 3rd ed. 1999. LC 00-362784. (Illus.). x, 242p. pap. (0-7487-3327-2) Nelson Thornes GBR. *Dist:* Intl Spec Bk.

Nursing, Communication & Education in an Information Age. Carolyn Anderson. 1990. (Nursing Education Ser.). pap., tchr. ed. 12.75 (0-8273-3434-6) Delmar.

Nursing Competence. (0-340-51841-3) E A GBR. *Dist:* Routldge.

Nursing Comprehensive Examination Review. George Horemis. 2nd ed. 1976. LC 76-14832. pap. 6.00 (0-668-02499-2) P-H.

Nursing Concepts: Mobility. Sylvia Durette. 2001. 200p. pap. text 24.00 (1-55642-520-1) SLACK Inc.

Nursing Curriculum: A Curricular Model. Fred Greaves. 1987. 108p. (Orig.). pap. (0-7099-3871-3) C Helm GBR. *Dist:* Routldge.

Nursing Curriculum Outline Study Guide. Peggy J. Walton. (C). 19.95 (0-911067-00-0) Health Ed Train.

Nursing Data Review - (Annual) 1997. 272p. 32.95 (0-88737-530-8, 19-2419) Natl League Nurse.

Nursing Data Review 1997. National League for Nursing Staff. 1997. (Illus.). 256p. pap. 41.95 (0-88737-732-7, 19-7327, NLN Pr) Natl League Nurse.

Nursing Datasource 1998. NLN Research Division Staff. 1999. (Illus.). 64p. (C). Vol. 2. pap. text 41.25 (0-7637-1114-4); Vol. 3. pap. text 41.25 (0-7637-1115-2) Jones & Bartlett.

Nursing Datasource 1997, Vol. 3. NLN Staff. 1999. (Illus.). (C). pap. text 41.25 (0-7637-0940-9) Jones & Bartlett.

Nursing Datasource 1997 Vol. II: Graduate Education in Nursing/Advanced Practice Nursing. NLN Staff. 1998. (Illus.). 48p. (C). pap. text 43.95 (0-7637-0939-5, 0939-5, N L N Bart) Jones & Bartlett.

Nursing DataSource 2000. NLN Research Division Staff. 2001. (Illus.). 64p. (C). pap. text 41.25 (0-7637-1113-6, 1113-6, N L N Bart) Jones & Bartlett.

Nursing Department Report, 1992-93. 1992. pap. 195.00 (0-939326-73-6) Hosp & Hlthcare.

Nursing Diagnoses: Definitions & Classification, 1999-2000. NANDA Staff. 1998. 136p. (C). pap. text 12.00 (0-9637042-5-7) Nursecom Inc.

Nursing Diagnoses in Psychiatric Nursing: Care Plans & Psychotropic Medications. Mary C. Townsend. 5th ed. 2000. LC 00-56953. (Illus.). 714p. 38.95 (0-8036-0703-2) Davis Co.

Nursing Diagnoses, Outcomes, & Interventions: Nanda, Noc & Nic Linkages. Marion Johnson et al. 2000. 415p. pap. 37.95 (0-323-01212-4) Mosby Inc.

Nursing Diagnosis. Kathy V. Gettrust & Paula D. Brabec. 1992. (C). pap. 37.50 (0-8273-4852-5) Delmar.

Nursing Diagnosis. Schonlau. 1999. pap. text (0-7216-4992-0) Saunders.

Nursing Diagnosis: Application to Clinical Practice. Lynda Juall Carpenito. 8th ed. 2000. LC 99-36287. 1,248p. pap. text 37.95 (0-7817-1970-4) Lppncott W & W.

Nursing Diagnosis: Process & Application. Marjorie Gordon. 3rd ed. 1993. LC 93-31601. (Illus.). 416p. (C). (gr. 13). text 42.00 (0-8016-6053-X, 06053) Mosby Inc.

Nursing Diagnosis & Care Planning. Barbara J. Taptich et al. 2nd ed. 1994. LC 93-33971. 336p. pap. text 18.95 (0-7216-5196-8) Saunders.

Nursing Diagnosis & Intervention. Gertrude K. McFarland & Elizabeth A. McFarlane. 3rd ed. 1996. LC 97-223430. (Illus.). 896p. (C). (gr. 13). pap. text 38.00 (0-8151-7026-2, 27464) Mosby Inc.

Nursing Diagnosis & Interventions for the Elderly. Meridean Maas et al. Ed. by Mark McCormick. 1991. 736p. (C). pap. text 45.25 (0-201-12679-6) Addison-Wesley.

Nursing Diagnosis & Process in Psychiatric Mental Health Nursing. Gertrude K. McFarland. 3rd ed. 1996. LC 96-41727. 528p. pap. text 26.95 (0-397-55317-X) Lppncott W & W.

Nursing Diagnosis for Wellness: Supporting Strengths. Houldin. 1987. (Illus.). 238p. pap. text 17.95 (0-397-54645-9) Lppncott W & W.

Nursing Diagnosis Handbook. Betty J. Ackley. 4th ed. 1999. LC 00-266184. xiii, 717p. (C). text 28.95 (0-323-00786-4) Mosby Inc.

Nursing Diagnosis Handbook. Judith M. Wilkinson. 7th ed. 1999. 664p. (C). spiral bd. 29.95 (0-8053-8094-9) Benjamin-Cummings.

Nursing Diagnosis Handbook: A Guide to Planning Care. Gail B. Ladwig. Ed. by Betty J. Ackley. 3rd ed. 1997. LC 96-47933. (Illus.). 528p. (C). (gr. 13). pap. text 27.00 (0-8151-0912-1, 28737) Mosby Inc.

***Nursing Diagnosis Handbook: A Guide to Planning Care.** Betty J. Ackley & Gail B. Ladwig. 5th ed. 2001. (Illus.). 845p. (0-323-01459-3) Mosby Inc.

Nursing Diagnosis Manual for the Well & Ill Client. T. Audean Duespohl. 1986. 312p. pap. text 26.00 (0-7216-1825-1) Saunders.

Nursing Diagnosis Pocket Manual. Sheila Sparks et al. 1995. 512p. spiral bd. 24.95 (0-87434-827-7) Springhouse Corp.

Nursing Diagnosis Reference Manual. Sheila M. Sparks & Cynthia M. Taylor. 5th ed. 2000. LC 00-56307. (Illus.). x, 741p. 39.95 (1-58255-072-7) Springhouse Corp.

Nursing Diagnosis, "Swallowing Impaired" The Bedside Assessment of Swallowing in Neurologically-Involved Cases. Jimmie R. Rankin. Date not set. 150p. pap. 19.95 (1-883938-06-6) Dry Bones Pr.

Nursing Documentation. Patricia W. Iyer & Nancy Camp. 3rd ed. 1999. LC 98-47696. (Illus.). 426p. pap. text 36.95 (0-323-00223-4) Mosby Inc.

Nursing Documentation: Charting, Recording, & Reporting. Ellen T. Eggland & Denise S. Heinemann. 1994. LC 93-6172. (Illus.). 272p. (C). pap. text 27.95 (0-397-55010-3, Lippnctt) Lppncott W & W.

Nursing Documentation: Legal Focus Across Practice Settings. Sue Meiner. 1999. LC 99-10239. 17p. 69.95 (0-7619-1071-9); xiii, 294p. pap. 34.95 (0-7619-1072-7, 81914) Sage.

Nursing Documentation Handbook. T. M. Marrelli. 3rd ed. 2000. LC 00-25398. 350p. spiral bd. 28.95 (0-323-01097-0) Mosby Inc.

Nursing Drug Handbook: 12 Copy Display, 11 Plus 1 Free. Springhouse Publishing Company Staff. 1995. 307.45 (0-87434-842-0) Springhouse Corp.

Nursing Drug Handbook 2001. Billie A. Wilson & Margaret Shannon. 2000. 1616p. 32.95 (0-13-028292-8) P-H.

Nursing Education. Cox. 1985. (International Journal of Nursing Studies). pap. 30.00 (0-08-031849-5, Pergamon Pr) Elsevier.

Nursing Education: An International Perspective. Ed. by T. G. Mashaba & H. I. Brink. 1994. 332p. (Orig.). (C). pap. text (0-7021-2620-9) Juta & Co ZAF. *Dist:* Intl Spec Bk.

Nursing Education in Thanatology: A Curriculum Continuum. Ed. by Florence E. Selder. 1991. LC 90-4470. (Loss, Grief & Care Ser.: Vol. 4, Nos. 1 & 2). 134p. text 39.95 (0-86656-996-0) Haworth Pr.

Nursing Education in the Middle East: Community Health Needs & Curriculum Development. Ed. by Myrna E. Mathia & Lorena S. Yamine. 1983. 244p. text 24.95 (0-8156-6066-9) Am U Beirut.

Nursing Elderly People. Ed. by Sally J. Redfern. 2nd ed. 1991. (Illus.). 600p. (Orig.). pap. text (0-443-04138-5) Church.

Nursing Ethics. Ian E. Thompson et al. 3rd ed. 1994. LC 94-5561. pap. text (0-443-04811-8) Church.

Nursing Ethics: Therapeutic Caring Presence. Bishop. 2000. (Philosophy Ser.). 152p. (C). pap. text 38.95 (0-534-54245-X) Wadsworth Pub.

Nursing Ethics: Therapeutic Caring Presence. John R. Scudder, Jr. & Anne Bishop. 1995. pap. 25.00 (0-86720-969-0) Jones & Bartlett.

Nursing Ethics & Law. Jacqulyn K. Hall. Ed. by Tom Eoyang. 1996. (Illus.). 516p. pap. text 29.50 (0-7216-4991-2) Saunders.

Nursing Ethics Through the Life Span. Elsie L. Bandman. 3rd ed. 1995. LC 95-1283. 312p. (C). pap. 45.00 (0-8385-6638-3, A6638-9) P-H.

Nursing Exam Review in Basic Sciences. George Horemis & Clemencia Matomors. 1973. LC 72-96307. 200p. (Orig.). pap. 4.00 (0-668-02946-3, Arc) Hungry Minds.

***Nursing Experience: Trends, Challenges & Transitions.** Lucille A. Joel & Lucie Young Kelly. 4th ed. 2001. LC 00-54886. (Illus.). 792p. pap. 34.95 (0-07-136315-7) McGraw-Hill Prof.

Nursing for a Multi-Ethnic Society. Gerrish et al. 1996. LC 96-24395. (Race, Health & Social Care Ser.). 192p. pap. (0-335-19615-2) OpUniv Pr.

Nursing for Continence. Katherine F. Jeter et al. 1990. 320p. text 42.00 (0-7216-2892-3) Saunders.

Nursing for Continence. Ed. by Christine Norton. 2nd ed. 1996. 400p. (0-906584-42-6) Beaconsfield GBR. *Dist:* Medicina Bio.

Nursing for Public Health. Ed. by Grace M. Lindsay & Pauline M. Craig. 2000. 300p. pap. text Price not set. (0-443-05942-X) Saunders.

Nursing for Women's Health see Caring for Women through the Life Cycle

Nursing Foundations: Canadian Perspectives. Beverly W. Dugas. 1993. text 73.33 (0-8385-7064-X) Appleton & Lange.

Nursing, from Whence to Where? Professorial Lecture. Alan Pearson. 1991. (C). pap. (0-7300-1448-7) Deakin Univ AUS. *Dist:* St Mut.

Nursing Frontiers: Accountability & the Boundaries of Care. Mike Walsh. 2000. LC 99-58096. (Illus.). 192p. pap. text 33.00 (0-7506-4316-1) Buttrwrth-Heinemann.

Nursing Fundamentals. Sharon Golub. 2nd ed. 1993. LC 93-25831. (Notes Ser.). 192p. pap. 18.95 (0-87434-615-0) Springhouse Corp.

***Nursing Fundamentals: Review & Rationales.** Mary A. Hogan & Donna Bowles. 2001. 468p. pap. 24.95 (0-13-030455-7) P-H.

Nursing Guide to Drugs. Margaret Havard. 3rd ed. 1990. (Illus.). 344p. pap. text (0-443-04142-3) Church.

Nursing Guide to Drugs. Havard. 4th ed. 1994. pap. text 19.95 (0-443-04762-6) Saunders.

Nursing, Health, & the Environment. Institute of Medicine Staff. Ed. by Andrew M. Pope et al. 1995. LC 95-39601. 304p. text 37.95 (0-309-05298-X) Natl Acad Pr.

Nursing Health Assessment: Concepts & Activities. Ed. by Margaret A. Fitzgerald et al. 1995. (Illus.). 359p. (C). pap. text 21.95 (0-8036-0118-2) Davis Co.

Nursing Health Care. Jack Rudman. (Regents External Degree Ser.: Vol. 19). 43.95 (0-8373-5669-5); (ACT Proficiency Examination Program Ser.: Vol. 46). 43.95 (0-8373-5596-6); 1994. (Regents External Degree Ser.: REDP-19). pap. 23.95 (0-8373-5619-9); 1994. (ACT Proficiency Examination Program Ser.: Vol. PEP-46). pap. 23.95 (0-8373-5546-X) Nat Learn.

Nursing Herbal Medicine Handbook. Lippincott, Williams and Wilkins Staff. 2001. LC 00-66120. (Illus.). 640p. 39.95 (1-58255-100-6) Springhouse Corp.

Nursing History: The State of the Art. Ed. by Christopher J. Maggs. LC 86-32802. 208p. pap. (0-7099-4637-6) C Helm GBR. *Dist:* Routldge.

Nursing History & the Politics of Welfare. Anne M. Rafferty et al. 1997. LC 96-19933. 296p. (C). 85.00 (*0-415-13835-3*); pap. 27.95 (*0-415-13836-1*) Routledge.

Nursing History Review, Vol. 1. 1992. 279p. pap. 35.00 (*0-8122-1450-1*) U of Pa Pr.

Nursing History Review: Official Journal of the American Association for the History of Nursing. Ed. by Joan E. Lynaugh. (Illus.). Vol. 2. 1993. 208p. pap. text 35.00 (*0-8122-1451-X*); Vol. 3. 1994. 312p. pap. text 35.00 (*0-8122-1452-8*); Vol. 4. 1995. 224p. pap. text 36.00 (*0-8122-1453-6*); Vol. 5. 1996. 256p. pap. text 36.00 (*0-8122-1454-4*) U of Pa Pr.

Nursing Home. Ira Eaton. l.t. ed. 1999. LC 98-96944. 332p. pap. 18.95 (*1-888725-23-0*, MacroPrintBks) Sci & Human Pr.

Nursing Home Activities Specialist. Jack Rudman. (Career Examination Ser.: C-3642). pap. 27.95 (*0-8373-3642-2*) Nat Learn.

Nursing Home Adjustment & Satisfaction. Charles M. Joiner. 1991. LC 91-808. (Studies on the Elderly in America). 174p. text 25.00 (*0-8153-0518-4*) Garland.

Nursing Home Administration. James E. Allen. 3rd ed. 1997. LC 96-33640. (Illus.). 632p. 69.95 (*0-8261-5392-5*) Springer Pub.

Nursing Home & Resident's Relatives. Marylou Hughes. 1987. 137p. (C). 18.50 (*1-877735-13-2*, 2119PP) Prof Prnting & Pub.

Nursing Home & You: Partners in Caring for a Relative with Alzheimer's Disease. Edna L. Blevins et al. 1987. 48p. (Orig.). pap. text 8.95 (*0-943774-37-3*) Am Assn Homes.

***Nursing Home Bankruptcies: What Caused Them? - Congressional Hearing.** Ed. by Chuck Grassley. 2001. 78p. pap. 25.00 (*0-7567-1181-9*) DIANE Pub.

Nursing Home Companion. Pauline B. Innis. 1993. 174p. 9.95 (*0-941402-10-X*) Devon Pub.

Nursing Home Connection: A Handbook for Visitors. Anne Sharp. 1990. LC 89-92775. (Illus.). 80p. (Orig.). pap. 4.95 (*0-9625382-0-5*) A Sharp.

Nursing Home Federal Requirements & Guidelines to Surveyors. James E. Allen. 3rd ed. 1997. LC 96-48423. 312p. 44.95 (*0-8261-8122-8*) Springer Pub.

Nursing Home Handbook: North Central Texas Region, 1992-1993 Edition. Amy Crawley & Cynthia O'Keafe. 1992. 300p. pap. 19.95 (*0-9634276-0-1*) Smart Choices.

Nursing Home Leadership. Wayne D. Ford. 1997. 317p. pap. 69.95 (*1-879876-00-0*, 30201) Mgmt Advantage.

Nursing Home Life: The Silver Lining. Helen F. Glazer. 1990. 160p. pap. 9.95 (*0-938823-05-1*) Pogment Pr.

Nursing Home Life: What It Is & What It Could Be. Clifford Bennett. 1980. LC 80-52650. (Illus.). 192p. pap. text 12.00 (*0-913292-19-2*) Tiresias Pr.

Nursing Home Ministry: A Manual. Ed. by Tom McCormick & Penny McCormick. 1982. (Orig.). pap. text 6.95 (*0-934688-08-7*) Great Comm Pubns.

Nursing Home Options: Getting Quality Care for the Elderly. James N. Fisher. Ed. by Betty McBride. 1991. LC 91-73498. 112p. (Orig.). pap. 9.25 (*0-9629201-7-7*) Collective Creations.

Nursing Home Regulations. 1995. LC 96-233538. 304p. pap. 35.00 (*0-8080-0066-7*, 4915) CCH INC.

Nursing Home Salary & Benefit Report, 1991. Zabka, John R., Associates Inc. Staff. 14th ed. 1992. 204p. pap. 250.00 (*0-939326-65-5*) Hosp & Hlthcare.

Nursing Home Salary & Benefits Report, 1992. Hospital Compensation Service Staff. 1992. pap. 250.00 (*0-939326-69-8*) Hosp & Hlthcare.

Nursing Home Salary & Benefits Report, 1993. 1994. 225p. pap. 250.00 (*0-939326-76-0*) Hosp & Hlthcare.

Nursing Home Task Force Report. Nursing Home Task Force National Hospice Organizat. 1998. LC 99-181747. 88p. (*0-931207-56-8*) Natl Hospice.

Nursing Home Volunteer Services Guide. Harold E. Knight, III & Carol J. Wortham. 1988. 60p. (Orig.). pap. 34.95 (*0-945253-03-6*) Thornsbury Bailey Brown.

Nursing Homes: Complaint Investigation Processes Often Inadequate to Protect Residents. Ed. by William J. Scanlon. 2000. (Illus.). 77p. (C). pap. text 20.00 (*0-7881-8644-2*) DIANE Pub.

Nursing Homes: Proposal to Enhance Oversight of Poorly Performing Homes Has Merit. William J. Scanlon. 2000. 68p. (C). pap. text 20.00 (*0-7881-8817-8*) DIANE Pub.

***Nursing Homes: Sustained Efforts Are Essential to Realize Potential of the Quality Initiatives.** Walter Ochinko. 2000. 83p. (C). pap. text 25.00 (*0-7567-0874-5*) DIANE Pub.

Nursing Homes & Nursing Care: Lessons from the Teaching Nursing Homes. Ed. by Mathy D. Mezey et al. 1988. 176p. 23.95 (*0-8261-6210-X*) Springer Pub.

Nursing Homes & Older People: Issues of Continuing Care. Ed. by Pauline Ford & Hazel Heath. 1996. 288p. pap. text 37.50 (*0-7506-2438-8*) Buttrwrth-Heinemann.

Nursing in a Violent Society: Issues & Research. Ed. by Harriet R. Feldman. 1995. LC 95-31624. 128p. 28.95 (*0-8261-9080-4*) Springer Pub.

Nursing in Action: Strengthening Nursing & Midwifery to Support Health for All. Jane Salvage. 1993. (WHO Regional Publications: No. 48). 128p. pap. text 21.60 (*92-890-1312-5*, 1310048) World Health.

Nursing in Ambulatory Care: The Future Is Here. American Nurses Association Staff & American Academy of Ambulatory Care Nursing Staff. 1997. LC 97-145420. 54p. 18.95 (*1-55810-135-7*, ST-2) Am Nurses Pub.

Nursing in America. Lewis Miller. 1989. (C). (*0-7223-2389-1*) A H S Ltd GBR. *Dist:* St Mut.

Nursing in Families. Suzanne L. Feetham et al. 1992. (Illus.). 320p. (C). pap. 34.95 (*0-8039-4716-X*, 4338) Sage.

Nursing in Gastroenterology. Bruce. 1997. text 33.00 (*0-443-05484-3*) Saunders.

***Nursing in General Practice: A Foundation Text.** 1995. (Illus.). pap. (*0-412-49840-5*) Chapman & Hall.

***Nursing in Haematological Oncology.** Maggie Grundy & Roslyne Bratt-Wyton. 2001. (Illus.). 320p. pap. (*0-7020-2323-X*) W B Saunders GBR. *Dist:* Saunders.

Nursing in Hospice & Terminal Care: Research & Practice. Ed. by Barbara M. Petrosino. 1986. LC 86-12015. (Hospice Journal: Vol. 2, No. 1). 138p. 39.95 (*0-86656-567-1*) Haworth Pr.

Nursing in Nursing Homes. Linda Nazarko. 1995. LC 94-49058. pap. 21.95 (*0-632-03987-6*) Blackwell Sci.

Nursing in the Community: Dimensions of Community Health Nursing. Mary Jo Dummer Clark. 3rd ed. 1998. 1103p. (C). pap. text 51.95 (*0-8385-6984-6*) Appleton & Lange.

Nursing in the Year 2000. Ed. by Joan Bilitski & Margaret C. Taylor. 1984. 70p. (Orig.). pap. 18.00 (*0-937058-20-3*) West Va U Pr.

Nursing in Today's World: Challenges, Issues, & Trends. Janice Rider Ellis & Celia Love Hartley. 7th ed. 2000. LC 00-42402. 592p. pap. text 32.95 (*0-7817-2455-4*) Lppncott W & W.

Nursing Informatics. Ed. by Paul Wainwright. 1994. LC 93-36803. pap. text (*0-443-04705-7*) Church.

Nursing Informatics: An International Overview for Nursing in a Technological Era; Proceedings of the Fifth IMIA International Conference on Nursing Use of Computers & Information Science, San Antonio, Texas, USA, June 17-22, 1994. International Conference on Nursing Use of Compute. Ed. by Susan J. Grobe & Elly S. Pluyter-Wenting. 1994. LC 94-16514. 876p. 279.50 (*0-444-81851-0*) Elsevier.

Nursing Informatics '97: The Impact of Nursing Knowledge on Health Care Information. Ed. by U. Gerdin et al. 1997. LC 97-75048. (Studies in Health Technology & Informatics: Vol. 46). 600p. 119.00 (*90-5199-362-5*, 362-5) IOS Press.

Nursing Interventions: Effective Nursing Treatments. Gloria M. Bulechek & Joanne C. McCloskey. Ed. by Thomas Eoyang. 3rd ed. 1999. LC 98-43443. (Illus.). xix, 747p. text (*0-7216-7724-X*) Saunders.

Nursing Interventions & Clinical Skills. Martha K. Elkin et al. (Illus.). 1996. 832p. (*0-8151-3043-0*); 1996. tchr. ed. (*0-8151-3030-9*); 1995. 832p. (C). (gr. 13). pap. text 50.00 (*0-8151-3045-7*, 24832) Mosby Inc.

Nursing Interventions & Clinical Skills. Martha K. Elkin. 2nd ed. 1999. tchr. ed. (*0-323-00803-8*); LC 00-267038. xx, 998p. (C). text (*0-323-00802-X*) Mosby Inc.

Nursing Interventions & Clinical Skills: Checklists. Martha K. Elkin et al. 1996. (*0-8151-3044-9*) Mosby Inc.

Nursing Interventions Classification (NIC) Joanne C. McCloskey et al. Ed. by Joanne C. McCloskey & Gloria M. Bulechek. 2nd ed. 1995. LC 95-25053. (Illus.). 768p. (C). (gr. 13). pap. text 37.95 (*0-8151-6302-9*, 26018) Mosby Inc.

Nursing Interventions Classification (NIC) Joanne Comi McCloskey & Gloria M. Bulechek. 3rd ed. 1999. LC 99-35032. xxxii, 911p. (*0-323-00894-1*) Mosby Inc.

Nursing Interventions for Infants & Children. Craft-Denehy. 1989. (Illus.). 416p. text 58.00 (*0-7216-2129-5*) Saunders.

Nursing Is My Bag. Marian George. 1989. (Illus.). 131p. (Orig.). pap. 9.95 (*0-9623843-0-5*) M George.

Nursing Issues for the Nineties & Beyond. Ed. by Bonnie Bullough & Vern Bullough. 1994. LC 92-49817. 248p. (C). text 29.95 (*0-8261-8050-7*) Springer Pub.

Nursing Issues in Leading & Managing Change. Jeanette Lancaster. 1998. LC 98-26134. 544p. pap. text 34.95 (*0-323-00250-1*) Mosby Inc.

Nursing Issues in the 21st Century: Perspectives from the Literature. Eleanor C. Hein. 2001. LC 00-63971. (Illus.). 560p. pap. text 31.95 (*0-7817-3017-1*) Lppncott W & W.

Nursing Issues, Trends & Portents. Castillo. 1997. (Nursing Education Ser.). pap. 26.50 (*0-8273-6270-6*) Delmar.

Nursing Knowledge & Practice: A Decision-Making Approach. Maggie Mallik. 1997. 644p. pap. text (*0-7020-1991-7*) W B Saunders GBR. *Dist:* Saunders.

Nursing Law & Ethics. John Tingle & A. Cribb. 1995. (Illus.). 256p. pap. 46.95 (*0-632-03617-6*) Blackwell Sci.

***Nursing Leaders Speak Out: Issues & Opinions.** Harriet R. Feldman. 2001. LC 00-69816. (*0-8261-1416-4*) Springer Pub.

Nursing Leadership & Management: An Experiential Approach. Elaine L. La Monica. 1983. LC 82-20193. (Illus.). 300p. (C). reprint ed. pap. text 43.95 (*0-86720-377-3*, 377-3) Jones & Bartlett.

Nursing Leadership & Management: Concepts & Practice. Ruth M. Tappen. 4th ed. 2000. LC 00-59041. (Illus.). 544p. pap. 38.95 (*0-8036-0609-5*) Davis Co.

Nursing Leadership & Management: Contemporary Strategies. Gertrude K. McFarland et al. 1989. LC 83-16724. 349p. (C). text 34.95 (*0-8273-4309-4*) Delmar.

Nursing Leadership, Management, & Professional Practice for the LPN/LVN. Mary Ann Anderson et al. 1997. LC 96-52836. (Illus.). 252p. (C). pap. text 22.95 (*0-8036-0209-X*) Davis Co.

Nursing Leadership, Management, & Professional Practice for the LPN/LVN. Mary Ann Anderson. 2nd ed. 2001. LC 00-47411. (Illus.). xvi, 320p. (C). pap. 24.95 (*0-8036-0794-6*) Davis Co.

Nursing Leadership, Management & Research. Ann B. Grant & Veta H. Massey. 1999. LC 98-49376. (Springhouse Notes Ser.). 256p. pap. 26.95 (*0-87434-968-0*) Springhouse Corp.

Nursing Made Easy. Sylvia Rayfield & Loretta Manning. 1997. (Illus.). 304p. pap. 24.95 (*0-9643622-2-8*) ICAN LA.

Nursing Malpractice: Implications for Clinical Practice & Nursing Education. J. Beckmann. 1994. LC 94-10802. 298p. pap. 22.50 (*0-295-97373-0*) U of Wash Pr.

Nursing Malpractice: Liability & Risk Management. Charles C. Sharpe. 1999. LC 98-31027. 240p. 65.00 (*0-86569-280-7*); pap. 22.95 (*0-86569-286-6*) Greenwood (Auburn Hse).

Nursing Management. Barter. 1998. (Nursing Education Ser.). 24.95 (*0-8273-7853-X*) Delmar.

Nursing Management: A Systems Approach. Dee A. Gillies. 3rd ed. 1994. (Illus.). 635p. pap., tchr. ed. (*0-7216-6597-7*); LC 93-23585. pap. text 33.00 (*0-7216-6588-8*) Saunders.

Nursing Management: An Experimental Skill Building Workbook. Eleanor J. Sullivan. 3rd ed. 1992. 272p. (C). pap. text 24.38 (*0-8053-7863-4*) Addison-Wesley.

Nursing Management: Concepts & Issues. Ed. by Katherine W. Vestal. 2nd ed. 1994. LC 94-9624. 400p. pap. text 32.95 (*0-397-55012-X*) Lppncott W & W.

Nursing Management: Issues & Ideas. Ed. by Montague Brown. 1992. (Health Care Management Review Ser.). 220p. pap. 55.00 (*0-8342-0301-4*, 20301) Aspen Pub.

Nursing Management Desk Reference: Concepts, Strategies & Skills. Ed. by Roxane Spitzer-Lehmann. 1994. LC 93-35928. (Illus.). 764p. text 55.00 (*0-7216-4346-9*) Saunders.

Nursing Management Handbook. Ken Hyett. 1988. (Illus.). 224p. (*0-443-03626-8*) Church.

Nursing Management in the 90's - An OBRA Guide for DON's. Mattie Locke. 1991. 224p. (C). 18.00 (*1-877735-31-0*, 2176PP) Prof Prnting & Pub.

Nursing Management of Diabetes Mellitus: A Guide to the Pattern Approach. Diana W. Guthrie & Richard A. Guthrie. 4th ed. 1997. LC 97-4384. (Illus.). 434p. 56.95 (*0-8261-7261-X*) Springer Pub.

Nursing Management of Multiple Birth Families: Preconception Through Postpartum. Joan E. Dauphinee et al. 1997. LC 96-40371. (*0-86525-076-6*) March of Dimes.

Nursing, Medicine & Primary Care. Anne Williams. 2000. LC 99-49874. 192p. pap. 27.95 (*0-335-20167-9*) Taylor & Francis.

Nursing Models for Practice. Alan Pearson & Barbara Vaughan. 2nd ed. 1996. 264p. pap. text 45.00 (*0-7506-1597-4*, Focal) Buttrwrth-Heinemann.

Nursing Mother's Companion. Kathleen Huggins. 4th rev. ed. 1999. LC 98-51793. (Illus.). 256p. 24.95 (*1-55832-151-9*) Harvard Common Pr.

Nursing Mother's Guide to Weaning. Kathleen Huggins & Linda Ziedrich. 1994. LC 94-30070. (Illus.). 208p. 18.95 (*1-55832-066-0*) Harvard Common Pr.

Nursing Mother's Guide to Weaning. Linda Ziedrich & Kathleen Huggins. 1994. LC 94-30070. (Illus.). 208p. pap. 11.95 (*1-55832-065-2*) Harvard Common Pr.

Nursing Mother's Problem Solver. Ed. by Claire Martin & Nancy Funnemark Krebs. 2000. LC 00-37198. (Illus.). 320p. pap. 13.00 (*0-684-85784-7*, Fireside) S&S Trade Pap.

Nursing NCLEX-RN Pearls of Wisdom: Over 2500 Questions. Gossman. 1998. (Pearls of Wisdom Ser.). pap. 26.00 (*1-890369-20-9*) Boston Medical.

Nursing Negligence: Analyzing Malpractice in the Hospital Setting. Janet P. Beckmann. 1996. LC 95-41787. (Illus.). 400p. 74.95 (*0-7619-0225-2*, 2089); pap. 38.95 (*0-7619-0226-0*, 2090) Sage.

Nursing 97 Drug Handbook. Springhouse Publishing Company Staff. Ed. by June Norris. 2nd rev. ed. 1996. (Illus.). 1360p. 31.95 incl. disk (*0-87434-867-6*) Springhouse Corp.

Nursing Now Notes. Deborah Stewart. Date not set. spiral bd. 14.00 (*0-9678177-0-6*) D L Stewart.

Nursing Outcomes Classification. Ed. by Marion Johnson & Meridean Maas. 1997. LC 96-50091. (Illus.). 448p. (C). (gr. 13). pap. text 37.95 (*0-8151-4546-2*, 30588) Mosby Inc.

Nursing Outcomes Classification (NOC) Iowa Outcomes Project Staff. Ed. by Marion Johnson & Meridean Maas. 2nd ed. 1999. LC 99-40690. text 37.95 (*0-323-00893-3*) Mosby Inc.

Nursing Partnership: A Model for Nursing Practice. Judith Christensen. 1993. LC 93-12698. 272p. pap. text (*0-443-04934-3*) Church.

Nursing Perspectives & Issues. Gloria M. Grippando. (Education Ser.). 3rd ed. 1986. pap., tchr. ed. 7.00 (*0-8273-2557-6*); 4th ed. 1989. 442p. (gr. 12). pap. 25.90 (*0-8273-3466-4*) Delmar.

Nursing Perspectives & Issues. Paula R. Mitchell & Gloria M. Grippando. 5th ed. 1992. (C). mass mkt. 31.25 (*0-8273-4983-1*) Delmar.

Nursing Perspectives & Issues. Gloria M. Grippando & Paula R. Mitchell. 6th ed. 2002. (C). text 25.50 net. (*0-7668-0271-X*) Delmar.

Nursing Perspectives & Issues: Instructor's Guide. Paula R. Mitchell & Gloria M. Grippando. 5th ed. 1993. pap., tchr. ed. 14.95 (*0-8273-4985-8*) Delmar.

Nursing Perspectives on Humor. Ed. by Karen Buxman & Ann LeMoine. 1995. LC 95-69075. (Illus.). pap. 19.95 (*0-9627246-5-3*) Power NY.

Nursing Perspectives on Radiation Oncology. Hassey. 1992. (C). text 34.95 (*0-8273-4650-6*) Delmar.

Nursing Pharmacology. Ed. by Norma L. Pinnell. 1996. (Illus.). 1149p. tchr. ed. (*0-7216-5154-2*) Saunders.

Nursing Pharmacology. Norma L. Pinnell. 1996. 1149p. pap., stu. ed. 17.95 (*0-7216-6783-X*) Saunders.

Nursing Pharmacology. Norma L. Pinnell. Ed. by Dan Ruth. 1996. LC 94-20441. (Illus.). 1248p. text 57.50 (*0-7216-6482-2*) Saunders.

Nursing Pharmacology. Paulette D. Rollant & Karen Hill. 2nd ed. 2001. LC 00-62483. (Rapid Review Ser.). (Illus.). xxvii, 370p. 24.95 (*0-323-01167-5*) Mosby Inc.

Nursing Pharmacology. Lane J. Wallace. 2nd ed. 1992. (Nursing-Health Science Ser.). (Illus.). 1120p. (C). text 59.95 (*0-86720-429-X*, 429-X) Jones & Bartlett.

Nursing Pharmacology. April H. Vallerand. 3rd ed. 1997. LC 96-48153. (Springhouse Notes Ser.). 304p. pap. 26.95 (*0-87434-903-6*) Springhouse Corp.

Nursing Pharmacology: A Comprehensive Approach to Drug Therapy. Sandra Wardell & Lorraine Bousard. 1985. (Illus.). 1200p. (C). text 46.25 (*0-534-01338-4*, 338-4) Jones & Bartlett.

Nursing Pharmacology: A Systems Approach to Drug Therapy & Nursing Practice. Alvin K. Swonger. 1978. 13.00 (*0-316-82553-0*, Little Brwn Med Div) Lppncott W & W.

Nursing Pharmacology: An Integrated Approach to Drug Therapy & Nursing Practice. Alvin K. Swonger & Myrtle P. Matejski. 1988. (C). text 62.33 (*0-673-39752-1*) Addson-Wesley Educ.

Nursing Pharmacology & Clinical Management. Leah Cleveland et al. 1998. LC 98-25822. 1,152p. text 54.95 (*0-397-55244-0*) Lppncott W & W.

Nursing Pharmacology Value Pack. Wallace. 1992. 57.50 (*0-86720-625-X*) Jones & Bartlett.

***Nursing, Physician Control & the Medical Monopoly: Historical Perspectives on Gendered Inequality in Roles, Rights & Range of Practice.** Thetis M. Group & Joan I. Roberts. 2001. LC 00-69714. 352p. 29.95 (*0-253-33926-X*) Ind U Pr.

Nursing Power & Social Judgement: An Interpretive Ethnography of a Hospital Ward. Martin Johnson. 1997. LC 97-71457. (Developments in Nursing & Health Care Ser.). (Illus.). 211p. text (*1-85972-651-8*) Ashgate Pub GBR. *Dist:* Ashgate Pub Co.

Nursing Practice: Hospital & Home; the Adult. Ed. by Margaret F. Alexander et al. 1995. LC 94-16626. pap. text (*0-443-04338-8*) Church.

Nursing Practice: Report of a WHO Expert Committee. 1996. (Technical Reports: Vol. 860).Tr. of Soins Infirmiers, Enfermeria. (ENG, FRE & SPA.). 33p. (Orig.). pap. 10.80 (*92-4-120860-0*, 1100860) World Health.

Nursing Practice & Health Care. 2nd ed. (*0-340-55788-5*) E A GBR. *Dist:* Routldge.

Nursing Practice & Health Care. Hinchcliffe. 2nd ed. 1993. 864p. pap. 63.75 (*1-56593-534-9*, 0538) Singular Publishing.

Nursing Practice & Health Care: A Foundation Text. Ed. by Sue Hinchliff et al. 3rd ed. 1998. (An Arnold Publication). (Illus.). 752p. pap. (*0-340-69230-8*) E A GBR. *Dist:* OUP.

Nursing Practice & Outcomes Measurement. Joint Commission on Accreditation of Healthcare Organizations. 1997. LC 96-43897. 193p. 50.00 (*0-86688-499-8*, OM-100) Joint Comm Hlthcare.

Nursing Practice & the Law. Milton Lesnik & Bernice E. Anderson. 2nd ed. 1976. LC 75-45453. 400p. reprint ed. lib. bdg. 75.00 (*0-8371-8729-X*, LENP, Greenwood Pr) Greenwood.

Nursing Practice & the Law: Avoiding Malpractice & Other Legal Risks. Mary E. O'Keefe. 2000. LC 00-22791. (Illus.). xxiv, 578p. 39.95 (*0-8036-0602-8*) Davis Co.

Nursing Practice in the U. K. & North America. Eugene Levine et al. 1993. LC 92-12312. 49.50 (*1-56593-024-X*, 0267) Thomson Learn.

***Nursing Practice, Policy & Change.** Ed. by Marjorie Gott. 2000. LC 2001-516014. 240p. pap. (*1-85775-351-8*) Radcliffe Med Pr GBR. *Dist:* Balogh.

***Nursing Practice Related to Spinal Cord Injury & Disorders: A Core Curriculum.** Ed. by Audrey Nelson et al. 2001. (Illus.). 550p. pap. text 75.00 (*0-9708873-1-0*) Estrn Prlyzed Vet.

Nursing Praxis: Knowledge & Action. Ed. by Sally Thorne & Virginia E. Hayes. 1997. LC 96-35661. 320p. 74.95 (*0-7619-0010-1*, 1549); pap. 37.95 (*0-7619-0011-X*, 1550) Sage.

M
N
O

Nursing Procedures. Springhouse Publishing Company Staff. 3rd ed. 2000. LC 99-50330. 832p. 49.95 (*0-87434-978-8*) Springhouse Corp.

*****Nursing Process.** Pearl Gardner. 2002. pap. text 33.95 (*0-7668-2225-7*) Delmar.

Nursing Process: Concepts & Applications. Seaback. 2000. (Illus.). 288p. (C). pap. text 35.95 (*0-7668-2045-9*) Delmar.

Nursing Process & Nursing Diagnosis. Patricia W. Iyer et al. 3rd ed. 1994. LC 94-17892. 576p. pap. text 24.00 (*0-7216-5614-5*) Saunders.

Nursing Process & Quality Care. 132p. pap. (*0-340-58112-3*) E A GBR. *Dist:* Routldge.

Nursing Process in Collaborative Practice. Carol V. Allen. 2nd ed. 1996. LC 96-8018. 240p. (Orig.). (C). pap. 36.60 (*0-8385-1467-7*, A1467-8) P-H.

Nursing Process in Psychiatry. Ward. 2nd ed. 1992. (Illus.). 256p. (Orig.). pap. text (*0-443-04225-X*) Church.

Nursing Quality Indicators: Definitions & Implications. American Nurses Association Staff et al. 1996. LC 96-19465. 88p. pap. 29.95 (*1-55810-125-X*, NP-108, Am Nurses Fnd) Am Nurses Pub.

Nursing Quality Indicators Beyond Acute Care: Literature Review. 2000. 156p. pap. 41.95 (*1-55810-149-7*) Am Nurses Pub.

Nursing Quality Indicators Beyond Acute Care: Measurement Instruments. 2000. 220p. pap. 58.95 (*1-55810-150-0*) Am Nurses Pub.

Nursing Quality Measurement: A Review of Nursing Studies. Marilyn J. Rantz. 1995. 198p. (Orig.). pap. 33.95 (*1-55810-105-5*, NP-93) Am Nurses Pub.

Nursing Reflections: A Century of Caring. C. V. Mosby Company Staff. 2000. LC 00-29218. 176p. pap. 34.95 (*0-323-01173-X*) Mosby Inc.

Nursing Research. 1996. (*92-871-3112-0*) Council of Europe FRA. *Dist:* Manhattan Pub Co.

Nursing Research. 240p. pap. (*0-340-66194-1*) E A GBR. *Dist:* Routldge.

Nursing Research. Carol T. Bush. 1985. (C). (*0-8359-5047-6*) P-H.

Nursing Research. Morse. 2nd ed. 1995. 208p. pap. 37.95 (*1-56593-586-1*, 1194) Singular Publishing.

Nursing Research: A Qualitative Perspective. Ed. by Patricia L. Munhall & Carolyn O. Boyd. 2nd ed. 1993. LC 93-20494. 506p. pap. 36.95 (*0-88737-590-1*) Natl League Nurse.

Nursing Research: A Qualitative Perspective. Patricia L. Munhall & NLN Staff. 3rd ed. 2001. LC 00-69418. (Illus.). 704p. (C). pap. text 44.95 (*0-7637-1135-7*, 1135-7, N L N Bart) Jones & Bartlett.

Nursing Research: A Quantitative & Qualitative Approach. Carol A. Roberts & Sharon O. Burke. 1989. (Illus.). 400p. text 49.95 (*0-86720-415-X*, 415-X) Jones & Bartlett.

Nursing Research: Ethical & Legal. De Raeve. 1996. pap. text 40.95 (*0-7020-1888-0*) Saunders.

Nursing Research: Methods, Critical Appraisal & Utilization. Geri Lobiondo-Wood & Judith Haber. 4th ed. (Illus.). 1998. tchr. ed. (*1-55664-431-0*); 1997. LC 97-33347. 624p. (C). (gr. 13). pap. text 36.00 (*0-8151-2390-6*, 31043) Mosby Inc.

*****Nursing Research: Methods, Critical Appraisal & Utilization.** Geri Lobiondo-Wood. 5th ed. 2001. (Illus.). 620p. (*0-323-01287-6*) Mosby Inc.

Nursing Research: Principles & Methods. Denise F. Polit & Bernadette P. Hungler. 6th ed. 1998. LC 98-39678. 816p. text 49.95 (*0-7817-1562-8*) Lppncott W & W.

*****Nursing Research: Theory & Practice.** 1994. (Illus.). pap. (*0-412-49850-2*) Chapman & Hall.

Nursing Research & Its Utilization: International State of the Science. Ed. by Joyce J. Fitzpatrick et al. 1994. LC 94-183. 256p. 41.95 (*0-8261-8090-6*) Springer Pub.

Nursing Research for Nursing Practice: An International Perspective. Ed. by Rebecca Bergman. 1990. 250p. pap. 37.50 (*0-412-33500-X*, A4439) Chapman & Hall.

Nursing Research in a Service Setting. Cheryl B. Stetler. 1984. (C). pap. text 33.50 (*0-8359-5045-X*) P-H.

Nursing Roles: Evolving or Recycled? Sue Moorhead & Diane G. Huber. 1997. LC 96-35619. (Series on Nursing Administration: Vol. 9). 245p. 78.95 (*0-7619-0149-3*) Sage.

Nursing School & Allied Health Entrance Exams. Marion Gooding. 14th ed. 1997. LC 97-80791. (Illus.). 423p. pap. 16.95 (*0-02-862193-X*, Arc) Hungry Minds.

Nursing School Entrance Examinations. Gooding. 13th ed. 1996. per. 15.95 (*0-671-52029-6*) S&S Trade.

Nursing School Entrance Examinations for Practical Nurse (PN) Jack Rudman. (Admission Test Ser.: Vol. 20). 47.95 (*0-8373-5120-0*); 1994. pap. 27.95 (*0-8373-5020-4*) Nat Learn.

Nursing School Entrance Examinations for Registered & Graduate Nurses (RN) Jack Rudman. 1994. (Admission Test Ser.: ATS-19). pap. 27.95 (*0-8373-5019-0*) Nat Learn.

Nursing School Entrance Exams. 1998. 29.95 incl. disk (*0-02-860603-5*) Macmillan.

Nursing Science: Major Paradigms, Theories & Critiques. Rosemarie Rizzo Parse. 1987. (Illus.). 224p. text 48.00 (*0-7216-1803-0*) Saunders.

Nursing Service in Transition: A Description of Organization for Classification & Utilization of Nurse Practitioners. Rachel Ayers. 1972. 124p. pap. 5.00 (*0-940876-03-5*) City Hope.

Nursing Service Procedure Manual. W. H. Heaton. 975p. ring bd. 149.95 (*1-881057-07-0*) Heaton Pubns.

Nursing Service Training Coordinator. Jack Rudman. 1994. (Career Examination Ser.: C-3398). pap. 39.95 (*0-8373-3398-9*) Nat Learn.

Nursing Shortage: New Approaches to an Old Problem. Melvin I. Krasner. 1989. (Papers: No. 12). 36p. 5.00 (*0-934459-61-4*) United Hosp Fund.

Nursing Skills for the Management of Head, Spinal, Chest, Abdominal & Orthopedic Trauma. Linda B. Chitwood. Ed. by Barbara Halliburton. 1991. 99p. (C). pap. text 24.95 (*1-878025-94-5*) Western Schls.

Nursing Spectrum of Lasers. Judith I. Pfister et al. 1988. (Illus.). 156p. (Orig.). (C). pap. text 32.50 (*0-9622255-0-9*) ED Inc.

Nursing Spinal Cord Injuries. Ed. by Nalzina M. Woll. 1986. LC 85-26285. (Nursing Research Ser.). 176p. (C). 46.50 (*0-8476-7380-4*); pap. 21.00 (*0-8476-7387-1*) Rowman.

Nursing, Sr. H. S. Jack Rudman. 1994. (Teachers License Examination Ser.: T-44). pap. 27.95 (*0-8373-8044-8*) Nat Learn.

Nursing Staff Development: A Component of Human Resource Development. Russell C. Swansburg. 1995. (Illus.). 416p. (C). text 52.95 (*0-86720-658-6*, 658-6) Jones & Bartlett.

Nursing Staff Development: Strategies for Success. Ed. by Roberta S. Abruzzese. 2nd ed. 1996. LC 95-49884. (Illus.). 368p. (C). (gr. 13). text 49.95 (*0-8151-0053-1*, 26131) Mosby Inc.

*****Nursing Staff Requirments & the Quality of Nusing Home Care: Nursing Home Care: A Report to the California State Legislature.** Brenda G. Klutz. 2001. 57p. (C). pap. text 20.00 (*0-7567-1439-7*) DIANE Pub.

Nursing Standards: The Guide to a Marker Model. Carolyn G. Smith-Marker. 1987. (*0-932491-81-2*) Res Appl Inc.

Nursing Student to Nursing Leader: The Critical Path To Leadership Development. Carol A. Fetters-Andersen. 1998. LC 98-2907. 323p. pap. text 32.95 (*0-7668-0255-8*) Delmar.

Nursing the Critically Ill Adult. Ed. by Nancy M. Holloway. 4th ed. 1993. LC 92-49611. 655p. (C). 84.00 (*0-8053-2544-1*) Addison-Wesley.

Nursing the Critically Ill Adult. Nancy M. Holloway. 2nd ed. 1984. LC 78-21153. (*0-201-12640-0*, 002665, Health Sci) Addison-Wesley.

Nursing, the Finest Art: An Illustrated History. M. Patricia Donahue. 2nd ed. 1996. (Illus.). 560p. (*84-7592-239-2*) Mosby-Doyma Libros ESP. *Dist:* Mosby Inc.

Nursing the Image: Media, Image & Professional Identity. Julia Hallam. 2000. (Illus.). 256p. 85.00 (*0-415-18454-1*); pap. 25.99 (*0-415-18455-X*) Routledge.

Nursing the Neonate. Helen Yeo. 1998. LC 98-5744. 324p. pap. 49.95 (*0-632-05049-7*) Blackwell Sci.

Nursing the Neurological & Neurotrauma Patient. Maria J. Kruse. 1986. LC 85-27837. (Nursing Research Ser.). 144p. 58.00 (*0-8476-7451-7*) Rowman.

Nursing the Orthopaedic Patient. Ed. by Peter S. Davis. 1995. LC 93-43058. pap. text (*0-443-04461-9*) Church.

Nursing the Psychiatric Emergency. Martin F. Ward. 1995. 224p. pap. text 35.00 (*0-7506-1592-3*) Buttrwrth-Heinemann.

Nursing the Whole Person. Dallalis. 1995. (LPN/LVN Nursing Ser.). text 59.95 (*0-8273-5459-2*) Delmar.

Nursing the Whole Person: Concept to Practice. White. 1997. (LPN/LVN Nursing Ser.). 36.75 (*0-8273-7453-4*); 16.95 (*0-8273-7447-X*); tchr. ed. 12.95 (*0-8273-7446-1*) Delmar.

Nursing Theories: Conceptual & Philosophical Foundations. Ed. by Hesook S. Kim & Ingrid Kollak. 1999. LC 99-27969. (Illus.). 208p. 34.95 (*0-8261-1287-0*) Springer Pub.

Nursing Theories: The Base for Professional Nursing Practice. Julia B. George. 4th ed. 1995. LC 94-41658. 460p. (C). pap. 52.00 (*0-8385-7056-9*, A7056-3) P-H.

Nursing Theories: The Base for Professional Nursing Practice. George. 5th ed. 2001. 624p. pap. 37.95 (*0-8385-7110-7*) P-H.

Nursing Theories & Models. Hugh McKenna. 1997. (Essentials for Nurses Ser.). (Illus.). 288p. (C). 85.00 (*0-415-14222-9*); pap. 27.95 (*0-415-14223-7*) Routledge.

Nursing Theories & Models. Ruby L. Wesley. 2nd ed. 1994. LC 94-22849. (Notes Ser.). 176p. pap. 18.95 (*0-87434-744-0*) Springhouse Corp.

Nursing Theories & Nursing Practice. Marilyn E. Parker. 2000. LC 00-30335. (Illus.). 512p. pap. text 39.95 (*0-8036-0604-4*) Davis Co.

Nursing Theories & Quality of Care. Hugh P. McKenna. 1994. LC 94-6399. (Developments in Nursing & Health Care Ser.: Vol. 23). 272p. (*1-85628-670-3*) Avebry GBR. *Dist:* Ashgate Pub Co.

Nursing Theories in Practice. Ed. by Marilyn E. Parker. 1991. 320p. pap. 32.95 (*0-88737-497-2*) Natl League Nurse.

Nursing Theorists & Their Work. Ann Marriner-Tomey & Martha Raile Alligood. 4th ed. 1997. LC 97-11533. (Illus.). 576p. (C). (gr. 13). pap. text 38.00 (*0-8151-4421-0*, 30903) Mosby Inc.

*****Nursing Theorists & Their Work.** Ann Marriner-Tomey & Martha Raile Alligood. 5th ed. 2001. LC 2001-44385. (*0-323-01193-4*) Mosby Inc.

Nursing Theory: Analysis, Application, Evaluation. Barbara J. S. Barnum. 3rd ed. 1990. (Illus.). 350p. text 32.50 (*0-673-39920-6*); 5th ed. 1998. LC 97-30274. 320p. pap. text 39.95 (*0-7817-1104-5*) Lppncott W & W.

Nursing Theory: Utilization & Application. Ed. by Martha Raile Alligood & Ann Marriner-Tomey. 1996. (Illus.). 256p. (C). (gr. 13). pap. text 35.00 (*0-8151-0812-5*, 27759) Mosby Inc.

*****Nursing Theory: Utilization & Application.** Martha Raile Alligood & Anne Marriner-Tomey. 2nd ed. 2001. LC 2001-31581. (Illus.). xviii, 507p. (*0-323-01194-2*) Mosby Inc.

Nursing Today: Transition & Trends. Ed. by JoAnn Zerwekh & Jo C. Claborn. (Illus.). 1994. pap., tchr. ed. (*0-7216-3646-2*); 2nd ed. 1997. pap., tchr. ed. (*0-7216-6901-8*) Saunders.

Nursing Today: Transition & Trends. JoAnn Zerwekh & Jo Carol Claborn. Ed. by Ilze Rader. 2nd ed. 1996. LC 96-15370. (Illus.). 544p. pap. text 26.00 (*0-7216-6899-2*) Saunders.

Nursing Today: Transition & Trends. JoAnn Zerwekh & Jo Carol Claborn. 3rd ed. Date not set. LC 99-51712. (Illus.). 575p. pap. text (*0-7216-8685-0*) Saunders.

Nursing Twenty-Twenty. 1988. 172p. pap. 7.95 (*0-88737-397-6*, 41-2217) Natl League Nurse.

Nursing 2000 Drug Handbook. Springhouse Publishing Company Staff. 1999. cd-rom 49.95 (*0-87434-994-X*) Springhouse Corp.

Nursing 2001 Drug Handbook. 22nd ed. 2000. (Nursing Drug Handbook Ser.). (Illus.). 1376p. pap. 36.95 incl. cd-rom (*1-58255-067-0*) Springhouse Corp.

Nursing with the "Third Ear" Reading What Patients Write - a Basic Course. Jimmie R. Rankin. 1994. (Literature of Patient Response Ser.). 100p. pap. 29.95 (*1-883938-16-3*) Dry Bones Pr.

Nursing Within a Faith Community: Promoting Health in Times of Transition. Margaret B. Clark & Joanne K. Olson. 2000. LC 00-8369. (Illus.). xxiv, 403p. 69.95 (*0-7619-1210-X*, 82089); pap. 37.95 (*0-7619-1211-8*, 82090) Sage.

Nursing Wounds: Nurse Practitioners, Doctors, Women Patients, & the Negotiation of Meaning. Sue Fisher. 1995. 275p. (C). text 45.00 (*0-8135-2180-7*); pap. text 17.00 (*0-8135-2181-5*) Rutgers U Pr.

Nursing Your Adopted Baby. Kathryn Anderson. 1986. (Illus.). 32p. pap. 2.50 (*0-912500-15-8*) La Leche.

Nursing 99 Drug Handbook (Australasian Edition) Springhouse Publishing Company Staff. 1998. 1019p. pap. 43.95 (*0-87434-963-X*) Springhouse Corp.

Nursing's Vision for Primary Care in the 21st Century. Lucy N. Marion & American Nurses Association Staff. 1996. LC 96-10795. 47p. (Orig.). pap. 23.95 (*1-55810-124-1*, CH-30) Am Nurses Pub.

Nurtrition: Pre- & Postnatal Development. M. Winick. 1979. LC 78-26941. (Human Nutrition Ser.). (Illus.). 516p. (C). text 110.00 (*0-306-40132-0*, Kluwer Plenum) Kluwer Academic.

Nurturing an Endangered Generation: Empowering Youth with Critical Social, Emotional, & Cognitive Skills. Rosemary Thompson. 1998. LC 97-30458. 358p. pap. 24.95 (*1-56032-669-7*) Hemisp Pub.

Nurturing the Nurse on the Path to Success. Carolyn T. Laskey. Ed. by Jerena B. Rezvan. 1994. LC 93-61664. 210p. pap. 16.95 (*1-880254-11-5*) Vista.

Nurturing the Premature Infant: Developmental Intervention in the Neonatal Intensive Care Nursery. Edward Goldson. 1999. LC 98-7850. (Illus.). 216p. text 49.95 (*0-19-508570-1*) OUP.

Nurturing Touch at Birth: A Labor Support Handbook. Paulina Perez. 1997. LC 97-91542. (Illus.). 84p. pap. 11.95 (*0-9641159-8-0*) Doubleday.

Nurturing Young Minds & Bodies. Judi Davis. 1995. 186p. pap. text 24.95 (*1-885477-16-3*) Fut Horizons.

Nutcracker Is Already Dancing: The HIVs & the HIV-Nots. Cary Savitch. Ed. by Ruth Orr et al. 1996. LC 96-90495. 204p. 23.95 (*0-9653697-5-7*) Teague Hse Pr.

*****Nutraceutical Revolution: 20 Cutting-Edge Nutrients to Help You Design Your Own Perfect Whole-Life Program.** Richard N. Firshein. 2001. 371p. reprint ed. 25.00 (*0-7567-5230-2*) DIANE Pub.

Nutraceuticals: The Complete Encyclopedia of Supplements, Herbs, Vitamins & Healing Foods. Arthur J. Roberts et al. 2001. LC 00-62435. xvi, 512p. pap. 21.95 (*0-399-52632-3*, Perigee Bks) Berkley Pub.

Nutricide: The Rise & Fall of Saturated Fat in the Affairs of Man. Michael D. Wagoner. 1991. LC 91-90351. 74p. (Orig.). pap. 7.95 (*0-9629675-0-5*) Low Fat Pr.

Nutrient Adequacy: Assessment Using Food Consumption Surveys. National Research Council Staff. 1986. 160p. pap. text 19.95 (*0-309-03634-8*) Natl Acad Pr.

Nutrient Deficiencies & Toxicities in Crop Plants. Ed. by William F. Bennett. 1993. LC 93-71744. (Illus.). 202p. 69.00 (*0-89054-151-5*) Am Phytopathol Soc.

Nutrient Elements & Toxicants. M. Rechcigl. 1977. (Comparative Animal Nutrition Ser.: Vol. 2). (Illus.). 85.25 (*3-8055-2351-3*) S Karger.

Nutrient Modulation of the Immune Response. Ed. by Susanna Cunningham-Rundle. 1992. LC 92-49727. (Illus.). 576p. text 225.00 (*0-8247-8448-0*) Dekker.

Nutrient Points of Common Foods: Nutrition for the Nation. Virginia T. Stucky & Clara L. Gerwick. rev. ed. 1991. 62p. pap. text 7.90 (*0-915187-01-9*) Nutrition Ed.

Nutrient Regulation During Pregnancy, Lactation & Infant Growth. L. Allen et al. 1994. LC 94-6848. (Advances in Experimental Medicine & Biology Ser.: Vol. 352). (Illus.). 308p. (C). text 89.50 (*0-306-44719-3*, Kluwer Plenum) Kluwer Academic.

Nutrient Regulation of Insulin Secretion. Ed. by P. R. Flatt. 1992. (Portland Press Research Monographs: Vol. 1). 415p. (*1-85578-004-6*) Portland Pr Ltd GBR. *Dist:* Ashgate Pub Co.

Nutrient Requirements of Dogs, 1985. National Research Council Staff. rev. ed. 1985. (Nutrient Requirements of Domestic Animals Ser.). 88p. reprint ed. pap. text 24.95 (*0-309-03496-5*) Natl Acad Pr.

Nutrient Requirements of Horses, Set. National Research Council Staff. 5th rev. ed. 1989. (Nutrient Requirements of Domestic Animals Ser.). 112p. pap. text 24.95 (*0-309-03989-4*) Natl Acad Pr.

Nutrient Requirements of Sheep. National Research Council Staff. 6th rev. ed. 1985. LC 85-21562. (Nutrient Requirements of Domestic Animals Ser.). 112p. pap. text 19.95 (*0-309-03596-1*) Natl Acad Pr.

Nutrients A-Z: A User's Guide to Foods, Herbs, Vitamins, Minerals & Supplements. Michael Sharon. 1998. 224p. pap. (*1-85375-261-4*) Prion GBR. *Dist:* Trafalgar.

Nutrients & Brain Function. Ed. by Walter B. Essman. 1987. (Illus.). viii, 252p. 190.50 (*3-8055-4566-5*) S Karger.

Nutrients & Cancer Prevention. Ed. by Kedar N. Prasad & Frank L. Meyskens, Jr. 1990. LC 90-4677. (Experimental Biology & Medicine Ser.: Vol. 23). (Illus.). 353p. 145.00 (*0-89603-171-3*) Humana.

Nutrients & Energy. Ed. by Geoffrey H. Bourne. 1983. (World Review of Nutrition & Dietetics Ser.: Vol. 42). (Illus.). xii, 228p. 172.25 (*3-8055-3710-7*) S Karger.

Nutrients & Foods in AIDS. Ronald R. Watson. 1998. LC 97-48635. (Series in Modern Nutrition). 256p. 94.95 (*0-8493-8561-X*) CRC Pr.

Nutrients As Ergogenic Aids for Sports & Exercise. Luke R. Bucci. 1993. 192p. 104.95 (*0-8493-4223-6*, QP176) CRC Pr.

Nutrients as Ergogenic Aids for Sports & Exercise. Luke R. Bucci. 2nd ed. 1999. (Nutrition in Exercise & Sport Ser.). 89.95 (*0-8493-7922-9*) CRC Pr.

Nutrients Catalog: Vitamins, Minerals, Amino Acids, Macronutrients - Beneficial Use, Helpers, Inhibitors, Food Sources, Intake Recommendations, & Symptoms of over or under Use. Harvey Newstrom. 1993. LC 92-56671. 558p. lib. bdg. 75.00 (*0-89950-784-0*) McFarland & Co.

Nutrients in Cancer Prevention & Treatment. Ed. by Kedar N. Prasad et al. 1995. LC 95-15205. (Experimental Biology & Medicine Ser.: Vol. 27). (Illus.). 405p. 160.00 (*0-89603-318-X*) Humana.

Nutrients in the Control of Metabolic Diseases. Ed. by A. P. Simopoulos. 1992. LC 92-49666. (World Review of Nutrition & Dietetics Ser.: Vol. 69). (Illus.). xii, 170p. 204.50 (*3-8055-5594-6*) S Karger.

Nutrifacts: A Quick Reference for Nutrition in HIV Care. Jeanette M. Dunn. Ed. by Camle A. Mutzabaugh et al. 1997. (Illus.). pap. (*1-891814-02-8*) Found Care Mgmt.

Nutrition. Carol C. Caldwell. 1992. (Illus.). 160p. 14.95 (*0-8442-8187-5*) NTC Contemp Pub Co.

Nutrition. Farrell & Nicoteri. 2000. (Quick Look Nursing Ser.). 18.95 (*1-889325-22-8*) Fence Crk Pubng.

*****Nutrition.** Insel et al. 2001. (Illus.). (C). 15.00 (*0-7637-1924-2*, 1924-2) Jones & Bartlett.

Nutrition. Tamara Shuttleworth. 1985. LC 85-99032. (Skills for Life Ser.). pap. text 10.95 (*0-7710-8154-5*) McCland & Stewart.

Nutrition. Dorothy Wenck et al. 1980. (Illus.). text 19.95 (*0-8359-5061-1*) P-H.

Nutrition. Smolin. 2nd ed. 1996. (C). pap. text, tchr. ed. 28.00 (*0-03-018633-1*) Harcourt.

Nutrition: A Development Approach. LaQuatra. 1990. (Nursing Education Ser.). pap., tchr. ed. 12.00 (*0-8273-3076-6*) Delmar.

Nutrition: A Health Promotion Approach. Webb P. Goffrey. 1996. 384p. pap. 34.95 (*0-340-61027-1*) Trafalgar.

Nutrition: A Health Promotion Approach. Geoffrey P. Webb. l.t. ed. 1995. 384p. pap. 34.95 (*1-56593-641-8*, 1330) Singular Publishing.

Nutrition: A Reference Handbook. David A. Bender & Arnold E. Bender. 1996. (Illus.). 612p. text 110.00 (*0-19-262368-0*) OUP.

Nutrition: Codata Directory of Data Sources for Science & Technology, Chapter Twelve. Ed. by CODATA Staff. 1985. (CODATA Bulletin Ser.). 93p. pap. (*0-08-032489-4*) PPL GBR. *Dist:* Elsevier.

Nutrition: Concepts & Controversies. California College for Health Sciences Staff. 1993. (Illus.). 226p. (C). spiral bd. 25.00 (*0-933195-04-4*) CA College Health Sci.

Nutrition: Concepts & Controversies. Frances S. Sizer & Eleanor Noss Whitney. Date not set. (Adaptable Courseware-Hardside Ser.). 34.25 (*0-534-15982-6*) Wadsworth Pub.

Nutrition: Concepts & Controversies. Eva M. Hamilton et al. Ed. by Marshall. 5th ed. 1991. 354p. (C). pap. text 49.25 (*0-314-81091-9*) West Pub.

Nutrition: Concepts & Controversies. Frances S. Sizer & Eleanor Noss Whitney. 7th ed. 1997. stu. ed. 17.50 (*0-314-20995-6*); 8th ed. 1999. pap. text, stu. ed. 19.75 net. (*0-534-56468-2*) Wadsworth Pub.

Nutrition: Eating for Good Health. 1995. lib. bdg. 251.95 (*0-8490-6686-7*) Gordon Pr.

Nutrition: Essentials & Diet Therapy. Nancy J. Peckenpaugh & Charlotte M. Poleman. 7th ed. 1995. (Illus.). 642p. pap., tchr. ed. (*0-7216-5131-3*); LC 94-21254. 560p. pap. text 31.00 (*0-7216-5130-5*) Saunders.

***Nutrition: Handbook for Community Nursing.** Judy Buttriss & Amanda Wyanne. 2001. 130p. (Orig.). (C). pap. (*1-86156-216-0*) Whurr Pub GBR. *Dist:* Taylor & Francis.

Nutrition: Metabolic & Clinical Applications, Vol. 4. R. E. Hodges et al. 1979. LC 78-27208. (Human Nutrition Ser.). (Illus.). 500p. (C). text 110.00 (*0-306-40203-3*, Kluwer Plenum) Kluwer Academic.

Nutrition: Proteins & Amino Acids. Ed. by A. Yoshida et al. 1990. (Illus.). 327p. 106.00 (*0-387-52223-9*) Spr-Verlag.

Nutrition: Science & Applications. Smolin. 1998. (C). pap. text 10.00 (*0-03-025702-6*) Harcourt Coll Pubs.

Nutrition: Science & Applications. Lori A. Smolin. 3rd ed. 1999. LC 99-62661. pap. text (*0-03-025893-6*) Harcourt CAN.

Nutrition: The Cancer Answer II. Maureen Kennedy Salaman. 1995. 19.95 (*0-913087-20-3*); pap. 16.95 (*0-913087-19-X*) MKS Inc.

Nutrition: The Challenge of Being Well Nourished. Dorothy Wenck. 2nd ed. 1983. (C). (*0-8359-5064-6*) P-H.

Nutrition Across the Life Span: The Life Cycle. Ed. by Mary Kay Mitchell. 1997. (Illus.). 512p. pap., tchr. ed. (*0-7216-5031-7*) Saunders.

Nutrition Across the Lifespan: The Life Cycle. Mary Kay Mitchell. Ed. by Maura Connor. 1997. 432p. pap. text 51.00 (*0-7216-3784-1*) Saunders.

Nutrition, Aging & the Elderly Vol. 6. H. N. Munro & D. B. Danford. 1989. LC 88-39816. (Human Nutrition Ser.). (Illus.). 414p. 110.00 (*0-306-43047-9*, Kluwer Plenum) Kluwer Academic.

Nutrition Almanac. John D. Kirschmann & Gayla J. Kirschmann. 4th ed. 1996. LC 96-13594. (Illus.). 494p. pap. 19.95 (*0-07-034922-3*) McGraw-Hill Educ Grp.

Nutrition & AIDS. 1994. lib. bdg. 250.75 (*0-8490-5632-2*) Gordon Pr.

Nutrition & Alcohol. Ronald R. Watson. 1992. 496p. 157.95 (*0-8493-7933-4*, RC565) CRC Pr.

Nutrition & Behavior. Ed. by S. A. Miller. 1981. 320p. pap. 65.00 (*0-89859-735-8*) L Erlbaum Assocs.

Nutrition & Behavior. Alexander G. Schauss. 1985. (Good Health Guides). (Orig.). pap. 2.95 (*0-87983-374-2*, Keats Pubng) McGraw-Hill Trade.

Nutrition & Behavior Vol. 5. J. R. Galler et al. 1984. LC 83-27035. (Human Nutrition Ser.). (Illus.). 532p. (C). text 132.00 (*0-306-41435-X*, Kluwer Plenum) Kluwer Academic.

Nutrition & Biotechnology in Heart Disease & Cancer: Proceedings of a Conference Held in Research Triangle Park, North Carolina, December 5-7, 1993. J. B. Longenecker et al. 1995. LC 95-7574. (Advances in Experimental Medicine & Biology Ser.: Vol. 369). (Illus.). 278p. (C). 95.00 (*0-306-44994-3*, Kluwer Plenum) Kluwer Academic.

Nutrition & Bone Development. Ed. by David J. Simmons. 1990. (Illus.). 400p. text 59.95 (*0-19-504376-6*) OUP.

Nutrition & Brain Development. Govind A. Dhopeshwarkar. 1983. LC 83-8139. (Illus.). 210p. 55.00 (*0-306-41060-5*, Plenum Trade) Perseus Pubng.

Nutrition & Cancer Prevention. Erica T. Goode et al. Ed. by Sheila Mahoney & Nancy Wiltsek. 1984. (Illus.). 17p. pap. 2.50 (*0-933161-01-8*) Better H Prog.

Nutrition & Cancer Prevention. Thomas E. Moon & Marc S. Micozzi. 1988. (Illus.). 608p. text 250.00 (*0-8247-7993-2*) Dekker.

Nutrition & Cancer Prevention. Ed. by Ronald R. Watson et al. 1995. LC 95-21177. (CRC Modern Nutrition Ser.). 384p. 149.95 (*0-8493-8503-2*, 8503) CRC Pr.

Nutrition & Candida Albicans. Galland. 1989. pap. 4.95 (*0-87983-446-3*, Keats Pubng) McGraw-Hill Trade.

Nutrition & Cardiovascular Disease. Ed. by Ruth J. Hegyeli. 1982. (Progress in Biochemical Pharmacology Ser.: Vol. 19). (Illus.). x, 316p. 201.00 (*3-8055-3571-6*) S Karger.

Nutrition & Cardiovascular Risks. Ed. by J. C. Somogyi et al. 1992. (Bibliotheca Nutritio et Dieta Ser.: No. 49). (Illus.). viii, 154p. 146.25 (*3-8055-5554-7*) S Karger.

Nutrition & Central Nervous System Function. John D. Fernstrom. 1993. 224p. 120.95 (*0-8493-4466-2*, QP136) CRC Pr.

Nutrition & Chronic Disease. Daphne A. Roe. 1997. LC 93-40740. pap. 59.95 (*0-412-07641-1*); 1993. text (*0-442-00974-7*) Chapman & Hall.

Nutrition & Dental Health. Ann Ehrlich. 2nd ed. 1994. LC 93-43043. 243p. (C). mass mkt. 29.75 (*0-8273-5716-8*) Delmar.

Nutrition & Diagnosis-Related Care. Sylvia Escott-Stump. 3rd ed. 1992. LC 91-42187. (Illus.). 617p. pap. text 39.95 (*0-8121-1556-2*); 4th ed. 1997. LC 97-6842. 785p. pap. 54.95 (*0-683-30120-9*) Lppncott W & W.

Nutrition & Diet Therapy. Wardlaw. Date not set. 53.25 net. (*0-07-234648-5*) McGraw.

Nutrition & Diet Therapy. Carroll A. Lutz & Karen R. Przytulski. 2nd ed. 1997. LC 97-4030. (Illus.). 630p. pap. 39.95 (*0-8036-0231-6*) Davis Co.

Nutrition & Diet Therapy. Susan M. Quillman. 2nd ed. 1993. (Notes Ser.). 208p. pap. 18.95 (*0-87434-612-6*) Springhouse Corp.

Nutrition & Diet Therapy. Carroll A. Lutz & Karen Rutherford Przytulski. 3rd ed. 2001. LC 2001-17385. (Illus.). 668p. pap. 49.95 (*0-8036-0804-7*) Davis Co.

Nutrition & Diet Therapy. Cataldo et al. 5th ed. 1998. LC 98-42478. (Health Sciences Ser.). 680p. pap. text 75.95 (*0-534-54594-7*) Wadsworth Pub.

Nutrition & Diet Therapy. Carolynn E. Townsend. 5th ed. 1989. 350p. (gr. 11-12). pap. 33.25 (*0-8273-3456-7*) Delmar.

Nutrition & Diet Therapy. E. Carolynn Townsend. 6th ed. 1994. LC 93-38517. (LPN/LVN Nursing Ser.). 519p. (C). mass mkt. 36.00 (*0-8273-5745-1*) Delmar.

Nutrition & Diet Therapy. Sue Rodwell Williams. 8th ed. 1998. tchr. ed. (*0-8151-9485-4*); 1997. (Illus.). 880p. (C). (gr. 13). text 64.00 (*0-8151-9273-8*, 28383) Mosby Inc.

Nutrition & Diet Therapy: A Nursing Approach. Michele Grodner et al. 1995. (Illus.). 768p. (C). (gr. 13). pap. text 43.00 (*0-8151-4041-X*, 24638) Mosby Inc.

Nutrition & Diet Therapy: Instructor's Guide. Carolynn E. Townsend. 6th ed. 1994. 39p. tchr. ed. 14.95 (*0-8273-6295-1*) Delmar.

Nutrition & Diet Therapy: Principles & Practice. Corinne B. Cataldo et al. Ed. by Marshall. 3rd ed. 1992. 613p. (C). pap. 52.50 (*0-314-93359-X*) West Pub.

Nutrition & Diet Therapy: Principles & Practice. Corinne B. Cataldo et al. 4th ed. 1995. LC 95-16288. 750p. (C). 57.95 (*0-314-04448-5*) West Pub.

Nutrition & Diet Therapy: Self-Instructional Modules. Peggy S. Stanfield & Y. H. Hui. 3rd ed. 1996. LC 96-28764. (Nursing Ser.). (Illus.). 576p. (C). pap. text 49.95 (*0-7637-0154-8*, 0154-8) Jones & Bartlett.

Nutrition & Diet Therapy Dictionary see Nutrition & Diet Therapy Reference Dictionary

Nutrition & Diet Therapy Dictionary. Virginia S. Claudio & Rosalinda T. Lagua. 3rd ed. 1991. (Illus.). 420p. pap. 69.00 (*0-442-00465-6*, VNR) Wiley.

Nutrition & Diet Therapy Reference Dictionary. Rosalinda T. Lagua & Virginia S. Claudio. 4th ed. 1995. LC 95-14630. Orig. Title: Nutrition & Diet Therapy Dictionary. 491p. (C). pap. 44.00 (*0-412-07061-8*); 80.00 (*0-412-07051-0*) Aspen Pub.

Nutrition & Diet Therapy Seven Prospectus. Sue Rodwell Williams. 1993. (*0-8016-8033-6*) Mosby Inc.

Nutrition & Dietary Advice in the Pharmacy. Pamela M. Mason. 1994. LC 93-42676. (Illus.). 304p. pap. 28.00 (*0-632-03427-0*) Blackwell Sci.

Nutrition & Dietetics for Health. Barker. 9th ed. 1996. pap. text 33.00 (*0-443-05252-2*) Saunders.

Nutrition & Dietetics for Nurses. Mary E. Beck. (Churchill Livingstone Nursing Text Ser.). (Illus.). 7th ed. 1984. pap. text (*0-443-03121-5*); 8th ed. 1991. 221p. pap. text (*0-443-03557-1*) Church.

Nutrition & Disease: An Annotated Bibliography. Karen Lieberman-Nissen. 1991. LC 90-14114. 190p. text 10.00 (*0-8240-7977-9*, 548) Garland.

Nutrition & Disease Update: Cancer. Ed. by David Kritchevsky & Kenneth K. Carroll. 1994. LC 93-49456. 304p. pap. 55.00 (*0-935315-49-7*) Am Oil Chemists.

Nutrition & Disease Update: Heart Disease. Ed. by David Kritchevsky & Kenneth K. Carroll. 1994. LC 93-49457. 288p. pap. 50.00 (*0-935315-50-0*) Am Oil Chemists.

Nutrition & Exercise Immunology. David C. Nieman & Bente Klarlund Pedersen. 2000. LC 00-21954. (Archives of the Holocaust Ser.). 208p. 89.95 (*0-8493-0741-4*) CRC Pr.

Nutrition & Feeding of Infants & Toddlers. Rosanne B. Howard & Harland S. Winter. 1984. 448p. 43.00 (*0-316-37473-3*, Little Brwn Med Div) Lppncott W & W.

***Nutrition & Fitness Pt. 2: Metabolic Studies in Health & Disease 4th International Conference on Nutrition & Fitness, Athens, May 2000.** Ed. by A. P. Simopoulos & K. N. Pavlou. 2001. (World Review of Nutrition & Dietetics Ser.: Vol. 90). (Illus.). xxiv, 200p. 198.25 (*3-8055-7211-5*) S Karger.

***Nutrition & Fitness, Diet, Genes, Physical Activity & Health Metabolic Studies in Health & Disease: 4th International conference on Nutrition & Fitness, Athens, May 2000.** Ed. by A. P. Simopoulos & K. N. Pavlou. 2nd abr. rev. ed. 2001. (World Review of Nutrition & Dietetics Ser.: Vol. 89). (Illus.). 198.25 (*3-8055-7190-9*) S Karger.

Nutrition & Fitness for Athletes, Pt. I. Ed. by Artemis P. Simopoulos & Konstantinos N. Pavlou. 1993. LC 93-18147. (World Review of Nutrition & Dietetics Ser.: Vol. 71). (Illus.). xvi, 200p. 257.50 (*3-8055-5707-8*) S Karger.

Nutrition & Fitness for Athletes, Nutrition & Fitness in Health & Disease & in Growth & Development Pts. I & II: Complete Set. Ed. by A. P. Simopoulos & Konstatinos N. Pavlou. 1993. (World Review of Nutrition & Dietetics Ser.: Vol. 71 & 72). (Illus.). xxx, 444p. 505.25 (*3-8055-5709-4*) S Karger.

Nutrition & Fitness in Health & Disease & in Growth & Development, Pt. II. Ed. by A. P. Simpoulos. 1993. (World Review of Nutrition & Dietetics Ser.: Vol. 72). (Illus.). xiv, 244p. 304.50 (*3-8055-5706-X*) S Karger.

Nutrition & Food Deficiencies Animals. Ed. by Miroslav Rechcigl. 1978. 307.00 (*0-8493-2797-0*, RC620); Vol. III. 388p. 70.50 (*0-8493-2798-9*) Franklin (CRC Reprint).

Nutrition & Food Preparation & Preventive Care & Maintenance. S. C. Lehman. 1981. (Lifeworks Ser.). text 13.96 (*0-07-037094-X*) McGraw.

Nutrition & Gene Expression. Ed. by Carolyn D. Berdanier & James L. Hargrove. 1992. 592p. 169.00 (*0-8493-6961-4*, QP144) CRC Pr.

Nutrition & Growth Vol. 2. D. B. Jelliffe & E. F. Jelliffe. 1979. LC 78-27076. (Human Nutrition Ser.). (Illus.). 472p. (C). text 110.00 (*0-306-40128-2*, Kluwer Plenum) Kluwer Academic.

Nutrition & Growth in Infancy & Early Childhood. Nancy E. Hitchcock et al. 1986. (Monographs in Pediatrics: Vol. 19). (Illus.). xii, 92p. 68.75 (*3-8055-4223-2*) S Karger.

***Nutrition & Health.** Ed. by Tanya Carr & Koen Descheemaeker. 2001. LC 2001-43889. (*0-632-05844-7*) Blackwell Sci.

Nutrition & Health: Topics & Controversies. Ed. by Felix Bronner. 1995. LC 95-16297. (CRC Series on Modern Nutrition Ser.). (Illus.). 272p. 74.95 (*0-8493-7849-4*, 7849) CRC Pr.

Nutrition & Health Campaign for Women Slide Set & Script Narratives. American Dietetic Association Staff. 1994. 66p. ring bd. 45.95 incl. sl. (*0-88091-141-7*) Am Dietetic Assn.

Nutrition & Health Dictionary. Percy J. Russell & Anita Williams. 3rd ed. 1995. LC 94-17804. 525p. (gr. 13). 55.00 (*0-412-98981-6*) Kluwer Academic.

Nutrition & Health Encyclopedia. David F. Tver. 2nd ed. 1989. pap. 55.95 (*0-442-23397-3*) Aspen Pub.

Nutrition & Health Encyclopedia. Percy J. Russell & Anita Williams. 3rd ed. 1995. LC 94-17804. 525p. pap. 41.00 (*0-412-98991-3*) Aspen Pub.

Nutrition & Health Habits: Discussion. Richard L. Crews & Richard L. Kozlenko. 1988. 80p. (C). stu. ed. (*0-945864-20-5*); pap. text (*0-945864-13-2*) Columbia Pacific U Pr.

Nutrition & Heart Disease. Ed. by H. Naito. 1982. (Monographs of the American College of Nutrition: Vol. 5). 365p. text 37.50 (*0-88331-168-2*) R B Luce.

Nutrition & HIV: A New Model for Treatment. Mary Romeyn. 1998. 353p. pap. text 19.00 (*0-7881-5711-6*) DIANE Pub.

Nutrition & HIV: A New Model for Treatment. Mary Romeyn. 2nd rev. ed. 1998. LC 97-41330. 448p. pap. 19.95 (*0-7879-3964-1*) Jossey-Bass.

Nutrition & Hydration in Hospice Care: Needs, Strategies, Ethics. Ed. by Charlette R. Gallagher-Allred & Madalon O. Amenta. LC 93-50675. (Hospice Journal: Vol. 9, Nos. 2/3). 157p. (C). 1997. pap. 14.95 (*0-7890-0216-7*); 1994. (Illus.). 39.95 (*1-56024-659-6*) Haworth Pr.

Nutrition & Immunology: Principles & Practice. Ed. by M. Eric Gershwin et al. 1999. LC 99-10901. 520p. 149.50 (*0-89603-719-3*) Humana.

Nutrition & Immunology Vol. 8, Vol. 8. D. M. Klurfeld. 1993. (Human Nutrition Ser.). (Illus.). 378p. (C). 110.00 (*0-306-44366-X*, Plenum Trade) Perseus Pubng.

Nutrition & Life. Robert C. Sandness. 1995. 300p. 17.95 (*0-9614076-3-8*) Sandness.

Nutrition & Managed Care Handbook. Ellyn C. Silverman. 1998. 250p. 55.00 (*0-8342-0985-3*, 09853) Aspen Pub.

Nutrition & Meal Planning in Child Care Programs: Practical Guide. Sari Edelstein. 1992. LC 92-355. spiral bd. 15.00 (*0-88091-103-4*) Am Dietetic Assn.

Nutrition & Mental Illness: An Orthomolecular Approach to Balancing Body Chemistry. Carl C. Pfeiffer. 1988. 128p. pap. 12.95 (*0-89281-226-5*, Heal Arts VT) Inner Tradit.

Nutrition & Metabolism in Patient Care. John M. Kinney et al. 1988. (Illus.). 736p. text 195.00 (*0-7216-1156-7*) Saunders.

Nutrition & Metabolism in Renal Disease. Ed. by Shaul G. Massry et al. 1992. (Journal: Vol. 18, Nos. 2-5, 1992). (Illus.). 268p. pap. 250.50 (*3-8055-5691-8*) S Karger.

Nutrition & Metabolism in Renal Disease: Proceedings of the 8th International Congress on Renal Nutrition & Metabolism, Naples, October, 1996. Ed. by J. D. Kopple et al. 1997. (Mineral & Electrolyte Metabolism Ser.: Vol. 23, Nos. 3-6, 1997). (Illus.). iv, 194p. pap. 86.25 (*3-8055-6586-0*) S Karger.

Nutrition & Metabolism in Renal Disease Vol. 22, No. 1-3: International Society of Renal Nutrition & Metabolism. Ed. by Shaul G. Massry et al. 1995. (Journal: Vol. 22, No. 1-3, 1996). (Illus.). 202p. pap. 129.75 (*3-8055-6249-7*) S Karger.

Nutrition & Metabolism in the Surgical Patient. Ed. by Josef E. Fischer. 2nd rev. ed. 1996. LC 95-31028. 704p. text 215.00 (*0-316-28390-8*) Lppncott W & W.

Nutrition & Metabolism of the Fetus & Infant. Ed. by H. K. Visser. 1979. (Nutricia Symposium Ser.: No. 5). text 171.00 (*90-247-2202-0*) Kluwer Academic.

Nutrition & Nervous System: Proceedings of the European Nutritionists Group Symposium, 9th, Chianciano, 1970. European Nutritionists Group Symposium Staff. Ed. by J. C. Somogyi & F. Fidanza. 1972. (Bibliotheca Nutritio et Dieta Ser.: No. 17). (Illus.). 202p. pap. 68.00 (*3-8055-1309-7*) S Karger.

Nutrition & Neurobiology. Ed. by J. C. Somogyi. 1986. (Bibliotheca Nutritio et Dieta Ser.: No. 38). (Illus.). viii, 224p. 155.75 (*3-8055-4246-1*) S Karger.

Nutrition & Performance, Vol 7/1-2. C. F. Consolazio. 1983. (Illus.). 200p. pap. 92.00 (*0-08-031013-3*, 38, Pergamon Pr) Elsevier.

Nutrition & Physical Degeneration. Weston A. Price. 6th ed. 1997. LC 97-41920. 528p. pap. 20.95 (*0-87983-816-7*, 38167K, Keats Pubng) McGraw-Hill Trade.

Nutrition & Physical Degeneration. Weston A. Price. 9th ed. 1977. (Illus.). 560p. 34.95 (*0-916764-00-1*) Price-Pottenger.

Nutrition & Pregnancy: A Complete Guide from Preconception to Postdelivery. Judith E. Brown. 1998. LC 97-38624. 240p. 25.00 (*1-56565-790-X*, 07909W, Anodyne) Lowell Hse.

Nutrition & Pregnancy: A Complete Guide from Preconception to Postdelivery. Judith E. Brown. 1998. LC 97-38624. (Illus.). 288p. reprint ed. pap. 16.00 (*0-7373-0018-3*, 00183W) NTC Contemp Pub Co.

Nutrition & Psychotropic Drugs in the Elderly. David A. Smith. Date not set. (Geriatric Psychopathology Ser.). (Orig.). pap. 29.95 (*1-884937-29-2*) Manisses Communs.

Nutrition & Reproduction. Ed. by George A. Bray & Donna H. Ryan. 1998. LC 98-10771. (Pennington Center Nutrition Ser.: Vol. 8). 460p. text 110.00 (*0-8071-2306-4*) La State U Pr.

Nutrition & Stress. Harold S. Rosenberg. Ed. by Richard A. Passwater & Earl R. Mindell. 1983. (Good Health Guides). 32p. pap. 3.95 (*0-87983-298-3*, 32983K, Keats Pubng) McGraw-Hill Trade.

Nutrition & Technology of Foods for Growing Humans: Proceedings of the European Nutritionists Group Symposium, Zurich, 1971. European Nutritionists Group Symposium Staff. Ed. by J. C. Somogyi. 1972. (Bibliotheca Nutritio et Dieta Ser.: No. 18). (Illus.). 200p. pap. 80.00 (*3-8055-1317-8*) S Karger.

Nutrition & the Adult: Macronutrients, Vol. 3A. R. B. Alfin-Slater & D. Kritchevsky. 1980. LC 79-25119. (Human Nutrition Ser.). (Illus.). 308p. (C). text 110.00 (*0-306-40287-4*, Kluwer Plenum) Kluwer Academic.

Nutrition & the Adult Vol. 3B: Micronutrients. R. B. Alfin-Slater & D. Kritchevsky. 1980. LC 79-25119. (Human Nutrition Ser.). (Illus.). 450p. (C). text 110.00 (*0-306-40288-2*, Kluwer Plenum) Kluwer Academic.

Nutrition & the Cancer Patient. Abby S. Bloch & Joyce D. Margie. 1983. LC 81-70351. 269p. pap. 11.95 (*0-8019-7120-9*) NP-Chilton.

Nutrition & the Diabetic Child: Proceedings of the 4th Beilinson Symposium, Herzlya, May 21-24, 1978. International Beilinson Symposium Staff. Ed. by Laron Zvi & Karp Moshe. 1980. (Pediatric & Adolescent Endocrinology Ser.: Vol. 7). pap. 159.25 (*3-8055-3019-6*) S Karger.

Nutrition & the Female Athlete. Jaime S. Ruud. 1996. LC 96-11966. (Nutrition in Exercise & Sport Ser.). 176p. 69.95 (*0-8493-7917-2*) CRC Pr.

Nutrition & the Immune Response. Ed. by J. Dwight Stinnett. 1983. LC 82-17708. 160p. 119.00 (*0-8493-5650-4*, RC623, CRC Reprint) Franklin.

Nutrition & the Quality of Life. Ed. by Geoffrey H. Bourne. 1987. (World Review of Nutrition & Dietetics Ser.: Vol. 49). (Illus.). x, 218p. 168.75 (*3-8055-4450-2*) S Karger.

Nutrition & Ventilatory Function. Ed. by R. D. Ferranti et al. 1992. LC 92-2313. (Current Topics in Rehabilitation Ser.). (Illus.). 200p. 69.95 (*0-387-19776-1*) Spr-Verlag.

Nutrition & Weight Control Study Guide. Patricia A. Eisenman et al. 1990. (American Coaching Effectiveness Program Ser.). (Illus.). 216p. spiral bd. 32.00 (*0-88011-385-5*, ACEP0207) Human Kinetics.

Nutrition & Women's Cancers. Barbara C. Pence & Dale M. Dunn. 1998. (Modern Nutrition Ser.). 192p. 84.95 (*0-8493-8562-8*) CRC Pr.

Nutrition Applied to Injury Rehabilitation & Sports Medicine. Luke R. Bucci. 1994. 304p. 131.95 (*0-8493-7913-X*, 7913) CRC Pr.

***Nutrition as Medicine.** Dharma Singh Khalsa. pap. (*0-7434-4228-8*) PB.

Nutrition, Cancer & You: What You Need to Know, & Where to Start. Susan Calhoun & Jane Bradley. Ed. by Michael McKenzie. 1996. LC 96-85765. 192p. pap. 12.95 (*1-886110-06-9*) Addax Pubng.

Nutrition Care. Moore. 4th ed. 2000. LC 00-45244. (Mosby's Pocket Guide Ser.). (Illus.). xii, 532p. 22.95 (*0-323-00843-7*) Mosby Inc.

Nutrition Care in Nursing Facilities. Clara L. Gerwick & Consultant Dietitians in Health Care Facilities St. 2nd rev. ed. 1992. LC 92-49942. pap. text 28.00 (*0-88091-105-0*) Am Dietetic Assn.

Nutrition Care of People with Diabetes Mellitus: A Nutrition Reference for Health Professionals. Penelope S. Easton et al. 1991. 89.95 (*1-56022-004-X*); LC 90-13936. 263p. pap. 39.95 (*1-56022-007-4*) Haworth Jrnl Co-Edits.

Nutrition Casebook on Developmental Disabilities. Ninfa S. Springer. 1982. LC 81-21383. 39.95 (*0-8156-2266-X*); pap. 16.95 (*0-8156-2259-7*) Syracuse U Pr.

Nutrition Challenge for Women. Louise Lambert-Lagace. 1990. 192p. pap. 12.95 (*0-923521-06-2*) Bull Pub.

Nutrition Chemistry & Biology. Julian F. Spallholz & Mallory Boylan. 2nd ed. 1998. LC 98-34621. (CRC Series in Modern Nutrition Ser.). 368p. 69.95 (*0-8493-8504-0*) CRC Pr.

Nutrition Counseling & Comunication Skills. Katharine Curry & Amy Jaffe. Ed. by Maura Connor. 1997. LC 97-34828. (Illus.). 384p. pap. text 32.95 (*0-7216-7298-1*) Saunders.

***Nutrition Counseling in Treatment of Eating Disorders.** Marcia Herrin. 2001. LC 2001-52573. 400p. (C). text 34.95 (*1-58391-031-X*) Brunner-Routledge.

Nutrition Counseling Skills for Medical Nutrition Therapy. Linda G. Snetselaar. 1997. LC 96-53385. 375p. 67.00 (*0-8342-0755-9*) Aspen Pub.

Nutrition Curriculum Activities Kit, Level 1. Paul E. Bell et al. 1986. LC 86-4203. (Illus.). 288p. pap., tchr. ed. 27.95 (*0-87628-617-1*, C-6171-7) Ctr Appl Res.

Nutrition Curriculum Activities Kits, Level 2. Paul E. Bell et al. 1987. (Illus.). 352p. pap., tchr. ed. 27.95 (*0-87628-618-X*, C-618X-3) Ctr Appl Res.

Nutrition Debate: Sorting Out Some Answers. Joan D. Gussow & Paul Thomas. 1986. LC 86-21616. 400p. (Orig.). pap. 8.00 (*0-915950-66-9*) Bull Pub.

Nutrition Desk Reference. Robert H. Garrison, Jr. & Elizabeth Somer. 1985. LC 84-26098. 264p. (C). 34.95 (*0-87983-523-0*, Keats Pubng) McGraw-Hill Trade.

Nutrition During Lactation. Institute of Medicine Staff. 1991. 326p. 34.95 (*0-309-04391-3*) Natl Acad Pr.

Nutrition During Pregnancy: Part I: Weight Gain, Part II: Nutrient Supplements, Pts. 1 & 2. Ed. by Committee on Nutritional Status During Pregnancy. 1990. 480p. 34.95 (*0-309-04138-4*) Natl Acad Pr.

Nutrition During Pregnancy & Lactation: An Implementation Guide. Institute of Medicine Staff. 1992. LC 92-19175. 144p. (Orig.). (C). pap. 14.95 (*0-309-04738-2*) Natl Acad Pr.

Nutrition Education: Study Guide. Ed. by Deakin University Press Staff. 1988. (C). pap. (*0-7300-0621-2*, SHN770) Deakin Univ AUS. *Dist:* St Mut.

Nutrition Education & Modern Concepts of Food Assimilation. Ed. by Geoffrey H. Bourne. 1982. (World Review of Nutrition & Dietetics Ser.: Vol. 40). (Illus.). xii, 192p. 141.75 (*3-8055-3519-8*) S Karger.

Nutrition Education Consultant. Jack Rudman. 1994. (Career Examination Ser.: C-2740). pap. 34.95 (*0-8373-2740-7*) Nat Learn.

Nutrition, Endocrinology & Disease. Ed. by George A. Bray & Donna H. Ryan. 1995. LC 95-18626. (Pennington Center Nutrition Ser.: Vol. 4). (Illus.). xiii, 232p. text 60.00 (*0-8071-1954-7*) La State U Pr.

Nutrition Essentials & Diet Therapy. Nancy J. Peckenpaugh & Charlotte M. Poleman. Ed. by Maura Connor. 8th ed. 1998. LC 98-48476. (Illus.). 635p. (C). pap. text 32.95 (*0-7216-7707-X*) Saunders.

Nutrition Factor: Its Role in National Development. Alan Berg. 1973. LC 73-1081. 290p. pap. 16.95 (*0-8157-0913-7*) Brookings.

Nutrition Facts for Better Bodies. Robert S. Wennik. 1995. LC 95-7324. (*1-56796-097-9*) WRS Group.

Nutrition for a Healthy Heart. Robert J. Peshek. 1979. (Illus.). 20.00 (*0-9605902-2-6*) Color Coded Charting.

Nutrition for a Healthy Pregnancy: The Complete Guide to Eating Before, During, & after Your Pregnancy. Elizabeth Somer. 1995. LC 94-42167. 256p. pap. 17.00 (*0-8050-3775-6*, Owl) H Holt & Co.

Nutrition for God's Temple. Dick Couey. 1993. LC 93-20409. (Studies in Health & Human Services: Vol. 22). 664p. pap. 109.95 (*0-7734-9288-7*); text 129.95 (*0-7734-9286-0*) E Mellen.

Nutrition for Health & Health Care. Eleanor N. Whitney et al. 2nd ed. 2000. LC 00-36513. (Health Sciences Ser.). (Illus.). 800p. 73.95 (*0-534-51552-5*) Wadsworth Pub.

***Nutrition for Health, Fitness, & Sport.** Melvin H. Williams. 6th ed. 2001. LC 2001-30629. (Illus.). xv, 509p. (*0-07-112288-5*) McGraw.

Nutrition for Nurses. O. L. Oke & Ojofeitimi. 1985. pap. text (*0-582-77705-4*) Addison-Wesley GBR. *Dist:* Trans-Atl Phila.

Nutrition for Pregnancy: Focus on Healthy Outcomes. Carol A. Hickey et al. 1994. LC 93-49591. (Maternal Nutrition Ser.: No. 3). (*0-86525-057-X*) March of Dimes.

Nutrition for Primary Care. Heber. 1999. text (*0-7216-4300-0*) Saunders.

Nutrition for Recovery: A Patient's Guide. Kathryn J. Reichert. 1993. 36.95 (*0-8493-8652-7*, RC552) CRC Pr.

Nutrition for Recovery: Eating Disorders. Kathryn J. Reichert. 1993. 144p. 65.00 (*0-8493-8651-9*, RC552) CRC Pr.

Nutrition for the Hospitalized Patient: Basic Science & Principles of Practice. Ed. by Michael H. Torosian. 1995. LC 94-43115. (Illus.). 712p. text 185.00 (*0-8247-9292-0*) Dekker.

Nutrition for the 90s. Judy Rainwater. 1992. pap., spiral bd. 13.50 (*0-9622066-1-X*) Ranrai Pub.

Nutrition for the Recreational Athlete. Ed. by Catherine G. Ratzin-Jackson. 1995. LC 94-19402. (Nutrition in Exercise & Sport Ser.). 272p. 94.95 (*0-8493-7914-8*) CRC Pr.

Nutrition for Vegetarians. Agatha Thrash & Calvin L. Thrash. 1982. (Illus.). 155p. pap. 7.95 (*0-942658-03-5*) NLB.

Nutrition, Genetics & Heart Disease. Ed. by George A. Bray & Donna H. Ryan. 1996. LC 96-9007. (Pennington Center Nutrition Ser.: Vol. 6). (Illus.). 408p. (C). text 75.00 (*0-8071-2051-0*) La State U Pr.

Nutrition, Genetics & Obesity. Ed. by George A. Bray & Donna H. Ryan. 1999. LC 98-50606. (Pennington Center Nutrition Ser.: Vol. 9). (Illus.). xviii, 568p. text 110.00 (*0-8071-2407-9*) La State U Pr.

Nutrition, Growth & Development: Proceedings of the International Symposium, Valencia, May, 1973. Ed. by C. A. Canosa et al. 1974. (Modern Problems in Pediatrics Ser.: Vol. 14). (Illus.). 85.25 (*3-8055-1757-2*) S Karger.

***Nutrition Handbook: A Guide to Assessment, Therapy & Education.** Patricia Worthington & Beth Wagner. 2001. (Illus.). 430p. pap. (*0-7216-6964-6*) Saunders.

Nutrition Handbook for AIDS. Jean E. Schreiner. 2nd ed. 1990. LC 91-118966. (Illus.). 134p. ring bd. 34.95 (*0-9622157-1-6*) Carrot Top Nutrition.

Nutrition Handbook for HIV/AIDS. Jean E. Schreiner. 3rd rev. ed. 1999. (Illus.). 165p. ring bd. 42.95 (*0-9622157-3-2*, HB301) Carrot Top Nutrition.

Nutrition Handbook for Nursing Practice. Susan G. Dudek. 4th ed. 2001. LC 00-41261. (Illus.). xv, 767p. pap. text 39.95 (*0-7817-2344-2*) Lppncott W & W.

***Nutrition, Immunity & Infections.** P. Shetty. 2001. 224p. pap. text 45.00 (*0-85199-531-4*) OUP.

Nutrition in Aging. Eleanor D. Schlenker. 3rd ed. 1997. LC 97-9477. (Illus.). 464p. pap. 48.44 (*0-8151-8504-9*, WCB McGr Hill) McGrw-H Hghr Educ.

Nutrition in Arabian Gulf Countries: Malnutrition & Minerals. Ed. by Geoffrey H. Bourne. 1987. (World Review of Nutrition & Dietetics Ser.: Vol. 54). (Illus.). xii, 292p. 226.75 (*3-8055-4682-3*) S Karger.

Nutrition in Cancer & Trauma-Sepsis. Ed. by F. Bozzetti & R. Dionigi. 1985. (Illus.). viii, 204p. pap. 64.50 (*3-8055-3959-2*) S Karger.

Nutrition in Cancer Care: A Quick Reference for Nutritional Oncology. Jeanette M. Dunn & Carole A. Mutzebaugh. Ed. by Brenda Garritson & Lizbeth Adams. 1997. (Illus.). viii, 132p. pap. (*1-891814-03-6*) Found Care Mgmt.

Nutrition in Clinical Care. Rosanne B. Howard. Ed. by Nancy H. Herbold. 2nd ed. 1982. (Illus.). 800p. (C). text 42.95 (*0-07-030514-5*) McGraw.

Nutrition in Clinical Dentistry. Abraham E. Nizel & Papas. 3rd ed. 1989. 400p. pap. text 48.50 (*0-7216-2423-5*) Saunders.

Nutrition in Clinical Nursing. Idamarie Laquatra. 1990. (Nursing Education Ser.). pap. 31.50 (*0-8273-3075-8*) Delmar.

Nutrition in Clinical Practice. Marion Nestle. 1986. LC 85-60806. 330p. (Orig.). pap. 19.95 (*0-930010-11-6*) Jones Med.

Nutrition in Clinical Practice: Proceedings of the Congress of the European Society of Parenteral & Enteral Nutrition (ESPEN), Leipzig, August 1988, 10th. Ed. by G. Dietze et al. 1989. (Illus.). x, 308p. 101.75 (*3-8055-4894-X*) S Karger.

Nutrition in Developmental Transition in South-East Asia. C. Gopalan. 1992. (SEARO Regional Health Papers: No. 21). xi, 130p. pap. text 10.00 (*92-9022-190-9*, 1580021) World Health.

Nutrition in Disease & Development. Ed. by Geoffrey H. Bourne. 1982. (World Review of Nutrition & Dietetics Ser.: Vol. 39). (Illus.). x, 194p. 139.25 (*3-8055-3459-0*) S Karger.

Nutrition in Early Childhood & Its Effects in Later Life. Ed. by J. C. Somogyi. 1982. (Bibliotheca Nutritio et Dieta Ser.: No. 31). (Illus.). viii, 144p. pap. 92.25 (*3-8055-3527-9*) S Karger.

Nutrition in Europe. Ed. by Leif Hambraeus. 1981. 150p. text 56.50 (*0-86598-059-4*) Rowman.

Nutrition in Exercise & Sport. Ed. by James F. Hickson, Jr. & Ira Wolinsky. 1989. 448p. 110.00 (*0-8493-4759-9*, TX361, CRC Reprint) Franklin.

Nutrition in General Practice: Giving Advice to Women. Nicola Seabrook. 1997. LC 97-24706. 208p. pap. text 37.50 (*0-7506-3464-2*) Buttrwrth-Heinemann.

Nutrition in Health Maintenance & Health Promotion for Primary Care Providers: A Self-Instructional Module. Yolanda M. Gutierrez. 1994. 262p. (Orig.). pap. 45.00 (*0-943671-10-8*) UCSF Schl Nursing.

Nutrition in Infancy & Childhood. Christine M. Trahms & Peggy L. Pipes. 6th ed. 1997. LC 97-70088. (Illus.). 480p. (C). pap. 48.44 (*0-8151-8455-7*) McGrw-H Hghr Educ.

Nutrition in Major Metabolic Diseases. Ed. by C. Gopalan & Kamala Krishnaswamy. 1997. (Illus.). 252p. text 29.95 (*0-19-564100-0*) OUP.

Nutrition in Pediatrics. W. Allan Walker & John B. Watkins. 2nd ed. 1996. LC 97-222636. 850p. 220.00 (*1-55009-026-7*) Blackwell Sci.

Nutrition in Pediatrics. W. Allan Walker & John B. Watkins. 1985. 830p. 120.00 (*0-316-91831-8*, Little Brwn Med Div) Lppncott W & W.

Nutrition in Pregnancy. Worthington. 7th ed. 2000. 32.25 net. (*0-07-230083-3*) McGraw.

Nutrition in Pregnancy & Growth. Ed. by P. J. Walter & M. Porrini. 1996. LC 96-19370. (Bibliotheca Nutritio et Dieta Ser.: No. 53, 1996). (Illus.). viii, 138p. 160.00 (*3-8055-6300-0*) S Karger.

Nutrition in Pregnancy & Lactation. Bonnie S. Worthington-Roberts & Sue Rodwell Williams. 6th ed. 1996. LC 96-32246. (Illus.). 576p. (C). pap. 48.44 (*0-8151-9522-2*) McGrw-H Hghr Educ.

Nutrition in Preventive Pediatrics. Ed. by R. Di Toro. 1989. (Contributions to Infusion Therapy Ser.: Vol. 22). (Illus.). vi, 168p. 65.25 (*3-8055-4852-4*) S Karger.

Nutrition in Primary Care. David L. Katz. 2000. LC 00-55875. 432p. (Orig.). pap. text 49.95 (*0-683-30638-3*) Lppncott W & W.

Nutrition in Primary Care. Briony Thomas. 1996. LC 96-30134. 256p. (Orig.). pap. 39.95 (*0-632-03981-7*) Blackwell Sci.

Nutrition in Public Health: A Handbook for Developing Programs & Services. Mildred Kaufman. 1990. LC 90-51. 592p. (C). 103.00 (*0-8342-0144-5*) Aspen Pub.

Nutrition in Sport. Ronald J. Maughan et al. 2000. LC 99-12066. (Encyclopedia of Sports Medicine Ser.: Vol. 7). (Illus.). 704p. 127.00 (*0-632-05094-2*) Blackwell Sci.

Nutrition in the Infant: Problems & Practical Procedures. Ed. by Victor Preedy et al. 2001. (Greenwich Medical Media Ser.). (Illus.). 448p. text (*1-900151-62-6*) Greenwich Med GBR. *Dist:* JAMCO Dist.

Nutrition in the 90s: Current Controversies & Analysis. Ed. by Gerald E. Gaull et al. 1991. (Illus.). 136p. text 49.50 (*0-8247-8525-8*) Dekker.

Nutrition in the 90s: Current Controversies in Nutrition. Frank N. Kotsonis & M. A. Mackey. Date not set. (*0-8247-9980-1*) Dekker.

Nutrition in the Prevention of Disease. Ed. by J. C. Somogyi & S. Hejda. 1989. (Bibliotheca Nutritio et Dieta Ser.: No. 44). (Illus.). v, 187p. 147.00 (*3-8055-4962-8*) S Karger.

Nutrition in Women's Health. Debra Krummel & Penny M. Kris-Etherton. 1995. LC 95-24231. 608p. 68.00 (*0-8342-0682-X*) Aspen Pub.

Nutrition Issues in Developing Countries: Part I: Diarrheal Diseases, Part II: Diet & Activity During Pregnancy & Lactation, Pts. 1 & 2. Ed. by Subcommittee on Nutrition and Diarrheal Control. 1992. 206p. pap. text 28.00 (*0-309-04092-2*) Natl Acad Pr.

Nutrition Labeling: Issues & Directions for the 1990s. Institute of Medicine Staff. 1990. 372p. pap. 34.95 (*0-309-04326-3*) Natl Acad Pr.

Nutrition Learning Packages: Joint WHO-UNICEF Nutrition Support Programme. 1989. (ENG, FRE & SPA.). vii, 170p. pap. text 30.00 (*92-4-154251-9*, 1150328) World Health.

Nutrition Management for Food Services. Leslie Cummings. (Food & Hospitality Ser.). 1990. pap., tchr. ed. 11.95 (*0-8273-3523-7*); 1989. text 44.25 (*0-8273-3522-9*) Delmar.

Nutrition Management of the Cancer Patient: A Practical Guide for Professionals. Abby S. Bloch. 1990. 431p. (C). 102.00 (*0-8342-0132-1*) Aspen Pub.

Nutrition Manual for At-Risk Infants & Toddlers. Ed. by Janice H. Cox. rev. ed. 1997. LC 96-49613. 248p. 59.95 (*0-944496-47-4*) Precept Pr.

Nutrition Matters: People, Food & Famine. Helen Young & Susanne Jaspers. 1995. LC 96-176128. 144p. pap. (*1-85339-243-X*) Intermed Tech GBR. *Dist:* Stylus Pub VA.

Nutrition Monitoring in the U. S., Chartbook: Selected Findings from the National Nutrition Monitoring & Related Research Program, No. 1. 1994. lib. bdg. 250.00 (*0-8490-8405-9*) Gordon Pr.

Nutrition Now. Judith E. Brown. 1995. LC 94-42869. 712p. (C). 49.95 (*0-314-04447-7*) West Pub.

***Nutrition Now.** Judy Brown. 3rd ed. 2001. 600p. (YA). pap. text 62.95 (*0-534-58007-6*) Wadsworth Pub.

Nutrition Nuggets & More: A Companion to Lowfat Lifestyle. Ronda Gates. 1990. (Illus.). 256p. (Orig.). pap. 10.95 (*1-878319-00-0*) Lifestyles Four.

Nutrition of Older Adults. 240p. pap. (*0-340-60156-6*) E A GBR. *Dist:* Routldge.

Nutrition of Older Adults. Geoffrey P. Webb & June Copeman. 1996. (Illus.). 238p. (Orig.). pap. 39.95 (*1-56593-768-6*, 1494) Singular Publishing.

Nutrition of the Rabbit. C. Blas & J. Wiseman. 1999. LC 98-7573. 352p. text 100.00 (*0-85199-279-X*) OUP.

Nutrition, Physical Activity, & Health in Early Life: Studies in Preschool Children. Jana Parizkova. 1996. LC 95-41134. (Nutrition in Exercise & Sport Ser.). 320p. 94.95 (*0-8493-7919-9*) CRC Pr.

Nutrition, Physiology & Obesity. Rachel Schemmel. 1980. 240p. 140.00 (*0-8493-5471-4*, RC628, CRC Reprint) Franklin.

Nutrition Policy Implementation: Issues & Experience. Ed. by Nevin S. Schrimshaw & Mitchel B. Wallerstein. 1982. (Illus.). 572p. 110.00 (*0-306-40858-9*, Plenum Trade) Perseus Pubng.

Nutrition Policy in Public Health. Ed. by Felix Bronner. 1997. LC 97-3392. (Illus.). 336p. 52.95 (*0-8261-9660-8*) Springer Pub.

Nutrition Power Talks: Over 1,000 Nutrition Ideas for Health Professionals. Linda Marcoux. Date not set. (Illus.). 157p. (Orig.). pap. (*0-9633536-0-8*) Hlth TREND.

***Nutrition Recommendations: The Report of the Scientific Review Committee.** 208p. pap. (*0-660-13417-9*) Can7 Govern Pub CAN. *Dist:* Intl Spec Bk.

Nutrition Research in South-East Asia: The Emerging Agenda of the Future. C. Gopalan. 1994. (WHO Regional Publications: No. 23). pap. text 15.00 (*92-9022-166-6*, 1560023) World Health.

Nutrition Screening, Assessment, & Guidance During Pregnancy. Carolyn O. Sharbaugh & Carol W. Suitor. 1994. LC 93-49497. (Maternal Nutrition Ser.: No. 7). (*0-86525-043-X*) March of Dimes.

Nutrition Second Metabolism in Pregnancy: Mother & Fetus. Pedro Rosso. 1990. (Illus.). 336p. text 59.95 (*0-19-503928-9*) OUP.

Nutrition Secrets: Questions You Will Be Asked in the Clinic, at the Bedside, on Exams. Charles W. Van Way. 1998. LC 98-21357. (Secrets Ser.). 275p. pap. 39.95 (*1-56053-206-8*) Hanley & Belfus.

Nutrition Services Consultant. Jack Rudman. 1994. (Career Examination Ser.: C-2836). pap. 34.95 (*0-8373-2836-5*) Nat Learn.

Nutrition Services in Perinatal Care. Institute of Medicine, Food and Nutrition Board. 2nd ed. 1992. LC 92-60920. 128p. (C). pap. text 19.00 (*0-309-04694-7*) Natl Acad Pr.

Nutrition, Stress & Aging: An Holistic Approach. Donald R. Morse & Robert L. Pollack. 1988. LC 87-45805. (Stress in Modern Society Ser.: No. 17). 32.50 (*0-404-63268-8*) AMS Pr.

Nutrition Support: Theory & Therapeutics. Scott A. Shikora. Ed. by George L. Blackburn. 1995. LC 96-28658. (Clinical Nutrition Ser.). 598p. 91.00 (*0-412-06681-5*) Aspen Pub.

Nutrition Support Handbook. Laura E. Matarese et al. 1997. (Illus.). 111p. (Orig.). 20.00 (*0-9615424-5-4*) Cleveland Clinic.

Nutrition Support in Home Health. Mindy Hermann-Zaidins & Riva Touger-Decker. 1989. LC 89-6701. 273p. (C). 74.00 (*0-8342-0059-7*) Aspen Pub.

Nutrition Support in the Critically Ill: A Handbook. Alexa Scott et al. 1997. 250p. 34.95 (*1-56593-874-7*, 1712) Singular Publishing.

Nutrition Support Policies, Procedures, Forms & Formulas. Annalynn Skipper. 1995. 500p. ring bd. 167.00 (*0-8342-0716-8*) Aspen Pub.

Nutrition Therapy: Advanced Counseling Skills. Ed. by Kathy K. Helm. 1995. (Illus.). 256p. (Orig.). (C). pap., wbk. ed. 14.95 (*0-9631033-3-4*); pap. text, stu. ed. 65.00 (*0-9631033-2-6*) Helm Seminars.

Nutrition Therapy: Advanced Counseling Skills. Ed. by Kathy K. Helm & Bridget Klawitter. 1995. (Illus.). 256p. (Orig.). (C). pap. 39.95 (*0-9631033-1-8*) Helm Seminars.

Nutrition Through the Life Cycle: Case Studies for the Dietary Manager. Litchford. 1997. 136p. spiral bd. 21.00 (*0-7872-3604-7*) Kendall-Hunt.

Nutrition Through the Lifecycle I: User's Guide. Mary D. Litchford et al. 1997. (C). pap., stu. ed. 7.00 (*1-880989-34-4*); 1994. 139.00 (*1-880989-31-X*); 1994. 139.00 (*1-880989-32-8*); 1994. 139.00 (*1-880989-33-6*); 1994. 139.00 (*1-880989-30-1*) Case Sftware.

Nutrition Through the Lifecycle II. Mary D. Litchford et al. 1995. 139.00 (*1-880989-46-8*); 139.00 (*1-880989-47-6*); 139.00 (*1-880989-48-4*); 139.00 (*1-880989-49-2*); (C). pap., stu. ed. 7.00 (*1-880989-50-6*) Case Sftware.

Nutrition Throughout the Life Cycle. Bonnie S. Worthington-Roberts & Sue R. Williams. 3rd ed. 1995. (Illus.). 528p. (C). pap. 72.19 (*0-8151-9427-7*) McGrw-H Hghr Educ.

Nutrition Throughout the Lifecycle. Roberts. 5th ed. 2002. 48.00 net. (*0-07-231615-2*) McGraw.

Nutrition, Toxicity & Cancer. Ian R. Rowland. 1991. 568p. 159.00 (*0-8493-8812-0*, QP141) CRC Pr.

Nutrition Two-Thousand Ed. by John A. Weyl. 1992. (Illus.). (Orig.). Set. 824p. pap. 69.90 (*0-9623293-9-8*); Vol. 1. 609p. pap. 39.95 (*0-9623293-5-5*); Vol. 2. 215p. pap. 29.95 (*0-9623293-6-3*) Pacific Odyssey.

Nutrition 2000-2001. Charlotte Cook-Fuller & Stephen Barrett. 12th ed. 2000. (Annual Editions Ser.). 240p. (C). pap. 17.50 (*0-07-236568-4*) McGrw-H Hghr Educ.

Nutritional Abnormalities in Infectious Diseases: Effects on Tuberculosis & AIDS. Ed. by Christopher E. Taylor. 1997. LC 96-51894. (Journal of Nutritional Immunology Ser.: Vol. 5, No. 1). 58p. (C). 17.95 (*0-7890-0019-9*) Haworth Pr.

Nutritional Adaptation to New Life Styles. Ed. by J. C. Somogyi & E. H. Koskinen. 1990. (Bibliotheca Nutritio et Dieta Ser.: No. 45). (Illus.). viii, 220p. 182.75 (*3-8055-5183-5*) S Karger.

Nutritional Ages of Women: A Lifetime Guide to Eating Right for Health, Beauty, & Well-Being. Patricia Long. 1986. 18.22 (*0-02-574760-6*) Macmillan.

Nutritional Anaemias: Proceedings of the WHO Scientific Group, Geneva, 1967. WHO Staff. 1968. (Technical Reports: No. 405). pap. text 5.00 (*92-4-120405-2*, 1100405) World Health.

Nutritional & Acid-Base Aspects of Amino Acid Metabolism: 7th International Ammoniagenesis Workshop, Galway, May 1996. Ed. by Daniel J. O'Donovan. 1997. LC 97-23206. (Contributions to Nephrology Ser.: Vol. 121, 1997). (Illus.). x, 172p. 198.25 (*3-8055-6490-2*) S Karger.

Nutritional & Environmental Influences on the Eye. Allen Taylor. 1999. LC 98-49170. (Modern Nutrition Ser.). (Illus.). 304p. 129.95 (*0-8493-8565-2*) CRC Pr.

Nutritional & Pharmacological Strategies in Chronic Renal Failure. Ed. by A. Albertazzi et al. 1991. (Contributions to Nephrology Ser.: Vol. 81). (Illus.). x, 290p. 29.75 (*3-8055-5189-4*) S Karger.

Nutritional & Toxicological Consequences of Food Processing. Ed. by M. Friedman. 1991. (Advances in Experimental Medicine & Biology Ser.: Vol. 289). (Illus.). 552p. (C). text 174.00 (0-306-43891-7, Kluwer Plenum) Kluwer Academic.

Nutritional Anemias. Usha Ramakrishnan. 2000. LC 00-45504. (Modern Nutrition Ser.). (Illus.). 280p. 89.95 (0-8493-8569-5) CRC Pr.

Nutritional Approaches to Aging Research. Gairdner B. Moment. 1982. 280p. 157.00 (0-8493-5831-0, QP86, CRC Reprint) Franklin.

Nutritional Aspects of Aging Linda H. Chen. 1986. LC 85-9720. Vol. 1. 336p. 171.00 (0-8493-5737-3, QP86); Vol. II. 288p. 144.00 (0-8493-5738-1, QP86) Franklin (CRC Reprint).

Nutritional Aspects of Fats. Ed. by J. C. Somogyi. 1977. (Bibliotheca Nutritio et Dieta Ser.: No. 25). (Illus.). 230p. 95.75 (3-8055-2655-5) S Karger.

Nutritional Aspects of HIV Infection. Tracie L. Miller & Sherwood L. Gorbach. 1998. LC 97-51261. pap. 49.95 (0-412-13601-5) Chapman & Hall.

Nutritional Aspects of HIV Infection. Ed. by Tracie L. Miller & Sherwood L. Gorbach. 1999. (Illus.). 224p. 69.50 (0-340-74195-3) OUP.

Nutritional Aspects of Osteoporosis. Ed. by P. Burckhardt et al. 1998. LC 98-13311. (Serono Symposia Ser.). (Illus.). 356p. 148.00 (0-387-98494-1) Spr-Verlag.

Nutritional Aspects of Physical Performance. Ed. by J. C. Somogyi. 1979. (Bibliotheca Nutritio et Dieta Ser.: No. 27). (Illus.). pap. 66.50 (3-8055-2913-9) S Karger.

Nutritional Assessment. Robert D. Lee & David C. Nieman. 2nd ed. 1995. LC 95-24647. (Illus.). 592p. (C). spiral bd. 64.38 (0-8151-5319-8) McGrw-H Hghr Educ.

Nutritional Assessment: A Laboratory Manual. Rosalind S. Gibson. 1993. (Illus.). 208p. (C). spiral bd., lab manual ed. 37.95 (0-19-508547-7) OUP.

Nutritional Assessment & Support. Anne Grant & Susan DeHoog. 1991. (Illus.). 400p. (C). pap. text 30.00 (0-9627678-0-8) Grant-DeHoog.

Nutritional Assessment & Support: A Primer. Carey P. Page & Thomas C. Hardin. 2nd ed. 1994. LC 93-23390. (Illus.). 256p. (Orig.). pap. 19.00 (0-683-06705-2) Lppncott W & W.

Nutritional Assessment in Health Programs. Ed. by George Christakos. 1973. LC 74-120960. 90p. 7.50 (0-87553-116-4, 070) Am Pub Health.

Nutritional Assessment in Malnutrition & Stress. Mary D. Litchford et al. 1994. 139.00 (1-880989-36-0); 139.00 (1-880989-37-9); 139.00 (1-880989-38-7); 139.00 (1-880989-39-5); (C). pap. 6.00 (1-880989-44-1) Case Sftware.

Nutritional Assessment of Elderly Populations: Measure & Function - Proceedings of the 13th Annual Bristol-Myers Squibb/Mead Johnson Symposium on Nutrition Research, Held in Boston on Oct. 11-13, 1993, No. 13. Ed. by Irwin H. Rosenberg. 1994. LC 94-26017. (Bristol-Meyers Squibb-Mead Johnson Nutrition Symposia Ser.: Vol. 13). 336p. 65.00 (0-7817-0232-1) Lppncott W & W.

Nutritional Assessment of Malnutrition & Stress User's Manual. Mary D. Litchford et al. 1994. (C). pap. 7.00 (1-880989-20-4) Case Sftware.

Nutritional Biochemistry. S. Ramakrishnan. 1995. LC 96-219803. x, 246p. 30.00 (81-85427-35-6) Intl Spec Bk.

Nutritional Biochemistry of the Vitamins. David A. Bender. 1992. (Illus.). 451p. (C). text 110.00 (0-521-38144-4) Cambridge U Pr.

Nutritional Care & the HIV Positive Persons: A Manual for Individuals & Their Caregivers. James F. Hickson Jr. 1995. (Modern Nutrition Ser.). 208p. 74.95 (0-8493-7843-5) CRC Pr.

Nutritional Care for High-Risk Newborns. Sharon Groh-Wargo et al. 3rd rev. ed. 2000. LC 00-106141. (Illus.). xx, 711p. 79.95 (1-56625-133-8) Bonus Books.

Nutritional Care of the Terminally Ill. Charlette R. Gallagher-Allred. 1989. LC 89-381. 304p. (C). 72.00 (0-8342-0060-0) Aspen Pub.

Nutritional Communications in Vitamin A Programs. International Vitamin A Consultative Group Staff. 1992. (Illus.). 124p. pap. 3.50 (0-944398-08-1) ILSI.

Nutritional Concerns for Women. Ed. by Ira Wolinsky et al. 1996. LC 95-42174. (Modern Nutrition Ser.). 352p. 69.95 (0-8493-8502-4) CRC Pr.

Nutritional Concerns Quarterly. 1994. (C). 223.75 (0-03-009364-3) Harcourt Coll Pubs.

Nutritional Conditions (Good, Bad & Diseased) Found in the Health of Americans: Index of Authors & Subjects. Onetta L. Stafford. 1993. 180p. 47.50 (1-55914-944-2); pap. 44.50 (1-55914-945-0) ABBE Pubs Assn.

Nutritional Considerations in a Changing World. Ed. by Geoffrey H. Bourne. 1984. (World Review of Nutrition & Dietetics Ser.: Vol. 44). (Illus.). x, 218p. 143.50 (3-8055-3837-5) S Karger.

Nutritional Deficiencies in Industrialized Countries. Ed. by J. C. Somogyi & G. Varela. 1981. (Bibliotheca Nutritio et Dieta Ser.: Vol. 30). (Illus.). viii, 172p. 111.50 (3-8055-1994-X) S Karger.

Nutritional Disorders & Requirements. Ed. by Geoffrey H. Bourne. 1987. (World Review of Nutrition & Dietetics Ser.: Vol. 50). (Illus.). xii, 272p. 208.75 (3-8055-4506-1) S Karger.

Nutritional Energetics. Leonard S. Bull. 1999. 60.00 (0-8493-8750-7) CRC Pr.

Nutritional Epidemiology. Walter Willett. 2nd ed. 1998. (Monographs in Epidemiology & Biostatistics: Vol. 30). (Illus.). 528p. text 67.50 (0-19-512297-6) OUP.

Nutritional Guide for the Problem Drinker. Ruth Guenther. 1983. (Good Health Guides). 32p. (Orig.). pap. 2.50 (0-87983-295-9, 32959K, Keats Pubng) McGraw-Hill Trade.

Nutritional Guide with Food Combining. Louise Tenney. 1991. 237p. (Orig.). pap. 14.95 (0-913923-90-7) Woodland UT.

Nutritional Guidelines for Correcting Behavior. Barbara Reed. rev. ed. 1984. pap. 10.00 (0-939956-07-1) Natural Pr.

Nutritional Healing: A Complete Guide to Vitamins, Minerals, Food Supplements & Herbs for over Two Hundred Common Ailments & Disorders. 1991. lib. bdg. 79.95 (0-8490-5121-5) Gordon Pr.

Nutritional Health: Strategies for Disease Prevention. Ed. by Ted Wilson & Norman J. Temple. 2001. LC 00-57513. (Nutrition & Health Ser.). 352p. 69.50 (0-89603-864-5) Humana.

Nutritional Health Premium Two. 1999. 9.95 (0-13-018394-6) P-H.

Nutritional Immunology. Jau-Fei Chen. Ed. by Taig D. Stewart et al. Date not set. pap. 9.95 (0-9651025-0-5) Bright Ideas Pr.

Nutritional Impact of Food Processing: Symposium Nutritional Impact of Food Processing, Reykjavik, September, 1987. Ed. by J. C. Somogyi. 1989. (Bibliotheca Nutritio et Dieta Ser.: No. 43). (Illus.). viii, 344p. 252.25 (3-8055-4848-6) S Karger.

Nutritional Implications of Macronutrient Substitutes. G. Harvey Anderson. 1999. (Annals of the New York Academy of Sciences Ser.). 272p. pap. text 24.95 (0-8018-6212-4) Johns Hopkins.

Nutritional Implications of Macronutrient Substitutes, Vol. 819. Ed. by G. Harvey Anderson et al. 1997. LC 97-19405. 95.00 (1-57331-084-0) NY Acad Sci.

Nutritional Influences on Illness: A Sourcebook of Clinical Research. Melvin R. Werbach. 1990. LC 89-2378. 508p. pap. 24.95 (0-87983-531-1, 35311K, Keats Pubng) McGraw-Hill Trade.

Nutritional Influences on Illness: A Sourcebook of Clinical Research. Melvyn R. Werbach. 2nd ed. 700p. 1996. LC 96-60020. pap. text 37.95 (0-9618550-5-3); 1993. text 64.95 (0-9618550-3-7) Third Line Pr.

Nutritional Influences on Mental Illness: A Sourcebook of Clinical Research. Melvyn R. Werbach. 1991. LC 91-65076. 360p. text 39.95 (0-9618550-1-0); 2nd ed. 1999. LC 99-70757. 454p. text 59.99 (0-9618550-8-8) Third Line Pr.

Nutritional Intervention in the Aging Process. Ed. by H. J. Armbrecht et al. 1984. (Illus.). 343p. 87.00 (0-387-96025-2) Spr-Verlag.

***Nutritional Issues.** Helen F. Galley. 2001. (Critical Care Focus Ser.: No. 7). (Illus.). 70p. pap. text (0-7279-1652-1) BMJ Pub GBR. Dist: AIDC.

Nutritional Management of Inflammatory Disorders: Assessing Toxic Susceptibility - Improving Glycemic Balance. 1998. (Illus.). 128p. pap. 45.00 (0-9624859-2-6) HealthComm Intl.

Nutritional Medicine: The Drug-Free Guide to Better Family Health. Stephen Davies & Alan Stewart. 1990. 640p. (Orig.). pap. 12.95 (0-380-70733-0, Avon Bks) Morrow Avon.

Nutritional Medicine: The Drug-Free Guide to Better Family Health. Stephen Davies & Alan Stewart. Ed. by Andrew Stanway. 1987. 543p. (Orig.). pap. (0-330-28833-4) Pan GBR. Dist: Trans-Atl Phila.

Nutritional Needs in Cold & High-Altitude Environments: Applications for Military Personnel in Field Operations. Institute of Medicine, Military Nutrition Research Staff. Ed. by Bernadette M. Marriott et al. 1996. 568p. (Orig.). pap. text 39.00 (0-309-05484-2) Natl Acad Pr.

Nutritional Needs in Hot Environments: Applications for Military Personnel in Field Operations. Institute of Medicine Staff. Ed. by Bernadette M. Mariott. 1993. 392p. (Orig.). (C). pap. text 39.00 (0-309-04840-0) Natl Acad Pr.

Nutritional Needs of the Preterm Infant. Ed. by Reginald C. Tsang et al. 1993. LC 92-49242. (Illus.). 450p. 55.00 (0-683-08425-9) Lppncott W & W.

Nutritional Oncology. Ed. by David Heber et al. 1998. LC 98-86561. (Illus.). xix, 632p. (C). text 149.95 (0-12-335960-0) Acad Pr.

Nutritional Outline for the Professional & the Wise Man. James F. Balch, Jr. & Phyllis Balch. 7th rev. ed. 1987. 329p. pap. 21.95 (0-942023-25-0) P A B Bks.

Nutritional Pathobiology. Ed. by E. Bajusz & C. Jasmin. 1972. (Methods & Achievements in Experimental Pathology Ser.: Vol. 6). (Illus.). 104.50 (3-8055-1343-7) S Karger.

Nutritional Pathology: Pathobiochemistry of Dietary Imbalances. Herschel Sidransky. 1985. (Biochemistry of Disease Ser.: Vol. 10). (Illus.). 416p. text 195.00 (0-8247-7303-9) Dekker.

Nutritional Physiology of Minerals. Richard C. Ewan. 1999. 65.00 (0-8493-8752-3) CRC Pr.

Nutritional Physiology of Vitamins. Ewan. 1994. (0-8493-8753-1) CRC Pr.

Nutritional Planning in India. Rajaram Dasgupta. 1989. (C). (81-7013-049-2) Navarang IND. Dist: S Asia.

Nutritional Problems & Education: Selected Topics. Ed. by Geoffrey H. Bourne. 1986. (World Review of Nutrition & Dietetics Ser.: Vol. 47). (Illus.). xii, 208p. 161.00 (3-8055-4214-3) S Karger.

Nutritional Problems of the Elderly. Ed. by J. C. Somogyi & F. Fidanza. 1983. (Bibliotheca Nutritio et Dieta Ser.: No. 33). (Illus.). viii, 200p. pap. 138.50 (3-8055-3700-X) S Karger.

Nutritional, Psychological & Social Aspects of Obesity. Ed. by J. C. Somogyi. 1977. (Bibliotheca Nutritio et Dieta Ser.: No. 26). (Illus.). 75.00 (3-8055-2764-0) S Karger.

Nutritional Requirements of Infants & Young Children: Practical Guidelines. Joyce M. Thompson & Gillian Howard. 1997. LC 97-22822. (Illus.). 224p. pap. 47.95 (0-632-04891-3) Blackwell Sci.

Nutritional Self Defense: A Reference Manual for the Health Professional & the Educated Layperson. Lily Splane. 4th rev. ed. 1993. (Illus.). 248p. (C). pap. text 27.95 (0-945962-04-5) Anaphase II.

Nutritional Status Assessment of the Individual. Ed. by G. E. Livingston. 1989. 479p. 125.00 (0-917678-25-7) Food & Nut Pr.

Nutritional Supplements & Chronic Fatigue Syndrome: A Guide. 1992. lib. bdg. 75.95 (0-8490-5315-3) Gordon Pr.

Nutritional Support for Sick Children. Ed. by R. Di Toro. 1988. (Contributions to Infusion Therapy Ser.: Vol. 19). (Illus.). vi, 150p. 51.50 (3-8055-4705-6) S Karger.

Nutritional Support in Nursing. Grant Staff & Kennedy-Caldwell. 1987. text 66.00 (0-8089-1889-3, Grune & Strat) Harcrt Hlth Sci Grp.

Nutritional Therapy: An Introductory Guide to the Healing Power of Food. Jeannette Ewim. 2000. (New Perspectives Ser.). (Illus.). 128p. pap. (1-86204-740-5) Oneworld.

Nutritional Therapy for Cat Diseases. Shawn Messonnier. 1998. (Pet Care Naturally Ser.). 64p. pap. 4.95 (0-87983-923-6, Keats Pubng) McGraw-Hill Trade.

Nutritional Therapy for Dog Diseases. Shawn Messonnier. 1998. (Pet Care Naturally Ser.). 64p. pap. 4.95 (0-87983-922-8, Keats Pubng) McGraw-Hill Trade.

Nutritional Treatment of Chronic Renal Failure. Ed. by Sergio Giovannetti. 1989. (Topics in Renal Medicine Ser.). (C). text 232.00 (0-7923-0086-6) Kluwer Academic.

Nutritional Triggers for Health & in Disease. Ed. by Artemis F. Simopoulos. 1991. (World Review of Nutrition & Dietetics Ser.: Vol. 67). (Illus.). x, 202p. 197.50 (3-8055-5265-3) S Karger.

Nutritional Value of Cereal Products, Beans & Starches. Ed. by Geoffrey H. Bourne. 1989. (World Review of Nutrition & Dietetics Ser.: Vol. 60). (Illus.). viii, 260p. 200.00 (3-8055-4992-X) S Karger.

Nutritional Value of Indigenous Wild Plants: An Annotated Bibliography. Compiled by Joel N. Elias & John R. K. Robson. 1978. LC 76-51040. vi, 232p. 38.50 (0-87875-112-2) Whitston Pub.

Nutritionist. Jack Rudman. 1994. (Career Examination Ser.: C-2326). pap. 27.95 (0-8373-2326-6) Nat Learn.

Nuts-&-Bolts Approach to Teaching Nursing. Victoria Schoolcraft. 1989. LC 89-11517. (Teaching of Nursing Ser.: Vol. 11). 224p. 32.95 (0-8261-6600-8) Springer Pub.

Nuts-&-Bolts Approach to Teaching Nursing. Victoria Schoolcraft & Jeanne Novotny. 2nd ed. 2000. LC 99-47510. (Teaching of Nursing Ser.). (Illus.). 212p. text 42.95 (0-8261-6601-6) Springer Pub.

Nystagmus As a Resultant in Accordance with the Theoretical Principals of the Physical Mechanisms of the Normal Human Labrinths. R. Grohmann. 1972. (Advances in OtoRhinoLaryngology Ser.: Vol. 18). (Illus.). 64.50 (3-8055-1357-7) S Karger.

O

O. R. Competencies. Johns Hopkins Hospital O.R. Nursing Staff. 1994. 180p. spiral bd. 125.00 (1-879575-52-3) Acad Med Sys.

O Rugged Land of Gold. Martha Martin. 1989. (Illus.). 226p. pap. 12.95 (0-940055-00-7) Vanessapress.

Oasis & Obqi: A Guide for Education & Implementation. Randa L. Sperling & Carolyn J. Humphrey. 1998. LC 98-36724. 272p. pap. text 37.95 (0-7817-1955-0) Lppncott W & W.

OAT - Optometry Admission Test: Comprehensive Manual Self Study. David M. Tarlow. 2nd rev. ed. 1999. 140p. (C). pap. text 19.95 (1-57732-100-6) Datar Pub.

OAT - Optometry Admission Test No. 1: Practice Exam Annotated Answers. David M. Tarlow. 2nd rev. ed. 1999. 20p. (C). pap. text 6.95 (1-57732-102-2) Datar Pub.

OAT - Optometry Admission Test No. 1: Practice Examination. David M. Tarlow. 2nd rev. ed. 1999. 40p. (C). pap. text 18.95 (1-57732-101-4) Datar Pub.

OAT - Optometry Admission Test No. 2: Practice Exam Annotated Answers. David M. Tarlow. 2nd rev. ed. 1999. 20p. (C). pap. text 6.95 (1-57732-104-9) Datar Pub.

OAT - Optometry Admission Test No. 2: Practice Examination, Vol. 2. David M. Tarlow. 2nd rev. ed. 1999. 40p. (C). pap. text 18.95 (1-57732-103-0) Datar Pub.

OAT - Optometry Admission Test No. 3: Practice Exam Annotated Answers. David M. Tarlow. 2nd rev. ed. 1999. 20p. (C). pap. text 6.95 (1-57732-106-5) Datar Pub.

OAT - Optometry Admission Test No. 3: Practice Examination. David M. Tarlow. 2nd rev. ed. 1999. (C). pap. text 18.95 (1-57732-105-7) Datar Pub.

OAT - Optometry Admission Test No. 4: Practice Exam Annotated Answers. David M. Tarlow. 2nd rev. ed. 1999. 20p. (C). pap. text 6.95 (1-57732-108-1) Datar Pub.

OAT - Optometry Admission Test No. 4: Practice Examination. David M. Tarlow. 2nd rev. ed. 1999. 40p. (C). pap. text 18.95 (1-57732-107-3) Datar Pub.

OAT - Optometry Admission Test No. 5: Practice Exam Annotated Answers. David M. Tarlow. 2nd rev. ed. 1999. 20p. (C). pap. text 6.95 (1-57732-110-3) Datar Pub.

OAT - Optometry Admission Test No. 5: Practice Examination. David M. Tarlow. 2nd rev. ed. 1999. 40p. (C). pap. text 18.95 (1-57732-109-X) Datar Pub.

OAT - Optometry Admission Test - Core Content. David M. Tarlow. 2nd rev. ed. 1999. (Illus.). 400p. pap. 49.95 (1-57774-007-6) Educ Tsting Cnslts.

OAT Exam No. 1: Annotated Answers (Optometry Admissions Test) David M. Tarlow. 7th ed. 1996. (Orig.). pap. 5.95 (1-57732-028-X) Datar Pub.

OAT Exam No. 1: (Optometry Admissions Test) David M. Tarlow. 7th ed. 1996. (Orig.). pap. 19.95 (1-57732-023-9) Datar Pub.

OAT Exam No. 2: Annotated Answers (Optometry Admissions Test) David M. Tarlow. 1996. pap. (1-57732-029-8) Datar Pub.

OAT Exam No. 2: (Optometry Admissions Test) David M. Tarlow. 7th ed. 1996. pap. 19.95 (1-57732-024-7) Datar Pub.

OAT Exam No. 3: Annotated Answers (Optometry Admissions Test) David M. Tarlow. 7th ed. 1996. (Illus.). (Orig.). pap. 5.95 (1-57732-030-1) Datar Pub.

OAT Exam No. 3: (Optometry Admissions Test) David M. Tarlow. 7th ed. 1996. (Orig.). pap. (1-57732-025-5) Datar Pub.

OAT Exam No. 4: Annotated Answers (Optometry Admissions Test) David M. Tarlow. 7th ed. 1996. (Orig.). pap. 5.95 (1-57732-031-X) Datar Pub.

OAT Exam No. 4: (Optometry Admissions Test) David M. Tarlow. 7th ed. 1996. (Orig.). pap. 19.95 (1-57732-026-3) Datar Pub.

OAT Exam No. 5: Annotated Answers (Optometry Admissions Test) David M. Tarlow. 7th ed. 1996. (Orig.). pap. 5.95 (1-57732-032-8) Datar Pub.

OAT Exam No. 5: (Optometry Admissions Test) David M. Tarlow. 7th ed. 1996. (Illus.). pap. 19.95 (1-57732-027-1) Datar Pub.

OAT (Optometry Admission Test) For Comprehensive Review. David M. Tarlow. 7th ed. 1996. (Orig.). pap., stu. ed. 19.95 (1-57732-022-0) Datar Pub.

OB Anaesthesia. Morgan. 1990. 160p. pap. text 32.50 (0-340-54108-3) Trafalgar.

Ob-Gyn Intern Pocket Survival Guide. Andrew Engel. 1998. 78p. (Orig.). (C). pap. 7.50 (1-883205-00-X) Intl Med Pub.

OB-GYN Secrets. Helen L. Frederickson & Louise Wilkins-Haug. 2nd ed. 1996. LC 96-79704. 375p. pap. 39.95 (1-56053-205-X) Hanley & Belfus.

Obagi Skin Health Restoration & Rejuvenation. Zein E. Obagi. 1999. LC 98-46307. (Illus.). 304p. 195.00 (0-387-98469-0) Spr-Verlag.

***Obase Medicine 3 Pt. III: MCQs for the MRCP.** McCrudden. 2003. 192p. pap. incl. cd-rom (1-84110-016-1) Greenwich Med GBR. Dist: JAMCO Dist.

Oberrheinisches Kardiologen-Symposium. Ed. by R. Voegtlin. 1981. (Cardiology Ser.: Vol. 68, Suppl. 1). (Illus.). 136p. pap. 35.75 (3-8055-3436-1) S Karger.

Oberrheinisches Kardiologen-Symposium, Freiburg, May, 1982: Journal: Cardiology, Vol. 70, Suppl. 1, 1983. Ed. by H. Loellgen. 1983. (Illus.). iv, 140p. pap. 41.75 (3-8055-3688-7) S Karger.

Obese Child. Ed. by P. L. Giorgi et al. 1992. (Pediatric & Adolescent Medicine Ser.: Vol. 2). (Illus.). viii, 256p. 201.00 (3-8055-5463-X) S Karger.

Obesidad Es un Problema Familiar. Judi Hollis. 1994.Tr. of Fat Is a Family Affair. (SPA.). 172p. pap. 15.00 (968-39-0517-X) Hazelden.

Obesities. J. Vague. rev. ed. 1998. 172p. pap. (0-86196-582-5) J Libbey Med GBR. Dist: Buttrwrth-Heinemann.

***Obesity.** Nick Finer. (British Medical Bulletin Ser.: Vol. 53, No. 2). pap. (1-85315-316-8) Royal Soc of Medicine Pr Ltd GBR. Dist: Balogh.

***Obesity.** Finer et al. 2003. (Fast Facts Ser.). (Illus.). 60p. pap. (1-899541-66-7) Health Pr GBR. Dist: JAMCO Dist.

Obesity. Barry Gumbiner. 2001. LC 00-69962. (ACP Expert Guide Ser.). (Illus.). pap. 35.00 (0-943126-93-2, 330301500) Amer Coll Phys.

Obesity: Advances in Understanding & Treatment. Leslie Weston. 1996. (Biomedical Library). 500p. pap. 795.00 (*1-57936-010-6*) Drug & Market Dev.

Obesity: Basic Concepts & Clinical Aspects. Ed. by F. Belfiore et al. 1991. (Frontiers in Diabetes Ser.: Vol. 11). (Illus.). viii, 220p. 214.00 (*3-8055-5405-2*) S Karger.

Obesity: Pathophysiology, Psychology & Treatment. Ed. by George L. Blackburn & Beatrice S. Kanders. 1995. (Clinical Nutrition Ser.). (Illus.). 368p. 85.00 (*0-412-98461-X*) Aspen Pub.

Obesity: The Report of the British Nutrition Foundation Task Force. British Nutrition Foundation Staff. 2000. LC 99-88087. pap. 69.95 (*0-632-05298-8*) Blackwell Sci.

***Obesity & Anti-Obesity Agents: Index of New Information & Guide-Book for Consumers, Reference & Research.** Joseph R. Richie. 2002. 180p. 57.50 (*0-7883-2432-2*); pap. 47.50 (*0-7883-2433-0*) ABBE Pubs Assn.

Obesity & Diabetes Mellitus. E. I. Sokolov. 1997. (Illus.). 331p. (*90-6764-212-6*) VSP NLD. *Dist:* Coronet Bks.

Obesity & Medical Student Education. Ed. by Walter Futterweit et al. 2000. 110p. (Orig.). pap. 18.95 (*0-930194-89-6*) Ctr Thanatology.

Obesity & Related Diseases. J. S. Garrow. 1988. LC 87-14631. (Illus.). 340p. text (*0-443-03798-1*) Church.

Obesity Assessment: Tools, Methods, Interpretations. Ed. by Sachiko T. St. Jeor. 1995. LC 96-35594. (Clinical Nutrition Ser.). 752p. (C). 121.00 (*0-412-07241-6*) Aspen Pub.

Obesity, Diabetes, & How to Eat to Live. Kevin Muhammad. 1997. LC 97-61410. (Within the Pulse Ser.: Vol. 1). (Illus.). 110p. pap. 10.95 (*0-9658864-0-9*) TechDoc.

Obesity Management. 124p. pap. text (*0-86471-068-2*) Adis Intl NZL. *Dist:* Lppncott W & W.

Obesity Sourcebook: Basic Consumer Health Information about Diseases & Other Problems Associated with Obesity. Ed. by Wilma Caldwell. 2001. LC 00-50122. (Health Reference Ser.). (Illus.). xii, 376p. lib. bdg. 48.00 (*0-7808-0333-7*) Omnigraphics Inc.

Obesity Treatment: Establishing Goals, Improving Outcomes & Reviewing the Research Agenda: Proceedings of a NATO ARW Held in New York City, June 2-5, 1993. Ed. by David B. Allison & Xavier F. Pi-Sunyer. 1995. (NATO Advanced Science Institutes Ser.: Vol. 278). (Illus.). 290p. (C). text 95.00 (*0-306-45115-8*, Kluwer Plenum) Kluwer Academic.

OB/GYN Medical Student Pearls of Wisdom. Smith. 1999. (Pearls of Wisdom Ser.). pap. 32.00 (*1-58409-001-4*) Boston Medical.

OB/GYN Nurse Practitioner. Jack Rudman. (Certified Nurse Examination Ser.: CN-19). pap. 27.95 (*0-8373-6119-2*) Nat Learn.

OB/GYN Pearls of Wisdom: Over 2500 Questions. Smith. 1999. (Pearls of Wisdom Ser.). pap. 88.00 (*1-890369-06-3*) Boston Medical.

***OB/GYN Recall PDA.** F. John Bourgeois et al. 2002. 29.95 (*0-7817-3303-0*) Lppncott W & W.

OB/GYN Ultrasound Triage & Evaluation for Advanced Practice Nurses. Cydney A. Menihan. 1997. LC 97-24741. 320p. spiral bd. 43.00 (*0-397-55383-8*) Lppncott W & W.

Object-Choice: All You Need Is Love. Klaus Theweleit. Tr. by Malcolm Green. 1994. LC 94-4665. 180p. (gr. 13). pap. 18.00 (*0-86091-642-1*) Verso.

Object Love & Reality: An Introduction to a Psychoanalytic Theory of Object Relations. Arnold H. Modell. 1968. LC 68-24219. 181p. 30.00 (*0-8236-3720-4*) Intl Univs Pr.

Object Relations & Self Psychology: An Introduction. Michael St. Clair. 1987. LC 86-8251. (Counseling-Psychology Ser.). 196p. (C). pap. 18.25 (*0-534-06708-5*) Brooks-Cole.

Object Relations Assessment in Younger Children: Rorschach & Tat Measures. Francis D. Kelly. 1996. LC 95-46127. 178p. text 43.95 (*0-398-06561-6*) C C Thomas.

Object Relations Brief Therapy: The Therapeutic Relationship in Short-Term Work. Michael Stadter. 1996. LC 95-20678. 376p. 60.00 (*1-56821-660-2*) Aronson.

Object Relations Couple Therapy. David E. Scharff & Jill S. Scharff. 1991. LC 90-19182. 328p. 60.00 (*0-87668-647-1*) Aronson.

Object Relations Family Therapy. David E. Scharff & Jill S. Scharff. 1987. LC 87-1755. 503p. 65.00 (*0-87668-938-1*) Aronson.

Object Relations in Psychoanalytic Theory. Jay R. Greenberg & Stephen A. Mitchell. 1983. 456p. 46.95 (*0-674-62975-2*) HUP.

Object Relations in Severe Trauma: Psychotherapy of the Sexually Abused Child. Stephen Prior. 1996. LC 95-32752. 200p. 40.00 (*1-56821-554-1*) Aronson.

Object Relations Individual Therapy. Jill S. Scharff & David E. Scharff. 1998. LC 97-23357. (Illus.). 656p. 70.00 (*0-7657-0117-0*) Aronson.

Object Relations Psychotherapy: An Individualized & Interactive Approach to Diagnosis & Treatment. Cheryl Glickauf-Hughes & Marolyn C. Wells. 1997. LC 97-8531. 504p. text 55.00 (*0-7657-0069-7*) Aronson.

Object Relations, the Self & the Group. Charles Ashbach & Victor L. Schermer. 1994. LC 94-9884. (International Library of Philosophy, Psychology, & Scientific Method). 328p. (C). pap. 29.95 (*0-415-11217-6*, B4262) Routledge.

Object Relations, the Self & the Group: A Conceptual Paradigm. Charles Asbach & Victor C. Schermer. 1987. 288p. 55.00 (*0-7100-9839-1*, Routledge Thoemms) Routledge.

Object Relations Theory & Clinical Psychoanalysis. Otto F. Kernberg. LC 75-42548. 304p. 1995. pap. 50.00 (*1-56821-612-2*); 1990. reprint ed. 55.00 (*0-87668-247-6*) Aronson.

Object Relations Theory & Psychopathology: A Comprehensive Text. Frank L. Summers. 1994. LC 93-39264. 424p. text 55.00 (*0-88163-155-8*) Analytic Pr.

Object Relations Therapy: Using the Relationship. Sheldon Cashdan. 1988. LC 88-12415. 198p. text 25.00 (*0-393-70059-3*) Norton.

Objective Diagnosis of Minimal Brain Dysfunction. Richard A. Gardner. 1979. LC 79-11054. xxvi, 452p. text 20.00 (*0-933812-00-0*) Creative Therapeutics.

Objective Measurement: Theory into Practice, Vol. 1. Ed. by Mark Wilson. 1992. 368p. 78.50 (*0-89391-727-3*); pap. 39.50 (*0-89391-814-8*) Greenwood (Ablex).

Objective Medical Decision Making: Systems Approach in Acute Disease. Ed. by J. E. Beneken & S. M. Lavelle. 1983. (Lecture Notes in Medical Informatics: Vol. 22). 243p. 42.95 (*0-387-12671-6*) Spr-Verlag.

Objective Mental Measurement: Individual & Program Evaluation Using the Rasch Model. Robert M. Hashway. 1978. LC 78-19739. 105p. 55.00 (*0-275-90297-8*, C0297, Praeger Pubs) Greenwood.

Objective Psychodiagnostic Inventories. Green & Henry A. Millon. 99th ed. 1995. 1.00 (*0-471-88315-8*) Wiley.

Objective Structured Clinical Examination in Obstetrics & Gynaecology. Justin C. Konje & D. J. Taylor. 1998. (Illus.). 100p. pap. 57.95 (*0-632-04764-X*) Blackwell Sci.

Objet de la Psychanalyse et l'Objet en Psychanalyse. Ed. by J. R. Freymann & A. Michels. 1989. (Apertura Ser.: Vol. 2). 200p. 34.95 (*0-387-18085-0*) Spr-Verlag.

OBRA Guidelines for Quality Improvement. Marie S. Jaffe. 3rd rev. ed. 1998. LC 98-232099. (Illus.). 400p. (C). ring bd. 155.95 (*1-56930-047-X*) Delmar.

OBRA Nurse Aide Skills Manual. Stephanie Vaughn & Sheila A. Sorrentino. 1992. 176p. pap. text 14.95 (*0-8016-6072-6*) Mosby Inc.

Obraized Quality Assurance Through Auditing. Linda Faber-Czingula & Virginia Toby. 1996. 133p. ring bd. 49.00 (*1-890118-04-4*, QualityCare Pub) Convalescnt Cnslts.

Observation & Inference: An Introduction to the Methods of Epidemiology. Alexander M. Walker. 1991. (Illus.). 173p. (Orig.). (C). pap. text 23.00 (*0-917227-07-7*) Epidemiology.

Observation Medicine. Louis G. Graff. 1992. (Illus.). 440p. text 84.00 (*1-56372-010-8*) Buttrwrth-Heinemann.

Observational Evaluation of Severely Multi-Handicapped Children. W. S. Curtis & E. T. Donlon. 1985. (Modern Approaches to the Diagnosis & Instruction of Multi-Handicapped Children Ser.: Vol. 18). viii, 204p. (*90-265-0595-7*) Swets.

Observations & Essays on the Statistics of Insanity. John Thurnam. 1976. LC 75-16734. (Classics in Psychiatry Ser.). reprint ed. 32.95 (*0-405-07455-7*) Ayer.

Observations by Mr. Dooley. Finley P. Dunne. 1973. 250.00 (*0-8490-0746-1*) Gordon Pr.

Observations on Madness & Melancholy: Including Practical Remarks on Those Diseases Together with Cases, & an Account of the Morbid Appearances on Dissection. John Haslam. 2nd enl. ed. 1976. LC 75-16707. (Classics in Psychiatry Ser.). reprint ed. 32.95 (*0-405-07432-8*) Ayer.

Observations on Maniacal Disorders: (1792) William Pargeter. Ed. by Stanley Jackson. 1989. (Tavistock Classic Reprints in the History of Psychiatry Ser.). 208p. 37.50 (*0-415-00638-4*) Routledge.

Observations on Mental Derangement: Being an Application of the Principles of Phrenology to the Elucidation of the Causes, Symptoms, Nature, Treatment of Insanity. Andrew Combe. 1972. LC 72-161928. (History of Psychology Ser.). 352p. reprint ed. 50.00 (*0-8201-1089-2*) Schol Facsimiles.

Observations on the Deranged Manifestations of the Mind, or Insanity. Johann C. Spurzheim. 1970. LC 78-81359. (History of Psychology Ser.). (Illus.). 268p. reprint ed. 50.00 (*0-8201-1078-7*) Schol Facsimiles.

Observations on the Growth of the Mind with Remarks on Other Subjects. Sampson Reed. 1970. LC 78-100126. 200p. reprint ed. 50.00 (*0-8201-1070-1*) Schol Facsimiles.

Observations on the Nature, Kinds, Causes, & Prevention of Insanity: Containing Observations on the Nature, & Various Kinds of Insanity & the Appearances on Dissection Thomas Arnold. 2nd ed. 1976. LC 75-16680. (Classics in Psychiatry Ser.). reprint ed. 56.95 (*0-405-07412-3*) Ayer.

Observations on the Soviet-Canadian Transporar Ski Trek. Ed. by R. J. Shephard & A. Rode. 1992. (Medicine & Sport Science Ser.: Vol. 33). (Illus.). x, 190p. 170.50 (*3-8055-5410-9*) S Karger.

Observing & Recording the Behavior of Young Children. Dorothy Cohen et al. 4th ed. 1996. LC 96-35584. 365p. (C). pap. 19.95 (*0-8077-3575-2*) Tchrs Coll.

Observing Children: A Practical Guide. Carole Sharman et al. 1995. LC 94-47130. xii, 114p. pap. 19.95 (*0-304-33261-5*); text 70.00 (*0-304-33263-1*) Continuum.

Observing Children in Their Natural Worlds: A Primer in Quantitative Observational Methods. Anthony D. Pellegrini. 1996. 272p. text 55.00 (*0-8058-2151-1*) L Erlbaum Assocs.

Observing Self: Mysticism & Psychotherapy. Arthur J. Deikman. 1983. LC 81-70486. 208p. reprint ed. pap. text 14.50 (*0-8070-2951-3*) Beacon Pr.

Observing Systems. Heinz Von Foerster. 1982. (Systems Inquiry Ser.). 425p. (Orig.). (C). pap. text 15.95 (*0-914105-19-1*) Intersystems Pubns.

Obsession. Arthur Guirdham. 186p. (Orig.). pap. 20.95 (*0-8464-4262-0*) Beekman Pubs.

Obsession. Arthur Guirdham. 1972. 109p. (Orig.). pap. (*0-85435-271-6*) C W Daniel GBR. *Dist:* Natl Bk Netwk.

Obsession & Possession. Torkom Saraydarian. 2000. LC 00-101975. (Illus.). 354p. per. 25.00 (*0-929874-29-3*) TSG Pub Found.

Obsessions et la Psychasthenie Pierre M. Janet. 1976. LC 75-16709. (Classics in Psychiatry Ser.). (FRE., Illus.). reprint ed. Set. 108.95 (*0-405-07434-4*); Vol. 1. 54.95 (*0-405-07435-2*); Vol. 1. 54.95 (*0-405-07436-0*) Ayer.

Obsessive-Compulsive & Related Disorders in Adults: A Comprehensive Clinical Guide. Lorrin M. Koran. 1999. LC 98-42347. (Illus.). 380p. (C). pap. text 59.95 (*0-521-55975-8*) Cambridge U Pr.

Obsessive-Compulsive Disorder. 1997. lib. bdg. 250.95 (*0-8490-8142-4*) Gordon Pr.

Obsessive-Compulsive Disorder. Maj. 2000. 322p. 95.00 (*0-471-87163-X*) Wiley.

Obsessive Compulsive Disorder: A Cognitive & Neuropsychological Perspective. Tallis. 1995. 222p. pap. 60.00 (*0-471-95772-0*) Wiley.

Obsessive Compulsive Disorder: A Guide. John H. Greist. 65p. rev. ed. 2000. pap. 4.95 (*1-890802-21-2*); 6th rev. ed. 1997. pap. 4.50 (*1-890802-03-4*) Madison Inst of Med.

Obsessive Compulsive Disorder: A Survival Guide for Family & Friends. Roy Cohen. 1993. LC 93-83800. 90p. pap. 9.95 (*0-9628066-1-7*) OCA.

Obsessive Compulsive Disorder: Contemporary Issues in Treatment. Ed. by Wayne K. Goodman et al. 1999. LC 98-56188. (Personality & Clinical Psychology Ser.). 661p. 69.95 (*0-8058-2837-0*) L Erlbaum Assocs.

Obsessive-Compulsive Disorder: Pastoral Care for the Road to Change. Robert M. Collie. 1999. LC 99-23094. xii, 267p. 49.95 (*0-7890-0707-X*); pap. 19.95 (*0-7890-0862-9*) Haworth Pr (Haworth Pastrl).

Obsessive-Compulsive Disorder: Psychological & Pharmacological Treatment. Ed. by Samuel M. Turner et al. 1985. (Illus.). 272p. (C). text 78.00 (*0-306-41850-9*, Kluwer Plenum) Kluwer Academic.

Obsessive-Compulsive Disorder: The Facts. Padmal De Silva & Stanley Rachman. 2nd ed. 1998. LC 98-155953. (Facts Ser.). (Illus.). 152p. pap. 19.95 (*0-19-262860-7*) OUP.

Obsessive-Compulsive Disorder: Theory, Research & Treatment. Ed. by Richard P. Swinson et al. 1998. LC 98-14388. 478p. 52.00 (*1-57230-335-2*, C0335) Guilford Pubns.

Obsessive-Compulsive Disorder Casebook. Ed. by John H. Greist & James W. Jefferson. 2nd rev. ed. 1995. LC 94-41299. 336p. text 41.95 (*0-88048-729-1*, 8729) Am Psychiatric.

Obsessive-Compulsive Disorder in Children & Adolescents. Ed. by Judith L. Rapoport. 1989. LC 88-24262. 355p. text 47.50 (*0-88048-282-6*, 8282) Am Psychiatric.

Obsessive Compulsive Disorder in Children & Adolescents: A Guide. Hugh F. Johnston. rev. ed. 1997. 58p. pap. 4.50 (*1-890802-13-1*) Madison Inst of Med.

Obsessive-Compulsive Disorder Spectrum: Pathogenesis, Diagnosis, & Treatment. Jose A. Yaryura-Tobias & Fugen A. Neziroglu. 1996. 337p. text 69.50 (*0-88048-707-0*, 8707) Am Psychiatric.

Obsessive-Compulsive Disorders. 1996. lib. bdg. 250.75 (*0-8490-5902-X*) Gordon Pr.

Obsessive-Compulsive Disorders. Ed. by Eric Hollander & Dan J. Stein. 1997. LC 97-11363. (Medical Psychiatry Ser.). (Illus.). 416p. text 155.00 (*0-8247-9856-2*) Dekker.

Obsessive-Compulsive Disorders. Michael A. Jenike. 3rd ed. 1998. LC 97-48499. (Illus.). 886p. (C). (gr. 13). text 75.00 (*0-8151-3840-7*, 30957) Mosby Inc.

***Obsessive-Compulsive Disorders: Personality Traits & Disorders, Autistic Traits & Biochemical Findings.** Susanne Bejerot. 2000. (Comprehensive Summaries of Uppsala Dissertations from the Faculty of Medicine Ser.: No. 915). 60p. pap. (*91-554-4680-9*) Uppsala Universitet SWE. *Dist:* Coronet Bks.

Obsessive-Compulsive-Related Disorders. Ed. by Eric Hollander. 1993. LC 92-10541. 286p. text 23.50 (*0-88048-402-0*, 8402) Am Psychiatric.

***Obstetric Anaesthesia.** P. Neville Robinson & David Vaughan. 2001. (Anaesthesia in a Nutshell Ser.). (Illus.). 160p. pap. 26.50 (*0-7506-5008-7*) Buttrwrth-Heinemann.

Obstetric Anaesthesia & Analgesia. Donald D. Moir. 2nd ed. 1980. text 49.95 (*0-02-858630-1*) Macmillan Info.

Obstetric & Gynecologic Care in Physical Therapy. Rebecca A. Stephenson & Linda J. O'Connor. 2nd ed. 2000. LC 99-59223. 352p. pap. text 35.00 (*1-55642-415-9*) SLACK Inc.

***Obstetric & Gynecologic Dermatology.** Martin M. Black et al. 2nd ed. 2001. (Illus.). 230p. pap. (*0-7234-3182-5*) Mosby Inc.

Obstetric & Gynecologic Milestones. Harold Speert. 1996. (Illus.). 702p. 159.95 (*1-85070-698-0*, Parthenon Pbng) CRC Pr.

Obstetric & Gynecologic Milestones. Harold Speert. 2nd ed. 1996. (Illus.). 145p. 145.00 (*0-930405-60-9*) Norman SF.

Obstetric & Gynecologic Nursing. Meg Gulanick et al. Ed. by Kathy V. Gettrust. 1993. LC 93-5045. (Plans of Care for Specialty Practice Ser.). 581p. (C). pap. 32.75 (*0-8273-5468-1*) Delmar.

Obstetric & Gynecology: A Problem Based Approach. M. C. James et al. 1999. LC 98-40973. (Illus.). 410p. pap. (*0-7020-2251-9*) W B Saunders.

Obstetric & Gynecology Oral Practice Handbook. D. Dawn. 1984. (C). (*0-7855-4657-X*) Current Dist IND. *Dist:* St Mut.

Obstetric & Neonatal Malpractice: Legal & Medical 1999. 2nd ed. 1999. pap. text, suppl. ed. 98.00 (*0-7355-0454-7*) Aspen Pub.

Obstetric & Neonatal Malpractice Vol. 2: Legal & Medical Handbook. Michael D. Volk. 2nd ed. 1996. LC 96-5646. (Medical Malpractice Library). 2272p. 265.00 (*0-471-12896-1*) Wiley.

Obstetric Anesthesia. Mark C. Norris. 2nd ed. 1998. LC 98-27543. 864p. text 149.00 (*0-7817-1017-0*) Lppncott W & W.

Obstetric Anesthesia: Principles & Practice. David H. Chestnut. 2nd ed. 1999. LC 99-25600. (Illus.). 1056p. (C). text (*0-323-00383-4*) Mosby Inc.

Obstetric Anesthesia & Uncommon Disorders. David R. Gambling & M. Joanne Douglas. Ed. by Leslie Day. 1997. LC 97-1435. (Illus.). 400p. text 89.00 (*0-7216-6157-2*) Saunders.

Obstetric Anesthesia Handbook, Vol. 2E. Sanjay Datta. 2nd ed. 1995. LC 95-788. (Illus.). 368p. (C). (gr. 13). pap. text 46.95 (*0-8151-2349-3*, 24719) Mosby Inc.

Obstetric Anesthesia Pearls. William E. Ackerman & Mushtaque M. Huneja. 1992. (Illus.). 280p. (C). pap. 37.95 (*0-8385-7173-5*, A7173-6) McGraw-Hill Prof.

Obstetric Anesthesia Pocket Reference. Edward T. Riley & Shelia E. Cohen. 2001. (Illus.). 144p. pap. 25.00 (*0-7506-7166-1*) Buttrwrth-Heinemann.

Obstetric Emergencies. Ed. by Guy I. Benrubi. 1989. (Illus.). 216p. text (*0-443-08614-1*) Church.

Obstetric Fistula. R. F. Zacharin. 1988. (Illus.). 286p. 196.00 (*0-387-82005-1*) Spr-Verlag.

Obstetric Forceps: Its History & Evolution. Kedarnath Das. 1993. (Illus.). 903p. 125.00 (*1-897849-00-1*) Norman SF.

Obstetric Genetics. Zoltan Papp & Richard H. Lindenbaum. 1990. 627p. (C). (*963-05-5689-8*) Akade Kiado HUN. *Dist:* Intl Spec Bk, St Mut.

Obstetric Infections: Amnionitis & Endometritis. Valerian A. Catanzarite & W. Patrick Duff. 1989. (*0-683-17956-X*) Lppncott W & W.

Obstetric Infections: Clinical Cases. Valerian A. Catanzarite & W. Patrick Duff. 1989. (*0-683-17958-6*) Lppncott W & W.

Obstetric Intensive Care: A Practice Manual. Michael R. Floey & Thomas H. Strong, Jr. Ed. by William Schmitt. 1997. LC 96-41406. 464p. pap. text 34.00 (*0-7216-1317-9*) Saunders.

Obstetric Litigation: A Trial Lawyer's Guide. Elliott B. Oppenheim. 1999. 300p. 300.00 (*1-930263-02-3*) Terra Firma NM.

Obstetric Myths vs. Research Realities: A Guide to the Medical Literature. Henci Goer. 1995. LC 94-17337. 400p. 82.50 (*0-89789-242-9*); pap. 31.50 (*0-89789-427-8*) Greenwood (Bergin & Garvey).

Obstetric Nursing. Yondell Masten. Ed. by Wendy Thompson. 2nd rev. ed. 1997. (Outline Ser.). 280p. (C). per. 22.95 (*1-56930-070-4*) Delmar.

Obstetric Survival Handbook. Yondel Masten. 2nd ed. 1998. LC 98-229378. (Illus.). 300p. per. 34.95 (*1-56930-083-6*) Delmar.

Obstetric Syndromes & Conditions. John P. O'Grady et al. 1998. LC 97-33562. (Clinical Handbook Ser.). (Illus.). 408p. lib. bdg. 85.95 (*1-85070-754-5*, O0243, Parthenon Pbng) CRC Pr.

Obstetric Ultrasound. Patricia Chudleigh. 2nd ed. 1992. 323p. (Orig.). pap. text (*0-443-04207-1*) Church.

Obstetric Ultrasound. Chudleigh. 3rd ed. 2000. pap. text 65.00 (*0-443-05471-1*) Saunders.

Obstetric Ultrasound. Ed. by James P. Neilson & S. E. Chambers. (Illus.). Vol. 1. 1993. 320p. 79.00 (*0-19-262224-2*); Vol. 2. 1995. 258p. text 79.00 (*0-19-262373-7*) OUP.

***Obstetric Ultrasound Made Easy.** Norman C. Smith & A. P. M. Smith. 2001. LC 2001-42215. (Illus.). 131p. pap. (*0-443-07013-X*) Church GBR. *Dist:* Saunders.

Obstetrical Emergencies. Denise Wjite & Judith H. Poole. Ed. by Karla Damus et al. 1996. LC 96-1652. (*0-86525-070-7*) March of Dimes.

Obstetrical Events & Developmental Sequelae. Ed. by Nergesh Tejani. 1989. 224p. lib. bdg. 142.00 (*0-8493-5762-4*, RG627); 2nd ed. 1994. 228p. 139.00 (*0-8493-4974-5*, 4974) CRC Pr.

Obstetrical Intervention & Technology in the 1980s. Ed. by Diony Young. 1983. LC 82-21301. (Women & Health Ser.: Vol. 7, Nos. 3-4). 203p. text 49.95 (*0-86656-143-9*) Haworth Pr.

Obstetrical Measurements: Used in a Routine Examination. A. B. Kurtz. 1997. pap. (*1-930047-40-1*, OBM) Am Inst Ultrasound.

Obstetrical Pearls: A Practical Guide for the Efficient Resident. Michael D. Benson. 3rd ed. 1999. LC 99-24043. (Illus.). 225p. pap. 21.95 (*0-8036-0432-7*) Davis Co.

Obstetrical Transfusion Practice. Ed. by Ronald A. Sacher & Mark E. Brecher. 1993. (Illus.). 138p. (C). text 35.00 (*1-56395-024-3*) Am Assn Blood.

Obstetrics. John Hare & Heather Greenway. 2000. (Medico-Legal Practitioner Ser.). 334p. (*1-85941-598-9*) Cavendish Pubng GBR. *Dist:* Gaunt.

Obstetrics. David K. James & Mary Pillai. 1994. LC 93-8274. (Colour Guide Ser.). (Illus.). 152p. pap. text 19.95 (*0-443-04777-4*) Harcrt Hlth Sci Grp.

Obstetrics. Ed. by Alec Turnbull & Geoffrey Chamberlain. 1989. (Illus.). 1201p. text (*0-443-03539-3*) Church.

Obstetrics. James. 2nd ed. 1999. (C). pap. text 16.95 (*0-443-05881-4*) Saunders.

Obstetrics. David K. James & Mary Pillai. 2nd ed. 2000. LC 97-22824. (Colour Guide Ser.). text (*0-443-05773-7*) Harcrt Hlth Sci Grp.

Obstetrics. Ed. by William F. Rayburn. 2nd ed. 1988. (House Officer Ser.). (Illus.). 272p. pap. text 20.00 (*0-683-07159-9*) Lppncott W & W.

Obstetrics: A Practical Manual. Roger Neuberg. 1995. (Illus.). 302p. pap. text 49.95 (*0-19-263007-5*) OUP.

Obstetrics: Colour Aids. David K. James & Mary Pillai. 1990. (Illus.). 144p. pap. text (*0-443-04011-7*) Church.

Obstetrics: Essentials of Clinical Practice. Kenneth R. Niswander. 2nd ed. 1981. 379p. 34.95 (*0-316-61147-6*, Little Brwn Med Div) Lppncott W & W.

Obstetrics: Normal & Problem Pregnancies. George J. Annas. Ed. by Steven G. Gabbe et al. 3rd ed. 1996. LC 96-20732. 1348p. text (*0-443-07690-1*) Church.

Obstetrics: Psychological & Psychiatric Syndromes. J. O'Grady & M. Rosenthal. 1991. (Current Topics in Obstetrics & Gynecology Ser.). (Illus.). 383p. (C). (gr. 13). text 74.95 (*0-412-04601-6*) Chapman & Hall.

Obstetrics: Textbook for Students & Practitioners. Whitridge J. Williams et al. abr. fac. collector's ed. 1997. LC 96-28900. 845p. (C). text 150.00 (*0-8385-7199-9*, A7199-1) McGraw-Hill Prof.

Obstetrics & Gyn on Call. Horowitz. 2nd ed. 1999. pap. text 28.95 (*0-8385-7141-7*, Medical Exam) Appleton & Lange.

Obstetrics & Gynaecology. Lawrence Impey. 1999. LC 98-28847. (*0-632-04901-4*) Blackwell Sci.

Obstetrics & Gynaecology. McCarthy. 1998. pap. text (*0-443-05244-1*) Church.

Obstetrics & Gynaecology. Stabile. 1998. (Illus.). 160p. pap. 29.95 (*0-412-60720-4*, Chap & Hall NY) Chapman & Hall.

Obstetrics & Gynaecology. James Willocks & Kevin Phillips. 5th ed. 1997. LC 97-2285. pap. (*0-443-04850-9*) Church.

Obstetrics & Gynaecology: A Critical Approach to the Clinical Problems. G. J. Jarvis. 1994. (Illus.). 744p. text 135.00 (*0-19-262058-4*) OUP.

Obstetrics & Gynaecology Vade-Mecum. Ed. by David K. James et al. 2000. (Arnold Publication). 352p. pap. 27.50 (*0-340-69274-X*) OUP.

Obstetrics & Gynecological Pharmaceutical Markets: New Delivery Systems for Changing Lifestyles. Market Intelligence Staff. 1993. 288p. 1995.00 (*1-56753-453-8*) Frost & Sullivan.

Obstetrics & Gynecology. Mark A. Frederiksen. 1999. LC 99-40518. (Rypins' Intensive Reviews Ser.). (Illus.). 302p. pap. text 23.00 (*0-397-51557-X*) Lppncott W & W.

Obstetrics & Gynecology. Lawrence Impey. 1997. LC 98-28847. (Illus.). 288p. pap. 57.95 (*0-86542-704-6*) Blackwell Sci.

Obstetrics & Gynecology. William F. Rayburn & J. Christopher Carey. 1996. LC 95-23109. (House Officer Ser.). (Illus.). 423p. pap. 27.95 (*0-683-07181-5*) Lppncott W & W.

Obstetrics & Gynecology. Arthur D. Sorosky. 1998. pap. text (*0-7216-5082-1*); pap. text (*0-7216-6345-1*) Saunders.

Obstetrics & Gynecology. Charles R. B. Beckmann et al. 2nd ed. 1995. LC 94-40390. (Illus.). 560p. (*0-683-00503-0*) Lppncott W & W.

Obstetrics & Gynecology. Mimi C. Berman & Harris L. Cohen. 2nd ed. 1997. LC 96-39954. (Diagnostic Medical Sonography Ser.). 736p. text 110.00 (*0-397-55261-0*, Lippnctt) Lppncott W & W.

Obstetrics & Gynecology. Pamela S. Miles et al. 2nd rev. ed. 1996. LC 96-7854. (Oklahoma Notes). (Illus.). 218p. pap. text 24.95 (*0-387-94632-2*) Spr-Verlag.

Obstetrics & Gynecology. William W. Beck, Jr. 3rd ed. 1993. LC 92-48888. (National Medical Series for Independent Study). (Illus.). 504p. pap. 27.00 (*0-683-06241-7*) Lppncott W & W.

Obstetrics & Gynecology. Charles R. B. Beckmann et al. 3rd ed. 1998. LC 97-49309. 675p. 40.00 (*0-683-30391-0*) Lppncott W & W.

Obstetrics & Gynecology. William W. Beck, Jr. 4th ed. 1996. LC 96-29165. (National Medical Series for Independent Study). 510p. pap. text 32.00 (*0-683-18015-0*) Lppncott W & W.

Obstetrics & Gynecology: A History & Iconography. Harold Speert. rev. ed. 1994. LC 93-44107.Tr. of Iconographia Gyniatrica. (Illus.). 540p. 245.00 (*0-930405-62-5*) Norman SF.

Obstetrics & Gynecology: Annual Review, 1989. Harrison H. Sheld. 1989. (Illus.). 321p. pap. 32.50 (*0-08-037906-0*) Alemany Pr.

Obstetrics & Gynecology: Digging up the Bones, Vol. 7. Nikos M. Linardakis & Sonia Lott. 1998. LC 98-10207. (Digging Up the Bones Ser.). (Illus.). 350p. pap. 19.95 (*0-07-038220-4*) McGraw-Hill Prof.

Obstetrics & Gynecology: PreTest Self-Assessment & Review. Ed. by Mark I. Evans. 8th ed. 1997. LC 97-26207. (Clinical Science Ser.). (Illus.). 200p. pap. 19.95 (*0-07-052529-3*) McGraw-Hill Educ Grp.

Obstetrics & Gynecology: PreTest Self Assessment & Review. Mark I. Evans. 9th ed. 2000. (Pretest Clinical Science Ser.). (Illus.). 263p. pap. 24.95 (*0-07-135961-3*) McGraw-Hill Prof.

***Obstetrics & Gynecology: Principles for Practice.** Ed. by Frank W. Ling & W. Patrick Duff. 2001. LC 00-60939. (Illus.). xv, 1387p. (*0-07-112013-0*) McGraw.

Obstetrics & Gynecology: Resident Survival Guide & Handbook for Clinicians. John D. Gordon et al. 4th ed. 1995. 177p. 12.95 (*0-9638338-0-4*) Stanford Bkstore.

Obstetrics & Gynecology: The Clinical Core. Ralph M. Wynn. 5th ed. 1992. (Illus.). 400p. text 36.00 (*0-8121-1565-1*) Lppncott W & W.

Obstetrics & Gynecology at a Glance. Errol R. Norwitz & John O. Schorge. 2001. LC 00-58500. (Illus.). 136p. pap. 22.95 (*0-632-04341-5*) Blackwell Sci.

Obstetrics & Gynecology Drug Handbook. Gerald I. Zatuchni & Ramona I. Slupik. 2nd ed. 1996. LC 95-224950. 560p. (C). (gr. 13). pap. text 33.95 (*0-8151-9894-9*, 24742) Mosby Inc.

Obstetrics & Gynecology for Medical Students. Charles R. B. Beckmann et al. 1992. (Illus.). 496p. pap. 33.00 (*0-683-00500-6*) Lppncott W & W.

Obstetrics & Gynecology On-Call. Ira R. Horowitz. 1996. (Illus.). 640p. (C). pap. text 32.95 (*0-8385-7174-3*, A7174-4) McGraw.

Obstetrics & Gynecology Recall. F. John Bourgeois et al. 1997. LC 97-10753. (Recall Ser.). (Illus.). 528p. pap. text 29.95 (*0-683-18214-5*) Lppncott W & W.

Obstetrics & Gynecology Review. Arthur D. Sorosky. 1998. pap. text (*0-7216-5083-X*) Saunders.

Obstetrics & Gynecology Review, 1996. Harrison H. Sheld. 1996. (Illus.). 656p. pap. text 48.00 (*0-07-057741-2*) McGraw-Hill Med Pub.

Obstetrics & Gynecology Two Thousand. Mishell. 2000. 79.00 (*0-8151-2200-4*, 31734) Mosby Inc.

Obstetrics & Newborn: Illustrated Text. Norman A. Beischer. 3rd ed. 1997. (Illus.). 794p. pap. text (*0-7020-2123-7*) Bailliere Tindall.

Obstetrics & Perinatology: Current Topics. V. I. Kulakov. 1990. 81.00 (*0-8493-7125-2*, RG572) CRC Pr.

Obstetrics Anesthesia. David J. Birnbach et al. 2000. LC 99-462024. (Illus.). xxiii, 830p. text (*0-443-06560-8*) Saunders.

Obstetrics by Ten Teachers. Ed. by Geoffrey V.P. Chamberlain. 16th ed. 1995. (Illus.). 384p. pap. text (*0-340-57313-9*) E A GBR. *Dist:* OUP.

Obstetrics by Ten Teachers. Ed. by Stuart Campbell & Christoph Lees. 17th ed. 2001. (Arnold Publication). (Illus.). 320p. (Orig.). pap. text 35.00 (*0-340-71986-9*) OUP.

Obstetrics, Contraception & Gynecology. David Brown. 1976. 208p. pap. 42.95 (*0-8464-1430-9*) Beekman Pubs.

Obstetrics-Gynecology: A Problem-Oriented Approach, Vol. 2. Richard L. Bernstine & Catherine Molloy. 1985. pap. 34.25 (*0-87488-801-8*) Elsevier.

Obstetrics, Gynecology & Infertility: Handbook for Clinicians - Resident Survival Guide. John David Gordon et al. 5th ed. 2000. (Illus.). 325p. pap. 14.95 (*0-9645467-6-0*) Scrub Hill.

Obstetrics Illustrated. Alistair W. Miller & Kevin P. Hanretty. 5th ed. 1997. LC 97-28645. pap. text (*0-443-05041-4*) Church.

Obstetrics/Gynecology Nutrition Handbook. Deborah Pesicka et al. 1996. LC 95-16241. (Nutrition Handbook Ser.: Vol. 1). 96p. (C). (gr. 13). spiral bd. 19.00 (*0-412-07501-6*) Kluwer Academic.

Obstructive Lung Disease. Ed. by Stephen G. Jenkinson. 1992. (Contemporary Management in Internal Medicine Ser.: Vol. 2, No. 3). (Illus.). 150p. text (*0-443-08872-1*) Church.

Obstructive Sleep Apnea Syndrome: Diagnosis & Treatment. B. Tucker Woodson et al. 1996. LC 96-28959. (Self-Instructional Package Ser.). (Illus.). 69p. (Orig.). pap. text 25.00 (*1-56772-050-1*) AAO-HNS.

***Obstructive Sleep Apnoea.** Johnson et al. 2001. (Illus.). 200p. (*1-901865-96-7*) Isis Med GBR. *Dist:* Bks Intl VA.

Obtaining & Using Medical Records in Massachusetts. Karen R. Stafford. 1994. LC 94-75468. 94p. pap. text 45.00 (*0-944490-62-X*) Mass CLE.

OCAT: Optometry College (Admission Test) Practice Examination, No. 3. David M. Tarlow. 1992. (Practice Examination Ser.). 40p. pap. text 16.95 (*0-931572-47-9*) Datar Pub.

OCAT (Optometry College Admission Test) Practice Examination. David M. Tarlow. 1992. (Practice Examination Ser.). 40p. No. 1. pap. 16.95 (*0-931572-19-3*); No. 2. pap. 16.95 (*0-931572-20-7*); No. 4. pap. 16.95 (*0-931572-17-7*); No. 5. pap. 16.95 (*0-931572-18-5*) Datar Pub.

OCAT Practice Examination: Annotated Master Answer Guide. David M. Tarlow. 1992. No. 1. 4.95 (*0-931572-42-8*); No. 2. 4.95 (*0-931572-43-6*); No. 3. 4.95 (*0-931572-44-4*); No. 4. 4.95 (*0-931572-45-2*); No. 5. 4.95 (*0-931572-46-0*) Datar Pub.

Occipital Seizures & Epilepsies in Children. Frederick Andermann. 1993. 256p. (*0-86196-385-7*) J Libbey Med GBR. *Dist:* Buttrwrth-Heinemann.

Occlusal Correction: Principles & Practice. Albert J. Solnit & Curnette. 1988. (Illus.). 413p. text 136.00 (*0-86715-161-7*) Quint Pub Co.

Occlusion. Hamish Thomson. 1975. 288p. pap. text (*0-7236-0401-0*) John Wright.

Occlusion. Margeaux Herman. unabr. ed. 1999. 219p. pap. 11.95 (*1-893667-02-2*) Sugar Mtn.

Occlusion. Sigurd P. Ramfjord & Major M. Ash. 4th ed. 1994. LC 94-7653. text 75.00 (*0-7216-5591-2*) Saunders.

Occlusion: Principles & Assessment. Iven Klineberg. 1992. (Illus.). 263p. pap. text 85.00 (*0-7236-0990-X*) Buttrwrth-Heinemann.

Ocular Pathology. Myron Yanoff & Ben S. Fine. 4th ed. 1995. text (*0-7234-2199-4*) Wolfe Publishing GBR. *Dist:* Mosby Inc.

Occult Family Physician & Botanic Guide to Health. Antonette Matteson. 1992. lib. bdg. 89.95 (*0-8490-8744-9*) Gordon Pr.

Occult Family Physician & Botanic Guide to Health. Antonette Matteson. 1996. 317p. reprint ed. spiral bd. 22.50 (*0-7873-0587-1*) Hlth Research.

Occult Family Physician & Botanic Guide to Health: A Description of American & Foreign Plants & Their Medical Virtues. Antonette Matteson. enl. rev. ed. 1993. (Illus.). 327p. reprint ed. pap. 12.50 (*0-916638-24-3*) Meyerbooks.

Occult Family Physician & Botanic Guide to Health, 1894. Antonette Matteson. 1996. 324p. reprint ed. pap. 24.95 (*1-56459-709-1*) Kessinger Pub.

Occult Nodal Metastasis in Solid Carcinomata: Second International Symposium on Celluar Oncology, 5. Ed. by Peter Moloy & Garth, L. Nicolson. 1987. LC 87-15764. 267p. 82.50 (*0-275-92665-6*, C2665, Praeger Pubs) Greenwood.

Occult Science in Medicine. Franz Hartmann. 1991. lib. bdg. 79.95 (*0-8490-4996-2*) Gordon Pr.

Occult Science in Medicine. Franz Hartmann. 1996. 100p. reprint ed. spiral bd. 11.00 (*0-7873-0380-1*) Hlth Research.

Occult Science in Medicine. Franz Hartmann. 1993. 100p. reprint ed. pap. 9.95 (*1-56459-355-X*) Kessinger Pub.

Occult Traumatic Lesions of the Cervical & Thoraco-Lumbar Vertebrae. Martin S. Abel. 2nd ed. 1983. 392p. 42.50 (*0-87527-312-2*) Green.

Occupation & Disease: How Social Factors Affect the Conception of Work-Related Disorders. Allard E. Dembe. 1996. LC 95-39781. 344p. 45.00 (*0-300-06436-5*) Yale U Pr.

Occupation & Ideology of the Salaried Employee. Carl Dreyfuss. Ed. by Leon Stein. 1977. LC 77-70490. reprint ed. lib. bdg. 46.95 (*0-405-10162-7*) Ayer.

Occupation As a Substitute for Restraint in the Treatment of the Mentally Ill: A History of the Passage of Two Bills Through the Massachusetts Legislature. L. Vernon Briggs. 1973. LC 72-2387. (Mental Illness & Social Policy; the American Experience Ser.). reprint ed. 21.95 (*0-405-05195-6*) Ayer.

Occupational & Environmental Cancers of the Urinary System. Wilhelm C. Hueper. 1969. LC 77-76741. (Illus.). 465p. 55.00 (*0-300-01126-1*) Yale U Pr.

Occupational & Environmental Chemical Hazards: Cellular & Biochemical Indices for Monitoring Toxicity. V. Foa et al. 1987. LC 86-27801. (Chemical Science Ser.). 588p. 92.95 (*0-470-20802-3*) P-H.

Occupational & Environmental Infectious Diseases: Epidemiology, Prevention & Clinical Management. Alain J. Couturier. 2000. LC 00-37443. (Illus.). xviii, 748p. (*1-883595-27-4*, OEM Pr) OEM Health.

Occupational & Environmental Medicine. Joseph Ladou. 2nd ed. 1997. 864p. (C). pap. text 54.95 (*0-8385-7216-2*, A-7216-3, Apple Lange Med) McGraw.

Occupational & Environmental Medicine. Composed by Ladou. 3rd ed. 2001. (C). 42.95 (*0-8385-7219-7*) Appleton & Lange.

Occupational & Environmental Medicine Self-Assessment & Review. Robert J. McCunney & Paul P. Rountree. 1998. LC 98-5990. 352p. pap. text 54.95 (*0-7817-1612-8*) Lppncott W & W.

Occupational & Environmental Neurotoxicology. Robert G. Feldman. 1998. LC 98-13524. (Illus.). 528p. text 110.00 (*0-7817-1739-6*) Lppncott W & W.

Occupational & Environmental Reproductive Hazards. Ed. by Maureen Paul. 1993. LC 92-13719. (Illus.). 448p. 95.00 (*0-683-06801-6*) Lppncott W & W.

Occupational & Environmental Respiratory Disease. Philip Harber et al. 1995. (Illus.). 1232p. (C). (gr. 13). text 155.00 (*0-8016-7728-9*, 07728) Mosby Inc.

Occupational & Industrial Hygiene: Concepts & Methods. Ed. by Nurtan A. Esmen & Myron A. Mehlman. 1984. (Advances in Modern Environmental Toxicology Ser.: Vol. 8). (Illus.). 259p. text 65.00 (*0-911131-09-4*) Specialist Journals.

Occupational & Physical Therapy in Educational Environments. Ed. by Irene R. McEwen. 1995. 39.95 (*1-56024-777-0*) Haworth Pr.

Occupational Asthma. Ed. by Emil J. Bardana, Jr. et al. 1991. LC 91-58457. 328p. 69.00 (*1-56053-017-0*) Hanley & Belfus.

Occupational Biomechanics 3e. Don B. Chaffin et al. 3rd ed. 1999. LC 98-28797. (Illus.). 600p. 89.95 (*0-471-24697-2*) Wiley.

Occupational Cancer in Developing Countries. Ed. by Harri Vainio et al. 1995. (IARC Scientific Publications Ser.: No. 129). (Illus.). 202p. pap. text 40.00 (*92-832-2129-X*) OUP.

Occupational Clinical Psychology. James S. Manuso. 1983. LC 82-19065. 336p. 70.00 (*0-275-91041-5*, C1041, Praeger Pubs) Greenwood.

Occupational Disease. 1987. 115p. 15.00 (*0-932387-14-4*) Insur Info.

Occupational Diseases: A Guide to Their Recognition 1991. lib. bdg. 995.00 (*0-8490-5110-X*) Gordon Pr.

Occupational Diseases in Relation to Compensation & Health Insurance. Rosamond W. Goldberg. LC 68-58581. (Columbia University. Studies in the Social Sciences: No. 345). reprint ed. 32.50 (*0-404-51345-X*) AMS Pr.

Occupational Disorders: A Treatment Guide for Therapists. Martin D. Kantor. 1997. LC 96-28536. 272p. 72.50 (*0-275-95529-X*, Praeger Pubs) Greenwood.

Occupational Disorders of the Upper Extremity. Ed. by Lewis H. Millender et al. 1991. (Illus.). 308p. text (*0-443-08797-0*) Church.

Occupational Electrical Injury Vol. 888: An International Symposium. Ed. by Chin-Tu Chen et al. 1999. LC 99-47060. (Annals of the New York Academy of Sciences Ser.: Vol. 888). (Illus.). xi, 372p. 120.00 (*1-57331-232-0*) NY Acad Sci.

Occupational Employee Assistance Programs for Substance Abuse & Mental Health Problems. Andrea E. Foote & John C. Erfurt. 1977. pap. 7.00 (*0-87736-327-7*) U of Mich Inst Labor.

Occupational Epidemiology. Richard R. Monson. 1986. 232p. 132.00 (*0-8493-5793-4*, RC964, CRC Reprint) Franklin.

Occupational Ergonomics: Work Related Musculoskeletal Disorders. Ed. by Francesco Violante & Asa Kilborn. 2000. 208p. (*0-7484-0933-5*) Tay Francis Ltd GBR. *Dist:* Taylor & Francis.

Occupational Exposure Limits for Airborne Toxic Substances. 3rd ed. 1991. (Occupational Safety & Health Ser.: No. 37). xiv, 455p. pap. 42.75 (*92-2-107293-2*) Intl Labour Office.

Occupational Exposure to Pesticides. K. Yoshida. 1999. text (*0-442-00458-3*, VNR) Wiley.

Occupational Exposure to Silica & Cancer Risk. Lorenzo Simonato et al. 1990. (IARC Scientific Publications Ser.: No. 97). (Illus.). 132p. pap. text 45.00 (*92-832-1197-9*) OUP.

Occupational Exposures in Insecticide Application & Some Pesticides. 1991. (IARC Scientific Publications Ser.: Vol. 53). 612p. pap. text 105.00 (*92-832-1253-3*, 1720053) World Health.

Occupational Exposures to Mists & Vapours from Strong Inorganic Acids, & Other Industrial Chemicals. 1992. (IARC Scientific Publications Ser.: Vol. 54). 336p. pap. text 72.00 (*92-832-1254-1*, 1720054) World Health.

Occupational Hand & Upper Extremity Injuries & Diseases. Morton L. Kasdan. 2nd ed. 1997. LC 97-27831. 556p. 88.00 (*1-56053-221-1*) Hanley & Belfus.

Occupational Hazards & Reproduction. Ed. by Kari Hemminki et al. 1985. LC 84-4545. (Illus.). 333p. 132.00 (*0-89116-281-X*) Hemisp Pub.

Occupational Hazards in the Health Professions. Ed. by Dag K. Brune & Christer Edling. 1989. 384p. 149.95 (*0-8493-6931-2*, RC965) CRC Pr.

Occupational Health. J. M. Harrington et al. 4th ed. 1998. LC 98-16050. (Pocket Consultant Ser.). (Illus.). pap. 52.95 (*0-632-04832-8*) Blackwell Sci.

Occupational Health: For the Nurse & Other Health Workers. Ed. by A. J. Kotze. 2nd ed. 1994. 278p. pap. text (*0-7021-2668-3*) Juta & Co ZAF. *Dist:* Intl Spec Bk.

Occupational Health: Recognizing & Preventing Work-Related Disease & Injury. Barry S. Levy & David H. Wegman. 4th ed. 1999. LC 99-35194. (Illus.). xxi, 842p. pap. text 69.95 (*0-7817-1954-2*) Lppncott W & W.

Occupational Health: Risk Assessment & Management. Stephen Sadhra & Krishna G. Rampal. 1999. LC 98-28848. xii, 492p. 187.95 (*0-632-04199-4*) Blackwell Sci.

Occupational Health & Hygiene: Physical, Chemical & Biological Hazards. Jeremy Stranks. 1994. (Health & Safety in Practice Ser.). 192p. (Orig.). pap. (*0-273-60908-4*) Pitman Pub GBR. *Dist:* Trans-Atl Phila.

Occupational Health & Safety in the Care & Use of Research Animals. NRC Committee on Occupational Health and Safety. 1997. LC 97-4794. 250p. (Orig.). pap. text 39.95 (*0-309-05299-8*) Natl Acad Pr.

Occupational Health & Safety in the Emergency Services. Angle. 1998. LC 98-28536. 282p. 50.95 (*0-8273-8359-2*) Delmar.

Occupational Health & Safety Management System: An AIHA Guidance Document. American Industrial Hygiene Association Staff. 1996. LC 96-231697. 31 p. (*0-932627-74-9*) Am Indus Hygiene.

Occupational Health & Safety Technologist Home Study Workbook, Set. Joseph LeBlanc. Ed. by Marvin Becker & James W. Watts. rev. ed. 2000. 352p. pap., wbk. ed. Not sold separately (*1-891017-32-2*) SPAN Intl Train.

Occupational Health & Safety Terms, Definitions, & Abbreviations. Ed. by Robert G. Confer & Thomas R. Confer. 1994. 224p. lib. bdg. 65.00 (*1-56670-077-9*, L1077) Lewis Pubs.

Occupational Health & Working Women in France: Phossy-Jaw & the Match Workers, 1890-1898. Bonnie Gordon. 1989. (Studies in Historical Demography). 200p. reprint ed. text 15.00 (*0-8240-3363-9*) Garland.

Occupational Health Aspects of Construction Work. P. Grandjean. 1983. (Euro Reports & Studies Ser.: No. 86). 28p. pap. text 4.00 (*92-890-1252-8*) World Health.

Occupational Health for the Nurse & Other Health Workers. A. J. Kotze. 2nd ed. 1997. LC 98-135328. x, 414p. (*0-7021-3557-7*) Juta & Co ZAF. *Dist:* Intl Spec Bk.

Occupational Health Hazards of Solvents. Ed. by Myron A. Mehlman et al. rev. ed. 1986. LC 86-61325. (Advances in Modern Environmental Toxicology Ser.: Vol. 2). (Illus.). 259p. pap. text 60.00 (*0-911131-02-7*) Specialist Journals.

Occupational Health in Aviation: Maintenance & Support Personnel. Ed. by Russell B. Rayman et al. 1995. LC 94-25272. (Illus.). 238p. text 63.00 (*0-12-583560-4*) Acad Pr.

Occupational Health in Developing Countries. J. Jeyaratnam. 1992. 576p. 93.00 (*0-19-262122-X*) OUP.

Occupational Health in National Development. 1994. LC 95-135376. 492p. text 43.00 (*981-02-1465-0*) World Scientific Pub.

Occupational Health in National Development. J. Jeyaratnam & Chia Kee Seng. 1994. 576p. text 109.00 (*981-02-1464-2*) World Scientific Pub.

Occupational Health Law. Diana M. Kloss. 3rd ed. 1999. LC 98-52410. 99.95 (*0-632-04263-X*) Blackwell Sci.

***Occupational Health Matters in General Practice.** Ruth Chambers et al. 2000. 208p. pap. (*1-85775-463-8*) Radcliffe Med Pr GBR. *Dist:* Balogh.

***Occupational Health Nursing.** Bannister. 2001. (Illus.). 552p. (*0-7020-2550-X*) W B Saunders GBR. *Dist:* Saunders.

Occupational Health Nursing: Concepts & Practice. Bonnie Rogers. 1994. LC 93-48841. (Illus.). 543p. text 60.00 (*0-7216-7588-3*) Saunders.

***Occupational Health Nursing: Concepts & Practice.** Bonnie Rogers. 2nd ed. 2001. (Illus.). 575p. (*0-7216-8511-0*) Saunders.

Occupational Health Nursing Care Guidelines. Ed. by Debra Daly-Gawenda et al. 1996. LC 96-8187. (Illus.). 336p. 49.95 (*0-8261-9350-1*) Springer Pub.

Occupational Health Pocket Consultant. J. M. Harrington & F. S. Gill. 3rd ed. 1992. (Pocket Consultant Ser.). (Illus.). 368p. pap. 39.95 (*0-632-03189-1*) Blackwell Sci.

Occupational Health Practice. H. A. Waldron & Christer Edling. 4th ed. 1997. LC 97-24662. 336p. (*0-7506-2720-4*) E A GBR. *Dist:* OUP.

Occupational Health Problems of Young Workers. S. Forssman & G. H. Coppee. 1984. (Occupational Safety & Health Ser.: No. 26). v, 143p. 9.00 (*92-2-101051-1*) Intl Labour Office.

Occupational Health Workbook. D. Jeff Burton. 1997. 300p. spiral bd., wbk. ed. 59.95 (*1-883992-10-9*) IVE Inc.

Occupational Hearing Loss. Robert T. Sataloff & Joseph Sataloff. 2nd rev. ed. 1993. LC 92-48421. (Occupational Safety & Health Ser.: Vol. 24). (Illus.). 856p. text 255.00 (*0-8247-8814-1*) Dekker.

Occupational Hygiene. Ed. by J. M. Harrington & K. Gardiner. 2nd ed. 1995. LC 94-45425. 576p. 135.00 (*0-632-03734-2*) Blackwell Sci.

Occupational Hygiene Management Guide. Stanley E. Jones et al. 1990. (Illus.). 145p. lib. bdg. 79.95 (*0-87371-255-2*, L255) Lewis Pubs.

Occupational, Industrial & Environmental Toxicology. Michael Greenberg. 1997. LC 96-44661. (Illus.). 624p. (C). (gr. 13). text 89.95 (*0-8151-3929-2*, 26883) Mosby Inc.

Occupational Injuries: Evaluation, Management & Prevention. Ed. by Thomas N. Herington & Linda H. Morse. 1994. (Illus.). 592p. (C). (gr. 13). text 98.00 (*0-8016-6805-0*, 06805) Mosby Inc.

Occupational Injuries & Illnesses: Counts, Rates & Characteristics, 1994. 1997. 374p. per. 34.00 (*0-16-049067-7*) USGPO.

Occupational Injuries & Illnesses: Counts, Rates & Characteristics, 1995. 2001. 406p. per. 45.00 (*0-16-061767-7*) USGPO.

Occupational Injuries & Illnesses: Counts, Rates & Characteristics, 1996. 1999. 517p. per. 53.00 (*0-16-050092-3*) USGPO.

Occupational Injury: Risk, Prevention & Injury. Ed. by Anne-Marie Feyer & Ann Williamson. 1998. LC 98-140392. 277p. text (*0-7484-0646-8*) Tay Francis Ltd GBR. *Dist:* Taylor & Francis.

Occupational Low Back Pain: Aggresive Nonsurgical Care. Ed. by Bryan D. Kaplansky. 1999. 288p. 69.95 (*0-8493-0089-4*) CRC Pr.

Occupational Low Back Pain: Assessment, Treatment & Prevention. Malcom H. Pope et al. 1990. (Illus.). 348p. (C). (gr. 13). text 94.00 (*0-8016-6252-4*, 06252) Mosby Inc.

Occupational Low Back Pain: Assessment, Treatment & Prevention. Malcolm H. Pope et al. 2nd ed. 2000. 395p. (C). (gr. 13). text 79.95 (*0-8151-4349-4*, 30028) Mosby Inc.

Occupational Low Back Pain Aggressive Nonsurgical Care. Bryan D. Kaplansky. 1999. 69.95 (*1-56670-244-5*) Lewis Pubs.

Occupational Lung Disease. Daniel E. Banks. 1999. LC 98-70535. (Illus.). 538p. text 110.00 (*0-412-73630-6*) OUP.

Occupational Lung Diseases. S. Keith Morgan & Anthony Seaton. 3rd ed. 1995. LC 94-19777. (Illus.). 624p. text 97.00 (*0-7216-4671-9*) Saunders.

Occupational Lung Diseases: Prevention & Control. 1991. (Occupational Safety & Health Ser.: No. 67). ix, 85p. (Orig.). pap. 15.75 (*92-2-106463-8*) Intl Labour Office.

Occupational Lung Diseases: Research Approaches & Methods. Margaret E. Turner-Warwick & Weill. 1981. (Lung Biology in Health & Disease Ser.: Vol. 18). (Illus.). 544p. text 199.00 (*0-8247-1362-1*) Dekker.

Occupational Lung Disorders. W. Raymond Parkes. 3rd ed. 1994. (Illus.). 912p. (*0-7506-1403-X*) E A GBR. *Dist:* OUP.

Occupational Medical Management. Jean Felton. 1989. 145.00 (*0-316-27775-4*, Little Brwn Med Div) Lppncott W & W.

Occupational Medicine: Principles & Practical A. Carl Zenz et al. 3rd ed. 1993. LC 93-40227. (Illus.). 1312p. (C). (gr. 13). text 200.00 (*0-8016-6676-7*, 06676) Mosby Inc.

Occupational Medicine: Quick Reference Guides for Family Physicians. James D. Lomax & Eckhardt Johanning. 2000. (Academy Collection). pap. text 29.95 (*0-7817-2053-2*) Lppncott W & W.

Occupational Medicine Practice Guidelines: A Quick Reference. Ed. by Jeffrey S. Harris. 1999. LC 99-14497. 262p. pap. text 55.00 (*1-883595-26-6*, OEM Pr) OEM Health.

Occupational Medicine Secrets. Ed. by James Cone & Rosemarie Bowler. 1999. LC 99-19893. (Secrets Ser.). (Illus.). 350p. pap. 39.95 (*1-56053-161-4*) Hanley & Belfus.

Occupational Musculoskeletal Disorders. Nortin M. Hadler. 2nd ed. 1999. LC 98-51593. 448p. text 79.95 (*0-7817-1495-8*) Lppncott W & W.

Occupational Neurotoxicology. Lucio G. Costa & Luigi Manzo. 1998. LC 98-5973. 296p. 139.95 (*0-8493-9231-4*) CRC Pr.

Occupational Orthopaedics. Gunnar B. J. Andersson et al. Ed. by Margareta Nordin. 1996. (Illus.). 688p. (C). (gr. 13). text 125.00 (*0-8016-7984-2*, 07984) Mosby Inc.

Occupational Perspective of Health. Ann Wilcock. 1998. LC 98-5746. (Illus.). 272p. pap. text 36.00 (*1-55642-358-6*, 33586) SLACK Inc.

Occupational Safety & Health: The Prevention & Control of Work-Related Hazards. Frank Goldsmith & Lorin E. Kerr. 1982. LC 81-20034. 320p. 45.95 (*0-89885-092-4*, Kluwer Acad Hman Sci) Kluwer Academic.

Occupational Safety & Health in the Emergency Services: Instructor's Guide. Angle. 1999. 128p. tchr. ed. 24.00 (*0-8273-8360-6*) Delmar.

Occupational Safety & Health Law. Mark A. Rothstein. 3rd ed. 1990. (Handbook Ser.). 722p. (C). text 66.30 net. (*0-314-76669-3*) West Pub.

Occupational Safety & Health Law, 1988, includes the 1999 supplement. Stephen A. Bokat & Horace A. Thompson, 2nd. 1988. LC 88-7252. 1034p. suppl. ed. 100.00 incl. trans. (*0-87179-527-2*, 9147-PR9) BNA Books.

Occupational Safety & Health Standards Course Guide Book. 1998. LC 98-83203. (Illus.). 660p. ring bd. 199.95 (*0-9669664-0-6*) Mangan Comns.

Occupational Science: The Evolving Discipline. Ruth Zemke. 1996. LC 96-10611. (Illus.). 466p. pap. 44.95 (*0-8036-0138-7*) Davis Co.

Occupational Science: The Foundation for New Models of Practice. Ed. by Jerry A. Johnson & Elizabeth J. Yerxal. 1990. LC 89-26933. (Occupational Therapy in Health Care Ser.: Vol. 6, No. 4). 112p. (C). text 39.95 (*0-86656-960-X*) Haworth Pr.

Occupational Skin Disease. Robert M. Adams. 2nd ed. 1990. 624p. text 156.00 (*0-7216-2926-1*, 790026) Saunders.

Occupational Skin Disease. Robert M. Adams. Ed. by Judy Fletcher. 3rd ed. 1999. LC 98-25698. (Illus.). 830p. text 125.00 (*0-7216-7037-7*) Saunders.

Occupational Skin Disorders. Daniel J. Hogan. 1994. LC 94-1678. (Topics in Clinical Dermatology Ser.). (Illus.). 184p. 82.50 (*0-89640-248-7*) Igaku-Shoin.

***Occupational Strain & Efficacy in Human Service Workers: When the Rescuer Becomes the Victim.** Maureen F. Dollard et al. 2001. 244p. pap. 47.00 (*0-7923-6853-3*) Kluwer Academic.

Occupational Strategy, Nursing. Jack Rudman. (ACT Proficiency Examination Program Ser.: Vol. 47). 43.95 (*0-8373-5597-4*); 1994. (ACT Proficiency Examination Program Ser.: PEP-47). pap. 23.95 (*0-8373-5547-8*); 1994. (Regents External Degree Ser.: REDP-20). pap. 23.95 (*0-8373-5620-2*) Nat Learn.

Occupational Stress: A Handbook. Ed. by Rick Crandall & Pamela L. Perrewe. 2nd ed. 1995. (Health Psychology & Behavioral Medicine Ser.). 280p. pap. 39.95 (*1-56032-367-1*) Taylor & Francis.

Occupational Stress: Proceedings of the Conference on Occupational Stress, 1977. Ed. by Rosalind M. Schwartz. 1993. 78p. reprint ed. 8.00 (*0-89215-096-3*) U Cal LA Indus Rel.

Occupational Stress & Organizational Effectiveness. Ed. by Anne W. Riley & Stephen J. Zaccaro. 1987. LC 86-25250. 287p. 59.95 (*0-275-92281-2*, C2281, Praeger Pubs) Greenwood.

Occupational Stress & Productivity. John Sweetland. 1979. (Studies in Productivity: Vol. 8). 44p. pap. 55.00 (*0-08-029489-8*) Work in Amer.

Occupational Stress & the Mental & Physical Health of Factory Workers. James S. House. 1980. 365p. (Orig.). pap. 20.00 (*0-87944-254-9*) Inst Soc Res.

Occupational Stress Management. 1986. 64p. pap. text 14.95 (*0-9610026-8-9*) Perf Resource Pr.

Occupational Therapist. Jack Rudman. 1994. (Career Examination Ser.: C-558). pap. 34.95 (*0-8373-0558-6*) Nat Learn.

Occupational Therapist Aide. Jack Rudman. 1994. (Career Examination Ser.: C-1380). pap. 27.95 (*0-8373-1380-5*) Nat Learn.

Occupational Therapist Assistant. Jack Rudman. 1994. (Career Examination Ser.: C-1381). pap. 29.95 (*0-8373-1381-3*) Nat Learn.

Occupational Therapy. Marguerite Abbott et al. (Opportunities in... Ser.). (Illus.). 160p. 1993. pap. 10.95 (*0-8442-6562-4*); 1990. 13.95 (*0-8442-6561-6*) McGraw-Hill Trade (VGM Career Bks).

Occupational Therapy. Simme Cynkin. 1979. 17.00 (*0-316-16610-3*, Little Brwn Med Div) Lppncott W & W.

Occupational Therapy. Simme Cynkin & Anne M. Robinson. 2nd ed. 1989. 304p. text 48.95 (*0-316-16611-1*) Lppncott W & W.

Occupational Therapy: Configuration of a Profession. Anne C. Mosey. 1986. 186p. text 50.00 (*0-89004-699-9*) Lppncott W & W.

Occupational Therapy: Enabling Function & Well-Being. Charles Christiansen & Carolyn Baum. 3rd ed. 2002. 80p. pap. text, tchr. ed. (*1-55642-532-5*) SLACK Inc.

Occupational Therapy: Enabling Function & Well-Being. Charles Christiansen & Carolyn M. Baum. 3rd ed. 2002. 650p. pap. text 52.00 (*1-55642-530-9*) SLACK Inc.

Occupational Therapy: Foundations for Practice. Hagedom. 2nd ed. 1996. pap. text (*0-443-05292-1*, H1258) Church.

Occupational Therapy: Perspectives & Processes. Rosemary Hagedorn. 1995. LC 95-20028. pap. text (*0-443-04978-5*) Church.

Occupational Therapy: Practice Skills for Physical Dysfunction. Lorraine W. Pedretti. 4th ed. 1995. (Illus.). 384p. (gr. 13). pap. text, stu. ed. 20.95 (*0-8151-7214-1*, 27650) Mosby Inc.

Occupational Therapy: Practice Skills for Physical Dysfunction. Ed. by Lorraine W. Pedretti. 4th ed. 1995. (Illus.). 896p. (C). (gr. 13). text 64.00 (*0-8151-6812-8*, 25289) Mosby Inc.

Occupational Therapy: Principles & Practice. Alice Punwar & Suzanne Peloquin. 3rd ed. 2000. LC 99-89084. 312p. pap. text 38.50 (*0-683-30453-4*) Lppncott W & W.

Occupational Therapy: Program Development for Health Promotion & Preventive Services. Ed. by Jerry A. Johnson & Evelyn Jaffe. 1989. LC 89-15460. (Occupational Therapy in Health Care Ser.: Vol. 5, No. 4). (Illus.). 135p. text 4.95 (*0-86656-952-9*) Haworth Pr.

Occupational Therapy: The First 30 Years 1900 to 1930. Virginia A. Quiroga. 1995. LC 95-161107. 290p. (C). pap. 25.00 (*1-56900-025-5*) Am Occup Therapy.

Occupational Therapy: Transition from Classroom to Clinic - Physical Disability Fieldwork Applications. Vicki Smith. 1994. LC 94-228038. (Illus.). 212p. (C). pap. text 42.00 (*1-56900-003-4*) Am Occup Therapy.

Occupational Therapy Across Cultural Boundaries: Theory, Practice & Professional Development. Ed. by Susan C. Merrill. 1992. LC 91-36744. (Occupational Therapy in Health Care Ser.). 116p. lib. bdg. 39.95 (*1-56024-223-X*) Haworth Pr.

Occupational Therapy Activities from Clay to Computers: Theory & Practice. Estelle B. Breines. (Illus.). 245p. 2001. pap. text 39.95 (*0-8036-0544-7*); 1994. LC 94-6968. pap. 41.95 (*0-8036-1145-5*) Davis Co.

Occupational Therapy & Adolescents with Disability. Ed. by Florence S. Cromwell. 1985. LC 85-13954. (Occupational Therapy in Health Care Ser.: Vol. 2, No. 3). 158p. text 39.95 (*0-86656-447-0*); pap. text 19.95 (*0-86656-455-1*) Haworth Pr.

Occupational Therapy & Mental Health: Principles, Skills & Practice. Ed. by Jennifer Creek. 1990. (Illus.). 569p. pap. text (*0-443-03758-2*) Church.

Occupational Therapy & Mental Health: Principles, Skills & Practice. Creek. 2nd ed. 1996. pap. text (*0-443-05202-6*, C8637) Church.

***Occupational Therapy & Physical Dysfunction: Principles, Skills & Practice.** Ann Warren Turner et al. 2001. (Illus.). 895p. pap. (*0-443-06224-2*) Church GBR. *Dist:* Saunders.

Occupational Therapy & Physical Dysfunction: Principles, Skills & Practice. Ed. by Ann Warren Turner et al. 4th ed. 1996. LC 95-40799. 896p. pap. text (*0-443-05177-1*) Church.

Occupational Therapy & Psychosocial Dysfunction. Intro. by Susan C. Merrill. 1993. LC 92-30263. (Occupational Therapy in Health Care Ser.: Vol. 8, Nos. 2 & 3). (Illus.). 247p. pap. text 19.95 (*1-56024-331-7*); lib. bdg. 39.95 (*1-56024-330-9*) Haworth Pr.

Occupational Therapy & the Elderly. Ed. by Marjorie Helm. 1987. (Illus.). 288p. (Orig.). pap. text (*0-443-03469-9*) Church.

Occupational Therapy & the Patient with Pain. Ed. by Florence S. Cromwell. LC 84-10496. (Occupational Therapy in Health Care Ser.: Vol. 1, No. 3). 135p. 1985. pap. text 19.95 (*0-86656-454-3*); 1984. text 39.95 (*0-86656-306-7*) Haworth Pr.

Occupational Therapy Approaches to Stroke. Anne A. Wilcock. 1985. (Illus.). 235p. (Orig.). pap. text (*0-443-03267-X*) Church.

Occupational Therapy Approaches to Traumatic Brain Injury. Ed. by Jerry A. Johnson & Laura Krefting. 1990. (Occupational Therapy in Health Care Ser.). 249p. text 39.95 (*1-56024-064-4*) Haworth Pr.

Occupational Therapy As a Career: An Introduction to the Field & a Structured Method for Observation. Laura Anderson & Christine Malaski. 1998. LC 98-28653. (Illus.). 156p. (C). pap. text 18.95 (*0-8036-0387-8*) Davis Co.

Occupational Therapy Assessment As the Keystone to Treatment Planning. Ed. by Florence Cromwell. LC 84-697. (Occupational Therapy in Health Care Ser.: Vol. 1, No. 2). 114p. 1985. pap. text 19.95 (*0-86656-453-5*); 1984. text 39.95 (*0-86656-305-9*) Haworth Pr.

Occupational Therapy Assessment Tools: An Annotated Index. Ina Asher. 2nd ed. 1996. LC 97-147652. 332p. pap. 40.00 (*1-56900-034-4*, 1020) Am Occup Therapy.

Occupational Therapy Assistant: A Primer. Haru Hirama. 1996. 297p. (Orig.). (C). pap. text 29.95 (*0-935273-00-X*) Chess Pub.

Occupational Therapy Assistant Career Profile. Naomi S. Greenberg. 1990. (Allied Health Professions Monograph). (Illus.). 236p. pap. 37.50 (*0-87527-270-3*) Green.

Occupational Therapy Assistant Management. Amy Solomon & Karen Jacobs. 2001. 250p. pap. text 28.00 (*1-55642-538-4*) SLACK Inc.

Occupational Therapy Consultation: Theory, Principles & Practice. Evelyn Jaffe-Epstein. 1992. (Illus.). 809p. (C). (gr. 13). text 54.00 (*0-8016-6204-4*, 06204) Mosby Inc.

Occupational Therapy Consultation: Theory, Principles & Practice. Evelyn Jaffe & Cynthia Epstein. 1992. 809p. (C). (gr. 13). text 49.95 (*0-8016-7509-X*) Mosby Inc.

Occupational Therapy Evaluation for Adults: A Pocket Guide. Maureen E. Neistadt. 2000. LC 00-42130. 288p. spiral bd. 34.95 (*0-7817-2495-3*) Lppncott W & W.

Occupational Therapy Examination Review Guide. Debra N. Anderson et al. 1996. LC 95-46117. (Illus.). 212p. (C). pap. text 28.95 (*0-8036-0029-1*) Davis Co.

Occupational Therapy for Children with Special Needs Elaine Wilson. 1998. LC 99-186943. 200p. pap. 39.95 (*1-86156-061-3*) Singular Publishing.

Occupational Therapy for Chronic Pain. Strong. 1997. pap. text (*0-443-05251-4*, S2269) Church.

Occupational Therapy for Orthopaedic Conditions. Dina Penrose. 1992. LC 92-49578. (Therapy in Practice Ser.: Vol. 36). 219p. 44.75 (*1-56593-044-4*, 0292) Singular Publishing.

Occupational Therapy for People with Eating Dysfunctions. Ed. by Florence S. Cromwell. 1986. LC 86-12016. (Occupational Therapy in Health Care Ser.: Vol. 3, No. 2). 161p. text 4.95 (*0-86656-588-4*) Haworth Pr.

Occupational Therapy for Physical Dysfunction. Ed. by Catherine A. Trombly. 4th ed. 1995. (Illus.). 941p. text 63.95 (*0-683-08390-2*) Lppncott W & W.

Occupational Therapy for Stroke Rehabilitation. Simon B. Thompson & Maryanne Morgan. Ed. by Jo Campling. 1990. (Therapy in Practice Ser.: No. 11). 192p. pap. 25.00 (*0-412-33530-1*, A4472) Chapman & Hall.

Occupational Therapy for the Brain Injured Adult. Jo Clark-Wilson & Gordon M. Giles. Ed. by Jo Campling. 1990. (Therapy in Practice Ser.). 200p. pap. (*0-412-33520-4*, A4409) Chapman & Hall.

Occupational Therapy for the Energy Deficient Patient. Ed. by Florence S. Cromwell. 1986. LC 85-27277. (Occupational Therapy in Health Care Ser.: Vol. 3, No. 1). 119p. text 39.95 (*0-86656-550-7*); pap. text 19.95 (*0-86656-551-5*) Haworth Pr.

Occupational Therapy Foundations for Practice: Models, Frames of Reference & Core Skills. Rosemary Hagedorn. 1991. (Illus.). 105p. (Orig.). pap. text (*0-443-04540-2*) Church.

Occupational Therapy in Long-Term Psychiatry. Moya Willson. 2nd ed. 1987. LC 86-29931. (Illus.). 222p. pap. text (*0-443-03565-2*) Church.

Occupational Therapy in Psychosocial Practice. Roann Barris et al. 1988. LC 88-43104. 150p. pap. 24.00 (*1-55642-072-2*) SLACK Inc.

Occupational Therapy in Rheumatology: An Holistic Approch. Lynne Sandles. 1990. (Therapy in Practice Ser.: No. 19). 172p. mass mkt. 26.00 (*0-412-31560-2*, A4426) Chapman & Hall.

Occupational Therapy in Short Term Psychiatry. Ed. by Moya Willson. 3rd ed. 1996. LC 96-1651. 269p. (Orig.). pap. text (*0-443-05396-0*) Church.

Occupational Therapy in the Treatment of Adult Hemiplegia. Ortrud Eggers et al. 1983. 160p. reprint ed. pap. text 47.50 (*0-7506-0128-0*) Buttrwrth-Heinemann.

Occupational Therapy Leadership: Marketing Yourself, Your Profession & Your Organization. Grace E. Gilkeson. 1997. LC 96-53182. (Illus.). 344p. pap. 28.95 (*0-8036-0253-7*) Davis Co.

Occupational Therapy Manager. American Occupational Therapy Association Staff. Ed. by Jeanette Bair. rev. ed. 1996. 685p. (C). pap. text 55.00 (*0-910317-76-3*) Am Occup Therapy.

Occupational Therapy Manager's Survival Handbook. Chestina Brollier & Florence S. Cromwell. 1988. LC 87-37486. (Occupational Therapy in Health Care Ser.: Vol. 5, No. 1). (Illus.). 221p. text 39.95 (*0-86656-686-4*) Haworth Pr.

Occupational Therapy Practice Guidelines for Adults with Alzheimer's Disease. AOTA Staff. 1999. (AOTA Practice Guidelines Ser.). (Illus.). 21p. pap. 22.00 (*1-56900-133-2*, 1191) Am Occup Therapy.

Occupational Therapy Practice Guidelines for Adults with Alzheimer's Disease. Mary Corcoran. Ed. by Deborah Lieberman. 2001. (AOTA Practice Guidelines Ser.). (Illus.). 24p. pap. 25.00 (*1-56900-146-4*) Am Occup Therapy.

Occupational Therapy Practice Guidelines for Adults with Carpal Tunnel Syndrome. AOTA Staff. 1999. (AOTA Practice Guidelines Ser.). (Illus.). 13p. pap. 22.00 (*1-56900-121-9*, 1188) Am Occup Therapy.

Occupational Therapy Practice Guidelines for Adults with Carpal Tunnel Syndrome. Deborah L. Rosman. Ed. by Deborah Lieberman. 3rd ed. 2001. (AOTA Practice Guidelines Ser.). (Illus.). 16p. pap. 25.00 (*1-56900-147-2*) Am Occup Therapy.

Occupational Therapy Practice Guidelines for Adults with Hip Fracture Replacement. Janet Verner Platt. Ed. by Deborah Lieberman. 3rd ed. 2001. (AOTA Practice Guidelines Ser.). (Illus.). 12p. pap. (*1-56900-148-0*) Am Occup Therapy.

Occupational Therapy Practice Guidelines for Adults with Hip Fracture/Replacement. AOTA Staff. 1999. (AOTA Practice Guidelines Ser.). (Illus.). 11p. pap. 22.00 (*1-56900-122-7*, 1153) Am Occup Therapy.

Occupational Therapy Practice Guidelines for Adults with Low Back Pain. AOTA Staff. 1999. (AOTA Practice Guidelines Ser.). (Illus.). 15p. pap. 22.00 (*1-56900-123-5*, 1155) Am Occup Therapy.

Occupational Therapy Practice Guidelines for Adults with Low Back Pain. Barbara L. Larson. Ed. by Deborah Lieberman. 3rd ed. 2001. (AOTA Practice Guidelines Ser.). (Illus.). 16p. pap. (*1-56900-149-9*) Am Occup Therapy.

Occupational Therapy Practice Guidelines for Adults with Low Vision. AOTA Staff. 1999. (AOTA Practice Guidelines Ser.). (Illus.). 25p. pap. 22.00 (*1-56900-124-3*, 1192) Am Occup Therapy.

Occupational Therapy Practice Guidelines for Adults with Low Vision. Mary Warren. Ed. by Deborah Lieberman. 3rd ed. 2001. (AOTA Practice Guidelines Ser.). (Illus.). 28p. pap. (*1-56900-150-2*) Am Occup Therapy.

Occupational Therapy Practice Guidelines for Adults with Mood Disorders. AOTA Staff. 2000. (AOTA Practice Guidelines Ser.). (Illus.). pap. (*1-56900-142-1*) Am Occup Therapy.

Occupational Therapy Practice Guidelines for Adults with Neurodegenerative Diseases. AOTA Staff. 1999. LC 00-500802. (AOTA Practice Guidelines Ser.). (Illus.). iv, 19p. pap. 22.00 (*1-56900-125-1*, 1194) Am Occup Therapy.

Occupational Therapy Practice Guidelines for Adults with Rheumatoid Arthritis. AOTA Staff. 2000. (AOTA Practice Guidelines Ser.). (Illus.). pap. (*1-56900-152-9*) Am Occup Therapy.

Occupational Therapy Practice Guidelines for Adults with Schizophrenia. AOTA Staff. 1999. (AOTA Practice Guidelines Ser.). (Illus.). 25p. pap. 22.00 (*1-56900-126-X*, 1189) Am Occup Therapy.

Occupational Therapy Practice Guidelines for Adults with Schizophrenia. Kathleen R. Kannenberg. Ed. by Deborah Lieberman. 3rd ed. 2001. (AOTA Practice Guidelines Ser.). (Illus.). 24p. pap. (*1-56900-153-7*) Am Occup Therapy.

Occupational Therapy Practice Guidelines for Adults with Spinal Cord Injury. AOTA Staff. 1999. (AOTA Practice Guidelines Ser.). (Illus.). 33p. pap. 22.00 (*1-56900-129-4*, 1154) Am Occup Therapy.

Occupational Therapy Practice Guidelines for Adults with Spinal Cord Injury. Cathy D. Dolhi. Ed. by Deborah Lieberman. 3rd ed. 2001. (AOTA Practice Guidelines Ser.). (Illus.). 32p. pap. (*1-56900-154-5*) Am Occup Therapy.

Occupational Therapy Practice Guidelines for Adults with Stroke. AOTA Staff. 1999. (AOTA Practice Guidelines Ser.). 15p. pap. 22.00 (*1-56900-127-8*, 1152) Am Occup Therapy.

Occupational Therapy Practice Guidelines for Adults with Stroke. Jane D. Acquaviva. Ed. by Deborah Lieberman. 3rd ed. 2001. (AOTA Practice Guidelines Ser.). (Illus.). 16p. pap. (*1-56900-155-3*) Am Occup Therapy.

Occupational Therapy Practice Guidelines for Adults with Traumatic Brain Injury. AOTA Staff. 1999. (AOTA Practice Guidelines Ser.). (Illus.). 18p. pap. 22.00 (*1-56900-128-6*, 1151) Am Occup Therapy.

Occupational Therapy Practice Guidelines for Adults with Traumatic Brain Injury. Mary Vining Radomski. Ed. by Deborah Lieberman. 3rd ed. 2001. (AOTA Practice Guidelines Ser.). (Illus.). 20p. pap. (*1-56900-156-1*) Am Occup Therapy.

Occupational Therapy Practice Guidelines for Attention-Deficit/Hyperactivity Disorders. AOTA Staff. 1999. (AOTA Practice Guidelines Ser.). (Illus.). 13p. pap. 22.00 (*1-56900-130-8*, 1159) Am Occup Therapy.

Occupational Therapy Practice Guidelines for Attention-Deficit/Hyperactivity Disorders. Barbara E. Hanft. Ed. by Deborah Lieberman. 3rd ed. 2001. (AOTA Practice Guidelines Ser.). (Illus.). 16p. pap. 25.00 (*1-56900-157-X*) Am Occup Therapy.

Occupational Therapy Practice Guidelines for Cerebral Palsy. AOTA Staff. 1999. (AOTA Practice Guidelines Ser.). (Illus.). 13p. (Orig.). pap. 22.00 (*1-56900-131-6*, 1156) Am Occup Therapy.

Occupational Therapy Practice Guidelines for Cerebral Palsy. Cheryl Colangelo & Delia Gorga. Ed. by Deborah Lieberman. 3rd ed. 2001. (AOTA Practice Guidelines Ser.). (Illus.). 12p. (Orig.). pap. 25.00 (*1-56900-158-8*) Am Occup Therapy.

Occupational Therapy Practice Guidelines for Chronic Pain. AOTA Staff. 1999. LC 00-697943. (AOTA Practice Guidelines Ser.). (Illus.). iv, 15p. pap. 22.00 (*1-56900-132-4*, 1193) Am Occup Therapy.

Occupational Therapy Practice Guidelines for Chronic Pain. Joyce Engel. Ed. by Deborah Lieberman. 2nd ed. 2001. (AOTA Practice Guidelines Ser.). (Illus.). 16p. pap. 25.00 (*1-56900-159-6*) Am Occup Therapy.

Occupational Therapy Practice Guidelines for Substance Use Disorders. AOTA Staff. 1999. (AOTA Practice Guidelines Ser.). (Illus.). 23p. pap. 22.00 (*1-56900-134-0*, 1190) Am Occup Therapy.

Occupational Therapy Practice Guidelines for Substance Use Disorders. AOTA Staff. Ed. by Deborah Lieberman. 3rd ed. 2001. (AOTA Practice Guidelines Ser.). (Illus.). pap. (*1-56900-160-X*) Am Occup Therapy.

Occupational Therapy Practice Guidelines for Tendon Injuries. AOTA Staff. 1999. (AOTA Practice Guidelines Ser.). (Illus.). 13p. pap. 22.00 (*1-56900-135-9*, 1157) Am Occup Therapy.

Occupational Therapy Practice Guidelines for Tendon Injuries. Lauren B. Rivet. 3rd ed. 2001. (AOTA Practice Guidelines Ser.). (Illus.). 16p. pap. (*1-56900-161-8*) Am Occup Therapy.

Occupational Therapy Practice Guidelines for Young Children with Delayed Development. AOTA Staff. 1999. (AOTA Practice Guidelines Ser.). (Illus.). 15p. pap. 22.00 (*1-56900-136-7*, 1158) Am Occup Therapy.

Occupational Therapy Practice Guidelines for Young Children with Delayed Development. Barbara E. Hanft. Ed. by Deborah Lieberman. 3rd ed. 2001. (AOTA Practice Guidelines Ser.). (Illus.). 16p. pap. (*1-56900-162-6*) Am Occup Therapy.

Occupational Therapy Protocol Management in Adult Physical Dysfunction. Marilyn S. Daniel & Randy Strickland. 1997. 464p. spiral bd. 110.00 (*0-8342-0314-6*, 20314) PRO-ED.

Occupational Therapy Quick Coding Guide. AOTA Staff. 1999. (Illus.). 20p. pap. 18.00 (*1-56900-115-4*, 1199) Am Occup Therapy.

Occupational Therapy Services for Children & Youth under the Individuals with Disabilities Education Act. Elizabeth Maruyama et al. 1997. LC 97-172030. iv, 240 p. 50.00 (*1-56900-069-7*) Am Occup Therapy.

Occupational Therapy Services for Children & Youth under the Individuals with Disabilities Education Act. AOTA Staff. 2nd ed. 1999. LC 00-265375. (Illus.). pap. (*1-56900-137-5*) Am Occup Therapy.

Occupational Therapy Stories: Psychosocial Interaction in Practice. Barbara Borg & Mary A. Bruce. 1997. LC 96-53891. 192p. (C). pap. 29.00 (*1-55642-313-6*, 33136) SLACK Inc.

Occupational Therapy Treatment Goals for the Physically & Cognitively Disabled. Claudia K. Allen et al. 1992. 350p. (C). pap. text 58.00 (*0-910317-72-0*) Am Occup Therapy.

Occupational Therapy with Borderline Patients. Ed. by Diane Gibson. 1983. LC 83-13008. (Occupational Therapy in Mental Health Ser.: Vol. 3, No. 3). 91p. text 39.95 (*0-86656-262-1*) Haworth Pr.

Occupational Therapy with Children. Helen Clancy. 1990. (Illus.). 320p. pap. text (*0-443-03437-0*) Church.

Occupational Therapy Workbook. Julie Bass Haugen. 2002. 150p. pap. text 22.00 (*1-55642-531-7*) SLACK Inc.

Occupational Toxicants: Critical Data Evaluation for MAK Values & Classification of Carcinogens. Ed. by Commission for the Investigation of Health Hazards & Dietrich Henschler. (Illus.). Vol. 1. 1990. 398p. 165.00 (*3-527-27019-1*); Vol. 2. 1991. 349p. 165.00 (*3-527-27022-1*); Vol. 3. 1992. 380p. 165.00 (*3-527-27023-X*); Vol. 4. 1992. 385p. 165.00 (*3-527-27025-6*) Wiley (Wiley-VCH).

Occupational Toxicology. Ed. by Neill H. Stacey. 1993. LC 93-13852. 420p. (*0-85066-830-1*); pap. (*0-85066-831-X*) Tay Francis Ltd GBR. *Dist:* Taylor & Francis.

Occurrence & Health Significance of Staphylococcus Aureus in a Pig Slaughter Line. Urszula J. Narucka. 1979. 96p. (*90-6191-070-6*) A A Balkema NLD. *Dist:* Ashgate Pub Co.

OCD in Children & Adolescents: A Cognitive-Behavioral Treatment Manual. John S. March & Karen Mulle. 1998. LC 98-2637. 298p. text 36.00 (*1-57230-242-9*, C0242) Guilford Pubns.

Oceanic Feeling: The Origins of Religious Sentiment in Ancient India. J. Moussaieff Masson. 1980. (Studies of Classical India: No. 3). 228p. text 140.50 (*90-277-1050-3*) Kluwer Academic.

Oceans Without Continents. Geoff Meads. 1997. LC 97-9200. (*1-85775-270-8*) Radcliffe Med Pr GBR. *Dist:* Balogh.

OClinical Gynecologic Endocrinology & Infertility. Leon Speroff et al. 6th ed. 1999. LC 98-36104. 1,170p. text 135.00 (*0-683-30379-1*) Lppncott W & W.

Octacosanol, Carnitine, & Other "Accessory" Nutrients, Vol. 2. Earl R. Mindell & Jeffrey S. Bland. 1982. (Good Health Guides: Vol. 2). 32p. pap. text 2.95 (*0-87983-316-5*, 33165K, Keats Pubng) McGraw-Hill Trade.

Ocular Accommodation, Convergence & Fixation Disparity: A Manual of Clinical Analysis. David A. Goss. 2nd ed. 1995. LC 95-13935. (Illus.). 222p. pap. text 44.99 (*0-7506-9497-1*) Buttrwrth-Heinemann.

***Ocular Adverse Reactions to Drugs: A Computer Database.** John Lawrenson. 2001. audio compact disk 159.00 (*0-7506-5421-X*) Buttrwrth-Heinemann.

Ocular Allergies. Barbara J. Jennings. 2001. 208p. pap. 45.00 (*0-7506-9794-6*) Buttrwrth-Heinemann.

Ocular Anatomy & Histology. David Pipe & Linda Rapley. 1989. (C). (*0-900099-19-4*) Assn Brit Dispen Opticians GBR. *Dist:* St Mut.

Ocular Anatomy & Physiology. Tammy Langley et al. 1999. LC 99-19851. (Basic Bookshelf for Eyecare Professionals Ser.). (Illus.). 160p. pap. 30.00 (*1-55642-348-9*, 63489) SLACK Inc.

Ocular Anatomy & Physiology. Trygve Saude. Tr. by Robert Fletcher. 1993. LC 92-48827. 184p. pap. 58.95 (*0-632-03599-4*) Blackwell Sci.

Ocular Anatomy & Physiology for Opticians. Jonathan I. Morris. 2001. 224p. 50.00 (*0-7506-9904-3*) Buttrwrth-Heinemann.

Ocular Anesthesia. Scott Greenbaum. Ed. by Richard Lampert. 1997. (Illus.). 256p. text 74.00 (*0-7216-5955-1*) Saunders.

Ocular Blood Flow. Ed. by H. J. Kaiser et al. 1996. (Illus.). viii, 226p. 145.25 (*3-8055-6238-1*) S Karger.

Ocular Blood Flow in Glaucoma: Means, Methods & Measurements. Ed. by G. N. Lambrou & E. L. Greve. 1989. LC 89-19833. (Illus.). 295p. lib. bdg. (*90-6299-053-3*) Kugler NLD. *Dist:* Lib Res.

Ocular Circulation & Neovascularization. Ed. by D. Benezra et al. 1987. (Documenta Ophthalmologica Proceedings Ser.). (C). lib. bdg. 285.50 (*0-89838-892-9*) Kluwer Academic.

Ocular Differential Diagnosis. Frederick H. Roy. 5th ed. 1992. LC 92-10384. 900p. pap. text 62.50 (*0-8121-1594-5*); 6th ed. 1996. LC 96-13229. (Illus.). 768p. pap. 85.00 (*0-683-07415-6*) Lppncott W & W.

Ocular Disease Manual. John Meyler & Geoffrey Roberson. 2001. (Manual Ser.). (Illus.). 224p. pap. 60.00 (*0-7506-1816-7*) Buttrwrth-Heinemann.

Ocular Disease Update Manual. Ed. by Louis J. Catania. 1991. 180p. 39.95 (*1-879040-12-3*) Scovill Paterson.

Ocular Disease Update 2. Ed. by Louis J. Catania. 1991. 296p. 49.95 (*1-879040-13-1*) Scovill Paterson.

Ocular Disorders Proven or Suspected to Be Hereditary in Dogs. American College of Veterinary Ophthalmologists, G. 1992. (Illus.). 296p. (Orig.). pap. text 10.00 (*0-9635163-0-2*) Canine Eye Reg.

Ocular Drug Handbook. Mosby Staff & Gaston Mauger. 1996. 320p. (C). (gr. 13). text 35.95 (*0-8151-6910-8*, 27119) Mosby Inc.

Ocular Examination: Measurements. Karla Zadnik. Ed. by Richard Lampert. 1996. LC 96-6968. 416p. pap. text 52.00 (*0-7216-5209-3*) Saunders.

Ocular Fluorophotometry & the Future. Ed. by J. G. Cunha-Vaz & E. B. Leite. 1989. LC 89-19845. (Illus.). 167p. pap. text (*90-6299-054-1*) Kugler NLD. *Dist:* Lib Res.

Ocular Histopathology: A Guide to Differential Diagnosis. Curtis Margo & Grossniklaus. 1990. (Illus.). 352p. text 130.00 (*0-7216-3291-2*) Saunders.

Ocular Immune Responses: Proceedings of the International Symposium on Immunology & Immunopathology of the Eye, 1st, Strasbourg, 1974. International Symposium on Immunology and Immunopath. Ed. by W. R. Boeke. 1976. (Modern Problems in Ophthalmology Ser.: Vol. 16). 300p. 86.25 (*3-8055-2192-8*) S Karger.

Ocular Immunology. Foster. 1999. text (*0-7216-6339-7*) Saunders.

Ocular Immunology in Health & Disease. Steven B. Koevary. 1998. 200p. pap. text 44.99 (*0-7506-9900-0*) Buttrwrth-Heinemann.

Ocular Infection: Investigation & Treatment in Practice. David V. Seal et al. 1998. (Illus.). 256p. (*1-85317-437-8*) Martin Dunitz GBR. *Dist:* Mosby Inc.

Ocular Infections & Immunity. Gary Holland et al. Ed. by Jay S. Pepose. 1995. (Illus.). 1584p. (C). (gr. 13). text 210.00 (*0-8016-6757-7*, 06757) Mosby Inc.

Ocular Inflammatory Disease. Foster. Date not set. text (*0-7216-6338-9*) Saunders.

Ocular Manifestations of Neurologic Disease. Bernard H. Blaustein. 1996. LC 95-50441. (Optometric Problem Solving Ser.). (Illus.). 304p. (C). (gr. 13). pap. text 39.95 (*0-8151-0507-X*, 24391) Mosby Inc.

Ocular Manifestations of Systemic Disease. Bernard H. Blaustein. 1994. 321p. (*0-443-08883-7*) Church.

Ocular Microsurgery. Ed. by Arthur S. Lim. 1981. (Developments in Ophthalmology Ser.: Vol. 1). (Illus.). viii, 96p. 43.50 (*3-8055-1106-X*) S Karger.

Ocular Needs in Africa. F. M. Mburu. 1984. 147p. pap. 25.00 (*0-08-031299-3*, Pergamon Pr) Elsevier.

Ocular Pathology. David J. Apple & Rabb. 5th ed. 1997. LC 97-41914. (Illus.). 718p. (C). (gr. 13). text 189.00 (*0-8151-0592-4*, 27523) Mosby Inc.

Ocular Pathology: A Color Atlas. Myron Yanoff & Ben S. Fine. 1988. LC 65-40033. text 95.00 (*0-397-44659-4*, Lippncott) Lppncott W & W.

Ocular Pharmacology & Therapeutics: A Primary & Shared Care Guide. Michael Doughty. 2001. LC 00-29259. (Illus.). 132p. pap. text 70.00 (*0-7506-4520-2*) Buttrwrth-Heinemann.

Ocular Prostheses. W. Warren. 1989. (C). (*0-89771-747-3*) Assn Brit Dispen Opticians GBR. *Dist:* St Mut.

***Ocular Surface Diseases.** Ed. by Edward J. Holland & Mark J. Mannis. 2001. LC 2001-31419. (Illus.). xiv, 283p. (*0-387-95161-X*) Springer Pub.

Ocular Surgery Comanagment. Paul M. Barney & Maynard L. Pohl. 2000. (Illus.). 500p. (C). 110.00 (*0-8385-7211-1*, Apple Lange Med) McGraw.

Ocular Therapeutics: Pharmacology & Clinical Application. Paul U. Fechner & Klaus D. Teichmann. 1997. LC 97-23207. (Illus.). 700p. pap. 55.00 (*1-55642-312-8*, 63128) SLACK Inc.

Ocular Therapeutics Handbook: A Clinical Manual. Bruce E. Onofrey et al. 1997. LC 97-25437. (Illus.). 640p. spiral bd. 59.95 (*0-397-51392-5*) Lppncott W & W.

Ocular Therapeutics Manual. Nizar K. Hirji. Date not set. 208p. pap. 52.50 (*0-7506-3910-5*) Buttrwrth-Heinemann.

Ocular Toxicity of Intraoperatively Used Drugs & Solutions. R. M. Nuijts. 1995. (Illus.). 150p. text (*90-6299-141-6*) Kugler NLD. *Dist:* Lib Res.

Ocular Toxicology: Proceedings of the 4th Congress of the International Society of Ocular Toxicology Held in Annecy, France, October 9-13, 1994. Ed. by Keith Green et al. 1995. 388p. 115.00 (*0-306-45133-6*, Kluwer Plenum) Kluwer Academic.

Ocular Tumors. Shields. 1993. 39.00 (*0-316-78579-2*, Little Brwn Med Div) Lppncott W & W.

Ocular Tumours. Bertil Damato. 2000. LC 00-20613. (Illus.). 249p. text 99.00 (*0-7506-2220-2*) Buttrwrth-Heinemann.

Oculo-Auditory Syndromes. Ed. by Lucian S. Regenbogen & Gabriel J. Coscas. 1985. (Illus.). 368p. (gr. 13). 86.50 (*0-89352-225-2*) Mosby Inc.

Oculocutaneous Manifestations of Rheumatic Diseases. George E. Ehrlich. 1973. (Rheumatology Ser.: Vol. 4). 150p. 52.25 (*3-8055-1594-4*) S Karger.

Oculoplastic & Orbital Emergencies. John V. Linberg. 1992. LC 89-15189. (Illus.). 237p. (C). pap. text 69.95 (*0-8385-3626-3*, A3626-7) McGraw.

Oculoplastic Surgery. Francis L. Tse. 1992. (Illus.). 528p. text 115.00 (*0-397-51070-5*) Lppncott W & W.

Oculoplastic Surgery: The Requisites in Ophthalmology. Jeffrey A. Nerad. 2001. LC 2001-18296. (Requisites in Ophthalmology Ser.). (Illus.). 600p. text 89.00 (*0-323-00174-2*) Mosby Inc.

***Oculoplastic Surgery Atlas.** Ed. by Geoffrey J. Gladstone. 2001. LC 2001-41111. (Illus.). xiv, 110p. 95.00 (*0-387-95316-7*) Spr-Verlag.

OD Source Book: A Practitioner's Guide. Robert M. Frame et al. 1986. LC 81-70786. 208p. pap. 95.00 (*0-88390-172-2*, Pffr & Co) Jossey-Bass.

Odontologia Pediatrica. Cameron. 1998. (C). text 42.50 (*84-8174-337-2*) Mosby Inc.

Odor Sensation & Memory. Trygg Engen. 1991. LC 91-21067. 168p. 55.00 (*0-275-94111-6*, C4111, Praeger Pubs) Greenwood.

Odoratus Sexualis: A Scientific & Literary Study of Sexual Scents & Erotic Perfumes. Iwan Bloch. LC 72-9620. reprint ed. 42.50 (*0-404-57414-9*) AMS Pr.

Odoratus Sexualis: Smell & Sex. I. Bloch. 1992. (Studies in the Psychopathology of Sex). lib. bdg. 88.00 (*0-8490-5365-X*) Gordon Pr.

Odyssey: A Psychotherapist's Journey along the Cutting Edge. Victor Bogart. 1993. LC 92-76171. 348p. (Orig.). pap. 24.95 (*0-9635500-1-2*) Baskin Pub OR.

Odyssey of a Nursing Home Administrator. Richard C. Schriever. Ed. by Oma Whitcomb. 1990. LC 90-70581. 15.95 (*0-9626978-1-8*) Whitcomb Pub.

Odyssey of Hearing Loss: Tales of Triumph. Michael A. Harvey. 1998. LC 98-8086. (Illus.). 240p. 23.95 (*1-58121-006-X*) Dawn Sign.

Odyssey of Primary Care Research: Historical Perspectives. Edward J. Bujold. Ed. by Thomas McGowen. 1997. LC 96-69743. 140p. pap. 24.95 (*0-9654202-0-5*) Speck Pub.

Odysseys in Psychotherapy. Ed. by Joseph J. Shay & Joan Wheelis. 2000. (Illus.). 416p. text 44.95 (*0-8290-5215-1*) Ardent Media.

***OECD Workshop on Genetic Testing: Vienna, 2000.** Ed. by E. Ronchi. 2001. (Community Genetics 2000 Ser.: Vol. 3, No. 4). (Illus.). 72p. 25.25 (*3-8055-7221-2*) S Karger.

Oedipal Paradigms in Collision: A Centennial Emendation of a Piece of Freudian Canon (1897-1997) Howard Covitz. 1998. LC 97-31584. (Reshaping of Psychoanalysis Ser.: Vol. 9). XVI, 385p. (C). text 59.95 (*0-8204-3921-5*) P Lang Pubng.

Oedipus & Beyond: A Clinical Theory. Jay Greenberg. 1993. 288p. pap. 19.50 (*0-674-63091-2*); 1992. LC 91-7078. 320p. (C). 42.50 (*0-674-63090-4*) HUP.

Oedipus Complex Today: Clinical Implications. Ronald Britton et al. 1989. 160p. reprint ed. pap. text (*0-946439-55-9*) Karnac Bks GBR. *Dist:* Other Pr LLC.

Oedipus in the Stone Age: A Psychoanalytic Study of Masculinization in Papua New Guinea. Theodore Lidz & Ruth W. Lidz. 1989. LC 88-25796. 215p. 35.00 (*0-8236-3727-1*) Intl Univs Pr.

Oedipus in the Trobriands. Melford E. Spiro. 1982. LC 82-7032. 224p. (C). pap. text 8.00 (*0-226-76989-5*); lib. bdg. 26.00 (*0-226-76988-7*) U Ch Pr.

Oedipus, Philosopher. Jean-Joseph Goux. Tr. by Catherine Porter. 1993. LC 92-40387. (Meridian: Crossing Aesthetics Ser.). 240p. 51.00 (*0-8047-2169-6*); pap. 17.95 (*0-8047-2171-8*) Stanford U Pr.

Oedipus Road: Searching for a Father in a Mother's Fading Memory. Tom Dodge. 1996. LC 95-26697. 212p. pap. 15.95 (*0-87565-153-4*) Tex Christian.

Oedipus Variations: Studies in Literature & Psychoanalysis. Karl Kerenyi & James Hillman. Tr. by Jon Solomon. 1990. LC 90-21611. (Dunquin Ser.: No. 19). 170p. (Orig.). pap. 14.50 (*0-88214-219-4*) Spring Pubns.

Oesophageal Atresia. Spencer W. Beasley et al. 1991. 424p. pap. 209.95 (*0-412-34820-9*) Chapman & Hall.

Oesterreichische Gesellschaft fuer Gynaekologie & Geburtshilfe, Bayerische Gesellschaft fuer Geburtshilfe & Frauenheilkunde, Jahrestagung, Salzburg, June 1993. Ed. by E. Reinold. 1993. (Journal: Vol. 33, Suppl. 1, 1993). (Illus.). x, 354p. pap. 158.50 (*3-8055-5916-X*) S Karger.

Oesterreichische Gesellschaft fuer Gynaekologie und Geburtshilfe: Jahrestagung, Mayrofen, 1988. Eduard Gitsch & E. Reinold. 1988. (Journal: Vol. 28, Suppl. 2, 1988). (Illus.). x, 278p. pap. 87.00 (*3-8055-4937-7*) S Karger.

Oesterreichische Gesellschaft fuer Gynaekologie und Geburtshilfe, Jahrestagung, Graz, Juni 1990: Journal: Gynaekologische Rundschau, Vol. 30, Suppl. 1, 1990. Ed. by Eduard Gitsch & E. Reinold. 1990. (Illus.). x, 260p. pap. 82.75 (*3-8055-5306-4*) S Karger.

***Oesterreichischer HNO-Kongress 2000 Band 10, Nr. 2: 44 Kongress, Wien, September 2000.** Ed. by M. C. Grasl & W. D. Baumgartner. 2000. (GER.). 54p. 25.25 (*3-8055-7160-7*) S Karger.

Oestrogen Deficiency: Causes & Consequences. Robert W. Shaw. 1996. LC 96-16860. (Advances in Reproductive Endocrinology Ser.: Vol. 8). 176p. lib. bdg. 74.95 (*1-85070-719-7*, Parthenon Pbng) CRC Pr.

Oestrogens: Physiological & Clinical Aspects. F. Bidlingmaier & D. Knorr. 1978. (Pediatric & Adolescent Endocrinology Ser.: Vol. 4). (Illus.). 59.25 (*3-8055-2845-0*) S Karger.

Oeuvres Completes de J. M. Charcot, Set. Jean M. Charcot. LC 70-169463. reprint ed. (*0-404-10000-7*) AMS Pr.

Of Children: An Introduction to Child Development. Guy R. Lefrancois. 5th ed. 1985. 606p. (C). pap. 28.00 net. (*0-534-05502-8*) Wadsworth Pub.

Of Course You Are Angry. Gayle Rosellini & Mark Worden. 1986. LC 86-45385. (Hazelden Book Ser.). (Orig.). pap. 12.00 (*0-06-255442-5*) Harper SF.

Of Diabetic Mothers & Their Babies: An Examination of the Impact of Maternal Diabetes on Offspring Prenatal Development & Survival. Harold Kalter. 2000. 260p. 58.00 (*90-5702-617-1*, Harwood Acad Pubs) Gordon & Breach.

Of Foxes & Hen Houses: Licensing & the Health Professions. Stanley J. Gross. 1984. LC 83-11218. (Illus.). 204p. 55.00 (*0-89930-059-6*, GFH/, Quorum Bks) Greenwood.

Of Love, Sex & Marriage. Robert Stein. 2000. 190p. pap. 19.00 (*1-882670-20-5*) Spring Jrnl.

Of Mice & Women: Aspects of Female Aggression. Ed. by Kaj Bjorkqvist & Pirkko Niemela. 1992. LC 92-8880. (Illus.). 414p. text 55.00 (*0-12-102590-X*) Acad Pr.

Of Power & Love & Sound Mind: Six Years with Undiagnosed Lyme Disease. Linda Hanner. 1989. 224p. 5.00 (*0-9622669-0-6*) Kashan Pub.

Of Primeval Steps & Future Leaps: An Essay on the Emergence of Human Beings, the Source of Women's Oppression, & the Road to Emancipation. Ardea Skybreak. 1985. LC 84-24448. 160p. (Orig.). pap. 8.95 (*0-916650-19-7*) Banner Pr Intl.

Of Rats, Sparrows & Flies: A Lifetime in China. Arthur Chung. 1994. LC 94-77656. 256p. (C). text 23.95 (*0-9623048-8-3*) Heritage West.

***Of Spirits & Madness: An American Psychiatrist in Africa.** Paul R. Linde. 2001. LC 2001-32656. 240p. text 24.95 (*0-07-136734-9*) McGraw-Hill Prof.

Off-Label Drug Use & FDA Review of Supplemental Drug Applications: Hearing Before the Subcommittee on Human Resources & Intergovernmental Relations of the Committee on Government Reform & Oversight, House of Representatives, One Hundred Fourth Congress, Second Session, September 12, 1996. Contrib. by U. S. Congress, House Committee on Government Reform & Oversight, Subcommittee on Human Resources and Intergovernmental Relations. 1997. LC 98-133428. (Illus.). (*0-16-055961-8*) USGPO.

Off the Beat: A Book about Abnormal Heart Rhythms. Julia A. Purcell. Ed. by Nancy R. Hull. 1996. LC 91-33673. (Illus.). 24p. pap. text 6.25 (*0-939838-32-X*) Pritchett & Hull.

Off the Pedestal: Transforming the Business of Medicine. Michael A. Greenberg. 1990. 167p. 14.95 (*0-942540-39-5*) Breakthru Pub.

Off the Pedestal: Transforming the Business of Medicine. Michael A. Greenberg. Ed. by Frank Reuter. 1992. 166p. pap. 9.95 (*0-9631700-0-7*) Making Med Wk.

Offender Profiling: Theory, Research & Practice. Ed. by Janet L. Jackson & Debra A. Bekerian. 1997. LC 97-17402. (Psychology of Crime, Policing, & Law Ser.). 254p. pap. 75.00 (*0-471-97565-6*) Wiley.

Offenders, Deviants or Patients? Herschel A. Prins. 2nd ed. 1995. LC 94-34150. (Illus.). 304p. (C). 84.95 (*0-415-10220-0*, C0116) Routledge.

Offending Women: A Study in Social Control & Its Resistance - Female Lawbreakers & the Criminal Justice System. Anne Worrall. 1996. (Sociology of Law & Crime Ser.). 208p. (C). pap. 26.95 (*0-415-03725-5*, A4076) Routledge.

Office & Bedside Procedures: Clinical Manual. Mary Chestnutt & Thomas Dewar. 1996. (Illus.). 483p. (C). pap. text 34.95 (*0-8385-1095-7*, A1095-7, Apple Lange Med) McGraw.

Office & Career Management for the Eyecare Paraprofessional. Bill Borover & Tammy Langley. 1997. LC 96-51005. (Basic Bookshelf for Eyecare Professionals Ser.). 144p. pap. text 30.00 (*1-55642-331-4*, 63314) SLACK Inc.

Office & Operative Hysteroscopy. B. Blanc et al. 1999. (Illus.). 260p. (C). (*2-287-59652-6*) Spl France Editions FRA. *Dist:* Spr-Verlag.

Office-Based Family Pharmacist. 1978. LC 78-58638. (Illus.). (Orig.). pap. text 10.95 (*0-9602034-1-9*) E V White.

Office-Based Infertility Practice. David B. Seifer & Robert L. Collins. 2001. LC 00-53200. (Illus.). 400p. 85.00 (*0-387-98390-2*) Spr-Verlag.

Office-Based Surgery in Otolaryngology. Ed. by Andrew Blitzer et al. 1998. LC 97-42732. (Illus.). 700p. 99.00 (*0-86577-739-X*) Thieme Med Pubs.

Office-Based Surgery in Otolaryngology. John H. Krouse et al. 1999. LC 98-26628. (Illus.). 300p. text (*0-7216-7674-X*) Saunders.

Office Emergencies. Scott. Date not set. pap. text (*0-7216-7779-7*) Saunders.

Office Endoscopy. Bergin F. Overholt & Sarkis J. Chobanian. 1990. 216p. 49.00 (*0-683-06660-9*) Lppncott W & W.

Office Gynecology. Ed. by Morton A. Stenchever. 2nd ed. 1996. (Illus.). 640p. (C). (gr. 13). text 59.95 (*0-8151-8225-2*, 27459) Mosby Inc.

Office Gynecology. Robert H. Glass. 4th ed. 1992. (Illus.). 448p. 95.00 (*0-683-03546-0*) Lppncott W & W.

Office Gynecology: Advanced Management Concepts. Ed. by John V. Knaus & John H. Isaacs. 1993. LC 93-18079. (*0-383-94032-X*); (Illus.). 384p. 89.00 (*0-387-94032-4*) Spr-Verlag.

Office Management of Digestive Diseases. Joseph Danzi & Joseph Scopelliti. 1992. (Illus.). 234p. text 49.00 (*0-8121-1436-1*) Lppncott W & W.

Office Management of the Colon & Rectal Disease. Guy L. Kratzer & Robert J. Demarest. 1985. (Illus.). 251p. text 115.00 (*0-7216-1189-3*) Saunders.

Office Orthopedics for Primary Care: Diagnosis & Treatment. Bruce C. Anderson. 1994. LC 94-25753. (Illus.). 208p. (C). pap. text 42.00 (*0-7216-4576-3*) Saunders.

Office Orthopedics for Primary Care: Diagnosis & Treatment. Bruce C. Anderson. Ed. by Ray Kersey. 2nd ed. 1998. LC 98-36303. (Illus.). 285p. (C). pap. text 42.00 (*0-7216-7089-X*) Saunders.

Office Practice of Medicine. Ed. by William T. Branch. 3rd ed. 1994. LC 93-20531. (Illus.). 1184p. text 115.00 (*0-7216-4338-8*) Saunders.

Office Practice of Medicine. Branch. 4th ed. 1999. text (*0-7216-7672-3*) Saunders.

Office Practice of Neurology. Ed. by Martin A. Samuels et al. 1995. 1280p. text (*0-443-08816-0*) Church.

Office Procedure Forms in the Academy Collection: Quick Reference Guides for Family Physicians. Thomas J. Zuber. 1998. LC 98-23693. (Academy Collection). 150p. spiral bd. 29.95 (*0-683-30580-8*) Lppncott W & W.

Office Procedures for Primary Care. John L. Pfenninger & Grant C. Fowler. 1994. LC 94-9013. (Mosby-Year Book Primary Care Ser.). (Illus.). 1200p. (C). (gr. 13). pap. text 71.95 (*0-8016-6384-9*, 06384) Mosby Inc.

Office Procedures in Managed Health Care with Data Disk for MediSoft for Windows. Patricia M. Boyd & Brent D. Boyd. 1999. LC 98-39160. 400p. text 35.00 incl. disk (*0-02-801222-4*) Glencoe.

Office Procedures in the Academy Collection: Quick Reference Guides for Family Physicians. Thomas J. Zuber & American Academy of Family Physicians Staff. 1998. LC 98-22560. (Academy Collection). 186p. pap. 29.95 (*0-683-30424-0*) Lppncott W & W.

Office Smart! Risk Management Techniques for Medical Office Professionals. Rosemary Gafner. 1993. 78p. stu. ed. 35.00 (*1-884269-01-X*) Med Risk Mgmt.

Office Sports Medicine. Ed. by Morris B. Mellion. 2nd ed. 1997. LC 95-35462. (Illus.). 400p. 54.00 (*1-56053-120-7*) Hanley & Belfus.

Office Staff Risk Management Resource: Audio Cassette & Handbook. RiskCare Staff. 1997. 38p. pap. text 29.00 incl. audio (*1-893929-09-4*) RiskCare.

Office Urgencies & Emergencies: Quick Reference Guides for Family Physicians. Richard B. Birrer. 2000. LC 2001-29059. (Academy Collection). (Illus.). xiii, 194p. pap. text 29.95 (*0-7817-2055-9*) Lppncott W & W.

Office Urology: The Clinician's Guide. Ed. by Elroy D. Kursh & James C. Ulchaker. 2000. LC 00-33560. (Current Clinical Urology Ser.: Vol. 3). 544p. 99.50 (*0-89603-789-4*) Humana.

Official ABMS Directory of Board Certified Medical Specialists, 1998 Ed. by Marquis Who's Who Staff & American Board of Medical Specialities Staff. 30th anniv. ed. 1997. 485.00 (*0-8379-0551-6*) Marquis.

Official ABMS Directory of Board Certified Medical Specialists 2000, 4 vols. Ed. by Marquis Who's Who Staff. 32nd ed. 1999. (Official ABMS Directory of Board Certified Medical Specialists Ser.). 11500p. 510.00 (*0-8379-0565-6*) Marquis.

Official ABMS Directory of Board Certified Medical Specialists 2001 Ed. by Marquis Who's Who Staff. 33rd ed. 2000. 11,500p. 525.00 (*0-8379-0571-0*) Marquis.

Official American Board of Medical Specialties (ABMS) Directory of Board Certified Colon & Rectal Surgeons. 1992. 34p. 79.95 (*0-8379-2500-2*) Marquis.

Official American Board of Medical Specialties (ABMS) Directory of Board Certified Dermatologists. 1992. 209p. 79.95 (*0-8379-2501-0*) Marquis.

Official American Board of Medical Specialties (ABMS) Directory of Board Certified Emergency Medicine Physicians. 1992. 248p. 79.95 (*0-8379-2503-7*) Marquis.

Official American Board of Medical Specialties (ABMS) Directory of Board Certified Medical Geneticists. 1992. 32p. 99.95 (*0-8379-2504-5*) Marquis.

Official American Board of Medical Specialties (ABMS) Directory of Board Certified Neurological Surgeons. 1992. 100p. 99.95 (*0-8379-2505-3*) Marquis.

Official American Board of Medical Specialties (ABMS) Directory of Board Certified Nuclear Medicine Specialists. 1992. 103p. 99.95 (*0-8379-2506-1*) Marquis.

Official American Board of Medical Specialties (ABMS) Directory of Board Certified Ophthalmologists. 1992. 389p. 79.95 (*0-8379-2507-X*) Marquis.

Official American Board of Medical Specialties (ABMS) Directory of Board Certified Plastic Surgeons. 1992. 121p. 79.95 (*0-8379-2508-8*) Marquis.

Official American Board of Medical Specialties (ABMS) Directory of Board Certified Thoracic Surgeons. 1992. 147p. 79.95 (*0-8379-2509-6*) Marquis.

Official American Board of Medical Specialties (ABMS) Directory of Board Certified Urologists. 1992. 227p. 99.95 (*0-8379-2510-X*) Marquis.

Official Annual Statement Blanks of the NAIC: Health Maintenance Organizations. Ed. by Patti Carli. 1998. 99p. ring bd. (*0-89382-523-9*, ASB-HU98) Nat Assn Insurance.

Official Annual Statement Blanks of the NAIC: Hospital, Medical, Dental & Indemnity Corporations. Patti Carli. rev. ed. 1999. 106p. ring bd. (*0-89382-529-8*, ASB-MU99) Nat Assn Insurance.

Official Disability Guidelines: Length of Disability Data by ICD-9-CM from CDC & OSHA Plus NHDS Hospital Length of Stay. Ed. by Philip L. Denniston. 1995. (Orig.). pap. 150.00 (*1-880891-21-2*) Work-Loss Data.

Official Guide to Caribbean Medical Schools. Salaish K. Sarin & Ravi K. Yalamanchi. 1997. (Illus.). 104p. pap. text 14.95 (*0-9663087-0-0*) CaribMed.

Official Guide to Graduate Nursing Schools. NLN Staff. 1999. (Illus.). 336p. (C). pap. text 27.95 (*0-7637-1060-1*, 1060-1, N L N Bart) Jones & Bartlett.

***Official Guide to Graduate Nursing Schools.** NLN Staff. 2nd ed. 2002. (C). pap. text 29.95 (*0-7637-1806-8*, 1806-8) Jones & Bartlett.

Official Guide to Undergraduate & Graduate Nursing Schools. NLN Research Division Staff. 1999. (Illus.). 1216p. (C). pap. text 34.95 (*0-7637-1107-1*, 1107-1, N L N Bart) Jones & Bartlett.

***Official Guide to Undergraduate & Graduate Nursing Schools.** National League for Nursing Staff. 2nd ed. 2002. (C). pap. text 37.95 (*0-7637-1807-6*, 1807-6, N L N Bart) Jones & Bartlett.

Official Guide to Undergraduate Nursing Schools. NLN Research Division Staff. 2000. (Illus.). 1024p. (C). pap. text 27.95 (*0-7637-1108-X*, 1108-X, N L N Bart) Jones & Bartlett.

Official Herbs: Botanical Substances in the United States Pharmacopoeias: 1820-1990. Wade Boyle. 1991. (Illus.). 97p. (Orig.). pap. 12.95 (*0-9623518-3-0*) Eclectic Med.

Official Laboratory Research Notebook. Jones and Bartlett Publishers Staff. 1998. (Illus.). 75p. (C). pap. text 9.95 (*0-7637-0904-2*, 0904-2) Jones & Bartlett.

Official Laboratory Research Notebook. Jones and Bartlett Publishers Staff. 1998. (Illus.). 50p. (C). spiral bd., lab manual ed. (*0-7637-0815-1*) Jones & Bartlett.

Official NAIC Annual Statement Blanks: Hospital, Medical, & Dental Service or Indemnity Corporation. Ed. by Patti Carli. 3rd rev. ed. 1996. 114p. ring bd. 75.00 (*0-89382-394-5*) Nat Assn Insurance.

Official Pocket Guide to Diabetic Exchanges. American Diabetes Association & American Dietetic Association Staff. 1997. LC 97-41452. (Illus.). 64p. pap. 5.95 (*1-58040-003-5*, 00035Q) Am Diabetes.

Official Study Guide for the Certified Occupational Therapy Assistant Cota Certification Examination. 1999. (C). pap. 35.00 (*0-9677436-0-5*) Natl Board Cert Occp Ther.

Official Study Guide for the CGFNS Qualifying Examination. Commission on Graduates of Foreign Nursing Schools. 3rd ed. 1995. 200p. (C). (*0-9630592-2-X*) Grads of For Nursing.

Official Study Guide for the Occupational Therapist Registered OTR Certification Examination. 1999. (C). pap. 35.00 (*0-9677436-1-3*) Natl Board Cert Occp Ther.

Official Wilderness First-Aid Guide. Wayne Merry. 1994. 408p. pap. 14.95 (*0-7710-8250-9*) McCland & Stewart.

Offshore Medicine. Ed. by R. A. Cox. 2nd ed. 1986. (Illus.). 258p. 102.00 (*0-387-16201-1*) Spr-Verlag.

Ofloxacin in Compromised Host: International Ofloxacin Symposium, July 12, 1990, Vancouver, Canada. Ed. by K. Shimizu. 1991. (Journal: Vol. 37, Suppl. 1, 1991). (Illus.). iv, 72p. pap. 50.50 (*3-8055-5423-0*) S Karger.

Ohio Health Care in Perspective, 1999. Ed. by Kathleen O'Leary Morgan & Scott E. Morgan. 1999. 21p. spiral bd. 19.00 (*0-7401-0084-X*) Morgan Quitno Corp.

Ohio Health Care in Perspective 2000. Ed. by Kathleen O'Leary Morgan & Scott E. Morgan. 2000. 21p. spiral bd. 19.00 (*0-7401-0234-6*) Morgan Quitno Corp.

Ohio Health Care Perspective, 1998. Ed. by Kathleen O'Leary Morgan & Scott E. Morgan. 1998. 20p. pap. 19.00 (*1-56692-834-6*) Morgan Quitno Corp.

Ohio Health Care Provider Law. Susan O. Scheutzow. 1994. LC 94-234100. 388p. (Orig.). pap. 52.50 (*0-8322-0381-5*) Banks-Baldwin.

Ohio Mental Health Law. Steven J. Eagle & Michael Kirkman. 2nd ed. 1990. (Baldwin's Ohio Handbook Ser.). 419p. pap. 53.00 (*0-8322-0305-X*) Banks-Baldwin.

Ohio Nursing Law. Sue D. Calloway. 1991. 536p. pap. text 48.50 (*0-8322-0371-8*) Banks-Baldwin.

OH's Intensive Care Manual. Andrew Bersten. 2002. 1024p. pap. 82.00 (*0-7506-5184-9*) Buttrwrth-Heinemann.

Okay, So I Don't Have a Headache: What I Learned (And What You Need to Know) about PMS, Hormones, Stress, Diet, Menopause - And Sex. Cristina Ferrare. 2000. 224p. pap. 12.95 (*0-312-26366-X*, St Martin Griffin) St Martin.

Oklahoma Elementary School Injury Prevention Eduation: The Subject-Integrated Safety Curriculum for Teachers - Grade Four. Ruth Azeredo. Ed. by Sue Mallonee & Shelli S. Stidham. 1995. (Illus.). 130p. (Orig.). pap. 7.50 (*1-889728-05-5*) OK St Dept Hlth Injury.

Oklahoma Elementary School Injury Prevention Education: The Subject-Integrated Safety Curriculum for Teachers - Grade Five. Ruth Azeredo. Ed. by Sue Mallonee & Shelli S. Stidham. 1995. (Illus.). 130p. (Orig.). pap. 7.50 (*1-889728-06-3*) OK St Dept Hlth Injury.

Oklahoma Elementary School Injury Prevention Education: The Subject-Integrated Safety Curriculum for Teachers - Grade One. Ruth Azeredo. Ed. by Sue Mallonee & Shelli S. Stidham. 1995. (Illus.). 130p. (Orig.). pap. 7.50 (*1-889728-02-0*) OK St Dept Hlth Injury.

Oklahoma Elementary School Injury Prevention Education: The Subject-Integrated Safety Curriculum for Teachers - Grade Three. Ruth Azeredo. Ed. by Sue Mallonee & Shelli S. Stidham. 1995. (Illus.). 130p. (Orig.). pap. 7.50 (*1-889728-04-7*) OK St Dept Hlth Injury.

Oklahoma Elementary School Injury Prevention Education: The Subject-Integrated Safety Curriculum for Teachers - Grade Two. Ruth Azeredo. Ed. by Sue Mallonee & Shelli S. Stidham. 1995. (Illus.). 130p. (Orig.). pap. 7.50 (*1-889728-03-9*) OK St Dept Hlth Injury.

Oklahoma Elementary School Injury Prevention Education: The Subject-Integrated Safety Curriculum for Teachers - Kindergarten. Ruth Azeredo. Ed. by Sue Mallonee & Shelli S. Stidham. 1995. (Illus.). 130p. (Orig.). pap. 7.50 (*1-889728-01-2*) OK St Dept Hlth Injury.

M N O

Oklahoma Elementary School Injury Prevention Education: The Subject-Integrated Safety Curriculum for Teachers - Kindergarten Through Grade Five. Ruth Azeredo. Ed. by Sue Mallonee & Shelli S. Stidham. 1995. (Illus.). 130p. (Orig.). pap. 40.50 (*1-889728-00-4*) OK St Dept Hlth Injury.

Oklahoma Health Care Perspective, 1998. Ed. by Kathleen O'Leary Morgan & Scott E. Morgan. 1998. 20p. pap. 19.00 (*1-56692-835-4*) Morgan Quitno Corp.

Oklahoma Notes: Pediatrics. A. E. Osburn. 1993. LC 92-49140. 280p. (*3-540-97955-7*) Spr-Verlag.

Oklahoma Notes: Study Skills & Test-Taking Strategies for Medical Students. Deborah D. Shain. 2nd ed. 1995. LC 95-18354. (Oklahoma Notes). (Illus.). 204p. 24.95 (*0-387-94396-X*) Spr-Verlag.

Old Age: Its Compensations & Rewards. A. L. Vischer. 1980. LC 79-8698. (Growing Old Ser.). (Illus.). reprint ed. lib. bdg. 21.95 (*0-405-12809-6*) Ayer.

Old Age: The Major Involution. Aldred Scott Warthin. Ed. by Robert J. Kastenbaum. 1979. LC 78-22224. (Aging & Old Age Ser.). (Illus.). reprint ed. lib. bdg. 19.95 (*0-405-11837-6*) Ayer.

Old Age & Finitude: A Contribution to Psychogerontology. Joep M. Munnichs. Ed. by Leon Stein. 1980. LC 79-8676. (Growing Old Ser.). reprint ed. lib. bdg. 19.95 (*0-405-12792-8*) Ayer.

Old Age Assistance Reports for Business, Consumers & Health Sciences: Index of New Information. Justin A. Kimberly. 1997. 160p. 57.50 (*0-7883-1694-X*); pap. 47.50 (*0-7883-1695-8*) ABBE Pubs Assn.

Old Age Challenge to the Biomedical Model: Paradigm Strain & Health Policy. Charles Longino & John Murphy. 1995. LC 94-30642. (Society & Aging Ser.). 184p. (C). 31.95 (*0-89503-165-5*) Baywood Pub.

Old Age in the Modern World: Report of the Third Congress of the International Association of Gerontology, London. International Association of Gerontology Staff. Ed. by Leon Stein. 1980. LC 79-8671. (Growing Old Ser.). reprint ed. lib. bdg. 63.95 (*0-405-12786-3*) Ayer.

Old Age in Transition: The Geriatric Ward. Peter Woolfson. 1997. LC 96-19120. 152p. 55.00 (*0-89789-497-9*, Bergin & Garvey) Greenwood.

Old & Ill. Ed. by Linda Challis & Helen Bartlett. 1989. (C). (*0-86242-059-8*) Age Concern Eng GBR. *Dist:* St Mut.

Old & New Dopamine Agonists in Parkinson's Disease. Ed. by U. Bonuccelli & J. M. Rabey. LC 95-37404. (Journals of Neural Transmission: No. 45). 1996. 300p. pap. 112.00 (*3-211-82717-X*); 1995. (*0-387-82717-X*) Spr-Verlag.

Old Dad Chiro: A Biography of D. D. Palmer Founder of Chiropractic. Vern Gielow. 1995. 142p. pap. 19.95 (*1-885048-07-6*) Barge Chiropract.

Old English Herbals. Eleanor S. Rhode. 1972. (Illus.). 248p. lib. bdg. 42.50 (*0-85636-003-1*) Lubrecht & Cramer.

Old Herb Doctor. Joseph E. Meyer. 2nd rev. ed. 1984. (Illus.). 176p. pap. 8.95 (*0-916638-08-1*) Meyerbooks.

Old Herb Doctor: Rare Herbal Formulas Which Have Healed Thousands Where Others Have Failed. 1991. lib. bdg. 79.95 (*0-8490-4995-4*) Gordon Pr.

Old Herb Doctor, His Secrets & Treatments. Ed. by Health Research Staff. 1996. 200p. reprint ed. spiral bd. 17.00 (*0-7873-0396-8*) Hlth Research.

Old Icelandic Medical Miscellany. Henning Larsen. LC 75-23736. reprint ed. 40.00 (*0-404-13293-6*) AMS Pr.

Old Law, New Medicine: Medical Ethics & Human Rights. Sheila McLean. 1999. 224p. (*0-86358-403-9*) Rivers Oram GBR. *Dist:* NYU Pr.

Old Loyalties, New Ties: Therapeutic Strategies with Stepfamilies. Emily B. Visher & John S. Visher. 1989. LC 87-23899. 272p. text 39.95 (*0-87630-489-7*) Brunner-Routledge.

Old People: Report of a Survey Committee on the Problems of Aging & the Care of Old People. B. Seebohm Rowntree. Ed. by Leon Stein. 1980. LC 79-8682. (Growing Old Ser.). (Illus.). reprint ed. lib. bdg. 23.95 (*0-405-12799-5*) Ayer.

Old Scapes, New Maps: A Training Program for Psychotherapy Supervisors. Ludmila W. Hoffman. LC 90-61678. iii, 223p. 1990. pap. text 7.95 (*0-9628475-0-X*); 1991. reprint ed. 15.95 (*0-9628475-1-8*) Milusik Pr.

Old Time Cures-Farmers Folklore. David J. Gerrick & Doreen Dietsche. 1980. 104p. (Orig.). pap. 3.95 (*0-916750-41-8*) Dayton Labs.

Old-Time Favorites. American Diabetes Association. 1998. (Month of Meals Menu Planning Ser.). 64p. pap. 14.95 (*1-58040-017-5*, 00175Q) Am Diabetes.

Old-Time Home Remedies. Ed. by Ken Tate. 1998. LC 97-72868. (Illus.). 160p. 24.95 (*1-882138-30-9*) Hse White Birches.

Old-Time Makers of Medicine. James J. Walsh. LC 75-23767. reprint ed. 36.00 (*0-404-13394-0*) AMS Pr.

Older Adult Psychotherapy Treatment Planner. Deborah Frazer & Arthur E. Jongsma, Jr. 1998. LC 98-42397. (Practice Planners Ser.). 288p. pap. 175.00 incl. disk, cd-rom (*0-471-29581-7*) Wiley.

Older Adult Resource Guide. SRG Publishing Staff. 1997. 216p. pap. text 5.95 (*0-8151-2208-X*) Mosby Inc.

Older Adults: Nutritional Interventions... For Major Chronic Conditions. Jonathan Silver. 1999. 75p. (C). spiral bd. 15.00 (*1-892870-07-X*) Best Years Inc.

Older Adults Coping with Cancer: Integrating Cancer into a Life Mostly Lived. Sarah H. Kagan. rev. ed. 1997. LC 96-30015. (Studies on the Elderly in America). (Illus.). 137p. text 44.00 (*0-8153-2859-1*) Garland.

Older Adults with Developmental Disabilities & Leisure: Issues, Policy, & Practice. Ed. by Ted Tedrick. 1997. LC 96-46303. (Activities, Adaptation & Aging Ser.: Vol. 21, No. 3). 116p. (C). 29.95 (*0-7890-0023-7*) Haworth Pr.

Older American's Medications Guide. Jonathan Silver. 1998. 45p. 20.00 (*1-892870-06-1*) Best Years Inc.

Older & Wiser. Richard Restack. 1997. LC 97-14232. 304p. 23.50 (*0-684-82976-2*) S&S Trade.

Older Deaf Child. P. Hoiberg et al. 1973. (Modern Approaches to the Diagnosis & Instruction of Multi-Handicapped Children Ser.: Vol. 12). viii, 64p. 17.75 (*90-237-4112-9*) Taylor & Francis.

Older Male Mortality & Cigarette Smoking, Vol. 6. Samuel H. Preston. 1976. LC 76-4875. (Population Monograph: No. 7). (Illus.). 150p. reprint ed. lib. bdg. 24.75 (*0-8371-8830-X*, PROM, Greenwood Pr) Greenwood.

Older Offenders: Perspectives in Criminology & Criminal Justice. Ed. by Belinda R. McCarthy & Robert J. Langworthy. 1988. LC 87-7147. 253p. 75.00 (*0-275-92734-2*, C2734, Praeger Pubs) Greenwood.

Older People & Community Care: Critical Theory & Practice. Beverley Hughes. 1995. LC 95-14731. (Rethinking Aging Ser.). 176p. (*0-335-19157-6*); pap. (*0-335-19156-8*) OpUniv Pr.

Older People, Nursing & Mental Health. Ed. by Stuart Darby et al. 1998. LC 98-29335. (Illus.). 192p. pap. text 35.00 (*0-7506-2440-X*) Buttrwrth-Heinemann.

Older Persons & Service Providers: An Instructor's Training Guide. Ed. by Glorian Sorensen. 1981. LC 80-22868. 366p. text 45.95 (*0-89885-020-7*, Kluwer Acad Hman Sci) Kluwer Academic.

Older Than My Mother: A Nurse's Life & Triumph over Breast Cancer. Augusta H. Gale. 1996. LC 96-18873. (Illus.). 144p. 18.00 (*0-9605670-8-9*) Ananse Pr.

Older Veterans: Linking VA & Community Resources. Ed. by Terrie Wetle & John Rowe. 1985. (Division of Health Policy Research & Education Ser.). 464p. 26.00 (*0-674-63275-3*) HUP.

Older Women in the City. Department for the Aging, City of New York. Ed. by Robert J. Kastenbaum. 1979. LC 78-73649. (Aging & Old Age Ser.). lib. bdg. 19.95 (*0-405-11839-2*) Ayer.

Older Women with Chronic Pain. Ed. & Intro. by Karen A. Roberto. 1994. LC 94-27471. (Journal of Women & Aging Ser.). (Illus.). 119p. pap. 9.95 (*1-56023-061-4*, Harrington Park); 128p. lib. bdg. 39.95 (*1-56024-706-1*) Haworth Pr.

Oldest Old in Everyday Life: Perception, Coping with Change & Stress. Ruth E. Dunkle et al. 2001. LC 00-64095. xii, 180p. (*0-8261-1385-0*) Springer Pub.

Oldtimers & Alzheimer's Vol. 1: The Descriptive Organization of Senility. Ed. by Jaber F. Gubrium. 1986. LC 86-10404. (Contemporary Ethnographic Studies). 219p. 73.25 (*0-89232-697-2*) Jai Pr.

Oleum Magistrale. George Baker. 1969. LC 72-171. (English Experience Ser.: No. 123). 104p. reprint ed. 16.00 (*90-221-0123-1*) Walter J Johnson.

Olfaction: A Model System for Computational Neuroscience. Ed. by Joel L. Davis & Howard Eichenbaum. 1991. LC 91-10563. (Illus.). 320p. 55.00 (*0-262-04124-3*) MIT Pr.

Olfaction & Taste: Proceedings of the 2nd International Symposium, Tokyo, Sept. 1965. T. Hayashi. 1967. LC 63-1222. (Wenner Gren Center International Symposium Ser.: Vol. 8). (*0-08-011695-7*) Pergamon Repr GBR. *Dist:* Franklin.

Oligodendroglia. Ed. by William T. Norton. 1984. (Advances in Neurochemistry Ser.: Vol. 5). 338p. 95.00 (*0-306-41547-X*, Plenum Trade) Perseus Pubng.

Oligonucleotide & Gene Therapy-Base Antisense Therapeutics. Ed. by Wendy Mori. 1997. (IBC Library Ser.). (Illus.). (Orig.). pap. (*1-57936-039-4*) Drug & Market Dev.

Oligonucleotides As Therapeutic Agents, Vol. 209. Derek J. Chadwick et al. 1997. LC 97-24989. (Oligonucleotides as Therapeutic Agents Ser.: Vol. 209). 260p. 128.00 (*0-471-97279-7*) Wiley.

Olive Leaf Extract. Morton Walker. 1997. LC 00-266637. 100p. mass mkt. 5.99 (*1-57566-226-4*, Knsington) Kensgtn Pub Corp.

Olive Oil Miracle. Jean Barilla. 1997. (Good Health Guides). 48p. pap. 3.95 (*0-87983-763-2*, 37632K, Keats Pubng) McGraw-Hill Trade.

Olsen Endomyocardial Biopsy. 1989. lib. bdg. (*0-85200-674-8*) Kluwer Academic.

Omaha Orange: A Popular History of EMS in America. Carl J. Post. 1992. (Illus.). (C). pap. text 28.95 (*0-86720-187-8*, 187-8) Jones & Bartlett.

Omaha System: Applications for Community Health Nursing. Ed. by Karen S. Martin & Nancy J. Scheet. 1991. (Illus.). 423p. pap. text 81.00 (*0-7216-6126-2*) Saunders.

Omega Solution: Unleash the Amazing, Scientifically Based Healing Power of Omega-3 & 6 Fatty Acids. Jonathan Goodman. 2001. LC 2001-21978. (Illus.). 256p. pap. 15.95 (*0-7615-1779-0*, Prima Health) Prima Pub.

***Omega 3 Connection.** Andrew Stoll. 2002. 304p. pap. 14.00 (*0-684-87139-4*, Fireside) S&S Trade Pap.

Omega-3 Fatty Acids: Metabolism & Biological Effcts. Ed. by Christian A. Drevon et al. 1993. LC 93-17079. (Advances in Life Sciences Ser.). ix, 389p. 103.00 (*0-8176-2884-3*) Birkhauser.

Omega-3 Fatty Acids & Health. Joyce A. Nettleton. 1995. LC 94-20759. 359p. (C). 97.00 (*0-412-98861-5*) Aspen Pub.

Omega-Three Fatty Acids in Health & Disease. Lees & Karel. 1990. (Food Science & Technology Ser.: Vol. 37). (Illus.). 328p. text 165.00 (*0-8247-8292-5*) Dekker.

Omens & Oracles: Collective Psychology in the Nuclear Age. Jerry Kroth. 1992. LC 90-27792. 240p. 64.00 (*0-275-93889-1*, C3889, Praeger Pubs) Greenwood.

Omentum: Proceedings of the First International Conference on the Omentum Held in Research Triangle Park, North Carolina, October 28-31, 1988. Ed. by H. S. Goldsmith. 1990. (Illus.). x, 252p. 108.00 (*0-387-97337-0*) Spr-Verlag.

Omentum Application to the Brain & Spinal Cord. Ed. by Harry S. Goldsmith. 2000. (Illus.). 250p. pap. text 59.95 (*0-9674933-0-7*) Forefront Pub.

Omeprazole & Acid Inhibition: The Essential Issues - Journal: Digestion, Vol. 47, Suppl. 1, 1990. Ed. by R. H. Hunt. 1991. (Illus.). iv, 84p. pap. 26.25 (*3-8055-5386-2*) S Karger.

Omni Book of Medicine. Ed. by Owen Davies. 1984. mass mkt. 3.95 (*0-8217-1364-7*, Zebra Kensgtn) Kensgtn Pub Corp.

Omnipotent Fantasies & the Vulnerable Self. Ed. by Carolyn S. Ellman & Joseph Reppen. 1997. LC 96-38978. (Library of Clinical Psychoanalysis). 50.00 (*0-7657-0046-8*) Aronson.

Omni's Future Medical Almanac. Dick Teresi & Patrice Adcroft. 1988. (McGraw-Hill Paperbacks). 372p. mass mkt. 7.95 (*0-07-063506-4*) McGraw.

On Adolescence: A Psychoanalytic Interpretation. Peter Blos. 1966. LC 61-14110. 269p. pap. 14.95 (*0-02-904330-1*) Free Pr.

On Aging: Revolt & Resignation. Jean Amery. Tr. by John D. Barlow. 1994. LC 93-41804. 160p. 19.95 (*0-253-30675-2*) Ind U Pr.

On Angiotensin - Degrading Aminopeptidases in the Rat Kidney. P. N. Kugler. Tr. by Terry C. Telger. 1982. (Advances in Anatomy, Embryology & Cell Biology Ser.: Vol. 76). (Illus.). 86p. 34.95 (*0-387-11452-1*) Spr-Verlag.

On Asthma. Moses Maimonides. Ed. by Gerrit Bos & Machael McVaugh. 2000. (Graeco-Arabic Sciences Ser.). (ARA & ENG.). 350p. 29.95 (*0-8425-2475-4*) Brigham.

On Astrocytes & Glutamate Neurotransmission: New Waves in Brain Information Processing. Elisabeth Hansson & Torsten Olsson. 1997. LC 97-13739. (Neuroscience Intelligence Unit Ser.). 209p. text 99.00 (*1-57059-446-5*) Landes Bioscience.

On Atmospheric Pollution: A Group of Contributions. J. H. Carter et al. 1951. (Meteorological Monograph: Vol. 1, No. 4). (Illus.). 55p. (Orig.). pap. 17.00 (*0-933876-00-9*) Am Meteorological.

***On Becoming a House Health Nurse: Practice Meets Theory in Home Care Nursing.** Leslie Jean Neal. 2000. LC 00-134221. (Illus.). 154p. (C). pap. (*1-930304-11-0*) Home Care Univ.

On Becoming a Person: A Therapist's View of Psychotherapy. Carl Ransom Rogers. 1995. 416p. pap. 16.00 (*0-395-75531-X*) HM.

On Becoming a Psychotherapist. Ed. by Wendy Dryden & Laurence Spurling. 1989. 272p. (C). pap. 27.95 (*0-415-03611-9*, A3643); 52.50 (*0-415-01933-8*, A3639) Routledge.

On Beginning an Analysis. Ed. by Theodore J. Jacobs & Arnold Rothstein. 1998. xviii, 309p. reprint ed. pap. 25.95 (*0-8236-8168-8*, BN 24440) Intl Univs Pr.

On Being a Client: Understanding the Process of Counselling & Psychotherapy. David Howe. 1993. (Illus.). 224p. (C). 69.95 (*0-8039-8888-5*, 9713); pap. 25.95 (*0-8039-8889-3*, 9714) Sage.

On Being a Doctor. Ed. & Intro. by Michael A. LaCombe. 1995. 192p. reprint ed. pap. 18.00 (*0-943126-65-7*) Amer Coll Phys.

On Being a Doctor II: Voices of Physicians & Patients. Michael A. LaCombe. 1999. LC 99-40565. 363p. 26.00 (*0-943126-82-7*) Amer Coll Phys.

On Being a Psychotherapist. Carl Goldberg. 1991. LC 90-14498. 424p. reprint ed. 55.00 (*0-87668-885-7*) Aronson.

On Being a Therapist. Jeffrey A. Kottler. 2nd rev. ed. 1993. LC 93-15864. (Social & Behavioral Science Ser.). 320p. pap. 22.00 (*1-55542-555-0*) Jossey-Bass.

On Call: Cardiology. Gabriel Khan. Ed. by William Schmitt. 1997. LC 96-14137. 336p. pap. text 21.95 (*0-7216-6848-8*) Saunders.

On Call: Neurology. Marshall. 1998. (C). text 5.63 (*0-8089-2099-5*, Grune & Strat) Harcrt Hlth Sci Grp.

On Call: Obstetrics & Gynecology. Chin. 1998. (C). text 5.00 (*0-8089-2076-6*, Grune & Strat) Harcrt Hlth Sci Grp.

On Call: Obstetrics & Gynecology. Homer G. Chin. Ed. by Williams Schmitt. 1997. LC 96-16716. 416p. pap. text 21.95 (*0-7216-1316-0*) Saunders.

On Call: Out-of-Hours Telephone Calls & Home Visits. James D. Knox. 1989. (Practical Guides for General Practice Ser.: No. 9). (Illus.). 76p. pap. text 14.95 (*0-19-261777-X*) OUP.

On Call: Pediatrics. Lewis. 1998. (C). text 5.50 (*0-8089-2096-0*, Grune & Strat) Harcrt Hlth Sci Grp.

On Call: Surgery. Adams. 1998. (C). text 5.00 (*0-8089-2070-7*, Grune & Strat) Harcrt Hlth Sci Grp.

On Call: Surgery. Gregg A. Adams & Stephen D. Bresnick. Ed. by William Schmitt. 1997. LC 96-29954. (Illus.). 320p. pap. text 21.95 (*0-7216-6432-6*) Saunders.

On Call in - Bone Marrow Transplantation. Ed. by Richard K. Burt et al. 1996. LC 96-6219. 580p. (gr. 13). pap. 49.95 (*0-412-10391-5*) Chapman & Hall.

On Call Laboratory Medicine & Pathology. John H. Henry & Sharad C. Mathur. Date not set. LC 00-23911. 415p. pap. text (*0-7216-9004-1*) Saunders.

On Call Neurology. Randolph S. Marshall & Stephan A. Mayer. 2nd ed. 2001. LC 2001-20108. (On Call Ser.). (Illus.). xx, 460p. text (*0-7216-9221-4*) Saunders.

On Call Neurology. Neurology. Randolph S. Marshall & Stephan A. Mayer. Ed. by William Schmitt. 1997. LC 96-36902. 352p. pap. text 21.95 (*0-7216-6523-3*) Saunders.

On Call Orthopedics. Douglas R. Dirschi & C. Michael LeCroy. Ed. by Bill Schmitt. 1998. LC 98-3606. (On Call in Ser.). (Illus.). 384p. (C). pap. text 21.95 (*0-7216-7990-0*) Saunders.

On Call Pediatrics. David Lewis & James J. Norton. Ed. by Bill Schmitt. 1997. LC 96-49867. (Illus.). 336p. pap. text 21.95 (*0-7216-6757-0*) Saunders.

On Call Principles & Protocols. Shane A. Marshall & John Ruedy. 2nd ed. 1993. (Illus.). 416p. pap. text 29.95 (*0-7216-3982-8*) Saunders.

On Call Principles & Protocols. Shane A. Marshall & John Ruedy. Ed. by Ray Kersey. 3rd ed. 1999. LC 98-32244. (On Call Ser.). (Illus.). xx, 478p. pap. text (*0-7216-5079-1*) Saunders.

On Call Procedures. Stephen D. Bresnick & Gregg A. Adams. Ed. by William Schmitt. 1999. LC 98-19200. (On Call Ser.). (Illus.). xxi, 253p. pap. 24.95 (*0-7216-7304-X*) Saunders.

On Call Psychiatry. Carol Bernstein et al. Ed. by William Schmitt. 1997. LC 96-42344. (Illus.). 272p. pap. text 21.95 (*0-7216-6526-8*) Saunders.

On Call Psychiatry. Carol A. Bernstein et al. 2nd ed. 2001. LC 2001-20322. (On Call Ser.). xxiii, 308p. text (*0-7216-9239-7*) Saunders.

On Children & Death. Elisabeth Kubler-Ross. 1997. 288p. pap. 12.00 (*0-684-83939-3*, Touchstone) S&S Trade Pap.

On Cogenic Herpesviruses. Ed. by Fred Rapp. 1980. Vol. 1. 208p. 120.00 (*0-8493-5619-9*, QR400); Vol. 2. 152p. 89.00 (*0-8493-5620-2*) Franklin (CRC Reprint).

On Death Without Dignity: The Human Impact of Technological Dying. David W. Moller. 1990. (Perspectives on Death & Dying Ser.). 134p. text 35.95 (*0-89503-067-5*) Baywood Pub.

On Defining Death: An Analytic Study of the Concept of Death in Philosophy & Medical Ethics. Douglas N. Walton. 1979. (*0-7735-0331-5*) McG-Queens Univ Pr CAN. *Dist:* CUP Services.

On Deployment of Health Resources in Rural Valle del Cauca, Colombia. David Eaton. 1979. (Working Papers Ser.: No. 11). 50p. pap. 2.50 (*0-89940-507-X*) LBJ Sch Pub Aff.

On Development: The Biology of Form. John T. Bonner. 1977. LC 73-88053. (Commonwealth Fund Publications). 224p. pap. 15.50 (*0-674-63412-8*) HUP.

On Doctoral Education in Nursing: The Voice of the Student. Dona R. Carpenter & Sharon Hudacek. 1996. 237p. pap. 36.95 (*0-88737-670-3*) Natl League Nurse.

On Dreams. Sigmund Freud. 1989. reprint ed. lib. bdg. 28.95 (*0-89966-633-7*) Buccaneer Bks.

On Dreams. Sigmund Freud. Ed. by James Strachey. 1990. pap. 8.95 (*0-393-00144-X*) Norton.

On Duty: A Nurse's Notes on Life & Death. Carolyn P. Fink. 1996. mass mkt. 5.99 (*0-449-14965-X*) Fawcett.

On Eagle's Wings: A Practical Guide for the Care of Terminally Ill Loved Ones. Connie C. Bobo. 1998. LC 98-93065. (Illus.). 136p. pap. 19.95 (*0-9665418-0-4*) Freefall Fact.

On Field Evaluation & Treatment of Sport Injuries. James R. Andrews. Ed. by William G. Clancy. 1997. LC 96-49798. (Illus.). 288p. (C). (gr. 13). pap. text 32.95 (*0-8151-0218-6*, 24095) Mosby Inc.

On Flirtation. Adam Phillips. 256p. 1996. pap. 15.95 (*0-674-63440-3*); 1994. LC 94-18821. text 19.95 (*0-674-63437-3*, PHIFLI) HUP.

On Freud's "A Child Is Being Beaten" Ethel S. Person et al. 1997. LC 97-8960. (Contemporary Freud). pap. (*0-300-07162-0*); (Contemporary Freud: Turning Points & Critical Issues Ser.: Vol. 5). 256p. 35.00 (*0-300-07161-2*) Yale U Pr.

On Freud's "Analysis Terminable & Interminable" Ed. by Joseph Sandler. 1991. (Contemporary Freud Ser.). 176p. (C). 50.00 (*0-300-04452-6*) Yale U Pr.

On Freud's Couch: Seven New Interpretations of Freud's Case Histories. Ed. by Irene Matthis & Imre Szecsody. 1998. LC 97-29931. (Library of Object Relations). (Illus.). 288p. 50.00 (*0-7657-0115-4*) Aronson.

On Freud's "Creative Writers & Day-Dreaming" Ed. by Ethel S. Person et al. 1995. LC 94-48270. (Contemporary Freud Ser.). xxi, 196p. 35.00 (*0-300-06266-4*) Yale U Pr.

On Holy Ground: The Impact of Psychotherapists' Spirituality on Their Practice. John P. Sullivan. 1998. LC 98-23788. 144p. (C). 46.00 (*0-7618-1176-1*); pap. 25.50 (*0-7618-1177-X*) U Pr of Amer.

On Human Nature. Edward O. Wilson. 1978. LC 78-17675. 260p. 33.95 (*0-674-63441-1*) HUP.

On Human Symbiosis & the Vicissitudes of Individuation Vol. 1: Infantile Psychoses. Margaret S. Mahler & Manuel Furer. 1968. LC 68-24453. 271p. 45.00 (*0-8236-3780-8*) Intl Univs Pr.

On Implementing a National Graduate Medical Education Trust Fund. Institute of Medicine Staff. 1997. LC 97-184448. xii, 74 p. (*0-309-05779-5*) Natl Acad Pr.

On Intelligence, 3. Hippolyte A. Taine. 1977. LC 77-72191. (Contributions to the History of Psychology Ser.: Vol. III, Pt. A). 320p. lib. bdg. 89.50 (*0-313-26927-0*, U6927, Greenwood Pr) Greenwood.

On Intimate Terms: The Psychology of Difference in Lesbian Relationships. Beverly Burch. 1993. LC 92-2631. 192p. (C). text 21.50 (*0-252-01801-X*) U of Ill Pr.

***On Keratin Mutations in Epidermolytic Hyperkeratotis & the Regulation of Keratin Expression by Retinoids.** Marie Virtanen. 2001. (Comprehensive Summaries of Uppsala Dissertations from the Faculty of Social Sciences Ser.: No. 1051). (Illus.). 45p. pap. (*91-554-5058-X*) Uppsala Universitet SWE. *Dist:* Coronet Bks.

On Kissing, Tickling & Being Bored: Psychoanalytic Essays on the Unexamined Life. Adam Phillips. 1993. LC 92-20662. 152p. text 19.95 (*0-674-63462-4*) HUP.

On Leading a Clinical Department: A Guide for Physicians. Harry W. Fritts, Jr. 1997. LC 97-15181. 216p. pap. text 18.95 (*0-8018-5781-3*) Johns Hopkins.

On Life & Death: The Edgar Cayce Readings. Compiled by Association for Research and Enlightenment, Readings Staff. 1973. (Library: Vol. 1). 188p. lib. bdg. 19.95 (*0-87604-065-2*, 1101) ARE Pr.

On-Line Database of Literature, Arts, & Medicine: An Annotated Bibliography. Ed. by Felice Aull. annot. ed. 1996. 445p. (Orig.). (C). pap. 35.00 (*0-9651593-1-0*) NY Univ Med Ctr.

On Looking Inward & Being Scientific: A Tribute to G. L. Engel, MD. Ed. by G. A. Fava. 2000. (Psychotherapy & Psychosomatics Ser.: Vol. 69). (Illus.). 64p. pap. 25.25 (*3-8055-7107-0*) S Karger.

On Losing the Soul: Essays in the Social Psychology of Religion. Ed. by Richard K. Fenn & Donald Capps. 1995. LC 94-31494. 249p. (C). text 21.50 (*0-7914-2493-6*); pap. text 20.95 (*0-7914-2494-4*) State U NY Pr.

On Love & Psychological Exercises A. R. Orage. 1998. LC 97-43968. (Illus.). 200p. reprint ed. pap. 14.95 (*1-57863-100-9*) Red Wheel ME.

On Loving, Hating, & Living Well: The Public Psychoanalytic Lectures of Ralph R. Greenson, M.D. Ed. by Robert A. Nemiroff et al. 1992. LC 92-1438. (Monograph Series of the Ralph R. Greenson Memorial Library of the San Diego Psychoanalytic Institute & Society). 382p. 55.00 (*0-8236-3790-5*) Intl Univs Pr.

On Moral Medicine: Theological Perspectives in Medical Ethics. Ed. by Stephen E. Lammers & Allen Verhey. 2nd exp. rev. ed. 1998. LC 97-35605. 1021p. pap. 52.00 (*0-8028-4249-6*) Eerdmans.

On Morphodynamics: Selected Papers. Ralph Abraham. 1986. (Illus.). 255p. pap. 25.00 (*0-942344-06-5*) Aerial Pr.

On Neuroses. Paul Schilder. Ed. by Lauretta Bender. 1979. LC 78-61181. 387p. 57.50 (*0-8236-3810-3*) Intl Univs Pr.

On Nursing: A Literary Celebration. Ed. by Margretta M. Styles & Patricia Moccia. 1993. 356p. (C). pap. text 34.95 (*0-88737-574-X*, 323); 59.95 (*0-88737-577-4*) Natl League Nurse.

On Obscure Diseases of the Brain & Disorders of the Mind: Their Incipient Symptoms, Pathology, Diagnosis, Treatment & Prophylaxis. Forbes Winslow. 1976. LC 75-16739. (Classics in Psychiatry Ser.). reprint ed. 49.95 (*0-405-07463-8*) Ayer.

***On Pathophysiological Mechanisms in Amyotrophic Lateral Sclerosis.** Eva Grundstrom. 2000. 52p. pap. (*91-554-4838-0*) Uppsala Universitet SWE. *Dist:* Coronet Bks.

On Perception & Event Structure, & the Psychological Environment: Selected Papers. Fritz Heider. 1959. (Psychological Issues Monographs: Vol. 1, No. 3). 123p. (Orig.). 27.50 (*0-8236-3840-5*) Intl Univs Pr.

On Private Madness. Andre Green. 1987. LC 86-27641. 390p. 57.50 (*0-8236-3853-7*) Intl Univs Pr.

On Psychotherapy. Clarkson. 1993. 266p. pap. 48.00 (*1-56593-247-1*, 0313) Singular Publishing.

On Psychotherapy. Petruska Clarkson. 1994. LC 94-71773. 266p. pap. 45.00 (*1-56821-310-7*) Aronson.

On Purpose: Collected Papers. Harold H. Mosak. 1977. LC 76-42942. pap. 14.95 (*0-918560-19-5*) Adler Sch Prof Psy.

On Purposeful Systems. Russell L. Ackoff & Fred Emery. 1982. (Systems Inquiry Ser.). 296p. (C). reprint ed. pap. text 15.95 (*0-914105-00-0*) Intersystems Pubns.

***"On Second Thought" & Other Essays in the History of Medicine & Science.** Owsei Temkin. 2001. LC 2001-29420. 288p. 42.00 (*0-8018-6774-6*) Johns Hopkins.

On Sensations from Pressure & Impact. Arnold Griffing. 1974. (Psychology Monographs General & Applied: Vol. 1). reprint ed. 55.00 (*0-8115-1400-5*) Periodicals Srv.

On Sex & Gender: Thoughts of Dr. Schenk. Roy U. Schenk. 1991. (Illus.). vii, 134p. (Orig.). pap. 6.00 (*0-9613177-2-8*) MPC Pr.

On Sexuality: Psychoanalytic Observations. Toksoz B. Karasu & Charles W. Socarides. 1979. LC 78-67478. 412p. 60.00 (*0-8236-3857-X*) Intl Univs Pr.

On-Site Drug Testing. Ed. by Amanda J. Jenkins & Bruce A. Goldberger. 2002. LC 2001-39632. (Forensic Science & Medicine Ser.). 304p. 89.50 (*0-89603-870-X*) Humana.

On-Site Occupational Health & Rehabilitation: A Model for the Manufacturing & Service Industries. Jane Pomper DeHart. 2000. LC 00-60194. (Illus.). 280p. text 150.00 (*0-8247-8986-5*) Dekker.

On Size & Life. Thomas McMahon & James Bonner. 1983. (Scientific American Library). (Illus.). 255p. text 32.95 (*0-7167-5000-7*) W H Freeman.

On Solitude. Francis Petrarch. Tr. by Jay Livernois. 2000. (Dunquin Ser.: Vol. 26). 316p. pap. 18.00 (*0-88214-228-3*) Spring Pubns.

On Soul & Conscience: Forensic Medicine in Glasgow, 1839-1989. M. A. Crowther & B. White. 1988. (Illus.). 248p. text (*0-08-036406-3*); pap. text (*0-08-036407-1*) Aberdeen U Pr GBR. *Dist:* Macmillan.

On Suicide: With Particular Reference to Suicide among Young Students. Ed. by Paul Friedman. 1967. LC 67-26190. 142p. 27.50 (*0-8236-3860-X*) Intl Univs Pr.

On Surgery & Instruments. Abu Al-Quasim Khalaf Ibn Abbuas Al-Zahrawi. 1997. 28p. (C). text 40.00 (*0-934905-81-9*, Library of Islam) Kazi Pubns.

On the Administrative Frontier of Medicine: The First Ten Years of the American Hospital Association, 1899-1908. Ed. by Charles E. Rosenberg. 1989. (Medical Care in the United States Ser.). 440p. text 25.00 (*0-8240-8330-X*) Garland.

On the Anatomy of Vertebrates Richard Owen. LC 72-1701. (Illus.). reprint ed. 225.00 (*0-404-08300-5*) AMS Pr.

On the Causes of Idiocy. Samuel G. Howe. 1979. LC 79-180578. (Medicine & Society in America Ser.). 100p. reprint ed. 23.95 (*0-405-03955-7*) Ayer.

***On the Cell Cycle of Escherichia Coli & Cell Division in Haloferax Mediterranei.** Bjorn Gullbrand. 2001. (Comprehensive Summaries of Uppsala Dissertations from the Faculty of Science & Technology Ser.: No. 640). (Illus.). 63p. pap. (*91-554-5056-3*) Uppsala Universitet SWE. *Dist:* Coronet Bks.

On the Centre of Gravity of the Human Body. W. Braune & Fischer. Tr. by P. G. Maquet et al from GER. 1984. (Illus.). 96p. 73.00 (*0-387-13216-3*) Spr-Verlag.

On the Circulation of the Blood: Latin Text of His Sixty-Fifth Letter to the Royal Society, 1688. Antoni Van Leeuwenhoek. 1962. (Illus.). 33p. reprint ed. text (*90-6004-098-8*) HES & DE GRAAF NLD. *Dist:* Coronet Bks.

On the Client's Path: A Manual for the Practice of Solution-Focused Therapy. A. J. Chevalier. 1995. LC 95-69483. 157p. 49.95 (*1-57224-021-0*) New Harbinger.

On the Construction, Organization, & General Arrangements of Hospitals for the Insane. Thomas S. Kirkbride. 2nd ed. 1973. LC 73-2405. (Mental Illness & Social Policy; the American Experience Ser.). reprint ed. 25.95 (*0-405-05215-4*) Ayer.

On the Contributions of Hugh Owen Thomas of Liverpool, Sir Robert Jones of Liverpool & London, John Ridlon, M. D. of New York & Chicago to Modern Orthopedic Surgery. H. Winnett Orr. Ed. by William R. Phillips & Janet Rosenberg. 1980. LC 79-6920. (Physically Handicapped in Society Ser.). reprint ed. lib. bdg. 26.95 (*0-405-13129-1*) Ayer.

On the Counselor's Path: A Guide to Teaching Brief Solution-Focused Therapy. A. J. Chevalier. 1996. 92p. pap. 24.95 (*1-57224-048-2*) New Harbinger.

On the Cutting Edge - A Great American Surgeon: Richard B. Cattell, M.D. Mary V. Dunmore. 1991. LC 91-60402. (Illus.). 256p. 29.95 (*0-9628738-0-2*) Jones Riv Pr.

On the Death of My Father: A Psychoanalyst's Memoir. Martin Silberberg. 1995. LC 94-28483. 164p. text 79.95 (*0-7734-9052-3*) E Mellen.

On the Development of Developmental Psychology. Ed. by J. A. Meacham & Deanna Kuhn. 1982. (Contributions to Human Development Ser.: Vol. 8). (Illus.). xii, 160p. pap. 42.75 (*3-8055-3568-6*) S Karger.

On the Difficulties Encountered by the Deaf & Dumb in Learning Language. Collins Stone. 1972. 250.00 (*0-8490-0764-X*) Gordon Pr.

On the Early Development of Mind: Selected Papers on Psychoanalysis, Vol. 1. Edward Glover. 1956. 483p. pap. 24.95 (*0-8236-8169-6*, 023760) Intl Univs Pr.

On the Edge Between Two Worlds: Ireland & the Ways of Healing. Kathleen Milner. Date not set. (Healing Arts Ser.). pap. (*1-886903-21-2*) K Milner.

On the Evaluation of Verbal Material in Parapsychology. J. G. Pratt. 1969. LC 70-94866. (Parapsychological Monographs: No. 10). pap. 5.00 (*0-912328-14-2*) Parapsych Foun.

On the Fabric of the Human Body Bk. 1: The Bones & Cartilages. Andreas Vesalius. Tr. by William F. Richardson & John B. Carman from LAT. 1998. LC 96-34817. (Norman Anatomy Ser.: No. 1). Orig. Title: De Humani Corporis Fabrica Libri Septem. (Illus.). lxiv, 416p. 250.00 (*0-930405-73-0*, NP32874) Norman SF.

On the Function of the Cerebrum. Shepherd I. Franz. 1974. (Psychology Monographs General & Applied: Vol. 19). reprint ed. 55.00 (*0-8115-1418-8*) Periodicals Srv.

On the Influence of Trades, Professions & Occupations in the United States in the Production of Disease. Benjamin W. McCready. 1980. LC 78-180583. (Medicine & Society in America Ser.). 144p. reprint ed. 19.95 (*0-405-03960-3*) Ayer.

***On-the-Job Training for Physicians: A Practical Guide.** David H. Hargreaves et al. 1997. 151p. pap. (*1-85315-325-7*) Royal Soc of Medicine Pr Ltd GBR. *Dist:* Balogh.

***On-the-Job Training for Surgeons.** David H. Hargreaves et al. 1997. 132p. pap. (*1-85315-314-1*) Royal Soc of Medicine Pr Ltd GBR. *Dist:* Balogh.

On the Monday Side of the Street: A Text on Alcoholism for Professional & Lay People. Corey A. Bohling. Tr. by Virginia Fieser. 1989. (Illus.). 100p. (Orig.). (C). pap. 5.95 (*0-9625478-3-2*, TXU-368-156) C Bohling Pub.

On the Motion of the Heart & Blood in Animals. William Harvey. 1993. LC 92-25948. (Great Minds Ser.). 91p. pap. 10.00 (*0-87975-854-6*) Prometheus Bks.

On the Mysterious Leap from the Mind to the Body: A Workshop Study on the Theory of Conversion. Ed. by Felix Deutsch. 1969. LC 59-8411. reprint ed. pap. 24.95 (*0-8236-8174-2*, 023800) Intl Univs Pr.

On the Nature of Health. Lennart Nordenfelt. 1987. (C). text 127.50 (*1-55608-032-8*) Kluwer Academic.

On the Nature of the Bilirubin Pigments in the Newborn Infant. Sina Aziz. 1995. (Acta Biomedica Lovaniensia Ser.). 194p. (Orig.). pap. (*90-6186-696-0*) Leuven Univ BEL. *Dist:* Coronet Bks.

On the Nature of the Psyche. Carl Gustav Jung. Ed. by G. Adler. Tr. by R. F. C. Hull. 1969. (Bollingen Ser.: Vol. 20). 184p. pap. 13.95 (*0-691-01751-4*) Princeton U Pr.

On the Notion of Mental Illness: Problematizing the Medical Model Conception of Abnormal Behavior & Mental Afflictions. Tommy Svensson. 1995. (Avebury Series in Philosophy). 160p. (*1-85972-160-5*) Avebry GBR. *Dist:* Ashgate Pub Co.

On the Origin of Species: A Facsimile of the First Edition. Charles Robert Darwin. 1964. LC 63-17196. (Harvard Paperbacks Ser.). 528p. pap. text 15.45 (*0-674-63752-6*) HUP.

On the Origins & Treatment of Homosexuality: A Psychoanalytic Reinterpretation. Gerald J. M. Van Den Aardweg. 1985. LC 85-9266. 320p. 42.95 (*0-275-90233-1*, C0233, Praeger Pubs) Greenwood.

On the Parts of the Animals. Aristotle. Tr. & Intro. by William Ogle. 1987. LC 86-29613. 263p. reprint ed. 40.00 (*0-8240-6925-0*) Garland.

***On the Pill: A Social History of Oral Contraceptives, 1950-1970.** Elizabeth Siegel Watkins. 2001. 208p. pap. text 14.95 (*0-8018-6821-1*) Johns Hopkins.

On the Self-Regulation of Behavior. Charles S. Carver & Michael F. Scheier. 1998. LC 98-15204. (Illus.). 464p. (C). text 52.95 (*0-521-57204-5*) Cambridge U Pr.

On the Shoulders of Freud: Freud, Lacan, & the Psychoanalysis of Phallic Ideology. Roberto Speziale-Bagliacca. 1991. 110p. (C). text 34.95 (*0-88738-409-9*) Transaction Pubs.

On the Shoulders of Women: The Feminization of Psychotherapy. Ilene J. Philipson. 1993. LC 93-25404. 177p. 24.95 (*0-89862-017-1*) Guilford Pubns.

On the Soul, Parva Naturalia, on Breath. Tr. by W. S. Hett. 1936. (Loeb Classical Library: No. 288). 546p. 18.95 (*0-674-99318-7*) HUP.

On the State of the Public Health, 1996. annuals HMSO Staff. 1997. 222p. pap. (*0-11-322097-9*, HM20979) Statnry Office GBR. *Dist:* Bernan Associates.

On the State of the Public Health, 1995. 1996. 222p. pap. (*0-11-321989-X*, HM1989X) Statnry Office GBR. *Dist:* Bernan Associates.

On the Texture of Brains: An Introduction to Neuroanatomy for the Cybernetically Minded. Tr. by E. H. Braitenbach from GER. 1977. LC 77-21851. (Illus.). 24.95 (*0-387-08391-X*) Spr-Verlag.

On the Trail of Heart Attacks in Seven Countries. Henry Blackburn. 1995. 180p. (*1-887268-00-6*) H Blackburn.

On the Use & Abuse of Alcoholic Liquors, in Health & Disease. William B. Carpenter. Ed. by Gerald N. Grob. 1981. LC 80-1216. (Addiction in America Ser.). reprint ed. lib. bdg. 19.95 (*0-405-13572-6*) Ayer.

On the Way to Individuality: Current Methodological Issues in Behavioral Genetics. Ed. by Michele C. LaBuda & Elena L. Grigorenko. 1998. 14p. (C). lib. bdg. 85.00 (*1-56072-427-7*) Nova Sci Pubs.

On the Way to Self: Ego & Early Oedipal Development. Johanna K. Tabin. 1985. LC 84-15558. 392p. text 57.50 (*0-231-05944-2*) Col U Pr.

On the Witness Stand: Essays on Psychology & Crime. Hugo Muensterberg. Ed. by Richard Moss. LC 70-156030. reprint ed. 35.00 (*0-404-09180-6*) AMS Pr.

On the Witness Stand: Essays on Psychology & Crime. Hugo Munsterberg. 1981. 269p. reprint ed. 38.00 (*0-8377-0840-0*, Rothman) W S Hein.

On Understanding Intervention in Psychology & Education. Howard S. Adelman & Linda Taylor. 1994. LC 94-2986. 296p. 68.00 (*0-275-94888-9*, Praeger Pubs) Greenwood.

On Wilhelm Reich & Orgonomy. Wilhelm Reich et al. Ed. by James DeMeo. 1994. (Illus.). 176p. (Orig.). (C). pap. text 20.00 (*0-9621855-3-1*) Natural Energy.

On Witchcraft: An Abridged Translation of Johann Weyer's "De Praestigiis Daemonum" Johann Weyer. Ed. by Benjamin G. Kohl & H. Erik Midelfort. Tr. by John Shea. abr. ed. 1998. LC 97-36160. 350p. pap. text 24.95 (*1-889818-02-X*, P34) Pegasus Pr.

On Women Healthsharing. Ed. by Enakshi Dua et al. 1994. 369p. pap. (*0-88961-201-3*) Womens Pr CAN. *Dist:* U of Toronto Pr.

On Wounds in the Head. in the Surgery. on Fractures, on Joints, Mochlikon, Vol. 3. Tr. by E. T. Withington. 1928. (On Wounds in the Head. in the Surgery. on Fractures, on Join Ser.: No.149). 484p. 19.95 (*0-674-99165-6*) HUP.

On Writing, Reading & Dyslexia. Arthur Linksz. 1973. LC 73-9978. (Illus.). 256p. text 55.50 (*0-8089-0789-1*, 792563, Grune & Strat) Harcrt Hlth Sci Grp.

On Your Own: Professional Growth Through Independent Nursing Practice. Mary L. Lynch. 1983. LC 81-19702. (Illus.). 250p. text 33.75 (*0-8185-0507-9*, 507-9) Jones & Bartlett.

Onboard Medical Handbook: First Aid & Emergency Medicine Afloat. Paul G. Gill. 1996. LC 96-22063. (Illus.). 230p. pap. 17.95 (*0-07-024274-7*) McGraw-Hill Prof.

Once a Doctor, Always a Doctor: The Memoirs of a German-Jewish Immigrant Physician. Heinz Hartmann. 1986. LC 86-42573. 189p. 31.00 (*0-87975-342-0*) Prometheus Bks.

Once a Month: Understanding & Treating PMS. Katharina Dalton. 6th ed. 1999. LC 99-10080. (Illus.). 320p. 25.95 (*0-89793-256-0*) Hunter Hse.

Once a Nurse, Always a Nurse? Exploring Your Career Alternatives. Betty Hafner. 1999. 200p. pap. 14.95 (*0-87576-223-9*) Pilot Bks.

Once Charitable Enterprise: Hospitals & Health Care in Brooklyn & New York, 1855-1915. David Rosner. 1982. LC 81-21725. (Interdisciplinary Perspectives on Modern History Ser.). 288p. text 54.95 (*0-521-24217-7*) Cambridge U Pr.

Once Daily Ceftriaxone vs. Multiple Comparative Drugs. Ed. by F. Fraschini. 1989. (Journal: Vol. 34, Suppl. 1). (Illus.). iv, 60p. pap. 19.25 (*3-8055-4961-X*) S Karger.

Once upon a Sound: Literature-Based Phonological Activities. Linda Smith-Kiewel & Tracy Claeys. 1998. LC 98-30856. 42.00 (*1-888222-31-X*) Thinking Pubns.

Once upon a Table: A Cookbook. Women's Auxiliary of the American Cancer Society Staff. Ed. by Anita Zebrovious. 1981. LC 81-69959. (Illus.). pap. 8.95 (*0-9607282-0-1*) Womens Auxiliary Cancer.

Onchocerciasis: Symptomatology, Pathology, Diagnosis. Ed. by A. A. Buck. 1974. pap. text 12.00 (*92-4-156041-X*, 1150123) World Health.

Onchocerciasis & Its Control: Report of a WHO Expert Committee on Onchocerciasis Control. 1995. (Technical Reports: No. 852). (ENG, FRE & SPA.). viii, 103p. (C). pap. text 15.00 (*92-4-120852-X*, 1100852) World Health.

Onchocerciasis & Mectizan: Training Activities for Community Health Workers. Helen Keller International Staff. 1995. LC 95-9921. 10.00 (*0-915173-33-6*); 10.00 (*0-915173-34-4*) Helen Keller Intl.

Onchocerciasis Control Programme in West Africa: An Example of Effective Public Health Management. E. M. Samba. 1994. LC 95-129803. (Public Health in Action Ser.). (ENG & FRE.). vii, 107p. pap. text 23.00 (*92-4-156168-8*, 1390001) World Health.

Oncogene & Transgenics Correlates of Cancer Risk Assessments. C. Zervos. 1992. LC 92-21812. (NATO Advanced Science Institutes Ser.: Vol. 232). (Illus.). 364p. (C). text 125.00 (*0-306-44242-6*, Kluwer Plenum) Kluwer Academic.

Oncogene & Tumour Supressor Gene Factsbook. Robin Hesketh. 2nd ed. 1997. LC 97-21738. (Factsbooks Ser.). (Illus.). 608p. pap. text 49.95 (*0-12-344548-5*) Morgan Kaufmann.

Oncogene Handbook. Robin T. Hesketh. 1994. (Illus.). 640p. text 115.00 (*0-12-344555-8*) Acad Pr.

Oncogenes. 1989. (Current Topics in Microbiology & Immunology Ser.: Vol. 147). (Illus.). 172p. 102.00 (*0-387-51050-8*) Spr-Verlag.

Oncogenes. Ed. by Christopher C. Benz. 1989. (Cancer Treatment & Research Ser.). (C). text 217.50 (*0-7923-0237-0*) Kluwer Academic.

Oncogenes. Enrique Pimentel. 1986. LC 85-28085. 224p. 125.00 (*0-8493-6566-X*, RC268, CRC Reprint) Franklin.

Oncogenes. Geoffrey M. Cooper. 2nd ed. 1995. LC 94-42582. (Biology Ser.). (Illus.). 400p. (C). text 61.95 (*0-86720-937-2*, 937-2) Jones & Bartlett.

Oncogenes, Vol. 1. Enrique Pimentel. 2nd ed. 1989. LC 85-28085. 528p. 206.00 (*0-8493-6505-8*, RC268) Franklin.

Oncogenes, Vol. II. Ed. by Enrique Pimentel. 2nd ed. 1989. 448p. 234.00 (*0-8493-6506-6*, RC268, CRC Reprint) Franklin.

Oncogenes: An Introduction to the Concept of Cancer Genes. K. B. Burck et al. 1989. (Illus.). 300p. reprint ed. 86.95 (*0-387-96423-1*) Spr-Verlag.

Oncogenes & Cancer: Proceedings of the Seventeenth International Symposium of the Princess Takamatsu Cancer Research Fund, June 1986. Ed. by Stuart A. Aaronson et al. 1987. 320p. lib. bdg. (*90-6764-101-4*) VSP NLD. *Dist:* Coronet Bks.

Oncogenes & Growth Control. Ed. by P. Kahn & T. Graf. 1986. (Illus.). 369p. 96.00 (*0-387-16839-7*) Spr-Verlag.

Oncogenes & Growth Factors. Ed. by Ralph A. Bradshaw & S. J. Prentis. 1987. xvi,306p. pap. 44.50 (*0-444-80827-2*) Elsevier.

Oncogenes & the Molecular Origins of Cancer. Ed. by Robert A. Weinberg. 1990. LC 89-23927. (Monographs: No. 18). 366p. 39.00 (*0-87969-336-3*) Cold Spring Harbor.

Oncogenes & Tumor Suppressor Genes. F. MacDonald & C. H. Ford. 1991. (Medical Perspectives Ser.). 112p. (Orig.). pap. (*1-872748-55-4*) Bios Sci GBR. *Dist:* Coronet Bks.

Oncogenes & Tumour Suppressors. Ed. by Gordon Peters & Karen H. Vousden. 1997. LC 97-855. (Frontiers in Molecular Biology Ser.: No. 19). (Illus.). 352p. pap. text 55.00 (*0-19-963594-3*) OUP.

Oncogenes As Transcriptional Regulators. Moshe Yaniv & J. Ghysdael. 1997. (Progress in Gene Expression Ser.). LC 97-8142. text 138.00 (*0-8176-5709-6*); LC 97-8142. (*0-8176-5486-0*); (*0-8176-5710-X*) Birkhauser.

Oncogenes in Cancer Diagnostics. Ed. by K. Munk et al. 1990. (Beitraege Zur Onkologie, Contributions to Oncology Ser.: Vol. 39). (Illus.). viii, 198p. 68.75 (*3-8055-5231-9*) S Karger.

Oncogenes in Pediatric Tumors. Ed. by L. Massimo et al. 1988. (Ettore Majorana International Life Sciences Ser.). xvii, 269p. text 195.00 (*3-7186-0469-8*) Gordon & Breach.

Oncogenes in the Development of Leukemia. Ed. by O. N. Witte. 1992. (Cancer Surveys Ser.: Vol. 15). (Illus.). 191p. (C). text 66.00 (*0-87969-406-8*) Cold Spring Harbor.

Oncogenesis & Herpesviruses I. Ed. by P. M. Biggs et al. 1986. (IARC Scientific Publications Ser.: No. 2). (Illus.). 515p. 65.00 (*0-19-723001-6*) OUP.

Oncogenesis & Molecular Biology of Pituitary Tumors. Shlomo Melmed. 1996. (Frontiers of Hormone Research Ser.: Vol. 20). (Illus.). vi, 198p. 198.25 (*3-8055-6254-3*) S Karger.

Oncogenesis & Natural Immunity in Syrian Hamsters. Ed. by F. Hombuger & J. J. Trentin. 1979. (Progress in Experimental Tumor Research Ser.: Vol. 23). (Illus.). 85.25 (*3-8055-2824-8*) S Karger.

Oncogenic Adenoviruses. Ed. by L. P. Merkow & M. Slifkin. 1973. (Progress in Experimental Tumor Research Ser.: Vol. 18). 85.25 (*3-8055-1348-8*) S Karger.

Oncogenic Virus Gross. 3rd ed. 1985. 120.00 (*0-08-032003-1*, Pergamon Pr) Elsevier.

Oncologic Imaging. Ed. by D. G. Bragg et al. 1985. (Illus.). 650p. 220.00 (*0-08-033653-1*, Pergamon Pr) Elsevier.

Oncologic Imaging. Rubin. 2nd ed. 1999. LC 2001-54245. text 139.00 (*0-7216-7494-1*) Saunders.

Oncologic Imaging: A Clinical Perspective. Claudia G. Berman et al. 1997. LC 96-32622. (Illus.). 512p. text 99.00 (*0-07-005114-3*) McGraw-Hill Prof.

Oncologic Therapies. Ed. by Everett E. Vokes & Harvey M. Golomb. 1998. (Illus.). 1259p. pap. 49.95 (*3-540-64052-5*) Spr-Verlag.

Oncological Nursing. JoAnn H. Eriksson. 2nd ed. 1993. LC 93-21898. (Springhouse Notes Ser.). (Illus.). 240p. pap. 18.95 (*0-87434-613-4*) Springhouse Corp.

Oncologists Managed Care Manual. Ed. by David B. Nash. 1997. (Illus.). 250p. (Orig.). spiral bd. 54.95 (*1-890045-02-0*) T L C Med Pub.

***Oncology.** Roy Spence & Patrick Johnston. 2001. LC 2001-277523. (Oxford Core Texts Ser.). (Illus.). 448p. (Orig.). pap. text 35.00 (*0-19-262982-4*) OUP.

Oncology. Hilmar M. Warenius. 1998. (Medico-Legal Practitioner Ser.). 208p. 72.00 (*1-85941-219-X*) Gaunt.

Oncology: A Multidisciplinary Textbook. Ed. by Alan Horwich. 1994. LC 94-71825. 728p. (gr. 13). 171.95 (*0-412-55250-7*) Chapman & Hall.

Oncology & Hematology 2000: An Internet Resource Guide. Ed. by Dan Goldenson. 2000. (Physician Ser.). 450p. pap. 24.95 (*0-9676811-0-3*) eMedguides.

Oncology Diet & Nutrition Patient Education Resource Manual. Simon B. Weavers et al. 2000. LC 00-38956. (ENG & SPA., Illus.). 528p. ring bd. 199.00 (*0-8342-1715-5*) Aspen Pub.

Oncology Fact Finder: The Johns Hopkins Manual of Oncology Nursing. Constance R. Ziegfeld. 1998. LC 98-11143. 512p. spiral bd. 32.50 (*0-7817-1480-X*) Lppncott W & W.

Oncology for Health-Care Professionals. V. Pervan. 1995. pap. (*0-7021-2669-1*) Juta & Co ZAF. *Dist:* Intl Spec Bk, Gaunt.

Oncology for Palliative Medicine. Peter Hoskin & Wendy Makin. 1998. LC 97-41041. (Illus.). 250p. text 48.50 (*0-19-262812-7*) OUP.

Oncology for the House Officer. Joseph F. O'Donnell et al. 1992. (Illus.). 352p. 21.95 (*0-683-06626-9*) Lppncott W & W.

Oncology Intern Pocket Survival Guide. Scott M. Tenner et al. 1993. 78p. (Orig.). (C). pap. text 7.50 (*0-9634063-9-6*) Intl Med Pub.

Oncology Nursing. Cynthia C. Snyder. 1986. (Illus.). 464p. (C). text 26.50 (*0-673-39406-9*) Lppncott W & W.

Oncology Nursing. Shirley E. Otto. 3rd ed. 1996. LC 96-23227. (Illus.). 928p. (C). (gr. 13). pap. text 54.95 (*0-8151-8955-9*, 29032) Mosby Inc.

Oncology Nursing: An Essential for Patient Care. Christine Miaskowski. Ed. by Barbara N. Cullen. 1996. (Illus.). 329p. pap. text 32.00 (*0-7216-6041-X*) Saunders.

Oncology Nursing: Assessment & Clinical Care. Christine Miaskowski & Patricia Buschsel. 1999. (Illus.). 1700p. text 95.00 (*0-8151-6990-6*, 27463) Mosby Inc.

Oncology Nursing Ambulatory Setting. Patricia C. Buchsel & Connie H. Yarbro. 1993. 275p. 64.95 (*0-86720-637-3*) Jones & Bartlett.

Oncology Nursing Care Plans. Danielle Gale & Jane Charette. 1995. 400p. (C). pap. 39.95 (*1-56930-004-6*) Delmar.

Oncology Nursing Homecare Handbook. Margaret Barton Burke. 1993. 285p. pap. text 39.95 (*0-86720-643-8*) Jones & Bartlett.

***Oncology Nursing in Ambulatory Setting.** Patricia Buchsel. 2nd ed. 2002. (Illus.). 384p. (C). text 66.95 (*0-7637-1474-7*, 1474-7) Jones & Bartlett.

Oncology Nursing Review. Connie H. Yarbro et al. 1999. LC 99-11078. (Illus.). 272p. (C). pap. text 43.95 (*0-7637-1040-7*, 1040-7) Jones & Bartlett.

Oncology Nursing Review. Connie Henke Yarbro et al. 1999. (Illus.). 272p. (C). pap. text (*0-7637-1127-6*) Jones & Bartlett.

Oncology Nursing Secrets. Rose A. Gates & Regina M. Fink. 1997. LC 97-3107. (Secrets Ser.). 37.95 (*1-56053-210-6*) Hanley & Belfus.

Oncology of the Eye & Adnexa: Atlas of Clinical Pathology. A. Brini et al. 1990. (Monographs in Ophthalmology). (C). text 304.50 (*0-7923-0409-8*) Kluwer Academic.

Oncology of the Nervous System. Michael D. Walker. 1983. text 187.00 (*0-89838-567-9*) Kluwer Academic.

Oncology Patient Education Manual. Aspen Reference Group Staff. Ed. by Kenneth E. Lawrence & Sara N. Di Lima. 1994. LC 94-1144. spiral bd. 249.00 (*0-8342-0543-2*, S125) Aspen Pub.

Oncology Policy & Procedures. Texas M. D. Anderson Cancer Center Staff. 1993. 140.00 (*1-879575-38-8*) Acad Med Sys.

Oncology Reviews, Vol. 3. Z. V. Pavlova & M. E. Isakova. 1989. (Soviet Scientific Reviews Ser.: Vol. 3, Pt. 3). 72, ivp. pap. text 61.00 (*3-7186-4913-6*) Gordon & Breach.

Oncology Reviews Vol. 3, Pt. 5: Poly-Radiomodification in the Radiotherapy of Tumors - Termoradio-Therapy in the U. S. S. R. - Oxybaro- & Hypoxyradiotherapy, Vol. 3. S. P. Yarmonenko. 1991. (Soviet Medical Reviews Ser.: Section F). 146p. pap. text 190.00 (*3-7186-5228-5*, Harwood Acad Pubs) Gordon & Breach.

Oncology Reviews Vol. 4, Pt. 2: Oropharyngeal Region Cancer - Modern Problems of Diagnosis, Treatment & Prognosis - the Oncological Service in the U. S. S. R., Vol. 4. E. G. Matyakin. 1991. (Soviet Medical Reviews Ser.: Section F). 108p. pap. text 130.00 (*3-7186-5230-7*, Harwood Acad Pubs) Gordon & Breach.

Oncology Reviews Vol. 4, Pt. 4.3: Review of Soviet Literature on the Problem of Esophageal Cancer for 1980-1990, Vol. 4. M. Davydov. 1992. (Soviet Medical Reviews Ser.: Section F). 98p. pap. text 96.00 (*3-7186-5360-5*, Harwood Acad Pubs) Gordon & Breach.

Oncology Reviews Vol. 4, Pt. 5: Hormonocytostatics - Antitumor Drugs with a Target Effect, Vol. 4. Z. Sof'ina. 1992. (Soviet Medical Reviews Ser.: Section F). 55p. pap. text 68.00 (*3-7186-5385-0*, Harwood Acad Pubs) Gordon & Breach.

Oncology Services Administration: Forms, Checklists & Guidelines. Aspen Health and Administration Development Group. 1998. LC 97-44161. ring bd. 219.00 (*0-8342-0906-3*, S468) Aspen Pub.

Oncology Services Policy & Procedure Guideline Manual. Diane Johnson. 1998. 198p. spiral bd. 110.00 (*1-879575-98-1*) Acad Med Sys.

Oncology Therapeutics: A Quick Reference Guide. Mark J. Ratain et al. 2000. LC 00-59064. (Illus.). 350p. pap. text 49.95 (*0-7216-8123-9*) Saunders.

Oncology/Hematology Handbook. Steven T. Rosen & Timothy M. Kuzel. 2001. (*1-891483-09-9*) PRR.

Oncotips. James Metz. 2001. pap. text 19.95 (*0-7817-2564-X*) Lppncott W & W.

Ondansetron - a New Concept in Anti-Emetic Therapy. Ed. by J. Smyth & K. Cunninghan. 1992. (Journal: Vol. 49, Vol. 4, 1992). (Illus.). 64p. pap. 88.75 (*3-8055-5656-X*) S Karger.

Ondansetron - Global Experience & Future Potential. Ed. by M. Soukop & K. Cunningham. 1993. (Journal: Vol. 50, No. 3, 1993). (Illus.). 48p. pap. 88.75 (*3-8055-5783-3*) S Karger.

Ondansetron & Chemotherapy Induced Emesis: 3rd International Congress on Neo-Adjuvant Chemotherapy. Ed. by M. Marty & M. Pappo. 1992. (Illus.). 77p. 49.95 (*0-387-54599-9*) Spr-Verlag.

One Cause One Cure Vol. VI: The Health & Life Philosophy of Chiropractic. Frederick H. Barge. 1996. LC 94-79233. 177p. reprint ed. text 38.95 (*1-885048-05-X*) Barge Chiropract.

One Couple, Four Realities: Multiple Perspectives on Couple Therapy. Ed. by Richard Chasin et al. LC 90-3037. 420p. 1990. 45.00 (*0-89862-437-1*); 1992. reprint ed. pap. 25.00 (*0-89862-029-5*, 2029) Guilford Pubns.

One Dark Mile: A Widower's Story. Eric Robinson. 1990. LC 89-32046. 200p. 30.00 (*0-87023-684-9*) U of Mass Pr.

One Day at a Time in Al-Anon. Al-Anon Family Group Headquarters, Inc. Staff. l.t. ed. 1989. LC 72-85153. 10.00 (*0-910034-63-X*) Al-Anon.

One-Day-at-a-Time Therapy. Christine A. Adams. 1990. LC 90-80719. (Illus.). 72p. (Orig.). pap. 4.95 (*0-87029-228-5*, 20204-4) Abbey.

One Degree Beyond: A Reiki Journey into Energy Medicine: Your 21-Day Step-by-Step Guide to Relax, Open & Celebrate. JaneAnne Narrin. 2nd rev. ed. 1999. (Illus.). 320p. (Orig.). pap. 18.95 (*0-9658545-4-X*) Little Whte Buffalo.

One Doctor Learns to Be a Patient. Kenneth B. Olson. Ed. by Susan E. Wills. 1993. LC 93-83044. (Illus.). 320p. 29.00 (*1-883122-00-7*) Pearce Pub.

One Earth One Mind. Michael W. Fox. 1984. LC 84-3929. 264p. (C). reprint ed. lib. bdg. 24.50 (*0-89874-752-X*) Krieger.

One-Eyed Doctor: Sigmund Freud. Ed. by Jay Harris & Jean Harris. 1984. LC 81-65787. (One Eyed Doctor Ser.). 260p. 50.00 (*0-87668-453-3*) Aronson.

One-Eyed Science: Occupational Health & Women Workers. karen Messing. 1998. LC 97-26885. (Labor & Social Change Ser.). (Illus.). 264p. 59.95 (*1-56639-597-6*) Temple U Pr.

One-Eyed Science: Occupational Health & Women Workers. Karen Messing. 1998. LC 97-26885. 264p. pap. 22.95 (*1-56639-598-4*) Temple U Pr.

One-Humped Camel in Eastern Africa: A Pictorial Guide to Diseases, Health Care & Management. Ed. by H. J. Schwartz & M. Dioli. 1992. (Illus.). 282p. (*3-8236-1218-2*) Backhuys Pubs NLD. *Dist:* Balogh.

One Hundred Alive & Stay Alive! Double Your Life Expectancy. Ed. by E. Masterdy. 1984. 162p. 12.95 (*0-8159-6415-3*) Devin.

***150 Practice ECGs: Interpretation & Review.** George Jesse Taylor. 2nd ed. 2001. LC 2001-3640. (Illus.). xii, 271p. pap. 32.95 (*0-632-04623-6*) Blackwell Sci.

101 Secrets of a High-Performance Optometric Practice. 2001. 160p. pap. 32.00 (*0-7506-7325-7*) Buttrwrth-Heinemann.

One Hundred & One Therapeutic Successes: Overcoming Transference & Resistance in Psychotherapy. Gerald Schoenewolf. 1989. LC 88-7612. 304p. 50.00 (*0-87668-869-5*) Aronson.

One Hundred & One Ways to Transform Your Life. Wayne W. Dyer. 1995. pap. text 5.95 (*1-56170-169-6*) Hay House.

100 Best Careers in Allied Health. Lois A. Mark. 1999. 304p. 15.95 (*0-02-862520-X*) Macmillan.

One Hundred Best Treatment Centers for Alcoholism & Drug Abuse. John W. Wright & Linda Sunshine. 1988. (Orig.). pap. 10.95 (*0-380-75489-4*, Avon Bks) Morrow Avon.

One Hundred Case Histories for the MRCP. Peter S. Sever et al. 3rd ed. 1993. LC 93-10622. pap. text (*0-443-04701-4*) Church.

One Hundred Case Histories in Obstetrics & Gynaecology. Michael D. Gillmer et al. 1991. 264p. (Orig.). pap. text (*0-443-02465-0*) Church.

100 Case Histories MRCP. Spalaton. 2nd ed. 1989. pap. text 19.00 (*0-443-02140-6*) Saunders.

***100 Chest X-Ray Problems.** Jonathan Corne et al. 2001. (Illus.). 205p. pap. (*0-443-07012-1*) Church GBR. *Dist:* Saunders.

***100 Data Interpretation Questions in Paediatrics for MRCP/MRCPCH.** Nagi Barakat. 1999. 128p. pap. (*1-85315-405-9*) Royal Soc of Medicine Pr Ltd GBR. *Dist:* Balogh.

100 Diseases for the MRCP Part 2. Timothy Gray & Miles Witham. 2001. LC 00-65682. (*0-443-06466-0*) Church.

One Hundred Drugs That Work: A Guide to Prescription & Non-Prescription Drugs. Mike Oppenheim. 1994. 348p. 22.95 (*1-56565-115-4*) Lowell Hse.

100 ECG Problems. John R. Hampton. 1997. LC 97-7204. pap. text (*0-443-05678-1*) Church.

100 Faces of Health Care. American Hospital Association Staff. 1999. LC 00-500765. (Illus.). pap. text (*1-55648-276-0*) AHPI.

150 Most-Asked Questions about Menopause: What Women Really Want to Know. Ruth S. Jacobowitz. 1996. LC 96-17715. 240p. pap. 12.00 (*0-688-14768-2*, Quil) HarperTrade.

150 Practice ECGs. George J. Taylor. 1997. (Illus.). 224p. 31.95 (*0-86542-511-6*) Blackwell Sci.

One Hundred Fifty Ways to Be a Savvy Medical Consumer. Charles B. Inlander. 1992. (Illus.). 96p. pap. 5.95 (*0-9627334-5-8*) Peoples Med Soc.

150 Years of British Psychiatry Vol. II: The Aftermath. Ed. by German E. Berrios & Hugh Freeman. 1996. LC 96-209910. 650p. (*0-485-11506-9*) Athlone Pr GBR. *Dist:* Humanities.

***150 Years of Caring: A Pictorial History of the American Pharmaceutical Association.** George B. Griffenhagen. 2000. LC 2001-53622. (*1-58212-040-4*) Am Pharm Assn.

100 Great Homeopaths. Jay Yasgur. 2000. LC 99-95147. (CHI, ENG, FRE, GER & SPA., Illus.). 220p. pap. text 16.00 (*1-886149-07-0*) Van Hoy Pubs.

100 Ideas for Better Patient Relations in Registration, Billing, & Collection. Chenyl Soburn. 1996. spiral bd. 41.00 (*0-8342-0909-8*, 20909) Aspen Pub.

One Hundred Maxims in Neurology: Behavioral Neurology. Porter. 1993. 384p. (gr. 13). 43.95 (*0-340-57720-7*) Mosby Inc.

100 Maxims in Neurology: Parkinson Disease. Porter. 1992. 169p. 42.95 (*0-340-58947-7*) Mosby Inc.

One Hundred Maxims in Neurology: Stroke, 3. Frank M. Yatsu et al. 1995. (Illus.). 178p. (C). (gr. 13). 47.95 (*0-8016-7281-3*, 07281) Mosby Inc.

100 Medical Milestones of World History. Ruth Dejauregui. 1997. pap. text 7.95 (*0-912517-31-X*) Bluewood Bks.

One Hundred Million Guinea Pigs: Dangers in Everyday Foods, Drugs, & Cosmetics. Arthur Kallet & F. J. Schlink. 1976. LC 75-39252. (Getting & Spending: The Consumer's Dilemma Ser.). reprint ed. 26.95 (*0-405-08025-5*) Ayer.

One Hundred One Common Therapeutic Blunders: Countertransference & Counterresistance in Psychotherapy. Richard C. Robertiello & Gerald Schoenewolf. 1987. LC 87-1406. 294p. 50.00 (*0-87668-960-8*) Aronson.

101 Interventions in Family Therapy. Ed. by Thorana S. Nelson & Terry S. Trepper. 1993. 428p. pap. 24.95 (*1-56024-193-4*); LC 91-22252. 452p. lib. bdg. 54.95 (*0-86656-902-2*) Haworth Pr.

101 More Interventions in Family Therapy. Ed. by Thorana S. Nelson & Terry S. Trepper. 1998. LC 97-51448. (Illus.). 511p. (C). 69.96 (*0-7890-0058-X*); pap. 39.95 (*0-7890-0570-0*) Haworth Pr.

One Hundred One Questions to Ask Your Heart Doctor: An Insider's View. Joy Hannah. 1988. LC 88-51511. 150p. (Orig.). pap. 9.95 (*0-9621546-3-6*) Tamarack Hse.

101 Secrets of a High-Performance Veterinary Practice. Bob Levoy. 1996. LC 96-60137. (Illus.). 101p. pap. 19.95 (*0-935078-60-6*) Veterinary Hlthcare.

101 Secrets of a High-Performance Dental Practice: From the Success Files of Bob Levoy. Robert P. Levoy. 1996. LC 96-51693. 44.95 (*0-87814-593-1*) PennWell Corp.

One Hundred One Simple Things You Can Do to Stay on a Diet & Lose Weight! Douglas Kirkpatrick. Ed. by Vikki Richards. 1992. LC 91-76748. 128p. (Orig.). pap. 4.95 (*0-913193-04-6*) Baker Pub.

101 Tips for Improving Your Blood Sugar: Feel Better Now & Avoid Complications Later. David S. Schade et al. 1996. LC 95-9922. (Illus.). 128p. pap. 12.50 (*0-945448-47-3*, 4805-01) Am Diabetes.

101 Tips for Staying Healthy with Diabetes: And Avoiding Complications. University of New Mexico Diabetes Care Group Staff. 1996. LC 96-18928. 112p. pap. 12.50 (*0-945448-71-6*, 4810-01) Am Diabetes.

101 Ways to Live 150 Years Young & Healthy. Betty Yulin Ho. Ed. by Amanda Elkan. 1992. (System of Government in the Living Body Ser.). 62p. pap. 15.00 (*0-9600148-6-1*) Juvenescent.

100 Orthopaedic Conditions Every Doctor Should Understand. Roy A. Meals. 1992. LC 92-6582. (Illus.). 328p. pap. 36.00 (*0-942219-37-6*) Quality Med Pub.

One Hundred Paediatrics Picture Tests. A. P. Winrow et al. 1994. LC 93-29088. pap. text (*0-443-04942-4*) Church.

***100 Questions & Answers about Breast Cancer.** Zora K Brown & Lasalle Leffall, Jr. 2002. (Illus.). (C). pap. text 16.95 (*0-7637-1853-X*, 1853-X) Jones & Bartlett.

100 Questions & Answers about Sleep Disorders. Sudhansu Chokroverty. 2001. (One Hundred Questions to Ask Your Doctor about Ser.). (Illus.). 112p. pap. 14.95 (*0-86542-583-3*) Blackwell Sci.

***100 Questions in Cardiology.** Hugh Montgomery & Diana Holdright. 2001. 240p. pap. (*0-7279-1489-8*) BMJ Pub GBR. *Dist:* AIDC.

100 Questions to Ask Your Doctor About: Hypertension. William M. Manger & Ray W. Gifford, Jr. 2000. LC 00-56422. (Illus.). xviii, 180p. pap. 14.95 (*0-632-04481-0*) Blackwell Sci.

One Hundred Secrets for a Six-Figure Private Practice Income. Ryan Elliott. Ed. by Beth Billstrom. 1994. (Your Six-Figure Private Practice Success Course Ser.). 120p. (Orig.). pap. text (*0-9615140-1-9*) Relaxed Bks.

100 Short Cases for the MRCP. Ed. by K. Gupta et al. 2nd ed. 1994. (An Arnold Publication). 304p. pap. (*0-412-54860-7*) E A GBR. *Dist:* OUP.

100 Top Hospitals: Benchmarks for Success, 1997. 1997. 80.00 (*1-57372-103-4*) Solucient.

125 Brain Games for Babies. Jackie Silberg. 1999. LC 99-17317. (125 Brain Games Ser.). (Illus.). 160p. (J). (ps). pap. 14.95 (*0-87659-199-3*, 19854) Gryphon Hse.

125 Things You Must Know about Being Pregnant. Nina Landi. 1998. LC 98-2644. (Illus.). 48p. pap. 11.00 (*0-8050-5860-5*, Owl) H Holt & Co.

One Hundred Twenty Years of Medicine in Los Angeles County, 1871-1991. Barbara B. Gray. 1991. 144p. 32.50 (*1-881547-11-6*) Pioneer Pubns.

100 Years of American Nursing: Celebrating a Century of Caring. Thelma M. Schorr & Maureen Shawn Kennedy. 1999. LC 99-10472. (Illus.). 240p. text 38.95 (*0-7817-1865-1*) Lppncott W & W.

One Hundred Years of Gynaecology. James Ricci. 2000. 651p. reprint ed. 85.00 (*1-57898-218-9*) Martino Pubng.

One Hundred Years of Public Health in Sutton. Ed. by Jennifer Bray & Michael J. Wilks. 1987. 54p. pap. (*0-907335-06-3*) Sutton Libs & Arts GBR. *Dist:* St Mut.

One Hundred Years of Pyrazolone Drugs. Ed. by Kay Brune. 1986. (Agents & Actions Supplements Ser.: Vol. 19). 356p. 85.00 (*0-8176-1814-7*) Spr-Verlag.

One Hundred Years of the National Formulary: A Symposium. Ed. by Gregory J. Higby. 1989. 112p. (Orig.). pap. 8.00 (*0-931292-21-2*) Am Inst Hist Pharm.

One Man's Odyssey. Pearce. 1986. 187p. pap. (*0-85207-179-5*) C W Daniel GBR. *Dist:* Natl Bk Netwk.

One Man's Opinion on a Cure for Chronic Back Pain. William C. Gagnon. Ed. by Norman Christenson. 1998. (Illus.). 62p. 19.95 (*0-9663568-0-2*) Our Earths.

One Medicine: A Tribute to Kurt Benirschke. Ed. by O. A. Ryder & M. L. Byrd. 1984. (Illus.). 373p. 86.95 (*0-387-13275-9*) Spr-Verlag.

One Nurse's Notes: A Personal Journal. Ed. by Creative Nursing Management Staff. 1988. 78p. (Orig.). pap. 5.00 (*0-9621520-6-4*) Creative Nursing.

One of the Boys: Masculinity, Homophobia & Modern Manhood. David Plummer. 1999. LC 99-34431. (Haworth Gay & Lesbian Studies). ix, 364p. (C). 49.95 (*1-56023-973-5*, Harrington Park) Haworth Pr.

One on One: Conversations with the Shapers of Family Therapy. Richard Simon. 1992. LC 91-43238. 192p. pap. 16.95 (*0-89862-269-7*) Guilford Pubns.

1, 1, 1-Trichloroethane. 1992. (Environmental Health Criteria Ser.: No. 136). (ENG, FRE & SPA.). 117p. pap. text 28.00 (*92-4-157136-5*, 1160136) World Health.

One Out of Three: Children Without Health Insurance, 1995-1996. Cynthia Costello & Cheryl Fish-Parcham. 1998. (Illus.). 41p. pap. text 20.00 (*0-7881-7057-0*) DIANE Pub.

One Particular Harbor. Janet L. James. 1994. LC 93-33479. 288p. (Orig.). pap. 13.95 (*1-879360-30-6*) Noble Pr.

1-Propanol. 1990. (Environmental Health Criteria Ser.: No. 102). 98p. pap. text 23.00 (*92-4-157102-0*, 1160102) World Health.

One Renegade Cell: How Cancer Begins. Robert A. Weinberg. 1999. (Science Masters Ser.). 176p. pap. 14.00 (*0-465-07276-3*) Basic.

One Revolution: Managing the Academic Medical Practice in an Era of Rapid Change. Ed. by David J. Bachrach & William R. Nicholas. 1997. 360p. pap. 75.00 (*1-56829-083-7*) M G M A.

One Sip at a Time: Making the Best of Swallowing Problems. Ed. by Anna Hollingsworth. 1995. (Illus.). 30p. (Orig.). pap. text 5.25 (*0-939838-39-7*) Pritchett & Hull.

One Size Fits All & Other Fables. Liz C. Higgs. 1993. LC 93-20672. 183p. 12.99 (*0-8407-6333-6*) Nelson.

One Split Second. Suzan B. Hoppe. 1993. (Illus.). 370p. (Orig.). pap. 15.00 (*0-9630608-3-X*) R Dean Pr.

One-Stage Prothrombin Time (PT) Test & Activated Partial Thromboplastin Time (APTT) Test: Approved Guideline (1996) 1996. 75.00 (*1-56238-301-9*, H47-A) NCCLS.

One Step at a Time: A Definitive Study of Alzheimer's Disease & a Practical Guide for Caregivers. Lorena S. Eaker. 1996. LC 96-69044. v, 207p. (Orig.). pap. 15.00 (*0-9653000-0-5*) S C K Pubns.

One Step at a Time: The Remarkable True Story of Bob Wieland. Bob Wieland. 1989. 192p. 12.99 (*0-310-51640-4*) Zondervan.

One Thousand C's for Better Living Diet Cookbook. Eleanor Welling. 1979. pap. 2.95 (*0-9602118-1-0*) CnE Varieties.

1000 MCQs for Davidson's Principles & Practice of Medicine. Michael J. Ford & A. T. Elder. 1997. LC 96-26058. (*0-443-05556-4*); 3rd ed. pap. text (*0-443-05462-2*) Church.

1000 MCQs for Davidson's Principles & Practice of Medicine. Ford. 4th ed. 1999. text 29.00 (*0-443-06399-0*) Harcrt Hlth Sci Grp.

1001 Multiple Choice Questions & Answers in Surgery. Ed. by H. Rains. 3rd ed. 1991. (Illus.). 200p. (Orig.). (C). (gr. 13). pap. text 27.00 (*0-412-40010-3*, Chap & Hall NY) Chapman & Hall.

1001 Multiple Choice Questions & Answers in Surgery: A Companion to Surgical Study Based on "Bailey & Love's Short Practice of Surgery" A. J. Rains. 4th ed. 1996. 240p. pap. (*0-412-55560-3*) E A GBR. *Dist:* OUP.

1001 Nursing Tips & Timesavers. Springhouse Publishing Company Staff. Ed. by June Norris. 3rd ed. 1996. LC 96-69628. (Illus.). 256p. (Orig.). pap. 22.95 (*0-87434-850-1*) Springhouse Corp.

1000 Questions about Women's Health. Jane Chihal & Nancy Brinker. 1997. 504p. pap. 16.99 (*1-56530-264-8*) Summit TX.

1000 Questions about Your Pregnancy. Jeffrey Thurston. 1997. LC 97-33880. (Illus.). 504p. (Orig.). pap. 16.99 (*1-56530-265-6*) Summit TX.

1, 3-Dichloropropene, 1, 2-Dichloropropane & Mixtures. 1993. (Environmental Health Criteria Ser.: No. 146). (ENG, FRE & SPA.). 261p. pap. text 50.00 (*92-4-157146-2*, 1160146) World Health.

One, Three-Dipolar Cycloaddition Chemistry, Vol. 2. Albert Padwa. 1984. (General Heterocyclic Chemistry Ser.: No. 1-128). 1521p. 925.00 (*0-471-08364-X*) Wiley.

1,2 Dichloroethane. 1995. (Environmental Health Criteria Ser.: Vol. 176). 148p. (C). pap. 30.00 (*92-4-157176-4*, 1160176) World Health.

One Woman's War: Letters Home from the Women's Army Corp, 1944-1946. Anne B. Green. 1989. LC 89-13000. (Illus.). xxiv, 308p. 22.50 (*0-87351-246-4*) Minn Hist.

One World, One Language: Paving the Way to Better Perspectives for Mental Health. World Congress of Psychiatry Staff. Ed. by Juan J. Lopez-Ibor et al. 1999. LC 99-17543. (Illus.). vi, 259p. pap. 39.00 (*0-88937-214-4*) Hogrefe & Huber Pubs.

One You Love Is Dying: 12 Ideas to Guide You on the Journey. James E. Miller. 1997. LC 97-60134. (Illus.). 64p. (Orig.). pap. text 6.95 (*1-885933-23-1*) Willowgreen Pubng.

1,25-Dihydroxyvitamin D3 & Its Analogues As Immunomodulators in Autoimmune Type 1 Diabetes: Mechanisms of Action & Preclinical Applications. Kristina Casteels. 1998. (Acta Biomedica Lovaniensia Ser.). (Illus.). 160p. pap. (*90-6186-876-9*) Leuven Univ BEL. *Dist:* Coronet Bks.

Ongoing Record Review: A Guide to JCAHO Compliance & Best Practice. Jean Clark. 1998. (Illus.). 120p. pap. text 87.00 (*1-57839-038-9*) Opus Communs.

Onions: Condiment, Nutrient, Medicine. Clarence Meyer. Ed. by David C. Meyer. 1993. (Illus.). 115p. (Orig.). pap. 8.95 (*0-916638-16-2*) Meyerbooks.

Online Consumer Guide to Healthcare & Wellness: The Best Online Sites, Resources & Services In: Health & Fitness, Diet & Weight Loss, Alternative Medicine, Family Health, Stress Management, Disease & Medical Conditions, Emergency Care & First Aid. Douglas E. Goldstein & Joyce Flory. 1996. LC 96-3034. (Best of the Net Ser.). 304p. pap. text 24.95 (*0-7863-0886-9*, Irwn Prfssnl) McGraw-Hill Educ Grp.

Online Drug Information Thesaurus. Martindale. 2nd ed. 1990. (*0-85369-229-7*) Pharmaceutical Pr GBR. *Dist:* Rittenhouse.

Online Guide to Healthcare Management & Medicine: The Best Online Sites, Resources & Services in Healthcare Management, Pharmaceuticals, Family Medicine, Patient Education, Emerging Healthcare Trends, Diagnostic Testing, Home Health Care, Financial Management & Telemedicine. Douglas E. Goldstein & Joyce Flory. 1996. LC 96-3033. (Best of the Net Ser.). 304p. pap. 24.95 (*0-7863-0885-0*, Irwn Prfssnl) McGraw-Hill Educ Grp.

Online Systems for Medical Professionals: How to Use & Access Computer Data Base. Harley Bjelland. Ed. by Jill Brittenham. 1992. 200p. 39.95 (*1-878487-44-2*, ME045) Practice Mgmt Info.

Only EKG Book You'll Ever Need. Ed. by Lippincott-Raven Staff. 3rd ed. 1999. LC 98-39871. 320p. pap. text 39.95 (*0-7817-1667-5*) Lppncott W & W.

Only Foolproof Way to Stop Smoking: Stop Smoking. Mary Lee. 1996. 75p. pap. 14.95 (*1-881242-01-3*) Pyramid Educ Inc.

Ontogenesis of Perception. Ed. by William Epstein. 1987. (Special Issue, Journal of Experimental Psychology: Human Perception & Performance Ser.: Vol. 13, No. 4). 107p. pap. 16.00 (*1-55798-008-X*) Am Psychol.

Ontogeny & Phylogeny of Hormone Receptors. G. Csaba. 1981. (Monographs in Developmental Biology: Vol. 15). (Illus.). xii, 172p. 125.25 (*3-8055-2174-X*) S Karger.

Ontogeny of Bonding Attachment. Ed. by P. O. Hubinont. 1984. (Progress in Reproductive Biology & Medicine Ser.: Vol. 11). (Illus.). vi, 178p. 126.25 (*3-8055-3862-6*) S Karger.

Ontogeny of Minerals. D. P. Grigor'ev. 1965. 256p. text 66.00 (*0-7065-0537-9*) Coronet Bks.

Ontogeny of the Immune System of the Gut. Thomas T. MacDonald. 1990. 128p. lib. bdg. 142.00 (*0-8493-6084-6*, QR185) CRC Pr.

Ontogeny of Transmitters & Peptides in the CNS. Anders T. Bjorklund et al. 1992. (Handbooks of Chemical Neuroanatomy: Vol. 10). 664p. 315.00 (*0-444-89283-4*) Elsevier.

Onychomycoses. Ed. by S. Nolting & H. C. Korting. 1990. (Illus.). 128p. 29.95 (*0-387-52132-1*) Spr-Verlag.

OP: Surgery. D. Das. 3rd ed. 1989. (C). (*0-7855-6115-3*) Current Dist IND. *Dist:* St Mut.

Open Airways: An Asthma Self-Management Program. 1991. lib. bdg. 74.95 (*0-8490-4339-5*) Gordon Pr.

Open Heart Surgery: A Second Chance. Nyles V. Reinfeld. 1983. 192p. 22.00 (*0-13-637520-0*); pap. 14.95 (*0-13-637512-X*) P-H.

Open Heart Surgery: Theory & Practice, 7. Ed. by John C. Callaghan & Joseph Wartak. 1986. LC 86-5005. (Surgical Science Ser.: Vol. 7). (Illus.). 190p. 62.50 (*0-275-92088-7*, C2088, Praeger Pubs) Greenwood.

Open Heart Therapy. Bob Mandel. 1995. LC 84-45360. 160p. (Orig.). text 8.95 (*0-89087-408-5*) Celestial Arts.

Open Learning for Nurses. Robinson. 1989. pap. text (*0-582-04616-5*) Addison-Wesley GBR. *Dist:* Trans-Atl Phila.

Open Learning in Nursing, Health & Welfare Education. Kate Robinson & Pam Shakespeare. 1995. LC 94-43323. 160p. (*0-335-19075-8*); pap. (*0-335-19074-X*) OpUniv Pr.

Open MRI. Peter Rothschild & Debra Reinking Rothschild. 1999. LC 99-42876. 400p. text 139.00 (*0-7817-2173-3*, Lippnctt) Lppncott W & W.

Open Rhinoplasty. Joseph Leach & Lanny Close. 1996. LC 96-14951. (Self-Instructional Package Ser.). pap. text 25.00 (*1-56772-021-8*) AAO-HNS.

Open Season: A Survival Guide for Natural Childbirth in the 1990s. Nancy W. Cohen. 1991. LC 91-10569. 464p. 29.95 (*0-89789-252-6*, H252); pap. 16.95 (*0-89789-272-0*, G272) Greenwood (Bergin & Garvey).

Open Season Guide: Federal Health Benefits & Premiums, 1993. National Association of Retired Federal Employees. Ed. by Gordon F. Brown. 1992. 152p. (Orig.). pap. 9.95 (*0-9631168-2-7*) Natl Ret Fed Emps.

Open Systems in Medicine: The Berlin Approach to Medical Information Processing. Ed. by Eckart Fleck. 1995. LC 92-51050. (Studies in Health Technology & Informatics: Vol. 8). 247p. (YA). (gr. 12 up). 117.00 (*90-5199-123-1*) IOS Press.

Open Water Dive Table Hardback. Jeppesen. 1987. 8.95 (*0-8016-9002-1*) Mosby Inc.

Open Wide . . . This Won't Hurt a Bit! A Dentist's Guide to Self-Discovery & Self-Management. Doug Siebert. 1991. (Illus.). 226p. 39.95 (*0-9631005-0-5*) D Siebert Co.

Open Your Mouth But Don't Say "Ah" Philip Thorek. 1994. LC 93-37682. (Illus.). 88p. pap. 14.95 (*0-89640-252-5*) Igaku-Shoin.

Opening a Dental Practice. R. H. Schaper. 1996. 29.95 (*0-87814-590-7*) PennWell Corp.

Opening Doors: What Happens in Gestalt Therapy. Daniel Rosenblatt. Date not set. pap. 20.00 (*0-939266-33-4*) Gestalt Journal.

Opening Doors to Public Health Nursing: A Guidebook. Joyce Zerwekh. 1998. (Illus.). 71p. pap. text 20.00 (*0-9662376-1-7*) WA Public Health.

Opening Gambits: The First Session of Psychotherapy. Peter S. Armstrong. 2000. LC 99-41431. 256p. 40.00 (*0-7657-0241-X*) Aronson.

Opening the Door: Improving the Healthy Families/Medi-Cal Application Process - Executive Summary. 1998. (Illus.). 48p. spiral bd. (*1-929008-22-8*) CA HlthCare Fnd.

Opening the Door: Improving the Healthy Families/Medi-Cal Application Process - Full Report. 1998. (Illus.). 98p. spiral bd. (*1-929008-23-6*) CA HlthCare Fnd.

Opening the Door to the Brain: Granular Cell Neuron Masses. Hyman Olken. (Illus.). 30p. (Orig.). pap. 12.00 (*0-934818-05-3*) Olken Pubns.

Opening the Doors to Canadian Medical Schools. Rod Elford. 1994. (Life Line Ser.). 112p. pap. 14.95 (*1-55059-084-7*) Temeron Bks.

Opening Up: The Healing Power of Expressing Emotions. James W. Pennebaker. 1997. LC 97-20544. 249p. pap. 15.95 (*1-57230-238-0*, 0238) Guilford Pubns.

***Operating on the Frontier: Memoirs of a Pioneer Canadian Neurosurgeon.** Frank Turnbull. 2nd ed. (Illus.). 307p. reprint ed. (*1-55017-135-6*); pap. (*1-55017-137-2*) Harbour Pub Co.

Operating Room Aide. Mary Virgilio. Ed. by Kay Cox. 1997. LC 97-67079. (Clinical Allied Healthcare Ser.). (Illus.). 256p. (C). pap. text 29.95 (*0-89262-433-7*) Career Pub.

Operating Room Aide: Instructor's Guide. Mary Virgilio. Ed. by Kay Cox. 1997. (Clinical Allied Healthcare Ser.). (Illus.). 283p. (C). tchr. ed., ring bd. 79.95 (*0-89262-441-8*) Career Pub.

Operating Room & Intensive Care Alarms: Information Transfer. Ed. by John Whyte-Hedley. 1992. LC 92-7225. (Special Technical Publications: No. 1152). (Illus.). 45p. text 19.00 (*0-8031-1449-4*, STP1152) ASTM.

Operating Room Management. Andrew P. Harris & William G. Zitzmann. 1997. LC 97-34545. (Illus.). 312p. (C). (gr. 13). pap. text 44.95 (*0-8151-4178-5*, 26867) Mosby Inc.

Operating Room Policy & Procedures. Nancy Meier. 1993. 145.00 (*1-879575-35-3*) Acad Med Sys.

Operating Room Risk Management, 1996, Set. Ed. by Ronni P. Solomon & Sharon Bayless. 1993. 1100p. ring bd. 595.00 (*0-941417-05-0*) ECRI.

Operation Desert Storm: Health Concerns of Selected Indiana Persian Gulf War Veterans. 1995. 43p. (Orig.). (C). pap. text 15.00 (*0-7881-2079-4*) DIANE Pub.

Operational Diagnostic Approaches in Psychosomatic Medicine & Psychotherapy. Ed. by H. J. Freyberger & W. Schneider. 1995. (Journal: Vol. 63, No. 2, 1995). (Illus.). 80p. pap. 42.75 (*3-8055-6133-4*) S Karger.

Operational Policy & Procedure Manual: Pharmaceutical Services. W. H. Heaton. 300p. ring bd. 125.00 (*1-881057-17-8*) Heaton Pubns.

Operational Radiation Safety Program. 1978. LC 79-62918. (Report Ser.: No. 59). 68p. pap. text 25.00 (*0-913392-43-X*) NCRP Pubns.

Operational Radiation Safety Program: Recommendations of the National Council on Radiation Protection & Measurements. National Council on Radiation Protection and Measure. 1998. LC 98-4407. (NCRP Reports: Vol. 127). pap. 30.00 (*0-929600-59-2*) NCRP Pubns.

Operational Radiation Safety-Training. Intro. by Warren K. Sinclair. 1983. LC 82-62031. (Report Ser.: No. 71). 54p. pap. text 25.00 (*0-913392-60-X*) NCRP Pubns.

Operations Committee Report: Training, Responsibilities, Staffing, Safety, Quality Assurance. Ed. by Patrick N. Kimbrell. 2000. 25p. pap. text 15.00 (*0-930406-16-8*) Undersea & Hyperbaric.

Operations Research: Applications in Health Care Planning. Ed. by No K. Kwak et al. 1984. (Illus.). 360p. (Orig.). pap. text 40.00 (*0-8191-4168-2*); lib. bdg. 79.00 (*0-8191-4167-4*) U Pr of Amer.

Operations Research: Helping Family Planning Programs Work Better. Ed. by Myrna Seidman & Marjorie Horn. 1991. (Progress in Clinical & Biological Research Ser.: No. 1922). 578p. 299.00 (*0-471-56161-4*, Wiley-Liss) Wiley.

Operative Arthroscopy. Ed. by John B. McGinty et al. 2nd ed. 1995. LC 95-15899. (Illus.). 1,296p. text 299.00 (*0-7817-0294-1*) Lppncott W & W.

Operative Atlas for Meningiomas. Ossama Al-Mefty. 1997. LC 97-2086. (Illus.). 480p. text 215.00 (*0-7817-0152-X*) Lppncott W & W.

Operative Challenges in Head & Neck Surgery. Pillsbury. 1991. (*0-8151-6707-5*) Mosby Inc.

Operative Colorectal Surgery. George E. Block & A. R. Moosa. 1994. LC 92-48340. (Illus.). 640p. text 155.00 (*0-7216-3366-8*) Saunders.

Operative Endoscopy of the Digestive Tract. G. Bedogni et al. 1984. 274p. text (*1-57235-014-8*) Piccin Nuova ITA. *Dist:* Gordon & Breach.

Operative Foot Surgery. John S. Gould. 1993. LC 93-1960. (Illus.). 992p. text 152.00 (*0-7216-3196-7*) Saunders.

Operative Gynecologic Endoscopy. Ed. by Joseph S. Sanfilippo & Ronald L. Levine. 2nd ed. 1996. LC 95-25735. (Clinical Perspectives in Obstetrics & Gynecology Ser.). 541p. 137.00 (*0-387-94467-2*) Spr-Verlag.

Operative Gynecologic Laparascopy: Principles & Techniques. Camran Nezhat et al. 1995. 352p. text 125.00 (*0-07-105422-7*) McGraw-Hill Med Pub.

Operative Gynecologic Laparoscopy: Principles & Techniques. Camran Nezhat. 2nd ed. 2000. LC 99-88759. (Illus.). 420p. text 150.00 (*0-07-105431-6*) McGraw-Hill Prof.

Operative Gynecology. David M. Gershenson et al. (Illus.). 1993. 672p. text 115.00 (*0-7216-3558-X*); 2nd ed. 1999. LC 00-32999. xx, 890p. text 139.00 (*0-7216-7987-0*) Saunders.

Operative Hand Surgery, Set. David P. Green. 3rd ed. 1993. (Illus.). 2512p. text (*0-443-08803-9*) Church.

Operative Hip Arthroscopy. J. W. Byrd. 1997. 149.00 (*0-86577-783-7*); LC 97-30914. (Illus.). 232p. 129.00 (*0-86577-679-2*) Thieme Med Pubs.

Operative Hysteroscopy: A Practical Guide. Thomas Roemer & Wolfgang Straube. 1997. (Illus.). viii, 96p. (C). pap. text 45.35 (*3-11-015667-9*) De Gruyter.

Operative Laparoscopy: The Masters' Techniques. Richard M. Soderstrom. 2nd ed. 1997. LC 97-14251. 320p. text 149.00 (*0-397-51797-1*) Lppncott W & W.

Operative Laparoscopy & Hysteroscopy. Ed. by Stephen M. Cohen. 1996. 320p. text (*0-443-08950-7*) Church.

Operative Laparoscopy & Thoracoscopy. Ed. by Bruce V. MacFadyen, Jr. & Jeffrey L. Ponsky. 1996. LC 95-20399. (Illus.). 992p. text 259.00 (*0-7817-0279-8*) Lppncott W & W.

Operative Laparoscopy for Gynecologists. David Hoffman et al. 1993. LC 95-37144. (Illus.). 207p. text 19.95 (*1-880906-05-8*) IDI Pub.

Operative Management of Breast Disease. R. Robinson Baker & John Niederhuber. 1992. (Illus.). 147p. text 179.00 (*0-7216-2960-1*) Saunders.

Operative Management of Lower Extremity Fractures in Children. Ed. by Robert N. Hensinger. 1992. 80p. pap. 38.00 (*0-89203-058-5*) Amer Acad Ortho Surg.

Operative Management of Upper Extremity Fractures in Children. Ed. by Kaye E. Wilkins. 1994. 112p. pap. 38.00 (*0-89203-085-2*) Amer Acad Ortho Surg.

Operative Manual of Endoscopic Surgery. Alfred Cuschieri et al. 1992. LC 92-2421. (Illus.). 353p. 175.00 (*0-387-53486-5*) Spr-Verlag.

Operative Manual of Endoscopic Surgery, Vol. 2. G. F. Buess & A. Cuschieki. 1994. (Illus.). 265p. 207.00 (*0-387-56810-7*) Spr-Verlag.

Operative Manual of Endoscopic Surgery, Vol. 2. J. Perissat. Ed. by Alfred Cuschieri & G. F. Buess. 1994. LC 92-2421. (Illus.). 265p. text 175.00 (*3-540-56810-7*) Spr-Verlag.

Operative Maxillofacial Surgery. Ed. by Mohan F. Patel & John D. Langdon. 1999. LC 97-69008. (Illus.). 536p. (*0-412-56000-3*) E A GBR. *Dist:* OUP.

Operative Nerve Repair & Reconstruction, In Two Volumes. Richard H. Gelberman. 1991. (Illus.). 1,699p. text 325.00 (*0-397-51074-8*) Lppncott W & W.

***Operative Neurosurgery**, Set. Andrew H. Kaye & Peter M. Black. 2000. (Illus.). 2349p. text (*0-443-05827-X*) Church GBR. *Dist:* Saunders.

Operative Neurosurgical Techniques: Indications, Methods, & Results, Set. Henry H. Schmidek & William H. Sweet. 3rd ed. 1995. LC 93-42522. (Illus.). 2112p. text 415.00 (*0-7216-5541-6*) Saunders.

Operative Obstetrics. Ed. by John P. O'Grady et al. 1995. LC 95-8734. (Illus.). 512p. (*0-683-06633-1*) Lppncott W & W.

Operative Obstetrics. Ed. by Leslie Iffy et al. 2nd ed. 1992. (Illus.). 488p. text 79.00 (*0-07-105395-6*) McGraw-Hill Educ Grp.

Operative Obstetrics. Gary D. Hankins et al. 5th ed. 1995. LC 95-1975. 782p. (C). text 160.00 (*0-8385-7409-2*, A7409-4, Apple Lange Med) McGraw.

M
N
O

Operative Orthopaedics Ed. by Michael W. Chapman & Michael Madison. 2nd ed. 1993. LC 92-49608. 1. 395.00 (*0-397-51304-6*); 2. (*0-397-51305-4*); 3. (*0-397-51306-2*); 4. (*0-397-51307-0*) Lppncott W & W.

Operative Orthopaedics Cd-Rom Library Institutional. A. W. Crenshaw. 1996. text 495.95 (*0-8151-1901-1*) Mosby Inc.

Operative Otolaryngology, Set. Eugene N. Myers. Ed. by Larry McGrew. 1997. LC 96-16724. (Illus.). 1408p. text 365.00 (*0-7216-3841-4*) Saunders.

Operative Otorhinolaryngology. Nigel Bleach et al. 1997. LC 95-47084. (Illus.). 512p. 299.95 (*0-632-03747-4*) Blackwell Sci.

Operative Paediatric Urology. Ed. by J. David Frank & J. H. Johnston. 1990. (Illus.). 256p. text (*0-443-03478-8*) Church.

Operative Pediatric Orthopaedics, No. 2. S. Terry Canale & James H. Beaty. 1994. (*0-8016-7990-7*) Mosby Inc.

Operative Pediatric Surgery. Ziegler. 1999. (C). pap. text 195.00 (*0-8385-7405-X*) Appleton & Lange.

Operative Pediatric Urology. Frank. 2nd ed. 1999. 292p. text 145.00 (*0-443-05358-8*) Saunders.

Operative Plastic Surgery. Ed. by Gregory R. Evans. 2000. LC 99-32189. (Illus.). 1020p. text 299.00 (*0-8385-7676-1*) McGraw-Hill Prof.

Operative Shoulder Surgery. Stephen Copeland. 1995. (Illus.). text (*0-443-04640-9*) Church.

Operative Spinal Surgery. Ed. by Michael J. Torrens & Robert A. Dickson. 1991. (Practice of Surgery Ser.). (Illus.). 333p. text (*0-443-03922-4*) Church.

Operative Spine Surgery. William C. Welch. 1999. LC 98-22965. 300p. text 159.00 (*0-8385-7393-2*) McGraw-Hill Educ Grp.

Operative Strategies in Inflammatory Bowel Disease. Ed. by Fabrizio Michelassi & Jeffrey W. Milsom. 1998. LC 97-20702. (Illus.). 535p. 165.00 (*0-387-94966-6*) Spr-Verlag.

Operative Strategies in Laparoscopic Surgery. Ed. by Edward H. Phillips & Raul J. Rosenthal. 1995. (*0-387-59214-8*); LC 95-24353. (Illus.). 288p. 115.00 (*3-540-59214-8*) Spr-Verlag.

Operative Strategy in General Surgery: An Expositive Atlas. J. L. Chassin. 2nd ed. 1997. LC 93-32984. (Illus.). 890p. reprint ed. 187.00 (*0-387-97968-9*) Spr-Verlag.

Operative Surgery. Shipman. 4th ed. 1987. (Illus.). 207p. (Orig.). (C). pap. 41.95 (*0-7186-0496-2*) Chapman & Hall.

Operative Surgery: Alimentary Tract & Abdominal Wall Part-1: General Principles, Oesophagus, Stomach, Duodenum, Small Intestine, Abdominal Wall, Hernia. Ed. by Hugh Dudley. 4th ed. 1983. (Rob & Smith's Operative Surgery Ser.). 512p. pap. text 155.00 (*0-407-00651-6*) Buttrwrth-Heinemann.

Operative Surgery: Alimentary Tract & Abdominal Wall-Part 3: Colon, Rectum & Anus. Ed. by Ian P. Todd & L. P. Fielding. 4th ed. 1993. (Health Sciences Ser.). (Illus.). 672p. text 175.00 (*0-407-00652-4*) Thomson Learn.

Operative Surgery: Cardiac Surgery. Ed. by Stuart W. Jamieson & Norman E. Shumway. 4th ed. 1986. (Rob & Smith's Operative Surgery Ser.). (Illus.). 624p. (gr. 13). pap. 475.95 (*0-407-00660-5*) Chapman & Hall.

Operative Surgery: Ear. Ed. by John Ballantyne & A. W. Morrison. 4th ed. 1986. (Rob & Smith's Operative Surgery Ser.). (Illus.). 232p. (gr. 13). text 353.95 (*0-407-00662-1*) Chapman & Hall.

Operative Surgery: General Principles, Breast & Extracranial Endocrines. Ed. by Hugh Dudley & Walter J. Pories. 4th ed. 1987. (Rob & Smith's Operative Surgery Ser.). 456p. (gr. 13). pap. 381.95 (*0-407-00650-8*) Chapman & Hall.

Operative Surgery: Gynecology & Obstetrics. Ed. by J. M. Monaghan. 4th ed. 1987. (Rob & Smith's Operative Surgery Ser.). (Illus.). 312p. (gr. 13). text 381.95 (*0-407-00680-X*) Chapman & Hall.

Operative Surgery: Nose & Throat. Ed. by John C. Ballantyne & D. F. Harrison. 4th ed. 1986. (Rob & Smith's Operative Surgery Ser.). (Illus.). 504p. pap. 184.95 (*0-407-00663-X*) Chapman & Hall.

Operative Surgery: Ophthalmic Surgery. Ed. by Thomas A. Rice et al. 4th ed. 1993. (Rob & Smith's Operative Surgery Ser.). (Illus.). 456p. (gr. 13). pap. 324.95 (*0-407-00657-5*) Chapman & Hall.

Operative Surgery: Orthopedics, Vol. 1. Bentley & Greer. 4th ed. 1993. 670p. (C). (gr. 13). pap. 262.95 (*0-7506-1480-3*) Chapman & Hall.

Operative Surgery: Plastic Surgery. Ed. by Thomas L. Barclay & Demond A. Kernahan. 4th ed. 1993. (Rob & Smith's Operative Surgery Ser.). (Illus.). 760p. (gr. 13). pap. 494.95 (*0-407-00664-8*) Chapman & Hall.

Operative Surgery: The Hand. Ed. by R. Birch & D. Brooks. 4th ed. 1993. (Rob & Smith's Operative Surgery Ser.). (Illus.). 552p. (gr. 13). pap. 381.95 (*0-407-00653-2*) Chapman & Hall.

Operative Surgery: Thoracic Surgery. Ed. by John W. Jackson & D. K. Cooper. 4th ed. 1986. (Rob & Smith's Operative Surgery Ser.). (Illus.). 408p. (gr. 13). pap. 343.95 (*0-407-00661-3*) Chapman & Hall.

Operative Surgery: Urology. Ed. by W. Scott McDoudal. 4th ed. 1993. (Rob & Smith's Operative Surgery Ser.). (Illus.). 804p. pap. 189.00 (*0-407-00658-3*) Chapman & Hall.

Operative Surgery: Vascular Surgery. Ed. by James A. DeWeese. 4th ed. 1985. (Rob & Smith's Operative Surgery Ser.). (Illus.). 552p. 180.00 (*0-407-00659-1*) Chapman & Hall.

Operative Surgery & Management. Keen & Farndon. 1998. pap. text (*0-7506-4238-6*) E A GBR. *Dist:* OUP.

Operative Surgery & Management. Ed. by Gerald Keen. 1981. (Illus.). 860p. text (*0-7236-0548-3*) John Wright.

Operative Surgery & Management. Keen. 2nd ed. 1987. 896p. (*0-7236-0836-9*) John Wright.

Operative Techniques & Surgical Topics for the FRCS: Viva Practice. K. M. Mokbel. 1995. 128p. (C). pap. text 22.00 (*0-7923-8881-X*) Kluwer Academic.

Operative Techniques in Pediatric Neurosurgery. Leland A. Albright. 2000. (Illus.). 352p. 179.00 (*0-86577-846-9*) Thieme Med Pubs.

Operative Trauma Management. Ed. by Erwin R. Thal et al. 2nd ed. 2001. 556p. text 250.00 (*0-8385-7388-6*) McGraw-Hill Prof.

Operative Trauma Management Atlas. Ed. by C. J. Carrico. 1998. LC 97-20619. (Illus.). 335p. (C). pap. text 189.00 (*0-8385-7401-7*, A-7401-1, Apple Lange Med) McGraw.

***Operative Treatment of Elbow Injuries.** Champ L. Baker & Kevin D. Plancher. 2001. LC 00-67910. (Illus.). 352p. 179.00 (*0-387-98905-6*, Copernicus) Spr-Verlag.

Operative Treatment of the Foot & Ankle. Armen S. Kelikian. 1998. LC 98-22076. 784p. text 199.00 (*0-8385-7386-X*) McGraw-Hill Prof.

Operative Urology Two, Vol. 13, Pt. 2. Ed. by C. E. Alken et al. 1970. (Illus.). 256p. 131.00 (*0-387-05142-2*) Spr-Verlag.

Operator Training for Medical & Other Solid Waste Incinerators. Doucet and Mainka Staff. 1992. (Illus.). 408p. (Orig.). pap. 169.00 (*0-87258-596-4*, 055210) Am Hospital.

Operator's Guide to Water Fluoridation. Glenn M. Tillman. 1993. 112p. lib. bdg. 45.00 (*0-87371-614-0*, L614) Lewis Pubs.

Ophthalmic Anesthesia. Caroline A. Carr et al. 2nd ed. 1996. (Illus.). 296p. pap. text (*0-340-56757-0*) E A GBR. *Dist:* OUP.

Ophthalmic Assistant: A Guide for Ophthalmic Medical Personnel. Harold A. Stein et al. 7th ed. 2000. LC 00-698636. (Illus.). xvi, 880p. pap. 63.00 (*0-323-00913-1*) Mosby Inc.

Ophthalmic Assistant: Fundamentals & Clinical Practices, Principles. Harold A. Stein & Bernard J. Slatt. 6th ed. 1994. LC 94-226814. (Illus.). 960p. (C). (gr. 13). pap. text 63.00 (*0-8151-7560-4*, 24208) Mosby Inc.

Ophthalmic Consultants of Boston. John J. Woog. Date not set. 224p. pap. 65.00 (*0-7506-7326-5*) Buttrwrth-Heinemann.

Ophthalmic Diagnostic Equipment Markets: Industry Focuses on Automated Equipment & Corneal Topography. Market Intelligence Staff. 1992. 343p. 1695.00 (*1-56753-414-7*) Frost & Sullivan.

Ophthalmic Disorders of Children. Ed. by David W. Kaplan. 1990. (Journal: Vol. 17, No. 3, 1990). (Illus.). 84p. pap. 48.00 (*3-8055-5209-2*) S Karger.

Ophthalmic Disorders Sourcebook: Basic Information about Glaucoma, Cataracts, Macular Degeneration, Strabismus, Refractive Disorders & More. Ed. by Allan R. Cook. 1996. LC 96-3345. (Health Reference Ser.: Vol. 17). lib. bdg. 78.00 (*0-7808-0081-8*) Omnigraphics Inc.

Ophthalmic Dispensing. Russell L. Stimson. 3rd ed. 1979. (Illus.). 720p. 94.95 (*0-398-03823-6*) C C Thomas.

Ophthalmic Dispensing: Present Day Realities. Ralph Drew. 1990. (Illus.). 304p. text 74.95 (*0-409-90225-X*) Buttrwrth-Heinemann.

Ophthalmic Drug Delivery: Biopharmaceutical, Technological & Clinical Aspects. Ed. by M. F. Saettone et al. 1988. (FIDIA Research Ser.: Vol. 11). 195p. 118.00 (*0-387-96599-8*) Spr-Verlag.

Ophthalmic Drug Delivery Systems. Ashim K. Mitra. 1993. (Drugs & the Pharmaceutical Sciences Ser.: Vol. 58). (Illus.). 536p. text 215.00 (*0-8247-8806-0*) Dekker.

***Ophthalmic Drug Facts 2002.** Ed. by Facts and Comparisons Staff. 2001. 430p. per. 59.95 (*1-57439-113-5*) Facts & Comparisons.

Ophthalmic Echography. Cynthia J. Kendall. 1990. LC 87-42952. (Ophthalmic Technical Skills Ser.: Vol. II). (Illus.). 200p. (C). pap. text 40.00 (*1-55642-027-7*) SLACK Inc.

Ophthalmic Echography. Ed. by K. C. Ossoinig. 1987. (Documenta Ophthalmologica Proceedings Ser.). (C). text 389.50 (*0-89838-873-2*) Kluwer Academic.

Ophthalmic Echography No. 13: Proceedings of the SIDUO Congress, 13th, Vienna, Austria, 1990. Ed. by P. Till. 1993. LC 92-19775. (Documenta Ophthalmologica Proceedings Ser.: Vol. 55). 560p. (C). text 264.50 (*0-7923-1808-0*) Kluwer Academic.

Ophthalmic Essentials. M. P. Vrabec. 1992. (Illus.). 464p. pap. 44.95 (*0-86542-202-8*) Blackwell Sci.

Ophthalmic Histopathology. W. R. Lee. 1993. (Illus.). 352p. 273.00 (*0-387-19686-2*) Spr-Verlag.

Ophthalmic Histopathology. William R. Lee. 1993. (Illus.). 352p. 250.00 (*3-540-19686-2*) Spr-Verlag.

Ophthalmic Laser Therapy. Kimiharu Noyori et al. 1992. (Illus.). 289p. 170.00 (*0-89640-199-5*) Igaku-Shoin.

Ophthalmic Lasers: A Primary Care Approach. Wormington. 2000. 304p. 49.95 (*0-7506-9572-2*) Buttrwrth-Heinemann.

Ophthalmic Lenses. H. H. Emsley. 1984. (Illus.). 340p. reprint ed. pap. 25.00 (*0-87556-375-9*) Saifer.

Ophthalmic Lenses & Dispensing. M. Jalie. 1999. LC 99-233330. 224p. pap. text 95.00 (*0-7506-4158-4*) Buttrwrth-Heinemann.

Ophthalmic Medical Assistant: An Independent Study Course. Ed. by Paul J. Wasson & Robert C. Allen. 1999. LC 99-35332. 270p. 110.00 (*1-56055-171-2*) Am Acad Ophthal.

Ophthalmic Medical Assisting: An Independent Study Course. Ed. by Robert L. Stamper & Paul J. Wasson. 2nd ed. 1994. LC 94-33317. pap. (*1-56055-025-2*) Am Acad Ophthal.

Ophthalmic Medical Assisting: An Independent Study Course. Tyree Carr. 3rd ed. 1999. LC 98-33325. (*1-56055-041-4*) Am Acad Ophthal.

Ophthalmic Medications & Pharmacology. Brian Duvall & Robert M. Kershner. 1997. LC 97-41938. (Basic Bookshelf for Eyecare Professionals Ser.). (Illus.). 144p. pap. 26.00 (*1-55642-328-4*, 63284) SLACK Inc.

Ophthalmic Microsurgery. Ed. by J. A. Draeger. 1986. (Illus.). xii, 184p. 149.75 (*3-8055-4028-0*) S Karger.

Ophthalmic Microsurgery: Proceedings of the Workshop on Microsurgery, Singapore, May 1977. S. Shan Ratnam & A. S. Lim. 1978. (Advances in Ophthalmology Ser.: Vol. 36). (Illus.). 102.75 (*3-8055-2782-9*) S Karger.

Ophthalmic Nursing. Rosalind Stollery. 2nd ed. 1996. LC 96-28897. 288p. pap. 50.95 (*0-632-03996-5*) Blackwell Sci.

Ophthalmic Optics. K. Kaushik. 1986. (C). (*0-89771-352-4*) Current Dist IND. *Dist:* St Mut.

Ophthalmic Optics & Clinical Refraction. David L. Guyton et al. 2nd rev. ed. 1999. 172p. spiral bd. 17.50 (*0-9665068-1-2*) Prism MD.

***Ophthalmic Pathology: An Atlas & Textbook**, Set. William H. Spencer. 1996. (Illus.). 3356p. 1625.00 incl. cd-rom (*0-7216-8196-4*) Saunders.

Ophthalmic Pathology: An Atlas & Textbook, Set. 4th ed. Ed. by William H. Spencer. Incl. Vol. One. Ophthalmic Pathology Vol. 1: An Atlas & Textbooks. 4th ed. LC 94-38768. 1995. (*0-7216-4909-2*); LC 94-38768. (Illus.). 3356p. 1996. Set text 699.00 (*0-7216-4908-4*) Saunders.

Ophthalmic Pathology Vol. 1: An Atlas & Textbooks, Vol. One. Ed. by William H. Spencer. 4th ed. 1995. LC 94-38768. (*0-7216-4909-2*) Saunders.

Ophthalmic Pathology - CD-ROM Single User Version: An Atlas & Textbook. William H. Spencer. Ed. by Richard Zorab. 4th ed. 1997. (Illus.). text 650.00 incl. cd-rom (*0-7216-8193-X*) Saunders.

Ophthalmic Pathology of Animals: An Atlas & Reference Book. L. Z. Saunders & L. F. Rubin. 1975. (Illus.). 250p. 141.75 (*3-8055-1580-4*) S Karger.

Ophthalmic Pathology with Clinical Correlations. Ed. by Joseph W. Sassani. 1997. (Illus.). 352p. text 129.00 (*0-397-51469-7*) Lppncott W & W.

Ophthalmic Pharmaceuticals: Successful Laboratory Results Equal Market Success. Market Intelligence Staff. 1992. 180p. (Orig.). 1895.00 (*1-56753-337-X*) Frost & Sullivan.

Ophthalmic Photography: A Textbook of Retinal Photography, Angiography, & Electronic Imaging. Patrick J. Saine et al. 1996. LC 96-25989. (Illus.). 334p. text 160.00 (*0-7506-9793-8*) Buttrwrth-Heinemann.

***Ophthalmic Photography: Retinal Photography, Angiography & Electronic Imaging.** Patrick J. Saine & Marshall E. Tyler. 2nd ed. 2001. LC 2001-46108. 424p. 150.00 (*0-7506-7372-9*) Buttrwrth-Heinemann.

Ophthalmic Plastic & Reconstructive Surgery. Nesi & Byron Smith. 2nd ed. 1997. LC 97-26132. (Illus.). 1248p. (C). (gr. 13). text 295.00 (*0-8151-6356-8*, 24723) Mosby Inc.

Ophthalmic, Plastic, Reconstructive & Orbital Surgery. Ed. by Charles M. Stephenson. 1997. LC 96-50457. (Illus.). 590p. text 215.00 (*0-7506-9081-X*) Buttrwrth-Heinemann.

Ophthalmic Plastic Surgery: Decision Making & Techniques. Robert C. Della Rocca & Maher. 2002. 300p. (C). 250.00 (*0-8385-7427-0*, Apple Lange Med) McGraw.

Ophthalmic Pocket Companion. Dean Dornic. 4th ed. 1995. LC 95-38750. 306p. pap. text 32.00 (*0-7506-9627-3*); 5th ed. 1998. LC 98-37681. 368p. pap. text 39.99 (*0-7506-7120-3*) Buttrwrth-Heinemann.

Ophthalmic Product Markets: Manufacturers Seek Ways to Penetrate Untapped Markets. Market Intelligence Staff. 1993. 400p. 1995.00 (*1-56753-572-0*) Frost & Sullivan.

Ophthalmic Research & Epidemiology: Evaluation & Application. Stanley W. Hatch. 1998. LC 97-45062. 312p. pap. text 54.99 (*0-7506-9914-0*) Buttrwrth-Heinemann.

Ophthalmic Surgery: Principles & Practice. George L. Spaeth. 3rd ed. 2002. text (*0-7216-6972-7*) Harcourt.

Ophthalmic Surgery: Principles & Techniques. Daniel M. Albert & Frederick S. Brightbill. 1998. LC 98-34615. (Illus.). 2080p. 418.95 (*0-632-04337-7*) Blackwell Sci.

Ophthalmic Surgical Anatomy: A Clinical Approach. David R. Jordan & Richard L. Anderson. 1995. (Ophthalmology Monographs: Vol. 9). 134p. 70.00 (*1-56055-029-5*) Am Acad Ophthal.

Ophthalmic Surgical Assistant. Regina Boess-Lott & Sharon Stecik. 1999. LC 98-45257. (Basic Bookshelf for Eyecare Professionals Ser.). 144p. pap. 30.00 (*1-55642-403-5*) SLACK Inc.

Ophthalmic Surgical Device Markets: New IDL Technology Improves Reimbursement Outlook. Market Intelligence Staff. 1992. 204p. 1695.00 (*1-56753-418-X*) Frost & Sullivan.

Ophthalmic Surgical Procedures. Peter Hersh. 1988. 280p. 87.95 (*0-316-35865-7*, Little Brwn Med Div) Lppncott W & W.

Ophthalmic Technologies II. Ed. by J. Parel. 1992. 85.00 (*0-8194-0790-9*, 1644) SPIE.

Ophthalmic Technologies VII, Vol. 2971. Ed. by Pascal O. Rol & Karen M. Joos. 1997. 226p. 80.00 (*0-8194-2382-3*) SPIE.

Ophthalmic Technologies VIII, Vol. 3246. Ed. by Pascal O. Rol et al. 1998. 324p. 89.00 (*0-8194-2685-7*) SPIE.

Ophthalmic Terminology: Speller & Vocabulary Builder. Harold A. Stein et al. 3rd ed. 1991. (Illus.). 384p. (C). (gr. 13). pap. text 39.00 (*0-8016-6438-1*, 06438) Mosby Inc.

Ophthalmic Toxicology. George C. Chiou. 2nd ed. 1999. LC 99-31971. (Target Organ Toxicology Ser.). (Illus.). xiv, 379p. 135.00 (*1-56032-722-7*) Taylor & Francis.

Ophthalmic Tumours. Ed. by Jendo A. Oosterhuis. 1985. (Monographs in Ophthalmology). text 233.50 (*90-6193-528-8*) Kluwer Academic.

Ophthalmic Ultrasonography. Ed. by Jeffrey S. Hillman & Malcolm M. Le May. 1983. (Documenta Ophthalmologica Proceedings Ser.). text 332.00 (*90-6193-734-5*) Kluwer Academic.

Ophthalmic Ultrasound: A Diagnostic Atlas. Cathy Dibernardo et al. 1998. LC 98-14389. 69.00 (*0-86577-765-9*) Thieme Med Pubs.

Ophthalmic Ultrasound: A Practical Guide. Atta. 1995. 156p. text (*0-443-04773-1*) Church.

Ophthalmology. Chawla. 1999. 354p. pap. text 37.50 (*0-7506-3963-6*) Buttrwrth-Heinemann.

Ophthalmology. N. R. Galloway & S. A. Vernon. 1988. 110p. 33.95 (*0-387-19516-5*) Spr-Verlag.

Ophthalmology. Jack J. Kanski. 1997. LC 96-39720. (Colour Guide Ser.). (*0-443-05804-0*) Harcrt Hlth Sci Grp.

Ophthalmology. Emanuel Rosen & William Rosen. 1997. LC 97-157872. (Medico-Legal Practitioner Ser.). 304p. (*1-85941-211-4*) Cavendish Pubng GBR. *Dist:* Gaunt.

Ophthalmology. Myron Yanoff. 1998. 265.00 (*0-323-00526-8*) Mosby Inc.

Ophthalmology. Myron Yanoff & Jay S. Duker. 1999. LC 98-20818. (Illus.). 1600p. 259.00 (*0-7234-2500-0*) Mosby Inc.

***Ophthalmology.** Myron Yanoff & Jay S. Duker. 1999. (Illus.). 1600p. 359.00 incl. cd-rom (*0-7234-3149-3*) Mosby Inc.

Ophthalmology. Hector Bryson Chawla. 2nd ed. 1993. LC 93-12292. 354p. pap. text (*0-443-04766-9*) Church.

Ophthalmology. Nicholas M. Sassani. 2nd ed. 1995. (Illus.). 296p. 98.50 (*0-19-262407-5*) OUP.

Ophthalmology. Fritz Hollwich. Tr. by Frederick C. Blodi from GER. 2nd ed. 1985. (Flexibook Ser.). (Illus.). 363p. pap. text 29.90 (*0-86577-184-7*) Thieme Med Pubs.

Ophthalmology. Kanski. 2nd ed. 1997. LC 98-14948. (Color Guide Ser.). 94p. (C). pap. text 16.95 (*0-443-05879-2*) Saunders.

Ophthalmology. Nicholas M. Evans. 2nd ed. 1996. (Illus.). 296p. reprint ed. pap. text 49.95 (*0-19-262406-7*) OUP.

Ophthalmology. Kenneth Wybar. 3rd ed. 1984. pap. text (*0-7216-0945-7*) Bailliere Tindall.

Ophthalmology: A Clinical Introduction. John W. Gittinger, Jr. 1984. 267p. 31.95 (*0-316-31470-6*, Little Brwn Med Div) Lppncott W & W.

Ophthalmology: A Diagnostic Text. William H. Coles. 1989. (Illus.). 424p. pap. text 35.00 (*0-683-02056-0*) Lppncott W & W.

Ophthalmology: A Pocket Textbook Atlas. G. K. Lang. 2000. LC 00-32597. (Illus.). 664p. pap. 39.00 (*0-86577-936-8*) Thieme Med Pubs.

Ophthalmology: A Symptom-Based Approach. Hector Bryson Chawla. 3rd ed. 1999. LC 99-19071. (Illus.). 215p. pap. text 40.00 (*0-7506-3979-2*) Buttrwrth-Heinemann.

Ophthalmology: An Illustration. Mark Batterbury. 1999. LC 99-27851. (Illus.). vii, 111p. text 32.00 (*0-443-05537-8*) Harcourt.

Ophthalmology: Clinical Signs & Differential Diagnosis. Jack J. Kanski & Ken K. Nischal. 1999. LC 98-20747. (*0-7234-3121-3*) Mosby Inc.

Ophthalmology: Clinical Signs & Differential Diagnosis. Jack J. Kanski & Ken K. Nischal. 1999. (Illus.). 496p. (*84-8174-395-X*) Mosby-Doyma Libros ESP. *Dist:* Mosby Inc.

Ophthalmology: Concise Medical Textbook. K. Wybar & M. Kerr Muir. 3rd ed. 1984. (Illus.). 375p. pap. text (*0-7020-1005-7*) W B Saunders GBR. *Dist:* Saunders.

Ophthalmology: Principles & Concepts. Frank W. Newell. 8th ed. 1996. (Illus.). 608p. (C). (gr. 13). text 75.00 (*0-8151-7093-9*, 27525) Mosby Inc.

Ophthalmology Companion. W. Happe. 1999. (Illus.). 304p. pap. text (*0-340-74093-0*) E A GBR. *Dist:* OUP.

Ophthalmology Examinations Review. Tien Yin Wong. 2000. 400p. 84.00 (*981-02-4399-5*); pap. 36.00 (*981-02-4400-2*) World Scientific Pub.

Ophthalmology for Medical Students & Primary Care Physicians. Ed. by Frank G. Berson. 6th ed. 1993. LC 93-21474. (1-56055-074-0) Am Acad Ophthal.

Ophthalmology for Primary Care. Gloria Wu. Ed. by Richard Lampert. 1997. LC 96-49580. (Illus.). 176p. pap. text 35.00 (0-7216-5078-3) Saunders.

Ophthalmology for the Pediatric Practitioner. Richard M. Robb. 1981. 31.50 (0-316-74894-3, Little Brwn Med Div) Lppncott W & W.

Ophthalmology for the Primary Care Practitioner. Palay. 1997. (Illus.). 331p. (C). (gr. 13). pap. text 59.95 (0-8151-8898-6, 30318) Mosby Inc.

Ophthalmology Made Ridiculously Simple. Stephen Goldberg. 1999. (Illus.). 84p. pap. text 13.95 (0-940780-01-1) MedMaster.

Ophthalmology Office Manual. Frank J. Weinstock. 1993. (Office Manual Ser.). 275p. 145.00 (1-890018-02-3) Anadem Pubng.

Ophthalmology Pearls of Wisdom. Mulrooney et al. 1999. (Pearls of Wisdom Ser.). pap. 88.00 (1-890369-18-7) Boston Medical.

Ophthalmology Resident Pocket Survival Guide. Shulpa Desai. 1999. 100p. (C). pap. 9.95 (1-883205-37-9) Intl Med Pub.

Ophthalmology Review. Myron Yanoff. 1999. (C). text 34.95 (0-323-00905-0) Mosby Inc.

Ophthalmology Review Manual. Kenneth C. Chern & Michael E. Zegans. 2000. LC 99-52560. (Illus.). 560p. pap. text 99.00 (0-683-30364-3) Lppncott W & W.

Ophthalmology Secrets. Ed. by James F. Vander. 1998. LC 97-52287. (Secrets Ser.). (Illus.). 375p. pap. 39.95 (1-56053-165-7) Hanley & Belfus.

Ophthalmology 2000: An Internet Resource Guide. Ed. by Dan Goldenson. 2001. 450p. pap. 24.95 (0-9700525-5-3) eMedguides.

Ophthamology. Van Heuven. 2nd ed. 1999. (C). text 79.95 (1-55664-454-X) Mosby Inc.

Opiate Addiction. Arthur Light et al. Ed. by Gerald N. Grob. 1981. LC 80-1257. (Addiction in America Ser.). reprint ed. lib. bdg. 16.95 (0-405-13604-8) Ayer.

Opiate Addiction: Its Handling & Treatment. Edward H. Williams. 1976. LC 75-17250. (Social Problems & Social Policy Ser.). reprint ed. 19.95 (0-405-07524-3) Ayer.

Opiate Receptors. Ed. by Gavril W. Pasternak. 1988. LC 87-3095. (Receptors Ser.). (Illus.). 520p. 145.00 (0-89603-120-9) Humana.

Opiate Receptors, Neurotransmitters, & Drug Dependence: Basic Science - Clinical Correlates. Ed. by Barry Stimmel. 1981. LC 81-7011. (Advances in Alcohol & Substance Abuse Ser.: Vol. 1, No. 1). 129p. text 39.95 (0-86656-103-X) Haworth Pr.

Opiates & Their Alternates for Pain & Cough Relief: Proceedings of the WHO Scientific Group, Geneva, 1971. WHO Staff. 1972. (Technical Reports: No. 495). pap. text 3.00 (92-4-120495-8, 1100495) World Health.

Opinion & Evidence: Disease Management. Ed. by Gordon Mallarkey. 200p. pap. text (0-86471-052-6) Adis Intl NZL. *Dist:* Lppncott W & W.

Opinion & Evidence: Drug Safety. I. Ralph Edwards. 168p. pap. text (0-86471-044-5); 2nd ed. 230p. pap. text (0-86471-065-8) Adis Intl NZL. *Dist:* Lppncott W & W.

Opinion & Evidence: Drug Treatment. 212p. pap. text (0-86471-051-8) Adis Intl NZL. *Dist:* Lppncott W & W.

Opinion & Evidence: Pharmacoeconomics. 208p. pap. text (0-86471-063-1) Adis Intl NZL. *Dist:* Lppncott W & W.

***Opinions of the Ethics Committee on the Principles of Medical Ethics with Annotations Especially Apllicable to Psychiatry 2001.** American Psychiatric Association Staff. 2001. 64p. pap. 10.00 (0-89042-144-7, 2144) Am Psychiatric.

Opinions of the Ethics Committee on the Principles of Medical Ethics with Annotations Especially Applicable to Psychiatry. APA Ethics Committee. 1995. 56p. pap. text 3.00 (0-89042-139-0, 2139) Am Psychiatric.

Opioid Addiction & Treatment: A 12-Year Follow-up. D. Dwayne Simpson. 1990. LC 88-29565. 288p. 32.50 (0-89464-309-6) Krieger.

Opioid Analgesics: Chemistry & Receptors. A. F. Casy & R. T. Parfitt. 1986. LC 86-1520. (Illus.). 534p. (C). text 145.00 (0-306-42130-5, Kluwer Plenum) Kluwer Academic.

Opioid Peptides: Pharmacology, Vol. II. Ed. by Jozsef I. Szekeley & Andras Z. Ronai. 1983. 256p. 144.00 (0-8493-6236-9, QP552, CRC Reprint) Franklin.

Opioid Peptides in Substance Abuse. Ed. by Jozsef I. Szekely. 1993. LC 93-9526. (Physiology of Drug Abuse Ser.). 288p. 141.95 (0-8493-7937-7, RC564) CRC Pr.

Opioids & Opioid Receptors: 2nd U.S.-Tawaiin Neuroscience Symposium, Miami, Fla., October 1999 - Proceedings Satellite Symposium of the 29th Annual Meeting of Neuroscience, Miami, Fla, October 1999. Ed. by L. F. Tseng et al. 2000. (Journal of Biomedical Science: Vol. 7). iv, 104p. pap. 34.00 (3-8055-7095-3) S Karger.

Opioids, Bulimia, & Alcohol Abuse & Alcoholism. Ed. by L. D. Reid. 1990. (Illus.). 393p. 99.00 (0-387-97242-0) Spr-Verlag.

Opioids Peptides: Opiate Receptors & Their Ligands-Experimental & Clinical Aspects, Vol. III. Ed. by Jozsef I. Szekely. 1983. 272p. 139.95 (0-8493-6237-7, QP552) CRC Pr.

Opioids 2. Ed. by G. V. Born et al. 1993. (Handbook of Experimental Pharmacology Ser.: Vol. 104/II). (Illus.). 840p. 510.00 (0-387-55517-X) Spr-Verlag.

Opiologia: or A Treatise Concerning the Nature & Safe Use of Opium. Angelo Sala. 1977. LC 77-7431. (English Experience Ser.: No. 892). reprint ed. lib. bdg. 20.00 (90-221-0892-9) Walter J Johnson.

Opium. John P. Gavit. Ed. by Gerald N. Grob. 1981. LC 80-1228. (Addiction in America Ser.). reprint ed. lib. bdg. 32.95 (0-405-13586-6) Ayer.

Opium: Its Use, Abuse, & Cure; or, from Bondage to Freedom. Leslie E. Keeley. Ed. by Gerald N. Grob. 1981. LC 80-1270. (Addiction in America Ser.). (Illus.). reprint ed. lib. bdg. 16.95 (0-405-13597-1) Ayer.

Opium Addiction in Chicago. Bingham Dai. 1970. LC 72-124503. (Criminology, Law Enforcement, & Social Problems Ser.: No. 126). 26.00 (0-87585-126-6) Patterson Smith.

Opium Addicts & Addiction. John A. Hawkins. Ed. by Gerald N. Grob. 1981. LC 80-1262. (Addiction in America Ser.). reprint ed. lib. bdg. 19.95 (0-405-13588-2) Ayer.

Opium & the Opium-Appetite. Alonzo Calkins. Ed. by Gerald N. Grob. 1981. LC 80-1215. (Addiction in America Ser.). reprint ed. lib. bdg. 40.95 (0-405-13571-8) Ayer.

Opium As an International Problem: The Geneva Conferences. Westel W. Willoughby. 1976. LC 75-17252. (Social Problems & Social Policy Ser.). reprint ed. 47.95 (0-405-07526-X) Ayer.

Opium Eating. Ed. by Gerald N. Grob. 1981. LC 80-1241. (Addiction in America Ser.). reprint ed. lib. bdg. 19.95 (0-405-13611-0) Ayer.

Opium Habit & Alcoholism. Fred H. Hubbard. Ed. by Gerald N. Grob. 1981. LC 80-1232. (Addiction in America Ser.). reprint ed. lib. bdg. 29.95 (0-405-13591-2) Ayer.

Opium Habit, with Suggestions As to the Remedy. Ed. by Horace Day & Gerald N. Grob. 1981. LC 80-1224. (Addiction in America Ser.). reprint ed. lib. bdg. 33.95 (0-405-13580-7) Ayer.

Opium Poppy: Botany, Chemistry, & Pharmacology. Ed. by L. D. Kapoor. 1997. LC 94-20779. 326p. (C). pap. 19.95 (0-7890-0202-7) Haworth Pr.

Opium Problem. Charles E. Terry & Mildred Pellens. 1970. LC 76-108232. (Criminology, Law Enforcement, & Social Problems Ser.: No. 115). (Illus.). reprint ed. 65.00 (0-87585-115-0) Patterson Smith.

Opium Smoking in America & China: A Study of Its Prevalence, & Effects, Immediate & Remote, on the Individual & the Nation. Harry H. Kane. 1976. LC 75-17227. (Social Problems & Social Policy Ser.). reprint ed. 18.95 (0-405-07497-2) Ayer.

Opium the Demon Flower. Sara Graham-Mulhall. Ed. by Gerald N. Grob. 1981. LC 80-1229. (Addiction in America Ser.). reprint ed. lib. bdg. 32.95 (0-405-13587-4) Ayer.

Oppenheimer's Diagnostic Neuropathology: A Practical Manual. Margaret M. Esiri. 2nd ed. 1996. (Illus.). 480p. 295.00 (0-86542-915-4) Blackwell Sci.

Opportunistic Infections. Vassil St. Georgiev. 2001. (Infectious Disease Ser.). 500p. 99.50 (1-58829-009-3) Humana.

Opportunistic Infections in Patients with the Acquired Immunodeficiency Syndrome. Leoung & Mills. 1989. (Infectious Disease & Therapy Ser.: Vol. 3). (Illus.). 476p. text 155.00 (0-8247-8080-9) Dekker.

Opportunistic Intracellular Bacteria & Immunity. Ed. by L. J. Paradise et al. 1998. LC 98-42016. (Infectious Agents & Pathogenesis Ser.). (Illus.). 302p. (C). text 125.00 (0-306-45894-2, Kluwer Plenum) Kluwer Academic.

Opportunities & Directions in Antisense & Other Oligonucleotide-Based Technologies. Market Intelligence Staff. 1993. 218p. 1495.00 (1-56753-603-4) Frost & Sullivan.

***Opportunities & Options in Medical Careers.** Ruth Chambers et al. 2000. 192p. pap. (1-85775-451-4) Radcliffe Med Pr GBR. *Dist:* Balogh.

Opportunities for Daily Choice Making. Linda M. Bambara & Freya Koger. Ed. by Diane M. Browder. 1996. LC 96-35425. (Innovations Ser.: Vol. 8). (Illus.). 48p. (Orig.). pap. 21.95 (0-940898-44-6) Am Assn Mental.

Opportunities in Animal & Pet Care. Mary P. Lee & Richard S. Lee. (Illus.). 160p. 1993. pap. 10.95 (0-8442-6245-5); 1991. 13.95 (0-8442-6244-7) McGraw-Hill Trade (VGM Career Bks).

Opportunities in Animal & Pet Care Careers. Mary P. Lee & Richard S. Lee. LC 93-17661. (Illus.). 1994. 160p. 14.95 (0-8442-4079-6, 40796); 1993. 205p. pap. 11.95 (0-8442-4081-8, 40818) McGraw-Hill Trade (VGM Career Bks).

Opportunities in Biotechnology Careers. Sheldon S. Brown. Ed. by Julie Han. 2nd ed. 1994. LC 93-47487. (Opportunities in... Ser.). (Illus.). 160p. pap. 11.95 (0-8442-4126-1, 41261, VGM Career Bks) McGraw-Hill Trade.

Opportunities in Chiropractic Careers. R. C. Schafer. 1994. 160p. pap. 10.95 (0-8442-4132-6, VGM Career Bks) McGraw-Hill Trade.

Opportunities in Chiropractic Health Careers. R. C. Shafer. (Opportunities in... Ser.). (Illus.). 160p. pap. 12.95 (0-8442-6566-7, 297OICHI); 1992. 14.95 (0-8442-6565-9) McGraw-Hill Trade (VGM Career Bks).

Opportunities in Dental Care. Bonnie Kendall. 1986. (Illus.). 160p. 13.95 (0-8442-6285-4); pap. 10.95 (0-8442-6286-2) McGraw-Hill Trade (VGM Career Bks).

Opportunities in Dental Care Careers. Noerper. 1992. (Illus.). 160p. 14.95 (0-8442-8575-7, 85757, VGM Career Bks) McGraw-Hill Trade.

Opportunities in Eye Care Careers. Kathleen Belikoff. 1998. LC 97-39478. (Opportunities in... Ser.). (Illus.). 160p. 14.95 (0-8442-2302-6, 23026); 206p. pap. 11.95 (0-8442-2303-4, 23034) McGraw-Hill Trade (VGM Career Bks).

Opportunities in Gerontology. Ellen Williams. 1988. (Illus.). 160p. 13.95 (0-8442-6166-1, VGM Career Bks) McGraw-Hill Trade.

Opportunities in Gerontology & Aging Services Careers. Ellen Williams. 1995. LC 95-3220. (Opportunities in... Ser.). (Illus.). 200p. pap. 11.95 (0-8442-4437-6, 44376, VGM Career Bks) McGraw-Hill Trade.

Opportunities in Health & Medical Careers. I. Donald Snook & Leo D'Orazio. (Illus.). 160p. 1993. 14.95 (0-8442-8573-0); 1991. pap. 12.95 (0-8442-8574-9, 297OIH&M) McGraw-Hill Trade (VGM Career Bks).

Opportunities in Health & Medical Careers. I. Donald Snook, Jr. & Leo D'Orazio. 1987. (Illus.). 149p. 13.95 (0-8442-6262-5); pap. 10.95 (0-8442-6263-3) McGraw-Hill Trade (VGM Career Bks).

Opportunities in Health & Medical Careers. I. Donald Snook et al. 1997. LC 97-17638. (Opportunities in... Ser.). (Illus.). 160p. 14.95 (0-8442-2317-4, 23174); 202p. pap. 11.95 (0-8442-2318-2, 23182) McGraw-Hill Trade (VGM Career Bks).

Opportunities in Holistic Health Care. Gillian Tierney. 1999. LC 98-21760. (Opportunities in... Ser.). 160p. 14.95 (0-8442-1846-4, 18464); 204p. pap. 11.95 (0-8442-1851-0, 18510) NTC Contemp Pub Co.

Opportunities in Hospital Administration Careers. Donald Snook. 1988. (Illus.). 160p. 14.95 (0-8442-6509-8, VGM Career Bks) McGraw-Hill Trade.

Opportunities in Hospital Administration Careers. I. Donald Snook. 1997. LC 96-40277. (Opportunities in... Ser.). (Illus.). 160p. 14.95 (0-8442-4562-3, 45623); 205p. pap. 11.95 (0-8442-4563-1, 45631) NTC Contemp Pub Co.

Opportunities in Medical Imaging Careers. Clifford Sherry. LC 93-19679. (Opportunities in... Ser.). pap. 12.95 (0-8442-4071-0, 297OIMI, VGM Career Bks) McGraw-Hill Trade.

Opportunities in Medical Imaging Careers. Clifford Sherry. 1993. LC 93-19679. (VGM Opportunities Ser.). 160p. 14.95 (0-8442-4070-2, Wiley-VCH) Wiley.

Opportunities in Medical Sales Careers. Chad Ellis. 1997. LC 96-45333. (Opportunities in... Ser.). (Illus.). 160p. 14.95 (0-8442-4560-7, 45607) NTC Contemp Pub Co.

Opportunities in Medical Technology Careers. Karen R. Karni & Jane S. Oliver. 1994. 160p. 13.95 (0-8442-8671-0, VGM Career Bks) McGraw-Hill Trade.

Opportunities in Medical Technology Careers. Karen Karni. rev. ed. 1996. (VGM Careers for You Ser.). (Illus.). LC 96-1133. 160p. 14.95 (0-8442-4637-9, 46379); 205p. pap. 11.95 (0-8442-4638-7, 46387) NTC Contemp Pub Co (Natl Textbk Co).

Opportunities in Mental Health Careers. Philip A. Perry. 1996. (VGM Opportunities Ser.). (Illus.). 160p. 14.95 (0-8442-4429-5, 44295, VGM Career Bks) McGraw-Hill Trade.

Opportunities in Mental Health Careers. Philip A. Perry & Virginia Simons. 1995. (Opportunities in... Ser.). (Illus.). 205p. pap. 11.95 (0-8442-4430-9, 44309, VGM Career Bks) McGraw-Hill Trade.

Opportunities in Nursing Assistant. Joan Fox-Rose. 1999. LC 99-31861. (Opportunities in... Ser.). 160p. 14.95 (0-8442-3431-1); 202p. pap. 11.95 (0-8442-3439-7) NTC Contemp Pub Co.

Opportunities in Nursing Careers. Keville Frederickson. rev. ed. 1995. LC 95-31374. (Opportunities in... Ser.). (Illus.). 205p. pap. 11.95 (0-8442-4576-3, 45763); 160p. 14.95 (0-8442-4575-5, 45755) McGraw-Hill Trade (VGM Career Bks).

Opportunities in Nutrition Careers. Carol C. Caldwell. (Illus.). 160p. 1993. pap. 10.95 (0-8442-6173-4); 1988. 13.95 (0-8442-6172-6) McGraw-Hill Trade (VGM Career Bks).

Opportunities in Nutrition Careers. Carol Coles Caldwell. 1992. (Opportunities in... Ser.). (Illus.). 160p. pap. 12.95 (0-8442-8188-3, 297OINT, VGM Career Bks) McGraw-Hill Trade.

Opportunities in Occupational Therapy Careers. Marie-Louis Franciscus et al. 1994. LC 94-19969. (VGM Opportunities Ser.). (Illus.). 160p. 14.95 (0-8442-4407-4, 44074); 200p. pap. 11.95 (0-8442-4408-2, 44082) McGraw-Hill Trade (VGM Career Bks).

Opportunities in Opticianry Today. Bacotti. LC 75-32613. (Illus.). 1995. lib. bdg. 13.95 (0-8442-6325-7); 1993. pap. text 10.95 (0-8442-6326-5) McGraw-Hill Trade (VGM Career Bks).

Opportunities in Osteopathic Medicine Careers. Terence J. Sacks. 2000. LC 00-44215. (Opportunities in... Ser.). xv, 143p. 15.95 (0-658-00184-1); pap. 12.95 (0-658-00186-8) McGraw-Hill Trade (VGM Career Bks).

Opportunities in Paramedical Careers. Alex Kacen. (Illus.). 160p. 1993. pap. 10.95 (0-8442-6507-1); 1991. 13.95 (0-8442-6506-3); 1994th rev. ed. 1995. LC 93-45609. 14.95 (0-8442-4095-8) McGraw-Hill Trade (VGM Career Bks).

Opportunities in Paramedical Careers. Alex Kacen. rev. ed. 1999. LC 99-26183. (Opportunities in... Ser.). 160p. 14.95 (0-8442-2906-7); 202p. pap. 11.95 (0-8442-2907-5) NTC Contemp Pub Co.

Opportunities in Pharmacy Careers. Fred B. Gable. (Opportunities in... Ser.). (Illus.). LC 97-35763. 160p. (YA). (gr. 8-12). pap. 12.95 (0-8442-8592-7, 297OIPHA); 1997. 160p. 14.95 (0-8442-2319-0, 23190); 1997. LC 97-35763. 200p. pap. 11.95 (0-8442-2320-4, 23204); 1993. LC 74-82639. 160p. (YA). (gr. 8-12). 14.95 (0-8442-8591-9) McGraw-Hill Trade (VGM Career Bks).

Opportunities in Physical Therapy Careers. Bernice R. Krumhansl. rev. ed. 1999. LC 99-34065. (Opportunities in... Ser.). 160p. 14.95 (0-8442-1804-9, 18049); 202p. pap. 11.95 (0-8442-1805-7, 18057) NTC Contemp Pub Co.

Opportunities in Physician Assistant Careers. Terence J. Sacks. 1994. LC 94-17799. (Opportunities in... Ser.). (Illus.). 160p. 14.95 (0-8442-4411-2, 44112); 205p. pap. 11.95 (0-8442-4412-0, 44120) McGraw-Hill Trade (VGM Career Bks).

Opportunities in Physician Careers. Jan Sugar-Webb. 1992. (Illus.). 160p. 14.95 (0-8442-8595-1, VGM Career Bks) McGraw-Hill Trade.

Opportunities in Physician Careers. Jan Sugar-Webb. rev. ed. 1999. LC 99-33038. (Opportunities in... Ser.). 160p. 14.95 (0-8442-2979-2); 204p. pap. 11.95 (0-8442-2984-9) NTC Contemp Pub Co.

Opportunities in Psychiatry. Fenton Keyes. LC 76-42885. (Illus.). (YA). (gr. 9 up). 1994. 160p. pap. 10.95 (0-8442-6368-0); 1988. 13.95 (0-8442-6367-2) McGraw-Hill Trade (VGM Career Bks).

Opportunities in Psychology Careers. Donald E. Super & Charles M. Super. (Illus.). 160p. 1995. pap. 10.95 (0-8442-6480-6); 1992. 13.95 (0-8442-6478-4) McGraw-Hill Trade (VGM Career Bks).

Opportunities in Public Health Careers. George E. Pickett & Terry W. Pickett. 2nd ed. (Opportunities in... Ser.). (Illus.). 200p. pap. 11.95 (0-8442-4416-3, 44163, VGM Career Bks) McGraw-Hill Trade.

Opportunities in Speech & Language Pathology Careers. Patricia L. Hicks. rev. ed. 1995. LC 95-30194. (Opportunities in... Ser.). (Illus.). 200p. pap. 11.95 (0-8442-4586-0, 45860, VGM Career Bks) McGraw-Hill Trade.

Opportunities in Sports Medicine Careers. William Ray Heitzmann. (Opportunities in... Ser.). (Illus.). 1995. 160p. 14.95 (0-8442-8168-9, 81689); 1991. 205p. pap. 11.95 (0-8442-8169-7, 81697) McGraw-Hill Trade (VGM Career Bks).

Opportunities in the Contraceptive & Fertility Markets: Demographic Changes Affect Market Dynamics. 1992. 248p. 1895.00 (1-56753-002-8) Frost & Sullivan.

Opportunities in the Nutrition & Food Sciences: Research Challenges & the Next Generation of Investigators. Ed. by Robert O. Earl et al. 1994. LC 93-41970. 328p. (C). pap. text 36.95 (0-309-04884-2) Natl Acad Pr.

Opportunities in Veterinary Medicine. Sarah Mikesell. LC 92-43493. (Opportunities in... Ser.). (Illus.). 1994. 160p. 14.95 (0-8442-4059-1, 40591); 1993. 200p. pap. 11.95 (0-8442-4060-5, 40605) McGraw-Hill Trade (VGM Career Bks).

Opsomer, Carmelia: Index de la Pharmacopee Latine du Ler Au Xe Siecle, Set. Carmelia Opsomer. 1989. (Alpha-Omega, Reihe A Ser.: Bd. CV). (GER.). lxxxviii, 824p. (3-487-09190-9) G Olms Pubs.

Optic Nerve Disorders. Lanning B. Kline. 1996. LC 96-28344. (Ophthalmology Monographs). (1-56055-037-6) Am Acad Ophthal.

Optic Nerve in Clinical Practice. Andrew S. Gurwood & Bruce G. Muchnick. 1997. LC 97-2671. 312p. text 95.00 (0-7506-9557-9) Buttrwrth-Heinemann.

Optic Nerve in Glaucoma. Ed. by Stephen M. Drance. 1995. LC 95-8861. (90-6299-123-8) Kugler NLD. *Dist:* Lib Res.

Optic Pathway Gliomas. Ed. by V. M. Riccardi. 1989. (Journal: Vol. 1, No. 4). (Illus.). 60p. pap. 33.25 (3-8055-4945-8) S Karger.

Optical & Imaging Techniques for Biomonitoring II. Ed. by Hans-Jochen Foth et al. 1996. (Europto Ser.: Vol. 2927). 236p. 66.00 (0-8194-2329-7) SPIE.

Optical & Imaging Techniques for Biomonitoring III. Ed. by Hans-Jochen Foth et al. 1998. LC 98-172805. (Europto Ser.: Vol. 3196). 244p. 69.00 (0-8194-2628-8) SPIE.

Optical & Imaging Techniques for Biomonitoring IV. Ed. by Marco D. Fante et al. 1999. (Europto Ser.: Vol. 3567). 80.00 (0-8194-3029-3) SPIE.

Optical Biopsies & Microscopic Techniques. Ed. by Irving J. Bigio et al. 1996. (Europto Ser.: Vol. 2926). 326p. 85.00 (0-8194-2328-9) SPIE.

Optical Biopsies & Microscopic Techniques II. Ed. by Irving J. Bigio et al. 1997. (Europto Ser.: Vol. 3197). 324p. 89.00 (*0-8194-2629-6*) SPIE.

Optical Biopsies & Microscopic Techniques III, Vol. 3568. Ed. by Irving J. Bigio et al. 1999. LC 99-226903. (Europto Ser.). 69.00 (*0-8194-3030-7*) SPIE.

Optical Biopsy II, Vol. 3250. Ed. by Robert R. Alfano. 1998. LC 98-227289. 226p. 69.00 (*0-8194-2689-X*) SPIE.

***Optical Biopsy III: 23-24 January 2000, San Jose, California.** Ed. by R. R. Alfano. 2000. LC 00-712000. (Progress in Biomedical Optics & Imaging Ser.: No. 1). (Illus.). ix, 268p. (*0-8194-3533-3*) SPIE.

Optical Coherence Tomography of Ocular Diseases. Carmen A. Puliafito et al. 1995. LC 95-20538. (Illus.). 384p. 175.00 (*1-55642-295-4*, 62954) SLACK Inc.

Optical Diagnostics of Biological Fluids & Advanced Techniques in Analytical Cytology, Vol. 2982. Ed. by Alexander V. Priezzhev et al. 1997. LC 97-175337. 510p. 107.00 (*0-8194-2393-9*) SPIE.

Optical Diagnostics of Biological Fluids III. Ed. by Alexander V. Priezzhev et al. 1998. LC 98-227283. (Proceedings of SPIE Ser.: Vol. 3252). 204p. 69.00 (*0-8194-2691-1*) SPIE.

***Optical Diagnostics of Living Cells III: 24-25 January 2000, San Jose, California.** Ed. by Daniel L. Farkas & Robert C. Leif. 2000. LC 00-711998. (Progress in Biomedical Optics & Imaging Ser.: No. 1). (Illus.). x, 344p. (*0-8194-3537-6*) SPIE.

Optical Fabrication & Testing. 1992. LC 92-60858. (Technical Digest Series, 1992: Vol. 24). 200p. pap. 66.00 (*1-55752-260-X*) Optical Soc.

Optical Fibers in Medicine. Ed. by A. Katzir. 1992. 66.00 (*0-8194-0795-X*, 1649) SPIE.

Optical Formulas Tutorial. Ellen D. Stoner et al. 1997. LC 97-14338. 232p. pap. text 39.99 (*0-7506-9913-2*) Buttrwrth-Heinemann.

Optical Imaging of Brain Function & Metabolism. U. Dirnagl et al. 1993. LC 93-24703. (Advances in Experimental Medicine & Biology Ser.: Vol. 333). (Illus.). 308p. (C). text 95.00 (*0-306-44528-X*, Kluwer Plenum) Kluwer Academic.

Optical Imaging of Brain Function & Metabolism No. 2: Physiological Basis & Comparison to Other Functional Neuroimaging Methods, Vol. 2. Ed. by A. Villringer & Ulrich Dirnagl. 1997. LC 97-7513. (Advances in Experimental Medicine & Biology Ser.: Vol. 413). (Illus.). 260p. (C). text 85.00 (*0-306-45585-4*, Kluwer Plenum) Kluwer Academic.

Optical Mapping of Cardiac Excitation & Arrhythmias. Ed. by David S. Rosenbaum & Jose Jalife. 2001. LC 00-54355. (Illus.). 480p. 99.00 (*0-87993-481-6*) Futura Pub.

Optical Methods for Tumor Treatment & Detection: Mechanisms & Techniques in Photodynamic Therapy. Ed. by T. J. Dougherty. 1992. 66.00 (*0-8194-0791-7*, 1645) SPIE.

Optical Methods for Tumor Treatment & Detection Vol. 2972: Mechanisms & Techniques in Photodynamic Therapy VI. Ed. by Thomas J. Dougherty. 1997. 194p. 69.00 (*0-8194-2383-1*) SPIE.

Optical Methods for Tumor Treatment & Detections Vol. 3247: Mechanisms & Techniques in Photodynamic Therapy VII. Ed. by Thomas J. Dougherty. 1998. 162p. 69.00 (*0-8194-2686-5*) SPIE.

Optical Methods in Biomedical & Environmental Sciences: Selected Contributions to the Third International Conference on Optics within Life Sciences, OWLS III, Tokyo, Japan, 10-14 April 1994. International Conference on Optics within Life Sciences Staff. Ed. by Hitoshi Ohzu & Shinichi Komatsu. 1994. LC 94-27064. (Series of the International Society on Optics Within Life Sciences: Vol. 3). 388p. 210.50 (*0-444-81817-0*) Elsevier.

Optical Performance of the Light Microscope. H. Wolfgang Zieler. 1974. LC 72-85238. (Illus.). 14. 25.00 (*0-904962-02-4*); 15. 30.00 (*0-904962-01-6*) Microscope Pubns.

Optical Principles of the Diffraction of X-Rays. R. W. James. 1982. LC 82-80706. reprint ed. 85.00 (*0-918024-23-4*) Ox Bow.

Optical Radiation & Visual Health. M. Waxler & V. Hitchins. 1986. LC 86-12933. 232p. 130.00 (*0-8493-5752-7*, CRC Reprint) Franklin.

Optical Radiations in Medicine. Edwin C. McCullough. 1997. (AAPM Reports: No. 3). 28p. (Orig.). pap. 10.00 (*1-888340-06-1*) AAPM.

Optical Resolution Procedures for Chemical Compounds Vol. 2: Acids Paul Newman. 1981. LC 78-61452. (*0-9601918-2-8*) Optical Resolution.

Optical Spanish Manual. Stanley S. Laburna. 1996. LC 96-36007. 176p. pap. text 19.99 (*0-7506-9674-5*) Buttrwrth-Heinemann.

Optical Systems for Soft X-Rays. A. G. Michette. 1986. (Illus.). 344p. (C). text 110.00 (*0-306-42320-0*, Kluwer Plenum) Kluwer Academic.

Optical Techniques for Industrial Inspection. Ed. by P. Cielo. 1988. 606p. text 138.00 (*0-12-174655-0*) Acad Pr.

Optical Tomography & Spectroscopy of Tissue Vol. 2979: Theory, Instrumentation Model, & Human Studies II. Ed. by Britton Chance & Robert R. Alfano. 1997. LC 98-122045. 878p. 149.00 (*0-8194-2390-4*) SPIE.

Optical Unconscious. Rosalind E. Krauss. 1994. (Illus.). 365p. pap. 24.95 (*0-262-61105-8*) MIT Pr.

Opticianry: The Practice & the Art, Set. William A. Borover. Incl. Vol. I. Introduction to Dispensing. (Illus.). 259p. 1981. per. 48.00 (*0-9606398-0-2*); Vol. II. Science of Opticianry. (Illus.). 300p. 1982. per. 48.00 (*0-9606398-2-9*); Vol. III. Dynamics of Dispensing. (Illus.). 1983. per. 48.00 (*0-9606398-3-7*); Vol. IV. Business of Opticianry. 1984. per. 48.00 (*0-9606398-4-5*); (Illus.). Set pap. 192.00 (*0-9606398-1-0*) Gracie Ent.

Opticrom Four Percent in Clinical Practice. Robert N. Ross. 1984. LC 84-72911. (Illus.). 43p. (*0-914132-05-9*) Fisons Corp.

Optics. Alan Tunnacliffe & Gordon Hirst. 1989. (C). (*0-900099-15-1*) Assn Brit Dispen Opticians GBR. *Dist:* St Mut.

Optics. Michael H. Freeman & Christopher Hull. 11th ed. 2001. (Illus.). 288p. 115.00 (*0-7506-4248-3*) Buttrwrth-Heinemann.

Optics for Clinicians. Melvin L. Rubin. 25th anniv. ed. 1993. LC 72-97862. (Illus.). 38.00 (*0-937404-34-9*) Triad Pub FL.

Optics in Biomedical Sciences: Graz Austria, 1981 Proceedings. G. V. Bally & P. Greguss. 1982. (Series in Optical Sciences: Vol. 31). (Illus.). 274p. 74.95 (*0-387-11666-4*) Spr-Verlag.

Optics in Medicine, Biology, & Environmental Research: Proceedings of the International Conference on Optics in Life Sciences, Partenkirchen, Germany, 12-16 August 1990. Ed. by Gert Von Bally & Shyam Hkanna. 1993. LC 93-24585. 392p. 238.50 (*0-444-89860-3*) Elsevier.

Optics in the Health Sciences: Index of New Information for Research & State of Current Progress. Fred O. Crowder. 1997. 150p. 57.50 (*0-7883-1380-0*); pap. 47.50 (*0-7883-1381-9*) ABBE Pubs Assn.

Optics of Contact Lenses. Ed. by Austin Bennett. 1989. (C). (*0-900099-22-4*) Assn Brit Dispen Opticians GBR. *Dist:* St Mut.

Optics of the Human Eye. David Atchinson & G. Smith. 2000. (Illus.). 288p. pap. text 60.00 (*0-7506-3775-7*) Buttrwrth-Heinemann.

Optics, Physiology & Vision. Ed. by Suzanne P. McKee. 1990. (Vision Research Ser.: No. VR 263). 400p. (*0-08-040692-0*) PPI GBR. *Dist:* Elsevier.

Optimal Control of Drug Administration in Cancer Chemotherapy. R. M. Martin & K. L. Teo. 1993. 204p. text 61.00 (*981 02 1428 6*) World Scientific Pub.

Optimal Experience: Psychological Studies of Flow in Consciousness. Ed. by Mihaly Csikszentmihalyi & Isabella S. Csikszentmihalyi. 1992. (Illus.). 430p. (C). pap. text 29.95 (*0-521-43809-8*) Cambridge U Pr.

Optimal Health Guidelines. John R. Lee. 4th rev. ed. 1999. (Illus.). xv, 211p. pap. 14.00 (*0-9643737-0-X*) BLL Pubng.

Optimal Implant Positioning & Soft Tissue Management for the Branemark System. Patrick Palacci. 1995. LC 95-15503. (Illus.). 83p. text 68.00 (*0-86715-308-3*) Quint Pub Co.

Optimal Surgical Approach for Elective Reconstruction of the Infra- & Juxta-Renal Abdominal Aorta: A Randomised Prospective Study. Hendrik Lacroix. 1997. (Acta Biomedica Lovaniensia Ser.: No. 157). 127p. pap. (*90-6186-841-6*) Almqvist & Wiksell SWE. *Dist:* Coronet Bks.

Optimal Use of Sandimmun in Endogenous Uveitis. D. Benezra et al. 1988. (Illus.). 32p. 39.95 (*0-387-18878-9*) Spr-Verlag.

Optimal Use of Sandimmun in Organ Transplantation. Ed. by W. Land. 1987. (Illus.). 32p. 41.95 (*0-387-17865-1*) Spr-Verlag.

Optimal Use of the Clinical Laboratory. Ed. by Oren Zinder. 1986. (Illus.). viii, 140p. 77.50 (*3-8055-4328-X*) S Karger.

***Optimising the Role of Herceptin in Breast Cancer.** Ed. by D. Khayat. 2001. (Illus.). 92p. pap. 34.00 (*3-8055-7327-8*) S Karger.

Optimistic Child: A Proven Program to Safeguard Children Against Depression & Build Lifelong Resilience. Martin E. Seligman et al. 600th ed. 1996. LC 96-16770. 352p. pap. 14.00 (*0-06-097709-4*, Perennial) HarperTrade.

Optimistic Organizations: How to Get, Grow, Keep Positive Power in Your Company. Jean A. Hollands. 1992. (Illus.). 152p. (Orig.). pap. 12.95 (*0-9632556-3-0*) Select Bks CA.

Optimization of Cancer Radiotherapy: Proceedings of the 2nd International Conference on Dose, Time Fractionation in Radiation Oncology Held at the University of Wisconsin, Madison, Wisconsin, September 12-14, 1984. Ed. by Bhudatt R. Paliwal et al. 1985. (American Association of Physicists in Medicine Symposium Ser.: No. 5). 560p. 45.00 (*0-88318-483-4*) Am Inst Physics.

Optimization of Image Quality & Patient Exposure in Diagnostic Radiology. Ed. by B. M. Moores. 1990. (BIR Reports Ser.: No. 20). pap. text (*0-905749-21-9*) Med Physics Pub.

Optimization of Radiotherapy, Particularly in Developing Countries: Report of a WHO Meeting of Investigators. 1980. (Technical Report Ser.: No. 644). 89p. pap. text 6.00 (*92-4-120644-6*, 1100644) World Health.

Optimizing Health Care for Turner Patients in the 21st Century: Proceedings of the 5th International Turner Syndrom Help in Naples on 23-25 March 2000. Paul Saenger & Anna-Maria Pasquino. 2000. LC 00-53536. (International Congress Ser.). 348p. 129.50 (*0-444-50583-0*, Excerpta Medica) Elsevier.

Optimizing Resources: A Manager's Guide to Success. AORN Staff. 1993. 107p. (Orig.). pap. text 43.75 (*0-939583-82-8*) AORN.

Optimizing the Clinical Devlopment of Antipsychotic Drugs. Neal R. Cutler et al. 1998. LC 97-3041. 216p. 79.95 (*0-471-97011-5*) Wiley.

Optimizing Theory & Experiments. Randall R. Robey & Martin C. Schultz. 1993. LC 92-25260. (Illus.). 186p. (Orig.). (C). pap. text 34.95 (*1-56593-078-9*, 0382) Thomson Learn.

***Optimizing Therapeutic Development in Diabetes.** G. Alexander Fleming et al. 1999. 193p. (*1-84110-038-2*) Greenwich Med GBR. *Dist:* JAMCO Dist.

Optimum Healing. Craig Brown. 1998. pap. (*0-7126-7107-2*) Random GBR. *Dist:* Trafalgar.

Optimum Health: A Cardiologist's Prescription. Stephen T. Sinatra. unabr. ed. 1996. LC 95-80607. (Illus.). 368p. 24.95 (*1-879111-81-0*) Lincoln-Bradley.

Optimum Physical Performance Capacity in Adults: Proceedings of the WHO Scientific Group, Geneva, 1968. WHO Staff. 1969. (Technical Reports: No. 436). pap. text 5.00 (*92-4-120436-2*, 1100436) World Health.

Options for Expanding the Health Families Program: Estimates. Elias Lopez & Richard A. Figueroa. 1999. 12p. pap. (*1-58703-101-9*, CRB-99-004) CA Res Bureau.

Optometric Case Analysis. Leonard C. Emery. Ed. by Sally M. Corngold. rev. ed. 1993. (Introduction to Behavioral Optometry Ser.). 117p. (C). lib. bdg. 18.00 (*0-943599-66-0*) OEPF.

Optometric Guide to Surgical Co-Management. Debra Bezan et al. 1992. LC 92-23818. (Illus.). 118p. spiral bd. 44.99 (*0-7506-9329-0*) Buttrwrth-Heinemann.

Optometric Management of Learning Related Vision D. Mitchell M. Scheiman & Michael Rouse. 1994. (Illus.). 606p. (C). (gr. 13). text 71.95 (*0-8016-6385-7*, 06385) Mosby Inc.

Optometric Management of Learning Related Vision Problems. Mitchell M. Scheiman & Michael W. Rouse. 1994. LC 94-3010. (*0-08-151638-X*) Mosby Inc.

Optometric Management of Nearpoint Vision Disorders. Martin H. Birnbaum. 1992. LC 92-16159. 416p. text 99.00 (*0-7506-9193-X*) Buttrwrth-Heinemann.

Optometric Management of Reading Disfunction. Ed. by John R. Griffin et al. 1996. LC 96-43032. 254p. pap. text 49.99 (*0-7506-9516-1*) Buttrwrth-Heinemann.

Optometric Vision Therapy. J. Baxter Swartwout. Ed. by Sally M. Corngold. rev. ed. 1988. (Introduction to Behavioral Optometry Ser.). (Illus.). 172p. reprint ed. pap. text 18.00 (*0-943599-03-2*) OEPF.

Optometric Vision Therapy Manual: Procedures & Forms. J. Baxter Swartwout. Ed. by Conkey et al. 1991. (Illus.). 419p. (C). spiral bd. 55.00 (*0-943599-20-2*) OEPF.

Optometrist. Jack Rudman. 1994. (Career Examination Ser.: C-557). pap. 29.95 (*0-8373-0557-8*) Nat Learn.

Optometrist's & Ophthalmologist's Guide to Pilot's Vision. Warren V. DeHaan. 1982. LC 81-69431. 200p. 33.00 (*0-941388-00-X*) Am Trend Pub.

Optometry. Frank M. Kitchell. (Opportunities in... Ser.). (Illus.). 160p. pap. 12.95 (*0-8442-6497-0*, 297OIO); 1988. 13.95 (*0-8442-6496-2*) McGraw-Hill Trade (VGM Career Bks).

Optometry A-Z. Nathan Efron. 2002. 560p. pap. 135.00 (*0-7506-4913-5*) Buttrwrth-Heinemann.

Optometry Admission Test (OAT) Jack Rudman. (Admission Test Ser.: Vol. 27). 47.95 (*0-8373-5127-8*) Nat Learn.

Optometry Admission Test Student Guide. David M. Tarlow. 1993. (Illus.). pap. 16.95 (*0-931572-04-5*) Datar Pub.

Optometry Admissions Test: Core Content. David M. Tarlow. 1996. (Medical Examinations Ser.). 592p. (Orig.). (C). pap. 49.95 (*1-57774-002-5*) Educ Tsting Cnslts.

Optometry & Health Sciences: Index of New Information with Authors & Subjects. Marshal D. Shantzman. 1997. 161p. 57.50 (*0-7883-1632-X*); pap. 47.50 (*0-7883-1633-8*) ABBE Pubs Assn.

Optometry & the Health Sciences: Index of New Information for Research & Clinical Practice. Fred O. Crowder. 1997. 150p. 57.50 (*0-7883-1378-9*); pap. 47.50 (*0-7883-1379-7*) ABBE Pubs Assn.

Optometry in America: A History of the Illinois College of Optometry (1872-1997) Anistatia R. Miller & Jared M. Brown. 1996. LC 96-77258. (Illus.). 160p. 45.00 (*0-9652759-1-4*) IL Coll Optometry.

OptoSource '94. Market Intelligence Staff. 1994. 396p. 595.00 (*1-56753-959-9*) Frost & Sullivan.

Optronic Techniques in Diagnostic & Therapeutic Medicine. Ed. by R. Pratesi. 1991. (Illus.). 328p. (C). text 114.00 (*0-306-43938-7*, Kluwer Plenum) Kluwer Academic.

Oral AIDS: Manifestations, Safety Measures & Questions of Transmissibility. Ed. by D. Ajdukovic. 1990. 256p. 95.00 (*0-444-01576-0*) P-H.

Oral Anatomy, Embryology & Histology. B. K. Berkovitz & B. J. Moxham. 1994. LC 94-46127. (Self-Assessment Picture Tests in Dentistry Ser.). 144p. (C). (gr. 13). text 25.50 (*0-7234-2007-6*) Mosby Inc.

***Oral Anatomy, Histology & Embryology.** B. Berkowitz & G. Holland. 3rd ed. 2001. (Illus.). 315p. (*0-7234-3181-7*) Mosby Inc.

Oral Anatomy 3. B. K. Berkovitz. 3rd ed. 2001. text 79.95 (*0-323-00873-9*) Mosby Inc.

Oral & Dental Trauma in Children & Adolescents. Graham Roberts & Peter Longhurst. 1996. (Illus.). 112p. (C). pap. text 59.95 (*0-19-262049-5*) OUP.

Oral & Maxillofacial Infections. Ed. by Richard G. Topazian & Morton H. Goldberg. 3rd ed. 1993. LC 92-48356. (Illus.). 672p. text 142.00 (*0-7216-4845-2*) Saunders.

Oral & Maxillofacial Pathology. Brad W. Neville et al. 1995. LC 94-20442. (Illus.). 688p. text 62.95 (*0-7216-6695-7*) Saunders.

***Oral & Maxillofacial Pathology.** Brad Neville et al. 2nd ed. 2001. LC 2001-54207. (Illus.). 760p. (*0-7216-9003-3*) Saunders.

Oral & Maxillofacial Radiology: Radiologic - Pathologic Correlations. Dale A. Miles et al. 1991. (Illus.). 352p. text 65.00 (*0-7216-3070-7*) Saunders.

Oral & Maxillofacial Radiology Today: Proceedings of the 12th International Congress of Dentomaxillofacial Radiology, Osaka, Japan, June 26-July 1, 1999. International Congress of Dento-Maxillo-Facial Radiology Staff et al. 2000. LC 00-28786. (International Congress Ser.: No. 1199). (Illus.). 680p. 214.50 (*0-444-50405-2*, Excerpta Medica) Elsevier.

Oral & Maxillofacial Surgery, Set. Raymond J. Fonseca. 7th ed. 2000. LC 99-11886. (Illus.). text 895.00 (*0-7216-9631-7*) Saunders.

***Oral & Maxillofacial Surgery Vol. 1: Anesthesia - Dentoalveolar Surgery - Office Management.** Raymond J. Fonseca. 2000. (Illus.). 706p. (*0-7216-9632-5*) Saunders.

***Oral & Maxillofacial Surgery Vol. 2: Orthognathic Surgery.** Raymond J. Fonseca. 2000. (Illus.). 596p. (*0-7216-9633-3*) Saunders.

***Oral & Maxillofacial Surgery Vol. 3: Trauma.** Raymond J. Fonseca. 2000. (Illus.). 500p. (*0-7216-9634-1*) Saunders.

***Oral & Maxillofacial Surgery Vol. 4: Temporomandibular Disorders.** Raymond J. Fonseca. 2000. (Illus.). 426p. (*0-7216-9635-X*) Saunders.

***Oral & Maxillofacial Surgery Vol. 5: Surgical Pathology.** Raymond J. Fonseca. 2000. (Illus.). 514p. (*0-7216-9636-8*) Saunders.

***Oral & Maxillofacial Surgery Vol. 6: Cleft - Craniofacial - Cosmetic Surgery.** Raymond J. Fonseca. 2000. (Illus.). 554p. (*0-7216-9637-6*) Saunders.

***Oral & Maxillofacial Surgery Vol. 7: Reconstructive & Implant Surgery.** Raymond J. Fonseca. 2000. (Illus.). 498p. (*0-7216-9638-4*) Saunders.

Oral & Maxillofacial Trauma. Raymond J. Fonseca & Robert V. Walker. Ed. by Larry McGrew. 2nd ed. 1997. LC 96-42342. (Illus.). 1376p. text 335.00 (*0-7216-6213-7*) Saunders.

Oral & Maxillofacial Traumatology, Vol. I. Eberhard Kruger & Wilfried Schilli. 1982. (Illus.). 402p. text 174.00 (*0-931386-68-3*) Quint Pub Co.

Oral & Maxillofacial Traumatology, Vol. 2. Wilfried Schilli. Ed. by Eberhard Kruger. 1986. (Illus.). 605p. text 194.00 (*0-931386-69-1*) Quint Pub Co.

Oral Antibiotics Education Course. Competence Assurance Systems Staff. 1984. (Illus.). pap. text 60.00 (*0-89147-061-1*) CAS.

Oral Anticoagulants: Chemical & Biological Properties & Clinical Applications. Ed. by Leon Poller & Jack Hirsch. 1996. (Arnold Publication). 356p. (C). 125.00 (*0-340-55266-2*) OUP.

Oral Antidiabetics. Ed. by Jochen Kuhlman & W. Puls. 1995. (Handbook of Experimental Pharmacology Ser.: Vol. 119). (Illus.). 732p. 515.00 (*3-540-58990-2*) Spr-Verlag.

Oral Biology for Dental Hygienist. Mary Bath-Balogh. 1997. (Illus.). 144p. pap. text, wbk. ed. 20.95 (*0-7216-6903-4*) Saunders.

Oral Biology for Dental Hygienists. Mary Bath-Balogh & Margaret J. Fehrenbach. Ed. by Selma Kaszczuk. 1996. LC 96-16729. (Illus.). 416p. pap. text 44.00 (*0-7216-6687-6*) Saunders.

Oral Bioscience. D. B. Ferguson. 1999. LC 98-32450. (*0-443-05373-1*) Church.

Oral Cancer. Date not set. 192p. pap. 52.00 (*0-7236-1086-X*) Buttrwrth-Heinemann.

Oral Cancer Sol Silverman & American Cancer Society Staff. 3rd ed. 1990. LC 90-199. xi, 148 p. (*0-944235-05-0*) Am Cancer NY.

Oral Cancer. Sol Silverman, Jr. 4th ed. 1998. LC 00-265097. 174p. pap. incl. cd-rom (*1-55009-050-X*) DEKR.

Oral Cancer: Epidemiology, Etiology & Pathology. Ed. by Colin J. Smith et al. 1990. 125p. 68.95 (*0-89116-541-X*) Hemisp Pub.

Oral Cancer: Synopsis of Pathology & Management. Dimitroulis & Avery. 1998. LC 98-4825. 176p. pap. text 42.50 (*0-7236-1022-3*) Buttrwrth-Heinemann.

Oral Cancer Clinical & Pathological Considerations: Clinical & Pathological Considerations. Ed. by Bruce A. Wright et al. 1988. LC 87-23892. 240p. 115.00 (*0-8493-6774-3*, RC280, CRC Reprint) Franklin.

M
N
O

Oral Care: The Mouth in Terminal & Critical Illness. Ed. by Austin H. Kutscher et al. 1980. LC 79-48046. lib. bdg. 23.95 (*0-405-12642-5*) Ayer.

Oral Cephalosporins. Ed. by Robert C. Moellering, Jr. 1995. LC 95-24188. (Antibiotics & Chemotherapy Ser.: Vol. 47). (Illus.). x, 190p. 188.00 (*3-8055-6163-6*) S Karger.

Oral Colon - Specific Drug Delivery. David R. Friend. 1992. 288p. 189.00 (*0-8493-6688-7*, RM355) CRC Pr.

Oral Communication Problems in Children & Adolescents. Sol Adler. 1987. text 24.50 (*0-8089-1887-7*, Grune & Strat) Harcrt Hlth Sci Grp.

Oral Complications of Cancer Chemotherapy. Ed. by Douglas E. Peterson. 1983. lib. bdg. 54.50 (*0-89838-563-6*) Kluwer Academic.

Oral Contraceptives: Technical & Safety Aspects. WHO Staff. 1982. (WHO Offset Publications: No. 64). 45p. 4.00 (*92-4-170064-5*) World Health.

Oral Contraceptives & Breast Cancer. Institute of Medicine Staff. 1991. 198p. text 24.95 (*0-309-04493-6*) Natl Acad Pr.

Oral Contraceptives & Breast Cancer: The Implications of the Present Findings for Informed Consent & Informed Choice. Ed. by R. D. Mann. 1990. (Illus.). 406p. lib. bdg. 71.95 (*1-85070-282-9*, Parthenon Pbng) CRC Pr.

Oral Contraceptives & Cardiovascular Disease: An Analysis of the Recent Discussions on the Safety of the Pill. Ed. by Jean Cohen. 1997. LC 96-39337. (Illus.). 88p. lib. bdg. 35.95 (*1-85070-787-1*, Parthenon Pbng) CRC Pr.

Oral Contraceptives & Neoplasia: Report of a WHO Scientific Group. 1992. (Technical Reports: No. 817). (CHI, ENG, FRE & SPA.). vi, 46p. pap. text 9.00 (*92-4-120817-1*, 1100817) World Health.

Oral Contraceptives Education Course. Competence Assurance Systems Staff. 1985. (Illus.). pap. text 85.00 (*0-89147-109-X*) CAS.

Oral Controlled Release Products. U. Gundert-Remey. 1990. 105.00 (*3-8047-1042-5*) CRC Pr.

Oral Development & Histology. James K. Avery. 2nd ed. 1996. LC 94-30332. (Illus.). 416p. 65.00 (*0-86577-553-2*) Thieme Med Pubs.

Oral Diagnosis: The Clinician's Guide. William S. Birnbaum et al. 2000. (Illus.). 320p. pap. text 35.00 (*0-7236-1040-1*) Buttrwrth-Heinemann.

Oral Diagnosis, Oral Medicine & Treatment Planning. Steven L. Bricker et al. 2nd ed. 1994. (Illus.). 868p. pap. text 64.00 (*0-8121-1605-4*) Lppncott W & W.

***Oral Disease.** Roderick Cawson et al. 2000. 379p. (*0-7234-3165-5*) Mosby Inc.

Oral Disease. Crispian Scully & R. A. Cawson. 2nd ed. 1999. LC 99-10154. (Colour Guide Ser.). (*0-443-06170-X*) Harcrt Hlth Sci Grp.

Oral Diseases in the Tropics. Ed. by S. R. Prabhu et al. 1992. (Illus.). 820p. text 175.00 (*0-19-262008-8*) OUP.

Oral Enteric Bacterial Vaccines: Proceedings of the WHO Scientific Group, Geneva, 1971. WHO Staff. 1972. (Technical Reports: No. 500). pap. text 4.00 (*92-4-120500-8*, 1100500) World Health.

Oral Enteric Vaccines: Report on a WHO Working Group. 1982. (Euro Reports & Studies Ser.: No. 63). 42p. pap. text 4.00 (*92-890-1229-3*) World Health.

Oral Examinations in Medical Specialty Board Certification. 1983. 29.95 (*0-934277-02-8*) Am Bd Med Spec.

Oral Health - Diet & Other Factors: The Report of the British Nutrition Foundation's Task Force. British Nutrition Foundation Staff. Ed. by Ursula Arens. 1998. LC 98-39770. 240p. 137.00 (*0-444-50025-1*) Elsevier.

Oral Health & the Older Adult. Kerschbaum. 1999. pap. text (*0-7216-4068-0*) Saunders.

Oral Health Care for the Geriatric Patient in a Long Term Care Facility. 11.13 (*0-934510-13-X*, J010) Am Dental.

Oral Health Promotion & Disease Prevention: Disease Prevention. Malvitz. 1996. pap. (*0-7216-4008-7*) Saunders.

Oral Health Services in Europe. J. Kostlan. 1979. (WHO Regional Publications, European Ser.). 141p. 16.00 (*92-9020-105-3*, 1310005) World Health.

Oral Health Sourcebook: Basic Information about Diseases & Conditions Affecting Oral Health. Ed. by Allan R. Cook. 1997. LC 97-28301. (Health Reference Ser.: Vol. 30). 600p. lib. bdg. 78.00 (*0-7808-0082-6*) Omnigraphics Inc.

Oral Health Surveys: Basic Methods. 1987. 51p. pap. text 12.60 (*92-4-154216-0*, 1150275) World Health.

Oral Histology & Embryology. Leslie P. Gartner. 1989. (Illus.). 246p. (C). pap. text 28.57 (*0-910841-06-3*) Jen Hse Pub Co.

Oral History of Gestalt Therapy: Interviews with Laura Perls, Isadore From, Erving Polster, Miriam Polster & Elliott Shapiro. Joe Wysong & Edward Rosenfeld. 2nd ed. 1989. 96p. pap. 10.00 (*0-939266-08-3*) Gestalt Journal.

Oral Hygiene for the Orthodontic Patient. Siegward D. Heintze et al. 1998. LC 98-8476. (Illus.). 170p. pap. text 58.00 (*0-86715-295-8*) Quint Pub Co.

Oral Implantology. S. Otobe. 1990. text (*1-57235-013-X*) Piccin Nuova.

Oral Implantology: Basic, ITI, Hollow Cylinder System. A. Schroeder. 2nd ed. 1996. (Illus.). 510p. pap. text 32.00 (*0-86577-545-1*) Thieme Med Pubs.

Oral Leukoplakia. J. Banoczy. 1982. text 137.50 (*90-247-2655-7*) Kluwer Academic.

Oral Manifestations of HIV Infection: Proceedings of the 2nd International Workshop on the Oral Manifestations of HIV Infection, January 31-February 3, 1993, San Francisco, California. International Workshop on the Oral Manifestation of HIV Infection Staff. Ed. by John S. Greenspan et al. 1995. LC 94-37145. (Illus.). 374p. pap. text 64.00 (*0-86715-286-9*) Quint Pub Co.

Oral Medicine. David Wray & J. Gibson. 1997. LC 97-10853. (Color Guide, Picture Tests Ser.). pap. text (*0-443-05301-4*) Church.

Oral Medicine. William R. Tyldesley & Anne E. Field. 4th ed. 1995. (Illus.). 178p. text 105.00 (*0-19-262626-4*); 180p. pap. text 61.50 (*0-19-262625-6*) OUP.

Oral Medicine: A Pocket Guide. Lewis R. Eversole. 1995. LC 94-47441. (Illus.). 208p. pap. text 36.00 (*0-7216-4973-4*) Saunders.

Oral Medicine: Diagnosis & Treatment. Drore Eisen & Denis P. Lynch. 1997. LC 97-4386. (Illus.). 320p. (C). (gr. 13). text 79.95 (*0-8151-3105-4*, 29157) Mosby Inc.

Oral Medicine & Hospital Practice. Peter Lockhart. 4th rev. ed. 1997. Orig. Title: A Practical Guide to Hospital Dental Practice. (Illus.). 550p. pap. text 30.00 (*0-9657191-0-3*) FSCOD.

Oral Microbiology & Immunology. Ed. by Russell J. Nisengard & Michael G. Newman. 2nd ed. 1993. LC 93-33973. (Illus.). 512p. pap. text 54.50 (*0-7216-6753-8*) Saunders.

Oral Morphine in Advanced Cancer. Robert Twycross. 3rd ed. 1997. 42p. pap. (*0-906584-45-0*) Beaconsfield GBR. *Dist:* Medicina Bio.

Oral Mucosal Drug Delivery. Michael J. Rathbone. 1996. LC 96-14719. (Drugs & the Pharmaceutical Sciences Ser.: Vol. 74). (Illus.). 464p. text 195.00 (*0-8247-9744-2*) Dekker.

Oral OB GYN Board Exam: How to Prepare for the Exam, How to Take the Exam, How to Pass the Exam. Anita K. Das. 1998. LC 98-24808. 91p. 22.95 (*1-56053-303-X*) Hanley & Belfus.

Oral Oncology. Gordon B. Snow & Isaac Van der Waal. 1984. (Developments in Oncology Ser.). text 161.00 (*0-89838-631-4*) Kluwer Academic.

Oral Pathology. R. A. Cawson & J. W. Odell. 1993. (Colour Guide Ser.). (Illus.). 152p. pap. text 16.95 (*0-443-04800-2*) Harcrt Hlth Sci Grp.

Oral Pathology. J. V. Soames & J. C. Southam. 2nd ed. 1993. LC 92-16493. (Oxford Medical Publications). (Illus.). 332p. pap. text 30.00 (*0-19-262214-5*) OUP.

Oral Pathology: Actual Diagnostic & Prognostic Aspects. Gerhard Seifert & Arne Burkhardt. 1997. LC 96-18025. (Current Topics in Pathology Ser.). (Illus.). 244p. 185.00 (*3-540-60987-3*) Spr-Verlag.

Oral Pathology: Clinical Pathology Correlations. Joseph A. Regezi & James Sciubba. Ed. by Judy Fletcher. 3rd ed. 1999. LC 97-51667. (Illus.). 688p. (C). text 63.95 (*0-7216-7731-2*) Saunders.

Oral Pathology Dental Hygienist. Ibsen. 2nd ed. 1995. 350.00 (*0-7216-6545-4*) Harcourt.

Oral Pathology for the Dental Hygienist. Olga A. Ibsen & Joan A. Phelan. Ed. by Selma Ozmat. 2nd ed. 1996. LC 95-30945. (Illus.). 560p. text 54.00 (*0-7216-6051-7*) Saunders.

Oral Pathology for the Dental Hygienist. Olga A. C. Ibsen. 3rd ed. 2000. LC 99-35202. (Illus.). 460p. text (*0-7216-8574-9*) Saunders.

Oral Pathology, Intestinal Pathology, Hypobaric Pathology: Proceedings of the International Society of Geographical Pathology, 11th Conference, Newcastle-upon-Tyne, August, 1972. International Society of Geographical Pathology St. Ed. by J. R. Ruettner. 1973. (Pathologia et Microbiologica Ser.: Vol. 39, No. 3-4). reprint ed. pap. 47.50 (*3-8055-1370-4*) S Karger.

Oral Presentation in Medicine. A. Fingerhut & F. Lacaine. 2000. 100p. pap. (*2-287-59686-0*) Spl France Editions FRA. *Dist:* Spr-Verlag.

Oral Psychophysiology: Stress, Pain & Behavior in Dental Care. Ilana Eli. 1992. 240p. lib. bdg. 89.95 (*0-8493-0159-9*, RK53) CRC Pr.

Oral Radiology: Principles & Interpretation. Paul W. Goaz & Stuart C. White. 4th ed. 1999. LC 98-53444. (Illus.). 752p. text 67.95 (*0-8151-9491-9*, 30605) Mosby Inc.

Oral Radiology: Principles & Interpretation. Stuart C. White & Michael J. Pharoah. 4th ed. 1999. (Illus.). 657p. (*84-8174-091-8*) Mosby-Doyma Libros ESP. *Dist:* Mosby Inc.

Oral Radiology No. 3: Principles & Interpretation. Paul W. Goaz & Stuart C. White. 3rd ed. 1994. LC 93-45306. (Illus.). 752p. (C). (gr. 13). text 74.00 (*0-8016-7295-3*, 07295) Mosby Inc.

Oral Rehabilitation: Clinical Determination of Occlusion. Sumiya Hobo & Hisao Takayama. 1997. 168p. text 55.00 (*4-87417-532-5*) Quint Pub Co.

Oral Retinoids in Dermatology Workshop Held on the 15th International Congress of Dermatology, Mexico City, October 1977. Ed. by C. E. Orfanos & R. Schuppli. 1978. pap. 22.75 (*3-8055-2950-3*) S Karger.

Oral Self Care: Strategies for Preventative Dentistry. Philip Weinstein et al. 1991. 230p. (C). pap. text 28.00 (*1-880291-00-2*) Cont Dental Educ.

Oral Sensory Mechanisms. Ed. by Yojiro Kawamura. 1983. (Frontiers of Oral Physiology Ser.: Vol. 4). (Illus.). x, 130p. 85.25 (*3-8055-3576-7*) S Karger.

Oral Surgery for the General Dentist. Hermann F. Sailer & Gion F. Pajarola. 1998. LC 98-8414. (Color Atlas of Dental Medicine Ser.). 199.00 (*3-13-108241-0*) Thieme Med Pubs.

Oral Surgery in General Dentistry: A Self-Instructional Guide, Set. James R. Hooley & Robert J. Whitacre. 1984. 1021p. pap. 129.50 (*0-89939-001-3*) Stoma Pr.

Oral Tolerance: Mechanisms & Applications. Ed. by Howard L. Weiner & Lloyd F. Mayer. 1996. (Annals of the New York Academy of Sciences Ser.: Vol. 778). 453p. pap. 115.00 (*0-89766-996-7*) NY Acad Sci.

Oral Tumoractivated Chemotherapy: A New Effective & Convenient Treatment in Oncology: Satellite Symposium Held at the 23rd ESMO Congress Athens, Greece, November 6, 1998. Ed. by Stan Kaye. 1999. (Oncology Ser.). iv,32p. (*3-8055-6877-0*) S Karger.

Oralpathologie I. 1996. 465.00 (*3-540-61036-7*) Spr-Verlag.

Orban's Oral Histology & Embryology. Bhaskar. 11th ed. 1990. (Illus.). 512p. (C). (gr. 13). text 61.95 (*0-8016-0239-4*, 00239) Mosby Inc.

Orbit & Oculoplasts. Ed. by Richard R. Tenzel. 1992. (Textbook of Ophthalmology Ser.). (Illus.). 208p. (gr. 13). text (*1-56375-096-1*) Gower-Mosby.

Orbit & the Visual Pathway: Anatomical & Pathological Aspects & Detailed Clinical Accounts. Ed. by Dieter Voth & Paul Glees. 1994. ix, 367p. (C). pap. text 190.80 (*3-11-012803-9*) De Gruyter.

Orbital Disorders. Ed. by G. M. Bleeker et al. 1978. (Illus.). text 268.50 (*90-6193-570-9*) Kluwer Academic.

Orbital Disorders: Proceedings of the International Symposium, 2nd, Amsterdam, May, 1973. International Symposium on Orbital Disorders Staff. Ed. by G. M. Bleeker et al. 1975. (Modern Problems in Ophthalmology Ser.: Vol. 14). 300p. 213.25 (*3-8055-2051-4*) S Karger.

Orbital Fractures: Diagnosis, Operative Treatment, Secondary Corrections. B. Hammer. 1995. (Illus.). 112p. text 112.00 (*0-88937-139-3*) Hogrefe & Huber Pubs.

Orbital Surgery: A Conceptual Approach. Jack Rootman et al. 1995. (Illus.). 416p. text 225.00 (*0-7817-0254-2*) Lppncott W & W.

Order & Life. Joseph Needham. 1968. pap. 15.95 (*0-262-64001-5*) MIT Pr.

Order or the Hospital of St. John of Jerusalem. William K. Bedford. LC 76-29831. reprint ed. 44.50 (*0-404-15412-3*) AMS Pr.

Order Restored: A Biblical Interpretation of Health, Medicine & Healing. Garth D. Ludwig. 1999. LC 99-21264. 272p. pap. 19.95 (*0-570-04272-0*) Concordia.

Ordered to Care: The Dilemma of American Nursing, 1850-1945. Susan M. Reverby. 1987. (Cambridge History of Medicine Ser.). (Illus.). 320p. pap. text 21.95 (*0-521-33565-5*) Cambridge U Pr.

Ordered to Return: My Life after Dying. George C. Ritchie, Jr. 2nd ed. 1998. LC 98-70607. 184p. reprint ed. pap. 12.95 (*1-57174-096-1*) Hampton Roads Pub Co.

Ordinal Methods for Behavioral Data Analysis. Norman Cliff. 1996. LC 96-22689. 224p. 45.00 (*0-8058-1333-0*) L Erlbaum Assocs.

Ordinary Life: A Memoir of Illness. Kathlyn Conway. 1996. LC 96-273316. 250p. text 22.95 (*0-7167-3036-7*) W H Freeman.

Ordinary Woman's Extraordinary Faith: The Autobiography of Patricia St. John. Patricia M. St. John. 1996. LC 95-44552. (North Wind Bks.). 312p. pap. 11.99 (*0-87788-751-9*, H Shaw Pubs) Waterbrook Pr.

Oregon Consumer Health Care Scorecard Project: Final Report. Pamela Hanes & Merwyn Greenlick. 1997. (Illus.). 129p. (Orig.). pap. text 30.00 (*0-7881-4490-1*) DIANE Pub.

Oregon Health Care Perspective, 1998. Ed. by Kathleen O'Leary Morgan & Scott E. Morgan. 1998. 20p. pap. 19.00 (*1-56692-836-2*) Morgan Quitno Corp.

Organ Allocation: Organized by Fondation Marcel Merieux & Universite Claude Bernard - Lyon 1 Proceedings of the 30th International Conference on Transplantation & Clinical Immunology, June 2-4, 1998. Ed. by Jean-Louis Touraine et al. 1998. (Transplantation & Clinical Immunology Ser.). 309p. 146.00 (*0-7923-5077-4*) Kluwer Academic.

***Organ & Tissue Donation: Reference Guide for Clergy.** Ed. by M. Lissa Cooper Hammon & Gloria J. Taylor. 4th ed. 2001. (Illus.). pap. 35.00 (*1-886651-40-X*) United Network.

Organ & Tissue Donation & Transplantation: A Humanities Curriculum for Medical Students. Phillip V. Davis & Bethany J. Speilman. 1997. 166p. ring bd. 25.00 incl. cd-rom (*0-931369-32-0*) Southern IL Univ Sch.

Organ & Tissue Donation for Transplantation. Ed. by Jeremy R. Chapman et al. 1997. LC 97-25104. (Arnold Publication). (Illus.). 488p. 115.00 (*0-340-61394-7*) OUP.

Organ & Tissue Transplantation: Nursing Care from Procurement Through Rehabilitation. M. K. Norris & Mary A. House. 1991. LC 90-14141. (Illus.). 346p. (C). 39.95 (*0-8036-6587-3*) Davis Co.

Organ Based Autoimmune Diseases. Ed. by J. M. Cruse & R. E. Lewis. 1985. (Concepts in Immunopathology Ser.: Vol. 2). (Illus.). x, 278p. 129.75 (*3-8055-3929-0*) S Karger.

Organ Behavior Moorhead. 5th ed. 1997. LC 97-72522. (C). text 72.76 (*0-395-84196-8*) HM.

Organ Conservation in Curative Cancer Treatment: Indications, Contraindications, Methods. Ed. by J. L. Meyer & J. M. Vaeth. 1993. (Frontiers of Radiation Therapy & Oncology Ser.: Vol. 27). (Illus.). xii, 256p. 216.75 (*3-8055-5663-2*) S Karger.

Organ Directed Toxicities of Anticance Drugs. Ed. by Miles P. Hacker & John Lazo. 1988. (Developments in Oncology Ser.). 272p. (C). text 130.50 (*0-89838-356-0*) Kluwer Academic.

Organ Donation & Transplantation: Psychological & Behavioral Factors. Ed. by James Shanteau & Richard J. Harris. 1990. 214p. 19.95 (*1-55798-079-9*) Am Psychol.

***Organ Donations: Congressional Hearing.** Ed. by Arlen Specter. 2001. 92p. (C). reprint ed. pap. text 25.00 (*0-7567-0467-7*) DIANE Pub.

Organ Donations & Procurements: Index of Authors & Subjects. American Health Research Institute Staff. 1993. 180p. 47.50 (*1-55914-936-1*); pap. 44.50 (*1-55914-937-X*) ABBE Pubs Assn.

Organ Farm: Pig to Human Transplants. Jenny Bryan & John Clare. 2001. (Illus.). 240p. (*1-84222-249-X*) Carlton Bks Ltd GBR. *Dist:* Natl Bk Netwk.

Organ Histology. 1997. LC 97-160089. 235p. 29.00 (*981-02-2612-8*); pap. 17.00 (*981-02-2613-6*) World Scientific Pub.

Organ Preservation Surgery For Laryngeal Cancer. Gregory S. Weinstein et al. 1999. LC 98-40983. (Illus.). 270p. text 366.95 (*1-56593-903-4*, 1788) Thomson Learn.

Organ Preservation Surgery of the Larynx: 1999 Singular Catalog. Weinstein. 1999. (*1-56593-956-5*) Thomson Learn.

Organ Procurement & Preservation. Goran B. Klintmalm & Marlon F. Levy. 1999. LC 98-55261. (Vademecum Ser.). 250p. spiral bd. 45.00 (*1-57059-498-8*) Landes Bioscience.

Organ Procurement & Preservation for Transplantation. Luis H. Toledo-Pereyra. 2nd ed. 1997. (Medical Intelligence Unit Ser.). 223p. pap. 89.95 (*0-412-11591-3*) Chapman & Hall.

Organ Procurement & Transplantation: Assessing Current Policies & the Potential Impact. Institute of Medicine Staff. 2000. LC 99-44515. (Illus.). 254p. pap. 53.00 (*0-309-06578-X*) Natl Acad Pr.

Organ Replacement Therapy: Ethics, Justice & Commerce: First Joint Meeting of ESOT & EDTA - ERA Munich, December 1990. Ed. by W. Land & J. B. Dossetor. 1991. (Illus.). 578p. 185.00 (*0-387-53687-6*) Spr-Verlag.

Organ-Selective Actions of Steroid Hormones. Ed. by D. T. Baird et al. 1995. LC 95-42665. (Ernst Schering Research Foundation Ser.: No. 16). (*0-387-60338-7*); (Illus.). 208p. 70.00 (*3-540-60338-7*) Spr-Verlag.

Organ Shortage - The Solutions: Proceedings of the 26th Conference on Transplantation & Clinical Immunology 13-15 June 1994. Ed. by J. L. Touraine et al. 1995. LC 94-37471. (Transplantation & Clinical Immunology Ser.: Vol. 26). 360p. (C). text 166.00 (*0-7923-3179-6*) Kluwer Academic.

Organ-Specific Autoantibodies in Addison's Disease & Autoimmune Polyendocrine Syndrome Type I. Annika Soderbergh. 2000. (Comprehensive Summaries of Uppsala Dissertations from the Faculty of Medicine Ser.: No. 944). (Illus.). 57p. (Orig.). pap. (*91-554-4779-1*) Uppsala Universitet SWE. *Dist:* Coronet Bks.

Organ Transplantation. Frank P. Stuart & Michael M. Abecassis. 2000. LC 99-57056. (Vademecum Ser.). (Illus.). 576p. spiral bd. 45.00 (*1-57059-529-1*) Landes Bioscience.

Organ Transplantation: A Manual for Nurses. Ed. by Barbara Williams et al. 1991. 376p. 49.95 (*0-8261-7230-X*) Springer Pub.

Organ Transplantation: Long-Term Results. Ed. by Paul & Kim Solez. 1992. LC 92-18547. (Illus.). 432p. text 190.00 (*0-8247-8599-1*) Dekker.

Organ Transplantation: Meanings & Realities. Ed. by Stuart J. Younger et al. 1996. LC 95-2995. 290p. pap. 22.95 (*0-299-14964-1*) U of Wis Pr.

Organ Transplantation & Tissue Grafting. Herve. 1996. 1600p. text 289.00 (*0-86196-383-0*) Buttrwrth-Heinemann.

Organ Transplantation in Religious, Ethical & Social Context: No Room for Death. Intro. by William R. DeLong. 1993. LC 93-29164. (Journal of Health Care Chaplaincy Ser.: Vol. 5, Nos. 1/2). (Illus.). 175p. lib. bdg. 39.95 (*1-56024-470-4*) Haworth Pr.

Organ Transplantation, 1990. Ed. by George M. Abouna et al. 1991. (Developments in Surgery Ser.). (C). text 341.00 (*0-7923-1191-4*) Kluwer Academic.

Organ Transplantation Policy: Issues & Prospects. Ed. by James F. Blumstein & Frank A. Sloan. 1989. LC 89-16928. 265p. (C). text 37.95 (*0-8223-0939-4*) Duke.

Organ Transplants: A Patient's Guide. Massachusetts General Hospital Organ Transplant Staff & H. F. Pizer. 1991. LC 91-7083. (Illus.). 256p. (C). text 24.95 (*0-674-64235-X*) HUP.

Organ Transplants: How to Boost Supply & Ensure Equitable Distribution. 1993. (Illus.). 94p. (Orig.). (C). pap. text 30.00 (*0-7881-0078-5*) DIANE Pub.

Organ Transplants: Making the Most of Your Gift of Life. Robert Finn. Ed. by Linda Lamb. 2000. LC 00-29837. (Patient-Centered Guides Ser.). (Illus.). 311p. pap. 19.95 (*1-56592-634-X*, Patient-Centered) OReilly & Assocs.

Organ Transplants & Ethics. David Lamb. 1996. (Avebury Series in Philosophy). 172p. text (*1-85972-507-4*) Avebury GBR. *Dist:* Ashgate Pub Co.

Organelle Diseases. Applegarth. 1997. 480p. (*0-412-54910-7*) E A GBR. *Dist:* OUP.

Organelles in Tumor Diagnosis: An Ultrastructural Atlas. Brian Eyden. 1996. LC 96-1857. (Illus.). 192p. 79.50 (*0-89640-311-4*) Igaku-Shoin.

Organic Acids in Man. R. A. Chalmers & A. M. Lawson. 1982. LC 81-11342. 82.50 (*0-412-14890-0*, NO. 6573) Chapman & Hall.

Organic Acidureas. Ed. by G. M. Addison et al. 1984. text 124.00 (*0-85200-875-9*) Kluwer Academic.

Organic Brain Pathology. Mary L. Marley. 1989. 264p. 99.00 (*0-205-10142-9*) P-H.

Organic Brain Pathology & the Bender-Gestalt Test: A Differential Diagnostic. Mary L. Marley. 1983. 264p. text 38.00 (*0-8089-1425-1*, 792683, Grune & Strat) Harcrt Hlth Sci Grp.

Organic C-Centered Radicals, Pt. 8. A. Berndt et al. 1977. LC 62-53136. (Illus.). 1248.95 (*0-387-08152-6*) Spr-Verlag.

Organic-Chemical Drugs & Their Synonyms: An International Survey, Set. Martin Negwer. 7th ed. 1994. LC 94-27326. 3952p. (*3-527-40040-0*) Akademie Verlag DEU. *Dist:* Wiley.

***Organic-Chemical Drugs & Their Synonyms 8th Edition.** Martin Negwer. 8th ed. 2001. 5500p. 1195.00 incl. cd-rom (*3-527-30247-6*) Wiley.

Organic Chemistry. Roger D. Barry. 1975. LC 74-79834. (Allied Health Ser.). stu. ed. 5.10 (*0-672-61379-4*, Bobbs) Macmillan.

Organic Chemistry. Ralph J. Fessenden & Joan S. Fessenden. 3rd ed. 1986. LC 86-17200. (Chemistry). 1100p. (C). mass mkt. 52.75 (*0-534-05088-3*) Brooks-Cole.

Organic Chemistry for Students of Health & Life Sciences. Paul W. Groundwater. 4th ed. 1997. 205p. (C). pap. text 40.00 (*0-582-29765-6*) P-H.

Organic Chemistry of Drug Design & Drug Action. Richard B. Silverman. 1992. LC 91-47041. (Illus.). 422p. text 65.00 (*0-12-643730-0*) Acad Pr.

Organic Chemistry of Drug Synthesis Daniel Lednicer & Lester A. Mitscher. 1996. 1856p. 450.00 (*0-471-16990-0*) Wiley.

Organic Chemistry of Drug Synthesis Daniel Lednicer & Lester A. Mitscher. Set. 1990. 1616p. 525.00 (*0-471-53176-6*); Vol. 1. 1977. LC 76-28387. (Organic Chemistry of Drug Synthesis Ser.: Vol. 1). 496p. 175.00 (*0-471-52141-8*); Vol. 2. 1980. LC 76-28387. (Organic Chemistry of Drug Synthesis Ser.: Vol. 2). 544p. 175.00 (*0-471-04392-3*); Vol. 3. 1984. 304p. 175.00 (*0-471-09250-9*); Vol. 4. 1990. LC 76-28387. (Organic Chemistry of Drug Synthesis Ser.: Vol. 4). 272p. 175.00 (*0-471-85548-0*) Wiley.

Organic Foundations of Animal Behavior. Joseph Altman. 1966. LC 65-18350. (Illus.). text 39.50 (*0-03-052230-7*) Irvington.

Organic Mental Disease. Frank R. Freemon. 1981. LC 79-23180. (Illus.). 248p. text 37.00 (*0-88331-169-0*) R B Luce.

Organic Psychiatry: The Psychological Consequences of Cerebral Disorder. William A. Lishman. 3rd ed. LC 97-7107. (Illus.). 1998. 99.95 (*0-86542-842-5*); 1997. 896p. pap. 115.95 (*0-86542-820-4*) Blackwell Sci.

Organic Reactions. Ed. by William G. Dauben. Vol. 21. 1974. 417p. 105.00 (*0-471-19622-3*); Vol. 22. 1975. 474p. 105.00 (*0-471-19623-1*); Vol. 23. 1976. 520p. 105.00 (*0-471-19624-X*); Vol. 25. 1977. 490p. 105.00 (*0-471-01741-8*); Vol. 26. 1979. 488p. 105.00 (*0-471-05209-4*) Wiley.

Organic Syntheses, Vol. 5, Vols. 40-49. Henry E. Baumgarten. 1973. (Organic Syntheses Ser.: Vol. 5). 1248p. 170.00 (*0-471-05707-X*) Wiley.

Organic Voice Disorders: Assessment & Treatment. Ed. by William S. Brown et al. 1996. LC 96-23807. (Illus.). 398p. (C). 55.00 (*1-56593-268-4*, 0590) Thomson Learn.

Organisation & Management of Intensive Care: A Prospective Study in 12 European Countries. D. Reis Miranda. Ed. by J. L. Vincent et al. 1997. LC 97-13204. (Update in Intensive Care & Emergency Medicine Ser.: Vol. 29). (Illus.). 286p. 112.00 (*3-540-62581-X*) Spr-Verlag.

Organisation of Maternity Care: A Guide to Evaluation. Campbell & Garcia. abr. ed. 1997. LC 97-224870. 160p. pap. text 34.99 (*1-898507-37-6*) Buttrwrth-Heinemann.

Organisational Culture. Andrew Brown. 2nd ed. 1998. 320p. pap. (*0-273-63147-0*) Pitman Pub GBR. *Dist:* Trans-Atl Phila.

Organisational Structure & the Care of the Mentally Retarded. Norma V. Raynes et al. 1979. LC 79-83740. (Praeger Special Studies). 240p. 66.00 (*0-275-90411-3*, C0411, Praeger Pubs) Greenwood.

Organising a Toy Library: A Description of the BJMH Toy Library. B. Wroe. 1985. 16p. 20.00 (*0-906054-38-9*) St Mut.

Organism & the Origins of Self. Ed. by Alfred I. Tauber. 1991. 400p. (C). lib. bdg. (*0-7923-1185-X*) Kluwer Academic NLD. *Dist:* Kluwer Academic.

Organism, Medicine, & Metaphysics. Ed. by Stuart F. Spicker. 1978. (Philosophy & Medicine Ser.: No. 7). 357p. text 98.50 (*90-277-0823-1*) Kluwer Academic.

Organization & Administration of Maternal & Child Health Services: Proceedings of the WHO Expert Committee on Maternal & Child Health, Geneva, 1968. WHO Staff. 1969. (Technical Reports: No. 428). pap. text 5.00 (*92-4-120428-1*, 1100428) World Health.

Organization & Methods for Endocrinology Laboratory Services: Report on a Working Group. 1981. (Euro Reports & Studies Ser.: No. 51). 18p. pap. text 4.00 (*92-890-1217-X*) World Health.

Organization & Replication of Viral DNA. Albert S. Kaplan. 1982. 208p. 124.95 (*0-8493-6405-1*, QR394) CRC Pr.

Organization Development in Health Care Settings: A Special Issue of Consultation: An International Journal. Ed. by R. Wayne Boss. 1988. 76p. pap. 12.95 (*0-89885-425-3*, Kluwer Acad Hman Sci) Kluwer Academic.

Organization for Radiation Protection: The Operations of the ICRP & NCRP, 1928. DOE Technical Information Center Staff & Lauriston S. Taylor. 1979. LC 79-607999. 2062p. lib. bdg. 59.75 (*0-87079-116-8*, DOE/TIC-10124) DOE.

Organization for the Care of Handicapped Children, National, State, Local. White House Conference on Child Health and Protectio. 1974. LC 74-1715. (Children & Youth Ser.: Vol. 14). 390p. reprint ed. 36.95 (*0-405-05990-6*) Ayer.

Organization of Afferents from the Brain Stem Nuclei to the Cerebellar Cortex in the Cat. B. Brown Gold. 1980. (Advances in Anatomy, Embryology & Cell Biology Ser.: Vol. 62). (Illus.). 90p. 37.00 (*0-387-09960-3*) Spr-Verlag.

Organization of Biochemical Systems: Structural & Regulatory Aspects. Ed. by Boris I. Kurganov & A. E. Lyubarev. 1994. 245p. (C). lib. bdg. 105.00 (*1-56072-092-1*) Nova Sci Pubs.

Organization of Health Workers & Labor Conflict. Ed. by Samuel Wolfe. 1978. LC 77-94410. (Policy, Politics, Health & Medicine Ser.: Vol. 2). 161p. pap. 25.00 (*0-89503-009-8*) Baywood Pub.

Organization of Local & Intermediate Health Administrations: Proceedings of the WHO Expert Committee, Geneva, 1971. WHO Staff. 1972. (Technical Reports: No. 499). pap. text 3.00 (*92-4-120499-0*, 1100499) World Health.

Organization of Mental Health Services in Developing Countries: Proceedings of the WHO Expert Committee on Mental Health, 16th, Geneva, 1974. WHO Staff. 1975. (Technical Reports: No. 564). pap. text 6.00 (*92-4-120564-4*, 1100564) World Health.

Organization of Prokaryotic Cell Membrane. Ed. by Bijan K. Ghosh. 1981. Vol. I. 272p. 119.00 (*0-8493-5653-9*, QR77); Vol. II. 224p. 127.00 (*0-8493-5654-7*) Franklin (CRC Reprint).

Organization of Prokaryotic Cell Membranes, Vol. III. Ed. by Bijan K. Ghosh. 1985. 280p. 159.00 (*0-8493-5659-8*, QR77, CRC Reprint) Franklin.

Organization of Public Health Care: An Economic Analysis of the Swedish Health Care System. Clas Rehnberg. 1991. (Linkoping Studies in Arts & Sciences: No. 58). 172p. (Orig.). pap. 60.50 (*91-7870-728-5*) Coronet Bks.

Organization of the Cerebral Cortex. Ed. by Francis O. Schmitt et al. 1981. (Illus.). 614p. 80.00 (*0-262-19189-X*) MIT Pr.

Organization of the Required Physical Education for Women in State Universities. Georgia B. Johnson. LC 73-176913. (Columbia University. Teachers College. Contributions to Education Ser.: No. 253). reprint ed. 37.50 (*0-404-55253-6*) AMS Pr.

Organization Research on Health Institutions. Ed. by Basil S. Georgopoulos. 1972. LC 72-619554. 429p. 20.00 (*0-87944-125-9*) Inst Soc Res.

Organizational Aspects of Health Communication Campaigns: What Works? Thomas E. Backer & Everett M. Rogers. 1993. (Illus.). 280p. (C). 64.95 (*0-8039-4997-9*, 4221); pap. 34.95 (*0-8039-4998-7*, 4222) Sage.

Organizational Aspects of Health Informatics: Managing Technological Change. Nancy M. Lorenzi & Robert T. Riley. 1994. LC 94-19977. (Computers in Health Care Ser.). (Illus.). 312p. 69.95 (*0-387-94226-2*) Spr-Verlag.

Organizational Behavior: Concepts & Experience. Charles G. Morris & Marshall Sashkin. 1984. (C). tchr. ed. (*0-8359-5294-0*); text (*0-8359-5293-2*) P-H.

Organizational Behavior in Chinese Society. Ed. by Sidney L. Greenblatt et al. 1981. LC 80-26728. 274p. 77.00 (*0-275-90638-8*, C0638, Praeger Pubs) Greenwood.

Organizational Behaviour: Text & Cases. M. Gangadhar Rao et al. 1990. 584p. text (*81-220-0040-1*) Konark Pubs Pvt Ltd IND. *Dist:* Advent Bks Div.

Organizational Culture. Karel De Witte. 2000. 112p. pap. (*0-86377-997-2*) Psychol Pr.

Organizational Culture, Rule-Governed Behavior & Organizational Behavior Management: Theoretical Foundations & Implications for Research & Practice. Ed. by Thomas C. Mawhinney. 1996. LC 92-30026. (Journal of Organizational Behavior Management: Vol. 12, No. 2). 137p. pap. 17.95 (*0-7890-0068-7*) Haworth Pr.

Organizational Development in Health Care. R. Wayne Boss. 1989. (Organization Development Ser.). (Illus.). 150p. (C). pap. text 26.95 (*0-201-18364-1*) Addison-Wesley.

***Organizational Ethics in Health Care: Principles, Cases & Practical Solutions.** Philip J. Boyle et al. 2001. LC 2001-1349. (Jossey-Bass Health Ser.). 448p. 59.00 (*0-7879-5558-2*) Jossey-Bass.

Organizational Ethics in the Compliance Context. John Abbott Worthley. 1999. LC 99-28710. 370p. pap. 48.00 (*1-56793-110-3*) Health Admin Pr.

***Organizational Leadership: Fire Services in the United States.** Charles H. Kime. 2001. LC 2001-50404. (Contemporary Studies in Applied Behavioral Science: Vol. 12). 134p. 82.00 (*0-7623-0796-X*) Jai Pr.

Organizational Paradoxes: Clinical Approaches to Management. Manfred F. De Vries. 2nd ed. 1994. LC 94-15858. (Illus.). 240p. (C). (gr. 13). pap. text 29.95 (*0-415-11073-4*, B4781) Thomson Learn.

Organizational Psychology. Ed. by Lynn R. Offermann & Marilyn K. Gowing. 1990. (Special Issue American Psychologist Ser.: Vol. 45, No. 2). 224p. pap. 16.00 (*1-55798-092-6*) Am Psychol.

Organizational Psychology: Foundations & Applications. Robert Lawson & Zheng Shen. 1997. LC 96-29599. (Illus.). 288p. (C). text 57.95 (*0-19-511069-2*) OUP.

Organizational Restructuring in the Emergency Department. Nancy S. Donatelli et al. Ed. by Linda Greenberg. 1995. 102p. pap. text 35.00 (*0-935890-53-X*) Emerg Nurses IL.

Organizational Risk Factors for Job Stress. Ed. by Steven L. Sauter & Lawrence R. Murphy. 1995. LC 95-31599. 400p. pap. 19.95 (*1-55798-297-X*) Am Psychol.

Organizations: Structure & Behavior. Joseph A. Litterer. 3rd ed. 1980. LC 80-15645. (Series in Management). 638p. pap. text 37.50 (*0-471-07786-0*) Krieger.

Organizations & Practitioners of Natural Hygiene & a Brief History of Natural Hygiene. Arthur M. Baker. 1994. 24p. (Orig.). pap. 5.95 (*1-883989-03-5*) Self Hlth Care.

Organized Religion & Seniors' Mental Health. Anthony J. Blasi. 1999. LC 99-11322. 118p. 39.00 (*0-7618-1347-0*) U Pr of Amer.

Organizing a Healthcare Financial Services Division. Russell A. Caruana. 3rd ed. 1989. 170p. 50.00 (*0-930228-69-3*) Hlthcare Fin Mgmt.

Organizing a Healthcare Financial Services Division. Russell A. Caruana. 1989. 225p. 50.00 (*0-930228-36-7*, Irwn Prfssnl) McGraw-Hill Educ Grp.

Organizing a Support Group. 1992. (*0-944093-19-1*) Am Brain Tumor.

Organizing Community Resources in Sexuality Counseling & Family Planning for the Retarded: A Community Workers' Manual. Karin Rolett. 1976. pap. 3.00 (*0-89055-118-9*) Carolina Pop Ctr.

Organizing Your Practice Through Automation: Managing Information & Data. American Psychological Association Staff. 1996. (APA Practitioner's Toolbox Ser.). 72p. pap. 29.95 (*1-55798-359-3*) Am Psychol.

Organogenesis of the Kidney. Lauri Saxen. 1987. (Developmental & Cell Biology Monographs: No. 19). (Illus.). 184p. text 59.95 (*0-521-30152-1*) Cambridge U Pr.

Organometallics in Cancer Chemotherapy, Vol. 1. Ionel Haiduc & Cristian Silvestru. 1989. 264p. 171.00 (*0-8493-5867-1*, RC271) CRC Pr.

Organometallics in Cancer Chemotherapy, Vol. 2. Ionel Haiduc. 1990. 384p. 230.00 (*0-8493-5868-X*, RC271) CRC Pr.

Organometals & Organometalloids: Occurrence & Fate in the Environment. Ed. by F. E. Brinckman & J. Michael Bellama. 1978. LC 78-24316. (ACS Symposium Ser.: No. 82). 49.95 (*0-8412-0461-6*) Am Chemical.

Organon of Medicine. Samuel Hahnemann. Tr. by Jost Kunzli et al from GER. 6th ed. 1993. 270p. reprint ed. pap. 16.95 (*0-9636312-0-9*) Cooper Pub.

Organon of Medicine. Samuel Hahnemann. Tr. by Naude Kunzli & Pendleton. 1980. (Illus.). 16.95 (*0-87477-223-0*) Formur Intl.

Organon of the Medical Art. Samuel Hahnemann. Ed. by Wenda Brewster O'Reilly. Tr. by Steven Decker. unabr. ed. 2001. 432p. 55.00 (*1-889613-01-0*); pap. 29.95 (*1-889613-00-2*) Birdcage Bks.

Organonitrogen Stereodynamics, Set, Pts. I & II. Ed. by Joseph B. Lambert & Yoshito Takeuchi. 1992. (Methods in Stereochemical Analysis Ser.). 692p. text 195.00 (*1-56081-556-6*, Wiley-VCH) Wiley.

Organophosphorus Pesticides Criteria (Dose-Effect Relationships) for Organophosphorus Compounds. Commission of the European Communities. Ed. by R. Derache. 1977. pap. 100.00 (*0-08-021993-4*) Pergamon Repr GBR. *Dist:* Franklin.

Organotransition Metal Chemistry: Applications to Organic Synthesis. Ed. by S. G. Davies. 1983. (Organic Chemistry Ser.: Vol. 2). (Illus.). 428p. text 190.00 (*0-08-026202-3*); pap. text 48.00 (*0-08-030714-0*) Franklin (CRC Reprint).

Organs of Equilibrium & Orientation As a Control System. Ed. by M. Valentinuzzi. 1980. (Biomedical Engineering & Computation Ser.: Vol. 2). xiv, 194p. text 322.00 (*3-7186-0014-5*) Gordon & Breach.

Organversagen in der Intensivmedizin. Ed. by W. Behrendt et al. 1983. (Beitraege zur Intensiv und Notfallmedizin Ser.: Vol. 1). (Illus.). xii, 182p. pap. 55.00 (*3-8055-3794-8*) S Karger.

Orgaran Extending the Frontiers of Venous Thrombosis Prophylaxis. Ed. by Jack Hirsh. 1992. (Journal: Vol. 22, No. 2, 1992). (Illus.). 60p. pap. 47.00 (*3-8055-5626-8*) S Karger.

Orgasms Vol. 2: Homosexual Encounters from First Hand. Ed. by Winston Leyland. 1985. (Illus.). 192p. pap. 14.95 (*0-917342-12-7*) Leyland Pubns.

Oriental Materia Medica. Hong-yen Hsu et al. 1986. 932p. 59.95 (*0-941942-22-8*) Orient Heal Arts.

Oriental Medicine: A Modern Interpretation. Tr. by Kihyon Kim from KOR. 1996. (Illus.). xii, 318p. (Orig.). pap. 29.95 (*0-915649-00-4*) Yuin Univ Pr.

Oriental Medicine: An Illustrated Guide to the Asian Arts of Healing. J. Van Alphen & A. Aris. 1997. pap. 39.95 (*1-57062-317-1*) Shambhala Pubns.

Oriental Medicine & Cancer. Myung C. Kim. 1997. LC 96-92634. (Illus.). 350p. (Orig.). pap. 19.95 (*1-890016-00-4*, 96-1001) Seven Galaxy.

Oriental Stories As Tools in Psychotherapy. N. Peseschkian. rev. ed. 1985. Orig. Title: The Merchant & the Parrot. (Illus.). 166p. reprint ed. 16.00 (*0-387-15765-4*) Spr-Verlag.

Orientation Manual for Long-Term Care Facilities: A Program for Developing & Retaining Vital Employees. Joan M. Iannone & Margaret G. Bye. 2nd ed. 1993. LC 93-25297. 216p. 33.95 (*0-8261-8280-1*) Springer Pub.

Orientation to Health Services. Ruth M. Lee. 1978. LC 77-15094. (gr. 11-12). tchr. ed. (*0-672-61435-9*); pap. (*0-672-61434-0*) Macmillan.

Orientation to Home Care Nursing. Carolyn J. Humphrey & Paula Milone-Nuzzo. 1995. LC 95-21181. 326p. pap. 57.00 (*0-8342-0706-0*, 20706) Aspen Pub.

Orientation to Inquiry in a Reflective Professional Psychology. Lisa L. Hoshmand. 1994. LC 93-39602. (SUNY Series, Alternatives in Psychology). 307p. (C). text 59.50 (*0-7914-2115-5*); pap. text 19.95 (*0-7914-2116-3*) State U NY Pr.

Orientation to Language & Learning Disorders in Children. Mitchell R. Burkowsky. 1973. LC 75-176182. 304p. 16.50 (*0-87527-098-0*) Green.

Origin & Development of Psychoanalysis. Sigmund Freud. 1960. 108p. pap. 8.95 (*0-89526-919-8*) Regnery Pub.

Origin & Education of a Doctor. Brooks Ranney. 1990. LC 90-92020. (Illus.). 396p. pap. 12.00 (*0-9618939-2-3*) B Ranney.

Origin & Evolution of Life: On the Theory of Action, Reaction & Interaction of Energy. Henry F. Osborn. Ed. by Stephen Jay Gould. 1980. LC 79-8340. (History of Paleontology Ser.). (Illus.). reprint ed. lib. bdg. 36.95 (*0-405-12728-6*) Ayer.

Origin & Evolution of the Vertebrate Immune System. Ed. by L. Du Pasquier & G. W. Litman. 2000. (Current Topics in Microbiology & Immunology Ser.: Vol. 248). (Illus.). 352p. 199.00 (*3-540-66414-9*) Spr-Verlag.

Origin & Evolution of Viruses. Esteban Domingo et al. 1999. LC 99-62165. (Illus.). viii, 499p. 120.00 (*0-12-220360-7*) Acad Pr.

Origin & Function of Human Feelings. Victor S. Johnston. 1998. (*0-201-36084-5*) Addison-Wesley.

Origin & Treatment of Schizophrenic Disorders. Theodore Lidz. 1990. 158p. reprint ed. pap. 26.95 (*0-8236-8206-4*, BN 23895) Intl Univs Pr.

Origin of Adaptations. Verne Grant. LC 63-11695. (Illus.). 606p. 1971. pap. text 34.50 (*0-231-08648-2*); 1963. text 111.50 (*0-231-02529-7*) Col U Pr.

Origin of Cells: Causes & Cures of Cancer: Bone, Face, Lungs, Prostate. Betty Zorotovich. 1980. (Illus.). 254p. (Orig.). pap. 19.95 (*0-9605084-0-6*) McCall-Faure.

Origin of Consciousness in the Breakdown of the Bicameral Mind. Julian Jaynes. 2000. (Illus.). 512p. pap. 18.00 (*0-618-05707-2*, Mariner Bks) HM.

Origin of Human Characteristics & Behavior. Charles W. Stiehl. (Enlightenment of Man Ser.). 128p. pap. text 29.95 (*0-9701997-0-8*, I) Scholars Libr.

Origin of the Fittest: Essays on Evolution & the Primary Factors of Organic Evolution Edward D. Cope. 1974. LC 73-17813. (Natural Sciences in America Ser.). 1066p. reprint ed. 76.95 (*0-405-05729-6*) Ayer.

Original Bassini Operation for Inguinal Hernia: Centenary Edition. A. Chinaglia. 1988. 116p. text (*1-57235-038-5*) Piccin Nuova.

***Original Intelligence: The Architecture of the Human Mind.** David Premack & Ann Premack. 2002. (Illus.). 304p. 24.95 (*0-07-138142-2*) McGraw-Hill Trade.

Original Writings of Edward Bach. Judy Howard & John Ramsell. 1990. 109p. pap. (*0-85207-230-9*) C W Daniel GBR. *Dist:* Natl Bk Netwk.

Original Writings of Edward Bach. Nora Weeks & Victor Bullen. (Illus.). 216p. (Orig.). pap. 20.95 (*0-8464-4264-7*) Beekman Pubs.

Origins: Brain & Self Organization. Ed. by Karl H. Pribram. 1994. (INNS Series of Texts, Monographs, & Proceedings). 728p. text 135.00 (*0-8058-1786-7*) L Erlbaum Assocs.

M
N
O

Origins & Career Consequences of Sex Differences in High School Mathematics Achievement. Lauress L. Wise et al. 1979. 128p. pap. 13.00 (*0-89785-656-2*) Am Inst Res.

Origins & Components of Behaviorology. Stephen F. Ledoux. 1997. LC 96-84449. 368p. 50.00 (*1-882508-07-6*) ABCs.

Origins & Consequences of Obesity: Symposium No. 201. CIBA Foundation Staff. 1996. LC 96-24161. (CIBA Foundation Symposia Ser.). 288p. 128.00 (*0-471-96506-5*) Wiley.

Origins & Development of Medical Imaging. T. Doby & G. Alker. 1996. LC 96-8134. (Medical Humanities Ser.). (Illus.). 176p. (C). 29.95 (*0-8093-2010-X*) S Ill U Pr.

Origins & Development of Schizophrenia: Advances in Experimental Psychopathology. Ed. by Mark F. Lenzenweger & Robert H. Dworkin. 1998. LC 97-52362. 557p. 49.95 (*1-55798-497-2*, 431-8730) Am Psychol.

Origins & Evolution of Behavior Disorders: From Infancy to Adult Life. Stella Chess & Alexander Thomas. 1987. LC 87-7582. 344p. pap. 20.50 (*0-674-64477-8*) HUP.

Origins & History of Consciousness. Erich Neumann & R. F. C. Hull. 1995. (Bollingen Ser.: Vol. 42). (Illus.). 520p. pap. 19.95 (*0-691-01761-1*, Bollingen) Princeton U Pr.

Origins & Psychodynamics of Creativity: A Psychoanalytic Perspective. Jerome D. Oremland. 1997. LC 96-43194. 224p. 32.50 (*0-8236-3905-3*, 03905) Intl Univs Pr.

Origins & Rise of Associate Degree Nursing Education. Patricia T. Haase. 1990. LC 89-13405. 210p. (Orig.). (C). text 49.95 (*0-8223-0978-5*); pap. text 16.95 (*0-8223-0991-2*) Duke.

Origins of Action: Interdisciplinary & International Perspectives. Ed. by L. Oppenheimer & Jaan Valsiner. 1991. (Illus.). 265p. 98.00 (*0-387-97510-1*) Spr-Verlag.

Origins of Aggression. Willard W. Hartup & Jan De Wit. 1978. (Psychological Studies: No. 10). (*90-279-7673-2*) Mouton.

Origins of Anatomically Modern Humans. M. H. Nitecki & D. V. Nitecki. 1994. (Interdisciplinary Contributions to Archaeology Ser.). (Illus.). 356p. (C). 52.50 (*0-306-44675-8*, Plenum Trade) Perseus Pubng.

Origins of Group Psychoanalysis. Ed. by Harold I. Kaplan & Benjamin J. Sadock. 1986. (Modern Group Book Ser.: Vol. 1). 160p. 30.00 (*0-87668-077-5*) Aronson.

Origins of Health & Disease, Vol. 1. Peter W. Nathanielsz. Date not set. text (*0-7167-2999-7*); pap. text (*0-7167-3024-3*) W H Freeman.

Origins of Human Diet & Medicine: Chemical Ecology. Timothy Johns. 1996. LC 96-20505. (Arizona Studies in Human Ecology). 356p. pap. 19.95 (*0-8165-1687-1*) U of Ariz Pr.

Origins of Human Potential: Evolution, Development, & Psychology. Ken Richardson. 1998. LC 97-14925. 240p. (C). 78.95 (*0-415-17369-8*) Routledge.

Origins of Indian Psychology. N. Ross Reat. 1990. LC 90-48484. 400p. (C). pap. 25.00 (*0-89581-924-4*) Asian Humanities.

Origins of Intelligence: Infancy & Early Childhood. Ed. by Michael Lewis. 2nd ed. 1983. 552p. 47.50 (*0-306-41225-X*, Plenum Trade) Perseus Pubng.

Origins of Intelligence in Children. Jean Piaget. 1974. 418p. (Orig.). pap. 27.95 (*0-8236-8207-2*, 23900) Intl Univs Pr.

Origins of Knowledge & Imagination. Jacob Bronowski. 1979. LC 77-13209. (Country Ser.: Vol. 44). pap. 14.00 (*0-300-02409-6*) Yale U Pr.

Origins of Language Disorders: A Special Issue of Developmental Neuropsychology. Ed. by Donna J. Thal & Judith S. Reilly. 1997. 248p. pap. 20.00 (*0-8058-9853-0*) L Erlbaum Assocs.

Origins of Medical Attitudes Toward Drug Addiction in America: Eight Studies, 1791 to 1858, an Original Anthology. Ed. by Gerald N. Grob. 1981. LC 80-1203. (Addiction in America Ser.). lib. bdg. 37.95 (*0-405-13563-7*) Ayer.

Origins of Mendelism. Robert C. Olby. 1996. LC 84-2491. (Illus.). xviii, 328p. pap. text 18.00 (*0-226-62592-3*) U Ch Pr.

Origins of Mental Illness: Temperament, Deviance & Disorder. Gordon Claridge. 2nd ed. 1995. 293p. pap. 15.00 (*1-883536-01-4*, Malor Bks) ISHK.

Origins of Modern Treatment & the Education of Physically Handicapped Children: An Original Anthology. Ed. by William R. Phillips & Janet Rosenberg. 1980. LC 79-6010. (Physically Handicapped in Society Ser.). lib. bdg. 44.95 (*0-405-13102-X*) Ayer.

Origins of Neuroscience: A History of Explorations into Brain Function. Stanley Finger. 2001. (Illus.). 462p. pap. 39.95 (*0-19-514694-8*) OUP.

Origins of Nurturance: Developmental, Biological & Cultural Perspectives on Caregiving. Ed. by Alan Fogel & Gail F. Melson. 1986. 304p. (C). text 69.95 (*0-89859-643-2*) L Erlbaum Assocs.

Origins of Public Health in America: Selected Essays, 1820-1855. 1977. 19.95 (*0-405-03963-8*, 15715) Ayer.

Origins of Sex: Three Billion Years of Genetic Recombination. Lynn Margulis & Dorion Sagan. 1990. 259p. (Orig.). (C). pap. 22.00 (*0-300-04619-7*) Yale U Pr.

Origins of Sexuality & Homosexuality. Michael G. Shively. Ed. by John P. De Cecco. 1994. LC 84-22563. (Journal of Homosexuality Ser.: Vol. 9, Nos. 2 & 3). 174p. reprint ed. pap. text 19.95 (*0-918393-00-0*, Harrington Park) Haworth Pr.

Origins of Specialization in American Medicine: An Anthology of Sources. Ed. by Charles E. Rosenberg. 1989. (Medical Care in the United States Ser.: Vol. 13). 200p. reprint ed. lib. bdg. 15.00 (*0-8240-8342-3*) Garland.

Origins of the Modern Mind: Three Stages in the Evolution of Culture & Cognition. Merlin Donald. 1991. (Illus.). 448p. (C). text 38.50 (*0-674-64483-2*) HUP.

Origins of the State Mental Hospital in America: Six Documentary Studies, 1837-1856. 1979. LC 73-2409. (Mental Illness & Social Policy; the American Experience Ser.). 29.95 (*0-405-05219-7*) Ayer.

Origins of Thoracic Anaesthesia. William W. Mushin & Leslie Rendell-Baker. 1991. Orig. Title: Principles of Thoracic Anaesthesia. (Illus.). xx, 172p. reprint ed. (*0-9614932-2-4*) Wood Lib-Mus.

Orofacial Myology: Beyond Tongue Thrust. Robert M. Mason et al. 1994. 63p. pap. text 40.00 (*0-910329-81-8*, 0111904) Am Speech Lang Hearing.

Orofacial Pain: Guidelines for Assessment, Classification, & Management. American Academy of Orofacial Pain Staff. Ed. by Jeffrey P. Okeson. 1996. LC 96-4651. (Illus.). 300p. pap. text 28.00 (*0-86715-312-1*) Quint Pub Co.

Orphaned Adult: Confronting the Death of a Parent. Marc Angel. 1987. LC 86-20161. 162p. 26.95 (*0-89885-334-6*, Kluwer Acad Hman Sci) Kluwer Academic.

Orphans & Incentives: Developing Technology to Address Emerging Infections. Ed. by Polly F. Harrison & Joshua Lederberg. 1997. LC 98-101323. 112p. (C). text 22.00 (*0-309-05941-0*) Natl Acad Pr.

Ortho Asia. Larry D. Iversen. 3rd ed. 1986. 10.95 (*0-316-43434-5*, Little Brwn Med Div) Lppncott W & W.

Ortho-Bionomy: A Practical Manual. Kathy Kain. 1997. LC 97-19837. (Illus.). 194p. (Orig.). pap. 19.95 (*1-55643-250-X*) North Atlantic.

Orthodontic Cephalometry. Athanasiou. 1995. 143.00 (*0-7234-2045-9*) Mosby Inc.

Orthodontic Diagnosis. Thomas Rakosi & Irmtrud Jonas. 1993. LC 92-49147. (Color Atlas of Dental Medicine Ser.). 179.00 (*0-86577-450-1*) Thieme Med Pubs.

Orthodontic Materials: Scientific & Clinical Aspects. William A. Brantley & Theodore Eliades. 2000. LC 00-5519. (Illus.). 256p. 79.00 (*0-86577-929-5*) Thieme Med Pubs.

Orthodontic Treatment: Management of Unfavorable Sequelae. Ed. by J. A. McNamara, Jr. & Carroll-Ann Trotman. 1996. (Craniofacial Growth Ser.: Vol. 31). (Illus.). 437p. 69.00 (*0-929921-27-5*) UM CHGD.

Orthodontic Treatment: Outcome & Effectiveness. Ed. by Carroll-Ann Trotman & James A. McNamara. 1995. (Craniofacial Growth Ser.: Vol. 30). (Illus.). 387p. 59.00 (*0-929921-26-7*) UM CHGD.

Orthodontic Treatment Mechanics & the Pre-Adjusted Appliance. John C. Bennett. 1993. (Illus.). 265p. (C). (gr. 13). text 142.00 (*0-8151-0673-4*, 23026) Mosby Inc.

Orthodontic Treatment Mechanics & the Pre-Adjusted Appliance. John C. Bennett & Richard B. McLaughlin. 1993. (Illus.). 265p. (*84-8086-086-3*) Mosby-Doyma Libros ESP. *Dist:* Mosby Inc.

Orthodontics. Spiro J. Chaconas. 2nd ed. 1989. (Illus.). 356p. (*0-8151-1612-8*) Mosby Inc.

Orthodontics: Current Principles & Techniques. 3rd ed. 1999. (Illus.). 976p. text 169.00 (*0-8151-9363-7*, 31746) Mosby Inc.

Orthodontics No. 2: Current Principles & Techniques. Thomas M. Graber et al. 2nd ed. 1994. LC 93-42589. (Illus.). 976p. (C). (gr. 13). text 180.00 (*0-8016-6590-6*, 06590) Mosby Inc.

Orthodontics & Paediatric Dentistry. Declan T. Millett & Richard Welbury. 1999. LC 99-53892. (Colour Guide Ser.). (Illus.). 167p. (*0-443-06287-0*) Church.

Orthodontics in an Aging Society. W. Andrew Achenbaum et al. Ed. by David S. Carlson. 1989. LC 88-71195. (Craniofacial Growth Ser.: Vol. 22). (Illus.). 199p. 49.00 (*0-929921-18-6*) UM CHGD.

Orthodontics Picture Test Atlas. Claire Nightingale & Jonathan Sandy. 2000. (Illus.). 192p. pap. text (*0-7236-1072-X*) John Wright GBR. *Dist:* Buttrwrth-Heinemann.

Orthodontics with Fixed Appliances. Frans P. Van der Linden. Tr. by John F. Jefferys. 1997. LC 97-3037. (Van der Linden Orthodontic Ser.). (Illus.). 567p. pap. text 120.00 (*1-85097-044-0*) Quint Pub Co.

Orthodox & Complementary Medicine: An Alliance for a Changing World. William H. Kirkaldy-Willis & A. A. Swartz. 2000. LC 00-32887. (Illus.). ix, 203p. (C). pap. 18.95 (*1-55643-355-7*) North Atlantic.

Orthoepic Dictionary of the Russian Language. S. N. Borunova et al. Ed. by R. I. Avanesova. 4th ed. 1988. (RUS.). 704p. reprint ed. 21.95 (*0-8285-5375-0*) Firebird NY.

Orthogeriatrics: Comprehensive Orthopedic Care for the Elderly Patient. Raymond J. Newman. 1992. (Illus.). 224p. text 150.00 (*0-7506-1371-8*) Buttrwrth-Heinemann.

Orthognathic Surgery: A Synopsis of Basis Principles & Surgical Techniques. George Dimitroulis et al. 1994. (Illus.). 198p. pap. text 52.50 (*0-7236-1017-7*) Buttrwrth-Heinemann.

Orthogonal Polarization Spectral Imaging a New Tool for the Observation & Measurement of the Human Microcirculation: 16th Bodensee Symposium on Microcirculation, Lindau, September 1999. Ed. by K. Messmer. 2000. LC 00-63324. (Progress in Applied Microcirculation Ser.: Vol. 24). (Illus.). x, 121p. 111.50 (*3-8055-7065-1*) S Karger.

Orthographies & Reading: Perspectives from Cognitive Psychology, Neuropsychology, & Linguistics. Ed. by Leslie Henderson. 1984. 144p. text 29.95 (*0-86377-009-6*) L Erlbaum Assocs.

Orthokeratology: A Practical Approach. David Ruston et al. 2001. (Illus.). 224p. pap. 52.50 (*0-7506-4007-3*) Buttrwrth-Heinemann.

Orthokeratology Handbook. Todd D. Winkler & Rodger T. Kame. 1994. LC 94-33552. (Illus.). 113p. spiral bd. 44.99 (*0-7506-9595-1*) Buttrwrth-Heinemann.

Orthomolecular Treatment for Schizophrenia. Abram Hoffer. 1999. (Good Health Guides). 48p. pap. 3.95 (*0-87983-910-4*, 39104K, Keats Pubng) McGraw-Hill Trade.

Orthopaedics 2001. Clement B. Sledge. 2001. 83.00 (*0-8151-1465-6*, 31715) Mosby Inc.

Orthopaed Physiother. Tidswell. 1998. 29.95 (*0-7234-2592-2*) Mosby Inc.

Orthopaedic. Brotzma. 1996. text 130.00 (*0-8151-1011-1*, 29167) Mosby Inc.

Orthopaedic Allograft Surgery. Andrei A. Czitrom & Heinz Winkler. 1996. LC 96-15022. (Illus.). 300p. 225.00 (*3-211-82647-5*) Spr-Verlag.

Orthopaedic Anaesthesia. A. Loach. 2nd ed. 1994. 192p. (*0-340-56438-5*) E A GBR. *Dist:* OUP.

Orthopaedic Anesthesia. Ed. by Denise J. Wedel. 1992. (Illus.). 441p. text (*0-443-08873-X*) Church.

Orthopaedic Assessment & Treatment of the Geriatric Patient. Carole B. Lewis & Karen A. Knortz. 1993. (Illus.). 424p. (C). (gr. 13). text 69.00 (*0-8016-6512-4*, 06512) Mosby Inc.

Orthopaedic Board Review. Ed. by Timothy S. Loth. 1992. LC 92-22708. (Illus.). 648p. (C). (gr. 13). pap. text 62.00 (*0-8016-2740-0*, 02740) Mosby Inc.

Orthopaedic Case Studies. Nancy Gann. 1995. LC 97-43309. 176p. pap. 31.00 (*0-8342-1077-0*) PRO-ED.

Orthopaedic Decision Making. Robert W. Bucholz. 2nd ed. 1996. (Illus.). 480p. (C). (gr. 13). text 92.95 (*0-8016-7356-9*, 07356) Mosby Inc.

Orthopaedic Diagnosis: Clinical, Radiological & Pathological Coordinates. H. A. Sissons et al. 1984. (Illus.). 420p. 84.95 (*0-387-12795-X*) Spr-Verlag.

Orthopaedic Diagnosis & Management: A Guide to the Care of Orthopaedic Patients. B. S. Goldie & D. C. Dunn. 1991. (Illus.). 272p. pap. 44.95 (*0-632-03043-7*) Blackwell Sci.

Orthopaedic Dictionary. Stanley Hoppenfeld. 1993. 456p. spiral bd. 110.00 (*0-397-51311-9*) Lppncott W & W.

Orthopaedic Infection: Diagnosis & Treatment. Ramon B. Gustilo. 1989. text 142.00 (*0-7216-2341-7*) Saunders.

Orthopaedic Knowledge Update, Vol. 5. Ed. by James R. Kasser. 1996. (Illus.). 720p. pap. 100.00 (*0-89203-114-X*) Amer Acad Ortho Surg.

Orthopaedic Knowledge Update: Foot & Ankle. Glenn B. Pfeffer & Mark S. Mizel. 1994. LC 94-77974. (Illus.). 324p. pap. 115.00 (*0-89203-112-3*) Amer Acad Ortho Surg.

Orthopaedic Knowledge Update: Hip & Knee Reconstruction. Ed. by John J. Callaghan. 1995. LC 95-39517. 334p. pap. 50.00 (*0-89203-117-4*) Amer Acad Ortho Surg.

Orthopaedic Knowledge Update: Pediatrics. Pediatric Orthopaedic Soc of North Amer. Ed. by B. Stephens Richards. 1996. 352p. pap. 115.00 (*0-89203-159-X*) Amer Acad Ortho Surg.

Orthopaedic Knowledge Update: Shoulder & Elbow. American Shoulder and Elbow Surgeons Staff. Ed. by Tom R. Norris. 1997. LC 97-43921. (OKU Specialty Ser.). (Illus.). 424p. pap. 115.00 (*0-89203-170-0*) Amer Acad Ortho Surg.

Orthopaedic Knowledge Update: Spine. North American Spine Society Staff. Ed. by Steven R. Garfin & Alexander R. Vaccaro. 1997. LC 97-3482. (OKU Specialty Ser.). (Illus.). 356p. pap. 115.00 (*0-89203-169-7*) Amer Acad Ortho Surg.

Orthopaedic Knowledge Update: Trauma. Alan M. Levine. 1996. LC 00-22812. 350p. pap. 50.00 (*0-89203-126-3*) Amer Acad Ortho Surg.

Orthopaedic Management in Childhood. Ed. by P. F. Williams & W. G. Cole. 2nd ed. 1991. LC 91-33901. 377p. 119.95 (*0-442-31496-5*); (Illus.). 392p. (gr. 13). pap. 209.95 (*0-412-34990-6*) Chapman & Hall.

Orthopaedic Medicine: A Practical Approach. Monica Kesson et al. 1998. LC 97-26142. 480p. pap. text 60.00 (*0-7506-2543-0*) Buttrwrth-Heinemann.

Orthopaedic Neurology: A Diagnostic Guide to Neurologic Levels. Stanley Hoppenfeld. 1977. LC 65-2199. (Illus.). 131p. text 69.95 (*0-397-50368-7*, Lippnctt) Lppncott W & W.

Orthopaedic Nursing. Leona A. Mourad. 1994. LC 94-16955. (Plans of Care for Specialty Practice Ser.). 360p. (C). pap. 32.75 (*0-8273-5944-6*) Delmar.

Orthopaedic Nursing. Ann B. Maher et al. 2nd ed. 1998. LC 97-37502. (Illus.). 944p. text 99.00 (*0-7216-6952-2*) Saunders.

Orthopaedic Nursing. Edward C. Pinney. 6th ed. 1983. (Illus.). 368p. text 22.00 (*0-7216-0933-3*) Saunders.

Orthopaedic Nursing & Rehabilitation. Mary Powell. 9th ed. 1986. (Illus.). 640p. (*0-443-03238-6*) Church.

Orthopaedic Nursing Care Competencies: Adult Acute Care. Gail A. Bryant et al. Ed. by Susan Smith. 1999. 102p. pap. 45.00 (*1-892665-04-2*) Natl Assn Ortho Nurse.

Orthopaedic Nursing in Developing Countries. M. Powell. 1977. (WHO Regional Publications, South-East Asia Ser.: No. 3). 147p. pap. text 16.00 (*92-9022-103-8*) World Health.

Orthopaedic Pathology. Vincent Vigorita. 1999. LC 98-26248. 736p. text 279.00 (*0-7817-0040-X*) Lppncott W & W.

Orthopaedic Physical Examination. Bruce Reider. Ed. by Richard Lampert. 1999. LC 98-38025. (Illus.). xiv, 402p. text (*0-7216-7437-2*) Saunders.

Orthopaedic Physical Therapy. Ed. by Robert A. Donatelli & Michael J. Wooden. 2nd ed. 1993. (Illus.). 864p. text (*0-443-08835-7*) Church.

Orthopaedic Physical Therapy. Robert A. Donatelli. 3rd ed. 1999. LC 00-46611. (Illus.). xv, 656p. (C). text (*0-443-07993-5*) Church.

Orthopaedic Physician's Assistant Techniques. Charles E. Lambert & Donald Stone. 1975. LC 74-77819. (Allied Health Ser.). pap. 7.05 (*0-672-61388-3*, Bobbs) Macmillan.

Orthopaedic Radiography. Bruce W. Long & John A. Rafert. 1994. LC 94-14941. (Illus.). 560p. text 75.00 (*0-7216-6649-3*) Saunders.

Orthopaedic Rehabilitation. Ed. by Vernon L. Nickel & Michael J. Botte. 2nd ed. 1992. (Illus.). 939p. text (*0-443-08726-1*) Church.

Orthopaedic Sports Medicine, Set. Ed. by Jesse C. DeLee, Jr. & David Drez. 1993. (Illus.). 1888p. text 280.00 (*0-7216-2836-2*) Saunders.

Orthopaedic Surgery: Basic Science & Clinical Science. Juan J. Rodrigo. 1985. 770p. 80.00 (*0-316-75369-6*, Little Brwn Med Div) Lppncott W & W.

Orthopaedic Surgical Pathology. Forest. 1998. (C). text (*0-443-05540-8*) Church.

Orthopaedic Testing: A Rational Approach to Diagnosis. Steven L. Kleinfield & Hanet A. Gerard. 1993. (Illus.). 688p. text (*0-443-08876-4*) Church.

Orthopaedic Trauma Protocols. Ed. by Sigvard T. Hansen, Jr. & Marc F. Swiontkowski. 1993. LC 92-48788. 416p. text 179.00 (*0-88167-994-1*) Lppncott W & W.

Orthopaedics. Fitzger. 2002. text 225.00 (*0-7234-2394-6*) Saunders.

***Orthopaedics.** Robert Fitzgerald et al. 2001. 1776p. 175.00 (*0-323-01318-X*) Mosby Inc.

Orthopaedics. Frank V. Aluisio et al. 2nd ed. 1998. LC 97-41655. (House Officer Ser.). (Illus.). 400p. 29.95 (*0-683-18213-7*) Lppncott W & W.

Orthopaedics. Hooper. 2nd ed. 1998. (Orig.). (C). pap. text 16.95 (*0-443-05888-1*) Saunders.

Orthopaedics Ed. by George Bentley & Robert B. Greer, III. 4th ed. 1993. (Rob & Smith's Operative Surgery Ser.). (Illus.). 1285p. (C). 754.95 (*0-7506-1029-8*) Chapman & Hall.

Orthopaedics. George Bentley & Robert B. Greer, III. 4th ed. 1993. (Rob & Smith's Operative Surgery Ser.). (Illus.). 1312p. pap. 125.00 (*0-7506-1680-6*) Chapman & Hall.

Orthopaedics, Vol. 2. Bentley & Greer. 4th ed. 1991. (Rob & Smith's Operative Surgery Ser.). 615p. pap. text 247.50 (*0-7506-1490-0*) Buttrwrth-Heinemann.

Orthopaedics. Ed. by Bentley & Greer. 4th ed. 1993. (Rob & Smith's Operative Surgery Ser.). (Illus.). 1285p. (C). (gr. 13). pap. 190.95 (*0-412-53790-7*, Chap & Hall NY) Chapman & Hall.

Orthopaedics: A Problem Solving Approach for Physiotherapists. K. Percival et al. 1998. (Illus.). 288p. (C). pap. (*0-443-05074-0*) Church.

Orthopaedics: A Review Book. Edward V. Craig. 2001. text 99.00 (*0-683-30243-4*) Lppncott W & W.

Orthopaedics: A Study Guide. Ed. by Jeffrey M. Spivak & Joseph D. Zuckerman. 1999. (Illus.). 936p. pap., stu. ed. 115.00 (*0-07-060355-3*) McGraw-Hill Prof.

Orthopaedics: Essentials of Diagnosis & Treatment. Ed. by Charles R. Clark & Michael Bonfiglio. 1994. (Illus.). text (*0-443-08807-1*) Church.

Orthopaedics: PreTest Self-Assessment & Review. Ed. by Frank C. Wilson et al. 1996. LC 95-21405. (Pretest Specialty Level Ser.). (Illus.). 314p. pap. 48.00 (*0-07-052076-3*) McGraw-Hill Prof.

Orthopaedics: Principles of Basic & Clinical Science. Felix Bronner & Richard V. Worrell. 1999. LC 99-20513. 312p. 79.95 (*0-8493-9237-3*) CRC Pr.

Orthopaedics: Problems in Primary Care. Randall E. Marcus. Ed. by Melanie C. Karaffa. 1991. (Illus.). 400p. (C). text 49.95 (*1-878487-33-7*, 5907M) Practice Mgmt Info.

Orthopaedics & Trauma. Ronald L. Huckstep & Eugene Sherry. 1994. LC 94-5218. (Color Guide Ser.). 158p. pap. text (*0-443-04980-7*) Church.

Orthopaedics & Trauma: An Illustrated Colour Text. Ronald K. McRae & A. W. Kinninmonth. 1997. LC 96-39211. (Illus.). 152p. pap. text (*0-443-05135-6*) Church.

Orthopaedics in General Practice. Andrew Carr & Anthony Hamden. 1997. LC 96-37668. (Illus.). 240p. pap. text 52.50 (*0-7506-2219-9*) Buttrwrth-Heinemann.

Orthopaedics in Primary Care. Gerald G. Steinberg et al. 3rd ed. 1998. LC 98-41147. (Illus.). 423p. text 79.95 (*0-683-30258-2*) Lppncott W & W.

Orthopaedics Two Thousand & Two. Sledge Clement. 2002. 83.00 (*0-8151-1555-5*, 31716) Mosby Inc.

Orthopedia: Spine, Back, & Neck. 1991. (Illus.). 928p. lib. bdg. 149.00 (*1-879952-01-7*) Inst Spine.

Orthopedic - Neurology Words & Phrases, 1994: A Quick Reference Guide. 1994. LC 94-176954. 630p. pap. 40.00 (*0-934385-55-6*) Hlth Prof Inst.

Orthopedic & Sports Physical Therapy. Terry Malone. Ed. by Thomas G. Mcpoil. 3rd ed. 1996. (Illus.). 656p. (C). (gr. 13). text 64.00 (*0-8151-5886-6*, 24514) Mosby Inc.

Orthopedic & Sports Physical Therapy. Terry Malone et al. 3rd ed. 1996. (Illus.). 656p. tchr. ed. (*0-8151-8908-7*) Mosby Inc.

Orthopedic Boards Review No. II: A Case Study Approach. Ed. by Timothy S. Loth. 1995. (Illus.). 480p. (C). (gr. 13). pap. text 80.00 (*0-8151-5322-8*, 24693) Mosby Inc.

Orthopedic Disability & Expert Testimony. Ed. by Harold Goodman. 4th ed. 1993. (Personal Injury Library). 254p. 160.00 (*0-471-59231-5*) Wiley.

Orthopedic Diseases of the Joints of the Dog. Robert L. Leighton. 2000. 230p. 22.50 (*1-58692-029-4*) Courier Custom.

Orthopedic Flash. Carole Lewis et al. 1997. 725p. text 249.00 (*0-9643582-4-7*) Learn Pubns.

Orthopedic Imaging: Techniques & Applications. Ed. by A. M. Davies et al. 1998. LC 97-49118. (Medical Radiology Ser.). (Illus.). 395p. 215.00 (*3-540-63187-9*) Spr-Verlag.

Orthopedic Infection. Ed. by David L. Schlossberg. 1988. (Clinical Topics in Infectious Disease Ser.). (Illus.). 182p. 115.00 (*0-387-96719-2*) Spr-Verlag.

Orthopedic Management of Cerebral Palsy. Eugene E. Bleck. 2nd ed. 1991. LC 65-80559. (Clinics in Developmental Medicine Ser.: No. 99-100). (Illus.). 497p. (C). text (*0-521-41218-8*) Mc Keith Pr GBR. *Dist:* Cambridge U Pr.

Orthopedic, Neurological & Chiropractic Physical Examinations. Barry Creighton. 1986. (Illus.). 80p. pap. 39.50 (*0-911110-57-7*, MICHIE) LEXIS Pub.

Orthopedic Nurse. Jack Rudman. (Certified Nurse Examination Ser.: Vol. 27). 47.97 (*0-8373-6177-X*); 1997. pap. 27.95 (*0-8373-6127-3*) Nat Learn.

Orthopedic Pathology. Michael J. Klein. Ed. by Debra S. Heller. 1995. (Blackwell Pathology CD-ROM Ser.: Vol. II). 299.95 (*0-86542-473-X*) Blackwell Sci.

Orthopedic Pathology. Schiller. 1997. text (*0-7216-4355-8*) Saunders.

Orthopedic Pathophysiology in Diagnosis & Treatment. Jonathan Cohen et al. 1989. (Illus.). 526p. text (*0-443-08070-4*) Church.

Orthopedic Pearls. Leon Benson & Jeffrey Visotsky. 1999. LC 99-14699. (Illus.). 402p. (C). pap. text 23.95 (*0-8036-0185-9*) Davis Co.

Orthopedic Physical Assessment. David J. Magee. 3rd ed. 1997. LC 96-41121. (Illus.). 815p. text 51.95 (*0-7216-6290-0*) Saunders.

Orthopedic Radiology. Adam Greenspan. 1988. LC 65-40140. (Illus.). 448p. text 210.00 (*0-397-44660-8*, Lippnctt) Lppncott W & W.

Orthopedic Radiology. Barbara Weissman. 2nd ed. 1999. text (*0-7216-3791-4*) Saunders.

Orthopedic Radiology: A Practical Approach. Adam Greenspan. 2nd ed. 1995. 728p. 236.50 (*0-563-75023-5*); 3rd ed. 1999. LC 99-10897. 976p. text 225.00 (*0-7817-1589-X*) Lppncott W & W.

Orthopedic Rehabilitation Review. Timothy S. Loth & Carolyn T. Wadsworth. 1997. LC 00-501974. (Illus.). 440p. (C). (gr. 13). pap. text 46.95 (*0-8151-2526-7*, 31050) Mosby Inc.

Orthopedic Rehabilitation Science: Principles for Clinical Management. Katie Lundon. 1999. LC 99-39419. (Illus.). 224p. pap. text 54.99 (*0-7506-7155-6*) Buttrwrth-Heinemann.

Orthopedic Research Procedures & Techniques Pt. 2: A Special Issue of the Journal Automedica. Ed. by M. H. Krag & M. H. Pope. 1989. 12p. text 306.00 (*0-677-25800-3*) Gordon & Breach.

Orthopedic Secrets. David E. Brown & Randall D. Neumann. 2nd rev. ed. 1999. LC 99-11421. (Secrets Ser.). (Illus.). 400p. pap. 39.95 (*1-56053-302-1*) Hanley & Belfus.

Orthopedic Sports Medicine Delee. 1993. text 320.00 (*0-7216-5602-1*) Harcourt.

Orthopedic Sports Medicine Delee. 1993. text 350.00 (*0-7216-4194-6*) Saunders.

Orthopedic Surgery: Elastic Compression. H. F. Boggiano. 2nd rev. ed. 1996. (Illus.). 650p. 85.00 (*0-9654469-0-5*) H F Boggiano.

Orthopedic Surgery! The Essentials. Mark E. Baratz et al. 1999. LC 98-45052. (Illus.). 992p. 99.00 (*0-86577-779-9*) Thieme Med Pubs.

Orthopedic Surgery Manual. Association of Surgical Technologists. 2000. (Allied Health Ser.). pap. 40.00 net. (*0-7668-1128-X*) Delmar.

Orthopedic Therapy of the Shoulder. Ed. by Martin J. Kelley & William A. Clark. 2nd ed. 1994. LC 94-28214. (Illus.). 480p. text 52.95 (*0-397-54830-3*) Lppncott W & W.

Orthopedic Transfusion Therapy. Ed. by Mark E. Brecher & Leigh C. Jefferies. 1995. LC 95-44616. (Illus.). 107p. (C). 40.00 (*1-56395-046-4*) Am Assn Blood.

Orthopedics. 1983. (Medical Ser.). (Illus.). 138p. pap. text 12.95 (*0-935920-06-4*, Ntl Pubs Blck) P-H.

Orthopedics. Geoffrey Hooper. 2nd ed. 1997. LC 96-29577. (Colour Guide Ser.). (*0-443-05806-7*) Harcrt Hlth Sci Grp.

Orthopedics. P. H. Regents. 3rd ed. 1993. 130p. pap. 20.17 (*0-13-156845-0*) P-H.

Orthopedics: A History & Iconography. Leonard F. Peltier. 1993. (Illus.). 305p. 225.00 (*0-930405-47-1*) Norman SF.

Orthopedics: An Essential Slide Collection. Michael M. Lewis & Lon Weiner. 1990. 95p. (gr. 13). text (*0-397-46469-X*, GM0087) Gower-Mosby.

Orthopedics in Infancy & Childhood. G. C. Lloyd-Roberts & John A. Fixsen. 2nd ed. 1990. 226p. pap. text 180.00 (*0-7506-1030-1*) Buttrwrth-Heinemann.

Orthopedist's Guide to Plain Film Imaging. Helene Pavlov. 1999. (Illus.). 336p. 65.00 (*0-86577-717-9*) Thieme Med Pubs.

Orthopsychiatry: Index of Modern Information. Peter J. Kasnevitch. 1990. LC 88-47972. 150p. 47.50 (*1-55914-028-3*); pap. 44.50 (*1-55914-029-1*) ABBE Pubs Assn.

Orthoptic Assessment & Management. David Stidwell. 1998. LC 97-51262. (Modern Optometry Ser.). pap. 85.00 (*0-632-05012-8*) Blackwell Sci.

Orthoptics: A Syllabus of Ocular Motility. Ed. by Paula M. Edelman. 2nd ed. 1992. LC 92-17635. (Illus.). (*1-56055-023-6*) Am Acad Ophthal.

Orthostatic Disorders of the Circulation: Mechanisms, Manifestations & Treatment. D. H. Streeten. 1986. LC 86-18748. (Illus.). 286p. (C). text 89.50 (*0-306-42322-7*, Kluwer Plenum) Kluwer Academic.

Orthotics: A Comprehensive Clinical Approach. Joan E. Edelstein & Jan Bruckner. 2001. 300p. (C). text 39.00 (*1-55642-416-7*) SLACK Inc.

Orthotics: Clinical Practice & Rehabilitation Technology. Ed. by John B. Redford et al. 1995. LC 95-35492. 337p. pap. text (*0-443-08992-2*) Church.

Orthotics & Prosthetics in Rehabilitation. Michelle M. Lusardi & Caroline Nielsen. 2000. 720p. text 99.00 (*0-7506-9807-1*) Buttrwrth-Heinemann.

Orthotics in Functional Rehabilitation of the Lower Limb. Deborah A. Nawoczenski & Marcia E. Epler. 1997. LC 96-25618. (Illus.). 315p. text 47.00 (*0-7216-6134-3*) Saunders.

Orthotics in Neurologic Rehabilitation. Ed. by Mindy L. Aisen. 1992. 160p. pap. 34.95 (*0-939957-47-7*) Demos Medical.

Orthotics in Rehabilitation: Splinting the Hand & Body. Pat McKee et al. 1998. LC 97-48427. (Illus.). 340p. pap. text 32.95 (*0-8036-0351-7*) Davis Co.

Orthotics, Prosthetics & Mobility Aids. 1994. lib. bdg. 250.00 (*0-8490-8406-7*) Gordon Pr.

Orthpaedic Knowledge Update: Sports Medicine. Ed. by Letha Y. Griffin. 1994. LC 94-77973. (Illus.). 400p. pap. 50.00 (*0-89203-113-1*) Amer Acad Ortho Surg.

OSCEs & MCQs in Obstetrics & Gynaecology: A Survival Guide. Contrib. by Joan Pitkin et al. 1999. LC 98-40977. (Illus.). vii, 404p. (*0-7020-2199-7*) Saunders Ents.

OSCE's in Paediatrics. A. Khan & H. Pandya. 1998. (Illus.). 192p. pap. (*0-443-05728-1*) Church.

Oscillatory Event-Related Brain Dynamics. C. Pantev et al. 1995. LC 94-48769. (NATO Advanced Science Institutes Ser.: Vol. 271). (Illus.). 478p. (C). text 130.00 (*0-306-44894-7*, Kluwer Plenum) Kluwer Academic.

OSHA & State Employee Hazard Communications Program, Vols. 1-2. H. G. Miller et al. Ed. by Knowles-McFarland. 1985. 622p. 395.00 (*0-940394-16-2*) Labelmaster.

OSHA & the Politics of Health Regulation: Organizational & Political Changes in a Regulatory Agency. Ed. by David P. McCaffrey. 1982. LC 82-11201. 210p. 42.50 (*0-306-41050-8*, Plenum Trade) Perseus Pubng.

OSHA Bloodborne Pathogens Exposure Control Plan. Neal Langerman. 1992. 382p. lib. bdg. 120.00 (*0-87371-802-X*, L802) Lewis Pubs.

OSHA Laboratory Standard Implementation Guide. Leo C. Hearn, Jr. et al. 1991. 152p. lib. bdg. 115.00 (*0-87371-532-2*, L532) Lewis Pubs.

OSHA Regulated Hazardous Substances: Health, Toxicity, Economic & Technological Data, Set. Occupational Safety and Health Administration Staff. 1990. LC 90-6751. (Illus.). 2294p. 195.00 (*0-8155-1240-6*) Noyes.

OSHA Regulations & Guidelines: A Guide for Health Care Providers. Ronald P. Neilsen. 1999. LC 99-11382. (Allied Health Ser.). 304p. (C). pap. text 43.95 (*0-7668-0478-X*) Delmar.

OSHA's Bloodborne Pathogen Procedures Made Cost Effective: FED-OSHA Mandated Exposure Control for Occupational Exposure Control to Bloodborne Pathogens. Med-Facts, Inc. Staff. rev. ed. 1993. 118p. stu. ed. 495.00 (*1-884006-25-6*) Med-Facts.

OSHA's Bloodborne Pathogens Standard: Compliance in Clinical Laboratory. Peggy P. Luebbert. 1992. 50.00 incl. VHS (*0-89189-349-0*) Am Soc Clinical.

OSHA's Final Bloodborne Pathogens Standard: Implications for Health Care Environmental Services. Pamela L. Blyth. 1993. 96p. (Orig.). pap. 40.00 (*0-87258-632-4*, 057014) Am Hospital.

OSHA's New Ergonomic Standard: A Cost-Effective Guide to Complying with the November 2000 Final Rule. Deborah Kearney. 2001. LC 00-54832. 184p. 95.00 (*0-86587-718-1*, 718) Gov Insts.

Osiris Complex: Case Studies in Multiple Personality Disorder. Colin A. Ross. 1994. LC 93-95100. (C). 470p. pap. 17.95 (*0-8020-7358-1*); 570p. text 50.00 (*0-8020-2858-6*) U of Toronto Pr.

Oski's Pediatrics: Principles & Practice. Julia A. McMillan & Frank A. Oski. 3rd ed. 1999. LC 98-50639. 2,848p. text 110.00 (*0-7817-1618-7*) Lppncott W & W.

Osler, & Other Papers. William S. Thayer. 1977. LC 78-84342. (Essay Index Reprint Ser.). 25.95 (*0-8369-1111-3*) Ayer.

Oslerian Pathology: An Assessment & Annotated Atlas of Museum Specimens. Intro. by Alvin E. Rodin. 1981. (Illus.). 250p. (C). 25.00 (*0-87291-144-6*) Coronado Pr.

Osler's Web: Inside the Labyrinth of the Chronic Fatigue Syndrome Epidemic. Hillary Johnson. 2000. 720p. reprint ed. text 30.00 (*0-7881-6980-7*) DIANE Pub.

Osmosis & Dialysis. Gayle N. Sauer & Conrad L. Stanitski. 1995. (Modular Laboratory Program in Chemistry Ser.). 12p. (C). pap. text 1.50 (*0-87540-454-5*, PROP 454-5) Chem Educ Res.

Osseo-Integrated Implants Vol. I: Basics, Materials, & Joint Replacements. Ed. by Gunther Heimke. 1990. 208p. 210.00 (*0-8493-5958-9*, RD132) CRC Pr.

Osseo-Integrated Implants Vol. II: Implants in Oral & Ent Surgery. Ed. by Gunther Heimke. 1990. 344p. 239.00 (*0-8493-5959-7*, RD132) CRC Pr.

Osseointegrated Dental Technology. Graham E. White. 1993. (Illus.). 233p. text 100.00 (*1-85097-031-9*, B8809) Quint Pub Co.

Osseointegration & Occlusal Rehabilitation. Sumiya Hobo et al. 1989. (Illus.). 478p. text 158.00 (*4-87417-274-1*) Quint Pub Co.

Osseointegration in Craniofacial Reconstruction. B. R. Anemark. Ed. by Per-Ingvar Branemark & Dan E. Tolman. 1998. LC 98-21397. (Illus.). 337p. text 156.00 (*0-86715-337-7*) Quint Pub Co.

Osseointegration in Dentistry: An Introduction. Ed. by Philip Worthington et al. 1994. LC 94-5464. (Illus.). 120p. pap. text 28.00 (*0-86715-281-8*) Quint Pub Co.

Osseointegration in Oral Rehabilitation: An Introductory Textbook. Ed. by Ignace Naert et al. 1993. (Illus.). 211p. (Orig.). pap. text 45.00 (*1-85097-030-0*, B8807) Quint Pub Co.

Osseointegration in Skeletal Reconstruction & Joint Replacement: 2nd International Workshop on Osseointegration in Skeletal Reconstruction & Joint Replacement, Rancho Santa Fe, California, October 27-29, 1994. Ingvar Branemark et al. 1997. LC 96-51486. 232p. pap. text 98.00 (*0-86715-325-3*) Quint Pub Co.

Osseous Development in the Hand As an Index of Skeletal Development. Charles D. Flory. 1936. (Society for Research in Child Development Monographs: Vol. 1, No. 3). 25.00 (*0-527-01488-5*) Periodicals Srv.

Osseous Reconstruction of the Maxilla & the Mandible: Surgical Techniques Using Titanium Mesh & Bone Mineral. Philip J. Boyne & Michael Peetz. 1996. LC 96-26147. (Illus.). 116p. text 68.00 (*0-86715-319-9*) Quint Pub Co.

Osteoarthritis. Ed. by Kenneth D. Brandt et al. 1998. LC 97-11747. (Illus.). 612p. (C). text 129.50 (*0-19-262735-X*) OUP.

Osteoarthritis: A Step-by-Step Sucess Story to Show Others They Can Help Themselves. Fred L. Savage. 1989. 96p. pap. 11.95 (*0-88268-086-2*) Station Hill Pr.

Osteoarthritis: Clinical & Experimental Aspects. Ed. by J. P. Pelletier et al. 1999. LC 98-33430. (Illus.). 539p. pap. 99.00 (*3-540-65127-6*) Spr-Verlag.

Osteoarthritis: Current Research & Prospects for Pharmacological Intervention. R. G. Russell & P. A. Dieppe. 1991. 232p. (C). (*1-85271-093-4*) IBC Tech Srvs GBR. *Dist:* St Mut.

***Osteoarthritis: Diagnosis & Medical/Surgical Management.** Roland W. Moskowitz et al. 3rd ed. (Illus.). 592p. 175.00 (*0-7216-8439-4*) Saunders.

Osteoarthritis: Fundamentals & Strategies for Joint-Preserving Treatment. Ed. by J. Grifka & D. J. Ogilvie-Harris. 2000. LC 99-58599. (Illus.). 240p. 89.00 (*3-540-66309-6*) Spr-Verlag.

Osteoarthritis: Public Health Implications for an Aging Population. Ed. by David Hamerman. 1997. LC 96-45259. 272p. 47.00 (*0-8018-5561-6*) Johns Hopkins.

Osteoarthritis in Rhesus Monkeys & Gibbons: A Locomotor Model of Joint Degeneration. C. J. DeRousseau. 1988. (Contributions to Primatology Ser.: Vol. 25). (Illus.). xiv, 146p. 83.50 (*3-8055-4700-5*) S Karger.

Osteochondral Allografts. Gary E. Friedlander et al. 1983. 403p. 120.00 (*0-316-29346-6*, Little Brwn Med Div) Lppncott W & W.

Osteolathyrismus: Quantitativ-Morphologische Untersuchungen der Experimentellen Skeletterkrankungen bei der Ratte. H. Plenk. Ed. by G. Wolf-Heidegger. 1976. (Bibliotheca Anatomica Ser.: No. 14). (Illus.). 104p. 41.75 (*3-8055-2306-8*) S Karger.

Osteology for Radiographers. Shillingford. 1985. (Illus.). 144p. pap. 29.95 (*0-632-01349-4*) Blackwell Sci.

Osteonecrosis: Etiology, Diagnosis, & Treatment. American Orthopaedic Association Staff. Ed. by James R. Urbaniak & John P. Jones, Jr. 1998. LC 97-41931. (Illus.). 453p. 120.00 (*0-89203-174-3*) Amer Acad Ortho Surg.

***Osteopathic Approach to Children.** Jane Carreiro. 2001. (Illus.). 320p. (*0-443-06360-5*) Church GBR. *Dist:* Saunders.

Osteopathic Approach to Diagnosis & Treatment. Eileen Digiovanna. 2nd ed. 1996. LC 96-41775. 512p. text 79.95 (*0-397-51581-2*, Lippnctt) Lppncott W & W.

Osteopathic Assessment: Anatomical Motion Testing. Caroline Stone. 2002. 192p. pap. 45.00 (*0-7506-4674-8*) Buttrwrth-Heinemann.

Osteopathic Athletic Health Care: Principles & Practice. W. Llewellyn McKone. 1996. LC 96-86087. (Illus.). pap. 43.95 (*0-412-59090-5*) Chapman & Hall.

Osteopathic Considerations in Systemic Dysfunction. Michael Kuchera & William Kuchera. 1996. (C). (*1-57074-348-7*) Greyden Pr.

Osteopathic Diagnosis. Emanuel Sammut & Patrick Searle-Barnes. 1998. (Illus.). 272p. pap. (*0-7487-3296-9*) Nelson Thornes GBR. *Dist:* Intl Spec Bk, Trans-Atl Phila.

Osteopathic Mechanics. Edythe F. Ashmore. 1996. 237p. reprint ed. pap. 22.00 (*0-7873-0043-8*) Hlth Research.

Osteopathic Mechanics: A Textbook. E. F. Ashmore. 1991. lib. bdg. 79.95 (*0-8490-4104-X*) Gordon Pr.

Osteopathic Medicine: Philosophy, Principles & Practice. W. Llewellyn McKone. 2001. LC 00-48550. (Illus.). 272p. pap. 83.95 (*0-632-05263-5*) Blackwell Sci.

Osteopathic Principles in Practice. Michael Kuchera & William Kuchera. 1996. (C). (*1-57074-347-9*) Greyden Pr.

Osteopathy: Index of New Developments & Modern Research. Stanley X. Garrett. 1993. 200p. 47.50 (*1-55914-514-5*); pap. 44.50 (*1-55914-515-3*) ABBE Pubs Assn.

Osteopathy (Original Osteopathic Moves As Taught by Still) Frederick W. Collins. 9th ed. 1997. 11p. reprint ed. spiral bd. 8.00 (*0-7873-0191-4*) Hlth Research.

Osteopathy Research & Practice. A. T. Still. 1992. LC 92-70915. 293p. (C). reprint ed. text 34.95 (*0-939616-14-9*) Eastland.

Osteoporose: Grundlagen, Diagnostik und Therapiekonzepte. Ed. by H. Broell & M. A. Dambacher. 1995. (Illus.). viii, 314p. 259.25 (*3-8055-6192-X*) S Karger.

Osteoporosis. Annemarie Colbin. 1999. 256p. pap. 23.95 (*0-525-94286-6*) NAL.

Osteoporosis. Ed. by Steven Cummings. 2001. (Women's Health Ser.). (Illus.). pap. text 35.00 (*0-943126-95-9*) Amer Coll Phys.

Osteoporosis. Ed. by Stanley G. Korenman & Robert Marcus. 1999. LC 99-34891. (Atlas of Clinical Endocrinology Ser.: Vol. 3). (Illus.). 198p. 131.95 (*0-632-04403-9*) Blackwell Sci.

Osteoporosis. Ed. by Robert Marcus et al. 1996. LC 95-33703. (Illus.). 1373p. text 149.95 (*0-12-470860-9*) Acad Pr.

Osteoporosis. Ed. by Robert Marcus. 1994. (Illus.). 352p. 99.95 (*0-86542-266-4*) Blackwell Sci.

Osteoporosis. Ed. by David J. Sartoris. 1996. (Illus.). 432p. text 175.00 (*0-8247-9507-5*) Dekker.

Osteoporosis. Ed. by John C. Stevenson & Robert Lindsay. 1999. (Illus.). 402p. (*0-412-48870-1*) E A GBR. *Dist:* OUP.

Osteoporosis. Woodland Publishing Staff. 1997. (Woodland Health Ser.). 32p. pap. 3.95 (*1-58054-006-6*) Woodland UT.

***Osteoporosis.** J. E. Compston & Rosen. 3rd ed. 2002. (Fast Facts Ser.). (Illus.). 64p. pap. (*1-899541-54-3*) Health Pr GBR. *Dist:* JAMCO Dist.

Osteoporosis: A Guide to Diagnostic & Treatment. Ed. by H. Broell & M. Dambacher. 1996. (Rheumatology Ser.: Vol. 18). (Illus.). viii, 292p. 259.25 (*3-8055-5624-1*) S Karger.

Osteoporosis: A Natural Approach to Prevention. Westeron Stephens, III. 1995. 57p. 12.95 (*0-9644215-1-8*) W Stephens.

Osteoporosis: A New Concept in Treatment & Prevention. John Papalia. 2000. (Illus.). 64p. spiral bd. 17.00 (*0-9704323-1-3*) Amer Bone.

Osteoporosis: A Source Guide. 1991. lib. bdg. 69.95 (*0-8490-4903-2*) Gordon Pr.

Osteoporosis: A Woman Doctor's Guide: Prevent & Reverse Bone Loss at Any Age. Yvonne R. Sherrer & Robin K. Levinson. 2001. (Illus.). 208p. mass mkt. 6.99 (*1-57566-578-6*, Knsington) Kensgtn Pub Corp.

Osteoporosis: An Exercise Guide. Margie Bissinger. 1998. (Illus.). 27p. pap., wbk. ed. 9.95 (*0-9668792-0-1*) Workfit Consult.

Osteoporosis: Diagnosis & Management. Pierre J. Meunier. 1997. 296p. (*1-85317-412-2*) Martin Dunitz GBR. *Dist:* Mosby Inc.

Osteoporosis: Diagnostic & Therapeutic Principles. Ed. by Clifford J. Rosen. 1996. (Current Clinical Practice Ser.). (Illus.). 312p. 69.50 (*0-89603-374-0*) Humana.

Osteoporosis: Etiology, Diagnosis & Management. Ed. by B. Lawrence Riggs & L. Joseph Melton, III. 2nd ed. 1995. LC 95-7020. 544p. text 139.00 (*0-7817-0275-5*) Lppncott W & W.

Osteoporosis: Genetics, Prevention & Treatment. John S. Adams & Barbara P. Lukert. 1999. LC 98-46837. (Endocrine Updates Ser.). 308p. (*0-7923-8366-4*) Kluwer Academic.

Osteoporosis: Medical Blunders & Treatment Strategies. William N. Taylor. 1996. LC 96-21046. 117p. per. 25.00 (*0-7864-0229-6*) McFarland & Co.

Osteoporosis: Nutritional Aspects. Ed. by A. P. Simopoulos & C. Galli. 1993. (World Review of Nutrition & Dietetics Ser.: Vol. 73). (Illus.). xii, 108p. 139.25 (*3-8055-5751-5*) S Karger.

Osteoporosis: Pathogenesis & Management. R. M. Francis. 1990. (C). text 89.50 (*0-7923-8933-6*) Kluwer Academic.

Osteoporosis: Pathophysiology & Clinical Management. Ed. by Eric S. Orwoll & Michael Bliziotes. 2001. (Contemporary Endocrinology Ser.). 425p. 99.50 (*0-89603-933-1*) Humana.

Osteoporosis: Pocketbook Edition. Woolf. 2nd ed. 2000. (*1-85317-678-8*) Martin Dunitz GBR. *Dist:* Blackwell Sci.

Osteoporosis: Prevention & Treatment. Felix Kolb et al. Ed. by Nancy Wiltsek. 1986. (Illus.). pap. 2.50 (*0-933161-07-7*) Better H Prog.

Osteoporosis: The Long Road Back. Pamela Horner. 1989. 210p. pap. 10.00 (*0-7766-0226-8*) Paul & Co Pubs.

Osteoporosis - Phases, Conditions & Therapy: Index of New Information with Authors, Subjects & References. Florence M. Connors. 1994. 150p. 47.50 (*1-55914-724-5*); pap. 44.50 (*1-55914-725-3*) ABBE Pubs Assn.

Osteoporosis - Questions & Answers. John Stevenson & Michael C. Ellerington. 1993. (Questions & Answers Ser.). (Illus.). 968p. 12.95 (*1-873413-50-5*); pap. 10.95 (*1-873413-55-6*) Merit Pub Intl.

Osteoporosis Book. Ed. by Nancy E. Lane. 1999. LC 98-19650. (Illus.). 224p. 27.50 (*0-19-511602-X*) OUP.

Osteoporosis Book: A Guide for Patients & Their Families. Nancy E. Lane. 2001. (Illus.). 224p. reprint ed. pap. 12.95 (*0-19-514238-1*) OUP.

Osteoporosis, Critique & Practicum. Richard D. Wasnich et al. 1989. (Illus.). 225p. (Orig.). pap. text 36.95 (*0-9623265-1-8*) Banyan Pr HI.

Osteoporosis Handbook. Sydney L. Bonnick. 2nd ed. 1997. LC 97-204669. (Illus.). 216p. (Orig.). pap. 14.95 (*0-87833-978-7*) Taylor Pub.

Osteoporosis in Asia: Crossing the Frontiers. 1997. LC 98-162311. 200p. lib. bdg. 34.00 (*981-02-2730-2*) World Scientific Pub.

***Osteoporosis in Chronic Liver Disease.** Sif Ormarsdottir. 2001. (Illus.). 60p. (*91-554-5021-0*) Uppsala Universitet SWE. *Dist:* Coronet Bks.

Osteoporosis in Clinical Practice: A Practical Guide for Diagnosis & Treatment. Ed. by Piet Geusens. 1997. LC 97-41383. (Illus.). 200p. pap. 48.00 (*3-540-76223-X*) Spr-Verlag.

Osteoporosis in Men. J. M. Kaufman. 2001. 200p. 75.00 (*1-84214-033-7*, Parthenon Pbng) CRC Pr.

Osteoporosis, 1996: Proceedings of the 1996 World Congress on Osteoporosis, Amsterdam, the Netherlands, 18-23 May 1996. World Congress on Osteoporosis Staff & S. Papapoulos. 1996. LC 96-38652. (International Congress Ser.). 422p. 165.00 (*0-444-82276-3*) Elsevier.

Osteoporosis Primer. Ed. by Janet E. Henderson & David Goltzman. 2000. LC 00-33695. (Illus.). 388p. pap. text 64.95 (*0-521-64446-1*) Cambridge U Pr.

Osteoporosis Research, Education & Health Promotion. 1993. 68p. (Orig.). (C). pap. text 30.00 (*0-7881-0063-7*) DIANE Pub.

Osteoporosis Solution. Carl Germano. 1999. LC 98-66722. 224p. text 22.00 (*1-57566-391-0*) Kensgtn Pub Corp.

Osteoporosis Sourcebook: Basic Consumer Health Information about Primary & Secondary Osteoporosis, Juvenile Osteoporosis & Related Conditions. Ed. by Allan R. Cook. 2001. LC 00-66907. (Health Reference Ser.). (Illus.). xiv, 584p. lib. bdg. 78.00 (*0-7808-0239-X*) Omnigraphics Inc.

Osteosarcoma in Adolescents & Young Adults: New Developments & Controversies. Ed. by G. Bennett Humphrey et al. 1993. LC 92-49668. (Cancer Treatment & Research Ser.: Vol. 62). (C). text 307.00 (*0-7923-1905-2*) Kluwer Academic.

Osteosynthesis in Spinal Surgery. Ed. by E. Ascani et al. 1990. (Progress in Spinal Pathology Ser.: Vol. 4). (Illus.). 185p. 62.95 (*0-387-82150-3*) Spr-Verlag.

Osterreichischer Hno-Kongress, 1999. 1999. 84p. 34.00 (*3-8055-6954-8*) S Karger.

Ostlere & Bryce-Smith's Anaesthetics for Medical Students. Thomas B. Boulton & Colin E. Blogg. 10th ed. 1989. (Illus.). 276p. pap. text (*0-443-02821-4*) Church.

Ostomies & Continent Diversions: Nursing Management. Beverly G. Hampton. 1992. (Illus.). 400p. (C). (gr. 13). text 45.00 (*0-8016-2041-4*, 02041) Mosby Inc.

Ostomy Book: Living Comfortably with Colostomies, Ileostomies & Urostomies. Barbara D. Mullen & Kerry A. McGinn. 2nd rev. ed. 1991. LC 91-36233. 252p. pap. 16.95 (*0-923521-12-7*) Bull Pub.

OT Aides: Guidelines for Training & Performance : a Manual for OT Practitioners. Contrib. by Ruth Ford. 1997. LC 97-175090. (*1-56900-075-1*) Am Occup Therapy.

OTC Medications: Symptoms & Treatment of Common Illnesses. A. Li Wan Po & G. Li Wan Po. 1991. (Illus.). 256p. pap. 31.95 (*0-632-02954-4*) Blackwell Sci.

OTC Medications: Symptoms & Treatments of Common Illnesses. Alain Wan Po Li & G. Wan Po Li. 2nd ed. 1997. LC 97-11878. pap. 49.95 (*0-632-04046-7*) Blackwell Sci.

Other Child - The Brain-Injured Child. Richard S. Lewis et al. 2nd ed. 1960. LC 60-6019. 160p. text 29.00 (*0-8089-0263-6*, 792527, Grune & Strat) Harcrt Hlth Sci Grp.

Other Diabetes: Living & Eating Well with Type 2 Diabetes. Elizabeth Hiser. 1999. LC 98-47490. (Illus.). x, 244p. 23.00 (*0-688-15329-1*, Wm Morrow) Morrow Avon.

Other Freud: Religion, Culture & Psychoanalysis. James DiCenso. 1999. LC 98-23772. 192p. (C). 80.00 (*0-415-19658-2*, D6252); pap. 26.95 (*0-415-19659-0*, D6256) Routledge.

Other Guy's Sperm: The Cause of Cancers & Other Diseases. Donald E. Tyler. 1994. LC 94-94234. 131p. pap. 14.95 (*1-884981-05-4*) Discov Bks.

Other Healers: Unorthodox Medicine in America. Ed. by Norman Gevitz. 1988. LC 88-6770. 324p. pap. text 19.95 (*0-8018-3710-3*) Johns Hopkins.

Other Lives, Other Selves: A Jungian Psychotherapist Discovers Past Lives. Roger J. Woolger. 1988. LC 88-47683. 408p. pap. 14.95 (*0-553-34595-8*) Bantam.

***Other People's Habits: How to Use Positive Reinforcement to Bring Out the Best in People Around You.** Aubrey C. Daniels. 2001. LC 00-60925. (Illus.). xi, 195p. pap. (*0-07-137374-8*) McGraw.

Other Side Makes Chocolate. Joan M. McCartney. 1981. (Illus.). 88p. (Orig.). pap. 2.95 (*0-9609788-0-1*) J M McCartney.

Other Side of Psychology. Denise D. Cummins. 1995. LC 95-8789. (Illus.). 272p. 22.95 (*0-312-13577-7*) St Martin.

Other Side of Psychology: How Experimental Psychologists Find Out about the Way We Think & Act. Denise D. Cummins. 2000. 240p. reprint ed. text 23.00 (*0-7881-6968-8*) DIANE Pub.

Other Side of Silence. Arden Neisser. 1990. LC 89-71507. 316p. pap. 15.95 (*0-930323-64-5*) Gallaudet Univ Pr.

Other Side of the Error Term: Aging & Development As Model Systems in Cognitive Neuroscience, Vol. 125. Naftali Raz. 1998. LC 98-3180. (Advances in Psychology Ser.). 472p. 113.00 (*0-444-82522-3*) Elsevier.

Other Side of War: On the Hospital Transports with the Army of the Potomac. Katharine P. Wormeley. Ed. by Christine T. Heidorf. 2nd unabr. ed. 1998. 244p. reprint ed. pap. 16.95 (*0-87928-118-9*) Corner Hse.

Other Times, Other Realities: Toward A Theory of Psychoanalytic Treatment. Arnold H. Modell. 1996. 192p. pap. text 18.50 (*0-674-64499-9*) HUP.

Other Times, Other Realities: Toward a Theory of Psychoanalytic Treatment. Arnold H. Modell. 1990. 208p. (C). 42.00 (*0-674-64498-0*) HUP.

Other Topics in Women's Health. 1998. (Ultrasound & Women's Health Ser.: Vol. 4). (*1-930047-53-3*, 98IV-P); pap. (*1-930047-49-5*, 98IV) Am Inst Ultrasound.

Other Women: Lesbian Experience & Psychoanalytic Theory of Women. Beverly Burch. 1997. LC 96-41400. 190p. 41.50 (*0-231-10602-5*); 192p. pap. 16.50 (*0-231-10603-3*) Col U Pr.

Otitis Media: Coping with the Effects in the Classroom. Dorinne S. Davis. 1989. 138p. (C). 26.20 (*0-9622326-0-2*) The Davis Ctr.

Otitis Media in Children: A Controversial Issue. Ed. by Jean-Philippe Guyot. 1999. (Oto-Rhino-Laryngologia Nova Ser.: Vol. 8, No. 3, Pt. 121-122, 1998). (Illus.). 48p. pap. 25.25 (*3-8055-6835-5*) S Karger.

Otitis Media in Infants & Children. Charles D. Bluestone & Jerome O. Klein. 2nd ed. 1994. LC 93-40646. (Illus.). 310p. text 69.00 (*0-7216-4818-5*) Saunders.

Otitis Media in Young Children: Medical, Developmental & Educational Considerations. Joanne E. Roberts et al. 1997. LC 96-42315. 336p. 48.95 (*1-55766-278-9*) P H Brookes.

Otitis Media with Effusion in Young Children. 1995. lib. bdg. 251.95 (*0-8490-6779-0*) Gordon Pr.

Otitis Media with Effusion in Young Children: Clinical Practice Guideline. 1997. lib. bdg. 250.95 (*0-8490-8141-6*) Gordon Pr.

Otitis Media with Effusion in Young Children: Clinical Practice Guideline. Sylvan E. Stool & Alfred O. Berg. 1998. (Illus.). 108p. (C). pap. text 30.00 (*0-7881-4822-2*) DIANE Pub.

Otitus Media with Effusion in Children. David Chalmers et al. 1991. (Clinics in Developmental Medicine Ser.: No. 108). (Illus.). 167p. (C). text (*0-521-41224-2*) Mc Keith Pr GBR. *Dist:* Cambridge U Pr.

Otoacoustic Emissions. Jan Maurer et al. 1997. LC 96-50973. (Self-Instructional Ser.). (Illus.). 60p. (Orig.). pap. text 25.00 (*1-56772-055-2*, 5506305) AAO-HNS.

***Otoacoustic Emissions.** Jan Maurer et al. 2nd ed. 2001. LC 2001-22730. (SIPac Ser.). (Illus.). 64p. (Orig.). pap. text 30.00 (*1-56772-035-8*) AAO-HNS.

Otoacoustic Emissions: A Manual for Clinical Applications. Brenda L. Lonsbury-Martin. 2000. 100p. pap. 49.95 (*1-56593-952-2*, 1882) Thomson Learn.

Otoacoustic Emissions: Clinical Applications. Martin S. Robinette & Theodore J. Glattke. 1997. (Illus.). 368p. 55.00 (*0-86577-579-6*) Thieme Med Pubs.

Otoendoscopically Guided Surgery. J. M. Thomassin. 1995. (Illus.). 103p. 104.00 (*3-540-59626-7*) Spr-Verlag.

Otogeny of the Immune System. Ed. by B. H. Waksman. 1981. (Progress in Allergy Ser.: Vol. 29). (Illus.). xii, 268p. 126.25 (*3-8055-2434-X*) S Karger.

Otoimmunology. Ed. by Jan E. Veldman & Brian F. McCabe. 1987. LC 87-17148. (Illus.). 196p. lib. bdg. (*90-6299-033-9*) Kugler NLD. *Dist:* Lib Res.

Otolaryngology English. 1993. (C). ring bd. 585.00 (*0-397-57244-1*) Lppncott W & W.

Otolaryngology Loose Leaf Reference Services Staff. Ed. by Gerald M. English. ring bd. 525.00 (*0-06-148010-X*) Lppncott W & W.

Otolaryngology 6th ed. Incl. Basic Sciences. Wright & Michael Gleeson. 804p. (*0-7506-0595-2*); Michael J. Cinnamond & David A. Adams. LC 97-148926. 640p. (*0-7506-0600-2*); Vol. 2. Adult Audiology. Dafydd Stephens. 640p. (*0-7506-0596-0*); Vol. 3. Booth. 778p. (*0-7506-0597-9*); Vol. 4. MacKay. 552p. (*0-7506-0598-7*); Vol. 5. Laryngology & Head & Neck Surgery. Hibbert. 608p. (*0-7506-0599-5*); 3928p. 1996. (*0-7506-1935-X*) E A GBR. *Dist:* OUP.

Otolaryngology. Michael J. Cinnamond & David A. Adams. 6th ed. 1996. LC 97-148926. (Scott Brown's Otolaryngology Ser.: Vol. 6). 640p. (*0-7506-0600-2*) E A GBR. *Dist:* OUP.

Otolaryngology Michael M. Paparella & Donald A. Shumrick. Ed. by William L. Meyerhoff. 3rd ed. 1990. LC 77-25566. (Illus.). 3536p. 1. 195.00 (*0-7216-1505-8*); 2. 195.00 (*0-7216-1506-6*); 3. 195.00 (*0-7216-1507-4*); 4. text 195.00 (*0-7216-3446-X*); Set. text 625.00 (*0-7216-1504-X*) Saunders.

Otolaryngology, Vol. 3. Booth. 6th ed. 1996. (Scott Brown's Otolaryngology Ser.: Vol. 3). 778p. (*0-7506-0597-9*) E A GBR. *Dist:* OUP.

Otolaryngology, Vol. 4. MacKay. 6th ed. 1996. (Scott Brown's Otolaryngology Ser.: Vol. 5). 552p. (*0-7506-0598-7*) E A GBR. *Dist:* OUP.

Otolaryngology: A Case Study Approach. Thomas A. Tami. 1998. LC 97-51988. pap. 69.00 (*0-86577-773-X*) Thieme Med Pubs.

Otolaryngology: Head & Neck Surgery. Charles W. Cummings. 1996. text 495.00 incl. cd-rom (*0-8151-2071-0*); text 895.00 incl. cd-rom (*0-8151-2076-1*) Mosby Inc.

Otolaryngology: Head & Neck Surgery. R. Slatin Pasha. 2000. LC 00-34509. (Illus.). 580p. pap. text 59.95 (*0-7693-0053-7*) Singular Publishing.

Otolaryngology: Head & Neck Surgery. Charles W. Cummings et al. 3rd ed. 1998. (Illus.). 3000p. (C). (gr. 13). text 495.00 (*0-8151-2067-2*, 29857) Mosby Inc.

Otolaryngology: Head & Neck Surgery Review. Charles W. Cummings, Jr. & Bruce Haughey. 1999. 320p. pap. 695.00 (*0-323-00503-9*) Mosby Inc.

Otolaryngology: Head & Neck Surgery Review. Charles W. Cummings, Jr. et al. 1998. 320p. (C). text (*0-323-00688-4*) Mosby Inc.

Otolaryngology: Pediatric Head & Neck Surgery, Vol. 3. Mark Richardson. 1998. (Illus.). 608p. (C). (gr. 13). text 150.00 (*0-8151-2135-0*, 29855) Mosby Inc.

Otolaryngology: Self-Assessment & Board Review. Charles A. Syms et al. 2001. (Illus.). 352p. pap. 49.00 (*0-86577-917-1*) Thieme Med Pubs.

Otolaryngology: The Essentials. Ed. by Allen M. Seiden et al. 2001. (Illus.). 1216p. pap. 69.00 (*0-86577-854-X*) Thieme Med Pubs.

Otolaryngology Head & Neck Surgery. John Jacob Ballenger. 16th ed. 2002. pap. 236.00 net. (*0-7693-0172-X*) Singular Publishing.

Otolaryngology Head & Neck Surgery Pocket Manual. John Jacob Ballenger. 16th ed. 2002. pap. 64.00 net. (*0-7693-0173-8*) Singular Publishing.

Otolaryngology in ASEAN Countries: 6th ASEAN Congress, Chiang, Rai, Thailand, November 1994. Ed. by Sujitra Prasansuk et al. 1996. LC 96-44296. (Advances in OtoRhinoLaryngology Ser.: Vol. 51, 1996). (Illus.). viii, 128p. 85.25 (*3-8055-6336-1*) S Karger.

Otolarynology. McCormick. 3rd ed. 1992. 240p. pap. text 19.95 (*0-340-39802-7*) Trafalgar.

Otolith Function in Spatial Orientation & Movement. Contrib. by Bernard Cohen & Bernhard J. M. Hess. 1999. LC 99-24766. (Annals of the New York Academy of Sciences Ser.: Vol. 871). (Illus.). xiv, 464p. (*1-57331-217-7*) NY Acad Sci.

Otolith Microstructure Examination & Analysis. Ed. by David K. Stevenson. 1992. 126p. (Orig.). pap. (*0-660-14747-5*) Can7 Govern Pub.

Otologic Surgery. Ed. by Derald E. Brackmann et al. 1994. LC 93-40738. (Illus.). text 173.00 (*0-7216-6639-6*) Saunders.

Otologic Surgery: Core Workbook & Update Service. Goin. 1991. (*0-8151-3707-9*) Mosby Inc.

Otologic Surgery: Manual of Oto-Surgical Techniques. Michel Portmann & Didier Portmann. 1998. LC 97-45064. (Illus.). 300p. 193.95 (*1-56593-939-5*, 1860) Thomson Learn.

Otological Significance of the Round Window. Y. Nomura. 1984. (Advances in OtoRhinoLaryngology Ser.: Vol. 33). (Illus.). x, 162p. 100.00 (*3-8055-3806-5*) S Karger.

Otology Today. Ed. by G. Babighian. 1987. (Advances in OtoRhinoLaryngology Ser.: Vol. 37). (Illus.). viii, 200p. 152.25 (*3-8055-4498-7*) S Karger.

Otoneurosurgery. W. Pellett et al. 1990. (Illus.). 220p. 238.00 (*0-387-50979-8*) Spr-Verlag.

Otoneurosurgery-Latral Skull Base. Salvinelli. 1996. text 93.00 (*0-7216-7051-2*) Saunders.

Otophysiology: Proceedings of the International Symposium, Ann Arbor, 1971. International Symposium on Otophysiology Staff. Ed. by J. E. Hawkins et al. 1973. (Advances in OtoRhinoLaryngology Ser.: Vol. 20). 182.75 (*3-8055-1338-0*) S Karger.

Otoplasty: Aesthetic & Reconstructive Techniques. Jack Davis. 2nd ed. 1997. LC 96-35161. (Illus.). 149p. 181.00 (*0-387-94878-3*) Spr-Verlag.

Otorhinolaryngology, Head & Neck Surgery: Proceedings of the XIV World Congress, Madrid, Spain, Sept. 10-15, 1989, Vols. 1 & 2. Ed. by T. Sacristan et al. 1991. LC 91-6998. (Illus.). lib. bdg. (*90-6299-071-1*) Kugler NLD. *Dist:* Lib Res.

Otorom, Interactive Middle Ear Pathology & Surgical Procedures, No. 1. Vincent. 1996. pap. 175.00 incl. audio compact disk (*0-7506-3063-9*) Buttrwrth-Heinemann.

Otosclerosis. Ed. by R. Filipo. 1990. LC 90-5230. (Illus.). 178p. lib. bdg. (*90-6299-061-4*) Kugler NLD. *Dist:* Lib Res.

Otosclerosis: Diagnosis & Treatment. Anthony F. Jahn & David M. Vernick. 2nd ed. 1993. (Self-Instructional Package Ser.). (Illus.). 79p. pap. text 25.00 (*1-56772-007-2*) AAO-HNS.

Otoscopy. Browning Staff. (*0-340-61376-9*) E A GBR. *Dist:* Routldge.

Otoscopy: A Structured Approach. P. J. Wormald & G. G. Browning. 1996. LC 96-115984. (Illus.). 104p. (Orig.). (C). pap. text 70.00 (*1-56593-706-6*, 1390) Singular Publishing.

Otto Gross, Freudian Psychoanalyst, 1877-1920: Literature & Ideas. Martin Green. 1999. LC 98-53713. 372p. text 99.95 (*0-7734-8164-8*) E Mellen.

Otto Selz: His Contribution to Psychology. Adriaan de Groot. Ed. by Nico H. Frijda. 1981. (Illus.). 306p. (*90-279-3438-X*) Mouton.

Ouderen in Het Jaar 2005 see Elderly in 2005: Health & Care: Updated Scenarios on Health & Aging, 1990-2005

Ounce of Prevention: Waste Reduction Strategies for Health Care Facilities. Glen McRae et al. 1993. (Illus.). 222p. (Orig.). pap. 50.00 (*0-87258-637-5*, 057007) Am Hospital.

Our Aging Brain: Changing & Growing. Harold W. Nash. Ed. by Timothy A. Nash. 1999. LC 98-92099. (Illus.). 162p. pap. 15.00 (*0-9666162-0-0*) Ontarolina.

Our Ailing Health Care System: Health Care Is Bankrupting America & Leaving Us Increasingly Diseased. Arthur M. Baker. 1994. LC 93-93556. 50p. (Orig.). pap. 8.95 (*1-883989-11-6*) Self Hlth Care.

Our Best Hope: Early Intervention with Prenatally Drug-Exposed Infants & Their Families. Jane Stump. 1992. pap. 9.95 (*0-87868-493-X*, 4930) Child Welfare.

Our Blind Children: Growing & Learning with Them. Berthold Lowenfeld. 3rd ed. 1977. (Illus.). 260p. 41.95 (*0-398-02200-3*) C C Thomas.

Our Bodies, Ourselves see Nuestros Cuerpos, Nuestras Vidas

Our Bodies, Ourselves for the New Century: A Book for & by Women. Boston Women's Health Book Collective Staff. rev. ed. 1998. LC 98-12725. (Illus.). 784p. 24.00 (*0-684-84231-9*, Touchstone) S&S Trade Pap.

Our Chemical Culture: Drug Use & Misuse. Marcia Summers et al. 1982. LC 81-5271. 120p. (gr. 10-12). text 18.95 (*0-87073-337-0*); pap. text 12.95 (*0-87073-336-2*) Schenkman Bks Inc.

Our Children Today: A Guide to Their Needs from Infancy Through Adolescence. Ed. by Child Study Association of America Staff. 1977. LC 72-4512. (Essay Index Reprint Ser.). reprint ed. 25.95 (*0-8369-2938-1*) Ayer.

Our Hands Are Tied: Legal Tensions & Medical Ethics. Marshall B. Kapp. 1998. LC 97-38581. 192p. 60.00 (*0-86569-276-9*, Auburn Hse) Greenwood.

Our Health, Our Lives: A Revolutionary Approach to Total Health Care for Women. Eileen Hoffman. Ed. by Julie Rubenstein. 1996. 448p. reprint ed. per. 16.00 (*0-671-88086-1*, PB Trade Paper) PB.

Our Healthier Nation: A Contract for Health, Command Paper 3852. 1998. (Command Papers: No. 81011068). pap. (*0-10-138522-6*, HM85226) Statnry Office GBR. *Dist:* Bernan Associates.

Our Inner Conflicts: A Constructive Theory of Neurosis. Karen Horney. 1992. 256p. pap. 13.95 (*0-393-30940-1*) Norton.

Our Journeys Through Life. Ruth D. Hadfield. 1988. LC 86-17331. pap. 13.95 (*0-87949-255-4*) Ashley Bks.

Our Man Sam: Making the Most Out of Life with Muscular Dystrophy. Susan C. Bayley. 1998. 112p. pap. 9.95 (*0-9667440-0-4*) S Bayle.

Our Medical Future: Breakthroughs in Health & Longevity by the Year 2000 & Beyond. Jeffrey A. Fisher. Ed. by Julie Rubenstein. 1993. LC 93-19867. Orig. Title: RX 2000. 272p. reprint ed. pap. 10.00 (*0-671-73845-3*) S&S Trade.

Our Need for Others & Its Roots in Infancy. Josephine Klein. 1987. 350p. (*0-422-61410-6*, A0811); pap. (*0-422-61420-3*, A0815) Tavistock GBR. *Dist:* Routldge.

Our Responses to a Deadly Virus: The Group-Analytic Approach. Angela Molnos. 1990. 220p. pap. text (*0-946439-80-X*) Karnac Bks GBR. *Dist:* Other Pr LLC.

Our Right to Drugs: The Case for a Free Market. Thomas Szasz. 1992. LC 91-30378. 232p. 30.00 (*0-275-94216-3*, C4216, Praeger Pubs) Greenwood.

Our Right to Drugs: The Case for a Free Market. Thomas Szasz. 1996. LC 95-46515. 229p. (C). pap. 19.95 (*0-8156-0333-9*, SZORP) Syracuse U Pr.

Our Secret Rules: Why We Do the Things We Do. Jordan Weiss. 2001. 164p. pap. 11.95 (*0-7570-0010-X*) Square One.

Our Sexuality. Robert Crooks. (Health Sciences Ser.). 5th ed. 1993. text 41.00 (*0-534-33939-5*); 6th ed. 1995. pap., stu. ed. 18.25 (*0-534-32096-1*) Brooks-Cole.

Our Sexuality. Crooks. 7th ed. 1998. (Psychology Ser.). pap. 29.95 (*0-534-36237-0*) Brooks-Cole.

Our Sexuality: Study Guide. Robert Crooks. 5th ed. 1993. (Health Sciences Ser.). pap., stu. ed. 17.95 (*0-534-33943-3*) Brooks-Cole.

Our Stolen Future: How We are Threatening Our Fertility Intelligence & Survival. Theo Colburn et al. 1997. LC 97-159794. 336p. pap. 13.95 (*0-452-27414-1*, Plume) Dutton Plume.

Our Stories of Miscarriage: Healing with Words. Rachel Faldet & Karen Fitton. 1997. LC 96-35348. 224p. pap. 13.95 (*1-57749-033-9*) Fairview Press.

Our Syndromes, Ourselves. Cathy Hamilton. 2000. LC 99-44000. 192p. pap. 9.95 (*0-7407-0665-9*) Andrews McMeel.

Out from the Inside: The Use of Creativity in Relationships. Larry R. Decker. 1985. LC 84-90461. 10.95 (*0-87212-186-0*) Libra.

Out of Bounds: Sexual Exploitation in Counselling & Therapy. Janice Russell. 1993. LC 92-59971. (Illus.). 160p. (C). 69.95 (*0-8039-8533-9*) Sage.

Out of Control: Family Therapy & Domestic Disorder. Jaber F. Gubrium. 1992. (Library of Social Research: Vol. 189). 272p. (C). 86.95 (*0-8039-4632-5*, 7765); pap. 37.95 (*0-8039-4633-3*, 7766) Sage.

Out of Control: The Addictive Behavioral Personality. Moses Calhoun. 1993. (Illus.). 250p. 29.95 (*0-9638949-0-0*) Winning Artist.

Out of Dr. Bill's Black Bag: From Northern Wisconsin . . . a Country Doctor Looks Back (1941-1991) William B. Bauer. 1994. LC 94-94225. 315p. (Orig.). pap. text 19.95 (*0-9640154-1-2*) Brother Bills.

Out-of-Hospital Transfusion Therapy. Ed. by Joy L. Fridey et al. 1994. (Illus.). 110p. (C). text 20.00 (*1-56395-029-4*) Am Assn Blood.

***Out of Its Mind: Psychiatry in Crisis.** Hobson. 2002. 304p. pap. text 17.00 (*0-7382-0685-7*) Perseus Bks Grp.

Out of Its Mind: Psychiatry in Crisis. J. Allan Hobson & Jonathan Leonard. 2001. 304p. text 26.00 (*0-7382-0251-7*) Perseus Bks Grp.

Out of My Head: An Experience of Neurosurgery. Viv Martin. 1997. 162p. pap. (*1-85776-179-0*) Book Guild Ltd GBR. *Dist:* Trans-Atl Phila.

Out of Order: Clinical Work & Unconscious Process. Martin Stanton. 1999. 140p. pap. 17.95 (*1-892746-18-2*, 46182) Other Pr LLC.

Out-of-Sync Child: Recognizing & Coping with Sensory Integration Dysfunction. Carol S. Kranowitz. 1998. LC 97-14601. 322p. pap. 14.00 (*0-399-52386-3*) Berkley Pub.

Out-of-the-Body Experiences. Celia Green. 1989. (C). 60.00 (*0-900076-01-1*) St Mut.

Out of the Corner of My Eye: Living with Vision Loss in Later Life. Nicolette P. Ringgold. l.t. ed. 1991. LC 91-3352. 120p. pap. 23.95 (*0-89128-193-2*) Am Foun Blind.

Out of the Dead House: 19th-Century Women Physicians & the Writing of Medicine. Susan Wells. 2001. LC 00-10614. (Illus.). xii, 312p. 57.95 (*0-299-17170-1*); pap. 22.95 (*0-299-17174-4*) U of Wis Pr.

Out of the Nightmare: Recovery from Depression & Suicidal Pain. David L. Conroy. 1991. LC 90-63398. 364p. (Orig.). reprint ed. pap. 12.95 (*1-879204-00-2*) New Liberty Pubns.

Out of the Shadows: Confronting America's Mental Illness Crisis. E. Fuller Torrey. LC 96-7716. 256p. 1996. 27.95 (*0-471-16161-6*); 2nd ed. 1998. pap. 16.95 (*0-471-24532-1*) Wiley.

Out of the Shadows, Emotions & the Enneagram see Emotions & the Enneagram: Working Through Your Shadow Life Script

Out of Wedlock: A Study of the Problems of the Unmarried Mother & Her Child. Leontine Young. 1978. LC 78-16486. 261p. reprint ed. lib. bdg. 62.50 (*0-313-20604-X*, YOWE, Greenwood Pr) Greenwood.

Out to Play: The Middle Years of Childhood. Alasdair Roberts. 1980. 175p. text 13.00 (*0-08-025719-4*, Pergamon Pr) Elsevier.

Outbreak Alert: Making Sense of Today's Infectious Diseases Threats. Jason Eberhart-Phillips. 2000. LC 99-75296. Orig. Title: Plagues on the Doorstep. 298p. pap. 15.95 (*1-57224-201-9*) New Harbinger.

Outcasts on Main Street: The Report of the Federal Task Force on Homelessness & Severe Mental Illness. 1993. (Illus.). 107p. (Orig.). pap. text 30.00 (*0-7881-0073-4*) DIANE Pub.

Outcome after Head, Neck, & Spinal Trauma: A Medico-Legal Guide. Ed. by Robert Macfarlane & David Hardy. 1997. 456p. text 135.00 (*0-7506-2178-8*) Buttrwrth-Heinemann.

Outcome & Innovation in Psychological Treatment of Schizophrenia. Til Wykes et al. 1999. LC 97-18366. 304p. pap. 49.95 (*0-471-97842-6*) Wiley.

Outcome Assessment in Residential Treatment. Ed. by Steven I. Pfeiffer. 1996. LC 96-20075. (Residential Treatment for Children & Youth Ser.: Vol. 13, No. 4). 99p. (C). 39.95 (*1-56024-839-4*) Haworth Pr.

Outcome Based Education: The State's Assault on Our Children's Value. Pamela Hoffecker & Peg Luksik. 1995. LC 94-78044. 208p. pap. 10.99 (*1-56384-025-1*) Huntington Hse.

Outcome-Based Quality Improvement for Long-Term Care: Using MDS, Process, & Outcome Measures. Marilyn Jean Rantz et al. rev. ed. 1998. LC 98-35896. 320p. ring bd. 179.00 (*0-8342-1147-5*, 11475) Aspen Pub.

Outcome Concept Systems: A Guide to the Measurement of Patient Outcomes. Alexis A. Wilson & Mary Hartnett. 2nd rev. ed. 1996. LC 95-62349. 58p. text 125.00 (*0-9633599-2-4*) Wilson & Assocs.

Outcome Management & Program Evaluation Made Easy: A Toolkit for Occupational Therapy Practitioners. Stephen Forer. 1996. 150p. (Orig.). pap. text 48.00 (*1-56900-038-7*, 1146) Am Occup Therapy.

Outcome Measures for Health Education & Other Health Care Interventions. John Lynch et al. 1996. LC 95-50181. (C). 168p. 66.95 (*0-7619-0066-7*, 1687); 99p. pap. 31.95 (*0-7619-0067-5*, 1688) Sage.

Outcome Measures in Home Care: Research, Vol. I. Ed. by Lynn T. Rinke & Alexis A. Wilson. 1987. 250p. (Orig.). pap. 22.95 (*0-88737-378-X*) Natl League Nurse.

Outcome Measures in Intensive Care. John Duncan Young. 2002. LC 2001-52527. 256p. pap. 49.99 (*0-7506-4982-8*) Buttrwrth-Heinemann.

Outcome Measures in Trauma. Ed. by P. B. Pynsent et al. 1994. LC 94-9397. (Illus.). 280p. text 95.00 (*0-7506-1653-9*) Buttrwrth-Heinemann.

Outcome of the Critically Ill: Medicine, Surgery & Trauma. R. B. Vukmir. 2001. LC 00-25525. 200p. pap. 43.95 (*1-85070-903-3*, Parthenon Pbng) CRC Pr.

Outcome Oriented Rehabilitation: Principles, Strategies & Tools for Effective Program Management. Pat K. Landrum et al. 1992. 340p. 68.00 (*0-8342-0665-X*) PRO-ED.

Outcome Oriented Therapeutic Massage. Carla-Krystin Andrade & Paul Clifford. 2000. LC 00-50677. (Illus.). 400p. pap. text 38.95 (*0-7817-1743-4*) Lppncott W & W.

Outcome Standards in Home Health Vol. III: State of the Art. 1987. 72p. 16.95 (*0-88737-389-5*) Natl League Nurse.

Outcomes & Incomes: How to Evaluate, Improve & Market Your Psychotherapy Practice by Measuring Outcomes. Paul W. Clement. 1999. LC 99-28874. (Clinician's Toolbox Ser.). 244p. 50.00 (*1-57230-486-3*) Guilford Pubns.

Outcomes & Technology Assessment in Nuclear Medicine. Leslee Shaw & Frank J. Papatheofanis. 1999. LC 99-16296. 124p. pap. 49.00 (*0-932004-71-7*) Soc Nuclear Med.

Outcomes Assessment in Clinical Practice. Ed. by Lloyd I. Sederer & Barbara Dickey. 1996. LC 95-4785. (Illus.). 384p. 55.00 (*0-683-07630-2*) Lppncott W & W.

Outcomes Effectiveness of Physical Therapy: An Annotated Bibliography. 1995. 551p. ring bd. 59.95 (*0-912452-94-3*, P-106) Am Phys Therapy Assn.

Outcomes for Children & Youth with Emotional & Behavioral Disorders & Their Families: Programs & Evaluation Best Practices. Albert J. Duchnowski. Ed. by Michael H. Epstein & Krista Kutash. 1998. LC 97-21294. 600p. 44.00 (*0-89079-750-1*, 8454) PRO-ED.

Outcomes in Neurological & Neurosurgical Disorders. Ed. by Michael Swash. 1998. (Illus.). 628p. (C). text 135.00 (*0-521-44327-X*) Cambridge U Pr.

Outcomes into Clinical Practice. Ed. by Tony Delamothe. 1994. 169p. (Orig.). pap. text (*0-7279-0888-X*) BMJ Pub GBR. *Dist:* AIDC.

Outcomes Management: Applications to Clinical Practice. Anne W. Wojner. 1999. (Illus.). 350p. 39.95 (*1-55664-411-6*) Mosby Inc.

Outcomes Management Resource Guide. Eric D. Joseph. 1995. 61p. (Orig.). pap. text 30.00 (*0-916499-63-4*) Care Educ Grp.

Outcomes Mandate: Case Management in Healthcare Today. Elaine L. Cohen & Vivien DeBack. 1998. LC 98-37881. 432p. text 42.95 (*0-323-00277-3*) Mosby Inc.

Outcomes of Effective Management Practice. Kathleen Kelly. 1996. (Series on Nursing Administration: Vol. 8). (Illus.). 265p. 78.95 (*0-8039-7175-3*, 7556) Sage.

Outcomes Research Resource Guide, 97-98: A Survey of Current Activities. Ed. by American Medical Association Staff. 1998. (Clinical Decision Making Ser.). 137p. pap. 49.95 (*0-89970-907-9*) AMA.

Outdoor Emergency Care. David Johe. Ed. by American Academy of Orthopaedic Surgeons Staff & National Ski Patrol Staff. 4th ed. 2002. (Illus.). (C). pap. text 64.95 (*0-7637-1715-0*, 1715-0) Jones & Bartlett.

Outdoor Emergency Care: Comprehensive First Aid for Nonurban Settings. Warren D. Bowman. Ed. by Rebecca W. Ayers. 2nd ed. 1993. LC 93-84167. (Illus.). 546p. pap. 30.00 (*0-929752-01-5*) Natl Ski Patrol.

Outdoor First-Aid: A Field Guide to Recognition & Treatment of Outdoor Injuries & Illnesses. Robert J. Koester. (Illus.). 1992. LC 91-72633. 104p. spiral bd. 13.95 (*1-879471-14-0*); 2nd ed. 1999. 136p. pap. 9.95 (*1-879471-27-2*); 2nd ed. 1997. 136p. 23.95 (*1-879471-26-4*); Waterproof. 2nd ed. 1999. 136p. pap. 13.95 (*1-879471-28-0*) DBS Prodns.

Outdoor First-Aid: Instructor's Manual. Robert J. Koester. 1996. 260p. (Orig.). pap. text, tchr. ed. 60.00 (*1-879471-23-X*) DBS Prodns.

Outer Shell: Skin. Sarah Angliss. 1999. (Human Machine Ser.). (Illus.). 32p. (J). lib. bdg. 16.95 (*1-929298-21-8*) Thameside Pr.

Outgrowing the Pain. Eliana Gil. 1988. 96p. (Orig.). pap. 10.95 (*0-440-50006-0*, Dell Trade Pbks) Dell.

Outline & General Principles of the History of Life: University of California Syllabus Series, Vol. 213. William D. Matthew. Ed. by Stephen Jay Gould. 1980. LC 79-8335. (History of Paleontology Ser.). (Illus.). reprint ed. lib. bdg. 24.95 (*0-405-12719-7*) Ayer.

Outline Guide to Chinese Herbal Patent Medicines in Pill Form - with Sample Pictures of the Boxes: An Introduction to Chinese Herbal Medicines. Margaret A. Naeser. 2nd ed. 1990. LC 90-80264. (Illus.). 372p. (Orig.). pap. 34.95 (*0-9625651-1-3*) Boston Chinese Med.

Outline of Animal Development. Richard Davenport. 1979. LC 78-62548. (Life Sciences Ser.). (Illus.). text (*0-201-01814-4*) Addison-Wesley.

Outline of Clinical Diagnosis. Brian J. Prout & John G. Cooper. 1987. 264p. pap. text 39.00 (*0-7506-2106-0*) Buttrwrth-Heinemann.

Outline of Clinical Diagnosis in the Horse. Date not set. pap. 59.95 (*0-8464-4164-0*) Beekman Pubs.

Outline of Clinical Diagnosis in the Horse. P. J. Pinsent. 1990. (Outline Ser.). 200p. pap. text 42.95 (*0-7236-0959-4*) Blackwell Sci.

Outline of Clinical Diagnosis in the Horse. P. J. Pinsent et al. 2nd ed. 1997. LC 96-52363. (Illus.). 202p. pap. 41.95 (*0-632-04136-6*) Blackwell Sci.

Outline of Fractures. John C. Adams & David L. Hamblen. 10th ed. 1992. (Illus.). 302p. pap. text (*0-443-04371-X*) Church.

Outline of Fractures, Including Joint Injuries. John C. Adams & David L. Hamblen. 11th ed. 1999. LC 98-32447. (*0-443-06027-4*) Church.

Outline of Hawaiian Physical Therapeutics. E. S. Handy et al. 1974. (BMB Ser.: No. 126). reprint ed. 25.00 (*0-527-02232-2*) Periodicals Srv.

Outline of Neurology. Christopher D. Ward. 2001. (John Wright Outline Ser.). (Illus.). 208p. pap. (*0-7506-1407-2*) Buttrwrth-Heinemann.

Outline of Opthalmology. Roger L. Coakes & Patrick Holmes Sellors. 2001. (Illus.). 192p. pap. 40.00 (*0-7506-4460-5*) Buttrwrth-Heinemann.

Outline of Oral Surgery. G. R. Seeward et al. 2nd ed. 2000. pap. text 22.95 (*0-7236-0996-9*) Buttrwrth-Heinemann.

Outline of Oral Surgery & Medicine. Malcolm Harris. Date not set. 256p. pap. 65.00 (*0-7236-1066-5*) Buttrwrth-Heinemann.

Outline of Orthopaedics. John C. Adams & David L. Hamblen. 12th ed. 1995. LC 95-6579. text (*0-443-05149-6*) Church.

Outline of Periodontics. B. M. Manson & J. D. Eley. 1999. LC 99-45299. (Illus.). 405p. pap. text 60.00 (*0-7236-1070-3*) Buttrwrth-Heinemann.

Outline of Psychoanalysis. Sigmund Freud. Ed. & Tr. by James Strachey. rev. ed. 1989. reprint ed. pap. 8.95 (*0-393-00151-2*) Norton.

Outline of Psychology as Applied to Medicine. 1987. text (*0-7506-2057-9*) E A GBR. *Dist:* OUP.

Outline of Psychology As Applied to Medicine. John Weinman. 1981. 288p. (C). pap. text (*0-7236-0591-2*) Buttrwrth-Heinemann.

Outline of Psychotherapy for Medical Students & Practitioners. Harold Maxwell. 1986. 107p. text 27.50 (*0-7236-0849-0*) Buttrwrth-Heinemann.

Outline of Sociology as Applied to Medicine. David Armstrong. 4th ed. 1997. LC 94-24686. 172p. pap. (*0-7506-1929-5*) E A GBR. *Dist:* OUP.

Outline of Swine Diseases: A Handbook. Ross P. Cowart. 1995. LC 95-22163. 152p. pap. text 24.95 (*0-8138-2899-6*) Iowa U Pr.

Outlines in Pathology. John H. Sinard. Ed. by Bill Schmitt. 1996. 256p. pap. text 44.00 (*0-7216-6341-9*) Saunders.

Outlines of Imperfect & Disordered Mental Action. Thomas C. Upham. 1973. LC 73-2426. (Mental Illness & Social Policy; the American Experience Ser.). reprint ed. 28.95 (*0-405-05235-9*) Ayer.

Outlines of Psychology. Harald Hoffding. 381p. 100.00 (*1-85506-670-X*) Thoemmes Pr.

Outlines of Psychology. Oswald Kulpe. 480p. 120.00 (*1-85506-682-3*) Thoemmes Pr.

Outlines of Psychology. Rudolf Hermann Lotze. 173p. 55.00 (*1-85506-668-8*) Thoemmes Pr.

Outlines of Psychology. Wilhelm M. Wundt. 1897. reprint ed. 39.00 (*0-403-00038-6*) Scholarly.

Outlines of Psychology. Wilhelm M. Wundt. 364p. 100.00 (*1-85506-686-6*) Thoemmes Pr.

Outlines of the Chief Camp Diseases of the United States Armies. Joseph Woodward. 1991. (American Civil War Medical Ser.: No. 11). 364p. reprint ed. 65.00 (*0-930405-43-9*) Norman SF.

Outlook for Managed Care, 1998: The National Picture. Efrem Sigel & Jondavid Klipp. 1997. 100p. 895.00 (*0-9662321-0-0*) Corp Res Grp.

Outpatient Antimicrobial Therapy: Recent Advances. Klein et al. 1989. 185p. 22.50 (*0-945986-12-2*) Health Care NJ.

Outpatient Behavior Therapy: A Clinical Guide. Michel Hersen. 1983. 414p. text 53.00 (*0-8089-1575-4*, 791974, Grune & Strat) Harcrt Hlth Sci Grp.

Outpatient Care Handbook. Peter A. Glassman et al. 2nd rev. ed. 1999. LC 98-41940. 400p. pap. 39.95 (*1-56053-260-2*) Hanley & Belfus.

Outpatient Case Management: Strategies for a New Reality. Ed. by Michelle R. Donovan & Theodore A. Matson. 1994. LC 94-9597. 320p. pap. 63.00 (*1-55648-119-5*, 027100) AHPI.

Outpatient Invasive Radiologic Procedures: Diagnostic & Therapeutic. Dublin. 1989. text 65.00 (*0-7216-1532-5*) Saunders.

Outpatient Management of HIV Infection. Joseph R. Masci. 2nd rev. ed. 1996. (Illus.). 448p. (C). (gr. 13). spiral bd. 39.95 (*0-8151-6144-1*, 25691) Mosby Inc.

Outpatient Medicine. Stephen D. Fihn. 2nd ed. 1997. LC 96-46544. 780p. pap. text 49.00 (*0-7216-6257-9*) Saunders.

Outpatient Medicine for PDAs & Desktops: 2001 Edition. Paul D. Chan & Michael Safani. rev. ed. 2000. (Current Clinical Strategies Ser.). 110p. pap. 28.95 incl. cd-rom (*1-881528-90-1*) Current Clin Strat.

Outpatient Medicine, 1997: Current Clinical Strategies. Paul D. Chan & Michael Safani. 1997. 110p. pap. 12.75 (*1-881528-29-4*) Current Clin Strat.

Outpatient Medicine Recall. John P. Franko & Steven A. Meixel. 1997. LC 97-34982. (Illus.). 350p. pap. text 29.95 (*0-683-18018-5*) Lppncott W & W.

Outpatient Parenteral Antimicrobial Therapy (OPAT) A Global Perspective Satellite Symposium Held at the 9th International Congress on Infectious Diseases (ICID), Buenos Aires, Argentina, April 2000. Ed. by A. Tice. 2000. (Chemotherapy Ser.: Vol. 47). (Illus.). iv, 40p. 25.25 (*3-8055-7168-2*) S Karger.

Outpatient Physical Therapy Policy & Procedure Manual. JoAnne Whipple. 1993. 110.00 (*1-879575-29-9*) Acad Med Sys.

Outpatient Psychiatry. Aaron Lazare. 2nd ed. 1988. (Illus.). 752p. lib. bdg. 79.00 (*0-683-04851-1*) Lppncott W & W.

Outpatient Services: Designing, Organizing & Managing Outpatient Resources. Duane C. Abbey. 1996. LC 97-41392. (HFMA Healthcare Financial Management Ser.). 250p. pap. text 60.00 (*0-7863-1085-5*, Irwn Prfssnl) McGraw-Hill Educ Grp.

Outpatient Surgery. George J. Hill. 3rd ed. 1988. (Illus.). 600p. text 105.00 (*0-7216-2104-X*) Saunders.

Outpatient Treatment of Child Molesters. Stan Friedman. Ed. by Harold H. Smith, Jr. 1991. LC 90-50824. (Practitioner's Resource Ser.). 64p. pap. 15.95 (*0-943158-65-6*, OTCBP, Prof Resc Pr) Pro Resource.

Outplacement of Older Psychiatric Patients into the Community. Robert D. Narkiewicz. 1992. LC 91-37479. (Studies on the Elderly in America). 96p. text 20.00 (*0-8153-0520-6*) Garland.

Output Measurements for Medical Ultrasound. Ed. by R. C Preston. 1991. (Illus.). 180p. 130.00 (*0-387-19692-7*) Spr-Verlag.

Outrageous Practices: The Alarming Truth about How Medicine Mistreats Women. Leslie Laurence & Beth Weinhouse. 1998. 434p. text 22.00 (*0-7881-5948-8*) DIANE Pub.

Outreach - Proceedings: Symposium Organised by the Pompidou Group & the World Health Organization - Bergen, 22-24 February, 1993. 1994. (*92-871-2601-1*) Council of Europe FRA. *Dist:* Manhattan Pub Co.

Outreach-Risk Reduction Strategies for Changing HIV-Related Risk Behaviors among Injection Drug Users. 1995. (Illus.). 77p. (Orig.). (C). pap. text 20.00 (*0-7881-2175-8*) DIANE Pub.

Outreach with the Elderly: Community Education, Assessment, & Therapy. Robert Knight. 1990. 320p. (C). pap. text 19.00 (*0-8147-4607-1*) NYU Pr.

Outreach Work with Drug Users: Principles & Practice. 1996. (*92-871-3110-4*) Council of Europe FRA. *Dist:* Manhattan Pub Co.

Outside Looking In: The Near-Death Experience. Rosemary S. Bahr. 1992. (Illus.). 180p. (Orig.). (C). pap. text 35.00 (*1-881604-00-4*) Scopcraeft.

Outsiders: Studies in the Sociology of Deviance. Howard S. Becker. 1966. LC 63-8413. 215p. pap. 14.95 (*0-02-902140-5*) Free Pr.

Outsiders in a Hearing World: A Sociology of Deafness. Paul C. Higgins. 1980. LC 80-12150. (Sociological Observations Ser.: Vol. 10). (Illus.). 205p. pap. 42.95 (*0-8039-1422-9*, 8741) Sage.

Outsmarting Diabetes: A Breakthrough Approach for Reducing the Effects of Insulin-Dependent Diabetes. Richard Beaser. 1994. 256p. pap. 14.95 (*0-471-34694-2*) Wiley.

Outsmarting Diabetes: A Breakthrough Approach for Reducing the Effects of Insulin-Dependent Diabetes. Richard S. Beaser. 1994. LC 94-11324. 256p. pap. 14.95 (*1-56561-051-2*) Wiley.

Outsmarting the Female Fat Cell: The First Weight-Control Program Designed Specifically for Women. Debra Waterhouse. 1994. 256p. reprint ed. mass mkt. (*0-446-60129-2*) Warner.

Outsourcing in Health Care: The Administrator's Guide. Jo Surpin et al. 1999. LC 98-47917. (Illus.). 142p. pap. 35.00 (*1-55648-251-5*) AHPI.

Outward Bound: Relocation & Community Care for People with Learning Difficulties. Tim Booth et al. 1990. 192p. (*0-335-15431-X*); pap. (*0-335-15430-1*) OpUniv Pr.

Outward Bound Wilderness First-Aid Handbook. Jeffrey Isaac. rev. ed. 1998. LC 97-43329. (Illus.). 272p. pap. 14.95 (*1-55821-682-0*, Lyons) Globe Pequot.

***Outwitting Poison Ivy: 101 Ways to Prevent & Treat the Effects of Poison Ivy, Poison Oak & Poison Sumac—For Hikers, Campers, Gardeners.** Susan C. Hauser. 2001. LC 00-102923. (Illus.). 128p. pap. 14.95 (*1-58574-273-2*, Lyons) Globe Pequot.

Outwitting Ticks. Susan C. Hauser. 2001. (Illus.). 160p. pap. 14.95 (*1-58574-021-7*, Lyons) Globe Pequot.

Ova-Dose: Australian Women & the New Reproductive Technology. 1992. (Illus.). 144p. (Orig.). pap. text (*1-86373-056-7*) Allen & Unwin Pty AUS. *Dist:* Paul & Co Pubs.

Ovarialkarzinom. Ed. by A. Pfleiderer. 1984. (Journal: Vol. 7, Suppl. 2). 70p. pap. 17.50 (*3-8055-3922-3*) S Karger.

Ovarian & Fallopian Tube Cancer. John J. Kavanagh et al. 1998. (Illus.). 95.00 (*0-632-04432-2*) Blackwell Sci.

Ovarian Apoptosis. Ed. by Benjamin K. Tsang. 2000. (Biological Signals & Receptors Ser.: Vol. 9, No. 2 (2000)). (Illus.). 56p. pap. 25.25 (*3-8055-7090-2*) S Karger.

Ovarian Cancer. 1997. lib. bdg. 250.95 (*0-8490-8155-6*) Gordon Pr.

Ovarian Cancer. Ed. by David S. Alberts & Earl A. Surwit. 1985. (Cancer Treatment & Research Ser.). text 153.00 (*0-89838-676-4*) Kluwer Academic.

Ovarian Cancer. Robert F. Ozols. 2000. (ACS Atlas of Clinical Oncology Ser.). 300p. incl. cd-rom (*1-55009-096-8*) DEKR.

Ovarian Cancer. Stephen C. Rubin. 2001. 464p. text 129.00 (*0-7817-2408-2*) Lppncott W & W.

Ovarian Cancer, Vol. 4. Ed. by Frank Sharp et al. 1996. (Illus.). 344p. (*0-412-72370-0*) E A GBR. *Dist:* OUP.

Ovarian Cancer: A Bibliography. 1995. lib. bdg. 250.95 (*0-8490-6707-3*) Gordon Pr.

Ovarian Cancer: Controversies in Management. David M. Gershenson & William P. McGuire. 1997. LC 97-34798. (Illus.). 464p. text (*0-443-07804-1*) Church.

Ovarian Cancer: Methods & Protocols. Ed. by John M. S. Bartlett. 2000. (Methods in Molecular Medicine Ser.: Vol. 39). (Illus.). 839p. 149.50 (*0-89603-583-2*) Humana.

Ovarian Cancer: Proceedings of the International Symposium on Ovarian Cancer, 24-25 September 1979, Birmingham. Ed. by C. E. Newman et al. 1980. LC 80-40166. (Illus.). 249p. 43.00 (*0-08-025532-9*, Pergamon Pr) Elsevier.

Ovarian Cancer 2: Biology, Diagnosis & Management. Ed. by Frank Sharp et al. 1993. LC 93-122540. (Illus.). 453p. (gr. 13). pap. 188.95 (*0-412-45190-5*) Chapman & Hall.

Ovarian Carcinoma: Etiology, Diagnosis & Treatments. H. R. Barber. 3rd ed. 1992. (Illus.). 362p. 130.00 (*0-387-97824-0*) Spr-Verlag.

Ovarian Cell Interactions: Genes to Physiology. Ed. by Aaron J. Hsueh & D. W. Schomberg. 1993. (Serono Symposia Ser.). (Illus.). 217p. 141.00 (*0-387-94052-9*) Spr-Verlag.

Ovarian Disorders: Pathology, Diganosis & Management. A. Altcheck & L. Deligdisch. 1996. (Illus.). 512p. 119.95 (*0-89640-263-0*) Igaku-Shoin.

Ovarian Tumors. Luther W. Brady et al. 1984. (Oncologic Ser.: Vol. 20). (Illus.). 232p. pap. 120.00 (*0-08-027472-2*, Pergamon Pr) Elsevier.

Ovary: Regulation, Dysfunction & Treatment. Ed. by M. Filicori & Carlo Flamigni. 1996. LC 96-20246. (International Congress Ser.: No. 1106). 450p. 165.00 (*0-444-82284-4*) Elsevier.

Over & over Again: Understanding Obsessive-Compulsive Disorder. Fugen A. Neziroglu & Jose A. Yaryura-Tobia. rev. ed. 1997. LC 97-12122. 240p. pap. 20.00 (*0-7879-0876-2*) Jossey-Bass.

Over 55: A Handbook on Health. Theodore G. Duncan. 1982. 668p. 99.95 (*0-89859-726-9*) L Erlbaum Assocs.

Over Forty & Fit: The Baby Boomer's Common Sense Guide for Staying Lean, Muscular, & Healthy. David Devon. 1995. LC 94-96747. (Illus.). 120p. (Orig.). pap. 9.99 (*0-9644558-0-3*) Grunt.

Over Half a Century of Michigan Pharmacology, 1942-2002. Ed. by E. F. Domino. 2001. (Illus.). 500p. 40.00 (*0-916182-12-6*) NPP Bks.

Over My Head: A Doctor's Account of Head Injury from the Inside Looking Out. Claudia L. Osborn. 1998. LC 97-67529. iv, 240p. pap. 16.00 (*0-9658750-0-8*) Peripatetic Pub.

Over My Head: A Doctor's Own Story of Head Injury from the Inside Looking Out. Claudia L. Osborn. 2000. 256p. pap. 12.95 (*0-7407-0598-9*) Andrews McMeel.

Doctors Book of Home Remedies for Dogs & Cats: Over 1000 Solutions to Your Pet's Problems. Prevention Magazine Editors. 1997. 496p. mass mkt. 6.99 (*0-553-57781-6*) Bantam.

Over-the-Counter Doctor. Charles B. Inlander. 1997. LC 97-16161. (Illus.). 352p. pap. 14.95 (*0-8362-3581-9*, Cader Bks) Andrews McMeel.

Over-the-Counter Pharmaceutical Formulations. David B. Braun. 1994. LC 94-2511. (Illus.). 443p. 129.00 (*0-8155-1347-X*) Noyes.

Over-the-Counter Pharmaceuticals in the European Union, No. R212. 1995. 1250.00 (*0-85058-830-8*) Economist Intell.

***Over-Weight, over Eating, Obeisty & Morbidity in America: Index of New Information & Guide-Book for Consumers, Reference & Research.** Tyrone T. Powers. 2002. 180p. pap. 47.50 (*0-7883-2491-8*) ABBE Pubs Assn.

***Over-Weight, over Eating, Obesity & Morbidity in America: Index of New Information & Guide-Book for Consumers, Reference & Research.** Tyrone T. Powers. 2002. 180p. 57.50 (*0-7883-2490-X*) ABBE Pubs Assn.

Overactive Child. Ed. by Eric A. Taylor. 1991. (Clinics in Developmental Medicine Ser.: No. 97). (Illus.). 269p. (C). text (*0-521-41216-1*) Mc Keith Pr GBR. *Dist:* Cambridge U Pr.

Overcoming AIDS: Case Histories of Those Who Conquered AIDS. 1992. lib. bdg. 79.95 (*0-8490-8799-6*) Gordon Pr.

Overcoming AIDS with Natural Medicine. Stephen C. Byrnes. 1997. LC 97-92719. (Illus.). ix, 224p. pap. 19.95 (*1-891530-04-6*) Centaur Bks.

***Overcoming Anorexia.** Chris Freeman. Date not set. LC 2001-51207. (Self-Help Overcoming Ser.). 230p. pap. 14.95 (*0-8147-2713-1*) NYU Pr.

***Overcoming Antimicrobial Resistance: World Health Organization Report on Infectious Diseases 2000.** Frwd. by Gro Harlem Brundtland. 2001. (Illus.). 67p. pap. 30.00 (*0-7567-1166-5*) DIANE Pub.

Overcoming Anxiety, Panic, Phobias Through a Support Group see You Have Choices: Recovering from Anxiety, Panic & Phobia

Overcoming Arthritis. Unofficial Panel of Experts Staff et al. 2nd ed. 1999. (Unofficial Guides Ser.). (Illus.). 384p. pap. 15.95 (*0-02-862714-8*, Unoffic Guide) Hungry Minds.

Overcoming Arthritis: See How Holistic Treatments Can Cure Arthritis, Fibromyalgia, Chronic Fatigue Syndrome & Other Conditions. David Brownstein. 2000. 256p. pap. 15.00 (*0-9660882-1-2*) Med Alternat.

Overcoming Arthritis & Other Rheumatic Diseases. Max Warmbrand. 1975. LC 75-13348. 220p. 15.00 (*0-8159-6311-4*) Devin.

Overcoming Barriers in Family Life & Sex Education from African Perspective Michael E. Akpan & Juliana M. Akpan. 1993. LC 93-71701. (Illus.). 114p. (Orig.). 1. pap. 13.95 (*0-9634998-2-3*); 2. pap. 15.00 (*0-9634998-5-8*) Ebewos Afr-Am.

Overcoming Binge Eating. Christopher G. Fairburn. 1995. (Illus.). 247p. pap. 16.95 (*0-89862-179-8*) Guilford Pubns.

Overcoming Bladder Disorders: Compassionate, Authoritative, Medical & Self-Help Solutions. Rebecca Chalker & Kristene E. Whitmore. 1991. LC 89-45789. 352p. pap. 14.00 (*0-06-092083-1*, Perennial) HarperTrade.

Overcoming Deficits of Aging: A Behavioral Approach. Roger L. Patterson. 1982. (Applied Clinical Psychology Ser.). 306p. 55.00 (*0-306-40947-X*, Plenum Trade) Perseus Pubng.

Overcoming Depression. Dennis Leonard. 1991. pap. 4.95 (*1-880809-01-X*) D Leonard Pubns.

***Overcoming Depression: A Five Areas Approach.** Chris Williams. 2001. (Arnold Publication). (Illus.). 240p. (Orig.). pap. text (*0-340-76383-3*) E A GBR. *Dist:* OUP.

Overcoming Depression: Get Rid of Depression Using This Practical Two-Part Programme. Dean Juniper. 2000. 144p. pap. (*1-85703-600-X*) How To Bks GBR. *Dist:* Midpt Trade.

Overcoming Depression: Therapist Protocol. Gary Emery. 1999. (Best Practices for Therapy Ser.). 116p. pap. 29.95 (*1-57224-160-8*) New Harbinger.

Overcoming Depressive Living Syndrome: How to Enjoy Life, Not Just Endure It. Earnie Larsen & Cara A. Macken. 1996. LC 95-46964. 208p. (Orig.). pap. 13.95 (*0-89243-868-1*, Liguori Triumph) Liguori Pubns.

Overcoming Doubt, Fear & Procrastination: Identifying the Symptoms, Overcoming the Obstacles. Barbara W. Sykes. 1996. 248p. pap. 24.95 (*0-9632857-7-7*) Collins Pubns.

Overcoming Eating Disorders: A Cognitive-Behavioral Treatment for Bulimia Nervosa & Binge Eating. W. Stewart Agras. 1997. pap. 37.50 (*0-15-813174-6*) Harcourt.

Overcoming Fear of Fat. Ed. by Laura S. Brown & Esther D. Rothblum. 1994. LC 89-19860. (Women & Therapy Ser.: Vol. 8, No. 3). 99p. pap. text 9.95 (*0-918393-71-X*, Harrington Park) Haworth Pr.

Overcoming Headaches: A Natural Approach. Pat Thomas. 2001. LC 00-50946. (Illus.). 128p. pap. 10.95 (*1-58091-105-6*) Crossing Pr.

Overcoming HIV Infection: Myths of HIV Testing & Test Results, the History of AIDS, Treatments for HIV Infection. 1991. lib. bdg. 79.95 (*0-8490-5138-X*) Gordon Pr.

Overcoming Hypertension. Kenneth H. Cooper. 1991. 464p. mass mkt. 6.99 (*0-553-28937-3*) Bantam.

Overcoming Infertility: 12 Couples Share Their Success Stories. Herbert A. Goldfarb. 1995. 252p. pap. 14.95 (*0-471-55706-4*) Wiley.

Overcoming Intestinal Disorders. Deepak Chopra. 1995. pap. 11.00 (*0-517-88492-5*) Random Hse Value.

Overcoming Jealousy & Possessiveness. Paul A. Hauck. 1981. LC 81-3040. 140p. pap. 15.95 (*0-664-24374-6*) Westminster John Knox.

Overcoming Jet Lag. Charles F. Ehret & Lynne Waller. 1987. (Illus.). 160p. (Orig.). pap. 11.95 (*0-425-09936-9*) Berkley Pub.

***Overcoming Low Self-Esteem.** Melanie Fennell. 2002. LC 2001-42708. (Self-Help Overcoming Ser.). (Illus.). 230p. pap. 14.95 (*0-8147-2714-X*) NYU Pr.

Overcoming Migraine: A Comprehensive Guide to Treatment & Prevention by a Survivor. Betsy Wyckoff. 1991. (Illus.). 112p. pap. 9.95 (*0-88268-126-5*); text 21.95 (*0-88268-110-9*) Station Hill Pr.

Overcoming Nervous Breakdown. Tony Lake. 1989. 107p. reprint ed. pap. 7.95 (*1-878290-01-0*) Intl Hlth MD.

Overcoming Panic Disorder. Lorna Weinstock & Eleanor Gilman. 1998. LC 97-42182. 288p. pap. 14.95 (*0-8092-3102-6*, 310260, Contemporary) McGraw-Hill Trade.

Overcoming Panic Disorder & Agoraphobia: Client Manual. Elke Zuercher-White. 1999. LC 00-502205. (Best Practices for Therapy Ser.). (Illus.). vi, 148p. pap. 15.95 (*1-57224-147-0*) New Harbinger.

Overcoming Panic Disorder & Agoraphobia: Therapist Protocol. Elke Zuercher-White. 1999. LC 00-502206. (Best Practices for Therapy Ser.). vi, 167p. pap. 29.95 (*1-57224-146-2*) New Harbinger.

Overcoming Post-Traumatic Stress Disorder: Client Manual. Larry Smyth. 1998. (Best Practices for Therapy Ser.). 95p. pap. 29.95 (*1-57224-163-2*) New Harbinger.

Overcoming Post-Traumatic Stress Disorder: Therapist Protocol. Larry Smyth. 1999. (Best Practices for Therapy Ser.). 190p. pap. 29.95 (*1-57224-162-4*) New Harbinger.

Overcoming Postpartum Depression: A Doctor's Own Story. Lois V. Nightingale. 1998. 128p. pap. 10.95 (*1-889755-26-5*) Nightngale Rose.

Overcoming Postpartum Depression & Anxiety. Linda Sebastian. 1998. LC 98-16262. (Illus.). 152p. pap. 12.95 (*1-886039-34-8*) Addicus Bks.

Overcoming Repetitive Motion Injuries the Rossiter Way. Richard H. Rossiter & Sue MacDonald. 1999. LC 98-68749. 256p. pap. 15.95 (*1-57224-134-9*) New Harbinger.

Overcoming Resistance: Rational-Emotive Therapy with Difficult Clients. Albert Ellis. 1985. 240p. 38.95 (*0-8261-4910-3*) Springer Pub.

Overcoming Resistance: Success in Counseling Men. George A. Harris. 1995. LC 95-35032. 156p. pap. 15.00 (*1-56991-032-4*) Am Correctional.

Overcoming Rheumatism & Arthritis. James G. Speight. 1984. 109p. pap. (*0-85207-166-3*) C W Daniel GBR. *Dist:* Natl Bk Netwk.

Overcoming Rheumatism & Arthritis. Phyllis Speight. 88p. (Orig.). pap. 8.95 (*0-8464-4265-5*) Beekman Pubs.

Overcoming Shyness & Social Phobia: A Step-by-Step Guide. Ronald M. Rapee. 1998. LC 97-27509. (Clinical Application of Evidence-Based Psychotherapy Ser.). 144p. pap. 25.00 (*0-7657-0120-0*) Aronson.

Overcoming Sleep Disorders: A Natural Approach. Brenda O'Hanlon. 2000. LC 00-30709. 110p. pap. 10.95 (*1-58091-014-9*) Crossing Pr.

Overcoming the Dark Side of Leadership: The Paradox of Personal Dysfunction. Gary L. McIntosh & Samuel D. Rima, Sr. 1997. LC 97-22265. 240p. (gr. 13). pap. 12.99 (*0-8010-9047-4*) Baker Bks.

Overcoming the Legacy of Overeating: How to Change Your Negative Eating Patterns. Nan K. Fuchs. rev. ed. 1996. 288p. pap. 16.00 (*1-56565-453-6*) Lowell Hse.

Overcoming the Legacy of Overeating: How Your Mother Influenced Your Eating Patterns & How You Can Change Them. Nan K. Fuchs. 1990. Orig. Title: My Mother Made Me Do It. 240p. reprint ed. pap. 9.95 (*0-929923-27-8*) Lowell Hse.

Overcoming the Legacy of Overeatings: How to Change Your Negative Eating Patterns. Nan K. Fuchs. 3rd ed. 1999. LC 99-41599. 288p. pap. 16.95 (*0-7373-0255-0*, 02550W) NTC Contemp Pub Co.

Overcoming the Rating Game: Beyond Self-Love - Beyond Self-Esteem. Paul A. Hauck. 1992. 112p. (Orig.). pap. 16.95 (*0-664-25310-5*) Westminster John Knox.

Overcoming the Recurring Nightmare of Schizophrenia. Jeanette Keil. 2nd ed. 21p. reprint ed. pap. 2.95 (*0-9616230-0-4*) K&A Pubns.

Overcoming Your Fear of the Dentist: A Dental Office Program Guide to Controlling Dental Anxiety. Leonard G. Horowitz. 2nd unabr. ed. 1987. (Freedom from Ser.). 20p. 19.95 incl. audio (*0-9609386-2-1*) Tetrahedron Pub.

Overdentures Made Easy: A Guide to Implant & Root Supported Prostheses. Harold W. Preiskel. 1996. 240p. text 98.00 (*1-85097-039-4*) Quint Pub Co.

Overdentures on Oral Implants. Ed. by E. Scherers. 1991. 173p. (Orig.). pap. (*90-6186-433-X*) Leuven Univ BEL. *Dist:* Coronet Bks.

Overexpression & Knockout of Cytokines in Transgenic Mice. Ed. by Chaim O. Jacob. 1994. (Illus.). 191p. text 69.00 (*0-12-378450-6*) Acad Pr.

Overseas Clinical Elective: A Survival Guide for Healthcare Workers. Renee Adomat. 1996. LC 96-25101. 176p. (Orig.). pap. text 29.95 (*0-632-04102-1*) Blackwell Sci.

Oversight of the Department of Education & the National Institute of Mental Health: Current Approaches to Attention Deficit/Hyperactivity Disorders : Hearing Before the Subcommittee on Human Resources & Intergovernmental Relations of the Committee on Government Reform & Oversight, House of Representatives, One Hundred Fourth Congress, Second Session, July 16, 1996. USGPO Staff. 1997. LC 98-159935. iii, 180 p. (*0-16-055847-6*) USGPO.

Overtraining in Sport. Ed. by Richard B. Kreider et al. 1997. LC 97-31205. (Illus.). 416p. text 49.00 (*0-88011-563-7*, BKRE0563) Human Kinetics.

Overuse Injuries of the Musculoskeletal System. Ivan Bojanic & Marko M. Pecina. 1993. LC 93-8061. 384p. 149.95 (*0-8493-4492-1*, RD97) CRC Pr.

Overview of Addiction Treatment Effectiveness. Mim J. Landry. 1996. (Illus.). 116p. (Orig.). (C). pap. text 35.00 (*0-7881-3656-9*) DIANE Pub.

Overview of Anesthesia for Nurses. Linda B. Chitwood. 1992. LC 94-60203. 81p. (C). pap. text 19.95 (*1-878025-40-6*) Western Schls.

Overview of Cardiac Surgery for the Cardiologist. Ed. by Richard T. Lee et al. 1993. LC 93-3832. (Illus.). 161p. 79.95 (*0-387-94066-9*) Spr-Verlag.

Overview of Cardiac Surgery for the Cardiologist. Richard T. Lee et al. 1993. LC 93-3832. (Illus.). 190p. (*3-540-94066-9*) Spr-Verlag.

Overview of Managerial Economics in the Health Care System. Shahram Heshmat. 2000. LC 00-60369. (Series in Health Services Administration). (Illus.). xiii, 158p. text 53.95 (*0-7668-1528-5*) Delmar.

Overview of Ocular Disorders. Nancy Gwin. 1998. (Basic Bookshelf for Eyecare Professionals Ser.). (Illus.). 112p. pap. 30.00 (*1-55642-336-5*, 63365) SLACK Inc.

Overview of Ocular Surgery & Surgical Counseling. Kim Pickett. 1999. LC 98-46244. (Basic Bookshelf for Eyecare Professionals Ser.). 128p. pap. 30.00 (*1-55642-332-2*, 63322) SLACK Inc.

Overview of the Indigent Health Care System in Texas. Don Brown & Andrew Cohen. 1992. (Working Papers Ser.: No. 67). 76p. pap. 5.50 (*0-89940-549-5*) LBJ Sch Pub Aff.

Overview of the New Age Movement. William A. Reck. 1995. LC 95-74802. 96p. pap. 4.50 (*1-877678-38-4*) Queenship Pub.

Overweight? It's All in Your Mind. John D. Hutto. 1987. LC 86-72988. (Illus.). (Orig.). pap. 5.00 (*0-940879-00-X*) All Amer Pr.

Overweight & Weight Management: The Health Professional's Guide to Understanding & Practice. Sharron Dalton. 1997. LC 97-6338. 550p. 68.00 (*0-8342-0636-6*) Aspen Pub.

Ovo-Implantation, Human Gonadotropines & Prolactin: Proceedings of the International Seminar on Reproductive Physiology & Sexual Endocrinology, 2nd, Brussels, 1968. International Seminar on Reproductive Physiology &. Ed. by P. O. Hubinont et al. 1970. (Illus.). 57.50 (*3-8055-0959-6*) S Karger.

Ovulation & Its Disorders. Ed. by W. M. Thompson et al. 1984. (Studies in Fertility & Sterility). lib. bdg. 114.50 (*0-85200-811-2*) Kluwer Academic.

Ovulation Induction. Ed. by R. L. Collins & Herbert J. Buchsbaum. 1990. (Clinical Perspectives in Obstetrics & Gynecology Ser.). (Illus.). 170p. 105.00 (*0-387-97351-6*) Spr-Verlag.

Ovulation Induction: Update '98. Ed. by M. Filicori & C. Flamigni. 1998. (Illus.). 246p. lib. bdg. 74.95 (*1-85070-025-7*, Parthenon Pbng) CRC Pr.

Ovulation Method Charting Booklet. Suzannah C. Doyle. 3rd rev. ed. 1991. (Illus.). 124p. pap. 10.00 (*0-9628284-0-8*) FA Services.

Ovulation Method of Natural Family Planning: A User Friendly Manual. Twin Cities Natural Family Planning Center, Inc. S. 1986. LC 86-50298. (Illus.). 130p. pap. 14.95 (*0-9616827-0-1*) TCNFPC.

Ovulation Method of Natural Family Planning: An Introductory Booklet for New Users. Thomas W. Hilgers. rev. ed. 1993. LC 92-81747. (Illus.). pap. text 4.80 (*0-9626485-2-3*) Pope Paul Sixth.

Own Your Own Body. Stan Malstrom. 1980. LC 76-58968. 414p. reprint ed. pap. 5.95 (*0-87983-215-0*, Keats Pubng) McGraw-Hill Trade.

Owner's Manual. Yogi Bhajan. Ed. & Illus. by Hari J. Khalsa. 1995. 50p. pap. 14.95 (*0-9639847-0-5*) KRI.

Owner's Manual: A Parent's Guide & Medical Record for a Child's First Two Years. James A. Waler. 1998. LC 98-93107. 115p. pap. 13.95 (*0-9664486-0-X*) Concpt Prodns.

Ownership of the Human Body: Philosophical Considerations on the Use of the Human Body & Its Parts in Healthcare. H. ten Have et al. 1998. LC 98-26395. (Philosophy & Medicine Ser.). 120.00 (*0-7923-5150-9*) Kluwer Academic.

Owning Your Own Shadow: Understanding the Dark Side of the Psyche. Robert A. Johnson. 1993. LC 90-56468. 128p. reprint ed. pap. 12.00 (*0-06-250754-0*) Harper SF.

Oxaliplatin: ASCO, May 2000. Ed. by H. J. Schmoll. 2000. (Onkologie Ser.: Vol. 23, Supp. 5). 32p. pap. 28.75 (*3-8055-7142-9*) S Karger.

Oxford Companion to the Mind. Ed. by Richard L. Gregory & O. L. Zangwill. 1987. (Illus.). 874p. 60.00 (*0-19-866124-X*) OUP.

Oxford Companion to the Mind. Ed. by Richard L. Gregory. 1999. LC 98-22974. (Illus.). 874p. reprint ed. pap. 26.50 (*0-19-860224-3*) OUP.

Oxford Dictionary of Sports Science & Medicine. Michael Kent. 2nd ed. 1998. LC 97-41377. (Illus.). 582p. text 39.95 (*0-19-262845-3*) OUP.

Oxford Handbook in Dental Patient Care. Crispian Scully. 1998. LC 98-9869. (Illus.). 456p. pap. 37.95 (*0-19-262915-8*) OUP.

Oxford Handbook of Accident & Emergency Medicine. Jonathan Wyatt et al. 1999. LC 98-4298. (Illus.). 800p. pap. 39.50 (*0-19-262751-1*) OUP.

Oxford Handbook of Acute Medicine. Punit s. Ramrakha & Kevin P. Moore. 1998. LC 97-26292. (Illus.). 892p. pap. 34.50 (*0-19-262682-5*) OUP.

Oxford Handbook of Clinical Dentistry. David A. Mitchell & Laura Mitchell. 3rd ed. 1999. LC 98-42398. (Illus.). 824p. pap. 39.95 (*0-19-262963-8*) OUP.

Oxford Handbook of Clinical Haematology. Drew Provan. 1998. LC 98-28128. 640p. pap. 39.95 (*0-19-262903-4*) OUP.

Oxford Handbook of Clinical Immunology. Gavin Spickett. 1999. LC 98-51592. (Oxford Medical Publications). 715p. pap. 34.50 (*0-19-262721-X*) OUP.

Oxford Handbook of Clinical Medicine. Ed. by David E. Thaler et al. 1999. LC 98-49082. (Illus.). 864p. pap. 29.95 (*0-19-512572-X*) OUP.

***Oxford Handbook of Clinical Surgery.** Ed. by Greg McLatchie & David Leaper. 2nd ed. 2002. (Illus.). 928p. pap. 32.50 (*0-19-262638-8*) OUP.

Oxford Handbook of Critical Care. Mervyn Singer & Andrew Webb. 1996. (Illus.). 560p. pap. 29.50 (*0-19-262542-X*) OUP.

***Oxford Handbook of General Practice.** Chantal Simon et al. 2002. LC 2001-52101. 848p. (Orig.). pap. text 29.95 (*0-19-263270-1*) OUP.

Oxford Handbook of Oncology. James Cassidy & D. Bissett. 2000. (Illus.). pap. text 29.95 (*0-19-263035-0*) OUP.

Oxford Handbook of Operative Surgery. Ed. by G. McLatchie & David J. Leaper. 1996. (Illus.). 734p. pap. 34.50 (*0-19-262097-5*) OUP.

Oxford Handbook of Sports Medicine. Ed. by Eugene Sherry & Stephen Wilson. 1998. LC 98-11503. (Illus.). 958p. pap. 34.50 (*0-19-262890-9*) OUP.

Oxford Handbook of Tropical Medicine. Michael Eddleston & Stephen Pierini. 1999. LC 98-50045. (Illus.). 666p. pap. 39.95 (*0-19-262772-4*) OUP.

Oxford Illustrated Companion to Medicine. Ed. by Stephen Lock et al. 3rd ed. 2001. LC 2001-21799. (Illus.). 1,008p. 60.00 (*0-19-262950-6*) OUP.

Oxford Textbook Of Clinical Hepatology Ed. by Johannes Bircher et al. 2nd ed. 1999. LC 98-30555. (Illus.). 2392p. text 350.00 (*0-19-262515-2*) OUP.

Oxford Textbook of Clinical Hepatology, Set. Ed. by N. McIntyre et al. 1992. 1772p. 295.00 (*0-19-261968-3*) OUP.

Oxford Textbook of Clinical Nephrology. Alex M. Davison et al. 2nd ed. 1998. 275.00 incl. disk (*0-19-268581-3*); 1997. LC 98-121868. (Illus.). 3,166p. text 495.00 (*0-19-262413-X*) OUP.

Oxford Textbook of Functional Anatomy, Vol. 1. Pamela C. B. MacKinnon & John B. Morris. 2nd rev. ed. 1994. LC 92-48317. (Oxford Medical Publications). (Illus.). 174p. (C). pap. text 24.95 (*0-19-262195-5*) OUP.

Oxford Textbook of Functional Anatomy Vol. 2: Thorax & Abdomen. Pamela C. B. MacKinnon & John B. Morris. 1988. (Illus.). 150p. pap. text 27.95 (*0-19-261518-1*) OUP.

Oxford Textbook of Functional Anatomy Vol. 3: Head & Neck, Vol. 2. Pamela C. B. MacKinnon & John F. Morris. rev. ed. 1991. (Illus.). 162p. pap. text 35.00 (*0-19-261519-X*) OUP.

Oxford Textbook of Geriatric Medicine. Ed. by John Grimley Evans et al. 2nd ed. 2000. LC 00-268634. (Oxford Medical Publications). (Illus.). 1,280p. text 198.00 (*0-19-262830-5*) OUP.

Oxford Textbook of Medicine David A. Warrell & D. J. Weatherall. 3rd ed. 1996. (Illus.). 5,024p. (C). text 299.00 (*0-19-262140-8*) OUP.

***Oxford Textbook of Oncology** Ed. by Robert L. Souhami et al. 2nd ed. 2002. (Illus.). 2368p. text 445.00 (*0-19-262926-3*) OUP.

Oxford Textbook of Oncology, Set. Ed. by Michael Peckham et al. 1995. (Illus.). text 275.00 (*0-19-261685-4*) OUP.

Oxford Textbook of Ophthalmology Ed. by David L. Easty & John M. Sparrow. 1999. LC 00-265153. (Oxford Medical Publications). (Illus.). 1,396p. text 295.00 (*0-19-262557-8*) OUP.

Oxford Textbook of Palliative Medicine. Ed. by Derek Doyle et al. 2nd ed. 1999. (Illus.). 1,309p. pap. text 95.00 (*0-19-263057-1*) OUP.

Oxford Textbook of Pathology Vol. 1: General Principles of Pathology, Vol. 1. Ed. by James O. McGee et al. 1992. (Illus.). 918p. pap. text 85.00 (*0-19-261972-1*) OUP.

Oxford Textbook of Pathology Vol. 2: Pathology of Systems, Vol. 2, Pts. 1 & 2. Ed. by James O. McGee et al. 1992. (Illus.). pap. text 160.00 (*0-19-261974-8*) OUP.

***Oxford Textbook of Public Health.** Ed. by Roger Detels et al. 2002. (Illus.). 1808p. text 475.00 (*0-19-263041-5*) OUP.

Oxford Textbook of Public Health, Set. Ed. by James McEwen et al. 3rd ed. 1997. (Illus.). 1,646p. text 475.00 (*0-19-262553-5*) OUP.

Oxford Textbook of Rheumatology Ed. by Peter J. Maddison et al. 2nd ed. 1998. LC 98-149774. (Illus.). text 375.00 (*0-19-262697-3*) OUP.

Oxford Textbook of Rheumatology, 2. Ed. by P. J. Maddison et al. 1993. LC 92-48994. (*0-19-262343-5*) OUP.

Oxford Textbook of Sports Medicine. Ed. by Mark Harries et al. 2nd ed. (Illus.). 2000. 960p. pap. text 98.50 (*0-19-263236-1*); 1998. LC 98-16976. 984p. text 115.00 (*0-19-262717-1*) OUP.

Oxford Textbook of Surgery. Ed. by Peter J. Morris & Ronald A. Malt. 1994. (Illus.). text 225.00 (*0-19-261800-8*) OUP.

Oxidant-Induced Stress & Antioxidant Defenses in Biology. Ed. by Sami Ahmad. 1995. LC 94-13342. 448p. (C). (gr. 13). pap. text 125.95 (*0-412-03971-0*) Chapman & Hall.

Oxidants & Antioxidants in Cutaneous Biology. Ed. by J. Thiele & P. Elsner. 2001. LC 00-48668. (Current Problems in Dermatology Ser.: 29). (Illus.). ix, 194p. 188.00 (*3-8055-7132-1*) S Karger.

Oxidants, Antioxidants & Free Radicals. Steven I. Baskin & Harry Salem. 1997. LC 97-13108. 450p. 135.00 (*1-56032-644-1*) Hemisp Pub.

Oxidation & Phosphorylation. Ed. by Ronald W. Estabrook et al. 1967. (Methods in Enzymology Ser.: Vol. 10). text 209.00 (*0-12-181850-0*) Acad Pr.

Oxidative Behavior of Materials by Thermal Analytical Techniques. Ed. by Alan T. Riga & Gerald H. Patterson. 1997. LC 97-39992. (STP Ser.: Vol. STP1326). (Illus.). 247p. 69.00 (*0-8031-2483-X*, STP1326) ASTM.

Oxidative Damage & Related Enzymes, Vol. 2. G. Rotilio. 1984. (Life Chemistry Reports). x, 436p. pap. text 225.00 (*3-7186-0221-0*) Gordon & Breach.

Oxidative Injury in Dermatopathology. J. Fuchs. 1992. (Illus.). 360p. 223.00 (*0-387-54355-4*) Spr-Verlag.

Oxidative Stress: Oxidants & Antioxidants. Ed. by Helmut Sies. 1991. (Illus.). 507p. (C). text 104.00 (*0-12-642762-3*) Acad Pr.

Oxidative Stress & Aging. R. G. Cutler et al. Ed. by Lester Packer. 1995. LC 95-105254. (Molecular & Cell Biology Updates Ser.: Vol. 12). 396p. 164.00 (*0-8176-5039-3*) Spr-Verlag.

***Oxidative Stress & Digestive Diseases.** Ed. by Toshikazu Yoshikawa & Yuji Naito. 2001. LC 2001-22536. (Illus.). x, 178p. 128.75 (*3-8055-7230-1*) S Karger.

Oxidative Stress & the Molecular Biology of Antioxidant Defenses. Ed. by John G. Scandalios. 1996. LC 96-92949. (Monographs: Vol. 34). (Illus.). 992p. (C). text 155.00 (*0-87969-502-1*) Cold Spring Harbor.

Oxidative Stress, Cell Activation & Viral Infection. Ed. by C Pasquier et al. 1993. LC 93-44396. (Molecular & Cell Biology Updates Ser.). (Illus.). 376p. 99.00 (*0-8176-2941-6*) Birkhauser.

Oxidative Stress in Cancer, AIDS & Neurodegenerative Diseases. Ed. by Luc Montagnier & C Pasquier. 1997. LC 97-41304. (Oxidative Stress & Disease Ser.). (Illus.). 578p. text 195.00 (*0-8247-9862-7*) Dekker.

Oxidative Stress in Dermatology. Ed. by Jurgen Fuchs & Lester Packer. 1993. (Basic & Clinical Dermatology Ser.: Vol. 8). (Illus.). 560p. text 250.00 (*0-8247-9049-9*) Dekker.

Oxidative Stress in Male Infertility. Ed. by Falk R. Ochsendorf & Jurgen Fuchs. 1995. 129.95 (*0-8493-4798-X*, 4798) CRC Pr.

Oxidative Stress in Neuronal Death. Irene Ceballos-Picot. 1997. LC 97-19204. (Medical Intelligence Unit Ser.). 196p. 99.00 (*1-57059-454-6*) Landes Bioscience.

Oxidative Stress in Neuronal Death: Role in Age-Related Neurodegenerative Disorders. Irene Ceballos-Picot. 1997. LC 97-19204. (Medical Intelligence Unit Ser.). 196p. pap. 89.95 (*0-412-13541-8*) Chapman & Hall.

Oxidative Stress in Skeletal Muscle. A. Z. Reznick. 1998. LC 98-6332. (Molecular & Cell Biology Updates Ser.). 140.00 (*0-8176-5820-3*) Birkhauser.

Oxidative Stress in Skeletal Muscle. Ed. by A. Z. Reznick et al. 1998. LC 98-6332. (Molecular & Cell Biology Updates Ser.). 500p. 140.00 (*3-7643-5820-3*) Birkhauser.

Oxidative Stress, Lipoproteins & Cardiovascular Dysfunction. Ed. by K. R. Bruckdorfer & Catherine A. Rice-Evans. 1995. (Portland Press Research Monographs: Vol. 6). 184p. (C). text (*1-85578-045-3*) Portland Pr Ltd GBR. *Dist:* Ashgate Pub Co.

Oxidative/Energy Metabolism in Neurodegenerative Disorders. Ed. by John P. Blass & Fletcher H. McDowell. 1999. (*1-57331-209-6*) NY Acad Sci.

Oxorn-Foote Human Labor & Birth. Harry Oxorn. 5th ed. 1998. (Illus.). 918p. (C). pap. text 59.95 (*0-8385-7665-6*, A7665-1, Apple Lange Med) McGraw.

Oxycal vs. Arthritis. Michael A. Cox. 1984. 171p. (Orig.). pap. 5.95 (*0-942078-07-1*) R Tanner Assocs Inc.

Oxygen: Basis of the Regulation of Vital Functions in the Fetus. Ed. by W. Kunzel & M. Kirschbaum. 1992. LC 92-20354. (Illus.). 190p. 129.00 (*0-387-55413-0*) Spr-Verlag.

Oxygen Administration. National Safety Council Staff. 1994. LC 94-215136. (Illus.). 60p. (C). pap. text 16.95 (*0-86720-983-6*, 983-6) Jones & Bartlett.

Oxygen & Living Processes: An Interdisciplinary Approach. Ed. by Daniel L. Gilbert. 1981. (Topics in Environmental Physiology & Medicine Ser.). (Illus.). 401p. 137.00 (*0-387-90554-5*) Spr-Verlag.

Oxygen Equipment. 1995. lib. bdg. 257.95 (*0-8490-6601-8*) Gordon Pr.

Oxygen-Free Radicals in Shock. Ed. by G. P. Novelli. 1986. (Illus.). xii, 248p. 139.25 (*3-8055-4233-X*) S Karger.

Oxygen, Gene Expression, & Cellular Function, Vol. 105. Donald Massaro & Linda B. Clerch. 1997. LC 97-11362. (Lung Biology in Health & Disease Ser.). (Illus.). 512p. text 225.00 (*0-8247-0062-7*) Dekker.

Oxygen Homeostasis & Its Dynamics. Ed. by Yuzuru Ishimura et al. 1998. LC 97-41378. (Keio University Symposia for Life Science & Medicine Ser.). (Illus.). 632p. 260.00 (*4-431-70202-4*) Spr-Verlag.

Oxygen Multistep Therapy: Physiological & Technical Foundations. Manfred Von Ardenne. Tr. by Paula Kirby & Winfried Kruger from GER. 1997. (Illus.). (C). text (*3-13-743501-3*) G Thieme DEU. *Dist:* Thieme Med Pubs.

Oxygen Multistep Therapy: Physiological & Technical Foundations. Manfred Von Ardenne. 1990. 69.00 (*0-86577-377-7*) Thieme Med Pubs.

Oxygen Radicals: Systemic Events & Disease Processes. Ed. by Dilip K. Das & Walter B. Essman. 1990. (Illus.). xii, 196p. 151.50 (*3-8055-5049-9*) S Karger.

Oxygen Radicals & the Disease Process. Ed. by Craig E. Thomas & Balaraman Kalyanaraman. 1998. 296p. text 60.00 (*90-5702-226-5*, Harwood Acad Pubs) Gordon & Breach.

Oxygen Radicals in Biological Systems. Sidney P. Colowick & Nathan O. Kaplan. 1984. (Methods in Enzymology Ser.: Vol. 105). text 188.00 (*0-12-182005-X*) Acad Pr.

Oxygen Radicals in Biology & Medicine. Ed. by Michael G. Simic et al. 1988. (Basic Life Sciences Ser.: Vol. 49). (Illus.). 1068p. 175.00 (*0-306-43021-5*, Plenum Trade) Perseus Pubng.

Oxygen Radicals in the Pathophysiology of Heart Disease. Ed. by Pawan K. Singal. 1988. (Developments in Cardiovascular Medicine Ser.). (C). text 150.00 (*0-89838-375-7*) Kluwer Academic.

Oxygen Regulation of Ion Channels & Gene Expression. Ed. by Jose Lopez-Barneo & E. Kenneth Weir. 1998. LC 97-50337. (Illus.). 288p. 120.00 (*0-87993-694-0*) Futura Pub.

Oxygen-Seventeen & Silicon-Twenty-Nine. J. P. Kintzinger & H. Marsmann. 1981. (NMR Ser.: Vol. 17). (Illus.). 235p. 79.95 (*0-387-10414-3*) Spr-Verlag.

Oxygen Status of Arterial Blood. Ed. by R. Zander & F. O. Mertzlufft. 1991. (Illus.). xii, 294p. 68.75 (*3-8055-5280-7*) S Karger.

Oxygen Stress & Tissue Damage. Ed. by J. Feher et al. 1994. LC 95-109779. 172p. pap. (*963-05-6657-5*) Akade Kiado HUN. *Dist:* Intl Spec Bk, St Mut.

Oxygen Therapies: A New Way of Approaching Disease. Ed McCabe. 1988. (Energy Publications Alternatives). (Illus.). 224p. (Orig.). (C). pap. 12.00 (*0-9620527-0-1*) Energy Pubns.

Oxygen Therapy. Lonny J. Ashworth. 1998. (CPG Mentor - Patient Cases in Respiratory Care Ser.: Unit 2). (*0-8151-2278-0*) Mosby Inc.

Oxygen Transport in Red Blood Cells: Proceedings of the Twelfth Aharon Katzie-Katchalsky Conference, Tours, France, 4-7 April 1984. Ed. by C. Nicolau. 1986. 204p. (*0-08-030800-7*) PPL.

Oxygen Transport in the Critically Ill Patient: Munster (FRG), 11-12 May, 1990. Ed. by M. Wendt et al. 1990. (Anaesthesiologie und Intensivmedizin Ser.). (Illus.). 240p. 33.95 (*0-387-52498-3*) Spr-Verlag.

Oxygen Transport to Tissue. Ed. by A. G. Hudetz & Duane F. Bruley. 1998. (Advances in Experimental Medicine & Biology Ser.: 454). (Illus.). 706p. (C). text 195.00 (*0-306-46043-2*, Kluwer Plenum) Kluwer Academic.

Oxygen Transport to Tissue, No. X. Ed. by M. Mochizuki et al. 1988. LC 87-32879. (Advances in Experimental Medicine & Biology Ser.: Vol. 222). (Illus.). 784p. 145.00 (*0-306-42795-8*, Plenum Trade) Perseus Pubng.

Oxygen Transport to Tissue, No. XI. Ed. by Karel Rakusan et al. 1989. (Advances in Experimental Medicine & Biology Ser.: Vol. 247). (Illus.). 812p. 165.00 (*0-306-43156-4*, Plenum Trade) Perseus Pubng.

Oxygen Transport to Tissue, Vol. 18. Ed. by Edwin M. Nemoto & Joseph C. LaManna. 1997. LC 97-4326. (Advances in Experimental Medicine & Biology Ser.: Vol. 411). (Illus.). 624p. (C). text 159.50 (*0-306-45516-1*, Kluwer Plenum) Kluwer Academic.

Oxygen Transport to Tissue, Vol. 115. Ed. by W. Erdmann & Duane F. Bruley. 1992. (Advances in Experimental Medicine & Biology Ser.: Vol. 317). (Illus.). 940p. (C). text 222.00 (*0-306-44232-9*, Kluwer Plenum) Kluwer Academic.

Oxygen Transport to Tissue: Proceedings of the 24th Annual Meeting of the International Society Held in Dundee, Scotland, August 19-23, 1996, Vol. 428. Ed. by David K. Harrison & David T. Delpy. 1998. LC 97-31219. (Advances in Experimental Medicine & Biology Ser.: Vol. XIX). (Illus.). 736p. 210.00 (*0-306-45711-3*, Kluwer Plenum) Kluwer Academic.

Oxygen Transport to Tissue. Ed. by T. K. Goldstick et al. 1992. (Advances in Experimental Medicine & Biology Ser.: Vol. 316). (Illus.). 504p. (C). text 174.00 (*0-306-44342-2*, Kluwer Plenum) Kluwer Academic.

Oxygen Transport to Tissue, Vol. 15. P. Vaupel et al. 1994. (Advances in Experimental Medicine & Biology Ser.: Vol. 345). (Illus.). 976p. (C). text 185.00 (*0-306-44632-4*, Kluwer Plenum) Kluwer Academic.

Oxygenation. Sheldon. 2000. (Nursing Concepts Ser.). 22.95 (*1-889325-55-4*) Fence Crk Pubng.

Oxygen/Nitrogen Radicals & Cellular Injury. Ed. by Kenneth B. Adler et al. 2000. (Illus.). 141p. (C). reprint ed. pap. text 30.00 (*0-7881-8538-1*) DIANE Pub.

Oxytocin: Cellular & Molecular Approaches in Medicine & Research. Ed. by Richard Ivell & John A. Russell. 1996. (Advances in Experimental Medicine & Biology Ser.: Vol. 395). (Illus.). 692p. (C). text 174.00 (*0-306-45290-1*, Kluwer Plenum) Kluwer Academic.

Ozone Chlorine-Dioxide Oxidation Products of Organic Materials. Ed. by Rip G. Rice & Joseph A. Cotruvo. 1978. LC 78-53924. (Illus.). text 50.00 (*0-918650-02-X*) Pan Am Intl Ozone.

Ozone Depletion & Health. Ed. by R. Russell Jones & T. M. Wigley. 1989. LC 89-16614. 302p. 375.00 (*0-471-92316-8*) Wiley.

P

P. A. T. H. Wellness Manual. Eric R. Braverman. 1993. (Illus.). 363p. pap. 25.00 (*0-9638869-0-8*) Pubns for Achieving.

P-ChIPS (Parent Version of ChIPS) Report Forms for P-ChIPS. Elizabeth B. Weller et al. 1999. pap. 19.95 (*0-88048-399-7*) Am Psychiatric.

P-ChIPS (Parent Version of ChIPS) Scoring Forms for P-ChIPS. Elizabeth B. Weller et al. 1999. pap. 24.95 (*0-88048-396-2*) Am Psychiatric.

P. Meera Khan Dedication Issue. Ed. by H. P. Klinger & P. L. Pearson. 1999. (Cytogenetics & Cell Genetics Ser.: Vol. 86, No. 2). (Illus.). 78p. pap. 25.25 (*3-8055-6989-0*) S Karger.

P. O. W. in the Pacific: Memoirs of an American Doctor in World War II. William N. Donovan. Ed. by Josephine Donovan. 1998. LC 97-48354. (Illus.). 176p. 22.95 (*0-8420-2725-4*) Scholarly Res Inc.

PACE System: An Expert Consulting System for Nursing. S. Evans. 1996. LC 96-12477. (Computers & Medicine Ser.). (Illus.). 167p. 59.95 (*0-387-94731-0*) Spr-Verlag.

Pacemaker Activity & Intercellular Communication. Ed. by Jan D. Huizinga. 1995. LC 94-28589. (Electronic Engineering Systems Ser.). 368p. 224.95 (*0-8493-7669-6*) CRC Pr.

Pacemaker Activity & Intercellular Communication, Set. Marvin Thompson. 1988. LC 87-18375. (Calcium Binding Proteins Ser.). 186.00 (*0-8493-4857-9*, QP552, CRC Reprint) Franklin.

Pacemaker Clinic of the 90's: Essentials in Brady-Pacing. Ed. by N. M. Van Hemel et al. 1995. LC 95-23889. (Developments in Cardiovascular Medicine Ser.: Vol. 175). 276p. text 95.50 (*0-7923-3688-7*) Kluwer Academic.

Pacemaker Emergency Intervention System. AAMI Staff. 1993. (Illus.). 8p. (Orig.). pap. 62.00 (*1-57020-009-2*, PAC49-209) Assn Adv Med Instrn.

Pacemaker Interpretation for Nurses. Carol J. Wallace. 1995. LC 95-69076. (Illus.). pap. 19.95 (*0-9627246-6-1*) Power NY.

Pacemaker Pocket Professor. Jonni Cooper. 1991. (C). (gr. 13). text 16.95 (*0-944132-47-2*) Mosby Inc.

Pacemaker Primer. Julie Ann Purcell. 2001. pap. text 39.95 (*0-7817-1900-3*) Lppncott W & W.

Pacemakers: Patient Care, Troubleshooting, Rhythm Analysis. Karen S. Kesten & Colleen K. Norton. 1985. 215p. (Orig.). pap. text 17.00 (*0-932491-22-7*) Res Appl Inc.

Pacific Partnerships for Health: Charting a New Course. Ed. by Jill C. Feasley & Robert S. Lawrence. 1998. LC 98-134880. 176p. pap. text 31.00 (*0-309-05948-8*) Natl Acad Pr.

Pacing Yourself: Steps to Help Save Your Energy. Diane Christy & Carol A. Sarafconn. 1990. (Illus.). 128p. (Orig.). pap. 10.95 (*0-915708-31-0*) Cheever Pub.

Package for Emergency Patient Care for the EMT-A. Janet Barber et al. 1982. (C). 25.00 (*0-8359-5412-9*) P-H.

Packaging Drugs & Pharmaceuticals. Wilmer Jenkins & Kenton R. Osborn. 1993. LC 93-60377. 368p. ring bd. 99.95 (*1-56676-014-3*) CRC Pr.

Packaging in the Medical & Pharmaceutical Industries: Market Demands Specialized Products. 1992. 210p. 1495.00 (*1-56753-025-7*) Frost & Sullivan.

Packaging of Pharmaceuticals & Healthcare Products. F. A. Paine & H. Lockhart. 1995. (Illus.). 211p. (*0-7514-0167-6*) B Acad & Prof GBR. *Dist:* Aspen Pub.

Paclitaxel in Cancer Treatment, No. 8. Ed. by William P. McGuire & Erick K. Rowinsky. 1995. LC 95-2352. (Basic & Clinical Oncology Ser.: Vol. 8). (Illus.). 368p. text 155.00 (*0-8247-9307-2*) Dekker.

PACS: Basics Principles & Applications. H. K. Huang. 1998. LC 98-23684. (Illus.). 519p. pap. 110.00 (*0-471-25393-6*, Wiley-Liss) Wiley.

PACS: Picture Archiving & Communication Systems in Biomedical Imaging. H. K. Huang. 1996. 489p. 195.00 (*0-471-18607-4*) Wiley.

PACU Policy & Procedure Guideline Manual: Policy & Procedure Guideline Manual. Diane I. Howery. 1994. 148p. spiral bd. 105.00 (*1-879575-08-6*) Acad Med Sys.

Paediatric Anaesthesia. Ed. by Edward Sumner & David Hatch. 2000. (Arnold Publication). (Illus.). 592p. 98.50 (*0-340-71942-7*) OUP.

Paediatric & Adolescent Gynecology. Ed. by A. S. Garden. 1998. LC 97-3430. (Illus.). 448p. text (*0-340-60764-5*) E A GBR. *Dist:* OUP.

***Paediatric Audiological Medicine.** Ed. by Valerie Newton. 2001. 300p. (Orig.). (C). pap. (*1-86156-228-4*) Whurr Pub GBR. *Dist:* Taylor & Francis.

Paediatric Audiology: Zero to Five Years. Barry McCormick. 2nd ed. 1993. 458p. 55.00 (*1-56593-239-0*, 0558) Singular Publishing.

Paediatric Cardiology. Robert H. Anderson. 2000. text 399.00 (*0-443-04517-8*) Saunders.

Paediatric Cases for Postgraduate Examinations. Simon Attard-Montalto & Vaskar Saha. 1994. 192p. pap. text (*0-7506-2096-X*) E A GBR. *Dist:* OUP.

Paediatric Chemical Pathology. B. E. Clayton. 1980. 176p. pap. 24.95 (*0-632-00564-5*) Blackwell Sci.

Paediatric Cholestasis: Novel Approaches to Treatment: Proceedings of the 63rd Falk Symposium Held in Titisee-Black Forest, Germany, October 9-10, 1992. Falk Symposium Staff. Ed. by M. Lentze & J. Reichen. 1992. LC 92-15070. 384p. (C). text 164.00 (*0-7923-8977-8*) Kluwer Academic.

Paediatric Clinical Examination. Denis Gill & Niall O'Brien. 2nd ed. 1993. LC 92-49185. (Illus.). 224p. pap. text (*0-443-04725-1*) Church.

Paediatric Endocrinology in Clinical Practice. A. Aynsley-Green. 1984. text 147.50 (*0-85200-864-3*) Kluwer Academic.

Paediatric Epilepsy Syndromes & Their Surgical Treatment. Tuxhom. 1997. 894p. (*0-86196-536-1*) J Libbey Med GBR. *Dist:* Buttrwrth-Heinemann.

Paediatric Exercise Science & Medicine. Ed. by Neil Armstrong & Willem Van Mechelen. 2000. LC 00-710815. (Oxford Medical Publications). (Illus.). xii, 472p. text 129.50 (*0-19-262977-8*) OUP.

Paediatric Forensic Medicine & Pathology. Ed. by J. K. Mason. 1989. (Illus.). 528p. (C). (gr. 13). text 188.95 (*0-412-29160-6*) Chapman & Hall.

Paediatric Gastroenterology. Ed. by J. Navarro & J. Schmitz. Tr. by Brian Barefoot. 1992. (Illus.). 560p. text 165.00 (*0-19-261771-0*) OUP.

Paediatric Gastroenterology, No. 2. Charlotte M. Anderson. 2nd ed. 1989. (gr. 13). 145.00 (*0-86793-176-0*) Mosby Inc.

***Paediatric Grey Cases for the MRCPCH.** Alan C. Fenton et al. 2001. (Illus.). 205p. pap. (*0-443-06444-X*) Church GBR. *Dist:* Saunders.

Paediatric History & Examination. Ian A. Laing & Neil McIntosh. 1994. (Illus.). 95p. text (*0-7020-1809-0*) W B Saunders GBR. *Dist:* Saunders.

Paediatric Intensive Care. Ed. by Neil S. Morton. 1997. (Illus.). 310p. text 65.00 (*0-19-262511-X*) OUP.

Paediatric Intensive Care Nursing. Carol Williams & Julie Asquith. 2000. LC 99-33459. viii, 442p. text (*0-443-05528-9*) Church.

Paediatric MCQ Revision for MRCP & MRCPCH. Jane Lucas & James Nicholson. 1997. 192p. pap. text (*0-7506-3014-0*) E A GBR. *Dist:* OUP.

Paediatric MCQs for Postgraduate Exams, Vol. 1. Simon Attard et al. 1996. 848p. pap. text (*0-7506-2769-7*) E A GBR. *Dist:* OUP.

Paediatric MCQs for Postgraduate Exams, Vol. 2. Simon Attard-Montalto et al. 1996. LC 96-197400. 112p. pap. text (*0-7506-2845-6*) E A GBR. *Dist:* OUP.

Paediatric Neoplasia: An Atlas & Text. S. Variend. 1993. LC 93-20356. (Current Histopathology Ser.: Vol. 22). 128p. (C). text 209.50 (*0-7923-8900-X*) Kluwer Academic.

Paediatric Nephrology: A Research Update. Ed. by D. Boda & S. Turi. 1988. (Contributions to Nephrology Ser.: Vol. 67). (Illus.). x, 238p. 29.75 (*3-8055-4689-0*) S Karger.

Paediatric Neurosurgery. Ed. by M. Choux et al. 1999. (Illus.). 700p. (C). text (*0-443-05630-7*) Church.

***Paediatric Neurosurgery.** Linda Mayes. 2001. 200p. (Orig.). (C). pap. (*1-86156-224-1*) Whurr Pub GBR. *Dist:* Taylor & Francis.

Paediatric Oncology. Ed. by W. Duncan. 1983. (Recent Results in Cancer Research Ser.: Vol. 88). (Illus.). 116p. 76.00 (*0-387-12349-0*) Spr-Verlag.

Paediatric Oncology: Acute Nursing Care Margaret Evans. 1998. 17p. pap. text 37.95 (*1-86156-047-8*) Singular Publishing.

Paediatric Oncology: Clinical Practice & Controversies. Ed. by P. N. Plowman & C. R. Pinkerton. 1992. (Illus.). 672p. 132.95 (*0-442-31595-3*) Chapman & Hall.

Paediatric Oncology: Clinical Practice & Controversies. P. W. Plowman & C. R. Pinkerton. 1991. (Illus.). 672p. (gr. 13). pap. 169.95 (*0-412-39780-3*) Chapman & Hall.

Paediatric Ophthalmology. David Conrad Taylor. 2nd ed. 1997. LC 96-24809. (Illus.). 1216p. 314.95 (*0-86542-831-X*) Blackwell Sci.

Paediatric Opthalmology. Ed. by Anthony Moore. 2001. (Fundamentals in Clinical Ophthalmology Ser.). 249p. text (*0-7279-1203-8*) BMJ Pub GBR. *Dist:* AIDC.

Paediatric Orthopaedics & Fractures, Set. W. J. Sharrard. 3rd ed. 1992. (Illus.). 1752p. 299.95 (*0-632-03457-2*) Blackwell Sci.

Paediatric Osteology: New Developments in Diagnostics & Therapy: Proceedings of the First International Workshop on Paediatric Osteology, Cologne, Germany, 5-7 October 1995. Ed. by Eckhard Schonau. 1996. LC 96-6146. (International Congress Ser.: No. 1105). 316p. 148.00 (*0-444-82277-1*, Excerpta Medica) Elsevier.

Paediatric Osteology: Prevention of Osteoporosis - A Paediatric Task?: Proceedings of the 2nd International Workshop on Paediatric Osteology, Cologne, October 3-5, 1997. Eckhardshop Sch Onau & V. Matkovic. 1998. LC 98-4052. (International Congress Ser.). 286p. 140.50 (*0-444-82840-0*) Elsevier.

Paediatric Pathology. Ed. by Colin L. Berry. 3rd ed. 1995. LC 95-33587. (Illus.). 942p. 225.00 (*3-540-19936-5*) Spr-Verlag.

Paediatric Perspectives on Epilepsy: A Symposium Held at the Grand Hotel, Eastbourne, December 1984, Vol. 198. Ed. by Euan Ross. 1985. LC 85-12009. 176p. 415.00 (*0-471-90817-7*) Wiley.

Paediatric Problems in General Practice. Michael Modell et al. 3rd ed. 1996. (Oxford General Practice Ser.: No. 36). (Illus.). 352p. pap. text 49.95 (*0-19-262512-8*) OUP.

Paediatric Research: Proceedings of the WHO Scientific Group, Geneva, 1967. WHO Staff. 1968. (Technical Reports: No. 400). pap. text 3.00 (*92-4-120400-1*, 1100400) World Health.

Paediatric Respiratory Disease. Ed. by M. H. Goetz & O. B. Stur. 1982. (Progress in Respiratory Research Ser.: Vol. 17). (Illus.). x, 306p. 152.00 (*3-8055-2658-X*) S Karger.

Paediatric Respiratory Physiology & Clinical Aspects of Paediatric Pneumology. Ed. by R. Kraemer. 1982. (Modern Problems in Pediatrics Ser.: Vol. 21). (Illus.). xii, 248p. pap. 143.50 (*3-8055-3505-8*) S Karger.

Paediatric Surgery. John D. Atwell. 1998. LC 98-12130. (Arnold Publication). (Illus.). 864p. 250.00 (*0-340-58608-7*) OUP.

Paediatric Surgical Disorders: An Illustrated Guide to Diagnosis. Spencer W. Beasley et al. 1994. LC 93-9269. 408p. (gr. 13). pap. 314.95 (*0-412-54420-2*) Chapman & Hall.

Paediatric Thoracic Surgery. Ed. by N. A. Myers & T. A. Angerpointner. 1991. (Progress in Pediatric Surgery Ser.: Vol. 27). (Illus.). 272p. 185.00 (*0-387-52525-4*) Spr-Verlag.

***Paediatric Ultrasound.** Ed. by Helen Carty et al. 2001. (Illus.). 216p. pap. text (*1-900151-17-0*) Greenwich Med GBR. *Dist:* JAMCO Dist.

Paediatrics. S. Attard-Montalto & V. Saha. 1998. LC 99-36782. (Illus.). 200p. pap. (*0-443-05516-5*) Church.

Paediatrics. A. Evans & C. McCarthy. 1986. (Management of Common Diseases in Family Practice Ser.). text 73.50 (*0-85200-759-0*) Kluwer Academic.

Paediatrics. Thomas. 2nd ed. 1998. (C). pap. text 16.95 (*0-443-05880-6*) Saunders.

Paediatrics: Key Questions Answered. Jonathan Round. 1999. LC 98-41105. (Key Questions Answered Ser.). 308p. pap. text 29.95 (*0-19-262904-2*) OUP.

Paediatrics: Understanding Child Health. Ed. by Tony Waterston et al. 1997. LC 97-218843. (Oxford Core Texts). (Illus.). 432p. (C). text 95.00 (*0-19-262564-0*) OUP.

Paediatrics & Blood Transfusion. Smith C. Sibinga. 1982. text 94.00 (*90-247-2619-0*) Kluwer Academic.

Paediatrics & Child Health. Malcolm I. Levene & Mary C. J. Rudolf. 1999. LC 98-24257. (Illus.). 10p. pap. 52.95 (*0-86542-957-X*) Blackwell Sci.

Paediatrics Revision. Kwei C. Chin & Michael J. Tarlow. 1989. (Illus.). 180p. pap. text (*0-443-03274-2*) Church.

Paediatrische Infektionskrankheiten IV. Ed. by U. B. Schaad. 1985. (Paediatrische Fortbildungskurse fuer die Praxis Ser.: Vol. 59). (Illus.). xii, 188p. pap. 34.00 (*3-8055-3954-1*) S Karger.

Paediatrische Infektionskrankheiten III. Ed. by U. B. Schaad. 1983. (Paediatrische Fortbildungskurse fuer die Praxis Ser.: Vol. 58). (Illus.). xvi, 132p. pap. 42.75 (*3-8055-3680-1*) S Karger.

Pagalami: Ethnopsychiatric Knowledge in Bengal. Deborah P. Bhattacharyya. 1986. (Foreign & Comparative Studies Program, South Asian Ser.: No. 11). (Orig.). (C). pap. 13.00 (*0-915984-89-X*) Syracuse U Foreign Comp.

Pages off the Doctor's Pad. Harold C. Klein. 1994. LC 93-79811. 104p. pap. 9.95 (*1-879653-07-9*) Lakeside Pr.

Paget's Disease of the Bone: Assessment & Management. R. C. Hamdy. 1981. 216p. 72.95 (*0-275-91344-9*, C1344, Praeger Pubs) Greenwood.

Pain. Ed. by J. Brihaye et al. 1987. (Acta Neurochirurgica Ser.: No. 38). (Illus.). 200p. 180.00 (*0-387-81990-8*) Spr-Verlag.

Pain. Kazanowski. 2000. (Nursing Concepts Ser.). 22.95 (*1-889325-56-2*) Fence Crk Pubng.

Pain. Dan Middleman. 1998. (Illus.). 226p. pap. 17.50 (*0-911521-52-6*) Tafnews.

Pain: A Handbook for Nurses. Beatrice Sofaer. 2nd ed. 1992. LC 92-49745. 35.00 (*1-56593-045-2*, 0293) Thomson Learn.

Pain: A Sourcebook for Nurses & Other Professionals. Ada K. Jacox. 1977. text 22.50 (*0-316-45590-3*, Little Brwn Med Div) Lppncott W & W.

Pain: Cause, Effect, Evaluation, Set. John P. Adams et al. 1987. (Illus.). 345.00 (*0-87473-463-0*, 62000-10, MICHIE) LEXIS Pub.

Pain: Clinical Manual. Margo McCaffery & Christine Pasero. 2nd ed. 1999. LC 99-462412. (Illus.). xvii, 795p. text 39.95 (*0-8151-5609-X*, 29563) Mosby Inc.

Pain: Its Modes & Functions. Frederik J. Buytendijk. Tr. by Eda O'Shiel. 1973. LC 72-12494. 189p. reprint ed. lib. bdg. 58.00 (*0-8371-6741-8*, BUPM, Greenwood Pr) Greenwood.

Pain: Its Nature & Management. Veronica Thomas. 1997. pap. text (*0-7020-2293-4*) W B Saunders GBR. *Dist:* Saunders.

Pain: Learning to Live Without It. David Corey. 1999. (Illus.). 211p. reprint ed. pap. text 14.00 (*0-7881-6796-0*) DIANE Pub.

Pain: Making Life Liveable. Dana S. DeBoskey. 1995. (Illus.). 80p. (Orig.). pap. 12.50 (*1-882855-36-1*) HDI Pubs.

Pain: Meaning & Management. Ed. by W. Lynn Smith et al. 1980. (Illus.). 182p. text 22.50 (*0-88331-170-4*) R B Luce.

Pain: Mechanisms & Management. Rene Cailliet. 1993. LC 93-9422. (Pain Ser.). (Illus.). 299p. (C). pap. text 24.95 (*0-8036-1635-X*) Davis Co.

Pain: Mechanisms & Management. Howard L. Fields. 2nd ed. 2001. (Illus.). 450p. text 55.00 (*0-07-020748-8*) McGraw-Hill Educ Grp.

Pain: Mechanisms & Management. Howard L. Fields. 1987. (Illus.). 354p. text 50.00 (*0-07-020701-1*) McGraw-Hill Med Pub.

Pain: Scientific Basis & Clin. Cousins. 2000. text (*0-7216-6220-X*) Saunders.

Pain: The Gift Nobody Wants. Paul Brand & Philip Yancey. 1999. 352p. reprint ed. text 22.00 (*0-7881-6372-8*) DIANE Pub.

Pain: Theory, Research & Intervention. Sandra Horn & Marcus Munafo. 1997. LC 96-29576. (Health Psychology Ser.). 152p. (*0-335-19689-6*); 160p. pap. (*0-335-19688-8*) OpUniv Pr.

Pain: What Psychiatrists Need to Know. Ed. by Mary Jane Massie. 2000. LC 00-23877. (Review of Psychiatry Ser.: Vol. 19, No. 2). (Illus.). xxi, 188p. pap. 28.50 (*0-88048-173-0*, 8173) Am Psychiatric.

Pain & Anxiety Control for the Conscious Dental Patient. John G. Meechan et al. 1998. LC 97-34665. (Illus.). 396p. pap. text 69.50 (*0-19-262848-8*) OUP.

Pain & Anxiety Control in Dentistry. Dionne. 2000. text (*0-7216-7278-7*) Saunders.

Pain & Behavioral Medicine: A Cognitive-Behavioral Perspective. Dennis C. Turk et al. LC 82-11695. (Clinical Psychology & Psychotherapy Ser.). 452p. 1987. pap. 35.00 (*0-89862-917-9*, 2917); 1983. text 40.00 (*0-89862-002-3*) Guilford Pubns.

Pain & Its Conquest. H. B. Gibson. 1982. 224p. 30.00 (*0-7206-0595-4*) Dufour.

Pain & Its Relief: An Exhibition at the National Museum of American History. Nancy Knight. 1983. (Illus.). 84p. (Orig.). pap. 5.50 (*0-929847-01-6*) Natl Mus Am.

Pain & Its Relief Without Addiction: Clinical Issues in the Use of Opioids & Other Analgesics. Barry Stimmel. 2nd ed. 1997. LC 96-8993. (Illus.). 420p. pap. 24.95 (*0-7890-0126-8*); (C). 49.95 (*1-56024-906-4*) Haworth Pr (Hawrth Medical).

Pain & Kampo: The Use of Japanese Herbal Medicine in Management of Pain. Ed. by T. Oyama & G. Smith. LC 93-47603. 1996. 105.00 (*4-431-70135-4*); 1994. (*3-540-70135-4*); 1994. (*0-387-70135-4*) Spr-Verlag.

Pain & Neurogenic Inflammation. Susan D. Brain & P. K. Moore. 1999. (Progress in Inflammation Research Ser.). LC 98-54474. (*0-8176-5875-0*); 330p. 175.00 (*3-7643-5875-0*) Birkhauser.

Pain & Neuroimmune Interactions. Suhayl J. Jabbur & A. Vania Apkarian. Ed. by Nayef E. Saade. 2000. LC 00-22562. 244p. 125.00 (*0-306-46371-7*, Kluwer Plenum) Kluwer Academic.

Pain & Passion: A Psychoanalyst Explores the World of S & M. R. J. Stoller. 1991. (Illus.). 316p. (C). 24.95 (*0-306-43770-8*) Da Capo.

Pain & Pleasure: A Study of Bodily Feelings. Thomas Szasz. 2nd ed. 1988. 368p. reprint ed. pap. 19.95 (*0-8156-0230-8*) Syracuse U Pr.

Pain & Suffering, Vols. 4, 4a, 4b & 4c. Loring F. Chapman. 1967. (Courtroom Medicine Ser.). ring bd. 888.00 (*0-8205-1242-7*) Bender.

Pain, Anesthesia & Analgesia in Common Laboratory Animals. 1995. lib. bdg. 250.95 (*0-8490-7587-4*) Gordon Pr.

Pain Assessment Instruments for Chronic Pain Evaluation a Valid Standardized Assessment Instrument. Rucker. 2000. pap. text 79.99 (*0-7506-7301-X*) Buttrwrth-Heinemann.

Pain Buster: Breakthrough 4-Step Program for Ending Pain. John Stamatos & Jane O'Boyle. 2001. LC 00-49900. (Illus.). xvi, 288p. 24.00 (*0-8050-6346-3*) H Holt & Co.

Pain Clinic No. I: Proceedings of the 1st International Symposium, Delft, the Netherlands, 1984, Vol. 1. Ed. by W. Erdmann et al. 1985. 378p. (*90-6764-039-5*) VSP NLD. *Dist:* Coronet Bks.

Pain Clinic No. IV: Proceedings of the 4th International Symposium, Kyoto, Japan, 1990, No. 4. Ed. by M. Hyodo et al. 1992. 368p. (*90-6764-147-2*) VSP NLD. *Dist:* Coronet Bks.

Pain Clinic Manual. Ed. by Simon J. Dolin et al. 1996. LC 95-43195. 320p. text 75.00 (*0-7506-2036-6*) Buttrwrth-Heinemann.

***Pain Control: An Open Learning Programme for Healthcare Workers.** Nan Stalker. 2000. 128p. wbk. ed. (*1-85775-436-0*) Radcliffe Med Pr GBR. *Dist:* Balogh.

Pain Control after Surgery: A Practical Guide. 1995. lib. bdg. 250.95 (*0-8490-6806-1*) Gordon Pr.

Pain Control with Transcutaneous Electrical Neuro Stimulation (TENS) Robert A. Ersek. 1981. LC 78-50175. 280p. 23.75 (*0-87527-168-5*) Green.

Pain, Distress, & the Newborn Baby. Margaret Sparshot. 1996. LC 96-23903. 224p. (Orig.). pap. 43.95 (*0-632-04077-7*) Blackwell Sci.

Pain Erasure: The Bonnie Prudden Way. Bonnie Prudden. 1985. 288p. pap. 14.00 (*0-345-33102-8*) Ballantine Pub Grp.

Pain Free: A Revolutionary Method for Stopping Chronic Pain. Pete Egoscue & Roger Gittines. 1998. LC 97-31745. (Illus.). 320p. 23.95 (*0-553-10630-9*) Bantam.

Pain Free: A Self-Help Guide & Program Description for Becoming Pain Free Again. Peter Migaly. Date not set. (Illus.). 100p. (Orig.). pap. 15.95 (*0-9647363-2-2*) P Migaly.

***Pain Free: In 6 Weeks.** Sherry A. Rogers. 2001. 415p. pap. text 19.95 (*1-887202-03-X*) SandKey.

Pain Free: The Definitive Guide to Healing Arthritis, Low-Back Pain, & Sports Injuries Through Nutrition & Supplements. Luke Bucci. 1995. LC 94-47120. 276p. 24.95 (*1-56530-161-7*) Summit TX.

Pain-Free Arthritis. Dvera Berson & Sander Roy. 1982. (Illus.). 130p. 23.50 (*0-9609608-0-5*) S & J Books.

***Pain Free for Women: The Revolutionary Progam for Ending Chronic Pain.** Pete Egoscue & Roger Gittnes. 2002. LC 2001-43938. 480p. 24.95 (*0-553-80105-8*) Bantam Dell.

Pain-Free Tryptophan Diet. Robert L. Polfack et al. 1987. 256p. 16.45 (*0-446-51317-2*); mass mkt. 3.95 (*0-446-34359-5*) Warner Bks.

Pain Imaging. Ed. by Kenneth L. Casey et al. 2000. LC 00-47139. (Progress in Pain Research & Management Ser.: 18). (Illus.). xvi, 256p. 89.00 (*0-931092-34-5*, PPRM4) Intl Assn Study Pain.

Pain in Animals. A. Iggo. 1988. 35.00 (*0-7855-1114-8*) St Mut.

Pain in Childbearing & Its Control. Rosemary Mander. 1998. LC 98-15544. xii, 252p. pap. 39.95 (*0-632-04097-1*) Blackwell Sci.

Pain in Children: Nature, Assessment & Treatment. Patricia A. McGrath. 1989. LC 89-11009. 466p. 52.00 (*0-89862-390-1*, 2390) Guilford Pubns.

Pain in Neonates. Ed. by K. J. S. Anand & Patrick J. McGrath. (Pain Research & Clinical Management Ser.: Vol. 5). 356p. 1995. pap. 92.00 (*0-444-82238-0*); 1993. LC 92-48284. 239.50 (*0-444-81226-1*) Elsevier.

Pain in Neonates. Contrib. by K. J. S. Anand et al. 2nd ed. 2000. LC 99-53891. (Pain Research & Clinical Management Ser.). 300p. 170.00 (*0-444-50348-X*) Elsevier.

Pain in Neonates. K. J. S. Anand et al. 2nd enl. rev. ed. 2000. LC 99-53891. (Pain Research & Clinical Management Ser.). xvi, 281p. pap. 68.00 (*0-444-50349-8*) Elsevier.

***Pain in Peripheral Nerve Diseases.** Ed. by C. Sommer. 2001. (Pain & Headache Ser.: Vol. 13). (Illus.). vi, 200p. 170.50 (*3-8055-7268-9*) S Karger.

Pain in Shoulder & Arm: An Integrated View. Ed. by J. M. Greep et al. 1979. (Developments in Surgery Ser.: No. 1). 306p. text 141.50 (*90-247-2146-6*) Kluwer Academic.

Pain in the Cancer Patient. Ed. by M. Zimmermann et al. 1983. (Recent Results in Cancer Research Ser.: Vol. 89). (Illus.). 238p. 83.00 (*0-387-12347-4*) Spr-Verlag.

Pain in the Elderly. Ed. by Betty R. Ferrell & Bruce A. Ferrell. 1996. LC 96-28282. (Illus.). 152p. pap. 25.00 (*0-931092-15-9*) Intl Assn Study Pain.

Pain in the Neck: The Latest Information on Causes, Therapies Prevention. Arthur Winter & Ruth Winter. Ed. by Craig Winter. 1997. LC 97-90874. (Illus.). 96p. pap. 11.95 (*0-9659599-0-2*) WiseGuide Pub.

Pain in the Neck - And How to Get Rid of It: Proven Techniques That Really Work. Rowlin L. Lichter. 2001. 224p. mass mkt. 5.99 (*1-57566-584-0*, Twin Streams) Kensgtn Pub Corp.

Pain-Its Neurosurgical Management: Part I: Procedures on Primary Afferent Neurons. 1977. (Progress in Neurological Surgery Ser.: Vol. 7). 166.50 (*3-8055-2317-3*) S Karger.

Pain-Its Neurosurgical Management Pt. II: Central Procedures. Ed. by H. Krayenbuehl et al. 1977. (Progress in Neurological Surgery Ser.: Vol. 8). 164.50 (*3-8055-2414-5*) S Karger.

Pain Journal. Bob Flanagan. 2000. LC 2001-271973. (Native Agents Ser.). 205p. pap. 11.95 (*1-58435-002-4*) Semiotexte.

Pain Management. Rebholz. 1998. (Professional Reference - Nursing Ser.). stu. ed. 31.50 (*0-8273-7382-1*) Delmar.

Pain Management. Ed. by Andrew D. Rosenberg et al. 1999. 436p. (C). text 126.00 (*0-7020-2285-3*) Harcourt Coll Pubs.

***Pain Management.** Ed. by David Rowbotham et al. 2002. (Principles & Practice Ser.). 250p. pap. (*0-7279-1576-2*) BMJ Pub GBR. *Dist:* AIDC.

Pain Management. C. C. Spanswick & C. J. Main. 1998. LC 00-57056. (Illus.). 304p. text (*0-443-05683-8*) Church.

Pain Management Ed. by Richard Weiner. 5th ed. 1994. (Illus.). 1408p. lib. bdg. 195.00 (*1-57444-045-4*) St Lucie Pr.

Pain Management: A Comprehensive Review. P. Prithvi Raj. 1995. (Illus.). 592p. (C). (gr. 13). pap. text 64.95 (*0-8016-7998-2*, 07998) Mosby Inc.

Pain Management: A Handbook of Psychological Treatment Approaches. Ed. by Arnold D. Holzman. 1986. (General Psychology Ser.: No. 136). (Illus.). 304p. 55.00 (*0-08-031931-9*, J115, Pergamon Pr) Elsevier.

Pain Management: Assessment & Treatment of Chronic & Acute Syndromes. Ed. by Wen-Hsien Wu. 1986. 397p. 45.95 (*0-89885-265-X*, Kluwer Acad Hman Sci) Kluwer Academic.

Pain Management: Expiring Patents Open OTC Markets. Market Intelligence Staff. 1993. 332p. 1995.00 (*1-56753-488-0*) Frost & Sullivan.

Pain Management: Nursing Perspective. Judith H. Watt-Watson & Marilee I. Donovan. 1992. (Illus.). 558p. (gr. 13). spiral bd. 35.95 (*1-55664-251-2*) Mosby Inc.

Pain Management: PreTest Self-Assessment & Review. Ed. by Cynthia Kahn. 1996. LC 95-25774. (Pretest Specialty Level Ser.). (Illus.). 162p. pap. 45.00 (*0-07-052079-8*) McGraw-Hill Prof.

Pain Management: Principles. Christine Miaskowski. 1999. text 65.00 (*0-7216-6040-1*) Saunders.

Pain Management: Theory & Practice. Ed. by Russell K. Portenoy & Ronald M. Kanner. 1996. LC 95-52200. (Contemporary Neurology Ser.: No. 48). (Illus.). 384p. 99.00 (*0-8036-0171-9*) OUP.

Pain Management & Anesthesiology. Ed. by Michael A. Ashburn et al. 1998. LC 98-9867. (Developments in Critical Care, Medicine, & Anesthesiology Ser.). 324p. 148.00 (*0-7923-4995-4*) Kluwer Academic.

***Pain Management & Improving End-of-Life Care: Congressional Hearing.** Ed. by James M. Jeffords. 2001. 136p. (C). reprint ed. pap. text 35.00 (*0-7567-1276-9*) DIANE Pub.

Pain Management, Anesthesia, & HIV/AIDS. Nedeljkovic. 2001. (Illus.). 336p. 74.99 (*0-7506-7167-X*) Buttrwrth-Heinemann.

Pain Management by Physical Therapy. Ed. by Peter E. Wells et al. 2nd ed. 1994. (Illus.). 326p. text 52.50 (*0-7506-0569-3*) Buttrwrth-Heinemann.

Pain Management for Health Professionals. P. O'Hara. 1996. (Illus.). 192p. (Orig.). pap. 39.95 (*1-56593-436-9*, 1105) Singular Publishing.

Pain Management for the Practicing Physician. Gordon A. Irving & Mark S. Wallace. 1996. LC 96-35129. pap. text (*0-443-07913-7*) Church.

Pain Management for the Small Animal Practitioner. William J. Tranquilli et al. 2000. (Made Easy Ser.). (Illus.). 130p. spiral bd. 65.00 incl. audio compact disk (*1-893441-16-4*) Teton New.

Pain Management Handbook. Evelyn Salerno & Joyce S. Willens. 1996. LC 95-43752. (Illus.). 544p. (C). (gr. 13). spiral bd. 34.95 (*0-8151-7924-3*, 26181) Mosby Inc.

Pain Management Handbook: A Concise Guide to Diagnosis & Treatment. Ed. by M. Eric Gershwin & Maurice E. Hamilton. 1998. LC 98-5986. (Current Clinical Practice Ser.). (Illus.). 390p. 99.50 (*0-89603-423-2*) Humana.

Pain Management in Animals. Ed. by Paul A. Flecknell & Avril Waterman-Pearson. 2000. (Illus.). 255p. pap. text (*0-7020-1767-1*) W B Saunders GBR. *Dist:* Saunders.

***Pain Management in Rehabilitation.** Ed. by Trilok Monga & Martin Grabors. 2002. 300p. 89.95 (*1-888799-63-3*) Demos Medical.

Pain Management in the Cancer Patient. 1994. lib. bdg. 260.95 (*0-8490-8526-8*) Gordon Pr.

Pain Management of AIDS Patients. Ed. by Thomas Janisse. 1991. (Current Management of Pain Ser.). (C). text 106.50 (*0-7923-1056-X*) Kluwer Academic.

Pain Management Practice Guide for Clinicians, Vol. 2. Richard S. Weiner. 5th ed. 1997. 616p. per. 99.00 (*1-57444-200-7*) St Lucie Pr.

Pain Management Psychotherapy: A Practical Guide. Bruce N. Eimer & Arthur M. Freeman. 1998. LC 97-15702. (Illus.). 528p. 100.00 (*0-471-15708-2*) Wiley.

Pain Management Secrets. Ed. by Ronald M. Kanner. 1997. LC 96-49764. (Secrets Ser.). (Illus.). 350p. pap. 39.95 (*1-56053-160-6*) Hanley & Belfus.

Pain Management Techniques for Older Adults. Sue V. Saxon. 1991. 114p. (C). text 33.95 (*0-398-05734-6*) C C Thomas.

Pain Mechanisms & Management. Ed. by J. C. Wells & Clifford Woolf. 1992. (British Medical Bulletin Ser.: Vol. 47, 3). (Illus.). 264p. text (*0-443-04491-0*) Church.

Pain of Premature Parents: A Psychological Guide for Coping. Michael T. Hynan & Lauren Leslie-Hynan. 1987. 106p. (Orig.). 40.00 (*0-8191-5808-9*) U Pr of Amer.

Pain, Pleasure, & American Childbirth: From the Twilight Sleep to the Read Method, 1914-1960, 13. Margarete Sandelowski. 1984. LC 83-18510. (Contributions in Medical History Ser.: No. 13). (Illus.). 152p. 50.00 (*0-313-24076-0*, SFC/) Greenwood.

Pain Procedure in Clinical Practice. Ed. by Ted A. Lennard. 2nd rev. ed. 2000. LC 99-42857. (Illus.). 434p. (C). 79.00 (*1-56053-367-6*) Hanley & Belfus.

Pain Relief Breakthrough: The Power of Magnets to Relieve Backaches, Arthritis, Menstrual Cramps, Carpal Tunnel Syndrome, Sports Injuries, & More. Julian Whitaker & Brenda Adderly. 1998. LC 97-76355. (Illus.). 224p. (gr. 8). 22.95 (*0-316-60193-4*) Little.

Pain Relief Handbook. C. Wells. 1996. pap. (*0-09-181371-9*) Random GBR. *Dist:* Trafalgar.

Pain Relief Handbook: Self-Help Methods for Managing Pain. Chris Wells & Graham Nown. 1998. (Illus.). 216p. pap. 14.95 (*1-55209-243-7*) Firefly Bks Limited.

Pain Relief in Anesthesia in Obstetrics. Andre Van Zundert. 1995. text (*0-443-04474-0*) Church.

Pain Relief in Far Advanced Cancer. Robert G. Twycross. 1994. pap. text (*0-443-04119-9*) Church.

Pain Relief in Labour. Contrib. by Robin Russell et al. 1997. 256p. pap. (*0-7279-1009-4*) BMJ Pub GBR. *Dist:* AIDC.

Pain Relief in Labour. Donald D. Moir. 5th ed. 1985. LC 85-11702. (Illus.). 196p. pap. text (*0-443-03389-7*) Church.

Pain Seeking Understanding: Suffering, Medicine & Faith. Ed. by Margaret E. Mohrmann & Mark J. Hanson. 1999. LC 99-34494. 224p. pap. 19.95 (*0-8298-1354-3*) Pilgrim OH.

Pain Sourcebook: Basic Information about Specific Forms of Acute & Chronic Pain. Ed. by Allan R. Cook. 1997. LC 97-37833. (Health Reference Ser.: Vol. 32). lib. bdg. 78.00 (*0-7808-0213-6*) Omnigraphics Inc.

Pain Specialist's Approach to the Headache Patient. Seymour Diamond. 1993. LC 93-13888. 162p. 27.50 (*0-8236-3930-4*) Intl Univs Pr.

Pain Surgery, Set. Kim J. Burchiel. 2001. (Illus.). 864p. 179.00 (*0-86577-912-0*) Thieme Med Pubs.

Pain System. W. D. Willis. 1985. (Pain & Headache Ser.: Vol. 8). (Illus.). x, 346p. 125.25 (*3-8055-3930-4*) S Karger.

Pain Treatment Centers at a Crossroads: A Practical & Conceptual Reappraisal. Ed. by Mitchell J. Cohen & James N. Campbell. 1996. LC 96-12622. (Progress in Pain Research & Management Ser.: Vol. 7). (Illus.). 352p. 39.00 (*0-931092-14-0*) Intl Assn Study Pain.

Painful Choices: Research & Essays on Health Care. David Mechanic. 1989. 320p. text 39.95 (*0-88738-258-4*) Transaction Pubs.

Painful Field: The Psychiatric Dimension of Modern War, 75. Richard A. Gabriel. 1988. LC 87-31789. (Contributions in Military Studies Ser.: No. 75). 207p. 62.50 (*0-313-24718-8*, GBP/, Greenwood Pr) Greenwood.

Painful Passages: Working with Children with Learning Disabilities. Elizabeth Dane. 1990. LC 90-6463. 221p. 24.95 (*0-87101-175-1*) Natl Assn Soc Wkrs.

Painful Prescription: Rationing Hospital Care. Henry J. Aaron & William B. Schwartz. 1984. LC 83-45962. (Studies in Social Economics). 161p. 11.95 (*0-8157-0034-2*) Brookings.

Painful Prescription: Rationing Hospital Care. Henry J. Aaron et al. 1984. LC 83-45962. (Studies in Social Economics). 161p. pap. 11.95 (*0-8157-0033-4*) Brookings.

Painless Guide to a Healthy Back. Ilan Horowitz. Tr. by Karen Gold from HEB. 1993. LC 93-11225. (Family Health Ser.). (Illus.). 93p. reprint ed. pap. 12.95 (*1-55643-168-6*) North Atlantic.

Painting Portraits: Families Groups & Systems. 1989. (Conference Proceedings Ser.). 141p. (Orig.). pap. 15.00 (*1-882147-07-3*) Am Art Therapy.

Paired Pulse Stimulation of the Heart. Ed. by Paul F. Cranefield & Brian F. Hoffman. 1968. (Illus.). 224p. 7.50 (*0-87470-009-4*) Rockefeller.

Palaeopathology of Aboriginal Australians: Health & Disease Across a Hunter-Gatherer Continent. Stephen Webb. 1995. (Illus.). 336p. (C). text 64.95 (*0-521-46044-1*) Cambridge U Pr.

Palaeopathology of Danish Skeletons: A Comparative Study of Demography, Disease, & Injury. Pia Bennike. 1985. (Illus.). 272p. (Orig.). pap. text 64.50 (*87-500-2571-6*) Coronet Bks.

Palaeoserology: Blood Typing with Fluorescent Antibody Method. I. A. Lengyel. 1975. 240p. (C). (*963-05-0355-7*) Akade Kiado HUN. *Dist:* St Mut.

Paleopathological & Paleoepidemiological: Study of Osseous Syphilis in Skulls of the Edo Period. Takao Suzuki. 1984. 50p. (*0-86008-358-6*) U of Tokyo JPN. *Dist:* Col U Pr.

Paleopathology: An Introduction to the Study of Ancient Evidences of Disease. Roy L. Moodie. LC 75-23744. reprint ed. 74.50 (*0-404-13350-9*) AMS Pr.

Paleopathology: Disease in the Fossil Record. Bruce M. Rothschild & Larry Martin. 1992. 400p. 148.95 (*0-8493-8897-X*, R134) CRC Pr.

Palliation in Malignant Disease. J. G. Mosley. 1988. (Illus.). 170p. text (*0-443-03690-X*) Church.

Palliative & Terminal Care: Health Care Needs Assessment: The Epidemiologically Based Needs Assessment Reviews, Second Series. Andrew Stevens et al. 1997. LC 97-13354. (*1-85775-206-6*) Radcliffe Med Pr GBR. *Dist:* Balogh.

Palliative Cancer Care: Policy Statement Based on the Recommendations of a WHO Consultation. 1989. 48p. pap. text 15.00 (*92-890-1059-2*) World Health.

Palliative Care: The Nurses's R. Jean Lugton & Margaret Kindlen. 1999. LC 98-48825. x, 306p. (C). pap. text (*0-443-05513-0*) Church.

***Palliative Care for Non-Cancer Patients.** Ed. by Julia Addington-Hall & Irene Higginson. 2001. LC 00-54848. (Illus.). 318p. text 55.00 (*0-19-262960-3*) OUP.

Palliative Care for People with Cancer. 2nd ed. 360p. pap. (*0-340-61391-2*) E A GBR. *Dist:* Routldge.

Palliative Care Formulary. Robert Twycross et al. 1998. 232p. pap. (*1-85775-264-3*) Radcliffe Med Pr GBR. *Dist:* Balogh.

Palliative Care Nursing: Quality Care to the End of Life. Marianne Matzo & Deborah Witt Shermann. 2001. LC 00-64094. (*0-8261-1384-2*) Springer Pub.

Palliative Care of the Cancer Patient: The Physician's Practical Guide. Ed. by Kristine E. Nelson. 2001. (Current Clinical Oncology Ser.). 400p. 89.50 (*0-89603-899-8*) Humana.

Palliative Care Patient & Family Couseling Manual. Aspen Reference Group Staff. 1996. ring bd. 179.00 (*0-8342-0762-1*, S289) Aspen Pub.

Palliative Day Care. 272p. pap. (*0-340-62521-X*) E A GBR. *Dist:* Routldge.

Palliative Medicine: A Case-Based Manual. Ed. by Neil MacDonald et al. 1998. (Illus.). 330p. pap. text 29.95 (*0-19-262657-4*) OUP.

Palliative Medicine: Problem Areas in Pain & Symptom Management. Ed. by G. W. Hanks. 1995. (Cancer Surveys Ser.: Vol. 21). 257p. 54.00 (*0-87969-435-1*) Cold Spring Harbor.

Palliative Medicine: Symptomatic & Supportive Care for Patients with Advanced Cancer & AIDS. Roger Woodruff. 3rd ed. 1999. LC 99-216273. 430p. pap. text 59.50 (*0-19-550647-2*) OUP.

Palliative Medicine Secrets. Suresh K. Joishy. 1998. LC 98-43418. (Secrets Ser.). (Illus.). 250p. pap. 39.95 (*1-56053-304-8*) Hanley & Belfus.

***Palliative Nursing: Bringing Comfort & Hope.** Shaun Kinghorn & Richard Gamlin. 2001. (Illus.). 255p. (*0-7020-2422-8*) W B Saunders GBR. *Dist:* Saunders.

Pallidotomy for the Treatment of Parkinson's Disease & Movement Disorders. Joachim K. Krauss & Robert G. Grossman. 1998. LC 98-19196. 352p. text 139.00 (*0-7817-1225-4*) Lppncott W & W.

Palm Beach: The Novel. Richard G. Hughes. 1984. LC 83-63232. pap. 9.95 (*0-88100-037-X*) Natl Writ Pr.

Palpation Skills: Assessment & Diagnosis Through Touch. Leon Chaitow. 1996. LC 96-37078. pap. text (*0-443-05320-0*) Church.

Palpitations & Arrhythmias: A Guide for Patients. Nora Goldschlanger. 1997. (Cardiology Ser.). 32p. pap. text 2.95 (*1-885274-50-5*) Health InfoNet Inc.

Panchakarma Treatment of Ayurveda. T. L. Devaraj. 1998. (*81-7030-591-8*) Sri Satguru Pubns IND. *Dist:* S Asia.

Panchakrma Therapy in Ayurveda. Divakar Ojha & Ashok Kumar. 1979. 219p. pap. 18.95 (*0-89744-057-9*) Auromere.

Pancreas. Ed. by Phillip P. Toskes. 1998. LC 97-5985. (Gastroenterology & Hepatology Ser.: Vol. 8). 185p. text (*0-443-07862-9*) Church GBR. *Dist:* Saunders.

Pancreas, Vol. 2. H. G. Beger et al. 1998. LC 97-7000. (Pancreas Ser.: Vol. 2). (Illus.). 1664p. 499.95 (*0-86542-420-9*) Blackwell Sci.

Pancreas: A Text & Atlas. Banks. 1998. text (*0-7216-6670-1*) Saunders.

Pancreas Transplantation. Ed. by Luis H. Toledo-Pereyra. 1988. (C). text 271.00 (*0-89838-369-2*) Kluwer Academic.

Pancreas Transplantation: Experimental & Clinical Studies. J. P. Squifflet. 1990. (Illus.). xvi, 188p. 128.00 (*3-8055-5102-9*) S Karger.

***Pancreatic Cancer.** D. B. Evans et al. 2001. (M. D. Anderson Solid Tumor Oncology Ser.). 416p. 169.00 (*0-387-95185-7*) Spr-Verlag.

Pancreatic Cancer: Advances in Molecular Pathology, Diagnosis & Clinical Management. Ed. by Fazlul H. Sarkar & Michael C. Dugan. 1998. LC 98-22363. (Illus.). 224p. 79.95 (*1-881299-12-0*, BioTechniques) Eaton Pub Co.

Pancreatic Cancer: Molecular & Clinical Advances. Ed. by John Neoptolemos et al. 1995. LC 95-35297. 360p. 150.00 (*0-86542-973-1*) Blackwell Sci.

Pancreatic Cancer: Pathogenesis, Diagnosis & Treatment. Ed. by Howard Reber. 1998. (Illus.). 360p. 135.00 (*0-89603-466-6*) Humana.

***Pancreatic Cancer - An Update.** P. Malfertheirner. 2001. (Digestive Diseases Ser.: Vol. 19). (Illus.). 94p. pap. 34.00 (*3-8055-7245-X*) S Karger.

Pancreatic Disease: State of the Art & Future Aspects of Research. Ed. by Paul G. Lankisch & Eugene P. DiMagno. 1999. LC 99-13105. (Illus.). 285p. pap. 82.00 (*3-540-65357-0*) Spr-Verlag.

Pancreatic Disease: Towards the Year 2000. C. D. Johnson & C. W. Imrie. 2nd ed. 1998. LC 98-17778. xviii, 468p. (C). (*1-85233-037-6*) Spr-Verlag GBR. *Dist:* Spr-Verlag.

Pancreatic Diseases: New Horizons. Ed. by M. W. Buechler et al. 1995. (Journal: Vol. 11, No. 3-6, 1994). (Illus.). vi, 342p. pap. 146.25 (*3-8055-6191-1*) S Karger.

***Pancreatic Enzyme Therapy Following Surgical Procedures in the Gastrointestinal Tract: EPC Associated Meeting, Luneburg, July 1999.** Ed. by P. G. Lankisch. 2001. vi, 72p. 25.25 (*3-8055-7184-4*) S Karger.

Pancreatic Enzymes in Health & Disease. Ed. by P. G. Lankisch. 1991. (Illus.). 224p. 100.00 (*0-387-53187-4*) Spr-Verlag.

Pancreatic Fistulas. Ed. by P. Pederzoli et al. 1992. LC 92-49618. 224p. 139.00 (*0-387-55338-X*) Spr-Verlag.

Pancreatic Growth & Regeneration. Nora Sarvetnick. 1997. (Tissue Engineering Intelligence Unit Ser.). 270p. 98.00 (*1-57059-500-3*) Landes Bioscience.

Pancreatic Growth & Regeneration. Ed. by Nora Sarvetnick. 1998. LC 97-41356. (Tissue Engineering Ser.). xiv, 250p. text 98.00 (*3-8055-6618-2*) S Karger.

Pancreatic Islet Cell Regeneration & Growth. A. I. Vinik. 1992. LC 92-49932. (Advances in Experimental Medicine & Biology Ser.: Vol. 321). (Illus.). 200p. (C). text 85.00 (*0-306-44259-0*, Kluwer Plenum) Kluwer Academic.

Pancreatic Transplantation. Ed. by C. C. Groth. 1988. 450p. text 142.00 (*0-7216-2637-8*, 791744, Grune & Strat) Harcrt Hlth Sci Grp.

Pancreatic Tumors in Children. G. Bennett Humphrey. 1982. text 191.50 (*90-247-2702-2*) Kluwer Academic.

Pancreatitis. P. G. Lankisch & Peter A. Banks. 1997. LC 97-21618. (Illus.). 377p. 104.00 (*3-540-61726-4*) Spr-Verlag.

Pancreatoduodenectomy. Ed. by F. Hanyu & K. Takasaki. 1997. LC 97-16186. (Illus.). 550p. 186.00 (*4-431-70194-X*) Spr-Verlag.

Pandemic Influcnza, 1700-1900: A Study in Historical Epidemiology. K. David Patterson. 1987. (Illus.). 128p. (C). 47.50 (*0-8476-7512-2*, R7512) Rowman.

Pandora's Box: Feminism Confronts Reproductive Technology. Nancy Lublin. 1998. LC 97-26354. (New Feminist Perspectives Ser.). 208p. pap. 14.95 (*0-8476-8637-X*) Rowman.

Panels of the Seventh World Sanskrit Conference Vol. 8: Medical Literature from India, Sri Lanka & Tibet, Rules & Remedies in Classical Indian Law, Vol. 9. Ed. by Johannes Bronkhorst. 1991. 90p. 91.00 (*90-04-09522-5*) Brill Academic Pubs.

Panic & Agoraphobia Scale (PAS) Borwin Bandelow. 1999. LC 99-71758. (Illus.). iii, 85p. pap. 49.00 (*0-88937-216-0*) Hogrefe & Huber Pubs.

Panic & Anxiety Attacks: Warning of a Physical Problem. Glenn M. Alger. 1990. 159p. (Orig.). pap. text 7.95 (*0-9626143-0-0*) Glendor Bks.

Panic & Phobias. Ed. by I. Hand & H. U. Wittchen. 1986. (Illus.). 130p. 51.00 (*0-387-16513-4*) Spr-Verlag.

Panic Anxiety & Its Treatment: A Publication of the World Psychiatric Association. Ed. by Gerald L. Klerman et al. 1993. LC 93-16381. 162p. text 12.95 (*0-88048-684-8*, 8684) Am Psychiatric.

Panic Buster: Learn to Conquer Panic Attacks & Agoraphobia. Bonnie Crandall. 1995. 67p. spiral bd., wbk. ed. 12.95 (*0-9663946-0-7*) Hatch Creek.

Panic Control after Surgery. 1995. lib. bdg. 250.75 (*0-8490-7580-7*) Gordon Pr.

Panic Disorder: Assessment & Treatment Through a Wide-Angle Lens. Frank M. Dattilio & Jesus A. Salas-Auvert. 2000. LC 99-27032. (Illus.). xvii, 313p. 38.50 (*1-891944-35-5*) Zeig Tucker Theisen.

Panic Disorder: The Great Pretender. H. M. Zal. LC 89-23176. (Illus.). 234p. (C). 22.95 (*0-306-43297-8*) Perseus Bks Grp.

Panic Disorder: The Medical Point of View. William D. Kerrode. Ed. by Anne Hill. 4th rev. ed. 1997. (Illus.). 209p. pap. 17.95 (*0-9631533-3-1*) W Kernodle.

Panic Disorder: Theory, Research & Therapy. R. Baker. 1992. (Clinical Psychology & Personality Ser.). 364p. pap. 145.00 (*0-471-93317-1*) Wiley.

Panic Disorder & Agoraphobia: A Comprehensive Guide for the Practitioner. Ed. by John R. Walker et al. 1991. 704p. (C). text 71.95 (*0-534-11286-2*) Brooks-Cole.

Panic Disorder & Agoraphobia: A Guide. John H. Greist & James W. Jefferson. rev. ed. 1998. 69p. pap. 4.95 (*1-890802-15-8*); 2nd rev. ed. 1993. 58p. pap. 4.50 (*1-890802-01-8*) Madison Inst of Med.

Panic Disorder in the Medical Setting. 1994. (Illus.). 135p. (Orig.). (C). pap. text 35.00 (*0-7881-0528-0*) DIANE Pub.

Panic Disorders: Causes & Cures. 1996. lib. bdg. 251.96 (*0-8490-5911-9*) Gordon Pr.

Panic Disorders in a Medical Setting. 1992. lib. bdg. 250.95 (*0-8490-8902-6*) Gordon Pr.

Panic No More: Your Guide to Overcome Panic Attacks. Jean Carlton. 1994. 288p. (Orig.). pap. 12.95 (*0-9639632-9-5*) Stonehorse.

Panic Psychological Perspectives. Ed. by Jack D. Maser & Stanley J. Rachman. 1988. 392p. text 89.95 (*0-8058-0091-3*) L Erlbaum Assocs.

Pankreas: Diagnostik, Therapie. Ed. by K. J. Paquet & W. A. Kozuschek. 1991. (Illus.). 584p. 178.50 (*3-8055-5545-8*) S Karger.

Pankreaserkrankungen. M. W. Buechler et al. 1996. (Illus.). x, 186p. 68.00 (*3-8055-6141-5*) S Karger.

Pao Zhi: An Introduction to Use of Processed Chinese Medicinals to Enhance Therapeutic Effects. Philippe Sionneau. Tr. by Bob Flaws. 1995. 350p. (Orig.). pap. 34.95 (*0-936185-62-7*) Blue Poppy Pr.

Pap Smear. Mathilde E. Boon & Albert J. Suurmeijer. 3rd ed. 1996. 384p. text 90.00 (*3-7186-5857-7*) Gordon & Breach.

Pap Test: The Procedure & Results. Mitchel S. Hoffman. Ed. by William Spellacy. 1996. (Women's Health Ser.). (Illus.). 24p. (Orig.). pap. 2.95 (*1-885274-20-3*) Health InfoNet Inc.

Papa Jim Medicinal Herbs: Commonly Used Herbs. Papa Jim, pseud. Ed. by Leticia M. Ayala. 1990. (Papa Jim Bks.: No. 4). (Illus.). 106p. pap. 3.95 (*1-878575-03-1*) El Rey Pub.

Papa Jim's Herbs for Illnesses: Herbs & Herbal Combinations. Papa Jim, pseud. Ed. by Leticia M. Ayala. 1990. (Papa Jim Bks.: No. 5). (Illus.). 78p. pap. 3.95 (*1-878575-02-3*) El Rey Pub.

Papanicolaou Technique: Approved Guideline, (1994) Kenneth D. McClatchy. 1994. 85.00 (*1-56238-238-1*, GP15-A) NCCLS.

Paper Dolls & Paper Airplanes: Therapeutic Exercises for Sexually Traumatized Children. Liana Lowenstein et al. 1997. (Illus.). 478p. 39.95 (*1-55864-048-7*) Kidsrights.

Paper Office: The Tools to Make Your Small Psychotherapy Practice Work Ethically, Legally, & Profitably. Edward Zukerman & Irvin P. Guyett. 1991. (Clinician's Toolbox Ser.). 252p. reprint ed. pap. text 39.95 incl. disk (*0-9622281-3-3*) Three Wishes.

Papers Dedicated to C.T.C. Wall, 145. Sylvain Cappell. 1999. LC 99-68088. (Annals of Mathematics Studies: Vol. 145). 448p. pap. 35.00 (*0-691-04938-6*) Princeton U Pr.

Papers Dedicated to Egil Amundsen: On the Occasion of his 60th Birthday March 18, 1984. Ed. by A. O. Aasen et al. 1984. (Journal: Vol. 16, Supp. 2). (Illus.). iv, 172p. pap. 45.25 (*3-8055-3889-8*) S Karger.

Papers of Alfred Blalock Ed. by Mark M. Ravitch. 1966. (Illus.). 2,047p. 250.00 (*0-8018-0544-9*) Johns Hopkins.

Papers of Wade Hampton Frost, M.D. A Contribution to Epidemiological Method. Wade H. Frost. Ed. by Barbara G. Rosenkrantz & Kenneth F. Maxcy. 1977. LC 76-40635. (Public Health in America Ser.). (Illus.). reprint ed. lib. bdg. 51.95 (*0-405-09826-X*) Ayer.

Papers on Psycho-Analysis. E. Jones. 5th ed. 1977. 510p. (*0-9501647-6-3*) Karnac Bks GBR. *Dist:* Other Pr LLC.

Papers on Psychoanalytic Psychology. Heinz Hartmann et al. 1964. LC 64-18532. (Psychological Issues Monographs: No. 14, Vol. 4, No. 2). 206p. 40.50 (*0-8236-3980-0*) Intl Univs Pr.

Papilloma Viruses & Human Cancer. Ed. by Herbert Pfister. 1990. 272p. lib. bdg. 229.00 (*0-8493-5860-4*, RC268) CRC Pr.

Papillomavirus Infections in Human Pathology. Kari J. Syrjanen. 2000. LC 98-54686. (Illus.). 630p. 360.00 (*0-471-97168-5*) Wiley.

Papillomaviruses. CIBA Foundation Staff. 1986. (CIBA Foundation Symposia Ser.: No. 120). 268p. 128.00 (*0-471-99837-0*) Wiley.

Papillomaviruses. Ed. by L. Gissmann. 1994. (Journal: Vol. 37, No. 3-4, 1994). (Illus.). 96p. pap. 78.25 (*3-8055-6096-6*) S Karger.

Papillomaviruses. Ed. by Bettie Steinberg et al. 1987. (Cancer Cells Ser.: No. 5). (Illus.). 480p. (Orig.). pap. text 80.00 (*0-87969-301-0*) Cold Spring Harbor.

Papovaviridae Vol. 2: The Papillomaviruses. N. P. Salzman. 1987. LC 86-15160. (Viruses Ser.). (Illus.). 408p. (C). text 120.00 (*0-306-42452-5*, Kluwer Plenum) Kluwer Academic.

Papyrus Eber: The First Medical Book in the World. Al I. Obaba. 1927. (Illus.). 167p. pap. text 24.00 (*0-916157-17-2*) African Islam Miss Pubns.

Para Emergency Care Exam Review. Richard A. Cherry & Bryan E. Bledsoe. 2nd ed. 1997. LC 97-145945. pap. text 35.00 (*0-8359-5103-0*) P-H.

***Para La Investigacion Sobre Sistemas De Salud**, Vol. 5. I. Parthmanathan et al. 1995. (Investigacisn en Sistemas De Salud Ser.). pap., instr.'s gde. ed. (*0-88936-746-9*) IDRC-CRDI CAN. *Dist:* Stylus Pub VA.

Paracelsus: His Mystical & Medical Philosophy. Manly P. Hall. pap. 5.95 (*0-89314-808-3*) Philos Res.

Paracelsus: Selected Writings. Jolande Jacobi. 2nd ed. 1995. LC 88-25569. (Bollingen Ser.: Vol. 28). (Illus.). 368p. pap. 19.95 (*0-691-01876-6*, Bollingen) Princeton U Pr.

***Paracetamol Acetaminophen: Critical Bibliographic Review.** Laurie F. Prescott. 2nd ed. 2001. (Illus.). 928p. (C). text 215.00 (*0-415-25845-6*) Routledge.

Paracoccidioidomycosis. Franco. 1993. 448p. 239.00 (*0-8493-4868-4*) CRC Pr.

Paradigms & Perspectives: Essays in Psychology. Hirsch L. Silverman. 1997. LC 97-25127. 208p. (C). 38.50 (*0-7618-0823-X*) U Pr of Amer.

Paradigms in Behavior Therapy: Present & Promise. Ed. by Daniel B. Fishman et al. 1988. (Behavior Therapy & Behavioral Medicine Ser.). 392p. (C). 49.95 (*0-8261-5130-2*) Springer Pub.

Paradigms of Clinical Social Work, 2. Rachelle A. Dorfman. 1998. (Paradigms of Clinical Social Work Ser.). 48.95 (*0-87630-882-5*) Brunner-Routledge.

Paradigms of Personality. Jane Loevinger. 1987. (Psychology Ser.). (Illus.). 269p. (C). pap. text 24.95 (*0-7167-1840-5*) W H Freeman.

Paradox & Counterparadox. Mara S. Palazzoli et al. Tr. by Elisabeth V. Burt from ITA. 1990. LC 84-45862. 208p. reprint ed. 45.00 (*0-87668-764-8*) Aronson.

Paradox & Healing: Medicine, Mythology, Transformation. Michael Greenwood & Peter Nunn. 3rd rev. ed. 1994. (Illus.). 247p. (C). pap. (*0-9695822-0-X*) Prdox Pubng CAN. *Dist:* New Centry Pr.

Paradox & Passion in Psychotherapy: An Existential Approach to Therapy & Counselling. Emmy Van Deurzen-Smith. 1998. LC 97-49908. 198p. 130.00 (*0-471-96191-4*); pap. 55.00 (*0-471-97390-4*) Wiley.

Paradox & the Family System. Camillo Loriedo & Gaspare Vella. 1992. LC 91-29684. 240p. 35.95 (*0-87630-635-0*) Brunner-Routledge.

Paradox of Power & Weakness: Levinas & an Alternative Paradigm for Psychology. George Kunz. 1998. LC 97-40917. (SUNY Series, Alternatives in Psychology). 224p. (C). text 21.50 (*0-7914-3889-9*); pap. text 20.95 (*0-7914-3890-2*) State U NY Pr.

Paradox of Progress. James Willis. 1998. LC 94-46871. 152p. pap. (*1-85775-063-2*) Radcliffe Med Pr GBR. *Dist:* Balogh.

Paradox of Sleep: The Story of Dreaming. Michel Jouvet. 1999. LC 98-50198. (Bradford Book Ser.). (Illus.). xiii, 211p. 25.00 (*0-262-10080-0*, Bradford Bks) MIT Pr.

Paradoxes of Delusion: Wittgenstein, Schreber, & the Schizophrenic Mind. Louis A. Sass. LC 93-24931. 208p. 1995. pap. 14.95 (*0-8014-9899-6*); 1993. 39.95 (*0-8014-2210-8*) Cornell U Pr.

Paradoxes of Longevity. Ed. by Jean-Marie Robine et al. 1999. LC 99-10782. (Research & Perspectives in Longevity Ser.). (Illus.). 147p. 95.00 (*3-540-65544-1*) Spr-Verlag.

Paradoxical Psychotherapy: Theory & Practice with Individuals, Couples, & Families. Gerald R. Weeks & Luciano L'Abate. 1982. LC 81-17083. 288p. text 41.95 (*0-87630-289-4*) Brunner-Routledge.

Paraganglia. P. Boeck. 1982. (Handbuch der Mikroskopischen Anatomie Des Menschen Ser.: Vol. 1-8). (Illus.). 315p. 228.00 (*0-387-10978-1*) Spr-Verlag.

Paraganglionic Chemoreceptor System: Physiology, Pathology, & Clinical Medicine. F. G. Zak & W. Lawson. 1982. (Illus.). 583p. 337.00 (*0-387-90621-5*) Spr-Verlag.

Parahippocampal Region: Implications for Neurological & Psychiatric Diseases. Helen E. Scharfman et al. 2000. LC 00-36153. (Annals of the New York Academy of Sciences Ser.: Vol. 911). (Illus.). xiii, 502p. (*1-57331-264-9*) NY Acad Sci.

Parahippocampal Region Vol. 911: Implications for Neurological & Psychiatric Diseases. Ed. by Helen E. Sharfman et al. 2000. LC 00-36153. (Annals of the New York Academy of Sciences Ser.: Vol. 911). (Illus.). xiii, 502p. 140.00 (*1-57331-263-0*) NY Acad Sci.

Parallel Architectures & Neural Networks: 2nd Italian Workshop. Ed. by E. R. Caianiello. 1990. 380p. (C). text 113.00 (*981-02-0146-X*) World Scientific Pub.

Parallel Distributed Processing: Explorations in the Microstructure of Cognition, Vol. 1: Foundations. PDP Research Group Staff et al. 1986. LC 85-24073. (Computational Models of Cognition & Perception Ser.). (Illus.). 567p. 90.00 (*0-262-18120-7*, Bradford Bks) MIT Pr.

Parallel Distributed Processing: Explorations in the Microstructure of Cognition, Vol. 2: Psychological & Biological Models. David E. Rumelhart et al. 1987. (Parallel Distributed Processing Ser.: Vol. 2). (Illus.). 623p. pap. 37.95 (*0-262-63110-5*, Bradford Bks) MIT Pr.

Parallel Models of Associative Memory. Ed. by Geoffrey E. Hinton & James A. Anderson. 1989. (Cognitive Science Ser.). 352p. pap. text 45.00 (*0-8058-0270-3*) L Erlbaum Assocs.

Parallel Models of Associative Memory. Ed. by Geoffrey E. Hinton & J. A. Anderson. enl. ed. 1989. 352p. text 79.95 (*0-8058-0269-X*) L Erlbaum Assocs.

Parallel Psychotherapy with Children & Parents. Barbara Piovano. 1998. LC 97-18427. 240p. 45.00 (*0-7657-0126-X*) Aronson.

Paralytic Shellfish Poisoning. B. Halstead & E. Schantz. 1984. (WHO Offset Publications: No. 79). 60p. 6.00 (*92-4-170079-3*) World Health.

Paralyzing Fear: The Triumph over Polio in America. Jane S. Smith et al. 1998. LC 00-709473. (Illus.). 288p. 29.95 (*1-57500-070-9*) TV Bks.

Paramedic. American College of Emergency Physicians Staff. 1997. LC 97-21620. (Illus.). 896p. (gr. 13). text 49.95 (*0-8016-6361-X*, 06361) Mosby Inc.

Paramedic. Peter Canning. 1998. mass mkt. 6.99 (*0-8041-1614-8*) Ivy Books.

Paramedic Care: Patient. Bryan E. Bledsoe & Robert S. Porter. 2000. 128p. wbk. ed. 31.33 (*0-13-021632-1*) P-H.

Paramedic Care: Principles & Practice, 3. Bryan E. Bledsoe et al. 2000. 737p. 50.67 (*0-13-021598-8*) P-H.

Paramedic Care: Principles Practice. Bledsoe. 4th ed. 2000. LC 99-59773. 660p. 50.67 (*0-8359-5033-6*) P-H.

Paramedic Care: Principles Practice, 5. Bryan Bledsoe & Robert Porter. 2000. 560p. 50.67 (*0-13-021599-6*) P-H.

Paramedic Care: Principles Practice, Vol.4. 2000. 518p. (C). 50.67 (*0-13-021613-5*) P-H.

Paramedic Care: Supplement Instructor's Resource Manual. Bryan E. Bledsoe & Robert S. Porter. 2000. pap., tchr. ed. 46.60 (*0-13-021631-3*) P-H.

***Paramedic Care Principles & Practice: Trauma Emergencies**, Vol. 4. Bledsoe & Porter. 2001. 224p. suppl. ed., wbk. ed. 20.00 (*0-13-021641-0*) P-H.

Paramedic Computerized Student Review. 4th ed. 1998. (C). 25.60 (*0-8359-5378-5*) P-H.

Paramedic Emergency Care. Bryan E. Bledsoe & Robert S. Porter. 3rd ed. 1996. LC 96-19776. 1136p. 82.00 (*0-8359-4987-7*) P-H.

Paramedic Emergency Care: Instructor's Resource Manual. Cherry. 3rd ed. 1996. pap., tchr. ed. 59.00 (*0-8359-5017-4*) P-H.

Paramedic Pocket Reference. Bryan E. Bledsoe & Dwayne E. Clayden. 2nd ed. 1997. LC 97-19809. 192p. pap. text 26.67 (*0-8359-5120-0*) P-H.

Paramedic Protocols. Ed. by Richard E. Westfal. 1996. LC 96-23226. (Illus.). 526p. pap. 29.95 (*0-07-069318-8*) McGraw-Hill Prof.

Paramedic Refresher Course: A Case-Based Approach. Alice Dalton. 1999. (Illus.). 280p. (gr. 13). pap. text 19.95 (*0-8151-1729-9*, 30352) Mosby Inc.

***Paramedic Review.** Bob Elling & Kirsten Elling. 2002. LC 2001-54381. 400p. text 34.95 (*0-7668-3118-3*) Delmar.

Paramedic Review Guide. Gail Walraven. 1997. LC 88-2488. 240p. (C). pap. 23.60 (*0-89303-751-6*) Brady Pub.

Paramedic Review Manual. Politis. 3rd ed. 1992. pap. text 26.00 (*0-7216-5041-4*) Saunders.

Paramedic Textbook with Pass Paramedic! Booklet. Sanders. 1995. (gr. 13). reprint ed. text 51.95 (*0-8151-7505-1*, 28790) Mosby Inc.

Paramedical Emergency Care. Porter. 3rd ed. 1996. LC 97-106333. pap., wbk. ed. 29.67 (*0-8359-5055-7*) P-H.

Paramyxoviruses. D. W. Kingsbury. 1990. (Viruses Ser.). (Illus.). 618p. (C). text 145.00 (*0-306-43553-5*, Kluwer Plenum) Kluwer Academic.

Paraneoplastic Syndromes. Ed. by Ursula Ruether et al. 1998. LC 97-46075. (Beitraege Zur Onkologie, Contributions to Oncology Ser.: Vol. 52, 1998). (Illus.). viii, 260p. 143.50 (*3-8055-6570-4*) S Karger.

Paranoia: New Psychoanalytic Perspectives. Ed. by John M. Oldham & Stanley Bone. 1994. LC 93-49081. 166p. 27.50 (*0-8236-3985-1*) Intl Univs Pr.

Parapharyngeal Space: Diagnosist & Management of Commonly Encountered Entities. Karen T. Pitman et al. 3rd ed. 1999. (Self-Instructional Package Ser.). (Illus.). 67p. pap. text 25.00 (*1-56772-070-6*, 5506115) AAO-HNS.

Paraprofessional in Home Health & Long-Term Care: Training Modules for Working with Older Adults. Ellen Cervantes et al. 1995. LC 95-11564. 272p. pap. text 30.00 (*1-878812-25-4*) Hlth Prof Pr.

Paraprofessionals in the Human Services. Ed. by Stanley Robin & Morton O. Wagenfeld. 1981. LC 80-18011. (Community Psychology Ser.: Vol. VI). 368p. 45.95 (*0-87705-490-8*, Kluwer Acad Hman Sci) Kluwer Academic.

Parapsychology & Self-Deception in Science. Ed. by R. A. McConnell. 1983. LC 81-90464. (Illus.). vii, 150p. pap. 10.00 (*0-9610232-2-8*) McConnell.

Parapsychology & the Experimental Method: Proceedings of an International Conference, New York, 1981. Ed. by Betty Shapin & Lisette Coly. 1982. LC 82-61144. 120p. (C). 16.00 (*0-912328-36-3*) Parapsych Foun.

Parasession on Clitics, Vol. 2. Ed. by Audra Dainora et al. 1995. 315p. pap. 16.00 (*0-914203-48-7*) Chicago Ling.

Parasite Menace: How to Prevent, Detect & Eradicate Parasites from Your Body. Skye Weintraub. 1998. 208p. pap. text 14.95 (*1-885670-88-5*) Woodland UT.

Parasites. Lisa Newman. 1999. LC 99-37373. (Crossing Press Pocket Ser.). 96p. mass mkt. 6.95 (*1-58091-006-8*) Crossing Pr.

Parasites. Stanley Weinberger. 1998. pap. 11.95 (*0-9616184-8-5*) Healing Within Prods.

Parasites. Woodland Publishing, Inc. Staff. 1997. (Woodland Health Ser.). 32p. pap. 3.95 (*1-885670-89-3*) Woodland UT.

Parasites & Pathogens of Insects Vol. 2: Pathogens. N. E. Beckage et al. 1993. LC 92-45034. (Illus.). 294p. text 100.00 (*0-12-084442-7*) Acad Pr.

Parasites & Skin Diseases. Peter Gray. 1995. 165p. pap. (*0-85131-624-7*) J A Allen GBR. *Dist:* Trafalgar, St Mut.

Parasites in Human Tissues. Lawrence R. Ash & Thomas C. Orihel. 1995. (Illus.). 300p. 165.00 (*0-89189-379-2*) Am Soc Clinical.

Parasitic & Infectious Diseases: Epidemiology & Ecology. Ed. by Marilyn E. Scott & Gary Smith. 1994. LC 93-39576. (Illus.). 398p. text 104.00 (*0-12-633325-4*) Acad Pr.

Parasitic & Related Diseases: Basic Mechanisms, Manifestations, & Control. Ed. by Thomas C. Cheng. 1986. LC 85-24447. (Comparative Pathobiology Ser.: Vol. 8). 176p. 65.00 (*0-306-42119-4*, Plenum Trade) Perseus Pubng.

Parasitic Diseases. M. B. Katz et al. (Illus.). 1986. 264p. 38.50 (*0-387-90689-4*); 2nd ed. 1988. 301p. 64.95 (*0-387-96800-8*) Spr-Verlag.

Parasitic Diseases: Treatment & Control. Ed. by Max J. Miller & Edgar J. Love. 1989. 360p. 195.00 (*0-8493-4922-2*, RC119) CRC Pr.

Parasitic Diseases in Water Resources Development: The Need for Intersectoral Negotiation. J. M. Hunter et al. 1993. (ENG, FRE & SPA.). x, 152p. pap. text 35.00 (*92-4-156155-6*, 1150396) World Health.

Parasitic Diseases International Nomenclature of Diseases Vol. II: Infectious Diseases, 2. 1987. (International Nomenclature of Diseases Ser.: No. 4). pap. text 20.00 (*92-4-154222-5*) World Health.

Parasitic Diseases of Wild Mammals. Ed. by William Samuel et al. 2nd ed. 2000. LC 00-47257. (Illus.). viii, 559p. 94.95 (*0-8138-2978-X*) Iowa U Pr.

Parasitic Disorders: Pathology, Diagnosis & Management. Tsieh Sun. 2nd ed. 1998. LC 98-10760. 328p. text 155.00 (*0-683-30566-2*) Lppncott W & W.

Parasitic Infections. Ed. by James H. Leech et al. 1988. (Contemporary Issues in Infectious Diseases Ser.: Vol. 7). (Illus.). 364p. text (*0-443-08561-7*) Church.

Parasitic Infections & the Immune System. Ed. by Felipe Kierszenbaum. 1993. LC 93-24095. (Illus.). 232p. text 63.00 (*0-12-406575-9*) Acad Pr.

Parasitic Infections in the Compromised Host. Peter D. Walzer & Robert M. Genta. 1988. (Infectious Disease & Therapy Ser.: Vol. 1). (Illus.). 552p. text 195.00 (*0-8247-7943-6*) Dekker.

Parasitic Infections of Domestic Animals: A Diagnostic Manual. Johannes Kaufmann. 1995. LC 95-39894. 423p. 69.50 (*0-8176-5115-2*) Birkhauser.

Parasitic Infections of Domestic Animals: A Diagnostic Manual. Johannes Kaufmann. 1996. LC 95-39894. 423p. 76.50 (*3-7643-5115-2*) Spr-Verlag.

Parasitic Lung Diseases. Adel A. Mahmoud. 1997. LC 96-39908. (Lung Biology in Health & Disease Ser.: Vol. 101). (Illus.). 256p. text 145.00 (*0-8247-9722-1*) Dekker.

Parasitic Nematodes - Antigens, Membranes & Genes. M. W. Kennedy. 1991. 250p. 110.00 (*0-85066-772-0*) Taylor & Francis.

Parasitic Protozoa, Vol. 1. Ed. by Julius P. Kreier & John R. Baker. 2nd ed. 1991. LC 91-19635. (Parasitic Protozoa Ser.: Vol. 1). (Illus.). 258p. (C). text 121.00 (*0-12-426011-X*) Acad Pr.

Parasitic Protozoa. Ed. by Julius P. Kreier. 2nd ed. 1993. (Parasitic Protozoa Ser.: Vol. 5). (Illus.). Vol. 5. 343p. text 121.00 (*0-12-426015-2*); Vol. 7. 314p. text 121.00 (*0-12-426017-9*) Acad Pr.

Parasitic Worms. D. W. Crompton & S. M. Joyner. 1980. 208p. pap. 18.00 (*0-85109-830-4*) Taylor & Francis.

Parasitic Zoonoses: Section C Ed. by Arambulo. 1982. (CRC Handbook Series in Zoonoses). Vol. I. 400p. 208.00 (*0-8493-2916-7*, RC113); Vol. II. 360p. 207.00 (*0-8493-2917-5*); Vol. III. 384p. 195.00 (*0-8493-2918-3*) Franklin (CRC Reprint).

Parasitology of Malaria: Proceedings of the WHO Scientific Group, Teheran, 1968. WHO Staff. 1969. (Technical Reports: No. 433). 70p. pap. text 5.00 (*92-4-120433-8*, 1100433) World Health.

Parathyroid Hormone. Ed. by Robert A. Nissenson & M. W. Draper. 1982. (Journal: Vol. 8, No. 3-4). (Illus.). vi, 124p. pap. 68.00 (*3-8055-3550-3*) S Karger.

Parathyroid Hormone in Kidney Failure: Proceedings of the International Symposium, 1st, New York, May, 1979. International Symposium on Parathyroid in Uremia Staff. Ed. by M. M. Avran & Geoffrey Merton Berlyne. 1980. (Contributions to Nephrology Ser.: Vol. 20). pap. 29.75 (*3-8055-0151-X*) S Karger.

Parathyroid Hormone-Related Protein: Normal Physiology & Its Role in Cancer. Bernard P. Halloran & Robert A. Nissenson. 1992. 224p. lib. bdg. 179.00 (*0-8493-4539-1*, QP572) CRC Pr.

Parathyroid Surgery. Ed. by M. Rothmund & S. A. Wells, Jr. 1986. (Progress in Surgery Ser.: Vol. 18). (Illus.). x, 250p. 154.00 (*3-8055-4217-8*) S Karger.

Paratuberculosis: Proceedings International Colloguium on Paratuberculosis, 6th, Melbourne, Australia, 1999. Ed. by Elizabeth J. B. Manning & Michael T. Collins. 1999. LC 99-48113. 720p. 225.00 (*0-9633043-4-8*) Intl Assn Paratuber.

Parent - Infant Communication: A Family-Centered Curriculum of Listening & Communication Skills Development for Children Birth - 4 Years of Age with Hearing Loss. Valerie Schuyler & Jayne Sowers. 4th rev. ed. 1998. 268p. ring bd. 55.00 (*1-883204-09-7*) Hearing & Speech.

Parent & Child. Ellyn Satter. Ed. by David Bull et al. 1985. (Illus.). 58p. pap. 2.50 (*0-933161-04-2*) Better H Prog.

Parent & the Fatally Ill Child: A Demonstration of Parent Participation in a Hospital Pediatric Department. Maurice B. Hamovitch. 1964. 152p. 12.00 (*0-940876-01-9*) City Hope.

Parent-Child Interaction & Parent-Child Relations. Ed. by Marion Perlmutter. 1984. (Minnesota Symposia on Child Psychology Ser.: Vol. 17). 208p. text 39.95 (*0-89859-380-8*) L Erlbaum Assocs.

Parent-Child Interaction Therapy: A Step-by-Step Guide for Clinicians. Toni L. Hembree-Kigin & Cheryl B. McNeil. 1995. (Clinical Child Psychology Library). (Illus.). 184p. (C). pap. 23.00 (*0-306-45024-0*, Kluwer Plenum) Kluwer Academic.

Parent-Child Play: Descriptions & Implications. Kevin MacDonald. 1993. LC 92-20562. (SUNY Series, Children's Play in Society). 389p. (C). pap. text 22.95 (*0-7914-1464-7*) State U NY Pr.

Parent-Child Play: Descriptions & Implications. Ed. by Kevin MacDonald. 1993. LC 92-20562. (SUNY Series, Children's Play in Society). 389p. (C). text 64.50 (*0-7914-1463-9*) State U NY Pr.

Parent-Child Separation: Psychosocial Effects on Development. Faren R. Akins et al. 1981. LC 81-7304. 368p. 95.00 (*0-306-65196-3*, Kluwer Plenum) Kluwer Academic.

Parent-Child Socialization in Diverse Cultures, 5. Ed. by Jaipaul L. Roopnarine et al. 1992. (Advances in Applied Developmental Psychology Ser.: Vol. 5). 336p. (C). 73.25 (*0-89391-849-0*, Ablex) Greenwood.

Parent Education As Early Childhood Intervention: Emerging Directions in Theory, Research & Practice, Vol. 3. Ed. by Purdue University Staff et al. 1988. (Advances in Applied Developmental Psychology Ser.: Vol. 3). 256p. (C). 77.00 (*0-89391-502-5*, Ablex) Greenwood.

Parent Guidance in the Nursery School. Margarete Ruben. 1970. LC 60-8066. 72p. reprint ed. 27.50 (*0-8236-4000-0*); pap. 24.95 (*0-8236-8180-7*, 24000) Intl Univs Pr.

Parent-Infant Intervention: Communication Disorders. A. Simmons-Martin & D. R. Calvert. 1979. 352p. text 29.95 (*0-8089-1185-6*, 794078, Grune & Strat) Harcrt Hlth Sci Grp.

Parent-Specific Adjustments for Assessment of Recumbent Length & Stature. Ed. by D. Thissen et al. 1981. (Monographs in Pediatrics: Vol. 13). (Illus.). x, 90p. pap. 57.50 (*3-8055-2594-X*) S Karger.

Parentage Testing Accreditation Requirements Manual. Ed. by Richard H. Walker. 2nd ed. 1995. 67p. (C). pap. text, lab manual ed. 30.00 (*1-56395-051-0*) Am Assn Blood.

Parental Bereavement. Lieberman. Date not set. 29.95 (*0-465-05444-7*) Basic.

Parental Concerns in College Student Mental Health. Ed. by Leighton C. Whitaker. LC 87-33625. (Journal of College Student Psychotherapy Ser.: Vol. 2, Nos. 1-2). (Illus.). 204p. 1989. text 6.95 (*0-86656-720-8*); 1988. pap. 3.95 (*0-86656-800-X*) Haworth Pr.

Parental Overprotection: A Risk Factor in Psychosocial Development. Gordon Parker. 1983. 352p. text 56.00 (*0-8089-1557-6*, 793246, Grune & Strat) Harcrt Hlth Sci Grp.

Parental Perspectives in Cases of Suspected Child Abuse. Hedy Cleaver. 1995. 230p. pap. (*0-11-321786-2*, HM17862) Statnry Office GBR. *Dist:* Bernan Associates.

Parental Presence: Reclaiming a Leadership Role in Bringing up Our Children. Haim Omer. 2000. LC 99-34352. xiv, 145p. pap. 19.95 (*1-891944-39-8*) Zeig Tucker Theisen.

Parental Psychiatric Disorder: Distressed Parents & Their Families. Ed. by Michael Gopfert et al. 1996. (Illus.). 382p. (C). text 130.00 (*0-521-45259-7*); pap. text 47.95 (*0-521-45892-7*) Cambridge U Pr.

Parenteral & Enteral Nutrition. Howard Silberman. 2nd ed. 1989. (Illus.). 458p. (C). pap. text 89.00 (*0-8385-7727-X*, A7727-9, Apple Lange Med) McGraw.

Parenteral Quality Control: Sterility, Pyrogen, Particulate, & Package Integrity Testing. Michael J. Akers. 2nd rev. ed. 1993. LC 93-25667. (Advances in Parenteral Sciences Ser.: Vol. 5). (Illus.). 400p. text 150.00 (*0-8247-9088-X*) Dekker.

Parenteral Therapy: Theory & Practices. Mansoor Khan & Indra K. Reddy. 1995. (Illus.). 102p. (Orig.). (C). pap., stu. ed. 17.50 (*1-878045-89-X*) Whittier Pubns.

Parenterale Ernaehrung (Forschung und Praxis) Deutsch-Skandinavisches Symposium, Kopenhagen, 197. Ed. by N. Zoellner. 1978. (Beitraege zur Infusionstherapie und Klinische Ernaehrung Ser.: Band 1). (Illus.). pap. 15.00 (*3-8055-2963-5*) S Karger.

Parenterals. Edwards. Date not set. (Pharmaceutical Engineering Ser.: No. 9). 170.00 (*0-7506-5143-1*) Buttrwrth-Heinemann.

Parenthood: Its Psychology & Psychopathology. Ed. by E. James Anthony & Therese Benedek. 1970. LC 75-112005. 650p. 33.00 (*0-316-04370-2*, Little Brwn Med Div) Lppncott W & W.

Parenting. Ed. by Betty Garee. 1989. LC 89-85623. 90p. (Orig.). pap. 7.95 (*0-915708-26-4*) Cheever Pub.

Parenting: Its Causes & Consequences. Ed. by L. Wladis Hoffman et al. 1982. 176p. text 29.95 (*0-89859-086-8*) L Erlbaum Assocs.

Parenting a Child with Arthritis: A Practical, Empathetic Guide to Help You & Your Child Live with Arthritis. Earl J. Brewer, Jr. & Kathy C. Angel. 1992. LC 91-36064. 224p. 21.95 (*0-929923-55-3*) Lowell Hse.

Parenting a Child with Diabetes. Gloria Loring. 2nd ed. 1999. LC 99-41048. 224p. pap. 14.95 (*0-7373-0301-8*, 03018W) Lowell Hse.

Parenting a Diabetic Child: A Practical, Empathetic Guide to Help You & Your Child Live with Diabetes. Gloria Loring. 1991. 240p. 19.95 (*0-929923-33-2*) Lowell Hse.

Parenting & Child Care Ed. by Joy D. Osofsky & Hiram E. Fitzgerald. 1999. LC 99-11893. (World Association for Infant Mental Health Ser.: Vol. 3). Orig. Title: Christian Parenting & Child Care. (Illus.). 425p. 220.00 (*0-471-18946-4*) Wiley.

Parenting & Children's Internalization of Values: A Handbook of Contemporary Theory. Joan E. Grusec & Leon Kuczynski. 1997. LC 97-1325. 439p. 170.00 (*0-471-12383-8*) Wiley.

Parenting & Teaching Young Children. Verna Hildebrand. Ed. by Carol Newman. 1981. (Illus.). 432p. (gr. 10-12). text 30.04 (*0-07-028775-9*) McGraw.

Parenting & You: A Guide for Parents with Seizure Disorders. Epilepsy Foundation of America Staff. 1994. 130p. pap. 12.95 (*0-916570-13-4*) Epilepsy Foundation of America.

Parenting Children with Disabilities. Peggy M. Miezo. 1983. (Pediatric Habilitation Ser.). 216p. text 75.00 (*0-8247-1090-8*) Dekker.

Parenting for Prevention: How to Raise a Child to Say No to Alcohol - Drugs for Parents, Teachers, & Other Concerned Adults. David J. Wilmes. rev. ed. 1995. 244p. (Orig.). pap. text 15.00 (*0-935908-46-3*, 3195, HazeldenJohnson Inst) Hazelden.

Parenting Guide to Pregnancy & Childbirth. Paula Spencer. Ed. by Parenting Magazine Staff. 1998. LC 97-35736. (Illus.). 384p. pap. 16.00 (*0-345-41179-X*, Ballantine) Ballantine Pub Grp.

Parenting Happy Healthy Children. Karen Olness. 1981. pap. 8.95 (*0-9602790-4-0*) Hlth Frontiers.

Parenting the Overactive Child: Alternatives to Drug Therapy. Paul Lavin. 1989. LC 89-2613. (Illus.). 160p. (Orig.). (C). 21.95 (*0-8191-7297-9*); pap. 10.95 (*0-8191-7315-0*) Madison Bks UPA.

Parents & Peers in Social Development: A Sullivan-Piaget Perspective. James Youniss. LC 79-25457. (Illus.). 320p. 1982. pap. text 11.95 (*0-226-96486-8*); 1980. lib. bdg. 28.00 (*0-226-96484-1*) U Ch Pr.

Parents & Teachers: Partners in Language Development. Audrey A. Simmons & Karen Glover-Rossi. 1990. (Centennial Celebration Ser.). 386p. (C). pap. text 27.95 (*0-88200-167-1*) Alexander Graham.

Parent's & Teacher's Handbook on Identifying & Preventing Child Abuse. James A. Monteleone. 1998. LC 98-22804. (Illus.). 256p. pap. 19.95 (*1-878060-27-9*, 31141) GW Medical.

Parents & Young Mentally Handicapped Children: A Review of Research Issues. Helen McConachie. 1986. 276p. text 29.95 (*0-914797-28-X*) Brookline Bks.

Parents as Therapeutic Partners: Listening to Your Child's Play. Arthur Kraft & Garry Landreth. 1998. LC 97-20340. 280p. pap. 40.00 (*0-7657-0106-5*) Aronson.

Parents, Children, & Adolescents: Interactive Relationships & Development in Context. Anne-Marie Ambert. 1997. LC 96-24646. 398p. (C). 59.95 (*0-7890-6034-5*);Incl. instr's. manual. pap. 24.95 (*0-7890-0181-0*) Haworth Pr.

Parents, Children & Sex. Ed. by John Robson. 1981. (Illus.). (Orig.). pap. 2.50 (*0-936098-31-7*) Intl Marriage.

Parent's Complete Guide to Ear Infections. Alan R. Greene. rev. ed. 1997. LC 97-8335. 256p. pap. 14.95 (*1-882606-29-9*) Peoples Med Soc.

Parents, Families, & the Stuttering Child. Lena Rustin. 1991. (Illus.). 130p. (Orig.). (C). pap. text 32.95 (*1-879105-16-0*, 0210) Thomson Learn.

***Parent's Guide to Asperger Syndrome & High-Functioning Autism: How to Meet the Challenges & Help Your Child Thrive.** James McPartland et al. 2002. 267p. 35.00 (*1-57230-767-6*) Guilford Pubns.

Parent's Guide to Asthma: How You Can Help Your Child Control Asthma at Home, School & Play. Nancy J. Sander. 1994. LC 93-49482. (Illus.). 336p. pap. 13.95 (*0-452-27216-5*) Dutton Plume.

Parent's Guide to Attention Deficit Disorders. Stephen B. McCarney & Angela M. Bauer. 1995. 408p. pap. 20.00 (*1-878372-01-7*, 840) Hawthorne Educ Servs.

Parent's Guide to Autism. Charles Hart. Ed. by Claire Zion. 1993. LC 93-9438. 256p. (Orig.). per. 14.00 (*0-671-75099-2*) S&S Trade.

Parents Guide to Baby & Child Medical Care. Ed. by Terril H. Hart. rev. ed. 1991. LC 89-29066. (Illus.). 240p. pap. 8.00 (*0-88166-132-5*) Meadowbrook.

Parent's Guide to Baby & Child Medical Care. Ed. by Terril H. Hart. rev. ed. 1990. 240p. 9.00 (*0-671-70157-6*) Meadowbrook.

Parent's Guide to Better Nutrition for Tots to Teenagers. Emory W. Thurston. 1979. LC 76-10041. pap. 4.95 (*0-87983-194-4*, Keats Pubng) McGraw-Hill Trade.

Parents' Guide to CFIDS: How to Be an Advocate for Your Child with Chronic Fatigue Immune Dysfunction Syndrome. David S. Bell et al. 1999. LC 98-21756. 162p. 39.95 (*0-7890-0631-6*); pap. 17.95 (*0-7890-0711-8*) Haworth Pr (Hawrth Medical).

Parents' Guide to Child Therapy. Richard Bush. 1994. LC 94-72054. (Master Work Ser.). 352p. pap. 40.00 (*1-56821-315-8*) Aronson.

***Parent's Guide to Childhood Eating Disorders: A Nutritional Approach to Solving Eating Disorders.** Marcia Herrin & Nancy Matsumoto. 2002. LC 2001-39837. 288p. pap. 16.00 (*0-8050-6649-7*, Owl) H Holt & Co.

***Parents Guide to Childhood Immunization.** 2001. 97p. pap. 7.50 (*0-16-050801-0*, Hlth & Human) USGPO.

***Parent's Guide to Children's Congenital Heart Defects: What They Are, How to Treat Them, How to Cope with Them.** Gerri Freid Kramer & Shari Maurer. 2001. LC 2001-27785. (Illus.). 288p. pap. 14.00 (*0-609-80775-7*, Three Riv Pr) Harmony Bks.

Parent's Guide to Cleft Lip & Palate. Sylvia Johnson et al. 1990. (University of Minnesota Guides to Birth & Childhood Disorders). 137p. 16.95 (*0-8166-1491-1*) U of Minn Pr.

Parent's Guide to Cystic Fibrosis. Burton L. Shapiro & Ralph C. Heussner, Jr. 1991. (University of Minnesota Guides to Birth & Childhood Disorders). (Illus.). 120p. 16.95 (*0-8166-1488-1*) U of Minn Pr.

Parent's Guide to Down Syndrome: Toward a Brighter Future. Ed. by Siegfried M. Pueschel. 1990. (Illus.). 336p. (C). text 22.95 (*1-55766-060-3*, 0603) P H Brookes.

Parent's Guide to Eating Disorders: Prevention & Treatment of Anorexia Nervosa & Bulimia. Brett Valette. 1990. 208p. mass mkt. 4.50 (*0-380-70834-5*, Avon Bks) Morrow Avon.

Parents' Guide to Feeding Your Kids Right. Childres Television Workshop Staff. 1989. 19.95 (*0-13-649922-8*) P-H.

Parents Guide to Food Allergies: Clear & Complete Advice from the Experts on Raising Your Food Allergic Child. Marianne Barber. 2001. LC 00-53920. (Illus.). xix, 384p. pap. 15.00 (*0-8050-6600-4*) St Martin.

Parent's Guide to Kidney Disorders. Glenn H. Bock et al. 1993. LC 92-35697. (University of Minnesota Guides to Birth & Childhood Disorders). (Illus.). 188p. (C). 18.95 (*0-8166-1745-7*) U of Minn Pr.

Parent's Guide to Raising Twins. Elizabeth Friedrich & Cherry Rowland. 1990. (Illus.). 320p. pap. 12.95 (*0-312-03906-9*) St Martin.

Parent's Guide to Spina Bifida. Beth-Ann Bloom & Edward L. Selijeskog. 1988. LC 88-10784. (Guides to Birth & Childhood Disorders Ser.). (Illus.). 96p. 16.95 (*0-8166-1486-5*) U of Minn Pr.

Parents' Guide to Teenage Pregnancy. Margaret Brownley. 1988. 36p. (Orig.). (gr. 10-12). pap. 3.95 (*0-945485-05-0*, 113P) Comm Intervention.

Parent's Handbook of Drug & Alcohol Prevention & Family Problem Solving. Telesis Corp. Staff. Tr. by Mary Ortega from ENG. 1985. 15p. (Orig.). 1.50 (*1-56117-008-9*) Telesis CA.

Parent's Helper: Who to Call on Health & Family Issues. Christine L. Williams & John J. Connolly. 1996. LC 95-70170. (Illus.). 409p. pap. 15.95 (*1-883769-72-8*) Castle Connolly Med.

Parents on Dyslexia. Van der Stoel. 1990. (*1-85359-077-0*); pap. (*1-85359-076-2*) Multilingual Matters GBR. *Dist:* Taylor & Francis.

Parent's Pipeline Guide: Plain Talk about Teens & Alcohol, Drugs, Sex, Eating Disorders & Depression. Sheila Fuller & Leigh Rudd. Ed. by Robert F. Fuller & Patty B. Walker. 1994. (Illus.). 175p. pap. 9.95 (*0-9631049-1-8*) Parents Pipeline.

Parents, Teenagers & Sex. Ed. by John Robson. 1982. (Illus.). 40p. (Orig.). pap. 2.50 (*0-936098-34-1*) Intl Marriage.

Parexel's Pharmaceutical R&D Statistical Sourcebook, 1996. Ed. by Mark Mathiew. 1996. 180p. 195.00 (*1-882615-26-3*) Parexel Intl.

Parish Nurse: Providing a Minister of Health for Your Congregation. Granger E. Westburg et al. 1990. LC 90-43206. 80p. (Orig.). pap. text 8.99 (*0-8066-2458-2*, 9-2458) Augsburg Fortress.

Parish Nursing: Promoting Whole Person Health Within Faith Communities. Phyllis A. Solari-Twadell & Mary A. McDermott. 1999. LC 98-25454. 316p. 72.95 (*0-7619-1182-0*, 81897) Sage.

Parish Nursing: Promoting Whole Person Health Within Faith Communities. Phyllis A. Solari-Twadell & Mary Ann McDermott. 1999. LC 98-25454. xxvii, 316p. pap. 31.95 (*0-7619-1183-9*, 81898) Sage.

Parity in Financing Mental Health Services: Managed Care Effects on Cost, Access & Quality. Harold E. Varmus. 1999. 112p. pap. text 25.00 (*0-7881-7630-7*) DIANE Pub.

Parkinson Predicament & a Spoonful of Sugar: My Life with Parkinson's Disease/A Prescription for Living with Parkinson's Disease. Barbara T. Coleman. Ed. by Barry Green. 1997. (Illus.). 112p. pap. text 24.95 (*0-9642109-2-4*) Parkinsonian.

Parkinsonian Syndromes. Ed. by Matthew B. Stern & William C. Koller. 1993. LC 93-6644. (Neurological Disease & Therapy Ser.: Vol. 18). (Illus.). 592p. text 255.00 (*0-8247-8838-9*) Dekker.

Parkinsonism. Calne. Date not set. (Pharmacology & Therapeutics Ser.). pap. (*0-08-034187-X*, Pergamon Pr) Elsevier.

Parkinsonism: Diagnosis & Treatment. 1989. 256p. pap. text 39.50 (*0-9621697-0-6*) Laurel Hse NJ.

Parkinsonism: Physiology, Pharmacology & Treatment. Donald B. Calne. 1970. LC 74-500723. xii, 136 p. (*0-7131-4175-1*) St Martin.

Parkinsonism-Symptoms, Syndrome & Tardive Dyskinesia: Index of New Information with Authors & Subjects. Roscoe J. Sacks. 1993. LC 92-54188. 180p. 47.50 (*1-55914-748-2*); pap. 44.50 (*1-55914-749-0*) ABBE Pubs Assn.

Parkinson's: A Patient's View. Sidney Dorros. 1989. LC 89-10122. pap. 12.95 (*0-929765-20-6*) Seven Locks Pr.

Parkinson's - A Personal Story of Acceptance. Sandi Gordon. 1993. (Illus.). 162p. pap. 12.95 (*0-8283-1949-9*) Branden Bks.

Parkinson's Challenge: A Beginner's Guide to a Good Life in the Slow Lane. Jan P. Stern. rev. ed. 1989. (Illus.). 60p. reprint ed. pap. 3.85 (*0-9623549-0-2*, TX2156483) DMS Pubs.

***Parkinson's Disease.** Clough et al. 2002. (Fast Facts Ser.). (Illus.). pap. (*1-899541-44-6*) Health Pr GBR. *Dist:* JAMCO Dist.

Parkinson's Disease. Porter. 1992. LC 92-49799. (One Hundred Maxims in Neurology Ser.). 169p. 35.95 (*0-8016-7279-1*) Mosby Inc.

Parkinson's Disease. F. Clifford Rose. 1987. (Current Problems in Neurology Ser.: Vol. 6). 224p. (*0-86196-110-2*) J Libbey Med GBR. *Dist:* Bks Intl VA.

Parkinson's Disease. Alvin Silverstein et al. 2002. LC 00-12073. (Diseases & People Ser.). (Illus.). 128p. (J). (gr. 6 up). lib. bdg. 20.95 (*0-7660-1593-9*) Enslow Pubs.

Parkinson's Disease: A Complete Guide for Patients & Families. William J. Weiner et al. 2001. LC 00-9630. (Health Bks.). (Illus.). 272p. pap. 15.95 (*0-8018-6556-5*) Johns Hopkins.

Parkinson's Disease: A Guide for Patient & Family. Roger C. Duvoisin & Jacob I. Sage. 4th ed. 1995. LC 95-4919. 192p. pap. text 32.95 (*0-7817-0312-3*) Lppncott W & W.

Parkinson's Disease: A Self-Help Guide. Marjan Jahanshahi et al. 2000. LC 00-35859. (Illus.). 400p. pap. 24.95 (*1-888799-38-2*) Demos Medical.

Parkinson's Disease: Biochemistry, Clinical Pathology, & Treatment. W. Birkmayer & P. Riederer. Tr. by G. Reynolds from GER. 1983. (Illus.). 194p. 82.95 (*0-387-81722-0*) Spr-Verlag.

Parkinson's Disease: Dianosis & Medical Management. Ed. by Stewart A. Factor & William J. Weiner. 2001. (Illus.). 600p. text 175.00 (*1-888799-50-1*) Demos Medical.

Parkinson's Disease: Experimental Models & Therapy. Contrib. by Riederer. 1996. (Illus.). 350p. pap. 190.00 (*3-211-82749-8*) Spr-Verlag.

Parkinson's Disease: From Clinical Aspects to Molecular Basis. Ed. by P. Riederer et al. 1992. (Key Topics in Brain Research Ser.). (Illus.). 240p. 92.00 (*0-387-82272-0*) Spr-Verlag.

Parkinson's Disease: Neurobehavioral Aspects. Steven J. Huber & Jeffrey L. Cummings. 1992. (Illus.). 384p. text 69.50 (*0-19-506969-2*) OUP.

Parkinson's Disease: Questions & Answers. Robert Hauser & Theresa Zesiewicz. 3rd ed. 2000. (Questions & Answers Ser.). (Illus.). 158p. pap. text 26.95 (*1-873413-92-0*) Merit Pub Intl.

Parkinson's Disease: The Complete Guide for Patients & Caregivers. Abraham N. Lieberman et al. 1993. LC 92-21419. 272p. (Orig.). pap. 12.00 (*0-671-76819-0*) S&S Trade Pap.

Parkinson's Disease: The Mystery, the Search & the Promise. Sue Dauphin. 1995. LC 92-93912. (Illus.). 229p. pap. 16.95 (*0-9620354-1-6*) Pixel Pr.

Parkinson's Disease: The Treatment Options. Ed. by Peter A. LeWitt & Wolfgang H. Oertel. 1999. 260p. (*1-85317-379-7*) Martin Dunitz.

Parkinson's Disease - Questions & Answers, 2nd Edition. Robert Hauser & Theresa Zesiewicz. 2nd rev. ed. 1998. (Illus.). 150p. pap. 15.95 (*1-873413-46-7*) Merit Pub Intl.

Parkinson's Disease & Its Management. J. Malcolm Pearce. 1992. (Illus.). 158p. text 39.95 (*0-19-262177-7*) OUP.

Parkinson's Disease & Movement Disorders. Ed. by Joseph Jankovic & Eduardo Tolosa. 2nd ed. 1993. LC 92-49846. (Illus.). 640p. 95.00 (*0-683-04380-3*) Lppncott W & W.

Parkinson's Disease & Movement Disorders. Joseph Jankovic & Eduardo Tolosa. 3rd ed. 1998. LC 97-45686. 720p. text 115.00 (*0-683-30016-4*) Lppncott W & W.

Parkinson's Disease & Movement Disorders: Diagnosis & Treatment Guidelines for the Practicing Physician. Ed. by Charles H. Adler & J. Eric Ahlskog. 2000. LC 00-27597. (Current Clinical Practice Ser.). (Illus.). xiv, 474p. 125.00 (*0-89603-607-3*) Humana.

Parkinson's Disease & Parkinsonism in the Elderly. Ed. by R. J. Meara & W. C. Koller. 2000. LC 99-57614. (Illus.). 262p. (C). pap. text 49.95 (*0-521-62884-9*) Cambridge U Pr.

Parkinson's Disease & Quality of Life. Ed. by Lucian Cote et al. 2000. LC 00-28034. 199p. pap. 19.95 (*0-7890-0810-6*); 49.95 (*0-7890-0763-0*) Haworth Pr (Hawrth Medical).

Parkinson's Disease & the Art of Moving. John Argue. 2000. LC 00-500901. (Illus.). vi, 220p. pap. 15.95 (*1-57224-183-7*) New Harbinger.

***Parkinson's Disease in Practice.** C. E. Clarke. 2001. (In Practice Ser.). 150p. pap. (*1-85315-486-5*) Royal Soc of Medicine Pr Ltd GBR. *Dist:* Balogh.

***Parkinson's Disease in the Older Patient.** Jeremy R. Playfer & John V. Hindle. 2001. (Arnold Publication). 256p. text (*0-340-75914-3*) E A GBR. *Dist:* OUP.

Parkinson's Disease Management Package. Kate Swinburn. 1996. pap. 125.00 (*1-56593-498-9*, 1154) Singular Publishing.

Parkinson's Handbook. Dwight C. McGoon. 1994. pap. 13.95 (*0-393-31143-0*) Norton.

Parkland Pocket Guide to HIV Care. Nassar. 1997. pap. text (*0-01-605400-8*) Collins.

Parkland Trauma Handbook, 2. Ed. by Fiemu Nwariaku & Erwin R. Thal. 2nd ed. 1999. LC 98-54476. (Illus.). 544p. (C). (gr. 13). pap. text 36.95 (*0-8151-2618-2*, 31645) Mosby Inc.

Parson's Diseases of the Eye. Stephen J. Miller. 18th ed. 1990. (Illus.). 442p. text (*0-443-04230-6*) Church.

Part B Billing Guide. James R. Lyle & Hoyt W. Torras. 1995. pap. 99.00 (*1-879249-16-2*) HlthCare Consult.

Part of Ourselves: Lament for Lives That Ended Too Soon. Ed. by Siobhan Parkinson. 1998. LC 98-120095. 188p. pap. (*1-899047-34-4*) A A Farmar IRL. *Dist:* Irish Bks Media.

Partera: Story of a Midwife. Fran Leeper Buss. 2001. LC 00-59984. (Ann Arbor Paperback Ser.). (SPA., Illus.). 152p. (C). pap. text 14.95 (*0-472-08712-6*, 08712) U of Mich Pr.

Partial Hospitalization: A Current Perspective. Ed. by R. F. Luber. 1979. LC 78-31915. (Illus.). 222p. 39.50 (*0-306-40201-7*, Plenum Trade) Perseus Pubng.

Partial Left Ventriculectomy: Its Theory, Results & Perspectives; Proceedings of the Cardiac Volume Reduction Forum '97, Tokyo, Japan, October 4, 1997. Ed. by Akira T. Kawaguchi & Leonard M. Linde. 1998. LC 98-40591. (International Congress Ser.). 128p. 105.00 (*0-444-50028-6*, Excerpta Medica) Elsevier.

Partial Left Ventriculectomy 2: Recent Evolution for Safe & Effective Application: Proceedings of the 2nd International Symposium on Partial Left Ventriculectomy, Tokyo, Japan, 12 December, 1998. Ed. by Akira T. Kawaguchi & Leonard M. Linde. 1999. LC 99-51724. 166p. 109.00 (*0-444-50279-3*) Elsevier.

Partial Removable Prosthodontics. F. James Kratochvil. 1988. (Illus.). 304p. pap. text 55.00 (*0-7216-2382-4*) Saunders.

Partial Seizure Disorders: A Guide for Parents & Families. Mitzi Waltz. 2001. LC 00-59823. (Patient-Centered Guides). (Illus.). xii, 274p. pap. 19.95 (*0-596-50003-3*) OReilly & Assocs.

Partial Seizures & Interictal Disorders: The Neuropsychiatric Elements. David P. Moore. 1997. LC 97-4329. 234p. text 74.99 (*0-7506-9931-0*) Buttrwrth-Heinemann.

Partially Halogenated Chlorofluorocarbons (Ethane Derivatives) 1992. (Environmental Health Criteria Ser.: No. 139). (ENG, FRE & SPA.). 130p. pap. text 29.00 (*92-4-157139-X*, 1160139) World Health.

Partially Halogenated Chlorofluorocarbons (Methane Derivatives) 1991. (Environmental Health Criteria Ser.: No. 126). (ENG, FRE & SPA.). 97p. pap. text 21.00 (*92-4-157126-8*, 1160126) World Health.

Participation by Families of Mentally Handicapped People in Policy Making & Planning. Alan Tyne. 1979. (*0-7855-0571-7*) Natl Inst Soc Work GBR. *Dist:* St Mut.

Participatory Approach to Rural AIDS Education: A Workshop Manual. Isaac Bekalo. ltd. ed. 1992. 94p. 4.00 (*0-942717-40-6*) Intl Inst Rural.

Participatory Planning in Community Health Education. Preston L. Schiller et al. 1987. LC 86-51164. 210p. pap. 15.95 (*0-89914-024-6*) Third Party Pub.

Participatory Plant Breeding: Proceedings of a Workshop. Ed. by P. Eyzaguirre & M. Iwanaga. 1997. (Illus.). 164p. (Orig.). (C). pap. text 35.00 (*0-7881-4550-9*) DIANE Pub.

Particle Interactions & Internal Tablet Structure: Factors Affecting the Mechanical Strength of Pharmaceutical Compacts. Helena Olsson. 2000. (Comprehensive Summaries of Uppsala Dissertations from the Faculty of Pharmacy Ser.: No. 228). (Illus.). 56p. pap. (*91-554-4725-2*) Uppsala Universitet SWE. *Dist:* Coronet Bks.

Particle-Lung Interactions. Ed. by Peter Gehrung & Joachim Heyder. Date not set. (Lung Biology in Health & Disease Ser.). (Illus.). 823p. text 225.00 (*0-8247-9891-0*) Dekker.

Particle Overload in the Rat Lung & Lung Cancer - Implications for Human Risk Assessment: Proceedings of MIT Conference Held March 29-30, 1995. Ed. by Robert J. McCunney & Joe L. Mauderly. 1996. LC 95-47904. 320p. 89.95 (*1-56032-543-7*) Hemisp Pub.

Particle-Particle Adhesion in Pharmaceutical Powder Handling. Fridrun Podczeck. 1998. 260p. (*1-86094-112-5*) Imperial College GBR. *Dist:* World Scientific Pub.

Particle Size - Selective Sampling for Particulate Air Contaminants. Ed. by James H. Vincent & American Conference of Governmental Industrial Hygienists Staff. 1998. LC 00-711864. (Illus.). 240p. text 39.00 (*1-882417-30-5*, 0830) Am Conf Govt Indus Hygienist.

Particles in Our Air: Exposures & Health Effects. Ed. by John D. Spengler & Richard Wilson. 1996. LC 96-79259. (Illus.). 300p. 20.00 (*0-674-24077-4*) HUP.

Particles of Reason: Medicine of the Eternal Self. Bahram Elahi. 2000. LC 00-52349. (Illus.). 159p. pap. 16.95 (*0-8453-4875-2*, Cornwall Bks) Assoc Univ Prs.

Particulate Air Pollution: Problems & Solutions. Louis Theodore et al. 1980. 112p. 70.00 (*0-8493-5541-9*, TD884, CRC Reprint) Franklin.

Particulate Debris from Medical Implants: Mechanisms of Formation & Biological Consequences. Ed. by Kenneth R. St. John. 1992. LC 91-47039. (Special Technical Publications: No. 1144). (Illus.). 215p. 59.00 (*0-8031-1441-9*, STP1144) ASTM.

Particulate Matter: Sources & Resources for Healthcare Manufacturers. Michael J. Groves. 1993. 299p. 86.95 (*0-935184-40-6*) IHS Health Grp.

***Parting the Fog: The Personal Side of Fibromyalgia/ Chronic Fatigue Syndrome.** Sue Jones. 2001. 120p. pap. 12.95 (*0-9712175-0-5*) LaMont Pubng.

Partitioned Representations: A Study in Mental Representation, Language Understanding & Linguistic Structure. John Dinsmore. 1991. 352p. (C). lib. bdg. 122.00 (*0-7923-1348-8*) Kluwer Academic.

Partners for the Dance: Forming Strategic Alliances in Health Care. Ed. by Arnold D. Kaluzny et al. 1995. LC 94-47387. pap. 19.50 (*1-56793-025-5*, 0955) Health Admin Pr.

Partners in Care? Hospices & Health Authorities. David Clark. 1993. (Occasional Papers on Social Administration). 176p. (*1-85628-227-9*) Avebry GBR. *Dist:* Ashgate Pub Co.

Partners in Caring Home Care Aid Video Series. 1994. 26p. tchr. ed. 15.00 (*0-8273-6542-X*) Delmar.

Partners in Healing: Healthcare Organizations & Parish Communities. Robert L. Kinast & Lawrence G. Seidl. 1996. LC 96-164009. 57p. pap. 5.00 (*0-87125-227-9*) Cath Health.

Partners in Healing: Redistributing Power in the Counselor-Client Relationship. Barbara Friedman. 1992. LC 92-3111. 200p. (Orig.). (C). pap. text 14.95 (*0-89390-226-8*) Resource Pubns.

Partners in Play: An Adlerian Approach to Play Therapy. Terry A. Kottman. 1995. LC 94-31001. 219p. pap. text 45.95 (*1-55620-141-9*, 72589) Am Coun Assn.

Partners of the Heart: Vivien Thomas & His Work with Alfred Blalock: An Autobiography. Vivien T. Thomas. 1998. LC 97-14222. 264p. (C). (gr. 13). pap. text 14.95 (*0-8122-1634-2*) U of Pa Pr.

Partnership & Pragmatism: Germany's Response to Aids Prevention & Care. Rolf Rosenbrock & Michael T. Wright. 2000. LC 00-31133. (Illus.). xvi, 254p. pap. (*0-415-24106-5*) Routledge.

Partnership & Pragmatism: Germany's Response to AIDS Prevention & Care. Ed. by Rolf Rosenbrock & Michael T. Wright. 2000. LC 00-31133. (Illus.). xvi, 254p. (*0-415-24105-7*) Routledge.

Partnership for Health: Building Relationships Between Women & Health Caregivers. Christina S. Beck et al. 1997. LC 96-54801. (Communication Ser.). 232p. pap. 21.50 (*0-8058-2445-6*); text 45.00 (*0-8058-2444-8*) L Erlbaum Assocs.

Partnership Games: The Musings of a Recently Retired Psychiatrist. Sanford L. Billet. 1997. LC 97-94034. 298p. 28.00 (*0-9659365-0-3*) Auth Village Pubns.

Partnership Way: New Tools for Living & Learning. Riane Eisler & David Loye. rev. ed. 1998. (Illus.). 214p. pap. 24.95 (*0-9627232-9-0*) Psychology Pr.

Partnerships in Healthcare: Transforming Relational Process. Ed. by Anthony L. Suchman et al. 1998. LC 97-45065. (Illus.). 368p. 95.00 (*1-878822-80-2*) Univ Rochester Pr.

Parts of Animals. A. L. Peck. 1968. (Loeb Classical Library: No. 323). (ENG & GRE.). (C). 15.50 (*0-674-99357-8*) HUP.

Parvoviruses. 1976. (Virology Monographs: Vol. 15). 47.00 (*0-387-81355-1*) Spr-Verlag.

Parvoviruses. Kenneth I. Berns. 1984. (Viruses Ser.). (Illus.). 424p. (C). text 115.00 (*0-306-41412-0*, Kluwer Plenum) Kluwer Academic.

Parvoviruses & Human Disease. Ed. by John R. Pattison. 1988. 208p. 117.00 (*0-8493-5956-2*, QR201, CRC Reprint) Franklin.

Pass CCRN! Robin D. Dennison. 1996. LC 95-47198. (Illus.). 752p. pap. text 37.95 (*0-8016-0128-2*, 00128) Mosby Inc.

Pass CCRN! A Comprehensive Critical Care Review. Robin D. Dennison. 2nd ed. 2000. LC 99-51958. 750p. pap. text 47.95 (*0-323-00999-9*) Mosby Inc.

Pass EMT-Basic: New Curriculum. American Safety Video Publishers, Inc. Staff. 1996. 32.95 (*0-8151-0883-4*, S2046) Mosby Inc.

Pass NCLEX-LPN Survival Kit. Melodie Chenevert & Martha Bramhall. 1994. (*0-8151-7881-6*) Mosby Inc.

Pass NCLEX-RN Survival Guide. Melodie Chenevert. 1994. (*0-8151-1535-0*) Mosby Inc.

***PASS Paramedic.** Mosby Inc. Staff. 2nd ed. 2001. (*0-323-01331-7*) Mosby Inc.

Pass the Micropsychology. Williams. 1996. pap. text 28.00 (*0-7020-2066-4*) Saunders.

Pass the MRC Psychology Essay. Christopher Williams & Peter Trigwell. 1996. (Illus.). 215p. pap. text (*0-7020-2154-7*) W B Saunders GBR. *Dist:* Saunders.

Pass the MRCP. Mark Elliot et al. 1996. (Illus.). 155p. pap. text (*0-7020-2198-9*) W B Saunders GBR. *Dist:* Saunders.

Pass the Summative Assessment & MRCGP: All the Techniques You Need. Peter Lindsay et al. 1996. 110p. pap. text (*0-7020-2194-6*) W B Saunders GBR. *Dist:* Saunders.

Passage Through Crisis: Polio Victims & Their Families. Fred Davis. 1991. 256p. (C). pap. text 24.95 (*0-88738-853-1*) Transaction Pubs.

Passage Through Menopause: Women's Life in Transition. Brenda Millette & Joellen Hawkins. 1983. pap. 17.95 (*0-8359-5461-7*) P-H.

Passage to Medicine Practical. A. Mukherji. 1989. (C). (*0-89771-357-5*) Current Dist IND. *Dist:* St Mut.

Passage to Medicine Practice. M. Mukherjee. 1990. (C). (*0-7855-4669-3*) Current Dist IND. *Dist:* St Mut.

Passage to Power: Natural Menopause Revolution. Leslie Kenton. 2nd rev. ed. 1998. LC 98-14278. 400p. pap. 14.95 (*1-56170-487-3*, 550) Hay House.

Passing: The Vision of Death in America, 2. Charles O. Jackson. 1977. LC 77-23794. (Contributions in Family Studies Ser.: No. 2). 258p. 67.00 (*0-8371-9757-0*, JPA/, Greenwood Pr) Greenwood.

Passing the USMLE: Step 1. Southland Staff. 1998. (C). Vol. I. 3rd rev. ed. 185p. pap., wbk. ed. 30.00 (*1-888628-00-6*); Vol. II. 3rd rev. ed. 171p. pap., wbk. ed. 30.00 (*1-888628-01-4*); Vol. III. 3rd rev. ed. 166p. pap., wbk. ed. 30.00 (*1-888628-02-2*); Vol. IV. rev. ed. 116p. pap., wbk. ed. 30.00 (*1-888628-03-0*) Southlnd Tutor.

Passing the USMLE: Step 2. Southland Staff. 1998. (C). Vol. I. 3rd rev. ed. 189p. pap., wbk. ed. 30.00 (*1-888628-06-5*); Vol. II. 3rd rev. ed. 273p. pap., wbk. ed. 30.00 (*1-888628-07-3*); Vol. III. 3rd rev. ed. 207p. pap., wbk. ed. 30.00 (*1-888628-08-1*); Vol. IV. rev. ed. pap., wbk. ed. 30.00 (*1-888628-09-X*) Southlnd Tutor.

Passing the USMLE: Step 3. Southland Staff. 1998. (C). Vol. II. 3rd rev. ed. 209p. pap., wbk. ed. 30.00 (*1-888628-14-6*); Vol. III. 3rd rev. ed. 223p. pap., wbk. ed. 30.00 (*1-888628-15-4*); Vol. IV. rev. ed. pap., wbk. ed. 30.00 (*1-888628-16-2*) Southlnd Tutor.

Passing the USMLE Case Clusters: Steps 2 & 3. Southland Staff. 3rd rev. ed. 1998. 163p. (C). pap., wbk. ed. 30.00 (*1-888628-21-9*) Southlnd Tutor.

Passing the USMLE Photo Diagnosis: Steps 1, 2 & 3. Southland Staff. 1998. Vol. I. 3rd ed. 77p. pap., wbk. ed. 30.00 (*1-888628-23-5*); Vol. II. pap., wbk. ed. 30.00 (*1-888628-24-3*) Southlnd Tutor.

Passing Through Transitions: A Guide for Practitioners. Naomi Golan. 1983. LC 83-70837. 330p. pap. 17.95 (*0-02-912080-2*) Free Pr.

Passion for the Possible: A Guide to Realizing Your True Potential. Jean Houston. 1998. LC 97-20406. 208p. pap. 11.00 (*0-06-251532-2*) Harper SF.

Passion in Theory: Conceptions of Freud & Lacan. Robyn Ferrell. 1996. LC 96-11543. (Warwick Studies in European Philosophy). (Illus.). 128p. (C). 70.00 (*0-415-09019-9*); pap. 19.95 (*0-415-09020-2*) Routledge.

Passion Play: Ancient Secrets for a Lifetime of Health & Happiness Through Sensational Sex. Felice Dunas & Philip Goldberg. 1997. LC 97-8420. (Illus.). 304p. 24.95 (*1-57322-076-0*, Riverhead Books) Putnam Pub Group.

Passionate Marriage: Sex, Love, & Intimacy in Emotionally Committed Relationships. David M. Schnarch. 1997. LC 96-40893. 484p. 25.00 (*0-393-04021-6*) Norton.

Passionate Technique: Strategic Psychodrama with Individuals, Families & Groups. Antony Williams. 1989. 256p. 49.50 (*0-415-00138-2*) Routledge.

Passions of the Human Soul, & Their Influence on Society & Civilization Francois M. Fourier. Tr. by H. Doherty. 1968. LC 67-29504. reprint ed. 95.00 (*0-678-00383-1*) Kelley.

Passivity: A Study of Its Development & Expression in Boys. Sylvia Brody. 1964. LC 64-18623. 184p. 28.50 (*0-8236-4020-5*) Intl Univs Pr.

Passkey for Health Insurance Licensing. 6th ed. 1999. LC 98-46492. 213p. pap. 26.00 (*0-7931-3537-0*) Dearborn.

Passport to Practical & Vocational Nursing. Linda Blair. 1998. (Illus.). 288p. tchr. ed. (*1-55664-438-8*) Mosby Inc.

Past Due: A Story of Disability, Pregnancy & Birth. Anne Finger. 1990. LC 89-70235. 200p. (Orig.). pap. 10.95 (*0-931188-87-3*) Seal Pr WA.

Past Imperfect: How Tracing Your Family Medical History Can Save Your Life. Carol Daus. 1999. LC 98-32131. 240p. pap. 12.95 (*1-891661-03-5*, 1035, Offbeat) Snta Monica.

Past, Present & Future Challenges in Renal Anaemia: Technical Forum, Organized by F. Hoffmann-La Roche Ltd. During the 36th ERA/EDTA Congress, Madrid, September 1999. Ed. by Fernando Valderrabano. 2000. (Nephron Ser.: Vol. 85, Suppl. 1). (Illus.). iv, 24p. pap. 25.25 (*3-8055-7069-4*) S Karger.

Past Trauma in Late Life: European Perspective on Therapeutic Work with Older People. Linda Hunt et al. 1997. LC 97-198033. 224p. pap. (*1-85302-446-5*) Jessica Kingsley GBR. *Dist:* Taylor & Francis.

Pasteur, Plagiarist, Impostor! The Germ Theory Exploded! R. B. Pearson. 1996. 148p. reprint ed. spiral bd. 18.00 (*0-7873-0662-2*) Hlth Research.

Pasteurellosis in Production Animals. B. E. Patten et al. 1993. 256p. (Orig.). pap. 159.00 (*1-86320-081-9*) St Mut.

Pastor & Patient: A Handbook for Clergy Who Visit the Sick. Ed. by Richard Dayringer. 1995. LC 80-70247. (Master Work Ser.). 292p. reprint ed. pap. 45.00 (*1-56821-512-6*) Aronson.

Pastor & the Patient. Kent D. Richmond & David L. Middleton. 1992. 144p. (Orig.). pap. 13.95 (*0-687-30352-4*) Abingdon.

Pastoral Care & Context. Ed. by Otto Stange. 1992. 160p. (Orig.). pap. text (*90-5383-041-3*) VU Univ Pr NLD. *Dist:* Paul & Co Pubs.

Pastoral Care for Survivors of Family Abuse. James Leehan. 1989. LC 89-5441. 156p. (Orig.). pap. 15.95 (*0-664-25025-4*) Westminster John Knox.

Pastoral Care in Emergencies. David K. Switzer. 2000. LC 00-27228. (Creative Pastoral Care & Counseling Ser.). (Illus.). ix, 191p. pap. 18.00 (*0-8006-3228-1*, Fortress Pr) Augsburg Fortress.

Pastoral Care in Hospitals. Neville Kirkwood. 1999. LC 98-35131. 288p. pap. 14.95 (*0-8192-1790-5*) Morehouse Pub.

Pastoral Care in Hospitals. Neville A. Kirkwood. 1995. 288p. pap. (*0-85574-405-7*) E J Dwyer AUS. *Dist:* Morehouse Pub.

Pastoral Care of Depression: A Guidebook. Binford W. Gilbert. 1997. LC 97-19563. 127p. 29.95 (*0-7890-0264-7*); pap. 19.95 (*0-7890-0265-5*) Haworth Pr (Haworth Pastrl).

Pastoral Care of the Mentally Disabled: Advancing Care of the Whole Person. Ed. by Sally K. Severino & Richard Liew. 1994. LC 94-17287. 116p. (C). 39.95 (*1-56024-665-0*) Haworth Pr.

Pastoral Care of the Sick: Rites of Anointing & Viaticum. 1983. 344p. 14.95 (*0-8146-1321-7*) Liturgical Pr.

Pastoral Medicine: The Collegial Working of Doctors & Priests. Rudolf Steiner. Tr. by Gladys Hahn from GER. 1987.Tr. of Pastoral-Medizinischer Kurs. 172p. pap. 16.95 (*0-88010-253-5*) Anthroposophic.

Pastoral-Medizinischer Kurs see Pastoral Medicine: The Collegial Working of Doctors & Priests

Pastoral Psychotherapy: Theory & Practice. Carroll Wise. 1983. LC 84-45025. 328p. 50.00 (*0-87668-661-7*) Aronson.

Pastoral Role in Caring for the Dying & Bereaved: Pragmatic & Ecumenical, 7. Ed. by Austin H. Kutscher et al. 1986. LC 86-545. (Foundation of Thanatology Ser.: Vol. 7). 245p. 78.00 (*0-275-92153-0*, C2153, Praeger Pubs) Greenwood.

Pastor's Guide to Psychiatric Disorders & Mental Health Resources. Ed. by W Brad Johnson & William L. Johnson. 2000. LC 99-462148. xii, 240p. 49.95 (*0-7890-0712-6*); pap. text 24.95 (*0-7890-1111-5*) Haworth Pr (Haworth Pastrl).

Pat Nixon of Texas: Autobiography of a Doctor. Pat I. Nixon. Ed. by Herbert H. Lang. 1979. LC 78-65575. 248p. 24.95 (*0-89096-072-0*) Tex A&M Univ Pr.

Pat, You Have Cancer: A Story of Hope. Robert Burtness & Patricia Burtness. 1994. 117p. (Orig.). pap. 8.95 (*0-9638111-0-X*) Riverhse Lit Creat.

Patch Testing: Test Concentrations & Vehicles for 3700 Chemicals. De Groot. 2nd ed. 1994. 334p. 167.00 (*0-444-81911-8*) Elsevier.

Patching the Safety Net: Shifting Health Care Costs & State Policies. Kala Ladenheim. 1997. LC 98-116504. 32p. 35.00 (*1-55516-751-9*, 6735) Natl Conf State Legis.

Patchwork. Koenemann Inc. Staff. 2000. (Take Up- Ser.). (Illus.). 72p. pap. text 3.95 (*3-8290-2783-4*, 520924) Konemann.

Pate: The Facts of Nature Underlying Pate Thinning Hair & Baldness-Its Causes & a Professional Program for Prevention (Also a Self-Help Book) Lawrence Holley. 1989. LC 89-92729. (Illus.). 140p. pap. 11.95 (*0-9625083-0-6*); lib. bdg. 14.95 (*0-9625083-1-4*) Pate Pub.

Patella. Giles R. Scuder. 1995. LC 94-29936. (*3-540-94371-4*); (Illus.). 351p. 132.00 (*0-387-94371-4*) Spr-Verlag.

Patella: A Team Approach. Ronald P. Grelsamer & Jenny McConnell. 1992. LC 97-46654. 273p. 70.00 (*0-8342-0753-2*, 20753) PRO-ED.

Patellofemoral Joint. Ed. by James M. Fox & Wilson Del Pizzo. 1993. LC 92-48244. (Illus.). 416p. text 110.00 (*0-07-021753-X*); VHS 95.00 (*0-07-021752-1*) McGraw-Hill Med Pub.

Patent Law in Biotechnology, Chemicals & Pharmaceuticals. Harold C. Wegner. 1992. 540p. 170.00 (*1-56159-048-7*) Groves Dictionaries.

Patenting of Human Genes & Living Organisms. Vogel F. Vogel. 1996. LC 94-3561. 244p. 66.95 (*0-387-58148-0*) Spr-Verlag.

Paternity—Disputed, Typing, PCR & DNA Tests: Index of New Information. Dexter Z. Franklin. 1998. 160p. 57.50 (*0-7883-1720-2*); pap. 47.50 (*0-7883-1721-0*) ABBE Pubs Assn.

Paternity in Primates: Tests & Theories: Implications of Human DNA Fingerprint. Ed. by R. D. Martin et al. 1991. (Illus.). xii, 288p. 215.75 (*3-8055-5494-X*) S Karger.

Paterson & Zderad: Humanistic Nursing Theory, No. 7. Nancy O'Connor. 1993. (Notes on Nursing Theories Ser.: Vol. 7). (Illus.). 64p. (C). pap. 14.95 (*0-8039-4489-6*, 3070) Sage.

Path. Health Related Profession. Damjano. 1996. 365.00 (*0-7216-6850-X*) Harcourt.

Path of Healing: Finding Your Soul's Potential. H. K. Challoner. 1976. LC 76-3660. 175p. pap. 9.95 (*0-8356-0662-7*, Quest) Theos Pub Hse.

***Path of Practice: A Woman's Book of Ayurvedic Healing.** Maya Tiwari. 2001. 432p. reprint ed. pap. 14.95 (*0-345-43484-6*, Ballantine) Ballantine Pub Grp.

Path of Practice: A Woman's Book of Healing with Food, Breath & Sound. Bri Maya Tiwari. 2000. LC 00-62121. (Illus.). 432p. 24.95 (*0-345-43030-1*, Ballantine) Ballantine Pub Grp.

Path of Pregnancy: A Handbook of Traditional Chinese Gestational & Birthing Disease, Vol. I. Bob Flaws. 1993. LC 92-75136. 235p. pap. 19.95 (*0-936185-39-2*) Blue Poppy Pr.

Path of Pregnancy Vol. II: A Handbook of Traditional Chinese Postpartum Diseases. Bob Flaws. 1993. LC 92-75136. 275p. pap. 19.95 (*0-936185-42-2*) Blue Poppy Pr.

Path of Psychotherapy: Matters of the Heart. David Ira Welch. 1997. LC 97-20314. (Counseling Ser.). 178p. pap. text 34.95 (*0-534-34411-9*) Brooks-Cole.

Path of Tumors of Oral Tissue. Cawson. 5th ed. 1998. (C). text (*0-443-03990-9*) Church.

Path to Mastery in Chiropractic: Seeking Excellence in Practice. James C. Smith. 1994. (Illus.). 450p. (C). pap. text (*0-9637924-5-8*) Chiropract Paradigm.

Path to Payment: The Guide for Effectively Using Your Health Insurance Plan to Save You Money. Fred P. Torres. 1996. 264p. (Orig.). mass mkt. 6.95 (*0-9651278-0-X*) Alverstone Med.

Path to Responsibility: A Comprehensive Therapist Treatment-Intervention Manual for Working with Sex Offenders. G. Richard Kishur. 1994. Vol. Unit 1. 396p. pap. text 39.95 (*1-885473-00-1*) Wood N Barnes.

Path We Tread: Blacks in Nursing Worldwide, 1854-1994. Mary E. Carnegie. 3rd ed. 1995. LC 94-49183. 325p. pap. 36.95 (*0-88737-640-1*) Natl League Nurse.

Path with a Heart: Ericksonian Utilization with Resistant & Chronic Clients. Yvonne M. Dolan. 1993. LC 85-4225. 224p. pap. text 28.95 (*0-87630-718-7*) Brunner-Routledge.

PathLab. Patrick C. Ward. 1994. text 400.00 (*1-56815-025-3*, 10025) Mosby Inc.

Pathlogy Pediatric Tumors. Atayde Perez. 1999. pap. text 195.00 (*0-8385-7802-0*, Medical Exam) Appleton & Lange.

Pathobiochemie: Ein Lehrbuch fur Studierende und Aerzte. Eckhart Buddecke. 2nd ed. 1983. (Illus.). 477p. 52.30 (*3-11-009658-7*) De Gruyter.

Pathobiochemistry, Vol. 5. Andrew H. Kang & Marcel E. Nimmi. rev. ed. 1992. LC 87-20946. (Collagen Ser.: Vol. V). 288p. 146.00 (*0-8493-4605-3*, QP552) Franklin.

Pathobiologie Oraler Strukturen: Zaehne, Pulpa, Parodont. H. E. Schroeder. (Illus.). 2nd rev. ed. 1991. xii, 266p. pap. 40.00 (*3-8055-5268-8*); 3rd ed. 1996. xiv, 256p. pap. 51.50 (*3-8055-6286-1*) S Karger.

Pathobiology & Clinics of Basal Ganglia Disorders. Ed. by P. Riederer & W. Wesemann. 1993. (Journals of Nonprofit & Public Sector Marketing: Suppl. 38). (Illus.). 155p. 72.95 (*0-387-82425-1*) Spr-Verlag.

Pathobiology of Cardiovascular Injury. Ed. by H. Lowell Stone & William B. Weglicki. 1985. (Developments in Cardiovascular Medicine Ser.). text 186.00 (*0-89838-743-4*) Kluwer Academic.

Pathobiology of Human Germ Cell Neoplasia. Ed. by J. W. Oosterhuis et al. 1991. (Recent Results in Cancer Research Ser.: Vol. 123). (Illus.). 192p. 106.00 (*0-387-53928-X*) Spr-Verlag.

Pathobiology of Malignant Melanoma. Ed. by D. E. Elder. 1987. (Pigment Cell Ser.: Vol. 8). (Illus.). viii, 224p. 151.50 (*3-8055-4348-4*) S Karger.

Pathobiology of Marine Mammal Diseases Edwin B. Howard. 1983. Vol. I. 248p. 143.00 (*0-8493-6311-X*, SF997); Vol. II. 240p. 140.00 (*0-8493-6312-8*, SF997) Franklin (CRC Reprint).

Pathobiology of Ocular Disease, Set. Ed. by Garner & Klintworth. 2nd exp. rev. ed. 1994. (Illus.). 1966p. text 250.00 (*0-8247-9136-3*) Dekker.

Pathobiology of Ocular Disease: A Dynamic Approach, Pt. B. Ed. by Garner & Klintworth. 2nd exp. rev. ed. 1994. (Illus.). 1966p. text 250.00 (*0-8247-9137-1*) Dekker.

Pathobiology of Soft Tissue Tumours. C. D. Fletcher & P. H. McKee. 1991. (Current Problems in Tumor Pathology Ser.). (Illus.). 358p. text (*0-443-03790-6*) Church.

Pathobiology of the Human Atherosclerotic Plaque. Ed. by S. Glagov et al. 1989. (Illus.). 923p. 160.00 (*0-387-97130-0*) Spr-Verlag.

Pathogenesis & Host Response in Helicobacter Pylori Infections. Ed. by A. P. Moran & C. A. O'Morain. 1997. pap. 30.00 (*0-926592-19-X*) Normed Verlag.

Pathogenesis & Immunity in Pertussis. Ed. by Alastair C. Wardlaw & Roger Parton. 1988. LC 88-125. 506p. 575.00 (*0-471-91820-2*) Wiley.

Pathogenesis & Risk Factors of Glaucoma. Ed. by E. Gramer & F. Grehn. 1999. LC 00-697747. (Illus.). 256p. 76.00 (*3-540-65912-9*) Spr-Verlag.

Pathogenesis & Treatment of Diabetes Mellitus. J. K. Radder et al. 1986. text 139.00 (*0-89838-828-7*) Kluwer Academic.

Pathogenesis & Treatment of Immunodeficiency. S. H. Horowitz & R. Hong. 1977. (Monographs in Allergy: Vol. 10). 65.25 (*3-8055-2624-5*) S Karger.

Pathogenesis & Treatment of Nephrolithiasis. Ed. by F. Linari et al. 1987. (Contributions to Nephrology Ser.: Vol. 58). x, 298p. 29.75 (*3-8055-4554-1*) S Karger.

Pathogenesis & Treatment of NIDDM & Its Related Problems: Proceedings of the 4th International Symposium on Treatment of Diabetes Melliuts, Nagoya, 23-26 October 1993. Ed. by N. Sakamoto et al. 1994. LC 94-10599. (International Congress Ser.: No. 1057). 532p. 256.25 (*0-444-81712-3*) Elsevier.

Pathogenesis & Treatment of Prostate Obstruction. Ed. by Christopher R. Chapple. 1994. LC 93-17266. (Illus.). 234p. 192.00 (*0-387-19681-1*) Spr-Verlag.

Pathogenesis, Complications & Treatment of Glomerulonephritis. Ed. by Shaul G. Massry & G. A. Cinotti. 1989. (American Journal of Nephrology: Vol. 9, Suppl. 1, 1989). (Illus.). iv, 84p. pap. 26.25 (*3-8055-4908-3*) S Karger.

***Pathogenesis of Alzheimer's Disease.** Jo Van Dorpe. 2001. (Acta Biomedical Lovaniensia Ser.: No. 230). (Illus.). 153p. (*90-5867-126-7*) Leuven Univ BEL. *Dist:* Coronet Bks.

Pathogenesis of Bacterial Infections. Ed. by George G. Jackson & H. Thomas. 1985. (Bayer Symposium Ser.: 8). (Illus.). 431p. 101.00 (*0-387-15304-7*) Spr-Verlag.

Pathogenesis of Functional Bowel Disease. W. J. Snape, Jr. 1989. (Topics in Gastroenterology Ser.). (Illus.). 388p. (C). text 95.00 (*0-306-43265-X*, Kluwer Plenum) Kluwer Academic.

Pathogenesis of Infectious Disease. Ed. by Cedric A. Mims et al. 4th ed. 1995. (Illus.). 414p. text 48.00 (*0-12-498262-X*) Acad Pr.

Pathogenesis of Intestinal Infections: Microbiological & Pathological Principles. M. V. Voino-Yasenetsky & T. Bakacs. 1977. 420p. (C). (*963-05-1131-2*) Akade Kiado HUN. *Dist:* St Mut.

Pathogenesis of Invertebrate Microbial Diseases. Ed. by Elizabeth W. Davidson. 1981. LC 81-65007. 576p. text 68.50 (*0-86598-014-4*) Rowman.

Pathogenesis of Neurodegenerative Disorders. Ed. by Mark P. Mattson. 2001. LC 00-63355. (Contemporary Neuroscience Ser.). (Illus.). x, 294p. 135.00 (*0-89603-838-6*) Humana.

Pathogenic & Therapeutic Aspects of Chronic Renal Failure. Ed. by K. M. Koch & Gunter Stein. 1997. (Illus.). 256p. text 125.00 (*0-8247-9894-5*) Dekker.

Pathogenic Yeasts & Yeast Infections. Segal & Gerald L. Baum. 1994. 256p. lib. bdg. 189.00 (*0-8493-6426-4*) CRC Pr.

Pathogenicity & Clinical Significance of Coagulase-Negative Staphylococci. Ed. by Gerhard Pulverer et al. 1987. (Zentralblatt fur Bakteriologie Ser.: Vol. 16). 290p. lib. bdg. (*0-89574-242-X*) Gustav Fischer DEU. *Dist:* Lubrecht & Cramer, Balogh.

Pathogenicity Islands & Other Mobile Virulence Elements. Ed. by James B. Kaper & Jorg Hacker. 1999. LC 99-24324. (Illus.). 320p. 99.95 (*1-55581-161-2*) ASM Pr.

Pathogenicity of Human Herpesviruses Due to Specific Pathogenicity Genes. Ed. by Yechiel Becker & G. Darai. 1994. LC 93-38678. (Illus.). 387p. 175.00 (*0-387-57127-2*) Spr-Verlag.

Pathogens of Invertebrates: Application in Biological Control & Transmission Mechanisms. Ed. by Thomas C. Cheng. 1984. (Comparative Pathobiology Ser.: Vol. 7). 286p. 79.50 (*0-306-41700-6*, Plenum Trade) Perseus Pubng.

Pathogens, Parasites & Predators of Medically Important Arthropods. D. W. Jenkins. 1964. (WHO Bulletin Supplement Ser.: Vol. 30). pap. text 9.00 (*92-4-168301-5*, 1033001) World Health.

Pathoghomonic Signs. Veerasamy K. Pillay. 2000. 80p. pap. 9.00 (*0-8059-4973-9*) Dorrance.

Pathologic Basis of Disease: A Self-Assessment & Review. Carolyn C. Compton. 4th ed. 1995. 250p. pap. text 23.00 (*0-7216-4041-9*) Saunders.

Pathological Basis Disease. Compton. 5th ed. 1999. pap. text (*0-7216-7857-2*) Saunders.

Pathological Basis of the Connective Tissue Diseases. (*0-340-57219-1*) E A GBR. *Dist:* Routldge.

Pathological Basis of the Connective Tissue Diseases. Dugald L. Gardner. 1992. LC 91-37878. 1050p. 175.00 (*0-8121-1563-5*) Lppncott W & W.

Pathological Cry, Stridor & Cough in Infants: A Clinical Acoustic Study. J. Hirschberg & T. Szende. 1982. 156p. (C). (*963-05-2820-7*) Akade Kiado HUN. *Dist:* St Mut.

Pathological Diagnosis of Acute Ischaemic Heart Disease: Proceedings of the WHO Scientific Group, Geneva, 1969. WHO Staff. 1970. (Technical Reports: No. 441). pap. text 3.00 (*92-4-120441-9*, 1100441) World Health.

Pathological Diagnosis of Vascular Diseases. B. Austin et al. 1999. 400p. 165.00 (*2-287-59660-7*) Spr-Verlag.

Pathological Effects of Oral Contraceptives. P. S. Boffa et al. 1973. LC 72-13565. (Illus.). 220p. (C). text 29.00 (*0-8422-7081-7*) Irvington.

Pathological Lying, Accusation & Swindling, a Study in Forensic Psychology. William Healy & Mary T. Healy. 1969. LC 69-14932. (Criminology, Law Enforcement, & Social Problems Ser.: No. 63). reprint ed. 24.00 (*0-87585-063-4*) Patterson Smith.

Pathological Ocular Conditions. Alan Tunnacliffe. 1989. (C). (*0-89771-746-5*) Assn Brit Dispen Opticians GBR. *Dist:* St Mut.

Pathological Self-Criticism: Assessment & Treatment. Raymond M. Bergner. 1995. (Series in Social/Clinical Psychology). 220p. 39.50 (*0-306-44961-7*, Kluwer Plenum) Kluwer Academic.

Pathologony of Tumours in Laboratory Animals Vol. 1: Tumours of the Rat, Pts. 1 & 2. Ed. by V. S. Turusov. 1987. (IARC Scientific Publications Ser.: Nos. 5 & 6). 533p. 120.00 (*92-832-1410-2*) OUP.

Pathology. L. A. Cree. 1997. (Illus.). 610p. pap. (*0-412-47200-7*) E A GBR. *Dist:* OUP.

Pathology. Ivan Damjanov et al. 1998. LC 98-2713. (Rypins' Intensive Reviews Ser.). 432p. pap. text 21.95 (*0-397-51555-3*) Lppncott W & W.

Pathology. N. K. Hall & D. L. Feeback. 1987. (Oklahoma Notes). (Illus.). 223p. (C). 12.95 (*0-387-96338-3*) Spr-Verlag.

Pathology. Heller & Klein. 1998. 664p. pap. (*0-7506-9584-6*) E A GBR. *Dist:* OUP.

Pathology. Emanuel Rubin et al. 1988. LC 65-8626. (Illus.). 1824p. text 62.50 (*0-397-50698-8*, Lippncott) Lppncott W & W.

Pathology. Arthur S. Schneider & Philip A. Szanto. 1993. LC 92-49705. (Board Review Ser.). (Illus.). 400p. pap. text 26.95 (*0-683-07608-6*) Lppncott W & W.

Pathology. Alan Stevens & James S. Lowe. 2000. LC 00-37254. xv, 652p. (*0-7234-3160-4*) Mosby Inc.

Pathology. Alan Stevens & Jim Lowe. 1994. (*84-8174-135-3*) Mosby-Doyma Libros ESP. *Dist:* Mosby Inc.

Pathology. J. B. Holliman et al. 2nd ed. 1991. 231p. 16.95 (*0-387-96718-4*) Spr-Verlag.

Pathology. Ed. by Virginia A. Livolsi et al. 3rd ed. 1994. LC 93-16371. (National Medical Series for Independent Study). (Illus.). 525p. pap. text 29.00 (*0-683-06243-3*) Lppncott W & W.

Pathology. Emanuel Rubin. 3rd ed. 1998. LC 98-3831. 1,648p. text 77.95 (*0-397-58422-9*) Lppncott W & W.

Pathology. John H. Holliman. 4th rev. ed. 1995. LC 94-47452. (Oklahoma Notes). 279p. 24.95 (*0-387-94390-0*) Spr-Verlag.

Pathology: Basic & Science. Woolf. 1998. pap. text 80.00 (*0-7020-2291-8*) Saunders.

Pathology: Digging up the Bones, Vol. 3. Linas M. Linardakis. 2nd ed. 1997. LC 97-49310. (Digging Up the Bones Ser.). (Illus.). 128p. pap. 19.95 (*0-07-038216-6*) McGraw-Hill Prof.

Pathology: Examination & Board Review. James R. Newland. 2nd ed. 1999. pap. 31.95 (*0-8385-8264-8*, Medical Exam) Appleton & Lange.

***Pathology: Illustrated Review in Color.** Alan Stevens & James Lowe. 2nd ed. 2000. (Illus.). 652p. (C). pap. 45.00 (*0-7234-3200-7*) Mosby Inc.

Pathology: Implications for the Physical Therapists. Catherine C. Goodman & William G. Bossonnault. Ed. by Margaret Biblis. 1997. LC 97-7701. (Illus.). 864p. text 65.00 (*0-7216-5636-6*) Saunders.

Pathology: International Edition. Goljan. 1998. (C). pap. text 17.50 (*0-8089-2061-8*, Grune & Strat) Harcrt Hlth Sci Grp.

Pathology: Pretest Self-Assessment & Review. Margaret H. Clements. 5th ed. 1988. pap. text 15.95 (*0-07-051965-X*) McGraw.

Pathology: Review for New National Boards. Frank N. Miller. 1993. (Illus.). 222p. pap. 25.00 (*0-8036-0714-8*) Davis Co.

Pathology: Review for New National Boards. Frank N. Miller. 1993. LC 93-79828. 222p. pap. text 25.00 (*0-9632873-3-8*) J & S Pub VA.

Pathology: Self-Assessment & Review. Earl J. Brown. 9th ed. 1998. (Pretest Basic Sciences Ser.). (Illus.). 465p. pap. 24.95 (*0-07-052686-9*) McGraw-Hill Educ Grp.

***Pathology: Self-Assessment & Review.** Earl J. Brown. 10th ed. 2001. (Pretest Self-Assessment & Review Ser.). (Illus.). 480p. pap. 24.95 (*0-07-137223-7*) McGraw-Hill Prof.

Pathology No. 2: The Mechanisms of Disease. Roderick A. Cawson et al. 2nd ed. 1989. (Illus.). 592p. (C). (gr. 13). pap. text 49.95 (*0-8016-1246-2*, 01246) Mosby Inc.

Pathology & Genetics of Tumours of the Nervous System. Ed. by P. Kleihues & W. K. Cavanee. 2nd ed. 2000. LC 00-698297. (World Health Organization Classification of Tumours Ser.). (Illus.). 316p. pap. text 75.00 (*92-832-2409-4*) OUP.

Pathology & Gynecology. Fos. 1991. 65.00 (*0-340-54444-9*) Trafalgar.

Pathology & Immunology of Transplantation & Rejection. Sathia Thiru & Herman Waldmann. 4th ed. 2001. LC 99-53903. (Illus.). x, 583p. 250.00 (*0-632-03676-1*) Blackwell Sci.

Pathology & Laboratory Medicine 2000. 2000. (Illus.). 500p. text 79.95 (*0-8151-2496-1*, 31768) Mosby Inc.

Pathology & Microbiology. Sharon S. Rowland. 1994. LC 94-14073. 416p. pap. text, lab manual ed. 33.00 (*0-316-76049-8*, Little Brwn Med Div) Lppncott W & W.

Pathology & Pathobiology of the Urinary Bladder & Prostate. Ronald S. Weinstein & William A. Gardner, Jr. 1992. LC 92-5499. (Monographs in Pathology: No. 34). (Illus.). 221p. 90.00 (*0-683-08911-0*) Lppncott W & W.

Pathology & Physiology of Allergic Reactions. Ed. by P. S. Norman. 1985. (Journal: Vol. 77, No. 1-2). (Illus.). 280p. pap. 101.00 (*3-8055-4056-6*) S Karger.

Pathology & Therapeutics for Pharmacists. Greene & Harris. 1994. (Illus.). 616p. (Orig.). mass mkt. 58.95 (*0-412-61100-7*, Chap & Hall NY) Chapman & Hall.

Pathology & Therapeutics for Pharmacists: A Basis for Clinical Pharmacy Practice. Russell J. Greene & Norman D. Harris. 1993. (Illus.). 736p. mass mkt. 164.95 (*0-412-36000-4*, A7510) Chapman & Hall.

***Pathology & Therapeutics for Pharmacists: A Basis for Clinical Pharmacy Practice.** Greene & Harris. 2nd ed. 2000. 788p. pap. (*0-85369-373-0*) Pharmaceutical Pr GBR. *Dist:* Rittenhouse.

Pathology & Trauma. J. K. Mason. 2nd ed. 1993. 384p. (*0-340-54820-7*) E A GBR. *Dist:* OUP.

Pathology Annual, 1988. Ed. by Paul P. Rosen & Robert E. Fechner. (Illus.). (C). Vol. 23, Pt. 1. 1988. 352p. pap. text 95.00 (*0-8385-7781-4*, A7781-6); Vol. 23, Pt. 2. 1992. 416p. pap. text 95.00 (*0-8385-7789-X*, A7789-9) McGraw (Apple Lange Med).

Pathology Annual, 1989, Vol. 24, Pt. 1. Ed. by Paul P. Rosen & Robert E. Fechner. 1989. (C). 400p. pap. text 95.00 (*0-8385-7733-4*, A7733-7); 2nd ed. 352p. pap. text 95.00 (*0-8385-7713-X*, A7713-9) McGraw (Apple Lange Med).

Pathology Annual, 1990. Paul P. Rosen & Robert E. Fechner. (Illus.). (C). Vol. 25, Pt. 1. 1989. 416p. pap. text 95.00 (*0-8385-7714-8*, A7714-7); Vol. 25, Pt. 2. 1990. 400p. pap. text 95.00 (*0-8385-7814-4*, A7814-5) McGraw (Apple Lange Med).

Pathology Annual, 1994. Paul P. Rosen & Robert E. Fechner. 1994. (C). Vol. 29, Pt. 1. (Illus.). 320p. pap. text 95.00 (*0-8385-7723-7*, A7723-8); Vol. 29, Pt. 2. pap. text 95.00 (*0-8385-7700-8*, A7700-6) McGraw (Apple Lange Med).

***Pathology at a Glance.** N. P. Mapstone. 2001. (At a Glance Ser.). (Illus.). 96p. pap. 19.95 (*0-632-04822-0*) Blackwell Sci.

Pathology for Health Sciences. Vardaxis. 1995. text 66.00 (*0-443-05324-3*) Saunders.

Pathology for Surgeons in Training. David Tweedle. 2nd ed. 1996. (Arnold Publication). (Illus.). 416p. pap. 45.00 (*0-340-60374-7*) OUP.

Pathology for the Health-Related Professions. Ivan Damjanov. 1996. (Illus.). 570p. pap., tchr. ed. (*0-7216-6473-3*) Saunders.

Pathology for the Health Related Professions: Instructor's Manual. Ivan Damjanov. 2nd ed. Date not set. 95p. pap. text, tchr. ed. (*0-7216-8119-0*) Saunders.

Pathology for the Physical Therapist Assistant. Penelope J. Lescher. 2001. (Illus.). 330p. pap. 33.00 (*0-8036-0786-5*) Davis Co.

Pathology for the Surgeon. Peter M. Banks & William G. Kraybill. Ed. by Larry McGrew. 1996. LC 95-11487. 416p. text 77.00 (*0-7216-5288-3*) Saunders.

Pathology Illustrated. Alasdair D. T. Govan et al. 4th ed. 1995. LC 94-20077. (Illus.). (Orig.). pap. text (*0-443-05068-6*) Church.

Pathology Illustrated. Peter S. Macfarlane et al. 5th ed. 2000. LC 99-28979. (Illus.). xi, 684p. (*0-443-05957-8*) Church.

Pathology Illustrated. Peter S. Macfarlane et al. 5th ed. 2000. LC 99-28979. (Illus.). xi, 684p. (*0-443-05956-X*) Harcrt Hlth Sci Grp.

Pathology in a Nutshell. Groysman. 2000. 356p. pap. 24.95 (*0-8385-8175-7*) McGraw-Hill Prof.

Pathology in Dentistry. Edward Sheffield. 1996. (Illus.). 292p. (C). pap. text 59.50 (*0-19-262421-0*) OUP.

Pathology in Gynecology & Obstetrics. Claude Gompel. 4th ed. 1993. 720p. (C). text 189.00 (*0-397-51226-0*) Lppncott W & W.

Pathology in Surgical Practice. Ed. by M. Hobsley et al. 1988. 512p. (*0-683-13033-1*) E A GBR. *Dist:* Williams & Wilkins.

***Pathology in the Urinary Bladder.** Christopher S. Foster & Jeffrey Ross. 2001. (Major Problems in Pathology Ser.). (Illus.). 365p. (*0-7216-9212-5*) Saunders.

Pathology Integrated: An A-Z of Disease & Its Pathologensis. Peter M. Lydyard et al. 2000. (An Arnold Publication). 304p. pap. (*0-340-74063-9*) E A GBR. *Dist:* OUP.

Pathology Medical Transcription: MDT 122. S. Turley. 1993. 142p. (C). stu. ed., ring bd. (*0-933195-53-2*) CA College Health Sci.

Pathology Occupational Lung Disease. Churg. 2nd ed. 1998. 416p. 120.00 (*0-683-30386-4*) Lppncott W & W.

Pathology of Adrenal & Extra-Adrenal Paragaglia. Ernest E. Lack. 1994. LC 93-32870. (Major Problems in Pathology Ser.: Vol. 29). text 79.00 (*0-7216-5263-8*) Saunders.

Pathology of Aging Syrian Hamsters. R. Schmidt & R. Eason. 1983. LC 82-20713. 256p. 145.00 (*0-8493-5099-9*, CRC Reprint) Franklin.

Pathology of AIDS: Textbook & Atlas of Diseases Associated with Acquired Immune Deficiency Syndrome. Harry L. Ioachim. 1989. (Illus.). 200p. (gr. 13). text (*0-397-44556-3*, GM0037) Gower-Mosby.

Pathology of Asbestos-Associated Diseases. Victor L. Roggli et al. 1992. LC 92-13417. 432p. text 199.00 (*0-316-75423-4*, Little Brwn Med Div) Lppncott W & W.

Pathology of Bladder Cancer Ed. by George T. Bryan & Samuel M. Cohen. 1983. Vol. I. 148p. 118.00 (*0-8493-6225-3*, RD755); Vol. II. 256p. 141.00 (*0-8493-6226-1*) Franklin (CRC Reprint).

Pathology of Bone. P. A. Revell. 1985. (Illus.). 302p. 204.00 (*0-387-15418-3*) Spr-Verlag.

Pathology of Bone & Joint Disorders: With Clinical & Radiographic Correlation. Edward F. McCarthy & Frank J. Frassica. Ed. by Alan Ross. 1998. LC 97-27845. (Illus.). 384p. (C). text 95.00 (*0-7216-6336-2*) Saunders.

Pathology of Bone & Joint Neoplasms. Timothy R. Helliwell & Allan Ross. 1998. LC 97-48343. (Major Problems in Pathology Ser.). (Illus.). xvi, 411p. (C). text 75.00 (*0-7216-6439-3*) Saunders.

Pathology of Bone Marrow. Faramarz Naeim. 1992. LC 91-35311. (Illus.). 376p. 175.00 (*0-89640-209-6*) Igaku-Shoin.

Pathology of Bone Marrow. Faramarz Naeim. 2nd ed. 1998. LC 97-42119. 400p. text 199.00 (*0-683-30336-8*) Lppncott W & W.

Pathology of Bone Tumors: Personal Experience. Andre Mazabraud. 1997. LC 97-29696. (Illus.). 567p. 185.00 (*3-540-62751-0*) Spr-Verlag.

Pathology of Congenital Heart Disease: A Personal Experience with More Than 6,300 Congenitally Malformed Hearts Saroja Bharati & Maurice Lev. 1996. (Illus.). 1608p. 395.00 (*0-87993-556-1*) Futura Pub.

Pathology of Devices. Ed. by C. L. Berry. 1994. LC 93-32868. (Current Topics in Pathology Ser.: Vol. 86). (Illus.). 336p. 237.00 (*0-387-54393-7*) Spr-Verlag.

Pathology of Domestic Animals. Ed. by K. V. Jubb et al. 4th ed. LC 92-12261. (Pathology of Domestic Animals Ser.: Vol. 1). (Illus.). 1992. 780p. text 104.00 (*0-12-391605-4*); Vol. 2. 1992. 747p. text 104.00 (*0-12-391606-2*); Vol. 3. 1993. 653p. text 104.00 (*0-12-391607-0*) Acad Pr.

Pathology of Drug Abuse. Steven B. Karch. 1993. 416p. lib. bdg. 80.95 (*0-8493-4418-2*, R); 2nd ed. 1996. LC 96-14757. (Illus.). 480p. 84.95 (*0-8493-9464-3*) CRC Pr.

Pathology of Early Cervical Neoplasia. Christopher P. Crum et al. 1996. LC 96-29476. (Contemporary Issues in Surgical Pathology Ser.). text (*0-443-07590-5*) Church.

Pathology of Eating: Psychology & Treatment. Sara Dulaney Gilbert. 1986. 256p. 37.50 (*0-7102-0271-7*, 02717, Routledge Thoemms) Routledge.

Pathology of Emerging Infections. C. Robert Horsburgh & Ann M. Nelson. 1997. LC 97-13857. (Illus.). 325p. 99.95 (*1-55581-120-5*) ASM Pr.

Pathology of Emerging Infections 2. Ed. by Ann M. Nelson & C. Robert Horsburgh. 1998. LC 98-8770. (Pathology of Emerging Infections Ser.: Vol. 2). (Illus.). 460p. 99.95 (*1-55581-140-X*) ASM Pr.

Pathology of Erythroblastic Mitosis in Occupational Benzenic Erythropathy & Erythremia. E. G. Rondanelli et al. 1969. (Bibliotheca Haematologica Ser.: No. 35). (Illus.). pap. 66.25 (*3-8055-0139-0*) S Karger.

Pathology of Fishes. Ed. by William E. Ribelin & George Migaki. 1975. LC 73-15261. (Illus.). 1016p. 75.00 (*0-299-06520-0*, 652) U of Wis Pr.

Pathology of Genetically Engineered Mice. Ed. by Jerrold Michael Ward et al. 2000. LC 00-38477. (Illus.). xi, 394p. 174.95 (*0-8138-2521-0*) Iowa U Pr.

Pathology of Heart Valve Replacement. A. G. Rose. 1987. text 229.00 (*0-85200-984-4*) Kluwer Academic.

Pathology of Homicide: A Vade Mecum for Pathologist, Prosecutor & Defense Counsel. Lester Adelson. fac. ed. 1974. (Illus.). 992p. 147.95 (*0-398-03000-6*) C C Thomas.

Pathology of Implanted Devices. Nir Kossovsky. 1993. (*0-397-51137-X*) Lppncott W & W.

Pathology of Incipient Neoplasia. Ed. by Donald Henson & Jorge Albores-Saavedra. 2nd ed. 1992. LC 92-11723. (Major Problems in Pathology Ser.: Vol. 28). (Illus.). 590p. text 99.00 (*0-7216-6457-1*) Saunders.

Pathology of Incipient Neoplasia. Ed. by Donald Earl Henson & Jorge Albores-Saavedra. 3rd ed. 2000. LC 99-52562. (Illus.). 856p. text 165.00 (*0-19-512338-7*) OUP.

Pathology of Limb Ischaema. Henry Dible. 1967. LC 67-27239. (Illus.). 110p. 9.00 (*0-87527-030-1*) Green.

Pathology of Lymph Nodes. Lawrence M. Weiss. 1996. LC 96-19840. (Contemporary Issues in Surgical Pathology Ser.). text (*0-443-07620-0*) Church.

Pathology of Melanocytic Nevi & Malignant Melanoma of the Skin. Raymond L. Barnhill. 1994. LC 94-33338. (Illus.). 312p. (*0-7506-9504-8*) E A GBR. *Dist:* OUP.

Pathology of Multiple Pregnancy. Virginia J. Baldwin. 1993. LC 92-48343. (Illus.). 400p. 225.00 (*0-387-94011-1*) Spr-Verlag.

Pathology of Neonatal Intensive Care: An Illustrated Reference. Derek J. Desa. 1994. (Illus.). 224p. (C). (gr. 13). 322.95 (*0-412-43490-3*, Chap & Hall NY) Chapman & Hall.

Pathology of Neoplasia in Children & Adolescents. Ed. by Milton Finegold. 1986. (Major Problems in Pathology Ser.). (Illus.). 481p. text 104.00 (*0-7216-1337-3*) Saunders.

Pathology of Neoplastic & Endocrine Induced Diseases of the Breast. R. Bassler & Hubner. 1987. 484p. (*0-89574-232-2*) Gustav Fischer DEU. *Dist:* Lubrecht & Cramer, Balogh.

Pathology of Occupational Lung Disease. Andrew M. Churg. 1988. LC 87-3296. (Illus.). 416p. 98.50 (*0-89640-121-9*) Igaku-Shoin.

Pathology of Occupational Lung Disease. Andrew Churg & Francis H. Green. 2nd ed. 1998. LC 97-33344. (*0-683-30342-2*) Lppncott W & W.

Pathology of Organ Transplantation. George E. Sale. 1990. (Illus.). 327p. pap. text (*0-409-90133-4*) E A GBR. *Dist:* OUP.

Pathology of Periodontal Disease. David M. Williams et al. 1992. (Illus.). 158p. text 75.00 (*0-19-261955-1*); pap. text 45.00 (*0-19-262120-3*) OUP.

Pathology of Pseudoneoplastic Lesions. Mark R. Wick et al. 1997. LC 96-43036. 704p. text 199.00 (*0-7817-0302-6*) Lppncott W & W.

Pathology of Pulmonary Disease. Saldana. 1993. 984p. (C). text 299.00 (*0-397-51257-0*) Lppncott W & W.

Pathology of Radiation Injury. Luis Felipe Fajardo. 1982. (C). (gr. 13). 87.00 (*0-89352-182-5*) Mosby Inc.

Pathology of Skeletal Muscle. Stirling Carpenter & George Karpati. 2nd ed. 2000. LC 99-45758. (Illus.). 704p. text 195.00 (*0-19-506364-3*) OUP.

Pathology of Solid Tumours in Children. Ed. by Stoker & Frederic B. Askin. 1997. LC 98-118515. 304p. (*0-412-40170-3*) E A GBR. *Dist:* OUP.

Pathology of the Aging Human Nervous System. Serge Duckett. 1991. LC 90-6638. (Illus.). 505p. text 99.00 (*0-8121-1355-1*) Lppncott W & W.

Pathology of the Appendix & Its Surgical Treatment. Richard A. Williams & Paul Myers. 1994. LC 93-32951. 192p. (gr. 13). pap. 150.95 (*0-412-54810-0*, Chap & Hall NY) Chapman & Hall.

Pathology of the Bone Marrow. Ed. by K. Lennert & K. Hubner. 1984. (Illus.). 426p. lib. bdg. (*0-89574-195-4*) Gustav Fischer DEU. *Dist:* Lubrecht & Cramer, Balogh.

Pathology of the Breast. Paul P. Rosen. 1996. LC 96-6385. 928p. text 299.00 (*0-397-51694-0*) Lppncott W & W.

Pathology of the Breast. Silverberg. 1997. text (*0-7216-5059-7*) Saunders.

Pathology of the Breast. Fatteneh A. Tavassoli. 2nd ed. 1999. LC 98-50680. (Illus.). 669p. text 250.00 (*0-8385-7704-0*) McGraw-Hill Prof.

Pathology of the Carotid Body & Sinus. D. Heath & P. Smith. 1988. 132p. (*0-683-13035-8*) E A GBR. *Dist:* Williams & Wilkins.

Pathology of the Colon, Small Intestine & Anus. Ed. by H. Thomas Norris. 2nd ed. 1991. (Contemporary Issues in Surgical Pathology Ser.: Vol. 17). (Illus.). 414p. text (*0-443-08729-6*) Church.

Pathology of the Ear. Harold F. Schuknecht. 2nd ed. 1993. LC 92-49497. (Illus.). 672p. text 155.00 (*0-8121-1562-7*) Lppncott W & W.

Pathology of the Ear & Temporal Bone. George T. Nager. 1993. LC 93-27739. (Illus.). 1408p. 295.00 (*0-683-63049-0*) Lppncott W & W.

Pathology of the Esophagus. H. T. Enterline & J. J. Thompson. 1984. (Illus.). 225p. 150.00 (*0-387-90896-X*) Spr-Verlag.

Pathology of the Eye. Gottfried O. Naumann & D. J. Apple. 1986. (Illus.). 998p. 533.00 (*0-387-96044-9*) Spr-Verlag.

Pathology of the Fischer Rat: Reference & Atlas. Ed. by Gary A. Boorman et al. 1990. 580p. text 167.00 (*0-12-115640-0*) Acad Pr.

Pathology of the Gallbladder, Biliary Tract & Pancreas. David A. Owen & James Kelly. 1998. LC 00-63498. (Illus.). x, 365p. text 79.00 (*0-7216-1910-X*) Saunders.

Pathology of the Gastro-Intestinal Tract. Ed. by Si-Chun Ming & Harvey Goldman. 1991. (Illus.). 975p. text 250.00 (*0-7216-6398-2*) Saunders.

Pathology of the Gastrointestinal Tract. Si-Chun Ming & Harvey Goldman. 2nd ed. 1997. LC 97-22939. 1,020p. text 299.00 (*0-683-18007-X*) Lppncott W & W.

Pathology of the Head & Neck. Armed Forces Institute of Pathology Staff. 1992. (C). 700.00 incl. disk (*1-56815-011-3*) Mosby Inc.

Pathology of the Head & Neck: With Clinical Correlations. Yao Shi Fu et al. 1998. LC 00-64377. (Illus.). 912p. text (*0-443-07558-1*) Church.

Pathology of the Human Embryo & Previable Fetus. Dagmar K. Kalousek. 1990. (Illus.). 241p. 156.00 (*0-387-97168-8*) Spr-Verlag.

Pathology of the Human Placenta. Kurt Benirschke & Peter Kaufmann. 4th ed. 2000. LC 99-32440. (Illus.). 968p. 189.00 (*0-387-98894-7*) Spr-Verlag.

Pathology of the Kidney Robert H. Heptinstall. 3rd ed. 1983. 225.00 (*0-316-35797-9*, Little Brwn Med Div) Lppncott W & W.

Pathology of the Liver. Ed. by Robert MacSween et al. 2nd ed. 1987. (Illus.). 717p. (*0-443-03049-9*) Church.

Pathology of the Liver. Ed. by Roderick N. MacSween et al. 3rd ed. 1994. LC 94-33377. text (*0-443-04454-6*) Church.

***Pathology of the Liver.** R. N. MacSween et al. 4th ed. 2001. (Illus.). 895p. (*0-443-06181-5*) Church GBR. *Dist:* Saunders.

Pathology of the Lung. Ed. by G. G. Pietra. 1987. (Journal: Vol. 4, No. 3, 1986). (Illus.). 96p. pap. 40.00 (*3-8055-4573-8*) S Karger.

Pathology of the Lung. Ed. by William M. Thurlbeck & Andrew M. Churg. 2nd ed. 1996. (Illus.). 1178p. 219.00 (*0-86577-534-6*) Thieme Med Pubs.

Pathology of the Mesothelium. Ed. by J. S. Jones. 1987. (Illus.). 268p. 167.00 (*0-387-16208-9*) Spr-Verlag.

Pathology of the Pancreas. A. H. Cruickshank & E. W. Benbow. 2nd ed. 1995. LC 95-33. (Illus.). 341p. 155.00 (*3-540-19923-3*) Spr-Verlag.

Pathology of the Parathyroid & Thyroid Glands. Ed. by Virginia A. Livolsi & Ronald A. DeLellis. 1993. LC 92-48313. (Monographs in Pathology: No. 35). (Illus.). 203p. 90.00 (*0-683-04817-1*) Lppncott W & W.

Pathology of the Peripheral Nerve. Edward P. Richardson, Jr. & Umberto DeGirolami. 1994. LC 94-20440. (Major Problems in Pathology Ser.: No. 32). 176p. text 64.00 (*0-7216-3298-X*) Saunders.

Pathology of the Placenta. Steven H. Lewis & Eugene Perrin. 2nd ed. 1998. LC 98-23008. (Contemporary Issues in Surgical Pathology Ser.: Vol. 23). (Illus.). 432p. (C). text (*0-443-07586-7*) Church.

Pathology of the Placenta MPP. Fox. 2nd ed. 1997. text (*0-7020-2196-2*) Bailliere Tindall.

Pathology of the Prostate. Christopher S. Foster & David G. Bostwick. Ed. by Lesley Day. 1997. LC 96-23370. (Major Problems in Pathology Ser.: Vol. 34). (Illus.). 464p. text 95.00 (*0-7216-6951-4*) Saunders.

Pathology of the Skin. Phillip H. McKee. 2nd ed. 1996. (*1-56375-588-2*) Gower-Mosby.

Pathology of the Skin. Evan R. Farmer. 2nd rev. ed. 1999. LC 98-18993. (Illus.). 987p. (C). text 225.00 (*0-8385-8079-3*) McGraw-Hill Prof.

Pathology of the Skin Atlas. Hurwitz & Hood. 1997. LC 97-37911. 535p. (C). text 199.00 (*0-8385-7689-3*, A-7689-1) McGraw-Hill Prof.

Pathology of the Syrian Hamster. Ed. by F. Homburger. 1972. (Progress in Experimental Tumor Research Ser.: Vol. 16). 163.50 (*3-8055-1367-4*) S Karger.

Pathology of the Testes. Reuter. 1997. text (*0-7216-4977-7*) Harcourt.

Pathology of the Thymus & Mediastinum. Michael J. Kornstein. 1995. LC 94-19417. (Illus.). 256p. text 68.00 (*0-7216-4337-X*) Saunders.

Pathology of the Thyroid. Virginia A. Livolsi. 2nd ed. 2002. text (*0-7216-6324-9*) Harcourt.

Pathology of the Thyroid MPP. Virginia A. Livolsi. 1990. (Illus.). 448p. text 92.00 (*0-7216-5782-6*) Saunders.

Pathology of the Urinary Bladder. Robert H. Young. 1989. (Contemporary Issues in Surgical Pathology Ser.: Vol. 13). (Illus.). 413p. text (*0-443-08603-6*) Church.

Pathology of the Vessel Wall: A Modern Appraisal. Ed. by Neville Woolf. 1983. 359p. 78.75 (*0-275-91419-4*, C1419, Praeger Pubs) Greenwood.

Pathology of Trauma. Ed. by Ken Mason & Basil Purdue. 3rd ed. 2000. LC 99-16933. (Illus.). 576p. text (*0-340-69189-1*) E A GBR. *Dist:* OUP.

Pathology of Tropical & Extraordinary Diseases 1994. lib. bdg. 750.95 (*0-8490-5629-2*) Gordon Pr.

Pathology of Tuberculosis in Old Age. L. Haranghy & C. Szemenyei. 1974. 210p. (C). (*963-05-0005-1*) Akade Kiado HUN. *Dist:* St Mut.

Pathology of Tumours in Laboratory Animals: Tumours of the Hamster, Vol. 3. Ed. by V. S.. Turusov & Ulrich Mohr. 2nd ed. 1996. LC 97-109979. (IARC Scientific Publications Ser.: No. 126). (Illus.). 496p. text 124.00 (*92-832-2126-5*) OUP.

Pathology of Tumours of the Nervous System. 5th ed. (*0-340-50905-8*) E A GBR. *Dist:* Routldge.

Pathology of Tumours of the Nervous System. Russell & Rubinstein. 5th ed. 1989. 974p. 249.00 (*0-683-07462-8*) Lppncott W & W.

Pathology of Viral Hepatitis. R. D. Goldin et al. 1998. LC 98-7631. (Arnold Publication). (Illus.). 192p. 125.00 (*0-340-59664-3*) OUP.

***Pathology of Viral Neuropathies in the Temporal Bone,** Vol.60. Ed. by R. R. Gacek & M. R. Gacek. 2001. (Advances in Oto-rhino-laryngology Ser.). (Illus.). 150p. 130.50 (*3-8055-7295-6*) S Karger.

Pathology of Zoo Animals: A Review of Necropsies Conducted over a Fourteen Year Period at the San Diego Zoo. Lynn A. Griner. 1983. LC 82-62698. (Illus.). 25.00 (*0-911461-11-6*) Zoological Soc.

Pathology Office Assistant. Jack Rudman. 1994. (Career Examination Ser.: C-3400). pap. 27.95 (*0-8373-3400-4*) Nat Learn.

Pathology Picture Tests. Alan Stevens & Jim Lowe. 1995. (C). (gr. 13). (*0-7234-2192-7*) Wolfe Publishing GBR. *Dist:* Mosby Inc.

Pathology Review. Goljan. 1998. (C). pap. text 13.50 (*0-8089-2062-6*, Grune & Strat) Harcrt Hlth Sci Grp.

Pathology Review. Ashraf M. Hassanein & Barbara F. Atkins. 1997. LC 97-33791. (USMLE Step 1 Review Ser.). 336p. pap. 39.95 (*0-7619-0517-0*, 80544) Sage.

Pathology Reviews - 1989. Ed. by Emanuel Rubin & Ivan Damjanov. 1989. (Illus.). 307p. 120.00 (*0-89603-162-4*) Humana.

Pathology Reviews - 1990. Ed. by Emanuel Rubin & Ivan Damjanov. 1990. (Illus.). 268p. 120.00 (*0-89603-195-0*) Humana.

Pathomechanism & Prevention of Sudden Cardiac Death Due to Coronary Insufficiency. Ed. by L. Szekeres et al. 1984. 319p. (C). (*963-05-3658-7*) Akade Kiado HUN. *Dist:* St Mut.

Pathophys Biological/Behaviora. Lee-Ellen C. Copstead & Jacquelyn L. Banasik. Ed. by Robin Carter. 2nd ed. 1999. LC 98-53145. (Illus.). xxi, 1337p. text 66.00 (*0-7216-7178-0*) Saunders.

Pathophysiologic Basis of Nuclear Medicine. Abdelhamid H. Elgazzar. 2001. LC 00-61892. (Illus.). 400p. 179.00 (*3-540-65914-5*) Spr-Verlag.

Pathophysiologic, Diagnostic & Therapeutic Aspects of Headache. Ed. by Mary E. Granger et al. 1976. (Pain & Headache Ser.: Vol. 4). 135p. 54.00 (*3-8055-2282-7*) S Karger.

Pathophysiologic Foundations of Critical Care. Michael R. Pinsky & Jean-Francois A. Dhainaut. 1993. LC 92-15867. (Illus.). 1008p. 125.00 (*0-683-06888-1*) Lppncott W & W.

Pathophysiological Aspects of Cancer Epidemiology. Ed. by G. Mathe & P. Reizenstein. 1985. (Advances in the Biosciences Ser.: No. 50). (Illus.). 276p. 83.50 (*0-08-030780-9*, Pergamon Pr) Elsevier.

Pathophysiological Phenomena in Nursing: Human Responses to Illness. Carrieri et al. 2nd ed. 1993. (Illus.). 622p. (C). text 79.00 (*0-7216-3494-X*) Saunders.

Pathophysiological Principles of Urology. Grannum R. Sant. 1993. LC 93-42937. 544p. pap. 55.00 (*0-86542-221-4*) Blackwell Sci.

Pathophysiological Problems in Clinical Nephrology: Proceedings of the Heidelberg Seminars in Nephrology, Heidelberg, September, 1978. Heidelberg Seminars in Nephrology Staff. Ed. by Eberhard Ritz et al. 1978. (Contributions to Nephrology Ser.: Vol. 14). (Illus.). 29.75 (*3-8055-2910-4*) S Karger.

Pathophysiologie. 5th ed. 1991. text 29.95 (*3-540-17831-7*) Spr-Verlag.

Pathophysiology. Chowdry. 1993. 53.75 (*0-697-09850-8*) McGraw.

Pathophysiology. Nowak. 1994. tchr. ed. 14.06 (*0-697-17438-7*) McGraw.

Pathophysiology. Catherine Paradiso. 2nd ed. 1999. LC 99-11784. (Lippincott's Review Ser.). 528p. pap. text 24.95 (*0-7817-1843-0*) Lppncott W & W.

Pathophysiology: A Physiological Approach. Kathryn L. McCance. 2nd ed. 1993. 1696p. (C). (gr. 13). text, tchr. ed. 34.00 (*0-8151-5749-5*, 24200) Mosby Inc.

Pathophysiology: A Self-Instructional Program. Mary Burns. 1998. LC 97-41936. 768p. (C). pap. 52.00 (*0-8385-8084-X*) P-H.

Pathophysiology: An Introduction to Mechanisms of Disease. Bernice L. Muir. 2nd ed. 1989. LC 87-25298. 685p. text 44.00 (*0-8273-4317-5*) Delmar.

Pathophysiology: Application to Clinical Practice. Maureen Groer. 2000. LC 00-38467. 512p. pap. text 49.95 (*0-7817-2336-1*) Lppncott W & W.

Pathophysiology: Biological & Behavioral Perspectives: Instructor's Manual. Jacquelyn L. Banasik. 2nd ed. Date not set. (Illus.). 335p. tchr. ed. (*0-7216-7179-9*) Saunders.

Pathophysiology: Biological & Behavioral: Study Guide for Copstead/Banasik. Lee-Ellen C. Copstead & Jacquelyn L. Banasik. 2nd ed. 1999. (Illus.). 350p. text, stu. ed. (*0-7216-7183-7*) Saunders.

Pathophysiology: Clinical Concepts of Disease Processes. Sylvia A. Price & Lorraine M. Wilson. 5th ed. (Illus.). tchr. ed. (*0-8151-2543-7*) Mosby Inc.

Pathophysiology: Clinical Concepts of Disease Processes. Sylvia Anderson Price. Ed. by Lorraine McCarty Wilson. 5th ed. 1996. LC 96-15023. (Illus.). 1232p. (C). (gr. 13). text 66.00 (*0-8151-6621-4*, 24418) Mosby Inc.

Pathophysiology: Concepts of Altered Health States. Carol M. Porth. 5th ed. 1998. LC 97-49116. 1,440p. text 68.95 (*0-397-55413-3*) Lppncott W & W.

Pathophysiology: Foundations of Disease & Clinical Intervention. Margie Hansen. Ed. by Barbara N. Cullen. 1998. LC 96-38014. (Illus.). 1152p. text 61.95 (*0-7216-4465-1*) Saunders.

***Pathophysiology: Foundations of Disease & Clinical Intervention - ExaMaster.** Margie Hansen. 1998. (*0-7216-7983-8*) Saunders.

***Pathophysiology: Foundations of Disease & Clinical Intervention - Test Manual.** Margie Hansen. 1998. (*0-7216-7982-X*) Saunders.

Pathophysiology: PreTest Self-Assessment & Review. Ed. by Maurice A. Mufson. 1998. LC 98-36684. (Pretest Basic Sciences Ser.). (Illus.). 250p. pap. 24.95 (*0-07-052692-3*) McGraw-Hill Educ Grp.

Pathophysiology: Principles of Disease. Martha J. Miller. 1983. (Illus.). 506p. tchr. ed. (*0-7216-2029-9*); 528p. 62.95 (*0-7216-6337-0*) Saunders.

***Pathophysiology: Self-Assessment & Review.** Maurice A. Mufson. 2nd ed. 2001. LC 2001-31230. (Pretest Self-Assessment & Review Ser.). (Illus.). 200p. pap. 24.95 (*0-07-137507-4*) McGraw-Hill Prof.

Pathophysiology: The Biological Basis for Disease in Adults & Children. Kathryn L. McCance & Sue E. Huether. 3rd ed. (Illus.). 1997. LC 97-22899. 1728p. (C). (gr. 13). text 66.00 (*0-8151-9481-1*, 29322); Includes Testbank. 1998. tchr. ed. (*1-55664-433-7*) Mosby Inc.

Pathophysiology & Pharmacology of Capillary Resistance. M. Gabor. 1974. 236p. (C). (*963-05-0238-0*) Akade Kiado HUN. *Dist:* St Mut.

Pathophysiology & Pharmacology of Erythropoietin. Ed. by Horst Pagel et al. 1992. LC 92-2312. (Illus.). 328p. 100.00 (*0-387-54777-0*) Spr-Verlag.

Pathophysiology & Pharmacology of Heart Disease: Proceedings of the Symposium Held at Chandigarh, India, Feb. 1988. Ed. by Inder S. Anand et al. 1989. (Developments in Cardiovascular Medicine Ser.). (C). text 131.50 (*0-7923-0367-9*) Kluwer Academic.

Pathophysiology & Rational Pharamacotherapy of Myocardial Ischemia. Ed. by G. Heusch. 1990. 300p. 66.00 (*0-387-91360-2*) Spr-Verlag.

Pathophysiology & Treatment of Inhalation Injuries. Ed. by Jacob Loke. 1987. (Lung Biology in Health & Disease Ser.: Vol. 34). (Illus.). 576p. text 250.00 (*0-8247-7795-6*) Dekker.

Pathophysiology & Treatment of Paget's Disease of Bone. John A. Kanis. 1991. LC 90-86388. (Illus.). 320p. lib. bdg. 110.00 (*0-89089-447-7*) Carolina Acad Pr.

Pathophysiology for the Boards & Wards: A Review of the USMLE Step 1. Carlos Ayala & Brad Spellberg. 3rd ed. 2000. LC 99-49378. (Boards & Wards Ser.). (Illus.). 305p. pap. 28.95 (*0-632-04485-3*) Blackwell Sci.

Pathophysiology for the Emt. Myers et al. 2002. LC 2001-47339. 480p. (C). text 31.95 (*0-7668-2548-5*) Delmar.

Pathophysiology for the Health-Related Professions. Barbara Gould. 1997. (Illus.). 493p. pap., tchr. ed. (*0-7216-7184-5*) Saunders.

Pathophysiology for the Health-Related Professions: Health Related Problems. Barbara Gould. Ed. by Selma Kaszczuk. 1997. LC 96-42341. (Illus.). 416p. pap. text 44.95 (*0-7216-5954-3*) Saunders.

Pathophysiology Made Incredibly Easy. Springhouse Publishing Company Staff. 1998. LC 97-46681. (Made Incredibly Easy Ser.). (Illus.). 408p. pap. 34.95 (*0-87434-935-4*) Springhouse Corp.

Pathophysiology of Blood Disorders. Ed. by Ch. Hershko & G. Izak. 1979. (Illus.). pap. 57.50 (*3-8055-3021-8*) S Karger.

***Pathophysiology of Calcification of Bioprosthetic Heart Valves: An Experimental Investigation.** Shigeyuki Ozaki. 2001. (Acta Biomedica Lovaniensia Ser.: No. 238). (Illus.). 116p. pap. (*90-5867-142-9*) Leuven Univ BEL. *Dist:* Coronet Bks.

Pathophysiology of Development & Rupture of Cerebral Aneurysms. H. J. Steiger. 1990. (Acta Neurochirurgica Ser.: Suppl. 48). 100p. 61.95 (*0-387-82192-9*) Spr-Verlag.

Pathophysiology of Disease: An Introduction to Clinical Medicine. Stephen J. McPhee & Ganong. 2nd ed. 1997. 624p. (C). pap. text 36.95 (*0-8385-7678-8*, A-7678-4, Apple Lange Med) McGraw.

Pathophysiology of Disease: An Introduction to Clinical Medicine. Stephen J. McPhee. 3rd ed. 1999. (Illus.). 662p. (C). pap. 44.95 (*0-8385-8160-9*) McGraw-Hill Prof.

Pathophysiology of Head & Neck Musculoskeletal Disorders. Ed. by D. B. Ferguson. 1990. (Frontiers of Oral Physiology Ser.: Vol. 7). (Illus.). viii, 180p. 208.75 (*3-8055-5123-1*) S Karger.

Pathophysiology of Heart Disease. Ed. by R. E. Beamish et al. 1987. (Developments in Cardiovascular Medicine Ser.). text 161.50 (*0-89838-864-3*) Kluwer Academic.

Pathophysiology of Heart Disease. Leonard Lilly. 1992. (Illus.). 300p. pap. 26.00 (*0-8121-1566-X*) Lppncott W & W.

Pathophysiology of Heart Disease: A Collaborative Project of Medical Students & Faculty. Harvard Medical School Staff. Ed. by Leonard S. Lilly. 2nd ed. 1997. LC 97-25006. 401p. pap. 34.95 (*0-683-30220-5*) Lppncott W & W.

Pathophysiology of Heart Failure. Ed. by Naranjan S. Dhalla et al. 1996. (Developments in Cardiovascular Medicine Ser.: No. DICM 168). 624p. (C). text 272.50 (*0-7923-3571-6*) Kluwer Academic.

Pathophysiology of Hypertension. A. Zanchetti & G. Mancia. 1996. LC 97-132210. (Handbooks of Hypertension: Vol. 17). 1122p. 315.00 (*0-444-82551-7*) Elsevier.

Pathophysiology of Hypertension. Alberto Zanchetti & Giuseppe Mancia. 1997. LC 97-132210. (Handbooks of Hypertension). xix, 1102p. (*0-444-90341-0*) Elsevier.

Pathophysiology of Hypertension in Blacks. John C. S. Fray & Janice G. Douglas. 1992. (Clinical Physiology Ser.). (Illus.). 320p. text 89.00 (*0-19-506720-7*) OUP.

Pathophysiology of Infantile Malnutrition: Protein Energy Malnutrition & Failure to Thrive. E. Kerpel-Fronius. 1983. 312p. (C). (*963-05-3222-0*) Akade Kiado HUN. *Dist:* St Mut.

Pathophysiology of Lipid Peroxides & Related Free Radicals: International Symposium on Physiology of Lipid Peroxides & Related Free Radicals, Inuyama, November 1996. Kunio Yagi. 1998. LC 98-145628. (Illus.). x, 182p. 173.25 (*3-8055-6590-9*) S Karger.

Pathophysiology of Lysosomel Transport. Bodie Thoene. 1992. 368p. 249.00 (*0-8493-6724-7*, RC632) CRC Pr.

Pathophysiology of Melanocytes: Proceedings of the International Pigment Cell Conference, 10th, Cambridge, Mass., October, 1977, Pt. 2. International Pigment Cell Conference Staff. Ed. by S. N. Klaus. 1979. (Pigment Cell Ser.: Vol. 5). (Illus.). 121.00 (*3-8055-2973-2*) S Karger.

Pathophysiology of Parasitic Infections. L. E. Symons. 1989. 300p. text 90.00 (*0-12-680125-8*) Acad Pr.

Pathophysiology of Plasma Protein Metabolism. Ed. by Giulian Mariant. 1985. 416p. 115.00 (*0-306-41771-5*, Plenum Trade) Perseus Pubng.

Pathophysiology of Pneumoperitoneum. Ed. by Raul J. Rosenthal et al. 1997. LC 97-20208. (Illus.). 187p. 102.00 (*3-540-63015-5*) Spr-Verlag.

Pathophysiology of Puberty. Ed. by E. Cacciari & A. Prader. 1981. LC 80-40928. (Serono Symposia Ser.: No. 36). text 167.00 (*0-12-154160-6*) Acad Pr.

Pathophysiology of Renal Disease. 1980. (Contributions to Nephrology Ser.: Vol. 23). (Illus.). vi, 234p. pap. 29.75 (*3-8055-0943-X*) S Karger.

Pathophysiology of Renal Disease. Shaul G. Massry & Eberhard Ritz. 1982. (Contributions to Nephrology Ser.: Vol. 33). (Illus.). viii, 276p. pap. 29.75 (*3-8055-3534-1*) S Karger.

Pathophysiology of Renal Disease. Burton D. Rose. 2nd ed. 1987. LC 86-33710. (Illus.). 623p. pap. 44.95 (*0-07-053629-5*) McGraw-Hill Prof.

Pathophysiology of Reperfusion Injury. DAS Staff. 1992. 528p. 219.00 (*0-8493-4555-3*, RB144) CRC Pr.

Pathophysiology of Severe Ischemic Myocardial Injury. Ed. by Hans M. Piper. 1990. 440p. text 294.00 (*0-7923-0459-4*) Kluwer Academic.

Pathophysiology of Shock, Sepsis, & Organ Failure. Ed. by Gunther O. Schlag & H. Redl. 1993. LC 93-10875. 1184p. 317.00 (*0-387-54223-X*) Spr-Verlag.

Pathophysiology of Splanchnic Circulation. Kvietys & Granger. 1987. Vol. I. 184p. 107.00 (*0-8493-4662-2*); Vol. II. 152p. 93.00 (*0-8493-4663-0*) Franklin (CRC Reprint).

Pathophysiology of Tachycardia-Induced Heart Failure. Ed. by Francis G. Spinale. 1996. LC 96-23241. (American Heart Association Monographs). (Illus.). 248p. 48.00 (*0-87993-649-5*) Futura Pub.

Pathophysiology of the Eye No. 1: The Preocular Tear Film. Feher Janos. 1993. (Pathophysiology of the Eye Ser.: No. 1). 142p. pap. (*963-05-6515-3*) Akade Kiado HUN. *Dist:* Intl Spec Bk, St Mut.

Pathophysiology of the Gut & Airways. P. L. Andrews & J. G. Widdicombe. 1993. 150p. (*1-85578-022-4*) Portland Pr Ltd GBR. *Dist:* Ashgate Pub Co.

Pathophysiology of the Microcirculation. Nicholas A. Mortillaro. 1994. 305p. lib. bdg. 239.00 (*0-8493-4547-2*, RC700) CRC Pr.

Pathophysiology of the Motor Systems: Principles & Clinical Presentations. Christopher M. Fredericks & Lisa K. Saladin. 1996. LC 95-37900. (Illus.). 594p. (C). text 44.95 (*0-8036-0093-3*) Davis Co.

Pathophysiology of the Nervous System. Lewis Sudarsky. 1990. 35.95 (*0-316-82117-9*, Little Brwn Med Div) Lppncott W & W.

Pathophysiology of the Visual System. Ed. by L. Maffei. 1981. (Documenta Ophthalmologica Proceedings Ser.: No. 30). 304p. text 171.00 (*90-6193-726-4*) Kluwer Academic.

Pathoschematics: From Disease to Nursing. Cook. 1992. (Education Ser.). pap. 19.95 (*0-8273-4415-5*) Delmar.

Paths Beyond Ego: The Transpersonal Vision. Ed. by Roger Walsh & Frances Vaughan. 1993. LC 93-6705. 288p. 15.95 (*0-87477-678-3*, Tarcher Putnam) Putnam Pub Group.

Paths to Asian Medical Knowledge. Ed. by Charles M. Leslie & Allan H. Young. 1992. LC 91-796. (Comparative Studies of Health Systems & Medical Care: Vol. 32). 296p. (C). text 50.00 (*0-520-07317-7*); pap. text 19.95 (*0-520-07318-5*) U CA Pr.

Paths to Asian Medical Knowledge. Ed. by Charles Leslie & Allan Young. 1993. 306p. (*81-215-0608-5*) M Manoharial IND. *Dist:* Coronet Bks.

Paths to Knowledge. Ed. by Barbara Sarter. 1988. 246p. pap. 16.50 (*0-88737-415-8*, 15-2233) Natl League Nurse.

Paths to Knowledge of Higher Worlds. Rudolf Steiner. 3rd ed. 1980. (GER.). 36p. reprint ed. pap. (*0-919924-13-1*) Steiner Book Centre CAN. *Dist:* Anthroposophic.

Paths to Mobility Checklist: Objectives for Teaching Gross Motor Skills to "Special Care" Children. John L. Presland. 1985. 20p. 35.00 (*0-906054-48-6*) St Mut.

Paths to Mobility in "Special Care" A Guide to Teaching Gross Motor Skills to Very Handicapped Children. John L. Presland. 1985. 59.00 (*0-906054-33-8*); pap. 39.00 (*0-906054-28-1*) St Mut.

Pathway for Oxygen. Ewald R. Weibel. 1984. (Illus.). 448p. 57.50 (*0-674-65791-8*); pap. 29.50 (*0-674-65790-X*) HUP.

Pathway for Patients & Families Facing Terminal Illness. 1997. 46p. pap. 11.85 (*0-931207-51-7*) Natl Hospice.

Pathways: From the Culture of Addiction to the Culture of Recovery: A Travel Guide for Addiction Professionals. William L. White. 2nd rev. ed. 1996. LC 96-2446. Orig. Title: The Culture of Addiction. 560p. 29.95 (*1-56838-123-9*) Hazelden.

Pathways: Moving Beyond Stroke & Aphasia. Susan A. Ewing & Beth Pfalzgraf. 1990. LC 90-12148. (William Beaumont Hospital Speech & Language Pathology Ser.). (Illus.). 198p. (C). pap. text 21.95 (*0-8143-2075-9*) Wayne St U Pr.

Pathways for Minorities into the Health Professions. Pedro J. Lecca & Thomas D. Watts. 1989. 98p. 39.00 (*0-8191-7552-8*) U Pr of Amer.

Pathways in Applied Immunology: In Memoriam Walter Brendel. Ed. by K. Messmer & M. Stein. 1991. (Illus.). 152p. 38.95 (*0-387-53989-1*) Spr-Verlag.

Pathways in Medical Ethics. Alan G. Johnson. 176p. pap. (*0-340-50720-9*) E A GBR. *Dist:* Routldge.

Pathways in Pediatrics. Brendan G. Loftus. 1995. 288p. (*0-340-59036-X*) E A GBR. *Dist:* OUP.

Pathways in Surgical Management see Arbeitsdiagnose - Neue Wege der Chirurgischen Diagnose und Therapie

Pathways of Addiction: Opportunities in Drug Abuse Research. Institute of Medicine, Committee on Opportunities. 1996. LC 96-30998. 328p. (Orig.). (C). pap. text 49.95 (*0-309-05533-4*) Natl Acad Pr.

Pathways of Care. Sue Johnson. 1997. LC 96-28014. 240p. (Orig.). pap. 49.95 (*0-632-04076-9*) Blackwell Sci.

Pathways of Growth: Essentials of Child Psychiatry, 1999 Edition, Vol. 1: Introduction to Child Psychiatry. Joseph D. Noshpitz & Robert King. 99th ed. 1991. LC 90-12693. (Child & Adolescent Mental Health Ser.: Vol. 1). 453p. 250.00 (*0-471-09917-1*) Wiley.

Pathways of Recovery: New Life for the Diminished Person. James A. Kitchens. 1991. 120p. (Orig.). (C). pap. 7.95 (*0-9624469-1-2*) Ads-Co.

Pathways of the Pulp. Stephen Cohen & Richard C. Burns. 7th ed. 1997. LC 98-184459. (Illus.). 912p. (C). (gr. 13). text 89.00 (*0-8151-8613-4*, 30606) Mosby Inc.

Pathways of the Pulp. Stephen Cohen & Richard C. Burns. 7th ed. 1998. (Illus.). 912p. (*84-8174-382-8*) Mosby-Doyma Libros ESP. *Dist:* Mosby Inc.

Pathways Through Adolescence: Individual Development in Relation to Social Contexts. Ed. by Lisa J. Crockett & Ann C. Crouter. 1995. (Penn State Series on Child & Adolescent Development). 280p. 49.95 (*0-8058-1500-7*) L Erlbaum Assocs.

Pathways Through Surgical Finals. J. A. Britto & M. J. Dalrymple-Hay. 1993. LC 93-12293. 200p. pap. text (*0-443-04806-1*) Church.

Pathways to Change: Brief Therapy Solutions with Difficult Adolescents. Matthew D. Selekman. 1993. LC 93-848. 186p. 29.00 (*0-89862-015-5*, 2015) Guilford Pubns.

Pathways to Healing: A Guide to Herbs, Ayurveda, Dreambody & Shamanism. Don Ollsin. 2000. LC 99-51552. (Illus.). 208p. pap. 14.95 (*1-58394-011-1*) Frog Ltd CA.

Pathways to Personal Growth: Adjustment in Today's World. George R. Goethals et al. 1998. LC 98-5941. 493p. pap. text 48.00 (*0-205-13955-8*) Allyn.

Pathways to Pregnancy & Parturition. Phillip L. Senger. 1997. LC 98-180612. (Illus.). x, 275p. (C). text (*0-9657648-0-X*) Current Concept.

***Pathways to Prominence: Reflections of Twentieth Century Neuropsychologists.** Ed. by Anthony Y. Stringer et al. 2001. 320p. (C). text (*0-86377-686-8*) Psychol Pr GBR. *Dist:* Taylor & Francis.

Pathways to Psychology. Sandra Scarry et al. 1997. LC 96-78389. 578p. (C). text 65.00 (*0-15-501047-6*) Harcourt Coll Pubs.

Pathways to Reality: Erickson-Inspired Treatment Approaches to Chemical Dependency. John D. Lovern. 1991. LC 91-13541. 240p. text 34.95 (*0-87630-633-4*) Brunner-Routledge.

Patience . . . Teach Me: Encounters along the Way with My Patients, Family & Friends. Roy R. Hall. 1997. 100p. (Orig.). pap. 11.95 (*1-57502-467-5*, P01398) Morris Pubng.

Patience in Islam: Sabr. Tallal Alie Turfe. 1996. LC 96-60267. (Illus.). 122p. (Orig.). (C). pap. text 7.95 (*1-879402-32-7*) Tahrike Tarsile Quran.

Patient: Biological, Psychological & Social Dimensions of Medical Practice. Hoyle Leigh & Morton F. Reiser. 3rd ed. 1992. (Illus.). 528p. (C). text 45.00 (*0-306-44142-X*, Kluwer Plenum) Kluwer Academic.

Patient Access to Alternative Treatments: Beyond the FDA: Hearings Before the Committee on Government Reform & Oversight, House of Representatives, 105th Congress, Second Session, February 4 & 12, 1998. 1998. LC 98-207020. iv, 337p. (*0-16-057168-5*) USGPO.

***Patient Access to Self-Injectable Prescription Drugs in the Medicare Program: Congressional Hearing.** Ed. by Michael Bilirakis. 2001. 70p. (C). reprint ed. pap. text 20.00 (*0-7567-1630-6*) DIANE Pub.

Patient Account Manager's 2000 Sourcebook. annuals Aspen Reference Group Staff. 2000. pap. 99.00 (*0-8342-1770-8*) Aspen Pub.

Patient Accounts Management Handbook. Allan P. DeKaye. 1997. LC 97-19454. 480p. 96.00 (*0-8342-0843-1*, 20843) Aspen Pub.

Patient Advocacy Strategies for Managed Care. Alex D'Alessandro. 1998. LC 98-49709. pap. text 89.00 (*0-935255-62-1*) Of Course Pubns.

Patient Alcohol Abuse: A Guide for Health Care Professionals. Faith S. Schaefer. Ed. by Milton E. Burglass. 1997. LC 97-167781. (Illus.). 174p. (Orig.). pap. text 38.00 (*1-879772-09-4*) Health Studies.

Patient & Decentralised Testing. Ed. by John P. Ashby. 1987. (C). text 102.50 (*0-7462-0036-6*) Kluwer Academic.

Patient & Family Education: A Compliance Guide to the JCAHO Standards. Joan Iacono & Ann Campbell. 1997. LC 97-170611. (Illus.). 124p. (Orig.). pap. text 67.00 (*1-57839-001-X*) Opus Communs.

Patient & Family Education: Teaching Programs for Managing Chronic Disease & Disability. Marcia Hanak. 1986. 272p. pap. 32.95 (*0-8261-5441-7*) Springer Pub.

Patient & Person: Developing Interpersonal Skills in Nursing. Jane Stein-Parbury. 1993. (Illus.). 280p. (Orig.). pap. text (*0-443-04253-5*) Church.

Patient & the Analyst. Joseph Sandler et al. 2nd ed. 1992. LC 92-1727. 250p. 40.00 (*0-8236-4031-0*) Intl Univs Pr.

Patient & the Plastic Surgeon. Robert M. Goldwyn. 1981. 32.50 (*0-316-31974-0*); 2nd ed. 1991. 75.00 (*0-316-31978-3*) Lppncott W & W (Little Brwn Med Div).

Patient As a Central Construct in Health Communication Research: A Special Issue of "Health Communication", Vol. 9, No. 1, 1997. Sharf & Street. 1996. pap. 20.00 (*0-8058-9880-8*) L Erlbaum Assocs.

Patient As Partner: A Theory of Human Experimentation Ethics. Robert M. Veatch. 1987. LC 86-45043. (Medical Ethics Ser.). (Illus.). 256p. 39.95 (*0-253-35725-X*) Ind U Pr.

Patient as Partner: The Cornerstone of Community Health Improvement. American Organization of Nurse Executives Staff. 1997. LC 97-1280. (AONE Leadership Ser.: Vol. 3). 86p. pap. 35.00 (*1-55648-200-0*, 054100) AHPI.

Patient Assessment: A Guide for Health Professionals. P. Barker. 2nd ed. 1997. (Illus.). 320p. pap. 49.95 (*1-56593-329-X*, 0659) Singular Publishing.

Patient Beware—Doctor Take Care! Edward Zebrowski. 1994. LC 94-61243. 303p. (Orig.). pap. 17.95 (*0-9640096-1-7*) Woodstock Books.

Patient Billing: Using Medisoft for Windows. Greg Harpole. 3rd ed. 1997. LC 97-51749. 39.89 (*0-02-801241-0*); 26.10 (*0-02-801242-9*) Glencoe.

***Patient Billing Using Medisoft for Windows.** Greg Harpole. 4th ed. 2002. LC 2001-53203. pap. (*0-07-827264-5*) Glencoe.

Patient Care. Erica K. Williams. Ed. by Stewart C. Bushong. 1998. LC 98-20597. (Essentials of Medical Imaging Ser.). (Illus.). vii, 147p. pap. 19.95 (*0-07-070632-8*) McGraw-Hill Prof.

Patient Care: Basic Skills for the Health Care Provider. Barbara Acello. 1998. 160p. pap. text, tchr. ed. 20.95 (*0-7668-0182-9*); 1997. LC 97-26953. 283p. (C). pap. text 33.95 (*0-8273-8423-8*) Delmar.

Patient Care Advisories. Donald K. Graves. 1995. (Illus.). 175p. spiral bd. 19.00 (*1-884135-23-4*) Mayer-Johnson.

Patient Care Decision-Making: A Legal Guide for Providers. annuals Claire C. Obade. rev. ed. 1991. LC 91-22470. (Health Law Ser.). ring bd. 125.00 (*0-87632-819-2*) West Group.

Patient Care During Operative & Invasive Procedures. Mark L. Phippen & Maryann P. Wells. Ed. by Maura Connor. 1999. LC 98-43363. (Illus.). 860p. text (*0-7216-7292-2*) Church.

Patient Care Emergency Handbook. Ed. by James Matheus & Joseph E. Scherger. 1991. 650p. (C). text 60.00 (*1-878487-30-2*, 5421M) Practice Mgmt Info.

Patient Care Flow Chart. Steven R. Alexander. 4th ed. 1988. (Illus.). 608p. (C). text 59.95 (*1-878487-27-2*, 4301M) Practice Mgmt Info.

Patient Care Guidelines for Nurse Practitioners. Axalla J. Hoole. 5th ed. 1999. LC 99-19760. 608p. spiral bd. 39.95 (*0-7817-1732-9*) Lppncott W & W.

Patient Care in Cardiac Surgery. Gus Vlahakes. 5th ed. 1994. LC 93-49425. 320p. pap. text 46.95 (*0-316-08779-3*) Lppncott W & W.

Patient Care in Colorectal Surgery. Beck & Well. 1991. 50.00 (*0-316-08653-3*, Little Brwn Med Div) Lppncott W & W.

Patient Care in Community Practice. Harman. 1989. pap. (*0-85369-209-2*) Pharmaceutical Pr GBR. *Dist:* Rittenhouse.

Patient Care in Interventional Radiology: A Resource Manual. Sonja A. Bartolomei & Constance A. Reifsnyder. 1997. LC 97-18581. ring bd. 169.00 (*0-8342-0816-4*, S306) Aspen Pub.

Patient Care in Neurology. Ed. by A. C. Williams. 1999. LC 98-39264. (Illus.). 512p. text 149.50 (*0-19-262857-7*) OUP.

Patient Care in Neurosurgery, No. 3. Ryan C. Amacher. 3rd ed. 1990. 45.00 (*0-316-03640-4*, Little Brwn Med Div) Lppncott W & W.

Patient Care in Pediatric Surgery. Lucian L. Leape. 1987. 448p. 52.95 (*0-316-51821-2*, Little Brwn Med Div) Lppncott W & W.

Patient Care in Plastic Surgery. Ed. by Bernard M. Barrett, Jr. 2nd ed. 1995. LC 95-44090. (Illus.). 528p. (C). (gr. 13). pap. text 54.00 (*0-8151-0563-0*, 25685) Mosby Inc.

Patient Care in Radiography. Ruth A. Ehrlich & Ellen D. McCloskey. 4th ed. 1993. tchr. ed. (*0-8151-4700-7*) Mosby Inc.

Patient Care in Radiography. Ruth A. Ehrlich et al. 5th ed. 1998. LC 99-180760. (Illus.). 352p. (C). (gr. 12). pap. text 36.00 (*0-8151-2856-8*, 31846) Mosby Inc.

Patient Care in Radiography with an Introduction to Medical Imaging. Ruth Ann Ehrlich et al. 5th ed. 1998. (Illus.). 352p. tchr. ed. (*0-323-00026-6*) Mosby Inc.

Patient Care in the Operating Room. Kaczmarowski. 1983. (Illus.). 258p. (*0-443-03911-9*) Church.

Patient Care Information Systems: Successful Design & Implementation. E. L. Drazen et al. 1996. LC 94-28728. (Computers in Health Care Ser.). (Illus.). 188p. 59.95 (*0-387-94255-6*) Spr-Verlag.

Patient Care Procedures for the Multi-Skilled Care Giver. Ed. by Perspective Press. 1996. (Illus.). 352p. (C). pap. text 35.95 (*0-89582-316-0*) Morton Pub.

Patient Care Procedures for Your Practice, 1991. Charles E. Driscoll & Robert E. Rakel. 2nd ed. 1991. (Illus.). 320p. (C). text (*1-878487-29-9*, 6584M) Practice Mgmt Info.

Patient Care Redesign: Lessons from the Field. American Organization of Nurse Executives Staff. Ed. by Diana Jane Weaver. 1999. LC 98-53882. (AONE Management Ser.). (Illus.). 192p. pap. 35.00 (*1-55648-248-5*) AHPI.

Patient Care Skills. Mary A. Minor & Scott D. Minor. 3rd ed. 1994. LC 94-20080. (Illus.). 512p. (C). pap. 42.61 (*0-8385-7709-1*, A7709-7) Appleton & Lange.

Patient Care Skills. Mary A. Minor & Scott D. Minor. 4th ed. 1998. LC 98-25824. 544p. (C). spiral bd. 51.00 (*0-8385-8157-9*) P-H.

Patient Care Standards. Virginia Mason Medical Center Department of Nursing Staff. 1999. LC 98-40590. 250p. ring bd. 199.00 (*0-8342-1222-6*, S15) Aspen Pub.

Patient Care Stds No. 7. Susan Martin Tucker et al. 7th ed. 2000. LC 99-43230. 967p. pap. text 46.95 (*0-323-00996-4*) Mosby Inc.

Patient Care Technician Manual. Total Renal Care, Inc., Educ. Dept. Staff. 1991. 315p. pap. 60.00 (*1-56488-004-4*) Dialyrn.

Patient Care Technician, Module 4 - Physical Therapy. University of Alabama Staff. 1997. (Illus.). 200p. (C). (gr. 13). pap. text 50.00 (*0-8151-9164-2*, 31213) Mosby Inc.

Patient Care Technician, Module 3 - Respiratory Care. University of Alabama Staff. 1997. (Illus.). 200p. (C). (gr. 13). pap. text 50.00 (*0-8151-9495-1*, 31212) Mosby Inc.

Patient Care Technician, Module 2 - EKG. University of Alabama Staff. 1997. (Illus.). 200p. (C). (gr. 13). pap. text 50.00 (*0-8151-9494-3*, 31211) Mosby Inc.

Patient Care Techniques. Dorothy J. Hicks. 1975. LC 74-18673. (Allied Health Ser.). pap. 7.75 (*0-672-61394-8*, Bobbs) Macmillan.

Patient Centered Audit. Christine G. Kruse. 1984. (Illus.). 69p. pap. 14.50 (*0-87527-247-9*) Green.

Patient Centered Care: A Model for Restructuring. Mickey L. Parsons. 1994. 7p. 114.00 (*0-8342-0573-4*, 20573) Aspen Pub.

Patient Centered Care: A Model for Restructuring. Mickey L. Parsons & Carolyn L. Murdaugh. 1997. 646p. pap. 54.00 (*0-8342-0983-7*, 20983) Aspen Pub.

Patient-Centered Care: Your Prescription for Maximum Patient Satisfaction & Loyalty. K. C. Warner. 1998. LC 98-71410. (How to Bks.). reprint ed. pap. 12.95 (*1-884926-87-8*, PATCA) Amer Media.

Patient-Centered Hospital Care: Reform from Within. Ed. by Kathryn J. McDonagh. 1993. LC 93-14569. 222p. text 44.00 (*1-56793-002-6*, 0936) Health Admin Pr.

Patient-Centered Medicine: Transforming the Clinical Method. Moira Stewart et al. 1995. LC 94-43063. (Illus.). 292p. pap. 39.95 (*0-8039-5689-4*, 4194) Sage.

Patient Children: Conditions of Poverty & the Use of Hospital-Based Ambulatory Care. Beth C. Weitzman. 1992. LC 92-33036. (Children of Poverty Ser.). 150p. text 15.00 (*0-8153-1121-4*) Garland.

Patient Comes First: A Nurse Speaks Out. Nancy Fox. 1988. LC 88-61282. (Illus.). 153p. pap. 21.00 (*0-87975-479-6*) Prometheus Bks.

Patient Compliance in Medical Practice & Clinical Trials. Ed. by Joyce A. Cramer & Bert Spilker. 1991. 432p. text 99.00 (*0-88167-735-3*) Lppncott W & W.

Patient Compliance with & Attitudes Towards Health Buddy. James H. Bigelow et al. 2000. (Illus.). 44p. pap. 10.00 (*0-8330-2894-4*) Rand Corp.

***Patient-Controlled Analgesia.** Michael Harmer. 2nd ed. 2001. (Illus.). 216p. 59.95 (*0-632-05275-9*) Blackwell Sci.

Patient-Controlled Analgesia: Confidence in Post-Operative Pain Control. Margaret Heath & Veronica J. Thomas. 1993. (Illus.). 224p. text 45.00 (*0-19-262165-3*) OUP.

Patient Controlled Epidural Analgesia. Ramon Pediani. 2003. 256p. pap. 25.00 (*0-7506-4299-8*) Buttrwrth-Heinemann.

Patient Counseling Handbook. U. S. Pharmacopeia Staff. 3rd rev. ed. 1998. 933p. pap. text 45.00 (*0-917330-91-9*) Am Pharm Assn.

Patient Data Management in Intensive Care, No. 6. Ed. by K. Lenz & A. N. Laggner. 1995. (Illus.). 157p. 39.00 (*0-387-82513-4*) Spr-Verlag.

Patient Drug Facts. Facts and Comparisons Staff. 2001. (ENG & SPA.). 1000p. ring bd. 169.00 incl. cd-rom (*1-57439-022-8*) Facts & Comparisons.

Patient Drug Facts. Bernie R. Olin et al. (C). 59.95 (*0-03-268636-6*) Lppncott W & W.

Patient Dumping in Hospital Emergency Rooms. Lauren Dame & Sidney M. Wolfe. 1996. 18p. (Orig.). pap. 10.00 (*0-937188-06-9*) Pub Citizen.

Patient Education. SPC Staff. 1997. LC 97-27722. (Healthcare Professional Guides: Vol. 4). 432p. spiral bd. 26.95 (*0-87434-914-1*) Springhouse Corp.

Patient Education: A Practical Approach. Richard D. Muma et al. 1996. LC 95-35463. (Illus.). 381p. (C). pap. text 37.95 (*0-8385-2039-1*, A2039-4, Apple Lange Med) McGraw.

Patient Education: A Practical Approach. Kate Lorig. 2nd ed. 1996. LC 95-36414. 81.95 (*0-7619-0073-X*, 1689); 2nd ed. 1996. LC 95-36414. 256p. pap. 39.95 (*0-7619-0074-8*, 1690); 3rd ed. 2000. LC 00-10036. pap. 32.95 (*0-7619-2290-3*) Sage.

Patient Education: Cardiovascular Disorders. Hurst. 1992. (*1-56375-024-4*) Gower-Mosby.

Patient Education: Nurses in Partnership with Other Health Care Professionals. Ed. by Carol E. Smith. 1986. 384p. text 55.00 (*0-8089-1833-8*, 794144, Grune & Strat) Harcrt Hlth Sci Grp.

Patient Education: Principles & Practice. Sally H. Rankin & Karen Duffy Stallings. 4th ed. 2000. LC 00-46433. (Illus.). 448p. pap. text 35.95 (*0-7817-2022-2*) Lppncott W & W.

Patient Education: Strategies & Skills for Living Well. Gretchen C. Peske et al. 1996. LC 95-76320. (Illus.). 300p. (Orig.). pap. 12.00 (*1-887109-00-5*) Blue Path Pr.

Patient Education & Discharge Planning for Rehabilitation. St. Joseph's Rehabilitation Hospital Staff. 1992. 816p. spiral bd. 305.00 (*0-8342-0715-X*, 20715) PRO-ED.

Patient Education for the Ill & the Well: Index of New Information. Judy A. Plaines. 1997. 160p. 57.50 (*0-7883-1774-1*); pap. 47.50 (*0-7883-1775-X*) ABBE Pubs Assn.

Patient Education Materials & Instructor's Guide: A Supplement to the Manual of Clinical Dietetics. Jo E. Shield & Mary C. Mullen. 1992. 15.00 (*0-88091-109-3*) Am Dietetic Assn.

Patient Elephant: More Exotic Cases from the World's Top Wildlife Vet. David Conrad Taylor. 1995. (Illus.). 194p. (*0-86051-835-3*) Robson Bks GBR. *Dist:* Parkwest Pubns.

Patient Emergencies. SPC Staff. 1997. LC 97-23888. (Healthcare Professional Guides: Vol. 5). 256p. spiral bd. 26.95 (*0-87434-915-X*) Springhouse Corp.

Patient Financial Services. Ed. by Allen G. Herkimer. 1993. 150p. (C). text 65.00 (*1-882198-14-X*) Hlthcare Fin Mgmt.

Patient GenRx. Mosby-Year Book Staff. 1999. (Illus.). 552p. ring bd. 89.00 (*0-8151-3752-4*) Mosby Inc.

Patient GenRx: Spanish Version. Mosby-Year Book Staff. 1999. (SPA., Illus.). 552p. ring bd. 89.00 (*0-8151-3754-0*) Mosby Inc.

Patient in the Family: An Ethics of Medicine & Families. Hilde Lindemann Nelson & James L. Nelson. 1995. LC 94-33652. 224p. (C). (gr. 13). pap. 19.95 (*0-415-91129-X*, B4914) Routledge.

Patient Instructions for the Emergency Physician. Stewart. 1993. text (*0-397-51166-3*) Lppncott W & W.

Patient Management Cluster. Ed. by L. Skrbic. rev. ed. 1991. (Illus.). 140p. (C). reprint ed. (*0-9626486-0-4*) Postgraduate Med Rev Ed.

Patient Management of Secondary Disability. Walker. 2000. pap. text Price not set. (*0-443-06117-3*) Church.

Patient Management Problems in Psychiatry: For the Mrcpsych Oral Examination. Parimala Moodley et al. 1991. (Illus.). 144p. (Orig.). pap. text (*0-443-04374-4*) Church.

Patient Management Skills for Dental Assistants. Barbara D. Ingersoll. 1986. (Illus.). 192p. pap. text 14.95 (*0-13-653718-9*) P-H.

Patient Monitoring Markets: Integrated Non-Invasive Products Enhance Manufacturer Opportunities. Market Intelligence Staff. 1992. 317p. (Orig.). 1995.00 (*1-56753-396-5*) Frost & Sullivan.

Patient or Person: Living with Chronic Pain. Penney Cowan. 1992. LC 91-25980. 196p. pap. 21.95 (*0-89876-186-7*) Gardner Pr.

Patient-Oriented Research. Edward H. Ahrens. 1992. LC 91-32064. (Illus.). 248p. text 39.95 (*0-19-505156-4*) OUP.

Patient Outcomes Research Teams (PORTS) Managing Conflict of Interest. Institute of Medicine Staff. Ed. by Molla S. Donaldson & Alexander M. Capron. 1991. 184p. pap. text 19.00 (*0-309-04482-0*) Natl Acad Pr.

Patient Participation in Program Planning. Mark Ozer et al. 2nd ed. 1999. LC 00-500770. (Illus.). 173p. pap. 29.95 (*0-07-077882-5*) McGraw-Hill Prof.

***Patient Persistence.** Adele M. Gill. 2000. (Illus.). 194p. pap. (*0-930958-00-4*, EP8004GN) Excptnl Parent.

Patient-Physician Relation Pt. 2: The Patient As Partner. Robert M. Veatch. 1991. LC 90-4261. (Medical Ethics Ser.). (Illus.). 320p. 28.95 (*0-253-36207-5*) Ind U Pr.

Patient Placement Criteria for the Treatment of Psychoactive Substance Use Disorders. Norman G. Hoffman et al. 1991. LC 91-74015. 170p. (Orig.). pap. 65.00 (*1-880425-01-7*) Am Soc Addict Med.

Patient Placement Criteria for the Treatment of Substance-Related Disorders: ASAM PPC-2. David Mee-Lee et al. Ed. by Bonnie B. Wilford. 2nd ed. 1996. LC 97-108914. 170p. 100.00 (*1-880425-03-3*) Am Soc Addict Med.

Patient Positioning. Mark J. Schubert. Ed. by Stewart C. Bushong. 1998. LC 98-35431. (Essentials of Medical Imaging Ser.). (Illus.). ix, 96p. pap. 19.95 (*0-07-058067-7*) McGraw-Hill Prof.

Patient Power: How to Protect Yourself From Medical Error. Richard N. Podell & William Proctor. 1996. LC 96-273. 416p. pap. 19.95 (*0-684-81515-X*, Fireside) S&S Trade Pap.

Patient Power: Overcoming Chronic Illness. James M. Galbraith. 1995. (Orig.). pap. 12.95 (*0-942246-02-0*) Benchmark Bks.

Patient Power: The Free-Enterprise Alternative to Clinton's Health Plan. John C. Goodman & Gerald L. Musgrave. 1993. LC 93-41604. 134p. pap. 4.95 (*1-882577-10-8*) Cato Inst.

Patient Power? The Politics of Patients' Associations in Britain & America. Contrib. by Bruce Wood. 2000. LC 99-41546. (*0-335-20368-X*) OpUniv Pr GBR. *Dist:* Taylor & Francis.

Patient Power! The Smart Patient's Guide to Health Care. Patricia Parsons. 1997. LC 97-139173. (Illus.). 320p. pap. 14.95 (*0-8020-7186-4*) U of Toronto Pr.

Patient Practitioner Interaction: An Experiential Manual for Developing the Art of Health Care. Carol M. Davis. 3rd ed. 1998. LC 98-3498. (Illus.). 352p. pap. text 32.00 (*1-55642-400-0*, 44000) SLACK Inc.

Patient Practitioner Interaction: Instructor's Manual. Carol M. Davis. 3rd ed. 1998. 26p. pap. text, tchr. ed. Price not set. (*1-55642-401-9*, 44019) SLACK Inc.

Patient Presentations in General Practice: A Comprehensive Guide to Diagnosis & Management. Ian D. Steven. 2000. (Illus.). 581p. pap. 79.95 (*0-07-470823-6*) McGraw-Hill Prof.

Patient Recruitment in Clinical Trials. Bert Spilker & Joyce A. Cramer. 1992. LC 92-12023. (Illus.). 368p. text 129.00 (*0-88167-931-3*) Lppncott W & W.

Patient Resources on the Internet: 1997 Guide to Health Care Professionals. Ed. by Lois Wingerson. 1997. (Illus.). 480p. pap. text 195.00 (*1-57987-000-7*) Faulkner & Gray.

Patient Safety Improvement Guidebook. Patrice L. Spath. 2000. 100p. 30.00 (*1-929955-07-3*) Brown Spath.

Patient Safety in Anesthetic Practice. Robert C. Morell & John H. Eichhorn. 1996. LC 96-30949. 527p. text (*0-443-07682-0*) Church.

Patient Satisfaction: A Guide to Practice Enhancement. Wendy Leebov et al. 1990. LC 89-8255. (Illus.). 380p. 49.95 (*0-87489-546-4*, ME003) Practice Mgmt Info.

Patient Satisfaction Pays: Quality Service for Practice Success. Stephen W. Brown et al. 1993. LC 93-20094. 432p. 88.00 (*0-8342-0394-4*) Aspen Pub.

Patient Self-Determination Act: Meeting the Challenges in Patient Care. Lawrence P. Ulrich. Ed. by Mark J. Hanson. 2001. LC 99-19307. (Hastings Center Studies in Ethics). 192p. 44.95 (*0-87840-747-2*); 304p. pap. 22.95 (*0-87840-748-0*) Georgetown U Pr.

Patient Self-Determination Act: Providers Offer Information on Advance Directives but Effectiveness Uncertain. 1996. (Illus.). 48p. (Orig.). (C). pap. text 20.00 (*0-7881-3038-2*) DIANE Pub.

Patient Self-Determination in Long-Term Care: Implementing the PSDA in Medical Decisions. Ed. by Marshall B. Kapp. 1994. (Illus.). 240p. 34.95 (*0-8261-8520-7*) Springer Pub.

Patient Teaching. Springhouse Publishing Company Staff. 1998. LC 98-36727. (Incredibly Easy Ser.). 320p. pap. 34.95 (*0-87434-959-1*) Springhouse Corp.

Patient Teaching Guides. Mosby Staff. 1996. 30p. text, suppl. ed. 19.95 (*0-8151-6907-8*) Mosby Inc.

Patient Teaching Guides on Disk. Mosby Staff. 1996. 200p. (C). (gr. 13). pap. 160.00 incl. disk (*0-8151-8557-X*, 28720); text 115.00 incl. cd-rom (*0-8151-8551-0*) Mosby Inc.

Patient Violence & the Clinician. Ed. by Burr S. Eichelman & Anne C. Hartwig. 1995. LC 94-36233. (Clinical Practice Ser.: No. 30). (Illus.). 200p. text 15.50 (*0-88048-454-3*, 8454) Am Psychiatric.

Patient Who Cured His Therapist: And Other Stories of Unconventional Therapy. Stanley Siegel & Ed Lowe. 2nd ed. 1999. LC 93-3435. 196p. pap. 12.95 (*1-56924-685-8*) Marlowe & Co.

Patients & Doctors: Life-Changing Stories from Primary Care. Ed. by Jeffrey M. Borkan et al. 1999. LC 99-19758. xii, 221p. text 24.95 (*0-299-16340-7*) U of Wis Pr.

Patients & Healers in the Context of Culture: An Exploration of the Borderland Between Anthropology, Medicine, & Psychiatry. Arthur Kleinman. 1979. LC 78-57311. (Comparative Studies of Health Systems & Medical Care: Vol. 5). pap. text 19.95 (*0-520-04511-4*) U CA Pr.

Patients & Methods. Douglas A. Gammon. 1991. (Illus.). 144p. pap. text 35.00 (*0-07-452733-9*) McGraw-Hill Med Pub.

Patients & Their Hospitals. Winifred Raphael. Ed. by King Edward's Hospital Fund Staff. 1977. 46p. pap. 19.95 (*0-8464-1297-7*) Beekman Pubs.

Patients As Effective Collaborators in Managing Chronic Conditions. Frwd. by Daniel M. Fox & Jessie Gruman. 1999. 32p. pap. (*1-887748-26-1*) Milbank Memorial.

Patients As People, Pt. 3. Esther L. Brown. 1965. 164p. pap. 14.95 (*0-87154-185-8*) Russell Sage.

Patients As Victims: Sexual Abuse in Psychotherapy & Counselling. Derek Jehu. 1995. LC 93-42345. (Psychotherapy & Counselling Ser.). 260p. pap. 100.00 (*0-471-94398-3*) Wiley.

Patients at Risk: AIDS in the Dentist's Office: Everything You Need to Know to Protect Yourself & Your Family! John P. Sullivan. 1993. LC 93-86275. (Illus.). 64p. (Orig.). pap. 9.95 (*0-9638856-1-8*) Pronet Pr.

Patients' Book: How to Survive in Today's Medical System. Sandra McCray & Diane Hartman. 2000. 150p. pap. 12.00 (*0-9678647-3-9*) Colorado Hlth.

Patients Build Your Practice: Word of Mouth Marketing for Healthcare Practitioners. Michael E. Cafferky. 1994. 170p. (Orig.). pap. text 29.95 (*0-07-600676-X*, ME114) Practice Mgmt Info.

Patients First: Experiences of a Patient-Focused Pioneer. William J. Leander et al. 1996. LC 95-46555. pap. 44.00 (*1-56793-039-5*, 0974) Health Admin Pr.

Patient's Guide to Anesthesia: Making the Right Choices. A. J. Hill. 1999. LC 00-500411. 288p. pap. 13.00 (*1-57566-405-4*, Knsington) Kensgtn Pub Corp.

Patient's Guide to Breast Cancer on the Internet. Ed. by Dan Goldenson. 2000. 450p. pap. 6.95 (*0-9700525-6-1*) eMedguides.

Patient's Guide to COPD & Lung Cancer. Tim Peters. 1991. (Humanatomy Board Bks.). (Illus.). 12p. bds. 9.95 (*1-879874-03-2*) T Peters & Co.

Patients Guide to Dialysis & Transplantation. R. Gabriel. 3rd ed. 1987. pap. text 29.00 (*0-85200-981-X*) Kluwer Academic.

Patient's Guide to Eye Care. Lawrence Winograd & Melvin L. Rubin. 2001. 272p. pap. (*0-937404-63-2*) Triad Pub FL.

Patient's Guide to Homeopathic Medicine. Robert W. Ullman & Judyth Reichenberg-Ullman. 1995. 96p. (Orig.). pap. 10.95 (*0-9640654-2-8*) Picnic Pt Pr.

***Patient's Guide to Infertility.** S. Bayer. 2002. 130p. ring bd. 29.95 (*1-84214-103-1*, Parthenon Pbng) CRC Pr.

Patient's Guide to Knee & Hip Replacement: Everything You Need to Know. Irwin Silber. 1999. LC 98-44423. (Illus.). 256p. per. 13.00 (*0-684-83920-2*, Fireside) S&S Trade Pap.

Patient's Guide to Medical Terminology. Charlotte Isler. 3rd rev. ed. 1997. LC 94-39738. 258p. (Orig.). reprint ed. pap. 12.95 (*1-885987-08-0*, ME080, Health Info Pr) Practice Mgmt Info.

Patient's Guide to Medical Tests. Yale University School of Medicine Staff. 1997. LC 96-53904. 448p. 40.00 (*0-395-76536-6*) HM.

Patient's Guide to Medical Tests: Everything You Need to Know about the Tests Your Doctor Prescribes. Joseph Stauffer & Joseph C. Segen. 4th ed. 1997. 432p. LC 97-37944. 29.95 (*0-8160-3471-0*); pap. 17.95 (*0-8160-3530-X*) Facts on File.

Patient's Guide to Prostate Cancer: An Expert's Successful Treatment Strategies & Options. Marc Garnick. 1996. 240p. pap. 12.95 (*0-452-27455-9*, Plume) Dutton Plume.

Patient's Guide to Radial Keratotomy. William Ellis. 1992. (Illus.). 80p. (Orig.). pap. text (*0-9633665-0-5*) Eye Ctr N CA.

Patient's Guide to Surgery. Edward L. Bradley, III. Ed. by Consumer Reports Books Editors. 1994. (Illus.). 256p. (C). text 26.50 (*0-8122-3280-1*) U of Pa Pr.

Patients Guide to Surgery. Weedwe. 1995. 22.95 (*0-02-624770-4*) Macmillan.

Patient's Guide to Understandng Hemodialysis. Regional Kidney Disease Program, Education Departm. rev. ed. 1986. 150p. reprint ed. ring bd. 30.00 (*1-56488-005-2*) Dialyrn.

Patient's Guide to Urology: Plumbing Problems in Layman's Terms. G. Mark Seal. 1995. (Illus.). 273p. text 21.95 (*0-9645773-0-5*); pap. text 12.95 (*0-9645773-1-3*) High Oaks Pub.

Patient's Interest Foremost: The Good Doctor's Ethics. 1996. 88p. pap. 10.00 (*981-02-2841-4*) World Scientific Pub.

***Patient's Internet Handbook.** R. Kiley & E. Graham. 2001. 100p. pap. (*1-85315-498-9*) Royal Soc of Medicine Pr Ltd GBR. *Dist:* Balogh.

Patient's Ordeal. William F. May. LC 90-45841. (Medical Ethics Ser.). 240p. 1994. pap. 11.95 (*0-253-20870-X*); 1991. 26.95 (*0-253-33717-8*) Ind U Pr.

Patients, Pain & Politics: Nursing Home Inspector's Shocking True Story & Expert Advice for You & Your Family. Mary R. Rollins. Ed. by Barbara Davis. 1994. 248p. (Orig.). pap. 11.95 (*1-884348-20-3*) N Century Pubng.

***Patient's Partner: The Only Health Planner That Organizes the Seriously Ill Patient's Medical & Personal Life.** Donna Wolf & Robin Levine. 2001. (Illus.). 212p. 29.95 (*0-9705937-0-8*) Bittersweet Bay.

Patients, Physicians, & Illness: A Sourcebook in Behavioral Science & Health. Ed. by E. Gartly Jaco. 3rd ed. 1979. LC 78-63407. text 29.95 (*0-02-915850-8*) Free Pr.

Patient's Point of View: Observations of a Chiropractic Advocate. William D. Esteb. 1992. 240p. pap. text 19.95 (*0-9631711-0-0*) Back Talk Systs.

Patients, Policies, & Politics: Before & after "Working for Patients" John Butler. 1992. LC 92-18762. (State of Health Ser.). 160p. pap. (*0-335-15647-9*) OpUniv Pr.

Patients, Policies, & Politics: Before & after "Working for Patients" John Butler. 1992. LC 92-18762. (State of Health Ser.). 160p. (*0-335-15648-7*) OpUniv Pr GBR. *Dist:* Taylor & Francis.

Patients, Power & the Poor in 18th Century Bristol. Mary E. Fissell. 1991. (Cambridge History of Medicine Ser.). (Illus.). 272p. (C). text 74.95 (*0-521-40047-3*) Cambridge U Pr.

Patients' Privacy: An Explanatory Study of Patients' Perception of Their Privacy in a German Acute Care Hospital. Irmgard L. Bauer. 1994. LC 94-16735. (Developments in Nursing & Health Care Ser.). 184p. (*1-85628-918-4*) Avebry GBR. *Dist:* Ashgate Pub Co.

Patient's Progress: Doctors & Doctoring in 18th-Century England. Dorothy Porter & Roy Porter. 1989. LC 89-60692. (Illus.). 313p. 51.00 (*0-8047-1744-3*) Stanford U Pr.

Patient's Progress: Sickness, Health & Medical Care in England, 1650-1850. Dorothy Porter & Roy Porter. (Medicine & Society Ser.: Vol. 4). 25.00 (*0-520-06661-8*) U CA Pr.

Patients, Psychiatrists & Lawyers: Law & the Mental Health System. Raymond L. Spring et al. 2nd ed. 1996. LC 99-188645. 938p. (C). 59.95 (*0-87084-797-X*); 3rd ed. 2000. text (*0-87084-311-7*) Anderson Pub Co.

Patient's Right to Know: Information Disclosure, the Doctor & the Law. Sheila A. McLean. 1989. 270p. pap. (*1-85521-021-5*); text (*1-85521-010-X*) Dartmth Pub GBR. *Dist:* Ashgate Pub Co.

Patients' Rights - Community Concerns. Ed. by Steven J. Friedman & Thomas M. Hughes. 1991. (Issues in Community Mental Health Ser.). 89p. (C). pap. text 6.95 (*0-88135-057-5*, Prodist) Watson Pub Intl.

Patients' Rights & Responsibilities: An Easy-to-Read Guide for People Taking Medicine. Michael G. Aman et al. 1999. (Project Med). (Illus.). pap. text (*0-9658966-1-7*, 1) OSU Nisonger.

Patients' Rights in the Age of Managed Health Care. Lisa Yount. 2001. (Library in a Book). 256p. 45.00 (*0-8160-4258-6*) Facts on File.

Patient's Story: Integrated Patient-Doctor Interviewing. Robert C. Smith. 1995. 232p. 29.95 (*0-316-80266-2*, Little Brwn Med Div) Lppncott W & W.

Patient's Voice: Experiences of Illness. Jeanine Young-Mason. 1996. LC 96-28901. (Illus.). 197p. (C). pap. text 25.95 (*0-8036-0162-X*) Davis Co.

Patients Who Deceive: Assessment & Management of Risk in Providing Health Care & Financial Benefits. Loren Pankratz. 1998. LC 98-12041. (American Series in Behavioral Science & Law). 274p. text 58.95 (*0-398-06866-6*); pap. text 43.95 (*0-398-06867-4*) C C Thomas.

Patients with Special Needs Vol. 39-1: Behavioral Aspects of Vision Care. 1998. (Illus.). 103p. pap. 20.00 (*0-943599-98-9*) OEPF.

Patients Without Frontiers: Negotiations on the Health Care Market. Ivan Wolffers. 1991. 70p. pap. (*90-6256-937-4*) VU Univ Pr NLD. *Dist:* Paul & Co Pubs.

Patologia Estructural y Funcional. Stanley L. Robbins. 4th ed. 1990. text 99.00 (*0-07-104001-3*) McGraw.

Patologie Vascolari Cerebrali Dell'Anziano. Ed. by W. Meier-Ruge. 1991. (Insegnamento E Formazione in Medicina Geriatrica Ser.: Vol. 2). viii, 188p. pap. 24.50 (*3-8055-5365-X*) S Karger.

Paton & Goldberg's Management of Ocular Injuries. Thomas A. Deutsch & Daniel B. Feller. 2nd ed. 1985. (Illus.). 248p. text 82.00 (*0-7216-1173-7*) Saunders.

Patriarchal Precedents: Sexuality & Social Relations. Rosalind Coward. 1983. 280p. (Orig.). pap. 14.95 (*0-7100-9324-1*, Routledge Thoemms) Routledge.

Patronage & Institutions: Science, Technology & Medicine at the European Court, 1500-1750. Ed. by Bruce T. Moran. 1991. (Illus.). 267p. (C). 75.00 (*0-85115-285-6*) Boydell & Brewer.

Pattern Electroretinogram, Circulatory Disturbances of the Visual System & Pattern Evoked Responses. Ed. by John R. Heckenlively & Theodore Lawwill. 1984. (Documenta Ophthalmologica Proceedings Ser.). text 219.50 (*90-6193-503-2*) Kluwer Academic.

Pattern of Health. Aubrey T. Westlake. 1963. 26.95 (*0-8159-6514-1*) Devin.

Pattern of Life. Alfred Adler. 2nd ed. LC 81-71160. pap. 10.95 (*0-918560-28-4*) Adler Sch Prof Psy.

Patterns: Sixteen Things You Should Know about Life. Mahlon Hoagland & Bert Dodson. 2nd ed. 1999. LC 99-10891. (Life Science Ser.). (Illus.). 64p. (C). pap. text 16.95 (*0-7637-0648-5*, 0648-5) Jones & Bartlett.

Patterns & Practice in Chinese Medicine. Xuemeii Li & Jingyi Zhao. 1998. LC 97-61504. (Illus.). 225p. 45.00 (*0-939616-27-0*) Eastland.

Pattern's Foundations of Embryology. Bruce M. Carlson. 5th ed. 1988. (C). text 77.25 net. (*0-07-009902-2*) McGraw.

Patterns in Forcible Rape. Menachem Amir. 1971. LC 79-14022. (C). lib. bdg. 35.00 (*0-226-01734-6*) U Ch Pr.

Patterns, Information & Chaos in Neuronal Systems. B. J. West. 1993. (Studies of Nonlinear Phenomena in Life). 248p. text 64.00 (*981-02-1377-8*) World Scientific Pub.

Patterns of Adoption. David Howe. 1997. LC 97-21647. (Working Together with Children, Young People, & Their Fami Ser.). 226p. pap. 47.95 (*0-632-04149-8*) Blackwell Sci.

Patterns of Attachment: A Psychological Study of the Strange Situation. M. D. Ainsworth et al. 1978. 416p. 99.95 (*0-89859-461-8*) L Erlbaum Assocs.

Patterns of Brief Family Therapy: An Ecosystemic Approach. Steve De Shazer. 1982. LC 81-7239. (Family Therapy Ser.). 157p. text 30.00 (*0-89862-038-4*, 2038) Guilford Pubns.

Patterns of Cancer in 5 Continents. Ed. by S. L. Whelan et al. 1990. (IARC Scientific Publications Ser.: No. 102). (Illus.). 186p. pap. text 67.50 (*92-832-2102-8*) OUP.

Patterns of Development. LC 95-176209. (*0-340-62511-2*) E A GBR. *Dist:* Routldge.

Patterns of Health Care Use among HIV-Infected Adults. 1996. lib. bdg. 263.99 (*0-8490-8353-2*) Gordon Pr.

Patterns of Hypnotic Techniques of Milton H. Erickson, M. D., Vol. 2. Richard Brandler et al. 1977. LC 75-24584. 22.95 (*0-916990-02-8*) META Pubns.

Patterns of Infidelity & Their Treatment. Emily M. Brown. 1991. LC 90-25925. (Frontiers in Couples & Family Therapy Ser.: No. 3). (Illus.). 304p. text 40.95 (*0-87630-631-8*) Brunner-Routledge.

***Patterns of Infidelity & Their Treatment.** Emily Brown. 2nd ed. 2001. 288p. (YA). (gr. 13 up). text 37.95 (*1-58391-017-4*) Brunner-Routledge.

***Patterns of Infidelity & Their Treatment.** Emily M. Brown. 2nd ed. 2001. LC 2001-18084. x, 359p. 34.95 (*1-58391-369-6*) Brunner-Routledge.

Patterns of Injury & Illness in Great Apes: A Skeletal Analysis. Nancy C. Lovell. 1990. LC 89-600389. (Illus.). 288p. 45.00 (*0-87474-678-7*) Smithsonian.

Patterns of Mothering: A Study of Maternal Influence During Infancy. Sylvia Brody. 1970. LC 56-8839. 446p. (Orig.). reprint ed. 65.00 (*0-8236-4040-X*) Intl Univs Pr.

Patterns of Nursing Theories in Practice. Ed. by Marilyn E. Parker. 1993. LC 93-3402. 330p. pap. 32.95 (*0-88737-600-2*, 15-2548) Natl League Nurse.

Patterns of Psychosexual Infantilism. Wilhelm Stekel. 1952. (C). 7.50 (*0-87140-840-6*) Liveright.

Patterns of Relating: An Adult Attachment Perspective. Malcolm L. West et al. 1994. LC 93-48128. 210p. 30.00 (*0-89862-671-4*) Guilford Pubns.

Patterns of Sexual Arousal: Psychophysiological Processes & Clinical Applications. Raymond C. Rosen & J. Gayle Beck. 1988. LC 87-19726. 404p. 49.95 (*0-89862-712-5*) Guilford Pubns.

Patterns of Time in Hospital Life: A Sociological Perspective. Eviatar Zerubavel. 1979. LC 78-11385. (Illus.). 182p. lib. bdg. 16.50 (*0-226-98160-6*) U Ch Pr.

Patty's Industrial Hygiene & Toxicology Vol. 1, Pt. A: General Principles, Vol. 1, Pt. A, General Principles. Ed. by George D. Clayton & Florence E. Clayton. 4th ed. 1991. LC 90-13080. (Patty's Industrial Hygiene & Toxicology Ser.: Vol. A). 1104p. 249.00 (*0-471-50197-2*) Wiley.

Patty's Industrial Hygiene & Toxicology Vol. 1, Pt. B: General Principles, Vol. 1, Pt. B, General Principles. Ed. by George D. Clayton & Florence E. Clayton. 4th ed. 1991. (Patty's Industrial Hygiene & Toxicology Ser.: Vol. B). 1120p. 249.00 (*0-471-50196-4*) Wiley.

Pau d'Arco: Immune Power from the Rainforest. Kenneth Jones. 1994. LC 94-1489. (Illus.). 160p. pap. 8.95 (*0-89281-497-7*, Heal Arts VT) Inner Tradit.

Paul Boeder, PhD: Teacher of Physiological Optics. Paul Boeder. 1992. (Ophthalmology Oral History Ser.). (Illus.). xxix, 194p. pap. 35.00 (*0-926866-04-4*) FAAO.

***Paul Ehrlich's Receptor Immunology: The Magnificent Obsession.** Arthur M. Silverstein. 2001. LC 2001-94613. 202p. 75.00 (*0-12-643765-3*) Acad Pr.

Paul Schilder - Mind Explorer. Donald A. Shashkan & William L. Roller. 1985. (Illus.). 316p. 43.95 (*0-89885-144-0*, Kluwer Acad Hman Sci) Kluwer Academic.

***Paulev/Guyton Package.** Paulev & Guyton. 1996. (*0-7020-2276-4*) W B Saunders GBR. *Dist:* Saunders.

Pauling Catalogue: Ava Helen & Linus Pauling Papers at Oregon State University. Ed. by Clifford S. Mead & Janet Wallace. 1991. (Illus.). 305p. 35.00 (*0-9629082-0-7*) Kerr Lib.

Pause: Positive Approaches to Perimenopause & Menopause. Lonnie G. Barbach. rev. ed. 2000. LC 99-32063. 320p. pap. 13.95 (*0-452-28110-5*, Plume) Dutton Plume.

Pavlov: A Biography. Boris P. Babkin. 1975. LC 49-11887. xiv, 366p. pap. text 4.25 (*0-226-03373-2*, P621) U Ch Pr.

Payer, Provider, Consumer: Industry Confronts Health Care Costs. R. H. Egdahl. 1977. LC 77-21020. (Springer Series in Industry & Health Care: No. 1). (Illus.). 117p. 63.00 (*0-387-90295-3*) Spr-Verlag.

Paying Attention to Children in a Changing Health Care System: Summaries of Workshops. Board on Children, Youth and Families Staff et al. 1996. LC 96-230003. 104p. (Orig.). pap. text 26.00 (*0-309-05588-1*, Joseph Henry Pr) Natl Acad Pr.

Paying for Health Care: Public Policy Choices for Illinois. Ed. by Lawrence B. Joseph. 1992. (Chicago Assembly Ser.). 304p. (C). pap. text 14.95 (*0-9626755-1-2*) UC Ctr UR&PS.

Paying for Health Care Trends. Kathleen O'Leary Morgan. 1999. 100p. per. 50.00 (*0-7401-0010-6*, M Quitno Pr) Morgan Quitno Corp.

Paying for India's Health Care. Peter Berman & M. E. Khan. 1993. LC 92-48184. (Illus.). 326p. 38.00 (*0-8039-9463-X*, 7505) Sage.

Paying for Long Term In-Home & Nursing Home Care, 1991: Washington State. Cheryl C. Mitchell & F. H. Mitchell, Jr. 1991. 120p. pap. text 25.00 (*1-879909-00-6*) Mitchell WA.

Paying for Medicare: The Politics of Reform. David G. Smith. 1992. (Social Institutions & Social Change Ser.). 284p. lib. bdg. 47.95 (*0-202-30393-4*) Aldine de Gruyter.

Paying Physicians: Choices for Medicare, Controlling Medicare Costs Through Competitive Consumer Choices. 1992. lib. bdg. 99.95 (*0-8490-5507-5*) Gordon Pr.

Paying the Doctor: Health Policy & Physician Reimbursement. Ed. by Jonathan D. Moreno. 1990. LC 90-37837. 208p. 60.00 (*0-86569-006-5*, T006, Auburn Hse) Greenwood.

Paying Your Sickness Bills. Michael M. Davis. 1972. LC 77-180572. (Medicine & Society in America Ser.). 292p. reprint ed. 21.95 (*0-405-03947-6*) Ayer.

Payment for Physicians Services: Strategies for Medicare. 1991. lib. bdg. 75.85 (*0-8490-4979-2*) Gordon Pr.

Payments for Care. A. Evers et al. 1994. 360p. pap. (*1-85972-008-0*) Avebry GBR. *Dist:* Ashgate Pub Co.

Paziente Anziano Nella Pratica Medica. Ed. by W. Meier-Ruge. 1990. viii, 256p. pap. 31.50 (*3-8055-5286-6*) S Karger.

PBMs: Reshaping the Pharmaceutical Distribution Network. Ed. by Sheila R. Shulman et al. 1998. LC 98-12622. (Journal of Pharmaceutical Marketing & Management Ser.: Vol. 12, Nos. 2-3). 189p. 49.95 (*0-7890-0512-3*, Pharmctl Prods) Haworth Pr.

PCAT: Pharmacy College Admission Test. D. B. Gourley. 3rd ed. 1997. LC 97-70060. (Arco PCAT: Pharmacy College Admission Test Ser.). (Illus.). 176p. pap. 19.95 (*0-02-861706-1*, Arc) Hungry Minds.

PCAT - Pharmacy College Admission Test: Comprehensive Review for Self Study. David M. Tarlow. 1999. 145p. (C). pap. text 19.95 (*1-57732-111-1*) Datar Pub.

PCAT - Pharmacy College Admission Test No. 1: Practice Exam Annotated Answers. David M. Tarlow. 2nd rev. ed. 1999. 20p. (C). pap. text 6.95 (*1-57732-113-8*) Datar Pub.

PCAT - Pharmacy College Admission Test No. 2: Practice Exam Annotated Answers. David M. Tarlow. 2nd rev. ed. 1999. (C). pap. text 6.95 (*1-57732-115-4*) Datar Pub.

PCAT - Pharmacy College Admission Test No. 2: Practice Examination. David M. Tarlow. 2nd rev. ed. 1999. 40p. (C). pap. text 18.95 (*1-57732-114-6*) Datar Pub.

PCAT - Pharmacy College Admission Test No. 3: Practice Exam Annotated Answers. David M. Tarlow. 2nd rev. ed. 1999. 20p. (C). pap. text 6.95 (*1-57732-117-0*) Datar Pub.

PCAT - Pharmacy College Admission Test No. 3: Practice Examination. David M. Tarlow. 2nd rev. ed. 1999. 40p. (C). pap. text 18.95 (*1-57732-116-2*) Datar Pub.

PCAT - Pharmacy College Admission Test No. 4: Practice Exam Annotated Answers. David M. Tarlow. 2nd rev. ed. 1999. 20p. (C). pap. text 6.95 (*1-57732-119-7*) Datar Pub.

PCAT - Pharmacy College Admission Test No. 4: Practice Examination. David M. Tarlow. 2nd rev. ed. 1999 40p. (C). pap. text 18.95 (*1-57732-118-9*) Datar Pub.

PCAT - Pharmacy College Admission Test No. 5: Practice Exam Annotated Answers. David M. Tarlow. 2nd rev. ed. 1999. 20p. (C). pap. text 6.95 (*1-57732-121-9*) Datar Pub.

PCAT - Pharmacy College Admission Test No. 5: Practice Examination. David M. Tarlow. 2nd rev. ed. 1999. 40p. (C). pap. text 18.95 (*1-57732-120-0*) Datar Pub.

PCAT - Pharmacy College Admission Test Vol. I: Practice Examination. David M. Tarlow. 2nd rev. ed. 1999. 40p. (C). pap. text 18.95 (*1-57732-112-X*) Datar Pub.

PCAT - Pharmacy College Admission Test - Core Content. David M. Tarlow. 2nd rev. ed. 1999. (Illus.). 400p. pap. 49.95 (*1-57774-008-4*) Educ Tsting Cnslts.

PCAT Exam No. 1: Annotated Answers (Pharmacy College Admission Test) David M. Tarlow. 7th ed. 1996. (Orig.). pap. 5.95 (*1-57732-039-5*) Datar Pub.

PCAT Exam No. 1: Pharmacy College Admissions Test. David M. Tarlow. 7th ed. 1996. (Illus.). (Orig.). pap. 19.95 (*1-57732-034-4*) Datar Pub.

PCAT Exam No. 2: Annotated Answers (Pharmacy College Admissions Test) David M. Tarlow. 7th ed. 1996. (Orig.). pap. 5.95 (*1-57732-040-9*) Datar Pub.

PCAT Exam No. 2: Pharmacy College Admission Test. David M. Tarlow. 7th ed. 1996. (Orig.). pap. 19.95 (*1-57732-035-2*) Datar Pub.

PCAT Exam No. 3: Annotated Answers (Pharmacy College Admissions Test) David M. Tarlow. 7th ed. 1996. (Orig.). pap. 5.95 (*1-57732-041-7*) Datar Pub.

PCAT Exam No. 3: Pharmacy College Admission Test. David M. Tarlow. 7th ed. 1996. (Illus.). (Orig.). pap. 19.95 (*1-57732-036-0*) Datar Pub.

PCAT Exam No. 4: Annotated Answers (Pharmacy College Admission Test) David M. Tarlow. 7th ed. 1996. pap. 5.95 (*1-57732-042-5*) Datar Pub.

PCAT Exam No. 4: Pharmacy College Admission Test. David M. Tarlow. 7th ed. 1996. (Illus.). (Orig.). pap. 19.95 (*1-57732-037-9*) Datar Pub.

PCAT Exam No. 5: Annotated Answers (Pharmacy College Admission Test) David M. Tarlow. 7th ed. 1996. (Illus.). pap. 5.95 (*1-57732-043-3*) Datar Pub.

PCAT Exam No. 5: Pharmacy College Admission Test. David M. Tarlow. 7th ed. 1996. (Illus.). (Orig.). pap. 19.95 (*1-57732-038-7*) Datar Pub.

PCAT (Pharmacy College Admission Test) Practice Examination. David M. Tarlow. 1992. (Practice Examination Ser.). 40p. No. 1. pap. 16.95 (*0-931572-22-3*); No. 2. pap. 16.95 (*0-931572-23-1*); No. 3. pap. 16.95 (*0-931572-24-X*); No. 4. pap. 16.95 (*0-931572-25-8*); No. 5. pap. 16.95 (*0-931572-26-6*) Datar Pub.

PCAT (Pharmacy College Admissions Test) For Comprehensive Review. David M. Tarlow. 7th ed. 1996. (Illus.). (Orig.). pap., stu. ed. 19.95 (*1-57732-033-6*) Datar Pub.

PCAT Practice Examination: Annotated Master Answer Guide. David M. Tarlow. 1992. No. 2. 4.95 (*0-931572-48-7*); No. 3. 4.95 (*0-931572-49-5*); No. 4. 4.95 (*0-931572-50-9*); No. 5. 4.95 (*0-931572-51-7*) Datar Pub.

PCMR 16th Annual Report to the President: Citizen With Mental Retardation—Equality Under the Law. 1987. 53p. (*1-55672-026-2*) US HHS.

PCP (Phencyclidine) Historical & Current Perspectives. Ed. by E. F. Domino. 1981. LC 80-81498. (Illus.). 537p. 95.00 (*0-916182-03-7*) NPP Bks.

PCP's Guide to Occupational/Environmental Medicine. Hodgson. 1999. (Illus.). 550p. text (*1-55664-467-1*) Mosby Inc.

PCR: Clinical Diagnostics & Research. A. Rolfs. 2nd ed. 1997. 300p. pap. text 68.00 (*3-540-59432-9*) Spr-Verlag.

PCR: Protocols for Diagnosis of Human & Animal Virus Diseases. Ed. by Gholamreza Darai & Yechiel Becker. 1995. LC 95-9546. (Illus.). 448p. 140.00 (*3-540-58899-X*) Spr-Verlag.

PCR Applications in Pathology: Principles & Practice. Ed. by David S. Latchman. 1995. (Modern Methods in Pathology Ser.). (Illus.). 284p. text 55.00 (*0-19-854835-4*) OUP.

PCR-Based Diagnostics in Infectious Diseases. Ed. by Garth D. Ehrlich & Steven J. Greenberg. 1993. LC 93-28476. (Illus.). 720p. 135.00 (*0-86542-252-4*) Blackwell Sci.

PCR in Situ Hybridization: Protocols & Applications. Gerard J. Nuovo. 3rd ed. 1996. LC 96-25449. 512p. text 99.00 (*0-397-58749-X*) Lppncott W & W.

PCR Protocols. Ed. by John M. Bartlett & David Stirling. 2nd ed. 2000. (Methods in Molecular Biology Ser.). 600p. 79.50 (*0-89603-627-8*) Humana.

PCR Protocols for Emerging Infectious Diseases. Ed. by David H. Persing. 1996. 180p. spiral bd., suppl. ed. 39.95 (*1-55581-108-6*) ASM Pr.

PCR Technology: Principles & Applications for DNA Amplification. Ed. by Henry A. Erlich. 1993. (Breakthroughs in Molecular Biology Ser.). (Illus.). 256p. pap. text 40.00 (*0-19-509875-7*) OUP.

PDA International Conference on Liquid Borne Particle Inspection & Metrology: Conference Proceedings. Parenteral Drug Association Incorporated Staff. Ed. by Marcy Feldman. 1987. (Illus.). 662p. pap. text 95.00 (*0-939459-12-4*) PDA.

PDQ Embryology. Moore. 1986. 27.95 (*0-8016-3533-0*) Mosby Inc.

PDQ Epidemiology. David L. Streiner & Geoffrey R. Norman. 2nd ed. 1998. (Illus.). 160p. pap. (*1-55009-077-1*) DEKR.

PDQ Evidence-Based Principles & Practice. Ann K. McKibbon et al. 1999. (Evidence-Based Ser.). 212p. text incl. cd-rom (*1-55009-118-2*) DEKR.

PDQ Statistics. Norman & David L. Steiner. 1986. 13.95 (*0-8016-3840-2*) Mosby Inc.

***PDR: Supplement A 2002.** Medical Economics Co. Staff. 56th rev. ed. 2002. (Illus.). 300p. pap. text 37.00 (*1-56363-414-7*) Med Econ.

PDR Companion Guide 2000. Ed. by Medical Economics Staff. 54th rev. ed. 2000. (Physicians' Desk Reference Companion Guide Ser.). (Illus.). 2000p. 60.00 (*1-56363-340-X*, PDR) Med Econ.

PDR Companion Guide, 2001, Vol. 55. Medical Economics Staff. 55th rev. ed. 2001. (Physicians' Desk Reference Companion Guide Ser.). (Illus.). 1900p. 63.00 (*1-56363-380-9*) Med Econ.

PD R Drug Interactions & Side Effects Data Card 2001. Medical Economics Staff. 2000. 100.00 (*1-56712-606-5*) Med Econ.

PDR Family Encyclopedia of Medical Care. PDR Staff. 1998. 640p. mass mkt. 6.99 (*0-345-42009-8*) Ballantine Pub Grp.

PDR Family Guide Encyclopedia of Medical Care. Medical Economics Staff. rev. ed. 1997. LC 97-170. 400p. pap. 23.00 (*0-609-80069-8*, Three Riv Pr) Harmony Bks.

PDR Pocket Guide to Prescription Drugs. Ed. by PDR Staff. 2nd ed. 1997. per. 6.99 (*0-671-01454-4*) PB.

PDR Family Guide to Natural Medicines & Healing Therapies. Medical Economics Staff. Ed. by David W. Sifton. 1999. LC 99-13367. (PDR Family Guides). (Illus.). 400p. pap. 23.00 (*0-609-80071-X*, Three Riv Pr) Harmony Bks.

PDR for Herbal Medicines. Medical Economics Staff & Joerg Gruenwalt. 2nd rev. ed. 2000. (Illus.). 1200p. 59.95 (*1-56363-361-2*, PDR) Med Econ.

PDR for Herbal Medicines Datacard 2001. Medical Economics Staff. 2000. 100.00 (*1-56712-541-7*) Med Econ.

PDR for Nonprescription Drugs & Dietary Supplements 2001. Medical Economics Staff. 22nd rev. ed. 2001. (Physicians' Desk Reference for Nonprescription Drugs Ser.: Vol. 22). 400p. 54.00 (*1-56363-381-7*, PDR) Med Econ.

PDR for Nutritional Supplements: Unbiased Profiles to Help You Separate Fact from Fiction. Medical Economics Staff et al. 2001. (Illus.). 700p. 59.95 (*1-56363-364-7*, PDR) Med Econ.

***PDR for Ophthalmic Medicines 2002.** Medical Economics Co. Staff. 30th rev. ed. 2001. 230p. 61.95 (*1-56363-410-4*, PDR) Med Econ.

P
Q
R

P
Q
R

PDR Guide to Over-the-Counter Drugs. Physicians Desk Reference. 1997. LC 97-97165. (Illus.). 688p. mass mkt. 6.99 (*0-345-41716-X*, Ballantine Epiphany) Ballantine Pub Grp.

PDR Medical Dictionary. Medical Economics Staff & Williams and Wilkins Staff. 2nd rev. ed. 2000. 2100p. 50.00 (*1-56363-338-8*, PDR) Med Econ.

PDR Nurse's Dictionary. 1996. LC 97-156486. 1900p. pap. text 15.00 (*1-56363-213-6*) Med Econ.

***PDR Nurse's Drug Handbook, 2002.** Medical Economics Staff et al. rev. ed. 2001. (Physicians' Desk Reference Nurse's Handbook Ser.). 1493p. pap. text 32.95 (*0-7668-3546-4*) Delmar.

PDR Nurses Drug Handbook, 2000. Ed. by Medical Economics Staff. 6th ed. 1999. (Physicians' Desk Reference Nurse's Handbook Ser.). 1536p. (C). pap. 29.95 (*0-7668-1086-0*) Thomson Learn.

PDR Nurses Handbook. George R. Spratto & Adrienne L. Woods. 4th ed. 1998. 1300p. (C). pap. text 29.95 (*0-7668-0913-7*) Delmar.

PDR Nurses Handbook Network CD-ROM 1999 Edition. George R. Spratto et al. 1998. 831.95 incl. cd-rom (*0-7668-0697-9*) Delmar.

***PDR Pharmacopoeia Pocket Dosing Guide.** Medical Economics Co. Staff. 2nd ed. 2001. pap. 99.50 (*1-56363-422-8*, PDR) Med Econ.

***PDR Pharmacopoeia Pocket Dosing Guide, 2002.** 2nd ed. 2001. 250p. pap. 9.95 (*1-56363-409-0*, PDR) Med Econ.

PDR Pharmacopoeia, Pocket Edition. Medical Economics Staff. 2000. (Illus.). 250p. pap. 10.00 (*1-56363-365-5*, PDR) Med Econ.

PDR Pocket Guide to Prescription Drugs. Medical Economics Staff. 1996. LC 96-213121. (TTL Ser.). pap. 6.99 (*0-671-52520-4*) PB.

PDR Pocket Guide to Prescription Drugs. Ed. by Physicians' Desk Reference Staff. 3rd rev. ed. 1998. (Illus.). 1480p. per. 6.99 (*0-671-02585-6*) PB.

PDR Pocket Guide to Prescription Drugs. Medical Economics Staff. 4th rev. ed. 2000. LC 00-708897. (Blackwell Anthologies Ser.). (Illus.). 1568p. per. 6.99 (*0-671-78643-1*, Pocket Books) PB.

***PDR Pocket Guide to Prescription Drugs.** Medical Economics Co. Staff. 5th ed. 2002. (Illus.). 1520p. reprint ed. mass mkt. 6.99 (*0-7434-3795-0*) PB.

PDR Supplement A. Medical Economics Staff. (Illus.). 300p. 54th rev. ed. 2000. pap. 30.00 (*1-56363-342-6*, PDR); Vol. 55. 55th rev. ed. 2001. pap. 35.00 (*1-56363-377-9*) Med Econ.

PDR Supplement B, Vol. 55. Medical Economics Staff. 55th rev. ed. 2001. (Illus.). 300p. pap. 35.00 (*1-56363-378-7*) Med Econ.

PDR Supplements, 2000: Combined Supplements A & B. Ed. by Medical Economics Staff. 54th rev. ed. 2000. (Physicians' Desk Reference Supplements A & B Ser.). (Illus.). 300p. 30.00 (*1-56363-344-2*, PDR) Med Econ.

PDR Supplements, 2001 Vol. 55: Combined Supps A & B. Medical Economics Staff. 55th rev. ed. 2001. (Physicians' Desk Reference Supplements A & B Ser.). (Illus.). 300p. pap. 35.00 (*1-56363-379-5*, PDR) Med Econ.

***PDR Supplements 2002: Supplement A.** Medical Economics Co. Staff. 56th rev. ed. 2002. 400p. pap. text 36.95 (*1-56363-413-9*, PDR) Med Econ.

PDR 3-Pack Configuration, 2001, Vol. 55. Medical Economics Staff. 55th rev. ed. 2000. (*1-56363-394-9*) Med Econ.

***PDR 2002: 3-Pack Configuration.** Ed. by Medical Economics Co. Staff. 2001. (Physicians' Desk Reference Ser.). (*1-56363-424-4*) Med Econ.

Peace after Abortion. Ava Torre-Bueno. 2nd rev. ed. 1997. LC 96-72071. 192p. (Orig.). pap. 9.95 (*0-9651383-1-3*) Pimpernel Pr.

Peace, Love & Healing: Bodymind Communication & the Path to Self-Healing: An Exploration. Bernie S. Siegel. 1998. LC 89-82587. (Illus.). 304p. pap. 14.00 (*0-06-091705-9*, Perennial) HarperTrade.

Peace, War, & Mental Health: Couples Therapists Look at the Dynamics. Ed. by Barbara J. Brothers. 1993. LC 93-18004. (Journal of Couples Therapy Ser.: Vol. 3, No. 4). (Illus.). 181p. lib. bdg. 39.95 (*1-56024-437-2*) Haworth Pr.

Peak Flow Meter Book: A Guide for People with Asthma. Nancy J. Sander & Guillermo R. Mendoza. Ed. by Martha White. rev. ed. 1995. (Illus.). 28p. pap. text 5.95 (*1-885543-01-8*) Allergy & Asthma.

Peak-Performance Living: Easy, Drug-Free Ways to Alter Your Own Brain Chemistry & Achieve Optimal Health. Joel C. Robertson & Tom Monte. 1997. LC 95-30971. (Illus.). 256p. pap. 13.00 (*0-06-251234-X*) Harper SF.

Peaks of Medical History. Charles L. Dana. 2nd ed. LC 75-23703. (Illus.). reprint ed. 55.00 (*0-404-13255-3*) AMS Pr.

Peanut Allergy Answer Book. Michael Young. 2000. 128p. pap. 8.95 (*1-86204-823-1*) Element MA.

Pearl Beyond Price: Integration of Personality into Being: an Object Relations Approach. A. H. Almaas. 2000. LC 00-40033. (Diamond Mind Ser.: Bk. 2). 506p. pap. 29.95 (*0-936713-02-X*) Diamond Bks CA.

Pearl Dictionary. Matthew Kurlan. 4th ed. 1999. LC 99-213905. (Illus.). 380p. ring bd. 27.00 (*0-9668187-1-7*) Pocket Brain.

Pearls & Pitfalls in Electrocardiography: Pithy Practical Pointers. Henry J. Marriott. 2nd ed. 1997. LC 97-13639. (*0-683-03017-5*) Lppncott W & W.

Pearls & Pitfalls in Electrocardiography: Pithy Practical Points. Henry J. Marriott. 1990. LC 90-5594. (Illus.). 157p. pap. text 29.00 (*0-8121-1334-9*) Lppncott W & W.

Pearls & Pitfalls in Electrocardiology. Henry J. Marriott. 2nd ed. 1997. (Illus.). 198p. pap. text 39.95 (*0-683-30170-5*) Lppncott W & W.

Pearls from a Pediatric Practice I. William Wadlington & Clifton K. Meador. 1998. 160p. pap. 17.95 (*1-56053-267-X*) Hanley & Belfus.

Pedi-Wheel: Pediatric Emergency Pocket Reference. Joseph Rose. 1995. (Illus.). 2p. 9.95 (*0-9658618-0-5*) EMS Advan.

Pedi-Wheel First Responder: Pediatric Emergency Pocket Reference. Joe Rose. 1997. (Illus.). 2p. 9.95 (*0-9658618-1-3*) EMS Advan.

Pediatric Acute Care Handbook. Mary Lieh-Lai. 1995. LC 95-9591. 258p. pap. text 34.95 (*0-316-09306-8*, Little Brwn Med Div) Lppncott W & W.

Pediatric Adapted Motor Development & Exercise: An Innovative Multisystem Approach for Professionals & Families. Jo E. Cowden et al. 1998. LC 97-46392. (Illus.). 346p. text 69.95 (*0-398-06848-8*) C C Thomas.

Pediatric Advanced Life Support. Barbara Aehlert. rev. ed. 1996. (Illus.). 240p. (C). (gr. 13). pap. text, stu. ed. 13.00 (*0-8151-1251-3*, 29598) Mosby Inc.

Pediatric Advanced Life Support, 1997-99. 1997. (Emergency Cardiovascular Care Programs Ser.). (Illus.). 198p. pap., tchr. ed. 25.00 (*0-87493-628-4*) Am Heart.

Pediatric Advanced Life Support, 1997-99. American Academy of Pediatrics Staff & American Heart Association Staff. Ed. by Leon Chameides & Mary Fran Hazinski. 1997. LC 99-179983. (Emergency Cardiovascular Care Programs Ser.). (Illus.). 150p. pap. 25.00 (*0-87493-619-5*) Am Heart.

Pediatric AIDS: The Challenge of HIV Infection in Infants, Children & Adolescents. Philip A. Pizzo & Catherine M. Wilfert. 2nd ed. 1994. (Illus.). 1088p. 99.00 (*0-683-06895-4*) Lppncott W & W.

Pediatric AIDS: The Challenge of HIV Infection in Infants, Children & Adolescents. Ed. by Philip A. Pizzo & Catherine M. Wilfert. 3rd ed. 1998. LC 98-6398. 1,000p. 110.00 (*0-683-30399-6*) Lppncott W & W.

Pediatric Airway. Borland. 1992. 39.00 (*0-316-10276-8*, Little Brwn Med Div) Lppncott W & W.

Pediatric Airway. Othersen. 1991. (Illus.). 256p. text 110.00 (*0-7216-2778-1*) Saunders.

Pediatric Airway: An Interdisciplinary Approach. Ed. by Charles M. Myer et al. 1994. (Illus.). 384p. text 89.00 (*0-397-51415-8*) Lppncott W & W.

***Pediatric Anaerobic Infections: Diagnosis & Management.** Brook. 3rd ed. 2001. LC 2001-53338. (Infectious Disease & Therapy Ser.: Vol. 29). (*0-8247-0615-3*) Dekker.

Pediatric Anaesthesia & Critical Care in the District Hospital. N. S. Norton & Jane M. Peutrell. 2000. (Illus.). 224p. pap. 50.00 (*0-7506-4302-1*) Buttrwrth-Heinemann.

Pediatric & Adolescent AIDS. Scott W. Henggler. 1992. 160p. (C). pap. 31.95 (*0-8039-3983-3*, 3292) Sage.

Pediatric & Adolescent Endocrinology, Vol. 10-11. 1983. (Illus.). xxvi, 458p. 235.00 (*3-8055-3681-X*) S Karger.

Pediatric & Adolescent Gynecology. Susan Pokorny. 1995. (Current Topics in Obstetrics & Gynecology Ser.). (Illus.). 160p. (*0-412-99471-2*) E A GBR. *Dist:* OUP.

Pediatric & Adolescent Gynecology. Ed. by Joseph S. Sanfilippo et al. 1993. LC 93-162. (Illus.). 744p. text 115.00 (*0-7216-3971-2*) Saunders.

Pediatric & Adolescent Gynecology. Sue Ellen Koehler Carpenter & John A. Rock. 2nd ed. 2000. LC 00-36096. 544p. text 99.00 (*0-7817-1781-7*) Lppncott W & W.

Pediatric & Adolescent Gynecology. S. Jean Emans & Donald P. Goldstein. 2nd ed. 1982. 42.50 (*0-316-23402-8*, Little Brwn Med Div) Lppncott W & W.

***Pediatric & Adolescent Gynecology.** Joseph S. Sanfilippo. 2nd ed. 2001. LC 00-58859. (Illus.). 608p. (*0-7216-8346-0*) Saunders.

Pediatric & Adolescent Gynecology. S. Jean Herriot Emans et al. 4th ed. 1997. LC 97-21996. (Illus.). 912p. pap. text 79.95 (*0-316-23395-1*, Little Brwn Med Div) Lppncott W & W.

Pediatric & Adolescent Obstetrics & Gynecology. Ed. by Joseph S. Sanfilippo & J. Patrick Lavery. 1985. (Clinical Perspectives in Obstetrics & Gynecology Ser.). (Illus.). 362p. 89.95 (*0-387-96073-2*) Spr-Verlag.

Pediatric & Adolescent Sports Medicine. Lyle J. Micheli. 1984. 218p. 62.95 (*0-316-56949-6*, Little Brwn Med Div) Lppncott W & W.

Pediatric & Adolescent Sports Medicine, Vol. 3. Ed. by Carl L. Stanitski et al. 1993. (Illus.). 560p. text 145.00 (*0-7216-3216-5*) Saunders.

Pediatric & Adult Electroencephalography. Michael R. Sperling & Martha J. Morrell. 1999. LC 93-27907. (Atlas of Electroencephalography Ser.: Vol. 2). 268p. pap. 102.00 (*0-444-81269-5*) Elsevier.

Pediatric & Fundamental Eletrocardiography. Ed. by Jerome Liebman et al. 1987. (Developments in Cardiovascular Medicine Ser.). text 242.00 (*0-89838-815-5*) Kluwer Academic.

Pediatric & Neonatal Critical Care Certification Review. M. K. Gaedeke. 1995. (Illus.). 560p. (C). (gr. 13). pap. text 36.95 (*0-8151-3455-X*, 27882) Mosby Inc.

Pediatric & Neonatal Tests & Procedures. H. William Taeusch et al. 1995. (Illus.). 560p. text 98.00 (*0-7216-5159-3*) Saunders.

Pediatric & Obstetrical Anesthesia. Ed. by Theodore H. Stanley & Patricia G. Schafer. 1995. LC 94-44630. (DCCA Ser.: Vol. 30). 384p. (C). text 144.00 (*0-7923-3346-2*) Kluwer Academic.

Pediatric & Post Partum Home Health Nursing: Assessment & Care Planning. Kathryn A. Melson & Maries S. Jaffe. 1996. LC 96-25620. (Illus.). 496p. (C). (gr. 13). spiral bd. 29.95 (*0-8151-4876-3*, 25760) Mosby Inc.

Pediatric & Reconstructive Urologic Surgery. John Libertino. 3rd ed. 1997. (Illus.). 800p. (C). (gr. 13). text 165.00 (*0-8016-7802-1*, 07802) Mosby Inc.

Pediatric Andrology. Ed. by S. J. Kogan & E. S. Hafez. 1981. 220p. text 220.00 (*90-247-2407-4*) Kluwer Academic.

Pediatric Anesthesia. George A. Gregory. 2001. LC 00-65825. (Illus.). 1100p. text Price not set. (*0-443-06561-6*) Church.

Pediatric Anesthesia. Ed. by George A. Gregory. 3rd ed. 1994. LC 94-2785. text (*0-443-08904-3*) Church.

Pediatric Anesthesia: A Pocket Companion. Edmond C. Bloch. 1994. LC 94-30840. 280p. 32.50 (*0-7506-9602-8*) Buttrwrth-Heinemann.

Pediatric Anesthesia: A Quick Pocket Reference. Edmond C. Bloch & Brian Ginsberg. 2nd ed. 1999. LC 99-19066. 365p. pap. text 34.99 (*0-7506-7142-4*) Buttrwrth-Heinemann.

Pediatric Anesthesia Handbook. Ed. by Charlotte Bell et al. 2nd ed. 1996. (Illus.). 720p. (C). (gr. 13). pap. text 44.95 (*0-8151-0659-9*, 25695) Mosby Inc.

Pediatric Anesthesia Handbook. Charlotte Bell et al. 2nd ed. 1997. (Illus.). 720p. pap. (*84-8174-307-0*) Mosby-Doyma Libros ESP. *Dist:* Mosby Inc.

Pediatric Applications of Transcranial Doppler Sonography. H. Bode. 1988. (Illus.). 150p. 49.95 (*0-387-82073-6*) Spr-Verlag.

Pediatric Associate, P.C. A Medical Office Simulation. Humphrey. 3rd ed. 1996. (KF -Office Education Ser.). 56p. stu. ed. 30.95 (*0-538-65376-0*) S-W Thomson.

Pediatric Asthma. H. William Kelly. Ed. by Shirley J. Murphy. 1999. LC 98-50991. (Lung Biology in Health & Disease Ser.). (Illus.). 608p. text 225.00 (*0-8247-0208-5*) Dekker.

Pediatric Basic Life Support, 1997-99. 1997. (Emergency Cardiovascular Care Programs Ser.). (Illus.). 115p. pap. 5.00 (*0-87493-622-5*); 58p. pap., tchr. ed. 25.00 (*0-87493-630-6*) Am Heart.

Pediatric Basic Life Support Plus, 1997-99: Emergency Cardiovascular Care Programs. 1998. 118p. pap. 7.50 (*0-87493-686-1*) Am Heart.

Pediatric Basic Trauma Life Support. Ann Marie Dietrich & Steven Shaner. Ed. by American College of Emergency Physicians Staff. 1995. (Illus.). (C). pap. text 24.95 (*0-9647418-0-6*) Basic Trauma.

Pediatric Basic Trauma Life Support Update. Ann Marie Dietrich & Steven Shaner. Ed. by John Campbell. 1998. (Illus.). (C). pap. text 24.95 (*0-9647418-1-4*) Basic Trauma.

Pediatric Behavioral Medicine. Ed. by Ben J. Williams et al. 1981. LC 81-5875. 277p. 62.95 (*0-275-90742-2*, C0742, Praeger Pubs) Greenwood.

Pediatric Behavioral Neurology. Ed. by Yitzchak Frank. 1996. LC 95-36119. 432p. 149.95 (*0-8493-2458-0*, 2458) CRC Pr.

Pediatric Bibliography. A. G. Mitchell. 1941. (SRCD M Ser.: Vol. 6, No. 1). 25.00 (*0-527-01517-2*) Periodicals Srv.

Pediatric Body CT. A. Daneman. 1986. (Illus.). 374p. 377.00 (*0-387-16217-8*) Spr-Verlag.

Pediatric Body CT. Ed. by Marilyn J. Siegel. 1987. (Contemporary Issues in Computed Tomography Ser.: Vol. 10). (Illus.). 426p. text (*0-443-08533-1*) Church.

Pediatric Bone Imaging: A Practical Approach. Soroosh Mahboubi. 1989. 120.00 (*0-316-54381-0*, Little Brwn Med Div) Lppncott W & W.

Pediatric Brain Death & Organ/Tissue Retrieval: Medical, Ethical & Legal Aspects. H. H. Kaufman. 1989. (Illus.). 384p. (C). text 75.00 (*0-306-42973-X*, Kluwer Plenum) Kluwer Academic.

Pediatric Brain Injury. Sellars. 1998. (C). pap. text 54.50 (*0-12-784582-8*) Acad Pr.

Pediatric Brain Injury: The Special Case of the Very Young Child. Carole W. Sellars et al. 1997. LC 97-3431. pap. 29.50 (*1-882855-55-8*) HDI Pubs.

Pediatric Cancer Sourcebook: Basic Consumer Health Information about Cancers in Children. Ed. by Edward Prucha. 1999. LC 99-41613. (Health Reference Ser.). (Illus.). xii, 587p. lib. bdg. 78.00 (*0-7808-0245-4*) Omnigraphics Inc.

Pediatric Cardiac Anesthesia. Lake. 3rd ed. 1998. LC 97-11876. 698p. (C). text 150.00 (*0-8385-7680-X*, A-7680-0) McGraw-Hill Educ Grp.

Pediatric Cardiac Imaging. William F. Friedman & Charles B. Higgins. 1984. (Illus.). 279p. text 82.00 (*0-7216-1287-3*) Saunders.

Pediatric Cardiac Intensive Care. Anthony C. Chang et al. 1998. LC 97-39558. (Illus.). 587p. 129.00 (*0-683-01508-7*) Lppncott W & W.

Pediatric Cardiac Pacing. Ed. by Paul C. Gillette & Vicki L. Zeigler. 1995. LC 95-12159. (Illus.). 264p. 45.00 (*0-87993-621-5*) Futura Pub.

Pediatric Cardiac Surgery. 2002. (C). 215.00 (*0-8385-8177-3*) Appleton & Lange.

Pediatric Cardiac Surgery. Ross Ungerleider & James Jaggers. 2001. (Vademecum Ser.). spiral bd. 45.00 (*1-57059-576-3*) Landes Bioscience.

Pediatric Cardiac Surgery: Current Issues. Ed. by Marshall L. Jacobs & William I. Norwood. 1992. (Illus.). 264p. text 125.00 (*0-7506-9061-5*) Buttrwrth-Heinemann.

Pediatric Cardiology. E. F. Doyle et al. 1985. (Illus.). I, 1340p. 198.00 (*0-387-96204-2*) Spr-Verlag.

Pediatric Cardiology. Karoly Lozsadi & Vilmos Kornyei. 2000. (Illus.). 966p. (*963-05-7702-X*) Akade Kiado HUN. *Dist:* Intl Spec Bk.

Pediatric Cardiology. Ed. by Milan Samanek. 1992. (Illus.). 464p. (*0-08-036860-3*) PPI GBR. *Dist:* McGraw.

Pediatric Cardiology. Anderson. 2nd ed. 2000. (Illus.). 1284p. text 375.00 (*0-443-07990-0*) Saunders.

Pediatric Cardiology: A Problem Oriented Approach. Ed. by Ira H. Gessner & Benjamin E. Victorica. 1993. LC 92-48475. (Illus.). 352p. text 58.00 (*0-7216-4564-X*) Saunders.

Pediatric Cardiology: An Introduction. N. Archer & M. Burch. 1999. (Illus.). 244p. (*0-412-73450-8*) E A GBR. *Dist:* OUP.

Pediatric Cardiology: Its Current Practice. Ed. by Timothy J. Bricker & Dan G. McNamara. 1988. (Illus.). 192p. (C). text 49.50 (*0-683-13007-2*) Lppncott W & W.

Pediatric Cardiology for Practitioners. Myung K. Park. 3rd ed. 1995. (Illus.). 560p. (C). (gr. 13). text 69.95 (*0-8151-6632-X*, 24218) Mosby Inc.

Pediatric Cardiology Handbook. Allan H. Rees et al. 1987. (Illus.). 194p. pap. 23.75 (*0-87527-348-3*) Green.

Pediatric Cardiology Handbook. Myung K. Park. 2nd ed. 1996. (Illus.). 368p. (C). (gr. 13). pap. text 29.95 (*0-8151-9005-0*, 29094) Mosby Inc.

Pediatric Cardiology Handbook. Myung K. Park. 2nd ed. 1997. (Illus.). 368p. pap. (*84-8174-429-8*) Mosby-Doyma Libros ESP. *Dist:* Mosby Inc.

Pediatric Cardiopulmonary Transplantation. Ed. by Kenneth L. Franco. 1997. LC 96-52001. (Illus.). 416p. 89.00 (*0-87993-397-6*) Futura Pub.

Pediatric Cardiovascular Imaging. Tonken. 1991. (Illus.). 320p. text 120.00 (*0-7216-3665-9*) Saunders.

Pediatric Cardiovascular Medicine. Moller. 1999. text 115.00 (*0-443-07677-4*) Saunders.

Pediatric Care of the ICN Graduate. Roberta A. Ballard. 1988. (Illus.). 368p. text 75.00 (*0-7216-1404-3*) Saunders.

Pediatric Care Planning. Speer. 3rd ed. 1998. LC 98-37811. 336p. pap. 39.95 (*0-87434-943-5*) Springhouse Corp.

Pediatric Care Plans. Sharon E. Axton & Terry Fugate. 1992. LC 92-49364. 496p. (C). spiral bd. 38.60 (*0-8053-0905-5*) Addison-Wesley.

Pediatric CheckMate. Angela G. Clarkson & Anne M. Larson. 3rd rev. ed. 2000. (Critical Care CheckMate Ser.). 112p. vinyl bd. (*0-9700484-8-3*) NNCC.

Pediatric Chiropractic. Claudia A. Anrig & Gregory Plaugher. 1997. LC 97-26950. (*1-68301-361-1*) Lppncott W & W.

Pediatric Chiropractic. Claudia Anrig & Gregory Plaugher. 1998. LC 97-26950. 848p. 89.00 (*0-683-00136-1*) Lppncott W & W.

Pediatric Chiropractic Practice Management. Jennifer B. Peet & Palmer M. Peet. 2nd ed. 1993. (Illus.). 187p. (C). 45.00 (*0-9638642-0-3*) Baby Adjusters.

Pediatric Clinical Advisor. Lynn Garfunkel. 2000. text 54.95 (*0-323-01049-0*) Mosby Inc.

Pediatric Clinical Gastroenterology. Ed. by Claude C. Roy et al. 4th ed. 1995. LC 94-12633. (Illus.). 960p. (C). (gr. 13). text 120.00 (*0-8151-7406-3*, 24171) Mosby Inc.

Pediatric Clinical Gastroenterology. Claude C. Roy. 4th ed. 1991. (Illus.). 970p. 89.95 (*0-8016-6216-8*) Mosby Inc.

Pediatric Clinical Skills. Richard B. Goldbloom. 2nd ed. 1997. LC 96-53606. pap. text (*0-443-07927-7*) Church.

Pediatric Companion. Harjit Singh. 1996. pap. (*81-85017-79-4*) Interprint IND. *Dist:* St Mut.

Pediatric Compliance: A Guide for the Primary Care Physician. Edward R. Christopherson. 1994. LC 93-41063. (Critical Issues in Developmental & Behavioral Pediatrics Ser.). (Illus.). 492p. (C). text 60.00 (*0-306-44454-2*, Kluwer Plenum) Kluwer Academic.

Pediatric Conscious Sedation Pt. I: Agents & Procedures, Package. Thomas J. Abramo. 1996. 36p. (*0-8151-0805-2*) Mosby Inc.

Pediatric Conscious Sedation Pt. II: Specific Procedures: Case Studies, Package. Thomas J. Abramo. 1996. 48p. (*0-8151-0808-7*) Mosby Inc.

Pediatric Consultation Liaison Psychiatry. Ed. by Charles E. Hollingsworth. 1983. LC 82-19744. 294p. text 29.95 (*0-88331-173-9*) R B Luce.

Pediatric Cranial MRI: An Atlas of Normal Development. John H. Bisese & Ay-Ming Wang. 1994. LC 93-47186. (Illus.). 183p. 192.00 (*0-387-94218-1*) Spr-Verlag.

Pediatric Critical Care. Bradley Fuhrman & Jerry J. Zimmerman. 2nd ed. 1997. LC 98-148809. (Illus.). 1520p. (C). (gr. 13). text 169.00 (*0-8151-2536-4*, 30772) Mosby Inc.

Pediatric Critical Care Nursing. Janis B. Smith. 1989. LC 83-10218. (Critical Care Nursing Ser.). (Illus.). 500p. (Orig.). (C). pap. text 36.95 (*0-8273-4374-4*) Delmar.

Pediatric Cytopathology. Kim Geissinger. 1995. (Illus.). 365p. 90.00 (*0-89189-378-4*) Am Soc Clinical.

Pediatric Day Case Surgery. Ed. by N. S. Morton & P. A. Raine. 1994. (Illus.). 130p. text 69.50 (*0-19-262256-0*) OUP.

Pediatric Decision Making. Al Pomeranz et al. 2000. LC 2001-32080. (Illus.). 415p. (C). pap. text (*0-7216-8246-4*) Saunders.

Pediatric Decision Making. Stephen Berman. 3rd ed. 1996. (Illus.). 704p. (C). (gr. 13). text 76.95 (*0-8151-0715-3*, 27677) Mosby Inc.

Pediatric Dental Care in CHIP & Medicaid: Paying for What Kids Need, Getting Value for State Payments. Frwd. by John M. Colmers et al. 1999. LC 00-708546. (Illus.). xi, 23p. pap. (*1-887748-28-8*) Milbank Memorial.

Pediatric Dentistry. Ed. by Angus C. Cameron & Richard P. Widmer. 1997. text 44.95 (*0-7234-3068-3*) Mosby Inc.

***Pediatric Dentistry: A Clinical Approach.** Gvran Koch. 2001. (Illus.). 484p. 112.00 (*87-16-12271-2*) Blackwell Sci.

Pediatric Dentistry: Infancy Through Adolescence. Ed. by James R. Pinkham et al. 2nd ed. 1993. LC 92-49086. (Illus.). 576p. text 70.00 (*0-7216-4695-6*) Saunders.

Pediatric Dentistry: Infancy Through Adolescence. J. R. Pinkham et al. Ed. by Judy Fletcher. 3rd ed. 1999. LC 99-24326. (Illus.). 670p. (C). text (*0-7216-8238-3*) Saunders.

Pediatric Dermatology. Bernard A. Cohen. 1993. LC 92-49298. (gr. 13). (*1-56375-019-8*) Gower-Mosby.

Pediatric Dermatology. Bernard Cohen. 2nd ed. 1999. LC 98-45704. (*0-7234-3010-1*) Mosby Inc.

Pediatric Dermatology Ed. by Lawrence A. Schachner & Ronald C. Hansen. 2nd ed. 1995. 1511p. text (*0-443-08921-3*); Set. 1988. (Illus.). 1674p. text (*0-443-08432-7*) Church.

Pediatric Dermatology - The World's Reality in the Children's Skin: Proceedings of the 7th International Congress of Pediatric Dermatology, Buenos Aires, September 27-October 1, 1994. International Congress of Pediatric Dermatology St. Ed. by Adrian-Martin Pierini et al. 1995. LC 95-37760. (International Congress Ser.: No. 1073). 372p. 191.50 (*0-444-81917-7*) Elsevier.

Pediatric Dermatology & Dermatopathology. Ruggero Caputo et al. 1995. (Illus.). Vol. 3. 516p. 165.00 (*0-683-01437-4*); Vol. 4. 476p. 165.00 (*0-683-01438-2*) Lppncott W & W.

Pediatric Dermatology & Dermatopathology: A Text & Atlas. Ruggero Caputo et al. LC 88-36885. (Illus.). 391p. (*0-8121-1166-4*); (*0-8121-1314-4*);IV. (*0-8121-1316-0*) Lppncott W & W.

Pediatric Dermatology & Internal Medicine: Internal Medicine & External Medicine, Proceedings. Congress of Pediatric Dermatology, 2nd, Mexico Cit. Ed. by Ramon Ruiz-Maldonado. 1978. (Modern Problems in Pediatrics Ser.: Vol. 20). (Illus.). 85.25 (*3-8055-2703-9*) S Karger.

Pediatric Dermatopathology: Clinical & Pathologic Correlations. Bernett L. Johnson et al. 1994. (Illus.). 334p. text (*0-7506-9264-2*) E A GBR. *Dist:* OUP.

Pediatric Diagnosis. Green. 6th ed. 1998. (C). text 6.25 (*0-8089-2086-3*, Grune & Strat) Harcrt Hlth Sci Grp.

Pediatric Diagnosis: Intrepretation of Symptoms & Signs in Children & Adolescent. Morris Green. Ed. by Judy Fletcher. 6th ed. 1998. LC 97-33312. (Illus.). 464p. (C). text 62.00 (*0-7216-7284-1*) Saunders.

Pediatric Disease (Fourth Series) Test & Syllabus. Marilyn J. Siegel et al. 1993. (Professional Self-Evaluation & Continuing Education Program Ser.: Vol. 35). (Illus.). 800p. 220.00 (*1-55903-035-6*) Am Coll Radiology.

Pediatric Disease (Third Series) Test & Syllabus. Thomas E. Sumner et al. 1989. (Professional Self-Evaluation & Continuing Education Program Ser.: Vol. 26). (Illus.). 800p. (C). 165.00 (*1-55903-026-7*) Am Coll Radiology.

Pediatric Disorders of Regulation in Affect & Behavior: A Therapist's Guide to Assessment & Treatment. Georgia A. Degangi. 2000. LC 00-101592. (Practical Resources for the Mental Health Professional Ser.). (Illus.). xiv, 371p. pap. 49.95 (*0-12-208770-4*) Acad Pr.

Pediatric Drug Formulations. Milap C. Nahata & Thomas F. Hipple. 3rd ed. 1997. LC 97-22898. xvi, 118p. (Orig.). pap. text 31.95 (*0-929375-19-X*) H W Bks.

Pediatric Drug Handbook. William E. Benitz & Davis S. Tatro. 3rd ed. 1995. LC 95-6862. (Illus.). 688p. (C). (gr. 13). pap. text 34.95 (*0-8151-0665-3*, 24727) Mosby Inc.

Pediatric Drug Reference: Current Clinical Strategies. Jane Gennrich. 1996. 80p. pap. 8.75 (*1-881528-22-7*) Current Clin Strat.

Pediatric Drugs & Nursing Implications. Ruth M. Bindler & Linda Berner Howry. 2nd rev. ed. 1996. LC 96-18530. 640p. (C). spiral bd. 57.00 (*0-8385-8085-8*, A8085-1) P-H.

Pediatric Drugs & Nursing Intervention. Helen Russell. 1979. (Illus.). text 20.95 (*0-07-054298-8*) McGraw.

Pediatric Dypshagia: Assessment & Intervention Considerations for Children & Young Adults. Joan C. Arvedson et al. 1998. 157p. 72.00 incl. audio (*1-58041-021-9*, 0112156) Am Speech Lang Hearing.

Pediatric Dysphagia: Management Challenges for the School-Based Speech-Language Pathologist. Joan C. Arvedson & Brian T. Rogers. 1998. 110.00 incl. VHS (*1-58041-018-9*, 0112094) Am Speech Lang Hearing.

Pediatric Dysphagia Resource Guide. Kelly Hall. 2000. LC 00-58847. 200p. pap. 49.95 (*0-7693-0063-4*) Singular Publishing.

Pediatric Echocardiographers Pocket Reference. Terry Reynolds. Ed. by Yeng Pan & Patricia Dubovec. 1999. (Illus.). 250p. 64.95 (*0-9635767-7-1*) AZ Heart Inst.

Pediatric Echocardiography. David T. Linker. 1998. LC 00-64372. (Illus.). xiv, 203p. text (*0-443-07640-5*) Church.

Pediatric Echocardiography. Norman H. Silverman. 1993. (Illus.). 640p. text 159.00 (*0-683-07713-9*) Lppncott W & W.

Pediatric Education for Prehospital Professionals. M. S. Aapro & AAP Staff. 2000. (Illus.). 360p. (C). pap. text 36.95 (*0-7637-1219-1*, 1219-1) Jones & Bartlett.

Pediatric EEG. American Journal of END Technology Staff. 1998. (Illus.). 267p. spiral bd. 28.00 (*1-57797-009-8*) ASET.

Pediatric Emergencies. Ed. by Stephen Ludwig. 1985. (Clinics in Emergency Medicine Ser.: Vol. 7). (Illus.). 266p. text (*0-443-08303-7*) Church.

Pediatric Emergencies: A Manual for Prehospital Care Providers. Pratsch. Ed. by Martin Eichelberger. 2nd ed. 1997. LC 97-6025. 272p. pap. text 60.00 (*0-8359-5123-5*) P-H.

Pediatric Emergency Management: Guidelines for Rapid Diagnosis. Ed. by Stanley Cohen. 1982. (Illus.). 416p. (C). text 32.95 (*0-87619-924-4*) P-H.

Pediatric Emergency Medicine. Earl J. Reisdorff et al. 1992. (Illus.). 1190p. text 164.00 (*0-7216-3281-5*) Saunders.

Pediatric Emergency Medicine: A Comprehensive Study Guide. Ed. by Gary R. Strange et al. 1995. LC 95-7448. (Illus.). 768p. pap. 69.00 (*0-07-062007-5*) McGraw-Hill Prof.

Pediatric Emergency Medicine: Companion Handbook. Ed. by Gary Strange et al. 1998. LC 98-21037. (Illus.). 976p. pap. 39.00 (*0-07-062008-3*) McGraw-Hill Prof.

Pediatric Emergency Medicine: Concepts & Clinical Practice. Roger M. Barkinq. 2nd ed. 1996. LC 97-106461. (Illus.). 1328p. (C). (gr. 13). text 169.00 (*0-8151-1002-2*, 29256) Mosby Inc.

Pediatric Emergency Medicine: Self-Assessment & Review. David H. Rubin & Roger M. Barkin. 2nd ed. 1998. LC 98-6926. 29.95 (*1-55664-453-1*) Mosby Inc.

Pediatric Emergency Medicine Package. Roger M. Barkin & Peter Rosen. 1997. 275.00 (*0-8151-2125-3*) Mosby Inc.

Pediatric Emergency Medicine Pearls of Wisdom: Over 3500 Questions. Turnstall Smith et al. 1999. (Pearls of Wisdom Ser.). pap. (*1-890369-14-4*) Boston Medical.

Pediatric Emergency Nursing. Susan J. Kelley. 2nd ed. 1995. LC 93-41701. (Illus.). 571p. (C). pap. text 64.95 (*0-8385-7705-9*, A7705-5, Apple Lange Med) McGraw.

Pediatric Emergency Nursing. Susan J. Kelley. 1984. (C). pap. text 27.50 (*0-8359-5478-1*) P-H.

Pediatric Emergency Nursing Manual. Ed. by Deborah Henderson & Dena Brownstein. 1994. (Illus.). 352p. (C). pap. text 49.95 (*0-8261-8330-1*) Springer Pub.

Pediatric Emergency Nursing Procedures. Lisa Marie Bernardo. 1992. (Nursing-Health Science Ser.). (Illus.). (C). pap. text 46.95 (*0-86720-330-7*, 330-7) Jones & Bartlett.

Pediatric Endocrine Disorders. Wales. 1995. text 92.95 (*0-7234-2137-4*) Mosby Inc.

Pediatric Endocrinology. 1986. (Journal: Vol. 22, No. 1-2, 1985). (Illus.). 128p. pap. 102.75 (*3-8055-4415-4*) S Karger.

Pediatric Endocrinology. Maria I. New. Ed. by C. Pintor et al. 1993. (Illus.). 256p. 242.00 (*0-387-54321-X*) Spr-Verlag.

Pediatric Endocrinology. Mark A. Sperling. Ed. by Lisette Bralow & Judy Fletcher. 1996. LC 95-37080. 608p. text 95.00 (*0-7216-5522-X*) Saunders.

Pediatric Endocrinology: A Clinical Guide. Ed. by Fima Lifshitz. 3rd exp. rev. ed. 1995. (Clinical Pediatrics Ser.: Vol. 8). (Illus.). 984p. text 235.00 (*0-8247-9369-2*) Dekker.

Pediatric Endocrinology: An Illustrated Reference. Warne & Crock. 1998. (Illus.). 256p. pap. 230.00 (*0-412-58560-X*, Chap & Hall NY) Chapman & Hall.

Pediatric Endocrinology: Physiology, Pathophysiolgy & Clinical Aspects. Ed. by Jean Bertrand et al. 2nd ed. 1993. LC 92-49159. (Illus.). 768p. 129.00 (*0-683-00609-6*) Lppncott W & W.

Pediatric Endoscopic Surgery. James W. Holcolmb, III. 1993. (Illus.). 180p. (C). pap. text 129.00 (*0-8385-8047-5*, A8047-1, Apple Lange Med) McGraw.

Pediatric Enteral Nutrition. Ed. by Robert D. Baker et al. 1995. (Clinical Nutrition Ser.). (Illus.). 545p. 91.00 (*0-412-98451-2*) Aspen Pub.

Pediatric Enteral Nutrition. Susan S. Baker & Anne Davis. 1993. text 69.95 (*0-442-01341-8*) Chapman & Hall.

Pediatric Epilepsy: Diagnosis & Therapy. Ed. by W. Edward Dodson & John M. Pellock. 1993. 464p. pap. 95.00 (*0-939957-33-7*) Demos Medical.

Pediatric Epilepsy: Diagnosis & Therapy. Ed. by John M. Pellock et al. 2000. 700p. 175.00 (*1-888799-30-7*) Demos Medical.

Pediatric Epilepsy & Epilepsy Surgery. Ed. by G. W. Mathern. 1999. (Developmental Neuroscience Ser.: Vol. 21, No. 3-5). (Illus.). 250p. pap. 48.75 (*3-8055-6925-4*) S Karger.

Pediatric Ethics - From Principles to Practice. Ed. by Robert C. Cassidy & Alan R. Fleischman. 1996. (Mongraphs in Clinical Pediatrics Ser). 224p. text 60.00 (*3-7186-5756-2*, Harwood Acad Pubs) Gordon & Breach.

Pediatric Examination. Gill. 3rd ed. 1998. (C). pap. text (*0-443-05961-6*) Church.

Pediatric Eye Care. Ed. by Simon Barnard & David Edgar. 1995. (Illus.). 288p. 157.95 (*0-632-03979-5*) Blackwell Sci.

Pediatric First Aid. National Safety Council Staff. 4th ed. 2001. (Illus.). 128p. (C). pap. text 11.95 (*0-7637-1336-8*, 1336-8) Jones & Bartlett.

Pediatric First Aid & CPR. National Safety Council Staff. 4th ed. 2001. (Illus.). 224p. (C). pap. text 25.95 (*0-7637-1322-8*, 1322-8) Jones & Bartlett.

***Pediatric First Aid & CPR: Instructor Toolkit.** National Safety Council Staff. 4th ed. 2001. (Illus.). (C). tchr. ed. 244.95 incl. audio compact disk (*0-7637-1906-4*, 1906-4) Jones & Bartlett.

Pediatric Foot & Ankle Surgery. Richard M. Jay. Ed. by Stephanie Donley. 1999. LC 98-31651. (Illus.). 395p. text (*0-7216-7445-3*) Saunders.

Pediatric Fractures: A Practical Approach to Assessment & Treatment. Ed. by G. Dean MacEwen et al. 1993. LC 92-48218. (Illus.). 464p. 120.00 (*0-683-05310-8*) Lppncott W & W.

Pediatric Gastroenterology. Ed. by D. Branski et al. 1986. (Frontiers of Gastrointestinal Research Ser.: Vol. 13). (Illus.). viii, 416p. 292.25 (*3-8055-4331-X*) S Karger.

Pediatric Gastroenterology & Clinical Nutrition. Donald Bentley et al. 2000. (Illus.). 304p. text 165.00 (*0-19-262808-9*) OUP.

Pediatric Gastroenterology & Hepatology. Michael Gracey & V. Burke. 3rd ed. 1993. (Illus.). 1168p. 265.00 (*0-86542-238-9*) Blackwell Sci.

***Pediatric Gastroenterology & Nutrition in Clinical Practice.** Lifschitz. 2001. LC 2001-53333. (*0-8247-0510-6*) Dekker.

Pediatric Gastrointestinal Diseases, Set. W. Allan Walker. 1990. 298.00 (*1-55664-209-1*) Mosby Inc.

Pediatric Gastrointestinal Diseases: Pathophysiology, Diagnosis, Management. Ed. by Robert Wyllie & Jeffrey S. Hyams. 1993. LC 92-11720. (Illus.). 1248p. text 210.00 (*0-7216-3128-2*) Saunders.

Pediatric Gastrointestinal Imaging & Intervention. David A. Stringer & Paul S. Babyn. 1999. (Illus.). 700p. incl. cd-rom (*1-55009-079-8*) DEKR.

Pediatric GI Problems. Ed. by Paul E. Hyman. 1996. LC 96-23054. (Gastroenterology & Hepatology Ser.: Vol. 4). (Illus.). 265p. text (*0-443-07852-1*) Church GBR. *Dist:* Saunders.

Pediatric Head Injuries Handbook. A. Loren Amacher. 1988. (Illus.). 138p. pap. 24.50 (*0-87527-337-8*) Green.

Pediatric Health Certification: Exam Review. Beverly Rothfeld. 1998. LC 98-22075. (Nurse Practitioner Certification Review Ser.). 296p. (C). pap. 40.00 (*0-8385-8137-4*, A-8137-0) P-H.

Pediatric Heart Surgeon & Facility Directory: Profiles of Individual Surgeons & Congenital Heart Programs. Ed. by James H. Myers. 1997. LC 97-68297. (Illus.). 128p. pap. 40.00 (*0-9658918-0-1*) CHASER.

Pediatric Hematology. John S. Lilleyman. 2nd ed. 1999. (C). text 225.00 (*0-443-05840-7*) Saunders.

***Pediatric Hematology - Oncology Secrets.** Ed. by Michael A. Weiner & Mitchell S. Cairo. 2001. (Secret Ser.). (Illus.). 400p. pap. 39.95 (*1-56053-444-3*) Hanley & Belfus.

Pediatric Hepatology. W. F. Balisterri & J. Thomas Stocker. 1990. 250.00 (*0-89116-738-2*) Hemisp Pub.

Pediatric History & Physical Examination, 2000: Current Clinical Strategies. Elizabeth K. Albright. 4th ed. 2000. (Current Clinical Strategies Ser.). 90p. pap. 12.95 (*1-881528-92-8*) Current Clin Strat.

Pediatric History & Physical Examination for PDAs & Desktops. Elizabeth K. Albright. 4th rev. ed. 2000. (Current Clinical Strategies Ser.). 90p. cd-rom 28.95 (*1-881528-93-6*) Current Clin Strat.

Pediatric HIV: Evaluation, Medical Management & Rehabilitation. Ed. by Jay P. Shah et al. 2001. (Infectious Disease Ser.). 425p. 99.50 (*0-89603-814-9*) Humana.

Pediatric Home Care. Wendy Votroubek & Julie L. Townsend. 2nd ed. 1997. LC 97-18624. 450p. 73.00 (*0-8342-0884-9*, 20884) Aspen Pub.

Pediatric Home Care Manual. Mary Ann Chestnut. 1997. LC 97-25843. 240p. pap. text 42.50 (*0-7817-1203-3*) Lppncott W & W.

Pediatric Home Companion: Commonsense Advice about Your Child's Health. Lisa Wiseman. 1997. LC 97-22119. 178p. 15.00 (*1-57626-036-4*) Quality Med Pub.

Pediatric Hospice Care: What Helps. Intro. by Belinda B. Martin. 1989. (Illus.). 400p. (C). (*0-9623727-0-6*) Child Hosp LA.

Pediatric Hospitalization: Family & Nurse Perspectives. Kathleen A. Knafl et al. 1988. 326p. (C). text 23.00 (*0-673-39732-7*) Lppncott W & W.

Pediatric Human Immunodeficiency Virus (HIV) Infection: A Compendium of AAP Guidelines on

Pediatric HIV Infection : a Compilation of AAP Policy Statements & Excerpts from Manuals Published Through February 1999. American Academy of Pediatrics Staff. 2nd ed. 1999. LC 99-72727. (Illus.). (*1-58110-027-2*) Am Acad Pediat.

Pediatric Hypertension. Ed. by Uri Alon & N. G. DeSanto. 1992. (Child Nephrology & Urology Journal: Vol. 12, No. 2-3, 1992). (Illus.). 112p. pap. 55.75 (*3-8055-5608-X*) S Karger.

Pediatric Imaging. Cecile Godderidge. 1995. LC 94-12234. (Contemporary Imaging Techniques Ser.). 256p. text 49.95 (*0-7216-4534-8*) Saunders.

Pediatric Imaging: Case Review. Hans Blickman. 1999. (Illus.). 224p. (C). pap. 39.95 (*0-323-00505-5*) Mosby Inc.

Pediatric Imaging for the Technologist. Ed. by D. M. Wilmot & G. A. Sharko. 1987. (Illus.). 285p. 144.00 (*0-387-96439-8*) Spr-Verlag.

Pediatric Immunology. Ed. by Z. Spirer et al. 1993. (Pediatric & Adolescent Medicine Ser.: Vol. 3). (Illus.). x, 228p. 233.25 (*3-8055-5647-0*) S Karger.

Pediatric Infectious Diseases. Ed. by D. Engelhard et al. 1993. LC 93-15434. (Pediatric & Adolescent Medicine Ser.: Vol. 4). (Illus.). viii, 226p. 233.25 (*3-8055-5697-7*) S Karger.

Pediatric Infectious Diseases. Ed. by Hal B. Jenson & Robert S. Baltimore. Date not set. LC 2001-32283. (C). text (*0-7216-8121-2*) Church.

Pediatric Infectious Diseases. Ed. by Gerald L. Mandell & Catherine M. Wilfert. 1999. (Atlas of Infectious Diseases Ser.: Vol. 11). (Illus.). 283p. (C). text (*0-443-06526-8*) Church GBR. *Dist:* Saunders.

Pediatric Infectious Diseases: A Comprehensive Guide to the Subspecialty. Gary J. Noel et al. 1997. LC 96-31925. (Illus.). 368p. pap. text 30.50 (*0-8018-5564-0*) Johns Hopkins.

Pediatric Infectious Diseases: Principles & Practices. Hal Jenson & Robert S. Baltimore. 1996. 1593p. (C). pap. text 199.00 (*0-8385-2474-5*, A2474-3, Apple Lange Med) McGraw.

Pediatric Infectious Diseases for the Practitioner. M. I. Marks. 1984. (Comprehensive Manuals in Pediatrics Ser.: Vol. 3). (Illus.). 845p. 185.00 (*0-387-96010-4*) Spr-Verlag.

Pediatric Intensive Care. Ed. by Alan Duncan et al. 1998. (Illus.). 288p. pap. (*0-7279-1073-6*) BMJ Pub GBR. *Dist:* AIDC.

Pediatric Intensive Care Unit. Carol Hurst. 1998. 208p. spiral bd. 125.00 (*1-879575-93-0*) Acad Med Sys.

Pediatric Interventional Radiology. Richard Towbin. 2000. (Illus.). 528p. 95.00 (*0-86577-617-2*) Thieme Med Pubs.

Pediatric Laparoscopy & Thoracoscopy. Thom E. Lobe & Kurt P. Schropp. 1993. (Illus.). 272p. text 102.00 (*0-7216-4610-7*) Saunders.

Pediatric Laryngology & Bronchoesophagology. Lauren Holinger. 1996. LC 96-8295. 424p. text 199.00 (*0-397-51650-9*) Lppncott W & W.

Pediatric Lung. Ed. by R. W. Wilmott. 1997. (Respiratory Pharmacology & Pharmacotherapy Ser.). 350p. text 175.00 (*3-7643-5703-7*) Birkhauser.

Pediatric Magnetic Resonance Imaging. Mervyn D. Cohen. 1986. (Illus.). 162p. text 86.00 (*0-7216-1396-9*) Saunders.

Pediatric Manual of Clinical Dietetics. American Dietetic Association Staff. 1997. LC 97-33561. (*0-88091-160-3*) Am Dietetic Assn.

Pediatric Massage. Kathy Fleming Drehobl. 1998. (Illus.). 127p. pap. 36.00 (*0-12-784569-0*) Acad Pr.

Pediatric Medical Student Pearls of Wisdom: Over 3000 Questions. Levin & Emblad. 1999. (Pearls of Wisdom Ser.). pap. 32.00 (*1-890369-24-1*) Boston Medical.

Pediatric Medication Education Text. Marcia L. Buck & Anne Hendrick. Tr. by Babel Communications Staff from SPA. 1997.Tr. of Texto Educativo de Medicamentos Pediatricos. 200p. (Orig.). pap. 35.00 (*1-880401-89-4*) Amer Coll of Clin.

Pediatric Medications: A Handbook for Nurses. Suanne Miller & Joanne Fioravanti. 1997. (Illus.). 864p. (C). text (*1-55664-482-5*) Mosby Inc.

Pediatric Molecular Pathology: Quantitation & Applications. Ed. by H. S. Rosenberg et al. 1992. (Perspectives in Pediatric Pathology Ser.: Vol. 16). (Illus.). xii, 170p. 182.75 (*3-8055-5496-6*) S Karger.

Pediatric-Neonatal Review Book. Hill et al. rev. ed. 1994. 468p. (C). pap. 49.95 (*0-933195-50-8*) CA College Health Sci.

Pediatric Neoplasia: Morphology & Biology. Ed. by David M. Parham. 1996. LC 95-42517. 576p. text 225.00 (*0-7817-0273-9*) Lppncott W & W.

Pediatric Nephrology. Ed. by A. Drukker & A. B. Gruskin. 1994. (Pediatric & Adolescent Medicine Ser.: Vol. 5). (Illus.). x, 242p. 238.50 (*3-8055-5835-X*) S Karger.

Pediatric Nephrology. Ed. by Howard Trachtman & Bernard Gauthier. 1998. (Monographs in Clinical Pediatrics: Vol. 10). 420p. text 110.00 (*90-5702-273-7*, Harwood Acad Pubs) Gordon & Breach.

Pediatric Nephrology. Ed. by Malcolm A. Holliday et al. 3rd ed. 1994. LC 93-451. (Illus.). 1520p. 190.00 (*0-683-04104-5*) Lppncott W & W.

Pediatric Nephrology. T. Martin Barratt et al. 4th ed. 1998. LC 97-48546. 1,416p. text 235.00 (*0-683-30055-5*) Lppncott W & W.

Pediatric Nephrology: Proceedings of the Pediatric Nephrology International Symposium, 5th, 1980, No.

3. Pediatric Nephrology International Symposium Staff. Ed. by Alan B. Gruskin & Michael E. Norman. 1981. 530p. text 211.50 (*90-247-2514-3*) Kluwer Academic.

Pediatric Neurimaging. William S. Ball. 1997. LC 97-7705. 816p. text 179.00 (*0-316-07987-1*) Lppncott W & W.

Pediatric Neuro-Oncology: New Trends in Clinical Research. Ed. by Roger J. Packer et al. 1991. LC 90-4990. (Monographs in Clinical Pediatrics: Vol. 3). 320p. text 143.00 (*3-7186-0524-4*) Gordon & Breach.

Pediatric Neuro-Ophthalmology. William Good. 1998. pap. 119.00 (*0-412-05671-2*) Chapman & Hall.

Pediatric Neuro-Ophthalmology. Robert L. Tomsak. 1994. LC 94-24894. (Illus.). 204p. text 105.00 (*0-7506-9315-0*) Buttrwrth-Heinemann.

Pediatric Neuroimaging: A Casebook Approach. Charles L. Truwit. 1992. (Illus.). 290p. 89.00 (*0-683-08400-3*) Lppncott W & W.

Pediatric Neurologic Physical Therapy. Ed. by Suzann K. Campbell. 2nd ed. 1991. (Clinics in Physical Therapy Ser.). (Illus.). 459p. text (*0-443-08764-4*) Church.

Pediatric Neurology. Edward M. Brett. 3rd ed. 1997. LC 97-3033. text (*0-443-05200-X*) Church.

Pediatric Neurology: Behavior & Cognition of the Child with Brain Dysfunction. Ed. by Naomi Amir et al. 1991. (Pediatric & Adolescent Medicine Ser.: Vol. 1). (Illus.). x, 186p. 151.50 (*3-8055-5223-8*) S Karger.

Pediatric Neurology: Principles & Practice Ed. by Kenneth F. Swaiman. 2nd ed. 1993. LC 93-25352. (Illus.). 1696p. (C). (gr. 13). text 263.00 (*0-8016-6695-3*, 06695) Mosby Inc.

Pediatric Neurology: Principles & Practice Ed. by Kenneth F. Swaiman & Stephen Ashwal. 3rd ed. 1999. LC 99-27972. (Illus.). xxviii, 1494p. text 250.00 (*0-8151-3097-X*, 31787) Mosby Inc.

Pediatric Neurology: Theory & Praxis. Ed. by C. P. Panteliadis & B. T. Darras. 1995. (Illus.). x, 684p. 170.50 (*3-8055-6287-X*) S Karger.

Pediatric Neuroophthalmology. Michael C. Brodsky et al. 1995. LC 95-16249. (Illus.). 491p. 185.00 (*0-387-94464-8*) Spr-Verlag.

Pediatric Neuropsychology. George W. Hynd & Willis. 1987. text 41.00 (*0-8089-1890-7*, Grune & Strat) Harcrt Hlth Sci Grp.

Pediatric Neurosonography: Clinical Tomographic & Neuropathologic Correlates. Asma Q. Fisher et al. 1985. 267p. (*0-471-89252-1*) Church.

Pediatric Neurosurgery. Ed. by M. Choux et al. 1998. LC 98-11502. (Illus.). 700p. (*0-443-06149-1*) Saunders.

Pediatric Neurosurgery: Proceedings. Congress of the European Society for Pediatric Neu. Ed. by R. Villani & M. Giovanelli. 1977. (Modern Problems in Pediatrics Ser.: Vol. 18). (Illus.). 121.75 (*3-8055-2668-7*) S Karger.

Pediatric Neurosurgery: Surgery of the Developing Nervous System. Ed. by William R. Checck & Arthur E. Marling. 3rd ed. 1994. LC 93-38501. (Illus.). 656p. text 230.00 (*0-7216-3767-1*) Saunders.

Pediatric Neurosurgery: Surgery of the Developing Nervous System. David G. McLone. 4th ed. 1999. LC 99-51711. 1275p. (C). text 350.00 (*0-7216-8209-X*) Saunders.

Pediatric Neurosurgery: Theoretical Principles. Art of Surgical Techniques. A. L. Schawlow & A. J. Raimondi. 2nd enl. rev. ed. 1998. LC 98-21390. (Illus.). 656p. 398.00 (*3-540-62777-4*) Spr-Verlag.

Pediatric Neurosurgical Intensive Care. Ed. by Brian T. Andrews & Gregory B. Hammer. 1997. (Neurosurgical Topics Ser.). (Illus.). 250p. 95.00 (*1-879284-45-6*) Am Assn Neuro.

Pediatric Neurosurgical Patient: A Cooperative Approach. Leslie P. Ivan et al. 1989. (Illus.). 340p. pap. 49.50 (*0-87527-352-1*) Green.

Pediatric Nuclear Imaging. Ed. by John H. Miller & Michael Gelfand. 1994. LC 93-38091. text 115.00 (*0-7216-3685-3*) Saunders.

Pediatric Nuclear Medicine. S. T. Treves. (Illus.). 1984. 338p. 156.00 (*0-387-96001-5*); 2nd ed. 1994. LC 94-9627. 598p. 162.00 (*0-387-94229-7*) Spr-Verlag.

Pediatric Nurse & the Life-Threatened Child. Ed. by Penelope Buschman et al. 1987. LC 86-82710. (Current Thanatology Ser.). 100p. pap. 14.95 (*0-930194-39-X*) Ctr Thanatology.

Pediatric Nurse Practioner Certification Study Question Book. Patricia Clinton. 1999. LC 99-22759. 300p. pap. text, stu. ed. 35.00 (*1-878028-21-9*) Hlth Lead Assoc.

Pediatric Nurse Practitioner. Jack Rudman. 1994. (Certified Nurse Examination Ser.: CN-8). pap. 27.95 (*0-8373-6108-7*) Nat Learn.

Pediatric Nurse Practitioner Certification Prep Exams. Amelie Hollier et al. 1999. 300p. (C). pap. text (*1-892418-03-7*) APEA.

Pediatric Nurse Practitioner Certification Review. JoAnn Zerwekh & Jo C. Claborn. Ed. by Robin Carter. 1999. LC 99-28365. 220p. pap. text (*0-7216-7745-2*) Saunders.

Pediatric Nurse Practitioner Certification Review Guide. Jane A. Fox & Linda Gilman. 2001. LC 00-48042. (Illus.). xxiv, 580p. pap. 59.95 (*0-323-00644-2*) Mosby Inc.

Pediatric Nurse Practitioner Certification Review Guide. Ed. by Virginia L. Millonig & Mary Baroni. 3rd ed. 1998. LC 98-29338. 600p. (C). pap. text 52.00 (*1-878028-17-0*) Hlth Lead Assoc.

Pediatric Nurse Practitioner Pearls of Wisdom: Over 3000 Questions. Krieger. 1999. (Pearls of Wisdom Ser.). pap. 32.00 (*1-58409-000-6*) Boston Medical.

***Pediatric Nurse Practitioner Reveiw & Resource Manual (PNP)** Nurse Practitioner Alternatives in Education, Inc. Staff. 2001. 650p. pap. text 90.00 (*1-55810-170-5*) Am Nurses Pub.

Pediatric Nurse's Survival Guide. Lisa Rebeschi & Mary Brown. 1996. (Nurse's Survival Guide Ser.). 300p. (Orig.). (C). per. 28.95 (*1-56930-018-6*) Delmar.

Pediatric Nursing. Blum-Condon & Gasparis. 1991. LC 91-5214. (Nursetest Ser.). 384p. pap. 21.95 (*0-87434-305-4*) Springhouse Corp.

Pediatric Nursing. Patricia A. Lesner. 1983. (LPN/LVN Nursing Ser.). pap., tchr. ed. 10.00 (*0-8273-1933-9*); LC 81-82910. (Illus.). 544p. text 35.95 (*0-8273-1932-0*) Delmar.

Pediatric Nursing. Paulette D. Rollant. 1995. LC 95-36764. (Mosby's Review Ser.). (Illus.). 432p. (C). (gr. 13). pap. text 24.95 incl. 3.5 hd (*0-8151-7248-6*, 24861) Mosby Inc.

Pediatric Nursing. Kathleen M. Speer. 1998. (Nursing Education Ser.). text 62.95 (*0-8273-6379-6*) Delmar.

Pediatric Nursing. Martha Velasco-Whetsell et al. 1999. LC 99-32630. (McGraw-Hill Nursing Core Ser.). (Illus.). 542p. pap. 49.95 (*0-07-070009-5*) McGraw-Hill Prof.

Pediatric Nursing. Anne Froese-Fretz et al. 2nd rev. ed. 1998. (Outline Ser.). (C). per. 23.95 (*1-56930-067-4*) Delmar.

Pediatric Nursing. Janice Selekman. 3rd ed. 1996. LC 96-29152. (Springhouse Notes Ser.). (Illus.). 740p. pap. 26.95 (*0-87434-863-3*) Springhouse Corp.

Pediatric Nursing: An Introductory Text. Eleanor D. Thompson & Jean W. Ashwill. 6th ed. 1992. (Illus.). pap., tchr. ed. (*0-7216-3126-6*) Saunders.

Pediatric Nursing: Caring for Children. Jane W. Ball & Ruth M. Bindler. 2nd ed. 1998. LC 98-25825. 1083p. (C). pap. text 62.95 (*0-8385-8123-4*) Appleton & Lange.

Pediatric Nursing & Drugs Package. Ball. 1996. pap. 75.95 (*0-8385-8105-6*, Prentice Hall) P-H.

Pediatric Nursing Care Plans. Marie S. Jaffe. 2nd rev. ed. 1998. (Illus.). 400p. (C). per. 37.95 (*1-56930-057-7*) Delmar.

Pediatric Nursing Media Edition: Caring for Children. Jane W. Ball & Ruth M. Bindler. 2nd ed. 2000. 1056p. 68.00 (*0-13-054923-1*, Prentice Hall) P-H.

Pediatric Nursing-Resource Manual. Homrighaus. 2nd rev. ed. 1999. 200p. (C). pap. 28.00 (*0-8385-8168-4*, Medical Exam) Appleton & Lange.

Pediatric Nursing Skills Manual. Betty J. Whitson & Judith M. McFarlane. 1990. LC 79-27079. 304p. (C). mass mkt. 27.50 (*0-8273-4384-1*) Delmar.

Pediatric Nutrition, No. 8. Ed. by R. Reifen et al. 1998. LC 98-12387. (Pediatric & Adolescent Medicine Ser.: Vol. 8 (1998)). (Illus.). viii, 262p. 275.00 (*3-8055-6652-2*) S Karger.

Pediatric Nutrition Handbook. Jill Feldhausen et al. 1995. (Nutrition Handbks.: Vol. 3). 126p. (C). spiral bd. 25.00 (*0-412-07511-3*) Aspen Pub.

Pediatric Nutrition Handbook. American Academy of Pediatrics Staff. 4th ed. 1998. LC 98-70031. 833p. pap. 69.95 (*1-58110-005-1*) Am Acad Pediat.

Pediatric Nutrition in Developmental Disorders & Chronic Diseases: Prevention, Assessment & Treatment. Shirley W. Ekvall. 1992. (Illus.). 568p. (C). text 65.00 (*0-19-507224-3*) OUP.

Pediatric Occupational Therapy: Facilitating Effective Service Provision. Winnie W. Dunn. 1990. LC 89-43515. 420p. pap. 42.00 (*1-55642-014-5*) SLACK Inc.

Pediatric Occupational Therapy & Early Intervention. Jane Case-Smith. 2nd ed. 1997. LC 97-18094. 280p. text 49.99 (*0-7506-9780-6*) Buttrwrth-Heinemann.

***Pediatric Occupational Therapy for the Occupational Therapy Assistant.** Claire Daffner & Sadako Vargas. 2001. (Illus.). 350p. pap. 39.00 (*0-8036-0781-4*) Davis Co.

Pediatric Oculoplastic Surgery. James A. Katowitz. 2000. LC 99-32438. (Illus.). 752p. 250.00 (*0-387-94961-5*) Spr-Verlag.

Pediatric Oncology: Clinical Practice & Controversies. C. R. Pinkerton & P. N. Plowman. 2nd ed. 1997. 824p. (*0-412-63080-X*) E A GBR. *Dist:* OUP.

Pediatric Oncology 1. Ed. by G. Bennett Humphrey & Louis P. Dehner. 1981. text 141.50 (*90-247-2408-2*) Kluwer Academic.

Pediatric Ophthalmology. Leonard B. Nelson. 1984. (Major Problems in Clinical Pediatrics Ser.: Vol. 25). (Illus.). 288p. text 84.00 (*0-7216-1191-5*) Saunders.

Pediatric Ophthalmology: A Text Atlas. Robert A. Catalano & Leonard B. Nelson. 1994. (Illus.). 1099p. (C). text 159.00 (*0-8385-7817-9*, A7817-8) McGraw-Hill Educ Grp.

Pediatric Ophthalmology: International Ophthalmology Clinics, No. 1, Winter 1992, Vol. 32, 1992. Frederick A. Jakobiec & Dimitri M.D. Azar. 1992. 39.00 (*0-316-45652-7*) Little.

Pediatric Optometry. Ray C. Wunderlich. Ed. by Sally M. Corngold. rev. ed. 1991. (Introduction to Behavioral Optometry Ser.). (Illus.). (C). lib. bdg. 18.00 (*0-943599-19-9*) OEPF.

Pediatric Optometry. Jerome Rosner & Joy Rosner. 2nd ed. 1990. (Illus.). 538p. text 65.00 (*0-409-90063-X*) Buttrwrth-Heinemann.

***Pediatric Orthopedic Deformities.** Frederic Shapiro. 2001. (Illus.). 169.95 (*0-12-638651-X*) Acad Pr.

Pediatric Orthopedic Radiology. M. B. Ozonoff. 2nd ed. 1991. (Illus.). 815p. text 179.00 (*0-7216-3618-7*) Saunders.

Pediatric Orthopedic Secrets. Lynn T. Staheli. 1997. LC 97-25774. (Secrets Ser.). 450p. pap. 39.95 (*1-56053-207-6*) Hanley & Belfus.

Pediatric Orthopedics. Ed. by Nigel S. Broughton. 1996. text 99.00 (*0-7020-1962-3*) Saunders.

Pediatric Orthopedics. Ed. by Harris & Knutson. 1992. 164p. pap. 30.00 (*0-912452-80-3*, P-83) Am Phys Therapy Assn.

Pediatric Orthopedics. Dennis S. Weiner. 1992. (Illus.). 170p. text (*0-443-08728-8*) Church.

Pediatric Orthopedics Mihran O. Tachdjian. 2nd ed. 1990. (Illus.). 3749p. 510.00 (*0-7216-8726-1*) Saunders.

Pediatric Orthopedics. Tachdjian. 3rd ed. 2000. text (*0-7216-5682-X*) Harcrt Hlth Sci Grp.

Pediatric Orthopedics: A Guide for the Primary Care Physician. R. J. Mier & T. J. Brower. 1994. (Illus.). 340p. (C). text 49.50 (*0-306-44796-7*, Kluwer Plenum) Kluwer Academic.

Pediatric Orthopedics in Primary Care. Vernon T. Tolo & Beverley Wood. 1993. LC 93-13960. (Illus.). 498p. 75.00 (*0-683-08330-9*) Lppncott W & W.

Pediatric Orthopedics in Primary Practice. Ed. by Peter D. Pizzutillo. 1995. LC 96-20621. (Illus.). 391p. text 65.00 (*0-07-050252-8*) McGraw-Hill Educ Grp.

Pediatric Otolaryngology for the General Otolaryngologist. Ed. by Andrew H. Hotaling & James A. Stankiewicz. 1996. LC 96-11914. (Illus.). 304p. 89.50 (*0-89640-312-2*) Igaku-Shoin.

Pediatric Otology. Ed. by C. Cremers & G. Hogland. 1988. (Advances in OtoRhinoLaryngology Ser.: Vol. 40). (Illus.). viii, 168p. 129.75 (*3-8055-4726-9*) S Karger.

Pediatric Otology & Neurotology. Ed. by Anil K. Lalwani & Kenneth M. Grundfast. 1997. LC 97-30730. (Illus.). 714p. text 169.00 (*0-397-51466-2*) Lppncott W & W.

Pediatric Otorhinolaryngology. Ed. by B. Jazbi. 1977. (Advances in OtoRhinoLaryngology Ser.: Vol. 23). (Illus.). 84.50 (*3-8055-2674-1*) S Karger.

Pediatric Otorhinolaryngology: An Update. D. Passali. 1998. (Illus.). x, 432p. (*90-6299-158-0*) Kugler NLD. *Dist:* Lib Res.

Pediatric Pain Pt. 1: A Special Issue of "Children's Health Care", Vol. 25, No. 4, 1996. Brown. 1996. pap. 20.00 (*0-8058-9887-5*) L Erlbaum Assocs.

Pediatric Pain Pt. 2: A Special Issue of "Children's Health Care", Vol. 26, No. 1, 1997. Ronald T. Brown. 1997. 64p. pap. 20.00 (*0-8058-9877-8*) L Erlbaum Assocs.

Pediatric Pain Handbook. Jayant K. Deshpande & Joseph D. Tobias. 1995. (Illus.). 384p. (C). (gr. 13). pap. text 36.95 (*0-8151-2431-7*, 25783) Mosby Inc.

Pediatric Pain Management. L. M. Dahlquist. 1999. LC 98-43928. (Clinical Child Psychology Library). (Illus.). 172p. (C). pap. text 24.95 (*0-306-46085-8*, Kluwer Plenum) Kluwer Academic.

Pediatric Pain Management. L. M. Dahlquist. 1999. LC 98-43928. (Clinical Child Psychology Library). (Illus.). 172p. (C). 75.00 (*0-306-46084-X*, Plenum Trade) Perseus Pubng.

Pediatric Pain Management & Sedation Handbook. Myron Yaster et al. 1997. (Illus.). 608p. (C). (gr. 13). pap. text 36.95 (*0-8151-9516-8*, 29479) Mosby Inc.

Pediatric Parenteral Nutrition. Robert D. Baker, Jr. et al. 2001. 465p. reprint ed. pap. 91.00 (*0-8342-1863-1*) Aspen Pub.

Pediatric Pathology. J. Thomas Stocker. 2nd ed. 2001. text 325.00 (*0-7817-1774-4*) Lppncott W & W.

Pediatric Patient Education Manual. Aspen Reference Group Staff. 1998. LC 98-21790. ring bd. 199.00 (*0-8342-1000-2*, 489S1) Aspen Pub.

Pediatric Pearls: The Handbook of Practical Pediatrics. Fossarelli & Beryl J. Rosenstein. 3rd ed. 1997. LC 96-34956. (Illus.). 496p. (C). (gr. 13). pap. text 36.95 (*0-8151-8682-7*, 28973) Mosby Inc.

Pediatric Pharmacopoeia. Lott. 1999. pap. text 15.00 (*0-7020-1833-3*) Harcourt.

Pediatric Physical Therapy. Harris. 2000. 52.00 (*0-07-134511-6*) McGraw.

Pediatric Physical Therapy. Jan S. Tecklin. 3rd ed. 1998. LC 98-18730. 624p. text 51.50 (*0-7817-1010-3*) Lppncott W & W.

Pediatric Physical Therapy for the Physical Therapist Assistant. Ratliffe. 1997. LC 97-29089. (Illus.). 464p. (gr. 13). text 39.00 (*0-8151-7088-2*, 27167) Mosby Inc.

Pediatric Plastic Surgery. Ed. by Michael L. Bentz. 1997. LC 96-53379. (Illus.). 1099p. (C). text 299.00 (*0-8385-7820-9*, A-7820-2) McGraw-Hill Prof.

Pediatric Pocket Guide. Cynthia A. Beard et al. unabr. ed. 1996. 22p. (Orig.). pap. 20.00 (*0-935890-07-6*, P31) Emerg Nurses IL.

Pediatric Primary Care: A Handbook for Nurse Practitioners. Catherine E. Burns et al. Ed. by Ilze Rader. 1996. (Illus.). 980p. text 68.00 (*0-7216-5013-9*) Saunders.

Pediatric Primary Care: A Handbook of Nurse Practitioners. Catherine E. Burns et al. 2nd ed. 2000. LC 99-47085. (Illus.). 990p. text 65.00 (*0-7216-8062-3*) Saunders.

Pediatric Primary Care: A Problem Oriented Approach. Ed. by M. Wiliam Schwartz & Thomas A. Curry. 3rd ed. 1997. LC 96-53905. (Illus.). 1040p. (C). (gr. 13). pap. text 64.95 (*0-8151-8054-3*, 27234) Mosby Inc.

Pediatric Primary Care: Spanish Edition. M. William Schwartz. 2nd ed. 1993. (SPA.). 144.45 (*0-8016-6713-5*) Mosby Inc.

Pediatric Primer: Answers to Questions Most Asked by Parents. Charles Ginsburg. 1996. LC 96-35679. (Illus.). 130p. pap. 8.95 (*1-56530-220-6*) Summit TX.

Pediatric Procedural Sedation & Analgesia. Baruch Krauss & Robert M. Brustowicz. 1999. LC 99-10331. 321p. pap. text 45.00 (*0-683-30558-1*) Lppncott W & W.

Pediatric Procedural Terminology - PPT. American Academy of Pediatrics Staff. 3rd ed. 1995. 184p. pap. 34.95 (*0-910761-67-1*) Am Acad Pediat.

Pediatric Psychology: An Introduction for Pediatricians & Psychologists. John V. Lavigne & William J. Burns. 1981. 375p. text 52.00 (*0-8089-1365-4*, 792451, Grune & Strat) Harcrt Hlth Sci Grp.

Pediatric Psychology: Psychological Interventions & Strategies for Pediatric Problems. Michael C. Roberts. 1986. (Psychology Practitioner Guidebooks). (Illus.). 128p. text 28.00 (*0-08-032412-6*, J115); pap. text 14.95 (*0-08-032411-8*) Elsevier (Pergamon Pr).

Pediatric Psychooncology: Psychological Perspectives on Children with Cancer. Ed. by David J. Bearison & Raymond K. Mulhern. 1994. LC 93-15993. (Illus.). 272p. text 60.00 (*0-19-507931-0*) OUP.

Pediatric Pulmonary Disease. J. Thomas Stocker. 1988. (Aspen Seminars on Pediatric Disease Ser.). 287p. 90.00 (*0-89116-830-3*) Hemisp Pub.

Pediatric Pulmonary Heart Disease. Harned. 1990. 125.00 (*0-316-34698-5*, Little Brwn Med Div) Lppncott W & W.

Pediatric Quick Reference. Donna L. Wong. 2nd ed. 1994. (Illus.). 64p. text 8.95 (*0-8151-9396-3*) Mosby Inc.

Pediatric Quick Reference. Donna Wong. 3rd ed. 2000. LC 00-268832. (Illus.). v, 88p. text 8.95 (*0-323-01056-3*) Mosby Inc.

Pediatric Radiation Oncology. Edward C. Halperin & Louis S. Constine. 3rd ed. 1998. LC 98-33919. 624p. text 149.00 (*0-7817-1500-8*) Lppncott W & W.

Pediatric Radiology. Johan G. Blickman. 2nd ed. 1997. LC 97-29332. (Requisites Ser.). (Illus.). 340p. (C). (gr. 13). text 79.00 (*0-8151-0993-8*, 29191) Mosby Inc.

Pediatric Radiology. Jack O. Haller & T. L. Slovis. 2nd ed. 1995. LC 95-32581. (Illus.). 217p. 88.95 (*3-540-59059-5*) Spr-Verlag.

Pediatric Radiology: A Teaching File. Susan John & Leonard E. Swischuk. 2003. 99.00 (*0-683-30043-1*) Lppncott W & W.

Pediatric Regional Anesthesia. Ed. by Bernard J. Dalens. 1989. 504p. 159.00 (*0-8493-5629-6*, RD84) CRC Pr.

Pediatric Rehabilitation. Gabriella E. Molnar. 2nd ed. 1991. (Illus.). 562p. 72.00 (*0-683-06118-6*) Lppncott W & W.

Pediatric Rehabilitation. Gabriella Molnar & Michael A. Alexander. 3rd rev. ed. 1998. LC 98-31219. (Illus.). 434p. 75.00 (*1-56053-306-4*) Hanley & Belfus.

Pediatric Rehabilitation Vol. 17, No. 4: Journal: Pediatrician. Ed. by David W. Kaplan. 1990. (Illus.). iv, 108p. pap. 61.00 (*3-8055-5270-X*) S Karger.

Pediatric Rehabilitation Nursing. Patricia A. Edwards et al. Ed. by Thomas Eoyang. 1999. LC 98-5825. (Illus.). 590p. (C). text 65.00 (*0-7216-5425-8*) Saunders.

Pediatric Renal Transplantation. Amir H. Tejani & Richard N. Fine. 1994. 572p. 174.00 (*0-471-59120-3*, Wiley-Liss) Wiley.

Pediatric Rheumatic Diseases. Ed. by Jeanne Melvin & Virginia Wright. (Rheumatologic Rehabilitation Ser.: Vol. 3). (Illus.). Date not set. pap. (*1-56900-087-5*); 2000. pap. (*1-56900-140-5*) Am Occup Therapy.

Pediatric Rheumatology for the Practitioner. J. C. Jacobs. 2nd ed. 1992. (Illus.). 714p. 141.00 (*0-387-97750-3*) Spr-Verlag.

***Pediatric Rhinosinusitis.** Scott R. Schoem & Andrew M. Shapiro. 2001. pap. text 30.00 (*1-56772-032-3*, 5506375) AAO-HNS.

Pediatric Risk Factors for Major Chronic Disease. Christine L. Williams. 1984. 176p. 22.50 (*0-87527-237-1*) Green.

Pediatric Secrets: Questions You Will Be Asked on Rounds, in the Clinic, on Oral Exams. Ed. by Richard A. Polin & Mark F. Ditmar. 2nd rev. ed. 1997. LC 96-29336. (Secrets Ser.). (Illus.). 575p. pap. 39.95 (*1-56053-171-1*) Hanley & Belfus.

Pediatric Skeletal Scintigraphy. Leonard P. Connolly & S. T. Treves. 1997. LC 96-29796. (Illus.). 286p. 152.00 (*0-387-94695-0*) Spr-Verlag.

Pediatric Skills for Occupational Therapy Assistants. Jean W. Solomon. 1999. LC 99-40705. xxii, 391p. text 49.95 (*0-323-00092-4*) Mosby Inc.

Pediatric Soft Tissue Tumors: A Clinical, Pathological, & Therapeutic Approach. Cheryl M. Coffin et al. 1997. LC 96-27565. (Illus.). 460p. text 129.00 (*0-683-02047-1*) Lppncott W & W.

***Pediatric Solid Organ Transplantation.** Amir H. Tejani & Richard N. Fine. 2000. (Illus.). 512p. 73.95 (*87-16-12273-9*) Blackwell Sci.

***Pediatric Sonography.** Ed. by Marilyn J. Siegel. 3rd ed. 2001. LC 2001-42276. (Illus.). 700p. text 199.00 (*0-7817-2753-7*) Lppncott W & W.

Pediatric Specialty Certification Examination Study Guide. Ed. by Jane Case-Smith & Caryl J. Semmler. 1991. 90p. (C). pap. text (*0-910317-70-4*) Am Occup Therapy.

Pediatric Spine. Ed. by Anthony J. Raimondi et al. 1989. (Principles of Pediatric Neurosurgery Ser.). (Illus.). Vol. 1. 238p. 195.00 (*0-387-96835-0*); Vol. 2. 297p. 210.00 (*0-387-96861-X*); Vol. 3. 215p. 165.00 (*0-387-96804-0*) Spr-Verlag.

Pediatric Splinting. Hogan et al. 1998. (Illus.). 181p. (C). pap. text 50.00 (*0-12-785071-6*) Acad Pr.

Pediatric Surgery. Robert M. Arensman. 2000. (Vademecum Ser.). spiral bd. 45.00 (*1-57059-499-6*) Landes Bioscience.

Pediatric Surgery. Keith W. Ashcraft & Thomas M. Holder. 2nd ed. 1992. (Illus.). 1080p. text 209.00 (*0-7216-3737-X*) Saunders.

Pediatric Surgery. Keith W. Ashcraft. Ed. by Richard Lampert. 3rd ed. 1999. LC 98-31214. (Illus.). xviii, 1091p. text (*0-7216-7312-0*) Saunders.

Pediatric Surgery. Lewis Spitz & H. H. Nixon. 4th ed. 1988. (Rob & Smith's Operative Surgery Ser.). 703p. pap. text 290.00 (*0-407-00666-4*) Buttrwrth-Heinemann.

Pediatric Surgery. Coran & Lewis Spitz. 5th ed. Date not set. (Operative Surgery Ser.). (*0-7506-1704-7*) Chapman & Hall.

Pediatric Surgery. O'Neil & Rowe. 5th ed. 1998. LC 97-51987. (Illus.). 2176p. (C). (gr. 13). text 295.00 (*0-8151-6518-8*, 26544) Mosby Inc.

Pediatric Surgery. Lewis Spitz & Arnold G. Coran. 5th ed. 1994. LC 94-68719. (Rob & Smith's Operative Surgery Ser.). (Illus.). 928p. (*0-412-59110-3*) E A GBR. *Dist:* OUP.

Pediatric Surgery: A Color Atlas. Ed. by Don K. Nakayama. 1991. (Illus.). 168p. (gr. 13). text (*1-56375-012-0*, GM0198) Gower-Mosby.

Pediatric Surgery of the Liver, Pancreas & Spleen. Schiller. 1991. (Illus.). 272p. text 134.00 (*0-7216-8014-3*) Saunders.

Pediatric Surgery Secrets. Ed. by Philip L Glick et al. 2000. LC 00-27594. (Secrets Ser.). (Illus.). 350p. pap. 39.95 (*1-56053-317-X*) Hanley & Belfus.

Pediatric Surgical Oncology. Richard J. Andrassy. Ed. by Richard Lampert. 1998. LC 96-53983. (Illus.). 400p. text 165.00 (*0-7216-6378-8*) Saunders.

Pediatric Swallowing & Feeding. Arvedson. 1997. 68.00 (*0-7616-1741-8*) Commun Skill.

Pediatric Swallowing & Feeding: Assessment & Management. Ed. by Joan C. Arvedson & Linda Brodsky. 1992. LC 92-49930. (Early Childhood Intervention Ser.). (Illus.). 486p. (Orig.). (C). pap. 59.95 (*1-56593-069-X*, 0376) Thomson Learn.

Pediatric Telephone Advice. Raymond C. Baker & Barton D. Schmitt. 2nd ed. 1998. LC 97-3048. 464p. spiral bd. 49.95 (*0-316-77390 5*) Lppncott W & W.

Pediatric Telephone Medicine: Principles, Triage & Advice. Jeffrey L. Brown. 320p. 2nd ed. 1994. (Illus.). pap. text 39.95 (*0-397-51379-8*); 3rd ed. 1998. spiral bd. 34.95 (*0-7817-1631-4*) Lppncott W & W.

Pediatric Therapy: A Systems Approach. Susan M. Porr et al. Ed. by Shelly J. Lane. 1999. LC 98-55693. (Pediatric Occupational Therapy Ser.). (Illus.). 607p. (C). pap. text 39.95 (*0-8036-0259-6*) Davis Co.

Pediatric Thoracic Surgery. James C. Fallis et al. Ed. by Georges Lemoine. 1991. (Current Topics in General Thoracic Surgery Ser.). 370p. 141.00 (*0-444-01605-8*) Elsevier.

Pediatric Thromboembolism & Stroke Protocols. Maureen Andrew & Gabrielle DeVebers. 1997. 72p. pap. (*1-55009-055-0*) DEKR.

Pediatric Thyroidology. Ed. by F. Delange et al. 1985. (Pediatric & Adolescent Endocrinology Ser.: Vol. 14). (Illus.). x, 412p. 239.25 (*3-8055-3968-1*) S Karger.

Pediatric Toxicology: Handbook of Poisoning in Children. Nicholas Edwards et al. 1997. 424p. 115.00 (*1-56159-162-9*) Groves Dictionaries.

Pediatric TPN: Standard Techniques. Keith Kanarek & Barbara Kellam. 1986. LC 85-62891. 128p. pap. 22.95 (*0-931028-75-2*) Precept Pr.

Pediatric Tracheostomy Home Care Guide. Cynthia M. Bissell. 2000. (Illus.). xiv, 66p. spiral bd. (*0-9704385-0-8*) Twin Enterp.

Pediatric Transfusion Medicine. Christina A. Kasprisin. 1987. Vol. 1. 224p. 219.00 (*0-8493-5593-1*); Vol. 2. 216p. 219.00 (*0-8493-5594-X*) CRC Pr.

Pediatric Trauma: Initial Assessment & Management. Edward G. Ford & Richard J. Andrassy. 1994. LC 94-6679. (Principles of the Pediatric Surgical Specialties Ser.). (Illus.). text 69.00 (*0-7216-2913-X*) Saunders.

Pediatric Trauma Anesthesia & Critical Care. Ed. by J. K. Hall & Jeffrey M. Berman. 1996. LC 96-23404. (Illus.). 528p. 98.00 (*0-87993-624-X*) Futura Pub.

Pediatric Traumatic Brain Injury. Jeffrey H. Snow & Stephen R. Hooper. 1994. (Developmental Clinical Psychology & Psychiatry Ser.: No. 31). 120p. 74.95 (*0-8039-5181-7*, 4329); pap. 34.95 (*0-8039-5182-5*, 4330) Sage.

Pediatric Traumatic Brain Injury: Proactive Intervention. Jean L Blosser & Roberta DePompei. 1994. LC 94-11315. (Neurogenic Communication Disorders Ser.). (Illus.). 280p. (Orig.). (C). pap. text 45.00 (*1-56593-168-8*, 0479) Thomson Learn.

Pediatric Triage Guidelines. Kathleen A. Murphy. 1996. (Illus.). 352p. (C). (gr. 13). text 35.95 (*0-8151-7333-4*, 27931) Mosby Inc.

Pediatric Tumor Boards, No. 1.1. R. Beverly Raney. 1997. cd-rom (*0-412-14411-5*) E A GBR. *Dist:* OUP.

Pediatric Tumors: Immunological & Molecular Markers. Ed. by John T. Kemshead. 1989. 200p. 153.00 (*0-8493-6752-2*, RC281) CRC Pr.

Pediatric Upper Extremity: Diagnosis & Management. F. William Bora. 1986. (Illus.). 429p. text 155.00 (*0-7216-1872-3*) Saunders.

Pediatric Urology. Keith W. Ashcraft. 1990. 544p. text 156.00 (*0-7216-2746-3*) Saunders.

Pediatric Urology. Ed. by Barry O'Donnell & Stephen A. Koff. 3rd ed. 1996. LC 96-44087. (Illus.). 848p. text (*0-7506-1365-3*) E A GBR. *Dist:* OUP.

Pediatric Urology for the General Urologist. Ed. by Jack S. Elder. 1996. LC 95-33163. (Topics in Clinical Urology Ser.). (Illus.). 248p. 75.00 (*0-89640-280-0*) Igaku-Shoin.

Pediatric Urology Practice. Edmond T. Gonzales & Stuart B. Bauer. 1998. LC 99-13237. 736p. text 175.00 (*0-397-51368-2*) Lppncott W & W.

Pediatric Videofluoroscopic Swallow Studies: A Professional Manual with Caregiver Guidelines. Joan C. Arvedson & Maureen A. Lefton-Greif. 1998. LC 98-5487. 69.00 (*0-7616-3228-X*) Commun Skill.

Pediatric Work Physiology. Ed. by E. Jokl et al. 1978. (Medicine & Sport Science Ser.: Vol. 11). (Illus.). 68.00 (*3-8055-2866-3*) S Karger.

Pediatricians, Families & Child Care. Audrey I. Brown & Toby Gross. Ed. by Janet B. McCracken. 1993. (Pediatric Round Table Ser.: No. 15). 110p. (Orig.). pap. text 10.00 (*0-931562-17-1*) J & J Consumer Prods.

Pediatrician's Guide to Managed Care. American Academy of Pediatrics Staff. 1995. 270p. ring bd. 49.95 (*0-910761-62-0*) Am Acad Pediat.

Pediatrics. Daniel Bernstein & Steven P. Shelov. 1996. (Illus.). 456p. pap. 37.95 (*0-683-00640-1*) Lppncott W & W.

Pediatrics. Oborn. Date not set. text (*0-323-01199-3*) Mosby Inc.

Pediatrics. Richard M. Heller et al. 2nd ed. 1987. (Exercises in Diagnostic Radiology Ser.). (Illus.). 256p. text 36.00 (*0-7216-1569-4*) Saunders.

Pediatrics. Ed. by Jane E. Puls & A. E. Osburn. 2nd ed. 1996. LC 96-13501. (Oklahoma Notes). 390p. 24.95 (*0-387-94634-9*) Spr-Verlag.

Pediatrics. Roslyn Thomas & David R. Harvey. 2nd ed. 1997. LC 96-39718. (Colour Guide Ser.). (*0-443-05776-1*) Harcrt Hlth Sci Grp.

Pediatrics. Mohsen Ziai. 3rd ed. 1983. 868p. 38.50 (*0-316-98753-0*); 4th ed. 1990. 49.95 (*0-316-98743-3*) Lppncott W & W (Little Brwn Med Div).

Pediatrics. Stockman. 2000th ed. 2000. (Illus.). 550p. text 67.95 (*0-8151-9038-7*, 29143) Mosby Inc.

Pediatrics: 2000 Edition. Paul D. Chan & Jane Gennrich. rev. ed. 2000. (Current Clinical Strategies Ser.). 104p. pap. 28.95 incl. cd-rom (*1-881528-86-3*) Current Clin Strat.

Pediatrics: A Clinical Guide for Nurse Practitioners. Katie Barnes. 2002. 256p. pap. 45.00 (*0-7506-4957-7*) Buttrwrth-Heinemann.

Pediatrics: A Primary Care Approach. Carol D. Berkowitz. (C). text (*0-8089-2074-X*); text (*0-8089-2118-5*) Harcrt Hlth Sci Grp (Grune & Strat).

Pediatrics: A Primary Care Approach. Carol D. Berkowitz. Ed. by Bill Schmitt. 1996. LC 95-23414. (STARS Ser.). (Illus.). 525p. pap. text 33.95 (*0-7216-5623-4*) Saunders.

Pediatrics: An Approach to Independent Learning. Ed. by C. William Daeschner, Jr. & C. Joan Richardson. 3rd ed. 1997. LC 96-36967. (Illus.). 440p. pap. text 38.95 (*0-8018-5604-3*) Johns Hopkins.

Pediatrics: An Essential Slide Collection. Ian W. Booth. 1984. 112p. (gr. 13). incl. sl. (*0-397-46359-6*, GM0019) Gower-Mosby.

Pediatrics: PreTest Self Assessment & Review. Robert J. Yetman. 9th ed. 2000. LC 00-36143. (Pretest Clinical Science Ser.). 295p. pap. 24.95 (*0-07-135955-9*) McGraw-Hill Prof.

Pediatrics: Review for USMLE, Step 2. Jerome A. Paulson. 2nd ed. 2000. (Illus.). 265p. (C). 25.00 (*0-8036-0761-X*) Davis Co.

Pediatrics: Review for USMLE, Step 2. Jerome A. Paulson. Ed. by Kurt E. Johnson. 2000. (Illus.). 250p. pap. text (*1-888308-08-7*) J Majors Co.

Pediatrics: Understanding Child Health. Ed. by Tony Waterston et al. 1997. LC 97-218843. (Oxford Core Texts). (Illus.). 432p. pap. text 49.95 (*0-19-262563-2*) OUP.

Pediatrics & Child Health. Ed. by Martin Bellman & Nigel Kennedy. 2000. 400p. 49.00 (*0-443-05901-2*) Harcrt Hlth Sci Grp.

Pediatrics & Neonatology 2000: An Internet Resource Guide. Ed. by Dan Goldenson. 2001. 450p. pap. 24.95 (*0-9700525-9-6*) eMedguides.

Pediatrics & Perinatology: The Scientific Basis. Peter D. Gluckman & Michael A. Heymann. 2nd ed. 1996. (Illus.). 1008p. 125.00 (*0-340-66190-9*) OUP.

Pediatrics at a Glance. Ed. by Steven Altschuler & Stephen Ludwig. 1998. LC 97-41516. 450p. (C). pap. 49.95 (*0-8385-8142-0*, A-8142-0) McGraw-Hill Prof.

Pediatrics 5-Minute Reviews: 2001-2002 Edition. Karen Scruggs. 2000. (Current Clinical Strategies Ser.). 250p. pap. 19.95 (*1-881528-98-7*); pap. 29.95 incl. cd-rom (*1-881528-62-6*) Current Clin Strat.

Pediatrics for Nurses. A. L. Speirs. 1981. (Illus.). 244p. 29.95 (*0-8464-1282-9*) Beekman Pubs.

Pediatrics for the Anesthesiologist. Ed. by Frederick A. Berry & David J. Steward. 1993. (Illus.). 400p. text (*0-443-08930-2*) Church.

Pediatrics Pearls of Wisdom: Over 4000 Questions. Michael Zevitz et al. 1998. (Pearls of Wisdom Ser.). pap. 88.00 (*1-890369-07-1*) Boston Medical.

Pediatrics Recall. Eugene D. McGahren & William G. Wilson. 1997. LC 96-29736. (Recall Ser.). 459p. pap. text 29.00 (*0-683-05855-X*) Lppncott W & W.

***Pediatrics Recall.** Eugene D. McGahren & William Wilson. 2nd ed. 2001. LC 2001-38525. (Recall Ser.). (Illus.). 475p. pap. text 29.95 (*0-7817-2611-5*) Lppncott W & W.

***Pediatrics Recall PDA.** Eugene D. McGahren, III & William Wilson. 2002. 29.95 (*0-7817-3302-2*) Lppncott W & W.

Pediatrics Through the Eyes of a Child. 2002. (C). (*0-8053-8182-1*) Benjamin-Cummings.

Pediatrics, Year 2000 Edition: Current Clinical Strategies. Paul D. Chan. rev. ed. 1999. (Current Clinical Strategies Ser.). 100p. pap. 12.95 (*1-881528-85-5*) Current Clin Strat.

Pedicle Flaps of the Upper Limb: Vascular Anatomy, Surgical Technique & Current Indications. Alain Gilbert et al. 1992. LC 92-2164. 248p. text 155.00 (*0-316-20772-1*, RD557, Little Brwn Med Div) Lppncott W & W.

Pedondontics. Das. 1985. (*0-7855-0823-6*); 1983. (*0-7855-0746-9*) Current Dist IND. *Dist:* St Mut.

Pedophilia: Biosocial Dimensions. Ed. by J. R. Feierman. 1990. (Illus.). 594p. 79.95 (*0-387-97243-9*) Spr-Verlag.

Pedophilia & Sex Behaviors: Index of New Information Including Analysis & Results. Arlene S. Shank. 1995. LC 95-16307. 151p. 57.50 (*0-7883-0462-3*); pap. 47.50 (*0-7883-0463-1*) ABBE Pubs Assn.

***Peer Appraisal Handbook for General Practitioners.** Hilary Haman et al. 2001. 152p. pap. (*1-85775-570-7*) Radcliffe Med Pr GBR. *Dist:* Balogh.

Peer Interaction of Young Children. Carollee Howes. 1988. (Monographs of the Society for Research in Child Development: No. 217 53.1). 100p. pap. text 15.00 (*0-226-35523-3*) U Ch Pr.

Peer Leadership: A Human Relations Process to Reduce Substance Abuse & Improve School Climate. Thomas Turney. 2nd ed. 1994. 232p. (Orig.). (gr. 8-12). pap. 23.95 (*0-9624365-1-8*) Accel Devel.

Peer Relationships in Child Development. Ed. by Thomas Berndt & Gary W. Ladd. 1989. LC 88-5779. (Personality Processes Ser.). 434p. 240.00 (*0-471-85131-0*) Wiley.

Peer Review Improvement Act of 1982: A Legislative History of Pub. Law No. 97-248. Ed. by Bernard D. Reams. 1990. LC 89-83917. (Federal Health Law Ser.: Part 2). 564p. lib. bdg. 58.00 (*0-89941-692-6*, 305930) W S Hein.

PEET: Pediatric Examination at Three. Melvin D. Levine. 1986. (Pediatric Assessment Systems Ser.). 64p. pap. 13.75 (*0-8388-1795-5*) Ed Pub Serv.

Pegasus: Providing Enrichment for the Gifted by Adapting Selected Units of Study. Christine L. Lewis et al. Ed. by Marjorie A. Cantor. 1980. 119p. pap., tchr. ed. 15.00 (*0-89824-017-4*) Trillium Pr.

Pelagonius - In Pelagonii Artem Veterinariam Concordantiae. Ed. by Klaus-Dietrich Fischer & Dietmar Najock. 1983. (Alpha-Omega, Reihe A Ser.: Bd. XLVIII). xiv, 482p. (*3-487-07409-5*) G Olms Pubs.

Pelagonius, Veterinary Treatises & the Language of Veterinary Medicine in Latin. J.N. Adams. 1995. LC 95-3754. (Studies in Ancient Medicine: Vol. 11). ix, 695p. 257.00 (*90-04-10281-7*) Brill Academic Pubs.

***Pelvic Floor.** Henry. 2000. 515p. (*0-7020-2307-8*) W B Saunders GBR. *Dist:* Saunders.

Pelvic Floor Anatomy & the Surgery of Pulsion Enterocoele. R. F. Zacharin. 1985. (Illus.). xvi, 170p. 93.95 (*0-387-81861-8*) Spr-Verlag.

Pelvic Floor Re-Education: Principles & Practice. Ed. by B. Schussler et al. 1994. LC 94-34927. (*3-540-19860-1*) Spr-Verlag.

Pelvic Girdle. Diane Lee. 1989. (Illus.). 149p. text (*0-443-03795-7*) Church.

Pelvic Girdle: An Approach to the Examination & Treatment of the Lumbo-Pelvic-Hip Region. Diane Lee. 2nd ed. 1999. LC 98-40027. text (*0-443-05814-8*) Church.

Pelvic Inflammatory Disease. Ed. by Daniel V. Landers & Richard L. Sweet. 1996. (Illus.). 222p. 71.95 (*0-387-94462-1*) Spr-Verlag.

Pelvic Injuries (Beckenverletzungen) Results of a Prospective Multicentre Study (Ergebnisse einer Prospektiven Multizentrischen Studie) Ed. by H. Tscherne et al. 1997. LC 97-39899. (Hefte zur Zeitschrift "Der Unfallchirurg" Ser.: Vol. 266). (Illus.). 320p. pap. text 90.00 (*3-540-63312-X*) Spr-Verlag.

Pelvic Locomotor Dysfunction. George De Franca. 256p. text (*0-443-08839-X*) Church.

***Pelvic Locomotor Dysfunction.** George G. Defranca. 1991. tchr. ed. (*0-8342-0835-0*) PRO-ED.

Pelvic Locomotor Dysfunction: A Clinical Approach. Geroge G. De Franca & Geroge G. De Franca. 1996. LC 95-47220. (Illus.). 464p. 87.00 (*0-8342-0756-7*, 20756) PRO-ED.

Pelvic Pain: Diagnosis & Management. Fred M. Howard et al. 2000. LC 00-27378. 544p. text 99.00 (*0-7817-1724-8*) Lppncott W & W.

Pelvic Surgery: Adhesion Formation & Prevention. Gere S. Dizerega. 1996. LC 96-35592. (Illus.). 269p. 159.00 (*0-387-94871-6*) Spr-Verlag.

Pelvic Ultrasound. Ali Shirkhoda & Beatrice Madrazo. 1992. LC 92-5835. (Illus.). 328p. 85.00 (*0-683-07697-3*) Lppncott W & W.

Pelvis, Vol. 4. 1972. (*0-443-00720-9*) Church.

Penem Antibiotics. Ed. by S. Mitsuhashi & G. Franceschi. 1991. (Illus.). 180p. 79.95 (*0-387-53142-4*) Spr-Verlag.

Penetrating Keratoplasty: Diagnosis & Treatment of Postoperative Complications. Maria Severino & Karl-Ulrich Bartz-Schmidt. 2000. LC 99-58766. (Illus.). 160p. 84.00 (*3-540-66491-2*) Spr-Verlag.

Penguin Guide to American Medical & Dental Schools. Harold R. Doughty. 1999. LC 98-45438. (Penguin Original Ser.). 312p. pap. 17.95 (*0-14-027515-0*) Penguin Putnam.

Penguin Passnotes Nursing. White & David. pap. (*0-14-077055-0*) Pnguin Bks Ltd GBR. *Dist:* Trafalgar.

Penicillin: A Paradigm for Biotechnology. Ed. by Richard I. Mateles. 1998. LC 98-70214. (Illus.). 114p. pap. 25.00 (*1-891545-01-9*) Candida.

Penicillin: Meeting the Challenge. Gladys L. Hobby. 1985. LC 84-19689. (Illus.). 319p. 50.00 (*0-300-03225-0*) Yale U Pr.

Penicillin in the Treatment of Syphilis: The Experience of Three Decades. O. Idse et al. 1972. (WHO Bulletin Supplement Ser.: Vol. 47). pap. text 12.00 (*92-4-068471-9*, 1034701) World Health.

Penicillium & Acremonium. J. F. Peberdy. 1987. LC 87-12328. (Biotechnology Handbooks Ser.: Vol. 1). (Illus.). 314p. (C). text 85.00 (*0-306-42345-6*, Kluwer Plenum) Kluwer Academic.

Penile Disorders. Symposium on Penile Disorder Staff. 1997. LC 96-53124. (Illus.). 299p. pap. 70.00 (*3-540-61674-8*) Spr-Verlag.

Penis. Azid Hashmat & Sakti Das. 1993. (Illus.). 350p. text 99.50 (*0-8121-1508-2*) Lppncott W & W.

Pennies from Heaven: 101 Meditations for Couples Trying to Get Pregnant. Frances Stone & Philip Stone. 1998. LC 97-45615. 176p. pap. 9.95 (*0-14-025529-X*) Penguin Putnam.

Pennsylvania Health Care in Perspective 2000. Ed. by Kathleen O'Leary Morgan & Scott E. Morgan. 2000. 21p. spiral bd. 19.00 (*0-7401-0237-0*) Morgan Quitno Corp.

Pennsylvania Health Care Perspective, 1998. Ed. by Kathleen O'Leary Morgan & Scott E. Morgan. 1998. 20p. pap. 19.00 (*1-56692-837-0*) Morgan Quitno Corp.

Penny Wonder Drug: What the Label on Your Aspirin Bottle Doesn't Tell You. Eugene Cisek & Robert S. Persky. Ed. by Susan P. Levy. 1993. 128p. (Orig.). pap. 9.95 (*0-913069-31-0*) Consultant Pr.

Pensamiento Salvaje. Claude Levi-Strauss. (Breviarios Ser.). (SPA.). pap. 9.99 (*968-16-0933-6*) Fondo CA.

Pension Plan Strategies: A Comprehensive Guide to Retirement Planning for Physicians & Other Professionals. C. Colburn Hardy & Howard J. Weiner. Ed. by Kathryn Swanson. 2nd ed. 1995. (Illus.). 153p. 44.95 (*1-878487-60-4*, ME055) Practice Mgmt Info.

Pentoxifylline, Pharmacological & Clinical Research. Ed. by J. L. Ambrus. 35.00 (*0-915340-06-2*) PJD Pubns.

People & Change: An Introduction to Counseling & Stress Management. Catherine M. Flanagan. 1990. 264p. LC 90-3074. 69.95 (*0-8058-0450-1*); pap. 39.95 (*0-8058-0451-X*) L Erlbaum Assocs.

People & Predicaments. Milton Mazer. 1976. (Illus.). 332p. 29.50 (*0-674-66075-7*) HUP.

People & Their Planet: A Textbook of Environmental Science. Miller. 1991. (Illus.). 640p. pap. text 39.95 (*0-8016-3301-X*) Mosby Inc.

People Are Not the Same: Leprosy & Identity in Twentieth-Century Mali. Eric Silla. 1998. LC 97-39954. (Social History of Africa Ser.). 272p. lib. bdg. 60.00 (*0-325-00005-0*); lib. bdg. 26.00 (*0-325-00004-2*) Greenwood.

People Care in Institutions: A Conceptual Schema & Its Application. Yochanan Wozner. 1990. LC 90-4609. (Child & Youth Services Ser.: Vol. 15, No. 1). 238p. text 7.95 (*1-56024-012-1*); pap. text 4.95 (*1-56024-082-2*) Haworth Pr.

People Detector: A Quick-Guide Handbook Revealing What People in Your Life Are Really Like...Their Hidden Motives & Emotions, Their Qualities & Quirks. Maryanna Korwitts & Jim Gash. 1994. 72p. pap. 15.95 (*1-887270-00-0*) Spiritpoint Pr.

People in Crisis: Strategic Therapeutic Interventions. Diana S. Everstine & Louis Everstine. 1987. LC 82-23969. 280p. text 36.95 (*0-87630-286-X*) Brunner-Routledge.

People in Crisis: Understanding & Helping. LeeAnn Hoff. 4th ed. 1995. LC 94-46309. (Health & Social & Behavioral Sciences Ser.). 512p. pap. 34.95 (*0-7879-0084-2*) Jossey-Bass.

People in Crisis: Understanding & Helping. Lee Ann Hoff. 5th ed. 2001. LC 2001-1538. (Jossey-Bass Health Care Ser.). (Illus.). 528p. pap. 39.00 (*0-7879-5421-7*) Jossey-Bass.

People of South East Asia: Biological Anthropology of India, Pakistan & Nepal. Ed. by John R. Lukacs. 1984. 458p. 110.00 (*0-306-41407-4*, Plenum Trade) Perseus Pubng.

People, Patients & Politics. Clark R. Cahow. Ed. by Gerald N. Grob. 1980. LC 78-22554. (Historical Issues in Mental Health Ser.). (Illus.). lib. bdg. 23.95 (*0-405-11908-9*) Ayer.

People Types & Tiger Stripes. Gordon Lawrence. 3rd ed. 1993. 430p. pap. 15.00 (*0-935652-16-7*) Ctr Applications Psych.

People Who Are Homeless: Mental Health Services: A Place in Mind: Commissioning & Providing Mental Health Services for People Who Are Homeless. H. M. S. O. Staff et al. 1995. LC 96-209757. 172p. pap. (*0-11-321925-3*, HM19253) Statnry Office GBR. *Dist:* Bernan Associates, Balogh.

***People with Disabilities: Community Action & Empowerment.** Ed. by Christopher B. Keys & Peter W. Dowrick. 2001. LC 2001-16698. (Journal of Prevention & Intervention in the Community Monograph: Vol. 21, No. 2). 117p. 59.95 (*0-7890-1310-X*, Haworth Info Pr); pap. text 29.95 (*0-7890-1311-8*) Haworth Pr.

People with HIV & Those Who Help Them: Challenges, Integration, Intervention. Dennis R. Shelby. 1995. LC 94-33087. 49.95 (*1-56024-922-6*); 245p. pap. 14.95 (*1-56023-865-8*) Haworth Pr.

People with Learning Disability & Severe Challenging Behavior: New Developments in Services & Therapy. Fleming & Biza Stenfert Kroese. 1993. LC 93-2706. (*0-7190-3690-9*) Manchester Univ Pr GBR. *Dist:* St Martin.

People with Mental Health Problems & Learning Disabilities, Report 1, No. RC1. 1993. pap. (*0-946088-41-1*) NCCL GBR. *Dist:* St Mut.

People's Animal Healthcare: An Annotated Bibliography of Ethnoveterinary Medicine. Ed. by Marina Martinetto et al. 2000. 480p. pap. (*1-85339-522-6*) Intermed Tech GBR. *Dist:* Stylus Pub VA.

People's Cancer Guide Book: Practical Information to Help You Understand Cancer: Its Causes, Early Detection, Prevention, Symptoms, Treatments, & Cure. Ronald E. Aigotti. 1995. LC 95-76465. 427p. (Orig.). pap. 29.95 (*0-9648656-0-2*) Belletrist.

People's Doctor: George Hatem & China's Revolution. Edgar A. Porter. 1997. LC 96-3401. text 60.00 (*0-8248-1840-7*); (Illus.). 360p. pap. text 29.95 (*0-8248-1905-5*) UH Pr.

People's Health, 1830-1910. F. B. Smith. 1993. (Modern Revivals in History Ser.). 442p. (*0-7512-0185-5*) Gregg Revivals GBR. *Dist:* Ashgate Pub Co.

People's Medical Answer Book: Plain Answers to One Thousand One Hundred Common Questions from Thirty-Six Leading Specialists. Richard I. Pyatt. 1984. 21.95 (*0-13-656596-4*); pap. 10.95 (*0-13-656588-3*) P-H.

People's Medical Society Men's Health & Wellness Encyclopedia. Charles B. Inlander & People's Medical Society Staff. 1998. LC 97-40601. (Illus.). 518p. 29.95 (*0-02-862295-2*) Mac Bks.

People's Needs for Nursing Care: A European Study. P. Ashworth & A. Bjorn. 1987. pap. text 22.00 (*92-890-1041-X*) World Health.

People's Pharmacy. Joe Graedon. 1998. 752p. mass mkt. 6.99 (*0-312-96416-1*) St Martin.

***People's Pharmacy Guide to Home & Herbal Remedies.** Joe Graedon & Teresa Graedon. 2002. reprint ed. mass mkt. 6.99 (*0-312-98139-2*) St Martin.

People's Remedy: The Struggle for Health Care in El Salvador's War of Liberation. Francisco Metzi. Tr. by Jean Carroll from SPA. 1988. 224p. (C). pap. 10.00 (*0-85345-775-1*) Monthly Rev.

People's Repertory: Your Guide to Jafe, Effective Homeopathic Remedies for First Aid, Cold & Flu, Women's Health, Emotional Upsets. Luc De Schepper. Ed. by Begabati Lennihan. 1998. (Illus.). 200p. pap. 9.95 (*0-942501-09-8*) Full of Life.

People's Representatives: Electoral Systems in the Asia-Pacific Region. Ed. by Graham Hassall & Cheryl Saunders. 1997. LC 97-157910. 272p. (*1-86448-258-3*) Allen & Unwin Pty AUS. *Dist:* Paul & Co Pubs.

Pep Talk: Inspiration from America's Great Coaches. Ed. by Mike Dowdall & Sheila Meehan. 1995. LC 94-33742. (Illus.). 88p. pap. 5.95 (*0-8118-0542-5*) Chronicle Bks.

Peptic Secretion. F. Di Mario et al. (Advances in Gastroenterology Ser.: No. 1). 116p. text (*1-57235-017-2*) Piccin Nuova.

Peptic Ulcer Disease: Investigation & Basis for Therapy. Ed. by Edward A. Swabb & Sandor Szabor. 1991. (Clinical Pharmacology Ser.: Vol. 17). (Illus.). 552p. text 230.00 (*0-8247-8226-7*) Dekker.

Peptic Ulcer Disease & Other Acid-Related Disorders. David Zakim & Andrew J. Dannenberg. 1991. (Illus.). 384p. pap. text (*0-9629180-0-8*) Acad Rsch Assocs.

Peptic Ulcer Diseases: Basic & Clinical Aspects. G. F. Nelis et al. 1985. (Developments in Gastroenterology Ser.). text 237.50 (*0-89838-759-0*) Kluwer Academic.

Peptide & Protein Drug Analysis. Contrib. by Ronald E. Reid et al. 1999. LC 99-51466. (Drugs & the Pharmaceutical Sciences Ser.: Vol. 101). (Illus.). 904p. text 235.00 (*0-8247-7859-6*) Dekker.

Peptide & Protein Drug Delivery. H. L. Vincent Lee. 1990. (Advances in Parenteral Sciences Ser.: Vol. 4). (Illus.). 912p. text 265.00 (*0-8247-7896-0*) Dekker.

Peptide Antibiotics. Ed. by Horst Kleinkauf & Hans Von Dohren. 1982. (Illus.). 479p. 173.10 (*3-11-008484-8*) De Gruyter.

***Peptide-Based Cancer Vaccines.** Ed. by W. Martin Kast. 2000. 239p. 119.00 (*1-58706-026-4*) Eurekah.

Peptide-Based Drug Design: Controlling Transport & Metabolism. Ed. by Michael D. Taylor & Gordon L. Amidon. 1995. LC 94-40969. (Professional Reference Book Ser.). (Illus.). 522p. 120.00 (*0-8412-3058-7*) Am Chemical.

Peptide Chemistry: A Practical Textbook. Miklos Bodanszky. 2nd rev. ed. 1993. LC 93-26806. (Illus.). 210p. 42.95 (*0-387-56675-9*) Spr-Verlag.

Peptide Growth Factors, Pt. A. Ed. by Sidney P. Colowick et al. 1987. (Methods in Enzymology Ser.: Vol. 146). 452p. text 157.00 (*0-12-182046-7*) Acad Pr.

Peptide Growth Factors & Their Receptors I. Ed. by Michael B. Sporn & A. B. Roberts. 1990. (Handbook of Experimental Pharmacology Ser.: Vol. 95). (Illus.). 794p. 292.90 (*0-387-51184-9*) Spr-Verlag.

Peptide Hormone Secreting Tumors. Ed. by Xavier Bertagna. 1990. (Journal: Vol. 32, 1-3, 1989). (Illus.). viii, 166p. pap. 101.00 (*3-8055-5167-3*) S Karger.

Peptide Hormones: Effects & Mechanisms of Action. Ed. by Andrea Negro-Vilar & P. Michael Conn. 1988. Vol. 1. LC 87-35530. 272p. 167.00 (*0-8493-6719-0*, QP572); Vol. II. 224p. 148.00 (*0-8493-6720-4*) Franklin (CRC Reprint).

Peptide Hormones: Effects & Mechanisms of Action, Vol. 3. Andrea Negro-Vilar & P. Michael Conn. 1988. 224p. 125.00 (*0-8493-6721-2*, CRC Reprint) Franklin.

Peptidergic Neuron. J. Joosse et al. 1992. (Progress in Brain Research Ser.: Vol. 92). 408p. 286.00 (*0-444-81457-4*) Elsevier.

Peptides: Design, Synthesis, & Biological Activity. C. Basava & G. M. Anantharamaiah. 1994. 352p. 92.00 (*0-8176-3703-6*) Birkhauser.

Peptides, Hormones & Behavior. Ed. by Charles B. Nemeroff & A. J. Dunn. 1984. (Illus.). 944p. text 150.00 (*0-88331-174-7*) R B Luce.

Peptides in Oncology 1. Ed. by K. Hoffken et al. 1992. (Recent Results in Cancer Research Ser.: Vol. 124). (Illus.). 141p. 72.00 (*0-387-55287-1*) Spr-Verlag.

Peptides in Oncology 2: Somatostatin Analogues & Bombesin Antagonists. Ed. by K. Hoffken. 1993. LC 93-13134. (Recent Results in Cancer Research Ser.: Vol. 129). (Illus.). 147p. 89.00 (*0-387-56669-4*) Spr-Verlag.

Peptidomimetics Protocols. Wieslaw M. Kazmierski. 1998. LC 98-26947. (Methods in Molecular Medicine Ser.: Vol. 23). (Illus.). 576p. 109.50 (*0-89603-517-4*) Humana.

Pequeno Diccionario Medico Practico: Small Practical Medical Dictionary. Pierre Neuville. 8th ed. 1987. (SPA.). 240p. pap. 10.95 (*0-7859-4945-3*) Fr & Eur.

Perceived Control, Motivation & Coping. Ellen A. Skinner. 1995. LC 94-23859. (Individual Differences & Development Ser.: 8). 192p. 76.95 (*0-8039-5560-X*, 4863); pap. 31.95 (*0-8039-5561-8*, 4864) Sage.

Perceived Self: Ecological & Interpersonal Sources of Self Knowledge. Ed. by Ulric Neisser. 1994. (Emory Symposia in Cognition Ser.: No. 5). (Illus.). 333p. (C). text 64.95 (*0-521-41509-8*) Cambridge U Pr.

Perceiving Events & Objects. Ed. by Gunnar Jansson et al. 1994. (Resources for Ecological Psychology Ser.). 544p. text 99.95 (*0-8058-1555-4*) L Erlbaum Assocs.

Perceiving Talking Faces: From Speech Perception to a Behavioral Principle. Dominic W. Massaro. 1997. LC 97-1575. (Cognitive Psychology: A Bradford Book Ser.). (Illus.). 507p. 65.00 (*0-262-13337-7*, Bradford Bks) MIT Pr.

Perceiving the Elephant: Essays on Eyesight. Ed. by Frances L. Neer. l.t. ed. 1998. LC 97-65992. 218p. pap. 14.95 (*0-88739-122-2*) Creat Arts Bk.

Perceptanalysis. Z. A. Piotrowski. 1957. 523p. text 49.95 (*0-8058-0102-2*) L Erlbaum Assocs.

Perception. Ed. by Kathleen Akins. 1996. (Vancouver Studies in Cognitive Science). 352p. pap. text 40.00 (*0-19-508462-4*) OUP.

Perception. Faith Hickman Brynie. 2001. LC 00-12022. (Amazing Brain Ser.). (Illus.). 64p. (YA). (gr. 6-10). 21.95 (*1-56711-423-7*, Blackbirch Pr) Gale.

Perception. Ed. by R. Held et al. 1978. (Handbook of Sensory Physiology Ser.: Vol. 8). (Illus.). 993p. 211.00 (*0-387-08300-6*) Spr-Verlag.

Perception. G. Robert Carlsen. 4th ed. 1985. (Themes & Writers Ser.). (Illus.). 640p. (gr. 8). text 27.60 (*0-07-009805-0*) McGraw.

Perception: Its Development & Recapitulation. Estelle Breines. 1981. LC 81-81244. (Illus.). 304p. (C). text 19.00 (*0-941930-01-7*) Geri-Rehab.

Perception & Action: Recent Advances in Cognitive Neuropsychology. Jean Decety. 1998. LC 99-187262. 481p. pap. text 64.95 (*0-86377-600-0*) Taylor & Francis.

Perception & Its Development: A Tribute to Eleanor J. Gibson. Ed. by A. D. Pick. 1979. 272p. text 49.95 (*0-89859-409-X*) L Erlbaum Assocs.

Perception & the Physical World: Psychological & Philosophical Issues in Perception. Mausfield. 2001. 416p. 125.00 (*0-471-49149-7*) Wiley.

Perception, Cognition & Development: Interactional Analyses. Ed. by Thomas J. Tighe & Bryan E. Shepp. 1983. 384p. (C). text 79.95 (*0-89859-254-2*) L Erlbaum Assocs.

Perception, Empathy & Judgment: An Inquiry into the Preconditions of Moral Performance. Arne J. Vetlesen. 1994. LC 92-43991. 668p. (C). pap. 23.95 (*0-271-01012-6*) Pa St U Pr.

Perception, Empathy, & Judgment: An Inquiry into the Preconditions of Moral Performance. Arne J. Vetlesen. 1994. LC 92-43991. 400p. (C). text 74.50 (*0-271-01056-8*) Pa St U Pr.

Perception, Memory & Emotion: Frontiers in Neuroscience. Taketoshi Ono. 1996. LC 96-2868. (Pergamon Studies in Neuroscience: Vol. 13). 632p. 196.50 (*0-08-042735-9*, Pergamon Pr) Elsevier.

Perception of Illusory Contours. Ed. by S. Petry & G. Meyer. 1987. (Illus.). 320p. 246.00 (*0-387-96518-1*) Spr-Verlag.

Perception of Self in Emotional Disorder & Psychotherapy. L. M. Hartman & K. R. Blankstein. 1986. (Advances in the Study of Communication & Affect Ser.: Vol. 11). (Illus.). 354p. (C). 90.00 (*0-306-42315-4*, Plenum Trade) Perseus Pubng.

Perception Without Awareness: Cognitive, Clinical, & Social Perspectives. Ed. by Robert F. Bornstein & Thane S. Pittman. 1992. LC 91-1547. 308p. text 42.00 (*0-89862-886-5*) Guilford Pubns.

Perceptions: The Book of Female Character Types. David Spencer & Donny Elliot. 1995. (Illus.). 150p. (Orig.). pap. 10.95 (*0-9645633-0-4*) Net Worth.

Perceptions & Interactions in a Medical Setting: A Sociological Study of a Woman's Hospital. Aneeta A. Minocha. 1996. (C). (*81-7075-043-1*) Hindustan IND. *Dist:* S Asia.

Perceptions of Health & Illness: Current Research & Applications. Ed. by Keith J. Petrie & John Weinman. 1997. 320p. pap. text 28.00 (*90-5702-103-X*, ECU20, Harwood Acad Pubs) Gordon & Breach.

Perceptions of Phobia & Phobics: The Quest for Control. Beulah McNab. 1993. (Illus.). 253p. text 115.00 (*0-12-485960-7*) Acad Pr.

Perceptive Types. Frank Jakubowsky. 1993. (Orig.). pap. 10.00 (*0-932588-17-4*) BOLD Bks.

Percepts, Concepts, & Categories: The Representation & Processing of Information. Ed. by Barbara Burns. 1992. LC 92-26533. xviii,696p. 192.00 (*0-444-88734-2*, North Holland) Elsevier.

Perceptual Adjustment Therapy: A Positive Approach to Addictions Treatment. James Holder & Thurman Williams. 1995. LC 95-14249. 150p. pap. 24.95 (*1-56032-393-0*) Accel Devel.

Perceptual & Cognitive Development. Ed. by Rochel Gelman et al. 2nd ed. 1996. LC 95-50891. (Handbook of Perception & Cognition Ser.). (Illus.). 454p. text 59.95 (*0-12-279660-8*) Acad Pr.

Perceptual Consequences of Cochlear Damage. Brian C. Moore. 1995. (Illus.). 246p. text 90.00 (*0-19-852330-0*) OUP.

Perceptual Constancy: Why Things Look As They Do. Ed. by Vincent Walsh & Janusz Kulikowski. 1998. LC 97-6655. (Illus.). 560p. (C). text 74.95 (*0-521-46061-1*) Cambridge U Pr.

Perceptual Development. Ed. by Seymour Wapner & Heinz Werner. 1957. LC 58-17798. (Monographs in Psychology & Related Disciplines: No. 2). 95p. pap. 6.00 (*0-914206-03-6*) Clark U Pr.

Perceptual Development: Visual, Auditory & Speech Perception. Alan Slater. 2000. (Studies of Developmental Psychology). 464p. pap. (*0-86377-851-8*) Psychol Pr.

Perceptual Development in Children. Ed. by Aline H. Kidd & Jeanne L. Rivoire. 1966. LC 66-25139. 548p. 80.00 (*0-8236-4060-4*) Intl Univs Pr.

Perceptual Motor Behavior: Developmental Assessment & Therapy. Judith I. Laszlo & Phillip J. Bairstow. 1985. 37.50 (*0-275-91650-2*, C1650, Praeger Pubs) Greenwood.

Perceptual-Motor Behavior in Down's Syndrome. Ed. by Daniel J. Weeks et al. 2000. LC 99-42474. (Illus.). 376p. text 47.00 (*0-88011-975-6*) Human Kinetics.

Perceptual Neuroscience: The Cerebral Cortex. Vernon B. Mountcastle. 1998. LC 98-15241. (Illus.). 448 p. 63.95 (*0-674-66188-5*) HUP.

Perceptual Organization & Visual Recognition. David Lowe. 1985. 176p. (C). reprint ed. text 122.00 (*0-89838-172-X*) Kluwer Academic.

Perchloroethylene (Carbon Dichloride, Tetrachloroethylene, Drycleaner, Fumigant) - Effects on Health & Work: Index of New Information. Michelle S. Leeds. 1995. 146p. 57.50 (*0-7883-0352-X*); pap. 47.50 (*0-7883-0353-8*) ABBE Pubs Assn.

Percival's Medical Ethics. Thomas Percival. Ed. by Chauncey D. Leake. LC 75-23750. reprint ed. 39.50 (*0-404-13356-8*) AMS Pr.

Percutaneous Absorption: Mechanisms - Methodology - Drug Delivery. Howard I. Maibach & Robert L. Bronaugh. 2nd ed. 1989. (Illus.). 632p. text 215.00 (*0-8247-8036-1*) Dekker.

***Percutaneous Central Venous & Arterial Catheterisation.** Ian P. Latto et al. 2001. (Illus.). 299p. (*0-7020-2509-7*) W B Saunders GBR. *Dist:* Saunders.

Percutaneous Lumbar Discectomy. Ed. by H. M. Mayer & M. Brock. 1989. (Illus.). 218p. 86.95 (*0-387-51032-X*) Spr-Verlag.

Percutaneous Prostate Cryoablation. Ed. by Gary M. Onik et al. 1994. LC 94-34029. (Illus.). 172p. text 75.00 (*0-942219-66-X*) Quality Med Pub.

Percutaneous Transluminal Angioscopy. Andreas Beck. 1993. LC 92-48747. (*3-540-51066-4*); (Illus.). 123p. 165.00 (*0-387-51066-4*) Spr-Verlag.

***Percutaneous Transluminal Endomyocardial Revascularization: Practical & Theoretical Approaches.** George S. Abela. 2001. 296p. 119.00 (*0-471-36166-6*) Wiley.

Percutaneous Venous Blood Sampling in Endocrine Diseases. Ed. by R. Sornesen & Renan Uflacker. 1992. (Illus.). 183p. 174.00 (*0-387-97681-7*) Spr-Verlag.

Perelandra Microbial Balancing Program Manual. Machaelle S. Wright. 1996. LC 95-92802. (Illus.). 167p. pap. 16.00 (*0-927978-21-0*) Perelandra Ltd.

Perez on Medicine. Jose Perez & Wayman R. Spence. 1993. (Illus.). 64p. 29.95 (*1-56796-005-7*) WRS Group.

Perfect Baby: A Pragmatic Approach to Genetics. Glenn McGee. 1997. LC 96-31064. 176p. 52.50 (*0-8476-8343-5*); pap. 14.95 (*0-8476-8344-3*) Rowman.

Perfect Baby: Parenthood in the New World of Cloning & Genetics. Glenn McGee. 2nd ed. 2000. LC 00-21041. x, 186p. pap. 16.95 (*0-8476-9759-2*); 57.00 (*0-8476-9758-4*) Rowman.

Perfect Daughters: Adult Daughters of Alcoholics. Robert J. Ackerman. 1989. 200p. pap. 8.95 (*1-55874-040-6*) Health Comm.

Perfect Digestion. Deepak Chopra. 1997. LC 95-30583. (Perfect Health Library). 144p. pap. 12.00 (*0-609-80076-0*) Harmony Bks.

Perfect Endings: A Conscious Approach to Dying & Death. Robert Sachs. 1998. LC 97-52064. 160p. pap. 12.95 (*0-89281-779-8*, Heal Arts VT) Inner Tradit.

Perfect Eyesight: The Art of Improving Vision Naturally. Robert A. Zuraw & Robert T. Lewanski. Ed. by Jack Goldstein. rev. ed. 1998. LC 98-60555. (Illus.). 122p. pap. 20.00 (*0-9608030-2-5*) Taoist Pubs.

Perfect Health: Accept No Substitutes. Elwood Babbitt. 1993. 300p. pap. 15.95 (*1-881343-01-4*) Channel One.

Perfect Health: How to Get It & How to Keep It. Charles C. Haskell. 1996. 209p. reprint ed. spiral bd. 16.00 (*0-7873-0383-6*) Hlth Research.

Perfect Ray-Free House: Concise Guide for Radiesthologists. Wilton Kullmann. 1994. (Illus.). 126p. pap. (*3-85068-440-7*) Ennsthaler AUT. *Dist:* Am Educ Systs.

***Perfect Smile: A Consumer's Guide to Dental Health & Cosmetic Dentistry.** James Doundoulakis & Warren Strugatch. 2002. 160p. pap. 14.95 (*1-57826-095-7*) Hatherleigh.

Perfect-Victim Factor: Taking Control of Destructive Personality Traits. Richard K. Nongard & Paula S. Nongard. 1997. LC 97-91576. 120p. (Orig.). pap. 12.95 (*0-9655979-1-1*, BO2PVF) Peachtree Prof.

Perfecta Salud (Perfect Health) La Guia Completa del Mente & Cuerpo (The Comlete Mind/Body Program) Deepak Chopra. 1997. (SPA., Illus.). 399p. pap. 14.00 (*0-609-80104-X*, Three Riv Pr) Harmony Bks.

Perfecting Social Skills: A Guide to Interpersonal Behavior Development. Richard M. Eisler & Lee W. Frederiksen. 1981. LC 80-21209. (Applied Clinical Psychology Ser.). 236p. 45.00 (*0-306-40592-X*, Plenum Trade) Perseus Pubng.

Perfectionism. Brian L. 1985. 20p. (Orig.). pap. 1.55 (*0-89486-259-6*, 1404B) Hazelden.

Perfectly Contented Meat-Eater's Guide to Vegetarianism: A Book for Those Who Really Don't Want to Be Hassled about Their Diet. Mark W. Reinhardt. 1998. LC 97-41023. (Illus.). 252p. pap. 17.95 (*0-8264-1082-0*) Continuum.

Perfluorinated Ionomer Membranes. Ed. by Adi Eisenberg & Howard L. Yeager. 1982. LC 81-20570. (ACS Symposium Ser.: No. 180). 60.95 (*0-8412-0698-8*) Am Chemical.

Performance Agreements from Standard Operating Procedures for All Dentists. Marsha Freeman. 2000. 145p. ring bd. 100.00 (*0-910167-61-3*, Dental Commun) Comm Unltd CA.

Performance Anxiety. Mitchell W. Robin & Rochelle Balter. 1994. 240p. pap. 12.00 (*1-55850-441-9*) Adams Media.

Performance Audit of the Regulation of Health Maintenance Organizations & Other Prepaid Health Service Plans (in Florida) Dorothy N. Gray. 1994. (Illus.). 43p. (Orig.). (C). pap. text 20.00 (*0-7881-1475-1*) DIANE Pub.

Performance Criteria & Measurements for Doppler Ultrasound Devices: Technical Discussion. 1993. (Illus.). pap. (*1-930047-41-X*, DU) Am Inst Ultrasound.

Performance Enhancement - Plans for LTC Employees. Margaret Christian. 1995. 309p. stu. ed. 39.50 (*0-929442-24-5*, 2237pp) Prof Prnting & Pub.

Performance Goals for the Internal Quality Control of Multichannel Hematology Analyzers. 1989. (Proposed Standard Ser.: Vol. 9). 75.00 (*1-56238-054-0*, H26-P) NCCLS.

Performance Goals for the Internal Quality Control of Multichannel Hematology Analyzers: Approved Standard (1996) 1996. 75.00 (*1-56238-312-4*, H26-A) NCCLS.

Performance Improvement: Winning Compliance Strategies for Your JCAHO Survey. Jodi Eisenberg & Cynthia Barnard. 1997. LC 98-132085. (Illus.). 197p. (Orig.). pap. text 87.00 (*1-57839-002-8*) Opus Communs.

Performance Improvement in Ambulatory Care. Joint Commission on Accreditation of Healthcare Organizations. 1997. LC 96-79557. iii, 212p. (*0-86688-528-5*) Joint Comm Hlthcare.

Performance Improvement in Health Information Services. William J. Rudman. Ed. by Lisa Biello. 1997. LC 96-46878. 224p. text 44.00 (*0-7216-6009-6*) Saunders.

Performance Improvement in Psychiatric & Substance Abuse Treatment Services. Patrice L. Spath. 1997. (Illus.). 190p. 40.00 (*1-929955-04-9*) Brown Spath.

Performance Indicators for Permanent Disability: Low-Back Injuries in New Jersey. Sara R. Pease. 1987. 35.00 (*0-935149-10-4*, WC-87-5) Workers Comp Res Inst.

Performance Indicators for Permanent Disability: Low-Back Injuries in Texas. Sara R. Pease. 1988. 35.00 (*0-935149-15-5*, WC-88-4) Workers Comp Res Inst.

Performance Indicators for Permanent Disability: Low-Back Injuries in Wisconsin. Sara R. Pease. 1987. 35.00 (*0-935149-09-0*, WC-87-4) Workers Comp Res Inst.

Performance Measures & Indicators for Managed Behavioral Health. 151p. spiral bd. 67.00 (*0-929156-64-1*) Atlantic Info Services Inc.

Performance of Healing. Ed. by Carol Laderman & Marina Roseman. LC 95-24568. 330p. (C). 1996. (gr. 13). 80.00 (*0-415-91199-0*); 1995. pap. 24.95 (*0-415-91200-8*) Routledge.

Performance Standards for Antimicrobial Disk & Dilution Susceptibility Tests for Bacteria Isolated from Animals: Proposed Standard (1994) Contrib. by Jeffrey L. Watts. 1994. 75.00 (*1-56238-258-6*, M31-P) NCCLS.

Performance Standards for Antimicrobial Disk & Dilution Susceptibility Tests for Bacteria Isolated from Animals: Tentative Standard (1997) 1997. 75.00 (*1-56238-330-2*, M31-T) NCCLS.

Performance Standards for Antimicrobial Disk Susceptibility Tests: Approved Standard (1997) Contrib. by James H. Jorgensen. 5th ed. 1997. (SPA.). 85.00 (*1-56238-308-6*, M2-A6) NCCLS.

Performance Standards for Antimicrobial Susceptibility Testing: Eighth International Supplement (1998) 1998. 115.00 (*1-56238-337-X*, M100-S8) NCCLS.

Performance Standards for Antimicrobial Susceptibility Testing: Seventh Informational Supplement (1997) Contrib. by James H. Jorgensen. 1997. 85.00 (*1-56238-309-4*, M100-S7) NCCLS.

Performance Without Pressure. Martin L. Seldman. 1988. 17.95 (*0-8027-1022-0*) Walker & Co.

Performing an Operational & Strategic Assessment for a Medical Practice. Reed Tinsley & Joey Havens. 1999. LC 98-42396. 256p. 105.00 (*0-471-29964-2*) Wiley.

Performing Arts Medicine. Robert T. Sataloff. 2nd ed. 1998. 49.95 (*1-56593-965-4*, 1910) Singular Publishing.

Performing Arts Medicine. Ed. by Robert T. Sataloff et al. 2nd ed. 1998. (Illus.). 454p. 279.95 (*1-56593-982-4*, 1944) Thomson Learn.

PeriAnesthesia CheckMate. Angela G. Clarkson & Anne M. Larson. 3rd ed. 2000. (Critical Care CheckMate Ser.). 144p. vinyl bd. (*0-9700484-7-5*) NNCC.

Pericardial Disease: New Insights & Old Dilemmas. Ed. by J. Soler-Soler et al. 1990. (Developments in Cardiovascular Medicine Ser.). (C). text 186.00 (*0-7923-0510-8*) Kluwer Academic.

Pericardial Tissue As a Cardiac Valve Substitute: Proceedings of a Symposium. Ed. & Illus. by Silent Partners, Inc. Staff. 1989. 221p. (Orig.). pap. (*1-878353-10-1*) Silent Partners.

Pericardium: A Comprehensive Textbook. David H. Spodick. 1996. LC 96-43173. (Fundamental & Clinical Oncology Ser.: Vol. 27). (Illus.). 496p. text 180.00 (*0-8247-9316-1*) Dekker.

Peridiniens Parasites: Morphologie, Reproduction, Ethologie. Edouard Chatton. 1975. (Archives de Zoologic Experimentale et Generale Ser.: Vol. 59, 1920). 475p. reprint ed. (*3-87429-100-6*, 002582) Koeltz Sci Bks DEU. *Dist:* Lubrecht & Cramer.

Peridontology & Its Origins up to 1980. Arthur J. Held. 1989. 240p. 87.50 (*0-8176-1955-0*) Birkhauser.

Peril to the Nerve: Glaucoma & Clinical Neuro-Ophthalmology, Proceedings of the 45th Annual Symposium, New Orleans, La, U. S. A., April 25-28, 1996. New Orleans Academy of Ophthalmology Staff et al. 1998. LC 97-13859. (Illus.). xiii, 283p. (*90-6299-153-X*) Kugler NLD. *Dist:* Lib Res.

Perilous Calling: The Hazards of Psychotherapy Practice. Michael B. Sussman. 1995. LC 94-34135. 332p. 110.00 (*0-471-05657-X*) Wiley.

Perilous Chastity: Women & Illness in Pre-Enlightenment Art & Medicine. Laurinda S. Dixon. 1995. LC 94-34911. (Illus.). 320p. 62.50 (*0-8014-3026-7*); pap. 26.50 (*0-8014-8215-1*) Cornell U Pr.

Perils of Progress: The Health & Environmental Hazards of Modern Technology, & What You Can Do about Them. John Ashton & Ron Laura. 1997. 350p. pap. (*0-86840-488-8*) New South Wales Univ Pr AUS. *Dist:* Intl Spec Bk.

Perimenopausal & Geriatric Gynecology. Hugh R. Barber. 1988. 640p. 75.00 (*0-02-305880-3*, Macmillan Coll) P-H.

Perimenopause. Bernard J. Cortese. 1998. LC 98-26905. (Vital Information Ser.). 112p. pap. 11.95 (*0-89594-914-8*) Crossing Pr.

Perimenopause. U. S. A. Serono Symposia Staff. Ed. by Rogerio Lobo. 1997. LC 97-16665. (Serono Symposia U. S. A. Ser.). (Illus.). 348p. 162.00 (*0-387-94967-4*) Spr-Verlag.

Perimenopause: Changes in Women's Health after 35. James E. Huston & L. Darlene Lanka. 1997. LC 97-66079. (Illus.). 416p. (Orig.). pap. 16.95 (*1-57224-085-7*) New Harbinger.

Perimenopause Handbook. Carol Turkington. 1998. LC 97-51584. 192p. pap. 14.95 (*0-8092-2935-8*, 293580, Contemporary) McGraw-Hill Trade.

Perimenopause the Natural Way. Deborah Gordon & Kerri Brenner. 2000. LC 00-35907. (Women's Natural Health Ser.). 240p. pap. 14.95 (*0-471-37960-3*) Wiley.

Perimetric Standards & Perimetric Glossary. Ed. by International Council of Ophthalmology Staff. 1979. text 85.50 (*90-6193-600-4*) Kluwer Academic.

Perimetry Update, 1988-1989. Ed. by A. Heijl. 1989. LC 89-2267. (Illus.). 477p. lib. bdg. (*90-6299-051-7*) Kugler NLD. *Dist:* Lib Res.

Perimetry Update, 1996 to 1997. Ed. by Michael Wall. 1997. (Illus.). xi, 477p. (*90-6299-139-4*) Kugler NLD. *Dist:* Lib Res.

Perimetry Update, 1990-1991. Ed. by R. P. Mills & A. Heijl. 1991. LC 91-14629. (Illus.). 585p. lib. bdg. (*90-6299-075-4*) Kugler NLD. *Dist:* Lib Res.

Perinatal & Multigeneration Carcinogenesis. Ed. by N. P. Napalkov et al. 1989. (IARC Scientific Publications Ser.: No. 96). (Illus.). 462p. pap. 110.00 (*92-832-1196-0*) OUP.

Perinatal & Pediatric HIV. Wara. 1998. text (*0-7216-6767-8*) Saunders.

Perinatal & Pediatric Respiratory Care. Barnhart. 1995. 450.00 (*0-7216-6742-2*) Harcourt.

Perinatal & Pediatric Respiratory Care. Ed. by Sherry L. Barnhart & Michael P. Czervinske. 1995. (Illus.). 731p. tchr. ed. (*0-7216-5942-X*) Saunders.

Perinatal & Pediatric Respiratory Care. Sherry L. Barnhart & Michael P. Czervinske. 1995. LC 94-25347. (Pediatric Respiratory Diseases Ser.). (Illus.). 656p. text 53.00 (*0-7216-6739-2*) Saunders.

Perinatal & Pediatric Respiratory Care. Ed. by Sherry L. Barnhart & Michael P. Czervinske. 1995. (Illus.). 731p. pap. text, wbk. ed. 16.95 (*0-7216-6741-4*) Saunders.

***Perinatal & Pediatric Respiratory Care.** Michael P. Czervinske & Sherry L. Barnhart. 2001. (Illus.). 700p. (*0-7216-8231-6*) Saunders.

Perinatal Asphyxia. Ed. by J. Haddad & E. Saliba. 1993. LC 92-48789. (Illus.). 267p. 149.00 (*0-387-56135-8*) Spr-Verlag.

Perinatal Asphyxia. A. Lacoius-Petruccelli. 1987. (Illus.). 188p. (C). text 65.00 (*0-306-42358-8*, Kluwer Plenum) Kluwer Academic.

Perinatal Audit: A Report Produced for The European Association of Perinatal Medicine. Ed. by P. M. Dunn & G. McIlwaine. 1996. 44p. lib. bdg. 19.95 (*1-85070-933-5*, Parthenon Pbng) CRC Pr.

Perinatal Autopsy Manual. Marie Valdes-Dapena & Dale Huff. 1993. (Illus.). 98p. (C). pap. text 40.00 (*0-7881-0176-5*) DIANE Pub.

Perinatal Autopsy Manual. Valdez-Depena & Huff. 2nd ed. 1983. (Illus.). 98p. reprint ed. pap. text 15.00 (*1-881041-38-7*) Am Registry Path.

Perinatal Biochemistry. Emilio Herrera. 1992. 288p. lib. bdg. 189.00 (*0-8493-6944-4*, PG615) CRC Pr.

***Perinatal Brain Injury: 2nd Hershey Conference on Developmental Cerebral Blood Flow & Metabolism, Hershey, Pa., June 2000: Proceedings & Abstracts.** Ed. by S. J. Vannucci et al. 2001. (Illus.). 98p. pap. 34.00 (*3-8055-7280-8*) S Karger.

Perinatal Endocrinology & Metabolism. Ed. by J. R. Girard. 1985. (Journal: Vol. 48, No. 4, 1985). (Illus.). 76p. pap. 38.50 (*3-8055-4235-6*) S Karger.

Perinatal Epidemiology. Michael B. Bracken. 1984. (Illus.). 550p. text 69.50 (*0-19-503389-2*) OUP.

Perinatal Epidemiology & Health Care Organisation: The Case of Belgium. Ed. by P. Buekens et al. 1989. (Journal: Vol. 55, No. 1,1989). (Illus.). iv, 72p. pap. 51.50 (*3-8055-4978-4*) S Karger.

Perinatal Haematological Problems. Ed. by Tom Turner. 1991. (Perinatal Practice Ser.). 252p. 340.00 (*0-471-91557-2*) Wiley.

Perinatal Hypoxia. Squier. 1999. (Illus.). 256p. pap. 138.00 (*0-412-70860-4*, Chap & Hall NY) Chapman & Hall.

Perinatal Impact of Alcohol, Tobacco & Other Drugs. Margaret Kearney et al. 1999. LC 99-22605. (*0-86525-083-9*) March of Dimes.

Perinatal Impact of Substance Abuse. Susan M. Weiner. Ed. by Beverly S. Raff & Ellen Fiore. 1992. LC 92-23656. (Nursing Issues for the Twenty-First Century Ser.: Series 4, Module 3). pap. (*0-86525-055-3*) March of Dimes.

Perinatal Medicine. Ed. by J. Clinch. 1985. text 225.00 (*0-85200-908-9*) Kluwer Academic.

Perinatal Medicine. Ed. by Johan Gentz et al. 1984. LC 83-2171. 558p. 83.50 (*0-275-91431-3*, C1431, Praeger Pubs) Greenwood.

Perinatal Medicine Manohar L. Rathi & Sudhir Kumar. 1982. text 39.50 (*0-07-051208-6*) McGraw.

Perinatal Medicine, Set. E. Kerpel-Fronius et al. 1978. 1448p. (C). (*963-05-1413-3*) Akade Kiado HUN. *Dist:* St Mut.

Perinatal Medicine, Vol. 1. Manohar L. Rathi & Sudhir Kumar. 1980. text 35.00 (*0-07-051204-3*) McGraw.

Perinatal Medicine: Proceedings. Congress on Perinatal Medicine, 2nd European, Lond. Ed. by P. J. Huntingford et al. 1971. 69.75 (*3-8055-1224-4*) S Karger.

Perinatal Mental Health. Diana Riley. 1994. (*1-870905-78-4*) Radcliffe Med Pr GBR. *Dist:* Balogh.

Perinatal Mortality & Morbidity Including Low Birth Weight: A South-East Asia Regional Profile. T. Perera & Khing. 1984. (SEARO Regional Health Papers: No. 3). 72p. pap. text 8.00 (*92-9022-172-0*) World Health.

Perinatal Mortality in the United States, 1985-91. 1995. LC 95-30868. (Vital & Health Statistics Ser.: Series 20, No. 26). (*0-8406-0508-0*) Natl Ctr Health Stats.

Perinatal Nephrology Journal: Biology of the Neonate, Vol. 53, No. 4, 1987. Ed. by J. P. Guignard. 1988. (Illus.). 80p. pap. 37.50 (*3-8055-4798-6*) S Karger.

Perinatal Nursing. Ballesteros. 1991. (Nursing Education Ser.). (C). pap. text 39.95 (*0-8273-3545-8*); pap. text, tchr. ed. 12.00 (*0-8273-3546-6*) Delmar.

Perinatal Nursing. Kathleen R. Simpson & Patricia A. Creehan. 2nd ed. 2001. LC 00-67266. (Illus.). xx, 726p. pap. text 44.00 (*0-7817-2510-0*) Lppncott W & W.

Perinatal Nursing: Care of the High Risk Infant. Janice Ouimette. 1986. (Illus.). 461p. (C). text 56.25 (*0-86720-356-0*, 356-0) Jones & Bartlett.

Perinatal Nursing: Legal Dimensions. Mahlmeiste. pap. text (*0-7216-5919-5*) Saunders.

Perinatal Pathology. Jonathan S. Wigglesworth. Ed. by Lesley Day. 2nd abr. ed. 1996. LC 95-42775. (Major Problems in Pathology Ser.: Vol. 15). 512p. text 74.00 (*0-7216-4252-7*) Saunders.

Perinatal-Pediatric Respiratory Therapeutics: RCP 306 Course. Wojciechowski et al. 1994. 213p. (C). ring bd. 43.95 (*0-933195-74-5*) CA College Health Sci.

Perinatal Practice in the Best Interest of Patients: Four Statements of Policy to Improve the Outcome of Pregnancy. Frwd. by Daniel M. Fox & Jennifer L. Howse. 1997. 48p. (Orig.). pap. (*1-887748-10-5*) Milbank Memorial.

Perinatal Thrombosis & Hemastasis. Ed. by S. Suzuki et al. 1991. (Illus.). 289p. 118.00 (*0-387-70055-2*) Spr-Verlag.

Perinatal Transfusion Medicine. Ed. by Melanie S. Kennedy. 1990. LC 90-14405. 218p. (C). text 7.00 (*0-915355-84-1*) Am Assn Blood.

Perinatologie. Ed. by E. Bern Rossi. 1975. (Paediatrische Fortbildungskurse fuer die Praxis Ser.: Band 41). 200p. 68.75 (*3-8055-2115-4*) S Karger.

Periodic Hemodynamics in Health & Disease. Jan A. Schmidt & Michael W. Parker. 1996. LC 96-9385. (Medical Intelligence Unit Ser.). 208p. 99.00 (*1-57059-366-3*) Landes Bioscience.

Periodontal & Prosthetic Management for Advanced Cases. Marvin M. Rosenberg et al. 1988. (Illus.). 375p. text 182.00 (*0-86715-162-5*, 1625) Quint Pub Co.

Periodontal Control. Grace & Smales. 1989. 144p. pap. text 34.00 (*1-85097-009-2*) Quint Pub Co.

Periodontal Disease: Immunological Factors, I. Irving Glickman et al. 1973. LC 72-10934. (Illus.). 220p. (C). text 32.50 (*0-8422-7061-2*) Irvington.

Periodontal Disease: Immunological Factors, II. L. Ivanyi et al. 1973. LC 72-10934. (Illus.). 193p. text 32.50 (*0-8422-7069-8*) Irvington.

Periodontal Disease Management. Ed. by M. McGuire & C. Townsend. 1994. (Illus.). 100p. (Orig.). pap. 65.00 (*0-9624699-5-5*) Amer Acad Periodontology.

Periodontal Diseases: Changing Concepts & Treatment Strategies. Peter N. Galgut et al. 2000. 240p. (*0-948269-84-7*) Martin Dunitz GBR. *Dist:* Thieme Med Pubs.

Periodontal Instrumentation. Anna Pattison & Gordon Pattison. 2nd ed. 1991. LC 91-25914. (Illus.). 496p. (C). pap. 57.00 (*0-8385-7804-7*, A7804-6) P-H.

Periodontal Instrumentation for the Practitioner. Jill S. Nield-Gehrig. 1998. LC 98-21882. 422p. pap. 30.95 (*0-683-30493-3*) Lppncott W & W.

Periodontal Ligament in Health & Disease. Ed. by B. K. Berkovitz et al. 1982. (Illus.). 472p. (*0-08-024412-2*) Pergamon Repr GBR. *Dist:* Franklin.

Periodontal Medicine. Louis F. Rose et al. 1999. 352p. incl. cd-rom (*1-55009-120-4*) DEKR.

Periodontal Regeneration: Current Status & Directions. Ed. by Alan Polson. 1994. LC 93-39373. (Illus.). 224p. text 72.00 (*0-86715-175-7*) Quint Pub Co.

Periodontal Therapy Vol. I: Clinical Approaches & Evidence of Success, Vol. 1. Ed. by Myron Nevins & James Mellonig. 1998. LC 97-42610. (Illus.). 412p. text 178.00 (*0-86715-309-1*) Quint Pub Co.

Periodontic Syllabus. Ed. by Peter F. Fedi, Jr. et al. 3rd ed. 1995. LC 94-33984. (Illus.). 231p. pap. 39.00 (*0-683-03104-X*) Lppncott W & W.

Periodontic Syllabus. Peter F. Fedi, Jr. et al. 4th ed. 1999. LC 99-32590. 272p. pap. text 40.95 (*0-683-30668-5*) Lppncott W & W.

Periodontics - The Scientific Way. Jan Egelberg. 1992. 272p. (C). (gr. 13). 75.95 (*87-16-11001-3*) Mosby Inc.

Periodontitis in Man & Other Animals. R. C. Page & H. E. Schroeder. 1982. (Illus.). x, 330p. 129.75 (*3-8055-2479-X*) S Karger.

Periodontium. H. E. Schroeder. 1986. (Handbook of Microscopic Anatomy Ser.: Vol. 5; Pt. 5). (Illus.). 418p. 471.00 (*0-387-16604-1*) Spr-Verlag.

Periodontology. Peter A. Heasman et al. 1997. LC 97-13822. (Colour Guide Ser.). 138p. pap. text 21.95 (*0-443-05705-2*) Harcrt Hlth Sci Grp.

Periodontology. Klaus H. Rateitschak et al. Tr. by Thomas Hassell from GER. 2nd rev. ed. 1989. (Dental Medicine Ser.). (Illus.). 400p. text 169.00 (*0-86577-318-1*) Thieme Med Pubs.

Periodontology for the Dental Hygienist. Dorothy A. Perry et al. Ed. by Selma Ozmat. 1995. LC 95-19487. (Illus.). 336p. pap. text 36.00 (*0-7216-4063-X*) Saunders.

Periodontology Today. Ed. by B. Guggenheim. 1989. (Illus.). viii, 350p. pap. 104.50 (*3-8055-4843-5*) S Karger.

Perioperative Autologous Transfusion (Transcripts from a Conference) Linda C. Stehling. 1991. LC 90-14536. 177p. (C). text 20.00 (*0-915355-91-4*) Am Assn Blood.

Perioperative Care. Ed. by Richard M. Peters & Jose Toledo. 1992. LC 92-49794. (Current Topics in General Thoracic Surgery Ser.: Vol. 2). 462p. 168.00 (*0-444-89660-0*) Elsevier.

Perioperative Care: Anesthesia, Medicine & Surgery. David J. Stone & Bogdonoff. 1997. LC 97-16896. (Illus.). 864p. (C). (gr. 13). text 59.95 (*0-8151-4639-6*, 29911) Mosby Inc.

***Perioperative Care, Anaesthesia, Pain Management & Intensive Care: An Illustrated Color Text.** Michael Avidan et al. 2001. (Illus.). 130p. pap. (*0-443-06410-5*) Church GBR. *Dist:* Saunders.

Perioperative Care in Cardiac Anesthesia & Surgery. Tirone E. David & Davy C. Cheng. 1999. LC 98-50222. (Vademecum Ser.). spiral bd. 45.00 (*1-57059-527-5*) Landes Bioscience.

Perioperative Care of the Eye Patient. Ed. by Gilli Vajidis et al. 2002. (Illus.). 70p. pap. text (*0-7279-1225-9*) BMJ Pub GBR. *Dist:* AIDC.

Perioperative Management: For House Surgeons. P. R. Hambly & M. C. Sainsbury. 1996. (Illus.). 288p. (Orig.). pap. text (*1-85996-185-1*) Bios Sci GBR. *Dist:* Bks Intl VA.

Perioperative Management of Pacemaker Patients. Ed. by J. L. Atlee, III et al. 1992. LC 92-49912. (Illus.). xi, 155p. (*3-540-53874-7*); 155p. pap. 59.00 (*0-387-53874-7*) Spr-Verlag.

Perioperative Management of the Patient with Congenital Heart Disease. William J. Greeley. 1996. (Society of Cardiovascular Anesthesiologists Monograph). (Illus.). 258p. 60.00 (*0-683-18302-8*) Lppncott W & W.

Perioperative Medicine: The Medical Care of the Surgical Patient. Ed. by David R. Goldmann et al. 2nd ed. 1993. LC 93-20975. (Illus.). 736p. text 99.00 (*0-07-023702-6*) McGraw-Hill Prof.

Perioperative Monitoring in Carotid Surgery: Methods, Limits, & Results, Long-Term Results in Carotid Surgery. Ed. by S. Horsch & K. Ktenidis. 1998. (Illus.). 202p. 54.00 (*3-7985-1074-1*) Spr-Verlag.

Perioperative Nursing. Linda B. Chitwood & Diane C. Swain. 1991. LC 91-4737. (Notes Ser.). 128p. pap. 16.95 (*0-87434-368-2*) Springhouse Corp.

Perioperative Nursing: Perioperative Practice. Linda K. Groah. 3rd rev. ed. 1996. LC 95-46563. 512p. (C). text 52.95 (*0-8385-7365-7*, A7365-8, Apple Lange Med) McGraw.

Perioperative Nursing: Principles & Practice. Ed. by Mark L. Phippen & Maryann P. Wells. 1993. LC 92-24341. (Illus.). 1088p. text 66.00 (*0-7216-7233-7*) Saunders.

Perioperative Nursing: Principles & Practice. Ed. by Susan S. Fairchild. 2nd ed. 1996. LC 95-50442. 652p. text 56.95 (*0-316-25969-1*, Little Brwn Med Div) Lppncott W & W.

Perioperative Nursing Care. Susan S. Fairchild. 1993. (Nut Shell Ser.). 900p. (C). 57.50 (*0-86720-432-X*) Jones & Bartlett.

Perioperative Nursing Care Planning. Jane C. Rothrock. 2nd ed. 1996. (Illus.). 656p. (C). (gr. 13). pap. text 42.95 (*0-8151-7147-1*, 24557) Mosby Inc.

Perioperative Nursing Core Curriculum: Achieving Competency in Clinical Practice. Ed. by Rosemary A. Roth. 1995. (Illus.). 392p. pap. text 41.00 (*0-7216-5197-6*) Saunders.

Perioperative Nursing Handbook. Maryann P. Wells. 1994. LC 94-25433. (Illus.). 345p. pap. text 25.00 (*0-7216-3412-5*) Saunders.

Perioperative Patient Care. Julia A. Kneedler & Gwen H. Dodge. 3rd ed. 1994. (Illus.). 552p. (C). text 63.95 (*0-86720-642-X*, 642-X) Jones & Bartlett.

Perioperative Services: Administration, Resource Management & Patient Care. Cynthia Spry & Cathy Frye. 2nd ed. 2000. ring bd. 249.00 (*0-8342-1664-7*) Aspen Pub.

Perioperative Transfusion Medicine. Bruce D. Spiess et al. 1997. LC 97-4138. 607p. text 115.00 (*0-683-07892-5*) Lppncott W & W.

Peripatetic Club, 1933-1993. Ed. by George Cahill, Jr. 1994. (Illus.). 211p. (Orig.). pap. (*0-9641132-0-1*) Peripat Club.

Peripheral & Spinal Mechanisms in the Neural Control of Movement. Ed. by M. D. Binder. 1999. LC 00-266346. (Progress in Brain Research Ser.: Vol. 123). (Illus.). 498p. 213.00 (*0-444-50288-2*, North Holland) Elsevier.

Peripheral Arterial Chemoreceptors & Cardiovascular Integration. M. De Burgh Daly. 1997. LC 96-9435. (Monographs of the Physiological Society: No. 46). (Illus.). 756p. text 225.00 (*0-19-857675-7*) OUP.

P
Q
R

Peripheral Blood Stem Cell Autografts. Ed. by E. W. Wunder & Philippe R. Henon. 1993. (Illus.). 240p. 125.00 (*0-387-52612-9*) Spr-Verlag.

Peripheral Blood Stem Cell Transplantation: Recommendations for Nursing Education & Practice. Wendy Holmes et al. Ed. by Susan Ezzone. 1997. (Illus.). 60p. (Orig.). pap. text 45.00 (*1-890504-03-3*) Oncology Nursing.

Peripheral Blood Stem Cells. Ed. by Douglas Smith et al. 1993. (Illus.). 99p. (C). text 35.00 (*1-56395-022-7*) Am Assn Blood.

Peripheral Dopamine Pathophysiology. Francesco Amenta. 1990. LC 89-7255. 408p. 205.00 (*0-8493-6949-5*, RC409, CRC Reprint) Franklin.

Peripheral Endovascular Interventions. Ed. by Rodney A. White & Thomas J. Fogarty. 1996. (Illus.). 576p. (C). (gr. 13). text 134.00 (*0-8151-9260-6*, 25194) Mosby Inc.

Peripheral Endovascular Interventions. Ed. by Rodney A. White & Thomas J. Fogarty. 2nd ed. 1999. LC 98-44697. (Illus.). 658p. 150.00 (*0-387-98444-5*) Spr-Verlag.

Peripheral Lymph: Formation & Immune Function. Waldemar L. Olszewski. 1985. 176p. 105.00 (*0-8493-6137-0*, QP115, CRC Reprint) Franklin.

Peripheral Manipulation. G. D. Maitland. 3rd ed. 1991. (Illus.). 336p. pap. text 60.00 (*0-7506-1031-X*) Buttrwrth-Heinemann.

Peripheral Musculoskeletal Ultrasound Atlas. Ed. by Robert Dondelinger et al. 1996. LC 95-39513. (Illus.). 224p. text 119.00 (*0-86577-592-3*) Thieme Med Pubs.

Peripheral Nerve Block. F. L. Jenkner. 1977. LC 77-8317. (Illus.). 36.95 (*0-387-81426-4*) Spr-Verlag.

Peripheral Nerve Blocks: A Color Atlas. Ed. by Jacques E. Chelly. 1999. LC 99-11892. 240p. text 129.00 (*0-7817-1626-8*) Lppncott W & W.

Peripheral Nerve Development & Regeneration. Ed. by E. Scarpini et al. 1990. (FIDIA Research Ser.: Vol. 19). 330p. 104.00 (*0-387-97110-6*) Spr-Verlag.

Peripheral Nerve Disease. Mark J. Brown. 1999. (*0-7506-9068-2*) Buttrwrth-Heinemann.

Peripheral Nerve Disorders 2, Vol. 2. Ed. by Arthur K. Asbury & P. K. Thomas. 1995. LC 95-11157. (Blue Books of Practical Neurology: Vol. 15). 328p. text 100.00 (*0-7506-1765-9*) Buttrwrth-Heinemann.

Peripheral Nerve Lesions. Ed. by Madjid Samii. 1990. (Illus.). 465p. 256.00 (*0-387-52432-0*) Spr-Verlag.

Peripheral Nerve Lesions: Diagnosis & Therapy. Ed. by Mark Mumenthaler & H. Schliack. 1991. (Illus.). 464p. text 119.00 (*0-86577-361-0*) Thieme Med Pubs.

Peripheral Nerve Surgery. Julia K. Terzis. 1987. text 155.00 (*0-7216-1268-7*) Saunders.

Peripheral Nervous System. Ed. by Anders T. Bjorklund et al. 1988. (Handbooks of Chemical Neuroanatomy: No. 6). 716p. 395.00 (*0-444-90431-X*) Elsevier.

Peripheral Nervous System: Structure, Function, & Clinical Correlations. Lawrence J. Mathers, Jr. 1984. (Illus.). 227p. (C). reprint ed. pap. text 39.95 (*0-409-90074-5*) Buttrwrth-Heinemann.

Peripheral Neurology: Case Studies in Electrodiagnosis. Jay Liveson. 3rd ed. 2000. LC 99-55262. (Illus.). 528p. pap. text 57.50 (*0-19-513563-6*) OUP.

Peripheral Neuropathies. 1980. (Technical Report Ser.: No. 654). 138p. pap. text 9.00 (*92-4-120654-3*) World Health.

Peripheral Neuropathies, 1988: What Is Significantly New? Ed. by J. P. Assal & C. Liniger. 1990. (FIDIA Research Ser.: Vol. 21). 600p. 139.00 (*0-387-97188-2*) Spr-Verlag.

Peripheral Neuropathy, Set. Peter J. Dyck et al. 3rd ed. 1992. LC 92-11721. (Illus.). 1845p. text 415.00 (*0-7216-3242-4*) Saunders.

Peripheral Neuropathy: A Practical Approach to Diagnosis & Management. Didier Cros. 1998. LC 00-48778. (Illus.). 448p. text 89.00 (*0-397-51781-5*) Lppncott W & W.

Peripheral Neuropathy in Childhood. R. A. Ouvrier et al. 2nd rev. ed. 1998. (International Review of Child Neurology Ser.). 300p. (C). text (*1-898683-17-4*) Mc Keith Pr GBR. *Dist:* Cambridge U Pr.

Peripheral Retina in Profile. Norman Byer. 1982. (Illus.). 159p. 295.00 incl. audio, sl. (*0-9609428-0-7*) Criterion Pr.

Peripheral Signaling of the Brain: Its Role in Neural-Immune Interactions, Learning & Memory. Ed. by James L. McGaugh & R. C. Frederickson. Tr. by D. L. Felton. 1991. (Nueronal Control of Bodily Function Ser.: Vol. 6). (Illus.). 550p. text 98.00 (*0-88937-035-4*) Hogrefe & Huber Pubs.

Peripheral Vascular Diseases. Ed. by Jess R. Young et al. 2nd ed. 1996. LC 95-48133. (Illus.). 768p. (C). (gr. 13). text 160.00 (*0-8151-9785-3*, 25864) Mosby Inc.

Peripheral Vascular Disorders. Merlin. 2001. text (*0-7216-8971-X*) Harcrt Hlth Sci Grp.

Peripheral Vascular Interventions for Cardiovascular Specialists. Ed. by Christopher J. White et al. 2002. (Illus.). (*0-87993-416-6*) Futura Pub.

Peripheral Vascular Sonography: A Practical Guide. Joseph F. Polak. 1992. (Illus.). 384p. 129.00 (*0-683-06914-4*) Lppncott W & W.

Peripheral Vascular Stenting for Cardiologists. Ed. by Richard R. Heuser. 1999. 174p. (*1-85317-621-4*) Martin Dunitz GBR. *Dist:* Mosby Inc.

Peripheral Vascular Ultrasound. Abigail Thrush & Timothy Hartshorne. 1999. LC 99-31336. 215p. text (*0-443-06049-5*) Saunders.

Perish the Thought: The Stress Connection. Herman Lubens & John C. Kiley. 1995. 129p. (Orig.). pap. 14.95 (*0-9633198-4-1*) Jason Pr.

Peritoneal Adhesions. Ed. by K. H. Treutner & V. Schumpelick. 1996. LC 96-28281. (Illus.). 360p. pap. 84.95 (*3-540-61192-4*) Spr-Verlag.

Peritoneal Carcinomatosis: Drugs & Diseases. Ed. by Paul H. Sugarbaker. 1996. (Cancer Treatment & Research Ser.). 288p. (C). text 224.00 (*0-7923-3726-3*) Kluwer Academic.

Peritoneal Carcinomatosis: Principles of Management. Ed. by Paul H. Sugarbaker. 1996. (Cancer Treatment & Research Ser.). 464p. (C). text 320.50 (*0-7923-3727-1*) Kluwer Academic.

Peritoneal Dialysis. Ed. by Karl D. Nolph. 2nd ed. 1985. text 326.50 (*0-89838-685-3*); 3rd ed. 1988. (C). text 315.00 (*0-89838-406-0*) Kluwer Academic.

Peritoneal, Ovarian & Recto-Vaginal Endometriosis: The Identification of Three Separate Diseases. M. Nisolle & J. Donnez. 1996. (Illus.). 190p. lib. bdg. 52.95 (*1-85070-941-6*, Parthenon Pbng) CRC Pr.

Peritoneal Surgery. Ed. by Gere S. Dizerega. 1999. LC 99-12449. (Illus.). 560p. 159.00 (*0-387-98610-3*) Spr-Verlag.

Peritoneum. Gere S. DiZerega & Kathleen E. Rodgers. LC 92-2221. (Illus.). 1994. 378p. 170.00 (*0-387-97830-5*); 1992. 340p. (*3-540-97830-5*) Spr-Verlag.

Peritonitis in CAPS. Ed. by R. Augustin. 1987. (Contributions to Nephrology Ser.: Vol. 57). (Illus.). viii, 256p. 29.75 (*3-8055-4519-3*) S Karger.

Peritrophic Membranes. W. Peters. 1992. LC 91-15512. (Zoophysiology & Ecology Ser.: Vol. 30). (Illus.). 238p. 208.00 (*0-387-53635-3*) Spr-Verlag.

Perkins & Hansell's Atlas of Diseases of the Eye. Damian O'Neill. 4th ed. 1993. LC 93-9993. 112p. text (*0-443-04822-3*) Church.

Permaculture Book of Ferment & Human Nutrition. Bill Mollison. 1997. (Illus.). 288p. (Orig.). pap. (*0-908228-06-6*) Tagari Pubns AUS. *Dist:* RDLE INST Bkstre.

Permar's Oral Embryology & Microscopic Anatomy: A Textbook for Students in Dental Hygiene. Rudy C. Melfi et al. 10th ed. 2000. LC 00-21829. (Illus.). xv, 297p. pap. text 40.95 (*0-683-30644-8*) Lppncott W & W.

Permethrin. 1990. (Environmental Health Criteria Ser.: No. 94). 125p. pap. text 24.00 (*92-4-154294-2*, 1160094) World Health.

Permissible Levels of Occupational Exposure to Airborne Toxic Substances: Report of the ILO-WHO Committee on Occupational Health, 6th, Geneva, 1968. ILO-WHO Committee on Occupational Health Staff. 1969. (Technical Reports: No. 415). pap. text 3.00 (*92-4-120415-X*, 1100415) World Health.

Peroxidizing Herbicides. R. Von Bothmer et al. Ed. by Peter Boger & Ko Wakabayashi. 1999. LC 98-40482. (Illus.). 418p. 150.00 (*3-540-64550-0*) Spr-Verlag.

Peroximones: A Personal Account, 001. Frank Roels. 1994. LC 94-182980. (Illus.). 151p. pap. (*90-70289-94-6*) VUB Univ Pr BEL. *Dist:* Paul & Co Pubs.

Peroxisome Proliferators: Unique Inducers of Drug-Metabolizing Enzymes. Ed. by David E. Moody. 1994. 200p. 199.00 (*0-8493-8305-6*, 8305) CRC Pr.

Peroxisomes. Ed. by N. Latruffe & M. Bugaut. 1994. (Illus.). 217p. stu. ed. 108.00 (*0-387-56860-3*) Spr-Verlag.

Peroxisomes: Biology & Importance in Toxicology & Medicine. Ed. by G. Gordan Gibson & Brian G. Lake. 1993. 734p. (*0-7484-0053-2*) Tay Francis Ltd GBR. *Dist:* Taylor & Francis.

Peroxisomes: Biology & Role in Toxicology & Disease. Janardan K. Reddy. 1997. LC 96-39418. (Annals of the New York Academy of Sciences Ser.). 801p. 150.00 (*0-89766-967-3*) NY Acad Sci.

Peroxisomes in Biology & Medicine. Ed. by H. D. Fahimi & Helmut Sies. 1987. (Proceedings in Life Sciences Ser.). (Illus.). 470p. 151.00 (*0-387-16689-0*) Spr-Verlag.

Persian Gulf Experience & Health: Current Bibliographies in Medicine: January 1971 Through March 1994. Jacqueline VandeKamp & John H. Ferguson. 1996. 24p. reprint ed. pap. text 20.00 (*0-7881-3345-4*) DIANE Pub.

Persian Gulf War Syndromes—Facts, Symptoms & Controversy: Index of New Information. Innis C. Haverhold. 1997. 160p. 57.50 (*0-7883-1768-7*); pap. 47.50 (*0-7883-1769-5*) ABBE Pubs Assn.

Persian Medical Manuscripts at the University of California, Los Angeles: A Descriptive Catalogue. Lutz Richter-Bernburg. 1978. LC 77-94986. (Humana Civilitas Ser.: Vol. 4). (Illus.). xxiv, 297p. 57.00 (*0-89003-026-X*) Undena Pubns.

Persistant Viral Infections. Rafi Ahmed et al. 1999. LC 98-24568. (Illus.). 738p. 380.00 (*0-471-98083-8*) Wiley.

Persistence & Change in Personality Patterns. Katherine E. Roberts. 1943. (SRCD M Ser.: Vol. 8, No. 3). 25.00 (*0-527-01528-8*) Periodicals Srv.

Persistence of Error: Essays in Developmental Epistemology. Robert Kalechofsky. 1987. LC 87-14224. 80p. 17.00 (*0-8191-6457-7*) U Pr of Amer.

Persistent & Slow Virus Infections. J. Hotchin. Ed. by Joseph L. Melnick. 1971. (Monographs in Virology: Vol. 3). (Illus.). 53.25 (*3-8055-1176-0*) S Karger.

Persistent Bacterial Infections. Ed. by James P. Nataro et al. 2000. LC 00-25074. (Illus.). xv, 453p. 115.95 (*1-55581-159-0*) ASM Pr.

Persistent Pain: Psychosocial Assessment & Intervention. Ed. by N. Timothy Lynch & Sridhar V. Vasudevan. 1988. (Current Management of Pain Ser.). (C). text 140.50 (*0-89838-363-3*) Kluwer Academic.

Persistent Renal-Genitourinary Disorders. Jose Strauss. 1986. (Developments in Nephrology Ser.). text 161.50 (*0-89838-845-7*) Kluwer Academic.

Person. McAdams. 2nd ed. 1994. (C). pap. text, tchr. ed. 35.00 (*0-15-501967-8*) Harcourt Coll Pubs.

Person: An Introduction to Personality Psychology. Dan P. McAdams. 2nd ed. 1994. LC 93-78992. (Illus.). 704p. (C). text 95.00 (*0-15-501274-6*) Harcourt Coll Pubs.

Person: His & Her Development Throughout the Life Cycle. Theodore Lidz. rev. ed. 1983. LC 76-22745. 625p. pap. 40.00 (*0-465-05541-9*) Basic.

Person Behind the Syndrome. Peter H. Beighton & Greta Beighton. 1996. LC 96-17384. (Illus.). 248p. 64.00 (*3-540-76044-X*) Spr-Verlag.

Person-Centred Therapy: A European Perspective. Brian Thorne & Elke Lambers. 1998. LC 98-61238. 243 p. 66.00 (*0-7619-5154-7*, 2395) Sage.

Person Identification by Means of the Teeth: A Practical Guide. S. Keiser-Nielsen. 1980. (Illus.). 124p. pap. text (*0-7236-0557-2*) John Wright.

Person-in-Distress: On the Biosocial Dynamics of Adaptation. Norris Hansell. 1976. LC 74-8096. 248p. 35.95 (*0-87705-213-1*, Kluwer Acad Hman Sci) Kluwer Academic.

Person-in-Environment System: The PIE Classification System for Social Functioning Problems. Ed. by James M. Karls & Karin E. Wandrei. 1994. LC 94-23170. (C). 204p. pap., stu. ed. 28.95 (*0-87101-254-5*, 2545); 442p. pap. 28.95 (*0-87101-240-5*, 2405A) Natl Assn Soc Wkrs.

Person Schemes & Maladaptive Interpersonal Patterns. Ed. by Mardi J. Horowitz. 1991. LC 90-49633. (John D. & Catherine T. MacArthur Foundation Series on Mental Health & Development). (Illus.). 444p. 41.95 (*0-226-35375-3*) U Ch Pr.

Persona: Social Role & Personality. Helen H. Perlman. LC 68-21892. 1992. lib. bdg. 16.00 (*0-226-66030-3*); 1986. 256p. pap. text 18.00 (*0-226-66028-1*) U Ch Pr.

Personal Adjustment in Old Age. Ruth S. Cavan et al. Ed. by Robert J. Kastenbaum. 1979. LC 78-22188. (Aging & Old Age Ser.). (Illus.). reprint ed. lib. bdg. 19.95 (*0-405-11806-6*) Ayer.

***Personal & Practice Development Plans in Primary Care: A Practical Guide to Getting Star.** Derek Gallen & Glynis Buckle. 2001. LC 2001-43580. 192p. pap. 29.99 (*0-7506-5289-6*) Buttrwrth-Heinemann.

Personal Assistance: The Future of Home Care. Robert Morris et al. 1998. LC 98-5933. 220p. pap. text 20.95 (*0-8018-5903-4*) Johns Hopkins.

Personal Being: A Theory for Individual Psychology. Rom Harre. (Illus.). 304p. 1986. pap. 14.95 (*0-674-66314-4*); 1984. 35.00 (*0-674-66313-6*) HUP.

Personal Care in the Home. Ed. by Perspective Press. 1995. (Illus.). 164p. pap. text 20.95 (*0-89582-315-2*) Morton Pub.

Personal Causation: The Internal Affective Determinants of Behavior. R. De Charms. 1983. 416p. pap. text 49.95 (*0-89859-336-0*) L Erlbaum Assocs.

Personal Choices & Public Commitments: Perspectives on the Medical Humanities. Ed. by William J. Winslade. 1989. (Orig.). pap. 12.00 (*0-9621294-0-2*) Univ TX Med Humanities.

Personal Computing for Health Professionals. Philip Burnard. 1993. 144p. pap. 49.50 (*1-56593-149-1*, 0461) Singular Publishing.

Personal Computing in Nuclear Medicine. D. P. Pretschner. 1982. (Lecture Notes in Medical Informatics: Vol. 18). 133p. 29.95 (*0-387-11598-6*) Spr-Verlag.

Personal Construct Counselling in Action. Fay Fransella & Peggy Dalton. 1990. 160p. (C). 57.95 (*0-8039-8280-1*, 9301); pap. 19.95 (*0-8039-8281-X*, 9302) Sage.

Personal Construct Psychology: Clinical & Personality Assessment. Alvin W. Landfield & Franz R. Epting. 1986. LC 86-10477. 327p. 51.95 (*0-89885-315-X*); pap. 24.95 (*0-89885-318-4*) Kluwer Academic (Kluwer Acad Hman Sci).

Personal Construct Psychology in Clinical Practice: Theory, Research & Applications. David Winter. 1994. LC 93-47681. 480p. (C). pap. 39.95 (*0-415-00601-5*, B3911) Routledge.

Personal Construct Theory & Mental Health: Theory, Research & Practice. Ed. by Eric Button. 1985. 404p. 20.00 (*0-914797-15-8*) Brookline Bks.

Personal Construct Therapy: A Handbook. Linda Viney. 1996. (Developments in Clinical Psychology Ser.). (Illus.). 250p. LC 96-19463. 77.00 (*1-56750-229-6*); pap. 39.50 (*1-56750-230-X*) Greenwood (Ablex).

Personal Coping: Theory, Research, & Application. Ed. by Bruce N. Carpenter. 1992. LC 92-8378. 276p. 72.50 (*0-275-93012-2*, C3012, Praeger Pubs) Greenwood.

Personal Counseling: A Practical Guie That Teaches Basic Counseling Skills. Elwood N. Chapman & Richard L. Knowdell. 3rd ed. 1993. LC 92-54366. (Fifty-Minute Ser.). 94p. pap. 12.95 (*1-56052-184-8*) Crisp Pubns.

Personal Disorder & the Family. Peter Lomas. 1998. LC 97-31564. 227p. text 36.95 (*1-56000-341-3*) Transaction Pubs.

Personal Footprints: A Swagger, a Limp & a Therapist's Journey from Alcoholism to Fundamentalism to Personal Use. Charles Griffin. 1991. (Illus.). 191p. (Orig.). pap. (*0-9627591-0-4*) Prsnl Footprint.

Personal Health. Vivian Bernstein. 1997. (Life Skills for Today's World Ser.). pap., stu. ed. 9.32 (*0-8114-1915-0*) Raintree Steck-V.

Personal Health Care & Social Security: A Report. ILO-WHO Joint Committee. 1971. (Technical Reports: No. 480). 74p. pap. text 5.00 (*92-4-120480-X*, 1100480) World Health.

Personal Health-Care Organizer: The Original Patient Management Workbook. Craig R. Perkins & Kelly A. Perkins. 1994. 110p. 39.95 (*0-9642711-1-7*); pap. 22.95 (*0-9642711-0-9*) Crakel Pubns.

Personal Health Choices. Christopher Smith & Sandra Lee Smith. 1990. pap. 25.00 (*0-86720-132-0*); (Illus.). (C). pap. text 48.95 (*0-86720-130-4*, 130-4) Jones & Bartlett.

Personal Health Notes. Joan Dwyer. 1999. 124p. pap. (*0-7392-0111-5*, PO3008) Morris Pubng.

Personal Health Record: Assuming Responsibility for One's Own Health Management. Arthur Kanowitz & Sandra Kanowitz. 1987. 36p. (Orig.). pap. 1.98 (*0-942933-00-1*) Premier Pub CO.

Personal Health Reporter. Albert E. Rees. 1992. 627p. 130.00 (*0-8103-8392-6*, 101230) Gale.

Personal Hygiene for College Students. Delbert Oberteuffer. LC 77-177126. (Columbia University. Teachers College. Contributions to Education Ser.: No. 407). (C). reprint ed. 37.50 (*0-404-55407-5*) AMS Pr.

Personal Identity. Ed. by John Perry. 1975. (Topics in Philosophy Ser.: Vol. 2). 246p. pap. text 18.95 (*0-520-02960-7*) U CA Pr.

Personal Immunization Record. Paula D. Golden. 1994. (Illus.). 32p. (Orig.). pap. 7.95 (*1-886730-60-1*) Romping Feet.

Personal Injury: Actions, Defenses, Damages Louis R. Frumer & R. L. Benoit. 1957. ring bd. 2889.00 (*0-8205-1530-2*) Bender.

Personal Injury Defense Techniques Mark A. Dombroff. 1987. ring bd. 653.00 (*0-8205-1542-6*) Bender.

Personal Injury Deskbook, 1961-1990. 1961. 1650.00 (*0-8377-9130-8*, Rothman) W S Hein.

Personal Injury Forms, 1981-1991. John J. Higgins. 1991. (Nebraska Legal Forms Ser.). 200p. ring bd. 69.95 (*0-86678-028-9*, 82009-10, MICHIE) LEXIS Pub.

Personal Injury Litigation: Legal Practice Course Guides. Denis Carey. rev. ed. Date not set. 200p. pap. (*1-85431-514-5*) Blackstone Pr GBR. *Dist:* Gaunt.

Personal Injury Practice Handbook. Lise A. Young. 1986. 120p. pap. 35.00 (*0-911110-56-9*, MICHIE) LEXIS Pub.

Personal Inventory/Medical Alert Kit. George Berrang. 2nd rev. ed. 1997. i, 10p. ring bd. 29.95 (*0-9663990-0-5*) Ancora Pubns.

Personal Meanings of Death. Ed. by Franz R. Epting & Robert A. Neimeyer. 1984. LC 83-8529. (Death Education, Aging & Health Care Ser.). (Illus.). 246p. text 59.95 (*0-89116-363-8*) Hemisp Pub.

Personal Medical Information Security, Engineering, & Ethics: Proceedings, Personal Information Workshop, Cambridge, U. K., June 21-22, 1996. Isaac Newton Institute for Mathematical Sciences S et al. Ed. by Ross Anderson. 1997. LC 97-27559. 251p. pap. 48.95 (*3-540-63244-1*) Spr-Verlag.

Personal Medical Records: A Reference & History Handbook. Beth B. O'Neill. 1996. (Illus.). 90p. wbk. ed. 15.00 (*0-9652930-0-9*) Sr Assist Essent.

Personal Medical Savings Accounts (Medical IRA's) An Idea Whose Time Has Come. John C. Goodman & Gerald L. Musgrave. 1993. 35p. pap. 5.00 (*1-56808-011-5*, BG128) Natl Ctr Pol.

Personal Memoirs of John H. Brinton, Major & Surgeon U. S. V., 1861-1865. John H. Brinton. 1996. LC 95-49078. (Shawnee Classics Ser.). (Illus.). 384p. (C). reprint ed. pap. 14.95 (*0-8093-2044-4*) S Ill U Pr.

Personal Myth in Psychoanalytic Theory. Ed. by Peter Hartocollis & Ian Graham. 1992. 420p. 75.00 (*0-8236-4065-5*) Intl Univs Pr.

Personal Nutrition. Marie A. Boyle & Gail Zyla. Ed. by Marshall. 2nd ed. 1992. 390p. (C). pap. 45.25 (*0-314-93333-6*) West Pub.

Personal Nutrition. Marie A. Boyle & Gail Zyla. 3rd ed. 1996. LC 95-45675. 450p. (C). 60.95 (*0-314-06380-3*) West Pub.

Personal Orientation Manual for the NHA. Steven V. Benson. 1991. 175p. (Orig.). (C). pap. text 34.50 (*1-877735-30-2*, 2175PP) Prof Prnting & Pub.

Personal Perspectives on Emotional Disturbance - Behavioral Disorders. Ed. by Benjamin L. Brooks & David A. Sabatino. 1996. LC 94-45064. 495p. (Orig.). (C). pap. text 38.00 (*0-89079-618-1*, 6929) PRO-ED.

Personal Psychopathology: Early Formulations. Harry Stack Sullivan. 1984. 416p. reprint ed. pap. 9.95 (*0-393-30184-2*) Norton.

Personal Relations Therapy: The Collected Papers of H. J. S. Guntrip. Ed. by Jeremy Hazell. 1994. LC 93-33868. (Library of Object Relations). 448p. 60.00 (*1-56821-164-3*) Aronson.

Personal Relationship Inventory (PRI) Manual for Scoring & Interpretation. Ronald L. Mann. 1994. 91p. (Orig.). pap. 18.00 (*1-879858-03-7*) Behaviordyne.

Personal Relationships Vol. 1: Studying Personal Relationships. Ed. by Steve Duck & Robin Gilmour. 1981. LC 80-41360. text 120.00 (*0-12-222801-4*) Acad Pr.

Personal Renewal: Your Guide to Vitality, Allure & a Joyful Life Using Healing, Herbs, Diet, Movement & Visualizations. Letha Hadady. 1999. (Illus.). 256p. pap. 13.00 (*0-609-80229-1*, Three Riv Pr) Crown Pub Group.

Personal Response Systems: An International Report of a New Home Care Service. Intro. by Andrew S. Dibner. 1993. LC 92-25580. (Home Health Care Services Quarterly Ser.: Vol. 13, Nos. 3 & 4, 1992). (Illus.). 280p. lib. bdg. 49.95 (*1-56024-272-8*) Haworth Pr.

Personal Responsibility & Therapy: An Integrative Approach. Richard Nelson-Jones. 1987. 214p. 49.95 (*0-89116-777-3*) Hemisp Pub.

Personal Stress Reduction Program. Jeffrey W. Forman & Dave Myers. 1987. (Illus.). 160p. 11.50 (*0-13-659277-5*) P-H.

Personal Wellness: How to Go the Distance. Alban Bacchus & Carol Bacchus. Ed. by Margaret Savage. 1999. (Illus.). 336p. pap. 24.95 (*0-9674834-0-9*, Medawellcom) Engin Systms Sol.

Personal Wellness: Your Most Profitable Investment. Rick Griggs. 1990. LC 89-81519. (Fifty-Minute Ser.). (Illus.). 104p. pap. 12.95 (*1-56052-021-3*, C021) Crisp Pubns.

Personality. Ed. by Lanning. 1999. (C). text (*0-321-01191-0*) Addson-Wesley Educ.

Personality. Jerry M. Burger. 2nd ed. 1989. 525p. (C). mass mkt. 51.50 (*0-534-11664-7*); 3rd ed. 1993. pap., stu. ed. 19.95 (*0-534-17222-9*) Brooks-Cole.

Personality. Seymour Feshbach & Bernard Weiner. 3rd ed. 1991. LC 90-82955. 650p. (C). text 67.56 (*0-669-20898-1*) HM Trade Div.

Personality: A Cognitive Approach. Jo Brunas-Wagstaff. 1998. LC 97-39541. (Psychology Focus Ser.). 176p. (C). pap. 15.95 (*0-415-16305-6*) Routledge.

Personality: A Systems Approach. Emmons. Date not set. (C). text 63.50 (*0-15-501985-6*) Harcourt Coll Pubs.

Personality: Analysis & Interpretation of Lives. David Winter. 1995. pap. text, tchr. ed., suppl. ed. (*0-07-071130-5*) McGraw.

Personality: Analysis & Interpretation of Lives. David G. Winter. 1995. LC 95-15697. 678p. (C). text 78.44 (*0-07-071129-1*) McGrw-H Hghr Educ.

Personality: Classic Theories & Modern Research. Friedman et al. 1998. LC 98-28088. 566p. 93.00 (*0-205-13953-1*) Allyn.

Personality: Critical Concepts in Psychology Cary L. Cooper & Lawrence A. Pervin. 1998. LC 97-32757. 1664p. (C). reprint ed. 735.00 (*0-415-13504-4*) Routledge.

Personality: Evolutionary Heritage & Human Distinctiveness. Arnold H. Buss. 1988. 280p. (C). text 49.95 (*0-8058-0298-3*) L Erlbaum Assocs.

Personality: In Search of Individuality. Nathan Brody. 1988. 270p. text 69.95 (*0-12-134845-8*) Acad Pr.

Personality: Inquiry & Application. Mark Sherman. 1979. LC 78-13540. (General Psychology Ser.: Vol. 74). 560p. 40.00 (*0-08-019585-7*, Pergamon Pr) Elsevier.

Personality: Selected Readings in Theory. Willard B. Frick. 1994. LC 93-86172. 323p. (C). pap. 37.00 (*0-87581-383-6*, PER) F E Peacock Pubs.

Personality: Strategies & Issues. Robert M. Liebert & Michael D. Spiegler. 5th ed. 1987. (C). pap. 39.00 (*0-534-10675-7*) Brooks-Cole.

Personality: The Individuation Process in the Light of C. G. Jung's Typology. C. A. Meier. 1995. 192p. pap. 16.95 (*0-385-63054-9*) Portunus Pubng.

Personality: Theories, Assessment, Research & Applications. Lewis R. Aiken. 2000. LC 00-44709. (Illus.). xiii, 461p. text 89.95 (*0-398-07110-1*); 4th ed. pap. text 64.95 (*0-398-07111-X*) C C Thomas.

Personality: Theory & Research. Jerry M. Burger. 4th ed. 1996. LC 96-3311. (Psychology Ser.). 590p. text 52.25 (*0-534-33924-7*) Brooks-Cole.

Personality: Theory & Research. Lawrence A. Pervin. 7th ed. 1996. LC 96-7678. 608p. 80.95 (*0-471-12804-X*) Wiley.

Personality & Ability: The Personality Assessment System. Charles J. Krauskopf & David R. Saunders. 1993. LC 93-26379. 282p. (Orig.). (C). 67.00 (*0-8191-9281-3*); pap. 35.00 (*0-8191-9282-1*) U Pr of Amer.

Personality & Adversity: Psychospiritual Aspects of Rehabilitation. Carolyn Vash. 1994. LC 94-1497. 304p. (C). text 37.95 (*0-8261-8040-X*) Springer Pub.

Personality & Depression: A Current View. Marjorie H. Klein. Ed. by David J. Kupfer et al. 1993. LC 92-48737. (Mental Health & Psychopathology Ser.). 195p. 35.00 (*0-89862-118-6*) Guilford Pubns.

Personality & Disease. Ed. by Howard S. Friedman. 1990. LC 90-11927. (Health Psychology & Behavioral Medicine Ser.). 315p. 205.00 (*0-471-61805-5*) Wiley.

Personality & Individual Differences: A Natural Science Approach. Hans J. Eysenck & M. W. Eysenck. 1985. (Perspectives on Individual Differences Ser.). (Illus.). 452p. (C). 49.50 (*0-306-41844-4*, Plenum Trade) Perseus Pubng.

Personality & Intelligence: Psychometric & Experimental Approaches. Ed. by Robert J. Sternberg & Patricia Ruzgis. 1994. LC 93-21757. (Illus.). 351p. (C). text 69.95 (*0-521-41790-2*); pap. text 24.95 (*0-521-42835-1*) Cambridge U Pr.

Personality & Its Disorders: A Biosocial Learning Approach. Theodore Millon & George S. Everly, Jr. 1985. LC 84-21995. 304p. (C). pap. 46.95 (*0-471-87816-2*) Wiley.

Personality & Persuasibility. Janis L. Irving. 1982. LC 82-11848. (Yale Studies in Attitude & Communication). 333p. reprint ed. lib. bdg. 78.50 (*0-313-23320-9*, JAPE, Greenwood Pr) Greenwood.

Personality & Psychological Assessment. Benjamin Kleinmuntz. 1985. LC 85-18142. 462p. (C). reprint ed. lib. bdg. 52.50 (*0-89874-893-3*) Krieger.

Personality & Psychopathology. Ed. by C. Robert Cloninger. 1999. LC 98-30095. (American Psychopathological Association Ser.). xv, 524p. 59.95 (*0-88048-923-5*, 8923) Am Psychiatric.

Personality & Sexuality in the Physically Handicapped Woman. Carney Landis & M. Marjorie Bolles. Ed. by William R. Phillips & Janet Rosebberg. 1980. LC 79-6912. (Physically Handicapped in Society Ser.). reprint ed. lib. bdg. 19.95 (*0-405-13121-6*) Ayer.

Personality & Social Adjustment. Charles A. Heidenreich. 1970. 9.95 (*0-9600428-4-9*) Heidenreich.

Personality & Social Behaviour. Adrian Furnham & Patrick C. Heaven. 1998. LC 98-37860. 352p. (*0-340-67724-4*); pap. (*0-340-67725-2*) E A GBR. *Dist:* OUP.

Personality & the Teaching of Composition. George H. Jensen & John K. DiTiberio. Ed. by Marcia Farr. 1989. LC 88-10446. (Writing Research Ser.: Vol. 20). 224p. (C). 77.00 (*0-89391-504-1*, Ablex) Greenwood.

Personality at the Crossroads. David Magnusson & Norman S. Endler. 1977. LC 77-4190. 464p. (C). text 79.95 (*0-89859-293-3*) L Erlbaum Assocs.

Personality Characteristics of Patients with Pain. Ed. by Robert J. Gatchel & James N. Weisberg. 2000. LC 99-52773. (Illus.). xii, 311p. 39.95 (*1-55798-646-0*) Am Psychol.

Personality, Cognition, & Social Interaction. Ed. by N. Cantor & John F. Kihlstrom. 1981. LC 81-208. 384p. text 79.95 (*0-89859-057-4*) L Erlbaum Assocs.

Personality Development: Theoretical, Empirical, & Clinical Investigations of Loevinger's Conception of Ego Development. P. Michiel Westenberg et al. 1998. LC 97-41407. 89.95 (*0-8058-1649-6*) L Erlbaum Assocs.

Personality Development & Deviation: A Textbook for Social Work. Ed. by George H. Wiedeman & Sumner Matison. 1974. LC 73-89439. 539p. 80.00 (*0-8236-4070-1*) Intl Univs Pr.

Personality Development & Psychopathology: A Dynamic Approach Norman Cameron & Joseph F. Rychlak. 2nd ed. 1984. LC 84-80710. 816p. (C). text 78.36 (*0-395-34387-9*) HM.

Personality Development & Psychotherapy in Our Diverse Society: A Sourcebook. Rafael A. Javier & William G. Herron. 1998. LC 98-5659. (Illus.). 728p. 65.00 (*0-7657-0167-7*) Aronson.

Personality Development in Adolescent Girls. Lawrence K. Frank et al. 1951. (SRCD M Ser.: Vol. 16). 25.00 (*0-527-01552-0*) Periodicals Srv.

Personality Differences & Biological Variations: A Study of Twins. Gordon S. Claridge et al. 1973. LC 72-10132. (C). (*0-08-017124-9*) Pergamon Repr GBR. *Dist:* Franklin.

Personality Disorder Interview IV: A Semistructured Interview for the Assessment of Personality Disorders. Thomas A. Widiger et al. 1995. LC 94-43676. 309p. 50.00 (*0-911907-21-1*) Psych Assess.

Personality Disorders: A Psychological Approach to Clinical Management. Ira D. Turkat. 1991. (Psychology Practitioner Guidebooks Ser.). 136p. text (*0-08-036124-2*); pap. text (*0-08-036123-4*) PPI GBR. *Dist:* Elsevier.

Personality Disorders: Diagnosis, Management & Course. Peter J. Tyrer. 2nd ed. 2000. LC 00-21641. (Illus.). 214p. pap. (*0-7506-3433-2*) E A GBR. *Dist:* OUP.

Personality Disorders: New Look at the Developmental Self & Object Relations Approach: Theory, Diagnosis & Treatment. James F. Masterson. 2000. LC 99-32777. (Illus.). 276p. 35.95 (*1-891944-33-9*) Zeig Tucker Theisen.

Personality Disorders: New Symptom-Focused Drug Therapy. Sonny Joseph. 1997. LC 96-28626. (Illus.). (C). 274p. 59.95 (*0-7890-0134-9*); 266p. pap. text 29.95 (*0-7890-0195-0*) Haworth Pr (Hawrth Medical).

Personality Disorders: Recognition & Clinical Management. Jonathan H. Dowson & Adrian T. Grounds. 1996. (Illus.). 414p. (C). text 95.00 (*0-521-45049-7*) Cambridge U Pr.

Personality Disorders & Culture: Clinical & Conceptual Interactions. Renato D. Alarcon et al. 1998. LC 97-46371. 310p. 100.00 (*0-471-14964-0*) Wiley.

Personality Disorders & the Five-Factor Model of Personality. Ed. by Paul T. Costa, Jr. & Thomas A. Widiger. 1994. LC 93-26795. 364p. text 39.95 (*1-55798-214-7*) Am Psychol.

Personality Disorders in Modern Life: Character Disorders. Theodore Millon & Roger D. Davis. 1999. LC 99-30334. (Illus.). 600p. 103.00 (*0-471-32355-1*) Wiley.

Personality Disorders in Older Adults: Emerging Issues in Diagnosis & Treatment. Ed. by Erlene Rosowsky et al. 1999. LC 98-49371. (Personality & Clinical Psychology Ser.). 328p. 39.95 (*0-8058-2683-1*) L Erlbaum Assocs.

Personality Dynamics. B. B. Wilman. 1991. (Illus.). 176p. (C). 39.50 (*0-306-43956-5*, Plenum Trade) Perseus Pubng.

Personality, Elevated Blood Pressure, & Essential Hypertension. Ed. by Ernest H. Johnson et al. 1992. LC 92-1480. (Series in Health Psychology & Behavioral Medicine). 69.95 (*1-56032-142-3*) Hemisp Pub.

Personality Factors in Mothers of Excessively Crying Infants. Martin Lakin. 1957. (SRCD M Ser.: Vol. 22, No. 1). pap. 25.00 (*0-527-01569-5*) Periodicals Srv.

Personality, Genetics, & Behavior: Selected Papers. Hans J. Eysenck. Ed. by Charles D. Speilberger. 1982. LC 81-15765. (Centennial Psychology Ser.). 340p. 55.00 (*0-275-90787-2*, C0787, Praeger Pubs) Greenwood.

Personality in Adulthood. Robert R. McCrae & Paul Costa. 1990. LC 89-78494. 198p. pap. 22.00 (*0-89862-528-9*, 2528) Guilford Pubns.

Personality in Adulthood. Robert R. McCrae & Paul T. Costa, Jr. 1990. LC 89-78494. 198p. text 45.00 (*0-89862-429-0*) Guilford Pubns.

Personality in Middle Life & Late Life: Empirical Studies. Bernice L. Neugarten et al. Ed. by Leon Stein. 1980. LC 79-8677. (Growing Old Ser.). (Illus.). reprint ed. lib. bdg. 25.95 (*0-405-12794-4*) Ayer.

Personality in the Social Process. Joel Aronoff & John P. Wilson. 1985. 408p. text 79.95 (*0-89859-526-6*) L Erlbaum Assocs.

Personality, Motivation & Action: Selected Papers. John W. Atkinson. Ed. by Charles D. Spielberger. 1983. LC 83-4261. (Centennial Psychology Ser.). 432p. 38.95 (*0-275-90937-9*, C0937, Praeger Pubs) Greenwood.

Personality Neurosurgery. 1988. 193p. 175.00 (*0-387-82088-4*) Spr-Verlag.

Personality Organization in Cognitive Controls & Intellectual Abilities. Riley W. Gardner et al. 1961. (Psychological Issues Monographs: No. 8, Vol. 2, No. 4). 148p. (Orig.). 27.50 (*0-8236-4080-9*) Intl Univs Pr.

Personality, Power & Authority: A View from the Behavioral Sciences, 1. Leonard William Doob. 1983. LC 83-1688. (Contributions in Psychology Ser.: No. 1). 218p. 60.00 (*0-313-23920-7*, DPA/, Greenwood Pr) Greenwood.

Personality Projection in the Drawing of the Human Figure: A Method of Personality Investigation. Karen Machover. 1980. (Illus.). 192p. 39.95 (*0-398-01184-2*) C C Thomas.

Personality Psychology. Ed. by D. M. Buss & Nancy Cantor. 1989. (Illus.). 352p. 89.95 (*0-387-96993-4*) Spr-Verlag.

Personality Psychology in Europe, Vol. 3. G. Van Heck et al. 1990. xiv, 242p. pap. (*90-265-1037-3*) Swets.

Personality Psychology in Europe Vol. 2: Current Trends & Controversies. Ed. by A. Angleitner et al. 1986. xii, 272p. pap. (*90-265-0597-3*) Swets.

Personality Puzzle. David C. Funder. 2nd ed. 2000. LC 00-33223. (Illus.). xxiv, 597p. (C). pap. 45.00 (*0-393-97541-X*, Norton Paperbks) Norton.

Personality, Roles & Social Behavior. Ed. by W. Ickes & E. S. Knowles. 1982. (Social Psychology Ser.). (Illus.). 362p. 105.00 (*0-387-90637-1*) Spr-Verlag.

Personality Self-Portrait see New Personality Self-Portrait: Why You Think, Work, Love & Act the Way You Do

Personality, Social, & Biological Perspectives on Personal Adjustment. Bem P. Allen. 1990. 550p. (C). text 48.95 (*0-534-13020-8*) Brooks-Cole.

Personality, Social Skills, & Psychopathology: An Individual Differences Approach. D. G. Gilbert & J. J. Connolly. 1991. (Perspectives on Individual Differences Ser.). (Illus.). 312p. (C). 59.50 (*0-306-43793-7*, Plenum Trade) Perseus Pubng.

Personality Structure & Human Interaction: The Developing Synthesis of Psychodynamic Theory. Harry Guntrip. 1964. LC 61-12135. 456p. 67.50 (*0-8236-4120-1*) Intl Univs Pr.

Personality Styles & Brief Psychotherapy. Mardi J. Horowitz. 1997. LC 97-23002. 368p. pap. 50.00 (*1-56821-870-2*) Aronson.

Personality Tests & Reviews II. Ed. by Oscar K. Buros. 1975. LC 74-13192. (Tests in Print Ser.). 841p. text 65.00 (*0-910674-19-1*) U of Nebr Pr.

Personality Theories Barbara O. Engler. 4th ed. 1994. LC 94-76501. (C). text 69.56 (*0-395-70835-4*) HM.

Personality Theory Barbara O. Engler. Date not set. LC 94-76501. (C). text, tchr. ed., suppl. ed. 69.56 (*0-395-71710-8*) HM.

Personality Theory & Clinical Practice. Peter Fonagy & Anna Higgitt. 1985. 194p. pap. 8.95 (*0-416-35630-3*, NO. 9182) Routledge.

Personality Theory in Action: Handbook for the Objective-Analytic (O-A) Battery. Raymond B. Cattell & James M. Schuerger. 1978. LC 78-50146. 58.75 (*0-918296-11-0*) Inst Personality & Ability.

Personality Traits. Gerald Matthews & Ian J. Deary. 1998. LC 97-14349. 319p. (C). text 54.95 (*0-521-49739-6*); pap. text 21.95 (*0-521-49759-0*) Cambridge U Pr.

Personality Type A: Index of New Information with Authors, Subjects, Research Categories & References. Lois A. Hutton. 1997. 150p. pap. 47.50 (*0-7883-1335-5*) ABBE Pubs Assn.

Personality Types. Don R. Riso & Russ Hudson. rev. ed. 1996. LC 96-22202. 456p. pap. 14.00 (*0-395-79867-1*) HM.

Personality Unfolded Through Script-Psychology. Rex Smith. unabr. ed. 1989. (Illus.). 414p. pap. text 24.95 (*0-9623117-0-7*) Writeway Servs.

Personalized Stress Management: A Manual for Everyday Life & Work. Joseph L. Gill. 1983. LC 82-90115. (Illus.). 175p. 14.95 (*0-910819-00-9*); pap. 9.95 (*0-910819-01-7*) Counsel & Consult.

***Personhood & Health Care.** Ed. by David C. Thomasma et al. 2001. LC 2001-50226. (International Library of Ethics, Law, & the New Medicine: Vol. 7). 462p. (*1-4020-0098-7*) Kluwer Academic NLD. *Dist:* Kluwer Academic.

Personhood in Advanced Old Age: Implications for Practice. Sheldon S. Tobin. 1991. LC 90-10444. 200p. 30.95 (*0-8261-7580-5*) Springer Pub.

Personhood of the Therapist. Ed. by Barbara Jo Brothers. 2000. LC 00-59674. 128p. 49.95 (*0-7890-1166-2*); pap. 29.95 (*0-7890-1167-0*) Haworth Pr.

Personnel for Health Care: Case Studies of Educational Programmes, Vol. 1. F. Katz. 1978. (Public Health Papers: No. 70). 260p. text 21.00 (*92-4-130070-1*, 1110070) World Health.

Personnel Law for Community Associations. William E. Stewart. 3rd ed. 1997. LC 97-187155. 76p. (C). pap. 18.95 (*0-941301-39-7*) CAI.

Personnel Management in the Medical Practice: The Physician's Handbook for Successful Management. American Medical Association Staff. 1996. (Practice Success Ser.). pap. 54.00 (*0-89970-756-4*, OP700995WE) AMA.

Personnel Management in the National Health Service. Maurice W. Cuming. 1978. pap. 17.95 (*0-434-90291-8*) Trafalgar.

Personnel Policies & Procedures for Health Care Facilities: A Manager's Manual & Guide. Eugene P. Buccini & Charles P. Mullaney. 1989. LC 88-36491. 311p. 89.50 (*0-89930-425-7*, BPQ, Quorum Bks) Greenwood.

Personnel Preparation in Disability & Community Life: Toward Universal Approaches to Support. Ed. by Julie Ann Racino. 2000. LC 00-37737. (Illus.). xx, 330p. 65.95 (*0-398-07077-6*) C C Thomas.

Personology: Method & Content in Personality Assessment & Psychobiography. Irving E. Alexander. 1990. LC 89-36230. 294p. (Orig.). (C). text 54.95 (*0-8223-0996-3*); pap. text 19.95 (*0-8223-1020-1*) Duke.

Persons, Animals, & Fetuses: An Essay in Practical Ethics. Mary G. Forrester. 1996. (Philosophical Studies: Vol. 66). 312p. (C). text 147.00 (*0-7923-3918-5*) Kluwer Academic.

Persons, Behavior, & the World: The Descriptive Psychology Approach. Mary M. Shideler. 1988. 362p. (Orig.). (C). pap. text 37.00 (*0-8191-6787-8*) U Pr of Amer.

Persons Handicapped by Rubella: Victors & Victims, a Follow-Up Study. Jan J. Van Dijk et al. 1991. 180p. (*90-265-1128-0*) Swets.

Perspective: A Conceptual, Ecological, Generic Model for Understanding Substance Use & Abuse: the Active Ingredients. Earl S. Shive. 2nd ed. 1994. (Illus.). 194p. (Orig.). (C). pap. text 22.25 (*0-9628229-2-2*) ESS Pubns.

Perspective in Zoosemiotics. Thomas A. Sebeok. 1972. LC 72-189708. (Janua Linguarum, Ser. Minor: No. 122). (Illus.). 188p. (Orig.). pap. text (*90-279-2121-0*) Mouton.

Perspective on New Techniques in Congenital & Acquired Heart Disease: Proceedings of the Cardiovascular Disease Conference, 4th, Snowmass at Aspen, Colorado, Jan. 1973. Cardiovascular Disease Conference Staff. Ed. by J. Vogel. 1974. (Advances in Cardiology Ser.: Vol. 11). 95.00 (*3-8055-1654-1*) S Karger.

Perspective on the Art of Chinese Healing Vol. II: Pathways to Wisdom. John Walter. 2001. 240p. pap. 15.95 (*1-58151-070-5*) BookPartners.

Perspectives & Issues in Health Care. Mitchell. (LPN/LVN Nursing Ser.). 1998. pap. 24.95 (*0-8273-6319-2*); 1996. tchr. ed. 14.95 (*0-8273-6320-6*) Delmar.

Perspectives & Promises of Clinical Psychology. A. Ehlers et al. 1992. (Applied Clinical Psychology Ser.). (Illus.). 262p. (C). 54.50 (*0-306-44098-9*, Plenum Trade) Perseus Pubng.

Perspectives in Ageing Research. Rameshwar Singh & G. S. Singhal. 1990. (Illus.). 395p. (*1-55528-219-9*) Today Tomorrow IND. *Dist:* Lubrecht & Cramer, Scholarly Pubns.

Perspectives in Applied Phonology. Barbara W. Hodson & Mary Louise Edwards. 1986. LC 96-43784. (Diagnostic & Management Strategies Ser.). pap. 51.00 (*0-8342-0881-4*) PRO-ED.

Perspectives in Asian Cross-Cultural Psychology. Ed. by J. L. Dawson et al. 1981. x, 198p. pap. (*90-265-0359-8*) Swets.

Perspectives in Avian Endocrinology. S. Harvey & R. Etches. 1996. 408p. 157.95 (*1-898099-09-X*) Blackwell Sci.

Perspectives in Behavioral Medicine: Eating Regulation & Discontrol. Ed. by Herbert Weiner & Andrew Baum. 1987. 248p. 49.95 (*0-89859-928-8*) L Erlbaum Assocs.

Perspectives in Bioethics. R. Lawler & W. May. Ed. by F. Lescoe & D. Liptak. 1983. (Pope John Paul II Lecture Series in Bioethics: Vol. I). 66p. (Orig.). pap. 3.75 (*0-910919-00-3*) Mariel Pubns.

Perspectives in Cellular Regulation: Bacteria to Cancer. Ed. by Judith Campisi et al. 1991. LC 90-26568. (MBL Lectures in Biology: Vol. 11). 370p. 215.00 (*0-471-56090-1*, Wiley-Interscience) Wiley.

Perspectives in Clinical Investigation. Ed. by Thomas P. Stossel. 1984. 72p. (Orig.). pap. 10.00 (*0-87470-040-X*) Rockefeller.

Perspectives in Dental Ceramics. Jack D. Preston. 1988. (Illus.). 472p. text 160.00 (*0-86715-136-6*, 1366) Quint Pub Co.

Perspectives in Ethology Vol. 4: Advantages of Diversity. Ed. by P. P. Bateson & Peter H. Klopfer. 1980. LC 73-79427. 276p. 65.00 (*0-306-40511-3*, Plenum Trade) Perseus Pubng.

Perspectives in Ethology Vol. 5: Ontogeny. Ed. by P. P. Bateson & Peter H. Klopfer. 1982. LC 73-79427. 536p. 79.50 (*0-306-41063-X*, Plenum Trade) Perseus Pubng.

Perspectives in Ethology Vol. 6: Mechanisms. Ed. by P. P. Bateson & Peter H. Klopfer. 1985. LC 73-79427. 324p. 69.50 (*0-306-41846-0*, Plenum Trade) Perseus Pubng.

Perspectives in Exercise Science & Sports Medicine. David R. Lamb et al. 1988. LC 88-70343. (*0-936157-34-8*) Brown & Benchmark.

Perspectives in Exercise Science & Sports Medicine: Energy Metabolism in Exercise & Sport, Vol. 5. Ed. by David Lamb & Carl V. Gisolfi. 1992. LC 91-73932. (Illus.). 495p. reprint ed. text 49.00 (*1-884125-36-0*) Cooper Pubng.

Perspectives in Exercise Science & Sports Medicine: Exercise, Heat, & Thermoregulation, Vol. 6. Ed. by David Lamb et al. 1993. LC 92-73445. (Illus.). 405p. text 49.00 (*1-884125-37-9*) Cooper Pubng.

Perspectives in Exercise Science & Sports Medicine: Prolonged Exercise, Vol. 1. Ed. by David R. Lamb & Robert Murray. 1988. LC 88-70343. (Illus.). 494p. reprint ed. text 49.00 (*1-884125-34-4*) Cooper Pubng.

Perspectives in Exercise Science & Sports Medicine: Youth, Exercise & Sport, Vol. 2. Ed. by Carl V. Gisolfi & David Lamb. 1989. LC 88-70343. (Illus.). 590p. reprint ed. text 49.00 (*1-884125-35-2*) Cooper Pubng.

Perspectives in Exercise Science & Sports Medicine Vol. 3: Fluid Homeostasis During Exercise. Ed. by Carl V. Gisolfi & David Lamb. 1990. LC 88-70343. (Illus.). 456p. reprint ed. text 49.00 (*1-884125-07-7*) Cooper Pubng.

Perspectives in Exercise Science & Sports Medicine Vol. 4: Ergogenics: Enhancement of Athletic Performance. Ed. by David Lamb & Melvin Williams. 1991. LC 88-70343. (Illus.). 444p. reprint ed. text 49.00 (*1-884125-08-5*) Cooper Pubng.

Perspectives in Exercise Science & Sports Medicine Vol. 7: Physiology & Nutrition of Competitive Sport. Ed. by David Lamb. 1994. LC 88-70343. (Illus.). 400p. (C). text 49.00 (*1-884125-09-3*) Cooper Pubng.

Perspectives in Exercise Science & Sports Medicine Vol. 8: Exercise in Older Adults. Ed. by David Lamb et al. 1995. LC 88-70343. (Illus.). 400p. text 49.00 (*1-884125-20-4*) Cooper Pubng.

Perspectives in Exercise Science & Sports Medicine Vol. 10: Optimizing Sport Performance. Ed. by David R. Lamb & Robert Murray. 1997. 450p. text 49.00 (*1-884125-63-8*) Cooper Pubng.

Perspectives in Exercise Science & Sports Medicine Vol. 11: Exercise, Nutrition, & Weight Control. Ed. by David R. Lamb & Robert Murray. 1998. LC 95-67366. 450p. text 49.00 (*1-884125-70-0*) Cooper Pubng.

Perspectives in Exercise Science & Sports Medicine Vol. 12: The Metabolic Basis of Performance in Sport & Exercise. Ed. by David R. Lamb & Robert Murray. 1999. 450p. (C). text 49.00 (*1-884125-73-5*) Cooper Pubng.

Perspectives in Exercise Science & Sports Medicine Vol. 12: The Metabolic Basis of Performance in Sport & Exercise. Douglas B. McKeag & David Hough. Ed. by David R. Lamb & Robert Murray. 1999. (Illus.). 450p. (C). 49.00 (*1-884125-68-9*) Cooper Pubng.

Perspectives in Experimental Gerontology. Ed. by Nathan W. Shock & Leon Stein. 1980. LC 79-8689. (Illus.). reprint ed. lib. bdg. 40.95 (*0-405-12805-3*) Ayer.

Perspectives in Glaucoma Research, Pt. I. Ed. by E. Luetjen-Drecoll. 1996. (Journal: Vol. 210, No. 5, 1996). (Illus.). 70p. pap. 69.75 (*3-8055-6378-7*) S Karger.

Perspectives in Glaucoma Research, Pt. II. Ed. by Elke Lutjen-Drecoll. 1997. (Journal: Vol. 211, No. 3, 1997). (Illus.). 84p. pap. 60.00 (*3-8055-6515-1*) S Karger.

Perspectives in Gynecology & Obstetrics: Selected Plenary Papers Presented at the XIV European Congress of Gynaecologists & Obstetricians, Granada, Spain, September, 1999. Ed. by F. Gonzalez Gomez & S. Palacios. 1999. LC 99-51628. (Illus.). 184p. lib. bdg. 71.95 (*1-85070-774-X*, Parthenon Pbng) CRC Pr.

Perspectives in Lung Cancer: Proceedings of the Frederick E. Jones Memorial Symposium in Thoracic Surgery, Columbus, Ohio, Oct. 1986. Jones, Frederick E., Memorial Symposium in Thoraci. Ed. by T. E. Williams et al. 1977. (Illus.). 38.50 (*3-8055-2649-0*) S Karger.

Perspectives in Medical Sociology. Ed. by Phil Brown. 3rd ed. 2000. LC 00-709570. (Illus.). xviii, 673p. (C). pap. 32.95 (*1-57766-134-6*) Waveland Pr.

Perspectives in Medicinal Chemistry. Ed. by B. Testa et al. 1993. (Illus.). 645p. (C). 230.00 (*3-527-28486-9*, Wiley-VCH) Wiley.

Perspectives in Medicine. New York Academy of Medicine Staff. 1977. LC 75-152204. (Essay Index Reprint Ser.). 19.95 (*0-8369-2813-X*) Ayer.

Perspectives in Memory Research. Ed. by Michael S. Gazzaniga. 1988. LC 88-8958. 336p. 40.00 (*0-262-07112-6*) MIT Pr.

Perspectives in Methodology for Study of the Microcirculation. Ed. by F. Hammersen et al. 1984. (Progress in Applied Microcirculation Ser.: Vol. 6). (Illus.). vi, 160p. pap. 64.50 (*3-8055-3988-6*) S Karger.

Perspectives in Nutrition. Wardlaw. 3rd ed. 1996. (*0-8151-9150-2*) Mosby Inc.

***Perspectives in Nutrition.** Gordon M. Wardlaw. 4th ed. 2000. stu. ed. 73.75 (*0-07-246816-5*) McGrw-H Hghr Educ.

Perspectives in Nutrition Study Guide. Gordon M. Wardlaw. (C). 1989. 352p. per. (*0-8016-5344-4*); 3rd ed. 1996. 368p. text, stu. ed. 21.87 (*0-8151-9073-5*) McGrw-H Hghr Educ (WCB McGr Hill).

Perspectives in Nutrition Study Guide & Software. Insel & Gordon M. Wardlaw. 1990. 16.95 (*0-8016-5322-3*) Mosby Inc.

Perspectives in Peptide Chemistry. Alex N. Eberle. Ed. by T. Wieland et al. 1980. (Illus.). xii, 444p. 126.25 (*3-8055-1297-X*) S Karger.

Perspectives in Personality Ed. by Robert T. Hogan & Warren H. Jones. 1991. Pt. A, set. 88.00 (*1-85302-086-9*); Pt. B. 88.00 (*1-85302-087-7*); set. 175.00 (*1-85302-085-0*) Taylor & Francis.

Perspectives in Psychological Experimentation: Toward the Year 2000. Ed. by Viktor Sarris & Allen Parducci. 1984. 384p. (C). text 79.95 (*0-89859-288-7*) L Erlbaum Assocs.

Perspectives in Public Health. Ed. by Sian Griffiths & David Hunter. 1999. LC 99-216545. 304p. pap. (*1-85775-209-0*) Radcliffe Med Pr GBR. *Dist:* Balogh.

Perspectives in Receptor Research. Ed. by D. Giardina et al. 1996. (Pharmacochemistry Library: Vol. 24). 422p. text 227.00 (*0-444-82204-6*) Elsevier.

Perspectives in Rehabilitation Ergonomics. Ed. by Shrawan Kumar. 1997. LC 97-171564. 408p. pap. (*0-7484-0673-5*); text (*0-7484-0644-1*) Tay Francis Ltd GBR. *Dist:* Taylor & Francis.

Perspectives in Transactional Analysis. Muriel James. 1998. LC 99-168604. (Illus.). 270p. pap. 25.00 (*0-89489-005-0*) Intl Transactional.

Perspectives of Antioxidant Treatment of Emphysema with N-Acetylcysteine: Journal: Respiration, Vol. 50, Suppl. 1, 1986. Ed. by V. Cichetti et al. 1986. vi, 74p. pap. 24.50 (*3-8055-4514-2*) S Karger.

Perspectives of Information Processing in Medical Application: Strategic Issues, Requirements & Options for the European Community. Ed. by F. Roger-France & G. Santucci. 1991. (Health Systems Research Ser.). (Illus.). 320p. 71.95 (*0-387-53856-9*) Spr-Verlag.

Perspectives of Motor Behavior & Its Neural Basis. Ed. by Marie-Claude Hepp-Reymond & Gabriella Marini. 1997. LC 97-3035. (Illus.). viii, 138p. 85.25 (*3-8055-6403-1*) S Karger.

***Perspectives of People with Dementia: Research Methods & Motivations.** Heather Wilkinson. 2001. LC 2001-53707. (*1-84310-001-0*) Jessica Kingsley.

Perspectives of Psychiatry. Paul R. Mchugh. 2nd ed. 1998. LC 98-26808. (Illus.). 375p. pap. text 18.95 (*0-8018-6046-6*) Johns Hopkins.

Perspectives on a Parent Movement: The Revolt of Parents of Children with Intellectual Limitations. Rosemary F. Dybwad. 1990. LC 90-35065. 186p. (Orig.). pap. text 17.95 (*0-914797-74-3*) Brookline Bks.

Perspectives on Abortion. Ed. by Paul Sachdev. 1984. LC 84-10573. 293p. 26.50 (*0-8108-1708-X*) Scarecrow.

Perspectives on Aids: Ethical & Social Issues. Ed. by Christine Overall & William P. Zion. 1991. 240p. pap. text 24.95 (*0-19-540749-0*) OUP.

Perspectives on Animal Research, Vol. 1. Ed. by Stephen R. Kaufman & Betsy Todd. 1989. 160p. pap. 10.00 (*0-9623858-1-6*) Med Res Modern.

Perspectives on Animal Research, 1989, Vol. 1. Ed. by Stephen R. Kaufman & Betsy Todd. 1989. 160p. 15.00 (*0-9623858-0-8*) Med Res Modern.

Perspectives on Autoimmunity. Ed. by Irun R. Cohen. 1987. 272p. 136.00 (*0-8493-6431-0*, RC600, CRC Reprint) Franklin.

Perspectives on Bacterial Pathogenesis & Host Defense. Ed. by Bernhard Urbaschek. 1988. 268p. lib. bdg. 42.00 (*0-226-84275-4*) U Ch Pr.

Perspectives on Behavioral Inhibition. Ed. by J. Steven Reznick. 1989. LC 89-32463. (John D. & Catherine T. MacArthur Foundation Series on Mental Health & Development). (Illus.). 326p. 39.95 (*0-226-71040-8*) U Ch Pr.

Perspectives on Bereavement. Irwin Gerber. 1979. 19.95 (*0-405-12481-3*) Ayer.

Perspectives on Bias in Mental Testing. Ed. by Cecil R. Reynolds & Robert T. Brown. 1984. (Perspectives on Individual Differences Ser.). 594p. 85.00 (*0-306-41529-1*, Plenum Trade) Perseus Pubng.

Perspectives on Biologically Based Cancer Risk Assessment. Vincent J. Cogliano et al. 1999. LC 99-30081. (NATO Challenges of Modern Society Ser.). 319p. (*0-306-46108-0*, Kluwer Plenum) Kluwer Academic.

Perspectives on Case Management Practice. Ed. by Carol D. Austin & Robert W. McClelland. 1996. LC 96-619. 278p. reprint ed. pap. 25.95 (*1-896918-12-3*, Manticore Europe) Manticore Pubs.

Perspectives on Cognitive Change in Adulthood & Aging. Fredda Blanchard-Fields & Thomas M. Hess. 1996. LC 95-81973. 528p. (C). pap. 51.88 (*0-07-028450-4*) McGrw-H Hghr Educ.

Perspectives on Cognitive Dissonance. R. A. Wicklund & J. W. Brehm. 1976. 349p. 79.95 (*0-89859-419-7*) L Erlbaum Assocs.

Perspectives on Community Health Education: A Series of Case Studies. Ed. by Raymond W. Carlaw. 1982. LC 80-54741. 224p. (C). pap. text 9.95 (*0-89914-007-6*) Third Party Pub.

Perspectives on Disability: Text & Readings on Disability. Ed. by Mark Nagler. 2nd ed. 1993. 460p. (C). text 45.00 (*0-9627640-3-5*) Hlth Mrkts Res.

Perspectives on Faculty Roles in Nursing Education. Ed. by Lynne B. Welch. 1992. LC 91-28999. 160p. 60.00 (*0-275-93789-5*, C3789, Praeger Pubs) Greenwood.

Perspectives on Fundamental Processes in Intellectual Functioning: A Survey of Research Approaches, 1. Sal Soraci & William J. McIlvane. 1998. LC 97-23866. 300p. 85.00 (*1-56750-358-6*, Ablex) Greenwood.

Perspectives on Fundamental Processes in Intellectual Functioning: A Survey of Research Approches. Sal Soraci & William J. McIlvane. 1998. LC 97-23866. 300p. pap. 39.50 (*1-56750-359-4*, Ablex) Greenwood.

Perspectives on Genetics: Anecdotal, Historical, & Critical Commentaries, 1987-1998. Ed. by James F. Crow & William F. Dove. 2000. LC 99-49567. (Illus.). xiii, 723p. pap. 19.95 (*0-299-16604-X*) U of Wis Pr.

Perspectives on Health Communication. Barbara C. Thornton & Gary L. Kreps. 1993. 237p. (C). pap. text 20.95 (*0-88133-711-0*) Waveland Pr.

Perspectives on Infant Development. 2001. (C). 66.00 (*0-205-28371-3*, Macmillan Coll) P-H.

Perspectives on Infant Mental Health Ed. by Joy D. Osofsky & Hiram E. Fitzgerald. 1999. LC 99-11893. (World Association for Infant Mental Health Ser.: Vol. 1). (Illus.). 403p. 220.00 (*0-471-18941-3*) Wiley.

Perspectives on Life-Threatening Illness for Allied Health Professionals: History, Approaches, Considerations. Ed. by Leslie M. Thompson et al. 1993. LC 92-49281. (Loss, Grief & Care Ser.: Vol. 7, Nos. 1 & 2). (Illus.). 220p. 49.95 (*1-56024-329-5*) Haworth Pr.

***Perspectives on Loss & Trauma: Assaults on the Self.** John H. Harvey. 2001. LC 2001-1021. ix, 317p. pap. 34.95 (*0-7619-2161-3*, 86500) Sage.

Perspectives on Medical Research, Vol. 3. Ed. by Stephen R. Kaufman. 1992. (Illus.). 91p. pap. 10.00 (*0-9623858-7-5*); text 15.00 (*0-9623858-6-7*) Med Res Modern.

Perspectives on Medical Research, Vol. 4, 1993. Ed. by Stephen R. Kaufman & Kathryn Hahner. 1993. 80p. pap. 10.00 (*0-9623858-9-1*); text 15.00 (*0-9623858-8-3*) Med Res Modern.

Perspectives on Memory Research. Ed. by L. G. Nilsson. 1979. 416p. text 79.95 (*0-89859-483-9*) L Erlbaum Assocs.

Perspectives on Mental Handicap in South Africa. Lea. Ed. by Don Foster. 1990. pap. text (*0-409-10919-3*) Buttrwrth-Heinemann.

Perspectives on Nursing Theory. Leslie H. Nicoll. 3rd ed. 1996. LC 96-33075. 816p. pap. text 42.95 (*0-397-55312-9*) Lppncott W & W.

Perspectives on Paedophilia. Brian Taylor. 1981. 160p. 38.50 (*0-7134-3718-9*); pap. 17.95 (*0-7134-3719-7*) Trafalgar.

Perspectives on Pathophysiology. Lee-Ellen C. Copstead. 1995. LC 94-21277. (Illus.). 1258p. text 65.00 (*0-7216-3846-5*) Saunders.

Perspectives on Person-Environment Interaction & Drug-Taking Behavior. Ed. & Intro. by Bernard Segal. 1988. LC 87-26268. (Drugs & Society Ser.: Vol. 2, No. 1). 170p. text 39.95 (*0-86656-716-X*) Haworth Pr.

Perspectives on Psychologism. Ed. by M. A. Notturno. 1989. LC 89-9849. (Brill's Studies in Epistemology, Psychology & Psychiatry). 504p. text 167.50 (*90-04-09182-3*) Brill Academic Pubs.

Perspectives on Rape & Sexual Assault. Ed. by June Hopkins. 1984. 160p. pap. (*0-335-09821-5*) OpUniv Pr GBR. *Dist:* Taylor & Francis.

Perspectives on Research in Emotional Stress. K. V. Sudakov et al. 1989. (Systems Research in Physiology Ser.: Vol. 3). xiv, 400p. text 367.00 (*2-88124-699-0*) Gordon & Breach.

Perspectives on the Classification of Specific Developmental Disorders. Ed. by Jan Rispens et al. 1998. LC 97-32490. (Neuropsychology & Cognition Ser.). 286p. 130.50 (*0-7923-4871-0*) Kluwer Academic.

Perspectives on the Educational Use of Animals. William Mayer et al. 1980. (Illus.). 77p. pap. 3.00 (*0-913098-38-8*) Orion Society.

Perspectives on the Molecular Biology & Immunology of the Pancreatic Beta Cell. Ed. by Douglas Hanahan et al. 1989. (Current Communications in Molecular Biology Ser.). (Illus.). 212p. (C). pap. text 24.00 (*0-87969-326-6*) Cold Spring Harbor.

Perspectives on the Study of Speech. Ed. by Peter D. Eimas & Joanne L. Miller. 1981. LC 80-39499. 464p. text 89.95 (*0-89859-052-3*) L Erlbaum Assocs.

Perspectives on Theory for the Practice of Occupational Therapy. Rosalie J. Miller & Kay F. Walker. 2nd ed. 1995. Orig. Title: Six Perspectives on Theory for the Practice of Occupational Therapy. 320p. 59.00 (*0-8342-0358-8*, 20358) PRO-ED.

Perspectives on 3rd World Workshop on Oral Medicine, 1998. Ed. by H. Dean Millard & David Mason. 2000. 392p. pap. text 65.00 (*0-9645852-1-9*) UMI Schl Dentsy.

Perspectives on Understanding & Working with Families. Kevin J. Swick. 1987. 130p. pap. text 7.80 (*0-87563-305-6*) Stipes.

Persuasion & Healing: A Comparative Study of Psychotherapy. Jerome D. Frank & Julia B. Frank. 3rd ed. 1993. 368p. reprint ed. pap. text 19.95 (*0-8018-4636-6*) Johns Hopkins.

Persuasion, Social Influence, & Compliance Gaining. Robert Gass et al. 1998. LC 98-7618. 354p. pap. text 54.00 (*0-205-26352-6*) Allyn.

Persuasive Communication & Drug Abuse Prevention. Ed. by L. Donohew et al. 1991. (Communication Ser.). 360p. (C). text 69.95 (*0-8058-0693-8*) L Erlbaum Assocs.

Persuasive Encounters. Gary C. Woodward. 1990. LC 90-32132. (Case Studies in Constructive Confrontation). 216p. 62.50 (*0-275-93091-2*, C3091); pap. 20.95 (*0-275-93092-0*, B3092) Greenwood (Praeger Pubs).

Pertinent Questions & Answers about Homeopathy. James G. Speight. 1984. 109p. pap. (*0-85207-164-7*) C W Daniel GBR. *Dist:* Natl Bk Netwk.

Pertinent Questions & Answers about Homoeopathy. Phyllis Speight. 28p. (Orig.). pap. 5.95 (*0-8464-4269-8*) Beekman Pubs.

Perturbing the Organism: The Biology of Successful Experience. Herbert Weiner. 1992. LC 91-838. (John D. & Catherine T. MacArthur Foundation Series on Mental Health & Development). (Illus.). 372p. 40.50 (*0-226-89041-4*) U Ch Pr.

Pertussis. Ed. by C. R. Manclark & W. Hennessen. 1986. (Developments in Biological Standardization Ser.: Vol. 61). (Illus.). xii, 600p. pap. 61.00 (*3-8055-4210-0*) S Karger.

Pertussis: Evaluation & Research on Acellular Pertussis Vaccines. Ed. by Y. Sato et al. 1991. (Developments in Biological Standardization Ser.: Vol. 73). (Illus.). xii, 386p. 61.00 (*3-8055-5457-5*) S Karger.

Pertussis Vaccine Trials: Symposium at the Istituto Superiore di Sanita, Rome, October/November 1995. Ed. by Fred Brown et al. 1997. LC 97-202571. (Developments in Biological Standardization Ser.: Vol. 89, 1997). (Illus.). xiv, 418p. pap. 339.25 (*3-8055-6481-3*) S Karger.

Peru: History of Coca, "the Divine Plant" of the Incas. William G. Mortimer. LC 74-15120. reprint ed. 69.50 (*0-404-11980-8*) AMS Pr.

Perugia Consensus Conference on Antiemetic Therapy. Ed. by R. J. Gralla et al. 1998. LC 98-22555. (Illus.). 200p. 54.00 (*3-540-64076-2*) Spr-Verlag.

Pervasive Developmental Disorders: Finding a Diagnosis & Getting Help. Mitzi Waltz. Ed. by Linda Lamb. 1999. LC 99-23708. (Patient-Centered Guides Ser.). (Illus.). xiii, 567p. pap. 24.95 (*1-56592-530-0*) OReilly & Assocs.

Perverse Economics of Health Care & How We Can Fix It. David R. Henderson. 1994. LC 94-34925. (Essays in Public Policy Ser.: No. 54). pap. 5.00 (*0-8179-5592-5*) Hoover Inst Pr.

Perversion: The Erotic Form of Hatred. Robert J. Stoller. 1994. 258p. pap. text (*0-946439-20-6*) Karnac Bks GBR. *Dist:* Other Pr LLC.

Perversion & Utopia: A Study in Psychoanalysis & Critical Theory. Joel Whitebook. (Studies in Contemporary German Social Thought). (Illus.). 1996. 360p. pap. 22.95 (*0-262-73117-7*); 1995. LC 94-22307. 368p. 35.00 (*0-262-23178-6*) MIT Pr.

Perversions of the Sex Instinct. Albert Moll. LC 72-11289.Tr. of Contraere Sexualempfindung. reprint ed. 38.50 (*0-404-57482-3*) AMS Pr.

Perversity. Ed. by Judith Squires. 1993. (New Formations Nineteen Ser.: No. 19). 192p. (C). pap. (*0-85315-760-X*) Lawrence & Wishart GBR. *Dist:* NYU Pr.

Pest Resistance to Pesticides. Ed. by G. P. Georghiou & Tetsuo Saito. 1983. LC 82-22369. 822p. 135.00 (*0-306-41246-2*, Plenum Trade) Perseus Pubng.

Pestalozzi's Educational Writings, 2. Johann H. Pestalozzi. Tr. by John A. Green from GER. 1977. LC 77-72191. (Contributions to the History of Psychology Ser.: Vol. II, Pt. B, Psychometrics). 424p. reprint ed. lib. bdg. 85.00 (*0-313-26937-8*, U6937, Greenwood Pr) Greenwood.

Pesticide Application Equipment for Vector Control. 1990. (Technical Reports: No. 791). (ENG, FRE & SPA.). 58p. pap. text 8.00 (*92-4-120791-4*, 1100791) World Health.

Pesticide Formulations & Applications Systems: 5th Symposium. Ed. by Thomas M. Kaneko & Larry D. Spicer. 1986. LC 86-22358. (Special Technical Publications: No. 915). (Illus.). 154p. text 32.00 (*0-8031-0481-2*, STP915) ASTM.

Pesticide Residues: Report of the 1967 Joint Meeting of the FAO Working Party & the WHO Expert Committee, 1968. 1968. (Technical Report Ser.: No. 391). 43p. pap. text 5.00 (*92-4-120391-9*, 1100391) World Health.

Pesticide Residues in Food: Joint Report of the FAO Working Party & the WHO Expert Committee on Pesticide, 1967. 1967. (Technical Report Ser.: No. 369). 19p. pap. text 3.00 (*92-4-120370-6*, 1100370) World Health.

Pesticide Residues in Food: Report, Geneva, 1975. FAO-WHO Experts on Pesticide Residues Staff. 1976. (Technical Reports: No. 592). pap. text 6.00 (*92-4-120592-X*, 1100592) World Health.

Pesticide Residues in Food: Report of the 1976 Joint FAO/WHO Meeting, 1977. 1977. (Technical Report Ser.: No. 612). 35p. pap. text 6.00 (*92-4-120612-8*, 1100612) World Health.

Pesticide Residues in Food: Report of the FAO-WHO Experts on Pesticide Residues, Geneva, 1968. FAO-WHO Experts on Pesticide Residues Staff. (Technical Reports: No. 574). 1975. pap. text 6.00 (*92-4-120574-1*, 1100574); 1974. pap. text 6.00 (*92-4-120545-8*, 1100545); 1972. pap. text 4.00 (*92-4-120502-4*, 1100502); 1971. pap. text 5.00 (*92-4-120474-5*, 1100474); 1970. pap. text 5.00 (*92-4-120458-3*, 1100458); 1969. pap. text 5.00 (*92-4-120417-6*, 1100417) World Health.

Pesticide Residues in Food & Human Bodies: Index of New Information. John C. Bartone. 1997. 160p. 57.50 (*0-7883-1670-2*); pap. 47.50 (*0-7883-1671-0*) ABBE Pubs Assn.

Pesticide Residues in Food, 1990 Pt. 2: Toxicology Evaluations. 1991. (Joint Meeting of the FAO Panel of Experts on Pesticide Residues in Food & the Environment & the WHO Expert Group on Pesticide Residues Ser.). x, 182p. pap. text 30.00 (*92-4-166506-8*, 1280006) World Health.

Pesticide Residues in Food, 1991 Pt. II: Toxicology Evaluations (WHO/PCS/9252) WHO Staff. 1992. (WHO Pesticides Residues in Food Ser.: No. 7). 318p. 35.00 (*92-4-166507-6*, 1280007) World Health.

Pesticide Use & Toxicology in Relation to Wildlife: Organophosphorus & Carbamate Compounds. Gregory J. Smith. 1992. LC 92-34055. 176p. 94.95 (*0-8493-8721-3*, QH545) CRC Pr.

Pesticides & Cancer: Index of New Information with Authors, Subjects, Research Categories & References. Bruce M. Brookline. 1995. 160p. 57.50 (*0-7883-0740-1*); pap. 47.50 (*0-7883-0741-X*) ABBE Pubs Assn.

Pesticides & Human Cancer Involvement: Index of New Information. John C. Bartone. 1997. 160p. 57.50 (*0-7883-1650-8*); pap. 47.50 (*0-7883-1651-6*) ABBE Pubs Assn.

Pesticides & Human Health. William H. Hallenbeck & K. M. Burns. 1984. 166p. 61.00 (*0-387-96050-3*) Spr-Verlag.

Pesticides & Neurological Diseases. Donald J. Ecobichon & Robert M. Joy. 2nd ed. 1993. LC 93-1125. 400p. lib. bdg. 169.00 (*0-8493-4361-5*, RC347) CRC Pr.

Pesticides & Neurological Diseases. Ed. by Donald J. Ecobichon & Robert M. Joy. 1982. 296p. 165.00 (*0-8493-5571-0*, RC346, CRC Reprint) Franklin.

Pesticides & Politics: The Life Cycle of a Public Issue. Christopher J. Bosso. LC 86-19245. (Series in Policy & Institutional Studies). (Illus.). 312p. reprint ed. 1988. pap. 16.95 (*0-8229-5418-4*); 1987. text 49.95 (*0-8229-3547-3*) U of Pittsburgh Pr.

Pesticides & the Immune System: The Public Health Risks. Robert C. Repetto & Sanjay S. Baliga. 1996. LC 96-12739. 100p. (Orig.). pap. 20.00 (*1-56973-087-3*) World Resources Inst.

Pesticides, Chemicals & Health. British Medical Association Staff. 1992. (Illus.). 224p. pap. text (*0-340-54924-6*, A6602) E A GBR. *Dist:* Routldge.

Pesticides in Food: A Guide for Professionals. 1991. LC 91-40494. pap. 5.50 (*0-88091-095-X*, 0155) Am Dietetic Assn.

Pesticides in the Diets of Infants & Children. National Research Council Staff. 1993. LC 93-14961. 408p. pap. text 47.95 (*0-309-04875-3*) Natl Acad Pr.

Pesticides in Urban Environments: Fate & Significance, Vol. 52. Ed. by Kenneth D. Racke & Anne R. Leslie. 1993. LC 92-42060. (ACS Symposium Ser.: Vol. 522). (Illus.). 385p. 94.95 (*0-8412-2627-X*) Am Chemical.

Pests of Paradise: First Aid & Medical Treatment of Injuries from Hawai'i's Animals. Susan Scott & Craig Thomas. 2000. LC 99-57565. (Latitude 20 Book Ser.). (Illus.). 204p. pap. 19.95 (*0-8248-2252-8*) UH Pr.

Pet Allergies: Remedies for an Epidemic. Alfred J. Plechner & Martin Zucker. 1986. LC 85-51341. 130p. (Orig.). pap. 6.95 (*0-9615452-0-8*) Very Healthy Ent.

***PET Applications in Schizophrenia: Functional & Pharmacological Dopamine Studies.** Ola Gefvert. 2000. (Comprehensive Summaries of Uppsala Dissertations from the Faculty of Medicine Ser.: No. 914). (Illus.). 48p. pap. (*91-554-4677-9*) Uppsala Universitet SWE. *Dist:* Coronet Bks.

***Pet Care in the New Century: Cutting-Edge Medicine for Dogs & Cats.** Amy D. Shojai. 2001. LC 2001-32627. pap. 14.00 (*0-451-20443-3*, Sig) NAL.

Pet First Aid: Cats & Dogs. American Red Cross Staff. 1997. (gr. 13). 10.00 (*0-8151-2318-3*) Mosby Inc.

Pet for Drug Development & Evaluation. Ed. by D. Comar. 1995. LC 95-24830. (Developments in Nuclear Medicine Ser.: Vol. 26). 384p. (C). text 144.00 (*0-7923-3716-6*) Kluwer Academic.

Pet Health Journal. Laurie Barranti-Teague. 1997. 105p. pap. (*0-9675257-0-5*) Bananknotcom.

***Pet Health Journal.** Laurie Barranti. rev. ed. 2001. 100p. spiral bd. 13.95 (*0-9675257-3-X*) Bananknotcom.

PET in Clinical Oncology. Ed. by H. J. Wieler & E. Coleman. 2000. 430p. (*3-7985-1219-1*) D Steinkopff DEU. *Dist:* Spr-Verlag.

PET in Oncology: Basics & Clinical Application. Ed. by Juergen Ruhlmann et al. Tr. by J. F. Leeson & M. W. Tannert. 1999. LC 99-26968. (Illus.). 224p. 89.00 (*3-540-65077-6*) Spr-Verlag.

Pet Loss & Human Emotion: Guiding Clients Through Grief. Cheri B. Ross & Jane B. Sorensen. 1998. LC 97-38965. (Falconguide Ser.). 164p. pap. 19.95 (*1-56032-652-2*) Hemisp Pub.

Pet-Oriented Child Psychotherapy. Boris M. Levinson & Gerald P. Mallon. 2nd ed. LC 96-8968. 242p. 1997. text 50.95 (*0-398-06673-6*); 1996. pap. text 35.95 (*0-398-06674-4*) C C Thomas.

Pet Studies on Amino Acid Metabolism & Protein Synthesis. Ed. by B. M. Mazoyer. 1993. (Developments in Nuclear Medicine Ser.). 288p. (C). text 145.50 (*0-7923-2076-X*) Kluwer Academic.

Peter Berner: On the Occasion of His 65th Birthday: Journal: Psychopathology, 1990, Vol. 23, No. 2. Ed. by H. G. Zapotoczky & E. Gabriel. 1990. (Illus.). 72p. 35.75 (*3-8055-5311-0*) S Karger.

Peterborough Symposium on Cardiology. F. J. Fawcet. 1975. pap. text 30.00 (*0-7855-2852-0*) St Mut.

Peterson's Game Plan for Getting into Medical School. Cathy S. Jewell. 2000. LC 99-87860. (Illus.). 196p. pap. 14.95 (*0-7689-0393-9*) Petersons.

Peterson's Guide to Medical Schools in the U. S. & Canada: M. D. & M. D. - Ph. D. Programs at Nearly 150 U. S. & Canadian Schools. Peterson's Guides Staff. Ed. by Jon Latimer. 2nd ed. 1997. 1000p. (C). pap. 21.95 (*1-56079-631-6*) Petersons.

Peterson's Guide to Nursing Programs: Baccalaureate & Graduate Nursing Education in the U. S. & Canada. 2nd ed. 1996. 688p. reprint ed. 24.95 (*1-56079-565-4*) Petersons.

Peterson's MCAT Success. Peterson's Guides Staff. 1997. (Peterson's Guides Ser.). 356p. pap. text 14.95 incl. cd-rom (*1-56079-929-3*) Petersons.

Peterson's MCAT Success 2001. Ed. by Peterson's Guides Staff. 5th ed. 2000. (Peterson's MCAT Success Ser.). 384p. pap. 16.95 incl. cd-rom (*0-7689-0444-7*) Petersons.

Petit Atlas des Champignons, Vols. 1 & 2. Henri Romagnesi. 1964. (Illus.). 25.00 (*0-934454-91-4*) Lubrecht & Cramer.

Petit Dictionnaire d'Anatomiem d'Embryologie et Histologie. Pierre Kamina. 1990. (FRE.). 775p. pap. 125.00 (*0-7859-7821-6*, 2224019009) Fr & Eur.

Petit Dictionnaire Droit des Malades. C. Evin. 1998. (FRE.). 37.95 (*0-320-00389-2*) Fr & Eur.

Petit Dictionnaire Medical. Alexandre Manuila. 4th ed. 1985. (FRE.). 566p. pap. 49.95 (*0-7859-4942-9*) Fr & Eur.

Petit Larousse de la Medecine. Jacques Bourneuf. Ed. by Andre Domart. 1976. (FRE.). 852p. 85.00 (*0-8288-5750-4*, F12060) Fr & Eur.

Petit Larousse de la Medecine, Vol. 1. Herve Negre. 1988. (FRE.). 975p. pap. 19.95 (*0-7859-4845-7*) Fr & Eur.

Petit Vianney Dictionnaire Medical Savant et Sympathetique. Yves-Marie Vianney. 1991. (FRE.). 70p. pap. 19.95 (*0-7859-8246-9*, 2908614049) Fr & Eur.

Pets & Mental Health. Intro. by Odean Cusack. 1988. LC 88-9671. 241p. text 39.95 (*0-86656-652-X*); pap. text 14.95 (*0-86656-801-8*) Haworth Pr.

Pets & the Elderly: The Therapeutic Bond. Ed. by Odean Cusack & Elaine Smith. 1984. LC 83-26409. (Activities, Adaptation & Aging Ser.: Vol. 4, Nos. 2 & 3). (Illus.). 257p. text 49.95 (*0-86656-259-1*, B259) Haworth Pr.

Pets in Therapy. Ed. by Margaret Abdill & Denise Juppe. 1997. LC 97-16973. (Illus.). 214p. pap. 15.00 (*1-882883-29-2*, 312) Idyll Arbor.

Pets Living with Cancer: A Pet Owner's Resource Guide. Robin Downing. 2000. LC 00-22489. (Illus.). xi, 142p. pap. 19.95 (*1-58326-022-6*, AAHA Pr) Am Animal Hosp Assoc.

Petticoat Surgeon. Bertha Van Hoosen. Ed. by Annette K. Baxter. 1980. LC 79-8820. (Signal Lives Ser.). reprint ed. lib. bdg. 37.95 (*0-405-12864-9*) Ayer.

PetVet: Dog First Aid. Sandra C. Mays & Michael P. Driscoll. 1995. (Illus.). 105p. (Orig.). pap. 16.95 (*1-878117-05-X*) Lagumo Corp.

Peyote Book: A Study of Native Medicine. Compiled by Guy Mount. 3rd ed. 1993. 144p. per. 9.95 (*0-9604462-3-0*) Sweetlight.

Peyronie's Disease: Induratio Penis Plastica. Ed. by A. Kelami & J. P. Pryor. 1983. (Progress in Reproductive Biology & Medicine Ser.: Vol. 9). (Illus.). viii, 116p. 98.50 (*3-8055-3513-9*) S Karger.

***p53 Alterations in Human Skin: A Molecular Study Based on Morphology.** Gao Ling. 2001. (Comprehensive Summaries of Uppsala Dissertations from the Faculty of Medicine Ser.: No. 1082). (Illus.). 60p. pap. (*91-554-5131-4*) Acta Univ SWE. *Dist:* Coronet Bks.

Pfizer Atlas of Veterinary Clinical Parasitology. Ed. by Byron L. Blagburn & Michael W. Dryden. 2000. (Illus.). 48p. (*0-9678005-3-6*) Gloyd Grp Inc.

Pfizer Focuses on High Growth Markets: Innovative Product Introductions Give Company Competitive Edge. 1992. 216p. 995.00 (*1-56753-022-2*) Frost & Sullivan.

Pfortaderhochdruck. Ed. by K. J. Paquet & J. Schoelmerich. 1994. (GER., Illus.). x, 702p. 181.75 (*3-8055-5659-4*) S Karger.

PH & Blood Gas. ring bd. 200.00 (*1-56238-247-0*, SC5-L) NCCLS.

PH & Brain Function. Ed. by Kai Kaila & Bruce R. Ransom. 1998. LC 97-40568. 688p. 236.00 (*0-471-11838-9*, Wiley-Liss) Wiley.

PH Health Human Sexuality, Vol. 94C. 1994. (gr. 9-12). pap. text, tchr. ed. 20.97 (*0-13-720996-7*) PH School.

Phacodynamics: Mastering the Tools & Techniques of Phacoemulsification Surgery. Barry Seibel. (Illus.). 304p. 1999. (SPA.). 125.00 (*1-55642-447-7*); 3rd ed. 1998. LC 98-29336. text 125.00 (*1-55642-388-8*, 63888) SLACK Inc.

Phacoemulsification: Principles & Techniques. Lucio Buratto. 1997. LC 97-34823. (Illus.). 544p. text 195.00 (*1-55642-360-8*, 63608) SLACK Inc.

Phacoemulsification in Difficult & Challenging Cases. Luisw Lu & Howard I. Fine. 1998. LC 98-4055. (Illus.). 200p. 99.00 (*0-86577-791-8*) Thieme Med Pubs.

Phacoemulsification Surgery. Ed. by T. M. Devine & William Banko. 1991. (Illus.). 144p. 125.00 (*0-08-036840-9*) McGraw.

Phacomatoses. Ed. by Pierre J. Vinken & George W. Bruyn. 1973. 300.50 (*0-444-10375-9*) Elsevier.

Phacomatosis in Japan: Epidemiology, Clinical Picture & Molecular Biology. Ed. by M. Niimura et al. 1999. (Gann Monographs on Cancer Research: Vol. 46). (Illus.). viii, 230p. 243.50 (*3-8055-6838-X*) S Karger.

Phaenomenologie und Psychotherapeutische Praxis Vol. 12, Nos. 1-4, 1995: Journal: Daseinsanalyse. Ed. by G. Condrau. 1995. (Journal: Vol. 12, No. 1-4, 1995). (Illus.). 250p. pap. 73.25 (*3-8055-6230-6*) S Karger.

Phagocytes & Cellular Immunity. Hans H. Gadebusch. 1979. 176p. 103.00 (*0-8493-5349-1*, QR185, CRC Reprint) Franklin.

Phagocytes & Disease. Ed. by M. S. Klempner et al. 1988. (Immunology & Medicine Ser.). (C). lib. bdg. 75.00 (*0-7462-0086-2*) Kluwer Academic.

Phakmatoses. Pierre J. Vinken & George W. Bruyn. 1972. (Handbooks of Clinical Neurology: Vol. 14). 824p. 451.00 (*0-7204-7214-8*) Elsevier.

Phallos: A Symbol & Its History in the Male World. Thorkil Vanggaard. 1972. LC 72-80553. (Illus.). 266p. pap. 24.95 (*0-8236-8192-0*, 24135) Intl Univs Pr.

Phantasy in Everyday Life: A Psychoanalytical Approach to Understanding Ourselves. Ed. by Julia Segal. 1995. LC 95-33577. 238p. pap. 45.00 (*1-56821-753-6*) Aronson.

Phantom of the Night: Overcome Sleep Apnea Syndrome - Win Your Hidden Struggle to Breathe, Sleep & Live. T. Scott Johnson et al. 3rd rev. ed. Date not set. (Illus.). 250p. pap. 29.95 (*1-882431-05-7*) New Technology.

Phantom of the Night: Overcome Sleep Apnea Syndrome—Win Your Hidden Struggle to Breathe, Sleep & Live. T. Scott Johnson & Jerry Halberstadt. rev. ed. 1998. (Illus.). 192p. (Orig.). pap. 29.95 (*1-882431-02-2*) New Technology.

Phantom Pain. Richard A. Sherman. 1996. LC 96-40883. (Series in Behavioral Psychophysiology & Medicine). (Illus.). 276p. 54.00 (*0-306-45339-8*, Kluwer Plenum) Kluwer Academic.

Phantoms for Performance Evaluation & Quality Assurance of CT Scanners. P. F. Purdy et al. 1977. (AAPM Reports: No. 1). 23p. (Orig.). pap. 10.00 (*1-888340-04-5*) AAPM.

Phantoms in the Brain: Probing the Mysteries of the Human Mind. V. S. Ramachandran & Sandra Blakeslee. 1998. LC 98-3953. (Illus.). 320p. 27.00 (*0-688-15247-3*, Wm Morrow) Morrow Avon.

Pharmaceutical Advertising: A Survey of Existing Legislation. rev. ed. 1968. (International Digest of Health Legislation Offprints: Vol. 19, No. 3). pap. text 14.00 (*92-4-169193-X*, 1956802) World Health.

Pharmaceutical & Biomedical Analysis: Development & Validation of Analytical Methods. Ed. by Christopher M. Riley & Thomas W. Rosanske. 1996. LC 96-33800. (Progress in Pharmaceutical & Biomedical Analysis Ser.: No. 3). 362p. 80.00 (*0-08-042792-8*, Pergamon Pr) Elsevier.

Pharmaceutical & Biomedical Applications of Liquid Chromatography. Christopher M. Riley. Ed. by W. John Lough et al. 1994. LC 94-20192. (Progress in Pharmacology & Clinical Pharmacology Ser.: No. 1). 380p. 150.00 (*0-08-041009-X*, Pergamon Pr) Elsevier.

Pharmaceutical Annual Register Pharm Chemists. 1990. (*0-85369-232-7*) Pharmaceutical Pr GBR. *Dist:* Rittenhouse.

Pharmaceutical Annual Register Pharm Chemists, 1991. 1991. (*0-85369-248-3*) Pharmaceutical Pr GBR. *Dist:* Rittenhouse.

Pharmaceutical Applications of Cell & Tissue Culture to Drug Transport. G. Wilson et al. 1992. (NATO Advanced Science Institutes Ser.: Vol. 218). (Illus.). 398p. (C). text 135.00 (*0-306-44082-2*, Kluwer Plenum) Kluwer Academic.

Pharmaceutical Applications of Membrane Sensors. Vaslie V. Casofret. 1992. 448p. lib. bdg. 129.00 (*0-8493-4406-9*, R857) CRC Pr.

Pharmaceutical Aspects of Cancer Care. Ed. by J. M. Vaeth. 1981. (Frontiers of Radiation Therapy & Oncology Ser.: Vol. 15). (Illus.). viii, 184p. 113.25 (*3-8055-1512-X*) S Karger.

Pharmaceutical Bioequivalence. Ed. by Peter G. Welling et al. 1991. (Drugs & the Pharmaceutical Sciences Ser.: Vol. 48). (Illus.). 488p. text 210.00 (*0-8247-8484-7*) Dekker.

Pharmaceutical Biotechnology: A Programmed Text. Ed. by S. William Zito. 2nd ed. 1998. LC 97-60885. 282p. 41.95 (*1-56676-519-6*) CRC Pr.

Pharmaceutical Biotechnology: An Introduction for Pharmacists & Pharmaceutical Scientists. 1997. 400p. text 110.00 (*90-5702-248-6*); pap. text 45.00 (*90-5702-249-4*) Gordon & Breach (Harwood Acad Pubs).

Pharmaceutical Biotechnology: Fundamentals & Essentials. Ed. by Melvin E. Klegerman & Michael J. Groves. 1992. 295p. 107.00 (*0-935184-37-6*) IHS Health Grp.

Pharmaceutical Calculations. Joel L. Zatz. 3rd ed. 1994. 368p. pap. 57.95 (*0-471-10623-2*) Wiley.

Pharmaceutical Calculations. Mitchell J. Stoklosa & Howard C. Ansel. 10th ed. 1996. LC 95-36483. 425p. 47.00 (*0-683-08001-6*) Lppncott W & W.

Pharmaceutical Calculations: A Self-Instructional Text. Werner Lowenthal. rev. ed. 1978. LC 74-9564. 460p. reprint ed. pap. 27.50 (*0-88275-573-0*) Krieger.

Pharmaceutical Care. Ed. by David H. Knowlton & Richard P. Penna. 1996. LC 95-14254. 360p. pap. (*0-412-06981-4*) E A GBR. *Dist:* OUP.

***Pharmaceutical Care: A Guide for Pharmacy.** William N. Tindall. 2002. 49.95 (*1-56676-953-1*) CRC Pr.

Pharmaceutical Care Practice. Robert J. Cipolle et al. 1998. LC 97-52763. (Illus.). 384p. text 49.95 (*0-07-012046-3*) McGraw-Hill Prof.

Pharmaceutical Chartbook. Ed. by Abraham G. Hartzema & Jean P. Gagnon. 1990. (Illus.). 344p. lib. bdg. 91.00 (*0-87371-173-4*, L173) Lewis Pubs.

Pharmaceutical Chartbook. Abraham G. Hartzema & C. Daniel Mullins. 2nd ed. 1995. LC 95-11616. (Illus.). 221p. (C). lib. bdg. 39.95 (*1-56024-956-0*) Haworth Pr.

Pharmaceutical Chemicals in Perspective. Harold A. Wittcoff. 1989. LC 88-36857. 518p. 185.00 (*0-471-84363-6*) Wiley.

Pharmaceutical Chemistry: Drug Synthesis. H. J. Roth & A. K. Kleeman. 1988. 328p. 62.95 (*0-470-21037-0*) P-H.

Pharmaceutical Chemistry of Adrenergic & Cholinergic Drugs. Ed. by Gyorgy D. Szasz. 1985. 192p. 92.00 (*0-8493-5158-8*, RS341, CRC Reprint) Franklin.

Pharmaceutical Chemistry of Antihypertensive Agents. Gyorgy Szasz & ZsuZsanna Budvari-Barany. 1990. 288p. lib. bdg. 202.00 (*0-8493-4724-6*, RS431) CRC Pr.

Pharmaceutical Corporate Presence in Developing Countries. Ed. by Lee A. Tavis & Oliver F. Williams. 1993. LC 92-56864. (Multinational Managers & Developing Country Concerns Ser.). xxii, 366p. (C). text 40.50 (*0-268-01511-2*) U of Notre Dame Pr.

Pharmaceutical Dictionary: English, French, German, Italian. Graa. 1964. (FRE, GER & SPA.). 124p. 45.00 (*0-7859-7497-0*) Fr & Eur.

***Pharmaceutical Dictionary: German, English, French, Espanol.** A. Maas & J. Brawley. 4th rev. ed. 2002. (ENG, FRE, GER & SPA.). (*3-87193-253-1*) Editio Cantor Verlag DEU. *Dist:* Balogh.

Pharmaceutical Dissolution Testing. Umesh V. Banakar. 1991. (Drugs & the Pharmaceutical Sciences Ser.: Vol. 49). (Illus.). 454p. text 215.00 (*0-8247-8567-3*) Dekker.

Pharmaceutical Dosage Forms: Disperse Systems, Vol. 1. Ed. by Herbert A. Lieberman et al. 2nd ed. 1996. LC 96-15604. (Illus.). 552p. text 175.00 (*0-8247-9387-0*) Dekker.

Pharmaceutical Dosage Forms: Parenteral Medication, Vol. 3. Kenneth E. Avis et al. Ed. by Leon Lieberman. 2nd exp. rev. ed. 1993. (Illus.). 592p. text 75.00 (*0-8247-9020-0*) Dekker.

Pharmaceutical Dosage Forms: Parenteral Medications, Vol. 2. Kenneth E. Avis et al. Ed. by Leon Liberman. 2nd ed. 1992. (Illus.). 616p. text 75.00 (*0-8247-8771-4*) Dekker.

Pharmaceutical Dosage Forms: Tablets, Vol. 1. H. A. Lieberman et al. 2nd ed. 1989. (Illus.). 576p. text 175.00 (*0-8247-8044-2*) Dekker.

Pharmaceutical Dosage Forms: Tablets, Vol. 2. Lieberman et al. 2nd ed. 1990. (Illus.). 640p. text 175.00 (*0-8247-8289-5*) Dekker.

Pharmaceutical Dosage Forms Vol. 1: Parental Medications, Vol. 1. Ed. by Kenneth E. Avis et al. 2nd exp. rev. ed. 1991. (Illus.). 689p. text 75.00 (*0-8247-8576-2*) Dekker.

Pharmaceutical Dosage Forms Vol. 2: Disperse Systems, Vol. 2. Ed. by Lieberman et al. 2nd ed. 1996. (Illus.). 528p. text 175.00 (*0-8247-9713-2*) Dekker.

Pharmaceutical Dosage Forms Vol. 3: Tablets. Herbert A. Lieberman et al. 2nd ed. 1990. (Illus.). 584p. text 69.75 (*0-8247-8300-X*) Dekker.

Pharmaceutical Dosage Forms & Drug Delivery Systems. Howard C. Ansel et al. 6th ed. 1994. LC 94-22471. (*0-683-01930-9*) Lppncott W & W.

Pharmaceutical Dosage Forms & Drug Delivery Systems. Howard Ansel et al. 7th ed. 1999. LC 99-17498. 608p. pap. text 48.00 (*0-683-30572-7*) Lppncott W & W.

Pharmaceutical Drugs. 1990. (IARC Scientific Publications Ser.: Vol. 50). 415p. pap. text 83.00 (*92-832-1250-9*, 1720050) World Health.

Pharmaceutical Education in the Queen City: 150 Years of Service, 1850-2000. Michael A. Flannery & Dennis B. Worthen. 2001. 353p. pap. 34.95 (*0-7890-1132-8*, Pharmctl Prods) Haworth Pr.

Pharmaceutical Enzymes. Albert Lauwers & Simon Scharpe. 1997. LC 97-15723. (Drugs & the Pharmaceutical Sciences Ser.: Vol. 84). (Illus.). 408p. text 165.00 (*0-8247-9375-7*) Dekker.

Pharmaceutical Equities: Evaluation & Trading. Andrew Porter. 1993. (International Equities Ser.). 208p. (*1-85573-090-1*) Woodhead Pubng GBR. *Dist:* Am Educ Systs.

Pharmaceutical Ethics. Salek. 2001. 300p. 90.00 (*0-471-49057-1*) Wiley.

Pharmaceutical Examiner. Jack Rudman. 1994. (Career Examination Ser.: C-1839). pap. 39.95 (*0-8373-1839-4*) Nat Learn.

Pharmaceutical Excipients: Characterization by IR & NMR Spectroscopy. David E. Bugay & W. Paul Findlay. 1999. LC 98-56652. (Drugs & the Pharmaceutical Sciences Ser.). (Illus.). 680p. text 250.00 (*0-8247-9373-0*) Dekker.

Pharmaceutical Excipients: Towards the Twenty-First Century. Christianah Adeyeye et al. 1998. 302p. ring bd. 159.95 (*1-56676-349-5*) CRC Pr.

***Pharmaceutical Excipients 2001.** Kibbe. 2001. cd-rom (*0-85369-497-4*) Pharmaceutical Pr GBR. *Dist:* Rittenhouse.

Pharmaceutical Experimental Design. Gareth Lewis & Didier Mathieu. 1998. LC 98-37068. (Drugs & the Pharmaceutical Sciences Ser.). (Illus.). 552p. text 195.00 (*0-8247-9860-0*) Dekker.

Pharmaceutical Industry. Ed. by Australian Industry Commission Staff. 1996. 912p. pap. (*0-644-36257-X*) Aust Gov Pub AUS. *Dist:* Accents Pubns.

Pharmaceutical Industry: Guide to Pollution Prevention. 1994. (Illus.). 74p. (Orig.). (C). pap. text 30.00 (*1-56806-082-3*) DIANE Pub.

Pharmaceutical Inhalation Aerosol Technology. Ed. by Anthony J. Hickey. 1992. (Drugs & the Pharmaceutical Sciences Ser.: Vol. 54). (Illus.). 384p. text 195.00 (*0-8247-8464-2*) Dekker.

Pharmaceutical Innovation: Revolutionizing Human Health. Ed. by Ralph Landau et al. 1999. LC 99-52121. (Chemical Heritage Foundation Series in Innovation & Entrepreneurship Ser.: Vol. 2). (Illus.). xxiii, 408p. 44.95 (*0-941901-21-1*) Chem Heritage Fnd.

Pharmaceutical Intervention in Apoptotic Pathways. J. F. Nagelkerke et al. 1998. 228p. pap. (*0-444-85823-7*) Royal Netherlands Acad NLD. *Dist:* Elsevier.

Pharmaceutical Manufactoring Change Control. Ed. by Simon Turner. 1999. LC 99-10444. (Illus.). xix, 180p. 179.00 (*1-57491-096-5*) IHS Health Grp.

Pharmaceutical Manufacturing Encyclopedia Marshall Sittig. 2nd ed. 1988. LC 87-31547. (Illus.). 1756p. 285.00 (*0-8155-1144-2*) Noyes.

Pharmaceutical Marketing: Strategy & Cases. Mickey C. Smith. 1991. LC 91-8047. (Illus.). 430p. (Orig.). pap. text 24.95 (*1-56024-110-1*); lib. bdg. 49.95 (*0-86656-861-1*) Haworth Pr.

Pharmaceutical Marketing in the 21st Century. Ed. by Mickey C. Smith. 1996. LC 95-26641. (Journal of Pharmaceutical Marketing & Management Ser.: Vol. 10, Nos. 2/3/4). 292p. (C). 49.95 (*1-56024-795-9*, Pharmctl Prods) Haworth Pr.

Pharmaceutical Markets: A Detailed Database on a 94 Billion Dollar Market. Market Intelligence Staff. 1992. 270p. 995.00 (*1-56753-083-4*) Frost & Sullivan.

Pharmaceutical Mass Spectra. Ed. by Ardrey. 1985. (*0-85369-172-X*) Pharmaceutical Pr GBR. *Dist:* Rittenhouse.

Pharmaceutical Medicine. Ed. by D. M. Burley et al. 2nd ed. 1993. 384p. (*0-340-52517-7*) E A GBR. *Dist:* OUP.

Pharmaceutical Medicine, Biotechnology & European Law. Ed. by Richard Goldberg & Julian Lonbay. 2001. LC 00-63011. 247p. text 74.95 (*0-521-79249-5*) Cambridge U Pr.

Pharmaceutical Medicines, Ethics, & Practice. No. 3. 1990. pap. (*0-85369-224-6*); No. 4. 1990. pap. (*0-85369-236-X*); No. 5. 1991. (*0-85369-239-4*); No. 6. 1991. pap. (*0-85369-261-0*) Pharmaceutical Pr GBR. *Dist:* Rittenhouse.

Pharmaceutical Microbiology. W. B. Hugo & A. D. Russell. (Illus.). 5th ed. 1992. 544p. pap. 75.00 (*0-632-03428-9*); 6th ed. 1998. LC 97-31976. 510p. pap. 104.95 (*0-632-04196-X*) Blackwell Sci.

Pharmaceutical Particulate Carriers: Therapeutic Applications. Ed. by Alain Rolland. 1993. (Drugs & the Pharmaceutical Sciences Ser.: Vol. 61). (Illus.). 448p. text 215.00 (*0-8247-9016-2*) Dekker.

Pharmaceutical Particulate Matter: Analysis & Control. Thomas Barber. 1993. (Illus.). 531p. 126.75 (*0-935184-29-5*) IHS Health Grp.

Pharmaceutical Pelletization Technology. Ghebre-Sellassie. 1989. (Drugs & the Pharmaceutical Sciences Ser.: Vol. 37). (Illus.). 296p. text 165.00 (*0-8247-8085-X*) Dekker.

Pharmaceutical Powder Compaction Technology. Ed. by Christer Nystrom & Goran Alderborn. 1995. (Drugs & the Pharmaceutical Sciences Ser.: Vol. 71). (Illus.). 624p. text 225.00 (*0-8247-9376-5*) Dekker.

Pharmaceutical Practice. Ed. by A. J. Winfield & R. M. Richards. 2nd ed. 1998. (Illus.). 544p. pap. (*0-443-05729-X*) Church.

Pharmaceutical Principles of Solid Dosage Forms. Jens T. Carstensen. 1993. LC 92-64420. 280p. 99.95 (*0-87762-955-2*) CRC Pr.

***Pharmaceutical Process Scale-Up.** Levin. 2001. (Drugs & the Pharmaceutical Sciences Ser.). (*0-8247-0625-0*) Dekker.

Pharmaceutical Process Validation. Ira A. Berry & Robert A. Nash. 2nd ed. 1993. (Drugs & the Pharmaceutical Sciences Ser.: Vol. 57). (Illus.). 648p. text 75.00 (*0-8247-8777-3*) Dekker.

Pharmaceutical Project Management. Tony Kennedy. 1997. LC 97-31537. (Drugs & the Pharmaceutical Sciences Ser.). (Illus.). 304p. text 135.00 (*0-8247-0111-9*) Dekker.

Pharmaceutical Quality Systems. Oliver Schmidt. 2000. LC 99-89315. 370p. 169.00 (*1-57491-109-0*) IHS Health Grp.

Pharmaceutical R&D: Costs, Risks & Rewards. 1994. (Illus.). 364p. (Orig.). (C). pap. text 50.00 (*0-7881-0468-3*) DIANE Pub.

Pharmaceutical Reformulation. James I. Wells. 1988. (Pharmaceutical Technology Ser.). 240p. 62.95 (*0-470-21114-8*) P-H.

Pharmaceutical Research & Development. 1995. lib. bdg. 275.99 (*0-8490-7581-5*) Gordon Pr.

Pharmaceutical Sales Management in a Changeable Market Place. Vincent F. Peters & Thomas B. Yeats. 2000. (Illus.). v, 220p. pap. 49.95 (*0-9656231-2-2*) Black Dog Pub.

Pharmaceutical Sector: Coordinated Sector Position on 31.12.1994. European Communities Staff. 1995. 363p. pap. text, lib. bdg. (*92-827-0020-8*) Comm Europ Commun BEL. *Dist:* Bernan Associates.

***Pharmaceutical Statistics.** Jones. 2002. 352p. pap. (*0-85369-425-7*) Pharmaceutical Pr GBR. *Dist:* Rittenhouse.

Pharmaceutical Substances: Syntheses, Patents, Applications. A. Kleemann. 1999. 999.00 incl. cd-rom (*0-86577-819-1*) Thieme Med Pubs.

Pharmaceutical Substances: Syntheses, Patents, Applications. Axel Kleemann & Jurgen Engel. 1999. LC 98-51303. (Illus.). 2304p. 399.00 (*0-86577-817-5*) Thieme Med Pubs.

Pharmaceutical Technology: Drug Stability. Ed. by M. H. Rubinstein. 1989. 167p. 69.95 (*0-470-21411-2*) P-H.

Pharmaceutical Thermal Analysis: Techniques & Applications. J. L. Ford & P. Timmins. 1989. 313p. 99.95 (*0-470-21219-5*) P-H.

***Pharmaceuticals: Classes, Therapeutic Agents & Areas of Application** John L. McGuire. 2000. 2300p. 975.00 (*3-527-29874-6*) Wiley.

Pharmaceuticals & Health Policy: International Perspectives on Provision & Control of Medicines. Ed. by Blum et al. 1981. LC 80-26498. 387p. 44.50 (*0-8419-0682-3*) Holmes & Meier.

Pharmaceuticals Market Outlook: U. S. Edition. Frost and Sullivan Staff. Date not set. 53p. (*0-7889-0416-7*, 2723-52) Frost & Sullivan.

Pharmaceuticals/Biotechnology Market Sourcebook - 1995 Edition. Ed. by Frost and Sullivan Staff. 1995. spiral bd. 1295.00 (*0-7889-0238-5*, 2724-59) Frost & Sullivan.

Pharmaceutics: The Science of Dosage Form Design. Michael E. Aulton. 1988. (Illus.). 774p. text (*0-443-03643-8*) Church.

Pharmaceutics Laboratory: Heterogeneous Systems. P. L. Madan. 1995. 69p. (Orig.). (C). pap., stu. ed. 12.50 (*1-878045-83-0*) Whittier Pubns.

Pharmaceutics Laboratory: Homogeneous Systems. P. L. Madan. 1995. 79p. (Orig.). (C). pap., stu. ed. 12.50 (*1-878045-82-2*) Whittier Pubns.

Pharmachology for the Psychotherapist. M. Goldenberg. 1990. LC 89-84338. xii, 388p. (C). 33.95 (*0-915202-97-2*) Accel Devel.

Pharmacie Bei Den Alten Culturvolkern. Julius Berendes. 1989. xxii, 528p. reprint ed. 120.00 (*3-487-00902-1*) G Olms Pubs.

Pharmacist. Jack Rudman. 1994. (Career Examination Ser.: C-580). pap. 34.95 (*0-8373-0580-2*) Nat Learn.

Pharmacist & the Challenge of New Social Trends. 1997. (*92-871-3317-4*) Council of Europe FRA. *Dist:* Manhattan Pub Co.

Pharmacist Disease Management Credentialing: Diabetes. American Pharmaceutical Association Staff. 2000. pap. 89.00 (*1-58212-027-7*) Am Pharm Assn.

Pharmacist I. Jack Rudman. 1994. (Career Examination Ser.: C-1836). pap. 34.95 (*0-8373-1836-X*) Nat Learn.

Pharmacist III. Jack Rudman. 1994. (Career Examination Ser.: C-1838). pap. 34.95 (*0-8373-1838-6*) Nat Learn.

Pharmacist Trainee. Jack Rudman. 1994. (Career Examination Ser.: C-649). pap. 27.95 (*0-8373-0649-3*) Nat Learn.

Pharmacist II. Jack Rudman. 1994. (Career Examination Ser.: C-1837). pap. 34.95 (*0-8373-1837-8*) Nat Learn.

***Pharmacist Workforce: A Study of the Supply & Demand for Pharmacists.** Judith Cooksey. 2001. (Illus.). 91p. (C). pap. 25.00 (*0-7567-0998-9*) DIANE Pub.

Pharmacist's Controlled Substances Regulatory Guide & Compliance Manual: A Complete Prescription Department Guide for Practicing Pharmacists. Ronald W. Buzzeo et al. 1995. 130p. 130.00 (*0-9648291-0-X*) Regulatory Info Ctr.

Pharmacist's Guide to Drug Eruptions & Interactions. J. Z. Litt. 2001. 558p. pap. 29.95 (*1-84214-063-9*, Parthenon Pbng) CRC Pr.

Pharmacist's Guide to Schools Offering Nontraditional Doctor of Pharmacy Degrees. D. S. Chan. 2000. 144p. (C). pap. 24.99 (*0-9663353-2-5*) Gratefuldeb.

Pharmacist's Guide to the Most Misused & Abused Drugs in America: Prescription Drugs - Over-the-Counter Drugs - Designer Drugs. Ken Liska. 1988. 23.99 (*0-02-572970-5*) Macmillan.

Pharmacist's Managed Care Manual. Ed. by David B. Nash. 1997. (Illus.). 250p. (Orig.). spiral bd. 54.95 (*1-890045-04-7*) T L C Med Pub.

Pharmacists Smart Guide to the Top 50 Herbs. Art Presser. 2000. LC 99-66309. (Smart Guide Ser.). (Illus.). 128p. pap. 9.95 (*1-890572-09-8*) Smart Pubns CA.

Pharmacists Talking with Patients: A Guide to Patient Couseling. Melanie J. Rantucci. 1997. LC 96-15264. (Illus.). 265p. 29.95 (*0-683-07127-0*) Lppncott W & W.

Pharmacoanglography in the Diagnosis of Tumours. G. Y. Vargha. 1981. 252p. (C). (*963-05-2912-2*) Akade Kiado HUN. *Dist:* St Mut.

***Pharmacodynamic Basis of Herbal Medicine.** Manuchair S. Ebadi. 2001. LC 2001-43781. 760p. 129.95 (*0-8493-0743-0*) CRC Pr.

Pharmacodynamic Models of Selected Toxic Chemicals in Man. A. D. Smith & M. C. Thorne. 1986. text 268.50 (*0-85200-953-4*) Kluwer Academic.

Pharmacodynamics: Perspectives in Clinical Pharmacology. Ed. by Neal R. Cutler & John J. Sramek. 1994. LC 94-6103. 508p. 334.95 (*0-471-95052-1*) Wiley.

Pharmacoeconomics: Unique Perspectives on Cost, Outcomes & Value. Fred M. Cox & Barbara L. Hesslegrave. 1998. (Illus.). 225p. 55.00 (*0-07-013404-9*) McGraw.

Pharmacoeconomics in Perspective: A Primer on Research, Techniques & Information. Robert J. Bonk. 1999. LC 98-47909. (Illus.). 116p. lib. bdg. 49.95 (*0-7890-0561-1*, Pharmctl Prods) Haworth Pr.

Pharmacoepidemiology. Ed. by Brian L. Strom. 1989. (Illus.). 424p. text (*0-443-08675-3*) Church.

Pharmacoepidemiology, Vol. I. Ed. by Stanley A. Edlavitch. 1989. (Illus.). 360p. lib. bdg. 110.00 (*0-87371-129-7*, L129) Lewis Pubs.

Pharmacogenetics. Wendell W. Weber. 1997. LC 96-36554. (Oxford Monographs on Medical Genetics: No. 32). (Illus.). 360p. text 59.50 (*0-19-506878-5*) OUP.

Pharmacogenetics: Bridging the Gap Between Basic Science & Clinical. Ed. by Wendy Hori & Johanna Schlegel. 1996. (Biomedical Library). pap. 795.00 (*1-57936-021-1*) Drug & Market Dev.

Pharmacogenetics: Proceedings of the WHO Scientific Group, Geneva, 1972. WHO Staff. 1973. (Technical Reports: No. 524). pap. text 4.00 (*92-4-120524-5*, 1100524) World Health.

Pharmacogenetics & Pharmacogenomics: Recent Conceptual & Technical Advances. Ed. by E. S. Vesell. 2000. (Pharmacology Ser.: Vol. 61). (Illus.). 116p. pap. 34.00 (*3-8055-7128-3*) S Karger.

Pharmacogenetics of Drug Metabolism. Werner Kalow. 1992. (International Encyclopedia of Pharmacology & Therapeutics Ser.: Vol. 137). 930p. 479.50 (*0-08-041175-4*, Pergamon Pr) Elsevier.

Pharmacognosy & Pharmacobiotechnology. James E. Robbers et al. 1996. (Illus.). 352p. 43.95 (*0-683-08500-X*) Lppncott W & W.

Pharmacokinetic Analysis: A Practical Approach. I-Der Lee & Gordon L. Amidon. 1996. LC 96-60272. 548p. 179.95 (*1-56676-425-4*) CRC Pr.

Pharmacokinetic & Pharmacodynamic Principles of Anticancer Therapy. Ed. by Roy B. Jones & Pablo J. Cagnoni. 2001. (Cancer Drug Discovery & Development Ser.). 400p. 135.00 (*0-89603-895-5*) Humana.

Pharmacokinetic Aspects of the Blood-Brain Barrier Transport & Equilibration of Opioids Studied with Microdialysis in Rats & Mice. Ruija Xie. 2000. (Comprehensive Summaries of Uppsala Dissertations from the Faculty of Pharmacy Ser.: 223). (Illus.). 60p. (Orig.). pap. (*91-554-4667-1*) Uppsala Universitet SWE. *Dist:* Coronet Bks.

Pharmacokinetic Profiles of Drugs. J. P. Labaune. 1996. (Pharmaceutical Sciences Ser.). 500p. 125.00 (*0-7484-0559-3*) Taylor & Francis.

Pharmacokinetic/Pharmacodynamic Analysis: Accelerating Drug Discovery & Development. Ed. by Johanna Schlegel. 1996. (Biomedical Library). 314p. pap. 795.00 (*1-57936-011-4*) Drug & Market Dev.

Pharmacokinetic/Pharmacodynamic Analysis II. Ed. by Wendy Mori. 1997. (Illus.). (Orig.). pap. (*1-57936-045-9*) Drug & Market Dev.

Pharmacokinetics. Ed. by H. Schoenfeld et al. 1978. (Antibiotics & Chemotherapy Ser.: Vol. 25). (Illus.). 138.50 (*3-8055-2752-7*) S Karger.

Pharmacokinetics: Classic & Modern. Ed. by J. H. Van Rossum & A. A. Maes. 1986. (Illus.). 63p. pap. 20.00 (*0-89573-542-3*, Wiley-VCH) Wiley.

Pharmacokinetics: Mathematical & Statistical Approaches. Ed. by A. Pecile & A. Rescigno. 1988. LC 87-36043. (NATO ASI Series A, Life Sciences: Vol. 145). (Illus.). 358p. 105.00 (*0-306-42806-7*, Plenum Trade) Perseus Pubng.

Pharmacokinetics: Processes & Mathematics. Peter G. Welling. 1986. LC 86-20644. (ACS Monograph: No. 185). (Illus.). xiv, 268p. 59.95 (*0-8412-0967-7*) Am Chemical.

Pharmacokinetics: Processes, Mathematics, & Applications. Peter G. Welling. 2nd ed. 1997. LC 97-12306. (Professional Reference Book Ser.). 400p. text 105.00 (*0-8412-3481-7*) Am Chemical.

Pharmacokinetics: Regulatory - Industrial - Academic Perspectives. Ed. by Peter G. Welling & Francis L. Tse. 2nd exp. rev. ed. 1995. (Drugs & the Pharmaceutical Sciences Ser.: Vol. 67). (Illus.). 528p. text 185.00 (*0-8247-9378-1*) Dekker.

Pharmacokinetics & Cancer Chemotherapy. Ed. by P. Workman & M. A. Graham. 1993. (Cancer Surveys Ser.: Vol. 17). (Illus.). 235p. (C). text 69.00 (*0-87969-390-8*) Cold Spring Harbor.

Pharmacokinetics & Clinical Pharmacology of Beta-Blockers in Hypertension. Ed. by P. M. Galletti. 1979. (Cardiology Ser.: Vol. 64, Suppl. 1). (Illus.). pap. 28.75 (*3-8055-3061-7*) S Karger.

Pharmacokinetics & Clinical Pharmacology of Cardiac Clyscosides. Ed. by K. Greeff. 1981. (Handbook of Experimental Pharmacology Ser.: Vol. 56). (Illus.). 394p. 216.00 (*0-387-10918-8*) Spr-Verlag.

Pharmacokinetics & Pharmacodynamics Vol. 1: Research Design & Analysis. Ed. by Randall B. Smith et al. 1986. LC 86-50775. (Illus.). viii, 104p. (Orig.). pap. text 2.00 (*0-9606488-4-4*) H W Bks.

Pharmacokinetics, Biodistribution & Mode of Action of Apomorphine: An In Vitro Study at Cellular Level & In Vivo Study Using Microdialysis. Exaud E. Sam. 1997. (Acta Biomedica Lovaniensia Ser.: No. 156). (Illus.). 182p. pap. (*90-6186-838-6*) Almqvist & Wiksell SWE. *Dist:* Coronet Bks.

Pharmacokinetics, Drug Metabolism & Clinical Effects of the Anti-malarial Artemisinin: Time-Dependencies & Modeling Aspects. Ulrika S.H. Svensson. 2000. (Illus.). 65p. (Orig.). pap. (*91-554-4672-8*) Uppsala Universitet SWE. *Dist:* Coronet Bks.

Pharmacokinetics for the Non-Mathematical. David W. Bourne et al. 1986. text 119.00 (*0-85200-712-4*) Kluwer Academic.

Pharmacokinetics for the Pharmaceutical Scientist. John Wagner. 1993. LC 93-60366. 336p. 116.95 (*1-56676-032-1*) CRC Pr.

Pharmacokinetics of Cardiovascular, Central Nervous System & Antimicrobial Drugs. Ed. by Peter G. Welling & F. L. Tse. 1985. 468p. (C). text (*0-85186-937-8*) Royal Soc Chem GBR. *Dist:* Spr-Verlag.

Pharmacokinetics of Drugs. Ed. by Peter G. Welling & Luc P. Balant. 1994. LC 93-43145. (Handbook of Experimental Pharmacology Ser.: Vol. 110). (Illus.). 5379p. 470.00 (*0-387-57506-5*) Spr-Verlag.

Pharmacokinetics of Psychoactive Drugs: Further Studies. Ed. by Louis Gottschalk. 1979. LC 79-9430. 140p. text 35.00 (*0-88331-176-3*) R B Luce.

Pharmacokinetics of Selected Antibacterial Agents. Axel Dalhoff. 1997. LC 97-33565. (Antibiotics & Chemotherapy Ser.: No. 49). (Illus.). vi, 148p. 148.00 (*3-8055-6576-3*) S Karger.

Pharmacokinetics of Sulfonamides Revisited. T. B. Vree et al. 1985. (Antibiotics & Chemotherapy Ser.: Vol. 34). (Illus.). x, 220p. 148.00 (*3-8055-3949-5*) S Karger.

Pharmacokinetics II. Ed. by H. Schoenfeld. 1981. (Antibiotics & Chemotherapy Ser.: Vol. 31). (Illus.). xiv, 226p. 128.75 (*3-8055-2448-X*) S Karger.

Pharmacologic Analysis of Drug-Receptor Interaction. Terry Kenakin. 3rd ed. 1997. LC 97-12942. 512p. text 120.00 (*0-397-51815-3*) Lppncott W & W.

Pharmacologic Approach to Gastrointestinal Disorders. James H. Lewis. 1994. LC 93-13185. (Illus.). 667p. 85.00 (*0-683-04970-4*) Lppncott W & W.

Pharmacologic Basis of Nursing Practice. Julia F. Clark & Sherry F. Queener. 5th ed. 1996. 96p. (C). (gr. 13). pap. text, stu. ed. (*0-8151-1510-5*, 28264) Mosby Inc.

Pharmacologic Basis of Nursing Practice. Julia F. Clark et al. 5th ed. 1997. tchr. ed., suppl. ed. (*0-8151-2124-5*); 5th ed. 1997. (C). text (*0-323-00701-5*); 6th ed. 1999. LC 99-35763. (Illus.). 848p. (C). pap. text 52.00 (*0-323-00684-1*) Mosby Inc.

Pharmacologic Basis of Nursing Practice: Instructor's Resources Manual with Testbank. Julia Freeman Clark et al. 6th ed. 2000. (Illus.). (C). tchr. ed. (*0-323-00722-8*) Mosby Inc.

Pharmacologic Basis of Nursing Practice: Text & Student Learning Guide Package. Set. Julia F. Clark et al. 5th ed. 1997. (C). text, stu. ed. (*0-8151-1511-3*) Mosby Inc.

Pharmacologic Basis of Patient Care. Mary K. Asperheim. 5th ed. 1985. (Illus.). 620p. tchr. ed. (*0-7216-2004-3*); text 65.00 (*0-7216-1229-6*) Saunders.

Pharmacologic Basis of Psychotherapeutics: An Introduction for Psychologists. Louis A. Pagliaro & Ann M. Pagliaro. 1997. LC 97-19994. (*1-56032-677-8*); pap. (*1-56032-678-6*) Hemisp Pub.

Pharmacologic Intervention in the Treatment of AIDS. Kirk R. Ryan. 1992. pap. 9.00 (*0-9623535-4-X*) Remco Inc.

Pharmacological & Chemical Synonyms. Compiled by E. E. Marler. 9th ed. 1990. 500p. reprint ed. 275.50 (*0-444-90487-5*) Elsevier.

Pharmacological & Therapeutic Aspects of Hypertension. Ardis Walker. 1980. Vol. 1. 224p. 130.00 (*0-8493-5385-8*, RC685); Vol. 2. 256p. 143.00 (*0-8493-5386-6*) Franklin (CRC Reprint).

Pharmacological Approaches to the Treatment of Brain & Spinal Cord Injury. Ed. by D. G. Stein & B. A. Sabel. 1988. LC 88-5942. (Illus.). 408p. 105.00 (*0-306-42732-X*, Plenum Trade) Perseus Pubng.

Pharmacological Approaches to the Treatment of Chronic Pain: New Concepts & Critical Issues. Ed. by Howard L. Fields & J. C. Liebeskind. 1994. LC 93-80786. (Progress in Pain Research & Management Ser.: Vol. 1). (Illus.). 326p. 36.00 (*0-931092-04-3*, PPRM1) Intl Assn Study Pain.

Pharmacological Aspect of Nursing Care. Barry S. Reiss & Mary E. Evans. 6th ed. 2001. LC 2001-28141. (Nursing Education Ser.). (C). pap. text 44.95 (*0-7668-0502-6*) Delmar.

Pharmacological Aspects & Neurological Potentials of Calcium Entry Blockers. Ed. by A. Hartmann & Pieter A. Van Zwieten. 1986. (Journal: Vol. 25, Suppl. 1, 1986). 128p. pap. 40.00 (*3-8055-4365-4*) S Karger.

Pharmacological Aspects of Drug Dependence: Toward an Integrated Neurobehavioral Approach. Ed. by Charles R. Schuster et al. 1996. LC 95-36826. (Handbook of Experimental Pharmacology Ser.: Vol. 118). (Illus.). 658p. 450.00 (*3-540-58989-9*) Spr-Verlag.

Pharmacological Aspects of Heart Disease. Ed. by Naranjan S. Dhalla et al. 1987. (Developments in Cardiovascular Medicine Ser.). text 176.50 (*0-89838-867-8*) Kluwer Academic.

Pharmacological Aspects of Nursing Care. Barry S. Reiss & Mary E. Evans. 4th ed. 1993. LC 92-49601. 766p. pap. 44.95 (*0-8273-4846-0*) Delmar.

Pharmacological Aspects of Nursing Care. Barry S. Reiss. 5th ed. 1996. (Nursing Education Ser.). 112p. tchr. ed. 10.50 (*0-8273-7669-3*) Delmar.

Pharmacological Aspects of Nursing Care. Barry S. Reiss & Mary E. Evans. 5th ed. 1995. (Nursing Education Ser.). 797p. (C). pap. text 68.95 (*0-8273-6662-0*) Delmar.

Pharmacological Aspects of Nursing Care: Instructor's Guide. Barry S. Reiss & Mary E. Evans. 4th ed. 1993. 139p. pap. 16.95 (*0-8273-5447-9*) Delmar.

Pharmacological Basis of Anesthesiology: Basic Science & Practical Applications. T. Andrew Bowdle. 1994. text (*0-443-08878-0*) Church.

Pharmacological Calculations for Nurses. Peggy H. Batastini. 2nd ed. 1991. 187p. (C). pap. 26.50 (*0-8273-4727-8*) Delmar.

Pharmacological Calculations for Nurses: A Worktext. Peggy H. Batastini & Judy K. Davidson. 1989. 202p. pap. text 24.95 (*0-8273-4202-0*) Delmar.

Pharmacological Calculations for Nurses: A Worktext 3E. Peggy H. Batastini & Judy K. Davidson. 3rd ed. 1999. LC 98-46290. 192p. (C). pap. text 23.95 (*0-7668-0166-7*) Delmar.

Pharmacological Control of Calcium & Potassium Homeostasis: Biological, Therapeutical & Clinical Aspects. Ed. by Theophile Godfraind et al. 1995. LC 95-19895. (Medical Science Symposia Ser.: Vol. 9). 292p. (C). text 125.00 (*0-7923-3604-6*) Kluwer Academic.

Pharmacological Denervation & Glaucoma. Philip F. Hoyng. 1981. text 127.50 (*90-6193-802-3*) Kluwer Academic.

Pharmacological Dictionary. Latin-Russian, Russian-Latin. 1977. (LAT & RUS.). 463p. 39.95 (*0-7859-0787-4*, M-9078) Fr & Eur.

Pharmacological Effects of Ethanol on the Nervous System. Ed. by Richard A. Deitrich et al. 1995. LC 95-9425. (Pharmacology & Toxicology Ser.). 480p. 139.95 (*0-8493-8389-7*, 8389) CRC Pr.

Pharmacological Effects of Lipids. Ed. by Jon J. Kabara. 1978. 228p. 40.00 (*0-935315-02-0*); Vol. II. 1985. 366p. 40.00 (*0-935315-10-1*) Am Oil Chemists.

Pharmacological Effects of Lipids III. Ed. by Jon J. Kabara. 1990. 366p. (C). 40.00 (*0-935315-28-4*) Am Oil Chemists.

Pharmacological Interventions on Central Cholinergic Mechanisms in Senile Dementia: Alzheimer's Disease. Ed. by H. Kewitz et al. 1989. (Clinical Pharmacology Ser.: Vol. 2). (Illus.). 328p. text (*3-88603-362-7*) W Zuckschwerdt DEU. *Dist:* Scholium Intl.

Pharmacological Issues in Alcohol & Substance Abuse. Ed. by Barry Stimmel. 1988. LC 87-36672. (Advances in Alcohol & Substance Abuse Ser.: Vol. 7, No. 1). (Illus.). 79p. text 39.95 (*0-86656-717-8*) Haworth Pr.

Pharmacological Management of Neurological & Psychiatric Disorders. Sam J. Enna & Joe Coyle. 1998. LC 98-16368. (Illus.). 736p. text 79.95 (*0-07-021764-5*) McGraw-Hill Prof.

Pharmacological Methods in Toxicology. Ed. by F. Gross & Gerhard Zbinden. 1979. (*0-08-021544-0*) Pergamon Repr GBR. *Dist:* Franklin.

Pharmacological Nutrition Immune Nutrition. L. Cynober et al. 1995. (Illus.). 147p. pap. text (*3-88603-543-3*) W Zuckschwerdt DEU. *Dist:* Scholium Intl.

Pharmacological Regulation of Gene Expression in the CNS: Towards An Understanding of Basal Ganglial Functions. Kalpana M. Merchant. 1996. LC 96-18410. (Pharmacology & Toxicology: Basic & Clinical Aspects Ser.). 224p. 139.95 (*0-8493-8550-4*) CRC Pr.

Pharmacological Research on Traditional Herbal Medicines. Hiroshi Watanabe. 1999. 248p. text 90.00 (*90-5702-054-8*, Harwood Acad Pubs) Gordon & Breach.

Pharmacological Sciences: Perspectives for Research & Therapy in the Late 1990s. Ed. by A. C. Cuello & B. Collier. 1995. LC 95-17107. xxi, 519p. 159.00 (*3-7643-5072-5*) Birkhauser.

Pharmacological Therapies for Drug & Alcohol Addictions. Ed. by Norman S. Miller & Mark S. Gold. 1994. LC 94-3755. (Illus.). 480p. text 175.00 (*0-8247-8979-2*) Dekker.

Pharmacological Treatment of Alzheimer's Disease: Molecular & Neurobiological Foundations. Ed. by Jorge D. Brioni & Micahel W. Decker. 1997. LC 96-30137. 549p. 130.00 (*0-471-16758-4*) Wiley.

Pharmacological Treatment of Endocrinopathies. Ed. by Charles Y. Pak. 1991. (Progress in Basic & Clinical Pharmacology Ser.: Vol. 5). (Illus.). x, 142p. 126.25 (*3-8055-5214-9*) S Karger.

Pharmacologist. Jack Rudman. 1994. (Career Examination Ser.: C-581). pap. 39.95 (*0-8373-0581-0*) Nat Learn.

Pharmacology. Donald C. Ahrens. 1996. (National Veterinary Medical Ser.). 360p. pap. text 29.95 (*0-683-00085-3*) Lppncott W & W.

Pharmacology. Daniel E. Becker. 1993. (C). stu. ed. 22.42 (*1-56870-094-6*) RonJon Pub.

Pharmacology. George M. Brenner. Date not set. LC 99-51716. 509p. pap. text (*0-7216-7757-6*) Saunders.

Pharmacology. Center for Emergency Medicine Staff. 1996. 96p. (gr. 13). pap. text 9.95 (*0-8151-7951-0*) Mosby Inc.

Pharmacology. Choca. 1996. (*0-7216-4579-8*) Saunders.

Pharmacology. Charles D. Ciccone. 1995. 158p. pap. 30.00 (*1-887759-00-X*, P-115) Am Phys Therapy Assn.

Pharmacology. Richard M. Kostrzewa. 1995. 380p. pap. 19.99 (*0-945819-48-X*) Sulzburger & Graham Pub.

Pharmacology. Ed. by J. I. Moore. 1988. (Oklahoma Notes). 247p. (C). 14.95 (*0-387-96332-4*) Spr-Verlag.

Pharmacology. Catherine Paradiso. 1997. LC 97-35555. (Lippincott's Review Ser.). 636p. pap. text 24.95 (*0-397-55327-7*) Lppncott W & W.

Pharmacology. Smolin. 1993. 39.00 (*0-316-80269-7*, Little Brwn Med Div) Lppncott W & W.

Pharmacology. Webster. 2000. (Quick Look Veterinary Ser.). 23.95 (*1-889325-47-3*) Fence Crk Pubng.

Pharmacology. Joyce L. Kee. 2nd ed. 1997. pap. text 61.00 (*0-7216-7573-5*) Saunders.

Pharmacology. Ed. by J. I. Moore. 2nd ed. 1991. (Oklahoma Notes). 251p. 15.95 (*0-387-97194-7*) Spr-Verlag.

Pharmacology. H. P. Rang & M. M. Dale. 2nd ed. 1991. (Illus.). 955p. pap. text (*0-443-04110-5*) Church.

Pharmacology. H. P. Rang et al. 3rd ed. 1995. LC 94-47182. pap. text (*0-443-07560-3*) Church.

Pharmacology. Gary C. Rosenfeld & David S. Loose-Mitchell. 3rd ed. 1997. LC 97-25644. (Board Review Ser.). (Illus.). 400p. pap. text 27.95 (*0-683-18050-9*) Lppncott W & W.

Pharmacology. Leonard S. Jacob. 4th ed. 1996. (National Medical Series for Independent Study). (Illus.). 385p. pap. text 29.00 (*0-683-06251-4*) Lppncott W & W.

Pharmacology. Ed. by Joanne I. Moore. 4th ed. 1995. LC 94-43678. (Oklahoma Notes). 235p. 24.95 (*0-387-94394-3*) Spr-Verlag.

Pharmacology. H. P. Rang. 4th ed. 1999. LC 98-31756. (*0-443-05974-8*) Church.

Pharmacology: A Comprehensive Guide to Drug Therapy. Sandra C. Wardell. 1979. text 14.95 P-H.

Pharmacology: A Nursing Process Approach. Ed. by Joyce L. Kee & Evelyn R. Hayes. 1993. (Illus.). pap., tchr. ed. (*0-7216-3661-6*); pap., stu. ed. (*0-7216-4613-1*) Saunders.

Pharmacology: A Nursing Process Approach. Joyce L. Kee & Evelyn R. Hayes. Ed. by Maura Connor. 2nd ed. 1996. LC 96-46545. 848p. pap. text 47.00 (*0-7216-6057-6*) Saunders.

Pharmacology: A Nursing Process Approach. Ed. by Joyce L. Kee & Evelyn R. Hayes. 2nd rev. ed. 1997. (Illus.). pap., tchr. ed. (*0-7216-6058-4*) Saunders.

Pharmacology: An Introductory Text. Mary K. Asperheim. 8th ed. 1996. (Illus.). pap., tchr. ed. (*0-7216-6039-8*) Saunders.

Pharmacology: An Introductory Text. Mary K. Asperheim. Ed. by Ilza Rader. 8th ed. 1996. LC 95-36451. (Illus.). 275p. pap. text 24.95 (*0-7216-6038-X*) Saunders.

***Pharmacology: An Open Learning Introduction for Healthcare Workers.** John Sneddon. 2000. 88p. pap., wbk. ed. (*1-85775-431-X*) Radcliffe Med Pr GBR. *Dist:* Balogh.

Pharmacology: Drug Actions & Reactions. Ruth R. Levine. 3rd ed. 1983. (Illus.). 24.50 (*0-316-52222-8*, Little Brwn Med Div) Lppncott W & W.

Pharmacology: Drug Actions & Reactions. Ruth R. Levine et al. 5th ed. 1996. LC 96-29172. (Illus.). 586p. ring bd. (*1-85070-780-4*, Parthenon Pbng) CRC Pr.

Pharmacology: Nursing Process Approach. Peery. 1990. (Education Ser.). pap., tchr. ed. 10.00 (*0-8273-3796-5*); pap., wbk. ed. 12.95 (*0-8273-3794-9*); (C). text 42.95 (*0-8273-3795-7*) Delmar.

Pharmacology: PreTest Self-Assessment & Review. Joseph R. Dipalma. 5th ed. 1988. pap. text 15.95 (*0-07-051966-8*) McGraw.

Pharmacology: PreTest Self-Assessment & Review. Ed. by Arnold Stern. 9th ed. 1998. (Pretest Basic Sciences Ser.). (Illus.). 259p. pap. 24.95 (*0-07-052694-X*) McGraw-Hill Educ Grp.

***Pharmacology: Review & Rationales.** Mary A. Hogan & Linda A. Silvestri. 2001. 468p. pap. 24.95 (*0-13-030462-X*) P-H.

Pharmacology: Review for New National Boards. Melvin L. Billingsley. 1995. (Illus.). 186p. pap. 25.00 (*0-8036-0716-4*) Davis Co.

Pharmacology: Review for New National Boards. Melvin L. Billingsley. 1995. LC 95-75271. (Illus.). 186p. pap. 25.00 (*0-9632873-7-0*) J & S Pub VA.

***Pharmacology: Self-Assessment & Review.** Arnold Stern. 10th ed. 2001. (Pretest Self-Assessment & Review Ser.). (Illus.). 272p. pap. 24.95 (*0-07-136704-7*) McGraw-Hill Prof.

Pharmacology & Applications of Chinese Materia Medica, Vol. 1. Ed. by H. M. Chang & P. P-H. But. 1986. 780p. text 114.00 (*9971-5-0121-X*) World Scientific Pub.

Pharmacology & Applications of Chinese Materia Medica, Vol. 2. Ed. by H. M. Chang & P. P-H. But. Tr. by L. L. Wang & S. C. Yeung. 1987. 556p. text 99.00 (*9971-5-0167-8*) World Scientific Pub.

Pharmacology & Dental Therapeutics. Robin Seymour et al. 3rd ed. 1999. LC 99-24161. (Illus.). 392p. pap. text 69.50 (*0-19-262952-2*) OUP.

Pharmacology & Drug Administration for Imaging Technologists. Jensen & Peppers. 1998. (Illus.). 192p. (gr. 13). pap. text 26.00 (*0-8151-4894-1*, 28605) Mosby Inc.

Pharmacology & Drug Administration for Imaging Technologists. Steven C. Jensen & Michael P. Peppers. 1998. tchr. ed. (*0-8151-4938-7*) Mosby Inc.

Pharmacology & Drug Management for Nurses. George Downie et al. 1995. LC 94-8716. pap. text (*0-443-04477-5*) Church.

Pharmacology & Drug Management for Nurses. George Downie. 2nd ed. 1999. (C). pap. text 30.00 (*0-443-05968-3*) Saunders.

Pharmacology & Natural Medicine Exam Review. Bertram G. Katzung. 4th ed. 1996. (C). pap. text 15.99 (*0-8385-8102-1*) P-H.

Pharmacology & Pharmacotherapeutics. R. S. Saroskar & S. D. Bhandarkar. 1989. (*0-86132-177-4*) Popular Prakashan IND. *Dist:* S Asia.

Pharmacology & Physiology in Anesthetic Practice. Robert K. Stoelting. 3rd ed. 1998. LC 98-29288. 848p. text 120.00 (*0-7817-1621-7*) Lppncott W & W.

Pharmacology & the Nursing Process. Linda Lane Lilley et al. (Illus.). tchr. ed. (*0-8151-5664-2*); 1996. text, stu. ed. 13.95 (*0-8016-8116-2*) Mosby Inc.

Pharmacology & the Nursing Process. Linda L. Lilley & Robert S. Aucker. 2nd ed. 1998. tchr. ed. (*1-55664-493-0*); (Illus.). stu. ed. (*1-55664-495-7*); LC 98-26135. (Illus.). 816p. pap. text 45.00 (*1-55664-492-2*) Mosby Inc.

Pharmacology & the Nursing Process. Gordon E. Johnson et al. 3rd ed. 1992. (Illus.). 799p. pap. (*0-920513-08-5*) Saunders.

***Pharmacology & the Nursing Process.** Linda Lilley & Robert Aucker. 3rd ed. 2001. LC 2001-31542. (Illus.). 255p. (*0-323-01267-1*) Mosby Inc.

***Pharmacology & the Nursing Process: Including Student Learning Guide.** Linda Lilley & Robert Aucker. 3rd ed. 2001. (*0-323-01266-3*) Mosby Inc.

***Pharmacology & the Nursing Process: Instructor's Resource Manual.** Linda Lilley & Robert Aucker. 3rd ed. 2001. (*0-323-01268-X*) Mosby Inc.

***Pharmacology & the Nursing Process: Student Learning Guide.** Linda Lilley & Robert Aucker. 3rd ed. 2001. stu. ed. (*0-323-01269-8*) Mosby Inc.

Pharmacology & the Nursing Process: Text & Student Learning Guide Package, Set. Linda L. Lilley & Robert S. Aucker. 2nd ed. 1998. (C). text, stu. ed. (*1-55664-494-9*) Mosby Inc.

Pharmacology & Therapeutics. Ed. by W. C. Bowman. 1981. (Illus.). Vol. 12, No. 1. LC 77-25743. 283p. pap. 73.00 (*0-08-026854-4*); Vol. 12, No. 2. 190p. pap. 73.00 (*0-08-026855-2*) Elsevier (Pergamon Pr).

Pharmacology & Therapeutics for Dentistry. John A. Yagiela et al. 4th ed. 1997. LC 97-229020. (Illus.). 752p. (C). text 64.00 (*0-8016-7962-1*, 07962) Mosby Inc.

***Pharmacology & Therapeutics in the New Millennium.** S. K. Gupta. 2001. 756p. 324.00 (*0-7923-7059-7*) Kluwer Academic.

Pharmacology & Toxicology of Amphetamine & Related Designer Drugs. 1993. lib. bdg. 261.95 (*0-8490-8913-1*); 1991. lib. bdg. 250.00 (*0-8490-4372-7*) Gordon Pr.

Pharmacology & Toxicology of Naturally Occurring Toxins Ed. by H. Raskova. 1971. LC 77-130797. (*0-08-016797-7*) Pergamon Repr GBR. *Dist:* Franklin.

Pharmacology at the Millennium: Past, Present & Future. R. J. Huxtable et al. 1999. vi, 76p. (C). pap. (*1-930061-00-5*) West Pharm Soc.

Pharmacology, Biology, & Clinical Applications of Androgens: Current Status & Future Prospects. Ed. by Shalender Bhasin et al. 1996. LC 95-46146. 529p. 145.00 (*0-471-13320-5*, Wiley-Interscience) Wiley.

Pharmacology Companion. Gary L. Gallia et al. Date not set. 250p. (Orig.). (C). pap. 25.95 (*0-9640124-3-X*) Alert & Oriented.

Pharmacology Essentials. Ed. by Jody A. Eckler & Judy M. Fair. 1996. (Illus.). pap., tchr. ed. (*0-7216-6811-9*) Saunders.

Pharmacology Essentials. Jody A. Eckler & Judy M. Fair. Ed. by Ilze Rader. 1996. LC 95-19853. (Illus.). 464p. pap. text 31.50 (*0-7216-6486-5*) Saunders.

Pharmacology Field Guide. Richard K. Beck. 1996. LC 95-50500. (Illus.). 122p. (C). pap. text 22.95 (*0-8036-0133-6*) Thomson Learn.

***Pharmacology for Anaesthesia & Intensive Care.** T. E. Peck & M Williams. 2000. 346p. incl. cd-rom (*1-84110-025-0*) Greenwich Med GBR. *Dist:* JAMCO Dist.

Pharmacology for Anaesthetists. Noel Cass & Linda Cass. 1995. LC 93-7322. 208p. pap. text (*0-443-04639-5*) Church.

Pharmacology for Athletic Trainers: Performance Enhancement & Social Drugs. Human Kinetics Staff. 1997. (Illus.). 96p. spiral bd. 69.00 (*0-88011-760-5*, COPS0760) Human Kinetics.

Pharmacology for Chemists. Joseph Cannon. 1998. LC 98-25069. (ACS Professional Reference Book Ser.). (Illus.). 288p. text 60.00 (*0-8412-3524-4*) Am Chemical.

Pharmacology for Dental Hygiene Practice. Elena B. Haveles. 1996. LC 96-17639. (Dental Assisting Procedures Ser.). 352p. (C). pap. text 68.95 (*0-8273-6602-7*) Delmar.

Pharmacology for Dental Hygiene Practice - IML. Haveles. 1996. tchr. ed. (*0-8273-8438-6*) Delmar.

Pharmacology for Health in Asia: Proceedings of Asian Congress of Pharmacology. Ed. by B. N. Dhawan. 1988. (C). (*0-8364-2336-4*) Allied Pubs IND. *Dist:* S Asia.

Pharmacology for Health Professionals. Evelyn Salerno. 1999. LC 00-500766. (Illus.). 816p. (C). (gr. 13). pap. text 39.00 (*0-8151-2711-1*, 31383) Mosby Inc.

Pharmacology for Health Professionals: Includes Testbank. Evelyn Salerno. 1999. (Illus.). tchr. ed. (*0-323-00257-9*) Mosby Inc.

Pharmacology for Medical Assistants. E. A. Watts. 1986. 100p. pap. text 12.95 (*0-935920-28-5*, Ntl Pubs Blck) P-H.

Pharmacology for Nurses. James Connechen. 5th ed. 1983. text 17.00 (*0-7216-0803-5*) Saunders.

Pharmacology for Nurses. James Connechen et al. 5th ed. 1983. 384p. pap. text (*0-7020-0868-0*) Bailliere Tindall.

Pharmacology for Nursing Care. Richard A. Lehne. 2nd ed. 1994. (Illus.). tchr. ed. (*0-7216-5167-4*); 3rd ed. 1998. (C). pap. text, stu. ed. 17.95 (*0-7216-7069-5*) Saunders.

Pharmacology for Nursing Care. Richard A. Lehne. Ed. by Maura Connor. 3rd ed. 1998. LC 97-39758. (Illus.). 1184p. pap. text 55.95 (*0-7216-7150-0*) Saunders.

Pharmacology for Nursing Care. Richard A. Lehne. 3rd ed. 1998. (Illus.). 1180p. tchr. ed. (*0-7216-7151-9*) Saunders.

***Pharmacology for Nursing Care.** Richard A. Lehne et al. 4th ed. 2001. (Illus.). tchr. ed. (*0-7216-8880-2*) Saunders.

***Pharmacology for Nursing Care: ExaMaster.** Richard A. Lehne. 3rd ed. 1998. (*0-7216-7153-5*) Saunders.

Pharmacology for Prehospital Emergency Care. Richard K. Beck. Ed. by James R. Vance. 2nd ed. 1994. LC 93-33629. 307p. (C). pap. 23.95 (*0-8036-0692-3*) Thomson Learn.

Pharmacology for Respiratory Care Practitioners. Gregory P. Cottrell. 1995. LC 94-41358. (Illus.). 414p. 37.95 (*0-8036-1989-8*) Davis Co.

Pharmacology for Surgical Technologists. Chris Keegan & Katherine Synder. Ed. by Maureen Pfeiffer et al. 1998. LC 98-33323. (Illus.). 255p. (C). pap. text 25.00 (*0-7216-6321-4*) Saunders.

***Pharmacology for Technicians.** Don A. Ballington & Mary M. Laughlin. 2nd ed. 2001. LC 2001-54476. (*0-7638-1527-6*) EMC-Paradigm.

Pharmacology for Technicians. Don A. Ballington & Mary M. Laughlin. 1998. LC 98-11383. (Illus.). vii, 470p. (*0-7638-0096-1*) Paradigm MN.

Pharmacology for Technicians: Instructor's Guide. Don A. Ballington & Mary M. Laughlin. 1999. LC 98-11383. (Illus.). vii, 470p. text 14.00 (*0-7638-0097-X*) EMC-Paradigm.

Pharmacology for the Primary Care Practitioner. Marilyn W. Edmunds. 1999. LC 00-268147. (Illus.). xxi, 1001p. (C). (gr. 13). text 89.00 (*0-8151-3092-9*, 28005) Mosby Inc.

Pharmacology for the Surgical Technologist. Slagle. 1996. pap. (*0-7216-4225-X*) Saunders.

Pharmacology for Veterinary Technicians. Robert Bill. 2nd ed. 1997. LC 97-11. (Illus.). 352p. (C). (gr. 13). pap. text 29.00 (*0-8151-0902-4*, 28335) Mosby Inc.

Pharmacology in Exercise & Sports. Ed. by Satu M. Somani & Mannfred Hollenger. 1995. LC 95-35490. (CRC Pharmacology & Toxicology: Basic & Clinical Aspects Ser.). 384p. 139.95 (*0-8493-8540-7*, 8540) CRC Pr.

Pharmacology in Medicine: Principles & Practice. Ed. by Sachin N. Pradhan et al. 1986. 1100p. (C). text 55.00 (*0-9617129-0-2*) SP Press Intl.

Pharmacology in Rehabilitation. Charles D. Ciccone. 2nd ed. 1995. LC 95-22130. (Contemporary Perspectives in Rehabilitation Ser.). (Illus.). 642p. (C). text 49.95 (0-8036-0030-5) Davis Co.

Pharmacology in the Practice of Anaesthesia. Ed. by Leon Kaufman & Peter Taberner. 1996. LC 96-4707. (Arnold Publication). (Illus.). 704p. pap. text 135.00 (0-340-55171-2) OUP.

Pharmacology Made Easy for NCLEX-PN. Linda L. Waide & Berta C. Roland. 1998. 242p. (C). pap. 23.95 (0-9659975-0-2) Learn Made.

*__Pharmacology Made Easy for NCLEX-PN: Review & Study Guide.__ Linda Waide & Berta Roland. 2001. LC 2001-42107. 240p. pap. 21.95 incl. disk (1-55652-392-0) Chicago Review.

Pharmacology Made Easy for NCLEX-RN. Linda L. Waide & Berta C. Roland. 1998. 242p. (Orig.). (C). pap. text 23.95 (0-9659975-1-0) Learn Made.

Pharmacology Math. Hocking Technical College Staff. 4th ed. 1996. 120p. (C). spiral bd. 21.95 (0-7872-2251-8, 41225101) Kendall-Hunt.

Pharmacology Nursing. Marshal Shlafer. Ed. by Debra Hunter. 1989. 1432p. (C). pap. text 9.95 (0-201-17839-7) Addison-Wesley.

Pharmacology of Aging Processes: Methods of Assessment & Potential Interventions. Ed. by Denham Harman et al. 1994. LC 94-15312. (Annals Ser.: Vol. 717). (0-89766-880-4); pap. 105.00 (0-89766-881-2) NY Acad Sci.

Pharmacology of Alcohol Abuse. R. F. Anton. Ed. by Henry R. Kranzler. 1994. LC 94-28586. (Handbook of Experimental Pharmacology Ser.: 114). (Illus.). 574p. 475.00 (0-387-57125-6) Spr-Verlag.

Pharmacology of Alcohol & Alcohol Dependence. Ed. by Henri Begleiter & Benjamin Kissin. 1996. (Alcohol & Alcoholism Ser.: No. 2). (Illus.). 536p. (C). text 99.50 (0-19-510094-8) OUP.

Pharmacology of Alcohol & Drugs of Abuse & Addiction. N. S. Miller. 1990. (Illus.). 365p. 121.00 (0-387-97383-4) Spr-Verlag.

Pharmacology of Antihypertensive Therapeutics. Ed. by D. Ganten & P. J Mulrow. 1990. (Handbook of Experimental Pharmacology Ser.: Vol. 93). (Illus.). 922p. 432.00 (0-387-50427-3) Spr-Verlag.

Pharmacology of Antimuscarinic Agents. Laszlo Gyermek. 1997. LC 97-24422. (Pharmacology & Toxicology Ser.). lib. bdg. 129.95 (0-8493-8559-8) CRC Pr.

Pharmacology of Anxiolytic Drugs. Luca Steardo et al. rev. ed. 1997. LC 96-3287. (WHO Expert Series on Neuroscience: Vol. 3). (Illus.). 144p. text 29.50 (0-88937-088-5) Hogrefe & Huber Pubs.

Pharmacology of Asthma. Ed. by John Morley & Kim D. Rainsford. 1983. (Agents & Actions Supplements Ser.: Vol. 13). 228p. 96.50 (0-8176-1503-2) Birkhauser.

Pharmacology of Asthma. Ed. by C. P. Page et al. 1991. (Handbook of Experimental Pharmacology Ser.: No. 98). (Illus.). 320p. 276.00 (0-387-52839-3) Spr-Verlag.

Pharmacology of Ayurvedic Medicinal Plants. C. R. Karnick. 1996. (81-7030-482-2) Sri Satguru Pubns IND. Dist: S Asia.

Pharmacology of Benzopyrone Derivatives & Related Compounds. Ed. by M. Gabor. 1988. pap. (963-05-4944-1) Akade Kiado HUN. Dist: St Mut.

Pharmacology of Cardiac & Vascular Remodelling: Antiproliferative Drugs. Ed. by J. G. De Mey et al. 1991. 200p. 47.95 (0-387-91391-2) Spr-Verlag.

Pharmacology of Cerebral Circulation. Ed. by Amilcare Carpi. 1972. LC 70-182263. 370p. (C). (0-08-016209-6) Pergamon Repr GBR. Dist: Franklin.

Pharmacology of Cerebral Ischemia. Gunter K. Krieglstein. 1989. 99.00 (3-8047-1036-0) CRC Pr.

Pharmacology of Chinese Herbs. Huang. Ed. by Kee Chang. 1992. 416p. 187.95 (0-8493-4915-X, RM666) CRC Pr.

Pharmacology of Chinese Herbs. Kee C. Huang & Walter M. Williams. 2nd ed. 1998. LC 98-13930. 544p. 149.95 (0-8493-1665-0) CRC Pr.

Pharmacology of Cytokines. Alberto Mantovani et al. 2000. LC 00-25524. (Illus.). 336p. pap. text 50.00 (0-19-850042-4) OUP.

Pharmacology of Diabetes: Present Practice & Future Perspectives. Ed. by C. E. Mogensen & E. Standl. 1991. (Illus.). xii, 374p. (C). pap. text 98.50 (3-11-012636-2) De Gruyter.

Pharmacology of Endogenous Neurotoxins. Andreas Moser. 1997. LC 97-12361. 120.00 (0-8176-3993-4) Birkhauser.

Pharmacology of Endogenous Neurotoxins. Andreas Moser. 1997. LC 97-12361. (Illus.). 328p. 99.95 (3-7643-3993-4) Spr-Verlag.

Pharmacology of Extrapyramidal Movement Disorders. Ed. by Harold L. Klawans, Jr. 1972. (Monographs in Neural Sciences: Vol. 2). 42.75 (3-8055-1421-2) S Karger.

Pharmacology of Fluorides. Ed. by F. A. Smith. (Handbook of Experimental Pharmacology Ser.: Vol. 20). (Illus.). Pt. 1. 1966. 608p. 140.00 (0-387-03537-0); Pt. 2. 1970. 451p. 131.00 (0-387-04846-4) Spr-Verlag.

Pharmacology of Ganglionic Transmission. Ed. by D. A. Kharkevich. 1979. LC 79-9406. (Handbook of Experimental Pharmacology Ser.: Vol. 53). (Illus.). 531p. 216.00 (0-387-09592-6) Spr-Verlag.

Pharmacology of Glaucoma. Stephen M. Drance et al. 1992. (Illus.). 356p. 125.00 (0-683-02655-0) Lppncott W & W.

Pharmacology of Ionic Channel Function: Activators & Inhibitors. Ed. by M. Endo et al. 2000. LC 00-26585. (Handbook of Experimental Pharmacology Ser.: Vol. 147). (Illus.). 650p. 369.00 (3-540-66127-1) Spr-Verlag.

Pharmacology of Lymphocytes. Ed. by M. A. Bray & J. Morley. 1988. (Handbook of Experimental Pharmacology Ser.: Vol. 85). (Illus.). 626p. 494.00 (0-387-18609-3) Spr-Verlag.

Pharmacology of Monoclonal Antibodies. Ed. by Martin Rosenberg & Gordon P. Moore. 1994. LC 93-44948. (Handbook of Experimental Pharmacology Ser.: Vol. 113). (Illus.). 406p. 385.00 (0-387-57123-X) Spr-Verlag.

Pharmacology of Opioid Peptides. Ed. by Leon F. Tseng. 1995. xiv, 524p. text 165.00 (3-7186-5632-9, Harwood Acad Pubs) Gordon & Breach.

Pharmacology of Pain. Ed. by A. H. Dickenson et al. 1997. LC 97-23531. (Handbook of Experimental Pharmacology Ser.: No. 130). (Illus.). 479p. 325.00 (3-540-62785-5) Spr-Verlag.

Pharmacology of Peptic Ulcer Disease: With Contributions by Numerous Experts. Ed. by M. J. Collen & S. B. Benjamin. 1991. (Handbook of Experimental Pharmacology Ser.: Vol. 99). (Illus.). 464p. 357.00 (0-387-52840-7) Spr-Verlag.

Pharmacology of Retinoids in the Skin: 8th CIRD Symposium on Advances in Skin Pharmacology, Cannes, September 1988. Ed. by U. Reichert & B. Shroot. 1989. (Pharmacology & the Skin Ser.: Vol. 3). (Illus.). x, 282p. 207.00 (3-8055-4909-1) S Karger.

Pharmacology of Sexual Function & Dysfunction. Ed. by J. Bancroft. 1995. LC 95-7067. (International Congress Ser.: Vol. 1075). 366p. 223.50 (0-444-82040-X, Excerpta Medica) Elsevier.

Pharmacology of Sleep. Ed. by Anthony Kales. 1995. (Handbook of Experimental Pharmacology Ser.: Vol. 116). (Illus.). 581p. 498.00 (3-540-58961-9) Spr-Verlag.

Pharmacology of Smooth Muscle. Ed. by Julius Gy. Papp & Laszlo Szekeres. 1994. LC 94-17635. (Handbook of Experimental Pharmacology Ser.: Vol. 111). (Illus.). 751p. 470.00 (0-387-57888-9) Spr-Verlag.

*__Pharmacology of the Critically Ill.__ Ed. by Gilbert Park & Maire Shelly. 2001. (Fundamentals of Anaesthesia & Acute Medicine Ser.). (Illus.). 192p. pap. (0-7279-1221-6) BMJ Pub GBR. Dist: AIDC.

Pharmacology of the Endocrine System & Related Drugs: Progesterone Progestational Drugs & Antifertility Agents. M. Tausk & L. Bengtsson. 1971. (International Encyclopedia of Pharmacology & Therapeutics Ser.: Vol. 1, Sect. 48). (0-08-015745-9) Pergamon Repr GBR. Dist: Franklin.

Pharmacology of the Eye. Ed. by M. L. Sears. 1983. (Handbook of Experimental Pharmacology Ser.: Vol. 69). (Illus.). 736p. 392.00 (0-387-12578-7) Spr-Verlag.

Pharmacology of the Respiratory Tract: Experimental & Clinical Research. Ed. by K. Fan Chung & Peter J. Barnes. 1993. (Lung Biology in Health & Disease Ser.: Vol. 67). (Illus.). 848p. text 275.00 (0-8247-8847-8) Dekker.

Pharmacology of the Skin. Hasan Mukhtar. 1991. (Illus.). 448p. 125.00 (0-8493-7292-5, RL801) CRC Pr.

Pharmacology of the Skin I. Ed. by S. Shuster & M. W. Greaves. 1988. (Handbook of Experimental Pharmacology Ser.: Vol. 87/1). (Illus.). 510p. 336.00 (0-387-19403-7) Spr-Verlag.

Pharmacology of the Skin II. Ed. by M. W. Greaves & S. Shuster. 1989. (Handbook of Experimental Pharmacology Ser.: Vol. 87-II). (Illus.). 7587p. 407.00 (0-387-50277-7) Spr-Verlag.

Pharmacology of the States of Alertness: Proceedings of the Satellite Symposium to the International Congress of Pharmacology, 7th, Paris, 1978. International Congress of Pharmacology Staff. Ed. by P. Passcuant & I. Oswald. 1979. (Illus.). 271p. 53.50 (0-08-023753-3, Pergamon Pr) Elsevier.

Pharmacology of the Urinary Tract: Clinical Practice in Urology. Ed. by M. Caine. 1984. (Illus.). 167p. 111.00 (0-387-13238-4) Spr-Verlag.

Pharmacology of Therapeutic Agents Used in Anesthesia: An Introduction. Robert I. Katz et al. 1994. LC 98-19098. 300p. 68.00 (0-9631310-2-8) Plexus Pub.

Pharmacology of Thermoregulation: Proceedings of a Satellite Symposium on the International Congress on Pharmacology, 5th, San Francisco, 1972. International Congress on Pharmacology Staff. Ed. by E. Schoenbaum & P. Lomax. 1973. 300p. 163.50 (3-8055-1391-7) S Karger.

Pharmacology of Topical Retinoids. U. Reichert. Ed. by H. Schaefer et al. 1994. (Journal: Vol. 6, Suppl. 1, 1993). (Illus.). vi, 84p. pap. 38.50 (3-8055-5922-4) S Karger.

Pharmacology of Vascular Smooth Muscle. Ed. by C. J. Garland & J. A. Angus. 1996. (Illus.). 448p. (C). text 125.00 (0-19-262387-7) OUP.

Pharmacology Recall. Anand Ramachandran. 1999. LC 99-20847. (Recall Ser.). (Illus.). 512p. pap. text 27.95 (0-683-30285-X) Lppncott W & W.

*__Pharmacology Recall PDA.__ Anand Ramachandran. 2001. 29.95 (0-7817-3342-1) Lppncott W & W.

Pharmacology Review. George M. Brenner. rev. ed. 1996. 255p. pap. text (0-7216-4604-2) Saunders.

Pharmacology Review Notes. Nikheel S. Kolatkar. 1997. 128p. (C). spiral bd. 19.95 (0-9665627-0-4) IatroSoft Corp.

*__Pharmacology Secrets.__ Patricia K. Anthony. 2001. (Secret Ser.). (Illus.). 400p. pap. 37.95 (1-56053-470-2) Hanley & Belfus.

*__Pharmacology Therapeutics: Principles & Practice.__ Derek Waller. 2001. 675p. (0-7020-2272-1) W B Saunders GBR. Dist: Saunders.

Pharmacophore Perception, Development & Use in Drug Design. Ed. by Osman F. Guner. 1999. LC 99-88143. (Biotechnology Ser.). (Illus.). xiii, 537p. (C). 109.95 (0-9636817-6-1) Intl Univ Line.

Pharmacopoeia of the People's Republic of China, 1992. 1993. 1100p. (7-5359-0945-0) HUWEI Cnslts CHN. Dist: Am Overseas Bk Co.

Pharmacopoeia of Tibetan Medicine. Vaidya B. Dash. 1994. LC 93-908824. (C). (81-7030-388-5) Sri Satguru Pubns IND. Dist: S Asia.

Pharmacopoeial Standards of Herbal Plants, Set, Vols. 1 & 2. C. R. Karnick. 1994. (C). text (81-7030-413-X) Sri Satguru Pubns IND. Dist: S Asia.

Pharmacotheon: Entheogenic Drugs, Their Plant Sources & History. Jonathan Ott & Albert Hofmann. rev. ed. 1997. 640p. LC 97-148651. 100.00 (0-9614234-8-X); pap. 40.00 (0-9614234-9-8) Natural Prod.

Pharmacotheon - Entheogenic Drugs, Their Plant Sources & History. Jonathan Ott. 1993. 640p. 70.00 (0-9614234-2-0) Natural Prod.

Pharmacotherapeutics: A Nursing Process Approach. Merrily Kuhn. 4th ed. 1997. (Illus.). 1093p. (C). text 59.95 (0-8036-0283-9) Davis Co.

Pharmacotherapeutics: A Primary Care Clinical Guide. Ellis Quinn Youngkin et al. 1998. LC 98-26172. 1500p. (C). pap. 92.00 (0-8385-7681-8) P-H.

Pharmacotherapeutics & Advanced Nursing Practice. Ed. by Laurel A. Eisenhauer & Margaret A. Murphy. 1998. LC 97-35644. (Illus.). 504p. pap. 44.95 (0-07-105485-5) McGraw-Hill Prof.

Pharmacotherapeutics for Nurses. Anita L. Wynne et al. 2001. LC 00-60152. (Illus.). 1264p. kivar 99.00 (0-8036-0535-8) Davis Co.

Pharmacotherapeutics for Nurses: Clinical Decision-Making in Nursing. Kathleen Gutierrez. Ed. by Maura Connor. 1999. LC 98-12900. (Illus.). 1435p. (C). text 50.00 (0-7216-5405-3) Saunders.

Pharmacotherapeutics of the Thyroid Gland. J. W. Barlow. Ed. by Anthony P. Weetman et al. 1997. (Handbook of Experimental Pharmacology Ser.: No. 128). (Illus.). 370p. 321.00 (3-540-62499-6) Spr-Verlag.

Pharmacotherapy. Joseph T. DiPiro. 3rd ed. 1998. text 175.00 (0-8385-7686-9) Appleton & Lange.

Pharmacotherapy: A Pathophysiologic Approach. Joseph T. DiPiro. 3rd ed. 1996. LC 95-25685. (C). pap. text 150.00 (0-8385-7892-6, A7892-1) Appleton & Lange.

*__Pharmacotherapy: A Pathophysiologic Approach Including Schwinghammer Case Book.__ Joseph T. DiPiro et al. 4th ed. 1999. (Illus.). 2700p. 175.00 (0-8385-8178-1, Apple Lange Med) McGraw.

Pharmacotherapy: A Patient Focused Approach. Terry Schwinghammer. 1996. (C). 416p. pap. text 39.95 (0-8385-8107-2, A8107-3); pap. text, tchr. ed. 24.95 (0-8385-8115-3, A8115-6) McGraw (Apple Lange Med).

*__Pharmacotherapy: Pathophysiologic Approach.__ Joseph T. DiPiro. 5th ed. 2002. LC 2001-31578. (0-07-136361-0) McGraw.

Pharmacotherapy & Management of Hypertension. John E. Bennett. 1994. text (0-443-08896-9) Church.

Pharmacotherapy Casebook: Patient Focused Approach. Schwinghammer & Dipiro. 2nd ed. 1999. pap. text, tchr. ed. 25.00 (0-8385-8155-2, Apple Lange Med) McGraw.

Pharmacotherapy for Child & Adolescent Psychiatric Disorders: An Updated Pocket Guide. Samuel Gershon et al. 1997. (0-87630-842-6) Brunner-Routledge.

Pharmacotherapy for Mood, Anxiety & Cognitive Disorders. Ed. by Uriel Halbreich & Stuart A. Montgomery. 2000. LC 99-13399. (Illus.). xxii, 804p. 79.00 (0-88048-885-9, 8885) Am Psychiatric.

Pharmacotherapy Handbook. Barbara G. Wells et al. 2nd ed. 1999. LC 99-73195. (Illus.). 1038p. pap. 44.95 (0-8385-8165-X) McGraw-Hill Prof.

Pharmacotherapy of Depression: Application for the Outpatient Practitioner. Jay D. Amsterdam. 1990. (Illus.). 496p. text 175.00 (0-8247-8209-7) Dekker.

Pharmacotherapy Self-Assessment Program 2nd ed. 1995. LC 94-72072. 2000p. pap. 395.00 (1-880401-13-4); 3rd rev. ed. 1998. LC 97-71255. 2800p. pap. 480.00 (1-880401-30-4) Amer Coll of Clin.

*__Pharmacotherapy Self-Assessment Program: Cardiovascular,__ Vols. 1-2. 4th rev. ed. 2001. LC 00-135886. 267p. pap. 70.00 (1-880401-54-1) Amer Coll of Clin.

Pharmacotherapy Self-Assessment Program: Cardiovascular Modules A & B, Vol. 1. 3rd rev. ed. 1998. LC 97-71255. 250p. pap. 150.00 (1-880401-31-2) Amer Coll of Clin.

Pharmacotherapy Self-Assessment Program: Cardiovascular Modules A & B, Answer Book. 3rd rev. ed. 1998. LC 97-71255. 250p. pap. (1-880401-32-0) Amer Coll of Clin.

Pharmacotherapy Self-Assessment Program: Critical Care Modules A & B, Vol. 2. 3rd rev. ed. 1998. LC 97-71255. 250p. pap. 150.00 (1-880401-33-9) Amer Coll of Clin.

Pharmacotherapy Self-Assessment Program: Critical Care Modules A & B, Answer Book, Vol 2. 3rd rev. ed. 1998. LC 97-71255. 250p. pap. (1-880401-34-7) Amer Coll of Clin.

Pharmacotherapy Self-Assessment Program: Gastroenterology, Nutrition. Modules A & B, Vol. 8. 3rd rev. ed. 1999. 250p. pap. 150.00 (1-880401-45-2) Amer Coll of Clin.

Pharmacotherapy Self-Assessment Program: Gastroenterology, Nutrition. Modules A & B, Answer Book, Vol. 8. 3rd rev. ed. 1999. LC 97-71255. 250p. pap. (1-880401-46-0) Amer Coll of Clin.

*__Pharmacotherapy Self-Assessment Program: Infectious Diseases,__ Vols. 1-2. 4th rev. ed. 2001. LC 00-135886. 351p. pap. 70.00 (1-880401-60-6) Amer Coll of Clin.

Pharmacotherapy Self-Assessment Program: Infectious Diseases Modules A & B, Answer Book, Vol. 3. 3rd rev. ed. 1998. LC 97-71255. 250p. pap. 150.00 (1-880401-35-5) Amer Coll of Clin.

Pharmacotherapy Self-Assessment Program: Nephrology, Immunology Modules A & B, Answer Book, Vol 7. 3rd rev. ed. 1999. LC 97-71255. 250p. pap. (1-880401-44-4) Amer Coll of Clin.

Pharmacotherapy Self-Assessment Program: Neurology, Psychiatry Modules A & B, Vol. 4. 3rd rev. ed. 1998. 250p. pap. 150.00 (1-880401-37-1) Amer Coll of Clin.

Pharmacotherapy Self-Assessment Program: Oncology Modules A & B, Vol. 10. 3rd rev. ed. 2000. LC 97-71255. 250p. pap. 150.00 (1-880401-49-5) Amer Coll of Clin.

Pharmacotherapy Self-Assessment Program: Oncology Modules A & B, Answer Book, Vol. 10. 3rd rev. ed. 2000. LC 97-71255. 250p. pap. (1-880401-50-9) Amer Coll of Clin.

Pharmacotherapy Self-Assessment Program: Pediatrics Modules A & B, Vol. 9. 3rd rev. ed. 2000. LC 97-71255. 250p. pap. 150.00 (1-880401-47-9) Amer Coll of Clin.

Pharmacotherapy Self-Assessment Program: Pediatrics Modules A & B, Answer Book, Vol. 9. 3rd rev. ed. 2000. LC 97-71255. 250p. pap. (1-880401-48-7) Amer Coll of Clin.

*__Pharmacotherapy Self-Assessment Program: Respiratory/Rheumatology/Endocrinology,__ Vol. 3. 4th rev. ed. 2001. LC 00-135886. 332p. pap. 70.00 (1-880401-58-4) Amer Coll of Clin.

Pharmacotherapy Self-Assessment Program: Women's Health Modules A & B, Vol. 11. 3rd rev. ed. 2000. LC 97-71255. 250p. pap. (1-880401-51-7) Amer Coll of Clin.

Pharmacotherapy Self-Assessment Program: Women's Health Modules A & B, Answer Book, Vol. 11. 3rd rev. ed. 2000. LC 97-71255. 250p. pap. (1-880401-52-5) Amer Coll of Clin.

Pharmacotherapy Self-Assessment Program Vol. 1: Cardiovascular Modules A & B. 1995. LC 94-72072. rev. ed. pap., stu. ed. Not sold separately (1-880401-15-0); 2nd rev. ed. 277p. pap. 150.00 (1-880401-14-2) Amer Coll of Clin.

Pharmacotherapy Self-Assessment Program Vol. 2: Critical Care Modules A & B. 1995. LC 94-72072. rev. ed. pap., stu. ed. Not sold separately (1-880401-17-7); 2nd rev. ed. 317p. pap. 150.00 (1-880401-16-9) Amer Coll of Clin.

Pharmacotherapy Self-Assessment Program Vol. 3: Infectious Diseases Modules A & B. 1995. LC 94-72072. rev. ed. pap., stu. ed. Not sold separately (1-880401-19-3); 2nd rev. ed. 169p. pap. 150.00 (1-880401-18-5) Amer Coll of Clin.

Pharmacotherapy Self-Assessment Program Vol. 4: Neurology/Psychiatry Modules A & B. 1995. rev. ed. pap., stu. ed. Not sold separately (1-880401-21-5); 2nd rev. ed. 195p. pap. 150.00 (1-880401-20-7) Amer Coll of Clin.

Pharmacotherapy Self-Assessment Program Vol. 5: Modules A & B. 1996. LC 94-72072. rev. ed. pap., tchr. ed. (1-880401-23-1); 2nd rev. ed. 142p. pap. 150.00 (1-880401-22-3) Amer Coll of Clin.

Pharmacotherapy Self-Assessment Program Vol. 6: Respiratory/Nephrology/Gastro A & B. 1996. LC 94-72072. rev. ed. pap., stu. ed. Not sold separately (1-880401-25-8); 2nd rev. ed. 323p. pap. 150.00 (1-880401-24-X) Amer Coll of Clin.

Pharmacotherapy Self-Assessment Program Vol. 7: Endocrinology/Immunology A & B. 1996. LC 94-72072. rev. ed. pap., stu. ed. Not sold separately (1-880401-27-4); 2nd rev. ed. 295p. pap. 150.00 (1-880401-26-6) Amer Coll of Clin.

Pharmacotherapy Self-Assessment Program Vol. 8: Nutrition/Oncology A & B. 1996. LC 94-7072. rev. ed. pap., stu. ed. Not sold separately (1-880401-29-0); 2nd rev. ed. 236p. pap. 150.00 (1-880401-28-2) Amer Coll of Clin.

*__Pharmacovigilance from A to Z.__ Cobert & Biron. 2001. (Illus.). pap. 49.95 (0-632-04586-8) Blackwell Sci.

Pharmacy: An Illustrated History. David L. Cowen & William H. Helfand. 1990. (Illus.). 272p. (gr. 13). 85.00 (0-8109-1498-0) Mosby Inc.

Pharmacy Aide. Jack Rudman. 1994. (Career Examination Ser.: C-2576). pap. 27.95 (0-8373-2576-5) Nat Learn.

Pharmacy & Medicine on the Air. Mickey C. Smith. 1989. (Illus.). 175p. 26.50 (0-8108-2279-2) Scarecrow.

Pharmacy & Pharmacotherapy of Asthma. Ed. by Patrick F. D'Arcy & James C. McElnay. 1989. 258p. 99.95 (*0-470-21522-4*) P-H.

Pharmacy & the U. S. Health Care System. Ed. by Jack E. Fincham & Albert I. Wertheimer. (Pharmaceutical Sciences Ser.). (Illus.). 1991. LC 90-5092. 336p. text 59.95 (*0-86656-849-2*); 1991. LC 90-5092. 336p. pap. text 29.95 (*1-56024-097-0*); 2nd ed. 1997. LC 97-33692. 557p. (C). 69.95 (*1-56024-998-6*, Pharmctl Prods); 2nd ed. 1997. LC 97-33692. 557p. (C). pap. 39.95 (*1-56024-999-4*, Pharmctl Prods) Haworth Pr.

Pharmacy Assistant. Jack Rudman. 1994. (Career Examination Ser.: C-1388). pap. 27.95 (*0-8373-1388-0*) Nat Learn.

Pharmacy Assistant II. Jack Rudman. 1994. (Career Examination Ser.: C-2943). pap. 29.95 (*0-8373-2943-4*) Nat Learn.

Pharmacy Assisting for the Technician, IML. Durgin & Hanan. 2nd ed. 1999. 80p. tchr. ed. 17.95 (*0-7668-0464-X*) Delmar.

Pharmacy Benefit Managers: Early Results on Ventures with Drug Manufacturers. 1996. (Illus.). 30p. reprint ed. pap. text 20.00 (*0-7881-3209-1*) DIANE Pub.

***Pharmacy Clerkship Manual: A Survival Manual for Students.** Ruth E. Nemire & Karen Kier. 2002. (Illus.). 304p. pap. 39.95 (*0-07-136195-2*) McGraw-Hill Med Pub.

Pharmacy College Admission Test. Jack Rudman. 1994. (Admission Test Ser.: ATS-52). pap. 27.95 (*0-8373-5052-2*) Nat Learn.

Pharmacy College Admission Test (PCAT) Jack Rudman. (Admission Test Ser.: Vol. 52). 47.95 (*0-8373-5152-9*) Nat Learn.

Pharmacy College Admission Test Student Guide. David M. Tarlow. 1993. (Illus.). pap. 16.95 (*0-931572-05-3*) Datar Pub.

Pharmacy College Admissions Test - Core Content. David M. Tarlow. 1996. (Medical Examinations Ser.). 575p. (Orig.). (C). pap. 49.95 (*1-57774-003-3*) Educ Tsting Cnslts.

Pharmacy Department Compliance Manual. Aspen Health Law and Compliance Center Staff. 3rd ed. 2001. LC 2001-22380. (AHLCC Compliance Ser.). 400p. pap. 145.00 (*0-8342-1958-1*) Aspen Pub.

Pharmacy Ethics. Ed. by Mickey C. Smith et al. 1991. LC 90-5011. (Pharmaceutical Sciences Ser.: Vol. 2). (Illus.). 297p. (C). pap. 29.95 (*1-56024-172-1*); text 69.95 (*0-86656-898-0*) Haworth Pr.

Pharmacy History: Pictoral. Tallis. 1991. (Illus.). pap. (*0-85369-241-6*) Pharmaceutical Pr GBR. *Dist:* Rittenhouse.

Pharmacy Inspector. Jack Rudman. 1994. (Career Examination Ser.: C-2536). pap. 34.95 (*0-8373-2536-6*) Nat Learn.

Pharmacy Law. Helen Wetherbee & Bruce D. White. 1980. LC 80-14608. (Paralegal). 592p. (C). mass mkt. 54.00 (*0-8299-2091-9*) West Pub.

***Pharmacy, Law & Ethics.** G. E. Appelbe & J. H. Wingfield. 7th ed. 2001. 688p. pap. (*0-85369-475-3*) Pharmaceutical Pr GBR. *Dist:* Rittenhouse.

Pharmacy Law & Practice. J. Merrills & J. Fisher. 1995. 384p. pap. (*0-632-03232-4*) Blckwell Science.

Pharmacy Law & Practice. Jonathan Merrills & Jonathan Fisher. 2nd ed. 1997. LC 97-25805. 400p. pap. 55.00 (*0-632-04809-3*) Blackwell Sci.

Pharmacy Law Digest. Fink. 59.50 (*0-03-268650-1*) Lppncott W & W.

Pharmacy Law Digest. Facts and Comparisons Staff. Ed. by Larry M. Simonsmeier & Joseph L. Fink. 27th rev. ed. Date not set. (C). ring bd. 110.00 (*0-932686-50-8*) Facts & Comparisons.

***Pharmacy Law Digest.** Ed. by Facts and Comparisons Staff. 36th ed. 2001. 900p. per. 59.95 (*1-57439-114-3*) Facts & Comparisons.

Pharmacy Legislation & Regulations, 1992. Intro. by American Society of Consultant Pharmacists Staff. rev. ed. 1992. 134p. pap. text 43.00 (*0-934322-09-0*) Am Soc Consult Phar.

Pharmacy Math for Technicians. Don A. Ballington & Mary M. Laughlin. 1998. LC 98-9872. 27.44 (*0-7638-0101-1*) Paradigm MN.

Pharmacy Math for Technicians: Instructor's Guide. Don A. Ballington & Mary M. Laughlin. text, tchr. ed. 14.00 (*0-7638-0102-X*) EMC-Paradigm.

Pharmacy Museums & Collections in the United States & Canada. George Griffenhagen & Ernst W. Stieb. rev. ed. 1988. 92p. pap. 9.00 (*0-931292-20-4*) Am Inst Hist Pharm.

Pharmacy Policy & Procedure Manual, 1992. Kathy D'Achilli. 1992. 350p. ring bd. 93.00 incl. disk (*0-934322-12-0*) Am Soc Consult Phar.

***Pharmacy Practice.** Stone & Curtis. 3rd ed. 2002. 224p. (*0-85369-482-6*) Uppsala Universitet SWE. *Dist:* Coronet Bks.

Pharmacy Practice: Social & Behavioral Aspects. Albert I. Wertheimer & Mickey C. Smith. 3rd ed. 1989. (Illus.). 472p. pap. text 39.95 (*0-683-08932-3*) Lppncott W & W.

Pharmacy Practice & the Law. Richard R. Abood & David B. Brushwood. 2nd ed. 1997. LC 97-18903. 448p. text 59.00 (*0-8342-0915-2*, 20915) Aspen Pub.

Pharmacy Practice & the Law. Richard R. Abood & David B. Brushwood. 3rd ed. 2000. LC 00-33162. 710p. pap. text 59.00 (*0-8342-1880-1*, 18801) Aspen Pub.

Pharmacy Practice for Technicians. Ed. by Jane Durgin & Zachary Hanan. 1993. LC 92-48679. 478p. (C). mass mkt. 33.50 (*0-8273-4660-3*) Delmar.

Pharmacy Practice for Technicians. Ed. by Jane M. Durgin et al. 2nd ed. 1999. LC 98-54627. (Allied Health Ser.). 544p. (C). pap. text 53.95 (*0-7668-0458-5*) Delmar.

Pharmacy Practice for Technicians: Instructor's Guide. Jane Durgin & Zachary Hanan. 1994. 96p. 16.00 (*0-8273-5905-5*) Delmar.

Pharmacy Practice Handbook of Medication Facts. Harold L. Kirschenbaum & Michelle K. Bazil. 2000. LC 99-67719. (Illus.). 783p. 49.95 (*1-56676-762-8*) CRC Pr.

***Pharmacy Practice Lab PDA.** Boh. 2nd ed. 2002. 40.00 (*0-7817-3713-3*) Lppncott W & W.

Pharmacy Practice Management: Forms, Checklists & Guidelines. Ed. by Sara N. Di Lima & Dwayne E. Eutsey. 1999. LC 98-30817. 400p. ring bd. 249.00 incl. cd-rom (*0-8342-1079-7*, S518) Aspen Pub.

Pharmacy Professional's Guide to Resumes, CVs & Interviewing. Thomas P. Reinders. 2001. 150p. pap. 25.00 (*1-58212-016-1*) Am Pharm Assn.

Pharmacy Student Companion: Your Road Map to Pharmacy Education & Careers. Daniel H. Albrant & Linda R. Harteker. Ed. by Vicki L. Meade. 3rd rev. ed. 1999. LC 00-689629. (Illus.). x, 157p. (C). pap. 20.00 (*0-917330-94-3*) Am Pharm Assn.

Pharmacy Tech: Basic Pharmacology & Calculations. Robert Reilly et al. 1994. (Illus.). 140p. (C). per. 29.95 (*1-56930-005-4*) Delmar.

Pharmacy Technician. Jack Rudman. 1997. (Career Examination Ser.: Vol. C-3822). pap. 27.95 (*0-8373-3822-0*) Nat Learn.

Pharmacy Technician. Marvin M. Stoogenke. 2nd ed. 1997. pap., tchr. ed. 17.67 (*0-8359-5154-5*); LC 97-13705. 416p. pap. 64.00 (*0-8359-5153-7*) P-H.

***Pharmacy Technician.** Marvin M. Stoogenke. 3rd ed. 2001. 496p. pap. 50.67 (*0-13-060629-4*) P-H.

Pharmacy Technician Certification Quick-Study Guide. Susan Moss Marks & William A. Hopkins, Jr. 2nd ed. 1999. 125p. pap. text 25.00 (*1-58212-000-5*) Am Pharm Assn.

Pharmacy Technician Certification Review & Practice Exam. 1998. LC 99-166176. 152p. 38.00 (*1-879907-80-1*) Am Soc Hlth-Syst.

Pharmacy Technician Companion: Your Road Map to Techinician Training & Careers. Linda R. Harteker. 1998. LC 98-23840. (Illus.). 102p. pap. text 20.00 (*0-917330-87-0*) Am Pharm Assn.

Pharmacy Technician's Pocket Drug Reference. Joyce A. Generali. 2000. LC 00-45114. vii, 131p. pap. 15.00 (*1-58212-020-X*) Am Pharm Assn.

Pharmacy Technology. Messler. 1999. pap. text (*0-7216-7432-1*) Saunders.

***Pharmako/Dynamis.** Dale Pendell. 2001. pap. 19.95 (*1-56279-125-7*) Mercury Hse.

Pharmako/Gnosis: Plant Teachers & the Poison Path. Dale Pendell. 1999. (Illus.). 304p. pap. 19.95 (*1-56279-104-4*) Mercury Hse.

Pharmako/Poeia: Plant Powers, Poisons & Herbcraft. Dale Pendell. 1995. LC 94-48573. (Illus.). 304p. pap. 19.95 (*1-56279-069-2*) Mercury Hse.

Pharmakotherapie der Depression: Bedeutung von Serotonin und Melatonin. Ed. by P. Kielholz & B. Muller-Oerlinghausen. 1987. (Advances in Pharmacotherapy Ser.: Band 3). (Illus.). x, 150p. 121.00 (*3-8055-4539-8*) S Karger.

Pharmasource, '94. Market Intelligence Staff. 1994. 311p. 595.00 (*1-56753-985-8*) Frost & Sullivan.

Pharmatecture 2nd Edition: Minimizing Medications to Maximize Results. Gideon Bosker. 2nd rev. ed. 1999. LC 99-205326. (Illus.). 484p. pap. 59.95 (*1-57439-047-3*) Facts & Comparisons.

Pharmazeutisches Medizinisches Terminologi. Beyer. 3rd ed. 1990. (GER.). 188p. 39.95 (*0-7859-7439-3*, 3804711197) Fr & Eur.

Pharmeceutical Skin Penetration Enhancement. Kenneth A. Walters & Jonathan Hadgraft. 1993. LC 92-48507. (Drugs & the Pharmaceutical Sciences Ser.: Vol. 59). (Illus.). 456p. text 199.00 (*0-8247-9017-0*) Dekker.

Pharmex Family Guide to Prescription Drugs. Pharmex Staff. Date not set. 310p. pap. text 5.95 (*0-89529-715-9*, Avery) Penguin Putnam.

PharmFacts for Nurses. Springhouse Publishing Company Staff. 1995. LC 95-36762. (Illus.). 736p. pap. 36.95 (*0-87434-803-X*) Springhouse Corp.

Pharmicist's Pick: The Non-Prescription Choices of a Pharmacist at Your Fingertips! Scott W. Holden. 1997. 101p. pap. 9.95 (*1-890622-07-9*) Leathers Pub.

Phase Resetting in Medicine & Biology: Stochastic Modelling & Data Analysis. Peter A. Tass. 1999. LC 99-25203. (Series in Synergetics). (Illus.). 368p. 99.00 (*3-540-65697-9*) Spr-Verlag.

PHC & Refugees. Ed. by Anke Van der Kwaak. 1995. LC 96-176946. (Primary Health Care Publications: No. 9). 160p. pap. (*90-5383-333-1*) VU Univ Pr NLD. *Dist:* Paul & Co Pubs.

Phencyclidine & Related Arylcyclohexylamines: Present & Future Applications. Ed. by J. M. Kamenka et al. 1983. LC 83-61728. (Illus.). 690p. 50.00 (*0-916182-04-5*) NPP Bks.

Phenol. 1994. (Environmental Health Criteria Ser.: No. 161). (ENG, FRE & SPA.). 151p. pap. text 30.00 (*92-4-157161-6*, 1160161) World Health.

Phenolic Compounds in Food & Their Effects on Health II: Antioxidants & Cancer Prevention. Ed. by Mou-Tuan Huang et al. 1992. LC 92-23283. (ACS Symposium Ser.: No. 507). (Illus.). 402p. text 95.00 (*0-8412-2476-5*) Am Chemical.

Phenols & Medicine: Subject, Reference & Research Guidebook. Mary S. Fayette. rev. ed. 1994. 149p. LC 87-47653. 57.50 (*0-7883-0668-5*); pap. 47.50 (*0-7883-0669-3*) ABBE Pubs Assn.

Phenomenological Inquiry in Psychology: Existential & Transpersonal Dimensions. R. Valle. 1998. LC 97-38473. (Illus.). 405p. (C). 75.00 (*0-306-45542-0*, Plenum Trade) Perseus Pubng.

Phenomenological Inquiry in Psychology: Existential & Transpersonal Dimensions. Ed. by Ron Valle. 1998. LC 97-38473. (Illus.). 464p. (C). pap. 42.50 (*0-306-45543-9*, Plenum Trade) Perseus Pubng.

Phenomenological Psychology. Ed. by Joseph J. Kockelmans. 1987. 266p. (C). lib. bdg. (*90-247-3501-7*) M Nijhoff NLD. *Dist:* Kluwer Academic.

Phenomenological Psychology: A Text for Beginners. Eugene M. DeRobertis. 1996. LC 96-33420. 88p. pap. text 19.50 (*0-7618-0500-1*) U Pr of Amer.

Phenomenological Research Methods. Clark Moustakas. 1994. LC 94-7355. 240p. pap. 36.95 (*0-8039-5799-8*, 9738) Sage.

Phenomenology & Nursing Research. Michael Crotty. 1996. 208p. pap. (*0-443-05432-0*) Church.

Phenomenology & Psychological Research. Amedeo Giorgi. 1985. LC 84-21168. 216p. pap. text 19.00 (*0-8207-0174-2*) Duquesne.

Phenomenology & Treatment of Alcoholism. Ed. by William E. Fann et al. 1980. LC 79-23224. (Illus.). 350p. text 40.00 (*0-88331-177-1*) R B Luce.

Phenomenology & Treatment of Anxiety. Ed. by William E. Fann et al. 1979. LC 78-32092. (Illus.). 455p. 40.00 (*0-88331-178-X*) R B Luce.

Phenomenology in Psychology & Psychiatry. Herbert Spiegelberg. 1972. LC 74-154833. (Studies in Phenomenology & Existential Philosophy). 411p. pap. 29.00 (*0-8101-0624-8*) Northwestern U Pr.

Phenomenology, Language, & Schizophrenia. Ed. by Manfred Spitzer et al. 1993. LC 92-48781. (Illus.). 389p. 71.95 (*0-387-97950-6*) Spr-Verlag.

Phenomenology of Depressive Illness. Ed. by J. John Mann. 1988. (Depressive Illness Ser.: Vol. 1). 263p. 42.95 (*0-89885-369-9*, Kluwer Plenum) Kluwer Academic.

Phenomenology of Everyday Life: Empirical Investigations of Human Experience. Howard R. Pollio et al. 1997. LC 96-40020. (Illus.). 412p. (C). text 59.95 (*0-521-46205-3*) Cambridge U Pr.

Phenomenology of Perception. Maurice Merleau-Ponty. Tr. by Colin J. Smith. 1981. (C). pap. 32.50 (*0-391-02551-1*) Routledge.

Phenotypic Mapping of Down Syndrome & Other Aneuploid Conditions: Proceedings of the National Down Syndrome Society Conference on the Phenotypic Mapping of Down Syndrome & Other Aneuploid Conditions, Held in New York, January 14 & 15, 1993. Ed. by Charles J. Epstein. 1993. (Progress in Clinical & Biological Research Ser.: Vol. 384). 254p. 245.00 (*0-471-30449-2*, Wiley-Interscience) Wiley.

Phenotypic Variation in Populations: Relevance to Risk Assessment. Ed. by Avril D. Woodhead et al. 1988. LC 87-35795. (Basic Life Sciences Ser.: Vol. 43). (Illus.). 316p. 75.00 (*0-306-42794-X*, Plenum Trade) Perseus Pubng.

Phenoxyalkanoic Herbicides: Chemistry, Analysis & Environmental Pollution, Vol. I. Shane S. Que Hee & Ronald G. Sutherland. 1981. 321p. 187.00 (*0-8493-5851-5*, SB952, CRC Reprint) Franklin.

Phenylpropanolamine: Risks, Benefits & Controversies, 5. Ed. by John P. Morgan & Doreen V. Kagan. 1985. LC 85-6590. (Clinical Pharmacology & Therapeutics Ser.: Vol. 5). 448p. 95.00 (*0-275-91336-8*, C1336, Praeger Pubs) Greenwood.

Phenytoin (Dilantin, Diphenylhydantoin) & Its Adverse Effects in the Human Body. American Health Research Institute Staff. 1990. LC 89-18673. 201p. 47.50 (*1-55914-120-4*); pap. 44.50 (*1-55914-121-2*) ABBE Pubs Assn.

Phenytoin (Dilantin, Diphenylhydantoin): Therapy & Clinical Uses: Index of New Information with Authors, Subjects & References. American Health Research Institute Staff. 1997. 150p. 57.50 (*0-7883-1356-8*); pap. 47.50 (*0-7883-1357-6*) ABBE Pubs Assn.

Pheochromocytoma: A Clinical & Experimental Overview. Ed. by William M. Manger. 2nd ed. 1995. 700p. (C). (*0-393-71028-9*) Norton.

Pheromones: Current Research U. Eugene Brady et al. 1974. 157p. text 31.50 (*0-8422-7212-7*) Irvington.

Pheromones: Current Research, Vol. 1. D. L. Struble et al. 1974. 176p. text 31.50 (*0-8422-7211-9*) Irvington.

Philadelphia Ghost Stories. Charles J. Adams, III. 1998. pap. text 11.95 (*1-880683-12-1*) Exeter Hse.

Philadelphia Magazines Guide to Healthcare in the Delaware Valley, 1994-1995. Carol Saline. 1994. pap. 6.95 (*0-9635666-2-8*) Phila Mag.

Philadelphia Police Department Annual Audit, Fiscal, 1994. Ed. by Donald R. Shopland et al. 1998. (Illus.). 564p. (Orig.). pap. text 50.00 (*0-7881-2843-4*) DIANE Pub.

Philanthropic Foundations & Resources for Health: An Anthology of Sources. Ed. by Rosenkrantz & Barbara S. Gutmann. 1990. (Medical Care in the United States Ser.: Vol. 14). 200p. text 15.00 (*0-8240-8343-1*) Garland.

Philanthropy & Gerontology: The Role of American Foundations, 12. Ann H. Sontz. 1989. LC 89-1679. (Contributions to the Study of Aging Ser.: No. 12). 159p. 55.00 (*0-313-26097-4*, SZF/, Greenwood Pr) Greenwood.

Philipp Franz von Siebold & His Era: Prerequisites, Developments, Consequences & Perspectives. Ed. by Arnulf Thiede et al. 1999. LC 99-39683. (Illus.). 160p. 58.00 (*3-540-64185-8*) Spr-Verlag.

Philippe Pinel et Son Oeuvre au Point de Vue de la Medecine Mentale. Rene Semelaigne. 1976. LC 75-16733. (Classics in Psychiatry Ser.). (FRE.). reprint ed. 18.95 (*0-405-07454-9*) Ayer.

Phillip's Science of Dental Mat. Kenneth J. Anusavice. 10th ed. 1996. 656p. text 61.95 (*0-7216-5741-9*) Saunders.

Phillips Thygeson, MD: External Eye Disease & the Proctor Foundation. Phillips Thygeson. 1988. (Ophthalmology Oral History Ser.). (Illus.). xxvi, 321p. (Orig.). (C). pap. 45.00 (*0-926866-01-X*) FAAO.

Philosophical & Theoretical Perspectives for Advanced Nursing Practice. Janet W. Kenney. 1996. (Nursing Ser.). (Illus.). 408p. (C). pap. text 48.75 (*0-86720-735-3*, 735-3) Jones & Bartlett.

***Philosophical & Theoretical Perspectives for Advanced Nursing Practice.** Janet W. Kenney. 3rd ed. 2001. (Illus.). (C). pap. text 54.95 (*0-7637-1858-0*, 1858-0, N L N Bart) Jones & Bartlett.

Philosophical Aspects of Thanatology, Vol. 1. Florence M. Hetzler & Austin H. Kutscher. 1979. 20.95 (*0-405-12515-1*) Ayer.

Philosophical Dimensions of Personal Construct Psychology. William Warren. 1998. LC 98-17308. 208p. 89.95 (*0-415-16850-3*) Routledge.

Philosophical Dimensions of the Neuro-Medical Sciences. Stuart F. Spicker & H. Tristram Engelhardt. 1976. LC 76-1204. (Philosophy & Medicine Ser.: Vol. 2). 280p. text 98.50 (*90-277-0672-7*) Kluwer Academic.

Philosophical Disease: Bioethics, Culture, & Identity. Carl Elliot. 1998. LC 98-7053. 256p. (C). pap. 20.95 (*0-415-91940-1*) Routledge.

Philosophical Examination of the History & Values of Western Medicine. Paul W. Sharkey. 1993. LC 92-49051. 200p. text 79.95 (*0-7734-9210-0*) E Mellen.

Philosophical Foundations of Gerontology. Ed. by Patrick L. McKee. 1982. LC 81-2922. 352p. 43.95 (*0-89885-040-1*); pap. 24.95 (*0-89885-041-X*) Kluwer Academic (Kluwer Acad Hman Sci).

Philosophical Issues in the Psychology of C. G. Jung. Marilyn Nagy. 1991. LC 89-26319. 252p. (C). text 22.50 (*0-7914-0451-X*) State U NY Pr.

Philosophical Medical Ethics. Raanan Gillon. 1986. LC 86-15749. (Medical Publications). 200p. pap. 74.95 (*0-471-91222-0*) Wiley.

Philosophical Medical Ethics: Its Nature & Significance. Ed. by Stuart F. Spicker & H. Tristram Englehardt, Jr. 1977. (Philosophy & Medicine Ser.: No. 3). 258p. text 96.00 (*90-277-0772-3*) Kluwer Academic.

Philosophical Perspectives on Psychiatric Diagnostic Classification. Ed. by John Z. Sadler et al. 1994. LC 93-15949. (Johns Hopkins Series in Psychiatry & Neuroscience Ser.). 416p. (C). pap. text 32.50 (*0-8018-4770-2*) Johns Hopkins.

Philosophical Problems in Health Care. Ed. by David Greaves & Hugh Upton. 1996. (Avebury Series in Philosophy). 215p. (*1-85972-222-9*) Avebury GBR. *Dist:* Ashgate Pub Co.

Philosophical Psychology & Interpretating Wittgenstein: How to Look at Words As Instruments. J. F. Hunter. 1990. 192p. (C). 78.00 (*0-389-20920-1*) Rowman.

Philosophical Psychopathology. Ed. by George Graham & G. Lynn Stephens. 1995. LC 94-31921. 344p. 50.00 (*0-262-07159-2*, Bradford Bks) MIT Pr.

Philosophical Works of Etienne Bonnot, Abbe de Condillac, Vol. II. Tr. by Franklin Philip & Harlan Lane from FRE. 1986. 192p. text 49.95 (*0-89859-616-5*) L Erlbaum Assocs.

Philosophie Zoologique Jean Baptiste Lamarck. 1960. reprint ed. 75.00 (*3-7682-0028-0*) Lubrecht & Cramer.

Philosophische Bemerkungen, 1. M. Nedo. 1994. (Ludwig Wittgenstein, Wiener Ausgabe Ser.). 196p. 98.00 (*0-387-82499-5*) Spr-Verlag.

Philosophy: Practice of Psychology. Philip J. Barker. 1999. 258p. pap. text 31.95 (*0-443-06004-5*) Mosby Inc.

Philosophy & Care of the Mentally Retarded: A Worldwide Status Report. Johnny L. Matson. 1983. 120p. pap. 15.25 (*0-08-028093-5*, Pergamon Pr) Elsevier.

Philosophy & Health Care. Michael A. Menlowe. 1992. 237p. (*1-85628-325-9*) Avebury GBR. *Dist:* Ashgate Pub Co.

Philosophy & Medical Welfare. Ed. by J. M. Bell & Susan Mendus. 1989. (Royal Institute of Philosophy Lectures: No. 23). 140p. (C). pap. text 24.95 (*0-521-36856-1*) Cambridge U Pr.

Philosophy & Medicine. E. K. Ledermann. 1986. (Avebury Series in the Philosophy of Science). 196p. text (*0-566-05062-5*) Avebury GBR. *Dist:* Ashgate Pub Co.

Philosophy & Medicine in Ancient Greece. W. H. Jones. 1980. 100p. pap. 15.00 (*0-89005-286-7*) Ares.

Philosophy & Medicine in Ancient Greece: With an Edition of Peri Archaiees Ieetrikees. William H. Jones. 1979. 16.95 (*0-405-10606-8*) Ayer.

Philosophy & Psychopathology. Ed. by Brendan A. Maher & Manfred Spitzer. 1990. 247p. 69.95 (*0-387-97303-6*) Spr-Verlag.

Philosophy & the Good Life: Reason & the Passions in Greek, Cartesian & Psychoanalytic Ethics. John Cottingham. 1998. LC 97-27898. (Illus.). 244p. (C). pap. text 17.95 (*0-521-47890-1*); text 49.95 (*0-521-47310-1*) Cambridge U Pr.

Philosophy & the Science of Behavior, Including Psychology & the Philosophy of Science. Merle B. Turner. 1967. LC 66-25267. (Century Psychology Ser.). (Illus.). 52.50 (*0-89197-341-9*); pap. text 12.95 (*0-89197-342-7*) Irvington.

Philosophy for Nursing. Jan Reed & Ian Ground. 1997. LC 96-167803. 176p. (Orig.). pap. (*0-340-61028-X*) E A GBR. *Dist:* Routldge.

Philosophy for Nursing. Jan Reed & Ian Ground. 1996. (Illus.). 192p. (Orig.). pap. 45.00 (*1-56593-757-0*, 1472) Singular Publishing.

Philosophy in Epidemiology & Public Health. Dale R. Tavris. 1997. 229p. (C). lib. bdg. 75.00 (*1-56072-426-9*) Nova Sci Pubs.

Philosophy Natural Therapeutics, Vol. I. Henry Lindlahr. 1975. (Natural Therapeutics Ser.). 327p. pap. (*0-85207-159-0*) C W Daniel GBR. *Dist:* Natl Bk Netwk.

Philosophy of Cognitive Science. B. Von Eckardt. 2002. (Dimensions of Philosophy Ser.). 256p. pap. text 23.00 (*0-8133-2490-4*) Westview.

Philosophy of Human Nature. Joseph Buchanan. 1969. LC 71-90941. (History of Psychology Ser.). (Illus.). 360p. reprint ed. 50.00 (*0-8201-1064-7*) Schol Facsimiles.

Philosophy of Medicine & Bioethicsa: Twenty-Year Retrospective & Critical Appraisal. Carson. 1997. LC 97-30020. text 117.50 (*0-7923-3545-7*) Kluwer Academic.

Philosophy of Mind. Alan R. White. 1978. LC 78-5722. 178p. reprint ed. lib. bdg. 38.50 (*0-313-20430-6*, WHPM, Greenwood Pr) Greenwood.

Philosophy of Nursing: A New Vision for Health Care. Janice M. Brencick & Glenn A. Webster. 1999. LC 99-11409. ix, 247p. (C). text 60.50 (*0-7914-4379-5*); pap. text 20.95 (*0-7914-4380-9*) State U NY Pr.

Philosophy of Oriental Medicine: Key to Your Personal Judging Ability. George Ohsawa. Ed. by Herman Aihara & Sandy Rothman. 1991. LC 91-76486. 153p. pap. 7.95 (*0-918860-52-0*) G Ohsawa.

Philosophy of Osteopathy. Andrew T. Still. LC 74-29302. reprint ed. 34.50 (*0-404-13426-2*) AMS Pr.

Philosophy of Psychology. Mario Bunge & R. Ardila. 1987. (Illus.). 327p. 112.00 (*0-387-96442-8*) Spr-Verlag.

Philosophy of Psychology. Daniel N. Robinson. 1989. 176p. pap. text 18.00 (*0-231-05923-X*) Col U Pr.

Philosophy of the Practice of Dentistry. Lindsey D. Pankey & William J. Davis. Ed. by Veronica Sanitate. 1987. (Illus.). 323p. text 69.50 (*0-944742-01-7*) Med Coll of OH Pr.

Philosophy of William James. Theodore Flournoy. 1977. LC 78-99658. (Select Bibliographies Reprint Ser.). 26.95 (*0-8369-5087-9*) Ayer.

Philosophy, Psychiatry & Neuroscience - Three Approaches to the Mind: A Synthetic Analysis of the Varieties of Human Experience. Edward M. Hundert. 1991. (Illus.). 360p. reprint ed. pap. text 28.00 (*0-19-824896-2*) OUP.

Philosophy, Psychology & Psychiatry. Ed. by A. Phillips Griffiths. 1995. (Royal Institute of Philosophy Supplements Ser.: No. 37). 249p. (C). pap. text 24.95 (*0-521-46902-3*) Cambridge U Pr.

PHJ: Personal Health Journal. Latrice Collins. 1999. 112p. 14.95 (*0-9660451-1-4*) Empower Press.

***Phlebography & Sonography of the Veins.** Hach. 1997. 288p. (C). 225.00 (*0-387-53772-4*) Spr-Verlag.

Phlebography & Sonography of the Veins. W. Hach & V. Hach-Wunderle. 1996. LC 96-13128. 288p. 225.00 (*3-540-53772-4*) Spr-Verlag.

Phlebologia Houston, 1991: Proceedings of the Intensive Practical Course in Phlebologia. Pauline Raymond-Martimbeau. 1991. 438p. (*1-880693-00-3*) P Ray-Mart.

Phlebology, '95: Proceedings of the XII World Congress Union Internationale de Phlebologie Ed. by David Negus et al. 1996. 1264p. 197.00 (*3-540-19999-3*) Spr-Verlag.

Phlebotomy. Kathleen Becan-McBride et al. 1993. 65.00 (*0-89189-328-8*) Am Soc Clinical.

Phlebotomy. Lynn B. Hoeltke. 1994. LC 93-46473. (Clinical Laboratory Manual Ser.). 139p. (C). mass mkt. 23.00 (*0-8273-5527-0*) Delmar.

Phlebotomy: A Client-Based Approach. Bonnie K. Davis. 1996. LC 95-45643. (Medical Lab Technician Ser.). (Illus.). 176p. (C). pap. text 38.95 (*0-8273-5453-3*) Delmar.

***Phlebotomy: A Customer Service Approach: A Textbook for Developing Phlebotomy & Customer Service Skills.** Bonnie K. Davis. 2nd ed. 2001. LC 2001-28991. 208p. text 33.95 (*0-7668-2518-3*) Delmar.

Phlebotomy Basics: With Other Laboratory Techniques. Bonnie F. Fremgen & Wendy Blume. 2000. LC 00-44109. (Illus.). 310p. pap. text 35.80 (*0-8359-6164-8*) P-H.

Phlebotomy Essentials. Ruth E. McCall & Cathee M. Tankersley. 2nd ed. 1997. LC 97-11637. 448p. pap. text 33.95 (*0-7817-9198-7*) Lppncott W & W.

Phlebotomy Exam Review. Ruth E. McCall. 1996. LC 96-19176. 256p. pap. text 29.95 (*0-397-55232-7*) Lppncott W & W.

Phlebotomy for Nurses & Nursing Personnel: What Every Nurse & Nursing Assistant Must Know about Blood Specimen Collection & Handling. Dennis J. Ernst & Catherine Ernst. 2000. LC 00-103918. (Illus.). 182p. pap. 29.95 (*0-9700588-9-6*) HealthStar Pr.

Phlebotomy Handbook. Diana Garza. 4th ed. 1996. (C). pap. text, tchr. ed. (*0-8385-8113-7*, A8113-1) Appleton & Lange.

Phlebotomy Handbook: Blood Collection Essentials. Garza et al. 5th ed. 1998. LC 98-22074. 525p. pap. 42.00 (*0-8385-8141-2*) P-H.

***Phlebotomy Handbook: Blood Collection Essentials.** Diana Garza & Kathleen Becan-McBride. 6th ed. 2001. 560p. pap. 40.00 (*0-13-092887-9*) P-H.

Phlebotomy Review Guide. Susan E. Phelan. 1998. LC 98-23247. 49.00 (*0-89189-433-0*) Am Soc Clinical.

Phlebotomy Techniques: A Laboratory Workbook. Susan Phelan. 1993. wbk. ed. 35.00 (*0-89189-343-1*) Am Soc Clinical.

Phlebotomy Techniques Curriculum Guide. Susan Phelan. 1993. 20.00 (*0-89189-359-8*) Am Soc Clinical.

Phlebotomy Workbook for the Multiskilled Healthcare Professional. Susan K. Strasinger & Marjorie A. Di Lorenzo. 1995. (Illus.). 382p. (C). pap. text 31.95 (*0-8036-8107-0*) Davis Co.

Phobia: Psychological & Pharmacological Treatment. Ed. by Matig Mavissaka & David H. Barlow. 1981. LC 80-15306. 256p. 35.00 (*0-89862-602-1*) Guilford Pubns.

Phobias: A Handbook of Theory, Research & Treatment. Graham C. L. Davey. 1997. LC 96-32895. 470p. 225.00 (*0-471-96983-4*) Wiley.

Phobic & Obsessive-Compulsive Disorders: Theory, Research, & Practice. Paul M. Emmelkamp. 1982. (Behavior Therapy Ser.). (Illus.). 366p. (C). 96.00 (*0-306-41044-3*, Plenum Trade) Perseus Pubng.

Phoenix: Therapeutic Patterns of Milton H. Erickson. David Gordon & Maribeth Meyers-Anderson. 1981. LC 81-85263. pap. 21.95 (*0-916990-10-9*) META Pubns.

Phoenix Rising V Vol. XIV: Proceedings of the 14th International Conference on the Study of Shamanism & Alternative Modes of Healing 1997, Santa Sabina Center, San Rafael, California, August 30-September 1, 1997. Ed. by Ruth-Inge Heinze. unabr. ed. 1997. LC 97-44898. (Illus.). 266p. (C). pap. text 21.75 (*0-945875-18-5*) Independent Scholars Asia Inc.

Phoenix Rising IV: Proceedings of the 13th International Conference on the Study of Shamanism & Alternate Modes of Healing Held at the Santa Sabina Center, San Rafael, California, August 31 to September 2, 1996. Ed. by Ruth-Inge Heinze. 1996. LC 96-29973. (Illus.). 392p. (C). pap. 21.75 (*0-945875-17-7*) Independent Scholars Asia Inc.

Pholosynthesis & Nitrogen Fixation, Pt. B. Ed. by Anthony San Pietro. 1972. (Methods in Enzymology Ser.: Vol. 24). text 199.00 (*0-12-181887-X*) Acad Pr.

Phonetics for Speech Pathology. Ball. 2nd ed. 1993. 314p. pap. 62.25 (*1-56593-240-4*, 0560) Singular Publishing.

Phonobuilding: Using Narratives to Facilitate Phonological Development. Jerry Vicino. 1993. LC 92-37172. (Illus.). 39.00 (*0-930599-80-2*) Thinking Pubns.

Phonological Disability in Children. Ed. by David Ingram. 2nd ed. 1990. 200p. pap. 45.00 (*1-56593-535-7*, 0034) Singular Publishing.

Phonology: Applications to Assessment & Intervention. Robert J. Lowe. 1994. (Illus.). 272p. 43.95 (*0-683-05205-5*) Lppncott W & W.

Phonology, Morphonology, Morphology. Olga Akhmanova. 1971. LC 72-159459. (Janua Linguarum, Ser. Minor: No. 101). 135p. pap. text (*90-279-1748-5*) Mouton.

Phonosurgery. N. Isshiki. 1989. (Illus.). 233p. 198.00 (*0-387-70037-4*) Spr-Verlag.

Phosphate in Pediatric Health & Disease. Ed. by Uri Alon & James C. Chan. 1993. 352p. lib. bdg. 219.00 (*0-8493-6785-9*, RJ399, CRC Reprint) Franklin.

Phosphates & Dental Caries. B. Lilienthal. 1977. (Monographs in Oral Science: Vol. 6). (Illus.). 60.00 (*3-8055-2677-6*) S Karger.

Phosphatidylcholine Metabolism. Ed. by Lipoprotein Research Group Staff & Dennis E. Vance. 1989. 264p. 191.00 (*0-8493-6338-1*, QP752) CRC Pr.

Phosphodiesterase Inhibitors. Ed. by Christian Schudt et al. 1996. (Handbook of Immunopharmacology Ser.). (Illus.). 228p. text 69.95 (*0-12-210720-9*) Acad Pr.

Phospholipase: Role & Function in Inflammation, Vol. A2. Ed. by P. Y. Wong & E. A. Dennis. 1990. (Illus.). 210p. (C). text 102.00 (*0-306-43611-6*, Kluwer Plenum) Kluwer Academic.

Phospholipase A2: Basic & Clinical Aspects in Inflammatory Diseases. Ed. by Waldemar H. Uhl et al. 1997. LC 97-261. (Progress in Surgery Ser.: Vol. 24, 1997). (Illus.). xii, 250p. 213.25 (*3-8055-6441-4*) S Karger.

Phospholipid Signaling Protocols. Ed. by Ian Bird. 1998. LC 98-3874. (Methods in Molecular Biology Ser.: Vol. 105). (Illus.). 400p. 99.50 (*0-89603-491-7*) Humana.

Phospholipid Transfer Proteins: Emerging Roles in Vesicle Trafficking, Signal Transduction & Metabolic Regulation. Vytas A. Bankaitis. 1995. (Molecular Biology Intelligence Unit Ser.). 163p. 99.00 (*1-57059-330-2*) Landes Bioscience.

Phospholipids: Biochemical, Pharmaceutical & Analytical Considerations. I. Hanin & G. Pepeu. 1990. (Illus.). 328p. (C). text 95.00 (*0-306-43698-1*, Kluwer Plenum) Kluwer Academic.

Phospholipids & Cellular Regulation, Vol. I. Ed. by Hyh-Fa Kuo. 1985. 256p. 149.00 (*0-8493-5537-0*, QH604, CRC Reprint) Franklin.

Phospholipids & Cellular Regulation, Vol. 2. J. F. Kuo. Ed. by Hyh-Fa Kuo. 1985. LC 84-28569. 256p. 147.00 (*0-8493-5538-9*, QH604, CRC Reprint) Franklin.

Phospholipids in the Nervous System. Ed. by Nicolas G. Bazan et al. 1989. (FIDIA Research Ser.: Vol. 17). (Illus.). 300p. 118.00 (*0-387-96994-2*) Spr-Verlag.

Photo Art Therapy: A Jungian Perspective. Jerry L. Fryrear & Irene E. Corbit. 1992. (Illus.). 220p. (C). text 51.95 (*0-398-05802-4*) C C Thomas.

Photobiology. Elli Kohen et al. 1995. LC 94-40230. (Illus.). 506p. text 74.00 (*0-12-417755-7*) Acad Pr.

Photobiology in Medicine. G. Jori et al. 1994. LC 94-24010. (NATO Advanced Science Institutes Ser.: Vol. 272). (Illus.). 200p. (C). text 85.00 (*0-306-44900-5*, Kluwer Plenum) Kluwer Academic.

Photobiology, 1984. Ed. by James W. Longworth et al. 1985. LC 85-604. 202p. 59.95 (*0-275-90189-0*, C0189, Praeger Pubs) Greenwood.

Photobiology of Low-Power Laser Therapy. T. I. Karu. 1989. (Laser Science & Technology Ser.: Vol. 8). xii, 190p. pap. text 192.00 (*3-7186-4970-5*) Gordon & Breach.

Photochemical Oxidants. 1978. (Environmental Health Criteria Ser.: No. 7). 110p. pap. text 16.00 (*92-4-154067-2*, 1160007) World Health.

Photochemical Stability of Drugs & Drug Formulations. Ed. by H. H. Tonnesen. 1996. 380p. 160.00 (*0-7484-0449-X*) Taylor & Francis.

Photochemotherapy: Photodynamic Therapy & Other Modalities II. Ed. by Stanley B. Brown et al. 1996. (Europto Ser.: Vol. 2924). 342p. 94.00 (*0-8194-2326-2*) SPIE.

Photochemotherapy: Photodynamic Therapy & Other Modalities III. Ed. by Kristian Berg et al. 1997. LC 98-164537. (Europto Ser.: Vol. 3191). 380p. 107.00 (*0-8194-2623-7*) SPIE.

Photochemotherapy in Dermatology. Elizabeth A. Abel. 1992. LC 91-7109. (Illus.). 352p. text 90.00 (*0-89640-186-3*) Igaku-Shoin.

Photochemotherapy of Cancer. Ed. by Benjamin Ehrenberg & Kristian Berg. 1999. LC 00-502175. (Europto Ser.: Vol. 3563). (Illus.). vii, 168p. 89.00 (*0-8194-3025-0*) SPIE.

Photodamage. Ed. by Barbara A. Gilchrest. 1995. LC 95-20981. 496p. 99.95 (*0-86542-343-1*) Blackwell Sci.

Photodamaged Skin: Clinical Signs, Causes & Management. Jean-Paul Ortonne & Ronald Marks. 1999. 149p. (*1-85317-345-2*) Martin Dunitz GBR. *Dist:* Mosby Inc.

Photodermatology. Ed. by J. L. M. Hawk. 1999. LC 97-69681. (Illus.). 328p. (*0-340-74094-9*) E A GBR. *Dist:* OUP.

Photodynamic Therapy, No. 271. C. J. Gomer. 1988. (Photochemistry & Photobiology Ser.: Vol. 46). 391p. 30.00 (*0-08-036081-5*, Pergamon Pr) Elsevier.

Photodynamic Therapy: Basic Principles & Clinical Applications. Ed. by Barbara W. Henderson & Thomas J. Dougherty. 1992. LC 92-14636. (Illus.). 480p. text 225.00 (*0-8247-8680-7*) Dekker.

Photodynamic Therapy of Intimal Hyperplasia. Glenn M. LaMuraglia. 1997. (Medical Intelligence Unit Ser.). 250p. 89.95 (*0-412-13051-3*) Chapman & Hall.

Photodynamic Therapy of Neoplastic Disease. David Kessel. 1990. Vol. I. 352p. lib. bdg. 159.00 (*0-8493-5816-7*, RC271); Vol. II. 280p. lib. bdg. 159.00 (*0-8493-5817-5*, RC271) CRC Pr.

Photographic Atlas of Civil War Injuries: Photographs of Surgical Cases & Specimens. Bradley P. Bengtson et al. 1996. (Illus.). 480p. LC 96-75434. 125.00 (*0-9635861-8-1*); lthr. 200.00 (*0-9653101-0-8*) Med Staff Pr.

Photographic Atlas of Practical Anatomy I: Abdomen, Lower Limb, Set. W. Thiel. Tr. by T. Telger. 1997. LC 97-7231. (Illus.). 868p. 325.00 (*3-540-61195-9*) Spr-Verlag.

Photographic Atlas of Practical Anatomy II: Neck, Head, Back, Chest, Upper Extremeties, Companion Volume Including Nomina Anatomica & Index. Walter Thiel. Tr. by T. C. Telger & U. Schumacher from GER. 1998. LC 97-7231. (Illus.). 431p. 299.00 (*3-540-62239-X*) Spr-Verlag.

Photographic Atlas of the Human Body. Gerard J. Tortora. 1999. LC 99-32135. (Illus.). 256p. pap. 37.95 (*0-471-37487-3*) Wiley.

Photographic Guide to Conformation. Robert Oliver & Bob Langrish. 1990. 250p. (*0-85131-522-4*) J A Allen GBR. *Dist:* Trafalgar, St Mut.

Photographic Manual of Regional Orthopaedic & Neurological Testing. Joseph J. Cipriano et al. 3rd ed. 1997. LC 96-43896. (Illus.). 480p. 67.00 (*0-683-18100-9*) Lppncott W & W.

Photographic Manual of Regional Orthopaedics & Neurological Testing. Joseph J. Cipriano. 2nd ed. 1991. (Illus.). 346p. 60.00 (*0-683-01701-2*) Lppncott W & W.

Photographic Techniques for Accident Investigation. 1984. 22p. 10.00 (*0-939874-60-1*) ASSE.

Photographing Medicine: Images & Power in Britain & America Since Eighteen Forty, 21. Daniel M. Fox & Christopher J. Lawrence. 1988. LC 87-25088. (Contributions in Medical Studies Ser.: No. 21). (Illus.). 357p. 90.00 (*0-313-23719-0*, FMC/) Greenwood.

Photography in Ophthalmology: Proceedings of the International Symposium, Miami, 1970. International Symposium on Photography in Ophthalmology Staff. Ed. by O. Ferrer. 1971. (Modern Problems in Ophthalmology Ser.: Vol. 9). 59.75 (*3-8055-1165-5*) S Karger.

Photoguide of Common Skin Disorders: Diagnosis & Management. Herbert P. Goodheart. 1998. LC 98-26292. (Illus.). 657p. text 99.00 (*0-683-30257-4*) Lppncott W & W.

Photoimmunology. Ed. by Jean Krutmann & Craig A. Elmets. 1995. LC 94-43729. (Illus.). 500p. 135.00 (*0-86542-826-3*) Blackwell Sci.

Photoimmunology. Ed. by John A. Parrish et al. 1983. LC 83-4216. 320p. 85.00 (*0-306-41280-2*, Plenum Trade) Perseus Pubng.

Photomedicine Ed. by Ehud Ben-Hur & Ionel Rosenthal. 1987. LC 86-34293. 361.00 (*0-8493-4673-8*, RM837, CRC Reprint) Franklin.

Photomicrography: A Comprehensive Treatise Roger P. Loveland. 1981. LC 80-12428. 1070p. reprint ed. lib. bdg. 119.50 (*0-89874-392-3*) Krieger.

Photon Propagation in Tissues IV. Ed. by David A. Benaron et al. 1998. LC 99-200353. (Europto Ser.: Vol. 3566). 80.00 (*0-8194-3028-5*) SPIE.

Photon Propagation in Tissues III. Ed. by David A. Benaron et al. 1998. (Europto Ser.: Vol. 3194). 546p. 107.00 (*0-8194-2626-1*) SPIE.

Photoreceptors: Their Role in Vision. Alan Fein & Ete Z. Szuts. 1982. LC 81-24209. (International Union of Pure & Applied Physics Biophysics Ser.: No. 5). (Illus.). 224p. pap. text 22.95 (*0-521-28684-0*) Cambridge U Pr.

Photosensitive Epilepsy. Graham F. A. Harding & Peter M. Jeavons. 2nd exp. ed. 1995. (Clinics in Developmental Medicine Ser.: No. 133). (Illus.). 182p. 59.95 (*0-521-68302-5*) Cambridge U Pr.

Photostatis & Related Phenomena. Ed. by Theodore P. Williams & Anne B. Thistle. 1998. LC 97-52808. (Illus.). 238p. (C). text 89.50 (*0-306-45806-3*, Kluwer Plenum) Kluwer Academic.

Photosynthesis, Pt. A. Ed. by Anthony San Pietro. 1971. (Methods in Enzymology Ser.: Vol. 23). text 209.00 (*0-12-181886-1*) Acad Pr.

Phototherapy & Photochemotherapy of Skin Disease. Warwick L. Morison. 2nd ed. 1990. 304p. text 99.00 (*0-88167-723-X*) Lppncott W & W.

Phototherapy in Mental Health. David A. Krauss & Jerry L. Fryrear. 1983. (Illus.). 260p. text 49.95 (*0-398-04785-5*) C C Thomas.

Phototherapy of Cancer. Ed. by George Morstyn & A. H. Kaye. 1990. x, 224p. text 198.00 (*3-7186-0510-4*) Gordon & Breach.

Phototherapy Treatment Protocols: For Psoriasis & Other Phototherapy Responsive Dermatoses. M. D. Zanolli et al. 2000. LC 99-46631. 168p. 43.95 (*1-85070-992-0*, Parthenon Pbng) CRC Pr.

Photothermal Therapies in Medicine. Ed. by Gaetano Bandieramonte et al. 1998. LC 98-164978. (Europto Ser.: Vol. 3193). 196p. 89.00 (*0-8194-2625-3*) SPIE.

Phrenological Dictionary of Nineteenth-Century Americans. Compiled by Madeleine B. Stern. 1982. LC 82-991. (Documentary Reference Collections). (Illus.). 430p. lib. bdg. 110.00 (*0-313-23286-5*, STN/, Greenwood Pr) Greenwood.

Phthalocyanines. Frank H. Moser & Arthur L. Thomas. 1983. Vol. I. 248p. 137.00 (*0-8493-5677-6*, QD441); Vol. II. 184p. 100.00 (*0-8493-5678-4*) Franklin (CRC Reprint).

Phunny Pharm. C. Ty Reidhead. 1996. LC 96-29285. (Illus.). 207p. (Orig.). pap. 21.00 (*1-56053-114-2*) Hanley & Belfus.

Phychotherapies for Black & Multicultured Communities. Sonia Stephen. 2000. 224p. pap. text (*0-7506-4313-7*) E A GBR. *Dist:* OUP.

Phylogenesis of Connective Tissue: Morphological Aspects & Biosynthesis of Sponge Intercellular Matrix. R. Garrone. Ed. by L. Robert. 1978. (Frontiers of Matrix Biology Ser.: Vol. 5). (Illus.). 135.00 (*3-8055-2767-5*) S Karger.

Phylogenesis of Immune Functions. Gregory W. Warr & Cohen. 1990. 344p. 239.00 (*0-8493-6434-5*, QR184) CRC Pr.

Phylogenetic Fantasy: An Overview of the Transference Neuroses. Sigmund Freud. Ed. by Ilse Grubrich-Simitis. Tr. by Axel Hoffer & Peter T. Hoffer from GER. 1987. LC 86-26468. (Illus.). 160p. 30.00 (*0-674-66635-6*, Belknap) HUP.

Phylogenetic Models in Functional Coupling of the CNS & the Cardiovascular System. Ed. by R. B. Hill et al. 1992. LC 92-20252. (Comparative Physiology Ser.: Vol. 11). (Illus.). xiv, 256p. 278.50 (*3-8055-5570-9*) S Karger.

Phylogenetic Perspectives on the Vertebrate Immune System. Ed. by Gregory Beck et al. 2001. LC 00-52732. (Advances in Experimental Medicine & Biology Ser.: Vol. 484). (Illus.). xii, 383p. 125.00 (*0-306-46431-4*, Kluwer Plenum) Kluwer Academic.

Phylogenetics: Theory & Practice of Phylogenetic Systematics. Edward O. Wiley. 1981. LC 81-5080. 456p. 195.00 (*0-471-05975-7*) Wiley.

Phylogeny & Development of Catecholamine Systems in the CNS of Vertebrates. Ed. by Wilhelmus J. Smeets & Anton Reiner. 1995. (Illus.). 504p. (C). text 110.00 (*0-521-44251-6*) Cambridge U Pr.

Phylogeny & Ontogeny. Piaget, Jean, Foundation Archives, Geneva Staff. 1984. (Human Development Ser.: Vol. 27, No. 5). (Illus.). vi, 134p. pap. 34.00 (*3-8055-3904-5*) S Karger.

Physcian ICD-9 CM Primer. Delmar Staff. 1998. 32.00 (*0-7668-0968-4*) Delmar.

Physicians GenRx 1997 Book Update. Physicians GenRx Staff Corporation. 1997. No. 1. rev. ed. (*0-8151-7222-2*); No. 2. 2nd rev. ed. (*0-8151-7223-0*) Mosby Inc.

Physical Activity, Aging & Sports Vol. III: Physiological & Biomedical Aspects Toward Health Aging-International Perspectives, Pt. 1. Ed. by Sara Harris et al. 1994. (Illus.). 320p. text 39.95 (*0-937829-06-4*) Ctr Study Aging.

Physical Activity, Aging & Sports Vol. IV: Psychology, Motivation & Programs Toward Health Aging-International Perspectives, Pt. 2. Ed. by Sara Harris et al. 1995. (Illus.). 400p. text 39.95 (*0-937829-07-2*) Ctr Study Aging.

Physical Activity, Aging & Sports Series, Vols. I-IV. Ed. by Raymond Harris et al. 1994. 1554p. 159.80 (*0-937829-05-6*) Ctr Study Aging.

Physical Activity & Behavioral Medicine. James F. Sallis & Neville Owen. 1998. LC 98-25362. pap. 34.95 (*0-8039-5997-4*, 1540); (Behavioral Medicine & Health Psychology Ser.: 3). 210p. 74.95 (*0-8039-5996-6*, 1539) Sage.

Physical Activity & Cancer. Laurie Hoffman-Goetz. 2000. (Exercise Physiology Ser.). 99.95 (*0-8493-8712-4*, 8712) CRC Pr.

Physical Activity & Coronary Heart Disease: Proceedings of the Paavo Nurmi Symposium, 2nd, Helsinki, 1975. Paavo Nurmi Symposium Staff. Ed. by V. Manninen. 1976. (Advances in Cardiology Ser.: Vol. 18). (Illus.). 240p. 104.50 (*3-8055-2356-4*) S Karger.

Physical Activity & Health. Ed. by N. G. Norgan. 1993. (Society for the Study of Human Biology Symposium Ser.: No. 34). (Illus.). 263p. (C). text 74.95 (*0-521-41551-9*) Cambridge U Pr.

Physical Activity & Health: A Report of the Surgeon General. Audrey F. Manley. 1996. (Illus.). 278p. (Orig.). (C). pap. text 40.00 (*0-7881-3496-5*) DIANE Pub.

Physical Activity & Health: A Report of the Surgeon General. U. S. Department of Health Staff. 1998. LC 98-27539. (Health Science Ser.). (Illus.). 306p. (C). pap. text 33.95 (*0-7637-0636-1*, 0636-1) Jones & Bartlett.

Physical Activity & Mental Health. Ed. by William P. Morgan. 1996. LC 96-20373. (Series in Health Psychology & Behavioral Medicine). 288p. 59.95 (*1-56032-365-5*) Taylor & Francis.

Physical Activity & Obesity. Ed. by Claude Bouchard. 2000. LC 99-88071. (Illus.). vii, 400p. text 52.00 (*0-88011-909-8*) Human Kinetics.

Physical Activity in Health & Disease. Per-Olof Astrand & Gunnar Grimby. 1986. (Acta Medica Scandinavica Symposium Ser.: No. 2). (Illus.). 228p. 96.50 (*91-22-00817-9*) Coronet Bks.

Physical Activity in Human Experience: Interdisciplinary Perspectives. James E. Curtis & Storm J. Russell. 1996. LC 96-8065. (Illus.). 304p. text 35.00 (*0-87322-765-4*, BCUR0765) Human Kinetics.

Physical Agent Modalities: Theory & Application for the Occupational Therapist. Alfred Bracciano. 2000. LC 00-25400. 176p. pap. 35.00 (*1-55642-376-4*, 33764) SLACK Inc.

Physical Agents: A Comprehensive Text for Physical Therapists. Bernadette Hecox et al. 1993. LC 93-4700. (Illus.). 496p. (C). 62.00 (*0-8385-8040-8*, A8040-6) P-H.

Physical Agents: A Comprehensive Text for Physical Therapists. Bernadette Hecox. 2nd ed. 2000. (C). 45.00 (*0-8385-8132-3*) Appleton & Lange.

Physical Agents: Theory & Practice for the Physical Therapist Assistant. Barbara J. Behrens & Susan L. Michlovitz. 1996. LC 95-26022. (Illus.). 438p. (C). text 39.95 (*0-8036-0111-5*) Davis Co.

Physical Agents for Physical Therapists. James E. Griffin & Terence C. Karselis. 3rd ed. 1988. (Illus.). 458p. 62.95 (*0-398-05384-7*) C C Thomas.

Physical Agents in Rehabilitation: From Research to Practice. Michelle H. Cameron. Ed. by Shirley Kuhn. 1998. LC 98-21395. (Illus.). 480p. (C). pap. text 39.00 (*0-7216-6244-7*) Saunders.

Physical Agents Laboratory Manual. Barbara Behrens. 1997. (Illus.). 172p. pap. text 21.95 (*0-8036-0275-8*) Davis Co.

***Physical & Biological Hazards of the Workplace.** Wald. 2nd ed. 2001. LC 2001-46816. 600p. 149.00 (*0-471-38647-2*) Wiley.

Physical & Mental Growth of Girls & Boys Age Six to Nineteen in Relation to Age at Maximum Growth. Frank K. Shuttleworth. 1939. (SRCD M Ser.: Vol. 4, No. 3). 25.00 (*0-527-01510-5*) Periodicals Srv.

Physical & Mental Issues in Aging Sourcebook: Basic Consumer Health Information on Physical & Mental Disorders Associated with the Aging Process. Ed. by Jenifer Swanson. 1999. LC 99-15540. (Health Reference Ser.). (Illus.). xiii, 660p. 78.00 (*0-7808-0233-0*) Omnigraphics Inc.

Physical & Motor Development in Persons with Mental Retardation. Ed. by A. Vermeer & W. E. Davis. 1995. LC 95-16242. (Medicine & Sport Science Ser.: Vol. 40). (Illus.). xii, 210p. 207.00 (*3-8055-6118-0*) S Karger.

Physical & Occupational Therapists' Job Search Handbook: Your Complete Job Search Strategy: How to Hire; How to Be Hired. Lynda Peringian. 1989. LC 89-50592. (Illus.). 160p. (C). text 25.00 (*0-9622773-0-4*) Peringian & Assocs.

Physical & the Moral: Anthropology, Physiology, & Philosophical Medicine in France, 1750-1850. Elizabeth A. Williams. 1994. (Cambridge History of Medicine Ser.). (Illus.). 300p. (C). text 80.00 (*0-521-43067-4*) Cambridge U Pr.

Physical Appearance, Stigma, & Social Behavior Vol. III: The Ontario Symposium on Personality & Social Psychology Bol. Ed. by E. Troy Higgins et al. 1986. 336p. (C). text 69.95 (*0-89859-638-6*) L Erlbaum Assocs.

Physical Aspect of the Living Cell: Proceedings of the Eugene Ernst Memorial Symposium Held in Pecs, Hungary, July 3-5, 1986. Ed. by J. Tigyi et al. 1991. (Illus.). 382p. (C). (*963-05-5926-9*) Akade Kiado HUN. *Dist:* Intl Spec Bk, St Mut.

Physical Aspects of Brachytherapy. T. J. Godden. 1988. (Medical Physics Handbook Ser.: No. 19). (Illus.). 304p. 21.00 (*0-85274-511-7*) Inst of Physics Pubng.

Physical Aspects of Hyperthermia: Proceedings of the AAPM Summer School Held at Dartmouth College, Hanover, New Hampshire, August 3-7, 1981. Ed. by Gilbert H. Nussbaum. 1982. (American Association of Physicists in Medicine Symposium Ser.: No. 8). 650p. 50.00 (*0-88318-414-1*) Am Inst Physics.

Physical Aspects of Stereotactic Radiosurgery. Ed. by M. H. Phillips. 1993. (Illus.). 312p. (C). text 75.00 (*0-306-44535-2*, Kluwer Plenum) Kluwer Academic.

Physical Assessment: A Guide for Evaluating Drug Therapy. R. Leon Longe & John C. Calvert. Ed. by Lloyd Y. Young. 1994. LC 94-76859. 486p. (Orig.). (C). pap. 44.50 (*0-915486-20-2*) Applied Therapeutics.

Physical Assessment of the Newborn. Ellen P. Tappero & Mary E. Honeyfield. 2nd rev. ed. 1996. LC 96-9065. (Illus.). 250p. pap. text 39.95 (*1-887571-00-0*) NICU Ink.

Physical Basis of Computed Tomography. Christopher Marshall. 1982. 171p. 37.50 (*0-87527-314-9*) Green.

Physical Basis of Organic Chemistry. Howard Maskill. 1986. (Illus.). 504p. (C). pap. text 44.95 (*0-19-855199-1*) OUP.

Physical Capacities Evaluation. Susan L. Smith & Patricia Baxter-Petralia. 1992. 130p. (C). pap. text 29.95 (*0-935273-02-6*) Chess Pub.

Physical Change & Aging: A Guide for the Helping Professions. Sue V. Saxon & Mary J. Etten. 3rd rev. ed. 1994. (Illus.). 448p. (Orig.). pap. text 24.90 (*0-913292-47-8*) Tiresias Pr.

Physical Characterization of Pharmaceutical Solids. Harry G. Brittain. 1995. LC 95-4852. (Drugs & the Pharmaceutical Sciences Ser.: Vol. 70). (Illus.). 440p. text 185.00 (*0-8247-9372-2*) Dekker.

Physical, Chemical, & Biological Properties of Radiocerium Relevant to Radiation Protection Guidelines. 1978. LC 79-84485. (Report Ser.: No. 60). 115p. pap. text 35.00 (*0-913392-44-8*) NCRP Pubns.

Physical Chemistry for the Biomedical Sciences. S. R. Logan. 1998. 250p. (*0-7484-0709-X*); pap. (*0-7484-0710-3*) Tay Francis Ltd GBR. *Dist:* Taylor & Francis.

Physical Chemistry of Lipids: From Alkanes to Phospholipids. D. M. Small. 1986. LC 85-19420. (Handbook of Lipid Research Ser.: Vol. 4). (Illus.). 682p. (C). text 145.00 (*0-306-41763-4*, Kluwer Plenum) Kluwer Academic.

Physical Chemistry of Membranes: An Introduction to the Structure & Dynamics of Biological Membranes. Brian L. Silver. 1985. (Illus.). 432p. (C). text 110.00 (*0-04-574028-3*) Routledge.

Physical Control of the Mind: Toward a Psychocivilized Society. Jose M. Delgado. Ed. by Ruth N. Anshen. 1971. (Illus.). 280p. (C). 29.50 (*0-8290-0574-9*); pap. text 12.95 (*0-8290-1765-8*) Irvington.

Physical Diagnosis. Jo-Ann Reteguiz & Beverly Cornel-Avendano. 4th ed. 2000. LC 00-33230. (Pretest Clinical Science Ser.). (Illus.). 328p. pap. 24.95 (*0-07-136098-0*) McGraw-Hill Prof.

Physical Diagnosis Secrets. Ed. by Salvatore Mangione. 1999. LC 98-43417. (Secrets Ser.). (Illus.). 350p. (Orig.). pap. 38.00 (*1-56053-164-9*) Hanley & Belfus.

Physical Dimensions of Aging. Waneen W. Spirduso. 1995. LC 94-43969. (Illus.). 448p. text 60.00 (*0-87322-323-3*, BSPI0323) Human Kinetics.

Physical Disability: A Psychosocial Approach. Beatrice A. Wright. 2nd ed. 1997. 544p. (C). pap. 80.00 (*0-06-047241-3*) Addson-Wesley Educ.

Physical Disability in Childhood. Ed. by Gillian T. McCarthy. 1992. (Interdisciplinary Approach to Management Ser.). (Illus.). 594p. text (*0-443-04288-8*) Church.

Physical Dysfunction Practice Skills for the Occupational Therapy Assistant. Early. 1997. LC 97-16858. (Illus.). 672p. (C). (gr. 13). text 49.95 (*0-8151-3091-0*, 27067) Mosby Inc.

Physical Dysfunction Practice Skills for the Occupational Therapy Assistant. Mary B. Early. 1998. (Illus.). 640p. tchr. ed. (*0-8151-2932-7*) Mosby Inc.

Physical Education. Jack Rudman. 1994. (Undergraduate Program Field Tests Ser.: Vol. UPFT-18). pap. 23.95 (*0-8373-6018-8*) Nat Learn.

Physical Education & Health: Selected Works of James H. Humphrey Ed. by Joy N. Humphrey & James H. Humphrey. LC 86-47843. (Studies in Education: No. 8). 75.00 (*0-404-12669-3*);Vol. 1. 37.50 (*0-404-12670-7*);Vol. 2. 37.50 (*0-404-12671-5*) AMS Pr.

Physical Education & the Study of Sport. Bob Davis. 4th ed. 2000. pap. text 34.00 (*0-7234-3175-2*) Saunders.

Physical Education for Exceptional Students: Theory to Practice. Douglas C. Wiseman. 1994. 80p. tchr. ed. 16.95 (*0-8273-5297-2*); LC 93-8387. 598p. (C). pap. 48.00 (*0-8273-5296-4*) Delmar.

Physical Environment & Behavior: An Annotated Bibliography & Guide to the Literature. J. F. Wohlwill & Gerald D. Weisman. 1981. LC 81-4840. 484p. 95.00 (*0-306-40739-6*, Plenum Trade) Perseus Pubng.

Physical Exam of the Neurologic System. Mosby Staff. 1995. 595.00 (*0-8151-6135-2*) Mosby Inc.

Physical Examination & Health Assessment. Ed. by Carolyn Jarvis. 2nd ed. 1996. (Illus.). tchr. ed. (*0-7216-6446-6*); pap. text, stu. ed. 17.95 (*0-7216-5986-1*) Saunders.

Physical Examination & Health Assessment. Carolyn Jarvis. Ed. by Barbara N. Cullen. 2nd ed. 1995. LC 95-3462. (Illus.). 954p. text 54.00 (*0-7216-5922-5*) Saunders.

***Physical Examination & Health Assessment.** Carolyn Jarvis. 3rd ed. 2000. tchr. ed. 45.00 (*0-7216-8430-0*) Saunders.

Physical Examination for the Spine & Extremities. Stanley Hoppenfeld. 1992. 288p. (C). pap. 12.15 (*0-8385-7867-5*) Appleton & Lange.

Physical Examination of the Heart & Circulation. Joseph K. Perloff. (Illus.). 2nd ed. 1989. 304p. pap. text 39.00 (*0-7216-7189-6*); 3rd ed. 2000. LC 99-49763. 300p. pap. text (*0-7216-8321-5*) Saunders.

Physical Examination of the Spine & Extremities. Stanley Hoppenfeld. 1976. (Illus.). 276p. (C). 63.00 (*0-8385-7853-5*, A7853-3) P-H.

Physical Examinations—Infants to Old Age & Body Parts: Index of New Information. Stanley B. Luray. 1999. (Illus.). 163p. 57.50 (*0-7883-1888-8*); pap. 47.50 (*0-7883-1889-6*) ABBE Pubs Assn.

Physical Exercise, Nutrition & Stress. Mary F. Asterita. 1985. LC 85-12261. 216p. 75.00 (*0-275-90044-4*, C0044, Praeger Pubs) Greenwood.

Physical Fitness: A Guide for Individuals with Lower Limb Loss. Ernest M. Burgess & Albert Rappoport. 1993. (Illus.). 245p. (Orig.). (C). pap. text 40.00 (*1-56806-432-2*) DIANE Pub.

Physical Fitness: A Guide for Individuals with Spinal Cord Injury. David F. Apple, Jr. 1996. (Illus.). 110p. (Orig.). pap. text 30.00 (*0-7881-3364-0*) DIANE Pub.

Physical Fitness: The Pathway to Healthful Ling. Robert V. Hockey. 2nd ed. 1973. LC 72-87646. ix, 194p. (*0-8016-2214-X*) Mosby Inc.

Physical Fitness & Nutrition During Growth: Studies in Children & Youth in Different Environments. Ed. by Jana Parizkova & Andrew Hills. 1998. LC 98-25054. (Medicine & Sport Science Ser.: Vol. 43, 1998). (Illus.). viii, 1672p. 169.75 (*3-8055-6679-4*) S Karger.

Physical Fitness for Adults. Bob Sharp & Danielle Kidder. 1995. (Illus.). 192p. (Orig.). pap. 12.95 (*1-886622-01-9*) Bayrock.

Physical Fitness-Sports Medicine Bibliography. 1994. lib. bdg. 260.95 (*0-8490-6431-7*) Gordon Pr.

Physical Forces & the Mammalian Cell. John Frangos. 1993. (Illus.). 400p. text 79.00 (*0-12-265330-0*) Acad Pr.

Physical Geology. F. Donald Bloss. 1991. (Illus.). 640p. 37.95 (*0-8016-0787-6*) Mosby Inc.

Physical Growth of Children: An Appraisal of Studies. Wilton M. Krogman. 1955. (SRCD M Ser.: Vol. 20, No. 1). pap. 25.00 (*0-527-01563-6*) Periodicals Srv.

Physical Growth of White Children. H. V. Meredith. 1936. (SRCD M Ser.: Vol. 1, No. 2). pap. 25.00 (*0-527-01487-7*) Periodicals Srv.

Physical Management for the Quadriplegic Patient. Jack R. Ford & Bridget Duckworth. 2nd ed. 1987. LC 87-479. (Illus.). 661p. text 59.00 (*0-8036-3676-8*) Davis Co.

Physical Management of Students Who Have Sustained a Traumatic Brain Injury: Guidelines & Strategies for School Personnel. Kathleen Q. Specht. 1996. 57p. (Orig.). tchr. ed., spiral bd. 16.50 (*1-882855-45-0*) HDI Pubs.

Physical Mechanisms in Radiation Biology: Proceedings. AEC Technical Information Center Staff. Ed. by Robert W. Wood & Raymond D. Cooper. 1974. LC 74-600124. 333p. fiche 9.00 (*0-87079-303-9*, CONF-721001) DOE.

Physical Medicine & Rehabilitation. Randall L. Braddom. 1995. LC 95-11493. 1168p. text 180.00 (*0-7216-5243-3*); 2nd ed. 2000. LC 00-25389. (Illus.). xxiii, 1435p. text 179.00 (*0-7216-8076-3*) Saunders.

Physical Medicine & Rehabilitation Secrets. Ed. by Mark Young & Bryan O'Young. 1996. LC 96-32242. (Secrets Ser.). (Illus.). 600p. (Orig.). pap. 39.95 (*1-56053-155-X*) Hanley & Belfus.

Physical Medicine Rehabilitation: The Complete Approach. Martin Grabois et al. 1999. LC 98-17785. (Illus.). 199.95 (*0-86542-536-1*) Blackwell Sci.

Physical Methods of Chemistry Bryant W. Rossiter & John F. Hamilton. 2nd ed. 1986. LC 85-6386. (Techniques of Chemistry Ser.). Vol. 1. 834p. 350.00 (*0-471-08034-9*); Vol. 2. 928p. 350.00 (*0-471-08027-6*) Wiley.

Physical Methods of Chemistry Pt. B: Determination of Chemical Composition & Molecular Structure, Vol. 3, Pt. B, Determination of Chemical Compositi. Bryant W. Rossiter & John F. Hamilton. 2nd ed. 1989. (Techniques of Chemistry Ser.). 992p. 350.00 (*0-471-85051-9*) Wiley.

Physical Nature of the Skin. Ed. by R. M. Marks et al. 1988. (C). text 144.00 (*0-85200-977-1*) Kluwer Academic.

Physical Optics Workbook. Vasudevan Lakshminarayanan. Date not set. 200p. pap. 35.00 (*0-7506-9859-4*) Buttrwrth-Heinemann.

Physical Pharmacy. Alfred Martin et al. 4th ed. 1993. (Illus.). 622p. text 62.00 (*0-8121-1438-8*) Lppncott W & W.

Physical Pharmacy: Text & Solutions Manual Set. Alfred Martin. 4th ed. 1993. 844p. 72.00 (*0-8121-1688-7*) Lppncott W & W.

Physical Pharmacy (book) Amiji. 2001. (*0-07-135076-4*) McGraw.

Physical Pharmacy (set 2) Amiji. 2001. 59.00 (*0-07-135075-6*) McGraw.

Physical Principles of Computed Tomography. William R. Hendee. 1983. 37.50 (*0-316-35594-1*, Little Brwn Med Div) Lppncott W & W.

Physical Principles of Medical Imaging. Perry Sprawls, Jr. 2nd ed. 1995. LC 95-14209. 656p. 69.95 (*0-944838-54-5*) Med Physics Pub.

Physical Principles of Medical Ultrasound. C. R. Hill et al. 2001. 600p. 120.00 (*0-471-97002-6*) Wiley.

Physical Properties of Plant & Animal Materials. Nuri N. Mohsenin. 1970. 758p. 150.00 (*0-677-02300-6*) Gordon & Breach.

Physical Rehabilitation: Assessment & Treatment. Susan B. O'Sullivan & Thomas J. Schmitz. 4th ed. 2000. LC 00-31700. (Illus.). 1152p. text 69.00 (*0-8036-0533-1*) Davis Co.

Physical Rehabilitation Laboratory Manual: Focus on Functional Training. Susan B. O'Sullivan & Thomas J. Schmitz. 1998. LC 98-205026. (Illus.). 388p. pap. 24.95 (*0-8036-0257-X*) Davis Co.

Physical Rehabilitation of the Injured Athlete. James R. Andrews & Gary L. Harrelson. Ed. by Richard Lampert. 2nd ed. 1997. LC 97-9769. (Illus.). 608p. text 75.00 (*0-7216-6549-7*) Saunders.

Physical Sensors for Biomedical Applications. Ed. by Michael R. Neuman et al. 1980. 168p. 101.00 (*0-8493-5975-9*, R857, CRC Reprint) Franklin.

Physical Signs in Child Abuse. Hobbs. 1995. text 89.00 (*0-7020-1778-7*) Saunders.

***Physical Signs in Dermatology.** Clifford M. Lawrence & Neil H. Cox. 2nd ed. 2001. (Illus.). 347p. pap. (*0-7234-3184-1*) Mosby Inc.

Physical Signs in Orthopaedics. Ed. by L. Klenerman. 1994. 104p. (Orig.). pap. text (*0-7279-0845-6*) BMJ Pub GBR. *Dist:* AIDC.

Physical Status - The Use & Interpretation of Anthropometry: Report of a WHO Expert Committee. 1995. LC 96-145907. (Technical Report Ser.: Vol. 854). (FRE & SPA.). 452p. (C). pap. 71.00 (*92-4-120854-6*, 1100854) World Health.

Physical Structure of Olympic Athletes. Ed. by J. E. Carter. 1984. (Medicine & Sport Science Ser.: Vol. 18). (Illus.). viii, 248p. 136.75 (*3-8055-3871-5*) S Karger.

Physical Therapist. Jack Rudman. 1994. (Career Examination Ser.: C-585). pap. 34.95 (*0-8373-0585-3*) Nat Learn.

Physical Therapist Assistant. 1997. (Career Examination Ser.). pap. 29.95 (*0-8373-3791-7*, C3791) Nat Learn.

Physical Therapy. Bernice Krumhansl. (Opportunities in... Ser.). (Illus.). 160p. 1993. pap. 10.95 (*0-8442-6159-9*); 1989. 13.95 (*0-8442-6158-0*) McGraw-Hill Trade (Passport Bks).

Physical Therapy. Crispian Scully & Marylou R. Barnes. 1989. (Illus.). 1,319p. text 60.00 (*0-397-50798-4*) Lppncott W & W.

Physical Therapy. John S. Coulter. LC 75-23658. (Clio Medica Ser.: 8). (Illus.). reprint ed. 29.50 (*0-404-58908-1*) AMS Pr.

Physical Therapy: A Survey of the Profession. Ron Scott. 2001. (Illus.). 300p. pap. 39.95 (*0-07-135590-1*) McGraw-Hill Prof.

Physical Therapy Aide: A Worktext. Roberta C. Weiss. 1993. LC 92-23403. 368p. (C). pap. 34.50 (*0-8273-5110-0*) Delmar.

Physical Therapy Aide: A Worktext Instructor's Guide. Roberta C. Weiss. 1993. 45p. pap., tchr. ed. 16.00 (*0-8273-5111-9*) Delmar.

Physical Therapy & Massage for the Horse: A Comprehensive Approach to Equine Kinesiology. Jean-Marie Denoux & Jean-Pierre Pailloux. 1996. LC 94-61970. (Illus.). 200p. 29.95 (*1-57076-021-7*, Trafalgar Sq Pub) Trafalgar.

Physical Therapy & Occupational Therapy in Schools Vol. 2: A Related Service. Bonnie Blossom et al. 1996. (Illus.). 317p. (C). pap. text 65.00 (*0-9630294-1-X*) Rehab P & T.

Physical Therapy & the Arthritis Patient: Clinical Aspects & Approaches to Management. Ed. by Eleanor F. Branch & Mary Singleton. 1988. LC 88-563. (Physical Therapy in Health Care Ser.: Vol. 2, Nos. 1-2). (Illus.). 78p. text 39.95 (*0-86656-728-3*) Haworth Pr.

Physical Therapy & the Pulmonary Patient: Aspects of Evaluation & Treatment. Ed. by Mary C. Singleton & Eleanor F. Branch. 1987. LC 87-21224. (Physical Therapy in Health Care Ser.: Vol. 1, Nos. 2-3). 99p. text 39.95 (*0-86656-705-4*) Haworth Pr.

Physical Therapy & the Stroke Patient: Pathologic Aspects & Clinical Management. Ed. by Eleanor F. Branch & Mary C. Singleton. 1987. LC 87-26668. (Physical Therapy in Health Care Ser.: Vol. 1, No. 4). 73p. text 39.95 (*0-86656-740-2*) Haworth Pr.

Physical Therapy Assistant License Exam. Rothman. 2000. (Physical Therapy Ser.). (C). 29.95 (*0-8273-8082-8*) Delmar.

Physical Therapy Evaluation in Early Infancy. Ed. by Irma J. Wilhelm. 1992. (Clinics in Physical Therapy Ser.). (Illus.). 316p. text (*0-443-08815-2*) Church.

Physical Therapy for Children. Suzann K. Campbell. Ed. by Robert Palisono & Darl W. Vander Linden. 1994. LC 94-10990. (Illus.). 880p. text 62.95 (*0-7216-6503-9*) Saunders.

Physical Therapy for Children. Ed. by Suzann Cambell et al. 2nd ed. Date not set. (Illus.). 1055p. text (*0-7216-8316-9*) Saunders.

Physical Therapy for Sports. Werner Kuprian. Tr. by Todd Konjte & Lynn Braunsdorf. 2nd ed. 1995. LC 94-7651. (Illus.). 464p. text 58.00 (*0-7216-3758-2*) Saunders.

Physical Therapy for the Cancer Patient. Ed. by Charles L. McGarvey, III. 1990. (Clinics in Physical Therapy Ser.). (Illus.). 188p. text (*0-443-08667-2*) Church.

Physical Therapy for Traumatic Head Injury. Jacqueline Montgomery. 1994. text (*0-443-08908-6*) Church.

Physical Therapy in Arthritis. Joan M. Walker & Antoine Helewa. Ed. by Margaret Biblis. 1996. (Illus.). 384p. text 58.00 (*0-7216-4999-8*) Saunders.

Physical Therapy in Craniomadibular Disorders. Tore L. Hansson et al. 1992. LC 92-1717. (Illus.). 80p. text 36.00 (*0-86715-192-7*) Quint Pub Co.

Physical Therapy in Public Schools Vol. 1: A Related Service. Bonnie Blossom & Fran Ford. 1991. LC 91-62293. (Illus.). 182p. (Orig.). (C). pap. text 45.00 (*0-9630294-0-1*) Rehab P & T.

Physical Therapy Licensure Examination Guide: Pretest Self-Assessment & Review. Theresa Nalty. 2000. 208p. pap. 24.95 (*0-07-134723-2*) McGraw-Hill Med Pub.

Physical Therapy Management of Arthritis, No. 16. Ed. by Barbara F. Banwell & Victoria Gall. 1987. (Clinics in Physical Therapy Ser.: Vol. 16). (Illus.). 212p. pap. text (*0-443-08438-6*) Church.

Physical Therapy of the Cervical & Thoracic Spine. Ed. by Ruth Grant. 1988. (Clinics in Physical Therapy Ser.: Vol. 17). (Illus.). 338p. text (*0-443-08507-2*) Church.

Physical Therapy of the Cervical & Thoracic Spine. Ruth Grant. 2nd ed. 1994. LC 94-12194. (Clinics in Physical Therapy Ser.). reprint ed. text (*0-443-08918-3*) Church.

Physical Therapy of the Foot & Ankle. Thomas G. McPoil. Ed. by Gary C. Hunt. 2nd ed. 1995. LC 95-7870. (Clinics in Physical Therapy Ser.). pap. text (*0-443-08925-6*) Church.

Physical Therapy of the Geriatric Patient. Ed. by Osa L. Jackson. 2nd ed. 1989. (Clinics in Physical Therapy Ser.: Vol. 21). (Illus.). 292p. text (*0-443-08619-2*) Church.

Physical Therapy of the Hip. Ed. by John L. Echternach. 1990. (Clinics in Physical Therapy Ser.). (Illus.). 221p. text (*0-443-08650-8*) Church.

Physical Therapy of the Knee. Ed. by Robert E. Mangine. 2nd ed. 1995. LC 95-12053. (Clinics in Physical Therapy Ser.). pap. text (*0-443-08916-7*) Church.

Physical Therapy of the Low Back. Ed. by Lance T. Twomey & James R. Taylor. 1987. (Clinics in Physical Therapy Ser.: Vol. 13). (Illus.). 328p. text (*0-443-08493-9*) Church.

Physical Therapy of the Low Back. Ed. by Lance T. Twomey & J. R. Taylor. 2nd ed. 1994. (Clinics in Physical Therapy Ser.). (Illus.). 384p. text (*0-443-08894-2*) Church.

Physical Therapy of the Low Back. Lance T. Twomey & James R. Taylor. 3rd ed. 2000. LC 00-22470. (Illus.). xii, 411p. text (*0-443-06552-7*) Saunders.

Physical Therapy of the Shoulder. Robert A. Donatelli. 3rd ed. 1996. LC 96-29475. (Clinics in Physical Therapy Ser.). pap. text (*0-443-07591-3*) Church.

Physical Therapy Pharmacology. Lynne Eddy. 1991. (Illus.). 208p. (gr. 13). pap. text 33.95 (*0-8151-3076-7*, 20946) Mosby Inc.

Physical Therapy Procedures: Selected Techniques. Ann H. Downer. 5th ed. 1995. LC 95-35460. (Illus.). 406p. (C). pap. 51.95 (*0-398-06556-X*) C C Thomas.

Physical Therapy Research: Principles & Applications. Elizabeth Domholdt. 1992. LC 92-13390. (Illus.). 464p. pap. text 43.00 (*0-7216-3611-X*) Saunders.

Physical Wisdom. Yogi Bhajan. Ed. & Illus. by Hari J. Khalsa. 1995. 50p. (Orig.). pap. 14.95 (*0-9639847-1-3*) KRI.

Physical Work Capacity in Organ Transplantation. Ed. by Michel Rieu. 1998. LC 97-51463. (Medicine & Sport Science Ser.: Vol. 42, 1998). (Illus.). viii, 188p. 194.00 (*3-8055-6610-7*) S Karger.

Physically & Sexually Abused Child: Evaluation & Treatment. C. Eugene Walker et al. 1988. 208p. 32.50 (*0-08-032769-9*); pap. 16.95 (*0-08-032768-0*) Elsevier (Pergamon Pr).

Physically Handicapped Children: A Medical Atlas for Teachers. Ed. by Eugene E. Bleck & Donald Nagel. 2nd ed. 1981. 560p. text 43.95 (*0-8089-1391-3*, 790623, Grune & Strat) Harcrt Hlth Sci Grp.

Physically Handicapped in India: Policy & Programme. Mani Rama. 1988. 223p. (C). (*81-7024-164-2*) Ashish Pub Hse IND. *Dist:* S Asia.

Physically Handicapped in Society Series Ed. by William R. Phillips & Janet Rosenberg. 1980. lib. bdg. 965.00 (*0-405-13100-3*) Ayer.

Physician. Jack Rudman. 1994. (Career Examination Ser.: C-1392). pap. 44.95 (*0-8373-1392-9*) Nat Learn.

Physician: Medicine & the Unsuspected Battle for Human Freedom. Richard Leviton. 2000. LC 99-95409. xi, 579p. pap. 16.95 (*1-57174-168-2*) Hampton Roads Pub Co.

Physician & Child-Rearing: Two Guides, 1809-1894. William Buchan & L. Emmett Holt, Jr. 1974. 19.95 (*0-405-03965-4*, 15717) Ayer.

Physician & Hospice Care: Roles, Attitudes, & Issues. Ed. by Wilma Bulkin et al. 1993. LC 92-49811. (Loss, Grief & Care Ser.: Vol. 6, Nos. 2 & 3). (Illus.). 200p. lib. bdg. 39.95 (*1-56024-320-1*) Haworth Pr.

Physician & Nurse Migration Analysis & Policy Implications. A. Mejia & H. Pizurki. 1979. 476p. 64.00 (*92-4-156059-2*) World Health.

Physician & Patient or a Practical View of the Mutual Duties, Relations & Interests of the Medical Profession & the Community. Worthington Hooker. 1972. LC 75-180577. (Medicine & Society in America Ser.). 456p. reprint ed. 28.95 (*0-405-03954-9*) Ayer.

***Physician & Philosopher: The Philosophical Fooundation of Medicine: Essays by Dr. Edmund Pellegrino.** Ed. by Roger J. Bulger et al. 2001. 344p. text (*1-891524-09-7*) Carden Jennings.

Physician & Sexuality in Victorian America. John S. Haller, Jr. & Robin M. Haller. 1995. LC 94-47384. 352p. (C). pap. 20.95 (*0-8093-2009-6*) S Ill U Pr.

Physician As Captain of the Ship: A Critical Appraisal. Ed. by Nancy M. King et al. 1988. 269p. text 153.00 (*1-55608-044-1*) Kluwer Academic.

Physician as Manager. J. J. Aluise. 2nd ed. 1986. (Illus.). 260p. 93.00 (*0-387-96381-2*) Spr-Verlag.

Physician Assistant: A Guide to Clinical Practice. Ed. by Ruth Ballweg et al. 1994. LC 93-12579. pap. text 72.50 (*0-7216-4586-0*) Saunders.

Physician Assistant: A Guide to Clinical Practice. Ruth Ballweg et al. Ed. by Edward M. Sullivan & Shirley Kuhn. 2nd ed. 1999. LC 98-24848. (Illus.). 860p. (C). text 71.00 (*0-7216-7653-7*) Harcourt.

Physician Assistant Legal Handbook. Aspen Health Law and Compliance Center Staff. 1997. LC 97-16412. 416p. 70.00 (*0-8342-0925-X*, 20925) Aspen Pub.

Physician Assistant Medical Handbook. James B. Labus. 1995. LC 94-17891. (Illus.). 752p. pap. text 41.00 (*0-7216-5169-0*) Saunders.

Physician Assistant Pearls of Wisdom: Over 3000 Questions. Gillian Lewke et al. 1998. (Pearls of Wisdom Ser.). pap. 32.00 (*1-890369-05-5*) Boston Medical.

Physician Assistant Protocols. Matthew M. Cohen & Anni Lanigan. 1994. 264p. pap. 55.00 (*0-924381-15-9*); ring bd. 85.00 (*0-924381-17-5*); disk (*0-924381-16-7*) Sunbelt Med Pubs.

Physician Assistant Surgical Handbook. James B. Labus. Ed. by Andrew Allen. 1997. LC 96-49868. (Illus.). 480p. pap. text 39.95 (*0-7216-6815-1*) Saunders.

Physician Assistants: Their Contribution to Health Care. Henry B. Perry & Bina Breitner. 1982. LC 81-6260. 331p. 45.95 (*0-89885-066-5*, Kluwer Acad Hman Sci) Kluwer Academic.

Physician Assistant's Clinical Companion. Springhouse Publishing Company Staff. 2000. LC 99-52569. 480p. 39.95 (*1-58255-005-0*) Springhouse Corp.

Physician Assistant's Drug Handbook. 1999. (Illus.). 1248p. 39.95 (*0-87434-975-3*) Springhouse Corp.

Physician Assistant's Emergency Medicine Handbook. Steven W. Salyer. Ed. by Lisa Biello. 1996. LC 96-7416. 656p. pap. text 41.00 (*0-7216-5869-5*) Saunders.

Physician Assistants in American Medicine. Roderick S. Hooker et al. 1997. LC 97-8216. pap. text (*0-443-05731-1*) Church.

Physician-Assisted Death. Ed. by James M. Humber et al. 1994. LC 84-640015. (Biomedical Ethics Reviews Ser.). 165p. 49.50 (*0-89603-265-5*) Humana.

Physician-Assisted Suicide. Ed. by Robert F. Weir. 1997. LC 96-49417. (Medical Ethics Ser.). 304p. 29.95 (*0-253-33282-6*) Ind U Pr.

Physician-Assisted Suicide: Pro & Con. David Mayo. 2000. (Point/Counterpoint Ser.). 53.00 (*0-8476-8815-1*) Rowman.

***Physician Assisted Suicide: Religious & Public Policy Perspectives.** Edwin R. DuBose. 2001. 90p. 6.95 (*0-945482-00-0*) Park Ridge Ctr.

Physician-Assisted Suicide & Euthanasia. Lisa Yount. 2000. LC 00-25775. (Library in a Book). 282p. lib. bdg. 39.95 (*0-8160-4021-4*) Facts on File.

Physician Compensation Systems. Max Reiboldt. Ed. by Kay Stanley. 1998. 54.00 (*0-89970-910-9*) AMA.

Physician-Computer Connection: A Practical Guide to Physician Involvement in Health Care Information Systems. William F. Bria & Richard L. Rydell. rev. ed. 1996. LC 96-26417. 124p. pap. 45.00 (*1-55648-166-7*, 093106) AHPI.

Physician Documentation for Reimbursement. Gabrielle M. Kotoski & Melinda Stegman. 1994. LC 94-7576. 254p. pap. 66.00 (*0-8342-0534-3*) Aspen Pub.

***Physician Documentation Handbook 2001 (Formerly Clinical Documentation Compliance Handbook)** Ingenix, Inc. Staff. pap. 64.95 (*1-56337-322-X*) Ingenix Inc.

Physician Empowerment Through Capitation. Clifford R. Frank & David Kibbe. 2000. LC 99-52792. 288p. pap. 68.00 (*0-8342-1212-9*) Aspen Pub.

Physician Equity Model. Keith M. Korenchuk. 1996. 229p. 45.00 (*1-56829-077-2*, 4908) M G M A.

Physician Executives & the Law: Issues & Trends in Liability. Ed. by Todd Sagin. 1996. LC 95-80572. 165p. (Orig.). pap. 48.00 (*0-924674-39-3*) Am Coll Phys Execs.

Physician Executives' Guide to Patient Management for the '90s & Beyond. Raymond J. Fabius. 1995. LC 95-76633. 107p. pap. 48.00 (*0-924674-33-4*) Am Coll Phys Execs.

Physician Fees, 1998. annuals rev. ed. 1998. 410p. pap. text 99.95 (*1-57066-080-8*, 9835) Practice Mgmt Info.

Physician Financial Planning in a Changing Environment. Russ A. Prince et al. 1996. 300p. (Orig.). reprint ed. pap. text 44.95 (*1-57066-104-9*, ME115) Practice Mgmt Info.

Physician, Heal Thyself. John Allegro. 1985. LC 85-43081. 93p. 28.00 (*0-87975-305-6*) Prometheus Bks.

Physician, Heal Thyself: A Doctor's Dietary Recovery from Incurable Cancer. Hugh Faulkner. 1993. 112p. pap. 7.95 (*0-9628528-6-4*) One Peaceful World.

Physician Heal Thyself: Medical Practitioner of Eighteenth-Century New York. Marynita A. Nolosco. 1994. LC 94-13012. (American University Studies: Vol. 170). (*0-8204-2580-X*) P Lang Pubng.

Physician Heal Thyself: What Every Practitioner Should Know about Alternative Medicine. Richard Sarnat. 1995. LC 95-77514. 112p. pap. 10.95 (*0-9639297-2-0*) Herbal Free.

Physician Himself & What He Should Add to His Scientific Acquirements. D. W. Cathell. 2nd ed. 1972. LC 70-180562. (Medicine & Society in America Ser.). 216p. reprint ed. 19.95 (*0-405-03941-7*) Ayer.

Physician Hospital Organizations. Keith M. Korenchuk. 1994. 209p. 45.00 (*1-56829-033-0*, 4541) M G M A.

Physician Hospital Organizations: Cases & Analysis. Thomas M. Gorey et al. 1997. LC 97-20196. 121p. pap. 18.20 (*1-56793-063-8*) Health Admin Pr.

Physician ICD 9 CM: 1999 Edition. Medicode, Med-Index Division Staff. 1999. (C). pap. 69.95 (*1-56337-283-5*) Thomson Learn.

Physician in Industry. William P. Shepard. Ed. by Leon Stein. 1977. LC 77-70532. reprint ed. lib. bdg. 33.95 (*0-405-10200-3*) Ayer.

Physician Interaction Style & Medication Management: Abstract, Executive Summary & Final Report. Betsy Sleath. 1998. (Illus.). 90p. (C). reprint ed. pap. text 25.00 (*0-7881-4502-9*) DIANE Pub.

Physician Interaction Systems Manual. M. Johnson. 1993. 32p. (C). pap., stu. ed. (*0-933195-63-X*) CA College Health Sci.

Physician Investigator Handbook: GCP Tools & Techniques. Deborah Rosenbaum & Fred O. Smith. 1997. LC 96-48071. (Practical Clinical Trials Ser.: Vol. 2). (Illus.). 300p. 145.00 (*1-57491-040-X*) IHS Health Grp.

***Physician Investigator Handbook: GCP Tools & Techniques.** Deborah Rosenbaum & Fred Smith. 2nd ed. 2002. LC 2001-39465. (Practical Clinical Trials Ser.). (*1-57491-124-4*) IHS Health Grp.

Physician Leader's Guide. Ed. by Jonathan T. Lord. 1992. 200p. pap. text 20.00 (*0-915963-10-8*, TPLG) Capitol Publns.

Physician Leader's Guide. 2nd ed. 1997. 104.00 (*1-56925-107-X*) Capitol VA.

Physician-Legislators of France: Medicine & Politics in the Early Third Republic, 1870-1914. Jack D. Ellis. 1990. (Cambridge History of Medicine Ser.). (Illus.). 317p. (C). text 85.00 (*0-521-38208-4*) Cambridge U Pr.

Physician Manager in Group Practice. John W. Pollard. 1994. 142p. pap. 36.00 (*1-56829-005-5*, 3931) M G M A.

Physician Manager's Handbook: Essential Skills for Succeeding in Health Care. Robert J. Solomon. 2nd ed. 1997. LC 96-24308. (Illus.). 464p. 98.00 (*0-8342-0768-0*) Aspen Pub.

Physician Networks: Strategy, Start-Up, & Operation. Richard Krohn. 1998. LC 98-21935. 46.00 (*1-56793-089-1*) Health Admin Pr.

Physician Office Health Records see Documentation & Reimbursement for Physician Offices

Physician Organizations: Cases & Analysis. Thomas M. Gorey. 1997. LC 97-20193. pap. 18.20 (*1-56793-064-6*) Health Admin Pr.

Physician Organizations & Medical Staff: Contracts, Rights & Liabilities Aspen Health Law Center Staff. 1996. ring bd. 260.00 (*0-8342-0792-3*, S287) Aspen Pub.

Physician Participation in Medicaid Managed Care. Sunday E. Ubokudom. 1997. LC 97-25938. (Health Care Policy in the United States Ser.). (Illus.). 224p. text 65.00 (*0-8153-2905-9*) Garland.

Physician-Patient Decision-Making: A Study in Medical Ethics, 27. Douglas N. Walton. 1985. LC 85-5412. (Contributions in Philosophy Ser.: No. 27). (Illus.). 265p. 65.00 (*0-313-24888-5*, WPH/, Greenwood Pr) Greenwood.

Physician-Patient Relationships: An Annotated Bibliography. Michael Glasser. 1991. LC 90-14126. (Applied Social Science Bibliographies Ser.: Vol. 4). 102p. text 28.00 (*0-8240-0688-7*, SS580) Garland.

Physician Payment Reform: Its Impact on Payers & Providers. Ed. by Richard Lauve. 1992. LC 92-81837. (Orig.). (C). pap. text 25.95 (*0-924674-15-6*) Am Coll Phys Execs.

Physician Performance Management: Tool for Survival & Success. Christine N. Micklitsch & Theresa A. Ryan-Mitlyng. 1996. (Illus.). 122p. (Orig.). pap. 75.00 (*1-56829-078-0*, 4928) M G M A.

Physician Practice Acquisition Resource Book. William O. Cleverley et al. 1995. (Illus.). 221p. pap. 995.00 (*1-882733-06-1*) Ctr Hlthcare IPS.

Physician Practice Compliance Resource Manual. Aspen Health Law and Compliance Center Staff. 2001. LC 00-67631. (Illus.). 500p. ring bd. 199.00 (*0-8342-1870-4*) Aspen Pub.

Physician Profiling: A Source Book for Health Care Administrators. Neill F. Piland. 1999. LC 99-11319. (Jossey-Bass Health Ser.). (Illus.). 166p. 46.00 (*0-7879-4601-X*) Jossey-Bass.

Physician Profiling: Background & Practical Experience. Ed. by Kenneth J. Pechman. 2000. 55.00 (*0-924674-74-1*) Am Coll Phys Execs.

Physician Profiling & Risk Adjustment. Norbert Goldfield. 2nd ed. 1999. LC 98-37565. 720p. 110.00 (*0-8342-1169-6*, 11696) Aspen Pub.

Physician Salary Survey Report, 1992. Hospital Compensation Service Staff. 1992. pap. 250.00 (*0-939326-68-X*) Hosp & Hlthcare.

Physician Socioeconomic Statistics Text 2000-2001. Ed. by AMA Staff. 2000. (Illus.). 210p. pap. 495.00 (*1-57947-088-2*) AMA.

Physician to the World: The Life of General William C. Gorgas. John M. Gibson. 1989. LC 89-33463. (Library of Alabama Classics). (Illus.). 352p. reprint ed. pap. text 19.95 (*0-8173-0457-6*) U of Ala Pr.

Physician Within: Practical Guide to Natural Healing. Ed. by Gross. 1999. 232p. 32.60 (*0-536-02687-4*) Pearson Custom.

Physician Within You: Medicine for the Millenium. Gladys Taylor McCarey & Jess Stearn. 2000. 295p. pap. 14.95 (*0-9658158-5-4*) Inkwell Prods.

Physicians & Hospitals: The Great Partnership at the Crossroads. Ed. by Duncan Yaggy & Patricia Hodgson. 1985. LC 84-25928. (Duke Press Policy Studies). xxiii, 202p. text 39.95 (*0-8223-0639-5*) Duke.

Physicians & Management in Health Care. Ed. by Montague Brown. 1992. (Health Care Management Review Ser.). 244p. pap. 55.00 (*0-8342-0300-6*, 20300) Aspen Pub.

Physicians & Surgeons Directory, 2001. American Business Directories Staff. rev. ed. 2000. 2,920p. 695.00 incl. cd-rom (*0-7687-0326-3*) Am Busn Direct.

Physicians & the Peace Movement. Nick Lewer. 1992. 140p. text (*0-7146-3438-7*) F Cass Pubs GBR. *Dist:* Intl Spec Bk.

Physicians As Employees. Aspen Health Law and Compliance Center Staff. 1998. LC 98-9397. (Current Issue Ser.). 160p. pap. 48.00 (*0-8342-1157-2*, 11572) Aspen Pub.

Physicians As Employees: Aspen Health Law Center Current Issues. Aspen Health Law Center Staff. 1998. LC 98-9397. 160p. pap. 39.00 (*0-8342-1121-1*) Aspen Pub.

Physician's Assistant. Jack Rudman. 1994. (Career Examination Ser.: C-2557). pap. 29.95 (*0-8373-2557-9*) Nat Learn.

Physicians at Teaching Hospitals (path) Audits: Hearing Before a Subcommittee of the Committee on Appropriations, United States Senate, One Hundred Fifth Congress, First Session, Special Hearing. U. S. Government Printing Office Staff. 1998. LC 98-160487. iii, 48p. (*0-16-056304-6*) USGPO.

***Physicians at Work, Patients in Pain.** Kaja Finkler. 2nd ed. 2001. 287p. (*0-89089-749-2*) Carolina Acad Pr.

Physicians' Attitudes Toward Elder Suicide. Lori M. Secouler. 1998. LC 97-32973. (Studies on the Elderly in America). 100p. text 35.00 (*0-8153-3005-7*) Garland.

Physicians' Book of Days. Marcia O. Levin. 1992. (Illus.). 128p. 10.95 (*0-88363-392-2*) H L Levin.

***Physician's Cancer Chemotherapy Drug Manual 2002.** Edward Chu & Vincent T. DeVita, Jr. rev. ed. 2001. pap. 59.95 (*0-7637-1973-0*, 1973-0) Jones & Bartlett.

Physicians, Colonial Racism & Diaspora in West Africa. Adell Patton. 1996. LC 95-45070. 296p. (C). 49.95 (*0-8130-1432-8*) U Press Fla.

Physician's Compass: A Navigation Guide to the Internet. Kevin W. Fergusson. 2000. 80p. pap. 7.00 (*0-615-11516-0*) DrPEN.

Physicians' Desk Reference for Nonprescription Drugs & Dietary Supplements. Ed. by Medical Economics Staff. 21st rev. ed. 2000. (Illus.). 1000p. 50.00 (*1-56363-341-8*, PDR) Med Econ.

***Physicians' Desk Reference 2002: Bookstore Edition.** Medical Economics Co. Staff. 56th rev. ed. 2001. 3,000p. 89.95 (*1-56363-412-0*, PDR) Med Econ.

***Physicians' Desk Reference 2002: Library/Hospital Version.** Medical Economics Co. Staff. 56th rev. ed. 2001. 3,000p. 89.95 (*1-56363-411-2*, PDR) Med Econ.

Physician's Desk Reference, 2001 Vol. 55: Library/Hospital Version. Medical Economics Staff. 55th rev. ed. 2000. (Illus.). 3000p. 87.00 (*1-56363-375-2*) Med Econ.

Physicians' Desk Reference, 2001: Bookstore Version, Vol. 55. Medical Economics Staff. 55th rev. ed. 2000. LC 82-642489. (Physicians' Desk Reference Ser.). 3,200 p. 87.00 (*1-56363-376-0*, PDR) Med Econ.

Physician's Drug Handbook. Springhouse Publishing Company Staff. 7th ed. 1997. (Illus.). 1232p. 39.95 (*0-87434-899-4*) Springhouse Corp.

Physicians Drug Handbook. 8th ed. 1999. LC 90-656192. (Illus.). 1312p. 39.95 (*0-87434-987-7*) Springhouse Corp.

Physicians' Drug Manual: 2001 Edition. Michael Safani & Paul D. Chan. rev. ed. 2000. (Current Clinical Strategies Ser.). 90p. pap. 9.95 (*1-881528-96-0*) Current Clin Strat.

Physicians' Drug Manual for PDAs & Desktops: 2001. Michael Safani, Pharmd. rev. ed. 2000. (Current Clinical Strategies Ser.). 90p. pap. 28.95 incl. cd-rom (*1-881528-97-9*) Current Clin Strat.

Physician's Eye. John Naish. 1997. LC 97-4009. (Mellen Lives Ser.: Vol. 6). (Illus.). 172p. text 79.95 (*0-7734-8662-3*) E Mellen.

Physician's Financial Sourcebook Vol. 1: Investment, Risk Management & Retirement Tools for a Balanced Life. Paul H. Sutherland. Ed. by Matthew F. Sutherland. 1998. LC 97-95333. (Illus.). 250p. pap. 29.95 (*0-9661060-0-8*) Finan Srcebk Pub.

Physicians for the 21st Century. Lawrence E. Stevens. 1997. vi, 171p. 14.95 (*0-9661514-0-2*, 1) White Bush Pub.

Physicians' Generix: The Official Drug Reference of FDA Prescribing Information & Therapeutic Equivalents, 1992. 1992. 2700p. 68.00 (*1-880891-02-6*) Work-Loss Data.

Physicians' Generix, 1993: The Official Drug Reference of FDA Prescribing Information & Therapeutic Equivalents. Ed. by Jonathan A. Epner. 1993. 2600p. 77.00 (*1-880891-03-4*) Work-Loss Data.

Physicians Genrix, 1995: The Complete Drug Reference of FDA Prescribing Information &... Philip L. Denniston. 1995. 77.00 (*1-880891-07-7*) Work-Loss Data.

Physician's Guide for Expert Witnessing. Reda A. Abdel-Fattah. 1993. 175p. 105.00 (*1-883865-01-8*) Biomed Pr.

Physician's Guide for the Collection & Handling of Bacteriogical & Viral Specimens. Stephen J. Cavalleri & Gilles R. G. Monif. 1995. (Illus.). 62p. pap. 6.95 (*1-880906-41-4*) IDI Pub.

Physician's Guide for the Collection of Bacteriogical & Viral Specimens. Gilles R. Monif. 55p. 7.95 (*1-880906-73-2*) IDI Pub.

Physician's Guide for the Handling of Gynecologic & Obstetric Tissue Specimens. Chhandra Bewtra. 1997. (Illus.). 78p. pap. 9.95 (*1-880906-15-5*) IDI Pub.

Physician's Guide to Advance Medical Directives. Alan D. Lieberson. Ed. by Melanie C. Karaffa. 1993. LC 92-48385. 350p. 69.95 (*1-878487-52-3*, ME223) Practice Mgmt Info.

Physician's Guide to Alternative Medicine, Vol. II. Ed. by Milo Falcon. 2000. 336p. 199.00 (*1-931107-00-9*) Am Health Consults.

Physician's Guide to Arthropods of Medical Importance. Jerome Goddard. 1993. 352p. lib. bdg. 126.95 (*0-8493-5160-X*, RA641); 2nd ed. 1996. LC 96-28904. 400p. lib. bdg. 139.00 (*0-8493-2662-1*) CRC Pr.

Physician's Guide to Disease Management. James B. Couch. 1997. LC 97-18244. 368p. pap. 56.00 (*0-8342-1003-7*) Aspen Pub.

Physician's Guide to Diving Medicine. C. W. Shilling et al. 1984. LC 84-14817. (Illus.). 768p. 165.00 (*0-306-41428-7*, Kluwer Plenum) Kluwer Academic.

Physician's Guide to Domestic Violence: How to Ask the Right Questions & Recognize Abuse. Patricia R. Salber & Ellen Taliaferro. 1995. LC 94-23000. 114p. pap. 10.95 (*1-884244-04-1*) Volcano Pr.

Physicians' Guide to Drug Eruptions. Jerome Z. Litt. 1997. LC 97-36824. 278p. lib. bdg. 74.95 (*1-85070-003-6*) CRC Pr.

***Physician's Guide to End-of-Life Care.** Ed. by Lois Snyder. 2001. LC 2001-22336. 267p. pap. 35.00 (*1-930513-28-3*) Amer Coll Phys.

Physician's Guide to Eye Care. Jonathan D. Trobe. 1993. LC 93-9068. 200p. pap. 59.95 (*1-56055-073-2*) Am Acad Ophthal.

Physicians' Guide to Free Radicals, Immunity & Aging. Lee-Benner. 1986. lib. bdg. 125.00 (*0-944213-00-6*) World Hlth Found.

Physician's Guide to Free Radicals, Immunity & Aging. Lord Lee-Benner. 1991. LC 90-71564. (Illus.). 301p. (C). deluxe ed. (*0-944213-27-8*); rev. ed. lib. bdg. 150.00 (*0-944213-26-X*); 2nd rev. ed. 125.00 (*0-944213-25-1*) World Hlth Found.

Physician's Guide to Internet Explorer. American Medical Association Staff. 1999. 29.95 (*0-89970-934-6*) AMA.

Physician's Guide to Managed Care. Ed. by David B. Nash. 1993. LC 93-24024. 272p. 88.00 (*0-8342-0393-6*, 20393) Aspen Pub.

Physician's Guide to Managed Care. James R. Lyle & Hoyt W. Torras. 2nd ed. 1995. pap. 49.95 (*1-879249-17-0*) HlthCare Consult.

Physician's Guide to Natural Remedies. D. Paul Barney. 1998. 406p. pap. text 19.95 (*1-885670-84-2*) Woodland UT.

Physicians' Guide to Nutriceuticals. Douglas L. Ringer. 1998. 290p. 39.99 (*0-9665665-0-5*) Nutrtnl Data Resces.

Physician's Guide to Pain & Symptom Management in Cancer Patients. Contrib. by J. Abrahm. 2000. LC 99-37061. (Illus.). 432p. 57.00 (*0-8018-6245-0*) Johns Hopkins.

Physician's Guide to Psychoactive Drugs. Richard Seymour & David E. Smith. 1987. LC 87-354. 186p. text 5.95 (*0-86656-382-2*) Haworth Pr.

Physicians' Guide to Rare Diseases. Ed. by Doris C. Smith. 1992. (Illus.). 1224p. 69.50 (*0-9628716-0-5*) Dowden Pub.

Physician's Guide to Rare Diseases: 1995 Edition. Ed. & Intro. by Jess G. Thoene. 2nd ed. 1995. (Illus.). 1200p. 129.99 (*0-9628716-1-3*) Dowden Pub.

Physician's Guide to Sunscreens. Nicholas Lowe. 1990. (Illus.). 232p. text 125.00 (*0-8247-8496-0*) Dekker.

Physician's Guide to the Laboratory Diagnosis of Inherited Metabolic Diseases. N. Blau et al. 1996. (Arnold Publication). (Illus.). 544p. text 69.00 (*0-412-57560-4*) OUP.

Physician's Guide to Thriving in the New Managed Care Environment: Selecting the Right Strategy for Your Practice. Richard V. Stenson. 2000. LC 99-22237. 320p. 49.95 (*1-58151-030-6*) BookPartners.

Physician's Guide to Transgendered Medicine. Sheila Kirk. Date not set. pap. 10.00 (*1-887796-03-7*) Together Lifeworks.

Physician's Hand. Barbara Melosh. 1982. (C). pap. text 22.95 (*0-87722-290-8*) Temple U Pr.

Physician's Handbook. Marcus A. Krupp. 20th ed. pap. text 12.00 (*0-87041-023-7*) Appleton & Lange.

Physician's Handbook of Clinical Nutrition. Henry Osiecki. 1990. 252p. (C). pap. (*1-875239-03-0*) Bio Concepts AUS. *Dist:* St Mut.

Physicians in Bureaucracy: A Case Study of Professional Pressures on Organizational Roles. Mary E. Goss. Ed. by Harriet Zuckerman & Robert K. Merton. 1980. LC 79-9002. (Dissertations on Sociology Ser.). lib. bdg. 19.95 (*0-405-12971-8*) Ayer.

Physicians in Corporations: Medicine As Management. Diana C. Walsh. 1987. LC 87-6096. 272p. 42.50 (*0-300-03902-6*) Yale U Pr.

Physicians in Managed Care: A Career Guide. Ed. by Mark Bloomberg & Steven Mohlie. 1994. LC 94-70991. 152p. (Orig.). pap. text 25.00 (*0-924674-25-3*) Am Coll Phys Execs.

Physicians in the Academic Marketplace, 53. Dolores L. Burke. 1991. LC 91-28327. (Contributions to the Study of Education Ser.: No. 53). 184p. 55.00 (*0-313-27850-4*, BYE/, Greenwood Pr) Greenwood.

Physician's Job-Search Rx: Marketing Yourself for the Position You Want. Javad H. Kashani et al. 1998. LC 97-38470. 229p. pap. 16.95 (*0-471-19336-4*) Wiley.

Physicians of Tomorrow: A Colloquium to Advance Medical Education in Alcohol & Other Drug Dependencies. 1989. pap. 4.00 (*0-911290-20-6*) Rutgers Ctr Alcohol.

Physicians of Western Medicine. Ed. by Robert A. Hahn & Atwood D. Gaines. 1984. pap. text 64.50 (*90-277-1881-4*); lib. bdg. 153.50 (*90-277-1790-7*) Kluwer Academic.

Physician's Office. Leif C. Beck. 1977. LC 77-87555. (Illus.). 14.95 (*90-219-0346-6*) Excerpta Princeton.

Physician's Office & Ambulatory Surgery: Detailed Survey Data of Value to Medical, Insurance & High Tech Industries. 1986. 277p. 1350.00 (*0-931634-63-6*) FIND-SVP.

Physician's Office Laboratory. Bernard D. Statland et al. 2nd ed. 1993. 468p. pap. 49.95 (*1-878487-49-3*, ME200) Practice Mgmt Info.

Physician's Office Laboratory Guidelines, Procedure Manual: Tentative Guideline. NCCLS Staff. 3rd ed. 1995. 200p. pap. text 150.00 (*1-56238-159-8*, POL1/2-T3) NCCLS.

Physician's Office 97: Coding Workbook. Covell. 4th ed. 1997. (Medical Assisting Ser.). (C). text, wbk. ed. 17.50 (*0-7668-0081-4*) Delmar.

Physician's Perspective on Medical Law. Ed. by Howard H. Kaufman & Jeffrey L. Lewin. 1997. (Neurosurgical Topics Ser.: Vol. 28). Vol. I. (Illus.). 202p. 95.00 (*1-879284-44-8*); Vol. II. 238p. 95.00 (*1-879284-53-7*) Am Assn Neuro.

Physicians Posy. Dorothy Shepard. 1993. 109p. pap. (*0-85207-272-4*) C W Daniel GBR. *Dist:* Natl Bk Netwk.

Physician's Posy. Dorothy Shepherd. 1993. 256p. (Orig.). pap. 19.95 (*0-8464-4177-2*) Beekman Pubs.

Physician's Practice. Ed. by John M. Eisenberg & Sankey V. Williams. 1984. LC 80-13691. 288p. reprint ed. 32.50 (*0-471-05469-0*) Krieger.

Physician's Reference Guide to Cardiology. Ed. by Dennis S. Reison. 1992. 935p. (*1-878212-00-1*) Prof & Tech Pub.

Physician's Reference Notebook. William A. McGarey. 2000. (Edgar Cayce Classics). 436p. pap. 19.95 (*0-87604-373-2*, 322) ARE Pr.

Physicians' Resume & Cover Letter Workbook. AMA Staff. 1998. LC 00-501890. (Career Development Ser.). 122p. 33.00 (*0-89970-888-9*) AMA.

Physician's Risk Management Desk Reference. Ed. by Grena G. Porto. 1997. xi, 176p. pap. 15.00 (*0-9629192-0-9*) V H A.

Physician's RX Shorthand. Stanley Jablonski. 1996. LC 97-102931. 40p. 9.95 (*1-56053-167-3*) Hanley & Belfus.

Physician's Socioeconomic Statistics, 1999-2000 Edition. American Medical Association Staff. 1999. 495.00 (*0-89970-974-5*) AMA.

Physician's Survival Guide to Business of Medicine. Robert W. Katz. 1994. LC 93-33907. 192p. ring bd. 123.00 (*0-8342-0532-7*) Aspen Pub.

Physician's Survival Guide to the Business of Medicine. Robert W. Katz. 2nd ed. 1998. 250p. 49.00 (*0-8342-1024-X*, 20124) Aspen Pub.

Physico-Chemical Factors of Biological Evolution. S. E. Shnol. 1981. (Soviet Scientific Reviews, Biology Reviews Supplement Ser.: Vol. 1). xvi, 280p. text 368.00 (*3-7186-0044-7*) Gordon & Breach.

Physico-Chemical Procedures for the Characterization of Vaccines: Les Pensieres, Veyrier-du-Lac, France, December 1999. Ed. by F. Brown et al. 2000. LC 2001-265391. (Developments in Biologicals Ser.: Vol. 103). (Illus.). x, 278p. 235.00 (*3-8055-7101-1*) S Karger.

Physicochemical Anthropology Pt. I: Human Behavioral Structure. N. R. Joseph. 1978. (Illus.). 68.00 (*3-8055-2793-4*) S Karger.

Physicochemical Anthropology Pt. II: Comparative Morphology & Behavior. N. R. Joseph. 1979. 85.25 (*3-8055-2951-1*) S Karger.

Physicochemical Aspects of Medicine Reviews: Affinity Chromatography in Artificial Detoxification Systems; Hemosorption in the Management of Atherosclerosis; Fertility Alpha2-Microglobulin (FAMG), Vol. 2. I. P. Andrianov et al. 1989. (Soviet Medical Reviews Ser.: Vol. 2, Pt. 1). ii, 84p. pap. text 63.00 (*3-7186-4966-7*) Gordon & Breach.

Physicochemical Aspects of Medicine Reviews: Electrochemical Methods of Detoxification for Medical Use, Vol. 2. V. I. Sergienko & Y. B. Vasiliev. 1989. (Soviet Medical Reviews Ser.: Vol. 2, Pt. 2). iv, 60p. pap. text 70.00 (*3-7186-4967-5*) Gordon & Breach.

Physicochemical Aspects of Medicine Reviews: The Rate of Myocardial Necrotization As a Major Criterion of Infarction Severity; Automated Analysis of Chromatin Structures in Interphase Cell Nuclei, Vol. 2. A. V. Vinogradov et al. 1989. (Soviet Medical Reviews Ser.: Vol. 2, Pt. 4.1 & Pt. 4.2). iv, 84p. pap. text 62.00 (*3-7186-4968-3*) Gordon & Breach.

Physicochemical Aspects of Medicine Reviews: Thymic Peptides As Immunoregulators, with Special Reference to T-Activin, Vol. 2. V. Y. Arion. 1989. (Soviet Medical Reviews Ser.: Vol. 2, Pt. 3). iv, 64p. pap. text 69.00 (*3-7186-4965-9*) Gordon & Breach.

Physicochemical Aspects of Medicine Reviews Vol. 3, Pt. 1.3: Methods for Evaluating Crystalline Lens Transparency, & Some Approaches to the Early Detection, Vol. 3. V. E. Formazyuk. 1991. (Soviet Medical Reviews Ser.: Section B). 528p. pap. text 177.00 (*3-7186-5231-5*, Harwood Acad Pubs) Gordon & Breach.

Physicochemical Aspects of Medicine Reviews Vol. 3, Pt. 2: Hydromechanics of the Eye, Vol. 3. A. Nesterov. 1992. (Soviet Medical Reviews Ser.: Section B). 68p. pap. text 71.00 (*3-7186-5256-0*, Harwood Acad Pubs) Gordon & Breach.

Physicochemical Aspects of Medicine Reviews Vol. 3, Pt. 3: Peroxidation of Blood Lipoproteins & the Development of Atherosclerosis, Vol. 3. O. Panosenko. 1992. (Soviet Medical Reviews Ser.: Section B). 76p. pap. text 92.00 (*3-7186-5290-0*, Harwood Acad Pubs) Gordon & Breach.

Physicochemical Aspects of Medicine Reviews Vol. 3, Pt. 4: The Skin & Atherosclerosis, a Three-Drop Test, Vol. 3. Y. M. Lopukhin. 1992. (Soviet Medical Reviews Ser.: Section B). 124p. pap. text 147.00 (*3-7186-5291-9*, Harwood Acad Pubs) Gordon & Breach.

Physicochemical Biology Reviews. Ed. by V. P. Skulachev. (Soviet Scientific Reviews Ser.: Section D). Vol. 4. 1984. xii, 334p. text 552.00 (*3-7186-0140-0*); Vol. 6. 1986. xi, 266p. text 503.00 (*3-7186-0268-7*) Gordon & Breach.

Physicochemical Principles of Pharmacy. Alexander T. Florence & D. Attwood. 3rd ed. 1998. (Illus.). 564p. (C). pap. text (*0-333-69081-8*) Macmillan Ed GBR. *Dist:* Scholium Intl.

Physics & Engineering of Medical Imaging. Ed. by Riccardo Guzzardi. 1987. text 529.00 (*90-247-3454-1*) Kluwer Academic.

Physics & Instrumentation of Diagnostic Medical Ultrasound. John Fish. 1990. 260p. pap. 165.00 (*0-471-92651-5*) Wiley.

Physics & Radiobiology of Nuclear Medicine. G. B. Saha. 2nd ed. 2000. LC 00-22559. (Illus.). 272p. 65.00 (*0-387-95021-4*) Spr-Verlag.

Physics & Technology of Hyperthermia. Ed. by Stanley B. Field & Cafiero Franconi. 1987. (C). text 306.50 (*90-247-3509-2*) Kluwer Academic.

Physics-Based Deformable Models: Applications to Computer Vision, Graphics & Medical Imaging. Dimitris N. Metaxas. 1996. LC 96-49366. 328p. (C). text 157.50 (*0-7923-9840-8*) Kluwer Academic.

Physics-Based Vision Shafer et al. (Illus.). (C). text 149.95 (*0-86720-452-4*) Jones & Bartlett.

Physics for Diagnostic Radiology. P. P. Dendy. 2nd ed. 1999. LC 99-24542. (Medical Science Ser.). (Illus.). xviii, 446p. 160.00 (*0-7503-0590-8*); pap. text 49.00 (*0-7503-0591-6*) Inst of Physics Pubng.

Physics for Medical Imaging. Farr. 1996. text 44.95 (*0-7020-1770-1*) Saunders.

Physics for Ophthalmologists. Ed. by Douglas J. Coster. 1994. LC 93-34293. 192p. text (*0-443-04935-1*) Church.

Physics for the Health Sciences. Carl R. Nave & Brenda C. Nave. 3rd ed. 1985. (Illus.). 430p. pap., tchr. ed. (*0-7216-2043-4*) Saunders.

Physics in Biology & Medicine. Paul Davidovits. 2nd ed. 2000. LC 00-107669. (Complementary Science Ser.). (Illus.). xv, 303p. pap. 34.95 (*0-12-204840-7*) Acad Pr.

Physics in Environmental & Biomedical Research: Rome, Italy, November 26-29, 1985. Ed. by S. Onori & E. Tabet. 1986. 608p. text 144.00 (*9971-5-0110-4*) World Scientific Pub.

Physics in Medicine. T. A. Delchar. 1997. (Illus.). 352p. (C). pap. text 99.95 (*0-412-61680-7*, Chap & Hall NY) Chapman & Hall.

Physics in Medicine & Biology, Vol. 1-2. T. F. McAinsh. 1986. 185.00 (*0-08-033930-1*); 135.00 (*0-08-033931-X*) Elsevier (Pergamon Pr).

Physics in Nuclear Medicine. Ed. by James A. Sorenson & Michael E. Phelps. 2nd ed. 1986. 608p. text 89.00 (*0-8089-1804-4*, 794189, Grune & Strat) Harcrt Hlth Sci Grp.

Physics of Cerebrovascular Diseases: Biophysical Mechanisms of Development, Diagnosis & Therapy. George J. Hademenos & Tarik F. Massoud. 1997. LC 97-30653. (Biological Physics Ser.: Vol. 2). (Illus.). 311p. 76.95 (*1-56396-558-5*, AIP Pr) Spr-Verlag.

Physics of Conformal Radiotherapy: Advances in Technology. S. Webb. 1997. (Medical Science Ser.). (Illus.). 272p. text 179.00 (*0-7503-0396-4*); pap. text 53.00 (*0-7503-0397-2*) Inst of Physics Pubng.

Physics of Diagnostic Imaging. D. Dowsett & P. Kennedy. 1997. (Illus.). 656p. (*0-412-46060-2*) E A GBR. *Dist:* OUP.

Physics of Medical Imaging. Ed. by Steve Webb. 1988. (Medical Science Ser.). (Illus.). 633p. 258.00 (*0-85274-361-0*); LC 88-4487. pap. 61.00 (*0-85274-349-1*) Inst of Physics Pubng.

Physics of Nuclear Medicine: Recent Advances: Proceedings of the AAPM 1983 Summer School Held at Farleigh Dickinson University, Madison, New Jersey, July 24-29, 1983. Ed. by Dandamudi V. Rao et al. 1984. (American Association of Physicists in Medicine Symposium Ser.: No. 10). 570p. 60.00 (*0-88318-440-0*) Am Inst Physics.

Physics of Radiation Therapy. Faiz M. Khan. 2nd ed. 1994. LC 92-18111. (Illus.). 608p. text 129.00 (*0-683-04502-4*) Lppncott W & W.

Physics of Radiology. Anthony B. Wolbarst. 1993. (Illus.). 576p. (C). pap. text 75.00 (*0-8385-5769-4*, A5769-3) Appleton & Lange.

Physics of Radiology. Anthony Brinton Wolbarst. 2000. 478p. pap. text 65.95 (*0-944838-95-2*) Med Physics Pub.

Physics of Radiology. Harold E. Johns & John R. Cunningham. 4th ed. 1983. (Illus.). 816p. (C). 82.95 (*0-398-04669-7*) C C Thomas.

Physics of Radiotherapy X-Rays from Linear Accelerators. Peter Metcalfe et al. 1997. LC 96-51445. (Illus.). 493p. pap. text 98.95 (*0-944838-76-6*) Med Physics Pub.

Physics of Speech. Dennis B. Fry. 1979. LC 78-56752. (Textbooks in Linguistics). (Illus.). 160p. pap. text 22.95 (*0-521-29379-0*) Cambridge U Pr.

Physics of the Body. John Cameron et al. 2nd ed. 1999. LC 99-26114. (Illus.). 410p. text 53.95 (*0-944838-90-1*); pap. text 45.95 (*0-944838-91-X*) Med Physics Pub.

Physics of Three Dimensional Radiation Therapy: Conformal Radiotherapy, Radiosurgery, & Treatment Planning. Steve Webb. 1993. LC 93-6665. (Medical Science Ser.). (Illus.). 373p. (C). 188.00 (*0-7503-0247-X*); pap. 48.00 (*0-7503-0254-2*) Inst of Physics Pubng.

***Physics 2000.** Elisha Huggins. 2001. (Illus.). 561p. 15.00 (*0-9707836-2-0*, P2K-2) Moose Moun.

Physics with Illustrative Examples from Medicine & Biology 2nd rev. ed. George B. Benedek & Felix M. H. Villars. Incl. Physics with Illustrative Examples from Medicine & Biology Vol. 1: Mechanics. 520p. 69.95 (*0-387-98769-X*, AIP Pr); Physics with Illustrative Examples from Medicine & Biology Vol. 2: Statistical Physics. 552p. 69.95 (*0-387-98754-1*); 2000. LC 99-33040. (Biological Physics Ser.). (Illus.). 2000. 169.00 (*0-387-98952-8*, AIP Pr) Spr-Verlag.

Physics with Illustrative Examples from Medicine & Biology G. B. Benedek & F. M. Villars. Vol. 2. 1974. 30.25 (*0-201-00551-4*); Vol. 3. 1979. pap. text 32.25 (*0-201-00559-X*) Addison-Wesley.

Physics with Illustrative Examples from Medicine & Biology Vol. 1: Mechanics George B. Benedek & Felix M. H. Villars. 2nd ed. 2000. LC 99-33040. (Biological Physics Ser.). (Illus.). 520p. 69.95 (*0-387-98769-X*, AIP Pr) Spr-Verlag.

Physics with Illustrative Examples from Medicine & Biology Vol. 2: Statistical Physics George B. Benedek & Felix M. H. Villars. 2nd ed. 2000. LC 99-33040. (Biological Physics Ser.). (Illus.). 552p. 69.95 (*0-387-98754-1*) Spr-Verlag.

Physiochemical Aspects of Medicine Reviews, Vol. 1. Yu. M. Lopukhin. 1987. xiii, 426p. text 500.00 (*3-7186-0316-0*) Gordon & Breach.

Physiognomy of Mental Diseases. Alexander Morison. 2nd ed. 1976. LC 75-16723. (Classics in Psychiatry Ser.). (Illus.). reprint ed. 25.95 (*0-405-07447-6*) Ayer.

Physiologic Basis of Obstetrics & Gynecology. David B. Seifer et al. 2001. LC 00-51990. 624p. text 110.00 (*0-683-30249-3*) Lppncott W & W.

Physiologic Basis of Surgery. Patrick J. O'Leary. Ed. by Lea R. Capote. 1993. LC 93-17306. (Illus.). 672p. 95.00 (*0-683-06634-X*) Lppncott W & W.

Physiologic Basis of Surgery. Ed. by J. Patrick O'Leary & Lea R. Capote. 2nd ed. 1996. LC 96-4702. (Illus.). 752p. 115.00 (*0-683-06616-1*) Lppncott W & W.

Physiologic Foundations of Perinatal Care. Ed. by Leo Stern et al. 1984. LC 84-24813. 398p. 78.75 (*0-275-91454-2*, C14541, Praeger Pubs) Greenwood.

Physiological Activity of the Speech Organs: An Analysis of the Speech-Organs During the Phonation of Sung, Spoken, & Whispered Czech Vowels on the Basis of X-Ray Methods. Jana Ondrackova. Tr. by D. Short from DUT. 1973. LC 72-94494. (Illus.). 105p. text (*90-279-2374-4*) Mouton.

Physiological Adaptability & Nutritional Status of the Japanese B, Vol. 4. Ed. by Asahina & R. Shigiya. 1975. (Japan International Biological Program Synthesis Ser.). 250p. (*0-86008-214-8*) U of Tokyo JPN. *Dist:* Col U Pr.

Physiological Adaptations in Vertebrates: Respiration, Circulation & Metabolism. Ed. by Stephen C. Wood et al. 1991. (Lung Biology in Health & Disease Ser.: Vol. 56). (Illus.). 432p. text 230.00 (*0-8247-8558-4*) Dekker.

Physiological & Biochemical Basis for Perinatal Medicine. Ed. by A. Minkowski & M. Monset-Couchard. 1981. (Illus.). xiv, 370p. 135.75 (*3-8055-1283-X*) S Karger.

Physiological & Biochemical Foundations of Therapeutics. Shirley D. Kraus. 1982. LC 80-67378. (Illus.). 259p. (Orig.). (C). pap. text 35.95 (*0-932126-33-2*) Graceway.

Physiological & Clinical Aspects of Short Chain Fatty Acids. Ed. by J. H. Cummings et al. 1995. (Illus.). 595p. (C). text 130.00 (*0-521-44048-3*) Cambridge U Pr.

Physiological & Medical Observations among the Indians of Southwestern United States & Northern Mexico. Ales Hrdlicka. 1995. (Bureau of American Ethnology Ser.). 460p. lib. bdg. 109.00 (*0-7812-4034-4*) Rprt Serv.

Physiological & Pathological Aspects of Eye Movements. A. Roucoux & M. Crommelinck. 1982. text 249.00 (*90-6193-730-2*) Kluwer Academic.

Physiological & Pharmacological Aspects of the Reticulo-rumen. Ed. by L. A. Ooms & A. D. Degryse. 1987. (Current Topics in Veterinary Medicine & Animal Science Ser.). (C). text 218.00 (*0-89838-878-3*) Kluwer Academic.

Physiological & Psychological Considerations in the Management of Stroke. Arnold S. Brown. 1976. LC 72-7682. 160p. 12.50 (*0-87527-094-8*) Green.

Physiological & Psychophysiological Bases for Jungian Concepts: An Annotated Bibliography. Katherine Benziger. 1996. (Illus.). 45p. pap. 15.00 (*1-880931-08-7*) KBA Pub.

Physiological Animal Ecology. Gideon N. Louw. 1992. 288p. (Orig.). (C). pap. text 48.00 net. (*0-582-05922-4*) Addison-Wesley GBR. *Dist:* Trans-Atl Phila, Longman.

Physiological Aspects of Digestion & Metabolism in Ruminants: Proceedings of the Seventh International Symposium on Ruminant Physiology. Ed. by T. Tsuda et al. 1991. (Illus.). 779p. (C). text 121.00 (*0-12-702290-2*) Acad Pr.

Physiological Aspects of Flight. Robert J. Del Vecchio. 1977. LC 77-82675. pap. 10.00 (*0-917428-05-6*, Dowling College) Global Pubns.

Physiological Aspects of the Liquor Problem John S. Billings & Wilbur O. Atwater. 1977. 42.95 (*0-8369-6965-0*, 7846) Ayer.

Physiological Assessment of Human Fitness. Ed. by Peter J. Maud & Carl Foster. 1995. LC 94-40072. (Illus.). 304p. text 52.00 (*0-87322-776-X*, BMAU0776) Human Kinetics.

Physiological Basis for Exercise & Sport. Edward L. Fox et al. 5th ed. 1993. 736p. (C). text 50.00 net. (*0-697-12626-9*) Brown & Benchmark.

Physiological Basis Musculoskeletal Therapy. David J. Magee. 1997. text (*0-7216-5982-9*) Saunders.

Physiological Basis of Aging & Geriatrics. Ed. by Paola S. Timiras. 2nd rev. ed. 1994. LC 93-44066. Orig. Title: Physiological Basis of Geriatrics. 336p. 104.95 (*0-8493-8979-8*) CRC Pr.

Physiological Basis of Anxiety. 1984. (Journal: Vol. 17, Suppl. 1). (Illus.). 120p. pap. 31.50 (*3-8055-3812-X*) S Karger.

Physiological Basis of Behaviour: Neural & Hormonal Processes. Kevin Silber. 1999. LC 98-33671. (Modular Psychology Ser.). (Illus.). xv, 144p. 50.00 (*0-415-18653-6*); pap. 13.95 (*0-415-18654-4*) Routledge.

Physiological Basis of Geriatrics see Physiological Basis of Aging & Geriatrics

Physiological Basis of Geriatrics. Paola S. Timiras. 1988. 448p. 62.95 (*0-02-420810-8*, Macmillan Coll) P-H.

Physiological Basis of Primary Care. Patrick Eggena. rev. ed. 1998. (Illus.). 734p. pap. text 59.95 (*0-9663441-0-3*) Novateur Med.

Physiological Basis of Ventilatory Support. Ed. by John J. Marini & Arthur S. Slutsky. 1998. LC 98-4262. (Lung Biology in Health & Disease Ser.). (Illus.). 1480p. text 295.00 (*0-8247-9861-9*) Dekker.

Physiological Chemistry of Domestic Animals. Rudolf Clarenburg. 1992. (Illus.). 448p. (gr. 13). pap. text 56.00 (*0-8016-6953-7*, 06953) Mosby Inc.

Physiological Chemistry of Exercise & Training. Ed. by P. E. Di Prampero & J. R. Poortmans. 1981. (Medicine & Sport Science Ser.: Vol. 13). (Illus.). viii, 216p. 85.25 (*3-8055-2028-X*) S Karger.

Physiological Chemistry of Training & Detraining. Ed. by J. R. Poortmans & P. Marconnet. 1984. (Medicine & Sport Science Ser.: Vol. 17). (Illus.). xii, 264p. 172.25 (*3-8055-3764-6*) S Karger.

Physiological Correlates of Human Behaviour, Vol. 3. Ed. by Anthony Gale & John A. Edwards. 1986. 308p. pap. text 55.00 (*0-12-273906-X*) Acad Pr.

Physiological Correspondences. John Worcester. 1987. (Illus.). 432p. reprint ed. 16.95 (*0-915221-64-0*) Swedenborg Sci Assn.

Physiological Measurements with Radionuclides in Clinical Practice. A. M. Peters & M. J. Myers. 1998. LC 97-21585. (Illus.). 318p. text 73.00 (*0-19-261994-2*) OUP.

Physiological Medicine. Vishwanath R. Lingappa. 2000. LC 00-29194. (Illus.). 1008p. pap. 49.95 (*0-07-038128-3*) McGraw-Hill Prof.

Physiological Origins of Heart Sounds & Murmurs CD-ROM. J. Michael Criley. 1995. 149.95 (*0-316-16154-3*, Little Brwn Med Div) Lppncott W & W.

Physiological Peptides & New Trends in Radioimmunology. Ed. by C. A. Bizollon. 1984. 370p. 136.25 (*0-444-80358-0*) Elsevier.

Physiological Pharmaceutics. Clive G. Wilson & Neena Washington. 1989. 186p. 69.95 (*0-470-21545-3*) P-H.

Physiological Psychology. Mark R. Rosenzweig & Arnold L. Leiman. 1989. 640p. (C). stu. ed. 10.50 (*0-394-37617-X*); text 32.95 (*0-394-37237-9*) Random.

Physiological Psychology: Neuroscience Approach. 1998. (*0-13-020570-2*) P-H.

Physiological Psychology: Study Guide. Robert B. Graham. 1990. (Psychology Ser.). mass mkt., stu. ed. 19.50 (*0-534-10105-4*) Brooks-Cole.

Physiological Psychology Dictionary: A Reference Guide for Students & Professionals. George S. Grosser & Carol S. Spafford. 1994. LC 94-18010. 368p. (C). pap. 20.00 (*0-07-059860-6*) McGrw-H Hghr Educ.

Physiological Researches on Life & Death. Marie F. Bichat. Ed. by Robert J. Kastenbaum. Tr. by F. Gold et al. 1977. LC 76-19561. (Death & Dying Ser.). reprint ed. lib. bdg. 33.95 (*0-405-09557-0*) Ayer.

Physiological Researches on Life & Death, 2. Xavier Bichat. Tr. by F. Gold from FRE. 1978. LC 77-72191. (Contributions to the History of Psychology Ser.: Vol. II, Pt. E, Physiological Psychology). 302p. reprint ed. lib. bdg. 89.50 (*0-313-26950-5*, U6950, Greenwood Pr) Greenwood.

Physiological Signal Processing, Modelling & System Implementation in Cardiography, Speech & Hearing. R. H. Mitchell. 1994. 201p. pap. text 196.00 (*2-88124-991-4*) Gordon & Breach.

Physiological Strategies for Gas Exchange & Metabolism. Ed. by A. J. Woakes et al. 1991. (Society for Experimental Biology Seminar Ser.: No. 41). (Illus.). 281p. (C). text 80.00 (*0-521-36602-X*) Cambridge U Pr.

Physiological Testing of the High-Performance Athlete. Ed. by J. Duncan MacDougall et al. 2nd ed. 1990. LC 90-35488. 448p. text 48.00 (*0-87322-300-4*, BMAC0300) Human Kinetics.

Physiological Tremor, Pathological Tremor & Clonus. Ed. by J. E. Desmedt. 1978. (Progress in Clinical Neurophysiology Ser.: Vol. 5). (Illus.). 85.25 (*3-8055-2713-6*) S Karger.

Physiological Variation & Its Genetic Basis. Ed. by J. S. Weiner. 1977. (Symposia of the Society for the Study of Human Biology Ser.: Vol. 17). 180p. 36.00 (*0-85066-108-0*) Taylor & Francis.

Physiology. Linda S. Costanzo. Ed. by William Schmitt. 1998. LC 97-28809. (Text & Review Ser.). (Illus.). 416p. pap. text 29.95 (*0-7216-6611-6*) Saunders.

Physiology. Montani. 1997. pap. text (*0-7216-5058-9*) Saunders.

Physiology. Ed. by R. Theis & Robert J. Person. 1991. (Oklahoma Notes). viii, 263p. pap. 17.95 (*0-387-97039-8*) Spr-Verlag.

Physiology. Ed. by R. Thies & Robert J. Person. 1988. (Oklahoma Notes). 237p. (C). 15.95 (*0-387-96340-5*) Spr-Verlag.

Physiology. John F. Fulton. LC 75-23655. (Clio Medica Ser.: 5). (Illus.). reprint ed. 34.50 (*0-404-58905-7*) AMS Pr.

Physiology. Paulev. rev. ed. 1996. pap. text, stu. ed. 26.00 (*0-7020-2043-5*) Saunders.

Physiology. J. Bullock et al. 2nd ed. 1991. (National Medical Ser.). (Illus.). 501p. 25.00 (*0-683-06258-1*) Lppncott W & W.

Physiology. Linda S. Costanzo. 2nd ed. 1998. LC 98-7540. (Board Review Ser.). 315p. pap. text 28.95 (*0-683-30396-1*) Lppncott W & W.

Physiology. Robert M. Berne et al. 4th ed. 1998. LC 97-38215. (Illus.). 1232p. (C). (gr. 13). text 60.00 (*0-8151-0952-0*, 31012) Mosby Inc.

Physiology. Roger Thies. 4th ed. 1995. LC 94-45261. (Oklahoma Notes). (Illus.). 280p. 24.95 (*0-387-94397-8*) Spr-Verlag.

Physiology. Ewald E. Selkurt. 5th ed. 1984. 691p. 34.00 (*0-316-78038-3*, Little Brwn Med Div) Lppncott W & W.

Physiology: 2000 Multiple-Choice Questions & Answers. 1999. 298p. spiral bd. 25.95 (*1-893720-02-0*) Biotest.

Physiology: Digging up the Bones, Vol. 8. Nikos M. Linardakis. 1998. LC 98-10208. (Digging Up the Bones Ser.). (Illus.). 350p. pap. 19.95 (*0-07-038221-2*) McGraw-Hill Prof.

Physiology: MEPC. David G. Penney. 9th ed. 1996. (Illus.). 255p. (C). pap. text 21.95 (*0-8385-6222-1*, A6222-2, Apple Lange Med) McGraw.

Physiology: Multiple Choice Questions for the FRCS. McDiarmid. 1995. 80p. pap. 14.95 (*0-340-59435-7*) Trafalgar.

Physiology: Review for New National Boards. Emma R. Jakoi & Ronald C. Bohn. 1994. LC 94-75277. (Illus.). 230p. pap. 25.00 (*0-9632873-4-6*) J & S Pub VA.

Physiology: Scientific Basis Physics. Bovell. 1995. pap. text 41.50 (*0-7020-1936-4*) Saunders.

***Physiology: Self-Assessment & Review.** Michael B. Wang & James P. Ryan. 10th ed. 2001. LC 2001-31483. (Pretest Self-Assessment & Review Ser.). (Illus.). 316p. pap. 24.95 (*0-07-137199-0*) McGraw-Hill Prof.

Physiology: The Basis of Clinical Practice. Glenn Irion. 2000. LC 00-26535. (Illus.). 432p. text 35.00 (*1-55642-380-2*) SLACK Inc.

Physiology: The Basis of Clinical Practice Instructor's Manual. Glenn Irion. 2000. 96p. pap. text, tchr. ed. (*1-55642-424-8*) SLACK Inc.

Physiology & Anatomy. 736p. pap. (*0-340-63190-2*) E A GBR. *Dist:* Routldge.

Physiology & Anatomy: A Basis for Nursing & Health Care. Sigrid Rutishauser. 1994. LC 94-27137. (C). pap. text (*0-443-04151-2*) Church.

Physiology & Anatomy: A Homeostatic Approach. John Clancy & Andrew McVicar. 1995. (Illus.). 736p. (Orig.). pap. text 47.99 (*1-56593-614-0*, 1274) Singular Publishing.

Physiology & Applied Anatomy for Veterinary Nurses. College of Animal Welfare Staff. 2005. (Illus.). 500p. pap. 49.50 (*0-7506-4802-3*) Buttrwrth-Heinemann.

Physiology & Behavior Therapy: Conceptual Guidelines for the Clinician. J. G. Hollandsworth, Jr. 1986. (Behavioral Psychophysiology Ser.). (Illus.). 256p. (C). 49.50 (*0-306-42180-1*, Plenum Trade) Perseus Pubng.

Physiology & Biochemistry of Exercise. Roy J. Shephard. 1982. LC 84-24862. 560p. 95.00 (*0-275-91380-5*, C1380, Praeger Pubs) Greenwood.

Physiology & Biochemistry of Plant-Pathogen Interactions. I. J. Misaghi. 1982. LC 82-18594. 304p. (C). 65.00 (*0-306-41059-1*, Plenum Trade) Perseus Pubng.

Physiology & Biochemistry of the Domestic Fowl, Vol. 4. Ed. by B. M. Freeman. 1983. text 157.00 (*0-12-267104-X*) Acad Pr.

Physiology & Biochemistry of the Uterus in Pregnancy & Labor. Ed. by Gabor Huszar. 1985. 328p. 187.00 (*0-8493-5997-X*, RG558, CRC Reprint) Franklin.

Physiology & Form of Fish Circulation. Geoffrey H. Satchell. 1991. (Illus.). 253p. (C). text 74.95 (*0-521-39519-4*) Cambridge U Pr.

Physiology & Growth, Vol. 1. Norman Kretchmer et al. 1987. x, 350p. text 195.00 (*3-7186-0344-6*) Gordon & Breach.

Physiology & Medicine of Diving. Peter B. Bennett & David H. Elliott. 1993. (Illus.). 613p. (C). pap. 84.00 (*0-941332-02-0*, D088) Best Pub Co.

Physiology & Medicine of Diving. Ed. by Peter B. Bennett & David H. Elliott. 4th ed. 1993. (Illus.). 624p. text (*0-7020-1589-X*) W B Saunders GBR. *Dist:* Saunders.

Physiology & Pathology of Interferon System. Ed. by L. Borecky & V. Lackovic. 1984. (Beitraege Zur Onkologie, Contributions to Oncology Ser.: Vol. 20). (Illus.). x, 390p. 68.75 (*3-8055-3839-1*) S Karger.

Physiology & Pathology of Mind Henry Maudsley. 3rd enl. rev. ed. LC 78-72810. reprint ed. 75.00 (*0-404-60878-7*) AMS Pr.

Physiology & Pathology of the Human Diencephalon. Ed. by N. I. Grashchenkov & G. N. Kasil. 1964. 424p. text 94.50 (*0-7065-0567-0*) Coronet Bks.

Physiology & Pathology of the Mind, 4. Henry Maudsley. 1977. LC 77-72191. (Contributions to the History of Psychology Ser.: Pt. C, Vol. IV, Medical Psychology). 442p. reprint ed. lib. bdg. 83.50 (*0-313-26943-2*, U6943, Greenwood Pr) Greenwood.

Physiology & Pathology of the Mucociliary System: Special Regards to Mucociliary Transport in Malignant Lesions of the Human Larynx. T. Deitmer. 1989. (Advances in OtoRhinoLaryngology Ser.: Vol. 43). (Illus.). x, 136p. 115.00 (*3-8055-4944-X*) S Karger.

Physiology & Pathology of the Newborn. A. N. Antonov. 1945. (SRCD M Ser.: Vol. 10, No. 2). 25.00 (*0-527-01535-0*) Periodicals Srv.

Physiology & Pathophysiology of Exercise Tolerance: Proceedings of an International Symposium Held in Ulm, Germany, September 21-24, 1994. Ed. by Jurgen M. Steinacker & Susan A. Ward. 1997. LC 96-39630. 346p. (C). text 95.00 (*0-306-45492-0*, Kluwer Plenum) Kluwer Academic.

Physiology & Pathophysiology of Leukcoyte Adhesion. Ed. by D. Neil Granger & Geert W. Schmid-Schonbein. 1995. LC 93-44619. (Illus.). 520p. text 89.50 (*0-19-508102-1*) OUP.

Physiology & Pathophysiology of the Endothelium: 15th Annual Meeting of the German Society for Clinical Microcirculation & Hemorheology, Dortmund, October 1996. Ed. by G. Siegel & Rolf K. Kinne. 1997. (International Journal of Microcirculation Ser.: Vol. 17, No. 5, 1997). (Illus.). 72p. pap. 38.25 (*3-8055-6607-7*) S Karger.

Physiology & Pathophysiology of the Heart. Ed. by Nicholas Sperelakis. (Developments in Cardiovascular Medicine Ser.). 1984. text 427.50 (*0-89838-615-2*); 2nd ed. 1988. 1040p. (C). text 427.50 (*0-89838-388-9*) Kluwer Academic.

Physiology & Pathophysiology of the Islets of Langerhans: Proceedings of the 1st International Meeting of the Pancreatic Islet Study Group Held in Alicante, Spain, November, 25-28, 1994. Ed. by Bernat Soria. 1998. LC 97-27991. (Advances in Experimental Medicine & Biology Ser.: Vol. 426). (Illus.). 468p. 150.00 (*0-306-45702-4*, Kluwer Plenum) Kluwer Academic.

Physiology & Pharmacology for the Anaesthetist. Kumar. 320p. pap. text (*0-340-56758-9*) E A GBR. *Dist:* Routldge.

Physiology & Pharmacology of Biological Rhythms. F. Andreotti et al. 1997. LC 96-2935. (Handbook of Experimental Pharmacology Ser.). (Illus.). 712p. 445.00 (*3-540-61525-3*) Spr-Verlag.

Physiology & Pharmacology of Bone. Ed. by Gregory R. Mundy & T. John Martin. 1993. LC 92-42565. (Handbook of Experimental Pharmacology Ser.: Vol. 107). (Illus.). 762p. 500.00 (*0-387-56293-1*) Spr-Verlag.

Physiology & Pharmacology of Cardio-Respiratory Control. Albert Dahan & Johannes H. Van Beek. Ed. by Luc Teppema. 1998. LC 98-22537. 59.00 (*0-7923-5135-5*) Kluwer Academic.

Physiology & Pharmacology of the Blood-Brain Barrier. Ed. by W. B. Bradury et al. 1992. LC 92-2227. (Handbook of Experimental Pharmacology Ser.: Vol. 103). (Illus.). 520p. 345.00 (*3-540-54492-5*); 549p. 369.00 (*0-387-54492-5*) Spr-Verlag.

Physiology & Pharmacology of the Heart. Hilary F. Brown & Roland Kozlowski. 1997. LC 96-18670. (Illus.). 126p. pap. 38.95 (*0-86542-722-4*) Blackwell Sci.

Physiology & Social Nutrition & Nutritional Education. Ed. by Geoffrey H. Bourne. 1982. (World Review of Nutrition & Dietetics Ser.: Vol. 38). (Illus.). x, 230p. 141.75 (*3-8055-3048-X*) S Karger.

Physiology & Technology of Reproduction in Female Domestic Animals. R. H. Hunter. 1981. text 178.00 (*0-12-361950-5*) Acad Pr.

***Physiology Cases & Problems.** Linda S. Costanzo. 2001. LC 2001-30010. (Board Review Ser.). (Illus.). xi, 338p. pap. text 22.00 (*0-7817-2482-1*) Lppncott W & W.

Physiology Coloring Book. Elson Kapit. 2nd ed. 1999. (Illus.). 320p. pap. text 19.99 (*0-321-03663-8*) Addison-Wesley.

Physiology for Health Care Students. Judy L. Hubbard & Derek J. Mechan. 1987. LC 86-23312. (Illus.). 344p. (Orig.). (C). pap. text (*0-443-02123-6*) Church.

Physiology for Nursing Practitioners. Hinchliff. 2nd ed. 1996. pap. text 44.00 (*0-7020-1638-1*) Saunders.

Physiology in Industry: Eval. Ind. Stresses Physiological Reactions of the Worker, Vol. 4. L. Brouha & J. Zapp. 2nd ed. 1960. LC 60-8058. (International Series of Monographs on Pure & Applied Mathematics). (*0-08-011703-1*) Pergamon Repr GBR. *Dist:* Franklin.

Physiology in Surgical Practice. 448p. (*0-7131-4558-7*) E A GBR. *Dist:* Routldge.

Physiology Monitor & Therapy of the Critically Ill Patient: Proceedings of the International Symposium on Acute Care, 5th, Rio de Janeiro, Sao Paulo, November, 1976. International Symposium on Acute Care Staff. Ed. by W. C. Shoemaker & B. M. Tavares. 1977. (Current Topics in Critical Care Medicine Ser.: Vol. 3). (Illus.). 49.75 (*3-8055-2652-0*) S Karger.

Physiology of Adrenocortical Secretion. T. Suzuki. 1983. (Frontiers of Hormone Research Ser.: Vol. 11). (Illus.). viii, 216p. 115.00 (*3-8055-3644-5*) S Karger.

Physiology of ALS & Related Diseases. Jun Kimura & Ryuji Kaji. 1997. LC 97-2859. 248p. 154.50 (*0-444-82557-6*); 252p. pap. 89.50 (*0-444-82668-8*) Elsevier.

Physiology of Behavior. 7th ed. 2000. 720p. (C). 0.00 (*0-205-32407-X*) Allyn.

Physiology of Blood & Lymph Vessels: Proceedings of the Symposia Angiologica Santoriana, 3rd International Symposium, Fribourg, 1970 Symposia Angiologica Santoriana Staff. Ed. by M. Comel & L. Lastz. 1972. 67.50 (*3-8055-1263-5*);Pt. 1. pap. text 52.75 (*3-8055-2472-2*);Pt. 2. pap. text 35.75 (*3-8055-1289-9*); (*3-8055-1726-2*) S Karger.

Physiology of Cell Aging. Ed. by V. V. Frolkis. 1984. (Interdisciplinary Topics in Gerontology Ser.: Vol. 18). (Illus.). viii, 208p. 142.75 (*3-8055-3866-9*) S Karger.

Physiology of Diuretic Action. Ed. by F. P. Lang. 1988. (Journal: Vol. 10, No. 3, 1987). 92p. pap. 49.75 (*3-8055-4769-2*) S Karger.

Physiology of Domestic Animals. William O. Reece. (Illus.). 1990. LC 90-5543. 372p. pap. text 39.50 (*0-8121-1307-1*); 2nd ed. 1997. LC 96-18088. 484p. 49.95 (*0-683-07240-4*) Lppncott W & W.

Physiology of Exercise & Sport, No. 2. Noble. 1991. (Illus.). 608p. 37.95 (*0-8016-3342-7*) Mosby Inc.

Physiology of Growth & Nutrition. Ed. by Miloslav Rechcigl, Jr. 1981. (Comparative Animal Nutrition Ser.: Vol. 4). (Illus.). xii, 344p. pap. 216.75 (*3-8055-1199-X*) S Karger.

Physiology of Health & Illness: With Related Anatomy. L. Hubbard & D. J. Mechan. 1999. 704p. pap. text (*0-7487-3173-3*) Nelson Thornes GBR. *Dist:* Intl Spec Bk, Trans-Atl Phila.

Physiology of Hemostasis. Derek Ogston. 1983. (Illus.). 390p. (C). 51.95 (*0-674-66660-7*) HUP.

Physiology of Human Placenta. Page. 1993. 192p. (*1-85728-065-2*); pap. (*1-85728-066-0*) UCL Pr Ltd GBR. *Dist:* Taylor & Francis.

Physiology of Immunity. Ed. by James A. Marsh & Marion D. Kendall. 1996. 464p. 139.95 (*0-8493-8033-2*) CRC Pr.

Physiology of Inflammation. Ed. by Klaus Ley. 2000. LC 00-35946. (Methods in Physiology Ser.). (Illus.). 560p. text 95.00 (*0-19-512829-X*) OUP.

Physiology of Joints, Vol. 1. I. A. Kapandji & Matthew J. Kandel. 5th ed. 1982. (Upper Limb Ser.: Vol. 1). 208p. pap. text (*0-443-02504-5*) Church.

Physiology of Joints, Vol. 3. I. A. Kapandji. Tr. by L. H. Honore. 2nd ed. 1974. (Trunk & Vertebral Column Ser.: Vol. 3). 256p. pap. text (*0-443-01209-1*) Church.

Physiology of Mammary Glands. Lewis G. Sheffield. 1999. 60.00 (*0-8493-8760-4*) CRC Pr.

Physiology of Marriage. William A. Alcott. 1972. LC 79-180551. (Medicine & Society in America Ser.). 266p. reprint ed. 20.95 (*0-405-03931-X*) Ayer.

Physiology of Membrane Disorders. Ed. by Thomas E. Andreoli et al. 2nd ed. 1986. LC 85-19367. (Illus.). 1094p. 234.00 (*0-306-41774-X*, Kluwer Plenum) Kluwer Academic.

Physiology of Membrane Fluidity Meir Shinitzky. 1984. 208p. 120.00 (*0-8493-6141-9*, QH601); Vol. II. 1985. 144p. 88.00 (*0-8493-6142-7*) Franklin (CRC Reprint).

Physiology of Oral Tissues. Ed. by Yojiro Kawamura. 1976. (Frontiers of Oral Physiology Ser.: Vol. 2). (Illus.). 350p. 101.00 (*3-8055-1360-7*) S Karger.

Physiology of Physical Stress: A Selective Bibliography, 1500-1964. Carl B. Chapman & Elinor C. Reinmiller. 1974. LC 74-15565. 376p. 51.95 (*0-674-66670-4*) HUP.

Physiology of Psychological Disorders: Schizophrenia, Depression, Anxiety, & Substance Abuse. J. G. Hollandsworth, Jr. 1990. LC 89-26559. (Behavioral Psychophysiology & Medicine Ser.). (Illus.). 336p. (C). 49.50 (*0-306-43353-2*, Plenum Trade) Perseus Pubng.

Physiology of Spinal Anesthesia. Nicholas M. Greene & Sorin J. Brull. 4th ed. 1993. LC 92-5578. (Illus.). 387p. 78.00 (*0-683-03555-X*) Lppncott W & W.

Physiology of Sport & Exercise Study Guide. Christine M. Drews & Jack H. Wilmore. 2nd ed. 1999. LC 99-22719. 368p. pap. text 18.00 (*0-7360-0090-9*) Human Kinetics.

Physiology of Stress: With Special Reference to the Neuroendocrine System. Mary F. Asterita. 1984. 240p. (C). pap. 22.95 (*0-89885-187-4*); text 42.95 (*0-89885-176-9*) Kluwer Academic (Kluwer Acad Hman Sci).

Physiology of Synapses. John C. Eccles. 1964. (Illus.). reprint ed. 61.95 (*0-387-03112-X*) Spr-Verlag.

Physiology of Taste: Or, Meditations on Transcendental Gastronomy. Jean Anthelme Brillat-Savarin. 1982. (Illus.). 350p. reprint ed. pap. 9.95 (*0-918172-11-X*) Leetes Isl.

Physiology of the Digestive Tract. Horace W. Davenport. 5th ed. 1982. (Illus.). 32.95 (*0-8151-2330-2*) Mosby Inc.

Physiology of the Eye. H. Davson. 5th ed. 1990. (Illus.). 750p. (*0-08-037907-9*) PPI GBR. *Dist:* McGraw.

Physiology of the Fetal & Neonatal Lung. Ed. by D. V. Walters et al. 1987. text 200.50 (*0-85200-948-8*) Kluwer Academic.

Physiology of the Gastrointestinal Tract Ed. by Leonard R. Johnson et al. 3rd ed. 1994. LC 93-6429. 2,320p. text 475.00 (*0-7817-0132-5*) Lppncott W & W.

Physiology of the Heart. Arnold M. Katz. 3rd ed. 2000. LC 00-57612. 736p. text 99.00 (*0-7817-1548-2*) Lppncott W & W.

Physiology of the Lower Urinary Tract. Ed. by M. J. Torrens & J. F. Morrison. 1987. (Illus.). 355p. 249.00 (*0-387-17486-9*) Spr-Verlag.

Physiology of Thirst & Sodium Appetite. Ed. by G. De Caro et al. 1986. LC 86-4982. (NATO ASI Series A, Life Sciences: Vol. 105). 586p. 125.00 (*0-306-42265-4*, Plenum Trade) Perseus Pubng.

Physiology, Pharmacology & Development of Epileptogenic Phenomena. Ed. by M. R. Klee et al. 1991. (Experimental Brain Research Ser.: Vol. 20). (Illus.). 288p. 79.95 (*0-387-53664-7*) Spr-Verlag.

Physiology Review Book. Montoni. Date not set. pap. text (*0-7216-5177-1*) Saunders.

Physiology, Stress & Malnutrition: Functional Correlates, Nutritional Intervention. John M. Kinney & Hugh N. Tucker. 1997. LC 96-51070. 688p. text 75.00 (*0-397-58763-5*) Lppncott W & W.

Physiology 250: A Study Guide. Patrick Dillon. 1993. (C). stu. ed. 12.00 (*1-881592-46-4*) Hayden-McNeil.

Physiopathological Processes of Aging: Towards a Multicasual Interpretation. Ed. by Nicola Fabris et al. 1992. LC 92-48196. (Annals Ser.: Vol. 673). (*0-89766-743-3*); pap. 90.00 (*0-89766-744-1*) NY Acad Sci.

Physiopathology of Cancer Vol. 2: Diagnosis, Treatment, Prevention. Ed. by H. Hamburger. 1976. 50.50 (*3-8055-1623-1*) S Karger.

Physiopathology of the Cardiovascular System. Joseph S. Alpert. 1984. 348p. 31.95 (*0-316-03504-1*, Little Brwn Med Div) Lppncott W & W.

Physiotherapy: A Psychosocial Approach. Sally French. 2nd ed. 1997. LC 96-37310. 464p. pap. text 45.00 (*0-7506-2608-9*) Buttrwrth-Heinemann.

Physiotherapy: Controlled Trials & Facts. Ed. by P. Schlapbach & N. Gerber. 1991. (Rheumatology, the Interdisciplinary Concept Ser.: Vol. 14). (Illus.). x, 252p. 85.25 (*3-8055-5234-3*) S Karger.

Physiotherapy & the Growing Child. Ed. by Yvonne R. Burns & Julie MacDonald. 1996. (Illus.). 529p. text (*0-7020-1942-9*) W B Saunders GBR. *Dist:* Saunders.

Physiotherapy Assessment. Anne Parry. 2nd ed. 1985. LC 85-4615. 168p. (Orig.). pap. (*0-7099-4009-2*) C Helm GBR. *Dist:* Routldge.

Physiotherapy for Amputees: The Roehampton Approach. Ed. by Barbara Engstrom & Catherine Van de Ven. 3rd ed. 1999. (C). text (*0-443-05975-6*) Church.

Physiotherapy for Respiratory & Cardiac Problems. Ed. by J. A. Pryor & B. A. Webber. 2nd ed. 1998. (Illus.). 556p. pap. (*0-443-05841-5*) Church.

Physiotherapy in Paediatrics. Roberta B. Shepherd. 3rd ed. 1995. (Illus.). 432p. pap. text 50.00 (*0-7506-0620-7*) Buttrwrth-Heinemann.

Physiotherapy in Respiratory Care: A Problem-Solving Approach to Respiratory & Cardiac Management. Alexandra Hough. 2nd ed. 1995. 352p. pap. 45.00 (*1-56593-131-9*, 1241) Singular Publishing.

Physiotherapy Management of Haemophilia. Brenda Buzzard & Karen Beeton. 2000. LC 00-39740. (Illus.). 168p. pap. 46.95 (*0-632-05764-5*) Blackwell Sci.

Physiotherapy with Older People. Pickles. 1995. pap. text 62.00 (*0-7020-1931-3*) Saunders.

Physique & Intellect. Donald G. Paterson. 1970. LC 73-98866. 304p. reprint ed. lib. bdg. 68.50 (*0-8371-2886-2*, PAPI, Greenwood Pr) Greenwood.

Physique et Physiciens en France, 1918-1940. D. Pestre. 2nd ed. 1992. (FRE.). xvi, 356p. pap. text 60.00 (*2-903928-08-8*) Gordon & Breach.

Physique, Fitness & Performance. Thomas Battinelli. 2000. LC 99-86251. (Exercise Physiology Ser.). 288p. 99.95 (*0-8493-0231-5*) CRC Pr.

Physique, Personality & Scholarship. N. R. Sanford et al. 1974. (Society for Research in Child Development Monographs: Vol. 8, No. 1). reprint ed. 65.00 (*0-527-01526-1*) Periodicals Srv.

Phyto-Aromatherapy in Clinical Practice. Gabriel Mojay. 2001. 256p. pap. 55.00 (*0-7506-4001-4*) Buttrwrth-Heinemann.

Phyto Paper No. 32: Status of Eutypa Lata as a Pathogen. M. V. Carter. 1991. (Illus.). 70p. (C). pap. text 38.00 (*0-85198-695-1*) C A B I Pub.

Phytochemical Resources for Medicine & Agriculture. H. N. Nigg & D. Seigler. 1992. LC 92-20152. (Illus.). 454p. (C). text 135.00 (*0-306-44245-0*, Kluwer Plenum) Kluwer Academic.

Phytochemicals in Human Health Protection, Nutrition & Plant Defense. Ed. by John T. Romeo. 1999. LC 99-37365. (Recent Advances in Phytochemistry Ser.). (C). text (*0-306-46203-6*, Kluwer Plenum) Kluwer Academic.

Phytochemistry of Plants Used in Traditional Medicine. Ed. by K. Hostettmann et al. 1995. (Proceedings of the Phytochemical Society of Europe Ser.: No. 37). (Illus.). 422p. text 145.00 (*0-19-857775-3*) OUP.

***Phytogenic Hormone Solution: Hormone Therapy the Natural Way.** Saundra Koke McKenna. 2002. 240p. pap. 12.95 (*0-8129-9196-6*) Random Trade.

Phytomedicines of Europe: Chemistry & Biological Activity. Ed. by Larry D. Lawson & Rudloph Bauer. 1998. (ACS Symposium Ser.: No. 691). (Illus.). 336p. text 125.00 (*0-8412-3559-7*) OUP.

Phytotherapy in Paediatrics: Handbook for Physicians & Pharmacists. Heinz Schilcher. Tr. by A.R. Meuss from GER. 2nd rev. ed. 1997. 181p. (C). pap. text (*3-88763-026-2*) Medpharm Sci Pubs DEU. *Dist:* Medicina Bio.

Phytotherapy of Chronic Fatigue Syndrome: Evidence-Based & Potentially Useful Botanicals in the Treatment of CFS. Roberto Patarca-Montero. 2000. LC 00-33544. viii, 94p. lib. bdg. 59.95 (*0-7890-0908-0*, Hawrth Medical) Haworth Pr.

Phytotherapy of Chronic Fatigue Syndrome: Evidence-Based & Potentially Useful Botanicals in the Treatment of CFS. Ed. by Roberto Patarca-Montero. 2000. LC 00-33544. viii, 94p. pap. 19.95 (*0-7890-0909-9*, Hawrth Medical) Haworth Pr.

Piaget & Knowledge: Theoretical Foundations. Hans G. Furth. 1995. LC 80-26284. 302p. pap. text 9.00 (*0-226-27420-9*) U Ch Pr.

Piaget & the Foundations of Knowledge. Ed. by Lynn Liben. 1984. 272p. text 59.95 (*0-89859-248-8*) L Erlbaum Assocs.

Piaget, Philosophy & the Human Sciences. Hugh J. Silverman. 1997. LC 97-2643. 185p. pap. 21.00 (*0-8101-1497-6*) Northwestern U Pr.

Piaget Primer: How a Child Thinks. Dorothy G. Singer & Tracey A. Revenson. var. ed. 1996. LC 96-1932. 160p. (C). pap. 12.95 (*0-452-27565-2*) Dutton Plume.

Piaget Systematized. Gilbert Voyat. 1982. (Illus.). 240p. text 49.95 (*0-89859-026-4*) L Erlbaum Assocs.

Piagetian Dimensions of Clinical Relevance. Hugh Rosen. 1985. LC 85-2608. 320p. text 64.50 (*0-231-06076-9*) Col U Pr.

Piaget's Babies: The First Two Years of Life: Child Development for the Intellectual. Joanne Burnett. 1995. 200p. (Orig.). pap. 21.95 (*0-9647389-0-2*) J Burnett.

Piaget's Construction of the Child's Reality. Susan Sugarman. 1990. (Illus.). 266p. (C). pap. text 18.95 (*0-521-37967-9*) Cambridge U Pr.

Piaget's Theory of Cognitive & Affective Development. Barry J. Wadsworth. 5th ed. 1995. 176p. (C). pap. text (*0-8013-1698-7*) Addison-Wesley.

Piaget's Theory of Cognitive & Affective Development: Foundations of Constructivism. Barry J. Wadsworth. 5th ed. 1995. LC 95-14394. 195p. (C). pap. 53.33 (*0-8013-0773-2*) Longman.

Picasso's Woman: A Breast Cancer Story. Rosalind MacPhee. Ed. by Deborah Baker. 1996. LC 95-42781. 288p. 20.00 (*1-56836-138-6*) Kodansha.

Pickard's Manual of Operative Dentistry. E. A. Kidd et al. 6th ed. 1990. (Illus.). 208p. pap. text 56.95 (*0-19-261808-3*) OUP.

Pickard's Manual of Operative Dentistry. E. A. Kidd & B. G. Smith. 7th ed. 1996. (Illus.). 208p. (C). text 124.50 (*0-19-262610-8*); pap. text 59.50 (*0-19-262609-4*) OUP.

Pick's Disease & Pick Complex. Andrew Kertesz & David G. Munoz. 1998. LC 97-34191. 301p. 105.00 (*0-471-17792-X*) Wiley.

Pickwells Binocular Vision Anomalies: Investigation & Treatment. Bruce J. W. Evans. 3rd ed. 1997. LC 96-24277. 280p. text 70.00 (*0-7506-2062-5*) Buttrwrth-Heinemann.

Pickwickian & Other Stories of Intensive Care: Medical & Ethical Challenges in the ICU. Lawrence Martin. 1991. LC 91-61828. 247p. pap. 10.95 (*1-879653-04-4*) Lakeside Pr.

Pictorial Anatomy of the Cat. Stephen G. Gilbert. rev. ed. 1975. LC 67-21200. (Illus.). 128p. (C). pap. 20.00 (*0-295-95454-X*) U of Wash Pr.

Pictorial Dogfish, Anatomy. S. Gilbert. 1973. LC 74-152331. (Illus.). 66p. (Orig.). (C). pap. 20.00 (*0-295-95148-6*) U of Wash Pr.

Pictorial Encyclopedia of Civil War Medical Instruments & Equipment. Gordon Dammann. (Illus.). 1983. LC 83-80357. 104p. pap. 9.95 (*0-933126-32-8*); Vol. II. 1988. LC 88-60472. 96p. pap. 8.95 (*0-933126-94-8*) Pictorial Hist.

Pictorial Fetal Pig Anatomy. S. Gilbert. 2nd rev. ed. 1966. LC 63-10797. (Illus.). 96p. (C). pap. 20.00 (*0-295-73877-4*) U of Wash Pr.

Pictorial Handbook of Anatomy & Physiology. James Bevan. 1994. (Illus.). 96p. pap. text 17.50 (*1-85732-392-0*) Buttrwrth-Heinemann.

Pictorial History, 1846-1966: School of Medicine & Biomedical Sciences, University at Buffalo. Ronald E. Batt et al. 1996. LC 95-47775. (*0-89865-963-9*) Donning Co.

Pictorial History of Blood Practices & Transfusion. A. Matthew Gottlieb. 1994. (Illus.). 399p. 99.00 (*0-9641510-0-6*) Arcane Publns.

Pictorial History of European Medicine & Pharmaceutics. J. Antall. 1981. 55.00 (*0-7855-1605-0*) St Mut.

Pictorial History of Medicine. Otto L. Bettmann. 1979. (Illus.). 336p. 50.95 (*0-398-00149-9*) C C Thomas.

Pictorial Information Systems in Medicine. Ed. by K. H. Hohne. 1986. (NATO ASI Ser.: Vol. 19). 525p. 217.00 (*0-387-13921-4*) Spr-Verlag.

Pictorial Review of Pediatrics: Acute Care & Emergency Medicine. Gary R. Fleisher et al. 1997. LC 97-28142. (Illus.). 390p. pap. 85.00 (*0-683-30267-1*) Lppncott W & W.

Picture Archiving & Communication Systems in Medical Imaging. H. K. Huang. 1995. LC 95-38928. (Illus.). 400p. 146.00 (*1-56081-685-6*, Wiley-VCH) Wiley.

Picture Archiving & Communication Systems (PACS) in Medicine. Ed. by H. K. Huang et al. 1991. (NATO ASI Ser.: Vol. 74). (Illus.). 438p. 123.00 (*0-387-53916-6*) Spr-Verlag.

Picture Test in Ophthalmology. Jack J. Kanski. 2nd ed. 1997. (Illus.). 166p. pap. text 16.95 (*0-443-06037-1*) Saunders.

Picture Tests & Short Cases for the MRCP. Debra King. 1996. (Illus.). 315p. pap. text (*0-7020-1815-5*) W B Saunders GBR. *Dist:* Saunders.

Picture Tests for the MRCP (Paediatrics) Adam Craig & Keith Brownlee. 1997. (Illus.). 235p. pap. text (*0-7020-2163-6*) W B Saunders GBR. *Dist:* Saunders.

Picture Tests in Anatomy. Robert M. McMinn et al. 1986. (Illus.). 128p. (C). (gr. 13). 15.95 (*0-8151-5836-X*, 09146) Mosby Inc.

Picture Tests in Haematology. Barbara J. Bain. 1999. LC 98-10014. (Colour Guide Ser.). pap. text (*0-443-05943-8*) Church.

Picture Tests in Obstetrics. Rymer. 1994. pap. text 16.95 (*0-443-04950-5*) Saunders.

Pictures at an Exhibition: Selected Essays on Art & Art Therapy. Ed. by Andrea Gilroy & Tessa Dalley. 1989. 240p. 48.00 (*0-415-00136-6*, A3500) Routledge.

Pictures of Health: A Photographic History of Health Care in Philadelphia, 1860-1945. Janet Golden & Charles E. Rosenberg. 1991. LC 90-22745. (Studies in Health, Illness, & Caregiving). (Illus.). 224p. (C). pap. 32.95 (*0-8122-1311-4*); text 52.50 (*0-8122-8237-X*) U of Pa Pr.

Pictures of the Body: Pain & Metamorphosis. James Elkins. 1999. LC 99-27632. (Illus.). xviii, 347p. pap. 29.95 (*0-8047-3024-5*) Stanford U Pr.

Picturing Health & Illness: Images of Identity & Difference. Sander L. Gilman. 1995. LC 95-75700. (Illus.). 200p. 36.95 (*0-8018-5197-1*) Johns Hopkins.

Pieces of Personality Puzzle. David C. Funder. 2nd ed. 2001. LC 00-52717. (Illus.). xiii, 537p. (C). pap. text (*0-393-97683-1*) Norton.

Piecing Together Hypertension. Anatomical Chart Company Staff. 2000. (Illus.). 9p. pap. 24.95 (*1-889241-05-9*, 9767FC) Anatomical Chart.

Piecing Together the Digestive System. Anatomical Chart Company Staff. 2000. (Illus.). 9p. pap. 24.95 (*1-889241-02-4*, 9859FC) Anatomical Chart.

Piecing Together the Heart. Anatomical Chart Company Staff. 2000. (Illus.). 9p. pap. 24.95 (*1-889241-01-6*, 8023FC) Anatomical Chart.

Piecing Together the Respiratory System. Anatomical Chart Company Staff. 2000. (Illus.). 9p. pap. 24.95 (*1-889241-03-2*, 9766FC) Anatomical Chart.

Piel y Alergia. R. Pelta & E. Vivas. 1997. (SPA.). 211p. pap. (*84-7978-298-6*) Ediciones Diaz ESP. *Dist:* IBD Ltd.

***Pierce's Disease: Congressional Hearing.** Ed. by Richard W. Pombo. 2001. 74p. (C). pap. 20.00 (*0-7567-1563-6*) DIANE Pub.

Pig Diseases. David Conrad Taylor. 6th ed. 1995. 300p. pap. 36.95 (*0-9506932-5-1*) Diamond Farm Bk.

Piggle. Donald Woods Winnicott. 1977. LC 76-46815. 201p. 35.00 (*0-8236-4137-6*); pap. 27.95 (*0-8236-8189-0*, BN 24137) Intl Univs Pr.

Pigment Microbiology. P. Z. Margalith. 1992. LC 92-38097. 176p. (C). (gr. 13). pap. text 119.95 (*0-412-41050-8*) Chapman & Hall.

Pigmentary System: Physiology & Pathophysiology. Ed. by James J. Nordlund et al. 1998. LC 97-28806. (Illus.). 1106p. text 225.00 (*0-19-509861-7*) OUP.

Pigmentation & Pigmentary Disorders. Norman Levine. 1993. (Dermatology). 576p. 210.00 (*0-8493-7353-0*, RL790) CRC Pr.

Pigs. George MacLeod. 1994. 129p. pap. (*0-85207-278-3*) C W Daniel GBR. *Dist:* Natl Bk Netwk.

Pigs: Homoeopathic Approach to the Treatment & Prevention. George MacLeod. 1994. pap. 29.95 (*0-8464-4336-8*) Beekman Pubs.

Pike's Illustrated Descriptive Catalogue of Optical, Mathematical, & Philosophical Instruments. Benjamin Pike, Jr. 1993. (Illus.). 755p. reprint ed. 125.00 (*0-930405-54-4*) Norman SF.

Pilgrimage & Service. Joseph Krimsky. Ed. by Moshe Davis. 1977. LC 77-70712. (America & the Holy Land Ser.). reprint ed. lib. bdg. 19.95 (*0-405-10261-5*) Ayer.

Pill Book. Harold M. Silverman. 1995. mass mkt. 8.99 (*0-553-85155-1*); 6th ed. 1995. mass mkt. 8.99 (*0-553-85146-2*); 7th ed. 1996. mass mkt. 8.99 (*0-553-85109-8*); 8th ed. 1998. 1248p. mass mkt. 25.95 (*0-553-57926-6*) Bantam.

Pill Book: The Illustrated Guide to the Most-Prescribed Drugs in the United States. Ed. by Harold M. Silverman. 9th exp. rev. ed. 2000. LC 00-268051. (Pill Bk.). (Illus.). 1168p. mass mkt. 6.99 (*0-553-57974-6*) Bantam.

Pill Book: The Illustrated Guide to the Most-Prescribed Drugs in the United States. Harold M. Silverman. 9th expurg. rev. ed. 2000. (Illus.). 1168p. pap. 25.95 (*0-553-37964-X*, Spectra) Bantam.

***Pill Book Guide to Alternative Medicines.** Michael Murray. 2002. mass mkt. (*0-553-58473-1*) Bantam.

***Pill Book Guide to Alternative Medicines.** Michael Murray. 2002. 1088p. mass mkt. 6.99 (*0-553-58194-5*) Bantam.

Pill Book Guide to Children's Medications. Michael D. Mitchell. 2nd rev. ed. 1990. LC 94-180836. 320p. mass mkt. 6.50 (*0-553-56927-9*) Bantam.

Pill Book Guide to Medication for Your Dog & Cat. Kate A. W. Roby & Lenny Southam. 1998. LC 99-159362. 624p. mass mkt. 6.99 (*0-553-57989-4*) Bantam.

Pill Peddlers: Essays on the History of the Pharmaceutical Industry. Ed. by Jonathan Liebenau et al. 1990. 133p. (Orig.). (C). pap. 10.95 (*0-931292-22-0*) Am Inst Hist Pharm.

PQR

Pillar of Salt: Gender, Memory, & the Perils of Looking Back. Janice Haaken. 1998. LC 97-45761. 336p. (C). 26.00 (*0-8135-2524-1*) Rutgers U Pr.

Pillar of Salt: Gender, Memory & the Perils of Looking Back. Janice Haaken. 2000. LC 97-45761. 336p. pap. 22.00 (*0-8135-2837-2*) Rutgers U Pr.

Pills-a-Go-Go: A Fiendish Investigation into Pill Marketing, Art, History & Consumption. Jim Hogshire. 1998. LC 2001-269493. (Illus.). viii, 247p. pap. 16.95 (*0-922915-53-9*) Feral Hse.

Pills, Potions, & Poisons: How Drugs Work. Trevor Stone & Gail Darlington. 2000. LC 99-52844. (Illus.). xvi, 476p. 27.50 (*0-19-850403-9*) OUP.

Pilot Review, 1992-1997. Joseph B. Strauss. 1997. 257p. (C). text 30.00 (*1-890419-09-5*) Fnd Chiropractic Educ.

Pilots, Personality, & Performance: Human Behavior & Stress in the Skies. Ed. by Sheila R. Deitz & William E. Thoms. 1991. LC 91-11427. 232p. 65.00 (*0-89930-577-6*, DPB/, Quorum Bks) Greenwood.

Pilots under Stress. S. J. Sloan & C. L. Cooper. 1987. 240p. 45.00 (*0-7102-0479-5*, 04795, Routledge Thoemms) Routledge.

Pima Indians: Pathfinders for Health. Ed. by Jane Demouy et al. 1998. (Illus.). 37p. pap. text 15.00 (*0-7881-7358-8*) DIANE Pub.

Pineal & Midbrain Lesions. G. Pendl. 1985. (Illus.). 280p. 126.00 (*0-387-81858-8*) Spr-Verlag.

Pineal & Reproduction. Ed. by Russell J. Reiter. 1978. (Progress in Reproductive Biology & Medicine Ser.: Vol. 4). (Illus.). 103.50 (*3-8055-2815-9*) S Karger.

Pineal Gland, Vol. I. Ed. by Russell J. Reiter. 1981. 186.00 (*0-8493-5714-4*, QP188, CRC Reprint) Franklin.

Pineal Gland: Extra-Reproductive Effects, Vol. III. Ed. by Russel J. Rieter. 1982. 248p. 144.00 (*0-8493-5717-9*, QP188, CRC Reprint) Franklin.

Pineal Gland: Proceedings of a Symposium with the 7th International Endocrinology Congress, Canada, April 1984. Ed. by G. M. Brown & S. D. Wainwright. 1985. LC 85-9571. (Advances in the Biosciences Ser.: Vol. 53). (Illus.). 390p. pap. (*0-08-031991-2*) Pergamon Repr.

Pineal Gland: Reproductive Effects, Vol. II. Ed. by Russell J. Reiter. 1981. 240p. 137.00 (*0-8493-5716-0*, QP188, CRC Reprint) Franklin.

Pineal Gland: Update 1996: From Molecular Mechanisms to Clinical Implications. Ed. by Russell J. Reiter & Susan M. Webb. 1996. LC 97-50031. 69.95 (*0-915340-19-4*) PJD Pubns.

Pineal Gland & Cancer: Neuroimmunoendocrine Mechanisms in Malignancy. Ed. by Christian Bartsch et al. 2000. LC 00-35760. (Illus.). 625p. 169.00 (*3-540-64051-7*) Spr-Verlag.

Pineal Gland & Its Endocrine Aspects: Proceedings of a Symposium with the 7th International Endocrinology Congress, Canada, April 1984. Ed. by G. Brown & S. D. Wainwright. 1985. LC 85-9571. (Advances in the Biosciences Ser.: Vol. 53). (Illus.). 390p. (*0-08-031992-0*) Pergamon Repr.

Pineal Gland & Its Hormones: Fundamentals & Clinical Perspectives: Proceedings of NATO ASI Held in Erice, Italy, June 7-13, 1994. Ed. by Russell J. Reiter et al. 1995. LC 95-33471. (NATO ASI Ser.: Series A, Vol. 277). (Illus.). 244p. (C). text 95.00 (*0-306-45105-0*) Plenum.

Pineal Gland Series Russell J. Reiter. 465.00 (*0-8493-5713-6*, CRC Reprint) Franklin.

Pineal Organ. L. E. Vollrath. 1981. (Handbuch der Mikroskopischen Anatomie Des Menschen Ser.: Vol. VI-7). (Illus.). 665p. 383.00 (*0-387-10313-9*) Spr-Verlag.

Pink Therapy: A Guide for Counsellors & Therapists Working with Lesbian, Gay, & Bisexual Clients. Ed. by Dominic Davies & Charles Neal. 1996. LC 95-26372. 256p. (*0-335-19657-8*); pap. (*0-335-19145-2*) OpUniv Pr.

Pinkus' Guide to Dermatohistopathology. Amir H. Mehregan et al. 6th ed. 1995. (Illus.). 816p. (C). pap. text 199.00 (*0-8385-8077-7*, A8077-8, Apple Lange Med) McGraw.

Pinpointing Student Behavioral Problems. Thomas McDonnell. 1988. (Orig.). pap. 9.95 (*1-55804-950-9*) Info Res Cons.

Pioneer Doctor in the Ozarks White River Country. Amy J. Miller. rev. ed. 1994. (Illus.). 165p. pap. 15.80 (*0-9643894-0-1*) Delphi Assocs.

Pioneer in Modern Medicine: David Linn Edsall of Harvard. Joseph C. Aub & Ruth K. Hapgood. 1970. LC 78-145896. (Illus.). 384p. 22.50 (*0-674-66875-8*) HUP.

Pioneer Programs in Palliative Care: Nine Case Studies. Frwd. by Daniel M. Fox & Rosemary Gibson. 2000. LC 2001-274279. (Illus.). vii, 225p. pap. (*1-887748-39-3*) Milbank Memorial.

Pioneer Recipes & Remedies: Enriched with Poetry : A Sesquicentennial Collection. Millie Foster Cheesman. 1997. LC 98-222646. xxiv, 402 p. (*0-9658406-0-3*) Daughters Utah.

Pioneer Work in Opening the Medical Profession to Women: Autobiographical Sketches. Elizabeth Blackwell. 1991. (American Biography Ser.). 264p. reprint ed. lib. bdg. 69.00 (*0-7812-8025-7*) Rprt Serv.

Pioneering Hematology: The Research & Treatment of Malignant Blood Disorders. William C. Maloney. 1997. LC 98-126281. xv, 196p. 24.95 (*0-88135-195-4*, Sci Hist) Watson Pub Intl.

Pioneering Research in Surgical Shock & Cardiovascular Surgery: Vivien Thomas & His Work with Alfred Blalock. Vivien T. Thomas. 1985. (Illus.). 304p. 47.95 (*0-8122-7989-1*) U of Pa Pr.

Pioneers in Invitro Fertilization: Proceedings of a Symposium Held in Oss, the Netherlands, November 5, 1993. Ed. by A. T. Alberda & Hendricus M. Vemer. 1995. LC 94-48589. (Studies in Profertility: Vol. 3). (Illus.). 122p. lib. bdg. 71.95 (*1-85070-566-6*, Parthenon Pbng) CRC Pr.

Pioneers in Jewish Medical Ethics. Fred Rosner. 1997. LC 97-12965. 280p. 40.00 (*0-7657-9968-5*) Aronson.

Pioneers in Medical Physics: A History of Hospital Physics. J. E. Roberts. 1998. LC 99-19619. (Illus.). 180p. 65.00 (*0-7503-0494-4*) Inst of Physics Pubng.

Pioneers in Pediatric Oncology. Ed. by Grant Taylor. 1990. xv, 355p. text 55.00 (*2-88124-508-0*) Gordon & Breach.

Pioneers of Interpersonal Psychoanalysis. Ed. by Donnel B. Stern et al. 1995. LC 95-30973. 272p. text 59.95 (*0-88163-177-9*); pap. text 29.95 (*0-88163-216-3*) Analytic Pr.

Pioneers of NMR & Magnetic Resonance in Medicine: The Story of MRI. James S. Mattson & Merrill Simon. 1996. (Illus.). 838p. lib. bdg. 75.00 (*0-9619243-1-4*) Dean Bks.

Pioneers of Public Health: The Story of Some Benefactors of the Human Race. M. E. Walker. 1977. LC 68-26483. (Essay Index Reprint Ser.). 25.95 (*0-8369-0965-8*) Ayer.

Piotr Gal'perin: A Lifetime of Searching for the Content of Psychology. Jacques Haenen. 1994. (Illus.). 267p. (C). lib. bdg. 95.00 (*1-56072-199-5*) Nova Sci Pubs.

PIP College "HELPS" - Handicapped & Exceptional Learners Programs & Services. P. M. Fielding. 1978. (College Handicapped & Exceptional Programs & Services Ser.: Vol. 3). pap. 8.95 (*0-937660-04-3*); Vol. 2. 1977. pap. 7.95 (*0-937660-03-5*) PIP.

Pitch Analysis: Journal: Phonetica, Vol. 39, No. 4-5, 1982. Ed. by K. J. Kohler. 1982. (Illus.). viii, 156p. pap. 81.75 (*3-8055-3670-4*) S Karger.

Pitfalls in Histopathologic Diagnosis of Malignant Melanoma. A. Bernard Ackerman & Kerl Delmut. rev. ed. 1993. (Illus.). 900p. text 195.00 (*0-8121-1352-7*) Lppncott W & W.

Pitfalls in Human Research: 10 Pivotal Points. Theodore X. Barber & A. Goldstein. 1976. LC 76-13488. (General Psychology Ser.: No. 67). 128p. (*0-08-020935-1*, BF76) Pergamon Repr GBR. *Dist:* Franklin.

Pitfalls, Variants & Artifacts in Body MR Imaging. Scott A. Mirowitz. 1996. (Illus.). 536p. (C). (gr. 13). text 155.00 (*0-8016-7670-3*, 07670) Mosby Inc.

Pituitary Adenomas. Glenn E. Sheline et al. 1981. (Oncologic Multidisciplinary Decisions in Onology Ser.). (Illus.). 248p. pap. 135.00 (*0-08-027463-3*, Pergamon Pr) Elsevier.

Pituitary Adenomas: From Basic Research to Diagnostic & Therapy, Proceedings of the 6th European Workshop on Pituitary Adenomas, Berlin, Germany, 24-27 July, 1996, Vol. 112. Klaus Von Werder & Rudolf Fahlbusch. 1996. LC 96-47748. (International Congress Ser.). 356p. 153.50 (*0-444-82425-1*) Elsevier.

Pituitary & Testis: Clinical & Experimental Studies. Ed. by David M. De Kretser et al. 1983. (Monographs in Endocrinology: Vol. 25). (Illus.). 186p. 100.00 (*0-387-11874-8*) Spr-Verlag.

Pituitary Diseases. Kalman Kovacs et al. 1980. 208p. 121.00 (*0-8493-5435-8*, RC658, CRC Reprint) Franklin.

Pituitary Function & Immunity. Ed. by Istvan Berczi. 1986. 336p. lib. bdg. 248.00 (*0-8493-6107-9*, QR182) CRC Pr.

Pituitary Gland. C. R. Kannan. 1987. (Clinical Surveys in Endocrinology Ser.: Vol. 1). (Illus.). 704p. (C). text 130.00 (*0-306-42506-8*, Kluwer Plenum) Kluwer Academic.

Pituitary Patient Resource Guide. Ed. by Shereen Ezzat. 2nd ed. 1997. (Illus.). 300p. pap. 39.95 (*0-9660141-0-3*) Pit Tumor Netwk.

Pituitaty Disorders: Comprehensive Management. Ed. by Ali F. Krisht & George T. Tindall. 1998. LC 98-3826. 422p. text 169.00 (*0-683-30143-8*) Lppncott W & W.

Pivotal Papers on Identification. Ed. by George H. Pollock. 1993. LC 93-9298. 508p. 72.50 (*0-8236-4130-9*) Intl Univs Pr.

PKD Patient's Manual: Understanding & Living with Autosomal Dominant Polycystic Kidney Disease. Irene Duley et al. Ed. by Wendy Rueb et al. 2nd rev. ed. 1995. (Illus.). 68p. tchr. ed. 15.00 (*0-9614567-4-4*) PKR Foundation.

***PLAB: 1000 Extended Matching Questions.** Una Coales. 2000. 282p. pap. (*1-85315-472-5*) Royal Soc of Medicine Pr Ltd GBR. *Dist:* Balogh.

***PLAB2: 100 Objective Structured Clinical Examinations.** Una Coales. 2001. 256p. pap. (*1-85315-503-9*) Royal Soc of Medicine Pr Ltd GBR. *Dist:* Balogh.

Place in Time: Caregivers for Their Elderly. Tom Koch. 1993. LC 92-1754. 244p. 40.00 (*0-275-94483-2*, C4483, Praeger Pubs) Greenwood.

Place of Connection: Expressive Counseling Techniques for Families & Individuals. Jackie S. Gerstein. 1998. (Illus.). 214p. pap. 27.95 (*1-885473-23-0*) Wood N Barnes.

Place of Herbs in Rational Therapy. Ellen Gould Harmon White. 1993. 40p. reprint ed. spiral bd. 8.00 (*0-7873-0958-3*) Hlth Research.

Place of the Humanities in Medicine. Eric J. Cassell. 1984. 7.00 (*0-916558-19-3*) Hastings Ctr.

Place to Live: Families & Child Health in a New Neighborhood of Cairo. Belgin Tekce et al. 1994. LC 94-204600. (Illus.). 272p. (*977-424-315-3*) Am Univ Cairo Pr EGY. *Dist:* Col U Pr.

Placebo Effect: An Interdisciplinary Exploration. Anne Harrington. 1997. LC 97-4324. (Illus.). 256p. 41.50 (*0-674-66984-3*) HUP.

Placebo Effect: An Interdisciplinary Exploration. Anne Harrington. 1999. 272p. pap. text 20.50 (*0-674-66986-X*) HUP.

Placebo Effects in Health & Disease: Index of New Information with Authors, Subjects & References. Joseph J. Hartwick. 1996. 150p. 57.50 (*0-7883-1256-1*); 1996. 150p. pap. 47.50 (*0-7883-1257-X*); 1997. 165p. 57.50 (*0-7883-1493-9*); 1997. 165p. pap. 47.50 (*0-7883-1494-7*) ABBE Pubs Assn.

Placebo or Panacea? Putting Psychiatric Drugs to the Test. Seymour Fisher & Roger P. Greenberg. 1997. LC 97-1074. 404p. 110.00 (*0-471-14848-2*) Wiley.

Placebo Response: How You Can Release the Body's Inner Pharmacy for Better Health. Howard Brody & Daralyn Brody. 336p. 2001. pap. 14.00 (*0-06-093297-X*); 2000. LC 00-708579. (Illus.). 25.00 (*0-06-019493-6*) HarperTrade (Cliff Street).

***Placebo Response: How You Can Release the Body's Inner Pharmacy For Better Health.** Howard Brody & Daralyn Brody. 2001. 312p. reprint ed. 25.00 (*0-7881-9968-4*) DIANE Pub.

Placement Handbook for Counseling Disabled Persons. Chrisann S. Geist & William A. Calzaretta. 1982. (Illus.). 346p. (C). text 63.95 (*0-398-04592-5*) C C Thomas.

Placenta: Basic Research for Clinical Application for the Next Decade. Ed. by Hiroaki Som. 1992. (Illus.). viii, 214p. 200.00 (*3-8055-5468-0*) S Karger.

Placenta: Human & Animal. Elizabeth M. Ramsey. 1982. LC 81-23372. 187p. 65.00 (*0-275-91378-3*, C1378, Praeger Pubs) Greenwood.

Placenta: Receptors, Pathology & Toxicology. R. K. Miller. Ed. by Henry A. Thiede. 1981. 390p. 99.75 (*0-275-91350-3*, C1350, Praeger Pubs) Greenwood.

Placenta: To Know Me Is to Love Me - A Reference Guide for Gross Placental Examination. Doris L. Schuler-Maloney & Steve S. Lee. 1998. (Illus.). xviii, 174p. spiral bd. 69.00 (*0-9670354-0-6*) D S M.

Placenta As a Model & a Source. Ed. by O. Genbacev et al. 1989. (Illus.). 162p. 65.00 (*0-306-43238-2*, Plenum Trade) Perseus Pubng.

Placenta in Clinical Practice. E. Jauniaux & R. K. Miller. 1998. (Illus.). 352p. text (*0-443-05604-8*) Church.

Placenta Transfer Methods & Interpretation. M. Young. 1981. 93.95 (*0-275-91357-0*, C1357, Praeger Pubs) Greenwood.

Placental & Fetal Doppler. K. H. Nicolaides & G. Rizzo. 2000. LC 00-25526. (Diploma in Fetal Medicine Ser.). (Illus.). 224p. 69.95 (*1-85070-757-X*, Parthenon Pbng) CRC Pr.

Placental Glucocorticoid Barrier & Adult Hypertension. C. R. Edwards. 1997. (Medical Intelligence Unit Ser.). 250p. 89.95 (*0-412-11651-0*) Chapman & Hall.

Placental Molecules in Hemodynamics, Vol. 9. Ed. by Toshio Hata et al. 1997. LC 97-28672. (Trophoblast Research Ser.: Vol. 9, Pt. 1). (Illus.). 600p. 150.00 (*1-58046-016-X*) Univ Rochester Pr.

Placental, Neonatal, & Pediatric Pathology: Based on the Proceedings of the 61st Annual Anatomic Pathology Slide Seminar of the American Society of Clinical Pathologists, New Orleans, Louisiana, September 21-22, 1995. Don B. Singer et al. 1996. LC 96-620. (*0-89189-404-7*) Am Soc Clinical.

Placental Pharmacology. B. V. Sastry. 1996. LC 97-106889. 224p. 139.95 (*0-8493-7811-7*) CRC Pr.

Placental Proteins. P. Bischof. 1984. (Contributions to Gynecology & Obstetrics Ser.: Vol. 12). (Illus.). viii, 96p. 57.50 (*3-8055-3853-7*) S Karger.

Placental Signals: Autocrine & Paracine Control of Pregnancy. Ed. by Lise Cedard & Anthony Firth. 1993. (Trophoblast Research Ser.: Vol. 6). (Illus.). 400p. (C). 90.00 (*1-878822-21-7*) Univ Rochester Pr.

Placental Toxology. Ed. by B. V. Sastry. 1995. LC 94-27711. 304p. 179.95 (*0-8493-7812-5*) CRC Pr.

Placing AIDS & HIV in Remission Vol. 1: A Guide to Aggressive Medical Therapy for People with HIV Infection. David Senechek. 1997. LC 97-91829. (Illus.). 202p. 24.95 (*0-9657466-0-7*) Senyczak Pubns.

Plague & Other Yersinia Infections. Thomas C. Butler. 1983. LC 83-17467. (Current Topics in Infectious Disease Ser.). 232p. 59.50 (*0-306-41414-7*, Plenum Trade) Perseus Pubng.

Plague Doctors: Responding to the AIDS Epidemic in France & America. Jamie L. Feldman. 1995. LC 94-43601. 288p. 67.00 (*0-89789-385-9*, Bergin & Garvey) Greenwood.

Plague in Sydney - The Anatomy of an Epidemic. Peter Curson & Kevin McCracken. 1990. 220p. pap. (*0-86840-219-2*) New South Wales Univ Pr AUS. *Dist:* Intl Spec Bk.

Plague Time: How Stealth Infections Cause Cancers, Heart Disease & Other Deadly Ailments. Paul W. Ewald. 2000. LC 00-44249. (Illus.). 288p. 25.00 (*0-684-86900-4*) Free Pr.

Plagues & Poxes: The Rise & Fall of Epidemic Disease. Alfred J. Bollet. 1987. LC 87-71319. 208p. pap. text 39.95 (*0-939957-06-X*) Demos Medical.

Plagues on the Doorstep see Outbreak Alert: Making Sense of Today's Infectious Diseases Threats

Plagues, Products, & Politics: Emergent Public Health Hazards & National Policymaking. Christopher H. Foreman, Jr. 1994. LC 94-15189. 210p. (C). text 34.95 (*0-8157-2876-X*); pap. text 14.95 (*0-8157-2875-1*) Brookings.

PLAID: Practical Lessons for Apraxia with Illustrated Drills. Brenda D. Whisonant. 1996. (Illus.). 168p. (Orig.). pap. text 22.95 (*0-937857-68-8*, 1424) Speech Bin.

Plain Concise Practical Remarks, on the Treatment of Wounds & Fractures. John Jones. 1979. 18.95 (*0-88143-147-8*); 1970. LC 77-140870. reprint ed. 18.00 (*0-405-01222-5*) Ayer.

Plain Pictures of Plain Doctoring: Vernacular Expression in New Deal Medicine & Photography. John D. Stoeckle. 1985. 274p. pap. text 17.50 (*0-262-69138-8*) MIT Pr.

Plain Talk about Acupuncture. Ellinor R. Mitchell. 1987. (Illus.). 123p. (Orig.). pap. 10.95 (*0-9617918-0-2*) Whalehall Inc.

Plain Talk about the Human Genome Project: A Tuskegee University Conference on Its Promise & Perils & Matters of Race. Ed. by Edward Smith & Walter Sapp. 1998. LC 97-61711. (Illus.). 292p. pap. 14.95 (*1-891196-01-4*) Tuskegee U CAENS.

Plain Treatise on the Peruvian Bark: The Stanitz Manuscript. Tr. & Intro. by Saul Jarcho. 1992. 116p. 19.95 (*0-88135-176-8*, Sci Hist) Watson Pub Intl.

Plain Words about AIDS: With a Glossary of Related Terms. W. Hovey Smith. 3rd ed. 1988. (Illus.). 200p. (Orig.). pap. 19.50 (*0-916565-11-4*) Whitehall Pr.

Plan Analysis: Toward Optimizing Therapy. Franz Caspar. 1995. LC 94-8571. (Illus.). 294p. text 35.00 (*0-88937-117-2*) Hogrefe & Huber Pubs.

Plan & Operation: National Nursing Home Survey Followup, 1987, 1988, 1990. Ilene B. Gottfried. 1993. LC 93-17510. (Vital & Health Statistics Ser.: Series 1, No. 30). (*0-8406-0481-5*) Natl Ctr Health Stats.

Plan & Operation of the National Hospital Ambulatory Medical Care Survey. Linda F. McCraig & Thomas McLemorel. 1994. LC 94-12448. (Vital & Health Statistics, Series 1, Programs & Collection Procedures: No. 34). 6.00 (*0-8406-0493-9*) Natl Ctr Health Stats.

Plan & Operation of the National Survey of Ambulatory Surgery (NSAS) Thomas McLemore et al. 1997. LC 97-36605. (Vital & Health Statistics Ser.: Series 1, No. 37). (*0-8406-0532-3*) Natl Ctr Health Stats.

Plan & Operation of the Nhanes II Mortality Study, 1992. Catherine M. Loria et al. 1999. LC 99-29384. (Vital & Health Statistics, Series 1, Programs & Collection Procedures). (*0-8406-0556-0*) Natl Ctr Health Stats.

Plan & Operation of the 1995 National Survey of Family Growth. Allen P. Duffer. 1997. LC 97-36607. (Vital & Health Statistics Ser.: Series 1, No. 37). (*0-8406-0531-5*) Natl Ctr Health Stats.

Plan & Operations of the NHANES I Epidemiologic Followup Study, 1992. National Center for Health Statistics Staff. 1998. LC 97-53305. (Vital & Health Statistics Ser.: Series 1, No. 35). (*0-8406-0542-0*) Natl Ctr Health Stats.

Plan Care Special Practice: Ambulatory Care. Bonnie Allbaugh. 1994. (Professional Reference - Nursing Ser.). pap. 20.95 (*0-8273-6121-1*) Delmar.

Plan for Managing the Costs of Biomedical Research. 1993. (Illus.). 34p. (Orig.). (C). pap. text 20.00 (*1-56806-425-X*) DIANE Pub.

Plan of Action for Implementing the Global Strategy for Health for All. 1982. text (*92-4-180007-0*) World Health.

Plan to Strengthen Public Health in the U. S. 1993. 86p. (Orig.). (C). pap. text 25.00 (*1-56806-557-4*) DIANE Pub.

Planet Medicine: From Stone Age Shamanism to Post-Industrial Healing. Richard Grossinger. 5th rev. ed. 1990. LC 82-50278. 496p. pap. 16.95 (*1-55643-093-0*) North Atlantic.

Planet Medicine Vol. I: Origins. Richard Grossinger. 6th rev. ed. 1995. LC 95-22428. (Illus.). 500p. (C). pap. 25.00 (*1-55643-179-1*) North Atlantic.

Planet Medicine Vol. II: Modalities. Richard Grossinger. 6th ed. 1995. LC 95-22428. (Illus.). 500p. pap. 25.00 (*1-55643-214-3*) North Atlantic.

Planetary Overload: Global Environmental Change & the Health of the Human Species. A. J. McMichael. 1993. LC 92-38292. (Illus.). 368p. (C). text 90.00 (*0-521-44138-2*) Cambridge U Pr.

Planned Approach to Community Health: Guide for the Local Coordinator. Byron Breedlove. 1998. (Illus.). 311p. (C). pap. text 50.00 (*0-7881-7262-X*) DIANE Pub.

Planned Approach to Community Health: Visual Aids. Byron Breedlove. 1998. (Illus.). 150p. (C). pap. text 25.00 (*0-7881-7261-1*) DIANE Pub.

Planned Change Theories for Nursing: Review, Analysis, & Implications. Constance R. Tiffany & Louette R. Johnson Lutjens. 1998. LC 97-33801. 320p. pap. 37.95 (*0-7619-0235-X*, 2150) Sage.

Planned Change Theories for Nursing: Review, Analysis & Implications. Constance R. Tiffany & Louette R. Johnson Lutjens. 1998. LC 97-33801. 320p. 74.95 (*0-7619-0234-1*, 2149) Sage.

Planned Markets & Public Competition: Strategic Reform in Northern European Health Systems. Richard B. Saltman & Casten Von Otter. 1992. (State of Health Ser.). 160p. (*0-335-09729-4*); pap. (*0-335-09728-6*) OpUniv Pr.

Planned Short-Term Psychotherapy: A Clinical Handbook. Bernard L. Bloom. 2nd ed. 1997. LC 96-48082. 309p. pap. text 52.00 (*0-205-19344-7*) Allyn.

Planned Short-Term Treatment. Richard A. Wells. 1982. 288p. 35.00 (*0-02-934650-9*); 2nd ed. 1994. LC 94-13229. 308p. 35.00 (*0-02-934655-X*) Free Pr.

Planning a Baby? A Complete Guide to Pre-Conceptual Care. Sarah Brewer. 1996. 296p. pap. (*0-09-181256-9*) Optima GBR. *Dist:* Trafalgar.

Planning a One-Day Geriatrics Retreat. 1998. 55p. ring bd. (*1-891539-00-0*) U Chi Pritzker Schl.

Planning an Endoscopy Suite for Office & Hospital. Jerome D. Waye & Martin Rich. 1990. LC 90-4105. (Illus.). 184p. 65.00 (*0-89640-173-1*) Igaku-Shoin.

Planning & Assessing Health Worker Activities Module 3: Facilitator's Guide. Martine Hilton. 1993. (Primary Health Care Management Advancement Programme Modules Ser.). 84p. pap. text (*1-882839-10-2*) Aga Khan Fnd.

Planning & Assessing Health Worker Activities Module 3: User's Guide. Khatidja Husein et al. 1993. (Primary Health Care Management Advancement Programme Modules Ser.). 136p. pap. text (*1-882839-02-1*) Aga Khan Fnd.

Planning & Evaluating Health Programs: A Primer. Charles D. Hale et al. 1993. LC 92-47070. 232p. (C). pap. 36.50 (*0-8273-5448-7*) Delmar.

Planning & Evaluation of Health Education Services: Proceedings of the WHO Expert Committee, Geneva, 1967. WHO Staff. 1969. (Technical Reports: No. 409). pap. text 6.00 (*92-4-120409-5*, 1100409) World Health.

Planning & Evaluation of Public Dental Health Services: Proceedings of the WHO Expert Committee, Geneva, 1975. WHO Staff. 1976. (Technical Reports: No. 589). pap. text 6.00 (*92-4-120589-X*, 1100589) World Health.

Planning & Making Crowns & Bridges. Bernard G. N. Smith. 3rd ed. 1998. 264p. (C). text (*1-85317-314-2*) Martin Dunitz GBR. *Dist:* Mosby Inc.

Planning & Managing Emergency Response. C. Calmbacher. 1993. text (*0-442-01647-6*, VNR) Wiley.

Planning & Organization of Health Laboratory Services: Proceedings of the WHO Expert Committee on Health Laboratory Services, 5th, Geneva, 1971. WHO Staff. 1972. (Technical Reports: No. 491). pap. text 4.00 (*92-4-120491-5*, 1100491) World Health.

Planning & Programming for Nursing Services. 1971. (Public Health Papers: No. 44). pap. text 7.00 (*92-4-130044-2*, 1110044) World Health.

Planning & Reduction Technique in Fracture Surgery. J. W. Mast et al. 1995. (Illus.). 270p. 265.00 (*0-387-16283-6*) Spr-Verlag.

Planning & Validating QC Procedures: Workshop Manual. James O. Westgard. 2nd ed. 1996. LC 95-90953. 154p. spiral bd. 75.00 (*1-886958-04-1*) Westgard Qual.

Planning Clinical Trials in the Pharmaceutical Industry: An Introduction to the Statistical Principles in the Planning & Design of Clinical Studies. William M. Wooding. 1993. LC 00-301. (Probability & Statistics Ser.). 560p. 150.00 (*0-471-62244-3*) Wiley.

Planning Community Mental Health Services for Women: A Multiprofessional Handbook. Ed. by Kathryn Abel et al. 1996. LC 95-38887. 280p. (C). 84.95 (*0-415-11455-1*); pap. 27.95 (*0-415-11456-X*) Routledge.

Planning Efficient Hospital Systems. Robert E. Coughlin & Walter Isard. 1963. (Discussion Papers: No. 1). pap. 10.00 (*1-55869-094-8*) Regional Sci Res Inst.

Planning Environmental Health Programs. Sanford M. Brown. 1986. LC 86-21267. 250p. 67.00 (*0-275-92237-5*, C2237, Praeger Pubs) Greenwood.

Planning for Alcohol & Other Drug Abuse Treatment for Adults in the Criminal Justice System. Ed. by Sandra Clunies. 1999. 116p. (C). pap. text 25.00 (*0-7881-7594-7*) DIANE Pub.

Planning for Community-Oriented Health Systems. James E. Rohrer. 1996. 168p. (Orig.). pap. 32.00 (*0-87553-230-6*) Am Pub Health.

Planning for Pharmacy Services, 1991, Level 2. 1991. 134p. ring bd. 63.00 (*1-879907-13-5*, P320) Am Soc Hlth-Syst.

Planning for Pregnancy, Birth, & Beyond. American College of Obstetricians and Gynecologists Staff. 2nd rev. ed. 1997. Orig. Title: ACOG Guide to Planning for Pregnancy, Birth, & Beyond. 352p. pap. 6.99 (*0-451-19175-7*, Sig) NAL.

Planning for the Future - Guidelines for Self Assessment & Service Planning. Resa Hall & Lori Hansherr. 1996. pap. 27.50 (*1-57654-006-5*, Creative Core) Creat Core.

Planning for the Needs of People with Dementia: The Development of a Profile for Use in Local Services. P. Spicker & D. S. Gordon. 1997. 184p. text (*1-85972-600-3*) Avebry GBR. *Dist:* Ashgate Pub Co.

Planning for Uncertainty: A Guide to Living Wills & Other Advance Directives for Health Care. David J. Doukas & William Reichel. 1993. LC 93-222. 168p. (C). pap. text 16.95 (*0-8018-4671-4*) Johns Hopkins.

Planning, Implementing & Evaluating Critical Pathways: A Guide for Health Care Survival into the 21st Century. Ed. by Patricia C. Dykes & Kathleen Wheeler. 1997. LC 97-16500. 184p. 34.95 (*0-8261-9790-6*) Springer Pub.

Planning, Implementing, & Evaluating Health Promotion Programs: A Primer. James F. McKenzie & Jan L. Smeltzer. 3rd ed. 2000. 381p. pap. 61.00 (*0-205-31915-7*) Allyn.

***Planning of District HIV/AIDS Programmes: A Practical Guide Based on Experiences in Tanzania.** Japheth Ng'weshemi. 2001. LC 2001-406667. (Illus.). 48p. pap. (*90-6832-139-0*) Royal Tropical NLD. *Dist:* Stylus Pub VA.

Planning of Health Services: Studies in 8 European Countries. G. McLachlan. 1980. (EURO Nonserial Publication Ser.). 252p. 20.00 (*92-9020-195-9*, 1340002) World Health.

Planning of Medical Education Programmes: Proceedings of the WHO Expert Committee, Geneva, 1973. WHO Staff. 1974. (Technical Reports: No. 547). pap. text 4.00 (*92-4-120547-4*, 1100547) World Health.

Planning Program Development & Evaluation. Thomas S. Timmreck. 1995. (Illus.). 240p. (C). pap. text 42.95 (*0-86720-787-6*, 787-6) Jones & Bartlett.

Planning Strategies of Intracranial Microsurgery. Wolfgang Seeger. 1986. (Illus.). 426p. 199.00 (*0-387-81916-9*) Spr-Verlag.

Planning Successful Practice Transitions. David W. Griggs. 1997. LC 97-42663. 59.95 (*0-87814-617-2*) PennWell Corp.

Planning Transportation Services for Handicapped Persons - User's Guide. 1983. (National Cooperative Highway Research Program Reports: No. 262). 74p. 8.00 (*0-309-03603-8*, NR262) Transport Res Bd.

Planning Your Career: A Business Decision Guide for the Ob-Gyn Resident. Ed. by Mark Dowden & Maria Kassberg. 2nd ed. 1995. 244p. pap. text (*0-9628716-2-1*) Dowden Pub.

Planning Your Veterinary Career. Ed. by John McCarthy. 1987. 115p. 15.00 (*0-941451-00-3*) Am Animal Hosp Assoc.

Plans & Provisions for the Mentally Handicapped. M. Bone et al. 1972. (*0-7855-0582-2*) Natl Inst Soc Work GBR. *Dist:* St Mut.

Plans of Care for Specialty Practice: Gerontological Nursing. Joan F. Needham. 1994. LC 94-25559. (Plans of Care for Specialty Practice Ser.). 384p. (C). pap. text 55.95 (*0-8273-6226-9*) Delmar.

Plans of Care for Specialty Practice: Oncology Nursing. Ed. by Christine Miaskowski. 1995. LC 94-32089. (Plans of Care for Specialty Practice Ser.). 416p. (C). pap. 45.95 (*0-8273-6118-1*) Delmar.

Plant Biochemical Regulators. Ed. by Harold W. Gausman. 1991. (Books in Soils, Plants & the Environment: Vol. 21). (Illus.). 368p. text 195.00 (*0-8247-8536-3*) Dekker.

Plant Disease Clinic & Field Diagnosis of Abiotic Diseases. Malcolm C. Shurtleff & Charles W. Averre, III. 1997. LC 96-85526. 256p. (C). text 89.00 (*0-89054-217-1*) Am Phytopathol Soc.

Plant Drug Analysis: A Thin Layer Chromatography Atlas, Vol. XII. Hildebert H. Wagner & Sabine Bladt. 2nd ed. 1996. (Illus.). 300p. 212.00 (*3-540-58676-8*) Spr-Verlag.

Plant Hormone Protocols. Ed. by Jeremy A. Roberts & Gregory A. Tucker. 2000. LC 99-58889. (Methods in Molecular Biology Ser.: Vol. 141). (Illus.). x, 199p. 79.50 (*0-89603-577-8*) Humana.

Plant Intoxicants: A Classic Text on the Use of Mind-Altering Plants. Ernst Von Bibra. 1995. LC 94-19230. (Illus.). 286p. pap. 16.95 (*0-89281-498-5*, Heal Arts VT) Inner Tradit.

Plant Nutrient Disorders Vol. 1: Temp & Sub. 1993. pap. text 46.95 (*0-909605-89-0*) Buttrwrth-Heinemann.

Plant Nutrition: Introduction to Current Concepts. Anthony D. Glass. 1989. (Illus.). (C). text 52.95 (*0-86720-080-4*, 080-4) Jones & Bartlett.

Plant Spirit Medicine: The Healing Power of Plants. Eliot Cowan. 1995. 175p. pap. 13.95 (*0-926524-09-7*) Granite Pub.

Plant Tissue Culture Manual B - W. Ed. by K. Lindsey. 1991. 585p. (C). lib. bdg. 143.00 (*0-7923-1115-9*) Kluwer Academic.

Plant Tumor Research. Ed. by A. C. Braun. 1972. (Progress in Experimental Tumor Research Ser.: Vol. 15). 54.00 (*3-8055-1262-7*) S Karger.

Plant Viruses Vol. 2: Pathology. Ed. by C. L. Mandahar. 1990. (Illus.). 368p. lib. bdg. 289.00 (*0-8493-6948-7*, QR351) CRC Pr.

Plantas Medicinales de Puerto Rico: Folklore y Fundamentos Cientificos. Esteban Nunez-Melendez. 2nd abr. rev. ed. 1989. LC 82-17321. (SPA., Illus.). xii, 498p. pap. 22.95 (*0-8477-2328-3*) U of PR Pr.

Plants for Malaria, Plants for Fever: Medicinal Species in Latin America - Bibliographic Study. W. Milliken. 1997. 150p. (*1-900347-29-6*) Royal Botnic Grdns GBR. *Dist:* Balogh.

Plants for Toxicity Assessment, STP 1115, Vol. 2. Kenneth R. St. John. Ed. by Joseph W. Gorsuch et al. 1991. (Special Technical Publications). 400p. text 95.00 (*0-8031-1422-2*, STP1115) ASTM.

Plants in Cardiology. Arthur Hollman. 1992. 49p. pap. text (*0-7279-0744-1*) BMJ Pub GBR. *Dist:* AIDC.

Plants in Hawaiian Medicine. Beatrice Krauss. 2001. (Illus.). 128p. pap. 11.21 (*1-57306-034-8*) Bess Pr.

Plants in Human Nutrition. A. P. Simopoulos. 1995. LC 94-42190. (World Review of Nutrition & Dietetics Ser.: Vol. 77). (Illus.). xiv, 160p. 172.25 (*3-8055-6101-6*) S Karger.

Plants in Indian Medicine, No. 4. Anthony R. Torkelson. 1999. (Cross Name Index to Medicinal Plants Ser.). 560p. 350.00 (*0-8493-1085-7*) CRC Pr.

Plants of the Gods: Their Sacred Healing, & Hallucinogenic Powers. Richard E. Schultes & Albert Hofmann. 1992. LC 92-16621. (Illus.). 192p. (Orig.). pap. 22.95 (*0-89281-406-3*, Heal Arts VT) Inner Tradit.

Plants Poisonous to People in Florida & Other Warm Areas. Julia F. Morton. 2nd rev. ed. 1982. LC 81-71614. (Illus.). 170p. pap. 19.75 (*0-9610184-0-2*) ECHO Inc.

Plants Used As Curatives by Certain Southeastern Tribes. Lyda A. Taylor. LC 76-43866. (Botanical Museum of Harvard University Ser.). reprint ed. 29.50 (*0-404-15725-4*) AMS Pr.

Planung & Verwirklichung Von Freizeitangeboten. Moeglichkeiten & Formen der Partizipation. S. Agricola & B. Von Schmettow. Ed. by R. Schmitz-Scherzer. 1976. (Psychologische Praxis Ser.: Band 50). 21.75 (*3-8055-2361-0*) S Karger.

Plaque & Calculus Removal: Considerations for the Professional. David L. Cochran et al. 1994. LC 94-17876. (Illus.). 109p. pap. text 32.00 (*0-86715-285-0*) Quint Pub Co.

Plasma Cell Dyscrasias. A. I. Pick. 1982. (Acta Haematologica Ser.: Vol. 68, No. 3). (Illus.). vi, 96p. pap. 51.50 (*3-8055-3549-X*) S Karger.

Plasma Chromatography. Ed. by Timothy W. Carr. 1984. (Illus.). 274p. (C). text 102.00 (*0-306-41432-5*, Kluwer Plenum) Kluwer Academic.

Plasma Fibronectin: Structure & Functions. J. McDonagh. 1985. (Hematology Ser.: Vol. 5). (Illus.). 288p. text 150.00 (*0-8247-7384-5*) Dekker.

Plasma Fractionation & Blood Transfusion. Ed. by C. T. Sibinga et al. 1985. (Developments in Hematology & Immunology Ser.). text 75.00 (*0-89838-761-2*) Kluwer Academic.

Plasma Homovanillic Acid in Schizophrenia: Implications for Presynaptic Dopamine Dysfunction. Ed. by Arnold J. Friedhoff & Farooq Amin. 1997. LC 96-30139. (Progress in Psychiatry Ser.: Vol. 52). 216p. text 34.00 (*0-88048-489-6*, 8489) Am Psychiatric.

Plasma Isoenzymes: The Current Status. Ed. by Victor H. Blaton & A. Van Steirteghem. 1986. (Advances in Clinical Enzymology Ser.: Vol. 3). (Illus.). viii, 208p. 155.75 (*3-8055-4321-2*) S Karger.

Plasma Products & European Self-Sufficiency: Collection, Preparation & Use. Council of Europe Staff. 1992. (*92-871-1925-2*) Council of Europe FRA. *Dist:* Manhattan Pub Co.

Plasma Proteins: An Introduction. M. W. Turner & B. Hulme. 1971. (Illus.). pap. 22.95 (*0-8464-0725-6*) Beekman Pubs.

Plasmapheresis in Immunology & Oncology: Beitraege zur Onkologie. Contributions to Oncology, Vol. 10. Ed. by G. A. Nagel et al. 1982. (Illus.). viii, 266p. pap. 50.50 (*3-8055-3467-1*) S Karger.

Plasmas & Fluids. National Research Council Staff. 1986. (Physics Through the 1990's Ser.). 336p. pap. text 31.50 (*0-309-03548-1*) Natl Acad Pr.

Plasminogen-Related Growth Factors, Vol. 212. Gregory Bock et al. 1998. LC 97-34811. (CIBA Foundation Symposia Ser.). 268p. 128.00 (*0-471-97456-0*) Wiley.

***Plastic & Orbital Surgery.** Collin et al. 2001. (Fundamentals in Clinical Ophthalmology Ser.). (Illus.). 200p. (*0-7279-1475-8*) BMJ Pub GBR. *Dist:* AIDC.

Plastic & Reconstructive Breast Surgery. G. Lemperle & J. Nievergelt. 1991. (Illus.). 192p. 262.00 (*0-387-52868-7*) Spr-Verlag.

Plastic & Reconstructive Breast Surgery John Bostwick, 3rd. 2nd ed. 1999. LC 99-46503. (Illus.). xxviii, 1606p. text 420.00 (*1-57626-104-2*) Quality Med Pub.

Plastic & Reconstructive Surgery. Nancymarie Fortunato & Susan M. McCullough. 1998. LC 98-155078. (Perioperative Nursing Ser.). (Illus.). 208p. (C). (gr. 13). text 54.95 (*0-8151-3305-7*, 27472) Mosby Inc.

Plastic & Reconstructive Surgery of the Breast: A Surgical Atlas. Heinz Bohmert. 1997. LC 96-33255. (Illus.). 2388p. text 199.00 (*0-86577-628-8*) Thieme Med Pubs.

Plastic & Reconstructive Surgery of the Head & Neck. Fred Stucker. 1990. 169.00 (*1-55664-211-3*) Mosby Inc.

Plastic & Reconstructive Surgery of the Orbitopalpebral Region. Denys Montandon et al. 1990. (Illus.). 360p. text (*0-443-04486-4*) Church.

Plastic Containers for Pharmaceuticals: Testing & Control. J. Cooper. 1974. (Offset Publications: No. 4). pap. text 28.80 (*92-4-170004-1*, 1120004) World Health.

Plastic, Reconstructive & Aesthetic Surgery. Ed. by Kiyonori Harii et al. 1995. (Illus.). 726p. text (*90-6299-118-1*) Kugler NLD. *Dist:* Lib Res.

Plastic Surgery. Ed. by William X. Grabb & James W. Smith. 3rd ed. 1980. 69.50 (*0-316-32269-5*, Little Brwn Med Div) Lppncott W & W.

Plastic Surgery McCarthy. 3rd ed. 1989. Set. (Illus.). 6448p. text 995.00 (*0-7216-1514-7*); Vol. 1. text 165.00 (*0-7216-2542-8*); Vol. 2. text 165.00 (*0-7216-2543-6*) Saunders.

***Plastic Surgery: Facts.** Stone. 2000. (Greenwich Medical Media Ser.). (Illus.). 488p. pap. (*1-84110-064-1*) Greenwich Med GBR. *Dist:* JAMCO Dist.

Plastic Surgery: Past & Present. J. Gabka & E. Vaubel. 1983. (Illus.). viii, 180p. 256.75 (*3-8055-3651-8*) S Karger.

Plastic Surgery Hopscotch: A Resource Guide for Those Considering Cosmetic Surgery. John McCabe. Ed. by Miriam Ingersoll. 1995. LC 93-74927. 384p. pap. 19.95 (*1-884702-32-5*) Carmania Bks.

Plastic Surgery in Pediatrics. Ian Muir. 1988. 116.00 (*0-316-58944-6*, Little Brwn Med Div) Lppncott W & W.

Plastic Surgery, Nerve Repair, Burns. Ed. by Gunther O. Schlag. 1995. LC 94-41582. (Fibrin Sealing in Surgical & Nonsurgical Fields Ser.: Vol. 3). (Illus.). 158p. 64.95 (*3-540-58550-8*) Spr-Verlag.

Plastic Surgery of the Breast. Maxwell. 1993. (Illus.). 900p. text 250.00 (*0-8016-5821-7*) Mosby Inc.

Plastic Surgery of the Facial Skeleton. S. Anthony Wolfe. 1989. 500p. 345.00 (*0-316-95105-6*, Little Brwn Med Div) Lppncott W & W.

Plastic Surgery of the Head & Neck Ed. by Richard B. Stark. 1986. (Illus.). 1580p. text (*0-443-08249-9*) Church.

Plastic Surgery of the Orbit & Eyelids. Caludia Tessier. 1981. (gr. 13). 82.50 (*0-89352-041-1*) Mosby Inc.

Plastic Surgery Sourcebook. Kimberly Henry & Penny Heckaman. 1996. LC 96-49696. (Illus.). 240p. 30.00 (*1-56565-464-1*) Lowell Hse.

Plastic Surgery Sourcebook. Kimberly A. Henry & Penny S. Heckaman. 2nd rev. ed. 1999. LC 99-24231. (Illus.). 272p. pap. 18.95 (*0-7373-0087-6*, 00876W) NTC Contemp Pub Co.

Plasticity & Morphology of the Central Nervous System. Ed. by C. L. Cazzulio et al. 1989. (C). text 152.50 (*0-7462-0094-3*) Kluwer Academic.

Plasticity & Regeneration of the Nervous System. Ed. by Paola S. Timiras et al. 1991. (Advances in Experimental Medicine & Biology Ser.: Vol. 296). (Illus.). 382p. (C). text 144.00 (*0-306-43933-6*, Kluwer Plenum) Kluwer Academic.

Plasticity in the Central Nervous System: Learning & Memory. Ed. by James L. McGaugh et al. 1995. 272p. text 39.95 (*0-8058-1573-2*) L Erlbaum Assocs.

Plasticity in the Nervous System. B. I. Kotlyar. 2nd ed. 1992. LC 92-1418. (Monographs in Neuroscience: Vol. 3). ix, 305p. text 141.00 (*2-88124-525-0*, QP376) Gordon & Breach.

Plasticity of Development. Ed. by Steven Brauth et al. 1991. 184p. 38.50 (*0-262-02326-1*, Bradford Bks) MIT Pr.

Plasticity of Muscle. Ed. by D. Pette. 1979. (C). 146.15 (*3-11-007961-5*) De Gruyter.

Plasticity of the Central Nervous System. Ed. by Susumu Ishii & Keiji Sano. 1987. (Acta Neurochirurgica Ser.: Supplementum 41). (Illus.). 140p. 131.00 (*0-387-82027-2*) Spr-Verlag.

Plasticity of the Neuromuscular System. 1988. LC 88-20780. (CIBA Foundation Symposia Ser.: No. 138). 284p. 128.00 (*0-471-91902-0*) Wiley.

Plastics for Medical Devices: What's Ahead? 1996. LC 97-120162. (Report Ser.: No. P-121R). 171p. 2950.00 (*1-56965-268-6*) BCC.

Plastics in Medical - Pharmaceutical Disposables: Driving Forces Creating New Opportunities. 1993. 2650.00 (*0-89336-958-6*, P-212) BCC.

Plastics in Medical Tubing. 1991. 108p. 1550.00 (*0-89336-861-X*, P-129) BCC.

Plastics in Non-Packaging Medical Applications. BCC Staff. 1990. 224p. 2350.00 (*0-89336-725-7*, P121) BCC.

Plastination: A Tool for Teaching & Research: The 8th International Conference on Plastination, Brisbane, July 1996. Ed. by Andreas H. Weiglein. 1997. (Acta Anatomica Ser.: Vol. 158, No. 1, 1997). (Illus.). 82p. pap. 75.00 (*3-8055-6572-0*) S Karger.

Platelet-Activating Factor & Cell Immunology. Ed. by Pierre Braquet. 1988. (New Trends in Lipid Mediators Research Ser.: Vol. 1). viii, 180p. 146.25 (*3-8055-4684-X*) S Karger.

Platelet Activating Factor & Human Disease. Ed. by P. Barnes et al. 1989. (Frontiers in Pharmacology & Therapeutics Ser.). (Illus.). 350p. 125.00 (*0-632-02684-7*) Blackwell Sci.

Platelet-Activating Factor & Related Lipid Mediators No. 2: Roles in Health & Disease. Ed. by Santosh Nigam et al. 1997. LC 97-3871. (Advances in Experimental Medicine & Biology Ser.: No. 416). (Illus.). 414p. (C). text 144.00 (*0-306-45506-4*, Kluwer Plenum) Kluwer Academic.

Platelet-Activating Factor Antagonists: New Developments for Clinical Application. Ed. by Joseph T. O'Flaherty & Peter W. Ramwell. 1990. (Advances in Applied Biotechnology Ser.: Vol. 9). (Illus.). 256p. (C). 55.00 (*0-943255-13-9*) Portfolio Pub.

Platelet Amine Storage Granule. Johnston. Ed. by Charles D. Barnes. 1992. 224p. 110.00 (*0-8493-8838-4*, QP97) CRC Pr.

Platelet-Dependent Vascular Occlusion. Ed. by Garret A. FitzGerald et al. 1994. LC 94-7321. (Annals of the New York Academy of Sciences Ser.: Vol. 714). 328p. pap. 90.00 (*0-89766-845-6*); pap. 90.00 (*0-89766-846-4*) NY Acad Sci.

Platelet Glycoprotein IIb/IIIa Inhibitors in Cardiovascular Disease. Ed. by A. Michael Lincoff & Eric J. Topol. 1999. LC 99-30220. (Contemporary Cardiology Ser.). (Illus.). 384p. 125.00 (*0-89603-727-4*) Humana.

Platelet Heterogeneity. Ed. by J. Martin & T. Trowbridge. 1990. (Illus.). 270p. 182.00 (*0-387-19602-1*) Spr-Verlag.

Platelet Immunology. Ed. by C. Kaplan et al. 1988. (Current Studies in Hematology & Blood Transfusion: No. 55). (Illus.). viii, 188p. 143.50 (*3-8055-4693-9*) S Karger.

Platelet Membrane in Transfusion Medicine. Ed. by Gail A. Rock & F. Decary. 1988. (Current Studies in Hematology & Blood Transfusion: No. 54). (Illus.). viii, 156p. 126.25 (*3-8055-4657-2*) S Karger.

Platelet Responses & Metabolism: Response-Metabolism Relationships, Vol. 3. Holm Holmsen. 1987. LC 86-135430. 336p. 185.00 (*0-8493-5899-X*, QP97) Franklin.

Platelet Responses & Metabolism Vol. 1: Responses. Holm Holmsen. 1986. LC 86-13543. 360p. 197.00 (*0-8493-5897-3*, CRC Reprint) Franklin.

Platelet Responses & Metabolism Vol. 2: Receptors & Metabolism. Holm Holmsen. 1986. LC 86-13543. 360p. 201.00 (*0-8493-5898-1*, CRC Reprint) Franklin.

Platelet Serology. Ed. by Francine Decary & Gail A. Rock. 1986. (Current Studies in Hematology & Blood Transfusion: No. 52). (Illus.). vii, 124p. 85.25 (*3-8055-4208-9*) S Karger.

Platelet-Vessel Wall Interaction. R. M. Pittilo & S. J. Machin. 1988. (Bloomsbury Series in Clinical Science). (Illus.). 189p. 103.00 (*0-387-17488-5*) Spr-Verlag.

Platelets, Analgesics & Asthma. Michael Schmitz-Schumann et al. 1987. (Agents & Actions Supplements Ser.: No. 21). 206p. 77.00 (*0-8176-1806-6*) Birkhauser.

Platelets & Atherosclerosis. Ed. by C. Kessler. 1990. (Illus.). 110p. 62.95 (*0-387-53006-1*) Spr-Verlag.

Platelets & Their Factors. Kalwant S. Authi et al. 1997. LC 96-39635. (Handbook of Experimental Pharmacology Ser.). (Illus.). 753p. 439.00 (*3-540-61997-6*) Spr-Verlag.

Platelets, Drugs & Thrombosis: Proceedings of the Symposium, Hamilton, Ont., Oct. 1972. Symposium, Hamilton, Ont. Staff et al. Ed. by Edward Schonbaum et al. 1974. 320p. 85.25 (*3-8055-1745-9*) S Karger.

***Platelets in Thrombotic & Non-thrombotic Disorders.** Ed. by P. Gresele et al. 2002. text 265.00 (*0-521-80261-X*) Cambridge U Pr.

Plates Illustrative of the Vocabulary for the Deaf & Dumb. Harvey Darton. 1972. 69.95 (*0-8490-0841-7*) Gordon Pr.

Platinum. 1991. (Environmental Health Criteria Ser.: No. 125). (ENG, FRE & SPA.). 167p. pap. text 29.00 (*92-4-157125-X*, 1160125) World Health.

Platinum & Other Metal Coordination Compounds in Cancer Chemotherapy. S. B. Howell. 1992. (Illus.). 558p. (C). text 174.00 (*0-306-44027-X*, Kluwer Plenum) Kluwer Academic.

Platinum & Other Metal Coordination Compounds in Cancer Chemotherapy. Ed. by Marino Nicolini. 1988. (Developments in Oncology Ser.). (C). text 330.00 (*0-89838-358-7*) Kluwer Academic.

Platinum & Other Metal Coornation Compounds in Cancer Chemotherapy 2: Proceeding of the 7th International Symposium Held in Amsterdam, The Netherlands, March 1-4, 1995, Vol. 2. Ed. by H. M. Pinedo & J. H. Schornagel. 1996. (Illus.). 368p. 102.00 (*0-306-45287-1*, Kluwer Plenum) Kluwer Academic.

Platinum-Based Drugs in Cancer Therapy. Lloyd R. Kelland & Nicholas P. Farrell. 2000. LC 99-32239. (Cancer Drug Discovery & Development Ser.: Vol. 7). (Illus.). xii, 341p. 145.00 (*0-89603-599-9*) Humana.

Platinum, Gold, & Other Metal Chemotherapeutic Agents. Ed. by Stephen J. Lippard. 1983. LC 82-24333. (ACS Symposium Ser.: No. 209). 453p. lib. bdg. 65.95 (*0-8412-0758-5*) Am Chemical.

***Plato of Praed Street: The Life & Times of Almroth Wright.** Michael S. Dunnill. 2000. (History of Medicine Ser.). 284p. pap. (*1-85315-477-6*) Royal Soc of Medicine Pr Ltd GBR. *Dist:* Balogh.

Platonism & Anti-Platonism in Mathematics. Mark Balaguer. 1998. 240p. text 45.00 (*0-19-512230-5*) OUP.

Play & Exploration in Children & Animals. Thomas G. Power. 1999. LC 99-30955. 497p. pap. (*0-8058-2242-9*) L Erlbaum Assocs.

Play & Intervention. Ed. by Joop Hellendoorn et al. 1994. LC 93-28930. (SUNY Series, Children's Play in Society). 369p. (C). text 21.50 (*0-7914-1933-9*); pap. text 20.95 (*0-7914-1934-7*) State U NY Pr.

Play & Mental Health. John E. Davis. 1982. 21.95 (*0-8434-0427-2*) McGrath NH.

Play & Playscapes Instructors Guide. Joe L. Frost. 1992. (Illus.). 320p. pap., tchr. ed. 10.50 (*0-8273-4700-6*) Delmar.

Play-Based Learning: A Module for Training Personnel Serving Families of Deaf & Hard of Hearing Infants & Young Children. Ed. by Valerie Schuyler. 1993. (Early Intervention Ser.). 37p. (C). tchr. ed. 89.00 incl. VHS (*0-9618297-5-3*) Hearing & Speech.

Play Behavior. Pref. by Joseph Levy. 1983. LC 83-6102. 250p. (C). reprint ed. text 29.50 (*0-89874-627-2*) Krieger.

Play Behavior & Choice of Play Materials of Pre-School Children. Dorothy Van Alstyne. 1976. LC 75-35083. (Studies in Play & Games). (Illus.). reprint ed. 16.95 (*0-405-07931-1*) Ayer.

Play Diagnosis & Assessment. Ed. by Karen Gitlin-Weiner et al. 2nd ed. 2000. LC 99-24905. (Illus.). 775p. 89.95 (*0-471-25457-6*) Wiley.

Play Hard, Eat Right! A Parent's Guide to Sports Nutrition for Their Children. American Dietetic Association Staff et al. 1995. 160p. pap. 10.95 (*0-471-34695-0*) Wiley.

Play Healthy, Stay Healthy: Your Guide to Managing & Treating 40 Common Sports Injuries. Gary N. Guten. 1991. LC 90-28365. (Illus.). 240p. pap. 15.95 (*0-88011-439-8*, PGUT0439) Human Kinetics.

Play in Childhood. Margaret Lowenfeld. 1991. (Classics in Developmental Medicine Ser.: No. 6). (Illus.). 242p. (C). text (*0-521-41331-1*) Mc Keith Pr GBR. *Dist:* Cambridge U Pr.

Play in Pediatric Occupational Therapy. Ed. by L. Diane Parham. 1996. (Illus.). 288p. (C). (gr. 13). text 47.00 (*0-8016-7838-2*, 07838) Mosby Inc.

Play Interviews for 4 Year Old Hospitilized Children. Florence H. Erickson. 1958. (SRCD M Ser.: Vol. 23, No. 3). pap. 25.00 (*0-527-01575-X*) Periodicals Srv.

Play of Animals. Karl Groos. 1976. LC 75-35072. (Studies in Play & Games). reprint ed. 31.95 (*0-405-07922-2*) Ayer.

Play Therapy. Virginia M. Axline. rev. ed. 1981. (Illus.). 384p. (C). mass mkt. 6.99 (*0-345-30335-0*) Ballantine Pub Grp.

Play Therapy: A Comprehensive Guide. O'Dessie O. James. 1997. LC 96-45165. 328p. 60.00 (*0-7657-0052-2*) Aronson.

Play Therapy: A Non-Directive Approach for Children & Adolescents. Kate Wilson et al. 1992. (Illus.). 245p. pap. text (*0-7020-1487-7*) W B Saunders GBR. *Dist:* Saunders.

Play Therapy: A Strategic Approach. Stanley Kissel. 1990. 108p. (C). text 31.95 (*0-398-05708-7*) C C Thomas.

Play Therapy: Dynamics of the Process of Counseling with Children. Garry L. Landreth. 1982. 380p. (C). text 58.95 (*0-398-04716-2*) C C Thomas.

Play Therapy Techniques. Ed. by Charles E. Schaefer & Donna M. Cangelosi. 1995. LC 92-49535. 304p. reprint ed. pap. 35.00 (*0-87668-176-3*) Aronson.

Play Therapy Theory & Practice: A Comparative Presentation. Ed. by Kevin O'Connor & Lisa M. Braverman. 1996. LC 96-21257. 432p. 80.00 (*0-471-10638-0*) Wiley.

Play Therapy with Children in Crisis: A Casebook for Practitioners. Ed. by Nancy B. Webb. 1991. LC 91-19756. 460p. text 45.00 (*0-89862-760-5*) Guilford Pubns.

Playful Approaches to Serious Problems: Narrative Therapy with Children & Their Families. Jennifer Freeman et al. 1997. LC 96-52874. 288p. 35.00 (*0-393-70229-4*) Norton.

Playground of Psychoanalytic Therapy. Jean Sanville. 2000. 312p. pap. 29.95 (*0-88163-331-3*) Analytic Pr.

Playing Ball on Running Water: Living Morita Psychotherapy - The Japanese Way to Building a Better Life. David K. Reynolds. 1984. LC 84-8399. 160p. pap. 8.95 (*0-688-03913-8*, Quil) HarperTrade.

Playing Cure: Individualized Play Therapy for Specific Childhood Problems. Ed. by Heidi G. Kaduson et al. 1997. LC 96-22725. 400p. 55.00 (*0-7657-0021-2*) Aronson.

Playing Doctor: Who Will Control Medical Practice in the Year 2000? Emily Friedman. 1989. (Papers: No. 9). 36p. 5.00 (*0-934459-57-6*) United Hosp Fund.

Playing for Real: Exploring the World of Child Therapy & the Inner Worlds of Children. Richard Bromfield. 1997. LC 97-13376. 256p. reprint ed. pap. 35.00 (*0-7657-0129-4*, RA1) Aronson.

Playing for Their Lives: Helping Troubled Children Through Play Therapy. Dorothy Singer. 1993. LC 92-38390. 240p. 27.95 (*0-02-928903-3*) Free Pr.

Playing God? Dissecting Biomedical Ethics & Manipulating the Body. Ed. by R. C. Sproul, Jr. 1997. LC 96-35213. 96p. (gr. 11). pap. 8.99 (*0-8010-5725-6*) Baker Bks.

Playing God? Genetic Determinism & Human Freedom. Ted Peters. 1996. 218p. (C). 80.00 (*0-415-91521-X*); LC 96-32892. pap. 22.95 (*0-415-91522-8*) Routledge.

Playing on the Mother-Ground: Cultural Routines for Children's Development. David F. Lancy. 1996. (Culture & Human Development Ser.). 240p. pap. 23.00 (*1-57230-215-1*, 0215) Guilford Pubns.

Playing the Hand Life Dealt & Winning the Jackpot! Auto-Immune Illness. Barbara Mascio & Richard Mascio. 1996. LC 96-230357. (Illus.). 100p. (Orig.). pap. 10.95 (*0-9653612-4-1*, AIBM-1) Harmony Publng.

Playing with Fire: Creative Conflict Resolution for Young Adults. Fiona Macbeth & Nic Fine. 1995. (Illus.). 192p. pap. 19.95 (*0-86571-306-5*) New Soc Pubs.

Play's the Thing: Exploring Text in Drama & Therapy. Marina Jenkins. 1996. 256p. (C). pap. 27.95 (*0-415-11498-5*) Routledge.

Playtherapy with Children. Sue Jennings. 1993. LC 93-5356. (Illus.). 224p. pap. 36.95 (*0-632-02442-9*) Blackwell Sci.

Plea for a Measure of Abnormality. Joyce McDougall. 1992. LC 92-29739. 493p. reprint ed. pap. text 39.95 (*0-87630-701-2*) Brunner-Routledge.

Pleasant Activities: COPE Program for Depression. John H. Greist et al. 1999. 56p. pap. (*0-9702974-3-2*) Healthcare Sys.

Please Ask. Cecelia Kroll. 1985. LC 85-90128. 241p. (Orig.). pap. 9.00 (*0-9614913-0-2*) C Kroll.

Please Don't Hurt Me, Doc! Humourous Experiences from 40 Years of Practice. Daniel L. Thomas, Jr. 1997. LC 97-35779. (Illus.). 79p. (Orig.). pap. 10.00 (*1-888683-57-0*) Wooster Bk.

Please Pass up the Salt. Lucy M. Williams. 1995. 48p. (J). (gr. k-4). 14.95 (*0-945080-18-2*) Sandridge Pub.

Pleasure & Frustration: A Resynthesis of Clinical & Theoretical Psychoanalysis. Leon Wallace. 1984. LC 84-3787. xiv, 193p. (C). 30.00 (*0-8236-4161-9*) Intl Univs Pr.

Pleasure Connection: How Endorphins Affect Our Health & Happiness. Deva Beck & James Beck. 1987. LC 87-60379. 235p. (Orig.). pap. 12.95 (*0-9617972-0-7*) Synthesis Pr.

Pleasure Prescription: To Love, to Work, to Play-Life in the Balance. Paul Pearsall. 1997. LC 96-28108. 288p. 23.95 (*0-89793-208-0*) Hunter Hse.

Pleneurethics: A New Concept of Healing, Vol. 2. Richard B. Collier. 2nd ed. 1993. xxvi, 288p. 17.95 (*1-882152-10-7*); pap. 11.95 (*1-882152-11-5*) R B Collier Pleneurethics.

Plethysmography: Safety, Effectiveness, & Clinical Utility in Diagnosing Vascular Disease. Thomas V. Holohan. 1998. 46p. (C). reprint ed. pap. text 20.00 (*0-7881-4191-0*) DIANE Pub.

Pleura in Health & Disease. Chretien et al. 1985. (Lung Biology in Health & Disease Ser.: Vol. 30). (Illus.). 906p. text 295.00 (*0-8247-7380-2*) Dekker.

Pleuropulmonary & Bronchial Infections. Ed. by Michael Simberkoff & Gerald L. Mandell. 1996. LC 95-45642. (Atlas of Infectious Diseases Ser.: Vol. 6). (Illus.). 283p. text (*0-443-07740-1*) Church GBR. *Dist:* Saunders.

Plexus Anesthesia: Perivascular Techniques of Brachial Plexus Block, Vol. 1. Alon P. Winnie. rev. ed. 1984. (Illus.). 272p. text 142.00 (*0-7216-1172-9*) Saunders.

Plugged Arteries & a Clogged Immune System. Milton G. Crane. 1998. LC 98-88032. (Illus.). 110p. per. 18.95 (*1-57258-145-X*) TEACH Servs.

Plumer's Principles & Practice of Intravenous Therapy. Ada L. Plumer & Cosentino. 4th ed. 1987. (Illus.). 567p. (C). text 31.50 (*0-673-39403-4*) Lppncott W & W.

Plumer's Principles & Practice of Intravenous Therapy. Sharon M. Weinstein. 7th ed. 2000. LC 00-44395. (Illus.). 784p. pap. text 39.95 (*0-7817-1988-7*) Lppncott W & W.

Plunging Through the Clouds: Constructive Living Currents. Ed. by David K. Reynolds. 1993. LC 91-45686. 199p. (C). text 20.50 (*0-7914-1313-6*) State U NY Pr.

Plunkett's Health Care Industry Almanac 2001-2002: The Only Complete Reference to the Health Care Industry. Jack W. Plunkett. rev. ed. 2001. 740p. pap. 199.95 incl. cd-rom (*1-891775-17-0*, PHCA01) Plunkett Res.

Plural Medical Systems in North-East Africa: The Legacy of "Sheikh" Hippocrates. Leendert J. Slikkerveer. 1989. (Monographs from the African Studies Centre). 200p. 69.50 (*0-7103-0203-7*) Routledge.

***Plural Medicine: Orthodox & Heterodox Medicine in Western & Colonial Countries During Nineteenth & Twentieth Centuries.** Waltraud Ernst. 2001. LC 2001-48501. (Studies in the Social History of Medicine). 224p. (C). (gr. 13). lib. bdg. 95.00 (*0-415-23122-1*) Routledge.

Plural Psyche: Personality, Morality & the Father. Andrew Samuels. 1989. 272p. 25.00 (*0-415-01759-9*, 9841) Routledge.

Pluralism & Personality: William James & Some Contemporary Cultures of Psychology. Don S. Browning. 1970. LC 78-75196. 280p. 38.50 (*0-8387-2265-2*) Bucknell U Pr.

Plutonium Files: America's Secret Medical Experiments in the Cold War. Eileen Welsome. 1999. LC 99-10991. (Illus.). ix, 580p. 26.95 (*0-385-31402-7*) Delacorte.

Plutonium Files: America's Secret Medical Experiments in the Cold War. Eileen Welsome. 2000. (Illus.). 592p. pap. 16.95 (*0-385-31954-1*, Dial Pr) Dell.

PMS: Self Help Book. Susan M. Lark. 1995. LC 89-25292. 240p. text 16.95 (*0-89087-587-1*) Celestial Arts.

PMS & Alcoholism. Therese Casey. 1984. 20p. (Orig.). (C). pap. 2.00 (*0-89486-247-2*, 1377B) Hazelden.

PMS & Perimenopause Sourcebook: A Guide to the Emotional, Mental & Physical Patterns of a Woman's Life. Lori A. Futterman & John E. Jones. 1998. 272p. pap. 16.00 (*1-56565-859-0*, 08590W) Lowell Hse.

PMS & You. Elizabeth K. White et al. 1994. (Illus.). 40p. pap. 3.60 (*0-910304-20-3*) Budlong.

PMS, Perimenopause & You: A Guide to the Physical, Mental & Emotional Patterns of a Woman' Lori A. Futterman. 2nd ed. 2000. LC 00-57934. (Illus.). 259p. pap. 16.95 (*0-7373-0511-8*) Lowell Hse.

PMS-Premenstrual Syndrome: The Cause & Cure of the Syndrome That Affects 5,000,000 American Women. Ronald V. Norris & Colleen Sullivan. 1983. LC 82-42700. 331p. 15.95 (*0-89256-238-2*, Rawson Assocs) Macmillan.

PMS Solution: A Nutritional Approach to Premenstrual Syndrome. Ann Nazzaro et al. 1985. 156p. (Orig.). 7.95 (*0-86683-793-0*, AY8554) Harper SF.

PMS Solving the Puzzle: Sixteen Causes of Premenstrual Syndrome & What to Do about It. Linaya Hahn. 1995. LC 95-160820. (Illus.). 176p. (Orig.). pap. 16.95 (*1-886094-15-2*) Chicago Spectrum.

PN-VN NCLEX Review Cards. 1999. (C). 32.95 (*1-56930-093-3*) Delmar.

Pneumatic Instrumentation. Dale R. Patrick & Steven R. Patrick. 3rd ed. 1993. LC 92-31773. 434p. mass mkt. 42.50 (*0-8273-5482-7*) Delmar.

Pneumococcus: Epidemiology, Prophylaxis, Treatment & Virulence. David A. Watson. 1997. (Medical Intelligence Unit Ser.). 250p. 89.95 (*0-412-13121-8*) Chapman & Hall.

Pneumocystis Carinii: Index of New Information. Jennifer G. Rescar. 1998. 57.50 (*0-7883-1814-4*); pap. 47.50 (*0-7883-1815-2*) ABBE Pubs Assn.

Pneumocystis Carinii, Vol. I. Walter T. Hughes, Jr. 1987. 144p. 86.00 (*0-8493-4665-7*, CRC Reprint) Franklin.

Pneumocystis Carinii, Vol. II. Hughes, Jr. 1987. 152p. 88.00 (*0-8493-4666-5*, CRC Reprint) Franklin.

Pneumocystis Carinii Pneumonia. Ed. by Peter D. Walzer. 2nd ed. 1993. LC 93-11338. (Lung Biology in Health & Disease Ser.: Vol. 69). (Illus.). 744p. text 255.00 (*0-8247-8854-0*) Dekker.

Pneumological Aspects of Gastroesophageal Reflux. L. Allegra & R. Dal Negro. 1999. LC 99-24353. 192p. (C). (*88-470-0049-1*) Spr-Verlag ITA. *Dist:* Spr-Verlag.

Pneumonias. Monroe Karetzky et al. 1993. xv, 328p. (*3-540-97945-X*); LC 92-49615. (Illus.). 328p. 128.00 (*0-387-97945-X*) Spr-Verlag.

Pneumonias. Hobart A. Reimann. 1971. LC 78-166458. (Illus.). 224p. 12.50 (*0-87527-119-7*) Green.

Pocket A-Z of Natural Healthcare. Belinda G. Viagas. 1997. (Orig.). mass mkt. (*0-7522-2126-4*) Boxtree GBR. *Dist:* Trans-Atl Phila.

Pocket Atlas of Acupuncture. Hans-Ulrich Hecker & Angelika Steveling. 2001. LC 2001-27470. (Illus.). xvi, 268p. pap. 29.00 (*0-86577-938-4*) Thieme Med Pubs.

Pocket Atlas of Cranial Magnetic Resonance Imaging. Victor M. Haughton & David L. Daniels. 1986. (Illus.). 64p. pap. text 19.95 (*0-88167-171-1*) Lppncott W & W.

Pocket Atlas of Cross-Sectional Anatomy: Computer Tomography & Magnetic Resonance Imaging Thorax, Abdomen & Pelvis, Vol. 2. Torsten B. Moeller & Emil Reif. 1994. LC 93-43883. 246p. pap. 32.00 (*0-86577-511-7*) Thieme Med Pubs.

Pocket Atlas of Cross-Sectional Anatomy Vol. 1: Head, Neck, Spine & Joints. Moeller. 2nd ed. 2000. pap. 32.00 (*0-86577-813-2*) Thieme Med Pubs.

Pocket Atlas of Cytology & Microscopic Anatomy. Wolfgang Kuhnel. 1981. 21.00 (*0-8151-5208-6*) Mosby Inc.

Pocket Atlas of Dermatology. G. K. Steigleder & Howard I. Maibach. 2nd rev. ed. 1993. (Flexibook Ser.). (Illus.). 304p. pap. text 32.00 (*0-86577-491-9*) Thieme Med Pubs.

Pocket Atlas of Emergency Medicine. Kevin Knoop et al. 1999. (Illus.). 334p. pap. 49.95 (*0-07-135807-2*) McGraw-Hill Prof.

Pocket Atlas of Hematology: Morphological Diagnosis for the Clinician. Theml. 1985. pap. 32.00 (*0-86577-210-X*) Thieme Med Pubs.

Pocket Atlas of Human Anatomy: Based on the International Nomenclature. Heinz Feneis & Wolfgang Dauber. 4th ed. 2000. LC 00-709227. (Illus.). vi, 500p. pap. 32.00 (*0-86577-928-7*) Thieme Med Pubs.

Pocket Atlas of MRI Body Anatomy. Thomas H. Bequist. 2nd ed. 1995. LC 95-17885. (Illus.). 112p. pap. text 19.95 (*0-7817-0336-0*) Lppncott W & W.

Pocket Atlas of MRI Musculoskeletal Anatomy. Thomas H. Berquist. 1995. LC 95-16479. (Illus.). 112p. pap. text 19.95 (*0-7817-0337-9*) Lppncott W & W.

Pocket Atlas of MRI of the Pelvis. Zella Campos et al. 1993. LC 92-49417. (Illus.). 128p. pap. text 19.95 (*0-88167-987-9*) Lppncott W & W.

Pocket Atlas of Normal CT Anatomy. James B. Weinstein et al. 1985. (Illus.). 88p. pap. text 19.95 (*0-88167-070-7*) Lppncott W & W.

Pocket Atlas of Obstetric Ultrasound. John C. Hobbins et al. 1996. LC 95-45314. (Illus.). 96p. pap. text 19.95 (*0-397-51623-1*) Lppncott W & W.

Pocket Atlas of Oral Diseases. George Laskaris. 1998. (Illus.). 444p. pap. text 29.00 (*0-86577-635-0*) Thieme Med Pubs.

Pocket Atlas of Pediatric Ultrasound. Carol M. Rumack et al. 1990. 120p. pap. text 19.95 (*0-88167-620-9*) Lppncott W & W.

Pocket Atlas of Radiographic Anatomy. Emil Reif & Toreten B. Moeller. 2nd ed. 2000. LC 99-40802. (Illus.). 391p. pap. 34.00 (*0-86577-874-4*) Thieme Med Pubs.

Pocket Atlas of Radiographic Positioning. Emil Reif & Therald B. Moeller. 1996. LC 97-110619. (Illus.). 290p. pap. text 19.90 (*0-86577-640-7*) Thieme Med Pubs.

Pocket Atlas of Rheumatology. Dieter Wessinghage. Tr. by Gottfried Stiasny. 1985. (Flexibook Ser.). (Illus.). 256p. pap. 32.00 (*0-86577-221-5*) Thieme Med Pubs.

Pocket Atlas of Sectional Anatomy Vol. 2: Computed Tomography & Magnetic Resonance Imaging. Torsten B. Moeller & Emil Reif. 2nd ed. 2001. LC 2001-268004. (Illus.). 264p. pap. 32.00 (*0-86577-872-8*) Thieme Med Pubs.

Pocket Book for Intensive Care. Tinker. 2nd ed. 176p. pap. (*0-340-51764-6*) E A GBR. *Dist:* Routldge.

Pocket Book Infectious Disease Therapy, 1997. John G. Bartlett. 8th ed. 1997. 379p. pap. 14.95 (*0-683-30357-0*) Lppncott W & W.

Pocket Book of Emergency & Disability Scores. Jonathan Handler. 1999. 40p. (C). pap. 6.00 (*1-883205-46-8*) Intl Med Pub.

Pocket Book of Pediatric Antimicrobial Therapy, 1995. John D. Nelson. 11th ed. 1995. LC 88-26186. (Illus.). 106p. pap. 13.95 (*0-683-06406-1*) Lppncott W & W.

***Pocket Brain of Clinical Pathophysiology.** Frank M. Griffin. 2001. LC 2001-1142. ix, 115p. pap. 17.95 (*0-632-04634-1*) Blackwell Sci.

Pocket Clinical & Drug Guide. Paul Debello. 672p. (Orig.). (C). 3rd ed. 1992. pap. text 25.00 (*0-9627160-2-2*); 4th ed. pap. text 25.00 (*0-9627160-3-0*) Tortoise NV.

Pocket Companion for Black & Matassarin-Jacobs Medical-Surgical Nursing: Clinical Management for Continuity of Care. Joyce M. Black & Esther Matassarin-Jacobs. 5th ed. 1997. (Illus.). 800p. pap. 23.00 (*0-7216-7287-6*) Saunders.

Pocket Companion for Cancer Nursing. Ed. by Ruth McCorkle & Marcia Grant. 1994. LC 94-6847. (Illus.). 537p. pap. text 38.95 (*0-7216-5410-X*) Saunders.

Pocket Companion for Critical Care Nursing. Sheila Melander & Linda Bucher. Ed. by Robin Carter. 1999. LC 98-43361. 475p. pap. text 23.95 (*0-7216-6919-0*) Saunders.

Pocket Companion for Home Health Nurses. Springhouse Publishing Company Staff. Ed. by June Norris. 1996. LC 96-17975. (Illus.). 512p. (Orig.). 28.95 (*0-87434-853-6*) Springhouse Corp.

Pocket Companion for Medical-Surgical Nursing. Donna D. Ignatavicius & Kathy A. Hausman. 2nd ed. 1994. (Illus.). 775p. pap. text 22.00 (*0-7216-4867-3*) Saunders.

Pocket Companion for Medical-Surgical Nursing: Foundations for Clinical Practice. Frances Donovan Monahan & Marianne Neighbors. 2nd ed. 1997. 514p. pap. 17.95 (*0-7216-7334-1*) Saunders.

Pocket Companion for Pharmacology: A Nursing Process Approach. Evelyn R. Hayes & Joyce L. Kee. 2nd ed. 1996. LC 96-43504. pap. text 20.95 (*0-7216-5957-8*) Saunders.

Pocket Companion for Physical Examination & Health Assessment. Carolyn Jarvis. 2nd ed. 1996. LC 95-24471. (Illus.). 329p. pap. text 24.00 (*0-7216-5899-7*) Saunders.

Pocket Companion for the Textbook of Physical Diagnosis. Mark H. Swartz. Ed. by William Schmitt. 2nd ed. 1997. LC 97-23179. (Illus.). 288p. pap. text 22.95 (*0-7216-7517-4*) Saunders.

Pocket Companion of Critical Care: Immediate Concerns. Robert R. Kirby et al. 1990. (Illus.). 760p. text 44.95 (*0-397-51030-6*) Lppncott W & W.

Pocket Companion to Cecil Textbook of Medicine. Lee Goldman & J. Claude Bennett. 21st ed. 2001. LC 00-34506. (Illus.). viii, 856p. 35.50 (*0-7216-8972-8*) Saunders.

Pocket Companion to Equine Medicine & Surgery. Christine King et al. 1999. LC 98-35658. (Illus.). 800p. (C). (gr. 13). pap. text 39.95 (*0-8151-1741-8*, 28581) Mosby Inc.

Pocket Companion to Home Health Nursing. Karen E. Monks. 2000. LC 99-44468. 475p. pap. text (*0-7216-8558-7*) Saunders.

Pocket Companion to Neurology in Clinical Practice. Walter G. Bradley et al. 3rd ed. 2000. (Illus.). 800p. pap. text 49.99 (*0-7506-7264-1*) Buttrwrth-Heinemann.

Pocket Companion to Obstetrics: Normal & Problem Pregnancies. J. Gabbe et al. 1998. LC 98-41893. (Illus.). 400p. (C). pap. text (*0-443-07982-X*) Church.

Pocket Companion to Pathologic Basis of Disease. Stanley L. Robbins et al. 5th ed. 1995. (Illus.). 630p. pap. text 26.95 (*0-7216-5742-7*) Saunders.

Pocket Companion to Principles & Practice of Medical Intensive Care. James A. Kruse et al. 1995. (Illus.). 608p. pap. text 44.00 (*0-7216-5633-1*) Saunders.

Pocket Companion to Textbook of Critical Care. William C. Shoemaker et al. 3rd ed. 1996. LC 95-31495. 608p. pap. text 43.00 (*0-7216-5833-4*) Saunders.

Pocket Companion to Textbook of Medical Physiology. Arthur C. Guyton & John E. Hall. 2nd ed. 2000. LC 00-58344. (Illus.). xiv, 730p. 24.95 (*0-7216-8729-6*) Saunders.

Pocket Companion to Textbook of Small Animal Surgery. Douglas H. Slatter. 2nd ed. 1995. LC 94-13110. 864p. pap. text 52.50 (*0-7216-5544-0*) Saunders.

Pocket Companion to Textbook of Veterinary Internal Medicine. Stephen J. Ettinger. 2nd ed. 1995. (Illus.). 900p. pap. text 43.00 (*0-7216-5766-4*) Saunders.

Pocket Consultant in Gastroenterology. S. P. Travis et al. 1991. (Pocket Consultant Ser.). (Illus.). 432p. pap. 36.95 (*0-632-01098-3*) Blackwell Sci.

***Pocket Diagnosis in General Surgery.** H. Ellis. 3rd ed. 2001. (Illus.). 320p. pap. 31.95 (*0-632-05479-4*) Blackwell Sci.

Pocket Dictionary/Nursing Assistant & Health Care. Hampton. 1995. (Home Care Aide Ser.). 12.95 (*0-8273-6475-X*) Delmar.

Pocket Dietitian (1918) J. H. Tilden. 1996. 112p. reprint ed. pap. 10.95 (*1-56459-871-3*) Kessinger Pub.

Pocket Doctor: A Passport to Healthy Travel. Stephen Bezruchka. 3rd ed. 1999. LC 98-52801. 127p. pap. 6.95 (*0-89886-614-6*) Mountaineers.

Pocket Doctor: Your Ticket to Good Health While Traveling. Stephen Bezruchka. 2nd ed. 1992. LC 92-19995. (Illus.). 96p. pap. 4.95 (*0-89886-345-7*) Mountaineers.

Pocket Doctor 1999. Michael S. Sherman & Edward S. Schulman. 1999. 176p. pap. 12.95 (*0-9672263-0-9*) Ed Commns NY.

Pocket Drug Guide. Constantine J. Gean et al. 1989. 257p. pap. text 25.00 (*0-683-03440-5*) Lppncott W & W.

Pocket Drug Guide. Frederick H. Meyers & Constantine J. Gean. 3rd ed. 1998. LC 98-13760. pap. 24.95 (*0-683-30597-2*) Lppncott W & W.

Pocket Enneagram: Understanding the 9 Types of people. Helen Palmer. 1995. LC 95-14044. (Illus.). 96p. pap. 9.00 (*0-06-251327-3*) Harper SF.

Pocket Essentials of Clinical Surgery. Ed. by S. Walker & C. Holcombe. 1997. (Illus.). 530p. (*0-7020-2064-8*) Saunders.

Pocket Examiner in Obstetrics & Gynaecology. Peter Bowen-Simpkins & David Pugh. 2nd ed. 1993. 260p. pap. text (*0-443-03929-1*) Church.

Pocket Examiner in Pathology. P. N. Cowen & F. G. Smiddy. 2nd ed. 1996. LC 95-33681. 148p. pap. text (*0-443-05418-5*) Church.

Pocket Examiner in Regional & Clinical Anatomy see Problem Solving for Tutorials in Anatomy

Pocket Examiner in Surgery. Tom Treasure et al. 2nd ed. 1999. LC 96-26055. pap. text (*0-443-04894-0*) Church GBR. *Dist:* Harcourt CAN.

Pocket Examiner Paediatrics. Lissauer. 1985. pap. text 22.00 (*0-443-03815-5*) Saunders.

Pocket Guide for Asthma Management & Prevention: A Pocket Guide for Physicians & Nurses. 1996. (Illus.). 28p. reprint ed. pap. text 15.00 (*0-7881-3543-0*) DIANE Pub.

Pocket Guide for Chiropractic Skeletal Radiography. Rhonda J. Boone. 2000. LC 00-32879. (Illus.). 321p. (C). pap. 34.95 (*0-8385-8130-7*) McGraw-Hill Prof.

Pocket Guide for the Home Care Aide. Barbara Stover Gingerich & Deborah Anne Ondeck. 1998. LC 98-26061. 350p. (gr. 6). pap. 35.00 (*0-8342-1161-0*, 11610) Aspen Pub.

Pocket Guide for the Textbook of Pharmacotherapy for Child & Adolescent Psychiatric Disorders. David Rosenberg et al. 1997. LC 97-33193. 192p. pap. 24.95 (*0-87630-871-X*) Brunner-Routledge.

Pocket Guide for Women & Cancer. Giselle Moore. 1998. (Nursing Ser.). (Illus.). 224p. (C). pap. text 37.95 (*0-7637-0548-9*, 0548-9) Jones & Bartlett.

Pocket Guide to Acne. Amrit Darvay & Anthony Chu. 2000. LC 00-22607. (Illus.). 50p. pap. 36.95 (*0-632-05437-9*) Blackwell Sci.

Pocket Guide to Acupressure Points for Women. Cathryn Bauer. 1997. LC 97-11570. (Crossing Press Pocket Ser.). (Illus.). 102p. (Orig.). pap. 6.95 (*0-89594-879-6*) Crossing Pr.

Pocket Guide to Ayurvedic Healing. Candis C. Packard. 1996. (Crossing Press Pocket Ser.). (Illus.). 144p. (Orig.). pap. text 6.95 (*0-89594-764-1*) Crossing Pr.

Pocket Guide to Bach Flower Essences. Rachelle Hasnas. 1997. LC 97-11517. (Crossing Press Pocket Ser.). 128p. pap. 6.95 (*0-89594-865-6*) Crossing Pr.

Pocket Guide to Basic Dysrhythmias: Interpretation & Management. Robert J. Huszar. 2nd ed. 1995. (Illus.). 126p. (*0-8151-4743-0*, 25903) Mosby Inc.

Pocket Guide to Basic Dysrhythmias Interpretation & Management. Robert J. Huszar. 1995. LC 95-221015. (Illus.). 128p. pap. text 9.95 (*0-8151-4746-5*) Mosby Inc.

Pocket Guide to Basic Skills & Procedures. Anne G. Perry & Patricia A. Potter. 4th ed. 1998. (Illus.). 576p. pap. (*84-8174-391-7*) Mosby-Doyma Libros ESP. *Dist:* Mosby Inc.

Pocket Guide to Basic Skills & Procedures, Vol. 4. Anne G. Perry. 4th ed. 1998. LC 99-187163. (Pocket Guide to Basic Skills & Procedures Ser.: Vol. 4). (Illus.). 576p. (YA). (gr. 13). text 22.95 (*0-8151-2714-6*, 31635) Mosby Inc.

Pocket Guide to Biotherapy. Paula Rieger. Date not set. (Nursing Ser.). 200p. pap. 31.25 (*0-7637-0543-8*) Jones & Bartlett.

Pocket Guide to Brain Injury, Cognitive' & Neurobehavioral Rehabilitation. Thomas J. Guilmette. 1997. LC 97-22897. (Illus.). 324p. (Orig.). pap. 45.00 (*1-56593-833-X*, 1628) Thomson Learn.

Pocket Guide to Breast Cancer. Karen Hassey Dow. 1999. LC 98-43153. (Nursing Ser.). (Illus.). 290p. (C). pap. text 34.95 (*0-7637-0683-3*, 0683-3) Jones & Bartlett.

***Pocket Guide to Breast Cancer.** Karen Hassey Dow. 2nd ed. 2001. (Illus.). (C). pap. text 35.95 (*0-7637-1814-9*, 1814-9, N L N Bart) Jones & Bartlett.

Pocket Guide to Breast Cancer - Genentech. Karen Hassey-Dow. 1998. (Illus.). (C). pap. text 33.95 (*0-7637-0988-3*, 0988-3) Jones & Bartlett.

Pocket Guide to Breastfeeding & Human Lactation. Kathleen G. Auerbach & Jan Riordan. 1996. LC 96-25990. (Illus.). 120p. (C). pap. text 24.95 (*0-7637-0258-7*, 0258-7) Jones & Bartlett.

Pocket Guide to Cardiovascular Disease. Edward K. Chung & Dennis A. Tighe. 1998. LC 98-45297. (Illus.). pap. 29.95 (*0-86542-508-6*) Blackwell Sci.

Pocket Guide to Cases of Medicine & Public Health Collaboration. Roz D. Lasker et al. 1998. LC 98-22071. (*0-924143-08-8*) NY Acad Med.

Pocket Guide to Chinese Patent Medicines. Bill Schoenbart. 1999. LC 98-47925. (Crossing Press Pocket Ser.). 111p. pap. 6.95 (*0-89594-978-4*) Crossing Pr.

Pocket Guide to Clinical Coding, 2001. M. Trayser Dunaway. 2000. 81p. spiral bd. 14.75 (*0-9664166-1-9*) Rebel Records.

Pocket Guide to Clinical Examination. Nicholas J. Talley. 1998. 204p. pap. 38.95 (*0-632-05152-3*) Blackwell Sci.

Pocket Guide to Clinical Examination. Owen Epstein et al. 2nd ed. 1998. 16.95 (*0-7234-2577-9*) Mosby Inc.

Pocket Guide to Clinical Microbiology. Patrick R. Murray. 2nd rev. ed. 1998. LC 98-21385. 350p. pap. 34.95 (*1-55581-137-X*) ASM Pr.

Pocket Guide to Common Drugs. Springhouse Publishing Company Staff. 1998. 336p. spiral bd. 22.95 (*0-87434-948-6*) Springhouse Corp.

Pocket Guide to Commonly Prescribed Drugs. Glenn N. Levine. 2nd ed. 1997. 422p. (C). pap. 19.95 (*0-8385-8099-8*, A8099-2, Apple Lange Med) McGraw.

Pocket Guide to Commonly Prescribed Drugs. Glenn N. Levine. 3rd ed. 1999. 480p. pap. 24.95 (*0-8385-8146-3*) McGraw-Hill Prof.

Pocket Guide to CPR for Infants & Children. Ed. by Gloria Blatti. 1998. LC 99-207577. (Illus.). 128p. per. 3.99 (*0-671-00975-3*) PB.

Pocket Guide to Critical Appraisal. Ed. by I. K. Crombie. 1996. 66p. pap. text (*0-7279-1099-X*) BMJ Pub GBR. *Dist:* AIDC.

Pocket Guide to Critical Care Assessment. Laura A. Talbot. 3rd ed. 1997. LC 96-44664. (Illus.). 400p. (C). (gr. 13). text 22.95 (*0-8151-5608-1*, 29562) Mosby Inc.

Pocket Guide to Critical Care Monitoring. Anna Owen. 2nd ed. 1996. (Illus.). 288p. (C). (gr. 13). text 22.95 (*0-8151-7374-1*, 28101) Mosby Inc.

Pocket Guide to Cultural Assessment. Elaine Marie Geissler. 2nd ed. 1998. LC 98-25821. (Mosby's Pocket Guide Ser.). (Illus.). 320p. (C). (gr. 12). spiral bd. 22.95 (*0-8151-3633-1*, 31285) Mosby Inc.

Pocket Guide to Cutaneous Medicine & Surgery. Philip E. LeBoit et al. 1995. (Illus.). 416p. pap. text 39.00 (*0-7216-5409-6*) Saunders.

Pocket Guide to Diagnostic Tests. Diana Nicoll et al. 2nd rev. ed. 1998. 457p. (C). pap. 24.95 (*0-8385-8100-5*, A8100-8) McGraw-Hill Educ Grp.

Pocket Guide to Diagnostic Tests. Diana Nicoll et al. 3rd ed. 2000. (Illus.). 511p. (C). pap. 34.95 (*0-8385-8135-8*) McGraw-Hill Prof.

Pocket Guide to ECG Diagnosis. Edward K. Chung. (Illus.). 1996. LC 96-3795. 495p. pap. text 34.95 (*0-86542-499-3*); 2nd ed. 2000. 528p. pap. 39.95 (*0-86542-589-2*) Blackwell Sci.

Pocket Guide to Eczema & Contact Dermatitis. Colin Holden & Lucy Ostlere. 2000. LC 00-23116. (Pocket Guide Ser.). (Illus.). 120p. pap. 36.95 (*0-632-05663-0*) Blackwell Sci.

Pocket Guide to Electrocardiography. Mary Boudreau Conover. 4th ed. 1997. LC 97-39597. (Illus.). 288p. (C). (gr. 13). text 22.95 (*0-8151-3695-1*, 31037) Mosby Inc.

Pocket Guide to Electrocardiography. Mary Boudreau Conover. 3rd ed. 1998. (Illus.). 288p. pap. (*84-8086-156-8*) Mosby-Doyma Libros ESP. *Dist:* Mosby Inc.

Pocket Guide to Emergency First Aid. Betty Cordes et al. 1993. (Illus.). 28p. spiral bd. 12.95 (*0-9633024-2-6*) Greycliff Pub.

Pocket Guide to Emergency Medicine. John M. Howell & B. Tilman Jolly. 2000. 782p. pap. 44.00 (*0-7216-5823-7*) Harcrt Hlth Sci Grp.

Pocket Guide to EMT Prehospital Care. Alice T. Dalton et al. 1994. LC 93-23587. (Illus.). 256p. pap. text 17.95 (*0-7216-3781-7*) Saunders.

Pocket Guide to Eponyms & Subtle Signs of Disease. Scott M. Tenner & Thomas M. Masterson. 1993. 78p. (Orig.). (C). pap. text 7.50 (*0-9634063-6-1*) Intl Med Pub.

Pocket Guide to Essential of Diagnosis & Treatment. Lawrence M. Tierney et al. 1997. 514p. (C). pap. 34.95 (*0-8385-3605-0*) McGraw-Hill Prof.

Pocket Guide to Evaluations of Drug Interactions. Ed. by Frederic J. Zucchero et al. 3rd rev. ed. 1999. 450p. pap. 35.00 (*0-917330-93-5*, T59-3) Am Pharm Assn.

***Pocket Guide to Evaluations of Drug Interactions.** Ed. by Frederic J. Zucchero. 4th ed. 2001. 500p. per. 39.00 (*1-58212-030-7*) Am Pharm Assn.

Pocket Guide to Examination of the Musculoskeletal System. Richard J. Hawkins & Kiefer. 1994. LC 94-28871. (Illus.). 304p. (C). (gr. 13). pap. text 27.00 (*0-8151-4162-9*, 20943) Mosby Inc.

Pocket Guide to Fetal Monitoring & Assessment. Susan M. Tucker. 4th ed. 2000. LC 99-88570. (Mosby's Pocket Guide Ser.). (Illus.). xx, 358p. pap. text 24.95 (*0-323-00884-4*) Mosby Inc.

Pocket Guide to Fluid, Electrolyte & Acid-Base Balance. Ursula Easterday Heitz et al. 4th ed. 2000. LC 00-46610. (Illus.). xvii, 332p. 24.95 (*0-323-01323-6*) Mosby Inc.

Pocket Guide to Fluids & Electrolytes. Mima M. Horne et al. 3rd ed. 1996. LC 96-10272. (Illus.). 320p. (C). (gr. 13). text 22.95 (*0-8151-4663-9*, 27461) Mosby Inc.

Pocket Guide to Fluids & Electrolytes. Mima M. Horne et al. 3rd ed. 1997. (Illus.). 320p. pap. (*84-8086-084-7*) Mosby-Doyma Libros ESP. *Dist:* Mosby Inc.

Pocket Guide to Fungal Infection. Malcolm Richardson & Elizabeth Johnson. 2000. LC 99-55311. (Illus.). vi, 114p. pap. 34.95 (*0-632-05325-9*) Blackwell Sci.

Pocket Guide to Gene Level Diagnostics in Clinical Practice. Victor A. Bernstam. 1992. 560p. lib. bdg. 69.95 (*0-8493-4485-9*, RB155) CRC Pr.

Pocket Guide to Gerontologic Assessment. Annette Lueckenotte. 3rd ed. 1997. LC 97-34218. (Illus.). 432p. (C). (gr. 13). text 22.95 (*0-8151-2799-5*, 31133); No. 2. 1994. 310p. (*0-08-151778-5*) Mosby Inc.

Pocket Guide to Healing Headaches. Pat Thomas. 2000. LC 00-30712. 128p. pap. 6.95 (*1-58091-083-1*) Crossing Pr.

Pocket Guide to Health Assessment. Patricia A. Potter. 4th ed. 1998. LC 97-47169. (Mosby's Pocket Guide Ser.). (Illus.). 416p. (C). (gr. 13). text 22.95 (*0-8151-8396-8*, 31696) Mosby Inc.

Pocket Guide to Health Assessment. Patricia A. Potter. 4th ed. 1998. (Illus.). 365p. (*84-8086-149-5*) Mosby-Doyma Libros ESP. *Dist:* Mosby Inc.

Pocket Guide to Herbal First Aid. Nancy Evelyn. 1998. LC 98-26032. (Pocket Ser.). 96p. pap. 6.95 (*0-89594-967-9*) Crossing Pr.

Pocket Guide to Home Care Standards: Complete Guidelines for Clinical Practice, Documentation, & Reimbursement. 2000. LC 00-41967. 704p. pap. 34.95 (*1-58255-039-5*) Springhouse Corp.

Pocket Guide to I. V. Drugs. Dawn N. Philp & Deborah L. Walz. 2000. LC 99-52578. vi, 234p. otabind 22.95 (*1-58255-044-1*) Springhouse Corp.

Pocket Guide to ICD - 10 Classification of Mental & Behavioural Disorders with Glossary & Diagnostic Criteria for Research DCR - 10. World Health Organization Staff. Ed. by J. E. Cooper. 1998. 419p. pap. (*0-443-04909-2*) Church.

Pocket Guide to Infection Prevention & Safe Practice. Susan D. Schaffer et al. 1995. LC 95-32784. (Illus.). 384p. (C). (gr. 13). 22.95 (*0-8151-7593-0*, 23641) Mosby Inc.

Pocket Guide to Injectable Chemotherapeutic Agents: Drug Information & Dosages. Byron G. Peters et al. 2nd rev. ed. 1998. xiii, 152p. pap. 24.95 (*0-9663138-0-1*) Oncology Educ.

Pocket Guide to Injectable Drugs: Companion to Handbook on Injectable Drugs. Lawrence A. Trissel. 8th rev. ed. 1994. 296p. pap. text 31.00 (*1-879907-50-X*); 9th ed. 1996. LC 97-116598. 300p. pap. text 31.00 (*1-879907-67-4*); 10th ed. 1998. LC 00-500797. 352p. pap. text 38.00 (*1-879907-89-5*); 11th ed. 2001. 400p. pap. (*1-58528-023-2*) Am Soc Hlth-Syst.

***Pocket Guide to Interpreting Lung Function Tests.** Robert John Hancox & Kenneth Frank Whyte. 2002. (Illus.). 120p. pap. 24.95 (*0-07-470979-8*) McGraw-Hill Prof.

Pocket Guide to Intravenous Therapy. Joanne C. LaRocca et al. 3rd ed. 1996. LC 96-14139. (Illus.). 464p. (C). (gr. 13). text 22.95 (*0-8151-5298-1*, 28205) Mosby Inc.

Pocket Guide to IV Therapy. Joanne C. Larocca. 4th ed. 1993. (Illus.). 213p. (C). (gr. 13). spiral bd. 28.95 (*0-8016-6910-3*, 06910) Mosby Inc.

Pocket Guide to Lymphoma Classification. D. Mason. 1998. (Illus.). pap. 34.94 (*0-632-05096-9*) Blackwell Sci.

Pocket Guide to Malignant Melanoma. John Buchan & Dafydd Lloyd Roberts. 2000. LC 99-53650. (Illus.). vii, 55p. pap. 36.95 (*0-632-05421-2*) Blackwell Sci.

Pocket Guide to Managing Contraception: 2000-2001 Edition. Robert A. Hatcher & Anita Nelson. 2000. (Illus.). 168p. pap. text 15.95 (*0-8290-5217-8*) Ardent Media.

Pocket Guide to Maternal & Neonatal Nursing. Kathryn A. May & Laura R. Mahlmeister. 1993. LC 93-30921. (*0-397-55125-8*) Lppncott W & W.

Pocket Guide to Medications Used in Dermatology. Andrew J. Scheman & David L. Severson. 4th ed. 1994. LC 94-21217. 16.00 (*0-683-07593-4*) Lppncott W & W.

Pocket Guide to Midwifery Care. Aviva J. Romm. 1998. LC 98-10584. (Crossing Press Pocket Ser.). (Illus.). 112p. pap. 6.95 (*0-89594-855-9*) Crossing Pr.

Pocket Guide to Musculoskeletal Assessment. Richard Baxter. Ed. by Margaret Biblis. 1998. LC 97-18626. (Illus.). 208p. pap. text 24.95 (*0-7216-3337-4*) Saunders.

Pocket Guide to Natural Health: The Essential A to Z Guide for Your Family. Stephen Langer & James F. Scheer. 2001. 400p. mass mkt. 6.99 (*1-57566-614-6*, Twin Streams) Kensgtn Pub Corp.

Pocket Guide to Naturopathic Medicine. Judith Boice. 1996. (Crossing Press Pocket Ser.). (Illus.). 128p. pap. 6.95 (*0-89594-821-4*) Crossing Pr.

***Pocket Guide to Neck Dissection Classification & TNM Staging of Head & Neck Cancer.** 2nd rev. ed. 2001. (Monograph). (Illus.). pap. text 10.00 (*1-56772-039-0*, 5206250) AAO-HNS.

Pocket Guide to Neonatal EKG Interpretation. Jobeth Pilcher. 1998. LC 97-26769. (Illus.). 53p. spiral bd. 17.95 (*1-887571-02-7*) NICU Ink.

P
Q
R

Pocket Guide to Nursing Diagnosis. MiJa Kim et al. 7th ed. 1997. 528p. (C). (gr. 13). text 24.00 (*0-8151-4989-1*, 28270) Mosby Inc.

Pocket Guide to Nutrition & Diet Therapy. Mary C. Moore. 3rd ed. 1996. LC 96-15024. (Illus.). 496p. (C). (gr. 13). text 22.95 (*0-8151-7370-9*, 28269) Mosby Inc.

Pocket Guide to Nutritional Care. Mary Courtney Moore. 3rd ed. 1997. (Illus.). 496p. (*84-8086-083-9*) Mosby-Doyma Libros ESP. *Dist:* Mosby Inc.

Pocket Guide to Oncology Nursing. Shirley E. Otto. 1995. LC 95-190710. (Illus.). 640p. (C). (gr. 13). text 22.95 (*0-8151-6547-1*, 23768) Mosby Inc.

Pocket Guide to Ophthalmology Review. Willie Y. W. Chen. 2000. LC 00-30109. 144p. (C). pap. text 29.00 (*1-55642-478-7*) SLACK Inc.

Pocket Guide to Pediatric Assessment. Joyce K. Engel. 3rd ed. 1996. LC 96-29197. (Illus.). 384p. (C). (gr. 13). pap. text 22.95 (*0-8151-3157-7*, 27512) Mosby Inc.

Pocket Guide to Physical Diagnosis. Janice L. Willms & Henry Schneiderman. 1996. (Illus.). 319p. pap. text 23.95 (*0-683-09116-6*) Lppncott W & W.

Pocket Guide to Prostate Cancer. Jeanne Held-Warmkessel. 2000. LC 00-62681. (Series in Oncology). (Illus.). 214p. (C). pap. text 32.95 (*0-7637-1476-3*, 1476-3) Jones & Bartlett.

Pocket Guide to Psoriasis. Simon Davison et al. 2000. LC 99-53651. (Illus.). 72p. pap. 36.95 (*0-632-05208-2*) Blackwell Sci.

Pocket Guide to Psychiatry. Allan Tasman. 1997. LC 97-226318. 631p. pap. text 36.95 (*0-7216-5241-7*) Saunders.

Pocket Guide to Radiography. Philip W. Ballinger. (Illus.). 400p. 3rd ed. 1995. LC 95-6295. (C). (gr. 13). spiral bd. 22.95 (*0-8151-0401-4*, 24273); 4th ed. 1999. spiral bd. 23.95 (*0-8151-2649-2*, 31647) Mosby Inc.

Pocket Guide to Regional Anesthesia Techniques. Eckhardt. 2001. 352p. pap. 35.00 (*0-7506-9851-9*) Buttrwrth-Heinemann.

Pocket Guide to Respiratory Disease. Robert L. Wilkins et al. 2001. LC 2001-17288. (Illus.). 192p. 16.95 (*0-8036-0566-8*) Davis Co.

Pocket Guide to Sectional Anatomy. Lorrie L. Kelley & Connie M. Petersen. 1997. (Illus.). 256p. spiral bd. 21.95 (*0-8151-8666-5*, 28945) Mosby Inc.

Pocket Guide to Stress Testing. Edward K. Chung & Dennis A. Tighe. 1997. LC 96-40175. (Illus.). 432p. pap. 40.95 (*0-86542-509-4*) Blackwell Sci.

Pocket Guide to Syndromes. Robert J. Shprintzen. 1999. LC 99-40684. (Illus.). xiv, 508p. pap. 65.00 net. (*0-7693-0019-7*) Singular Publishing.

Pocket Guide to the Oesophagus. David Evans. 1998. (Illus.). 128p. pap. text 29.95 (*0-632-05085-3*) Blackwell Sci.

Pocket Guide to the Operating Room. Maxine A. Goldman. 2nd ed. 1995. LC 95-21883. (Illus.). 655p. (C). pap. text 34.95 (*0-8036-0033-X*) Davis Co.

Pocket Guide to the 12 Steps. Kathleen S. 1997. LC 97-11609. (Crossing Press Pocket Ser.). (Illus.). 128p. pap. 6.95 (*0-89594-864-8*) Crossing Pr.

Pocket Guide to Treatment in Speech-Language Pathology. M. N. Hegde. 1995. LC 95-39127. (Illus.). 320p. (Orig.). (C). pap. text 45.00 (*1-56593-274-9*, 0596) Thomson Learn.

Pocket Guide to 12 Lead ECG Interpretation. Gerry C. Mulholland. 1998. LC 97-42698. pap. text 29.95 (*0-683-40235-8*) Lppncott W & W.

Pocket Guide to Vaccination & Prophylaxis. Hal B. Jenson. Ed. by Lisette Bralow. 1998. LC 98-38330. (Illus.). 270p. (C). pap. text 19.95 (*0-7216-7993-5*) Saunders.

Pocket Guide to Vitamins. Susan K. Podell. 1994. LC 93-2344. 56p. pap. 2.99 (*0-385-46823-7*) Doubleday.

Pocket Handbook: Radiographic Positioning & Techniques. Kenneth L. Bontrager. 2nd ed. 1995. (Illus.). 294p. pap. text 27.75 (*0-9641723-1-3*) Bontrager Pub.

Pocket Handbook of Chinese Herbal Medicine Vol. 1: 300 Individual Herbs. Zong Lan Xu. 2000. LC 00-90259. 328p. pap. 24.95 (*0-9679935-0-4*) Waclion.

Pocket Handbook of Clinical Psychiatry. Harold I. Kaplan & Benjamin J. Sadock. 1990. 352p. 33.00 (*0-683-04523-7*) Lppncott W & W.

Pocket Handbook of Emergency Psychiatric Medicine. Harold I. Kaplan & Benjamin J. Sadock. 1993. LC 93-18379. 376p. 49.95 (*0-683-04539-3*) Lppncott W & W.

Pocket Handbook of Primary Care Psychiatry. Harold I. Kaplan & Benjamin J. Sadock. 1996. LC 96-32243. (Illus.). 528p. pap. 49.95 (*0-683-30017-2*) Lppncott W & W.

Pocket Handbook of Psychiatric Drug Treatment. Harold I. Kaplan & Benjamin J. Sadock. 1992. LC 92-22846. (Illus.). 288p. pap. 33.00 (*0-683-04538-5*) Lppncott W & W.

Pocket Handbook, Radiographic Positioning & Techniques: Student Edition. Kenneth L. Bontrager. 1994. (Illus.). 290p. (Orig.). (C). pap. text 24.00 (*0-9641723-0-5*) Bontrager Pub.

***Pocket Health Guide.** Snow White. 2001. (Illus.). 191p. pap. (*1-895919-67-3*) Hushion Hse.

Pocket Herbal Reference. Rita Elkins. 1997. 160p. pap. 6.95 (*1-885670-37-0*) Woodland UT.

Pocket Herbal Reference Guide. Debra N. St. Claire. 1992. LC 93-104037. (Pocket Ser.). (Illus.). 144p. pap. 6.95 (*0-89594-568-1*) Crossing Pr.

Pocket Idiot's Guide to First Aid. Stephen J. Rosenberg & Karla Dougherty. 1997. LC 97-73179. (Pocket Idiot's Guide Ser.). (Illus.). 192p. pap. 9.95 (*0-02-862015-1*) Hungry Minds.

***Pocket Labs.** Annette M. Matthews. 2001. (Pocket Card Ser.). (Illus.). 80p. pap. text 15.95 (*0-7817-2772-3*) Lppncott W & W.

Pocket Manual of Basic Surgical Skills. Charles W. Van Way & Buerk. 1986. (Illus.). 240p. (C). (gr. 13). spiral bd. 29.00 (*0-8016-5231-6*, 05231) Mosby Inc.

Pocket Manual of Differential Diagnosis. Stephen N. Adler et al. 4th ed. 1999. LC 99-42878. (Illus.). 464p. pap. text 29.95 (*0-7817-1943-7*) Lppncott W & W.

Pocket Medical Dictionary: English - Arabic. K. A. Shihabi. enl. rev. ed. 1983. (ARA & ENG.). 343p. pap. 14.95 (*0-86685-342-1*, LDL3421) Intl Bk Ctr.

Pocket Medical French. Russell Dollinger. 1995. (ENG & FRE.). 262p. spiral bd. 11.95 (*0-945585-03-9*) Booksmythe.

Pocket Medical Russian. Russell Dollinger. 1995. LC 99-183184. (ENG & FRE.). spiral bd. 11.95 (*0-945585-04-7*) Booksmythe.

Pocket Medical Spanish. Russell Dollinger. 1991. (Medical Interpreting Aid Ser.). (ENG & SPA.). 262p. spiral bd. 11.95 (*0-945585-02-0*) Booksmythe.

Pocket Medicinal Herbs. Penelope Ody. 1997. LC 96-30991. (Illus.). 96p. pap. 9.95 (*0-7894-1616-6*) DK Pub Inc.

Pocket Medicinal Herbs. Storey Publishing Staff. 1997. 9.95 (*0-676-57029-1*) Random.

Pocket Neonatology. Terence Stephenson. 2000. LC 00-46273. (*0-443-04992-0*) Church.

Pocket OB/GYN. C. Scott Naylor. 1999. LC 99-44469. 88p. 27.95 (*0-7817-1770-1*, Lippnctt) Lppncott W & W.

Pocket Obstetrics & Gynecology. Ed. by Stanley G. Clayton & John R. Newton. 11th ed. 1988. (Illus.). 392p. pap. text (*0-443-03777-9*) Church.

***Pocket Paediatrics.** C. O'Callaghan. 2nd ed. 2001. (Illus.). 443p. pap. (*0-443-06011-8*) Church GBR. *Dist:* Saunders.

Pocket Pathology. Ivan Damjanov & Emanuel Rubin. 7th ed. 1999. LC 98-21735. (Illus.). 1,648p. text 56.95 (*0-7817-1636-5*) Lppncott W & W.

Pocket PDR. 1997. 129.95 (*1-56712-353-8*, F0987) Franklin Elect.

Pocket PDR Datacard, 2000. Medical Economics Staff. rev. ed. 2000. disk 130.00 (*1-56712-544-1*) Med Econ.

Pocket Pediatrician: The BC Children's Hospital Manual. Ed. by M. Seear. 1996. (Illus.). 644p. (C). pap. text 42.95 (*0-521-56881-1*) Cambridge U Pr.

Pocket Pediatrics. Mary Lieh-Lai. 2001. LC 00-61848. (Illus.). xxii, 307p. 27.95 (*0-7817-2567-4*) Lppncott W & W.

Pocket Pediatrics. Terence Stephenson & Chris O'Callaghan. 1992. (Illus.). 394p. (Orig.). pap. text (*0-443-04360-4*) Church.

Pocket Picture Guide in Limb Injuries. E. J. Burge. 1989. LC 65-40108. (Illus.). 88p. (gr. 13). text (*0-397-44576-8*, GM0026) Gower-Mosby.

Pocket Picture Guide to Cancer. Jeffrey S. Tobias. 1993. 99p. (gr. 13). (*1-56375-616-1*) Gower-Mosby.

Pocket Picture Guide to Cardiology. Adam D. Timmis. 3rd ed. 1995. text (*0-7234-2443-8*) Martin Dunitz GBR. *Dist:* Mosby Inc.

Pocket Picture Guide to Head Injuries. Peter J. Teddy & Philip Anslow. 1989. LC 65-40322. (Illus.). 96p. (gr. 13). text (*0-397-44569-5*, GM0041) Gower-Mosby.

Pocket Power No. 1: Medical. Joseph M. Leonard. 1988. 48p. (Orig.). pap. 2.95 (*0-945893-00-0*) Pocket Power.

Pocket Power No. 4: Dental. Wayne A. Brannon & Joseph M. Leonard. 1988. 48p. (Orig.). pap. 2.95 (*0-945893-03-5*) Pocket Power.

Pocket Power No. 5: Veterinary. John L. Augustine & Joseph M. Leonard. 1988. 48p. (Orig.). pap. 2.95 (*0-945893-04-3*) Pocket Power.

Pocket Pre-Hospital Spanish. Russell Dollinger. Date not set. (SPA.). spiral bd. (*0-945585-07-1*) Booksmythe.

Pocket Protein Counter. Natow Annette B. et al. 1997. 96p. per. 3.99 (*0-671-00380-1*) PB.

Pocket Rad Tech. Mary J. Hagler. 1992. (Illus.). 608p. pap. text 30.00 (*0-7216-3981-X*) Saunders.

Pocket Reference for Long Term Care Nursing Assistant. Barbara R. Hegner & Joan F. Needham. 1992. pap. 14.95 (*0-8273-4840-1*) Delmar.

Pocket Reference for Pediatric ECG's. Susan Duszynski. 3rd rev. ed. 2000. (Illus.). 76p. pap. 13.00 (*1-930605-00-5*, 104001) Maxishare.

Pocket Reference for Psychiatrists. Susan C. Jenkins & Mark R. Hansen. 2nd ed. 1995. LC 95-2541. 240p. pap. text 24.50 (*0-88048-721-6*, 8721) Am Psychiatric.

Pocket Reference for Psychiatrists. Susan C. Jenkins et al. 3rd ed. 2001. LC 00-29740. (Illus.). xiii, 332p. pap. 29.50 (*1-58562-008-4*, 62008) Am Psychiatric.

Pocket Reference of Diagnosis & Management for the Speech-Language Pathologist. Patricia F. White. 2000. 528p. pap. text 39.99 (*0-7506-7248-X*) Buttrwrth-Heinemann.

Pocket Reference of Medical Abbreviations & Acronyms. Healeye. 1995. (C). pap. text 11.95 (*0-8273-6081-9*) Delmar.

Pocket Reference to Radiographic Exposure Techniques. Kathleen Kath. 1993. (Illus.). 97p. (C). (gr. 13). spiral bd. 19.95 (*0-8016-6907-3*, 06907) Mosby Inc.

Pocket Reference to Sensible Analysis of the ECG. Kathryn Monica Lewis & Kathleen A. Handal. 2000. LC 99-89617. (Allied Health Ser.). 304p. (C). spiral bd. 27.95 (*0-7668-0522-0*) Delmar.

Pocket Review of Surgery. Sergio Huerta. 2000. (Illus.). 200p. pap. 36.00 (*0-8036-0759-8*) Davis Co.

Pocketbook in Vascular Surgery. 1997. pap. (*0-7020-2062-1*) W B Saunders GBR. *Dist:* Saunders.

Pocketbook of Drug Eruptions & Interactions. J. Z. Litt. 2nd ed. 2001. 544p. 29.95 (*1-84214-031-0*, Parthenon Pbng) CRC Pr.

Pocketbook of Drug Eruptions & Interactions: Millennium Edition. J. Z. Litt. 1999. 328p. 35.95 (*1-85070-077-X*, Parthenon Pbng) CRC Pr.

***Pocketbook of Drug Eruptions & Interactions for Palm Pilot (or Palm Os)** J. Z. Litt. 2001. 44.95 (*1-84214-099-X*, Parthenon Pbng) CRC Pr.

***Pocketbook of Drug Eruptions & Interactions on Disk.** J. Z. Litt. 2001. 29.95 (*1-84214-096-5*, Parthenon Pbng) CRC Pr.

Pocketbook of Hair & Scalp Disorders: An Illustrated Guide. John Gray & R. P. Dawber. 1998. LC 98-26852. (Illus.). pap. 38.95 (*0-632-05189-2*) Blackwell Sci.

Pocketbook of Infectious Disease Therapy, 1994. John G. Bartlett. 1994. (Illus.). 272p. 13.95 (*0-683-00444-1*) Lppncott W & W.

Pocketbook of Palliative Care. Robin Hull. 1994. (Illus.). 118p. pap. 26.00 (*0-07-470138-X*) McGraw-Hill Educ Grp.

Pocketbook of Prostatic Disease. 2001. 55.00 (*1-84214-064-7*, Parthenon Pbng) CRC Pr.

Pocketful of Prevention: Preventive Care Guidelines. Ed. by Thomas Masterson. 1998. 40p. (C). pap. 7.50 (*1-883205-44-1*) Intl Med Pub.

PocketGuide for Family Planning Service Providers. Paul D. Blumenthal & Noel McIntosh. Ed. by Elizabeth Oliveras. 2nd ed. 1996. (Illus.). (Orig.). pap. text 15.00 (*0-929817-45-1*) JHPIEGO.

PocketGuide for Family Planning Service Providers. Noel McIntosh & Paul Blumenthal. Ed. by Elizabeth Oliveras. 2nd rev. ed. 1998. (POR., Illus.). 200p. (Orig.). pap. 15.00 (*0-929817-53-2*) JHPIEGO.

Podiatric Medical Assisting. Ed. by Leonard A. Levy & Anne K. Thompson. 2nd ed. 1992. (Illus.). 295p. pap. text (*0-443-08760-1*) Church.

Podiatric Radiology. Mandraachi. 2001. text (*0-7216-9123-4*) Harcrt Hlth Sci Grp.

Podiatry: Index of Modern Information. Victor A. Chandra. 1989. LC 88-48010. 150p. 47.50 (*1-55914-054-2*); pap. 44.50 (*1-55914-055-0*) ABBE Pubs Assn.

Podiatry Office Manual. Robert D. Sowell & William F. Munsey. 1994. (Office Manual Ser.). 201p. 89.00 (*1-890018-03-1*) Anadem Pubng.

Podiatry Sourcebook: Basic Consumer Health Information about Foot Conditions, Diseases & Injuries. Ed. by M. Lisa Weatherford. 2001. LC 2001-36477. (Health Reference Ser.). (Illus.). 380p. lib. bdg. 78.00 (*0-7808-0215-2*) Omnigraphics Inc.

Podos: External Diseases. Chandler. 1993. (*1-56375-101-1*) Gower-Mosby.

Podos: Glaucoma. Paul Kaufman. 1993. (C). (gr. 13). (*1-56375-098-8*) Gower-Mosby.

Podos: Strabismus & Pediatric Ophthalmology. Gary R. Diamond. 1993. (C). (gr. 13). (*1-56375-097-X*) Gower-Mosby.

Podros: Neuro-Ophthalmology. Thomas L. Slamovits. 1993. (C). (gr. 13). (*1-56375-099-6*) Gower-Mosby.

Poems for Old Geezers & Young Whippersnappers. Jefferson D. Bates. 1990. (Poetry Ser.: No. 4). (Illus.). 96p. (Orig.). pap. 6.95 (*0-938823-04-3*) Pogment Pr.

Poems in Persons: An Introduction to the Psychoanalysis of Literature. Norman N. Holland. 1989. (Morningside Bk.). 192p. pap. text 18.00 (*0-231-06983-9*) Col U Pr.

Poetic Expressions in Nursing... Sharing the Caring. Susan J. Farese. Ed. by Nursing A. Liotta. 1993. LC 93-61138. 128p. pap. 9.95 (*1-880254-10-7*) Vista.

Poetic Wisdom: Poetic Wisdom: Revealing & Healing. Susan R. Makin. 1998. LC 98-16987. 246p. text 49.95 (*0-398-06878-X*); pap. text 36.95 (*0-398-06879-8*) C C Thomas.

Poetry as Therapy. Morris R. Morrison. 1987. LC 86-15281. 229p. 35.95 (*0-89885-312-5*, Kluwer Acad Hman Sci) Kluwer Academic.

Point of Care Testing: Principles, Management, & Clinical Practice. Gerald J. Kost. 1999. (Illus.). 288p. (*0-07-038306-5*) McGraw-Hill Med Pub.

Pointers to Cancer Prognosis. Ed. by Basil A. Stoll. 1987. (Developments in Oncology Ser.). pap. text 101.50 (*0-89838-876-7*); lib. bdg. 222.00 (*0-89838-841-4*) Kluwer Academic.

Points of View: Stories of Psychopathology. James E. Mitchell. 2000. LC 00-41355. xix, 222p. pap. 29.95 (*1-58391-005-0*) Brunner-Routledge.

Poison Conspiracy. Karl Grossman. 1983. 281p. 28.00 (*0-932966-26-8*) Permanent Pr.

Poison Detection in Human Organs. Alan S. Curry. 4th ed. 1988. (Illus.). 358p. 82.95 (*0-398-05425-8*) C C Thomas.

Poison in the Pot: The Legacy of Lead. Curtus. 1984. LC 84-2296. 287p. 31.95 (*0-8093-1156-9*) S Ill U Pr.

Poison in the Pot: The Legacy of Lead. Richard P. Wedeen. 2000. (Illus.). 274p. reprint ed. text 30.00 (*0-7881-9172-1*) DIANE Pub.

Poison Ivy, Poison Oak, Poison Sumac & their Relatives. Edward Frankel. 1991. 9.95 (*0-940168-18-9*) Boxwood.

Poisoning & Drug Overdose: A Lange Clinical Manual. Kent R. Olson. 4th ed. 1998. pap. text 36.95 (*0-8385-8172-2*) Appleton & Lange.

Poisoning & Drug Overdose: Clinical Manual. Kent R. Olson. 3rd ed. 1998. LC 90-51. (Illus.). 569p. spiral bd. 44.95 (*0-8385-0260-1*) McGraw-Hill Prof.

Poisoning & Toxicology Compendium. Jerrold Leikin. 1998. (Lexi-Comp's Clinical Reference Library). 1465p. 74.75 (*0-916589-61-7*) Lexi-Comp.

***Poisonous Pastime: The Health Risks of Shooting Ranges & Lead to Children, Families & the Environment.** Tom Diaz. Ed. by Aimee Stenzel. 2001. (Illus.). 71p. pap. 15.00 (*0-927291-31-2*) Violence Policy Ctr.

Poisonous Plants. Richard A. Howard & Gordon P. DeWolf. (Illus.). 48p. reprint ed. pap. text 3.95 (*1-878297-01-5*) Arnold Arboretum.

Poisonous Plants: A Source Guide. 1991. lib. bdg. 75.00 (*0-8490-4825-7*) Gordon Pr.

Poisonous Plants & Venomous Animals of Alabama & Adjoining States. Whit Gibbons et al. 1990. LC 88-34003. (Illus.). 368p. pap. 24.95 (*0-8173-0442-8*) U of Ala Pr.

Poisonous Plants of India. R. N. Chopra et al. 1984. 762p. (C). (*0-7855-2270-0*) Scientific GBR. *Dist:* St Mut.

Poisonous Plants of Paradise: First Aid & Medical Treatment of Injuries from Hawai'i's Plants. Susan Scott & Craig Thomas. 2000. LC 99-50088. (Latitude 20 Book Ser.). (Illus.). 200p. pap. 19.95 (*0-8248-2251-X*) UH Pr.

Poisonous Plants of the Central United States. H. A. Stephens. 1980. LC 79-28161. (Illus.). xiv, 166p. pap. 15.95 (*0-7006-0204-6*) U Pr of KS.

Poisons of the Past: Molds, Epidemics, & History. Mary K. Matossian. 1991. (Illus.). 208p. (C). reprint ed. pap. 15.00 (*0-300-05121-2*) Yale U Pr.

Polarity Therapy: The Complete Collected Works, Vol. 2. Randolph Stone. 1987. LC 84-71548. (Illus.). 240p. pap. 35.00 (*0-916360-25-3*) CRCS Pubns CA.

Polarity Therapy: The Power That Heals. Alan Siegel. Ed. by Phil Young. 1987. (Illus.). 129p. pap. (*0-907061-85-0*) Prism Pr GBR. *Dist:* Assoc Pubs Grp.

Polarity Therapy Workbook. John Beaulou. 1994. 225p. (*0-9640604-0-X*) Bio Sonic Ent.

Polarographic Oxygen Sensor: Its Theory of Operation & Its Application in Biology, Medicine & Technology. Irving Fatt. 1982. LC 82-6581. 290p. (Orig.). reprint ed. 59.95 (*0-89874-511-X*) Krieger.

Police, Firefighter & Paramedic Stress: An Annotated Bibliography, 6. Compiled by John J. Miletich. 1990. LC 89-28649. (Bibliographies & Indexes in Psychology Ser.: No. 6). 239p. lib. bdg. 68.50 (*0-313-26682-4*, MPF, Greenwood Pr) Greenwood.

Police Officer's Guide to Survival, Health & Fitness. John F. Reintzell. 1990. 152p. 38.95 (*0-398-05711-7*) C C Thomas.

Police Psychology into the 21st Century. Ed. by Martin I. Kurke & Ellen M. Scrivner. 1995. (Applied Psychology Ser.). 544p. text 39.95 (*0-8058-1344-6*) L Erlbaum Assocs.

Police Surgeon. Jack Rudman. 1994. (Career Examination Ser.: C-596). pap. 49.95 (*0-8373-0596-9*) Nat Learn.

Policies & Procedures for Long-Term Care Dietetic Services. Ann P. Hunter. 1989. 320p. ring bd. 182.00 (*0-8342-0128-3*, 20128) Aspen Pub.

Policies & Procedures for the Electroneurodiagnostic Laboratory: A Reference Manual. ASET Committee. 1999. 150p. spiral bd. 80.00 (*1-57797-039-X*) ASET.

Policies, Plans & People: Culture & Health Development in Nepal. Judith Justice. 1986. pap. text 18.95 (*0-520-06788-6*) U CA Pr.

Policing & Prescribing: The British System of Drug Control. Ed. by David K. Whynes & Philip T. Bean. 1991. 270p. 76.00 (*0-333-52229-X*) Intl Spec Bk.

***Policy Alternatives in Transfusion Medicine.** Ed. by J. P. AuBuchon et al. 2001. text (*1-56395-146-0*) Am Assn Blood.

Policy & Politics in Nursing & Health Care. Diana J. Mason & Judith K. Leavitt. 3rd ed. 1998. LC 98-21520. (Illus.). 784p. (C). pap. text 42.00 (*0-7216-7038-5*) Saunders.

Policy & Practice: Certified Home Health Care in New York City. Kimberley S. Fox. 1990. (Papers: No. 11). 48p. 5.00 (*0-934459-59-2*) United Hosp Fund.

Policy Choices & Practical Problems in Health Economics: Cases from Latin America & the Caribbean. Ed. by Catherine A. Overholt & Margaret K. Saunders. 1997. LC 94-29559. (EDI Learning Resources Ser.: Vol. 3). 242p. pap. 22.00 (*0-8213-3012-8*, 13012) World Bank.

Policy Issues in Nursing. Ed. by Jane Robinson et al. 1991. 192p. pap. (*0-335-09466-X*) OpUniv Pr.

Policy Options in Long-Term Care. Ed. by Judith Meltzer et al. 1995. LC 81-10445. (C). pap. text 15.00 (*0-226-51974-0*); lib. bdg. 34.00 (*0-226-51973-2*) U Ch Pr.

Policy Reference Guide of the American Academy of Pediatrics: A Comprehensive Guide to AAP Statements Issued Through December 1997. American Academy of Pediatrics Staff. 11th ed. 1998. pap. 79.95 (0-910761-98-1) Am Acad Pediat.

Policy Report of the Physician Consortium on Substance Abuse Education. 1993. (Illus.). 24p. (Orig.). (C). pap. text 20.00 (1-56806-433-0) DIANE Pub.

Polio. Ed. by Thomas M. Daniel & Frederick C. Robbins. 1997. LC 97-18522. (Illus.). 216p. 29.95 (1-878822-90-X) Univ Rochester Pr.

Polio. Alvin Silverstein et al. 2001. LC 00-10993. (Diseases & People Ser.). (Illus.). 128p. (YA). (gr. 6-12). lib. bdg. 20.95 (0-7660-1592-0) Enslow Pubs.

Poliomyelitis: Essential of Surgical Management. J. I. James. 1988. 182p. (0-683-13045-5) E A GBR. *Dist:* Williams & Wilkins.

Polio's Legacy: An Oral History. Edmund J. Sass et al. 296p. (C). 2002. pap. text 35.00 (0-7618-0144-8); 1996. lib. bdg. 63.00 (0-7618-0143-X) U Pr of Amer.

Poliovirus Attenuation: Molecular Mechanisms & Practical Aspects. Ed. by F. Brown & B. P. Lewis. 1993. (Developments in Biological Standardization Ser.: Vol. 78). (Illus.). viii, 192p. pap. 156.75 (3-8055-5744-2) S Karger.

Polish-English Medical Dictionary. Przemyslaw Slomski. 2nd ed. 1991. (ENG & POL.). 802p. 150.00 (0-7859-9335-5) Fr & Eur.

Polish-English Medical Dictionary: Slownik Lekarski Polsko-Angielski. Przemyslaw Stomski. 1986. (ENG & POL.). 899p. 75.00 (0-8288-0576-8, F 105610) Fr & Eur.

Polish-French Medical Dictionary: Dictionnaire Medical Polonais-Francais. Brunon Neuman. 2nd ed. 1984. 50.00 (0-8288-1854-1, M15407) Fr & Eur.

Polish School of Philosophy of Medicine: From Tytus Chalubinski (1820-1889) to Ludwick Fleck (1896-1961) Iklana Lowey & Inserm. 1990. (Philosophy & Medicine Ser.). 296p. lib. bdg. (0-7923-0958-8) Kluwer Academic NLD. *Dist:* Kluwer Academic.

Polish/English-English/Polish Medical Dictionary. Przemyslaw Slomski. 1996. (ENG & POL.). 83.00 (0-7859-9703-2) Fr & Eur.

Political Action Handbook for Nurses. Diana J. Mason & Susan W. Talbott. 1985. 640p. (C). pap. text 29.75 (0-201-16368-3, Health Sci) Addison-Wesley.

Political Approaches to Injury Control at the State Level. Ed. by Abraham B. Bergman. 1992. LC 91-40227. 128p. pap. text 9.95 (0-295-97176-2) U of Wash Pr.

Political Cognition: The 19th Annual Carnegie Mellon Symposium on Cognition. Ed. by Richard R. Lau & David O. Sears. 1986. (Carnegie Symposium on Cognition Ser., 19th Annual). 424p. (C). text 79.95 (0-89859-652-1) L Erlbaum Assocs.

Political Economy of Diet & Health. Ben Fine. 1998. LC 99-163026. 192p. (C). 90.00 (0-415-16366-8) Routledge.

Political Economy of Health in Africa. Ed. by Toyin Falola & Dennis Ityavyar. 1991. LC 91-39117. (Monographs in International Studies, Africa: No. 60A). 258p. (Orig.). (C). pap. text 20.00 (0-89680-168-3) Ohio U Pr.

Political Structure of the Federal Health Planning Program. Lawrence D. Brown. 1982. LC 81-70468. 47p. pap. 7.95 (0-8157-1159-X) Brookings.

Political Values on Health Care: The German Experience. Ed. by Donald W. Light & Alexander Schuller. 1986. (Humanistic & Social Dimensions of Medicine Ser.). (Illus.). 550p. 65.00 (0-262-12109-3) MIT Pr.

Politicized Medicine. Intro. by Hans F. Sennholz. 1993. (Freeman Classics Ser.). 161p. (Orig.). pap. 9.95 (0-910614-87-3) Foun Econ Ed.

Politics & Health Care Organization: HMO's As Federal Policy. Lawrence D. Brown. 1983. LC 81-70466. 540p. 44.95 (0-8157-1158-1); pap. 19.95 (0-8157-1157-3) Brookings.

Politics & Morality of Deviance: Moral Panics, Drug Abuse, Deviant Science, & Reversed Stigmatization. Nachman Ben-Yehuda. 1989. LC 89-4201. (SUNY Series in Deviance & Social Control). 348p. (C). pap. text 25.95 (0-7914-0123-5) State U NY Pr.

Politics & Planning in the NHS. Neil Small. 1989. 224p. pap. (0-335-09259-4) OpUniv Pr.

Politics & Primary Medical Care: Dehumanization & Overutilization. Zeev Ben-Sira. 1988. 232p. text (0-566-05566-X) Avebry GBR. *Dist:* Ashgate Pub Co.

Politics & the Expanding Physician Supply. Michael L. Millman. 1980. LC 78-73591. (Conservation of Human Resources Ser.: No. 11). (Illus.). 176p. text 34.50 (0-916672-84-0) Rowman.

Politics of Breast Cancer Screening. Alison Mann. 1996. (Developments in Nursing & Health Care Ser.: Vol. 8). 176p. (1-85972-323-3) Avebry GBR. *Dist:* Ashgate Pub Co.

Politics of Cancer Revisited. Samuel S. Epstein. 1998. LC 98-41094. 790p. 34.95 (0-914896-46-6) East Ridge Pr.

Politics of Community Conflict: The Fluoridation Decision. Robert L. Crain et al. 1969. LC 68-31777. pap. text 6.95 (0-672-60840-5) Irvington.

Politics of Emerging & Resurgent Infectious Diseases. Jim Whitman. 2000. LC 99-58996. xiii, 223p. 69.95 (0-312-22854-6) St Martin.

Politics of Evolution: Morphology, Medicine, & Reform in Radical London. Adrian Desmond. 1992. LC 89-5137. (Science & Its Conceptual Foundations Ser.). (Illus.). 514p. pap. text 22.95 (0-226-14374-0) U Ch Pr.

Politics of Exemption: Tax Revenue vs. Community Benefit - Not-for-Profit Hospitals. 1999. 84p. pap. 70.00 (0-9667828-3-6) VHA Inc.

Politics of Fat: Food & Nutrition Policy in America. Laura S. Sims. 1998. LC 97-26608. (Bureaucracies, Public Administration, & Public Policy Ser.). 328p. text 70.95 (0-7656-0193-1); (gr. 13). pap. text 32.95 (0-7656-0194-X) M E Sharpe.

Politics of Health. Gardner. 2nd ed. 1995. LC 96-118212. text 41.00 (0-443-04775-8) Saunders.

Politics of Health Care Reform: Lessons from the Past, Prospects for the Future. Ed. by James A. Morone & Gary S. Belkin. 1994. LC 94-10005. 552p. text 54.95 (0-8223-1461-4); pap. text 21.95 (0-8223-1489-4) Duke.

Politics of Health in Europe. Richard Freeman. 2000. LC 00-21462. (European Policy Studies). (0-7190-4213-5) Manchester Univ Pr GBR. *Dist:* St Martin.

Politics of Health Legislation: An Economic Perspective. Paul J. Feldstein. 2nd ed. 1996. LC 96-11238. pap. 48.00 (1-56793-045-X) Health Admin Pr.

Politics of Health Policy: The U. S. Reforms, 1980-1993. Vicente Navarro. 1994. LC 93-40683. 260p. pap. 29.95 (1-55786-318-0) Blackwell Pubs.

Politics of International Health: The Children's Vaccine Initiative & the Struggle to Develop Vaccines for the Third World. William Muraskin. 1998. LC 97-51725. 288p. (C). text 23.50 (0-7914-3999-2); pap. text 22.95 (0-7914-4000-1) State U NY Pr.

Politics of Knowledge: Activist Movements in Medicine & Planning. Lily M. Hoffman. 1989. LC 88-17447. (SUNY Series in the Sociology of Work). 290p. (C). text 67.50 (0-88706-948-7); pap. text 25.95 (0-88706-949-5) State U NY Pr.

Politics of Madness: A Theory of the Function of Madness in a Stratified Society. Hope Landrine. 1992. LC 91-16889. (American University Studies: Ser. VIII, Vol. 22). XVI, 217p. 44.95 (0-8204-1571-5) P Lang Pubng.

Politics of Medical Encounters: How Patients & Doctors Deal with Social Problems. Howard B. Waitzkin. LC 90-45611. 320p. (C). 1991. 42.50 (0-300-04949-8); 1993. reprint ed. pap. 21.00 (0-300-05511-0) Yale U Pr.

Politics of Medicare. Theodore R. Marmor. 2nd ed. 2000. LC 99-52364. (Social Institutions & Social Change Ser.). 228p. pap. text 16.95 (0-202-30425-6); 253p. lib. bdg. 35.95 (0-202-30399-3) Aldine de Gruyter.

Politics of Nursing in Victorian, 1987. Fay Marles. 1989. (C). pap. (0-7300-0691-3, NPR803) Deakin Univ AUS. *Dist:* St Mut.

Politics of Psychiatry in Revolutionary Cuba. Charles J. Brown & Armando M. Lago. 1992. LC 91-7537. 215p. (C). text 39.95 (1-56000-020-1) Transaction Pubs.

Politics of Public Health. Meredeth Turshen. 1989. LC 88-36976. 300p. (C). text 45.00 (0-8135-1421-5); pap. text 19.00 (0-8135-1422-3) Rutgers U Pr.

Politics of Reform in Medical Education & Health Services: The Negev Project, No. 14. Basil Porter & William E. Seidelman. 1991. LC 91-4826. (Medical Education Ser.). 144p. (C). text 29.95 (0-8261-7730-1) Springer Pub.

Politics of Uncertainty: Attachment in Private & Public Life. Peter Marris. 1996. LC 95-43632. 208p. (C). 78.95 (0-415-13171-5); pap. 26.95 (0-415-13172-3) Routledge.

Politics of Women's Health: Exploring Agency & Autonomy. Susan Sherwin. 1998. LC 98-16025. 320p. (C). pap. 19.95 (1-56639-633-6); (Illus.). text 59.95 (1-56639-632-8) Temple U Pr.

Politics of Women's Health Care: Medicalization As a Form of Social Control. Karen B. Levy. 1992. LC 92-39492. (Woman in History Ser.: Vol. 60). (Illus.). 133p. pap. 10.00 (0-86663-201-8) Ide Hse.

Politics, Power & Policy Making: The Case of Health Care Reform in the 1990s. Mark E. Rushefsky & Kant Patel. 1998. LC 97-33625. 316p. (C). (gr. 13). text 74.95 (1-56324-955-3) M E Sharpe.

Politics, Power & Policy Making: The Case of Health Care Reform in the 1990s. Mark E. Rushefsky et al. 1998. LC 97-33625. 316p. (C). (gr. 13). pap. text 30.95 (1-56324-956-1) M E Sharpe.

Politics, Science, & Dread Disease: A Short History of the United States Medical Research Policy. Stephen P. Strickland. 1972. LC 72-78427. (Commonwealth Fund Publications). 345p. 44.50 (0-674-68955-0) HUP.

Pollen Biotechnology: Gene Expression & Allergen Characterization. Ed. by Shyam S. Mohapatra & R. Bruce Knox. 1995. LC 94-42327. 288p. (C). (gr. 13). pap. text 107.95 (0-412-03521-9) Chapman & Hall.

Pollinosis. Ed. by Paolo Falagiani. 1989. 272p. lib. bdg. 191.00 (0-8493-6482-5, RC589) CRC Pr.

Pollutant Transfer & Transport in the Sea Gunnar Kullenberg. 1982. Vol. I. 240p. 150.00 (0-8493-5601-6, GC1085); Vol. II. 248p. 142.00 (0-8493-5602-4, GC1085) Franklin (CRC Reprint).

Polly's Birth Book: Obstetrics for the Home. Polly Block. 1996. LC 96-68998. (Illus.). 563p. reprint ed. pap. 21.95 (1-57636-019-9) SunRise Pbl.

Polyamines. Ed. by Herbert Tabor & Celia W. Tabor. 1983. (Methods in Enzymology Ser.: Vol. 94). text 188.00 (0-12-181994-9) Acad Pr.

Polyamines in Cancer: Basic Mechanisms & Clinical Approaches. K. Nishioka. 1996. (Medical Intelligence Unit Ser.). 228p. (C). pap. 89.95 (0-412-11051-2) Chapman & Hall.

Polyamines in Cancer: Basic Mechanisms & Clinical Approaches. Kenji Nishioka. 1996. LC 96-15935. (Medical Intelligence Unit Ser.). 278p. 99.00 (1-57059-346-9) Landes Bioscience.

Polyamines in Health & Nutrition. Susan Bardocz & Ann White. 1999. LC 99-31741. (Illus.). vii, 335p. (0-412-82220-2) Kluwer Academic.

Polybrominated Biphenyls. Ed. by World Health Organization Staff. 1994. (Environmental Health Criteria Ser.: No. 152). (ENG, FRE & SPA.). 577p. pap. text 103.00 (92-4-157152-7, 1160152) World Health.

Polycarbonate-Workshop Amsterdam, September 1985. Ed. by L. W. Henderson et al. 1986. (Journal: Vol. 4, No. 1-3, 1986). (Illus.). 184p. pap. 128.00 (3-8055-4352-2) S Karger.

Polychaeta from Hawaii. M. Holly. 1974. (BMB Ser.: No. 129). reprint ed. pap. 25.00 (0-527-02235-7) Periodicals Srv.

Polychlorinated Biphenyls & Terphenyls. 2nd ed. 1993. (Environmental Health Criteria Ser.: No. 140). (ENG, FRE & SPA.). 682p. pap. text 110.00 (92-4-157140-3, 1160140) World Health.

Polychlorinated Dibenzo-Paradioxins & Dibenzofurans. 1990. (Environmental Health Criteria Ser.: No. 88). 409p. pap. text 63.00 (92-4-154288-8, 1160088) World Health.

Polychromatic Layering Technique. Ludwig A. Rinn. 1990. (Illus.). 155p. text 88.00 (0-86715-225-7) Quint Pub Co.

Polycyclic Aromatic Hydrocarbon Carcinogenesis: Structure-Activity Relationships. Ed. by Shen K. Yang & B. D. Silverman. 1988. 256p. Vol. I. 129.00 (0-8493-6730-1, RC268); Vol. II. 128.00 (0-8493-6731-X) Franklin (CRC Reprint).

Polycystic Kidney Disease. Ed. by M. H. Breuning et al. 1992. (Contributions to Nephrology Ser.: Vol. 97). (Illus.). vi, 142p. 49.75 (3-8055-5586-5) S Karger.

Polycystic Kidney Disease. Ed. by Michael L. Watson & Vicente E. Torres. 1996. LC 95-31363. (Oxford Clinical Nephrology Ser.). (Illus.). 606p. (C). text 125.00 (0-19-262578-0) OUP.

Polycystic Ovarian Disease. W. Futterweit. 1984. (Clinical Perspectives in Obstetrics & Gynecology Ser.). (Illus.). 210p. 87.00 (0-387-90981-8) Spr-Verlag.

Polycystic Ovaries: A Disorder or a Symptom?, Vol. 3. Ed. by Robert W. Shaw. 1991. (Advances in Reproductive Endocrinology Ser.). (Illus.). 222p. (C). 74.95 (1-85070-343-4, Parthenon Pbng) CRC Pr.

Polycystic Ovary Syndrome. Gabor Kovacs. 2000. LC 99-52561. (Illus.). 240p. text 90.00 (0-521-66073-4) Cambridge U Pr.

Polycystic Ovary Syndrome: Proceedings of the Symposium, Sponsored by Serono Symposia U S A, Inc., Held in Boston, Massachusetts, May 18-21, 1995. Ed. by R. Jeffrey Chang. 1996. LC 96-11919. (Illus.). 370p. 148.00 (0-387-94741-8) Spr-Verlag.

Polycystic Ovary Syndrome - Fighting Back! A PCOS Lifestyle Manual. Angela Kay Dotson. Ed. by Michael Cioffi. 2000. 138p. pap. 17.95 (0-9705025-0-8) Sparhawk Health.

Polycythemia Vera & the Myleoproliferative Disorders. Louis R. Wasserman et al. 1994. LC 94-1680. (Illus.). 416p. text 115.00 (0-7216-4213-6) Saunders.

Polydiagnostic Approach in Psychiatry. Ed. by G. Lenz & G. Pakesch. 1987. (Journal: Vol. 19, No. 5, 1986). (Illus.). 76p. pap. 38.50 (3-8055-4540-1) S Karger.

Polyether Antibiotics Vol. 2: Naturally Occurring Acid Ionophores: Chemistry. J. Westley. 1983. (Illus.). 432p. text 175.00 (0-8247-1888-7) Dekker.

Poly(ethylene Glycol) Chemistry: Biotechnical & Biomedical Applications. J. M. Harris. 1992. (Topics in Applied Chemistry Ser.). (Illus.). 408p. (C). text 110.00 (0-306-44078-4, Kluwer Plenum) Kluwer Academic.

Polyfunctional Cytokines: IL-6 & LIF. Ed. by Gregory R. Bock & Kate Widdows. 1992. LC 92-5732. (CIBA Foundation Symposia Ser.: Vol. 167). 290p. 128.00 (0-471-93439-9) Wiley.

Polyfunctionality of Hematopoietic Regulators Vol. 12, Supplement 2: The Metcalf Forum. Ed. by Martin J. Murphy, Jr. 1994. LC 94-73349. (Illus.). 326p. (C). text 69.00 (1-880854-19-8); pap. text 49.00 (1-880854-20-1) AlphaMed Pr.

Polymer Gels: Fundamentals & Biomedical Applications. D. DeRossi et al. 1991. LC 91-2631. (Illus.). 354p. (C). text 110.00 (0-306-43805-4, Kluwer Plenum) Kluwer Academic.

Polymerase Chain Reaction (PCR) The Technique & Its Application. Rosalind A. Eeles & Alasdair Stamps. 1993. LC 93-4961. (Molecular Biology Intelligence Unit Ser.). 99.00 (1-879702-58-4) Landes Bioscience.

Polymerase Chain Reaction (PCR) for Human Viral Diagnosis. Jonathan P. Clewley. 1994. 240p. lib. bdg. 79.95 (0-8493-4833-1) CRC Pr.

Polymeric Biomaterials. Ed. by Erhan Piskin & Allan S. Hoffman. 1986. text 175.00 (90-247-3303-0) Kluwer Academic.

***Polymeric Biomaterials.** Dumitriu. 2nd ed. 2001. LC 2001-55548. (0-8247-0569-6) Dekker.

Polymeric Delivery Systems Vol. 52: Properties & Applications. Ed. by Magda A. El-Nokaly et al. 1993. LC 92-40099. (ACS Symposium Ser.: Vol. 520). (Illus.). 430p. 120.00 (0-8412-2624-5) Am Chemical.

Polymeric Dental Materials, Vol. XIV. Michael Braden et al. 1997. LC 97-457. (Macromolecular Systems, Materials Approach Ser.). (Illus.). 164p. 149.00 (3-540-61646-2) Spr-Verlag.

Polymeric Drugs & Drug Administration, Vol. 54. Ed. by Raphael M. Ottenbrite. 1994. LC 93-48086. (ACS Symposium Ser.: No. 545). 254p. 100.00 (0-8412-2744-6) Am Chemical.

Polymeric Drugs & Drug Delivery Systems. Ed. by Richard L. Dunn & Raphael M. Ottenbrite. 1991. LC 91-23423. (ACS Symposium Ser.: No. 469). (Illus.). 313p. text 90.00 (0-8412-2105-7) Am Chemical.

Polymeric Materials & Artificial Organs. Ed. by Charles G. Gebelein. 1984. LC 84-9297. (ACS Symposium Ser.: No. 256). 208p. lib. bdg. 40.95 (0-8412-0854-9) Am Chemical.

Polymeric Nanoparticles & Microspheres. Ed. by Pierre Guiot & Patrick Couvreur. 1986. 216p. 126.00 (0-8493-5696-2, RS201, CRC Reprint) Franklin.

Polymers: Their Properties & Blood Compatibility. Ed. by Steen Dawids. 1989. (Developments in Hematology & Immunology Ser.). (C). text 251.00 (0-7923-0491-8) Kluwer Academic.

Polymers As Biomaterials. Ed. by Shalaby W. Shalaby et al. 1985. 400p. 105.00 (0-306-41886-X, Plenum Trade) Perseus Pubng.

Polymers, Biomaterials & Medical Applications: Biomaterials & Medical Applications. Ed. by Jacqueline I. Kroschwitz. 1989. LC 89-32479. (Encyclopedia Reprints Ser.). 555p. 220.00 (0-471-51207-9) Wiley.

Polymers for Controlled Drug Delivery. Peter J. Tarcha. 1990. 296p. 295.00 (0-8493-5652-0, RS201) CRC Pr.

Polymers in Medicine. Ed. by G. E. Zaikov. 1995. LC 95-24679. 207p. 125.00 (1-56072-252-5) Nova Sci Pubs.

Polymers in Medicine: Biomedical & Pharmaceutical Applications. Ed. by Raphael M. Ottenbrite & Emo Chiellini. 1992. LC 92-60021. 272p. 69.95 (0-87762-929-3) CRC Pr.

Polymers in Medicine & Pharmacy: Materials Research Society Symposium Proceedings. Ed. by Antonios G. Mikos et al. 1995. (MRS Symposium Proceedings Ser.: Vol. 394). 208p. text 90.00 (1-55899-297-9, 394) Materials Res.

Polymers in Medicine I: Biomedical & Pharmacological Applications. Ed. by Emo Chiellini & P. Giusti. 1983. 425p. 105.00 (0-306-41360-4, Plenum Trade) Perseus Pubng.

Polymers in Medicine II: Biomedical & Pharmaceutical Applications. Ed. by Luigi Nicolais et al. 1986. (Polymer Science & Technology Ser.: Vol. 34). 440p. 105.00 (0-306-42390-1, Plenum Trade) Perseus Pubng.

Polymethylmethacrylate: A Flexible Membrane for a Tailored Dialysis. Ed. by Claudio V. Ronco. 1998. LC 98-42558. (Contributions to Nephrology Ser.: Vol. 125). (Illus.). viii, 246p. 198.25 (3-8055-6760-X) S Karger.

Polymodal Receptor: A Gateway to Pathological Pain. Takao Kumazawa et al. 1996. LC 96-41062. (Progress in Brain Research Ser.). 560p. 204.50 (0-444-82473-1) Elsevier.

Polymorphisms & Fertility. Ed. by M. Adinolfi. 1985. (Journal: Vol. 2, No. 2). (Illus.). 88p. pap. 35.00 (3-8055-4066-3) S Karger.

Polynesian Herbal Medicine. W. Arthur Whistler. 1993. (Illus.). 238p. pap. text 33.00 (0-915809-16-8) Natl Trop Bot.

Polynuclear Aromatic Hydrocarbons: Chemical Analysis & Biological Fate. Ed. by Marcus Cooke & Anthony J. Dennis. 1981. LC 81-3669. (Fifth International Symposium on Polynuclear Aromatic Hydrocarbons Ser.). 770p. 65.00 (0-935470-09-3) Battelle.

Polynuclear Aromatic Hydrocarbons: Chemistry, Characterization & Carcinogenesis. M. Cooke & A. J. Dennis. 1986. LC 86-18430. (Ninth International Symposium on Polynuclear Aromatic Hydrocarbons Ser.). 987p. 75.00 (0-935470-25-5) Battelle.

Polyol Paradigm & Complications of Diabetes. M. P. Cohen. 1986. (Illus.). xii, 143p. 99.00 (0-387-96418-5) Spr-Verlag.

Polyoma Virus. B. E. Eddy. 1969. (Virology Monographs: Vol. 7). (Illus.). iv, 174p. 51.00 (0-387-80934-1) Spr-Verlag.

Polypropylene. H. P. Frank. 1968. LC 68-24786. (Polymer Monographs: Vol. 2). (Illus.). x, 134p. text 156.00 (0-677-01540-2) Gordon & Breach.

***Polyps of the Human Body: Index of New Information for Reference & Research.** Ed. by Research and Development Division Staff & John C. Bartone. 2001. (Illus.). 180p. 47.50 (0-7883-2468-3); pap. 44.50 (0-7883-2469-1) ABBE Pubs Assn.

Polytene Chromosomes in Genetic Research. V. Sorsa. 1988. 272p. 57.95 (0-470-21215-2) P-H.

Polytrauma: Diagnostik, Therapie. Ed. by W. A. Kozuschek & H. B. Reith. 1993. (Illus.). xii, 540p. 115.00 (3-8055-5796-5) S Karger.

Polyunsaturated Fatty Acids. Ed. by Wolf H. Kunau & R. T. Holman. 1977. 272p. 30.00 (0-935315-01-2) Am Oil Chemists.

Polyunsaturated Fatty Acids in Nutrition: Proceedings of a Round Table in Polyunsaturated Fatty Acids in Nutrition, Milan, Italy, April 1979. Ed. by Corraldo L. Galli & P. Avogaro. 1980. (Progress in Food & Nutrition Science Ser.: Vol. 4, No. 5). (Illus.). 80p. pap. 32.00 (0-08-027362-9, Pergamon Pr) Elsevier.

P Q R

Polyurethanes in Biomedical Devices. Stuart L. Cooper et al. 1997. LC 97-41911. 288p. 139.95 (*0-8493-4517-0*) CRC Pr.

Polyurethanes in Medicine. Michael D. Lelah & Stuart L. Cooper. 1986. 256p. 136.00 (*0-8493-6307-1*, R857, CRC Reprint) Franklin.

Pomo Doctors & Poisoners. L. S. Freeland. fac. ed. 1923. (University of California Publications in American Archaeology & Ethnology: Vol. 20: 4). 18p. (C). reprint ed. pap. text 2.19 (*1-55567-240-X*) Coyote Press.

Poor & Minority Health Care. Ed. by Gary E. McCuen. 1988. LC 87-91953. (Ideas in Conflict Ser.). (Illus.). 202p. (YA). (gr. 7-12). lib. bdg. 15.95 (*0-86596-065-8*) G E M.

Poor Eaters: Helping Children Who Refuse to Eat. J. Macht. LC 89-26514. (Illus.). 328p. (C). 19.95 (*0-306-43451-2*) Da Capo.

Poore-Mans Plaster-Box, No. 664. Richard Hawes. 1974. LC 74-80183. 44p. reprint ed. 10.00 (*90-221-0664-0*) Walter J Johnson.

Popper & the Human Sciences. Ed. by Gregory Currie & Alan E. Musgrave. 1985. 225p. pap. text (*90-247-3141-0*) M Nijhoff NLD. *Dist:* Kluwer Academic.

Poppy Flower: A Journey Thru Addiction. Penny Jones. Ed. by Barbara McCaig. 1987. (Illus.). 40p. (Orig.). pap. text 4.95 (*0-935201-18-1*) Affordable Adven.

Popular Interset in Psychiatric Remedies: A Study in Social Control. Egon Bittner. Ed. by Harriet Zuckerman & Robert K. Merton. 1980. LC 79-8977. (Dissertations on Sociology Ser.). lib. bdg. 26.95 (*0-405-12953-X*) Ayer.

Popular Medical Encyclopedia. B. V. Petrovskih. 1984. (RUS.). 704p. 85.00 (*0-8288-1860-6*, M15422) Fr & Eur.

Popular Medicine in Seventeenth-Century England. Doreen E. Nagy. 1988. LC 88-70523. 140p. (C). 26.95 (*0-87972-435-8*); pap. 13.95 (*0-87972-436-6*) Bowling Grn St Univ.

Popular Medicine in Thirteenth - Century England: Introduction & Texts. Tony Hunt. 1994. (Illus.). 478p. (C). reprint ed. 99.00 (*0-85991-290-6*) Boydell & Brewer.

Popular Physiology: An Application to the Preservation of Health (1884) R. T. Trall. 1996. 223p. reprint ed. pap. 17.95 (*1-56459-813-6*) Kessinger Pub.

Population - Control, Density, Dynamics, Growth, & Surveillance: Index of New Information with Authors, Subjects & Bibliography. James N. Palmerson. rev. ed. 1994. LC 94-34027. 136p. 57.50 (*0-7883-0382-1*); pap. 47.50 (*0-7883-0383-X*) ABBE Pubs Assn.

Population & Community Ecology: Principles & Methods. E. C. Pielou. 1974. LC 72-86334. (Illus.). viii, 429p. text 225.00 (*0-677-03580-2*) Gordon & Breach.

Population & Development Planning. 285p. 20.00 (*92-1-151249-2*, E.92.XIII.13) UN.

Population-Based Medicine. Ed. by Mack Lipkin, Jr. & William A. Lybrand. 1982. LC 81-21116. 198p. 55.00 (*0-275-91370-8*, C1370, Praeger Pubs) Greenwood.

Population Biology & Evolution of Clonal Organisms. Jeremy B. Jackson. Ed. by Leo W. Buss & Robert E. Cook. 1986. LC 85-14186. 608p. (C). 80.00 (*0-300-03379-6*) Yale U Pr.

Population Biology of Infectious Diseases: Berlin, 1982. Ed. by R. C. Anderson & Raoul M. May. 1982. (Dahlem Workshop Reports Ser.: Vol. 25). (Illus.). 315p. 35.00 (*0-387-11650-8*) Spr-Verlag.

Population Dynamics, Reproduction, & Activities of the Kangaroo Rat, Dipodomys ordii, in Western Texas. Herschel W. Garner. 1974. (Graduate Studies: No. 7). (Illus.). 28p. pap. 2.00 (*0-89672-014-4*) Tex Tech Univ Pr.

Population, Environment & Resources, & Third World Development, 5. Ed. by Pradip K. Ghosh. 1984. LC 83-26430. (International Development Resource Bks.: No. 5). (Illus.). 634p. lib. bdg. 110.00 (*0-313-24141-4*, GPL/, Greenwood Pr) Greenwood.

Population Genetics: A Concise Guide. John H. Gillespie. 1997. LC 97-19509. (Illus.). 190p. pap. text 21.95 (*0-8018-5755-4*) Johns Hopkins.

Population Genetics in Animal Breeding. Franz Pirchner. Tr. by D. L. Frape from GER. 2nd ed. 1983. LC 83-2164. 424p. 95.00 (*0-306-41201-2*, Plenum Trade) Perseus Pubng.

Population Health: Concepts & Methods. T. Kue Young. 1998. LC 97-46851. (Illus.). 328p. text 39.95 (*0-19-511972-X*) OUP.

***Population Health & Aging: Strengthening the Dialogue Between Epidemiology & Demography.** Ed. by Maxine Weinstein et al. 2001. LC 2001-55878. (Annals of the New York Academy of Sciences Ser.: Vol. 954). 475p. 145.00 (*1-57331-372-6*) NY Acad Sci.

Population Health Research: Linking Theory & Methods. Ed. by Kathryn Dean. 1993. (Illus.). 256p. (C). 69.95 (*0-8039-8751-X*, 9573); pap. 26.50 (*0-8039-8752-8*, 9574) Sage.

Population, Labor Force & Long Swings in Economic Growth: The American Experience. Richard A. Easterlin. 1968. (General Ser.: No. 86). (Illus.). 318p. 82.70 (*0-87014-474-X*) Natl Bur Econ Res.

Population of Selves: A Therapeutic Exploration of Personal Diversity. Erving Polster. 1995. LC 94-42595. (Social & Behavioral Sciences Ser.). 251p. 35.00 (*0-7879-0076-1*) Jossey-Bass.

Population-Oriented Psychiatry. Gerald Caplan. 1989. LC 87-30985. 244p. 38.95 (*0-89885-418-0*, Kluwer Acad Hman Sci) Kluwer Academic.

Population Planning in India: Policy Issues & Research Priorities. Ed. by Ashish Bose & P. B. Desai. 1990. (*81-7018-575-0*) BR Pub IND. *Dist:* S Asia.

Population Policy. Ed. by Mark Schneider & Michael E. Kraft. 1977. (C). pap. 15.00 (*0-918592-23-2*) Pol Studies.

Population Research, Policy & Related Studies in Puerto Rico: An Inventory. Kent C. Earnhardt. 1984. LC 77-16466. (Planning Ser.: No. S-6). 132p. pap. 5.00 (*0-8477-2447-6*) U of PR Pr.

Populations, Species, & Evolution: An Abridgment of Animal Species & Evolution. Ernst W. Mayr. abr. ed. 1970. LC 79-111486. (Belknap Press Ser.). 453p. pap. 18.50 (*0-674-69013-3*, Belknap) HUP.

Porcelain & Composite Inlays & Onlays: Esthetic Posterior Restorations. David Garber & Ronald E. Goldstein. 1993. (Illus.). 158p. text 68.00 (*0-86715-171-4*) Quint Pub Co.

Pornography & Sexual Aggression. Neil M. Malamuth & Edward Donnerstein. 1986. pap. text 55.00 (*0-12-466281-1*); 1984. text 84.95 (*0-12-466280-3*) Acad Pr.

Porose Integumental Organs of Oribatid Mites: Acari, Oribatida. Ed. by Gerd Alberti & Roy A. Norton. 1997. (Zoologica Ser.: Vol. 146). (Illus.). 143p. pap. 122.00 (*3-510-55033-1*) Lubrecht & Cramer.

Porphyrins in Human Diseases: Proceedings of the International Porphyrin Meeting, 1st, Freiburg, Germany, May, 1975. International Porphyrin Meeting Staff. Ed. by M. Doss. 1976. (Illus.). 400p. 167.00 (*3-8055-2259-2*) S Karger.

Porpoises & Sonar. Winthrop N. Kellogg. 1992. LC 61-11294. (Illus.). xiv, 178p. pap. text 2.25 (*0-226-43005-7*, P518) U Ch Pr.

Port-Site & Wound Recurrences in Cancer Surgery: Incidence - Pathogenesis - Prevention. Ed. by M. A. Reymond et al. Tr. by A. Jack from GER. 2000. (Illus.). 208p. 104.00 (*3-540-66929-9*) Spr-Verlag.

Portable Internist. Ed. by Anthony J. Zollo, Jr. 1994. (Illus.). 704p. pap. 49.95 (*1-56053-066-9*) Hanley & Belfus.

Portable Jung. Carl Gustav Jung. Ed. by Joseph Campbell. Tr. by R. F. C. Hull. 1976. LC 76-44022. (Viking Portable Library: No. 70). 659p. pap. 17.00 (*0-14-015070-6*, Penguin Bks) Penguin Putnam.

Portable Kristeva. Kelly Oliver & Julia Kristeva. 1997. LC 96-34403. (European Perspectives; A Series in Social Thought & Culturall Criticism Ser.). 464p. (C). pap. 18.50 (*0-231-10505-3*) Col U Pr.

Portable Lawyer for Mental Health Professionals: An A-Z Guide to Protecting Your Clients, Your Practice & Yourself. Barton E. Bernstein & Thomas L. Hartsell. 1998. LC 98-10048. 288p. pap. 49.95 (*0-471-24869-X*) Wiley.

Portable Pediatrician for Parents. Laura W. Nathanson. 1994. LC 93-24395. (Illus.). 544p. pap. 23.00 (*0-06-273176-9*, Harper Ref) HarperCollins Pubs.

Portable Skeletal X-Ray Library: An Atlas of Correlative Radiology. Marshall N. Deltoff & Peter L. Kogon. 1997. LC 97-3246. (Illus.). 384p. (gr. 13). text 67.95 (*0-8151-2244-6*, 24846) Mosby Inc.

Portable Stein. Fred F. Ferri. 1993. (Illus.). 368p. (C). (gr. 13). pap. text 32.95 (*0-8016-7825-0*, 07825) Mosby Inc.

Portable Therapist. Donald C. Doyle. Ed. by Betty Doyle. 1995. LC 95-92394. 280p. (Orig.). (C). pap. 14.95 (*0-9648370-0-5*) D&D Publns.

Portable Therapist. Susanna McMahon. 1994. LC 93-30957. 256p. pap. 11.95 (*0-440-50603-4*) Dell.

Portal Design in Radiation Therapy. B. Dasher et al. 1994. 168p. pap. text 45.00 (*0-9642715-0-8*) D W V.

Portal Hypertension: A Multidisciplinary Approach to Current Clinical Management. Ed. by Stuart J. Knechtle. 1998. LC 98-25898. (Illus.). 298p. 150.00 (*0-87993-414-X*) Futura Pub.

Portal Hypertension: Clinical & Physiological Aspects. Ed. by Kunio Okuda & J. P. Benhamou. 1991. (Illus.). 592p. 336.00 (*0-387-70054-4*) Spr-Verlag.

Portal Hypertension: Diagnostic Imaging & Imaging-Guided Therapy. Ed. by Plinio Rossi et al. 2000. LC 99-55309. (Medical Radiology Ser.). (Illus.). 352p. 199.00 (*3-540-65797-5*) Spr-Verlag.

Portal Hypertension: Pathophysiology & Treatment. Ed. by Jaime Bosch & Roberto J. Groszmann. 1994. LC 94-5895. (Illus.). 190p. 70.00 (*0-86542-846-8*) Blackwell Sci.

Portal Hypertension: Proceedings of the 79th Falk Symposium (Part III of the Gastroenterology Week Freiburg 1994), Held in Freiburg-in-Breisgau, Germany, June 17-19, 1994. Falk Symposium 79 Staff. Ed. by A. Holstege et al. 1995. LC 95-20105. text 184.00 (*0-7923-8879-8*) Kluwer Academic.

Portal Hypertension II: Definitions, Methodology & Therapeutic Strategies, 2. Ed. by Roberto De Franchis. 1995. 336p. pap. 90.00 (*0-86542-614-7*) Blackwell Sci.

Portal Hypertension III: Proceedings of the Third Baveno International Consensus Workshop on Definitions, Methodology & Therapeutic Strategies. Baveno International Consensus Workshop on Definitions Methodology Staff & Roberto De Franchis. 2000. LC 00-45448. (Illus.). xvii, 247p. 90.00 (*0-632-05918-4*) Blackwell Sci.

Portale Hypertension. K. J. Paquet et al. Ed. by H. Denck & R. Berchtold. 1982. x, 282p. pap. 56.75 (*3-8055-3480-9*) S Karger.

Porter's EMS Protocols. William Porter. 1997. 164p. ring bd. 595.00 (*1-882740-08-4*) Porter & Assocs.

***Porter's Pocket Guide to Nursing.** 2002. 18.95 (*1-882740-09-2*) Porter & Assocs.

Porter's Pocket Guide to Nursing. William Porter. 1999. (Illus.). pap. 18.95 (*1-882740-21-1*) Porter & Assocs.

Portfolio Guidance for Veterinary Nurses. Ed. by College of Animal Welfare Staff. 2000. 128p. pap. text 29.99 (*0-7506-4809-0*) Buttrwrth-Heinemann.

Portrait & Story: Dramaturgical Approaches to the Study of Persons, 7. Larry Cochran. 1986. LC 85-12708. (Contributions in Psychology Ser.: No. 7). 203p. 60.00 (*0-313-24966-0*, CPS/, Greenwood Pr) Greenwood.

Portrait Catalog New York Academy of Medicine Staff. 1971. suppl. ed. 160.00 (*0-8161-0900-1*); 1970. suppl. ed. 175.00 (*0-8161-0733-5*) Gale (Macmillan Ref).

Portrait of Aphasia. David Knox. 1985. LC 85-8958. 124p. (Orig.). reprint ed. pap. 14.95 (*0-8143-1800-2*) Wayne St U Pr.

Portrait of the Immune System: Scientific Publications of Niels Kaj Jerne. Ivan Lefkovits. 1996. pap. text 48.00 (*981-02-2614-4*) World Scientific Pub.

Portrait of the Immune System Scientific Publications of Niels Kaj Jerne. 1996. 878p. 97.00 (*981-02-2605-5*) World Scientific Pub.

Portrait of the Menopause: Expert Reports on Medical & Therapeutic Strategies for the 1990's. Ed. by H. Burger & M. Boulet. 1991. (Illus.). 110p. (C). lib. bdg. 49.95 (*1-85070-357-4*, Parthenon Pbng) CRC Pr.

Portrait of the Person: A Personality Theory for the Clinician. Zoltan Gross. 1992. 275p. 29.95 (*0-9632977-0-8*) Global Vil CA.

Portrait of the Psychopath As a Young Woman. Edward Lee & Elizabeth Steffen. 1998. pap. 12.95 (*1-889186-09-0*) Necro Publns.

Portraits in Homoeopathic Medicines Vol. 3: Expanding Views of the Materia Medica. Catherine R. Coulter. 1998. LC 97-30347. 338p. 33.00 (*1-57626-091-7*, QMP) Quality Med Pub.

Portraits of Adjustment. Heesacker & Washington Post Writers Staff. 1994. LC 94-173813. 352p. pap. text 31.00 (*0-205-15808-0*) Allyn.

Portraits of Homoeopathic Medicines Vol. 1: Psychophysical Analyses of Selected Constitutional Types. Catherine R. Coulter. 1997. LC 97-222920. 422p. 33.00 (*1-57626-089-5*) Quality Med Pub.

Portraits of Homoeopathic Medicines Vol. 2: Psychophysical Analyses of Selected Constitutional Types. Catherine R. Coulter. 1997. LC 97-30347. 300p. 33.00 (*1-57626-090-9*) Quality Med Pub.

Portraits of Pioneers in Psychology, Vol. II. Ed. by Gregory A. Kimble et al. 1996. LC 91-7226. (Illus.). 351p. (C). text 79.95 (*1-55798-344-5*, 431-7630); pap. text 29.95 (*1-55798-345-3*, 431-7631) Am Psychol.

Portraits of Pioneers in Psychology. Ed. by Gregory A. Kimble et al. 1991. LC 91-7226. (Portraits of Pioneers in Psychology Ser.: Vol. 1). (Illus.). 384p. 79.95 (*0-8058-0620-2*); 1991. (Portraits of Pioneers in Psychology Ser.: Vol. 1). (Illus.). 384p. pap. 29.95 (*0-8058-1136-2*); Vol. 2. 1996. 300p. text 79.95 (*0-8058-2197-X*); Vol. 2. 1996. (Portraits of Pioneers in Psychology Ser.: Vol. 2). 300p. pap. text 29.95 (*0-8058-2198-8*) L Erlbaum Assocs.

Portraits of Spirituality in Recovery: The Use of Art in Recovery from Co-Dependency and/or Chemical Dependency. Nancy Barrett Chickerneo. 1993. LC 92-42194. (Illus.). 254p. text 57.95 (*0-398-05845-8*) C C Thomas.

Portraits of the Artist: Psychoanalysis of Creativity & Its Vicissitudes. John E. Gedo. 1989. 336p. pap. 29.95 (*0-88163-097-7*) Analytic Pr.

Portraits of Viruses: A History of Virology. Ed. by Frank Fenner & Adrian J. Gibbs. 1988. (Illus.). viii, 344p. 128.00 (*3-8055-4819-2*) S Karger.

Ports Designated in Application of the International Health Regulations: Situation As on 1 April 1992. 1992. (ENG & FRE.). 40p. pap. text 10.00 (*92-4-058013-1*, 0150387) World Health.

Portuguese-English Medical Pocket Translator: Continantal, Brazilian, & Cape Verdean Dialects. Christopher Harding. 2000. (Medical Pocket Translator Ser.). pap. 9.95 (*0-9649425-2-6*) Intl Med Volntrs.

Portuguese Pioneers in India: Spotlight on Medicine. P. D. Gaitonde. 1983. (*0-8364-1052-1*) Popular Prakashan IND. *Dist:* S Asia.

Pos Parenting: A Guide to Greatness. Art Fettig. 1986. LC 85-80482. (Illus.). 128p. pap. 5.95 (*0-916927-01-6*) Growth Unltd.

Position for Success! Strategic Marketing for Group Practices. Andrea T. Eliscu. 1994. 148p. 49.00 (*1-56829-044-6*, 4812) M G M A.

Position of Modern Science on the Beginning of Human Life. Scientists for Life Staff. 1983. 45p. (Orig.). pap. 1.75 (*0-937930-02-4*) Sun Life.

Positional Release Technique. Chaitow. 1998. (C). pap. text (*0-443-06129-7*) Church.

Positional Release Techniques. Chaitow. 1996. text 38.95 (*0-443-05299-9*) Saunders.

Positional Release Techniques: From a Dynamic Systems Perspective. Denise Deig. 2000. LC 00-26041. (Illus.). 248p. text 59.99 (*0-7506-7225-0*) Buttrwrth-Heinemann.

Positional Release Therapy: Assessment & Treatment of Musculoskeletol Dysfunction. Kerry J. D'Ambrogio et al. 1997. LC 96-25538. (Illus.). 280p. (C). (gr. 13). text 79.95 (*0-8151-0096-5*, 26559) Mosby Inc.

***Positioning & Technique for Diagnostic Imaging.** Louise Smith et al. 2001. (Illus.). 843p. (*0-443-06212-9*) Church GBR. *Dist:* Saunders.

Positioning for Function: The Wheelchair & Other Assistive Technologies. Adrienne F. Bergen et al. 1990. (Illus.). (Orig.). (C). pap. text 49.95 (*0-911681-04-3*) Valhalla Rehab.

Positioning in a Wheelchair: A Guide for Professional Caregivers of the Disabled Adult. Jan K. Mayall & Guylaine Desharnais. 2nd ed. 1995. LC 94-27090. 176p. pap. 23.00 (*1-55642-251-2*, 42512) SLACK Inc.

Positioning in Anesthesia & Surgery. John T. Martin & Mark A. Warner. Ed. by Lesley Day. 3rd ed. 1996. 352p. text 79.00 (*0-7216-6674-4*) Saunders.

***Positioning Patients for Surgery.** Servant & Purkiss. 2002. (Illus.). 180p. pap. (*1-84110-052-8*) Greenwich Med GBR. *Dist:* JAMCO Dist.

Positive: HIV Affirmative Counseling. Craig Kain. 1996. 270p. pap. text 45.95 (*1-55620-147-8*, 72573) Am Coun Assn.

Positive & Negative Symptoms in Psychosis: Description, Research & Future Directions. Ed. by Philip D. Harvey & Elaine Walker. 1987. 351p. (C). text 49.95 (*0-89859-880-X*) L Erlbaum Assocs.

Positive & Negative Syndromes in Schizophrenia. Stanley R. Kay. 1991. LC 90-15113. (Einstein Clinical & Experimental Psychiatry Monograph Ser.: No. 5). 288p. text 45.95 (*0-87630-608-3*) Brunner-Routledge.

Positive Approaches to Dementia Care. U. P. Holden & R. T. Woods. 3rd ed. 1995. (Illus.). 240p. pap. (*0-443-04970-X*) Church.

Positive Approaches to Living with End Stage Renal Disease: Psychosocial & Thanatalogic Aspects, 6. Ed. by Michael A. Hardy. 1986. LC 85-28334. 239p. 57.75 (*0-275-92019-4*, C2019, Praeger Pubs) Greenwood.

Positive Attitudes for the Physically Challenged. Hoyt Anderson. 1986. 20p. (Orig.). pap. 3.95 (*0-937743-00-3*) Successful Living.

Positive Behavior Support in People with Developmental Disabilities: A Research Synthesis. Edward G. Carr. 1999. LC 99-22505. 108p. 31.95 (*0-940898-60-8*) Am Assn Mental.

Positive Caregiver Attitudes. James R. Sherman. 1994. (Illus.). 80p. pap. 9.95 (*0-935538-18-6*) Pathway Bks.

Positive Deviance in Child Nutrition. 153p. 30.00 (*92-808-0697-1*, 89.III.A.7) UN.

Positive Discipline. Jane Nelsen. 2nd ed. 1987. 242p. pap. 7.95 (*0-9606896-1-3*) Ballantine Pub Grp.

Positive Environment: Physical & Social Influences on People with Senile Dementia in Residential Care. Ann Netten. 1993. LC 92-44396. 110p. (*1-85742-107-8*); pap. (*1-85742-112-4*) Arena GBR. *Dist:* Ashgate Pub Co.

Positive Life: Portraits of Women Living with HIV. Photos by Mary Berridge. 1997. LC 96-72481. (Illus.). 128p. 27.50 (*0-7624-0198-2*) Running Pr.

Positive Lives - Responses to HIV: A Photodocumentary. Ed. by Stephen Mayes & Lyndall Stein. 1993. LC 93-40472. text 60.00 (*0-304-32846-4*) Continuum.

Positive Nutrition for HIV Infection & AIDS: A Medically Sound Take Charge Plan to Maintain. Stacey J. Bell. 1996. 192p. pap. 12.95 (*1-56561-089-X*) Wiley.

Positive Nutrition for HIV Infection & AIDS: A Medically Sound Take Charge Plan to Maintain. Stacy Jane Bell. 1996. 192p. pap. 12.95 (*0-471-34696-9*) Wiley.

Positive Options: A Handbook for People Living with HIV. Karin Timour & Kevin Armington. 1995. (Illus.). 152p. (Orig.). pap. 15.00 (*0-9653952-0-0*) Body Positive.

Positive Options for Crohn's Disease: Self-Help & Treatment. Joan Gomez. 2000. LC 00-21084. 182p. 22.95 (*0-89793-279-X*); pap. 12.95 (*0-89793-278-1*) Hunter Hse.

***Positive Options for Living with a Stoma: Self-Help & Treatment.** Craig A. White. 2002. LC 2001-43083. 12.95 (*0-89793-358-3*) Hunter House.

Positive Peer Culture: A Selected Bibliography. Larry K. Brendtro et al. 1994. xxi, 172p. (Orig.). (C). pap. text 19.95 (*0-9639084-1-3*) S D A Pub.

Positive Pregnancy Fitness: A Guide to a More Comfortable Pregnancy & Easier Birth Through Exercise & Relaxation. Sylvia K. Olkin. 1987. LC 87-18844. (Illus.). 272p. pap. 12.95 (*0-89529-373-0*, Avery) Penguin Putnam.

Positive Regard: Carl Rogers & Other Notables He Inspired. Mel Suhd. 1994. LC 93-87337. 457p. 26.95 (*0-8314-0081-1*) Sci & Behavior.

Positive-Strand RNA Viruses. Ed. by M. A. Brinton et al. 1996. LC 94-3138. (Archives of Virology Ser.: Suppl. 9). (Illus.). 234.00 (*0-387-82522-3*) Spr-Verlag.

Positive Women: Voices of Women Living with AIDS. Ed. by Andrea Rudd & Darien Taylor. 1992. (Illus.). 510p. pap. (*0-929005-30-9*) Sec Story Pr CAN. *Dist:* LPC InBook.

Positively False: Exposing the Myths around HIV & AIDS. Joan Shenton. 1998. LC 99-202560. 278p. *(1-86064-333-7)* I B T GBR. *Dist:* St Martin.

Positively Women: Living with AIDS. Sue O'Sullivan. 1996. LC 98-212253. 336p. pap. *(0-04-440943-5)* Pandora GBR. *Dist:* NYU Pr.

Positron Emission Tomography: Applications in Oncology. Ed. by Nielson Tse & Carl Hoh. 1994. 123p. 89.95 *(1-57059-128-8,* LN9128) CRC Pr.

Positron Emission Tomography: Research & Clinical Applications. R. E. Coleman. Date not set. *(0-8247-9486-9)* Dekker.

Positron Emission Tomography in Clinical Research: Tracer Modelling & Radioreceptors. Ed. by C. Beckers et al. 1989. (C). text 171.00 *(0-7923-0254-0)* Kluwer Academic.

Positron Emission Tomography in the Millennium: Proceedings of the International PET Symposium Held in Hokkaido, Japan, 24-26th September, 1999. International PET Symposium Staff & Nagara Tamaki. 2000. LC 00-34075. 342p. 145.00 *(0-444-50385-4,* North Holland) Elsevier.

Possibility of Joy: Chronic Depression & Recovery-Thirty Healthy Minded Things to Do. James Drey. 2000. 128p. pap. 14.95 *(0-9675060-1-8)* Stone House Pr Inc.

Possible Health Effects of Exposure to Residential Electric & Magnetic Fields. Ed. by John B. Little. 1997. (Illus.). 356p. (Orig.). (C). text 60.00 *(0-7881-4516-9)* DIANE Pub.

Possible Health Effects of Exposure to Residential Electric & Magnetic Fields. NRC, Possible Effects of Electromagnetic Fields on. 1997. LC 96-51230. 384p. text 39.95 *(0-309-05447-8)* Natl Acad Pr.

***Possible Health Effects of Pyridostigmine Bromide on Persian Gulf War Veterans: Congressional Hearing.** Ed. by Cliff Stearns. 2001. 135p. reprint ed. pap. text 30.00 *(0-7567-1767-1)* DIANE Pub.

Possible Vision: Holistic New Age Education. George A. Jones. 1981. LC 80-52612. 104p. pap. 5.00 *(0-917610-02-4)* Peacehaven.

Possible Worlds: And Other Papers. John Burdon Sanderson Haldane. 1977. LC 75-167351. (Essay Index Reprint Ser.). reprint ed. 22.95 *(0-8369-2452-5)* Ayer.

Post-Abortion Aftermath: A Comprehensive Consideration. Michael T. Mannion. 1994. LC 94-21556. 190p. (Orig.). pap. 12.95 *(1-55612-708-1)* Sheed & Ward WI.

Post Acute Care Reimbursement Manual. Cherilyn G. Murer et al. 1997. LC 97-36013. *(0-7863-1248-3)* McGraw.

Post-Anaesthetic Recovery. R. J. Eltringham et al. 2nd ed. 1990. (Illus.). 193p. 51.95 *(0-387-19555-6)* Spr-Verlag.

Post Anesthesia Care Unit: A Critical Care Approach to Post Anesthesia Nursing. Cecil B. Drain. 3rd ed. 1994. LC 93-8029. (Illus.). 640p. text 52.50 *(0-7216-4571-2)* Saunders.

Post Anesthesia Care Unit Competencies. Barbara Godden. 1996. 126p. ring bd. 115.00 *(1-879575-37-X)* Acad Med Sys.

Post-Basic Nursing Education Programmes for Foreign Students. 1960. (Technical Report Ser.: No. 199). 48p. pap. text 3.00 *(92-4-120199-1)* World Health.

Post-Imperative Negative Variation in Schizophrenic Patients & Healthy Subjects. Christoph Klein. (Psychophysiologie in Labor und Feld Ser.: Bd. 3). (Illus.). 386p. 1997. pap. 63.95 *(3-631-31078-1)*; 1996. LC 96-53386. pap. text 63.95 *(0-8204-3233-4,* RC514) P Lang Pubng.

Post-Jungians Today: Key Papers in Contemporary Analytical Psychology. Ann Casement. 1998. LC 98-9829. 248p. (C). 94.95 *(0-415-16154-1)*; pap. 27.95 *(0-415-16155-X)* Routledge.

Post-Lesion Neural Plasticity. Ed. by H. Flohr. 1988. (Illus.). 708p. 133.00 *(0-387-19455-X)* Spr-Verlag.

Post-Natal Depression: Psychology, Science, & the Transition to Motherhood. Paula Nicolson. 1998. LC 97-49218. (Women & Psychology Ser.). 160p. (C). 63.95 *(0-415-16362-5)*; pap. 19.95 *(0-415-16363-3)* Routledge.

Post-Operative Care of Ophtalmic Surgery. Epstein. 1999. pap. text *(0-7216-1911-8)* Saunders.

Post Operative Complications in Intracranial Neurosurgery. Ed. by Emily Friedman et al. 1993. LC 92-49908. 99.00 *(0-86577-438-2)* Thieme Med Pubs.

Post-Operative Recovery & Pain Relief. Ed. by Roger J. Eltringham et al. 1997. LC 97-14221. (Illus.). 240p. pap. 54.00 *(3-540-76078-4)* Spr-Verlag.

Post-Polio. Betty Garee. 1987. LC 87-71476. 48p. (Orig.). reprint ed. pap. text 3.95 *(0-915708-21-3)* Cheever Pub.

Post-Polio Syndrome. Ed. by Lauro S. Halstead & Gunnar Grimby. 1995. LC 94-42418. (Illus.). 230p. 44.95 *(1-56053-117-7)* Hanley & Belfus.

Post-Polio Syndrome. Theodore L. Munsat. 1990. (Illus.). 144p. text 80.00 *(0-409-90153-9)* Buttrwrth-Heinemann.

Post-Stroke Rehabilitation: Clinical Practice Guideline. Glen E. Gresham et al. 1997. (Illus.). 248p. (C). reprint ed. pap. text 50.00 *(0-7881-4144-9)* DIANE Pub.

Post-Stroke Rehabilitation Clinical Practice Guideline. Post-Stroke Rehabilitation Guideline Panel Staff et al. 1993. LC 95-44619. 250p. pap. 26.00 *(0-8342-0811-3)* PRO-ED.

Post-Therapeutic Neurodiagnostic Imaging. J. Randy Jinkins. 1996. LC 96-42057. 320p. text 149.00 *(0-397-58406-7)* Lppncott W & W.

Post-Trauma Stress: Reduce Long-Term Effects & Hidden Emotional Damage Caused by Violence & Disaster. Frank Parkinson. 2000. LC 00-20658. 208p. pap. 14.00 *(1-55561-249-0)* Fisher Bks.

Post-Traumatic Stress Disorder: A Clinician's Guide. K. Peterson et al. 1990. LC 90-14309. (Stress & Coping Ser.). (Illus.). 276p. (C). 42.50 *(0-306-43542-X,* Plenum Trade) Perseus Pubng.

Post-Traumatic Stress Disorder: A Complete Treatment Guide. Aphrodite Matasakis. 1994. LC 93-87082. 384p. 49.95 *(1-879237-68-7)* New Harbinger.

Post-Traumatic Stress Disorder: A Lifespan Developmental Perspective. A. Maercker et al. 1998. LC 98-36649. viii, 264p. 39.00 *(0-88937-187-3)* Hogrefe & Huber Pubs.

Post Traumatic Stress Disorder: A Police Officers Report. L. Ken Rogers. 2000. LC 99-75954. 272p. pap. 14.95 *(1-882792-83-1)* Proctor Pubns.

Post-Traumatic Stress Disorder: Assessment, Differential Diagnosis, & Forensic Evaluation. Ed. by Carroll L. Meek. 1990. LC 89-43413. 264p. 31.45 *(0-943158-35-4,* PTSDBP, Prof Resc Pr) Pro Resource.

Post-Traumatic Stress Disorder: Defining, Examining, Preventing & Treating. Charles R. Figley. 1994. (Innovations in Psychology Ser.). 200p. lib. bdg. 39.95 *(1-57444-166-3,* SL1663) St Lucie Pr.

Post-Traumatic Stress Disorder: Diagnosis, Treatment, & Legal Issues. C. B. Scrignar. 2nd ed. 1988. (Illus.). 344p. (C). pap. 32.95 *(0-945032-01-3)*; 2nd l.t. ed. 1988. (Illus.). 344p. (C). 49.95 *(0-945032-00-5)*; 3rd ed. 1996. text 59.95 *(0-945032-05-6)*; 3rd ed. 1996. pap. text 39.95 *(0-945032-06-4)* Bruno Pr.

Post Traumatic Stress Disorder: The Latest Assessment & Treatment Strategies. Matthew J. Friedman. 2000. LC 00-21872. (Illus.). 108p. pap. 14.95 *(1-887537-14-7)* Compact Clinicals.

Post-Traumatic Stress Disorder: The Victim's Guide to Healing & Recovery. Raymond B. Flannery, Jr. 1995. 240p. reprint ed. pap. 19.95 *(0-8245-1445-9)* Crossroad NY.

Post Traumatic Stress Disorder & Dramatherapy. Linda Winn. 1993. 160p. 36.00 *(1-85302-183-0)* Taylor & Francis.

Post-Traumatic Stress Disorder Sourcebook: A Guide to Healing, Recovery & Growth. Glenn R Schiraldi. 2000. LC 99-47837. (Illus.). 446p. pap. 18.95 *(0-7373-0265-8,* 02658W, Contemporary) McGraw-Hill Trade.

Post-Traumatic Stress Disorders: Concepts & Therapy. William Yule. 1999. LC 98-24146. (Clinical Psychology & Personality Ser.). (Illus.). 344p. pap. 55.00 *(0-471-97080-8)* Wiley.

Post-Traumatic Therapy & Victims of Violence. Frank M. Ochberg. 1988. LC 87-26877. (Psychosocial Stress Ser.: No. 11). 384p. text 47.95 *(0-87630-490-0)* Brunner-Routledge.

Post Viral Fatigue Syndrome. James F. Mowbray. Ed. by Rachel Jenkins. 1993. LC 90-13138. 502p. pap. 215.00 *(0-471-93879-3,* Wiley-Liss) Wiley.

Postabortion Care: A Reference Manual for Improving the Quality of Care. Ed. by Judith Winkler et al. 1995. (Illus.). (Orig.). pap. text 15.00 *(0-929817-08-7)* JHPIEGO.

Postabortion Care: Lessons from Operations Research. Ed. by Dale Huntington & Nancy J. Piet-Pelon. 1999. LC 99-49051. *(0-87834-100-5)* Population Coun.

***Postal Work - Work Organizational Changes as Tools to Improve Health.** Kurt Wahlstedt. 2001. (Comprehensive Summaries of Uppsala Dissertations from the Faculty of Medicine Ser.: No. 1022). 87p. *(91-554-4994-8)* Uppsala Universitet SWE. *Dist:* Coronet Bks.

Posterior Capsule Opacification: An Experiemental Study in Vitro & in Vivo. Niklas Wallentin. 2000. (Comprehensive Summaries of Uppsala Dissertations from the Faculty of Pharmacy Ser.: No. 230). (Illus.). 52p. pap. *(91-554-4753-8)* Uppsala Universitet SWE. *Dist:* Coronet Bks.

Posterior Circulation Disease: Clinical Findings, Diagnosis, & Management. Louis R. Caplan. 1996. LC 96-3448. (Illus.). 700p. 175.00 *(0-86542-298-2)* Blackwell Sci.

Posterior Fossa, Spinal Cord & Peripheral Nerve Disease, Vol. 2. Ed. by L. G. Kempe. 1986. (Illus.). 281p. 368.00 *(0-387-04890-1)* Spr-Verlag.

Posterior Fossa Tumors. Ed. by Anthony J. Raimondi et al. 1993. LC 92-49986. (Principles of Pediatric Neurosurgery Ser.). (Illus.). 214p. 239.00 *(0-387-97915-8)* Spr-Verlag.

Posterior Segment Intraocular Inflammation - Guidelines. John V. Forrester et al. Ed. by Shigeaki Ohno. 1998. (Illus.). xiii, 202p. *(90-6299-167-X)* Kugler NLD. *Dist:* Lib Res.

Posterior Uveitis, Pt. 2. Tabbara. 1995. 39.00 *(0-316-06077-1,* Little Brwn Med Div) Lppncott W & W.

Posterior Uveitis: Diagnosis & Management. Khalid F. Tabbara & Robert B. Nussenblatt. 1994. LC 94-32315. (Illus.). 199p. text 120.00 *(0-7506-9599-4)* Buttrwrth-Heinemann.

Postgastrectomy & Postvagatomy Syndromes. H. D. Becker & W. F. Caspary. 1980. (Illus.). 500p. 108.00 *(0-387-09445-8)* Spr-Verlag.

Postgraduate Education & Training in Public Health: Proceedings of the WHO Expert Committee, Geneva, 1973. WHO Staff. 1973. (Technical Reports: No. 533). pap. text 5.00 *(92-4-120533-4,* 1100533) World Health.

Postgraduate Education for Medical Personnel in the U. S. S. R. Report Prepared by the Participants in a Study Tour Organized by the World Health Organization. 1970. (Public Health Papers: No. 39). 52p. pap. text 4.00 *(92-4-130039-6,* 1110039) World Health.

Postgraduate Haematology. Ed. by A. Victor Hoffbrand et al. 4th ed. 1998. LC 97-18995. 734p. *(0-7506-0583-9)* E A GBR. *Dist:* OUP.

Postgraduate Psychiatry: Clinical & Scientific Foundations. David Forshaw & Louis Appleby. 1990. 192p. pap. text *(0-7506-0448-4)* E A GBR. *Dist:* OUP.

Postgraduate Psychiatry: Clinical & Scientific Foundations. Lois Appleby et al. 2nd ed. 2000. (Illus.). 624p. pap. *(0-7506-3503-7)* E A GBR. *Dist:* OUP.

Postgraduate Surgery: The Candidate's Guide. M. A. R. Al-Fallouji. 2nd ed. 1998. LC 97-22534. 688p. pap. text *(0-7506-1591-5)* E A GBR. *Dist:* OUP.

Postgraduate Textbook of Clinical Orthopaedics. N. H. Harris & R. Birch. 2nd ed. 1995. 1120p. 250.00 *(0-632-02902-1)* Blackwell Sci.

Postinfectious Glomerulonephritis. Karin Sorger. 1986. (Progress in Pathology Ser.: Band 125). 110p. pap. *(0-89574-223-3)* Gustav Fischer DEU. *Dist:* Lubrecht & Cramer, Balogh.

Postmodern Nursing Redefining Nursing. Jean Watson. 1998. LC 99-36289. (C). pap. text *(0-443-05744-3)* Church.

Postmodernism, Sociology & Health. Nicholas J. Fox. 1993. LC 93-4286. 192p. 37.50 *(0-335-19046-4)*; pap. 12.99 *(0-335-19045-6)* U of Toronto Pr.

Postnatal Care. Ed. by Jo Alexander et al. 1993. 290p. pap. text 17.95 *(0-8020-7452-9)* U of Toronto Pr.

Postnatal Development, Aging & Degeneration of the TMJ. Hans U. Luder. 1996. (Craniofacial Growth Ser.: Vol. 32). (Illus.). 270p. 55.00 *(0-929921-28-3)* UM CHGD.

Postnatal Growth Vol. 2: Neurobiology. F. Falkner & J. M. Tanner. 2nd ed. 1986. LC 85-19397. (Human Growth Ser.). (Illus.). 578p. (C). text 125.00 *(0-306-41952-1)* Kluwer Academic.

Postoperative Critical Care Procedures of the Massachusetts General Hospital. W. Andrew Kofke & Gerold H. Levy. 1986. 544p. 27.00 *(0-316-50098-4,* Little Brwn Med Div) Lppncott W & W.

Postoperative Epidural Opioids. J. Chrubasik et al. 1993. (Illus.). 115p. pap. *(3-540-56871-9)*; LC 93-25591. 131p. 35.00 *(0-387-56871-9)* Spr-Verlag.

Postoperative Management of the Cardiac Surgical Patient. Ed. by John P. Williams. 1995. 435p. text *(0-443-08932-9)* Church.

Postoperative Pain Management. Ed. by F. Michael Ferrante & Timothy R. VadeBoncouer. 1992. (Illus.). 300p. (Orig.). pap. text *(0-443-08766-0)* Church.

Postoperative Thromboembolism: Frequency, Etiology, Prophylaxis. David Bergqvist. 1983. (Illus.). 234p. 71.95 *(0-387-12062-9)* Spr-Verlag.

Postpartum Depression. Sharon Roan. 1993. *(0-471-54678-X)* Wiley.

Postpartum Depression: A Research Guide & International Bibliography. Laurence Kruckman & Chris Asmann-Finch. 1986. LC 85-31136. (Reference Books on Family Issues: Vol. 8). 200p. text 52.00 *(0-8240-9121-3,* SS335) Garland.

Postpartum Depression: Causes & Consequences. M. W. O'Hara & Lauren B. Alloy. 1994. (Series in Psychopathology). (Illus.). 222p. 99.00 *(0-387-94261-0)* Spr-Verlag.

Postpartum Depression & Child Development. Ed. by Lynne Murray & Peter J. Cooper. 1997. LC 96-39987. 322p. text 40.00 *(1-57230-197-X,* 0197) Guilford Pubns.

Postpartum Mood Disorders. Ed. by Laura J. Miller. 1998. LC 98-24929. (Clinical Practice Ser.). 280p. text 39.50 *(0-88048-929-4,* 8929) Am Psychiatric.

Postpartum Nursing: Health Care of Women. Joellen W. Hawkins & Beverly Gorvine. 1984. (Illus.). 192p. pap. 25.95 *(0-8261-4690-2)* Springer Pub.

Postpartum Psychiatric Illness: A Picture Puzzle. Ed. by James A. Hamilton & Patricia N. Harberger. 1992. LC 91-30386. (Illus.). 384p. (C). text 35.00 *(0-8122-3137-6)* U of Pa Pr.

Postpartum Survival Guide. Ann Dunnewald & Diane G. Sanford. 1994. LC 94-67045. (Illus.). 288p. pap. 14.95 *(1-879237-80-6)* New Harbinger.

Postreproductive Gynecology. Ed. by Hugh M. Shingleton & W. Glenn Hurt. 1990. (Illus.). 590p. text *(0-443-08641-9)* Church.

Posttramatic Stress Intervention: Challenges, Issues, & Perspectives. Ed. by John M. Violanti et al. 2000. LC 00-25323. (Illus.). xvii, 244p. text 44.95 *(0-398-07066-0)* C C Thomas.

Posttraumatic Nightmares: Psychodynamic Explorations. Melvin R. Lansky & Carol R. Bley. 1995. LC 94-43415. 208p. 37.50 *(0-88163-193-0)* Analytic Pr.

Posttraumatic Stress Disorder: A Behavioral Approach to Assessment & Treatment. Ed. by Philip A. Saigh. 1991. (Psychology Practitioner Guidebooks Ser.). 212p. text *(0-08-036830-1)*; pap. text *(0-08-036829-8)* PPI GBR. *Dist:* Elsevier.

Posttraumatic Stress Disorder: A Comprehensive Text. Ed. by Philip A. Saigh et al. 1998. LC 98-38799. 434p. 73.00 *(0-205-26734-3)* Allyn.

Posttraumatic Stress Disorder: A Guide. John H. Greist et al. 2000. 69p. pap. 4.95 *(1-890802-22-0)* Madison Inst of Med.

Posttraumatic Stress Disorder: Acute & Long-Term Responses to Trauma & Disaster. Ed. by Carol S. Fullerton & Robert J. Ursano. 1997. LC 96-24027. (Progress in Psychiatry Ser.: Vol. 51). 308p. text 42.50 *(0-88048-751-8,* 8751) Am Psychiatric.

Posttraumatic Stress Disorder: Additional Perspectives. Merrill I. Lipton. 1994. LC 93-37142. 258p. (C). text 55.95 *(0-398-05899-7)* C C Thomas.

Posttraumatic Stress Disorder: DSM-IV & Beyond. Ed. by Jonathan R. Davidson & Edna B. Foa. 1992. LC 92-7052. 262p. text 35.00 *(0-88048-502-7,* 8502) Am Psychiatric.

Posttraumatic Stress Disorder: Etiology, Phenomenology, & Treatment. Ed. by Marion E. Wolf & Aron D. Mosnaim. 1990. LC 90-68. 270p. text 19.95 *(0-88048-299-0,* 8299) Am Psychiatric.

Posttraumatic Stress Disorder in Children. Spencer Eth & Robert S. Pynoos. 1985. LC 85-15762. (Progress in Psychiatry Ser.: No. 4). 186p. 19.95 *(0-88048-067-X,* 8067) Am Psychiatric.

Posttraumatic Stress Disorder in Litigation: Guidelines for Forensic Assessment. Ed. by Robert I. Simon. 1994. LC 94-30643. 192p. text 29.50 *(0-88048-687-2,* 8687) Am Psychiatric.

Postulates of Re-Evaluation Counseling: Arabic Translation. Harvey Jackins. 1987. pap. 1.00 *(0-913937-21-5)* Rational Isl.

Postulates of Re-Evaluation Counseling: Chinese Translation. Harvey Jackins. Tr. by Sun Jian-Min from ENG. 1987. pap. 1.00 *(0-913937-27-4)* Rational Isl.

Postulates of Re-Evaluation Counseling: Hungarian Translation. Harvey Jackins. Tr. by Molnar Gabriella. 1981. pap. 1.00 *(0-911214-93-3)* Rational Isl.

Postural Behavior in Newborn Infants. Paul Casear. 1991. (Clinics in Developmental Medicine Ser.: Vol. 72). (Illus.). 112p. (C). text *(0-521-41201-3)* Mc Keith Pr GBR. *Dist:* Cambridge U Pr.

Posture & Motility in Preterm Infants: A Clinical Approach. Laila De Groot. 1994. 160p. pap. *(90-5383-239-4)* VU Univ Pr NLD. *Dist:* Paul & Co Pubs.

Posture Makes Perfect Health. Victor Barker. 1993. (Illus.). 206p. (Orig.). pap. 22.00 *(0-87040-871-2)* Japan Pubns USA.

Posture Prescription: A Doctor's Rx For Eliminating Back, Muscle & Joint Pain; Achieving Optimum Strength & Mobility; Living a Lifetime of Fitness & Well-Being. Arthur White & Kate Kelly. 2002. LC 00-34419. (Illus.). 256p. pap. 15.00 *(0-609-80631-9,* Three Riv Pr) Harmony Bks.

Postviral Fatigue Syndrome. Ed. by Peter Behan et al. 1992. (British Medical Bulletin Ser.: Vol. 47, No. 4). (Illus.). 264p. text *(0-443-04490-2)* Church.

Pot: New Facts, Old Fictions. Jim Parker. rev. ed. 1999. pap. 0.50 *(0-89230-162-7)* Do It Now.

Potassium. Horacio J. Adrogue & Donald E. Wesson. 1994. LC 94-17877. (Basics of Medicine Ser.). (Illus.). 248p. pap. 10.95 *(0-86542-427-6)* Blackwell Sci.

Potassium. Horacio J. Adrogue & Donald E. Wesson. 1992. (& W Basics in Medicine Ser.). 250p. text 29.95 *(0-9630670-1-X)* Libra & Gemini.

Potassium Channel Modulators, Pharmacological, Molecular & Clinical Aspects. A. H. Weston & T. C. Hamilton. 1992. (Frontiers in Pharmacology & Therapeutics Ser.). (Illus.). 528p. 175.00 *(0-632-03044-5)* Blackwell Sci.

Potassium Channels in Normal & Pathological Conditions. Ed. by J. Vereecke et al. 1995. (Illus.). 447p. (Orig.). pap. *(90-6186-701-0)* Leuven Univ BEL. *Dist:* Coronet Bks.

Potatoes As Food & Medicine. H. Valentine Knaggs. 1991. lib. bdg. 72.00 *(0-8490-4963-6)* Gordon Pr.

Potatoes As Food & Medicine: Epsom Salt, Its Value & Use & the Cleansing Saline Fast. H. Valentine Knaggs. 1996. 15p. reprint ed. spiral bd. 9.50 *(0-7873-0503-0)* Hlth Research.

Potential Health Hazards of Existing Chemicals. Ed. by B. G. Chemie. 1990. LC 90-10020. (Toxicological Evaluations Ser.: Vol. 1). (Illus.). 341p. 67.95 *(0-387-52577-7)* Spr-Verlag.

Potential of Fantasy & Imagination. A. A. Sheikh & John T. Shaffer. 1979. LC 79-88092. lib. bdg. 15.00 *(0-913412-31-7)* Brandon Hse.

Potential Radiation Exposure in Military Operations: Protecting the Soldier Before, During & After. Institute of Medicine Staff. 1999. LC 99-227398. xvii, 139p. pap. 34.75 *(0-309-06439-2)* Natl Acad Pr.

Potential Transmission of Spongiform Encephalopathies to Humans: The Food & Drug Administration's (FDA) Ruminant to Ruminant Feed Ban & the Safety of Other Products. Ed. by Christopher Shays. 1998. 131p. (C). pap. text 30.00 *(0-7881-7300-6)* DIANE Pub.

Potentiating Health & the Crisis of the Immune System: Integrative Approaches to the Prevention & Treatment of Modern Diseases. Ed. by Avshalom Mizrahi et al. 1997. LC 97-16693. (Illus.). 300p. (C). text 114.00 (*0-306-45602-8*, Kluwer Plenum) Kluwer Academic.

Pottenger Portfolio: Fifty-Five Reprints of Medical Papers of Dr. Francis M. Pottenger, Jr. 1974. 35.00 (*0-916764-03-6*) Price-Pottenger.

Pottengers' Cats: A Study in Nutrition. Francis M. Pottenger, Jr. 1983. LC 83-80360. (Illus.). 126p. 5.95 (*0-916764-06-0*) Price-Pottenger.

Potter. Iowa Valley Community College Staff. 1996. (Nursing Texts Ser.). (C). (gr. 13). text 87.00 (*0-8151-4455-5*, 30719) Mosby Inc.

Potter's Atlas of Fetal & Infant Pathology. Edith L. Potter & Enid Gilbert-Barness. 1998. LC 98-23495. 398p. text 149.00 (*0-323-00126-2*) Mosby Inc.

Potter's New Cyclopaedia of Botanical Drugs & Preparations. R. C. Wren. rev. ed. 1994. (C). pap. 32.50 (*0-8464-1039-7*) Beekman Pubs.

Potter's New Cyclopaedia of Botanical Drugs & Preparations. R. C. Wren. 1988. 376p. pap. (*0-85207-197-3*) C W Daniel GBR. *Dist:* Natl Bk Netwk.

Potter's New Cyclopaedia of Botanical Drugs & Preparations. R. C. Wren. 1980. 50.00 (*0-85032-176-X*) St Mut.

Potter's Pathology of the Fetus & Infant Ed. by Enid Gilbert-Barnes. 1996. (Illus.). 1776p. (C). (gr. 13). text 310.00 (*0-8016-7870-6*, 07870) Mosby Inc.

Potter's Perinatal Pathology. Alan Blanc. 1991. (*0-8151-0868-0*) Mosby Inc.

Potyviridae. D. D. Shukla et al. 1994. LC 96-170505. (Illus.). 448p. text 150.00 (*0-85198-864-4*) OUP.

Potyvirus Taxonomy. Ed. by O. W. Barnett. 1992. LC 92-25228. (Archives of Virology Ser.: Suppl. 5). (Illus.). 400p. 207.00 (*0-387-82353-0*) Spr-Verlag.

Poultry Diseases. Jordan. 4th ed. 1996. text 74.00 (*0-7020-1912-7*) Saunders.

Poultry Diseases & Meat Hygiene: A Color Atlas. Drago C. Herenda & Don A. Franco. 1996. LC 96-5731. (Illus.). 356p. text 99.95 (*0-8138-2463-X*) Iowa U Pr.

Pound of Prevention: The Case for Universal Maternity Care in the U. S. Ed. by Jonathan Kotch et al. 1992. 275p. 30.00 (*0-87553-206-3*) Am Pub Health.

Pour une Naissance sans Violence see Birth Without Violence: The Book that Revolutionized the Way We Bring Our Children into the World

***Poverty & Child Health.** Nick Spencer. 2nd exp. ed. 2000. 368p. pap. (*1-85775-477-8*) Radcliffe Med Pr GBR. *Dist:* Balogh.

Poverty & Health: Working with Families. Clare Blackburn. 1991. 160p. pap. (*0-335-09734-0*) OpUniv Pr.

Poverty & Health in New York City. United Hospital Fund Staff. Ed. by Melvin I. Krasner. 1989. 224p. 40.00 (*0-934459-52-5*) United Hosp Fund.

Poverty, Development & Health Policy. B. Abel-Smith & A. Leiserson. 1978. (Public Health Papers: No. 69). 109p. pap. text 10.00 (*92-4-130069-8*, 1110069) World Health.

Poverty, Vulnerability, & the Value of Human Life: A Global Agenda for Bioethics. Ed. by Z. Bankowski & J. H. Bryant. 1994. (Highlights & Papers of the XXVIIIth CIOMS Conference, Ixtapa, Guerrero State, Mexico). xi, 246p. pap. text 25.00 (*92-9036-060-7*, 1830028) World Health.

Powder Technology & Pharmaceutical Processes. Dominique Chulia et al. 1993. LC 93-41271. (Handbook of Powder Technology Ser.: 9). 584p. 262.50 (*0-444-81533-3*) Elsevier.

Power & Community: Organizational & Cultural Responses to AIDS. Dennis Altman. 1994. LC 94-5754. 69.95 (*0-7484-0193-8*); pap. 24.95 (*0-7484-0194-6*) Taylor & Francis.

Power & Compassion: Working with Difficult Adolescents & Abused Parents. Jerome A. Price. 1996. LC 96-29012. (Guilford Family Therapy Ser.). 196p. 35.00 (*1-57230-141-4*, 0141) Guilford Pubns.

Power & Family Therapy: A Special Issue of Contemporary Family Therapy. Ed. by William C. Nichols. 1988. 75p. pap. 14.95 (*0-89885-430-X*, Kluwer Acad Hman Sci) Kluwer Academic.

Power & Illness: The Failure & Future of American Health Policy. Daniel M. Fox. 1995. pap. text 15.95 (*0-520-20151-5*); 1993. LC 93-2977. text 30.00 (*0-520-08409-8*) U CA Pr.

Power & the Profession of Obstetrics. William R. Arney. LC 82-8410. (Illus.). (C). 1993. xii, 290p. pap. text 10.95 (*0-226-02729-5*); 1983. xii, 304p. lib. bdg. 30.00 (*0-226-02728-7*) U Ch Pr.

Power Behind Your Eyes: Improving Your Eyesight with Integrated Vision Therapy. Robert-Michael Kaplan. 1995. LC 95-24981. (Illus.). 192p. pap. 16.95 (*0-89281-536-1*, Heal Arts VT) Inner Tradit.

Power Building in Documentation. Deborah Montone. Ed. by Adrianne Williams. 1998. LC 97-34986. 320p. (C). pap. text 18.95 (*0-7216-6933-6*) Saunders.

Power Building in the Money Trail. Deborah Montone. Ed. by Adrianne Williams. 1998. LC 98-25996. (Illus.). 430p. (C). pap. text 24.95 (*0-7216-6931-X*) Saunders.

Power Building Medical Coding. Deborah Montone. 1998. LC 98-4061. (C). pap. text 21.00 (*0-7216-6930-1*) Harcourt.

Power Dreamers: The Jocasta Complex. Ursule Molinaro. 1994. 128p. 16.00 (*0-929701-44-5*) McPherson & Co.

Power Eating. Susan M. Kleiner & Maggie Greenwood-Robinson. 1998. LC 97-43566. (Illus.). 240p. pap. 15.95 (*0-88011-702-8*, PKLE0702) Human Kinetics.

Power Healing: Use the New Integrated Medicine to Cure Yourself. Leo Galland. 1998. 352p. pap. 14.95 (*0-375-75139-4*) Random.

Power in Psychotherapeutic Practice. David Heller. 1985. 197p. 29.95 (*0-89885-228-5*, Kluwer Acad Hman Sci) Kluwer Academic.

Power in the Helping Professions. Adolf Guggenbuhl-Craig. Tr. by Myron B. Gubitz from GER. 1971. LC 86-17901. 158p. (C). pap. 15.00 (*0-88214-304-2*) Spring Pubns.

Power Nutrition for Your Chronic Illness. Kristine Napier. 1998. LC 98-5192. 320p. pap. 19.95 (*0-02-862059-3*) Hungry Minds.

Power of Clan: The Influence of Human Relationships on Heart Disease. Stewart G. Wolf & John G. Bruhn. 1998. 192p. (C). text 34.95 (*1-56000-043-0*) Transaction Pubs.

Power of Family Therapy. Michael Nichols. rev. ed. 1993. 464p. (C). reprint ed. pap. text 29.95 (*0-89876-204-9*, RC488.5.N5345) Gardner Pr.

Power of 5: Hundreds of 5-Second to 5-Minute Techniques to Improve All of Your Life Without Wasting Any of Your Time. Harold H. Bloomfield. 1994. LC 94-33084. 24.95 (*0-87596-201-7*) Rodale Pr Inc.

Power of Form. Gilbert J. Rose & Andrew Farge. 1980. LC 79-53592. (Psychological Issues Monographs: No. 49, Vol. 13, No. 1). (Illus.). 252p. 35.00 (*0-8236-4171-6*) Intl Univs Pr.

Power of Hope: A Doctor's Perspective. Howard Spiro. 1998. LC 98-18731. 320p. 45.00 (*0-300-07410-7*); pap. 17.95 (*0-300-07632-0*) Yale U Pr.

Power of Human Imagination: New Methods in Psychotherapy. J. L. Singer & K. S. Pope. 1978. LC 78-15392. (Emotions, Personality, & Psychotherapy Ser.). (Illus.). 426p. (C). 70.00 (*0-306-31140-2*, Plenum Trade) Perseus Pubng.

Power of Images: Studies in the History & Theory of Response. David Freedberg. 1998. LC 88-27638. (Illus.). 560p. 47.95 (*0-226-26144-1*) U Ch Pr.

Power of Knowing Who I Am in Christ. J. R. Reinhart. 1983. LC 82-73254. 220p. pap. 8.95 (*0-918060-04-4*) Burn Hart.

Power of Language in the Clinical Process. RoseMarie P. Foster. 1998. LC 98-7632. 40.00 (*0-7657-0179-0*) Aronson.

Power of Natural Healing. Hua-Ching Ni. 1991. LC 90-60823. 143p. pap. 14.95 (*0-937064-31-9*, Yo San Bks) SevenStar Comm.

Power of Self-Management: Achieving Success in Your Healthcare Career. Michael H. Cohen. 1992. (Illus.). 196p. (Orig.). pap. 7.95 (*0-9613768-1-3*) Canoe Press.

Power of Sound: How to Manage Your Personal Soundscape for a Vital, Productive, & Healthy Life. Joshua Leeds. 2001. LC 00-50573. x, 325p. pap. 25.00 incl. audio (*0-89281-768-2*, Heal Arts VT) Inner Tradit.

Power of the Image: Essays on Representation & Sexuality. Annette Kuhn. 1985. (Illus.). 176p. pap. 10.95 (*0-7100-9731-X*, Routledge Thoemms) Routledge.

Power of the Inner Judge: Psychodynamic Treatment of the Severe Neuroses. Leon Wurmser. 2000. LC 99-46506. 376p. 55.00 (*0-7657-0177-4*) Aronson.

Power of Your Own Medicine. Robert G. Chaney. 1995. LC 95-75540. 192p. pap. 15.95 (*0-918936-30-6*) Astara.

Power over Headaches. Linda Fowler. 1997. (Orig.). pap. 15.95 (*0-9654001-0-7*) Life Style Prods.

***Power over Panic.** Bronwyn Fox. 2nd ed. 2001. 110p. pap. 12.95 (*1-74009-487-5*) Mac USA.

Power, Pain & Dentistry. Sarah Nettleton. 1992. 192p. (*0-335-09723-5*); pap. (*0-335-09722-7*) OpUniv Pr.

Power Plays: Their Uses & Abuses in Human Relations. Gerald Alper. 1998. LC 97-51293. 294p. 34.95 (*1-57309-267-3*); pap. 16.95 (*1-57309-259-2*) Intl Scholars.

Power, Politics & Policy in Nursing. Rita R. Wieczorek. 1984. 288p. 29.95 (*0-8261-4630-9*) Springer Pub.

Power, Politics, & Public Policy: A Matter of Caring. Ed. by Anne Boykin. 1995. 260p. 32.95 (*0-88737-644-4*, 14-2684, NLN Pr) Natl League Nurse.

Power to Communicate: Gender Differences As Barriers. Deborah Borisoff & Lisa Merrill. 3rd rev. ed. 1998. LC 99-195446. 151p. pap. text 14.95 (*0-88133-989-X*) Waveland Pr.

Power to Heal. H. B. Wilson. 1991. lib. bdg. 75.00 (*0-8490-4519-3*) Gordon Pr.

***Power to the Patient: The Treatments to Insist on When You're Sick.** Isadore Rosenfeld. 2002. LC 2001-46645. 480p. 25.95 (*0-446-52694-0*) Warner Bks.

Powered Endoscopic Sinus Surgery. John H. Krouse & Dewey A. Christmas. 1997. LC 97-677. 225.00 (*4-260-14347-6*); (*0-89640-347-5*) Igaku-Shoin.

Powered Instrumentation in Otolaryngology: Head & Neck Surgery. Eiji Yanagisawa et al. 2001. LC 00-47001. 356p. text 174.95 (*0-7693-0123-1*) Singular Publishing.

Powermind System: Twelve Lessons on the Psychology of Success. Michael M. Kiefer. Ed. by Carol A. Kennedy. 1995. LC 95-94200. (Illus.). 435p. (Orig.). pap. 13.95 (*0-9645934-0-8*) Kiefer Enterprises.

Powerplay: Toys as Popular Culture. Dan Fleming. 1997. LC 95-43362. (Illus.). 224p. pap. 27.95 (*0-7190-4717-X*) St Martin.

Powers of Hypnosis. Jean Dauven. 1980. LC 71-87948. (Illus.). 254p. pap. 5.95 (*0-8128-1391-X*, Scrbrough Hse) Madison Bks UPA.

Powers That Make Us Human: The Foundations of Medical Ethics. Ed. by Kenneth Vaux. 1986. LC 84-28028. 152p. text 21.95 (*0-252-01187-2*) U of Ill Pr.

***PowerWeb: Drugs & Substance Abuse.** 2001. 16.55 (*0-07-246368-6*) McGrw-H Hghr Educ.

***PowerWeb: Health.** Richard Yarian. 2000. 3.75 (*0-07-243175-X*) McGrw-H Hghr Educ.

***PowerWeb: Psychology.** 2000. 16.55 (*0-07-247075-5*) McGrw-H Hghr Educ.

Powwowing in Union County: A Study of Pennsylvania German Folk Medicine in Context. Barbara L. Reimensnyder. 1989. LC 88-35082. (Immigrant Communities & Ethnic Minorities in the U. S. & Canada Ser.: No. 31). 55.00 (*0-404-19441-9*) AMS Pr.

PQQ & Quinoproteins. Ed. by J. A. Jongejan & J. A. Duine. 1989. (C). text 202.50 (*0-7923-0248-6*) Kluwer Academic.

Prac Quantitative Doppler John H. Phillips. 1991. (Illus.). 152p. 99.95 (*0-8493-4921-4*, RC683) CRC Pr.

Practica Forense Federal. 1992. suppl. ed. 22.00 (*1-56257-114-1*, 84263-10, MICHIE) LEXIS Pub.

Practica Forense Federal. Ed. by Butterworth Staff. 1992. 390p. 40.00 (*0-88063-506-1*, MICHIE) LEXIS Pub.

Practica Forense Puertorriquena Tomo 3: Evidencia. 2000. (SPA.). 800p. (*0-327-11138-0*, 4752313) LEXIS Pub.

Practical Account of General Paralysis, Its Mental & Physical Symptoms, Statistics, Causes, Seat, & Treatment. Thomas J. Austin. 1976. LC 75-16681. (Classics in Psychiatry Ser.). reprint ed. 22.95 (*0-405-07413-1*) Ayer.

Practical Algorithms in Pediatric Endocrinology. Ed. by Ze'va Hochberg. 1998. LC 98-29290. (Illus.). iv, 104p. pap. 48.00 (*3-8055-6693-X*) S Karger.

Practical Allergy. Milgrom. 2001. pap. text (*0-323-01236-1*) Mosby Inc.

Practical Anaesthesia & Analgesia for Day Surgery. J. Millar et al. 1997. (Illus.). 256p. (Orig.). pap. (*1-85996-081-2*) Bios Sci GBR. *Dist:* Bks Intl VA.

Practical & Theoretical Aspects of Psychoanalysis. Lawrence S. Kubie. rev. ed. 1975. LC 74-6433. 361p. 55.00 (*0-8236-4181-3*); pap. 24.95 (*0-8236-8193-9*, 24180) Intl Univs Pr.

Practical Anesthesia Information Guide. Raymond Jerome. 1992. 127p. pap. 12.95 (*0-929240-21-9*) EMIS.

Practical Animal Handling. Andrew T. Edney. 1991. (Veterinary Handbook Ser.). (Illus.). 300p. text 130.00 (*0-08-036151-X*); pap. text 45.00 (*0-08-036152-8*) Elsevier (Pergamon Pr).

Practical Animal Husbandry. T. K. Ewer. 1982. (Illus.). 272p. text 85.00 (*0-85608-026-8*) Blackwell Sci.

Practical Answers to Common Questions about Sex in Marriage. Tim F. LaHaye & Beverly LaHaye. 1984. 72p. (Orig.). pap. 1.70 (*0-310-27042-1*, 18340P) Zondervan.

Practical Anthropometry. Ales Hrdlicka. 2nd ed. LC 71-137243. reprint ed. 41.50 (*0-404-03372-5*) AMS Pr.

Practical Application of Computer-Aided Drug Design. Paul S. Charifson. 1997. LC 97-20897. (Illus.). 564p. text 185.00 (*0-8247-9885-6*) Dekker.

Practical Application of Meridian-Style Acupuncture. John E. Pirog. 1996. LC 95-69801. (Illus.). 392p. (Orig.). pap. 70.00 (*1-881896-13-7*) Pacific View Pr.

Practical Applications of Clinical Neurophysiological Testing. Thoru Yamada & Mark Ross. 1999. (Advances In Pulp & Paper Chemistry Ser.). 89.95 (*0-8493-7692-0*) CRC Pr.

Practical Applications of Fiberoptics in Critical Care Monitoring. Ed. by F. R. Lewis & U. J. Pfeiffer. 1990. (Illus.). 190p. 64.00 (*0-387-51718-9*) Spr-Verlag.

Practical Applications of Quantitative Structure- Activity Relationships (QSAR) in Environmental Chemistry & Toxicology. Ed. by Walter Karcher & J. Devillers. 1990. (C). text 248.50 (*0-7923-0827-1*) Kluwer Academic.

Practical Applied Optometry. A. M. Skeffington. Ed. by Sally M. Coringold. 1991. (Illus.). 114p. (C). reprint ed. lib. bdg. 18.00 (*0-943599-18-0*) OEPF.

Practical Approach Pediatric I. Isaacs. 1996. text 83.00 (*0-443-05142-9*) Saunders.

Practical Approach to Acupuncture. Prabha Borwanker. 1988. (C). (*0-8364-2396-8*) Popular Prakashan IND. *Dist:* S Asia.

Practical Approach to Cardiac Anesthesia. Ed. by Frederick A. Hensley, Jr. & Donald E. Martin. 2nd rev. ed. 1995. LC 94-42512. 736p. pap. text 79.00 (*0-316-35786-3*) Lppncott W & W.

Practical Approach to Cardiac Arrhythmias. Stephen C. Vlay. 2nd rev. ed. 1995. 464p. pap. text 59.95 (*0-316-91483-5*, Little Brwn Med Div) Lppncott W & W.

Practical Approach to Clinical Paediatrics. J. M. Gupta & D. W. O'Gorman-Hughes. 1996. 250p. text 53.00 (*981-02-1849-4*) World Scientific Pub.

Practical Approach to Clinical Pediatrics. J. M. Gupta & D. W. O'Gorman-Hughes. 1996. 250p. pap. text 30.00 (*981-02-2136-3*) World Scientific Pub.

Practical Approach to Epilepsy. Ed. by Mogens Dam. 1991. 300p. (*0-08-041171-1*) PPI GBR. *Dist:* McGraw.

Practical Approach to Head & Neck Tumors. Jack Gluckman et al. 1994. LC 94-26061. 224p. text 99.00 (*0-7817-0228-3*) Lppncott W & W.

Practical Approach to Infectious Diseases. Ed. by Richard E. Reese & Robert F. Betts. 4th ed. 1996. LC 96-11889. 1,482p. pap. text 99.00 (*0-316-73721-6*, Little Brwn Med Div) Lppncott W & W.

Practical Approach to Neuro-Oncology: A Guide. Leslie D. McAllister et al. 5th ed. 2001. LC 2001-35367. (Illus.). 320p. pap. 39.99 (*0-7506-7180-7*) Buttrwrth-Heinemann.

Practical Approach to Occupational & Environmental Medicine. Ed. by Robert J. McCunney. 2nd exp. rev. ed. Orig. Title: Handbook of Occupational Medicine. 850p. pap. 59.95 (*0-88048-736-4*, OP915995WE) Am Psychiatric.

Practical Approach to Occupational & Environmental Medicine. Ed. by Robert J. McCunney & Paul W. Brandt-Rauf. 2nd rev. ed. 1994. LC 94-11269. Orig. Title: Handbook of Occupational Medicine. 856p. reprint ed. pap. text 79.95 (*0-316-55534-7*, Little Brwn Med Div) Lppncott W & W.

Practical Approach to Pain Management. Ed. by Mathew Lefkowitz et al. 1996. 310p. pap. text 45.00 (*0-316-51958-8*, Little Brwn Med Div) Lppncott W & W.

Practical Approach to Permanent Pacemaker Implantation, Set. Peter H. Belott. 1996. LC 94-39121. (Illus.). 152p. wbk. ed. 95.00 incl. VHS (*0-87993-594-4*) Futura Pub.

Practical Approach to Pulmonary Medicine. Ronald H. Goldstein et al. 1997. LC 97-9420. 624p. text 69.95 (*0-7817-1237-8*) Lppncott W & W.

Practical Approach to Pulmonary Medicine. Joel Karlinsky et al. 1997. 600p. text 69.95 (*0-316-54884-7*) Lppncott W & W.

Practical Approach to Quality Improvement. Karen Parsley & Philomena Corrigan. 1993. LC 93-36305. (*0-412-48360-2*) Chapman & Hall.

Practical Approach to Quality Improvement. Karen Parsley & Philomena Corrigan. 1993. LC 93-36305. 176p. pap. 54.25 (*1-56593-236-6*, 0556) Singular Publishing.

Practical Approaches in Treating Adolescent Chemical Dependency: A Guide to Clinical Assessment & Intervention. Ed. by Paul B. Henry. 1989. LC 89-1660. (Journal of Chemical Dependency Treatment Ser.: Vol. 2, No. 1). 284p. text 49.95 (*0-86656-709-7*); pap. text 17.95 (*0-86656-813-1*) Haworth Pr.

Practical Approaches to Alcoholism Psychotherapy. Ed. by Sheldon Zimberg et al. 2nd ed. 1985. LC 84-24922. (Illus.). 432p. 39.50 (*0-306-41762-6*, Kluwer Plenum) Kluwer Academic.

Practical Approaches to Cancer Invasion & Metastases: A Compendium of Radiation Oncologists' Responses to 40 Histories. Ed. by A. Robert Kagan & Richard J. Steckel. 1994. LC 93-42006. (Medical Radiology Ser.). (Illus.). 155p. 123.00 (*0-387-56375-X*) Spr-Verlag.

Practical Approaches to Mental Health Care. Patricia Jacobs et al. 1990. 400p. (*0-7329-0229-0*) Intl Spec Bk.

Practical Approaches to the Treatment of Heart Failure. Roger M. Mills, Jr. & James B. Young. 1997. LC 97-41999. 250p. 49.95 (*0-683-18104-1*) Lppncott W & W.

Practical Aspects of Gynaecourology: Proceedings of the 9th Annual Meeting of IUGA, Budapest, Hungary, 9-11 Sept. 1985. Ed. by Attila Tanko et al. 1986. (Illus.). 469p. (*963-05-4440-7*) Akade Kiado HUN. *Dist:* St Mut.

Practical Aspects of Intravenous Drug Administration: Principles for Nurses, Pharmacists, & Physicians. Richard D. Leff & Robert J. Roberts. 1992. 64p. (C). pap. text 15.00 (*1-879907-23-2*) Am Soc Hlth-Syst.

Practical Aspects of Memory - Current Research & Issues Vol. 1: Memory of Everyday Life, Vol. 1, Memory of Everyday Life. Ed. by Michael M. Gruneberg et al. 1988. 580p. 165.00 (*0-471-91234-4*) Wiley.

Practical Aspects of Memory - Current Research & Issues Vol. 2: Clinical & Educational Implications, Vol. 2, Clinical and Educational Implications. Ed. by Michael M. Gruneberg et al. 1988. 584p. 750.00 (*0-471-91867-9*) Wiley.

Practical Aspects of Munchausen by Proxy & Munchausen Syndrome Investigation. Kathryn Artingstall. 1998. LC 98-13159. (CRC Series in Practical Aspects of Criminal & Forensic Inv Ser.). 384p. 74.95 (*0-8493-8162-2*, 8162) CRC Pr.

Practical Aspects of Ophthalmic Optics. Margaret Dowaliby. 4th ed. 2000. LC 00-60890. (Illus.). 296p. text 54.99 (*0-7506-7189-0*) Buttrwrth-Heinemann.

Practical Aspects of Staged Therapy Defibrillators. Ed. by Lukas Kappenberger & Fred W. Lindemans. 1992. LC 92-14637. (Bakken Research Center Ser.: Vol. 5). (Illus.). 156p. 35.00 (*0-87993-531-6*) Futura Pub.

Practical Aspects of the Transfusion Service. Harold B. Anstall & Robert C. Blylock. 1996. LC 95-40102. 335p. pap. 55.00 (*0-89189-396-2*) Am Soc Clinical.

Practical Aspects of Urinary Incontinence. Ed. by F. M. Debruyne & E. V. Van Kerrebroeck. 1986. (Developments in Surgery Ser.). text 111.00 (*0-89838-752-3*) Kluwer Academic.

Practical Atlas of Pseudomalignancy. Ed. by S. Al-Sam & Sunil R. Lakhani. 1998. LC 98-3605. (Illus.). 384p. 195.00 (*0-340-64616-0*) OUP.

Practical Atlas of Retinal Disease & Therapy. Ed. by William R. Freeman. 2nd ed. 1997. LC 97-14106. (Illus.). 416p. text 225.00 (*0-397-51841-2*) Lppncott W & W.

Practical Avian Medicine. Ed. by Heidi L. Hoefer. 1997. (Illus.). 240p. pap. text 48.00 (*1-884254-34-9*) Vet Lrn Syst.

Practical Ayurveda: Secrets to Physical, Sexual & Spiritual Health. Atreya. 1998. LC 97-48967. (Illus.). 256p. pap. 14.95 (*1-57863-029-0*) Red Wheel ME.

Practical Bazar Medicines with over 200 Useful Prescriptions. G. T. Birdwood. 1986. 220p. reprint ed. (*0-8364-1768-2*) Manohar IND. *Dist:* S Asia.

Practical Biomechanics for the Orthopaedic Surgeon. Eric L. Radin et al. 2nd ed. 1991. (Illus.). 216p. text (*0-443-08702-4*) Church.

Practical Blood Transfusion. Douglas W. Huestis et al. 4th ed. 1988. 489p. 85.00 (*0-316-37953-0*, Little Brwn Med Div) Lppncott W & W.

Practical Cardiovascular Pathology. Mary N. Sheppard & Michael J. Davies. 1998. LC 98-3645. (Arnold Publication). (Illus.). 240p. text 125.00 (*0-340-67749-X*) OUP.

Practical Care of the Ambulatory Patient. Kenneth Stults & Dere. 1989. 592p. text 80.00 (*0-7216-2474-X*) Saunders.

Practical Chemotherapy of Malaria: Report of a WHO Scientific Group. 1990. (Technical Reports: No. 805). (ENG, FRE & SPA.). 158p. pap. text 16.00 (*92-4-120805-8*, 1100805) World Health.

Practical Clinical Biochemistry. Alan H. Gowenlock Varley. 6th ed. 1988. 105.00 (*0-8493-0156-4*) CRC Pr.

Practical Clinical Medicine. John Davies. 1992. (Illus.). 384p. pap. text (*0-7506-0026-8*) E A GBR. *Dist:* OUP.

Practical Clinical Psychopharmacology. William Appleton. 3rd ed. 1988. 224p. pap. 33.00 (*0-683-00239-2*) Lppncott W & W.

Practical Clinical Ultrasonic Diagnosis. 1997. 300p. 54.00 (*981-02-2922-4*) World Scientific Pub.

Practical Compendium of Colorpuncture. Peter Mandel. Tr. by Christopher Baker from GER. 1986. (Illus.). 269p. text 98.00 (*3-925806-08-3*) Medicina Bio.

Practical Critical Care in Cardiology. Zab Mohsenifar & P. K. Shah. 1997. LC 97-45024. (Fundamental & Clinical Cardiology Ser.). (Illus.). 472p. text 195.00 (*0-8247-0097-X*) Dekker.

Practical Cross Infection Control in Dentistry. Peter R. Wood. 1992. (Illus.). 207p. (C). (gr. 13). text 55.95 (*0-8151-9439-0*, 21903) Mosby Inc.

Practical Cytopathology. Robert W. Astarita. 1989. (Illus.). 472p. text (*0-443-08469-6*) Church.

Practical Delivery of Sports Medicine Services: A Conceptual Approach. Jerald D. Hawkins. Ed. by PRC Publishing, Inc. Staff. 1993. (Illus.). 425p. (Orig.). pap. text 39.95 (*0-944183-16-6*) PRC Pub.

Practical Dementia Care. Peter V. Rabins et al. 1999. LC 98-49715. (Illus.). 304p. text 34.95 (*0-19-510625-3*) OUP.

Practical Dentofacial Orthopedics. Frans Van der Linden. 1997. LC 96-205290. (Illus.). 708p. pap. text 120.00 (*1-85097-041-6*) Quint Pub Co.

Practical Dermatology. Beth G. Goldstein. 2nd ed. 1997. LC 96-28852. (Illus.). 448p. (C). (gr. 13). pap. text 59.95 (*0-8151-3764-8*, 26815) Mosby Inc.

Practical Developments in Inherited Metabolic Diseases. Ed. by G. M. Addison et al. 1986. text 206.50 (*0-85200-690-X*) Kluwer Academic.

Practical Diabetes Care. Rowan Hillson. 1996. LC 95-36166. (Illus.). 236p. pap. text 49.50 (*0-19-261859-8*) OUP.

Practical Diagnosis in Traditional Chinese Medicine. Tieh-Tao Teng & Kevin Ergil. 1999. LC 98-37012. xiv, 549p. (*0-443-04582-8*) Church.

Practical Diagnosis of Hematologic Disorders. Ed. by Carl R. Kjeldsberg. 4th ed. 1995. LC 95-15075. 75.00 (*0-89189-442-X*) Am Soc Clinical.

Practical Dictionary of Acupuncture & Accupressure see Dictionnaire Pratique de l'Acupuncture et de l'Acupressure

Practical Dictionary of Adult Emergency Medicine: Diccionario Practico de Urgencias Medicas del Adulto. Arnaud Cenac et al. 1982. (SPA.). 368p. 69.95 (*0-8288-1864-9*, S39898) Fr & Eur.

Practical Dictionary of Cardiology: Dizionario Pratico Di Cardiologia. Giuseppe Folli & Erminio Vitolo. 1986. (ITA.). 432p. 125.00 (*0-8288-1847-9*, F45090) Fr & Eur.

Practical Dictionary of Chinese Medicine. Nigel Wiseman & Feng Ye. 1998. LC 94-18575. 944p. (C). 125.00 (*0-912111-54-2*) Ashgate Pub Co.

Practical Dictionary of Clinical Medicine: Dictionnaire Pratique de Medecine Clinique. Leon Perlemuter. 2nd ed. 1982. (FRE.). 1856p. 195.00 (*0-8288-1821-5*, M6440) Fr & Eur.

Practical Dictionary of English for Biologists, Chemists & Doctors: Dictionnaire Pratique de l'Anglais pour les Biologistes, Chimistes, Medecins. J. G. Bieth et al. 1983. (ENG & FRE.). 272p. 89.95 (*0-8288-0560-1*, M14532) Fr & Eur.

Practical Dictionary of Medical Therapy (Dictionnaire Pratique de Therapeutique Medicale) Leon Perlemuter. 6th ed. 1990. (FRE.). 1824p. ring bd. 150.00 (*0-7859-4566-0*) Fr & Eur.

Practical Dictionary of Odontology & Stomatology: Dictionnaire Pratique d'Odontologie et de Stomatologie. Michel Goudaert & Michel Danhiez. 1983. 342p. 65.00 (*0-8288-1807-X*, M886) Fr & Eur.

Practical Dictionary of Pediatric Therapeutics see Dictionnaire Pratique de Therapeutique Pediatrique

Practical Dictionary of Therapeutic Pediatrics: Diccionario Practico de Terapeutica Pediatrica. Robert Steinschneider. 1982. 768p. 85.00 (*0-8288-1879-7*, S39897) Fr & Eur.

Practical Dictionary to Understand the Study of Cancer: Dictionnaire Pratique du Cancer: Pour Comprendre le Langage du Cancerologue. Philippe Lagarde. 1984. (FRE.). 59.95 (*0-8288-1812-6*, M404) Fr & Eur.

Practical Differential Diagnosis in Surgical Neuropathology. Ed. by Richard A. Prayson & Mark L. Cohen. 2000. LC 00-38925. (Illus.). 192p. 89.50 (*0-89603-817-3*) Humana.

Practical Digital Imaging & PACs: 1999 AAPM Summer School Proceedings. Ed. by J. Anthony Seibert et al. 2000. (Illus.). 562p. pap. text 65.00 (*0-944838-92-8*) Med Physics Pub.

Practical Doppler Ultrasound for the Clinician. Raymond L. Powis & Robert A. Schwartz. 1991. (Illus.). 208p. 60.00 (*0-683-06958-6*) Lppncott W & W.

Practical Echocardiography & Doppler. Mark J. Monaghan. 1990. 154p. 284.95 (*0-471-92069-X*) Wiley.

Practical Echocardiography in the Adult: With Doppler & Color-Doppler Flow Imaging. J. P. Hamer. 1990. (C). text 221.50 (*0-7923-0670-8*) Kluwer Academic.

Practical Electromyography. Ernest W. Johnson. 2nd ed. 1988. 620p. 75.00 (*0-683-04463-X*) Lppncott W & W.

Practical Electrosurgery. S. Duffy & G. V. Cobb. 1994. 144p. (gr. 13). 112.95 (*0-412-47580-4*) Chapman & Hall.

Practical Encyclopedia of Natural Healing. Mark Bricklin. 1992. 10.98 (*1-56731-005-2*, MJF Bks) Fine Comms.

Practical Encyclopedia of Sex & Health: From Aphrodisiacs & Hormones to Potency, Stress, Vasectomy, & Yeast Infection. Prevention Magazine Editors & Stefan Bechtel. 1993. LC 92-35043. 352p. 27.95 (*0-87596-163-0*) Rodale Pr Inc.

Practical Endocrinology & Diabetes in Childhood. J. Raine et al. 2001. LC 00-48614. (Illus.). x, 206p. 99.95 (*0-632-05161-2*) Blackwell Sci.

Practical Endodontics: A Clinical Atlas. Edward Besner et al. 1993. LC 93-7003. (Illus.). 296p. (C). (gr. 13). text 77.95 (*0-8016-7798-X*, 07798) Mosby Inc.

Practical Endoscopic Sinus Surgery. Ed. by Vijay K. Anand & William R. Panje. 1992. LC 92-49884. (Illus.). 186p. text 139.00 (*0-07-105419-7*) McGraw-Hill Educ Grp.

Practical Endoscopy. Ed. by Shephard & J. Mason. 1997. LC 97-224771. (Illus.). 464p. pap. (*0-412-54000-2*) E A GBR. *Dist:* OUP.

Practical Epidemiology. D. J. Barker & A. J. Hall. 4th ed. 1991. (Illus.). 176p. pap. text (*0-443-03787-6*) Church.

Practical Equine Dermatology. David Lloyd et al. 2001. (Illus.). 160p. pap. text (*0-632-04807-7*) Blckwell Science GBR. *Dist:* Iowa U Pr.

Practical Ethics for Students, Interns, & Residents: A Short Reference Manual. C. Junkerman & D. Schiedermayer. 2nd rev. ed. 1998. 77p. pap. text 6.95 (*1-55572-054-4*) Univ Pub Group.

Practical Evaluation & Management of the Shoulder. Fredrick A. Matsen, III et al. 1994. LC 93-41664. text 85.00 (*0-7216-4819-3*) Saunders.

Practical Exercise Therapy. Margaret Hollis & Phil F. Cook. 4th ed. 1999. LC 98-53120. pap. 50.95 (*0-632-04973-1*) Blackwell Sci.

Practical Exotic Animal Medicine. 1997. LC 97-178478. (Illus.). 275p. pap. text 51.00 (*1-884254-33-0*) Vet Lrn Syst.

Practical Feeding of Horses & Ponies. Sarah Pilliner. 1998. LC 97-27543. (Illus.). 192p. pap. 29.95 (*0-632-04828-X*) Blackwell Sci.

Practical Fiberoptic Intubation. Mansukh Popat. 2001. 208p. pap. text 63.00 (*0-7506-4496-6*) Buttrwrth-Heinemann.

Practical Flexible Sigmoidoscopy. Basuk Cohen & Waye Cohen. 1995. (Illus.). 192p. 54.95 (*0-89640-272-X*) Igaku-Shoin.

Practical Flow Cytometry: Clinical Applications. Marion G. Macey. 1994. LC 93-42963. (Illus.). 320p. 115.00 (*0-632-03673-7*) Blackwell Sci.

Practical Folk Medicine of Hawaii. L. R. McBride. 1975. (Illus.). 104p. pap. 8.95 (*0-912180-27-7*) Petroglyph.

Practical Footcare for Nurse Practitioners: A Training Manual & Clinical Handbook. Ronald A. Nicholson. 1994. LC 94-66314. (Illus.). 192p. (Orig.). (C). pap. text 69.95 (*1-885421-01-X*) Practical Footcare.

Practical Footcare for Physician Assistants: A Training Manual & Clinical Handbook. Ronald A. Nicholson. 1994. LC 94-66313. (Illus.). 192p. (Orig.). (C). pap. text 69.95 (*1-885421-00-1*) Practical Footcare.

Practical Footcare for Primary Care Physicians: A Training Manual & Clinical Handbook. Ronald A. Nicholson. 1994. LC 94-66215. (Illus.). 192p. (Orig.). (C). pap. text 69.95 (*1-885421-02-8*) Practical Footcare.

Practical Forensic Anthropology of Human Skeletal Remains Recovery Analysis & Resolution. William D. Haglund et al. 1999. 54.95 (*0-8493-8157-6*, 8157) CRC Pr.

Practical Forensic Pathology. Charles V. Wetli. 1988. LC 87-35275. (Illus.). 160p. 63.00 (*0-89640-144-8*) Igaku-Shoin.

Practical Fracture Treatment. Ronald K. McRae. 3rd ed. 1994. LC 93-7651. 384p. pap. text (*0-443-04809-6*) Church.

Practical Gastrointestinal Endoscopy. Ed. by P. B. Cotton & Christopher Blake Williams. 3rd ed. 1990. (Illus.). 288p. 54.95 (*0-632-02435-6*) Mosby Inc.

Practical Gastrointestinal Endoscopy. Peter B. Cotton & Christopher Blake Williams. 4th ed. 1996. LC 95-25737. (Illus.). 352p. 160.95 (*0-86542-851-4*) Blackwell Sci.

Practical General Practice: Guidelines for Effective Clinical Management. Contrib. by Alex Khot & Andrew Polmear. 3rd ed. 1999. LC 99-202782. 424p. pap. text 63.00 (*0-7506-3462-6*) Buttrwrth-Heinemann.

Practical Genetic Counselling. Peter S. Harper. 5th ed. 1998. LC 98-28065. 376p. pap., suppl. ed. (*0-7506-3368-9*) E A GBR. *Dist:* OUP.

Practical Genetic Counselling. Peter S. Harper. 4th ed. 1988. (Illus.). 306p. (*0-7506-0342-9*) John Wright GBR. *Dist:* Buttrwrth-Heinemann.

Practical Geriatrics. Ed. by H. P. Hahn. 1975. (Illus.). 448p. 28.00 (*3-8055-1768-8*) S Karger.

***Practical Guide: Identification, Evaluation & Treatment of Overweight & Obesity in Adults.** F. Xavier Pi-Sunyer. 2002. (Illus.). 80p. (C). reprint ed. pap. text 20.00 (*0-7567-1918-6*) DIANE Pub.

Practical Guide for Experimental Microvascular Surgery: A Practical Guide. Kenneth E. Korber & Jeanne G. Halpern. 1990. (Illus.). 311p. (C). pap. 47.50 (*0-87527-470-6*) Green.

***Practical Guide for Medical Teachers.** Ronald Harden & John Dent. 2001. (Illus.). 335p. pap. (*0-443-06273-0*) Church GBR. *Dist:* Saunders.

***Practical Guide for the Diagnosis & Management of Asthma.** Ed. by Barry Leonard. 2002. (Illus.). 52p. (C). reprint ed. pap. text 15.00 (*0-7567-1920-8*) DIANE Pub.

Practical Guide Medical & Surgical Procedures. Alan Dudley. 1989. 179p. pap. text 49.50 (*0-433-00058-9*) Buttrwrth-Heinemann.

Practical Guide to Alternative Assessment. Joan L. Herman et al. 1992. LC 92-30244. pap. 13.95 (*0-87120-197-6*) ASCD.

Practical Guide to Anorectal Testing. Ed. by Lee E. Smith. 2nd ed. 1995. LC 95-1315. (Illus.). 344p. pap. 69.50 (*0-89640-278-9*) Igaku-Shoin.

Practical Guide to Applying Treatment Outcomes & Efficacy Research. Ed. by Roberta Kreb. 1997. LC 98-114042. 28.00 (*0-910329-99-0*, 0112030) Am Speech Lang Hearing.

Practical Guide to Art Therapy Groups. Diane Fausek. 1997. LC 96-34526. 115p. pap. 22.95 (*0-7890-0186-1*); 39.95 (*0-7890-0136-5*) Haworth Pr.

Practical Guide to Cardiac Pacing. H. Weston Moses et al. 5th ed. 2000. LC 99-46283. 224p. pap. text 49.95 (*0-7817-1956-9*) Lppncott W & W.

Practical Guide to Child Nutrition. Angela Dare & Margaret O'Donovan. 1996. 128p. pap. (*0-7487-2375-7*) Nelson Thornes GBR. *Dist:* Trans-Atl Phila.

Practical Guide to Clinical Data Management. Susanne Prokscha. 1999. LC 99-21232. 189.00 (*1-57491-100-7*) IHS Health Grp.

Practical Guide to Clinical Teaching in Medicine. Karen Douglas et al. 1988. (Medical Education Ser.). 208p. 29.95 (*0-8261-5940-0*) Springer Pub.

Practical Guide to Clinical Virology. Ed. by G. C. Haukenes et al. 1989. LC 89-14767. 218p. pap. 59.95 (*0-471-91978-0*) Wiley.

***Practical Guide to Clinical Virology.** Ed. by Lars R. Haaheim et al. 2nd ed. 2002. 200p. 95.00 (*0-470-84429-9*) Halsted Pr.

Practical Guide to Cognitive Therapy. Dean Schuyler. 1991. 180p. 22.95 (*0-393-70105-0*) Norton.

Practical Guide to Contemporary Pharmacy Practice. Judith E. Thompson. 1998. LC 98-15843. 350p. pap. 35.95 (*0-683-30538-7*) Lppncott W & W.

Practical Guide to Cranial Adjustment. Harvey Getzoff. 1996. LC 98-10405. (Illus.). 85p. pap., spiral bd. 39.95 (*0-938198-02-5*) Weidner & Sons.

Practical Guide to Creative Senility. Donovan Bess. 1988. LC 88-9551. (Illus.). 176p. (Orig.). pap. 9.95 (*0-931892-16-3*) B Dolphin Pub.

Practical Guide to Dental Equipment. Nicholas M. Jedyakiewicz. 1992. LC 92-12792. (Illus.). 193p. (C). (gr. 13). text 29.95 (*0-8151-4867-4*, 21945) Mosby Inc.

Practical Guide to Diagnostic Imaging. Connie M. Han et al. 1994. pap. (*84-8174-197-3*) Mosby-Doyma Libros ESP. *Dist:* Mosby Inc.

Practical Guide to Diagnostic Imaging. Ed. by Neil T. Specht. 1997. LC 97-23636. (Illus.). 650p. (C). (gr. 13). spiral bd. 32.95 (*0-8151-9356-4*, 29194) Mosby Inc.

Practical Guide to Diagnostic Imaging: Radiography & Ultrasonography. C. M. Ham et al. 1994. LC 94-71186. 300p. pap. text 31.00 (*0-939674-54-8*) Am Vet Pubns.

Practical Guide to Diagnostic Imaging for the Veterinary Technician. Connie M. Han & Cheryl D. Hurd. 2nd ed. 2000. LC 99-55179. (Illus.). xii, 282p. pap. 39.00 (*0-323-00475-X*) Mosby Inc.

Practical Guide to ECG Interpretation. Ken Grauer. 2nd ed. 1998. (Illus.). 576p. pap. text 34.95 (*1-55664-557-0*) Mosby Inc.

Practical Guide to Echocardiography & Cardiac Doppler Ultrasound. Ibrahim A. Jawad. 2nd ed. 1996. LC 95-43199. 432p. pap. text 59.95 (*0-316-45837-6*) Lppncott W & W.

Practical Guide to ELISA. D. M. Kemeny. 1991. (Illus.). 128p. 51.00 (*0-08-037508-1*); pap. 29.50 (*0-08-037507-3*) Elsevier (Pergamon Pr).

Practical Guide to Emergency & Protective Crisis Intervention: Dealing with the Violent & Self-Destructive Person. Joel Foxman. 1990. 320p. (C). text 69.95 (*0-398-05621-8*) C C Thomas.

Practical Guide to Fetal Echocardiography. Alfred Abuhamad. 1997. LC 97-2780. (Illus.). 144p. text 69.00 (*0-397-51674-6*) Lppncott W & W.

Practical Guide to Fundholding. Rod Smith et al. 1994. LC 93-39133. (Illus.). 320p. pap. 34.95 (*0-632-03869-1*) Blackwell Sci.

Practical Guide to Gastrointestinal Function Testing. C. Stendal. 1997. (Illus.). 320p. 90.00 (*0-632-04918-9*) Blackwell Sci.

Practical Guide to Head Injury Management. Ed. by Paul V. Marks & Christopher B. Lavy. 1992. (Illus.). 168p. text (*0-7020-1615-2*) W B Saunders GBR. *Dist:* Saunders.

Practical Guide to Head Injury Rehabilitation: A Focus on Postacute Residential Treatment. Michael D. Wesolowski & Arnie H. Zencius. 1994. LC 93-30642. (Critical Issues in Neuropsychology Ser.). 254p. 39.50 (*0-306-44427-5*, Kluwer Plenum) Kluwer Academic.

Practical Guide to Health & Diseases: Health Is Bliss. Alice K. Wong & Gary C. Lee. (CHI., Illus.). 375p. (Orig.). pap. (*0-9641190-1-3*) Beacon Hlth.

Practical Guide to Health Assessment. Shelly Leasia. Ed. by Barbara N. Cullen. 1997. LC 96-41703. (Illus.). 464p. pap. text 24.95 (*0-7216-1468-X*) Saunders.

Practical Guide to Health Assessment Through the Life Span. Mildred O. Hogstel & Linda Cox-Curry. 3rd ed. 2001. LC 2001-17246. (Illus.). xxi, 512p. (C). pap. 27.95 (*0-8036-0803-9*) Davis Co.

Practical Guide to Health Assessment Through the Lifespan. Mildred O. Hogstel. 2nd ed. 1996. (Illus.). 411p. pap. 22.95 (*0-8036-0130-1*) Davis Co.

Practical Guide to Health Promotion after Spinal Cord Injury. Indira S. Lanig & Teresa Chase. 1988. 300p. spiral bd. 72.00 (*0-8342-0628-5*) PRO-ED.

Practical Guide to High-Risk Pregnancy & Delivery. Fernando Arias. 2nd ed. 1992. (Illus.). 496p. (C). (gr. 13). pap. text 62.00 (*0-8016-0057-X*, 00057) Mosby Inc.

Practical Guide to Holistic Health. Swami Rama. rev. ed. 1999. LC 99-35677. 110p. pap. 14.95 (*0-89389-174-6*) Himalayan Inst.

Practical Guide to Hospital Dental Practice see Oral Medicine & Hospital Practice

Practical Guide to Human Cancer Genetics. S. V. Hodgson & E. R. Maher. 1993. LC 92-49932. (Illus.). 258p. (C). text 105.00 (*0-521-40128-3*); pap. text 42.95 (*0-521-40951-9*) Cambridge U Pr.

Practical Guide to Human Cancer Genetics. Shirley V. Hodgson & Eamonn R. Maher. 2nd exp. rev. ed. (Illus.). (C). 1999. LC 00-500460. 354p. pap. text 54.95 (*0-521-64961-7*); 1998. 260p. text 100.00 (*0-521-64025-3*) Cambridge U Pr.

Practical Guide to Implementing the Family & Medical Leave Act, 1996 Supplement. Robert L. Duston & Scott Robins. 1997. 65.00 (*1-878240-56-0*) CUPA-HR.

***Practical Guide to Magnet Therapy.** Peter Rose. 2001. (Illus.). 128p. pap. 16.95 (*0-8069-2777-1*) Sterling.

Practical Guide to Medical Billing. Denna L. Holmes. 155p. pap. 89.00 (*0-934213-53-4*, PB98-114374) Natl Tech Info.

Practical Guide to Medical Mycology: Diagnosis & Patient Management. Alan M. Sugar. 1996. 224p. pap. text 49.00 (*0-397-51772-6*) Lppncott W & W.

Practical Guide to Medically Important Fungi & the Diseases They Cause. Alan M. Sugar & Caron A. Lyman. 1997. LC 96-29896. 170p. pap. text 62.00 (*0-397-51686-X*, Lippnctt) Lppncott W & W.

Practical Guide to Medicine & the Law. Ed. by J. P. Jackson. 1991. (Illus.). 320p. 54.95 (*0-387-19677-3*) Spr-Verlag.

Practical Guide to Monoclonal Antibodies. J. Eryl Liddell & A. Cryer. 1991. LC 90-13056. 206p. pap. 147.00 (*0-471-92905-0*) Wiley.

Practical Guide to Movement Disorders: Diagnosis, Investigation & Treatment. Roger A. Barker. 2001. (Illus.). 224p. pap. 57.50 (*0-7506-4469-9*) Buttrwrth-Heinemann.

Practical Guide to Multiple Sclerosis: Diagnosis, Investigation & Treatment. Alasdair J. Coles. 2001. 224p. pap. 59.00 (*0-7506-4800-7*) Buttrwrth-Heinemann.

Practical Guide to Nursing Home Advocacy. Legal Counsel for the Elderly Staff. 1991. 245p. pap. 30.00 (*0-933945-02-7*) Legal Coun Elderly.

Practical Guide to Pediatric Intensive Care, 3. Jeffery L. Blumer. 3rd ed. 1990. (Illus.). 1120p. (C). (gr. 13). pap. text 69.00 (*0-8016-2854-7*, 02854) Mosby Inc.

Practical Guide to Pediatric Respiratory Diseases. Ed. by Daniel V. Schidlow & David S. Smith. 1994. LC 94-14803. (Illus.). 330p. 57.00 (*1-56053-009-X*) Hanley & Belfus.

Practical Guide to Peripheral Nerve & Neuromuscular Disorders. David J. Dick. 2002. (Illus.). 320p. pap. 67.50 (*0-7506-4895-3*) Buttrwrth-Heinemann.

Practical Guide to Pharmaceutical Care. Ed. by John P. Rovers. 1998. LC 98-8812. 242p. pap. 40.00 (*0-917330-90-0*) Am Pharm Assn.

Practical Guide to Psychic Self-Defense: Strengthen Your Aura. Melita Denning & Osborne Phillips. 3rd enl. ed. 1999. LC 00-49760. (Practical Guides to Personal Power). (Illus.). xx, 235p. pap. 9.95 (*0-87542-190-3*) Llewellyn Pubns.

Practical Guide to Rapid High Efficiency Dialysis. Prakash Keshaviah et al. rev. ed. 1989. 132p. reprint ed. spiral bd. 75.00 (*1-56488-001-X*) Dialyrn.

Practical Guide to Real-Time Office Sonography in Obstetrics & Gynecology. Robert V. Giglia et al. 1986. LC 85-12033. (Illus.). 236p. (C). spiral bd. 78.00 (*0-306-41865-7*, Kluwer Plenum) Kluwer Academic.

Practical Guide to Respirator Usage in Industry. David S. Blackwell & Gyan S. Rajhans. 1985. (Illus.). 144p. 42.95 (*0-7506-9232-4*) Buttrwrth-Heinemann.

Practical Guide to Setting up & Running an IVF Unit. N. G. Nargund & S. Kelly. 2002. (Illus.). 300p. 89.95 (*1-85070-699-9*, Parthenon Pbng) CRC Pr.

Practical Guide to Sports Injuries. Malcolm Read. 2000. LC 00-40398. (Illus.). 336p. pap. text 45.00 (*0-7506-3251-8*) Buttrwrth-Heinemann.

Practical Guide to Stroke, Diagnosis, Investigation & Treatment. Liz Warburton. 2001. 224p. pap. 60.00 (*0-7506-4753-1*) Buttrwrth-Heinemann.

Practical Guide to Surgical Pathology with Cytologic Correlation: A Text & Color Atlas. K. Kim & B. Naylor. 1991. (Illus.). 359p. 217.00 (*0-387-97538-1*) Spr-Verlag.

Practical Guide to the Care of Geriatric Patient. Fred F. Ferri et al. 2nd ed. 1996. LC 97-106715. (Illus.). 624p. (C). (gr. 13). spiral bd. 29.95 (*0-8151-3194-1*, 29178) Mosby Inc.

Practical Guide to the Care of the Ambulatory Patient. Tom J. Wachtel & Michael D. Stein. 1995. LC 95-195344. (Practical Guide Ser.). (Illus.). 560p. (C). (gr. 13). spiral bd. 32.95 (*0-8016-8063-8*, 08063) Mosby Inc.

Practical Guide to the Care of the Ambulatory Patient. 2nd ed. 1999. (Illus.). 625p. spiral bd. 29.95 (*0-8151-7888-3*, 30954) Mosby Inc.

Practical Guide to the Care of the Critically Ill Parent. Joseph Varon. 1994. LC 94-19744. (Illus.). 424p. (C). (gr. 13). spiral bd. 32.00 (*0-8016-8106-5*, 08106) Mosby Inc.

Practical Guide to the Care of the Gynecologic-Obstetric Patient. George T. Danakas. 1996. (Illus.). 1072p. (C). (gr. 13). pap. text 39.95 (*0-8151-2316-7*, 25553) Mosby Inc.

Practical Guide to the Care of the Medical Patient, No. 4. Fred F. Ferri. 4th ed. 1998. LC 97-22493. (Practical Guide to the Care of the Medical Patient Ser.: Vol. 4). (Illus.). 1168p. (C). (gr. 13). spiral bd. 32.95 (*0-8151-3668-4*, 32806) Mosby Inc.

Practical Guide to the Care of the Pediatric Patient. Anthony J. Alario. 1997. (Illus.). 800p. (C). (gr. 13). spiral bd. 35.95 (*0-8151-0150-3*, 26341) Mosby Inc.

Practical Guide to the Care of the Psychiatric Patient. Richard J. Goldberg. 2nd ed. 1998. LC 99-181154. (Illus.). 496p. (C). (gr. 13). spiral bd. 29.95 (*0-8151-7892-1*, 30955) Mosby Inc.

Practical Guide to the Determination of Human Exposure to Radio Frequency Fields. Intro. by Charles B. Meinhold. 1993. LC 93-45910. (Report Ser.: No. 119). 233p. (Orig.). pap. 40.00 (*0-929600-35-5*) NCRP Pubns.

Practical Guide to the Evaluation of Child Physical Abuse & Neglect. Angelo P. Giardino et al. 1997. LC 96-35623. 352p. 117.95 (*0-8039-5426-3*, 4815) Sage.

Practical Guide to the Evaluation of Sexual Abuse in the Prepubertal Child. Angelo P. Giardino et al. 1992. (Illus.). 128p. (C). 74.95 (*0-8039-4815-8*, 3955) Sage.

Practical Guide to the MPI Clean-Up: Step One in Creating Your Enterprise MPI. Maida R. Herbst & June Muniz. 1998. LC 00-500200. (Illus.). viii, 136p. pap. text (*1-57839-037-0*) Opus Communs.

Practical Guide to the Treatment of Bulimia Nervosa. Johan Vanderlinden et al. 1992. LC 91-40876. (Brunner-Mazel Eating Disorders Monographs: No. 6). 224p. text 33.95 (*0-87630-656-3*) Brunner-Routledge.

Practical Guide to the Use of the High-Resolution Electrocardiogram. Edward J. Berbari & Jonathan S. Steinberg. 1999. LC 99-52567. (Illus.). vii, 182p. 52.00 (*0-87993-445-X*) Futura Pub.

Practical Guide to Therapeutic Plasma Exchange. Andre A. Kaplan. 1998. LC 98-33622. (Illus.). 253p. pap. 48.95 (*0-632-04395-4*) Blackwell Sci.

Practical Guide to Ultrasound in Obstetrics & Gynecology. Eric E. Sauerbrei et al. 2nd ed. 1997. LC 97-11902. (Illus.). 608p. pap. text 69.95 (*0-397-51698-3*) Lppncott W & W.

Practical Guide to Using Video in the Behavioral Sciences. Peter W. Dowrick. 1991. LC 90-19418. 335p. 180.00 (*0-471-63613-4*) Wiley.

Practical Guide to Veterinary Microbiology. Quinn. 1993. 112.00 (*0-8151-6975-2*) Mosby Inc.

Practical Guide to Vibrational Medicine: Energy Healing & Spiritual Transformation. Richard Gerber. 2001. 464p. pap. 15.00 (*0-06-095937-1*, Quil) HarperTrade.

Practical Guidelines for Reducing the Risk of Communicable Disease in a School Setting. MESD School Health Services Staff. 1992. 7.50 (*1-880118-06-8*) MESD Pr.

Practical Guidelines for Transfusion Medicine. 2000. (Illus.). pap. text (*1-56395-128-2*) Am Assn Blood.

Practical Gynecologic Oncology. Jonathan S. Berek & Neville F. Hacker. 3rd ed. 2000. LC 99-57484. 960p. text 159.00 (*0-683-30719-3*) Lppncott W & W.

Practical Gynecology. Farook Al-Azzawi. 2001. 250p. 85.00 (*1-84214-062-0*, Parthenon Pbng) CRC Pr.

Practical Gynecology. Janice Ryden & Paul Blumenthal. 2001. (ACP Women's Health Ser.). (Illus.). pap. text 50.00 (*0-943126-94-0*, 330300900) Amer Coll Phys.

Practical Gynecology: Clinical Manual. Allan Jacobs & Michael Gast. 1994. (Illus.). 528p. (C). pap. text 29.95 (*0-8385-1336-0*, A1336-5, Apple Lange Med) McGraw.

Practical Handbook for Hospital Epidemiologists. Loreen Herwaldt & Michael Decker. 1998. LC 97-10168. (Illus.). 448p. pap. text 65.00 (*1-55642-302-0*, 13020) SLACK Inc.

Practical Handbook of Clinical Gerontology. Laura L. Carstensen et al. 1996. LC 96-9986. 688p. 98.95 (*0-8039-5237-6*, 4313) Sage.

Practical Handbook of Human Biologic Age Determination. Ed. by Arthur K. Balin. 1994. 544p. lib. bdg. 165.00 (*0-8493-0129-7*, QP86) CRC Pr.

Practical Handbook of Joint Fluid Analysis. Robert A. Gatter & H. Ralph Schumacher. 2nd ed. 1991. (Illus.). 122p. text 44.50 (*0-8121-1377-2*) Lppncott W & W.

Practical Handbook of Medical Physics. Robert G. Waggener. 1990. 49.95 (*0-8493-3701-1*) CRC Pr.

Practical Handbook of Nutrition in Clinical Practice. Ed. by Donald F. Kirby & Stanley J. Dudrick. 1994. LC 93-45906. (Modern Nutrition Ser.). 320p. 104.95 (*0-8493-7847-8*) CRC Pr.

Practical Handbook of Plant Alchemy: An Herbalist's Guide to Preparing Medicinal Essences, Tinctures, & Elixirs. Manfred M. Junivs. 2nd ed. 1993. LC 92-47111. (Illus.). 272p. pap. 19.95 (*0-89281-485-3*, Heal Arts VT) Inner Tradit.

Practical Handbook of Psychophanmacology. Edward A. Workman. 1993. 192p. per. 73.95 (*0-8493-8638-1*, RC483) CRC Pr.

Practical Handbook of Sample Size Guidelines for Clinical Trials. Jonathan J. Shuster. 1992. 224p. 115.95 (*0-8493-4487-5*, R853); 115.95 (*0-8493-8678-0*, R853) CRC Pr.

Practical Head & Neck Ultrasound. Ed. by Rhodri Evans & Anil Ahuja. 2000. (Greenwich Medical Media Ser.). (Illus.). 172p. pap. text (*1-900151-99-5*) Greenwich Med GBR. *Dist:* JAMCO Dist.

Practical Hematology. Ed. by John Vivian Dacie & S. M. Lewis. 7th ed. 1991. (Illus.). 556p. text (*0-443-03952-6*) Church.

Practical Hematology. John Vivian Dacie & S. M. Lewis. 8th ed. 1995. pap. text (*0-443-04931-9*) Church.

Practical Home Care Medicine: A Natural Approach. Ed. by Christine Murphy. 2000. LC 00-48798. (Illus.). 96p. pap. 10.00 (*1-930051-09-3*) Lantern Books.

Practical Homeopathy: A Beginner's Guide. Vinton McCabe. 2000. LC 99-26936. xxxi, 592p. pap. 19.95 (*0-312-20669-0*) St Martin.

Practical House Officer. Imogen Mitchell & G. R. Teale. 2nd ed. 1997. LC 96-31455. (Illus.). 352p. pap. 37.95 (*0-86542-769-0*) Blackwell Sci.

Practical How-Tos of Dental Infection Control. R. R. Runnells. 1987. 82p. (C). pap. text (*0-936751-03-7*) Infection Control.

Practical HRT. P. G. H. M. Van der Weijer. 2001. 300p. 78.00 (*1-84214-028-0*, Parthenon Pbng) CRC Pr.

Practical Hypnotism, Theories & Experiments. Comte C. De Saint-Germain. 1996. reprint ed. spiral bd. 17.00 (*0-7873-0268-6*) Hlth Research.

Practical Hysteroscopy. P. J. Taylor & A. G. Gordon. 1993. (Illus.). 128p. 65.00 (*0-632-03672-9*) Blackwell Sci.

Practical Imaging in Orthopaedics. Stoker. 1999. 200p. pap. 109.00 (*0-412-54900-X*) Chapman & Hall.

Practical Immunisation. G. Dick. 1986. text 82.00 (*0-85200-925-9*) Kluwer Academic.

Practical Immunoassay. Wilfrid Butt. 1984. (Clinical & Biochemical Analysis Ser.: Vol. 14). (Illus.). 328p. text 175.00 (*0-8247-7094-3*) Dekker.

***Practical Immunology.** Frank C. Hay et al. 4th ed. 2001. LC 2001-35417. pap. (*0-86542-961-8*) Blackwell Sci.

Practical Implications of the Health Care Quality Improvement Act: Antitrust Analysis. 1994. LC 94-70083. 80p. pap. 40.00 (*0-89707-929-9*, 503-0235, ABA Antitrust) Amer Bar Assn.

Practical Infection Control in Dentistry. James A. Cottone et al. (Illus.). 1990. LC 90-5643. 286p. pap. 36.95 (*0-8121-1326-8*); 2nd ed. 1996. LC 95-2678. 456p. pap. 37.50 (*0-683-02138-9*) Lppncott W & W.

Practical Intensive Care Medicine: Problem Solving in the ICU. Charlie Corke. 2000. LC 00-41440. (Illus.). 192p. pap. text 34.99 (*0-7506-4752-3*) Buttrwrth-Heinemann.

Practical Interventional Radiology of the Hepatobiliary System & Gastrointestinal Tract. Ed. by Andy Adam & Robert Gibson. 1994. 224p. (*0-340-55166-6*) E A GBR. *Dist:* OUP.

Practical Interventional Radiology of the Musculoskeletal System. David Wilson. 1995. (Practical Interventional Radiology Series). (Illus.). 160p. (*0-340-57645-6*) E A GBR. *Dist:* OUP.

Practical Interventional Radiology of the Peripheral Vascular System. Ed. by Anna-Maria Belli. 1994. 136p. (*0-340-55865-2*) E A GBR. *Dist:* OUP.

Practical Introduction: Reflexology. Inge Dougans. 1998. LC 98-24940. (Illus.). 208p. pap. 14.95 (*1-86204-160-1*) Element MA.

Practical Introduction to ENT Disease. N. B. Solomons. 1990. (Illus.). 82p. 21.95 (*0-387-19566-1*) Spr-Verlag.

Practical Introduction to Major Chinese Herbal Formulas. Hong-yen Hsu. 1993. pap. 4.95 (*0-941942-00-7*) Orient Heal Arts.

Practical Introduction to Research Methods. Eugene B. Zechmeister & John J. Shaughnessy. 2nd ed. 1993. LC 94-117668. (C). pap. text 18.50 net. (*0-07-072703-1*) McGraw.

Practical Introduction to Research Methods in Psychology. John J. Shaughnessy & Eugene B. Zechmeister. 3rd ed. 1996. LC 97-104644. 276p. (C). pap. 29.38 (*0-07-072705-8*) McGrw-H Hghr Educ.

Practical Joint Assessment: Upper Quadrant. Anne Hartley. 2nd ed. 1994. LC 94-11608. (Illus.). 368p. (C). (gr. 13). spiral bd. 46.00 (*0-8151-4238-2*, 24264) Mosby Inc.

Practical Joint Assessment Upper Quadrant: A Sports Medicine Manual. Anne Hartley. 2nd ed. 1994. LC 94-18031. (Illus.). 368p. (C). (gr. 13). spiral bd. 46.00 (*0-8151-4237-4*, 24265) Mosby Inc.

Practical Jung: Nuts & Bolts of Jungian Psychotherapy. Harry A. Wilmer. 1987. LC 87-18233. 640p. pap. 19.95 (*0-933029-16-0*) Chiron Pubns.

Practical Kinesiology for Physical Therapist Assistant: Laboratory Manual. Jeff G. Konin. 1999. (Illus.). 80p. pap. text 12.00 (*1-55642-419-1*) SLACK Inc.

Practical Kinesiology for the Physical Therapist Assistant. Jeff Konin. 1999. LC 99-20311. (Illus.). xx, 212p. pap. 35.00 (*1-55642-299-7*, 42997) SLACK Inc.

Practical Laboratory Andrology. David Mortimer. 1994. LC 92-48921. (Illus.). 416p. text 75.00 (*0-19-506595-6*) OUP.

Practical Laparoscopy. A. G. Gordon & P. J. Taylor. 1993. (Illus.). 160p. 65.00 (*0-632-03658-3*) Blackwell Sci.

Practical Lessons in Endodontic Surgery. Donald E. Arens et al. 1998. LC 98-15844. (Illus.). 216p. spiral bd. 82.00 (*0-86715-333-4*) Quint Pub Co.

Practical Liver Biopsy Interpretation: A Manual of Diagnostic Tables. Jurgen Ludwig. 1992. 248p. 75.00 (*0-89189-347-4*) Am Soc Clinical.

Practical Liver Biopsy Interpretation: Diagnostic Algorithms. Jurgen Ludwig & Kenneth P. Batts. 2nd ed. 1998. LC 98-9870. 105.00 (*0-89189-431-4*) Am Soc Clinical.

Practical Management. Tim Clark & John Rees. 3rd ed. 1998. 176p. (C). text (*1-85317-587-0*) Martin Dunitz GBR. *Dist:* Mosby Inc.

Practical Management for the Dental Team. Betty Ladley Finkbeiner. 5th ed. 2000. (Illus.). 595p. spiral bd. 49.95 (*0-323-00886-0*) Mosby Inc.

Practical Management of Asthma. T. Clark & J. Rees. 1985. (Practical Problems in Medicine Ser.). (Illus.). 174p. lib. bdg. 45.00 (*0-906348-74-9*, Wiley-VCH) Wiley.

Practical Management of Asthma. Tim Clark. 2nd ed. 1996. 176p. (C). text (*1-85317-199-9*) Martin Dunitz GBR. *Dist:* Mosby Inc.

***Practical Management of Depression in Older People.** Ed. by Stephen Curran et al. 2001. (Arnold Publication). 200p. (Orig.). pap. text (*0-340-76386-8*) E A GBR. *Dist:* OUP.

Practical Management of Hypertension. Ed. by William H. Birkenhager. 1991. (Developments in Cardiovascular Medicine Ser.). (C). lib. bdg. 124.50 (*0-7923-0918-9*) Kluwer Academic.

Practical Management of Hypertension. Francisco Leyva-Leon & Andrew J. Coats. 1999. LC 98-32240. (*0-632-05045-4*) Blackwell Sci.

Practical Management of Hypertension. Ed. by William H. Birkenhager. 2nd ed. 1996. LC 96-115. (Developments in Cardiovascular Medicine Ser.: Vol. 184). 224p. text 100.50 (*0-7923-3952-5*) Kluwer Academic.

Practical Management of Low-Grade Primary Brain Tumors. Jack P. Rock. 1999. LC 98-44542. (Illus.). 256p. text 139.00 (*0-7817-1101-0*) Lppncott W & W.

***Practical Management of Oesophageal Disease.** Ed. by William J. Owen, Sr. et al. 2000. (Illus.). 180p. (*1-899066-94-2*) Isis Med.

Practical Management of Pain. P. Prithvi Raj. (Illus.). (C). (gr. 13). 2nd ed. 1991. 1120p. text 190.00 (*0-8151-7012-2*, 22126); Vol. 3. 3rd ed. 2000. LC 00-28753. xviii, 1070p. text 190.00 (*0-8151-2569-0*, 31308) Mosby Inc.

Practical Management of Pediatric Cardiac Arrhythmias. Ed. by Vicki L. Zeigler & Paul C. Gillette. 2001. (Illus.). 432p. 69.00 (*0-87993-466-2*) Futura Pub.

Practical Management of Spasticity in Children & Adults. Mel B. Glenn & John Whyte. 1990. LC 89-13414. 325p. text 49.50 (*0-8121-1297-0*) Lppncott W & W.

Practical Management of the Balance Disorder Patient. Ed. by Neil T. Shepard & Steven A. Telian. 1996. 240p. (Orig.). pap. 55.00 (*1-879105-84-5*, 0347) Thomson Learn.

Practical Management of the Dizzy Patient. Joel A. Goebel. 2000. LC 00-44814. 432p. text 99.00 (*0-7817-1820-1*) Lppncott W & W.

Practical Management of the Newborn. I. M. Balfour-Lynn & H. B. Valman. 5th ed. 1993. LC 92-49491. 304p. pap. (*0-632-03571-4*) Blckwell Science.

Practical Management of the Side Effects of Psychotropic Drugs. Ed. by Richard Balon. 1998. LC 98-44760. (Medical Psychiatry Ser.: Vol. 12). (Illus.). 304p. text 150.00 (*0-8247-1926-3*) Dekker.

Practical Manual for a Basic Approach to Clinical Electrodynography. Sheldon Langer et al. 1988. 68p. pap. text 24.00 (*0-936445-02-5*) Langer Found BSMR.

Practical Manual of Brachytherapy. Ed. by Bernard Pierquin & Ginette Marinello. Tr. by Frank Wilson et al from FRE. 1997. LC 96-49909.Tr. of Manuel Pratique de Curietherapie. (Illus.). 300p. text 109.95 (*0-944838-73-1*) Med Physics Pub.

Practical Manual of Laparoscopy. R. R. Levine & R. Pasic. 2001. (Illus.). 250p. lib. bdg. 99.95 (*1-84214-077-9*, Parthenon Pbng) CRC Pr.

Practical Manual of Medical Translation English-French. Hoof. 1996. Orig. Title: Precis Pratique de Traduction Medicale. 309p. (*2-224-01183-0*) Maloine FRA. *Dist:* IBD Ltd.

Practical Manual of Operative Laparoscopy & Hysteroscopy. Ricardo Azziz & Ana A. Murphy. 2nd ed. 1996. LC 96-21229. (Illus.). 366p. 104.00 (*0-387-94696-9*) Spr-Verlag.

Practical Mastitis Control in Dairy Herds. W. H. Giesecke et al. 1999. (Illus.). 328p. pap. 39.95 (*0-409-10923-1*) Buttrwrth-Heinemann.

Practical Math for Respiratory Care. Ray Sibberson. 1995. (Illus.). 304p. (gr. 13). pap. text, wbk. ed. 22.00 (*0-8151-8001-2*, 25934) Mosby Inc.

Practical Mathematics in Nuclear Medicine Technology. Patricia C. Wells. 1999. LC 99-34617. 373p. 63.00 (*0-932004-67-9*) Soc Nuclear Med.

Practical Measurement in Physical Education & Sport. Harold M. Barrow et al. 4th ed. 1989. LC 88-34035. (Illus.). 364p. text 39.95 (*0-8121-1216-4*) Lppncott W & W.

Practical Meat Inspection. Andrew Wilson & William Wilson. 6th ed. 1997. LC 97-20711. (Illus.). 320p. 62.95 (*0-632-04898-0*) Blackwell Sci.

Practical Medical Ethics. David Seedhouse & Lisetta Lovett. 1993. 142p. pap. 65.00 (*0-471-92843-7*, Wiley-Liss) Wiley.

Practical Medical Halakhah. Fred Rosner & Moshe Tendler. 3rd ed. 1997. LC 97-28714. 192p. pap. 40.00 (*0-7657-9990-1*) Aronson.

Practical Medicine from Salerno to the Black Death. Luis G. Ballester et al. 1994. LC 92-49013. (Illus.). 416p. (C). text 100.00 (*0-521-43101-8*) Cambridge U Pr.

Practical Methodology of Forensic Photography. David R. Redsicker. 1992. (Practical Aspects of Criminal & Forensic Investigation Ser.). 304p. 69.95 (*0-8493-9519-4*) CRC Pr.

Practical Microscopic Hematology. Fritz Heckner. 4th ed. 1994. (Illus.). 124p. 34.95 (*0-8121-1711-5*) Lppncott W & W.

Practical Minor Surgery. David Crawford & Chris Khoo. 1996. (Illus.). incl. audio compact disk (*90-5702-006-8*); pap. incl. audio compact disk (*90-5702-007-6*) GBSP NLD. *Dist:* Gordon & Breach.

Practical, Moral, & Personal Sense of Nursing: A Phenomenological Philosophy of Practice. Anne H. Bishop & John R. Scudder, Jr. 1990. LC 89-11480. 185p. (C). pap. text 22.95 (*0-7914-0252-5*) State U NY Pr.

Practical MRI: A Teaching File. Jeffrey J. Brown & Franz J. Wippold, II. 1995. (Illus.). 544p. text 145.00 (*0-7817-0200-3*) Lppncott W & W.

Practical Neuro-Urology: Genitourinary Complications in Neurologic Disease. Michael B. Chancellor & Jerry G. Blaivas. 1995. LC 95-2117. 390p. text 99.00 (*0-7506-9556-0*, Focal) Buttrwrth-Heinemann.

Practical Neuroangiography. Pearse Morris. 1997. LC 97-3874. (Illus.). 400p. 110.00 (*0-683-30020-2*) Lppncott W & W.

Practical Neurology. Jose Biller. 1997. LC 97-4327. 752p. pap. text 69.95 (*0-316-09483-8*) Lppncott W & W.

Practical Neurology of the Elderly. Ed. by Jacob I. Sage & Margery H. Mark. 1996. (Neurological Disease & Therapy Ser.: Vol. 41). (Illus.). 1176p. text 275.00 (*0-8247-9506-7*) Dekker.

Practical Nuclear Medicine. Edwin L. Palmer et al. 1992. (Illus.). 409p. text 94.00 (*0-7216-7030-X*) Saunders.

Practical Nuclear Medicine. Ed. by Peter F. Sharp et al. 2nd ed. 1998. LC 97-34661. (Illus.). 362p. pap. text 59.50 (*0-19-262841-0*) OUP.

Practical Nurse. Jack Rudman. 1994. (Career Examination Ser.: C-642). pap. 27.95 (*0-8373-0642-6*) Nat Learn.

Practical Nursing. M. Clark. 14th ed. 1991. (Illus.). 416p. pap. text (*0-7020-1411-7*) Bailliere Tindall.

Practical Nursing Philosophy: The Universal Ethical Code. David Seedhouse. 2000. LC 00-43437. 234p. pap. 35.00 (*0-471-49012-1*) Wiley.

Practical Obstetric Anesthesia. David M. Dewan. Ed. by David D. Hood & Lesley Day. 1996. 320p. text 58.00 (*0-7216-3658-6*) Saunders.

P
Q
R

***Practice Management for the Dental Team: Instructor's Manual.** Betty Ladley Finkbeiner & Charles Allan Finkbeiner. 5th ed. 2001. (Illus.). tchr. ed., spiral bd. (0-323-00887-9) Mosby Inc.

Practice Manager's Law Handbook: A Ready Reference to the Law for Managers of Medical General Practices. Arthur Brown. 2000. LC 00-34258. pap. 52.95 (0-632-05549-9) Blackwell Sci.

Practice of Anaesthesia & Resuscitation. P. K. Gupta. 1985. (0-7855-0747-7) Current Dist IND. Dist: St Mut.

Practice of Anasthesia. P. K. Gupta. 1989. (C). (0-89771-351-6) Current Dist IND. Dist: St Mut.

Practice of Anesthesia & Resuscitation. A. K. Gupta. 2nd ed. 1989. (C). (0-7855-4664-2) Current Dist IND. Dist: St Mut.

Practice of Anesthesia for Infants & Children. Charles J. Cote et al. 2nd ed. 1992. (Illus.). 558p. text 96.00 (0-7216-3198-3) Saunders.

Practice of Aromatherapy: A Classic Compendium of Plant Medicines & Their Healing Properties. Jean Valnet. Ed. by Robert Tisserand. 1990. 280p. pap. 14.95 (0-89281-398-9, Heal Arts VT) Inner Tradit.

Practice of Autonomy: Patients, Doctors & Medical Decisions. Carl E. Schneider. 1998. LC 98-12178. 336p. text 39.95 (0-19-511397-7) OUP.

Practice of Autosuggestion by the Method of Emile Coue. C. Harry Brooks. 1981. 120p. pap. 12.00 (0-89540-076-6, SB-076) Sun Pub.

Practice of Behavior Therapy. Joseph Wolpe. 3rd ed. 1982. (Illus.). 425p. text 96.00 (0-08-027165-0, J115); pap. text 31.00 (0-08-027164-2) Elsevier (Pergamon Pr).

Practice of Behavior Therapy. Joseph Wolpe. 4th ed. 1991. (General Psychology Ser.). 450p. text (0-08-036455-1); pap. text (0-08-036454-3) PPI GBR. Dist: Elsevier.

Practice of Behavioral & Cognitive Psychotherapy. Richard Stern & Lynne M. Drummond. 1991. (Illus.). 264p. (C). pap. text 42.95 (0-521-38742-6) Cambridge U Pr.

Practice of Breast Ultrasound: Techniques, Findings, Differential Diagnosis. Contrib. by H. Madjar & Jack Jellins. 2000. LC 99-52543. (Illus.). xi, 254p. (3-13-124341-4) G Thieme.

Practice of Breast Ultrasound: Techniques, Findings, Differential Diagnosis. H. Madjar & Jack Jellins. 2000. LC 99-52543. (Illus.). xi, 254p. 99.00 (0-86577-898-1) Thieme Med Pubs.

Practice of Brief Psychotherapy. S. L. Garfield. 1989. (Psychology Practitioner Guidebooks). 176p. text 30.00 (0-08-035890-X); pap. text 15.95 (0-08-035889-6) Elsevier (Pergamon Pr).

Practice of Brief Psychotherapy. Sol L. Garfield. 2nd ed. 1998. LC 98-9987. 320p. 85.00 (0-471-24251-9) Wiley.

Practice of Cardiac Pacing. Seymour Furman & David L. Hayes. Ed. by David R. Holmes, Jr. 3rd enl. rev. ed. 1993. (Illus.). 816p. 95.00 (0-87993-538-3) Futura Pub.

Practice of Cardiology. Ed. by Robert A. Johnson et al. 1980. 82.00 (0-316-46945-9, Little Brwn Med Div) Lppncott W & W.

Practice of Child Therapy. Ed. by Richard J. Morris & Thomas R. Kratochwill. 1983. (General Psychology Ser.: No. 124). (Illus.). 360p. text 100.00 (0-08-028033-1); pap. text 40.00 (0-08-028032-3) Elsevier (Pergamon Pr).

Practice of Child Therapy. Thomas R. Kratochwill & Richard J. Morris. 2nd ed. 1991. (General Psychology Ser.). 504p. text (0-08-036430-6); pap. text (0-08-036429-2) PPI GBR. Dist: Elsevier.

Practice of Clinical Child Psychology. Alan O. Ross. 1959. LC 59-9399. (Illus.). 288p. text 55.00 (0-8089-0390-X, 793662, Grune & Strat) Harcrt Hlth Sci Grp.

***Practice of Clinical Echocardiography.** Ed. by Catherine M. Otto. 2nd ed. 2002. LC 2001-49709. (0-7216-9204-4) Saunders.

Practice of Clinical Health Psychology. Cynthia D. Belar et al. 1987. (Psychology Practitioner Guidebooks). 160p. text 30.00 (0-08-034678-2); pap. text 15.95 (0-08-034677-4) Elsevier (Pergamon Pr).

Practice of Clinical Neuropsychiatry & Behavioural Neurology. Moore. 2001. (Illus.). 450p. (0-7506-4940-2) E A GBR. Dist: OUP.

Practice of Coronary Disease Prevention. Michael Miller & Robert A. Vogel. 1996. LC 95-45490. (Illus.). 352p. pap. 29.95 (0-683-18045-2) Lppncott W & W.

Practice of Counselling in Primary Care. Robert Bor & Damian McCann. 1999. LC 99-71216. (Clinical & Counseling Ser.). (Illus.). 251p. 74.00 (0-7619-5879-7, 84815) Sage.

Practice of Counselling in Primary Care. Contrib. by Robert Bor & Damian McCann. 1999. LC 99-71216. (Clinical & Counseling Ser.). (Illus.). 251p. pap. 27.95 (0-7619-5880-0, 81567) Sage.

Practice of Electrocardiography: A Problem-Solving Guide to Confident Interpretation. Thomas M. Blake. 5th ed. 1994. LC 93-39587. (Illus.). 336p. pap. 49.00 (0-89603-261-2) Humana.

Practice of Electroconvulsive Therapy: Recommendations for Treatment, Training & Privileging. American Psychiatric Association Staff. 2nd ed. 2001. LC 00-32794. (Illus.). viii, 355p. 52.00 (0-89042-206-0, 2206) Am Psychiatric.

Practice of Emergency Care. James H. Cosgriff, Jr. & Diann L. Anderson. 2nd ed. 1984. (Illus.). 652p. text 39.75 (0-397-54357-3, 64-02994, Lippncott) Lppncott W & W.

Practice of Family Therapy: Key Elements Across Models. Suzanne M. Hanna & Joseph H. Brown. 1994. LC 94-16803. 248p. 51.75 (0-534-25098-X) Brooks-Cole.

Practice of Forensic Neuropsychology: Meeting Challenges in the Courtroom. Robert J. McCaffrey et al. 1996. LC 96-37015. (Critical Issues in Neuropsychology Ser.). (Illus.). 235p. (C). text 47.00 (0-306-45256-1, Kluwer Plenum) Kluwer Academic.

Practice of Geriatrics. Edmund H. Duthie, Jr. & Paul R. Katz. Ed. by Ray Kersey. 3rd ed. 1998. LC 97-22941. (Illus.). 544p. (C). text 85.00 (0-7216-6599-3) Saunders.

Practice of Group Therapy. Ed. by S. R. Slavson. 1965. 272p. 40.00 (0-8236-4200-3) Intl Univs Pr.

***Practice of Health Program Evaluation.** David Grembowski. 2001. LC 00-12866. (Illus.). xx, 323p. 79.95 (0-7619-1846-9, 84505) Sage.

Practice of Health Services Research. Ong. 1993. 174p. pap. 54.25 (1-56593-214-5, 0567) Singular Publishing.

Practice of Hypnotism Andre M. Weitzenhoffer. 1989. 800p. 400.00 (0-471-62199-4) Wiley.

Practice of Inpatient Behavior Therapy: A Clinical Guide. Ed. by Michel Hersen. 1985. 304p. text 44.00 (0-8089-1715-3, 791976, Grune & Strat) Harcrt Hlth Sci Grp.

Practice of Interventional Cardiology. King, III et al. Ed. by Morton J. Kern. 1998. (Illus.). 1000p. (C). (gr. 13). text 159.00 (0-8151-4945-X, 30379) Mosby Inc.

Practice of Interventional Neuroradiology. J. J. Connors & Joan C. Wojak. 1999. LC 97-28810. (Illus.). xxiv, 795p. (C). text 190.00 (0-7216-7147-0) Saunders.

Practice of Love: Lesbian Sexuality & Perverse Desire. Teresa De Lauretis. 1994. LC 93-44453. 352p. 36.95 (0-253-31681-2); pap. 15.95 (0-253-20878-5) Ind U Pr.

Practice of M-Mode & Two-Dimensional Echocardiagraphy. Jos R. Roelandt. 1983. text 191.50 (90-247-2745-6) Kluwer Academic.

Practice of Medical Radiesthesia. Vernon D. Wethered. 1977. 160p. (C). 14.95 (0-8464-1040-0) Beekman Pubs.

Practice of Medicine among the Burmese. Keith N. MacDonald. LC 77-87505. reprint ed. 42.50 (0-404-16837-X) AMS Pr.

Practice of Mental Health Consultation. Fortune V. Mannino. 1975. 24.95 (0-89876-082-8) Gardner Pr.

Practice of Multimodal Therapy: Systematic, Comprehensive, & Effective Psychotherapy. Arnold A. Lazarus. 1989. LC 88-46076. (Illus.). 304p. reprint ed. pap. text 18.95 (0-8018-3811-8) Johns Hopkins.

Practice of Neural Science. John C. Brunst. 1999. LC 99-43399. (Illus.). 296p. (C). pap. 29.95 (0-8385-8117-X, A-8117-2) McGraw-Hill Prof.

Practice of Neurosurgery, In Three Volumes. George B. Tindall et al. 1995. 4,000p. (0-683-30003-2) Lppncott W & W.

Practice of Neurosurgery, In Three Volumes. George N. Tindall et al. 1996. (Illus.). 4,000p. text 699.00 (0-683-08266-3) Lppncott W & W.

Practice of Nursing Research. Nancy Burns. 3rd ed. 1997. text 59.00 (0-7216-7572-7) Saunders.

Practice of Nursing Research: Conduct, Critique & Utilization. Nancy Burns & Susan K. Grove. 3rd ed. 1997. (Illus.). 848p. tchr. ed. (0-7216-3057-X) Saunders.

Practice of Nursing Research: Conduct, Critique & Utilization. Nancy Burns & Susan K. Grove. Ed. by Thomas Eoyang. 3rd ed. 1997. (Illus.). 715p. text 47.00 (0-7216-3054-5) Saunders.

Practice of Nursing Research: Conduct, Critique & Utilization. Nancy Burns & Susan K. Grove. 4th ed. 2001. LC 00-47072. (Illus.). xx, 840p. 49.00 (0-7216-9177-3) Saunders.

***Practice of Nursing Research: Conduct, Critique & Utilization.** Nancy Burns & Susan K. Grove. 4th ed. 2001. (Illus.). tchr. ed. 250.00 (0-7216-9314-8) Saunders.

Practice of Obstetrics & Gynecology. Geoffrey V.P. Chamberlain & C. J. Dewhurst. 1977. (Illus.). 271p. 34.95 (0-8464-1120-2) Beekman Pubs.

Practice of Obstetrics & Gynecology. Geoffrey Chamberlain & J. Friend. 3rd ed. 1998. LC 98-32449. (Illus.). 266p. pap. (0-443-05103-8) Church.

Practice of Oxygen Measurement for Divers. J. S. Lamb. 1999. LC 98-86313. (Illus.). 120p. pap. 19.95 (0-941332-68-3, B0990) Best Pub Co.

Practice of Patient Education. Barbara K. Redman & Barbara Klug. 8th ed. 1996. LC 96-20571. (Illus.). 304p. (C). (gr. 13). pap. text 34.00 (0-8151-9357-2, 29203) Mosby Inc.

Practice of Patient Education. Barbara Klug Redman. 9th ed. 2000. LC 00-46297. (Illus.). xi, 314p. 35.00 (0-323-01279-5) Mosby Inc.

Practice of Pharmacy: Institutional & Ambulatory Pharmaceutical Services. Ed. by Donald C. McLeod & William A. Miller. 1981. LC 81-51777. (Illus.). 502p. text 9.00 (0-9606488-0-1) H W Bks.

Practice of Primary Nursing. Marie Manthey. 1980. LC 79-92975. 96p. 10.00 (1-886624-10-0, B240) Creative Nursing.

Practice of Psycho-Social Occupational Therapy. Linda Finlay. 2nd ed. 1997. 224p. 39.95 (1-56593-931-X, 1848) Singular Publishing.

Practice of Quality. Donald Irvine & Sally Irvine. 1996. LC 95-51478. 206p. (1-85775-073-X) Radcliffe Med Pr GBR. Dist: Balogh.

Practice of Rational Emotive Behavior Therapy. Albert Ellis & Windy Dryden. 2nd ed. 1997. LC 96-32061. 280p. 42.95 (0-8261-5471-9) Springer Pub.

Practice of Supportive Psychotherapy. David S. Werman. 1988. LC 84-12740. 208p. text 32.95 (0-87630-365-3) Brunner-Routledge.

Practice of Surgery. Ronald A. Malt. 1993. LC 92-22929. (Illus.). 512p. text 240.00 (0-7216-1811-1) Saunders.

Practice of Therapeutic Endoscopy. Guido Tytgat. 2nd ed. 2000. 315p. text (0-7020-2561-5) W B Saunders GBR. Dist: Saunders.

Practice of Uncertainty: Medicine & Malpractice Claims Through the Voices of Physicians & Patients. Stephen L. Fielding. 1999. LC 98-31028. 256p. 68.00 (0-86569-284-X, Auburn Hse) Greenwood.

Practice of Urology. Barry Stein. Date not set. Vol. 1. (0-393-71002-5); Vol. 2. (0-393-71003-3) Norton.

Practice of Veterinary Dentistry: A Team Effort. Jan Bellows. 1998. LC 98-33711. (Illus.). 216p. (C). text 64.95 (0-8138-2617-9) Iowa U Pr.

Practice Oriented Nutrition Research: An Outcomes Measurement Guide. Carol S. Ireton-Jones et al. 1997. LC 97-23618. 272p. 62.00 (0-8342-0885-7, 20885) Aspen Pub.

Practice Parameters from the American Academy of Pediatrics: A Compilation of Evidence-Based Guidelines for Pediatric Practice. American Academy of Pediatrics Staff. 1997. 396p. pap. 39.95 (0-910761-78-7) Am Acad Pediat.

Practice Parameters in Medicine & Primary Care: 1999-2000 Edition. Paul D. Chan. rev. ed. 1999. (Current Clinical Strategies Ser.). 235p. pap. 36.95 incl. cd-rom (1-881528-64-2) Current Clin Strat.

***Practice Patterns of General/Family Practice 2000-2002.** 2001. 40p. pap. 95.00 (1-57947-255-9) AMA.

***Practice Patterns of Internal Medicine 2000-2002.** 2001. 40p. pap. 95.00 (1-57947-256-7) AMA.

***Practice Patterns of Obstetrics/Gynecology 2000-2002.** 2001. 40p. pap. 95.00 (1-57947-257-5) AMA.

***Practice Patterns of Surgery 2000-2002.** 2001. 40p. pap. 95.00 (1-57947-258-3) AMA.

Practice Problems for Dosage Calculations. Kathryn A. Melson. 1991. pap., tchr. ed. 11.00 (0-8273-4401-5) Delmar.

Practice Standards of ASHP, 1997-1998. Professional Practice Division Staff. 1997. 424p. reprint ed. pap. text 38.00 (1-879907-75-5, P510) Am Soc Hlth-Syst.

Practice Standards of ASHP, 1995-1996. Ed. by Wanda E. Hicks. rev. ed. 1995. (Illus.). 364p. pap. 20.00 (1-879907-58-5) Am Soc Hlth-Syst.

Practice Success! The Physician's Guide to Survival & Success in the Medical Practice. Coker Group Staff. Ed. by Kay B. Stanley. 3rd ed. 1997. 500p. 195.00 (0-9655304-0-X) Coker Publishing.

Practice Tests for Nursing Students. Bourque. 1990. 160p. (C). (gr. 13). pap. text 15.95 (0-8016-0737-X, 00737) Mosby Inc.

Practice Therapeutic Endoscopy. Ed. by Guido N. J. Tytgat. 1995. text 166.00 (0-443-04832-0) Saunders.

Practice Tips. John Murtagh. 2nd ed. 1995. (Illus.). 224p. pap. 49.00 (0-07-470180-0, Apple Lange Med) McGraw.

Practices of Freedom: Selected Writings on HIV-AIDS. Simon Watney. 1994. LC 94-11033. (Series Q). 312p. pap. 16.95 (0-8223-1564-5); text 49.95 (0-8223-1553-X) Duke.

Practices of Human Genetics Michael Fortun & Everett Mendelsohn. 1999. LC 98-49927. (Sociology of the Sciences Ser.). 17p. (0-7923-5333-1) Kluwer Academic.

Practicing Adolescent Medicine: A Collection of Resources. American Academy of Pediatrics Staff. 1994. LC 94-70994. 362p. pap. 44.95 (0-910761-56-6) Am Acad Pediat.

Practicing Cognitive Therapy: A Guide to Interventions. Ed. by Robert L. Leahy. 1997. LC 97-5689. 504p. text 60.00 (1-56821-824-9) Aronson.

Practicing Desire: Homosexual Sex in Era of AIDS. Gary W. Dowsett. 1996. LC 96-10879. viii, 322p. 56.00 (0-8047-2711-2); pap. 19.95 (0-8047-2712-0) Stanford U Pr.

Practicing Family Therapy in Diverse Settings. Michael Berger & Gregory J. Jurkovic. 1994. LC 94-70555. (Master Work Ser.). 396p. pap. 50.00 (1-56821-238-0) Aronson.

Practicing Feminisms, Reconstructing Psychology: Notes on a Liminal Science. Jill G. Morawski. 1994. LC 94-10786. (Critical Perspectives on Women & Gender Ser.). 288p. (C). text 47.50 (0-472-09481-5, 09481); pap. text 19.95 (0-472-06481-9, 06481) U of Mich Pr.

Practicing Harm Reduction Psychotherapy: An Alternative Approach to Addictions. Patt Denning. 2000. LC 00-25503. 246p. pap. 32.50 (1-57230-555-X, 8R0555) Guilford Pubns.

Practicing in the New Mental Health Marketplace: Ethical, Legal & Moral Issues. Ed. by Richard F. Small & Laurence R. Barnhill. 1998. LC 98-15627. 277p. 39.95 (1-55798-494-8, 431-709A) Am Psychol.

Practicing Psychiatry in the Community: A Manual. Ed. by Jerome V. Vaccaro & Gordon H. Clark, Jr. 1996. 560p. text 69.50 (0-88048-663-5, 8663) Am Psychiatric.

Practicing Psychology in Hospitals & Other Health Care Facilities. American Psychological Association Staff. 1998. LC 97-51278. (Illus.). 156p. pap. 29.95 (1-55798-491-3) Am Psychol.

Practicing Psychology in Rural Settings: Hospital Privileges & Collaborative Care. Jerry A. Morris. 1997. LC 97-25216. (Illus.). 159p. pap. text 19.95 (1-55798-452-2) Am Psychol.

Practicing Psychotherapy: A Casebook. Michael F. Basch. 1992. LC 91-55601. 224p. 48.00 (0-465-06175-3) Basic.

Practicing Rehabilitation with Geriatric Clients. Ed. by J. Dermot Frengley et al. 1990. 256p. 36.95 (0-8261-6980-5) Springer Pub.

Practicing Therapy: Exercises for Growing Therapists. Anne H. Rambo et al. 1993. LC 93-4152. 180p. (C). pap. 14.95 (0-393-70161-1) Norton.

Practicing to Take the GRE Psychology Test. 1983. (Orig.). pap. 6.95 (0-88685-006-1) Educ Testing Serv.

Practicum & Internship: Textbook for Counseling & Psychotherapy. John C. Boylan et al. 2nd ed. 1995. 350p. pap. 34.95 (1-56032-392-2) Accel Devel.

Practicum in Healthcare Management: HSM 489. California College for Health Sciences Staff. 1994. 10p. (C). pap., stu. ed. (0-933195-56-7) CA College Health Sci.

Practicum in Healthcare Management: HSM 489. M. Cronin. rev. ed. 1994. 10p. (C). spiral bd. (0-933195-71-0) CA College Health Sci.

Practising Health Promotion. Naidoo. 1998. (C). pap. text 35.00 (0-7020-2122-9) Saunders.

Practitioner Manual for Introductory Patterns of Neuro Linguistic Programming. Maryann Reese & Carol L. Yancar. 1986. 245p. 30.00 (0-9615502-1-X) Southern Inst Pr.

Practitioner Research: Critical Appreciation of Practice As a Basis for Professional Development. Della Fish. 1998. LC 98-20551. (Illus.). 288p. pap. text 32.00 (0-7506-3001-9) Buttrwrth-Heinemann.

Practitioner's Guide to Clinical Neuropsychology. Robert M. Anderson, Jr. 1994. LC 94-2057. (Critical Issues in Neuropsychology Ser.). 406p. (C). spiral bd. 49.50 (0-306-44616-2, Kluwer Plenum) Kluwer Academic.

Practitioner's Guide to Developmental & Psychological Testing. G. P. Aylward. 1994. (Critical Issues in Developmental & Behavioral Pediatrics Ser.). (Illus.). 276p. (C). spiral bd. 39.50 (0-306-44689-8, Kluwer Plenum) Kluwer Academic.

***Practitioner's Guide to Empirically Based Measures of Anxiety.** Ed. by Martin M. Antony et al. 2001. LC 2001-23683. (AABT Clinical Assessment Ser.). xxi, 512p. 69.95 (0-306-46582-5, Kluwer Plenum) Kluwer Academic.

Practitioner's Guide to Empirically-Based Measures of Depression. Ed. by Arthur M. Nezu et al. 2000. LC 00-39073. (AABT Clinical Assessment Ser.). 362p. 69.95 (0-306-46246-X, Kluwer Plenum) Kluwer Academic.

Practitioner's Guide to Evaluating Change with Neuropsychological Assessment Instruments. Holly James Westervelt. Ed. by Robert J. McCaffrey & Kevin Duff. 2000. LC 99-57688. (Critical Issues in Neuropsychology Ser.). 552p. pap. 69.95 (0-306-46361-X, Kluwer Plenum) Kluwer Academic.

Practitioner's Guide to Psychoactive Drugs. Ed. by Alan J. Gelenberg et al. 3rd ed. 1991. 486p. spiral bd. 45.00 (0-306-43461-X, Plenum Trade) Perseus Pubng.

Practitioner's Guide to Psychoactive Drugs. Ed. by Alan J. Gelenberg & Ellen L. Bassuk. 4th rev. ed. 1997. LC 97-29885. 568p. spiral bd. 49.50 (0-306-45468-8, Kluwer Plenum) Kluwer Academic.

Practitioner's Guide to Psychoactive Drugs for Children & Adolescents. Ed. by John S. Werry & Michael G. Aman. (Illus.). (C). 1993. LC 93-7044. 472p. spiral bd. 39.50 (0-306-44389-9); 2nd ed. 1998. LC 98-29332. 528p. spiral bd. 39.50 (0-306-45885-3) Kluwer Academic (Kluwer Plenum).

Practitioner's Guide to Rational-Emotive Therapy. Windy Dryden et al. 2nd ed. 1992. (Illus.). 400p. (C). pap. text 33.95 (0-19-507169-7) OUP.

Practitioner's Guide to the Neuropsychiatry of HIV/AIDS. Ed. by Wilfred G. Van Gorp & Stephan L. Buckingham. 1998. LC 97-42478. 341p. text 40.00 (1-57230-309-3, C0309) Guilford Pubns.

Practitioner's Guide to Understanding Indigenous & Foreign Cultures: An Analysis of Relationships Between Ethnicity, Social Class & Therapeutic Intervention Strategies. George Henderson & Dorscine Spigner-Littles. 2nd ed. 1996. 262p. 61.95 (0-398-06593-4); pap. 42.95 (0-398-06594-2) C C Thomas.

Practitioner's Guide to Veterinary Dentistry. Anthony D. Shipp & Peter Fahrenkrug. 1992. (Illus.). 288p. text 69.00 (0-9635578-0-7) Dr Shipps Lab.

Practitioner's Pocket Pal: Ultra Rapid Medical Reference. Jim Hancock. 2000. (Illus.). 96p. pap. text 15.95 (0-940780-43-7) MedMaster.

Practitioner's Power of Choice in Staff-Development & Inservice Training. Ed. by H. K. Letiche et al. 1991. 184p. pap. (90-265-1124-8) Swets.

***Prader-Wili Syndrome: Effect of Human Growth Hormone Treatment.** Urs Eiholzer. 2001. (Endocrine Development Ser.: Vol. 3). (Illus.). xii, 118p. 76.50 (3-8055-7256-5) S Karger.

Prader-Willi Syndrome. Ed. by M. L. Caldwell & R. L. Taylor. 1988. (Illus.). 110p. 115.00 (0-387-96699-4) Spr-Verlag.

Prader Willi Syndrome. James et al. 1992. LC 92-49609. 240p. pap. 44.75 (*1-56593-046-0*, 0294) Singular Publishing.

Prader-Willi Syndrome & Other Chromosome 15q Deletion Disorders. Ed. by S. B. Cassidy. 1992. (NATO ASI Ser.: Vol. 61). (Illus.). 265p. 182.00 (*0-387-53095-9*) Spr-Verlag.

Praeventive Aspekte in der Paediatrie. Ed. by G. Stalder & C. P. Fliegel. 1981. (Paediatrische Fortbildungskurse fuer die Praxis Ser.: Vol. 52). (Illus.). vi, 182p. 64.50 (*3-8055-1980-X*) S Karger.

Pragmatic Approach to Group Psychotherapy. Henry I. Spitz & Susan T. Spitz. 1998. LC 98-18652. 34.95 (*0-87630-896-5*) Brunner-Routledge.

Pragmatic Approaches to Aphasia Therapy. Sergio Carlomagno. 1994. (Illus.). 170p. (Orig.). (C). pap. text 42.50 (*1-56593-244-7*, 0568) Singular Publishing.

Pragmatic Disability in Children: Studies in Disorders of Communication. Ed. by Michael F. McTear & Gina Conti-Ramsden. 1991. (Illus.). 246p. (C). pap. 45.00 (*1-879105-56-X*, 0237) Thomson Learn.

Pragmatic-Existential Psychotherapy with Personality Disorders. Herbert M. Potash. 1993. 300p. (C). text 35.00 (*0-940524-05-8*) G Handwerk.

Pragmatic Women & Body Politics. Ed. by Margaret Lock & Patricia Kaufert. 1998. LC 97-10263. (Cambridge Studies in Medical Anthropology: No. 5). 376p. (C). text 74.95 (*0-521-62099-6*); pap. text 24.95 (*0-521-62929-2*) Cambridge U Pr.

Pragmatics: From Theory to Practice. Ed. by Judith F. Duchan et al. 1993. LC 93-10009. 214p. pap. 60.00 (*0-13-678988-9*) P-H.

Pragmatics in Neurogenic Communication Disorders. Michel Paradis & International Association of Logopedics and Phoniatr. 1998. LC 98-6486. 270p. 106.00 (*0-08-043065-1*, Pergamon Pr) Elsevier.

Pragmatics of Psychotherapy: A Survey of Theories & Practices. William Schofield. 1988. 272p. text 34.95 (*0-88738-174-X*) Transaction Pubs.

Pragmatism. William James. Ed. by Bruce Kuklick. 1980. LC 80-21788. (HPC Classics Ser.). 152p. (C). pap. text 5.95 (*0-915145-05-7*); lib. bdg. 24.95 (*0-915145-04-9*) Hackett Pub.

Pragmatism & the Meaning of Truth. William James. 1978. LC 77-28535. 400p. pap. 18.00 (*0-674-69737-5*) HUP.

Prairie Practitioners: 20th Century South Dakota Veterinarians. Janice L. Kitzler. Ed. & Intro. by Thomas B. Ludgate. 1996. 288p. (Orig.). pap. (*1-57579-033-5*) Pine Hill Pr.

Prairie Voices: Process Anthropology in Family Medicine. Howard F. Stein. 1996. LC 95-44321. 160p. 57.95 (*0-89789-429-4*, Bergin & Garvey) Greenwood.

Prakriti: Your Ayurvedic Constitution. Robert E. Suoboda. Ed. by Margaret Mahan & John Clancy. 2nd rev. ed. 1988. (Illus.). 208p. pap. 15.00 (*0-9656208-3-2*) Sadhana Pubns.

Prakruti: Your Ayurvedic Constitution. Robert E. Svoboda. 1988. (Illus.). 206p. (Orig.). pap. 12.00 (*0-945669-00-3*) Geocom Ltd.

Praktische Aspekte der Onkologie. Ed. by U. R. Kleeberg. 1984. (Journal: Vol. 7, Suppl. 1). (Illus.). 64p. pap. 77.50 (*3-8055-3918-5*) S Karger.

Praktische Lexikon der Naturheilkunde: Practical Lexicon of Natural Healing. Ernst Meyer-Camberg. 1977. (GER.). pap. 45.00 (*0-8288-5514-5*, M7594) Fr & Eur.

Praktische Neonatologie. Ed. by E. Bossi. 1983. (Paediatrische Fortbildungskurse fuer die Praxis Ser.: Vol. 57). (Illus.). xii, 208p. pap. 85.25 (*3-8055-3657-7*) S Karger.

Praktischer Leitfaden fuer die Therapeutische Anwendung von Cefotiam. Ed. by H. C. Neu & L. D. Sabath. 1983. (Pharmanual Ser.: Vol. 3). (Illus.). vi, 182p. pap. 48.75 (*3-8055-3694-1*) S Karger.

Pratt Institute Creative Arts Therapy Review, Vol. 16. Ed. by Arthur Robbins. 1995. (Orig.). pap. text 8.00 (*1-884870-01-5*) Pratt Inst.

Prayer Is Good Medicine: How to Reap Healing Benefits of Prayer. Larry Dossey. 1997. LC 96-12273. 272p. pap. 13.00 (*0-06-251424-5*) Harper SF.

Prayer That Heals: Praying for Healing in the Family. Francis S. MacNutt. 1981. LC 80-69770. 120p. pap. 7.95 (*0-87793-219-0*) Ave Maria.

Praying for a Cure: When Medical & Religious Practices Conflict. Peggy DesAutels et al. 1999. LC 98-45358. (Point/Counterpoint Ser.). 160p. 57.00 (*0-8476-9262-0*) Rowman.

***Praying in the Wesleyan Spirit: 52 Prayers for Today.** Paul Wesley Chilcote et al. 2001. LC 2001-17373. xii, 172p. pap. 12.00 (*0-8358-0950-1*) Upper Room Bks.

Praying with One Another for Healing. Dennis Linn et al. 1984. pap. 11.95 (*0-8091-2619-2*) Paulist Pr.

Praywell: A Holistic Guide to Health & Renewal. Walter L. Weston. 1996. (Illus.). 442p. (Orig.). pap. 19.95 (*1-884537-06-5*) Transit Press.

Pre- & Perinatal Psychology: An Introduction. Thomas R. Verny. 1986. LC 86-27222. 296p. text 44.95 (*0-89885-327-3*, Kluwer Acad Hman Sci) Kluwer Academic.

Pre- & Post-Anesthesia Nursing Knowledge Base & Clinical Competencies. Ed. by Deborah B. Atsberger & Monica T. Zichuhr. 1994. (Illus.). 158p. pap. text 47.00 (*0-7216-5645-5*) Saunders.

Pre- & Post-Operative Care of the Cataract Patient. Paul C. Ajamian. 1992. LC 92-16080. (Illus.). 134p. spiral bd. 47.50 (*0-7506-9073-9*) Buttrwrth-Heinemann.

Pre & Post-Natal Development of the Human Brain: Proceedings of the 1972 International Children's Center Conference, Vol. 13. International Children's Center Conference Staff. Ed. by Samuel R. Berenberg & N. P. Masse. 1974. (Illus.). 300p. 112.25 (*3-8055-1667-3*) S Karger.

Pre-Clinical Assessment Manual. California College for Health Sciences Staff. 1985. 106p. (C). (*0-933195-52-4*) CA College Health Sci.

Pre-Employment Screening for Psychopathology: A Guide to Professional Practice. Rodney L. Lowman. Ed. by Harold H. Smith, Jr. 1989. LC 88-43546. (Practitioner's Resource Ser.). 86p. pap. 16.95 (*0-943158-34-6*, PESPB, Prof Resc Pr) Pro Resource.

Pre End Stage Renal Disease: A Guide for the Professional Nutritionist. Mary Denny et al. 218p. (C). pap. text 22.50 (*1-883146-52-6*) Coun Renal Nutrit.

Pre-Exam for Nursing Home Administrator Examinees Preparing for the Licensure Examination. Edmond Boudreaux. 4th ed. 1991. 44p. (C). pap. text 10.00 (*1-878199-01-3*) Pro Exam Review.

Pre-Feeding Skills. Morris. 1998. (Illus.). 413p. pap. 65.00 (*0-12-784568-2*) Acad Pr.

Pre-Hospital Emergency Care by Ambulance Services. Dorothy J. Douglas & Julian A. Roth. 1989. 300p. text 39.50 (*0-8290-2391-7*) Irvington.

Pre-Malthusian Doctrines of Population. Charles E. Stangeland. (Columbia University. Studies in the Social Sciences: No. 56). reprint ed. 32.50 (*0-404-51056-6*) AMS Pr.

Pre-Med Handbook. Howard Levitin. 1986. 336p. (Orig.). mass mkt. 12.95 (*0-446-38291-4*) Warner Bks.

Pre-Nursing Reviews in Arithmetic. Mary E. Stehman. 2nd ed. 1961. 33p. pap. 3.95 (*0-8036-8140-2*) Davis Co.

Pre-Object Relatedness: Early Attachment & the Psychoanalytic Situation. Ivri Kumin. 1995. LC 95-19657. (Guilford Psychoanalysis Ser.). 240p. text 40.00 (*1-57230-015-9*, 0015) Guilford Pubns.

Pre-Production Quality Assurance for Healthcare Manufacturers. G. W. Hough et al. 1997. LC 97-2869. (Illus.). 308p. 169.00 (*1-57491-045-0*) IHS Health Grp.

Pre-Prosthetic Surgery: A Self-Instructional Guide, Bk. 7. James R. Hooley & Robert J. Whitacre. 3rd rev. ed. 1983. (Illus.). 58p. pap. 5.95 (*0-89939-071-4*) Stoma Pr.

***Pre-Psychoanalytic Writings of Sigmund Freud.** Ed. by Gertrudis Van De Vijver & Filip Geerardyn. 2001. 270p. (*1-85575-285-9*) Karnac Bks GBR. *Dist:* Other Pr LLC.

Pre-Referral Intervention Manual: The Most Common Learning & Behavior Problems Encountered in the Educational Environment. Stephen B. McCarney et al. 1993. 504p. pap. 36.00 (*1-878372-11-4*) Hawthorne Educ Servs.

Pre-Test Clinical Vignettes for USML: Step I. McGraw-Hill Editors. 1999. LC 99-13440. 280p. pap. 24.95 (*0-07-135133-7*) McGraw-Hill Educ Grp.

Preadmissions Policy & Procedures. Olga Cotera. 1993. 70.00 (*1-879575-32-9*) Acad Med Sys.

Preanesthetic Assessment, Vol. 4. Ed. by Elizabeth Frost. 1994. 366p. 29.95 (*0-9641623-0-X*) McMahon Grp.

Precancer: Biology, Importance & Possible Prevention. Ed. by J. Ponten. 1998. (Cancer Surveys Ser.: No. 32). (Illus.). 238p. (C). text 93.00 (*0-87969-540-4*) Cold Spring Harbor.

Precautions in the Management of Patients Who Have Received Therapeutic Amounts of Radionuclides. 1970. LC 76-125343. (Report Ser.: No. 37). 66p. pap. text 25.00 (*0-913392-19-7*) NCRP Pubns.

Precepting Medical Students in the Office. Paul M. Paulman. 2000. LC 99-52722. (Illus.). 232p. pap. text 20.95 (*0-8018-6366-X*) Johns Hopkins.

Preceptors As Teachers: A Guide to Clinical Teaching. Neal A. Whitman & Thomas L. Schwenk. 1995. 30p. (Orig.). (C). reprint ed. pap. text 10.00 (*0-940193-04-3*) Univ UT Sch Med.

***Preceptorship & Clinical Supervision.** 2001. 224p. pap. (*0-7487-5690-6*) Nelson Thornes GBR. *Dist:* Intl Spec Bk.

Precis: An Update in Obstetrics & Gynecology. American College of Obstetrics and Gynecology. 1978. text 27.50 (*0-07-001134-6*) McGraw.

Precis: An Update in Obstetrics & Gynecology. American College of Obstetricians and Gynecologists Staff. 2nd ed. 1999. LC 99-15357. (*0-915473-51-8*) Am Coll Obstetric.

Precis de Terminologie Medicale. J. Chevalier. 4th ed. 1983. 280p. 35.00 (*0-8288-1795-2*, M6070) Fr & Eur.

Precis, Oncology: An Update in Obstetrics & Gynceology. American College of Obstetricians and Gynecologists Staff. 1998. LC 97-51748. pap. (*0-915473-42-9*, A2841) American College of Emergency Physicians.

Precis Pratique de Psychiatrie. R. Duguay. 2nd ed. 1984. (FRE.). 756p. 125.00 (*0-8288-1802-9*, M15382) Fr & Eur.

Precis Pratique de Traduction Medicale see Practical Manual of Medical Translation English-French

Precis, Reproductive Endocrinology: An Update in Obstetrics & Gynecology. American College of Obstetricians and Gynecologists Staff. 1998. LC 97-51260. 39.00 (*0-915473-43-7*) Am Coll Obstetric.

Precision Radiotherapy Planning. James M. Slater. 1984. (Oncologic Ser.: Vol. 19). pap. 120.00 (*0-08-027470-6*, Pergamon Pr) Elsevier.

Precision Therapy: A Professional Manual of Fast & Effective Hypnoanalysis Techniques. Duncan McColl. 1995. 224p. pap. text (*1-85398-069-2*) Ashgrove Pr GBR. *Dist:* Words Distrib.

Preclinical & Clinical Development of New Vaccines: Symposium, Institut Pasteur, Paris, May, 1997, Vol.95. Ed. by Stanley A. Plotkin et al. 1998. LC 99-166529. (Developments in Biological Standardization Ser.: Vol. 95). (Illus.). xii, 284p. pap. 235.00 (*3-8055-6734-0*) S Karger.

Preclinical & Clinical Modulation of Anticancer Drugs. Kenneth D. Tew. 1993. (Pharmacology & Toxicology Ser.). 384p. 140.00 (*0-8493-7291-7*, RC271) CRC Pr.

Preclinical & Clinical Strategies for the Treatment of Neurodegenerative, Cerebrovascular & Mental Disorders: Workshop, Tokyo, October/November 1994. Ed. by T. K. Shibuya. 1996. (International Academy for Biomedical & Drug Research Ser.: Vol. 11). (Illus.). xiv, 302p. 291.50 (*3-8055-6244-6*) S Karger.

Preclinical Drug Disposition: A Laboratory Handbook. Francis L. Tse & James M. Jaffe. 1991. (Drugs & the Pharmaceutical Sciences Ser.: Vol. 46). (Illus.). 184p. text 130.00 (*0-8247-8500-2*) Dekker.

Preclinical Hyperthermia. Ed. by W. Hinkelbein et al. 1988. (Recent Results in Cancer Research Ser.). (Illus.). 261p. 120.00 (*0-387-18487-2*) Spr-Verlag.

Preclinical Sciences. Matthew T. Wood & E. Jeff Burkes, Jr. 3rd ed. 1980. (Dental Assisting Manuals Ser.: No. 3). ix, 92p. (C). pap. text 17.95 (*0-8078-1377-X*) U of NC Pr.

Preconceptional Health Care: A Practical Guide. Robert C. Cefalo & Merry K. Moos. 2nd ed. 1994. LC 94-10569. (Illus.). 276p. (C). (gr. 13). pap. text 50.95 (*0-8151-1638-1*, 24064) Mosby Inc.

Preconceptional Health Promotion. Merry K. Moos & Margaret C. Freda. Ed. by Karla Damus. 1994. LC 94-37837. (*0-86525-061-8*) March of Dimes.

Preconscious Stimulation in Dreams, Associations & Images: Classical Studies. Otto Potzl et al. 1961. (Psychological Issues Monographs: No. 7, Vol. 2, No. 3). 156p. (Orig.). 27.50 (*0-8236-4260-7*) Intl Univs Pr.

Precursor & Essential Chemicals in Illicit Drug Production: Approaches to Enforcement. James R. Sevick. l.t. ed. 1994. (Illus.). 68p. (Orig.). (C). pap. text 25.00 (*0-7881-0789-5*) DIANE Pub.

Precursors & Chemicals Frequently Used in the Illicit MAnufacture of Narcotic Drugs & Psychotropic Substances: Chemicals Frequently Used in the Illicit Manufacture of Narcotic Drugs. International Narcotics Board Staff. 100p. pap. 18.00 (*92-1-148097-3*) UN.

Precursors of Gastric Cancer. Ed. by Si-Chun Ming. 1984. LC 83-27025. 334p. 89.95 (*0-275-91444-5*, C1444, Praeger Pubs) Greenwood.

Precursors of Prostatic Adenocarcinoma: Recent Findings & New Concepts. Ed. by R. Montironi & C. C. Schulman. 1996. (Journal: Vol. 30, No. 2, 1996). (Illus.). iv, 148p. reprint ed. 77.50 (*3-8055-6367-1*) S Karger.

Predatory Behavior among Wild Chimpanzees. Geza Teleki. 1975. LC 70-124442. (Illus.). 232p. 40.00 (*0-8387-7747-3*) Bucknell U Pr.

Prediabetes. Ed. by R. A. Camerini-Davalos & H. S. Cole. 1989. (Illus.). 418p. 110.00 (*0-306-43105-X*, Plenum Trade) Perseus Pubng.

Prediabetes - Are We Ready to Intervene? Ed. by Z. Laron & M. Karp. 1993. (Pediatric & Adolescent Endocrinology Ser.: Vol. 23). (Illus.). x, 192p. 213.25 (*3-8055-5665-9*) S Karger.

Predicting Adult Stature for Individuals. Ed. by Alex F. Roche. 1975. (Monographs in Pediatrics: Vol. 3). 42.75 (*3-8055-1843-9*) S Karger.

Predicting Health Behaviour: Research & Practice with Social Cognition Models. Ed. by Mark Connor & Paul Norman. 1995. LC 95-14732. 240p. pap. (*0-335-19320-X*) OpUniv Pr.

Predicting Successful Hospital Mergers & Acquisitions: A Financial & Marketing Analytical Tool. David P. Angrisani & Robert L. Goldman. 1997. LC 96-24638. (Illus.). 132p. (C). pap. 22.95 (*0-7890-0182-9*) Haworth Pr.

Prediction in Psychotherapy Research: A Method for the Transformation of Clinical Judgments into Testable Hypotheses. Helen D. Sargent et al. 1968. LC 68-18496. (Psychological Issues Monographs: No. 21, Vol. 6, No. 1). 154p. (Orig.). 27.50 (*0-8236-4285-2*) Intl Univs Pr.

Prediction of Neuroleptic Treatment Outcome in Schizophrenia: Concepts & Methods. Ed. by W. Gaebel & A. G. Awad. 1994. LC 95-10013. (Illus.). 224p. pap. 59.00 (*0-387-82602-5*) Spr-Verlag.

Prediction of Percutaneous Penetration: Methods, Measurement, Modelling. R. C. Scott et al. 1990. 450p. (C). (*1-85271-117-5*) IBC Tech Srvs GBR. *Dist:* St Mut.

Prediction of Performance in Clinical Psychology. Everett L. Kelly & Donald W. Fiske. 1969. LC 69-10113. (Illus.). reprint ed. lib. bdg. 90.00 (*0-8371-0914-0*, KECP, Greenwood Pr) Greenwood.

Prediction of Suicide. Ed. by Aaron T. Beck et al. 1987. LC 86-71588. 256p. reprint ed. pap. 19.95 (*0-914783-16-5*) Charles.

Prediction of Tumor Treatment Response. J. D. Chapman et al. 1988. (Illus.). 336p. 58.00 (*0-08-034689-8*, Pergamon Pr) Elsevier.

Predictors of Treatment Response in Mood Disorders. Ed. by Paul J. Goodnick. 1995. LC 95-15494. (Clinical Practice Ser.: No. 34). 224p. text 32.00 (*0-88048-494-2*, 8494) Am Psychiatric.

Preemies: A Companion Guide for Parents of Premature Babies. Dana Wechsler Linden et al. 2000. pap. (*0-671-02413-2*, PB Trade Paper) PB.

Preferred Provider's Handbook: Building a Successful Private Therapy Practice in the Managed Care Marketplace. William L. Poynter. 1994. LC 93-38869. 184p. pap. text 23.95 (*0-87630-708-X*, 708X) Brunner-Routledge.

Prefrontal Cortex. Diamond. 1997. 220p. pap. text 15.00 (*0-226-14477-1*) U Ch Pr.

Prefrontal Cortex: Its Structure, Function & Pathology: Proceedings of the 16th International Summer School of Brain Research, Amsterdam, The Netherlands, 28 Aug.-1 Sept., 1989. Ed. by H. B. Uylings et al. 1991. (Progress in Brain Research Ser.: No. 85). 574p. 297.75 (*0-444-81124-9*) Elsevier.

Pregnancy. Gordon Bourne. rev. ed. 1996. (Illus.). (Orig.). pap. (*0-330-33912-5*) Pan GBR. *Dist:* Trans-Atl Phila.

Pregnancy: The Authoritative Guide to Pregnancy, Labor & Motherhood. Gordon Bourne. 4th ed. 1989. (Illus.). 576p. (Orig.). pap. (*0-330-30865-3*) Pan GBR. *Dist:* Trans-Atl Phila.

Pregnancy: The Complete Guide from Planning to Birth. Heather Welford. Ed. by Reader's Digest Editorial Staff. 1998. LC 97-38730. (Illus.). 224p. 19.95 (*0-7621-0040-0*) RD Assn.

Pregnancy: The Inside Story. Joan Raphael-Leff. 1995. LC 95-32293. (Master Work Ser.). 224p. 40.00 (*1-56821-579-7*) Aronson.

Pregnancy - The Time to Develop the Child's Awareness. Eunice J. Bernard. 1997. 15p. (Orig.). pap. text 5.00 (*0-9629950-8-8*) Ashbrook Pub.

Pregnancy & Abortion in Adolescence: Proceedings of the WHO Expert Committee, Geneva, 1974. WHO Staff. 1975. (Technical Reports: No. 583). pap. text 6.00 (*92-4-120583-0*, 1100583) World Health.

Pregnancy & Birth: Your Questions Answered. Christopher C. Lees et al. 1998. LC 96-33518. (Illus.). 240p. pap. 19.95 (*0-7894-1470-8*) DK Pub Inc.

Pregnancy & Birth Sourcebook: Basic Information about Planning for Pregnancy, Maternal Health, Fetal Growth & Development & More. Ed. by Heather E. Aldred. 1997. LC 97-36154. (Health Reference Ser.: Vol. 31). xiii, 737p. lib. bdg. 78.00 (*0-7808-0216-0*) Omnigraphics Inc.

Pregnancy & Childbirth. Jan De Vries. 1996. 144p. pap. (*1-85158-657-1*) Mainstream Pubng GBR. *Dist:* Trafalgar.

Pregnancy & Childbirth. Tracy Hotchner. rev. ed. 1997. LC 96-23748. pap. 12.50 (*0-380-78039-9*, Avon Bks) Morrow Avon.

Pregnancy & Childbirth: The Complete Guide for a New Life. Tracy Hotchner. 1990. (Orig.). pap. 11.00 (*0-380-75946-2*, Avon Bks) Morrow Avon.

Pregnancy & Diabetes: An Annotated Bibliography. 1996. 54p. reprint ed. pap. text 30.00 (*0-7881-2760-8*) DIANE Pub.

***Pregnancy & Drug Misuse.** Ed. by Catherine Siney. 2nd ed. 2001. 168p. pap. (*1-898507-77-5*) Books For Midwives Pr GBR. *Dist:* Buttrwrth-Heinemann.

Pregnancy & Infertility. 1998. (Ultrasound & Women's Health Ser.: Pt. I). (*1-930047-46-0*, 98I); pap. (*1-930047-50-9*, 98 I-P) Am Inst Ultrasound.

Pregnancy & Parenting. Phyllis N. Stern. 1988. (Health Care for Women International Publication). 201p. 32.95 (*0-89116-846-X*) Hemisp Pub.

Pregnancy & Parenting Program. Kathy M. Johnson. 1987. (Illus.). 423p. tchr. ed. 250.00 (*0-9616488-2-1*) Alef Bet Comns.

Pregnancy & Renal Disorders. Ed. by Graeme R. Catto. 1988. (New Clinical Applications in Nephrology Ser.). (C). text 95.50 (*0-7462-0057-9*) Kluwer Academic.

Pregnancy & Work. Jean G. Fitzpatrick. 1984. 256p. pap. 7.95 (*0-380-88666-9*, Avon Bks) Morrow Avon.

Pregnancy, Birth, & the Early Months. Richard I. Feinbloom. 3rd ed. Date not set. pap. (*0-201-36099-3*) Addison-Wesley.

Pregnancy, Birth & the Early Months: The Thinking Woman's Guide. Richard I. Feinbloom. 3rd rev. ed. 2000. (Illus.). 400p. reprint ed. pap. 17.50 (*0-7382-0181-2*) Perseus Bks Grp.

Pregnancy Book. Linda H. Holt et al. 1997. LC 96-48905. (Illus.). 448p. pap. 21.95 (*0-316-77914-8*, Back Bay) Little.

Pregnancy Book for Today's Woman. Harold I. Shapiro. 2nd ed. 1993. LC 92-53284. 544p. pap. 20.00 (*0-06-273030-4*, Harper Ref) HarperCollins Pubs.

Pregnancy-Care & Physiology: Index of Modern Authors & Subjects with Guide for Rapid Research. Scott W. Towers. rev. ed. 1994. 57.50 (*0-7883-0188-8*); pap. 47.50 (*0-7883-0189-6*) ABBE Pubs Assn.

Pregnancy, Childbirth & the Newborn: The Complete Guide. Penny Simkin et al. rev. ed. 1991. LC 91-29224. 311p. pap. 12.00 (*0-88166-177-5*) Meadowbrook.

Pregnancy Counseling for Success: A Guide to Effective Counseling. Bethany Productions Staff. 1990. 80p. (Orig.). pap. 16.95 (*1-879058-02-2*) Bethany Prods.

Pregnancy Diary. Tracy Hotchner. 1992. (Illus.). 240p. pap. 14.00 (*0-380-76543-8*, Avon Bks) Morrow Avon.

Pregnancy Exclusions in State Living Will & Medical Proxy Statutes. Kathleen D. Stoll. 1992. (Law & Pregnancy Ser.). (C). pap. 8.00 (*1-877966-14-2*) Ctr Women Policy.

Pregnancy for Older Women: Assessing the Medical Risks. Phyllis K. Mansfield. 1986. LC 86-9440. 230p. 67.00 (*0-275-92184-0*, C2184, Praeger Pubs) Greenwood.

Pregnancy in a High-Tech Age: Paradoxes of Choice. Robin Gregg. 1995. 232p. (C). text 45.00 (*0-8147-3067-1*); LC 94-39520. pap. text 18.50 (*0-8147-3075-2*) NYU Pr.

Pregnancy Journal. James Dalley & Tamara Dalley. 1994. 136p. 18.95 (*0-9642259-0-5*) Castle Peak.

Pregnancy Journal: A Day-to-Day Guide to a Happy and Healthy Pregnancy. A. Christine Harris. 1996. LC 95-12870. (Illus.). 176p. spiral bd. 18.95 (*0-8118-1156-5*) Chronicle Bks.

Pregnancy-Mayo Clinic Co. Mayo Foundation for Medical Education and Research. 1994. LC 94-7264. (Illus.). 750p. 33.00 (*0-688-11761-9*, Wm Morrow) Morrow Avon.

Pregnancy Myths: An Obstetrician Demystifies Pregnancy from Conception to Birth. Michael D. Benson. 1998. LC 98-28523. 352p. pap. 14.95 (*1-56924-695-5*) Marlowe & Co.

Pregnancy Nutrition: Good Health for You & Your Baby. American Dietetic Association Staff. 1998. 96p. pap. 8.95 (*0-471-34697-7*) Wiley.

Pregnancy Prescription: The Success-Oriented Approach to Overcoming Infertility. Hugh D. Melnick & Nancy Intrator. 1998. LC 97-94304. (Illus.). 184p. (Orig.). pap. 17.95 (*0-9660419-0-9*, JO) Josara Pub.

Pregnancy Pure & Simple: Everything Expectant Parents Need to Know. Tracy Hotchner. 1995. LC 94-34817. (Orig.). pap. 12.50 (*0-380-77434-8*, Avon Bks) Morrow Avon.

Pregnancy, Sex Hormones, & the Liver: Proceedings of the 89th Falk Symposium, Held in Santiago, Chile, 10-11 November 1995. Ed. by H. B. Reyes et al. 1996. LC 96-17382. text 147.00 (*0-7923-8704-X*) Kluwer Academic.

Pregnancy Sickness: Protecting Your Baby to Be. Margie Profet. 2000. LC 97-7307. 320p. pap. 10.00 (*0-201-15492-7*) Perseus Bks Grp.

Pregnancy Sourcebook. M Sara Rosenthal. 2nd rev. ed. 1997. 288p. pap. 15.00 (*1-56565-804-3*, Anodyne) Lowell Hse.

Pregnancy Sourcebook. M Sara Rosenthal. 3rd ed. 1999. (Illus.). 336p. pap. 17.95 (*0-7373-0105-8*, 01058W) NTC Contemp Pub Co.

Pregnancy the Natural Way. Sarah Brewer. 2000. 256p. pap. (*0-285-63511-5*) Souvenir Pr Ltd.

Pregnancy Week-by-Week. Amanda Roberts. 1997. LC 97-177472. (Illus.). 96p. pap. 21.95 (*0-06-273483-0*, Perennial) HarperTrade.

Pregnancy Workbook. Ellen K. Anderson. 1983. (Illus.). 96p. (Orig.). pap. 8.95 (*0-939374-01-3*) Homefront Graphics.

Pregnant Husband's Handbook. Jeff Justice. Ed. by Diane Pfeifer. 1989. (Illus.). 96p. (Orig.). pap. 5.95 (*0-9618306-8-9*) Strawberry GA.

Pregnant, Substance-Using Women: A Treatment Improvement Protocol. (Orig.). 1994. (Illus.). 92p. (C). pap. text 40.00 (*0-7881-1165-5*); 1993. 98p. pap. text 45.00 (*1-57979-153-0*) DIANE Pub.

Pregnant Woman's Comfort Book: A Self-Nurturing Guide to Your Emotional Well-Being During Pregnancy & Early Motherhood. Jennifer Louden. 1995. LC 94-47638. 240p. pap. 16.00 (*0-06-251165-3*) Harper SF.

***Pregnant Women - Violent Men: What Midwives Need to Know.** Sheila C. Hunt & Ann M. Martin. 2001. 204p. pap. text 29.95 (*0-7506-5203-9*) Buttrwrth-Heinemann.

Pregnant Women on Drugs: Combating Stereotypes & Stigma. Sheigla Murphy & Marsha Rosenbaum. 1999. LC 98-20130. 192p. (C). text 49.00 (*0-8135-2602-7*) Rutgers U Pr.

Prehistoric Tuberculosis in the Americas. Ed. by Jane E. Buikstra. 1981. LC 80-28660. (Scientific Papers Ser.: No. 5). (Illus.). 194p. (Orig.). pap. 7.25 (*0-942118-10-3*) Ctr Amer Arche.

Prehospital Care Administration: Issues, Readings, Cases. Joseph J. Fitch. 1995. (C). (gr. 13). text 46.95 (*0-8151-3391-X*, 25879) Mosby Inc.

Prehospital Care for the EMT-Intermediate Assessment & Intervention. Stephen LaFevers & Loren Marshall. 1984. (C). tchr. ed. (*0-8359-5603-2*); pap. text 33.00 (*0-8359-5579-6*) P-H.

Prehospital Care of Pediatric Emergencies. James S. Seidel & Deborah P. Henderson. (Nursing-Health Science Ser.). (Illus.). (C). 1987. 109p. pap. text 35.00 (*0-86720-680-2*, 680-2); 2nd ed. 1996. LC 96-32245. 312p. pap. text 40.00 (*0-86720-505-9*, 505-9) Jones & Bartlett.

Prehospital Drug Therapy. Sheryl M. Gonsoulin & William Raynovich. 1993. LC 93-120. (Illus.). 336p. (gr. 13). pap. text 35.95 (*0-8016-1969-6*, 01969) Mosby Inc.

Prehospital Drug Therapy 2. Sheryl M. Gonsoulin et al. 2nd ed. 2000. 416p. (C). pap. text 30.95 (*0-8151-2965-3*, 31834) Mosby Inc.

Prehospital Emergency Care. Brent Q. Hafen & Keith J. Karren. 5th ed. 1996. (C). pap. text, tchr. ed. 15.00 (*0-89303-771-0*); 1995. LC 99-23560. 896p. pap. 46.00 (*0-89303-763-X*) P-H.

Prehospital Emergency Care. Hafen & Karren. 6th ed. 1999. pap. text, tchr. ed. 45.00 net. (*0-8359-5739-X*) Globe Fearon.

Prehospital Emergency Care. Joseph J. Mistovich et al. Ed. by Howard A. Werman. 6th ed. 1999. LC 99-23560. 970p. pap. 59.00 (*0-8359-5705-5*) P-H.

Prehospital Emergency Care: A Guide for Paramedics. Jean T. Abbott & Marilyn J. Gifford. 3rd ed. 1996. LC 95-49532. (Clinical Handbook Ser.). (Illus.). 382p. 26.95 (*1-85070-636-0*, Parthenon Pbng) CRC Pr.

Prehospital Emergency Care Secrets: Questions You Will Be Asked—at the Scene, in the ER, on Oral Exams. Peter T. Pons & V. Markovchick. 1998. LC 97-51462. (Secrets Ser.). 300p. pap. 39.95 (*1-56053-250-5*) Hanley & Belfus.

Prehospital Emergency Medicine: Challenges & Options in Emergency Services. Ed. by John Schou. 2nd ed. 1997. 448p. text (*90-5702-003-3*) GBSP NLD. *Dist:* Gordon & Breach.

Prehospital Emergency Pharmacology. Bryan E. Bledsoe et al. LC 83-15893. 336p. pap. text 19.95 (*0-89303-765-6*) P-H.

Prehospital Emergency Pharmacology. Bryan E. Bledsoe. 2nd ed. 1988. (Illus.). 304p. pap. text 31.00 (*0-89303-797-4*) P-H.

Prehospital Medicine: The Art of on-Line Medical Command. Ed. by Paul M. Paris & Ronald N. Roth. 1996. (Illus.). 288p. (C). (gr. 13). pap. text 50.95 (*0-8151-6849-7*, 24810) Mosby Inc.

Prehospital Medicine & the Law. Date not set. (C). 42.67 (*0-13-021220-2*) P-H.

Prehospital Nursing: A Collaborative Approach. Renee S. Holleran. 1994. (Illus.). 394p. (C). (gr. 13). text 59.95 (*0-8016-7894-3*, 07894) Mosby Inc.

Prehospital Pediatric Emergencies. Martin R. Eichelberger et al. 1991. pap. 22.00 (*0-89303-802-4*, 740801) P-H.

Prehospital Providers' Guide to Medication. Alan J. Azzara. 1998. LC 99-21429. (Illus.). 255p. pap. (*0-7216-1136-2*) Saunders.

Prehospital Trauma Life Support. National Association of Emergency Medical Technicians Staff. 4th ed. 1998. LC 98-27270. (Illus.). 384p. (gr. 13). pap. text 36.95 (*0-8151-4569-1*, 30219) Mosby Inc.

Prehospital Trauma Life Support. National Association of Emergency Technicians Staff. 4th ed. 1998. tchr. ed. (*0-323-00300-1*) Mosby Inc.

Preimplantation Diagnosis of Genetic Disease: A New Technique in Assisted Reproduction. Ed. by Yuri Verlinsky & Anver Kuliev. 1992. 166p. 150.00 (*0-471-58824-5*, Wiley-Liss) Wiley.

Preimplantation Diagnosis of Human Genetic Disease. Ed. by Robert G. Edwards. 1993. (Illus.). 352p. (C). text 110.00 (*0-521-40425-8*) Cambridge U Pr.

Preimplantation Embryo Development. Ed. by Barry D. Bavister. 1993. LC 92-49441. 352p. (*3-540-97934-4*); (Illus.). 354p. 129.00 (*0-387-97934-4*) Spr-Verlag.

Preimplantation Genetic Diagnosis. Harper. 2001. LC 00-43470. (Illus.). 278p. 95.00 (*0-471-98500-7*) Wiley.

Prejudice & Your Child. Kenneth B. Clark. 1988. LC 85-17862. 327p. reprint ed. per. 19.95 (*0-8195-6155-X*, Wesleyan Univ Pr) U Pr of New Eng.

Prelevements en Biologie Medicale. C. Perez. 1991. 82p. pap. 27.50 (*2-906077-17-8*) Elsevier.

Preliminary Estimates from the Drug Abuse Warning Network, 1995. Linda McCaig. 1998. 75p. pap. text 30.00 (*0-7881-4034-5*) DIANE Pub.

Preliminary Evaluation of Quantitative Clinical Laboratory Methods. 1993. (Tentative Guideline Ser.: Vol. 9). 85.00 (*1-56238-022-2*, EP10-T2) NCCLS.

Prelinguistic Communication in Infancy. Alan Ziajka. 1981. LC 81-379. 178p. 58.00 (*0-275-90747-3*, C0747, Praeger Pubs) Greenwood.

Prelude to Strategic Planning: Making Your Organization & Community Fit for Success. American Hospital Association Staff. 1989. (Illus.). 52p. (Orig.). pap. 35.00 (*0-87258-521-2*, 184206) Am Hospital.

Premalignancy & Early Cancer: In General Surgery. J. W. Fielding & W. L. Allum. 1996. (Illus.). 206p. text 115.00 (*0-19-263028-8*) OUP.

Premalignancy & Tumor Dormancy. Eitan Yefenof. 1996. (Medicine Ser.). pap. 89.95 (*0-412-10441-5*, VNR) Wiley.

Premature Baby Book: A Parents Guide to Coping & Caring in the First Years. Helen Harrison & Ann Kositsky. 1983. (Illus.). 320p. pap. 19.95 (*0-312-63649-0*) St Martin.

Premature in Context. Max Sugar. 1982. 141p. text 20.00 (*0-88331-183-6*) R B Luce.

Premature Infant: Nursing Assessment & Management. Lyn E. Vargo et al. 1998. LC 98-42498. (*0-86525-082-0*) March of Dimes.

Premature Infants & Their Families: Developmental Interventions. M. Virginia Wyly et al. 1995. LC 95-271. (Early Childhood Intervention Ser.). (Illus.). 276p. (Orig.). (C). pap. text 45.00 (*1-879105-87-X*, 0350) Thomson Learn.

Premature Menopause Book: When the "Change of Life" Comes Too Early. Kathryn Petras. 1999. LC 99-94866. 416p. pap. 14.00 (*0-380-80541-3*, Avon Bks) Morrow Avon.

Premature Vascular Disease in Homocystinaemia. Ed. by S. Coccheri. 1989. (Journal: Vol. 19, Suppl. 1, 1989). (Illus.). iv, 50p. pap. 77.50 (*3-8055-4998-9*) S Karger.

PreMed: Who Makes It & Why. Mary Ann Maguire. 1999. LC 98-48715. (Sociology of Education Ser.). 256p. pap. 21.95 (*0-8077-3832-8*); xiii, 161p. text 44.00 (*0-8077-3833-6*) Tchrs Coll.

Premenstrual Dysphorias: Myths & Realities. Ed. by Judith H. Gold & Sally K. Severino. 1994. LC 93-47479. 262p. text 19.95 (*0-88048-666-X*, 8666) Am Psychiatric.

Premenstrual Solution: How to Tame the Shrew in You. Jo Ann C. Friedrich. 1987. 168p. pap. 14.95 (*0-9617317-0-2*) Bright Bks CA.

Premenstrual Syndrome. Keye. 1988. pap. text 55.00 (*0-7216-2560-6*, Grune & Strat) Harcrt Hlth Sci Grp.

***Premenstrual Syndrome.** Caroline Shreeve. 1992. pap. (*0-7225-2684-9*) Thorsons GBR. *Dist:* Natl Bk Netwk.

Premenstrual Syndrome: A Clinician's Guide. Sally K. Severino & Margaret L. Moline. 1997. (Illus.). 340p. reprint ed. text 15.00 (*0-7881-5054-5*) DIANE Pub.

Premenstrual Syndrome: A Nutritional Approach. Louise Tenney. 1997. (Woodland Health Ser.: No. 3). 32p. pap. 3.95 (*0-913923-30-3*) Woodland UT.

Premenstrual Syndrome: A Self Help Guide. Wendy V. Rappoport. 1984. (Illus.). 96p. (Orig.). pap. 4.95 (*0-936320-19-2*) Compact Books.

Premenstrual Syndrome: Ethical & Legal Implications in a Biomedical Perspective. Ed. by Benson E. Ginsburg & Bonnie F. Carter. 1987. LC 86-30562. 452p. 79.50 (*0-306-42498-3*, Plenum Trade) Perseus Pubng.

Premenstrual Syndrome: How You Can Benefit from Diet, Vitamins, Minerals, Herbs, Exercise & Other Natural Methods. Michael T. Murray. 1997. LC 97-5744. (Getting Well Naturally Ser.). 176p. pap. 11.00 (*0-7615-0820-1*, Prima Health) Prima Pub.

Premenstrual Syndrome: Index of Modern Information. Jacob L. Liehaus. 1990. LC 88-47618. 150p. 47.50 (*1-55914-138-7*); pap. 44.50 (*1-55914-139-5*) ABBE Pubs Assn.

Premenstrual Tension: A Multidisciplinary Approach. Ed. by Charles M. Debrovner. 1982. LC 81-6653. 111p. 30.95 (*0-89885-019-3*, Kluwer Acad Hman Sci) Kluwer Academic.

Premier ICD-9-CM Code Book, 1999-2000. St. Anthony's Publishing Staff. 1999. (C). pap. 72.00 (*1-56329-667-5*) Thomson Learn.

Prenatal & Obstetric Care in Los Angeles County, 1990. Toni Richards et al. 1993. LC 93-20333. pap. text 9.00 (*0-8330-1343-2*, MR-182-NHF) Rand Corp.

Prenatal & Perinatal Factors in the Development of Childhood Reading Disorders. A. A. Kawi. 1959. (SRCD M Ser.: Vol. 24, No. 4). 25.00 (*0-527-01580-6*) Periodicals Srv.

Prenatal & Perinatal Infections. 1985. (EURO Reports & Studies: No. 93). 147p. pap. text 12.00 (*92-890-1259-5*, 1330093) World Health.

Prenatal & Perinatal Psychology & Medicine: Encounter with the Unborn. Ed. by P. G. Fedor-Freybergh & M. L. Vogel. 1987. (Illus.). 699p. 68.00 (*1-85070-181-4*, Parthenon Pbng) CRC Pr.

Prenatal Antecedents of Postnatal Growth. Stanley Garn. Date not set. (Illus.). 224p. text 25.00 (*0-472-10074-2*) U of Mich Pr.

Prenatal Care. Miriam Stoppard. 1998. LC 97-48451. (DK Healthcare Ser.). (Illus.). 80p. pap. 7.95 (*0-7894-3097-5*) DK Pub Inc.

Prenatal Care: Reaching Mothers, Reaching Infants. Institute of Medicine Staff. 1988. 264p. pap. text 27.95 (*0-309-03892-8*) Natl Acad Pr.

Prenatal Care for Hispanic Women: Opportunities for Improvement. Helen M. Wallace et al. 1994. (Illus.). 130p. (Orig.). pap. 19.95 (*0-89914-046-7*) Third Party Pub.

Prenatal Care in the United States, 1980-94. National Center For Health Statistics Staff. 1996. LC 96-9472. (Vital & Health Statistics Ser.: Series 21, No. 54). (*0-8406-0518-8*) Natl Ctr Health Stats.

Prenatal Cocaine Exposures. Ed. by Richard J. Konkol & George D. Olsen. 1996. LC 95-48362. 208p. 134.95 (*0-8493-9465-1*) CRC Pr.

Prenatal Diagnosis. Curry. text (*0-7216-6813-5*) Saunders.

Prenatal Diagnosis. Ed. by Jack Fitzsimmons. 1993. (Current Topics in Obstetrics & Gynecology Ser.). 266p. (gr. 13). pap. 88.95 (*0-412-04671-7*) Chapman & Hall.

Prenatal Diagnosis: Methods & Protocols. Ed. by Gordon W. Lowther. 2001. (Methods in Molecular Medicine Ser.). 350p. 99.50 (*0-89603-784-3*) Humana.

***Prenatal Diagnosis & Management of Fetal Anomalies.** Frank A. Manning & Harman. 2001. (Illus.). 605p. (*0-7216-8068-2*) Saunders.

Prenatal Diagnosis & Reproductive Genetics. Jeffrey A. Kuller & Robert C. Cefalo. 1995. (Illus.). 320p. (C). (gr. 13). text 45.95 (*0-8151-5209-4*, 24021) Mosby Inc.

Prenatal Diagnosis & Screening. Ed. by M. A. Ferguson-Smith et al. 1992. (Illus.). 785p. text (*0-443-04379-5*) Church.

Prenatal Diagnosis & Selective Abortion. Harry Harris. 1975. LC 75-3847. (Rock Carling Fellowship Ser.). 101p. 23.50 (*0-674-70080-5*) HUP.

Prenatal Diagnosis in Obstetric Practice. Ed. by M. J. Whittle & J. M. Connor. 2nd ed. 1995. LC 94-26804. 360p. 145.95 (*0-632-03838-1*) Blackwell Sci.

Prenatal Diagnosis of Congenital Anomalies. Roberto Romero et al. 1997. (Illus.). 466p. (C). pap. text 135.00 (*0-8385-7921-3*, A7921-8, Apple Lange Med) McGraw.

Prenatal Diagnosis of Foetal Malformations & Diseases: Teaching Atlas of Amniofoetography. Lothar Abet et al. 1991. 88p. (*3-05-500611-9*) Akademie Verlag DEU. *Dist:* Wiley.

Prenatal Diagnosis of Heritable Skin Diseases. Ed. by Tobias Gedde-Dahl & K. D. Wuepper. 1987. (Current Problems in Dermatology Ser.: Vol. 16). (Illus.). viii, 216p. 189.75 (*3-8055-4397-2*) S Karger.

Prenatal Diagnosis of Thalassemia & the Hemoglobinopathies. Ed. by Dimitris Loukopoulos. 1988. 272p. 151.00 (*0-8493-5972-4*, RJ416, CRC Reprint) Franklin.

Prenatal Drug Exposure: Kinetics & Dynamics. 1992. lib. bdg. 88.00 (*0-8490-5496-6*) Gordon Pr.

Prenatal Exposure to Drugs - Alcohol: Characteristics & Educational Implications of Fetal Alcohol Syndrome & Cocaine - Polydrug Effects. Jeanette M. Soby. 1994. LC 93-23234. (Illus.). 138p. (C). text 37.95 (*0-398-05891-1*) C C Thomas.

Prenatal Exposure to Toxicants: Developmental Consequences. Ed. by Herbert L. Needleman & David Bellinger. 1994. LC 93-34394. (Series in Environmental Toxicology). 336p. 99.00 (*0-8018-4704-4*) Johns Hopkins.

Prenatal Exposures in Schizophrenia. Ed. by Ezra S. Susser et al. 1999. LC 97-41045. (Progress in Psychiatry Ser.: Vol. 56). 352p. text 38.00 (*0-88048-499-3*, 8499) Am Psychiatric.

Prenatal Growth Reduction & Postnatal Endocrinopathies. Inge Francois. 1999. (Acta Biomedica Lovaniensia Ser.: Vol. 197). (Illus.). 131p. pap. (*90-6186-962-5*) Leuven Univ BEL. *Dist:* Coronet Bks.

Prenatal Person: Frank Lake's Maternal-Fetal Distress Syndrome. Stephen M. Maret. 1997. LC 97-3170. 224p. (C). 43.00 (*0-7618-0768-3*) U Pr of Amer.

Prenatal Screening for Major Fetal Disorders Vol. II: Screening for Down Syndrome. James E. Haddow et al. 1998. (Illus.). 296p. ring bd. 90.00 (*0-9653655-4-9*) Fnd Blood Res.

Prenatal Screening, Policies, & Values: The Example of Neural Tube Defects. Ed. by Elena O. Nightingale & Susan B. Meister. 1987. (Illus.). 160p. pap. 10.95 (*0-674-70075-9*) HUP.

Prenatal Testing: A Sociological Perspective. Aliza Kolker & B. Burke. 1994. LC 93-43731. 248p. 62.95 (*0-89789-337-9*, Bergin & Garvey) Greenwood.

Prenatal Testing: A Sociological Perspective with new Afterword. Aliza Meredith Kolker & B. Burke. 1998. LC 93-43731. 280p. pap. 23.95 (*0-89789-633-5*, Bergin & Garvey) Greenwood.

Prenatal Testing & Disability Rights. Ed. by Erik Parens & Adrienne Asch. 2000. LC 00-26361. (Hastings Center Studies in Ethics). xvi, 371p. pap. 23.95 (*0-87840-804-5*); text 65.00 (*0-87840-803-7*) Georgetown U Pr.

Prenatal Yoga & Natural Birth. Jeannine P. Baker. 2nd exp. ed. 1986. LC 74-19553. (Illus.). reprint ed. pap. text 10.00 (*0-913512-52-4*) Freestone Pub Co.

***Prentice Hall Health Professional's Drug Guide 2002.** Margaret Shannon et al. 2nd ed. 2001. 1568p. 32.95 (*0-13-042036-0*, Prentice Hall) P-H.

Preoedipal Origin & Psychoanalytic Therapy of Sexual Perversions. Charles W. Socarides. 1988. 80.00 (*0-8236-4287-9*) Intl Univs Pr.

Preoperative & Postoperative Dermatologic Surgical Care. Ed. by Hubert T. Greenway, Jr. & Terry L. Barrett. 1995. LC 94-22504. (Illus.). 224p. 69.50 (*0-89640-261-4*) Igaku-Shoin.

Preoperative Cardiac Assessment: A Society of Cardiovascular Anesthesiologists Mono. Dennis T. Mangano. 1990. (Illus.). 200p. text 38.00 (*0-397-51089-6*) Lppncott W & W.

Preoperative Events: Their Effects on Behavior Following Brain Damage. J. Schulkin. 1989. 368p. 79.95 (*0-8058-0021-2*); pap. 39.95 (*0-8058-0535-4*) L Erlbaum Assocs.

Preoperative (Neoadjuvant) Chemotherapy. Ed. by J. Ragaz et al. 1986. (Recent Results in Cancer Research Ser.: Vol. 103). (Illus.). 162p. 76.00 (*0-387-16129-5*) Spr-Verlag.

Preoperative Preparation & Intraoperative Monitoring. 1997. LC 96-53605. (Atlas of Anesthesia Ser.). text (*0-443-07902-1*) Church.

Preparation & Assay of Enzymes. Ed. by Sidney P. Colowick & Nathan O. Kaplan. (Methods in Enzymology Ser.: Vol. 6). 1963. text 209.00 (*0-12-181806-3*); 1961. text 209.00 (*0-12-181805-5*); 1955. text 209.00 (*0-12-181801-2*); 1955. text 209.00 (*0-12-181802-0*) Acad Pr.

Preparation & Assay of Substrates. Ed. by Sidney P. Colowick & Nathan O. Kaplan. 1957. (Methods in Enzymology Ser.: Vol. 3). text 209.00 (*0-12-181803-9*) Acad Pr.

Preparation & Revision for DRCOG. Janice Rymer et al. 1990. (Illus.). 258p. pap. text (*0-443-04248-9*) Church.

Preparation & Revision for the Diploma of the Royal College of Obstetricians & Gynaecologists. Janice Rymer. 2nd ed. 1998. LC 97-18740. (*0-443-05097-X*) Church.

Preparation & Revision for the MRCPCH, Pt. 1. R. Skinner et al. 1998. (Illus.). 400p. pap. (0-443-06139-4) Church.

Preparation & Revision for the MRCS & AFRCS Examinations. W. E. Thomas. 2nd ed. 1998. (Illus.). 220p. pap. (0-443-05046-5) Church.

Preparation & Testing of Reagent Water in the Clinical Laboratory. National Committee for Clinical Laboratory Standards. 3rd ed. 1991. (Approved Guideline Ser.: Vol. 8). 75.00 (1-56238-127-X, C3-A2) NCCLS.

Preparation for Aging: Proceedings of the Seventeenth International Congress of IAUTA Held in Jyvaskyla, Finland, August 12-14, 1994. Ed. by Eino Heikkinen et al. 1995. (Illus.). 306p. 95.00 (0-306-45068-2, Kluwer Plenum) Kluwer Academic.

Preparation for Birth: The Complete Guide to the Lamaze Method. Beverly Savage & Diana Simkin. 1987. 496p. (Orig.). pap. 14.00 (0-345-31230-9, Ballantine) Ballantine Pub Grp.

Preparation for Board Certification & Licensing Examinations in Psychology: The Professional, Legal & Ethical Components. Robert G. Meyer. 1992. 184p. 29.00 (0-9634417-0-1) Monkestee Pr.

Preparation for Credentialing in Radiography. Mary A. Sherer. 9th ed. 1992. LC 92-13350. (Illus.). 255p. pap. text 26.00 (0-7216-3282-3) Saunders.

Preparation for Examinations in Nuclear Medicine Technology. Ann M. Steves. 1997. LC 97-5945. pap. text 25.00 (0-932004-49-0) Soc Nuclear Med.

Preparation for NCLEX-RN: Saunders Nursing Review & Practice Tests. Dee A. Gillies. 4th ed. 1987. 416p. pap. text 36.00 (0-7216-1454-X) Saunders.

Preparation for the DCH. N. J. Gilbertson & S. Walker. 1993. (Illus.). 256p. (Orig.). pap. text (0-443-04375-2) Church.

Preparation for the MCAT: The Medical College Admission Test, Bklet. B. Northwestern Learning Center Staff. 1997. 80p. pap. 15.00 (1-884083-97-8) Maval Pub.

Preparation for the MCAT Test: The Medical College Admission Test, Booklet A. Johan Eptekar & Northwestern Learning Center Staff. 1997. (Illus.). 100p. pap. text 15.00 (1-884083-95-1) Maval Pub.

Preparation for the Toddler Years: The Next Step. Gary Ezzo & Anne M. Ezzo. 1994. (Illus.). 118p. stu. ed. 25.00 (1-883035-19-8) Grow Families.

Preparation for the United States Medical Licensing Examinations, Step 1, Bk. F. Medical Education Board. 1997. (USMLE Ser.). (Illus.). 150p. (C). 18.00 (1-884083-08-0) Maval Pub.

Preparation for the United States Medical Licensing Examinations, Step 1, Bklt. C. Mauricio L. Waintrub & Medical Education Board Staff. 1998. 76p. (C). lib. bdg., stu. ed. 15.00 (1-884708-15-3) Maval Pub.

Preparation for the United States Medical Licensing Examinations, Step 1, Bklt. C. Hobart Walling et al. 1998. (USMLE Ser.). (Illus.). 278p. (C). stu. ed. 18.00 (1-884083-21-8) Maval Pub.

Preparation for the United States Medical Licensing Examinations, Step 1, Bklt. D/E. Mauricio L. Waintrub et al. 4th ed. 1998. (USMLE Ser.). (Illus.). 76p. (C). pap. text 15.00 (1-884083-16-1) Maval Pub.

Preparation for the United States Medical Licensing Examinations, Step 1, Bklt. A. Valentin Waintrub & Maria Luder. Ed. by Mauricio L. Waintrub & Maval Medical Education Staff. 4th ed. 1998. (USMLE Ser.). (Illus.). 76p. (C). pap. text 15.00 (1-884083-13-7) Maval Pub.

Preparation for the United States Medical Licensing Examinations, Step 1, Bklt. B. Mauricio L. Waintrub et al. 4th ed. 1998. (USMLE Ser.). (Illus.). 76p. (C). pap. text, stu. ed. 15.00 (1-884083-14-5) Maval Pub.

Preparation for the United States Medical Licensing Examinations. Mauricio W. Waintrub & Medical Education Board Staff. 3rd ed. 1995. 76p. (C). Step 2, Bklt. 2. pap. 15.00 (1-884083-58-7); Step 2, Bklt. 3. pap. 15.00 (1-884083-59-5) Maval Pub.

Preparation for the United States Medical Licensing Examinations, Step 3, Bklet. C. Mauricio L. Waintrub & Medical Education Board Staff. 3rd ed. 1995. 76p. (C). lib. bdg. 15.00 (1-884083-81-1) Maval Pub.

Preparation for the United States Medical Licensing Examinations. Mauricio L. Waintrub & Medical Education Board. 3rd ed. 1995. 76p. (C). Step 3, Bklt. C. lib. bdg. 15.00 (1-884083-83-8); Step 3, Bklt. A. lib. bdg. 15.00 (1-884083-80-3) Maval Pub.

Preparation for the United States Medical Licensing Examinations: English Test 1, Booklet 1. Mauricio W. Waintrub. 2nd ed. 1997. 44p. (C). pap. 15.00 incl. audio (1-884083-28-5) Maval Pub.

Preparation for the United States Medical Licensing Examinations: English Test 2, Booklet 2. Mauricio W. Waintrub. 2nd ed. 1997. 44p. (C). pap. 15.00 incl. audio (1-884083-29-3) Maval Pub.

Preparation for the United States Medical Licensing Examinations: English Test 3, Bklet. 3. Mauricio L. Waintrub. 2nd ed. 1997. 44p. (C). pap. 15.00 incl. audio (1-884083-30-7) Maval Pub.

Preparation for the USMLE: Step 1 Booklet C, Booklet C. Mauricio L. Waintrub et al. 4th ed. 1998. (USMLE Ser.). 76p. (C). pap. text 15.00 (1-884083-15-3) Maval Pub.

Preparation of Formula for Infants: Guidelines for Health Care Facilities. American Dietetic Association Staff et al. 1991. LC 91-26127. pap. 10.95 (0-88091-089-5, 0164) Am Dietetic Assn.

Preparation to Care: A Foundation NVQ Text for Health Care Assistants. Ed. by Aileen Richardson. 1995. (Illus.). 246p. pap. (0-7020-1793-0) W B Saunders GBR. *Dist:* Saunders.

Preparatory States & Processes. Ed. by Sylvan Kornblum & Jean Requin. 1984. 400p. text 79.95 (0-89859-325-5) L Erlbaum Assocs.

Prepare & Enjoy Creative Dental Retirement. Armen Z. Mesrobian. 1992. LC 92-81607. (Illus.). 196p. spiral bd. 29.95 (0-9632735-0-7) EPS Excel Pub.

Prepare for Surgery, Heal Faster: A Guide of Mind-Body Techniques. Peggy Huddleston. 1996. 276p. pap. 14.95 (0-9645757-4-4) Angel River Pr.

Preparing a Drug Information Response: Module 3. Kimberly A. Galt et al. 1995. (Clincial Skills Program Drug Information Ser.). (C). 50.00 (1-879907-55-0) Am Soc Hlth-Syst.

Preparing Adolescents for Life After Foster Care: The Central Role of Foster Parents. Ed. by Anthony N. Maluccio et al. 1990. pap. 24.95 (0-87868-433-6, 3526) Child Welfare.

Preparing & Passing the Primary FRCA. Steven M. Yentis. 2002. 320p. pap. 39.95 (0-7506-5220-9) Buttrwrth-Heinemann.

Preparing & Winning Medical Negligence: 1990 Supplement, Vol. 2. Cyril H. Wecht. 1992. (0-87473-724-9, 66054-10, MICHIE) LEXIS Pub.

Preparing for a Career in Medicine. Kent Shih. 1998. LC 98-67821. 142p. (0-9666809-0-1) Christ Med & Dental Assns.

Preparing for Birth with Yoga: Exercises for Pregnancy & Childbirth. Janet Balaskas. 1994. LC 94-27152. (Home Library of Alternative Medicine). (Illus.). 192p. pap. 18.95 (1-85230-431-6) Element MA.

Preparing for Childbirth: Relaxing for Labor, Learning for Life. Betty Parsons. 1997. LC 97-7177. (Illus.). 112p. pap. 9.95 (1-55561-128-1) Fisher Bks.

Preparing for Client Change in Rational Emotive Behavior Therapy. Dryden. 1994. 149p. pap. 32.95 (1-56593-511-X, 1180) Singular Publishing.

Preparing for Crises in the Schools: Manual for Building School Crisis Response Teams. Stephen E. Brock et al. 1995. LC 95-4474. (0-88422-156-3) Clinical Psych.

Preparing for FDA Pre-Approval Inspections. Ed. by Martin D. Hynes, III. 1998. LC 98-27750. (Drugs & the Pharmaceutical Sciences Ser.). (Illus.). 304p. text 165.00 (0-8247-0218-2, 0218-2) Dekker.

Preparing for Medical Practice Made Ridiculously Simple. Daniel Lichtstein. 1998. 70p. pap. text 12.95 (0-940780-38-0) MedMaster.

Preparing for Surgery: A Mind-Body Approach to Enhance Healing & Recovery. William W. Deardorff & John Reeves. 1997. LC 96-71159. 252p. pap. 17.95 (1-57224-071-7) New Harbinger.

Preparing for Your Deposition: A Comprehensive Guide to the Deposition Process for Physicians & Other Professionals. Raymond M. Fish et al. Ed. by Gregg Rogers. 2nd rev. ed. 1995. LC 94-9088. 160p. (C). 29.95 (1-878487-19-1, 5588M) Practice Mgmt Info.

Preparing Nursing Research for the 21st Century: Evolution, Methodologies, Challenges. Faye G. Abdellah & Eugene Levine. 1994. LC 94-6045. 288p. 39.95 (0-8261-8440-5) Springer Pub.

Preparing Orthopedic Disability Cases. Mikel A. Rothenberg. 5th ed. 1995. LC 98-51350. (Illus.). 820p. 150.00 (1-56706-983-5) Aspen Law.

Preparing the Pharmacy for a Joint Commission Survey. Charles P. Coe. 3rd ed. 1996. LC 97-132864. 185p. pap. 40.50 (1-879907-70-4); 4th rev. ed. 1998. LC 00-265544. 336p. pap. 69.00 (1-879907-86-0) Am Soc Hlth-Syst.

Preparing to Enter Medical School. Shailer A. Peterson. 1980. text 14.95 (0-13-697342-6, Spectrm) Hungry Minds.

Preparing to Sit for the PT Licensure Examination. Patricia R. Evans. 1999. LC 99-22839. 161p. pap. 29.95 (0-8036-0251-0) Davis Co.

Preparticipation Physical Evaluation. American Academy of Family Physicians Staff & Preparticipation Physical Evaluation Task Force. 2nd ed. 1996. LC 96-27879. text 29.95 (0-07-001627-5) McGraw.

Presbyopia Research: From Molecular Biology to Visual Adaptation. G. Obrecht & L. W. Stark. 1990. (Illus.). 318p. (C). text 85.00 (0-306-43659-0, Kluwer Plenum) Kluwer Academic.

Preschool Child: Assessment, Diagnosis, & Treatment. Paul V. Trad. 1989. LC 88-20731. (Child & Adolescent Mental Health Ser.). 672p. 275.00 (0-471-61757-1) Wiley.

Preschool Children with Special Health Care Needs. Mary T. Urbano. 1992. LC 91-5140. (Illus.). 240p. (Orig.). (C). pap. 34.95 (1-879105-41-1, 0225) Thomson Learn.

Preschool Issues in Autism. Ed. by Eric Schopler et al. 1993. LC 93-20597. (Current Issues in Autism Ser.). (Illus.). 294p. (C). 54.00 (0-306-44440-2, Plenum Trade) Perseus Pubng.

Preschool Screening: Identifying Young Children with Developmental & Educational Problems. Robert Lichtenstein & Harold Ireton. 1984. 336p. text 31.00 (0-8089-1625-4, 792532, Grune & Strat) Harcrt Hlth Sci Grp.

Preschoolers & Substance Abuse: Strategies for Prevention & Intervention. Pedro J. Lecca & Thomas D. Watts. 1993. LC 91-35921. 112p. pap. 14.95 (1-56024-235-3); 118p. lib. bdg. 39.95 (1-56024-234-5) Haworth Pr.

Preschoolers with Special Needs: Children-At-Risk or Who have Disabilities. Janet Lerner et al. 1998. LC 97-33961. 400p. 65.00 (0-205-26735-1) P-H.

Prescribed Drugs & the Alternative Practitioner: The Essential Guide. Stephen Gascoigne. 1992. pap. (1-85398-022-6) Ashgrove Pr GBR. *Dist:* Words Distrib.

Prescribed Usage. Roger Brown. Date not set. 19.95 (0-465-06271-7); pap. 18.00 (0-465-06270-9) Basic.

Prescriber. John Henrik Clarke. 11th ed. 1972. 382p. (C). pap. 31.95 (0-8464-1041-9) Beekman Pubs.

Prescriber. John Henrik Clarke. 1972. 109p. (0-85032-088-7) C W Daniel GBR. *Dist:* Natl Bk Netwk.

Prescriber. John Henrik Clarke. 1980. 29.00 (0-85032-050-X) St Mut.

Prescriber's Guide to Hormone Replacement Therapy. Ed. by M. I. Whitehead. 1998. LC 98-10869. (Illus.). 220p. lib. bdg. 115.95 (1-85070-974-2, Parthenon Pbng) CRC Pr.

Prescribing Hemodialysis: A Guide to Urea Modeling, No. 29. D. A. Depner. 1990. (Developments in Nephrology Ser.). (C). text 152.00 (0-7923-0833-6) Kluwer Academic.

Prescribing in General Practice. Ed. by Conrad M. Harris. 1995. (1-85775-042-X) Radcliffe Med Pr GBR. *Dist:* Balogh.

Prescribing in Pregnancy. Ed. by Peter Rubin. 2nd ed. 1995. 168p. (C). pap. text (0-7279-0949-5); 3rd ed. 2002. 198p. pap. text (0-7279-1449-9) BMJ Pub GBR. *Dist:* AIDC.

Prescribing in Primary Care. Ed. by Colin P. Bradley. 1998. (Oxford General Practice Ser.: No. 42). (Illus.). 228p. pap. text 52.95 (0-19-262687-6) OUP.

Prescribing Narcotics: Physician Implementation of Pain Management Guidelines. Patricia D. Salvato et al. 1998. LC 99-70499. (Illus.). 292p. pap. 169.95 (0-9665067-1-5) Prefer Pub Co.

Prescribing Our Future: Ethical Challenges in Genetic Counseling. Ed. by Dianne M. Bartels et al. 1993. LC 92-21469. 208p. pap. text 23.95 (0-202-30453-1); lib. bdg. 47.95 (0-202-30452-3) Aldine de Gruyter.

Prescribing the Price of Pharmaceuticals. W. Duncan Reekie. 1995. (Choice in Welfare Ser.: No. 26). 120p. pap. (0-255-36363-X) Inst Economic Affairs GBR. *Dist:* Coronet Bks.

Prescription & Over-the-Counter Dermatology Markets: An Analysis of U. S. Worldwide Revenues, 1995-2000. Feedback Research Services Staff. 1996. 127p. spiral bd. 495.00 (1-889713-00-7) Feedback Rsch.

***Prescription & Over-the-Counter Drugs.** Contrib. by Reader's Digest Editorial Staff. rev. ed. 2001. (Illus.). 896p. 39.95 (0-7621-0323-X) RD Assn.

Prescription Drug Abuse: The Hidden Epidemic; A Guide to Coping & Understanding. Rod Colvin. 1995. 196p. (Orig.). pap. 14.95 (1-886039-22-4) Addicus Bks.

Prescription Drug Abuse & Dependence: How Prescription Drug Abuse Contributes to the Drug Abuse Epidemic. Daniel P. Greenfield. Ed. by Ralph Slovenko. 1994. LC 94-30116. (American Series Behavioral Science & Law: No. 1088). (Illus.). 184p. (C). pap. 33.95 (0-398-05954-3); text 45.95 (0-398-05931-4) C C Thomas.

***Prescription Drug Addiction: The Hidden Epidemic.** Rod Colvin. 2001. LC 2001-4894. (Illus.). 200p. pap. 15.95 (1-886039-52-6) Addicus Bks.

***Prescription Drug Expenditures in 2000: The Upward Trend Continues.** Barry Leonard. 2001. (Illus.). 51p. (C). pap. text 15.00 (0-7567-1344-7) DIANE Pub.

Prescription Drug Market: International Perspectives & Challenges for the Future. Ed. by Christine Huttin & Nick Bosanquet. 1995. LC 92-16413. (Advanced Series in Management: Vol. 17). 308p. 108.00 (0-444-89559-0, North Holland) Elsevier.

Prescription Drug Prices: Price Gouging by Pharmaceutical Companies? 1993. (Illus.). 70p. (Orig.). (C). pap. text 30.00 (1-56806-217-6) DIANE Pub.

Prescription Drugs. Consumer Guide Editors. 1997. mass mkt. 7.99 (0-451-19240-0); 4th rev. ed. 1998. 1024p. pap. 8.99 (0-451-19435-7) NAL (Sig).

Prescription Drugs. Consumer Guide Editors. 1993. (Illus.). 384p. pap. 9.95 (1-56173-452-7, 4005200) Pubns Intl Ltd.

Prescription Drugs: An Indispensable Guide for People over 50. Brian S. Katcher. 1989. 400p. mass mkt. 4.95 (0-380-70670-9, Avon Bks) Morrow Avon.

***Prescription Drugs: Modernizing Medicare fro the 21st Century: Congressional Hearing.** Ed. by Michael Bilirakis. 2001. (Illus.). 155p. (C). reprint ed. pap. text 35.00 (0-7567-1195-9) DIANE Pub.

***Prescription Drugs: What We Know & Don't Know about Seniors' Access to Coverage: Congressional Hearing.** Ed. by Michael Bilirakis. 2001. 132p. (C). reprint ed. pap. text 30.00 (0-7567-1147-9) DIANE Pub.

Prescription Drugs & Medicaid: Automated Review Systems Can Help Promote Safety, Save Money. 1996. (Illus.). 31p. (Orig.). (C). pap. text 25.00 (0-7881-3468-X) DIANE Pub.

Prescription Drugs & Their Side Effects. Edward L. Stern. 1987. 192p. pap. 7.95 (0-399-51357-4) Berkley Pub.

Prescription Drugs for People over 50. Center for the Study of Pharmacy and Therapeutics for the Elderly Staff et al. 1997. LC 98-119623. 576p. (0-7853-2465-8) Pubns Intl Ltd.

Prescription Drugs over 40. Consumer Guide Editors. 1997. 400p. pap. 6.99 (0-451-19273-7, Sig) NAL.

***Prescription Drugs under Medicare: The Legacy of the Task Force on Prescription Drugs.** Ed. by Mickey C. Smith. 2001. LC 00-68834. (Journal of Research in Pharmaceutical Economics: Vol. 10, Nos. 2-4). (Illus.). 235p. 69.95 (0-7890-1306-1, Pharmctl Prods) Haworth Pr.

***Prescription Drugs under Medicare: The Legacy of the Task Force on Prescription Drugs.** Mickey C. Smith. 2000. LC 00-68834. (Journal of Research in Pharmaceutical Economics: Vol. 10, Nos. 2-4). (Illus.). 235p. pap. text 34.95 (0-7890-1307-X, Pharmctl Prods) Haworth Pr.

Prescription Filled. James R. Lincoln. 1981. LC 81-51752. (Illus.). 202p. 12.50 (0-88492-039-9) W S Sullwold.

Prescription for Addiction? The Arizona & California Medical Drug Use Initiatives: Congressional Hearing. Ed. by Orrin G. Hatch. 2000. (Illus.). 133p. pap. text 30.00 (0-7567-0063-9) DIANE Pub.

Prescription for Anger: Coping with Angry Feelings & Angry People. Gary D. Hankins. 1988. LC 88-19896. pap. 14.95 (0-943367-01-8) Princess Pub.

Prescription for Disaster: The Hidden Dangers in Your Medicine Cabinet. Thomas J. Moore. 1998. LC 97-47081. 272p. 25.00 (0-684-82998-3) S&S Trade.

Prescription for Health Care. John R. Krismer. 1996. 324p. (Orig.). pap. 17.95 (1-57502-113-7) Morris Pubng.

Prescription for Health Care Policy: The Case for Retargeting Tax Subsidies to Health Care. Walter M. Cadette. 1997. (Public Policy Briefs Ser.: Vol. 30). (Illus.). 40p. (Orig.). pap. text 3.00 (0-941276-23-6, Levy Econ Inst Bard) Bard Coll Pubns.

Prescription for Life: The Jason Winters Story, a Cancer Survivor. John Perkins. 1997. 290p. (Orig.). pap. 16.95 (1-57901-016-4) Intl Promotions.

Prescription for Preventing AIDS: Cure the Body Politic of Prejudice. Neal A. Dickerson. 1993. LC 93-5232. (Politics of AIDS Ser.: Vol. 3). (Illus.). xii, 183p. pap. 12.00 (0-930383-35-4) Monument Pr.

Prescription for Profit: How Doctors Defraud Medicaid. Paul Jesilow et al. 1993. LC 91-36944. 247p. 50.00 (0-520-07614-1) U CA Pr.

Prescription for Profits: How the Pharmaceutical Industry Bankrolled the Unholy Marriage between Science & State. Linda Marsa. 1997. LC 96-48440. 304p. 24.50 (0-684-80002-0, Macmillan Ref) Gale.

Prescription Medicide: The Goodness of Planned Death. Jack Kevorkian. 1991. LC 89-92751. (Illus.). 268p. 36.00 (0-87975-677-2); pap. 23.00 (0-87975-872-4) Prometheus Bks.

***Prescription Medicines Side Effects & Natural Alternatives.** Joseph Longfellow. 2001. 212p. pap. 19.95 (1-884350-76-3) Alpha Pubng.

Prescription Narcotics: The Addictive Painkillers. Michael Bunsey & Paul Sanberg. 1986. (Encyclopedia of Psychoactive Drugs Ser.: No. 1). (Illus.). 124p. (YA). (gr. 7 up). lib. bdg. 19.95 (0-87754-770-X) Chelsea Hse.

Prescription Pads. Travell. 1992. pap. text 23.95 (0-683-17536-X) Lppncott W & W.

Prescription Privileges for Psychologist: A Critical Appraisal. Ed. by Steven C. Hayes & Elaine M. Heiby. 1998. LC 98-39199. 282p. (C). 34.95 (1-878978-30-6) Context Pr.

Prescription Writing. A. Mukherji. 1989. (C). (0-89771-356-7) Current Dist IND. *Dist:* St Mut.

Prescriptions: The Dissemination of Medical Authority, 27. Ed. by Gayle L. Ormiston & Raphael Sassower. 1990. LC 89-17183. (Contributions in Medical Studies Ser.: No. 27). 200p. 57.50 (0-313-26625-5, OPR/, Greenwood Pr) Greenwood.

Prescriptions for Child Mental Health. Goldstein. 1978. (C). 52.95 (0-205-14356-3, H4356); pap. 25.95 (0-205-14355-5, H4355) Allyn.

Prescriptions for Child Mental Health & Education. Arnold P. Goldstein. 1978. text 80.00 (0-08-022250-1); pap. text 25.00 (0-08-022249-8) Elsevier (Pergamon Pr).

Prescriptions for Children with Learning & Adjustment Problems: A Consultant's Desk Reference. Ralph F. Blanco & David F. Bogacki. 3rd ed. 1988. 264p. 45.95 (0-398-05390-1) C C Thomas.

Prescriptions for Good Taste. Walgreen Drug Stores Historical Foundation Staff. 1995. 464p. 19.95 (0-9648458-0-6) Walgrn Drug.

Prescriptions for Life with Cancer. Eric Fairbank. 1996. pap. text (0-85572-269-X) Hill Content Pubng AUS. *Dist:* Seven Hills Bk.

Prescriptive Seating for Wheeled Mobility: Theory, Application, & Terminology, Vol. I. Diane E. Ward. 1994. LC 93-78396. (Illus.). 214p. per. 43.95 (0-9614029-1-1) Healthwealth.

Presence in the Flesh: The Body in Medicine. Katharine G. Young. 1997. LC 96-39721. (Illus.). 224p. 30.00 (0-674-70181-X) HUP.

P Q R

Presence of Care: The History of St. Luke's Hospital. Edward T. Matheny, Jr. Ed. by Frederic J. Hron. 1997. (Illus.). 456p. 24.95 (*0-9657425-0-4*) St Lukes Hosp.

Presence of Caring in Nursing. Ed. by Delores A. Gaut. 1992. 292p. (C). pap. text 12.95 (*0-88737-547-2*) Natl League Nurse.

Presence of Mind: Literary & Philosophical Roots of a Wise Psychotherapy. Stephen Schoen. 1993. 312p. 28.50 (*0-939266-19-9*) Gestalt Journal.

Presenilins & Alzheimer's Disease. Ed. by S. G. Youkin et al. 1998. LC 97-52014. (Research & Perspectives in Alzheimer's Disease Ser.). (Illus.). 116p. 99.00 (*3-540-63997-7*) Spr-Verlag.

Present & Future Aspects in Endocrinology: Thirteenth International Symposium on Endocrinology & Development, Rome, October 1994. Ed. by A. Attansio & S. Bernasconi. 1995. (Journal: Vol. 43, No. 4, 1995). (Illus.). 60p. pap. 47.00 (*3-8055-6139-3*) S Karger.

Present & Future of Prevention: Essays in Honor of George W. Albee. Marc Kessler et al. 1992. LC 92-2244. (Primary Prevention of Psychopathology Ser.: Vol. 15). 288p. (C). 74.95 (*0-8039-4590-6*, 3935) Sage.

Present & Future Role of Monoclonal Antibodies in the Management of Cancer: 24th Annual San Francisco Cancer Symposium, San Francisco, Calif., February 1989. Ed. by J. M. Vaeth & J. L. Meyer. 1990. (Frontiers of Radiation Therapy & Oncology Ser.: Vol. 24). (Illus.). x, 266p. 221.00 (*3-8055-5029-4*) S Karger.

Present-Day Concepts in the Treatment of Chronic Renal Failure: Dialysis & Transplantation. Ed. by J. E. Traeger et al. 1989. (Contributions to Nephrology Ser.: Vol. 71). (Illus.). viii, 184p. 29.75 (*3-8055-4946-6*) S Karger.

Present State of Leptospirosis Diagnosis & Control. Ed. by W. A. Ellis & T. W. Little. 1986. (Current Topics in Veterinary Medicine & Animal Science Ser.). text 145.50 (*0-89838-777-9*) Kluwer Academic.

Present State of Thoracic Surgery. Ed. by J. A. Dyde & R. E. Smih. 1981. 300p. pap. 59.00 (*0-8464-1218-7*) Beekman Pubs.

Present Status of Non-Toxic Concepts in Cancer. Ed. by K. F. Klippel & E. Macher. 1987. (Illus.). xii, 288p. pap. 61.75 (*3-8055-4437-5*) S Karger.

Presentation of Clinical Data. Bert Spilker & John Schoenfelder. 1989. 576p. text 110.00 (*0-88167-566-0*, 2035) Lppncott W & W.

Presenter's Survival Kit: It's a Jungle Out There. Lori Backer. 1994. LC 95-171568. 432p. (C). (gr. 13). spiral bd. 28.95 (*0-8151-0373-5*, 26258) Mosby Inc.

Presenting Past: The Core of Psychodynamic Counselling & Therapy. Michael Jacobs. 2nd ed. 1998. LC 98-18440. xii, 242p. (*0-335-20197-0*); pap. (*0-335-20196-2*) OpUniv Pr.

Presenting the Past: Psychoanalysis & Sociology of Misremembering. Jeffrey Prager. 1999. LC 97-49904. 240p. text 32.50 (*0-674-56641-6*) HUP.

Preservation & Restoration of Tooth Structure. Graham J. Mount & W. R. Hume. 1998. (Illus.). 384p. 81.00 (*0-7234-3102-7*) Mosby Inc.

Preservation & Restoration of Tooth Structure. Graham J. Mount & W. R. Hume. 2nd ed. 1998. (Illus.). 384p. (*84-8174-390-9*) Mosby-Doyma Libros ESP. *Dist:* Mosby Inc.

Preservation of Fruits & Vegtables Foods Products. S. D. Holdsworth. 1984. (Science in Horticulture Ser.). (Illus.). 171p. (C). pap. text 35.00 (*0-333-32292-4*) Scholium Intl.

Preservation of the Self in the Oldest Years: With Implications for Practice. Sheldon S. Tobin. 2nd ed. 1999. LC 98-31378. 256p. 41.95 (*0-8261-7581-3*) Springer Pub.

Preserve Your Love for Science: Life of William Hammond, American Neurologist. Bonnie E. Blustein. 1991. (History of Medicine Ser.). (Illus.). 301p. (C). text 85.00 (*0-521-39262-4*) Cambridge U Pr.

Preserving Dignity for People in Your Care. Suzanne A. Rymer. 2000. LC 00-709005. (Illus.). 76p. pap. 29.95 (*1-888343-32-X*) Hartman Pub.

Presidential Advisory Committee on Gulf War Veterans' Illnesses: Final Report. Ed. by Joyce C. Laslof et al. 1997. (Illus.). 174p. (Orig.). pap. text 40.00 (*0-7881-4271-2*) DIANE Pub.

Presidential Advisory Committee on Gulf War Veterans' Illnesses: Interim Report. 1996. 60p. (Orig.). pap. text 30.00 (*0-7881-3279-2*) DIANE Pub.

Presidential Forum: Citizens with Mental Retardation & Community Integration. 1988. 250p. (*1-55672-036-X*) US HHS.

President's Cancer Panel Meeting: Evaluating the National Cancer Program: Transcript of Proceedings, September 22, 1993. 1995. 281p. (Orig.). (C). pap. text 50.00 (*0-7881-1951-6*) DIANE Pub.

President's Commission for the Study of Ethical Problems in Medicine & Biomedical & Behavioral Research, Set. Ed. by President's Commission for the Study of Ethical Pr. 1997. LC 97-80015. reprint ed. 595.00 (*1-57588-391-0*, 311430) W S Hein.

***Presidents of the Royal Society of Medicine.** J. H. Moll. (History of Medicine Ser.). (Illus.). 552p. (*1-85315-264-1*); lthr. (*1-85315-265-X*) Royal Soc of Medicine Pr Ltd GBR. *Dist:* Balogh.

***President's Proposal to Reform Medicare: Congressional Hearing.** Ed. by William V. Roth, Jr. 2001. (Illus.). 147p. (C). reprint ed. pap. 30.00 (*0-7567-0986-5*) DIANE Pub.

Pressure at Work. Tanya Arroba & Kim James. 1989. 208p. pap. 11.95 (*0-07-084931-5*) McGraw.

Pressure Point Therapy: The Complete Do-It-Yourself. Michael Pinkus. 1994. LC 94-94008. (At Home Treatment Manual Ser.). (Illus.). 58p. (Orig.). pap. 29.90 (*0-9640393-0-3*) Alternat Hlth.

Pressure Point Therapy System: The Complete Book, Video & Chart Pack. Michael Pinkus. 1995. (Illus.). 65p. pap. 79.90 incl. VHS (*0-9640393-3-8*) Alternat Hlth.

Pressure Points. Peggy Overstein. 1999. (*0-679-45288-5*) McKay.

Pressure Sore Prevention. Dickson Weir-Hughes et al. 1996. (Illus.). 118p. (Orig.). pap. 24.95 (*1-56593-818-6*, 1608) Singular Publishing.

Pressure Sores. Jenny Phillips. 1997. LC 97-17573. (Access to Clinical Education Ser.). text (*0-443-05532-7*) Church.

Pressure Sores: Clinical Practice & Scientific Approach. Ed. by Dan Bader. 1989. text 74.00 (*0-333-48628-5*) Intl Spec Bk.

Pressure Ulcer in Adults. 1995. lib. bdg. 251.95 (*0-8490-6778-2*) Gordon Pr.

Pressure Ulcers: Guidelines for Prevention & Management. JoAnn Maklebust & Mary Sieggreen. 3rd ed. 2000. LC 00-44625. (Illus.). xiv, 322p. 39.95 (*1-58255-035-2*) Springhouse Corp.

Pressure Ulcers: Principles & Techniques of Management. Ed. by Mark B. Constantian. 1980. 320p. text 50.00 (*0-316-15330-3*, Little Brwn Med Div) Lppncott W & W.

Pressure Ulcers in Adults: Prediction & Prevention. 1994. (Illus.). 73p. (Orig.). (C). pap. text 20.00 (*0-7881-0469-1*) DIANE Pub.

Presurgical Evaluation of Epileptics. Ed. by H. G. Wieser & C. E. Elger. 1987. (Illus.). 389p. 206.00 (*0-387-16344-1*) Spr-Verlag.

Presurgical Psychological Screening in Chronic Pain Syndromes: A Guide for the Behavioral Health Practitioner. Andrew R. Block. 1996. LC 96-18082. 150p. 49.95 (*0-8058-2407-3*); pap. 24.50 (*0-8058-2408-1*) L Erlbaum Assocs.

Presynadtic Receptors: Proceedings of the Satellite Symposium, Paris, July 22-23 1978, 7th International Congress of Pharmacology. S. Z. Langer et al. 1979. (Illus.). 340p. 69.50 (*0-08-023190-X*, Pergamon Pr) Elsevier.

Presynaptic Receptors & Neuronal Transporters: Proceedings of the Official Satellite Symposium to the IUPHAR 1990 Congress Held in Rouen, France, 26-29 June 1990. Ed. by S. Z. Langer et al. 1992. (Advances in the Biosciences Ser.: No. 82). (Illus.). 372p. 181.50 (*0-08-041165-7*, Pergamon Pr) Elsevier.

Pretend Play Among Three-Year-Olds. Mira Stambak & Hermine Sinclair. 1993. 144p. text 39.95 (*0-8058-1243-1*) L Erlbaum Assocs.

Preterm Labor. M. G. Elder et al. 1997. LC 97-18582. text (*0-443-05857-1*) Church.

Preterm Labor: Prevention & Nursing Management. Margaret Comerford Freda & Ellen T. Patterson. Ed. by Karla Damus. 1994. (*0-86525-062-6*) March of Dimes.

Preterm Prelabour Amniorrhexis. S. G. Carroll et al. 1995. LC 95-15963. (Frontiers in Fetal Medicine Ser.). (Illus.). 176p. lib. bdg. 71.95 (*1-85070-692-1*, C1302, Parthenon Pbng) CRC Pr.

Pretest & Review for Acupuncture Examination. Sidong Chen. Ed. by Sidong Chen & Elizabeth Jones. 1995. (Illus.). 275p. (C). pap. text 109.00 (*0-9645339-0-1*) Dr Chens.

Pretest, EMT-Intermediate. Richard E. Westfal. 1998. LC 98-36143. (Pretest Clincial Science Ser.). (Illus.). 168p. pap. 29.95 (*0-07-069636-5*) McGraw-Hill Prof.

Pretest Step 2 Simulated Exam. Ed. by John R. Thornborough. 1992. (Pretest Simulated Exam Ser.). (Illus.). 176p. text 30.00 (*0-07-064521-3*) McGraw-Hill Med Pub.

Pretty-Shield: Medicine Woman of the Crows. Frank B. Linderman. 1973. LC 72-3273. (Illus.). 256p. reprint ed. pap. 10.95 (*0-8032-5791-0*, Bison Books) U of Nebr Pr.

Prevalence & Characteristics of Persons with Hearing Trouble: United States, 1990-91. 1993. LC 93-4737. (Vital & Health Statistics Ser. 10: Data from the National Health Interview Survey: No. 188). (*0-8406-0483-1*) Natl Ctr Health Stats.

Prevalence of Back Pain in Great Britain in 1996: A Report on Research for the Department of Health Using the ONS Omnibus Survey. Tricia Dodd. 1997. (Omnibus Survey Publications Report: No. OS 8). 15p. (*0-11-620968-2*) Statnry Office GBR. *Dist:* Balogh.

Prevalence of Psychiatric Morbidity among Adults Living in Private Households Report 1: OPCS Surveys of Psychiatric Morbidity in Great Britain. Howard Meltzer. 1995. xii, 174p. (*0-11-691627-3*, HM16273) Statnry Office GBR. *Dist:* Bernan Associates, Balogh.

Prevalence of Selected Chronic Conditions: United States, 1986-88. U. S. Department of Health & Human Services Staff et al. 1992. LC 92-38011. (*0-8406-0472-6*) Natl Ctr Health Stats.

Prevalence of Selected Chronic Conditions: United States, 1990-1992. John Gary Collins. 1996. LC 96-50061. (Vital & Health Statistics Ser.: Series 10, No. 194). (*0-8406-0522-6*) Natl Ctr Health Stats.

Prevent Cancer Now. Michael Colgan. 2nd ed. 1992. (Illus.). 140p. pap. text 9.95 (*0-9624840-3-2*, C I Pubns CA) Colgan Inst.

Prevent Cancer Now! Arm Yourself with Powerful Weapons Against Cancer. Michael Colgan. 2000. 140p. pap. text (*1-896817-07-6*) ApPubng.

Prevent Cancer Now: Your Guide to Self Protection, 2nd Edition. Michael Colgan. 1992. (Illus.). 140p. 19.50 (*0-9624840-2-4*) Colgan Inst.

Prevent Gas on Stomach. Max. 1997. (Illus.). 50p. pap. 40.00 (*0-922070-89-X*) M Tecton Pub.

Prevent Hemorrhoids/How To. Max. 1997. 50p. pap. 32.00 (*0-922070-36-9*) M Tecton Pub.

Prevent the Common Cold: It's Ridiculous to Catch a Cold in This Modern Age. Max. 1997. 50p. pap. 40.00 (*0-922070-34-2*) M Tecton Pub.

Prevent Tooth Decay. Max. 1997. 50p. pap. 40.00 (*0-922070-42-3*) M Tecton Pub.

Preventative Health Care in Companion Animals. Ed. by Caroline Jevring & Thomas E. Catanzaro. 1998. (Illus.). 255p. pap. (*0-7020-2393-0*) W B Saunders.

Preventative Management of Children with Congenital Anomalies & Syndromes. Golder N. Wilson & W. Carl Cooley. 2000. LC 99-40520. (Illus.). 566p. (C). pap. text 74.95 (*0-521-77673-2*) Cambridge U Pr.

Preventing a Crisis: AIDS & Family Planning Work. Gill Gordon & Tony Klouda. rev. ed. 1989. (Illus.). 200p. reprint ed. pap. text 12.00 (*0-333-51721-0*) Scholium Intl.

Preventing Adolescent Drug Abuse: From Theory to Practice. 1992. lib. bdg. 88.00 (*0-8490-8819-4*) Gordon Pr.

Preventing Adverse Events in Behavioral Health Care: A Systems Approach to Sentinel Events. Joint Commission on Accreditation of Healthcare Organizations. 1999. LC 99-73029. (Illus.). 254p. pap. 45.00 (*0-86688-640-0*, BHSE-50) Joint Comm Hlthcare.

Preventing AIDS: A Guide to Effective Education for the Prevention of HIV Infection. Nicholas Freudenberg. 1989. 236p. 28.50 (*0-87553-166-0*) Am Pub Health.

Preventing AIDS.. A Practical Guide for Everyone. Joseph F. Benza, Jr. & Ralph D. Zumwalde. 1987. 85p. (Orig.). 18.95 (*0-9617818-0-7*) Jalsco Inc.

Preventing AIDS: A Programmatic Perspective. Ed. by Ronald O. Valdiserri. 1989. LC 88-36573. 350p. (C). text 38.00 (*0-8135-1433-9*); pap. text 17.00 (*0-8135-1434-7*) Rutgers U Pr.

Preventing AIDS: A Sourcebook for Behavioral Interventions. Seth C. Kalichman. 1998. LC 97-39257. 275p. (*0-8058-2490-1*); pap. (*0-8058-2491-X*) L Erlbaum Assocs.

Preventing AIDS: Theories & Methods of Behavioral Interventions. Ed. by Ralph J. DiClemente & J. L. Peterson. 1994. (AIDS Prevention & Mental Health Ser.). (Illus.). 356p. (C). text 59.00 (*0-306-44606-5*, Kluwer Plenum) Kluwer Academic.

Preventing AIDS among Industrial Workers in India: Special Reference to the Third World Countries. R. M. Kalra. 1999. LC 98-917866. 108 p. (*81-259-0275-9*) S Asia.

Preventing AIDS in Drug Users & Their Sexual Partners. James L. Sorensen et al. 1991. LC 91-24707. (Substance Abuse Ser.). 220p. 28.95 (*0-89862-173-9*) Guilford Pubns.

Preventing Alcohol & Tobacco Problems: Manipulating Consumption: Information, Law & Voluntary Controls, Vol. 2. Ed. by Christine Godfrey & David Robinson. 1990. (Illus.). 226p. text (*0-566-05702-6*) Avebry GBR. *Dist:* Ashgate Pub Co.

Preventing Alcohol & Tobacco Problems: The Addiction Market: Consumption, Production & Policy Development, Vol. 1. Ed. by Alan Maynard & Philip Tether. 1990. (Illus.). 270p. text (*0-566-05701-8*) Avebry GBR. *Dist:* Ashgate Pub Co.

Preventing & Controlling Cancer in North America: A Cross-Cultural Perspective. Diane Weiner. 1999. LC 99-19202. (Illus.). 264p. 72.50 (*0-275-96180-X*, Praeger Pubs) Greenwood.

Preventing & Controlling Drug Abuse. M. Gossop & M. Grant. 1990. 138p. 24.00 (*92-4-156134-3*) World Health.

Preventing & Controlling Iron Deficiency Anaemia through Primary Health Care: A Guide for Health Administrators & Programme Managers. E. DeMaeyer & P. Dallman. 1989. 58p. 11.00 (*92-4-154249-7*) World Health.

Preventing & Mitigating AIDS in Sub-Saharan Africa: Research & Data Priorities for the Social & Behavioral Science. National Research Council Staff. Ed. by Barney Cohen & James Trussell. 1996. LC 96-11347. 368p. (Orig.). pap. text 39.00 (*0-309-05480-X*) Natl Acad Pr.

Preventing & Reversing Osteoporosis: Every Woman's Essential Guide. Alan Gaby. 1995. 320p. pap. 15.95 (*0-7615-0022-7*, Prima Health) Prima Pub.

Preventing & Treating Carpal Tunnel Syndrome. Roger Williams. 1994. LC 95-135684. (Illus.). 32p. pap. text 6.00 (*1-56900-012-3*) Am Occup Therapy.

Preventing Antisocial Behavior: Interventions from Birth Through Adolescence. Ed. by Joan McCord & Richard E. Tremblay. 1992. LC 92-1444. 391p. 50.00 (*0-89862-882-2*, 2882) Guilford Pubns.

***Preventing Arthritis: A Holistic Approach to Life Without Pain.** Ronald Melvin Lawrence & Martin Zucker. 2001. LC 00-68857. (Illus.). 272p. 22.95 (*0-399-14742-X*) Penguin Putnam.

Preventing Breast Cancer: The Politics of an Epidemic. Cathy Read. 1995. LC 98-212239. 264p. pap. text 13.00 (*0-04-440909-5*) NYU Pr.

Preventing Breast Cancer: The Story of a Major, Proven, Preventable Cause of This Disease. John W. Gofman. 2nd ed. 1996. LC 96-2453. (Illus.). 422p. (Orig.). pap. 17.00 (*0-932682-96-0*) Comm Nuclear Respon.

Preventing Cancers. Ed. by Tom Heller et al. 1992. 208p. (*0-335-19004-9*) OpUniv.

Preventing Cancers. Ed. by Tom Heller et al. 1992. 208p. pap. (*0-335-19003-0*) OpUniv Pr GBR. *Dist:* Taylor & Francis.

Preventing Caregiver Burnout. James R. Sherman. Ed. by Merlene T. Sherman & Christopher J. Sherman. 1994. (Illus.). 80p. (Orig.). pap. 9.95 (*0-935538-16-X*) Pathway Bks.

Preventing Childhood Disorders, Substance Abuse, & Delinquency. Ray D. Peters & Robert J. McMahon. 1996. LC 96-4477. (Banff International Behavioral Science Ser.: Vol. 3). (Illus.). 344p. 86.95 (*0-7619-0014-4*, 1537) Sage.

Preventing Childhood Disorders, Substance Abuse, & Delinquency. Ed. by Ray D. Peters & Robert J. McMahon. 1996. LC 96-4477. (Banff International Behavioral Science Ser.: Vol. 3). (Illus.). 344p. pap. 37.95 (*0-7619-0015-2*, 1538) Sage.

Preventing Childhood Eating Problems. Jane R. Hirschmann & Lela Zaphiropoulos. 3rd ed. 1993. LC 89-91514. 176p. pap. 10.95 (*0-936077-25-5*) Gurze Bks.

Preventing Computer Injury: The HAND Book with KeyMoves Software. Stephanie Brown. 1993. 100p. pap. 49.95 incl. 3.5 hd (*1-884388-01-9*) Ergonome.

Preventing Coronary Heart Disease: The Role of Antioxidants, Vegetables & Fruit. TSO Staff. 1997. 86p. pap. (*0-11-322001-4*, HM20014) Statnry Office GBR. *Dist:* Bernan Associates.

Preventing Diabetes: Theory, Practice & New Approaches. Dan Cheta. 1999. LC 99-14783. (Illus.). 198p. 80.00 (*0-471-99914-8*) Wiley.

Preventing Disability in the Elderly: Report on a WHO Working Group. 1982. (Euro Reports & Studies Ser.: No. 65). 55p. pap. text 4.00 (*92-890-1231-5*) World Health.

Preventing Disease: Beyond the Rhetoric. Ed. by R. B. Goldbloom & R. S. Lawrence. 1991. (Frontiers of Primary Care Ser.). (Illus.). 478p. 69.00 (*0-387-97063-0*) Spr-Verlag.

Preventing Drug Abuse: What Do We Know? National Research Council Staff. Ed. by Dean R. Gerstein & Lawrence W. Green. 1993. LC 93-7333. 176p. text 32.95 (*0-309-04627-0*) Natl Acad Pr.

Preventing Elderly Suicide: Overcoming Personal Despair, Professional Indifference, & Social Bias. Joseph Richman. 1993. LC 92-35995. (Death & Suicide Ser.: Vol. 11). 176p. 29.95 (*0-8261-7480-9*) Springer Pub.

Preventing Falls: A Defensive Approach. J. Thomas Hutton. 2000. LC 99-40082. pap. 22.00 incl. VHS (*1-57392-762-7*); (Illus.). 145p. pap. 19.00 (*1-57392-761-9*) Prometheus Bks.

Preventing Falls in the Elderly. Kathlene Benson. 2000. (Illus.). 77p. pap. 29.95 (*1-888343-28-1*) Hartman Pub.

Preventing Family Violence. Kevin Browne & Martin Herbert. LC 96-28875. (Family Psychology Ser.). 402p. 1999. pap. 35.00 (*0-471-94140-9*); 1997. 135.00 (*0-471-92771-6*) Wiley.

Preventing Heart Disease: What Every Woman Should Know. Rita Baron-Faust. 2000. 280p. text 20.00 (*0-7881-9141-1*) DIANE Pub.

Preventing Heat Stress & Human Heat Strain: Recognition, Evaluation, & Control. Roger L. Wabeke. 1998. LC 98-18177. (*1-885581-16-5*) ASSE.

Preventing HIV in Developing Countries: Biomedical & Behavioral Approaches. Ed. by L. Gibney et al. 1999. LC 98-44310. (AIDS Prevention & Mental Health Ser.). (Illus.). 424p. (C). text 75.00 (*0-306-45961-2*, Kluwer Plenum) Kluwer Academic.

Preventing HIV Transmission: The Role of Sterile Needles & Bleach. Institute of Medicine Staff. Ed. by Jacques Normand et al. 1995. LC 95-35458. 352p. 37.95 (*0-309-05296-3*) Natl Acad Pr.

Preventing Illness among People with Coronary Heart Disease. Ed. by John D. Piette et al. 1996. LC 96-27430. (Prevention & Intervention in the Community Ser.: Vol. 13, Nos. 1/2). 200p. (C). 34.95 (*0-7890-0006-7*) Haworth Pr.

Preventing Injury & Death of Firefighters. 1995. lib. bdg. 251.99 (*0-8490-6679-4*) Gordon Pr.

Preventing Lead Poisoning in Young Children. 1993. (Illus.). 107p. (Orig.). (C). pap. text 30.00 (*0-7881-0076-9*) DIANE Pub.

Preventing Low Birthweight. Institute of Medicine Staff. 1985. 296p. pap. text 27.95 (*0-309-03530-9*) Natl Acad Pr.

Preventing Low Birthweight: Summary. Institute of Medicine Staff. 1985. 41p. (C). pap. text 5.00 (*0-309-03535-X*) Natl Acad Pr.

Preventing Maladjustment from Infancy Through Adolescence. Annette U. Rickel & La Rue Allen. 1988. (Developmental Clinical Psychology & Psychiatry Ser.: Vol. 11). 160p. 74.95 (*0-8039-2868-8*, 5953); pap. 34.95 (*0-8039-2869-6*, 5954) Sage.

Preventing Malpractice: The Co-Active Solution. T. L. Leaman & J. W. Saxton. 1993. (Illus.). 254p. (C). text 39.50 (*0-306-44441-0*, Kluwer Plenum) Kluwer Academic.

Preventing Maternal Deaths. E. Royston & S. Armstrong. 1989. 233p. 40.00 (*92-4-156128-9*) World Health.

Preventing Medical Malpractice Suits: A Handbook for Doctors & Those Who Work with Them. James E. Schutte. 1995. LC 94-78608. (Illus.). 230p. text 39.00 (*0-88937-135-0*) Hogrefe & Huber Pubs.

Preventing Mental Illness. Jennifer Newton. 1988. 272p. text 65.00 (*0-7102-0930-4*, Routledge Thoemms) Routledge.

Preventing Mental Illness: Mental Health Promotion in Primary Care. Rachel Jenkins et al. 1998. LC 97-16272. 518p. 175.00 (*0-471-97562-1*) Wiley.

Preventing Miscarriage: The Good News. Jonathan Scher & Carol Dix. 1991. LC 89-45063. (Illus.). 256p. reprint ed. pap. 13.00 (*0-06-092056-4*, Perennial) HarperTrade.

Preventing Misdiagnosis of Women: A Guide to Physical Disorders That Have Psychiatric Symptoms. Elizabeth A. Klonoff & Hope Landrine. 1997. LC 96-25183. (Women's Mental Health & Development Ser.: Vol. 1). 190p. 86.95 (*0-7619-0046-2*, 1659) Sage.

Preventing Misdiagnosis of Women: A Guide to Recognizing Physiological Disorders That Have Psychiatric Symptoms. Elizabeth A. Klonoff & Hope Landrine. 1997. LC 96-25183. (Women's Mental Health & Development Ser.: Vol. 1). 190p. pap. 32.95 (*0-7619-0047-0*, 1660) Sage.

Preventing Occupational Disease & Injury. Ed. by James L. Weeks et al. 1991. 750p. 28.50 (*0-87553-172-5*) Am Pub Health.

Preventing Organic Dust Toxic Syndrome. 1995. lib. bdg. 251.75 (*0-8490-6678-6*) Gordon Pr.

Preventing Patient Falls. Janice M. Morse. 1996. 200p. 61.95 (*0-7619-0592-8*, 80611); pap. 31.95 (*0-7619-0593-6*, 80612) Sage.

Preventing Physical & Emotional Abuse of Children. David A. Wolfe. 1991. LC 91-24679. (Treatment Manuals for Practitioners Ser.). 168p. 49.95 (*0-89862-208-5*); pap. 21.00 (*0-89862-219-0*, 2219) Guilford Pubns.

Preventing Prenatal Harm: Should the State Intervene? Deborah R. Mathieu. 2nd ed. 1996. LC 95-36923. (Clinical Medical Ethics Ser.). 208p. pap. 19.95 (*0-87840-600-X*) Georgetown U Pr.

Preventing Prenatal Harm: Should the State Intervene? Deborah R. Mathieu. 1991. 168p. lib. bdg. (*0-7923-0984-7*) Kluwer Academic NLD. *Dist:* Kluwer Academic.

Preventing Pressure Ulcers: A Patient's Guide. 1994. lib. bdg. 250.00 (*0-8490-8407-5*) Gordon Pr.

Preventing Reactive Hypoglycemia: The Great Dilemma. Fred D. Hofeldt. 1983. 144p. 18.50 (*0-87527-214-2*) Green.

Preventing Relapse in the Addictions: A Biopsychosocial Approach. Emil Chiauzzi. 1991. (Psychology Practitioner Guidebooks Ser.). 192p. text (*0-08-037919-2*); pap. text (*0-08-037918-4*) PPI GBR. *Dist:* Elsevier.

Preventing Substance Abuse among Children & Adolescents. Jean E. Rhodes & Leonard Jason. 1988. 160p. text 30.00 (*0-08-035753-9*); pap. text 15.95 (*0-08-035752-0*) Elsevier (Pergamon Pr).

Preventing Teenage Pregnancy: What Educators Need to Know. 1994. 49p. (Orig.). pap. text 20.00 (*1-56806-162-5*) DIANE Pub.

Preventing Teenage Suicide: The Living Alternative Handbook. Polly Joan. 1985. LC 84-27872. (Illus.). 153p. 30.95 (*0-89885-247-1*); pap. 18.95 (*0-89885-349-4*) Kluwer Academic (Kluwer Acad Hman Sci).

Preventing TMJ & OS6's Injuries in Dental Practice. Reda A. Abdel-Fattah. 1993. 352p. 207.00 (*0-8493-4725-4*) CRC Pr.

Preventing Tobacco Use Among Young People: A Report of the Surgeon General 1994. (Illus.). 326p. pap. text 60.00 (*1-57979-061-5*) DIANE Pub.

Preventing Tobacco Use Among Young People: A Report of the Surgeon General. M. Jocelyn Elders. 1994. (Illus.). 314p. (Orig.). (C). pap. text 50.00 (*0-7881-0569-8*) DIANE Pub.

Preventing Unknown Barriers from Creeping into Your Treatment. Mary-Kim Arnold. 1995. (Orig.). pap. 39.95 (*1-884937-32-2*) Manisses Communs.

Preventing Youth Suicide. Sandra McKillop. 1992. (Australian Institute Conference Proceedings Ser.: Vol. 13). pap. (*0-642-17512-8*) Aust Inst Criminology AUS. *Dist:* Advent Bks Div.

Prevention: Basic & Clinical Aspects. Ed. by G. Nikiforuk. 1985. (Understanding Dental Caries Ser.: Vol. 2). (Illus.). xiv, 290p. 50.50 (*3-8055-3905-3*) S Karger.

Prevention: The Michigan Experience. Ed. by Betty Tableman & Robert Hess. 1985. LC 85-8071. (Prevention in Human Services Ser.: Vol. 3, No. 4). 121p. text 29.95 (*0-86656-458-6*) Haworth Pr.

Prevention Across the Life Span: Healthy People for the Twenty-First Century. Ed. by Ruth N. Knollmueller. 1994. 120p. (C). pap. text 14.95 (*1-55810-091-1*, CH-27) Am Nurses Pub.

Prevention & Care of Pressure Sores. Jetta Fuzy. 1997. (Illus.). 68p. pap. 29.95 (*1-888343-05-2*) Hartman Pub.

Prevention & Control of Aggression Principles, Practices & Research. Center for Research of Aggression Staff. 1983. 384p. 75.00 (*0-08-029375-1*, Pergamon Pr) Elsevier.

Prevention & Control of Cardiovascular Diseases. 1995. (EMRO Technical Publications, Eastern Mediterranean Ser.: Vol. 22). 65p. (Orig.). pap. 5.00 (*92-9021-205-5*, 1450022) World Health.

Prevention & Control of Nosocomial Infections. Richard P. Wenzel. 2nd ed. 1992. LC 92-18119. (Illus.). 1072p. 115.00 (*0-683-08921-8*); 3rd ed. 1997. LC 96-17731. 1,000p. text 149.00 (*0-683-08916-1*) Lppncott W & W.

Prevention & Control of Yellow Fever in Africa. 1986. 99p. pap. text 17.00 (*92-4-156091-6*, 1150242) World Health.

Prevention & Cure: The London School of Hygiene & Tropical Medicine, a 20th Century Quest. Lise Wilkinson & Anne Hardy. 2000. LC 99-22748. (Illus.). 350p. (*0-7103-0624-5*) Kegan Paul Intl GBR. *Dist:* Col U Pr.

Prevention & Detection of Gynecologic & Breast Cancer. Istvan Nyirjesy. 1994. 150p. pap. text (*0-9642179-0-2*) Intl Fnd Gynecol.

Prevention & Early Detection of Colorectal Cancer. Ed. by Graeme P. Young et al. 1996. (Illus.). 399p. text (*0-7020-2018-4*) W B Saunders GBR. *Dist:* Saunders.

Prevention & Early Intervention: Individual Differences As Risk Factors for the Mental Health of Children - A Festschrift for Stella Chess & Alexander Thomas. Ed. by William B. Carey & Sean C. McDevitt. 1994. LC 93-25940. 328p. text 47.95 (*0-87630-723-3*) Brunner-Routledge.

Prevention & Health: Directions for Policy & Practice. Ed. by Alfred Katz et al. 1987. LC 87-17634. (Prevention in Human Services Ser.: Vol. 5, No. 1). 136p. text 39.95 (*0-86656-668-6*) Haworth Pr.

Prevention & Management of Complications in Minimally Invasive Surgery. Ed. by Raymond J. Lanzafame. 1996. LC 96-1928. (Illus.). 348p. 148.50 (*0-89640-296-7*) Igaku-Shoin.

Prevention & Management of Hypertension. 1996. (EMRO Technical Publications Ser.: No. 23). 49p. pap. 9.00 (*92-9021-218-7*, 1450023) Am Soc Clinical.

Prevention & Management of Laparoendoscopic Surgical Complications. Society of Laparoendoscopic Surgeons Inc. 1999. LC 98-61024. (Illus.). text 145.00 (*0-9663768-0-3*) Soc Laparo Surg.

Prevention & Screening in Office Practice. Andrew K. Diehl. 1991. (Contemporary Management in Internal Medicine Ser.: Vol. 1, No. 4). (Illus.). 169p. text (*0-443-08826-8*) Church.

Prevention & Social Medicine. Ed. by P. Park. 12th ed. 1989. (C). (*0-7855-4677-4*) Current Dist IND. *Dist:* St Mut.

Prevention & Treatment of Alcohol Problems: Research Opportunities. Institute of Medicine Staff. 1989. 354p. (C). pap. text 30.00 (*0-309-04182-1*) Natl Acad Pr.

Prevention & Treatment of Cancer. Robert Bell. 1996. 88p. reprint ed. spiral bd. 10.00 (*0-7873-0089-6*) Hlth Research.

Prevention & Treatment of Cancer. Robert Bell. 1996. 88p. reprint ed. pap. 8.95 (*1-56459-890-X*) Kessinger Pub.

Prevention & Treatment of Complications of Diabetes: A Guide for Primary Care Practitioners. Frwd. by Charles M. Clark, Jr. 1992. 93p. (Orig.). (C). pap. text 20.00 (*1-56806-015-7*) DIANE Pub.

Prevention & Treatment of Contraceptive Failure. Ed. by S. Shan Ratnam & Uta Landy. 1986. LC 86-25318. 256p. 69.50 (*0-306-42477-0*, Plenum Trade) Perseus Pubng.

Prevention & Treatment of Diabetic Nephropathy. Harry Keen & M. Legrain. 1983. 400p. text 164.00 (*0-85200-744-2*) Kluwer Academic.

***Prevention & Treatment of HIV Infection in Infants & Children.** Arthur J. Ammann & Eun Seong Hwang. 2001. (Annals of the New York Academy of Sciences Ser.). 390p. pap. text 31.50 (*0-8018-6831-9*) NY Acad Sci.

Prevention & Treatment of HIV Infection in Infants & Children. Arthur J. Ammann & Arye Rubinstein. 2000. LC 00-61301. (Annals Ser.: Vol. 918). (Illus.). 390p. (*1-57331-268-1*) NY Acad Sci.

Prevention & Treatment of HIV Infection in Infants & Children. Ed. by Arthur J. Ammann & Arye Rubinstein. 2000. LC 00-61301. (Annals of the New York Academy of Sciences Ser.: Vol. 918). (Illus.). 390p. 140.00 (*1-57331-267-3*) NY Acad Sci.

Prevention & Treatment of Osteoporosis. Ed. by Lawrence B. Riggs. 1993. LC 92-48734. (Illus.). 50p. 19.90 (*0-88937-098-2*) Hogrefe & Huber Pubs.

***Prevention des Infections: Guide de Reference a l'Intention des Prestataires de Soins de Sante.** Engender Health Staff. 2001.Tr. of Infection Prevention: A Reference Booklet for Health Care Providers. (FRE., Illus.). 81p. pap. text (*1-885063-29-6*) EngenderHlth.

Prevention, Detection & Diagnosis of Cancer. Susan L. Groenwald. 1991. (Illus.). pap. text 24.95 (*0-86720-301-3*, 301-3) Jones & Bartlett.

Prevention Effectiveness: A Guide to Decision Analysis & Economic Evaluation, Vol.2. Ed. by Anne C. Haddix et al. 1996. (Illus.). 248p. (C). text 36.00 (*0-19-510063-8*) OUP.

Prevention Funding Information Bulletin: A Compendium of State, Federal & Private Funding Sources for Prevention & Children's Programs. 1993. 63p. (Orig.). (C). pap. text 20.00 (*0-7881-0178-1*) DIANE Pub.

Prevention, Health, & British Politics. Michael P. Mills. 1993. 200p. (*1-85628-190-6*) Avebry GBR. *Dist:* Ashgate Pub Co.

Prevention "How-To Dictionary of Healing Remedies & Techniques" Prevention Magazine Editors. 1996. 672p. mass mkt. 7.99 (*0-425-15191-3*) Berkley Pub.

Prevention in Childhood & Youth of Adult Cardiovascular Diseases - Time for Action: Report of a WHO Expert Committee. 1990. (Technical Reports: No. 792). (CHI, ENG, FRE, RUS & SPA.). 105p. pap. text 12.00 (*92-4-120792-2*, 1100792) World Health.

Prevention in Clinical Practice. D. H. Becker & L. B. Gardner. 1988. LC 88-12568. (Illus.). 468p. (C). text 85.00 (*0-306-42624-2*, Kluwer Plenum) Kluwer Academic.

Prevention in Community Mental Health Centers. Robert E. Hess & John Morgan. 1990. LC 90-4418. (Prevention in Human Services Ser.). 171p. text 4.95 (*0-86656-999-5*) Haworth Pr.

Prevention in Community Mental Health Practice. Jeffery J. Haugaard & N. Dickon Reppucci. 1991. pap. 27.95 (*0-914797-70-0*) Brookline Bks.

Prevention in Mental Health. Ed. by Henri Parens & Selma Kramer. 1993. LC 93-19429. 232p. pap. 27.50 (*1-56821-027-2*) Aronson.

Prevention in Nephrology. Ed. by Marc E. De Broe. 1991. (Developments in Nephrology Ser.). 120p. text 102.00 (*0-7923-0951-0*) Kluwer Academic.

Prevention Methods & Programmes for Oral Diseases: Report of a WHO Expert Committee, 1984. WHO Staff. 1984. (Technical Report Ser.: No. 713). 46p. 5.00 (*92-4-120713-2*) World Health.

Prevention of Alcohol Abuse. Ed. by Peter M. Miller & Ted D. Nirenberg. 1984. 536p. 100.00 (*0-306-41328-0*, Plenum Trade) Perseus Pubng.

Prevention of Atherosclerosis & Hypertension Beginning in Youth. Lloyd J. Filer et al. 1994. (Illus.). 270p. text 48.50 (*0-8121-1641-0*) Lppncott W & W.

Prevention of Blindness: Proceedings of the WHO Scientific Group, Geneva, 1972. WHO Staff. 1973. (Technical Reports: No. 518). pap. text 3.00 (*92-4-120518-0*, 1100518) World Health.

Prevention of Cancer. 1964. (Technical Report Ser.: No. 276). 53p. pap. text 3.00 (*92-4-120276-9*) World Health.

Prevention of Cardiovascular Disease in Primary Care: An Evidence-Based Approach. Ed. by Andrew Neil et al. 1996. (General Practice Ser.). (Illus.). 352p. pap. text 59.50 (*0-19-262397-4*) OUP.

Prevention of Child Sexual Abuse in Ireland: The Development & Evaluation of the Stay Safe Programme. Deirdre MacIntyre & Alan Carr. 2000. LC 00-34864. (Studies in Health & Human Services: Vol. 38). x, 191p. text 89.95 (*0-7734-7715-2*) E Mellen.

Prevention of Childhood Blindness. 1992. vii, 51p. pap. text 15.00 (*92-4-156151-3*, 1150378) World Health.

Prevention of Clinical Parasitology. Tsieh Sun. 1989. 56.00 (*0-938607-23-5*) Field & Wood Inc Medical.

Prevention of Contact Dermatitis. Ed. by Howard I. Maibach et al. 1996. LC 96-20543. (Current Problems in Dermatology Ser.: Vol. 25, 1996). (Illus.). x, 226p. text 240.00 (*3-8055-6311-6*) S Karger.

Prevention of Coronary Heart Disease. 1982. (Technical Report Ser.: No. 678). 53p. pap. text 5.00 (*92-4-120678-0*) World Health.

Prevention of Coronary Heart Disease. Ed. by Ira S. Ockene & Judith Ockene. 1992. LC 92-10336. 85.00 (*0-316-62214-1*, Little Brwn Med Div) Lppncott W & W.

Prevention of Dental Disease. John J. Murray. 2nd ed. 1989. (Illus.). 528p. pap. 49.95 (*0-19-261806-7*); 520p. 95.00 (*0-19-261807-5*) OUP.

Prevention of Diabetes Mellitus: Report of a WHO Study Group. 1994. LC 95-103034. (Technical Reports: No. 844). (CHI, ENG, FRE & SPA.). viii, 100p. pap. text 15.00 (*92-4-120844-9*, 1100844) World Health.

Prevention of Disabilities in Patients with Leprosy: A Practical Guide. H. Srinivasan. 1993. (ENG, FRE & SPA.). viii, 140p. pap. text 29.00 (*92-4-154456-2*, 1150401) World Health.

Prevention of Eating Disorders. Walter Vandereycken & Greta Noordenbos. 1998. LC 98-4537. (Studies in Eating Disorders). 224p. text 50.00 (*0-8147-8798-3*); pap. text 18.50 (*0-8147-8799-1*) NYU Pr.

Prevention of Eye Disease. Ed. by Mitchell H. Friedlaender. 1988. 208p. 156.00 (*0-913113-17-4*) M Liebert.

Prevention of Falls & Hip Fractures in the Elderly. Ed. by David F. Apple, Jr. & Wilson C. Hayes. 1994. 148p. pap. 45.00 (*0-89203-101-8*) Amer Acad Ortho Surg.

Prevention of Food Poisoning. Jill Trickett. 3rd ed. 1999. 137p. pap. (*0-7487-1522-3*) Nelson Thornes GBR. *Dist:* Trans-Atl Phila.

***Prevention of Food Poisoning.** Jill Trickett. 4th ed. 2001. (Illus.). 192p. pap. (*0-7487-5893-3*) Nelson Thornes GBR. *Dist:* Intl Spec Bk.

Prevention of Infant Mortality & Morbidity. Ed. by Frank Falkner. 1985. (Child Health & Development Ser.: Vol. 4). (Illus.). viii, 176p. 77.50 (*3-8055-3989-4*) S Karger.

Prevention of Liver Cancer: Report of a WHO Meeting, 1983. 1983. (Technical Report Ser.: No. 691). 30p. pap. text 3.00 (*92-4-120691-8*, 1100691) World Health.

Prevention of Mental Handicap: Proceedings of the British Institute of Mental Handicap. M. J. Griffiths et al. 1985. 63p. 40.00 (*0-906054-29-X*) St Mut.

Prevention of Mental Illness in Primary Care. 1996. 414p. pap. text 54.95 (*0-521-57648-2*) Cambridge U Pr.

Prevention of Mental Illness in Primary Care. Ed. by Tony Kendrick et al. 1996. LC 95-38679. (Illus.). 414p. (C). text 150.00 (*0-521-47057-9*) Cambridge U Pr.

Prevention of Micronutrient Deficiencies: Tools for Policymakers & Public Health Workers. Ed. by Institute of Medicine Staff et al. 1998. LC 98-133582. 207p. pap. 30.00 (*0-309-06029-X*) Natl Acad Pr.

Prevention of Myocardial Infraction. Ed. by Joann E. Manson et al. 1996. (Illus.). 584p. text 65.00 (*0-19-508582-5*) OUP.

Prevention of Obstruction of Coronary & Vital Arteries. William Dock. 1983. LC 79-50185. 200p. (C). 42.50 (*0-87527-202-9*) Green.

Prevention of Occupational Cancer. Ed. by Charles R. Shaw. 1981. 256p. 145.00 (*0-8493-5625-3*, RC628, CRC Reprint) Franklin.

Prevention of Occupational Cancer International Symposium: Proceedings of the International Symposium on the Prevention of Occupational Cancer, Helsinki, April 21-24. International Agency for Research on Cancer Staff. 1982. (Occupational Safety & Health Ser.: No. 46). viii, 658p. (Orig.). pap. 42.75 (*92-2-002907-3*) Intl Labour Office.

Prevention of Occupationally-Acquired Blood-Borne Infections. Ed. by C. H. Collins & D. A. Kennedy. 1998. (CAB International Publication). 320p. text 100.00 (*0-85199-167-X*) OUP.

Prevention of Oral Disease. Ed. by John J. Murray. 3rd ed. 1996. (Illus.). 294p. pap. text 59.95 (*0-19-262457-1*) OUP.

Prevention of Oral Diseases. WHO Staff. 1987. (WHO Offset Publications: No. 103). 88p. 14.00 (*92-4-170103-X*) World Health.

Prevention of Perinatal Mortality & Morbidity. Frank Falkner. 1984. (Child Health & Development Ser.: Vol. 3). (Illus.). vi, 182p. 64.50 (*3-8055-3854-5*) S Karger.

Prevention of Perinatal Mortality & Morbidity: Proceedings of the WHO Expert Committee, Geneva, 1970. WHO Staff. 1970. (Technical Reports: No. 457). 60p. pap. text 6.00 (*92-4-120457-5*, 1100457) World Health.

Prevention of Perinatal Mortality & Morbidity: Proceedings of the WHO Seminar, Tours, 1969. WHO Staff. 1972. (Public Health Papers: No. 42). 97p. pap. text 5.40 (*92-4-130042-6*, 1110042) World Health.

Prevention of Perioperative Infections. H. Schoenfeld. 1985. (Antibiotics & Chemotherapy Ser.: Vol. 33). (Illus.). viii, 208p. 129.75 (*3-8055-3936-3*) S Karger.

Prevention of Pressure Sores: Engineering & Clinical Aspects. Ed. by J. G. Webster. 1991. (Biomedical Engineering Ser.). (Illus.). 250p. 116.00 (*0-7503-0099-X*) Inst of Physics Pubng.

***Prevention of Pressure Ulcers in Patients with Hip Fractures: Definition, Measurement & Improvement of the Quality of Care.** Lena Gunningberg. 2000. (Comprehensive Summaries of Uppsala Disertations from the Faculty of Medicine: No. 979). (Illus.). 44p. (Orig.). pap. (*91-554-4889-5*) Uppsala Universitet SWE. *Dist:* Coronet Bks.

Prevention of Progressive Chronic Renal Failure. Ed. by A. Meguid El Nahas et al. 1993. LC 92-48906. (Oxford Clinical Nephrology Ser.). (Illus.). 350p. text 65.00 (*0-19-262237-4*) OUP.

Prevention of Progressive Uremia Eli Friedman. 1990. 125.00 (*0-938607-28-6*); 1989. 65.00 (*0-938607-07-3*); Vol. 2. 1989. 75.00 (*0-938607-15-4*) Field & Wood Inc Medical.

Prevention of Progressive Uremia, Vol. 3. Friedman. Date not set. (*0-938607-41-3*) Field & Wood Inc Medical.

Prevention of Respiratory Diseases. Ed. by Albert Hirsch et al. 1993. (Lung Biology in Health & Disease Ser.: Vol. 68). (Illus.). 728p. text 245.00 (*0-8247-8850-8*) Dekker.

Prevention of Rh Sensitization: Proceedings of the WHO Scientific Group, Geneva, 1970. WHO Staff. 1971. (Technical Reports: No. 468). pap. text 5.00 (*92-4-120468-0*, 1100468) World Health.

Prevention of Rheumatic Fever. 1957. (Technical Report Ser.: No. 126). 27p. pap. text 3.00 (*92-4-120126-6*) World Health.

Prevention of Sexual Transmission of Human Immunodeficiency Virus. 1990. (WHO AIDS Ser.: No. 6). (ARA, ENG, FRE & SPA.). iii, 27p. pap. text 8.00 (*92-4-121006-0*, 1870006) World Health.

Prevention of Sexually Transmitted Diseases. Ed. by Lawrence R. Stanberry & David I. Bernstein. 2000. (Illus.). 424p. 112.50 (*0-12-663330-4*) Acad Pr.

Prevention of Spina Bifida & Other Neural Tube Defects. Ed. by John Dobbing. 1983. text 99.00 (*0-12-218860-8*) Acad Pr.

Prevention of Sports Injuries: A Biomechanical Approach. Carole J. Zebas & Mike Chapman. 1990. 200p. pap. 24.95 (*0-945483-01-5*) E Bowers Pub.

Prevention of Stroke. Ed. by J. W. Norris & Vladimir C. Hachinski. 1991. (Illus.). 280p. 159.00 (*0-387-97442-3*) Spr-Verlag.

Prevention of Suicide. 1968. (Public Health Papers: No. 35). 84p. pap. text 4.00 (*92-4-130035-3*, 1110035) World Health.

Prevention of Tachyarrhythmias with Cardiac Pacing. Ed. by J. Claude Daubert et al. 1996. LC 96-46589. (Illus.). 224p. 39.50 (*0-87993-651-7*) Futura Pub.

Prevention of the Re-Introduction of Malaria: Report of a WHO Meeting, 1967. 1967. (Technical Report Ser.: No. 375). 32p. pap. text 3.00 (*92-4-120374-9*, 1100374) World Health.

Prevention of Traffic Accidents in Childhood: Report on a WHO Study. J. P. Deschamps. 1981. (EURO Reports & Studies: No. 26). 54p. pap. text 4.00 (*92-9020-165-7*, 1330026) World Health.

***Prevention of Type 1 Diabetes Mellitus in Experimental Studies.** Maria Holstad. 2001. (Comprehensive Summaries of Uppsala Dissertations from the Faculty of Medicine Ser.: No. 1014). (Illus.). 48p. (*91-554-4972-7*) Uppsala Universitet SWE. *Dist:* Coronet Bks.

Prevention of Venous Thromboembolism. Ed. by Samuel Z. Goldhaber. 1992. LC 92-49981. (Fundamental & Clinical Cardiology Ser.: Vol. 12). (Illus.). 632p. text 140.00 (*0-8247-8757-9*) Dekker.

Prevention Plus III: Assessing Alcohol & Other Drug Prevention Programs at the School & Community Level: A Four-Step Guide to Useful Program Assessment. Jean A. Linney & Abraham Wandersman. 1993. (Illus.). 461p. (Orig.). (C). pap. text 50.00 (*0-7881-0085-8*) DIANE Pub.

Prevention Practice. Rothman. 1992. text 78.95 (*0-7216-3261-0*) Saunders.

Prevention Practice in Substance Abuse. Ed. by Carl G. Leukefeld et al. 1995. LC 95-13748. (Drugs & Society Ser.: Vol. 8, No. 3 & 4). 141p. 39.95 (*1-56024-734-7*) Haworth Pr.

Prevention Primer: An Encyclopedia of Alcohol, Tobacco, & Other Drug Prevention Terms. 1995. 134p. (Orig.). pap. text 25.00 (*0-7881-2136-7*) DIANE Pub.

Prevention Research: Determining Drug Abuse among Children & Adolescents. 1986. lib. bdg. 175.00 (*0-8490-3498-1*) Gordon Pr.

Preventions & Treatments of Alcohol & Drug Abuse: A Socio-Epidemiological Sourcebook. Brenda Forster & Jeffrey C. Salloway. 1991. LC 91-22618. (Interdisciplinary Studies in Alcohol & Drug Use & Abuse: Vol. 7). 596p. lib. bdg. 119.95 (*0-7734-9714-5*) E Mellen.

Prevention's Best: Complementary Cures. Health Prevention Staff. 2000. LC 00-702298. xii, 276p. mass mkt. 5.99 (*0-312-97480-9*) St Martin.

Prevention's Best: Healing Herbs. Prevention Magazine Health Book Staff. 2000. 288p. mass mkt. 5.99 (*0-312-97584-8*, St Martins Paperbacks) St Martin.

Prevention's Healing with Vitamins. Prevention Magazine Health Book Staff. 1996. LC 96-10202. 608p. 27.95 (*0-87596-292-0*) Rodale Pr Inc.

Prevention's Symptom Solver for Dogs & Cats: From Arfs & Arthritis to Whimpers & Worms, an Owner's Cure Finder. Ed. by Matthew Hoffman. 1999. LC 98-39964. (Illus.). 512p. 29.95 (*0-87596-523-7*) Rodale Pr Inc.

Preventive & Community Medicine. Ed. by Duncan W. Clark & Brian Macmahon. 2nd ed. 1981. 65.00 (*0-316-14596-3*, Little Brwn Med Div) Lppncott W & W.

Preventive & Therapeutic Nutrition Handbook. Cynthia Thomson et al. 1996. LC 95-14999. 128p. (C). (gr. 13). spiral bd. 19.00 (*0-412-07491-5*) Kluwer Academic.

Preventive Approaches to Couples Therapy. Rony Berger. 1999. LC 99-14074. 410p. text 39.95 (*0-87630-876-0*) Brunner-Routledge.

Preventive Cardiology. Ed. by Eugene I. Chazov et al. 1987. (Soviet Medical Reviews Supplement, Cardiology Ser.: No. 1). xviii, 680p. text 436.00 (*3-7186-0338-1*) Gordon & Breach.

Preventive Cardiology. Ed. by Eugene I. Chazov & Raphael G. Oganov. 1989. LC 89-15394. 320p. 45.00 (*0-8236-4293-3*) Intl Univs Pr.

Preventive Cardiology. Nathan D. Wong et al. 1999. LC 99-34769. (Illus.). 630p. text 69.00 (*0-07-071856-3*) McGraw-Hill Prof.

Preventive Cardiology: A Guide for Clinical Practice. Ed. by Killian Robinson. 1998. LC 98-6277. (Illus.). 432p. 69.00 (*0-87993-692-4*) Futura Pub.

Preventive Cardiology: An Introduction. Ed. by H. S. Wasir. 1992. (Illus.). xxx, 409p. (C). (*0-7069-5891-8*) Vikas IND. *Dist:* S Asia.

Preventive Cardiology: Strategies for the Prevention & Treatment of Coronary Artery Disease. Ed. by Joanne Micale Foody & Eugene Braunwald. 2000. LC 00-37004 (Contemporary Cardiology Ser.). (Illus.). 376p. 99.50 (*0-89603-811-4*) Humana.

Preventive Cardiology Vol. 2, Pt. B: Metabolism of Ischemic Myocardium. Vol. 2. E. I. Chazov et al. Ed. by V. N. Smirnov. 1989. (Soviet Medical Reviews Supplement Ser.). xii, 304p. pap. text 437.00 (*3-7186-4925-X*) Gordon & Breach.

Preventive Care for Elderly People. David C. Kennie. 1993. 335p. (C). text 90.00 (*0-521-43044-5*); pap. text 31.95 (*0-521-43629-X*) Cambridge U Pr.

Preventive Care Sourcebook 1999. Aspen Reference Group Staff. 1998. 200p. pap. 89.00 (*0-8342-1056-8*, 10568) Aspen Pub.

Preventive Diet for Heart & Overweight: Transition to Vegetarian Diet. Edmond B. Szekely. 1977. (Illus.). 48p. pap. 3.50 (*0-89564-040-6*) IBS Intl.

Preventive Family Therapy: Patterns of Change in the Family, Bk. 6. Rose A. Parvin. 1995. LC 95-35697. 288p. (*1-885917-05-8*) Univrsl Pubng.

Preventive Health Care. Robert S. Chang. 1981. LC 80-24183. 35.00 (*0-8161-2165-6*, Macmillan Ref) Gale.

Preventive Health Care for Children: Experience from Selected Foreign Countries. 1994. (Illus.). 37p. (Orig.). (C). pap. text 30.00 (*0-7881-0198-6*) DIANE Pub.

Preventive Health Care for Young Children: Findings from a 10-Country Study & Directions for United States Policy. C. Arden Miller & Bret C. Williams. 1991. LC 91-61824. 80p. (Orig.). pap. 9.50 (*0-943657-16-4*) ZERO TO THREE.

***Preventive Interventions under Managed Care: Mental Health & Substance Abuse Services.** Sharon Dorfman. 2001. 87p. (C). pap. text 25.00 (*0-7567-1107-X*) DIANE Pub.

Preventive Medicine: Natural Options for Keeping Well. Time-Life Books Editors. 1997. LC 96-43447. (Illus.). 144p. pap. 16.95 (*0-7835-4916-4*) Time-Life.

Preventive Medicine & Public Health. B. Cassens. 2nd ed. 1992. (National Medical Series for Independent Study). (Illus.). 497p. pap. text 32.00 (*0-683-06262-X*) Lppncott W & W.

Preventive Medicine & Public Health: PreTest Self-Assessment & Review. Ed. by Sylvie Ratelle. 8th ed. 1998. LC 97-22240. (Clinical Science Ser.). (Illus.). 200p. pap. 19.95 (*0-07-052534-X*) McGraw-Hill Educ Grp.

Preventive Medicine & Public Health: PreTest Self-Assessment & Review. Sylvie Ratelle. 9th ed. 2000. LC 00-41564. (Pretest Clinical Science Ser.). (Illus.). 238p. pap. 24.95 (*0-07-135962-1*) McGraw-Hill Med Pub.

Preventive Medicine Between Obligation & Aspiration. M. F. Verweij. 2000. LC 00-49317. (International Library of Ethics, Law, & the New Medicine: Vol. 4). (Illus.). viii, 190p. 62.00 (*0-7923-6691-3*) Kluwer Academic.

Preventive Medicine in the United States, 1900-1975, Trends & Interpretations. George Rosen. 1976. LC 75-35978. (Illus.). 128p. lib. bdg. 15.00 (*0-88202-103-6*, Sci Hist) Watson Pub Intl.

Preventive Medicine in the United States 1900-1990: Trends & Interpretations. Bonnie Bullough & George Rosen. 1992. LC 92-20428. 15.95 (*0-88135-180-6*); pap. 11.95 (*0-88135-177-6*) Watson Pub Intl (Sci Hist).

Preventive Nutrition: The Comprehensive Guide for Health Professionals. Ed. by Adrianne Bendich & Richard J. Deckelbaum. 2nd ed. 2001. LC 00-50030. (Nutrition & Health Ser.). (Illus.). 520p. 99.50 (*0-89603-911-0*) Humana.

Preventive Nutrition: The Comprehensive Guide for the Health Professionals. Ed. by Adrianne Bendich & Richard J. Deckelbaum. 1997. LC 96-37937. (Nutrition & Health Ser.). (Illus.). 616p. 129.50 (*0-89603-351-1*) Humana.

Preventive Psychiatry: Early Intervention & Situational Crisis Management. Ed. by Samuel C. Klagsbrun et al. 1989. LC 88-663414. 272p. text 38.95 (*0-914783-28-9*); pap. text 23.95 (*0-914783-29-7*) Charles.

Preventive Psychology: Theory, Research & Practice. Ed. by Robert D. Felner et al. 1983. 475p. 39.50 (*0-08-026340-2*, Pergamon Pr) Elsevier.

Preventive Services for School-Age Children. Ed. by O. Jeanneret. 1988. (Journal: Vol. 15, No. 3, 1988). (Illus.). 68p. pap. 35.00 (*3-8055-4824-9*) S Karger.

Preventive Services in the Clinical Setting: What Works & What It Costs. 1994. lib. bdg. 250.95 (*0-8490-5823-6*) Gordon Pr.

Preventive Therapy in Asthma. Ed. by John Morley. 1991. (Perspectives in Asthma Ser.: Vol. 5). (Illus.). 300p. (C). text 83.00 (*0-12-506448-9*) Acad Pr.

Preventv Treatmnt Athers. D. H. Blankenhorn. 1984. (C). text 39.95 (*0-201-10638-8*, Health Sci) Addison-Wesley.

Price of Greatness: Resolving the Creativity & Madness Controversy. Arnold M. Ludwig. 1995. LC 94-44905. 310p. 41.00 (*0-89862-839-3*) Guilford Pubns.

Price of Health. Ed. by George J. Agich & Charles E. Begley. 1986. 312p. (C). text 126.50 (*90-277-2285-4*) Kluwer Academic.

Price of Health: Australian Governments & Medical Politics, 1910-1960. James A. Gillespie. 1991. (Studies in Australian History). (Illus.). 376p. (C). text 74.95 (*0-521-38183-5*) Cambridge U Pr.

Price Portfolio: Forty-Six Reprints of Medical Papers of Dr. Weston A. Price. 1978. 35.00 (*0-916764-04-4*) Price-Pottenger.

Pricing Life: Why It's Time for Health Care Rationing. Peter A. Ubel. 2000. LC 99-20664. (Basic Bioethics Ser.). (Illus.). xix, 208p. 25.00 (*0-262-21016-9*) MIT Pr.

Pride. Mel B. 1985. 24p. (Orig.). pap. 2.00 (*0-89486-267-7*, 1397B) Hazelden.

Pride of Women: An Illustrated Book of Days. 1987. (Archives & Special Collections on Women in Medicine Ser.). (Illus.). 110p. (Orig.). 10.00 (*0-944542-02-6*) Med Coll PA ASCWM.

Primacy of Caring: Stress & Coping in Health & Illness. Patricia E. Benner & Judith Wrubel. 1989. 406p. (C). pap. text 52.00 (*0-201-12002-X*) Addison-Wesley.

Primacy of Structure: Psychotherapy of Underlying Character Pathology. Althea J. Horner. 1991. LC 90-41165. 328p. 55.00 (*0-87668-748-6*) Aronson.

Primal Wound: A Transpersonal View of Trauma, Addiction, & Growth. John Firman & Ann Gila. 1997. LC 96-43767. (SUNY Series in the Philosophy of Psychology). (Illus.). 284p. (C). text 59.50 (*0-7914-3293-9*); pap. text 22.95 (*0-7914-3294-7*) State U NY Pr.

Primal Wound: Understanding the Adopted Child. Nancy N. Verrier. 1993. 252p. (Orig.). pap. 15.00 (*0-9636480-0-4*) Verrier Pub.

Primary Abilities at Mental Age Six. C. E. Meyers et al. 1962. (SRCD M Ser.: Vol. 27, No. 1). pap. 25.00 (*0-527-01592-X*) Periodicals Srv.

Primary Afferent Neuron: A Survey of Recent Morpho-Functional Aspects. Ed. by W. Zenker & W. L. Neuhuber. 1990. LC 89-70967. (Illus.). 270p. 85.00 (*0-306-43480-6*, Plenum Trade) Perseus Pubng.

Primary Anatomy. John V. Basmajian. 1998. (Illus.). 404p. (C). pap. text 19.80 (*0-87563-806-6*) Stipes.

Primary & Emergency Dental Care: A Practitioner's Guide. Keith H. Figures & David J. Lamb. 1995. LC 96-115807. 176p. pap. text 45.00 (*0-7236-1013-4*) Buttrwrth-Heinemann.

Primary & Secondary Brain Stem Lesions. G. Csecsei et al. 1987. (Illus.). 150p. 131.00 (*0-387-82025-6*) Spr-Verlag.

Primary & Secondary Eating Disorders: A Psychoneuroendocrine & Metabolic Approach. Ed. by E. Ferrari et al. 1994. (Advances in the Biosciences Ser.: Vol. 90). 532p. 174.00 (*0-08-042192-X*, Pergamon Pr) Elsevier.

Primary & Secondary Prevention of Malignant Melanoma. Ed. by Rona M. MacKie. 1996. (Pigment Cell Ser.: Vol. 11, 1996). (Illus.). viii, 130p. 158.25 (*3-8055-6273-X*) S Karger.

Primary & Secondary Preventive Nutrition. Ed. by Adrianne Bendich & Richard J. Deckelbaum. 2001. LC 00-53891. (Nutrition & Health Ser.). (Illus.). 480p. 125.00 (*0-89603-758-4*) Humana.

Primary & Team Health Care Education. Ed. by Troy L. Thompson & Richard L. Byny. 1983. LC 83-2156. 245p. 68.50 (*0-275-91416-X*, C1416, Praeger Pubs) Greenwood.

Primary Angioplasty in Acute Myocardial Infarction. James E. Tcheng. 2001. (Contemporary Cardiology Ser.). 350p. 125.00 (*0-89603-904-8*) Humana.

Primary Biliary Cirrhosis: From Pathogenesis to Clinical Treatment. Ed. by Keith D. Lindor et al. 1998. 192p. 86.00 (*0-7923-8740-6*) Kluwer Academic.

Primary Bone Cancer: The Multidiscipline Disease: Proceedings of the Annual West Coast Cancer Symposium, 10th, San Francisco, CA, September 1974. Annual West Coast Cancer Symposium. Ed. by J. M. Vaeth. 1975. (Frontiers of Radiation Therapy & Oncology Ser.: Vol. 10). viii, 243p. 82.75 (*3-8055-2185-5*) S Karger.

Primary Brain Tumors. Ed. by William S. Fields. 1989. (Illus.). 286p. 55.00 (*0-387-97055-X*) Spr-Verlag.

Primary Cardiology. Lee Goldman & Eugene Braunwald. Ed. by Richard Zorab. 1998. LC 97-50317. (Illus.). 496p. text 60.00 (*0-7216-6402-4*) Saunders.

Primary Cardiology: International Edition. Goldman. 1998. (C). text 50.00 (*0-8089-2060-X*, Grune & Strat) Harcrt Hlth Sci Grp.

Primary Cardiology (Cardiologia en Atencion Primaria) Lee Goldman & Eugene Braunwald. 21st ed. 2000. (ENG & SPA., Illus.). 541p. (*84-8174-432-8*) Mosby-Doyma Libros ESP. *Dist:* Mosby Inc.

Primary Care. John Noble. 1987. 142.00 (*0-316-61150-6*, Little Brwn Med Div) Lppncott W & W.

Primary Care. Joanne K. Singleton & Robert V. Digregorio. 1998. LC 98-42214. 944p. text 67.95 (*0-7817-1041-3*) Lppncott W & W.

Primary Care: A Collaborative Approach. Ed. by Terry Mahan Buttaro et al. 1999. LC 99-26596. (Illus.). 1450p. text 84.95 (*0-8151-3823-7*, 31844) Mosby Inc.

Primary Care: America's Health in a New Era. Institute of Medicine Staff. Ed. by Molla S. Donaldson et al. 1996. LC 96-25823. 416p. text 42.95 (*0-309-05399-4*) Natl Acad Pr.

Primary Care: Balancing Health Needs, Services, & Technology. Barbara Starfield. 1998. LC 98-10794. (Illus.). 448p. text 49.95 (*0-19-512542-8*); pap. text 27.50 (*0-19-512543-6*) OUP.

Primary Care: The Art & Science of Advanced Practice Nursing. Lynn M. Dunphy & Jill E. Winland-Brown. 2001. LC 00-64528. (Illus.). 1328p. kivar 99.00 (*0-8036-0589-7*) Davis Co.

Primary Care: Understanding Health Need & Demand. Anne Rogers & Heather Elliott. 1997. LC 97-14955. (National Primary Care Research & Development Centre Ser.). 88p. pap. (*1-85775-237-6*) Radcliffe Med Pr GBR. *Dist:* Balogh.

Primary Care Across the Life Span. Denise Robinson & Pamela Kidd. 1999. LC 99-37349. (Illus.). xviii, 1470p. (*0-323-00148-3*) Mosby Inc.

Primary Care & Home Care Scenarios, 1990-2005: Scenario Report Commissioned by the Steering Committee on Future Health Scenarios. E. Schade. 1994. LC 94-2258. 253p. pap. text 106.00 (*0-7923-2658-X*) Kluwer Academic.

Primary Care Annotated Bibliography & Reference List Joyce J. Fitzpatrick. 1996. LC 97-205908. 570p. pap. 39.95 (*1-55810-130-6*); LC 97-204882. 49p. pap. 39.95 (*1-55810-131-4*) Am Nurses Pub (Am Acad Nursing).

Primary Care Cardiology. Glenn N. Levine. 2000. LC 99-42866. 224p. pap. text 35.00 (*0-683-30688-X*) Lppncott W & W.

Primary Care Cardiology: A Board Review for Internists & Family Practitioners. George J. Taylor. 1994. LC 94-15573. (Illus.). 256p. pap. 49.95 (*0-86542-358-X*) Blackwell Sci.

Primary Care Challenge. Robinson. 1999. (C). pap. text (*0-443-05634-X*) Church.

Primary Care Consultant. Shelia A. Dunn. 1998. LC 97-42363. (Illus.). 704p. (C). (gr. 13). text 49.95 (*0-8151-2950-5*, 29682) Mosby Inc.

Primary Care Dermatology Kenneth A. Arndt et al. Ed. by Judy Fletcher. 1997. LC 96-44227. (Illus.). 352p. pap. text 49.95 (*0-7216-6096-7*) Saunders.

Primary Care for Older Americans: A Primer. Tim M. Henderson & Linda R. Lipson. 1997. 75p. 20.00 (*1-55516-706-3*, 6715) Natl Conf State Legis.

Primary Care for Physician Assistants. Ed. by Rodney L. Moser. 2nd ed. 1998. LC 97-50437. (Illus.). 744p. text 65.00 (*0-07-043491-3*) McGraw-Hill Educ Grp.

Primary Care for Physician Assistants. Rodney L. Moser. 2nd ed. 2001. LC 00-49622. (Illus.). 745p. text 74.95 (*0-07-137014-5*) McGraw-Hill Prof.

Primary Care for Physician Assistants: Companion Handbook. Ed. by Rick Dehn. 1998. LC 98-22423. (Illus.). 608p. pap. 34.95 (*0-07-016151-8*) McGraw-Hill Educ Grp.

***Primary Care for Physician Assistants: Pretest Self-Assessment & Review.** Rodney Moser. 2nd ed. 2001. (Pretest Self-Assessment & Review Ser.). (Illus.). 292p. pap. 34.95 (*0-07-137015-3*) McGraw-Hill Prof.

Primary Care for the Obstetrician & Gynecologist. Thomas E. Nolan. 1996. LC 95-46498. (Illus.). 349p. pap. 62.95 (*0-471-12279-3*) Wiley.

Primary Care for the Obstetrician & Gynecologist. Ed. by Yvonne S. Thornton. 1996. LC 96-31525. (Illus.). 288p. pap. 69.50 (*0-89640-324-6*) Igaku-Shoin.

Primary Care for the Older Adult. Mary Burke. 1999. (Illus.). 550p. text 54.95 (*0-8151-8916-8*, 31744) Mosby Inc.

Primary Care for Women. Phyllis Leppert. 1996. LC 96-30176. 998p. text 110.00 (*0-397-51523-5*) Lppncott W & W.

Primary Care Geriatrics: A Case-Based Approach. Ed. by Richard J. Ham & Philip D. Sloane. 3rd ed. 1996. LC 96-12932. (Illus.). 640p. (C). (gr. 13). pap. text 64.95 (*0-8151-4188-2*, 25866) Mosby Inc.

Primary Care Geriatrics: A Case-Based Approach. Richard J. Ham & Philip D. Sloane. 3rd ed. 1996. (Illus.). 640p. pap. (*84-8086-111-8*) Mosby-Doyma Libros ESP. *Dist:* Mosby Inc.

Primary Care Geriatrics: A Case-Based Approach. Richard J. Ham et al. 4th ed. 2001. (Illus.). 635p. text 69.95 (*0-323-01450-X*) Mosby Inc.

Primary Care in Obstetrics & Gynecology: A Handbook for Clinicians. Roger P. Smith & Joseph S. Sanfilippo. 1997. LC 96-29795. (Illus.). 666p. pap. 46.95 (*0-387-94739-6*) Spr-Verlag.

Primary Care Making Connection: Making Connections. P. Boaden. 1997. LC 97-13905. (State of Health Ser.). (*0-335-19749-3*); pap. (*0-335-19748-5*) OpUniv Pr.

Primary Care Management: Cases & Discussions. Goutham Rao. 1999. LC 98-25307. 79.95 (*0-7619-1204-5*, 82071); pap. 39.95 (*0-7619-1205-3*, 82072) Sage.

Primary Care Management of Heart Disease. Contrib. by George Jesse Taylor. 2000. LC 99-42879. 658p. 69.00 (*0-323-00256-0*) Mosby Inc.

Primary Care Medicine. Allan H. Goroll et al. 1997. 99.00 (*0-397-58410-5*) Lppncott W & W.

Primary Care Medicine: Office Evaluation & Management of the Adult Patient. Allan H. Goroll et al. 4th ed. 2000. LC 00-27376. 1,344p. text 75.00 (*0-7817-1248-3*) Lppncott W & W.

Primary Care Medicine for Psychiatrists: A Practitioner's Guide. Ed. by John R. Hubbard & Delmar Short. 1997. LC 97-23366. (Illus.). 372p. (C). spiral bd. 45.00 (*0-306-45533-1*, Kluwer Plenum) Kluwer Academic.

Primary Care Medicine Package. John Noble. 3rd ed. 2000. 165.00 (*0-323-00832-1*) Mosby Inc.

***Primary Care Medicine Recommendations PDA.** Allan H. Goroll & Albert G. Mulley. 2001. (*0-7817-3489-4*) Lppncott W & W.

Primary Care Meets Mental Health "Tools for the 21st Century" Ed. by Joel D. Haber & Grant E. Mitchell. 1997. 97.50 (*1-887452-12-5*) Manisses Communs.

Primary Care of Children. Patricia Ludder Jackson & Judith A. Vessey. 3rd ed. 1999. LC 99-48131. xvi, 876p. text 69.95 (*0-323-00883-6*) Mosby Inc.

Primary Care of Landmine Injuries in Africa. Ian Maddocks et al. 2000. (Illus.). 72p. pap. 10.00 (*1-893368-03-3*) Intl Phys PONW.

Primary Care of the Anterior Segment. Louis J. Catania. 2nd ed. 1996. (Illus.). 552p. (C). text 129.95 (*0-8385-7911-6*, A7911-9) McGraw-Hill Educ Grp.

Primary Care of the Cataract Patient. Cynthia A. Murrill et al. 1994. (Illus.). 267p. (C). pap. text 110.00 (*0-8385-7899-3*, A7899-6, Apple Lange Med) McGraw.

Primary Care of the Glaucomas. Ed. by Murray Fingeret & Thomas L. Lewis. 2nd ed. 2000. LC 99-87835. 555p. (C). text 135.00 (*0-8385-8158-7*) McGraw-Hill Prof.

Primary Care of the Newborn. Beryl J. Rosenstein & Henry M. Seidel. 2nd ed. 1996. LC 96-23663. (Illus.). 664p. (C). (gr. 13). pap. text 32.95 (*0-8151-8681-9*, 28972) Mosby Inc.

Primary Care of the Newborn. Henry M. Seidel et al. 2nd ed. 1997. (Illus.). 664p. pap. (*84-8174-292-9*) Mosby-Doyma Libros ESP. *Dist:* Mosby Inc.

Primary Care of the Posterior Segment. Larry L. Alexander. 2nd ed. 1993. (Illus.). 495p. (C). text 125.00 (*0-8385-7970-1*, A7970-5) McGraw-Hill Prof.

Primary Care of Women. Karen J. Carlson et al. 1995. LC 95-3983. (Illus.). 608p. (C). (gr. 13). text 79.95 (*0-8016-7677-0*, 07677) Mosby Inc.

Primary Care of Women. Dawn P. Lemcke et al. 1996. (Illus.). 624p. (C). pap. text 44.95 (*0-8385-9813-7*, A9813-5, Apple Lange Med) McGraw.

Primary Care of Women & Children with HIV: A Multidisciplinary Approach. Susan Holman. Ed. by Patricia Kelly. 1995. LC 94-34337. (Series in Oncology & HIV-Related Illnesses). (Illus.). 328p. (C). pap. text 42.95 (*0-86720-709-4*, 709-4) Jones & Bartlett.

Primary Care Oncology. Kathryn L. Boyer et al. Ed. by Shirley Kuhn. 1998. LC 98-5822. (Illus.). 416p. (C). pap. text 45.00 (*0-7216-7316-3*) Saunders.

Primary Care Optometry. Theodore Grosvenor. 4th ed. 2001. LC 2001-25465. (Illus.). 688p. 89.99 (*0-7506-7308-7*) Buttrwrth-Heinemann.

Primary Care Orthopaedics. Royce C. Lewis, Jr. 1987. (Illus.). 328p. text (*0-443-08356-8*) Church.

Primary Care Orthopaedics in Chiropractic. Steven Brier. 1999. LC 00-500848. (Illus.). 494p. (C). (gr. 13). text 59.00 (*0-8016-6381-4*, 06381) Mosby Inc.

Primary Care Orthopedics. Victoria R. Masear. 1995. (Illus.). 336p. text 60.00 (*0-7216-5436-3*) Saunders.

Primary Care Orthopedics. Scott W. Shiffer & William McDaniel. 2001. (Illus.). 170p. pap. 29.95 (*0-8290-5214-3*) Ardent Media.

Primary Care Patient Education Manual. annuals Ed. by Sara N. Di Lima et al. 1999. LC 98-45294. 500p. ring bd. 175.00 (*0-8342-1015-0*, S498) Aspen Pub.

Primary Care Pediatric Otolaryngology. Patrick S. Pasquariello, Jr. et al. 1995. 244p. text 35.00 (*1-887064-00-1*) J M Ryan.

Primary Care Pediatrics. Carol Green-Hernandez & Joanne K. Singleton. 2001. LC 00-56915. (Illus.). xiii, 933p. text 69.95 (*0-7817-2008-7*) Lppncott W & W.

Primary Care Physicians: Financing Their Graduate Medical Education in Ambulatory Settings. Institute of Medicine Staff. 1989. 274p. pap. text 33.00 (*0-309-04134-1*) Natl Acad Pr.

Primary Care Podiatry. Ed. by Jeffrey M. Robbins. 1994. LC 93-17926. text 69.00 (*0-7216-4363-9*) Saunders.

Primary Care Provider's Guide to Compensation & Quality. Carolyn Buppert. 2000. LC 00-21640. (Illus.). 304p. pap. 99.00 (*0-8342-1744-9*) Aspen Pub.

Primary Care Psychiatry. Knesper. 1997. LC 96-43966. 350p. pap. text 41.00 (*0-7216-6509-8*) Saunders.

Primary Care Psychiatry & Behavioral Medicine: Brief Office Treatment & Management Pathways. Ed. by Robert E. Feinstein & Anne A. Brewer. 1998. LC 98-42017. 528p. 59.95 (*0-8261-1224-2*) Springer Pub.

Primary Care Research: Encounter Records & the Denominator Problem. S. J. Kilpatrick, Jr. & Russell Boyle. 1984. LC 83-24744. 156p. 55.00 (*0-275-91439-9*, C1439, Praeger Pubs) Greenwood.

Primary Care Secrets. Jeanette Mladenovic. 2nd rev. ed. 1998. LC 98-42098. (Secrets Ser.). (Illus.). 525p. pap. 39.95 (*1-56053-305-6*) Hanley & Belfus.

Primary Care Urology: A Practitioner's Guide. Larry I. Lipshultz & Isaac Kleinman. 2nd ed. 1996. 43.95 (*0-7234-2482-9*) Mosby Inc.

Primary Care Women No. 2. Carlson. 2nd ed. 2001. LC 2001-52183. pap. text (*0-323-01065-2*) Mosby Inc.

Primary Dermatologic Care. Bonnie J. Hooper & Mitchel P. Goldman. 1998. LC 98-29425. 368p. pap. text 49.95 (*1-55664-412-4*) Mosby Inc.

Primary Eye Care Manual. 1985. (PAHO Scientific Publication Ser.). 63p. pap. text 15.00 (*92-75-11490-0*) World Health.

***Primary Eyecare in Systemic Disease.** Kelly H. Thomann et al. 2nd ed. 2001. (Illus.). 736p. text 120.00 (*0-8385-8176-5*) McGraw-Hill Prof.

Primary Headache Disorders. Alan M. Rapoport & Fred D. Sheftell. Ed. by Bill Schmitt. 1996. 176p. text 41.00 (*0-7216-4051-6*) Saunders.

Primary Health Care: Report of the International Conference on Primary Health Care, 1978. 1978. text (*92-4-180001-1*) World Health.

Primary Health Care: The African Experience. Ed. by Raymond W. Carlaw & William B. Ward. 1988. LC 80-54741. (Case Studies in Community Health Education: Vol. 2). 472p. pap. 19.95 (*0-89914-025-4*) Third Party Pub.

Primary Health Care - From Theory to Action: Report on a WHO Symposium. 1982. (Euro Reports & Studies Ser.: No. 69). 29p. pap. text 4.00 (*92-890-1235-8*) World Health.

Primary Health Care & Local Health Systems in the Caribbean. 1989. 206p. text 25.00 (*92-75-12022-6*) World Health.

Primary Health Care & Psychiatric Epidemiology. Brian Cooper & Robin Eastwood. 1992. 320p. (C). text 110.00 (*0-415-07073-2*, A6619) Routledge.

Primary Health Care & the Private Sector. Maureen Devlin. 1998. LC 98-198177. (National Primary Care Research & Development Centre Ser.). 104p. pap. (*1-85775-244-9*) Radcliffe Med Pr GBR. *Dist:* Balogh.

Primary Health Care Buildings. Gordon Staff. 1997. (Briefing & Design Guides Ser.). (Illus.). 128p. pap. text (*0-419-20130-0*, Spon) Routledge.

***Primary Health Care for the Working Population.** Carol Love. 2002. (Illus.). (C). pap. text 34.95 (*0-7637-1881-5*, 1881-5) Jones & Bartlett.

Primary Health Care in Industrialized Countries. 1985. (EURO Reports & Studies: No. 95). 60p. pap. text 6.30 (*92-890-1261-7*, 1330095) World Health.

Primary Health Care in Omaha Nebraska: A Case Study of Nine Primary Health Care Centers. Stella G. Limson. 1986. (Illus.). 50p. (Orig.). pap. 3.50 (*1-55719-025-9*) U NE CPAR.

Primary Health Care in Undergraduate Medical Education: Summaries in French, German & Russian. 1984. pap. text 9.00 (*92-890-1027-4*) World Health.

Primary Health Care in Urban Communities. Ed. by Beverly J. McElmurry et al. 1997. 25.95 (*0-88737-734-3*, 14-7343, NLN Pr) Natl League Nurse.

Primary Health Care of the Young. Jane A. Fox. 1981. (Illus.). 1024p. text 51.95 (*0-07-021741-6*) McGraw.

Primary Health Care Pioneer: The Selected Works of Dr. Cicely D. Williams. Ed. by Naomi Baumslag. 1986. 12.00 (*0-87553-140-7*) Am Pub Health.

Primary Health Care Provision in Nepal. Shailendra Sigdel. 1998. pap. (*0-7855-7480-8*) Ratna Pustak Bhandar NPL. *Dist:* St Mut.

Primary Health Care Reviews: Guidelines & Methods. A. El Bindari-Hammad & D. L. Smith. 1992. (ENG & FRE.). xiv, 226p. pap. text 40.00 (*92-4-154437-6*, 1150374) World Health.

Primary Health Care Sciences: A Reader. Jane Sims. 1999. LC 00-500887. 220p. pap. text (*1-86156-103-2*) Whurr Pub.

Primary Healthcare of Children. Ed. by Jane A. Fox. 1997. LC 97-187475. (Illus.). 1120p. (C). (gr. 13). text 72.00 (*0-8151-3310-3*, 28202) Mosby Inc.

Primary Hematology. Ed. by Ayalew Tefferi. 2001. LC 00-53982. (Illus.). xiv, 472p. 99.00 (*0-89603-664-2*) Humana.

***Primary Hyperparathyroidism: A Study of Cardiovascular Dysfunction & Its Reversibility after Parathyroidectomy.** Inga-Lena Nilsson. 2001. (Comprehensive Summaries of Uppsala Dissertations from the Faculty of Medicine Ser.: No. 1066). (Illus.). 58p. pap. (*91-554-5090-3*) Acta Univ SWE. *Dist:* Coronet Bks.

Primary Hyperparathyroidism: Report Presented at the 93rd French Surgical Congress, Paris, September 1991. Ed. by J. Barbier & J. F. Henry. 1993. 168p. 97.00 (*0-387-59578-3*) Spr-Verlag.

Primary Liver Cancer. Ed. by Z. Tang & M. Wu. 1989. (Illus.). 495p. 368.00 (*0-387-50228-9*) Spr-Verlag.

Primary Liver Cancer: Etiology & Progression Factors. Christian Brechot. 1994. 320p. lib. bdg. 195.00 (*0-8493-4913-3*) CRC Pr.

Primary Liver Cancer in Japan. Ed. by T. Tobe. 1993. (Illus.). 466p. 331.00 (*0-387-70089-7*) Spr-Verlag.

Primary Low Vision Care. Rodney W. Nowakowski. 1995. LC 94-8438. 300p. (C). pap. text 75.00 (*0-8385-7980-9*, A7980-4, Apple Lange Med) McGraw.

Primary Management of Musculoskeletal Trauma. David Seligson & Kurt Voos. 1996. LC 96-42532. 256p. pap. text 42.00 (*0-397-51389-5*) Lppncott W & W.

Primary Medical Practice: A Psychiatric Evaluation. Lucy M. Zabarenko et al. 1968. LC 67-26018. (Illus.). 272p. 11.75 (*0-87527-090-5*) Green.

Primary Mental Health Care. James Behrman. 1992. 161p. (Orig.). pap. 12.95 (*0-929240-48-0*) EMIS.

Primary Neurologic Care. Jeannine Millette Petit. 2000. LC 00-41137. (Illus.). xi, 307p. text 49.95 (*0-8151-5304-X*, 29742) Mosby Inc.

Primary Nursing: Nursing in the Burford & Oxford Nursing Development Units. Ed. by Alan Pearson. 1988. 160p. pap. text (*0-7099-4066-1*) C Helm GBR. *Dist:* Routldge.

Primary Nursing Practice. Gloria Caliandro & Barbara L. Judkins. 1988. 663p. (C). text 50.00 (*0-673-39731-9*) Lppncott W & W.

Primary Orthopedic Care. Christy Crowther. 1999. LC 99-36528. (Illus.). 450p. (C). (gr. 13). pap. text 54.95 (*0-8151-1376-5*, 29560) Mosby Inc.

Primary Pediatric Care. Robert A. Hoekelman. 3rd ed. 1996. (Illus.). 1936p. (C). (gr. 13). text 99.95 (*0-8151-4547-0*, 24922) Mosby Inc.

Primary Pediatric Care. Robert A. Hoekelman et al. 4th ed. 2000. pap. 199.00 incl. cd-rom (*0-323-00829-1*) Mosby Inc.

Primary Pediatric Care Package. Robert A. Hoekelman. 1996. (*0-8151-2396-5*) Mosby Inc.

Primary Pediatric Pulmonolgy. Ed. by Allen J. Dozor. 2000. LC 00-34098. (Illus.). 450p. 88.00 (*0-87993-464-6*) Futura Pub.

Primary Prevention & Cancer. Ed. by Willy J. Eylenbosch et al. 1991. (Recent Results in Cancer Research Ser.). (Illus.). 130p. 69.00 (*0-387-53704-X*) Spr-Verlag.

Primary Prevention for Children & Families. Ed. by Mary Frank. 1982. LC 81-17858. (Journal of Children in Contemporary Society: Vol. 14, Nos. 2-3). 119p. text 39.95 (*0-86656-107-2*) Haworth Pr.

Primary Prevention of Coronary Heart Disease. 1985. (Euro Reports & Studies Ser.: No. 97). 96p. pap. text 10.00 (*92-890-1264-1*) World Health.

Primary Prevention of Essential Hypertension. 1983. (Technical Report Ser.: No. 686). 40p. pap. text 4.00 (*92-4-120686-1*) World Health.

Primary Prevention of Rheumatic Diseases. R. D. Wigley. 1993. (Illus.). 370p. lib. bdg. 93.95 (*1-85070-366-3*, Parthenon Pbng) CRC Pr.

Primary Prevention Practices. Martin Bloom. 1996. LC 95-41736. (Issues in Children's & Families' Lives Ser.: Vol. 5). (Illus.). 512p. 86.95 (*0-8039-7151-6*, 2677); xiv, 442p. pap. 37.95 (*0-8039-7152-4*, 2676) Sage.

Primary Preventive Counseling. Robert Conyne. 1987. LC 87-70757. xvi, 272p. 23.95 (*0-915202-70-0*) Accel Devel.

Primary Pulmonary Hypertension. Ed. by Lewis J. Rubin & Stuart Rich. 1996. LC 96-36758. (Lung Biology in Health & Disease Ser.: Vol. 99). (Illus.). 384p. text 185.00 (*0-8247-9505-9*) Dekker.

Primary Pulmonary Hypertension: Proceedings of the WHO Expert Committee, Geneva, Oct. 15-17, 1973. WHO Staff. Ed. by S. Hatano & T. Strasser. 1975. pap. text 9.00 (*92-4-156044-4*, 1150131) World Health.

Primary Reference Preparations Used to Standardize Calibration of Immunochemical Assays for Serum Prostate Specific Antigen (PSA) Approved Guideline (1996) Contrib. by Robert M. Nakamura. 1996. 75.00 (*1-56238-263-2*, I/LA19-A) NCCLS.

Primary Reference Preparations Used to Standardize Calibration of Immunochemical Assys for Serum Prostate Specific Antigen (PSA) Approved Guideline (1997) 1997. 75.00 (*1-56238-323-X*, I/LA19-A) NCCLS.

Primary Repair of Soft Tissue Injuries: With Special Reference to the Head & Extremities. R. V. Thompson. 1969. 39.95 (*0-522-83924-X*) Intl Spec Bk.

Primary Rhinoplasty. John B. Tebbetts. 1998. LC 98-20961. (Illus.). 368p. (C). (gr. 13). text 275.00 (*0-8151-8892-7*, 28888) Mosby Inc.

Primary Sclerosing Cholangitis. R. W. Chapman et al. Ed. by M. P. Manns. 1998. 144p. 108.00 (*0-7923-8745-7*) Kluwer Academic.

***Primary Sjogren's Syndrome: Clinical Studies with Reference to Hormonal Status, Psychiatric Symptoms & Well-Being.** Sigridur Th. Valtysdottir. 2001. (Comprehensive Summaries of Uppsala Disertations from the Faculty of Medicine: No. 984). (Illus.). 50p. (Orig.). pap. (*91-554-4903-4*) Uppsala Universitet SWE. *Dist:* Coronet Bks.

Primary Tumors of the Brain & Spinal Cord. S. Clifford Schold, Jr. et al. 1996. LC 96-45076. 181p. text 59.99 (*0-7506-9060-7*) Buttrwrth-Heinemann.

***Primary Tumours of the Central Nervous System.** Posner et al. 2001. (Illus.). 256p. (*1-901865-37-1*) Isis Med GBR. *Dist:* Bks Intl VA.

Primary Veterinary Anatomy. Ranajit Kumar Ghosh. 1999. 350p. pap. (*81-86793-34-8*) Current Bks Intl.

Primate Atherosclerosis. G. A. Gresham. Ed. by David Kritchevsky et al. 1976. (Monographs on Atherosclerosis: Vol. 7). 42.75 (*3-8055-2270-3*) S Karger.

Primate Brain Evolution: Methods & Concepts. Ed. by Este Armstrong & Dean Falk. 1982. LC 81-21150. 346p. (C). 79.50 (*0-306-40914-3*, Plenum Trade) Perseus Pubng.

Primate Laterality: Current Behavioral Evidence of Primate Asymmetrics. Ed. by J. P. Ward & W. D. Hopkins. 1993. (Recent Research in Psychology Ser.). (Illus.). 356p. 86.95 (*0-387-97961-1*) Spr-Verlag.

Primate Model for the Study of Colitis & Colonic Carcinoma: The Cotton Top Tamarin (Saguinus Oedipus) Neal K. Clapp. 1993. 352p. 225.00 (*0-8493-5363-7*, RC862) CRC Pr.

Primate Nervous System Pt. II. F. E. Bloom et al. 1998. (Handbooks of Chemical Neuroanatomy: Vol. 14). 448p. 211.50 (*0-444-82912-1*) Elsevier.

Primate Ovary. Ed. by Richard L. Stouffer. 1988. LC 88-2545. (Serono Symposia U. S. A. Ser.). (Illus.). 288p. 75.00 (*0-306-42824-5*, Plenum Trade) Perseus Pubng.

Primate Responses to Environmental Change. Ed. by Hilary O. Box. 1991. (Illus.). 430p. (C). (gr. 13). pap. text 179.95 (*0-412-29940-2*, A1630) Chapman & Hall.

Primate Societies: Group Techniques of Ecological Adaptations. Hans Kummer. 1971. LC 78-140010. (Worlds of Man Ser.). (C). pap. text 12.95 (*0-88295-613-2*) Harlan Davidson.

Primer Drug Action. Julien. 8th ed. 2000. pap. 24.00 (*0-7167-3365-X*) W H Freeman.

Primer for Beginning Psychotherapy. William N. Goldstein. (Basic Principles into Practice Ser.). 1997. LC 97-25327. 101p. pap. (*0-87630-859-0*); 2nd ed. 2001. LC 00-46675. 138p. 19.95 (*1-58391-074-3*) Brunner-Routledge.

Primer for Health Care Ethics. Ed. by Kevin D. O'Rourke. 2nd ed. 2000. LC 00-25273. xiii, 323p. pap. text 21.95 (*0-87840-802-9*) Georgetown U Pr.

Primer for Health Care Ethics: Essays for a Pluralistic Society. Patrick Norris et al. 1994. LC 94-11005. 255p. pap. 19.95 (*0-87840-562-3*) Georgetown U Pr.

Primer for Health Care, Health Education & All Disciplines Amidst Change. Ed. by Joseph S. DiPietro. 1999. LC 99-21013. (Studies in Health & Human Services: Vol. 33). 156p. 69.95 (*0-7734-7958-9*) E Mellen.

Primer for Heart Disease: For Patients & Their Families. Joe R. Wise. 2000. LC 00-102173. (Illus.). 112p. pap. 9.95 (*1-890437-28-X*) Western Reflections.

Primer for Impairment Evaluations. Gabriel E. Sella. 1995. 397p. (C). pap. text 120.00 (*1-884325-10-6*) G E Sella.

Primer for Prevention. Paul Terry et al. 1991. stu. ed. (*1-884153-05-4*) Prk Nicollet.

Primer for Psychiatric Nurses. Ed. by Ed Lister & A. Silva. 1990. 159p. (Orig.). (C). pap. text 24.95 (*0-9627287-9-9*) Cnslts Psych Nursing.

Primer for Stuttering Therapy. Howard D. Schwartz. 1998. LC 98-23833. 226p. (C). pap. text 87.00 (*0-205-27556-7*) Allyn.

Primer for Today's Substance Abuse Counselors. Rostyslaw Roback. 1991. 152p. 23.95 (*0-669-26935-2*) Lxngtn Bks.

Primer for Treating Substance Abusers. Jerome D. Levin. 1998. LC 98-6397. (Library of Substance Abuse & Addiction Treatment). 312p. 30.00 (*0-7657-0078-6*) Aronson.

Primer for Working with Child Abuse & Neglect. Vernon R. Wiehe. 1996. (Interpersonal Violence Ser.: Vol. 15). 208p. 79.95 (*0-7619-0348-8*, 2541); pap. 31.95 (*0-7619-0349-6*, 2542) Sage.

Primer in Phenomenological Psychology. Ernest Keen. 1982. LC 81-40901. (Illus.). 192p. reprint ed. pap. text 19.50 (*0-8191-2262-9*) U Pr of Amer.

Primer in Preventive Cardiology. T. A. Pearson et al. 1994. (Illus.). 290p. (C). pap. (*0-87493-006-5*) Am Heart.

Primer of Applied Radiation Physics. F. A. Smith. 1999. 460p. pap. text 46.00 (*981-02-3713-8*) World Scientific Pub.

Primer of Biomechanics. George L. Lucas et al. 1998. LC 97-48865. (Illus.). 314p. pap. 49.95 (*0-387-98456-9*) Spr-Verlag.

Primer of Biostatistics. Stanton A. Glantz. 4th ed. 1997. LC 96-26907. (Illus.). 473p. pap. 34.95 (*0-07-024268-2*) McGraw-Hill Educ Grp.

Primer of Biostatistics. Stanton A. Glantz. 3rd ed. 1992. (Illus.). 416p. pap. text 68.00 incl. disk (*0-07-864124-1*) McGraw-Hill Med Pub.

Primer of Brain Tumors. American Brain Tumors Association Staff. 7th ed. 1998. (Illus.). 132p. pap. (*0-944093-52-3*) Am Brain Tumor.

Primer of Brief Psychotherapy. John F. Cooper. 1995. LC 94-45948. 160p. (C). 23.00 (*0-393-70189-1*) Norton.

Primer of Cardiac Diagnosis: The Physical & Technical Study of the Cardiac Patient. Aldo A. Luisada & Gurmukh S. Sainani. 1968. LC 68-20943. (Illus.). 262p. 12.75 (*0-87527-049-2*) Green.

Primer of Chemical Pathology. E. S. Koay & R. N. Walmsley. 1997. 360p. text 48.00 (*981-02-2449-4*, QBcQm-UTB2921) World Scientific Pub.

Primer of Child Psychology. Paul L. Adams. 2nd ed. 1982. 19.00 (*0-316-03726-5*, Little Brwn Med Div) Lppncott W & W.

Primer of Clinical Intersubjectivity. Joseph M. Natterson & Raymond J. Friedman. 1995. LC 94-43799. 184p. pap. 35.00 (*1-56821-446-4*) Aronson.

Primer of Clinical Radiology. Thomas T. Thompson. 2nd ed. 1980. 19.95 (*0-316-84184-6*, Little Brwn Med Div) Lppncott W & W.

Primer of Dermatopathology. Antoinette F. Hood. 2nd ed. 1993. 496p. pap. text 105.00 (*0-316-37233-1*) Lppncott W & W.

Primer of Diagnostic Imaging. Jack Wittenberg & H. Weissleder. 2nd ed. 1996. (Illus.). 992p. (C). (gr. 13). pap. text 89.95 (*0-8151-9478-1*, 29192) Mosby Inc.

Primer of Drug Action. Robert M. Julien. 8th ed. 1997. LC 97-17171. 528p. text 29.95 (*0-7167-3112-6*) W H Freeman.

Primer of Epidemiology. Gary D. Friedman. 4th ed. 1994. LC 93-47357. 366p. pap. 29.00 (*0-07-022454-4*) McGraw-Hill Prof.

Primer of Experimental Psychology. Werner. 1992. (C). text 21.00 net. (*0-07-069547-4*) McGraw.

Primer of Freudian Psychology. Calvin S. Hall. 1999. LC 98-34780. 144p. pap. 13.95 (*0-452-01183-3*, Plume) NAL.

Primer of Freudian Psychology: Twenty-Fifth Anniversary Edition. Calvin S. Hall. 1955. pap. 6.99 (*0-451-62625-7*, ME2253, Ment) NAL.

Primer of Group Psychotherapy. Ray Naar. 1982. LC 81-4244. 215p. 35.95 (*0-89885-027-4*); pap. 22.95 (*0-89885-289-7*) Kluwer Academic (Kluwer Acad Hman Sci).

Primer of Human Behavioral Pharmacology. Alan D. Poling. 1986. (Applied Clinical Psychology Ser.). (Illus.). 262p. (C). 65.00 (*0-306-42186-0*, Plenum Trade) Perseus Pubng.

Primer of Immunology. Lyndon E. Mansfield. 1991. 25.00 (*0-07-039919-0*) McGraw.

Primer of Intraoperative Neurophysiologic Monitoring. Garfield B. Russell & Lawrence D. Rodichok. 1995. LC 95-12875. 331p. text 69.99 (*0-7506-9553-6*) Buttrwrth-Heinemann.

Primer of Jungian Psychology. Calvin S. Hall. 1999. LC 98-34779. 144p. pap. 13.95 (*0-452-01186-8*, Plume) NAL.

Primer of Jungian Psychology. Calvin S. Hall & Vernon J. Nordby. 1973. 144p. pap. 6.99 (*0-451-62578-1*, ME2233, Ment) NAL.

Primer of Kleinian Therapy. Irving Solomon. 1995. LC 94-36578. 240p. pap. text 45.00 (*1-56821-391-3*) Aronson.

Primer of Medical RadioBiology. E. L. Travis. 2nd ed. 1989. 320p. (gr. 13). pap. text 41.95 (*0-8151-8837-4*, 20123) Mosby Inc.

Primer of Misbehavior: An Introduction to Abnormal Psychology. George R. Wesley. 1975. (Quality Paperback Ser.: No. 262). 203p. reprint ed. pap. 3.95 (*0-8226-0262-8*) Littlefield.

Primer of Nursing Research. Mary R. Castles. 1987. (Illus.). 208p. pap. text 29.00 (*0-7216-1713-1*) Saunders.

Primer of Nursing Research. Divina Grossman. 1999. (C). pap. text (*0-8053-3240-5*) Benjamin-Cummings.

Primer of Palliative Care. Porter Storey. 1994. 57p. (Orig.). pap. 4.95 (*1-889296-00-7*) Am Acad Hospice.

Primer of Pancreatitis. P. G. Lankisch et al. 1997. LC 97-28507. (Illus.). 68p. pap. 17.00 (*3-540-63259-X*) Spr-Verlag.

Primer of Population Biology. Edward O. Wilson & William H. Bossert. 1971. LC 73-155365. (Illus.). 192p. (C). pap. text 21.95 (*0-87893-926-1*) Sinauer Assocs.

Primer of Projective Techniques of Psychological Assessment. Ed. by James C. Crumbaugh. 1989. LC 87-92178. 20.00 (*0-87212-215-8*) Libra.

Primer of Psychotherapy. Robert J. Langs. 1993. LC 86-22869. 256p. (C). reprint ed. pap. text 29.50 (*0-89876-197-2*) Gardner Pr.

Primer of Sectional Anatomy with MRI & CT Correlation. Charles P. Barrett et al. 2nd ed. 1994. LC 93-34302. (Illus.). 160p. pap. 29.00 (*0-683-00472-7*) Lppncott W & W.

Primer of Supportive Psychotherapy. Henry Pinsker. 1997. LC 97-41400. 296p. 49.95 (*0-88163-274-0*) Analytic Pr.

***Primer of Transference Focused Psychotherapy for the Borderline Patient.** Frank Yeomans et al. 2001. pap. 45.00 (*0-7657-0355-6*) Aronson.

Primer of Veterinary Anatomic. Dunstan. 1993. (*0-397-51102-7*) Lppncott W & W.

Primer of Water, Electrolyte & Acid-Base Syndromes. Jeffrey M. Brensilver & Emanuel Goldberger. 8th ed. 1996. LC 95-11650. (Illus.). 416p. (C). pap. 32.50 (*0-8036-0054-2*) OUP.

Primer on Amputations & Artificial Limbs. George Murdoch & A. Bennett Wilson, Jr. 1997. LC 97-22982. (Illus.). 314p. text 66.95 (*0-398-06800-3*); pap. text 51.95 (*0-398-06801-1*) C C Thomas.

Primer on Cerebrovascular Diseases. Ed. by K. M. Welch et al. 1997. LC 96-49201. (Illus.). 823p. text 159.00 (*0-12-743170-5*); pap. text 87.00 (*0-12-743171-3*) Morgan Kaufmann.

Primer on Corticosteroid-Induced Osteoporosis. Jonathan D. Adachi & George Ioannidis. 1999. 54p. pap. text 49.95 (*0-7817-2443-0*) Lppncott W & W.

Primer on Death & Dying for Medical Students. Richard M. Blacher et al. rev. ed. 2000. 60p. reprint ed. 8.95 (*0-930194-91-8*) Ctr Thanatology.

Primer on Integrating Psychotherapies for Children & Adolescents. Sebastiano Santostefano. 1998. LC 97-29509. 352p. pap. 50.00 (*0-7657-0109-X*) Aronson.

Primer on Kidney Diseases. Greenberg. 2nd ed. 1998. (C). 49.95 (*0-12-299095-1*) Acad Pr.

Primer on Kidney Diseases. Ed. by Arthur Greenberg. 2nd ed. 1997. LC 98-106530. (Illus.). 542p. pap. text 57.95 (*0-12-299090-0*) Morgan Kaufmann.

***Primer on Lymphedema.** Deborah G. Kelly. 2001. 176p. pap. 30.67 (*0-13-022410-3*) P-H.

Primer on Measurement: An Introductory Guide to Measurement Issues. 1993. 146p. pap. 36.75 (*0-912452-92-7*, P-98) Am Phys Therapy Assn.

Primer on Medical Malpractice. Harry Rein. 1988. 400p. stu. ed. 100.00 (*1-55917-569-9*, 132B) Natl Prac Inst.

Primer on Neural Nets. Jack D. Cowan & David H. Sharp. 1995. 150p. 17.50 (*0-262-03146-9*) MIT Pr.

Primer on Public & Private Juridic Persons: Applications to the Healthcare Ministry. Jordan F. Hite. 2000. 43p. pap. 18.00 (*0-87125-257-0*) Cath Health.

Primer on Rational-Emotive Therapy. Windy Dryden & Raymond DiGiuseppe. 1990. LC 89-69838. 108p. (Orig.). pap. text 11.95 (*0-87822-319-3*, 4420) Res Press.

Primer on Soft Tissue Injuries. Harry Rein. 1988. 272p. stu. ed. 25.00 (*1-55917-566-4*, 131B) Natl Prac Inst.

Primer on the Autonomic Nervous System. Ed. by David Robertson et al. 1996. LC 95-25734. (Illus.). 343p. text 79.95 (*0-12-589760-X*); pap. text 47.00 (*0-12-589761-8*) Acad Pr.

Primer on the Complexities of Traumatic Memory of Childhood Sexual Abuse: A Psychological Approach. Fay H. Knopp & Anna Benson. Ed. by Euan Bear. 1997. 320p. (C). text 20.00 (*1-884444-20-2*) Safer Soc.

Primer on the Rheumatic Diseases. John H. Klippel et al. Ed. by Arthritis Foundation Staff. 11th ed. 1998. LC 97-25311. 528p. pap. 39.95 (*0-912423-16-1*) Longstreet.

Primer on Theory & Operation of Linear Accelerators in Radiation Therapy. C. J. Karmark & Robert J. Morton. 2nd ed. 1997. LC 96-24382. pap. text 26.95 (*0-944838-66-9*) Med Physics Pub.

Primer on Transplantation. Douglas J. Norman et al. 1997. LC 97-50158. (Illus.). xxii, 586p. text 120.00 (*0-9660150-0-2*) ASTP.

Primer on Working with Resistance. Martha Stark. 1994. LC 93-32471. 280p. pap. 45.00 (*1-56821-093-0*) Aronson.

Primeros Auxilios y RCP. National Safety Council Staff. 1994. (Emergency Care Ser.). (Illus.). 96p. (C). pap. text 16.95 (*0-86720-847-3*, 847-3) Jones & Bartlett.

Primeval Forest: Including on the Edge of the Primeval Forest; And, More from the Primeval Forest. Albert Schweitzer & Albert Schweitzer Institute for the Humanities Staff. 1998. LC 98-6946. (Albert Schweitzer Library). pap. (*0-8018-6034-2*) Johns Hopkins.

Priming the Anabolic Environment: A Practical, Scientific Guide to the Art & Science of Building Muscle. William D. Brink. 1996. (Illus.). viii, 120p. pap. (*1-55210-003-0*) MuscleMag Intl CAN. *Dist:* BookWorld.

Primitive & Ancient Medicine, Vol. 1. Plinio Prioreschi. 1991. LC 91-29934. 672p. lib. bdg. 129.95 (*0-7734-9661-0*) E Mellen.

Primitive Drinking: A Study of the Uses & Functions of Alcohol in Preliterate Societies. Chandler Washburne. 1961. 25.95 (*0-8084-0253-6*) NCUP.

Primitive Edge of Experience see Limita Primitiva a Experientei

Primitive Edge of Experience. Thomas H. Ogden. LC 89-6878. 256p. 1993. pap. 40.00 (*0-87668-290-5*); 1989. 40.00 (*0-87668-982-9*) Aronson.

***Primitive Experiences of Loss: Working with the Paranoid-Schizoid Patient.** Robert Waska. 2001. pap. (*1-85575-260-3*) Karnac Bks GBR. *Dist:* Other Pr LLC.

Primitive Internalized Object Relations: A Clinical Study of Schizophrenic, Borderline, & Narcissistic Patients. Vamik D. Volkan. 1976. LC 75-18608. 304p. 52.50 (*0-8236-4995-4*) Intl Univs Pr.

Primitive Mental States: Across the Lifespan, Ed. by Shelley Alhanati & Katina Kostoulas. 1997. LC 10-901949. (Primitive Mental States Ser.: Vol. I). 296p. 52.00 (*1-56821-685-8*) Aronson.

Primitive Mental States & the Rorschach Test. Ed. by Howard D. Lerner & Paul M. Lerner. 1988. 80.00 (*0-8236-4295-X*) Intl Univs Pr.

Primordial Breath Vol. I: An Ancient Chinese Way of Prolonging Life Through Breath Control. Tr. by Jane Lu Huang & Michael Wurmbrand from CHI. 1987. 170p. (C). 22.50 (*0-944558-00-3*) Original Bks.

Primordial Immunity: Foundations for the Verterbrate Immune System. Ed. by Gregory Beck. 1994. LC 94-4703. (Annals Ser.). pap. 100.00 (*0-89766-840-5*) NY Acad Sci.

Primordial VRM System & Evolution of Vertebrate Immunity. J. Stewart. 1994. (Molecular Biology Intelligence Unit Ser.). 99.00 (*1-57059-119-9*) Landes Bioscience.

Primum Non Nocere Today - a Symposium on Pediatric Bioethics: Proceedings of the International Symposium on Pediatric Bioethics, Pavia, 26-28 May 1994. Ed. by G. Roberto Burgio et al. 1994. LC 94-40670. (International Congress Ser.: Vol. 1071). 186p. 158.50 (*0-444-81920-7*) Elsevier.

Princes & Peasants: Smallpox in History. Donald R. Hopkins. LC 83-6472. (Illus.). 1985. xx, 380p. pap. 12.95 (*0-226-35177-7*); 1983. 384p. 25.00 (*0-226-35176-9*) U Ch Pr.

Principal Addiction Specialist. Jack Rudman. 1994. (Career Examination Ser.: C-1398). pap. 34.95 (*0-8373-1398-8*) Nat Learn.

Principal Alcoholism Rehabilitaion Counselor. Jack Rudman. 1994. (Career Examination Ser.: C-2796). pap. 34.95 (*0-8373-2796-2*) Nat Learn.

Principal Diseases of Marine Fish & Shellfish, Vol. 1. Ed. by Carl J. Sindermann. 2nd ed. 1990. 521p. text 126.00 (*0-12-645851-0*) Acad Pr.

Principal Diseases of Marine Fish & Shellfish: Diseases of Marine Shellfish, Vol. 2. Carl J. Sindermann. 2nd ed. 1990. 516p. text 126.00 (*0-12-645852-9*) Acad Pr.

Principal Drug & Alcohol Counselor. Jack Rudman. 1994. (Career Examination Ser.: C-2743). pap. 34.95 (*0-8373-2743-1*) Nat Learn.

Principal Hospital Care Investigator. Jack Rudman. 1994. (Career Examination Ser.: C-612). pap. 34.95 (*0-8373-0612-4*) Nat Learn.

Principal Housing Inspector. Jack Rudman. 1994. (Career Examination Ser.: C-1426). reprint ed. pap. 39.95 (*0-8373-1426-7*) Nat Learn.

Principal Program Research Analyst. Jack Rudman. 1994. (Career Examination Ser.: C-2218). reprint ed. pap. 39.95 (*0-8373-2218-9*) Nat Learn.

Principal Public Health Nutritionist. Jack Rudman. 1994. (Career Examination Ser.: C-1566). pap. 34.95 (*0-8373-1566-2*) Nat Learn.

Principal Public Health Representative. Jack Rudman. 1994. (Career Examination Ser.: C-3025). pap. 34.95 (*0-8373-3025-4*) Nat Learn.

Principal Public Health Sanitarian. Jack Rudman. 1994. (Career Examination Ser.: C-3347). pap. 34.95 (*0-8373-3347-4*) Nat Learn.

Principal Safety Coordinator. Jack Rudman. 1994. (Career Examination Ser.: C-2669). pap. 39.95 (*0-8373-2669-9*) Nat Learn.

Principal Senior Citizens' Program Coordinator. Jack Rudman. 1994. (Career Examination Ser.: C-2799). pap. 34.95 (*0-8373-2799-7*) Nat Learn.

Principal X-Ray Technician. Jack Rudman. 1994. (Career Examination Ser.: C-979). pap. 34.95 (*0-8373-0979-4*) Nat Learn.

Principalization of Plastic Surgery. D. Ralph Millard, Jr. 1986. 235.00 (*0-316-57153-9*, Little Brwn Med Div) Lppncott W & W.

Principal's Guide to Attention Deficit Hyperactivity Disorder. Elaine K. McEwan. 1998. (Principals Ser.). 240p. 69.95 (*0-8039-6531-1*, 80771) Corwin Pr.

Principals of Medical Biology Vol. 12: Reproductive Endocrinology & Biology. E. Edward Bittar & Neville Bittar. 1998. LC 98-18709. 354p. 90.00 (*1-55938-817-X*) Jai Pr.

Principals of Pharmacology: Basic Concepts & Clinical Applications. Ed. by Paul L. Munson et al. 1994. LC 94-41659. 1800p. (gr. 13). text 92.00 (*0-412-04701-2*) Chapman & Hall.

Principle Aspects of Clinical Nutrition. Ed. by J. C. Somogyi. 1985. (Bibliotheca Nutritio et Dieta Ser.: No. 35). (Illus.). viii, 132p. 98.50 (*3-8055-3950-9*) S Karger.

Principle of Autologous, Allogenic & Cyropreserved Venous Transplantation. Ed. by Kevin G. Brockbank. 1995. LC 95-19008. (Medical Intelligence Unit Ser.). 110p. text 79.00 (*1-57059-221-7*) Landes Bioscience.

Principled Practice: A Comprehensive Guide to the Non-Clinical Aspects of Dentistry. Cheryl A. Matschek. 1995. LC 94-47411. 389p. (*0-943367-05-0*) Princess Pub.

Principles: Practice of Mechanical Ventilation. John J. Marini & Sue A. Ravenscraft. 1994. (Illus.). 544p. (*0-683-05556-9*) Lppncott W & W.

Principles & Application of Collective Dose in Radiation Protection. Intro. by Charles B. Meinhold. 1995. LC 95-26030. (NCRP Reports: No. 121). 106p. (Orig.). pap. 25.00 (*0-929600-46-0*) NCRP Pubns.

Principles & Applications of Biomedical Magnetic Resonance Imaging. Ed. by Felix W. Wehrli et al. 1988. LC 87-29566. 601p. 115.00 (*0-89573-349-8*, Wiley-VCH) Wiley.

Principles & Applications of Cardiorespiratory Equipment. Ed. by David Eubanks & Roger C. Bone. 1994. LC 93-30441. (Illus.). 394p. (C). (gr. 13). text 56.00 (*0-8016-7448-4*, 01534) Mosby Inc.

Principles & Applications of Hydrochemistry. Erik Eriksson. 1986. 200p. (gr. 13). pap. 119.95 (*0-412-25040-3*, 9671) Chapman & Hall.

Principles & Applications of Intraocular Gas. Marc M. Whitacre. 1997. LC 97-21509. (Illus.). 400p. text 95.00 (*0-7506-9713-X*) Buttrwrth-Heinemann.

Principles & Art of Cure by Homoeopathy. 1942. 14.95 (*0-85032-049-6*) Formur Intl.

Principles & Art of Cure by Homoeopathy. Herbert A. Roberts. 1942. 286p. (C). pap. 38.95 (*0-8464-1042-7*) Beekman Pubs.

Principles & Art of Cure by Homoeopathy. Herbert A. Roberts. 1980. 30.00 (*0-85032-181-6*) St Mut.

Principles & Dynamics of Local Skin Flaps. Terence M. Davidson et al. 4th rev. ed. 1998. LC 98-3832. (Self-Instructional Package Ser.). (Illus.). 110p. pap. text 25.00 (*1-56772-062-5*) AAO-HNS.

Principles & General Procedures for Handling Emergency & Accidental Exposure of Workers. ICRP Staff. 1978. (International Commission on Radiological Protection Ser.: Vol. 28). 22p. pap. 13.50 (*0-08-022636-1*, Pergamon Pr) Elsevier.

Principles & Issues in Nutrition. Yiu H. Hui. 1985. LC 84-27051. (Nursing-Health Science Ser.). (Illus.). 700p. (C). pap. text, tchr. ed. 10.00 (*0-534-04375-5*, 375-5) Jones & Bartlett.

Principles & Management of Adrenal Cancer. Ed. by Nasser Javadpour. 1987. (Illus.). 180p. 110.00 (*0-387-16210-0*) Spr-Verlag.

Principles & Methods for Assessing Direct Immunotoxicity Associated with Exposure to Chemicals. Date not set. (Environmental Health Criteria Ser.: No. 180). 379p. (Orig.). pap. text 64.80 (*92-4-157180-2*, 1160180) Am Soc Clinical.

Principles & Methods for the Assessment of Nephrotoxicity Associated with Exposure to Chemicals. 1991. (Environmental Health Criteria Ser.: No. 119). (ENG, FRE & SPA.). 266p. pap. text 46.00 (*92-4-157119-5*, 1160119) World Health.

Principles & Methods of Quality Management in Health Care. Donald E. Lighter & Douglas C. Fair. 2000. LC 00-29976. (Illus.). xiii, 458p. 64.00 (*0-8342-1861-5*) Aspen Pub.

Principles & Methods of Social Psychology. Edwin P. Hollander. 4th ed. 1981. (Illus.). 574p. (C). text 38.95 (*0-19-502822-8*) OUP.

Principles & Methods of Sterilization in Health Sciences. John J. Perkins. 2nd ed. 1983. (Illus.). 580p. 83.95 (*0-398-01478-7*) C C Thomas.

Principles & Methods of Toxicology. A. Wallace Hayes. 4th ed. 2000. LC 00-37719. (Illus.). xix, 1887p. (gr. 13). text 110.00 (*1-56032-814-2*) Taylor & Francis.

Principles & Perspective in Drug Bioavailability. J. Blanchard et al. 1978. 85.25 (*3-8055-2440-4*) S Karger.

Principles & Positioning for MRI. Noyes. 2001. (Allied Health Ser.). (Illus.). 448p. (C). pap. 40.00 net. (*0-7668-1204-9*) Delmar.

Principles & Positioning for MRI-Exam Review. Noyes. 2001. (Allied Health Ser.). 224p. (C). pap. 20.00 net. (*0-7668-1205-7*) Delmar.

Principles & Positioning For Ultrasound. Noyes. 2002. (C). pap. 45.00 net. (*0-7668-1304-5*) Delmar.

Principles & Practice for Nursing Research. Laura A. Talbot. 1995. 752p. (C). text, tchr. ed. (*0-8151-8925-7*) Mosby Inc.

Principles & Practice of Addictions in Psychitry. Ed. by Norman S. Miller. 1997. LC 95-20662. (Illus.). 589p. 73.00 (*0-7216-5211-5*) Saunders.

Principles & Practice of Adult Health Nursing. Patricia G. Beare & Judith L. Myers. 1990. 50p. 75.00 (*0-8016-0389-7*); 3rd ed. 1998. 168p. pap. text, stu. ed. (*0-8151-1012-X*, 29579) Mosby Inc.

Principles & Practice of Adult Health Nursing. Ed. by Patricia G. Beare & Judith L. Myers. 3rd ed. 1997. LC 97-35022. (Illus.). 1920p. (C). (gr. 13). text 67.00 (*0-8151-1006-5*, 29567) Mosby Inc.

Principles & Practice of Adult Health Nursing: With Study Guide. Patricia G. Beare & Myers. 3rd ed. 1997. (Illus.). 2048p. (C). (gr. 13). text, stu. ed. 74.00 (*0-8151-1032-4*, 29577) Mosby Inc.

Principles & Practice of Ambulatory Pediatrics. S. Rajkumar & C. Toback. 1988. (Illus.). 856p. (C). text 210.00 (*0-306-42500-9*, Kluwer Plenum) Kluwer Academic.

Principles & Practice of Anesthesiology. John H. Tinker. Ed. by David E. Longnecker. 2nd ed. 1997. LC 97-24668. (Illus.). 2720p. (C). (gr. 13). text 225.00 (*0-8151-5479-8*, 29082) Mosby Inc.

Principles & Practice of Assisted Human Reproduction. Robert G. Edwards & Steven A. Brody. 1995. LC 94-25781. (Illus.). 702p. text 149.00 (*0-7216-3626-8*) Saunders.

Principles & Practice of Biologic Therapy of Cancer. Steven A. Rosenberg. 3rd ed. 2000. 944p. text 179.00 (*0-7817-2272-1*) Lppncott W & W.

Principles & Practice of Brachytherapy. Ed. by Subir Nag. 1997. LC 96-46939. (Illus.). 752p. 160.00 (*0-87993-654-1*) Futura Pub.

Principles & Practice of Burn Management. Settle. 1996. text (*0-443-04476-7*, S3611) Church.

Principles & Practice of Cardiopulmonary Physical Therapy. Donna L. Frownfelter & Dean. 3rd ed. 1996. (Illus.). 864p. (C). (gr. 13). text 66.00 (*0-8151-3340-5*, 24124) Mosby Inc.

Principles & Practice of Cardiopulmonary Physical Therapy: Clinical Case. Dean & Donna L. Frownfelter. 3rd ed. 1996. (Illus.). 256p. (C). (gr. 13). pap. text, stu. ed. 19.95 (*0-8151-2243-8*, 24873) Mosby Inc.

Principles & Practice of Cardiovascular Imaging. Gerald M. Pohost. 1990. 135.00 (*0-316-71247-7*, Little Brwn Med Div) Lppncott W & W.

Principles & Practice of Cardiovascular Medicine. Ed. by James T. Willerson & Jay N. Cohn. 1994. (Illus.). 1976p. text (*0-443-08781-4*) Church.

Principles & Practice of Child Psychiatry. Stella Chess & Mahin Hassibi. 2nd ed. 1986. (Illus.). 550p. (C). text 78.00 (*0-306-42167-4*, Kluwer Plenum) Kluwer Academic.

Principles & Practice of Clinical Anaerobic Bacteriology. Paul Engelkirk et al. 1992. (Illus.). 450p. pap. text 49.95 (*0-89863-160-2*) Star Pub CA.

Principles & Practice of Clinical Mycology. Christopher C. Kibbler et al. 1996. 288p. 285.00 (*0-471-96104-3*, Wiley-Interscience) Wiley.

Principles & Practice of Clinical Parasitology. Stephen Gillespie. 2001. LC 00-47755. 752p. 240.00 (*0-471-97729-2*) Wiley.

Principles & Practice of Clinical Virology. Arie J. Zuckerman et al. 4th ed. 1999. LC 98-50139. 800p. 325.00 (*0-471-97340-8*) Wiley.

Principles & Practice of Critical Care. Ed. by Christopher G. Garrard et al. 1997. LC 96-31346. (Illus.). 880p. 309.95 (*0-632-03283-9*) Blackwell Sci.

Principles & Practice of Day Surgery Nursing. Sarah Penn & Tony Davenport. 1996. LC 96-34126. (Illus.). 244p. (Orig.). pap. 46.95 (*0-632-03973-6*) Blackwell Sci.

Principles & Practice of Dentofacial Orthopaedics. Hugo Stockfisch. 1995.Tr. of Rationelle Kieferorthop Adie. (Illus.). 527p. text 98.00 (*1-85097-029-7*) Quint Pub Co.

Principles & Practice of Dermatology. Ed. by W. Mitchell Sams & Peter J. Lynch. 2nd ed. 1996. LC 95-38678. text (*0-443-08988-4*) Church.

Principles & Practice of Diagnostic Immunology. David E. Normansell. 1994. LC 94-3583. (Analytical Techniques in Clinical Chemistry & Laboratory Medicine Ser.). 60.00 (*1-56081-534-5*, Wiley-VCH) Wiley.

Principles & Practice of Dialysis. Ed. by William L. Henrich. 1994. LC 93-14146. (Illus.). 496p. 129.00 (*0-683-03973-3*) Lppncott W & W.

Principles & Practice of Dialysis. William L. Henrich. 2nd ed. 1998. LC 98-10017. 554p. text 129.00 (*0-683-30241-8*) Lppncott W & W.

Principles & Practice of Disinfection, Preservation & Sterilisation. A. D. Russell et al. 3rd ed. 1999. LC 98-14781. (Illus.). 826p. 208.95 (*0-632-04194-3*) Blackwell Sci.

Principles & Practice of Disinfection, Preservation & Sterilization. Ed. by A. D. Russell et al. 2nd ed. 1992. (Illus.). 656p. 165.00 (*0-632-02625-1*) Blackwell Sci.

Principles & Practice of Echocardiography. Arthur E. Weyman. 2nd ed. 1993. LC 90-13578. (Illus.). 1,335p. text 229.00 (*0-8121-1207-5*) Lppncott W & W.

Principles & Practice of Electron Microscope Operation. A. W. Agar et al. 1974. (Practical Methods in Electron Microscopy Ser.: Vol. 2). 346p. pap. 58.00 (*0-7204-4255-9*) Elsevier.

Principles & Practice of Electrotherapy. Joseph Kahn. (Illus.). 2nd ed. 1991. 170p. pap. text (*0-443-08730-X*); 3rd ed. 1994. pap. text (*0-443-08919-1*) Church.

Principles & Practice of Electrotherapy. Joseph Kahn. 4th ed. 1999. LC 99-51477. (Illus.). 220p. pap. text (*0-443-06553-5*) Saunders.

Principles & Practice of Emergency Medicine. George R. Schwartz et al. 4th ed. 1998. LC 98-3827. (Illus.). 2,100p. text 249.00 (*0-683-07646-9*) Lppncott W & W.

Principles & Practice of Emergency Medicine, Set. C. Gene Cayten et al. Ed. by Thom Mayer & Mary A. Mangelsen. 3rd ed. 1992. (Illus.). text 199.00 (*0-8121-1373-X*) Lppncott W & W.

Principles & Practice of Emergency Medicine: The Essential Update. George R. Schwartz. 1989. 250p. text 49.55 (*0-7216-2459-6*) Saunders.

Principles & Practice of Endocrinology & Metabolism. Kenneth L. Becker et al. 3rd ed. 2001. 2,512p. text 235.00 (*0-7817-1750-7*) Lppncott W & W.

***Principles & Practice of Endodontics.** Richard E. Walton & Mahmoud Torabinejad. 3rd ed. 2001. LC 2001-42814. (Illus.). 575p. (*0-7216-9160-9*) Saunders.

Principles & Practice of Environmental Medicine. Ed. by A. B. Tarcher. 1992. (Illus.). 648p. (C). text 114.00 (*0-306-42893-8*, Kluwer Plenum) Kluwer Academic.

Principles & Practice of Family Medicine: An Asian-Pacific Perspective of Primary Health Care. Ed. by John Fry & Nat Yuen. 1994. (*1-85775-045-4*) Radcliffe Med Pr GBR. *Dist:* Balogh.

Principles & Practice of Forensic Psychiatry. Ed. by Richard Rosner. 1999. LC 93-20238. (Arnold Publication). (Illus.). 656p. 145.00 (*0-442-01118-0*) OUP.

Principles & Practice of Gastroenterology & Hepatology. Ed. by Gary Gitnick et al. 2nd ed. 1994. LC 93-45496. (Illus.). 1162p. (C). pap. text 159.00 (*0-8385-8064-5*, A8064-6, Apple Lange Med) McGraw.

Principles & Practice of Genitourinary Oncology. Derek Raghavan. 1996. LC 96-8893. 1,184p. text 165.00 (*0-397-51458-1*) Lppncott W & W.

Principles & Practice of Geriatric Medicine, Set. Ed. by M. S. Pathy & Emeritus. 3rd ed. 1998. LC 96-37118. 1688p. 595.00 (*0-471-96348-8*) Wiley.

Principles & Practice of Geriatric Psychiatry. John R. Copeland et al. 1994. LC 92-48920. 1084p. 575.00 (*0-471-92654-X*, Wiley-Interscience) Wiley.

Principles & Practice of Geriatric Surgery. Ed. by Ronnie A. Rosenthal et al. 2000. LC 99-55303. (Illus.). 1224p. 195.00 (*0-387-98393-7*) Spr-Verlag.

Principles & Practice of Gynecologic Laser Surgery. Joseph H. Bellina & Gaetano Bandieramonte. 1984. LC 84-3434. 308p. 75.00 (*0-306-41543-7*, Plenum Trade) Perseus Pubng.

Principles & Practice of Gynecologic Oncology. William J. Hoskins et al. 3rd ed. 2000. LC 00-22097. 1,296p. text 199.00 (*0-7817-1978-X*) Lppncott W & W.

Principles & Practice of Hemodialysis. Total Renal Care, Inc., Educ. Dept. Staff. 1982. 214p. ring bd. 95.00 (*1-56488-000-1*) Dialyrn.

Principles & Practice of Hormone Therapy in Gynaecology & Obstetrics. Joachim Ufer. 1969. (C). 49.25 (*3-11-000614-6*) De Gruyter.

Principles & Practice of Immunoassay. Ed. by Christopher/P. Price & David J. Newman. 2nd ed. 1997. 650p. 140.00 (*1-56159-175-0*) Groves Dictionaries.

Principles & Practice of Immunotoxicology. K. Miller et al. 1991. (Illus.). 392p. 204.95 (*0-632-02563-8*) Blackwell Sci.

Principles & Practice of Infectious Diseases. Ed. by Gerald L. Mandell et al. 3rd ed. 1990. (Illus.). 2340p. text (*0-443-08686-9*); 4th ed. 1994. text (*0-443-08935-3*) Church.

***Principles & Practice of Infectious Diseases.** Gerald Mandell. 5th ed. 2000. 395.00 incl. cd-rom (*0-443-06581-0*) Harcrt Hlth Sci Grp.

Principles & Practice of Infectious Diseases: Antimicrobial Therapy 1996/1997. G. L. Mandell et al. 1996. 200p. pap. (*0-443-07844-0*) Church.

Principles & Practice of Infectious Diseases: Handbook of Antimicrobial Therapy. Gerald L. Mandell et al. 1992. 166p. (Orig.). (*0-443-08818-7*) Church.

Principles & Practice of Intensive Care Monitoring. Ed. by Martin Tobin. 1997. LC 97-42653. (Illus.). 1560p. (C). text 159.00 (*0-07-065094-2*) McGraw-Hill Prof.

Principles & Practice of Interventional Cardiology. M. Sue Apple. 1998. LC 99-38188. 320p. pap. text 32.95 (*0-7817-1020-0*) Lppncott W & W.

Principles & Practice of Maternal Nutrition. B. Luke & Louis G. Keith. 1992. LC 92-14082. (Illus.). 161p. lib. bdg. 42.95 (*1-85070-324-8*, Parthenon Pbng) CRC Pr.

Principles & Practice of Mechanical Ventilation. Ed. by Martin J. Tobin. 1994. LC 93-37105. 1328p. text 159.00 (*0-07-064943-X*) McGraw-Hill Prof.

Principles & Practice of Medical Intensive Care. Ed. by Richard W. Carlson & Michael A. Geheb. 1993. (Illus.). 1824p. text 220.00 (*0-7216-3396-X*) Saunders.

Principles & Practice of Medical Laboratory Science Vol. 1: Basic Histotechnology. Anthony S. Y. Leong. 1996. (Illus.). 179p. pap. (*0-443-05369-3*) Church GBR. *Dist:* Saunders.

Principles & Practice of Medical Laboratory Science Vol. 2: Medical Microbiology, Virology & Molecular Technology. Ed. by A. S. Leong. 1997. (Illus.). 252p. pap. (*0-443-05982-9*) Church.

Principles & Practice of Medical Therapy in Pregnancy. Louis Buttino, Jr. 3rd ed. 1998. 200p. pap., stu. ed. 55.00 (*0-8385-6296-5*) McGraw-Hill Prof.

Principles & Practice of Medical Therapy in Pregnancy. Norbert Gleicher. 3rd ed. 1998. LC 97-46683. (Illus.). 1600p. (C). text 159.00 (*0-8385-7677-X*, A-7677-6) McGraw-Hill Prof.

Principles & Practice of Medicine. John D. Stobo. 23rd ed. 1996. LC 96-23756. 1064p. (C). text 54.95 (*0-8385-7963-9*, A7963-0) McGraw-Hill Prof.

Principles & Practice of Medicine. Composed by Stobo. 24th ed. 2001. (Lange Medical Bks.). (Illus.). 1200p. (C). pap. 49.95 (*0-8385-8128-5*, Apple Lange Med) McGraw.

Principles & Practice of Military Forensic Psychiatry. Ed. by R. Gregory Lande & David T. Armitage. 1997. LC 96-52386. 554p. text 103.95 (*0-398-06752-X*) C C Thomas.

Principles & Practice of Movement Disorders. Ed. by S. Fahn et al. 1998. (Illus.). 600p. text (*0-443-07941-2*) Church.

Principles & Practice of Neuroanaesthesia. N. Edwards. 1990. (Illus.). 544p. (C). (gr. 13). pap. 169.95 (*0-412-37220-7*) Chapman & Hall.

Principles & Practice of Nuclear Medicine. Early & Sodee. 2nd ed. 1994. (Illus.). 896p. (gr. 13). text 99.00 (*0-8016-2577-7*, 02577) Mosby Inc.

***Principles & Practice of Nuclear Medicine.** Paul J. Early et al. 3rd ed. 2001. (Illus.). 860p. (*0-323-01204-3*) Mosby Inc.

***Principles & Practice of Nurse Anesthesia.** Wynne R. Waugaman & Scot D. Foster. 3rd ed. 2001. 899p. 60.00 (*0-13-098020-X*) P-H.

Principles & Practice of Nurse Anesthesia. Wynne R. Waugaman et al. 3rd ed. 1998. LC 97-46159. (Illus.). 912p. 106.67 (*0-8385-8118-8*) P-H.

Principles & Practice of Nurse Education. F. M. Quinn. 3rd ed. 1999. 496p. pap. (*0-7487-3170-9*); 4th ed. 2000. (Illus.). 656p. pap. (*0-7487-3895-9*) Nelson Thornes GBR. *Dist:* Intl Spec Bk, Trans-Atl Phila.

Principles & Practice of Nursing Research. Laura A. Talbot. 1994. (Illus.). 752p. (C). (gr. 13). text 46.00 (*0-8016-6450-0*, 06450) Mosby Inc.

Principles & Practice of Obstetric Anaesthesia & Analgesia. A. Holdcroft & T. Thomas. 2000. LC 99-21230. (Illus.). 466p. 157.95 (*0-86542-828-X*) Blackwell Sci.

Principles & Practice of Obstetrics. V. Padubidri. 2000. (Illus.). 400p. text 39.95 (*0-19-564951-6*) OUP.

Principles & Practice of Ophthalmic Plastic & Reconstructive Surgery, Set. Stephen Bosniak. 1995. LC 95-12616. (Illus.). 1152p. text 375.00 (*0-7216-3559-8*) Saunders.

Principles & Practice of Ophthalmology, Set. Ed. by Daniel M. Albert & Frederick A. Jakobiec. 1993. (Illus.). text 825.00 (*0-7216-6592-6*) Saunders.

***Principles & Practice of Ophthalmology**, Set. Daniel M. Albert & Frederick A. Jakobiec. 2nd ed. 2000. (Illus.). 5583p. 1295.00 incl. cd-rom (*0-7216-8618-4*) Saunders.

Principles & Practice of Ophthalmology, Set. Daniel M. Albert & Frederick A. Jakobiec. 2nd ed. 2000. LC 99-29496. (Illus.). 5583p. (C). text 950.00 (*0-7216-7500-X*) Saunders.

Principles & Practice of Ophthalmology: Basic Sciences, Vol. 1. Ed. by Daniel M. Albert & Frederick A. Jokobiec. 1993. LC 93-12658. (Illus.). 1435p. text 195.00 (*0-7216-3416-8*) Saunders.

Principles & Practice of Ophthalmology: Clinical Practice, Set. Ed. by Daniel M. Albert & Frederick A. Jakobiec. 1993. LC 93-7247. (Illus.). text 695.00 (*0-7216-3418-4*) Saunders.

Principles & Practice of Opthalmology. Daniel M. Albert & Frederick A. Jakobiec. cd-rom (*0-7216-8614-1*) Saunders.

Principles & Practice of Oral Medicine. Stephen T. Sonis et al. 2nd ed. 1994. (Illus.). 512p. text 72.00 (*0-7216-8449-1*) Saunders.

Principles & Practice of Orthodontics. J. R. Mills. 2nd ed. 1987. LC 87-10291. (Dental Ser.). (Illus.). 294p. pap. text (*0-443-03608-X*) Church.

Principles & Practice of Orthopaedic Sports Medicine. William E. Garrett, Jr. et al. 2000. 976p. text 169.00 (*0-7817-2578-X*) Lppncott W & W.

Principles & Practice of Pain Management. Ed. by Carol A. Warfield. 1992. LC 92-20392. (Illus.). 552p. text 89.00 (*0-07-068291-7*) McGraw-Hill Educ Grp.

Principles & Practice of Pediatric Anesthesia. Bruno Bissonnette & Bernard J. Dalens. 2001. LC 2001-31484. (Illus.). 1200p. text 195.00 (*0-07-135454-9*) McGraw-Hill Prof.

Principles & Practice of Pediatric Infectious Diseases. Sarah S Long et al. 1996. LC 96-19019. text (*0-443-08943-4*) Church.

Principles & Practice of Pediatric Neurosurgery. A. Leland Albright et al. 1999. LC 98-29770. (Illus.). 1472p. 249.00 (*0-86577-799-3*) Thieme Med Pubs.

Principles & Practice of Pediatric Optometry. David Rosenbloom & Meredith W. Morgan. 1990. (Illus.). 496p. text 75.00 (*0-397-50917-0*) Lppncott W & W.

Principles & Practice of Pharmaceutical Medicine. Andrew Fletcher et al. 2001. LC 2001-24251. 584p. 150.00 (*0-471-98655-0*) Wiley.

Principles & Practice of Pharmacology for Anaesthetists. T. Norman Calvey & N. E. Williams. 3rd ed. 1997. LC 96-20973. (Illus.). 608p. 165.00 (*0-632-04156-0*) Blackwell Sci.

Principles & Practice of Phycology. Simon Mills & Kerry Bone. 1999. 643p. (C). text 75.00 (*0-443-06016-9*) Harcourt Coll Pubs.

Principles & Practice of Physical Therapy. W. E. Arnould-Taylor. 3rd ed. 1991. (Illus.). 224p. pap. (*0-7487-1250-X*) Nelson Thornes GBR. *Dist:* Trans-Atl Phila.

Principles & Practice of Physiologic Acupuncture. George A. Ulett. 1982. 232p. 42.50 (*0-87527-309-2*) Green.

Principles & Practice of Podiatric Medicine. L. A. Levy & V. J. Hetherington. 2nd ed. 1998. (Illus.). 854p. text (*0-443-07940-4*) Church.

***Principles & Practice of Psychiatric Nursing: Instructor's Electronic Resource.** Gail W. Stuart & Michele T. Laraia. 2001. (*0-323-01255-8*) Mosby Inc.

Principles & Practice of Psychopharmacotherapy. Philip G. Janicak et al. 2nd ed. 1997. LC 97-13497. 668p. 105.00 (*0-683-30266-3*) Lppncott W & W.

Principles & Practice of Public Health Surveillance. 1993. 380p. (Orig.). (C). pap. text 65.00 (*1-56806-516-7*) DIANE Pub.

Principles & Practice of Pulmonary Rehabilitation. Ed. by Richard Casaburi & Thomas L. Petty. 1993. LC 92-13386. (Illus.). 528p. text 92.00 (*0-7216-3304-8*) Saunders.

Principles & Practice of Radiation Oncology. Ed. by Carlos A. Perez & Luther Brady. 3rd ed. 1997. (Illus.). 2,368p. text 299.00 (*0-397-58416-4*) Lppncott W & W.

Principles & Practice of Radiation Oncology. Carlos A. Perez & Luther W. Brady. 3rd ed. 1997. 2,368p. 325.00 (*0-7817-1691-8*) Lppncott W & W.

Principles & Practice of Radiation Therapy: Physics, Simulation, & Treatment Planning. Charles M. Washington & Dennis T. Leaver. 2nd ed. 1996. (Illus.). 320p. (C). (gr. 13). text 61.00 (*0-8151-9136-7*, 24803) Mosby Inc.

Principles & Practice of Radiation Therapy: Practical Applications. Charles M. Washington & Dennis T. Leaver. (Illus.). 384p. 3. 3rd ed. 1996. (C). (gr. 13). text 59.00 (*0-8151-9137-5*, 24804); Vol. 3. 1997. tchr. ed. (*0-8151-9253-3*) Mosby Inc.

Principles & Practice of Radiotherapy Treatment Planning. Euan Thomson et al. 2000. (Illus.). 300p. pap. text 49.50 (*1-900151-89-8*) OUP.

Principles & Practice of Refractive Surgery. Richard E. Elander et al. Ed. by Richard Lampert. 1997. LC 96-17646. 640p. text 236.00 (*0-7216-6552-7*) Saunders.

Principles & Practice of Regional Anesthesia. J. A. Wildsmith & Edward N. Armitage. 1987. (Illus.). 288p. (*0-443-03128-2*) Church.

Principles & Practice of Regional Anesthesia. Ed. by J. A. Wildsmith & Edward N. Armitage. 2nd ed. 1993. LC 92-49107. (Illus.). 272p. text (*0-443-04475-9*) Church.

Principles & Practice of Renal Nursing. Paul Challinor & John Sedgewick. 1998. (Illus.). pap. (*0-7487-3331-0*) Nelson Thornes GBR. *Dist:* Intl Spec Bk, Trans-Atl Phila.

Principles & Practice of Research in Midwifery. Contrib. by Elizabeth R. Cluett & Rosalind Bluff. 2000. LC 99-53490. (*0-7020-2425-2*) Bailliere Tindall.

Principles & Practice of Sedation. J. G. Whitwam & M. R. Vinik. 1998. LC 97-46160. (Illus.). 300p. 99.95 (*0-86542-678-3*) Blackwell Sci.

Principles & Practice of Sedation. J. G. Whitwam. 2nd rev. ed. 1998. 115.95 (*0-632-05219-8*) Blackwell Sci.

Principles & Practice of Skin Excisions. Borut I. Jemec & Gregor B. Jemec. 1995. 308p. 117.50 (*0-444-82341-7*) Elsevier.

Principles & Practice of Sleep Medicine. Ed. by Meir H. Kryger et al. 2nd ed. 1993. LC 92-48200. (Illus.). 1008p. text 140.00 (*0-7216-4217-9*) Saunders.

Principles & Practice of Sleep Medicine in the Child. Richard Ferber & Meir H. Kryger. 1995. (Illus.). 320p. text 52.00 (*0-7216-4761-8*) Saunders.

Principles & Practice of Supportive Oncology. Ann Berger et al. 1997. LC 97-41365. 976p. text 139.00 (*0-397-51559-6*) Lppncott W & W.

Principles & Practice of Surgery. Ed. by A. P. Forrest et al. 2nd ed. 1990. (Illus.). 729p. text (*0-443-03909-7*) Church.

Principles & Practice of Surgical & Cytopathology. Steven G. Silverberg et al. 3rd ed. 1997. LC 97-2455. text (*0-443-07541-7*) Church.

Principles & Practice of Surgical Laparoscopy. Ed. by Simon Paterson-Brown & James Garden. 1994. (Illus.). 619p. pap. text 76.00 (*0-7020-1712-4*) Saunders.

Principles & Practice of Travel Medicine. Jane N. Zuckerman. 2001. LC 2001-26216. 488p. 225.00 (*0-471-49079-2*) Wiley.

Principles & Practice of Veterinary Technology. James Pratt. 1997. LC 97-14020. (Illus.). 730p. (gr. 13). text 56.00 (*0-8151-7308-3*, 27767) Mosby Inc.

Principles & Practice of Veterinary Technology. Paul W. Pratt. 1998. (Illus.). tchr. ed. (*0-323-00051-7*) Mosby Inc.

Principles & Practices in Cardio Pulmonary Phy. 2nd ed. 1996. text 75.00 (*0-8151-3313-8*, 28997) Mosby Inc.

Principles & Practices in Diagnosing Schizophrenia. A. Pakaslahti. 1986. 173p. (Orig.). pap. 38.50 (*951-669-202-8*) Coronet Bks.

Principles & Practices of Chiropractic Techniques. Scott Haldeman. 2nd ed. 1993. (Illus.). 641p. (C). pap. text 95.00 (*0-8385-6360-0*, A6360-0, Apple Lange Med) McGraw.

Principles & Practices of Cholera Control. J. De Araoz et al. 1970. (Public Health Papers: No. 40). 139p. pap. text 13.00 (*92-4-130040-X*, 1110040) World Health.

Principles & Practices of Contemporary Acupuncture. Sung J. Liao et al. 1994. LC 94-21951. (Illus.). 472p. text 79.75 (*0-8247-9291-2*) Dekker.

Principles & Practices of Isokinetics in Sports Medicine & Rehabilitation. Kai-Ming Chan et al. (Illus.). 1997. (CHI.). 500p. (*962-356-027-3*); 1996. 232p. (*962-356-016-8*) Lppncott W & W.

***Principles & Practices of Pharmacology for Anaesthetists.** T. Norman Calvey. 2001. LC 00-57950. (Illus.). 368p. 167.95 (*0-632-05605-3*) Blackwell Sci.

Principles & Practices of Psychology Nursing I. Laraia. (C). text (*981-4033-14-6*) Harcourt Coll Pubs.

***Principles & Practices of Regional Anaesthesia.** Ed. by J. A. W. Wildsmith et al. 3rd ed. 2001. (Illus.). 315p. text (*0-443-06226-9*) Church GBR. *Dist:* Saunders.

Principles & Practices of Rehabilitation. Henry H. Kessler. Ed. by William R. Phillips & Janet Rosenberg. 1980. LC 79-6909. (Physically Handicapped in Society Ser.). (Illus.). reprint ed. lib. bdg. 44.95 (*0-405-13119-4*) Ayer.

Principles & Practices of Surgery. Forrest. 3rd ed. 1995. text 55.00 (*0-443-04860-6*) Saunders.

Principles & Practices of the College-Based Radiography Program. Gary Lauer. Ed. by Alvin F. Gardner. 1984. (Allied Health Professions Monograph). 294p. (C). 37.50 (*0-87527-310-6*) Green.

***Principles & Practices of Unbiased Stereology: A Manual for Biomedical Scientists.** Peter R. Mouton. 2001. LC 2001-967. 304p. pap. text 34.95 (*0-8018-6797-5*) Johns Hopkins.

Principles & Techniques of Cutaneous Surgery. Ed. by Gary P. Lask & Ronald L. Moy. 1995. 637p. text 199.00 (*0-07-036471-0*) McGraw-Hill Educ Grp.

Principles & Techniques of Nerve Regeneration: Alzheimer's Disease & the Dementias: Based on the Readings of Edgar Cayce. David McMillin. 1997. LC 97-4120. (Edgar Cayce Health Ser.). 164p. pap. 14.95 (*0-87604-381-3*, 496) ARE Pr.

Principles & Techniques of Patient Care. Frank M. Pierson. Ed. by Shirley Kuhn. 2nd ed. 1998. LC 98-5492. (Illus.). 384p. (C). pap. text 39.95 (*0-7216-7524-7*) Saunders.

Principles & Techniques of Spine Surgery. Howard S. An. 1997. LC 97-5525. (Illus.). 816p. text 175.00 (*0-683-30260-4*) Lppncott W & W.

Principles & Techniques of Surgical Pathology. Waldemar A. Schmidt. 1986. 746p. (*0-409-90085-0*) E A GBR. *Dist:* OUP.

Principles & Treatment of Lipoprotein Disorders. Ed. by F. Gotthard Schettler & Andreas J. Habenicht. 1994. LC 93-6449. (Handbook of Experimental Pharmacology Ser.: Vol. 109). (Illus.). 502p. 450.00 (*0-387-57121-3*) Spr-Verlag.

Principles Behavioral Neurosciences. Beatty. 3rd ed. 2000. pap. text, stu. ed. 14.30 (*0-697-36165-9*) McGraw.

Principles for Evaluating Chemical Effects on the Aged Population. 1993. (Environmental Health Criteria Ser.: No. 144). (ENG, FRE & SPA.). 159p. pap. text 30.00 (*92-4-157144-6*, 1160144) World Health.

Principles for Evaluating Epidemiologic Data in Regulatory Risk Assessment. Ed. by William Kelly. 1996. LC 96-88998. 115p. (Orig.). pap. (*0-9654148-0-9*) Fed Focus.

Principles for Evaluating Health Risks from Chemicals During Infancy & Early Childhood: The Need for a Special Approach. 1986. (Environmental Health Criteria Ser.: No. 59). 73p. pap. text 15.00 (*92-4-154259-4*, 1160059) World Health.

Principles for Health Care Reform. Debra L. Miller. 1994. (CSIS Panel Report Ser.). 34p. (Orig.). (C). pap. 10.95 (*0-89206-269-X*) CSIS.

Principles for Management Health Care Professionals. Toot. 1998. text (*0-7216-3259-9*) Saunders.

Principles for Nurse Staffing with Annotated Bibliography. Compiled by Rita Munley Gallagher & Katherine A. Kany. 1999. LC 99-19077. 56p. pap. 19.95 (*1-55810-144-6*, 9902AB) Am Nurses Pub.

Principles for Pre-Clinical Testing of Drug Safety: Report of a WHO Scientific Group, 1966. 1966. (Technical Report Ser.). 22p. pap. 3.00 (*92-4-120341-2*, 1100341) World Health.

Principles for the Safety Assessment of Food Additives & Contaminants in Food. 1987. (Environmental Health Criteria Ser.: No. 70). (RUS.). 174p. pap. text 23.00 (*92-4-154270-5*, 1160070) World Health.

Principles for the Testing & Evaluation of Drugs for Carcinogenicity: Proceedings of the WHO Scientific Group, Geneva, 1968. WHO Staff. 1969. (Technical Reports: No. 426). pap. text 3.00 (*92-4-120426-5*, 1100426) World Health.

Principles for the Testing of Drugs for Teratogenicity: Report of a WHO Scientific Group, 1967. 1967. (Technical Report Ser.: No. 350). 18p. pap. text 3.00 (*92-4-120364-1*, 1100364) World Health.

Principles for the Toxicological Assessment of Pesticide Residues in Food. 1990. (Environmental Health Criteria Ser.: No. 104). (CHI, ENG & RUS.). 117p. pap. text 24.00 (*92-4-157104-7*, 1160104) World Health.

Principles, Guidelines & Guarantees for the Protection of Persons Detained on Grounds of Mental Ill-Health or Suffering from Mental Disorder. 1986. 38p. mass mkt. 7.00 (*92-1-154056-9*, E.85.XIV.9) UN.

Principles in General Pharmacology. Ronald J. Tallarida et al. 1988. (Pharmacologic Science Ser.). (Illus.). 243p. 113.00 (*0-387-96602-1*) Spr-Verlag.

Principles of Acupuncture. A. Hicks. 1998. pap. (*0-7225-3409-4*) Thorsons GBR. *Dist:* Natl Bk Netwk.

Principles of Adaptive Behavior. 1999. LC 99-73324. 126p. 24.95 (*0-8187-0326-1*) Harlo Press.

Principles of Addiction Medicine: ASAM Review Course Syllabus. Ed. by Norman Miller et al. 1994. 1000p. 140.00 (*1-880425-02-5*) Am Soc Addict Med.

Principles of Administration Applied to Nursing Service. H. A. Goddard. 1958. (Monographs: No. 41). pap. text 12.00 (*92-4-140041-2*, 1140041) World Health.

Principles of Advanced Trauma Care. Michael W. Hubble & Johnsie P. Hubble. 2001. LC 2001-28448. (Illus.). 800p. (C). text 55.95 (*0-7668-1987-6*) Delmar.

Principles of Airway Management. Brendan T. Finucane & Albert H. Santora. 2nd ed. 1995. LC 95-32783. (Illus.). 368p. (C). (gr. 13). pap. text 39.95 (*0-8151-3337-5*, 24020) Mosby Inc.

Principles of Ambulatory Medicine. L. Randol Barker et al. 3rd ed. 1990. 1487p. 109.00 (*0-683-00437-9*) Lppncott W & W.

Principles of Ambulatory Medicine. Ed. by L. Randol Barker et al. 4th ed. 1995. LC 93-46869. (Illus.). 1584p. 115.00 (*0-683-00438-7*) Lppncott W & W.

Principles of Ambulatory Medicine. L. Randol Barker et al. 5th ed. 1998. LC 97-40570. (Illus.). 1660p. 110.00 (*0-683-30352-X*) Lppncott W & W.

Principles of Amino Acid Nutrition for Ruminants. Ed. by John Malcolm Asplund. 1994. 224p. 169.00 (*0-8493-4910-9*, SF98) CRC Pr.

Principles of Anatomy & Physiology. Gerard J. Tortora. 8th ed. 1996. 987p. (C). pap. 88.13 (*0-321-40297-9*) Addson-Wesley Educ.

Principles of Anatomy & Physiology: Cat Lab Manual. George A. Wistreich & Patricia J. Donnelly. 5th ed. 1997. LC 95-49973. 704p. (C). pap. text, lab manual ed. 73.00 (*0-673-99939-4*) Addson-Wesley Educ.

Principles of Anatomy & Physiology: Learning Guide. Gerard J. Tortora & Sandra R. Grabowski. 7th ed. 1993. (C). pap. 28.13 (*0-06-501197-X*) Addson-Wesley Educ.

Principles of Anatomy & Physiology with Atlas of Human Skeleton. Gerard J. Tortora. 8th ed. 1998. pap. 88.13 (*0-321-03733-2*) Addison-Wesley.

Principles of Anesthesiology: General & Regional Anesthesia. Vincent J. Collins. 3rd ed. 1992. LC 91-7038. (Illus.). 850p. 198.50 (*0-8121-1322-5*) Lppncott W & W.

Principles of Anesthetic Techniques & Anesthetic Emergencies. Kevin K. Tremper. 1998. LC 97-28243. (Atlas of Anesthesia Ser.). text (*0-443-07903-X*) Church.

Principles of Animal Extrapolation. Edward J. Calabrese. 1991. 616p. lib. bdg. 119.00 (*0-87371-410-5*, L410) Lewis Pubs.

Principles of Applied Biomedical Instrumentation. Leslie A. Geddes & L. E. Baker. 3rd ed. 1989. LC 88-27915. 992p. 200.00 (*0-471-60899-8*) Wiley.

Principles of Arterial Blood Gases. Vincent C. Madama. (Respiratory Care Ser.). 1997. pap. 46.95 (*0-8273-5559-9*); 1994. tchr. ed. 12.00 (*0-8273-5560-2*) Delmar.

Principles of Aural Rehabilitation. Mark Ross. 1972. LC 78-183116. (Studies in Communicative Disorders). (C). pap. (*0-672-61283-6*, Bobbs) Macmillan.

Principles of Ayurveda. Anne Green. 2000. pap. (*0-7225-3745-X*) Thorsons GBR. *Dist:* Natl Bk Netwk.

Principles of Ayurvedic Therapeutics. Atmakuri V. Kumar. 1995. LC 95-904683. (C). (*81-7030-463-6*) Sri Satguru Pubns IND. *Dist:* S Asia.

Principles of Bach Flower Remedies: The Only Introduction You'll Ever Need. Stefan Ball. 2000. pap. (*0-7225-3919-3*) Thorsons GBR. *Dist:* Natl Bk Netwk.

Principles of Basic Trauma Nursing Skills. Brita M. O'Carroll. 2000. (Illus.). 320p. pap. (*1-57801-044-6*) Western Schls.

Principles of Behavior Neuroscience: Student Study Art Notebook. Beatty. 1995. 15.74 net. (*0-697-29192-8*, WCB McGr Hill) McGrw-H Hghr Educ.

Principles of Behavior Therapy. G. Terence Wilson & K. Daniel O'Leary. 1980. (Social Learning Theory Ser.). (Illus.). text 24.95 (*0-13-701102-4*) P-H.

Principles of Behavioral Neuroscience. Beatty. 1995. 78.75 (*0-697-22876-2*, WCB McGr Hill) McGrw-H Hghr Educ.

Principles of Behavioral Neuroscience. Jackson Beatty. 1995. LC 93-74861. 224p. (C). text, stu. ed. 23.12 (*0-697-12743-5*) Brown & Benchmark.

Principles of Behavioral Neuroscience. Jackson Beatty. 1994. LC 93-74861. 576p. (C). text 81.25 (*0-697-12741-9*) McGrw-H Hghr Educ.

Principles of Biochemistry Vol. 1: Energy, Proteins & Catalysis, Vol. 1. Geoffrey L. Zubay et al. 1994. 352p. (C). text 25.00 net. (*0-697-24169-6*, WCB McGr Hill) McGrw-H Hghr Educ.

Principles of Biochemistry Vol. 2: Metabolism, Vol. 2. Geoffrey L. Zubay et al. 1994. 528p. (C). text 31.00 net. (*0-697-24170-X*, WCB McGr Hill) McGrw-H Hghr Educ.

Principles of Biological Autonomy. Francisco J. Varela. 1979. (North Holland Series in General Systems Research: Vol. 2). 336p. 76.00 (*0-444-00321-5*) P-H.

Principles of Biomedical Engineering for Nursing Staff. Hans A. Von Der Mosel. 1994. LC 93-46212. (Illus.). 192p. pap. 39.95 (*0-632-03788-1*) Blackwell Sci.

Principles of Biomedical Instrumentation & Monitoring. Robert J. Traister. 1981. 300p. (C). text 32.00 (*0-8359-5611-3*) P-H.

Principles of Biopsy: A Self-Instructional Guide, Bk. 8. Thomas H. Morton, Jr. et al. 3rd rev. ed. 1983. (Illus.). 94p. pap. 14.95 (*0-89939-081-1*) Stoma Pr.

Principles of Biopsychology. Simon Green. Ed. by Michael W. Eysenck et al. 1994. (Principles of Psychology Ser.). 224p. 29.95 (*0-86377-281-1*) L Erlbaum Assocs.

Principles of Bone Biology. Ed. by John P. Bilezikian et al. 1996. LC 96-32323. (Illus.). 1398p. text 165.00 (*0-12-098650-7*) Acad Pr.

Principles of Brain Functioning: A Synergetic Approach to Brain Activity, Behavior, & Cognition. Hermann Haken. 1995. LC 95-41276. (Series in Synergetics: Vol. 67). (Illus.). 347p. 75.95 (*3-540-58967-8*) Spr-Verlag.

Principles of Brain Stimulation. John S. Yeomans. 1990. (Illus.). 192p. text 45.00 (*0-19-506138-1*) OUP.

Principles of Cancer Biotherapy. Ed. by Robert K. Oldham. 3rd ed. 1997. LC 97-2588. 892p. lib. bdg. 380.00 (*0-7923-3507-4*) Kluwer Academic.

Principles of Cardiac Diagnosis & Treatment: A Surgeon's Guide. D. N. Ross et al. 2nd ed. 1991. (Illus.). 269p. 144.00 (*0-387-17494-X*) Spr-Verlag.

Principles of Cardiac Toxicology. Steven I. Baskin. 1991. (Illus.). 704p. 159.00 (*0-8493-8809-0*, RC682) CRC Pr.

Principles of Cell Proliferation. J. K. Heath. 2001. LC 00-56483. (Illus.). x, 137p. pap. 39.95 (*0-632-04886-7*) Blackwell Sci.

Principles of Cellular, Molecular & Developmental Neuroscience. O. Steward. 1989. (Illus.). 257p. 71.95 (*0-387-96803-2*) Spr-Verlag.

Principles of Chemoprevention. Ed. by Paul Kleihues et al. 1997. (IARC Scientific Publications Ser.: No. 139). (Illus.). 370p. pap. text 89.50 (*92-832-2139-7*) OUP.

Principles of Chest Roentgenology: A Programmed Text. Benjamin Felson et al. 1965. LC 65-23091. (Illus.). text 49.00 (*0-7216-3605-5*) Saunders.

Principles of Child Neurology. Ed. by Bruce O. Berg. 1996. LC 91-55399. (Illus.). 1799p. text 139.00 (*0-07-005193-3*) McGraw-Hill Prof.

***Principles of Chiropractic Orthopedics.** Keith B. Konowitz & James Herzog. 2001. (Illus.). 795p. (*0-443-06590-X*) Church GBR. *Dist:* Saunders.

Principles of Clinical Anatomy. Lawrence H. Mathers, Jr. et al. 1995. (Illus.). 816p. (C). (gr. 13). text 57.00 (*0-8016-6356-3*, 06356) Mosby Inc.

Principles of Clinical Electromyography: Case Studies. Shin J. Oh. 1998. LC 98-10426. 352p. pap. 75.00 (*0-683-18106-8*) Lppncott W & W.

Principles of Clinical Medicine. Ed. by D. G. Williams & P. John Rees. 1995. (Illus.). 984p. pap. (*0-340-56300-1*) E A GBR. *Dist:* OUP.

***Principles of Clinical Pharmacology.** Ed. by Arthur J. Atkinson, Jr. 2001. LC 2001-93791. (Illus.). 460p. 79.95 (*0-12-066060-1*) Acad Pr.

Principles of Clinical Practice: An Introductory Textbook. Ed. by Mark B. Mengel. 1991. (Illus.). 432p. (C). text 45.00 (*0-306-43847-X*, Kluwer Plenum) Kluwer Academic.

Principles of Colonic Irrigation: The Only Introduction You'll Ever Need. Jillie Collings. 1996. 160p. pap. (*0-7225-3029-3*) Thorsons GBR. *Dist:* Natl Bk Netwk.

Principles of Colour Healing. Ambika Wauters & Gerry Thompson. 1998. pap. (*0-7225-3340-3*) Thorsons GBR. *Dist:* Natl Bk Netwk.

Principles of Community Health Promotion. Marlene Tappe & Regina Galer-Unti. 2000. (Illus.). 480p. (C). pap. text 54.95 (*0-7637-1077-6*, 1077-6) Jones & Bartlett.

Principles of Community Psychology: Perspectives & Trends. Murray Levine & David V. Perkins. 2nd ed. 1996. LC 95-46425. (Illus.). 512p. (C). text 54.95 (*0-19-509844-7*) OUP.

Principles of Comparative Anatomy of Invertebrates V. N. Beklemishev. Ed. by Z. Kabata. Tr. by J. M. McLennan. 1970. LC 70-97749. lib. bdg. 72.00 (*0-226-04175-1*) U Ch Pr.

Principles of CPT Coding. American Medical Association Staff. 1999. (Coding Ser.). (Illus.). 325p. pap. 49.95 (*0-89970-996-6*) AMA.

Principles of Critical Care. Jesse B. Hall et al. 1992. (Illus.). 2432p. text 155.00 (*0-07-071589-0*) McGraw-Hill Med Pub.

Principles of Critical Care. Janet K. Ihde et al. 1987. (Illus.). 456p. pap. text 45.00 (*0-7216-1802-2*) Saunders.

Principles of Critical Care. Farokh E. Udwadia. 1996. (Illus.). 696p. text 62.50 (*0-19-563728-3*) OUP.

Principles of Critical Care. 2nd ed. 1999. pap. 8.90 (*0-07-135735-1*) McGraw-Hill Educ Grp.

Principles of Critical Care. Jesse B. Hall et al. 2nd ed. 1998. LC 99-22444. (Illus.). 1767p. (C). text 199.00 (*0-07-025934-8*) McGraw-Hill Prof.

Principles of Critical Care. Jesse B. Hall. 1. (*0-07-025874-0*); 2. (*0-07-025875-9*) McGraw.

Principles of Critical Care: Companion Handbook. Ed. by Jesse B. Hall et al. 1993. LC 92-48941. (Companion Handbook Ser.). (Illus.). 608p. pap. text 32.00 (*0-07-025828-7*) McGraw-Hill Med Pub.

Principles of Critical Care: Companion Handbook. Ed. by Jesse B. Hall et al. 2nd ed. 1999. (Illus.). 1075p. pap. 49.00 (*0-07-026029-X*) McGraw-Hill Prof.

Principles of Critical Care: Noseworthy Chapter. 1999. pap. 3.35 (*0-07-135748-3*) McGraw-Hill Educ Grp.

Principles of Critical Care: PreTest Self-Assessment & Review. Jesse B. Hall et al. 2nd ed. 1997. (Pretest Specialty Level Ser.). (Illus.). 256p. pap. 45.00 (*0-07-052294-4*) McGraw-Hill Prof.

Principles of Dental Imaging. Olaf E. Langland & Robert P. Langlais. 1997. LC 97-2361. (Illus.). 300p. pap. 40.95 (*0-683-18241-2*) Lppncott W & W.

Principles of Dental Suturing: The Complete Guide to Surgical Closure. Lee M. Silverstein. Ed. by Allison Loperfido. 2000. (Illus.). 80p. pap. text 45.00 (*0-9673009-0-8*) Montage Media Corp.

Principles of Dermatology. Donald P. Lookingbill & James G. Marks, Jr. 2nd ed. 1993. LC 92-48750. (Illus.). 384p. pap. text 55.00 (*0-7216-4290-X*) Saunders.

Principles of Dermatology. Donald P. Lookingbill & James G. Marks. 3rd ed. Date not set. LC 99-57051. 335p. pap. text (*0-7216-7971-4*) Saunders.

Principles of Design & Operation of the Brain: Proceedings of a Study Week Organized by the Pontifical Academy of Sciences Casina Pius IV, Vatican City. Ed. by John C. Eccles & O. Creutzfeldt. 1991. (Experimental Brain Research Ser.: Vol. 21). (Illus.). 600p. 115.00 (*0-387-53416-4*) Spr-Verlag.

Principles of Development of Model Health Care Programmes. 1985. (EURO Reports & Studies: No. 96). 41p. pap. text 6.00 (*92-890-1262-5*, 1330096) World Health.

Principles of Doppler & Color Doppler Imaging. R. Haerten & M. Muck-Weymann. 2nd ed. 1994. 50p. pap. 89.95 (*3-8009-4212-7*) Wiley.

Principles of Drug Action. Ed. by William B. Pratt & Palmer Taylor. 3rd ed. 1990. (Illus.). 834p. text (*0-443-08676-1*) Church.

Principles of Drug Addiction Treatment: A Research - Based Guide. Pref. by Alan I. Leshner. 2000. 54p. pap. text 20.00 (*0-7567-0065-5*) DIANE Pub.

Principles of Drug Design. Ed. by Miller. 1996. (Illus.). 352p. (C). (gr. 13). pap. 49.95 (*0-412-03051-9*) Chapman & Hall.

Principles of Drug Development in Transplantation & Autoimmunity. Ronald Lieberman & Asoke Mukherjee. 1996. LC 95-37929. (Medical Intelligence Unit Ser.). 874p. 130.00 (*1-57059-283-7*) Landes Bioscience.

Principles of Drug Information & Scientific Literature Evaluation. Frank J. Ascione et al. 1994. LC 93-41705. 236p. (C). pap. text 30.00 (*0-914768-52-2*, T169) Am Pharm Assn.

Principles of Educational & Psychological Measurement & Evaluation. Gilbert Sax. 3rd ed. 1989. 678p. (C). pap. 46.00 (*0-534-09978-5*) Wadsworth Pub.

Principles of Eidetics: Outline of a Theory. A. Arduini. 1991. 251p. 108.00 (*0-387-54506-9*) Spr-Verlag.

Principles of Electrosurgery: Practical Overview of R. F. Electrosurgical Generators. Ronald L. Bussiere. 1997. (Illus.). 33p. 45.00 (*0-9661128-0-6*) Tektran.

Principles of Emergency Medical Dispatch. Jeff J. Clawson & Kate B. Dernocoeur. Ed. by Gordon W. Cottle & Robert L. Martin. 2nd ed. 1997. (Illus.). ix, 250p. (C). 44.99 (*0-9658890-0-9*); LC 97-74551. pap. 36.99 (*0-9658890-1-7*) Medical Priority.

Principles of Emergency Medical Dispatch. Jeff J. Clawson et al. Ed. by Bob Sinclair. 3rd ed. 2000. (Illus.). 450p. (*0-9658890-2-5*) Medical Priority.

Principles of EMS Systems. American College of Emergency Physicians Staff. 2nd ed. 1994. 95.00 (*0-07-000213-4*) McGraw.

Principles of Endocrine Pharmacology. John A. Thomas & Edward J. Keenan. 1986. LC 85-28251. (Illus.). 310p. (C). pap. text 47.00 (*0-306-42143-7*, Kluwer Plenum) Kluwer Academic.

Principles of Endodontics. Mumford & Jedynakiewicz. 1988. pap. text 54.00 (*1-85097-006-8*, 1569) Quint Pub Co.

Principles of Endosurgery. Kevin R. Loughlin et al. 1995. LC 95-41190. (Illus.). 352p. pap. 59.95 (*0-86542-264-8*) Blackwell Sci.

Principles of Environmental Health Science. Douglas Crawford-Brown. 1998. 350p. 49.95 (*0-8342-0656-0*) Aspen Pub.

Principles of Environmental Medicine. Jacques G. Descotes. 2000. 400p. 120.00 (*0-471-97245-2*) Wiley.

Principles of Environmental Toxicology, Vol. 190. Sigmund F. Zakrzewski. 2nd ed. 1997. LC 96-52362. (ACS Monographs). 352p. text 95.00 (*0-8412-3380-2*) Am Chemical.

Principles of Equine Osteosynthesis. G. E. Fackelman. 2000. (Illus.). 380p. 189.00 incl. cd-rom (*0-86577-826-4*) Thieme Med Pubs.

Principles of Everyday Behavior Analysis. L. Keith Miller. 2nd ed. 1980. LC 79-27797. 512p. (C). pap. 30.75 (*0-8185-0373-4*) Brooks-Cole.

Principles of Everyday Behavior Analysis. L. Keith MIller. 3rd ed. 1996. LC 96-2625. (Psychology Ser.). 624p. (C). pap. text 65.95 (*0-534-16146-4*) Brooks-Cole.

Principles of Exercise Biochemistry. Ed. by J. R. Poortmans. (Medicine & Sport Science Ser.: Vol. 27). (Illus.). 1988. viii, 260p. 195.00 (*3-8055-4790-0*); 2nd rev. ed. 1993. viii, 304p. 135.75 (*3-8055-5778-7*) S Karger.

Principles of Exercise Prescription. Mark R. Bookhout & Philip E. Greenman. 2001. (Illus.). 368p. 49.95 (*0-7506-9885-3*) Buttrwrth-Heinemann.

Principles of Exercise Testing & Interpretation: Including Pathophysiology & Clinical Applications. Karlman Wasserman. 3rd ed. 1999. LC 98-43362. 550p. text 85.00 (*0-683-30646-4*) Lppncott W & W.

Principles of Experimental Design for the Life Sciences. Murray R. Selwyn. 1996. LC 96-321. 176p. 59.95 (*0-8493-9461-9*) CRC Pr.

Principles of Experimental Phonetics. Ed. by Norman J. Lass. 1995. (Illus.). 600p. (C). (gr. 13). text 69.00 (*0-8016-7975-3*, 07975) Mosby Inc.

Principles of Experimental Psychology: Instructor's Course Planner. Levin. 1994. 14.68 (*0-697-12795-8*) McGraw.

Principles of Exposure Measurement in Epidemiology. Bruce Armstrong et al. 1994. (Monographs in Epidemiology & Biostatistics: No. 21). (Illus.). 360p. reprint ed. pap. text 59.95 (*0-19-262020-7*) OUP.

Principles of Facial Reconstruction. Wayne Larrabee, Jr. 1995. (Illus.). 272p. text 120.00 (*0-7817-0150-3*) Lppncott W & W.

Principles of Fluoroscopic Image Intensification & Television Systems: Workbook & Laboratory Manual. Robert J. Parelli. 1996. (Illus.). 256p. per. 45.00 (*1-57444-082-9*) St Lucie Pr.

Principles of Forensic Medicine. William A. Guy. 3rd enl. rev. ed. LC 75-23715. (Illus.). reprint ed. 54.00 (*0-404-13268-5*) AMS Pr.

Principles of Forensic Toxicology. Barry Levine. 1998. 370p. pap. 57.00 (*1-890883-07-7*, 202024) Am Assn Clinical Chem.

***Principles of Genetics.** Robert H. Tamarin et al. 6th ed. 2000. (C). stu. ed. 74.38 incl. cd-rom (*0-07-242485-0*) McGrw-H Hghr Educ.

Principles of Genetics. Eldon J. Gardner et al. 8th ed. 1991. LC 90-48758. 736p. text 78.95 (*0-471-50487-4*) Wiley.

Principles of Genitourinary Radiology. Z. L. Barbaric. 2nd rev. ed. 1994. (Flexibook Ser.). (Illus.). 520p. 99.00 (*0-86577-493-5*) Thieme Med Pubs.

Principles of Geriatric Medicine & Gerontology. Ed. by William R. Hazzard et al. 4th ed. 1998. LC 98-3613. (Illus.). xxxiii, 1668p. text 149.00 (*0-07-027502-5*) McGraw-Hill Prof.

Principles of Gestalt Family Therapy. Walter Kempler. 1973. LC 74-26006. pap. 10.00 (*0-9600808-1-3*) Kempler Inst.

Principles of Grammar & Learning. William D. O'Grady. 1987. LC 86-11402. 248p. (C). 33.00 (*0-226-62074-3*) U Ch Pr.

Principles of Gynaecological Surgery. Ed. by S. L. Stanton. 1987. (Illus.). 306p. 49.50 (*0-387-17485-0*) Spr-Verlag.

Principles of Hand Surgery. Ed. by F. D. Burke et al. 1989. (Illus.). 392p. text (*0-443-03466-4*) Church.

Principles of Health & Disability Insurance Selling. Contrib. by Scholarly Resources. 3rd rev. ed. 1992. 180p. pap. text 24.95 (*0-7931-0585-4*, 5403-043A) Dearborn.

Principles of Health Care Ethics. Ann Lloyd. Ed. by Raanan Gillon. 1994. LC 92-23746. 1152p. 477.50 (*0-471-93033-4*) Wiley.

Principles of Health Education & Health Promotion. J. Thomas Butler. 3rd ed. 2000. LC 00-63418. (Physical Education Ser.). (Illus.). 384p. pap. text 51.95 (*0-534-52374-9*) Wadsworth Pub.

Principles of Health Maintenance. Paul R. Schnurrenberger. Ed. by Robert S. Sharman. 1983. LC 82-18067. 291p. 72.50 (*0-275-91413-5*, C1413, Praeger Pubs) Greenwood.

Principles of Health Planning in the U. S. S. R. G. A. Popov. 1971. (Public Health Papers: No. 43). pap. text 9.00 (*92-4-130043-4*, 1110043) World Health.

Principles of Hematology. Peter J. Haen. 1995. LC 94-70283. 472p. (C). pap. 89.38 (*0-697-13301-X*, WCB McGr Hill) McGrw-H Hghr Educ.

Principles of Holistic Therapy with Herbal Essences. Dietrich Gumbel. Tr. by Ritva Abao from GER. 2nd ed. 1993. (Illus.). 268p. pap. text (*2-8043-4002-3*) K F Haug Pubs DEU. *Dist:* Medicina Bio.

Principles of Homeopathic Philosophy. Margaret Roy. 1993. LC 93-14982. 150p. pap. text (*0-344-30482-5*) Church.

Principles of Human Anatomy. Gerard J. Tortora. 8th ed. 1999. LC 98-7560. (Illus.). 916p. (C). 88.13 (*0-321-00037-4*) Addison-Wesley.

Principles of Human Anatomy: Lab Manual for Human Cadavers. Victor P. Eroschenko. 2nd ed. 1995. (C). tchr. ed. (*0-673-55986-6*) Addson-Wesley Educ.

***Principles of Human Neuropsychology.** G. Dennis Rains. 2001. LC 2001-31489. (*1-55934-623-X*) McGraw.

Principles of Hypnotherapy. Vera Peiffer. 1997. pap. (*0-7225-3242-3*) Thorsons GBR. *Dist:* Natl Bk Netwk.

Principles of Imaging Science & Protection. Michael A. Thompson et al. 1994. LC 93-12638. text 59.00 (*0-7216-3428-1*) Saunders.

Principles of Imaging Science & Protection. Ed. by Michael A. Thompson et al. 1994. (Illus.). Solutions to the Exercises. 531p. (*0-7216-3430-3*); Vol. 2. 485.00 (*0-7216-4221-7*) Saunders.

Principles of Imaging Science & Protection: Science & Protection. Thompson. 1994. 531p. (C). pap., tchr. ed., wbk. ed. 21.00 (*0-7216-3429-X*) Harcrt Hlth Sci Grp.

Principles of Immunopharmacology. Franciscus P. Nijkamp & Michael J. Parnham. 1999. LC 99-10441. xvi, 497p. pap. (*0-8176-5780-0*) Birkhauser.

Principles of Industrial Therapy for the Mentally Ill. Bertram J. Black. 1970. LC 73-88017. 200p. text 60.00 (*0-8089-0062-5*, 790600, Grune & Strat) Harcrt Hlth Sci Grp.

Principles of Infertility Nursing. Catherine H. Garner. 1991. 224p. 69.95 (*0-8493-4652-5*, RC889) CRC Pr.

Principles of Instrumented Spinal Surgery. Harms. 1999. (Illus.). 208p. 149.00 (*0-86577-744-6*) Thieme Med Pubs.

Principles of Intensive Psychotherapy. Frieda Fromm-Reichmann. 1960. LC 50-9782. 263p. pap. text 12.95 (*0-226-26599-4*, P49) U Ch Pr.

Principles of Interpretation: Mastering Clear & Concise... pap. 45.00 (*1-56821-798-6*) Aronson.

Principles of Joint Replacement Surgery. Clement B. Sledge & Myron B. Spector. 1993. text 125.00 (*0-07-058173-8*) McGraw.

Principles of Laboratory Animal Science: A Contribution to the Humane Use & Care of Animals & to the Quality of Experimental Results. Ed. by L. F. Van Zutphen et al. 1993. LC 93-7467. 404p. 227.00 (*0-444-81270-9*) Elsevier.

Principles of Laparoscopic Surgery: Basic & Advanced Techniques. Ed. by Maurice E. Arregui. 1995. LC 94-22505. (*3-540-94236-X*) Spr-Verlag.

Principles of Laparoscopic Surgery: Basic & Advanced Techniques. Ed. by Maurice E. Arregui et al. 1995. LC 94-22505. (Illus.). 852p. 258.00 (*0-387-94236-X*) Spr-Verlag.

Principles of Laryngeal Videostroboscopy. Joseph C. Stemple & Leslie E. Glaze. 1997. 110.00 incl. VHS (*1-58041-016-2*, 0112090) Am Speech Lang Hearing.

Principles of Long-Term Health Care Administration. Peter J. Buttaro. 1995. LC 99-14786. 326p. pap. 114.00 (*0-8342-1371-0*) Aspen Pub.

Principles of Magnetic Resonance Imaging. Robert J. Parelli. 1997. (Illus.). 28p. (Orig.). pap., wbk. ed. 15.00 (*1-880359-12-X*) Par Rad.

Principles of Magnetic Resonance Imaging: Student Workbook. Ritenour. 1985. (gr. 13). spiral bd. 13.95 (*0-8016-4532-8*, 04532) Mosby Inc.

Principles of Management of Health Laboratories. L. Houang & M. M. El-Nageh. 1993. (WHO Regional Publications: No. 3). x, 120p. pap. text 10.00 (*92-9021-180-6*, 1440003) World Health.

Principles of Manual Medicine. Philip E. Greenman. (Illus.). 1989. 364p. text 62.00 (*0-683-03556-8*); 2nd ed. 1996. LC 95-9178. 584p. 120.00 (*0-683-03558-4*) Lppncott W & W.

Principles of Medical Biochemistry. Gerhard Meisenberg & William H. Simmons. 1998. LC 98-2505. (Illus.). 768p. (C). (gr. 13). pap. text 38.95 (*0-8151-4410-5*, 30897) Mosby Inc.

Principles of Medical Biology Vol. 1A: Bioethics. Ed. by E. Edward Bittar & Neville Bittar. 1994. LC 94-15763. 224p. 90.00 (*1-55938-801-3*) Jai Pr.

Principles of Medical Biology Vol. 2: Cellular Organelles. Ed. by E. Edward Bittar & Neville Bittar. 1995. LC 95-16568. 298p. 90.00 (*1-55938-803-X*) Jai Pr.

Principles of Medical Biology Vol. 3: Cellular Organelles & the Extracellular Matrix. Ed. by E. Edward Bittar & Neville Bittar. 1995. LC 95-24345. (Principles of Medical Biology Ser.). 304p. 90.00 (*1-55938-804-8*) Jai Pr.

Principles of Medical Biology Vol. 4, Pt. II: Cell Chemistry & Physiology. Ed. by E. Edward Bittar & Neville Bittar. 1996. 322p. 90.00 (*1-55938-806-4*) Jai Pr.

Principles of Medical Biology Vol. 4, Pt. III: Cell Chemistry & Physiology. Ed. by E. Edward Bittar & Neville Bittar. 1996. 359p. 90.00 (*1-55938-807-2*) Jai Pr.

Principles of Medical Biology Vol. 4, Pt. IV: Cell Chemistry & Physiology. Ed. by E. Edward Bittar & Neville Bittar. 1996. 508p. 90.00 (*1-55938-808-0*) Jai Pr.

Principles of Medical Biology Vol. 6: Immunobiology. Ed. by E. Edward Bittar & Neville Bittar. 1996. LC 96-35160. 350p. 90.00 (*1-55938-811-0*) Jai Pr.

Principles of Medical Biology Vol. 8A, B & C: Molecular & Cellular Pharmacology. Ed. by E. Edward Bittar & Neville Bittar. 1997. LC 97-15195. 1208p. 375.00 (*1-55938-813-7*) Jai Pr.

Principles of Medical Biology Vol. 9A & B: Microbiology. Ed. by E. Edward Bittar & Neville Bittar. 1998. LC 97-36100. 404p. 90.00 (*1-55938-814-5*) Jai Pr.

Principles of Medical Biology Vol. 10A & B: Molecular & Cellular Endocrinology. Ed. by E. Edward Bittar & Neville Bittar. 1998. LC 97-41660. 684p. 257.00 (*1-55938-815-3*) Jai Pr.

Principles of Medical Biology Vol. 11: Developmental Biology. E. Edward Bittar & Neville Bittar. 1998. LC 98-18490. 90.00 (*1-55938-816-1*) Jai Pr.

Principles of Medical Biology Vol. 13: Cell Injury, Vol. 13. E. Edward Bittar & Neville Bittar. 1998. LC 98-16467. 314p. 90.00 (*1-55938-818-8*) Jai Pr.

Principles of Medical Biology Vol. 14: Psychiatry. Ed. by E. Edward Bittar & Neville Bittar. 2000. LC 99-88148. 662p. 86.00 (*1-55938-819-6*) Jai Pr.

Principles of Medical Ethics Relevant to the Protection of Prisoners Against Torture. 1983. (CIOMS Nonserial Publication Ser.). pap. text 4.00 (*92-9036-015-1*) World Health.

Principles of Medical Ethics with Annotations Especially Applicable to Psychiatry: 1998 Edition. American Psychiatric Association Ethics Committee. 1998. 38p. pap. text 3.00 (*0-89042-140-4*, 2140) Am Psychiatric.

Principles of Medical Genetics. Thomas D. Gelehrter. 1990. (Illus.). 300p. pap. 38.00 (*0-683-03447-2*) Lppncott W & W.

Principles of Medical Genetics. Thomas F. Gelehrter et al. 2nd ed. 1997. (Illus.). 432p. pap. 44.00 (*0-683-03445-6*) Lppncott W & W.

Principles of Medical Imaging. K. Kirk Shung et al. 1992. LC 92-7143. (Illus.). 289p. text 73.00 (*0-12-640970-6*) Acad Pr.

***Principles of Medical Law: Fourth Cumulative Supplement.** Andrew Grubb. 2001. 160p. (Orig.). pap. text 65.00 (*0-19-924582-7*) OUP.

***Principles of Medical Law: Main Volume & Fourth Cumulative Supplement.** Ian Kennedy. Ed. by Ian Kennedy & Andrew Grubb. 2002. 1050p. text 265.00 (*0-19-924583-5*) OUP.

Principles of Medical Law: Second Cumulative Supplement. Andrew Grubb. 2000. 104p. pap. text 45.00 (*0-19-829882-X*) OUP.

Principles of Medical Pharmacology. Derek Waller & Andrew Renwick. 1994. (Illus.). 409p. pap. text (*0-7020-1613-6*) W B Saunders GBR. *Dist:* Saunders.

Principles of Medical Pharmacology. Ed. by Harold Kalant & Walter H. Roschlau. 6th ed. 1997. LC 96-29399. (Illus.). 976p. text 59.95 (*0-19-510024-7*) OUP.

Principles of Medical Psychology: Being the Outlines of a Course of Lectures. Ernst F. Von Feuchtersleben. Ed. by B. G. Babington. Tr. by H. Evans Lloyd from GER. 1976. LC 75-16704. (Classics in Psychiatry Ser.). reprint ed. 36.95 (*0-405-07430-1*) Ayer.

Principles of Medical Therapy in Pregnancy. Norbert Gleicher. 1985. LC 84-24903. (Illus.). 1320p. (C). text 250.00 (*0-306-41845-2*, Kluwer Plenum) Kluwer Academic.

Principles of Medicinal Chemistry. Ed. by William O. Foye. 3rd ed. 1988. LC 87-21395. 950p. (C). text 60.00 (*0-8121-1098-6*) Lppncott W & W.

Principles of Medicinal Chemistry. Ed. by William O. Foye et al. 4th ed. 1995. LC 94-29481. (Illus.). 1,024p. text 70.00 (*0-683-03323-9*) Lppncott W & W.

Principles of Medicinal Chemistry. William O. Foye et al. 4th ed. 1995. 1,024p. 85.00 (*0-683-30621-9*) Lppncott W & W.

***Principles of Medicinal Chemistry.** William O. Foye et al. 5th ed. 2002. LC 2001-50327. text 75.00 (*0-683-30737-1*) Lppncott W & W.

Principles of Mental Hygiene. William A. White. 1972. LC 76-180596. (Medicine & Society in America Ser.). 344p. reprint ed. 25.95 (*0-405-03979-4*) Ayer.

Principles of Microsurgical Techniques in Infertility. Ed. by J. Victor Reyniak & Niels H. Lauersen. 1982. LC 81-3045. 310p. 65.00 (*0-306-40781-7*, Kluwer Plenum) Kluwer Academic.

Principles of Modern Microbiology. Mark Wheelis. 2003. (Illus.). 832p. (C). text 76.95 (*0-7637-1075-X*, 1075-X) Jones & Bartlett.

Principles of Modern Psychological Measurement: A Festschrift for Frederic M. Lord. Ed. by Howard Wainer & Samuel Messick. 1983. 416p. text 79.95 (*0-89859-277-1*) L Erlbaum Assocs.

Principles of Molecular Medicine. Ed. by J. Larry Jameson. 1998. LC 98-17729. (Illus.). 1156p. 175.00 (*0-89603-529-8*) Humana.

Principles of Molecular Oncology. Ed. by Miguel H. Bronchud et al. 2000. LC 99-16733. 468p. 125.00 (*0-89603-581-6*) Humana.

Principles of Molecular Regulation. Ed. by P. Michael Conn & Anthony R. Means. 2000. LC 00-27312. (Illus.). 476p. 135.00 (*0-89603-630-8*) Humana.

Principles of Molecular Rheumatology. Ed. by George C. Tsokos. 2000. LC 00-24930. (Current Molecular Medicine Ser.: Vol. 1). 542p. 165.00 (*0-89603-773-8*) Humana.

Principles of Neural Development. Dale Purves & Jeff W. Lichtman. 1985. LC 84-10566. (Illus.). 433p. text 67.95 (*0-87893-744-7*) Sinauer Assocs.

Principles of Neuroanatomy. Jay B. Angevine, Jr. & Carl W. Cotman. 1981. (Illus.). 393p. text 29.95 (*0-19-502885-6*) OUP.

Principles of Neuroepidemiology. Tracy Batchelor & Merit E. Cudkowicz. 2000. LC 00-56439. (Illus.). 464p. text 99.00 (*0-7506-7042-8*) Buttrwrth-Heinemann.

Principles of Neurologic Rehabilitation. Ed. by Richard B. Lazar. 1997. (Illus.). 709p. text 89.00 (*0-07-036794-9*) McGraw-Hill Prof.

Principles of Neurology. Raymond D. Adams & Maurice Victor. 5th ed. 1993. LC 92-48805. (Illus.). 1402p. text 79.00 (*0-07-000341-6*) McGraw-Hill Med Pub.

Principles of Neurology: Companion Handbook. Raymond D. Adams et al. 6th ed. 1997. LC 98-132505. (Illus.). 512p. pap. 32.00 (*0-07-000514-1*) McGraw-Hill Prof.

Principles of Neuropsychological Rehabilitation. George P. Prigatano. 1999. LC 98-50681. (Illus.). 374p. text 49.95 (*0-19-508143-9*) OUP.

Principles of Neuropsychology. Eric A. Zillmer & Mary V. Spiers. 2000. LC 00-49954. (Psychology Ser.). 640p. 83.95 (*0-534-34144-6*) Brooks-Cole.

Principles of Neuropsychopharmacology. Robert S. Feldman et al. 1996. LC 96-3306. (Illus.). 909p. (C). text 87.95 (*0-87893-175-9*) Sinauer Assocs.

Principles of Neurosurgery. Setti S. Rengachary & Robert H. Wilkins. 1994. LC 93-10153. (C). 210.00 (*1-56375-022-8*) Mosby Inc.

Principles of Neurosurgery. Ed. by Robert G. Grossman & Christopher M. Loftus. 2nd ed. 1998. LC 98-27638. (Illus.). 864p. text 179.00 (*0-397-51840-4*) Lppncott W & W.

Principles of Neurotoxicology, No. 26. Louis W. Chang. 1994. LC 94-7435. (Neurological Disease & Therapy Ser.: Vol. 26). (Illus.). 824p. text 265.00 (*0-8247-8836-2*) Dekker.

Principles of Nuclear Medicine. Ed. by Henry N. Wagner, Jr. et al. 2nd ed. 1995. LC 95-10051. (Illus.). 1248p. text 249.00 (*0-7216-9091-2*) Saunders.

Principles of Nucleic Acid Structure. W. Saenger. 1995. (Advanced Texts in Chemistry Ser.). (Illus.). 576p. 59.95 (*0-387-90761-0*) Spr-Verlag.

Principles of Nursing in Process Context. Nancy Roper. 4th ed. 1988. (Illus.). 336p. (Orig.). text (*0-443-03576-8*) Church.

Principles of Nutrition: Study Guide. Ed. by Deakin University Press Staff. 1986. (C). pap. (*0-7300-0751-0*, SHN710) Deakin Univ AUS. *Dist:* St Mut.

Principles of Nutritional Assessment. Ed. by Rosalind S. Gibson. 1990. (Illus.). 712p. text 67.95 (*0-19-505838-0*) OUP.

Principles of Ocular Pharmacology. 2002. (Illus.). 256p. pap. 80.00 (*0-7506-4326-9*) Buttrwrth-Heinemann.

Principles of Oocyte & Embryo Donation. Ed. by M. V. Sauer. 1998. LC 97-17443. (Illus.). 385p. 104.00 (*0-387-94960-7*) Spr-Verlag.

Principles of Ophthalmic Lenses. Mohammed Jalie. 1989. (C). (*0-900099-20-8*) Assn Brit Dispen Opticians GBR. *Dist:* St Mut.

***Principles of Oral & Maxillofacial Surgery.** U.J. Moore et al. 5th ed. 2001. LC 2001-18129. (Illus.). 288p. pap. 334.00 (*0-632-05438-7*) Blackwell Sci.

Principles of Organ Transplantation. M. Wayne Flye. 1989. (Illus.). 688p. text 205.00 (*0-7216-1323-3*) Saunders.

Principles of Organ Transplantation. Flye. 2nd ed. 2000. text (*0-7216-6907-7*) Harcrt Hlth Sci Grp.

Principles of Orthopedic Practice. Ed. by Roger Dee et al. 2nd ed. 1996. LC 96-38647. (Illus.). 1552p. text 199.95 (*0-07-016356-1*) McGraw-Hill Prof.

Principles of Pediatric Fluid Therapy. Robert W. Winters. 2nd ed. 1982. 22.00 (*0-316-94738-5*, Little Brwn Med Div) Lppncott W & W.

Principles of Pediatric Nursing. Rosa M. Sacharin. 2nd ed. 1986. LC 85-11685. (Illus.). 617p. (C). text (*0-443-03301-3*) Church.

Principles of Perinatal-Neonatal Metabolism. Ed. by Richard M. Cowett. 2nd ed. 1998. LC 97-24816. (Illus.). 1298p. 275.00 (*0-387-94965-8*) Spr-Verlag.

Principles of Personality. Jerry S. Wiggins et al. 1976. LC 75-28729. (Illus.). 549p. (C). text 21.00 (*0-394-34784-6*) Random.

Principles of Pharmacoeconomics. J. Lyle Bootman et al. 2nd ed. 1996. 312p. pap. 54.75 (*0-929375-17-3*) H W Bks.

Principles of Pharmacology. Bills. 1997. 96p. text, tchr. ed. 19.95 (*0-8273-8300-2*) Delmar.

Principles of Pharmacology: A Tropical Approach. David T. Okpako. 1991. (Illus.). 590p. (C). text 130.00 (*0-521-34095-0*) Cambridge U Pr.

Principles of Pharmacology: Basic Concepts & Clinical Applications. Paul L. Munson et al. 2nd ed. 1996. (Arnold Publication). (Illus.). 1808p. 93.95 (*0-412-12231-6*) OUP.

Principles of Pharmacology for Medical Assistants. Rice. 1989. (Medical Assisting Ser.). pap., tchr. ed. 14.00 (*0-8273-3093-6*) Delmar.

Principles of Pharmacology for Medical Assisting. Jane Rice. (C). 2nd ed. 1994. LC 93-26739. 548p. pap. 32.00 (*0-8273-5744-3*); 3rd ed. 1998. LC 98-21887. 560p. pap. text 49.95 (*0-7668-0325-2*) Delmar.

Principles of Pharmacology for Medical Assisting: Instructor's Guide. Jane Rice. 2nd ed. 1994. 89p. 16.00 (*0-8273-6353-2*) Delmar.

Principles of Pharmacology for Medical Assisting - IML. Rice. 3rd ed. 1998. 112p. tchr. ed. 19.95 (*0-7668-0326-0*) Delmar.

Principles of Pharmacology for Respiratory Care. Georgine W. Bills & Robert C. Soderberg. 1994. LC 93-48582. 333p. pap. 34.95 (*0-8273-5274-3*) Delmar.

Principles Of Pharmacology For Respiratory Care. Georgine W. Bills & Robert C. Soderberg. 2nd ed. 1997. LC 97-22776. 384p. pap. text 54.95 (*0-8273-8299-5*) Delmar.

Principles of Pharmacology for Respiratory Care Workbook. Georgine W. Bills & Robert C. Soderberg. 1994. 111p. 17.95 (*0-8273-5275-1*) Delmar.

Principles of Pharmacy for Respiratory Care. Bills. 1994. (Respiratory Care Ser.). 15.00 (*0-8273-6360-5*) Delmar.

Principles of Physical Medicine & Rehabilitation in the Musculoskeletal Diseases. Ed. by James C. Leek et al. 1986. 544p. text 129.00 (*0-8089-1773-0*, 792502, Grune & Strat) Harcrt Hlth Sci Grp.

Principles of Physiology. Robert M. Berne & Matthew N. Levy. 2nd ed. 1996. (Illus.). 816p. pap. (*84-8174-211-2*) Mosby-Doyma Libros ESP. *Dist:* Mosby Inc.

Principles of Primary Wound Management: A Guide to the Fundamentals. Michael D. Mortiere. 1996. LC 96-94515. (Illus.). 96p. (Orig.). pap. text 16.00 (*0-9652878-0-7*) Clifton Pub.

Principles of Process Research & Chemical Development in the Pharmaceutical Industry. Oljan Repic. 1997. LC 97-13904. 240p. 89.95 (*0-471-16516-6*) Wiley.

Principles of Protein Structure. G. E. Schulz & R. H. Schirmer. LC 78-11500. (Advanced Texts in Chemistry Ser.). (Illus.). 314p. 1996. 59.95 (*0-387-90334-8*); 1979. 29.95 (*0-387-90386-0*) Spr-Verlag.

Principles of Psychoanalysis: Their Application to the Neuroses. Herman Nunberg. 1969. LC 55-11549. 382p. (Orig.). reprint ed. 57.50 (*0-8236-4300-X*); pap. 24.95 (*0-8236-8198-X*, 24300) Intl Univs Pr.

Principles of Psychoanalytic Psychotherapy: A Manual for Supportive-Expressive Treatment. Lester Luborsky. 1984. LC 83-54377. 292p. pap. 37.50 (*0-465-06328-4*) Basic.

Principles of Psychology William James. 1950. pap. text 14.95 (*0-486-20381-6*) Dover.

Principles of Psychology William James. 714p. 1260.00 (*1-85506-679-3*) Thoemmes Pr.

Principles of Psychology. Intro. by William James & George A. Miller. 1983. 1312p. pap. text 34.50 (*0-674-70625-0*) HUP.

Principles of Psychology. Herbert Spencer. 632p. 145.00 (*1-85506-655-6*) Thoemmes Pr.

Principles of Psychology. Engle. 9th ed. 1989. (gr. 11-12). pap. text, tchr. ed. 45.00 (*0-15-374801-X*); pap. text, wbk. ed. 12.25 (*0-15-374802-8*) Holt R&W.

Principles of Psychology, Vol. 2. William James. 1950. pap. text 16.95 (*0-486-20382-4*) Dover.

Principles of Psychology, Set. William James. 1990. 56.50 (*0-8446-2310-5*) Peter Smith.

Principles of Psychology: A Systematic Text in the Science of Behavior. Fred S. Keller & William N. Schoenfeld. 1995. (R. F. Skinner Reprint Ser.). 431p. (C). pap. text 20.00 (*0-87411-765-8*) Copley Pub.

Principles of Psychology: Tests. Engle. 9th ed. 1989. (gr. 11-12). pap. 11.25 (*0-15-374803-6*) Holt R&W.

Principles of Psychopathology: Two Worlds - Two Minds - Two Hemispheres. John C. Cutting. 1997. LC 96-29144. (Illus.). 604p. (C). text 120.00 (*0-19-262240-4*) OUP.

Principles of Psychophysiology: A Survey of Modern Scientific Psychology Leonard T. Troland. 1970. LC 68-57643. (Illus.). reprint ed. lib. bdg. 145.00 (*0-8371-9954-9*, TRPS);Vol. 1. lib. bdg. 60.00 (*0-8371-1007-6*, TRPT);Vol. 2. lib. bdg. 60.00 (*0-8371-1008-4*, TRPU);Vol. 3. lib. bdg. 55.00 (*0-8371-1009-2*, TRPV) Greenwood.

Principles of Psychophysiology: Physical, Social & Inferential Elements. Ed. by John T. Cacioppo & Louis G. Tassinary. 1990. (Illus.). 926p. (C). pap. text 47.95 (*0-521-34885-4*) Cambridge U Pr.

Principles of Psychotherapy. Brice Avery. 1997. pap. (*0-7225-3348-9*) Thorsons GBR. *Dist:* Natl Bk Netwk.

Principles of Psychotherapy. Pierre M. Janet. Tr. by H. M. Guthrie & Edwin R. Guthrie. 1977. (Select Bibliographies Reprint Ser.). reprint ed. 26.95 (*0-8369-5894-2*) Ayer.

Principles of Psychotherapy with Children. John M. Reisman & Shelia Ribordy. 2nd ed. 1993. LC 93-1430. (Scientific Foundations of Clinical & Counseling Psychology Ser.). 49.95 (*0-669-28055-0*) Free Pr.

Principles Of Public Health Care Practice. Keck Scutchfield & C. William Keck. 1996. LC 96-14785. (Health Services Administration Ser.). 432p. (C). 91.95 (*0-8273-6271-4*) Delmar.

Principles of Pulmonary Medicine. Steven E. Weinberger. Ed. by Judy Fletcher. 3rd ed. 1998. LC 97-4388. (Illus.). 432p. pap. text 39.00 (*0-7216-8668-0*) Saunders.

Principles of Radiation Oncology for Cancer of the Head & Neck. Robert M. Kellman & Chung T. Chung. 1993. (Self-Instruction Package Ser.). (Illus.). 85p. (Orig.). pap. text 25.00 (*1-56772-003-X*) AAO-HNS.

Principles of Radiographic Imaging. Richard R. Carlton & Arlene M. Adler. 1990. text 53.50 (*0-8273-3605-5*) Delmar.

Principles of Radiographic Imaging. Carlton. 2nd ed. 1996. (Radiographic Technology Ser.). 96p. tchr. ed. 18.00 (*0-8273-6865-8*); (C). lab manual ed. 23.00 (*0-8273-6866-6*) Delmar.

Principles of Radiographic Imaging: An Art & a Science. Richard R. Carlton. (Radiographic Technology Ser.). (Illus.). 2nd ed. 1996. 736p. (C). mass mkt. 77.95 (*0-8273-6864-X*); 3rd ed. 2000. LC 00-43193. 752p. 83.95 (*0-7668-1300-2*) Delmar.

Principles of Radiographic Imaging: Instructor's Guide. Richard R. Carlton & Arlene M. Adler. 1991. pap., tchr. ed. 18.00 (*0-8273-3606-3*) Delmar.

Principles of Radiographic Positioning & Procedures Pocket Guide. Richard R. Carlton. 2nd ed. 1999. LC 98-43726. 448p. (C). pap. 21.95 (*0-8273-6372-9*) Delmar.

Principles of Radiological Physics. Robin J. Wilks. 2nd ed. 1987. LC 86-17526. (Illus.). 608p. (Orig.). (C). pap. text (*0-443-03780-9*) Church.

Principles of Radiological Physics. D. T. Graham. 3rd ed. 1996. (Illus.). 667p. pap. (*0-443-04816-9*) Church.

Principles of Radiopharmacology Ed. by Lelio G. Columbetti. 1979. Vol. 1. 304p. 165.00 (*0-8493-5465-X*, RM858); Vol. 2. 288p. 158.00 (*0-8493-5466-8*); Vol. 3. 352p. 194.00 (*0-8493-5467-6*) Franklin (CRC Reprint).

Principles of Recepterology. Ed. by M. K. Agarwal. 1983. LC 83-15441. (Illus.). vii, 677p. 196.15 (*3-11-009558-0*) De Gruyter.

Principles of Reflexology: The Only Introduction You'll Ever Need. Nicola M. Hall. 2nd ed. 1996. pap. (*0-7225-3352-7*) Thorsons GBR. *Dist:* Natl Bk Netwk.

Principles of Reiki. Kasja K. Borang. 1997. pap. (*0-7225-3406-X*) Thorsons GBR. *Dist:* Natl Bk Netwk.

Principles of Renal Physiology. Christopher J. Lote. 3rd ed. 1994. LC 93-35421. 216p. (C). (gr. 13). pap. text 59.95 (*0-412-55520-4*, Chap & Hall NY) Chapman & Hall.

Principles of Research in Behavioral Science. Bernard E. Whitley, Jr. 1995. LC 95-24593. 692p. (C). text 68.95 (*1-55934-249-8*, 1249) Mayfield Pub.

*__Principles of Research in Behavioral Science.__ Bernard E. Whitley. 2nd ed. 2001. LC 2001-18329. xix, 668p. (*0-7674-2175-2*) Mayfield Pub.

Principles of Respiratory Care. Robert Kacmarek & David J. Pierson. 1999. (Illus.). 864p. (*0-07-034379-9*) McGraw-Hill Med Pub.

Principles of Scientific Literature Evaluation: Critiquing Clinical Drug Trials. Frank J. Ascione. 2001. LC 00-45333. (Illus.). viii, 198p. (C). pap. 42.00 (*1-58212-008-0*) Am Pharm Assn.

Principles of Seating the Disabled. R. Mervyn Letts. 1991. (Illus.). 384p. lib. bdg. 139.00 (*0-8493-6021-8*, RD757) CRC Pr.

Principles of Self-Damage. Edmund Bergler. 1992. LC 92-1423. 506p. (C). reprint ed. 70.00 (*0-8236-4315-8*) Intl Univs Pr.

Principles of Social Psychiatry. Dinesh K. L. Bhugra & Julian P. Leff. 1993. (Illus.). 600p. 165.00 (*0-632-03336-3*) Blackwell Sci.

Principles of Social Psychology. Kelly G. Shaver. 3rd ed. 1987. 656p. text 39.95 (*0-89859-592-4*); 210p. pap. text, tchr. ed. (*0-8058-0041-7*) L Erlbaum Assocs.

Principles of Spinal Surgery Ed. by Arnold H. Menezes & Volker K. Sonntag. 1995. LC 95-30569. 1520p. text 295.00 (*0-07-912043-1*) McGraw-Hill Med Pub.

*__Principles of Sterile Product Preparation.__ Barbara T. McKinnon et al. Ed. by E. Clyde Buchanan. rev. ed. 2001. (*1-58528-026-7*) Am Soc Hlth-Syst.

Principles of Stress Management Vera Peiffer. 1997. pap. (*0-7225-3243-1*) Thorsons GBR. *Dist:* Natl Bk Netwk.

Principles of Surgery. Seymour I. Schwartz. 6th ed. Date not set. 1. (*0-07-055929-5*); 2. (*0-07-055930-9*) McGraw.

Principles of Surgery. Ed. by Seymour I. Schwartz et al. 7th ed. 1998. (Illus.). 2176p. LC 98-28061. text 129.00 (*0-07-054256-2*);Set. pap. 159.00 (*0-07-912318-X*) McGraw-Hill Prof.

Principles of Surgery: Companion Handbook. Ed. by Seymour I. Schwartz et al. 7th ed. 1998. LC 98-45752. (Illus.). 1118p. pap. 39.95 (*0-07-058085-5*) McGraw-Hill Prof.

Principles of Surgery Self-Assessment & Review. Ed. by Seymour I. Schwartz. 7th ed. 1998. LC 98-45751. (Illus.). 250p. pap. 45.00 (*0-07-057964-4*) McGraw-Hill Prof.

*__Principles of Surgical Practice.__ Kingsnorth & Majid. 2001. (Illus.). 344p. (*1-84110-019-6*) Greenwich Med GBR. *Dist:* JAMCO Dist.

Principles of Surgical Technique: The Art of Surgery. Gary G. Wind & Norman M. Rich. 2nd ed. 1987. LC 86-15910. (Illus.). 224p. text 69.95 (*0-683-09133-6*) Lppncott W & W.

Principles of the Human Mind. Alfred Smee. 1980. LC 80-68665. (Illus.). 96p. pap. 5.95 (*0-89708-030-0*) And Bks.

*__Principles of Thics with Annotations Especially Applicable to Psychiatry 2001.__ American Psychiatric Association Staff. 2001. 48p. pap. 10.00 (*0-89042-143-9*, 2143) Am Psychiatric.

Principles of Thoracic Anaesthesia see Origins of Thoracic Anaesthesia

Principles of Toxicokinetic Studies. 1986. (Environmental Health Criteria Ser.: No. 57). 167p. pap. text 23.00 (*92-4-154257-8*, 1160057) World Health.

Principles of Toxicology. Phillip L. Williams et al. 2nd ed. 1998. 560p. 51.95 (*0-442-23738-3*, VNR) Wiley.

*__Principles of Traditional Chinese Medicine.__ Xu Xiangcai. 2001. pap. 18.95 (*1-886969-99-X*) YMAA Pubn.

Principles of Transfusion Medicine. Ennio C. Rossi et al. 1990. (Illus.). 816p. 115.00 (*0-683-07385-0*) Lppncott W & W.

Principles of Transfusion Medicine. Toby L. Simon et al. Ed. by Ennio C. Rossi. 2nd ed. 1995. LC 95-11651. (Illus.). 953p. text 169.00 (*0-683-07386-9*) Lppncott W & W.

Principles of Trauma Surgery. Ed. by Joseph A. Moylan. 2nd ed. 1991. (Illus.). 446p. (gr. 13). text (*1-56375-013-9*, GM0199) Gower-Mosby.

Principles of Treatment in Multiple Sclerosis. Clive Hawkins. 2000. LC 00-700047. (Illus.). 352p. text 75.00 (*0-7506-4270-X*) Buttrwrth-Heinemann.

Principles of Veterinary Therapeutics. R. Einstein et al. 1996. (Illus.). 598p. (*0-582-02963-5*) Addison-Wesley GBR. *Dist:* Trans-Atl Phila, Longman.

Principles of Warmwater Aquaculture. Robert R. Stickney. 1979. LC 78-25642. 375p. 160.00 (*0-471-03388-X*) Wiley.

Principles of Wound Management. Richard F. Edlich. 1988. (Illus.). 400p. pap. text 45.00 (*0-07-019018-6*) McGraw.

Principles of Zoology, Touching the Structure, Development, Distribution, & Natural Arrangement of the Races of Animals Living & Extinct. Louis Agassiz & Augustus Gould. 1974. LC 76-125729. (American Environmental Studies). (Illus.). reprint ed. 19.95 (*0-405-02654-4*) Ayer.

Principles Operative Surgery. Poston. 2nd ed. 1996. pap. text 24.95 (*0-443-05019-8*) Saunders.

Principles, Practice & Patients. Beatrice Sofaer. 3rd ed. 1998. (Illus.). 144p. pap. (*0-7487-3329-9*) Nelson Thornes GBR. *Dist:* Aspen Pub.

Principles, Techniques & Applications in Microsurgery. Ed. by T. S. Chang & Peter C. Leung. 1986. 400p. text 130.00 (*9971-978-08-3*); pap. text 49.00 (*9971-978-09-1*) World Scientific Pub.

Princples & Practice of Endodontics. Richard E. Walton & Mahmoud Torabinejad. 2nd ed. 1995. LC 94-43383. (Illus.). 512p. text 62.95 (*0-7216-4924-6*) Saunders.

Prion Biology & Diseases. Ed. by Stanley B. Prusiner. 1999. LC 99-72366. (Monographs). (Illus.). xiii, 794p. (C). 125.00 (*0-87969-547-1*) Cold Spring Harbor.

Prion Diseases. Ed. by Harry F. Baker & Rosalind M. Ridley. 1996. LC 96-3408. (Methods in Molecular Medicine Ser.: Vol. 3). (Illus.). 336p. 119.00 (*0-89603-342-2*) Humana.

Prion Diseases. Ed. by John Collinge & Mark Palmer. 1997. LC 96-30984. (Illus.). 212p. text 59.50 (*0-19-854789-7*) OUP.

Prion Diseases: Diagnosis & Pathogenesis. Ed. by M. H. Groschup et al. 2001. LC 2001-265762. (Special Edition of Archives of Virology Ser.). (Illus.). ix, 290p. 129.00 (*3-211-83530-X*) Spr-Verlag.

Prions: Molecular & Cellular Biology. Ed. by David A. Harris. 1999. LC 99-206578. (Illus.). x, 217p. (*1-898486-07-7*) Horizon Sci GBR. *Dist:* Intl Spec Bk.

Prions & Brain Diseases in Animals & Humans. Ed. by Douglas R. Morrison. 1998. LC 98-12133. (NATO Advanced Science Institutes Ser.: No. 295). (Illus.). 372p. (C). text 125.00 (*0-306-45825-X*, Kluwer Plenum) Kluwer Academic.

Prions (Prusiner's Particles) Index of New Information. Science and Life Consultants Association Staff. 1998. 160p. 57.50 (*0-7883-1866-7*); pap. 47.50 (*0-7883-1867-5*) ABBE Pubs Assn.

Priorities for Critical Care Nursing. Linda D. Urden et al. 2nd ed. 1997. (Illus.). 552p. (*84-8174-304-6*) Mosby-Doyma Libros ESP. *Dist:* Mosby Inc.

Priorities for Health Promotion & Disease Prevention. Gerald C. Hyner & Christopher L. Melby. 1987. 178p. pap. text 19.95 (*0-912855-74-6*) E Bowers Pub.

Priorities in Critical Care Nursing. Linda D. Urden et al. Ed. by Mary E. Lough. 2nd rev. ed. 1995. LC 95-20589. (Illus.). 552p. (C). (gr. 13). text 48.00 (*0-8151-8947-8*, 26419) Mosby Inc.

Priorities in Critical Care Nursing. Stacey Urden. 3rd ed. 1999. LC 00-265423. 543p. pap. text 57.95 (*0-323-01000-8*) Mosby Inc.

*__Priorities in Critical Care Nursing: Instructor's Resource Manual.__ Linda D. Urden & Kathleen M. Stacy. 3rd ed. 2000. (Illus.). pap. (*0-323-01071-7*) Mosby Inc.

Priority Health Conditions: An Integrated Strategy to Evaluate the Relationship Between Illness & Exposure to Hazardous Substances. Ed. by Jeffrey A. Lybarger et al. 1994. 214p. (Orig.). (C). pap. text 50.00 (*0-7881-0530-2*) DIANE Pub.

Priority Research for Health for All. 1988. (European Health for All Ser.: No. 3). pap. text 15.00 (*92-890-1054-1*) World Health.

Priority Setting in Action: Purchasing Dilemmas. Frank Honigsbaum et al. 1995. LC 95-23267. 200p. pap. (*1-85775-100-0*) Radcliffe Med Pr GBR. *Dist:* Balogh.

Prism Workbook. David B. Wexler. 1991. LC 91-9530. 73p. (Orig.). pap. 12.95 (*0-393-70119-0*) Norton.

Prison Crowding: A Psychological Perspective. P. B. Paulus. 1988. (Research in Criminology Ser.). (Illus.). 115p. 116.00 (*0-387-96650-1*) Spr-Verlag.

Prison Madness: The Mental Health Crisis Behind Bars & What We Must Do about It. Terry A. Kupers & Hans Toch. 1999. LC 98-25505. 336p. 25.00 (*0-7879-4361-4*) Jossey-Bass.

Prisoner of Fear: My Long Road to Freedom from Anxiety Disease, Panic Attacks & Agoraphobia. Richard Maro. 1990. 250p. (Orig.). pap. 12.95 (*0-9628509-0-X*) Hickory Grove Pr.

Prisoner's Dilemma. Anatol Rapoport et al. 1965. (Illus.). 270p. pap. text 18.95 (*0-472-06165-8*, 06165, Ann Arbor Bks) U of Mich Pr.

Prisoners of Childhood. Alice Miller. 1996. 128p. reprint ed. 22.00 (*0-465-06287-3*) Basic.

Prisoners of Ritual: An Odyssey into Female Genital Circumcision in Africa. Pref. by Hanny Lightfoot-Klein. 1989. LC 89-15639. (Haworth Series on Women: No. 2). (Illus.). 306p. text 39.95 (*0-86656-877-8*) Haworth Pr.

Prisonhouse of Psychoanalysis. Arnold Goldberg. 1990. 184p. text 29.95 (*0-88163-121-3*) Analytic Pr.

Prisons & AIDS: A Public Health Opportunity. Ronald L. Braithwaite et al. 1996. LC 96-22690. (Jossey-Bass Health Ser.). 247p. 39.00 (*0-7879-0308-6*) Jossey-Bass.

Pristina Medicamenta: Ancient & Medieval Botany. Jerry Stannard. Ed. by Katherine E. Stannard & Richard Kay. 1999. LC 98-74833. (Variorum Collected Studies Ser.). xx, 367p. text 110.95 (*0-86078-773-7*) Ashgate Pub Co.

Pritikin Promise. Nathan Pritikin. 1991. mass mkt. 5.99 (*0-671-73267-6*) PB.

Privacy: A Vanishing Value? Ed. by William C. Bier. 1980. LC 79-56138. (Pastoral Psychology Ser.: No. 10). xii, 398p. 70.00 (*0-8232-1044-8*) Fordham.

Privacy & Confidentiality in Mental Health Care. John J. Gates & Bernard S. Arons. 1999. LC 99-45960. xxiv, 242p. pap. 34.00 (*1-55766-426-9*) P H Brookes.

Privacy & Health Care. Ed. by James M. Humber & Robert F. Almeder. 2001. (Biomedical Ethics Reviews Ser.). (Illus.). 195p. 44.50 (*0-89603-878-5*) Humana.

Privacy Issues in Biomedical & Clinical Research: Privacy Issues in Biomedical & Clinical Research Proceedings of Forum on November 1, 1997, National Academy of Sciences, Washington, D. C. National Research Council Staff. 1998. LC 99-183451. (Compass Ser.). ix, 48 p. (*0-309-06328-0*) Natl Acad Pr.

Privacy under a Microscope: Balancing the Needs of Research & Confidentiality: Hearing of the Committee on Health, Education, Labor & Pensions, United States Senate, One Hundred Sixth Congress, First Session... February 24, 1999. Contrib. by U. S. Congress, Senate Committee on Health, Education, Labor and Pensions. 1999. LC 99-216803. (*0-16-058379-9*) USGPO.

Private Acts, Social Consequences: AIDS & the Politics of Public Health. Ronald Bayer. 1989. 280p. 35.00 (*0-02-901961-3*) Free Pr.

Private Acts, Social Consequences: AIDS & the Politics of Public Health. Ronald Bayer. 1991. LC 90-42039. 282p. pap. 17.95 (*0-8135-1624-2*) Rutgers U Pr.

Private & Public Initiatives: Working Together for Health & Education. Jacques Van der Gaag. 1995. LC 95-222718. (Directions in Development Ser.). 76p. pap. 22.00 (*0-8213-3417-4*, 13417) World Bank.

Private Choices & Public Health: The AIDS Epidemic in an Economic Perspective. Tomas J. Philipson & Richard A. Posner. 1993. LC 93-17417. (Illus.). 272p. 39.50 (*0-674-70738-9*) HUP.

Private Choices, Social Costs, & Public Policy: An Economic Analysis of Public Health Issues. Nancy Hammerle. 1992. LC 92-3459. 248p. 67.00 (*0-275-94172-8*, C4172, Praeger Pubs) Greenwood.

Private Eye, Heart & Hip. Yates. 1995. (C). pap. text 21.95 (*0-443-05466-5*) Saunders.

Private Health Care in India: A Sociological Inquiry. Rama V. Baru. 1998. LC 98-28220. 39.95 (*0-7619-9286-3*, 84727) Sage.

Private Health Insurance: Progress & Challenges in Implementing 1996 Federal Standards. Ed. by William J. Scanlon. 2000. (Illus.). 52p. (C). pap. text 20.00 (*0-7881-8810-0*) DIANE Pub.

Private Health Providers in Developing Countries: Serving the Public Interest? Sara Bennett et al. 1997. LC 97-6650. (*1-85649-495-0*); pap. 25.00 (*1-85649-496-9*) Brill Academic Pubs.

Private Health Sector Growth in Asia. William C. Newbrander & Asian Development Bank Staff. 1997. LC 96-47180. 272p. 130.00 (*0-471-97236-3*) Wiley.

Private Lives & Professional Identity of Medical Students. Robert S. Broadhead. 1983. LC 82-19502. 140p. text 34.95 (*0-87855-478-5*) Transaction Pubs.

Private Markets in Health & Welfare: An International Perspective. Ed. by Norman Johnson. 1995. LC 94-34789. xiv, 249p. 47.50 (*0-85496-822-9*); pap. 19.50 (*1-85973-097-3*) Berg Pubs.

Private Medical Practice: Getting Started & Making It Work. Debi Carey. 1997. LC 97-10674. (HFMA Healthcare Financial Management Ser.). 320p. 175.00 (*0-7863-1118-5*, Irwn Prfssnl) McGraw-Hill Educ Grp.

Private Medicine & Public Health: Profit, Politics & Prejudice in the American Health Care Enterprise. Lawrence D. Weiss. 1997. LC 96-40916. 240p. (C). pap. text 29.00 (*0-8133-3351-2*) Westview.

Private Myths: Dreams & Dreaming. Anthony Stevens. 1996. LC 95-45926. 400p. 27.95 (*0-674-21638-5*) HUP.

Private Practice. McCue. 1991. 32.95 (*0-316-55531-2*, Little Brwn Med Div) Lppncott W & W.

Private Practice in Communication Disorders. Mary L. Wood. 1991. (Illus.). 390p. (C). reprint ed. pap. 45.00 (*1-879105-30-6*, A072) Thomson Learn.

Private Practice in Occupational Therapy. Ed. by Florence S. Cromwell. 1985. LC 85-5513. (Occupational Therapy in Health Care Ser.: Vol. 2, No. 2). 138p. pap. text 19.95 (*0-86656-412-8*); text 39.95 (*0-86656-411-X*) Haworth Pr.

Private Practice of Behavior Therapy: A Guide for Behavioral Practitioners. S. J. Kaplan. 1986. LC 86-51165. (Applied Clinical Psychology Ser.). (Illus.). 306p. (C). 59.50 (*0-306-42193-3*, Plenum Trade) Perseus Pubng.

Private Practice, Public Payment: Canadian Medicine & the Politics of Health Insurance, 1911-1966. C. David Naylor. 1986. 320p. (C). pap. (*0-7735-0568-7*); text (*0-7735-0557-1*) McG-Queens Univ Pr CAN. *Dist:* CUP Services.

Private Regulation of American Health Care. Betty Leyerle. 1994. LC 93-42516. 240p. pap. 34.95 (*1-56324-289-3*); (gr. 13). 74.95 (*1-56324-288-5*) M E Sharpe.

Private Sector Involvement in Health Care: Implications for Access, Cost, & Quality, Vol. 9. Ed. by Richard M. Scheffler et al. 1988. (Advances in Health Economics & Health Services Research Ser.). 265p. 73.25 (*0-89232-937-8*) Jai Pr.

Private Versus Public Sector Insurance Coverage for Drug Abuse. Jeannette A. Rogowski. 1993. LC 93-12592. pap. text 13.00 (*0-8330-1345-9*, MR-166-DPRC) Rand Corp.

Privatisation & the National Health Service: The Scope for Collaboration. Ed. by Jeffrey Chandra & Andrew Kakabadse. 1985. LC 85-16857. 120p. text (*0-566-00813-0*) Dartmth Pub GBR. *Dist:* Ashgate Pub Co.

Privatization & Mental Health Care: A Fragile Balance. Robert A. Dorwart & Sherrie S. Epstein. 1993. LC 92-38615. 208p. 60.00 (*0-86569-002-2*, T002, Auburn Hse) Greenwood.

Privatization & Restructuring of Health Services in Singapore. Phua K. Hong. 1991. (Institute for Policy Studies Ser.: No. 5). 48p. pap. (*981-210-002-4*) Times Academic SGP. *Dist:* Intl Spec Bk.

Privatizing Health Services in Africa. Meredeth Turshen. 1999. LC 98-23537. 200p. (C). text 50.00 (*0-8135-2580-2*); pap. text 23.00 (*0-8135-2581-0*) Rutgers U Pr.

Privilege & the Responsibility: Working in a Nursing Home. Michael Jacobs. 1999. 150p. pap. 19.00 (*0-929442-49-0*, 2118PP) Prof Prnting & Pub.

Privilege in the Medical Academy: A Feminist Examines Gender, Race & Power. Delse Wear. 1997. LC 97-11213. (Athene Ser.). 42.00 (*0-8077-6290-3*); 144p. pap. 18.95 (*0-8077-6288-1*) Tchrs Coll.

Privileging Quick Reference Guide. Ed. by Beverly E. Pybus. 1998. 130p. pap. text 97.00 (*1-57839-022-2*) Opus Communs.

Pro-Choice-Pro-Life: An Annotated, Selected Bibliography (1972-1989), 20. Ed. by Joan P. Diana. 1991. LC 91-12625. (Bibliographies & Indexes in Sociology Ser.: No. 20). 264p. lib. bdg. 62.95 (*0-313-27579-3*, FPJ, Greenwood Pr) Greenwood.

Pro-Protein & Pro-Hormone Convertases: Reprint from Journal Enzyme, Vol. 45, Nos. 5 & 6, 1991. Ed. by N. G. Seidah. 1992. (Illus.). iv, 88p. 85.25 (*3-8055-5705-1*) S Karger.

Pro-Vita! Plan: For Optimal Nutrition. Jack Tips. 2nd rev. ed. 1992. LC 92-70715. (Illus.). 235p. pap. text 19.95 (*0-929167-05-8*) Apple-a-Day.

Proactive Approaches in Psychosocial Occupational Therapy. Rita P. Cottrell. 2000. LC 00-29178. (Illus.). 576p. pap. text 42.00 (*1-55642-455-8*) SLACK Inc.

Proactive Responses to the Assisted Suicide/Euthanasia Debate. Ed. by National Hospice Organization Ethics Committee. 1996. 96p. (Orig.). pap., per. 11.85 (*0-931207-45-2*, 713438) Natl Hospice.

Probabilistic Models for Some Intelligence & Attainment Tests. Georg Rasch. 1993. LC 80-16546. (Illus.). 222p. (C). reprint ed. pap. text 20.00 (*0-941938-05-0*) Mesa Pr.

Probabilistic Models for Some Intelligence & Attainment Tests. Georg Rasch. 1980. LC 80-16546. 208p. pap. text 9.00 (*0-226-70554-4*) U Ch Pr.

Probability of Addiction: Legal, Medical & Social Implications. David A. Peters. 1997. LC 96-46207. 166p. pap. 49.95 (*1-57292-052-1*) Austin & Winfield.

Probability Without Equations: Concepts for Clinicians. Bert K. Holland. 1997. LC 97-18994. (Illus.). 128p. 49.00 (*0-8018-5759-7*); pap. text 18.95 (*0-8018-5760-0*) Johns Hopkins.

Probe Microphone Measurements: Hearing Aid Selection & Assessment. H. Gustav Mueller et al. 1992. (Illus.). 256p. (C). pap. 65.00 (*1-879105-68-3*, 0323) Thomson Learn.

Probing Bioactive Mechanisms. Ed. by John H. Block et al. 1989. LC 89-17998. (ACS Symposium Ser.: No. 413). (Illus.). 400p. text 65.00 (*0-8412-1702-5*) Am Chemical.

Probiotics: The Scientific Basis. Ed. by Ray Fuller. Date not set. (Illus.). 416p. (C). (gr. 13). text 80.95 (*0-412-40850-3*, Chap & Hall NY) Chapman & Hall.

Probiotics 3: Immunomodulation by the Gut Microflora & Probiotics. G. Perdigon. Ed. by R. Fuller. 2000. 280p. 132.50 (*0-7923-6244-6*) Kluwer Academic.

Problem-Based Learning Applied to Medical Education. Howard S. Barrows. 2000. 25.00 (*0-931369-34-7*) Southern IL Univ Sch.

Problem-Based Learning in a Health Sciences Curriculum. Ed. by Christine Alavi. 1995. LC 94-35357. 224p. (C). 85.00 (*0-415-11207-9*, C0059); pap. 29.95 (*0-415-11208-7*, C0060) Routledge.

***Problem-Based Learning in Medicine: A Practical Guide for Students & Teachers.** Tim David et al. 1999. 104p. pap. (*1-85315-430-X*) Royal Soc of Medicine Pr Ltd GBR. *Dist:* Balogh.

***Problem-Based Obstetrics & Gynaecology.** J. J. Walker & L. A. Greer. 2001. (Illus.). 190p. pap. (*0-443-05305-7*) Church GBR. *Dist:* Saunders.

Problem Based Pediatrics. David J. Field. 1997. LC 97-19288. pap. text (*0-443-05254-9*) Church.

Problem-Based Psychiatry. Ben Green. 1996. LC 95-40795. pap. text (*0-443-05198-4*) Church.

Problem Behaviors in Long-Term Care: Recognition, Diagnosis, & Treatment. Ed. by Peggy A. Szwabo & George T. Grossberg. 1992. LC 92-2232. 320p. 39.95 (*0-8261-7820-0*) Springer Pub.

Problem Drinkers: Guided Self-Change Treatment. Mark B. Sobell & Linda C. Sobell. 1993. LC 92-48479. (Treatment Manuals for Practitioners Ser.). 187p. 42.00 (*0-89862-212-3*) Guilford Pubns.

Problem Drinkers Seeking Treatment. Eileen M. Corrigan. 1974. LC 73-620006. (Monographs: No. 8). 5.00 (*0-911290-39-7*) Rutgers Ctr Alcohol.

Problem Drinking: How to Help a Friend. Charles Downs. 2000. 128p. (Orig.). pap. 7.99 (*0-87788-662-8*, H Shaw Pubs) Waterbrook Pr.

Problem Drinking Among American Men. Don Cahalan & Robin Room. 1974. 25.95 (*0-8084-0380-X*) NCUP.

Problem Drinking Among American Men. Don Cahalan & Robin Room. 1974. LC 72-619570. (Monographs: No. 7). 8.25 (*0-911290-38-9*) Rutgers Ctr Alcohol.

Problem Foods. Walter Last. 1987. LC 86-18130. (*0-943920-54-X*) Metamorphous Pr.

Problem Knee. Macricol. 1998. 224p. pap. text (*0-7506-4044-8*) E A GBR. *Dist:* OUP.

Problem Knee. Malcolm F. Macnicol. 2nd ed. 1995. LC 94-45158. (Illus.). 224p. 100.00 (*0-7506-0487-5*) Buttrwrth-Heinemann.

Problem of Age, Growth, & Death. Charles S. Minot. Ed. by Robert J. Kastenbaum. 1979. LC 78-22211. (Aging & Old Age Ser.). (Illus.). reprint ed. lib. bdg. 27.95 (*0-405-11824-4*) Ayer.

Problem of Evil: Disturbance & Its Resolution in Modern Psychotherapy. Eric Greenleaf. 2000. LC 00-712096. xviii, 298p. text 34.95 (*1-891944-41-X*) Zeig Tucker Theisen.

Problem of Loss & Mourning: Psychoanalytic Perspectives. Ed. by David R. Dietrich & Peter Shabad. 1989. 500p. 67.50 (*0-8236-4349-2*, BN 04349) Intl Univs Pr.

Problem of Meaning: Behavioral & Cognitive Perspectives. Charlotte Mandell & Allyssa McCabe. 1997. LC 97-25320. (Advances in Psychology Ser.: Vol. 122). 486p. 125.00 (*0-444-82479-0*) Elsevier.

Problem of Mental Disorder. National Research Council Staff. Ed. by Gerald N. Grob. 1980. LC 78-22580. (Historical Issues in Mental Health Ser.). reprint ed. lib. bdg. 30.95 (*0-405-11932-1*) Ayer.

Problem of Perversion: The View from Self Psychology. Arnold Goldberg. 1994. LC 94-28556. 40.00 (*0-300-06030-0*) Yale U Pr.

Problem of Rationality in Science & Its Philosophy: On Popper vs. Polanyi, the Polish Conferences 1988-89. Ed. by Jozef Misiek. 1995. LC 94-17897. (Boston Studies in the Philosophy of Science: Vol. 160). 280p. (C). lib. bdg. (*0-7923-2925-2*) Kluwer Academic NLD. *Dist:* Kluwer Academic.

Problem of the Medical Profession: A Political Primer for Patients & Doctors. B. Monahan. 1991. lib. bdg. 69.00 (*0-8490-4404-9*) Gordon Pr.

Problem-Oriented Clinical Microbiology & Infection. H. Humphreys & W. I. Irving. 1996. (Illus.). 168p. pap. (*0-443-04914-9*) Church.

Problem-Oriented Medical Diagnosis. Ed. by H. Harold Friedman. 4th ed. 1987. (Spiral Manual Ser.). (C). spiral bd. 22.50 (*0-316-29378-4*, Little Brwn Med Div) Lppncott W & W.

Problem-Oriented Medical Diagnosis. H. Harold Friedman. 5th ed. 1991. LC 95-31027. 29.95 (*0-316-29387-3*, Little Brwn Med Div); 7th ed. 2000. LC 00-41235. (Illus.). xv, 441p. per. (*0-7817-2955-6*) Lppncott W & W.

Problem-oriented Medical Diagnosis. Ed. by H. Harold Friedman. 7th ed. 2000. LC 00-41235. (Illus.). 464p. spiral bd. 39.95 (*0-7817-2909-2*) Lppncott W & W.

Problem-Oriented Medical Record for High-Risk Obstetrics. Ed. by Curtis L. Cetrulo et al. 1984. LC 83-17712. 510p. 110.00 (*0-306-41325-6*, Plenum Trade) Perseus Pubng.

Problem-Oriented Nursing Assessment. Patricia Larkin & Barbara Backer. 1977. (C). text 17.95 (*0-07-036450-8*) McGraw.

Problem-Oriented Pediatric Diagnosis. Roger M. Barkin. 1990. 320p. spiral bd. 34.95 (*0-316-08102-7*) Lppncott W & W.

Problem-Oriented Record in Psychiatry & Mental Health Care. Ralph S. Ryback et al. Ed. by Richard Longabaugh & Robert D. Fowler. 2nd ed. 1981. 270p. pap. text 56.00 (*0-8089-1308-5*, 793701, Grune & Strat) Harcrt Hlth Sci Grp.

Problem Oriented with Pediatric Diagnosis. Roger M. Barkin. 1990. 10.95 (*0-316-08103-5*); 15.95 (*0-316-08104-3*) Lppncott W & W (Little Brwn Med Div).

Problem Solving: Manager's Guide. Martine Hilton et al. 1993. (Primary Health Care Management Advancement Programme Modules Ser.). 54p. pap. text (*1-882839-19-6*) Aga Khan Fnd.

Problem-Solving Exercises for Nutrition. Betty A. Clamp et al. 5th rev. ed. 1997. (Illus.). pap. text 23.95 (*1-890871-00-1*) Holcomb Hath.

Problem Solving for Health Care Quality Improvement: The Basics & Beyond. Barbara Katz. 1994. (Illus.). 202p. (Orig.). pap. 29.95 (*0-9640405-0-6*) Hlth Interact.

Problem Solving for Tutorials in Anatomy. Peter H. Abrahams et al. 1995. LC 95-11349. Orig. Title: Pocket Examiner in Regional & Clinical Anatomy. reprint ed. pap. text (*0-443-05285-9*) Church.

Problem Solving in Blood Banking. Robert R. Harr & Deirdre DeSantis. 1997. (C). 51.95 (*0-8036-0277-4*) Davis Co.

Problem Solving in Clinical Medicine: From Data to Diagnosis. Paul Cutler. 1997. 2nd ed. (Illus.). 550p. pap. text 35.00 (*0-683-02252-0*); 3rd ed. 531p. 49.95 (*0-683-30377-5*) Lppncott W & W.

Problem Solving in Endodontics. James L. Gutmann et al. 3rd ed. 1996. LC 97-106504. (Illus.). 384p. (C). (gr. 13). text 81.95 (*0-8151-4044-4*, 25551) Mosby Inc.

Problem Solving in Families: Research & Practice. Samuel Vuchinich. 1999. LC 98-25540. (Understanding Families Ser.). 238p. 89.95 (*0-7619-0877-3*, 81309); x, 238p. pap. 31.95 (*0-7619-0878-1*, 81310) Sage.

Problem Solving in Medicine, Vol. 1. Ed. by William Rosenberg & E. Edward Bittar. Date not set. 128.50 (*0-7623-0397-2*) Jai Pr.

Problem Solving, Physical Pharmacy IV. Alfred Martin. 1993. 222p. pap. text 19.50 (*0-8121-1642-9*) Lppncott W & W.

Problem-Solving Therapy. Jay Haley. 2nd ed. 1991. LC 87-45413. (Social & Behavioral Science Ser.). 288p. pap. 28.00 (*1-55542-362-0*) Jossey-Bass.

Problem-Solving Therapy for Depression: Theory, Research & Clinical Guidelines. Arthur M. Nezu et al. 1989. LC 88-17287. (Personality Processes Ser.). 274p. 160.00 (*0-471-62885-9*) Wiley.

Problem That Won't Go Away: Reforming U. S. Health Care Financing. Ed. by Henry J. Aaron. 1995. LC 95-37621. 298p. (C). text 42.95 (*0-8157-0010-5*) Brookings.

Problematic Pigmented Lesions: A Case Method Approach. Martin C. Mihm, Jr. & Paul Googe. 1990. LC 89-12216. (Illus.). 543p. text 98.00 (*0-8121-1261-X*) Lppncott W & W.

Probleme de la Sexualite Chez les Champignons: Recherches sur le Genre Coprinus. A. Quintanilha. 1968. (Illus.). reprint ed. pap. 24.00 (*3-7682-0556-8*) Lubrecht & Cramer.

Probleme der Krebsnachsorge. Ed. by A. Pfleiderer. 1980. (Beitraege Zur Onkologie, Contributions to Oncology Ser.: Band 4). (Illus.). 112p. pap. 28.75 (*3-8055-1378-X*) S Karger.

Problems & Cases in Health Information Management. Susan P. Bailey. 1997. (Illus.). v, 93p. (Orig.). (C). pap. text 22.95 (*0-9657783-0-4*) Lenox Pub Co.

Problems & Cases in Health Information Management: Instructor Guide. Susan P. Bailey. 1997. (Illus.). v, 93p. (Orig.). (C). pap. text, tchr. ed. 26.95 (*0-9657783-1-2*) Lenox Pub Co.

Problems & Methods in the History of Medicine. Roy Porter & Andrew Wear. 1987. (Welcome Institute Series in the History of Medicine). 256p. (*0-7099-3687-7*) C Helm GBR. *Dist:* Routldge.

Problems & Procedures in Dentofacial Orthopedics, Vol. 4. Frans P. G. M. Van der Linden. 1990. (Illus.). 382p. pap. text 70.00 (*0-86715-212-5*) Quint Pub Co.

Problems & Programmes Related to Alcohol & Drug Dependence in 33 Countries. J. Moser. 1974. (Offset Publications: No. 6). pap. text 20.00 (*92-4-170006-8*, 1120006) World Health.

Problems & Solutions: A Guide to Psychotherapy for the Beginning Psychotherapist. Martin D. Kantor. 1990. LC 89-72198. 216p. 62.50 (*0-275-93490-X*, C3490, Praeger Pubs) Greenwood.

Problems & Solutions in Complete Denture Fabrication. D. J. Lamb. 1993. (Illus.). 168p. text 52.00 (*1-85097-021-1*) Quint Pub Co.

Problems & Solutions in Radiation Protection. James E. Turner et al. 1988. (Illus.). 320p. pap. 30.00 (*0-08-035552-8*, Pergamon Pr) Elsevier.

Problems & Solutions in Radiation Protection. James E. Turner et al. 1991. 316p. text 30.00 (*0-07-105322-0*) McGraw-Hill Med Pub.

Problems in Biology. Carol Knox & Katheryn Rowsey. 1980. (Illus.). 90p. (Orig.). (gr. 10-11). stu. ed. 13.60 (*0-88334-132-8*); 9.28 (*0-8013-0095-9*) Longman.

Problems in Cardiothoracic Anaesthesia. John Gothard. 1998. LC 98-52023. 224p. pap. text 40.00 (*0-7506-2033-1*) Buttrwrth-Heinemann.

Problems in Diagnosis & Management of Polycystic Kidney Disease: Proceedings of the First International Workshop on PKD. Ed. by Jared J. Grantham & Kenneth D. Gardner, Jr. 1985. (Illus.). 216p. 14.95 (*0-9614567-0-1*) PKR Foundation.

Problems in Equine Medicine. Christopher M. Brown. 1989. LC 88-27255. (Illus.). 302p. text 50.00 (*0-8121-1171-0*) Lppncott W & W.

Problems in General Surgery. Ed. by Jack Pickleman. 1982. LC 81-22702. (Reviewing Surgical Topics Ser.). 382p. (C). 75.00 (*0-306-40765-5*, Kluwer Plenum) Kluwer Academic.

Problems in Gynaecology. E. P. Tatford. 1986. (Problems in Practice Ser.). text 164.00 (*0-85200-278-5*) Kluwer Academic.

Problems in Health Care Law. Robert D. Miller & Rebecca C. Hutton. 8th ed. 1999. LC 99-47599. 700p. 70.00 (*0-8342-1602-7*) Aspen Pub.

Problems in Intrahepatic Cholestasis: Proceedings of the International Symposium, 2nd, Florence, October 13-14, 1978. International Symposium on Intrahepatic Cholestasis Staff. Ed. by Paolo Gentilini et al. 1979. (Illus.). 101.00 (*3-8055-3009-9*) S Karger.

Problems in Pediatric Drug Therapy. Ed. by Louis A. Pagliaro & Ann Marie Pagliaro. 3rd rev. ed. 1995. LC 94-37762. 1145p. pap. 60.00 (*0-914768-53-0*, T168); 4th rev. ed. 2002. 600p. 80.00 (*1-58212-001-3*) Am Pharm Assn.

Problems in Personal Identity. James Baillie. 1992. 176p. pap. 16.95 (*1-55778-521-X*) Paragon Hse.

Problems in Small Animal Neurology. Cheryl L. Chrisman. 2nd ed. 1991. LC 90-5881. (Illus.). 526p. text 70.00 (*0-8121-1349-7*) Lppncott W & W.

Problems in the Psychology of Reading. J. Q. Quantz. 1974. (Psychology Monographs General & Applied: Vol. 2). reprint ed. pap. 55.00 (*0-8115-1401-3*) Periodicals Srv.

Problems, Issues & Concepts in Therapeutic Recreation. Ronald P. Reynolds & Gerald S. O'Morrow. 1985. 304p. (C). text 39.00 (*0-13-717430-6*) P-H.

Problems of Adrenergic Mechanisms in Blood Vessel. Ed. by W. Osswald. 1984. (Journal: Vol. 21, No. 3, 1984). (Illus.). 44p. pap. 35.00 (*3-8055-3927-4*) S Karger.

Problems of Aging: Biological & Medical Aspects. Ed. by E. V. Cowdry & Robert J. Kastenbaum. 1979. LC 78-22196. (Aging & Old Age Ser.). (Illus.). reprint ed. lib. bdg. 52.95 (*0-405-11813-9*) Ayer.

Problems of Antiviral Therapy. Ed. by John S. Oxford & Charles H. Stuart-Harris. 1984. (Beecham Colloquia Ser.). 360p. text 94.00 (*0-12-674760-1*) Acad Pr.

Problems of Autistic Behavior: Experimental Analysis of Autism, Vol. 1. O. Ivar Lovaas et al. 300p. text (*0-8290-0740-7*) Irvington.

Problems of Human Pleasure & Behavior. Michael Balint. 1973. pap. 3.95 (*0-87140-279-3*) Liveright.

Problems of Intracranial Pressure in Childhood. Ed. by Robert A. Minns. 1991. (Clinics in Developmental Medicine Ser.: Nos. 113-114). (Illus.). 458p. (C). text (*0-521-41272-2*) Mc Keith Pr GBR. *Dist:* Cambridge U Pr.

Problems of Modern Living: Psychology of Adjustment. Benjamin B. Wolman. 1987. (Illus.). 217p. (Orig.). (C). pap. text 19.95 (*0-89641-145-1*) American Pr.

Problems of Normal & Genetically Abnormal Retinas. Ed. by R. M. Clayton et al. 1983. text 104.00 (*0-12-176180-0*) Acad Pr.

Problems of Pain & Stress: Twenty-Sixth Annual Conference of the Society for Psychosomatic Research. Ed. by Andrew Steptoe. 1984. 96p. pap. 32.00 (*0-08-031301-9*, Pergamon Pr) Elsevier.

Problems of Parents. Benjamin M. Spock. 1979. LC 78-13982. 308p. reprint ed. lib. bdg. 35.00 (*0-313-21000-4*, SPPPA, Greenwood Pr) Greenwood.

Problems of Physiology & Pathology of Digestion & Metabolism. 1964. 756p. text 143.50 (*0-7065-0271-X*) Coronet Bks.

Problems of Psychiatry & Neuropathology 1961. 672p. text 135.00 (*0-7065-0128-4*) Coronet Bks.

Problems of Psychiatry in General Practice: Neurasthenia, Obsessive-Compulsive Disorder, Advances in Treatment of Depression, Teaching & Training of the GP. Ed. by Markus Gastpar & Paul Kielholz. 1993. LC 92-48275. (Illus.). 168p. text 21.00 (*0-88937-084-2*) Hogrefe & Huber Pubs.

Problems of Psychoanalytic Technique. Otto Fenichel. 1969. pap. 16.00 (*0-911194-00-2*) Psych Qtly.

Problems of Psychoanalytic Training, Diagnosis, & the Technique of Therapy. Anna Freud. 1971. LC 67-9514. (Writings of Anna Freud: Vol. 7). 311p. 47.50 (*0-8236-6876-2*) Intl Univs Pr.

Problems of Psychopharmacology. Ed. by L. L. Rokhlin et al. 1964. 336p. text 77.75 (*0-7065-0532-8*) Coronet Bks.

Problems of Radiobiology, Set. 1962. 1170p. text 335.00 (*0-7065-0180-2*) Coronet Bks.

Problems of the Gastrointestinal Tract in Anaesthesia, the Perioperative Period & Intensive Care: International Symposium in Wurzburg, Germany, 1-3 October, 1998. Ed. by M. K. Herbert et al. 1999. LC 99-39685. (Illus.). 416p. 93.00 (*3-540-65901-3*) Spr-Verlag.

Problems of the Innermost Self: A Psychological & Conceptanalytical Study Along with Some Parapsychological Reflections. Svante Bohman. 1988. 114p. (Orig.). pap. 31.50 (*91-22-01270-2*) Coronet Bks.

Problems of the Keimbahn. W. Hilscher. 1983. (Bibliotheca Anatomica Ser.: No. 24). (Illus.). viii, 128p. pap. 85.25 (*3-8055-3614-3*) S Karger.

Problems of Vision: An Inquiry into the Causal Theory of Perception. Gerald Vision. 1997. LC 96-23100. (Illus.). 288p. text 45.00 (*0-19-510498-6*) OUP.

Problems Related to Alcohol Consumption. 1980. (Technical Report Ser.: No. 650). 72p. pap. text 5.00 (*92-4-120650-0*) World Health.

Problems with Patients: Managing Complicated Transactions. Kingsley Norton & Samuel P. Smith. 1994. (Illus.). 192p. (C). text 59.95 (*0-521-43043-7*); pap. text 21.95 (*0-521-43628-1*) Cambridge U Pr.

Problems with Protease Inhibitor Development Plans. David Barr et al. 1995. 21p. (Orig.). (C). pap. text 15.00 (*0-7881-2364-5*) DIANE Pub.

Procedimentos DIU para Programas de Servicos de Planejamento Familiar: Un Manual de Referencia para la Solucion de Problemas. Ed. by Noel McIntosh et al. 2nd ed. Date not set. (POR., Illus.). pap. text 15.00 (*0-929817-37-0*) JHPIEGO.

Procedural Coding Crosswalk, 2000. Medicode, Med-Index Division Staff. 1999. (C). 80.00 (*1-56337-309-2*) Thomson Learn.

Procedural Skills: Instructor's Manual. Wigton. 1996. (Illus.). 148p. (C). (gr. 13). tchr. ed., spiral bd. 22.95 (*0-8151-9278-9*, 25693) Mosby Inc.

Procedure Cards for Clinical Use. Rebecca J. Rayman et al. 3rd ed. 1997. (C). 23.95 (*1-56930-054-2*) Delmar.

Procedure Checklist to Accompany Caroline Bunker Rosdahl's Textbook of Basic Nursing, 7th Ed. Vicki V. Earnest & Caroline B. Rosdahl. 1999. LC 98-32440. (*0-7817-1856-2*, Lippnctt) Lppncott W & W.

Procedure Coding for Cardiologists: The American College of Cardiology Guide to CPT-4. American College of Cardiology Staff. 1992. 100p. pap. text 55.00 (*1-882764-00-5*) Am Coll Cardiology.

Procedure Documentation for Advanced Imaging: Mammography & Quality Management. Erica Williams. 1999. LC 00-267123. (Illus.). 168p. text 34.95 (*0-07-135398-4*) McGraw-Hill Prof.

Procedure for Determining Packed Cell Volume by the Microhematocrit Method. 2nd ed. 1993. (Approved Standard Ser.: Vol. 5). 75.00 (*1-56238-038-9*, H7-A2) NCCLS.

Procedure for the Determination of Fibrinogen in Plasma: Approved Guidelines (1994) Contrib. by H. James Day. 1994. 75.00 (*1-56238 221-7*, H30-A) NCCLS.

Procedure Manual for the Diagnosis of Intestinal Parasites. Donald L. Price. 1994. LC 93-7450. 288p. 78.95 (*0-8493-8654-3*, RC862) CRC Pr.

Procedures, Vol. 3. 1996. (*1-57372-026-7*); 1995. (*1-880678-89-6*) Solucient.

Procedures & Guidelines for Disaster Preparedness Planning. W. Nick Carter. 1985. viii, 195p. pap. 12.25 (*0-86638-063-9*) EW Ctr HI.

Procedures & Techniques in Intensive Care Medicine. Richard S. Irwin et al. 2nd ed. 1999. LC 99-20295. 336p. pap. text 59.95 (*0-7817-2047-8*) Lppncott W & W.

Procedures for Investigating Intentional & Unintentional Food Additives: Report of a WHO Scientific Group, 1967. 1967. (Technical Report Ser.: No. 348). 25p. pap. text 3.00 (*92-4-120348-X*, 1100348) World Health.

Procedures for Primary Care Physicians. John L. Pfenninger. 2nd ed. 2000. (Illus.). 1204p. 79.95 (*0-323-00506-3*) Mosby Inc.

Procedures for the Collection of Diagnostic Blood Specimens by Skin Puncture. 3rd ed. 1991. (Approved Standard Ser.: Vol. 6). 95.00 (*1-56238-111-3*, H4-A3) NCCLS.

Procedures for the Collection of Diagnostic Blood Specimens by Venipuncture: Approved Standard. 3rd ed. 1991. (Approved Standard Ser.: Vol. 6). 95.00 (*1-56238-108-3*, H3-A3) NCCLS.

Procedures for the Handling & Transport of Diagnostic Specimens & Etiologic Agents: Approved Standard (1994) Contrib. by Joan D. Wiseman. 3rd ed. 1994. 75.00 (*1-56238-232-2*, H5-A3) NCCLS.

Procedures for the Primary Care Practitioner. Ed. by Marilyn W. Edmunds & Maren S. Mayhew. 1996. LC 95-40072. (Illus.). 320p. (C). (gr. 13). spiral bd. 38.95 (*0-8151-3034-1*, 27060) Mosby Inc.

Procedures for the Recovery & Identification of Parasites from the Intestinal Tract: Approved Guideline (1997) 1997. 85.00 (*1-56238-342-6*, M28-A) NCCLS.

Procedures for the Recovery & Identification of Parasites from the Intestinal Tract: Proposed Guideline (1993) Contrib. by Lynne S. Garcia. 1993. 85.00 (*1-56238-212-8*, M28-P) NCCLS.

Procedures in Diagnostic Radiology. Terence Doyle et al. 1989. (Illus.). 248p. pap. text (*0-443-02982-2*) Church.

Procedures in Hepatogastroenterology. G. N. Tytgat & C. J. Mulder. 2nd ed. 1997. LC 97-2359. (Developments in Gastroenterology Ser.). text 257.50 (*0-7923-4352-2*) Kluwer Academic.

Procedures in Infants & Children. Michele Walsh-Sukys & Steven E. Krug. Ed. by Lisette Bralow. 1997. LC 96-48725. 384p. text 69.00 (*0-7216-3789-2*) Saunders.

Procedures in Marriage & Family Therapy. Gregory W. Brock & Charles P. Barnard. 3rd ed. 1998. LC 98-13583. 228p. pap. text 60.00 (*0-205-28782-4*) Allyn.

Procedures in Phlebotomy. Ed. by John C. Flynn, Jr. 1993. (Illus.). 256p. pap. text 25.00 (*0-7216-4685-9*) Saunders.

P
Q
R

Procedures in Phlebotomy. John C. Flynn, Jr. Ed. by Adrianne Williams. 2nd ed. 1998. LC 98-43926. 255p. pap. text 23.00 (*0-7216-7583-2*) Saunders.

Procedures in Plastic & Reconconstructive Surgery: How They Do It. Vistnes. 1991. 325.00 (*0-316-90437-6*, Little Brwn Med Div) Lppncott W & W.

Procedures in Practice. Ed. by Nigel A. Scott. 3rd ed. 1994. (Illus.). 296p. pap. text (*0-7279-0823-5*) BMJ Pub GBR. *Dist:* AIDC.

Procedures in Vascular Surgery. Chilton Crane & Richard Warren. 2nd ed. 1976. LC 75-22597. 47.00 (*0-316-16014-8*, Little Brwn Med Div) Lppncott W & W.

Procedures Manual to Accompany Fundamentals of Nursing, Fifth edition. Barbara Kozier et al. 5th ed. 1995. LC 94-33383. (C). pap. text 27.19 (*0-8053-3503-X*) Benjamin-Cummings.

Procedures Resource Book. Center for Healthcare Industry Performance Studies. 1995. 235p. pap. 295.00 (*1-882733-03-7*) Ctr Hlthcare IPS.

Procedures Update. Ed. by Patricia Schull. 1996. LC 96-31994. (Illus.). 768p. (Orig.). 100.00 (*0-87434-869-2*) Springhouse Corp.

Proceed with Care: Final Report of the Royal Commission on New Reproductive Technologies. Royal Commission on New Reproductive Technologies. 1993. (Orig.). 26p. pap. (*0-660-58996-6*); (Illus.). 1275p. pap. (*0-660-15359-9*) Can7 Govern Pub CAN. *Dist:* Intl Spec Bk.

Proceedings of the 18th Annual International Conference of the IEEE Engineering in Medicine & Biology Society. IEEE, Engineering in Medicine and Biology Staff. Ed. by Institute of Electrical and Electronics Engineers, Inc. Staff. 1997. 2435p. lib. bdg. (*0-7803-3812-X*, 96CH36036) Inst Electrical.

Proceeding Without Anecdotal Details of Imagery. Pat Merchant. 1992. (Orig.). pap. 16.00 (*0-913412-62-7*) Brandon Hse.

Proceedings. Ambulatory ECG Monitoring, First National Conferen. Ed. by Nancy K. Jacobsen & Stephen R. Yarnall. 1976. (Illus.). 150p. 16.50 (*0-917054-08-3*) Med Communications.

Proceedings. Conference on Information Processing of Medical Re. Ed. by J. Anderson & J. M. Forsythe. LC 76-126497. text (*0-7204-2042-3*) Brill Academic Pubs.

Proceedings. Workshop on Advances in Experimental Pharmacology Staff. Ed. by W. Meier-Ruge. 1977. (Gerontology Ser.: Vol. 24, Suppl. 1). (Illus.). 42.75 (*3-8055-2687-3*) S Karger.

Proceedings: FEBS Meeting, 11th, Set. Ed. by Per Schambye. 1978. (Illus.). (*0-08-021527-0*) Pergamon Repr GBR. *Dist:* Franklin.

Proceedings: International Symposium on Bifonazole, Kopenhagen, June 1984. Ed. by Hamburg Rieth. 1985. (Journal: Vol. 169, Suppl. 1). iv, 148p. pap. 40.00 (*3-8055-4021-3*) S Karger.

Proceedings - First International Symposium on the Artificial Insemination of Poultry. M. R. Bakst & G. J. Wishart. 1995. (Illus.). 300p. (Orig.). (C). pap. text 35.00 (*0-9649811-0-6*) Poultry Sci.

Proceedings - KSO XIVth International Symposium on Medicinal Chem: Maastricht, 8-12 September 1996. Frans M. Awouters. 1997. LC 97-22116. (Pharmacochemistry Library). 576p. 170.00 (*0-444-82798-6*) Elsevier.

Proceedings - XVII International Congress of Allergology & Clinical Immunology: Sidney, October 15-20, 2000. Ed. by C. Katelaris & Janet Rimmer. 2000. (Illus.). viii, 139p. 49.00 (*0-88937-230-6*) Hogrefe & Huber Pubs.

Proceedings A Symposium of the Bell Museum, Univ. of Minn. Med. School see Death & Attitudes Towards Death

Proceedings Eighteenth European Conference Microcirculation, ESM, Rome, September 1994 No. 14, Supplement 1, No. 14. Ed. by C. Allegra & A. Carlizza. 1994. (International Journal of Microcirculation Ser.). (Illus.). iv, 262p. pap. 77.50 (*3-8055-6035-4*) S Karger.

Proceedings from the Annual Meeting of the Association for Equine Sports Medicine, 10th. 1992. LC 92-60324. (Illus.). 48p. (Orig.). (C). pap. text 10.00 (*0-9603534-1-0*) Vet Practice.

Proceedings from the Eleventh Annual Meeting of the Association for Equine Sports Medicine. 1993. LC 93-60278. (Illus.). 96p. (Orig.). pap. text 25.00 (*0-9603534-4-5*) Vet Practice.

Proceedings from the Scientific Conference on Omega-3 Fatty Acids in Nutrition, Vascular Biology, & Medicine. Ed. by Henry J. Pownall & Arthur A. Spector. (Illus.). 275p. pap. text (*0-87493-007-3*) Am Heart.

Proceedings from the Twelfth Meeting of the Association for Equine Sports Medicine. Ed. by Jonathan Foreman. 1994. (Illus.). 94p. (Orig.). pap. 25.00 (*0-9603534-5-3*) Vet Practice.

Proceedings High Plains Disease Symposium. Charles M. Rush & Gerald J. Michels, Jr. 1995. (Illus.). 77p. (Orig.). pap. text 10.00 (*0-926195-01-8*, AREC 96-19) TX AES.

Proceedings in Gastrointestinal Radiology. J. Dobranowski et al. 1990. (Illus.). 231p. 110.00 (*0-387-97113-0*) Spr-Verlag.

Proceedings of a Symposium on Quality Assurance of Radiotherapy Equipment: Held at the University of Kansas, Kansas City, Missouri, June 4-5, 1982. Ed. by George Starkschall. 1983. (American Association of Physicists in Medicine Symposium Ser.: No. 3). 240p. 45.00 (*0-88318-422-2*) Am Inst Physics.

Proceedings of an Institute on the Roles of Psychology & Psychologists in Rehabilitation Held at Princeton, New Jersey, February 3-7, 1958. Beatrice A. Wright. Ed. by Janet Rosenberg. 1980. LC 79-6929. (Physically Handicapped in Society Ser.). reprint ed. lib. bdg. 19.95 (*0-405-13136-4*) Ayer.

Proceedings of an International Symposium Jointly Organized by IAEA & WHO, Parts 27-31 October 1980. International Atomic Energy Agency Staff. 1981. (Proceedings Ser.). (Illus.). 596p. pap. (*92-0-010281-6*, ISP567, IAEA) IAEA AUT. *Dist:* Bernan Associates.

Proceedings of European Dialysis & Transplant. Date not set. Vol. 17. 39.95 (*0-8464-4465-8*); Vol. 18. 39.95 (*0-8464-4466-6*); Vol. 19. 39.95 (*0-8464-4467-4*) Beekman Pubs.

Proceedings of G. I. N. I.'s Third International Polio & Independent Living Conference, May 10-12, 1985, St. Louis, Missouri. Ed. by G. Laurie & J. Raymond. 1986. 68p. (Orig.). pap. 4.00 (*0-931301-02-5*) Gazette Intl.

Proceedings of International Symposium on the Chemical Mediators on Skin Inflammation, Sendai, August 1988. Ed. by H. Tagami & Tosio Kato. 1989. (Journal: Vol. 179, Suppl. 1, 1989). (Illus.). vi, 146p. pap. 66.25 (*3-8055-5065-0*) S Karger.

Proceedings of Rehabilitation Gazette's Second International Post-Polio Conference & Symposium on Living Independently with Severe Disability. Ed. by G. Laurie & J. Raymond. 1984. 74p. (Orig.). pap. 4.00 (*0-931301-01-7*) Gazette Intl.

Proceedings of 2nd European Workshop on Periodontology: Chemicals in Periodontics. Ed. by Niklaus P. Lang et al. 1997. (Illus.). 428p. pap. 68.00 (*3-87652-423-7*) Quint Pub Co.

Proceedings of the 11th Meeting of the World Society for Stereotactic & Functional Neurosurgery, Ixtapa, Mexico, October 1993, Pt. I. Ed. by Philip L. Gildenberg et al. 1995. (Journal: Vol. 62, No. 1-4, 1994). (Illus.). viii, 320p. pap. 201.75 (*3-8055-6159-8*) S Karger.

Proceedings of the Advanced Medicine Symposia, 10th, 1974. Advanced Medicine Symposia Staff & Royal College of Physicians Staff. Ed. by J. G. Ledingham. 1974. (Illus.). pap. text 50.00 (*0-7855-7130-2*) St Mut.

Proceedings of the Advanced Medicine Symposia, 11th, 1975. Advanced Medicine Symposia Staff & Royal College of Physicians Staff. Ed. by A. F. Lant. 1975. (Illus.). pap. text 40.00 (*0-7855-7131-0*) St Mut.

Proceedings of the Advanced Medicine Symposia, 7th, 1971. Advanced Medicine Symposia Staff. Ed. by I. A. Boucher. 1971. pap. text 30.00 (*0-7855-7129-9*) St Mut.

Proceedings of the American Association for the Study & Cure of Inebriates: 1870 to 1875. American Association for the Study and Cure of Inebr. Ed. by Gerald N. Grob. 1981. LC 80-1271. (Addiction in America Ser.). lib. bdg. 49.95 (*0-405-13565-3*) Ayer.

Proceedings of the Annual Meeting of the International Continence Society, 6th, Antwerp, Sept. 1976. Annual Meeting of the International Continence Society. Ed. by B. Coolsaet. 1978. (Urologia Internationalis Ser.: Vol. 33, No. 1-3). pap. 64.50 (*3-8055-2898-1*) S Karger.

Proceedings of the Arthur Purdy Stout Society Symposium, "Current Problems in the Surgical Pathology of Infectious Disease" & the Gastrointestinal Pathology Society Symposium, "Gastrointestinal Endocrine Pathology" Ed. by Stephen S. Sternberg. 1987. (American Journal of Surgical Pathology Ser.: Vol. 11, Supplement 1). (Illus.). 104p. pap. 37.00 (*0-88167-503-2*) Lppncott W & W.

Proceedings of the Arthur Purdy Stout Society Symposium on Neoplasia. Ed. by Stephen S. Sternberg. 1986. (American Journal of Surgical Pathology Ser.: Vol. 10, Supplement 1). (Illus.). 116p. pap. 33.50 (*0-88167-658-6*) Lppncott W & W.

Proceedings of the Asthma & Chronic Bronchitis in Children & Their Prognosis into Adult Life Symposium, 3rd, Davos, 1969. Asthma and Chronic Bronchitis in Children and Their Prognosis into Adult Life Symposium. Ed. by F. Suter & R. E. Altounyan. 1970. pap. 73.25 (*3-8055-0754-2*) S Karger.

Proceedings of the Bioflow Small Diameter Graft Symposium. Ed. & Illus. by Silent Partners, Inc. Staff. 1989. 98p. (Orig.). pap. (*1-878353-09-8*) Silent Partners.

Proceedings of the Carpentier-Edwards Pericardial Prostheses Mini-Symposium. Ed. & Illus. by Silent Partners, Inc. Staff. 1994. 142p. pap. (*1-878353-30-6*) Silent Partners.

Proceedings of the Conference on Measuring Chaos in the Human Brain, April 3-5, 1991, at the Supercomputer Computations Research Institute, Florida State University, Tallahassee, FL. Ed. by D. W. Duke et al. 1991. LC 92-23707. 250p. (C). text 89.00 (*981-02-0701-8*) World Scientific Pub.

Proceedings of the Conference on Simulation in Health Care & Social Services. Anderson. 1992. 120p. pap. 48.00 (*1-56555-010-2*, MC92-4) Soc Computer Sim.

Proceedings of the Conference on the Capabilities & Needs of Disabled Persons in the ESCWA Region. 1990. 535p. 60.00 (*92-1-128119-9*, 90.II.L.9) UN.

Proceedings of the Conference on Training Clinician Child Psychologists. Ed. by June M. Tuma. 1989. 175p. pap. 29.95 (*0-8058-0591-5*) L Erlbaum Assocs.

Proceedings of the Eleventh International Conference on the Study of Shamanism & Alternate Modes of Healing, Held at the Santa Sabina Center, San Rafael, California, September 3-5, 1994. Ed. by Ruth-Inge Heinze. 1995. LC 95-43549. (Illus.). vi, 352p. (C). pap. 21.75 (*0-945875-12-6*) Independent Scholars Asia Inc.

Proceedings of the Eleventh International Congress on Hyperbaric Medicine. Ed. by Wen-Ren Li & Frederick S. Cramer. 1995. LC 95-77069. (Illus.). 306p. 49.50 (*0-941332-44-6*, B0787) Best Pub Co.

Proceedings of the European Workshop on Mechanical Plaque Control. Ed. by Niklaus P. Lang et al. 2000. 314p. pap. (*3-87652-428-8*) Quintessenz Verlags DEU. *Dist:* Quint Pub Co.

Proceedings of the FAO-WHO Expert Committee on Nutrition, 8th. FAO-WHO Joint Committee Expert Committee on Nutrit. 1971. (Technical Reports: No. 477). 80p. pap. text 5.00 (*92-4-120477-X*, 1100477) World Health.

Proceedings of the FAO-WHO Joint Expert Committee on Brucellosis, 4th, Geneva, 1963. FAO-WHO Joint Expert Committee on Brucellosis. 1964. (Technical Reports: No. 289). 65p. pap. text 5.00 (*92-4-120289-0*, 1100289) World Health.

Proceedings of the FAO-WHO Joint Expert Committee on Brucellosis, 5th, Geneva, 1970. FAO-WHO Joint Expert Committee on Brucellosis. 1971. (Technical Reports: No. 464). 76p. pap. text 5.00 (*92-4-120464-8*, 1100464) World Health.

Proceedings of the 15th International Pig Veterinary Society Congress, Set. Ed. by S. T. Done et al. 1999. pap. incl. cd-rom (*1-897676-84-0*) Nottingham Univ Pr GBR. *Dist:* St Mut.

Proceedings of the Fifth Annual Cardiac Residents' Program on Cardiovascular Surgery. Ed. & Illus. by Silent Partners, Inc. Staff. 1989. 92p. (Orig.). pap. (*1-878353-08-X*) Silent Partners.

Proceedings of the Fifth International Colloquium on Paratuberculosis, September 29-October 4, 1996: A Meeting of the International Association for Paratuberculosis, Madison, Wisconsin, U. S. A. Ed. by Michael T. Collins & Elizabeth J. B. Manning. 1997. LC 97-25264. pap. (*0-9633043-3-X*) Intl Assn Paratuber.

Proceedings of the Fifth International Conference on the Study of Shamanism & Alternate Modes of Healing, 1988, Santa Sabina Center, San Rafael, California, September 3-5, 1988. Ed. by Ruth-Inge Heinze. 1989. LC 89-2092. (Illus.). 432p. (C). pap. 21.75 (*0-945875-02-9*) Independent Scholars Asia Inc.

Proceedings of the First International Clinical Symposium on the CarboMedics Prosthetic Heart Valve. Ed. & Illus. by Silent Partners, Inc. Staff. 1989. 105p. (Orig.). pap. (*1-878353-11-X*) Silent Partners.

Proceedings of the First International Congress on Cataract Surgery, Florence, 1978. International Congress on Cataract Surgery Staff. Ed. by J. Francois et al. 1979. (Documenta Ophthalmologica Proceedings Ser.: No. 21). (Illus.). text 366.50 (*90-6193-162-2*) Kluwer Academic.

Proceedings of the First National Scientific Meeting of the Royal College of Obstetricians & Gynaecologists, Singapore, 20-23 September 1990. Ed. by F. H. Tsakok et al. 1992. LC 92-18105. 275p. (C). text 81.00 (*981-02-0794-8*) World Scientific Pub.

Proceedings of the 1st Seattle Symposium in Biostatistics, Vol. 123. D. Mposium Lin & Thomas R. Fleming. 1997. LC 97-13962. (Lecture Notes in Statistics). 309p. pap. 39.95 (*0-387-94992-5*) Spr-Verlag.

Proceedings of the 14th Symposium: or Neuroadiologicum: London, June, 17-23, 1990. Ed. by George Du Boulay et al. 1991. (Illus.). 680p. 278.00 (*0-387-53726-0*) Spr-Verlag.

Proceedings of the Fourth International Conference on Coccidioidomycosis. Ed. by Einstein & Catanzaro. 1985. LC 85-60255. 532p. 40.00 (*0-9614520-0-5*) NFID.

Proceedings of the Fourth International Conference on Myopia, Sponsored by the Myopia International Research Foundation, Inc. March 14, 15 & 16, 1990, Singapore. Ed. by Joel Weintraub. 1990. (Illus.). 438p. pap. (*1-879037-00-9*) Myopia Internatl Res Fndtn.

Proceedings of the Fourth International Conference on the Study of Shamanism & Alternate Modes of Healing, 1987, Santa Sabina Center, San Rafael, California, September 5-7, 1987. Ed. by Ruth-Inge Heinze. 1988. (Illus.). 258p. (C). pap. 21.75 (*0-945875-01-0*) Independent Scholars Asia Inc.

Proceedings of the Fourth Meeting of the World Federation for Ultrasound in Medicine & Biology. Ed. by Australian Society of Ultrasound in Medicine Staff. 1986. 500p. pap. 155.00 (*0-08-032792-3*) Elsevier.

Proceedings of the Heartworm Symposium, '89. Ed. by Gilbert Otto. 1990. text 43.00 (*0-940275-01-5*) Am Heartworm Soc.

Proceedings of the Heartworm Symposium '92. Ed. by Mark D. Soll. 1993. (Illus.). 341p. (*1-878353-29-2*) Silent Partners.

Proceedings of the International Conference on Environmental Epidemiology & Exposure Analysis: I, Health Hazards from Toxic Pollutants & Biological Monitoring; II, Ethics & Law in Environmental Epidemiology. Ed. by Michael D. Lebowitz. 1993. (Journal of Exposure Analysis & Environmental Epidemiology Ser.: Vol. 1, No. 1). (Illus.). pap. text 60.00 (*0-911131-71-X*) Specialist Journals.

Proceedings of the International Conference on Spinal Manipulation, 1992. Intro. by Deborah L. Callahan. 1992. (Annual ICSM Proceedings Ser.). (Illus.). 210p. pap. 35.00 (*0-9631715-1-8*) Fnd Chiro Educ Res.

Proceedings of the International Conference on the Individual & the Community in the Research, Development: And Use of Biologicals. 1977. (Bulletin Supplement Ser.: No. 55). 177p. pap. text 18.00 (*92-4-068552-9*) World Health.

Proceedings of the International Congress on Pharmacognosy & Phytochemistry, Munich, 1970. International Congress on Pharmacognosy and Phytoche. Ed. by H. Wagner & L. Hoerhammer. 1971. LC 79-149122. (Illus.). 386p. 68.95 (*0-387-05316-6*) Spr-Verlag.

Proceedings of the Meeting of the American Society for Stereotactic & Functional Neurosurgery, Pittsburgh, PA, June 1991, Pt. 1: Journal: Stereotactic & Functional Neurosurgery, Vol. 58, Nos. 1-4, 1992. Ed. by L. D. Lunsford et al. 1992. (Illus.). vi, 214p. pap. 188.00 (*3-8055-5684-5*) S Karger.

Proceedings of the Meeting of the American Society for Stereotactic & Functional Neurosurgery, Pittsburgh, PA, June 1991, Pt. 2: Journal: Stereotactic & Functional Neurosurgery, Vol. 59, Nos. 1-4, 1992. Ed. by L. D. Lunsford et al. 1992. (Illus.). vi, 210p. pap. 188.00 (*3-8055-5688-8*) S Karger.

Proceedings of the Meeting of the Leksell Gamma Knife Society, Buenos Aires, March 1992: Journal: Stereotactic & Functional Neurosurgery, Vol. 61, Suppl. 1, 1993. Ed. by J. C. Ganz et al. 1993. (Illus.). iv, 188p. pap. 59.25 (*3-8055-5945-3*) S Karger.

Proceedings of the Michigan Morphometrics Workshop. Ed. by Fred L. Bookstein. 1990. (Special Publications: No. 2). viii, 380p. (C). pap. text 17.50 (*0-9628499-0-1*) U MI Mus Zool.

Proceedings of the Myopia International Conference, 3rd, Copenhagen, 1980. Myopia International Conference Staff. Ed. by H. C. Fledelius et al. 1981. (Documenta Ophthalmologica Proceedings Ser.: No. 28). 266p. text 191.50 (*90-6193-725-6*) Kluwer Academic.

Proceedings of the National Heart, Lung & Blood Institute Symposium on Rapid Identification & Treatment of Acute Myocardial Infarction: Issues & Answers. Ed. by Judith H. LaRosa et al. 1996. (Illus.). 157p. (Orig.). pap. text 25.00 (*0-7881-2825-6*) DIANE Pub.

Proceedings of the National Quarantine & Sanitary Convention, 1st-4th: Original Anthology. National Quarantine and Sanitary Convention Staff. Ed. by Barbara G. Rosenkrantz. 1977. LC 76-40668. (Public Health in America Ser.). reprint ed. lib. bdg. 89.95 (*0-405-09877-4*) Ayer.

Proceedings of the 1995 21st Annual Northeast Bioengineering Conference. IEEE, Engineering in Medicine and Biology Staff. Ed. by IEEE, Institute of Electrical and Electronics Engineers, Inc. Staff. 1995. LC 88-646567. 150p. pap. text (*0-7803-2692-X*, 95CH35807); 150p. lib. bdg. (*0-7803-2693-8*, 95CH35807); mic. film (*0-7803-2694-6*, 95CH35807) Inst Electrical.

Proceedings of the 1993 Connectionist Models Summer School. Ed. by David S. Touretzky et al. 1994. 424p. text 89.95 (*0-8058-1590-2*) L Erlbaum Assocs.

Proceedings of the Ninth International Conference on the Study of Shamanism & Alternate Modes of Healing: Held at the St. Sabina Center, San Rafael, California, September 5-7, 1992. Ed. by Ruth-Inge Heinze. 1993. LC 92-47429. (Illus.). 340p. (C). pap. 21.75 (*0-945875-09-6*) Independent Scholars Asia Inc.

Proceedings of the Ninth International Congress on Hyperbaric Medicine. Ed. by Ian P. Unsworth & Frederick S. Cramer. 1998. LC 93-70913. (Illus.). 228p. 38.00 (*0-941332-34-9*, B0485) Best Pub Co.

Proceedings of the Ninth International Symposium Trace Elements in Man & Animals (Tema-9) Ed. by P. W. Fischer et al. 1997. 677p. (*0-660-16404-3*) NRC Pr.

Proceedings of the 9th RID National Convention, 1985: Interpreting: The Art of Cross-Cultural Mediation. Ed. by Marina L. McIntire. 1990. 192p. (C). reprint ed. pap. 10.95 (*0-916883-05-1*) RID Pubns.

Proceedings of the Ninth World Congress on Pain. Ed. by Marshall Devor et al. 2000. (Progress in Pain Research & Management Ser.: No. 16). (Illus.). xxiv, 1154p. 80.00 (*0-931092-31-0*) Intl Assn Study Pain.

Proceedings of the Protein-Ligand Interactions Symposium, University of Konstanz, Germany, Sept. 1974. Protein-Ligand Interactions Symposium Staff. Ed. by Gideon Blauer & Horst Sund. 1975. (C). 188.50 (*3-11-004881-7*) De Gruyter.

Proceedings of the Regional Workshop on Environmental Health Management in Refugee Areas. 1994. (WHO/EMRO Technical Publication Ser.: No. 19). pap. text 18.00 (*92-9021-185-7*) World Health.

Proceedings of the RPA, NIDDK Meeting 1994 Joint Annual Meeting in Conjunction with Renal Physicians, Association Annual Membership Meeting. Ed. by M. J. Scherbenske et al. 1994. (Journal: Vol. 12 No. 1, 1994). (Illus.). 84p. pap. 47.00 (*3-8055-6029-X*) S Karger.

Proceedings of the Scandinavian Clinical Symposium on the CarboMedics Prosthetic Heart Valve. Ed. & Illus. by Silent Partners, Inc. Staff. 1991. 147p. (Orig.). pap. (*1-878353-20-9*) Silent Partners.

Proceedings of the Second International Clinical Symposium (CarboMedics) Ed. & Illus. by Silent Partners, Inc. Staff. 1990. 145p. (Orig.). pap. (*1-878353-12-8*) Silent Partners.

Proceedings of the Second International Scientific Meeting Microwaves in Medicine 1993. IEEE, Italy Section Staff. Ed. by Institute of Electrical and Electronics Engineers, Inc. Staff. 1993. LC 93-61233. 320p. pap. (*0-7803-1468-9*, 93TH0591-8); fiche (*0-7803-1469-7*) Inst Electrical.

Proceedings of the Second National Conference on Citizens with Mental Retardation & the Law. 1987. 52p. (*1-55672-050-5*) US HHS.

Proceedings of the Seventeenth Annual Conference of the Cognitive Science Society. Cognitive Science Society Staff. Ed. by Jill F. Lehman & Johanna D. Moore. 1995. 824p. pap. 150.00 (*0-8058-2159-7*) L Erlbaum Assocs.

Proceedings of the Seventh International Conference of Racing Analysts & Veterinarians. Ed. by Thomas Tobin et al. 1990. 95.00 (*0-9626367-0-3*) Univ KY Vet Sci.

Proceedings of the Seventh Scientific Meeting of the Inter-American Society. Ed. by Edgar Haber. 1988. LC 73-2001. (Hypertension Ser.: No. 4). 235p. 16.80 (*0-87493-653-5*) Am Heart.

Proceedings of the Sixth Complement Genetics Workshop & Conference, Mainz, July 1989. Ed. by C. Rittner et al. 1990. (Illus.). vi, 142p. reprint ed. 113.25 (*3-8055-5342-0*) S Karger.

Proceedings of the 6th European Society of Contraception. Ed. by E. Aubeny & H. Meden-Vrtovec. 2001. LC 2001-36287. (International Congress, Symposium, & Seminar Ser.: Vol. 16). (Illus.). 120p. lib. bdg. 84.95 (*1-84214-021-3*, Parthenon Pbng) CRC Pr.

Proceedings of the Sixth International Conference on the Study of Shamanism & Alternate Modes of Healing, 1989, Santa Sabina Center, San Rafel, California, September 2-4, 1989. Ed. by Ruth-Inge Heinze. 1990. LC 90-4220. (Illus.). 402p. (C). pap. 21.75 (*0-945875-04-5*) Independent Scholars Asia Inc.

Proceedings of the 6th International Symposium on Artificial Heart & Assist Devices, July 30-31, 1996 Tokyo, Japan No. 6. Contrib. by E. Asan. 1998. LC 97-41992. (Illus.). 400p. 260.00 (*4-431-70209-1*) Spr-Verlag.

Proceedings of the Symposium of the International Society for Corneal Research. Ed. by J. Francois et al. 1979. (Documenta Ophthalmologica Proceedings Ser.: No. 20). text 141.50 (*90-6193-157-6*) Kluwer Academic.

Proceedings of the Symposium on Compatability of Biomedical Implants. Ed. by P. K. Kovacs & N. S. Istephanous. 1994. LC 94-70847. (Proceedings Ser.: Vol. 94-15). 390p. 50.00 (*1-56677-047-5*) Electrochem Soc.

Proceedings of the 10th International Conference on Mechanics in Medicine & Biology, Honolulu, Hawaii, March 2-5, 1998. Ed. by J. A. Ashton-Miller. 1998. (*0-9652469-5-7*) Pac Ctr Thermal.

Proceedings of the Tenth International Conference on the Study of Shamanism & Alternate Modes of Healing, 1993, Santa Sabina Center, San Rafael, California, September 4-6, 1998. Ed. by Ruth-Inge Heinze. 1994. LC 94-2722. (Illus.). 381p. (C). pap. 21.75 (*0-945875-10-X*) Independent Scholars Asia Inc.

Proceedings of the 3rd International Congress on Neo-Adjuvant Chemotherapy. Ed. by P. Banzet et al. 1992. (Illus.). 477p. 174.00 (*0-387-55039-9*) Spr-Verlag.

Proceedings of the Third International Clinical Symposium (CarboMedics) Ed. & Illus. by Silent Partners, Inc. Staff. 1992. 156p. (Orig.). pap. (*1-878353-24-1*) Silent Partners.

Proceedings of the Third International Colloquium on Paratuberculosis. Rodrick J. Chiodini & J. Kreeger. 1992. (C). pap. text 145.00 (*0-9633043-0-5*) Intl Assn Paratuber.

Proceedings of the Third International Conference on the Study of Shamanism & Alternate Modes of Healing, 1986, Santa Sabina Center, San Rafael, California, August 30-September 1, 1986. Ed. by Ruth-Inge Heinze. 1987. (Illus.). 349p. (C). pap. 21.75 (*0-945875-00-2*) Independent Scholars Asia Inc.

Proceedings of the Third International Symposium on the Edwards Duromedics Bileaflet Valve. Ed. & Illus. by Silent Partners, Inc. Staff. 1987. 123p. (Orig.). pap. (*1-878353-05-5*) Silent Partners.

Proceedings of the Transgenic Animal Research Workshop. Ed. by Joan Hopper et al. 1989. (Studies in Technology & Social Change: No. 10). 167p. (Orig.). (C). pap. 15.00 (*0-945271-14-X*) ISU-CIKARD.

Proceedings of the 12th International Congress on Hyperbaric Medicine. Ed. by G. Oriani & F. Wattel. 1998. LC 97-73095. (Illus.). 320p. 64.00 (*0-941332-63-2*, D938) Best Pub Co.

Proceedings of the Twelfth International Conference on the Study of Shamanism & Alternate Modes of Healing 1995, Santa Sabina Center, San Rafael, California, September 2-4, 1990, Vol. XII. Ed. by Ruth-Inge Heinze. 1995. LC 95-50127. (Illus.). 327p. (C). pap. 21.75 (*0-945875-15-0*) Independent Scholars Asia Inc.

Proceedings of the 25th Annual International Congress on Veterinary Acupuncture. Gary Allen et al. 1999. (Illus.). 240p. spiral bd. 30.00 (*0-9616627-0-0*) Intl Vet Acup.

***Proceedings of the 27th Annual International Congress on Veterinary Acupuncture.** Elaine Cebuliak et al. 2001. (Illus.). 240p. spiral bd. 30.00 (*0-9616627-1-9*) Intl Vet Acup.

Proceedings of the Workshop on Advances in Experimental Pharmacology of Hydergine Basel, December 1976. Workshop on Advances in Experimental Pharmacology Staff. 1977. LC 71-114908. (Select Bibliographies Reprint Ser.). 33.95 (*0-8369-5313-4*) Ayer.

Proceedings of the Workshop on General Population Exposure to Gasoline: (Gasoline Assessment of Human Exposure) Ed. by Edo Pellizari. 1992. (Journal of Exposure Analysis & Environmental Epidemiology Ser.: Vol. 2, No. 1). (Illus.). pap. text 65.00 (*0-911131-28-0*) Specialist Journals.

Proceedings of the XV Symposium Neuroradiologicum. M. Takahashi & Y. Korogi. 1995. (Illus.). 624p. suppl. ed. 310.00 (*3-540-58755-1*) Spr-Verlag.

Proceedings of XI European Congress of Perinatal Medicine. Ed. by Ermelando V. Cosmi & G. C. Di Renzo. 1989. xvi, 874p. pap. text 249.00 (*3-7186-4919-5*) Gordon & Breach.

Proceedings Sixth International Congress of Pharmacology, Helsinki 1975, Set. J. Tuomisto & M. Paasonen. 1976. (*0-08-020458-9*) Pergamon Repr GBR. *Dist:* Franklin.

Proceedings-Workshop on Needle Exchange & Bleach Distribution Programs. National Research Council Staff et al. 1994. LC 94-67632. 320p. (Orig.). (C). pap. text 39.00 (*0-309-05084-7*) Natl Acad Pr.

Process-Centered Health Care Organizations. Suzanne P. Smith & Dominick L. Flarey. 1999. LC 99-18270. 400p. 62.00 (*0-8342-1249-8*, 12498) Aspen Pub.

Process in Neurobiology, Vol. 21. Ed. by G. A. Kerkut & J. W. Phillis. 1985. (Illus.). 360p. 150.00 (*0-08-032321-9*, Pergamon Pr) Elsevier.

Process of Change. Peggy Papp. 1983. LC 83-12814. (Guilford Family Therapy Ser.). 248p. 42.00 (*0-89862-052-X*) Guilford Pubns.

Process of Counseling & Therapy. Janet Moursund. 3rd ed. 1992. LC 92-12024. 240p. (C). pap. 36.60 (*0-13-720657-7*) P-H.

Process of Human Development: A Holistic Life-Span Approach. Clara S. Schuster & Shirley S. Ashburn. 3rd ed. 1992. (Illus.). 992p. text 51.95 (*0-397-54881-8*) Lppncott W & W.

Process of Neurologic Care in Medical Practice. Thomas H. Glick. 1984. LC 83-12899. (Illus.). 373p. 54.50 (*0-674-71080-0*) HUP.

Process of New Drug Discovery & Development. Charles G. Smith. 1992. 160p. 131.95 (*0-8493-4211-2*, RM301) CRC Pr.

Process of Psychotherapy: An Integration of Clinical Experiences & Empirical Research. John R. Thompson. 1987. 424p. (Orig.). 68.00 (*0-8191-6602-2*); 40.00 (*0-8191-6603-0*) U Pr of Amer.

Process of Regeneration: Change. Oletha M. Pinkston. 1991. LC 90-82451. 112p. (Orig.). pap. 9.95 (*0-9627055-0-0*) Pinkston.

Process Skills Development in Ambulatory Family Practice. CSOF Staff. 1999. 246p. ring bd. 47.96 (*0-7872-5591-2*, 41559101) Kendall-Hunt.

Process Theory of Medicine: Problems in Contemporary Philosophy. Ed. by Marcus P. Ford. 1987. LC 87-7865. (Problems in Contemporary Philosophy Ser.: Vol. 5). 240p. lib. bdg. 89.95 (*0-88946-328-X*) E Mellen.

Processes in Cutaneous Epidermal Differentiation. Ed. by I. A. Bernstein. 1987. LC 87-10327. 400p. 110.00 (*0-275-92406-8*, C2406, Praeger Pubs) Greenwood.

Processes in Individual Differences. Colin Cooper & Ved P. Varma. 1997. LC 96-52970. (Illus.). 192p. (C). 75.00 (*0-415-14119-2*) Routledge.

Processes of Cognitive Growth: Infancy. Jerome S. Bruner. 1968. LC 68-27831. (Heinz Werner Lectures: No. 3). 9.00 (*0-8271-6810-1*) Clark U Pr.

Processes of the Cranial Midline: International Symposium Vienna, Austria, May 21-25, 1990. Ed. by Wolfgang T. Koos & B. Richling. 1991. (Acta Neurochirurgica Ser.: Supplement 53). (Illus.). 205p. 168.00 (*0-387-82309-3*) Spr-Verlag.

Processing Medical Documents. Robert P. Poland. 2nd ed. 1998. LC 98-49590. 256p. 38.95 (*0-02-804745-1*) Glencoe.

Processing Medical Documents Using WordPerfect. Robert P. Poland. 1995. LC 94-12977. (*0-02-802536-9*) Glencoe.

Processing of Medical Information in Aging Patients: Cognitive & Human Factors Perspectives. Ed. by Denise C. Park et al. 1999. LC 98-30256. 344p. 69.95 (*0-8058-2889-3*) L Erlbaum Assocs.

Processing of Reusable Surgical Textiles for Use in Health Care Facilities: ANSI/AAMI ST65:2000. 2000. (Illus.). pap. 100.00 incl. cd-rom (*1-57020-128-5*) Assn Adv Med Instrn.

Procudural Skills for Internal Medicine, Individual Version. Robert S. Wigton & Thomas G. Tape. 1997. 148p. (C). (*0-8151-9410-2*) Mosby Inc.

Procurement of Human Fetal Tissue. Lili Wong. 1997. (Medical Intelligence Unit Ser.). 200p. (C). 89.95 (*0-412-10871-2*) Chapman & Hall.

Procurement of Pancreatic Islets, Vol. I. Ed. by Robert P. Lanza & William L. Chick. 1994. 130p. 94.00 (*1-57059-133-4*, LN9133) CRC Pr.

Procurement, Preservation & Allocation of Vascularized Organs. Ed. by G. M. Collins et al. 1997. LC 96-38863. 384p. lib. bdg. 275.00 (*0-7923-4299-2*) Kluwer Academic.

Procuring Organs for Transplant: The Debate over Non-Heart-Beating Cadaver Protocols. Ed. by Stuart J. Youngner et al. 1995. LC 94-44011. 270p. 59.00 (*0-8018-5100-9*) Johns Hopkins.

Prodrugs: Topical & Ocular Drug Delivery. Ed. by Kenneth B. Sloan. 1992. (Drugs & the Pharmaceutical Sciences Ser.: Vol. 53). (Illus.). 336p. text 165.00 (*0-8247-8629-7*) Dekker.

Producing a Quality Plan: Pharmaceutical Automation: A Systems-Based Approach. Tony Simmons. Date not set. (Illus.). 49.50 (*1-930114-21-4*) Davis Horwood Intl.

Producing Patient-Centered Health Care: Patient Perspectives about Health & Illness & the Physician/Patient Relationship. James Monroe Smith. 1999. LC 99-12474. (Illus.). 240p. 68.00 (*0-86569-293-9*, Auburn Hse) Greenwood.

Producing Quality Radiographs. Angeline Cullinan. 1987. (Illus.). 289p. text 41.50 (*0-397-50778-X*, Lippnctt); 2nd ed. 1993. 352p. text 52.95 (*0-397-55031-6*) Lppncott W & W.

Product Development Planning for Healthcare Products Regulated by the FDA. Elaine Whitmore. 1997. LC 96-48101. 159p. 35.00 (*0-87389-416-2*, H0957) ASQ Qual Pr.

Product Safety Evaluation. Ed. by Alan M. Goldberg. 1983. (Alternative Methods in Toxicology Ser.: Vol. 1). 376p. text 191.00 (*0-913113-00-X*) M Liebert.

Product Safety Evaluation Handbook. Ed. by Shayne C. Gad. 2nd ed. 1999. LC 99-30388. (Illus.). 712p. text 195.00 (*0-8247-1971-9*) Dekker.

Production & Utilization of Radiation Vaccines Against Helminthic Diseases. 1964. (Technical Reports: No. 30). (Illus.). 84p. pap. (*92-0-115164-0*, IDC30) IAEA AUT. *Dist:* Bernan Associates.

Production Line: Reproduction & Growing Up. Sarah Angliss. 1999. (Human Machine Ser.). (Illus.). 32p. (J). lib. bdg. 16.95 (*1-929298-20-X*) Thameside Pr.

Production of Basic Diagnostic Laboratory Reagents. M. El-Nageh & C. Heuck. 1995. LC 96-168047. (WHO Regional Publications, Eastern Mediterranean Series: No. 11). pap. text 15.00 (*92-9021-189-X*) World Health.

Production of Speech. Ed. by P. F. MacNeilage. 1983. (Illus.). 302p. 107.00 (*0-387-90735-1*) Spr-Verlag.

Production, Pollution, Protection. Ed. by J. S. Weiner et al. 1972. (Wykeham Science Ser.: No. 19). 368p. pap. 18.00 (*0-85109-250-0*) Taylor & Francis.

Productive Living Strategies for People with AIDS. Ed. by Jerry A. Johnson & Michael Pizzi. (Occupational Therapy in Health Care Ser.). 249p. 1994. pap. text 19.95 (*0-918393-83-3*); 1991. 39.95 (*1-56024-024-5*) Haworth Pr.

Productive Thinking. Max Wertheimer. enl. ed. 1996. LC 82-10913. (Phoenix Ser.). 318p. (C). pap. text 11.00 (*0-226-89376-6*) U Ch Pr.

Productivity Management. Ed. by Vana Prewitt. 1991. (ACCRUE Ser.: Level II). 175p. ring bd. 63.00 (*1-879907-01-1*) Am Soc Hlth-Syst.

Productivity Measurement System for Administrators of Social Work Programs in Health Care. Shirley M. Keller et al. 1993. LC 92-48852. 72p. (Orig.). pap. text 37.50 (*0-87258-625-1*, 187151) Am Hospital.

Productivity of Health Care & Pharmaceuticals: An International Comparison. H. E. Frech, III & Richard D. Miller. 1999. LC 98-48714. xi, 97p. pap. 14.95 (*0-8447-7124-4*, AEI Pr) Am Enterprise.

Profession & Practice of Educational Psychology: Future Directions. Ed. by Sheila Wolfendale et al. 1992. 208p. pap. text 31.95 (*0-304-32347-0*) Continuum.

Profession of Conscience: The Making & Meaning of Life-Sciences Liberalism. Robert H. Sprinkle. 1994. LC 94-9662. 272p. 40.00 (*0-691-03365-X*) Princeton U Pr.

Profession of Dietetics. Ester A. Winterfeldt et al. 1998. LC 97-42006. 352p. 59.00 (*0-8342-0888-1*) Aspen Pub.

Profession of Dietetics: A Team Approach. Deborah D. Canter et al. 2nd ed. 1999. LC 99-32799. (Illus.). 192p. pap. text 36.40 (*0-13-646886-1*) P-H.

Profession of Medicine: A Study of the Sociology of Applied Knowledge. Eliot Freidson. 1988. LC 88-1328. 440p. pap. text 16.95 (*0-226-26228-6*) U Ch Pr.

Profession of One's Own: Organized Medicine's Opposition to Chiropractic. Susan L. Smith-Cunnien. 1997. LC 97-38181. 224p. (C). 43.00 (*0-7618-0943-0*) U Pr of Amer.

Professional Accident Investigation: Methods & Techniques. Raymond L. Kuhlman. 1977. LC 77-77275. (Illus.). 262p. ring bd. 75.00 (*0-88061-012-3*) Intl Loss Cntrl.

Professional Aspects of Nurse Anesthesia Practice. American Association of Nurse Anesthetists Educati. Ed. by Scot D. Foster & Lorraine M. Jordan. 1993. LC 93-31370. (Illus.). 412p. (C). 53.00 (*0-8036-0134-4*) Davis Co.

Professional Burnout in Medicine & the Helping Professions. T. Wessells, Jr. et al. 1989. LC 88-28409. (Loss, Grief & Care Ser.: Vol. 3, Nos. 1 & 2). (Illus.). 123p. text 39.95 (*0-86656-785-2*) Haworth Pr.

***Professional Care for the Elderly & Mental.** 1995. pap. (*0-412-58990-7*) Chapman & Hall.

Professional Care for the Elderly Mentally Ill. Ed. by L. Matthew. 1995. 288p. pap. 44.75 (*1-56593-327-3*, 0657) Singular Publishing.

Professional Chaplaincy: What Is Happening to It During Health Care Reform? Larry VandeCreek. 2000. LC 00-39661. xv, 85p. (C). 49.95 (*0-7890-1172-7*); pap. text 22.95 (*0-7890-1173-5*, Haworth Pastrl) Haworth Pr.

Professional Collaboration: A Team Approach to Health Care. Carol M. Frattali. Ed. by Leah C. Lorendo. Date not set. (Clinical Ser.: Vol. 11). 84p. (Orig.). pap. text 9.00 (*0-910329-80-X*, 0111969) Am Speech Lang Hearing.

Professional Commitment: Issues & Ethics in Nursing. Carroll A. Quinn & Michael D. Smith. 1987. 208p. pap. text 32.00 (*0-7216-1098-6*) Saunders.

Professional Communications in Eye Care. Ellen R. Ettinger. 1993. LC 93-6134. (Illus.). 272p. pap. text 54.99 (*0-7506-9306-1*) Buttrwrth-Heinemann.

Professional Competence & Quality Assurance in the Caring Professions. Ed. by Roger Ellis. 1988. 280p. lib. bdg. (*0-7099-5313-5*) C Helm GBR. *Dist:* Routldge.

Professional Competence & Quality Assurance in the Caring Professions. Ed. by Roger Ellis. 1990. 256p. 29.95 (*0-412-34080-1*, A4447) Chapman & Hall.

Professional Conduct Manual. National Association of School Psychologists. 2nd ed. 1992. pap. text 12.00 (*0-932955-12-6*) Natl Assn Schl Psych.

Professional Counseling: Transitioning into the Next Millennium. Ed. by Charlotte G. Dixon & William G. Emener. 1999. LC 99-30363. (Illus.). 194p. pap. 25.95 (*0-398-06986-7*) C C Thomas.

Professional Dental Hygiene. Gurenlian. Date not set. text (*0-7216-5005-8*) Harcourt.

Professional Development for Quality Care. Paul Shanahan. 1996. LC 96-21185. pap. text (*0-443-05331-6*) Church.

Professional Development in General Practice. Ed. by David Pendleton & John Hasler. 1996. (Oxford General Practice Ser.: No. 37). (Illus.). 188p. pap. text 55.95 (*0-19-262532-2*) OUP.

Professional Development in Nursing: A Handbook for Practice. Ed. by Frank Quinn & John Humphreys. 1998. pap. (*0-7487-3333-7*) Nelson Thornes GBR. *Dist:* Intl Spec Bk, Trans-Atl Phila.

Professional Dietitian's Natural Fiber Diet. Margaret B. Salmon. 1981. LC 79-1262. pap. 4.95 (*0-13-725341-9*) Techkits.

Professional Discipline in Nursing, Midwifery, & Health Visiting: Including a Treatise on Professional Regulation. Reginald H. Pyne. 3rd ed. 1997. LC 97-23059. 224p. pap. 41.95 (*0-632-04086-6*) Blackwell Sci.

Professional Dispensing for Opticianry. Opticians Association of America Staff. 2nd ed. 1996. text 80.00 (*0-7506-9889-6*) Buttrwrth-Heinemann.

Professional Education for General Practice. Peter Havelock et al. 1995. (Oxford General Practice Ser.: No. 31). (Illus.). 200p. pap. text 49.95 (*0-19-262607-8*) OUP.

Professional Ethics: A Guide for Rehabilitation Professionals. Scott. 1998. LC 98-9244. (Illus.). 240p. (C). (gr. 13). pap. text 29.95 (*0-8151-2525-9*, 31051) Mosby Inc.

Professional Ethics & Primary Care Medicine: Beyond Dilemmas & Decorum. Harmon L. Smith & Larry R. Churchill. 1986. LC 85-16098. viii, 118p. (Orig.). text 39.95 (*0-8223-0521-6*); pap. text 16.95 (*0-8223-0540-2*) Duke.

Professional Ethics for Audiologists & Speech-Language Pathologists. David M. Resnick. 1993. LC 92-34723. (Illus.). 196p. (Orig.). (C). pap. text 39.95 (*1-56593-087-8*, 0392) Thomson Learn.

Professional Ethics in Health Care Services. Ed. by Eugene W. Kelly. 1989. LC 88-27691. (Illus.). 230p. (Orig.). (C). 53.00 (*0-8191-7210-3*); 26.00 (*0-8191-7211-1*) U Pr of Amer.

Professional Ethics in Nursing. Joyce E. Thompson. 1990. LC 89-2667. 232p. (Orig.). 23.50 (*0-89464-352-5*) Krieger.

***Professional Guide to Complementary & Alternative Therapies.** Contrib. by Springhouse Corporation Staff. 2001. LC 2001-49079. 736p. 42.95 (*1-58255-127-8*) Springhouse Corp.

Professional Guide to Diseases. Springhouse Publishing Company Staff. 6th ed. 1998. LC 97-42712. (Professional Guide to Diseases Ser.). 1360p. 39.95 (*0-87434-926-5*) Springhouse Corp.

Professional Guide to Diseases. Lippincott, Williams and Wilkins Staff. 7th ed. 2001. LC 00-49226. (Professional Guide to Diseases Ser.). (Illus.). xiv, 1376p. 42.95 (*1-58255-073-5*) Springhouse Corp.

Professional Guide to Signs & Symptoms. 3rd ed. 2001. LC 00-30053. (Illus.). xi, 852p. 42.95 (*1-58255-074-3*) Springhouse Corp.

Professional Handbook of Diagnostic Tests. Matt Cahill. 1995. LC 94-39918. (Illus.). 704p. 32.95 (*0-87434-775-0*) Springhouse Corp.

Professional Hypnotism Manual. John G. Kappas. rev. ed. 1999. LC 78-107043. (Illus.). 276p. pap. 27.95 (0-937671-53-3) Panorama Van Nuys.

Professional Hypnotism Manual: Introducing Physical & Emotional Suggestibility & Sexuality. John G. Kappas. rev. ed. 1978. pap. 17.95 (0-87505-250-9) Panorama Van Nuys.

Professional ICD-9-CM Code Bk,1999-2000, Vols.1-3. St. Anthony's Publishing Staff. 1999. (Medical Assisting Ser). (C). pap. 56.00 (1-56329-656-X) Thomson Learn.

Professional Issues in Speech Language Pathology & Audiology. Ed. by Rosemary Lubinski & Carol Frattali. 2nd ed. 2000. LC 00-35775. 504p. pap. text 57.95 (0-7693-0002-2) Singular Publishing.

Professional Judgment: A Reader in Clinical Decision Making. Ed. by J. Dowie & Arthur S. Elstein. 1988. (Illus.). 584p. pap. text 41.95 (0-521-34696-7) Cambridge U Pr.

Professional Liability: Guidelines in Obstetrics & Gynecology. Roberts. 1991. 275.00 (0-8016-3357-5) Mosby Inc.

Professional Liability: Medical Text & Course Guide 1997. Robert A. Bregman et al. 1997. (Registered Professional Liability Underwriter Ser.: Vol. IV). 374p. ring bd. 115.00 (1-886813-28-0) Intl Risk Mgt.

Professional Liability & Risk Management. Ed. by Bruce E. Bennett et al. 1990. LC 90-1199. 128p. (Orig.). pap. text 19.95 (1-55798-101-9) Am Psychol.

Professional Liability-Risk Management: A Manual for Surgeons. Ed. by Paul F. Nora. 1991. 240p. pap. text (0-9620370-8-7) Am Coll Surgeons.

Professional Liability-Risk Management: A Manual for Surgeons. Paul F. Nora & American College of Surgeons Staff. 2nd ed. 1997. LC 96-35880. pap. (1-880696-08-8) Am Coll Surgeons.

Professional Lifeguard Textbook. American Red Cross Staff. 1994. 96p. (C). (gr. 13). pap. text 10.00 (0-8016-7554-5) Mosby Inc.

Professional Manual of Botanical Medicines Used in Western Clinical Practice: Teaching Guide. Mark William McDermott. 2000. 28p. pap., tchr. ed. 12.00 (0-9653431-4-6) Design to Prnt.

Professional Medical Assistant: Clinical Practice. Bonnie J. Lindsey & Francis M. Rayburn. 1990. LC 92-18589. 316p. pap. 34.95 (0-8273-4150-4) Delmar.

Professional Medical Assistant: Clinical Practice CTB. Bonnie J. Lindsey. 1993. (Medical Assisting Ser.). 62.95 (0-8273-5901-2) Delmar.

Professional Medical Assistant Clinical Practice: Instructor's Resource Guide. Bonnie J. Lindsey & Francis M. Rayburn. 1990. 216p. pap., tchr. ed. 18.00 (0-8273-4151-2) Delmar.

Professional Medical Assistant Clinical Practice: Workbook. Bonnie J. Lindsey & Francis M. Rayburn. 1991. 134p. pap., wbk. ed. 16.95 (0-8273-4155-5) Delmar.

Professional Medical Secretary. Aurandt. 1989. text 29.95 (0-87350-333-3) Milady Pub.

Professional Medical Secretary. Aurandt. 1984. instr.'s gde. ed. 30.95 (0-87350-336-8) Milady Pub.

Professional Medical Secretary Student Transcripts. Aurandt. 1986. (General Business & Business Education Ser.). pap. 28.00 (0-87350-608-1, VNR) Wiley.

Professional Nurse. Jack Rudman. 1994. (Career Examination Ser.: C-624). pap. 29.95 (0-8373-0624-8) Nat Learn.

Professional-Nurse Handbook. Melodie Chenevert. 3rd ed. 1996. LC 96-24753. (Illus.). 192p. (C). (gr. 13). pap. text 22.00 (0-8151-1215-7, 29588) Mosby Inc.

Professional Nursing: Concepts & Challenges. Kay K. Chitty. 2nd ed. 1997. (Illus.). 575p. pap., tchr. ed. (0-7216-6883-6) Saunders.

Professional Nursing: Concepts & Challenges. Kay K. Chitty. Ed. by Maura Connor. 2nd ed. 1996. (Illus.). 576p. pap. text 32.00 (0-7216-6882-8) Saunders.

***Professional Nursing: Concepts & Challenges.** Kay Kittrell Chitty. 3rd ed. 2001. (Illus.). 640p. pap., tchr. ed. 75.00 (0-7216-8714-8) Saunders.

Professional Nursing: Concepts & Challenges. Kay Kittrell Chitty. 3rd ed. 2000. LC 00-24856. (Illus.). xviii, 622p. (0-7216-8711-3) Saunders.

Professional Nursing Practice. Marilyn H. Oermann. 1996. LC 96-24608. 288p. (Orig.). (C). pap. 45.00 (0-8385-8114-5, A8114-9) P-H.

Professional Nursing Practice: Concepts & Perspectives. Barbara Kozier et al. 3rd ed. 1996. LC 96-17922. 470p. (C). pap. text 52.00 (0-8053-3523-4) Addison-Wesley.

***Professional Nursing Practice: Concepts & Perspectives.** Kathy Blais et al. 4th ed. 2001. LC 2001-51033. 432p. pap. 45.33 (0-13-028288-X) P-H.

Professional Orientation to Counseling. Nicholas A. Vacc & Larry C. Loesch. 1994. LC 93-27363. 560p. (C). 36.95 (1-55959-051-3) Accel Devel.

Professional Orientation to Counseling. Nicolas Vacc. 3rd ed. 2000. LC 00-34294. (Accelerated Development Ser.). (Illus.). xiv, 381p. 45.95 (1-56032-851-7) Taylor & Francis.

Professional Power & the Need for Health Care. Ian Rees Jones. 1999. LC 99-72601. (Developments in Nursing & Health Care Ser.). 174p. text (1-85972-626-7) Ashgate Pub GBR. *Dist:* Ashgate Pub Co.

Professional Practice: A South African Nursing Perspective. Charlotte Searle. 1987. 346p. pap. text 45.00 (0-409-10906-1) Buttrwrth-Heinemann.

Professional Practice in Health Care Marketing. Ed. by William J. Winston. 1986. LC 85-22036. (Health Marketing Quarterly Ser.: Vol. 3, Nos. 2 & 3). 224p. 49.95 (0-86656-549-3) Haworth Pr.

Professional Practice of Nursing Administration. Lillian M. Simms et al. 1989. LC 84-2209. 379p. text 36.95 (0-8273-4364-7) Delmar.

Professional Practice of Nursing Administration. Lillian M. Simms et al. 3rd ed. 2000. 685p. text 66.95 (0-7668-0790-8) Delmar.

Professional Practice of Psychology. Georgiana S. Tryon. Ed. by Glenn R. Caddy. 1986. LC 85-13433. (Developments in Clinical Psychology Ser.). 320p. 77.00 (0-89391-163-1, Ablex) Greenwood.

Professional Psychologist's Handbook. Ed. by Bruce D. Sales. 1983. 780p. 110.00 (0-306-40934-8, Plenum Trade) Perseus Pubng.

Professional Psychology in Canada. Ed. by Keith S. Dobson & D. Dobson. 1993. (Illus.). 480p. text 49.00 (0-88937-043-5) Hogrefe & Huber Pubs.

Professional Rescuer. Amercian Red Cross Staff. 2nd ed. 1997. (C). (0-8151-1253-X) Mosby Inc.

Professional Social Work Education & Health Care: Challenges for the Future. Ed. by Mildred D. Mailick & Phyllis Caroff. 1996. LC 96-30654. (Social Work in Health Care Ser.: Vol. 24, Nos. 1/2). 158p. (C). 39.95 (0-7890-0010-5) Haworth Pr.

Professional Strategies, Nursing. Jack Rudman. (ACT Proficiency Examination Program Ser.: Vol. 50). 43.95 (0-8373-5925-2) Nat Learn.

Professional Strategies (Nursing) Jack Rudman. (Regents External Degree Ser.: Vol. 26). 43.95 (0-8373-5676-8) Nat Learn.

Professional Training for Feminist Therapists: Personal Memoirs. Esther D. Rothblum & Ellen Cole. 1991. LC 90-26555. (Women & Therapy Ser.). 129p. text 39.95 (1-56024-123-3) Haworth Pr.

Professional Turnover: The Case of Nurses. James L. Price & Charles W. Mueller. 1980. (Health Systems Management Ser.). 218p. (C). 25.00 (0-88331-184-4) R B Luce.

Professional Voice: Science & Art of Clinic Care. Sataloff. 3rd ed. 2002. pap. 316.75 net. (0-7693-0166-5) Singular Publishing.

Professional Voice: The Science & Art of Clinical Care. Ed. by Robert T. Sataloff. 2nd ed. 1997. (Illus.). 1094p. 417.95 (1-56593-728-7, 1416) Singular Publishing.

***Professionalism & Ethics in Complementary & Alternative Medicine.** John K. Crellin & Fernando Ania. 2002. LC 2001-39102. (Illus.). 256p. pap. text 24.95 (0-7890-1226-X); lib. bdg. 49.95 (0-7890-1225-1) Haworth Pr (Integrative Healing Pr).

Professionalism in Basic Nursing. Lois Harrion. 1991. (C). mass mkt. 24.50 (0-8273-3680-2); pap. text 8.00 (0-8273-3681-0) Delmar.

Professionalism in Practice. 1988. (Conference Proceedings Ser.). 128p. (Orig.). pap. 15.00 (1-882147-08-1) Am Art Therapy.

Professionalization of Dental Students. M. L. Helfrich & E. L. Quarantelli. 1974. pap. 16.95 (0-8084-0382-6) NCUP.

Professionalization of Nursing: Current Issues & Trends. Patricia M. Schwirian. 3rd ed. 1998. LC 97-45687. 368p. pap. text 34.95 (0-7817-1045-6) Lppncott W & W.

Professionalization of Psychology in Nazi Germany. Ulfried Geuter. Tr. by Richard Holmes. 1992. (Cambridge Studies in the History of Psychology). (Illus.). 359p. (C). text 64.95 (0-521-33297-4) Cambridge U Pr.

Professionalizing Modern Medicine: Paris Surgeons & Medical Science & Institutions in the Eighteenth Century, 6. Toby Gelfand. 1980. LC 79-8955. (Contributions in Medical History Ser.: No. 6). (Illus.). 271p. 70.00 (0-313-21488-3, GPM/) Greenwood.

Professionally Speaking: A Marketing & Management Handbook for Dental & Medical Professionals. Neil H. Shulkin & Glenn H. Shulkin. 1994. (Illus.). 182p. (Orig.). pap. 79.95 (0-9640863-0-1) Dental Store.

Professional's Handbook of Complementary & Alternative Medicines. C. W. Fetrow & Juan R. Avila. 1999. LC 99-179767. 784p. spiral bd. 39.95 (0-87434-971-0) Springhouse Corp.

Professional's Handbook of Drug Therapy for Pain. Springhouse Publishing Company Staff. 2001. LC 00-50986. (Illus.). 768p. 39.95 (1-58255-102-2) Springhouse Corp.

Professional's Handbook of Psychotropic Drugs. Springhouse Publishing Company Staff. 2001. LC 00-47624. (Illus.). x, 502p. pap. 39.95 (1-58255-066-2) Springhouse Corp.

Professionals in Distress: Issues, Syndromes, & Solutions in Psychology. Ed. by Richard R. Kilburg et al. 1986. LC 85-18487. 299p. 29.95 (0-912704-43-8) Am Psychol.

Professions & Patriarchy. Anne Witz. 1992. (International Library of Sociology). 224p. (C). pap. 26.95 (0-415-07044-9); text 85.00 (0-415-05008-1) Routledge.

Professions & the Public Interest: Medical Power, Altruism & Alternative Medicine. Mike Saks. 1994. LC 94-9582. 272p. (C). 95.00 (0-415-01805-6, B4657) Routledge.

Professions, Information Technology & Management in Hospitals. Mike Dent. 1996. LC 96-84597. xii, 212 p. pap. (1-85628-869-2) Avebry GBR. *Dist:* Ashgate Pub Co.

Professor Dirk Durrer: 35 Years of Cardiology in Amsterdam. Ed. by F. L. Meijler & H. B. Burchell. 1986. 648p. (0-444-85656-0); pap. (0-444-85654-4) Royal Netherlands Acad NLD. *Dist:* Elsevier.

Professor Hein J. J. Wellens: 33 Years of Cardiology & Arrhythmology. J. Smeets et al. 2000. LC 00-24700. (Illus.). xv, 679p. 160.00 (0-7923-6209-8, Kluwer Plenum) Kluwer Academic.

Professor James Beart Simonds: A Great British Veterinarian Forgotten. Iain Pattison. 1990. 172p. (0-85131-491-0) J A Allen GBR. *Dist:* St Mut.

Professor, the Institute, & DNA. Rene Jules Dubos. 1976. LC 76-26812. (Illus.). 262p. 15.00 (0-87470-022-1) Rockefeller.

Profile in Alternative Medicine: The Eclectic Medical College of Cincinnati, 1835-1942. John S. Haller, Jr. 1999. LC 98-43302. (Illus.). 224p. text 35.00 (0-87338-610-8) Kent St U Pr.

Profile of the Negro in American Dentistry. Foster Kidd. 1979. LC 79-16159. (Illus.). 224p. 16.95 (0-88258-034-5) Howard U Pr.

Profiles: Giants in Medicine. Frederick Eberson. 1980. LC 80-53139. (Illus.). 116p. (Orig.). pap. 10.00 (0-934616-11-6) Valkyrie Pub Hse.

Profiles & Trends: Hospital Inpatient & Ambulatory Care in Southern New York, Vol. II. Compiled by Division of Research, Analysis, and Planning Staff. 1985. 43p. 15.00 (0-934459-07-X) United Hosp Fund.

Profiles in Caregiving: The Unexpected Career. Leonard I. Pearlin et al. 1995. LC 95-3498. (Illus.). 408p. pap. text 42.00 (0-12-059540-0) Acad Pr.

Profiles in Medical History, Vol. I. Glenn M. Bruss. 1997. (Illus.). 120p. pap. 12.00 (0-8059-4215-7) Dorrance.

Profiles in Stress. James H. Humphrey. 1986. LC 86-48066. (Stress in Modern Society Ser.: No. 2). 32.50 (0-404-63252-1) AMS Pr.

Profiles of Activities to Reduce Perinatal Transmission of HIV: Assessing the Response. Michelle Renaud & Elizabeth Kresse. 1998. (Illus.). 115p. (C). pap. text 25.00 (0-7881-7379-0) DIANE Pub.

Profiles of European Hospital Disposable Suppliers. Ed. by Frost and Sullivan Staff. 1997. 594p. spiral bd. 1995.00 (0-7889-0688-7, 3333-51) Frost & Sullivan.

Profiles of European Patient Monitoring Equipment Manufacturers. Ed. by Frost and Sullivan Staff. 1996. 542p. spiral bd. 1995.00 (0-7889-0409-4, 3206-56) Frost & Sullivan.

Profiles of Leading Biotechnology Companies. 1996. 665p. spiral bd. 1995.00 (0-7889-0562-7, 3332-43) Frost & Sullivan.

Profit Fever: The Drive to Corporatize Health Care & How to Stop It. Charles Andrews. 1995. 150p. LC 95-14883. pap. text 11.95 (1-56751-056-6); text 29.95 (1-56751-057-4) Common Courage.

Profit Motive & Patient Care: The Changing Accountability of Doctors & Hospitals. Bradford H. Gray. 1991. 456p. pap. 24.95 (0-674-71338-9); LC 90-5119. (Illus.). 448p. 54.00 (0-674-71337-0, GRAPRM) HUP.

Profitable & Necessarie Booke of Observations. William Clowes. 1971. LC 73-171740. (English Experience Ser.: No. 366). reprint ed. 33.50 (90-221-0366-8) Walter J Johnson.

Profitable Promises: Essays on Women, Science & Health. Ruth Hubbard. 1994. LC 94-37839. 150p. (Orig.). pap. 11.95 (1-56751-040-X) Common Courage.

Profiting from Quality: Outcomes Strategies for Medical Practice. Steven F. Isenberg & Richard E. Gliklich. 1999. LC 99-12557. (Jossey-Bass Health Ser.). (Illus.). 222p. 53.00 (0-7879-4624-9) Jossey-Bass.

Profits, Politics & Drugs. Duncan W. Reekie & Michael H. Weber. 1979. LC 78-24496. 185p. 49.50 (0-8419-0461-8) Holmes & Meier.

Profound Retardation & Multiple Impairment Vol. 3: Medical & Physical Care & Management. Ed. by James C. Hogg et al. 1990. 250p. pap. 36.95 (0-412-34630-3, A4456) Chapman & Hall.

Progesterone in Orthomolecular Medicine. Raymond Peat. 2001. LC 00-191564. 64p. pap. 7.00 (0-9702913-1-0, 200) R Peat.

Progestins & Antiprogestins in Clinical Practice. Ed. by Regine Sitruk-Ware & Daniel R. Mishell. 1999. LC 99-47752. (Illus.). 424p. text 165.00 (0-8247-8291-7) Dekker.

Progno 1.0: Prognostic Models in Fertility Practice. M. A. Wiegerinck. 1996. 165.95 incl. disk (1-85070-794-4, Parthenon Pbng) CRC Pr.

Prognose und Verlauf Ersthospitalisierter Schizophrener: Unter Mitarbeit von Wolfgang Brauer, Dagmar Laubenstein, Michael Handel & Martin Volz. Eibe-Rudolf Rey & Josef Bailer. 1997. (Illus.). 199p. 38.95 (3-631-30074-3) P Lang Pubng.

Prognoserechung. 5th ed. 1995. 91.00 (0-387-00758-X) Spr-Verlag.

Prognosis & Risk Assessment in Cardiovascular Disease. Ed. by Amar S. Kapoor & Bramah N. Singh. 1992. (Illus.). 578p. text (0-443-08768-7) Church.

Prognosis & Treatment of Cardiomyopathies & Myocarditis: Cardiomyopathy Update 5. Ed. by Morie Sekiguchi & Peter J. Richardson. 1995. 412p. (0-86008-511-2) U of Tokyo JPN. *Dist:* Col U Pr.

Prognosis in Neurology. James M. Gilchrist. 1998. LC 97-52638. 496p. text 95.00 (0-7506-9888-8) Buttrwrth-Heinemann.

Prognosis in the Rheumatic Diseases. Ed. by Nicholas Bellamy. 1991. 528p. text 279.50 (0-7923-8958-1) Kluwer Academic.

Prognosis of Coronary Heart Disease-Progression of Coronary Arteriosclerosis. Ed. by H. Roskamm. 1983. (Illus.). 248p. 48.95 (0-387-12367-9) Spr-Verlag.

Prognosis of Diabetes in Children. Ed. by Z. Laron. 1989. (Pediatric & Adolescent Endocrinology Ser.: Vol. 18). xiv, 304p. 216.75 (3-8055-4702-1) S Karger.

Prognostic & Predictive Value of p53: European School of Oncology Scientific Updates, Vol. 1. Ed. by J. G. Klijn. 1997. LC 97-29349. (Prognostic & Predictive Value of P53 Ser.: Vol. 1). 174p. 83.50 (0-444-82832-X) Elsevier.

Prognostic Factors in Cancer. International Union Against Cancer Staff & M. K. Gospodarowicz. Ed. by D. E. Henson et al. 1995. LC 95-19216. (Illus.). 272p. 72.00 (3-540-58688-1) Spr-Verlag.

Program Administration, Vol. 1. Larry Cooper & Yvonne Harrison. 1994. (Restorative Nursing for Long Term Care Ser.). 544p. ring bd. 60.00 (1-885506-02-3) Cooper & Harrison.

Program & Abstract Book. Paul A. Anderson et al. 1990. 180p. (C). pap. 22.00 (0-9627560-0-8) U of MD Physical Therapy.

Program Evaluation: A Compilation of Articles from the Journal of Health Education. Des. by Randall R. Cottrell et al. 1997. (Illus.). 124p. pap. 15.95 (0-88314-607-X) AAHPERD.

Program Evaluation & Family Violence Research. Ed. by Sally K. Ward & David Finkelhor. 2000. LC 00-58208. (Journal of Aggression, Maltreatment & Trauma Ser.: Vol. 4, Nos. 1, 7). xvi, 317p. (C). 69.95 (0-7890-1184-0); pap. 29.95 (0-7890-1185-9) Haworth Pr (Maltreatment & Trauma Pr).

Program Evaluation for Mental Health: Methods, Strategies & Participants. Ed. by Robert D. Coursey. 1977. LC 77-5634. 432p. text 72.00 (0-8089-1019-1, 790920, Grune & Strat) Harcrt Hlth Sci Grp.

Program Evaluation in the Health Fields, Vol. II. Ed. by Herbert C. Schulberg et al. 1979. LC 78-102679. 467p. 54.95 (0-87705-339-1, Kluwer Acad Hman Sci) Kluwer Academic.

Program for Personal & Cultural Change: Modules on Smoking, Nutrition, Weight Control, Physical Fitness, & Stress Robert F. Allen. 1981. (Illus.). 60p. (C). reprint ed. pap. 8.95 (0-941703-03-7) Healthyculture.

Program for Personal & Cultural Change on Nutrition. Robert F. Allen. 1990. LC 81-17569. (Illus.). 40p. (C). reprint ed. pap., stu. ed. 8.95 (0-941703-07-X) Healthyculture.

Program for Personal Change on Smoking. Robert F. Allen. 1990. LC 81-15025. (Illus.). 40p. (C). reprint ed. pap., stu. ed. 8.95 (0-941703-04-5) Healthyculture.

Program for Personal Change on Stress Resolution. Robert F. Allen. 1990. LC 81-15041. (Illus.). 40p. (C). reprint ed. pap., stu. ed. 8.95 (0-941703-05-3) Healthyculture.

Program for Personal Change on Weight Control. Robert F. Allen. 1990. LC 81-15026. 40p. reprint ed. pap., stu. ed. 8.95 (0-941703-06-1) Healthyculture.

Program for Research in Military Nursing: Progress & Future Direction. Contrib. by Institute of Medicine Staff. 1996. 128p. (Orig.). (C). pap. text 19.00 (0-309-05490-7) Natl Acad Pr.

Program for Staying Fit after Chelation. Arline Brecher. Ed. by Harold Brecher. 1989. 80p. (Orig.). pap. 29.95 (0-927839-13-X) HlthSavers Pr.

Program for the Assessment & Instruction of Swallowing (PAIS) Virginia A. Mulpeter & Judith F. Rosenfield. 1993. 24p. (Orig.). (C). tchr. ed. 55.00 (0-937857-39-4, 1529) Speech Bin.

Program Guide for Infants & Toddlers with Neuromotor & Other Developmental Disabilities. Frances P. Connor et al. 1978. LC 77-28188. 408p. pap. 21.95 (0-8077-2546-3) Tchrs Coll.

Program Implementation in Preventive Trials. Joseph A. Durlak. Ed. by Joseph R. Ferrari. 1998. LC 98-3323. 94p. 29.95 (0-7890-0523-9) Haworth Pr.

Program Planning for Health Education & Promotion. Mark Dignan & Patricia A. Carr. 2nd ed. 1993. (Illus.). 176p. pap. 37.95 (0-8121-1554-6) Lppncott W & W.

Program Your Baby's Health: The Pregnancy Diet for Your Child's Lifelong Well-Being. Barbara Luke & Tamara Eberlein. 2001. LC 00-68067. (Illus.). 432p. pap. 14.00 (0-345-44199-0) Ball Well.

Programa para Ti: Una Guia Disenada del Libro Grande. Tr. of Guide to the Big Book's Design for Living. (SPA.). 190p. pap. 10.00 (0-89486-874-8) Hazelden.

Programmable Hearing Aids: The Art & Science. H. Gustav Mueller & Dennis Hampton. 1997. 38.00 incl. audio (1-58041-009-X, 0112074) Am Speech Lang Hearing.

Programmed Approach to the Circulatory System. George I. Sackheim. 1960. (Illus.). pap. 10.80 (0-87563-014-6) Stipes.

Programmed Cell Death: The Cellular & Molecular Biology of Apoptosis. Ed. by Martin Lavin & Dianne Watters. 1993. LC 93-27865. xviii, 331p. text 129.00 (3-7186-5461-X) Gordon & Breach.

Programmed Cell Death in Tumours & Tissues. I. D. Bowen & S. M. Bowen. 1990. (Illus.). 200p. (C). (gr. 13). pap. text 179.95 (0-412-27970-3, A9835) Chapman & Hall.

Programmed Instruction: Radiation Therapy. Pilapil & Studva. 1980. (gr. 13). 11.00 (*0-89352-099-3*) Mosby Inc.

Programmed Introduction to Upper Gastrointestinal Radiology. Stephen L. Gammill. 1977. pap. text 22.00 (*0-316-30294-5*, Little Brwn Med Div) Lppncott W & W.

Programmed Mathematics for Nurses. George I. Sackheim & Lewis Robins. 8th ed. 1995. LC 95-26302. (Illus.). 313p. pap. 24.95 (*0-07-105398-0*) McGraw-Hill Prof.

Programmed Medical Language. Myrna LaFleur Brooks & Danielle LaFleur. 1998. (*0-8151-5417-8*); 1998. text incl. audio (*0-323-00113-0*); 1996. tchr. ed. (*0-8151-7852-2*) Mosby Inc.

Programmed Medical Language. Myrna LaFleur Brooks et al. 1995. LC 95-673. (Illus.). 352p. (C). (gr. 13). spiral bd. 27.00 (*0-8016-7835-8*, 07835) Mosby Inc.

Programmed Medical Language: Text/Dictionary. Myrna LaFleur Brooks & Danielle LaFleur. 1996. text (*0-323-00112-2*) Mosby Inc.

Programmed Therapy for Stuttering in Children & Adults. Bruce P. Ryan. (Illus.). 1980. 200p. spiral bd. 28.25 (*0-398-03104-5*); 2nd ed. 2000. LC 00-50901. 338p. 79.95 (*0-398-07106-3*); 2nd ed. 2000. LC 00-50901. 338p. pap. 54.95 (*0-398-07107-1*) C C Thomas.

Programmes of Analysis of Mortality Trends & Levels: Proceedings of the U. N.-WHO Meeting, Geneva, 1968. United Nations Staff & World Health Organization Staff. 1970. (Technical Reports: No. 440). pap. text 5.00 (*92-4-120440-0*, 1100440) World Health.

Programmes to Promote Breastfeeding. Ed. by Derrick B. Jelliffe & Patrice E. Jelliffe. 1988. (Illus.). 514p. pap. 60.00 (*0-19-261457-6*) OUP.

Programming & Design for Dementia: Development of a 50 Person Residential Environment. Gerald D. Weisman et al. 1992. (Publications in Architecture & Urban Planning: No. R90-3). (Illus.). 107p. (C). reprint ed. per. 12.00 (*0-938744-72-0*) U of Wis Ctr Arch-Urban.

Progress & Perspectives in the Treatment of Lung Cancer. Ed. by P. Van Houtte & P. Rocmans. 1999. LC 98-35108. (Medical Radiology Ser.). (Illus.). 290p. 199.00 (*3-540-62548-8*) Spr-Verlag.

Progress in AIDS Pathology. Heidrum Rotterdam. 1989. 75.00 (*0-938607-21-9*); Vol. 2. 1990. 109.00 (*0-938607-35-9*) Field & Wood Inc Medical.

Progress in Alcohol Research Vol. 1: Alcohol Nutrition & the Nervous System. Ed. by S. H. Parvez et al. 1985. 340p. lib. bdg. (*90-6764-050-6*) VSP NLD. *Dist:* Coronet Bks.

Progress in Alcohol Research Vol. 2: Alcohol & Behaviour: Basic & Clinical Aspects. Ed. by H. Parvez et al. 1990. 285p. (*90-6764-124-3*) VSP NLD. *Dist:* Coronet Bks.

Progress in Allergy see Idiotypes in Biology & Medicine

Progress in Allergy. Ed. by P. Kallos et al. (Illus.). 26. 1979. 86.25 (*3-8055-2934-1*); 27. 1979. 100.00 (*3-8055-3053-6*); Vol. 13. 1969. 300p. 94.00 (*3-8055-0378-4*) S Karger.

Progress in Allergy. Ed. by P. Kallos & B. H. Waksman. Vol. 14. 1970. 74.00 (*3-8055-0379-2*); Vol. 15. 1971. 95.75 (*3-8055-1238-4*) S Karger.

Progress in Allergy. Ed. by P. Kallos et al. Vol. 16. 1972. (Illus.). 111.50 (*3-8055-1335-6*); Vol. 17. 1973. (Illus.). 300p. 84.50 (*3-8055-1539-1*); Vol. 18. 1974. 300p. 162.75 (*3-8055-1660-6*) S Karger.

Progress in Allergy, Vol. 19. Ed. by P. Kallos. 1975. (Illus.). 300p. 111.50 (*3-8055-2033-6*) S Karger.

Progress in Allergy, Vol. 20. Ed. by P. Kallos & B. H. Waksman. 1975. (Illus.). 111.50 (*3-8055-2189-8*) S Karger.

Progress in Allergy. Ed. by P. Kallos et al. Vol. 21. 1976. (Illus.). 133.25 (*3-8055-2342-4*); Vol. 22. 1977. 82.75 (*3-8055-2419-6*); Vol. 23. 1977. (Illus.). 128.75 (*3-8055-2665-2*); Vol. 24. 1977. (Illus.). 129.75 (*3-8055-2781-0*); Vol. 25. 1978. (Illus.). 86.25 (*3-8055-2849-3*) S Karger.

Progress in Allergy & Clinical Immunology: Kyoto, Vol. 2. Minoru Okuda. Ed. by Terumasa Miyamoto. 1992. LC 92-53196. (Illus.). 747p. text 50.00 (*0-88937-087-7*) Hogrefe & Huber Pubs.

Progress in Allergy & Clinical Immunology Vol. 1: Montreux. Ed. by W. J. Pichler et al. 1989. LC 89-1678. 580p. 48.00 (*0-920887-45-7*) Hogrefe & Huber Pubs.

Progress in Allergy & Clinical Immunology Vol. 3: Stockholm Proceedings of the 15th International Congress of Allergology & Clinical Immunology, & the 1994 Annual Meeting of the European Academy of Allergology & Clinical Immunology Stockholm, June 7-July 1, 1994. Ed. by S. G. Johansson. 1995. LC 94-74177. 352p. text 56.00 (*0-88937-122-9*) Hogrefe & Huber Pubs.

Progress in Allergy & Clinical Immunology Vol. 4: Cancun. A. Oehling. 1997. LC 97-73937. 436p. 58.00 (*0-88937-179-2*) Hogrefe & Huber Pubs.

Progress in Alzheimer's & Parkinson's Diseases: Proceedings of the 4th International Conference Held in Eilat, Israel, May 18-23, 1997. Ed. by Abraham Fisher et al. 1998. LC 98-26174. (Advances in Behavioral Biology Ser.: Vol. 49). (Illus.). 912p. 175.00 (*0-306-45903-5*, Kluwer Plenum) Kluwer Academic.

Progress in Alzheimer's Disease & Similar Conditions. Ed. by Leonard L. Heston. 1997. LC 96-26156. (American Psychopathological Association Ser.). (Illus.). 326p. text 49.50 (*0-88048-760-7*, 8760) Am Psychiatric.

Progress in Ambulatory Assessment. Ed. by Jochen Fahrenberg. 2001. (Illus.). x, 640p. 49.50 (*0-88937-225-X*) Hogrefe & Huber Pubs.

Progress in Animal Retroviruses. Ed. by D. Gaudry & W. Hennessen. 1990. (Developments in Biological Standardization Ser.: Vol. 72). (Illus.). x, 394p. pap. 61.00 (*3-8055-5271-8*) S Karger.

Progress in Anterior Eye Segment: Research & Practice. Ed. by Otto Hockwin & W. B. Rathbun. 1979. (Documenta Ophthalmologica Proceedings Ser.: No. 18). (Illus.). pap. text 239.50 (*90-6193-158-4*) Kluwer Academic.

Progress in Anti-Cancer Chemotherapy. Ed. by Gabriel N. Hortobagyi & David Khayat. (Illus.). 1997. LC 97-15125. 224p. 89.95 (*0-86542-564-7*); Vol. 2. 1998. 322p. 99.95 (*0-632-04408-X*) Blackwell Sci.

Progress in Anti-Cancer Chemotherapy. Ed. by Gabriel N. Hortobagyi & David Khayat. Vol. 3. 1999. 200p. (C). (*2-287-59666-6*); Vol. 4. 2000. x, 269p. pap. (*2-287-59692-5*) Spl France Editions FRA. *Dist:* Spr-Verlag.

Progress in Assessment of Morbidity Due to Schistosomiasis: Reviews of Recent Literature. K. Mott & M. Chen. 1989. (Document Published by WHO Parasitic Diseases Programme Ser.). 56p. pap. text 20.00 (*0-9510869-4-4*) World Health.

Progress in Behavior Modification, Vol. 29. Ed. by Michel Hersen et al. 1993. 250p. (C). text 34.95 (*0-9625233-6-4*) Sycamore Pub.

Progress in Behavioral Studies, Vol. I. Ed. by Aaron J. Brownstein et al. 1989. 144p. 29.95 (*0-89859-511-8*) L Erlbaum Assocs.

Progress in Biomedical Polymers. Ed. by Charles G. Gebelein & R. L. Dunn. 1990. LC 90-7298. (Illus.). 420p. 115.00 (*0-306-43523-3*, Plenum Trade) Perseus Pubng.

Progress in Biophysics & Molecular Biology, Vol. 34. D. Noble. 1979. 76.00 (*0-08-024858-6*, Pergamon Pr) Elsevier.

Progress in Biophysics & Molecular Biology, Vol. 35. Ed. by D. Noble & T. L. Blundell. 1981. (Illus.). 206p. 76.00 (*0-08-027122-7*, Pergamon Pr) Elsevier.

Progress in Biophysics & Molecular Biology, Vol. 36, Nos. 1-3 Complete. D. Noble & T. L. Blundell. 1981. (Illus.). 130p. 83.00 (*0-08-028394-2*, Pergamon Pr) Elsevier.

Progress in Biophysics & Molecular Biology, Vol. 43. Ed. by D. Noble & T. L. Blundell. 1985. (Illus.). 268p. 110.00 (*0-08-032324-3*, Pergamon Pr) Elsevier.

Progress in Caries Prevention: European Organization for Caries Research (ORCA) - 25th Anniversary. Ed. by Y. Ericsson. 1978. (Caries Research Ser.: Vol. 12, Suppl. 1). (Illus.). pap. 27.00 (*3-8055-2920-1*) S Karger.

Progress in Cell Cycle Research, Vol. 1. Ed. by Laurent Meijer & Silvana Guidet. 1996. (Illus.). 384p. 95.00 (*0-306-45280-4*, Kluwer Plenum) Kluwer Academic.

Progress in Cerebrovascular Disease: Papers Presented at the XIVth World Congress of Neurology, New Delhi, 22-27 Oct., 1989. Ed. by H. Lechner et al. 1990. 142p. 110.50 (*0-444-81421-3*) Elsevier.

Progress in Clinical Biochemistry. 1989. (Illus.). 106p. 95.00 (*0-387-51097-4*) Spr-Verlag.

Progress in Clinical Biochemistry & Medicine Vol. 11: Immobilized Enzymes in Medicine. V. P. Torchilin. Ed. by International Board of Experts Staff & John A. Kellen. 1991. (Illus.). 206p. 159.00 (*0-387-52778-8*) Spr-Verlag.

Progress in Clinical Immunology. Ed. by Gianni Marone & M. Ricci. 1983. (Monographs in Allergy: Vol. 18). (Illus.). x, 314p. 142.75 (*3-8055-3697-6*) S Karger.

Progress in Clinical Pacing 1990: Proceedings of the International Symposium on Progress in Clinical Pacing, Rome, Italy, 5-8 December, 1990. Ed. by M. Santini et al. 1990. (Current Clinical Practice Ser.: No. 55). 516p. 223.00 (*90-219-9885-8*, Excerpta Medica) Elsevier.

Progress in Clinical Parasitology, Vol. 2. Tsieh Sun. 1990. 110.00 (*0-938607-36-7*) Field & Wood Inc Medical.

Progress in Clinical Parasitology, Vol. 3. Ed. by T. Sun. 1992. (Illus.). 209p. 163.00 (*0-387-97860-7*) Spr-Verlag.

Progress in Clinical Parasitology, Vol. 4. Ed. by Tsieh Sun. 1994. 192p. lib. bdg. 149.00 (*0-8493-7647-5*, 7647) CRC Pr.

Progress in Clinical Psychiatry. Ed. by Malcolm P. Weller & Daniel P. Van Kammen. 1997. (Illus.). 361p. pap. (*0-7020-2270-5*) W B Saunders GBR. *Dist:* Saunders.

Progress in Community Child Health Care. Spencer. 2nd ed. 1997. (C). pap. text (*0-443-05584-X*) Church.

Progress in Community Child Health Care, Vol. 1. Ed. by N. Spencer. 1995. (C). pap. text 46.00 (*0-443-05197-6*) Saunders.

Progress in Community Mental Health, Vol. 1. Ed. by Leopold Bellak & Harvey H. Barten. 1969. LC 69-15739. 280p. text 63.00 (*0-8089-0047-1*, 790501, Grune & Strat) Harcrt Hlth Sci Grp.

Progress in Comparative Placentology. Ed. by K. S. Ludwig & H. Hartels. 1973. (Illus.). 35.00 (*3-8055-1365-8*) S Karger.

Progress in Diagnostics & Therapy of Prostatic Cancer. Ed. by W. B. Peeling et al. 1996. (Illus.). 80p. pap. 52.95 (*3-540-60195-3*) Spr-Verlag.

Progress in Diet & Nutrition. Ed. by C. Horwitz & P. Rozen. 1988. (Frontiers of Gastrointestinal Research Ser.: Vol. 14). (Illus.). x, 226p. 168.75 (*3-8055-4608-4*) S Karger.

Progress in Digital Angiocardiography. Ed. by Paul H. Heintzen & J. H. Bursch. 1988. (Developments in Cardiovascular Medicine Ser.). (C). text 282.00 (*0-89838-965-8*) Kluwer Academic.

Progress in Drug Metabolism, Vol. 13. Ed. by G. Gordon Gibson. 1992. 360p. (*0-7484-0012-5*) Tay Francis Ltd GBR. *Dist:* Taylor & Francis.

Progress in Drug Research. Ed. by Ernst Jucker. 1983. (Progress in Drug Research Ser.: Vol. 27). 400p. (C). text 164.95 (*3-7643-1365-X*); Vol. 4. 1994. vii, 322p. 276.50 (*0-8176-5042-3*); Vol. 14. 1993. 408p. 357.00 (*0-8176-2925-4*) Birkhauser.

Progress in Drug Research, Vol. 23. Ernst Jucker. 1980. 320p. 214.50 (*0-8176-1070-7*) Birkhauser.

Progress in Drug Research. Ed. by Ernst Jucker. Vol. 24. 1980. 300p. 265.50 (*0-8176-1148-7*); Vol. 26. 1982. 412p. 296.50 (*0-8176-1261-0*) Birkhauser.

Progress in Drug Research, Vol. 28. Ernst Jucker. 1984. 255.50 (*0-8176-1556-3*) Birkhauser.

Progress in Drug Research. Ed. by Ernst Jucker. Vol. 29. 1986. 503p. 329.00 (*0-8176-1672-1*); Vol. 30. 1986. 580p. 491.50 (*0-8176-1752-3*); Vol. 31. 1988. 480p. 542.00 (*0-8176-1837-6*) Birkhauser.

Progress in Drug Research. Ernst Jucker & Urs A. Meyer. Vol. 32. 1988. 500p. 439.00 (*0-8176-1943-7*); Vol. 33. 1989. 550p. 439.00 (*0-8176-2306-X*) Birkhauser.

Progress in Drug Research, Vol. 34. Ernst Jucker. 1990. 544p. 439.00 (*0-8176-2351-5*) Birkhauser.

Progress in Drug Research. Ed. by Ernst Jucker. Vol. 35. 1990. 600p. 461.00 (*0-8176-2499-6*); Vol. 36. 1991. vii, 475p. 378.00 (*0-8176-2582-8*); Vol. 37. 1991. ix, 410p. 357.00 (*0-8176-2626-3*); Vol. 38. 1992. 380p. 326.50 (*0-8176-2705-7*); Vol. 39. 1992. ix, 398p. 357.00 (*0-8176-2717-0*); Vol. 40. 1993. vii, 204p. 258.00 (*0-8176-2850-9*) Birkhauser.

Progress in Drug Research, Vol. 42. Ernst Jucker. 1994. 464p. 349.00 (*0-8176-2995-5*) Birkhauser.

Progress in Drug Research, Vol. 44. Ed. by Ernst Jucker. 1995. (Illus.). 352p. 269.00 (*0-8176-5149-7*) Birkhauser.

***Progress in Drug Research**, Vol. 46. Ed. by Ernst Jucker. 1996. 336p. 313.50 (*3-7643-5298-1*) Birkhauser.

Progress in Drug Research. Ed. by Ernst Jucker. Vol. 49. 1997. 373p. text 267.00 (*3-7643-5672-3*); Vol. 50. 1998. (Progress in Drug Research Ser.: Vol. 50). 300p. stu. ed. 250.00 (*3-7643-5821-1*); Vol. 54. 2000. (Illus.). 250p. 249.00 (*3-7643-6113-1*) Birkhauser.

Progress in Drug Research, Vol. 48. Ed. by Ernst Jucker. 1997. (Illus.). 288p. 249.00 (*3-7643-5671-5*) Spr-Verlag.

***Progress in Drug Research**, Vol. 56. Ed. by E. Jucker. 2001. 300p. (*3-7643-6265-0*) Birkhauser CHE. *Dist:* Spr-Verlag.

Progress in Electrodermal Research. J. C. Roy et al. 1993. LC 93-11397. (NATO Advanced Science Institutes Ser.: Vol. 249). (Illus.). 360p. (C). text 110.00 (*0-306-44536-0*, Kluwer Plenum) Kluwer Academic.

Progress in Ergometry: Quality Control & Test Criteria, Fifth International Seminar on Ergometry. Ed. by H. Loellgen & H. Mellerowicz. 1984. (Illus.). 275p. 54.95 (*0-387-13570-7*) Spr-Verlag.

Progress in Experimental Personality & Psychopathology Research, Vol. 15. Ed. by Elaine F. Walker et al. 1992. 336p. 49.95 (*0-8261-6090-5*) Springer Pub.

Progress in Experimental Personality & Psychopathology Research, Vol. 16. Ed. by Loren J. Chapman et al. 1992. 304p. 49.95 (*0-8261-6091-3*) Springer Pub.

Progress in Experimental Personality & Psychopathology Research, Vol. 17. Ed. by Don C. Fowles et al. 1994. (Special Focus on Antisocial Personality Ser.). 344p. 49.95 (*0-8261-6092-1*) Springer Pub.

Progress in Experimental Tumor Research, Vols. 27-28. 1984. (Illus.). xxxii, 500p. 204.50 (*3-8055-3857-X*) S Karger.

Progress in Fibrin Sealing. Ed. by H. W. Waclawiczek. 1989. (Illus.). 180p. 103.00 (*0-387-50797-3*) Spr-Verlag.

Progress in Food & Nutrition Science. Ed. by R. K. Chandra. 1984. (Illus.). 198p. pap. 92.00 (*0-08-030928-3*, Pergamon Pr) Elsevier.

Progress in Food & Nutrition Science, Vol. 2, No. 11-12. H. M. Sinclair. 1979. LC 75-7734. (Illus.). 70p. pap. 28.00 (*0-08-023758-4*, Pergamon Pr) Elsevier.

Progress in Forensic Genetics B: Proceedings of the 18th International ISFH Congress, San Francisco, 17-21 August 1999. Ed. by G. F. Sansabaugh et al. 2000. (International Congress Ser.: Vol. 1193). 656p. 183.50 (*0-444-50303-X*, Excerpta Medica) Elsevier.

Progress in Functional Psychoses. Ed. by Robert Cancro et al. 1979. LC 78-31828. (Illus.). 250p. 44.95 (*0-88331-185-2*) R B Luce.

Progress in Gastroenterology, Vol. 4. Ed. by George B. Glass & Paul Sherlock. 1983. 624p. text 190.00 (*0-8089-1555-X*, 791564, Grune & Strat) Harcrt Hlth Sci Grp.

Progress in Gynecology & Endocrinology. Ed. by Andrea R. Genazzani et al. 1990. 944p. (C). 125.00 (*1-85070-299-3*, Parthenon Pbng) CRC Pr.

Progress in Haematology No. 2. Ed. by C. Pallister & C. Dunn. 2nd ed. 1999. (Illus.). 208p. pap. text (*1-900151-79-0*) Greenwich Med.

Progress in Hemostasis & Thrombosis, Vol. 10. Barry S. Coller. 1990. (Illus.). 368p. text 180.00 (*0-7216-3445-1*) Saunders.

Progress in Hepatic Encephalopathy & Metabolic Nitrogen Exchange Proceedings: Seventh International Symposium on Ammonia. Finn Bengtsson et al. 1991. (Illus.). 576p. 324.00 (*0-8493-0180-7*, 180FV, CRC Reprint) Franklin.

Progress in Hepatocellular Carcinoma Treatment. Ed. by K. Okita. 1999. LC 99-48955. 124p. 79.00 (*4-431-70257-1*) Spr-Verlag.

Progress in Hepatology Vol. 4: Liver Cirrhosis Update; Proceedings. Takahashi Memorial Forum on Progress in Hepatology, Liver Cirrhosis Update (1997: Tokyo, Japan) Ed. by Masami Yamanaka. 1998. (International Congress Ser.: Vol. 1163). 152p. 110.00 (*0-444-82940-7*) Elsevier.

Progress in HPLC Vol. 2: Electromechanical Detection in Medicine & Chemistry. Ed. by S. H. Parvez et al. 1987. 480p. lib. bdg. (*90-6764-062-X*) VSP NLD. *Dist:* Coronet Bks.

Progress in HPLC Vol. 4: Supercritical Fluid Chromatography & Microbore-HPLC. Ed. by M. Yoshioka et al. 1988. 300p. (*90-6764-113-8*) VSP NLD. *Dist:* Coronet Bks.

Progress in Human African Trypanosomiasis, Sleeping Sickness. Michael Dumas. 1999. LC 98-31567. (Illus.). 350p. 159.00 (*2-287-59655-0*) Spr-Verlag.

Progress in Human Auditory & Vestibular Histopathology. Salvatore Iurato & Jan E. Veldman. 1997. LC 96-38655. (*90-6299-151-3*) Kugler NLD. *Dist:* Lib Res.

Progress in Hypertension: Antihypertensive Drugs Today, Vol. 2. Ed. by H. Saito et al. 1992. 383p. 140.00 (*90-6764-140-5*) Coronet Bks.

Progress in Hypertension Vol. 1: Neurotransmitters As Modulators of Blood Pressure. Ed. by H. Saito et al. 1987. 380p. lib. bdg. (*90-6764-100-6*) VSP NLD. *Dist:* Coronet Bks.

Progress in Hypertension Vol. 3: New Advances in SHR Research. Pathophysiology & Pharmacology. Ed. by H. Saito et al. 1995. 240p. (*90-6764-198-7*) VSP NLD. *Dist:* Coronet Bks.

Progress in Immunodeficiency: Proceedings of the 7th Meeting of the European Society of Immunodeficiencies, June 6-9, 1996, Goteborg, Sweden, Vol. 1. European Society of Immunodeficiencies Staff et al. 1996. LC 96-49576. (Advances in the Biosciences Ser.). 140p. 112.50 (*0-444-82462-6*) Elsevier.

Progress in Immunology, Vol. VII. Ed. by F. Melchers et al. 1989. (Illus.). 1318p. 207.00 (*0-387-51053-2*) Spr-Verlag.

Progress in Immunology 8: Proceedings of the 8th International Congress of Immunology, Budapest 1992. Ed. by J. Gergely. 1993. (Illus.). 987p. 181.00 (*0-387-56401-2*) Spr-Verlag.

Progress in In Vitro Toxicology, Vol. 6. 1988. (Alternative Methods in Toxicology Ser.). 350p. 191.00 (*0-913113-16-6*) M Liebert.

Progress in Inflammation Research & Therapy. Ed. by N. R. Ackerman et al. 1991. (Agents & Actions Supplements Ser.: Vol. 35). (Illus.). 208p. 141.50 (*0-8176-2529-1*) Birkhauser.

Progress in Iron Research. C. Hershko et al. 1994. (Advances in Experimental Medicine & Biology Ser.: Vol. 356). (Illus.). 412p. (C). text 125.00 (*0-306-44729-0*, Kluwer Plenum) Kluwer Academic.

Progress in Laboratory Diagnosis. 1997. text 19.00 (*3-540-99546-3*) Spr-Verlag.

Progress in Learning Disabilities. Ed. by Helmer R. Myklebust. Vol. 3. 1975. 240p. text 54.00 (*0-8089-0911-8*, 793033); Vol. 4. 1978. 272p. text 47.00 (*0-8089-1128-7*, 793034) Harcrt Hlth Sci Grp (Grune & Strat).

Progress in Lipid Research, Vol. 18. Ed. by Ralph T. Holman. 1981. (Illus.). 180p. 91.00 (*0-08-027129-4*, Pergamon Pr) Elsevier.

Progress in Lipid Research: Golden Jubilee International Conference, Minnesota, May 4-7, 1980, Vol. 20. Ed. by R. J. Holman. 1982. (Illus.). 968p. (*0-08-028011-0*, H115, H125) Pergamon Repr GBR. *Dist:* Franklin.

Progress in Liver Diseases, Vol. 9. Fenton Schaffner & Arthur N. Popper. 1990. (Illus.). 736p. text 235.00 (*0-7216-2940-7*) Saunders.

Progress in Liver Transplantation. Ed. by Chris H. Gips. 1985. (Developments in Gastroenterology Ser.). text 215.00 (*0-89838-726-4*) Kluwer Academic.

Progress in Medical Radiation Physics, Vol. 1. Ed. by Colin G. Orton. 1982. 402p. 95.00 (*0-306-40713-2*, Plenum Trade) Perseus Pubng.

Progress in Medical Radioisotope Scanning: Proceedings. Ed. by Ralph M. Kniseley & Gould A. Andrews. 1963. (AEC Symposium Ser.). 539p. fiche 9.00 (*0-87079-314-4*, TID-7673) DOE.

Progress in Medical Terminology. Ed. by Alexandre Manuila. 1981. (Illus.). xii, 116p. pap. 68.75 (*3-8055-2112-X*) S Karger.

Progress in Medical Virology. Ed. by Joseph L. Melnick. Vol. 12. 1970. 75.00 (*3-8055-0409-8*); Vol. 13. 1971. 95.75 (*3-8055-1181-7*); Vol. 14. 1972. 82.75 (*3-8055-1291-0*); Vol. 16. 1973. (Illus.). 85.25 (*3-8055-1601-0*); Vol. 17. 1974. 400p. 85.25 (*3-8055-1642-8*); Vol. 20. 1975. (Illus.). 400p. 86.25

P
Q
R

P
Q
R

(*3-8055-2161-8*); Vol. 22. 1976. 250p. 103.50 (*3-8055-2315-7*); Vol. 23. 1977. (Illus.). 95.75 (*3-8055-2423-4*); Vol. 24. 1978. (Illus.). 94.00 (*3-8055-2810-8*); Vol. 25. 1979. (Illus.). 77.50 (*3-8055-2978-3*); Vol. 26. 1980. (Illus.). viii, 240p. 129.75 (*3-8055-0702-X*); Vol. 28. 1982. (Illus.). x, 234p. 128.75 (*3-8055-2983-X*); Vol. 29. 1984. (Illus.). x, 246p. 128.75 (*3-8055-3618-6*) S Karger.

Progress in Medical Virology, Vol. 30. Ed. by Joseph L. Melnick & K. Hummeler. 1984. (Illus.). viii, 212p. 135.00 (*3-8055-3851-0*) S Karger.

Progress in Medical Virology. Ed. by Joseph L. Melnick. (Illus.). Vol. 31. 1984. x, 234p. 142.75 (*3-8055-3909-6*); Vol. 33. 1986. viii, 182p. 129.75 (*3-8055-4155-4*); Vol. 34. 1987. x, 206p. 150.50 (*3-8055-4468-5*); Vol. 35. 1988. viii, 220p. 173.25 (*3-8055-4711-0*); Vol. 36. 1989. viii, 210p. 164.50 (*3-8055-4834-6*); Vol. 37. 1990. x, 250p. 197.50 (*3-8055-5077-4*); Vol. 39. 1992. x, 270p. 231.50 (*3-8055-5428-1*); Vol. 40. 1993. viii, 224p. 230.50 (*3-8055-5600-4*) S Karger.

Progress in Medicinal Chemistry. Ed. by F. D. King & A. W. Oxford. 1999. 310p. 166.00 (*0-444-50090-1*) Elsevier.

Progress in Medicinal Chemistry, 33. Ed. by G. P. Ellis & D. K. Luscombe. 1995. 362p. 187.00 (*0-444-82057-4*) Elsevier.

Progress in Medicinal Chemistry, Vol. 29. G. P. Ellis & D. K. Luscombe. 1992. 350p. 187.50 (*0-444-89472-1*) Elsevier.

Progress in Medicinal Chemistry, Vol. 31. Ed. by G. P. Ellis et al. 1994. 474p. 217.00 (*0-444-81807-3*) Elsevier.

Progress in Medicinal Chemistry, Vol. 34. Ed. by D. K. Luscombe et al. 1997. 286p. 170.00 (*0-444-82632-7*) Elsevier.

Progress in Medicinal Chemistry, Vol. 35. Ed. by G. P. Ellis et al. 1998. 268p. 172.00 (*0-444-82909-1*) Elsevier.

Progress in Medicinal Chemistry 30, 31. Ed. by G. P. Ellis & D. K. Luscombe. 1993. 474p. 216.00 (*0-444-89989-8*) Elsevier.

Progress in Medicine. Iago Galdston. 1977. LC 76-39166. (Essay Index Reprint Ser.). 25.95 (*0-8369-2689-7*) Ayer.

Progress in Microcirculation Research. Niimi. 1994. LC 94-26568. 540p. 173.00 (*0-08-042503-8*, Pergamon Pr) Elsevier.

Progress in Molecular & Subcellular Biology, Vol. 4. 1976. (Illus.). 251p. 61.95 (*0-387-07487-2*) Spr-Verlag.

Progress in Molecular & Subcellular Biology: Biological Response Modifiers Interferone, Double-Stranded RNA & 2-5 Adenylate, Vol. 14. Ed. by W. E. G. Muller et al. 1994. (Illus.). 275p. 136.00 (*0-387-57285-6*) Spr-Verlag.

Progress in Motor Control: Bernstein's Traditions in Movement Studies. Ed. by Mark L. Latash. 1998. LC 97-44950. (Illus.). 408p. text 52.00 (*0-88011-674-9*, BLAT0674) Human Kinetics.

Progress in Multiple Sclerosis Research. Ed. by H. J. Bauer. 1980. (Illus.). 677p. 68.95 (*0-387-09867-4*) Spr-Verlag.

Progress in Neurobiology. G. A. Kerkut. 1975. Vol. 2. 125.00 (*0-08-017882-0*); Vol. 3. 125.00 (*0-08-017963-0*) Elsevier (Pergamon Pr).

Progress in Neurobiology, Vol. 11. Ed. by G. A. Kerkut & J. W. Phillis. 1979. 125.00 (*0-08-024857-8*, Pergamon Pr) Elsevier.

Progress in Neurobiology, Vol. 12. G. A. Kerkut. 1980. (Illus.). 312p. 125.00 (*0-08-024888-8*, Pergamon Pr) Elsevier.

Progress in Neurobiology, Vol. 13, Complete. Ed. by G. A. Kerkut. 1980. (Illus.). 440p. 125.00 (*0-08-026039-X*, Pergamon Pr) Elsevier.

Progress in Neurobiology, Vol. 14 Complete. Ed. by G. A. Kerkut & J. W. Phillis. 1980. 344p. 125.00 (*0-08-027114-6*, Pergamon Pr) Elsevier.

Progress in Neurobiology, Vol. 15, No.4. 1981. pap. 32.00 (*0-08-027148-0*, Pergamon Pr) Elsevier.

Progress in Neurobiology. Ed. by G. A. Kerkut & J. W. Phillis. Vol. 16. 1982. (Illus.). 320p. 125.00 (*0-08-029105-8*); Vol. 17. 1983. 289p. 125.00 (*0-08-029697-1*, Pergamon Pr); Vol. 18. 1983. (Illus.). 338p. 130.00 (*0-08-031046-X*, Pergamon Pr); Vol. 19. 1984. (Illus.). 370p. 130.00 (*0-08-031508-9*, Pergamon Pr); Vol. 20. 1984. LC 72-12616. (Illus.). 348p. 130.00 (*0-08-031706-5*, Pergamon Pr) Elsevier.

Progress in Neurobiology, Vol. 24. Ed. by G. A. Kerkut & J. W. Phillis. (Illus.). 350p. (*0-08-033679-5*, H140, H110) PPL GBR. *Dist:* Elsevier.

Progress in Neuroendocrinology Vol. 1: Neuroendricrinology of Hormone-Transmitter Interactions. Ed. by H. Parvez et al. 1985. 315p. lib. bdg. (*90-6764-049-2*) VSP NLD. *Dist:* Coronet Bks.

Progress in Neurological Surgery, Vol. 5. H. Krayenbuehl et al. 1973. (Illus.). 500p. 149.75 (*3-8055-1499-9*) S Karger.

Progress in Neuropeptide Research. K. D. Dohler & M. Pawlikowski. 1989. (Congress Reports: No. 3). 185p. 57.50 (*0-8176-2268-3*) Birkhauser.

Progress in Neuropsychopharmacology, Vol. 4, No. 6. Ed. by C. Radouco-Thomas & F. Garcin. 1981. (Illus.). 110p. pap. 31.00 (*0-08-027157-X*, Pergamon Pr) Elsevier.

Progress in Neuroscience. Ed. by Richard F. Thompson. 1985. LC 85-16120. (Scientific American Reader Ser.). (Illus.). 151p. (C). pap. 16.95 (*0-7167-1727-1*) W H Freeman.

Progress in Neutron Capture Therapy for Cancer. Ed. by B. J. Allen et al. 1992. (Illus.). 702p. (C). text 186.00 (*0-306-44104-7*, Kluwer Plenum) Kluwer Academic.

Progress in Non-Histone Protein Research. Ed. by Isaac Bekhor. 1985. Vol. I. 224p. 130.00 (*0-8493-5528-1*, QP552); Vol. II. 240p. 137.00 (*0-8493-5529-X*) Franklin (CRC Reprint).

Progress in Nonmammalian Brain Research Ed. by Giuseppe Nistico & Liana Bolis. 1983. III. 146.00 (*0-8493-6352-7*); Vol. I. 208p. 114.00 (*0-8493-6350-0*, QP376); Vol. II. 240p. 135.00 (*0-8493-6351-9*) Franklin (CRC Reprint).

Progress in Nuclear Magnetic Resonance Spectroscopy, Vol. 15. Ed. by James W. Emsley et al. 1984. (Illus.). 430p. 130.00 (*0-08-031510-0*, Pergamon Pr) Elsevier.

***Progress in Nucleic Acid Research Vol. 68: Base Excision Repair.** Ed. by Kivie Moldave. 2001. (Progress in Nucleic Acid Research & Molecular Biology Ser.: Vol. 68). (Illus.). 403p. 119.95 (*0-12-540068-3*) Acad Pr.

Progress in Nucleic Acid Research & Molecular Biology, Vol. 5. Ed. by Kivie Moldave. 1997. (Illus.). 404p. (C). text 89.95 (*0-12-540058-6*) Morgan Kaufmann.

Progress in Nucleic Acid Research & Molecular Biology, Vol. 48. Ed. by Waldo E. Cohn & Kivie Moldave. 1994. (Illus.). 379p. (C). text 104.00 (*0-12-540048-9*) Acad Pr.

Progress in Nucleic Acid Research & Molecular Biology, Vol. 59. Ed. by Kivie Moldave. 1997. (Illus.). 373p. (C). text 89.95 (*0-12-540059-4*) Morgan Kaufmann.

Progress in Obesity, No. 7. A. Angel. 1996. 788p. (*0-86196-532-9*) J Libbey Med GBR. *Dist:* Buttrwrth-Heinemann.

Progress in Obstetrics & Gynaecology. Ed. by John W. Studd. (Illus.). No. 7. 1989. 412p. pap. text (*0-443-03885-6*); Vol. 6. 1987. LC 81-21699. 456p. pap. text (*0-443-03572-5*); Vol. 8. 1990. 416p. pap. text (*0-443-04170-9*); Vol. 9. 1991. 412p. pap. text (*0-443-04412-0*) Church.

Progress in Obstetrics/Gynecology. Studd. 13th ed. 1999. (C). text 60.00 (*0-443-05868-7*) Saunders.

Progress in Occupational Epidemiology: Proceedings of the 6th International Symposium on Epidemiology in Occupational Health, Stockholm, Sweden, 16-19 Aug., 1988. Ed. by C. Hogstedt & C. Reuterwall. 1991. (International Congress Ser.: No. 829). 400p. 153.50 (*0-444-81057-9*, Excerpta Medica) Elsevier.

Progress in Oncology. David Khayat & Gabriel N. Hortobagyi. 1999. LC 99-19801. (Progress in Anti-Cancer Chemotherapy Ser.). (*3-540-59666-6*) Spr-Verlag.

***Progress in Oncology 2001.** Ed. by Vincent T. DeVita, Jr. et al. 2001. LC 2001-25720. (Illus.). 376p. (C). text 99.95 (*0-7637-1589-1*, 1589-1) Jones & Bartlett.

Progress in Parkinson Research. Ed. by F. Hefti & William J. Weiner. 1989. (Illus.). 238p. 69.50 (*0-306-43096-7*, Plenum Trade) Perseus Pubng.

Progress in Pathology, Vol. 4. Nigel Kirkham. 271p. 62.00 (*0-443-06032-0*) Harcrt Hlth Sci Grp.

***Progress in Pathology**, Vol. 5. Kirkham. 2001. (Illus.). 208p. (*1-84110-050-1*) Greenwich Med GBR. *Dist:* JAMCO Dist.

Progress in Pediatric Neurology I. J. Gordon Millichap. 1991. LC 91-90076. 598p. text 57.95 (*0-9629115-0-X*) PNB Pub.

Progress in Pediatric Neurology III. J. Gordon Millichap. 1997. LC 94-1233. 611p. (C). 64.95 (*0-9629115-6-9*) PNB Pub.

Progress in Pediatric Neurology II. J. Gordon Millichap. 1994. LC 94-66683. (Illus.). 550p. 64.95 (*0-9629115-8-5*) PNB Pub.

Progress in Peptic Ulcer. T. Javor & Gy Mozsik. 1976. 774p. (C). (*963-05-1210-6*) Akade Kiado HUN. *Dist:* St Mut.

Progress in Peptide Research, Vol. 2. Ed. by Saul Lande. 1972. LC 76-153298. x, 394p. text 510.00 (*0-677-13610-2*) Gordon & Breach.

Progress in Perinatal Medicine, Vol. 9. D. F. Hawkins. 1990. (Ettore Majorana International Life Sciences Ser.). 350p. text 160.00 (*3-7186-5054-1*, Harwood Acad Pubs) Gordon & Breach.

Progress in Phycological Research, Vol. 9. Ed. by F. E. Round & D. J. Chapman. 1993. (Illus.). 376p. lib. bdg. (*0-948737-19-0*) Biopress GBR. *Dist:* Balogh.

Progress in Physical Organic Chemistry, Vol. 19. Ed. by Robert W. Taft. 1993. LC 63-19364. 349p. 240.00 (*0-471-52442-5*) Wiley.

Progress in Preventing AIDS? Dogma, Dissent & Innovation - Global Perspectives. Ed. by David Buchanan & George Cernada. 1998. LC 97-1804. (Health Services Ser.). 368p. pap. text 49.95 (*0-89503-176-0*) Baywood Pub.

Progress in Psychobiology & Physiological Psychology, Vol. 15. Ed. by Alan N. Epstein & Adrian R. Morrison. 1992. (Illus.). 309p. (C). text 115.00 (*0-12-542115-X*) Acad Pr.

Progress in Psychobiology & Physiological Psychology, Vol. 16. Ed. by Steven J. Fluharty et al. 1995. (Illus.). 231p. (C). text 99.95 (*0-12-542116-8*) Acad Pr.

Progress in Quantitative Coronary Arteriography. Ed. by Johan H. Reiber & Patrick W. Serruys. 1994. LC 94-13374. (Developments in Cardiovascular Medicine Ser.: Vol. 155). 432p. (C). text 251.00 (*0-7923-2814-0*) Kluwer Academic.

Progress in Radiopharmacology, 1985. Ed. by Peter H. Cox et al. 1985. LC 85-13774. (Developments in Nuclear Medicine Ser.). text 191.00 (*0-89838-745-0*) Kluwer Academic.

Progress in Radiopharmacology 3. Peter H. Cox. 1982. text 141.50 (*90-247-2768-5*) Kluwer Academic.

Progress in Radiopharmacy. Ed. by Peter H. Cox et al. 1986. (Developments in Nuclear Medicine Ser.). lib. bdg. 314.00 (*0-89838-823-6*) Kluwer Academic.

Progress in Radiopharmacy. Ed. by P. August Schubiger & Gerrit Westera. 1992. (Developments in Nuclear Medicine Ser.). 256p. (C). text 137.50 (*0-7923-1525-1*) Kluwer Academic.

Progress in Reaction Kinetics, Vol. 12. Ed. by K. R. Jennings et al. 1985. (Illus.). 268p. 130.00 (*0-08-032326-X*, Pergamon Pr) Elsevier.

Progress in Regional Cancer Therapy. Ed. by R. Jakesz & H. Rainer. 1990. (Illus.). 322p. 118.00 (*0-387-51259-4*) Spr-Verlag.

Progress in Reproductive & Urinary Tract Pathology. Ivan Damjanov. 1989. 70.00 (*0-938607-13-8*) Field & Wood Inc Medical.

Progress in Reproductive Medicine, Vol. 2. Ed. by Richard H. Asch & John W. Studd. 1995. (Illus.). 304p. lib. bdg. 71.95 (*1-85070-574-7*, Parthenon Pbng) CRC Pr.

Progress in Retinal Research, Vol. 1. Ed. by Neville N. Osborne & Gerald J. Chader. 1982. (Illus.). 245p. 107.00 (*0-08-028901-0*, Pergamon Pr) Elsevier.

Progress in Retinal Research, Vol. 2. Ed. by Neville N. Osborne. 1983. (Illus.). 337p. 95.00 (*0-08-030773-6*, 07, Pergamon Pr) Elsevier.

Progress in Retinal Research. Ed. by Neville N. Osborne & Gerald J. Chader. (Illus.). Vol. 3. 1984. 358p. 69.50 (*0-08-031701-4*); Vol. 4. 1985. 330p. 116.00 (*0-08-031738-3*) Elsevier (Pergamon Pr).

Progress in Sensory Physiology, Vol. 5. 1985. (Illus.). 175p. 79.95 (*0-387-15339-X*) Spr-Verlag.

Progress in Sensory Physiology, Vol. 12. Ed. by H. Autrum et al. 1991. (Illus.). 260p. 136.00 (*0-387-52985-3*) Spr-Verlag.

Progress in Sensory Physiology: Ionic & Volume Changes in the Microenvironment of Nerve & Receptor Cells, Vol. 13. Ed. by H. Autrum et al. 1992. (Illus.). 167p. 123.00 (*0-387-54553-0*) Spr-Verlag.

Progress in Social Psychology, Vol. 1. M. Fishbein. 1980. LC 79-67453. (Illus.). 240p. text 49.95 (*0-89859-005-1*) L Erlbaum Assocs.

Progress in Standardization in Health Care Informatics. Ed. by Georges J. E. De Moor et al. 1993. (Studies in Health Technology & Informatics: Vol. 6). 215p. (YA). (gr. 12 up). 98.00 (*90-5199-114-2*) IOS Press.

Progress in Surgery Ed. by M. Allgoewer et al. 11. 1972. (Illus.). 57.50 (*3-8055-1379-8*); 12. 1973. (Illus.). 85.25 (*3-8055-1617-7*); Vol. 10. 1971. (Illus.). x, 132p. 48.00 (*3-8055-1285-6*); Vol. 13. 1974. 300p. 121.00 (*3-8055-1741-6*); Vol. 14. 1975. x, 192p. 80.00 (*3-8055-2181-2*) S Karger.

Progress in Surgery, Vol. 15. Ed. by U. F. Gruber et al. 1977. 60.00 (*3-8055-2365-3*) S Karger.

Progress in Surgery of the Liver, Pancreas & Biliary System. Ed. by Stig Bengmark. 1988. (Developments in Surgery Ser.). (C). text 271.50 (*0-89838-956-9*) Kluwer Academic.

Progress in Surgical Pathology. 1992. 149.00 (*0-387-54130-6*) Spr-Verlag.

Progress in Surgical Pathology, Vol. 6. Cecilia M. Fenoglio-Preiser et al. 1988. 400p. (C). text (*0-938607-00-6*) Macmillan.

Progress in Surgical Pathology. Cecilia M. Fenoglio-Preiser. Vol. 9. 1989. 75.00 (*0-938607-11-1*); Vol. 10. 1989. 75.00 (*0-938607-14-6*); Vol. 11. 1990. 85.00 (*0-938607-31-6*) Field & Wood Inc Medical.

Progress in the Characterization of Venoms & Standardization of Antivenoms. WHO Staff. 1981. (WHO Offset Publications: No. 58). 44p. 6.00 (*92-4-170058-0*) World Health.

Progress in the Chemistry of Organic Natural Products, Vol. 36. Ed. by W. Herz et al. 1979. (Illus.). 157.95 (*0-387-81472-8*) Spr-Verlag.

Progress in the Development & Use of Antiviral Drugs & Interferon. 1987. (Technical Reports: No. 754). 25p. pap. 5.00 (*92-4-120754-X*, 1100754) World Health.

Progress in the Development of Cost-Effective Treatment for Drug Abusers. 1986. lib. bdg. 175.00 (*0-8490-3517-1*) Gordon Pr.

Progress in the Management of Endometriosis: The Proceedings of the 4th World Congress on Endometriosis, 1994. Ed. by E. M. Coutinho et al. 1995. (Illus.). 459p. 93.95 (*1-85070-651-4*, Parthenon Pbng) CRC Pr.

Progress in the Management of the Menopause: Proceedings of the 8th International Congress on the Menopause, Sydney, Australia, November, 1996. Ed. by Barry G. Wren. 1997. LC 97-34442. (Illus.). 508p. lib. bdg. 99.95 (*1-85070-799-5*, Parthenon Pbng) CRC Pr.

Progress in the Treatment of Fluency Disorders. Ed. by Lena Rustin et al. 1987. 330p. 62.25 (*1-56593-545-4*, 0066) Singular Publishing.

Progress in Thyroid Research: Proceedings of the 10th International Thyroid Conference, the Hague, 4-8 February 1991. Ed. by A. Gordon et al. 1991. 930p. (*90-5410-028-1*) A A Balkema NLD. *Dist:* Ashgate Pub Co.

Progress in Transfusion Medicine, No. 3. Ed. by John D. Cash. 1988. (Illus.). 232p. text (*0-443-03721-3*) Church.

Progress in Transplantation. A. Munakata. 2000. (International Congress Ser.). 132p. 72.50 (*0-444-50570-9*) Elsevier.

Progress in Tryptophan & Serotonin Research: Proceedings - Fourth Meeting of the International Study Group for Tryptophan Research (ISTRY) Ed. by H. G. Schlossberger et al. 1984. LC 84-1719. xix, 889p. 219.25 (*3-11-009760-5*) De Gruyter.

Progress in Vaccinology, Vol. 2. Ed. by Gursaran P. Talwar. 1989. (Illus.). 483p. 265.00 (*0-387-96734-6*) Spr-Verlag.

Progress Notes. Laskin. 1994. text 65.00 (*0-7216-5964-0*) Saunders.

Progress of Experiment: Science & Therapeutic Reform in the United States, 1900-1990. Harry M. Marks. 1997. LC 96-38997. (Cambridge History of Medicine Ser.). 271p. (C). text 64.95 (*0-521-58142-7*) Cambridge U Pr.

Progress on Biomechanics. Nuri Akkas. 1979. (NATO Advanced Study Institutes Ser.). 395p. text 122.00 (*90-286-0479-0*) Kluwer Academic.

Progress Report: An Investigation to Determine Whether the Built Environment Affects Patient's Medical Outcomes. Haya R. Rubin & Amanda J. Owens. 1996. 48p. (C). pap. text 19.00 (*0-9638938-3-1*) Ctr for Hlth.

Progress to Improved Movement: For Handicapped Children & Adults with Poor Posture. K. Hollis. 1985. 36p. 50.00 (*0-906054-17-6*) St Mut.

Progress to Standing: For Children with Severe Physical Handicap. K. Hollis. 1985. 24p. 50.00 (*0-906054-16-8*) St Mut.

Progress with Nucleic Acid Research & Molecular Biology, Vol. 49. Ed. by Waldo E. Cohn & Kivie Moldave. 1994. (Illus.). 394p. (C). text 100.00 (*0-12-540049-7*) Acad Pr.

Progresses of Aging: Social & Psychological Perspectives Ed. by Richard H. Williams et al. 1980. LC 79-8692. (Growing Old Ser.). reprint ed. lib. bdg. 113.95 (*0-405-12811-8*) Ayer.

Progression & Regression in Language: Sociocultural, Neuropsychological, & Linguistic Perspectives. Ed. by Kenneth Hyltenstam & Ake Viberg. 1994. LC 92-46241. 501p. (C). pap. text 34.95 (*0-521-43874-8*) Cambridge U Pr.

Progression of Chronic Renal Diseases. Ed. by H. Koide. 1996. LC 95-49917. (Contributions to Nephrology Ser.: Vol. 118). (Illus.). x, 270p. 198.25 (*3-8055-6243-8*) S Karger.

Progressive Casting & Splinting. Cusick. 1998. 58.00 (*0-12-784576-3*) Acad Pr.

Progressive Myoclonus Epilepsies. Frederick Andermann. Date not set. 19.95 (*0-7506-9199-9*) Buttrwrth-Heinemann.

Progressive Nature of Epileptogenesis. U. Heinemann. 1996. LC 96-41409. (Epilepsy Research Ser.). 408p. 238.50 (*0-444-82270-4*) Elsevier.

Progressive Nature of Renal Disease. William E. Mitch. 2nd ed. 1992. (Contemporary Issues in Nephrology Ser.: Vol. 26). 288p. text (*0-443-08819-5*) Church.

Progressive Nature of Renal Diseases: Myths & Facts. Ed. by L. Oldrizzi. 1989. (Contributions to Nephrology Ser.: Vol. 75). (Illus.). viii, 218p. 29.75 (*3-8055-5021-9*) S Karger.

Progressive Neuromuscular Diseases. Ed. by M. R. Dimitrijevic et al. 1986. (Limited Volume Ser.: Vol. 2). (Illus.). xii, 360p. 242.75 (*3-8055-4222-4*) S Karger.

Progressive Relaxation: A Physiological & Clinical Investigation of Muscular States & Their Significance in Psychology & Medical Practice. Edmund Jacobson. 3rd rev. ed. 1993. LC 38-13310. (Midway Reprint Ser.). xvii, 494p. reprint ed. pap. text 22.00 (*0-226-39059-4*) U Ch Pr.

Progressive Supranuclear Palsy: Clinical & Research Approaches. Ed. by Irene Litvan & Yves Agid. 1992. (Illus.). 304p. text 67.50 (*0-19-507229-4*) OUP.

Progressive Vitality & Dynamic Posture. J. Lawson-Wood & Denis Lawson-Wood. 1980. 50.00 (*0-85032-135-2*) St Mut.

Proinflammatory & Antiinflammatory Peptides. Sami Said & Federation of American Societies for Experimentation Staff. 1998. LC 97-47124. (Lung Biology in Health & Disease Ser.). (Illus.). 760p. text 215.00 (*0-8247-0120-8*) Dekker.

Project Based Group Work Facilitator's Manual: Participation in Practice. Andy Gibson. 1994. 200p. text 27.00 (*1-85302-169-5*) Taylor & Francis.

Project Focus, '93: Conference on Work-Related Injury. 1994. 77p. pap. 30.00 (*0-912452-96-X*, P-107) Am Phys Therapy Assn.

Project Focus, '96: The Conference on Sports Related Injury. Ed. by Holtzman, Robert, and Assoc, Inc. Staff. 1997. (Illus.). 84p. pap. 17.95 (*0-9628807-1-X*) FPT VA.

Project Management for Clinical Trials. Nancy J. Stark. 1999. (Safety, Efficacy & Performance of Medical Devices Ser.). 300p. ring bd. 200.00 (*1-889160-05-9*) Clinical Design.

Project SAEFP Workbook. Society of Teachers of Family Medicine Staff. 2nd ed. 1991. (Illus.). 489p. 75.00 (*0-942295-24-2*, 80) Soc Tchrs Fam Med.

Projection, Identification, Projective Identification. Ed. by Joseph Sandler. 1987. 35.00 (*0-8236-4370-0*) Intl Univs Pr.

Projections & Interface Conditions: Essays on Modularity. Ed. by Anna-Maria Di Sciullo. 1997. (Illus.). 272p. text 65.00 (*0-19-510414-5*) OUP.

Projections of National Health Expenditures. 1993. (Illus.). 57p. (Orig.). (C). pap. text 20.00 (*1-56806-367-9*) DIANE Pub.

Projections to the Spinal Cord of the Rat During Development: A Time-Table of Descent. E. A. Lakke. 1997. LC 96-39080. (Advances in Anatomy, Embryology & Cell Biology Ser.). (Illus.). 80p. pap. 78.00 (*3-540-61878-3*) Spr-Verlag.

Projective & Introjective Identification & the Use of the Therapist's Self. Jill S. Scharff. 1992. LC 91-26070. 344p. 50.00 (*0-87668-530-0*) Aronson.

Projective Identification & Psychotherapeutic Technique. Thomas H. Ogden. 1982. LC 81-67124. 256p. 45.00 (*0-87668-446-0*) Aronson.

Projective Psychodiagnostic Assessment. H. Stephen Caldwell & Stacey L. Dixon. 1992. 185p. (Orig.). pap. text 12.95 (*0-929240-49-9*) EMIS.

Projective Techniques & Cross-Cultural Research. Gardner Lindzey. 1976. LC 61-15951. (Century Psychology Ser.). reprint ed. 32.75 (*0-89197-361-3*); pap. text 12.95 (*0-89197-908-5*) Irvington.

Projective Techniques for Adolescents & Children. Albert I. Rabin. 1986. (Illus.). 384p. 44.95 (*0-8261-4920-0*) Springer Pub.

Projective Testing & Psychoanalysis. Roy Schafer. 1967. LC 67-15418. 229p. 34.50 (*0-8236-4380-8*) Intl Univs Pr.

Projective Use of Mother-&-Child Drawings: A Manual for Clinicians. Jacquelyn Gillespie. 1994. LC 94-11439. (Illus.). 168p. text 32.95 (*0-87630-736-5*) Brunner-Routledge.

Prokaryotic Genetics: Gene Transfer in Prokaryotes. F. Joset & J. Guespin. 1993. (Illus.). 416p. pap. 54.95 (*0-632-02728-2*) Blackwell Sci.

Prolactin Lesions in Breasts, Uterus, Prostate. Ed. by Hiroshi Nagasawa. 1988. 272p. 138.00 (*0-8493-6836-7*, RC280, CRC Reprint) Franklin.

Prolactinomas. Ed. by Jerrold M. Olefsky & Richard J. Robbins. 1985. (Contemporary Issues in Endocrinology & Metabolism Ser.: Vol. 2). (Illus.). 230p. text (*0-443-08406-8*) Church.

Prolegomena to the Psychological Study of Religion. Benjamin Beit-Hallahmi. 1989. LC 88-48020. 128p. 28.50 (*0-8387-5159-8*) Bucknell U Pr.

Proliferative Vitreoretinopathy - Epidemiology of Glaucoma. Ed. by W. Straub. 1989. (Developments in Ophthalmology Ser.: Vol. 16). (Illus.). viii, 118p. 99.25 (*3-8055-4853-2*) S Karger.

Proliferative Vitreoretinopathy (PVR) Ed. by H. M. Freeman & F. I. Tolentio. 1988. (Illus.). 197p. 140.00 (*0-387-96806-7*) Spr-Verlag.

Prolo Your Pain Away: Curing Chronic Pain with Prolotherapy. Ross A. Hauser et al. 1997. LC 99-166478. (Illus.). 252p. (Orig.). pap. 24.95 (*0-9661010-0-6*) Mann Daniel.

Prolo Your Sports Injuries Away! Curing Sports Injuries & Enhancing Athletic Performance with Prolotherapy. Ross A. Hauser & Marion A. Hauser. 2001. (Illus.). 800p. 99.00 (*0-9661010-1-4*) Mann Daniel.

Prolongation of Life: Optimistic Studies. Elie Metchnikoff. Ed. by Robert J. Kastenbaum. Tr. by P. Chalmers Mitchell. 1977. LC 76-19583. (Death & Dying Ser.). (Illus.). reprint ed. lib. bdg. 34.95 (*0-405-09579-1*) Ayer.

Promethean Fire: Reflections on the Origin of Mind. Charles J. Lumsden & Edward O. Wilson. 1983. (Illus.). 224p. 30.00 (*0-674-71445-8*) HUP.

Promise & the Power: Public Policy Analysis & the AIDS Movement. Neal A. Dickerson. 1993. LC 93-2597. (Politics of AIDS Ser.: Vol. 1). (Illus.). xii, 153p. (Orig.). pap. 12.00 (*0-930383-33-8*) Monument Pr.

Promise Is. Kip Zegers. 1985. LC 84-14. (Vox Humana Ser.). 96p. 14.95 (*0-89603-081-4*); pap. 11.95 (*0-89603-087-3*) Humana.

Promise of a New Day. Karen Casey & Martha Vanceburg. 2nd ed. 1996. (Meditation Ser.). (Illus.). 400p. (Orig.). pap. 10.00 (*0-89486-203-0*) Hazelden.

Promise of Cognitive Psychology. Richard E. Mayer. 1990. (Illus.). 136p. (C). reprint ed. pap. text 20.50 (*0-8191-7653-2*) U Pr of Amer.

Promise of the Fountain: Health Secrets for Life, Longevity & Freedom from Fear of Disease. Michael Capria. 1993. (Illus.). 264p. (Orig.). pap. text 15.95 (*0-9638492-0-4*) Plumosa Pr.

Promise of Youth: Follow-up Studies of a Thousand Gifted Children. Barbara S. Burks et al. 1930. (Genetic Studies of Genius: Vol. III). xiv, 508p. 72.00 (*0-8047-0011-7*) Stanford U Pr.

Promises to Keep: The Family's Role in Nursing Home Care. Katherine L. Karr. 1991. LC 91-7990. (Golden Age Bks.). (Illus.). 127p. (C). pap. 21.00 (*0-87975-661-6*) Prometheus Bks.

Promising (Drug) Prevention Strategies: A Look at What Works. 1992. (Illus.). 54p. (Orig.). pap. text 20.00 (*1-56806-092-0*) DIANE Pub.

***Promising Practices in Children's Mental Health Vol. I: Cultural Strengths & Challenges in Implementing a System of Care Model in American Indian Communities.** Terry L. Cross. 2001. 94p. (C). pap. text 20.00 (*0-7567-1363-3*) DIANE Pub.

***Promising Practices in Children's Mental Health Vol. II: Using Evaluation Data to Manage, Improve, Market & Sustain Children's Services.** Michelle W. Woodbridge & Larke N. Huang. 2001. (Illus.). 145p. (C). pap. text 30.00 (*0-7567-1364-1*) DIANE Pub.

***Promising Practices in Children's Mental Health Vol. III: For the Long Haul: Maintaining Systems of Care Beyond the Federal Investment.** Chris Koyanagi & Darienne Feres-Merchant. 2001. 83p. (C). pap. text 20.00 (*0-7567-1365-X*) DIANE Pub.

***Promising Practices in Children's Mental Health Vol. V: Training Strategies for Serving Children with Serious Emotional Disturbance & Their Families in a System of Care.** Judith Meyers et al. 2002. 112p. reprint ed. pap. text 30.00 (*0-7567-1366-8*) DIANE Pub.

***Promising Practices in Children's Mental Health Vol. VI: Building Collaboration in Systems of Care.** Sharon Hodges et al. 2002. 88p. (C). reprint ed. pap. text 20.00 (*0-7567-1367-6*) DIANE Pub.

***Promising Practices in Children's Mental Health Vol. VII: A Compilation of Lessons Learned from the 22 Grantees of the 1997 Comprehensive Community Mental Health Services for Children & Their Families Program.** Frwd. by Nelba Chavez & Bernard Arons. 2002. (Illus.). 124p. (C). reprint ed. pap. text 30.00 (*0-7567-1368-4*) DIANE Pub.

Promocion de la Salud y la Educacion para la Salud en America Latina: Un Analisis Sectorial. Hiram V. Arroyo & Maria T. Cerqueira. 1997. 330p. pap. 16.95 (*0-8477-0295-2*) U of PR Pr.

Promoting a Fighting Spirit: Psychotherapy for Cancer Patients, Survivors & Their Families. Linda Seligman. 1996. LC 95-32119. (Health Ser.). 360p. 39.00 (*0-7879-0190-3*) Jossey-Bass.

Promoting Change Through Brief Therapy in Christian Counseling. Gary J. Oliver et al. 1997. LC 97-25133. (AACC Counseling Library Ser.). 287p. 24.99 (*0-8423-5059-4*) Tyndale Hse.

Promoting Change Through Paradoxical Therapy. Ed. by Gerald R. Weeks. rev. ed. 1991. LC 91-10961. 336p. pap. text 39.95 (*0-87630-645-8*) Brunner-Routledge.

Promoting Children's Health: Progress Report of the Child Health Workgroup Board of Scientific Counselors with New Guidance for Toxilogical Profiles. Frwd. by Jeffrey P. Koplan. 2000. 127p. pap. 25.00 (*0-7881-8924-7*) DIANE Pub.

Promoting Cognitive Growth over the Life Span. Ed. by M. Schwebel et al. 1990. 256p. text 69.95 (*0-8058-0663-6*) L Erlbaum Assocs.

Promoting Community Health. Sidney Kark & Emily Kark. 1999. LC 99-225076. (*1-86814-316-3*) Witwatersrand U.

Promoting Community Health: The Role of the Academic Health Center. Ed. by W. Douglas Skelton & Marian Osterweis. 1993. LC 92-75185. 306p. (Orig.). pap. 25.00 (*1-879694-05-0*) AAH Ctrs.

Promoting Continence. Kathryn Getliffe. 1996. (C). pap. text 69.95 (*0-7020-1963-1*) Harcourt.

***Promoting Creativity Across the Life Span.** Ed. by Martin Bloom & Thomas Gullotta. 2001. LC 2001-25530. (Illus.). vii, 321p. (*0-87868-811-0*, CWLA Pr) Child Welfare.

Promoting Cultural Competence in Systems of Care. Ed. by Mario Hernandez & Mareasa Isaacs. 1998. LC 98-8149. (Systems of Care for Children's Mental Health Ser.). text 32.95 (*1-55766-287-8*, 2878) P H Brookes.

Promoting Cultural Diversity: Strategies for Health Care Professionals. Kathryn H. Kavanagh & Patricia H. Kennedy. 1992. 175p. (C). pap. 26.95 (*0-8039-4657-0*, 3416) Sage.

Promoting Early Communication 1 - Prelinguistics Communication: A Module for Training Personnel Serving Families of Deaf & Hard of Hearing Infants & Young Children. Ed. by Valerie Schuyler. 1993. (Early Intervention Ser.). 31p. (C). 89.00 incl. VHS (*0-9618297-6-1*) Hearing & Speech.

Promoting Early Communication 2, The Role of the Family: A Module for Training Personnel Serving Families of Deaf & Hard of Hearing Infants & Young Children. Ed. by Valerie Schuyler. 1993. (Early Intervention Ser.). 36p. (C). 89.00 incl. VHS (*0-9618297-7-X*) Hearing & Speech.

Promoting Employee Health: A Guide for Worksite Wellness. Rebecca Anderson. 1986. 73p. 20.00 (*0-939874-74-1*) ASSE.

Promoting Health: A Practical Guide. Ewles. 4th ed. 1999. (C). pap. text 29.00 (*0-7020-2308-6*) Harcourt.

Promoting Health & Mental Health in Children, Youth, & Families. Ed. by David S. Glenwick & Leonard A. Jason. 1993. LC 93-14539. (Behavior Therapy & Behavioral Medicine Ser.). 280p. 39.95 (*0-8261-7310-1*) Springer Pub.

Promoting Health & Preventing Disease. Ed. by Marian Osterweis et al. 1992. LC 92-7351. (Health Policy Annual Ser.: Vol. II). 250p. (Orig.). 20.00 (*1-879694-04-2*) AAH Ctrs.

Promoting Health in Multicultural Populations: A Handbook for Practitioners. Robert M. Huff & Michael V. Kline. LC 98-25455. xvii, 554p. 1999. 96.95 (*0-7619-0182-5*, 1997); 1998. pap. 44.95 (*0-7619-0183-3*, 1998) Sage.

Promoting Health in Old Age: Critical Issues in Self Health Care. Miriam Bernard. 2000. LC 99-42447. (Rethinking Ageing Ser.). 224p. pap. (*0-335-19247-5*) OpUniv Pr.

Promoting Health in the Workplace. Patricia A. McPartland. 1991. xiv, 266p. (C). text 58.00 (*3-7186-0528-7*) Gordon & Breach.

Promoting Health Promotion: Anatomy of a Hospital-Based Approach. Ed. & Tr. by Norbert Reinstein. 2nd ed. 2000. (Illus.). 180p. pap. 15.95 (*1-888822-09-0*) Singlish Pub.

Promoting Health Systems Research as a Management Tool. Ann Brownlee. 1992. 145p. pap. (*0-88936-583-0*) IDRC-CRDI CAN. *Dist:* Stylus Pub VA.

Promoting Health Through Part H: Promoting the Health of Infants & Toddlers with Disabilities Through Part H of the Individuals with Disabilities Evaluation Act. NEC-TAS Health Focus Group Staff & Emily Fenichel. 1991. 49p. (Orig.). pap. 7.00 (*0-943657-17-2*) ZERO TO THREE.

Promoting Health Through the Schools: A Challenge for the Eighties: A Special Issue of Health Education Quarterly, Vol. 8, No. 1. Ed. by Donald C. Iverson. 1981. LC 80-81022. 120p. pap. 16.95 (*0-89885-104-1*, Kluwer Acad Hman Sci) Kluwer Academic.

Promoting Healthy Aging: A Nursing & Community Perspective. Ann C. Beckingham. 1993. 496p. (C). (gr. 13). pap. text 30.00 (*0-8016-0916-X*, 00916) Mosby Inc.

***Promoting Healthy Behavior: How Much Freedom? Whose Responsibility?** Ed. by Daniel Callahan. 2001. (Hastings Center Studies in Ethics). 192p. pap. 19.95 (*0-87840-853-3*) Georgetown U Pr.

Promoting Healthy Diets & Active Lifestyles to Lower-Ses Adults: Market Research for Public Education. 1994. lib. bdg. 250.00 (*0-8490-5747-7*) Gordon Pr.

Promoting Human Wellness: New Frontiers for Research, Practice & Policy. Ed. by Margaret S. Jamner & Daniel Stokols. 2000. LC 99-87690. (Illus.). xii, 737p. pap. 35.00 (*0-520-22609-7*) U CA Pr.

Promoting Human Wellness: New Frontiers for Research, Practice & Policy. Ed. by Margaret Schneider Jamner & Daniel Stokols. 2000. LC 99-87690. (Illus.). 749p. text 60.00 (*0-520-22608-9*) U CA Pr.

Promoting Legal Awareness in Physical & Occupational Therapy. Ron Scott. 1996. LC 96-33589. (Illus.). 328p. (gr. 13). text 35.00 (*0-8151-7996-0*, 26653) Mosby Inc.

Promoting Men's Health. Ed. by Neil Davidson & Trefor Lloyd. 2000. (Illus.). 304p. pap. text (*0-7020-2416-3*) W B Saunders GBR. *Dist:* Saunders.

Promoting Palliative Care: Sociological & Policy Perspectives. P. Clark. 1999. LC 98-28627. (Facing Death Ser.). viii, 213p. (*0-335-19455-9*) OpUniv Pr.

Promoting Safer Sex. Ed. by M. Paalman. 1990. x, 252p. (*90-265-1012-8*) Swets.

Promoting Social/Emotional Development: The PATHS Project. Greenberg. 1993. LC 93-15605. 240p. 50.00 (*0-295-97227-0*) U of Wash Pr.

Promoting Speech Development: A Module for Training Personnel Serving Families of Deaf & Hard of Hearing Infants & Young Children. Ed. by Valerie Schuyler. 1993. (Early Intervention Ser.). 40p. (C). 89.00 incl. VHS (*0-9618297-8-8*) Hearing & Speech.

Promoting Successful Breastfeeding. Marie Comberford Biancuzzo. 1998. LC 98-42525. (Illus.). 480p. (C). (gr. 13). pap. text 26.95 (*0-8151-2453-8*, 31178) Mosby Inc.

Promoting Teamwork in Primary Care. 240p. pap. (*0-340-65244-6*) E A GBR. *Dist:* Routldge.

Promoting the Health of the Nation. Kendall. 1995. (C). pap. text 50.00 (*0-443-05225-5*) Saunders.

Promoting the Profession: A Resource Guide for Marketing & Publicizing Occupational Therapy. Ed. by Suzanne Carlton & Crystal W. Brockington. 1993. 129p. (Orig.). pap. text 16.00 (*1-56900-002-6*) Am Occup Therapy.

Promoting Tissue Regeneration Potency & Mechanism of Natural Products: Muscle Regeneration. Xuhui Wang & Sophie Chen. 1993. (CHI., Illus.). (Orig.). pap. 65.00 (*0-9636432-0-7*) Int Med Res.

Promotion & Development of Traditional Medicine: Report of a WHO Meeting, 1978. 1978. (Technical Report Ser.: No. 622). 40p. pap. text 5.00 (*92-4-120622-5*, 1100622) World Health.

Promotion of Medical Practitioners' Interest in Preventive Medicine. 1964. (Technical Report Ser.: No. 269). 22p. pap. text 3.00 (*92-4-120269-6*) World Health.

Promotion of Mental Health, 1995. Ed. by Colin Reed & Dennis R. Trent. 1996. (Mental Health Promotion Unit Ser.: No. 5). 429p. pap. (*1-85972-284-9*) Avebry GBR. *Dist:* Ashgate Pub Co.

Promotion of Mental Health, 1996. Ed. by Denis R. Trent & Colin A. Reed. 1997. 368p. text (*1-85972-652-6*) Avebry GBR. *Dist:* Ashgate Pub Co.

Promotion of Mental Health, 1991, Vol. 1. Dennis R. Trent. 1992. (Mental Health Promotion Unit Ser.). 356p. (*1-85628-307-0*) Avebry GBR. *Dist:* Ashgate Pub Co.

Promotion of Mental Health, 1992, Vol. 2. Dennis R. Trent & Colin Reed. 1993. 662p. (*1-85628-430-1*) Avebry GBR. *Dist:* Ashgate Pub Co.

Promotion of Mental Health, 1994, Vol. 4. Ed. by Colin Reed & Dennis R. Trent. 1995. (Mental Health Promotion Unit Ser.). 560p. (*1-85972-065-X*) Avebry GBR. *Dist:* Ashgate Pub Co.

Promotion of Pharmaceuticals: Issues, Trends, Options. Ed. by Dev S. Pathak et al. 1993. LC 92-49617. (Journal of Pharmaceutical Marketing & Management Ser.: Vol. 7, No. 1). (Illus.). 203p. pap. text 19.95 (*1-56024-384-8*); lib. bdg. 49.95 (*1-56024-383-X*) Haworth Pr.

Promotion of Physical Activity in the Community: A Manual for Community Health Professionals. Health Promotion Resource Center Staff. Ed. by Abby C. King et al. 2nd ed. 1991. 86p. reprint ed. pap. 19.50 (*1-879552-19-1*) SCRDP.

Promotion of Wellness in Children & Adolescents. Ed. by Dante Cicchetti et al. 2000. LC 00-30364. (Illus.). xxvi, 515p. pap. 28.95 (*0-87868-791-2*, CWLA Pr) Child Welfare.

Proof, Herbs Against Cancer. Cynthia J. Sommers. 1993. LC 93-85420. (Illus.). 140p. (Orig.). pap. 13.95 (*0-9640193-0-2*) Red Wing Pubng.

Proof Positive: How to Reliably Combat Diseases & Achieve Optimal Health. Neil Nedley. Ed. by David De Rose. 1998. (Illus.). 560p. text 49.00 (*0-9661979-3-3*) Nedley Publishing.

Propachlor. 1993. (Environmental Health Criteria Ser.: No. 147). (ENG, FRE & SPA.). 110p. pap. text 26.00 (*92-4-157147-0*, 1160147) World Health.

Propagation of Mammalian Cells in Culture, Vol. I. J. D. Roth et al. 1976. text 39.50 (*0-8422-7290-9*) Irvington.

Propagations: Thirty Years of Influence from the Mental Research Institute. Ed. by Wendel A. Ray & John H. Weakland. 1995. LC 94-32743. 310p. (C). lib. bdg. 49.95 (*1-56024-936-6*) Haworth Pr.

Propecia: The Hair-Growth Breakthrough. Othneil J. Seiden. 1998. LC 98-12168. (Illus.). 256p. pap. 14.00 (*0-7615-1536-4*, Prima Health) Prima Pub.

Propedeutics of Children's Diseases. V. Molchanov et al. Tr. by Mir Publishers Staff from RUS. 1975. (Illus.). 392p. (C). 29.00 (*0-8464-0768-X*) Beekman Pubs.

Properties of Biomaterials in the Physiological Environment. Stephen D. Bruck. 1980. 160p. 110.00 (*0-8493-5685-7*, R857, CRC Reprint) Franklin.

Properties of Water in Foods in Relation to Quality & Stability. Ed. by D. Simatos & J. L. Multon. 1985. text 344.50 (*90-247-3153-4*) Kluwer Academic.

Prophetess of Health see Prophetess of Health: Ellen G. White & the Origins of Seventh-Day Adventist Health Reform

Prophetess of Health: Ellen G. White & the Origins of Seventh-Day Adventist Health Reform. Ed. by Ronald L. Numbers. 1992. LC 91-22807. Orig. Title: Prophetess of Health. (Illus.). 408p. (C). reprint ed. 49.95 (*0-87049-712-X*); pap. text 19.95 (*0-87049-713-8*) U of Tenn Pr.

Prophetic Analyst: Erich Fromm's Contributions to Psychoanalysis. Ed. by Maruicio Cortina & Michael Maccoby. 1996. LC 95-16850. 480p. 50.00 (*1-56821-621-1*) Aronson.

Prophetic Medical Sciences. Sehban Ul-Hind. Tr. by Badr Azimabadi. 1989. 350p. 29.00 (*1-56744-360-5*) Kazi Pubns.

Prophylaxis of Infectious & Other Diseases by Means of Vaccination & the Use of Immunoglobulins. Ed. by T. M. Inderbitzin. 1975. (Monographs in Allergy: Vol. 9). (Illus.). 300p. 66.25 (*3-8055-1779-3*) S Karger.

Propolis: Nature's Energizer. Carlson Wade. 1987. (Good Health Guides). 32p. (Orig.). pap. 2.95 (*0-87983-329-7*, Keats Pubng) McGraw-Hill Trade.

Propolis Power-Plus. Joan A. Friedrich & Carlson Wade. Ed. by Don R. Bensen. 1996. (Good Health Guides). 48p. pap. 3.95 (*0-87983-698-9*, 36989K, Keats Pubng) McGraw-Hill Trade.

Proposed National Strategies for the Prevention of Leading Work-Related Diseases & Injuries: 1988 Edition. 1994. 196p. (C). reprint ed. pap. text 50.00 (*0-7881-0452-7*) DIANE Pub.

Proposed Standard International Acupuncture Nomenclature: Report of a WHO Scientific Group. WHO Staff. 1991. 30p. 9.00 (*92-4-154417-1*) World Health.

Propositional Attitudes: An Essay on Thoughts & How We Ascribe Them. Mark Richard. 1990. (Cambridge Studies in Philosophy). (Illus.). 285p. (C). pap. text 28.95 (*0-521-38819-8*) Cambridge U Pr.

Proprioceptive Neuromuscular Facilitation. Dorothy E. Voss & Marjorie K. Ionta. 3rd ed. 1985. LC 84-25958. (Illus.). 370p. text 47.00 (*0-06-142595-8*, Lppncott) Lppncott W & W.

Propylene Oxide. 1986. (Environmental Health Criteria Ser.: No. 56). 53p. pap. text 11.70 (*92-4-154196-2*, 1160056) World Health.

Prosecution of False Memory. Makram K. Girgis. 2000. pap. 22.95 (*0-87527-528-1*) Green.

Prosecution of the Mentally Disturbed: Dilemmas of Identification & Discretion. D. Chiswick et al. 1984. 192p. text 35.90 (*0-08-028481-7*, Pergamon Pr) Elsevier.

Prosecutorial Response to Heavy Drug Caseloads: Comprehensive Problem-Reduction Strategies. Kerry M. Healey & Barbara Boland. 1994. (Illus.). 106p. (Orig.). (C). pap. text 35.00 (*0-7881-1304-6*) DIANE Pub.

Prosody Management of Communicative Disorders. Patricia M. Hargrove & Nancy S. McGarr. 1993. (Illus.). 332p. (Orig.). (C). pap. text 49.95 (*1-879105-88-8*, 0351) Thomson Learn.

Prospecting for Drugs in Ancient & Medieval European Texts: A Scientific Approach. Ed. by Bart K. Holland. 1996. 182p. text 65.00 (*3-7186-5928-X*, Harwood Acad Pubs) Gordon & Breach.

Prospective Community Studies in Developing Countries. Ed. by Monica Das Gupta et al. 1998. (International Studies in Demography). (Illus.). 358p. text 85.00 (*0-19-829209-0*) OUP.

Prospective Issues in Infancy Research. Ed. by Kathleen Bloom. 1981. LC 80-17479. 208p. text 39.95 (*0-89859-059-0*) L Erlbaum Assocs.

Prospective Memory: Theory & Applications. Ed. by Maria Brandimonte et al. 1996. 432p. text 79.95 (*0-8058-1536-8*) L Erlbaum Assocs.

Prospective Payment for Home Health Agencies. Judith J. Baker. 1998. LC 98-38051. 300p. 69.00 (*0-8342-1111-4*, 11114) Aspen Pub.

Prospective Payment for Long Term Care 2001-2002. Judith J. Baker. 2000. 479p. ring bd. 145.00 (*0-8342-1799-6*) Aspen Pub.

Prospective Payment Systems for Inpatient Hospital Services Fiscal Year 1998 Regulations & Rates: Final Rule with Provider Reimbursement Provisions from the Balanced Budget Act of 1997. Ed. by CCH Editorial Staff. 1997. LC 98-170465. 256p. pap. 18.00 (*0-8080-0158-2*) CCH INC.

Prospective Payments & Hospital Discharge Planning with Older Adults. Cynthia Stuen. rev. ed. 1991. LC 91-30937. (Studies on the Elderly in America). 208p. text 30.00 (*0-8153-0516-8*) Garland.

Prospective Studies of Crime & Deliquency. Katherine Teilmann Van Dusen & Sarnoff A. Mednick. 1983. LC 83-178. (Longitudinal Research in the Behavioral, Social, & Medical Sciences Ser.). lib. bdg. 139.50 (*0-89838-131-2*) Kluwer Academic.

Prospectives: Celebrating 40 Years of AD Nursing Education. Ed. by Jean A. Simmons. 1993. 9.95 (*0-88737-576-6*, 23-2517) Natl League Nurse.

Prospects in Diagnosis & Treatment of Breast Cancer. Ed. by Manfred Schmitt et al. 1994. LC 94-13767. (International Congress Ser.: No. 1050). 252p. 183.00 (*0-444-81707-7*, Excerpta Medica) Elsevier.

Prospects of Eternity. Russell. 1982. 188p. (*0-85435-394-1*) C W Daniel GBR. *Dist:* Natl Bk Netwk.

Prospects of Heart Surgery. Alan Radley. 1988. (Contributions to Psychology & Medicine Ser.). (Illus.). 246p. 116.00 (*0-387-96721-4*) Spr-Verlag.

Prosper Lucas's "On the Heredity of Mental Illness" (1850) Prosper Lucas. Ed. by Charles D. Mellon. Tr. by Linda F. Mellon from FRE. 1996. LC 96-94516. (Illus.). 83p. 29.50 (*0-9653362-1-2*) Genetics Heritage.

Prostacyclin & Hypertension. Gerd Bonner & K. H. Rahn. 1990. (Illus.). 104p. 17.95 (*0-387-52140-2*) Spr-Verlag.

Prostacyclin & Its Receptors. Helen D. Wise & Robert L. Jones. 1999. LC 99-52122. ix, 310p. (*0-306-46308-3*, Kluwer Plenum) Kluwer Academic.

Prostaglandin. 1988. 69.95 (*0-387-50098-7*) Spr-Verlag.

Prostaglandin & Fertility Regulation. Ed. by M. Toppozada et al. 1984. (Advances in Reproductive Health Care Ser.). text 225.00 (*0-85200-804-X*) Kluwer Academic.

Prostaglandin & Lipid Metabolism in Radiation Injury. Ed. by T. L. Walden, Jr. & H. N. Hughes. 1988. LC 87-32663. (Illus.). 434p. 110.00 (*0-306-42793-1*, Plenum Trade) Perseus Pubng.

Prostaglandin Inhibitors in Tumor Immunology & Immunotherapy. Jules E. Harris. 1994. 256p. 249.00 (*0-8493-6903-7*, QR188) CRC Pr.

Prostaglandins: Biology & Chemistry of Prostaglandins & Related Eicosanoids. Ed. by P. B. Curtis-Prior. 1988. (Illus.). 720p. text (*0-443-02519-3*) Church.

Prostaglandins & Arachidonate Metabolites. Ed. by Sidney P. Colowick & William E. Lands. 1982. LC 82-6791. (Methods in Enzymology Ser.: Vol. 86). text 188.00 (*0-12-181986-8*) Acad Pr.

Prostaglandins & Control of Vascular Smooth Muscle Cell Proliferation. Ed. by K. Schror et al. 1997. (Agents & Actions Supplements Ser.: Vol. 48). 129p. 56.50 (*3-7643-5689-8*) Birkhauser.

Prostaglandins & Eicosanoids. Curtis. text (*0-471-48984-0*) Wiley.

Prostaglandins & Immunity. Ed. by James S. Goodwin. 1985. LC 85-4989. (Prostaglandins, Leukotrienes, & Cancer Ser.: No. 4). text 113.50 (*0-89838-723-X*) Kluwer Academic.

Prostaglandins & Inflammation. Ed. by Kim D. Rainsford & A. Ford-Hutchinson. 1980. (Agents & Actions Supplements Ser.: No. 6). (Illus.). 242p. 69.50 (*0-8176-1132-0*) Birkhauser.

Prostaglandins & Other Eicosanoids in the Cardiovascular System. Ed. by K. Schroer. 1985. (Illus.). xiv, 570p. pap. 143.50 (*3-8055-4007-8*) S Karger.

Prostaglandins & the Kidney. Ed. by R. Horton & M. J. Dunn. 1981. (Journal: Vol. 6, No. 1-2). (Illus.). 104p. pap. 61.00 (*3-8055-3406-X*) S Karger.

Prostaglandins & the Kidney: Biochemistry, Physiology, Pharmacology & Clinical Applications. Ed. by Michael J. Dunn et al. 1982. LC 82-18117. 438p. 95.00 (*0-306-41054-0*, Kluwer Plenum) Kluwer Academic.

Prostaglandins & the Uterus. Ed. by J. O. Drife & A. A. Calder. 1992. (Illus.). 301p. 172.00 (*0-387-19719-2*) Spr-Verlag.

Prostaglandins in Bone Resorption. Ed. by Wilson Harvey. 1987. 144p. 87.00 (*0-8493-5591-5*, QP88, CRC Reprint) Franklin.

Prostaglandins in Cancer Research: Proceedings. Ed. by E. Garaci et al. 1987. (Life Sciences Ser.). (Illus.). 288p. 108.00 (*0-387-17548-2*) Spr-Verlag.

Prostaglandins in Cardiovascular & Renal Function. Ed. by Alexander Scriabine et al. 1980. (Monographs of the Physiology. Soc. of Phila.: Vol. 6). (Illus.). 481p. text 75.00 (*0-88331-186-0*) R B Luce.

Prostaglandins in the Cardiovascular System. Ed. by K. Schror & Helmet F. Sinzinger. 1992. (Agents & Actions Supplements Ser.: Vol. 37). 390p. 120.50 (*0-8176-2701-4*) Birkhauser.

Prostaglandins, Leukotrienes, & Lipoxins. Ed. by J. Martyn Bailey. 1985. LC 85-16941. (GWUMC Department of Biochemistry & Molecular Biology Annual Spring Symposium Ser.). 722p. 150.00 (*0-306-41980-7*, Plenum Trade) Perseus Pubng.

Prostaglandins, Leukotrienes, & the Immune Response. John L. Ninneman. 1988. (Illus.). 240p. text 69.95 (*0-521-33483-7*) Cambridge U Pr.

Prostaglandins, Leukotrienes, Lipoxins & PAF: Mechanisms of Action, Molecular Biology & Clinical Applications. J. M. Bailey. 1992. (GWUMC Department of Biochemistry & Molecular Biology Annual Spring Symposium Ser.). (Illus.). 448p. (C). text 123.00 (*0-306-44055-5*, Kluwer Plenum) Kluwer Academic.

Prostaglandins, Prostacyclin, Thromboxanes Measurement. Ed. by J. M. Boeynaems & A. G. Herman. 1980. (Developments in Pharmacology Ser.: No. 1.). (Illus.). 209p. text 101.50 (*90-247-2417-1*) Kluwer Academic.

Prostanoids & Drugs. Ed. by Bengt Samuelsson et al. 1990. LC 89-22775. (NATO ASI Series A, Life Sciences: Vol. 177). (Illus.). 270p. 89.50 (*0-306-43330-3*, Plenum Trade) Perseus Pubng.

Prostate. Ed. by John M. Fitzpatrick & Robert J. Kane. 1989. (Illus.). 464p. text (*0-443-03558-X*) Church.

Prostate: A Guide for Men & the Women Who Love Them. Patrick C. Walsh & Janet F. Worthington. 1995. LC 94-33397. (Health Bks.). (Illus.). 344p. 45.00 (*0-8018-4988-8*) Johns Hopkins.

Prostate: A Guide for Men & the Women Who Love Them. Patrick C. Walsh & Janet F. Worthington. 1997. (Illus.). 464p. mass mkt. (*0-446-60432-1*) Warner.

Prostate: A Guide for Men & the Women Who Love Them. Janet F. Worthington & Patrick C. Walsh. 1995. LC 94-33397. (Health Bks.). (Illus.). 344p. pap. 16.95 (*0-8018-4989-6*) Johns Hopkins.

Prostate: Basic & Clinical Aspects. Rajesh K. Naz. 1997. LC 96-49184. 400p. 104.95 (*0-8493-3159-5*) CRC Pr.

Prostate: Guides to Clinical Aspiration Biopsy. Tilde S. Kline. 1985. LC 84-12957. (Illus.). 200p. 72.50 (*0-89640-106-5*) Igaku-Shoin.

Prostate: Questions You Have, Answers You Need. Sandra Salmans. 2nd rev. ed. 1996. LC 96-28223. (Illus.). 192p. pap. 12.95 (*1-882606-63-9*) Peoples Med Soc.

***Prostate - Small Gland, Big Problem.** Roger S. Kirby. 2001. 92p. pap. (*1-899541-74-8*) Health Pr GBR. *Dist:* JAMCO Dist.

Prostate Accessory Male Sex Gland. S. Battaglia. 1986. (Journal: Vol. 3, No. 4). (Illus.). iv, 72p. pap. 52.25 (*3-8055-4464-2*) S Karger.

Prostate & Cancer: A Family Guide to Diagnosis, Treatment & Survival. Sheldon Marks. 3rd rev. ed. LC 99-37432. (Illus.). 2000. 343p. pap. 18.50 (*1-55561-262-8*); 1999. 360p. pap. 14.95 (*1-55561-206-7*) Fisher Bks.

Prostate & Finasteride: Index of New Information with Authors, Subjects, & References. Patrick J. Mullin. 1996. LC 96-12486. 57.50 (*0-7883-1040-2*); pap. 47.50 (*0-7883-1041-0*) ABBE Pubs Assn.

Prostate & Male Health: Index of New Information with Authors & Subjects. Virginia L. Jensen. 1992. 180p. 47.50 (*1-55914-702-4*); pap. 44.50 (*1-55914-703-2*) ABBE Pubs Assn.

Prostate Answer Book. Roberta Altman. 1993. 176p. (Orig.). mass mkt. 5.50 (*0-446-36408-8*) Warner Bks.

Prostate As an Endocrine Gland. Ed. by Richard J. Ablin. 1989. 232p. 129.00 (*0-8493-5364-5*, QP257) CRC Pr.

Prostate Book. Stephen Rous. 3rd rev. ed. 2001. LC 00-52714. (Illus.). 288p. 26.95 (*0-393-05010-6*) Norton.

Prostate Brachtherapy Made Complicated. Kent Wallner et al. l.t. ed. 1997. (Illus.). 325p. text 155.00 (*0-9648991-1-6*) SmartMedicine.

Prostate Cancer. Colin Buck. 1995. (Questions & Answers Ser.). (Illus.). 120p. pap. 10.95 (*1-873413-85-8*) Merit Pub Intl.

Prostate Cancer. Peter R. Carroll. 2000. (ACS Atlas of Clinical Oncology Ser.). 400p. incl. cd-rom (*1-55009-130-1*) DEKR.

Prostate Cancer. Ed. by Nancy A. Dawson & Nicholas J. Vogelzang. 1994. LC 93-44295. (Current Clinical Oncology Ser.). 300p. 142.00 (*0-471-58834-2*, Wiley-Liss) Wiley.

Prostate Cancer. Richard E. Peschel. Ed. by Marc S. Ernstoff et al. 1998. LC 98-119236. 240p. 75.00 (*0-632-04317-2*) Blackwell Sci.

***Prostate Cancer.** Kirby et al. 3rd ed. 2000. (Fast Facts Ser.). (Illus.). 76p. pap. (*1-899541-14-4*) Health Pr GBR. *Dist:* JAMCO Dist.

Prostate Cancer: A Multidisciplinary Guide. Philip W. Kantoff et al. 1996. LC 96-39071. (Illus.). 281p. (Orig.). pap. 54.95 (*0-86542-456-X*) Blackwell Sci.

Prostate Cancer: A Non-Surgical Perspective. Kent Wallner. LC 95-90687. (Illus.). (Orig.). l.t. ed. 1996. 172p. pap. 15.95 (*0-9648991-0-8*); 2nd l.t. rev. ed. 2000. 230p. pap. 18.95 (*0-9648991-3-2*) SmartMedicine.

Prostate Cancer: A Survivor's Guide. Donald F. Kaltenbach & Tim Richards. 3rd rev. ed. 1996. (Illus.). 296p. pap. 16.95 (*0-9640088-2-3*) Seneca Hse.

Prostate Cancer: All You Need to Know to Take an Active Part in Your Treatment. S. Larry Goldenberg. 2nd rev. ed. 1997. (Illus.). 197p. pap. text (*0-9696125-3-2*) ITPG.

Prostate Cancer: Biology, Genetics & the New Therapeutics. Ed. by Leland W. K. Chung et al. 2001. LC 00-40712. (Contemporary Cancer Research Ser.). (Illus.). xviii, 531p. 145.00 (*0-89603-868-8*) Humana.

Prostate Cancer: Cell & Molecular Mechanisms in Diagnosis & Treatment. Ed. by J. T. Isaacs. 1991. (Cancer Surveys Ser.: Vol. 11). (Illus.). 287p. (C). text 60.00 (*0-87969-368-1*) Cold Spring Harbor.

Prostate Cancer: Current Issues, New Approaches. Ed. by R. S. Kirby. 1996. (Journal: Vol. 29, No. 2, 1996). (Illus.). iv, 136p. pap., suppl. ed. 50.50 (*3-8055-6314-0*) S Karger.

***Prostate Cancer: Diagnosis & Surgical Treatment.** Ed. by R. Hofmann et al. 2001. (Illus.). 300p. pap. 99.00 incl. cd-rom (*3-540-42019-3*) Spr-Verlag.

Prostate Cancer: Hormonal Treatment & Treatment of Advanced Disease. Ed. by Donald W. Newling. 1994. (Journal: Vol. 26, Suppl. 1, 1994). (Illus.). iv, 34p. pap. 21.75 (*3-8055-6111-3*) S Karger.

Prostate Cancer: Making Survival Decisions. Sylvan Meyer & Seymour C. Nash. 1994. LC 94-25487. 284p. 19.95 (*0-226-56857-1*) U Ch Pr.

Prostate Cancer: New Approaches to Endocrine Therapy. Ed. by P. H. Smith. 1990. (Journal: Vol. 18, Supplement 3, 1990). (Illus.). iv, 68p. pap. 21.75 (*3-8055-5336-6*) S Karger.

Prostate Cancer: Overcoming Denial with Action: A Guide to Screening, Treatment & Healing. Allen E. Salowe. 1998. 224p. pap. 14.95 (*0-312-18159-0*, St Martin Griffin) St Martin.

Prostate Cancer: Overcoming Denial with Action: A Guide to Screening, Treatment & Healing. Allen E. Salowe & Leon M. Lessinge. 1997. LC 96-50460. 205p. 15.00 (*1-57626-023-2*) Quality Med Pub.

Prostate Cancer: Potraits of Empowerment. Ed. by Nadine Jelsing. 1999. LC 98-45154. 304p. (ps-3). pap. text 14.00 (*0-8133-6657-7*) Westview.

Prostate Cancer: Principles & Practice. Philip Kantoff et al. 2001. text 159.00 (*0-7817-2006-0*) Lppncott W & W.

Prostate Cancer: Treatment & Recovery. Richard Y. Handy. 1996. LC 96-18737. 251p. pap. text 21.00 (*1-57392-074-6*) Prometheus Bks.

***Prostate Cancer - Second Opinions: A Survey of Treatment Specialists.** 2002. 251p. pap. 16.95 (*0-9651827-6-2*) Proste Cancer.

Prostate Cancer & Bone Metastasis. J. P. Karr & H. Yamanaka. 1992. (Advances in Experimental Medicine & Biology Ser.: Vol. 324). (Illus.). 334p. (C). text 95.00 (*0-306-44314-7*, Kluwer Plenum) Kluwer Academic.

Prostate Cancer Answer Book. Marion Morra & Eve Potts. 1996. LC 96-5684. pap. 12.50 (*0-380-78564-1*, Avon Bks) Morrow Avon.

Prostate Cancer Detection & Cure. A. M. Durrani. Ed. by Pete Billac. 1997. LC 97-66581. (Illus.). 120p. (Orig.). pap. 9.95 (*0-943629-30-6*) Swan Pub.

Prostate Cancer, '96. Kirby. 1996. text (*0-7234-2050-5*) Wolfe Publishing GBR. *Dist:* Mosby Inc.

Prostate Cancer Patient Outcomes & Choice of Providers: Development of an Infrastructure for Quality Assessment. Mark Litwin et al. 2000. LC 00-709332. (Illus.). ix, 248p. (C). pap. 37.50 (*0-8330-2873-1*) Rand Corp.

Prostate Cancer Protection Plan: The Powerful Foods, Supplements & Drugs That Could Save Your Life. Robert Burns Arnot. l.t. ed. 2000. LC 00-61587. (Basic Ser.). 485p. 29.95 (*0-7862-2926-8*, Thorndike) Gale.

Prostate Cancer Screening. Ed. by Ian M. Thompson et al. 2001. LC 00-44884. (Current Clinical Urology Ser.). 328p. 99.50 (*0-89603-901-3*) Humana.

Prostate Cancer Sourcebook: How to Make Informed Treatment Choices. Marcus H. Loo & Marian Betancourt. 1998. LC 97-33001. 256p. pap. 15.95 (*0-471-15927-1*) Wiley.

Prostate Cancer Treatment Options: A Guide to the Basics. Will Connell. 2000. LC 99-95100. (Illus.). xiv, 220p. pap. 19.95 (*0-9673892-1-6*) Edconco Pr.

Prostate Cancer 2000. Ed. by L. Denis. 1994. LC 94-30517. (Monographs of the European School of Oncology). (Illus.). 101p. 89.00 (*0-387-58296-7*); (*3-540-58296-7*) Spr-Verlag.

Prostate Cancers: Prevention & Control: Index of New Information for Medicine, Science, & Research with Update of Progress. Patrick J. Mullins. 1996. LC 96-12484. 57.50 (*0-7883-1150-6*); pap. 47.50 (*0-7883-1151-4*) ABBE Pubs Assn.

Prostate Cancers - Prevention & Control: Index of New Information for Medicine Science & Research with New Update of Progress. Patrick J. Mullins. rev. ed. 1997. 151p. 57.50 (*0-7883-1616-8*); pap. 47.50 (*0-7883-1617-6*) ABBE Pubs Assn.

Prostate Cure: The Revolutionary natural Approach to Treating Enlarged Prostates. Harry G. Preuss & Brenda D. Adderly. 1998. LC 98-29437. 288p. 23.00 (*0-609-60323-X*) Crown Pub Group.

Prostate Diet Cookbook: Cancer-Fighting Foods for a Healthy Prostate. Buffy Sanders. 2001. LC 00-63375. (Illus.). xix, 304p. 23.95 (*0-936197-42-0*) Harbor Pr.

Prostate Disease: A Massachusetts General Hospital Book. W. Scott McDougal & Pat Skerrett. 1996. LC 95-15175. (Illus.). 368p. pap. 14.00 (*0-8129-2319-7*, Crown) Crown Pub Group.

Prostate Diseases. Ed. by Herbert Lepor & Russell K. Lawson. 1993. LC 92-49620. (Illus.). 512p. text 115.00 (*0-7216-4545-3*) Saunders.

Prostate Enlargement: Symptoms, Causes, Treatment & Recovery. 1991. lib. bdg. 79.00 (*0-8490-5155-X*) Gordon Pr.

Prostate Gland & Seminal Vesicle. G. Aumueller. 1979. (Handbuch der Mikroskopischen Anatomie Des Menschen Ser.: Vol. 7, Pt. 6). (Illus.). 380p. 191.00 (*0-387-09191-2*) Spr-Verlag.

Prostate Gland Troubles. Ed. by Health Research Staff. 1994. 24p. reprint ed. spiral bd. 10.00 (*0-7873-1261-4*) Hlth Research.

Prostate Guidebook. Date not set. pap. (*1-884350-65-8*) Alpha Pubng.

Prostate Miracle: New Natural Therapies That Can Save Your Life! Jesse A. Stoff & Dallas Clouatre. 2000. LC 2001-274887. (Illus.). xvi, 272p. pap. 12.00 (*1-57566-544-1*, Knsington) Kensgtn Pub Corp.

Prostate Problem. Chet Cunningham. 1995. pap. 8.95 (*0-8217-4892-0*) NAL.

Prostate Problems: Every Man's Fear: What Everyone Should Know About the Prostate. Martin K. Gelbard & William Bentley. 1995. LC 94-26400. (Illus.). 272p. per. 12.00 (*0-671-88465-4*, Fireside) S&S Trade Pap.

Prostate Problems & Elective Surgery. 1994. lib. bdg. 250.95 (*0-8490-5665-9*) Gordon Pr.

Prostate Problems & Their Treatment: Information & Advice for Sufferers. Jeremy Hamand. 1991. pap. (*0-7225-2252-5*) Thorsons.

Prostate Research: Index of New Information with Authors & Subjects. Virginia L. Jensen. rev. ed. 1994. LC 94-33829. 163p. 57.50 (*0-7883-0248-5*); LC 94-33829. 163p. pap. text 47.50 (*0-7883-0249-3*); 57.50 (*0-7883-0152-7*); pap. 47.50 (*0-7883-0153-5*) ABBE Pubs Assn.

Prostate Sourcebook. Steven Morganstern & Allen Abrahams. 3rd ed. 1998. LC 99-188320. 272p. pap. 16.00 (*1-56565-871-X*, 0871XW) Lowell Hse.

***Prostate-Specific Antigen.** Michael K. Brawer. 2001. LC 2001-28928. (Illus.). 327p. 150.00 (*0-8247-0555-6*) Dekker.

Prostatic Carcinoma: Biology & Diagnosis. Ed. by E. S. Hafez & E. Spring-Mills. 1980. (Clinics in Andrology Ser.: No. 6). (Illus.). 200p. text 211.50 (*90-247-2379-5*) Kluwer Academic.

Prostatic Disease. Herbert Lepor. 1999. LC 99-48130. (Illus.). xvii, 586p. text (*0-7216-7416-X*) Saunders.

Prostatic Diseases. George S. White. 3rd ed. 1996. 127p. reprint ed. spiral bd. 12.00 (*0-7873-0962-1*) Hlth Research.

Prostatic Hyperplasia: Etiology, Surgical & Conservative Management. Ed. by R. Ackermann & F. H. Schroder. 1989. (New Developments in Biosciences Ser.: No. 5). x, 154p. (C). pap. text 41.45 (*0-89925-528-0*) De Gruyter.

Prostatic Outflow Obstructions. Julian Shah. 1994. LC 93-45851. (Illus.). 192p. (*0-632-03557-9*) Blckwell Science.

Prostatitis: Etiopathology, Diagnosis & Therapy. Ed. by Wolfgang Weidner et al. 1994. LC 93-29539. (Illus.). 269p. 150.00 (*0-387-56624-4*) Spr-Verlag.

Prostesis Sobre Implantes see Implant-Supported Prostheses: Occlusion, Clinical Cases, & Laboratory Procedures

Prostheses & Abdominal Wall Hernias. Ed. by Robert Bendavid. 1994. 500p. 205.00 (*1-879702-70-3*, R) CRC Pr.

Prosthetic Dentistry: Principles & Treatment Strategies. Bengt Owall et al. 1995. (Illus.). 256p. text (*0-7234-2046-7*) Martin Dunitz GBR. *Dist:* Mosby Inc.

Prosthetic Dentistry: Principles & Treatment Strategies. Bengt Owall et al. 1996. (Illus.). 256p. (*84-8174-186-8*) Mosby-Doyma Libros ESP. *Dist:* Mosby Inc.

Prosthetic Gait Training Program for Lower Extremity Amputees. Robert S. Gailey & Ann M. Gailey. 1989. (Rehabilitation Series for Lower Extremity Amputees: Vol. 1). (Illus.). 36p. (C). pap. text 7.00 (*1-888131-00-4*) Adv Rehab Therapy.

Prosthetic Knee Ligament Reconstruction. Marc J. Friedman & Richard D. Ferkel. 1988. text 115.00 (*0-7216-2559-2*, Grune & Strat) Harcrt Hlth Sci Grp.

Prosthetic Rehabilitation. Keith F. Thomas. 1994. (Illus.). 280p. text 130.00 (*1-85097-032-7*, B8810) Quint Pub Co.

***Prosthetic Treatment of the Edentulous Patient.** Basker. 2002. text 26.95 (*0-632-05998-2*) Blackwell Sci.

Prosthetics: Methods of Producing Facial & Body Restorations. Carl D. Clarke. 1965. (Illus.). 336p. 40.00 (*0-911426-07-8*) Standard Arts.

Prosthetics - Amputations - Orthotics - Orthopedics & Spinal Cord Injury & Other Neurological Disorders. Ed. by Mindy L. Aisen. 2000. (Illus.). 59p. (C). pap. text 20.00 (*0-7881-8674-4*) DIANE Pub.

Prosthetics & Orthotics. Donald G. Shurr. 1990. LC 89-17650. (Illus.). 240p. (C). 59.00 (*0-8385-7977-9*, A7977-0) P-H.

Prosthodontic Treatment for Edentulous Patients. Boucher & George A. Zarb. 11th ed. 1997. LC 96-51006. (Illus.). 576p. (C). (gr. 13). text 76.00 (*0-8151-9899-X*, 24125) Mosby Inc.

***Prosthodontics: A Case-Based Learning Approach.** Hugh Devlin. 2001. (Illus.). 130p. 54.95 (*3-540-42183-1*) Spr-Verlag.

Prosthodontics for the Elderly: Diagnosis & Treatment. Ejvind Budtz-Jorgensen. 1999. LC 99-38079. 266p. text 89.00 (*0-86715-368-7*) Quint Pub Co.

Prosthondontics for the Elderly: Diagnosis & Treatment. Ejvind Budtz-Jergensen. 2000. (Illus.). 255p. (*4-87417-607-0*) QPC JPN. *Dist:* Quint Pub Co.

Prostitutes in Medical Literature: An Annotated Bibliography, 6. Compiled by Sachi S. Kantha. 1991. LC 91-3211. (Bibliographies & Indexes in Medical Studies: No. 6). 256p. lib. bdg. 68.50 (*0-313-27491-6*, KPQ, Greenwood Pr) Greenwood.

Protean Gate Structure & Plasticity of the Primary Nociceptive Analyzer: Structure & Plasticity of the Primary Nociceptive Analyzer. B. Csillik & E. Csillik-Knyihar. 1986. 294p. (C). (*963-05-3928-4*) Akade Kiado HUN. *Dist:* Intl Spec Bk, St Mut.

Protease Inhibitors: Therapeutic Application & Development. Ed. by Norra Macready. 1997. (Biomedical Library). pap. 795.00 (*1-57936-022-X*) Drug & Market Dev.

Protease Inhibitors As Cancer Chemopreventive Agents. W. Troll & A. R. Kennedy. 1993. LC 93-24959. (Illus.). 334p. (C). text 95.00 (*0-306-44390-2*, Kluwer Plenum) Kluwer Academic.

Protease Inhibitors of Human Plasma-Biochemistry & Pathophysiology. Genesio Murano. 1985. (Reviews of Hematology: Vol. II). 69.95 (*0-915340-14-3*) PJD Pubns.

Proteases: Potential Role in Health & Disease, Vol. 2. Ed. by Walter H. Horl & August Heidland. 1988. (Advances in Experimental Medicine & Biology Ser.: Vol. 240). (Illus.). 572p. 135.00 (*0-306-43018-5*, Plenum Trade) Perseus Pubng.

Proteases of Infectious Agents. Ben Dunn. 1999. LC 98-89642. (Illus.). 282p. 69.95 (*0-12-420510-0*) Acad Pr.

Proteases, Protease Inhibitors & Protease-Derived Peptides: Importance in Human Pathophysiology & Therapeutics. Ed. by J. C. Cheronis & J. E. Repine. 1993. LC 93-15611. (Agents & Actions Supplements Ser.: Vol. 42). viii, 248p. 93.00 (*0-8176-2868-1*) Birkhauser.

Proteasomes: Multicatalytic Proteinase Complexes. Ed. by S. Wilk. 1994. (Journal: Vol. 47, No. 4-6, 1993). (Illus.). 192p. pap. 59.25 (*3-8055-6081-8*) S Karger.

Protect Your Assets: The Nurses Self Defense Guide. Audrey Stephan. Ed. by Diane Dettmore. 1993. LC 93-60935. 104p. (C). pap. 12.95 (*1-880254-09-3*) Vista.

Protect Your Life in the Sun: How to Minimize Your Exposure to Ultraviolet Sunlight & Prevent Skin Cancer & Eye Disorders. Paul L. Gourley & Gail M. Gourley. 1993. LC 93-77915. (Illus.). 104p. (Orig.). pap. 9.95 (*0-9636297-1-9*) High Light Pub.

Protect Your Prostate: The World-Renowned Colgan Institute Reveals Its Program for a Healthy Prostate. Michael Colgan. 2000. 105p. 12.95 (*1-896817-17-3*) Apple Pubg Co.

Protect Yourself Against Tuberculosis: A Respiratory Protection Guide for Health Care Workers. 1997. lib. bdg. 251.95 (*0-8490-8147-5*) Gordon Pr.

Protecting Children & Young People. Colin Findlay & Anne P. Salter. 1992. LC 92-49353. (Skills for Caring Ser.). (Illus.). 48p. pap. text (*0-443-04618-2*) Church.

Protecting Children in Substance-Abusing Families. Vickie Kropenske & Judy Howard. 1995. (Illus.). 128p. (C). pap. text 30.00 (*0-7881-1826-9*) DIANE Pub.

Protecting Health Care Workers from HIV Infection. 1990. (State Legislative Reports: Vol. 15, No. 11). 9p. 15.00 (*1-55516-267-3*, 7302-1511) Natl Conf State Legis.

Protecting Human Subjects: Departmental Subject Pools & Institutional Review Boards. Ed. by Garvin Chastain & R. Eric Landrum. 1999. LC 99-22348. 228p. pap. 29.95 (*1-55798-575-8*, 431-617A) Am Psychol.

Protecting Judgment-Impaired Adults: Issues, Interventions & Policies. Ed. by Edmund F. Dejowski. 1990. LC 90-45236. (Journal of Elder Abuse & Neglect Ser.). 178p. text 39.95 (*1-56024-054-7*) Haworth Pr.

Protecting Privacy in Computerized Medical Information. 1994. (Illus.). 168p. (Orig.). (C). pap. text 40.00 (*0-7881-0446-2*) DIANE Pub.

Protecting Privacy in Computerized Medical Information. 1994. (Orig.). lib. bdg. 250.00 (*0-8490-5769-8*) Gordon Pr.

Protecting, Promoting, & Supporting Breast-Feeding: The Special Role of Maternity Services, a Joint WHO-UNICEF Statement. 1989. (ARA, ENG, FRE & SPA.). iv, 32p. pap. text 6.00 (*92-4-156130-0*) World Health.

Protecting the Children: Strategies for Optimizing Emotional & Behavioral Development. Ed. by Raymond P. Lorion. 1990. LC 89-28933. (Prevention in Human Services Ser.: Vol. 7, No. 1). (Illus.). 275p. text 49.95 (*0-86656-970-7*) Haworth Pr.

Protecting the Emotional Development of the Ill Child: The Essence of the Child Life Profession. Evelyn K. Oremland. Ed. by Jerome D. Oremland. 2000. LC 99-17720. (Illus.). xi, 266p. 45.00 (*1-887841-20-2*, 64385, Psychosocial) Intl Univs Pr.

Protecting the Health of the Elderly: A Review of WHO Activities. M. Skeet. 1983. (Public Health in Europe Ser.: No. 18). 125p. pap. text 11.00 (*92-890-1154-8*) World Health.

Protecting Workers' Health in the Third World: National & International Strategies. Ed. by Michael R. Reich & Toshiteru Okubo. 1992. LC 92-6991. 328p. 68.00 (*0-86569-026-X*, T026, Auburn Hse) Greenwood.

Protecting Your Baby-to-Be: Preventing Birth Defects in the First Trimester. Margie Profet. 1995. LC 95-4873. (Illus.). 168p. 20.00 (*0-201-40768-X*) Addison-Wesley.

Protection Against Ionizing Radiations: A Survey of Current World Legislation. 1972. (International Digest of Health Legislation Offprints: Vol. 22, No. 4). 328p. pap. text 28.00 (*92-4-169224-3*, 1957201) World Health.

Protection Against Ischemia Reperfusion Damage of the Heart. Yasushi Abiko & M. Karmazyn. 1998. LC 98-6390. 250p. 129.00 (*4-431-70226-1*) Spr-Verlag.

Protection Against Neutron Radiation. 1971. LC 73-138550. (Report Ser.: No. 38). 161p. pap. text 25.00 (*0-913392-20-0*) NCRP Pubns.

Protection in Nuclear Medicine & Ultrasound Diagnostic Procedures in Children. Intro. by Warren K. Sinclair. 1983. LC 83-61834. (Report Ser.: No. 73). 81p. pap. text 30.00 (*0-913392-63-4*) NCRP Pubns.

Protection of Brain from Ischemia, Vol. 3. Philip R. Weinstein & Alan I. Faden. 1990. 307p. 87.00 (*0-683-08908-0*) Lppncott W & W.

Protection of Human Research Subjects: A Practical Guide to Federal Laws & Regulations. Dennis M. Maloney. 1984. LC 84-4873. (Illus.). 442p. 107.00 (*0-306-41522-4*, Kluwer Plenum) Kluwer Academic.

Protection of Human Rights in the Light of Scientific & Technological Progress in Biology & Medicine: 8th CIOMS Round Table Conference. 1974. pap. text 27.90 (*92-4-056007-6*, 0830008) World Health.

Protection of the Patient in Diagnostic Radiology. Ed. by International Commission on Radiological Protection et al. 1983. (International Commission on Radiological Protection Ser.: No. 34). 88p. pap. 28.00 (*0-08-029797-8*, Pergamon Pr) Elsevier.

Protection of the Patient in Nuclear Medicine. International Commission on Radiological Protection. 1988. (International Commission on Radiological Protection Ser.: No. 52). (Illus.). 46p. pap. 32.00 (*0-08-033188-2*, Pergamon Pr) Elsevier.

Protection of the Patient in Radiation Therapy. Ed. by F. D. Sowby. 1985. (International Commission on Radiological Protection Ser.: No. 44). (Illus.). 58p. pap. 32.00 (*0-08-032336-7*, Pergamon Pr) Elsevier.

Protection of the Patient in Radionuclide Investigations. International Commission on Radiological Protection. 1971. (International Commission on Radiological Protection Ser.: No. 17). pap. 11.00 (*0-08-016773-X*, Pergamon Pr) Elsevier.

Protection of the Public in the Event of Radiation Accidents: Proceedings. United Nations Food and Agriculture Organization Staff et al. 1965. (ENG, FRE & RUS., Illus.). 370p. pap. text 34.00 (*92-4-156025-8*, 1150128) World Health.

Protection of the Thyroid Gland in the Event of Releases of Radioiodine. 1977. LC 77-82607. (Report Ser.: No. 55). 66p. pap. text 20.00 (*0-913392-37-5*) NCRP Pubns.

Protective Effect of BCG in Experimental Tuberculosis. Donald W. Smith. 1985. (Advances in Tuberculosis Research Ser.: Vol. 22). (Illus.). viii, 100p. 77.50 (*3-8055-4089-2*) S Karger.

Protective Shell in Children & Adults. Frances Tustin. 1990. 256p. pap. text (*0-946439-81-8*) Karnac Bks GBR. *Dist:* Other Pr LLC.

Protein - DNA Interactions. Ed. by John N. Abelson et al. 1991. (Methods in Enzymology Ser.: Vol. 208). (Illus.). 700p. text 125.00 (*0-12-182109-9*) Acad Pr.

Protein & Amino Acid Metabolism in Cancer. Peter W. Pisters. 1996. (Medicine Ser.). pap. 89.95 (*0-412-10031-2*, VNR) Wiley.

Protein & Amino Acid Metabolism in Cancer Cachexia. Murray F. Brennan & Peter W. Pisters. 1995. LC 95-24641. (Medical Intelligence Unit Ser.). 213p. 99.00 (*1-57059-291-8*) Landes Bioscience.

Protein & Energy: A Study of Changing Ideas in Nutrition. Kenneth J. Carpenter. 1994. LC 93-32130. (Illus.). 296p. (C). text 47.95 (*0-521-45209-0*) Cambridge U Pr.

Protein Based Materials. David Kaplan & Kevin Mcgrath. 1996. LC 96-28021. (*3-7643-3848-2*) Birkhauser.

Protein Compartmentalization. Ed. by A. W. Strauss et al. 1986. (Molecular Biology, Biochemistry & Biophysics Ser.). (Illus.). 140p. 68.00 (*0-387-96292-1*) Spr-Verlag.

Protein Delivery: Physical Systems. Ed. by Lynda M. Sanders & R. Wayne Hendron. 1997. LC 97-176. (Pharmaceutical Biotechnology Ser.: No. 10). (Illus.). 455p. (C). text 114.00 (*0-306-45359-2*, Kluwer Plenum) Kluwer Academic.

Protein Design & the Development of New Therapeutics & Vaccines. J. B. Hook & G. Poste. 1990. (Illus.). 512p. (C). text 120.00 (*0-306-43463-6*, Kluwer Plenum) Kluwer Academic.

Protein Dynamics Using NMR Relaxation. Kevin H. Mayo & Vladimir A. Daragan. 1998. 300p. (*1-86094-076-5*) Imperial College GBR. *Dist:* World Scientific Pub.

Protein-Energy Malnutrition. Waterlow. 1992. 352p. 80.00 (*0-340-50127-8*) Trafalgar.

Protein Evolution. Laszio Patthy. 4th ed. 1999. LC 00-58501. (Illus.). x, 512p. pap. 68.95 (*0-632-04774-7*) Blackwell Sci.

Protein Formulation & Delivery. Eugene J. McNally. 1999. LC 99-40675. (Drugs & the Pharmaceutical Sciences Ser.). (Illus.). 278p. text 150.00 (*0-8247-7883-9*) Dekker.

Protein Functionality in Foods. Ed. by John P. Cherry. 1981. LC 81-97. (ACS Symposium Ser.: No. 147). 49.95 (*0-8412-0605-8*) Am Chemical.

***Protein Interactions Involved in Viral Replication Characterized by T7 Phage Display.** Hamid Houshmand. 2001. (Comprehensive Summaries of Uppsala Dissertations from the Faculty of Medicine Ser.: No. 995). (Illus.). 60p. pap. (*91-554-4927-1*) Uppsala Universitet SWE. *Dist:* Coronet Bks.

Protein Kinases. Ed. by Hsien-Jien Kung. 1998. (Journal of Biomedical Science: Vol. 5, No. 2). (Illus.). 86p. pap. 21.00 (*3-8055-6704-9*) S Karger.

Protein Kinases in Blood Cell Function. Chi-Kuang Huang. 1993. 320p. lib. bdg. 199.00 (*0-8493-6353-5*, QP606) CRC Pr.

Protein Metabolism in Renal Diseases. Ed. by Bradley J. Maroni. 1997. (Mineral & Electrolyte Metabolism Ser.: Vol. 24, No. 1, 1998). (Illus.). 102p. pap. 52.25 (*3-8055-6573-9*) S Karger.

Protein Methylation. Ed. by Woon K. Paik & Sangduk Kim. 1989. 464p. 254.00 (*0-8493-6818-9*, QP551) CRC Pr.

Protein Motions. S. Subbiah. 1996. (Medicine Ser.). pap. 89.95 (*0-412-10651-5*) Wiley.

Protein Nutrition & Mineral Absorption. Raul A. Wapnir. 1990. (Illus.). 352p. 239.00 (*0-8493-5227-4*, QP533) CRC Pr.

Protein Pharmacokinetics & Metabolism. B. L. Ferraiolo et al. 1992. (Pharmaceutical Biotechnology Ser.: Vol. 1). (Illus.). 292p. (C). text 75.00 (*0-306-44151-9*, Kluwer Plenum) Kluwer Academic.

Protein Phosphorylation. Ed. by Bartholomew M. Sefton & Tony Hunter. 1998. LC 98-149611. (Selected Methods in Enzymology Ser.). (Illus.). 675p. (C). 69.95 (*0-12-634490-6*) Acad Pr.

Protein Phosphorylation & Bio-Regulation. Ed. by J Gordon et al. 1980. (Illus.). x, 234p. 71.50 (*3-8055-1168-X*) S Karger.

Protein Phosphorylation in Heart Muscle. R. John Solaro. 1986. 192p. 102.00 (*0-8493-5133-2*, QP113, CRC Reprint) Franklin.

***Protein Protocols Handbook.** Ed. by John M. Walker. 2nd ed. 2002. 1200p. pap. 125.00 (*0-89603-941-2*) Humana.

Protein-Sparing Diets: A Special Issue of Journal of Obesity & Weight Regulation. Ed. by Robert S. Sherwin & Jonathan K. Wise. 1984. 80p. pap. 14.95 (*0-89885-220-X*, Kluwer Acad Hman Sci) Kluwer Academic.

Protein Structural Biology in Biomedical Research, Set. Ed. by E. Edward Bittar. 1997. (Advances in Molecular & Cell Biology Ser.: Vol. 22). 627p. 257.00 (*0-7623-0283-6*) Jai Pr.

Protein Synthesis: Translational & Post-Translational Events. Ed. by Abraham K. Abraham et al. 1984. LC 83-26463. 477p. 145.00 (*0-89603-060-1*) Humana.

Proteins: Major Non-Immune System Proteins of Blood Plasma, Vol. 5. Ed. by Geoffrey Allen. Date not set. 128.50 (*1-55938-675-4*) Jai Pr.

Proteins: Protein & the Immune System, Vol. 4. Ed. by Geoffrey Allen. Date not set. 128.50 (*1-55938-674-6*) Jai Pr.

Proteins & Non-Protein Nitrogen in Human Milk. Ed. by Stephanie A. Atkinson. 1989. 256p. lib. bdg. 210.00 (*0-8493-6795-6*, QP246) CRC Pr.

Proteins & Steroids in Early Pregnancy. Ed. by H. M. Beier & P. Karlson. 1982. (Illus.). 346p. 65.95 (*0-387-10457-7*) Spr-Verlag.

Proteins at Low Temperatures. Ed. by Owen R. Fennema. 1979. LC 79-16561. (Advances in Chemistry Ser.: No. 180). 43.95 (*0-8412-0484-5*) Am Chemical.

Proteins, Peptides & Amino Acids in Enternal Nutrition. Ed. by P. Furst & V. Young. 2000. LC 00-43438. (Nestle Nutrition Workshop Ser.: Vol. 3). (Illus.). xvi, 284p. 198.25 (*3-8055-7108-9*) S Karger.

Proteinuria. Ed. by J. Brod et al. 1975. (Contributions to Nephrology Ser.: Vol. 1). (Illus.). 250p. 29.75 (*3-8055-2183-9*) S Karger.

Proteinuria: American Journal of Nephrology, Vol. 10, Suppl. 1. Ed. by Shaul G. Massry et al. 1990. (Illus.). iv, 166p. pap. 35.00 (*3-8055-5245-9*) S Karger.

Proteolytic & Cellular Mechanisms in Prohormone Processing. Vivian Y. Hook. 1998. LC 98-28730. (Molecular Biology Intelligence Unit Ser.). 215p. 99.00 (*1-57059-553-4*) Landes Bioscience.

Proteolytic Enzymes. Ed. by Gertrude E. Perlmann & Laszlo Lorand. 1970. (Methods in Enzymology Ser.: Vol. 19). text 209.00 (*0-12-181881-0*) Acad Pr.

Proteolytic Enzymes: Aspartic & Metallo Peptidases. Ed. by John N. Abelson et al. 1995. (Methods in Enzymology Ser.: Vol. 248). (Illus.). 873p. text 121.00 (*0-12-182149-8*) Acad Pr.

Proteolytic Enzymes: Tools & Targets. Ed. by Erwin E. Sterchi & Walter Stocker. 1999. LC 99-20523. (Lab Manual Ser.). (Illus.). 375p. ring bd. 82.00 (*3-540-61233-5*) Spr-Verlag.

Proteolytic Enzymes in Cancer Invasion. Ed. by Liliana Ossowski & R. M. Lopez. 1996. (Journal: Vol. 49, No. 1-3, 1996). (Illus.). 182p. pap. 62.75 (*3-8055-6318-3*) S Karger.

Proteolytic Enzymes in Coagulation, Fibrinolysis, & Complement Activation Pt. B: Complement Activation, Fibrinolysis, & Nonmammalian Blood Coagulation Factors & Inhibitors. Ed. by Laszlo Lorand et al. 1993. (Methods in Enzymology Ser.: Vol. 223). (Illus.). 433p. text 94.00 (*0-12-182124-2*) Acad Pr.

Prothrombin & Other Vitamin K Proteins, Vol. I. Ed. by Walter H. Seegers & Daniel A. Walz. 1986. LC 85-7869. 208p. 104.00 (*0-8493-6308-X*, QP93, CRC Reprint) Franklin.

Prothrombin & Other Vitamin K Proteins, Vol. II. Ed. by Daniel A. Walz & Walter H. Seegers. 1986. 192p. 94.00 (*0-8493-6309-8*, QP93) CRC Pr.

Prothrombin & Related Coagulation Factors. H. Coenraad Hemker. 1975. text 141.50 (*90-6021-236-3*) Kluwer Academic.

Proto-Oncogenes in Cell Development - Symposium No. 150. CIBA Foundation Staff. 1990. LC 90-11986. (CIBA Foundation Symposia Ser.: No. 150). 306p. 128.00 (*0-471-92686-8*) Wiley.

Protocol Analysis: Verbal Reports As Data. K. Anders Ericsson & Herbert A. Simon. rev. ed. 1993. LC 92-33817. (Illus.). 420p. 45.00 (*0-262-05047-1*); 496p. pap. 32.00 (*0-262-55023-7*) MIT Pr.

Protocol & Guidelines for Monotoring & Evaluation Procedures. Ed. by E. Leparsky & F. E. Nussel. 1987. xiii, 60p. pap. 32.70 (*0-387-18458-9*) Spr-Verlag.

Protocol & Procedures for Quality Assurance of Linear Accelerators. Chris Constantinou. 1993. (Illus.). (Orig.). (C). pap. (*0-9638266-0-3*); text (*0-9638266-1-1*) CNC Med Physics.

Protocol for a Plague: AIDS Research, Access to Life-Saving Therapies, & Drug Approval. Neal A. Dickerson. 1993. LC 93-2606. (Politics of AIDS Ser.: Vol. 5). (Illus.). xii, 157p. pap. 12.00 (*0-930383-37-0*) Monument Pr.

Protocol for Phallometric Assessment: A Clinician's Guide. Deloris T. Roys & Pat Roys. Ed. by Euan Bear. 1999. 78p. (Orig.). pap., stu. ed. 10.00 (*1-884444-11-3*) Safer Soc.

Protocol Techniques in Cardiology. Simpson. 1998. (Illus.). 200p. pap. text (*0-7020-1902-X*) Saunders.

Protocol to the Convention on the Elaboration of a European Pharmacopoeia. Council of Europe Staff. 1989. (Conventions & Agreements Ser.: No. 134). (ENG & FRE.). (*92-871-1781-0*) Council of Europe FRA. *Dist:* Manhattan Pub Co.

Protocols for Adapting Activities to the Changing Needs of People with Dementia. Ruth M. Griffin. 1996. 58p. (C). pap. text 11.00 (*0-935273-09-3*) Chess Pub.

Protocols for Evaluating Dehydrated Mueller-Hinton Agar: Tentative Standard, 1993. Contrib. by George L. Evans. 1993. 75.00 (*1-56238-215-2*, M6-T) NCCLS.

Protocols for Gene Transfer in Neuroscience: Towards Gene Therapy of Neurological Disorders. Ed. by P. R. Lowenstein & Lynn W. Enquist. 1996. LC 95-45487. 446p. pap. 229.95 (*0-471-95766-6*) Wiley.

Protocols for Gynecologic & Obstetric Health Care. Barger et al. 1987. pap. text 43.00 (*0-8089-1897-4*, Grune & Strat) Harcrt Hlth Sci Grp.

Protocols for Health Care Executive Behavior: A Factor for Success. Carson F. Dye. 1993. LC 93-14057. 231p. text 42.00 (*1-56793-000-X*, 0934) Health Admin Pr.

Protocols for High-Risk Pregnancies. John T. Queenan et al. 3rd ed. 1995. LC 95-33220. (Protocols in Obstetrics & Gynecology Ser.). 512p. 54.95 (*0-86542-444-6*) Blackwell Sci.

Protocols for Infectious Diseases in Obstetrics & Gynecology. Philip B. Mead et al. 2nd ed. 1999. LC 99-30332. (Protocols in Obstetrics & Gynecology Ser.). (Illus.). xxvi, 605p. pap. 52.95 (*0-632-04324-5*) Blackwell Sci.

Protocols for Neural Cell Culture. Ed. by Sergey Fedoroff & Arleen Richardson. 3rd ed. 2001. 352p. spiral bd. 79.50 (*0-89603-902-1*) Humana.

Protocols for Office Gynecologic Surgery. Ed. by Philip D. Darney et al. 1996. LC 95-41188. (Protocols in Obstetrics & Gynecology Ser.). 400p. 52.95 (*0-86542-374-1*) Blackwell Sci.

Protocols for Recreation Therapy Programs. Alberta Hospital Edmonton, Recreation Therapy Staff. Ed. by Jill Kelland. 1995. LC 95-60642. 132p. (C). pap. 24.95 (*0-910251-73-8*, PRT79) Venture Pub PA.

***Protocols for the Breast Care Center.** Robert Caplan. 2002. (Illus.). (C). text 64.95 (*0-7637-1813-0*, 1813-0) Jones & Bartlett.

Protocols for the Sex Abuse Evaluation. Richard A. Gardner. 1995. LC 94-39476. 431p. pap. text 40.00 (*0-933812-38-8*) Creative Therapeutics.

Protocols in Neonatal Nursing: Physiological Perspective. Carole A. Kenner. Ed. by Maura Connor. 2nd ed. 1998. LC 97-48248. (Illus.). 704p. (C). pap. text 35.00 (*0-7216-6117-3*) Saunders.

Protocols in Primary Care Geriatrics. J. P. Sloan. 2nd ed. 1996. 221p. pap. 46.95 (*0-387-94690-X*) Spr-Verlag.

Protoctista Glossary. Lynn Margulis. 1993. (Illus.). 288p. (C). text 54.95 (*0-86720-081-2*, 081-2) Jones & Bartlett.

Proton Passage Across Cell Membranes. CIBA Foundation Staff. 1988. LC 88-25026. (CIBA Foundation Symposia Ser.: No. 139). 278p. 128.00 (*0-471-91903-9*) Wiley.

Proton Pump Inhibitors: Milestones in Drug Therapy. Ed. by L. Olbe. 1999. 250p. 160.00 (*3-7643-5897-1*) Birkhauser.

P
Q
R

Proton Therapy & Radiosurgery. Hans Breuer & Berend J. Smit. 2000. LC 99-35197. (Illus.). 304p. 146.00 (*3-540-64100-9*) Spr-Verlag.

Protooncogenes & Growth Factors in Steroid Hormone-Induced Growth & Differentiation. Ed. by Sohaib A. Khan & George M. Stancel. 1993. 288p. 115.00 (*0-8493-8672-1*, SF105) CRC Pr.

Prototype Action-Oriented School Health Curriculum for Primary Schools: National Guidelines. 1990. text, tchr. ed. 43.20 (*92-9021-014-1*) World Health.

Protozoal Diseases: A Comprehensive Guide. Herbert M. Gilles. 2000. LC 98-55680. (Illus.). 740p. (*0-340-74090-6*) E A GBR. *Dist:* OUP.

Proven Health Tips Encyclopedia. Michael Allen. 1997. 433p. (Orig.). pap. 18.95 (*0-9638596-6-8*) Amer Pubng.

Proven Practice, Vol. 2. 1994. 48.00 (*1-56925-005-7*, PP2) Capitol Publns.

Provider-Patient Partnerships. Mary L. Hardy & Helen Meldrum. 2001. LC 00-65133. 168p. pap. text 21.95 (*0-7506-7334-6*) Buttrwrth-Heinemann.

Provider Report Cards: A Guide for Promoting Health Care Quality to the Public. Patrice L. Spath. 1999. LC 99-20309. (Illus.). 174p. pap. 36.00 (*1-55648-250-7*) AHPI.

Provider Sponsored Organizations: Emerging Opportunities for Growth. Allan Fine & Colleen E. Dowd. 1998. LC 98-28499. 190p. pap. 96.00 (*0-8342-1177-7*, 11777) Aspen Pub.

Providing & Receiving Consultation in Long-Term Care. Marylou Hughes. 1998. 29.50 (*0-929442-31-8*, 2137PP) Prof Prnting & Pub.

Providing Comprehensive Sexual Health Care in Spinal Cord Injury Rehabilitation: Continuing Education & Training for Health Care Professionals. Mitchell S. Tepper. 1997. 143p. ring bd. 95.00 (*0-9659185-0-5*) Sexual Hlth.

Providing Health Care Benefits in Retirement. Ed. by Judith F. Mazo et al. 1994. LC 94-13655. (Ralph H. Blanchard Memorial Endowment Ser.). 280p. (C). text 42.50 (*0-8122-3270-4*) U of Pa Pr.

Providing Home Care: A Textbook for Home Care Aides. William Leahy. Ed. by Jetta Fuzy & Julie Grafe. 1998. LC 00-500438. (Illus.). 368p. (C). pap. text 34.95 (*1-888343-22-2*, TEXT22-2) Hartman Pub.

Providing Out-of-Hospital Care to Infants & Children. Elizabeth M. Wertz. 2001. LC 00-52284. (Illus.). xxvii, 332p. (C). pap. text 44.95 (*0-7668-1986-8*) Delmar.

Providing Services for People with Vision Loss: A Multidisciplinary Perspective. Ed. by Susan L. Greenblatt. 1989. pap. 19.95 (*0-929718-02-X*) Resc Rehab.

Proving Medical Diagnosis & Prognosis Marshall Houts & Leonard Marmor. 1970. ring bd. 1669.00 (*0-8205-1564-7*) Bender.

Provision of Primary Experience: Winnicottian Work with Children & Adolescents. Barbara Dockar-Drysdale. 1991. LC 91-4536. 232p. 45.00 (*0-87668-525-4*) Aronson.

Provocation Testing in Clinical Practice. Ed. by Sheldon L. Spector. 1994. (Clinical Allergy & Immunology Ser.: Vol. 5). (Illus.). 816p. text 250.00 (*0-8247-9249-1*) Dekker.

Provocative Challenge Procedures: Bronchial Oral Nasal & Exercise. Sheldon L. Spector. 1983. LC 82-22655. 224p. 129.00 (*0-8493-6325-X*, CRC Reprint) Franklin.

Provocative Challenge Procedures Vol. 2: Bronchial Oral Nasal & Exercise. Sheldon L. Spector. 1983. LC 82-22655. 208p. 118.00 (*0-8493-6326-8*, CRC Reprint) Franklin.

Prozac: Panacea or Pandora?: "The Rest of the Story" on the New Class of SSRI Antidepressants (Prozac, Zoloft, Paxil, Lovan, Luvox, & More) Ann B. Tracy. 1994. (Illus.). 424p. pap. 15.95 (*0-916095-59-2*) Pubs Pr UT.

Prozac: Questions & Answers. Ronald R. Fieve. 1994. LC 94-179140. pap. 5.99 (*0-380-77718-5*, Avon Bks) Morrow Avon.

Prozac Alternative: Natural Relief from Depression with St. John's Wort, Kava, Ginkgo, 5-HTP, Homeopathy & Other Alternative Therapies. Ran Knishinsky. 1998. LC 98-25770. 176p. pap. 12.95 (*0-89281-791-7*, Heal Arts VT) Inner Tradit.

Prozac (Fluoxetine) - Side Effects & Harmful Reactions: New Information with Authors & Subjects. American Health Research Institute Staff. rev. ed. 1994. 57.50 (*0-7883-0172-1*) ABBE Pubs Assn.

Pruritis in Clinical Medicine: Pathology & Treatment. Stefano Gatti & Ferdinando Serri. 1990. 112p. pap. 45.00 (*0-07-038776-1*) McGraw-Hill Prof.

PSA: How a Simple Blood Test Can Save Your Life. Don Kaltenbach. 1998. 32p. pap. 5.00 (*0-9651827-5-4*) Proste Cancer.

Psychologies of 1930. Ed. by Carl Murchison. 1976. LC 73-2980. (Classics in Psychology Ser.). reprint ed. 34.95 (*0-405-05152-2*) Ayer.

Pseudoepileptic Seizures. Ed. by Lennart Gram et al. 1993. 192p. (*1-871816-18-1*) Wrightson Biomed GBR. *Dist:* Taylor & Francis.

Pseudoepileptic Seizures. Rowan & Gates. 1991. 69.95 (*0-939957-41-8*) Demos Medical.

Pseudomonas Aeruginosa. Ed. by D. P. Speert & R. E. Hancock. 1985. (Antibiotics & Chemotherapy Ser.: Vol. 36). (Illus.). viii, 176p. 128.75 (*3-8055-3966-5*) S Karger.

Pseudomonas Aeruginosa - Infections & Treatment, No. 12. Ed. by Aldona L. Baltch & Raymond P. Smith. 1994. (Infectious Disease & Therapy Ser.: Vol. 12). (ITA., Illus.). 640p. text 225.00 (*0-8247-9210-6*) Dekker.

Pseudomonas Aeruginosa As an Opportunistic Pathogen. M. Campa et al. 1993. (Infectious Agents & Pathogenesis Ser.). (Illus.). 440p. (C). text 110.00 (*0-306-44265-5*, Kluwer Plenum) Kluwer Academic.

Pseudomonas Aeruginosa in Human Diseases. Ed. by J. Y. Homma et al. 1991. (Antibiotics & Chemotherapy Ser.: Vol. 44). (Illus.). x, 250p. 189.75 (*3-8055-5385-4*) S Karger.

Pseudomonas Aeruginosa Infection, 1988. Ed. by N. Hoiby et al. 1989. (Antibiotics & Chemotherapy Ser.: Vol. 42). (Illus.). 308p. 208.75 (*3-8055-5002-2*) S Karger.

Pseudomonas Aeruginosa the Opportunist: Pathogenesis & Disease. Ed. by Robert B. Fick, Jr. 1992. LC 92-23816. 272p. 184.00 (*0-8493-4811-0*, QR201) CRC Pr.

Pseudoscience in Biological Psychiatry: Blaming the Body. Ross Conlin et al. 1994. LC 94-27307. (General & Clinical Psychology Ser.). 304p. 140.00 (*0-471-00776-5*) Wiley.

PSI & Psychoanalysis. Jule Eisenbud. 1970. LC 71-75145. 368p. text 70.00 (*0-8089-0126-5*, 791150, Grune & Strat) Harcrt Hlth Sci Grp.

PSI & States of Awareness. Proceedings of the International Conference, Paris, France, Aug. 24-26, 1977. International Conference, Paris Staff. Ed. by Betty Shapin & Lisette Coly. 1978. LC 78-50167. 17.00 (*0-912328-30-4*) Parapsych Foun.

Psicoanalisis. C. Thompson. (Breviarios Ser.). (SPA.). pap. 8.99 (*968-16-0298-6*) Fondo CA.

Psicoanalisis y Existencialismo. Viktor E. Frankl. (Breviarios Ser.). (SPA.). pap. 9.99 (*968-16-0072-X*) Fondo CA.

Psicologia de la Comunicacion. Ana M. O'Neill. 1987. (SPA.). 541p. reprint ed. 11.75 (*0-8477-2907-9*) U of PR Pr.

Psicologia de los Sentimientos (Psychology of Feelings) Pierre Janet. 1997. (Fondo 2000 Ser.). (SPA.). 87p. pap. 2.99 (*968-16-5193-6*) Fondo CA.

Psilocybin Mushrooms of the World: An Identification Guide. Paul Stamets. 1996. LC 96-15717. (Illus.). 245p. pap. 24.95 (*0-89815-839-7*) Ten Speed Pr.

***Psionic Medicine: The Study & Treatment of the Causative Factors in Illness.** J. H. Reyner. 2001. pap. (*0-85207-342-9*) C W Daniel GBR. *Dist:* Natl Bk Netwk.

***Psiquiatria Nino y Adolescente (Child & Adolescent Psychiatry)** Dean X. Parmelee. Ed. by Ronald B. David. 1996. (Mosby's Neurology - Psychiatry Access Ser.). (SPA., Illus.). 360p. (*84-8174-329-1*) Mosby-Doyma Libros ESP. *Dist:* Mosby Inc.

Psoraisis & Eczema Solution: New Hope for Physical & Emotional Relief. Michael F. Holick et al. 1999. LC 98-87931. (Illus.). 200p. 21.95 (*1-890819-06-9*) TransMedia Group.

Psoriasis. Charles Camisa. 1993. LC 93-11762. (Illus.). 368p. 99.95 (*0-86542-247-8*) Blackwell Sci.

***Psoriasis.** Menter et al. 2002. (Fast Facts Ser.). (Illus.). 60p. pap. (*1-899541-98-5*) Health Pr GBR. *Dist:* JAMCO Dist.

Psoriasis. Henry H. Roenigk & Howard I. Maibach. 3rd ed. 1998. LC 98-16975. (Basic & Clinical Dermatology Ser.). (Illus.). 880p. text 225.00 (*0-8247-0108-9*) Dekker.

Psoriasis Handbook: A Self-Help Guide. Muriel K. MacFarlane. 1995. LC 95-61640. (Illus.). 224p. (Orig.). pap. 12.95 (*1-887053-01-8*) United Res CA.

Psoriatic Arthritis. Ed. by Lynn H. Gerber. 1985. 224p. text 72.00 (*0-8089-1709-9*, 791544, Grune & Strat) Harcrt Hlth Sci Grp.

Psych Symptoms & Their Treatment in Alzheimers Disease: Pocketbook Edition. Devanand. 2000. (*1-85317-918-3*) Martin Dunitz GBR. *Dist:* Blackwell Sci.

Psych Tech Notes. Eugene Galanter. Ed. by John Van Laer. 1988. (Illus.). 210p. (Orig.). (C). pap. 11.95 (*0-937431-02-8*) Adams Bannister Cox.

Psych Tech Notes, Version 2.1. Eugene Galanter & Alicia Walton. 2nd rev. ed. 1994. LC 94-22644. (Illus.). 249p. (C). pap. text 19.95 (*0-937431-05-2*) Adams Bannister Cox.

Psychanalyse du Feu. Gaston Bachelard. 1985. (FRE.). pap. 12.95 (*0-7859-2799-9*) Fr & Eur.

***Psyche & Brain: The Biology of Talking Cures.** Fred M. Levin. unabr. ed. 2001. 295p. pap. text 34.95 (*0-8236-5259-9*, 25259) Intl Univs Pr.

Psyche & Cerebrum. John N. Findlay. 1972. LC 72-76593. (Aquinas Lectures). 52p. 15.00 (*0-87462-137-2*) Marquette.

Psyche & Eros: Mind & Gender in the Life Course. Gisela Labouvie-Vief. 1994. LC 93-21292. 345p. (C). text 64.95 (*0-521-43340-1*); pap. text 22.95 (*0-521-46824-8*) Cambridge U Pr.

Psyche & Family: Jungian Applications to Family Therapy. Ed. by Laura S. Dodson & Terrill L. Gibson. 1997. LC 96-25236. 164p. pap. 17.95 (*1-888602-02-3*, 023) Chiron Pubns.

Psyche & Helix: Psychological Aspects of Genetic Counseling. Seymour Kessler. 2000. LC 00-20717. (Illus.). 192p. 79.95 (*0-471-35055-9*) Wiley.

Psyche & Matter. Marie-Louise Von Franz. 1992. LC 91-53229. (C. G. Jung Foundation Bks.). 352p. pap. 18.00 (*0-87773-902-1*) Shambhala Pubns.

Psyche & Schizophrenia: The Bond Between Affect & Logic. Luc Ciompi. Tr. by Deborah L. Schneider. 1988. LC 88-6768. (Illus.). 320p. 55.00 (*0-674-71990-5*) HUP.

Psyche & Society: Explorations in Psychoanalytic Sociology. Robert Endleman. 1981. LC 81-1646. 448p. text 69.50 (*0-231-04992-7*) Col U Pr.

Psyche & Sports: Baseball, Hockey, Martial Arts, Running, Swimming, Tennis & Others. Ed. by Murray Stein & John Hollwitz. 1994. LC 94-28089. (Illus.). 248p. (Orig.). pap. 16.95 (*0-933029-79-9*) Chiron Pubns.

Psyche & Substance: Essays on Homeopathy in the Light of Jungian Psychology. Edward C. Whitmont. 3rd rev. ed. 1991. LC 82-22322. 300p. pap. 16.95 (*1-55643-106-6*) North Atlantic.

Psyche & Symbol: A Selection from the Writings from C. G. Jung. Carl Gustav Jung. Tr. by R. F. C. Hull from GER. 1991. LC 90-36021. (Bollingen Ser.). (Illus.). 384p. (C). pap. 18.95 (*0-691-01903-7*) Princeton U Pr.

Psyche & the Social World: Developments in Group-Analytic Theory. Ed. by Dennis G. Brown & Louis Zinkin. LC 93-3918. (International Library of Philosophy, Psychology, & Scientific Method). (C). 1994. 288p. pap. 27.99 (*0-415-08709-0*, B0881); 1993. 272p. text 79.95 (*0-415-08708-2*, B0877) Routledge.

Psyche & the Split-Brain. Jenny L. Yates. (Illus.). 106p. (Orig.). (C). 49.50 (*0-8191-9446-8*); pap. 23.00 (*0-8191-9447-6*) U Pr of Amer.

Psyche at Work: Workplace Applications of Jungian Analytical Psychology. Ed. by Murray Stein & John Hollwitz. 1992. LC 92-12176. 248p. (Orig.). pap. 16.95 (*0-933029-61-6*) Chiron Pubns.

Psyche in Medicine. Arthur Guirdham. 1978. 109p. (*0-85978-031-7*) C W Daniel GBR. *Dist:* Natl Bk Netwk.

Psyche Speaks: A Jungian Approach to Self & World. Russell A. Lockhart. 1987. LC 87-18260. 130p. 29.95 (*0-933029-28-4*); pap. 15.95 (*0-933029-22-5*) Chiron Pubns.

Psyche-Therapy: How to Master Your Mind(s) & Emotions. I. Lovejoy. 1991. 250p. (Orig.). pap. 19.95 (*0-9601978-7-7*) Health Res Las Vegas.

Psychedelic Drugs Reconsidered. Lester Grinspoon & James B. Bakalar. 3rd ed. 1997. (Drug Policy Classics Reprints Ser.: No. 1). 385p. reprint ed. pap. 12.95 (*0-9641568-5-7*) Open Soc Inst.

Psychedelic Shamanism: The Cultivation, Preparation & Shamanic Use of Psychoactive Plants. Jim DeKorne. 1994. LC 94-75331. (Illus.). 155p. (C). pap. text 19.95 (*1-55950-110-3*, 85182) Loompanics.

Psychedelics. Compiled by Thomas Lyttle. 1993. LC 93-19655. 272p. pap. 14.95 (*0-9623032-2-4*) Barricade Bks.

Psyche's Stories: Modern Jungian Interpretations of Fairy Tales, Vol. 1. Ed. by Murray Stein & Lionel Corbett. 1991. LC 90-26108. (Illus.). 184p. (Orig.). pap. 17.95 (*0-933029-39-X*) Chiron Pubns.

Psycheye. Akhter Ahsen. 1977. 288p. 30.00 (*0-913412-47-3*) Brandon Hse.

Psychiatric - Mental Health Nursing. Jack Rudman. (Regents College Proficiency Examination Ser.: Vol. 34). 43.95 (*0-8373-5484-6*); (ACT Proficiency Examination Program Ser.: Vol. 40). 43.95 (*0-8373-5590-7*) Nat Learn.

Psychiatric Administration: A Comprehensive Text for the Clinician-Executive. Ed. by John A. Talbott & Seymour R. Kaplan. 1982. 410p. text 56.00 (*0-8089-1529-0*, 794501, Grune & Strat) Harcrt Hlth Sci Grp.

***Psychiatric & Cognitive Disorders in Parkinsons Disease.** Sergio E. Starkstein & Marcelo Merello. 2002. 200p. text 64.95 (*0-521-66305-9*) Cambridge U Pr.

Psychiatric & Mental Health Nurse. Jack Rudman. 1994. (Certified Nurse Examination Ser.: CN-12). pap. 27.95 (*0-8373-6112-5*) Nat Learn.

Psychiatric & Mental Health Nursing CTB. Frisch. 1998. (Nursing Education Ser.). 47.95 (*0-8273-7235-3*) Delmar.

Psychiatric Aspects of Cancer. Ed. by R. J. Goldberg. 1988. (Advances in Psychosomatic Medicine Ser.: Vol. 18). (Illus.). viii, 160p. 60.00 (*3-8055-4745-5*) S Karger.

Psychiatric Aspects of Chronic Pulmonary Disease. Ed. by Wendy L. Thompson & T. L. Thompson. 1985. (Advances in Psychosomatic Medicine Ser.: Vol. 14). (Illus.). x, 174p. 95.75 (*3-8055-4088-4*) S Karger.

Psychiatric Aspects of General Patient Care. Bonnie Fossett. Ed. by Barbara Halliburton. 3rd rev. ed. 1996. 186p. (C). pap. text 49.95 (*1-878025-92-9*) Western Schls.

Psychiatric Aspects of Juvenile Delinquency. L. Bovet. 1951. (WHO Monograph Ser.: No. 1). 90p. 5.00 (*92-4-140001-3*) World Health.

Psychiatric Aspects of Juvenile Delinquency. Lucien Bovet. 1970. LC 74-98747. 90p. reprint ed. lib. bdg. 58.00 (*0-8371-3019-0*, BOPA, Greenwood Pr) Greenwood.

Psychiatric Aspects of Minimal Brain Dysfunction in Adults. Ed. by Leopold Bellak. 1979. 224p. text 40.00 (*0-8089-1192-9*, 790513, Grune & Strat) Harcrt Hlth Sci Grp.

Psychiatric Aspects of Neurologic Disease. Ed. by D. Frank Benson & Dietrich Blumer. 1975. (Seminars in Psychiatry Ser.). (Illus.). 336p. text 55.00 (*0-8089-0860-X*, 790542, Grune & Strat) Harcrt Hlth Sci Grp.

Psychiatric Aspects of Neurologic Disease, Vol. 2. Ed. by Frank Benson & Diedrich Blumer. 1982. (Seminars in Psychiatry Ser.). 352p. text 39.00 (*0-8089-1477-4*, 790543, Grune & Strat) Harcrt Hlth Sci Grp.

Psychiatric Aspects of Organ Transplantation. John Craven. Ed. by Gary M. Rodin. 1992. (Illus.). 254p. text 55.00 (*0-19-262073-8*) OUP.

Psychiatric Aspects of Personal Injury Claims. George Mendelson. 1988. (Illus.). 296p. (C). text 61.95 (*0-398-05411-8*) C C Thomas.

Psychiatric Aspects of Reproductive Technology. Ed. by Nada L. Stotland. 1990. LC 90-266. (Issues in Psychiatry Ser.). 168p. text 9.95 (*0-88048-316-4*, 8316) Am Psychiatric.

Psychiatric Aspects of Symptom Management in Cancer Patients. Ed. by William Breitbart & Jimmie C. Holland. 1993. LC 92-6969. (Clinical Practice Ser.: No. 25). 278p. text 14.95 (*0-88048-193-5*, 8193) Am Psychiatric.

Psychiatric Aspects of Terminal Illness. Ed. by Samuel C. Klagsbrun et al. 1988. LC 87-72173. 216p. pap. text 21.95 (*0-914783-23-8*) Charles.

Psychiatric Aspects of Trauma. Ed. by Linda G. Peterson & G. J. O'Shanick. 1986. (Advances in Psychosomatic Medicine Ser.: Vol. 16). (Illus.). x, 238p. 66.75 (*3-8055-4219-4*) S Karger.

Psychiatric Assessment: Pre & Post Admission. Valerie A. Brown. 1997. LC 97-222449. (Forensic Focus Ser.: Vol. 8). 48p. pap. (*1-85302-575-5*) Jessica Kingsley GBR. *Dist:* Taylor & Francis.

Psychiatric Attendant. Jack Rudman. 1994. (Career Examination Ser.: C-1434). pap. 27.95 (*0-8373-1434-8*) Nat Learn.

Psychiatric Care in the Nursing Home. Ed. by William E. Reichman & Paul R. Katz. 1996. (Illus.). 328p. text 49.95 (*0-19-508515-9*) OUP.

Psychiatric Care Planning. Susan L. Krupnick & Andrew J. Wade. 1992. LC 92-2365. 320p. pap. 32.95 (*0-87434-399-2*) Springhouse Corp.

Psychiatric Care Planning. Susan Krupnick & Andrew J. Wade. 2nd rev. ed. 1998. LC 98-38122. 336p. pap. 37.95 (*0-87434-953-2*) Springhouse Corp.

Psychiatric Care Plans: Guidelines for Planning & Documenting Client Care. Marilynn E. Doenges et al. 3rd ed. 1997. LC 97-24117. (Illus.). 532p. (C). pap. text 36.95 (*0-8036-0322-3*) Davis Co.

Psychiatric Claims in Workers' Compensation & Civil Actions, Vol. 2. Herbert Lasky. 1993. (Personal Injury Library). 592p. 255.00 (*0-471-58490-8*) Wiley.

Psychiatric Clinical Pathways: An Interdisciplinary Approach. Patricia C. Dykes. 1998. LC 98-5909. 400p. pap. 74.00 (*0-8342-1156-4*, 11564) Aspen Pub.

Psychiatric Comorbidity in Epilepsy: Basic Mechanisms, Diagnosis, & Treatment. Ed. by Harry W. McConnell & Peter J. Snyder. 1998. LC 97-2319. 416p. text 56.00 (*0-88048-853-0*, 8853) Am Psychiatric.

Psychiatric Consequences of Brain Disease in the Elderly: A Focus on Management. Ed. by D. K. Conn et al. 1989. (Illus.). 224p. 65.00 (*0-306-43216-1*, Plenum Trade) Perseus Pubng.

Psychiatric Consultation in Childbirth Settings: Parent- & Child-Oriented Approaches. R. L. Cohen. 1988. LC 88-6005. (Illus.). 298p. (C). text 57.50 (*0-306-42758-3*, Kluwer Plenum) Kluwer Academic.

Psychiatric Consultation in Schools: A Report of the American Psychiatric Association. APA Committee on Psychiatry and Mental Health in Schools. 1993. LC 93-6913. 96p. text 9.95 (*0-89042-243-5*, 2243) Am Psychiatric.

Psychiatric Diagnosis. Donald W. Goodwin & Samuel B. Guze. 5th ed. 1996. 384p. (C). text 39.95 (*0-19-510421-8*); pap. text 29.50 (*0-19-510422-6*) OUP.

Psychiatric Diagnosis: A World Perspective. Ed. by Juan E. Mezzich et al. 1994. LC 93-46006. (Illus.). 336p. 148.00 (*0-387-94221-1*) Spr-Verlag.

***Psychiatric Diagnosis & Classification.** Maj. 2002. LC 2001-57370. 264p. 92.00 (*0-471-49681-2*) Wiley.

Psychiatric Dictionary. Robert J. Campbell. 7th ed. 1996. LC 95-17720. 840p. (C). text 67.50 (*0-19-510259-2*) OUP.

Psychiatric Differential Diagnosis. Jeremy M. Pfeffer & Gillian Waldron. 1987. LC 86-26356. (Illus.). 192p. (Orig.). (C). text (*0-443-03703-5*) Church.

Psychiatric Dilemma of Adolescence. James F. Masterson. 2nd ed. 1986. LC 83-24039. 232p. reprint ed. text 38.95 (*0-87630-356-4*) Brunner-Routledge.

Psychiatric Dimensions of Medical Practice: What Primary-Care Physicians Should Know about Delirium, Demoralization, Suicidal Thinking, & Competence to Refuse Medical Advice. Phillip R. Slavney. 1998. LC 97-52406. 140p. pap. text 17.95 (*0-8018-5906-9*) Johns Hopkins.

Psychiatric Disabilities, Employment, & the Americans with Disabilities Act. 1997. lib. bdg. 251.95 (*0-8490-8213-7*) Gordon Pr.

Psychiatric Disabilities, Employment & the Americans with Disabilities Act (ADA) 1994. (Illus.). 136p. (Orig.). (YA). (gr. 12 up). pap. text 20.00 (*0-7881-0860-3*) DIANE Pub.

Psychiatric Disorders. 1995. LC 94-33379. (Professional Care Guides Ser.). 224p. 24.95 (*0-87434-781-5*) Springhouse Corp.

Psychiatric Disorders in America. Ed. by Lee N. Robins & Darrel A. Regier. 1990. LC 90-3168. (Illus.). 400p. 60.00 (*0-02-926571-1*) Free Pr.

Psychiatric Disorders with a Biochemical Basis: Including Pharmacology, Toxicology & Nutritional Aspects. David Donaldson. 1998. LC 97-7656. (Illus.). 252p. lib. bdg. 49.95 (*1-85070-789-8*, Parthenon Pbng) CRC Pr.

Psychiatric Drugs. Jeffrey Leiberman & Allan Tasman. 2000. LC 99-44546. (Illus.). 255p. pap. text (*0-7216-5884-9*) Saunders.

Psychiatric Emergencies. Ed. by William R. Dubin et al. 1984. (Clinics in Emergency Medicine Ser.: Vol. 4). (Illus.). 268p. text (*0-443-08288-X*) Church.

Psychiatric Emergencies. Ed. by J. D. Pollitt. 1987. (C). text 82.00 (*0-85200-676-4*) Kluwer Academic.

Psychiatric Emergencies, No. 11. Stephen Merson & David Baldwin. 1995. (Oxford Handbooks in Emergency Medicine Ser.: Vol. 11). 134p. text 69.50 (*0-19-262478-4*); pap. text 35.00 (*0-19-262477-6*) OUP.

Psychiatric Emergencies: Crisis Intervention Booklet, Part 1. Pamela Marcus. 1995. 32p. (C). (gr. 13). pap. text 16.95 (*0-8151-7287-7*, 27739) Mosby Inc.

Psychiatric Emergencies Pt. 1: Crisis Intervention. Pamela E. Marcus & John J. Hanlon. 1995. incl. VHS (*0-8151-7286-9*) Mosby Inc.

Psychiatric Emergencies, Three-Part Video Series Module 3: Violence, Aggression, Suicide & Post-Traumatic Stress Disorder (PTSD) Pamela E. Marcus. 1995. (Illus.). 20p. (C). (gr. 13). text 39.95 incl. VHS (*0-8151-7290-7*, 27742) Mosby Inc.

Psychiatric Emergencies Video Series Pamela E. Marcus. 1995. 96p. incl. VHS (*0-8151-5699-5*) Mosby Inc.

Psychiatric Emergency: Its Recognition & Management. Ed. by Eugene S. O'Neill. 1986. LC 85-21986. (Emergency Health Services Review Ser.: Vol. 3, No. 1). 128p. text 4.95 (*0-86656-518-3*) Haworth Pr.

Psychiatric Ethics Primer. American Psychiatric Association Staff. 2001. LC 00-58662. xiv, 101p. pap. 24.00 (*0-89042-317-2*, 2317) Am Psychiatric.

Psychiatric Factors in Drug Abuse. Roy W. Pickens & Leonard Heston. 1979. 400p. text 52.00 (*0-8089-1214-3*, 793289, Grune & Strat) Harcrt Hlth Sci Grp.

Psychiatric Genetics. John I. Nurnberger & Berrettini. 1997. (Illus.). 176p. 45.00 (*0-412-53580-7*) OUP.

Psychiatric Home Care. Anita W. Finkelman. 1997. LC 96-48674. 607p. 68.00 (*0-8342-0928-4*) Aspen Pub.

Psychiatric Home Care. Barry Menikoff 1999. LC 99-62666. (Practical Resources for the Mental Health Professional Ser.). (Illus.). 288p. (C). text 59.95 (*0-12-490940-X*) Acad Pr.

Psychiatric Home Care & Care Paths: Step by Step. LeeAnn Blazek. 1995. (Orig.). pap. (*0-9649995-0-1*) L A Blazek.

Psychiatric Hospital: Context, Values & Therapeutic Process. Ed. by Henry L. Lennard & Alexander Gralnick. 1986. 221p. 35.95 (*0-89885-297-8*, Kluwer Acad Hman Sci) Kluwer Academic.

Psychiatric Hospital Closure: Myths & Realities. Shulamit Ramon. 1992. 224p. pap. 47.75 (*1-56593-048-7*, 0296) Thomson Learn.

Psychiatric Ideologies & Institutions. Anselm L. Strauss et al. 1981. LC 80-20225. 418p. pap. text 29.95 (*0-87855-785-7*) Transaction Pubs.

***Psychiatric Intensive Care.** M. Dominic Beer et al. 2000. (Greenwich Medical Media Ser.). (Illus.). 354p. pap. text (*1-900151-87-1*) Greenwich Med GBR. *Dist:* JAMCO Dist.

Psychiatric Interview. Harry Stack Sullivan. 1970. 256p. reprint ed. pap. 11.95 (*0-393-00506-2*) Norton.

Psychiatric Interview: A Guide to History Taking & the Mental State Examination. Saxby Pridmore. 2000. 176p. 38.00 (*90-5823-072-4*); pap. 22.00 (*90-5823-106-2*) Gordon & Breach (Harwood Acad Pubs).

Psychiatric Interview in Clinical Practice. Roger A. MacKinnon & Robert Michels. 1971. LC 70-151680. text 52.00 (*0-7216-5973-X*) Saunders.

Psychiatric Interviewing: The Art of Understanding. Shawn C. Shea. 2nd ed. 1998. LC 97-36788. (Illus.). 656p. (C). text 37.50 (*0-7216-7011-3*) Saunders.

Psychiatric Issues in Epilepsy: A Practical Guide to Diagnosis & Treatment. Alan B. Ettinger & Andres M. Kanner. 2001. LC 00-67143. 416p. text 110.00 (*0-7817-2176-8*) Lppncott W & W.

Psychiatric Justice. Thomas Szasz. 1988. 304p. reprint ed. pap. 17.95 (*0-8156-0231-6*) Syracuse U Pr.

Psychiatric-Legal Decision Making by the Mental Health Practitioner: The Clinician As de Facto Magistrate. Ed. by Harvey Bluestone et al. 1994. LC 93-5998. (Einstein Psychiatry Publication Ser.: Vol. 9). 310p. 180.00 (*0-471-00431-6*) Wiley.

Psychiatric Length of Stay by Diagnosis, 1997: North Central. 1997. pap. 195.00 (*1-57372-077-1*) Solucient.

Psychiatric Length of Stay by Diagnosis, 1997: Northeastern. 1997. pap. 195.00 (*1-57372-076-3*) Solucient.

Psychiatric Length of Stay by Diagnosis, 1997: Southern. 1997. pap. 195.00 (*1-57372-078-X*) Solucient.

Psychiatric Length of Stay by Diagnosis, 1997: United States. 1997. pap. 195.00 (*1-57372-075-5*) Solucient.

Psychiatric Length of Stay by Diagnosis, 1997: Western. 1997. pap. 195.00 (*1-57372-079-8*) Solucient.

Psychiatric Length of Stay by Diagnosis, United States. 1996. (*1-57372-042-9*) Solucient.

Psychiatric Malpractice: Cases & Comments for Clinicians. Robert I. Simon & Robert L. Sadoff. 1992. LC 91-4540. 309p. text 44.00 (*0-88048-107-2*, 8107) Am Psychiatric.

Psychiatric Malpractice: Stories of Patients, Psychiatrists, & the Law. James L. Kelley. 1996. LC 95-52270. 240p. (C). 29.95 (*0-8135-2323-0*) Rutgers U Pr.

Psychiatric Management for Medical Practitioners. D. S. Kornfeld & Finkel. 1982. 496p. text 36.00 (*0-8089-1420-0*, 792373, Grune & Strat) Harcrt Hlth Sci Grp.

Psychiatric Medications: A Guide for Mental Health Professionals. Kenneth J. Bender. 1990. (Human Services Guides Ser.: Vol. 61). (Illus.). 120p. (C). pap. 34.95 (*0-8039-3337-1*, 6334) Sage.

Psychiatric Medicine: A Handbook. James L. Mathis. Ed. by James F. Gardner. 1984. (Allied Health Professions Monograph). 212p. (C). 22.50 (*0-87527-320-3*) Green.

Psychiatric Mental Health Nursing. Mary Ann Boyd & Mary Ann Nihart. 1998. LC 97-30272. 1,200p. text 52.95 (*0-397-55178-9*) Lppncott W & W.

Psychiatric-Mental Health Nursing. Marga S. Coler & Karen G. Vincent. 1995. LC 94-29976. (Plans of Care for Specialty Practice Ser.). 288p. (C). pap. 28.00 (*0-8273-6102-5*) Delmar.

Psychiatric-Mental Health Nursing. Ed. by Katherine M. Fortinash & Patricia A. Holoday-Worret. 1995. LC 95-39307. (Illus.). 816p. (C). (gr. 13). text 55.00 (*0-8151-3348-0*, 23765) Mosby Inc.

Psychiatric-Mental Health Nursing. Katherine M. Fortinash & Patricia A. Holoday-Worret. 1992. (Illus.). tchr. ed. (*0-8151-3349-9*) Mosby Inc.

Psychiatric Mental Health Nursing. Frisch-Griffin. 1998. (C). stu. ed. 16.75 net. (*0-7668-1006-2*) Delmar.

Psychiatric Mental Health Nursing. Frisch et al. 1998. LC 97-42749. (Nursing Education Ser.). 862p. (C). 75.95 (*0-8273-7233-7*) Delmar.

Psychiatric Mental Health Nursing. Ellen H. Janosik & Janet L. Davies. 1986. (Illus.). 761p. (C). text 42.50 (*0-86720-352-8*, 352-8) Jones & Bartlett.

Psychiatric Mental Health Nursing. Joan Norris et al. 1989. text 49.95 (*0-8273-4324-8*) Delmar.

Psychiatric-Mental Health Nursing. Jack Rudman. 1994. (Regents College Proficiency Examination Ser.: CPEP-34). pap. 23.95 (*0-8373-5434-X*); (ACT Proficiency Examination Program Ser.: Vol. PEP-40). pap. 23.95 (*0-8373-5540-0*) Nat Learn.

Psychiatric Mental Health Nursing. Katherine M. Fortinash & Patricia A. Holoday-Worret. (C). 1999. reprint ed. text (*0-323-00788-0*); 2nd ed. 2000. LC 99-43208. (Illus.). 854p. text 54.00 (*0-323-00648-5*) Mosby Inc.

Psychiatric Mental Health Nursing. Ellen H. Janosik & Janet L. Davies. 2nd ed. 1989. 1024p. pap., tchr. ed. 10.00 (*0-86720-425-7*); (Illus.). text 78.95 (*0-86720-420-6*, 420-6);Supplement. tchr. ed. 97.50 (*0-86720-426-5*) Jones & Bartlett.

Psychiatric Mental Health Nursing: Adaptation & Growth. Barbara Johnson. 4th ed. 1996. LC 96-32247. 1,120p. text 56.95 (*0-397-55243-2*) Lppncott W & W.

***Psychiatric Mental Health Nursing: Computerized Test Bank.** Katherine M. Fortinash & Patricia A. Holoday-Worret. 2nd ed. 2000. 500.00 (*0-323-01115-2*) Mosby Inc.

***Psychiatric Mental Health Nursing: Instructor's Resource Manual.** Katherine M. Fortinash & Patricia A. Holoday-Worret. 2nd ed. 2000. 250.00 (*0-323-01112-8*) Mosby Inc.

Psychiatric-Mental Health Nursing: Integrating the Behavioral & Biological Sciences. Ed. by Angela B. McBride & Joan K. Austin. 1995. LC 95-10059. (Illus.). 471p. text 56.00 (*0-7216-4038-9*) Saunders.

Psychiatric Mental Health Nursing Care Plans. Deborah Antai-Otong. 2002. (C). pap. 27.75 (*0-7668-1141-7*) Thomson Learn.

Psychiatric Mental Health Nursing Psychopharmacology Project. American Nurses Association Staff. 1994. 88p. (Orig.). pap. text 25.95 (*1-55810-104-7*, PMH-13) Am Nurses Pub.

***Psychiatric Mental Health Nursing Research Digest.** Ed. by Joyce J. Fitzpatrick & Patricia A. Wilke. 2001. LC 2001-17013. xiii, 305p. (*0-8261-1393-1*) Springer Pub.

Psychiatric Mental Health Readings. Barbara A. Backer et al. 1985. LC 84-29937. (Contemporary Readings Ser.). (Illus.). 300p. (C). pap. text 36.25 (*0-534-04644-4*, 644-4) Jones & Bartlett.

Psychiatric Mental Status Examination. Paula T. Trzepacz & Robert W. Baker. 1993. LC 92-48947. (Illus.). 216p. text 42.50 (*0-19-506251-5*) OUP.

Psychiatric Music Therapy: Origins & Development. Florence Tyson. 1982. (Illus.). 24.95 (*0-9606876-0-2*); pap. 14.95 (*0-9606876-1-0*) CARC.

Psychiatric Neuroimaging Research: Contemporary Strategies. Ed. by Drain D. Dougherty & Scott L. Rauch. 2001. LC 00-61073. 448p. 79.95 (*0-88048-844-1*, 8844) Am Psychiatric.

Psychiatric Nurse. Jack Rudman. 1994. (Career Examination Ser.: C-986). pap. 29.95 (*0-8373-0986-7*) Nat Learn.

Psychiatric Nursing. 384p. pap. (*0-340-62523-6*) E A GBR. *Dist:* Routldge.

***Psychiatric Nursing.** pap. (*0-7021-2979-8*) Juta & Co ZAF. *Dist:* Intl Spec Bk.

Psychiatric Nursing. 2000. 37.00 (*0-07-135482-4*); 1999. (*0-07-135483-2*); 1999. (*0-07-135485-9*) McGraw.

Psychiatric Nursing. Deborah Antai-Otong. 1995. 125.00 (*0-7216-6225-0*) Harcourt.

Psychiatric Nursing. Brooking. 1992. (Illus.). 640p. (Orig.). pap. text (*0-443-03461-3*) Church.

Psychiatric Nursing. Nardi. 1992. (Nursing Education Ser.). (C). text 35.95 (*0-8273-3654-3*) Delmar.

Psychiatric Nursing. Visual Education Corporation Staff. 1992. (NSNA Review Ser.). tchr. ed. 12.00 (*0-8273-3655-1*) Delmar.

Psychiatric Nursing. Ed. by Christine A. Grant. 2nd ed. 1992. LC 93-37961. (NSNA Review Ser.). 165.00 (*0-8273-5372-3*) Delmar.

Psychiatric Nursing. Holly S. Wilson & Carol R. Kneisl. 2nd ed. 1983. stu. ed. (*0-201-11703-7*, Health Sci) Addison-Wesley.

Psychiatric Nursing. Norman L. Keltner et al. 3rd ed. 1998. LC 98-38935. (Illus.). 816p. 39.00 (*0-323-00399-0*) Mosby Inc.

Psychiatric Nursing. Kools. 3rd ed. 1998. (Illus.). 304p. (C). pap. text, stu. ed. (*0-8151-5285-X*, 28747) Mosby Inc.

Psychiatric Nursing. 5th ed. 1995. 256p. (C). text 22.50 (*0-8053-9409-5*) Benjamin-Cummings.

Psychiatric Nursing. Holly S. Wilson. 5th ed. 1995. LC 95-37750. 920p. (C). 81.00 (*0-8053-9408-7*) Addison-Wesley.

Psychiatric Nursing: A Comprehensive Reference. Ed. by Suzanne Lego. 2nd ed. 1996. LC 95-26303. 688p. text 63.95 (*0-397-55266-1*) Lppncott W & W.

Psychiatric Nursing: Biological & Behavioral Concepts. Deborah Anai-Otong. 1995. LC 94-25346. (Illus.). 1008p. text 51.00 (*0-7216-3778-7*) Saunders.

Psychiatric Nursing: Biological & Behavioral Concepts. Ed. by Deborah Antai-Otong. 1995. (Illus.). 820p. tchr. ed. (*0-7216-4925-4*);Assessment & Medications Booklet. (C). pap. text (*0-7216-6231-5*) Saunders.

Psychiatric Nursing: Ethical Strife. Ed. by Philip J. Barker & Ben Davidson. 1997. (Illus.). 272p. (Orig.). pap. 38.25 (*1-56593-762-7*, 1482) Singular Publishing.

Psychiatric Nursing: Includes Testbank. Norman L. Keltner et al. 3rd ed. 1998. (Illus.). tchr. ed. (*0-323-00400-8*) Mosby Inc.

Psychiatric Nursing: Promoting Mental Health. Ann Burgess. 1996. LC 96-8408. 912p. (C). 64.00 (*0-8385-8087-4*, A8087-7) P-H.

Psychiatric Nursing: Review & Study Guide. Elaine Zimbler. 1996. 368p. (C). pap., stu. ed. 25.60 (*0-8385-8121-8*, A8121-4) Appleton & Lange.

Psychiatric Nursing: Theory & Application. Lucille A. Joel & Doris L. Collins. 1978. (Illus.). text 32.00 (*0-07-032537-5*) McGraw.

Psychiatric Nursing Administration Manual. Anita W. Finkelman. 1994. LC 94-12892. ring bd. 129.00 (*0-8342-0582-3*, S146) Aspen Pub.

Psychiatric Nursing As a Human Experience. Lisa Robinson. 3rd ed. 1983. (Illus.). text 58.00 (*0-7216-7622-7*) Saunders.

Psychiatric Nursing Care Plans. Katherine M. Fortinash & Patricia A. Holoday-Worret. 3rd ed. 1998. LC 98-29832. (Illus.). 368p. 34.95 (*0-323-00403-2*) Mosby Inc.

Psychiatric Nursing (cd-rom) 1999. cd-rom (*0-07-135484-0*) McGraw.

Psychiatric Nursing Certification Review Guide for the Generalist & Clinical Specialist in Adult, Child, & Adolescent Psychiatric & Mental Health Nursing. Ed. by Clare Houseman. 2nd ed. 1998. LC 98-12134. 600p. (C). pap. 52.00 (*1-878028-19-7*) Hlth Lead Assoc.

Psychiatric Nursing Clinical Guide: Assessment Tools & Diagnoses. Elizabeth M. Varcarolis. 2000. LC 99-49759. (Illus.). 495p. pap. text (*0-7216-8336-3*) Saunders.

Psychiatric Nursing Diagnosis Care Plans. Mary F. Paquette. 1991. pap. text 40.00 (*0-86720-310-2*) Jones & Bartlett.

Psychiatric Nursing Diagnosis Care Plans for DSM IV. Mary Paquette & Christine Rodemich. 4th ed. 1997. LC 96-45656. (Nursing Ser.). (Illus.). 224p. (C). pap. text 45.00 (*0-7637-0255-2*, 0255-2) Jones & Bartlett.

Psychiatric Nursing Handbook. Lloyd A. Wells. 1989. (Allied Health Professions Monograph). 440p. 47.50 (*0-87527-295-9*) Green.

Psychiatric Nursing Skills. G. Dexter & Michael Wash. 2nd ed. 1994. (Illus.). 336p. pap. text 45.95 (*1-56593-098-3*, 0431) Singular Publishing.

Psychiatric Nursing Skills: A Patient-Centered Approach. Graham Dexter & Michael Wash. 1985. LC 85-13252. 320p. (C). pap. (*0-7099-3617-6*) C Helm GBR. *Dist:* Routldge.

Psychiatric Nursing Value Package. Davies. 1991. 71.25 (*0-86720-311-0*) Jones & Bartlett.

Psychiatric Occupational Therapy: A Workbook of Practical Skills. Peggy Denton. 1986. 208p. (Orig.). pap. text 40.00 (*0-316-18088-2*) Lppncott W & W.

Psychiatric Occupational Therapy in the Army. Ed. by Paul D. Ellsworth & Diane Gibson. 1983. LC 83-10859. (Occupational Therapy in Mental Health Ser.: Vol. 3, No. 2). 88p. text 39.95 (*0-86656-234-6*) Haworth Pr.

Psychiatric Pearls. Jeffrey M. Lyness. 1997. LC 96-29495. (Illus.). 328p. pap. 21.95 (*0-8036-0280-4*) Davis Co.

Psychiatric Rehabilitation. William A. Anthony et al. 1990. LC 89-62415. 283p. text 39.95 (*1-878512-00-5*) Boston Univ Ctr Psy Rehab.

Psychiatric Rehabilitation. Carlos Pratt et al. 1999. LC 98-89453. (Illus.). 350p. 59.95 (*0-12-564245-8*) Acad Pr.

Psychiatric Rehabilitation: A Handbook for Practitioners. Lynda Katz. 1992. (Illus.). 407p. pap. 55.00 (*0-87527-500-1*) Green.

Psychiatric Rehabilitation: A Practical Guide. Mounir Y. Ekdawi et al. 1994. 154p. 44.50 (*1-56593-299-4*, 0623) Singular Publishing.

Psychiatric Rehabilitation in Practice. Robert W. Flexor & Phyllis L. Solomon. 1993. LC 92-49873. 268p. text 63.00 (*1-56372-025-6*) Buttrwrth-Heinemann.

Psychiatric Rehabilitation of Chronic Mental Patients. Ed. by Robert P. Liberman. 1988. LC 87-1492. 319p. pap. text 28.00 (*0-88048-201-X*, 8201) Am Psychiatric.

Psychiatric Research in America: Two Studies, Nineteen Thirty-Six to Nineteen Forty-One Ed. by Gerald N. Grob. 1980. LC 78-22583. (Historical Issues in Mental Health Ser.). reprint ed. lib. bdg. 31.95 (*0-405-11935-6*) Ayer.

Psychiatric Secrets: Questions You Will Be Asked on Rounds in the Clinic, on Oral Exams. Ed. by James L. Jacobson & Alan Jacobson. 2nd ed. 2000. LC 00-37043. (Secrets Ser.). 500p. pap. 39.95 (*1-56053-418-4*) Hanley & Belfus.

Psychiatric Self-Assessment & Review (PSA-R) American Psychiatric Association Staff. 1999. pap. 225.00 (*0-89042-285-0*) Am Psychiatric.

Psychiatric Self-Help. Gordon R. Forrer. 1973. LC 72-85870. 10.00 (*0-87212-029-5*) Libra.

Psychiatric Senior Attendant. Jack Rudman. 1994. (Career Examination Ser.: C-1435). pap. 29.95 (*0-8373-1435-6*) Nat Learn.

Psychiatric Services in Jails & Prisons. American Psychiatric Association Staff. 2nd ed. 2000. LC 99-50098. 96p. pap. 19.00 (*0-89042-287-7*, 2287) Am Psychiatric.

Psychiatric Side Effects of Prescription & Over-the-Counter Medications: Recognition & Management. Thomas M. Brown & Alan Stoudemire. 1998. LC 97-42717. 417p. text 79.00 (*0-88048-868-9*, 8868) Am Psychiatric.

Psychiatric Social Work Assistant. Jack Rudman. 1994. (Career Examination Ser.: C-2414). pap. 27.95 (*0-8373-2414-9*) Nat Learn.

Psychiatric Social Work in India. Ratna Verma. 1991. (Illus.). 244p. 29.95 (*0-8039-9103-7*, 9193) Sage.

Psychiatric Social Work Supervisor. Jack Rudman. 1994. (Career Examination Ser.: C-2357). pap. 34.95 (*0-8373-2357-6*) Nat Learn.

Psychiatric Social Worker. Jack Rudman. 1994. (Career Examination Ser.: C-987). pap. 29.95 (*0-8373-0987-5*) Nat Learn.

Psychiatric Social Worker Trainee. Jack Rudman. 1994. (Career Examination Ser.: C-988). pap. 23.95 (*0-8373-0988-3*) Nat Learn.

Psychiatric Society. Francoise Castel et al. Tr. by Arthur Goldhammer from FRE. 1982. LC 81-15504. (European Perspectives; A Series in Social Thought & Culturall Criticism Ser.). 368p. text 67.00 (*0-231-05244-8*) Col U Pr.

Psychiatric Staff Attendant. Jack Rudman. 1994. (Career Examination Ser.: C-1436). pap. 27.95 (*0-8373-1436-4*) Nat Learn.

Psychiatric Staffing Crisis in Community Mental Health: A Report of Findings. Goplerud, Knight, and McGuire Staff. 1990. 20p. pap. 20.00 (*1-883066-06-9*) Natl Comm Mental.

Psychiatric Status Rating Scales: Index & Reference Book of New Information. Jacob L. Liehaus. 1996. 150p. 57.50 (*0-7883-0826-2*); pap. 47.50 (*0-7883-0827-0*) ABBE Pubs Assn.

Psychiatric Status Rating Scales: Index of New Information for Medicine, Science, Research with New Update of Progress. Waldlow A. Harrington. rev. ed. 1997. 187p. 57.50 (*0-7883-1558-7*); pap. 47.50 (*0-7883-1559-5*) ABBE Pubs Assn.

Psychiatric Syndromes & Drug Treatment. Nathan S. Kline & Jules Angst. 1979. LC 79-5193. 320p. 65.00 (*0-87668-379-0*) Aronson.

Psychiatric Team & the Social Definition of Schizophrenia: An Anthropological Study of Person & Illness. Rob Barrett. 1996. (Studies in Social & Community Psychiatry). (Illus.). 359p. (C). text 90.00 (*0-521-41653-1*) Cambridge U Pr.

Psychiatric Therapy Aide. Jack Rudman. 1994. (Career Examination Ser.: C-2124). reprint ed. pap. 27.95 (*0-8373-2124-7*) Nat Learn.

Psychiatric Treatment Is Much More Than Psychotherapy. John D. Moriarty. 1993. 300p. 24.00 (*0-9633747-0-2*); LC 92-82596. pap. 16.95 (*0-9633747-1-0*) SoCal Med Pr.

Psychiatric Treatment of Adolescents. Ed. by Aaron H. Esman. 1982. LC 83-208. xiii, 543p. 80.00 (*0-8236-5595-4*) Intl Univs Pr.

Psychiatric Treatment of Alzheimer's Disease. Group for the Advancement of Psychiatry Staff. 1988. (GAP Reports: No. 125). 160p. text 28.95 (*0-87630-519-2*) Brunner-Routledge.

Psychiatric Treatment of Neurological Illness. J. Schwartz & N. Speed. Date not set. (Medical Psychiatry Ser.). (*0-8247-9413-3*) Dekker.

Psychiatric Unit in a General Hospital: Its Current & Future Role. Ed. by M. Ralph Kaufman. 1965. LC 65-24003. 482p. 72.50 (*0-8236-5600-4*) Intl Univs Pr.

Psychiatric Update: American Psychiatric Association Annual Review, Vol. 5. Ed. by Allen J. Frances & Robert E. Hales. 1986. 791p. text 15.00 (*0-88048-241-9*, 8241); pap. text 10.00 (*0-88048-240-0*, 8240) Am Psychiatric.

Psychiatric Vade-Mecum. Basant Puri & Heather McKee. 1998. (An Arnold Publication). (Illus.). 352p. pap. (*0-340-69171-9*) E A GBR. *Dist:* OUP.

Psychiatric Words & Phrases. Mary A. D'Onofrio & Elizabeth D'Onofrio. 2nd ed. 1997. LC 99-159101. Orig. Title: Psychiatric Words & Phrases: A Quick Reference Guide. 12p. pap. 36.00 (*0-934385-70-X*) Hlth Prof Inst.

Psychiatric Words & Phrases: A Quick Reference Guide see Psychiatric Words & Phrases

Psychiatrie: Ein Lehrbuch Fur Studirende und Aerzte. Emil Kraepelin. 5th ed. 1976. LC 75-16713. (Classics in Psychiatry Ser.). (GER.). reprint ed. 69.95 (*0-405-07442-5*) Ayer.

Psychiatrist. Jack Rudman. 1994. (Career Examination Ser.: C-626). pap. 49.95 (*0-8373-0626-4*) Nat Learn.

Psychiatrist & the Dying Patient. K. R. Eissler. 1970. pap. 24.95 (*0-8236-8265-X*, 25720) Intl Univs Pr.

Psychiatrist As an Expert Witness. Thomas G. Gutheil. 1998. LC 97-29246. 176p. 26.00 (*0-88048-763-1*, 8763) Am Psychiatric.

Psychiatrist in Court: A Survival Guide. Thomas G. Gutheil. 1998. LC 97-34483. 126p. 26.00 (*0-88048-764-X*, 8764) Am Psychiatric.

Psychiatrist in the Courtroom: Selected Papers of Bernard L. Diamond, M.D. Ed. by Jacques M. Quen. 1994. LC 94-33422. 376p. 47.50 (*0-88163-160-4*) Analytic Pr.

Psychiatrist of America: The Life of Harry Stack Sullivan. Helen S. Perry. 1987. 474p. pap. 16.95 (*0-674-72077-6*); 1982. LC 81-7066. (Illus.). 74p. 36.50 (*0-674-72076-8*) HUP (Belknap).

Psychiatrist Recollects: Stories from the Lives of Psychiatric Patients. Malcolm B. Bowers, Jr. 1989. LC 88-2791. (Insight Bk.). 150p. 21.95 (*0-89885-433-4*, Kluwer Acad Hman Sci) Kluwer Academic.

Psychiatrist Speaks Out: Psychiatry, Sexuality & Maturity. J. Dennis Freund. 1991. LC 90-3848. 256p. 26.95 (*0-89876-179-4*) Gardner Pr.

Psychiatrist's Guide to Capitation & Risk-Based Contracting. American Psychiatric Association Staff. 1997. LC 97-12762. 114p. pap. text 27.00 incl. disk (*0-89042-453-5*, 2453) Am Psychiatric.

Psychiatrist's Guide to Managed Care Contracting. American Psychiatric Association Staff. 1997. LC 97-12315. 96p. pap. text 27.00 (*0-89042-454-3*, 2454) Am Psychiatric.

Psychiatrist's Guide to Practice Management. American Psychiatric Association Staff. 1997. LC 97-8762. 104p. pap. text 27.00 (*0-89042-451-9*, 2451) Am Psychiatric.

Psychiatrist's Managed Care Primer. American Psychiatric Association Staff. 1997. LC 97-11404. 111p. pap. text 26.00 (*0-89042-450-0*, 2450) Am Psychiatric.

Psychiatrist's Search for God: Back to God - Finding Joy in Divine Union. Adrian Finkelstein. 1996. 232p. pap. 15.95 (*0-9647831-0-X*) Fifty Gates.

Psychiatry. Dilling. 1990. 23.95 (*0-387-51980-7*) Spr-Verlag.

Psychiatry. Joan Gomez. 1997. (Medico-Legal Practitioner Ser.). ix, 135p. (*1-85941-017-0*) Cavendish Pubng GBR. *Dist:* Gaunt.

Psychiatry. Michael Gelder et al. 2nd ed. 1998. LC 98-22504. (Oxford Core Texts). (Illus.). 502p. pap. text 35.00 (*0-19-262888-7*) OUP.

Psychiatry. J. Scully et al. 2nd ed. 1990. (National Medical Ser.). 355p. 27.00 (*0-683-06264-6*) Lppncott W & W.

Psychiatry. L. B. Shaffer & Ronald S. Krug. 2nd ed. 1996. LC 96-13741. (Oklahoma Notes). 249p. pap. 24.95 (*0-387-94633-0*) Spr-Verlag.

Psychiatry. David A. Tomb. 4th ed. 1992. (House Officer Ser.). 265p. pap. 21.95 (*0-683-08342-2*) Lppncott W & W.

Psychiatry. A. Mezzacappa. 9th ed. 2000. LC 00-41871. (Pretest Clinical Science Ser.). (Illus.). 255p. pap. 24.95 (*0-07-136155-3*) McGraw-Hill Prof.

Psychiatry, Set. Allan Tasman et al. Ed. by Judy Fletcher. 1996. 1856p. 239.00 (*0-7216-5255-7*) Saunders.

Psychiatry: A Textbook for Students & Physicians Emil Kraepelin. 1991. (Resources in Medical History Ser.). 750p. (C). (*0-88135-086-9*);Set. 59.95 (*0-88135-087-7*) Watson Pub Intl (Sci Hist).

Psychiatry: An Illustrated Colour Text. L. Stevens. 1998. LC 2001-17071. (Illus.). 112p. pap. (*0-443-05703-6*) Church.

Psychiatry: Behavioral Science & Clinical Essentials. Jerald Kay et al. Ed. by Judy Fletcher. 1999. LC 98-31267. (Illus.). xii, 707p. pap. (*0-7216-5846-6*) Saunders.

Psychiatry: Common Drug Treatments. R. Spector et al. 1984. (Practical Problems in Medicine Ser.). (Illus.). 192p. lib. bdg. 45.00 (*0-906348-64-1*, Wiley-VCH) Wiley.

Psychiatry: Help or Betrayal?: An Authoritative Text on the History & Development of Psychiatry. Carlynn L. McCormick & J. Allen Chamberlin. 1991. pap. 12.95 (*0-9631117-0-1*) Gavilan Hills.

Psychiatry: Past Reflections - Future Visions. Ed. by B. T. Taylor & I. Taylor. 1992. 280p. 118.00 (*0-444-01583-3*) Elsevier.

Psychiatry: Review & Assessment. David H. Taylor et al. Ed. by Lesley Day & Judy Fletcher. 1996. LC 96-29396. 352p. pap. text 36.00 (*0-7216-5242-5*) Saunders.

Psychiatry & Applied Mental Health, 2000. Talbott. 2000. (Illus.). 575p. text 73.00 (*0-8151-2739-1*, 31322) Mosby Inc.

Psychiatry & Biological Factors. E. Kurstak. 1991. (Illus.). 322p. (C). text 85.00 (*0-306-43621-3*, Kluwer Plenum) Kluwer Academic.

Psychiatry & Criminal Culpability. Ralph Slovenko. 1995. 436p. 200.00 (*0-471-05425-9*) Wiley.

Psychiatry & General Practice. Ed. by A. W. Clare & Malcolm H. Lader. 1982. text 104.00 (*0-12-174720-4*) Acad Pr.

Psychiatry & Health: A Comprehensive Integration. Jules H. Masserman. 1986. 253p. 35.95 (*0-89885-256-0*, Kluwer Acad Hman Sci) Kluwer Academic.

Psychiatry & Medical Education: Two Studies Ed. by Gerald N. Grob. 1980. LC 78-22582. (Historical Issues in Mental Health Ser.). (Illus.). reprint ed. lib. bdg. 53.95 (*0-405-11934-8*) Ayer.

Psychiatry & Medical Practice in a General Hospital. Ed. by Norman E. Zinberg. 1964. LC 64-24868. 364p. 55.00 (*0-8236-5540-7*) Intl Univs Pr.

Psychiatry & Mental Health Science Handbook. Claudewell S. Thomas & Jacob J. Lindenthal. 1988. (Illus.). 267p. pap. 29.50 (*0-87527-370-X*) Green.

Psychiatry & Primary Health Care. Sean E. Baumann. 1999. 525p. pap. (*0-7021-4207-7*) Juta & Co ZAF. *Dist:* Intl Spec Bk.

Psychiatry & Religion: Context Consensus & Controversies. Ed. by Dinesh K. L. Bhugra. 1997. 256p. (C). pap. 27.95 (*0-415-16512-1*) Routledge.

Psychiatry & the Cinema. Krin Gabbard & Glen O. Gabbard. 1995. LC 86-25000. (Illus.). xx, 304p. (C). pap. 16.95 (*0-226-27791-7*) U Ch Pr.

Psychiatry & the Criminal Process. Ed. by Ronald D. Mckay & Kenneth V. Russell. 1986. (Leicester Polytechnic Law School Monograph Ser.). 48p. pap. (*0-948997-28-1*) Milltak Ltd.

***Psychiatry & the Human Condition.** Bruce Charlton. 2000. LC 00-421526. 264p. pap. (*1-85775-314-3*) Radcliffe Med Pr GBR. *Dist:* Balogh.

Psychiatry As Medicine: Contemporary Psychotherapies. Yehuda Fried & Joseph Agassi. 1983. 202p. lib. bdg. (*90-247-2837-1*) M Nijhoff NLD. *Dist:* Kluwer Academic.

Psychiatry at a Glance. Cornelius L. Katona. 1995. LC 95-4482. (At a Glance Ser.). (Illus.). 80p. pap. 22.95 (*0-86542-873-5*) Blackwell Sci.

Psychiatry at a Glance. Cornelius L. Katona & M. Robertson. 2nd ed. 2000. (At a Glance Ser.). (Illus.). 96p. pap. 22.95 (*0-632-05554-5*) Blackwell Sci.

Psychiatry Between the Wars, 1918-1945: A Recollection. 10. Walter Bromberg. 1982. LC 82-6153. (Contributions in Medical History Ser.: No. 10). 184p. 60.00 (*0-313-23460-4*, BWN/, Greenwood Pr) Greenwood.

Psychiatry, Communication & Awareness Training: Journal: Biosciences Communications, Vol. 3, No. 2. Ed. by R. Shaw. 1977. (Illus.). 16.75 (*3-8055-2709-8*) S Karger.

Psychiatry Education Today. Ives Hendrick. 1965. LC 65-15705. 110p. 27.50 (*0-8236-5500-8*, BN05500) Intl Univs Pr.

Psychiatry Exam Douglas A. Bernstein. Date not set. (C). text 65.96 (*0-395-69045-5*) HM.

Psychiatry for Beginners. Illus. by Bernard Canavan. 1986. (Writers & Readers Documentary Comic Bks.). 176p. pap. 6.95 (*0-86316-029-8*) Writers & Readers.

Psychiatry for Beginners. David A. Brizer. 2nd ed. 1993. (Illus.). 176p. pap. 9.95 (*0-86316-166-9*) Writers & Readers.

Psychiatry for Lawyers. Andrew S. Watson. rev. ed. 1978. LC 77-92183. 488p. 72.50 (*0-8236-5521-0*) Intl Univs Pr.

Psychiatry for Medical Students. Robert J. Waldinger. 3rd ed. 1997. 632p. LC 96-46911. text 58.00 (*0-88048-770-4*, 8770); pap. text 44.95 (*0-88048-789-5*, 8789) Am Psychiatric.

Psychiatry for Primary Care Physicians. Larry S. Goldman et al. 1997. LC 97-36835. 49.95 (*0-89970-892-7*) AMA.

Psychiatry for the Rich: A History of Ticehurst Private Asylum, 1792-1917. Charlotte MacKenzie. 1993. LC 92-49160. (Wellcome Institute Series in the History of Medicine). (Illus.). 224p. (C). 89.95 (*0-415-08891-7*, A9941) Routledge.

Psychiatry in a General Hospital: The First Fifty Years. Ed. by Thomas P. Hackett et al. 1987. (Illus.). 176p. 56.00 (*0-88416-570-1*) Mosby Inc.

Psychiatry in American Life. Ed. by Charles J. Rolo. 1977. LC 76-156711. (Essay Index Reprint Ser.). reprint ed. 22.95 (*0-8369-2424-X*) Ayer.

Psychiatry in Anthropological & Biomedical Context. Gerlof Verwey. 1984. lib. bdg. 154.50 (*90-277-1713-3*) Kluwer Academic.

Psychiatry in Court: The Use of Psychiatric Reports in Court Proceedings. Peter Shea. 1993. (Institute of Criminology Monographs: No. 3). xvii, 156p. pap. 30.00 (*0-86758-673-7*) Gaunt.

Psychiatry in Court: The Use(Fulness) of Psychiatric Reports & Psychiatric Evidence in Court Proceedings. Peter Shey. 2nd ed. 1996. LC 97-205448. 195p. pap. (*1-876067-03-9*, Hawkins Pr) Federation Pr AUS. *Dist:* Gaunt.

Psychiatry in Crisis. Ed. by Richard C. Hall. 1982. LC 80-22379. 156p. text 29.00 (*0-88331-188-7*) R B Luce.

Psychiatry in General Practice. Ed. by Ben Green. 1994. LC 94-39091. pap. (*0-7923-8852-6*) Kluwer Academic.

Psychiatry in Industry. V. V. Anderson. Ed. by Leon Stein. 1977. LC 77-70477. reprint ed. lib. bdg. 35.95 (*0-405-10151-1*) Ayer.

Psychiatry in Learning Disability. Read Staff. 1997. pap. text (*0-7020-2119-9*) Bailliere Tindall.

Psychiatry in Russia & Spain: An Original Anthology. Desmaisons. 1976. LC 75-16729. (Classics in Psychiatry Ser.). (FRE & GER.). 28.95 (*0-405-07452-2*) Ayer.

Psychiatry in the American Community. H. G. Whittington. 1969. LC 66-24393. 476p. reprint ed. pap. 24.95 (*0-8236-8250-1*, 25460) Intl Univs Pr.

Psychiatry in the Elderly. Robin Jacoby & Catherine Oppenheimer. 2nd ed. 1997. (Illus.). 814p. text 189.50 (*0-19-262789-9*) OUP.

Psychiatry in the Nursing Home: Assessment, Evaluation, & Intervention. D. Peter Birkett. 1991. 192p. text 49.95 (*1-56024-068-7*); pap. text 19.95 (*1-56024-069-5*) Haworth Pr.

Psychiatry in Transition. Ramon. 1990. 288p. (C). pap. (*0-7453-0470-2*) Pluto GBR GBR. *Dist:* Stylus Pub VA.

Psychiatry in Transition. Judd Marmor. 2nd ed. 1994. LC 94-3844. 464p. (C). pap. text 24.95 (*1-56000-736-2*) Transaction Pubs.

Psychiatry in Transition: The British & Italian Experiences. Ramon. 1990. 288p. (C). (*0-7453-0177-0*) Pluto GBR GBR. *Dist:* Stylus Pub VA.

Psychiatry Made Ridiculously Simple. William V. Good & Jefferson E. Nelson. 3rd ed. 1999. (Illus.). 96p. pap. text 12.95 (*0-940780-22-4*) MedMaster.

Psychiatry Made Simple. Hoslam. Date not set. 384p. pap. text (*0-7506-0725-4*) Buttrwrth-Heinemann.

Psychiatry Medical Student Pearls of Wisdom: Over 2000 Questions. (*1-58409-013-8*) Boston Medical.

Psychiatry, 1982: The American Psychiatric Association Annual Review Psychiatry Update, Vol. 1. Ed. by Lester Grinspoon. Incl. Vol. 2. Psychiatry Update: The American Psychiatric Association Annual Review. 604p. 1983. text 15.00 (*0-88048-007-6*, 8007); Vol. 3. Psychiatry Update: The American Psychiatric Association Annual Review. 648p. 1984. text 15.00 (*0-88048-015-7*, 8015); (Illus.). 552p. 1982. 15.00 (*0-88048-000-9*, 8000) Am Psychiatric.

Psychiatry, 1995: Digging up the Bones, Vol. 6. Medical Review Staff. 1998. (Medical Review Ser.). (Illus.). 108p. pap. 19.95 (*0-07-038219-0*) McGraw-Hill Prof.

Psychiatry of Stroke. Ed. by D. Peter Birkett. 1996. LC 95-17692. 416p. 56.00 (*0-88048-540-X*, 8540) Am Psychiatric.

Psychiatry Pearls of Wisdom: Over 2500 Questions. Schmidt. 1999. (Pearls of Wisdom Ser.). pap. 88.00 (*1-890369-13-6*) Boston Medical.

Psychiatry, Psychoimmunology & Viruses. Ed. by Norbert Mueller. 1999. (Key Topics in Brain Research Ser.). (Illus.). 180p. pap. 84.00 (*3-211-83249-1*) Spr-Verlag.

Psychiatry Recall. Barbara Fadem & Steven S. Simring. 1997. LC 96-41667. 250p. pap. text 29.95 (*0-683-18004-5*) Lppncott W & W.

Psychiatry Review. Cutler. 1999. pap. text (*0-7216-6053-3*) Saunders.

Psychiatry Specialty Board Review for the DSM-IV. John C. Duffy & J. Bryce McLaulin. 1996. (Brunner/Mazel Continuing Education in Psychiatry & Psychology Ser.: No. 5). 128p. pap. 22.95 (*0-87630-788-8*) Brunner-Routledge.

***Psychiatry Survival & God.** Stephen Edward Stevens. 2001. 112p. 19.99 (*0-9711095-0-8*) Temple Univ Schl Med.

Psychiatry Takes to the Streets: Outreach & Crisis Intervention for the Mentally Ill. Ed. by Neal L. Cohen. 1990. LC 89-23741. 306p. 42.00 (*0-89862-426-6*, 2426) Guilford Pubns.

Psychiatry 2000: An Internet Resource Guide. Ed. by Dan Goldenson. 2000. 450p. pap. 24.95 (*0-9676811-2-X*) eMedguides.

Psychiatry Update: American Psychiatric Association Annual Review. Ed. by Robert E. Hales & Allen J. Frances. Vol. 4. 1985. 671p. text 15.00 (*0-88048-239-7*, 8239); Vol. 4. 1985. 671p. pap. text 10.00 (*0-88048-039-4*, 8039); Vol. 6. 1987. (Illus.). 852p. text 15.00 (*0-88048-243-5*, 8243); Vol. 6. 1987. (Illus.). 852p. pap. text 10.00 (*0-88048-242-7*, 8242) Am Psychiatric.

Psychiatry Update: The American Psychiatric Association Annual Review. Ed. by Lester Grinspoon. (Illus.). Vol. 2. 1983. 604p. text 15.00 (*0-88048-007-6*, 8007); Vol. 3. 1984. 648p. text 15.00 (*0-88048-015-7*, 8015) Am Psychiatric.

Psychiatry/Neurology: PreTest Self-Assessment & Review. Ed. by Joseph Friedman & James Duffy. 3rd rev. ed. 1997. LC 97-72. (Pretest Specialty Level Ser.). (Illus.). 326p. pap. 45.00 (*0-07-052535-8*) McGraw-Hill Educ Grp.

Psychic Deadness. Michael Eigen. 1996. LC 95-24825. xxv, 233p. 50.00 (*1-56821-735-8*) Aronson.

Psychic Empowerment for Health & Fitness. Joe H. Slate. 1999. LC 96-12237. (Strategies for Success Ser.). 256p. pap. 12.95 (*1-56718-634-3*) Llewellyn Pubns.

Psychic Energy: The Magic Power of the Mind. Lloyd K. Ulery. 1978. LC 77-91279. 150p. 9.45 (*0-930984-02-1*) Psychic Bks.

Psychic Equilibrium & Psychic Change: Selected Papers of Betty Joseph. Ed. by Michael Feldman & Elizabeth B. Spillius. 1989. 240p. (C). pap. 29.99 (*0-415-04117-1*, A3644) Routledge.

Psychic Healing. Yogi Ramacharaka. reprint ed. 15.00 (*0-911662-07-3*) Yoga.

Psychic Healing Book. Amy Wallace & Bill Henkin. 1982. LC 77-16019. 224p. reprint ed. pap. 14.95 (*0-914728-34-2*) Wingbow Pr.

Psychic Healing with Spirit Guides & Angels. Diane Stein. 1996. LC 95-53703. (Illus.). 256p. (Orig.). pap. 18.95 (*0-89594-807-9*) Crossing Pr.

Psychic Injuries, Vols. 12, 12a & 12b. Marvin E. Lewis & Robert L. Sadoff. 1975. (Courtroom Medicine Ser.). 621.00 (*0-8205-1256-7*) Bender.

Psychic Retreats: Pathological Organisations in Psychotic, Neurotic, & Borderline Patients. John Steiner. 1993. LC 92-48548. (New Library of Psychoanalysis : No. 19). 176p. (C). pap. 25.99 (*0-415-09924-2*, B0889) Routledge.

Psychic Side of Sports. Michael Murphy & Rhea White. 1978. (Illus.). 10.95 (*0-201-04728-4*) Addison-Wesley.

Psychic Structure & Psychic Change: Essays in Honor of Robert S. Wallerstein, M.D. Ed. by Mardi J. Horowitz et al. 1993. LC 93-16491. 384p. 55.00 (*0-8236-5253-X*) Intl Univs Pr.

Psychic Wholeness & Healing: Using All the Powers of the Human Psyche. Conrad W. Baars & Anna A. Terruwe. 1981. LC 81-4964. 278p. (Orig.). pap. 12.95 (*0-8189-0410-0*) Alba.

Psyching Out Diabetes. Richard Rubin et al. 2nd rev. ed. 1997. LC 98-149742. 312p. pap. 16.00 (*1-56565-808-6*, Anodyne) Lowell Hse.

Psyching Out Diabetes: A Positive Approach to Your Negative Emotions. Richard Rubin et al. 1993. 312p. pap. 16.00 (*1-56565-088-3*, Anodyne); 1992. 288p. 22.95 (*0-929923-97-9*) Lowell Hse.

Psyching Out Diabetes: A Positive Approach to Your Negative Emotions. Richard R. Rubin et al. 3rd ed. 1999. LC 00-267412. (Illus.). xxvi, 277p. pap. 16.95 (*0-7373-0258-5*, 02585W) NTC Contemp Pub Co.

Psychischen Schadigungen Durch Kopfschuss im Kriege, 1914-16 see Disturbances of Lower & Higher Visual Capacities Caused by Occipital Damage: With Special Reference to the Psychopathological, Pedagogical, Industrial, & Social Implications

Psychischen Storungen des Kindesalters. Hermann Emminghaus. 1976. LC 75-16701. (Classics in Psychiatry Ser.). (GER., Illus.). reprint ed. 27.95 (*0-405-07428-X*) Ayer.

Psycho-Analysis As History: Negation & Freedom in Freud. Michael S. Roth. 1987. LC 86-29192. 208p. 35.00 (*0-8014-1957-3*) Cornell U Pr.

Psycho-Analytic Explorations. Donald Woods Winnicott. Ed. by Clare Winnicott et al. 1992. (Illus.). 624p. pap. 25.50 (*0-674-72091-1*) HUP.

Psycho-Analytic Explorations. Donald Woods Winnicott et al. Ed. by Clare Winnicott et al. 1989. LC 88-21465. (Illus.). 616p. 50.00 (*0-674-72090-3*) HUP.

Psycho-Economics: Managed Care in Mental Health in the New Millennium. Ed. by Robert D. Weitz. 1999. LC 99-47992. (Critical Strategies Ser.: Vol. 1, No. 1). 165p. (C). 39.95 (*0-7890-0780-0*); pap. text 19.95 (*0-7890-0815-7*) Haworth Pr.

Psycho-Immune-Neuroendocrine Integrative Mechanisms. Ed. by D. P. Cardinali & F. Fraschini. 1998. (Biological Signals & Receptors Ser.: Vol. 7, No. 1, 1998). (Illus.). 74p. pap. 33.25 (*3-8055-6685-9*) S Karger.

Psycho-Logic. J. Smedslund. 1988. 112p. 45.00 (*0-387-18518-6*) Spr-Verlag.

Psycho-Marxism: Marxism & Psychoanalysis Late in the 20th Century. Robert Miklitsch. 1998. 250p. pap. 12.00 (*0-8223-6460-3*) Duke.

Psycho-Oncology. Ed. by Jimmie C. Holland. 1998. (Illus.). 1216p. text 139.50 (*0-19-510614-8*) OUP.

Psycho-Politics & Cultural Desires. Jan Campbell. 1998. pap. text 24.95 (*1-85728-807-6*) Taylor & Francis.

Psycho Surgery. Mark A. J. O'Callaghan. 1983. lib. bdg. 124.00 (*0-942068-06-8*) Kluwer Academic.

Psycho-Therapeutics. Charles Lloyd Tuckey. 96p. 55.00 (*1-85506-678-5*) Thoemmes Pr.

Psychoacoustics. J. Donald Harris. reprint ed. pap. text 5.95 (*0-8290-0327-4*) Irvington.

Psychoacoustics. J. Donald Harris. 1974. LC 74-10512. (Studies in Communicative Disorders). (C). pap. text (*0-672-61332-8*, Bobbs) Macmillan.

Psychoacoustics: Facts & Models. E. Zwicker & H. Fastl. Ed. by T. S. Huang et al. 1990. (Information Sciences Ser.: Vol. 22). (Illus.). 352p. text 59.50 (*0-387-52600-5*) Spr-Verlag.

Psychoacoustics, Speech, & Hearing Aids: Proceedings of the Summer School & International Symposium, Bad Zwischenahn, 31 Aug-5 Sep 95. Ed. by B. Kollmeier. 1996. LC 96-6736. 372p. (*981-02-2561-X*) World Scientific Pub.

Psychoactive Drugs: Improving Prescribing Practices. H. Ghodse & I. Khan. 1988. 108p. 18.00 (*92-4-156112-2*) World Health.

Psychoactive Drugs: Including Combinations. Ed. by F. Wider. 1974. (Data Processing in Medicine Ser.: Vol. 3). 260p. 104.50 (*3-8055-1740-8*) S Karger.

Psychoactive Drugs: The Street Pharmacopoeia. Alasdair J. M. Forsyth. 2000. 192p. pap. (*0-11-702475-9*) Statnry Office GBR. *Dist:* Balogh.

Psychoactive Drugs: Tolerance & Sensitization. Ed. by A. J. Goudie & M. W. Emmett-Oglesby. 1989. LC 89-11094. (Contemporary Neuroscience Ser.). 608p. 145.00 (*0-89603-148-9*) Humana.

Psychoactive Drugs & Harm Reduction: From Faith to Science. Heather. 1993. 366p. pap. 34.95 (*1-56593-246-3*, 0520) Singular Publishing.

Psychoactive Medications in the Treatment of Adults & Adolescents. Frederick M. Jacobsen & Robert Golden. 1996. 400p. 45.00 (*0-471-55074-4*) Wiley.

Psychoanalysis. Toews. 1997. 26.95 (*0-8057-8642-2*); pap. 14.95 (*0-8057-8643-0*) Gale (Macmillan Ref).

Psychoanalysis. Eli Zaretsky. 1999. (*0-679-44654-0*) Knopf.

Psychoanalysis: A Contemporary Introduction. Robert M. Galatzer-Levy. 1998. 212p. pap. (*0-465-06492-2*) Basic.

Psychoanalysis: Clinical & Theoretical. Robert S. Wallerstein. 1999. LC 98-31872. 446p. 70.00 (*0-8236-5219-X*, 05219) Intl Univs Pr.

Psychoanalysis: Clinical Theory & Practice. Jacob A. Arlow. 1991. LC 91-20811. 450p. (C). 65.00 (*0-8236-5202-5*) Intl Univs Pr.

Psychoanalysis: Observation, Theory, Application: Selected Papers of Robert Waelder. Ed. by Samuel A. Guttman. 1976. LC 75-6432. 709p. 85.00 (*0-8236-5250-5*) Intl Univs Pr.

Psychoanalysis: Science & Profession. Maxwell Gitelson. 1973. LC 72-8789. xiv, 439p. 65.00 (*0-8236-5255-6*) Intl Univs Pr.

Psychoanalysis: The Impossible Profession. Janet Malcolm. 1994. LC 94-72518. (Master Work Ser.). 184p. 30.00 (*1-56821-342-5*) Aronson.

Psychoanalysis: The Impossible Profession. Janet Malcolm. 1982. LC 82-40036. 192p. pap. 13.00 (*0-394-71034-7*) Vin Bks.

Psychoanalysis: The Major Concepts. Burness E. Moore & Bernard D. Fine. 1995. LC 95-173. 562p. 75.00 (*0-300-06329-6*) Yale U Pr.

Psychoanalysis: The Possible Profession. Ed. by Herbert S. Strean. 1986. LC 85-24757. (Current Issues in Psychoanalytic Practice Ser.: Vol. 2, No. 2). 102p. text 39.95 (*0-86656-509-4*) Haworth Pr.

Psychoanalysis: The Science of Mental Conflict - Essays in Honor of Charles Brenner. Ed. by Arnold D. Richards & Martin S. Willick. 1986. (Essays in Honor of Chas Brenner Ser.). 439p. text 55.00 (*0-88163-054-3*) Analytic Pr.

Psychoanalysis: The Vital Issues Ed. by John E. Gedo & George H. Pollock. LC 83-26429. (Emotions & Behavior Monographs: Nos. 2 & 3). Vol. 1. 1983. 448p. 65.00 (*0-8236-5385-4*); Vol. 2. 1985. 498p. 75.00 (*0-8236-5386-2*) Intl Univs Pr.

Psychoanalysis: Toward the Second Century. Arnold Cooper. 1990. 248p. (C). 50.00 (*0-300-04558-1*) Yale U Pr.

Psychoanalysis - A Theory in Crisis. Marshall Edelson. 1998. (Illus.). 416p. 39.95 (*0-226-18437-4*); 1990. LC 88-1142. xxxvi, 428p. pap. text 22.00 (*0-226-18429-3*) U Ch Pr.

Psychoanalysis & ... Ed. by Richard Feldstein & Henry Sussman. 1989. 256p. 45.00 (*0-415-90152-9*, A3423) Routledge.

Psychoanalysis & American Medicine, 1894-1918: Medicine, Science, & Culture. John C. Burnham. 1967. LC 67-31293. (Psychological Issues Monographs: No. 20, Vol. 5, No. 4). 249p. (Orig.). 37.50 (*0-8236-5100-2*) Intl Univs Pr.

Psychoanalysis & Anthropology. Geza Roheim. 1968. 496p. reprint ed. pap. 24.95 (*0-8236-8234-X*, 25120) Intl Univs Pr.

***Psychoanalysis & Art: The Artistic Representation of the Parent/Child Relationship.** Ed. by Elsa Blum et al. unabr. ed. 2001. LC 2001-51718. 340p. pap. text 49.95 (*0-8236-5115-0*, 05115) Intl Univs Pr.

Psychoanalysis & Beyond. Charles Rycroft. 1995. 316p. (C). pap. text 15.00 (*0-226-73289-4*) U Ch Pr.

Psychoanalysis & Catholicism. Benjamin B. Wolman. 1995. LC 95-32605. (Master Work Ser.). 234p. 40.00 (*1-56821-715-3*) Aronson.

Psychoanalysis & Cinema: AFI Film Readers. Ed. by E. Ann Kaplan. 1989. 256p. (C). pap. 23.95 (*0-415-90029-8*); 39.50 (*0-415-90028-X*) Routledge.

Psychoanalysis & Civilization. Paul Rosenfels. 1963. LC 62-18668. 10.95 (*0-87212-016-3*) Libra.

Psychoanalysis & Cognitive Science: A Multiple Code Theory. Wilma Bucci. 1997. LC 96-52825. (Illus.). 362p. text 45.00 (*1-57230-213-5*, 0213) Guilford Pubns.

Psychoanalysis & Contemporary Thought. Ed. by John D. Sutherland. 1977. LC 75-134139. (Essay Index Reprint Ser.). reprint ed. 19.95 (*0-8369-2373-1*) Ayer.

Psychoanalysis & Culture. Ed. by Lesley Caldwell. 1997. (New Formations Twenty-Six Ser.). 192p. (C). pap. (*0-85315-813-4*) Lawrence & Wishart GBR. *Dist:* NYU Pr.

Psychoanalysis & Culture: Contemporary States of Mind. Rosalind Minsky. 1998. LC 98-23538. (C). text 50.00 (*0-8135-2585-3*); 245p. pap. text 20.00 (*0-8135-2586-1*) Rutgers U Pr.

Psychoanalysis & Development: Representations & Narratives. Ed. by Massimo Ammaniti & Daniel N. Stern. 1994. LC 94-14618. (Psychoanalytic Crosscurrents Ser.). 208p. (C). text 55.00 (*0-8147-0616-9*) NYU Pr.

Psychoanalysis & Developmental Therapy. Anne Hurry. 1998. 256p. pap. (*1-85575-213-1*) Karnac Bks GBR. *Dist:* Other Pr LLC.

Psychoanalysis & Discourse. Patrick Mahony. Ed. by David Tuckett. 1987. (New Library of Psychoanalysis). 250p. (C). pap. (*0-422-61720-2*); lib. bdg. (*0-422-61030-5*) Tavistock GBR. *Dist:* Routldge.

Psychoanalysis & Eating Disorders. Ed. by Jules R. Bemporad & David B. Herzog. 1989. 174p. 30.00 (*0-89862-388-X*, 2388) Guilford Pubns.

Psychoanalysis & Ethics. Ernest Wallwork. 1994. 360p. pap. 21.00 (*0-300-06167-6*); 1991. LC 91-15276. 392p. 55.00 (*0-300-04878-5*) Yale U Pr.

Psychoanalysis & Ethics. Lewis S. Feuer. 1973. LC 73-1433. 134p. reprint ed. lib. bdg. 59.75 (*0-8371-6795-7*, FEPE, Greenwood Pr) Greenwood.

Psychoanalysis & Family Therapy. Helm Stierlin. 1987. LC 77-2275. 355p. reprint ed. 50.00 (*0-87668-257-3*) Aronson.

***Psychoanalysis & Film.** Ed. by Glenn O. Gabbard. 2001. 239p. pap. (*1-85575-275-1*) Karnac Bks GBR. *Dist:* Other Pr LLC.

Psychoanalysis & Gender: An Introductory Reader. Rosalind Minsky. 1996. LC 95-16457. (Critical Readers in Theory & Practice Ser.). 336p. (C). 94.95 (*0-415-09220-5*); pap. 25.99 (*0-415-09221-3*) Routledge.

Psychoanalysis & Group Behavior: A Study of Freudian Group Psychology. Saul Scheidlinger. 1971. LC 77-141267. 245p. reprint ed. lib. bdg. 95.00 (*0-8371-5838-9*, SCPS, Greenwood Pr) Greenwood.

Psychoanalysis & Groups: History & Dialectics. David Rosenfeld. 1989. 212p. reprint ed. pap. text (*0-946439-48-6*) Karnac Bks GBR. *Dist:* Other Pr LLC.

Psychoanalysis & Hypnosis. Erika Fromm & Michael Nash. 1997. LC 96-43561. (Mental Health Library Ser.: Monograph 5). 318p. 50.00 (*0-8236-5181-9*, BN 05181) Intl Univs Pr.

Psychoanalysis & Infant Research. Joseph D. Lichtenberg. 1991. (Psychoanalytic Inquiry Bk.: Vol. 2). 280p. (C). reprint ed. pap. 29.95 (*0-88163-145-0*) Analytic Pr.

Psychoanalysis & Male Sexuality. Ed. by Hendrik M. Ruitenbeek. 1966. pap. 15.95 (*0-8084-0256-0*) NCUP.

Psychoanalysis & Moral Values. Heinz Hartmann. 1960. LC 58-9230. (New York Psychoanalytic Institute Freud Anniversary Lecture Ser.). 121p. 27.50 (*0-8236-5240-8*) Intl Univs Pr.

Psychoanalysis & Philosophy. Ed. by Charles Hanly & Morris Lazerowitz. 1971. LC 73-138247. 362p. 55.00 (*0-8236-5185-1*) Intl Univs Pr.

Psychoanalysis & Psychology: Minding the Gap. Stephen Frosh. 1989. 304p. (C). text 18.00 (*0-8147-2595-3*) NYU Pr.

Psychoanalysis & Psychopathology. Philip S. Holzman. 1995. LC 95-15115. (Master Work Ser.). 224p. pap. 45.00 (*1-56821-588-6*) Aronson.

Psychoanalysis & Psychosis. Ed. by Ann-Louise S. Silver. 1989. (Illus.). 600p. 87.50 (*0-8236-5183-5*) Intl Univs Pr.

Psychoanalysis & Psychotherapy: Selected Papers. Frieda Fromm-Reichmann. Ed. by Dexter M. Bullard. 1997. LC 59-10746. 368p. reprint ed. pap. 15.95 (*0-226-26597-8*, P580) U Ch Pr.

Psychoanalysis & Religion. Erich Fromm. 1959. (Terry Lectures). pap. 12.00 (*0-300-00089-8*, Y12) Yale U Pr.

Psychoanalysis & Religion. Neville Symington. 1994. LC 93-37975. 20.95 (*0-304-32887-1*) Continuum.

Psychoanalysis & Religious Experience. William W. Meissner. 1986. LC 83-51296. 254p. pap. 19.00 (*0-300-03751-1*, Y-599) Yale U Pr.

Psychoanalysis & Religious Mysticism. David C. McMelland. 1959. (C). pap. 4.00 (*0-87574-104-5*) Pendle Hill.

Psychoanalysis & Severe Emotional Illness Vol. 18, No. 1: Journal of the American Academy of Psychoanalysis. Ed. by Ann-Louise S. Silver & Morton B. Cantor. 1990. 208p. 30.00 (*0-89862-435-5*) Guilford Pubns.

Psychoanalysis & Social Theory: The Limits of Sociology. Ian Craib. 1989. LC 89-20163. 224p. (C). pap. 15.95 (*0-87023-702-0*); lib. bdg. 35.00 (*0-87023-701-2*) U of Mass Pr.

Psychoanalysis & Spiritual Psychology. Rudolf Steiner. Tr. by May Laird-Brown from GER. 1990. 128p. 24.95 (*0-88010-351-5*) Anthroposophic.

Psychoanalysis & Spiritual Psychology. Rudolf Steiner & Robert J. Sardello. Tr. by May Laird-Brown from GER. 1990. LC 90-43423. 128p. pap. 12.95 (*0-88010-290-X*) Anthroposophic.

Psychoanalysis & the Bible: A Study in Depth of Seven Leaders. Dorothy F. Zeligs. 1988. 372p. 45.95 (*0-89885-389-3*, Kluwer Acad Hman Sci) Kluwer Academic.

Psychoanalysis & the Concept of a Rule: An Essay in the Philosophy of Psychoanalysis. A. Mooij. Tr. by S. Firth & J. H. Scheffer from DUT. 1991. 100p. 31.95 (*0-387-53573-X*) Spr-Verlag.

Psychoanalysis & the Future of Theory. Malcolm Bowie. 1993. LC 93-25937. (Bucknell Lectures in Literary Theory: Vol. 9). (Illus.). 192p. pap. text 18.95 (*0-631-18926-2*) Blackwell Pubs.

Psychoanalysis & the Humanities. Ed. by Laurie Schneider Adams & Jacques Szaluta. 1996. LC 95-50330. (Psychoanalytic Practice Monographs: No. 6). (Illus.). 176p. text 26.95 (*0-87630-743-8*) Brunner-Routledge.

Psychoanalysis & the Occult. Ed. by George Devereux. 1970. 432p. pap. 24.95 (*0-8236-8240-4*, 25180) Intl Univs Pr.

Psychoanalysis & the Philosophy of Science: Collected Papers of Benjamin B. Rubinstein, M. D., Vol. 1. Ed. by Robert R. Holt. 1997. LC 96-42969. (Psychological Issues Ser.: Nos. 62 & 63). 715p. 95.00 (*0-8236-5245-9*) Intl Univs Pr.

Psychoanalysis & the Sciences. Andre Haynal. Tr. by Elizabeth Holder from FRE. 1993. LC 92-48742. xii, 290p. (C). 35.00 (*0-520-08299-0*) U CA Pr.

Psychoanalysis & Women: Contemporary Reappraisals. Ed. by Judith L. Alpert. 1994. 360p. reprint ed. pap. 29.95 (*0-88163-191-4*) Analytic Pr.

Psychoanalysis As a Human Science: Beyond Foundationalism. Bhargavi V. Davar & Parameshwar R. Bhat. LC 94-39606. 1995. 212p. 22.50 (*0-8039-9196-7*, 7762); 1994. (*81-7036-424-8*); 1994. pap. text (*81-7036-425-6*) Sage.

Psychoanalysis As a Science. Leopold Bellack. 1992. LC 92-10471. 208p. (C). 77.00 (*0-205-13904-3*, Longwood Div) Allyn.

Psychoanalysis As Science: The Hixon Lectures on the Scientific Status of Psychoanalysis. Ed. by Eugene Pumpian-Mindlin. 1970. LC 70-106692. 174p. reprint ed. lib. bdg. 62.50 (*0-8371-3365-3*, PUMP, Greenwood Pr) Greenwood.

Psychoanalysis at Its Limits: Navigating the Postmodern Turn. Ed. by Anthony Elliott & Charles Spezzano. 1999. LC 00-268904. x, 306p. (*1-85343-464-7*) Free Assoc Bks GBR. *Dist:* Intl Spec Bk.

Psychoanalysis at One Hundred: An Issues in Ego Psychology Book. Ed. by Gerd H. Fenchel. 1993. (Commemorating the Thirtieth Anniversary of Washington Square Institute for Psychotherapy & Mental Health Ser.). 288p. (Orig.). (C). 69.00 (*0-8191-9242-2*); pap. 42.00 (*0-8191-9243-0*) U Pr of Amer.

Psychoanalysis, Behavior Therapy, & the Relational World. Paul L. Wachtel. 1997. LC 96-53417. (APA Psychotherapy Integration Book Ser.: Vol. 1). 485p. 39.95 (*1-55798-409-3*, 4317850) Am Psychol.

Psychoanalysis for Our Time: Exploring the Blindness of the Seeing I. Jeffrey B. Rubin. 1998. LC 98-58002. 230p. text 35.00 (*0-8147-7491-1*) NYU Pr.

Psychoanalysis for Teachers & Parents. Anna Freud. Tr. by Barbara Low from GER. 1979. 119p. reprint ed. pap. 8.95 (*0-393-00918-1*) Norton.

Psychoanalysis in a New Context. Arnold H. Modell. 1985. LC 84-12965. xii, 294p. 45.00 (*0-8236-5212-2*, 05212) Intl Univs Pr.

Psychoanalysis in Art History. Margaret Iversen. 160p. pap. text 19.95 (*0-631-19475-4*) Futura Pub.

Psychoanalysis in Childhood & Adolescence. Ed. by K. Von Klitzing et al. 2000. LC 00-23280. (Illus.). viii, 156p. 51.25 (*3-8055-6993-9*) S Karger.

Psychoanalysis in China: Literary Transformations, 1919-1949. Jingyuan Zhang. 1992. (Cornell East Asia Ser.: No. 55). 210p. (Orig.). (C). pap. 11.90 (*0-939657-55-4*) Cornell East Asia Pgm.

Psychoanalysis in Contexts: Paths Between Theory & Modern Culture. Ed. by Anthony Elliott & Stephen Frosh. 1994. LC 94-14823. 288p. (Orig.). (C). 70.00 (*0-415-09703-7*, B7002) Routledge.

Psychoanalysis in France. Ed. by Serge Lebovici & K. Widlocher. Tr. by J. Diamanti from FRE. 1980. LC 79-2483. 620p. 70.00 (*0-8236-5210-6*) Intl Univs Pr.

Psychoanalysis in Our Time. Stefi Pedersen. 1973. LC 70-173220. 5.95 (*0-672-51411-7*, Bobbs) Macmillan.

Psychoanalysis in the Americas. Ed. by Robert E. Litman. 1966. LC 66-24394. 328p. 50.00 (*0-8236-5200-9*) Intl Univs Pr.

Psychoanalysis in Transition: A Personal View. Merton M. Gill. 2000. LC 94-17701. 200p. 29.95 (*0-88163-112-4*) Analytic Pr.

Psychoanalysis International: A Guide to Psychoanalysis Throughout the World, Vol. 1. Ed. by Peter Kutter. 1992. 344p. text 49.95 (*0-88163-119-1*) Analytic Pr.

Psychoanalysis, Its Theories & Practical Application. Abraham Arden Brill. 1972. LC 78-180559. (Medicine & Society in America Ser.). 346p. reprint ed. 23.95 (*0-405-03939-5*) Ayer.

Psychoanalysis, Literature & War: Papers 1972-1995. Hanna Segal. Ed. & Intro. by John Steiner. 1997. LC 96-7559. (New Library of Psychoanalysis : Vol. 27). 192p. (C). 78.95 (*0-415-15328-X*); pap. 26.95 (*0-415-15329-8*) Routledge.

Psychoanalysis of Children. Melanie Klein. 1984. LC 84-13774. (Writings of Melanie Klein Ser.: Vol. 2). 352p. (C). 45.00 (*0-02-918430-4*) Free Pr.

Psychoanalysis of Developmental Arrests: Theory & Treatment. Robert D. Stolorow & Frank M. Lachman. 1980. LC 79-53593. 211p. 32.50 (*0-8236-5146-0*) Intl Univs Pr.

Psychoanalysis of Drug Dependence. Winstead Adams. 1978. 352p. text 62.50 (*0-8089-1148-1*, 790025, Grune & Strat) Harcrt Hlth Sci Grp.

Psychoanalysis of Fire. Gaston Bachelard. Tr. by A. C. Ross. 1964. pap. text 15.50 (*0-8070-6461-0*) Beacon Pr.

Psychoanalysis of Organizations: A Psychoanalytic Approach to Behaviour in Groups & Organizations. Robert De Board. 1978. 158p. pap. (*0-422-76530-9*, NO. 2731) Tavistock GBR. *Dist:* Routldge.

Psychoanalysis of Race. Christopher Lane. 1998. LC 97-38840. (Illus.). 1p. 52.00 (*0-231-10946-6*); 432p. pap. 19.50 (*0-231-10947-4*) Col U Pr.

Psychoanalysis of the Sexual Functions of Women. Helene Deutsch. Ed. by P. Roazen. 1991. 148p. pap. text (*0-946439-95-8*) Karnac Bks GBR. *Dist:* Other Pr LLC.

Psychoanalysis of War. Franco Fornari. Tr. by Alenka Pfeifer from ITA. 1975. LC 74-17458. 20.00 (*0-253-34632-0*) Ind U Pr.

Psychoanalysis, Psychotherapy, & the New England Medical Scene, 1894-1944. Ed. by George E. Gifford. 1978. 40.00 (*0-88202-169-9*) Watson Pub Intl.

***Psychoanalysis, Science, & Politics.** Michael Rustin. 2001. LC 2001-45372. (Disseminations: Psychoanalysis in Contexts Ser.). 240p. pap. 24.95 (*0-8195-6479-6*); lib. bdg. 60.00 (*0-8195-6478-8*) U Pr of New Eng (Wesleyan Univ Pr).

Psychoanalysis, Scientific Method & Philosophy. Ed. by Sidney Hook. 1990. 370p. pap. text 24.95 (*0-88738-834-5*) Transaction Pubs.

Psychoanalyst in Psychiatry. Thomas Freeman. 1988. LC 87-10684. 208p. (C). 40.00 (*0-300-04071-7*) Yale U Pr.

Psychoanalysts Talk. Virginia Hunter. 1994. LC 93-40502. 456p. 55.00 (*0-89862-373-1*, 2373) Guilford Pubns.

Psychoanalytic Anthropology after Freud: Essays on the 50th Anniversary of Freud's Death. Ed. by David H. Spain. 1992. 340p. (C). text 40.00 (*0-9622885-4-3*) Psyche Pr NY.

Psychoanalytic Approaches to Addiction. Ed. by Angelo Smaldino. 1991. LC 91-357. (Current Issues in Psychoanalytic Practice Ser.: No. 3). 128p. text 31.95 (*0-87630-644-X*) Brunner-Routledge.

Psychoanalytic Approaches to Supervision. Ed. by Robert C. Lane. 1990. LC 90-1971. (Current Issues in Psychoanalytic Practice Ser.: No. 2). 224p. text 35.95 (*0-87630-603-2*) Brunner-Routledge.

Psychoanalytic Approaches to the Resistant & Difficult Patient. Ed. by Herbert S. Strean. 1985. LC 84-25210. (Current Issues in Psychoanalytic Practice Ser.: Vol. 1, No. 4). 140p. text 4.95 (*0-86656-340-7*) Haworth Pr.

Psychoanalytic Approaches to the Very Troubled Child: Therapeutic Practice Innovations in Residential & Educational Settings. Ed. by Barry L. Childress. 1989. LC 89-11010. (Residential Treatment for Children & Youth Ser.: Vol. 6, No. 4). 88p. text 39.95 (*0-86656-928-6*) Haworth Pr.

Psychoanalytic Approaches with the Hostile & Violent Patient. Ed. by Herbert S. Strean. 1984. LC 84-3784. (Current Issues in Psychoanalytic Practice Ser.: Vol. 1, No. 2). 83p. text 29.95 (*0-86656-319-9*) Haworth Pr.

Psychoanalytic Case Formulation. Nancy McWilliams. 1999. LC 98-56044. 240p. pap. 36.00 (*1-57230-462-6*, 8R0462) Guilford Pubns.

Psychoanalytic Case Studies. Ed. by G. Pirooz Sholevar & Jules Glenn. 1991. LC 90-36401. xiv, 286p. 42.50 (*0-8236-4405-7*, BN 04405) Intl Univs Pr.

Psychoanalytic Clinical Practice. Richard D. Chessick. 2000. 300p. (*1-85343-479-5*) Free Assoc Bks GBR. *Dist:* Intl Spec Bk.

Psychoanalytic Concepts & the Structural Theory. Jacob A. Arlow & Charles Brenner. 1964. LC 64-16190. (Journal of the American Psychoanalytic Association Monograph Ser.: No. 3). 216p. (Orig.). 32.50 (*0-8236-5060-X*) Intl Univs Pr.

Psychoanalytic Conversations: Interviews with Clinicians, Commentators & Critics. Ed. by Peter Rudnytsky. 2000. LC 00-63985. 376p. 55.00 (*0-88163-328-3*) Analytic Pr.

Psychoanalytic Core: Essays in Honor of Leo Rangell, M. D. Ed. by Harold P. Blum et al. 1989. LC 89-36104. 550p. 70.00 (*0-8236-4409-X*) Intl Univs Pr.

Psychoanalytic Criticism: Theory to Practice. Elizabeth Wright. 1985. (New Accents Ser.). 224p. (C). pap. 13.95 (*0-416-32660-9*, NO. 9253) Routledge.

Psychoanalytic Culture: Psychoanalytic Discourse in Western Society. Ian Parker. 1997. 304p. 74.50 (*0-7619-5642-5*, 81889); LC 97-67536. pap. 25.95 (*0-7619-5643-3*, 81890) Sage.

Psychoanalytic Diagnosis: Understanding Personality Structure in the Clinical Process. Nancy McWilliams. 1994. LC 94-8549. 398p. 45.00 (*0-89862-199-2*, 2199) Guilford Pubns.

Psychoanalytic Dialogue. Stanley A. Leavy. 1987. LC 79-21796. 141p. pap. 15.00 (*0-300-04037-7*, Y-683) Yale U Pr.

Psychoanalytic Education & Research: The Current Situation & Future Possibilities. Stanley Goodman. 1977. LC 76-44638. 424p. 62.50 (*0-8236-4410-3*) Intl Univs Pr.

Psychoanalytic Explorations in Art. Ernst Kris. Date not set. (Illus.). 377p. 55.00 (*0-8236-4440-5*, 04440) Intl Univs Pr.

Psychoanalytic Explorations in Music. Ed. by Stuart Feder et al. 1990. (Applied Psychoanalysis Monographs: No. 1). 540p. 77.50 (*0-8236-4407-3*); Second Series. 1993. LC 93-575. 324p. 47.50 (*0-8236-4408-1*) Intl Univs Pr.

Psychoanalytic Explorations of Technique: Discourse on the Theory of Therapy. Ed. by Harold P. Blum. 1980. LC 79-22349. 468p. 70.00 (*0-8236-5053-7*) Intl Univs Pr.

Psychoanalytic Group Dynamics: Basic Reading. Ed. by Saul Scheidlinger. 1980. LC 79-20604. 315p. 47.50 (*0-8236-4445-6*, 04445) Intl Univs Pr.

Psychoanalytic Group Theory & Therapy: Essays in Honor of Saul Scheidlinger, Ph.D. Ed. by Saul Tuttman. 1991. LC 90-5324. (American Group Psychotherapy Association Monographs: No. 7). 500p. 65.00 (*0-8236-4433-2*) Intl Univs Pr.

Psychoanalytic Group Therapy. Karl Konig & Wolf-Volker Lindnerer. 1994. LC 93-32905. 216p. 40.00 (*1-56821-119-8*) Aronson.

Psychoanalytic Interpretation in Rorschach Testing. R. Schafer. 1954. LC 54-9030. 460p. text 39.00 (*0-8089-0404-3*, 793820, Grune & Strat) Harcrt Hlth Sci Grp.

Psychoanalytic Knowledge. Eugene B. Brody. 1990. 250p. 35.00 (*0-8236-4447-2*) Intl Univs Pr.

Psychoanalytic Mind. Marcia Cavell. 1996. 288p. pap. text 17.50 (*0-674-72096-2*) HUP.

Psychoanalytic Mind: From Freud to Philosophy. Marcia Cavell. 1993. LC 93-7325. 288p. 39.50 (*0-674-72095-4*) HUP.

Psychoanalytic Model of Attention & Learning. Fred Schwartz & Peter H. Schiller. 1970. LC 79-105070. (Psychological Issues Monographs: No. 23, Vol. 6, No. 3). 134p. (Orig.). 27.50 (*0-8236-4450-2*) Intl Univs Pr.

Psychoanalytic Object Relations Theory & the Study of Religion: On Faith & the Imaging of God. John McDargh. 1983. 296p. (C). pap. text 28.00 (*0-8191-3511-9*); lib. bdg. 62.00 (*0-8191-3510-0*) U Pr of Amer.

Psychoanalytic Object Relations Therapy. Althea J. Horner. 304p. 1995. pap. text 40.00 (*1-56821-637-8*); 1992. LC 91-3132. 50.00 (*0-87668-534-3*) Aronson.

Psychoanalytic Perspectives of Movement: An Original Anthology. Ed. by Martha Davis. 1975. LC 74-9161. (Body Movement Perspectives in Research Ser.). 164p. reprint ed. 35.95 (*0-405-06199-4*) Ayer.

Psychoanalytic Perspectives on Art. Ed. by Mary M. Gedo. Vol. 2. 1987. 360p. text 49.95 (*0-88163-058-6*); Vol. 3. 1988. 331p. text 49.95 (*0-88163-078-0*) Analytic Pr.

Psychoanalytic Perspectives on Developmental Psychology. Ed. by Joseph M. Masling & Robert F. Bornstein. 1996. LC 96-30399. (Empirical Studies of Psychoanalytic Theories: Vol. 6). 351p. 49.95 (*1-55798-385-2*, 431-6810) Am Psychol.

Psychoanalytic Perspectives on Psychopathology. Ed. by Joseph M. Masling & Robert F. Bornstein. 1993. LC 93-26281. (Empirical Studies of Psychoanalytic Theories: Vol. 4). 309p. text 34.95 (*1-55798-211-2*) Am Psychol.

Psychoanalytic Perspectives on the Rorschach. Paul M. Lerner. 1998. LC 97-51640. 512p. 59.95 (*0-88163-234-1*) Analytic Pr.

Psychoanalytic Perspectives on Women. Ed. by Elaine V. Siegel. 1992. LC 91-43418. (Current Issues in Psychoanalytic Practice Ser.: No. 4). 160p. text 29.95 (*0-87630-655-5*) Brunner-Routledge.

Psychoanalytic Pioneers. Ed. by Franz Gabriel Alexander et al. 1995. LC 94-41115. xxxi, 616p. pap. text 34.95 (*1-56000-815-6*) Transaction Pubs.

Psychoanalytic Practice, Set. Helmut Thoma & Horst Kachele. 1994. LC 94-72375. (Master Work Ser.). 1116p. pap. text 140.00 (*1-56821-344-1*) Aronson.

Psychoanalytic Practice: Principles, Vol. 1. H. Kachele & Helmut Thoma. 1987. 421p. 87.95 (*0-387-16876-1*) Spr-Verlag.

Psychoanalytic Practice Vol. 1: Principles. Helmut Thoma & Horst Kachele. 1994. LC 94-72375. 448p. pap. 47.50 (*1-56821-346-8*) Aronson.

Psychoanalytic Practice Vol. 2: Clinical Studies. Helmut Thoma & H. Kachele. Tr. by M. Wilson from GER. 1991. 540p. 94.00 (*0-387-17515-6*) Spr-Verlag.

Psychoanalytic Practice Vol. 2: Clinical Studies. Helmut Thoma & Horst Kachele. 1994. LC 94-72375. 568p. pap. 47.50 (*1-56821-347-6*) Aronson.

Psychoanalytic Process: Theory, Clinical Observation & Empirical Research. Joseph Weiss et al. 1986. LC 85-30548. 423p. 58.00 (*0-89862-670-6*, 2670) Guilford Pubns.

Psychoanalytic Psychology: The Development of Freud's Thought. Raymond E. Fancher. 1973. LC 73-1273. (Illus.). 241p. (C). pap. text 12.00 (*0-393-09356-5*) Norton.

Psychoanalytic Psychology of Normal Development (1970-1980) Anna Freud. 1981. LC 81-11809. (Writings of Anna Freud: Vol. 8). 389p. 57.50 (*0-8236-6877-0*) Intl Univs Pr.

Psychoanalytic Psychotherapy in a College Context. Ed. by Robert May. 1988. LC 87-2836. 214p. 62.50 (*0-275-92733-4*, C2733, Praeger Pubs) Greenwood.

Psychoanalytic Psychotherapy in Institutional Settings. Julia Pestalozzi et al. 1998. 256p. pap. (*1-85575-198-4*) Karnac Bks GBR. *Dist:* Other Pr LLC.

Psychoanalytic Psychotherapy in the Independent Tradition. Sue Johnson & Stanley Ruszczynski. 1999. 204p. pap. (*1-85575-176-3*) Karnac Bks GBR. *Dist:* Other Pr LLC.

Psychoanalytic Psychotherapy in the Kleinian Tradition. Ed. by Stanley Ruszczynski & Sue Johnson. 1999. 216p. pap. (*1-85575-175-5*) Karnac Bks GBR. *Dist:* Other Pr LLC.

Psychoanalytic Psychotherapy of the Severely Disturbed Adolescent. Ed. by Dimitris Anastopoulos et al. 1999. (EFPP Clinical Monograph Ser.). 216p. pap. (*1-85575-214-X*) Karnac Bks GBR. *Dist:* Other Pr LLC.

Psychoanalytic Quarterly Cumulative Index, 1967-1976, Vols. XXXVI-XLV. 1977. LC 36-12164. 60.00 (*0-911194-03-7*) Psych Qtly.

Psychoanalytic Quarterly Cumulative Index, 1977-1986, Vols. LV-LXIV. 1990. LC 36-12164. 60.00 (*0-911194-04-5*) Psych Qtly.

Psychoanalytic Reader: An Anthology of Essential Papers with Critical Introductions. Ed. by Robert Fliess. 1969. 358p. (Orig.). reprint ed. 52.50 (*0-8236-4480-4*) Intl Univs Pr.

Psychoanalytic Reflections on Current Issues. Ed. by Judith Lasky et al. 1991. 228p. (C). text 45.00 (*0-8147-7909-3*) NYU Pr.

Psychoanalytic Research: Three Approaches to the Experimental Study of Subliminal Processes. Ed. by Martin Mayman & Herbert J. Schlesinger. 1975. LC 73-2848. (Psychological Issues Monographs: 30, Vol. 8, No. 2). 116p. (C). 27.50 (*0-8236-4490-1*) Intl Univs Pr.

Psychoanalytic Situation. Leo Stone. 1961. LC 61-18794. (New York Psychoanalytic Institute Freud Anniversary Lecture Ser.). 160p. 30.00 (*0-8236-4500-2*) Intl Univs Pr.

Psychoanalytic Studies of Biography. Ed. by George Moraitis & George H. Pollock. 1987. LC 86-27750. (Emotions & Behavior Monographs: No. 4). 85.00 (*0-8236-4515-0*, BN#04515) Intl Univs Pr.

Psychoanalytic Studies of Religion: A Critical Assessment & Annotated Bibliography, 39. 1996. LC 96-18524. (Bibliographies & Indexes in Religious Studies: Vol. 39). 208p. lib. bdg. 72.95 (*0-313-27362-6*, Greenwood Pr) Greenwood.

Psychoanalytic Studies of the Personality. W. Ronald Fairbairn. 1994. LC 94-8493. 336p. (C). pap. 25.99 (*0-415-10737-7*, B4304); 1974. reprint ed. 37.50 (*0-7100-1361-2*, Routledge Thoemms) Routledge.

Psychoanalytic Study of Society, Vol. 10. Ed. by Werner L. Muensterberger et al. 1984. (Muensterberger Ser.). 400p. text 39.95 (*0-88163-004-7*) Analytic Pr.

Psychoanalytic Study of Society, Vol. 8. Ed. by Werner L. Muensterberger et al. 1979. LC 61-486. (Illus.). 50.00 (*0-300-02257-3*) Yale U Pr.

Psychoanalytic Study of Society: Essays in Honor of George A. De Vos, Vol. 19. Ed. by L. Bryce Boyer et al. 1994. 392p. text 45.00 (*0-88163-183-3*) Analytic Pr.

Psychoanalytic Study of Society: Essays in Honor of George Devereux, Vol. 12. Ed. by L. Bryce Boyer & Simon A. Grolnick. 1987. (Muensterberger Ser.). 248p. (C). text 29.95 (*0-88163-069-1*) Analytic Pr.

Psychoanalytic Study of Society: Essays in Honor of Melford E. Spiro, Vol. 15. Ed. by L. Bryce Boyer & Simon A. Grolnick. 1990. (Muensterberger Ser.). 416p. text 39.95 (*0-88163-115-9*) Analytic Pr.

Psychoanalytic Study of Society: Essays in Honor of Werner Muensterberger, Vol. 11. Ed. by L. Bryce Boyer & Simon A. Grolnick. 1985. (Muensterberger Ser.). 264p. (C). text 29.95 (*0-88163-032-2*) Analytic Pr.

Psychoanalytic Study of Society: Essays in Honor of Westo LaBarre, Vol. 13. Ed. by L. Bryce Boyer & Simon A. Grolnick. 1988. (Muensterberger Ser.). 224p. text 29.95 (*0-88163-079-9*) Analytic Pr.

Psychoanalytic Study of Society Vol. 17: Essays in Honor of George D. & Louise A. Spindler. Ed. by L. Bryce Boyer & Ruth Boyer. 1992. 384p. text 36.00 (*0-88163-151-5*) Analytic Pr.

Psychoanalytic Study of Society Vol. 18: Essays in Honor of Alan Dundes. L. Bryce Boyer et al. 1993. 522p. 45.00 (*0-88163-161-2*) Analytic Pr.

Psychoanalytic Study of the Child. Albert J. Solnit. 1995. 65.00 (*0-300-06471-3*) Yale U Pr.

Psychoanalytic Study of the Child. Ed. by Ruth S. Eissler et al. LC 45-11304. Vol. 1. 1945. text 65.00 (*0-8236-4520-7*); Vol. 2. 1946. text 65.00 (*0-8236-4540-1*); Vol. 5. 1949. text 65.00 (*0-8236-4580-0*); Vol. 6. 1950. text 65.00 (*0-8236-4600-9*); Vol. 7. 1951. text 65.00 (*0-8236-4620-3*); Vol. 8. 1952. text 65.00 (*0-8236-4640-8*); Vol. 10. 1954. text 65.00 (*0-8236-4700-5*); Vol. 11. 1995. text 65.00 (*0-8236-4720-X*); Vol. 12. 1956. text 65.00 (*0-8236-4740-4*); Vol. 13. 1957. text 65.00 (*0-8236-4760-9*); Vol. 14. 1958. text 65.00 (*0-8236-4780-3*); Vol. 15. 1959. text 65.00 (*0-8236-4800-1*); Vol. 16. 1960. text 65.00 (*0-8236-4820-6*); Vol. 17. 1961. text 65.00 (*0-8236-4840-0*); Vol. 18. 1962. text 65.00 (*0-8236-4860-5*); Vol. 19. 1963. text 65.00 (*0-8236-4880-X*); Vol. 21. 1965. text 65.00 (*0-8236-4920-2*); Vol. 22. 1967. text 65.00 (*0-8236-4940-7*); Vol. 23. 1968. text 65.00 (*0-8236-4960-1*); Vol. 24. 1969. text 65.00 (*0-8236-4961-X*); Vol. 25. 1970. text 65.00 (*0-8236-4962-8*); Vols. 3-4. 1947. text 65.00 (*0-8236-4560-6*) Intl Univs Pr.

Psychoanalytic Study of the Child, Vol. 27. Ed. by Ruth S. Eissler. 1974. 55.00 (*0-300-01780-4*) Yale U Pr.

Psychoanalytic Study of the Child. Ed. by Ruth S. Eissler et al. Vol. 28. 1973. 70.00 (*0-300-01703-0*); Vol. 29. 1974. LC 45-11304. 500p. 70.00 (*0-300-01796-0*); Vol. 30. 1975. LC 75-1934. (Psychoanalytic Study of the Child Ser.: Vol. 30). 800p. 70.00 (*0-300-01916-5*); Vol. 32. 1977. LC 45-11304. 70.00 (*0-300-02159-3*) Yale U Pr.

Psychoanalytic Study of the Child, Vol. 34. Ed. by Ruth S. Eissler. 1979. 65.00 (*0-300-02419-3*) Yale U Pr.

Psychoanalytic Study of the Child. Ed. by Ruth S. Eissler et al. Vol. 35. 1980. LC 45-11304. 600p. 65.00 (*0-300-02607-2*); Vol. 36. 1981. LC 45-11304. 468p. 65.00 (*0-300-02762-1*); Vol. 37. 1982. LC 45-11304. 562p. 65.00 (*0-300-02909-8*); Vol. 38. 1983. LC 45-11304. 800p. 60.00 (*0-300-03127-0*); Vol. 39. 1984. LC 45-11304. 65.00 (*0-300-03260-9*); Vol. 40. 1986. LC 45-11304. 608p. 65.00 (*0-300-03503-9*); Vol. 42. 1987. LC 45-11304. 609p. 65.00 (*0-300-04057-1*); Vol. 43. 1988. (C). 65.00 (*0-300-04341-4*); Vol. 44. 1989. LC 45-11304. (C). 65.00 (*0-300-04594-8*); Vol. 45. 1990. 544p. (C). 65.00 (*0-300-04908-0*); Vol. 47. 1992. LC 45-11304. 432p. (C). 65.00 (*0-300-05249-9*); Vol. 48. 1993. 416p. 65.00 (*0-300-05780-6*); Vol. 49. 1994. 544p. 65.00 (*0-300-06131-5*); Vol. 53. 1998. 464p. 65.00 (*0-300-07556-1*) Yale U Pr.

Psychoanalytic Study of the Child: Abstracts & Index, Vols. 1-25. Ed. by Ruth S. Eissler. 1975. LC 74-79973. 280p. 70.00 (*0-300-01778-2*) Yale U Pr.

Psychoanalytic Study of the Child Vol. 51: Anna Freud Anniversary Issue. Ed. by Albert J. Solnit et al. 1996. 464p. 65.00 (*0-300-06579-5*) Yale U Pr.

Psychoanalytic Study of the Child, 52, Vol. 52. Ed. by Albert J. Solnit et al. 1997. (Illus.). 464p. 65.00 (*0-300-07136-1*) Yale U Pr.

Psychoanalytic Supervision. Joan Fleming & Therese Benedek. Ed. by Chicago Institute for Psychanalysis Staff. 1983. LC 83-22763. (Classics in Psychoanalysis Monographs: No. 1). xii, 252p. (C). reprint ed. 37.50 (*0-8236-5041-3*) Intl Univs Pr.

Psychoanalytic Technique. Ed. by Herbert S. Strean. 1988. LC 87-30436. (Current Issues in Psychoanalytic Practice Ser.: Vol. 4, Nos. 3-4). (Illus.). 139p. text 39.95 (*0-86656-689-9*) Haworth Pr.

Psychoanalytic Technique & Psychic Conflict. Charles Brenner. 1976. LC 76-15047. 126p. (Orig.). 32.50 (*0-8236-5054-5*) Intl Univs Pr.

Psychoanalytic Technique & the Creation of Analytic Patients. A. Rothstein. 1998. 184p. pap. (*1-85575-205-0*) Karnac Bks GBR. *Dist:* Other Pr LLC.

Psychoanalytic Technique & the Creation of Analytic Patients. Arnold Rothstein. 1995. LC 95-46202. 137p. 27.50 (*0-8236-5057-X*, RC506); 2nd ed. 1997. LC 97-42836. 165p. 29.95 (*0-8236-5058-8*) Intl Univs Pr.

Psychoanalytic Terms & Concepts. Ed. by Burness E. Moore & Bernard D. Fine. 1990. LC 89-36223. 225p. (C). pap. 19.00 (*0-300-04701-0*) Yale U Pr.

Psychoanalytic Theories of Affect. Ruth Stein. 1991. LC 91-2762. 240p. 75.00 (*0-275-93984-7*, C3984, Praeger Pubs) Greenwood.

Psychoanalytic Theories of Affect. Ruth Stein. 1999. 240p. pap. (*1-85575-231-X*) Karnac Bks GBR. *Dist:* Other Pr LLC.

Psychoanalytic Theories of Development: An Integration. Phyllis Tyson & Robert L. Tyson. 1993. 414p. (C). reprint ed. pap. 22.00 (*0-300-05510-2*) Yale U Pr.

Psychoanalytic Theory: An Introduction. Anthony Elliott. 1994. 240p. pap. 27.95 (*0-631-18847-9*) Blackwell Pubs.

Psychoanalytic Theory & Clinical Relevance: What Makes a Theory Consequential for Practice? Louis S. Berger. 1985. 213p. 29.95 (*0-88163-042-X*) Analytic Pr.

Psychoanalytic Theory of Neurosis. Otto Fenichel. 1945. 39.95 (*0-393-01019-8*); 50th annot. ed. 1995. LC 95-20907. 730p. 42.50 (*0-393-03890-4*) Norton.

Psychoanalytic Theory, Therapy & the Self. Harry Guntrip. 1973. LC 79-135563. 224p. pap. 24.00 (*0-465-09511-9*) Basic.

Psychoanalytic Therapy & Behavior Therapy: Is Integration Possible? Ed. by Hal Arkowitz & Stanley Messer. 1984. 370p. 62.50 (*0-306-41578-X*, Plenum Trade) Perseus Pubng.

Psychoanalytic Therapy in the Hospital Setting. Paul Janssen. Tr. by Dinah Cannell. 1994. LC 93-20497. (ENG & GER.). 224p. (C). text 74.95 (*0-415-07295-6*) Routledge.

Psychoanalytic Understanding of the Dream. Paul Sloane. 1990. LC 79-50290. 288p. reprint ed. 40.00 (*0-87668-362-6*) Aronson.

Psychoanalytic Understanding of Violence & Suicide. Ed. by Rosine J. Perelberg. 1999. LC 98-25639. (New Library of Psychoanalysis). 200p. (C). 95.00 (*0-415-19931-X*, D6659); pap. 29.99 (*0-415-19932-8*, D6663) Routledge.

Psychoanalytic Vocation: Rank, Winnicott, & the Legacy of Freud. Peter L. Rudnytsky. 1991. 224p. (C). 40.00 (*0-300-05067-4*) Yale U Pr.

Psychoanalytical Approaches to Sexual Problems. Ed. by Herbert S. Strean. 1984. LC 84-12961. (Current Issues in Psychoanalytic Practice Ser.: Vol. 1, No. 3). 100p. text 29.95 (*0-86656-341-5*) Haworth Pr.

Psychoanalytical Method & the Doctrine of Freud Roland Dalbiez. Tr. by T. F. Lindsay from FRE. 1977. (Select Bibliographies Reprint Ser.). reprint ed. 52.95 (*0-8369-6715-1*) Ayer.

Psychoanalyzing: On the Order of the Unconscious & the Practice of the Letter. Serge Leclaire. Tr. by Peggy Kamauf from ENG. 1998. LC 97-21856. (Meridian: Crossing Aesthetics Ser.). 125p. 37.00 (*0-8047-2910-7*) Stanford U Pr.

Psychoanalyzing: On the Order of the Unconscious & the Practice of the Letter. Serge Leclaire. Tr. by Peggy Kamuf from ENG. 1998. LC 97-21856. (Meridian: Crossing Aesthetics Ser.). 125p. pap. 13.95 (*0-8047-2911-5*) Stanford U Pr.

***Psychoanlysis & Psychotherapy: The Controversies & the Future.** Ed. by Serge Frisch. 2001. 200p. pap. (*1-85575-266-2*) Karnac Bks GBR. *Dist:* Other Pr LLC.

Psychobabbl Biobank. Wade. 4th ed. 1997. (C). 13.00 (*0-673-97467-7*) Addison-Wesley.

Psychobiographic Approach to Psychotherapy: A Study of the Power Structure of Psychotherapy. Herzel Yerushalmi. 1998. LC 97-21398. 298p. 45.00 (*1-887841-12-1*, Psychosocial) Intl Univs Pr.

Psychobiological Approaches to Social Behavior. Ed. by P. Herbert Leiderman & David Shapiro. 1964. xv, 203p. 27.50 (*0-8047-0202-0*) Stanford U Pr.

Psychobiological Aspects of Allergic Disorders. Ed. by Stuart H. Young et al. 1985. LC 85-19390. 399p. 78.75 (*0-275-91301-5*, C1301, Praeger Pubs) Greenwood.

Psychobiological Foundations of Psychiatric Care. Norman L. Keltner et al. 1997. LC 97-262. (Illus.). 368p. (C). (gr. 13). pap. text 36.95 (*0-8151-5658-8*, 28786) Mosby Inc.

Psychobiology. Sdorow. 1999. 17.50 net. (*0-697-10912-7*) McGraw.

Psychobiology: Psychophysiological & Psychohumoral Processes Combined. Ed. by P. Netter. 1993. (Journal: Vol. 28, No. 1-2, 1993). (Illus.). 112p. pap. 117.50 (*3-8055-5853-8*) S Karger.

Psychobiology: The Neuron & Behavior. Katherine B. Hoyenga & Kermit T. Hoyenga. 1988. LC 86-26837. 513p. (C). text 83.95 (*0-534-06978-9*) Brooks-Cole.

Psychobiology & Treatment of Anorexia Nervosa & Bulimia Nervosa. Ed. by Katherine A. Halmi. 1992. LC 92-17984. (American Psychopathological Association Ser.). 356p. text 49.50 (*0-88048-506-X*, 8506) Am Psychiatric.

Psychobiology of Affective Development. Ed. by Nathan A. Fox & Richard J. Davidson. 1984. 424p. (C). text 99.95 (*0-89859-269-0*) L Erlbaum Assocs.

Psychobiology of Affective Disorders. Ed. by J. Mendels. 1981. (Illus.). viii, 220p. pap. 34.00 (*3-8055-1400-X*) S Karger.

Psychobiology of Aggression: Engines, Measurement, Control. Ed. by Marc Hillbrand & Nathaniel J. Pallone. 1994. LC 94-45057. (Journal of Offender Rehabilitation: Vol. 21, No. 3-4). (Illus.). 260p. lib. bdg. 49.95 (*1-56024-715-0*) Haworth Pr.

Psychobiology of Alcohol. Blum. 1983. (Substance & Alcohol Actions & Misuse Ser.). pap. 46.00 (*0-08-030949-6*, Pergamon Pr) Elsevier.

Psychobiology of Behavioral Development. Ronald Gandelman. 1992. (Illus.). 352p. (C). text 54.95 (*0-19-503941-6*) OUP.

Psychobiology of Bulimia Nervosa. Ed. by K. M. Pirke et al. 1988. (Illus.). 181p. 53.00 (*0-387-18670-0*) Spr-Verlag.

Psychobiology of Cancer: Automatization & Boredom in Health & Disease. Augustin De la Pena. 1983. 240p. 49.95 (*0-275-90968-9*, C0968, Praeger Pubs) Greenwood.

Psychobiology of Consciousness. Ed. by Richard J. Davidson & Julian M. Davidson. 1980. LC 79-316. 508p. 80.00 (*0-306-40138-X*, Plenum Trade) Perseus Pubng.

Psychobiology of Down Syndrome. Ed. by Lynn Nadel. 1988. LC 88-12999. (Issues in the Biology of Language & Cognition Ser.). 496p. 52.95 (*0-262-14043-8*, Bradford Bks) MIT Pr.

Psychobiology of Emotions. J. G. Thompson. 1988. LC 88-5937. (Emotions, Personality, & Psychotherapy Ser.). (Illus.). 418p. (C). 59.50 (*0-306-42843-1*, Plenum Trade) Perseus Pubng.

Psychobiology of Human Motivation. Hugh Wagner. 1999. LC 98-41034. (Psychology Focus Ser.). xiii, 189p. (*0-415-19274-9*) Routledge.

Psychobiology of Language. Ed. by Michael Studdert-Kennedy & David N. Caplan. 1983. LC 83-972. (Mit Press Studies in Neuropsychology & Neurolinguistics). (Illus.). 272p. 30.50 (*0-262-19217-9*) MIT Pr.

Psychobiology of Parkinson's Disease. Keith F. Tipton. 1993. 64.95 (*3-211-82483-9*) Spr-Verlag.

Psychobiology of Parkinson's Disease. Keith F. Tipton & M. B. Youndim. 1993. LC 93-44011. (Journals of Neural Transmission: Suppl. 40). (Illus.). 122p. 69.95 (*0-387-82483-9*) Spr-Verlag.

Psychobiology of Personality. Marvin Zuckerman. 1991. (Problems in the Behavioral Sciences Ser.: No. 10). (Illus.). 498p. (C). pap. text 42.95 (*0-521-35942-2*) Cambridge U Pr.

Psychobiology of Post-Traumatic Stress Disorder. 1997. LC 97-21354. (Annual Academy of Sciences Ser.: Vol. 821). pap. 110.00 (*1-57331-079-4*) NY Acad Sci.

Psychobiology of Post-Traumatic Stress Disorder, Vol. 821. Ed. by Rachel Yehuda & Alexander C. McFarlane. 1997. LC 97-21354. 550p. 110.00 (*1-57331-078-6*) NY Acad Sci.

Psychobiology of Stress: Proceedings of the NATO Advanced Research Workshop Held in Sorrento, Italy, August 28 - September 2, 1988. Ed. by Stefan Puglisi-Allegra. 1990. (C). text 195.50 (*0-7923-0682-1*) Kluwer Academic.

Psychobiology of the Hand. Ed. by Kevin J. Connolly. 1999. (Clinics in Developmental Medicine Ser.: No. 147). (Illus.). 250p. (C). text (*1-898683-14-X*) Mc Keith Pr GBR. *Dist:* Cambridge U Pr.

Psychocutaneous Diseases. Ed. by Caroline Koblenzer. 1987. text 82.00 (*0-8089-1865-6*, 792329, Grune & Strat) Harcrt Hlth Sci Grp.

Psychocybernetic Model of Art Therapy. Aina O. Nucho. 1987. (Illus.). 248p. 54.95 (*0-398-05339-1*); pap. 37.95 (*0-398-06646-9*) C C Thomas.

Psychodiagnostic Evaluation of Children: A Casebook Approach. Barbara R. Slater & John M. Thomas. 1983. 402p. (C). pap. text 30.95 (*0-8077-2734-2*) Tchrs Coll.

Psychodiagnostics & Personality Assessment: A Handbook. Donald P. Ogdon. 2nd ed. 1975. LC 66-29866. (Professional Handbook Ser.). 144p. (C). pap. 39.50 (*0-87424-095-6*, W-95) Western Psych.

Psychodietetics: Food As the Key to Emotional Health. Emanuel Cheraskin et al. 1989. LC 86-43196. 228p. pap. 7.95 (*0-8128-6266-X*, Scrbrough Hse) Madison Bks UPA.

Psychodrama: Group Psychotherapy as Experimental Theater. Eva Roine. 1997. LC 98-137745. 224p. pap. (*1-85302-494-5*) Jessica Kingsley GBR. *Dist:* Taylor & Francis.

Psychodrama & Audience Attitude Change. Ira A. Greenberg. 1968. LC 68-54532. 10.00 (*0-911958-00-2*) Behavioral Studies.

Psychodrama & Systemic Therapy. Chris Farmer. 1995. 136p. pap. (*1-85575-089-9*) Karnac Bks GBR. *Dist:* Other Pr LLC.

Psychodrama for the Timid Clinician see Clinician's Guide to Psychodrama

Psychodrama Since Moreno: Innovations in Theory & Practice. Ed. by Paul Holmes et al. 1994. LC 93-44657. (Lifeskills Library). (Illus.). 272p. (C). pap. 29.95 (*0-415-09351-1*, B4312) Routledge.

Psychodrama Since Moreno: Innovations in Theory & Practice. Ed. by William Dean Howells et al. 1994. LC 93-44657. (Lifeskills Library). (Illus.). 324p. (C). 84.95 (*0-415-09350-3*, B4308) Routledge.

Psychodynamic Approaches to Sexual Problems. Brian Daines & Angelina Perrett. 2000. LC 99-39401. 144p. pap. (*0-335-20159-8*) OpUniv Pr GBR. *Dist:* Taylor & Francis.

Psychodynamic Approaches to Sexual Problems. Contrib. by Brian Daines & Angelina Perrett. 2000. LC 99-39401. 177p. (*0-335-20160-1*) OpUniv Pr GBR. *Dist:* Taylor & Francis.

Psychodynamic Concepts in General Psychiatry. Ed. by Harvey J. Schwartz et al. 1995. LC 94-34974. 544p. text 69.50 (*0-88048-536-1*, 8536) Am Psychiatric.

Psychodynamic Group Psychotherapy. J. Scott Rutan & Walter N. Stone. 2nd ed. 1993. LC 93-15055. 274p. text 35.00 (*0-89862-096-1*); 3rd ed. 2000. LC 00-61756. 386p. text 42.00 (*1-57230-518-5*, C0518) Guilford Pubns.

Psychodynamic Perspectives on Sickness & Health. Paul Raphael Duberstein & Joseph M. Masling. 2000. LC 99-58549. (Empirical Studies of Psychoanalytic Theories: Vol. 9). 408p. 49.95 (*1-55798-668-1*) Am Psychol.

Psychodynamic Psychiatry in Clinical Practice. Glen O. Gabbard. 3rd ed. 2000. LC 99-54484. 616p. 79.95 (*1-58562-002-5*, 62002) Am Psychiatric.

Psychodynamic Psychiatry in Clinical Practice: The DSM-IV Edition. Glen O. Gabbard. 2nd ed. 1994. LC 93-27939. 656p. text 75.00 (*0-88048-658-9*, 8658) Am Psychiatric.

Psychodynamic Psychiatry, Theory & Practice John Frosch. 1990. 1. 55.00 (*0-8236-5645-4*, BN 05645); 2. 75.00 (*0-8236-5646-2*, BN 05646) Intl Univs Pr.

Psychodynamic Psycho Therapy: Supervisory Process. Rosemary M. Balsam. 2001. LC 2001-39627. 250p. pap. 39.95 (*0-8236-5642-X*, 05642) Intl Univs Pr.

Psychodynamic Psychotherapy: Learning to Listen from Multiple Perspectives. Jon Frederickson. 1998. LC 98-47697. 262p. pap. 31.95 (*0-87630-962-7*) Brunner-Routledge.

Psychodynamic Psychotherapy of Borderline Patients. Otto F. Kernberg et al. 1989. 224p. pap. 45.00 (*0-465-06643-7*) Basic.

Psychodynamic Psychotherapy of Children. Henry P. Coppolillo. 1987. 60.00 (*0-8236-4455-3*, BN#04455) Intl Univs Pr.

Psychodynamic Studies on Aging: Creativity, Reminiscing & Dying. Ed. by Sidney Levin & Ralph J. Kahana. 1967. LC 67-27427. 345p. 50.00 (*0-8236-5640-3*) Intl Univs Pr.

Psychodynamic Supervision: Perspectives for the Supervisor & the Supervisee. Martin H. Rock. 2000. LC 96-5634. 420p. 50.00 (*1-56821-693-9*) Aronson.

Psychodynamic Technique in the Treatment of the Eating Disorders. Ed. by C. Philip Wilson et al. 1992. LC 91-17197. 440p. 60.00 (*0-87668-622-6*) Aronson.

Psychodynamic Treatment of Anorexia Nervosa & Bulimia. Ed. by Craig L. Johnson. 1990. LC 90-13867. 404p. 48.00 (*0-89862-550-5*, 2550) Guilford Pubns.

Psychodynamics & Cognition. Mardi J. Horowitz. 1988. LC 87-25505. (Illus.). xii, 402p. 33.00 (*0-226-35368-0*) U Ch Pr.

Psychodynamics of Culture: Abram Kardiner & Neo-Freudian Anthropology, 3. William C. Manson. 1988. LC 88-17778. (Contributions to the Study of Anthropology Ser.: No. 3). 162p. 57.50 (*0-313-26267-5*, MDY/, Greenwood Pr) Greenwood.

Psychodynamics of Drug Dependence. Ed. by Jack D. Blaine & Demetrios A. Julius. 1994. LC 93-35969. 196p. pap. 40.00 (*1-56821-157-0*) Aronson.

Psychodynamics of Family Life: Diagnosis & Treatment of Family Relationships. Nathan W. Ackerman. 1995. LC 94-72519. (Master Work Ser.). 396p. pap. text 50.00 (*1-56821-341-7*) Aronson.

Psychodynamics of Work & Organizations: Theory & Application. William M. Czander. 1993. LC 93-13405. 408p. 48.00 (*0-89862-284-0*, 2284) Guilford Pubns.

Psychodynamics, Training & Outcome in Brief Psychotherapy. David H. Malan & Ferruccio Osimo. 2000. (Illus.). 336p. text (*0-7506-1545-1*) E A GBR. *Dist:* OUP.

Psychoeducational Assessment: Integrating Concepts & Techniques. George B. Helton et al. 1982. 364p. text 38.00 (*0-8089-1482-0*, 791963, Grune & Strat) Harcrt Hlth Sci Grp.

Psychoeducational Assessment of Minority Group Children: A Casebook. Ed. by Reginald L. Jones. 1988. LC 87-20861. 429p. pap. text 20.00 (*0-943539-00-5*) Cobb & Henry Pubs.

Psychoeducational Assessment of Students Who Are Visually Impaired or Blind: Infancy Through High School. Sharon Bradley-Johnson. 2nd rev. ed. 1994. LC 93-23211. (Illus.). 253p. (C). pap. 29.00 (*0-89079-599-1*, 6693) PRO-ED.

Psychoeducational Evaluation of Children & Adolescents with Low Incidence Handicaps. Philip J. Lazarus & Stephen S. Strichart. 1986. 336p. text 42.00 (*0-8089-1779-X*, 794415, Grune & Strat) Harcrt Hlth Sci Grp.

Psychoeducational Evaluation of the Preschool Child: A Manual Utilizing the Haeussermann Approach. Eleonora Jedrysek et al. 1972. LC 75-168848. (Illus.). 160p. (C). pap. text 45.00 (*0-8089-0735-2*, 792175, Grune & Strat) Harcrt Hlth Sci Grp.

Psychoeducational Groups for Patients with Schizophrenia: A Guide for Practitioners. Haya Ascher-Svanum & Audrey A. Krause. 1991. LC 90-14474. 308p. spiral bd. 104.00 (*0-8342-0197-6*) PRO-ED.

Psychoeducational Interventions in the Schools: Methods & Procedures for Enhancing Student Competence. Ed. by Charles A. Maher. 1987. (General Psychology Ser.: No. 150). 240p. text 35.00 (*0-08-033632-9*); pap. text 19.95 (*0-08-033631-0*) Elsevier (Pergamon Pr).

Psychoeducational Profile-Revised (PEP-R) Manual, Vol. I. Eric Schopler et al. 1979. LC 78-13415. (Illus.). 256p. 62.00 (*0-89079-238-0*, 1492) PRO-ED.

Psychoendocrine Aspects of Epilepsy. Harold E. Simmons. 1974. pap. 5.00 (*0-87312-004-3*) Psychogenic Disease.

Psychoendocrinology of Human Sexual Behavior, 6. Harold Persky. 1987. LC 87-6976. (Sexual Medicine Ser.: Vol. 6). 280p. 105.00 (*0-275-92526-9*, C2526, Praeger Pubs) Greenwood.

Psychofraud & Ethical Therapy. John D. Garcia. 1974. LC 73-92028. 200p. 6.95 (*0-87426-032-9*) Whitmore.

Psychogalvanic Reactions of Exceptional & Normal School Children. Robin D. Collmann. LC 79-176664. (Columbia University. Teachers College. Contributions to Education Ser.: No. 469). reprint ed. 37.50 (*0-404-55469-5*) AMS Pr.

Psychogenesis: The Early Development of Gender Identity. Elizabeth R. Moberly. 1983. 120p. 29.95 (*0-7100-9271-7*, Routledge Thoemms) Routledge.

Psychogenic Biochemical Aspects of Cancer. Harold E. Simmons. 1979. pap. 15.00 (*0-87312-010-8*) Psychogenic Disease.

Psychogenic Theory of Disease: A New Approach to Cancer Research. Harold E. Simmons. 1966. pap. 15.00 (*0-87312-000-0*) Gen Welfare Pubns.

Psychogeriatric Care in the Community. 1979. (Public Health in Europe Ser.: No. 10). 119p. 11.00 (*92-9020-129-0*, 1320010) World Health.

Psychogeriatrics: An Introduction to the Psychiatry of Old Age. Brice Pitt. 2nd ed. 1982. (Illus.). 224p. pap. text (*0-443-01598-8*) Church.

Psychographics in Personal Growth. George Burtt. 1972. LC 72-95846. pap. 3.50 (*0-913596-00-0*) Vector Counsel.

PsychoHeresy: The Psychological Seduction of Christianity. Martin M. Bobgan & Deidre N. Bobgan. 1987. LC 87-80001. 272p. (Orig.). pap. 15.00 (*0-941717-00-3*) EastGate Pubs.

Psychoimmunology: CNS-Immune Interactions. Alan J. Husband. 1993. 192p. 139.00 (*0-8493-4879-X*, QP356) CRC Pr.

Psychoimmunology of Human Cancer: Mind & Body in the Fight for Survival? Ed. by Jennifer Barraclough et al. 1995. LC 94-8027. (Illus.). 452p. text 89.50 (*0-19-262365-6*) OUP.

Psychokinesiology: Doorway to the Subconscious. Alexander S. Holub & Evelyn B. Michaels. 1999. LC 99-38726. 288p. pap. 16.95 (*1-893157-06-7*) Bridger Hse.

Psycholinguistic Learning Disabilities: Diagnosis & Remediation. Samuel A. Kirk & Winifred D. Kirk. 1971. LC 70-139805. 208p. pap. 12.50 (*0-252-00142-7*) U of Ill Pr.

Psycholinguistic Study of Phonological Interference. Eugene J. Briere. 1968. LC 68-13339. (Janua Linguarum, Ser. Minor: No. 66). pap. text (*90-279-0594-0*) Mouton.

Psycholinguistics. Joseph A. DeVito. 1971. LC 73-183112. (Studies in Communicative Disorders). 36p. (C). pap. (*0-672-61277-1*, Bobbs) Macmillan.

Psycholinguistics. Michael Garman. 1990. (Textbooks in Linguistics). (Illus.). 532p. (C). pap. text 34.95 (*0-521-27641-1*) Cambridge U Pr.

Psycholinguistics. Glea Berko. 2nd ed. 1997. (C). text 81.00 (*0-15-504106-1*) Harcourt.

Psycholinguistics: An Introduction. 2nd ed. 1979. (Illus.). 342p. 96.00 (*0-387-90417-4*) Spr-Verlag.

***Psycholinguistics: Critical Concepts.** Ed. by Gerry T. M. Altmann. 2001. LC 2001-48584. (Critical Concepts Ser.). 1600p. (C). (gr. 13). lib. bdg. 1010.00 (*0-415-22990-1*) Routledge.

Psychologcl Science: Historicl Fndtns Science Research. 2nd ed. 2000. 348p. (C). 25.00 (*0-536-61399-0*) Pearson Custom.

Psychological Abuse of Children in Health Care: The Issues. Ed. by Pat Azarnoff & Patricia Lindquist. 2nd rev. ed. 1997. (Issues in Pediatric Mental Health Ser.: No. 2). 130p. (C). spiral bd. 28.00 (*0-912599-06-5*) Pediatric Projects.

Psychological & Behavioral Aspects of Physical Disability: A Manual for Health Practitioners. James E. Lindemann et al. 1981. LC 81-17885. 452p. (C). 59.50 (*0-306-40776-0*, Plenum Trade) Perseus Pubng.

Psychological & Behavioral Assessment: Impact on Pediatric Care. Ed. by Phyllis R. Magrab. 1984. 384p. 70.00 (*0-306-41697-2*, Plenum Trade) Perseus Pubng.

Psychological & Biological Approaches to Emotion. Ed. by N. L. Stein et al. 1990. 456p. (C). pap. 55.00 (*0-8058-0150-2*); text 115.00 (*0-8058-0149-9*) L Erlbaum Assocs.

Psychological & Biological Assessment at the Turn of the Century. Ed. by John F. Clarkin & John P. Docherty. 1997. (Review of Psychiatry Ser.: Vol. 16, Sect. V). 144p. (Orig.). pap. text 25.00 (*0-88048-449-7*, 8449) Am Psychiatric.

Psychological & Human Reproduction. James W. Selby et al. 1980. LC 80-1641. 24.95 (*0-02-928690-5*) Free Pr.

Psychological & Medical Aspects of Induced Abortion: A Selective, Annotated Bibliography, 1970-1986, 7. Compiled by Eugenia B. Winter. annot. ed. 1988. LC 88-194. (Bibliographies & Indexes in Women's Studies: No. 7). 177p. lib. bdg. 62.95 (*0-313-26100-8*, WPY/) Greenwood.

***Psychological & Medical Effects of Concentration Camps & Related Persecutions on Survivors of the Holocaust: A Research Bibliography.** Leo Eitinger & Robert Krell. 1985. 180p. (Orig.). pap. (*0-7748-0220-0*) UBC Pr.

Psychological & Medical Well-Being & Their Relation in Adults with Insulin-Dependent Diabetes Mellitus. Bjorn Karlson. 1997. (Studia Psychologica et Pedagogica Ser.: Altera CXXVII). 106p. (Orig.). pap. (*91-22-01746-1*) Almqvist & Wiksell SWE. *Dist:* Coronet Bks.

Psychological & Neuropsychological Testing Terms: A Glossary in Nontechnical Language Version 1.0. Paul R. Lees-Haley. 1998. 19.95 (*0-9668410-0-X*) Lees-Haley Psych.

Psychological & Psychiatric Problems in Men. Joan Gomez. 1993. LC 93-7214. pap. (*0-415-09713-4*) Routledge.

Psychological & Psychosocial Consequences of Combat & Deployment with Special Emphasis on the Gulf War. David H. Marlowe. 2001. LC 2001-18159. (Gulf War Illnesses Ser.). xxxi, 181p. pap. 15.00 (*0-8330-2685-2*) Rand Corp.

Psychological & Social Impact of Disability. Ed. by Robert P. Marinelli & Arthur E. Dell Orto. 384p. 3rd ed. 1991. LC 91-4809. (C). 39.95 (*0-8261-2212-4*); 4th ed. 1999. 49.95 (*0-8261-2213-2*) Springer Pub.

Psychological Androgyny. Ellen Piel Cook. 1985. (General Psychology Ser.: No. 133). 256p. pap. text 25.00 (*0-08-031612-3*, Pergamon Pr) Elsevier.

Psychological Anthropology & Education: A Delineation of a Field of Inquiry. Charles Harrington. 1979. LC 78-18943. (Studies in Education: No. 5). 32.50 (*0-404-16012-3*) AMS Pr.

Psychological Anthropology Reconsidered. John M. Ingham. 1996. (Publications of the Society for Psychological Anthropology: No. 8). 320p. (C). text 74.95 (*0-521-55107-2*); pap. text 29.95 (*0-521-55918-9*) Cambridge U Pr.

Psychological Approach to Hospital-Acquired Infections. C. A. Bartzokas et al. 1995. LC 94-27126. 164p. text 79.95 (*0-7734-9030-2*) E Mellen.

Psychological Approaches in Psychiatric Nursing. Breda Kingston. 1987. 150p. pap. (*0-7099-1521-7*) C Helm GBR. *Dist:* Routldge.

Psychological Approaches to Pain Management: A Practitioner's Handbook. Ed. by Robert J. Gatchel & Dennis C. Turk. 1996. LC 95-26230. (Illus.). 519p. pap. 65.00 (*0-89862-292-1*, 2292) Guilford Pubns.

Psychological Approaches to Sports Injury Rehabilitation. Jim Taylor & Shel Taylor. 1998. LC 97-20420. 302p. 55.00 (*0-8342-0973-X*) PRO-ED.

Psychological Approaches to the Care of the Elderly. John Hodge. Ed. by Ian Hanley. 1984. 250p. 35.00 (*0-416-00941-7*, NO. 5077) Routledge.

Psychological Aspects of Abortion. Ed. by David Mall & Walter F. Watts. 1979. LC 79-88679. 156p. pap. 20.95 (*0-313-27053-8*, P7053, Greenwood Pr) Greenwood.

Psychological Aspects of Balance of Diabetes in Juvenile: Proceedings of the 3rd Beilinson Symposium, Pt. 2, Herzlyg, 1875. International Beilinson Symposium Staff. Ed. by Zvi Laron. 1977. (Pediatric & Adolescent Endocrinology Ser.: Vol. 3). (Illus.). 42.75 (*3-8055-2631-8*) S Karger.

Psychological Aspects of Cancer. Ed. by M. Watson & T. Morris. 1985. (Advances in the Biosciences Ser.: No. 49). (Illus.). 112p. pap. 28.50 (*0-08-030791-4*, Pergamon Pr) Elsevier.

Psychological Aspects of Cancer Care. Lawrence Goldie. 1996. 160p. pap. text (*1-85302-358-2*) Jessica Kingsley GBR. *Dist:* Taylor & Francis.

Psychological Aspects of Caring in a Mixed Economy. Open Learning Foundation Staff. 1996. 130p. pap. (*0-443-05733-8*) Church.

Psychological Aspects of Diabetes in Children & Adolescents. Ed. by Z. Laron & A. Galatzer. 1983. (Pediatric & Adolescent Endocrinology Ser.: Vol. 10). xvi, 248p. 160.00 (*3-8055-3575-9*) S Karger.

Psychological Aspects of Early Breast Cancer. C. Ray & M Baum. 1985. (Contributions to Psychology & Medicine Ser.). (Illus.). 133p. 75.95 (*0-387-96122-4*) Spr-Verlag.

Psychological Aspects of Genetic Counselling. Ed. by Alan E. Emery & Ian Pullen. 1984. text 104.00 (*0-12-238220-X*) Acad Pr.

Psychological Aspects of Geriatric Rehabilitation. Robert Hartke. 1991. LC 90-14530. 304p. 84.00 (*0-8342-0211-5*) Aspen Pub.

Psychological Aspects of Health & Illness: A Life-Span Perspective. Ed. by Thomas L. Whitman et al. 1998. LC 98-21788. 300p. (*0-8058-2771-4*); pap. (*0-8058-2772-2*) L Erlbaum Assocs.

Psychological Aspects of Illness & Disease. California College for Health Sciences Staff. 1992. 166p. (C). spiral bd. 155.00 (*0-933195-16-8*) CA College Health Sci.

Psychological Aspects of Infertility. Ed. by Anthony Reading. 220p. 34.95 (*0-471-52792-0*) Wiley.

Psychological Aspects of Modernity. Ed. by Jerome Braun. 1993. LC 93-20297. 288p. 77.00 (*0-275-94262-7*, C4262, Praeger Pubs) Greenwood.

Psychological Aspects of Pregnancy, Birthing, & Bonding. Barbara L. Blum. 1980. LC 80-14227. (New Directions in Psychotherapy Ser.: Vol. IV). 380p. 49.00 (*0-87705-210-7*, Kluwer Acad Hman Sci) Kluwer Academic.

Psychological Aspects of Radiation Therapy: The Patient, the Family & the Staff. Patricia Tretter & Lillian G. Kutscher. 1981. 21.95 (*0-405-13096-1*) Ayer.

Psychological Aspects of Rheumatoid Arthritis. M. L. Pritchard. 1989. (Recent Research in Psychology Ser.). (Illus.). 208p. 59.95 (*0-387-97116-5*) Spr-Verlag.

Psychological Aspects of Serious Illness: Chronic Conditions, Fatal Diseases, & Clinical Care. Ed. by Paul T. Costa, Jr. & Gary R. VandenBos. 1990. 172p. pap. text 19.95 (*1-55798-105-1*) Am Psychol.

Psychological Aspects of Surgery. Ed. by Frederick G. Guggenheim. 1986. (Advances in Psychosomatic Medicine Ser.: Vol. 15). (Illus.). viii, 232p. 121.00 (*3-8055-4090-6*) S Karger.

Psychological Aspects of Terminal Care. Owens. pap. 30.00 (*0-471-96621-5*) Wiley.

Psychological Aspects of Terminal Care. Glynn R. Ownes. 1998. (Clinical Psychology & Personality Ser.). 300p. 65.00 (*0-471-95291-5*) Wiley.

Psychological Aspects of Women's Health Care: The Interface Between Psychiatry & Obstetrics & Gynecology. Ed. by Donna E. Stewart & Nada L. Stotland. 1993. LC 92-48771. 572p. text 74.50 (*0-88048-421-7*, 8421) Am Psychiatric.

Psychological Aspects of Women's Reproductive Health. Ed. by Michael O'Hara et al. 1995. LC 94-36163. 368p. 43.95 (*0-8261-8660-2*) Springer Pub.

Psychological Assessment: A Conceptual Approach. Michael P. Maloney & Michael P. Ward. 1976. (Illus.). 422p. text 41.95 (*0-19-502027-8*) OUP.

Psychological Assessment: A Theory Systems Approach. James R. Barclay. 1991. LC 89-37230. 458p. (C). lib. bdg. 47.00 (*0-89464-405-X*) Krieger.

***Psychological Assessment & Treatment of Anxiety Disorders.** Vimala Veeraraghavan & Shalini Singh. 2002. LC 2001-48290. (*0-7619-9558-7*); (*81-7829-065-0*) Sage.

Psychological Assessment in Medical Rehabilitation. Ed. by Laura A. Cushman & Marcia J. Scherer. 1995. LC 95-11109. (Measurement & Instrumentation in Psychology Ser.). 471p. text 29.95 (*1-55798-299-6*) Am Psychol.

Psychological Assessment in Medical Settings. Ronald H. Rozensky et al. 1997. LC 97-24814. (Applied Clinical Psychology Ser.). (Illus.). 340p. (C). 49.50 (*0-306-45551-X*, Plenum Trade) Perseus Pubng.

P
Q
R

PQR

Psychological Assessment in Medicine. Ed. by Samuel E. Krug. 1977. LC 77-71889. 15.00 (*0-918296-07-2*) Inst Personality & Ability.

Psychological Assessment of Abused & Traumatized Children. Francis D. Kelly. 1999. LC 98-31089. (Lea Series in Personality & Clinical Psychology Ser.). 272p. 29.95 (*0-8058-2973-3*) L Erlbaum Assocs.

Psychological Assessment of Adult Posttraumatic States. John Briere. 1997. LC 96-52132. (Psychotherapy Practitioner Resource Bks.). 251p. pap. text 24.95 (*1-55798-403-4*, 431-7840) Am Psychol.

Psychological Assessment of Mental & Physical Handicaps. Ed. by Peter Mittler. 1974. 886p. pap. (*0-422-75600-8*, NO. 2819) Tavistock GBR. *Dist:* Routldge.

Psychological Assessment of Presidential Candidates. Stanley A. Renshon. 1998. LC 98-11839. 528p. (C). reprint ed. pap. 26.95 (*0-415-92146-5*) Routledge.

Psychological Assessment, Psychiatric Diagnosis, & Treatment Planning. Stephen Hurt et al. 1991. LC 90-15146. 512p. text 61.95 (*0-87630-607-5*) Brunner-Routledge.

Psychological Assessment with the Millon Clinical Multiaxial Inventory (II) No. II: An Interpretive Guide. Robert J. Craig. 1993. LC 93-11583. 120p. pap. 29.00 (*0-911907-10-6*) Psych Assess.

Psychological Assessment with the MMPI. Alan Friedman et al. 1989. (C). 424p. text 55.00 (*0-8058-0310-6*); text, stu. ed. 65.00 (*0-8058-1066-8*) L Erlbaum Assocs.

Psychological Assessment with the MMPI-2. Alan F. Friedman. 2000. LC 99-87193. (Illus.). xxxiii, 688p. (*0-8058-1444-2*) L Erlbaum Assocs.

Psychological Atlas. David Katz. Tr. by Frank Gaynor. 1968. LC 68-28587. 142p. reprint ed. lib. bdg. 69.50 (*0-8371-0123-9*, KAPA, Greenwood Pr) Greenwood.

Psychological Autopsy in the Courtroom: Contributions of the Social Sciences to Resolving Issues Surrounding Equivocal Deaths. James Selkin. 1987. LC 87-90140. 112p. 19.95 (*0-8377-1150-9*, Rothman) W S Hein.

Psychological Bases of Sport Injuries. Ed. by David Pargman. 1993. LC 92-73668. 315p. (C). 38.00 (*0-9627926-3-2*) Fit Info Tech.

Psychological Birth of the Human Infant. Margaret S. Mahler et al. 1975. LC 74-77255. 320p. pap. 47.00 (*0-465-06659-3*) Basic.

Psychological Care in Physical Illness. Keith A. Nichols. 1984. LC 84-71617. 204p. pap. text 21.95 (*0-914783-06-8*) Charles.

Psychological Care in Physical Illness. Nichols. 2nd ed. 1993. 248p. pap. 41.50 (*1-56593-134-3*, 0446) Singular Publishing.

Psychological Care in Physical Illness. Keith A. Nichols. 2nd ed. 1993. LC 92-49595. pap. (*0-412-43560-8*) Chapman & Hall.

Psychological Care of Infant & Child. John B. Watson. 1976. LC 75-169399. (Family in America Ser.). 206p. reprint ed. 14.95 (*0-405-03876-3*) Ayer.

Psychological Case Formulation in Clinical Practice. Glenn Waller & Liz Offen. 2000. 250p. 49.95 (*0-471-97568-0*); pap. 49.95 (*0-471-95726-7*) Wiley.

Psychological Classification of the Adult Male Prison Inmate. Patricia Van Voorhis. 1994. LC 93-13292. (Series in New Directions in Crime & Justice Studies). 364p. text 64.50 (*0-7914-1793-X*) State U NY Pr.

Psychological Commentaries on the Teaching of Gurdjieff & Ouspensky, No. 1. Maurice Nicoll. 1996. LC 96-16548. 384p. reprint ed. 30.00 (*0-87728-899-2*) Red Wheel ME.

Psychological Concepts & Biological Psychiatry: A Philosophical Analysis. Peter Zachar. 2000. LC 00-56430. (Advances in Consciousness Research Ser.: Vol. 28). xix, 340p. pap. 39.95 (*1-55619-991-0*) J Benjamins Pubng Co.

Psychological Concepts & Dissociative Disorders. Ed. by Raymond Klein & Benjamin Doane. 1994. 384p. text 89.95 (*0-8058-0516-8*) L Erlbaum Assocs.

Psychological Concomitants of Illness, Vol. 2. 155p. pap. (*0-89970-008-X*, OP-079) AMA.

Psychological Consequences of Crowding. Uday Jain. 1987. 160p. (C). 17.95 (*0-8039-9546-6*, 7087) Sage.

Psychological Consultation: Introduction to Theory & Practice. Duane Brown & Walter B. Pryzwansky. 5th ed. 2000. LC 00-40138. 384p. 68.00 (*0-205-32210-7*) Allyn.

Psychological Consultation: Perspectives & Applications. William A. Wallace & Donald L. Hall. 1995. (Counseling Ser.). 361p. spiral bd. 86.95 (*0-534-23094-6*) Brooks-Cole.

Psychological Consultation & Collaboration in School & Community Settings. A. Michael Dougherty. 3rd ed. 1999. LC 99-28748. (Counseling Ser.). 416p. text 69.95 (*0-534-35555-2*) Brooks-Cole.

Psychological Consulting to Management: A Clinician's Perspective. Lester R. Tobias. 1990. LC 89-22098. 208p. text 29.95 (*0-87630-564-8*) Brunner-Routledge.

Psychological Contracts in Employment: Cross Cultural Perspectives. Ed. by Denise M. Rousseau & Renae Schalk. 2000. LC 00-8446. ix, 324p. 79.95 (*0-7619-1680-6*, 82887) Sage.

Psychological Debriefing: Theory, Practice & Evidence. Ed. by Beverley Raphael & John P. Wilson. 2000. LC 99-52565. (Illus.). 386p. pap. text 59.95 (*0-521-64700-2*) Cambridge U Pr.

Psychological Decision Theory. Jozef Kozielecki. 1982. lib. bdg. 176.50 (*90-277-1051-1*) Kluwer Academic.

Psychological Defenses in Everyday Life. Robert W. Firestone & Joyce Catlett. rev. ed. 1989. 264p. pap. 16.95 (*0-9676684-1-7*) Glendon Assn.

Psychological Defenses in Everyday Life. Robert W. Firestone & Joyce Catlett. 1989. (Insight Bk.). 256p. pap. 22.95 (*0-89885-454-7*, Kluwer Acad Hman Sci) Kluwer Academic.

Psychological Deprivation: Index of New Information, with Authors, Subjects & Bibliography. Susanna L. Warren. 1995. LC 95-14594. 57.50 (*0-7883-0700-2*); pap. 47.50 (*0-7883-0707-X*) ABBE Pubs Assn.

Psychological Deprivation: Index of New Information with Authors, Subjects & Bibliography. S. L. Warren. rev. ed. 1994. 143p. 57.50 (*0-7883-0176-4*); 57.50 (*0-7883-0262-0*); pap. 47.50 (*0-7883-0177-2*); pap. 47.50 (*0-7883-0263-9*) ABBE Pubs Assn.

Psychological Development. Kathleen M. Speer. 1998. (C). pap. text, tchr. ed. 28.00 (*0-15-500924-9*); pap. text, tchr. ed., suppl. ed. 28.00 (*0-15-500926-5*) Harcourt Coll Pubs.

Psychological Development: A Life-Span Approach. Paul H. Mussen et al. 1979. LC 78-11977. (C). text 30.33 (*0-06-044692-7*) Addson-Wesley Educ.

Psychological Development of Deaf Children. Marc Marschark. 1997. (Illus.). 288p. reprint ed. pap. text 24.95 (*0-19-511575-9*) OUP.

Psychological Development of Low-Birthweight Children, 6. Ed. by National Institutes of Child Health and Human Development Staff et al. 1992. (Advances in Applied Developmental Psychology Ser.: Vol. 6). 505p. (C). 87.50 (*0-89391-855-5*, Ablex) Greenwood.

Psychological Development of the Child. Paul H. Mussen. 3rd ed. 1979. (Foundations of Modern Psychology Ser.). (Illus.). text 17.95 (*0-13-732420-0*) P-H.

Psychological Dimensions of Organizational Behavior. Ed. by Barry M. Staw. 2nd ed. 1994. LC 94-19440. 528p. 67.00 (*0-02-416153-5*, Macmillan Coll) P-H.

Psychological Disorders in General Medical Settings. Ed. by Norman Sartorius et al. 1990. LC 89-24611. 220p. (C). text 39.00 (*0-920887-59-7*) Hogrefe & Huber Pubs.

Psychological Disturbance in Adolescence. Irving B. Weiner. 2nd ed. 1992. LC 91-18344. (Personality Processes Ser.: No. 1341). 496p. 150.00 (*0-471-82596-4*) Wiley.

Psychological Disturbances in Epilepsy. Ed. by J. Chris Sackellares et al. 1995. LC 95-40942. 272p. text 89.99 (*0-7506-9605-2*) Buttrwrth-Heinemann.

Psychological Disturbances in Y. Ed. by Micheal Rutter. 1997. 425p. pap. text 24.95 (*0-521-59873-7*) Cambridge U Pr.

Psychological Dynamics of Religious Experience. Andre Godin. Tr. by Mary Turton from FRE. 1985. LC 85-2354. Orig. Title: Psychologie des Experiences Religieuses. 279p. pap. 18.95 (*0-89135-039-X*) Religious Educ.

Psychological Effects of Aerobic Fitness Training: Research & Theory. D. G. McDonald & J. A. Hodgdon. 1991. 224p. 72.95 (*0-387-97603-5*) Spr-Verlag.

Psychological Effects of Cocaine & Crack Addiction. Ann Holmes & Claire E. Reinburg. Ed. by Carol C. Nadelson. 1998. LC 98-30975. (Encyclopedia of Psychological Disorders Ser.). 144p. 22.95 (*0-7910-4898-5*) Chelsea Hse.

Psychological Effects of Motherhood: A Study of First Pregnancy. Myra Leifer. 1980. LC 79-26179. 304p. 14.95 (*0-275-91691-X*, C1691, Praeger Pubs) Greenwood.

Psychological Effects of Police Work: A Psychodynamic Approach. P. Bonifacio. 1991. (Criminal Justice & Public Safety Ser.). (Illus.). 220p. (C). 42.50 (*0-306-43955-7*, Plenum Trade) Perseus Pubng.

Psychological Effects of War & Violence on Children. Ed. by Lewis A. Leavitt & Nathan A. Fox. 1993. 392p. pap. 36.00 (*0-8058-1172-9*); text 89.95 (*0-8058-1171-0*) L Erlbaum Assocs.

Psychological Evaluation of Children's Human Figure Drawings. Elizabeth M. Koppitz. 1967. (Illus.). 352p. text 35.95 (*0-8089-0240-7*, 792355, Grune & Strat) Harcrt Hlth Sci Grp.

Psychological Evaluation of Human Figure Drawings by Middle School Students. Elizabeth M. Koppitz. 1984. 208p. text 25.00 (*0-8089-1682-3*, 792355, Grune & Strat) Harcrt Hlth Sci Grp.

Psychological Evaluation of the Developmentally & Physically Handicapped. V. B. Van Hasselt & M. Hersen. 1987. LC 87-15275. (Illus.). 348p. (C). 80.00 (*0-306-42514-9*, Plenum Trade) Perseus Pubng.

Psychological Evaluations for the Courts: A Handbook for Mental Health Professionals & Lawyers. Gary B. Melton et al. 2nd ed. 1997. LC 97-10163. (Law & Behavior Ser.). (Illus.). 794p. text 75.00 (*1-57230-236-4*, 0236) Guilford Pubns.

Psychological Examination: A Guide for Clinicians. Paul W. Pruyser. 1979. LC 78-70234. 311p. 47.50 (*0-8236-5605-5*) Intl Univs Pr.

Psychological Examination of the Child. Theodore H. Blau. 1991. LC 90-39091. (Personality Processes Ser.). 279p. 160.00 (*0-471-63559-6*) Wiley.

Psychological Experts in Divorce Actions. Marc J. Ackerman & Andrew W. Kane. 3rd ed. 1998. LC 98-194251. xxxiii, 1190p. 165.00 (*1-56706-922-3*) Aspen Law.

Psychological Explanations of Crime. Ed. by David P. Farrington. 1994. (International Library of Criminology, Criminal Justice, & Penology). 484p. (*1-85521-447-4*) Dartmth Pub GBR. *Dist:* Ashgate Pub Co.

Psychological Factors Affecting Medical Conditions. Alan Stoudemire. 1995. LC 94-27559. 240p. text 32.00 (*0-88048-708-9*, 8708) Am Psychiatric.

Psychological Factors in Competitive Sport. Don Davies & Malcom Armstrong. 1989. 180p. pap. 34.95 (*1-85000-607-5*, Falmer Pr) Taylor & Francis.

Psychological Factors of Peace & War. Tom H. Pear. 1977. 262p. 19.95 (*0-8369-2290-5*) Ayer.

Psychological Foundations of Criminal Justice: Contemporary Perpectives on Forensic Psychiartry & Psychology, Vol. 2. Ed. by Harold J. Vetter & Robert W. Rieber. 1980. LC 78-18781. (Illus.). 416p. (C). 20.00 (*0-89444-025-X*) John Jay Pr.

Psychological Foundations of Criminal Justice: Historical Perspectives on Forensic Psychology, Vol. 1. Ed. by Robert W. Rieber & Harold J. Vetter. 1978. LC 78-18781. (Illus.). (C). 20.00 (*0-89444-009-8*) John Jay Pr.

Psychological Foundations of Education. Jack Rudman. (National Teacher Examination Ser.: NC-1). pap. 23.95 (*0-8373-8401-X*) Nat Learn.

Psychological Foundations of the Curriculum (UNESCO) 1974. (Education Studies & Documents: No. 26). reprint ed. pap. 25.00 (*0-8115-1350-5*) Periodicals Srv.

Psychological Healing: A Historical & Clinical Study Pierre M. Janet. LC 75-16710. (Classics in Psychiatry Ser.). reprint ed. Set. 1976. 101.95 (*0-405-07437-9*); Vol. 1. 1977. 51.95 (*0-405-07438-7*); Vol. 2. 1977. 51.95 (*0-405-07439-5*) Ayer.

Psychological Impact of Unemployment. N. T. Feather. 1989. (Illus.). 285p. 98.00 (*0-387-97027-4*) Spr-Verlag.

Psychological Interventions: A Guide to Strategies. Ed. by Mary Ballou. 1995. LC 95-6939. 232p. 59.95 (*0-275-94851-X*, Praeger Pubs) Greenwood.

Psychological Issues in Biblical Lore: Explorations in the Old Testament. Albert I. Rabin. 1998. LC 98-17874. (Series on Social Work). 34.95 (*0-8261-1212-9*) Springer Pub.

Psychological Issues Related to Child Maltreatment Vol. 24: Working Group Report by the Coordinating Committee on Child Abuse & Neglect, American Psychological Association. Ed. by Diane J. Willis. 1996. 101p. pap., suppl. ed. 20.00 (*0-8058-9924-3*) L Erlbaum Assocs.

Psychological Kinesiology: Changing the Body's Beliefs. William F. Whisenant. rev. ed. 1994. (Illus.). 400p. (Orig.). pap. 49.95 (*1-880790-55-6*) Monarch Butterfly.

Psychological Maltreatment of Children & Youth. Ed. by Marla R. Brassard et al. 1987. (General Psychology Ser.: No. 143). 400p. 55.00 (*0-08-032775-3*, J115, Pergamon Pr) Elsevier.

Psychological Management of Chronic Headaches. Paul R. Martin. LC 92-48225. (Treatment Manuals for Practitioners Ser.). 266p. 1996. pap. 24.00 (*1-57230-122-8*, 0122); 1993. text 42.00 (*0-89862-211-5*) Guilford Pubns.

Psychological Management of Chronic Pain, set. 2nd ed. H. Clare Philips & Stanley J. Rachman. Incl. Psychological Management of Chronic Pain: Patient Manual. 80p. tchr. ed. 14.95 (*0-8261-6112-X*); Set. Psychological Management of Chronic Pain: A Treatment Manual. LC 95-39060. 304p. 42.95 (*0-8261-6111-1*); (Illus.). (Behavior Therapy & Behavioral Medicine Ser.). 1996. 52.00 (*0-8261-6113-8*, P4821) Springer Pub.

Psychological Management of Chronic Pain: A Treatment Manual, Set. H. Clare Philips & Stanley J. Rachman. 2nd ed. 1996. LC 95-39060. (Behavior Therapy & Behavioral Medicine Ser.). (Illus.). 304p. 42.95 (*0-8261-6111-1*) Springer Pub.

Psychological Management of Chronic Pain: Patient Manual. H. Clare Philips & Stanley J. Rachman. 2nd ed. 1996. (Behavior Therapy & Behavioral Medicine Ser.). (Illus.). 80p. tchr. ed. 14.95 (*0-8261-6112-X*) Springer Pub.

Psychological Managements for Psychosomatic Disorders. J. W. Paulley & H. E. Pelser. 1989. (Illus.). 335p. 86.95 (*0-387-19298-0*) Spr-Verlag.

Psychological Meaning of Chaos: Translating Theory into Practice. Ed. by Frank Masterpasqua & Phyllis A. Perna. 1997. LC 97-12954. 323p. text 39.95 (*1-55798-429-8*, 431-7910) Am Psychol.

Psychological Measurements in Psychopharmacology. Ed. by P. Pichot & R. Olivier-Martin. 1974. (Modern Problems of Pharmacopsychiatry Ser.: Vol. 7). (Illus.). 85.25 (*3-8055-1630-4*) S Karger.

Psychological Medicine Insights: Treating Patients' Medical Psychological Problems. Harry Ireton. 1985. LC 85-73695. 80p. (Orig.). pap. text 15.00 (*0-936787-00-7*) Behavior Sci Systs.

Psychological Medicine of HIV Infection. Ed. by J. Catalan et al. 1996. (Illus.). 316p. text 85.00 (*0-19-262202-1*) OUP.

Psychological Methods in Criminal Investigation & Evidence. Ed. by David Raskin. 1989. 416p. 46.95 (*0-8261-6450-1*) Springer Pub.

Psychological Methods of Child Assessment. Jacquelin Goldman et al. 1984. LC 83-20889. 416p. text 47.95 (*0-87630-348-3*) Brunner-Routledge.

Psychological Methods of Testing Intelligence, 4. William L. Stern. Tr. by G. M. Whipple from GER. 1977. LC 77-72191. (Contributions to the History of Psychology Ser.). 494p. reprint ed. lib. bdg. 85.00 (*0-313-26939-4*, U6939, Greenwood Pr) Greenwood.

Psychological Mindedness: A Contemporary Understanding. Ed. by Mary McCallum & William E. Piper. 1997. LC 97-2440. (Lea Series in Personality & Clinical Psychology Ser.). (Illus.). 375p. text 39.95 (*0-8058-1722-0*) L Erlbaum Assocs.

Psychological, Neuropsychiatric, & Substance Abuse Aspects of AIDS. 1990. lib. bdg. 79.95 (*0-87700-892-2*) Revisionist Pr.

Psychological Operations & Political Warfare in Long-Term Strategic Planning. Janos Radvanyi. 1990. LC 90-31183. 168p. 58.00 (*0-275-93623-6*, C3623, Praeger Pubs) Greenwood.

Psychological Perspectives & the Religious Quest: Essays in Honor of Orlo Strunk, Jr. Ed. by Lallene J. Rector & Weaver Santaniello. 1998. LC 98-31582. 208p. 51.00 (*0-7618-1292-X*); pap. 27.50 (*0-7618-1293-8*) U Pr of Amer.

Psychological Perspectives of Essential Hypertension. W. Linden. 1984. (Biobehavioral Medicine Ser.: Vol. 3). (Illus.). x, 130p. pap. 60.00 (*3-8055-3662-3*) S Karger.

Psychological Perspectives on Deafness. Ed. by Marc Marschark & M. Diane Clark. 1993. 400p. text 79.95 (*0-8058-1054-4*) L Erlbaum Assocs.

Psychological Perspectives on Lesbian & Gay Male Experiences. Ed. by Linda D. Garnets & Douglas C. Kimmel. 1993. LC 93-35562. (Between Men-Between Women: Lesbian & Gay Studies). 512p. pap. 31.50 (*0-231-07885-4*) Col U Pr.

Psychological Perspectives on Pregnancy & Childbirth. Sarah Clement. 1998. LC 97-36826. 273p. pap. text (*0-443-05760-5*) Church.

Psychological Perspectives on Self & Identity. Ed. by Abraham Tesser et al. 2000. LC 00-21139. (Illus.). x, 252p. text 39.95 (*1-55798-678-9*, 431-8940) Am Psychol.

Psychological Perspectives on Sexual Problems: New Directions in Theory & Practice. Ed. by Jane M. Ussher & Christine D. Baker. 1993. LC 92-13346. (Illus.). (C). 256p. 89.95 (*0-415-05508-3*, A7777); 224p. pap. 27.99 (*0-415-05509-1*, A7781) Routledge.

Psychological Perspectives on the Self. Ed. by Jerry Suls. 1993. 248p. 59.95 (*0-8058-1181-8*) L Erlbaum Assocs.

Psychological Perspectives on the Self, Vol. 2. Ed. by Jerry Suls & Anthony G. Greenwald. 1983. 408p. text 79.95 (*0-89859-276-3*) L Erlbaum Assocs.

Psychological Perspectives on Women's Health. Vincent J. Adesso. 1994. 360p. 27.95 (*1-56032-335-3*) Hemisp Pub.

Psychological Practice in a Changing Health Care System: Issues & New Directions. Ed. by Robert L. Glueckauf et al. 1996. LC 96-26099. (Illus.). 224p. 43.95 (*0-8261-9280-7*) Springer Pub.

Psychological Practice in Small Towns & Rural Areas. Intro. by Robert D. Weitz. 1992. LC 91-35398. (Psychotherapy in Private Practice Ser.: Vol. 10, No. 3, 1992). 137p. 39.95 (*1-56024-280-9*) Haworth Pr.

Psychological Principles & the Black Experience. Lawrence N. Houston. 1990. 194p. (C). pap. text 25.50 (*0-8191-7957-4*); lib. bdg. 47.50 (*0-8191-7956-6*) U Pr of Amer.

Psychological Problems Before & after Myocardial Infarction. Ed. by H. Denolin. 1982. (Advances in Cardiology Ser.: Vol. 29). viii, 156p. 85.25 (*3-8055-3424-8*) S Karger.

Psychological Problems in the Father-Son Relationship. Harold A. Abramson. 1969. LC 71-81849. 7.50 (*0-8079-0154-7*) October.

Psychological Problems of Aging Assessment Treatment Care. Robert T. Woods. 1999. LC 98-46227. (Clinical Psychology & Personality Ser.). (Illus.). 368p. pap. 60.00 (*0-471-97434-X*) Wiley.

Psychological Processes & Advertising Effects: Theory, Research, & Applications. Ed. by Linda F. Alwitt & Andrew A. Mitchell. 1991. 320p. pap. 34.00 (*0-89859-515-0*) L Erlbaum Assocs.

Psychological Profiles of Conjoined Twins: Heredity, Environment, & Identity. J. David Smith. 1988. LC 88-1592. 171p. 60.00 (*0-275-92965-5*, C2965, Praeger Pubs) Greenwood.

Psychological Reflections: A New Anthology of His Writings, 1905-1961. Carl Gustav Jung. Ed. by Jolande Jacobi & R. F. C. Hull. 1973. LC 88-177442. (Bollingen Ser.: Vol. 31). 332p. pap. 19.95 (*0-691-01786-7*) Princeton U Pr.

Psychological Research: Innovative Methods & Strategies. John Haworth. 1995. (Illus.). 304p. (C). pap. 27.95 (*0-415-11790-9*) Routledge.

Psychological Research: Innovative Methods & Strategies. Ed. by John Haworth. 1995. (Illus.). 304p. (C). 80.00 (*0-415-11789-5*) Routledge.

Psychological Research: The Ideas Behind the Methods. Douglas Mook. 2001. LC 00-48079. (Illus.). xv, 573p. (C). 50.00 (*0-393-97620-3*, Norton Paperbks) Norton.

Psychological Risks of Coronary Bypass Surgery. June B. Pimm & Joseph R. Feist. 1984. 226p. 59.50 (*0-306-41586-0*, Plenum Trade) Perseus Pubng.

Psychological Services for Law Enforcement. Theodore H. Blau. 1994. LC 93-28411. 464p. 200.00 (*0-471-55950-4*) Wiley.

Psychological Studies. Theodor Lipps. 2nd ed. 1974. LC 73-2972. (Classics in Psychology Ser.). reprint ed. 23.95 (*0-405-05145-X*) Ayer.

Psychological Studies on Religious Man. T. Kallstad. 1978. 252p. pap. text 47.50 (*91-554-0801-X*) Coronet Bks.

Psychological Study of Immigrant Children at Ellis Island. Bertha M. Boody. 1970. LC 79-129391. (American Immigration Collection. Series 2). reprint ed. 17.95 (*0-405-00546-6*) Ayer.

Psychological Symptoms. Frank J. Bruno. 1994. LC 92-28510. 288p. pap. 27.95 (*0-471-01610-1*) Wiley.

Psychological Techniques for Teachers. Don C. Locke & Joseph C. Ciechalski. 2nd ed. 1995. LC 95-10447. 286p. 69.95 (*1-56032-388-4*); pap. 34.95 (*1-56032-389-2*) Accel Devel.

Psychological Territories. Andrea F. Litkei. 1992. 176p. 14.95 (*1-880165-00-7*) Hanlit Pubns.

Psychological Testing: An Introduction. George Domino. 1999. LC 99-19524. 657p. (C). 97.00 (*0-13-020143-X*) P-H.

Psychological Testing: History, Principles, & Applications. Robert J. Gregory. 1992. 768p. (C). text 32.95 (*0-205-13264-2*); 3rd ed. 1999. LC 99-25926. 697p. 99.00 (*0-205-30479-6*) Allyn.

Psychological Testing: Principles, Applications, & Issues. Robert M. Kaplan & Dennis P. Saccuzzo. (Psychology Ser.). (C). 1982. LC 81-38461. 1150p. mass mkt. 34.00 (*0-8185-0494-3*); 2nd ed. 1988. LC 88-18755. 618p. mass mkt. 52.25 (*0-534-09516-X*); 4th ed. 1996. LC 96-16325. 736p. mass mkt. 95.95 (*0-534-26364-X*) Brooks-Cole.

Psychological Testing: Theory & Applications. Louis H. Janda. 1997. LC 97-33720. 455p. (C). 94.00 (*0-205-19434-6*) Allyn.

Psychological Testing & Assessment. Lewis R. Aiken. 10th ed. 1999. LC 99-13723. 501p. (C). 99.00 (*0-205-29567-3*) Allyn.

Psychological Testing & Assessment: An Introduction to Tests & Measurement. Ronald J. Cohen et al. 4th ed. 1998. LC 98-20417. xxvii, 769p. (C). text 71.95 (*0-7674-0509-9*, 0509-9) Mayfield Pub.

***Psychological Testing & Assessment: An Introduction to Tests & Measurement.** Ronald Jay Cohen & Mark E. Swerdlik. 5th ed. 2001. LC 2001-41015. (Illus.). xx, 667p. (*0-7674-2157-4*) McGraw.

***Psychological Testing at Work: How to Use, Interpret & Get the Most Out of the Newest Tests in Personality, Learning Style, Aptitudes, Interests & More!** Edward Hoffman. 2001. 224p. pap. 16.95 (*0-07-136079-4*) McGraw-Hill Prof.

Psychological Testing of Children from Early Childhood through Adolescence: A Psychodynamic Approach. Miriam G. Siegel. 1987. 530p. 77.50 (*0-8236-5615-2*) Intl Univs Pr.

Psychological Testing, Theory, & Applications: Instructor's Manual with Test Bank, with Test Bank. Louis Janda. 1997. 128p. (C). text, tchr. ed. (*0-205-28142-7*, T8142-6) Allyn.

Psychological Tests & Testing: Index of New Information with Authors, Subjects & Bibliography. Rosalie F. Zoltano. rev. ed. 1994. 179p. 57.50 (*0-7883-0180-2*); LC 94-34893. 57.50 (*0-7883-0252-3*); pap. 47.50 (*0-7883-0181-0*); LC 94-34893. pap. 47.50 (*0-7883-0253-1*) ABBE Pubs Assn.

Psychological Theories from a Structuralist Point of View. Ed. by H. Westmeyer. 1989. (Recent Research in Psychology Ser.). (Illus.). 213p. 56.95 (*0-387-51904-1*) Spr-Verlag.

Psychological Theories of Drinking & Alcoholism. Ed. by Howard T. Blane & Kenneth E. Leonard. 1986. LC 86-18472. (Guilford Alcohol & Drug Abuse Ser.). 403p. text 47.50 (*0-89862-166-6*) Guilford Pubns.

Psychological Theories of Human Learning. Guy R. Lefrancois. 2nd ed. 1982. LC 81-15511. (Psychology Ser.). 348p. (C). 39.95 (*0-8185-0501-X*) Brooks-Cole.

Psychological Theories of Learning. Guy R. Lefrancois. 3rd rev. ed. 1994. LC 94-30411. (Psychology Ser.). (Illus.). 380p. pap. 54.75 (*0-534-23202-7*) Brooks-Cole.

Psychological Theories of Learning & Teaching: An Analysis of the Use of the Psychology. David C. Payne. Ed. by Don Y. Lee. 1988. LC 87-82508. 270p. (C). 43.50 (*0-939758-18-0*) Eastern Pr.

Psychological Time & Mental Illness. Matthew Edlund. 1987. LC 85-20577. 137p. text 29.95 (*0-89876-122-0*) Gardner Pr.

Psychological Tools: A Sociocultural Approach to Education. Alex Kozulin. 1998. LC 98-23168. (Illus.). 192p. 36.50 (*0-674-72141-1*) HUP.

Psychological Transactions & Other Posthumous Tracts, 1734-1744. Emanuel Swedenborg. Ed. & Pref. by Alfred Acton. 2nd ed. 1984. 282p. reprint ed. 14.95 (*0-915221-62-4*) Swedenborg Sci Assn.

Psychological Trauma. Bessel A. Van der Kolk. 1986. LC 86-14149. 237p. text 34.00 (*0-88048-233-8*, 8233) Am Psychiatric.

Psychological Trauma. Ed. by Rachel Yehuda. 1998. LC 98-10614. (Review of Psychiatry Ser.). 206p. pap. text 29.00 (*0-88048-837-9*, 8837) Am Psychiatric.

Psychological Trauma & the Adult Survivor: Theory, Therapy, & Transformation. I. Lisa McCann & Laurie A. Pearlman. 1990. LC 90-2336. (Psychosocial Stress Ser.: No. 21). 320p. text 43.95 (*0-87630-594-X*) Brunner-Routledge.

Psychological Treatment of Cancer Patients: A Cognitive-Behavioral Approach. William L. Golden et al. 1991. (Psychology Practitioner Guidebooks Ser.). 188p. text (*0-08-037909-5*); pap. text (*0-08-037908-7*) PPI GBR. *Dist:* Elsevier.

Psychological Treatment of Depression: A Guide to the Theory & Practice of Cognitive Behaviour Therapy. J. Mark Williams. 2nd ed. 1993. LC 92-49155. pap. (*0-415-06744-8*) Routledge.

Psychological Treatment of Depression: A Guide to Theory & Practice of Cognitive Behavior. J. Mark & G. Williams. 2nd ed. 1995. LC 94-44552. 312p. (C). pap. 26.95 (*0-415-12874-9*, A7433) Routledge.

Psychological Treatment of Mental Illness. Ed. by R. J. Daly & E. A. Sand. 1987. (Illus.). 155p. 79.95 (*0-387-17596-2*) Spr-Verlag.

Psychological Treatment of Older Adults: An Introductory Text. Ed. by Michel Hersen & Vincent B. Van Hasselt. 1996. LC 96-25547. (Adult Development & Aging Ser.). (Illus.). 333p. (C). 47.00 (*0-306-45234-0*, Kluwer Plenum) Kluwer Academic.

Psychological Treatment of Panic. David H. Barlow & Jerome A. Cerny. 1988. LC 87-19682. (Treatment Manuals for Practitioners Ser.). 227p. pap. 23.00 (*0-89862-507-6*, 2507); text 45.00 (*0-89862-203-4*) Guilford Pubns.

Psychological Type: An Introduction. Alan W. Brownsword. 1988. 46p. (Orig.). (C). pap. text 8.00 (*0-944393-01-2*) Baytree Pubn.

Psychological Types & the Seven Rays, Vol. 1. Kurt B. Abraham. 1983. LC 82-81863. 163p. (Orig.). pap. 15.00 (*0-9609002-0-9*) Lampus Pr.

Psychological View of the Legal System. Linda A. Foley. 1992. 400p. (C). text 40.50 net. (*0-697-12982-9*) Brown & Benchmark.

Psychological Vulnerability to Chronic Pain. Ed. by Roy C. Grzesiak & Donald Ciccone. 1994. LC 94-6565. 248p. 38.95 (*0-8261-8070-1*) Springer Pub.

Psychological Warfare. Paul M. Linebarger. 1977. LC 72-4671. (International Propaganda & Communications Ser.). (Illus.). 318p. reprint ed. 27.95 (*0-405-04755-X*) Ayer.

Psychological Warfare & Propaganda: Irgun Documentation. Ed. by Eli Tavin & Yonah Alexander. 1982. LC 81-52469. 265p. (C). pap. 17.95 (*0-8420-2189-2*); lib. bdg. 45.00 (*0-8420-2188-4*) Scholarly Res Inc.

Psychological Work & Human Performance: Case Book. Robert D. Smithers. 2nd ed. 1997. (C). pap., stu. ed. 24.00 (*0-06-502060-X*) Addson-Wesley Educ.

Psychological Writings & Letters of Freud. Sigmund Freud. Ed. by Sander L. Gilman. 1995. LC 93-47191. (German Library). 324p. (C). text 39.50 (*0-8264-0722-6*) Continuum.

Psychologiche Perspektiven des Bluthochdrucks. W. Linden. 1983. (Illus.). vii, 132p. 58.50 (*3-8055-3642-9*) S Karger.

Psychologie. Jean Piaget. 1987. (FRE.). lib. bdg. 165.00 (*0-7859-3854-0*) Fr & Eur.

Psychologie des Experiences Religieuses see Psychological Dynamics of Religious Experience

Psychologie Genetique et Didactique des Sciences. Ed. by Andre Giordan et al. 2nd ed. 1997. (Exploration Ser.). (FRE., Illus.). 322p. (*3-906759-34-2*) P Lang CHE. *Dist:* P Lang Pubng.

Psychologie-Lexikon. Uwe Tewes. 1992. (GER.). 428p. 75.00 (*0-7859-8399-6*, 3486209477) Fr & Eur.

Psychologie Sociale: Une Discipline en Mouvement. Denise Jodelet. 1970. (Textes de Sciences Sociales Ser.: No. 3). pap. (*90-279-6309-6*) Mouton.

Psychologie Sociale et Experimentation. Gerard Lemaine & Jean-Marie Lemaine. 1969. (Textes de Sciences Sociales Ser.: No. 2). pap. (*90-279-6308-8*) Mouton.

Psychologie Sociale Theorique et Experimentale. Claude Faucheux. 1971. (Recueil de Textes Choisis & Presentes Textes de Sciences Sociales Ser.: No. 8). pap. (*90-279-6920-5*) Mouton.

Psychologisches Woerterbuch. Friedrich Dorsch. 9th ed. 1976. (GER.). 784p. 95.00 (*0-8288-5752-0*, M7595) Fr & Eur.

Psychologisches Woerterbuch. Dorsch. 11th ed. 1992. (GER.). 921p. 135.00 (*0-7859-7546-2*, 3456816146) Fr & Eur.

Psychologism & Psychoaesthetics: A Historical & Critical View of Their Relations. John Fizer. 1981. (Linguistic & Literary Studies in Eastern Europe: Vol. 6). xvi, 278p. 65.00 (*90-272-1506-5*) J Benjamins Pubng Co.

Psychologist As Expert Witness. Theodore H. Blau. 2nd ed. 1998. LC 98-2523. 596p. 160.00 (*0-471-17870-5*) Wiley.

***Psychologist as Expert Witness.** Theodore H. Blau. 2nd ed. 2001. 608p. pap. 55.00 (*0-471-11366-2*) Wiley.

Psychologist at Work. Mary R. Harrower. 1977. LC 71-102243. (Select Bibliographies Reprint Ser.). 28.95 (*0-8369-5128-X*) Ayer.

Psychologist of Sorts: The Autobiography & Publications of the Inventor of the Porteus Maze Tests. Stanley D. Porteus. 1969. LC 68-31287. (Illus.). x, 325p. 27.95 (*0-87015-174-6*) Pacific Bks.

Psychologist Trainee. Jack Rudman. 1994. (Career Examination Ser.: C-2621). pap. 29.95 (*0-8373-2621-4*) Nat Learn.

Psychologist's Book of Personality Tests: 24 Revealing Tests to Identify & Overcome Your Personal... Louis Janda. 2000. LC 00-43397. 224p. pap. 12.95 (*0-471-37102-5*) Wiley.

Psychologist's Companion: A Guide to Scientific Writing for Students & Researchers. Robert J. Sternberg. 3rd ed. 1993. 234p. (C). text 49.95 (*0-521-45123-X*) Cambridge U Pr.

Psychologists' Desk Reference. Gerald P. Koocher et al. 1998. LC 98-5781. (Illus.). 648p. text 65.00 (*0-19-511186-9*) OUP.

Psychologist's Guide to an Academic Career. Harriet L. Rheingold. 1994. LC 94-532. 203p. pap. text 19.95 (*1-55798-227-9*) Am Psychol.

Psychologist's Imagination & the Fantastic World of Imagery: A Handbook of Psycho-Imagination Therapy. Joseph E. Shorr. 1998. LC 98-23084. 240p. pap. 22.50 (*1-56474-285-7*) Fithian Pr.

Psychologists' Neuropsychotropic Drug Reference. Louis A. Pagliaro. 1999. LC 98-32463. xxvii, 456p. 64.95 (*0-87630-956-2*) Brunner-Routledge.

Psychologists on the March: Science, Practice, & Professional Identity in America, 1929-1969. James H. Capshew. 1999. LC 97-47526. (Cambridge Studies in the History of Psychology). 288p. (C). text 59.95 (*0-521-56267-8*); pap. text 21.95 (*0-521-56585-5*) Cambridge U Pr.

Psychologist's Proactive Guide to Managed Mental Health Care. Ed. by Alan J. Kent & Michel Hersen. 2000. LC 99-16478. (Illus.). viii, 171p. (*0-8058-2910-5*) L Erlbaum Assocs.

Psychologist's Proactve Guide to Managed Mental Health Care. Ed. by Alan J. Kent & Michel Hensen. 2000. LC 99-16478. 171p. 19.95 (*0-8058-3488-5*) L Erlbaum Assocs.

Psychology. 2000. 496p. tchr. ed. (*0-205-31816-9*) Allyn.

***Psychology.** Lewis M. Barker. 2001. stu. ed., suppl. ed. 22.67 (*0-13-094603-6*) P-H.

Psychology. Don Baucum. 1996. LC 95-43647. (Barron's EZ-101 Study Keys Ser.). pap. 6.95 (*0-8120-9580-4*) Barron.

Psychology Douglas A. Bernstein. (C). Date not set. (*0-395-78965-6*); 1993. pap., tchr. ed. 6.76 (*0-395-69046-3*); 1993. pap., tchr. ed., suppl. ed. 6.76 (*0-395-69047-1*) HM.

Psychology Lynne A. Bond et al. Ed. by Arthur W. Biddle. 2000. LC 86-82608. (Writer's Guide Ser.). 222p. (C). pap. text 24.36 (*0-669-12004-9*) HM Trade Div.

Psychology. Center for Learning Network Staff. 1998. (Social Studies). 268p. (gr. 9-12). tchr. ed., spiral bd. 37.95 (*1-56077-547-5*) Ctr Learning.

Psychology. Stephen F. Davis & Joseph J. Palladino. 1994. (Illus.). 700p. (C). text 47.00 (*0-02-327851-X*, Macmillan Coll) P-H.

Psychology. Ed. by Stephen Everson. 1991. (Companions to Ancient Thought Ser.: No. 2). 277p. (C). text 80.00 (*0-521-35338-6*); pap. text 28.95 (*0-521-35861-2*) Cambridge U Pr.

Psychology. Saul M. Kassin. (C). Date not set. pap., stu. ed. 20.36 (*0-395-72053-2*); 1994. LC 94-76518. text 65.96 (*0-395-52681-7*) HM.

Psychology. Kelley. 2000. pap. text 11.97 net. (*0-395-97204-3*) HM.

Psychology. Laird. 1992. (C). pap. 59.56 (*0-395-63342-7*) HM.

Psychology. Donald A. Laird. (C). 1992. pap. text, tchr. ed., suppl. ed. 5.96 (*0-395-59233-X*); 1991. pap. text, stu. ed. 21.16 (*0-395-59231-3*) HM.

Psychology. James D. Laird & Nicholas S. Thompson. 1991. (C). text 65.96 (*0-395-47090-0*) HM.

Psychology. Olf. 1994. pap. text 34.00 (*0-443-05274-3*) Saunders.

Psychology. Rubin. Date not set. (C). pap. 59.16 (*0-395-65554-4*) HM.

Psychology. Z. Rubin. 1992. (C). text 65.96 (*0-395-60550-4*) HM.

Psychology. Jack Rudman. (Graduate Record Examination Ser.: Vol. 17). 47.95 (*0-8373-5267-3*); (Undergraduate Program Field Tests Ser.: Vol. 21). 43.95 (*0-8373-6071-4*); 1994. (National Teacher Examination Ser.: Vol. NT-42). pap. 23.95 (*0-8373-8452-4*); 1994. (Undergraduate Program Field Tests Ser.: Vol. UPFT-21). pap. 23.95 (*0-8373-6021-8*) Nat Learn.

Psychology. Schultz & Hailstorks. 1995. pap. text, stu. ed. 27.00 (*0-205-17418-3*) Allyn.

Psychology. Smith. Date not set. pap. text, tchr. ed. (*0-314-02076-4*) West Pub.

Psychology. Smith & Philip G. Zimbardo. 1994. pap., tchr. ed. 11.00 (*0-06-502354-4*) Addson-Wesley Educ.

Psychology. Camille B. Wortman. 1987. 51.50 (*0-394-36537-2*) Knopf.

Psychology. Aristotle. 1976. LC 75-13253. (History of Ideas in Ancient Greece Ser.). (ENG & GRE.). reprint ed. 30.95 (*0-405-07290-2*) Ayer.

Psychology. 2nd ed. 2000. (C). 22.20 (*0-8087-1494-5*) Pearson Custom.

Psychology. Henry Gleitman. 2nd ed. Date not set. (C). pap., tchr. ed. (*0-393-95534-6*) Norton.

Psychology. Don H. Hockenbury & Sandra E. Hockenbury. 2nd ed. 1999. LC 99-15582. text 69.95 (*1-57259-423-3*) W H Freeman.

Psychology. Kassin. 2nd ed. 1998. pap. text, stu. ed. 20.00 (*0-13-884388-0*) P-H.

Psychology. K. Martin. 2nd ed. 1997. (Illus.). 256p. pap. text (*0-7506-3472-3*) Buttrwrth-Heinemann.

Psychology. Margaret W. Matlin. 2nd ed. 1994. (C). pap. text, stu. ed. 26.50 (*0-15-502108-7*) Harcourt Coll Pubs.

Psychology. Christopher Peterson. 2nd ed. 1997. 400p. (C). pap. text, stu. ed. 26.00 (*0-673-52546-5*) Addison-Wesley.

Psychology. Wayne Weiten. 2nd ed. 1993. (Psychology Ser.). pap. 47.50 (*0-534-19977-1*) Brooks-Cole.

Psychology. 3rd ed. 2000. (C). text (*0-13-025953-5*) P-H.

Psychology. Robert Baron & Bruce Earhard. 3rd ed. 2000. 398p. pap. 26.60 (*0-205-30745-0*) P-H.

Psychology. Ludy T. Benjamin, Jr. et al. 3rd ed. 1993. LC 93-5036. 880p. (C). text 52.00 (*0-02-308290-9*, Macmillan Coll) P-H.

Psychology Douglas A. Bernstein. 3rd ed. 1993. LC 93-78678. (C). text 65.96 (*0-395-64955-2*) HM.

Psychology. Stephen F. Davis. 3rd ed. 1999. LC 99-21562. 807p. 62.00 (*0-13-932583-2*) P-H.

Psychology. Saul Kassin. 3rd ed. 2000. LC 00-38541. (Illus.). 848p. stu. ed. 90.00 (*0-13-026926-3*) P-H.

Psychology. Matlin. 3rd ed. 1998. (C). pap. text, tchr. ed. 26.75 (*0-15-508401-1*); pap. text, stu. ed. 32.50 (*0-15-508400-3*) Harcourt Coll Pubs.

Psychology. Margaret W. Matlin. 3rd ed. 1998. LC 98-71493. 800p. (C). text 96.95 (*0-15-505495-3*) Wadsworth Pub.

Psychology. David G. Myers. 3rd ed. 1991. LC 91-72014. 636p. (gr. 11-12). text 65.95 (*0-87901-506-3*, 2319) Worth.

Psychology. Sdorow. 3rd ed. 1995. pap. 30.62 (*0-697-15064-X*) McGraw.

Psychology. Lester M. Sdorow. 3rd ed. (C). 1995. text, stu. ed. 15.62 (*0-697-26756-3*); 1995. text, stu. ed. 15.62 (*0-697-26758-X*); 1994. 792p. (gr. 10-12). text 38.50 net. (*0-697-15062-3*) Brown & Benchmark.

Psychology. Carole Wade & Carol Tavris. 3rd ed. 1997. (C). pap., stu. ed. 29.00 (*0-06-500519-8*) Addson-Wesley Educ.

Psychology. Wayne Weiten & Wasden. 3rd ed. 1994. (Psychology Ser.). mass mkt., stu. ed. 18.75 (*0-534-24668-0*) Brooks-Cole.

Psychology. WGBH Educational Foundation Staff. 3rd ed. 1994. (C). pap. text, stu. ed. 31.00 (*0-15-502092-7*) Harcourt Coll Pubs.

Psychology. Baron & Kalsher. 4th ed. 1997. pap. text, stu. ed. 19.00 (*0-205-27290-8*) P-H.

Psychology. Bentley. 4th ed. 1992. 320p. (C). pap. text, stu. ed., wbk. ed. 18.80 (*0-13-735176-3*) P-H.

Psychology. Henry Gleitman. 4th ed. Date not set. (C). text 50.00 incl. 5.25 hd (*0-393-96690-9*); text 52.00 incl. mac hd (*0-393-96778-6*); pap. (*0-393-96950-9*); pap. (*0-393-96951-7*); pap. (*0-393-96952-5*); pap. (*0-393-96953-3*) Norton.

Psychology. Gray. 4th ed. 2001. pap. text, stu. ed. 18.00 (*0-7167-5163-1*) Worth.

Psychology. Peter Gray. 4th ed. 2001. LC 2001-26103. text 63.00 (*0-7167-5162-3*) Worth.

Psychology. Spencer A. Rathus. 4th ed. 1990. 768p. (C). text 76.00 (*0-03-034597-9*) Harcourt Coll Pubs.

Psychology. Henry L. Roediger, III et al. 4th ed. 1997. LC 95-43775. 750p. (C). spiral bd. 90.95 (*0-314-06160-6*) Thomson Learn.

Psychology. Santrock. 4th rev. ed. 1994. 22.50 (*0-697-22460-0*) McGraw.

Psychology. John P. Dworetzky. Ed. by Clyde Perlee. 5th ed. 1994. LC 93-41549. 650p. (C). text 60.00 (*0-314-02478-6*) West Pub.

Psychology. Alan J. Fridlund et al. 5th ed. 1999. LC 98-29515. 848p. text 61.00 (*0-393-97364-6*) Norton.

Psychology. Lester M. Sdorow & Cheryl A. Rickabaugh. 5th ed. 2000. LC 2001-31481. (Illus.). 50.00 (*0-07-235832-7*) McGraw.

Psychology. Camille B. Wortman et al. 5th ed. 1998. LC 98-14650. (*0-07-115869-3*) McGraw.

Psychology. Camille B. Wortman et al. 5th ed. 1998. LC 98-14650. 768p. text 83.75 (*0-07-071931-4*) McGrw-H Hghr Educ.

Psychology. John M. Darley et al. 5th enl. rev. ed. 1990. 752p. (C). text 66.00 (*0-13-734377-9*, 670106) P-H.

Psychology. 6th ed. 2000. (C). (*0-13-018521-3*); (*0-13-018522-1*); (*0-13-018523-X*); (*0-13-088012-4*); (*0-13-028799-7*); text (*0-13-026422-9*) P-H.

Psychology. 6th ed. 2000. (C). text (*0-321-05979-4*) S&S Trade.

Psychology. Myers. 6th ed. 2001. pap. text, stu. ed. 16.50 (*0-7167-5147-X*); 2000. pap. text, stu. ed. 19.95 (*1-57259-958-8*) Worth.

Psychology. Spencer A. Rathus. 6th ed. 1995. LC 94-79633. (C). text 81.00 (*0-15-501699-7*) Harcourt Coll Pubs.

Psychology. Benjamin B. Lahey. 7th ed. 2000. 768p. (C). pap. 65.00 incl. cd-rom (*0-07-240731-X*) McGrw-H Hghr Educ.

Psychology. Bishop. 9th ed. 1996. pap. text, stu. ed. 21.00 (*0-13-443243-6*) P-H.

Psychology. Brent D. Slife. 9th ed. 1996. tchr. ed. 1.56 (*0-697-31397-2*, WCB McGr Hill) McGrw-H Hghr Educ.

P
Q
R

Psychology. 10th ed. 1999. 752p. 53.97 (*0-13-436104-0*); 1998. (C). (*0-13-095703-8*, Macmillan Coll) P-H.

Psychology. Duffy. 24th ed. 1994. 12.74 net. (*1-56134-286-6*) McGraw.

Psychology. Duffy. 25th ed. 1995. (*1-56134-368-4*, Dshkn McG-Hill) McGrw-H Hghr Educ.

Psychology: A Behavioral Overview. A. Poling et al. 1989. (Applied Clinical Psychology Ser.). (Illus.). 412p. (C). 45.00 (*0-306-43432-6*, Plenum Trade) Perseus Pubng.

Psychology: A Biopsychosocial Approach. Chris Peterson. 2nd ed. 1997. LC 96-24666. 779p. (C). 84.00 (*0-673-52414-0*) Addison-Wesley.

Psychology: A Connectext. Terry F. Pettijohn. 4th ed. 1998. 250p. (C). pap., stu. ed. 39.69 (*0-07-292904-9*) McGrw-H Hghr Educ.

Psychology: A Contemporary Introduction. Peter Scott & Christopher Spencer. 1998. LC 97-16961. (Illus.). 736p. (C). pap. 50.95 (*0-631-19235-2*); 98.95 (*0-631-19234-4*) Blackwell Pubs.

*__Psychology: A Journey.__ Dennis Coon. 2001. 608p. pap. text 52.95 (*0-534-56888-2*) Wadsworth Pub.

Psychology: A Very Short Introduction. 2000. 160p. 8.95 (*0-19-285381-3*) OUP.

Psychology: An Elementary Text-Book. Hermann Ebbinghaus. Ed. & Tr. by Max Meyer. 1977. LC 73-2965. (Classics in Psychology Ser.). reprint ed. 19.95 (*0-405-05138-7*) Ayer.

Psychology: An Evolutionary Approach. A. Gaulin. 2000. LC 00-20213. (Illus.). 416p. pap. 43.00 (*0-13-759994-3*) P-H.

Psychology: An Integrated Approach. Eysenck. 1998. 829p. pap. 64.00 (*0-582-29884-9*) Longman.

Psychology: An Introduction. Lahey. 5th ed. 1994. 86.87 (*0-697-22875-4*, WCB McGr Hill) McGrw-H Hghr Educ.

Psychology: An Introduction. Benjamin B. Lahey. 6th ed. 1997. LC 96-78737. 752p. (C). text 43.00 net. (*0-697-25310-4*, WCB McGr Hill) McGrw-H Hghr Educ.

Psychology: An Introduction. Lahey & Schneider. 7th ed. 2000. 329p. (C). pap., stu. ed. 24.06 (*0-697-36246-9*) McGrw-H Hghr Educ.

Psychology: An Introduction. Kagan. 8th ed. 1994. (C). pap. text, tchr. ed. 44.50 (*0-15-502508-2*) Harcourt Coll Pubs.

Psychology: An Introduction. Jerome Kagan & Julius Segal. 8th ed. 1994. LC 94-35276. 771p. (C). pap. text 25.95 (*0-15-501476-5*) Harcourt.

Psychology: An Introduction. Kagan. 9th ed. 2001. (C). pap. text 22.50 (*0-15-508114-4*) Harcourt Coll Pubs.

Psychology: An Introduction, Study Guide. Benjamin B. Lahey. 5th ed. 1994. 400p. (C). text, stu. ed. 18.75 (*0-697-14521-2*) Brown & Benchmark.

Psychology: An Introduction - Test Bank. Kagan. 8th ed. 1995. (C). pap. text, tchr. ed., suppl. ed. 44.50 (*0-15-502509-0*) Harcourt Coll Pubs.

Psychology: An Introduction - Text Index File, No. 2. Lahey. 5th ed. 1995. 20.62 (*0-697-26612-5*, WCB McGr Hill) McGrw-H Hghr Educ.

Psychology: An Introduction S-Cart. Morris. 10th ed. 1999. 63.00 (*0-13-020663-6*) P-H.

Psychology: An Introduction with Student Study Guide. Lahey. 5th ed. 1994. 59.74 net. (*0-697-23285-9*) McGraw.

Psychology: An Introductory Bibliography. Salem Press Staff. Ed. by Susan E. Beers. 1996. LC 95-48933. (Magill Bibliographies Ser.). 440p. 55.00 (*0-8108-3119-8*) Scarecrow.

Psychology: Another View. Harold F. Sorensen. 1990. LC 88-62824. 240p. (C). text 18.00 (*0-9622100-0-5*) Pawprint Pr.

Psychology: Briefer Course. William James. 1985. (Works of William James). (Illus.). 512p. 50.00 (*0-674-72102-0*) HUP.

Psychology: Coast Telecourse. Carole Wade & Carol Tavris. 3rd ed. 1997. (C). pap., stu. ed. 24.33 (*0-06-501642-4*) Addison-Wesley Educ.

Psychology: Contexts & Applications. Jane S. Halonen & John W. Santrock. 3rd ed. 1998. LC 98-15014. 736p. pap. 65.94 (*0-697-37648-6*, WCB McGr Hill) McGrw-H Hghr Educ.

Psychology: Contexts & Applications. Jane S. Halonen & Steven A. Schneider. 3rd ed. 1998. 364p. (C). pap., stu. ed. 28.13 (*0-697-37667-2*, WCB McGr Hill) McGrw-H Hghr Educ.

Psychology: Contexts of Behavior. Halonen & Santrock. 2nd ed. 1995. tchr. ed. 17.81 (*0-697-14910-2*) McGraw.

Psychology: Instructor's Resources. Peter Gray. 2nd ed. 1994. tchr. ed., ring bd. (*0-87901-696-5*) Worth.

Psychology: Introduction. Josh R. Gerow. 4th ed. 1995. LC 94-16489. (C). (gr. 7-12). text 40.75 (*0-673-46869-0*) HarperCollins Pubs.

Psychology: Learning & Behavior: Test Item File. Schwartz. 4th ed. 1995. pap. text, tchr. ed. (*0-393-96662-3*) Norton.

Psychology: Mind, Brain & Culture. Drew Westen. 2nd ed. 1998. LC 97-51291. (Illus.). 1024p. 82.95 (*0-471-24049-4*) Wiley.

Psychology: Mind, Brain & Culture. Drew Westen. 3rd ed. 2001. LC 2001-33245. 800p. 83.95 (*0-471-38754-1*) Wiley.

Psychology: Perspective Readings. Carol Tavis & Carole Wade. 1995. (C). text 15.00 (*0-06-502529-6*) Addson-Wesley Educ.

Psychology: Principles & Applications. Stephen Worchel & Wayne J. Shebilski. 5th ed. 1995. LC 94-31006. 715p. 99.00 (*0-13-556474-3*) P-H.

Psychology: Realizing Human Potential. Rene V. Dawis & Rosemary T. Fruehling. 8th ed. 1994. LC 94-20886. text 34.95 (*1-56118-341-5*, 01131) Paradigm MN.

Psychology: Science & Application. Mark G. McGee & David W. Wilson. 1984. (Illus.). 666p. (C). text 60.00 (*0-314-77927-2*) West Pub.

Psychology: Science & Understanding. Barry D. Smith. 1998. LC 97-25300. 832p. (C). text 83.75 (*0-07-058652-7*) McGrw-H Hghr Educ.

Psychology: Science, Behavior. Stephen J. Ettinger. 3rd ed. 1994. (C). pap. text, tchr. ed. 35.00 (*0-15-501358-0*) Harcourt Coll Pubs.

Psychology: Science, Behavior - TB. Stephen J. Ettinger. 3rd ed. 1994. (C). pap. text, tchr. ed., suppl. ed. 44.50 (*0-15-501360-2*) Harcourt Coll Pubs.

Psychology: Science, Behavior & Life. Robert L. Crooks et al. 3rd ed. 1993. LC 92-75742. (Illus.). 750p. (C). text 91.50 (*0-15-500998-2*) Harcourt Coll Pubs.

Psychology: Study Guide. Gleitman & Reisberg. 5th ed. 1999. pap. text, stu. ed. 16.00 (*0-393-97366-2*) Norton.

Psychology: Study Guide: Canadian Edition. Baron. 3rd ed. 2000. pap. 20.00 (*0-205-32290-5*) Allyn.

Psychology: Telecourse Study Guide. Spencer A. Rathus. 6th ed. 1995. (C). pap. text, stu. ed. 28.50 (*0-15-503654-8*) Harcourt Coll Pubs.

Psychology: Test Bank. Margaret W. Matlin. 2nd ed. 1994. (C). pap. text 44.50 (*0-15-502109-5*) Harcourt Coll Pubs.

Psychology: The Adaptive Mind. James S. Nairne. 1996. LC 96-28954. (Psychology Ser.). 659p. (C). mass mkt. 52.50 (*0-534-20682-4*) Brooks-Cole.

Psychology: The Adaptive Mind. Narine. 1996. (Psychology Ser.). pap., stu. ed. 17.25 (*0-534-33853-4*) Brooks-Cole.

Psychology: The Brain, the Person, & the World. 2000. 784p. (C). (*0-205-32436-3*) Allyn.

Psychology: The Briefer Course. William James. Ed. by Gordon W. Allport. 1985. LC 84-40821. (Notre Dame Series in the Great Bks.). 360p. (C). reprint ed. pap. text 15.00 (*0-268-01557-0*) U of Notre Dame Pr.

Psychology: The Essential Science. Robert A. Baron. 1989. 630p. 48.00 (*0-205-11432-6*, H14327) Allyn.

Psychology: The Hope of a Science. Gregory A. Kimble. 1995. LC 95-21458. (Illus.). 176p. 29.95 (*0-262-11204-3*, Bradford Bks) MIT Pr.

Psychology: The Science of Behavior. Neil R. Carlson. 3rd ed. 1989. 800p. text 48.00 (*0-205-12166-7*, H21660) Allyn.

Psychology: The Science of Behavior. Neil H. Carlson & William Buskist. 5th ed. 1996. LC 96-3411. 683p. 91.00 (*0-205-19345-5*) Allyn.

Psychology: The Science of Behaviour European Adaptation. Neil R. Carlson. 2000. 744p. (*0-13-021228-8*) P-H.

Psychology: The Science of Mental Life. George A. Miller. 3rd ed. 1998. LC 98-12443. (Illus.). 388p. reprint ed. pap. text 29.95 (*0-937431-06-0*) Adams Bannister Cox.

Psychology: The Science of Mind & Behavior. John W. Santrock. 4th rev. ed. 1995. 326p. (C). pap. text (*0-697-20890-7*) Brown & Benchmark.

Psychology: The Science of Mind & Behaviour: Study Guide. Richard D. Gross & Paul Humphreys. 2nd ed. 1993. (Illus.). 192p. pap. (*0-340-58736-9*, B2218) E A GBR. *Dist:* Routldge.

Psychology: Themes & Variation Brief. Wayne Weiten. 3rd ed. 1996. (Psychology Ser.). (C). mass mkt., stu. ed. 17.75 (*0-534-34187-X*); stu. ed. 17.00 (*0-534-34193-4*); stu. ed. 17.00 (*0-534-34194-2*); stu. ed. 17.00 (*0-534-34195-0*) Brooks-Cole.

Psychology: Themes & Variations. Wayne Weiten. 1989. LC 88-26207. 697p. (C). mass mkt. 45.50 (*0-534-08760-4*) Brooks-Cole.

Psychology: Themes & Variations. Richard B. Stalling & Wayne Weiten. 2nd ed. 1993. (Psychology Ser.). mass mkt. 18.00 (*0-534-19969-0*) Brooks-Cole.

Psychology: Themes & Variations. Wayne Weiten. 2nd ed. 1991. LC 91-6752. 752p. (C). pap., stu. ed. 17.95 (*0-534-15331-3*); 2nd ed. 1991. LC 91-6752. 752p. (C). text 53.95 (*0-534-15330-5*); 3rd ed. 1996. LC 96-6003. 564p. (C). pap. 41.00 (*0-534-33926-3*); 3rd ed. 1994. LC 94-30585. 784p. text 54.50 (*0-534-24666-4*) Brooks-Cole.

Psychology: Themes & Variations. Wayne Weiten. 3rd ed. 1996. pap. 74.95 (*0-534-34653-7*) Thomson Learn.

Psychology: Themes & Variations. Wayne Weiten. 3rd ed. text 47.00 net. (*0-534-33730-9*) Wadsworth Pub.

Psychology: Themes & Variations. Wayne Weiten & Wasden. 3rd exp. ed. 1995. (Psychology Ser.). stu. ed. 18.50 (*0-534-24670-2*) Brooks-Cole.

Psychology: Themes & Variations. Wayne Weiten. 4th ed. 1997. LC 97-26784. (Psychology Ser.). 809p. pap. 79.95 (*0-534-34014-8*) Brooks-Cole.

Psychology: Themes & Variations, Briefer Version. Wayne Weiten. 2nd ed. 1993. LC 93-19857. mass mkt. 40.25 (*0-534-19968-2*) Brooks-Cole.

*__Psychology: Themes & Variations, Briefer Version.__ Wayne Weiten. 5th ed. 2001. 640p. pap. 56.95 (*0-534-59319-4*) Duxbury.

Psychology: Themes & Variations, Briefer Version (Paperbound) Wayne Weiten. 4th ed. 1999. LC 98-32260. (Psychology Ser.). 640p. pap. text 58.95 (*0-534-36379-2*) Brooks-Cole.

Psychology: Themes & Various brief Cases with Infotrac. Wayne Weiten. 3rd ed. 1998. (Psychology Ser.). 48.50 (*0-534-36371-7*) Brooks-Cole.

Psychology: Theoretical-Historical Perspectives. Ed. by Robert W. Rieber & Kurt D. Salzinger. 2nd rev. ed. 1998. LC 98-28447. 509p. 49.95 (*1-55798-524-3*) Am Psychol.

Psychology: Theory & Application. Phillip Banyard & Nicky Hayes. 1995. (Illus.). 576p. (Orig.). (YA). (gr. 13 up). pap. 34.95 (*0-412-46440-3*) Chapman & Hall.

Psychology & Adult Learning. Mark Tennant. 1990. 186p. (C). pap. 19.95 (*0-415-05032-4*, A4563) Routledge.

Psychology & AIDS. Ed. by Thomas E. Backer et al. 1988. (Special Issue, American Psychologist Ser.: Vol. 43, No. 11). 156p. pap. 16.00 (*1-55798-053-5*) Am Psychol.

Psychology & A.I.D.S. Index of Modern Information. Roth Polinski. 1990. LC 88-47613. 150p. 47.50 (*1-55914-232-4*); pap. 44.50 (*1-55914-233-2*) ABBE Pubs Assn.

Psychology & American Law. Curt R. Bartol. 1983. 373p. (C). mass mkt. 44.00 (*0-534-01217-5*) Brooks-Cole.

Psychology & Cognitive Therapy of the Neuroses. Hans Lungwitz. Ed. by Reinhold Becker. Tr. by Norman Maclean from GER. rev. ed. 1993. LC 93-17037.Tr. of Systematik der Neurosen. (Illus.). 200p. 48.50 (*0-8176-2866-5*) Birkhauser.

Psychology & Communication in Deaf Children. R. D. Savage et al. 1981. 304p. text 47.00 (*0-8089-1339-5*, 793798, Grune & Strat) Harcrt Hlth Sci Grp.

Psychology & Community Change: Challenges of the Future. Kenneth Heller et al. 2nd rev. ed. 1989. 421p. (C). mass mkt. 40.00 (*0-534-10561-0*) Brooks-Cole.

Psychology & Crime: An Introduction to Criminological Psychology. Clive R. Hollin. 1989. 240p. 49.95 (*0-415-01806-4*, A3249); 288p. (C). pap. 27.95 (*0-415-01807-2*, A3253) Routledge.

Psychology & Education: The State of the Union. Ed. by Frank Farley & Neal J. Gordon. 1981. LC 80-82902. (National Society for the Study of Education Publication Ser.). 400p. (C). 40.00 (*0-8211-0506-X*) McCutchan.

Psychology & Education of the Gifted. Ed. by Walter B. Barbe & Joseph S. Renzulli. 3rd ed. 1981. LC 80-11174. 544p. pap. text 22.95 (*0-8290-0234-0*) Irvington.

Psychology & Family Law: A New Zealand Perspective. M. E. Pipe & Fred Seymour. 1997. LC 98-168648. 176p. pap. (*1-877133-22-1*) Univ Otago Pr NZL. *Dist:* Intl Spec Bk.

Psychology & General Sociology Reviews: Future Prospects for Population Phenogenetics, Vol. 4. V. M. Zakharov. Ed. by E. T. Turpaev & A. V. Yaslokov. 1989. (Soviet Scientific Reviews Ser.: Vol. 4, Pt. 3). iv, 84p. text 92.00 (*3-7186-5012-6*) Gordon & Breach.

Psychology & General Sociology Reviews: Neuronal Basis of Associative Learning; Neuronal Mechanisms of Short-Term Memory, Vol. 4. V. M. Storozhuk & A. S. Batuev. Ed. by E. T. Turpaev & A. V. Yaslokov. 1990. (Soviet Scientific Reviews Ser.: Vol. 4, Pt. 4). 188p. pap. text 89.00 (*3-7186-5013-4*) Gordon & Breach.

Psychology & General Sociology Reviews: The Problems of Higher Nervous Activity, Vol. 4. P. V. Simonov. Ed. by E. T. Turpaev & A. V. Yaslokov. 1990. (Soviet Scientific Reviews Ser.: Vol. 4, Pt. 5). iv, 108p. text 123.00 (*3-7186-5014-2*) Gordon & Breach.

Psychology & Gynaecological Problems. Annabel K. Broome & Louise Wallace. 1984. 320p. (Orig.). pap. (*0-422-78590-3*, 9251) Tavistock GBR. *Dist:* Routldge.

Psychology & Health. Donald A. Bakal. 2nd ed. 1992. LC 91-5241. Orig. Title: Psychology & Medicine, 1979. 256p. (C). text 36.95 (*0-8261-7900-2*) Springer Pub.

Psychology & Health: Index of Modern Information with Bibliography. Manfred J. Robineault. 1990. LC 89-78054. 150p. 47.50 (*1-55914-228-6*); pap. 44.50 (*1-55914-229-4*) ABBE Pubs Assn.

Psychology & Health Promotion. P. Bennett. 1997. LC 97-9042. pap. (*0-335-19765-5*) OpUniv Pr.

Psychology & Health Promotion. Paul Bennett & Simon Murphy. 1997. LC 97-9042. (*0-335-19766-3*) OpUniv Pr.

Psychology & Its Allied Disciplines. Ed. by Marc H. Bornstein. 1984. (Cross Currents in Contemporary Psychology Bornstein Ser.). 992p. (C). lib. bdg. 145.00 (*0-89859-318-2*);Set. pap. 79.95 (*0-89859-319-0*) L Erlbaum Assocs.

Psychology & Its Allied Disciplines Vol. 1: Psychology & the Humanities. Ed. by Marc H. Bornstein. 1984. 352p. 34.50 (*0-89859-320-4*) L Erlbaum Assocs.

Psychology & Its Allied Disciplines Vol. 2: Psychology & the Social Sciences. Ed. by Marc H. Bornstein. 1984. 304p. pap. 32.50 (*0-89859-321-2*) L Erlbaum Assocs.

Psychology & Its Practice: Index of Modern Information. Althea Y. Peltier. 1990. LC 89-78057. 150p. 47.50 (*1-55914-202-2*); pap. 44.50 (*1-55914-203-0*) ABBE Pubs Assn.

Psychology & Law: A Critical Introduction. Andreas Kapardis. 1997. (Illus.). 395p. (C). text 85.00 (*0-521-55321-0*); LC 96-40439. pap. text 29.95 (*0-521-55738-0*) Cambridge U Pr.

Psychology & Law: International Perspectives. Ed. by Freidrich Losel et al. 1992. LC 92-30454. xxviii, 557p. lib. bdg. 144.65 (*3-11-013725-9*) De Gruyter.

Psychology & Law: Research & Application. Curt R. Bartol & Anne M. Bartol. 2nd ed. 1993. LC 93-39459. mass mkt. 48.00 (*0-534-16320-3*) Brooks-Cole.

Psychology & Law for the Helping Professions. Leland C. Swenson. 2nd ed. 1996. LC 96-9241. (Counseling Ser.). 456p. (C). spiral bd. 80.95 (*0-534-34285-X*) Brooks-Cole.

Psychology & Life: With SuperSite & MindMatters CD-ROM. Philip G. Zimbardo. 15th ed. 1998. LC 98-34502. 848p. (C). text 88.00 incl. cd-rom (*0-321-01650-5*) Allyn.

Psychology & Life Study Guide. Philip G. Zimbardo. 15th ed. 1999. (C). pap. text, stu. ed. 22.50 (*0-321-03505-4*) Addson-Wesley Educ.

Psychology & Life Telecourse Study Guide. Philip G. Zimbardo. 15th ed. 1998. 352p. (C). pap. text, stu. ed. 26.00 (*0-321-03517-8*) Addson-Wesley Educ.

Psychology & Medical Research of Self Concepts: Index of New Information & Research Bible. Bakus G. Francis. 1994. 160p. 57.50 (*0-7883-0212-4*); 1994. 160p. pap. 47.50 (*0-7883-0213-2*); 1996. LC 96-3123. 159p. 57.50 (*0-7883-1036-4*); 1996. LC 96-3123. 159p. pap. 47.50 (*0-7883-1037-2*) ABBE Pubs Assn.

Psychology & Medicine, 1979 see Psychology & Health

Psychology & Mental Health, Set. Ed. by Jaclyn Rodriguez. 2000. LC 00-46312. (Magill's Choice Ser.). (Illus.). xx, 729p. 95.00 (*0-89356-066-9*, Magills Choice) Salem Pr.

Psychology & Mental Health of Afro-American Women: A Selected Bibliography. Ed. by Glenell S. Young & Janet Sims-Wood. 1984. LC 83-51604. (Resources on Afro-American Women Ser.: No. 1). 102p. pap. 6.95 (*0-915549-00-X*) Afro Res Inc.

Psychology & Military Proficiency. Charles W. Bray. 1969. LC 69-13837. 242p. reprint ed. lib. bdg. 59.75 (*0-8371-1444-6*, BRMI, Greenwood Pr) Greenwood.

Psychology & Modern Problems. Ed. by James A. Hadfield. 1977. LC 72-10844. (Essay Index Reprint Ser.). reprint ed. 22.95 (*0-8369-7220-1*) Ayer.

Psychology & Nihilism: A Genealogical Critique of the Computational Model of Mind. Fred J. Evans. 1992. LC 91-42019. (SUNY Series in the Philosophy of the Social Sciences). 303p. (C). text 20.50 (*0-7914-1249-0*) State U NY Pr.

Psychology & Performing Arts. Ed. by Glenn D. Wilson. 1991. 324p. (*90-265-1119-1*) Swets.

Psychology & Personal Growth. Abe Arkoff. 3rd ed. 1987. text 36.00 (*0-205-10533-5*, H05333) Allyn.

Psychology & Physiology of Breathing: In Behavioral Medicine, Clinical Psychology, & Psychiatry. R. Fried. 1993. LC 93-512. (Behavioral Psychophysiology & Medicine Ser.). (Illus.). 398p. (C). 54.50 (*0-306-44278-7*, Plenum Trade) Perseus Pubng.

Psychology & Policing. Ed. by Neil Brewer & Carlene Wilson. 1995. LC 95-1425. 504p. text 89.95 (*0-8058-1418-3*) L Erlbaum Assocs.

Psychology & Postmodernism. Steiner Kvale. 1992. (Inquiries in Social Construction Ser.). (Illus.). (C). 340p. 74.50 (*0-8039-8603-3*, 9413); 240p. pap. 26.50 (*0-8039-8604-1*, 9414) Sage.

Psychology & Practice. Andrew B. Crider et al. 4th ed. 1997. LC 92-30213. (C). pap. text 93.00 (*0-673-46835-6*) Addson-Wesley Educ.

Psychology & Productivity. Ed. by P. Whitney & R. B. Ochsman. 1989. (Illus.). 212p. 75.00 (*0-306-42937-3*, Plenum Trade) Perseus Pubng.

Psychology & Professional Practice: The Interface of Psychology & the Law. Ed. by Francis R. Fields & Rudy J. Horwitz. 1982. LC 81-19899. (Illus.). 210p. 62.95 (*0-89930-015-4*, FIH/, Quorum Bks) Greenwood.

Psychology & Promotion of Health. Ed. by Jean-Pierre Dauwalder. 1994. LC 93-46517. (Swiss Monographs in Psychology: Vol. 2). (Illus.). 250p. pap. text 36.00 (*0-88937-089-3*) Hogrefe & Huber Pubs.

Psychology & Psychiatry Serials: A Bibliographic Aid for Collection Development. Ed. by Dorothy M. Persson & Michael F. Winter. 1990. LC 90-39559. (Behavioral & Social Sciences Librarian Ser.: Vol. 9, No. 2). 121p. text 39.95 (*1-56024-048-2*) Haworth Pr.

Psychology & Psychological Principles, 8. James Ward. 1977. LC 77-72191. (Contributions to the History of Psychology Ser.: Vol. 8, Pt. A, Orientations). 504p. lib. bdg. 99.75 (*0-313-26932-7*, U6932, Greenwood Pr) Greenwood.

Psychology & Psychology Study Guide, 2 bks. Baron. 4th ed. 1997. text, stu. ed. 77.00 net. (*0-205-28706-9*) A&B Bks.

Psychology & Psychotherapy of Otto Rank: An Historical & Comparative Introduction. Fay B. Karpf. 1970. LC 70-90539. 132p. reprint ed. lib. bdg. 58.00 (*0-8371-3029-8*, KAOR, Greenwood Pr) Greenwood.

Psychology & Public Policy: Balancing Public Service & Professional Need. Ed. by Raymond P. Lorion et al. 1996. LC 95-26810. 417p. pap. text 19.95 (*1-55798-347-X*, 431-6700) Am Psychol.

Psychology & Religion: Eight Points of View. Andrew R. Fuller. 2nd ed. 1986. 286p. pap. text 28.50 (*0-8191-5336-2*) U Pr of Amer.

Psychology & Sexual Orientation: Coming to Terms. Janis S. Bohan. 1996. LC 96-2187. 256p. (C). pap. 22.95 (*0-415-91514-7*); 2nd ed. 70.00 (*0-415-91513-9*) Routledge.

Psychology & Social Issues: A Tutorial Text. Ed. by Raymond Cochrane & Douglas Carroll. 1991. (Contemporary Psychology Ser.). 224p. 79.95 (*1-85000-835-3*); pap. 29.95 (*1-85000-836-1*) Taylor & Francis (Falmer Pr).

Psychology & the Critical Revolution. Anton G. Hardy. 1988. 145p. 18.50 (*0-9615267-0-X*) James Pubns NY.

Psychology & the East. Carl Gustav Jung. Ed. by G. Adler. Tr. by R. F. C. Hull. 1978. LC 77-92815. (Bollingen Ser.: Vol. 438). (Illus.). 232p. pap. 14.95 (*0-691-01806-5*) Princeton U Pr.

Psychology & the Legal System. Lawrence S. Wrightsman. 2nd ed. 1990. LC 90-41445. 464p. (C). mass mkt. 48.50 (*0-534-14634-1*) Brooks-Cole.

Psychology & the Legal System. Lawrence S. Wrightsman & Michael T. Nietzel. 4th ed. 1997. LC 97-19080. (Psychology Ser.). 590p. spiral bd. 77.95 (*0-534-34085-7*) Brooks-Cole.

Psychology & the Legal System. Lawrence S. Wrightsman. 5th ed. 2001. LC 2001-26526. (Illus.). 608p. 74.95 (*0-534-36544-2*) Duxbury.

Psychology & the Notes: A Visual Companion. 6th ed. 1999. (C). pap., stu. ed. 68.13 (*0-07-240001-3*) McGrw-H Hghr Educ.

Psychology & the Occult. Carl Gustav Jung. Ed. by G. Adler. Tr. by R. F. C. Hull. 1978. LC 75-34810. (Bollingen Ser.). (Illus.). 177p. pap. 13.95 (*0-691-01791-3*) Princeton U Pr.

Psychology & the Poetics of Growth: Figurative Language in Psychology, Psychotherapy, & Education. Howard R. Pollio et al. 1977. 272p. text 49.95 (*0-89859-484-7*) L Erlbaum Assocs.

Psychology & the Teacher. Dennis Child. 5th ed. 1993. (Education Ser.). 416p. pap. 39.95 (*0-304-32649-6*) Continuum.

Psychology & Treatment of Addictive Behavior, No. 8. Ed. by Scott Dowling. 1995. (Workshop Series of the American Psychoanalytic Association: Monograph 8). 207p. 35.00 (*0-8236-5562-8*) Intl Univs Pr.

Psychology & Work: Productivity, Change, & Employment. Ed. by Michael S. Pallak & Robert Perloff. 1986. LC 86-7952. (Master Lectures: Vol. 5). 220p. (Orig.). pap. 24.95 (*0-912704-48-9*) Am Psychol.

Psychology & You. Frank B. McMahon et al. 2nd ed. 1994. LC 93-41159. (gr. 10-12). mass mkt. 47.25 (*0-314-02772-6*) West Pub.

Psychology Applied to Life & Work. Harry W. Hepner. 6th ed. 1979. LC 78-11923. (Illus.). text 54.00 (*0-13-732461-8*) P-H.

Psychology Applied to Modern Life: Adjustment at the Turn of the Century. Wayne Weiten & Margaret A. Lloyd. 6th ed. 1999. LC 99-24198. (Counseling Ser.). 624p. text 85.95 (*0-534-35553-6*) Brooks-Cole.

Psychology Applied to Modern Life: Adjustment in the 80's. Wayne Weiten. 2nd ed. 1985. LC 85-11645. (Psychology Ser.). 566p. (C). pap. 14.75 (*0-534-05413-7*); pap. 37.75 (*0-534-05412-9*) Brooks-Cole.

Psychology Applied to Modern Life: Adjustment in the 90s. Margaret A. Lloyd et al. 3rd ed. 1990. 500p. (C). pap. 46.00 (*0-534-09708-1*) Brooks-Cole.

Psychology Applied to Modern Life: Adjustment in the 90s. Wayne Weiten & Sosulski. 3rd ed. 1990. (Counseling Ser.). pap. text, stu. ed. 18.00 (*0-534-09709-X*) Brooks-Cole.

Psychology Applied to Modern Life: Adjustment in the 90s. Wayne Weiten. 4th ed. 1993. (Counseling Ser.). pap., stu. ed. 17.00 (*0-534-19892-9*) Wadsworth Pub.

Psychology Applied to Modern Life: Adjustment in the 90s. Wayne Weiten & Margaret A. Lloyd. 4th ed. 1993. LC 93-19884. (Illus.). 607p. pap. 50.00 (*0-534-19890-2*) Brooks-Cole.

Psychology Applied to Modern Life: Adjustment in the 90s. Wayne Weiten et al. 4th ed. 1993. (Counseling-Psychology Ser.). pap. text, tchr. ed. (*0-534-19893-7*) Brooks-Cole.

Psychology Applied to Modern Life: Adjustment in the '90s. Wayne Weiten & Margaret A. Lloyd. 5th ed. 1996. (C). pap., tchr. ed. (*0-534-34358-9*) Brooks-Cole.

Psychology Applied to Modern Life: Adjustment in the 90's. Wayne Weiten & Margaret A. Lloyd. 5th ed. 1996. LC 96-34649. (Psychology). 630p. (C). pap. 50.25 (*0-534-33938-7*) Brooks-Cole.

Psychology Applied to Modern Life: Adjustment in the 90s, Personal Explorations Workbook. Wayne Weiten & Margaret A. Lloyd. 5th ed. 1996. pap., wbk. ed. 2.00 (*0-534-34359-7*) Brooks-Cole.

Psychology Applied to Modern Life: Adjustment in the '90s, Test Items. Wayne Weiten & Margaret A. Lloyd. 5th ed. 1996. pap. 2.56 (*0-534-34360-0*) Brooks-Cole.

Psychology Applied to Teaching. Robert F. Biehler & Jack Snowman. (C). 5th ed. 1985. LC 85-60849. 752p. 47.96 (*0-395-40820-2*); 5th ed. 1985. LC 85-60849. 752p. 47.96 (*0-395-40822-9*); 5th ed. 1985. LC 85-60849. 752p. 47.96 (*0-395-40821-0*); 6th ed. 1990. pap. text 9.96 (*0-395-53286-8*); 6th ed. 1990. 80.36 (*0-395-52906-9*); 6th ed. 1989. pap. text 2.76 (*0-395-52634-5*); 6th ed. 1989. pap. text 3.16 (*0-395-52636-1*) HM.

Psychology Applied to Work. Paul M. Muchinsky. 2nd ed. 1989. 602p. (C). mass mkt. 38.50 (*0-534-10729-X*) Brooks-Cole.

Psychology Applied to Work. Muchinsky. 6th ed. 1999. (Psychology Ser.). mass mkt., wbk. ed. 14.00 (*0-534-36254-0*) Brooks-Cole.

Psychology Applied to Work: An Introduction to Industrial & Organizational Psychology. Paul M. Muchinsky. (C). 3rd ed. 1990. 650p. mass mkt. 50.00 (*0-534-13032-1*); 5th ed. 1996. LC 96-20143. 538p. pap. 53.25 (*0-534-33876-3*) Brooks-Cole.

Psychology Applied to Work: Student Exercise Book. Paul M. Muchinsky. 5th ed. 1996. (Psychology Ser.). mass mkt., wbk. ed. 18.00 (*0-534-34237-X*) Brooks-Cole.

Psychology Applied to Work: Student Workbook. Paul M. Muchunsky. 4th ed. 1993. (Psychology Ser.). pap., wbk. ed. 19.95 (*0-534-16623-7*) Brooks-Cole.

Psychology As a Profession: Foundations of Practice. Walter B. Pryzwansky & Robert N. Wendt. 1987. (Psychology Practitioner Guidebooks). 170p. text 32.50 (*0-08-033129-7*); pap. text 16.95 (*0-08-033128-9*) Elsevier (Pergamon Pr).

Psychology As Applied to Nursing. Andrew McGhie. 8th ed. 1986. LC 83-7753. (Illus.). 329p. pap. text (*0-443-02836-2*) Church.

Psychology Assistant I. Jack Rudman. 1994. (Career Examination Ser.: C-919). pap. 29.95 (*0-8373-0919-0*) Nat Learn.

Psychology Assistant III. Jack Rudman. 1994. (Career Examination Ser.: C-922). pap. 34.95 (*0-8373-0922-0*) Nat Learn.

Psychology Assistant II. Jack Rudman. 1994. (Career Examination Ser.: C-921). pap. 34.95 (*0-8373-0921-2*) Nat Learn.

Psychology Astray: Fallacies in Studies of "Repressed Memory" & Childhood Trauma. Harrison G. Pope, Jr. 1997. LC 97-9022. 140p. pap. 12.95 (*0-89777-149-4*, 070397, Upton Bks) SIRS Pubng.

Psychology at Iowa: Centennial Essays. Ed. by J. H. Cantor. 1991. 176p. (C). text 39.95 (*0-8058-0761-6*) L Erlbaum Assocs.

Psychology at Work. Ed. by Paul S. Achilles. 1977. LC 74-156602. (Essay Index Reprint Ser.). reprint ed. 22.95 (*0-8369-2262-X*) Ayer.

Psychology at Work. Peter E. Warr. 4th ed. 1996. 480p. pap. (*0-14-024648-7*) Pnguin Bks Ltd GBR. *Dist:* Trafalgar.

Psychology at Work: An Introduction to Industrial & Organizational Psychology. Lilly M. Berry. 2nd ed. 1997. LC 97-13527. 592p. text 77.50 (*0-697-20173-2*, WCB McGr Hill) McGrw-H Hghr Educ.

Psychology Aweigh! A History of Clinical Psychology in the United States Navy, 1900-1988. Frederick L. McGuire. 1990. LC 90-279. 249p. 19.95 (*1-55798-086-1*) Am Psychol.

Psychology Boundries & Froniters. William Buskist & David Gerbing. 1989. LC 93-22902. (C). reprint ed. pap. 83.44 (*0-673-38023-8*) Addson-Wesley Educ.

Psychology Brief. 2000. (C). pap., stu. ed. 20.31 (*0-07-240378-0*) McGrw-H Hghr Educ.

***Psychology CATs 2 & 3, 1999: Review Questions with Answers.** Maren Rawlings. 2001. 240p. pap. text 12.95 (*0-521-65916-7*) Cambridge U Pr.

Psychology Experimenter. Microteac Staff. 1986. (C). 340.00 (*0-15-572674-9*) Harcourt Coll Pubs.

Psychology Exposed or, the Emperor's New Clothes. Paul Kline. 1988. 208p. text 45.00 (*0-415-00643-0*); pap. text 13.95 (*0-415-00644-9*) Routledge.

***Psychology for Christian Ministry.** Fraser Watts et al. 2001. LC 2001-34798. 224p. (C). (gr. 13). lib. bdg. 80.00 (*0-415-24036-0*) Routledge.

Psychology for Living: Adjustment, Growth, & Behavior Today. Eastwood Atwater & Karen G. Duffy. 6th ed. 1998. LC 98-15321. 507p. (C). pap. text 70.00 (*0-13-958778-0*) P-H.

Psychology for Medicine. 310p. pap. (*0-7131-4543-9*) E A GBR. *Dist:* Routldge.

Psychology for Nurses & the Caring Professions. Sheila Payne & Janet Walker. 1995. LC 95-14761. (Social Science for Nurses & the Caring Professions Ser.). 192p. (*0-335-19411-7*); 240p. pap. (*0-335-19410-9*) OpUniv Pr.

Psychology for Parents & Teachers. Mark F. Sohn. 2nd ed. 1991. 13.00 (*0-9616911-7-4*) M F Sohn Pubns.

Psychology for Teaching: A Bear Will Not Commit Himself Just Now. Guy R. Lefrancois. 7th ed. 1990. 448p. (C). pap. 45.95 (*0-534-14412-8*) Wadsworth Pub.

***Psychology for the Christian Ministry.** Fraser Watts et al. 2001. LC 2001-34798. 224p. (Orig.). (C). (gr. 13). pap. 24.95 (*0-415-24037-9*) Routledge.

Psychology from an Empirical Standpoint. Franz Brentano. Tr. by Linda L. McAlister et al. 1995. LC 95-7729. (International Library of Philosophy, Psychology, & Scientific Method). 448p. (C). pap. 29.95 (*0-415-10661-3*, B4322) Routledge.

Psychology, Humanism, & Scientific Inquiry: The Selected Essays of Hadley Cantril. Ed. by Albert H. Cantril. 1988. 288p. text 44.95 (*0-88738-176-6*) Transaction Pubs.

Psychology I. 2000. (Super Reviews Ser.). 144p. pap. 8.95 (*0-87891-089-1*) Res & Educ.

Psychology II. 2000. (Super Reviews Ser.). 144p. pap. 8.95 (*0-87891-090-5*) Res & Educ.

Psychology in a Physical World: Forty Years of Just Thinking About Science. Art Z. Orzeck. 1995. 108p. (Orig.). (C). pap. 21.50 (*0-8191-9799-8*) U Pr of Amer.

Psychology in Action. Ed. by David V. Canter. 1995. (Dartmouth Benchmark Ser.). (Illus.). 340p. text (*1-85521-365-6*) Dartmth Pub GBR. *Dist:* Ashgate Pub Co.

Psychology in Action. Karen Huffman et al. 4th ed. 1997. pap. 28.95 incl. cd-rom (*0-471-16773-8*); 1996. 636p. text 109.90 incl. cd-rom (*0-471-18961-8*) Wiley.

Psychology in Action, Chapter 17. Huffman. 5th ed. 1999. 40p. text 1.00 net. (*0-471-35902-5*) Wiley.

Psychology in Childbearing. Nora Tisdall. 1997. LC 97-200218. 54p. pap. text 24.99 (*1-898507-28-7*) Buttrwrth-Heinemann.

Psychology in Context: Voices & Perspectives. David N. Sattler & Virginia Shabatay. 1996. (C). text, tchr. ed. 11.96 (*0-395-83513-5*) HM.

Psychology in Foreign Language Teaching. Steven H. McDonough. 2nd ed. 1987. (Illus.). 192p. pap. text 16.95 (*0-04-418006-3*) Routledge.

Psychology in Industrial Organizations Norman R. Maier & Trudy G. Verser. 5th ed. 1982. LC 81-81702. (Illus.). 672p. (C). text 75.96 (*0-395-31740-1*) HM.

Psychology in International Perspective. Ed. by Uwe P. Gielen et al. 1992. LC 92-9057. xii, 340p. pap. (*90-265-1236-8*) Swets.

Psychology in New Millennium. Rathus. 7th ed. 1998. (C). pap. text, stu. ed. 28.00 (*0-15-508221-3*) Harcourt.

Psychology in Organizations: Integrating Science & Practice. Ed. by Kevin R. Murphy & Frank E. Saal. 1990. 304p. (C). text 75.00 (*0-8058-0477-3*) L Erlbaum Assocs.

Psychology in Practice with Young People, Families, & Schools. Ed. by Allan Sigston et al. 1996. LC 96-141650. 256p. pap. (*1-85346-390-6*) David Fulton GBR. *Dist:* Taylor & Francis.

Psychology in Prisons. David J. Cooke et al. 1993. LC 92-47425. pap. (*0-04-159414-2*); 160p. (C). pap. 24.99 (*0-415-09714-2*, B2537) Routledge.

Psychology in Questions & Answers. Hilarion Duerk. 2000. 256p. reprint ed. 20.75 (*0-9661325-5-6*) R A McCaffrey.

Psychology in Sports Performance: Applying Principles to Practice. Ed. by Richard Butler. 1997. LC 96-51509. 288p. pap. (*0-7506-2437-X*) E A GBR. *Dist:* OUP.

Psychology in Teaching, Learning & Growth. Don E. Hamachek. 5th ed. 1994. LC 94-6126. 640p. pap. text 86.00 (*0-205-15269-4*) Allyn.

Psychology in the Dental Office. Ann Ehrlich. 1983. (Illus.). 7.95 (*0-940012-15-4*) Colwell Syst.

Psychology in Utopia: Toward a Social History of Soviet Psychology. Alex Kozulin. 1984. 180p. 30.00 (*0-262-11087-3*) MIT Pr.

Psychology Is Social. Edward Krupat. 3rd ed. 1994. (C). text 32.81 (*0-673-46918-2*) Addson-Wesley Educ.

Psychology Law. Ed. by Horowitz. 2nd ed. 1997. (C). pap. text 50.00 (*0-673-46689-2*) Addison-Wesley.

Psychology, Law, & Eyewitness Testimony. Peter B. Ainsworth. 1999. LC 98-19886. (Psychology of Crime, Policing, & Law Ser.). 208p. pap. 49.95 (*0-471-98238-5*) Wiley.

Psychology Lectures & Study Guide. 4th ed. 2000. 312p. (C). 35.80 (*0-536-61346-X*) Pearson Custom.

Psychology, 1995. David G. Myers. 4th ed. 1994. 864p. pap. text, stu. ed. 16.95 (*0-87901-645-0*); LC 94-60649. text 67.95 (*0-87901-644-2*) Worth.

Psychology 1999-2000. Karen Duffy. 29th ed. 1998. (Annual Editions Ser.). (C). pap., stu. ed. 17.50 (*0-07-041372-X*) McGrw-H Hghr Educ.

Psychology 1996/97. Duffy. 26th annot. ed. 1996. tchr. ed. (*0-697-31677-7*, WCB McGr Hill) McGrw-H Hghr Educ.

Psychology of a Musical Prodigy. Geza Revesz. 1970. LC 78-100832. 180p. reprint ed. lib. bdg. 49.75 (*0-8371-4004-8*, REMP, Greenwood Pr) Greenwood.

Psychology of a Musical Prodigy. Geza Revesz. 1972. LC 77-173178. (Illus.). reprint ed. 22.95 (*0-405-08879-5*) Ayer.

Psychology of Abnormality. Peterson. 1995. (C). pap. text, tchr. ed. 35.00 (*0-15-503029-9*); pap. text, stu. ed. 29.50 (*0-15-503030-2*) Harcourt Coll Pubs.

Psychology of Abnormality. Christopher Peterson. 1995. LC 94-74222. 656p. (C). text 90.00 (*0-15-500092-6*) Harcourt Coll Pubs.

Psychology of Abnormality: Computerized Test Bank. Christopher Peterson. 1996. (C). disk 279.50 (*0-15-503034-5*) Harcourt Coll Pubs.

Psychology of Abnormality: Test Bank. Christopher Peterson. 1995. (C). pap. text 44.50 (*0-15-503031-0*) Harcourt.

Psychology of Adaptation to Absurdity: Tactics of Make-Believe. Seymour Fisher & Rhoda L. Fisher. 1993. 248p. text 59.95 (*0-8058-1205-9*) L Erlbaum Assocs.

Psychology of Addiction. Mary McMurran. 1994. LC 94-16356. (Contemporary Psychology Ser.). xiv, 182p. (*0-7484-0187-3*); pap. (*0-7484-0188-1*) Tay Francis Ltd GBR. *Dist:* Taylor & Francis.

Psychology of Adjustment & Human Relations. James F. Calhoun & Joan R. Acocella. 3rd ed. 1990. 512p. (C). text 71.56 (*0-07-557738-0*) McGrw-H Hghr Educ.

Psychology of Adjustment & Well-Being. Stanley L. Brodsky. 1988. 480p. (C). pap. text 67.00 (*0-03-013368-8*) Harcourt Coll Pubs.

Psychology of Adolescence. Marvin Powell. 2nd ed. 1971. 678p. text 13.15 (*0-672-60782-4*, Bobbs) Macmillan.

Psychology of Adolescence: Essential Readings. Ed. by Aaron H. Esman. 1975. LC 74-21177. 425p. (Orig.). 85.00 (*0-8236-5565-2*) Intl Univs Pr.

Psychology of Adolescent Satanism: A Guide for Parents, Counselors, Clergy, & Teachers. Anthony Moriarty. 1992. LC 92-12731. 168p. 39.95 (*0-275-94307-0*, C4307, Praeger Pubs) Greenwood.

Psychology of Aging: An Annotated Bibliography, 28. Ed. by Bert Hayslip et al. 1995. LC 95-6291. (Bibliographies & Indexes in Gerontology Ser.: No. 28). 152p. lib. bdg. 59.95 (*0-313-29376-7*, Greenwood Pr) Greenwood.

Psychology of Aging: An Introduction. Ian Stuart-Hamilton. 2nd ed. 1994. LC 93-39928. 27.00 (*1-85302-233-0*) Taylor & Francis.

Psychology of Aging: Theory, Research & Intervention. Janet K. Belsky. 2nd ed. 1989. (Psychology Ser.). 460p. (C). pap. 49.75 (*0-534-12114-4*) Brooks-Cole.

Psychology of Aging: Theory, Research, & Interventions. Belsky. 3rd ed. 1998. LC 98-17981. (Psychology Ser.). 655p. spiral bd. 81.95 (*0-534-35912-4*) Brooks-Cole.

Psychology of Aging: Theory, Research & Practice. Janet K. Belsky. 1984. LC 83-20923. (Psychology Ser.). 550p. (C). mass mkt. 32.25 (*0-534-02868-3*) Brooks-Cole.

Psychology of Alcoholism. George B. Cutten. Ed. by Gerald N. Grob. 1981. LC 80-1223. (Addiction in America Ser.). reprint ed. lib. bdg. 37.95 (*0-405-13579-3*) Ayer.

Psychology of Animal Learning. N. J. Mackintosh. 1974. text 125.00 (*0-12-464650-6*) Acad Pr.

Psychology of Anxiety. Eugene E. Levitt. 2nd ed. 1980. LC 80-107. 188p. text 29.95 (*0-89859-040-X*) L Erlbaum Assocs.

Psychology of Anxiety, Worry & Troublesome Problems: Index of New Information with Authors & Subjects. Frances B. Lopez. rev. ed. 1994. LC 94-24769. 157p. 57.50 (*0-7883-0370-8*); pap. 47.50 (*0-7883-0371-6*) ABBE Pubs Assn.

Psychology of Asthma Management. Hyland. 1998. (C). pap. text (*0-443-05682-X*) Church.

Psychology of Attempted Suicide: A Medical Subject Analysis with Reference Bibliography. Harold P. Drummond. rev. ed. 1992. 163p. (Orig.). 47.50 (*1-55914-952-3*); pap. 44.50 (*1-55914-953-1*) ABBE Pubs Assn.

Psychology of Attention. Harold E. Pashler. 1997. LC 96-29300. (Illus.). 510p. 49.50 (*0-262-16165-6*, Bradford Bks) MIT Pr.

Psychology of Attention. Elizabeth A. Styles. 1997. 304p. pap. 26.95 (*0-86377-465-2*) L Erlbaum Assocs.

Psychology of Attitude Change & Social Influence. Philip G. Zimbardo & Michael R. Leippe. 3rd ed. 1991. 288p. (C). pap. 38.13 (*0-07-072877-1*) McGrw-H Hghr Educ.

Psychology of Attitudes. Alice Eagly & Shelly Chaiken. Ed. by Dawn Youngblood. 1993. LC 92-52667. (Illus.). 800p. (C). text 100.00 (*0-15-500097-7*) Harcourt Coll Pubs.

Psychology of Back Pain: A Clinical & Legal Handbook. Albert M. Drukteinis. 1996. (American Behavioral Science & Law Ser.). (Illus.). 208p. (C). text 43.95 (*0-398-06559-4*); pap. text 28.95 (*0-398-06560-8*) C C Thomas.

Psychology of Behaviour at Work: The Individual in the Organization. Adrian Furnham. 1997. 500p. (*1-85728-668-5*); pap. (*1-85728-278-7*) UCL Pr Ltd GBR. *Dist:* Taylor & Francis.

Psychology of Birth. Leslie Feher. 1985. 224p. reprint ed. pap. text 27.00 (*0-9612182-1-5*) Assn Birth Psych.

Psychology of Body, Soul & Spirit. Rudolf Steiner. Tr. by Marjorie Spock et al from GER. 1999. LC 99-11939. (Illus.). 320p. pap. 24.95 (*0-88010-397-3*) Anthroposophic.

Psychology of C. G. Jung. Jolande Jacobi. Tr. by Ralph Manheim. 1973. (Illus.). (C). pap. 14.95 (*0-300-01674-3*, Y75) Yale U Pr.

Psychology of C. G. Jung: The Meaning & Significance of Dreams, Vol. II. Carl A. Meier. 1987. 163p. 40.00 (*0-938434-11-X*); pap. 16.95 (*0-938434-69-1*) Sigo Pr.

Psychology of C. G. Jung, Vol. III: Consciousness, Vol. III. Carl A. Meier. Tr. by David Roscoe from GER. 1989. (Illus.). 128p. (C). 40.00 (*0-938434-12-8*); pap. 16.95 (*0-938434-70-5*) Sigo Pr.

Psychology of Call-Reluctance: How to Overcome the Fear of Self-Promotion. George W. Dudley & Shannon L. Goodson. 1986. LC 85-73334. 208p. (Orig.). reprint ed. 26.95 (*0-935907-00-9*); pap. 18.95 (*0-935907-01-7*) Behavioral Sci.

Psychology of Carl Jung: Essays in Application & Deconstruction. David Holt. 1992. LC 92-5417. 536p. lib. bdg. 119.95 (*0-7734-9481-2*) E Mellen.

Psychology of Childbirth. Aidan MacFarlane. 1977. (Developing Child Ser.). (Illus.). 160p. pap. text 9.50 (*0-674-72106-3*) HUP.

Psychology of Childhood Illness. Christine Eiser. 1985. (Contributions to Psychology & Medicine Ser.). (Illus.). 212p. 87.95 (*0-387-96096-1*) Spr-Verlag.

Psychology of Chronic Illness: The Healing Work of Patients, Therapists, & Families. Robert Shuman. 1996. LC 96-10957. 288p. 35.00 (*0-465-09534-8*) Basic.

Psychology of Cognition. Gillian Cohen. 2nd ed. 1983. pap. text 44.95 (*0-12-178762-1*) Acad Pr.

Psychology of Computer Use. Ed. by Thomas Green et al. 1983. (Computers & People Ser.). text 67.00 (*0-12-297420-4*) Acad Pr.

Psychology of Consciousness. G. William Farthing, Jr. 1991. LC 91-7185. 480p. (C). text 47.20 (*0-13-728668-6*) P-H.

Psychology of Consciousness: An Intelligent Guide to Psychic Liberation. Charles Spaegel & Ruth E. Norman. 1985. (Illus.). 375p. (Orig.). (C). stu. ed., spiral bd. 90.00 (*0-932642-97-7*) Unarius Acad Sci.

Psychology of Cosmetic Treatments. Jean A. Graham & Albert M. Klingman. 1985. LC 84-26651. 272p. 82.50 (*0-275-91315-5*, C1315, Praeger Pubs) Greenwood.

Psychology of Couples & Illness: Theory, Research & Practice. Ed. by Karen B. Schmaling & Tamara Goldman Sher. 2000. LC 99-59782. xvi, 407p. 49.95 (*1-55798-649-5*) Am Psychol.

Psychology of Creativity. Margaret Gilchrist. 1972. (Second Century in Australian Education Ser.: Vol. 4). 102p. pap. 14.95 (*0-522-84024-8*) Intl Spec Bk.

Psychology of Criminal Conduct. D. A. Andrews & James Bonta. 2nd ed. 1998. LC 98-6867. 423p. (C). per. 39.95 (*0-87084-712-0*) Anderson Pub Co.

Psychology of Culture: A Course of Lectures. Edward Sapir. Ed. by Judith T. Irvine. 1993. LC 93-38287. (Illus.). x, 266p. (C). pap. text (*3-11-012920-5*) Mouton.

Psychology of Deafness: Senory Deprivation, Learning & Adjustment. Helmer R. Myklebust. 2nd ed. 1965. (Illus.). 436p. text 47.00 (*0-8089-0339-X*, 793027, Grune & Strat) Harcrt Hlth Sci Grp.

Psychology of Deafness: Understanding Deaf & Hard-of-Hearing People. McCay Vernon & Jean F. Andrews. 1990. 304p. (C). text 52.33 (*0-8013-0322-2*, 78090) Longman.

Psychology of Death. Robert J. Kastenbaum. 3rd ed. 2000. 320p. pap. (*1-85343-502-3*) Free Assoc Bks GBR. *Dist:* Intl Spec Bk.

Psychology of Death. Robert J. Kastenbaum. 2nd rev. ed. 1992. LC 91-33877. 280p. (C). text 36.95 (*0-8261-1922-0*); 3rd ed. 1999. LC 99-43555. (Illus.). 288p. text 36.95 (*0-8261-1300-1*) Springer Pub.

Psychology of Dementia. Edgar Miller & Robin Morris. 1994. LC 93-5046. (Clinical Psychology & Personality Ser.). 216p. 180.00 (*0-471-92776-7*) Wiley.

Psychology of Dental Care. G. Kent & Anthony S. Blinkhorn. 2nd rev. ed. 1991. (Dental Handbook Ser.). (Illus.). 176p. pap. text 45.00 (*0-7236-2339-2*) Buttrwrth-Heinemann.

Psychology of Difference: The American Lectures. Otto Rank. Ed. & Intro. by Robert Kramer. 1996. LC 95-43758. 416p. 57.50 (*0-691-04470-8*) Princeton U Pr.

Psychology of Disability. Toot. 1994. (*0-8151-8824-2*) Mosby Inc.

Psychology of Disability. Carolyn L. Vash. 1981. (Series on Rehabilitation: Vol. 1). 288p. (C). 39.95 (*0-8261-3340-1*) Springer Pub.

Psychology of Discipline: Six Approaches to Discipline. Darwin Dorr et al. 1981. LC 81-20775. xi, 253p. 40.00 (*0-8236-5581-4*) Intl Univs Pr.

Psychology of Dreams. Paul R. Robbins. 1988. LC 87-29889. (Illus.). 184p. lib. bdg. 29.95 (*0-89950-270-9*) McFarland & Co.

Psychology of Early Childhood up to the Sixth Year of Age. William L. Stern. 1979. LC 74-21428. (Classics in Child Development Ser.). (Illus.). 566p. reprint ed. 56.95 (*0-405-06477-2*) Ayer.

Psychology of Eating & Drinking. Alexandra W. Logue. 2nd ed. 1991. (Series of Books in Psychology). (Illus.). 352p. (C). pap. text 22.95 (*0-7167-2197-X*) W H Freeman.

Psychology of Educational Technology & Instructional Media. Ken Spencer. 1988. 208p. (C). lib. bdg. 45.00 (*0-415-00567-1*) Routledge.

Psychology of Emotion. John G. Carlson & Elaine Hatfield. 1992. LC 91-13622. (Illus.). 519p. (C). text 87.50 (*0-03-055419-5*) Harcourt Coll Pubs.

Psychology of Emotion: Theories of Emotion in Perspective. K. T. Strongman. 4th ed. 1996. LC 96-20324. 266p. pap. 80.00 (*0-471-96619-3*) Wiley.

Psychology of Emotions. C. E. Izard. 1991. (Emotions, Personality, & Psychotherapy Ser.). (Illus.). 472p. (C). 42.50 (*0-306-43865-8*, Plenum Trade) Perseus Pubng.

Psychology of Everyday Things. Donald A. Norman. 1930. LC 87-47782. (Illus.). 288p. 28.00 (*0-465-06709-3*) Basic.

Psychology of Existence: An Integrative, Clinical Perspective. Kirk J. Schneider & Rollo May. 1994. LC 94-19497. 416p. (C). text 60.63 (*0-07-041017-8*) McGrw-H Hghr Educ.

Psychology of Expertise: Cognitive Research & Empirical AI. Ed. by Robert R. Hoffman. 1994. 408p. text 79.95 (*0-8058-1900-2*) L Erlbaum Assocs.

Psychology of Facial Expression. Ed. by James A. Russell & Jose-Miguel Fernandez-Dols. 1997. LC 96-36250. (Studies in Emotion & Social Interaction). (Illus.). 415p. (C). text 90.00 (*0-521-49667-5*); pap. text 31.95 (*0-521-58796-4*) Cambridge U Pr.

Psychology of Gender. Ed. by Anne E. Beall & Robert J. Sternberg. 278p. 1995. pap. 22.00 (*0-89862-283-2*, 2283); 1993. LC 93-11508. 42.00 (*0-89862-286-7*) Guilford Pubns.

Psychology of Gender. Smith. 2000. (C). text 39.00 (*0-15-501995-3*) Harcourt Coll Pubs.

Psychology of Growing Old: Looking Forward. Robert Slater. 1995. LC 95-5368. (Rethinking Aging Ser.). 160p. (*0-335-19319-6*); pap. text (*0-335-19318-8*) OpUniv Pr.

Psychology of Health. Salovey. Date not set. (C). text (*0-395-79686-5*) HM.

Psychology of Health: An Introduction. Marian Pitts & Keith Phillips. 2nd ed. 1998. LC 97-40283. (Illus.). 432p. (C). 89.95 (*0-415-15023-X*); pap. 29.95 (*0-415-15024-8*) Routledge.

Psychology of Health: Application of Psychology for Health Professionals. Beth Alder. 1995. 208p. text 48.00 (*3-7186-5761-9*); 224p. pap. text 20.00 (*3-7186-5762-7*) Gordon & Breach (Harwood Acad Pubs).

Psychology of Human Behavior. Richard A. Kalish. 5th ed. 1983. LC 82-12851. (Psychology Ser.). (C). 144p. pap., stu. ed. 17.95 (*0-534-01220-5*); 465p. text 47.95 (*0-534-01219-1*) Brooks-Cole.

Psychology of Human Cognition: Mainstream & Genevan Traditions. Mary Howes. 1990. (General Psychology Ser.). 550p. text 55.00 (*0-08-035554-4*); pap. text 27.50 (*0-08-035553-6*) Elsevier (Pergamon Pr).

Psychology of Human-Computer Interaction. Stuart K. Card et al. 1983. 488p. (C). pap. 55.00 (*0-89859-859-1*) L Erlbaum Assocs.

Psychology of Human Control: A General Theory of Purposeful Behavior. Myles I. Friedman & George H. Lackey, Jr. 1991. LC 90-43301. 264p. 68.00 (*0-275-93811-5*, C3811, Praeger Pubs) Greenwood.

Psychology of Human Freedom. M. R. Westcott. 1988. (Illus.). 227p. 47.00 (*0-387-96809-1*) Spr-Verlag.

Psychology of Human Possibility & Constraint. Jack Martin & Jeff Sugarman. 1999. LC 98-21999. (SUNY Series, Alternatives in Psychology). (C). 192p. text 60.50 (*0-7914-4123-7*); 160p. pap. text 20.95 (*0-7914-4124-5*) State U NY Pr.

Psychology of Hypertension: Medical Analysis Index with Research Bibliography. Rosetta R. Hardine. rev. ed. 1994. 145p. LC 85-47583. 57.50 (*0-7883-0676-6*); pap. 47.50 (*0-7883-0677-4*) ABBE Pubs Assn.

Psychology of Illness: In Sickness & in Health. Richard G. Druss. 1995. LC 94-23688. 144p. text 23.50 (*0-88048-661-9*, 8661) Am Psychiatric.

Psychology of Illustration. Ed. by H. A. Houghton & D. M. Willows. 1987. (Instructional Issues Ser.: Vol. 2). (Illus.). 196p. 128.00 (*0-387-96453-3*) Spr-Verlag.

Psychology of Imagination. Jean-Paul Sartre. 1978. LC 78-6632. 282p. lib. bdg. 35.00 (*0-313-20498-5*, SAPI, Greenwood Pr) Greenwood.

Psychology of Interpersonal Behaviour. Michael Argyle. 1994. 368p. pap. (*0-14-017274-2*) Pnguin Bks Ltd GBR. *Dist:* Trafalgar.

Psychology of Intimacy. Karen J. Prager. LC 95-37284. (Guilford Series on Personal Relationships Ser.). 367p. 1997. pap. 25.00 (*1-57230-267-4*, C0267); 1995. 45.00 (*1-57230-006-X*, 0006) Guilford Pubns.

Psychology of Jealousy & Envy. Ed. by Peter Salovey. 1991. LC 90-23329. 293p. 42.00 (*0-89862-555-6*, 2555) Guilford Pubns.

Psychology of Juvenile Crime. Amy Lamson. 1982. 123p. 32.95 (*0-89885-060-6*); pap. 18.95 (*0-89885-290-0*) Kluwer Academic (Kluwer Acad Hman Sci).

Psychology of Language. David W. Carroll. 1985. LC 85-22393. (Psychology Ser.). 467p. (C). mass mkt. 44.00 (*0-534-05640-7*) Brooks-Cole.

Psychology of Language. Whitney. Date not set. (C). pap. 11.96 (*0-395-75751-7*) HM.

Psychology of Language. David W. Carroll. 2nd ed. 1993. LC 93-26969. pap. 45.75 (*0-534-21300-6*) Brooks-Cole.

Psychology of Language: An Introduction to Sentence & Discourse Processes. Ed. by Murray Singer. 1990. 320p. (C). text 29.95 (*0-8058-0005-0*) L Erlbaum Assocs.

Psychology of Language & Communication. Andrew W. Ellis & Geoffrey Beattie. 1993. LC 86-14828. 374p. pap. 23.95 (*0-89862-046-5*) Guilford Pubns.

Psychology of Learning. Edwin R. Guthrie. rev. ed. 1952. 18.75 (*0-8446-1213-8*) Peter Smith.

Psychology of Learning & Behavior. Barry Schwartz et al. 5th ed. 2001. LC 2001-30036. (C). 55.00 (*0-393-97591-6*, Norton Paperbks) Norton.

Psychology of Learning & Motivation. Ed. by Douglas L. Medin. (Illus.). Vol. 30. 1993. 328p. text 99.95 (*0-12-543330-1*); Vol. 31. 1994. 366p. text 99.95 (*0-12-543331-X*); Vol. 35. 1996. 337p. text 69.95 (*0-12-543335-2*) Acad Pr.

Psychology of Learning & Motivation, Vol. 38. Ed. by Douglas L. Medin. 1998. (Illus.). 306p. (C). 89.95 (*0-12-543338-7*) Acad Pr.

Psychology of Learning & Motivation Vol. 27: Advances in Research & Theory. Ed. by Gordon H. Bower. 1991. (Illus.). 349p. (C). text 99.95 (*0-12-543327-1*) Acad Pr.

Psychology of Learning & Motivation Vol. 28: Advances in Research & Theory. Ed. by Douglas L. Medin. 1992. (Illus.). 296p. text 99.95 (*0-12-543328-X*) Acad Pr.

Psychology of Learning & Motivation Vol. 34: Causal Learning. Ed. by Douglas L. Medin et al. 1996. (Illus.). 442p. text 74.95 (*0-12-543334-4*) Acad Pr.

Psychology of Learning & Motivation- Advances in Research & Theory: Categorization by Human & Machines, Vol. 29. Ed. by Doug L. Medin et al. 1993. (Illus.). 552p. text 99.95 (*0-12-543329-8*) Acad Pr.

Psychology of Learning Science. Ed. by Shawn M. Glynn et al. 1991. 280p. (C). text 49.95 (*0-8058-0668-7*) L Erlbaum Assocs.

Psychology of Left & Right. Michael C. Corballis & Ivan L. Beale. 1976. 240p. text 49.95 (*0-89859-114-7*) L Erlbaum Assocs.

Psychology of Man's Possible Evolution. P.D. Ouspensky. 2nd ed. 1973. 128p. pap. 8.00 (*0-394-71943-3*) Knopf.

Psychology of Mathematics for Instruction. Lauren B. Resnick & Wendy W. Ford. 1981. LC 80-29106. 288p. text 59.95 (*0-89859-029-9*) L Erlbaum Assocs.

Psychology of Medicine & Surgery. Peter Salmon. 2000. LC 99-59484. (Clinical Psychology & Personality Ser.). (Illus.). 328p. 75.00 (*0-471-97597-4*, Wiley Heyden) Wiley.

Psychology of Memory Ed. by Peter E. Morris & Martin E. Conway. 1993. LC 92-45221. (International Library of Critical Writings in Business History). (C). lib. bdg. 375.00 (*0-8147-5496-1*) NYU Pr.

Psychology of Men: Psychoanalytic Perspectives. Gerald I. Fogel. 1996. LC 95-62214. 310p. pap. 20.00 (*0-300-06620-1*) Yale U Pr.

Psychology of Mental Retardation. I. Biler & Manny Sternlicht. 1977. LC 77-4137. 800p. 39.95 (*0-88437-013-5*) Psych Dimensions.

Psychology of Mind-Body Healing: New Concepts of Therapeutic Hypnosis. Ernest L. Rossi. 2nd rev. ed. 1993. LC 93-23757. 304p. (C). 39.00 (*0-393-70168-9*) Norton.

Psychology of Motor Behavior. Ed. by Leonard Zaichkowsky & C. Zvi Fuchs. 1989. (Illus.). 300p. pap. 34.95 (*0-932392-24-5*) Mouvement Pubns.

Psychology of Music. James L. Mursell. 1991. lib. bdg. 45.00 (*0-403-01750-5*) Scholarly.

Psychology of Music. James L. Mursell. 1971. LC 77-110274. (Illus.). 389p. reprint ed. lib. bdg. 72.50 (*0-8371-4500-7*, MUPM, Greenwood Pr) Greenwood.

Psychology of Music. H. P. Rao. 1986. (Illus.). 80p. reprint ed. (*0-8364-1765-8*) Abhinav IND. *Dist:* S Asia.

Psychology of Music. Carl E. Seashore. 1967. 408p. reprint ed. pap. 10.95 (*0-486-21851-1*) Dover.

Psychology of Music. Diana Deutsch. 2nd ed. 1998. LC 98-85210. (Academic Press Ser.). (Illus.). 807p. (C). pap. text 69.95 (*0-12-213565-2*) Acad Pr.

Psychology of Music: A Survey for Teacher & Musician. Max Schoen. 1940. LC 73-181248. 258p. reprint ed. 39.00 (*0-403-01673-8*) Scholarly.

Psychology of Nursery Education. Ivan Ward. 1998. 96p. pap. (*1-85575-206-9*) Karnac Bks GBR. *Dist:* Other Pr LLC.

Psychology of Nursing: Coping with Anxiety. Oliver. 1997. (Professional Reference - Nursing Ser.). (C). pap. text 24.95 (*0-8273-6967-0*) Delmar.

Psychology of Nutrition. David Booth. 1994. LC 93-45603. 264p. pap. (*0-7484-0159-8*) Tay Francis Ltd GBR. *Dist:* Taylor & Francis.

Psychology of Nutrition. David Booth. 1994. LC 93-45603. 264p. 85.00 (*0-7484-0158-X*) Taylor & Francis.

Psychology of Occupations. Anne Roe. Ed. by Leon Stein. 1977. LC 77-70529. (Work Ser.). (Illus.). reprint ed. lib. bdg. 35.95 (*0-405-10197-X*) Ayer.

Psychology of Perceptions: Index of Modern Information. Roth Polinski. rev. ed. 1991. LC 88-47983. 150p. 47.50 (*1-55914-486-6*); pap. 44.50 (*1-55914-487-4*) ABBE Pubs Assn.

Psychology of Personality. David C. Funder. Date not set. (C). pap. 16.00 (*0-393-96744-1*, Norton Paperbks) Norton.

Psychology of Personality: An Epistemological Inquiry. James T. Lamiell. 1987. (Critical Assessments of Contemporary Psychology Ser.). (Illus.). 256p. text 57.50 (*0-231-06020-3*) Col U Pr.

***Psychology of Physical Activity: Determinants, Well-Being & Interventions.** Stuart J. H. Biddle & Nanette Murtie. 2001. 368p. pap. 40.95 (*0-415-23252-X*) Routledge.

Psychology of Physical Symptoms. James W. Pennebaker. 1982. (Illus.). 197p. 52.95 (*0-387-90730-0*) Spr-Verlag.

Psychology of Play. Brian Sutton-Smith. 1978. LC 75-35082. (Studies in Play & Games). (Illus.). reprint ed. 35.95 (*0-405-07930-3*) Ayer.

Psychology of Play Activities. Harvey C. Lehman & Paul A. Witty. 1976. LC 75-35074. (Studies in Play & Games). (Illus.). reprint ed. 23.95 (*0-405-07924-9*) Ayer.

Psychology of Politics. Hans J. Eysenck. 1998. LC 98-24888. 343p. pap. text 29.95 (*0-7658-0430-1*) Transaction Pubs.

Psychology of Pregnancy & Childbirth. L. Sherr. 1995. LC 94-48263. (Illus.). 256p. pap. (*0-632-03388-6*) Blckwell Science.

Psychology of Questions. Ed. by Arthur C. Graesser & John B. Black. 1985. 392p. text 79.95 (*0-89859-444-8*) L Erlbaum Assocs.

Psychology of Reading: An Interdisciplinary Approach. Mildred C. Robeck & Randall R. Wallace. 2nd ed. 1990. pap., tchr. ed. (*0-8058-0885-X*) L Erlbaum Assocs.

Psychology of Reading: An Interdisciplinary Approach. Ed. by R. R. Wallace & Mildred C. Robeck. 2nd ed. 1990. 456p. (C). pap. 49.95 (*0-8058-0374-2*); text 99.95 (*0-8058-0373-4*) L Erlbaum Assocs.

Psychology of Reading & Spelling Disabilities. Anthony F. Jorm. 1983. (International Library of Philosophy, Psychology, & Scientific Method). 150p. pap. 14.95 (*0-7100-9344-6*, Routledge Thoemms) Routledge.

Psychology of Religion. Joseph F. Byrnes. 1984. LC 84-47854. 320p. (C). 35.00 (*0-02-905380-5*) Free Pr.

Psychology of Religion: A Short Introduction. Kate M. Loewenthal. 2000. 192p. pap. (*1-85168-212-0*) Oneworld.

Psychology of Religion: An Empirical Approach. Ralph W. Hood, Jr. et al. 2nd ed. 1996. LC 96-22625. 546p. text 62.00 (*1-57230-116-3*, 0116) Guilford Pubns.

Psychology of Religion & Coping: Theory, Research, Practice. Kenneth I. Pargament. 1997. LC 97-9599. 548p. 55.00 (*1-57230-214-3*, 0214) Guilford Pubns.

Psychology of Religious Behaviour, Belief, & Experience. Benjamin Beit-Hallahmi & Michael Argyle. 1997. LC 97-205504. 336p. (C). 80.00 (*0-415-12330-5*); pap. 26.95 (*0-415-12331-3*) Routledge.

Psychology of Religious Belief. L. B. Brown. 1988. text 100.00 (*0-12-136355-4*) Acad Pr.

Psychology of Self-Affirmation with an Assertiveness Attitude: Index of New Information with Authors & Subjects. Rosetta R. Hardine. 1993. 180p. 47.50 (*1-55914-862-4*); pap. 44.50 (*1-55914-863-2*) ABBE Pubs Assn.

Psychology of Self & Other. Elizabeth R. Moberly. 1985. 112p. (*0-422-79740-5*, 9417) Tavistock GBR. *Dist:* Routldge.

Psychology of Self-Esteem: How Our Judgments about Ourselves Affect Our Success in Love & Human Relationships. Nathaniel Branden. 32nd anniv. ed. 2001. LC 00-10734. 304p. (Orig.). pap. 19.95 (*0-7879-4526-9*) Jossey-Bass.

Psychology of Sex Differences Eleanor E. Maccoby & Carol N. Jacklin. 1974. LC 73-94488. xv, 634p. Vol. I. pap. 24.95 (*0-8047-0974-2*); Vol. II. pap. 18.95 (*0-8047-0975-0*) Stanford U Pr.

Psychology of Sex Relations. Theodor Reik. 1975. LC 74-28525. 243p. reprint ed. lib. bdg. 65.00 (*0-8371-7916-5*, RESR, Greenwood Pr) Greenwood.

Psychology of Sexual Emotion: The Basis of Selective Attraction. Vernon W. Grant. 1979. LC 75-36356. 270p. reprint ed. lib. bdg. 38.50 (*0-8371-8631-5*, GRPS, Greenwood Pr) Greenwood.

Psychology of Soccer. Massimo Cabrini. 1999. (Illus.). 137p. pap. 12.95 (*1-890946-25-7*) Reedswain.

Psychology of Sports, Exercise & Fitness: Social & Adjustmental Issues. Louis Diamant. 1991. 256p. 79.95 (*1-56032-170-9*) Hemisp Pub.

Psychology of Stalking. Ed. by J. Reid Meloy. 1998. LC 98-84369. (Illus.). xvii, 327p. (C). text 59.95 (*0-12-490560-9*) Acad Pr.

Psychology of Status. Herbert H. Hyman. Ed. by Harriet Zuckerman & Robert K. Merton. 1980. LC 79-9005. (Dissertations on Sociology Ser.). lib. bdg. 16.95 (*0-405-12974-2*) Ayer.

Psychology of Suggestion: A Research into the Subconscious Nature of Man & Society. Boris Sidis. 1973. LC 73-2415. (Mental Illness & Social Policy; the American Experience Ser.). reprint ed. 25.95 (*0-405-05225-1*) Ayer.

Psychology of Suicide. Edwin S. Shneidman et al. 1983. LC 84-2818. 744p. 45.00 (*0-87668-668-4*) Aronson.

Psychology of Synergy: A Guide to Personal Power. Madeleine Singer. 1991. (Illus.). 176p. (Orig.). pap. 9.95 (*0-941404-03-X*) New Falcon Pubns.

Psychology of Tactical Communication. Ed. by Michael J. Cody & Margaret L. MacLaughlin. 1989. 576p. (*1-85359-040-1*); 350p. pap. (*1-85359-039-8*) Multilingual Matters GBR. *Dist:* Taylor & Francis.

Psychology of Temperament: Index of New Information with Authors, Subjects & References. Lorna S. Collett. rev. ed. 1998. 150p. 57.50 (*0-7883-1944-2*); pap. 47.50 (*0-7883-1945-0*) ABBE Pubs Assn.

Psychology of the Afro-American: A Humanistic Approach. Adelbert H. Jenkins. 1982. (General Psychology Ser.: No. 103). (Illus.). 270p. text 50.00 (*0-08-027206-1*); pap. text 22.00 (*0-08-027205-3*) Elsevier (Pergamon Pr).

Psychology of the Child. Jean Piaget & Barbel Inhelder. Tr. by Helen Weaver. 1972. LC 73-78449. 192p. pap. 20.00 (*0-465-09500-3*) Basic.

Psychology of the Dentist-Patient Relationship. S. Bochner. 1988. (Contributions to Psychology & Medicine Ser.). (Illus.). 187p. 112.00 (*0-387-96642-0*) Spr-Verlag.

Psychology of the Family in Health, Stress & Disease: Index of New Information. Valerie N. Hullinger. 1997. 149p. 57.50 (*0-7883-1538-2*); 1997. 149p. pap. 47.50 (*0-7883-1539-0*); 1994. 150p. 57.50 (*0-7883-0066-0*); 1994. 150p. pap. 47.50 (*0-7883-0067-9*) ABBE Pubs Assn.

Psychology of the Female Body. Jane M. Ussher. 1989. 200p. 45.00 (*0-415-01556-1*, A1686) Routledge.

Psychology of the Future: Lessons from Modern Consciousness Research. Stanislav Grof. 2000. LC 00-25255. (Suny Series, Transpersonal & Humanistic Psychology Ser.). (Illus.). xv, 345p. pap. text 20.95 (*0-7914-4622-0*) State U NY Pr.

Psychology of the Negro: An Experimental Study. George O. Ferguson. 1970. LC 74-107481. 138p. reprint ed. lib. bdg. 55.00 (*0-8371-3783-7*, FEP&, Greenwood Pr) Greenwood.

Psychology of the Physically Handicapped. Jon Eisenson et al. Ed. by William R. Phillips & Janet Rosenberg. 1980. LC 79-6922. (Physically Handicapped in Society Ser.). reprint ed. lib. bdg. 37.95 (*0-405-13130-5*) Ayer.

Psychology of the Physically Ill Patient: A Clinician's Guide. M. E. Backman. 1989. LC 88-39667. (Illus.). 252p. (C). 49.50 (*0-306-43051-7*, Plenum Trade) Perseus Pubng.

Psychology of the Psalms. Maralene Wesner & Miles E. Wesner. 1997. 63p. pap. 5.95 (*0-936715-49-9*, 127) Diversity Okla.

Psychology of the Self: A Casebook. Ed. by Arnold Goldberg. 1992. 468p. reprint ed. pap. 24.95 (*0-8236-8262-5*) Intl Univs Pr.

Psychology of the Social. Ed. by Uwe Flick. 1998. LC 97-42130. 299p. (C). text 64.95 (*0-521-58159-1*) Cambridge U Pr.

Psychology of the Unconscious: A Study of the Transformations & Symbolisms of the Libido: A Contribution to the History of the Evolution of Thought. Carl Gustav Jung. Tr. by Beatrice M. Hinkle. 1992. LC 91-17591. (Bollingen Ser.: Vol. XX: B). (Illus.). 420p. 72.50 (*0-691-09973-1*) Princeton U Pr.

Psychology of the Youthful Offender. Robert N. Walker. 3rd ed. 1995. LC 95-16135. 130p. (C). text 42.95 (*0-398-06529-2*); pap. text 28.95 (*0-398-06530-6*) C C Thomas.

Psychology of Today's Woman. Ed. by Toni Bernay & Dorothy W. Cantor. 1989. LC 89-31197. 400p. pap. text 15.95 (*0-674-72109-8*) HUP.

Psychology of Today's Woman: New Psychoanalytic Visions. Ed. by Toni Bernay & Dorothy W. Cantor. 1986. 377p. (C). text 45.00 (*0-88163-036-5*) Analytic Pr.

Psychology of Touch. Ed. by Morton Heller & William Schiff. 1991. 408p. (C). pap. 45.00 (*0-8058-0751-9*) L Erlbaum Assocs.

Psychology of Touch: A Special Issue of Journal of Nonverbal Behavior. Ed. by Stephen Thayer. 1986. LC 80-649435. 80p. pap. 16.95 (*0-89885-321-4*, Kluwer Acad Hman Sci) Kluwer Academic.

***Psychology of Travel: How Study Abroad & Positive Regression Affect Personal Growth.** Greta E. Couper. 2001. 205p. cd-rom 15.00 (*0-9620635-1-7*) TreCavalli Pr.

Psychology of Underachievement: Differential Diagnosis & Differential Treatment. Harvey P. Mandel & Sander I. Marcus. 1988. LC 87-37127. (Personality Processes Ser.). 397p. 215.00 (*0-471-84855-7*) Wiley.

Psychology of Voice Disorders. Deborah C. Rosen & Robert T. Sataloff. 1997. LC 96-50038. (Illus.). 302p. text 73.95 (*1-56593-839-9*, 1638) Thomson Learn.

Psychology of Women. Michele A. Paludi. 1998. LC 97-41464. 406p. (C). pap. text 52.00 (*0-13-955840-3*) P-H.

Psychology of Women. Mary R. Walsh. 1987. LC 87-6167. 480p. pap. 25.00 (*0-300-03966-2*) Yale U Pr.

Psychology of Women. Margaret W. Matlin. 4th ed. 2000. LC 99-61163. 704p. (C). pap. 74.00 (*0-15-507896-8*) Harcourt Coll Pubs.

Psychology of Women: Future Directions in Research. J. A. Sherman & F. L. Denmark. 1979. LC 78-31824. 800p. 59.95 (*0-88437-009-7*) Psych Dimensions.

Psychology of Women: Psychoanalytic Perpectives. Ed. by Arnold Richards & Phyllis Tyson. 2001. LC 97-784. (Books-on-Demand Ser.). (Illus.). xii, 592p. pap. 39.95 (*0-8236-5588-1*, No. 05588) Intl Univs Pr.

Psychology of Women: Selected Readings. Ed. by Juanita H. Williams. 2nd ed. 1985. 579p. (C). pap. text 25.00 (*0-393-95379-3*) Norton.

Psychology of Women's Health: Progress & Challenges in Research & Application. Ed. by Annette L. Stanton & Sheryle J. Gallant. 1995. LC 95-10460. 651p. text 24.95 (*1-55798-296-1*, 431-7530) Am Psychol.

Psychology Office Manual. Donald J. Weinstein. 1994. (Office Manual Ser.). 155p. 89.00 (*1-890018-06-6*) Anadem Pubng.

Psychology 101 Supplement: Getting Familiar with the Study of Behavior. Bruce B. Svore. 1998. 100p. (C). pap. text 26.00 (*0-9666323-1-1*, 100-2) Bordalice.

Psychology Online: Social & Applied Psychology. Patricia M. Wallace. 1996. 50p. (C). pap. 13.13 (*0-697-37485-8*, WCB McGr Hill) McGrw-H Hghr Educ.

Psychology: or A View of the Human Soul, Including Anthropology. Friedrich Rauch. 1975. LC 74-22335. (History of Psychology Ser.). 416p. 60.00 (*0-8201-1142-2*) Schol Facsimiles.

Psychology, Pain & Anaesthesia. Ed. by Hamilton B. Gibson. 1993. LC 93-32615. 220p. 54.25 (*1-56593-129-7*, 0441) Thomson Learn.

Psychology, Pain & Anaesthesia. Ed. by Robert J. Smith & Karen H. Simpson. 1990. LC 93-32615. 220p. (*0-412-33650-2*, A4410) Chapman & Hall.

Psychology, Phenomenology, & Chinese Philosophy: Chinese Philosophical Studies VI. Vincent Shen et al. 1994. LC 94-7728. (Cultural Heritage & Contemporary Change Series III: Vol. 6). 185p. pap. 17.50 (*1-56518-045-3*) Coun Res Values.

Psychology Place Sticker One. 1999. (*0-321-06042-3*) Addison-Wesley.

Psychology Problem Solver. M. Fogiel. rev. ed. 1999. LC 80-53174. (REA Problem Solvers Ser.). (Illus.). 1056p. (C). pap. text 23.95 (*0-87891-523-0*) Res & Educ.

Psychology, Psychiatry, & the Law: A Clinical & Forensic Handbook. Charles P. Ewing. 1985. LC 85-60449. 576p. (C). pap. 39.95 (*0-943158-11-7*, PPL-BBP, Prof Resc Pr) Pro Resource.

Psychology Readings Catalogue of the North East London Polytechnic, London, England, Set. North East London Polytechnic Staff. 1976. 180.00 (*0-8161-1179-0*, Macmillan Ref) Gale.

Psychology Research & Public Policy. Richard A. Kasschau. 1985. LC 85-3600. 55.00 (*0-275-90126-2*, C0126, Praeger Pubs) Greenwood.

Psychology Research Handbook: A Primer for Graduate Students & Research Assistants. Frederick T. Leong & James T. Austin. 1996. LC 96-10017. 408p. 89.95 (*0-8039-7048-X*, 2773) Sage.

Psychology, Society & Subjectivity: An Introduction to German Critical Psychology. Charles W. Tolman. 1994. LC 94-3934. (Critical Psychology Ser.). 184p. (C). pap. 27.95 (*0-415-08976-X*, B3200); text 62.95 (*0-415-08975-1*, B3196) Routledge.

Psychology Student Writer's Manual. Jill M. Scott et al. 1998. LC 98-21462. (Illus.). 221p. pap. text, stu. ed. 27.60 (*0-13-633041-X*) P-H.

Psychology the Search for Understanding. Janet Simons et al. 1987. (Psychology). (Illus.). 716p. (C). mass mkt. 50.75 (*0-314-26213-X*) West Pub.

Psychology Today. Richard R. Bootzin et al. 5th ed. 1982. LC 82-20450. (C). text (*0-394-32581-8*) Random.

Psychology Versus Metapsychology: Psychoanalytic Essays in Memory of George S. Klein. Ed. by Merton M. Gill & Philip S. Holzman. 1975. LC 75-23354. (Psychological Issues Monographs: No. 36, Vol. 9, No. 4). 376p. 55.00 (*0-8236-5586-5*) Intl Univs Pr.

Psychology with Machiavellianism: Index of New Information for Reference & Research. Lois A. Hutton. 1997. 150p. 57.50 (*0-7883-1240-5*); pap. text 47.50 (*0-7883-1241-3*) ABBE Pubs Assn.

***Psychology with Making the Grade & Power Web.** Passer. 2000. 703p. text 80.63 (*0-07-247975-2*) McGrw-H Hghr Educ.

Psychology with Psychplace. Wade. 5th ed. 1998. (C). text 77.00 (*0-321-04937-3*) Addison-Wesley.

Psychology with Supersite Pin Code. Robert A. Baron. 5th ed. 2000. 768p. 86.00 (*0-205-32404-5*) Allyn.

Psychology's Crisis of Disunity: Philosophy & Method for a Unified Science. Arthur W. Staats. 1983. LC 83-2154. 401p. 75.00 (*0-275-91082-2*, C1082, Praeger Pubs) Greenwood.

Psychology's Myths & Misconceptions. Dawes. 23.00 (*0-465-06700-X*) Basic.

Psychology's Second Century: Enduring Issues, Vol. 2. Richard A. Kasschau & Charles N. Cofer. 1981. LC 81-11882. 303p. 67.00 (*0-275-90659-0*, C06592, Praeger Pubs) Greenwood.

Psycholytic & Psychedelic Therapy Research, 1931-1995: A Complete International Bibliography. Torsten Passie. 1997. LC 97-195979. (Kleine Bibliographische Reihe Ser.). 102p. (*0-393-61483-2*) Norton.

Psychometric Foundations & Behavioral Assessment. Fernando Silva. 1993. LC 93-7506. (Illus.). 160p. (C). pap. 26.95 (*0-8039-5267-8*, 4944) Sage.

Psychometric Methods: Item Response Theory for Psychologists. Susan E. Embretson & Steve Reise. 2000. LC 99-48454. (Multivariate Applications Ser.). (Illus.). xi, 371p. 39.95 (*0-8058-2819-2*) L Erlbaum Assocs.

Psychometric Properties of Fourteen Latent Constructs from the Oregon Youth Society. D. Capaldi & G. R. Patterson. 1988. (Recent Research in Psychology Ser.). (Illus.). 287p. 78.95 (*0-387-96845-8*) Spr-Verlag.

Psychometric Theory. Jim C. Nunnally & Ira H. Bernstein. 3rd ed. 1994. LC 93-22756. (Series in Social Psychology). 736p. (C). text 96.25 (*0-07-047849-X*) McGrw-H Hghr Educ.

Psychomotor Domain & the Seriously Handicapped. Ed. by Paul Jansma. 3rd ed. 1989. (Illus.). 520p. 49.00 (*0-8191-7240-5*) U Pr of Amer.

Psychomotor Domain Training & Serious Disabilities. Paul Jansma. 4th ed. 1993. LC 93-19856. (Illus.). 408p. (C). pap. 46.00 (*0-8191-9163-9*) U Pr of Amer.

Psychonephrology Vol. 1: Psychological Factors in Hemodialysis & Transplantation. Ed. by Norman B. Levy. 1981. LC 80-20681. 306p. 75.00 (*0-306-40586-5*, Plenum Trade) Perseus Pubng.

Psychonephrology Vol. 2: Psychological Problems in Kidney Failure & Their Treatment. Ed. by Norman B. Levy. 1983. LC 83-8015. 312p. 85.00 (*0-306-41154-7*, Plenum Trade) Perseus Pubng.

Psychoneural Reduction: The New Wave. John Bickle. 1998. LC 97-28252. (Bradford Book Ser.). (Illus.). 372p. 45.00 (*0-262-02432-2*, Bradford Bks) MIT Pr.

Psychoneuroendocrine Dysfunction. Ed. by Nandkumar S. Shah & Alexander G. Donald. 1984. LC 83-19202. 660p. 140.00 (*0-306-41320-5*, Plenum Trade) Perseus Pubng.

Psychoneuroendocrinology. Ed. by C. S. Holmes. 1989. (Illus.). 359p. 137.00 (*0-387-97112-2*) Spr-Verlag.

Psychoneuroendocrinology: Proceedings. Conference of the International Society for Psycho. Ed. by Noboru Hatotani. 1974. (Illus.). 450p. 116.75 (*3-8055-1711-4*) S Karger.

Psychoneuroendocrinology & Abnormal Behavior. Ed. by Julien Mendlewicz. 1980. (Advances in Biological Psychiatry Ser.: Vol. 5). (Illus.). vi, 130p. pap. 50.50 (*3-8055-0599-X*) S Karger.

Psychoneuroendocrinology of Aging. Ed. by G. Valenti. 1989. (FIDIA Research Ser.: Vol. 16). 175p. 70.00 (*0-387-96943-8*) Spr-Verlag.

***Psychoneuroimmunolgy,** Vol. 2. David L. Felton. Ed. by Robert Ader & Nicholas Cohen. 3rd ed. 2001. LC 00-102888. (Illus.). (*0-12-044316-3*) Acad Pr.

Psychoneuroimmunology. Ed. by Robert Ader et al. 2nd ed. 1990. LC 90-216. 1218p. text 210.00 (*0-12-043782-1*) Acad Pr.

Psychoneuroimmunology: An Interdisciplinary Introduction. Manfred Schedlowski & Uwe Tewes. 1999. LC 99-38184. pap. (*0-306-45975-2*); 535p. pap. (*0-306-45976-0*) Kluwer Academic (Kluwer Plenum).

Psychoneuroimmunology: Interactions Between Brain, Nervous System, Behavior, Endocrine & Immune System. Ed. by H. J. Schmoll et al. 1992. LC 91-35385. (Illus.). 276p. text 34.00 (*0-88937-066-4*) Hogrefe & Huber Pubs.

Psychoneuroimmunology: Stress, Mental Disorders & Health. Ed. by Karl Goodkin & Adriaan P. Visser. 2000. LC 98-51393. (Progress in Psychiatry Ser.: No. 59). (Illus.). xxiii, 444p. 55.00 (*0-88048-171-4*, 8171) Am Psychiatric.

Psychoneuroimmunology, Stress, & Infection. Ed. by Herman Friedman et al. 1995. LC 95-41098. 304p. 179.95 (*0-8493-7638-6*, 7638) CRC Pr.

Psychoneuroses & Their Treatment by Psychotherapy. Joseph J. Dejerine & E. Gauckler. Tr. by Smith E. Jelliffe. 1976. LC 75-16697. (Classics in Psychiatry Ser.). reprint ed. 36.95 (*0-405-07425-5*) Ayer.

Psychopathia Sexualis. Richard Von Krafft-Ebing. Tr. by Franklin S. Klaf from GER. 1998. LC 98-13156. 464p. pap. 40.00 (*1-55970-426-8*) Arcade Pub Inc.

Psychopathic Mind: Origins, Dynamics, & Treatment. J. Reid Meloy. 1992. LC 88-3454. 496p. reprint ed. pap. 45.00 (*0-87668-311-1*) Aronson.

Psychopathic Personality Commitment Law: A Study of Its Implementation in Minnesota. Marlys McPherson. 1997. (Illus.). 48p. reprint ed. pap. text 25.00 (*0-7881-4707-2*) DIANE Pub.

Psychopathological & Neurological Dysfunctions Following Open-Heart Surgery, Milwaukee 1980: Proceedings. Ed. by R. Becker et al. 1983. (Illus.). 384p. 103.00 (*0-387-11621-4*) Spr-Verlag.

Psychopathological Disorders of Childhood. Ed. by Herbert C. Quay & John S. Werry. 3rd ed. 1986. LC 86-11105. 704p. 80.95 (*0-471-88974-1*) Wiley.

Psychopathologie de la Vie Quotidienne. Sigmund Freud. 1989. (FRE.). pap. 24.95 (*0-7859-3039-6*) Fr & Eur.

Psychopathology. John D. Stirling. 1999. LC 98-33124. (Modular Psychology Ser.). xv, 174p. 40.00 (*0-415-19270-6*); pap. 13.95 (*0-415-19271-4*) Routledge.

Psychopathology. L. Willerman & D. B. Cohen. 1989. (C). pap. text 21.87 (*0-07-070312-4*) McGraw.

Psychopathology. L. Willerman & D. B. Cohen. 1989. 350p. (C). text 64.06 (*0-07-070311-6*) McGrw-H Hghr Educ.

Psychopathology. Edward J. Kempf. 1976. LC 75-16711. (Classics in Psychiatry Ser.). (Illus.). reprint ed. 65.95 (*0-405-07440-9*) Ayer.

Psychopathology: A Case Book. Robert L. Spitzer et al. 1983. (Illus.). 352p. (C). 61.25 (*0-07-060350-2*) McGrw-H Hghr Educ.

Psychopathology: A Source Book. Ed. by Charles F. Reed et al. 1958. LC 58-10405. (Illus.). 815p. 77.50 (*0-674-72200-0*) HUP.

Psychopathology: Contemporary Jungian Perspectives. Ed. by A. Samuels. 1989. 355p. pap. (*0-946439-67-2*) Karnac Bks GBR. *Dist:* Other Pr LLC.

Psychopathology: Contemporary Jungian Perspectives. Ed. by Andrew Samuels. LC 91-12646. 355p. reprint ed. 1992. pap. 26.00 (*0-89862-473-8*, 2473); 1991. text 42.00 (*0-89862-765-6*) Guilford Pubns.

Psychopathology: The Evolving Sciences of Mental Disorder. Ed. by Steven Matthysse et al. 1996. (Illus.). 608p. (C). text 74.95 (*0-521-44469-1*) Cambridge U Pr.

Psychopathology & Adaptation in Infancy & Early Childhood. Stanley I. Greenspan. 1983. LC 81-19282. (Clinical Infant Reports: No. 1). 263p. 42.00 (*0-8236-5660-8*) Intl Univs Pr.

Psychopathology & Addictive Disorders. Ed. by Roger E. Meyer. 1986. LC 85-30547. 384p. 47.50 (*0-89862-680-3*) Guilford Pubns.

Psychopathology & Cognition. Ed. by Keith S. Dobson & Philip C. Kendall. 1993. LC 93-19571. (Personality, Psychopathology, & Psychotherapy Ser.). (Illus.). 492p. text 65.00 (*0-12-404175-2*) Acad Pr.

Psychopathology & Differential Diagnosis: A Primer, Set. Henry Kellerman & Anthony Burry. 1989. (Personality, Psychopathology & Psychotherapy: Theoretical & Clinical Perspectives Ser.). text 87.50 (*0-231-06702-X*) Col U Pr.

Psychopathology & Differential Diagnosis - A Primer Vol. 2: Diagnosis. Henry Kellerman & Anthony Burry. 1989. (Personality, Psychopathology & Psychotherapy: Theoretical & Clinical Perspectives Ser.). 250p. text 52.50 (*0-231-06704-6*) Col U Pr.

Psychopathology & Nosology. Ed. by E. Gabriel & H. G. Zapotoczky. 1985. (Journal: Vol. 8, No. 2-3, 1985). 124p. pap. 65.25 (*3-8055-4218-6*) S Karger.

Psychopathology & Pictorial Expression, Vol. IV. Ed. by Sandoz. 1978. (Series 19-22, & 25). (Illus.). 104.50 (*3-8055-2929-5*) S Karger.

Psychopathology & Politics. Harold D. Lasswell. 1986. xxvi, 368p. pap. text 23.00 (*0-226-46919-0*) U Ch Pr.

Psychopathology & Psychiatry. Anna Pavlova. 1993. LC 93-5454. 550p. (C). pap. text 29.95 (*1-56000-707-9*) Transaction Pubs.

Psychopathology & Psychotherapy: From Diagnosis to Treatment. Len Sperry & Jon Carlson. 1993. LC 91-72222. xx, 664p. (C). 44.95 (*1-55959-032-7*) Accel Devel.

Psychopathology & Psychotherapy: From DSM-IV Diagnosis to Treatment. Len Sperry & Jon Carlson. 2nd ed. 1996. 704p. 44.95 (*1-56032-492-9*) Accel Devel.

Psychopathology & Psychotherapy in Homosexuality. Ed. by Michael Ross. 1988. LC 87-29894. (Journal of Homosexuality Ser.: Vol. 15, Nos. 1-2). 222p. text 49.95 (*0-86656-499-3*) Haworth Pr.

Psychopathology & Violent Crime. Ed. by Andrew E. Skodol. 1998. LC 97-51790. (Review Ser.). 156p. pap. text 27.00 (*0-88048-834-4*, 8834) Am Psychiatric.

Psychopathology in Adulthood. Ed. by Michel Hersen & Alan S. Bellack. 2nd ed. 1999. LC 99-25834. 481p. (C). 65.00 (*0-205-20027-3*) Allyn.

Psychopathology in the Mentally Retarded. Ed. by Johnny L. Matson. 1991. 312p. (C). (*0-205-13463-7*) Allyn.

Psychopathology in the Mentally Retarded. Ed. by Johnny L. Matson & Rowland P. Barrett. 1982. text 41.95 (*0-8089-1511-8*, 792808, Grune & Strat) Harcrt Hlth Sci Grp.

Psychopathology of Adolescence: Proceedings, Vol. 26. American Psychopathological Association Staff. Ed. by Joseph Zubin & Alfred Freedman. 1969. 354p. text 79.50 (*0-8089-0558-9*, 794986, Grune & Strat) Harcrt Hlth Sci Grp.

Psychopathology of Childhood: A Clinical-Experimental Approach. Steven Schwartz & James H. Johnson. 2nd ed. 1985. (General Psychology Ser.: No. 95). 464p. text 29.50 (*0-08-030935-6*, Pergamon Pr) Elsevier.

Psychopathology of Crime: Criminal Behavior As a Clinical Disorder. Adrian Raine. 1993. LC 93-911. (Illus.). 377p. text 69.95 (*0-12-576160-0*) Acad Pr.

Psychopathology of Crime: Criminal Behavior As a Clinical Disorder. Adrian Raine. 1997. (Illus.). 377p. reprint ed. pap. text 44.95 (*0-12-576155-4*) Morgan Kaufmann.

Psychopathology of Everyday Life. Sigmund Freud. Ed. by James Strachey. Tr. by Alan Tyson. 1990. (Standard Edition of the Complete Psychological Works of Sigmund Freud). 395p. pap. 13.95 (*0-393-00611-5*) Norton.

Psychopathology of Language & Cognition. Harold J. Vetter & R. W. Rieber. 1995. LC 94-44347. (Cognition & Language Ser.). (Illus.). 212p. (C). 49.50 (*0-306-44757-6*, Plenum Trade) Perseus Pubng.

Psychopathology of Perception: Proceedings of the Third Leeds Psychopathology Symposium, September 1988 - Psychopathology Journal, Vol. 24, No. 6. Ed. by A. M. Mortimer & K. J. Rix. 1991. (Illus.). 36p. pap. 55.00 (*3-8055-5536-9*) S Karger.

Psychopathy: A History of the Concepts. Henry Werlinder. 1978. 218p. pap. text 37.50 (*91-554-0782-X*) Coronet Bks.

Psychopathy: Antisocial, Criminal & Violent Behavior. Ed. by Theodore Millon et al. 1998. LC 98-6845. 476p. 60.00 (*1-57230-344-1*, C0344) Guilford Pubns.

Psychopathy: Theory, Research & Implications for Society, Alvor, Portugal, November 29-December 7, 1995. Ed. by David J. Cooke et al. 1998. LC 97-49859. (NATO Advanced Science Institutes Ser.). 428p. 194.00 (*0-7923-4919-9*) Kluwer Academic.

Psychopharmaco-Endocrinology & Depression Research. G. Laakmann. 1990. (Illus.). 219p. 79.95 (*0-387-52075-9*) Spr-Verlag.

Psychopharmacologists, Vol. 2. David Healy. 1998. 672p. pap. (*1-86036-010-6*) E A GBR. *Dist:* OUP.

Psychopharmacologists III. David Healy. 3rd ed. 2000. 640p. text (*0-340-76110-5*) E A GBR. *Dist:* OUP.

Psychopharmacology. Ed. by Alan A. Boulton et al. 1989. LC 88-32813. (Neuromethods Ser.: Vol. 13). (Illus.). 836p. 149.50 (*0-89603-129-2*) Humana.

Psychopharmacology. Ed. by Geroge. 1999. (C). text (*0-321-01394-8*) Addson-Wesley Educ.

Psychopharmacology: An Introduction. Rene Spiegel. Tr. by Terry Watson from GER. 3rd ed. 1996. LC 95-32202. (Medical Publications).Tr. of Einfuhrung in die Psychopharmakologie. 312p. 190.00 (*0-471-95729-1*) Wiley.

Psychopharmacology: Basic Mechanisms & Applied Interventions. Ed. by John Grabowski & Gary R. VandenBos. 1992. 207p. (Orig.). pap. 24.95 (*1-55798-158-2*) Am Psychol.

Psychopharmacology: Basics for Counselors. Gregory L. Little. 1996. (Illus.). 279p. (C). pap. text 24.95 (*0-9655392-0-2*) Advanced Trnging.

Psychopharmacology: The Fourth Generation of Progress. Ed. by David J. Kupfer & Floyd E. Bloom. 4th ed. 1994. LC 94-7409. 2,048p. text 250.00 (*0-7817-0166-X*) Lppncott W & W.

Psychopharmacology & Psychobiology of Ethnicity. Ed. by Keh-Ming Lin et al. 1993. LC 92-49996. (Progress in Psychiatry Ser.: No. 39). 276p. text 29.95 (*0-88048-471-3*, 8471) Am Psychiatric.

Psychopharmacology & Psychotherapy: Strategies for Maximizing Treatment Outcomes. Len Sperry. 1995. LC 95-21881. (Mental Health Practice under Managed Care Ser.: No. 1). 208p. text 22.95 (*0-87630-787-X*) Brunner-Routledge.

P Q R

Psychopharmacology & Psychotherapy: Synthesis or Antithesis? Ed. by Norman Rosenzweig & Hilda Griscon. 1978. LC 78-4088. 256p. 35.95 (*0-87705-354-5*, Kluwer Acad Hman Sci) Kluwer Academic.

Psychopharmacology & Women: Sex, Gender, & Hormones. Ed. by Margaret F. Jensvold et al. 1996. 615p. text 69.95 (*0-88048-545-0*, 8545) Am Psychiatric.

Psychopharmacology Desktop Reference. Ed. by Stephen Saklad. 1999. pap. 149.00 (*1-884937-61-6*) Manisses Communs.

Psychopharmacology for Everyday Practice. T. A. Ban & M. H. Hollender. 1981. x, 198p. pap. 32.75 (*3-8055-2241-X*) S Karger.

Psychopharmacology for the Aged. Ed. by T. H. Ban. 1980. xii, 216p. pap. 34.00 (*3-8055-1204-X*) S Karger.

Psychopharmacology from a Feminist Perspective. Ed. by Jean A. Hamilton et al. 1995. 137p. LC 95-14408. 39.95 (*1-56024-684-7*); pap. 14.95 (*1-56023-059-2*, Harrington Park) Haworth Pr.

Psychopharmacology of Aggression. Ed. by F. A. Freyhan et al. 1978. (Modern Problems of Pharmacopsychiatry Ser.: Vol. 13). (Illus.). 68.00 (*3-8055-2751-9*) S Karger.

Psychopharmacology of Aging. Carl Eisdorfer. Ed. by W. E. Fann. 1980. (Illus.). 327p. text 55.00 (*0-88331-190-9*) R B Luce.

Psychopharmacology of Animal Behavior Disorders. Nicholas H. Dodman & Louis Shuster. 1998. LC 97-27824. (Illus.). 300p. 78.95 (*0-632-04358-X*) Blackwell Sci.

Psychopharmacology of Antipsychotics. Stephen M. Stahl. 1999. 148p. (*1-85317-601-X*) Martin Dunitz.

Psychopharmacology of Anxiolytics & Antidepressants. Ed. by Sandra E. File. 1991. (International Encyclopedia of Pharmacology & Therapeutics Ser.: 136). (Illus.). 284p. 134.50 (*0-08-040698-X*, North Holland) Elsevier.

Psychopharmacology of Childhood. Ed. by D. Siva Sankar. 1976. LC 74-27253. 49.95 (*0-915340-00-3*) PJD Pubns.

Psychopharmacology of Cognitive & Psychiatric Disorders in the Elderly. D. Wheatley. 2nd ed. 1997. LC 97-69680. (Illus.). 240p. text (*0-412-82470-1*) E A GBR. *Dist:* OUP.

Psychopharmacology of Depression. Ed. by Stuart A. Montgomery & Tim H. Corn. 1994. LC 93-44896. (British Association for Psychopharmacology Monographs: No. 13). (Illus.). 270p. (C). text 98.50 (*0-19-262278-1*) OUP.

Psychopharmacology of Herbal Medicine: Plant Drugs That Alter Mind, Brain & Behavior. Marcello Spinella. 2001. LC 00-52535. (Illus.). 500p. pap. 24.95 (*0-262-69265-1*) MIT Pr.

Psychopharmacology of Panic. Ed. by Stuart A. Montgomery. 1993. LC 92-16486. (British Association for Psychopharmacology Monographs: No. 12). (Illus.). 160p. text 47.50 (*0-19-262087-8*) OUP.

Psychopharmacology of Schizophrenia. Ed. by Michael A. Reveley & J. F. William Deakin. 2000. (An Arnold Publication). 288p. (*0-340-75912-7*) E A GBR. *Dist:* OUP.

Psychopharmacology of the Developmental Disabilities. Ed. by Michael G. Aman & N. N. Singh. 1988. (Disorders of Human Learning, Behavior, & Communication Ser.). (Illus.). 277p. 108.00 (*0-387-96679-X*) Spr-Verlag.

Psychopharmacology of the Limbic System. Ed. by Michael R. Trimble & E. Zarifian. 1985. (Illus.). 280p. pap. 29.95 (*0-19-261575-0*) OUP.

Psychopharmacology Sourcebook. Mark Zetin. 2000. LC 99-51478. xix, 364p. pap. 17.95 (*0-7373-0266-6*, 02666W) NTC Contemp Pub Co.

Psychophysical Approaches to Cognition. Ed. by Daniel Algom. 1992. LC 92-19503. (Advances in Psychology Ser.: Vol. 92). 628p. 192.00 (*0-444-88978-7*, North Holland) Elsevier.

Psychophysical Elements in Parapsychological Traditions. A. Tanagras. 1967. LC 67-19168. (Parapsychological Monographs: No. 7). pap. 6.00 (*0-912328-10-X*) Parapsych Foun.

Psychophysical Explorations of Mental Structures: Selected Papers of the Centennial Symposium in Honor of Gustav Theodor Fechner. Ed. by Hans-Georg Geissler et al. 1990. LC 90-4265. (Illus.). 560p. text 79.00 (*0-88937-031-1*) Hogrefe & Huber Pubs.

Psychophysical Physiological & Behavioral Studies in Hearing: Proceedings of the International Symposium on Hearing, 5th, Noordwijkerhout, the Netherlands, April 8-12, 1980. International Symposium on Hearing Staff. Ed. by G. Van den Brink & F. A. Bilsen. 1980. 480p. lib. bdg. 132.00 (*90-286-0780-3*) Kluwer Academic.

Psychophysics: Introduction to Its Perceptual, Neural, & Social Prospects. S. S. Stevens. 1986. 335p. reprint ed. pap. text 24.95 (*0-88738-643-1*) Transaction Pubs.

Psychophysics: Method, Theory, & Application. George A. Gescheider. 2nd ed. 1984. 304p. (C). text 49.95 (*0-89859-375-1*) L Erlbaum Assocs.

Psychophysiological Aspects of Reading & Learning. Victor Rentel et al. 1985. (Monographs in Psychobiology). xx, 352p. text 174.00 (*2-88124-000-3*); 390p. pap. text 83.00 (*2-88124-025-9*) Gordon & Breach.

Psychophysiological Disorders: Research & Clinical Applications. Ed. by Robert J. Gatchel & Edward B. Blanchard. 1993. (Application & Practice in Health Psychology Ser.). (Illus.). 483p. pap. 29.95 (*1-55798-523-5*) Am Psychol.

Psychophysiology: Human Behavior & Physiological Response. John L. Andreassi. 2nd ed. 1989. 488p. pap. 34.50 (*0-8058-0180-4*); 3rd ed. 1995. 400p. pap. 55.00 (*0-8058-1104-4*); 3rd ed. 1995. 400p. text 99.95 (*0-8058-1103-6*) L Erlbaum Assocs.

Psychophysiology: The Mind-Body Perspective. Kenneth Hugdahl. 1996. LC 95-21933. (Perspectives in Cognitive Neuroscience Ser.). (Illus.). 448p. (C). 58.50 (*0-674-72207-8*) HUP.

Psychophysiology for Clinical Psychologists. Walter W. Surwillo. Ed. by Glenn R. Caddy. 1990. LC 90-37389. (Developments in Clinical Psychology Ser.). 192p. (C). 77.00 (*0-89391-679-X*, Ablex) Greenwood.

Psychophysiology of Low Back Pain. Adams. 1997. text 36.95 (*0-443-05259-X*) Saunders.

Psychophysiology of Mental Imagery: Theory, Research, & Application. Ed. by Robert G. Kunzendorf & Anees A. Sheikh. 1990. (Imagery & Human Development Ser.). 236p. text 38.95 (*0-89503-063-2*); pap. text 30.00 (*0-89503-062-4*) Baywood Pub.

Psychophysiology of the Gastrointestinal Tract: Experimental & Clinical Applications. Ed. by Rupert Holzl & William E. Whitehead. 1983. 390p. 85.00 (*0-306-41089-3*, Plenum Trade) Perseus Pubng.

Psychophysiology of Visual Masking: The Fine Structure of Conscious Experience, Horizons in Psychology. T. Bachmann. 1994. LC 93-19895. 191p. (C). pap. text 125.00 (*1-56072-066-2*) Nova Sci Pubs.

Psychophysiology Today & Tomorrow. N. P. Bechtereva. 1981. (*0-08-025930-8*) Pergamon Repr GBR. *Dist:* Franklin.

Psychopolitics. Milton Greenblatt. 1978. 352p. text 49.00 (*0-8089-1062-0*, 791729, Grune & Strat) Harcrt Hlth Sci Grp.

Psychoses. Jacques Lacan. Date not set. (*0-393-01925-X*) Norton.

Psychoses & Pervasive Developmental Disorders in Childhood & Adolescence. Ed. by Fred R. Volkmar. 1996. LC 95-38068. 368p. text 48.50 (*1-882103-01-7*, 0301) Am Psychiatric.

Psychoses of the Schizophrenic Spectrum in Twins: A Discussion on the Nature-Nurture Debate in the Etiology of "Endogenous" Psychoses. Ernest Franzek & Helmut Beckmann. 1999. LC 99-25477. (Illus.). 200p. pap. 49.95 (*3-211-83298-X*) Spr-Verlag.

Psychosexual Imperatives: Their Role in Identity Formation. Ed. by Marie C. Nelson & Jean Ikenberry. 1979. LC 78-17739. (Self-in-Process Ser.: Vol. 2). 397p. 45.95 (*0-87705-302-2*, Kluwer Acad Hman Sci) Kluwer Academic.

Psychosexual Medicine: A Study of Underlying Themes. Lincoln. 1992. 230p. pap. 47.75 (*1-56593-049-5*, 0297) Thomson Learn.

*__Psychosexual Medicine: An Introduction.__ Ed. by Ruth L. Skrine & A. Heather Montford. 2nd ed. 2001. (Arnold Publication). 288p. (Orig.). pap. text, suppl. ed. 49.50 (*0-340-76142-3*) OUP.

Psychosexual Training & the Doctor/Patient Relationship: Edited Transcripts of Leaders Workshops. Ruth L. Skrine. 1995. (Illus.). 390p. pap. 34.95 (*1-56593-785-6*, 1532) Singular Publishing.

Psychosis: Understanding & Treatment. Ed. by Jane Ellwood. 1994. LC 95-6606. 224p. pap. 34.95 (*1-85302-265-9*) Taylor & Francis.

Psychosis & Civilization. Herbert Goldhamer & Andrew W. Marshall. Ed. by Gerald N. Grob. 1980. LC 78-22560. (Historical Issues in Mental Health Ser.). (Illus.). reprint ed. lib. bdg. 18.95 (*0-405-11914-3*) Ayer.

Psychosis & Near Psychosis: Ego Function, Symbol Structure & Treatment. Eric R. Marcus. 1993. 308p. 123.00 (*0-387-97765-1*) Spr-Verlag.

Psychosis & Sexual Identity: Toward a Post-Analytic View of the Schreber Case. Ed. by David B. Allison et al. 1988. LC 87-10077. (SUNY Series, Intersections). (Illus.). 343p. pap. text 25.95 (*0-88706-617-8*) State U NY Pr.

Psychosocial Adaptation in Pregnancy: Assessment of Seven Dimensions of Maternal Development. Regina P. Lederman. 2nd rev. ed. 1996. (Illus.). 49.95 (*0-8261-6710-1*) Springer Pub.

Psychosocial Adaptation to Chronic Illness & Disability. Hanoch Livneh & Richard F. Antonak. 2000. LC 97-14138. 576p. 55.00 (*0-8342-0967-5*) PRO-ED.

Psychosocial & Public Health Impacts of New HIV Therapies. Ed. by D. G. Ostrow & S. C. Kalichman. 1999. LC 98-56536. (AIDS Prevention & Mental Health Ser.). (Illus.). 240p. (C). text 75.00 (*0-306-45973-6*, Kluwer Plenum) Kluwer Academic.

Psychosocial Approach to Alcoholism. Noble. 1984. (Substance & Alcohol Actions & Misuse Ser.). pap. 20.00 (*0-08-031611-5*, Pergamon Pr) Elsevier.

Psychosocial Approaches to Deeply Disturbed Persons. Ed. by Peter R. Breggin & E. Mark Stern. 1996. LC 96-12677. 231p. (C). 39.95 (*1-56024-841-6*) Haworth Pr.

Psychosocial Aspects of AIDS. 1997. lib. bdg. 250.95 (*0-8490-6078-8*) Gordon Pr.

Psychosocial Aspects of AIDS: A Bibliography & Sourcebook. 1996. lib. bdg. 252.75 (*0-8490-5985-2*) Gordon Pr.

Psychosocial Aspects of Cardiovascular Disease. Ed. by James Reiffel et al. 1980. LC 79-27765. 365p. 12.50 (*0-930194-32-2*) Ctr Thanatology.

Psychosocial Aspects of Chemotherapy in Cancer Care: The Patient, Family, & Staff. Ed. by Robert DeBellis et al. 1987. LC 86-33623. (Loss, Grief & Care Ser.: Vol. 1, No. 3 & 4). 136p. text 39.95 (*0-86656-627-9*) Haworth Pr.

Psychosocial Aspects of Chronic Illness & Disability among African Americans. Faye Z. Belgrave. 1998. LC 98-9635. 176p. 62.50 (*0-86569-242-4*, Auburn Hse) Greenwood.

Psychosocial Aspects of Cystic Fibrosis: A Model for Chronic Lung Disease. Ed. by Paul Patterson et al. 1973. LC 72-9893. 234p. 12.50 (*0-930194-33-0*) Ctr Thanatology.

Psychosocial Aspects of Depression. Ed. by Joseph Becker & Arthur Kleinman. 1990. 272p. (C). text 89.95 (*0-8058-0079-4*) L Erlbaum Assocs.

Psychosocial Aspects of Disability. George Henderson & Willie V. Bryan. 2nd ed. 1997. LC 96-34655. 342p. text 67.95 (*0-398-06678-7*); pap. text 51.95 (*0-398-06679-5*) C C Thomas.

Psychosocial Aspects of Disaster. Gist. 1989. LC 88-33898. (Personality Processes Ser.). 357p. 240.00 (*0-471-84894-8*) Wiley.

Psychosocial Aspects of End-Stage Renal Disease: Issues of Our Times. Mark A. Hardy et al. 1991. (Loss, Grief & Care Ser.: Vol. 5 Nos. 1 & 2). (Illus.). 216p. text 49.95 (*1-56024-149-7*) Haworth Pr.

Psychosocial Aspects of HIV & AIDS & the Evaluation of Preventive Strategies: Report on a WHO Meeting. 1991. (WHO Regional Publications, European Ser.: No. 36). 45p. pap. text 10.00 (*92-890-1127-0*) World Health.

Psychosocial Aspects of Narcolepsy. Ed. by Meeta Goswami et al. 1992. LC 92-1525. (Loss, Grief & Care Ser.: Vol. 5, Nos. 3-4). 203p. 49.95 (*1-56024-222-1*) Haworth Pr.

*__Psychosocial Aspects of Pediatric Oncology.__ Shulamith Kreitler & Myriam Arush. 2001. 300p. pap. 115.00 (*0-471-49939-0*) Wiley.

Psychosocial Aspects of Sickle Cell Disease: Past, Present, & Future Directions of Research. Ed. by Kermit B. Nash. 1994. LC 94-12367. (Journal of Health & Social Policy: Vol. 5, Nos. 3 & 4). (Illus.). 282p. 49.95 (*1-56024-578-6*) Haworth Pr.

Psychosocial Assessment in Terminal Care. David M. Dush et al. 1987. LC 86-22801. (Hospice Journal: Vol. 2, No. 3). 150p. text 39.95 (*0-86656-461-6*) Haworth Pr.

Psychosocial Care of Children & Families in HC Settings. Rosemary Bolig & Judy A. Rollins. 2001. 350p. 54.00 (*0-8342-1677-9*) Aspen Pub.

Psychosocial Components of Occupational Therapy. Anne C. Mosey. 1986. 624p. text 53.00 (*0-89004-334-5*) Lppncott W & W.

Psychosocial Development of Puerto Rican Women. Ed. by Cynthia G. Coll & Marie D. Mattei. 1989. LC 88-26047. (Illus.). 290p. 55.00 (*0-275-92345-2*, C2345, Praeger Pubs) Greenwood.

Psychosocial Dimensions of Cancer. Susan L. Groenwald. 1991. (Illus.). pap. text 19.95 (*0-86720-303-X*, 303-X) Jones & Bartlett.

Psychosocial Dimensions of Oncology Nursing Care. Ed. by Catherine Burke. 1998. LC 98-68085. 218p. pap. text 18.00 (*1-890504-06-8*) Oncology Nursing.

Psychosocial Disorders in Young People: Time Trends & Their Causes. Ed. by Michael E. Rutter & David J. Smith. 1995. LC 95-1906. (Clinical Psychology & Personality Ser.). 864p. 270.00 (*0-471-95054-8*) Wiley.

Psychosocial Disturbances in Young People: Challenges for Prevention. Ed. by Michael Rutter. 1995. (Illus.). 425p. (C). text 69.95 (*0-521-46187-1*) Cambridge U Pr.

Psychosocial Education of Nurses: The Interpersonal Dimension. Josephine Gregory. 1996. (Nursing Ser.). 320p. (*1-85972-345-4*) Avebry GBR. *Dist:* Ashgate Pub Co.

Psychosocial Effects of Screening for Disease Prevention & Detection. Robert T. Croyle. 1995. LC 94-22279. (Illus.). 232p. text 45.00 (*0-19-507556-0*) OUP.

Psychosocial Factors Affecting Health. Mack Lipkin, Jr. 1982. LC 82-11249. 374p. 78.75 (*0-275-91371-6*, C1371, Praeger Pubs) Greenwood.

Psychosocial Factors & Metabolic Control in Insulin-Dependent Diabetes Mellitus. Ulf Stenstrom. 1997. (Studia Psychologica et Paedagogica: No. 126). 102p. pap. (*91-22-01739-9*) Almqvist & Wiksell SWE. *Dist:* Coronet Bks.

Psychosocial Factors at Work & Their Relation to Health. C. L. Cooper. Ed. by R. Kalimo et al. 1987. 254p. pap. text 39.00 (*92-4-156102-5*, 1150264) World Health.

Psychosocial Intervention in HIV Disease: A Stage Focused & Culture Specific Approach. Baruch Fishman & Isiah Crawford. 1995. LC 96-14097. (Cognitive-Behavioral Therapy Ser.). 240p. 40.00 (*1-56821-825-7*) Aronson.

Psychosocial Intervention in Long-Term Care: An Advanced Guide. Gary W. Hartz & D. Michael Splain. 1997. LC 96-48819. (Illus.). 219p. 49.95 (*0-7890-0114-4*); pap. 22.95 (*0-7890-0189-6*) Haworth Pr.

Psychosocial Intervention with Aged African Americans—A Primer. James H. Carter. 2000. LC 99-93821. pap. 10.95 (*0-533-13157-X*) Vantage.

Psychosocial Interventions for Cardiopulmonary Patients. Wayne M. Sotile. 1996. LC 95-35146. (Illus.). 424p. text 39.00 (*0-87322-766-2*, BSOT0766) Human Kinetics.

Psychosocial Interventions in Patients with Cancer & Coronary Heart Disease: Examples of Field Studies & Methodological Considerations. Ed. by C. L. Mulder & E. J. De Bruin. 1993. LC 93-19354. 96p. pap. (*90-265-1349-6*) Swets.

Psychosocial Interventions with Physically Disabled Persons. Ed. by Bruce W. Heller et al. 1989. (Mind & Medicine Ser.). 336p. (C). text 38.00 (*0-8135-1423-1*); pap. text 17.00 (*0-8135-1424-X*) Rutgers U Pr.

Psychosocial Interventions with Sensorially Disabled Persons. Ed. by Bruce W. Heller et al. 1986. (Mind & Medicine Ser.: No. III). 288p. text 49.95 (*0-8089-1826-5*, 791962, Grune & Strat) Harcrt Hlth Sci Grp.

Psychosocial Issues in Day Care. Ed. by Shahla S. Chehrazi. 1990. LC 90-561. 292p. text 14.95 (*0-88048-310-5*, 8310) Am Psychiatric.

Psychosocial Issues in Health. Ramsden. 1999. (C). text (*0-7020-2230-6*) W B Saunders GBR. *Dist:* Saunders.

Psychosocial Issues in Malignant Disease: Proceedings of the First Annual Conference of the British Psychosocial Oncology Group, London, 7-8 November, 1984. Ed. by M. Watson & S. Greer. 1986. LC 85-26043. 100p. (*0-08-032010-4*) Pergamon Repr GBR. *Dist:* Franklin.

Psychosocial Issues in the Treatment of Alcoholism. Ed. by David Cook et al. 1985. LC 84-28966. (Alcoholism Treatment Quarterly Ser.: Vol. 2, No. 1). 134p. pap. text 14.95 (*0-86656-401-2*); text 39.95 (*0-86656-363-6*) Haworth Pr.

Psychosocial Nursing: Care of Physically Ill Patients & Their Families. Patricia D. Barry. 3rd ed. 1996. LC 95-40125. 624p. pap. text 34.95 (*0-397-55146-0*) Lppncott W & W.

Psychosocial Nursing Care along the Cancer Continuum. Ed. by Rose Mary Carroll-Johnson et al. 1998. LC 98-65615. (Illus.). 502p. pap. text 36.00 (*1-890504-04-1*) Oncology Nursing.

Psychosocial Nursing for General Patient Care. Linda M. Gorman et al. 2nd ed. 2002. LC 2001-47637. 448p. pap. 31.95 (*0-8036-0802-0*) Davis Co.

Psychosocial Nursing Handbook for the Nonpsychiatric Nurse. Linda Gorman et al. 1989. 304p. pap. text 26.00 (*0-683-03666-1*) Lppncott W & W.

Psychosocial Occupational Therapy: A Clinical Practice. Cara MacRae. 1997. LC 97-46388. (Teaching Methods Ser.). 688p. (C). pap. text 40.95 (*0-8273-6283-8*) Delmar.

Psychosocial Occupational Therapy: A Holistic Approach. Franklin Stein & Susan K. Cutler. 1998. LC 97-51710. (Illus.). 601p. pap. text 61.95 (*1-56593-925-5*, 1832) Thomson Learn.

Psychosocial Occupational Therapy: A Holistic Approach. Stein. 2nd ed. 2001. 650p. pap. text 55.95 (*0-7693-0032-4*) Thomson Learn.

Psychosocial Occupational Therapy: Frames of Reference for Intervention. Mary Ann Bruce & Barbara Borg. (C). 2nd ed. 1993. LC 91-52849. (Illus.). 450p. pap. 37.00 (*1-55642-203-2*); 3rd ed. 2001. 400p. pap. text 37.00 (*1-55642-494-9*) SLACK Inc.

Psychosocial Occupational Therapy: Proactive Approaches. Rita P. Cottrell. 1993. 600p. (C). pap. text 60.00 (*0-910317-96-8*) Am Occup Therapy.

Psychosocial Oncology & Palliative Care in Hong Kong: The First Decade. Ed. by Richard Fielding & Cecilia Lai-wan Chan. 2000. 298p. pap. (*962-209-503-8*) HK Univ Pr HKG. *Dist:* Intl Spec Bk, Coronet Bks.

Psychosocial Origins of Mental Retardation. Harold E. Simmons. 1980. pap. 10.00 (*0-87312-011-6*) Psychogenic Disease.

Psychosocial Perspectives on AIDS: Etiology, Prevention & Treatment. Ed. by Lydia Temoshok & Andrew Baum. 1990. 336p. 89.95 (*0-8058-0207-X*) L Erlbaum Assocs.

Psychosocial Perspectives on Donor Insemination: International Social Science Perspectives. Ed. by Ken Daniels & Erica Haimes. 1998. LC 97-40984. 197p. (C). text 54.95 (*0-521-49709-4*) Cambridge U Pr.

Psychosocial Perspectives on Health: Implications for Research & Developing Services. Ed. by David A. Hamburg & Norman Sartorius. 1989. (Illus.). 240p. (C). text 69.95 (*0-521-36352-7*) Cambridge U Pr.

Psychosocial Processes & Health: A Reader. Ed. by Andrew Steptoe & Jane Wardle. 1995. (Illus.). 537p. (C). text 125.00 (*0-521-41610-8*); pap. text 47.95 (*0-521-42618-9*) Cambridge U Pr.

Psychosocial Research on Pediatric Hospitalization & Health Care: A Review of the Literature. Richard H. Thompson. 1985. (Illus.). 364p. (C). 59.95 (*0-398-05070-8*) C C Thomas.

Psychosocial Resource Variables in Cancer Studies: Conceptual & Measurement Issues. Ed. by Barbara Curlow & Mark R. Somerfield. 1995. LC 95-23013. (Journal of Psychosocial Oncology Ser.: Vol. 13, No. 1-2). 216p. pap. 39.95 (*1-56024-758-4*, Hawrth Medical) Haworth Pr.

Psychosocial Stress. A. J. J. M. Vingerhoets. 1985. xiv, 146p. pap. (*90-265-0629-5*) Swets.

Psychosocial Stress: Perspectives on Structure, Theory, Life-Course, & Methods. Ed. by Howard B. Kaplan. 1996. LC 95-41461. (Illus.). 428p. text 59.95 (*0-12-397565-4*) Acad Pr.

Psychosocial Studies. Ed. by Phyllis Caroff & Mary Gottesfeld. 1987. LC 86-22806. 185p. text 32.50 (*0-89876-100-X*) Gardner Pr.

Psychosocial Theories of the Self. Benjamin Lee. 1982. (PATH in Psychology Ser.). 230p. 55.00 (*0-306-41117-2*, Plenum Trade) Perseus Pubng.

Psychosocial Treatments. Ed. by David Reiss. 1994. 104p. pap. 14.95 (*0-89862-298-0*, 2298) Guilford Pubns.

Psychosocial Treatments for Child & Adolescent Disorders: Empirically Based Strategies for Clinical Practice. Ed. by Euthymia D. Hibbs & Peter S. Jensen. 1996. LC 96-1003. 761p. 59.95 (*1-55798-330-5*) Am Psychol.

Psychosocial Worlds of the Adolescent: Public & Private. Vivian C. Seltzer. 1989. LC 89-5710. 336p. 185.00 (*0-471-63258-9*) Wiley.

Psychosoical Scenarios for Pediatrics. Paul V. Trad. 1987. 276p. 86.95 (*0-387-96586-6*) Spr-Verlag.

Psychosomatic Approach to Prevention of Disease: Proceedings of the 20th Annual Conference for Psychosomatic Research, London, Nov. 15-16, 1976. Annual Conference for Psychosomatic Research Staff. Ed. by M. Carruthers & R. Priest. 1978. pap. 26.00 (*0-08-022253-6*, Pergamon Pr) Elsevier.

Psychosomatic Classics: Selected Papers from Psychosomatic Medicine, 1939-1958. Psychosomatic Medicine, Editorial Committee. 1971. pap. 31.00 (*3-8055-1232-5*) S Karger.

Psychosomatic Concepts. Roy R. Grinker. 1983. LC 84-451254. 228p. 40.00 (*0-87668-698-6*) Aronson.

Psychosomatic Delusion: Why the Mind Is Not the Source of All Our Ills. Robert Dantzer. LC 93-19682. 247p. 1998. (Illus.). per. 16.00 (*0-684-86346-4*); 1993. 24.95 (*0-02-906937-8*) Free Pr.

Psychosomatic Disorders. 1964. (Technical Report Ser.: No. 275). 27p. pap. text 3.00 (*92-4-120275-0*) World Health.

Psychosomatic Disorders. B. B. Wolman. 1988. LC 88-22555. (Illus.). 326p. (C). text 57.50 (*0-306-42945-4*, Kluwer Plenum) Kluwer Academic.

Psychosomatic Disorders: A Psychological Approach to Etiology & Treatment. Ed. by Stephen N. Haynes et al. 1981. LC 81-10754. 546p. 55.50 (*0-275-90640-X*, C0640, Praeger Pubs) Greenwood.

Psychosomatic Disorders: Theoretical & Clinical Aspects, No. 7. Ghazi Asaad. 1996. (Basic Principles into Practice Ser.: Vol.67). 147p. pap. text 21.95 (*0-87630-803-5*) Brunner-Routledge.

Psychosomatic Disorders in Childhood. Melitta Sperling. 1978. LC 76-22870. 35.00 (*0-87668-274-3*) Aronson.

Psychosomatic Disorders in General Practice. Fred Kroger et al. Tr. by G. Blythe from GER. 3rd enl. rev. ed. 1992. (Illus.). 296p. 64.95 (*0-387-54556-5*) Spr-Verlag.

Psychosomatic Families: Anorexia Nervosa in Context. Salvador Minuchin et al. 1978. 351p. 40.50 (*0-674-72220-5*) HUP.

Psychosomatic Illnesses. Brian Broom. 1997. pap. (*1-85343-381-0*) Free Assoc Bks GBR. *Dist:* Intl Spec Bk, NYU Pr.

Psychosomatic Medicine: A Core Approach to Clinical Medicine. Ed. by Y. Ikemi & H. Ishikawa. 1979. (Illus.). pap. 113.25 (*3-8055-3022-6*) S Karger.

Psychosomatic Medicine: Past & Future. Ed. by G. N. Christodoulou. 1988. LC 87-29075. (Illus.). 396p. 95.00 (*0-306-42780-X*, Plenum Trade) Perseus Pubng.

Psychosomatic Medicine: Theory, Physiology, & Practice. Ed. by Stanley Cheren. 1989. (Stress & Health Ser.: No. 1-2). 1000p. 62.50 (*0-8236-5725-6*, BN#05725); 75.00 (*0-8236-5726-4*, BN#05726) Intl Univs Pr.

Psychosomatic Medicine & Contemporary Psychoanalysis. Graeme J. Taylor. 1987. LC 86-27698. (Stress & Health Ser.: No. 3). 60.00 (*0-8236-5723-X*, BN#05723) Intl Univs Pr.

Psychosomatic Medicine & Liaison Psychiatry: Selected Papers. Zbigniew J. Lipowski. 1985. LC 85-12474. (Illus.). 470p. (C). text 108.00 (*0-306-42038-4*, Kluwer Plenum) Kluwer Academic.

Psychosomatic Medicine & Logotherapy. Hiroshi Takashima. 1977. (Illus.). 91p. (Orig.). pap. 6.95 (*0-917867-03-3*) V Frankl Inst.

Psychosomatic Medicine in a Changing World: Theoretical, Clinical & Transcultural Aspects. Ed. by Adam J. Krakowski & C. P. Kimball. 1982. (Journal: Vol. 38, No. 1-4). (Illus.). 310p. pap. 115.00 (*3-8055-3544-9*) S Karger.

Psychosomatic Medicine in Obstetrics & Gynecology: Proceedings of the International Congress, 3rd, London, 1971. International Congress of Psychosomatic Obstetrics. Ed. by Norman Morris. 1972. (Illus.). 130.50 (*3-8055-1314-3*) S Karger.

Psychosomatic Medicine: New Facts & Old Controversies: Proceedings of the World Congress of the International College of Psychosomatic Medicine Held in Sydney-Australia, 9th, August-September, 1987, Pt. 1. Ed. by D. G. Byrne et al. 1988. (Journal: Vol. 47, No. 3-4, 1987). (Illus.). iv, 108p. pap. 99.25 (*3-8055-4845-1*) S Karger.

Psychosomatic Medicine: New Facts & Old Controversies: Proceedings of the World Congress of the International College of Psychosomatic Medicine Held in Sydney-Australia, 9th, August-September, 1987, Pt. II. Adam J. Krakowski. 1988. (Journal: Vol. 48, No. 1-4, 1987). (Illus.). 3p. pap. 124.50 (*3-8055-4847-8*) S Karger.

Psychosomatic Obstetrics & Gynecology. Ed. by Miriam B. Rosenthal & D. H. Smith. 1985. (Advances in Psychosomatic Medicine Ser.: Vol. 12). (Illus.). vi, 190p. 71.50 (*3-8055-3967-3*) S Karger.

Psychosomatic Research: Proceedings of the European Conference on Psychosomatic Research, 12th, Bodo, July 1978. European Conference on Psychosomatic Research Staff. Ed. by H. Freyberger. 1980. (Psychotherapy & Psychosomatics Ser.: Vol. 32, No. 1-4). (Illus.). 113.25 (*3-8055-3044-7*) S Karger.

Psychosomatic Symptoms: Psychodynamic Treatment of The Underlying Personality Disorder. Ed. by C. Philip Wilson & Ira L. Mintz. 1989. LC 88-19470. 460p. 65.00 (*0-87668-877-6*) Aronson.

Psychosomatic Syndromes & Somatic Symptoms. Robert Kellner. 1991. LC 91-4867. 260p. text 14.95 (*0-88048-110-2*, 8110) Am Psychiatric.

Psychosomatics, Bk. 1. Oluremilekun A. Oke. 1996. LC 92-96858. 200p. 15.00 (*0-533-10441-6*) Vantage.

Psychosomatics - A Challenge to Health Care: Journal: Psychotherapy & Psychosomatics. Ed. by P. Tienari & G. A. Fava. 1991. (Illus.). Pt. 1. iv, 152p. pap. 121.75 (*3-8055-5412-5*); Pt. 2. 112p. pap. 81.00 (*3-8055-5415-X*) S Karger.

Psychosomatics & Pleasure: Proceedings of the Twenty-Third Annual Conference of the Society for Psychosomatic Research Held at the Royal College of Physicians, London, 19-20 November 1979. Ed. by C. Aitken. 1981. 88p. pap. 24.00 (*0-08-026797-1*, Pergamon Pr) Elsevier.

Psychosomatics in War & Peace: Proceedings of the Society for Psychosomatic Research, 22nd, Royal College of Physicians, London, Nov. 27-28, 1978. Society for Psychosomatic Research Staff. Ed. by P. Williams. 1980. 112p. pap. 26.00 (*0-08-026064-0*, Pergamon Pr) Elsevier.

Psychosomatics, Psychoanalysis, & Inflammatory Disease of the Colon. Charles C. Hogan. 1995. (Stress & Health Ser.: Monograph 5). 312p. 46.50 (*0-8236-5732-9*) Intl Univs Pr.

Psychosomatische Medizin: Grundlagen und Anwendungsgebiete. Franz Gabriel Alexander. 4th rev. ed. 1985. (GER., Illus.). xvi, 244p. pap. text 44.65 (*3-11-010192-0*) De Gruyter.

Psychosomatische Rehabilitation und Sozialmedizin. Ed. by Dieter Olbrich & Reinhard Plassmann. 1997. (Illus.). 210p. pap. 37.95 (*3-631-31866-9*) P Lang Pubng.

Psychosoziale Aspekte in der Betreuung von Kindern und Jugendlichen mit Diabetes. Ed. by Roswitha Roth & H. M. Borkenstein. 1991. (Illus.). x, 202p. 35.00 (*3-8055-5414-1*) S Karger.

Psychotherapeutic Action of the Physician: Proceedings of the International Congress of Psychosomatic Medicine, 4th, Paris, Sept., 1970, Vol. 21, Nos. 1-6. International Congress of Psychosomatic Obstetrics. Ed. by Leon Chertok & M. Sapir. 1973. (Illus.). reprint ed. 75.00 (*3-8055-1482-4*) S Karger.

Psychotherapeutic Approaches to the Resistant Child. Richard A. Gardner. 2nd ed. 1990. LC 90-462. 408p. 60.00 (*0-87668-770-2*) Aronson.

Psychotherapeutic Conspiracy. Robert J. Langs. 1995. 356p. pap. text 50.00 (*1-56821-731-5*) Aronson.

Psychotherapeutic Instrument. Stanley L. Olinick. 1980. LC 80-620. 216p. 40.00 (*0-87668-403-7*) Aronson.

Psychotherapeutic Intervention in Hysterical Disorders. William J. Mueller & Albert S. Aniskiewicz. 1986. LC 85-15. 300p. 50.00 (*0-87668-913-6*) Aronson.

Psychotherapeutic Intervention in Schizophrenia. Lewis B. Hill. 1994. LC 94-71837. (Master Work Ser.). 224p. pap. 40.00 (*1-56821-313-1*) Aronson.

Psychotherapeutic Interventions for Adults with Brain Injury or Stroke: A Clinician's Treatment Resource. Ed. by Karen G. Langer et al. 1999. LC 99-24556. 257p. 35.00 (*1-887841-23-7*, 65433, Psychosocial) Intl Univs Pr.

Psychotherapeutic Interventions in Life-Threatening Illness. Ed. by H. Freyberger. 1980. (Advances in Psychosomatic Medicine Ser.: Vol. 10). (Illus.). xviii, 206p. 82.75 (*3-8055-3066-8*) S Karger.

Psychotherapeutic Metaphors: A Guide to Theory & Practice. Philip Barker. 1996. LC 95-20643. (Basic Principles Into Practice Ser.: Vol. 5). 176p. pap. text 21.95 (*0-87630-776-4*) Brunner-Routledge.

Psychotherapeutic Process: A Research Handbook. Ed. by Leslie S. Greenberg & William M. Pinsof. 1986. LC 85-30596. 734p. 85.00 (*0-89862-651-X*) Guilford Pubns.

Psychotherapeutic Process: Proceedings of the International Congress of Psychotherapy, 10th, Paris, July, 1976. International Congress of Psychotherapy Staff. Ed. by J. C. Benoit et al. 1978. (Psychotherapy & Psychosomatics Ser.: Vol. 29, Nos. 1-4). 123.50 (*3-8055-2762-4*) S Karger.

Psychotherapeutic Strategies in Late Latency Through Early Adolescence. Charles A. Sarnoff. 1987. LC 87-19474. 275p. 40.00 (*0-87668-937-3*) Aronson.

Psychotherapeutic Strategies in the Latency Years. Charles A. Sarnoff. 1987. LC 87-24194. 550p. 50.00 (*0-87668-936-5*) Aronson.

Psychotherapeutic Techniques of Richard A. Gardner. Richard A. Gardner. 1992. LC 86-11531. 893p. 45.00 (*0-933812-14-0*) Creative Therapeutics.

Psychotherapeutic Treatment of Cancer Patients. Intro. by Jane Goldberg. 1990. 396p. pap. text 24.95 (*0-88738-829-9*) Transaction Pubs.

Psychotherapeutics: A Symposium. Morton Prince et al. 1976. LC 75-16728. (Classics in Psychiatry Ser.). reprint ed. 19.95 (*0-405-07451-4*) Ayer.

Psychotheraphy & Multiple Personality: Selected Essays. Morton Prince. Ed. by Nathan G. Hale, Jr. 1975. LC 74-82574. 336p. 43.00 (*0-674-72225-6*) HUP.

Psychotheraphy for Borderline Personality. John F. Clarkin et al. 1998. LC 98-28270. (Illus.). 400p. 69.95 (*0-471-17042-9*, J320-Y2T) Wiley.

Psychotheraphy of Everyday Life. N. Peseschkian. 1986. (Illus.). 247p. 16.00 (*0-387-15767-0*) Spr-Verlag.

Psychotherapie - Heilkunst Oder Heilslehre? Reprint from Journal: Daseinsanalyse, Vol. 9, No. 2-3, 1992. Ed. by G. Condrau. 1992. (Illus.). 212p. reprint ed. pap. 47.00 (*3-8055-5681-0*) S Karger.

Psychotherapies with Children & Adolescents: Adapting the Psychodynamic Process. Ed. by John D. O'Brien et al. 1992. LC 91-44051. 346p. text 49.50 (*0-88048-406-3*, 8406) Am Psychiatric.

Psychotherapies with Children & Adolescents: Adapting the Psychodynamic Process. Contrib. by John D. O'Brien et al. 2000. LC 99-57474. pap. 35.00 (*0-7657-0253-3*) Aronson.

Psychotherapist: Use & Abuse of Psychological Influences. Gordon Warme. 1996. LC 95-24831. 218p. pap. 40.00 (*1-56821-736-6*) Aronson.

Psychotherapist's Book Guide. Ed. by Aronson, Jason, Inc. Staff. 1994. 208p. pap. 3.95 (*1-56821-277-1*) Aronson.

Psychotherapist's Guide to Cost Containment: How to Survive & Thrive in an Age of Managed Care. Bernard D. Beitman. 1998. LC 97-33921. 91.95 (*0-8039-7381-0*, 1379); pap. 46.95 (*0-8039-7382-9*, 1380) Sage.

Psychotherapists' Guide to Managed Care in the 21st Century: Surviving Big Brother. Sondra Tuckfelt et al. 1997. LC 96-40915. Orig. Title: How to Get Along with Big Brother. 416p. text 50.00 (*0-7657-0002-6*) Aronson.

Psychotherapist's Guide to Neuropsychiatry: Diagnostic & Treatment Issues. Ed. by James M. Ellison et al. 1994. LC 93-48516. 684p. text 82.95 (*0-88048-566-3*, 8566) Am Psychiatric.

Psychotherapist's Guide to Psychopharmacology. Michael J. Gitlin. 1990. LC 90-1734. (Illus.). 432p. 40.00 (*0-02-911781-X*) Free Pr.

Psychotherapist's Guide to Psychopharmacology. Michael J. Gitlin. 2nd ed. 1996. LC 95-43353. (Illus.). 560p. 39.95 (*0-684-82737-9*) Free Pr.

Psychotherapists in Action. Hans H. Strupp. 1960. LC 60-6020. (Illus.). 352p. text 62.00 (*0-8089-0490-6*, 794430, Grune & Strat) Harcrt Hlth Sci Grp.

Psychotherapist's Interventions: Integrating Psychodynamic Perspectives in Clinical Practice. T. Byram Karasu. 1998. LC 97-42382. 360p. 45.00 (*1-56821-689-0*) Aronson.

Psychotherapist's Resource on Psychiatric Medications: Issues of Treatment & Referral. Hebert Buelow. 2nd ed. 1999. LC 99-33331. 192p. pap. text 47.95 (*0-534-35703-2*) Thomson Learn.

Psychotherapists' Sexual Involvement with Clients: Intervention & Prevention. Gary R. Schoener et al. 1989. (Illus.). 850p. (C). lib. bdg. 69.95 (*0-9624337-0-5*) Walk-In Counseling.

Psychotherapy. Simon and Schuster Staff. 1994. LC 94-1141. 248p. 72.50 (*0-275-94690-8*, Praeger Pubs) Greenwood.

Psychotherapy. Marie-Louise Von Franz. 1993. LC 92-56454. (C. G. Jung Foundation Bks.). 312p. pap. 20.00 (*0-87773-879-3*) Shambhala Pubns.

Psychotherapy: A Basic Text. Robert J. Langs. 1982. LC 81-17663. 800p. 70.00 (*0-87668-466-5*) Aronson.

Psychotherapy: An Eclectic-Integrative Approach. Sol L. Garfield. 2nd ed. 1995. LC 94-38838. (Personality Processes Ser.). 290p. 45.00 (*0-471-59556-X*) Wiley.

Psychotherapy: An Erotic Relationship. David Mann. 1997. LC 96-27225. 224p. (C). 80.00 (*0-415-14851-0*); pap. 27.99 (*0-415-14852-9*) Routledge.

Psychotherapy: Impact on Psychoanalytic Training. Ed. by Edward D. Joseph & Robert S. Wallerstein. 1983. LC 82-12719. xvi, 174p. 40.00 (*0-8236-5405-2*) Intl Univs Pr.

Psychotherapy: Processes & Techniques. Christiane Brems. 1998. LC 98-13488. 352p. 73.00 (*0-205-27532-X*) Allyn.

Psychotherapy: The Analytic Approach. Ed. by Morton J. Aronson & Melvin A. Scharfman. 1992. LC 92-10540. 400p. 60.00 (*0-87668-508-4*) Aronson.

Psychotherapy: The Art of Wooing Nature. Sheldon Roth. 1987. LC 86-28763. 304p. pap. 35.00 (*0-87668-945-4*) Aronson.

Psychotherapy: The Mystery Solved. Charles W. Patterson. (Orig.). 1984. LC 84-61941. 118p. pap. 8.00 (*0-9614334-1-8*); 2nd ed. 1995. LC 95-68732. 187p. pap. text 17.95 (*0-9614334-3-4*) Passages.

Psychotherapy: The Purchase of Friendship. William Schofield. 1986. 212p. reprint ed. pap. text 24.95 (*0-88738-659-8*) Transaction Pubs.

Psychotherapy Abbreviation: A Practical Guide. Gene Pekarik. 1996. LC 95-42382. (Illus.). 191p. 39.95 (*1-56024-934-X*) Haworth Pr.

Psychotherapy, Adolescents, & Self-Psychology. Gustavo A. Lage & Harvey K. Nathan. 1991. LC 90-4924. 500p. 67.50 (*0-8236-5403-6*) Intl Univs Pr.

Psychotherapy after Kohut: A Textbook of Self Psychology. Ronald R. Lee & J. Colby Martin. 1991. 352p. 45.00 (*0-88163-129-9*) Analytic Pr.

Psychotherapy & a Christian View of Man. David E. Roberts. 1990. LC 88-21391. 162p. reprint ed. lib. bdg. 57.50 (*0-313-25326-9*, RPSY, Greenwood Pr) Greenwood.

Psychotherapy & AIDS: The Human Dimension. Lucy A. Wicks. 1997. LC 97-1721. (*1-56032-617-4*); pap. (*1-56032-618-2*) Hemisp Pub.

Psychotherapy & Behavior Change: Social, Cultural & Methodological Perspectives. H. N. Higginbotham et al. 1988. (General Psychology Ser.: No. 152). 416p. text 60.00 (*0-08-028089-7*); pap. text 25.00 (*0-08-028088-9*) Elsevier (Pergamon Pr).

Psychotherapy & Buddhism: Toward an Integration. Jeffrey B. Rubin. 1996. LC 96-34822. (Issues in the Practice of Psychology Ser.). (Illus.). 197p. (C). 47.00 (*0-306-45441-6*, Plenum Trade) Perseus Pubng.

Psychotherapy & Character Structure: How to Recognize & Treat Particular Character Types. Mary Ahern & Abraham J. Malerstein. 1993. 260p. (C). text 22.50 (*0-9644089-2-9*) Cole Valley Pr.

Psychotherapy & Confidentiality: Testimonial Privileged Communication, Breach of Confidentiality, & Reporting Duties. Ralph Slovenko. 1998. LC 97-39505. (Illus.). 660p. text 83.95 (*0-398-06827-5*) C C Thomas.

Psychotherapy & Counseling in the Treatment of Drug Abuse. 1993. lib. bdg. 254.95 (*0-8490-8500-4*); 1992. lib. bdg. 75.00 (*0-8490-8820-8*) Gordon Pr.

Psychotherapy & Counseling with Minorities: A Cognitive Approach to Individual & Cultural Differences. M. Ramirez, III. 1991. (Psychology Practitioner Guidebooks Ser.). 208p. text (*0-08-036443-8*); pap. text (*0-08-036442-X*) PPI GBR. *Dist:* Elsevier.

***Psychotherapy & Counselling in Practice.** Digby Tantam. 2001. LC 2001-35261. 240p. pap. text 28.95 (*0-521-47963-0*) Cambridge U Pr.

Psychotherapy & Its Discontents. Ed. by Wendy Dryden & Colin Feltham. 1992. 256p. (*0-335-09678-6*); pap. (*0-335-09677-8*) OpUniv Pr.

Psychotherapy & Managed Care: Reconciling Research & Reality. Catherine H. Chambliss. 1999. LC 98-56528. 368p. (C). 39.00 (*0-205-27950-3*) Allyn.

Psychotherapy & Medication: A Dynamic Integration. Ed. by Meri Schachter. 1993. LC 92-49162. 352p. 65.00 (*0-87668-296-4*) Aronson.

Psychotherapy & Mental Handicap. Alexis Waitman & Suzanne Conboy-Hill. 1991. LC 91-51055. 224p. (C). pap. 27.95 (*0-8039-8373-5*, 9930) Sage.

Psychotherapy & Process: The Fundamentals of an Existential-Humanistic Approach. James F. Bugental. 1978. 163p. (C). pap. text 28.25 net. (*0-07-554827-5*) McGraw.

Psychotherapy & Psychoanalysis: Theory, Practice, Research. Robert S. Wallerstein. 1975. LC 73-16854. 400p. (C). 70.00 (*0-8236-5410-9*) Intl Univs Pr.

Psychotherapy & Substance Abuse: A Practitioner's Handbook. Ed. by Arnold M. Washton. LC 95-183. (Substance Abuse Ser.). 500p. 1996. pap. 27.00 (*1-57230-202-X*, C0202); 1995. 46.95 (*0-89862-838-5*) Guilford Pubns.

Psychotherapy & the Abrasive Patient. Ed. by E. Mark Stern. 1984. LC 84-6644. (Psychotherapy Patient Ser.: Vol. 1, No. 1). 140p. text 4.95 (*0-86656-325-3*) Haworth Pr.

Psychotherapy & the Behavioral Sciences. Lewis R. Wolberg. 1966. LC 66-78287. 206p. text 59.00 (*0-8089-0535-X*, 794869, Grune & Strat) Harcrt Hlth Sci Grp.

Psychotherapy & the Bored Patient. Ed. by E. Mark Stern. 1988. LC 87-31085. (Psychotherapy Patient Ser.: Vol. 3, Nos. 3-4). (Illus.). 164p. text 39.95 (*0-86656-641-4*) Haworth Pr.

Psychotherapy & the Confrontation Problem-Solving Technique. Harry H. Garner. 1971. LC 74-110426. 362p. 18.50 (*0-87527-011-5*) Green.

Psychotherapy & the Creative Patient. Ed. by E. Mark Stern. 1988. LC 88-2694. (Psychotherapy Patient Ser.: Vol. 4, No. 1). (Illus.). 174p. text 39.95 (*0-86656-642-2*); pap. text 19.95 (*0-86656-831-X*) Haworth Pr.

Psychotherapy & the Dangerous Patient. Ed. by E. Mark Stern & Jerome A. Travers. 1995. LC 94-44247. (Psychotherapy Patient Ser.). (Illus.). 219p. 39.95 (*1-56024-719-3*) Haworth Pr.

Psychotherapy & the Grandiose Patient. Frwd. by E. Mark Stern. 1989. LC 89-24438. (Psychotherapy Patient Ser.: Vol. 5, Nos. 3-4). (Illus.). 205p. text 6.95 (*0-86656-946-4*) Haworth Pr.

Psychotherapy & the Grieving Patient. Ed. by E. Mark Stern. 1986. (Psychotherapy Patient Ser.: Vol. 2, No. 1). 138p. LC 85-17618. text 4.95 (*0-86656-514-0*); LC 85-17619. reprint ed. pap. text 29.95 (*0-918393-24-8*, Harrington Park) Haworth Pr.

Psychotherapy & the Law. Ed. by Louis Everstine & Diana Sullivan-Everstine. 1986. 288p. text 38.00 (*0-8089-1780-3*, 791172, Grune & Strat) Harcrt Hlth Sci Grp.

PQR

Psychotherapy & the Lonely Patient. Ed. by Samuel M. Natale. 1986. (Psychotherapy Patient Ser.: Vol. 2, No. 3). 120p. LC 86-12108. (C). text 3.95 (*0-86656-517-5*); LC 86-12101. reprint ed. pap. 29.95 (*0-918393-26-4*, Harrington Park) Haworth Pr.

Psychotherapy & the Memorable Patient. Ed. by William Kir-Stimon & Mark Stern. 1986. LC 86-25648. (Psychotherapy Patient Ser.: Vol. 2, No. 4). 152p. text 4.95 (*0-86656-516-7*) Haworth Pr.

Psychotherapy & the Memorable Patient. William Kir-Stimon. 1986. LC 86-22852. (Psychotherapy Patient Ser.: Vol. 2, No. 4). 152p. (C). reprint ed. pap. 29.95 (*0-918393-25-6*, Harrington Park) Haworth Pr.

Psychotherapy & the Paranoid Process. William W. Meissner. 1994. LC 85-15614. 432p. 60.00 (*0-87668-752-4*) Aronson.

Psychotherapy & the Poverty Patient. Intro. by E. Mark Stern. 1991. (Psychotherapy Patient Ser.). 198p. text 39.95 (*1-56024-066-0*) Haworth Pr.

Psychotherapy & the Promiscuous Patient. Intro. by E. Mark Stern. LC 92-49176. (Psychotherapy Patient Ser.: Vol. 8, Nos. 1-2). (Illus.). 192p. 1993. pap. text 14.95 (*1-56024-317-1*); 1992. lib. bdg. 39.95 (*1-56024-316-3*) Haworth Pr.

Psychotherapy & the Religiously Committed Patient. Ed. by E. Mark Stern. 1985. LC 84-25276. (Psychotherapy Patient Ser.: Vol. 1, No. 3). 158p. text 4.95 (*0-86656-394-6*); pap. text 19.95 (*0-86656-396-2*) Haworth Pr.

Psychotherapy & the Remorseful Patient. Ed. by E. Mark Stern. 1989. 330p. 49.95 (*0-86656-755-0*) Haworth Pr.

Psychotherapy & the Remote Patient. Intro. by Jerome A. Travers. 1990. LC 89-26686. (Psychotherapy Patient Ser.: Vol. 6, Nos. 1-2). (Illus.). 280p. text 39.95 (*0-86656-971-5*) Haworth Pr.

Psychotherapy & the Sacred: Religious Experience & Religious Resources in Psychotherapy. C. Michael Smith. 1995. LC 92-74688. (Studies in Religion, Society & Personality). 201p. text 32.95 (*0-913348-28-7*) Ctr Sci Study.

Psychotherapy & the Self-Contained Patient. Ed. by E. Mark Stern. 1989. LC 88-37929. (Psychotherapy Patient Ser.: Vol. 4, Nos. 3-4). (Illus.). 360p. text 6.95 (*0-86656-754-2*) Haworth Pr.

Psychotherapy & the Self-Less Patient. Ed. by Jerome A. Travers. 1986. LC 85-24817. (Psychotherapy Patient Ser.: Vol. 2, No. 2). 109p. text 3.95 (*0-86656-515-9*) Haworth Pr.

Psychotherapy & the Self-Righteous Patient. Ed. by E. Mark Stern & Jerome A. Travers. 1991. LC 91-17950. (Psychotherapy Patient Ser.). 168p. lib. bdg. 5.95 (*1-56024-169-1*) Haworth Pr.

Psychotherapy & the Selfless. Jerome A. Travers. 1986. pap. 14.95 (*0-918393-27-2*, Harrington Park) Haworth Pr.

Psychotherapy & the Somatizing Patient. Ed. by E. Mark Stern & Virginia F. Stern. 1989. LC 88-16476. (Psychotherapy Patient Ser.: Vol. 4, No. 2). 208p. text 6.95 (*0-86656-753-4*) Haworth Pr.

Psychotherapy & the Terrorized Patient. Ed. by E. Mark Stern. 1985. LC 85-8468. (Psychotherapy Patient Ser.: Vol. 1, No. 4). 116p. text 3.95 (*0-86656-442-X*) Haworth Pr.

Psychotherapy & the Uncommitted Patient. Ed. by Jerome A. Travers & E. Mark Stern. 1985. LC 84-19754. (Psychotherapy Patient Ser.: Vol. 1, No. 2). 105p. text 3.95 (*0-86656-371-7*) Haworth Pr.

Psychotherapy & the Widowed Patient. E. Mark Stern. 1990. LC 90-4502. (Psychotherapy Patient Ser.: Vol. 6, Nos. 3-4). 257p. text 39.95 (*1-56024-016-4*) Haworth Pr.

Psychotherapy As a Mutual Process. J. Marvin Spiegelman. 1996. LC 96-164991. 208p. pap. 14.95 (*1-56184-063-7*) New Falcon Pubns.

Psychotherapy As a Personal Relationship. Valerian J. Derlega et al. 1991. LC 90-3997. 227p. 31.50 (*0-89862-554-8*) Guilford Pubns.

Psychotherapy As If Life Really Mattered. Christopher A. Anderson. 1995. LC 95-76211. (Illus.). 147p. (Orig.). pap. 12.00 (*0-931353-39-4*) Andersons Pubns.

Psychotherapy by Reciprocal Inhibition. Joseph Wolpe. 1958. xiv, 239p. 32.50 (*0-8047-0509-7*) Stanford U Pr.

Psychotherapy by Structured Learning Theory. Raymond B. Cattell. 1987. (Illus.). 192p. 37.95 (*0-8261-5080-2*) Springer Pub.

Psychotherapy, Counselling & Primary Mental Health Care: Assessment for Brief or Longer-Term Treatment. Mary Burton. 1998. LC 98-13952. 270p. 125.00 (*0-471-97657-1*); pap. 65.00 (*0-471-98228-8*) Wiley.

Psychotherapy Documentation Primer. Donald E. Wiger. 1998. LC 98-18229. (Practice Planners Ser.). (Illus.). 224p. pap. 45.00 (*0-471-28990-6*) Wiley.

Psychotherapy East & West: A Unifying Paradigm. Swami Ajaya. 1984. LC 83-22608. (Illus.). 340p. pap. 15.95 (*0-89389-087-1*) Himalayan Inst.

Psychotherapy for Depression. Byram Karasu. 1990. LC 90-1103. 200p. 40.00 (*0-87668-691-9*) Aronson.

Psychotherapy for Mothers & Infants: Interventions for Dyads at Risk. Eva R. G. Gochman. 1995. LC 94-24215. 160p. 62.50 (*0-275-94927-3*, Praeger Pubs) Greenwood.

Psychotherapy for Women: Treatment Toward Equality. Edna I. Rawlings & Dianne K. Carter. 1977. (Illus.). 500p. text 77.95 (*0-398-03584-9*) C C Thomas.

Psychotherapy Grounded in the Feminine Principle. Barbara S. Sullivan. 1989. LC 89-9713. (Illus.). 224p. (Orig.). pap. 24.95 (*0-933029-43-8*) Chiron Pubns.

Psychotherapy in a New Key: A Guide to Time-Limited Dynamic Psychotherapy. Hans H. Strupp & Jeffrey L. Binder. 1985. LC 83-46075. 352p. pap. 49.00 (*0-465-06747-6*) Basic.

Psychotherapy in a Religious Framework: Spirituality in the Emotional Healing Process. Rebecca L. Propst. 1987. LC 86-27582. 209p. 38.95 (*0-89885-350-8*, Kluwer Acad Hman Sci) Kluwer Academic.

Psychotherapy in Independent Practice: Current Issues for Clinicians. Ed. by Robert D. Weitz. 1992. LC 92-1537. (Psychotherapy in Private Practice Ser.). (Illus.). 207p. text 39.95 (*1-56024-232-9*) Haworth Pr.

Psychotherapy in Managed Health Care: The Optimal Use of Time & Resources. Ed. by Carol S. Austad & William H. Berman. 1991. 285p. pap. text 19.95 (*1-55798-314-3*) Am Psychol.

Psychotherapy in Practice: A Life in the Mind. Jennifer Stein & Samuel Stein. 1999. LC 99-22362. 368p. pap. (*0-7506-3002-7*) E A GBR. *Dist:* OUP.

Psychotherapy in the Community: A Psychoanalytically Based Guide to the Treatment of the Adult. Eric Lager & Isreal Zwerling. Ed. by Alvin F. Gardner. 1983. (Allied Health Professions Monograph). 208p. (C). 22.50 (*0-87527-315-7*) Green.

Psychotherapy Indications & Outcomes. Ed. by David S. Janowsky. 1999. LC 98-43413. (American Psychopathological Association Ser.). 416p. 51.95 (*0-88048-761-5*, 8761) Am Psychiatric.

Psychotherapy Insight & Style: The Existential Moment. Len Bergantino. 1986. LC 86-71119. 288p. 45.00 (*0-87668-906-3*) Aronson.

Psychotherapy Isn't What You Think: Bringing the Psychotherapeutic Engagement into the Living Moment. James F. Bugental. 1999. LC 98-41823. xix, 278p. 38.95 (*1-891944-13-4*) Zeig Tucker Theisen.

Psychotherapy Maze: A Consumer's Guide to Getting in & Out of Therapy. Otto Ehrenberg & Miriam Ehrenberg. rev. ed. 1986. LC 86-28748. 240p. 30.00 (*0-87668-959-4*) Aronson.

Psychotherapy of Abused & Neglected Children. John W. Pearce & Terry D. Pezzot-Pearce. 1997. LC 96-43650. 368p. text 40.00 (*1-57230-163-5*, 0163) Guilford Pubns.

Psychotherapy of Antisocial Behavior & Depression in Adolescence. Richard A. Gardner. 1999. 9176p. pap. 22.00 (*0-7657-0208-8*) Aronson.

Psychotherapy of Carl Rogers: Cases & Commentary. Ed. by Barry A. Farber et al. 1998. 383p. pap. 24.00 (*1-57230-377-8*, C0377) Guilford Pubns.

Psychotherapy of Cocaine Addiction: Entering the Interpersonal World of the Cocaine Addict. David Mark & Jeffrey Faude. 1997. LC 97-6518. 288p. 50.00 (*0-7657-0072-7*) Aronson.

*__Psychotherapy of Difficult Cases.__ Arnold W. Rachman. 2001. 348p. pap. (*1-887841-40-7*, Psychosocial) Intl Univs Pr.

Psychotherapy of Everyday Life. Peter Lomas. 1993. LC 92-456. 168p. (C). pap. text 24.95 (*1-56000-629-3*) Transaction Pubs.

Psychotherapy of Preoedipal Conditions. Hyman Spotnitz. 1987. LC 75-37489. 448p. 65.00 (*0-87668-242-5*) Aronson.

Psychotherapy of Schizophrenia. Gaetano Benedetti. 1996. 274p. pap. 50.00 (*1-56821-756-0*) Aronson.

Psychotherapy of Schizophrenia: Effective Clinical Approaches - Controversies, Critiques & Recommendations. Ed. by Gaetano Benedetti & Pier Furlan. 1993. LC 91-20852. (Illus.). 429p. text 39.90 (*0-88937-077-X*) Hogrefe & Huber Pubs.

Psychotherapy of Sexually Abused Children & Their Families. William N. Friedrich. 1990. 318p. 34.95 (*0-393-70079-8*) Norton.

Psychotherapy of the Adolescent: At Different Levels of Psychiatric Practice with Special Emphasis on the Role of the School. Ed. by Benjamin H. Balser. 1959. LC 57-9326. 270p. (Orig.). reprint ed. pap. 24.95 (*0-8236-8249-8*, 225400) Intl Univs Pr.

Psychotherapy of the Borderline Adult: A Developmental Approach. James F. Masterson. 1988. LC 76-16564. 377p. text 38.95 (*0-87630-127-8*) Brunner-Routledge.

Psychotherapy of the Brain-Injured Patient: Reclaiming the Shattered Self. Laurence Miller. 1993. LC 92-48297. 256p. (C). 29.95 (*0-393-70158-1*) Norton.

Psychotherapy of the Disorders of the Self: The Masterson Approach. Ed. by James F. Masterson & Ralph Klein. 1988. LC 88-19341. 480p. text 45.95 (*0-87630-533-8*) Brunner-Routledge.

Psychotherapy of the Elderly Self. Hyman L. Muslin. 1992. LC 91-43419. 240p. text 31.95 (*0-87630-657-1*) Brunner-Routledge.

Psychotherapy of the Quiet Borderline Patient: The As-If Personality Revisited. Vance R. Sherwood & Charles P. Cohen. 1994. LC 93-46522. 320p. 50.00 (*1-56821-060-4*) Aronson.

Psychotherapy of the Religious Patient. Ed. by Moshe H. Spero. 1996. LC 96-10343. 256p. pap. 50.00 (*1-56821-811-7*) Aronson.

Psychotherapy of the Submerged Personality. Ed. by Alexander Wolf & Irwin L. Kutash. 1991. LC 90-1234. 304p. 50.00 (*0-87668-644-7*) Aronson.

Psychotherapy Process Research: Paradigmatic & Narrative Approaches. Shake G. Toukmanian & David L. Rennie. 1992. LC 92-12391. (Focus Editions Ser.: Vol. 143). 320p. (C). 86.95 (*0-8039-4354-7*, 8095); (Illus.). pap. 38.95 (*0-8039-4355-5*, 8096) Sage.

Psychotherapy, Psychological Treatments & the Addictions. Ed. by Griffith Edwards & Christopher Dare. 1996. (Illus.). 284p. (C). pap. text 28.95 (*0-521-55675-9*); text 80.00 (*0-521-55357-1*) Cambridge U Pr.

Psychotherapy Relationship Theory, Research, & Practice. Charles J. Gelso & Jeffrey A. Hayes. 1998. LC 98-10212. 304p. 60.00 (*0-471-12720-5*) Wiley.

Psychotherapy Research: An International Review of Programmatic Studies. Ed. by Larry E. Beutler & Marjorie Crago. 1991. 334p. pap. 19.95 (*1-55798-090-X*) Am Psychol.

Psychotherapy Revised: New Frontiers in Research & Practice. E. Lakin Phillips. 1985. 264p. (C). text 49.95 (*0-89859-571-1*) L Erlbaum Assocs.

Psychotherapy Through Imagery. Joseph E. Shorr. 1994. LC 82-51144. 476p. pap. 35.00 (*1-56474-121-4*) Fithian Pr.

Psychotherapy to Go: 14 Mind-Expanding Comedies & Dramas That Have Nothing at All to Do with Sigmund Freud. Steve Trott. 1997. LC 97-173140. (Drama Topics Ser.). pap. 16.99 (*0-8341-9602-6*) Lillenas.

Psychotherapy Tradecraft: The Technique & Style of Doing Therapy. Theodore H. Blau. 1988. LC 87-21786. 328p. text 38.95 (*0-87630-479-X*) Brunner-Routledge.

Psychotherapy Training: Contextual & Developmental Influences in Settings, Stages & Mind Sets. Thomas H. Peake & John D. Ball. 1991. (Clinical Supervisor Ser.). (Illus.). 230p. text 6.95 (*1-56024-133-0*); pap. text 19.95 (*1-56024-134-9*) Haworth Pr.

Psychotherapy with Adolescent Girls. D. Lamb. 2nd ed. 1986. LC 86-12211. (Illus.). 278p. (C). 54.50 (*0-306-42242-5*, Plenum Trade) Perseus Pubng.

Psychotherapy with Adolescents. Richard A. Gardner. 1988. LC 88-20280. xxvi, 806p. 45.00 (*0-933812-18-3*) Creative Therapeutics.

Psychotherapy with African American Women: Innovations in Psychodynamic Perspectives & Practice. Ed. by Leslie C. Jackson & Beverly Greene. 2000. LC 00-30870. 298p. 36.00 (*1-57230-585-1*, 8R0585) Guilford Pubns.

Psychotherapy with Children. Richard A. Gardner. 1993. LC 93-708. 360p. reprint ed. pap. 40.00 (*1-56821-030-2*) Aronson.

Psychotherapy with Couples: Theory & Practice at the Tavistock Institute of Marital Studies. Ed. by Stanley Ruszczynski. 1993. LC 93-41900. 256p. pap. text (*1-85575-045-7*) Karnac Bks GBR. *Dist:* Other Pr LLC.

Psychotherapy with Deaf & Hard of Hearing Persons: A Systemic Model. Michael A. Harvey. 1989. 288p. 59.95 (*0-8058-0204-5*) L Erlbaum Assocs.

Psychotherapy with Deaf Clients from Diverse Groups. Ed. by Irene W. Leigh. 1999. LC 99-40434. (Illus.). xxiii, 384p. 65.00 (*1-56368-083-1*) Gallaudet Univ Pr.

Psychotherapy with High-Risk Clients: Legal & Professional Standards. Richard L. Bednar et al. 1991. 226p. (C). text 45.95 (*0-534-15408-5*) Brooks-Cole.

Psychotherapy with Impossible Cases: The Efficient Treatment of Therapy Veterans. Barry L. Duncan et al. 1997. LC 96-35581. 256p. (C). 35.00 (*0-393-70246-4*) Norton.

Psychotherapy with Lesbian Clients: Theory into Practice. Kristine L. Falco. 1991. LC 90-15083. 208p. text 30.95 (*0-87630-622-9*) Brunner-Routledge.

Psychotherapy with Older Adults. Bob G. Knight. 1996. LC 95-50151. (Illus.). 192p. 74.95 (*0-8039-5401-8*, 3707); 2nd ed. pap. 39.95 (*0-8039-5402-6*, 3708) Sage.

Psychotherapy with Priests, Protestant Clergy & Catholic Religious: A Practical Guide. Joseph W. Ciarrocchi & Robert J. Wicks. 2000. LC 99-88813. (Illus.). 211p. 40.00 (*1-887841-22-9*, 65430, Psychosocial) Intl Univs Pr.

Psychotherapy with Psychotherapists. Ed. by Florence W. Kaslow. 1994. LC 94-72278. 218p. pap. 45.00 (*1-56821-326-3*) Aronson.

Psychotherapy with Psychotherapists. Florence W. Kaslow. 1984. LC 83-18655. 202p. text 39.95 (*0-86656-207-9*) Haworth Pr.

Psychotherapy with Schizophrenics. Ed. by Eugene B. Brody & Frederick C. Redlich. 1964. (Monograph Series on Schizophrenia: No. 3). 246p. (Orig.). 35.00 (*0-8236-5420-6*) Intl Univs Pr.

Psychotherapy with Severely Deprived Children. Ed. by Mary Boston & Rolene Szur. 1990. 158p. reprint ed. pap. text (*0-946439-97-4*) Karnac Bks GBR. *Dist:* Other Pr LLC.

Psychotherapy with Severely Deprived Children. Ed. by Mary Boston & Rolene Szur. 1983. 176p. pap. 11.95 (*0-7100-9536-8*, Routledge Thoemms) Routledge.

Psychotherapy with Sex-Abuse Victims: True, False, & Hysterical. Richard A. Gardner. 1996. LC 95-47817. (Dr. Richard A. Gardner's Books on Psychology & Psychiatry). xxiii, 512p. pap. 40.00 (*0-933812-41-8*) Creative Therapeutics.

Psychotherapy with Sexually Abused Boys: An Integrated Approach, Vol. IV. William N. Friedrich. 1995. LC 95-3736. (Interpersonal Violence Ser.: Vol. 12). (Illus.). 249p. 79.95 (*0-8039-5694-0*, 4893); 264p. pap. 31.95 (*0-8039-5695-9*, 4894) Sage.

Psychotherapy with the Arab Patient. Kutaiba S. Chaleby & John C. Racy. 1999. LC 98-89893. pap. 25.00 (*0-9669830-0-9*) Q S O V.

Psychotherapy with the Elderly: Becoming Methuselah's Echo. George Bouklas. 1997. LC 96-46668. 392p. 60.00 (*0-7657-0051-4*) Aronson.

Psychotherapy Workbook: A Home-Study Guide for Growth & Change. Kathleen Cairns. 1997. 255p. pap. 19.95 (*1-891409-00-X*) Life Goes On.

Psychotic: Aspects of the Personality. David Rosenfeld. 1991. 336p. pap. text (*0-946439-96-6*) Karnac Bks GBR. *Dist:* Other Pr LLC.

Psychotic Conflict & Reality. Edith Jacobson. 1967. LC 67-29736. (New York Psychoanalytic Institute Freud Anniversary Lecture Ser.). 80p. 27.50 (*0-8236-5680-2*) Intl Univs Pr.

Psychotic Core. Michael Eigen. 1986. LC 85-3956. 387p. 50.00 (*0-87668-895-4*) Aronson.

Psychotic Disorders in Children & Adolescents. Robert L. Findling. 2000. LC 00-9512. (Developmental Clinical Psychology & Psychiatry Ser.). pap. 26.95 (*0-7619-2237-7*, 85706) Sage.

Psychotic Disorders in Children & Adolescents. Robert L. Findling & Charles Schulz. 2000. LC 00-9512. 49.95 (*0-7619-2019-6*, 85705) Sage.

Psychotic Patient: Medication & Psychotherapy. David Greenfield. 1994. LC 94-72516. (Master Work Ser.). 206p. pap. text 40.00 (*1-56821-343-3*) Aronson.

Psychotic Process. John Frosch. 1983. LC 82-21392. xiii, 521p. 77.50 (*0-8236-5690-X*) Intl Univs Pr.

Psychotic States in Children. Margaret Rustin. 1998. LC 97-50306. (Tavistock Clinic Ser.). 304p. (C). 85.00 (*0-415-92082-5*); pap. 25.95 (*0-415-92083-3*) Routledge.

Psychotrauma. Ed. by W. S. De Loos & W. Op den Velde. 1992. (Psychotherapy & Psychosomatics Ser.: Vol. 57, No. 4, 1992). (Illus.). iv, 72p. pap. 22.75 (*3-8055-5662-4*) S Karger.

Psychotraumatology: Key Papers & Core Concepts in Post-Traumatic Stress. Ed. by George S. Everly, Jr. & J. M. Lating. 1994. (Plenum Series on Stress & Coping). (Illus.). 440p. (C). pap. text 65.00 (*0-306-44783-5*, Kluwer Plenum) Kluwer Academic.

Psychotrends: What Sort of People Are We Becoming? Shervert Frazier. 1994. LC 93-35897. 272p. 23.00 (*0-671-75159-X*) S&S Trade.

Psychotronics: A Primer on Instruments Using Variable Capacity Tuning. Ed. & Intro. by Peter J. Kelly. rev. ed. 1986. 106p. pap. text 15.00 (*0-943975-01-8*) Interdimens Sci.

Psychotropic Agents: Part I, Antipsychotics & Antidepressants. Ed. by G. Stille & F. Hoffmeister. 1980. (Handbook of Experimental Pharmacology Ser.: Vol. 55, Pt. 1). (Illus.). 734p. 256.00 (*0-387-09858-5*) Spr-Verlag.

Psychotropic Drug Development: Social, Economic & Pharmacological Aspects. D. Healy. 1995. (Illus.). 128p. (*0-412-71220-2*) E A GBR. *Dist:* OUP.

Psychotropic Drug Handbook. Paul J. Perry et al. 7th ed. 1997. LC 96-26095. 757p. spiral bd. 44.50 (*0-88048-851-4*, 8851) Am Psychiatric.

Psychotropic Drug Handbook. Paul J. Perry et al. 6th ed. 1991. LC 90-71835. (Illus.). vi, 358p. pap. text 4.00 (*0-929375-06-8*) H W Bks.

Psychotropic Drug Use in the Medically Ill. Ed. by P. Silver. 1994. (Advances in Psychosomatic Medicine Ser.: Vol. 21). (Illus.). viii, 170p. 107.00 (*3-8055-5969-0*) S Karger.

Psychotropic Drugs. Norman L. Keltner & David G. Folks. 2nd ed. 1996. LC 96-10647. (Illus.). 624p. (C). (gr. 13). pap. text 32.95 (*0-8151-4968-9*, 28187); 3rd ed. 2000. LC 00-45565. 638p. pap. text 32.95 (*0-323-01003-2*) Mosby Inc.

Psychotropic Drugs: Fast Facts. Jerrold S. Maxmen & Nicholas G. Ward. 2nd ed. 1995. LC 95-32578. 320p. pap. 35.00 (*0-393-70181-6*) Norton.

Psychotropic Drugs: Fast Facts. Maxmen et al. 3rd ed. 1999. (Professional Book Ser.). 480p. 45.00 (*0-393-70301-0*) Norton.

Psychotropic Drugs: Understanding Adverse Reactions. F. Gary Mears. 1999. 352p. 42.00 (*0-393-70284-7*) Norton.

Psychotropic Drugs & Nursing Intervention. Patricia Irons. 1978. (Illus.). text 20.95 (*0-07-032052-7*) McGraw.

Psychotropic Drugs & the Human EEG. Ed. by M. Itil Turan et al. 1974. (Modern Problems of Pharmacopsychiatry Ser.: Vol. 8). (Illus.). 300p. 130.50 (*3-8055-1419-0*) S Karger.

Psychotropic Drugs in Psychiatry. Michael Shepherd. 1979. LC 77-17731. (Psychotropic Drugs in Psychiatry C Ser.). 288p. 30.00 (*0-87668-273-5*) Aronson.

Psychotropic Drugs of Abuse. D. J. K. Balfour. 1990. (International Encyclopedia of Pharmacology & Therapeutics Ser.). (Illus.). 384p. 203.00 (*0-08-036851-4*, Pergamon Pr) Elsevier.

Psychotropic Medication Compliance by Elders. David A. Smith. 1995. (Geriatric Psychopathology Ser.). (Orig.). pap. text 29.95 (*1-884937-30-6*) Manisses Communs.

Psychotropic Medications Pt. II: A Desktop Reference for Mental Health Practitioners. Ed. by John J. Sramek et al. 2nd ed. 1997. 400p. ring bd. 149.00 (*1-884937-45-4*) Manisses Communs.

Psychotropic Substances: Assessments of Medical & Scientific Requirements for Substances in Schedules II, III & IV. Requirement of Import Authorization for Substances in Schedules III & IV. International Narcotics Board Staff. 252p. 40.00 (*92-1-048062-7*) UN.

Psychotropic Substances in Europe: Trends in Licit Use. 1990. 76p. 12.00 (*92-1-148081-7*, 90.XI.2) UN.

Psychovenereology: Personality & Lifestyle Factors in Sexually Transmitted Diseases in Homosexual Men. 3. Michael W. Ross. 1986. LC 85-25683. (Sexual Medicine Ser.). 258p. 55.00 (*0-275-92122-0*, C2122, Praeger Pubs) Greenwood.

Psychrotrophic Microorganisms in Spoilage & Pathogenicity. Ed. by Terence A. Roberts et al. 1982. LC 81-67902. 552p. text 157.00 (*0-12-589720-0*) Acad Pr.

PsychState MAX 2.2. Tobey K. Koop. 1994. LC 93-92566. 136p. 59.95 incl. disk (*0-9631763-1-5*) PsychStat.

Psychware Sourcebook. Samuel Krug. 4th ed. 1993. 37.00 (*0-9635895-0-4*) MetriTech.

Psycles: Using Your Circadian Rhythms to Control Accidents, Illness, & Psychological Problems. Dwight H. Bulkley. 1981. LC 80-692. 224p. 10.95 (*0-672-52651-4*, Bobbs) Macmillan.

Psycology & Sociology Applied to Medicine. M. Porter. 1998. LC 98-44803. (Illustrated Colour Text Ser.). (*0-443-04971-8*) Church.

PSYOP (Psychological Operations Warfare) Waging Warfare for the Mind. 1995. (Illus.). 54p. (Orig.). (C). pap. text 15.00 (*0-7881-2548-6*) DIANE Pub.

Pszichologiai Ertelmezo Szotar: Explanatory Psychological Dictionary. B. Lajos. 1981. (HUN.). 24.95 (*0-8288-2220-4*, M172) Fr & Eur.

PT Activities for Pediatric Groups. Karen L. Kane. 1998. (Illus.). 128p. pap. text 45.00 (*0-12-784595-X*) Acad Pr.

PTCA - An Investigational Tool & a Non-Operative Treatment of Acute Ischemia. Ed. by Patrick W. Serruys et al. 1990. (Developments in Cardiovascular Medicine Ser.). (C). text 257.50 (*0-7923-0346-6*) Kluwer Academic.

Pterygium Surgery. Lucio Buratto et al. 2000. 200p. (C). pap. text 59.00 (*1-55642-492-2*) SLACK Inc.

PTSD-Borderlines in Therapy: Finding the Balance. Jerome Kroll. 1993. LC 93-6841. 240p. (C). 35.00 (*0-393-70157-3*) Norton.

***PTSD in Children & Adolescents: Review of Psychiatry,** Vol 20. Ed. by Spencer Eth. 2001. LC 00-67404. (Review of Psychiatry Ser.: Vol. 20). 208p. pap. 29.95 (*1-58562-026-2*, 62026) Am Psychiatric.

Pubertal Maturation in Female Development. Ed. by Haken Stattin & David Magnusson. 1990. (Paths Through Life Ser.). 408p. 99.95 (*0-8058-0595-8*) L Erlbaum Assocs.

Public & Community Health Nurse's Consultant: A Health Promotion Guide. Marcia Stanhope & Ruth N. Knollmueller. 1996. LC 96-219771. (Illus.). 800p. (C). (gr. 13). pap. text 32.95 (*0-8151-9003-4*, 29089) Mosby Inc.

Public Awareness of the Nebraska Regional Poison Control Center. Michael A. Montwill et al. 1979. 14p. (Orig.). pap. 1.50 (*1-55719-023-2*) U NE CPAR.

Public Concerns, Community Initiatives: The Successful Management of Nursing Home Consumer Information Programs. United Hospital Fund Staff. Ed. by Carol Ewig & John Griggs. 1985. 268p. 25.00 (*0-934459-25-8*) United Hosp Fund.

Public Enemy Number 1 Stress: A Practical Guide to the Effects of Stress & Nutrition on the Aging Process & Life Extension. Herman Todorov et al. 1999. LC 99-54397. x, 234p. (*1-56072-752-7*) Nova Sci Pubs.

Public Environments. Ed. by Joan Harvey & Don Henning. 1987. 36.00 (*0-939922-10-X*) EDRA.

Public Health. 1991. 58.95 (*0-387-53185-8*) Spr-Verlag.

Public Health: Index of New Information of Advances, Practices, Problems, Risks, & Research Development. Henrick H. Hoffstaetter. 1995. LC 95-18252. 57.50 (*0-7883-0242-6*); pap. 47.50 (*0-7883-0243-4*) ABBE Pubs Assn.

Public Health: Index of New Information of Advances, Practices, Problems, Risks & Research Development. Henrick H. Hoffstaetter. 2000. 187p. 57.50 (*0-7883-2450-0*); 2000. 187p. pap. 47.50 (*0-7883-2451-9*); 1994. 159p. 57.50 (*0-7883-0198-5*); 1994. 159p. pap. 47.50 (*0-7883-0199-3*) ABBE Pubs Assn.

Public Health: Its Promise for the Future. Wilson G. Smillie. 1976. LC 75-22841. (America in Two Centuries Ser.). (Illus.). reprint ed. 43.95 (*0-405-07712-2*) Ayer.

Public Health: Myth, Mysticism & Reality. U. Ko Ko. 1986. (SEARO Regional Health Papers: No. 14). 72p. pap. text 12.00 (*92-9022-183-6*, 1580014) World Health.

Public Health: Policy & Politics. Rob Baggott. 2000. LC 00-33319. (*0-312-23814-2*) St Martin.

Public Health Action in Emergencies Caused by Epidemics: A Practical Guide. P. Bres. 1986. 299p. pap. text 49.00 (*92-4-154207-1*, 1150253) World Health.

Public Health Administrator. Jack Rudman. 1994. (Career Examination Ser.: C-2082). reprint ed. pap. 39.95 (*0-8373-2082-8*) Nat Learn.

Public Health Advocacy: Creating Community Change to Improve Health. David G. Altman et al. 1994. (Illus.). 150p. (Orig.). pap. 24.00 (*1-879552-12-4*) SCRDP.

Public Health Aide. Jack Rudman. 1994. (Career Examination Ser.: C-1441). pap. 23.95 (*0-8373-1441-0*) Nat Learn.

Public Health Aide I. Jack Rudman. 1994. (Career Examination Ser.: C-2334). pap. 27.95 (*0-8373-2334-7*) Nat Learn.

Public Health Aide II. Jack Rudman. 1994. (Career Examination Ser.: C-1812). pap. 29.95 (*0-8373-1812-2*) Nat Learn.

Public Health & Aging. Ed. by Tom Hickey et al. 1997. LC 96-2928. 360p. pap. text 25.95 (*0-8018-5559-4*) Johns Hopkins.

***Public Health & Health Care.** Ed. by Gudrun Lindberg & Mans Rosen. 2001. 128p. 99.50 (*91-87760-49-5*) Coronet Bks.

Public Health & Insurance. Arthur Newsholme. 1979. LC 78-19270. 28.95 (*0-405-10617-3*) Ayer.

***Public Health & Municipal Policy Making: Britain & Sweden, 1900-1940.** Marjaana Niemi. 2002. (Historical Urban Studies). 250p. (*0-7546-0334-2*) Ashgate Pub GBR. *Dist:* Ashgate Pub Co.

Public Health & Preventive Medicine. Robert B. Wallace. 14th ed. 1998. LC 97-53116. 1200p. (C). text 139.00 (*0-8385-6185-3*) McGraw-Hill Prof.

Public Health & Social Justice in the Age of Chadwick: Britain, 1800-1854. Christopher Hamlin. 1998. LC 97-20658. (Cambridge Studies in the History of Medicine). (Illus.). 379p. (C). text 64.95 (*0-521-58363-2*) Cambridge U Pr.

Public Health & the Medical Use of Ionizing Radiation. 1965. (Technical Report Ser.: No. 306). 41p. pap. text 5.00 (*92-4-120306-4*) World Health.

Public Health & the State: Changing Views in Massachusetts, 1842-1936. Barbara G. Rosenkrantz. 1972. LC 70-172321. (Illus.). 271p. pap. 18.50 (*0-674-72236-1*); 37.50 (*0-674-72235-3*) HUP.

Public Health Approaches to Violence Prevention. Mary Haug. 1999. (Illus.). 64p. reprint ed. pap. text 25.00 (*0-7881-7530-0*) DIANE Pub.

Public Health Aspects of Criminal Prosecution of Workplace-Related Deaths, Injury, & Disease. Ed. by Eula Bingham et al. 1994. (International Journal of Occupational Medicine, Immunology, & Toxicology Ser.: Vol. 3, No. 4). (Illus.). pap. text 50.00 (*0-911131-79-5*) Specialist Journals.

Public Health Aspects of Low Birth Weight. 1961. (Technical Report Ser.: No. 217). 16p. pap. text 3.00 (*92-4-120217-3*) World Health.

Public Health Aspects of the Use of Antibiotics in Food & Feedstuffs. 1963. (Technical Report Ser.: No. 260). 30p. pap. text 3.00 (*92-4-120260-2*) World Health.

Public Health Assistant. Jack Rudman. 1994. (Career Examination Ser.: C-629). pap. 23.95 (*0-8373-0629-9*) Nat Learn.

Public Health at the Crossroads: Achievements & Prospects. Robert Beaglehole & Ruth Bonita. 1997. (Illus.). 261p. (C). text 100.00 (*0-521-58373-X*); pap. text 35.95 (*0-521-58665-8*) Cambridge U Pr.

Public Health Australia: An Introduction. James S. Lawson. 1991. (Illus.). 225p. pap. text 24.00 (*0-07-452913-7*) McGraw-Hill Med Pub.

Public Health Communication Interventions: Values & Ethical Dilemmas. Nurit Guttman. 2000. LC 99-50602. (Health Communication & Promotion Ser.). (Illus.). 286p. pap. 31.95 (*0-7619-0260-0*, 2172) Sage.

Public Health Consequences of Disasters. 1990. lib. bdg. 74.00 (*0-8490-4013-2*) Gordon Pr.

Public Health Consequences of Disasters. Ed. by Eric K. Noji. 1996. LC 96-25497. (Illus.). 488p. text 59.95 (*0-19-509570-7*) OUP.

Public Health Director. Jack Rudman. 1994. (Career Examination Ser.: C-2240). pap. 39.95 (*0-8373-2240-5*) Nat Learn.

Public Health Education Trainee. Jack Rudman. 1994. (Career Examination Ser.: C-983). pap. 27.95 (*0-8373-0983-2*) Nat Learn.

Public Health Educator. Jack Rudman. 1994. (Career Examination Ser.: C-630). pap. 29.95 (*0-8373-0630-2*) Nat Learn.

Public Health Educator I. Jack Rudman. 1994. (Career Examination Ser.: C-2354). pap. 34.95 (*0-8373-2354-1*) Nat Learn.

***Public Health Effects of Toxic Mold: California Senate Hearing.** Ed. by Deborah V. Ortiz. 2002. 210p. (C). pap. text 35.00 (*0-7567-1921-6*) DIANE Pub.

Public Health Engineer. Jack Rudman. 1994. (Career Examination Ser.: C-1979). pap. 34.95 (*0-8373-1979-X*) Nat Learn.

Public Health Engineer Trainee. Jack Rudman. 1994. (Career Examination Ser.: C-1881). pap. 27.95 (*0-8373-1881-5*) Nat Learn.

Public Health Epidemiologist. Jack Rudman. 1994. (Career Examination Ser.: C-2246). pap. 34.95 (*0-8373-2246-4*) Nat Learn.

Public Health Impact of Mental Disorders. Ed. by David Goldberg & Digby Tantam. 1990. LC 90-4355. (Illus.). 250p. text 48.00 (*0-920887-65-1*) Hogrefe & Huber Pubs.

Public Health Impact of Pesticides Used in Agriculture. 1990. (ENG, FRE, RUS & SPA.). 128p. pap. text 21.00 (*92-4-156139-4*, 1150348) World Health.

Public Health Implications of Medical Waste. 1995. lib. bdg. 252.75 (*0-8490-7545-9*) Gordon Pr.

Public Health Implications of Medical Waste: A Report to Congress. 1993. (Illus.). 225p. (Orig.). (C). pap. text 40.00 (*0-7881-0161-7*) DIANE Pub.

Public Health Implications of Radioactive Waste Releases. C. W. Straub. 1970. 61p. pap. text 9.00 (*92-4-156006-1*, 1150129) World Health.

Public Health in America Ed. by Barbara G. Rosenkrantz. 1977. (Public Health in America Ser.). reprint ed. lib. bdg. 1242.00 (*0-405-09804-9*) Ayer.

Public Health in British India: Anglo-Indian Preventive Medicine, 1859-1914. Mark Harrison. 1994. (Cambridge History of Medicine Ser.). (Illus.). 344p. (C). text 90.00 (*0-521-44127-7*); pap. text 31.95 (*0-521-46688-1*) Cambridge U Pr.

Public Health in Europe. European Commission Staff. 1997. LC 98-125524. (Employment & Social Affairs Ser.). 193 p. (*92-828-0390-2*) Comm Europ Commun.

Public Health in Europe. McKee & Dickens. 56.95 (*1-85972-634-8*) Ashgate Pub Co.

Public Health in the Town of Boston, 1630-1822. John B. Blake. 1959. LC 59-10314. (Harvard Historical Studies: No. 72). (Illus.). 288p. 20.00 (*0-674-72250-7*) HUP.

Public Health Informatics: Current Bibliographies in Medicine: January 1980 Through December 1995. Catherine Selden et al. 1996. 21p. (Orig.). pap. text 15.00 (*0-7881-3346-2*) DIANE Pub.

Public Health Inspector. Jack Rudman. 1994. (Career Examination Ser.: C-1753). pap. 29.95 (*0-8373-1753-3*) Nat Learn.

***Public Health Issues in Disaster Preparedness: Focus on Bioterrorism.** Novick. 2001. 120p. pap. 54.00 (*0-8342-2117-9*) Aspen Pub.

***Public Health Issues in Infant & Child Nutrition,** Vol. 48. Ed. by Robert E. Black & Kim Fleischer Michaelsen. 2002. LC 2001-50414. (Nestle Nutrition Workshop: Vol. 48). text 89.00 (*0-7817-3751-6*) Lppncott W & W.

Public Health Laboratory Service. 1957. (Technical Report Ser.: No 128). 49p. pap. text 3.00 (*92-4-120128-2*) World Health.

Public Health Law: Power, Duty, Restraint. Larry O. Gostin. 2001. LC 00-37773. (California/Milbank Series on Health & the Public : Vol. 3). (Illus.). xxviii, 491p. pap. text 24.95 (*0-520-22648-8*) U CA Pr.

Public Health Law: Power, Duty, Restraint. Lawrence O. Gostin. 2001. LC 00-37773. (California/Milbank Series on Health & the Public : Vol. 3). (Illus.). 517p. text 60.00 (*0-520-22646-1*) U CA Pr.

Public Health Law Manual. Frank P. Grad. 2nd ed. 1990. 337p. 45.00 (*0-87553-167-9*) Am Pub Health.

Public Health Leaders Tell Their Stories. Lloyd F. Novick. 1997. LC 97-15629. 192p. pap. 43.00 (*0-8342-0961-6*) Aspen Pub.

***Public Health Leadership & Management.** Capper. 2001. 69.00 (*0-7619-2318-7*) Sage.

Public Health Nurse. Jack Rudman. 1994. (Career Examination Ser.: C-631). pap. 27.95 (*0-8373-0631-0*) Nat Learn.

Public Health Nursing. Mary S. Gardner. Ed. by Barbara G. Rosenkrantz. 1977. LC 76-25664. (Public Health in America Ser.). reprint ed. lib. bdg. 26.95 (*0-405-09819-7*) Ayer.

***Public Health Nursing Leadership: A Guide to Managing the Core Functions.** Bobbie Berkowitz et al. 2001. LC 2001-22078. xi, 104p. pap. text 34.95 (*1-55810-155-1*) Am Nurses Pub.

Public Health Nutritionist. Jack Rudman. 1994. (Career Examination Ser.: C-632). pap. 27.95 (*0-8373-0632-9*) Nat Learn.

Public Health Policies & Social Inequality. Charles F. Andrain. 1998. LC 97-48835. 292p. text 50.00 (*0-8147-0676-2*) NYU Pr.

Public Health, Preventive Medicine & Social Services. Davies. 6th ed. LC 96-218055. 432p. pap. (*0-340-61373-4*) E A GBR. *Dist:* Routldge.

Public Health, Preventive Medicine & Social Services. Brian M. Davies. 6th ed. 1995. 368p. pap. text 29.95 (*1-56593-503-9*, 1164) Singular Publishing.

Public Health Progress. John A. R. Miles. 1984. lib. bdg. 107.50 (*90-277-9085-X*) Kluwer Academic.

Public Health Representative. Jack Rudman. 1994. (Career Examination Ser.: C-2369). pap. 29.95 (*0-8373-2369-X*) Nat Learn.

Public Health Responsibilities in Radiation Protection. 1963. (Technical Report Ser.: No. 254). 23p. pap. text 3.00 (*92-4-120254-8*) World Health.

Public Health Scientist. Jack Rudman. 1994. (Career Examination Ser.: C-634). pap. 34.95 (*0-8373-0634-5*) Nat Learn.

Public Health Service: Its History, Activities & Organization. Laurence F. Schmeckebier. LC 72-3023. (Brookings Institution. Institute for Government Research. Service Monographs of the U. S. Government: No. 10). reprint ed. 49.50 (*0-404-57110-7*) AMS Pr.

Public Health Services for All: Revitalizing a Shattered Plan. Colin Erickson & Harold M. Erickson, Sr. 1993. (Illus.). 275p. (Orig.). pap. 8.95 (*0-9640626-0-7*) H M Erickson.

Public Health Social Work Assistant. Jack Rudman. 1994. (Career Examination Ser.: C-1442). pap. 27.95 (*0-8373-1442-9*) Nat Learn.

Public Health Sourcebook: Basic Information about Government Health Agencies, along with Full Contact Information for Each Agency. Ed. by Wendy Wilcox. 1998. LC 98-15705. (Health Reference Ser.). 700p. lib. bdg. 78.00 (*0-7808-0220-9*) Omnigraphics Inc.

Public Health Surveillance. Ed. by William Halperin et al. 1992. 264p. 49.95 (*0-471-28432-7*, VNR) Wiley.

Public Health Surveillance. Ed. by William Halperin & Edward L. Baker. 1992. (Illus.). 272p. pap. 34.95 (*0-442-00762-0*, VNR) Wiley.

Public Health System in Texas. Barbara N. Samuels. 1992. (Working Papers Ser.: No. 66). 127p. pap. 5.50 (*0-89940-548-7*) LBJ Sch Pub Aff.

Public Health Systems & Emerging Infections: Assessing the Capabilities of the Public & Private Sectors. Johnathan R. Davis et al. 2000. LC 00-699205. 128p. pap. 23.00 (*0-309-06829-0*) Natl Acad Pr.

Public Health Technician. Jack Rudman. 1994. (Career Examination Ser.: C-2226). pap. 29.95 (*0-8373-2226-X*) Nat Learn.

Public Hospital Systems in New York & Paris. Ed. by Victor G. Rodwin et al. 1992. LC 92-6083. 320p. (C). text 50.00 (*0-8147-7422-9*) NYU Pr.

Public Hygiene in America. Henry I. Bowditch. 1972. LC 70-180557. (Medicine & Society in America Ser.). (Illus.). 415p. reprint ed. 29.95 (*0-405-03937-9*) Ayer.

Public Information about Osteoporosis: What's Available, What's Needed? 1995. (Illus.). 62p. (Orig.). pap. text 25.00 (*0-7881-2499-4*) DIANE Pub.

Public Information Specialist. Jack Rudman. 1994. (Career Examination Ser.: C-2111). pap. 29.95 (*0-8373-2111-5*) Nat Learn.

Public Interest in Conversions of Nonprofit Health Charities. Judith E. Bell et al. 1997. LC 98-124762. 60p. pap. (*1-887748-15-6*) Milbank Memorial.

***Public Law & Health Care.** Nigel Pleming et al. 2001. 320p. (*1-84113-155-5*) Hart Pub GBR. *Dist:* Intl Spec Bk.

Public Law & Health Service Accountability. Diane Longley. 1993. LC 92-13011. (State of Health Ser.). (*0-335-09686-7*); pap. (*0-335-09685-9*) OpUniv Pr.

Public Law 99-457 & the Basics of Family-Centered Intervention: A Module for Training Personnel Serving Families of Deaf & Hard of Hearing Infants & Young Children. Ed. by Valerie Schuyler. 1993. (Early Intervention Ser.). 40p. (C). 89.00 incl. VHS (*0-9618297-0-2*) Hearing & Speech.

Public Mental Health: A Changing System in an Era of Managed Care. American Psychiatric Association Staff. 1997. LC 97-11029. 74p. pap. text 26.00 (*0-89042-452-7*, 2452) Am Psychiatric.

Public Mental Health Marketing: Developing a Consumer Attitude. Ed. by Donald R. Self. 1993. LC 91-41001. (Journal of Nonprofit & Public Sector Marketing Ser.). 212p. lib. bdg. 49.95 (*1-56024-189-6*) Haworth Pr.

Public Oversight of Managed Health Care Entities: Issues for State Policymakers. Patricia A. Butler. 1996. 31p. pap. 33.00 (*1-55877-254-5*) Natl Governor.

Public Places & Spaces. I. Altman & E. H. Zube. 1989. (Human Behavior & Environment Ser.: Vol. 10). (Illus.). 334p. (C). 60.00 (*0-306-43079-7*, Plenum Trade) Perseus Pubng.

Public Policy & Mental Illness: Four Investigations, 1915-1939, an Original Anthology. Ed. by Gerald N. Grob. 1980. LC 78-22585. (Historical Issues in Mental Health Ser.). (Illus.). lib. bdg. 55.95 (*0-405-11936-4*) Ayer.

Public Policy & the Problem of Addiction: Four Studies, 1914 to 1924, an Original Anthology. Ed. by Gerald N. Grob. 1981. LC 70-1208. (Addiction in America Ser.). lib. bdg. 19.95 (*0-405-13564-5*) Ayer.

Public Pricing of Nursing Home Care. Howard Birnbaum et al. 1984. (Illus.). 222p. reprint ed. lib. bdg. 61.00 (*0-8191-4065-1*) U Pr of Amer.

Public-Private Collaboration in Health Information Policy. Frwd. by John M. Colmers et al. 1999. LC 00-699166. viii, 23p. pap. (*1-887748-29-6*) Milbank Memorial.

Public Privates: Performing Gynecology from Both Ends of the Speculum. Terri Kapsalis. 1997. LC 92-29409. (Illus.). 272p. pap. 16.95 (*0-8223-1921-7*); lib. bdg. 49.95 (*0-8223-1928-4*) Duke.

Public Relations for Pharmacists. Tina L. Pugliese. 2000. LC 00-38958. x, 166p. pap. 28.00 (*1-58212-011-0*) Am Pharm Assn.

Public Relations in the Emergency Department. Cyril T. Cameron. 1980. LC 80-15894. 126p. text 18.95 (*0-87619-746-2*) P-H.

Public Relations Manual for Healthcare Facilities. Lisa Gardner. 2000. 148p. pap. 29.50 (*0-929442-60-1*) Prof Prnting & Pub.

Public Self & Private Self. Ed. by Roy F. Baumeister. 1986. (Social Psychology Ser.). (Illus.). 257p. 63.00 (*0-387-96303-0*) Spr-Verlag.

Public Support for Private Residential Care. Jonathan Bradshaw & Ian Gibbs. 1988. 187p. text (*0-566-05661-5*) Avebry GBR. *Dist:* Ashgate Pub Co.

Publication Manual of the American Psychological Association. American Psychological Association Staff. 4th ed. 1994. LC 94-11498. 368p. text 31.95 (*1-55798-243-0*, 420-0041); pap. text 21.95 (*1-55798-241-4*, 4200040) Am Psychol.

Publications of the World Health Organization, 1963-1967: A Bibliography. 1969. (ENG & FRE.). 152p. pap. text 16.20 (*92-4-152002-7*, 1150010) World Health.

Publications of the World Health Organization, 1968-1972: A Bibliography. 1974. pap. text 18.00 (*92-4-152004-3*, 1150009) World Health.

Publicity Guide for Nutrition Education. 1985. 21p. pap. 8.00 (*0-910869-22-7*) Soc Nutrition Ed.

Publishing & Presenting Clinical Research. Warren S. Browner. 1998. LC 98-36024. 194p. pap. 49.95 (*0-683-30745-2*) Lppncott W & W.

Publishing in the Life Sciences: Index of Modern Authors & Subjects with Guide for Rapid Research. Science and Life Consultants Association Staff. 1991. LC 90-56272. 200p. pap. 44.50 (*1-55914-319-3*) ABBE Pubs Assn.

Publishing Your Medical Research Paper: What They Don't Teach in Medical School. Daniel W. Byrne. 1997. LC 97-29896. 288p. pap. 26.95 (*0-683-30074-1*) Lppncott W & W.

Puddephatt's Primers. Puddephatt. 1976. 110p. pap. (*0-85032-136-0*) C W Daniel GBR. *Dist:* Natl Bk Netwk.

Puer Aeternus. Marie-Louise Von Franz. 2nd ed. 1981. LC 80-28090. (Illus.). 292p. pap. 17.95 (*0-938434-01-2*) Sigo Pr.

Pulmonar Metastas Order. Weiss. 1979. lib. bdg. (*90-247-2157-1*) M Nijhoff NLD. *Dist:* Kluwer Academic.

Pulmonary Actions of the Endothelins. R. G. Goldie & Douglas W. Hay. 1999. LC 99-11900. (Respiratory Pharmacology & Pharmacotherapy Ser.). 350p. 265.00 (*3-7643-5859-9*) Birkhauser.

Pulmonary & Cardiac Imaging. Caroline Chiles & Charles E. Putman. 1997. LC 97-722. (Lung Biology in Health & Disease Ser.: Vol. 103). (Illus.). 680p. text 235.00 (*0-8247-9743-4*) Dekker.

Pulmonary & Critical Care Medicine: Update 5. Roger C. Bone. 5th ed. 1997. (Illus.). 950p. (C). (gr. 13). text 128.00 (*0-8151-1371-4*, 29725) Mosby Inc.

Pulmonary & Critical Care Medicine on CD-ROM, 1999. Roger C. Bone. rev. ed. 1998. (C). (gr. 13). spiral bd. 125.00 (*0-8151-2083-4*) Mosby Inc.

Pulmonary & Critical Care Pharmacology & Therapeutics. Ed. by Alan R. Leff. 1996. LC 96-12852. (Illus.). 1219p. text 159.00 (*0-07-037096-6*) McGraw-Hill Prof.

Pulmonary & Peripheral Gas Exchange in Health & Disease. Josep Roca et al. 2000. LC 00-31585. (Lung Biology in Health & Disease Ser.: Vol. 148). (Illus.). 824p. text 225.00 (*0-8247-0335-9*) Dekker.

Pulmonary Artery Catheter in Critical Care: A Concise Handbook. Claude Perret et al. 2nd ed. 1997. (Illus.). 360p. 125.00 (*0-632-04212-5*) Blackwell Sci.

Pulmonary Blood Vessels in Lung Disease. Ed. by J. Widimsky. 1990. (Progress in Respiratory Research Ser.: Vol. 26). (Illus.). viii, 150p. 117.50 (*3-8055-5155-X*) S Karger.

Pulmonary Circulation. Ed. by M. Morpurgo et al. 1990. (Current Topics in Rehabilitation Ser.). 159p. 69.95 (*0-387-19542-4*) Spr-Verlag.

Pulmonary Circulation: A Handbook for Clinicians. A. J. Peacock. 1999. (Illus.). 536p. (*0-412-56870-5*) E A GBR. *Dist:* OUP.

Pulmonary Circulation: Moving from Passive to Active Control. Ed. by Michael R. Pinsky et al. 1996. (Illus.). 275p. text (*0-7020-2201-2*) W B Saunders GBR. *Dist:* Saunders.

Pulmonary Circulation: Normal & Abnormal: Mechanisms, Management, & the National Registry. Ed. by Alfred P. Fishman. 1990. LC 89-40403. (Illus.). 578p. (C). text 99.95 (*0-8122-8110-1*) U of Pa Pr.

Pulmonary Circulation: Proceedings of the Symposium, Prague, 1969. Pulmonary Circulation Symposium Staff. Ed. by J. Widimsky et al. 1971. (Progress in Respiratory Research Ser.: Vol. 5). 125.25 (*3-8055-1152-3*) S Karger.

Pulmonary Circulation & Gas Exchange. Ed. by Wiltz W. Wagner, Jr. & E. Kenneth Weir. 1994. LC 93-38017. (Illus.). 440p. 75.00 (*0-87993-572-3*) Futura Pub.

Pulmonary Complications of Systemic Disease. Ed. by John F. Murray. 1992. LC 92-18424. (Lung Biology in Health & Disease Ser.: Vol. 59). (Illus.). 708p. text 250.00 (*0-8247-8707-2*) Dekker.

Pulmonary Defences. Robert A. Stockley. 1997. LC 96-35098. 364p. 215.00 (*0-471-97000-X*) Wiley.

Pulmonary Disease Diagnosis & Therapy: A Practical Approach. M. Gabriel Kahn & Joseph P. Lynch, III. 1997. LC 96-43620. (Illus.). 691p. pap. 53.95 (*0-683-04613-6*) Lppncott W & W.

Pulmonary Disease in the Elderly Patient. Ed. by Donald A. Mahler. 1992. LC 92-49321. (Lung Biology in Health & Disease Ser.: Vol. 63). (Illus.). 528p. text 225.00 (*0-8247-8752-8*) Dekker.

Pulmonary Diseases. Ed. by F. B. Askin et al. 1995. (Perspectives in Pediatric Pathology Ser.: Vol. 18). (Illus.). x, 234p. 248.75 (*3-8055-6049-4*) S Karger.

Pulmonary Diseases. Ed. by Carlo Grassi et al. 1999. (Clinical Medicine Ser.). (Illus.). 7580p. pap. 79.95 (*0-07-709521-9*) McGraw-Hill Prof.

Pulmonary Diseases: Mechanisms of Altered Structure & Function. Adam Wanner & Marvin A. Sackner. 1983. 282p. (C). 36.95 (*0-316-92150-5*, Little Brwn Med Div) Lppncott W & W.

Pulmonary Diseases & Disorders. Alfred P. Fishman. 3rd ed. 2001. (Illus.). 600p. pap. (*0-07-022002-6*) McGraw-Hill Med Pub.

Pulmonary Diseases & Disorders: Companion Handbook. Ed. by Alfred P. Fishman. 2nd ed. 1993. LC 93-27563. (Companion Handbook Ser.). (Illus.). 519p. pap., suppl. ed. 32.00 (*0-07-021157-4*) McGraw-Hill Prof.

Pulmonary Disorders. Anthony A. Gal & Michael N. Koss. 1997. LC 96-40066. (Differential Diagnosis in Pathology Ser.). (Illus.). 192p. (*0-89640-329-7*) Igaku-Shoin.

Pulmonary Edema. Michael A. Matthay & David H. Ingbar. 1998. LC 98-3647. (Lung Biology in Health & Disease Ser.). (Illus.). 688p. text 225.00 (*0-8247-0150-X*) Dekker.

Pulmonary Edema. E. Kenneth Weir & John T. Reeven. 1998. LC 97-34820. (American Heart Association Monograph Ser.). (Illus.). 432p. 98.00 (*0-87993-689-4*) Futura Pub.

Pulmonary Edema in Man & Animals. Aldo A. Luisada. 1970. LC 71-96988. (Illus.). 168p. 15.00 (*0-87527-050-6*) Green.

Pulmonary Embolism. Mario Morpurgo. 1994. LC 93-46951. (Lung Biology in Health & Disease Ser.: Vol. 75). (Illus.). 360p. text 180.00 (*0-8247-9178-9*) Dekker.

Pulmonary Embolism. T. Nakano & Samuel Z. Goldhaber. 1999. LC 99-24991. (Illus.). 208p. 132.00 (*4-431-70238-5*) Spr-Verlag.

Pulmonary Embolism. Ed. by J. Widimsky. 1980. (Progress in Respiratory Research Ser.: Vol. 13). (Illus.). viii, 192p. 126.25 (*3-8055-0487-X*) S Karger.

Pulmonary Embolism: Epidemiology, Diagnosis & Treatment. Matthijs Oudkerk et al. 1998. (Illus.). 430p. 188.95 (*0-632-04223-0*) Blackwell Sci.

Pulmonary Embolism & Deep Venous Thrombosis. Contrib. by Samuel Z. Goldhaber. 1985. (Illus.). 295p. text 105.00 (*0-7216-4151-2*) Saunders.

Pulmonary Emergencies. Ed. by Alan Fein et al. 1994. LC 94-25020. 224p. text (*0-7506-9529-3*) E A GBR. *Dist:* OUP.

Pulmonary Emphysema: Proceedings. International Symposium on Pathophysiology Staff. Ed. by G. L. Scarpa. 1976. (Progress in Respiratory Research Ser.: Vol. 10). 85.25 (*3-8055-2273-8*) S Karger.

Pulmonary Endothelium in Health & Disease. Ed. by Una S. Ryan. 1987. (Lung Biology in Health & Disease Ser.: Vol. 32). (Illus.). 520p. text 255.00 (*0-8247-7758-1*) Dekker.

Pulmonary Eosinophilia. F. E. Udwadia. Ed. by H. Herzog. 1975. (Progress in Respiratory Research Ser.: Vol. 7). (Illus.). xi, 286p. 121.75 (*3-8055-1739-4*) S Karger.

Pulmonary Fibroblast Heterogeneity. Richard P. Phipps. 1992. 352p. 194.00 (*0-8493-6038-2*, RC776, CRC Reprint) Franklin.

Pulmonary Fibrosis. Ed. by Sem H. Phan & Roger S. Thrall. 1995. LC 94-43568. (Lung Biology in Health & Disease Ser.: Vol. 80). (Illus.). 1008p. text 275.00 (*0-8247-8851-6*) Dekker.

Pulmonary Fibrosis. Ed. by Tamotsu Takishima. 1994. 544p. lib. bdg. 129.00 (*0-8493-8927-5*, RC776) CRC Pr.

Pulmonary Function: A Guide for Clinicians. Gabriel Laszlo. 1994. (Illus.). (C). 259p. text 110.00 (*0-521-43050-X*); 261p. pap. text 45.95 (*0-521-44679-1*) Cambridge U Pr.

Pulmonary Function Indices in Critical Care Patients. J. Brunner & G. Wolff. 1988. (Illus.). 171p. 77.95 (*0-387-18432-5*) Spr-Verlag.

Pulmonary Function Testing. Costa. 1995. (*0-8493-8859-7*) CRC Pr.

Pulmonary Function Testing: A Practical Approach. Jack Wanger. 1992. 248p. 29.00 (*0-683-08607-3*) Lppncott W & W.

Pulmonary Function Testing: Principles & Practice. Ed. by Stephen A. Conrad et al. 1984. (Illus.). 378p. pap. text (*0-443-08182-4*) Church.

Pulmonary Function Testing & Cardiopulmonary Stress Testing. Vince Madama. 2nd ed. 1997. LC 97-37682. 512p. (C). pap. text 49.95 (*0-8273-8410-6*) Delmar.

Pulmonary Function Testing & Cardiopulmonary Stress Testing - IML. Madama. 2nd ed. 1997. 76p. tchr. ed. 14.95 (*0-8273-8411-4*) Delmar.

Pulmonary Function Testing & Cardiopulmonary Stress Testing Transparency Masters. Vincent C. Madama. 1990. 126p. pap. 26.25 (*0-8273-3864-3*) Delmar.

Pulmonary Function Testing & Cardiovascular Stress Testing. Vincent C. Madama. 1993. LC 92-18604. (Respiratory Care Ser.). 590p. (C). mass mkt. 33.00 (*0-8273-3863-5*) Delmar.

Pulmonary Function Tests: A Practical Guide. Robert E. Hyatt & Paul D. Scanlon. 1997. LC 97-2778. (Illus.). 224p. pap. text 44.95 (*0-316-26261-7*, Little Brwn Med Div) Lppncott W & W.

Pulmonary Gas Exchange. Ed. by M. Meyer & J. Piiper. 1986. (Progress in Respiratory Research Ser.: Vol. 21). (Illus.). xiv, 274p. 216.75 (*3-8055-4330-1*) S Karger.

Pulmonary Health - Rehab & Exercise Testing. Jody C. Heggestad. 1999. 435p. per. 150.00 (*1-879575-05-1*) Acad Med Sys.

Pulmonary Heart Disease. Ed. by Lewis J. Rubin. 1984. text 200.00 (*0-89838-632-2*) Kluwer Academic.

Pulmonary Hypertension: Proceedings of the International Symposium on Pulmonary Circulation, 2nd, Prague, June, 1974. International Symposium on Pulmonary Circulation S. Ed. by J. Widimsky. 1975. (Progress in Respiratory Research Ser.: Vol. 9). (Illus.). 320p. 155.00 (*3-8055-2171-5*) S Karger.

Pulmonary Infections & Immunity. H. Chmel et al. 1994. (Infectious Agents & Pathogenesis Ser.). (Illus.). 378p. (C). text 95.00 (*0-306-44609-X*, Kluwer Plenum) Kluwer Academic.

Pulmonary Macrophage & Epithelial Cells: Proceedings. Ed. by Charles L. Sanders & Richard P. Schneider. 1977. LC 77-12024. (ERDA Symposium Ser.). 629p. pap. 23.75 (*0-87079-204-0*, CONF-760927); fiche 9.00 (*0-87079-316-0*, CONF-760927) DOE.

Pulmonary Management in Physical Therapy. Ed. by Cynthia C. Zadai. 1992. (Clinics in Physical Therapy Ser.). (Illus.). 234p. text (*0-443-08741-5*) Church.

***Pulmonary Medicine & Critical Care: Board Preparation Question Book - 500 Questions & Answers.** Eddy Jean-Baptiste. 2001. (Illus.). xii, 201p. 45.00 (*0-9715079-0-2*) J B Universal.

Pulmonary Nuclear Medicine: Techniques in Diagnosis of Lung Disease. Harold L. Atkins. 1984. (Lung Biology in Health & Disease Ser.: Vol. 23). (Illus.). 386p. text 175.00 (*0-8247-7233-4*) Dekker.

Pulmonary Nursing Care. Patricia A. Dettenmeier. 1991. (Illus.). 465p. (C). (gr. 13). pap. text 31.95 (*0-8016-5876-4*, 05876) Mosby Inc.

Pulmonary Pathology. Ed. by D. H. Dail & Samuel P. Hammar. 1987. (Illus.). 1200p. 267.00 (*0-387-96491-6*) Spr-Verlag.

Pulmonary Pathology. Dail. 2nd ed. 1993. LC 92-2383. (Illus.). 1640p. 350.00 (*0-387-97897-6*) Spr-Verlag.

Pulmonary Pathology. David H. Dail et al. 2nd ed. 1995. LC 94-17331. (Illus.). 530p. 192.00 (*0-387-94315-3*) Spr-Verlag.

Pulmonary Pathology: Proceedings of the 46th Annual Anatomic Pathology Slide Seminar. Merle A. Legg & Lynne M. Reid. 1986. LC 86-7992. 156p. pap. text 35.00 (*0-89189-178-1*) Am Soc Clinical.

Pulmonary Pathophysiology. G. Criner & G. D'Alonzo. 1998. (Pathophysiology Ser.). pap. 30.95 (*1-889325-05-8*) Blackwell Sci.

Pulmonary Pathophysiology: A Problem-Oriented Approach. Michael A. Grippi. 1995. LC 94-41688. (Lippincott's Pathophysiology Ser.). (Illus.). 352p. pap. text 27.95 (*0-397-51329-1*) Lppncott W & W.

Pulmonary Pathophysiology: The Essentials. John B. West. 4th ed. 1991. 229p. 26.00 (*0-683-08936-6*); 5th ed. 1997. LC 99-12450. (Illus.). 198p. pap. 31.00 (*0-683-30225-6*) Lppncott W & W.

Pulmonary Pearls. Ed. by Steven A. Sahn & John E. Heffner. 1988. LC 88-81283. (Pearls Ser.). (Illus.). 242p. pap. 45.00 (*0-932883-16-8*) Hanley & Belfus.

Pulmonary Pearls of Wisdom: Over 3000 Questions. Richard Lenhardt. 1998. (Pearls of Wisdom Ser.). pap. 88.00 (*1-890369-17-9*) Boston Medical.

Pulmonary Pearls II, Vol. II. Ed. by John Heffner & Steven A. Sahn. 2nd ed. 1994. LC 94-23207. (Pearls Ser.). (Illus.). 306p. (Orig.). pap. 45.00 (*1-56053-121-5*) Hanley & Belfus.

Pulmonary Physiology. Michael G. Levitsky. 5th ed. 1999. (Illus.). 320p. pap. 29.95 (*0-07-134543-4*) McGraw-Hill Prof.

Pulmonary Physiology & Pathophysiology: An Integrated, Case-Based Approach. John B. West. 2000. LC 00-56542. (Illus.). 166p. pap. text 31.95 (*0-7817-2910-6*) Lppncott W & W.

Pulmonary Physiology Fetus, Newborn, Child, Adolescent. Ed. by Emile M. Scarpelli. 2nd ed. 1989. LC 89-2361. (Illus.). 500p. text 98.00 (*0-8121-1225-3*) Lppncott W & W.

Pulmonary Radiology. Manuel Cardoso Ramon. 1998. LC 98-52914. 448p. pap. text 80.00 (*0-7817-1449-4*) Lppncott W & W.

Pulmonary Radiology: By Members of the Fleischner Society. Ed. by James Potchen et al. 1993. LC 93-3835. 600p. text 91.00 (*0-7216-4821-5*) Saunders.

Pulmonary Rehabilitation. Ed. by John R. Bach. 1995. 430p. 75.00 (*1-56053-109-6*) Hanley & Belfus.

Pulmonary Rehabilitation. Alfred P. Fishman. 1996. (Lung Biology in Health & Disease Ser.: Vol. 91). (Illus.). 864p. text 295.00 (*0-8247-9673-X*) Dekker.

Pulmonary Rehabilitation. Ed. by J. F. Muir et al. 1996. 261p. pap. text (*0-7279-1022-1*) BMJ Pub GBR. *Dist:* AIDC.

Pulmonary Rehabilitation: Guidelines to Success. John E. Hodgkin et al. 3rd ed. 2000. LC 00-35743. (Illus.). 744p. text 64.00 (*0-7817-1989-5*) Lppncott W & W.

Pulmonary Rehabilitation Program Administration & Patient Education Manual. Kathleen V. Morris & John E. Hodgkin. 1993. LC 96-3798. 432p. spiral bd. 155.00 (*0-8342-0754-0*) PRO-ED.

Pulmonary Science & Medicine: A Review of Fundamental Principles. Michael A. Grippi et al. 2000. LC 00-30738. (USMLE Step 1 Review Ser.). (Illus.). 168p. pap. text 17.95 (*0-7817-1650-0*) Lppncott W & W.

Pulmonary Surfactant: Biochemical, Functional, Regulatory, & Clinical Concepts. Jacques R. Bourbon. 1991. (Illus.). 448p. 271.95 (*0-8493-6924-X*, QP752) CRC Pr.

Pulmonary Surfactant: From Molecular Biology to Clinical Practice. Ed. by Bengt D. Robertson et al. 1992. LC 92-48791. 754p. 346.00 (*0-444-89475-6*) Elsevier.

Pulmonary Therapy & Rehabilitation. Francois Haas & Kenneth Axen. 2nd ed. 1991. (Illus.). 424p. 68.00 (*0-683-03887-7*) Lppncott W & W.

Pulmonary Toxicology of Respirable Particles: Proceedings. Ed. by Charles L. Sanders et al. 1980. (DOE Symposium Ser.). 687p. pap. 25.25 (*0-87079-121-4*, CONF-791002); fiche 9.00 (*0-87079-404-3*, CONF-791002) DOE.

Pulmonary Vascular Diseases. K. Moser. 1979. (Lung Biology in Health & Disease Ser.: Vol. 14). (Illus.). 728p. text 275.00 (*0-8247-6609-1*) Dekker.

Pulmonary Vascular Physiology & Pathophysiology. Kenneth E. Weir. Ed. by John T. Reeves. 1988. (Lung Biology in Health & Disease Ser.: Vol. 38). (Illus.). 784p. text 235.00 (*0-8247-7972-X*) Dekker.

Pulmonary Vascular Remodelling. Ed. by J. E. Bishop et al. 1995. (Portland Press Research Monographs: Vol. 7). 288p. (C). (*1-85578-041-0*) Portland Pr Ltd GBR. *Dist:* Ashgate Pub Co.

Pulmonary/Respiratory Therapy Secrets. Ed. by Polly E. Parsons & John E. Heffner. 1996. LC 96-47624. (Secrets Ser.). (Illus.). 500p. (Orig.). pap. 38.00 (*1-56053-163-0*) Hanley & Belfus.

Pulmonary Disease 2000. Jett. 2000. (Illus.). 450p. text 87.00 (*0-8151-2735-9*, 31318) Mosby Inc.

Pulsatile Drug Delivery/Current Applications, Future Trends. Robert Gurny & Junginger. 1993. 63.00 (*3-8047-1257-6*) CRC Pr.

Pulsatile Flow Velocity of the Central Arterial Blood. D. Scheu. 1972. (Bibliotheca Cardiologica Ser.: No. 28). (Illus.). vi, 74p. pap. 22.75 (*3-8055-1259-7*) S Karger.

Pulsatility in Neuroendocrine Systems. Ed. by Gareth Leng. 1988. 272p. 155.00 (*0-8493-4944-3*, QP356, CRC Reprint) Franklin.

Pulse Check: National Trends in Drug Abuse. Lee P. Brown. 1995. (Illus.). 36p. (Orig.). (C). pap. text 20.00 (*0-7881-1842-0*) DIANE Pub.

***Pulse Check: Trends in Drug Abuse - Mid-Year 2000 Ecstasy & Other Drugs.** Marcia Meth et al. 2001. (Illus.). 69p. (C). pap. 20.00 (*0-7567-1186-X*) DIANE Pub.

Pulse Classic: A Translation of the Mai Jing. Wang Shu-He. Ed. by Bob Flaws. Tr. by Yang Shou-Zhong from CHI. 1997. LC 96-86688. (Great Masters Ser.).Tr. of Mai Jing. 400p. 54.95 (*0-936185-75-9*) Blue Poppy Pr.

Pulse Diagnosis. Li Sh Zhen. Ed. by Garry Seifert. Tr. by Hoc Ku Huynh from CHI. 1993. LC 85-3506. 128p. (Orig.). pap. text 14.00 (*0-912111-06-2*) Paradigm Publns.

Pulse Diagnosis: Detailed Interpretations for Eastern & Western Treatments. Rueben Amber & A. M. Babey-Brooke. 1993. 228p. pap. 14.95 (*0-943358-41-8*) Aurora Press.

Pulse Oximetry. Ed. by J. P. Payne & J. W. Severinghaus. 1986. (Illus.). 197p. 69.95 (*0-387-16857-5*) Spr-Verlag.

Pulsed & Self Regulated Drug Delivery. Hans-Peter Kost. 1990. 232p. lib. bdg. 195.00 (*0-8493-4546-4*, RS199) CRC Pr.

Pump Operations. J. Steven Kidd & John Czajkowski. 1995. pap. text, wbk. ed. (*0-8151-5085-7*) Mosby Inc.

Pumpkin - A Young Woman's Struggle with Lupus. Patricia M. Fagan. Ed. by Adolfo Caso. 1994. 190p. text 12.95 (*0-8283-1961-8*) Branden Bks.

Pupil. E. Alexandridis. Tr. by Terry C. Telger from GER. 1985. (Illus.). 117p. 105.00 (*0-387-96109-7*) Spr-Verlag.

Pupil: Anatomy, Physiology & Clinical Applications Irene E. Loewenfeld & Otto Lowenstein. 1999. LC 98-53982. (Illus.). 2312p. text 275.00 (*0-7506-7143-2*) Buttrwrth-Heinemann.

Puppet of Desire: The Psychology of Hysteria, Possession & Hypnosis. Jean-Michel Oughourlian. Tr. by Eugene Webb from FRE. 1991. LC 90-42448. 289p. 51.00 (*0-8047-1823-7*) Stanford U Pr.

Puppy's First Year: A Guide to Veterinary Care for Your Puppy. Race Foster & Marty Smith. 1999. LC 98-52387. (Illus.). 256p. 19.95 (*1-58245-052-8*, Howell) Hungry Minds.

Purchase of Medical Care Through Fixed Periodic Payment. Pierce Williams. 1976. LC 75-17251. (National Bureau of Economic Research Ser.). reprint ed. 26.95 (*0-405-07525-1*) Ayer.

Purchase of Medical Care Through Fixed Periodic Payment. Pierce Williams & Isabel C. Chamberlain. 1932. (General Ser.). 328p. reprint ed. 85.30 (*0-87014-019-1*) Natl Bur Econ Res.

Purchasing & Inventory Control, 1990. 1990. 224p. ring bd. 63.00 (*0-930530-97-7*, P308) Am Soc Hlth-Syst.

Purchasing & Provide Costs. Drummond. 1994. (C). pap. text 33.50 (*0-443-04946-7*) Saunders.

Purchasing for Health: A Multidisciplinary Introduction to the Theory & Practice of Health Purchasing. John Vretveit. 1994. LC 94-27592. 224p. (Orig.). text (*0-335-19333-1*) OpUniv Pr.

Purchasing for Health: A Multidisciplinary Introduction to the Theory & Practice of Health Purchasing. John Vretveit. 1994. LC 94-27592. 224p. (Orig.). pap. text 38.95 (*0-335-19332-3*) Taylor & Francis.

Purchasing Managed Care Services for Alcohol & Other Drug Treatment: Essential Elements & Policy Issues. Stephen Moss & Jeffrey N. Kushner. 1997. (Illus.). 58p. (C). reprint ed. pap. text 30.00 (*0-7881-4035-3*) DIANE Pub.

***Purchasing of Health Care Primary Care Organizations: An Evaluation & Guide to Future Policy.** Ed. by Nicholas Mays et al. 2001. LC 00-68923. (State of Health Ser.). 288p. pap. (*0-335-20900-9*); text (*0-335-20901-7*) OpUniv Pr GBR. *Dist:* Taylor & Francis.

Purchasing Power in Health: Business, the State, & Health Care Politics. Linda A. Bergthold. 1990. LC 89-37778. 264p. (C). text 40.00 (*0-8135-1487-8*) Rutgers U Pr.

Purdue Pharmacy: The First Century. Robert B. Eckles. 1979. LC 78-58099. (Illus.). 114p. 10.00 (*0-931682-01-0*) Purdue U Pubns.

Pure & Simple Natural Weight Control. Norman W. Walker. rev. ed. 1995. LC 81-11080. 132p. pap. 7.95 (*0-89019-078-X*) Norwalk Pr.

Pure Cure for Arthritis & Other Auto-Immune & Inflammatory Diseases. Bob L. Owen & Thomas Johnson. 1997. LC 97-93664. (Illus.). 112p. (Orig.). pap. 14.00 (*1-882657-14-4*) Health Digest.

Pure Practice for ECG's. Louise Smith. 1995. 452p. pap. text 27.95 (*0-8151-7923-5*, 25711) Mosby Inc.

Pure Practice for ECGs Instructor's Kit. Louise Smith & Frank Fish. 1995. (Illus.). 290p. tchr. ed. (*0-8151-7873-5*, 25726) Mosby Inc.

Pure Practice in 12-Lead ECG's. Robin B. Purdie & Sam L. Earnest. 1997. (Illus.). 576p. pap. text 34.95 (*0-8151-4669-8*) Mosby Inc.

Pure Practice in 12-Lead ECGS Instructor's Kit. Robin B. Purdie & Sam L. Earnest. 1997. (Illus.). 576p. (C). text, tchr. ed. (*0-8151-4670-1*) Mosby Inc.

Purged see My Experience with Clinical Depression

Purification of Fermentation Products: Applications to Large-Scale Processes. Ed. by Derek LeRoith et al. 1985. LC 84-24316. (ACS Symposium Ser.: No. 271). 198p. lib. bdg. 49.95 (*0-8412-0890-5*) Am Chemical.

Purification of Laboratory Chemicals. D. D. Perrin et al. 2nd ed. 1980. LC 79-41708. 580p. 110.00 (*0-08-022961-1*, Pergamon Pr) Elsevier.

Purification Tools for Monoclonal Antibodies. Peter S. Gagnon. 1996. LC 96-90448. (Illus.). 254p. (Orig.). pap. 89.00 (*0-9653515-9-9*) Validated Biosysts.

Purine & Pyrimidine Metabolism in Man: Second Europeon Symposium, Chiemsee, Sept. 1989. Ed. by N. Zoellner et al. 1989. (Journal: Vol. 33, No. 4 1989). (Illus.). 48p. pap. 35.00 (*3-8055-5072-3*) S Karger.

Purine & Pyrimidine Metabolism in Man 11. Ed. by Andrea Griesmacher et al. 1998. LC 97-52565. (Advances in Experimental Medicine & Biology Ser.: No. 431). (Illus.). 892p. (C). text 185.00 (*0-306-45778-4*, Kluwer Plenum) Kluwer Academic.

Purine & Pyrimidine Metabolism in Man Vol. 7B: Structural Biochemistry, Pathogenesis & Metabolism. R. A. Harkness et al. 1991. (Advances in Experimental Medicine & Biology Ser.: Vol. 309B). (Illus.). 416p. (C). text 125.00 (*0-306-44093-8*, Kluwer Plenum) Kluwer Academic.

Purine & Pyrimidine Metabolism in Man Vol. 7A: Chemotherapy, ATP Depletion & Gout. R. A. Harkness et al. 1991. (Advances in Experimental Medicine & Biology Ser.: Vol. 309A). (Illus.). 496p. (C). text 140.00 (*0-306-44092-X*, Kluwer Plenum) Kluwer Academic.

Purine & Pyrimidine Metabolism in Man VI Ed. by K. Mikanagi et al. 1989. (Illus.). Pt. A. 574p. 120.00 (*0-306-43233-1*); Pt. B. 566p. 120.00 (*0-306-43234-X*) Perseus Pubng (Plenum Trade).

Purine & Pyrimidine Metabolism in Man VIII: Proceedings of the Eighth International Symposium Held in Bloomington, Indiana, May 22-27, 1994. Ed. by Amerik Sahota & Milton W. Taylor. 1995. (Advances in Experimental Medicine & Biology Ser.: Vol. 370). (Illus.). 858p. (C). text 169.50 (*0-306-44997-8*, Kluwer Plenum) Kluwer Academic.

Purinergic Approaches in Experimental Therapeutics. Kennethalan Jacobson & Michael F. Jarvis. 1997. LC 96-38941. 581p. 170.00 (*0-471-14071-6*) Wiley.

Purines: Basic & Clinical Aspects. Trevor W. Stone. 1991. 264p. text 174.50 (*0-7923-8925-5*) Kluwer Academic.

Purines & Myocardial Protection. Ed. by Anwar-Saad A. Abd-Elfattah & Andrew S. Wechsler. 1995. (Developments in Cardiovascular Medicine Ser.: Vol. 161). 592p. (C). text 272.50 (*0-7923-3831-6*) Kluwer Academic.

Purity & Pollution: Gender, Embodiment & Victorian Medicine. Bashford. 1998. LC 97-28323. 208p. 59.95 (*0-312-21038-8*) St Martin.

Purloined Self: Interpersonal Perspective in Psychoanalysis. Edgar A. Levenson. 1991. 266p. 30.95 (*0-9629993-0-X*); 288p. pap. 24.95 (*0-9629993-1-8*) Contemp Psycho.

Purposive Behaviour & Teleological Explanations. Ed. by Frank George & Les Johnson. 1985. (Studies in Cybernetics: Vol. 8). xxii, 310p. text 137.00 (*2-88124-110-7*) Gordon & Breach.

Put Prevention Into Practice: Clinician's Handbook of Preventive Services. 1998. LC 98-121900. 571p. per. 35.00 (*0-16-049227-0*) USGPO.

Put Prevention into Practice: Clinician's Handbook of Preventive Services. 1994. 419p. per. 23.00 (*0-16-043115-8*) USGPO.

Putative Melatonin Receptors in Peripheral Tissues. Ed. by S. F. Pang et al. 1994. (Journal: Vol. 2, No. 4, 1993). (Illus.). 64p. pap. 28.75 (*3-8055-5947-X*) S Karger.

Putting Children First: State-Level Collaboration Between Education & Health. National Health & Education Consortium Staff. 1995. 50p. 10.00 (*0-937846-43-0*) Inst Educ Lead.

Putting Health Care on the National Agenda. Arnold Birenbaum. 1995. LC 95-3861. 256p. 68.00 (*0-275-95163-4*); pap. 22.00 (*0-275-95164-2*) Greenwood (Praeger Pubs).

Putting Health into Place: Landscape, Identity, & Well-Being. Robin A. Kearns & Wilbert M. Gesler. 1998. LC 97-36239. (Space, Place, & Society Ser.). 49.95 (*0-8156-2767-X*) Syracuse U Pr.

Putting Health into Place: Landscape, Identity, & Well-Being. Robin A. Kearns & Wilbert N. Gesler. 1998. LC 97-36239. (Space, Place, & Society Ser.). (Illus.). 272p. pap. 24.95 (*0-8156-2768-8*) Syracuse U Pr.

Putting Healthcare Promises into Practice: Strategies for Empowerment & Innovation in Managing Care. Dennis A. Robbins. 2000. LC 00-697775. 274p. text 37.95 (*0-7668-1972-8*) Delmar.

Putting It All Together: The New Orthomolecular Nutrition. Abram Hoffer & Morton Walker. Ed. by Don R. Bensen. rev. ed. 1996. 224p. pap. 17.95 (*0-87983-633-4*, 36334K, Keats Pubng) McGraw-Hill Trade.

***Putting Patients FIrst: Increasing Organ Supply for Transplantation: Congressional Hearing.** Ed. by Michael Bilirakis. 2001. (Illus.). 126p. (C). reprint ed. pap. text 25.00 (*0-7567-1604-7*) DIANE Pub.

Putting Patients First: Resolving Allocation of Transplant Organs: Joint Hearing Before the Subcommittee on Health & Environment of the Committee on Commerce, House of Representatives & the Committee on Labor & Human Resources, U.S. Senate, One Hundred Fifth Congress, Second Session, June 18, 1998. Contrib. by U. S. Congress, House Committee on Commerce, Subcommittee on Health and the Environment & U. S. Congress, Senate Committee on Labor and Human Resources. 1998. LC 99-172383. (Illus.). (*0-16-057534-6*) USGPO.

Putting Patients First: Resolving Allocations of Transplant Organs: Congressional Hearings. Ed. by Michael Bilirakis. 1999. 240p. (C). reprint ed. pap. text 40.00 (*0-7881-8452-0*) DIANE Pub.

Putting Practice Guidelines to Work in the Department of Defense Medical System: A Guide for Action. Will Nicholas et al. 2001. LC 00-65315. 110p. pap. 15.00 (*0-8330-2944-4*) Rand Corp.

Putting Prevention into Practice: Problem Solving in Clinical Prevention. Richard K. Riegelman & Gail J. Povar. 1988. 432p. 32.95 (*0-316-74519-7*, Little Brwn Med Div) Lppncott W & W.

Putting Psychology in Its Place: An Introduction from a Critical Historical Perspective. Graham Richards. 1996. 208p. (C). 73.95 (*0-415-12862-5*); pap. 26.95 (*0-415-12863-3*) Routledge.

Putting the Patient First: Up Front with Advocacy & Community Service. Bob Richards & Jeanan Yasiri. 1997. 149p. (Orig.). pap. 90.00 (*1-56829-082-9*, 5001) M G M A.

Putting the Pieces Together Vol. 4: A Linguistically Based Cognitive Retraining Manual. Kathryn Kilpatrick. 1985. (Illus.). 389p. stu. ed. 37.00 (*1-880504-04-9*) Visit Nurse.

Putting the Pieces Together Again: A Physicians Guide to Thriving on Stress. Frederic F. Flach. rev. ed. 1995. LC 95-50894. 212p. pap. 8.95 (*1-886330-03-4*) Hatherleigh.

Puzzle of Heart Failure - Putting the Pieces Together: For Heart Failure Patients. Susan D. Allen et al. 1991. (Illus.). 64p. pap. text 3.25 (*0-916999-09-2*) HERC Pubng.

Puzzle People: Memoirs of a Transplant Surgeon. Thomas E. Starzl. 1992. LC 92-455. (Illus.). 400p. (C). text 24.95 (*0-8229-3714-X*) U of Pittsburgh Pr.

Puzzling Child: From Recognition to Treatment. Ed. by Mary Frank. 1982. LC 82-11692. (Journal of Children in Contemporary Society: Vol. 14, No. 4). 109p. text 39.95 (*0-86656-119-6*) Haworth Pr.

PVP: A Critical Review of the Kinetics & Toxicology of Polyvinylpyrrolidone (Povidone) B. V. Robinson et al. 1990. (Illus.). 232p. lib. bdg. 159.00 (*0-87371-288-9*, L288) Lewis Pubs.

Pycnogenol: Miracle Antioxidant. 1996. lib. bdg. 250.95 (*0-8490-5908-9*) Gordon Pr.

Pyelonephritis. F. Renyi-Vamos & F. Balogh. 1979. 190p. (C). (*963-05-1724-8*) Akade Kiado HUN. *Dist:* St Mut.

Pyloric Sphincteric Cylinder in Health & Disease. A. D. Keet. 1993. LC 92-48803. (Illus.). 432p. 217.00 (*0-387-55814-4*) Spr-Verlag.

Pyongyang Conference: Primary Health Care in Action. 1985. (SEARO Regional Health Papers: No. 6). 352p. pap. text 20.00 (*92-9022-175-5*, 1580006) World Health.

***Pyramid Approach to Education in Autism.** Andrew S. Bondy & Beth Sulzer-Azaroff. 2001. 200p. text 32.00 (*1-928598-03-X*) PEPI.

Pyretics & Antipyretics. Ed. by A. S. Milton. 1982. (Handbook of Experimental Pharmacology Ser.: Vol. 60). (Illus.). 691p. 392.00 (*0-387-11511-0*) Spr-Verlag.

Pyrogens: Endotoxins & LAL Testing & Depyrogenation. F. C. Pearson. 1985. (Advances in Parenteral Science Ser.: Vol. 2). (Illus.). 288p. text 145.00 (*0-8247-7436-1*) Dekker.

Pyrogens: Endotoxins, LAL Testing & Depyrogenation. F. C. Pearson. 2nd exp. rev. ed. Date not set. (Advances in Parenteral Science Ser.). (Illus.). 384p. text 150.00 (*0-8247-9362-5*, 9362-5) Dekker.

Pyrroles: The Synthesis, Reactivity, & Physical Properties of Substituted Pyrroles, Vol. 48. Ed. by R. Alan Jones. 1992. (Chemistry of Heterocyclic Compounds Monographs: Vol. 48, Pt. 2). 640p. 550.00 (*0-471-51306-7*) Wiley.

Pyruvate Carboxylase. John C. Wallace & D. Bruce Keech. 1985. 280p. 155.00 (*0-8493-6552-X*, QP619, CRC Reprint) Franklin.

Q

Q & A about the Silva Method. 3.95 (*0-913343-45-5*) Inst Psych Inc.

Q & A on PKD, Vol. 3. PKR Foundation Scientific Advisors Staff. Ed. by Jared J. Grantham et al. rev. ed. 1995. 96p. (C). pap. 15.00 (*0-9614567-2-8*) PKR Foundation.

Q & A on Reporting Periodontal Services. American Academy of Periodontology Staff. 1992. 32p. pap. 25.00 (*0-9624699-4-7*) Amer Acad Periodontology.

Q Book: The Physics of Radiotherapy X-Rays: Problems & Solutions. Peter Metcalfe et al. 1998. (Illus.). 100p. (C). pap. text, wbk. ed. 33.95 (*0-944838-86-3*) Med Physics Pub.

Q Fever: The Biology of Coxiella Burnetii. Jim C. Williams & Herbert A. Thompson. 1991. (Illus.). 368p. 189.95 (*0-8493-5983-X*, QR201) CRC Pr.

Q Fever Vol. 1: The Disease, Vol. 1. Ed. by Thomas J. Marrie. 1990. LC 96-3686. (Illus.). 264p. 179.00 (*0-8493-5984-8*, RC182) CRC Pr.

QA-CQI Manual for Clinical Lab. M. Cronin. 1994. (C). 208p. 99.95 (*0-933195-67-2*); 115p. (*0-933195-70-2*) CA College Health Sci.

QA-CQI Manual for Home Care. M. Cronin. rev. ed. 1994. 122p. (C). ring bd. 99.95 (*0-933195-39-7*) CA College Health Sci.

QA-CQI Manual for Physical Therapy. M. Cronin. rev. ed. 1994. 110p. (C). ring bd. 99.95 (*0-933195-38-9*) CA College Health Sci.

QA-CQI Manual for Respiratory Care. M. Cronin. rev. ed. 1994. 208p. (C). ring bd. 99.95 (*0-933195-32-X*) CA College Health Sci.

QA Issues in Clinical Toxicology. Ed. by Shirley Welch. 1996. 70p. pap. 11.00 (*0-915274-86-8*, 202687, AACC Pr) Am Assn Clinical Chem.

***Qbase Anaesthesia 4: MCQs for the Primary FRCA.** Henry P. W. Paw. 1997. (Illus.). 208p. pap. text incl. cd-rom (*1-900151-98-7*) Greenwich Med GBR. *Dist:* JAMCO Dist.

***Qbase for the Undergraduate.** E. Hammond. 2003. 192p. pap. incl. cd-rom (*1-84110-061-7*) Greenwich Med GBR. *Dist:* JAMCO Dist.

***Qbase Medicine 1: MCQs for the MRCP.** Punit S. Ramrakha. 1997. 192p. pap. text incl. cd-rom (*1-900151-33-2*) Greenwich Med GBR. *Dist:* JAMCO Dist.

***Qbase Medicine 2: MCQs for the MRCP Part I.** McCrudden. 2000. (Greenwich Medical Media Ser.). 230p. pap. text incl. cd-rom (*1-900151-59-6*) Greenwich Med GBR. *Dist:* JAMCO Dist.

***Qbase Paediatrics 1: MCQs for the MRCPCH.** Sidwell & Thompson. 2001. (Greenwich Medical Media Ser.). 140p. pap. incl. cd-rom (*1-84110-044-7*) Greenwich Med GBR. *Dist:* JAMCO Dist.

***Qbase Radiology 1: MCQs for the FRCR.** Misra et al. 2001. (Greenwich Medical Media Ser.). 218p. pap. incl. cd-rom (*1-84110-032-3*) Greenwich Med GBR. *Dist:* JAMCO Dist.

***Qbase Radiology 2: MCQs for the FRCR.** Misra et al. 2001. (Greenwich Medical Media Ser.). 208p. pap. incl. cd-rom (*1-84110-040-4*) Greenwich Med GBR. *Dist:* JAMCO Dist.

***Qbase Surgery 1: MCQs for the MRCS.** James Green & Wajed. 2001. (Greenwich Medical Media Ser.). 208p. pap. text incl. cd-rom (*1-900151-37-5*) Greenwich Med GBR. *Dist:* JAMCO Dist.

QDT, 1997: Quintessence of Dental Technology, Vol. 20. Ed. by John Sorensen. 1997. (Illus.). 190p. pap. text 56.00 (*0-86715-322-9*) Quint Pub Co.

QDT, 1993. Ed. by Robert Renner. 1993. (Illus.). 188p. (Orig.). pap. text 54.00 (*0-86715-186-2*) Quint Pub Co.

Qi Gong for Health & Longevity: The Ancient Chinese Art of Relaxation-Meditation-Physical Fitness. Simon Wang & Julius L. Liu. 1994. LC 94-32135. 285p. (Orig.). 29.98 (*0-9641605-0-1*); pap. 24.98 (*0-9641605-2-8*) East Hlth Dev.

Qi Gong Therapy: The Chinese Art of Healing with Energy. Tsu Kuo Shih. 1992. (Illus.). 160p. pap. 15.95 (*0-88268-138-9*) Station Hill Pr.

Qigone for Arthritis see Arthritis: The Chinese Way of Healing & Prevention

Qigong: Chinese Medicine or Pseudoscience? Lin Zixin et al. 2000. LC 99-36666. (Illus.). 155p. 25.00 (*1-57392-232-3*) Prometheus Bks.

Qigong for Treating Common Ailments: The Essential Guide to Self Healing. Xu Xiancai. 2nd ed. 2000. LC 00-101607. (Practical TCM Ser.). (Illus.). xiv, 128p. pap. 15.95 (*1-886969-70-1*) YMAA Pubn.

Qin Bowei Anthology. Qin Bowei. Ed. by Robert L. Felt, Jr. Tr. by Charles Chace. 1997. LC 97-4783. 220p. (C). pap. text 35.00 (*0-912111-41-0*) Paradigm Publns.

QSAR & Drug Design: New Developments & Applications. Ed. by Toshio Fujita & H. Timmerman. 1995. LC 95-45138. (Pharmacochemistry Library: No. 23). 508p. 238.00 (*0-444-88615-X*) Elsevier.

QT Dispersion. Ed. by Marek Malik et al. 2000. LC 00-28825. (Clinical Approaches to Tachyarrhythmias Ser.: Vol. 12). (Illus.). 160p. pap. 69.00 (*0-87993-456-5*) Futura Pub.

Quackery & You. William T. Jarvis. 1983. (Illus.). (Orig.). pap. 1.49 (*0-8280-0148-0*) Review & Herald.

Quacks: Fakers & Charlatans in English Medicine. Roy Porter. 2000. (Illus.). 224p. (*0-7524-1776-2*) Tempus Pubng GBR. *Dist:* Arcadia Publng.

Quadrilingual Dictionary of the Press & Media (Dictionnaire Quadrilingue de la Presse et des Medias) CILF Staff. 1990. (FRE, ITA, POR & SPA.). 304p. 95.00 (*0-7859-4580-6*, 2853192210) Fr & Eur.

Quadruplets & Higher Multiple Births. Marie M. Clay. 1991. (Clinics in Developmental Medicine Ser.: No. 107). (Illus.). 186p. (C). text (*0-521-41223-4*) Mc Keith Pr GBR. *Dist:* Cambridge U Pr.

Qualitative Analysis of Human Movement. Duane Knudson & Craig Morrison. 1997. LC 96-48347. (Illus.). 216p. text 34.00 (*0-88011-523-8*, BKNU0523) Human Kinetics.

Qualitative Gerontology. Ed. by Shulamit Reinharz & Graham D. Rowles. 1987. 336p. (C). 36.95 (*0-8261-5230-9*) Springer Pub.

Qualitative Health Research. Janice M. Morse. 1992. LC 92-20585. (Illus.). 272p. (C). pap. 36.95 (*0-8039-4775-5*, 4556) Sage.

***Qualitative Inquiry: The Path of Sciencing.** Rosemarie Rizzo Parse. 2001. LC 00-65652. (Illus.). 368p. (C). pap. text 34.95 (*0-7637-1565-4*, 1565-4) Jones & Bartlett.

***Qualitative Methods in Organizational Research & Practice.** Gillian Symon et al. 2001. 160p. (C). pap. (*0-86377-623-X*) Psychol Pr GBR. *Dist:* Taylor & Francis.

Qualitative Methods in Psychology: A Research Guide. Peter Banister et al. 1994. LC 94-25724. 160p. pap. (*0-335-19181-9*) OpUniv Pr.

Qualitative Nursing Research: A Contemporary Dialogue. Janice M. Morse. rev. ed. 1991. (Illus.). 360p. (C). pap. 34.95 (*0-8039-4079-3*, 3668) Sage.

Qualitative Research & Evaluation in Group Care. Ed. by Rivka A. Eisikovits & Yitzhak Kashti. 1987. LC 86-14848. (Child & Youth Services Ser.: Vol. 8, Nos. 3 & 4). 132p. text 4.95 (*0-86656-608-2*) Haworth Pr.

Qualitative Research for Nurses. Immy Holloway & Stephanie Wheeler. 1996. LC 95-26498. x, 214p. pap. 38.95 (*0-632-03765-2*) Blackwell Sci.

Qualitative Research in Health: An Introduction. Carol Grbich. 1998. LC 99-214296. viii, 312p. pap. 27.95 (*0-7619-6104-6*, 84630) Sage.

Qualitative Research in Nursing: Methods in Context. J. Lawler. 1998. 176p. pap. (*0-443-05207-7*) Church.

Qualitative Research in Pharmacy Practice. Ed. by Sheila Phillips et al. 1996. (Cardiff Papers in Qualitative Research). 224p. (*1-85972-211-3*) Avebry GBR. *Dist:* Ashgate Pub Co.

Qualitative Research Methodology in Nursing & Health Care. Open Learning Foundation Staff. 1997. 120p. pap. (*0-443-05738-9*) Church.

Qualitative Research Methods in Nursing. Ed. by Madeleine M. Leininger. 1985. 384p. text 64.00 (*0-8089-1676-9*, 792508, Grune & Strat) Harcrt Hlth Sci Grp.

Qualitative Studies in Health & Medicine. Ed. by Michael Bloor & Patricia Taraborrelli. 1994. (Cardiff Papers in Qualitative Research). 139p. (*1-85628-579-0*) Avebry GBR. *Dist:* Ashgate Pub Co.

Qualitative Study of the Co-Construction of Therapeutic Reality: A Process & Outcome Model. Jon L. Winek. 1998. LC 98-30820. (Studies in Sociology: Vol. 20). 143p. text 79.95 (*0-7734-8236-9*) E Mellen.

Qualitatssicherung in der Gerontopsychiatrischen Tagesklinik: Ergebnisse Einer Begleitstudie Mit Einer Einleitung von Holger K. Schneider, Direktor des Bezirkskrankenhauses Erlangen. Krista Stosberg & Harald J. Losch. 1997. (GER.). xi, 187p. 42.95 (*3-631-49869-1*) P Lang Pubng.

Quality Acceleration in Hygiene & Operative. Michael J. Segerdal. 1995. (Illus.). 52p. incl. VHS (*1-883558-04-2*) PIBL.

Quality Advantage: A Strategic Guide for Health Care Leaders. Julianne M. Morath. 1998. LC 98-36020. (Illus.). 264p. 42.00 (*1-55648-256-6*) AHPI.

Quality & Cost-Containment in Care of the Elderly: Health Services Research Perspectives. Ed. by James C. Romeis & Rodney Coe. 1990. LC 90-10439. 248p. 42.95 (*0-8261-7170-2*) Springer Pub.

Quality & Cost in Health Care Choice in Developing Countries. Victor Lavy & Jean-Marc Germain. 1994. LC 94-12590. (LSMS Working Papers: No. 105). 48p. pap. 22.00 (*0-8213-2854-9*, 12854) World Bank.

Quality & Quantity: The Quest for Biological Regeneration in Twentieth Century France. William H. Schneider. 1990. (History of Medicine Ser.). (Illus.). 402p. (C). text 69.95 (*0-521-37498-7*) Cambridge U Pr.

Quality Around the World. 1997. LC 97-52055. x, 92p. pap. (*1-56395-091-X*) Am Assn Blood.

Quality Assessment & Assurance in Long-Term Care Facilities. Charlotte K. Eliopoulos. 2nd ed. 2001. 97p. pap. 25.00 (*1-882515-01-3*) Hlth Educ Netwk.

Quality Assessment & Improvement in Long Term Care: A Continuous Process. Barbara A. Vitale & Stella M. Vengroski. 1993. LC 92-48816. (Illus.). 346p. (C). pap. text 90.00 (*0-8036-8960-8*) Davis Co.

Quality Assessment for Healthcare: A Baldrige-Based Handbook. Ned Barber. 1995. LC 95-41103. 204p. pap. 29.95 (*0-527-76305-5*) Product Pr.

Quality Assessment for Primary Care Centers. Dale S. Benson & Jane A. Miller. 3rd rev. ed. 1993. (Quality Primary Care Ser.). pap. 28.00 (*0-9603164-9-3*) Clarian Hlth.

Quality Assurance & Assessment in Primary Health Care. M. Roemer & C. Montoya-Aguilar. 1988. (WHO Offset Publications: No. 105). 82p. 15.00 (*92-4-170105-6*) World Health.

Quality Assurance & Image Artifacts in Magnetic Resonance Imaging. James R. Knowles & John A. Markisz. 1987. (Illus.). 160p. 36.95 (*0-316-49974-9*, Little Brwn Med Div) Lppncott W & W.

Quality Assurance Compliance: Procedures for Pharmaceutical & Biotechnology Manufacturers. Ira Peine. 1994. 279p. ring bd. 199.00 (*0-935184-51-1*) IHS Health Grp.

Quality Assurance Criteria Sets for Pediatric Nutrition Conditions: A Model. 1988. LC 88-72200. ring bd. 24.00 (*0-88091-039-9*, 0109) Am Dietetic Assn.

Quality Assurance for Biopharmaceuticals. Jean F. Huxsoll. 1994. LC 93-46160. 216p. 99.95 (*0-471-03656-0*) Wiley.

Quality Assurance for Clinical Radiotherapy Treatment Planning: Report of the AAPM Radiation Therapy Committee TG#53. Benedick A. Fraass et al. 1998. (Report Ser.: No. 62). 57p. 10.00 (*1-888340-18-5*, TG#53) AAPM.

Quality Assurance for Diagnostic Imaging. 1988. LC 88-25435. (Report Ser.: No. 99). 252p. (C). pap. text 50.00 (*0-929600-00-2*) NCRP Pubns.

Quality Assurance for Pharmacy-Prepared Sterile Products Workbook: A Multi-Media Self-Instructional Program. Ed. by Gergory A. Snyder et al. 1994. 112p. (Orig.). pap. 15.00 (*1-879907-46-1*) Am Soc Hlth-Syst.

Quality Assurance for the Indirect Immunofluorescence Test for Autoantibodies to Nuclear Antigen (IF-ANA) Approved Guideline (1996) 1996. 75.00 (*1-56238-311-6*, I/LA2-A) NCCLS.

Quality Assurance for the Indirect Immunofluorescence Test for Autoantibodies to Nuclear Antigen (IF-ANA) Tentative Guideline (1993) Contrib. by Robert M. Nakamura. 1993. 75.00 (*1-56238-187-3*, I/LA2-T) NCCLS.

Quality Assurance Handbook for Veterinary Laboratories. James E. C. Bellamy & Dennis W. Olexson. 2000. LC 00-22038. (Illus.). x, 101p. pap. 32.95 (*0-8138-0276-8*) Iowa U Pr.

Quality Assurance in Diagnostic Radiology. 1982. (Nonserial Publication). 65p. pap. text 11.00 (*92-4-154164-4*, 1150204) World Health.

Quality Assurance in Dialysis. Ed. by Lee W. Henderson & Richard S. Thuma. 1994. LC 94-970. (Developments in Nephrology Ser.: Vol. 36). 272p. (C). text 161.50 (*0-7923-2723-3*) Kluwer Academic.

Quality Assurance in Health Care. 286p. pap. (*0-340-55273-5*) E A GBR. *Dist:* Routldge.

Quality Assurance in Nuclear Medicine. 1982. (Nonserial Publication). 72p. pap. text 11.00 (*92-4-154165-2*, 1150203) World Health.

Quality Assurance in Prehospital Care. National Association of EMS Physicians Staff. Ed. by Robert A. Swor et al. 1992. LC 92-49237. (Illus.). 272p. (gr. 13). pap. text 19.95 (*0-8016-6579-5*, 06579) Mosby Inc.

Quality Assurance in Radiotherapy. WHO Staff. 1988. 52p. 11.00 (*92-4-154224-1*) World Health.

Quality Assurance in Transfusion Medicine, Vol. I. M. J. Seghatchian. 1992. LC 92-9276. 544p. 295.00 (*0-8493-4938-9*, RM171, CRC Reprint) Franklin.

***Quality Assurance of Aseptic Preparation Services.** Beaney. 3rd ed. 2001. 144p. pap. (*0-85369-487-7*) Pharmaceutical Pr GBR. *Dist:* Rittenhouse.

Quality Assurance of Pharmaceuticals: A Compendium of Guidelines & Related Materials, Vol. 1. WHO Staff. 1997. LC 98-130399. (*92-4-154504-6*) World Health.

Quality Assurance Policies & Procedures for Ambulatory Health Care. Judith M. Bulau. 1990. 368p. ring bd. 184.00 (*0-8342-0138-0*, 20138) Aspen Pub.

Quality Assurance Program on Stereotactic Radiosurgery: Report From a Quality Assurance Task Group. Gunther H. Hartmann et al. 1995. LC 95-32580. (Illus.). 96p. 48.95 (*3-540-59199-0*) Spr-Verlag.

Quality Assurance Through Credentialing Vol. 1: Global Perspectives. Ed. by Ann H. Cary & Chris Wharton. 1999. 79p. (*1-55810-146-2*) Am Nurses Pub.

Quality Assurance Through Credentialing Vol. 2: Concepts, Issues, & Trends. Ed. by Ann H. Cary & Chris Wharton. 1999. 85p. (*1-55810-147-0*) Am Nurses Pub.

Quality Assurance with Care Planning. Mattie Locke. 1992. 290p. (C). 42.00 (*1-877735-36-1*, 2185PP) Prof Prnting & Pub.

Quality Audit Systems for Primary Care Centers. Dale S. Benson & William R. Van Osdol. 3rd rev. ed. 1993. (Quality Primary Care Ser.). x, 451p. pap. 85.00 (*1-884742-01-7*) Clarian Hlth.

Quality Care: Prescription for Injecting Quality into Health Care Systems. Marlene Caroselli. 1997. LC 97-163014. (Illus.). 304p. 69.95 (*1-57444-043-8*) St Lucie Pr.

Quality Care: Prescription for Injecting Quality into Healthcare Systems. Marlene Caroselli & Linda Edison. 1998. tchr. ed., spiral bd. 39.95 (*1-57444-138-8*, SL1388) St Lucie Pr.

Quality Care for Elderly People. Ed. by Peter P. Mayer et al. 1997. LC 97-65432. (Illus.). 312p. (*0-412-61830-3*) E A GBR. *Dist:* OUP.

Quality Care in the Nursing Home. John Morris et al. 1996. LC 96-17375. 900p. (gr. 13). text 54.95 (*0-8151-4222-6*, 26266) Mosby Inc.

Quality Control: A Component of Process Control in Blood Banking & Transfusion Medicine. American Association of Blood Banks Staff. Ed. by Katherine Garnier Kavemeier & Leane Watanabe Ziebell. 1999. (Illus.). 132p. pap. (*3-8055-7059-7*) S Karger.

Quality Control of Diabetes Care & Chronic Compications in Young People after St. Vincent & Kos: 4th International Workshop "Diabetic Angiopathy in Children (DAC)", Berlin, September 4 - 6, 1997. Ed. by Thomas Danne & Bruno Weber. 1998. (Hormone Research Ser.: Vol. 50, Suppl. 1). (Illus.). vi, 108p. pap. 48.75 (*3-8055-6720-0*) S Karger.

Quality Control of Pharmaceutical Preparations. 1962. (Technical Report Ser.: No. 249). 35p. pap. text 3.00 (*92-4-120249-1*) World Health.

Quality Control Testing of Rinderpest Cell Culture Vaccine - Standard Operating Procedure. M. Rweyemamu et al. 1994. LC 95-131051. (Animal Production & Health Papers: No. 118). 112p. pap. (*92-5-103444-3*, F34443) FAO ITA. *Dist:* Bernan Associates.

Quality Determinants of Mammography. 1995. lib. bdg. 251.95 (*0-8490-6845-2*) Gordon Pr.

Quality Evaluation of Dental Restorations. Ed. by Kenneth J. Anusavice. 1989. (Illus.). 424p. text 106.00 (*0-86715-202-8*) Quint Pub Co.

Quality, Evidence, & Effectiveness in Health Promotion. John K. Davies & Gordon MacDonald. 1998. LC 98-22995. (C). 240p. pap. 27.95 (*0-415-17967-X*); (Illus.). 248p. 90.00 (*0-415-17966-1*) Routledge.

Quality First: Better Health Care for All Americans: Final Report to the President of the United States. Ed. by Janet Corrigan. 1999. 315p. (C). pap. text 35.00 (*0-7881-7796-6*) DIANE Pub.

Quality Health Care for the Elderly: A Manual for Instructors for Nurses & Other Health Workers. 1995. (Western Pacific Education in Action Ser.: No. 6). 256p. (C). pap. text 22.00 (*92-9061-136-7*, 1500006) World Health.

Quality Imperative: Measurement & Mangement of Quality in Healthcare. John R. Kimberly. 1999. LC 99-88946. 224p. (*1-86094-173-7*) Imperial College GBR. *Dist:* World Scientific Pub.

Quality Improvement in Health Care: Putting Evidence into Practice. Karen Parsley & Philomena Corrigan. 2nd ed. 1999. (Illus.). 448p. pap. (*0-7487-3355-8*) Nelson Thornes GBR. *Dist:* Intl Spec Bk.

Quality Improvement Projects in Health Care: Problem Solving in the Workplace. Eleanor G. Gilpatrick. 1998. LC 98-25380. 84.95 (*0-7619-1166-9*, 81639); pap. 46.95 (*0-7619-1167-7*, 81640) Sage.

Quality Improvement Techniques for Hospital Safety. Hugh Greeley & Jennifer I. Cofer. 1993. (Health Care Quality Improvement Ser.). 246p. pap. text 57.00 (*1-885829-08-6*) Opus Communs.

Quality Improvement Techniques for Medical Records. Jennifer I. Cofer & Hugh Greeley. 1996. (Health Care Quality Improvement Ser.). 217p. pap. text 47.00 (*1-885829-04-3*) Opus Communs.

Quality Improvement Techniques for Radiology. Jennifer I. Cofer & Hugh Greeley. 1994. (Health Care Quality Improvement Ser.). 230p. pap. text 47.00 (*1-885829-06-X*) Opus Communs.

Quality Improvement Techniques for Respiratory Care. Jennifer L. Cofer & Hugh Greeley. 1993. (Health Care Quality Improvement Ser.). 220p. pap. text 42.00 (*1-885829-05-1*) Opus Communs.

Quality in Action. Ed. by Judy B. Duckett et al. 1996. (Illus.). 90p. pap. text 55.00 (*1-56395-063-4*, PC97-960016) Am Assn Blood.

Quality in Health Care: Theory, Application & Evolution. Nancy D. Graham. 3rd ed. 1997. 384p. 75.00 (*0-8342-0625-0*, 20625) Aspen Pub.

***Quality in Helath Care: Strategic Issues in Health Care Management.** Ed. by H. T. O. Davies et al. 2001. 246p. text (*0-7546-1613-4*) Ashgate Pub GBR. *Dist:* Ashgate Pub Co.

Quality in Nursing Services. Beyers. 1997. text (*0-7216-4255-1*) Saunders.

***Quality Indicators for General Practice: A Practical Guide for Primary Health Care Professionals & Managers.** M. Marshall et al. 2001. 100p. pap. (*1-85315-488-1*) Royal Soc of Medicine Pr Ltd GBR. *Dist:* Balogh.

Quality Management: A Guide for Health Care Managers. Marylane Wade Koch. 1991. (Illus.). 352p. 36.95 (*0-8016-2731-1*) Mosby Inc.

Quality Management for Chemical Safety Testing. 1992. (Environmental Health Criteria Ser.: No. 141). (ENG, FRE & SPA.). 112p. pap. text 26.00 (*92-4-157141-1*, 1160141) World Health.

Quality Management in Health Care. Peter Goldschmidt & Lionel Wilson. 1995. (Illus.). 520p. pap. 99.95 (*0-07-470247-5*) McGraw-Hill Prof.

Quality Management In Radiography: A Technologist's Guide. Andrea Trigg Stevens. 2000. LC 00-55042. (Illus.). 448p. (C). pap. 39.95 (*0-8385-8249-4*) McGraw-Hill Prof.

Quality Management Integration in Long-Term Care: Guidelines for Excellence. Maryjane G. Bradley & Nancy R. Thompson. 1999. LC 99-27315. 174p. 31.95 (*1-878812-61-0*) Hlth Prof Pr.

Quality Management, 2000: Preparing the Quality Improvement Professional for the Future. Deborah K. Wall & Mitchell M. Proyect. 1997. LC 97-23808. (Illus.). 192p. pap. 40.00 (*0-944496-51-2*) Precept Pr.

Quality Managment in the Imaging Sciences. Jeffrey Papp. 1998. LC 97-46903. (Illus.). 320p. (C). text 38.00 (*0-8151-2968-8*, 31848) Mosby Inc.

Quality of Care: Selections from the New England Journal of Medicine. Ed. by Jerome P. Kassirer & Marcia Angell. 1997. LC 97-71084. 77p. pap. 15.00 (*0-910133-40-9*) Mass Med Pub Div.

Quality of Death Rates by Race & Hispanic-Origin. Harry M. Rosenberg. 1999. LC 99-41288. (Vital & Health Statistics Ser.). pap. (*0-8406-0559-5*) Natl Ctr Health Stats.

Quality of Life: From Nursing & Patient Perspectives. Cynthia King. 1998. LC 98-14252. (Nursing Ser.). (Illus.). 416p. (C). text 52.95 (*0-7637-0628-0*, 0628-0) Jones & Bartlett.

Quality of Life: The New Medical Dilemma. Thomas A. Shannon. Ed. by James J. Walter. 1991. LC 90-41235. 368p. pap. 14.95 (*0-8091-3191-9*) Paulist Pr.

Quality of Life Vol. II: Application to Persons with Disabilities Ed. by Robert L. Schalock. 1997. LC 95-50087. (Illus.). 267p. (Orig.). pap. 35.00 (*0-940898-41-1*) Am Assn Mental.

Quality of Life & Health. I. Guggenmoos-Holzman et al. 1996. (Illus.). 200p. (Orig.). (C). pap. text 75.00 (*0-86542-668-6*) Blackwell Sci.

Quality of Life & Mental Health Services. J. P. Oliver. 1997. LC 96-44152. (Illus.). 256p. (C). pap. 29.95 (*0-415-16151-7*) Routledge.

Quality of Life & Pharmacoeconomics in Clinical Trials. Joyce Cramer. 2nd abr. ed. 1997. LC 97-37999. (Illus.). 288p. pap. text 49.95 (*0-397-51845-5*) Lppncott W & W.

Quality of Life & Pharmacoeconomics in Clinical Trials. Ed. by Bert Spilker. 2nd rev. ed. 1995. LC 95-17690. (Illus.). 1,312p. text 175.00 (*0-7817-0332-8*) Lppncott W & W.

Quality of Life & Psychosomatics: In Mechanical Circulation in Heart Transplantation. Ed. by W. Albert et al. 1998. (Illus.). 118p. 38.00 (*3-7985-0991-3*) Spr-Verlag.

Quality of Life Assessment - International Perspectives: Proceedings of the Joint Meeting Organized by the World Health Organization & the Foundation IPSEN in Paris, July 2-3,1993. Ed. by J. Orley & W. Kuyken. 1994. LC 94-26934. (Illus.). 215p. 97.00 (*0-387-58205-3*) Spr-Verlag.

Quality of Life Assessment in Clinical Trials: Methods & Practice. Ed. by Maurice J. Staquet et al. 1998. (Illus.). 370p. text 47.50 (*0-19-262785-6*) OUP.

Quality of Life Following Renal Failure: Psychosocial Challenges Accompanying High Technology Medicine. Hannah McGee. 1994. pap. (*3-7186-5522-5*) Gordon & Breach.

Quality of Life Following Renal Failure: Psychosocial Challenges Accompanying High Technology Medicine. Ed. by Hannah M. McGee & Clare Bradley. 1994. 312p. text 59.00 (*3-7186-5501-2*) Gordon & Breach.

Quality of Life in Behavioral Medicine Research. Ed. by Joel E. Dimsdale & Andrew S. Baum. 1995. (Perspectives on Behavioral Medicine Ser.). 304p. text 59.95 (*0-8058-1653-4*) L Erlbaum Assocs.

***Quality of Life in Child & Adolescent Illness: Concepts, Methods & Findings.** Hans Koot. 2001. 398p. 69.00 (*90-5823-218-2*); pap. 35.00 (*90-5823-219-0*) Gordon & Breach (Harwood Acad Pubs).

Quality of Life in Epilepsy: Beyond Seizure Counts in Assessment & Treatment. Ed. by Gus A. Baker & Ann Jacoby. 2000. 235p. 58.00 (*90-5823-121-6*, Harwood Acad Pubs) Gordon & Breach.

Quality of Life in Health Care. Ed. by Gary L. Albrecht & Ray Fitzpatrick. 1994. (Advances in Medical Sociology Ser.: Vol. 5). 311p. 78.50 (*1-55938-838-2*) Jai Pr.

Quality of Life in Health Promotion & Rehabilitation: Conceptual Approaches, Issues, & Applications. Rebecca Renwick et al. 1996. LC 95-41770. (Illus.). 320p. 76.95 (*0-8039-5913-3*, 2943); pap. 38.95 (*0-8039-5914-1*, 2942) Sage.

Quality of Life in Mental Disorders. Heinz Katschnig et al. 1997. LC 97-23241. 402p. 170.00 (*0-471-96643-6*) Wiley.

***Quality of Life in Patients with Endocrine Gastrointestinal Tumours.** Gunnel Larsson. 2001. (Comprehensive Summaries of Uppsala Dissertations from the Faculty of Medicine Ser.: No. 989). (Illus.). 67p. pap. (*91-554-4916-6*) Uppsala Universitet SWE. *Dist:* Coronet Bks.

Quality of Life Measurement among Persons with Chronic Mental Illness: A Critique of Measures & Methods. Mark J. Atkinson & Sharon Zibin. 1996. iv, 65p. (*0-662-25002-8*) Intl Spec Bk.

Quality of Medical Care: Evaluation & Improvement. Beverly C. Payne. 1976. LC 75-27157. 10.00 (*0-87914-029-1*, 669153) Hosp Res & Educ.

Quality Point of Care Testing: A Joint Commission Handbook. Joint Commission on Accreditation of Healthcare Organizations. 1999. (Illus.). 142p. pap. 47.00 (*0-86688-604-4*, POC-100) Joint Comm Hlthcare.

Quality Program: Quality Plan Manual. Ed. by Jenni L. Robbins. 1994. LC 94-27478. (Illus.). (C). ring bd. 175.00 (*1-56395-040-5*) Am Assn Blood.

Quality Program: Self-Assessment Manual. Ed. by Jenni L. Robbins. 1994. LC 94-27478. (Illus.). (C). ring bd. 175.00 (*1-56395-039-1*) Am Assn Blood.

Quality Reengineering in Healthcare: A Case Study from the Clinical Laboratory of the University of Wisconsin Hospital & Clinics. Russel H. Tomar et al. 1998. LC 98-7848. 35.00 (*0-89189-435-7*) Am Soc Clinical.

Quality Resource Packet for Trustees. American Hospital Association Staff. 1992. 78p. (Orig.). pap. 100.00 (*0-87258-629-4*, 196300) Am Hospital.

Quality System Compendium: GMP Requirements & Industry Practice. Susan S. Reilly et al. 1996. (Orig.). pap. 295.00 (*1-57020-076-9*, GMPS-209) Assn Adv Med Instrn.

Quality System for European Orthodontic Professionals: The EURO-QUAL - European Orthodontic Quality Manual. Ed. by B. J. Njio et al. 1999. (Biomedical & Health Research Ser.: Vol. 31). 98p. pap., wbk. ed. 62.00 (*90-5199-478-8*) IOS Press.

Quality System for European Orthodontic Professionals (Info Book) Ed. by B. J. Njio. 2000. (Biomedical & Health Research Ser.: Vol. 32). (*90-5199-479-6*) IOS Press.

Quality Systems in the Blood Bank & Laboratory Environment. David E. Nevalainen & Marjana F. Callery. 1994. (Illus.). (C). pap. text 89.00 (*1-56395-038-3*) Am Assn Blood.

Quality Systems in the Blood Bank Environment. American Association of Blood Banks Staff. 2nd ed. 1998. 410p. pap. (*3-8055-6902-5*) S Karger.

Quality Systems in the Blood Bank Environment. Ed. by Leane Ziebel & Kathy Keuemeir. 2nd ed. 1999. LC 99-182220. text (*1-56395-098-7*) Am Assn Blood.

Quality Team Workbook. Barbara Katz. 1999. 112p. ring bd. 9.95 (*0-9640405-2-2*) Hlth Interact.

Quality Use of Medicines. Andrea Mant. 1999. (Illus.). 249p. pap. 44.95 (*0-07-470769-8*) McGraw-Hill Prof.

Quantification & the Quest for Medical Certainty. J. Rosser Matthews. 1995. LC 94-24091. 200p. 50.00 (*0-691-03794-9*) Princeton U Pr.

Quantification of Brain Function: Tracer Kinetics & Image Analysis in Brain PET. Ed. by K. Uemura et al. 1993. LC 93-6089. (International Congress Ser.: No. 1030). 720p. 289.00 (*0-444-89859-X*, Excerpta Medica) Elsevier.

Quantification of Circulating Proteins. W. T. Hermens. 1982. text 141.50 (*90-247-2755-3*) Kluwer Academic.

Quantification of Human Defense Mechanisms. Ed. by M. Olff et al. 1991. (Recent Research in Psychology Ser.). (Illus.). 327p. 79.95 (*0-387-53821-6*) Spr-Verlag.

Quantification of Neurologic Deficit. Theodore L. Munsat. 1989. (Illus.). 372p. text 89.95 (*0-409-90152-0*) Buttrwrth-Heinemann.

Quantification of Occupational Cancer. Ed. by Richard Peto & Marvin Schneiderman. 1981. LC 81-10218. (Banbury Reports: Vol. 9). 756p. (C). 99.00 (*0-87969-208-1*) Cold Spring Harbor.

Quantification of the Effects of Air Pollution on Health in the United Kingdom. 1998. (*0-11-322102-9*, HM221029) Statnry Office GBR. *Dist:* Bernan Associates.

Quantitative Anaesthesia. Ed. by K. Van Ackern et al. 1989. (Anaesthesiologie und Intensivmedizin Ser.: Vol. 204). (Illus.). 170p. 38.95 (*0-387-50436-2*) Spr-Verlag.

Quantitative Analysis for Health Services Administration. Charles J. Austin & Stuart B. Boxerman. 1995. 333p. 60.00 (*1-56793-032-8*, 0964) Health Admin Pr.

***Quantitative Analysis of Disease Associated Mutations & Sequence Variants.** Charlotta Olsson. 2001. (Comprehensive Summaries of Uppsala Dissertations from the Faculty of Medicine Ser.: No. 1036). (Illus.). 55p. (*91-554-5018-0*) Uppsala Universitet SWE. *Dist:* Coronet Bks.

Quantitative & Dynamic Thermal Imaging in Medical Diagnosis. Michael Anbar. 1994. 288p. lib. bdg. 110.00 (*0-8493-4409-3*) CRC Pr.

Quantitative Assessment in Epilepsy Care. H. Meinardi et al. 1993. LC 93-26823. (NATO ASI Series A, Life Sciences: Series A, Vol. 255). (Illus.). 222p. (C). text 85.00 (*0-306-44620-0*) Plenum.

Quantitative Auriculotherapy. Meyer R. Rosen. 1994. LC 94-76974. 52p. pap. 35.00 (*0-9641617-1-0*) Interact Cnslting.

Quantitative Calculations in Pharmaceutical Practice & Research. Themistocles P. Hadjioannou et al. 1993. LC 93-3446. (Analytical Techniques in Clinical Chemistry & Laboratory Medicine Ser.). 120.00 (*0-89573-282-3*); pap. 59.95 (*1-56081-654-6*) Wiley (Wiley-VCH).

Quantitative Cerebral Blood Flow Measurements Using Stable Xenon/CT: Clinical Applications. Ed. by Masamichi Tomonaga et al. 1995. LC 94-42191. (Illus.). 368p. 75.00 (*0-87993-609-6*) Futura Pub.

Quantitative Coronary Angiography in Clinical Practice. Ed. by Patrick W. Serruys et al. 1994. LC 93-22792. (Developments in Cardiovascular Medicine Ser.: Vol. 145). text 402.50 (*0-7923-2368-8*) Kluwer Academic.

Quantitative Coronary Arteriography. Ed. by Johan H. Reiber & Patrick W. Serruys. 1991. (Developments in Cardiovascular Medicine Ser.). (C). text 272.50 (*0-7923-0913-8*) Kluwer Academic.

Quantitative Examination of Neurologic Functions Ed. by Alfred R. Potvin & Wallace W. Tourtellotte. 1985. Vol. I. 272p. 147.00 (*0-8493-5926-0*, RC348); Vol. II. 224p. 125.00 (*0-8493-5927-9*) Franklin (CRC Reprint).

Quantitative Explorations in Drug Abuse Policy. Ed. by Irving Leveson. 1980. LC 79-21399. 183p. 45.00 (*0-88331-192-5*) R B Luce.

Quantitative Foundations of Counseling Psychology Research. Ed. by Bruce E. Wampold. 1987. (Special Issue, Journal of Counseling Psychology Ser.: Vol. 34, No. 4). 133p. pap. 16.00 (*1-55798-007-1*) Am Psychol.

Quantitative Functional Brain Imaging with Positron Tomography. Ed. by Richard E. Carson et al. 1998. LC 98-85439. (Illus.). 504p. (C). 139.95 (*0-12-161340-2*) Acad Pr.

***Quantitative Imaging with PET: Performance & Application of 76Br, 52Fe, 110mIn, 134La.** Mark Lubberink. 2001. (Illus.). 70p. (*91-554-5015-6*) Uppsala Universitet SWE. *Dist:* Coronet Bks.

Quantitative Industrial Hygiene: A Formula Workbook. Jack Caravanos. Ed. by American Conference of Governmental Industrial Hygenists Staff. 1991. (Illus.). 214p. (C). pap. text 37.00 (*0-936712-95-3*) Am Conf Govt Indus Hygienist.

Quantitative Methods. Lapin. 6th ed. 1995. tchr. ed. 9.25 net. (*0-534-51055-8*) Brooks-Cole.

Quantitative Methods for Behavioral Sciences: Introduction to Statistics. Steven Haggbloom. 1998. 226p. (C). pap. 25.63 (*0-07-154125-X*) McGrw-H Hghr Educ.

Quantitative Methods for Health Sciences. Gary Lawler. 1996. (Illus.). 332p. pap. 24.50 (*0-8273-5968-3*) Delmar.

Quantitative Methods for the Evaluation of Cancer Screening. Ed. by Stephen Duffy et al. 2000. (An Arnold Publication). 320p. (*0-340-74125-2*) E A GBR. *Dist:* OUP.

Quantitative Methods in Biological & Medical Sciences: A Historical Essay. H. O. Lancaster. 1994. LC 94-8063. 297p. 110.00 (*0-387-94279-3*) Spr-Verlag.

Quantitative Methods in Bone Densitometry. Alan Huddleston. 1988. (C). text 179.50 (*0-89838-362-5*) Kluwer Academic.

Quantitative Nursing Research. Thomas R. Knapp. 1998. LC 97-45338. (Education Ser.). 287p. 79.95 (*0-7619-1362-9*, 82303); pap. 39.95 (*0-7619-1363-7*, 82304) Sage.

Quantitative PCR Protocols. Bernd Kochanowski & Udo Reischl. 1999. LC 99-10332. (Methods in Molecular Medicine Ser.: Vol. 26). (Illus.). 320p. 99.50 (*0-89603-518-2*) Humana.

Quantitative Problem Solving in Maternal, Child, & Adolescent Health. Ed. by Jeffrey B. Gould. 1994. (Illus.). 222p. (Orig.). pap. 19.95 (*0-89914-042-4*) Third Party Pub.

Quantitative Psychology. J. Drosler. 1989. LC 89-7457. (Illus.). 200p. (C). text 38.00 (*0-88937-028-1*) Hogrefe & Huber Pubs.

Quantitative Risk Assessment. Ed. by Robert F. Almeder & James M. Humber. 1987. LC 84-640015. (Biomedical Ethics Reviews Ser.: No. 1986). 278p. 59.50 (*0-89603-056-3*) Humana.

Quantitative Risk Assessment for Environmental & Occupational Health. William H. Hallenbeck. 2nd ed. 1993. 240p. lib. bdg. 75.00 (*0-87371-801-1*, L801) Lewis Pubs.

Quantitative Risk Assessment in Regulation. Ed. by Lester B. Lave. 1983. LC 82-22603. (Studies in the Regulation of Economic Activity). 264p. text 34.95 (*0-8157-5164-8*); pap. text 14.95 (*0-8157-5163-X*) Brookings.

Quantitative Structure-Activity Relations in Environmental Toxicology. Klaus L. Kaiser. 1984. text 185.50 (*90-277-1776-1*) Kluwer Academic.

Quantities & Units In Radiation Protection Dosimetry. ICRU Staff. Ed. by W. Roger Ney. 1993. (ICRU Report Ser.: No. 51). 19p. pap. 30.00 (*0-913394-50-5*) Intl Comm Rad Meas.

Quantities, Symbols, Units andbbreviations in the Life Sciences: A Guide for Authors & Editors. Arnost Kotyk. 1999. LC 98-31182. 152p. pap. 24.95 (*0-89603-649-9*) Humana.

Quantum Brain Dynamics & Consciousness: An Introduction. Mari Jibu & Kunio Yasue. 1995. LC 95-35756. (Advances in Consciousness Research Ser.: Vol. 3). xvi, 244p. 38.95 (*1-55619-183-9*) J Benjamins Pubng Co.

***Quantum Change: When Epiphanies & Sudden Insights Transform Ordinary Lives.** William R. Miller & Janet C'Debaca. 2001. LC 00-66340. 212p. 35.00 (*1-57230-667-X*) Guilford Pubns.

Quantum Field Theory & Parastatistics. Y. Ohnuki & S. Kamefuchi. 1982. (Illus.). 489p. 123.00 (*0-387-11643-5*) Spr-Verlag.

Quantum Healing: Exploring the Frontiers of Body, Mind, Medicine. Deepak Chopra. 1990. LC 88-7761. 272p. pap. 14.95 (*0-553-34869-8*) Bantam.

Quantum Mind: The Edge Between Physics & Psychology. Arnold Mindell. 2000. LC 99-66088. (Illus.). 629p. pap. 26.95 (*1-887078-64-9*) Lao Tse Pr.

Quantum Psychology: How Brain Software Programs You & Your World. Robert A. Wilson. 2nd ed. 1993. LC 92-63046. 256p. (Orig.). pap. 14.95 (*1-56184-071-8*) New Falcon Pubns.

Quantum Psychology: Steps to a Postmodern Ecology of Being. Stephen T. DeBerry. 1993. LC 92-28474. 224p. 62.50 (*0-275-94171-X*, C4171, Praeger Pubs) Greenwood.

Quarreling. Gail Hudson. 1997. LC 98-220779. (Child's Magazine Guide to Ser.). 208p. per. 5.99 (*0-671-88040-3*) PB.

Quarry. Jeffery D. Phillips. 1998. 24.95 (*1-891128-54-X*) Chapel & Croft.

Que Deberia Hacer? Cuidado de Emergencia Y Sequridad. Judith Schneider. 1997. (SPA.). 57p. pap. 10.95 (*0-944454-20-8*) CAPE Center.

Que Dice Usted Despues de Decir Hola? Eric Berne. 1997. (SPA.). pap. text (*968-419-610-5*) Grijalbo Edit.

Que Gordita! A Study of Weight among Women in a Puerto Rican Community. Emily B. Massara. 1989. LC 88-35144. (Immigrant Communities & Ethnic Minorities in the U. S. & Canada Ser.: No. 46). 57.50 (*0-404-19456-7*) AMS Pr.

Que Hacer Cuando Su Nino Se Enferme: Facil de Leer & Facil de Usar. Gloria G. Mayer & Ann Kuklierus. 2000. (SPA., Illus.). 181p. pap. 14.95 (*0-9701245-1-1*) IHA.

Que Hacer Para la Salud de las Personas de Edad. Albert Barnett et al. 2000. (SPA., Illus.). pap. 14.95 (*0-9701245-5-4*) IHA.

Que Hacer Para la Salud de los Adolescentes. Gloria G. Mayer & Ann Kuklierus. 2000. (Illus.). pap. 14.95 (*0-9701245-3-8*) IHA.

Que Paso? An English-Spanish Guide for Medical Personnel. Martin P. Kantrowitz et al. 4th rev. ed. 1984. LC 83-14670. 77p. pap. 7.95 (*0-8263-0725-6*) U of NM Pr.

Que se Puede Esperar Cuando se Esta Esperando (What to Expect When You're Expecting) Arlene Eisenberg et al. 1997. LC 97-25464. (SPA., Illus.). 576p. pap. 13.95 (*0-7611-0949-8*) Workman Pub.

Queen Victoria's Gene: Haemophilia & the Royal Family. D. M. Potts. 1997. LC 96-143392. xi, 160p. (*0-7509-0868-8*) Sutton Pub Ltd GBR. *Dist:* Intl Pubs Mktg.

Queer Blood: The Secret AIDS Genocide Plot. Alan Cantwell, Jr. Ed. by Sallie Fiske. 1993. 168p. (Orig.). pap. 12.95 (*0-917211-26-X*) Aries Rising.

Quest for Answers: A Primer of Understanding & Treating Severe Personality Disorders. Salman Akhtar. 1995. LC 94-22794. 240p. pap. 40.00 (*1-56821-364-6*) Aronson.

Quest for Common Learning: The Aims of General Education. Ernest L. Boyer & Arthur Levine. 1981. LC 81-66307. 68p. pap. 12.00 (*0-931050-18-9*) Carnegie Fnd Advan Teach.

Quest for Conception: Gender, Infertility, & Egyptian Medical Traditions. Marcia C. Inhorn. 1994. LC 94-10899. (Illus.). 472p. (Orig.). (C). text 49.95 (*0-8122-3221-6*) U of Pa Pr.

Quest for Cost-Effectiveness in Health Care: Achieving Clinical Excellence While Controlling Costs. Jeffrey P. Trotter. 1995. LC 94-43404. 114p. pap. 35.00 (*1-55648-130-6*, 061171) AHPI.

Quest for Cure: Restoring Function after Spinal Cord Injury. Sam Maddox. 1993. LC 92-50575. (Illus.). 200p. (Orig.). pap. 22.45 (*0-929819-03-9*) Paralyzed Vets.

Quest for Fruition Through Ngoma: The Political Aspects of Healing in South Africa. Ed. by Rijk Van Dijk et al. 1999. LC 99-45652. 172p. text 44.95 (*0-8214-1303-1*); pap. text 22.95 (*0-8214-1304-X*) Ohio U Pr.

Quest for Immortality: Science at the Frontiers of Aging. S. Jay Olshansky et al. 2000. LC 00-58391. 176p. 25.95 (*0-393-04836-5*) Norton.

Quest for Mental Health in America, Eighteen Eighty to Nineteen Seventeen. Barbara Sicherman. Ed. by Gerald N. Grob. 1980. LC 78-22589. (Historical Issues in Mental Health Ser.). lib. bdg. 37.95 (*0-405-11940-2*) Ayer.

Quest for Mercy: The Forgotten Ingredient in Health Care Reform. Roger J. Bulger. 1997. 120p. pap. text 10.00 (*1-891524-01-1*) Carden Jennings.

Quest for Mind: Piaget, Levi-Strauss & the Structuralist Movement. Howard Gardner. 2nd ed. 1981. 320p. pap. text 9.00 (*0-226-28332-1*) U Ch Pr.

***Quest for Personal Power: Transforming Stress into Strength.** Phil Nuernberger. 2001. 286p. reprint ed. 24.00 (*0-7881-9868-8*) DIANE Pub.

Quest for the Father: A Study of the Darwin-Butler Controversy. Phyllis Greenacre. 1963. LC 63-13193. (New York Psychoanalytic Institute Freud Anniversary Lecture Ser.). 27.50 (*0-8236-5760-4*) Intl Univs Pr.

Quest for Therapy in Lower Zaire. John M. Janzen. 1978. (Comparative Studies of Health Systems & Medical Care: Vol. 1). pap. text 22.00 (*0-520-04633-1*) U CA Pr.

Quest for Voice in Contemporary Psychoanalysis. Carlo Strenger. 2001. 270p. pap. text 39.95 (*0-8236-5762-0*) Intl Univs Pr.

Question & Answer Book: American Journal of Nursing. American Journal of Nursing Staff et al. 5th ed. 1996. 320p. (C). (gr. 13). pap. text 28.95 (*0-8151-0081-7*, 27083) Mosby Inc.

***Question & Answer Review for Dental Hygiene.** Barnes. 5th ed. 2001. 406p. pap. 38.67 (*0-8385-0342-X*) P-H.

Question & Answer Review of Medical Assisting. Tom Palko & Hilda Palko. 6th ed. 2000. LC 00-61133. (Success Across the Boards Ser.). (Illus.). 469p. pap. 43.33 (*0-13-088189-9*) P-H.

Question of AIDS. Ed. by Richard Liebmann-Smith. 1985. 89p. pap. text 6.00 (*0-89766-302-0*) NY Acad Sci.

Question of Choice: Bioethical Reflections on a Spiritual Response to the Technological Imperative. Pamela McGrath. 1997. LC 97-74821. (Series in Philosophy). 256p. text (*1-84014-166-2*) Ashgate Pub GBR. *Dist:* Ashgate Pub Co.

Question of Guidance. White. 1988. 188p. pap. (*0-85207-193-0*) C W Daniel GBR. *Dist:* Natl Bk Netwk.

Question of Lay Analysis. Sigmund Freud. Ed. & Tr. by James Strachey. 1990. reprint ed. pap. 6.95 (*0-393-00503-8*) Norton.

Question Review for Fleisher & Ludwig's Textbook of Pediatric Emergency Medicine. Sujit Sharma et al. 4th ed. 2000. 496p. pap. text 49.95 (*0-7817-2467-8*) Lppncott W & W.

Questioning Chemotherapy: A Critique of the Use of Toxic Drugs in the Treatment of Cancer. Ralph W. Moss. 1995. LC 95-11440. pap. 19.95 (*1-881025-25-X*) Equinox Pr.

Questioning Misfortune: The Pragmatics of Uncertainty in Eastern Uganda. Susan R. Whyte. 1998. LC 97-10235. (Cambridge Studies in Medical Anthropology: No. 4). (Illus.). 272p. (C). text 74.95 (*0-521-59402-2*) Cambridge U Pr.

Questioning the Solution: The Politics of Primary Health Care & Child Survival. David Werner et al. 1997. LC 96-79528. (Illus.). 206p. 25.00 (*0-9655585-1-7*); pap. 18.00 (*0-9655585-2-5*, RJ103) HealthWrights.

Questionnaires: Design & Use. John F. Anderson et al. 2nd ed. 1986. LC 86-1783. 344p. 34.50 (*0-8108-1884-1*) Scarecrow.

Questionnaires & Inventories: Surveying Opinions & Assessing Personality. Lewis R. Aiken. 1997. LC 96-53659. (Illus.). 319p. 105.00 incl. disk (*0-471-16871-8*) Wiley.

Questionnaires from the National Health Interview Survey, 1985-89. U. S. Department of Health & Human Services Staff et al. 1993. LC 93-854. (Vital & Health Statistics Ser. 1: Programs & Collection Procedures: No. 31). (*0-8406-0480-7*) Natl Ctr Health Stats.

Questions & Answers. John Ramsell. 128p. pap. 13.95 (*0-8464-4277-9*) Beekman Pubs.

Questions & Answers. John Ramsell. 1991. 110p. pap. (*0-85207-240-6*) C W Daniel GBR. *Dist:* Natl Bk Netwk.

Questions & Answers about Depression & Its Treatment: A Consultation with a Leading Psychiatrist. Ivan K. Goldberg. 1993. LC 93-9430. 160p. (Orig.). pap. 16.95 (*0-914783-68-8*) Charles.

Questions & Answers about Electric & Magnetic Fields (EMF) Associated with the Use of Electric Power. 1997. (Illus.). 66p. (C). reprint ed. pap. text 25.00 (*0-7881-4622-X*) DIANE Pub.

Questions & Answers about Pain Control: A Guide for People with Cancer & Their Families. 1994. (Illus.). 76p. (Orig.). pap. text 20.00 (*0-7881-1157-4*) DIANE Pub.

Questions & Answers about Suicide. David Lester. 1989. LC 89-60683. 184p. (Orig.). (C). pap. text 17.95 (*0-914783-31-9*) Charles.

Questions & Answers for Dental Nurses. Hollins. 1997. 160p. 24.95 (*0-632-04283-4*) Blackwell Sci.

Questions & Answers for Medical Nurses. A. Zzizinga. 1983. pap. text (*0-582-77702-X*) Addison-Wesley GBR. *Dist:* Trans-Atl Phila.

Questions & Answers for Symptoms & Signs in Clinical Medicine. Colin Ogilvie & J. E. Earls. 1987. (Illus.). 268p. pap. text 32.50 (*0-7236-0865-2*) Buttrwrth-Heinemann.

Questions & Answers in Magnetic Resonance Imaging. Allen D. Elster & Jonathan Burdette. 2nd ed. 2001. LC 00-48043. (Illus.). xiv, 333p. (*0-323-01184-5*) Mosby Inc.

Questions & Answers in Nuclear Medicine. Stephen M. Karesh et al. 1998. LC 98-22425. (Illus.). 288p. (C). text (*1-55664-428-0*) Mosby Inc.

Questions & Answers on AIDS. Lyn Frumkin & John Leonard. 1987. 192p. (Orig.). pap. 3.95 (*0-380-75467-3*, Avon Bks) Morrow Avon.

Questions & Answers on AIDS. Lyn Frumkin & John Leonard. (PMIC Consumer Health Ser.). (Orig.). 2nd ed. 1995. 206p. pap. 6.99 (*1-878487-86-8*, ME224); 3rd rev. ed. 1997. LC 96-78924. (Illus.). 292p. pap. 12.95 (*1-885987-07-2*, ME079, Health Info Pr) Practice Mgmt Info.

Questions & Answers on Apley's Concise System of Orthopedics. Christopher Lavy & David S. Barrett. 1991. 192p. pap. text 30.00 (*0-7506-1170-7*) Buttrwrth-Heinemann.

Questions & Answers on the Science of Mind. Ernest Holmes & Alberta Smith. 1981. 176p. pap. 10.95 (*0-911336-88-5*) Sci of Mind.

Questions & Answers on Tropical Medicine & Infectious Diseases. Contrib. by S. K. Owusu. 1997. LC 98-982046. (*9964-3-0204-5*) Ghana U Pr.

Questions & Uncertainties in Prostate Cancer. Ed. by W. B. Peeling. 1996. LC 95-39904. 320p. pap. 79.95 (*0-86542-965-0*) Blackwell Sci.

Questions for Freud: The Secret History of Psychoanalysis. Nicholas Rand. 1997. LC 97-15084. 240p. 24.95 (*0-674-74325-3*) HUP.

Questions from the Heart: Answers to 100 Questions about Chelation Therapy, a Safe Alternative to Bypas Surgery. Terry Chappell. 1996. LC 97-111497. 136p. pap. text 10.95 (*1-57174-026-0*) Hampton Roads Pub Co.

Questions in Human Anatomy. Whitmore. 1995. mass mkt. (*0-7234-2055-6*) Wolfe Publishing GBR. *Dist:* Mosby Inc.

Questions in Physiology. Bindman. 2nd ed. 1993. pap. text 14.95 (*0-340-57926-9*) Trafalgar.

Questions Most Asked about Anxiety & Phobias: A Lively, Down to Earth Guide for Overcoming Panic. J. D. Miller. 1996. 166p. (Orig.). pap. 10.50 (*0-9654873-0-X*) Pretext Pr.

Questions of Consciousness. Ed. by Anthony P. Cohen & Nigel Rapport. 1995. LC 95-15785. (ASA Monographs: Vol. 33). 256p. (C). pap. 29.95 (*0-415-12396-8*) Routledge.

Questions of Destiny: Mental Retardation & Curative Education. Carlo Pietzner. 1988. (Illus.). 60p. (Orig.). pap. 6.95 (*0-88010-264-0*) Anthroposophic.

Questions of Life: Diary of an Old Physician. Nikolai I. Pirogov. 1992. LC 89-24332. (Resources in Medical History Ser.). (Illus.). xxii, 480p. 29.95 (*0-88135-061-3*, Sci Hist) Watson Pub Intl.

Quick & Accurate 12-Lead ECG Interpretation. Dale Davis. 3rd ed. 2000. LC 00-29047. (Illus.). 464p. pap. text 39.95 (*0-7817-2327-2*) Lppncott W & W.

Quick & Easy Dosage Calculations: Using Dimensional Analysis. Christina Nasrawi & Judith Ann Allender. Ed. by Maura Conner et al. 1999. LC 98-24851. (Illus.). 285p. (C). pap. text 29.95 (*0-7216-7133-0*) Harcourt.

Quick & Easy Medical Terminology. Peggy C. Leonard. 2nd ed. 1995. (Illus.). 369p. pap., tchr. ed. (*0-7216-5687-0*); 352p. pap. text 30.00 (*0-7216-5686-2*) Saunders.

Quick & Easy Nutrition Counter for Pregnancy. Lynn Sonberg. 1994. 352p. (Orig.). mass mkt. 5.99 (*0-380-77418-6*, Avon Bks) Morrow Avon.

Quick-Consult Manual of Evidence Based Medicine. Burton W. Lee et al. 1997. LC 97-3306. (Illus.). 762p. pap. text 55.00 (*0-316-51887-5*) Lppncott W & W.

Quick Consult Manual of Primary Care Medicine. Gideon Bosker & Paul Stander. 1996. LC 96-27078. 320p. spiral bd. 39.95 (*0-316-10312-8*) Lppncott W & W.

Quick Critical Care Reference. Susan B. Stillwell. 3rd ed. 1998. (Illus.). 80p. (C). (gr. 13). pap. text 8.95 (*0-8151-3694-3*, 31036) Mosby Inc.

Quick Emergency Care Reference. Gennell Lee. 1991. (Illus.). 60p. (C). (gr. 13). pap. text 8.95 (*0-8016-6584-1*, 06584) Mosby Inc.

Quick IV Therapy Reference. Cynthia L. Hermey. 1995. (Illus.). 88p. (C). pap. text 8.95 (*0-8151-4236-6*, 24616) Mosby Inc.

***Quick Guide to Physician Fraud & Abuse.** Ingenix, Inc. Staff. pap. 59.95 (*1-56337-371-8*) Ingenix Inc.

Quick Guide to Solving Common Health Conditions with Commercial Herb Formulas. Steven H. Horne & Steven R. Johnson. 1997. (Illus.). 100p. pap. 9.95 (*1-890855-01-4*) Tree of Light.

Quick Index to R. O. P. Long-Term Care Facilities. W. H. Heaton. 1991. 277p. ring bd. 89.95 (*1-881057-01-1*) Heaton Pubns.

Quick Look Books in Immunology. Mark Mamula. 1999. pap. 23.95 (*1-889325-40-6*) Blackwell Sci.

Quick Look Drug Book. 1994. 600p. 24.95 (*0-683-07047-9*); 1991. (*0-683-07053-3*) Lppncott W & W.

Quick Look Drug Book, 1998. Leonard L. Lance. 1998. (*0-683-40174-2*) Lppncott W & W.

Quick Look Drug Book, 1997. Leonard L. Lance et al. 1997. 719p. pap. 34.95 (*0-683-40057-6*) Lppncott W & W.

Quick Look Drug Book, 1996. Leonard L. Lance et al. 1996. 787p. (Orig.). pap. 34.95 (*0-683-07045-2*) Lppncott W & W.

Quick Look Nursing: Pharmacology. Nancy A. Craig-Williams et al. 2002. 112p. pap. text 21.95 (*1-55642-502-3*) SLACK Inc.

Quick Medical Spanish. Peter T. Rogers & Olga Ruiz-Rogers. 2nd ed. 1996. LC 96-31450. 183p. (C). pap. 24.95 (*0-8385-8258-3*, A8258-4) McGraw-Hill Prof.

Quick Medical Terminology. Genevieve L. Smith et al. 3rd ed. 1992. LC 91-37703. (Self-Teaching Guides: No. 1581). 304p. pap. 19.95 (*0-471-54267-9*) Wiley.

Quick Pediatric Reference. Donna L. Wong. 1991. (Illus.). 64p. (C). (gr. 13). pap. text 8.95 (*0-8016-6362-8*, 06362) Mosby Inc.

Quick Psychopharmacology Reference. Michele T. Laraia. 2nd ed. 1994. (Illus.). 64p. (C). (gr. 13). pap. text 8.95 (*0-8016-8064-6*, 08064) Mosby Inc.

Quick Reference: Lab & Diagnostic Tests. McFarland. 1995. (Nursing Education Ser.). 23.95 (*0-8273-6169-6*) Delmar.

Quick Reference Dictionary for Physical Therapy. Jennifer M. Bottomley. 2000. 592p. pap. text 24.00 (*1-55642-426-4*) SLACK Inc.

Quick Reference for Advanced Cardiac Life Support. Karen Fenstemacher & Barbara D. Hudson. 1995. (Illus.). 205p. pap. text 19.95 (*0-7216-4637-9*) Saunders.

Quick Reference for Clinical Nursing. June M. Thompson. 2nd ed. 1997. (Illus.). 96p. (C). (gr. 13). pap. text 8.95 (*0-8151-3721-4*, 31299) Mosby Inc.

Quick Reference for Emergency Nursing. Beverley Tipsord-Klinkhammer & Coleen P. Andreoni. Ed. by Barbara N. Cullen. 1997. LC 96-53896. (Illus.). 230p. pap. text 29.00 (*0-7216-6889-5*) Saunders.

Quick Reference for Maternity & Gynecologic Nursing. Irene M. Bobak. 1992. 93p. (C). (gr. 13). pap. text 8.95 (*0-8016-6666-X*, 06666) Mosby Inc.

Quick Reference for Pediatric Emergency Nursing. Colleen Andreoni. 2000. LC 99-35201. (Illus.). 445p. pap. text (*0-7216-8327-4*) Saunders.

Quick Reference for Psychiatric Nursing. Marianne W. Miles. 1994. 64p. pap. text 8.95 (*0-8151-8919-2*) Mosby Inc.

Quick Reference for Psychopharmacology. Elizabeth A. Rankin. 2000. LC 99-38317. 558p. pap. text 33.95 (*0-7668-0631-6*) Delmar.

Quick Reference Glossary of Eyecare Terminology. Joseph Hoffman. 2nd ed. 1997. LC 97-42375. (Basic Bookshelf for Eyecare Professionals Ser.). 240p. pap. text 22.00 (*1-55642-370-5*, 63705) SLACK Inc.

Quick Reference Guide to Using Early Recollections in Treating Personality Disorders. Michael Meier. 1988. LC 87-92202. (Orig.). (C). pap. text 9.95 (*0-945628-00-5*) Diagnostic Solns.

Quick Reference Handbook of Oncology. Bay Area Hospital Staff. 1996. (Illus.). 181p. pap. text 23.00 (*0-7216-6894-1*) Saunders.

Quick Reference Health Care Guide: For Busy Families, Young Adults & Seniors: Professional Medical Advice in Clear Easy Steps. Health Education Resources Staff et al. 3rd rev. ed. 1997. LC 97-76970. Orig. Title: Health Care Recipak. (Illus.). 312p. reprint ed. pap. 15.95 (*0-9653928-4-8*, QRHCG-3) Hlth Educ Res.

Quick Reference System for Basic Medication & Fluid Administration. Jane A. Sennett. 1999. (Illus.). 7p. spiral bd. 9.99 (*0-9670164-2-8*) Jalor Med.

Quick Reference to Anatomy & Physiology. Patton & Gary A. Thibodeau. 1992. (Illus.). 64p. (C). (gr. 13). pap. text 9.95 (*0-8016-7530-8*, 07530) Mosby Inc.

Quick Reference to Cardiovascular Diseases. Edward K. Chung. 2nd ed. 1982. (Illus.). 672p. text 39.50 (*0-397-50482-9*, 65-06232, Lippnctt) Lppncott W & W.

***Quick Reference to Cardiovascular Pharmacotherapy.** Judy W. M. Cheng. 2002. 59.95 (*1-58716-044-7*) CRC Pr.

Quick Reference to Clinical Dietetics. Ed. by Lucinda K. Lysen. 1997. LC 96-50455. 292p. pap. 41.00 (*0-8342-0629-3*) Aspen Pub.

Quick Reference to Community Health Nursing. Marcia Stanhope & Jeanette Lancaster. 2nd ed. 1995. 64p. (C). (gr. 13). pap. text 8.95 (*0-8151-8335-6*, 28197) Mosby Inc.

Quick Reference to Critical Care. Nancy H. Diepenbrock. 1999. LC 98-44543. 336p. pap. text 26.95 (*0-7817-1862-7*) Lppncott W & W.

Quick Reference to Internal Medicine. Ed. by Roger C. Bone & Robert L. Rosen. 1994. LC 93-25286. (Illus.). 1568p. 49.50 (*0-89640-229-0*) Igaku-Shoin.

Quick Reference to Nursing Assessment. Phelps. 1998. (Nursing Education Ser.). (C). pap. text 26.95 (*0-8273-7893-9*) Delmar.

Quick Reference to Occupational Therapy. Kathlyn L. Reed. 2nd ed. 1993. LC 99-44008. 640p. pap. 49.00 (*0-8342-1631-0*, 16310) PRO-ED.

Quick Reference to Outbreak Investigation & Control in Health Care Facilities. Kathleen Meehan Arias. 1999. LC 99-33381. 300p. pap. 72.00 (*0-8342-1179-3*) Aspen Pub.

***Quick Reference to Pharmacokinetics.** Ronald D. Schoenwald. 2002. LC 2001-52887. 59.95 (*1-56676-973-6*) CRC Pr.

Quick Reference to Physical Therapy. Julie A. Pauls & Kathlyn L. Reed. 1995. 688p. pap. 53.00 (*0-8342-0654-4*, 20654) PRO-ED.

***Quick Reference to Physical Therapy.** Julie A. Pauls. 2nd ed. 1989. 55.00 (*0-8342-1940-9*) PRO-ED.

Quick Reference to Radiology. Ed. by John C. Lipman. 1995. LC 94-33452. 447p. (C). pap. text 44.95 (*0-8385-8196-X*, A8196-6, Apple Lange Med) McGraw.

Quick Reference to the Diagnostic Criteria from DSM-IV-TR. American Psychiatric Association Staff. 2000. 496p. pap. 23.00 (*0-89042-026-2*, 2026) Am Psychiatric.

Quick Reference to Triage. Valerie G. Grossman. 1999. LC 98-38546. 240p. spiral bd. 32.95 (*0-7817-1861-9*) Lppncott W & W.

Quick Reference to Veterinary Medicine. Ed. by William R. Fenner & Terence A. Olive. 3rd ed. 1998. LC 00-35223. (Illus.). 752p. pap. text 49.95 (*0-397-51608-8*) Lppncott W & W.

Quick Reference to Wound Care. Pamela Brown et al. 2000. LC 00-61849. 259p. pap. 54.00 (*0-8342-1665-5*, 16655) Aspen Pub.

Quick Response Therapy: A Time-Limited Treatment Approach. Judith Goldring. 1997. LC 97-16481. 144p. pap. text 30.00 (*0-7657-0092-1*) Aronson.

Quick Review: Dental Assistant. Emily Andujo. 1998. LC 97-30650. (Quick Review Ser.). 272p. (C). pap. 27.51 (*0-8385-1526-6*, A-1526-1) P-H.

Quick Tests: The Life & Work of Dr. Armand J. Quick. Edith M. Ebel. 1995. (Illus.). 464p. (Orig.). 21.95 (*0-936015-60-8*); pap. 16.95 (*0-936015-57-8*) Pocahontas Pr.

Quick Workouts. 1987. (Fitness, Health & Nutrition Ser.). (Illus.). 144p. 17.27 (*0-8094-6179-X*) Time-Life.

QuickCalc Med Dosage Calculations. Merrilee T. McDuffie. 1994. LC 93-39298. 273p. (C). spiral bd. 39.40 (*0-8053-1366-4*) Benjamin-Cummings.

Quid Pro Quo: Studies in the History of Drugs. John M. Riddle. 1992. (Collected Studies: No. CS367). 320p. (*0-86078-319-7*) Variorum GBR. *Dist:* Ashgate Pub Co.

Quiet Haven: Quakers, Moral Treatment & Asylum Reform. Charles L. Cherry. 1990. LC 88-48019. (Illus.). 240p. 38.50 (*0-8386-3341-2*) Fairleigh Dickinson.

Quiet, Healing Zone! Herbert L. Beierle. 1980. (C). pap. 14.95 (*0-940480-10-7*) UNIPress.

Quiet Mind: Techniques for Transforming Stress. Ed. by John Harvey. 1989. LC 88-12055. (Techniques for Transforming Stress Ser.). (Illus.). 305p. pap. 15.95 (*0-89389-096-0*) Himalayan Inst.

Quiet Therapies: Japanese Pathways to Personal Growth. David K. Reynolds. 1982. LC 80-17611. 144p. reprint ed. pap. 9.95 (*0-8248-0801-0*) UH Pr.

Quinine & Quarantine: Missouri Medicine Through the Years. Loren Humphrey. 2000. LC 99-54575. (Missouri Heritage Readers Ser.). (Illus.). xi, 128p. pap. text 9.95 (*0-8262-1269-7*) U of Mo Pr.

Quinolone Antibacterials. D. Beermann. Ed. by J. Kuhlmann et al. 1997. LC 97-455. (Handbook of Experimental Pharmacology Ser.: No. 127). (Illus.). 491p. 359.00 (*3-540-62512-7*) Spr-Verlag.

Quinolone Antimicrobial Agents. Ed. by David C. Hooper & John S. Wolfson. 2nd ed. 1993. LC 93-10990. (Illus.). 563p. 79.00 (*1-55581-059-4*) ASM Pr.

Quinolones. Vincent T. Andriole. 3rd ed. 2000. LC 00-106606. (Illus.). xx, 517p. 125.00 (*0-12-059517-6*) Acad Pr.

Quinolones in Everyday Clinical Practice. Ed. by W. Graninger. 1996. (Journal: Vol. 42, Suppl. 1, 1996). (Illus.). iv, 62p. pap. 21.75 (*3-8055-6299-3*) S Karger.

Quinolones in Pulmonary Tuberculosis Management. Len J. LaScolea, Jr. & Ramzan Rangoonwala. 1996. LC 96-13283. (Illus.). 120p. text 55.00 (*0-8247-9740-X*) Dekker.

Quintessence of Dental Technology, 1995, Vol. 18. Ed. by John A. Sorenson. 1995. (Illus.). 217p. (Orig.). pap. text 56.00 (*0-86715-289-3*, B0606) Quint Pub Co.

Quintessence of Dental Technology 1998, Vol. 21. John Sorenson. 1998. 208p. pap. 60.00 (*0-86715-344-X*) Quint Pub Co.

Quintessence Tantras of Tibetan Medicine. Dalai Lama XIV, pseud. Tr. by Barry Clark. 1995. LC 93-40282. 260p. (Orig.). pap. 22.95 (*1-55939-009-3*) Snow Lion Pubns.

Quit for Life: The Sensational New Program for Smokers. Robert S. Sobel. 2nd ed. 1989. LC 88-90751. 164p. (Orig.). pap. 11.50 (*0-929517-03-2*) MDTA Pr.

Quit Smart Leader Manual: Scientific Foundations & Implementation Guidelines for the Quit Smart Stop Smoking Method. Robert H. Shipley. 1994. (Illus.). 175p. ring bd. 75.00 (*1-880781-95-6*) Quit Smart.

Quit Smart Stop Smoking Kit: Stop Smoking Guide, Hypnosis Type, & Cigarette Substitute. Robert H. Shipley & Jed Rose. rev. ed. 1994. pap. 24.95 (*1-880781-94-8*) Quit Smart.

Quitters Are Winners: New 30 Day Stop Smoking Plan. Yvon Morris. 1996. 51p. pap. 9.98 (*1-888139-04-8*) Y Morris Carib.

Quittin' Time: An Ex-Smoker's Step-by-Step Plan for Beating Your Cigarette Addiction, Vol. 1. Jenny N. Duffey. Ed. by Bonnie Welch. 1993. (Orig.). 14.95 (*0-9642103-0-4*, TX3-677-725) Duffey Pubng.

Quitting Cocaine. Arnold M. Washton. 1996. pap. 4.00 (*0-89486-677-X*) Hazelden.

Quitting Cocaine: The Struggle Against Impulse. Howard J. Shafer et al. 1990. LC 87-45977. 198p. pap. 15.95 (*0-669-19690-8*) Lxngtn Bks.

Qusta Ibn Luqa on Numbness: A Book on Numbness, Its Kinds, Causes & Treatment According to the Opinion of Galen & Hippocrates. Ed. by Lena Ambjorn. 2000. (ARA & ENG.). 178p. pap. (*91-22-01879-4*) Almqvist & Wiksell SWE. *Dist:* Coronet Bks.

R

R. B. E. for High-LET Radiations with Respect to Mutagenesis. International Commission on Radiological Protection. 1972. (International Commission on Radiological Protection Ser.: No. 18). 50p. pap. 12.50 (*0-08-017008-0*, Pergamon Pr) Elsevier.

R. D. Laing: A Biography. Adrian C. Laing. 1995. LC 95-118981. 248p. (*0-7206-0934-8*) P Owen Ltd GBR. *Dist:* Dufour.

R-Factors: Their Properties & Possible Control: Symposium, Baden Near Vienna, April 27-29, 1977. Ed. by J. Drews. 1978. (Topics in Infectious Diseases Ser.: Vol. 2). (Illus.). 362p. 53.95 (*0-387-81455-8*) Spr-Verlag.

R. N., 1997. Princeton Review Publishing Staff. Date not set. pap. (*0-679-76916-1*) Random Ref & Info.

R. V. H. Manual on Palliative-Hospice Care: A Resource Book. Ed. by Ina Ajemian & Balfour M. Mount. pap. 37.95 (*0-405-13934-9*) Ayer.

Rabbit Dissection Manual. Bruce D. Wingerd. 1985. LC 84-15761. 80p. pap. text 13.95 (*0-8018-2470-2*) Johns Hopkins.

Rabies. Ed. by J. B. Campbell & K. M. Charlton. 1988. (Developments in Veterinary Virology Ser.). (C). text 249.50 (*0-89838-390-0*) Kluwer Academic.

Rabies in Bats: Natural History & Public Health Implications. Danny A. Brass. 1994. LC 93-78291. (Illus.). 335p. 49.95 (*0-9637045-1-6*) Livia Pr CT.

Rabies in the Tropics. Ed. by E. Kuwert et al. 1985. (Illus.). 786p. 118.00 (*0-387-13826-9*) Spr-Verlag.

Rabies, Lyme Disease, & Hanta Virus: And Other Animal-Borne Human Diseases in the United States & Canada. E. Lendell Cockrum. 1997. LC 98-151852. (Illus.). 160p. pap. 14.95 (*1-55561-138-9*) Fisher Bks.

Race Against Time: Psychotherapy & Psychoanalysis in the Second Half of Life. Robert A. Nemiroff & Calvin A. Colarusso. 1985. LC 84-17683. (Critical Issues in Psychiatry Ser.). (Illus.). 350p. (C). 55.00 (*0-306-41753-7*, Plenum Trade) Perseus Pubng.

Race & Childbirth. Savita Katbamna. 2000. LC 99-30674. (Race, Health & Social Care Ser.). 176p. pap. (*0-335-19946-1*) OpUniv Pr.

Race & Childbirth. Contrib. by Savita Katbamna. 2000. LC 99-30674. 151p. (*0-335-19947-X*) OpUniv Pr GBR. *Dist:* Taylor & Francis.

Race & Culture in Psychiatry. Suman Fernando. 1988. 200p. lib. bdg. (*0-7099-4912-X*) C Helm GBR. *Dist:* Routldge.

Race & Excellence: My Dialogue with Chester Pierce. Ezra E. H. Griffith. 1998. LC 97-46429. (Illus.). 190p. text 24.95 (*0-87745-628-3*) U of Iowa Pr.

Race & Health in Contemporary Britain. Ed. by Waqar I. Ahmad. 1993. LC 93-25331. 192p. pap. (*0-335-15697-5*) OpUniv Pr.

Race & Health Policy. Allan McNaught. 1987. 160p. lib. bdg. (*0-7099-4673-2*) C Helm GBR. *Dist:* Routldge.

Race & Sex Effects in the Conformity Behavior of Children. Gordon N. Cantor. 1978. (Augustana College Library Occasional Papers, Wallin Lecture: No. 14). 16p. pap. 1.00 (*0-910182-37-X*) Augustana Coll.

Race & the Subject of Masculinities. Ed. by Harry Stecopoulos & Michael Uebel. 1997. LC 96-49942. (New Americanists Ser.). (Illus.). 418p. pap. text 18.95 (*0-8223-1966-7*); 448p. lib. bdg. 54.95 (*0-8223-1958-6*) Duke.

Race, Culture, & Counselling. Colin Lago & Joyce Thompson. 1996. LC 95-24920. 192p. pap. (*0-335-19294-7*) OpUniv Pr.

Race, Culture, & Mental Disorder. Philip Rack. 1982. 300p. (*0-422-78160-6*, NO. 3801) Tavistock GBR. *Dist:* Routldge.

Race Equality in Health Care. Baxter Staff. 1997. pap. text (*0-7020-2031-1*) Bailliere Tindall.

Race, Ethnicity & Treatment of Children & Adolescents in Hospitals by Diagnosis. D. Robert Harris et al. 1997. (Illus.). 107p. (Orig.). (C). pap. text 35.00 (*0-7881-3852-9*) DIANE Pub.

Race, Folk, Individuality & Mankind. Albert Steffen. Tr. by Arvia MacKaye. 1982. 30p. pap. 3.50 (*0-932776-04-3*) Adonis Pr.

Race for Consciousness. John G. Taylor. 1999. LC 98-37294. (Illus.). 522p. 39.95 (*0-262-20115-1*) MIT Pr.

Race for Life: From Cancer to the Ironman. Ruth Heidrich. 1990. (Illus.). 200p. (Orig.). pap. 14.95 (*0-9604190-1-2*) Hawaii Hlth Pubs.

Race, Gender, & Health. Marcia Bayne-Smith. 1996. LC 95-35483. (Sage Series on Race & Ethnic Relations: Vol. 15). (Illus.). 240p. pap. 36.95 (*0-8039-5505-7*, 4852) Sage.

Race, I. Q. & Jensen. James R. Flynn. 1980. 320p. 32.50 (*0-7100-0651-9*, Routledge Thoemms) Routledge.

Race in the Making: Cognition, Culture, & the Child's Construction of Human Kinds. Lawrence A. Hirschfeld. 1996. LC 95-40230. (Learning, Development, & Conceptual Change Ser.). (Illus.). 243p. (C). 50.00 (*0-262-08247-0*, Bradford Bks) MIT Pr.

Race Is Run One Step at a Time: Every Woman's Guide to Taking Charge of Breast Cancer. Nancy Brinker & Catherine M. Harris. 1995. LC 95-24204. 224p. pap. 13.95 (*1-56530-182-X*) Summit TX.

Race, Place, & Medicine: The Idea of the Tropics in Nineteenth-Century Brazil. Julyan G. Peard. 1999. LC 99-34867. x, 315p. 49.95 (*0-8223-2376-1*) Duke.

Race, Place & Medicine: The Idea of the Tropics in Nineteenth-Century Brazil. Julyan G Peard. 1999. LC 99-34867. x, 315p. pap. text 17.95 (*0-8223-2397-4*) Duke.

Race, Science & Medicine, 1700-1960. Bernard Harris & Waltraud Ernst. 1999. LC 98-55200. (Illus.). ix, 300p. text 95.00 (*0-415-18152-6*) Routledge.

Racewalking for Fun & Fitness. John Gray. 1985. 176p. 15.95 (*0-13-944711-3*); pap. 7.95 (*0-13-944703-2*) P-H.

Rachel Weeping: And Other Essays on Abortion. James T. Burtchaell. 1991. 383p. (C). reprint ed. pap. 11.95 (*0-919225-34-9*) Life Cycle Bks.

RACI National Convention, 8th, August 1987, Vol. 13, No. 2. Ed. by P. R. Andrews & J. S. Morley. 1988. (Drug Design & Delivery Ser.: Vol. 3, No. 2). 108p. pap. text 218.00 (*3-7186-4836-9*) Gordon & Breach.

Racial & Ethnic Differences in Disease. Anthony P. Polednak. 1989. (Illus.). 376p. text 59.95 (*0-19-505970-0*) OUP.

Racial Characteristics of Syrians & Armenians. Carl C. Seltzer. 1936. (HU PMP Ser.). 25.00 (*0-527-01230-0*) Periodicals Srv.

Racial Differences in Perceptions of Access to Health Care among the Elderly. Shulamit L. Bernard. rev. ed. 1997. LC 96-39994. (Studies on the Elderly in America). (Illus.). 183p. text 58.00 (*0-8153-2646-7*) Garland.

Racial Hygiene: Medicine under the Nazis. Robert N. Proctor. 1988. (Illus.). 496p. pap. text 19.50 (*0-674-74578-7*) HUP.

Racial/Ethnic Patterns of Cancer in the United States, 1988-1992. Ed. by Barry A. Miller. 1997. (Illus.). 138p. (C). pap. text 25.00 (*0-7881-4592-4*) DIANE Pub.

Racing to the Beginning of the Road: The Search for the Origin of Cancer. Robert A. Weinberg. 1998. (Illus.). 263p. pap. text 14.95 (*0-7167-3283-1*) W H Freeman.

Racism, Health, & Post-Industrialism: A Theory of African-American Health. Clovis E. Semmes. 1996. LC 95-34440. 200p. pap. 20.95 (*0-275-95428-5*, Greenwood Pr) Greenwood.

***Rad Tech's Guide to Mammography: Physics, Instrumentation, & Quality Control.** Donald R. Jacobson. 2001. LC 2001-1217. (Rad Tech's Guide Ser.). (Illus.). xiii, 120p. pap. 19.95 (*0-632-04499-3*) Blackwell Sci.

Radar Imaging of Airborne Targets: A Primer for Applied Mathematicians & Physicists. Brett Borden. 1999. LC 99-19620. (Illus.). 25p. 85.00 (*0-7503-0617-3*) Inst of Physics Pubng.

***Radiant Beauty: Your Healthy & Organic Guide to Total Body Well-Being.** Mary Beth Janssen. 2001. LC 2001-3703. (*0-87596-926-7*) Rodale Pr Inc.

Radiant Child. Thomas Armstrong. 1985. LC 85-40409. 220p. pap. 8.95 (*0-8356-0600-7*, Quest) Theos Pub Hse.

***Radiant Health Without Prescription: Perfect Health Through Prevention.** Dele Aderara. Ed. by Merille Weithers. unabr. ed. 2001. LC 00-91028. (Radiant Health Ser.). 272p. pap. 17.95 (*0-942307-05-4*, Newbreed) Adebara & Honeycomb.

Radiation. Davidson. 1986. 110p. pap. (*0-85207-180-9*) C W Daniel GBR. *Dist:* Natl Bk Netwk.

Radiation: Cells & People. Ernest C. Pollard. 1991. (Illus.). 133p. (Orig.). (C). pap. 12.00 (*0-9612798-3-4*) Woodburn Pr.

Radiation: The Hidden Enemy. Rita H. Awana. 1994. pap. text 12.95 (*1-881116-22-0*) Black Forest Pr.

Radiation & Cancer Risk. Ed. by Tor Brustad et al. 1989. (Cancer Ser.). 300p. 94.95 (*0-89116-978-4*) Hemisp Pub.

Radiation & Gut. Ed. by C. S. Potten & J. H. Hendry. 1995. LC 96-105368. 328p. 296.00 (*0-444-89053-X*) Elsevier.

Radiation & Human Health Proposal from Nagasaki: Proceedings of the Nagasaki Symposium '95, 50th Anniversary Meeting of the Atomic Bombing in Nagasaki, Nagasaki, Japan, 19 September 1995. Ed. by Shigenobu Nagataki & Shunichi Yamashita. 1996. (International Congress Ser.: No. 1103). 306p. 172.00 (*0-444-82287-9*, Excerpta Medica) Elsevier.

Radiation & Life. Eric J. Hall. 2nd ed. 1984. 42.00 (*0-08-028819-7*, Pergamon Pr) Elsevier.

Radiation & Medicine. Lentle. 1985. (Radiation Physics & Chemistry Ser.). pap. 61.00 (*0-08-032402-9*, Pergamon Pr) Elsevier.

Radiation & Public Perception: Benefits & Risks, Vol. 24. Ed. by Jack P. Young & Rosalyn S. Yalow. 1995. LC 94-35190. (Advances in Chemistry Ser.: No. 243). (Illus.). 360p. 80.00 (*0-8412-2932-5*); pap. 40.00 (*0-8412-3037-4*) Am Chemical.

Radiation & Society Vol. 1: Comprehending Radiation Risk: Report to the IAEA. International Atomic Energy Agency Staff. 1994. LC 95-131989. 196p. pap. (*92-0-102194-1*, STI/PUB/959) IAEA AUT. *Dist:* Bernan Associates.

Radiation & the Gastrointestinal Tract. Andre Dubois et al. 1994. LC 94-27144. 304p. lib. bdg. 175.00 (*0-8493-7667-X*, 7667) CRC Pr.

Radiation & the Lymphatic System: Proceedings. Ed. by John E. Ballou. 1976. LC 75-38685. (ERDA Symposium Ser.). 265p. pap. 14.50 (*0-87079-030-7*, CONF-740930); fiche 9.00 (*0-87079-317-9*, CONF-740930) DOE.

Radiation Biochemistry. A. M. Kuzin. 1964. 288p. text 72.00 (*0-7065-0534-4*) Coronet Bks.

Radiation Bioeffects & Management Test & Syllabus, Vol. 32. Louis K. Wagner et al. 1991. (Professional Self-Evaluation & Continuing Education Program Ser.). (Illus.). 500p. 190.00 (*1-55903-032-1*) Am Coll Radiology.

Radiation Biology. 1983. (Advanced Health Physics Training Ser.). (Illus.). 255p. ring bd. 110.00 (*0-87683-203-6*) GP Courseware.

Radiation Biology. Ed. by Donald J. Pizzarello. 1982. 312p. 139.95 (*0-8493-6011-0*, QP82, CRC Reprint) Franklin.

Radiation Biology Ed. by A. Zuppinger. 1966. (Handbook of Medical Radiology Ser.: Vol. 2, Pts. 1 & 2). (Illus.). Pt. 1. 304.00 (*0-387-03544-3*); Pt. 2. 304.00 (*0-387-03545-1*) Spr-Verlag.

Radiation Biology of the Fetal & Juvenile Mammal: Proceedings. Ed. by Melvin R. Sikov & D. Dennis Mahlum. 1969. LC 74-603748. (AEC Symposium Ser.). 1026p. pap. 33.75 (*0-87079-318-7*, CONF-690501); fiche 9.00 (*0-87079-319-5*, CONF-690501) DOE.

Radiation Damage to Skin: British Journal of Radiology Supplement 19. 1986. pap. text (*0-905749-13-8*) Med Physics Pub.

Radiation-Dose Reconstruction for Epidemiologic Uses. National Research Council Staff. 1995. LC 95-10524. 140p. (C). text 34.95 (*0-309-05099-5*) Natl Acad Pr.

Radiation Dose to Patients from Radiopharmaceuticals. International Commission on Radiological Protectio. 1988. (International Commission on Radiological Protection Ser.: No. 53). (Illus.). 388p. 125.50 (*0-08-035591-9*, Pergamon Pr) Elsevier.

Radiation Doses, Effects, Risks. 1986. 64p. 12.00 (*92-807-1104-0*, E.86.III.D.4) UN.

Radiation Dosimetry: Physical & Biological Aspects. Ed. by Colin G. Orton. 1986. (Illus.). 340p. (C). text 107.00 (*0-306-42056-2*, Kluwer Plenum) Kluwer Academic.

Radiation Dosimetry: X Rays Generated at Potentials of 5 to 150 kV, No. 17. International Commission on Radiation Units and Measurements Staff. 1970. LC 74-126755. 35.00 (*0-913394-10-6*) Intl Comm Rad Meas.

Radiation Exposure & Occupational Risks. Ed. by E. Scherer et al. 1990. (Medical Radiology Ser.). (Illus.). 150p. 149.00 (*0-387-51174-1*) Spr-Verlag.

Radiation from Medical Procedures in the Pathogenesis of Cancer & Ischemic Heart Disease: Dose-Response Studies with Physicians per 100,000 Population. John W. Gofman. Ed. by Egan O'Connor. 1999. LC 99-45096. 699p. 35.00 (*0-932682-97-9*); (Illus.). pap. 27.00 (*0-932682-98-7*) Comm Nuclear Respon.

Radiation Hazards in Perspective. 1962. (Technical Report Ser.: No. 248). 37p. pap. text 3.00 (*92-4-120248-3*) World Health.

***Radiation Health.** Thormod Henriksen & David Maillie. 2001. 234p. (*90-5699-345-3*); pap. (*90-5699-346-1*) GBSP NLD. *Dist:* Gordon & Breach.

Radiation, Health & Society. Bjorn Wahlstrom. 1998. (Illus.). 56p. pap. text 20.00 (*0-7881-4953-9*) DIANE Pub.

Radiation Histopathology, Vol. 2. George W. Casarett. 1981. 176p. 89.00 (*0-8493-5358-0*, RA1231) CRC Pr.

Radiation Histopathology, Vol. 1. George W. Casarett. 1981. 160p. 90.00 (*0-8493-5357-2*, RA1231, CRC Reprint) Franklin.

Radiation in Medicine. Robert C. Reno. 2nd ed. 1994. LC 94-73544. (Illus.). 104p. (C). pap. text 27.95 (*0-916615-05-7*) Bks of Sci.

Radiation in Medicine: A Need for Regulatory Reform. Institute of Medicine Staff. Ed. by Kate-Louise D. Gottfried & Gary Penn. 1996. LC 95-72801. 328p. text 49.95 (*0-309-05386-2*) Natl Acad Pr.

Radiation-Induced Cancer. International Atomic Energy Agency Staff. 1969. (Proceedings Ser.). (Illus.). 498p. pap. (*92-0-010269-7*, ISP228) IAEA AUT. *Dist:* Bernan Associates.

Radiation-Induced Cancer from Low-Dose Exposure: An Independent Analysis. John W. Gofman. 1990. LC 89-62431. 480p. (Orig.). (C). pap. 29.95 (*0-932682-89-8*) Comm Nuclear Respon.

Radiation Injury: Advances in Management & Prevention, 32nd San Francisco Cancer Symposium, San Francisco, Calif., March 1997. Ed. by John L. Meyer. 1999. LC 99-24336. (Frontiers of Radiation Therapy & Oncology Ser.: Vol. 32). (Illus.). x, 200p. pap. 174.00 (*3-8055-6802-9*) S Karger.

Radiation Injury & the Chernobyl Catastrophe, Vol. 15, Supplement 2. N. Dainiak et al. 1997. LC 97-73747. 336p. pap. text 49.00 (*1-880854-22-8*) AlphaMed Pr.

Radiation Monitoring: A Programmed Instruction Book. AEC Technical Information Center Staff et al. 1967. 287p. pap. 36.50 (*0-87079-322-5*, EDM-123) DOE.

Radiation Oncology. Stewart M. Jackson et al. 1985. (Illus.). 264p. pap. 37.50 (*0-87527-334-3*) Green.

Radiation Oncology: Management Decisions. Carlos A. Perez et al. 1998. LC 98-22422. 768p. pap. text 59.95 (*0-397-58468-7*) Lppncott W & W.

Radiation Oncology: Technology & Biology. Ed. by Peter Mauch & Jay Loeffler. 1994. LC 93-31650. text 125.00 (*0-7216-6724-4*) Saunders.

Radiation Oncology - Radiobiological & Physiological Perspectives: The Boundary-Zone Between Clinical Radiotherapy & Fundamental Radiobiology & Physiology. Hassan K. Awwad. 1990. (Developments in Oncology Ser.). (C). text 309.50 (*0-7923-0783-6*) Kluwer Academic.

Radiation Oncology of Gynecological Cancers. I. A. Adamietz. 1997. LC 96-29741. (Medical Radiology Ser.). (*3-540-56768-2*) Spr-Verlag.

Radiation Oncology Physics, 1986: Proceedings of the AAPM 1986 Summer School Held at Miami University, Oxford, Ohio, July 27-August 1, 1986. Ed. by James G. Kereiakes et al. 1987. (American Association of Physicists in Medicine Symposium Ser.: No. 15). 820p. 75.00 (*0-88318-533-4*) Am Inst Physics.

Radiation Pathology. Luis Felipe Fajardo et al. 2000. LC 99-57488. (Illus.). 472p. text 165.00 (*0-19-511023-4*) OUP.

Radiation Physics, Lessons 1-7. William R. Hendee. 1985. 200p. (C). (gr. 13). stu. ed., spiral bd. 27.95 (*0-8016-4552-2*, 04552) Mosby Inc.

Radiation Preservation of Foods. International Atomic Energy Agency Staff. 1973. (Proceedings Ser.). (Illus.). 774p. pap. (*92-0-010373-1*, ISP317) IAEA AUT. *Dist:* Bernan Associates.

Radiation Protection. Ed. by Steward C. Bushong. 1998. (Essentials of Medical Imaging Ser.). (Illus.). 288p. pap. 19.95 (*0-07-012013-7*) McGraw-Hill Prof.

Radiation Protection. Ronald L. Kathren. 1985. (Medical Physics Handbook Ser.: No. 16). (Illus.). 212p. 19.00 (*0-85274-554-0*) Inst of Physics Pubng.

Radiation Protection. Euclid Seeram. 1996. LC 96-25440. 320p. pap. text 33.95 (*0-397-55032-4*) Lppncott W & W.

Radiation Protection. rev. ed. 1981. (Illus.). 184p. text 79.50 (*0-87683-173-0*) GP Courseware.

Radiation Protection: A Systematic Approach to Safety: Proceedings of the 5th Congress of the International Radiation Protection Society, March 1980, Jerusalem Ed. by Ronald L. Eisenberg. 1980. (Illus.). 1055p. (*0-08-025912-X*) Pergamon Repr GBR. *Dist:* Franklin.

Radiation Protection - In the Health Sciences. G. Q. Macguire & Marilyn E. Noz. 1995. 300p. text 66.00 (*981-02-2406-0*) World Scientific Pub.

Radiation Protection - In the Health Sciences. Gerald Q. Maguire, Jr. & Marilyn E. Noz. 1995. LC 95-49066. 300p. pap. text 32.00 (*981-02-2407-9*) World Scientific Pub.

Radiation Protection - Recommendations of the ICRP. International Commission on Radiological Protection. 2nd ed. 1977. (International Commission on Radiological Protection Ser.: No. 26). pap. 17.25 (*0-08-021511-4*, Pergamon Pr) Elsevier.

Radiation Protection & Biology. Ritenour. 1985. 128p. (C). (gr. 13). stu. ed., spiral bd., wbk. ed. 17.95 (*0 8016 4013 X*, 04013) Mosby Inc.

Radiation Protection & Measurement for Low-Voltage Neutron Generators. Intro. by Warren K. Sinclair. 1983. LC 83-62802. (Report Ser.: No. 72). 82p. pap. text 30.00 (*0-913392-61-8*) NCRP Pubns.

Radiation Protection & the Internal Emitter Saga. J. Newell Stonnard. 1990. LC 90-13334. (Taylor Lectures: No. 14). (Orig.). pap. text 25.00 (*0-929600-13-4*) NCRP Pubns.

Radiation Protection Concepts & Trade Offs. Hymer L. Friedell. 1979. LC 79-90466. (Taylor Lectures: No. 3). 20.00 (*0-913392-50-2*) NCRP Pubns.

Radiation Protection Dose Limit Standards & Regulations. 1983. (Advanced Health Physics Training Ser.). (Illus.). 70p. 59.50 (*0-87683-353-9*) GP Courseware.

Radiation Protection Dosimetry: A Radical Reappraisal. J. A. Simmons & D. E. Watt. 1999. LC 98-52973. (Illus.). 160p. (C). pap. text 35.95 (*0-944838-87-1*) Med Physics Pub.

Radiation Protection for Medical & Allied Health Personnel. 1989. LC 89-23872. (Report Ser.: No. 105). 129p. pap. text 40.00 (*0-929600-09-6*) NCRP Pubns.

Radiation Protection for Radiologic Technologists. Robert Frankel. 1976. (Illus.). text 36.95 (*0-07-021875-7*) McGraw.

Radiation Protection for Student Radiographers. Mary A. Statkiewicz. 1985. (Orig.). 18.95 (*0-8016-4738-X*) Mosby Inc.

Radiation Protection in Educational Institutions. 1966. LC 66-25710. (Report Ser.: No. 32). 56p. pap. text 25.00 (*0-913392-14-6*) NCRP Pubns.

Radiation Protection in Hospitals. Richard F. Mould. 1985. (Medical Science Ser.). (Illus.). 224p. 100.00 (*0-85274-802-7*) Inst of Physics Pubng.

Radiation Protection in Medical Radiography. Mary Alice Statkiewicz-Sherer et al. 3rd ed. 1998. LC 98-13312. 320p. (C). (gr. 13). pap. text 32.00 (*0-8151-2896-7*, 30088) Mosby Inc.

Radiation Protection in Medicine: Proceeding of the 28th Annual Meeting. Ed. by Andrew K. Poznanski. 1993. LC 92-48318. (Annual Meeting Proceedings Ser.: No. 14). 250p. (Orig.). pap. text 40.00 (*0-929600-29-0*) NCRP Pubns.

Radiation Protection in Pediatric Radiology. 1978. LC 81-80187. (Report Ser.: No. 68). 143p. pap. text 40.00 (*0-913392-54-5*) NCRP Pubns.

Radiation Protection in Veterinary Medicine. 1970. LC 77-121706. (Report Ser.: No. 36). 60p. pap. text 20.00 (*0-913392-18-9*) NCRP Pubns.

Radiation Protection Instrumentation & Its Application, No. 20. International Commission on Radiation Units and Measurements Staff. 1971. LC 70-177297. (Illus.). v, 60p. 30.00 (*0-913394-13-0*) Intl Comm Rad Meas.

Radiation Protection Manual. Lita Lee. 3rd rev. ed. 1991. (Illus.). 150p. pap. 6.95 (*1-880358-00-X*) Lita Lee.

Radiation Protection of Patients. Ed. by R. J. Wootton. 1993. LC 92-49743. (Postgraduate Medical Science Ser.: No. 1). (Illus.). 166p. (C). pap. text 31.95 (*0-521-42669-3*) Cambridge U Pr.

Radiation Protection Progress Reports, 1979. Ed. by C. E. C. Staff. 1980. (Commission of the European Communities Ser.). xvi, 910p. text 688.00 (*3-7186-0047-1*) Gordon & Breach.

Radiation Protection Quantities for External Exposure, Vol. 9. G. Burger et al. 1981. (Commission of the European Communities Ser.). viii, 260p. text 277.00 (*3-7186-0063-3*) Gordon & Breach.

Radiation Protection Standards. Lauriston S. Taylor. 1971. (Monotopic Reprint Ser.). 112p. 29.00 (*0-8493-0111-4*, CRC Reprint) Franklin.

Radiation Protection Theory & Practice: Proceedings of the Fourth International Symposium of the Society for Radiation Protection, Malvern, 4-9 June 1989. Ed. by E. P. Goldfinch. 1989. (Illus.). 512p. 232.00 (*0-85498-052-0*) Inst of Physics Pubng.

Radiation, Radiobiology & Nuclear Medicine: English-German-French-Russian. Ed. by Ralf Sube. rev. ed. 1985. (ENG, FRE, GER & RUS.). 476p. text 50.00 (*3-86117-024-8*) Paul & Co Pubs.

Radiation Risks to the Developing Nervous System. Gerber et al. 1986. LC 86-7703. 435p. pap. (*0-89574-225-X*) Gustav Fischer DEU. *Dist:* Lubrecht & Cramer, Balogh.

Radiation Safety for Laboratory Technicians. Charles A. Kelsey. Ed. by Alvin F. Gardner. 1983. (Allied Health Professions Monograph). 42p. (C). pap. 5.00 (*0-87527-319-X*) Green.

Radiation Safety in Hot Facilities. International Atomic Energy Agency Staff. 1970. (Proceedings Ser.: No. 238). (Illus.). 754p. pap. (*92-0-020070-2*, ISP238) IAEA AUT. *Dist:* Bernan Associates.

Radiation Safety in Nuclear Medicine. Max H. Lombardi. 1998. LC 98-25760. (Illus.). 216p. 84.95 (*0-8493-1897-1*) CRC Pr.

Radiation Safety Training Criteria for Industrial Radiography. 1978. LC 78-61401. (Report Ser.: No. 61). 38p. pap. text 25.00 (*0-913392-45-6*) NCRP Pubns.

Radiation Science & Societal Decision Making. Ed. by Leonard A. Sagan. 1994. LC 94-3423. (NCRP Annual Meeting Proceedings Ser.: No. 15). 329p. (Orig.). pap. text 45.00 (*0-929600-37-1*) NCRP Pubns.

Radiation Science for Physicians & Public Health Workers. Marco Zaider & Harald H. Rossi. 2000. LC 00-34895. (Illus.). 224p. 55.00 (*0-306-46403-9*, Kluwer Plenum) Kluwer Academic.

Radiation Sterilization of Plastic Medical Devices: Seminar under the Auspices of the University of Lowell, Mass., March 1979. H. K. Mann. 1980. 128p. pap. 25.00 (*0-08-025067-X*, Pergamon Pr) Elsevier.

Radiation Technician. Jack Rudman. 1994. (Career Examination Ser.: C-681). pap. 29.95 (*0-8373-0681-7*) Nat Learn.

Radiation Technology Clinical Manual. Robert J. Parelli. 1997. (Illus.). 248p. per. 49.95 (*1-57444-147-7*) St Lucie Pr.

Radiation Therapy & You: A Guide to Self-Help During Cancer Treatment. Ed. by Barry Leonard. rev. ed. 2000. (Illus.). 60p. pap. text 20.00 (*0-7567-0517-7*) DIANE Pub.

Radiation Therapy & You: A Guide to Self-Help During Treatment. 1992. (Illus.). 52p. (Orig.). pap. text 20.00 (*1-56806-113-7*) DIANE Pub.

Radiation Therapy for Head & Neck Neoplasms. C. C. Wang. 3rd ed. 1996. LC 96-16482. 400p. 160.00 (*0-471-14971-3*) Wiley.

Radiation Therapy in Pediatric Oncology. K. Kian Ang et al. Ed. by J. Robert Cassady. 1995. LC 94-2790. (Medical Radiology Ser.). (Illus.). 388p. 123.00 (*0-387-54105-5*) Spr-Verlag.

Radiation Therapy of Benign Diseases: A Clinical Guide. S. E. Order & S. S. Donaldson. 2nd rev. ed. 1998. LC 97-30099. (Medical Radiology Ser.). 269p. 129.00 (*3-540-58865-5*) Spr-Verlag.

Radiation Therapy of Benign Diseases: Current Indications & Techniques 33rd San Francisco Cancer Symposium, San Francisco, Calif., April 1999. Ed. by J. L. Meyer. 1999. LC 00-51994. (Frontiers of Radiation Therapy & Oncology Ser.: Vol. 35). (Illus.). xii, 221p. 170.50 (*3-8055-7063-5*) S Karger.

Radiation Therapy of Brain Tumors. rev. ed. Pt. I. 1989. (*0-944093-06-X*); Pt. II. 1990. (*0-944093-07-8*) Am Brain Tumor.

Radiation Therapy of Brain Tumors: A Basic Guide, Pt. I. 1994. (*0-944093-28-0*) Am Brain Tumor.

Radiation Therapy of Head & Neck Cancer. 1989. (Medical Radiology Ser.). (Illus.). 237p. 198.00 (*0-387-19360-X*) Spr-Verlag.

Radiation Therapy Package Charles M. Washington & Dennis T. Leaver. 1998. 150.00 (*0-323-00785-6*) Mosby Inc.

Radiation Therapy Physics. M. D. Altschuler. Ed. by A. R. Smith et al. 1996. (Illus.). 465p. 149.00 (*0-387-55430-0*) Spr-Verlag.

Radiation Therapy Physics. Ed. by M. D. Altschuler et al. 1994. LC 94-25784. (*3-540-55430-0*) Spr-Verlag.

Radiation Therapy Physics, Simulation, & Treatment Planning, Vol. 2. Charles M. Washington & Dennis T. Leaver. 1997. (Illus.). 320p. tchr. ed. (*0-8151-9252-5*) Mosby Inc.

Radiation Therapy Simulation Workbook. Sue Mizer et al. 1986. 192p. 65.00 (*0-08-033652-3*, Pergamon Pr) Elsevier.

Radiation Toxicology. Lorris G. Cockerham. 1988. 76p. text 107.00 (*2-88124-413-0*) Gordon & Breach.

Radicals in Biochemistry. Ed. by M. J. Dewar et al. 1982. (Topics in Current Chemistry Ser.: Vol. 108). (Illus.). 140p. 61.95 (*0-387-11864-0*) Spr-Verlag.

Radicals in Clinical Medicine: Radical Reactivity & DNA Damage: (Third Biennial Meeting of the Society for Free Radical Research, West Germany, 1986) Helmut Sies & H. De Groot. Ed. by J. V. Bannister. 1987. (Free Radical Research Communications Ser.: Vol. 2). 330p. pap. text 498.00 (*3-7186-0395-0*) Gordon & Breach.

Radicals, Ions & Tissue Damage. B. Matkovics et al. 1990. (Illus.). 323p. (C). (*963-05-5879-3*) Akade Kiado HUN. *Dist:* Intl Spec Bk.

Radio Contrast Agents P. R. Knoefel. 1971. (*0-08-016144-8*) Pergamon Repr GBR. *Dist:* Franklin.

Radio-Frequency & ELF Electromagnetic Energies: A Handbook for Health Professionals. Timothy R. Hitchcock & Robert M. Patterson. 1995. (Industrial Health & Safety Ser.). 552p. 140.00 (*0-471-28454-8*, VNR) Wiley.

Radio Nutrician Service Provider's Kit: A Nutrition Education Program for the Hispanic Community. 1996. (SPA.). incl. audio (*1-886567-08-5*) Assn Farmwrker.

Radioactive & Stable Isotope Tracers in Biomedicine: Principles & Practice of Kinetic Analysis. Robert R. Wolfe. 1992. 480p. 205.00 (*0-471-56131-2*, Wiley-Liss) Wiley.

Radioactive Fallout from Nuclear Weapons Tests: Proceedings. Ed. by Alfred W. Klement, Jr. 1965. LC 65-62945. (AEC Symposium Ser.). 953p. pap. 32.25 (*0-87079-323-3*, CONF-765); fiche 9.00 (*0-87079-324-1*, CONF-765) DOE.

Radioactive Isotopes in Clinical Medicine & Research. Ed. by H. Bergmann et al. 1995. LC 94-42695. (Advances in Pharmacological Sciences Ser.). 480p. 120.00 (*0-8176-5082-2*) Birkhauser.

Radioactive Isotopes in Clinical Medicine & Research. Ed. by Helmet F. Sinzinger & H. Bergmann. 1995. LC 94-42695. (Advances in Pharmacological Sciences Ser.). (*3-7643-5082-2*) Birkhauser.

Radioactive Isotopes in Clinical Medicine & Research: Proceedings of the 22nd Badgastein Symposium. Ed. by H. Bergmann et al. 1997. LC 96-39717. (Advances in Pharmacological Sciences Ser.: Vol. XXIV). (Illus.). 528p. 155.00 (*3-7643-5645-6*) Spr-Verlag.

Radioactive Isotopes in Clinical Medicine & Research: Proceedings of the 22nd Badgastein Symposium. H. Bergmann & A. Kroiss. 1997. LC 96-39717. (Advances in Pharmacological Sciences Ser.). (*0-8176-5645-6*) Birkhauser.

Radioactive Isotopes in Clinical Medicine & Research: Proceedings of the 23rd International Badgastein Symposium. H. Bergmann et al. 1998. LC 98-43515. 600p. 159.00 (*3-7643-5967-6*) Birkhauser.

Radioactive Isotopes in Clinical Medicine & Research XXIII: Proceedings of the 23rd International Badgastein Symposium. H. Bergmann. 1999. LC 98-43515. xxix, 561p. (*0-8176-5967-6*) Birkhauser.

Radioactive Pharmaceuticals: Proceedings. Ed. by Gould A. Andrews et al. 1966. LC 66-60068. (AEC Symposium Ser.). 702p. pap. 25.50 (*0-87079-325-X*, CONF-651111); fiche 9.00 (*0-87079-326-8*, CONF-651111) DOE.

Radioactivity: A Science in Its Historical & Social Context. Edgar N. Jenkins. 1979. (Wykeham Science Ser.: No. 48). 200p. pap. 18.00 (*0-85109-730-8*) Taylor & Francis.

Radioactivity: A Science in Its Historical & Social Context. Edgar N. Jenkins & I. Lewis. 1979. LC 78-11959. (Wykeham Science Ser.: No. 52). 197p. (C). pap. 18.00 (*0-8448-1371-0*, Crane Russak) Taylor & Francis.

Radioactivity & Atomic Theory. Ed. by Thaddeus J. Trenn. 1975. 536p. 55.00 (*0-85066-077-7*) Taylor & Francis.

Radioactivity & Health: A History J. Newell Stannard. 1989. LC 88-600371. 2010p. 97.50 (*0-87079-590-2*) Battelle.

Radiobiology & Radiation Pro. Mosby Staff. 1998. tchr. ed. (*0-8151-5402-X*) Mosby Inc.

***Radiobiology & Radiation Protection.** Mosby Inc. Staff. 1999. (Mosby's Radiographic Instructional Ser.). 1350.00 incl. cd-rom (*0-8151-6949-3*) Mosby Inc.

Radiobiology & Radiation Protection Study Guide. Mosby Staff. 1998. (Radiographic Instructional Ser.). (Illus.). 200p. stu. ed. (*0-8151-5423-2*) Mosby Inc.

Radiobiology for the Radiologist. Eric J. Hall. 5th ed. 2000. LC 00-39105. 608p. text 95.00 (*0-7817-2649-2*) Lppncott W & W.

Radiochemistry: Theory & Experiment. T. A. Peacocke. 1978. (Wykeham Science Ser.: No. 50). 274p. pap. 18.00 (*0-85109-690-5*) Taylor & Francis.

Radiodiagnosis of Endophytic Gastric Cancer. L. M. Portnoi & M. P. Dibirov. 1995. LC 95-12084.Tr. of Luchevaia Diagnostika Endofitnogo Raka Zheludka. (*1-56700-028-2*) Begell Hse.

Radiodiagnosis of the Skull. J. L. Dietmann. Tr. by M. T. Wackenheim from FRE. 1985. (Exercises in Radiological Diagnosis Ser.). (Illus.). 200p. 35.95 (*0-387-13266-X*) Spr-Verlag.

P Q R

Radiofrequency & Microwaves. 1981. (Environmental Health Criteria Ser.: No. 16). 134p. pap. text 15.00 (*92-4-154076-1*, 1160016) World Health.

Radiofrequency Catheter Ablation of Cardiac Arrhythmias: Basic Concepts & Clinical Applications. Ed. by Shoei K. Stephen Huang & David J. Wilber. 2nd ed. 2000. LC 99-36034. (Illus.). 902p. 135.00 (*0-87993-438-7*) Futura Pub.

Radiograhic Critique. Kathy McQuillen-Martensen. 1996. (Illus.). 320p. text 52.50 (*0-7216-4978-5*) Saunders.

Radiographer's Pocket Companion. Bown. 1998. (C). pap. text (*0-7020-2166-0*) Bailliere Tindall.

Radiographic Anatomy: A Gallery of Images. Raskin. 1996. (Illus.). pap. text 24.95 (*0-9655384-0-0*) Scholar Educ Systs.

Radiographic Anatomy & Positioning. Alan B. Evantash et al. 1991. (C). text 700.00 incl. disk (*1-56815-004-0*) Mosby Inc.

Radiographic Anatomy & Positioning. Miller. 1999. (C). 40.00 (*0-8385-8251-6*, Apple Lange Med) McGraw.

Radiographic Anatomy & Positioning: An Integrated Approach. Andrea G. Cornuelle & Dinae H. Gronefeld. 1997. LC 96-46591. 565p. (C). pap. 98.00 (*0-8385-8238-9*, A8238-6) McGraw-Hill Prof.

Radiographic Anatomy & Positioning Instructor's Ma... Bontrager. 1985. spiral bd. 60.00 (*0-8016-4494-1*); spiral bd. 21.95 (*0-8016-4505-0*) Mosby Inc.

Radiographic Anatomy & Positioning Instructor's Manual. Bontrager. 1985. spiral bd. 23.95 (*0-8016-4524-7*) Mosby Inc.

Radiographic Anatomy, Positioning & Procedures Workbook. Steven G. Hayes, Sr. 2nd ed. 1999. (Illus.). 736p. (C). text, wbk. ed. (*0-323-00230-7*) Mosby Inc.

Radiographic Atlas of Skeletal Development of the Hand & Wrist. William W. Greulich & S. Idell Pyle. 2nd ed. 1950. (Illus.). xvi, 256p. 125.00 (*0-8047-0398-1*) Stanford U Pr.

Radiographic Cephalometry: From Basics to Videoimaging. Ed. by Alexander Jacobson. 1995. LC 95-19432. (Illus.). 336p. text 88.00 (*0-86715-294-X*) Quint Pub Co.

Radiographic Critique: Text & Exercises Package. Kathy McQuillen-Martensen. 1996. (Illus.). 465p. text 94.00 (*0-7216-6179-3*) Saunders.

Radiographic Evaluation of the Spine. Post. 1980. (gr. 13). 169.00 (*0-89352-050-0*) Mosby Inc.

Radiographic Exposure: Principles & Practice. Jerry E. Wallace. 1995. LC 95-741. (Illus.). 574p. (C). pap. text 49.95 (*0-8036-0051-8*) Davis Co.

Radiographic Exposure & Technique. Kathleen D. Euganeo & Alan B. Evantash. 1992. (C). text 700.00 incl. disk (*1-56815-003-2*) Mosby Inc.

Radiographic Image & Its Evaluation. Stewart C. Bushong. 2002. (Illus.). 160p. text 19.95 (*0-07-012015-3*) McGraw-Hill Educ Grp.

Radiographic Imaging. Evelyn F. Burns. 1992. pap. text, lab manual ed. 16.95 (*0-7216-3245-9*) Saunders.

Radiographic Imaging. John Ball. Ed. by Tony Price. 6th rev. ed. 1995. LC 95-5293. xiv, 429p. pap. 58.95 (*0-632-03901-9*) Blackwell Sci.

Radiographic Imaging: A Guide for Producing Quality Radiographs. Evelyn F. Burns. 1992. (Illus.). 223p. tchr. ed. (*0-7216-3247-5*); LC 92-19465. text 39.50 (*0-7216-3246-7*) Saunders.

Radiographic Imaging: A Practical Approach. Derrick P. Roberts & Nigel L. Smith. (Orig.). 1988. (Illus.). 368p. pap. (*0-443-03061-8*); 2nd ed. 1994. LC 94-4029. text (*0-443-04397-3*) Church.

Radiographic Imaging & Exposure. Terri Fauber & Barry Burns. 2000. LC 99-89531. (Illus.). 415p. 35.00 (*0-323-00405-9*) Mosby Inc.

***Radiographic Imaging & Exposure.** Terri L. Fauber. 2000. (Illus.). pap., tchr. ed. 250.00 (*0-323-00457-1*) Mosby Inc.

Radiographic Imaging for Dental Auxiliaries. Dale A. Miles et al. 2nd ed. 1993. LC 92-17230. (Illus.). 336p. pap. text 43.00 (*0-7216-6729-5*) Saunders.

Radiographic Imaging for Dental Auxiliaries. Dale A. Miles et al. Ed. by Shirley Kuhn. 3rd ed. 1999. LC 98-27545. (Illus.). 380p. pap. text 35.00 (*0-7216-8016-X*) Saunders.

Radiographic Imaging Study Guide. Mosby Staff. 1998. (Radiographic Instructional Ser.). (Illus.). 176p. (C). stu. ed. (*0-8151-5408-9*) Mosby Inc.

Radiographic Interpretation for the Dental Hygienist. Joen I. Haring & Laura J. Lind. 1993. (Illus.). 208p. pap. text 39.50 (*0-7216-3704-3*) Saunders.

Radiographic Interpretation for the Small Animal Clinician. Jerry M. Owens et al. 2nd ed. 1998. LC 98-41669. (Illus.). 400p. 49.95 (*0-683-06684-6*) Lppncott W & W.

Radiographic Pathology. TerriAnn Linn-Watson. (Illus.). 1996. 315p. tchr. ed. (*0-7216-4134-2*); 1995. LC 95-13455. 256p. text 45.00 (*0-7216-4129-6*) Saunders.

Radiographic Pathology. Manning & Weber. 2001. (C). pap., wbk. ed. 14.50 net. (*0-7668-1282-0*) Delmar.

Radiographic Pathology Exams. TerriAnn Linn-Watson. 1996. 195.00 (*0-7216-4172-5*) Saunders.

Radiographic Pathology Workbook. TerriAnn Linn-Watson. 1995. 315p. pap. text, wbk. ed. 22.00 (*0-7216-4169-5*) Saunders.

Radiographic Planning & Assessment of Endosseous Oral Implants. Reinhilde Jacobs & D. Van Steenberghe. 1997. LC 97-21358. (Illus.). 115p. 89.00 (*3-540-63087-2*) Spr-Verlag.

Radiographic Positioning. Dowd. 1995. (C). pap. text (*0-7216-5566-1*) Saunders.

Radiographic Positioning. Ronald L. Eisenberg et al. 2nd ed. 1995. LC 94-24133. 432p. text 78.00 (*0-316-22499-5*) Lppncott W & W.

Radiographic Positioning, Vol. 1. Greathouse. 1998. (Radiographic Technology Ser.). tchr. ed. 16.00 (*0-8273-6783-X*) Delmar.

Radiographic Positioning, Vol. II. Cowling. 1998. (Radiographic Positioning Ser.: Vol. II). tchr. ed. 14.00 (*0-8273-6994-8*) Delmar.

Radiographic Positioning & Related Anatomy Slide Set & IM. Kenneth L. Bontrager & John P. Lampignano. 1998. (Illus.). tchr. ed. (*0-8151-4377-X*) Mosby Inc.

Radiographic Positioning & Related Anatomy Workbook & Laboratory Manual. Kenneth L. Bontrager & John P. Lampignano. 4th ed. 1997. (Illus.). 624p. wbk. ed., lab manual ed. (*0-8151-1373-0*) Mosby Inc.

Radiographic Positioning Competency: Based Applications. James Barba & William Leonard. 1993. 340p. (C). mass mkt., stu. ed. 32.75 (*0-8273-4456-2*) Delmar.

Radiographic Positioning Competency-Based Applications: Instructor's Guide. James Barba & William Leonard. 1992. 48p. pap., tchr. ed. 14.00 (*0-8273-4457-0*) Delmar.

Radiographic Positioning CTB, Vol. II. Cowling. 1998. (Radiographic Technology Ser.). 49.95 (*0-8273-6996-4*) Delmar.

Radiographic Techniques: Dog. Joe Morgan et al. 268p. (*3-87706-524-4*) Schlutersche Verlags DEU. *Dist:* Iowa U Pr.

Radiography: Program Review & Exam Preparation (PREP) Dorothy A. Saia. 2nd ed. 1999. LC 99-17638. (Illus.). 480p. (C). pap. 39.95 (*0-8385-8262-1*) McGraw-Hill Prof.

Radiography: Technology, Environment, Professionalism. Frances Campeau. 1998. LC 98-24217. 230p. pap. text 29.95 (*0-397-55196-7*) Lppncott W & W.

Radiography Dental Auxiliary. Frommer's Staff. 1995. (Illus.). 384p. pap. text 49.00 (*0-8151-3379-0*, 27998) Mosby Inc.

Radiography Examination Review. William L. Leonard. (Illus.). 174p. (C). 8th ed. 29.95 (*0-9644624-0-0*); 9th rev. ed. 1997. pap. text 29.95 (*0-9644624-2-7*) JLW Pub.

***Radiography in a Flash!** Cynthia Griffiths et al. 2002. 39.95 (*0-7668-4346-7*) Delmar.

Radiography in Veterinary Technology. Lisa M. Lavin. Ed. by Adrianne Williams. 2nd ed. 1998. LC 98-3626. (Illus.). 440p. (C). text 44.00 (*0-7216-7552-2*) Saunders.

Radiography of Spine Injury. Phyllis Kornguth et al. 1992. (C). 400.00 incl. disk (*1-56815-007-5*) Mosby Inc.

Radiography Procedure & Competency Manual. Anita Biedrzycki. 2000. LC 00-20849. (Illus.). 449p. (C). pap. text 29.00 (*0-8036-0672-9*) Davis Co.

Radiography Study Guide & Registry Review. Ruth S. Widmer & Kenneth W. Van Soelen. Ed. by Andrew Allen. 1998. LC 98-13364. (Illus.). 304p. (C). text 39.95 (*0-7216-7289-2*) Saunders.

Radioimmunoassay & Reproductive Endocrinology, Pt. 1. Ed. by H. Baum & J. Gergely. 1977. pap. 12.75 (*0-08-021518-1*) Elsevier.

Radioimmunoassay of Hormones for Clinical Trials of Fertility Regulating Agents in Developing Countries: Report. 1975. (Technical Reports: No. 578). pap. text 5.00 (*92-4-120578-4*, 1100578) World Health.

Radioiodination: Theory Practice & Biomedical Application. Mrinal K. Dewanjee. 1992. (Developments in Nuclear Medicine Ser.). 658p. (C). text 265.00 (*0-7923-1491-3*) Kluwer Academic.

Radioisotope X-Ray Fluorescence Spectrometry. 1970. (Technical Reports Ser.: No. 115). (Illus.). 102p. (Orig.). pap. (*92-0-165170-8*, IDC115) IAEA AUT. *Dist:* Bernan Associates.

Radioisotopes & Radiation: Recent Advances in Medicine, Agriculture, & Industry. J. H. Lawrence et al. 1990. (Illus.). 18.75 (*0-8446-0765-7*) Peter Smith.

Radioisotopes in Medicine-In Vitro Studies: Proceedings. Ed. by Raymond L. Hayes et al. 1968. LC 68-60071. (AEC Symposium Ser.). 753p. pap. 26.75 (*0-87079-327-6*, CONF-671111); fiche 9.00 (*0-87079-328-4*, CONF-671111) DOE.

Radioisotopic Methods for Biological & Medical Research. Herman W. Knoche. 1991. (Illus.). 448p. (C). text 58.00 (*0-19-505806-2*) OUP.

Radiolabeled Blood Elements: Recent Advances in Techniques & Applications. J. Martin-Comin et al. 1994. (NATO Advanced Science Institutes Ser.: Vol. 262). (Illus.). 382p. (C). text 125.00 (*0-306-44700-2*, Kluwer Plenum) Kluwer Academic.

Radiolabeled Monoclonal Antibodies for Imaging & Therapy. Ed. by S. C. Srivastava. 1988. LC 88-19623. (NATO ASI Series A, Life Sciences: Vol. 152). (Illus.). 890p. 175.00 (*0-306-42982-9*, Plenum Trade) Perseus Pubng.

Radiologia Pediatrica. Johan G. Blickman. 2nd ed. 1999. (Illus.). 340p. (C). text (*84-8174-370-4*) Mosby-Doyma Libros ESP. *Dist:* Mosby Inc.

Radiologic A & P: A Self-Paced Multimedia Learning S. Bontrager. 1995. (*0-8016-6851-4*); (*0-8016-6852-2*) Mosby Inc.

Radiologic Anatomy of the Brain. G. Salamon & Y. P. Huang. 1976. LC 75-45294. (Illus.). 199.00 (*3-540-07528-3*) Spr-Verlag.

Radiologic Anatomy of the Jaws. Harrison M. Berry, Jr. 1982. LC 82-60263. (Illus.). 144p. (Orig.). pap. text 29.95 (*0-8122-1130-8*) U of Pa Pr.

Radiologic & Histologic Pathology of Nontumorous Diseases of Bones & Joints James W. Milgram. Ed. by John G. Gruhn. 1990. (Illus.). 1382p. 199.00 (*0-9614018-1-8*) Northbrook Pub.

Radiologic Approach to Diseases of the Chest. Irwin M. Freundlich & David G. Bragg. (Illus.). 1991. 572p. 99.00 (*0-683-03373-5*); 2nd ed. 1997. LC 96-13796. 866p. text 150.00 (*0-683-03372-7*) Lppncott W & W.

Radiologic Atlas of Bone Tumors. H. M. Kroon et al. 1993. LC 92-49602. 762p. 338.50 (*0-444-81293-8*) Elsevier.

Radiologic Atlas of Brain Tumors. Glenn S. Forbes. 1991. (C). 700.00 incl. disk (*1-56815-005-9*) Mosby Inc.

Radiologic Atlas of Pulmonary Abnormalities in Children. David B. Singleton et al. 2nd ed. 1988. (Illus.). 368p. text 126.00 (*0-7216-2062-0*) Saunders.

***Radiologic Diagnosis of Chest Disease.** Ed. by Miriam Sperber. 2nd ed. 2001. LC 00-38603. 608p. 210.00 (*1-85233-298-0*) Spr-Verlag.

***Radiologic Diagnosis of Diseases of the Chest.** Nestor L. Muller et al. 2001. LC 00-66129. (Illus.). 845p. (*0-7216-8808-X*) Saunders.

Radiologic Oral Examination: Questions & Guide. Richard B. Rafal. 1994. LC 93-26566. 464p. pap. 59.50 (*0-89640-246-0*) Igaku-Shoin.

Radiologic Physics Study Guide: Study Guide. Mosby Staff. 1997. (Radiographic Instructional Ser.). (Illus.). 208p. stu. ed. (*0-8151-5405-4*) Mosby Inc.

Radiologic Science for Technologists. Stewart C. Bushong. 6th ed. 1997. LC 96-29488. (Illus.). 608p. (C). (gr. 13). text 59.00 (*0-8151-1579-2*, 30086) Mosby Inc.

Radiologic Technologist. Jack Rudman. 1994. (Career Examination Ser.: C-1544). pap. 34.95 (*0-8373-1544-1*) Nat Learn.

Radiologic Tumor Localization. John C. Rathe & Paul Elliott. 1982. 71p. (C). pap. 12.50 (*0-87527-249-5*) Green.

Radiological Anatomy of the Abdomen. Weill. 1997. text (*0-443-05238-7*, W0383) Church.

Radiological Anatomy of the Cranial Nerves. C. Zacchi et al. 1981. 154p. text (*1-57235-063-6*) Piccin Nuova.

Radiological Aspects of Renal Transplantation: Proceedings of the Microsymposium, Nymegen, 1977. Microsymposium Staff. Ed. by William Penn. 1977. (Radiologia Clinica et Biologica Ser.: Vol. 47, No. 1). (Illus.). 17.00 (*3-8055-2844-2*) S Karger.

Radiological Atlas of Common Diseases of the Small Bowel. J. L. Sellink. 1976. pap. text 282.00 (*90-207-0476-1*) Kluwer Academic.

Radiological, Clinical & Biomechanical Aspects of Chest Trauma. Stuart A. Groskin. 1991. (Illus.). 172p. 158.00 (*0-387-53712-0*) Spr-Verlag.

Radiological Contamination & Public Health. 1996. LC 98-106850. (Hazardous, Nuclear & Solid Waste Environmental Management Ser.: No. 3). pap. 10.00 (*1-55516-513-3*, 4660) Natl Conf State Legis.

Radiological Diagnosis of Breast Diseases. Ed. by M. Friedrich & Edward A. Sickles. 1996. LC 96-80070. (Medical Radiology Ser.). (Illus.). 387p. 259.00 (*3-540-58863-9*) Spr-Verlag.

Radiological Diagnosis of Breast Diseases. Ed. by Michael Friedrich & Edward A. Sickles. 1999. LC 96-8070. (Medical Radiology Ser.). (Illus.). 400p. reprint ed. pap. 75.00 (*3-540-66339-8*) Spr-Verlag.

Radiological Effect of Nuclear War: British Journal of Radiology Reprint. 1983. 50p. pap. text (*0-444-40823-1*) Elsevier.

Radiological Emergencies: A Handbook for Emergency Responders. Nicholas A. Klimenko & James F. Redington. 1988. (Illus.). 200p. (Orig.). (C). tchr. ed. 19.95 (*0-913019-01-1*); pap. text 18.95 (*0-913019-00-3*) BRADCOMM.

Radiological Evaluation of the Spinal Cord Milosh Perovitch. 1981. Vol. 1. 256p. 145.00 (*0-8493-5041-7*, RC402); Vol. 2. 192p. 108.00 (*0-8493-5043-3*) Franklin (CRC Reprint).

Radiological Examination of the Colon. R. E. Miller & Jovitas Skucas. 1983. text 380.00 (*90-247-2666-2*) Kluwer Academic.

Radiological Imaging of Sports Injuries. C. Masciocchi & A. Barile. 1997. LC 97-12401. (Medical Radiology Ser.). (Illus.). 255p. 198.00 (*3-540-60870-2*) Spr-Verlag.

Radiological Officer. Jack Rudman. 1994. (Career Examination Ser.: C-3406). pap. 34.95 (*0-8373-3406-3*) Nat Learn.

Radiological Protection in Biomedical Research. ICRP Staff. 1993. (International Commission on Radiological Protection Ser.: Vol. 62). 72p. pap. 62.50 (*0-08-042203-9*, Pergamon Pr) Elsevier.

Radiologist. Jack Rudman. 1994. (Career Examination Ser.: C-1447). pap. 44.95 (*0-8373-1447-X*) Nat Learn.

Radiology. Friedrich A. Pasler. Tr. by Thomas M. Hassell & Arthur F. Hefti. 1993. LC 92-49748. (Color Atlas of Dental Medicine Ser.). 159.00 (*0-86577-460-9*) Thieme Med Pubs.

Radiology. Bradford J. Wood & Sangeeta D. Wood. 1997. LC 97-27521. (House Officer Ser.). 352p. pap. 29.95 (*0-683-30363-5*) Lppncott W & W.

Radiology: An Illustrated History. Ronald L. Eisenberg. 1992. (Illus.). 620p. text 115.00 (*0-8016-1526-7*) Mosby Inc.

Radiology: MGH Clinical Review. Felix S. M. Chew et al. Ed. by Daniel I. Rosenthal et al. 1994. LC 93-20747. (Illus.). 464p. pap. text 58.00 (*0-7216-4609-3*) Saunders.

Radiology: Pre-Test Self-Assessment & Review. Ed. by David M. Hovsepian. 1993. LC 92-48942. (Pretest Specialty Level Ser.). (Illus.). 268p. pap. 45.00 (*0-07-052007-0*) McGraw-Hill Prof.

Radiology Administration Forms, Checklists & Guidelines. Aspen Reference Group Staff. Ed. by Kenneth E. Lawrence & Dwayne E. Eutsey. 1994. LC 93-35879. ring bd. 249.00 (*0-8342-0546-7*) Aspen Pub.

Radiology an Illustrated History. Ronald L. Eisenberg. 1995. 240p. 99.00 (*0-8151-1526-1*) Mosby Inc.

Radiology & Imaging for Medical Students. David Sutton. 6th ed. 1994. LC 93-19864. pap. text (*0-443-04883-5*) Church.

Radiology & Physics. Mosby Staff. 1997. text 1150.00 (*0-8151-6947-7*) Mosby Inc.

Radiology & the Kidney: Some Present Concepts. Ed. by C. J. Hodson. 1977. (Contributions to Nephrology Ser.: Vol. 5). (Illus.). 29.75 (*3-8055-2385-8*) S Karger.

Radiology Dictionary: Radiologisches Woerterbuch. Kurt Freye & Wayne P. Lammers. 1982. (GER.). 556p. 125.00 (*0-8288-1837-1*, M15426) Fr & Eur.

Radiology for Anaesthetists. Conrad Wittram & Graham H. Whitehouse. 1996. (Illus.). 176p. pap. (*0-340-55790-7*) E A GBR. *Dist:* OUP.

Radiology for Dental Auxiliaries. Herbert H. Frommer. 6th ed. 1996. (Illus.). 416p. stu. ed. (*0-8151-3378-2*); 6th ed. 1995. (Illus.). 416p. (C). (gr. 13). pap. text 44.00 (*0-8151-3229-8*, 24203); 7th ed. 2000. LC 00-61674. 464p. 48.00 (*0-323-00520-9*); 7th ed. 2000. 112p. stu. ed. 13.95 (*0-323-00649-3*) Mosby Inc.

***Radiology for Dental Auxiliaries: Instructor's Manual.** Herbert H. Frommer. 7th ed. 2001. (Illus.). pap. 250.00 (*0-323-00523-3*) Mosby Inc.

***Radiology for Surgeons.** Misra et al. 2002. (Illus.). 288p. pap. (*1-84110-033-1*) Greenwich Med GBR. *Dist:* JAMCO Dist.

Radiology for the MRCP. John Curtis & Graham Whitehouse. 1998. (Arnold Publication). (Illus.). 400p. pap. text 42.50 (*0-340-71886-2*) OUP.

Radiology for the MRCP. Nicola Strickland. 1997. (Illus.). 260p. (*0-7020-2220-9*) W B Saunders GBR. *Dist:* Saunders.

Radiology for the MRCP. Zezulka. 1997. (Illus.). 304p. (Orig.). pap. text (*0-412-58120-5*, Chap & Hall NY) Chapman & Hall.

Radiology Imaging Words & Phrases. Sally C. Pitman. 1997. LC 98-234809. vii, 617p. (Orig.). pap. 46.25 (*0-934385-68-8*) Hlth Prof Inst.

Radiology in Medical Diagnostics: Evolution of X-Ray Applications 1895-1995. Gerd Rosenbusch et al. 1995. 570p. 110.00 (*0-86542-899-9*) Blackwell Sci.

Radiology in Oto-Rhino-Laryngology. Ed. by S. Brunner. 1974. (Advances in OtoRhinoLaryngology Ser.: Vol. 21). (Illus.). 162p. 80.00 (*3-8055-1632-0*) S Karger.

Radiology in the Management of Cancer. Ed. by R. J. Johnson et al. 1990. (Illus.). 484p. text (*0-443-03732-9*) Church.

Radiology Life Support (Rad-Ls) A Practical Approach. William H. Bush & Bernard F. King. 1998. LC 97-42700. 208p. pap. 39.95 (*0-412-13591-4*) Chapman & Hall.

Radiology Life Support (RAD-LS) A Practical Approach. William H. Bush et al. 1999. (Illus.). 208p. pap. 35.00 (*0-340-74158-9*) OUP.

Radiology Made Easy. Arpan Banerjee. 1999. (Illus.). 184p. pap. text 39.95 (*1-84110-014-5*) OUP.

Radiology Management: A Guide for Administrators, Supervisors, & Students Eric Bouchard. 1993. (Orig.). (C). LC 94-21553. pap. text 49.95 (*1-881795-06-3*);Vol. 1. 269p. pap. text 27.95 (*1-881795-04-7*) Bellwether-Cross.

Radiology Medical Transcription: MDT 130. S. Turley. 1993. 120p. (C). stu. ed. (*0-933915-51-9*) CA College Health Sci.

Radiology of Acute Cervical Spine Trauma. John H. Harris, Jr. et al. 2nd ed. 1986. (Illus.). 296p. 68.00 (*0-683-03928-8*) Lppncott W & W.

Radiology of Acute Cervical Spine Trauma. John H. Harris, Jr. & Stuart E. Mirvis. 3rd ed. 1996. LC 95-17806. (Illus.). 560p. text 115.00 (*0-683-03929-6*) Lppncott W & W.

Radiology of Aids. Ed. by Jacques W. A. J. Reeders & Philip C. Goodman. 2001. LC 00-48254. (Medical Radiology Ser.). (Illus.). 350p. 169.00 (*3-540-66510-2*) Spr-Verlag.

Radiology of Blunt Trauma of the Chest. P. Schnyder & M. Wintermark. Ed. by A. L. Baert et al. 2000. (Medical Radiology Ser.). (Illus.). 160p. 89.00 (*3-540-66217-0*) Spr-Verlag.

Radiology of Bone Diseases. George B. Greenfield. 5th ed. 1990. (Illus.). 962p. text 175.00 (*0-397-50979-0*) Lppncott W & W.

Radiology of Carpal Instability: A Practical Approach. W. R. Obermann. 1994. LC 95-119769. 200p. 233.50 (*0-444-82080-9*) Elsevier.

Radiology of Chest Diseases. Ed. by Sebastian Lange. Tr. by Terry Telger. 2nd rev. ed. 1997. LC 97-28204. (Illus.). 370p. 79.00 (*0-86577-637-7*) Thieme Med Pubs.

Radiology of Childhood Leukemia & Its Therapy. Nancy S. Rosenfield. 1981. (Illus.). 128p. (C). pap. text 22.50 (*0-87527-173-1*) Green.

Radiology of Congenital Heart Disease. Kurt Amplatz et al. 1992. LC 92-49972. (*0-8016-0329-3*) Mosby Inc.

Radiology of Diabetes. B. Eyes & I. A. MacFarlane. 1986. text 59.00 (*0-85200-936-4*) Kluwer Academic.

Radiology of Emergency Medicine. John H. Harris et al. 4th ed. 1999. LC 99-35711. (Illus.). 1,600p. text 199.00 (*0-683-30679-0*) Lppncott W & W.

Radiology of Haemophilic. Jeno Forrai. 1979. text 85.50 (*90-247-2130-X*) Kluwer Academic.

Radiology of Joint Disease, Vol. 2. D. M. Forrester & J. C. Brown. 3rd ed. 1987. (Monographs in Clinical Radiology Ser.). (Illus.). 608p. text 105.00 (*0-7216-3827-9*) Saunders.

Radiology of Liver Circulation. C. L'Hermine. 1985. LC 85-8905. (Radiology Ser.). text 215.00 (*0-89838-715-9*) Kluwer Academic.

Radiology of Occupational Chest Disease. Ed. by A. Solomon & L. Kreel. 1989. (Illus.). 212p. 147.00 (*0-387-96877-6*) Spr-Verlag.

Radiology of Orthopaedic Implants: An Atlas of Techniques & Assessment. Ed. by Andrew A. Freiberg. 2000. LC 2001-18323. (Illus.). xvi, 255p. 99.00 (*0-323-00222-6*) Mosby Inc.

Radiology of Orthopedic Procedures. Martin I. Gelman. 1984. (Monographs in Clinical Radiology Ser.: Vol. 24). (Illus.). 300p. text 99.00 (*0-7216-4079-6*) Saunders.

Radiology of Peripheral Vascular Diseases. Ernst Ammann. Ed. by E. Zeitler. 2000. LC 97-50385. (Medical Radiology Ser.). (Illus.). 400p. 289.00 (*3-540-58758-6*) Spr-Verlag.

Radiology of Renal Failure. Harry J. Griffiths. 2nd ed. 1990. (Illus.). 272p. text 75.00 (*0-7216-4289-6*) Saunders.

Radiology of Skeletal Disorders Ronald O. Murray et al. 3rd ed. 1989. (Illus.). 2368p. text (*0-443-01980-0*) Church.

Radiology of Skeletal Trauma Lee F. Rogers. 2nd ed. 1992. LC 92-9204. (Illus.). 1619p. text (*0-443-08550-1*) Church.

***Radiology of Skeletal Trauma,** Set. Lee F. Rogers. 3rd rev. ed. 2001. (Illus.). 1595p. (*0-443-06563-2*) Church GBR. *Dist:* Saunders.

Radiology of Small Animal Fracture Management. Joe P. Morgan et al. 1994. LC 94-13109. (Illus.). 400p. text 83.00 (*0-7216-5455-X*) Saunders.

Radiology of Sports Injuries. I. F. Anderson et al. 1999. (Illus.). 248p. text 139.00 (*0-07-470497-4*) McGraw-Hill Prof.

Radiology of Syndromes, Metabolic Disorders, & Skeletal Dysplasias. Hooshang Tabyi & Ralph S. Lachman. 4th ed. 1995. LC 95-40103. (Illus.). 1162p. (C). text 230.00 (*0-8151-8709-2*, 25694) Mosby Inc.

Radiology of the Arthritides: A Clinical Perspective. Adam Greenspan & Eric E. Gershwin. 1990. (Illus.). 272p. (gr. 13). text (*0-397-44675-6*, GM0083) Gower-Mosby.

Radiology of the Cat. Charles S. Farrow. 1993. LC 93-39041. (Illus.). 280p. (C). text 105.00 (*1-55664-129-X*); 480p. 80.00 (*0-8016-8062-X*) Mosby Inc.

Radiology of the Esophagus. Levine. 1989. text 155.00 (*0-7216-2906-7*) Saunders.

Radiology of the Extremities. Nancy Baker. 1991. (Illus.). 144p. (gr. 13). text (*1-56375-005-8*, GM0007) Gower-Mosby.

Radiology of the Female Pelvic Organs. Ed. by Erich K. Lang & Susan Ascher. 1998. LC 97-50319. (Medical Radiology Ser.). (Illus.). 250p. 180.00 (*3-540-61119-3*) Spr-Verlag.

Radiology of the Foot. Stephen D. Weissman. 2nd ed. 1999. (Illus.). 512p. reprint ed. (*0-9670506-0-X*) Diagnostic X-Ray.

Radiology of the Foot & Ankle. Thomas H. Berquist. 2nd ed. 1999. LC 99-30529. (Illus.). 608p. text 189.00 (*0-7817-2009-5*) Lppncott W & W.

Radiology of the Hand. P. Bourjat. 1987. (Exercises in Radiological Diagnosis Ser.). (Illus.). 204p. 40.00 (*0-387-16537-1*) Spr-Verlag.

Radiology of the Hand. C. J. Thijn. 1986. (Illus.). 302p. 216.00 (*0-387-15345-4*) Spr-Verlag.

Radiology of the Heart. H. Spindola-Franco & B. G. Fish. 1985. (Illus.). 700p. 561.00 (*0-387-90742-4*) Spr-Verlag.

Radiology of the Kidney & Genitourinary Tract. Alan J. Davidson et al. Ed. by Lisette Bralow. 3rd ed. 1998. LC 98-9758. (Illus.). x, 761p. (C). text 195.00 (*0-7216-7144-6*) Saunders.

Radiology of the Kidney & Urinary Tract. Ed. by Alan J. Davidson & David S. Hartman. 2nd ed. 1993. (Illus.). 864p. text 159.00 (*0-7216-3552-0*) Saunders.

Radiology of the Lower Urinary Tract. Ed. by Erich K. Lang. 1994. LC 93-49790. (Medical Radiology Ser.). (Illus.). 350p. 306.00 (*0-387-53720-1*) Spr-Verlag.

Radiology of the Pancreas. Ed. by Albert L. Baert et al. 2nd rev. ed. 1999. LC 98-50337. (Medical Radiology Ser.). (Illus.). 351p. 249.00 (*3-540-63479-7*) Spr-Verlag.

Radiology of the Sella Turcica. J. F. Bonneville et al. 1980. (Illus.). 262p. 181.00 (*0-387-10319-8*) Spr-Verlag.

Radiology of the Small Intestine. P. Bret et al. 1989. (Illus.). 314p. 370.00 (*0-387-59508-2*) Spr-Verlag.

Radiology of the Spine. L. J. Rowe. 1998. (Illus.). 800p. (*0-443-08968-X*) Church.

Radiology of the Stomach. Richard H. Marshak et al. 1983. (Illus.). 656p. text 180.00 (*0-7216-6124-6*) Saunders.

Radiology of the Upper Urinary Tract. Ed. by E. K. Lang et al. 1991. (Medical Radiology Ser.). (Illus.). 370p. 316.00 (*0-387-52546-7*) Spr-Verlag.

Radiology of the Urinary System. Ed. by Milton Elkin. 1980. 1. 135.00 (*0-316-23275-0*); 2. 135.00 (*0-316-23276-9*) Lppncott W & W (Little Brwn Med Div).

Radiology of Thoracic Trauma. Paul Stark. 1992. (Illus.). 160p. text (*1-56372-004-3*) E A GBR. *Dist:* OUP.

Radiology of Trauma. Ed. by M. Heller & A. Fink. 1996. LC 95-46532. (Medical Radiology Ser.). (Illus.). 400p. 259.00 (*3-540-59324-1*) Spr-Verlag.

Radiology of Trauma. Ed. by Martin Heller & A. Fink. 1999. (Medical Radiology Ser.). (Illus.). 416p. pap. 75.00 (*3-540-66338-X*) Spr-Verlag.

Radiology of Trauma Vol. I: Skeletal Trauma. Salvatore J. Sclafoni. 1991. LC 65-40272. (Illus.). 176p. (gr. 13). text (*1-56375-007-4*, GM0196) Gower-Mosby.

Radiology of Trauma Vol. II: Soft-Tissue Trauma. Salvatore J. Sclafani. 1992. LC 65-40280. (Illus.). 112p. (*0-397-44665-9*) Gower-Mosby.

Radiology of Veterinary Orthopedics: Features of Diagnosis. Joe P. Morgan. 2000. (Illus.). 320p. pap. 44.95 (*0-8138-0312-8*) Iowa U Pr.

Radiology on Call: A Survival Handbook. O'Kane & Kranis. 1999. (Illus.). 320p. (C). (gr. 13). pap. text 39.00 (*0-8151-4487-3*, 29953) Mosby Inc.

Radiology On-Call Survival Guide. Brian Funaki & Martin J. Lipton. 1996. LC 96-45213. 194p. pap. text 39.95 (*0-316-28237-5*) Lppncott W & W.

***Radiology Picture Tests.** Misra et al. 2000. (Greenwich Medical Media Ser.). (Illus.). 320p. pap. (*1-84110-039-0*) Greenwich Med GBR. *Dist:* JAMCO Dist.

Radiology Recall. Ed. by Spencer Gay & Richard Woodcock. 1999. LC 99-40820. 636p. pap. text 29.95 (*0-683-30663-4*) Lppncott W & W.

***Radiology Reference Manual: A Practical Guide to Training in Diagnostic Radiology.** Ed. by Douglas P. Beall. 2002. 250p. 69.50 (*1-58829-126-X*) Humana.

Radiology Review Manual. Wolfgang F. Dahnert. 2nd ed. 1993. LC 92-49039. (Illus.). 742p. 76.00 (*0-683-02340-3*); 3rd ed. 1997. 139.00 incl. cd-rom (*0-683-30083-0*, D1128); 3rd ed. 1997. 139.00 incl. cd-rom (*0-683-30082-2*, D0788); 3rd ed. 1997. 139.00 incl. cd-rom (*0-683-30081-4*, D0789); 3rd ed. 1996. LC 95-21072. (Illus.). 871p. 85.00 (*0-683-02338-1*); 4th ed. 1998. 952p. 160.00 (*0-7817-2169-5*); 4th ed. 1998. LC 98-27272. 952p. pap. 99.00 (*0-683-30623-5*) Lppncott W & W.

Radiology Secrets. Ed. by Douglas S. Katz et al. 1997. LC 97-31327. (Secrets Ser.). (Illus.). 575p. (Orig.). pap. 39.95 (*1-56053-158-4*) Hanley & Belfus.

Radiology Word Book. Theresa Indovina & Wilburta Q. Lindh. 1990. LC 89-25983. (Illus.). 504p. (C). pap. text 29.95 (*0-8036-4856-1*) Davis Co.

Radionics & the Subtle Anatomy of Man. David V. Tansley. (C). pap. 12.95 (*0-8464-1044-3*) Beekman Pubs.

Radionics & the Subtle Anatomy of Man. David V. Tansley. 1980. (*0-85032-193-X*); 1972. 110p. pap. (*0-85032-089-5*) C W Daniel GBR. *Dist:* Natl Bk Netwk.

Radionics Interface with the Ether Fields. David V. Tansley. 1979. 112p. (C). pap. 16.95 (*0-8464-1045-1*) Beekman Pubs.

Radionics Interface with the Ether Fields. David V. Tansley. 1975. 110p. pap. (*0-85032-129-8*) C W Daniel GBR. *Dist:* Natl Bk Netwk.

Radionuclide Bone Imaging & Densitometry. Ed. by Fred A. Mettler. 1987. (Contemporary Issues in Nuclear Imaging Ser.: Vol. 4). (Illus.). 344p. text (*0-443-08546-3*) Church.

Radionuclide Carcinogenesis: Proceedings. Ed. by Charles L. Sanders & R. H. Bush. 1973. LC 73-600127. (AEC Symposium Ser.). 500p. pap. 20.75 (*0-87079-329-2*, CONF-720505); fiche 9.00 (*0-87079-330-6*, CONF-720505) DOE.

Radionuclide Exposure of the Embryo/Fetus. National Council on Radiation Protection and Measure. 1998. LC 98-27800. (NCRP Reports: No. 128). pap. 35.00 (*0-929600-60-6*) NCRP Pubns.

Radionuclide Generators: New Systems for Nuclear Medicine Applications. Ed. by Fern F. Knapp & Thomas A. Butler. 1984. LC 83-25875. (ACS Symposium Ser.: No. 241). 238p. lib. bdg. 87.95 (*0-8412-0822-0*) Am Chemical.

Radionuclide Imaging of the Breast. Ed. by Raymond Taillefer & Iraj Khalkhali. 1998. LC 98-29128. (Illus.). 536p. text 225.00 (*0-8247-0202-6*) Dekker.

***Radionuclide Targeting with Particular Emphasis on Urinary Bladder Carcinoma.** Anna Sjostrom. 2001. (Comprehensive Summaries of Uppsala Dissertations from the Faculty of Medicine Ser.: No. 1042). (Illus.). 51p. (*91-554-5035-0*) Uppsala Universitet SWE. *Dist:* Coronet Bks.

Radionuclide Tracers. Michael F. L'Annunziata. 1987. 485p. text 217.00 (*0-12-436252-4*) Acad Pr.

Radionuclide Ventricular Function Studies: Correlation with ECG, Echo & X-ray Data. P. J. Ell et al. 1982. text 321.50 (*90-247-2639-5*) Kluwer Academic.

Radionuclides in Brachytherapy Radium & after Effects: British Journal of Radiology Supplement 21. 1988. pap. text (*0-905749-14-6*) Med Physics Pub.

Radionuclides in Medicine & Health. Yanch. 2002. 900p. (*0-471-32206-7*) Wiley.

Radionuclides in Nephro-Urology. Ed. by M. Donald Blaufox. 1990. (Contributions to Nephrology Ser.: Vol. 79). (Illus.). xii, 232p. 29.75 (*3-8055-5073-1*) S Karger.

Radionuclides in Nephrology. Ed. by A. Bischof-Delaloye & M. Donald Blaufox. 1987. (Contributions to Nephrology Ser.: Vol. 56). (Illus.). x, 278p. 29.75 (*3-8055-4445-6*) S Karger.

Radionuclides in Nephrourology. Andrew Taylor et al. 1997. LC 97-3057. pap. 70.00 (*0-932004-48-2*) Soc Nuclear Med.

Radionuclides in Therapy. Richard P. Spencer. 1987. 216p. 123.00 (*0-8493-5843-4*, CRC Reprint) Franklin.

Radiopharmaceuticals: Chemistry & Pharmacology. Ed. by Adrian D. Nunn. 1992. LC 92-18394. (Drugs & the Pharmaceutical Sciences Ser.: Vol. 55). (Illus.). 460p. text 215.00 (*0-8247-8624-6*) Dekker.

Radiopharmaceuticals: Progress & Clinical Perspectives. Ed. by Alan R. Fritzberg. 1986. Vol. I. 208p. 102.00 (*0-8493-6335-7*, RM852); Vol. II. 176p. 95.00 (*0-8493-6336-5*) Franklin (CRC Reprint).

Radiopharmaceuticals & Brain Path Studied with Pet & Spect. Mirko Diksic. Ed. by Richard C. Reba. 1990. 464p. lib. bdg. 249.95 (*0-8493-4863-3*, RC386) CRC Pr.

Radiopharmaceuticals & Labelled Compounds. International Atomic Energy Agency Staff. 1973. (Proceedings Ser.). (Illus.). 847p. Vol. 1. pap. (*92-0-040073-6*, ISP344-1); Vol. 2. pap. (*92-0-040173-2*, ISP344-2) IAEA AUT. *Dist:* Bernan Associates.

Radiopharmaceuticals & Other Compounds Labelled with Short-Lived Radionuclides. Ed. by Michael J. Welch. 1977. LC 76-26764. pap. 48.00 (*0-08-021344-8*, Pergamon Pr) Elsevier.

Radiopharmaceuticals for Positron Emission Tomography: Methodological Aspects. Ed. by G. Stocklin & V. W. Pike. 1993. LC 93-1703. (Developments in Nuclear Medicine Ser.). 194p. (C). text 98.50 (*0-7923-2340-8*) Kluwer Academic.

Radiopharmaceuticals from Generator-Produced Radionuclides. 1971. (Panel Proceedings Ser.). 205p. pap. (*92-0-111471-0*, ISP294) IAEA AUT. *Dist:* Bernan Associates.

Radiopharmaceutics: Using Radioactive Compounds in Pharmaceutics & Medicine. Ed. by A. E. Theobald. 1989. 184p. 74.95 (*0-470-21510-0*) P-H.

Radiopharmacy & Radiopharmacology: Yearbook 1. Peter H. Cox & Christine M. King. 1985. xii, 376p. text 157.00 (*2-88124-114-X*); 376p. pap. text 58.00 (*2-88124-113-1*) Gordon & Breach.

Radiopharmacy & Radiopharmacology: Yearbook 2. Ed. by Peter H. Cox. 1987. (C). xii, 434p. text 190.00 (*2-88124-167-0*); 434p. pap. text 74.00 (*2-88124-168-9*) Gordon & Breach.

Radiopharmacy & Radiopharmacology: Yearbook 3. P. Cox. 1988. xii, 348p. kivar 282.00 (*2-88124-670-2*) Gordon & Breach.

Radioprotectors: Chemical, Biological, & Clincial Perspectives. Edward A. Bump & Kamal Malaker. 1997. LC 97-22136. 448p. 159.95 (*0-8493-4756-4*) CRC Pr.

Radiosurgery: Enhancement of Clinical Excellence. Ed. by E. Alexander, III et al. 1992. (Illus.). 112p. pap. 69.75 (*3-8055-5546-6*) S Karger.

Radiosurgery 1999: 4th International Stereotactic Radiosurgery Society Meeting, Sydney, February 1999. Ed. by Douglas Kondziolka. 2000. LC 99-4844. (Radiosurgery Ser.: Vol. 3). (Illus.). xii, 294p. 248.00 (*3-8055-6922-X*) S Karger.

Radiosurgery, 1997 Vol. 2: 3rd International Stereotactic Radiosurgery Society Meeting, Madrid, June 1997. Ed. by Douglas Kondziolka. 1997. LC 97-46316. (Radiosurgery Ser.: Vol. 2, 1998). xii, 268p. text 224.50 (*3-8055-6547-X*) S Karger.

Radiotherapeutic Management of Prostate Adenocarcinoma. Anthony V. D'Amico & Gerald E. Hanks. 1999. LC 00-500852. (An Arnold Publication). (Illus.). 224p. (*0-340-74110-4*) E A GBR. *Dist:* OUP.

Radiotherapy & Cancer Immunology. Ed. by Naresh Prasad. 1981. 216p. 98.95 (*0-8493-5901-5*, RC268) CRC Pr.

Radiotherapy for Head & Neck Cancers: Indications & Techniques. K. Kian Ang et al. 1993. LC 93-6754. (Illus.). 300p. 80.00 (*0-8121-1678-X*) Lppncott W & W.

Radiotherapy in Cancer Management: A Practical Manual. Ed. by G. P. Hanson & J. Stjernsward. 1997. LC 97-65556. (Illus.). 312p. pap. (*0-412-63580-1*) E A GBR. *Dist:* OUP.

Radiotherapy of Intraocular & Orbital Tumors. Ed. by W. E. Alberti & Robert H. Sagerman. 1993. LC 92-48365. (Medical Radiology Ser.). (*3-540-17686-1*); (Illus.). 424p. 307.00 (*0-387-17686-1*) Spr-Verlag.

***Radiotherapy of Intraocular & Orbital Tumors.** Ed. by W. E. Alberti & R. H. Sagerman. 2nd rev. ed. 2001. (Medical Radiology Ser.). 300p. (*3-540-67373-3*) Spr-Verlag.

Radiotherapy of Malignant Disease. Ed. by E. C. Easson & R. C. Pointon. 1985. (Illus.). 474p. 166.00 (*0-387-13104-3*) Spr-Verlag.

Radiotherapy of Malignant Disease: Founded by Easson. Ed. by R. C. Pointon. 2nd ed. 1991. (Illus.). 496p. 215.00 (*0-387-19622-6*) Spr-Verlag.

Radiotherapy of Ocular Disease: 1st International Symposium on Special Aspects of Radiotherapy, Berlin, May 1996. Ed. by W. Hinkelbein et al. 1997. LC 97-3528. (Frontiers of Radiation Therapy & Oncology Ser.: Vol. 30, 1997). (Illus.). x, 302p. 191.50 (*3-8055-6392-2*) S Karger.

Radiotherapy Principles & Practices. Griffiths. 1994. text 83.00 (*0-443-04783-9*) Saunders.

Radiotherapy Safety: Proceedings of a Short Course Held at the University of Wisconsin, Madison, Wisconsin, March 25-26, 1982. Ed. by Bruce Thomadsen. 1984. (American Association of Physicists in Medicine Symposium Ser.: No. 4). 175p. 45.00 (*0-88318-443-5*) Am Inst Physics.

Radiotracers for Medical Applications, Vol. I. Ed. by Garimella V. Rayudu. 1983. 320p. 155.00 (*0-8493-6015-3*, R895) CRC Pr.

Radiotracers for Medical Applications, Vol. II. Ed. by Garimella V. Rayudu. 1983. 304p. 154.00 (*0-8493-6016-1*, R895, CRC Reprint) Franklin.

Radius & Ulna. Jesse Jupiter & Margaret M. McQueen. 1999. LC 98-52736. (Arnold Publication). 188p. 75.00 (*0-7506-0835-8*) OUP.

Radographic Pathology for Technologists. James D. Mace. 3rd ed. 1997. LC 97-23176. (Illus.). 352p. (C). (gr. 13). pap. text 39.00 (*0-8151-4568-3*, 30347) Mosby Inc.

Radon Exposure of the U. S. Population - Status of the Problem. Intro. by Warren K. Sinclair. 1991. (Commentary Ser.: No. 6). 27p. (Orig.). pap. text 20.00 (*0-929600-17-7*) NCRP Pubns.

Radon, Radium, & Uranium in Drinking Water. Ed. by C. Richard Cothern & Paul A. Rebers. 1990. (Illus.). 296p. lib. bdg. 99.95 (*0-87371-207-2*, L207) Lewis Pubs.

Radurization of Scampi, Shrimp & Cod. 1971. (Technical Reports: No. 124). (Illus.). 93p. (Orig.). pap. (*92-0-115171-3*, IDC124) IAEA AUT. *Dist:* Bernan Associates.

Rage, Power, & Aggression. Ed. by Robert A. Glick & Steven T. Roose. 1993. LC 92-49297. (Role of Affect in Development, Motiv Ser.: No. 2). 288p. (C). 55.00 (*0-300-05271-5*) Yale U Pr.

Ragged Mountain Press Pocket Guide to Wilderness Medicine & First Aid. Paul G. Gill, Jr. 1997. LC 96-49971. (Illus.). 232p. pap. 14.95 (*0-07-024552-5*) McGraw-Hill Prof.

Raging Hormones: Do They Rule Our Lives? Gail Vines. 1994. LC 93-44921. (C). text 35.00 (*0-520-08776-3*); pap. text 25.00 (*0-520-08777-1*) U CA Pr.

Rain-Forest Remedies: 100 Healing Herbs of Belize. Rosita Arvigo & Michael J. Balick. 2nd rev. ed. 1993. LC 93-80280. 336p. (Orig.). pap. 15.95 (*0-914955-13-6*) Lotus Pr.

Rainbow for Patti. Carol West. 1992. (Illus.). 46p. (Orig.). pap. 9.95 (*0-938837-11-7*) Behav Sci Ctr Pubs.

Rainbow Man. Richard G. Rockman, Jr. Ed. by Dean C. Ouellette. rev. ed. 1992. (Illus.). 201p. (Orig.). pap. 9.95 (*0-9630916-1-1*) R G Rockman.

Rainbow Reiki: Expanding the Reiki System with Powerful Spiritual Abilities. Walter Luebeck. 1997. LC 97-71446. (Illus.). 192p. (Orig.). pap. 14.95 (*0-914955-28-4*) Lotus Pr.

Rainbow Stress Reduction: Play Your Stress Away with Colorful Healing Art & Stress Reducing Games. Venu. 1991. LC 93-147454. (Illus.). 84p. pap. 19.95 (*0-87877-167-0*) Red Rose Pr.

Raising a Healthy Athlete. Theresa Foy DiGeronimo & Douglas A. Avella. 1990. 200p. (*0-945167-37-7*) British Amer Pub.

Raising & Educating a Deaf Child. Marc Marschark. 1998. (Illus.). 256p. reprint ed. pap. 13.95 (*0-19-512658-0*) OUP.

Raising Happy Healthy Children. Karen Olness. 1981. pap. 3.95 (*0-9602790-5-9*) Hlth Frontiers.

Raising Happy, Healthy, Weight-Wise Kids. Judy Toews & Nicole Parton. 2000. (Illus.). 184p. pap. (*1-55263-179-6*) Key Porter CAN. *Dist:* Firefly Bks Limited.

Raising Healthy Children in an Alcoholic Home. Barbara L. Wood. 1992. LC 92-15532. 192p. (Orig.). pap. 11.95 (*0-8245-1205-7*) Crossroad NY.

Raising Healthy Pets: Insights of a Holistic Veterinarian. Norman Ralston & Gale Jack. 1996. LC 97-158266. 128p. (Orig.). pap. 10.95 (*1-882984-22-6*) One Peaceful World.

Raising of Intelligence: A Selected History of Attempts to Raise Retarded Intelligence. Herman H. Spitz. 1986. 288p. text 59.95 (*0-89859-836-2*) L Erlbaum Assocs.

Raising Standards in American Health Care: Best People, Best Practices, Best Results. V. Clayton Sherman. 1999. LC 98-53278. 332p. 45.00 (*0-7879-4621-4*) Jossey-Bass.

Raising the Dead. Scott A. Isard & Stuart H. Gage. 2001. LC 00-64605. (Illus.). 118p. pap. text 16.95 (*0-87013-550-3*) Mich St U Pr.

Raising the Young Blind Child: A Guide for Parents & Educators. Shulamith Kastein et al. 1980. LC 79-17820. 208p. 35.95 (*0-87705-422-3*); pap. 20.95 (*0-89885-288-9*) Kluwer Academic (Kluwer Acad Hman Sci).

Rakhma Story: Unconditional Love & Caring for People with Alzheimer's & Dementia. Shirley J. Shaw & Lynn Baskfield. 1998. LC 98-54693. pap. 16.95 (*1-880090-83-X*) Galde Pr.

Raman & Infrared Chemical Imaging. Morris. 400p. (*0-471-24674-3*) Wiley.

Rambles in the Mammoth Cave During the Year 1844 by a Visiter. Alexander C. Bullitt. 1985. LC 85-6698. (Illus.). 134p. pap. 5.95 (*0-939748-16-9*) Cave Bks MO.

Rambo's Nursing Skills for Clinical Practice. Ed. by Susan C. DeWit. 4th ed. 1994. (Illus.). pap., tchr. ed. (*0-7216-4178-4*); pap. text, stu. ed. 18.00 (*0-7216-4324-8*) Saunders.

Rambo's Nursing Skills for Clinical Practice. Susan C. DeWit. 4th rev. ed. 1994. LC 93-36409. (Illus.). 1200p. pap. text 37.00 (*0-7216-3642-X*) Saunders.

Rancho Santa Fe Coloring Book. Louise Rogers. 1997. LC 97-24463. (Illus.). 40p. (Orig.). (J). (gr. k-6). pap. 3.00 (*0-938711-48-2*) Tecolote Pubns.

Random House Handbook: Diagnostic Tests. Frederick C. Crews. 4th ed. Date not set. pap. text (*0-07-013643-2*) McGraw.

Random House Health & Medicine Dictionary. Random House Staff. 2nd ed. 1997. 432p. pap. 6.99 (*0-679-77709-1*) Random Ref & Info.

Random House Webster's American Sign Language Medical Dictionary. Elaine Costello. 2000. (Illus.). 256p. 34.95 (*0-375-42554-3*) Random Ref & Info.

Random House Webster's Medical Dictionary. Random House Editors. 1997. mass mkt. (*0-345-41442-X*) Ballantine Pub Grp.

Randomised Controlled Clinical Trials. Christopher J. Bulpitt. LC 96-41439. 1983. text 139.50 (*90-247-2749-9*); 2nd ed. 1996. 448p. (C). text 205.50 (*0-7923-4257-7*) Kluwer Academic.

Randomised Controlled Trials. Ed. by A. R. Jadad. 1998. 123p. pap. (*0-7279-1208-9*) BMJ Pub GBR. *Dist:* AIDC.

Randomised Controlled Trials versus Real Life Practice in BPH: Satellite Symposium Held at the XVth Congress of the European Association of Urology, Brussels, April 2000. Ed. by C. R. Chapple. 2000. (European Urology Ser.: 38). (Illus.). iv, 60p. 25.25 (*3-8055-7181-X*) S Karger.

Randomized Clinical Trial & Therapeutic Decisions. Niels Tygstrup et al. 1982. (Statistics: Textbooks & Monographs: Vol. 43). (Illus.). 320p. text 145.00 (*0-8247-1856-9*) Dekker.

Rand/U. C. L. A. Appropriateness Method User's Manual. Kathryn Fitch et al. 2001. LC 00-45830. (Illus.). xiii, 109p. pap. 15.00 (*0-8330-2918-5*) Rand Corp.

Ranks of Death: A Medical History of the Conquest of America. Percy M. Ashburn. Ed. by Frank D. Ashburn. 1980. LC 80-24672. (Perspectives in Latin American History Ser.: No. 2). xix, 298p. reprint ed. lib. bdg. 45.00 (*0-87991-599-4*) Porcupine Pr.

Ransoming the Mind: An Integration of Yoga & Modern Therapy. Charles Bates. 1986. LC 86-50084. (Illus.). 329p. (Orig.). pap. 11.95 (*0-936663-00-6*) Yes Intl Pubs.

Rape: Social Facts from England & America. Donna I. Qureshi. 1979. 293p. pap. text 8.60 (*0-87563-178-9*) Stipes.

Rape & Violence: Index of New Information with Authors, Subjects, Research Categories & References. Richard B. Zarkado. 1995. 160p. 57.50 (*0-7883-0730-4*); pap. 47.50 (*0-7883-0731-2*) ABBE Pubs Assn.

Rape Crisis Intervention Handbook: A Guide for Victim Care. S. L. McCombie. 1980. LC 80-14191. (Illus.). 250p. 47.50 (*0-306-40401-X*, Kluwer Plenum) Kluwer Academic.

Rape, Incest, & Sexual Harassment: A Guide for Helping Survivors. Kathryn Quina & Nancy Carlson. 1989. LC 89-16160. 275p. 70.00 (*0-275-92533-1*, C2533, Praeger Pubs) Greenwood.

***Rape of the Soul: How the Chemical Imbalance Model of Modern Psychiatry Has Failed its Patients.** Ty Colbert. 2001. 279p. per. 17.95 (*0-9643635-2-6*) Kevco Pubg.

Rape Plots: A Feminist Cultural Study of Genesis 34. Susanne Scholz. 2000. LC 98-40740. (Studies in Biblical Literature: Vol. 13). 232p. (C). text 50.95 (*0-8204-4154-6*) P Lang Pubng.

Rape Victim: Clinical & Community Interventions. Mary P. Koss & Mary R. Harvey. 2nd ed. 1991. (Library of Social Research: Vol. 185). (Illus.). 288p. pap. 37.95 (*0-8039-3895-0*, 7734) Sage.

Rapha's Twelve-Step Program for Overcoming Eating Disorders. Robert S. McGee & William D. Mountcastle. 1990. pap. 15.99 (*0-945276-19-2*) Rapha Pub.

Rapid Access Guide to Internal Medicine. Paul L. Fine. 2nd ed. 2000. LC 00-42035. (Illus.). 429p. pap. text 29.95 (*0-7817-2357-4*) Lppncott W & W.

Rapid Access Guide to the Physical Examination. Don Novey. 2nd ed. 1998. LC 98-3979. (Illus.). 783p. spiral bd. 29.95 (*0-323-00128-9*) Mosby Inc.

Rapid Access Pediatrics: Companion Handbook to Oski's Pediatrics. Loren JD. Walensky et al. 1999. LC 98-32462. x, 593p. pap. text 29.95 (*0-7817-1914-3*) Lppncott W & W.

Rapid Analysis of Arrhythmias: A Self-Study Program. Contrib. by Emanuel Stein. 3rd ed. 1999. LC 99-30300. (Illus.). 272p. pap. text 45.00 (*0-683-30655-3*) Lppncott W & W.

Rapid Assessment Procedures for Nutrition & Primary Health Care. Susan C. Scrimshaw & Elena Hurtado. 1987. LC 87-3193. (Reference Ser.). 69p. (Orig.). pap. 10.95 (*0-87903-111-5*) UCLA Lat Am Ctr.

Rapid Cognitive Therapy: The Professional Therapists' Guide to Rapid Change Work. Georges Philips & Terence Watts. 1999. (Professional Therapist's Guide to Rapid Change Work Ser.: Vol. 1). 246p. pap. (*1-899836-37-3*) Crown Hse GBR. *Dist:* LPC Group.

Rapid Detection of Infectious Agents. Ed. by Steven Specter et al. 1999. (Infectious Agents & Pathogenesis Ser.). xxiii, 216p. (C). text 69.50 (*0-306-45848-9*, Kluwer Plenum) Kluwer Academic.

Rapid Diagnosis of Mycoplasmas. Ed. by I. Kahane & A. Adoni. 1994. (FEMS Symposium Ser.: No. 62). (Illus.). 246p. (C). text 95.00 (*0-306-44621-9*, Kluwer Plenum) Kluwer Academic.

Rapid ECG Interpretation. Khan. 1997. LC 97-12030. pap. text 20.95 (*0-7216-7468-2*) Saunders.

Rapid ECG Interpretation: A Self-Teaching Manual. Ann E. Norman. 1991. 300p. pap. 29.00 (*0-07-105302-6*) McGraw-Hill Prof.

Rapid Guide to Hazardous Air Pollutants. Howard J. Beim et al. 1997. 582p. pap. 52.95 (*0-471-29234-6*, VNR) Wiley.

Rapid Interpretation of Heart Sounds & Murmurs. Emanuel Stein & Abner J. Delman. 4th ed. 1996. 168p. pap. 37.95 incl. audio (*0-683-30084-9*) Lppncott W & W.

Rapid Interpretation of Heart Sounds, Murmurs & Arrhythmias: A Guide to Cardiac Auscultation in Dogs & Cats. Larry P. Tilley & Frances W. Smith, Jr. 1992. (Illus.). pap. text 36.00 incl. audio (*0-8121-1568-6*) Lppncott W & W.

Rapid Methods & Automation in Microbiology & Immunology. Ed. by A. Vaheri et al. 1991. (Illus.). 573p. 130.00 (*0-387-53983-2*) Spr-Verlag.

Rapid Methods in Clinical Microbiology: Present Status & Future Trends. Ed. by B. Kleger et al. 1989. LC 90-6776. (Advances in Experimental Medicine & Biology Ser.: Vol. 263). (Illus.). 158p. 69.50 (*0-306-43507-1*, Plenum Trade) Perseus Pubng.

Rapid Nursing Intervention. Delmar Publishing Staff & Suzan J. Watanabe. rev. ed. 1995. LC 95-23118. (Rapid Nursing Interventions Ser.). 224p. (C). mass mkt. 21.50 (*0-8273-7092-X*) Delmar.

Rapid Psychological Assessment. Jason T. Olin & Carolyn Keatinge. 1998. LC 97-45506. 336p. 85.00 (*0-471-18181-1*) Wiley.

Rapid Reference to Clinical Dentistry 1997, Vol. 1. Constant Crohin & Michele Crohin. 1997. (Illus.). 49p. pap. 10.00 (*0-9662831-0-4*) Boabab Pub.

Rapid-Sequence Review of Anesthesiology: With Time-Limited Pressure. Won K. Chee. 1997. LC 96-50977. 168p. pap. text 44.99 (*0-7506-9933-7*) Buttrwrth-Heinemann.

Rapidly Progressive Glomerulonephritis. Ed. by Charles D. Pusey & Andrew J. Reese. 1998. LC 97-16817. (Oxford Clinical Nephrology Ser.). (Illus.). 290p. text 129.50 (*0-19-262636-1*) OUP.

Rapprochement: The Critical Subphase of Separation-Individuation. Ruth Lax et al. 1980. LC 80-66351. 528p. pap. 45.00 (*0-87668-409-6*) Aronson.

Rapprochment: The Critical Subphase of Separation-Individuation. Ed. by Ruth F. Lax et al. 1994. LC 80-66351. 528p. pap. 50.00 (*1-56821-103-1*) Aronson.

Raptor Biomedicine III: Including Bibliography of Diseases of Birds of Prey. Ed. by J. T. Lumeij et al. 2001. LC 00-105874. 476p. (C). text 99.00 (*0-9636996-1-X*) Zoological Educ.

Raquela: A Woman of Israel. Ruth Gruber. 2000. LC 00-34417. (Illus.). 456p. pap. 16.00 (*0-8129-3153-X*, Three Riv Pr) Crown Pub Group.

***Rare Kidney Diseases**, Vol.136. Ed. by A. Schieppati et al. 2001. (Contributions to Nephrology Ser.). (Illus.). x, 340p. 198.25 (*3-8055-7278-6*) S Karger.

Ras-MAPK Signaling on Differentiating SH-SY5Y Human Neuroblastoma Cells. Anna-Karin Olsson. 2000. (Comprehensive Summaries of Uppsala Dissertations from the Faculty of Medicine Ser.: No. 950). (Illus.). 66p. (Orig.). pap. (*91-554-4793-7*) Uppsala Universitet SWE. *Dist:* Coronet Bks.

Ras Oncogenes. Ed. by D. A. Spandidos. 1989. (NATO ASI Series A, Life Sciences: Vol. 170). (Illus.). 332p. 95.00 (*0-306-43228-5*, Plenum Trade) Perseus Pubng.

Rasch Models: Foundations, Recent Developments, & Applications. Ed. by Gerhard H. Fischer & Ivo W. Molenaar. 1996. LC 95-3740. (Illus.). 436p. 82.95 (*0-387-94499-0*) Spr-Verlag.

Rashes of Childhood Diseases. Nancy J. Denke et al. 1999. (Illus.). 92p. ring bd. 55.00 (*0-935890-47-5*) Emerg Nurses IL.

Rat: A Study in Behavior. S. A. Barnett. rev. ed. 1981. LC 74-33509. xiv, 336p. pap. text 13.50 (*0-226-03742-8*) U Ch Pr.

Rat As an Animal Model in Breast Cancer Research. Matthew J. Van Zwieten. 1984. (Developments in Oncology Ser.). 300p. text 179.50 (*0-89838-624-1*) Kluwer Academic.

Rat Histopathology: A Glossary for Use in Toxicity & Carcinogenicity Studies. P. Greaves & J. M. Faccini. 2nd rev. ed. 1992. LC 92-41672. 302p. 178.50 (*0-444-88361-4*) Elsevier.

Rat Hybrodimas & Rat Monoclonal Antibodies. Ed. by Herve Bazin. 1990. 480p. lib. bdg. 299.00 (*0-8493-5438-2*, QR185) CRC Pr.

Rat Nervous System. Ed. by George T. Paxinos. 2nd ed. 1994. LC 94-26442. (Illus.). 1136p. text 207.00 (*0-12-547635-3*) Acad Pr.

Rate Adaptive Cardiac Pacing. Ed. by E. U. Alt et al. 1993. LC 92-48249. (Illus.). 331p. 120.00 (*0-387-54051-2*) Spr-Verlag.

Rate-Controlled Drug Administraton & Action. Harry A. Struyker-Boudier. 1986. 296p. 168.00 (*0-8493-6151-6*, RS201, CRC Reprint) Franklin.

Rates of Protein Synthesis During Aging. Ed. by James R. Florini et al. 1974. 253p. text 34.50 (*0-8422-7221-6*) Irvington.

Rating Scale of Communication in Cognitive Decline RSCCD. Rick Bollinger & Carole J. Hardiman. 1996. 50p. pap. 30.00 (*0-937857-66-1*, 1655) Speech Bin.

Rating Scales & Assessment Instruments for Use in Pediatric Psychopharmacology Research. Ed. by C. Keith Conners et al. 1995. 415p. (Orig.). (C). pap. text 60.00 (*0-7881-2518-4*) DIANE Pub.

Rating Scales & Checklists: Evaluating Behavior, Personality, & Attitudes. Lewis A. Aiken. 1996. LC 95-39106. 320p. 105.00 incl. disk (*0-471-12787-6*) Wiley.

Rating Scales for Psychoneuropharmacology: A Comprehensive Database for the Rapid Selection of Relevant Scales for Clinical Trials. Ed. by H. Van Riezen & M. C. Vrijmoed-de Vries. 2000. audio compact disk 385.50 (*0-444-82805-2*) Elsevier.

Rating Scales for Psychopathology, Health Status, & Quality of Life: A Compendium on Documentation in Accordance with the DSM-III-R & WHO Systems. Per Bech. 1993. LC 92-49556. (Illus.). 503p. 159.00 (*0-387-55903-5*) Spr-Verlag.

Rational Approach to Radiodiagnostic Investigations. 1983. (Technical Report Ser.: No. 689). 52p. pap. text 5.00 (*92-4-120689-6*) World Health.

Rational Basis for Anesthesiology. G. Dal Santo. 1990. 934p. text (*1-57235-010-5*) Piccin Nuova.

Rational Basis for the Surgical Treatment of Epilepsy. Giovanni Broggi. 1986. (Current Problems in Epilepsy Ser.: Vol. 5). 350p. (*0-86196-099-8*) J Libbey Med GBR. *Dist:* Bks Intl VA.

Rational Behavior Therapy. Maxie C. Maultsby, Jr. 1984. (Illus.). 288p. (C). pap. 28.95 (*0-13-752907-4*) P-H.

Rational Behavior Therapy: The Self-Help Psychotherapy. Maxie C. Maultsby, Jr. 1990. (Illus.). 254p. reprint ed. pap. 18.95 (*0-932838-08-1*) Tangrm Bks.

Rational Choice: The Contrast Between Economics & Psychology. Robin M. Hogarth & Melvin W. Reder. 1987. LC 86-27241. 344p. pap. text 15.95 (*0-226-34859-8*) U Ch Pr.

Rational Counseling with School Aged Populations: A Practical Guide. Jerry Wilde. 1992. LC 92-53190. xvi, 200p. pap. text 17.95 (*1-55959-040-8*) Accel Devel.

Rational Diagnosis & Treatment: Evidence-Based Clinical Decision Making. Henrik R. Wulff & Peter C. Gotzsche. 3rd ed. 2000. (Illus.). 232p. 89.95 (*0-632-03197-2*) Blackwell Sci.

Rational-Emotive Approaches to the Problems of Childhood. A. Ellis & M. E. Bernard. 1983. (Illus.). 560p. (C). 100.00 (*0-306-41331-0*, Plenum Trade) Perseus Pubng.

Rational Emotive Behavior Therapy: A Reader. Windy Dryden. 1995. LC 94-74902. 304p. 69.95 (*0-8039-7858-8*, 9823); pap. 31.50 (*0-8039-7859-6*, 9824) Sage.

Rational Emotive Behavior Therapy: A Therapist's Guide. Albert Ellis & Catharine MacLaren. 1998. LC 98-7505. (Practical Therapist Ser.: Vol. 2). 176p. 24.95 (*1-886230-12-9*) Impact Pubs CA.

***Rational Emotive Behavior Therapy with Children & Adolescents: Verbatim Case Studies.** Albert Ellis & Jerry Wilde. 2001. LC 2001-44990. 160p. pap. 18.00 (*0-13-087281-4*) P-H.

Rational Emotive Consultation in Applied Settings. Ed. by Michael Bernard & Raymond DiGuiseppe. 1993. (School Psychology Ser.). 224p. text 49.95 (*0-8058-0578-8*) L Erlbaum Assocs.

Rational-Emotive Counselling in Action. Windy Dryden. 1989. (Counselling in Action Ser.: Vol. 9). 112p. (C). 65.00 (*0-8039-8269-0*, 9297); pap. 22.95 (*0-8039-8270-4*, 9298) Sage.

Rational-Emotive Couple Counseling: A Special Issue of Journal of Rational Emotive Therapy. Russell M. Grieger. 1986. 109p. pap. 16.95 (*0-89885-300-1*, Kluwer Acad Hman Sci) Kluwer Academic.

Rational-Emotive Couples Therapy. A. Ellis et al. 1989. (PPG Psychology Practitioner Guidebooks Ser.). 144p. 23.50 (*0-08-035759-8*); pap. 13.95 (*0-08-035758-X*) Alemany Pr.

Rational-Emotive Family Therapy: A Systems Perspective. Charles H. Huber & Leroy G. Baruth. 1989. 208p. 27.95 (*0-8261-6100-6*) Springer Pub.

Rational-Emotive Theraphy with Alcoholics & Substances Abusers. Albert Ellis et al. 1988. (Psychology Practitioner Guidebooks). 180p. text 30.00 (*0-08-033975-1*, Pergamon Pr) Elsevier.

Rational-Emotive Therapy with Children & Adolescents. M. E. Bernard. 2nd ed. 1994. 352p. 45.00 (*0-471-57670-0*) Wiley.

Rational Health Care. Maxwell. 1995. text 92.00 (*0-443-05336-7*) Saunders.

Rational Models of Cognition. Ed. by M Oaksford & N. Chater. 1999. (Illus.). 496p. text 115.00 (*0-19-852415-3*) OUP.

Rational Option for a National Health Program. John Canham-Clyne et al. 1995. LC 94-74595. 112p. 17.95 (*0-9630587-2-X*); pap. 9.95 (*0-9630587-1-1*) Pamphleteers.

Rational Phytotherapy: A Physician's Guide to Herbal Medicine. Volker Schulz et al. 3rd ed. 1997. LC 97-27399. 49.95 (*0-387-62648-4*) Spr-Verlag.

Rational Phytotherapy: A Physician's Guide to Herbal Medicine. Volker Schulz et al. Tr. by T. C. Telger from GER. 4th ed. 2000. LC 00-44010. (Illus.). 350p. 49.95 (*3-540-67096-3*) Spr-Verlag.

Rational Plypharmacy. Ed. by Ilo E. Leppik. 1996. LC 96-43598. (Epilepsy Research Ser.: No. 11). 274p. 143.50 (*0-444-82455-3*) Elsevier.

Rational Suicide? Implications for Mental Health Professionals. James L. Werth, Jr. 1996. LC 95-38733. (Series in Death Education, Aging, & Health Care). 200p. 69.95 (*1-56032-424-4*); pap. 22.95 (*1-56032-450-3*) Hemisp Pub.

Rational Therapeutics: A Clinical Pharmacologic Guide for the Health Professional. D. Craig Brater et al. Ed. by Roger Lawrence Williams. 1989. (Clinical Pharmacology Ser.: Vol. 16). (Illus.). 808p. text 250.00 (*0-8247-7946-0*) Dekker.

Rational Use of Diagnostic Imaging in Paediatrics: Report of a WHO Study Group, 1987. WHO Staff. 1987. (Technical Report Ser.: No. 757). 102p. 14.00 (*92-4-120757-4*) World Health.

Rational Use of Drugs: Report of the Conference of Experts, Nairobi. WHO Staff. 1987. 329p. 52.00 (*92-4-156105-X*) World Health.

Rational Use of Drugs in the Management of Acute Diarrhoea in Children. 1990. (ENG, FRE, RUS & SPA.). iv, 71p. pap. text 14.00 (*92-4-156142-4*, 1150355) World Health.

Rational Use of Drugs Report of the Conference of Experts, Nairobi (25-29 November 1985) 1987. 329p. pap. text 29.00 (*92-4-156104-1*, 1150271) World Health.

Rational Use of Magnetic Resonance Imaging. Peter A. Rinck. 1996. (Illus.). 300p. 135.00 (*0-86542-823-9*) Blackwell Sci.

Rational Use of Medicines: Resolution AP (94) 1 & Explanatory Memorandum. 1995. LC 96-118345. (ENG & FRE.). (*92-871-2702-6*) Council of Europe FRA. *Dist:* Manhattan Pub Co.

Rationale for the Terminology of the Fundamentals of Chinese Medicine: The Case for Literal Translation. Nigel Wiseman. 1998. LC 98-7652. (*0-912111-58-5*) Paradigm Publns.

Rationale of Estrogen Dose Reduction: The Justification for 20 mg Ethinylestradiol. European Society of Contraception Staff. Ed. by Mary Ann Short. 1998. LC 97-20954. (Illus.). 76p. lib. bdg. 35.95 (*1-85070-785-5*, Parthenon Pbng) CRC Pr.

Rationale of Operative Fracture Care. Joseph Schatzker & Marvin Tile. 2nd enl. rev. ed. 1997. LC 95-39615. (Illus.). 656p. 250.00 (*3-540-59388-8*) Spr-Verlag.

Rationality: An Essay Towards an Analysis. Jonathan Bennett. 1989. LC 88-30267. 134p. (C). reprint ed. pap. 7.95 (*0-87220-066-3*); lib. bdg. 24.95 (*0-87220-067-1*) Hackett Pub.

Rationalizing Acute Care Services. Pauline Mistry. 1996. LC 96-33576. 120p. pap. (*1-85775-125-6*) Radcliffe Med Pr GBR. *Dist:* Balogh.

Rationalizing Medical Work: Decision-Support Techniques & Medical Practices. Marc Berg. 1997. LC 96-2928. (Inside Technology Ser.). 250p. 38.00 (*0-262-02417-9*) MIT Pr.

Rationelle Kieferorthop Adie see Principles & Practice of Dentofacial Orthopaedics

Rationing America's Medical Care: The Oregon Plan & Beyond. Ed. by Martin A. Strosberg et al. 1992. LC 91-77958. (Brookings Dialogues on Public Policy Ser.). 240p. (C). pap. 16.95 (*0-8157-8197-0*) Brookings.

Rationing Health Care in America: Perceptions & Principles of Justice. Larry R. Churchill. 1987. LC 86-40582. (C). pap. text 13.00 (*0-268-01631-3*) U of Notre Dame Pr.

Rationing in Action. 1993. 160p. pap. text (*0-7279-0813-8*) BMJ Pub GBR. *Dist:* AIDC.

Rationing Medical Care for the Critically Ill. Ed. by Martin A. Strosberg et al. 1989. LC 88-63909. (Brookings Dialogues on Public Policy Ser.). 98p. pap. 11.95 (*0-8157-8199-7*) Brookings.

Rationing Medicine. Robert H. Blank. 1989. 290p. pap. text 20.00 (*0-231-06537-X*); 1988. (Illus.). 288p. text 52.50 (*0-231-06536-1*) Col U Pr.

Raumliches Horen see Spatial Hearing: The Psychophysics of Human Sound Localization

Raven - Johnson: Understanding Biology Test Bank. Van Norman. 1991. 512p. pap. 100.00 (*0-8016-4692-8*) Mosby Inc.

Raw Food Treatment of Cancer. Kristine Holfi. 1995. LC 95-61547. 50p. 3.95 (*1-57258-057-7*) TEACH Servs.

Raw Material: Producing Pathology in Victorian Culture. Erin O'Conner. 2000. LC 00-30308. (Body, Commodity, Text Ser.). (Illus.). 280p. lib. bdg. 54.95 (*0-8223-2608-6*) Duke.

Raw Material: Producing Pathology in Victorian Culture. Erin O'Connor. 2001. LC 00-30308. (Body, Commodity, Text Ser.). (Illus.). 280p. pap. 18.95 (0-8223-2616-7) Duke.

Raynaud Update: Pathophysiology & Treatment. Ed. by E. Davis. 1985. (Advances in Microcirculation Ser.: Vol. 12). (Illus.). vi, 162p. 120.00 (3-8055-3992-4) S Karger.

Raynaud's Disease: Index of New Information & Bibliography. Steven Y. Garrison. 1996. 150p. 57.50 (0-7883-0982-X); pap. 47.50 (0-7883-0983-8) ABBE Pubs Assn.

Raynaud's Phenomenon. Jay D. Coffman. 1989. (Illus.). 200p. text 39.95 (0-19-505756-2) OUP.

Rays of Hope: How One Man's Personal War with Cancer Could Save Your Life. Arianne Wing-Miller. 2000. 176p. 24.95 (0-942540-24-7) Breakthru Pub.

Raystede Handbook of Homeopathic Remedies for Animals. M. Raymonde Hawkins & George Macleod. 72p. (Orig.). pap. 11.95 (0-8464-4281-7) Beekman Pubs.

Razonamiento Medico. C. Corral Corral. 1994. (SPA.). 204p. pap. (84-7978-125-4) Ediciones Diaz ESP. Dist: IBD Ltd.

RBE for Deterministic Effects, ICRP Publication: A Report of a Task Group of Committee 1 of the International Commission on Radiological Protection. ICRP Staff. 1990. (International Commission on Radiological Protection Ser.: Vol. 20, No. 58). (Illus.). 64p. pap. 40.00 (0-08-040173-2, Pergamon Pr) Elsevier.

RBRVS: Untangling the Web. Paul L. Grimaldi. 1992. 50p. 20.00 (0-930228-92-8) Hlthcare Fin Mgmt.

R.D. Laing & the Paths of Anti-Psychiatry. Zbigniew Kotowicz. 1997. LC 96-3254. (Makers of Modern Psychotherapy Ser.). 160p. (C). 68.95 (0-415-11610-4); pap. 26.95 (0-415-11611-2) Routledge.

RDA: Rats, Drugs & Assumptions. Majid Ali. 1995. (Illus.). 670p. pap. 21.00 (1-879131-07-2) Inst of Prev Med.

Re-Aligning African Heads: Yoruba Curatives for Maafa-Related Ailments. Adetokunbo F. Borishade. 1996. (Illus.). xxi, 101p. (Orig.). pap. text 10.00 (0-9654009-0-5) Sankofa Pr.

Re-Biographing & Deviance: Psychotherapeutic Narrativism & the Midrash. Mordechai Rotenberg. 1987. LC 87-2451. 256p. 68.00 (0-275-92391-6, C2391, Praeger Pubs) Greenwood.

Re-Creating Medicine: Ethical Issues at the Frontiers of Medicine. Gregory E. Pence. 2000. LC 99-86178. 192p. 22.95 (0-8476-9690-1) Rowman.

Re-Education in a Nursery Group: A Study in Clinical Psychology. Ruth W. Washburn. 1944. (SRCD Ser.: Vol. 9, No. 2). 25.00 (0-527-01531-8) Periodicals Srv.

Re-Envisioning Medicare: Facts on Medicare & Congressional Proposals to Change It. League of Women Voters Education Fund Staff. 1995. 15p. 3.99 (0-89959-398-4, 1037) LWVUS.

Re-Envisioning Psychology: Moral Dimensions of Theory & Practice. Frank C. Richardson et al. 1999. LC 98-40146. 368p. 45.00 (0-7879-4384-3) Jossey-Bass.

Re-Parenting the Adult Child: Leader Guide. 1991. tchr. ed. 12.00 (0-9622150-2-3) Aurora VA.

Re-Visioning Family Therapy: Race, Culture & Gender in Clinical Practice. Ed. by Monica McGoldrick. 1998. LC 98-6174. 444p. text 46.00 (1-57230-027-2, C0027) Guilford Pubns.

Re-Visioning Psychology. James Hillman. 1997. LC 91-50502. 304p. pap. 14.50 (0-06-090563-8, CN563, Perennial) HarperTrade.

Reach for the Dream! Developing Individual Service Plans for Persons with Disabilities. Dale DiLeo. 2nd ed. 1994. LC 95-119994. 50p. pap. 20.00 (1-883302-01-3) Trning Res.

Reach for the Rainbow: Advanced Healing for Survivors of Sexual Abuse. Lynne D. Finney. rev. ed. 1992. LC 91-45486. 336p. pap. 15.95 (0-399-51745-6, Body Pr-Perigree) Berkley Pub.

Reach Out & Teach: Meeting the Training Needs of Parents of Visually & Multiply Handicapped Young Children, Set. Kay A. Ferrell. 1985. (Illus.). 49.95 (0-89128-128-2) Am Foun Blind.

Reaching Across Boundaries of Culture & Class: Widening the Scope of Psychotherapy. Ed. by RoseMarie P. Foster et al. 1996. LC 95-52039. 296p. 50.00 (1-56821-487-1) Aronson.

Reaching Health for All. Ed. by Jon E. Rohde et al. 1993. (Illus.). 540p. pap. text 19.95 (0-19-563236-2) OUP.

Reaching India's Poor: Non-Governmental Approaches to Community Health. Ed. by Saroj Pachauri. 1994. LC 94-4731. 420p. 29.95 (0-8039-9172-X, 3743) Sage.

Reaching New Highs: Alternative Therapies for Drug Addicts. H. K. Heggenhougen. 1997. LC 96-35037. 224p. 39.95 (0-7657-0036-0) Aronson.

Reaching Out: A Directory of National Organizations Related to Maternal & Child Health. 1994. LC 94-68294. 208p. pap. text (1-57285-001-9) Nat Ctr Educ.

Reaching Out: The Prevention of Drug Abuse Through Increased Human Interaction. Gerald D. Edwards. 1985. 217p. reprint ed. pap. 12.00 (0-88268-029-3) Station Hill Pr.

Reaching Out in Family Therapy: Home-Based, School & Community Interventions. Nancy Boyd-Franklin & Brenna Hafer Bry. 2000. LC 99-49066. 244p. 35.00 (1-57230-519-3, O519) Guilford Pubns.

Reaching Out to Others. 1985. (Pocket Power Ser.). 16p. (Orig.). pap. 1.25 (0-89486-311-8, 5400B) Hazelden.

Reaching Teens Through Film & Music. Michael Scully. 1999. (Jesus in Modern Media Ser.: Vol. 2000). 128p. (YA). pap. 19.95 (0-937997-60-9, 3700) Pflaum Pubng Grp.

Reaching the Affect: Style in the Psychodynamic Therapies. Emanuel F. Hammer. 1990. LC 89-38897. 232p. 50.00 (0-87668-818-0) Aronson.

Reaching the Autistic Child: A Parent Training Program. Martin A. Kozloff. 1983. LC 83-25228. 250p. reprint ed. pap. text 14.95 (0-914797-02-6) Brookline Bks.

Reaching the Young Autistic Child. Sybille Janert. 2000. 200p. pap. (1-85343-498-1) Free Assoc Bks GBR. Dist: Intl Spec Bk.

Reaching Women Who Need Prenatal Care: Strategies for Improving State Perinatal Programs. Ian T. Hill. Ed. by Gerry R. Feinstein. 1988. 126p. (Orig.). pap. text 15.00 (1-55877-008-9) Natl Governor.

Reaction Patterns in Human Teeth. Ivar A. Mjor. 1983. 248p. 143.00 (0-8493-6645-3, RK280) CRC Pr.

Reaction Patterns of the Lymph Node Pt. 1: Cell Types & Functions. Ed. by Ekkehard Grundmann et al. 1990. (Current Topics in Pathology Ser.). (Illus.). 288p. 214.00 (0-387-52287-5) Spr-Verlag.

Reaction Patterns of the Lymph Node Pt. 2: Reactions Associated with Neoplasia & Immune Deficient States. Ed. by Ekkehard Grundmann & E. Vollmer. 1991. (Current Topics in Pathology Ser.: Vol. 84/2). (Illus.). 225p. 135.00 (0-387-52288-3) Spr-Verlag.

Reactions on Polymers: Proceedings of the NATO Advanced Study Institute, No. C-4, Troy, N. Y., July, 1973. NATO Advanced Study Institute Staff. Ed. by James A. Moore. 1973. LC 73-91207. text 171.00 (90-277-0416-3) Kluwer Academic.

Reactions to Critical Life Events: A Social Psychological Analysis. Marita Inglehart. 1991. LC 90-27790. 240p. 67.00 (0-275-93875-1, C3875, Praeger Pubs) Greenwood.

***Reactivation of the Cell Cycle in Terminally Differentiated Cells.** Marco Crescenzi. 2002. LC 2001-4700. (Molecular Biology Intelligence Unit Ser.: Vol. 17). 100p. 119.00 (1-58706-071-X); pap. 69.00 (1-58706-100-7) Eurekah.

Reactive Arthritis. Ed. by Auli Toivanen & Paavo Toivanen. 1988. LC 87-27648. 192p. 115.00 (0-8493-6118-4, RC933, CRC Reprint) Franklin.

Reactor Dosimetry: Methods, Applications, & Standardization. Ed. by Harry Farrar, IV & E. P. Lippincott. 1989. LC 88-36726. (Special Technical Publications: No. STP 1001). (Illus.). 820p. text 142.00 (0-8031-1184-3, STP1001) ASTM.

Read My Desire: Lacan Against the Historicists. Joan Copjec. 1994. LC 94-383. (October Bk.). (Illus.). 288p. 32.00 (0-262-03219-8) MIT Pr.

Read to Work: Health Occupations. Phyllis Dutwin. text 12.25 (0-8359-4687-8) Globe Fearon.

Reader: History & Systems of Psychology. James F. Brennan. 2nd ed. 1997. LC 97-7923. 280p. pap. text 38.00 (0-13-626797-1) P-H.

Reader in Medical Librarianship. Ed. by Winifred Sewell. 1983. LC 72-86634. 382p. lib. bdg. 83.50 (0-313-24043-4, ZRK/, Greenwood Pr) Greenwood.

Reading after Freud: Essays on Goethe, Holderlin, Habermas, Nietzsche, Brecht, Celan, & Freud. Rainer Nagele. 1987. LC 86-20730. 216p. text 57.50 (0-231-06286-9) Col U Pr.

Reading & Deafness. C. M. King & Stephen P. Quigley. 1985. 326p. (0-85066-585-X) Taylor & Francis.

Reading & Deafness. Cynthia M. King & Stephen P. Quigley. 1985. LC 85-5694. 422p. (C). text 39.00 (0-88744-107-6, 1718) PRO-ED.

Reading & Language Processing. Ed. by John M. Henderson et al. 1995. 360p. pap. 45.00 (0-8058-1903-7) L Erlbaum Assocs.

Reading & Reviewing Research: A Guide for the Perioperative Nurse (MILs) Susan V. Kleinbeck et al. 1989. 99p. (Orig.). pap. 18.75 (0-939583-47-X) AORN.

Reading & Understanding: An Introduction to the Psychology of Reading. Geoffrey Underwood & Vivienne Batt. 1996. (Illus.). 288p. (C). 60.95 (0-631-17949-6); pap. 33.95 (0-631-17951-8) Blackwell Pubs.

Reading & Writing about Health Careers. Ralph Cappell & Ethel M. Howard. 1984. (Career Ser.). 79p. stu. ed. 4.25 (0-910307-02-4) Comp Pr.

Reading Between the Lines. Lucille H. Blum. 1972. LC 79-182040. 183p. 28.50 (0-8236-5770-1); pap. 24.95 (0-8236-8268-4, 25770) Intl Univs Pr.

Reading Birth & Death: A History of Obstetric Thinking. Jo Murphy-Lawless. 1998. 288p. (1-85918-176-7); pap. (1-85918-177-5) Cork Univ IRL. Dist: Intl Spec Bk.

Reading Birth & Death: A History of Obstetric Thinking. Jo Murphy-Lawless. LC 99-185712. 352p. 1999. text 39.95 (0-253-33475-6); 1998. pap. 19.95 (0-253-21258-8) Ind U Pr.

Reading Development & Dyslexia. Charles Hulme & Margaret Snowling. 1994. (Illus.). 252p. (Orig.). (C). pap. text 42.50 (1-56593-368-0, 0745) Singular Publishing.

Reading Disabilities: Genetic & Neurological Influences. Ed. by Bruce F. Pennington. 1992. 240p. (C). lib. bdg. 153.00 (0-7923-1606-1) Kluwer Academic.

Reading Disabilities in College & High School: Diagnosis & Management. P. G. Aaron & Catherine Baker. 1991. LC 90-72124. (Illus.). 207p. pap. text 22.00 (0-912752-23-8) York Pr.

Reading Engelhardt: Essays on the Thought of H. Tristram Engelhardt, Jr. Ed. by Brendan P. Minogue et al. 1997. LC 97-16317. 330p. text 120.50 (0-7923-4572-X) Kluwer Academic.

Reading Faces: Window to the Soul? Leslie A. Zebrowitz. 1997. LC 96-52663. (New Directions in Social Psychology Ser.). 288p. (C). pap. text 28.00 (0-8133-2747-4) Westview.

Reading Freud: Explorations & Entertainments. Peter Gay. 1990. LC 89-28615. 240p. (C). 35.00 (0-300-04681-2) Yale U Pr.

Reading Freud's Reading. Ed. by Sander L. Gilman et al. 1993. LC 93-11102. (Literature & Psychoanalysis Ser.: Vol. 5). 320p. (C). text 45.00 (0-8147-3051-5) NYU Pr.

Reading Medical Records: The McQuade System. J. Stanley McQuade. Ed. by Luis A. Davila-Lizardi. 1999. (Illus.). iv, 333p. per. 49.95 (0-941787-00-1) Davila Assocs.

Reading Medical Records - The McQuade Method: Computer Based Training. J. Stanley McQuade et al. 1999. (Illus.). 333p. per. 89.95 incl. cd-rom (0-941787-01-X) Davila Assocs.

Reading Melanie Klein. John Phillips & Lyndsey Stonebridge. 1998. LC 97-47651. (Illus.). 280p. (C). 85.00 (0-415-16236-X); pap. 25.99 (0-415-16237-8) Routledge.

Reading Nursing Texts. A. Faulkner. Date not set. (C). pap. 11.96 (0-395-77037-8) HM.

Reading Nursing Texts. Ann Faulkner & Dana K. Stahl. 1998. LC 97-72465. xvi, 297 p. (C). pap. text 32.36 (0-395-77036-X) HM.

Reading of Silence: Virginia Woolf in the English Tradition. Patricia O. Laurence. 1993. 253p. (C). pap. 19.95 (0-8047-2179-3) Stanford U Pr.

Reading Problems: Consultation & Remediation. P. G. Aaron & R. Malatesha Joshi. 1992. LC 92-3124. (Guilford School Practitioner Ser.). 285p. 35.00 (0-89862-365-0, 2365) Guilford Pubns.

Reading Seminar XI: Lacan's Four Fundamental Concepts of Psychoanalysis: The Paris Seminars in English. Ed. by Richard Feldstein et al. 1995. LC 93-50120. (Series in Psychoanalysis & Culture). 291p. (C). text 23.50 (0-7914-2147-3) State U NY Pr.

Reading Seminars I & II: Lacan's Return to Freud. Ed. by Richard Feldstein et al. 1996. LC 94-12517. (Series in Psychoanalysis & Culture). 444p. (C). text 24.50 (0-7914-2779-X); pap. text 23.95 (0-7914-2780-3) State U NY Pr.

Reading the Body: Ohashi's Book of Oriental Diagnosis. Watari Ohashi & Tom Monte. 1991. LC 91-9902. 156p. pap. 21.00 (0-14-019362-6, Penguin Compass) Penguin Putnam.

Reading the Book of Nature: The Other Side of the Scientific Revolution. Allen G. Debus & Michael T. Walton. 1997. LC 97-33101. (Sixteenth Century Essays & Studies Ser.: Vol. 41). 268p. 40.00 (0-940474-47-6, SCJP) Truman St Univ.

Reading the Eye, Pulse & Tongue for the Indicated Remedy. Eli G. Jones. Ed. by Wade Boyle. 1990. 99p. (Orig.). pap. 10.00 (0-9623518-2-2) Eclectic Med.

Reading the Medical Record. Mary D. Litchford & Laura Yordy. 1995. 139.00 (1-880989-40-9); 139.00 (1-880989-41-7); 139.00 (1-880989-42-5); 139.00 (1-880989-43-3); pap. 6.00 (1-880989-45-X) Case Sftware.

Reading the Medical Record User's Manual. Mary D. Litchford et al. rev. ed. 1995. (C). pap. 7.00 (1-880989-26-3) Case Sftware.

Reading Toes. Date not set. pap. 19.95 (0-8464-4570-0) Beekman Pubs.

Reading Toes: Your Feet As Reflections of Your Personality. Imre Somogyi. 1997. (Illus.). 128p. pap. (0-85207-310-0) C W Daniel GBR. Dist: Natl Bk Netwk.

Readings: Child Psychology. Ed. by George R. Smrtic & Victor P. Garlock. 1973. LC 73-4447. 145p. pap. text 12.00 (0-8422-5094-8) Irvington.

Readings for a New Public Health. Ed. by Claudia J. Martin & David V. McQueen. 1991. 336p. pap. text (0-85224-616-1); 1988. 250p. (0-85224-598-X) Edinburgh U Pr GBR. Dist: Col U Pr.

Readings for General Psychology. Holmes. 1998. (C). pap. text 32.00 (0-201-45682-6) Addison-Wesley.

Readings in Abnormal Psychology. Jill M. Giiket et al. 1989. LC 88-26796. 624p. pap. 33.95 (0-471-63107-8) Wiley.

Readings in American Health Care: Current Issues in Socio-Historical Perspective. Ed. by William G. Rothstein. 1995. LC 95-12317. 426p. 49.95 (0-299-14530-1); pap. 22.95 (0-299-14534-4) U of Wis Pr.

Readings in Behavior. Ed. by William G. Van der Kloot et al. 1974. LC 73-15700. (Illus.). pap. text 19.50 (0-03-084077-5) Irvington.

Readings in Behavior Modification. Marilyn T. Erickson et al. 1973. LC 73-8528. 29.75 (0-8422-5106-5); pap. 32.75 (0-8422-0312-5) Irvington.

Readings in Behavior Modification Research with Children. Marilyn T. Erickson et al. 1973. LC 73-8536. pap. text 27.95 (0-8422-0313-3) Irvington.

Readings in Biological Science. Ed. by Irving W. Knobloch. 3rd ed. 1973. LC 72-93743. (C). pap. text 17.95 (0-89197-371-0) Irvington.

Readings in Child Development. A. Lynn Scoresby & Alvin H. Price. 2nd ed. 1992. (C). text 12.25 net. (0-07-055963-5) McGraw.

Readings in Clinical Spectrography in Speech. Ed. by Ronald J. Baken & Raymond G. Daniloff. 1990. (Illus.). 576p. (Orig.). (C). pap. text 55.00 (1-879105-04-7, 0005) Thomson Learn.

Readings in Cognitive Science: A Perspective from Psychology & Artificial Intelligence. Ed. by Alan Collins & Edward Smith. 1998. 630p. (C). pap. text 46.95 (1-55860-013-2) Morgan Kaufmann.

Readings in Community Based Nursing. Roberta Hunt. 2000. LC 99-58099. 352p. pap. text 21.00 (0-7817-2081-8) Lppncott W & W.

Readings in Community Health Nursing. Barbara W. Spradley & Judith Ann Allender. 5th ed. 1996. LC 96-31654. 672p. pap. text 34.95 (0-397-55436-2) Lppncott W & W.

Readings in Comparative Health Law & Bioethics. Timothy Stoltzfus Jost. 2001. 418p. pap. 40.00 (0-89089-615-1) Carolina Acad Pr.

Readings in Controversial Issues in Education of the Mentally Retarded. Ed. by Frank Warner & Robert Thrapp. 1972. 29.50 (0-8422-5007-7) Irvington.

Readings in Educational Psychology. Anita Woolfolk. 2nd ed. 1997. LC 97-31589. 209p. pap. text 24.00 (0-205-27889-2) P-H.

Readings in Emotional Disturbance. Ed. by Phyllis L. Newcomer. 1994. LC 93-5040. 313p. pap. text 19.00 (0-89079-588-6, 6666) PRO-ED.

Readings in Environmental Psychology Series. David V. Canter. 1995. pap. text 106.24 (0-12-158810-6) Acad Pr.

Readings in Ethnic Psychology. Ed. by Pamela Balls-Organista et al. 1998. LC 97-44675. 384p. (C). (gr. 13). pap. 34.95 (0-415-91963-0) Routledge.

Readings in Ethnic Psychology. Ed. by Pamela Balls Organista & Kevin M. Chun. 1998. LC 97-44675. 432p. (C). (gr. 13). 90.00 (0-415-91962-2) Routledge.

Readings in Existential Psychology & Psychiatry. Ed. by Keith Hoeller. 1992. LC 93-24311. (Studies in Existential Psychology & Psychiatry). 362p. (Orig.). (C). pap. 22.50 (0-391-03781-1) Brill Academic Pubs.

Readings in General Psychology. Ed. by Wayne Dennis. 1977. LC 71-167334. (Essay Index Reprint Ser.). reprint ed. 36.95 (0-8369-2493-2) Ayer.

Readings in Gerontological Nursing. Judith Ann Allender & Cherie Rector. 1998. LC 97-33646. 608p. pap. text 33.95 (0-7817-9201-0) Lppncott W & W.

Readings in Health Care Ethics. Ed. by Elisabeth Airini Boetzkes & Wilfred J. Waluchow. 2000. LC 00-710786. viii, 605p. pap. (1-55111-258-2) Broadview.

Readings in Pediatric Psychology. Ed. by Michael Roberts et al. 1993. LC 93-7736. (Illus.). 402p. (C). pap. 54.00 (0-306-44423-2, Plenum Trade) Perseus Pubng.

Readings in Personality: Classic Theories & Modern Research. Howard S. Friedman & Miriam W. Schustack. 2000. LC 00-64606. 338p. pap. 45.00 (0-205-32149-6) Allyn.

Readings in Philosophy of Psychology, Vol. I. Ed. by Ned J. Block et al. 1983. (Readings in Philosophy of Psychology Ser.: Vol. I). 318p. pap. 19.50 (0-674-74876-X) HUP.

Readings in Philosophy of Psychology, Vol. 2. Ed. by Ned J. Block. 1985. (Language & Thought Ser.). (Illus.). 372p. pap. 16.95 (0-674-74878-6) HUP.

Readings in Psychiatric Rehabilitation. Ed. by William A. Anthony & LeRoy Spaniol. 1994. LC 94-72719. 552p. (C). pap. text 34.95 (1-878512-02-1) Boston Univ Ctr Psy Rehab.

Readings in Rehabilitation Counseling. C. H. Patterson & H. Moses. 1971. pap. 8.60 (0-87563-034-0) Stipes.

Readings in Strategies & Tactics in Behavioral Research: Text. James M. Johnston & Henry S. Pennypacker. 2nd ed. 1993. 408p. text 45.00 (0-8058-0905-8) L Erlbaum Assocs.

Readings in the Philosophy of Psychology, Vol. 2. Ed. by Ned J. Block. 1981. LC 79-25593. (Language & Thought Ser.: Vol. 2). (Illus.). 372p. 41.50 (0-674-74877-8) HUP.

Readings in the Psychology of Perception. Ed. by Thomas L. Bennett. 1971. 179p. (C). pap. text 11.95 (0-8422-0160-2) Irvington.

Readings on Cognitive Ergonomics: Mind & Computers. Ed. by G. C. Van der Veer et al. 1984. (Lecture Notes in Computer Science: Vol. 178). 269p. 35.95 (0-387-13394-1) Spr-Verlag.

Readings on Diarrhoea. 1992. (ENG & FRE.). vii, 147p. pap. text, stu. ed. 20.00 (92-4-154444-9, 1150386) World Health.

Readings on Induced Abortion Vol. 1: Politics & Policies. Alan Guttmacher Institute Staff. 2000. 392p. pap. 20.00 (0-939253-54-2) Guttmacher Inst.

Readings on Teenage Pregnancy from Family Planning Perspectives, 1985-1989. 1989. 386p. pap. 15.00 (0-939253-16-X) Guttmacher Inst.

Readjustment Counseling Service: Vet Centers Address Multiple Client Problems, but Improvement Is Needed. 1996. (Illus.). 42p. (Orig.). (C). pap. text 25.00 (0-7881-3461-2) DIANE Pub.

Ready for Any Challenge: An Advanced Training Guide for Getting a Good Systemic Handle on Change. Lutz

P Q R

H. Schlicke & Heinz M. Schlicke. 1994. LC 94-15997. (Illus.). 384p. pap. 19.95 (*0-942963-43-1*) Distinctive Pub.

Ready Reference for Critical Care. Rhonda M. Strawn & Bonnie P. Stewart. 1992. (Nursing-Health Science Ser.). (Illus.). 376p. (C). spiral bd. 33.75 (*0-86720-327-7*, 327-7) Jones & Bartlett.

Ready Reference for Critical Care. Rhonda M. Strawn & Bonnie Stewart. 2nd ed. 1997. LC 96-37503. (Nursing Ser.). (Illus.). 448p. (C). pap. text 42.95 (*0-7637-0251-X*, 0251-X) Jones & Bartlett.

Ready Reference for Critical Care Drugs with Nursing Care Plans. Bonnie P. Stewart & Rhonda M. Strawn. 2nd ed. 1996. (Illus.). 352p. (C). pap. text 42.95 (*0-86720-455-9*, 455-9) Jones & Bartlett.

Reagents for Organic Synthesis, Vol. 10. Fieser and Fieser's Staff. 1982. (Fieser's Reagents for Organic Synthesis Ser.: Vol. 10). 536p. 115.00 (*0-471-86636-9*) Wiley.

Real Estate Issues in the Health Care Industry: Proceedings of the First Annual Conference of the Health Care Real Estate Institute. Ed. by Ronald S. Barak. 1996. LC 95-50404. (Current Topics in Real Estate Finance & Economics Ser.). 184p. (C). lib. bdg. 78.50 (*0-7923-9696-0*) Kluwer Academic.

Real Food. Joann Grohman. 1992. (Illus.). 179p. (Orig.). pap. 18.95 (*0-9631814-0-8*) Coburn Pr.

Real People Working in Health Care. Blythe Camenson & Jan Goldberg. 1996. LC 96-26671. (On the Job Ser.). (Illus.). 396p. pap. 14.25 (*0-8442-4727-8*, NT7278, Natl Textbk Co) NTC Contemp Pub Co.

Real-Resumes for Medical Jobs. Ed. by Anne McKinney. 2001. LC 2001-18562. (Real-Resumes Ser.). (Illus.). 192p. pap. 16.95 (*1-885288-14-X*) PREP Pubng.

Real Self: A Developmental, Self, & Object Relations Approach. James F. Masterson. 1985. LC 85-12824. 192p. text 34.95 (*0-87630-400-5*) Brunner-Routledge.

Real Solids & Radiation. A. E. Hughes & D. Pooley. 1975. (Wykeham Science Ser.: No. 35). 208p. pap. 18.00 (*0-85109-011-7*) Taylor & Francis.

Real Solution Anxiety - Panic Workbook. Richard H. Pfeiffer. 1998. 138p. pap., wbk. ed. 54.00 (*1-893505-02-2*, 1904) Growth Publ.

Real-Time Ultrasound: A Manual for Physician & Technical Personnel. Royal J. Bartrum, Jr. & Harte C. Crow. 2nd ed. 1983. LC 77-72802. (Illus.). text 65.00 (*0-7216-1552-X*) Saunders.

Real-Time Ultrasound Imaging in the Abdomen. M. Leon Skolnick. 1981. (Illus.). 241p. 120.00 (*0-387-90570-7*) Spr-Verlag.

Real Time Ultrasound in Perinatal Medicine. Ed. by R. Chef. 1979. (Contributions to Gynecology & Obstetrics Ser.: Vol. 6). (Illus.). pap. 68.75 (*3-8055-2976-7*) S Karger.

Real to Real in Exposing Radiology: True Stories in Radiologic Technology. Ricardo Scott. 1999. (Ricardo Relates True Life Experiences Ser.). (Illus.). 150p. pap. (*1-58470-030-0*) Crnerstone GA.

Real World Calculations. Messler. 1999. pap. text 26.95 (*0-7216-7556-5*) Saunders.

Real-World Nursing Survival Guide Pathophysiology. Contrib. by Saunders, W.B., Publishing Staff. 2001. LC 2001-49985. (Real World Nursing Survival Guide Ser.). (Illus.). 416p. pap. 26.95 (*0-7216-9046-7*) Saunders.

Realignments in the Welfare State: Health Policy in the United States, Britain, & Canada. Mary Ruggie. 1996. LC 96-10966. (Illus.). 336p. 47.50 (*0-231-10484-7*); 298p. pap. 19.50 (*0-231-10485-5*) Col U Pr.

***Realising Participation: Elderly People as Active Users of Health & Social Care.** 2001. 264p. text 69.95 (*0-7546-1773-4*) Ashgate Pub Co.

Realities in Childbearing. Mary Lou Moore. 2nd ed. 1983. 1160p. 79.00 (*0-7216-6498-9*) Saunders.

Realities in Coping with Progressive Neuromuscular Diseases. Ed. by Leon I. Charash et al. 1987. LC 87-71168. 228p. (C). text 34.95 (*0-914783-20-3*) Charles.

Realities of Contemporary Nursing. Persis M. Hamilton. 2nd ed. 1995. LC 95-8827. 440p. (C). pap. 50.00 (*0-8053-2020-2*) Addison-Wesley.

Realities of Contemporary Nursing. 3rd ed. 2000. (C). (*0-8053-2781-9*) Benjamin-Cummings.

Realities of Dental Therapy: A Detailed Review of Periodontal Prosthetic Treatment. Ronald L. Moloff & Stephen D. Stein. 1982. (Illus.). 471p. text 110.00 (*0-931386-42-X*) Quint Pub Co.

Realities of Transference. Arnold Goldberg. 1990. (Progress in Self Psychology Ser.: Vol. 6). 288p. text 45.00 (*0-88163-114-0*) Analytic Pr.

Reality Game: A Guide to Humanistic Counselling & Therapy. John Rowan. 2nd rev. ed. 1998. LC 97-46440. 256p. (C). 84.95 (*0-415-16433-8*); pap. 26.95 (*0-415-16434-6*) Routledge.

Reality Gap: Global Access to Health Care & the Legislative Impact of the World Health Organization's "HEA2000" David R. Schanker. Ed. by Victoria J. Cuffel. 1993. LC 93-655022. (MacArthur Scholar Series, Occasional Paper: No. 19). 141p. (Orig.). (C). pap. 4.50 (*1-881157-16-4*) In Ctr Global.

Reality of Dyslexia. John Osmond. rev. ed. 1995. LC 95-41696. 150p. pap. text 14.95 (*1-57129-017-6*) Brookline Bks.

Reality of the Psyche. Ed. by Joseph B. Wheelwright. 1968. LC 68-15614. (Illus.). 16.00 (*0-913430-16-1*) C G Jung Foun.

Reality Orientation: Psychological Approaches to the 'Confused' Elderly. Una P. Holden & Robert T. Woods. 2nd ed. 1988. (Illus.). 264p. pap. text (*0-443-03460-5*) Church.

Reality Therapy: A New Approach to Psychiatry. William Glasser. 1989. LC 89-45657. 192p. pap. 12.00 (*0-06-090414-3*, CN414, Perennial) HarperTrade.

Reality Therapy for the 21st Century. Robert E. Wubbolding. 2000. LC 00-35561. (Illus.). 352p. (gr. 13). pap. 24.95 (*1-56032-886-X*) Routledge.

Reality Therapy with Dr. Robert Wubbolding: Psychotherapy with the Experts. 1998. (C). 89.95 (*0-205-28176-1*, Macmillan Coll) P-H.

Realizing Mental Health. Roger C. Mills. 1995. 207p. (Orig.). (C). pap. text 14.99 (*0-945819-78-1*) Sulzburger & Graham Pub.

Really Essential Medical Immunology. Arthur Rabson & Ivan Roitt. 2000. LC 00-23045. (Illus.). 192p. (C). pap. 34.95 (*0-632-05506-5*) Blackwell Sci.

Really Governing: How Health System & Hospital Boards Can Make More of a Difference. Dennis D. Pointer & Charles M. Ewell. 1994. LC 94-25555. (Health & Life Science Ser.). 240p. mass mkt. 42.50 (*0-8273-5577-7*) Delmar.

Really Managing Health Care. V. Iles. 1996. LC 96-17866. (Health Services Management Ser.). 224p. pap. (*0-335-19414-1*) OpUniv Pr.

Realm of Tolerance. Ed. by P. Ivanyi. 1989. (Illus.). 314p. 46.95 (*0-387-51056-7*) Spr-Verlag.

Realtime Ophthalmic Ultrasonography & Biometry. Richard S. Koplin et al. 1984. 134p. 41.95 (*0-316-50169-7*, Little Brwn Med Div) Lppncott W & W.

Reanimacion Cardiopulmonar Avanzada (Advanced Cardiac Life Support), 1997-99. Date not set. (Emergency Cardiovascular Care Programs Ser.). (SPA.). 386p. pap. text 25.00 (*0-87493-633-0*) Am Heart.

REA's Authoritative Guide to Medical/Dental School. Research and Education Association Staff. 1997. 592p. pap. 21.95 (*0-87891-479-X*) Res & Educ.

Reason & Rationality in Health & Human Services Delivery. Charles F. Langino, Jr. & John W. Murphy. Ed. by John T. Pardeck. 1998. LC 98-10498. 120p. 29.95 (*0-7890-0509-3*) Haworth Pr.

Reason for Optimism: Treating Cancer with a Bone Marrow Transplant. Barbara J. Munson. 1996. LC 96-60273. (Illus.). 110p. (Orig.). pap. 13.95 (*0-9648754-0-3*) Two Pillars.

Reasonable Insanity: A True Story of the Seventies. Carol L. Mithers. 1994. LC 93-30571. ix, 419p. 23.00 (*0-201-57071-8*) Addison-Wesley.

Reasoning & Concepts. Daniel N. Osherson. 1976. (Child Psychology Ser.: Vol. 4). 256p. text 29.95 (*0-89859-503-7*) L Erlbaum Assocs.

Reasoning & Decision Making in Hematology. Benjamin C. Djulbegovic. 1992. 253p. pap. text (*0-443-08858-6*) Church.

***Reasoning & Decision Making in Hematology & Oncology: Evidence-Based Management.** Benjamin Djulbegovic et al. 2001. (Illus.). 605p. pap. (*0-443-06578-0*) Church GBR. *Dist:* Saunders.

Reasoning & Discourse Processes. Ed. by Terry Myers et al. 1986. (Cognitive Science Ser.). 312p. text 160.00 (*0-12-512320-5*) Acad Pr.

Reasoning, Necessity & Logic: Developmental Perspectives. Ed. by W. F. Overton. 1990. (Jean Piaget Symposia Ser.). 344p. (C). text 89.95 (*0-8058-0090-5*) L Erlbaum Assocs.

Reassessing Community Care. Ed. by Nigel A. Malin. 1987. (C). (*0-7099-1738-4*) C Helm GBR. *Dist:* Routldge.

Reassessing Psychotherapy Research. Ed. by Robert L. Russell. 1994. LC 94-8548. 240p. 40.00 (*0-89862-755-9*, C2755) Guilford Pubns.

Reassessment in Psychology: The Interbehavioral Alternative. Ed. by Noel W. Smith et al. 1983. LC 83-1234. 550p. (C). pap. text 42.00 (*0-8191-3082-6*) U Pr of Amer.

Reassessment of Inactivated Poliomyelitis Vaccine. Ed. by W. Hennessen & Antonius L. Van Wezel. 1981. (Developments in Biological Standardization Ser.: Vol. 47). (Illus.). viii, 364p. pap. 61.00 (*3-8055-1820-X*) S Karger.

Reauthorization of the Prescription Drug User Fee Act & FDA Reform: Hearing Before the Subcommittee on Health & Environment of the Committee on Commerce, House of Representatives, One Hundred Fifth Congress, First Session, April 23, 1997. Contrib. by U. S. Congress, House Committee on Commerce, Subcommittee on Health and the Environment. 1997. LC 97-215042. (Illus.). (*0-16-055213-3*) USGPO.

Reauthorization of the Substance Abuse & Mental Health Services Administration: Hearing Before the Subcommittee on Public Health & Safety of the Committee on Labor & Human Resources, United States Senate, One Hundred Fifth Congress, First Session, on Taking a Close Look at the Current Needs of Individuals Who Are Substance Abusers, Those with Mental Illness & the Providers of Services to These Individuals, in Addition, Focusing on Areas Which Can Alter SAMSHSA to Help the Age. Contrib. by U. S. Congress, Senate Committee on Labor and Human Resources, Subcommittee on Public Health and Safety. 1997. LC 98-115917. (Illus.). (*0-16-055338-5*) USGPO.

Rebellious Body: Reclaim Your Life from Environmental Illness or Chronic Fatigue Syndrome. Janice S. Wittenberg. 1996. (Illus.). 308p. (C). 20.95 (*0-306-45402-5*) Perseus Bks Grp.

Rebels Within the Ranks: Psychologists' Critique of Scientific Authority & Democratic Realities in New Deal America. Katherine Pandora. 1997. (Cambridge Studies in the History of Psychology). 272p. (C). text 64.95 (*0-521-58358-6*) Cambridge U Pr.

Rebirth: My Transplant Experience. Nancy Cassell. 1993. 64p. (Orig.). pap. 4.95 (*0-9625402-3-4*) Altan Pub.

Rebounding from Childbirth: Toward Emotional Recovery. Lynn Madsen. 1994. LC 93-40162. 192p. pap. 14.95 (*0-89789-348-4*, Bergin & Garvey) Greenwood.

Rebuilding Shattered Lives: The Responsible Treatment of Complex Post-Traumatic & Dissociative Disorders. James A. Chu. 1998. LC 97-32847. 288p. 55.00 (*0-471-24732-4*) Wiley.

Rebuilding Therapy: Incorporating the Past for a More Effective Future. Michael A. Gass. 1997. LC 96-36360. 352p. 70.00 (*0-275-95329-7*, Praeger Pubs) Greenwood.

Recalled by Life. Anthony J. Sattilaro & Tom Monte. 1994. 240p. mass mkt. 5.99 (*0-380-65573-X*, Avon Bks) Morrow Avon.

Recasting Ritual: Performance, Media, Identity. Ed. by Felicia Hughes-Freeland & Mary M. Crain. 1998. LC 98-29700. (European Association of Social Anthropologists Ser.). (C). 184p. pap. 26.95 (*0-415-18280-8*, D6291); 176p. 80.00 (*0-415-18279-4*, D6287) Routledge.

Recent Advances & Future Directions in Bone Marrow Transplantation. Ed. by S. J. Baum et al. 1987. (Experimental Hematology Today 1987 Ser.). (Illus.). 199p. 108.00 (*0-387-96582-3*) Spr-Verlag.

Recent Advances & New Developments in Hemostaseology: Abstracts. Ed. by H. K. Breddin et al. 1986. (Journal: Vol. 16, Suppl. 5, 1986). iv, 148p. pap. 39.25 (*3-8055-4505-3*) S Karger.

Recent Advances Hematology, Vol. 7. Brenner. 1993. text 66.00 (*0-443-04689-1*) Saunders.

Recent Advances in Aerospace Medicine: Proceedings of the International Congress of Aviation & Space Medicine, 18th, Amderstderdam, 1969. International Congress of Aviation and Space Medicine Staff. Ed. by D. E. Busby. 1970. LC 74-131264. 358p. text 121.50 (*90-277-0162-8*) Kluwer Academic.

Recent Advances in AIDS & Kaposi's Sarcoma. Ed. by G. Giraldo et al. 1987. (Antibiotics & Chemotherapy Ser.: Vol. 38). (Illus.). vii, 196p. 148.00 (*3-8055-4512-6*) S Karger.

Recent Advances in Anaesthesia. A. P. Adams. 19th ed. 1996. pap. text 76.00 (*0-443-05306-5*) Saunders.

Recent Advances in Anaesthesia & Analgesia, Vol. 20. Ed. by A. P. Adams & J. N. Cashman. 1998. (Illus.). 224p. pap. (*0-443-05988-8*) Church.

Recent Advances in Animal Nutrition, 1989. Ed. by W. Haresign. 1989. 298p. 185.00 (*0-408-04149-8*) Buttrwrth-Heinemann.

Recent Advances in Basic Microcirculatory Research: Proceedings. Conference of the European Society for Microcircul. Ed. by G. Wolf-Heidegger & D. H. Lewis. 1977. (Bibliotheca Anatomica Ser.: No. 15). (Illus.). Pt. 1. 172.25 (*3-8055-2757-8*); Pt. 2. 172.25 (*3-8055-2758-6*) S Karger.

Recent Advances in Beta Blockade, 1986. Ed. by Shaul G. Massry et al. 1986. (American Journal of Nephrology: Vol. 6, Suppl. 2). (Illus.). iv, 116p. pap. 36.75 (*3-8055-4442-1*) S Karger.

Recent Advances in Biomedical Imaging: Proceedings of the International Workshop on Biomedical Imaging: MR & Pet Spect, Fukui, Japan, 28-30 August 1996. Ishii, Yasushi, Workshop on Biomedical Imaging: MR. 1997. LC 97-12193. (International Congress Ser.). 260p. 148.00 (*0-444-82539-8*) Elsevier.

Recent Advances in Blood Coagulants. Poller. 7th ed. 1996. text 68.00 (*0-443-05316-2*) Saunders.

Recent Advances in Blood Coagulation, No. 5. Ed. by L. Poller. 5th ed. 1991. (Illus.). 312p. text (*0-443-04343-4*) Church.

Recent Advances in Brain Tumor Research. Ed. by W. G. Bingham. 1972. (Progress in Experimental Tumor Research Ser.: Vol. 17). 121.75 (*3-8055-1402-6*) S Karger.

Recent Advances in Burns & Plastic Surgery: The Chinese Experience. Ed. by Tishen Chang et al. 1985. text 445.50 (*0-85200-814-7*) Kluwer Academic.

Recent Advances in Canadian Neuropsychopharmacology. Ed. by P. Grof & B. Saxena. 1981. x, 238p. pap. 85.25 (*3-8055-1459-X*) S Karger.

Recent Advances in Cardiac Pacing: Goals for the 21st Century. S. Serge Barold & Jacques Mugica. 1997. LC 97-19572. (Illus.). 464p. 98.00 (*0-87993-639-8*) Futura Pub.

Recent Advances in Cardiology, Vol. 12. Rowlands. 12th ed. 1995. text 89.00 (*0-443-05199-2*) Saunders.

Recent Advances in Cardiology - 11. Ed. by Derek J. Rowlands. 1993. (Illus.). 224p. (Orig.). pap. text (*0-443-04565-8*) Church.

Recent Advances in Cell Biology of Acute Leukemia: Impact on Clinical Diagnosis & Therapy. Ed. by W. D. Ludwig & E. Thiel. 1993. LC 93-16157. (Recent Results in Cancer Research Ser.: Vol. 131). (Illus.). 407p. 150.00 (*0-387-56417-9*) Spr-Verlag.

Recent Advances in Cellular & Molecular Aspects of Angiotensin Receptors. Ed. by Mohan K. Raizada et al. 1996. (Advances in Experimental Medicine & Biology Ser.: Vol. 396). (Illus.). 262p. (C). text 102.00 (*0-306-45209-X*, Kluwer Plenum) Kluwer Academic.

Recent Advances in Chemical Information II. Ed. by H. Collier. 1993. (Special Publications). 330p. (C). (*0-85186-235-7*) Royal Soc Chem GBR. *Dist:* Spr-Verlag.

Recent Advances in Chemotherapy: Proceedings of the 18th International Congress of Chemotherapy, Stockholm, Sweden, June 27-July 2, 1993. Ed. by Jerzy Einhorn et al. 1994. LC 94-6905. 1120p. 129.95 (*1-55581-074-8*) ASM Pr.

Recent Advances in Clinical Neurology, No. 6. Ed. by Christopher Kennard. 1990. (Illus.). 276p. text (*0-443-04116-4*) Church.

Recent Advances in Clinical Neurology - 7. Christopher Kennard. 1993. (Illus.). 224p. (Orig.). text (*0-443-04570-4*) Church.

Recent Advances in Clinical Psychiatry - 7. Ed. by Kenneth L. Granville-Grossman. 7th ed. 1992. (Illus.). 200p. text (*0-443-04499-6*) Church.

Recent Advances in Clinical Psychiatry - 8. Ed. by Kenneth Granville-Grossman. 1993. (Illus.). 224p. text (*0-443-04696-4*) Church.

Recent Advances in Clinical Trial Design & Analysis. Ed. by Peter F. Thall. 1995. LC 94-41111. (Cancer Treatment & Research Ser.: No. 75). 272p. (C). text 212.00 (*0-7923-3235-0*) Kluwer Academic.

Recent Advances in Clinical Virology. Gueh-Djen Hsiung. 1981. LC 80-25926. 120p. 47.50 (*0-275-90647-7*, C0647, Praeger Pubs) Greenwood.

Recent Advances in Cognitive-Developmental Theory, Progress in Cognitive Developmental Research. Ed. by Charles J. Brainerd. 1983. (Cognitive Development Ser.). (Illus.). 270p. 121.00 (*0-387-90767-X*) Spr-Verlag.

Recent Advances in Coloproctology. Ed. by J. Beynon & Nicholas D. Carr. 1999. LC 99-24162. 255p. (*1-85233-169-0*) Spr-Verlag GBR. *Dist:* Spr-Verlag.

Recent Advances in Coronary Circulation. Ed. by E. Maruyama et al. 1994. (Illus.). 336p. 199.00 (*0-387-70130-3*) Spr-Verlag.

Recent Advances in Critical Care. Evans. 4th ed. 1996. text 52.00 (*0-443-04711-1*) Saunders.

Recent Advances in Critical Microcirculatory Research: Proceedings of the European Conference on Microcirculation, 8th le Touguet, 1974. European Conference on Microcirculation Staff. Ed. by D. H. Lewis. 1975. (Bibliotheca Anatomica Ser.: No. 13). (Illus.). 380p. 122.75 (*3-8055-2277-0*) S Karger.

Recent Advances in Crohn's Disease: Developments in Gastroenterology One. Ed. by A. S. Pena. 1981. 549p. text 229.00 (*90-247-2475-9*) Kluwer Academic.

Recent Advances in Dermatology, No. 8. Ed. by Robert H. Champion & Richard J. Pye. 8th ed. 1990. (Illus.). 248p. text (*0-443-04168-7*) Church.

Recent Advances in Dermatology 9. Ed. by Robert H. Champion & Richard J. Pye. 1992. (Illus.). 226p. text (*0-443-04451-1*) Church.

Recent Advances in Diagnosis & Treatment of Infections: Special Issue of Journal of Medicine. Ed. by Thomas R. Beam, Jr. 1983. 35.00 (*0-915340-12-7*) PJD Pubns.

Recent Advances in Diagnostic Neuroradiology. Ed. by Philippe Demaerel. 2000. LC 00-20834. (Medical Radiology Ser.). (Illus.). 500p. 279.00 (*3-540-65723-1*) Spr-Verlag.

Recent Advances in Diseases of the Esophagus: Selected Papers in the 5th World Congress of the International Society for Diseases of the Esophagus, Kyoto, Japan, 1992. Fifth World Congress of the International Society for Diseases of the Esophagus Staff. Ed. by K. Nabeya et al. 1993. LC 93-5883. (Illus.). 1107p. 378.00 (*0-387-70121-4*) Spr-Verlag.

Recent Advances in Endocrinology & Metabolism, No. 3. Ed. by Christopher R. Edwards & Dennis W. Lincoln. 1989. (Illus.). 324p. text (*0-443-03951-8*) Church.

Recent Advances in Endocrinology & Metabolism 4. Ed. by Christopher R. Edwards & Dennis W. Lincoln. 4th ed. 1992. (Illus.). 208p. text (*0-443-04518-6*) Church.

Recent Advances in Event-Related Brain Potential Research: Proceedings of the 11th International Conference on Event-Related Potentials (EPIC), Okinawa, Japan, 25-30 June 1995. Ed. by C. Ogura et al. 1996. LC 96-25000. (International Congress Ser.: No. 1099). 1118p. 262.50 (*0-444-82280-1*, Excerpta Medica) Elsevier.

Recent Advances in Fertility Control: Proceedings of the 2nd International Symposium on Recent Advances in Fertility Control, Tokyo, Japan, Oct. 24, 1987, Vol. 2. Ed. by Shoichi Matsumoto. 1989. (Current Clinical Practice Ser.: No. 50). 40p. 25.75 (*90-219-1676-2*, Excerpta Medica) Elsevier.

Recent Advances in Gastroenteritis. Pounder. 10th ed. 1994. pap. text 69.95 (*0-443-05021-X*) Saunders.

Recent Advances in Gastroenterology, Vol. 8. Ed. by Roy Pounder. 1990. (Illus.). 280p. text (*0-443-04324-8*) Church.

Recent Developments in Psychoanalysis: A Critical Evaluation. Morris N. Eagle. 1987. LC 87-196. 272p. pap. 18.00 (*0-674-75080-2*) HUP.

Recent Developments in the Field of Thrombin Inhibitors. Ed. by Jorg Struzebecher. 1995. 110p. pap. text 253.00 (*3-7186-5783-X*, Harwood Acad Pubs) Gordon & Breach.

Recent Developments in the Pharmacology of Inflammatory Mediators. Ed. by I. L. Bonta. 1980. (Agents & Actions Supplements Ser.: No. 2). 178p. 55.00 (*0-8176-0914-8*) Birkhauser.

Recent Developments in the Study of Benign Breast Disease: The Proceedings of the 4th International Benign Symposium, Manchester, April 1991. R. E. Mansel. 4th ed. 1991. (Illus.). 233p. lib. bdg. 74.95 (*1-85070-386-8*, Parthenon Pbng) CRC Pr.

Recent Developments in the Study of Benign Breast Disease: The Proceedings of the 5th International Symposium on Benign Breast Disease. Ed. by R. E. Mansel. 5th ed. 1993. LC 93-41022. (Illus.). 280p. (C). lib. bdg. 49.95 (*1-85070-532-1*, Parthenon Pbng) CRC Pr.

Recent Developments in the Study of Benign Breast Disease: The Proceedings of the 6th International Symposium on Benign Breast Disease. Ed. by R. E. Mansel. 1997. LC 97-3902. (Illus.). 158p. lib. bdg. 63.95 (*1-85070-775-8*, Parthenon Pbng) CRC Pr.

Recent Developments in Therapeutic Drug Monitoring & Clinical Toxicology. Ed. by Irving Sunshine. 1992. (Illus.). 824p. text 250.00 (*0-8247-8586-X*) Dekker.

Recent Developments in Toxicology: Trends, Methods & Problems: Proceedings of the European Society of Toxicology Meeting Held in Leipzig, September 12-14, 1990. Ed. by P. L. Chambers et al. 1991. (Archives of Toxicology Ser.: Suppl. 14). (Illus.). 323p. 158.00 (*0-387-51422-8*) Spr-Verlag.

Recent Health Policy Innovations in Social Security. Ed. by Aviva Ron & Xenia Scheil Adlung. 2000. LC 00-54382. (International Social Security Ser.: Vol. 5). (Illus.). 350p. pap. 29.95 (*0-7658-0753-X*) Transaction Pubs.

Recent Perspectives on American Sign Language. Ed. by Harlan Lane & Francois Grosjean. 1989. 176p. reprint ed. pap. 34.50 (*0-8058-0560-5*) L Erlbaum Assocs.

Recent Progress in Atherosclerosis Research. Ed. by E. Vollmer & A. Roessner. 1994. LC 93-31211. (Current Topics in Pathology Ser.: Vol. 87). (Illus.). 255p. 199.00 (*0-387-54394-5*) Spr-Verlag.

Recent Progress in Blood Coagulation & Fibrinolysis: Proceedings of the International Symposium 'Clot Formation & Lysis' Held on March 21-22, 1997, Hamamatsu, Japan, As a Satellite Symposium of the 74th Annual Meeting of the Japanese Society of Physiology. Akikazu Takada et al. 1997. LC 97-41913. (International Congress Ser.). 272p. 142.50 (*0-444-82602-5*) Elsevier.

Recent Progress in Blood Coagulation & Thrombosis Research. Ed. by O. N. Ulutin. 1978. (Bibliotheca Haematologica Ser.: No. 44). (Illus.). 85.25 (*3-8055-2896-5*) S Karger.

Recent Progress in Cardiovsacular Mechanics. Ed. by Saichi Hosada et al. 1994. LC 93-43890. xv, 400p. text 85.00 (*3-7186-5417-2*) Gordon & Breach.

Recent Progress in Cell Biology: Leukocytes & Platelets. Ed. by O. N. Ulutin. 1978. (Bibliotheca Haemotologica Ser.: No. 45). (Illus.). pap. 81.75 (*3-8055-2897-3*) S Karger.

Recent Progress in Child & Adolescent Psychiatry. Ed. by M. Shimizu. 1996. (Illus.). 214p. pap. 95.00 (*4-431-70172-9*) Spr-Verlag.

Recent Progress in Child & Adolescent Psychiatry, Vol. 2. Ed. by M. Hanada. 1999. (Illus.). 300p. pap. 79.00 (*4-431-70243-1*) Spr-Verlag.

Recent Progress in Electropharmacology of the Heart. Ed. by Junji Toyama et al. 1995. LC 95-36118. 240p. 179.95 (*0-8493-7691-2*, 7691) CRC Pr.

Recent Progress in Failing Heart Syndrome. Ed. by S. Sasayama & Hiroyuki Suga. 1992. (Illus.). 336p. 205.00 (*0-387-70073-0*) Spr-Verlag.

Recent Progress in Hormone Research, Vol. 49. Ed. by C. Wayne Bardin. 1994. (Illus.). 400p. text 94.00 (*0-12-571149-2*) Acad Pr.

Recent Progress in Mathematical Psychology. Ed. by Cornelia E. Dowling et al. 1998. LC 97-31138. (Scientific Psychology Ser.). 350p. (*0-8058-1975-4*) L Erlbaum Assocs.

Recent Progress in Medico-Social Problems in Juvenile Diabetics, Pt. II. Ed. by Z. Laron & A. Galatzer. 1983. (Pediatric & Adolescent Endocrinology Ser.: Vol. 11). (Illus.). x, 210p. 133.25 (*3-8055-3594-5*) S Karger.

Recent Progress in the Chemical Synthesis of Antibiotics. Ed. by Gabor Lukacs & M. Ohno. 1990. (Illus.). 803p. 291.00 (*0-387-52444-4*) Spr-Verlag.

Recent Progress in the Genetic Epidemiology of Cancer. Ed. by Henry T. Lynch & P. Tautu. 1991. (Illus.). 162p. 79.95 (*0-387-53022-3*) Spr-Verlag.

Recent Progress of Pineal Research - 40 Years after Discovery of Melatonin: Asia Pacific Meeting, Hamamatsu, March, 1997: Proceedings. Ed. by Y. Morita. 1998. (Biological Signals Ser.: Vol. 6, Nos. 4-6, 1997). (Illus.). 139p. pap. 50.50 (*3-8055-6638-7*) S Karger.

Recent Research in Developmental Psychopathology. Ed. by J. E. Stevenson. 1984. (Illus.). 261p. 31.50 (*0-08-030828-7*, Pergamon Pr) Elsevier.

Recent Research in Psychosomatics. Ed. by R. A. Pierloot. 1971. (Psychotherapy & Psychosomatics Ser.: Vol. 18, No. 1-6). (Illus.). viii, 376p. reprint ed. 99.25 (*3-8055-1219-8*) S Karger.

Recent Research on European Sign Languages. Ed. by F. Loncke et al. 1984. vi, 166p. pap. (*90-265-0465-9*) Swets.

Recent Research on Gynecological Endocrinology. Ed. by A. R. Genazzani & F. Petraglia. 2001. (Illus.). 276p. lib. bdg. 76.95 (*1-84214-073-6*, Parthenon Pbng) CRC Pr.

Recent Research on Gynecological Endocrinology, Set. Ed. by Andrea R. Genazzani et al. 1989. (Illus.). 110.00 (*1-85070-209-8*, Parthenon Pbng) CRC Pr.

Recent Results of Research on Arteriosclerosis. Ed. by F. Gotthard Schettler. 1989. (Sitzungsberichte der Heidelberger Akademie der Wissenschaften Ser., Mathematisch-Naturwissenschaftliche Klasse, Jahrgang 1991: Suppl. 4). (Illus.). 34p. 19.95 (*0-387-50288-2*) Spr-Verlag.

Recent Soviet Psychology. Ed. by N. O'Connor. 1961. (C). 8.00 (*0-87140-864-3*) Liveright.

Recent Strategies for the Study of Invasive & Metastatic Cancer. 1985. (Journal: Vol. 4, Suppl. 1, 1984). (Illus.). iv, 68p. pap. 24.50 (*3-8055-4008-6*) S Karger.

Recent Studies of Hypothalamic Function: Proceedings of the Symposium, Calgary, Alberta, May 1973. Symposium, Calgary, Alberta Staff. Ed. by K. Lederis & K. E. Cooper. 1974. (Illus.). 450p. 50.50 (*3-8055-1694-0*) S Karger.

Recent Studies on the Human Thalamus: Proceedings of the Annual Meeting of the Japanese Society for Sterotactic 8, Functional Neurosurgery, 15th, Maebashi, October 1976. Annual Meeting of the Japanese Society for Stereotactic 8. Ed. by P. L. Gildenberg & Chihiro Ohye. 1977. (Applied Neurophysiology Ser.: Vol. 39, No. 3-4). (Illus.). 50.50 (*3-8055-2847-7*) S Karger.

Recent TCM Research From China. Ed. & Tr. by Bob Flaws from CHI. Tr. by Charles Chace from CHI. 1994. LC 94-70761. 200p. (Orig.). pap. 18.95 (*0-936185-56-2*) Blue Poppy Pr.

Recent Theories of Human Development. R. Murray Thomas. 2000. LC 00-10059. (Illus.). xi, 311p. pap. 34.95 (*0-7619-2247-4*, 87220) Sage.

Recent Trends in Aerobiology, Allergy & Immunology. Ed. by S. N. Agashe. 1994. (Illus.). 332p. text 90.00 (*1-886106-02-9*) Science Pubs.

Recent Trends in Allergen & Complement Research. Ed. by K. Ishizaka et al. 1982. (Progress in Allergy Ser.: Vol. 30). (Illus.). xiv, 234p. 115.75 (*3-8055-2580-X*) S Karger.

Recent Trends in Diabetes Research. Ed. by H. Bostrom. 1982. 308p. (Orig.). text 42.50 (*91-22-00566-8*) Coronet Bks.

Recent Trends in Medical Genetics: Proceedings of the Conference on Recent Trends in Medical Genetics, Madras, India, 8-10 December, 1983. Ed. by K. M. Marimuthu & P. M. Gopinath. 1986. (Illus.). 370p. 128.00 (*0-08-031993-9*, Pergamon Pr) Elsevier.

Recent Trends in Plant Disease Control: National Symposium Proceedings. Ed. by H. B. Singh. 1992. (Current Trends in Life Sciences Ser.: Vol. XIX). (Illus.). 286p. (*1-55528-274-1*) Today Tomorrow IND. *Dist:* Lubrecht & Cramer, Scholarly Pubns.

Recent Trends in Regeneration Research. Ed. by V. Kiortsis et al. 1989. (NATO Advanced Science Institutes Ser.: Vol. 172). (Illus.). 514p. (C). text 174.00 (*0-306-43232-3*, Kluwer Plenum) Kluwer Academic.

Recent Trends in Theoretical Psychology. Ed. by W. J. Baker et al. 1988. (Recent Research in Psychology Ser.). (Illus.). 380p. 61.95 (*0-387-96757-5*) Spr-Verlag.

Recent Trends in Theoretical Psychology: Proceedings of the Fourth Biennial Conference of the International Society for Theoretical Psychology, June 24-28, 1991. Ed. by J. Stam Henderikus et al. 1993. LC 92-21112. (Recent Research in Psychology Ser.: Vol. 3). (Illus.). 537p. 92.00 (*0-387-97963-8*) Spr-Verlag.

Recent Trends in Theoretical Psychology: Proceedings of the Third Biennial Conference of the International Society for Theoretical Psychology April 17-21, 1989, Vol. 2. Ed. by W. J. Baker et al. 1990. (Illus.). 465p. 86.95 (*0-387-97311-7*) Spr-Verlag.

Recent Views on Hypertrophic Cardiomyopathy. Ed. by Ernst E. Van der Wall & K. I. Lie. 1985. (Developments in Cardiovascular Medicine Ser.). text 118.00 (*0-89838-694-2*) Kluwer Academic.

Recent Vitamin Research. Ed. by M. H. Briggs. 1984. 224p. 130.00 (*0-8493-5618-0*, QP771, CRC Reprint) Franklin.

Receptivity to Malaria & Other Parasitic Diseases: Report on a WHO Working Group. 1979. (EURO Reports & Studies: No. 15). 103p. 10.00 (*92-9020-154-1*, 1330015) World Health.

Receptor - Based Drug Design. Ed. by Leff. 1998. LC 98-13320. (Illus.). 400p. text 185.00 (*0-8247-0162-3*) Dekker.

Receptor Agonists & Blockers: Products, Applications, Medical Sales & New Developments. 1996. (Report Ser.: No. B-102). 255p. 3450.00 (*1-56965-020-9*) BCC.

Receptor & Non-Receptor Mediated Actions of Melatonin: International Symposium Held in Hong Kong, China, November 1999: Selected Papers. Ed. by S. Y. W. Shiu & S. F. Pang. 2000. (Biological Signals & Receptors Ser.: Vol. 9). (Illus.). 82p. pap. 34.00 (*3-8055-7125-9*) S Karger.

Receptor Autoradiography: Principles & Practice. Ed. by John Wharton & Julia M. Polak. 1994. LC 93-6952. (Modern Methods in Pathology Ser.). (Illus.). 352p. spiral bd. 64.00 (*0-19-262209-9*) OUP.

Receptor Binding in Drug Research. A. O'Brien. 1986. (Clinical Pharmacology Ser.: Vol. 5). (Illus.). 544p. text 225.00 (*0-8247-7548-1*) Dekker.

Receptor Binding Radiotracers. William C. Eckelman. 1982. Vol. I. 200p. 112.00 (*0-8493-6019-6*, QP519); Vol. II. 248p. 138.00 (*0-8493-6020-X*, QP519) Franklin (CRC Reprint).

Receptor Classification: The Integration of Operational, Structural, & Transductional Information. D. G. Trist. 1997. LC 97-6552. (Annals of the New York Academy of Sciences Ser.). 90.00 (*0-89766-987-8*) NY Acad Sci.

Receptor Desensitization & Ca2+-Signaling: Cellular Aspects of Possible Molecular Dynamics. Ed. by M. K. Uchida. 1996. (Illus.). viii, 214p. 231.50 (*3-8055-6283-7*) S Karger.

Receptor Dynamics in Neural Development. Ed. by Christopher A. Shaw. 1996. LC 95-42841. (Pharmacology & Toxicology Ser.). 368p. 169.95 (*0-8493-7817-6*) CRC Pr.

Receptor Localization: Laboratory Methods & Procedures. Marjorie Ariano. 1998. LC 97-17105. (Receptor Biochemistry & Methodology Ser.). 264p. 179.00 (*0-471-16571-9*) Wiley.

Receptor Mediated Endocytosis. P. Cuatrecasas & T. Roth. 1984. (Receptors & Recognition Series B: Vol. 15). (Illus.). 77.00 (*0-412-24820-4*, NO. 6827) Chapman & Hall.

Receptor Research Methods. Ben Greenstein. 1995. 352p. text 127.00 (*3-7186-5670-1*); spiral bd. 53.00 (*3-7186-5671-X*) Gordon & Breach (Harwood Acad Pubs).

Receptors & Ligands in Neurological Disorders. Ed. by Amartya K. Sen & Tyrone Lee. 1988. (Intercellular & Intracellular Communications Ser.: No. 4). (Illus.). 352p. text 90.00 (*0-521-30720-1*) Cambridge U Pr.

Receptors & Ligands in Psychiatry. Ed. by Amartya K. Sen & Tyrone Lee. 1988. (Intercellular & Intracellular Communications Ser.: No. 3). (Illus.). 608p. text 130.00 (*0-521-30719-8*) Cambridge U Pr.

Receptors As Surramolecular Entities: Proceedings of the Biannual Capo Bio Conference, Cagliari, Italy, 7-10 June, 1981. Ed. by Giovanni Biggio et al. 1983. (Advances in the Biosciences Ser.: Vol. 44). (Illus.). 476p. 92.50 (*0-08-029804-4*, Pergamon Pr) Elsevier.

Receptors for CNS Agents, Growth Factors, Hormones & Related Substances. Ed. by Gerald Litwack. 1990. LC 90-4689. (Receptor Purification Ser.: Vol. 1). (Illus.). 514p. 159.50 (*0-89603-167-5*) Humana.

Receptors for Steroid Hormones, Thyroid Hormones, Water-Balancing Hormones & Others. Ed. by Gerald Litwack. 1990. LC 90-4689. (Receptor Purification Ser.: Vol. 2). (Illus.). 430p. 159.50 (*0-89603-183-7*) Humana.

Receptors in the Developing Nervous System. Ed. by Ian S. Zagon & Patricia J. McLaughlin. 1993. LC 92-49100. (gr. 13). Set. 264p. pap. 263.95 (*0-412-54520-9*); Vol. 1. 272p. (C). pap. text 161.95 (*0-412-45240-5*); Vol. 2. 276p. (C). pap. text 161.95 (*0-412-49400-0*) Chapman & Hall.

Recertification: New Evaluation Methods & Strategies. Ed. by Elliott L. Mancall & Philip G. Bashook. 1994. LC 94-70217. 195p. lib. bdg. 44.95 (*0-934277-19-2*) Am Bd Med Spec.

Recertification for Medical Specialists. Ed. by Donald G. Langsley & John S. Lloyd. 1987. LC 87-72510. 276p. lib. bdg. 39.95 (*0-934277-10-9*) Am Bd Med Spec.

Recessive Oncogenes & Tumor Suppression. Ed. by Webster Cavenee et al. 1989. (Current Communications in Molecular Biology Ser.). (Illus.). 234p. (C). pap. text 24.00 (*0-87969-332-0*) Cold Spring Harbor.

Recetas: Biblioteca Universitaria, Salamanca MS.2262. Ed. by Maria Carmen De La Cal. 1987. (Medieval Spanish Medical Texts Ser.: No. 20). (SPA.). 6p. 10.00 incl. fiche (*0-940639-16-5*) Hispanic Seminary.

Rechtschreibungs-Woerterbuch der Medizin. Klaus P. Eschenbach. 1985. (ENG & GER.). 206p. 39.95 (*0-8288-1836-3*, M15433) Fr & Eur.

Rechtsphilosophische Aspekte Moderner Medizintechniken Am Beispiel der Organtransplantation und der Intensivmedizin. Nikolaus J. Kufner. 1997. (Europaische Hochschulschriften Ser.: Reihe 2, Bd. 2119). (GER.). 196p. 42.95 (*3-631-31729-8*) P Lang Pubng.

Recipes for a Healthy Lifestyle: Low Fat, Low Cholesterol, Low Sodium. Virginia Defendorf. 1994. 128p. ring bd. 6.95 (*0-914846-95-7*) Golden West Pub.

Recipes for Fat Free Living Cookbook. Jyl Steinback. 1993. 193p. pap. 14.95 (*0-9636876-6-2*) Fat Free Living.

Recipes for Kids to Lower Their Fat Thermostats. LaRene Gaunt & Edward A. Parent. 1994. LC 93-61785. (Illus.). 192p. pap. 15.95 (*0-912547-14-6*) Vitality Hse Int Inc.

Recipes to Lower Your Fat Thermostat. LaRene Gaunt. 2nd ed. 1992. LC 84-52705. (Fat Thermostat Program Ser.). (Illus.). 456p. pap. 15.95 (*0-912547-10-3*) Vitality Hse Int Inc.

Reclaim Your Health. David Frahm & Anne Frahm. 1995. LC 94-24442. 240p. pap. 14.00 (*0-89109-869-0*) Pinon Press.

Reclaim Your Health: Nutritional Strategies for Conquering Chronic Ailments. David Frahm & Anne Frahm. 1998. LC 98-36126. 240p. reprint ed. 12.95 (*0-87477-951-0*, Tarcher Putnam) Putnam Pub Group.

Reclaimed Powers: Men & Women in Later Life. David Gutmann. 1994. LC 94-3892. (Psychosocial Issues Ser.). 300p. reprint ed. pap. 22.00 (*0-8101-1120-9*) Northwestern U Pr.

Reclaiming Our Lives after Breast & Gynecologic Cancer. Kristine Falco. 1998. LC 97-16795. Orig. Title: Women & Women's Cancer. (Illus.). 248p. 40.00 (*0-7657-0099-9*) Aronson.

Reclaiming Soul in Health Care: Practical Strategies for Revitalizing Providers of Care. Linda G. Henry & James D. Henry. 1999. LC 98-45909. 202p. pap. 33.00 (*1-55648-263-9*) AHPI.

Reclaiming the Authentic Self: Dynamic Psychotherapy with Gay Men. Carlton Cornett. 1995. LC 94-24827. 224p. text 45.00 (*1-56821-395-6*) Aronson.

Reclaiming the Inner Child. Ed. by Jeremiah Abrams. 1990. (New Consciousness Reader Ser.). 336p. (Orig.). pap. 15.95 (*0-87477-551-5*, Tarcher Putnam) Putnam Pub Group.

Reclaiming the Menstrual Matrix: Evolving Feminine Wisdom. Tamara Slayton. 2001. 224p. pap. 18.00 (*1-930051-01-8*) Lantern Books.

Reclaiming the Wisdom of the Body. S. Hill. 1997. pap. (*0-09-477340-8*) Constable & Co GBR. *Dist:* Trafalgar.

Reclaiming Your Life: A Step-by-Step Guide to Using Regression Therapy to Overcome the Effects of Childhood Abuse. Jean C. Jenson. 1996. 224p. pap. 14.00 (*0-452-01169-8*, Mer) NAL.

Reclaiming Your Life: A Step-by-Step Guide to Using Regression Therapy to Overcome the Effects of Childhood Abuse. Jean C. Jenson. 1999. pap. 11.95 (*0-452-27545-8*) Viking Penguin.

Reclaiming Your Life: A Step-by-Step Guide to Using Regression Therapy to Overcome the Effects of Childhood Abuse. Jean Jenson. 1999. 202p. reprint ed. pap. text 21.00 (*0-7881-6308-6*) DIANE Pub.

Recognition & Alleviation of Pain & Distress in Laboratory Animals. National Research Council Staff. 1992. 160p. text 29.95 (*0-309-04275-5*) Natl Acad Pr.

Recognition & Interpretation of ECG Rhythms. Ginger Ochs et al. 3rd rev. ed. 1997. LC 96-29695. 375p. (C). pap. 52.00 (*0-8385-4323-5*, A4323-0) P-H.

Recognition & Management of Nursing Home Infections. 1992. (Illus.). 89p. pap. 6.00 (*0-9614520-1-3*) NFID.

Recognition & Management of Pesticide Poisonings. Donald P. Morgan. 4th ed. 1996. (Illus.). 207p. (C). pap. text 30.00 (*0-7881-3176-1*) DIANE Pub.

Recognition, Identification & Prevention of Acute Viral Infections. Donald H. McLean. 1991. 389p. pap. 42.50 (*0-87527-480-3*) Green.

Recognition of Child Abuse for the Mandated Reporter. Ed. by James A. Monteleone. 2nd rev. ed. 1996. LC 96-32412. (Illus.). 300p. (Orig.). (C). pap. 42.95 (*1-878060-24-4*, 30961) GW Medical.

Recognition of M. Leprae Antigens. Tom Ottenhoff & Rene De Vries. 1987. (Developments in Hematology & Immunology Ser.). (C). text 122.00 (*0-89838-887-2*) Kluwer Academic.

Recognize & Manage Your Allergies. Doris J. Rapp. 1987. (Self-Care Health Library). 32p. (Orig.). pap. 2.50 (*0-87983-396-3*, 33963K, Keats Pubng) McGraw-Hill Trade.

Recognizing Alcoholism & Its Effects: A Mini-Guide. H. R. St. Clair. 1991. x, 106p. pap. 21.75 (*3-8055-5395-1*) S Karger.

Recognizing & Managing Children with Fetal Alcohol Syndrome - Fetal Alcohol Effects: A Guidebook. Brenda McCreight. 1997. LC 97-9039. pap. 16.95 (*0-87868-607-X*) Child Welfare.

Recognizing & Monitoring Classroom Psychopharmacology. Gregg F. Wright. 1998. 109p. 48.00 incl. audio (*1-58041-027-8*, 0112142) Am Speech Lang Hearing.

Recognizing Brain Dysfunction: A Guide for Mental Health Professionals. Cooper B. Holmes. 1992. 114p. (Orig.). pap. text 15.95 (*0-88422-116-4*) Clinical Psych.

Recognizing Child Abuse: A Guide for the Concerned. Douglas J. Besharov. 1990. LC 89-25638. 270p. pap. 14.95 (*0-02-903082-X*) Free Pr.

Recollections of a Medical Doctor in Jerusalem: From the Notebooks of Professor Julius J. Kleeberg, 1930-1988. P. Gillon. 1992. (Illus.). vi, 174p. 61.00 (*3-8055-5522-9*) S Karger.

Recollections of My Life. Santiago R. Cajal. Tr. by E. Horne Craigie & Juan Cano from SPA. 1989. LC 89-8087. (Illus.). 664p. reprint ed. pap. 27.95 (*0-262-68060-2*) MIT Pr.

Recollections of Richard Dewey: Pioneer in American Psychiatry. Richard Dewey. Ed. by Ethel L. Dewey. 1973. LC 73-2395. (Mental Illness & Social Policy; the American Experience Ser.). reprint ed. 23.95 (*0-405-05203-0*) Ayer.

Recollections of Sexual Abuse: Treatment Principles & Guidelines. Christine A. Courtois. 1999. LC 98-42100. 448p. text 45.00 (*0-393-70281-2*) Norton.

Recombinant Bovine Growth Hormone: FDA Approval Should Be Withheld until the Mastitis Issue Is Resolved. 1993. 64p. (Orig.). (C). pap. text 20.00 (*1-56806-394-6*) DIANE Pub.

Recombinant DNA. Ed. by Sidney P. Colowick & Nathan O. Kaplan. 1983. LC 79-26584. (Methods in Enzymology Ser.: Vol. 101). Pt. C. text 188.00 (*0-12-182001-7*); Pt. B. text 188.00 (*0-12-182000-9*) Acad Pr.

Recombinant DNA Products: Insulin, Interferon & Growth Hormone. Arthur P. Bollon. 1985. 208p. 118.00 (*0-8493-5542-7*, QH442, CRC Reprint) Franklin.

Recombinant DNA Research & Viruses. Ed. by Yechiel Becker. 1984. (Developments in Molecular Virology Ser.). text 161.00 (*0-89838-683-7*) Kluwer Academic.

Recombinant DNA Technologies in Neuroendocrinology. Ed. by Hirro Imura. 1992. LC 92-48664. (Current Topics in Neuroendocrinology Ser.: Vol. 11). (Illus.). 232p. 217.00 (*0-387-55455-6*) Spr-Verlag.

Recombinant DNA Vaccines: Rationale & Strategy. Ed. by Richard E. Issacson. 1992. LC 92-17708. (Illus.). 432p. text 155.00 (*0-8247-8699-8*) Dekker.

Recombinant FSH (Puregon) Preclinical & Clinical Experience. Ed. by H. J. Out & H. J. Bennink. 1996. LC 96-20463. (Studies in Profertility: Vol. 5). 190p. lib. bdg. 71.95 (*1-85070-746-4*, O0242, Parthenon Pbng) CRC Pr.

Recombinant Inteferons: New Aspects in Research & Therapy. Ed. by S. Eckhardt. 1985. (Journal: Vol. 42, Suppl. 1, 1985). iv, 46p. pap. 24.50 (*3-8055-4238-0*) S Karger.

Recombinant Poxviruses. Mathew M. Binns. 1992. 368p. 229.00 (*0-8493-6179-6*, QR412) CRC Pr.

Recombinant Technology in Hemostasis & Thrombosis. Ed. by Leon W. Hoyer & W. N. Drohan. 1991. (Advances in Experimental Medicine & Biology Ser.). (Illus.). 270p. (C). text 102.00 (*0-306-43893-3*, Kluwer Plenum) Kluwer Academic.

Recombinant Vectors in Vaccine Development. Ed. by F. Brown. 1994. (Developments in Biological Standardization Ser.: Vol. 82). (Illus.). viii, 272p. pap. 217.50 (*3-8055-5997-6*) S Karger.

Recombinational Repair of Damage. Andrei Kuzminov. 1996. (Medicine Ser.). pap. 89.95 (*0-412-10671-X*, VNR) Wiley.

Recommendations for Improving Cholesterol Measurement. Ed. by Barry Leonard. 2000. 84p. (C). reprint ed. pap. text 20.00 (*0-7567-0069-8*) DIANE Pub.

Recommendations for Stroke Management: European Stroke Initiative (EUSI) on Behalf of the European Stroke Council (ESC), the European Neurological Society (ENS), the European Federation of Neurological Societies (EFNS) S. Karger Staff. 2000. (Cerebrovascular Diseases Ser.: Vol. 10). (Illus.). iv, 34p. pap. 25.25 (*3-8055-7123-2*) S Karger.

Recommendations for the Practice of Clinical Neurophysiology: Guidelines of the International Federation of Clinical Neurophysiology. Ed. by Geunther Deuschl & Andrew Eisen. 2nd rev. ed. 1999. LC 99-37656. 320p. 92.50 (*0-444-50295-5*) Elsevier.

Recommendations of the International Commission on Radiological Protection, 1990. ICRP Staff. 1991. (International Commission on Radiological Protection Ser.: No. 60). (Illus.). 215p. pap. 152.00 (*0-08-041144-4*, Pergamon Pr) Elsevier.

Recommendations Regarding the Use of Advanced Telecommunications Technologies to Improve Rural Health Education & Health Care Delivery in Minnesota. 1995. (Illus.). 141p. (Orig.). (C). pap. text 30.00 (*0-7881-1962-1*) DIANE Pub.

Recommended Dietary Allowances: Tenth Edition. Institute of Medicine Staff & National Research Council, Subcommittee on Metabolism Staff. 10th ed. 1992. 302p. pap. 19.95 (*0-309-04633-5*) Natl Acad Pr.

Recommended Dietary Allowances: Tenth Edition. Institute of Medicine Staff et al. 10th ed. 1989. 302p. 24.95 (*0-309-04041-8*) Natl Acad Pr.

Recommended Health-Based Limits in Occupational Exposure to Selected Mineral Dusts (Silica, Coal) 1986. (Technical Reports: No. 734). 82p. pap. text 12.00 (*92-4-120734-5*, 1100734) World Health.

Recommended Health-Based Limits in Occupational Exposure to Selected Organic Solvents. 1981. (Technical Report Ser.: No. 664). 84p. pap. text 6.00 (*92-4-120664-0*) World Health.

Recommended Health-Based Occupational Exposure Limits for Selected Vegetable Dusts. 1983. (Technical Report Ser.: No. 684). 78p. pap. text 6.00 (*92-4-120684-5*) World Health.

Recommended Infection-Control Practices for Dentistry. Ed. by Barbara F. Gooch. 1998. (Illus.). 82p. (C). pap. text 25.00 (*0-7881-4011-6*) DIANE Pub.

Recommended Nomenclature for Physical Quantities in Medical Application of Light. M. Patterson et al. 1996. (Report Ser.: No. 57). 10p. (Orig.). (*1-888340-02-9*) AAPM.

Recommended Procedures for Disease & Serological Surveillance, As Part of the Global Rinderpest Eradication Programme. 1995. (Illus.). 51p. (Orig.). (C). pap. text 25.00 (*0-7881-1950-8*) DIANE Pub.

Recommended Ultrasound Terminology. 2nd ed. 1997. (Illus.). 119p. pap. 40.00 (*1-930047-15-0*, RT) Am Inst Ultrasound.

Reconciling Empirical Knowledge & Clinical Experience: The Art & Science of Psychotherapy. Ed. by Stephen Soldz & Leigh McCullough. 1999. LC 99-16810. 286p. text 39.95 (*1-55798-603-7*, 431-734A) Am Psychol.

Reconnecting. Susan D. Allen & Colleen A. Holloran. 1991. (Illus.). 32p. pap. text 2.75 (*0-916999-11-4*) HERC Pubng.

Reconsideration of Health Behavior Change Models, Vol. 4. Ed. by Gary L. Albrecht. 1994. (Advances in Medical Sociology Ser.). 280p. 78.50 (*1-55938-758-0*) Jai Pr.

Reconstructed Human Skin, 1990: Journal: Skin Pharmacology, Vol. 3, No. 2. Ed. by R. Schmidt. 1990. (Illus.). 88p. pap. 41.75 (*3-8055-5283-1*) S Karger.

Reconstructing Illness: Studies in Pathography. Anne Hunsaker Hawkins. 1993. LC 92-49892. 200p. (C). 30.95 (*1-55753-030-0*); pap. 18.95 (*1-55753-038-6*) Purdue U Pr.

Reconstructing Illness: Studies in Pathography. Anne Hunsaker Hawkins. 2nd ed. 1998. LC 98-30170. 289p. pap. 18.95 (*1-55753-126-9*) Purdue U Pr.

Reconstructing Nursing: Beyond. Diane Marks-Maran. 1996. pap. text 28.00 (*0-7020-2000-1*) Saunders.

Reconstructing the Body. David Williams. 2000. 1098p. Vol. 1 & 2. pap. (*0-85323-675-5*); Vol. I & 2. (*0-85323-665-8*) Liverpool Univ Pr GBR. *Dist:* Intl Spec Bk.

Reconstructing the Mind: Replicability in Research on Human Development. Ed. by Rene Van der Veer et al. 1994. 296p. (C). 85.00 (*0-89391-871-7*, Ablex) Greenwood.

Reconstruction in Psychoanalysis: Childhood Revisited & Recreated. Harold P. Blum. 1994. LC 93-38933. 206p. 32.00 (*0-8236-5783-3*) Intl Univs Pr.

Reconstruction of Cell Evolution: A Periodic System. Werner Schwemmler. 1984. LC 83-26280. 256p. 148.00 (*0-8493-5532-X*, QH371, CRC Reprint) Franklin.

Reconstruction of Life from the Skeleton. Ed. by M. Yasar Iscan & Kenneth A. Kennedy. 1989. 332p. 125.00 (*0-471-56229-7*) Wiley.

Reconstruction of Nasal Tissue Deficits. Joseph Leach. 1998. LC 98-4650. (Self-Instructional Package Ser.). (Illus.). 88p. pap. text 25.00 (*1-56772-061-7*, 5506325) AAO-HNS.

Reconstruction of the Child's Hand. Peter R. Carter. 1990. LC 90-6068. (Illus.). 321p. text 89.00 (*0 8121 1350 0*) Lppncott W & W.

Reconstruction of the Knee Joint, Vol. XII. Ed. by S. Niwa et al. 1997. (Illus.). 432p. 218.00 (*4-431-70170-2*) Spr-Verlag.

***Reconstruction of the Nose.** Shan R. Baker. 2001. LC 2001-44975. (Illus.). 395p. (*0-323-01147-0*) Mosby Inc.

Reconstruction of the Oral Cavity. Jonas T. Johnson et al. 2nd rev. ed. 1994. LC 94-31837. (Self-Instructional Package Ser.). (Illus.). 75p. pap. text 25.00 (*1-56772-014-5*) AAO-HNS.

Reconstruction Surgery & Traumatology, Vol. 12. Ed. by G. Chapchal. 1971. 85.25 (*3-8055-1183-3*) S Karger.

Reconstruction Surgery & Traumatology, Vol. 14. G. Chapchal. 1974. (Illus.). 200p. 85.25 (*3-8055-1563-4*) S Karger.

Reconstruction Surgery & Traumatology. Ed. by G. Chapchal. Vol. 15. 1976. 42.75 (*3-8055-2250-9*); Vol. 16. 1977. (Illus.). 50.50 (*3-8055-2696-2*) S Karger.

Reconstruction Surgery & Traumatology Vol. 13: Operative Treatment of Cerebral Palsy. Ed. by G. Chapchal. 1972. (Illus.). 85.25 (*3-8055-1385-2*) S Karger.

Reconstructive & Cosmetic Surgery Sourcebook: Basic Consumer Health Information on Cosmetic & Reconstructive Plastic Surgery. Ed. by M. Lisa Weatherford. 2001. LC 00-66880. (Health Reference Ser.). (Illus.). xii, 374p. lib. bdg. 48.00 (*0-7808-0214-4*) Omnigraphics Inc.

Reconstructive & Esthetic Mammoplasty. Guthrie & Schwartz. 1989. 848p. text 177.00 (*0-7216-2806-0*) Saunders.

Reconstructive & Plastic Surgery of the External Genitalia: Adult & Pediatric. Richard M. Ehrlich & Gary J. Alter. Ed. by Richard Zorab. 1998. LC 96-27738. (Illus.). 480p. (C). text 225.00 (*0-7216-6328-1*) Saunders.

Reconstructive Flaps in the Head & Neck. Hayden. 1999. (Illus.). 350p. (C). (gr. 13). text 195.00 (*0-8151-4453-9*, 29485) Mosby Inc.

Reconstructive Knee Surgery. Ed. by Douglas W. Jackson. 1994. LC 94-2265. (Master Techniques in Orthopaedic Surgery Ser.). (Illus.). 336p. text 199.00 (*0-7817-0031-0*) Lppncott W & W.

Reconstructive Microsurgery. Bernard M. O'Brien & Wayne A. Morrison. 1987. (Illus.). 540p. text (*0-443-02557-6*) Church.

Reconstructive Plastic Surgery: Principles & Procedures in Correction Reconstruction & Transplantation Ed. by John M. Converse. 2nd ed. 1977. LC 74-21010. (Illus.). 1. text 140.00 (*0-7216-2680-7*); 2. text 140.00 (*0-7216-2681-5*); 3. text 140.00 (*0-7216-2682-3*); 4. text 140.00 (*0-7216-2683-1*); 5. text 140.00 (*0-7216-2684-X*); 6. text 140.00 (*0-7216-2685-8*); 7. text 140.00 (*0-7216-2686-6*); Set. text 900.00 (*0-7216-2691-2*) Saunders.

Reconstructive Preprosthetic Oral & Maxillofacial Surgery Raymond J. Fonseca & W. Howard Davis. 2nd ed. 1995. LC 94-31809. (Illus.). 1040p. text 280.00 (*0-7216-3307-2*) Saunders.

Reconstructive Surgery: Principles, Anatomy & Technique Stephen J. Mathes & Foad Nahai. 1997. LC 96-29462. text (*0-443-07981-1*) Church.

Reconstructive Surgery: Principles, Anatomy & Technique, Set. Stephen J. Mathes & Foad Nahai. 1996. LC 96-29462. (Illus.). 1625p. 499.00 (*0-942219-02-3*) Quality Med Pub.

***Reconstructive Surgery of the Esophagus.** Mark K. Ferguson. 2001. LC 2001-40911. (Illus.). (*0-87993-494-8*) Futura Pub.

Reconstructive Surgery of the Joints, Set. Ed. by Bernard F. Morrey. 2nd rev. ed. 1995. LC 95-44399. Orig. Title: Joint Replacement Arthroplasty. 1876p. text (*0-443-08982-5*) Church.

Reconstructive Surgery of the Long Bones with Autogenous & Homogenous Grafts. O. Verbeek et al. 1973. text 135.00 (*90-207-0343-9*) Kluwer Academic.

Reconstructive Surgery of the Middle Ear. J. I. Suzuki et al. 1999. 200p. 135.00 (*0-444-50207-6*) Elsevier.

***Reconstructive Urethral Surgery.** Ed. by F. Schreiter & J. Jordan. 2002. (Illus.). 200p. 119.00 incl. cd-rom (*3-540-41226-3*) Spr-Verlag.

Reconstructive Urology George Webster et al. 1992. (Illus.). 1152p. 350.00 (*0-86542-229-X*) Blackwell Sci.

Record That Serves & Protects. Eric D. Joseph. Ed. by Nancy Webster. 1999. 20p. pap. 4.00 (*0-916499-76-6*) Care Educ Grp.

Recording & Notification of Occupational Accidents & Diseases: An ILO Code of Practice. 1996. LC 97-169647. xxii, 96p. pap. 18.00 (*92-2-109451-0*) Intl Labour Office.

Records of the American Women's Hospitals, 1917-1982: An Inventory. Nancy A. Hewitt. 1987. (Illus.). 55p. (Orig.). (C). 5.00 (*0-944542-01-8*) Med Coll PA ASCWM.

Recovered: Absolute Victory over Alcoholism. Ed. by Amy Crozier et al. 2000. LC 99-75781. (Recovered Ser.: Vol. 1). 272p. pap. 15.95 (*1-893808-00-9*) Ursa Pub Co Inc.

Recovered Memories & False Memories. Ed. by Martin A. Conway. 1997. (Debates in Psychology Ser.). (Illus.). 312p. pap. text 29.95 (*0-19-852386-6*) OUP.

Recovered Memories of Abuse: Assessment, Therapy, Forensics. Kenneth S. Pope & Laura S. Brown. 1996. LC 96-33009. (Psychotherapy Practitioner Resource Bks.). 315p. pap. 24.95 (*1-55798-395-X*) Am Psychol.

Recovered Memories of Abuse: True or False? Ed. by Joseph Sandler & Peter Fonagy. 1997. (Psychoanalytic Monograph Ser.). 272p. pap. (*1-85575-166-6*) Karnac Bks GBR. *Dist:* Other Pr LLC.

Recovered Memories of Child Sexual Abuse: Psychological, Social & Legal Perspectives on a Contemporary Mental Health Controversy. Sheila Taub. 1999. LC 99-37927. (American Series in Behavioral Science & Law: Vol. 1098). (Illus.). 234p. pap. text 33.95 (*0-398-07006-7*) C C Thomas.

Recovered Memories of Child Sexual Abuse: Psychological, Social & Legal Perspectives on a Contemporary Mental Health Controversy. Ed. by Sheila Taub. 1999. LC 99-37927. (Illus.). 234p. text 46.95 (*0-398-07005-9*) C C Thomas.

Recovered Memories of Trauma: Transferring the Present to the Past. C. Brooks Brenneis. 1997. LC 96-39645. 220p. 31.50 (*0-8236-5788-4*, BN05788) Intl Univs Pr.

Recovered Memory & Other Assaults upon the Mysteries of Consciousness: Hypnosis, Psychotherapy, Fraud & the Mass Media. William Rogers. 1995. LC 95-15794. 152p. lib. bdg. 30.00 (*0-7864-0109-5*) McFarland & Co.

Recovering Bodies: Illness, Disability, & Life-Writing. G. Thomas Couser. 1997. LC 97-11952. (Wisconsin Studies in American Autobiography). 334p. pap. 24.95 (*0-299-15564-1*) U of Wis Pr.

Recovering Couples Anonymous: Big Book. 2nd ed. 1992. 122p. pap. 18.00 (*0-9637495-1-X*) Recov Couples.

***Recovering Damages for Psychiatric Injury.** Michael Napier & Kay Wheat. 2001. pap. (*1-84174-133-7*) Blackstone Pr.

Recovering for Psychological Injuries. William A. Barton. Ed. by Christine M. Griffith & Arnett J. Holloway. 2nd ed. 1990. LC 90-30974. 417p. 80.00 (*0-941916-51-0*) West Group.

Recovering from a Heart Attack. Elizabeth S. Weiss. 1980. 12.95 (*0-02-625830-7*) Macmillan.

Recovering from Breast Surgery: Exercises to Strengthen Your Body & Relieve Pain. Diana Stumm. 1995. LC 95-3153. (Illus.). 128p. pap. 11.95 (*0-89793-180-7*) Hunter Hse.

Recovering from Incest: Imagination & the Healing Process. Evangeline Kane. 1989. 232p. (Orig.). pap. 16.95 (*0-938434-42-X*) Sigo Pr.

Recovering Love: Codependency to CoRecovery. J. Richard Cookerly. 1992. 192p. pap. (*0-8306-3837-7*, 4121) McGraw-Hill Educ Grp.

Recovering the Nation's Body: Cultural Memory, Medicine, & the Politics of Redemption. Linda F. Hogle. 1999. LC 98-45601. 256p. (C). pap. 22.00 (*0-8135-2645-0*); text 50.00 (*0-8135-2644-2*) Rutgers U Pr.

Recovery: How to Survive Sexual Assault for Women, Men, Teenagers, Their Friends & Families. Helen Benedict. rev. ed. 1994. LC 94-15856. 46.00 (*0-231-09674-7*); 365p. pap. 18.00 (*0-231-09675-5*) Col U Pr.

Recovery: Loss & Return of Vision. 1991. (Illus.). 16.95 (*0-9628434-0-7*) J Grubb Taylor.

Recovery after Acute Stroke: Symposium to the 8th European Stroke Conference, Venice, April 7-10, 1999. Ed. by J. Bogousslavsky & C. Fieschi. 1999. (Cerebrovascular Diseases Ser.). iv, 32p. (*3-8055-6955-6*) S Karger.

Recovery after Traumatic Brain Injury. Ed. by Barbara P. Uzzell & Henry H. Stonnington. 1996. (Institute for Research in Behavioral Neuroscience Ser.). 336p. 79.95 (*0-8058-1823-5*); pap. 34.50 (*0-8058-1824-3*) L Erlbaum Assocs.

Recovery & Relapse Prevention for Parents of Chemically Dependent Children. Dennis Daley & Judy Miller. 1993. pap. 4.95 (*1-56246-027-7*, P183, HazeldenJohnson Inst) Hazelden.

Recovery Dynamics: Client Guide Book. Joe McQuany. 1989. 104p. pap. text 15.00 (*1-883094-02-X*) Kelly Fnd.

Recovery Dynamics: Counselors Manual. Joe McQuany. 1989. 400p. text 60.00 (*1-883094-01-1*) Kelly Fnd.

Recovery Dynamics: Individual Evaluation Packet. Joe McQuany. 1989. 96p. pap. text 14.00 (*1-883094-03-8*) Kelly Fnd.

Recovery Education: A Guide for Teaching Chemically Dependent People. Merlene Miller. 1992. pap. 4.00 (*0-8309-0565-0*) Herald Pub Hse.

Recovery from Abuse. Dale Ryan & Juanita Ryan. 1990. (Life Recovery Guides Ser.). 64p. pap., wbk. ed. 4.99 (*0-8308-1158-3*, 1158) InterVarsity.

Recovery from Addiction. John Finnegan & Daphne Gray. 1995. LC 90-1941. 264p. (Orig.). text 14.00 (*0-89087-599-5*) Celestial Arts.

Recovery from AIDS by Natural Methods & Restoring the Immune System. 1991. (AIDS Ser.). lib. bdg. 79.95 (*0-8490-4804-4*) Gordon Pr.

Recovery from Alcoholism: Beyond Your Wildest Dreams. Jerome D. Levin. 1991. LC 90-1232. 296p. 50.00 (*0-87668-625-0*) Aronson.

Recovery from Brain Damage: Reflections & Directions. Francis D. Rose & D. A. Johnson. 1993. (Advances in Experimental Medicine & Biology Ser.: Vol. 325). (Illus.). 224p. (C). text 102.00 (*0-306-44344-9*, Kluwer Plenum) Kluwer Academic.

***Recovery from Schizophrenia.** Ornstein. 2001. 552p. pap. 66.00 (*1-887841-39-3*, Psychosocial) Intl Univs Pr.

Recovery from Schizophrenia. Richard Wagner. 2nd rev. ed. 1994. LC 93-38556. 336p. (C). pap. 31.95 (*0-415-09261-2*, B7010) Routledge.

Recovery from Schizophrenia: Psychiatry & Political Economy. Richard Warner. 1988. 416p. pap. text 18.95 (*0-7102-1395-6*, Routledge Thoemms) Routledge.

Recovery in Aphasics. Ed. by Y. Lebrun & R. Hoops. 1976. (Neurolinguistics Ser.: Vol. 4). 270p. (*90-265-0228-1*) Swets.

Recovery of a Cancer Patient: A Personal Diary. Barbara A. Arpante. Ed. by Aaron Melenski. 1992. (Illus.). 54p. (Orig.). pap. text 7.95 (*0-9625313-2-4*) Mntn Pr MA.

Recovery of Function in the Nervous System. Ed. by F. Cohadon & J. Lobo Antunes. 1988. (FIDIA Research Ser.: Vol. 13). 191p. 90.00 (*0-387-96785-0*) Spr-Verlag.

Recovery of Unconscious Memories: Hypermnesia & Reminiscence. Matthew H. Erdelyi. (John D. & Catherine T. MacArthur Foundation Series on Mental Health & Development). (Illus.). 264p. 1998. pap. text 17.00 (*0-226-21661-6*); 1996. LC 96-914. 28.95 (*0-226-21660-8*) U Ch Pr.

Recovery of Your Inner Child. Lucia Capacchione. 1991. (Illus.). 288p. (Orig.). pap. 15.00 (*0-671-70135-5*, Fireside) S&S Trade Pap.

Recovery Room! A Nurse's Guide to Care of the Patient, Post Anesthesia. Jimmie R. Rankin. 1994. 150p. pap. 24.95 (*1-883938-15-5*) Dry Bones Pr.

Recovery Workbook: Practical Coping & EM Powerment Strategies for People with Psychiatric Disability. LeRoy Spaniol et al. 1994. 120p. pap. text 29.95 (*1-878512-01-3*) Boston Univ Ctr Psy Rehab.

***Recrafting Life: Coping with Chronic Illness & Pain.** Johnson. 2001. 300p. text 39.95 (*0-87630-969-4*) Brunner-Routledge.

Recreating Brief Therapy: Preferences & Possibilities. John Walter. 2000. LC 00-20986. (Professional Book Ser.). (Illus.). xiii, 191p. 32.00 (*0-393-70325-8*) Norton.

Recreating Partnership. Phillip Ziegler. 2001. LC 2001-30352. (Professional Book Ser.). 384p. 32.00 (*0-393-70349-5*) Norton.

Recreation Experiences for the Severely Impaired or Nonambulatory Child. Susan P. Levine et al. 1983. (Illus.). 96p. spiral bd. 21.95 (*0-398-04783-9*) C C Thomas.

Recreation for the Disabled Child. Ed. by Donna B. Bernhardt. 1985. LC 84-19330. (Physical & Occupational Therapy in Pediatrics Ser.: Vol. 4, No. 3). 110p. text 39.95 (*0-86656-263-X*) Haworth Pr.

Recreation, Leisure, & Chronic Illness: Therapeutic Rehabilitation As Intervention in Health Care. Miriam P. Lahey et al. 1993. LC 93-16983. (Loss, Grief & Care Ser.: Vol. 6, No. 4). (Illus.). 162p. lib. bdg. 39.95 (*1-56024-418-6*) Haworth Pr.

P
Q
R

Rectal Bleeding & Colon Polyps. John M. MacKeigan & Kathleen M. Hillary. Ed. by Oliver D. Grin & Dorothy L. Bouwman. 1990. (Patient Education Ser.). (Illus.). 26p. pap. text 4.00 (*0-929689-43-7*) Ludann Co.

Rectal Cancer: Surgical Management, Basic & Clinical Research. Ed. by P. M. Schlag. 1998. LC 97-38313. (Recent Results in Cancer Research Ser.: Vol. 146). (Illus.). 200p. 125.00 (*3-540-63544-0*) Spr-Verlag.

Rectal Cancer Surgery: Optimisation, Standardisation & Documentation. Ed. by O. Soreide & J. Norstein. 1996. LC 96-38509. (Illus.). 472p. 139.00 (*3-540-61566-0*) Spr-Verlag.

Recueil des Cours, 1983, Vol. 183. Academic de Droit International de la Haye Staff. 1985. lib. bdg. 129.00 (*90-247-3248-4*) Kluwer Academic.

Recurrent Education, Earnings & Well-Being: A Fifty-Year Longitudinal Study of a Cohort of Swedish Men. Albert Tuijnman. 1989. (Stockholm Studies in Education & Psychology: No. 24). 284p. (Orig.). pap. (*91-22-01317-2*) Umea U Bibl SWE. *Dist:* Coronet Bks.

Recurrent Mood Disorders: New Perspectives in Therapy. Ed. by G. F. Placidi et al. 1993. LC 92-48355. 178.00 (*3-540-54046-6*); (Illus.). 321p. 143.00 (*0-387-54046-6*) Spr-Verlag.

Recurrent Spontaneous Abortion. Salim Daya. 1999. 179.95 (*0-8493-5852-3*) CRC Pr.

Red Blood Cell Aging. Ed. by M. Magnani & A. De Flora. 1991. (Advances in Experimental Medicine & Biology Ser.). (Illus.). 400p. (C). text 156.00 (*0-306-44021-0*, Kluwer Plenum) Kluwer Academic.

Red Blood Cell Membranes: Structure, Function, Clinical Implications. Peter Agre & John C. Parker. 1989. (Hematology Ser.: Vol. 11). (Illus.). 760p. text 250.00 (*0-8247-8022-1*) Dekker.

Red Blood Cells As Carriers for Drugs. Ed. by DeLoach et al. 1985. (Current Studies in Hematology & Blood Transfusion: No. 51). (Illus.). viii, 162p. 90.50 (*3-8055-3940-1*) S Karger.

Red Blood Cells As Carriers for Drugs: Potential Therapeutic Applications. Ed. by C. Ropars et al. 1987. (Illus.). 272p. 100.50 (*0-08-036137-4*, Pergamon Pr) Elsevier.

Red Book of Ophthalmology, 1992. 1992. 320p. pap. text 95.00 (*0-7506-9296-0*) Buttrwrth-Heinemann.

Red Book 2000. Ed. by Medical Economics Staff. 104th rev. ed. 2000. (Red Book: Pharmacy's Fundamental Reference Ser.). (Illus.). 800p. pap. 62.00 (*1-56363-357-4*, PDR) Med Econ.

Red Book, 2001, Vol. 105. Medical Economics Staff. 105th rev. ed. 2001. (Red Book: Pharmacy's Fundamental Reference Ser.). (Illus.). 800p. pap. 65.00 (*1-56363-392-2*, PDR) Med Econ.

***Red Book 2002.** Medical Economics Co. Staff. 106th rev. ed. 2002. (Illus.). 800p. pap. text 69.95 (*1-56363-418-X*) Med Econ.

Red Book Update, 2001, Vol. 105. Medical Economics Staff. 105th rev. ed. 50p. 99.00 (*1-56363-393-0*, PDR) Med Econ.

Red Book Updates, 2000. Medical Economics Staff. 104th rev. ed. 1999. (Illus.). 50p. pap. 99.00 (*1-56363-358-2*, PDR) Med Econ.

Red Cell: Production, Metabolism, Destruction, Normal & Abnormal. John W. Harris & Robert Kellermeyer. rev. ed. 1970. (Commonwealth Fund Publications). 815p. pap. 29.50 (*0-674-75102-7*) HUP.

Red Cell Deformability & Filterability. Ed. by John A. Dormandy. 1983. (Developments in Hematology & Immunology Ser.). text 141.50 (*0-89838-578-4*) Kluwer Academic.

Red Cell Manual. Robert S. Hillman. 7th ed. 1996. LC 96-7350. (Illus.). 190p. (C). pap. text 26.95 (*0-8036-0145-X*) Davis Co.

Red Cell Membrane: A Model for Solute Transport. Ed. by Beat U. Raess & G. Tunnicliff. 1990. LC 89-15438. (Contemporary Biomedicine Ser.: Vol. 10). (Illus.). 495p. 139.50 (*0-89603-158-6*) Humana.

Red Cell Shape: Physiology, Pathology, Ultrastructure. Ed. by M. Bessis et al. 1973. LC 73-77351. (Illus.). 180p. 50.00 (*0-387-06257-2*) Spr-Verlag.

Red Cell Transfusion: A Practical Guide. Ed. by Marion E. Reid & Sandra J. Nance. 1997. LC 97-39691. (Contemporary Hematology Ser.). (Illus.). 240p. 120.00 (*0-89603-412-7*) Humana.

Red Devil: A Memoir about Beating the Odds. Katherine Russell Rich. 2000. LC 00-61564. 256p. pap. 12.95 (*0-609-80324-7*, Three Riv Pr) Harmony Bks.

Red Face & Other Facial Rashes. Marks. 1998. (Illus.). 160p. (C). pap. 149.95 (*0-412-63520-8*, Chap & Hall NY) Chapman & Hall.

Red Manual for the Surgery Boars. Hratch L. Karamanoukian. 1998. 460p. spiral bd. 49.00 (*0-9663292-1-X*) Magalhaes Sci Pr.

Red Miracle. Edward Podolsky. 1977. LC 70-167402. (Essay Index Reprint Ser.). 26.95 (*0-8369-2818-0*) Ayer.

Red Moon Passage: The Power & Wisdom of Menopause. Ed. by Bonnie J. Horrigan. 2000. 242p. reprint ed. text 24.00 (*0-7881-6906-8*) DIANE Pub.

Red Vienna & the Golden Age of Psychology, 1918-1938. Sheldon Gardner & Gwendolyn Stevens. 1992. LC 91-36401. 304p. 68.50 (*0-275-94013-6*, C4013, Praeger Pubs) Greenwood.

Redecision Therapy: A Brief, Action-Oriented Approach. Ed. by Carolyn E. Lennox. 1997. LC 96-41624. 336p. 40.00 (*0-7657-0043-3*) Aronson.

Redeeming Marketplace Medicine: A Theology of Health Care. Abigail Rian Evans. 1999. LC 98-50597. 208p. pap. 16.95 (*0-8298-1310-1*) Pilgrim OH.

Redefining AIDS: The Dead & the Disposessed Neal A. Dickerson. 1993. LC 93-2599. (Politics of AIDS Ser.: Vol. 4). (Illus.). xii, 159p. pap. 12.00 (*0-930383-36-2*) Monument Pr.

Redesigning Health Care Delivery. Peter Boland. 1996. (Illus.). 926p. 79.00 (*0-9652717-1-4*, 71714) Boland Hlthcare.

Redesigning Life? The Worldwide Challenge to Genetic Engineering. Brian Tokar. 2001. LC 00-43431. 440p. (*1-85649-834-4*) Zed Books.

Redesigning Life? The Worldwide Challenge to Genetic Engineering. Brian Tokar. 2001. LC 00-43431. 440p. pap. (*1-85649-835-2*) Zed Books GBR. *Dist:* St Martin.

Redesigning School Health Services. Annette Lynch. 1983. LC 82-12178. (Illus.). 351p. 45.95 (*0-89885-102-5*, Kluwer Acad Hman Sci) Kluwer Academic.

Redgrave, Fife & Machin: Health & Safety. John Hendy & Michael Ford. 2nd ed. 1997. pap., suppl. ed. (*0-406-99990-2*, RFMH2S3, MICHIE) LEXIS Pub.

Redgrave, Fife & Machin's: Health & Safety in Factories. Ian Fife & E. Anthony Machin. 2nd ed. 1982. reprint ed. 170.00 (*0-406-14601-2*, MICHIE) LEXIS Pub.

Redirecting Boards: A New Vision of Governance for Planned Parenthood. R. James LeFevre. 1993. LC 92-46519. 134p. 11.95 (*0-934586-73-X*) Plan Parent.

Rediscovering Midwifery. Ed. by Lesley Ann Page & Pat Percival. 1998. LC 99-48228. 418p. (C). pap. text (*0-443-05572-6*) Church.

Rediscovering Nursing: An Up-Date for the Returning Nurse. Martin Johnson et al. 1990. 172p. pap. 24.95 (*0-412-35440-3*, A5044) Chapman & Hall.

Rediscovering Real Medicine: The New Horizons of Homeopathy. Jean Elmigar. 1998. LC 97-46813. 256p. pap. 16.95 (*1-86204-199-7*) Element MA.

Reduced Dose Mammography. Wende W. Logan & E. Phillip Muntz. 1979. LC 79-63202. (Illus.). 576p. (gr. 13). 62.00 (*0-89352-060-8*) Mosby Inc.

Reducing Benzodiazepine Consumption. M. A. Cormack et al. 1989. (Recent Research in Psychology Ser.). 96p. 59.95 (*0-387-97035-5*) Spr-Verlag.

Reducing Breast Cancer in Women. Ed. by Basil A. Stoll. 1995. LC 94-29394. 248p. lib. bdg. 100.00 (*0-7923-3064-1*) Kluwer Academic.

Reducing Cesarean Section Rates While Maintaining Maternal & Infant Outcomes. Bruce L. Flamm & Institute for Healthcare Improvement Staff. 1997. LC 97-71063. (Breakthrough Guide Ser.). xvii, 179p. (*1-890070-01-7*) Inst for Hlthcare.

Reducing Drug Abuse in America. 1997. 52p. pap. 6.00 (*0-16-061876-2*) USGPO.

Reducing Drug Abuse in America. Ed. by Barry R. McCaffrey. 1998. (Illus.). 52p. (C). pap. text 20.00 (*0-7881-7463-0*) DIANE Pub.

Reducing Hazardous Waste Generation: An Evaluation & a Call for Action. National Research Council Staff. 1985. 76p. pap. text 9.95 (*0-309-03498-1*) Natl Acad Pr.

Reducing Litigation: Using Disability Guidelines & State Evaluators in Oregon. Leslie I. Boden et al. 1991. LC 91-33586. 35.00 (*0-935149-29-5*, WC-91-3) Workers Comp Res Inst.

Reducing Spouse/Partner Abuse: A Psychoeducational Approach for Individuals & Couples Robert Geffner. Ed. by Carol Mantooth. 1999. pap., wbk. ed. 75.00 (*0-8261-1274-9*); (SPA.). pap., wbk. ed. 75.00 (*0-8261-1275-7*) Springer Pub.

Reducing Spouse/Partner Abuse: A Psychoeducational Approach for Individuals & Couples, Incl. Manual. Ed. by Robert Geffner & Carol Mantooth. 1999. (Illus.). pap., wbk. ed. 38.95 (*0-8261-1269-2*) Springer Pub.

Reducing Stigma Through Education: Post Traumatic Stress Disorder. Dushka Crane-Ross. Ed. by Terence M. Keane. 1998. 175.00 (*1-889022-06-3*) Mental Hlth KY.

Reducing Stress Fracture in Physically Active Military Women. Institute of Medicine Staff. 1998. 132p. pap. text 29.00 (*0-309-06091-5*) Natl Acad Pr.

Reducing Stress in Young Children's Lives. Ed. by Janet B. McCracken. 1986. LC 86-62564. (Illus.). 170p. pap. 7.00 (*0-935989-03-X*, NAEYC 216) Natl Assn Child Ed.

Reducing the Health Consequences of Smoking: 25 Years of Progress: A Report of the Surgeon General. 1995. (Illus.). 703p. (Orig.). (C). pap. text 50.00 (*0-7881-2313-0*) DIANE Pub.

Reducing the Odds: Preventing Perinatal Transmission of HIV. Michael A. Stoto. 1999. LC 98-40214. 416p. 39.95 (*0-309-06286-1*) Natl Acad Pr.

Reducing the Risk: Building Skills to Prevent Pregnancy, STD & HIV. Richard P. Barth. 2nd ed. 1993. LC 92-39092. 34.95 (*1-56071-147-7*) ETR Assocs.

Reducing the Risks for Substance Abuse: A Lifespan Approach. Raymond P. Daugherty & Carl Leukefeld. 1998. LC 98-29801. (Prevention in Practice Library). (Illus.). 192p. (C). pap. 22.50 (*0-306-45899-3*, Kluwer Plenum) Kluwer Academic.

Reducing the Storm to a Whisper: The Story of a Breakdown. Patrick J. Howell. 2000. LC 99-69850. 228p. pap. 14.95 (*0-9645727-7-X*, Ulyssian Pubns) Pine Orchard.

Reduction Mammaplasty. Robert M. Goldwyn. 1989. 220.00 (*0-316-31977-5*, Little Brwn Med Div) Lppncott W & W.

Reduction of Anticancer Drug Toxicity: Pharmacologic, Biologic, Immunologic & Molecular Genetic Approaches. Gerhard Eisenbrand. Ed. by K. Hellmmann et al. 1995. (Beitraege Zur Onkologie, Contributions to Oncology Ser.: Vol. 48). (Illus.). viii, 210p. 174.00 (*3-8055-6042-7*) S Karger.

Redux Revolution: Everything You Need to Know about the Most Important Weight Loss Discovery of the Century. Sheldon Levine. 1996. LC 96-26000. 192p. 20.00 (*0-688-15153-1*, Wm Morrow) Morrow Avon.

Redy-Refs for Critical Care Nurses. Deborah Borelli. 1996. (Illus.). 50p. text 12.95 (*0-943202-57-4*) H & H Pub.

Redy-Refs for Medical - Surgical Nurses. Deborah Borelli. 1996. (Illus.). 40p. text 12.95 (*0-943202-56-6*) H & H Pub.

Reeder & Felson's Gamuts in Bone, Joint, & Spine Radiology: Comprehensive Lists of Roentgen Differential Diagnosis. Maurice M. Reeder. 1993. 501p. 39.95 (*0-387-94016-2*) Spr-Verlag.

Reeder & Felson's Gamuts in Cardiovascular Radiology: Comprehensive Lists of Radiographic & Angiographic Differential Diagnosis. Maurice M. Reeder. 1994. LC 93-46633. 141p. 36.95 (*0-387-94219-X*) Spr-Verlag.

Reeder & Felson's Gamuts in Neuroradiology: Comprehensive Lists of Roentgen & MRI Differential Diagnosis. Maurice M. Reeder & William G. Bradley, Jr. 1993. LC 93-10195. 357p. 41.95 (*0-387-94034-0*) Spr-Verlag.

Reeder & Felson's Gamuts in Radiology: Comprehensive Lists of Roentgen Differential Diagnosis. Maurice M. Reeder & William G. Bradley. 1997. 24p. pap. 210.00 incl. audio compact disk (*0-387-14228-2*) Spr-Verlag.

Reeder & Felson's Gamuts in Radiology: Comprehensive Lists of Roentgen Differential Diagnosis. Maurice M. Reeder & William G. Bradley, Jr. 3rd ed. LC 92-49707. 1993. 706p. 121.00 (*0-387-97891-7*); 1992. 640p. (*3-540-97891-7*) Spr-Verlag.

Reenchanted Science: Holism in German Culture from Wilhelm II to Hitler. Anne Harrington. 1996. LC 95-48463. (Illus.). 368p. 55.00 (*0-691-02142-2*) Princeton U Pr.

Reengineering Health Care: Building on CQI. John R. Griffith et al. 1995. LC 94-42697. 300p. 50.00 (*1-56793-022-0*, 0952) Health Admin Pr.

Reengineering Healthcare Liability Litigation. Miles J. Zaremski & Frank D. Heckman. 1997. 110.00 (*1-55834-547-7*, 61235) LEXIS Pub.

Reengineering Healthcare Liability Litigation: 1998 Supplement. Miles J. Zaremski & Frank D. Heckman. 1998. LC 97-73330. 132p. suppl. ed. 40.00 (*0-327-00213-1*, 61236-10) LEXIS Pub.

Reengineering Nursing & Health Care Delivery: The Handbook for Organizational Transformation. Suzanne S. Blancett & Dominick L. Flarey. 1995. 416p. 87.00 (*0-8342-0660-9*, 20660) Aspen Pub.

Reengineering of Operative & Invasive Services: Preparing for the Capitated Dollar. Mae Taylor Moss. 1996. LC 96-2940. 240p. 105.00 (*0-8342-0850-4*, 20850) Aspen Pub.

Reengineering Verbal Orders: New Team-Based Strategies. Jennifer I. Coper et al. 1999. LC 00-698735. (Illus.). x, 83p. pap. text 87.00 (*1-57839-074-5*) Opus Communs.

Reexamining Family Stress: New Theory & Research. Wesley R. Burr & Shirley Klein. (Library of Social Research: Vol. 193). (Illus.). 224p. (C). 1994. 86.95 (*0-8039-4929-4*, 4281); 1993. pap. 37.95 (*0-8039-4930-8*, 4282) Sage.

Reference & Information Services in Health Sciences Librarianship. Ed. by Sandra Wood & Alison Bunting. 1994. LC 94-5665. (Current Practice in Health Sciences Librarianship Ser.: Vol. 1). 394p. 41.50 (*0-8108-2765-4*) Scarecrow.

Reference & Selected Procedures for the Quantitative Determination of Hemoglobin in Blood: Approved Standard (1994) Contrib. by A. Richardson Jones. 1994. 75.00 (*1-56238-237-3*, H15-A2) NCCLS.

Reference Companion to the History of Abnormal Psychology John G. Howells & M. Livia Osborn. 1984. LC 80-27163. 1141p. lib. bdg. 250.00 (*0-313-22183-9*, HOL/);Vol. 1. xviii, 1141p. lib. bdg. 150.00 (*0-313-24261-5*, HOL/01);Vol. 2. xviii, 1141p. lib. bdg. 150.00 (*0-313-24262-3*, HOL/02) Greenwood.

Reference Guide to First Aid Procedures. Tel-A-Train, Inc. Staff. 1988. stu. ed. 3.50 (*1-56355-231-0*) Tel-A-Train.

Reference Guide to Medicinal Plants. John K. Crellin & Jane Philpott. 1997. LC 97-17089. (Illus.). 560p. (Orig.). pap. 22.95 (*0-8223-1019-8*) Duke.

Reference Guide to Medicinal Plants: Herbal Medicine Past & Present. J. K. Crellin & Jane Philpott. 1997. LC 97-17089. pap. (*0-8223-2068-1*) Duke.

Reference Manual for Communicative Sciences & Disorders: Speech & Language. Raymond D. Kent. 1994. 393p. (C). pap. text 54.00 (*0-89079-419-7*, 1578) PRO-ED.

Reference Manual for Growth & Development. John M. Buckler. 2nd ed. 1997. LC 96-30415. (Illus.). 128p. pap. 49.95 (*0-86542-680-5*) Blackwell Sci.

Reference Manual for Writing Rehabilitation Therapy Treatment Plans. Penny Hogberg & Mary Johnson. 1994. LC 94-61216. 112p. pap. 16.95 (*0-910251-67-3*) Venture Pub PA.

Reference Materials of the European Communities: Results of Hemocompatibility Tests. Ed. by W. Lemm. 1992. LC 92-30458. 272p. (C). text 148.50 (*0-7923-2002-6*) Kluwer Academic.

Reference Method for Broth Dilution Antifungal Susceptibility Testing of Yeasts: Tentative Guideline (1992) Contrib. by John N. Galgiani. 1995. 100.00 (*1-56238-186-5*, M27-T) NCCLS.

Reference 2000: Health Care Info Source. Jerry Gill. 3rd rev. ed. 1998. 350p. 19.95 (*1-889823-03-1*) GLB Worldwide.

Reference Values in Human Chemistry: Proceedings of the 2nd Symposium of the Internal Colloquium on Automatisation & Prospective Biology Pont-a-Mousson, Oct, 1972. International Colloquium, Automatisation and Prospec. Ed. by G. Siest. 1973. 112.25 (*3-8055-1622-3*) S Karger.

References en Biologie Clinique. G. Henry Siest & F. Schiele. 1991. 680p. pap. 102.00 (*2-906077-16-X*) Elsevier.

Refiguring Self & Psychology. Kenneth J. Gergen. 1993. (Benchmark Ser.). 288p. (*1-85521-369-9*) Dartmth Pub GBR. *Dist:* Ashgate Pub Co.

Refined by Fire: The Evolution of Straight Chiropractic. Joseph B. Strauss. 1994. (Illus.). 315p. text 30.00 (*1-890419-06-0*) Fnd Chiropractic Educ.

Refinements in Facial & Body Contouring. Luiz S. Toledo. 1998. LC 98-17731. 384p. text 225.00 (*0-397-51600-2*) Lppncott W & W.

Reflecting on the Past, Envisioning the Future. 1994. (Conference Proceedings Ser.). 172p. 20.00 (*1-882147-24-3*) Am Art Therapy.

Reflecting Team in Action: Collaborative Practice in Family Therapy. Ed. by Steven Friedman. 1995. LC 95-14307. (Guilford Family Therapy Ser.). 366p. text 40.00 (*1-57230-003-5*, 0003) Guilford Pubns.

Reflection, Recollection & Change: The Nevada State Board of Medical Examiners. Anita E. Watson. 1996. 124p. lib. bdg. 25.00 (*1-56475-370-0*) U NV Oral Hist.

Reflections. Jose Silva. 5.95 (*0-913343-30-7*) Inst Psych Inc.

Reflections of a Country Doctor. Barry Ladd. Ed. by James A. Keene. 1995. LC 95-77536. 200p. 20.95 (*0-944435-37-8*) Glenbridge Pub.

Reflections of a Family Doctor: Writings of Herbert J. Levin, M.D. Herbert J. Levin. 1994. 185p. (Orig.). (C). pap. text 19.95 (*0-9642777-0-0*) Levin Family.

Reflections on Biochemistry. Arthur Kornberg et al. 1976. (*0-08-021011-2*) Pergamon Repr GBR. *Dist:* Franklin.

Reflections on Biologic Research. Giulio Gabbiani et al. 1967. LC 67-26012. (Illus.). 256p. 10.50 (*0-87527-035-2*) Green.

Reflections on Contemporary Nursing Practice. Judith Townshend & Margaret McMillan. 1995. LC 95-186879. 352p. pap. text 54.99 (*0-7506-8911-0*) Buttrwrth-Heinemann.

Reflections on Counseling. Dryden. 1993. 118p. pap. 48.00 (*1-56593-262-5*, 0552) Singular Publishing.

Reflections on Diabetes. Richard R. Rubin et al. 1996. LC 96-6157. 104p. pap. 9.95 (*0-945448-65-1*, 00651Q) Am Diabetes.

Reflections on Healing: A Central Nursing Construct. Ed. by Phyllis Beck Kritek. 1996. LC 96-50950. 606p. pap. 34.95 (*0-88737-725-4*) Natl League Nurse.

Reflections on Mary's Help Hospital & Seton Medical Center, 1893-1985. Marie M. Mahoney. 1986. 180p. 25.00 (*0-9616516-0-1*) Seton Med Ctr.

Reflections on Midwifery. Kirkham. 1997. pap. text (*0-7020-2125-3*) Bailliere Tindall.

Reflections on Palliative Care: Sociological & Policy Perspectives. David Clark & Jane Seymour. 1999. LC 98-28627. (Facing Death Ser.). 224p. pap. (*0-335-19454-0*) OpUniv Pr.

Reflections on Relaxation. Judy Loosmore. 1994. (Life Line Ser.). (Illus.). 160p. pap. (*1-55059-081-2*) Detselig Ents CAN. *Dist:* Temeron Bks.

Reflections on Renal Function. James Roper Robinson. 2nd ed. 1988. LC 88-212127. ix, 310 p. (*0-632-02102-0*) Blackwell Sci.

Reflections on Self Psychology. Ed. by Joseph D. Lichtenberg & Samuel Kaplan. 1983. LC 83-12293. (Psychoanalytic Inquiry Ser.: Vol. 1). 448p. text 59.95 (*0-88163-001-2*) Analytic Pr.

Reflections on Suicide. Madame de Stael. LC 77-37724. reprint ed. 39.50 (*0-404-56838-6*) AMS Pr.

Reflections on the Principles of Psychology: William James after a Century. Ed. by Michael G. Johnson & Tracy B. Henley. 1990. 344p. 89.95 (*0-8058-0205-3*) L Erlbaum Assocs.

Reflective Helping in HIV & AIDS. Ed. by Charles Anderson & Patricia Wilkie. 1991. 256p. (*0-335-15632-0*); pap. (*0-335-15631-2*) OpUniv Pr.

Reflective Practice in Nursing: The Growth of the Professional Practitioner. Ed. by Anthony M. Palmer et al. 1994. LC 93-38307. (Illus.). 193p. pap. 28.95 (*0-632-03597-8*) Blackwell Sci.

Reflective Teaching & Learning in The Health Professions. David Kember. 2001. LC 00-52963. (Illus.). 192p. pap. 35.95 (*0-632-05739-4*) Blackwell Sci.

Reflex & Bone Structure. Clarence Major. 1996. LC 96-11532. 144p. reprint ed. pap. 12.95 (*1-56279-084-6*) Mercury Hse.

Reflex Control of the Circulation. Irving H. Zucker & Joseph P. Gilmore. 1991. (Telford Press Ser.). 1073p. 225.00 (*0-8493-8801-5*, QP109) CRC Pr.

Reflex Sympathetic Dystrophy: A Reappraisal. Ed. by Wilfrid Janig & Michael D. Stanton-Hicks. 1996. LC 95-45160. (Progress in Pain Research & Management Ser.: Vol. 6). (Illus.). 268p. 55.00 (*0-931092-13-2*) Intl Assn Study Pain.

Reflex Sympathetic Dystrophy: Pathophysiological Mechanisms & Clinical Implications. Ed. by Robert F. Schmidt & Wilfrid Janig. 1992. LC 92-49653. 306p. 97.00 (*1-56081-284-2*, Wiley-VCH) Wiley.

Reflex Testing Methods for Evaluating CNS Development. Mary R. Fiorentino. 2nd ed. 1981. (Illus.). 72p. 29.95 (*0-398-02584-3*) C C Thomas.

Reflex Zone Therapy for Health Professionals. Ann Lett. 2nd ed. 2000. 184p. pap. (*0-443-06015-0*) Church.

Reflex Zone Therapy of the Feet. Hanne Marquardt. 1984. LC 88-30052. 160p. pap. 16.95 (*0-89281-234-6*, Heal Arts VT) Inner Tradit.

Reflexes & Motor Integration: Sherrington's Concept of Integrative Action. Judith P. Swazey. 1969. LC 69-13768. (Harvard Monographs in the History of Science). (Illus.). 448p. 30.50 (*0-674-75240-6*) HUP.

Reflexology. 2001. (Gem Ser.). (Illus.). 192p. pap. (*0-00-710145-7*) HarpC GBR. *Dist:* Trafalgar.

Reflexology. Maybelle Segal. 1976. pap. 7.00 (*0-87980-358-4*) Wilshire.

Reflexology. Chris Stormer. 1995. (Headway Lifeguides Ser.). (Illus.). 128p. pap. (*0-340-55594-7*) Hodder & Stought Ltd GBR. *Dist:* Lubrecht & Cramer, Trafalgar.

Reflexology: A Definitive Guide to Self-Treatment. Chris Stormer. 1995. 160p. pap. (*0-340-62038-2*) Hodder & Stought Ltd GBR. *Dist:* Lubrecht & Cramer, Trafalgar.

Reflexology: A Practical Approach. Vicki Pitman et al. 1998. (Illus.). 288p. (Orig.). pap. (*0-7487-2867-8*) Nelson Thornes GBR. *Dist:* Trans-Atl Phila.

Reflexology: A Step-by-Step Guide. Ed. by Caro Ness. 1997. (In a Nutshell Ser.). (Illus.). 64p. pap. 7.95 (*1-86204-010-9*) Element MA.

Reflexology: Art, Science & History. Christine Issel. 1990. (Illus.). 204p. (Orig.). pap. 14.95 (*0-9625448-0-9*) New Frntr Pub.

Reflexology: Guide to Herbalism. Beryl Crane. 1999. LC 98-41259. (Illustrated Guides Ser.). (Illus.). 144p. pap. 19.95 (*1-86204-169-5*) Element MA.

Reflexology: The Definitive Practitioner's Manual: Recommended by the International Therapy Examination Council for Students & Practitioners. Beryl Crane. 1998. LC 97-29169. (Illus.). 448p. 59.95 (*1-86204-125-3*) Element MA.

Reflexology & Acupressure: Pressure Points for Healing. Janet Wright. 2000. LC 00-45424. (Illus.). 130p. pap. 17.95 (*1-57067-108-7*) Book Pub Co.

Reflexology Manual: An Easy-to-Use Illustrated Guide to Healing Zones of the Hands & Feet. Pauline Wills. 1995. LC 95-12387. (Illus.). 144p. pap. 19.95 (*0-89281-547-7*, Heal Arts VT) Inner Tradit.

Reflexology Partnership: A Healing Bond. Suzanne Adamson & Eilish Harris. 1996. (Illus.). 160p. pap. (*1-85626-149-2*) Cathie Kyle GBR. *Dist:* Trafalgar.

Reflexology Today: The Stimulation of the Body's Healing Forces Through Foot Massage. Doreen E. Bayly. 1984. 64p. pap. 9.95 (*0-89281-284-2*) Inner Tradit.

Reflexology Today - A Family Affair: A Self-Help Guide for Family Wellness. Njideka N. Olatunde. 1999. (Illus.). 116p. pap. (*0-7392-0171-9*, PO3132) Morris Pubng.

Reflexotherapy of the Feet. H. Marquardt. 2000. (Illus.). 232p. 35.00 (*0-86577-931-7*) Thieme Med Pubs.

Reflextherapy. Christine B. Jones. 2000. 224p. pap. 50.00 (*0-7506-4051-0*) Buttrwrth-Heinemann.

Reflux Nephropathy Update, 1983. Ed. by C. J. Hodson et al. 1984. (Contributions to Nephrology Ser.: Vol. 39). (Illus.). xvi, 388p. 29.75 (*3-8055-3807-3*) S Karger.

Refocusing Educational Psychology. Ed. by Neville Jones & Norah Frederickson. 1990. 255p. pap. 43.95 (*1-85000-493-5*, Falmer Pr) Taylor & Francis.

Reform & Regulation in Long Term Care. Ed. by Valerie LaPorte & Jeffrey Rubin. 1979. LC 79-9761. 216p. 65.00 (*0-275-90379-6*, C0379, Praeger Pubs) Greenwood.

Reformatory Schools for the Children of the Perishing & Dangerous Classes & for Juvenile Offenders: With Index Added. Mary Carpenter. 1970. LC 72-108223. (Criminology, Law Enforcement, & Social Problems Ser.: No. 106). reprint ed. lib. bdg. 15.00 (*0-87585-106-1*) Patterson Smith.

Reforming Health Care: A Market Prescription. 1987. (CED Statement on National Policy Ser.). 114p. pap. 9.50 (*0-87186-084-8*); lib. bdg. 11.50 (*0-87186-784-2*) Comm Econ Dev.

Reforming Health Care: The Philosophy & Practice of International Health Reform. Ed. by David Seedhouse. 1995. LC 94-44374. 252p. pap. 61.95 (*0-471-95325-3*) Wiley.

Reforming Health Care Systems: Experiments with the NHS. Ed. by A. J. Culyer & Adam Wagstaff. 1996. LC 95-42419. (Section F Series, British Association for the Advancement of Science). (Illus.). 192p. 90.00 (*1-85898-329-0*) E Elgar.

Reforming Private Health Insurance. Mark A. Hall. 1994. LC 94-14779. 150p. 19.95 (*0-8447-3862-X*); pap. 12.95 (*0-8447-3863-8*) Am Enterprise (AEI Pr).

Reforming the Health Care Market: An Interpretive Economic History. David F. Drake. 1994. LC 94-13475. 240p. 42.50 (*0-87840-567-4*); pap. 16.95 (*0-87840-568-2*) Georgetown U Pr.

Reforming the Schools—for Teachers. John W. Friesen. 1987. LC 87-13361. 164p. (Orig.). 51.00 (*0-8191-6479-8*) U Pr of Amer.

Reforming the Schools for Teachers. John W. Friesen. 1987. LC 87-13361. 164p. (Orig.). pap. 22.50 (*0-8191-6480-1*) U Pr of Amer.

Refraction: A Programmed Text. Robert D. Reinecke & Robert Herm. 3rd ed. 1983. (Illus.). 373p. (C). pap. text 39.95 (*0-8385-8300-8*, A8300-4) Appleton & Lange.

Refractive Anomalies. Theodore Grosvenor & Merton C. Flom. 1990. (Illus.). 464p. text 99.95 (*0-409-90149-0*) Buttrwrth-Heinemann.

Refractive Cataract Surgery & Multifocal IOLS. R. Bruce Wallace, III. 2000. LC 00-45027. (Illus.). 243p. (C). text 110.00 (*1-55642-460-4*) SLACK Inc.

Refractive Eye Surgery. Leo S. Bores. 2nd ed. 2001. LC 00-56420. (Illus.). 592p. 362.95 (*0-632-04364-4*) Blackwell Sci.

Refractive Management of Ametropia. Ed. by Kenneth E. Brookman. 1996. LC 95-45065. (Illus.). 222p. pap. text 44.99 (*0-7506-9569-2*) Buttrwrth-Heinemann.

Refractive Surgery. Sunita Agarwal & Ioannis Pallikaris. 1999. 500p. (C). text (*81-7179-700-8*) Jaypee Brothers IND. *Dist:* SLACK Inc.

Refractive Surgery. Dimitri Azar. 1997. LC 97-126370. 691p. (C). pap. text 179.00 (*0-8385-8276-1*, A8276-6, Apple Lange Med) McGraw.

Refractive Surgery. Olivia N. Serdarevic. 1994. 39.00 (*0-316-78067-7*, Little Brwn Med Div) Lppncott W & W.

Refractive Surgery. Helen K. Wu. 1998. (Illus.). 624p. 175.00 (*0-86577-759-4*) Thieme Med Pubs.

Refractive Surgery: Current Techniques & Management. Olivia N. Serdarevic. 1996. LC 96-29391. (Illus.). 368p. 158.50 (*0-89640-325-4*) Igaku-Shoin.

Refractive Surgery & Optometric Practice. Emanuel Rosen et al. 2001. (Illus.). 256p. 90.00 (*0-7506-3959-8*) Buttrwrth-Heinemann.

Refractive Surgery for Eyecare Paraprofessionals. Johnny L. Gayton & Robert M. Kerstner. 1997. LC 97-10167. (Basic Bookshelf for Eyecare Professionals Ser.). (Illus.). 112p. pap. text 21.00 (*1 55642-337-3*, 63373) SLACK Inc.

Refractory Depression: Current Strategies & Future Directions. William A. Nolen et al. 1994. LC 93-49532. 252p. 230.00 (*0-471-94315-0*) Wiley.

Refractory Glaucomas. Ed. by Fathi El-Sayyad et al. 1995. LC 95-7750. (Illus.). 320p. 95.00 (*0-89640-284-3*) Igaku-Shoin.

Reframing Women's Health: Multidisciplinary Research & Practice. Ed. by Alice Dan. 1994. LC 94-7456. 78.95 (*0-8039-5773-4*, 3903); pap. 39.95 (*0-8039-5860-9*, 9496) Sage.

Refresher: Emergency Care & Transportation of the Sick & Injured. American Academy of Orthopaedic Surgeons Staff. 1999. LC 99-40846. (Illus.). 488p. (C). pap. text 36.95 (*0-7637-0912-3*, 0912-3) Jones & Bartlett.

Refrigerated Medical Equipment, UL 416. 4th ed. 1993. (C). pap. text 175.00 (*1-55989-466-0*) Underwrtrs Labs.

Refugee Mental Health in Resettlement Countries. Ed. by Carolyn L. Williams & Joseph Westermeyer. 1986. (Clinical & Community Psychology Ser.). 267p. text 73.95 (*0-89116-445-6*) Hemisp Pub.

Refugee Women & Reproductive Health Care: Reassessing Priorities. Deirdre Wulf. 1994. 77p. pap. (*0-9637711-1-6*) Intl Rescue Comm.

Refugee Women & Reproductive Health Care: Reassessing Priorities. Deirdre Wulf et al. 1997. 77p. pap. text 30.00 (*0-7881-3841-3*) DIANE Pub.

Refusal Skills: Preventing Drug Use in Adolescents. Arnold P. Goldstein et al. 1990. LC 90-60924. 176p. (Orig.). pap. text Price not set. (*0-87822-323-1*, 4422) Res Press.

Regaining the Power of Youth. Kenneth H. Cooper. 1999. LC 98-45029. 288p. 19.99 (*0-7852-7142-2*) Nelson.

Regaining Wholeness Through the Subtle Dimensions: Where Science Meets Magic. Don Paris. 1993. (Illus.). 160p. (Orig.). pap. 12.95 (*1-884246-00-1*) Liv from Vis.

Regeneration & Transplantation Eugene Korschelt. 1991. (Resources in Medical History Ser.). (Illus.). 1300p. (C). (*0-88135-095-8*); (*0-88135-096-6*);Set. 85.00 (*0-88135-097-4*) Watson Pub Intl (Sci Hist).

Regeneration of Vertebrate Sensory Receptor Cells - Symposium No. 160. CIBA Foundation Staff. 1991. LC 91-21619. (CIBA Foundation Symposia Ser.: No. 160). 352p. 128.00 (*0-471-92960-3*, Wiley-Interscience) Wiley.

Regenerative Diet. John R. Christopher. 1982. LC 90-205281. 275p. per. 9.95 (*1-879436-00-0*, 99111) Christopher Pubns.

Regents: Prentice-Hall Medical Assisting Kit. Regents Staff. 3rd ed. 1998. pap. 240.67 (*0-13-614736-4*) P-H.

Regents College Clinical Performance in Nursing Examination Video Workbook. 1997. (Illus.). 130p. pap. text, wbk. ed. (*1-889403-09-1*) Regnts College.

Regimen for Weight Control in Retired Couples & Others Who Want to Control Weight Happily. Charles N. Aronson. 1973. LC 73-88985. (Illus.). (C). 5.00 (*0-915736-03-9*) C N Aronson.

Regimiento Contra la Peste: Biblioteca Nacional de Madrid I-51. Fernando Alvarez. Ed. by Maria Purificacion Zabia. 1987. (Medieval Spanish Medical Texts Ser.: No. 18). (SPA.). 6p. 10.00 incl. fiche (*0-940639-14-9*) Hispanic Seminary.

Regional Anaesthesia for Babies & Children. Jane M. Peutrell & Stephen J. Mather. 1997. (Illus.). 270p. (C). text 69.50 (*0-19-262425-3*) OUP.

Regional Anesthesia: An Atlas of Anatomy & Techniques. Ed. by Marc B. Hahn et al. 1995. LC 95-31275. (Illus.). 336p. (C). (gr. 13). text 145.00 (*0-8151-4121-1*, 23613) Mosby Inc.

Regional Anesthesia: An Illustrated Procedural Guide. Michael F. Mulroy. 2nd ed. 1995. LC 95-4493. (Illus.). 327p. pap. text 79.95 (*0-316-58906-3*, Little Brwn Med Div) Lppncott W & W.

Regional Anesthesia & Analgesia. David L. Brown. Ed. by Richard Zorab. 1996. (Illus.). 800p. text 146.00 (*0-7216-5654-4*) Saunders.

Regional Atlas of Bone Disease: A Guide to Pathologic & Normal Variation in the Human Skeleton. Robert W. Mann & Sean P. Murphy. 1990. (Illus.). 224p. (C). text 49.95 (*0-398-05675-7*) C C Thomas.

Regional Block: A Handbook for Use in the Clinical Practice of Medicine & Surgery. Daniel C. Moore. 4th ed. 1981. (Illus.). 532p. 56.95 (*0-398-01337-3*) C C Thomas.

Regional Blood Flow & Clinical Considerations. Ed. by B. M. Altura & S. Halevy. 1987. (Cardiovascular Actions of Anesthetics & Drugs Used in Anesthesia Ser.: Vol. 2). (Illus.). viii, 296p. 187.00 (*3-8055-4158-9*) S Karger.

Regional Cancer Treatment. Ed. by K. R. Aigner et al. 1988. (Beitraege Zur Onkologie, Contributions to Oncology Ser.: Vol. 29). (Illus.). viii, 312p. 65.25 (*3-8055-4762-5*) S Karger.

Regional Chemotherapy. Ed. by U. Laffer. 1988. (Antibiotics & Chemotherapy Ser.: Vol. 40). (Illus.). viii, 100p. 77.50 (*3-8055-4670-X*) S Karger.

Regional Chemotherapy: Clinical Research & Practice. Ed. by Maurie Markman. 2000. LC 99-22882. (Current Clinical Oncology Ser.: Vol. 2). (Illus.). 376p. 149.50 (*0-89603-729-0*) Humana.

Regional Dermatology. Gary M. White. 2nd ed. 1997. 39.95 (*0-7234-3003-9*) Mosby Inc.

Regional Health Facility System Planning: An Access Opportunity Approach. Jerry B. Schneider & John G. Symons, Jr. 1971. (Discussion Papers: No. 48). pap. 10.00 (*1-55869-106-5*) Regional Sci Res Inst.

Regional Nerve Blocks. Danilo Jankovic & Chris Wells. 2nd ed. 2001. (Illus.). 348p. 140.00 (*0-632-05557-X*) Blackwell Sci.

Regional Network for Latin America on Animal Disease Diagnosis Using Immunoassay & Labelled DNA Probe Techniques. 1993. (Illus.). 196p. (Orig.). (C). pap. text 50.00 (*1-56806-391-1*) DIANE Pub.

Regional Opioid Analgesia. J. De Castro et al. 1990. (Developments in Anesthesiology & Critical Care Ser.). (C). text 385.50 (*0-7923-0162-5*) Kluwer Academic.

Regional Pulmonary Function in Health & Disease. Ed. by B. L. Holman & J. F. Lindeman. 1973. (Progress in Nuclear Medicine Ser.: Vol. 3). 196p. 61.00 (*3-8055-1425-5*) S Karger.

Regional Review of the Stock of Hospital Floorspace. G. Samuelsson-Brown & S. Whittome. 1992. (*0-86022-321-3*) Build Servs Info Assn GBR. *Dist:* St Mut.

Regional Strategy for Health Care of the Elderly in the Eastern Mediterranean Region, 1992-2001. 1994. LC 96-138362. (Regional Advisory Panel on Health Care of the Elderly Ser.). 22p. pap. text 6.00 (*92-9021-188-1*, 1440009) World Health.

Regionale Chemotherapie der Leber. Ed. by K. Aigner. 1985. (Beitraege Zur Onkologie, Contributions to Oncology Ser.: Vol. 21). (Illus.). viii, 140p. 68.75 (*3-8055-4014-0*) S Karger.

Regionalization: Issues in Intensive Care for High Risk Newborns & their Families. Claire S. Rudolph & Susan R. Borker. 1987. LC 87-15136. 216p. 72.50 (*0-275-92547-1*, C2547, Praeger Pubs) Greenwood.

Regions, Bones, Ligaments & Muscles, Vol. 1. Johannes Sobotta. Ed. by Frank H. Figge & Walter J. Hild. 1978. 290p. text 39.50 (*0-8067-1719-X*) Lppncott W & W.

Regions of the Mind: Brain Research & the Quest for Scientific Certainty. Susan Leigh Star. 1989. LC 89-4432. (Illus.). 304p. 51.00 (*0-8047-1673-0*) Stanford U Pr.

Registered Professional Nurse. Jack Rudman. 1994. (Career Examination Ser.: C-671). pap. 29.95 (*0-8373-0671-X*) Nat Learn.

Registered Professional Nurses & Unlicensed Assistive Personnel. American Nurses Association Staff. 2nd ed. 1996. LC 97-147045. 96p. (Orig.). 16.95 (*1-55810-132-2*, NP-89A) Am Nurses Pub.

Registered Technologist, R. T. (AR-RT) Jack Rudman. 1994. (Career Examination Ser.: C-680). pap. 29.95 (*0-8373-0680-9*) Nat Learn.

Registration Examination for Dieticians (RED) Jack Rudman. 1994. (Admission Test Ser.: ATS-41). pap. 39.95 (*0-8373-5041-7*) Nat Learn.

Registration Examination for Dietitians (RED) Jack Rudman. (Admission Test Ser.: Vol. 41). 59.95 (*0-8373-5141-3*) Nat Learn.

Registry of Toxic Effects of Chemical Substances, RTECS: A Comprehensive Guide. Ed. by Doris V. Sweet. 1994. 70p. (Orig.). (C). pap. text 25.00 (*0-7881-0565-5*) DIANE Pub.

Registry Review for Computed Tomography. Daniel N. DeMaio. Ed. by Lisa Biello. 1996. LC 95-49210. 240p. pap. text 26.00 (*0-7216-6285-4*) Saunders.

Regreso al Eden. Jethro Kloss. rev. ed. 2000. LC 99-96483.Tr. of Back to Eden. (SPA., Illus.). 882p. pap. 19.95 (*0-940985-05-5*) Lotus Pr.

Regression Analysis of Survival Data in Cancer Chemotherapy. Walter H. Carter & Galen L. Wampler. 1983. (Statistics Ser.: 44). (Illus.). 224p. text 125.00 (*0-8247-1736-8*) Dekker.

Regression, Stress, & Readjustment in Aging: A Structured, Bio-Psychosocial Perspective on Coping & Professional Support. Zeev Ben-Sira. 1991. LC 91-17302. 184p. 60.00 (*0-275-94078-0*, C4078, Praeger Pubs) Greenwood.

Regression Therapy Using Hypnosis: How Reliving Early Experiences Can Improve Your Life. Ursula Markham. 1996. 126p. (Orig.). pap. text (*0-7499-1032-1*) Piatkus Bks GBR. *Dist:* London Brdge.

Regular Exercise: A Handbook for Clinical Practice. Steven Jonas. 1995. LC 94-42548. 264p. 34.95 (*0-8261-8860-5*) Springer Pub.

Regulating America, Regulating Sweden: A Comparative Study of Occupational Safety & Health Policy. Steven Kelman. 1981. 280p. 32.50 (*0-262-11076-8*) MIT Pr.

Regulating Birth see Making Midwives Legal: Childbirth, Medicine, & the Law

Regulating HMO's. Walter M. Cadette. 1998. (Public Policy Brief Highlights Ser.: Vol. 47A). 6p. pap. (*0-941276-60-0*, Levy Econ Inst Bard) Bard Coll Pubns.

Regulating HMO's: An Ethical Framework for Cost-Effective Medicine. Walter M. Cadette. 1998. (Public Policy Briefs Ser.: Vol. 47). 44p. pap. (*0-941276-59-7*, Levy Econ Inst Bard) Bard Coll Pubns.

Regulating How We Die: The Ethical, Medical, & Legal Issues Surrounding Physician-Assisted Suicide. Linda L. Emanuel. 1999. LC 97-38892. 304p. 41.50 (*0-674-66653-4*) HUP.

Regulating Managed Care: Theory, Practice & Future Options. Stuart Altman. 1999. LC 99-24496. (Jossey-Bass Health Ser.). 400p. 50.00 (*0-7879-4783-0*) Jossey-Bass.

Regulating Medical Work: Formal & Informal Controls. J. Allsop. 1996. (Health Services Management Ser.). 224p. (*0-335-19405-2*); LC 96-17728. pap. (*0-335-19404-4*) OpUniv Pr.

Regulating Medicines in Europe: Competition, Experts & Public Health. John Abraham & Graham Lewis. 2000. LC 00-28615. 248p. 90.00 (*0-415-20877-7*); pap. 29.99 (*0-415-20878-5*) Routledge.

Regulating Reproduction. Robert H. Blank. 1992. 272p. (C). pap. text 19.00 (*0-231-07017-9*) Col U Pr.

***Regulating Reproduction: Law, Technology & Autonomy.** Emily Jackson. 2001. 224p. pap. (*1-84113-301-9*) Hart Pub GBR. *Dist:* Intl Spec Bk.

Regulating Residential Care: A Case Study of a Voluntary Home. Sally Sainsbury. 1989. (Occasional Papers on Social Administration). 172p. text (*0-566-07039-1*) Avebry GBR. *Dist:* Ashgate Pub Co.

Regulation & Functional Significance of T-Cell Subsets. Ed. by R. L. Coffman. 1992. (Chemical Immunology Ser.: Vol. 54). (Illus.). x, 218p. 182.75 (*3-8055-5577-6*) S Karger.

Regulation of Adenovirus Alternative Pre-mRNA Splicing: Functional Characterization of Exotic & Intronic Splicing Enhancer Elements. Bai-Gong Yue. 2000. (Comprehensive Summaries of Uppsala Dissertations from the Faculty of Medicine Ser.: vol. 926). (Illus.). 55p. pap. (*91-554-4712-0*) Uppsala Universitet SWE. *Dist:* Coronet Bks.

Regulation of Aldostorone Biosynthesis. J. Muller. 2nd rev. ed. 1987. (Monographs in Endocrinology: Vol. 29). (Illus.). 364p. 158.00 (*0-387-17907-0*) Spr-Verlag.

Regulation of Angiogenesis. I. D. Goldberg & E. M. Rosen. 1996. LC 97-126063. (Experientia Supplementum Ser.: Vol. 79). (Illus.). 430p. 185.00 (*3-7643-5309-0*) Birkhauser.

Regulation of Body Fluid Volumes by the Kidney: Proceedings of the Natriuretic Hormone Symposium, Czechoslovakia, June, 1969. Natriuretic Hormone Symposium Staff. Ed. by J. H. Cort & B. Lichardus. 1970. (Illus.). 192p. 59.25 (*3-8055-0772-0*) S Karger.

Regulation of Breathing. Ed. by Jerome A. Dempsey & Allan I. Pack. 2nd exp. rev. ed. 1994. LC 94-3562. (Lung Biology in Health & Disease Ser.: Vol. 79). (Illus.). 1250p. text 235.00 (*0-8247-9227-0*) Dekker.

Regulation of Carbohydrate Metabolism, Vol. 1. Rivka Beitner. 1985. LC 84-12060. 176p. 105.00 (*0-8493-5262-2*, QP701, CRC Reprint) Franklin.

Regulation of Carbohydrate Metabolism, Vol. 2. Ed. by Rivka Beitner. 1985. LC 84-12060. 224p. 132.00 (*0-8493-5263-0*, QP701, CRC Reprint) Franklin.

Regulation of Carbon & Nitrogen Reduction & Utilization in Maize. Ed. by Jack C. Shannon et al. 1986. LC 86-72906. 382p. (Orig.). pap. text 20.00 (*0-943088-09-7*) Am Soc of Plan.

P Q R

Regulation of Carcinogens: Are Animal Tests a Sound Foundation? Aaron Wildavsky. 44p. pap. 5.95 (*0-945999-57-7*, 1009) Independent Inst.

Regulation of Cardiac Function: Molecular, Cellular, & Pathophysiological Aspects. International Society and Federation of Cardiology S. Ed. by Lionel H. Opie et al. 1984. 342p. lib. bdg. (*90-6764-035-2*) VSP NLD. *Dist:* Coronet Bks.

Regulation of Cerebral Blood Flow. John W. Phillis. 1993. 448p. 225.00 (*0-8493-5096-4*, QP108) CRC Pr.

Regulation of Cerebral Circulation: Proceedings of the 4th Tbilisi Symposium on Cerebral Circulation, Tbilist, 19-21 April, 1978. G. I. Mchedlishvili et al. 1979. 266p. (C). (*963-05-2209-8*) Akade Kiado HUN. *Dist:* St Mut.

Regulation of Coronary Blood Flow. Ed. by M. Inoue et al. 1992. (Illus.). 336p. 108.00 (*0-387-70072-2*) Spr-Verlag.

Regulation of DNA Replication & Transcription. M. Beljanski. 1983. (Experimental Biology & Medicine Ser.: Vol. 8). (Illus.). x, 190p. pap. 108.00 (*3-8055-3631-3*) S Karger.

Regulation of Gene Expression & Brain Function. Ed. & Contrib. by Paul J. Harrison. 1994. LC 93-26907. (Basic & Clinical Aspects of Neuroscience Ser.: Vol. 6). (Illus.). 64p. 39.95 (*0-387-57156-6*) Spr-Verlag.

Regulation of Gene Expression in Animal Viruses. L. Carrasco et al. 1993. (NATO Advanced Science Institutes Ser.: Vol. 240). (Illus.). 334p. (C). text 115.00 (*0-306-44408-9*, Kluwer Plenum) Kluwer Academic.

Regulation of Growth in Neoplasia. Ed. by G. V. Sherbet. 1981. (Illus.). x, 202p. 101.00 (*3-8055-2305-X*) S Karger.

Regulation of Health: Case Studies of Sweden & Switzerland. Peter Zweifel et al. 1998. LC 98-37468. (Developments in Health Economics & Public Policy Ser.). 9p. (*0-7923-8342-7*) Kluwer Academic.

Regulation of Health Risk - Bearing Entities. 1997. 70p. (C). lib. bdg. 25.00 (*0-89382-502-6*, RBE-OP) Nat Assn Insurance.

Regulation of Heme Protein Synthesis. Ed. by Hiroyoshi Fujita. 1994. LC 93-50106. 139p. 49.00 (*1-880854-18-X*) AlphaMed Pr.

Regulation of Hemoglobin Synthesis. J. Neuwirt & P. Ponka. 1977. text 85.50 (*90-247-1999-2*) Kluwer Academic.

Regulation of Hepatic Metabolism: Intra- & Intercellular Compartmentation. Ed. by Ronald G. Thurman et al. 1986. LC 85-30084. (Illus.). 510p. (C). text 162.00 (*0-306-42137-2*, Kluwer Plenum) Kluwer Academic.

*__Regulation of Human Eosinophil Transmigration Across Lung Epithelium.__ Lixin Liu. 2001. (Comprehensive Summaries of Uppsala Dissertations from the Faculty of Medicine Ser.: No. 1044). (Illus.). 48p. (*91-554-5042-3*) Uppsala Universitet SWE. *Dist:* Coronet Bks.

*__Regulation of Human Mast Cell Development.__ Malin Hjertson. 2000. (Comprehensive Summaries of Uppsala Dissertations from the Faculty of Medicine Ser.: No. 905). (Illus.). 49p. pap. (*91-554-4652-3*) Uppsala Universitet SWE. *Dist:* Coronet Bks.

Regulation of Immune Response Dynamics Ed. by Charles Delisi & Jacques R. Hiernaux. 1982. Vol. I. 176p. 104.00 (*0-8493-6632-1*, QR186); Vol. II. 184p. 107.00 (*0-8493-6633-X*) Franklin.

Regulation of Male Fertility. Ed. by G. R. Cunningham et al. 1980. (Clinics in Andrology Ser.: No. 5). (Illus.). 245p. text 206.50 (*90-247-2373-6*) Kluwer Academic.

Regulation of Membrane Lipid Metabolism. Guy A. Thompson, Jr. 1980. 256p. 132.00 (*0-8493-5427-7*, QH601, CRC Reprint) Franklin.

Regulation of Neuroendocrine Aging. Ed. by A. V. Everitt & Judie R. Walton. 1988. (Interdisciplinary Topics in Gerontology Ser.: Vol. 24). (Illus.). viii, 156p. 121.75 (*3-8055-4770-6*) S Karger.

Regulation of Ovarian & Testicular Function. Ed. by Virendra B. Mahesh et al. 1987. LC 87-22073. (Advances in Experimental Medicine & Biology Ser.: Vol. 219). (Illus.). 774p. 135.00 (*0-306-42676-5*, Plenum Trade) Perseus Pubng.

Regulation of Pharmaceuticals in Developing Countries: Legal Issues & Approaches. D. C. Jayasuriya. 1985. 118p. pap. text 14.00 (*92-4-156089-4*, 1150236) World Health.

Regulation of Pituitary Function. Ed. by T. Van Wimersma Greidanus & W. J. Lamberts. 1985. (Frontiers of Hormone Research Ser.: Vol. 14). (Illus.). vi, 218p. 155.75 (*3-8055-4061-2*) S Karger.

Regulation of Porphyrin & Heme Biosynthesis: Proceedings of the International Research Conference, Marburg an der Lahn, June 28-July 1, 1973. International Research Conference Staff. Ed. by Manfred Doss. rev. ed. 1974. (Enzyme Ser.: Vol. 16, No. 1-6 & Vol. 17, No. 1-2). 384p. reprint ed. 123.50 (*3-8055-1652-5*) S Karger.

Regulation of Provider Risk Sharing & Other Limitations on Risk Bearing Provider Networks. Randolph S. Jordan. 1996. (Health Law & Business Ser.: No. 2300). 125.00 (*1-55871-336-0*) BNA.

Regulation of Secondary Metabolism in Actinomycetes. Ed. by Stuart Shapiro. 1989. 304p. lib. bdg. 259.00 (*0-8493-6927-4*, QR82) CRC Pr.

Regulation of Serum Lipids by Physical Exercise. Eino Hietanen. 1982. 192p. 109.00 (*0-8493-6330-6*, QP99, CRC Reprint) Franklin.

Regulation of Smooth Muscle Contraction. Ed. by R. S. Moreland. 1991. (Advances in Experimental Medicine & Biology Ser.: Vol. 304). (Illus.). 576p. (C). text 180.00 (*0-306-44041-5*, Kluwer Plenum) Kluwer Academic.

Regulation of Target Cell Responsiveness, Vol. 1. International Foundation for Biochemical Endocrino. Ed. by Kenneth W. McKerns et al. 1984. LC 83-24773. (Biochemical Endocrinology Ser.). 550p. 125.00 (*0-306-41500-3*, Plenum Trade) Perseus Pubng.

Regulation of Target Cell Responsiveness, Vol. 2. Ed. by International Foundation for Biochemical Endocrino et al. 1984. LC 83-24773. (Biochemical Endocrinology Ser.). 564p. 125.00 (*0-306-41501-1*, Plenum Trade) Perseus Pubng.

Regulation of the Contractile Cycle in Smooth Muscle. Ed. by T. Nakano & D. J. Hartshorne. 1996. 133.00 (*0-387-70149-4*); 247p. 103.00 (*3-540-70149-4*) Spr-Verlag.

Regulation of the Healthcare Professions. Ed. by Timothy Stoltzfus Jost. 1997. LC 97-2634. 216p. (Orig.). pap. 44.00 (*1-56793-058-1*) Health Admin Pr.

Regulation of the IGE Antibody Response. Ed. by K. Ishizaka. 1982. (Progress in Allergy Ser.: Vol. 32). (Illus.). x, 346p. 185.25 (*3-8055-3470-1*) S Karger.

Regulation of the Vascular Endothelium: Signals & Transduction Mechanisms. J. M. Boeynaems & S. Pirotton. 1994. (Molecular Biology Intelligence Unit Ser.). 118p. 99.00 (*1-57059-026-5*, LN9026) Landes Bioscience.

Regulation of Vertebrate Limb Regeneration. Ed. by Raymond E. Sicard. 1985. (Illus.). 195p. text 45.00 (*0-19-503604-2*) OUP.

Regulations for the Medical Department of the Army. 1989. 96p. reprint ed. 18.75 (*1-877791-00-8*) Bohemian Brigade.

Regulatory Control & Standardization of Allergenic Extracts. Ed. by Reinhard Kurth & Gerhard Siefert. 2nd ed. 1988. (Arbeiten aus dem Paul-Ehrlich Institut Ser.: Vol. 82). 269p. pap. 75.00 (*0-89574-268-3*, Wiley-VCH) Wiley.

Regulatory Gut Peptides in Paediatric Gastroenterology & Nutrition. Ed. by P. Heinz-Erian et al. 1992. (Frontiers of Gastrointestinal Research Ser.: Vol. 21). (Illus.). viii, 264p. 215.75 (*3-8055-5549-0*) S Karger.

Regulatory Mechanisms for Nursing Training & Practice: Meeting Primary Health Care Needs. 1986. (Technical Reports: No. 738). 71p. pap. text 10.00 (*92-4-120738-8*, 1100738) World Health.

Regulatory Mechanisms in Breast Cancer: Advances in Cellular & Molecular Biology of Breast Cancer. Ed. by Marc E. Lippman & Robert B. Dickson. 1991. (Cancer Treatment & Research Ser.). (C). text 237.00 (*0-7923-0868-9*) Kluwer Academic.

Regulatory Mechanisms in Gastrointestinal Function. Ed. by Timothy S. Gaginella. 1995. LC 95-8329. 352p. 169.95 (*0-8493-9439-2*, 9439) CRC Pr.

Regulatory Mechanisms of Human Neoplastic Cell Growth by Cytokines: Past & Future Prospect. Ed. by Fumimaro Takaku & Takeshi Ogura. 1993. LC 93-4563. (Gann Monographs on Cancer Research: No. 40). 79.95 (*0-8493-7747-1*) CRC Pr.

Regulatory Mechanisms of Neuron to Vessel Communication in the Brain. Ed. by S. Govoni et al. 1989. (NATO ASI Ser.: Vol. 33). (Illus.). 416p. 151.00 (*0-387-50379-X*) Spr-Verlag.

Regulatory Practice for Biopharmaceutical Production. Ed. by Anthony S. Lubiniecki & Susan A. Vargo. 1994. 566p. 205.00 (*0-471-04900-X*) Wiley.

Regulatory Process in Allergy & Asthma. Ed. by K. Blaser. 1990. (Journal: Vol. 90, Suppl. 1). (Illus.). iv, 76p. pap. text 33.25 (*3-8055-5152-5*) S Karger.

Regulatory Processes in Clinical Endocrinology. Ed. by Walter B. Essman. 1982. 300p. text 40.00 (*0-88331-193-3*) R B Luce.

Regulatory Protein Modification: Techniques & Protocols. Ed. by Hugh C. Hemmings. 1996. (Neuromethods Ser.: Vol. 30). (Illus.). 480p. 145.00 (*0-89603-415-1*) Humana.

Regulatory References. 1998. 184p. pap. 80.00 (*0-9663593-2-1*); 2nd rev. ed. 2000. 300p. pap. text 95.00 (*0-9663593-5-6*) Ctr for Clin Res.

Regulatory Role of the Nervous System in Aging. Ed. by H. T. Blumenthal. 1970. (Interdisciplinary Topics in Gerontology Ser.: Vol. 7). 45.25 (*3-8055-0508-6*) S Karger.

Rehabilitating Blind & Visually Impaired People: A Psychological Approach. Dodds. 1993. 218p. pap. 47.75 (*1-56593-153-X*, 0465) Singular Publishing.

Rehabilitating Blind & Visually Impaired People: A Psychological Approach. Allan Dodds. 1993. LC 93-16158. 224p. pap. 34.95 (*0-412-46970-7*) Chapman & Hall.

Rehabilitation. Fuzy. 1996. (C). pap. text, tchr. ed. 12.00 (*0-8273-7932-3*) Delmar.

Rehabilitation: A Component of Comprehensive Cardiac Care. Ed. by Nanette K. Wenger. 1986. (Bibliotheca Cardiologica Ser.: No. 40). (Illus.). xii, 132p. 115.75 (*3-8055-4359-X*) S Karger.

Rehabilitation: The Federal Government's Response to Disability, 1935 to 1954. Edward D. Berkowitz. Ed. by William R. Phillips & Janet Rosenberg. 1980. LC 79-6896. (Physically Handicapped in Society Ser.). lib. bdg. 36.95 (*0-405-13107-0*) Ayer.

Rehabilitation: Twenty-Five Years of Concepts, Principles, Perspectives. Ed. by Stephen J. Regnier & Marian Petkovsek. 1985. (Illus.). 192p. (Orig.). pap. 9.95 (*0-933851-00-6*) Natl Easter Seal.

Rehabilitation Activities Profile. G. J. Lankhorst et al. 1996. 80p. pap. (*90-5383-398-6*) VUB Univ Pr BEL. *Dist:* Paul & Co Pubs.

Rehabilitation after Cardiovascular Diseases, with Special Emphasis on Developing Countries: Report of a WHO Expert Committee. 1993. (Technical Reports: No. 831). (CHI, ENG, FRE & SPA.). viii, 122p. pap. text 17.00 (*92-4-120831-7*, 1100831) World Health.

Rehabilitation after Myocardial Infarction: The European Experience. Ed. by Veikko Kallio & Elizabeth Clay. 1985. (Public Health in Europe Ser.: No. 24). 148p. pap. text 13.00 (*92-890-1160-2*, 1320024) World Health.

Rehabilitation & Comprehensive Secondary Prevention after Acute Myocardial Infarction. D. Dorossiev. 1983. (Euro Reports & Studies Ser.: No. 84). 99p. pap. text 8.00 (*92-890-1250-1*) World Health.

Rehabilitation & Disability: Psychosocial Case Studies. E. Davis Martin, Jr. & Gerald L. Gandy. 1990. 200p. (C). text 43.95 (*0-398-05698-6*) C C Thomas.

Rehabilitation & Handicapped Literature, 1982-1985 Update: A Bibliographic Guide to the Microfiche Collection. Ed. by Mary E. Morrison. 1987. (Orig.). 20.00 (*0-8357-0732-6*) Univ Microfilms.

Rehabilitation & Restorative Care in the Community. Shirley P. Hoeman. 1990. (Illus.). 368p. (C). (gr. 13). pap. text 27.95 (*0-8016-2415-0*, 02415) Mosby Inc.

Rehabilitation & the Law: Liability & the OT Practitioner. Steve Long & Rita Burghardt. 1996. 60p. (Orig.). pap. text 21.00 (*1-56900-040-9*, 1145) Am Occup Therapy.

Rehabilitation Approaches to Drug & Alcohol Dependence. Behrouz Shahandeh. 1988. viii, 91p. pap. 13.50 (*92-2-100526-7*) Intl Labour Office.

Rehabilitation Aspects of Drug Dependence. Ed. by Arnold J. Schecter. 1977. 192p. 112.00 (*0-8493-5475-7*, RC566, CRC Reprint) Franklin.

Rehabilitation Assistant. Jack Rudman. 1994. (Career Examination Ser.: C-545). pap. 29.95 (*0-8373-0545-4*) Nat Learn.

Rehabilitation Audiology: Children & Adults. Ed. by Jerome G. Alpiner & Patricia A. McCarthy. 3rd ed. 1999. LC 99-32657. 690p. text 60.00 (*0-683-30652-9*) Lppncott W & W.

Rehabilitation Caseload Management: Concepts & Practice. Jack L. Cassell & S. Wayne Mulkey. 1985. LC 85-3385. 350p. pap. text 34.00 (*0-936104-67-8*, 1275) PRO-ED.

Rehabilitation Center: Role Play Peacegames. David W. Felder. 1996. 44p. pap. text 8.95 (*0-910959-68-4*, B&G 13D) Wellington Pr.

Rehabilitation Counseling: Basics & Beyond. Ed. by Edna Szymanski & Randall M. Parker. 2nd ed. 1992. LC 97-10241. 444p. (Orig.). pap. text 36.00 (*0-89079-518-5*, 1409) PRO-ED.

Rehabilitation Counseling: Basics & Beyond. Randall M. Parker & Edna Szymanski. 3rd ed. 1997. LC 97-10241. 348p. (Orig.). pap. 39.00 (*0-89079-723-4*, 7807) PRO-ED.

Rehabilitation Counseling: Collected Papers. C. H. Patterson. 1969. pap. 7.80 (*0-87563-015-4*) Stipes.

Rehabilitation Counselor. Jack Rudman. 1994. (Career Examination Ser.: C-672). pap. 29.95 (*0-8373-0672-8*) Nat Learn.

Rehabilitation Counselor Trainee. Jack Rudman. 1994. (Career Examination Ser.: C-1783). pap. 27.95 (*0-8373-1783-5*) Nat Learn.

Rehabilitation Engineering. Ed. by Raymond V. Smith. 1990. 576p. 289.00 (*0-8493-6951-7*, RM950) CRC Pr.

Rehabilitation Engineering Applied to Mobility & Manipulation. Rory A. Cooper. 1995. LC 95-38066. (Medical Science Ser.). (Illus.). 516p. 200.00 (*0-7503-0343-3*, RM950) Inst of Physics Pubng.

Rehabilitation Equipment & Product Market—1995 Update: Effective Technology Leads to Improved Patient Compliance. Frost and Sullivan Staff. 1996. 381p. spiral bd. 1995.00 (*0-7889-0418-3*, 5313-58) Frost & Sullivan.

Rehabilitation Evaluation: Some Application Guidelines. Ed. by James A. Bitter & Don L. Goodyear. 1975. LC 75-9719. text 32.50 (*0-8422-5223-1*); pap. text 12.95 (*0-8422-0502-0*) Irvington.

Rehabilitation for Mental Health Problems: An Introduction Handbook. Clephane A. Hume & Ian Pullen. 2nd ed. 1993. LC 93-18261. 288p. pap. text (*0-443-04554-2*) Church.

Rehabilitation for the Post-Surgical Patient: Procedures & Protocols. Lisa Maxey & Jim Magnusson. 1999. LC 00-51100. (Illus.). 416p. (C). text 59.00 (*0-323-00166-1*) Mosby Inc.

Rehabilitation for Traumatic Brain Injury. Baontke et al. Date not set. 40.00 (*0-7506-9581-1*) Buttrwrth-Heinemann.

Rehabilitation for Traumatic Brain Injury. Ed. by Randall M. Chestnut. 1999. 176p. (C). pap. text 35.00 (*0-7881-8376-1*) DIANE Pub.

Rehabilitation in Managed Care: Controlling Cost, Ensuring Quality. Chris Hagen. 1997. LC 99-12291. 300p. pap. 45.00 (*0-8342-0923-3*, 20923) PRO-ED.

Rehabilitation in Mental Health Goals & Objectives for Independent Living. Barbara J. Hemphill et al. 1991. LC 89-43121. 160p. pap. 29.00 (*1-55642-143-5*) SLACK Inc.

Rehabilitation in Parkinson's Disease. F. I. Caird. 1991. (Therapy in Practice Ser.: No. 25). pap. 33.95 (*0-412-34600-1*) Chapman & Hall.

Rehabilitation in Parkinson's Disease. F. I. Caird. 1991. 144p. pap. 54.50 (*1-56593-561-6*, 0707) Singular Publishing.

Rehabilitation in Psychiatry: An Introductory Handbook. Clephane Hume & Ian Pullen. 1986. LC 85-11677. (Illus.). 256p. (Orig.). pap. text (*0-443-02509-6*) Church.

Rehabilitation in Sports Medicine. Ed. by Paul K. Canavan. 10th ed. 1997. LC 97-17095. 600p. (C). text 69.95 (*0-8385-8313-X*, A-8313-7) McGraw-Hill Prof.

Rehabilitation Inspector. Jack Rudman. 1994. (Career Examination Ser.: C-2639). pap. 34.95 (*0-8373-2639-7*) Nat Learn.

Rehabilitation Interventions for the Institutionalized Elderly. Ed. by Ellen D. Taira. 1989. LC 88-18065. (Physical & Occupational Therapy in Geriatrics Ser.: Vol. 6, No. 2). (Illus.). 77p. text 39.95 (*0-86656-833-6*) Haworth Pr.

Rehabilitation Literature, 1950 to 1955: A Bibliographic Review of the Medical Care, Education, Employment, Welfare & Psychology of Handicapped Children & Adults. Earl C. Graham & Marjorie Mullen. Ed. by William R. Phillips & Janet Rosenberg. 1980. LC 79-6901. (Physically Handicapped in Society Ser.). reprint ed. lib. bdg. 61.95 (*0-405-13112-7*) Ayer.

Rehabilitation Medicine: Principles & Practice. Joel A. Delisa & Bruce M. Gans. 3rd ed. 1998. LC 97-49687. (Illus.). 1,856p. text 199.00 (*0-7817-1015-4*) Lppncott W & W.

Rehabilitation Methods in Neuropsychiatry. Nicholas L. Rock et al. 1996. LC 95-48870. (Illus.). 314p. (Orig.). pap. 49.95 (*1-56593-632-9*, 1310) Thomson Learn.

Rehabilitation Model of Substance Abuse Counseling. John J. Benshoff & Timothy P. Janikowski. 1999. LC 99-50374. (Counseling Ser.). (Illus.). 300p. pap. text 57.95 (*0-534-34223-X*) Brooks-Cole.

Rehabilitation, Music & Human Well-Being. Ed. by Mathew H.M. Lee. 1989. (Illus.). 263p. pap. 29.95 (*0-918812-59-3*, ST 190) MMB Music.

Rehabilitation Nurse's Survival Guide. Roslyn Heffner. 1994. (Illus.). 360p. (Orig.). pap. 20.00 (*0-9653317-0-9*) R Heffner Vocat.

Rehabilitation Nursing: Process & Application. Shirley P. Hoeman. 2nd ed. 1995. LC 94-49100. (Illus.). 752p. (C). (gr. 13). text 64.00 (*0-8016-7766-1*, 07766) Mosby Inc.

Rehabilitation Nursing: Process & Application. Ed. by Shirley P. Hoeman. 3rd ed. 2001. 862p. text (*0-323-01190-X*) Mosby Inc.

Rehabilitation Nursing for the Neurological Patient. Marcia Hanak. 1992. LC 91-5189. 240p. (C). 32.95 (*0-8261-7660-7*) Springer Pub.

Rehabilitation Nursing Procedures Manual. Therese Alexander et al. 2nd ed. 1999. LC 99-10684. (Illus.). 448p. pap. 59.95 (*0-07-048266-7*) McGraw-Hill Prof.

Rehabilitation of Arthritic Hand & Wrist. Mackin. 2000. (*0-443-08997-3*) Church.

Rehabilitation of Cognitive Disabilities. Ed. by J. Michael Williams & Charles J. Long. 1987. (Illus.). 246p. (C). 102.00 (*0-306-42594-7*, Plenum Trade) Perseus Pubng.

Rehabilitation of Movement. Pitt-Brook. 1997. pap. text 69.00 (*0-7020-2157-1*) Saunders.

Rehabilitation of Older People: A Handbook for the Multidisciplinary Team. Ed. by Ananda J. Squires. 2nd ed. 1996. (Illus.). 316p. (Orig.). pap. 49.95 (*1-56593-735-X*, 1430) Singular Publishing.

Rehabilitation of People with Traumatic Brain Injury. Shanker Nesathurai. 2000. (Illus.). 128p. pap. 16.95 (*0-632-04517-5*) Blackwell Sci.

Rehabilitation of Persons with Rheumatoid Arthritis. Rouland W. Chang et al. 1996. 300p. 79.00 (*0-8342-0679-X*, 20679) PRO-ED.

Rehabilitation of the Adult & Child with Traumatic Brain Injury. Ed. by M. Rosenthal et al. 3rd ed. 1999. LC 98-37319. (Illus.). 620p. (C). text 89.00 (*0-8036-0391-6*) Davis Co.

Rehabilitation of the Aging & Elderly Patient. Susan J. Garrison. Ed. by Gerald Felsenthal et al. 1993. LC 92-48558. (Illus.). 592p. 91.00 (*0-683-03125-2*) Lppncott W & W.

Rehabilitation of the Brain-Damaged Adult. Gerald Goldstein & Leslie Ruthven. 1983. (Applied Clinical Psychology Ser.). 280p. 54.50 (*0-306-40498-2*, Plenum Trade) Perseus Pubng.

Rehabilitation of the Brain Injured Adult. Gordon M. Giles & Jo Clark-Watson. 2nd ed. 1999. (Illus.). 352p. pap. (*0-7487-3352-3*) Nelson Thornes GBR. *Dist:* Intl Spec Bk.

Rehabilitation of the Cardiac Patient. Ed. by Nanette K. Wenger et al. 1987. (Advances in Cardiology Ser.: Vol. 33). (Illus.). xvi, 192p. 142.75 (*3-8055-4339-5*) S Karger.

Rehabilitation of the Foot. Anthony Sammarco. 1994. (Illus.). 402p. (C). (gr. 13). text 84.00 (*0-8016-7771-8*, 07771) Mosby Inc.

Rehabilitation of the Hand. James M. Hunter. 4th ed. 1995. (Illus.). 2080p. (C). (gr. 13). text 225.00 (*0-8016-7125-6*, 07125) Mosby Inc.

Rehabilitation of the Knee: A Problem Solving Approach. Ed. by Bruce H. Greenfield et al. 1993. LC 93-324. (Contemporary Perspectives in Rehabilitation Ser.: Vol. 11). (Illus.). 467p. (C). text 45.95 (*0-8036-4335-7*) Davis Co.

Rehabilitation of the Older Adult. Andrews. (*0-340-54825-8*) E A.

Rehabilitation of the Older Adult. Keith Andrews. 1988. (Illus.). 388p. (C). text (*0-683-13002-1*) E A GBR. *Dist:* Williams & Wilkins.

Rehabilitation of the Patient with Respiratory Disease. annuals Neil S. Cherniack et al. 1998. LC 99-10475. (Illus.). 1100p. text 129.00 (*0-07-011649-0*) McGraw-Hill Prof.

Rehabilitation of the Physically Disabled Adult. C. John Goodwill. Ed. by M. Anne Chamberlain & Chris Evans. 2nd ed. 1997. (Illus.). 580p. pap. 125.00 (*1-56593-320-6*, 0650) Singular Publishing.

Rehabilitation of the Spine: A Practitioner's Manual. Ed. by Craig Liebenson. 1996. (Illus.). 464p. 82.00 (*0-683-05032-X*) Lppncott W & W.

Rehabilitation of the Surgical Knee. Ed. by George J. Davies. 1984. (Illus.). 100p. (Orig.). pap. 25.00 (*0-930269-00-4*) CyPr NY.

Rehabilitation of the TBI Patient in the ICU: Integrating Critical Care & Early Rehabilitation. Linda E. Mackay et al. 1997. LC 97-21586. 622p. 86.00 (*0-8342-0655-2*) PRO-ED.

Rehabilitation of the Wounded. Ed. by Carl Kelsy et al. 1980. LC 79-6910. (Physically Handicapped in Society Ser.). reprint ed. lib. bdg. 19.95 (*0-405-13120-8*) Ayer.

Rehabilitation R & D Progress Reports (1997) Ed. by Tamara T. Sowell. 1998. 357p. (C). pap. text 50.00 (*0-7881-7330-8*) DIANE Pub.

Rehabilitation R&D Progress Reports, 1995. 1997. 359p. reprint ed. pap. text 50.00 (*0-7881-4696-3*) DIANE Pub.

Rehabilitation Series for Lower Extremity Amputees Robert S. Gailey & Ann M. Gailey. 1995. (Illus.). 201p. pap. text 25.00 (*1-888131-04-7*) Adv Rehab Therapy.

Rehabilitation Sourcebook: Basic Consumer Health Information about Rehabilitation & the Recovery & Therapy Processes. Ed. by Theresa Murray. 1999. LC 99-45827. (Health Reference Ser.). (Illus.). xii, 531p. lib. bdg. 78.00 (*0-7808-0236-5*) Omnigraphics Inc.

Rehabilitation Specialist's Handbook. Jules M. Rothstein et al. 2nd ed. 1997. LC 97-18584. (Illus.). 1267p. (C). pap. text 41.95 (*0-8036-0047-X*) Davis Co.

Rehabilitation Strategies for Sensorineural Hearing Loss: Proceedings of the 2nd Conference on Auditory Techniques. Ed. by Paul Yanick, Jr. 1979. 240p. text 29.50 (*0-8089-1215-1*, 794946, Grune & Strat) Harcrt Hlth Sci Grp.

Rehabilitation Studies Handbook. Ed. by Barbara A. Wilson & D. L. McLellan. 1997. LC 96-22502. (Illus.). 425p. (C). pap. text 54.95 (*0-521-43713-X*) Cambridge U Pr.

Rehabilitation Surgery for Deformities Due to Poliomyelitis: Techniques for the District Hospital. Ed. by Edwin J. Krol & World Health Organization Staff. 1993. (CHI, ENG & FRE., Illus.). 112p. pap. text 25.00 (*92-4-154457-0*, 1150403) World Health.

Rehabilitation Teaching: For Persons Experiencing Vision Loss. Diane S. Weiss et al. Ed. by Irene Ludwig. 2nd ed. 1998. (CIL Publications & Audiobks.). 118p. (C). pap. text 24.00 (*1-890786-07-1*) Visions-Srvs.

Rehabilitation Techniques in Sports Medicine. William E. Prentice. 1993. (C). pap. text 79.38 (*0-8016-7819-6*); 1993. (C). pap. text 79.38 (*0-8016-7820-X*); 3rd ed. 1998. LC 98-6338. (Illus.). 624p. text 74.69 (*0-07-289470-9*) McGrw-H Hghr Educ.

Rehabilitation Technology. Glenn Hedman. 1990. LC 90-4593. (Physical & Occupational Therapy in Pediatrics Ser.: Vol. 10, No. 2). (Illus.). 181p. text 39.95 (*1-56024-033-4*) Haworth Pr.

Rehabilitation Technology: Strategies for the European Union: Proceedings of the First Tide Congress, Apr 6-7, 1993, Brussels. Ed. by E. Ballabio et al. 1993. LC 93-78138. (Studies in Health Technology & Informatics: Vol. 9). 261p. 105.00 (*90-5199-131-2*) IOS Press.

***Rehabilitation und Nachsorge von Patienten nach Stammzellentransplantation.** Ed. by H. H. Bartsch. 2001. (GER.). viii, 180p. 65.75 (*3-8055-7234-4*) S Karger.

Rehabilitative & Restorative Nursing in LTC. Marguerite A. Bouvette. 1988. (Illus.). 122p. (C). 17.50 (*1-877735-24-8*, 2141PP) Prof Prnting & Pub.

Rehabilitative Audiology. Ed. by Raymond Hull. 1982. 542p. text 47.00 (*0-8089-1434-0*, 792079, Grune & Strat) Harcrt Hlth Sci Grp.

Rehabilitative Audiology: Children & Adults. Jerome G. Alpiner & Patricia A. McCarthy. 2nd ed. 1993. (Illus.). 544p. 49.00 (*0-683-00078-0*) Lppncott W & W.

Rehearsals for Growth: Theater Improvisation for Psychotherapists. Daniel J. Wiener. 1994. LC 94-20894. 288p. 32.00 (*0-393-70187-5*) Norton.

Reich for Beginners. David Z. Mairowitz. 1986. (Writers & Readers Documentary Comic Bks.). (Illus.). 176p. pap. 6.95 (*0-86316-031-X*) Writers & Readers.

Reid's Controversy in Obstetrics & Gynecology 3. Frederick P. Zuspan & C. Donald Christian. 3rd ed. 1983. (Illus.). 672p. text 145.00 (*0-7216-2565-7*) Saunders.

Reiki: A Practical Guide. Bill Liaites et al. 1998. (Healing Ser.). (Illus.). 128p. pap. (*965-494-046-9*) Astrolog Pub ISR. *Dist:* Assoc Pubs Grp, IPG Chicago.

Reiki: A Torch in Daylight. Karyn K. Mitchell. 1994. LC 94-75679. 128p. pap., stu. ed. 14.95 (*0-9640822-1-7*) Mind Rivers.

Reiki: Beyond the Usui System. Karyn K. Mitchell. 1994. 256p. (Orig.). pap., stu. ed. 19.96 (*0-9640822-2-5*) Mind Rivers.

Reiki: The Healer's Touch. Elizabeth F. Severino. 1995. (Illus.). 202p. pap. 19.95 (*1-888674-08-3*) Healing Connect.

Reiki - for First Aid: Reiki Treatment As Accompanying Therapy for Over 40 Types of Illness. With a Supplement on Natural Healing. Walter Lubeck. 1995. 160p. (Orig.). pap. 14.95 (*0-914955-26-8*) Lotus Pr.

Reiki - Hands That Heal. Joyce J. Morris. rev. ed. 1996. (Illus.). 200p. (Orig.). pap. 22.00 (*1-888196-22-X*) Ctr Bkstore.

Reiki - Universal Life Energy: Heals Body, Mind & Spirit - A Holistic Method Suitable for Self-Treatment & the Home, Professional Practice, Teleotherapeutics-Spiritual Healing. Bodo Baginski & Shalila Sharamon. Tr. by Chris Baker & Judith Harrison from GER. 2001. (Illus.). 211p. (Orig.). reprint ed. pap. 12.95 (*0-940795-02-7*) LifeRhythm.

Reiki & Medicine. Nancy Eos. 1995. LC 95-90006. (Illus.). 108p. (Orig.). pap. 14.95 (*0-9644923-0-X*) Nancy Eos.

Reiki Class. William L. Rand. 1994. pap. Price not set. incl. audio (*1-886785-01-5*) Vision Pub.

Reiki Energy Medicine: Bringing the Healing Touch into Home, Hospital, & Hospice. Libby Barnett et al. 1996. LC 96-3962. (Illus.). 192p. pap. 12.95 (*0-89281-633-3*, Heal Arts VT) Inner Tradit.

Reiki Fire: New Information about the Origin of the Reiki Power a Complete Method. Frank A. Petter. 1997. LC 97-71444. (Shangri-La Ser.). (Illus.). 144p. (Orig.). pap. 12.95 (*0-914955-50-0*) Lotus Pr.

Reiki Handbook. Larry Arnold & Sandy Nevius. 4th ed. 1982. 160p. pap. 13.50 (*0-9625500-1-9*) PSI Pr PA.

Reiki II Manual. Karen Miller. 2nd ed. 1993. (Illus.). 124p. (Orig.). spiral bd. 12.95 (*0-9630439-6-X*) Bayrock.

Reiki in Everyday Living: How Universal Energy Is a Natural Part of Life, Medicine, & Personal Growth. Earlene F. Gleisner. 4th ed. 1993. (ENG, IND, POR & SWE.). 104p. (Orig.). pap. 12.95 (*1-880357-07-0*) WFP.

Reiki Plus Natural Healing: A Manual for First Degree Reiki Natural Healing. David G. Jarrell. Ed. by Richard Levitt. 5th rev. ed. 1983. (Illus.). 96p. per. 15.00 (*0-9634690-0-2*) Reiki Plus.

Reiki Plus Professional Practitioner's Manual for Second Degree: A Spiritual & Practitioner's Guide for Reiki Natural Healing & Holistic Healthcare Providers. David G. Jarrell & Richelle M. Jarrell. 3rd rev. ed. 2000. (Illus.). 176p. pap. 22.00 (*0-9634690-3-7*) Reiki Plus.

Reiki Practical Ways to Harmony. Mari Hall. 2001. (*0-00-710124-4*) Thorsons GBR. *Dist:* Natl Bk Netwk.

Reimbursement for Athletic Trainers. Marjorie Albohm et al. 2001. LC 2001-20075. (Athletic Training Library). 148p. (C). pap. text 24.00 (*1-55642-408-6*) SLACK Inc.

Reimbursement Manual for the Medical Office. James B. Davis. 3rd ed. 1996. 316p. pap. text 49.95 (*1-57066-025-5*, ME064) Practice Mgmt Info.

Reimbursement Manual for the Medical Office. James B. Davis. Ed. by Kathryn Swanson. 4th rev. ed. 2000. LC 00-34001. 460p. pap. text 49.95 (*1-57066-147-2*, ME123) Practice Mgmt Info.

Reimbursement Strategies for Medical Equipment in Managed Care. Brian Rasmussen. 1997. LC 97-16282. ring bd. 159.00 (*0-8342-0868-7*, S440) Aspen Pub.

Reintegration Resource: Compensatory Bridges to Independence. Donna Miazga. 1995. pap. 35.00 (*0-930599-42-X*) Thinking Pubns.

Reintegration to School after Hospital Treatment: Needs & Services. Isobel Larcombe. 1995. 137p. (C). (*1-85628-990-7*) Avebry GBR. *Dist:* Ashgate Pub Co.

Reinterpreting Menopause. Ed. by Paul Komesaroff et al. 1997. LC 96-28892. 288p. (C). 75.00 (*0-415-91564-3*); pap. 22.95 (*0-415-91565-1*) Routledge.

Reinventing Eve: Modern Woman in Search of Herself. Kim Chernin. 2nd ed. 1994. LC 93-40772. 224p. reprint ed. pap. 14.00 (*0-06-092503-5*, Perennial) HarperTrade.

Reinventing Healthcare. Jack J. Tawil & F. C. Bold. 1994. vii, 310p. 23.95 (*1-883021-12-X*) Research Ent.

Reinventing Hospitals: On Target for the 21st Century. Isabel Milton et al. 1998. 257p. pap. (*0-919292-03-8*) Stoddart Publ CAN. *Dist:* General Distrib Services.

Reinventing Medicine: Beyond Mind-Body to a New Era of Healing. Larry Dossey. LC 99-27970. 288p. 2000. pap. 14.00 (*0-06-251644-2*); 1999. 24.00 (*0-06-251622-1*) Harper SF.

Reinventing the Sexes: Biomedical Construction of Femininity & Masculinity. Marianne Van den Wijngaard. 1997. LC 96-41378. (Race, Gender & Science Ser.). 29.95 (*0-253-33250-8*); 184p. pap. 12.95 (*0-253-21087-9*) Ind U Pr.

Reinventing Your Nursing Career: A Handbook for Success in the Age of Managed Care. Michael Newell & Mario Pinardo. 1997. LC 97-30346. 272p. pap. 37.00 (*0-8342-1007-X*, 21007) Aspen Pub.

Reinventing Your Practice as a Business Psychologist: A Step-by-Step Guide. Louis A. Perrott. 1999. LC 98-40286. (Jossey-Bass Psychology Ser.). 224p. 40.00 (*0-7879-4349-5*) Jossey-Bass.

Reishi: Ancient Herb for Modern Times. Kenneth Jones. 1992. (Illus.). 34p. (Orig.). pap. 5.95 (*0-9625638-1-1*) Sylvan Pr WA.

Reiter Treponeme: A Review of the Literature. A. L. Wallace & A. D. Harris. 1967. pap. text 12.00 (*92-4-068362-3*, 1033602) World Health.

Rejection. James R. Sherman. 1982. LC 81-86079. 87p. (Orig.). pap. 4.95 (*0-935538-02-X*) Pathway Bks.

Rejection & Tolerance: Proceedings of the 25th Conference on Transplantation & Clinical Immunology 24-26 May 1993. Ed. by J. L. Touraine. 1994. (Transplantation & Clinical Immunology Ser.: No. 25). 472p. (C). text 200.50 (*0-7923-2671-7*) Kluwer Academic.

Rejuvenating Plants of Tropical Africa: Aphrodisiacs, Sterility, Impotence, Infertility. Albert A. Enti. Ed. & Intro. by Anthony K. Andoh. 1988. LC 88-63959. (Illus.). 56p. (Orig.). pap. 9.95 (*0-916299-07-4*) North Scale Co.

Rejuvenation: A Wellness Guide for Women & Men. Horst Rechelbacher. 1987. (Illus.). 224p. pap. 14.95 (*0-89281-248-6*, Heal Arts VT) Inner Tradit.

Rejuvenator's Bible: Winning the Anti-Aging Revolution - Working Ways to Create Perpetual Youth Naturally. Jesse Anson Dawn. 1999. LC 99-71085. (Illus.). 238p. pap. (*0-9636589-1-3*) Wrld Changing.

Relacion Hospedante-Parasito Mecanismo de Patogenicidad de los Microorganismos. Manuel R. Leiva. 1981. (Serie de Biologia: No. 14). 91p. (C). pap. 3.50 (*0-8270-1322-1*) OAS.

Relapse: A Guide to Successful Recovery. Dennis C. Daley. Ed. by Lee M. Joiner. 1987. LC 87-24385. 48p. (Orig.). pap. text 4.25 (*0-943519-02-0*, B1902) Sulzburger & Graham Pub.

Relapse: Conceptual, Research & Clinical Perspectives. Pref. by Dennis C. Daley. LC 89-15611. (Journal of Chemical Dependency Treatment Ser.: Vol. 2, No. 2). (Illus.). 257p. 1994. text 49.95 (*0-86656-919-7*); 1989. pap. text 19.95 (*0-86656-976-6*) Haworth Pr.

Relapse & Addictive Behaviour. Michael Gossop. 1989. 224p. 35.00 (*0-415-02354-8*) Routledge.

Relapse & Recovery in Drug Abuse. 1991. lib. bdg. 77.95 (*0-8490-4356-5*) Gordon Pr.

Relapse Prevention. Dennis C. Daley. 1989. pap. 14.95 (*0-8306-9004-2*) Sulzburger & Graham Pub.

Relapse Prevention. Gregory L. Little. 1996. 40p. pap., wbk. ed. 10.00 (*0-9655392-1-0*) Advanced Trnging.

Relapse Prevention: Maintenance Strategies in the Treatment of Addiction. Ed. by G. Alan Marlatt & Judith R. Gordon. 1985. LC 84-19319. (Guilford Clinical Psychology & Psychotherapy Ser.). 558p. text 58.00 (*0-89862-009-0*, 2009) Guilford Pubns.

Relapse Prevention: Treatment Alternatives & Counseling Aids. Dennis C. Daley. Ed. by Lee M. Joiner. 1988. LC 88-873. 144p. (Orig.). pap. text 14.95 (*0-943519-06-3*, B1906) Sulzburger & Graham Pub.

Relapse Prevention Counseling for African Americans: A Culturally Specific Model. Roland Williams & Terence T. Gorski. 1997. LC 97-228815. 112p. pap. text 9.00 (*0-8309-0774-2*) Herald Pub Hse.

Relapse Prevention Counseling Workbook: Managing High-Risk Situations. Terence T. Gorski. 1996. LC 95-48376. 4.50 (*0-8309-0739-4*) Herald Pub Hse.

Relapse Prevention with REBT. F. Michler Bishop. wbk. ed. 22.95 incl. audio (*0-917476-26-3*, C050) Inst Rational-Emotive.

Relapse Prevention Workbook for Women. Karen Mattson. 1992. 48p. pap. 5.50 (*1-56246-030-7*, 3227, HazeldenJohnson Inst) Hazelden.

Relapse Prevention Workbook for Youth in Treatment. Charlene Steen. Ed. by Euan Bear et al. 1993. 160p. (Orig.). pap. 15.00 (*1-884444-02-4*) Safer Soc.

Relating: Dialogues & Dialectics. Leslie A. Baxter & Barbara M. Montgomery. 1996. LC 96-18281. 285p. 42.00 (*1-57230-099-X*) Guilford Pubns.

Relating & Interacting: An Introduction to Interpersonal Communication. Raymond S. Ross & Mark Ross. 1982. (Illus.). 320p. (C). pap. text 33.05 (*0-13-771923-X*) P-H.

Relating in Psychotherapy: The Application of a New Theory. John Birtchnell. 1999. LC 98-38281. (Human Evolution, Behavior, & Intelligence Ser.). 288p. 68.00 (*0-275-96376-4*, Praeger Pubs) Greenwood.

Relating Theory & Data: Essays on Human Memory in Honor of Bennet B. Murdock. Ed. by William Hockley & Stephen Lewandowsky. 1991. 576p. pap. 49.95 (*0-8058-0733-0*); text 99.95 (*0-8058-0732-2*) L Erlbaum Assocs.

Relating to the Relatives: Breaking Bad News, Communication & Support. Thurstan B. Brewin & Margaret Sparshott. 1996. LC 96-42946. 192p. (*1-85775-081-0*) Radcliffe Med Pr GBR. *Dist:* Balogh.

Relation of Accelerated Normal & Retarded Puberty to the Height & Weight of School Children. Herman G. Richard. 1937. (SRCD M Ser.: Vol. 2, No. 1). pap. 25.00 (*0-527-01494-X*) Periodicals Srv.

Relation of Aging to Immunity. R. L. Walford et al. 1973. (Illus.). 220p. (C). text 32.75 (*0-8422-7106-6*) Irvington.

Relation of Certain Anomalies of Vision & Lateral Dominance to Reading Disability. Philip W. Johnston. 1942. (SRCD M Ser.: Vol. 7, No. 2). 25.00 (*0-527-01523-7*) Periodicals Srv.

Relation of Certain Formal Attributes of Siblings to Attitudes Held Toward Each Other & Toward Their Parents. H. L. Koch. 1960. (SRCD M Ser.: Vol. 25, No. 4). 25.00 (*0-527-01586-5*) Periodicals Srv.

Relation of Parental Authority to Children's Behavior & Attitudes, Vol. 22. Marian J. Yarrow. 1969. LC 76-92312. 123p. reprint ed. lib. bdg. 48.00 (*0-8371-2701-7*, YAPA, Greenwood Pr) Greenwood.

Relation of Sensation to Other Categories in Contemporary Psychology. Carl Rahn. 1974. (Psychology Monographs General & Applied: Vol. 16). reprint ed. pap. 55.00 (*0-8115-1415-3*) Periodicals Srv.

Relation of Theory to Practice in Psychotherapy. Ed. by Leonard D. Eron & Robert Callahan. 1969. LC 69-13705. 42.50 (*0-202-26017-8*) Irvington.

Relational Concepts in Psychoanalysis: An Integration. Stephen A. Mitchell. 1988. LC 88-11168. 312p. 48.95 (*0-674-75411-5*) HUP.

Relational Perspectives in Psychoanalysis. Ed. by Neil J. Skolnick & Susan C. Warshaw. 1992. LC 92-49413. 392p. 49.95 (*0-88163-107-8*) Analytic Pr.

Relational Psychoanalysis: The Emergence of a Tradition. Ed. by Stephen A. Mitchell & Lewis Aron. 1999. LC 99-228505. (Relational Perspectives Bks.: Vol. 14). 536p. pap. 39.95 (*0-88163-270-8*) Analytic Pr.

Relational Self: Theoretical Convergences in Psychoanalysis & Social Psychology. Ed. by Rebecca C. Curtis. 1991. LC 90-15734. 319p. 41.95 (*0-89862-558-0*) Guilford Pubns.

Relational Systems Model for Family Therapy: Living in the Four Realities. Donald R. Bardill. 1996. LC 96-4072. (Illus.). 294p. (C). 49.95 (*0-7890-0074-1*) Haworth Pr.

Relational Therapy for Personality Disorders. Jeffrey J. Magnavita. 1999. LC 99-11517. (Couples & Family Dynamics & Treatment Ser.). 291p. 45.00 (*0-471-29566-3*) Wiley.

Relations Between Psychopathological & Socio-Professional Factors in Out-Patient Department Psychiatry. Ed. by G. Leresche & J. Bovet. 1986. (Journal: Vol. 19, Suppl. 1, 1986). (Illus.). 260p. pap. 68.00 (*3-8055-4332-8*) S Karger.

Relations of Development & Aging. Ed. by James E. Birren & Leon Stein. 1980. LC 79-8659. (Growing Old Ser.). (Illus.). reprint ed. lib. bdg. 30.95 (*0-405-12775-8*) Ayer.

Relationship Between Emotional Expression, Treatment, & Outcome in Psychotherapy: An Empirical Study. Rita Rosner. 1996. LC 96-41164. (European University Studies: Series 6, Vol. 565). (Illus.). 138p. pap. text 35.95 (*0-8204-2983-X*) P Lang Pubng.

Relationship Between HIV & Other Conditions. (*0-340-58715-6*) E A GBR. *Dist:* Routldge.

Relationship Between Homosexuality & Psychological Functioning in a Perspective of Personality Types. Lena N. Schonnesson. 1983. 283p. (Orig.). 33.50 (*91-22-00634-6*) Coronet Bks.

Relationship Between Inflammation & Structural Changes in the Airways of the Lower & Upper Respiratory Tract: Studies in Patients with Asthma, Sjogren's Syndrome, Rhinitis & Children with Otitis Media with Effusion. Kawa Amin. 2000. (Comprehensive Summaries of Uppsala Dissertations from the Faculty of Medicine Ser.: No. 932). (Illus.). 66p. pap. (*91-554-4727-9*) Uppsala Universitet SWE. *Dist:* Coronet Bks.

Relationship Between Mental Health & Substance Abuse among Adolescents. Ed. by Dena R. Gerstein & Janet Greenblatt. 2000. (Illus.). 216p. (C). pap. text 30.00 (*0-7881-8841-0*) DIANE Pub.

Relationship Between Prefrontal & Limbic Cortex: A Comparative Anatomical Review. Ed. by R. Reep. 1985. (Journal: Vol. 25, Nos. 1-2). (Illus.). 80p. pap. 48.00 (*3-8055-4033-7*) S Karger.

Relationship Between Social & Cognitive Development. Ed. by Willis F. Overton. 1983. (Jean Piaget Symposia Ser.). 272p. (C). text 49.95 (*0-89859-249-6*) L Erlbaum Assocs.

Relationship Enhancement Family Therapy. Barry G. Ginsberg. 1997. LC 96-46033. (Couples & Family Dynamics & Treatment Ser.). 286p. 95.00 (*0-471-04955-7*) Wiley.

Relationship Management of the Borderline Patient: From Understanding to Treatment. David L. Dawson & Harriet L. MacMillan. 1993. LC 93-18886. (Illus.). 240p. text 30.95 (*0-87630-714-4*) Brunner-Routledge.

Relationship of Histology to Cancer Treatment: Proceedings of the West Coast Cancer Symposium, 9th Annual, San Francisco, 1973. West Coast Cancer Symposium Staff. Ed. by J. M. Vaeth. 1974. (Frontiers of Radiation Therapy & Oncology Ser.: Vol. 9). 200p. 123.50 (*3-8055-1748-3*) S Karger.

Relationship of Verbal & Non-Verbal Communication. Ed. by Mary R. Key. 1981. (Contributions to the Sociology of Language Ser.: No. 25). pap. text (*90-279-7637-6*) Mouton DEU. *Dist:* De Gruyter.

Relationships: Adult Children of Alcoholics. Joseph F. Perez. 1989. LC 87-21105. 23.95 (*0-89876-150-6*) Gardner Pr.

Relationships & Development. Ed. by William W. Hartup & Z. Rubin. 1986. 240p. text 49.95 (*0-89859-621-1*) L Erlbaum Assocs.

Relationships at Risk: Assessing Your Kid's Drug Abuse Potential. Timothy Titus. 1990. LC 90-81091. (Illus.). 49p. stu. ed. 6.95 (*0-925190-02-0*) Fairview Press.

P
Q
R

Relationships Between Women in Later Life. Ed. by Karen A. Roberto. 1996. LC 96-30653. (Journal of Women & Aging Ser.: Vol. 8, Nos. 3/4). 204p. (C). pap. 14.95 (*1-56023-091-6*, Harrington Park) Haworth Pr.

Relationships, Chronic Illness, & Disability. Renee F. Lyons et al. 1995. LC 95-4428. (Series on Close Relationships: Vol. 11). 176p. 64.95 (*0-8039-4703-8*, 1769); pap. 36.95 (*0-8039-4704-6*, 1770) Sage.

Relationships in Dermatology: The Skin & Mouth, Eye, Sarcoidosis, Porphyria. Ed. by Julian L. Verbov. 1988. (New Clinical Applications in Dermatology Ser.). (C). text 95.50 (*0-7462-0097-8*) Kluwer Academic.

Relationships in Marriage & Family. Nick Stinnet & Nancy Stinnet. 3rd ed. 1990. LC 90-32511. 496p. (C). 120.00 (*0-02-417580-3*, Macmillan Coll) P-H.

Relationships in Old Age: Coping with the Challenge of Transition. Robert O. Hansson & Bruce N. Carpenter. 1994. LC 93-46488. (Guilford Series on Personal Relationships Ser.). 180p. text 30.00 (*0-89862-198-4*, 2198) Guilford Pubns.

Relationships in Recovery: Healing Strategies for Couples & Families. Emily Marlin. 1990. LC 89-45687. 288p. pap. 8.95 (*0-00-001645-4*, Perennial) HarperTrade.

Relative Risk Analysis in Regulating the Use of Radiation-Emitting Medical Devices. 1996. lib. bdg. 254.99 (*0-8490-6379-5*) Gordon Pr.

Relative Value Studies: Includes RBRVS, 1999 (ASCII) Ed. by Mark N. Painter & Stacy Louck Sturgeon. 1999. 189.95 incl. disk (*1-929061-01-3*) Relative Val.

Relative Value Studies, Inc. 's Complete RBRVS 2000. Ed. by Stacy Louck Sturgeon & Mark N. Painter. 1999. 560p. pap. 89.00 (*1-929061-02-1*) Relative Val.

Relative Value Studies, Inc.'s Complete RBRVS, 1999. Ed. by Mark N. Painter & Stacy Louck Sturgeon. 1999. 560p. pap. 99.95 (*1-929061-00-5*) Relative Val.

Relative Values for Dentists, 2000. Ed. by Stacy Louck Sturgeon & Mark N. Painter. 1999. 200p. 99.00 (*1-929061-12-9*) Relative Val.

Relative Values for Physicians. Relative Value Studies, Inc. Staff. 1995. incl. disk (*0-07-810178-6*) Healthcare Pr.

Relative Values for Physicians, 1996-1997. Relative Value Studies, Inc. Staff. 1996. 249.00 (*0-07-600822-3*) McGraw.

Relative Values for Therapists, 1999 (ASCII) Ed. by Stacy Louck Sturgeon & Mark N. Painter. 1998. disk 99.00 (*1-929061-26-9*) Relative Val.

Relative Values for Therapists, 1999. Ed. by Stacy Louck Sturgeon & Mark N. Painter. 1998. 175p. 79.00 (*1-929061-25-0*) Relative Val.

Relax & Renew: Restful Yoga for Stressful Times. Judith Lasater. 1995. LC 95-68875. (Illus.). 240p. (Orig.). pap. 21.95 (*0-9627138-4-8*) Rodmell Pr.

Relax, This Won't Hurt: Painless Answers to Women's Most Pressing Health Questions. Judith Reichman. 2001. 384p. pap. 13.00 (*0-06-095932-0*, Quil) HarperTrade.

Relaxation: A Comprehensive Manual for Adults, Children, & Children with Special Needs. Joseph R. Cautela & June Groden. 1978. LC 78-62906. (Illus.). 108p. spiral bd. Price not set. (*0-87822-186-7*, 1867) Res Press.

Relaxation: An Illustrated Programme of Exercises, Techniques & Meditations. Nitya Lacroix & Chrissie Gallagher-Mundy. 2000. (Illus.). 128p. reprint ed. pap. text 17.00 (*0-7881-9135-7*) DIANE Pub.

Relaxation & De-Sensitization Training. Set-RD. Russell E. Mason. 1975. (Train-Ascendance Cassettes Ser.). pap. 45.00 incl. audio (*0-89533-006-7*, 55.GT-RD) F I Comm.

Relaxation Sensation: The Number One Success Factor in Life. Lorenzo. 1981. (Illus.). 128p. (Orig.). pap. 9.95 (*0-941122-00-X*) Lorenzo Prema.

Relaxation Techniques: A Practical Handbook for the Health Care Professional. Rosemary A. Payne. 1995. LC 94-33408. pap. text (*0-443-04933-5*) Church.

Relaxation Techniques: A Practical Handbook for the Health Care Professional. Rosemary A. Payne. 2nd ed. 2000. 264p. pap. text 35.00 (*0-443-06263-3*) Saunders.

Relaxing & Contracting Factors: Biological & Clinical Research. Ed. by Paul M. Vanhoutte. 1988. LC 87-22541. (Endothelium Ser.). 543p. 145.00 (*0-89603-128-4*) Humana.

Release & Disclosure: Guidelines Regarding Maintenance & Disclosure of Health Information. Mary D. Brandt. 1997. 116p. pap. text 35.00 (*1-58426-007-6*, AB101197) Am Hlth Info.

Release & Transport of Drugs in Some Complex & Interacting Systems. Hans Sjoberg. 2000. (Comprehensive Summaries of Uppsala Dissertations from the Faculty of Pharmacy Ser.: No. 229). (Illus.). 46p. pap. (*91-554-4731-7*) Uppsala Universitet SWE. *Dist:* Coronet Bks.

Releasing Anger. S. Richard. 1985. 20p. pap. 2.00 (*0-89486-249-9*, 1420B) Hazelden.

Releasing Arthritis: The Seven Year Plan. Linda F. Fleming. Ed. by Mary Abrams. 1990. LC 89-92230. 200p. (Orig.). pap. 11.00 (*1-877631-02-7*) LF Pub VA.

Releasing Resources to Achieve Health Gain. Ed. by Christopher Riley et al. 1995. (*1-85775-018-7*) Radcliffe Med Pr GBR. *Dist:* Balogh.

Relevance of Animal Studies to the Evaluation of Human Cancer Risk. R. D'Amato et al. 1992. (Progress in Clinical & Biological Research Ser.). 482p. 385.00 (*0-471-56183-5*, Wiley-Interscience) Wiley.

Relevance of Ethnic Factors in the Clinical Evaluation of Medicines. Ed. by Stuart Walker et al. 1994. LC 94-1681. (CMR Workshop Ser.). text 154.50 (*0-7923-8843-7*) Kluwer Academic.

Relevance of the Family to Psychoanalytic Theory. Theodore Lidz. 1992. LC 92-1477. ix, 228p. (C). 37.50 (*0-8236-5784-1*) Intl Univs Pr.

Relevance of the Use of the Couch in Contemporary Psychoanalysis. Moraitis. 1995. (Psychoanalytic Inquiry Ser.: Vol. 15, No. 3). pap. 20.00 (*0-88163-994-X*) Analytic Pr.

Relevance of Tumor Models for Anticancer Drug Development. Ed. by Heinz-Herbert Fiebig. 1999. (Contributions to Oncology Ser.: Vol. 54). (Illus.). viii, 462p. 172.25 (*3-8055-6786-3*) S Karger.

Relevance to Human Cancer of N-Nitroso Compounds, Tobacco Smoke & Mycotoxins. Ed. by I. K. O'Neill et al. 1991. (IARC Scientific Publications Ser.: No. 105). (Illus.). 634p. pap. text 150.00 (*92-832-2105-2*) OUP.

Reliability & Validity in Neuropsychological Assessment. M. D. Franzen. 1989. (Critical Issues in Neuropsychology Ser.). (Illus.). 320p. (C). 54.50 (*0-306-43065-7*, Plenum Trade) Perseus Pubng.

Reliable Design of Medical Devices. Richard C. Fries. 1997. LC 96-49203. (Illus.). 728p. text 235.00 (*0-8247-9843-0*) Dekker.

Reliable Healthcare Companions: Understanding & Managing Arthritis. Ed. by John L. Decker. 1987. 192p. (Orig.). mass mkt. 6.95 (*0-380-75011-2*, Avon Bks) Morrow Avon.

Reliable Healthcare Companions: Understanding & Managing Asthma. John L. Decker. Ed. by Michael A. Kaliner. 1988. 192p. mass mkt. 6.95 (*0-380-75427-4*, Avon Bks) Morrow Avon.

Reliable Healthcare Companions: Understanding & Managing Diabetes. Ed. by John L. Decker & Phillip Gorden. 1987. 192p. mass mkt. 6.95 (*0-380-75247-6*, Avon Bks) Morrow Avon.

Reliable Healthcare Companions: Understanding & Managing Hypertension. John L. Decker & Harry R. Keiser. 1987. 224p. mass mkt. 6.95 (*0-380-75248-4*, Avon Bks) Morrow Avon.

Reliable Healthcare Companions: Understanding & Managing Osteoporosis. Ed. by John L. Decker. 1988. 176p. mass mkt. 6.95 (*0-380-75429-0*, Avon Bks) Morrow Avon.

Reliable Healthcare Companions: Understanding & Managing Ulcers. John L. Decker & Paul N. Maton. 1988. mass mkt. 6.95 (*0-380-75428-2*, Avon Bks) Morrow Avon.

Relief at Last: Neutralization for Food Allergy & Other Illnesses. Joseph B. Miller. 1987. (Illus.). 352p. (C). text 63.95 (*0-398-05283-2*) C C Thomas.

Relief for the Body, Renewal for the Soul. G. Scott Morris. 2001. LC 00-12094. xxiv, 144p. pap. 13.95 (*1-55725-269-6*) Paraclete MA.

Relief from Back Pain: The Tollison Program. C. David Tollison. 1987. 253p. text 24.95 (*0-89876-140-9*) Gardner Pr.

Relief from Candida: Allergies & Ill Health. Greta Sichel. 1994. pap. text (*1-86351-001-X*) Sally Milner AUS. *Dist:* Seven Hills Bk.

Relief from Headache. Donald I. Peterson. 2nd ed. 1990. LC 83-71941. (Illus.). 226p. pap. 9.95 (*0-913657-00-X*) D E Donel.

Relief from IBS (Irritable Bowel Syndrome) Elaine F. Shimberg. 1991. 240p. mass mkt. 6.99 (*0-345-36712-X*) Ballantine Pub Grp.

Relief of Pain from Headaches & TMJ. Paula Mackowiak. 1989. LC 89-927914. (Illus.). 200p. (Orig.). pap. 11.95 (*0-9625508-2-5*) Solomon Bks.

Relief Veterinarian's Manual: (And Survival Guide) Carin A. Smith. rev. ed. 1999. 100p. ring bd., wbk. ed. 79.00 (*1-885780-09-5*) Smith Vet Srvs.

Relieve Your Aching Head: Secrets for Soothing Head & Neck Aches. Anne E. Hunt. Ed. by Eric A. Mein. 1991. (Natural Remedies for Common Ailments & Conditions Ser.). 85p. (Orig.). pap. 4.95 (*0-87604-280-9*, 365) ARE Pr.

Relieving Pain: A Basic Hypotherapeutic Approach. Donald W. Schaefer. 1995. LC 95-21426. 312p. pap. 50.00 (*1-56821-481-2*) Aronson.

Religio Medici: Medicine & Religion in Seventeenth-Century England. Ed. by Ole P. Grell & Andrew Cunningham. 1996. LC 96-2822. (Illus.). 356p. (C). (*1-85928-339-X*) Scolar Pr GBR. *Dist:* Ashgate Pub Co.

Religion, Aging & Health: A Global Perspective. Ed. by William M. Clements. 1989. LC 88-16357. (Journal of Religion & Aging: Vol. 4, Nos. 3-4). (Illus.). 146p. text 39.95 (*0-86656-803-4*) Haworth Pr.

Religion & Mental Illness. Carol R. Murphy. 1955. (C). pap. 4.00 (*0-87574-082-0*) Pendle Hill.

Religion & Neoplatonism in Renaissance Medicine. Walter Pagel. Ed. by Marianne Winder. 1985. (Collected Studies: No. CS226). (Illus.). 346p. (C). reprint ed. text (*0-86078-174-7*) Variorum GBR. *Dist:* Ashgate Pub Co.

Religion & Prevention in Mental Health: Research, Vision & Action. Kenneth I. Pargament et al. 1992. LC 92-5887. (Prevention in Human Services Ser.: Vol. 9, No.2). (Illus.). 232p. text 59.95 (*1-56024-225-6*); pap. text 24.95 (*1-56024-226-4*) Haworth Pr.

Religion & Psychology: A Dialogical Approach. Maurice Friedman. 1992. LC 91-30769. 240p. (C). pap. 16.95 (*1-55778-346-2*) Paragon Hse.

Religion & Psychology in Transition: Psychoanalysis, Feminism & Theology. James W. Jones. 1996. LC 96-15777. (Illus.). 224p. 32.00 (*0-300-06769-0*) Yale U Pr.

Religion & the HIV-AIDS Community: Index of New Information with Authors & Subjects. American Health Research Institute Staff. rev. ed. 1994. LC 94-34806. 109p. 57.50 (*0-7883-0448-8*); pap. 47.50 (*0-7883-0449-6*) ABBE Pubs Assn.

Religion, Belief & Unbelief: A Psychological Study. A. Vergote. 1996. 344p. (Orig.). pap. (*90-6186-751-7*) Leuven Univ BEL. *Dist:* Coronet Bks.

Religion, Health & Suffering: A Cross-Cultural Study of Attitudes to Suffering & the Implications for Medicine in a Multi-Religious Society. John R. Hinnells & Roy Porter. 1998. LC 97-50133. 280p. (*0-7103-0611-3*) Kegan Paul Intl GBR. *Dist:* Col U Pr.

Religion, Personality & Mental Health. Ed. by L. B. Brown. 1993. (Recent Research in Psychology Ser.). (Illus.). 225p. (*3-540-97773-2*) Spr-Verlag.

Religion, Personality & Mental Health. Ed. by Laurence B. Brown. 1994. LC 93-15258. (Recent Research in Psychology Ser.). (Illus.). 217p. 107.00 (*0-387-97773-2*) Spr-Verlag.

Religion, Society & Psychoanalysis: Readings in Contemporary Theory. Donald Capps. Ed. by Janet L. Jacobs. 1997. LC 97-573. 288p. (C). pap. text 31.00 (*0-8133-2648-6*) Westview.

Religion with Medical, Psychological & Philosophical Aspects: Index of New Information & Bible of Progress. Gersten G. Panopolos. 1996. 160p. 57.50 (*0-7883-0226-4*); pap. 47.50 (*0-7883-0227-2*) ABBE Pubs Assn.

Religious & Ethical Factors in Psychiatric Practice. Ed. by Don S. Browning et al. 1990. 313p. text 36.95 (*0-8304-1225-5*) Burnham Inc.

Religious Commitment, Personal Narrative & Healthcare Ethics: Caring Well. David H. Smith. 2000. LC 00-36671. 276p. pap. 24.95 (*0-664-22256-0*) Westminster John Knox.

Religious Diagnosis in a Secular Society: A Staff for the Journey. Donald D. Denton, Jr. 1997. 158p. (C). pap. 29.00 (*0-7618-0965-1*) U Pr of Amer.

Religious Function of the Psyche. Lionel Corbett. 1996. LC 95-25778. 272p. (C). 89.95 (*0-415-14400-0*); pap. 27.95 (*0-415-14401-9*) Routledge.

Religious Medicine: The History & Evolution of Indian Medicine. Kenneth G. Zysk. 1993. LC 92-20088. 340p. (C). text 49.95 (*1-56000-076-7*) Transaction Pubs.

Religious Methods & Resources in Bioethics. Ed. by Paul F. Camenisch. 1993. LC 93-24817. (Theory & Medicine Ser.: Vol. 2). 356p. (C). lib. bdg. (*0-7923-2102-2*) Kluwer Academic NLD. *Dist:* Kluwer Academic.

Religious Therapeutics: Body & Health in Yoga, Ayurveda, & Tantra. Gregory P. Fields. 2001. LC 00-49234. (SUNY Series in Religious Studies). (Illus.). xv, 222p. (C). pap. text 17.95 (*0-7914-4916-5*) State U NY Pr.

Religious Values of the Terminally Ill: A Handbook for Health Professionals. Delfi Mondragon. 1997. LC 97-16793. 148p. pap. text 15.00 (*0-940866-64-1*) U Scranton Pr.

Reluctant Exhibitionist. Martin Shepard. 1985. LC 83-63255. 280p. pap. 5.95 (*0-932966-57-8*) Permanent Pr.

Reluctant Treasures: The Practice of Analytic Psychotherapy. Gordon Warme. 1994. LC 93-47136. 288p. 50.00 (*1-56821-217-8*) Aronson.

Remaking Health Care in America: The Evolution of Organized Delivery Systems. Stephen M. Shortell et al. 2nd ed. 2000. LC 00-8904. (Jossey-Bass Health Care Ser.). (Illus.). 368p. 45.00 (*0-7879-4823-3*) Jossey-Bass.

Remaking Men: Jung Spirituality & Social Change. David Tacey. 1997. LC 97-186867. 240p. (C). 78.95 (*0-415-14240-7*); pap. 26.95 (*0-415-14241-5*) Routledge.

Remaking the Body: Explorations in Embodiment. Wendy Seymour. 1998. LC 97-46633. 224p. (C). 80.00 (*0-415-18601-3*); pap. 27.95 (*0-415-18602-1*) Routledge.

Remarkable Healings: A Psychiatrist Discovers Unsuspected Roots of Mental & Physical Illness. Shakuntala Modi. 1997. LC 98-72108. 632p. pap. text 18.95 (*1-57174-079-1*) Hampton Roads Pub Co.

Remarkable Lives of 100 Women Healers & Scientists. Brooke Bailey. 1997. 208p. reprint ed. pap. text 12.00 (*0-7881-5061-8*) DIANE Pub.

Remarkable Surgical Practice of John Benjamin Murphy. Ed. by Robert L. Schmitz & Timothy T. Oh. 1993. LC 92-524. (Illus.). 256p. text 39.95 (*0-252-01958-X*) U of Ill Pr.

Remarks on the Philosophy of Psychology, Vol. 1. Ludwig Josef Johann Wittgenstein. Ed. & Tr. by G. E. Anscombe. Ed. by George H. Von Wright. 1988. (Remarks on the Philosophy of Psychology Ser.: Vol. 1). 424p. pap. text 22.50 (*0-226-90436-9*) U Ch Pr.

Remarks on the Philosophy of Psychology, Vol. 1. Ludwig Josef Johann Wittgenstein. Ed. by G. E. Anscombe & George H. Von Wright. 1980. LC 80-52781. (Remarks on the Philosophy of Psychology Ser.: Vol. 1). 424p. (C). lib. bdg. 48.00 (*0-226-90433-4*) U Ch Pr.

Remarks on the Philosophy of Psychology, Vol. 2. Ludwig Josef Johann Wittgenstein. Ed. by George H. Von Wright & Heikki Nyman. Tr. by C. G. Luckhardt & A. E. Aue. LC 80-52781. (Remarks on the Philosophy of Psychology Ser.: Vol. 2). (C). 1988. 269p. pap. text 17.95 (*0-226-90437-7*); 1980. 271p. lib. bdg. 33.00 (*0-226-90434-2*) U Ch Pr.

Remediation & Management of Low Vision. Ed. by Roy G. Cole & Bruce P. Rosenthal. 1995. LC 95-39180. (Mosby's Optometric Problem Solving Ser.). (Illus.). 320p. (C). (gr. 13). pap. text 39.95 (*0-8151-5204-3*, 26454) Mosby Inc.

Remediation of Articulation Disorders (RAD) A Pragmatic Approach. Jan Bieniosek. 1996. (Illus.). 92p. (Orig.). pap. text 18.95 (*0-937857-69-6*, 1420) Speech Bin.

Remedies Against the Plague. Arnold C. Klebs & Eugene Droz. LC 75-23732. reprint ed. 35.00 (*0-404-13290-1*) AMS Pr.

Remedies & Rackets: The Truth about Patent Medicines Today. James Cook. 1976. LC 75-39284. (Getting & Spending: The Consumer's Dilemma Ser.). reprint ed. 23.95 (*0-405-08059-X*) Ayer.

Remedies, Potions & Razzmatazz. Ed. by Donald L. Roberts. 1991. (Illus.). 510p. (Orig.). reprint ed. pap. 15.95 (*0-9628676-0-8*) Nostalgia CA.

Remedios: Traditional Herbal Remedies of the Southwest. Michael Moore. 1990. LC 90-61682. (SPA., Illus.). 120p. (Orig.). pap. 9.95 (*1-878610-06-6*) Red Crane Bks.

Remedios Caseros para Proteger su Salud. Ed. by Atenedor Rojas. deluxe ed. 1999. (SPA., Illus.). 192p. pap. 5.95 (*0-939193-32-9*) Edit Concepts.

Remedios de la Naturaleza: Desde la Aromaterapia Hasta Layoga, la Gu la Maxima de Los Mejores Tratamientos Sin Medicamentos Todos Comprobados. Michael Castleman. 1997. LC 97-24241. 29.95 (*0-87596-502-4*) Rodale Pr Inc.

Remedy Box. Amy J. Conway. 1994. LC 94-7706. 56p. 24.95 (*0-8048-3015-0*) Tuttle Pubng.

Remembered Present: A Biological Theory of Consciousness. Gerald M. Edelman. 1990. LC 89-42907. (Illus.). 384p. pap. 50.00 (*0-465-06910-X*) Basic.

Remembered Self: Emotion & Memory in Personality. Jefferson A. Singer & Peter Salovey. 1993. LC 93-8017. xi, 257p. 40.00 (*0-02-901581-2*) Free Pr.

Remembering. F. C. Bartlett. 1995. (Illus.). 337p. (C). pap. text 21.95 (*0-521-48356-5*) Cambridge U Pr.

Remembering Anna O. Mikkel Borch-Jacobsen. 1996. 144p. (C). 65.00 (*0-415-91776-X*); LC 96-21013. pap. 18.95 (*0-415-91777-8*) Routledge.

Remembering Self: Construction & Accuracy in the Self-Narrative. Ed. by Ulric Neisser & Robyn Fivush. 1994. LC 93-40556. (Emory Symposia in Cognition Ser.: Vol. 6). 315p. (C). text 59.95 (*0-521-43194-8*) Cambridge U Pr.

Remembering to Live: Illness at the Intersection of Anxiety & Knowledge. M. C. Hays. 2001. LC 2001-2486. (Southeast Asia Ser.). (Illus.). 360p. (C). text 49.50 (*0-472-09785-7*, 09785) U of Mich Pr.

Remembrance of Patients Past: Patient Life at the Toronto Hospital for the Insane, 1870-1940. Geoffrey Reaume. 2000. (Canadian Social History Ser.). (Illus.). 376p. pap. text 19.95 (*0-19-541538-8*) OUP.

Remembrances in Endocrinology: An Endocrine Society History of the Study of Endocrinology & Its Practitioners. 1993. (Illus.). 113p. (C). 20.00 (*1-879225-09-3*) Endocrine Soc.

Remington: The Science & Practice of Pharmacy. Alfonso R. Gennaro. 10th ed. 2000. 2,100p. pap. text 110.00 (*0-683-30647-2*) Lppncott W & W.

Remington: The Science & Practice of Pharmacy Ed. by Alfonso R. Gennaro. 19th ed. 1995. LC 60-53334. 2000p. pap. 125.00 (*0-912734-05-1*) Mack Pub.

Reminiscence & Nursing Home Life. Donna E. Schafer. 1994. LC 93-48154. (Studies on the Elderly in America). (Illus.). 204p. text 30.00 (*0-8153-1614-3*) Garland.

Reminiscence Reviewed: Perspectives, Evaluations, Achievements. Ed. by Joanna Bornat. 1993. LC 93-22968. (Rethinking Aging Ser.). 160p. pap. (*0-335-19041-3*) OpUniv Pr.

Reminiscence Work with Old People. Clare Gillies & Anne James. 1994. LC 94-71059. 144p. pap. 26.95 (*0-412-58070-5*) Chapman & Hall.

Reminiscences of a Viennese Psychoanalyst. Richard F. Sterba. 1982. LC 82-11149. (Illus.). 186p. 34.95 (*0-8143-1716-2*) Wayne St U Pr.

Remote Sensing & Geographical Information Systems in Epidemiology. Ed. by Simon I. Hay & Sarah E. Randolph. 2000. (Advances in Parasitology Ser.: Vol. 47). (Illus.). 340p. pap. 69.95 (*0-12-333560-4*) Acad Pr.

Remote Sensing Laboratory Manual. Floyd F. Sabins. 1996. 240p. (C). spiral bd. 53.95 (*0-7872-2543-6*, 41254301) Kendall-Hunt.

Removable Appliance Fabrication. Emil Witt et al. 1988. (Illus.). 266p. text 79.00 (*0-86715-180-3*, 1803) Quint Pub Co.

Removable Orthodontic Appliances. K. G. Isaacson et al. 2002. (Illus.). 256p. 64.99 (*0-7236-1053-3*) Buttrwrth-Heinemann.

Removable Partial Dentures. George Graber. 1988. (Color Atlas of Dental Medicine Ser.). (Illus.). 224p. 159.00 (*0-86577-276-2*) Thieme Med Pubs.

Removable Partial Dentures. Robert P. Renner & Louis J. Boucher. 1987. (Illus.). 416p. text 62.00 (*0-86715-189-7*, 1897) Quint Pub Co.

Removable Partial Dentures on Osseointegrated Implants: Principles of Treatment Planning & Prosthetic Rehabilitation in Edentulous Mandible. Christian Besimo. Tr. by Thomas M. Hassel from GER. 1997. LC 97-3822. 232p. text 98.00 (*0-86715-329-6*) Quint Pub Co.

Removable Partial Prosthodontics. Alastair R. MacGregory & Sybille K. Lechner. 1994. LC 93-2006. (Case Oriented Manual of Treatment). 160p. (gr. 13). 51.95 (*0-7234-1960-4*) Mosby Inc.

Removable Prosthodontic Techniques. John B. Sowter. Ed. by Roger E. Barton. 1987. LC 86-7065. (Dental Laboratory Technology Manuals Ser.). (Illus.). viii, 248p. pap. 42.50 (*0-8078-4166-8*) U of NC Pr.

Removal of Teeth: A Self-Instructional Guide, Bk. 2. James R. Hooley & Robert J. Whitacre. 3rd rev. ed. 1983. (Illus.). 117p. pap. 19.95 (*0-89939-021-8*) Stoma Pr.

Removing Barriers Improving Choices: A Case Study in Reproductive Health Services & Managed Care. Shirley Gordon. 1996. 98p. pap. text 5.00 (*1-890671-12-6*) Center Reprod.

Removing the Roadblocks: Group Psychotherapy with Substance Abusers & Family Members. Marsha Vannicelli. 1992. LC 91-35427. (GSAS Ser.). 325p. 40.00 (*0-89862-174-7*) Guilford Pubns.

Remunerating General Practitioners in Western Europe. Peter P. Groerewegen et al. 1991. 131p. text (*1-85628-162-0*) Avebry GBR. *Dist:* Ashgate Pub Co.

Remyelination in the Central Nervous System. Ed. by S. E. Pfeiffer & E. Barbares. 1989. (Journal: Vol. 11, No. 2, 1989). (Illus.). 72p. pap. 31.50 (*3-8055-5033-2*) S Karger.

Renaissance des Hausarztes. Erdmann Strum. 1983. (Patient Allgemeinmedizin Ser.: Band 1). (Illus.). 290p. 29.00 (*3-540-12374-1*) Spr-Verlag.

Renaissance Medical Learning: Evolution of Tradition. Michael R. McVaugh & Nancy G. Siraisi. 1994. (Osiris Ser.: Vol. 6). 244p. pap. text 25.00 (*0-934235-17-1*); lib. bdg. 39.00 (*0-934235-18-X*) U Ch Pr.

Renaissance of American Medicine: A Century of New Learning & Caring. Alan C. Mermann. 2000. LC 00-46672. 248p. 56.00 (*0-7618-1864-2*) U Pr of Amer.

Renaissance of Interstitial Brachytherapy: Proceedings of the Annual San Francisco Cancer Symposium, 12th, March 4-5, 1977. Annual San Francisco Cancer Symposium. Ed. by J. M. Vaeth. 1977. (Frontiers of Radiation Therapy & Oncology Ser.: Vol. 12). (Illus.). 102.75 (*3-8055-2706-3*) S Karger.

Renaissance of Medicine in Italy. Arturo Castiglioni. 1979. LC 79-114967. 18.95 (*0-405-10587-8*) Ayer.

Renaissance of the State Psychiatric System: A Special Issue of Psychiatric Quarterly. Ed. by Stephen L. Katz. 1985. 102p. 16.95 (*0-89885-346-X*, Kluwer Acad Hman Sci) Kluwer Academic.

Renal Ammonia Metabolism. Ed. by R. L. Tannen et al. 1982. (Contributions to Nephrology Ser.: Vol. 31). (Illus.). x, 154p. 29.75 (*3-8055-3481-7*) S Karger.

Renal Ammoniagenesis: Journal: Mineral & Electrolyte Metabolism, Vol. 16, Nos. 5 & 6, 1990. Ed. by Ira Kurtz. 1990. (Illus.). iv, 100p. pap. 55.00 (*3-8055-5238-6*) S Karger.

Renal Ammoniagenesis & Interorgan Cooperation in Acid-Base Homeostasis. Ed. by A. Tizianello et al. 1994. (Contributions to Nephrology Ser.: Vol. 110). (Illus.). xii, 184p. 49.75 (*3-8055-5915-1*) S Karger.

Renal & Electrolyte Disorders. Ed. by Robert W. Schrier. 3rd ed. 1986. 37.50 (*0-316-77479-0*, Little Brwn Med Div) Lppncott W & W.

Renal & Electrolyte Disorders. Robert W. Schrier. 5th ed. 1997. LC 97-5943. (Illus.). 784p. pap. text 67.00 (*0-316-77454-5*, Little Brwn Med Div) Lppncott W & W.

Renal & Urologic Aspects of HIV Infection. Ed. by Paul L. Kimmel & Jeffrey S. Berns. 1995. LC 94-48435. (Contemporary Issues in Nephrology Ser.: Vol. 29). text (*0-443-08952-3*) Church.

Renal Biopsy. Vivette D. D'Agati et al. Ed. by Leslely Day. 3rd ed. 1997. 336p. text 84.00 (*0-7216-6412-1*) Saunders.

Renal Biopsy in Glomerular Diseases. Edit Beregi et al. 1978. 334p. (C). 110.00 (*963-05-1356-0*) St Mut.

Renal Biopsy in Glomerular Diseases: Clinical Histological, Immunohistological & Electron-Microscopic Studies. F. Antoni & M. Staub. 1978. 164p. (C). (*963-05-1562-8*) Akade Kiado HUN. *Dist:* St Mut.

Renal Biopsy Interpretation. Fred G. Silva et al. 1996. LC 96-18700. text (*0-443-07784-3*) Church.

Renal Cell Carcinoma. Eric A. Klein et al. 1993. (Illus.). 368p. text 195.00 (*0-8247-9033-2*) Dekker.

Renal Cell Carcinoma: Molecular Biology, Immunology & Clinical Management. Ed. by Ronald M. Bukowski & Andrew Novick. 2000. LC 99-53889. (Current Clinical Oncology Ser.). (Illus.). 448p. 145.00 (*0-89603-781-9*) Humana.

Renal Cells in Culture: Journal: Mineral & Electrolyte Metabolism, Vol. 12, No. 1, 1986. Ed. by Leon G. Fine. 1986. (Illus.). 84p. pap. 81.75 (*3-8055-4160-0*) S Karger.

Renal Complications of Neoplasia. Ed. by Thurman D. McKinney. 1985. 270p. 75.00 (*0-275-92031-3*, C2031, Praeger Pubs) Greenwood.

Renal Cortical Necrosis. F. A. Laszlo. 1981. (Contributions to Nephrology Ser.: Vol. 28). (Illus.). viii, 216p. pap. 29.75 (*3-8055-2109-X*) S Karger.

Renal Cystic Disease. Hartman. 2nd ed. 1989. 240p. pap. text 1.50 (*0-7216-2343-3*) Saunders.

Renal Dialysis. Ed. by J. D. Briggs et al. 1994. (Illus.). 488p. (gr. 13). 188.95 (*0-412-31310-3*) Chapman & Hall.

Renal Disease. G. Venkat Raman. 1997. (Illus.). 496p. (*0-412-45700-8*) E A GBR. *Dist:* OUP.

Renal Disease: Classification & Atlas of Glomerular Diseases. Jacob Churg et al. 2nd ed. 1995. LC 94-22200. (Illus.). 541p. 159.95 (*0-89640-257-6*) Igaku-Shoin.

Renal Disease: Classification & Atlas of Tubulo-Interstitial & Vascular Diseases. Surya V. Seshan et al. 1998. LC 98-15851. 384p. text 179.00 (*0-683-30677-4*) Lppncott W & W.

Renal Disease in the Aged. Saubert Porush. 1991. 82.95 (*0-316-71401-1*, Little Brwn Med Div) Lppncott W & W.

Renal Disease in the Elderly. Pierre F. Faubert & Jerome G. Porush. 2nd ed. 1998. LC 98-36838. (Illus.). 448p. text 195.00 (*0-8247-9900-3*) Dekker.

Renal Disease Progression & Management: Role of Vasoactive Agents, Cytokines, Lipids & Nutrition. Ed. by Morrell M. Avram & Saulo Klahr. 1996. (Illus.). 372p. text 99.00 (*0-7216-3833-3*) Saunders.

Renal Disorders. Dorothy Brundage. 1991. (Illus.). 256p. (C). (gr. 13). text 32.95 (*0-8016-1685-9*, 01685) Mosby Inc.

***Renal Drug Handbook.** Ed. by Ray Bunn & Caroline Ashley. 1999. 392p. pap. (*1-85775-115-9*) Radcliffe Med Pr GBR. *Dist:* Balogh.

Renal Dysfunction: Mechanisms Involved in Fluid & Solute Imbalance. Heinz Valtin. 1979. 30.95 (*0-316-89554-7*, Little Brwn Med Div) Lppncott W & W.

Renal Effects of Petroleum Hydrocarbons. Ed. by Myron A. Mehlman et al. 1984. (Advances in Modern Environmental Toxicology Ser.: Vol. 7). (Illus.). 320p. pap. text 65.00 (*0-911131-08-6*) Specialist Journals.

Renal Eicosanoids. Ed. by Michael J. Dunn. 1989. (Illus.). 438p. 105.00 (*0-306-43320-6*, Plenum Trade) Perseus Pubng.

Renal Failure. Horacio J. Adrogue & Donald E. Wesson. 1995. 224p. pap. 24.95 (*0-86542-430-6*) Blackwell Sci.

Renal Failure: Diagnosis & Treatment. Ed. by J. Gary Abuelo. 1995. LC 95-7920. (Developments in Nephrology Ser.: Vol. 37). 284p. (C). text 173.50 (*0-7923-3438-8*) Kluwer Academic.

Renal Function. Heinz Valtin. 3rd ed. 1994. LC 94-13503. 336p. pap. text 37.95 (*0-316-89560-1*) Lppncott W & W.

Renal Immunology. G. Lubec. 1983. (Contributions to Nephrology Ser.: Vol. 35). (Illus.). vi, 194p. pap. 29.75 (*3-8055-3587-2*) S Karger.

Renal Involvement in Systemic Vasculitis: Seminar, 1st, Vimercate, September 22, 1990. Ed. by Adalberto Sessa. 1991. (Contributions to Nephrology Ser.: Vol. 94). (Illus.). x, 206p. 49.75 (*3-8055-5422-2*) S Karger.

Renal Ion Channels: Function & Regulation. Ed. by R. V. Thakker. 2000. (Experimental Nephrology Ser.: Vol. 8, No. 6). (Illus.). iv, 66p. pap. 25.25 (*3-8055-7143-7*) S Karger.

Renal Lifestyles Manual: The Renal Diet Guidebook for Professionals & Patients. Peggy Harum. Ed. by Edward J. Doherty. 3rd rev. ed. 1999. 338p. 29.95 (*0-9670439-0-5*) R & D.

Renal Medicine: Concise Medical Textbook. Roger Gabriel. 3rd ed. 1988. (Illus.). 288p. text (*0-7020-1267-X*) Bailliere Tindall.

Renal Nerves: Journal: Mineral & Electrolyte Metabolism, Vol. 15, Nos. 1 & 2. Ed. by G. F. DiBona. 1989. (Illus.). 96p. pap. 73.25 (*3-8055-4887-7*) S Karger.

Renal Nuclear Magnetic Resonance. Ed. by Z. H. Endre & A. Iaina. 1989. (Journal: Vol. 12, No. 3, 1989). (Illus.). 76p. pap. 51.50 (*3-8055-5063-4*) S Karger.

Renal Nursing. Ed. by P. R. Uldall. 3rd ed. 1987. (Illus.). 440p. pap. 39.95 (*0-632-01728-7*) Blackwell Sci.

Renal Nutrition Case Study. Helen Sanders & Hamid Rabb. 1992. 115p. (Orig.). (C). pap. text 100.00 (*1-880864-03-7*) F S H.

Renal Osteodystrophy. Ed. by David A. Bushinsky. 1998. LC 97-46074. (Illus.). 528p. text 119.00 (*0-397-51836-6*) Lppncott W & W.

Renal Pathology. Ed. by Frederick Dische. 2nd ed. 1995. (Illus.). 230p. text 125.00 (*0-19-263032-6*) OUP.

Renal Pathology: With Clinical & Functional Correlations. Ed. by C. Craig Tisher et al. 1989. LC 65-9434. (Illus.). 1728p. text 225.00 (*0-397-50779-8*, Lippnctt) Lppncott W & W.

Renal Pathology with Clinical & Functional Correlations Ed. by C. Craig Tisher & Barry M. Brenner. 2nd ed. 1993. 1. (*0-397-51238-4*); 2. (*0-397-51239-2*); In Two Volumes. 1,856p. text 325.00 (*0-397-51240-6*) Lppncott W & W.

Renal Pathophysiology. L. Riley, Jr. 1998. (Pathophysiology Ser.). pap. 24.95 (*1-889325-03-1*) Fence Crk Pubng.

Renal Pathophysiology. Burton D. Rose & Helmut G. Rennke. 1994. LC 93-13959. (Illus.). 344p. 28.00 (*0-683-07354-0*) Lppncott W & W.

Renal Pathophysiology. Alexander Leaf & Ramzi Cotran. 3rd ed. 1985. (Illus.). 432p. pap. text 26.95 (*0-19-503488-0*) OUP.

Renal Pathophysiology: A Problem-Oriented Approach. James A. Shayman. 1995. (Illus.). 208p. pap. text 24.95 (*0-397-51372-0*) Lppncott W & W.

Renal Patient's Guide to Good Eating. Judith A. Curtis. 1989. (Illus.). 214p. (C). text 40.95 (*0-398-05611-0*) C C Thomas.

Renal Physiology. Bruce M. Koeppen & Bruce A. Stanton. 2nd ed. 1996. LC 96-16798. (Illus.). 272p. (C). (gr. 13). pap. text 30.00 (*0-8151-5202-7*, 28157) Mosby Inc.

Renal Physiology. E. Koushanpour & Wilhelm Kriz. 2nd ed. 1986. (Illus.). 390p. 152.00 (*0-387-96304-9*) Spr-Verlag.

Renal Physiology. Bruce M. Koeppen & Bruce A. Stanton. 3rd ed. 2000. LC 00-41839. (Mosby Physiology Monograph Ser.). (Illus.). xiv, 258p. (*0-323-01242-6*) Mosby Inc.

Renal Physiology. Arthur L. Vander. 5th ed. 1994. LC 94-27777. (Illus.). 238p. pap. 29.95 (*0-07-067009-9*) McGraw-Hill Prof.

Renal Physiology: People & Ideas. Ed. by Carl W. Gottschalk et al. 1988. (American Physiological Society Book). (Illus.). 520p. text 87.50 (*0-19-520702-5*) OUP.

Renal Physiology in Health & Disease. Barry M. Brenner et al. 1987. (Illus.). 190p. pap. text 36.00 (*0-7216-1973-8*) Saunders.

Renal Problems in Critical Care. Ed. by Lynn Schoengrund & Pamela Balzer. 1989. LC 84-27075. (Critical Care Nursing Ser.). 309p. pap. text 32.20 (*0-8273-4358-2*) Delmar.

Renal Protective Effect of ACE Inhibition & Angiotensin II Blockade. Ed. by Giuseppe Remuzzi. 1996. (Journal: Vol. 4, Supplement 1, 1996). (Illus.). iv, 62p. pap. 28.75 (*3-8055-6442-2*) S Karger.

Renal Radiology & Imaging. O. P. Fitzgerald-Finch. 1981. (Topics in Renal Disease Ser.). 96p. text 59.00 (*0-85200-423-0*) Kluwer Academic.

Renal Research: Clinical & Experimental Contributions from Japan. Ed. by K. Kobayashi et al. 1977. (Contributions to Nephrology Ser.: Vol. 6). 29.75 (*3-8055-2402-1*) S Karger.

Renal Scarring: A Multi-Organ Approach to Fibrosis. Ed. by A. Mequid El Nahas. 1995. (Journal: Vol. 3, No. 2-3, 1995). (Illus.). 84p. pap. 54.00 (*3-8055-6149-0*) S Karger.

Renal Sonography. E. Bihr et al. 2nd rev. ed. 1986. (Illus.). 210p. 171.00 (*0-387-15343-8*) Spr-Verlag.

Renal Stone Disease: Pathogenesis, Prevention, & Treatment. Ed. by Charles Y. Pak. 1987. (Topics in Renal Medicine Ser.). (C). text 162.50 (*0-89838-886-4*) Kluwer Academic.

Renal Stones: Etiology, Management, & Treatment. U. Backman et al. 1985. 206p. (Orig.). 71.50 (*91-22-00764-4*) Coronet Bks.

***Renal System.** Michael Field et al. 2001. 180p. pap. (*0-443-06478-4*) Church GBR. *Dist:* Saunders.

Renal System. B. Jackson et al. 1998. (Integrated Medical Sciences Ser.). (C). pap. 29.95 (*1-889325-31-7*) Blackwell Sci.

Renal Tract Stone: Metabolic Basis & Clinical Practice. Ed. by J. E. Wickham & A. Colin Buck. 1990. (Illus.). 462p. text (*0-443-03803-1*) Church.

Renal Transplant Tolerance: Molecular Mechanisms of T Cell Regulation. Ed. by Giuseppe Remuzzi. 1992. (Journal: Vol. 1, No. 2, 1993). (Illus.). 76p. pap. 40.00 (*3-8055-5699-3*) S Karger.

Renal Transplantation. Ed. by Marvin R. Garovoy & Ronald D. Guttmann. 1986. (Illus.). 446p. text (*0-443-08263-4*) Church.

Renal Transplantation. Ron Shapiro et al. 1998. LC 96-28894. 572p. (C). text 110.00 (*0-8385-8383-0*, A8383-0) McGraw-Hill Prof.

Renal Transplantation: Sense & Sensitization. S. M. Gore & B. A. Bradley. 1988. (Developments in Nephrology Ser.). (C). text 218.00 (*0-89838-370-6*) Kluwer Academic.

Renal Transport of Organic Substances. Ed. by R. Greger et al. 1981. (Proceedings in Life Sciences Ser.). (Illus.). 314p. 64.95 (*0-387-10904-8*) Spr-Verlag.

Renal Vascular Disease. Novick. 1995. text 107.00 (*0-7020-1814-7*) Saunders.

Rene Spitz: Dialogues from Infancy. Ed. by Robert N. Emde. 1984. LC 83-26461. 495p. 72.50 (*0-8236-5787-6*) Intl Univs Pr.

Renegade Psychiatrist's Story: An Introduction to the Science of Human Nature. Paul Rosenfels. 1979. LC 86-142970. (Ninth Street Center Monographs). (Orig.). pap. 3.95 (*0-932961-05-3*) Ninth St Ctr.

Renegotiating Health Care: Resolving Conflict to Build Collaboration. Leonard Marcus. 2nd ed. 1999. 496p. pap. 38.00 (*0-7879-5021-1*) Jossey-Bass.

Renew Your Heart One Beat at a Time. Maureen Maloof & Catherine Maloof. 1998. 127p. pap. 9.95 (*1-891361-00-7*, 27252) Maloof Enter.

Renewable Fuels & the Future Security of U. S. Energy Supplies: Hearing Before the Committee on Agriculture, Nutrition, & Forestry, U. S. Senate. Ed. by Richard G. Lugar. 1999. (Illus.). 117p. (C). reprint ed. pap. text 25.00 (*0-7881-3572-4*) DIANE Pub.

Renewing Female Balance: PMS, Breast, Uterine Fibroids, Ovarian Cysts, Endometriosis, Yeast Infections & More. Linda R. Page. 4th exp. ed. 1997. (Library Ser.). (Illus.). 48p. per. 4.50 (*1-884334-64-4*) Hlthy Healing.

Renewing Male Health & Energy with Herbs. Linda R. Page. 2nd rev. ed. 1995. (Healthy Healing Library). (Illus.). 32p. pap. 3.50 (*1-884334-30-X*) Hlthy Healing.

Renewing the Promise: Medicare & Its Reform. Ed. by David Blumenthal et al. 1988. (Illus.). 238p. text 37.95 (*0-19-504304-9*) OUP.

Renin-Angiotensin System: Biochemistry, Physiology, Pathophysiology & Therapeutics. Ed. by J. Ian Robertson & Gary S. Nicholls. 1992. (Illus.). 1200p. (*1-56375-519-X*) Gower-Mosby.

Renin-Angiotensin System Textbook. J. Ians Robertson. 1992. (C). (gr. 13). text (*1-56375-550-5*) Gower-Mosby.

Renovascular & Renal Parenchymatous Hypertension. Ed. by Thomas F. Luscher & N. M. Kaplan. 1992. (Illus.). 574p. 187.00 (*0-387-53324-9*) Spr-Verlag.

Renovascular Hypertension. Ed. by J. Ian Robertson et al. 1986. (Journal: Vol. 44, Suppl. 1, 1986). (Illus.). iv, 116p. pap. 36.75 (*3-8055-4387-5*) S Karger.

Renunciemos a Falsas Expectativas y "Desilusiones" see Give up False Expectations & "Disappointment"

Reoperations in Cardiac Surgery. Ed. by J. Stark. 1989. (Illus.). 390p. 385.00 (*0-387-19552-1*) Spr-Verlag.

Reoperative Aesthetic & Reconstructive Plastic Surgery, Set. Ed. by James C. Grotting. 1995. LC 94-39605. (Illus.). 1661p. (C). text 395.00 (*0-942219-25-2*) Quality Med Pub.

Reoperative General Surgery. Donald G. McQuarrie. Ed. by Edward N. Humphrey. 2nd ed. 1996. LC 96-46310. (Illus.). 960p. (C). (gr. 13). text 180.00 (*0-8151-7028-9*, 27465) Mosby Inc.

Reoperative Gynecologic & Obstetrics Surgery. David Nichols. 2nd ed. 1997. (Illus.). 464p. (C). (gr. 13). text 95.00 (*0-8151-6452-1*, 26542) Mosby Inc.

Reorganization & Renewal: Strategies for Healthcare Leaders. Donald N. Lombardi. 1997. LC 97-18702. pap. 44.00 (*1-56793-062-X*) Health Admin Pr.

Reorientation of Medical Education: Goal, Strategies & Targets, 2. 1989. (SEARO Regional Publications Ser.: No. 18). 19p. pap. text 3.00 (*92-9022-121-6*) World Health.

Reorientation of Medical Education: Indicators for Monitoring & Evaluation, 3. 1989. (SEARO Regional Publications Ser.: No. 18). 101p. pap. text 5.00 (*92-9022-122-4*) World Health.

Reorientation of Medical Education: The Rationale & Vision - A Springboard for Change, 1. 1989. (SEARO Regional Publications Ser.: No. 18). 45p. pap. text 3.00 (*92-9022-120-8*) World Health.

Reorientation of Medical Education Pt. 4: Guidelines for Developing National Plans for Action. 1991. (WHO Regional Publications, South-East Asia Ser.: No. 18). ii, 16p. pap. text 3.00 (*92-9022-160-7*, 1564018) World Health.

Reorientation of Medical Education Pt. 5: Introducing Problem-Based Learning in the South-East Asia Region. P. Abeykoon et al. 1992. (WHO Regional Publications, South-East Asia Ser.: No. 18). viii, 42p. pap. 4.00 (*92-9022-164-X*, 1565018) World Health.

Reoviruses II: Cytopathogenicity & Pathogenesis. Ed. by K. L. Tyler et al. 1998. (Current Topics in Microbiology & Immunology Ser.: Vol. 233, Vol. 2). (Illus.). 220p. 129.00 (*3-540-63947-0*) Spr-Verlag.

Reoviruses I: Structure, Proteins, & Genetics. Ed. by K. L. Tyler et al. 1998. (Current Topics in Microbiology & Immunology Ser.: Vol. 233, Vol. I). (Illus.). 241p. 139.00 (*3-540-63946-2*) Spr-Verlag.

Repair & Regeneration of the Nervous System: Berlin, 1981 Proceedings. J. G. Nicholls. 1982. (Dahlem Workshop Reports Ser.: Vol. 24). (Illus.). 411p. 42.95 (*0-387-11649-4*) Spr-Verlag.

Repair & Renewal: Journey Through the Mind & Body. Ed. by Robert Somerville. 1994. LC 94-18844. (Journey Through the Mind & Body Ser.). (Illus.). 144p. lib. bdg. 17.99 (*0-7835-1049-7*) Time-Life.

Repairing Body Fluids: Principles & Practice. Kassirer et al. 1989. 176p. text 62.00 (*0-7216-1149-4*) Saunders.

Repairing Intimacy: An Object Relations Approach to Couples Therapy. Judith Siegel. 1993. LC 92-11152. 288p. 30.00 (*0-87668-459-2*) Aronson.

Reparation: Restoring the Damaged Self in Child & Adult Psychotherapy. Hugh G. Clegg. 1995. LC 95-13022. Orig. Title: The Reparative Motif in Child & Adult Therapy. 244p. reprint ed. pap. 45.00 (*1-56821-527-6*) Aronson.

Reparative Motif in Child & Adult Therapy see Reparation: Restoring the Damaged Self in Child & Adult Psychotherapy

Reparative Therapy of Male Homosexuality: A New Clinical Approach. annuals Joseph Nicolosi. 1997th ed. 1997. LC 97-37093. 384p. pap. 40.00 (*0-7657-0142-1*) Aronson.

Repentance. Archbishop Chrysostomos of Etna. 2nd ed. 1997. (Themes in Orthodox Patristic Psychology: Vol. III). 50p. per. 5.00 (*0-911165-09-6*) Ctr Trad Orthodox.

Reperfusion-Induced Arrhythmias: Control & Mechanisms. Arpad Tosaki. 1995. 105p. pap. (*963-05-6851-9*) Akade Kiado HUN. *Dist:* Intl Spec Bk.

Reperfusion-Induced Arrhythmias: Control & Mechanisms. Arpad Tosaki. 1995. 105p. pap. 18.00 (*963-8326-03-4*) Pendragon NY.

Reperfusion Injuries & Clinical Capillary Leak Syndrome. Ed. by B. A. Zikria et al. 1994. LC 94-5629. (Illus.). 480p. 85.00 (*0-87993-583-9*) Futura Pub.

P
Q
R

Repertory Additions from Kent's Lectures on Homeopathic Materia Medica. Linda Johnston. 1990. 554p. (C). stu. ed. 55.00 (*1-877691-24-0*) C Kent Agency.

Repertory of the Homoeopathic Materia Medica. J. T. Kent. 6th ed. 1992. reprint ed. (*81-7021-083-6*) Sarat IND. *Dist:* S Asia.

Repetition & Trauma: Toward a Teleonomic Theory of Psychoanalysis. Max M. Stern. Ed. by Liselotte B. Stern. 1988. 192p. text 29.95 (*0-88163-073-X*) Analytic Pr.

Repetition Strain Injuries: Index of New Information with Authors, Subjects, References, & Research Categories. Sidney M. Hobwell. 1996. LC 96-12513. 57.50 (*0-7883-1186-7*); pap. 47.50 (*0-7883-1187-5*) ABBE Pubs Assn.

Repetitive Motion Disorders of the Upper Extremity. Ed. by Stephen L. Gordon et al. 1995. 554p. 105.00 (*0-89203-143-3*) Amer Acad Ortho Surg.

Repetitive Strain Injuries. Timothy J. Jameson. 1998. LC 98-15967. (Illus.). 280p. pap. 14.95 (*0-87983-802-7*, 38027K, Keats Pubng) McGraw-Hill Trade.

Repetitive Strain Injury: A Computer User's Guide. Emil Pascarelli & Deborah Quilter. 1994. LC 93-31758. 240p. pap. 17.95 (*0-471-59533-0*) Wiley.

Repetitive Strain Injury Handbook: A Complete Guide to Prevention, Related Issues & an 8-Step Recovery Plan. Ruth Aleskovsky & Robert M. Simon. 2000. LC 99-36203. (Illus.). 244p. pap. 15.00 (*0-8050-5930-X*, Owlet Pbks) H Holt Bks Young Read.

Repetitive Strain Injury Recovery Book. Deborah Quitter. 1998. LC 97-36007. 240p. (Orig.). pap. 14.95 (*0-8027-7514-4*) Walker & Co.

Repetitive Strain Injury Sourcebook. Sandra Peddie et al. 1998. LC 97-34717. (Illus.). 384p. reprint ed. pap. 17.00 (*0-7373-0022-1*, 00221W) NTC Contemp Pub Co.

Repetitive Strain Injury Sourcebook. Sandra Peddle et al. 1998. LC 97-34717. 224p. reprint ed. 30.00 (*1-56565-791-8*, 07918W, Anodyne) Lowell Hse.

Replacement Cardiac Valves. Endre Bodnar & Robert W. Frater. 1991. (Illus.). 480p. (*0-08-035773-3*) PPI GBR. *Dist:* McGraw.

Replacement of Renal Function by Dialysis. Ed. by Claude Jacobs. 4th ed. 1996. LC 95-31081. 1480p. (C). lib. bdg. 325.00 (*0-7923-3610-0*) Kluwer Academic.

Replacement of Renal Function by Dialysis: A Textbook of Dialysis. Ed. by John F. Maher. 3rd enl. ed. 1989. (C). text 420.50 (*0-89838-414-1*) Kluwer Academic.

Replication of Anterior Teeth in the Four Seasons of Life. Klaus Muterthies. 1991. (Illus.). 92p. text 66.00 (*1-85097-023-8*) Quint Pub Co.

Replication of DNA & RNA. 1979. (Landmark Ser.). 25.50 (*0-8422-4124-8*) Irvington.

Replication of Viral & Cellular Genomes. Ed. by Yechiel Becker. 1983. (Developments in Molecular Virology Ser.). text 163.50 (*0-89838-589-X*) Kluwer Academic.

Report. American Psychological Association Staff. Ed. by R.S. Woodworth. 1974. (Psychology Monographs General & Applied: Vol. 13). reprint ed. pap. 55.00 (*0-8115-1412-9*) Periodicals Srv.

Report: 15th Report, Geneva, 1970. WHO Expert Committee on Malaria. 1971. (Technical Reports: No. 467). (ENG, FRE & SPA.). 59p. pap. 2.00 (*92-4-120467-2*, 1078) World Health.

Report: Proceedings of the WHO Expert Committee on Biological Standardization, 21st, Geneva, 1968. WHO Staff. (Technical Reports: No. 463). 1971. 91p. pap. text 7.00 (*92-4-120463-X*, 1100463); 1970. 132p. pap. text 7.00 (*92-4-120444-3*, 1100444); 1969. (ENG, FRE, RUS & SPA.). 106p. pap. text 7.00 (*92-4-120413-3*, 1100413); 1968. (ENG, FRE, RUS & SPA.). 384p. pap. 7.00 (*92-4-120384-6*, 1100384); 1964. (ENG, FRE, RUS & SPA.). 86p. pap. text 5.00 (*92-4-120293-9*, 1100293) World Health.

Report: Proceedings of the WHO Expert Committee on Filariais, 16th, Geneva, 1961. WHO Staff. 1962. (Technical Reports: No. 233). (ENG, FRE, RUS & SPA.). 49p. pap. text 3.00 (*92-4-120233-5*, 1100233) World Health.

Report: Proceedings of the WHO Expert Committee on Gonococcal Infections, 1st, Geneva, 1962. WHO Staff. 1963. (Technical Reports: No. 262). (ENG, FRE, RUS & SPA.). 70p. pap. text 5.00 (*92-4-120262-9*, 1100262) World Health.

Report: Proceedings of the WHO Expert Committee on Onchocerciasis, 2nd, Geneva, 1965. WHO Staff. 1966. (Technical Reports: No. 335). (ENG, FRE, RUS & SPA.). 96p. pap. text 5.00 (*92-4-120335-8*, 1100335) World Health.

Report: Proceedings of the WHO Expert Committee on Respiratory Virus Diseases, 1st, Stockholm, 1958. WHO Staff. 1959. (Technical Reports: No. 170). (ENG, FRE & SPA.). 59p. pap. text 3.00 (*92-4-120170-3*, 1100170) World Health.

Report: Proceedings of the WHO Expert Committee on Smallpox, Eradication, 2nd, 1972. WHO Staff. 1972. (Technical Reports: No. 493). 64p. pap. 7.00 (*92-4-120493-1*, 1100493) World Health.

Report: Proceedings of the WHO Expert Committee on Yellow Fever, 3rd, 1971. WHO Staff. 1971. (Technical Reports: No. 479). 56p. pap. 5.00 (*92-4-120479-6*, 1100479) World Health.

Report of a General Plan for the Promotion of Public & Personal Health. Nathaniel P. Banks et al. 1972. LC 70-180589. (Medicine & Society in America Ser.). 554p. reprint ed. 31.95 (*0-405-03971-9*) Ayer.

Report of a Working Party of the Standing Medical Advisory Committee on Sickle Cell, Thalassaemia & Other Haemoglobinopathies. HMSO Staff. 1994. 125p. pap. (*0-11-321699-8*, HM16998) Statnry Office GBR. *Dist:* Bernan Associates, Balogh.

Report of Infant Mortality Study in San Diego County. Helen M. Wallace et al. 1993. (Illus.). 124p. (Orig.). pap. 19.95 (*0-89914-038-6*) Third Party Pub.

Report of the Committee of Inquiry into the Personality Disorder Unit, Ashworth. 1999. (Command Papers: No. 4194-II). (*0-10-141943-0*, HM19430) Statnry Office GBR. *Dist:* Bernan Associates.

Report of the Council of Hygiene & Public Health of the Citizens' Association of New York Upon the Sanitary Condition of the City. Citizens' Association of New York Staff. 1976. LC 77-112532. (Rise of Urban America Ser.). (Illus.). reprint ed. 51.95 (*0-405-02443-6*) Ayer.

Report of the Experiments on Animal Magnetism: Proceedings of the Committee of the Medical Section of the French Royal Academy of Sciences, June 21-28, 1831. French Royal Academy of Sciences, Medical Section Staff & J. C. Colquhoun. 1975. LC 75-7371. (Perspectives in Psychical Research Ser.). reprint ed. 25.95 (*0-405-07022-5*) Ayer.

Report of the Expert Panel on Blood Cholesterol Levels in Children & Adolescents. 1996. (Illus.). 119p. (Orig.). pap. text 25.00 (*0-7881-2817-5*) DIANE Pub.

Report of the Expert Panel on Detection, Evaluation, & Treatment of High Blood Cholesterol in Adults. Scott M. Grundy. 1997. (Illus.). 170p. pap. text 35.00 (*0-7881-4680-7*) DIANE Pub.

Report of the Expert Panel on Population Strategies for Blood Cholesterol Reduction. 1996. (Illus.). 139p. reprint ed. pap. text 25.00 (*0-7881-2816-7*) DIANE Pub.

***Report of the Expert Panel Workshop on the Psychological Responses to Hazardous Substances.** Pamela D. Tucker. 2001. 87p. (C). pap. text 25.00 (*0-7567-0414-6*) DIANE Pub.

Report of the Fluoroquinolone Working Group. 1998. 54p. (C). reprint ed. pap. text 25.00 (*0-7881-3909-6*) DIANE Pub.

Report of the International Narcotics Control Board for 1988. 1988. 12.00 (*92-1-148076-0*, E.88.XI.4) UN.

Report of the Select Committee of the Senate of the U. S. on the Sickness & Mortality on Board Emigrant Ships. Hamilton Fish. Ed. by Barbara G. Rosenkrantz. 1977. LC 76-25663. (Public Health in America Ser.). (Illus.). reprint ed. lib. bdg. 18.95 (*0-405-09818-9*) Ayer.

Report of the State Commission to Investigate Provision for the Mentally Deficient. New York State Commission to Investigate Provision. 1976. LC 75-17234. (Social Problems & Social Policy Ser.). (Illus.). reprint ed. 96.95 (*0-405-07503-0*) Ayer.

***Report of the Surgeon General's Conference on Children's Mental Health: A National Action Agenda.** Ed. by S. Serene Olin. 2001. 52p. (C). pap. 25.00 (*0-7567-0975-X*) DIANE Pub.

Report of the Task Force on Child Abuse - Neglect System Safeguards. 1992. 40p. (Orig.). (C). pap. text 20.00 (*1-56806-094-7*) DIANE Pub.

Report on Carcinogens: Carcinogen Profiles 2000. Ed. by Barry Leonard. 9th ed. 2000. (Illus.). 1000p. pap. text 95.00 (*0-7567-0215-1*) DIANE Pub.

Report on Confidential Enquiries into Maternal Deaths in the United Kingdom, 1988-1990. 1994. 164p. pap. (*0-11-321691-2*, HM16912) Statnry Office GBR. *Dist:* Bernan Associates.

Report on Confidential Enquiries into Maternal Deaths in the United Kingdom, 1991-1993. HMSO Staff. 1996. 164p. pap. (*0-11-321983-0*, HM19830) Statnry Office GBR. *Dist:* Bernan Associates.

Report on Effective Psychotherapy: Legislative Testimony. Roberta Russell. Ed. by Suzanne Smith. 1981. LC 81-90112. 81p. (C). 30.00 (*0-940106-00-0*) Hillgarth Pr.

Report on Effective Psychotherapy: Legislative Testimony & Recommendations for Therapeutic Relationships in a Caring World. Roberta Russell. Ed. by Suzanne Smith. rev. ed. 120p. pap. text 14.95 (*0-940106-54-X*) Hillgarth Pr.

***Report on Evaluation of the Azoospermic Male: An American Urological Association Best Practice Policy & American Society for Reproductive Medicine Practice Committee Report.** Ira Sharlip et al. 2001. (Reports on Male Infertility). pap. (*0-9649702-8-7*) Am Urological.

***Report on Management of Obstructive Azoospermia Vol. 4: An American Urological Association Best Practice Policy & American Society for Reproductive Medicine Practice Committee Report.** Ira Sharlip et al. 2001. (Reports on Male Infertility). pap. (*0-9709327-0-7*) Am Urological.

***Report on Optimal Evaluation of the Infertile Male: An American Urological Association Best Practice Policy & American Society for Reproductive Medicine Practice Committee Report.** Ira Sharlip et al. 2001. (Reports on Male Infertility). pap. (*0-9649702-7-9*) Am Urological.

Report on Radionics. Edward W. Russell. 6th ed. (Illus.). 256p. pap. 26.95 (*0-8464-4283-3*) Beekman Pubs.

Report on Radionics. Edward W. Russell. 1973. LC 73-88197. 110p. pap. (*0-85435-002-0*) C W Daniel GBR. *Dist:* Natl Bk Netwk.

Report on State Public Health Work, Based on a Survey of State Boards of Health. Charles V. Chapin. Ed. by Barbara G. Rosenkrantz. 1977. LC 76-25657. (Public Health in America Ser.). (Illus.). reprint ed. lib. bdg. 23.95 (*0-405-09807-3*) Ayer.

Report on the Condition of the Insane Poor in the County Poor Houses of New York. Sylvester D. Willard. 1973. LC 73-2430. (Mental Illness & Social Policy; the American Experience Ser.). reprint ed. 17.95 (*0-405-05238-3*) Ayer.

Report on the Perinatal Drug Exposure Task Force in Virginia. 1993. 48p. (Orig.). (C). pap. text 20.00 (*0-7881-0151-X*) DIANE Pub.

Report on the Poor & Insane in Rhode-Island. Thomas R. Hazard. 1973. LC 73-2403. (Mental Illness & Social Policy; the American Experience Ser.). reprint ed. 17.95 (*0-405-05209-X*) Ayer.

***Report on Varicocele & Infertility Vol. 4: An American Urological Association Best Practice Policy & American Society for Reproductive Medicine Practice Committee Report.** 2001. (Reports on Male Infertility). pap. (*0-9709327-1-5*) Am Urological.

Report Writing for Speech-Language Pathologists. Grace Middleton et al. 1998. 173p. pap. text 44.00 (*0-12-784563-1*) Acad Pr.

Report Writing for Speech-Language Pathologists. Grace Middleton et al. 1992. 173p. pap. text 46.00 (*0-7616-7797-6*) Commun Skill.

Reporting Chronic Pain Episodes on Health Surveys. 1993. 71p. (Orig.). (C). pap. text 25.00 (*1-56806-503-5*) DIANE Pub.

Reporting Chronic Pain Episodes on Health Surveys. 1992. LC 92-49423. (Vital & Health Statistics Ser.: Series 6, No. 6). (Orig.). (*0-8406-0466-1*) Natl Ctr Health Stats.

Reporting Histopathology Sections. Ed. by D. G. Lowe. 1997. (Illus.). 440p. pap. (*0-412-43040-1*) E A GBR. *Dist:* OUP.

Reporting on Risks: The Practice & Ethics of Health & Safety Communication. William J. Willis & Albert A. Okunade. 1997. LC 96-37692. 240p. 72.50 (*0-275-95296-7*); pap. 25.95 (*0-275-95298-3*) Greenwood (Praeger Pubs).

Reports of ORCA on Water Fluoridation. Ed. by European Organization for Caries Research, Board. 1974. (Journal: Vol. 8, Suppl. 1). 36p. 15.00 (*3-8055-1707-6*) S Karger.

Reports on AIDS in the African Press: An Annotated Bibliography. Nancy J. Schmidt. 1988. 47p. 5.00 (*0-941934-60-8*) Indiana Africa.

Reports on Ceftriaxone (RocephinR) Ed. by H. Schoenfeld. 1981. (Journal: Vol. 27, Suppl. 1). (Illus.). iv, 104p. pap. 25.25 (*3-8055-3034-X*) S Karger.

Reports on the Committee on Vision, 1947-1990. Committee on Vision, National Research Council Sta. 1990. 124p. pap. text 15.00 (*0-309-04148-1*) Natl Acad Pr.

Reports Regarding Medicare Payment Policies: Hearing Before the Subcommittee on Health of the Committee on Ways & Means, House of Representatives, One Hundred Fifth Congress, Second Session, March 3, 1998. U. S. Government Printing Office Staff. 1998. LC 98-211672. iii, 114p. (*0-16-057342-4*) USGPO.

Repossessions: Psychoanalysis & the Phantasms of Early Modern Culture. Timothy Murray. 1998. LC 98-2998. 256p. pap. 21.95 (*0-8166-2961-7*) U of Minn Pr.

Representation of Complex Stimuli in the Primate Visual Cortex. Martin Tovee. 1997. 200p. 89.95 (*0-412-14101-9*) Landes Bioscience.

Representations: Social Constructions of Gender. Ed. by R. Unger. 1989. 336p. text 47.95 (*0-89503-057-8*); pap. text 36.00 (*0-89503-052-7*) Baywood Pub.

Representations of Old Age (DINROO) Notes Towards a Critique & Revision of Ageism in Nursing Practice. Heather Gibbs. 1990. (Research Monographs: No. 2). (C). pap. (*0-7300-1447-9*) Deakin Univ AUS. *Dist:* St Mut.

Repressed Memories. Ed. by David Spiegel. 1997. (Review of Psychiatry Ser.: Vol. 16, Sect. II). 176p. (Orig.). pap. text 25.00 (*0-88048-446-2*, 8446) Am Psychiatric.

Repression & Dissociation: Implications for Personality Theory, Psychopathology & Health. Ed. by Jerome L. Singer. 1999. (John D. & Catherine T. MacArthur Foundation Series on Mental Health & Development). (Illus.). 544p. 34.95 (*0-226-76105-3*) U Ch Pr.

Repression & Fear: New Approaches to Resolve the Crisis in Psychopathology. Yacov Rofe. 1989. 500p. 78.95 (*0-89116-056-6*) Hemisp Pub.

Repression of Psychoanalysis: Otto Fenichel & the Political Freudians. Russell Jacoby. 1986. LC 86-11358. xiv, 218p. (C). reprint ed. pap. 13.50 (*0-226-39069-1*) U Ch Pr.

Reprinted Selected Top Articles Published, 1976-1977. Ed. by G. H. Berlyne. 1978. (Nephrology One Ser.). (Illus.). pap. 13.25 (*3-8055-2938-4*) S Karger.

Reprinted Selected Top Articles Published, 1977, No. 1. Compiled by H. M. Myers. 1979. (Oral Science One Ser.). 13.25 (*3-8055-3028-5*) S Karger.

Repro Lab: A Laboratory Manual for Animal Reproduction. A. M. Sorensen, Jr. 4th ed. 1979. (Illus.). 151p. pap. text 17.95 (*0-89641-011-0*) American Pr.

***Reprocessing of Single-Use Medical Devices: Congressional Hearing.** Ed. by James M. Jeffords. 2001. 215p. (C). pap. text 35.00 (*0-7567-1286-6*) DIANE Pub.

Reproducing Reproduction: Kinship, Power, & Technological Innovation. Ed. by Sarah Franklin & Helena Ragone. 1998. LC 97-36945. 264p. (C). pap. 18.50 (*0-8122-1584-2*) U of Pa Pr.

Reproduction. N. T. Adler et al. 1985. (Handbook of Behavioral Neurobiology Ser.: Vol. 7). (Illus.). 820p. (C). text 175.00 (*0-306-41768-5*, Kluwer Plenum) Kluwer Academic.

Reproduction: Endocrinology & Infertility. Samuel S. Yen. 2000. text (*0-7216-4454-6*) Saunders.

Reproduction & Aging. Andras Balazs et al. 1974. 331p. (C). text 32.50 (*0-8422-7159-7*) Irvington.

Reproduction & Environment. R. L. Holmes. 1971. (Contemporary Science Library). (Illus.). (C). reprint ed. pap. 1.50 (*0-393-00588-7*) Norton.

Reproduction & Man. Richard J. Harrison. 1971. (Contemporary Science Library). (Illus.). (C). reprint ed. pap. 1.50 (*0-393-00581-X*) Norton.

Reproduction in Farm Animals. E. Hafez. 7th ed. 2000. LC 99-53783. (Illus.). 528p. text 59.95 (*0-683-30577-8*) Lppncott W & W.

Reproduction of Mothering: Psychoanalysis & the Sociology of Gender. Nancy Julia Chodorow. 1978. 263p. pap. 17.95 (*0-520-03892-4*) U CA Pr.

Reproduction, Technology & Rights. Ed. by James M. Humber & Robert F. Almeder. 1996. LC 84-640015. (Biomedical Ethics Reviews Ser.). 168p. 59.50 (*0-89603-326-0*) Humana.

Reproductive & Developmental Behavior in Sheep: An Anthology from "Applied Animal Ethology" Ed. by A. F. Fraser. 1985. (Developments in Animal & Veterinary Science Ser.: Vol. 18). x,440p. 154.50 (*0-444-42444-X*) Elsevier.

Reproductive & Perinatal Epidemiology. Michele Kiely. 1990. 624p. lib. bdg. 195.00 (*0-8493-5379-3*, RG627) CRC Pr.

Reproductive Biology. Hing-Sing Yu. 1994. 304p. 94.95 (*0-8493-4439-5*) CRC Pr.

Reproductive Biology of Invertebrates Vol. 8: Progress in Developmental Biology. Ed. by K. G. Adiyodi & Rita G. Adiyodi. 1998. 382p. 250.00 (*0-471-96808-0*) Wiley.

Reproductive Biology of the Mare: Basic & Applied Aspects. O. J. Ginther. 2nd rev. ed. 1992. LC 91-75595. 642p. 93.00 (*0-9640072-1-5*) Equisrvs Pubng.

Reproductive Biology of the Primates. Ed. by P. Luckett. 1974. (Contributions to Primatology Ser.: Vol. 3). 284p. pap. 112.25 (*3-8055-1671-1*) S Karger.

Reproductive Endocrinology. Ed. by Bryan D. Cowan. 1996. LC 96-28717. 304p. text 110.00 (*0-397-51186-8*) Lppncott W & W.

Reproductive Endocrinology: Physiology, Pathophysiology & Clinical Management. Yen. 3rd ed. 1991. (Illus.). 1024p. text 185.00 (*0-7216-3206-8*) Saunders.

Reproductive Endocrinology: Physiology, Pathophysiology & Clinical Management. Samuel S. Yen et al. Ed. by Lisette Bralow. 4th ed. 1999. LC 97-36836. (Illus.). viii, 839p. (C). text 185.00 (*0-7216-6897-6*) Saunders.

Reproductive Endocrinology, Surgery, & Technology Ed. by Eli Y. Adashi et al. 1995. (Illus.). 2,544p. text 339.00 (*0-7817-0203-8*) Lppncott W & W.

Reproductive Endocrinology/Infertility Nursing. Jack Rudman. (Certified Nurse Examination Ser.: CN-23). pap. 27.95 (*0-8373-6123-0*) Nat Learn.

Reproductive Fitness. Ed. by C. R. Austin & R. V. Short. 2nd ed. 1985. (Reproduction in Mammals Ser.: Bk. 4). (Illus.). 256p. pap. text 27.95 (*0-521-31984-6*) Cambridge U Pr.

Reproductive Genetic Testing: Impact upon Women. Ed. by M. I. Evans. 1993. (Journal: Vol. 8, Suppl. 1, 1993). (Illus.). vi, 246p. pap. 42.75 (*3-8055-5715-9*) S Karger.

Reproductive Hazards in the Workplace: Bibliography. 1996. 166p. (C). reprint ed. pap. text 30.00 (*0-7881-3380-2*) DIANE Pub.

Reproductive Hazards in the Workplace: Mending Jobs, Managing Pregnancies. Regina Kenen. 1992. LC 91-34582. (Illus.). 302p. lib. bdg. 49.95 (*1-56024-154-3*) Haworth Pr.

Reproductive Hazards of the Workplace. Linda M. Frazier et al. 1997. 600p. 110.00 (*0-471-28698-2*, VNR) Wiley.

Reproductive Health: A Key to a Brighter Future: Special Programme of Research, Development, & Research Training in Human Reproduction Biennial Report 1990-1991. Ed. by J. Khanna et al. 20th anniv. ed. 1992. xiii, 171p. pap. text 35.00 (*92-4-156153-X*, 1150385) World Health.

Reproductive Health & Infectious Disease in the Middle East. Ed. by Robin Barlow & Joseph W. Brown. 1998. LC 98-72620. 228p. text (*1-84014-384-3*) Ashgate Pub GBR. *Dist:* Ashgate Pub Co.

Reproductive Health of Adolescents: A Strategy for Action: A Joint WHO - UNFPA - UNICEF Statement. WHO Staff. 1989. 18p. 3.00 (*92-4-156125-4*) World Health.

Reproductive Heatlh Trends. Kathleen O'Leary Morgan. 1999. 100p. per. 50.00 (*0-7401-0008-4*, M Quitno Pr) Morgan Quitno Corp.

Reproductive Immunology. Richard Bronson et al. 1996. 1000p. 235.00 (*0-86542-367-9*) Blackwell Sci.

Reproductive Immunology. Ed. by L. B. Olding. 1997. (Current Topics in Microbiology & Immunology Ser.: Vol. 222). (Illus.). 219p. 155.00 (*3-540-61888-0*) Spr-Verlag.

Reproductive Life: Advances in Research in Psychosomatic Obstetrics & Gynaecology. Ed. by K. Wijma & B. Von Schoultz. 1992. 708p. (C). lib. bdg. 85.95 (*1-85070-446-5*, Parthenon Pbng) CRC Pr.

Reproductive Medicine. Carr & Blackwell. 2nd ed. 1998. 223p. (C). pap., stu. ed. 55.00 (*0-8385-8894-8*) McGraw-Hill Prof.

Reproductive Medicine: From A to Z. Herbert Reiss. 1998. LC 97-35789. (Illus.). 162p. pap. text 49.95 (*0-19-262901-8*) OUP.

Reproductive Medicine: Molecular, Cellular & Genetic Fundamentals. B. C. J. M. Fauser. 2002. (Illus.). 450p. 119.95 (*1-84214-019-1*, Parthenon Pbng) CRC Pr.

Reproductive Medicine & the Law. Ed. by A. Templeton & Douglas J. Cusine. 1990. (Illus.). 167p. text (*0-443-04410-4*) Church.

Reproductive Neureoendocrinology of Aging & Drug Abuse. Ed. by Dipak K. Sarkar & Charles D. Barnes. 1994. 416p. 99.50 (*0-8493-2451-3*, 2451) CRC Pr.

Reproductive Pathology of Domestic Mammals. Kenneth McEntee. 1990. 401p. text 125.00 (*0-12-483375-6*) Acad Pr.

Reproductive Physiology. Ed. by Luigi Mastroianni, Jr. & C. Coutifaris. 1989. (F. I. G. O. Manual of Human Reproduction Ser.: Vol. 1). (Illus.). 114p. text 35.00 (*1-85070-192-X*, Parthenon Pbng) CRC Pr.

Reproductive Physiology of Domestic Lab Primate Animals. Charles O. Woody, Jr. et al. 1999. (*0-8493-8764-7*, BW8764) CRC Pr.

Reproductive Physiology of Vertebrates. Ari Van Tienhoven. 2nd ed. 1983. (Comstock Bk.). (Illus.). 491p. 65.00 (*0-8014-1281-1*) Cornell U Pr.

Reproductive Potential & Fertility Control. Ed. by Anne Walker & Catherine A. Niven. 1995. (Psychology of Reproduction Ser.: Vol. 1). 208p. pap. text (*0-7506-2249-0*) E A GBR. *Dist:* OUP.

Reproductive Processes & Contraception. Ed. by Kenneth W. McKerns. 1981. LC 80-20744. (Biochemical Endocrinology Ser.). 752p. 120.00 (*0-306-40534-2*, Plenum Trade) Perseus Pubng.

Reproductive Science, Genetics, & Birth Control. Ed. by Philip K. Wilson. 1996. LC 96-794. (Childbirth Ser.: Vol. 4). (Illus.). 448p. reprint ed. text 88.00 (*0-8153-2233-X*) Garland.

Reproductive System. Thomas Braem. 1994. (Organs of the Human Anatomy: Vol. 7). 88p. (C). spiral bd. 15.95 (*1-878576-32-1*) Flash Anatomy Inc.

Reproductive System. Kerri O'Donnell. 2000. LC 00-9754. (Insider's Guide to the Body Ser.). (Illus.). 48p. (J). lib. bdg. 19.95 (*0-8239-3334-2*) Rosen Group.

***Reproductive System.** John Sladek. 2001. 192p. pap. (*0-575-07116-8*) V Gollancz GBR. *Dist:* Sterling.

Reproductive System Course. Competence Assurance Systems Staff. 1984. (Illus.). pap. text 45.00 (*0-89147-107-3*) CAS.

Reproductive Technologies. Annette Burfoot. Date not set. 800p. text 100.00 (*0-8153-0148-0*) Garland.

Reproductive Technology: A Research Guide to the Legal Status of the Frozen Human Embryo. Timothy Coppo. 1996. LC 95-33288. (Legal Research Guides Ser.: Vol. 25). (9) 40 (12)p. 42.00 (*0-89941-982-8*, 308900) W S Hein.

Reproductive Toxicology: In Vitro Germ Cell Developmental Toxicology from Science to Social. Ed. by J. Del Mazo. 1998. (Advances in Experimental Medicine & Biology Ser.: 444). (Illus.). 236p. (C). text 130.00 (*0-306-46025-4*, Kluwer Plenum) Kluwer Academic.

Reproductive Tract Infections. A. Germain et al. 1992. (Reproductive Biology Ser.). (Illus.). 408p. (C). text 115.00 (*0-306-44241-8*, Kluwer Plenum) Kluwer Academic.

Reproductively Active Chemicals. Richard J. Lewis. 1991. 864p. text 167.95 (*0-442-31878-2*, VNR) Wiley.

Reproductively Active Chemicals: A Reference Guide. Richard J. Lewis. 1991. (Sax/Lewis Program Ser.). 841p. 195.00 (*0-471-28973-6*, VNR) Wiley.

Reptile Clinician's Handbook: A Compact Clinical & Surgical Reference. Fredric L. Frye. rev. ed. 1998. pap. 29.50 (*1-57524-100-5*) Krieger.

Reptile Diseases. Rolf Hackbarth. Tr. by U. Erich Friese from GER. 1990. (KW Ser.). (Illus.). 96p. lib. bdg. 9.95 (*0-86622-824-1*, KW-197) TFH Pubns.

Reptile Medicine & Surgery. Douglas R. Mader. 1995. LC 95-9672. (Illus.). 624p. text 98.00 (*0-7216-5208-5*) Saunders.

Reptilia & Batrachia. John Anderson. 1965. (Zoologica Ser.: No. 1). (Illus.). reprint ed. 180.00 (*3-7682-0240-2*) Lubrecht & Cramer.

Requirements for Biological Substances: 5 Requirements for Smallpox Vaccine. 1959. (Technical Report Ser.: No. 180). 24p. pap. text 3.00 (*92-4-120180-0*) World Health.

Requirements for Biological Substances: 7 Requirements for Poliomyelitis Vaccine. 1962. (Technical Report Ser.: No. 237). 29p. pap. text 3.00 (*92-4-120237-8*) World Health.

Requirements for Poultry Virus Vaccines: Proceedings of the International Symposium, Lyon, 1973. International Symposium on Requirements for Poultry Viruses Vaccines Staff. Ed. by Ch Merieux et al. 1976. (Developments in Biological Standardization Ser.: Vol. 25). 61.00 (*3-8055-2413-7*) S Karger.

Requirements of Ascorbic Acid, Vitamin D, Vitamin B12, Folate & Iron: Proceedings of the WHO Expert Committee, Geneva, 1969. WHO Staff. 1970. (Technical Reports: No. 452). 75p. pap. text 7.00 (*92-4-120452-4*, 1100452) World Health.

Requisites in Ophthalmology: Glaucoma. Wallace L. M. Alward. 1999. (Illus.). 350p. (C). text (*0-323-00106-8*) Mosby Inc.

Requisites in Ophthalmology: Neuro-Ophthalmology. Timothy J. Martin & James J. Corbett. 1999. (Illus.). 300p. (C). text 89.00 (*0-323-00182-3*) Mosby Inc.

Requisites in Ophthalmology: Pathology, Physiology & Refraction. Morton E. Smith et al. 1999. (Illus.). 425p. (C). text (*0-323-00236-6*) Mosby Inc.

Requisites in Ophthalmology: Pediatric Ophthalmology & Strabismus. Kenneth W. Wright & Peter Spiegel. 1999. LC 99-34127. (Illus.). 350p. (C). text (*0-323-00181-5*) Mosby Inc.

Requisites in Ophthalmology: Retina, Choroid & Vitreous. Jose Pulido. 1999. (Illus.). 475p. (C). text (*0-323-00237-4*) Mosby Inc.

Requisites in Ophthalmology: The Anterior Segment. Christopher J. Rapuano et al. 1999. LC 99-35199. (Illus.). 425p. (C). text 89.00 (*0-323-00173-4*) Mosby Inc.

Rescue 911 Family First Aid & Emergency Care Book: Simple Step-by-Step Guide. Julie Motz. 1996. mass mkt. 5.99 (*0-671-52514-X*, PB Trade Paper) PB.

Rescue Technician: Operational Readiness for Rescue Providers. Maryland Fire and Rescue Institute Staff. 1997. (Illus.). 240p. (gr. 13). pap. text 32.95 (*0-8151-8390-9*, 31690) Mosby Inc.

Rescuers in Action. Barry D. Smith. 1995. LC 95-77713. (Illus.). 224p. (C). (gr. 13). text 14.95 (*0-8151-7902-2*, 25773) Mosby Inc.

Rescuing Brain Injured Children. Keith Pennock. 1998. (*1-85398-111-7*) Ashgrove Pr GBR. *Dist:* Words Distrib.

Rescuing the "Inner Child" Therapy for Adults Sexually Abused As Children. Penny Parks. 194p. (*0-285-65084-X*) Souvenir Pr Ltd GBR. *Dist:* IPG Chicago.

Research: Developments & Progress in Science, Life & Medicine Including Concerns & World-Wide Criticisms. John C. Bartone. 1997. 185p. 57.50 (*0-7883-1020-8*); pap. 47.50 (*0-7883-1021-6*) ABBE Pubs Assn.

Research: Some Ground Rules. J. S. Lumley & W. Benjimen. 1995. LC 94-23261. (Illus.). 260p. text 70.00 (*0-19-854823-0*); pap. text 35.00 (*0-19-854822-2*) OUP.

Research: Successful Approaches. Elaine R. Monsen. 1991. LC 91-31303. pap. 29.95 (*0-88091-092-5*, 0180) Am Dietetic Assn.

Research: The Validation of Clinical Practice. Otto D. Payton. 3rd ed. 1993. LC 93-26828. (Illus.). 355p. (C). pap. text 24.95 (*0-8036-6800-7*) Davis Co.

Research: The Validation of Clinical Practice. Otto D. Payton & Scott Sullivan. 4th ed. 2000. LC 93-26828. (Illus.). 355p. (C). pap. text 24.95 (*0-8036-0458-0*) Davis Co.

Research—World Developments in Health, Science, Life & Work: Index of New Information. American Health Research Institute Staff. 1997. 160p. 57.50 (*0-7883-1722-9*); pap. 47.50 (*0-7883-1723-7*) ABBE Pubs Assn.

Research Abstracts: Southeast Asia Region, 4. 1994. (WHO Regional Publications, South-East Asia Ser.: No. 16). 102p. pap. text 10.00 (*92-9022-165-8*) World Health.

Research Abstracts Vol. 3: South-East Asia Region. 1991. (WHO Regional Publications, South-East Asia Ser.: No. 16). iv, 109p. pap. text 10.00 (*92-9022-161-5*, 1560016) World Health.

Research Advances in Alcohol & Drug Problems, Vol. 6. Ed. by Yedi Israel et al. 1981. LC 73-18088. 536p. 95.00 (*0-306-40672-1*, Plenum Trade) Perseus Pubng.

Research Advances in Alcohol & Drug Problems, Vol. 8. Ed. by Reginald G. Smart et al. 1984. 328p. 85.00 (*0-306-41551-8*, Plenum Trade) Perseus Pubng.

Research Advances in Alcohol & Drug Problems, Vol. 9. Ed. by Howard D. Cappell et al. 1986. 315p. 79.50 (*0-306-42426-6*, Plenum Trade) Perseus Pubng.

Research Advances in Alcohol & Drug Problems, Vol. 10. L. T. Kozlowski et al. 1990. LC 73-18088. (Illus.). 424p. (C). 100.00 (*0-306-43295-1*, Plenum Trade) Perseus Pubng.

Research Advances in Alcohol & Drug Problems Vol. 5: Alcohol & Drug Problems in Women. Oriana J. Kalant. 1980. LC 73-18088. 784p. 110.00 (*0-306-40394-3*, Plenum Trade) Perseus Pubng.

Research Advances in Alcohol & Drug Problems Vol. 11: Drug Testing in the Workplace. Scott MacDonald & Paul Roman. 1994. (Research Advances in Alcohol & Drug Problems: Vol. 11). (Illus.). 356p. (C). 100.00 (*0-306-44557-3*, Plenum Trade) Perseus Pubng.

Research Advances in Alzheimer's Disease & Related Disorders. Ed. by Khalid Iqbal et al. 1995. LC 94-36061. 828p. 475.00 (*0-471-95236-2*) Wiley.

Research Adventures Across the Life Span. Ed. by Matthew R. Merrens & Gary G. Brannigan. 1995. (Developmental Psychology Ser.). 310p. (C). pap. 27.50 (*0-07-007259-0*) McGrw-H Hghr Educ.

Research Agendas in the Sociology of Emotions. Ed. by Theodore D. Kemper. 1990. LC 89-26193. (SUNY Series in the Sociology of Emotions). 335p. (C). pap. text 25.95 (*0-7914-0270-3*) State U NY Pr.

Research & Change in Urban Community Health. Ed. by Bruce Nigel. 1995. 464p. (*1-85972-159-1*) Avebry GBR. *Dist:* Ashgate Pub Co.

***Research & Design Methods: A Process Approach.** Kenneth S. Bordens & Bruce B. Abbott. 5th ed. 2001. LC 2001-18697. (Illus.). xv, 490p. (*0-7674-2152-3*) Mayfield Pub.

Research & Development & School Change. Ed. by R. Glaser. 1978. 128p. 19.95 (*0-89859-449-9*) L Erlbaum Assocs.

Research & Evaluation Methodology. Louise Gresham. 1993. 114p. (C). spiral bd. Price not set. (*0-933195-09-5*) CA College Health Sci.

Research & Intervention: Preventing Substance Abuse in Higher Education. Ed. by Gerardo M. Gonzalez & Vonnie V. Clement. 1997. (Illus.). 125p. (C). reprint ed. pap. text 30.00 (*0-7881-4595-9*) DIANE Pub.

Research & Its Application. Ed. by James P. Smith. 1994. LC 94-2693. (Advanced Nursing Ser.). (Illus.). 224p. pap. 37.95 (*0-632-03867-5*) Blackwell Sci.

Research & Methodology in General Pediatrics: A Swiss Experience. Ed. by P. Girardet. 1981. (Journal: Vol. 9, Nos. 5-6). (Illus.). 128p. pap. 61.00 (*3-8055-2661-X*) S Karger.

Research & Practice in Alzheimer's Disease. Bruno J. Vellas. 1998. 463p. pap. text 46.95 (*0-8261-1194-7*) Springer Pub.

Research & Recipes on Dementia, Heart Disease, Osteoporosis & Cancer. Rosemary C. Fisher. 1997. LC 97-170609. pap. 9.95 (*0-87527-530-3*) Green.

Research & Service Programs in the PHS: Challenges in Organization. Institute of Medicine Staff. 1991. 156p. pap. text 19.00 (*0-309-04581-9*) Natl Acad Pr.

Research & Source Guide for Students in Speech Pathology & Audiology. Gordon F. Holloway & L. Michael Webster. 1978. LC 73-571. 112p. 9.50 (*0-87527-154-5*) Green.

Research Animals & Concepts of Applicability to Clinical Medicine Vol. 7: Experimental Biology & Medicine. Ed. by K. Gaertner et al. 1982. (Illus.). x, 234p. pap. 128.75 (*3-8055-3492-2*) S Karger.

Research Animals & Experimental Design in Nephrology. H. Stolte & Jeannette Alt. 1980. (Contributions to Nephrology Ser.: Vol. 19). (Illus.). x, 250p. pap. 29.75 (*3-8055-3075-7*) S Karger.

Research Approaches to Movement & Personality. Philip Eisenberg et al. 1979. 28.95 (*0-405-03146-7*, 11041) Ayer.

Research at the Hampstead Child-Therapy Clinic & Other Papers. Anna Freud. 1969. LC 67-9514. (Writings of Anna Freud: Vol. 5). 575p. 85.00 (*0-8236-6874-6*) Intl Univs Pr.

***Research Basis for Autism Intervention.** Ed. by Eric Schopler. 2001. LC 2001-25357. 254p. 55.00 (*0-306-46585-X*, Kluwer Plenum) Kluwer Academic.

Research, Design & Analysis. Ed. by Mark E. Brecher & Michael Paul Busch. 1998. LC 99-172014. text (*1-56395-100-2*) Am Assn Blood.

Research Design & Evaluation in Speech-Language Pathology & Audiology. Franklin H. Silverman. 4th ed. 1997. LC 97-6601. 392p. 84.00 (*0-205-19799-X*) Allyn.

Research Design & Methods: A Process Approach. Kenneth S. Bordens & Bruce B. Abbott. 4th ed. 1998. LC 98-4480. xix, 583p. text 66.95 (*0-7674-0507-2*, 0507-2) Mayfield Pub.

Research Design in Clinical Psychology. Alan E. Kazdin. 3rd ed. 1997. LC 97-37711. 524p. (C). pap. 70.00 (*0-205-26088-8*) Allyn.

Research Designs & Methods in Psychiatry. Ed. by Mathilde Fava & J. F. Rosenbaum. 1992. LC 92-49613. (Techniques in the Behavioral & Neural Sciences Ser.: Vol. 9). xvi,324p. 224.00 (*0-444-89595-7*); 324p. pap. 120.50 (*0-444-89594-9*) Elsevier.

Research Directions of Black Psychologists. Anderson J. Franklin & J. Frank Yates. Ed. by A. Wade Boykin et al. 1980. LC 79-7348. 440p. 50.00 (*0-87154-254-4*) Russell Sage.

Research Directory: Research Activities Within Medical Groups & Research Centers. Ed. by Suzanne S. White & Donna L. Burman. 1996. 350p. (Orig.). pap. text 35.00 (*1-56829-012-8*) M G M A.

Research Ethics: A Psychological Approach. Ed. by Barbara Stanley et al. 1996. LC 95-22886. 273p. text 45.00 (*0-8032-4188-7*) U of Nebr Pr.

Research Experience for Nurses: Realities of Studies into Nursing. Jill Buckeldee. Ed. by Richard McMahon. 1994. LC 93-35414. 144p. pap. 41.50 (*1-56593-193-9*, 0508) Singular Publishing.

Research Explorations in Adult Attachments. Intro. by Karl Pottharst. 1991. (American University Studies: Ser. VIII, Vol. 14). (Illus.). XIV, 353p. (C). text 53.95 (*0-8204-1050-0*) P Lang Pubng.

Research Findings on Smoking of Abused Substances. Ed. by C. Nora Chiang & Richard L. Hawks. 1994. (Illus.). 178p. (Orig.). (C). pap. text 30.00 (*0-7881-0372-5*) DIANE Pub.

Research for Clinical Therapis. Carolyn Hicks et al. 3rd ed. 1999. LC 98-52975. (C). pap. text 39.00 (*0-443-06266-8*) Saunders.

Research for Health Professionals: Concepts, Designs & Methods. Julius Sim & Chris Wright. 2000. (Illus.). 320p. pap. (*0-7487-3718-9*) Nelson Thornes GBR. *Dist:* Intl Spec Bk, Trans-Atl Phila.

Research for Physiotherapists: Project Design & Analysis. Carolyn M. Hicks. 2nd ed. 1995. LC 94-25780. 253p. pap. text (*0-443-04999-8*) Church.

Research for the Health Professional: A Practical Guide. Diana M. Bailey. 2nd ed. 1997. LC 96-36840. (Illus.). 278p. (C). pap. text 26.95 (*0-8036-0151-4*) Davis Co.

Research for the Reorientation of National Health Systems. 1983. (Technical Report Ser.: No. 694). 71p. pap. text 7.00 (*92-4-120694-2*) World Health.

Research Foundations for Psychology & Behavior Sciences. Frank M. Loos. 1995. (C). text 63.50 (*0-673-99481-3*) Addson-Wesley Educ.

Research Foundations for Psychotherapy Practice. Ed. by Mark Aveline & David A. Shapiro. 1995. LC 95-127070. (Computational Methods in Applied Sciences Ser.). 346p. 230.00 (*0-471-95219-2*) Wiley.

Research Fraud in the Behavioral & Biomedical Sciences. Ed. by David J. Miller & Michel Hersen. 1992. LC 91-21625. 272p. 185.00 (*0-471-52068-3*) Wiley.

Research Frontiers: Implantable Defibrillator Surgery. Henry M. Spotnitz. 1992. 120p. 94.00 (*1-879702-41-X*) CRC Pr.

Research Guide for Psychology, 1. Raymond G. McInnis. 1982. LC 81-1377. (Reference Sources for the Social Sciences & Humanities Ser.: No. 1). (Illus.). 604p. lib. bdg. 120.00 (*0-313-21399-2*, MCR/, Greenwood Pr) Greenwood.

Research Guide to Human Sexuality. Kara Lichtenberg. 1994. LC 93-37236. 527p. text 20.00 (*0-8153-0867-1*, SS836) Garland.

Research Guide to the Health Sciences: Medical, Nutritional, & Environmental, 4. Kathleen J. Haselbauer. 1987. LC 87-17592. (Reference Sources for the Social Sciences & Humanities Ser.: No. 4). 672p. lib. bdg. 110.00 (*0-313-23530-9*, HHS/, Greenwood Pr) Greenwood.

Research Guidelines for Evaluating the Safety & Efficacy of Herbal Medicines. 1993. v, 86p. pap. text 7.50 (*92-9061-110-3*, 1520003) World Health.

Research in Addiction: An Update. Ed. by Hanns Hippius et al. 1995. LC 94-26617. (Psychiatry in Progress Ser.: Vol. 2). (Illus.). 160p. text 32.00 (*0-88937-134-2*) Hogrefe & Huber Pubs.

Research in Chronic Viral Hepatitis. Ed. by Wolfram H. Gerlich. 1994. (Archives of Virology Ser.: No. 8). (Illus.). 315p. 214.00 (*0-387-82497-9*) Spr-Verlag.

Research in Community & Mental Health, Vol. 2. Ed. by James R. Greenley & Roberta G. Simmons. 1981. 357p. 73.25 (*0-89232-152-0*) Jai Pr.

Research in Community & Mental Health. Ed. by James R. Greenley. Vol. 3. 1983. 317p. 73.25 (*0-89232-299-3*); Vol. 4. 1984. 370p. 73.25 (*0-89232-489-9*); Vol. 5. 1995. 350p. 73.25 (*0-89232-548-8*); Vol. 7. 1992. 325p. 73.25 (*1-55938-441-7*); Vol. 8. 1995. 73.25 (*1-55938-139-6*) Jai Pr.

Research in Community & Mental Health, Vol. 9. Joseph Morrissey. Ed. by James R. Greenley. 1998. 73.25 (*1-55938-140-X*) Jai Pr.

Research in Community & Mental Health Vol. 6: Mental Disorders in Social Context. Ed. by James R. Greenley. 1991. 436p. 73.25 (*0-89232-726-X*) Jai Pr.

Research in Congenital Hypothyroidism. Ed. by F. Delange et al. 1989. (NATO ASI Series A, Life Sciences: Vol. 161). (Illus.). 380p. 105.00 (*0-306-43141-6*, Plenum Trade) Perseus Pubng.

Research in Counseling. Ed. by C. Edward Watkins, Jr. & Lawrence J. Schneider. 1991. 328p. text 69.95 (*0-8058-0689-X*) L Erlbaum Assocs.

Research in Counseling & Psychotherapy: Practical Applications. Windy Dryden. 1996. LC 96-67700. 272p. pap. 27.95 (*0-8039-7841-3*, 9736) Sage.

Research in Dementia Precox. Nolan D. Lewis. Ed. by Gerald N. Grob. 1980. LC 78-22572. (Historical Issues in Mental Health Ser.). reprint ed. lib. bdg. 25.95 (*0-405-11925-9*) Ayer.

Research in Family Planning. Ed. by J. Bonnar et al. 1984. (Studies in Fertility & Sterility). lib. bdg. 163.50 (*0-85200-813-9*) Kluwer Academic.

Research in General Practice. J. G. Howie. 2nd ed. 1989. 256p. 36.95 (*0-412-33730-4*, A4444) Chapman & Hall.

Research in Health Care: Design, Conduct & Interpretation of Health Services Research. I. K. Crombie & H. T. Davies. 1996. LC 95-42359. 302p. pap. 59.95 (*0-471-96259-7*) Wiley.

Research in Health Care Settings. Kathleen E. Grady & Barbara Strudler-Wallston. 1988. LC 88-3154. (Applied Social Research Methods Ser.: Vol. 14). 160p. (C). pap. 26.95 (*0-8039-2875-0*, 5694) Sage.

Research in Human Capital & Development: Public Health & Development. Ed. by Richard Frank et al. 1988. (Research in Human Capital & Development Ser.: Vol. 5). 293p. 78.50 (*0-89232-508-9*) Jai Pr.

Research in Human Reproduction: Biennial Report, 1986-1987. E. Diczfalusy & P. Griffin. 1988. 346p. 25.00 (*92-4-156120-3*) World Health.

Research in Human Reproduction: Biennial Report, 1988-1989. WHO Staff. 1990. 191p. 31.00 (*92-4-156140-8*) World Health.

PQR

Research in Immunology: Report of 5 Scientific Groups Convened by the Director-General of the World Health Organization, Geneva, 1962. 1964. (Technical Reports: No. 286). (ENG, FRE, RUS & SPA.). 97p. pap. text 7.00 (*92-4-120286-6*, 1100286) World Health.

Research in Mental Health Computing: The Next Five Years. Ed. by John H. Greist et al. 1988. LC 87-35269. (Computers in Human Services Ser.: Vol. 2, Nos. 3-4). 176p. text 5.95 (*0-86656-648-1*) Haworth Pr.

Research in Organizational Behavior, Vol. 2. Ed. by Barry M. Staw & L. L. Cummings. 1980. 368p. 78.50 (*0-89232-099-0*) Jai Pr.

Research in Organizational Behavior. Ed. by Barry M. Staw & Larry L. Cummings. Vol. 3. 1981. 356p. 78.50 (*0-89232-151-2*); Vol. 4. 1982. 364p. 78.50 (*0-89232-147-4*); Vol. 7. 1985. 408p. 78.50 (*0-89232-497-X*) Jai Pr.

Research in Parapsychology, 1980: Abstracts & Papers from the 23rd Annual Convention of the Parapsychological Association, 1980. Ed. by Parapsychological Association Staff et al. 1981. LC 66-28580. 173p. 30.00 (*0-8108-1425-0*) Scarecrow.

Research in Parapsychology, 1982: Jubilee Centenary Issue: Abstracts & Papers from the 25th Annual Convention of the Parapsychological Association, 1982. Ed. by Parapsychological Association Staff et al. 1983. LC 66-28580. 382p. 30.00 (*0-8108-1627-X*) Scarecrow.

Research in Parapsychology, 1977: Abstracts & Papers from the 20th Annual Convention of the Parapsychological Association, 1977. Parapsychological Association Staff. Ed. by William G. Roll. 1978. LC 66-28580. 279p. lib. bdg. 30.00 (*0-8108-1131-6*) Scarecrow.

Research in Parapsychology, 1979: Abstracts & Papers from the 22nd Annual Convention of the Parapsychological Association. Parapsychological Association Staff. Ed. by William G. Roll. 1980. LC 66-2858. 238p. 30.00 (*0-8108-1327-0*) Scarecrow.

Research in Population Genetics of Primitive Groups. 1964. (Technical Report Ser.: No. 279). 26p. pap. text 3.00 (*92-4-120279-3*) World Health.

Research in Psychiatry: Issues, Strategies & Methods. L. K. Hsu & M. Hersen. 1992. (Critical Issues in Psychiatry Ser.). (Illus.). 504p. (C). text 75.00 (*0-306-44162-4*, Kluwer Plenum) Kluwer Academic.

Research in Psychoanalysis: Process, Development, Outcome. Ed. by Theodore Shapiro & Robert N. Emde. 1995. LC 94-3704. 447p. 65.00 (*0-8236-5795-7*) Intl Univs Pr.

Research in Psychology: Methods & Design. C. James Goodwin. 2nd ed. 1998. LC 98-23943. 560p. 80.95 (*0-471-19986-9*) Wiley.

Research in Rehabilitation Counseling: A Guide to Design, Methodology & Utilization. James L. Bellini & Phillip D. Rumrill, Jr. 1999. LC 99-37751. 252p. 47.95 (*0-398-06993-X*); pap. 34.95 (*0-398-06994-8*) C C Thomas.

Research in Soviet Social Psychology. Ed. by L. H. Strickland et al. 1986. (Recent Research in Psychology Ser.). (Illus.). 99p. 59.95 (*0-387-96317-0*) Spr-Verlag.

Research in the Economics of Mental Health. Ed. by Richard M. Scheffler et al. 1994. (Advances in Health Economics & Health Services Research Ser.: Vol. 14). 264p. 73.25 (*1-55938-612-6*) Jai Pr.

Research in the Sociology of Health Care. Ed. by Jennie J. Kronenfeld & Rose Weitz. Supp. 1: Organizational Constraints on Psychiatric. 1981. (Research in the Sociology of Health Care Ser.: Supplement No. 1). 164p. 78.50 (*0-89232-176-8*); Vol. 2: Changing Struct. of Hlth Serv. Occupations. 1982. 352p. 78.50 (*0-89232-199-7*); Vol. 3: The Control of Costs & Performance of Med. 1984. (Research in the Sociology of Health Care Ser.: Vol. 3). 350p. 78.50 (*0-89232-310-8*); Vol. 5: International Comparisons of Hlth Services. 1987. (Research in the Sociology of Health Care Ser.: Vol. 5). 301p. 78.50 (*0-89232-597-6*); Vol. 6: The Experience & Mgmt. of Chronic Illness. 1987. 321p. 78.50 (*0-89232-834-7*); Vol. 7. 1988. 333p. 78.50 (*0-89232-883-5*); Vol. 8. 1989. 341p. 78.50 (*1-55938-043-8*); Vol. 9. 1991. 353p. 78.50 (*1-55938-098-5*); Vol. 10. 1993. 287p. 78.50 (*1-55938-444-1*); Vol. 11: Agents of Health & Illness. 1994. 208p. 78.50 (*1-55938-840-4*); Vol. 12. 1995. 355p. 78.50 (*1-55938-894-3*) Jai Pr.

Research in the Sociology of Health Care, Vol. 13. Ed. by Jennie J. Kronenfeld. 1996. 157.00 (*0-7623-0049-3*) Jai Pr.

Research in the Sociology of Health Care Vol. 1: Professional Control of Health Services & Chal. Ed. by Jennie J. Kronenfeld & Rose Weitz. 1980. 377p. 78.50 (*0-89232-145-8*) Jai Pr.

Research in the Sociology of Health Care Vol. 4: The Adoption & Social Consequences of Medical Technologies. Ed. by Jennie J. Kronenfeld & Rose Weitz. 1986. 317p. 78.50 (*0-89232-492-9*) Jai Pr.

Research into Environmental Pollution: A Report of 5 WHO Scientific Groups. 1968. (Technical Reports: No. 406). 83p. pap. text 6.00 (*92-4-120406-0*, 1100406) World Health.

Research into Nurse Education. Ed. by Bryn D. Davis. 1983. 208p. pap. (*0-7099-0825-3*) C Helm GBR. *Dist:* Routldge.

Research into Practice. Crookes. 1998. (C). pap. text 21.00 (*0-7020-2068-0*) Saunders.

Research into Practice: A Reader for Nurses & the Caring Professions. Ed. by Roger Sapsford & Pamela Abbott. 1992. 160p. pap. (*0-335-09742-1*) OpUniv Pr.

Research into Practice: A Reader for Nurses & the Caring Professions. P. Abbott. 2nd ed. 1997. LC 96-49631. (Social Science for Nurses & the Caring Professions Ser.). (*0-335-19696-9*); pap. (*0-335-19695-0*) OpUniv Pr.

Research into Spinal Deformities. Ed. by J. A. Sevastik & K. M. Diab. 1997. LC 96-79139. (Studies in Health Technology & Informatics: Vol. 37). 524p. 122.00 (*90-5199-308-0*, 308-0) IOS Press.

Research Issues in Human Behavior & Sexually Transmitted Diseases in the AIDS Era. Ed. by Judith N. Wasserheit et al. 1991. (Illus.). 401p. 99.95 (*1-55581-036-5*) ASM Pr.

Research Meth Nurses. P. Abbott. 2nd ed. 1998. LC 97-42886. 200p. pap. (*0-335-19698-5*) OpUniv Pr.

Research Methodologies in Human Diabetes. Ed. by C. E. Mogensen & E. Standl. 1994. LC 93-50659. 470p. 129.25 (*3-11-014248-1*) De Gruyter.

Research Methodology in Nursing & Health Care. Open Learning Foundation Staff. 1996. 144p. pap. (*0-443-05737-0*) Church.

Research Methods. Donald H. McBurney. 3rd ed. 1993. LC 93-5651. 410p. mass mkt. 54.25 (*0-534-17646-1*) Brooks-Cole.

Research Methods & Audit in General Practice. David Armstrong & John Grace. 3rd ed. 2000. LC 00-36754. (Oxford General Practice Ser.: No. 46). (Illus.). 192p. pap. text 59.95 (*0-19-263191-8*) OUP.

Research Methods & Statistics in Health Care. 144p. pap. (*0-7131-4522-6*) E A GBR. *Dist:* Routldge.

Research Methods for Clinical Social Workers: Empirical Practice. John S. Wodarski. 1997. LC 96-40362. (Social Work Ser.). (Illus.). 288p. 39.95 (*0-8261-9650-0*) Springer Pub.

Research Methods for Community Health & Welfare: An Introduction. Karl E. Bauman. 1980. 160p. pap. text 19.95 (*0-19-502699-3*) OUP.

Research Methods for Health Sciences. David A. Brodie et al. 1994. LC 94-1258. xii, 210p. pap. text 27.00 (*3-7186-5527-6*) Gordon & Breach.

Research Methods for Nurses & the Caring Professions. Roger Sapsford & Pamela Abbott. 1992. 160p. (*0-335-09621-2*); pap. (*0-335-09620-4*) OpUniv Pr.

Research Methods for Nurses & the Caring Professions. Pamela Abbott. 2nd ed. 1998. (Social Science for Nurses & the Caring Professions Ser.). 200p. pap. (*0-335-19697-7*) OpUniv Pr.

Research Methods for the Health Sciences. David A. Brodie. 1994. xii, 210p. text 52.00 (*3-7186-5609-4*, Harwood Acad Pubs) Gordon & Breach.

Research Methods for Therapists. A. Drummond. 1996. LC 96-83981. (Illus.). 176p. (Orig.). pap. 47.75 (*1-56593-207-2*, 0521) Singular Publishing.

Research Methods in Applied Behavior Analysis: Issues & Advances. A. Poling & R. W. Fuqua. 1986. (Applied Clinical Psychology Ser.). (Illus.). 352p. (C). 65.00 (*0-306-42127-5*, Plenum Trade) Perseus Pubng.

Research Methods in Clinical Psychology. Ed. by Alan S. Bellack & M. Hersen. 1984. (General Psychology Ser.: No. 130). (Illus.). 416p. text 75.00 (*0-08-029410-3*); pap. text 29.50 (*0-08-029409-X*) Elsevier (Pergamon Pr).

Research Methods in Family Therapy. Ed. by Douglas H. Sprenkle & Sidney M. Moon. 1996. LC 96-21297. 514p. text 58.00 (*1-57230-111-2*, 0111) Guilford Pubns.

Research Methods in Health: Investigating Health & Health Services. D. Bowling. 1997. LC 97-7997. pap. (*0-335-19885-6*) OpUniv Pr.

Research Methods In Neurochemistry, Vol. 5. Ed. by Neville Marks & Richard Rodnight. 1981. LC 72-222263. 334p. 79.50 (*0-306-40583-0*, Plenum Trade) Perseus Pubng.

Research Methods in Occupational Epidemiology. Harvey Checkoway et al. 1989. (Monographs in Epidemiology & Biostatistics: No. 13). (Illus.). 368p. text 52.50 (*0-19-505224-2*) OUP.

Research Methods in Primary Care. Ed. by Yvonne Carter & Cathryn Thomas. 1997. LC 96-53628. 200p. pap. (*1-85775-198-1*) Radcliffe Med Pr GBR. *Dist:* Balogh.

Research Methods in Psychology. Glynis M. Breakwell et al. 1994. 432p. pap. 24.95 (*0-8039-7765-4*, 4150) Sage.

Research Methods in Psychology. Gary W. Heiman. 1994. (C). tchr. ed. 11.96 (*0-395-64620-0*) HM.

Research Methods in Psychology. John J. Shaughnessy & Eugene B. Zechmeister. 2nd ed. 1990. (C). text 59.74 net. (*0-07-072859-3*) McGraw.

Research Methods in Psychology. David G. Elmes et al. Ed. by Schiller. 4th ed. 1992. 400p. (C). text 54.25 (*0-314-92999-1*) West Pub.

Research Methods in Psychology. John J. Shaughnessy & Eugene B. Zechmeister. 4th ed. 1996. LC 96-22572. 544p. (C). text 80.31 (*0-07-057272-0*) McGrw-H Hghr Educ.

Research Methods in Psychology. David G. Elmes & Kantowitz. 5th ed. 1995. (Psychology Ser.). pap., stu. ed. 18.00 net. (*0-314-05880-X*) Brooks-Cole.

Research Methods in Psychology. David G. Elmes et al. 6th ed. 1998. LC 98-22497. (Psychology Ser.). 24p. pap. 50.00 (*0-534-35811-X*) Brooks-Cole.

Research Methods in Psychology. David G. Elmes et al. 5th ed. 1995. LC 94-34602. 496p. (C). pap. 49.75 (*0-314-04458-2*) West Pub.

Research Methods in Psychology: A Primer. Siu L. Chow. 1992. 320p. (Orig.). (C). pap. text 25.95 (*1-55059-031-6*) Temeron Bks.

***Research Methods in Social Relations.** Rick H. Hoyle et al. 7th ed. 2001. LC 2001-95096. (Illus.). 573p. text 98.95 (*0-15-506139-9*) Wadsworth Pub.

Research Mindedness for Practice: An Interactive Approach for Nursing & Health Care. Ed. by P. Smith. 1997. (Illus.). 304p. pap. (*0-443-05293-X*) Church.

Research of Infectious Diseases at the University of Maryland, 1807-2000. Theodore E. Woodward. 2000. (Illus.). 286p. 23.80 (*0-9619119-2-1*) Medical Alumni Association of Univ.

Research on Adulthood & Aging: The Human Science Approach. Ed. by L. Eugene Thomas. 1989. LC 88-31873. (SUNY Series in Aging). 249p. (C). pap. text 21.95 (*0-7914-0069-7*) State U NY Pr.

Research on Alcohol & Alcoholism. 1993. (Illus.). 105p. (Orig.). (C). pap. text 30.00 (*0-7881-0021-1*) DIANE Pub.

Research on Alcoholics Anonymous: Opportunities & Alternatives. Barbara S. McCrady & William R. Miller. 1993. LC 92-63233. 440p. (Orig.). (C). pap. 25.95 (*0-911290-24-9*, BBK-139) Rutgers Ctr Alcohol.

Research on Genetics in Psychiatry: Report of a WHO Scientific Group, 1966. 1966. (Technical Report Ser.). 20p. pap. text 3.00 (*92-4-120346-3*, 1100346) World Health.

Research on Group Treatment Methods: A Selectively Annotated Bibliography, 9. Bernard Lubin & C. Wilson. 1996. LC 96-23114. (Bibliographies & Indexes in Psychology Ser.: No. 9). 264p. lib. bdg. 78.75 (*0-313-28339-7*, Greenwood Pr) Greenwood.

Research on Human Population Genetics: Report of a WHO Scientific Group, 1968. 1968. (Technical Report Ser.: No. 387). 32p. pap. text 3.00 (*92-4-120387-0*, 1100387) World Health.

Research on Human Subjects: Ethics, Law & Social Policy. David N. Weisstub. 1998. LC 98-38306. 684p. 135.00 (*0-08-043434-7*, Pergamon Pr) Elsevier.

Research on Human Subjects: Problems of Social Control in Medical Experimentation. Bernard Barber et al. 1973. LC 70-83831. 264p. 40.00 (*0-87154-090-8*) Russell Sage.

Research on Human Subjects: Problems of Social Control in Medical Experimentation. Bernard Barber et al. 1979. LC 78-55938. 263p. reprint ed. pap. text 24.95 (*0-87855-649-4*) Transaction Pubs.

Research on Steroids, Vol. 3. Ed. by C. Cassano et al. text (*0-7204-4042-4*) Brill Academic Pubs.

Research on the Menopause. 1981. (Technical Report Ser.: No. 670). 120p. pap. text 8.00 (*92-4-120670-5*) World Health.

Research on the Menopause in the 1990s: Report of a WHO Scientific Group. 1996. LC 97-119614. (WHO Technical Reports: Vol. 866). 106p. pap. 18.00 (*92-4-120866-X*, 1100866) World Health.

Research on the Treatment of Narcotic Addiction. 1990. 250.00 (*0-87700-888-4*) Revisionist Pr.

Research on the Viral Hypothesis of Mental Disorders. Ed. by P. V. Morozov. 1983. (Advances in Biological Psychiatry Ser.: Vol. 12). (Illus.). x, 178p. pap. 79.25 (*3-8055-3706-9*) S Karger.

Research Opportunities in Primary Care. Ed. by Cathryn Thomas & Yvonne Carter. 1999. LC 99-200484. (Illus.). 256p. pap. (*1-85775-242-2*) Radcliffe Med Pr GBR. *Dist:* Balogh.

Research Paradigms in Psychosomatic Medicine. Ed. by T. N. Wise & G. A. Fava. 1987. (Advances in Psychosomatic Medicine Ser.: Vol. 17). (Illus.). viii, 272p. 152.25 (*3-8055-4484-7*) S Karger.

Research Policies for Health for All. 1988. (European Health for All Ser.: No. 2). pap. text 8.00 (*92-890-1053-3*) World Health.

Research Primer for Occupational & Physical Therapy. Charlotte B. Royeen. 1997. 360p. (Orig.). (C). pap. text 55.00 (*1-56900-063-8*); lib. bdg. 60.00 (*1-56900-062-X*) Am Occup Therapy.

Research Priorities: Proceedings of the 4th National Title V Maternal & Child Health Research Priorities Conference. Ed. by G. Lamberty et al. 1996. LC 96-70894. 144p. pap. (*1-57285-037-X*) Nat Ctr Educ.

Research Priorities on Alcohol: Proceedings of a Symposium. Ed. by Mark Keller. 1979. (Journal of Studies on Alcohol: Suppl. No. 8). 10.00 (*0-911290-03-6*) Rutgers Ctr Alcohol.

Research Process in Nursing. Patricia A. Dempsey & Arthur D. Dempsey. 2nd ed. 1986. (Nursing-Health Science Ser.). (Illus.). 320p. (C). pap. text 32.50 (*0-86720-350-1*, 350-1) Jones & Bartlett.

Research Process in Nursing. Desmond F. Cormack. 3rd ed. 1996. 432p. pap. 34.95 (*0-632-04019-X*) Blackwell Sci.

Research Process in Nursing. Patricia Ann Dempsey. 3rd ed. 1992. (Nursing-Health Science Ser.). 336p. (C). 42.50 (*0-86720-449-4*) Jones & Bartlett.

Research Process in Nursing. Desmond Cormack. 4th ed. 2000. LC 99-33656. pap. 38.95 (*0-632-05158-2*) Blackwell Sci.

Research Projects: Research Projects Within Medical Groups & Research Centers. Ed. by Suzanne S. White & Donna L. Burman. 1996. 137p. (Orig.). pap. text 20.00 (*1-56829-013-6*) M G M A.

Research Stories for Introductory Psychology. Lary Shaffer & Matthew R. Merrens. 2000. LC 00-25330. 347p. pap. text 28.00 (*0-205-29929-6*) Allyn.

Research Strategies for Nurses in Advanced Practice. Susan L. Norwood. 1999. LC 99-26913. 499p. (C). 48.00 (*0-8385-8406-3*) P-H.

Research Strategies in Alcoholism Treatment Assessment. Pref. by Dan J. Lettieri. 1989. LC 88-7212. (Drugs & Society Ser.: Vol. 2, No. 2). (Illus.). 123p. text 39.95 (*0-86656-782-8*) Haworth Pr.

Research Strategies in Human Communication Disorders. Donald G. Doehring. 2nd ed. 1996. LC 90-22481. 261p. (C). pap. text 29.00 (*0-89079-644-0*, 7803) PRO-ED.

Research Symposium on the Male Adolescent Voice. Ed. by Maria Runfola & Lee Bash. 1984. (Proceedings Ser.). (Illus.). 182p. (Orig.). pap. 14.95 (*0-931111-00-5*) SUNY Buff Music.

Research Teachings in Health Science. James J. Neutens & Laurna Rubinson. 2nd ed. 1996. LC 96-30361. 352p. 88.00 (*0-205-17924-X*) Allyn.

Research, Training & Practice in Clinical Medicine of Aging. Ed. by Lawrence J. Gitman & E. Woodford-Williams. 1970. (Interdisciplinary Topics in Gerontology Ser.: Vol. 5). 30.50 (*3-8055-0505-1*) S Karger.

Research with Disabled Children: Issues & Methods. Stationery Office Staff & Bryony Beresford. 1997. LC 98-217988. pap. (*0-11-702148-2*, HM021482) Statnry Office GBR. *Dist:* Bernan Associates.

Researcher Experience in Qualitative Research. Susan Diemert Moch & Marie F. Gates. 1999. LC 99-6666. 193p. 64.95 (*0-7619-1341-6*, 82221) Sage.

Researches on Acupuncture & Moxibustion & Acupuncture Anaesthesia. Ed. by X. Zhang. 1986. (Illus.). 1179p. 112.00 (*0-387-10901-3*) Spr-Verlag.

Researching Community Psychology: Issues of Theory & Methods. Ed. by Patrick Tolan et al. 1990. 259p. pap. text 19.95 (*1-55798-234-1*) Am Psychol.

Researching Cultural Differences in Health. Ed. by David Kelleher & Sheila Hillier. 1996. LC 95-25980. (*0-04-151118-2*) Routledge.

Researching Health Risks. 1995. lib. bdg. 251.95 (*0-8490-6693-X*); 1994. lib. bdg. 252.75 (*0-8490-5819-8*) Gordon Pr.

Researching Persons with Mental Illness. Rosalind J. Dworkin. 1992. (Applied Social Research Methods Ser.: Vol. 30). 160p. (C). 69.95 (*0-8039-3603-6*, 7405); LC 92-11719. pap. 26.95 (*0-8039-3604-4*, 74062) Sage.

Researching Sexual Violence Against Women: Methodological & Personal Perspectives. Martin D. Schwartz. 1997. LC 96-51226. 272p. 74.95 (*0-8039-7369-1*, 1361); pap. 32.95 (*0-8039-7370-5*, 1362) Sage.

Researching Social Gerontology: Concepts, Methods & Issues. Sheila M. Peace. Ed. by Peter G. Norton et al. 1990. 224p. (C). pap. 26.50 (*0-8039-8285-2*, 9390) Sage.

Researching Therapist: A Practical Guide to Planning, Performing & Communicating Research. Sue Jenkins et al. 1998. LC 97-20081. pap. text (*0-443-05761-3*) Church.

Resection & Plastic Surgery of Bronchi. Boris Petrovsky et al. Tr. by Mir Publishers Staff from RUS. 1975. (Illus.). 375p. (C). 27.95 (*0-8464-0790-6*) Beekman Pubs.

Resetting the Clock: 5 Anti-Aging Hormones That Are Revolutionizing the Quality & Length of Life. Elmer M. Cranton & William Fryer. 1996. LC 96-23750. 272p. 21.95 (*0-87131-801-6*) M Evans.

Resettlement from Large Psychiatric Hospital to Small Community Residence: One Step to Freedom? R. V. Forrester-Jones & Gordon Grant. 1997. (Avebury Studies in Care in the Community). 232p. text (*1-85972-363-2*) Avebury GBR. *Dist:* Ashgate Pub Co.

Reshaping Dementia Care: Issues in Nursing Home Care. Ed. by Miriam K. Aronson & Donna C. Post. 1994. 176p. 47.95 (*0-8039-5159-0*, 3399); pap. 26.95 (*0-8039-5160-4*, 3400) Sage.

***Reshaping Health Care in Latin America: A Comparative Analysis of Health Care Reform in Argentina, Brazil, & Mexico.** Ed. by Sonia Fleury et al. 2001. 292p. pap. (*0-88936-923-2*) IDRC-CRDI CAN. *Dist:* Stylus Pub VA.

Reshaping Inpatient Care: Efficiency & Quality in New York City Hospitals. Lynn Rogut. 1996. LC 96-45277. (Papers). 44p. 12.00 (*1-881277-29-1*) United Hosp Fund.

Reshaping the Female Body: The Dilemma of Cosmetic Surgery. Kathy Davis. 1994. LC 94-19290. 256p. (C). (gr. 13). pap. 22.95 (*0-415-90632-6*, A7456) Routledge.

Reshaping the National Health Service, Vol. II. Ed. by Robert Maxwell. 1988. (Reshaping the Public Sector Ser.). 256p. text 34.95 (*0-946967-18-0*); pap. text 21.95 (*0-946967-30-X*) Transaction Pubs.

Reshaping the Psychoanalytic Domain: The Work of Melanie Klein, W. R. D. Fairbairn, & D. W. Winnicott. Judith M. Hughes. 1989. 256p. (C). text 45.00 (*0-520-06480-1*) U CA Pr.

Residency Director's Role in Specialty Certification. Ed. by John S. Lloyd. 1985. LC 85-70465. (Illus.). 255p. lib. bdg. 34.95 (*0-934277-05-2*) Am Bd Med Spec.

Residency Handbook. Lyle D. Victor. 1994. LC 94-34495. (Clinical Handbook Ser.). (Illus.). 216p. (Orig.). (C). 21.95 (*1-85070-583-6*, Parthenon Pbng) CRC Pr.

Residential & Inpatient Treatment of Children & Adolescents. R. D. Lyman et al. 1989. (Illus.). 390p. (C). text 75.00 (*0-306-43161-0*, Kluwer Plenum) Kluwer Academic.

Residential Care: The Provision of Quality Care in Residential & Educational Group Care Setting. Alan Davison. 1995. 432p. (*1-85742-309-7*) Arena GBR. *Dist:* Ashgate Pub Co.

Residential Care for the Elderly: Critical Issues in Public Policy. 13. Sharon A. Baggett. 1989. LC 89-2152. (Contributions to the Study of Aging Ser.: No. 13). 185p. 62.50 (*0-313-26759-6*, BRZ/, Greenwood Pr) Greenwood.

Residential Care Handbook: A Practical Guide to Caring & Staying in Business. Ray Schwartz. 2nd ed. 1997. LC 97-67326. 250p. ring bd. 30.00 (*0-89089-920-7*) Carolina Acad Pr.

Residential Care Services for the Elderly: Business Guide for Home-Based Eldercare. Doris K. Williams. 1996. LC 91-34626. (Journal of Housing for the Elderly: Vol. 8, No. 2). 106p. pap. 14.95 (*0-7890-0066-0*) Haworth Pr.

Residential Child Care: Team Development Programme. Joan Walton. 1994. (*0-902789-90-2*) Natl Inst Soc Work GBR. *Dist:* St Mut.

Residential Education As an Option for At-Risk Youth. Ed. by Jerome Beker & Douglas Magnuson. 1996. LC 96-12415. 133p. text 39.95 (*1-56024-818-1*) Haworth Pr.

Residential Group Care in Community Context: Insights from the Israeli Experience. Zvi C. Eisikovits. Ed. by Jerome Beker. 1986. LC 85-7682. (Child & Youth Services Ser.: Vol. 7, Nos. 3 & 4). 167p. text 39.95 (*0-86656-186-2*) Haworth Pr.

Residential School or Mainstreaming? A Guide for Parents of the Visually Impaired Child. Richard W. Webster. 1989. LC 89-83520. 116p. (Orig.). pap. text 8.00 (*0-9622460-0-X*) Katan Pubns.

Residential Services & Developmental Disabilities in the U.S. A National Survey of Staff Compensation, Turnover & Related Issues. David Braddock & Dale Mitchell. 1992. (Orig.). (C). pap. 38.95 (*0-940898-28-4*) Am Assn Mental.

Residential Treatment: A Cooperative, Competency-Based Approach to Therapy & Program Design. Michael Durrant. 1993. LC 93-9476. 240p. (C). 27.95 (*0-393-70154-9*) Norton.

Residents As Teachers: A Guide to Educational Practice. Thomas L. Schwenk & Neal A. Whitman. 1984. 84p. (Orig.). (C). reprint ed. pap. text 15.00 (*0-940193-03-5*) Univ UT Sch Med.

Resident's Guide to Ambulatory Care: Frequently Encountered & Commonly Confused Clinical Conditions. Michael B. Weinstock & Daniel M. Neides. 4th ed. 2000. 448p. per. 32.50 (*1-890018-35-X*) Anadem Pubng.

Resident's Guide to Starting in Medical Practice. Ed. by C. James Holliman. 1994. LC 94-36733. (Illus.). 320p. 25.00 (*0-683-04125-8*) Lppncott W & W.

Resident's Guide to Treatment of People with Chronic Mental Illness. Group for Advancement of Psychiatry Staff. 1993. LC 92-48698. (GAP Reports: No. 136). 230p. text 16.95 (*0-87318-204-9*, 7204) Am Psychiatric.

Residents Handbook of Neonatology. Max Perlman et al. 2nd ed. 1999. 500p. pap. (*1-55009-071-2*) DEKR.

Resident's Neurology Book. Orrin Devinsky et al. 1997. LC 96-48408. (Illus.). 282p. (C). pap. text 26.95 (*0-8036-0186-7*) Davis Co.

***Residents' Teaching Skills.** Ed. by Janine C. Edwards et al. 2001. LC 2001-49142. (Springer Series on Medical Education). (Illus.). xxi, 254p. (*0-8261-1436-9*) Springer Pub.

Residue Reviews, Vol. 72. Ed. by Francis A. Gunther & J. Davies Gunther. 1979. (Illus.). 154p. 75.95 (*0-387-90418-2*) Spr-Verlag.

Residue Reviews, Vol. 74. 1980. (Illus.). 138p. 96.00 (*0-387-90503-0*) Spr-Verlag.

Residue Reviews. Ed. by Francis A. Gunther. (Illus.). Vol. 75. 1980. 189p. 104.00 (*0-387-90534-0*); Vol. 76. 1980. 218p. 104.00 (*0-387-90535-9*); Vol. 79. 1981. 270p. 89.95 (*0-387-90539-1*); Vol. 97. 1986. 151p. 89.95 (*0-387-96294-8*) Spr-Verlag.

Residue Reviews: Residues of Pesticides & Other Contaminants in the Total Environment, Vol. 73. Ed. by Francis A. Gunther & J. Davies Gunther. 1980. (Illus.). 140p. 35.00 (*3-540-90470-0*) Spr-Verlag.

Residues of Pesticides & Other Contaminants in the Total Environment. Ed. by Francis A. Gunther. 1984. (Residue Reviews Ser.: Vol. 92). (Illus.). 210p. 81.95 (*0-387-96018-X*); 207p. 81.95 (*0-387-96019-8*) Spr-Verlag.

Residues of Pesticides & Other Contaminants in the Total Environment. M. Spindler et al. 1983. (Residue Reviews Ser.: Vol. 90). 124p. 89.95 (*0-387-90905-2*) Spr-Verlag.

Residues of Some Veterinary Drugs in Animals & Foods: Albendazole, Dimetridazole, Diminazene Aceturate, Ipronidazole, Isometamidium Chloride, Metronidazole, Ronidazole, Sulfadimidine, Sulfathiazole, Trenbolone Acetate, 34th Meeting of JECFA, Geneva, 1989. 1990. 112p. (*92-5-102933-4*, F0293) FAO ITA. *Dist:* Bernan Associates.

Residues of Some Veterinary Drugs in Animals & Foods: Azaperone, Carazolol, Febantel, Fenbendazole, Oxfendazole, Propionylpromazine, Spiramycin, Tylosin. 1991. (Monographs, 38th Meeting of JECFA, Rome, 1991). 148p. (*92-5-103096-0*) FAO ITA. *Dist:* Bernan Associates.

Residues of Some Veterinary Drugs in Animals & Foods: Benzyl Penicillin, Carbadox, Closantel, Ivermectin, Levamisole, Olaquindox, Oxytetracycline, 36th Meeting of JECFA, Rome, 1990. 1991. 129p. (*92-5-103061-8*, F0618) FAO ITA. *Dist:* Bernan Associates.

Residues of Some Veterinary Drugs in Animals & Foods: Chloramphenicol, Dexamethasone, Diminazene, Levamisole, Olaquindox, Spectinomycin, 42nd Meeting of JECFA, Rome, 1994. 1994. 97p. (*92-5-103553-9*, F35539) FAO ITA. *Dist:* Bernan Associates.

Residues of Some Veterinary Drugs in Animals & Foods: Food & Nut Paper. Prod. by Food and Agriculture Organization of the United Nations Staff. 1997. LC 98-110871. (Abamectin Chlortetracycline & Tetracycline, Clenbuterol, Cypermethrin Ser.: No. 9). 140p. pap. (*92-5-103972-0*, F39720) FAO ITA. *Dist:* Bernan Associates.

Residues of Some Veterinary Drugs in Animals & Foods - Food & Nut Paper: Abamectin, Ceftiofur Sodium, Chlorte Tracycline, Diclazuril Doramectin, Vol. 8. Prod. by Food and Agriculture Organization of the United Nations Staff. 1996. 130p. pap. (*92-5-103839-2*, F38392) FAO ITA. *Dist:* Bernan Associates.

Resilience: Stories of a Family Therapist. Moshe Lang & Tesse Land. 1996. LC 97-160525. 258p. (*1-86330-459-2*) Mdrin Au.

Resilience Enhancement for the Resident Physician. Edward Messner. 1993. 163p. pap. 7.95 (*0-929240-57-X*) EMIS.

Resilient Adults: Overcoming a Cruel Past. Gina O. Higgins. 1996. (Psychology Ser.). 400p. reprint ed. pap. 26.00 (*0-7879-0253-5*) Jossey-Bass.

Resipiratory Care Calculations. David W. Chang. 1994. LC 93-38719. 276p. (C). mass mkt. 33.25 (*0-8273-6148-3*) Delmar.

Resistance: Psychodynamic & Behavioral Approaches. Ed. by Paul L. Wachtel. 1982. LC 81-23494. 288p. 42.50 (*0-306-40769-8*, Plenum Trade) Perseus Pubng.

Resistance Arteries: Integration of the Regulatory Pathways. Ed. by William Halpern et al. 1994. LC 94-34398. (Experimental Biology & Medicine Ser.: Vol. 26). 384p. 135.00 (*0-89603-303-1*) Humana.

Resistance of Vectors of Disease to Pesticides. 1980. (Technical Report Ser.: No. 655). 82p. pap. text 6.00 (*92-4-120655-1*) World Health.

Resistance to Antineoplastic Drugs. Ed. by David Kessel. 1989. LC 87-33744. 432p. 254.00 (*0-8493-4800-5*, RC271, CRC Reprint) Franklin.

Resistance to Antitumor Agents: Laboratory & Clinical Studies. Ed. by M. Ghione et al. 1989. (Ettore Majorana International Life Sciences Ser.: Vol. 7). x, 322p. pap. text 189.00 (*3-7186-4956-X*) Gordon & Breach.

Resistance to Multiculturalism: Issues & Interventions. Jeffrey Scott Mio & Gene I. Awakuni. 1999. LC 99-45387. xvii, 177p. (*0-87630-955-4*) Brunner-Routledge.

Resistance to Tuberculosis: Experimental Studies in Native & Acquired Defense Mechanisms. Max B. Lurie. 1965. LC 64-25055. (Commonwealth Fund Publications). (Illus.). 410p. 40.00 (*0-674-76516-8*) HUP.

Resistance Vessels: Physiology, Pharmacology & Hypertensive Pathology. Ed. by M. J. Mulvany et al. 1985. (Mikrozirkulation in Forschung und Klinik Ser.: Vol. 8). (Illus.). x, 236p. pap. 121.75 (*3-8055-4052-3*) S Karger.

Resistances of Psychoanalysis. Jacques Derrida. 1998. LC 97-45151. (Meridian: Crossing Aesthetics Ser.). ix, 130p. 42.00 (*0-8047-3018-0*); 200p. pap. 15.95 (*0-8047-3019-9*) Stanford U Pr.

Resistenzproblem Bei der Chemo- und Radiotherapie Maligner Tumoren. Ed. by S. Seeber et al. 1984. (Beitraege Zur Onkologie, Contributions to Oncology Ser.: Vol. 18). (Illus.). viii, 474p. 120.00 (*3-8055-3801-4*) S Karger.

Resisting Reform: A Policy Analysis of the Israeli Health Care Delivery System. Gerald Steinberg & Etta Bick. 1992. 260p. (C). lib. bdg. 65.00 (*0-8191-8654-6*) U Pr of Amer.

Resisting 12-Step Coercion: How to Fight Forced Participation in AA, NA or 12-Step Treatment. Stanton Peele et al. 2000. LC 99-91322. 204p. pap. 14.95 (*1-884365-17-5*) See Sharp Pr.

Resolution of Inner Conflict: An Introduction to Psychoanalytic Therapy. Frank Auld & Marvin Hyman. 1991. 267p. text 29.95 (*1-55798-116-7*) Am Psychol.

Resolving Conflict in Your Marriage. Bob Horner & Jan Horner. 1993. (Homebuilders Couples Ser.). stu. ed., spiral bd. 9.99 (*0-8307-1618-1*) Gospel Lght.

Resolving Counterresistances in Psychotherapy. Herbert S. Strean. 1993. LC 92-49095. 240p. text 33.95 (*0-87630-713-6*) Brunner-Routledge.

Resolving Disputes over Life-Sustaining Treatment: A Health Care Provider's Guide. Thomas L. Hafemeister & Paula L. Hannaford. 1996. LC 96-70341. 170p. (Orig.). pap. 20.00 (*0-89656-167-4*, R-186) Natl Ctr St Courts.

Resolving Ethical Dilemmas: A Guide for Clinicians. Bernard Lo. 2nd ed. 2000. LC 99-59588. 384p. pap. text 45.00 (*0-7817-2219-5*) Lppncott W & W.

Resolving Grievances in the Nursing Home: A Study of the Ombudsman Program. Abraham Monk et al. 1984. (Social Work & Social Issues Ser.). text 57.50 (*0-231-05702-4*) Col U Pr.

Resolving Impasses in Therapeutic Relationships. Sue N. Elkind. 1992. LC 92-1692. 335p. 40.00 (*0-89862-892-X*, 2892) Guilford Pubns.

Resolving Infertility. Resolve Staff & Diane Aronson. 2001. LC 00-47270. (Illus.). 384p. pap. 18.00 (*0-06-095799-9*, Quil) HarperTrade.

Resolving Infertility: Understanding the Options & Choosing Solutions When You Want to Have a Baby. Diane Aronson & Resolve Staff. 1999. LC 00-266484. (Illus.). 384p. 27.50 (*0-06-273522-5*) HarperCollins Pubs.

Resolving Patient Complaints: A Step-by-Step Guide to Effective Service Recovery. Liz Osborne. 1995. 212p. ring bd. 138.00 (*0-8342-0674-9*) Aspen Pub.

Resolving Resistance in Group Psychotherapy. Leslie Rosenthal. 1987. LC 85-19940. 216p. 50.00 (*0-87668-914-4*) Aronson.

Resolving Sexual Abuse. Yvonne M. Dolan. 1991. 256p. 29.95 (*0-393-70112-3*) Norton.

Resolving the Antibiotic Paradox: Progress in Understanding Drug Resistance & Development of New Antibiotics. Ed. by S. Mobashery. 1999. LC 98-46308. (Advances in Experimental Medicine & Biology Ser.: 456). (Illus.). 294p. (C). text 97.50 (*0-306-46039-4*, Kluwer Plenum) Kluwer Academic.

Resolving the Dilemmas of the Difficult to Serve: Innovative Strategies & Training Techniques. Margaret Walsh & Ann Berson. 2nd ed. 1999. 52p. pap. (*1-930304-05-6*) Home Care Univ.

Resolving Treatment Impasses: The Difficult Patient. Theodore Saretsky. 1997. LC 97-16893. (Master Work Ser.). 288p. 40.00 (*0-7657-0095-6*) Aronson.

Resolving Treatment Impasses: The Difficult Patient. Theodore Saretsky. 1981. LC 80-24661. 267p. 34.95 (*0-87705-088-0*, Kluwer Acad Hman Sci) Kluwer Academic.

Resonance of Emptiness: A Buddhist Inspiration for Contemporary Psychotherapy. Gay Watson. 1998. (Critical Studies in Buddhism: Vol. 5). 288p. text (*0-7007-1057-4*) Curzon Pr Ltd GBR. *Dist:* UH Pr.

***Resonancia Magnetica y Artroscopia (MRI-Arthroscopy Correlative Atlas)** Mark D. Miller et al. 1997. (SPA., Illus.). 243p. (*84-8174-323-2*) Mosby-Doyma Libros ESP. *Dist:* Saunders.

Resonant Ultrasound Spectroscopy: Applications to Physics, Materials Measurements & Non-Destructive Evaluation. Albert Migliori & John L. Sarrao. 1997. LC 96-29930. 201p. 94.95 (*0-471-12360-9*) Wiley.

Resource Allocation Model for Public Health Planning: A Case Study of Tuberculosis Control. M. S. Feldstein et al. 1973. (WHO Bulletin Supplement Ser.: Vol. 48). pap. text 16.00 (*92-4-068481-6*, 1034801) World Health.

Resource Book: Directory of Organizations, Associations, Self Help Groups & Hotlines for Mental Health & Human Services Professionals & Their Clients. Robert L. Barker. 1987. LC 86-25765. 165p. text 4.95 (*0-86656-622-8*) Haworth Pr.

Resource Book on Progressive Pharmaceutical Services. 2nd ed. 1992. 200p. (Orig.). pap. text (*1-879907-17-8*) Am Soc Hlth-Syst.

Resource for Optimal Care of the Injured Patient, 1993. American College of Surgeons, Committee on the Imp. rev. ed. 1993. LC 93-11972. (Illus.). pap. text 12.00 (*1-880696-03-7*) Am Coll Surgeons.

Resource Guide for Injury Control Programs for Older Persons. 1987. 48p. (*1-55672-023-8*) US HHS.

Resource Guide for the Alzheimer's Caregiver. 1995. (Illus.). 73p. pap. 4.00 (*1-930181-07-8*) A H A F.

Resource Guide of Continence Products & Services. 1991. (Incontinence Ser.). lib. bdg. 75.00 (*0-87700-962-7*) Revisionist Pr.

Resource Guide to Accompany Breastfeeding & Human Lactation. Jan Riordan & Kathleen G. Auerbach. 1996. LC 96-175925. (Illus.). 232p. (C). pap. text 42.95 (*0-7637-0220-X*, 0220-X) Jones & Bartlett.

Resource Guide to Chiropractic: A Bibliography of Chiropractic & Related Areas, 1895-1981. Matthew J. Brennan. 1981. 155p. (C). pap. text 18.00 (*0-9606618-0-8*, K-12) Am Chiro Assn.

Resource Manual: Social Workers & Social Work Services As Defined in Medicare Law & Regulation. Ed. by Madeleine Golde. 2nd ed. 1992. 420p. pap. text 70.00 (*0-87101-216-2*) Natl Assn Soc Wkrs.

Resource Manual for Providing Hospice Care to People Living with AIDS. National Hospice Organization AIDS Resource Commit. 1996. 109p. (Orig.). pap., per. 11.85 (*0-931207-44-4*) Natl Hospice.

Resource of Objectives for Training in Family Medicine: An Atlas. Compiled by STFM Task Force on Objectives Staff. 1979. 160p. 5.00 (*0-942295-10-2*) Soc Tchrs Fam Med.

Resource Protection & Long-Term Healthcare Planning: A Guide to MassHealth. (*1-57589-180-8*) Mass CLE.

Resource Sharing in Biomedical Research. Institute of Medicine Staff. Ed. by Kenneth I. Berns et al. 1996. LC 96-71100. 104p. (Orig.). pap. text 29.00 (*0-309-05582-2*, Joseph Henry Pr) Natl Acad Pr.

Resource Utilization in Cardiac Disease. Lloyd W. Klein & James E. Calvin. 1999. LC 99-24723. (Developments in Cardiovascular Medicine Ser.). 314p. (*0-7923-8509-8*) Kluwer Academic.

Resourceful Caregiver: Helping Family Caregivers Help Themselves. National Family Caregivers Association Staff. 1996. 168p. (C). (gr. 13). pap. text 12.95 (*0-8151-5556-5*, 30587) Mosby Inc.

Resources: Handbook of Aid & Benefits for People with AIDS - ARC - HIV-Positive in Syracuse & Onondaga County. Compiled by Michael Welch. 1991. 90p. (Orig.). pap. text 10.00 (*0-936826-36-3*) PS Assocs Croton.

Resources for Health: Technology Assessment for Policy Makings. Ed. by H. David Banta. 1982. LC 81-21079. 235p. 62.95 (*0-275-91358-9*, C1358, Praeger Pubs) Greenwood.

Resources for Health, Fitness & Learning. Ed. by David I. Weiss. 1990. LC 90-70268. viii, 216p. pap. 9.95 (*0-9618049-2-0*) D I Weiss.

Resources for Nursing Research: An Annotated Bibliography. Cynthia G. L. Clamp & Stephen Gough. 3rd ed. 1999. LC 99-71274. 92.00 (*0-7619-6065-1*, 85233) Sage.

Resources for Reproductive Rights Research. Intro. by Stephanie Aronson. 1993. LC 93-77744. (Orig.). pap. (*1-878428-10-1*) Inst Womens Policy Rsch.

Resources for Teaching Gerontology. Ed. by Verle Waters. 1994. 82p. pap. 32.95 (*0-88737-605-3*, 14-2608, NLN Pr) Natl League Nurse.

Resources, Needs & Outcomes in Community-Based Care. Andrew Bebbington & Davies Bleddyn. 1990. 497p. text (*1-85628-130-2*) Avebry GBR. *Dist:* Ashgate Pub Co.

Resources of the Southern Fields & Forests, Medical, Economical & Agricultural. Francis P. Porcher. 1991. (American Civil War Medical Ser.: No. 4). 601p. reprint ed. 75.00 (*0-930405-33-1*) Norman SF.

Respecting Patient Autonomy. Benjamin H. Levi. 1999. LC 98-25360. (Illus.). 296p. 45.95 (*0-252-02441-9*); pap. 19.95 (*0-252-06749-5*) U of Ill Pr.

Respirando Bien: Su Guia Para Vivir con Asma & Alergias. Elizabeth Lykins. 1999. (SPA., Illus.). 118p. pap. 18.95 (*0-9701963-1-8*) B L Enter.

Respiration. Paul Berghuis et al. 1992. (Biophysical Measurement Ser.). (Illus.). 170p. (Orig.). (C). 28.00 (*0-9627449-3-X*) SpaceLabs.

Respiration & Metabolism of Embryonic Vertebrates. Ed. by Roger Seymour. 1984. LC 84-9751. (Perspectives in Vertebrate Science Ser.). text 321.50 (*90-6193-053-7*) Kluwer Academic.

Respiration in Health & Disease. Reuben M. Cherniack & Louis Cherniack. 3rd ed. 1983. (Illus.). 480p. text 57.00 (*0-7216-2527-4*) Saunders.

Respiratory & Alimentary Tract Disease. Ed. by H. S. Rosenberg & J. Bernstein. 1987. (Perspectives in Pediatric Pathology Ser.: Vol. 11). (Illus.). x, 218p. 191.50 (*3-8055-4435-9*) S Karger.

Respiratory & Pulmonary Medicine: An Internet Resource Guide. Ed. by Dan Goldenson. 2000. 450p. pap. 24.95 (*0-9676811-6-2*) eMedguides.

Respiratory Autogenic Training & Obstetric Psychoprophylaxis. U. Piscicelli. 1987. 292p. pap. text (*1-57235-026-1*) Piccin Nuova.

Respiratory Burst & Its Physiological Significance. A. J. Sbarra & R. R. Strauss. 1988. (Illus.). 500p. (C). text 130.00 (*0-306-42883-0*, Kluwer Plenum) Kluwer Academic.

Respiratory Care. Ed. by Jennifer A. Pryor. 1991. (International Perspectives in Physical Therapy Ser.: Vol. 7). (Illus.). 244p. pap. text (*0-443-03611-X*) Church.

Respiratory Care: A Guide to Clinical Practice. George G. Burton. 4th ed. 1997. LC 96-40216. 1,264p. text 71.95 (*0-397-55165-7*) Lppncott W & W.

Respiratory Care: Comprehensive Workbook. Mosby Staff. 1995. (Respiratory Care Workbook Ser.). (C). (*0-8151-6313-4*, 26030) Mosby Inc.

Respiratory Care: Evolution of a Profession. Gary A. Smith et al. 1989. LC 89-81413. 233p. (Orig.). (C). 35.00 (*0-9624754-1-6*); pap. 17.50 (*0-9624754-0-8*) Applied Measurement.

Respiratory Care Anatomy & Physiology: Foundations for Clinical Practice. Will Beachey. 1997. (Illus.). wbk. ed. (*0-8151-2582-8*) Mosby Inc.

Respiratory Care Assistant: Performance Evaluation Guide. California College for Health Sciences Staff. 1992. 60p. (C). (*0-933195-34-6*) CA College Health Sci.

Respiratory Care Assistant Program. M. Jouett. 2nd ed. 1993. LC 82-74058. 676p. (C). reprint ed. ring bd. (*0-933195-02-8*) CA College Health Sci.

Respiratory Care Calculations. David W. Chang. 2nd ed. 1998. LC 98-43498. (Allied Health Ser.). 304p. (C). pap. text 37.95 (*0-7668-0517-4*) Delmar.

Respiratory Care Certification Guide: Complete Review Resource for Entry Level E. James R. Sills. 3rd ed. 1999. LC 00-21453. (Illus.). xv, 398p. text 44.95 (*0-323-00739-2*) Mosby Inc.

***Respiratory Care CRRT Exam Review.** James B. Hiers, Jr. 2000. (Illus.). 336p. pap. 39.00 (*0-07-135592-8*, Apple Lange Med) McGraw.

Respiratory Care Drug Reference. Fred Hill. 1998. LC 00-502183. 575p. (C). text 24.95 (*0-8273-9066-1*) Delmar.

Respiratory Care Drug Reference. Joseph L. Rau. 1996. LC 96-31552. (Illus.). 464p. (C). (gr. 13). pap. text 19.95 (*0-8151-8456-5*, 28390) Mosby Inc.

Respiratory Care Equipment. Richard D. Branson et al. 1993. (Illus.). 750p. text (*0-397-50856-5*) Lppncott W & W.

Respiratory Care Equipment. Goulet. 1997. text (*0-7216-5193-3*) Saunders.

Respiratory Care Exam Guide: Review for the Entry-Level & Advanced Exams. Gary Persing. 3rd ed. 2000. LC 99-462366. (Illus.). 510p. (C). pap. Price not set. (*0-7216-8288-X*) Saunders.

Respiratory Care in Alternate Sites. Wyka. 1997. 80p. text, tchr. ed. 15.95 (*0-7668-0145-4*) Delmar.

Respiratory Care of the Newborn & Child. Clarie A. Aloan. 2nd ed. 1997. LC 96-39478. 608p. pap. text 45.50 (*0-397-54925-3*) Lppncott W & W.

Respiratory Care Pearls. Ed. by Frank A. Mazzagatti & Leon C. Lebowitz. 1997. LC 97-3043. (Pearls Ser.). (Illus.). 200p. pap. 45.00 (*1-56053-204-1*) Hanley & Belfus.

Respiratory Care Pharmacology. Crystal Dunlevy. 5th ed. 1998. (Illus.). 146p. wbk. ed. (*0-8151-2004-4*) Mosby Inc.

Respiratory Care Pharmacology. Joseph L. Rau. 5th ed. 1997. LC 97-18095. (Illus.). 432p. (C). (gr. 13). pap. text 39.00 (*0-8151-2337-X*, 31046) Mosby Inc.

Respiratory Care Pharmacology: Includes Testbank. Joseph L. Rau, Jr. 5th ed. 1998. tchr. ed. (*0-323-00358-3*) Mosby Inc.

Respiratory Care Sciences: An Integrated Approach. William V. Wojciechowski. 3rd ed. 1999. LC 99-29382. (Respiratory Care Ser.). 640p. (C). pap. text 58.95 (*0-7668-0780-0*) Delmar.

Respiratory Care Workbook. Howard B. Surkin & Anna W. Parkman. 1990. LC 89-16982. (Illus.). 372p. pap. text, wbk. ed. 27.95 (*0-8036-8229-8*) Davis Co.

Respiratory Control: A Modeling Perspective. Ed. by G. D. Swanson & Fred S. Grodins. 1990. (Illus.). 460p. (C). text 162.00 (*0-306-43366-4*, Kluwer Plenum) Kluwer Academic.

Respiratory Control: Peripheral & Central Mechanisms. Ed. by Dexter F. Speck et al. 1993. LC 92-13720. (Illus.). 248p. text 80.00 (*0-8131-1788-7*) U Pr of KY.

Respiratory Disease. Gray. 2000. pap. (*0-85131-570-4*) J A Allen GBR. *Dist:* Trafalgar.

Respiratory Disease: Principles of Patient Care. Ed. by Robert L. Wilkins & James R. Dexter. 2nd ed. 1997. LC 97-9419. (Illus.). 513p. (C). text 45.95 (*0-8036-0155-7*) Davis Co.

Respiratory Disease in the Elderly Patient. Martin J. Connolly. 1995. 344p. (C). (gr. 13). 150.95 (*0-412-56830-6*) Chapman & Hall.

Respiratory Diseases & Disorders Sourcebook: Basic Information about Respiratory Diseases & Disorders, Including Asthma, Cystic Fibrosis, Influenza & Others. Ed. by Allan R. Cook & Peter D. Dresser. 1995. LC 95-19214. (Health Reference Ser.: Vol. 6). 771p. lib. bdg. 78.00 (*0-7808-0037-0*) Omnigraphics Inc.

***Respiratory Disorders & Behavioral Research.** Ed. by Adrian A. Kaptein & Thomas L. Creer. 2001. 412p. 64.00 (*90-5823-240-9*) Gordon & Breach.

Respiratory Distress Syndrome. 1979. (Landmark Ser.). 25.50 (*0-8422-4121-3*) Irvington.

Respiratory Distress Syndrome. Ed. by Kari O. Raivio et al. 1984. text 125.00 (*0-12-576180-5*) Acad Pr.

Respiratory Drug Delivery. Ed. by Peter R. Byron. 1989. 3304p. 158.00 (*0-8493-5344-0*, RM161, CRC Reprint) Franklin.

Respiratory Drug Delivery VII. Ed. by Peter R. Byron et al. 2000. (Illus.). Vol. 1. 274p. 150.00 (*1-930114-14-1*); Vol. 2. 382p. 150.00 (*1-930114-16-8*) Davis Horwood Intl.

Respiratory Drug Delivery VI. Ed. by Peter Byron et al. 1998. (Illus.). 354p. 200.00 (*1-57491-076-0*) IHS Health Grp.

Respiratory Facts. John H. Riggs. 1989. LC 88-2057. (Illus.). 327p. (C). text 18.95 (*0-8036-7333-7*) Davis Co.

Respiratory Failure. Horacio J. Adrogue & Martin J. Tobin. 1997. LC 96-9846. (Basics of Medicine Ser.). (Illus.). 248p. pap. 42.95 (*0-86542-478-0*) Blackwell Sci.

Respiratory Function in Disease. David V. Bates. 3rd ed. 1989. 560p. text 77.00 (*0-7216-1592-9*) Saunders.

Respiratory Function in Speech & Song. Thomas J. Hixon. 1991. (Illus.). 448p. (C). reprint ed. pap. text 45.00 (*1-879105-24-1*, A032) Singular Publishing.

Respiratory Function of the Upper Airway. Oommen P. Matthew & Sant'Ambrogio. 1988. (Lung Biology in Health & Disease Ser.: Vol. 35). (Illus.). 672p. text 215.00 (*0-8247-7802-2*) Dekker.

Respiratory Health Effects of Passive Smoking: Lung Cancer & Other Disorders. 1993. (Illus.). 364p. (Orig.). (C). pap. text 55.00 (*1-56806-738-0*) DIANE Pub.

Respiratory Health Effects of Passive Smoking: Lung Cancer & Other Disorders (Orig.). 1997. lib. bdg. 600.95 (*0-8490-8144-0*); Set. 1995. lib. bdg. 603.99 (*0-8490-6687-5*) Gordon Pr.

Respiratory Home Care. Patrick J. Dunne & Susan L. McInturff. 1997. LC 97-18412. (Illus.). 207p. (C). pap. text 24.95 (*0-8036-0154-9*) Davis Co.

Respiratory Illness in Children. Peter D. Phelan et al. 4th ed. 1994. LC 93-51012. (Illus.). 424p. 149.00 (*0-632-03764-4*) Blackwell Sci.

Respiratory Immune Defense in Children: Current Knowledge & Possible Therapeutic Interventions. Ed. by J. A. Bellanti & J. P. Boissel. 1994. (Journal: Vol. 61, Suppl. 1, 1994). (Illus.). iv, 32p. pap. 15.75 (*3-8055-6077-X*) S Karger.

Respiratory Infections: Diagnosis & Management. Ed. by James E. Pennington. 3rd ed. 1994. LC 93-48578. 832p. spiral bd. 110.00 (*0-7817-0173-2*) Lppncott W & W.

Respiratory Intensive Care. Kenneth F. MacDonnell et al. 1987. 478p. 100.00 (*0-316-54193-1*, Little Brwn Med Div) Lppncott W & W.

Respiratory Measurement. Ed. by Goran Hedenstierna. 1998. (Illus.). 172p. pap. (*0-7279-1207-0*) BMJ Pub GBR. *Dist:* AIDC.

Respiratory Medicine R. A. Brewis. 2nd ed. 1995. text 275.00 (*0-7020-1641-1*) Saunders.

Respiratory Medicine. David C. Flenley & Douglas. 2nd ed. 1990. (Illus.). 392p. (Orig.). pap. text (*0-7020-1342-0*) Bailliere Tindall.

***Respiratory Medicine: An Illustrated Color Text.** Colin Selby. 2001. (Illus.). 95p. pap. (*0-443-05949-7*) Church GBR. *Dist:* Saunders.

Respiratory Monitoring. Martin J. Tobin. 1992. (Contemporary Management in Critical Care Ser.: Vol. 1, No. 4). (Illus.). 253p. text (*0-443-08831-4*) Church.

Respiratory Muscles in Chronic Obstructive Pulmonary Disease. Ed. by A. Grassino et al. 1988. (Current Topics in Rehabilitation Ser.). 178p. 65.95 (*0-387-19509-2*) Spr-Verlag.

Respiratory Pharmaceuticals Market: Demand for Non-Sedating Antihistamines Drives Market Growth. 1992. 210p. 1995.00 (*1-56753-010-9*) Frost & Sullivan.

Respiratory Pharmacology & Toxicology. Mannfred A. Hollinger. 1985. (Illus.). 202p. text 46.00 (*0-7216-1617-8*) Saunders.

Respiratory Physiology. J. A. Jacques. 1979. text 35.00 (*0-07-032247-3*) McGraw.

Respiratory Physiology. Widdicomb. 1991. 14.95 (*0-340-55253-0*) Trafalgar.

Respiratory Physiology. Allan H. Mines. 3rd ed. 1992. LC 92-49692. (Series in Physiology). 192p. text 78.00 (*0-88167-963-1*) Lppncott W & W.

Respiratory Physiology: An Analytical Approach. H. K. Chang. Ed. by Manuel Paiva. 1988. (Lung Biology in Health & Disease Ser.: Vol. 40). (Illus.). 896p. text 275.00 (*0-8247-7855-3*) Dekker.

Respiratory Physiology: Basics & Applications. Alan R. Leff & Paul T. Schumacker. 1993. LC 93-6718. (Illus.). 224p. pap. text 27.00 (*0-7216-3952-6*) Saunders.

Respiratory Physiology: People & Ideas. Ed. by John B. West. 1996. (Illus.). 448p. (C). text 85.00 (*0-19-508081-5*) OUP.

Respiratory Physiology: The Essentials. John B. West. 4th ed. 1989. (Illus.). 195p. 26.00 (*0-683-08942-0*); 5th ed. 1994. LC 94-7758. (Illus.). 224p. 27.00 (*0-683-08937-4*); 6th ed. 2000. LC 99-12450. 192p. pap. text 31.00 (*0-683-30734-7*) Lppncott W & W.

Respiratory Physiology: Understanding Gas Exchange from Basic Principles to Applications. Henry D. Prange. 1995. LC 95-24639. 224p. (C). (gr. 13). pap. text 35.95 (*0-412-05211-3*) Chapman & Hall.

Respiratory Physiology of Animals. James N. Cameron. 1989. (Illus.). 368p. text 70.00 (*0-19-506019-9*) OUP.

Respiratory Protection: A Manual & Guideline. Ed. by C. E. Colton et al. 2nd ed. 1991. 146p. 50.00 (*0-932627-45-5*) Am Indus Hygiene.

Respiratory Protection Handbook. William H. Revoir. 1997. LC 96-47080. 464p. lib. bdg. 75.00 (*0-87371-281-1*, L281) Lewis Pubs.

Respiratory Protection Program. Mark M. Moran. 1992. (OSHA Written Compliance Programs Ser.: No. 23). (Illus.). 50p. ring bd. 169.00 (*1-890966-17-7*) SafetyCertified.

Respiratory Sensation. Ed. by Lewis Adams & Abraham Guz. 1996. (Lung Biology in Health & Disease Ser.: Vol. 90). (Illus.). 464p. text 195.00 (*0-8247-8846-X*) Dekker.

Respiratory Support. Ed. by Keith Sykes. 1995. 256p. (Orig.). (C). pap. text (*0-7279-0830-8*) BMJ Pub GBR. *Dist:* AIDC.

Respiratory Support in Intensive Care. Ed. by Keith Sykes et al. 2nd ed. 1999. 305p. pap. (*0-7279-1379-4*) BMJ Pub GBR. *Dist:* AIDC.

Respiratory Surveillance. P. Harber. 1994. text (*0-442-01519-4*, VNR) Wiley.

Respiratory System. 1983. (Medical Ser.). (Illus.). 52p. pap. text 9.95 (*0-935920-12-9*, Ntl Pubs Blck) P-H.

Respiratory System. Thomas Braem. 1994. (Organs of the Human Anatomy: Vol. 6). 80p. (C). spiral bd. 15.95 (*1-878576-31-3*) Flash Anatomy Inc.

Respiratory System. Ed. by Thomas C. Jones et al. 1985. (Monographs in Pathology of Laboratory Animals). (Illus.). 240p. 288.00 (*0-387-13521-9*) Spr-Verlag.

Respiratory System. Ed. by Ulrich Mohr et al. 1993. LC 93-178961. (Illus.). 68p. pap. text 30.00 (*92-832-0121-3*) OUP.

Respiratory System. Ed. by T. C. Jones et al. 2nd ed. 1996. LC 95-45938. (Monographs on Pathology of Laboratory Animals). (Illus.). 357p. 320.00 (*0-944398-69-3*) ILSI.

Respiratory System. Ed. by T. C. Jones et al. 2nd ed. 1996. LC 95-45938. (Monographs in Pathology of Laboratory Animals). (Illus.). 357p. 330.00 (*3-540-60383-2*) Spr-Verlag.

Respiratory System. 3rd ed. 1993. LC 92-48260. (Regents - Prentice-Hall Medical Assistant Kit Ser.). 64p. pap. 16.00 (*0-13-227026-9*) P-H.

***Respiratory System: Systems of the Body.** Andrew Davies & Carl Moores. 2001. (Illus.). 220p. pap. (*0-443-06231-5*) Church GBR. *Dist:* Saunders.

Respiratory System Course. Competence Assurance Systems Staff. 1981. (Illus.). pap. text 45.00 (*0-89147-105-7*) CAS.

Respiratory Systems Symposium. Ed. by M. A. Epstein & J. R. Ligas. 1990. (Illus.). 201p. 69.95 (*0-387-97404-0*) Spr-Verlag.

Respiratory Technology: Procedure & Equipment Manual. Doris L. Hunsinger. 3rd ed. 1980. (Illus.). 448p. pap. text 34.50 (*0-8359-6670-4*) P-H.

Respiratory Therapist Manual. Stanley Pincus. 1975. LC 74-79838. (Allied Health Ser.). pap. 7.05 (*0-672-61389-1*, Bobbs) Macmillan.

Respiratory Therapy Competency Evaluation Manual. Craig D. Scanlan. 1984. 432p. (C). (gr. 13). pap. text 40.95 (*0-86542-015-7*, A-4324-4) Mosby Inc.

Respiratory Therapy Equipment. Charles E. Spearman & McPherson. 4th ed. 1990. (Illus.). 512p. pap. text, stu. ed. 17.95 (*0-8016-3378-8*) Mosby Inc.

Respiratory Therapy Technician. Jack Rudman. 1994. (Career Examination Ser.: C-3422). pap. 29.95 (*0-8373-3422-5*) Nat Learn.

Respiratory Viruses: Proceedings of the WHO Scientific Group, Geneva, 1967. WHO Staff. 1969. (Technical Reports: No. 408). 100p. pap. text 7.00 (*92-4-120408-7*, 1100408) World Health.

Respite Care: Programs, Problems & Solutions. Ed. by Lynn M. Tepper & John A. Toner. 1993. LC 92-48396. 240p. (Orig.). (C). pap. text 19.95 (*0-914783-67-X*) Charles.

Respite Care: Time Out for Families. Epilepsy Foundation of America Staff. 1992. 66p. pap. 9.95 (*0-916570-06-1*) Epilepsy Foundation of America.

Respite for Caregivers of Alzheimer's Patients: Research & Practice. M. Powell Lawton et al. 1991. 176p. 27.95 (*0-8261-6610-5*) Springer Pub.

Respite Resource Guide. National Council on the Aging, Inc. Staff. 1990. 40p. pap. 8.00 (*0-910883-51-3*, 2040) Natl Coun Aging.

Respond to the AIDS Challenge. Pye. Date not set. pap. text (*0-582-06434-1*) Addison-Wesley GBR. *Dist:* Trans-Atl Phila.

Responding to AIDS: Psychosocial Initiatives. Ed. by Carl G. Leukefeld & Manuel F. Fimbres. 1987. LC 87-15211. 162p. pap. text 12.95 (*0-87101-148-4*) Natl Assn Soc Wkrs.

Responding to AIDS: The Healthcare Professional's Guide to Legal Issues & Responsibilities. Jonathan P. Tomes. 1994. 225p. text 42.50 (*1-55738-613-7*, Irwn Prfssnl) McGraw-Hill Educ Grp.

Responding to Disaster: A Guide for Mental Health Professionals. Ed. by Linda S. Austin. 1992. LC 91-44366. (Clinical Practice Ser.: No. 24). 256p. 12.95 (*0-88048-464-0*, 8464) Am Psychiatric.

Responding to Emergencies. American Red Cross Staff. 2nd ed. 1996. (gr. 13). pap. text 25.00 (*0-8151-0351-4*) Mosby Inc.

Responding to the Sexual Abuse of Adults with Learning Disabilities. Hilary Brown & Ann Craft. 1996. 200p. pap. (*1-85302-204-7*) Jessica Kingsley GBR. *Dist:* Taylor & Francis.

Response & Adaptation to Hypoxia: Organ to Organelle. Ed. by Sukhamay Lahiri et al. 1991. (Clinical Physiology Ser.). (Illus.). 272p. text 68.00 (*0-19-506244-2*) OUP.

Response Errors in Surveys of Children's Immunizations. Roger Tourangeau & National Center for Health Statistics Staff. 1998. LC 98-37770. (Vital & Health Statistics Ser.). 48p. (*0-8406-0549-8*) Natl Ctr Health Stats.

Response of Different Species to Total Body Irradiation. Ed. by J. J. Broerse & T. J. MacVittie. 1984. (Radiology Ser.). text 141.50 (*0-89838-678-0*) Kluwer Academic.

Response of Rav Moshe Feinstein: Translation & Commentary. Moses Feinstein & Moshe D. Tendler. 1996. LC 96-11212. 22.95 (*0-88125-444-4*) Ktav.

Response Set in Personality Assessment. Ed. by Irwin A. Berg. 1967. LC 66-28342. 42.75 (*0-202-25019-9*) Irvington.

Response to Disaster: Psychosocial, Community & Ecological Approaches. Richard Gist & Bernard Lubin. 1999. LC 99-28627. (Series in Clinical & Community Psychology, Ser.). (Illus.). xix, 363p. pap. 24.95 (*0-87630-999-6*) Brunner-Routledge.

Response to Disasters: Psychosocial, Community & Ecological Approaches. Ed. by Richard Gist & Bernard Lubin. 1999. LC 99-28627. (Series in Clinical & Community Psychology). (Illus.). xix, 363p. 59.95 (*0-87630-998-8*) Brunner-Routledge.

Response to the National Research Council's Assessment of Rand's "Controlling Cocaine" Study. Jonathan P. Caulkins et al. 2000. LC 00-45727. (Illus.). ix, 27p. pap. 8.00 (*0-8330-2911-8*) Rand Corp.

Responsibilities of Health Authorities in the Field of Blood Transfusion (Recommendation), No. R(88)4. Council of Europe Staff. 1989. (*92-871-1688-1*) Council of Europe FRA. *Dist:* Manhattan Pub Co.

Responsibility for Drug Induced Injury (RISK) A Reference Book for Lawyers, the Health Profession & Manufacturers. Ed. by Graham Dukes et al. 1998. LC 97-78442. 537p. (YA). (gr. 12 up). 125.00 (*90-5199-387-0*) IOS Press.

Responsibility in Health Care. George J. Agich. 1982. 318p. text 126.50 (*90-277-1417-7*) Kluwer Academic.

Responsibility in Mental Disease, 3. Henry Maudsley. 1977. LC 77-72191. (Contributions to the History of Psychology Ser.: Vol. III, Pt. C, Medical Psychology). 603p. reprint ed. lib. bdg. 99.75 (*0-313-26942-4*, U6942, Greenwood Pr) Greenwood.

Responsibility Trap: A Blueprint for Treating the Alcoholic Family. Claudia Bepko & Jo-Ann Krestan. 1985. LC 85-1588. (Illus.). 320p. (C). 35.00 (*0-02-902880-9*) Free Pr.

Responsible Conduct with Animals in Research. Ed. by Lynette A. Hart. 1998. (Illus.). 208p. text 65.00 (*0-19-510511-7*); pap. text 27.50 (*0-19-510512-5*) OUP.

Responsible Test Use: Case Studies for Assessing Human Behavior. Lorraine D. Eyde et al. 1993. LC 93-1786. 244p. (Orig.). pap. 24.95 (*1-55798-203-1*) Am Psychol.

Responsive Therapy: A Systematic Approach to Counseling Skills. Sterling K. Gerber. 1986. LC 85-21869. 250p. 35.95 (*0-89885-267-6*); pap. 22.95 (*0-89885-269-2*) Kluwer Academic (Kluwer Acad Hman Sci).

Rest of Your Life Is the Best of Your Life: David Brown's Guide to Growing Gray Disgracefully. David Brown. 1991. LC 91-19324. 128p. 14.95 (*0-942637-35-6*) Barricade Bks.

Rest Principle: A Neurophysiological Theory of Behavior. John D. Sinclair. 1981. LC 80-17396. 240p. text 39.95 (*0-89859-065-5*) L Erlbaum Assocs.

Restaurants - Conditions & Syndromes: Index of Actions & Reports. David S. Lehigh. 1991. LC 90-56273. 160p. 47.50 (*1-55914-328-2*); pap. 44.50 (*1-55914-329-0*) ABBE Pubs Assn.

Restenosis after Intervention with New Mechanical Devices. Ed. by Patrick W. Serruys. 1992. (Developments in Cardiovascular Medicine Ser.). 528p. (C). text 350.00 (*0-7923-1555-3*) Kluwer Academic.

Restitutional Ear Surgery. M. E. Wigand. 2000. (Illus.). 304p. 149.00 (*0-86577-934-1*) Thieme Med Pubs.

Restoration of Brain Function by Tissue Transplantation. Ed. by O. Lindvall. 1993. LC 92-49462. (Basic & Clinical Aspects of Neuroscience Ser.: Vol. 5). (Illus.). 74p. 38.95 (*0-387-55823-3*) Spr-Verlag.

Restoration of Dialogue: Readings in the Philosophy of Clinical Psychology. Ed. by Ronald B. Miller. 1992. 654p. 29.95 (*1-55798-157-4*); pap. 29.95 (*1-55798-166-3*) Am Psychol.

Restoration of Function after Brain Injury. Aleksandr R. Luria & B. Haigh. 1963. LC 63-10016. (*0-08-010130-5*) Pergamon Repr GBR. *Dist:* Franklin.

Restoration of Motor Function in the Stroke Patient: A Physiotherapist's Approach. Margaret Johnstone. 3rd ed. 1987. LC 86-9554. (Illus.). 240p. (Orig.). pap. text (*0-443-03398-6*) Church.

Restoration of Normal Movement after Stroke. Margaret Johnstone. 1995. LC 94-41153. (Illus.). text (*0-443-05247-6*) Church.

Restoration of Teeth. T. R. Ford. 2nd ed. 1992. (Illus.). 312p. pap. 49.95 (*0-632-03252-9*) Blackwell Sci.

Restoration of the Self. Heinz Kohut. 1977. LC 76-45545. 345p. 55.00 (*0-8236-5810-4*) Intl Univs Pr.

Restoration of Walking for Paraplegics: Recent Advancements & Trends. Ed. by Maurizio Ferrarin & Antonio Pedotti. 1992. LC 92-53259. (Commission of the European Communities Ser.). 373p. pap. (*90-5199-094-4*) IOS Pr NLD. *Dist:* IOS Press.

Restorative & Rehabilitation Programs: A Three Phase Approach with Application to Medicare PPS. Diane P. Atchinson. Ed. by Dorothy Turrieta et al. 1999. LC 99-90700. (Illus.). 181p. ring bd. 125.00 (*1-929162-03-0*, ResM005) DPA Assocs.

Restorative Care: Fundamentals for the Certified Nursing Assistant. Barbara Acello. 1999. LC 99-17380. 368p. pap. text 27.95 (*0-8273-8141-7*) Delmar.

Restorative Dental Materials. Robert G. Craig. 10th ed. 1996. (Illus.). 608p. (C). (gr. 13). pap. text 60.00 (*0-8151-1920-8*, 25552) Mosby Inc.

Restorative Dental Materials. Robert G. Craig. 10th ed. 1997. (Illus.). 608p. pap. (*84-8174-287-2*) Mosby-Doyma Libros ESP. *Dist:* Mosby Inc.

***Restorative Dental Materials.** Robert Craig & John Powers. 11th ed. 2001. (Illus.). 670p. (*0-323-01442-9*) Mosby Inc.

Restorative Dentistry: A Resume. Jerome M. Schweitzer. 1985. LC 85-70279. (Illus.). 367p. 85.00 (*0-9614591-0-7*) Garson Associates.

Restorative Dentistry: An Integrated Approach. P. H. Jacobsen. 1998. LC 98-15937. 304p. pap. text 60.00 (*0-7236-1742-2*) Buttrwrth-Heinemann.

Restorative Neurology: Advances in Pharmacotherapy for Recovery after Stroke. Ed. by Larry B. Goldstein. 1998. LC 98-12046. (Illus.). 336p. 90.00 (*0-87993-407-7*, Futura Media) Futura Pub.

Restorative Nursing: A Training Manual for Nursing Assistants. Illus. by Catherine A. Tracey. Date not set. (*1-884278-10-8*) Rehab Nursing.

Restorative Proctocolectomy. David C. Bartolo et al. 1993. LC 92-48681. (Illus.). 176p. 99.95 (*0-632-03333-9*) Blackwell Sci.

Restorative Techniques in Paediatric Dentistry: An Illustrated Guide to the Restoration of Extensively Carious Primary Teeth. Monty S. Duggal et al. 1995. (Illus.). 134p. text 49.00 (*0-7216-6007-X*) Saunders.

Restorative Techniques in Paediatric Dentistry: An Illustrated Guide to the Restoration of Extensively Carious Primary Teeth. M. S. Duggal et al. rev. ed. 2000. (Illus.). 136p. (*1-85317-592-7*) Martin Dunitz GBR. *Dist:* Thieme Med Pubs.

***Restore Yourself: A Woman's Guide to Reviving Her Sexual Desire & Passion for Life.** James A. Simon & Victoria Houston. 2001. LC 2001-35407. 208p. pap. 14.00 (*0-425-18179-0*) Berkley Pub.

Restoring Balance: Community-Directed Health Promotion for American Indians & Native Alaskans. Beth Howard-Pitney et al. Ed. by Prudence Breitrose. 1992. (Illus.). 131p. (Orig.). pap. 15.00 (*1-879552-39-6*) SCRDP.

Restoring Vision: An Ethical Perspective on Doctors Curing Blindness Around the World. Tela Zasloff. 1995. 232p. (C). text 60.00 (*0-7618-0116-2*); pap. text 33.00 (*0-7618-0117-0*) U Pr of Amer.

Restraint-Free Care: Individualized Approaches for Frail Elders. Neville E. Strumpf et al. 1998. LC 98-29833. (Series on Geriatric Nursing). (Illus.). 168p. 32.95 (*0-8261-1215-3*) Springer Pub.

Restraint of Domestic Animals. T. F. Sonsthagen. 1994. LC 90-813235. (Illus.). 250p. pap. 27.00 (*0-939674-28-9*) Am Vet Pubns.

Restricted Environmental Stimulation: Research & Commentary. Ed. by John W. Turner, Jr. & Thomas H. Fine. 1990. (Illus.). 273p. lib. bdg. 30.00 (*0-944742-03-3*) Med Coll of OH Pr.

Restricted Environmental Stimulation: Theoretical & Empirical Developments in Flotation REST. Ed. by Peter Suedfeld et al. 1990. (Recent Research in Psychology Ser.). (Illus.). 216p. 79.95 (*0-387-97348-6*) Spr-Verlag.

Restriction Fragment Length Polymorphism. Marie-Paule LeFranc & G. LeFranc. 1989. (Experimental & Clinical Immunogenetics Ser.: Vol. 7, No. 1, 1990). (Illus.). 88p. pap. 41.00 (*3-8055-5113-4*) S Karger.

Restructuring: The Impact on Leadership in Hospitals. Joyce C. Clifford & American Organization of Nurse Executives Staff. 1998. LC 98-10015. 154p. 43.00 (*1-55648-229-9*) AHPI.

Restructuring & Resizing: Strategies for Social Work & Other Human Services Administrators in Health Care. Candyce Berger. 1993. LC 92-33264. (Illus.). 84p. (Orig.). pap. 57.00 (*0-87258-626-X*, 187150) Am Hospital.

Restructuring Canada's Health Service System: How Do We Get There from Here? Ed. by Raisa B. Deber & Gail G. Thompson. 1992. 640p. (Orig.). pap. text 25.00 (*0-8020-6005-6*) U of Toronto Pr.

Restructuring Chronic Disease Management: Best Practices & Innovations in Team-Based Treatment. Jon B. Christianson et al. 1998. LC 97-46162. 228p. 55.00 (*0-7879-4070-4*) Jossey-Bass.

Restructuring Health Care: The Patient-Focused Paradigm. J. Philip Lathrop. 1993. LC 93-29550. (Health Ser.). 218p. 46.00 (*1-55542-594-1*) Jossey-Bass.

Restructuring Health Policy: An International Challenge. Ed. by John M. Virgo. 1986. 500p. (Orig.). pap. 25.00 (*0-914943-02-2*) IHEMI.

Restructuring Personality Disorders: A Short-Term Dynamic Approach. Jeffrey J. Magnavita. 1997. LC 96-44159. (Assessment of Personality & Psychopathology Ser.). 345p. text 42.00 (*1-57230-185-6*, 0185) Guilford Pubns.

Restructuring Professional Organisation: Accounting Healthcare & Law. Ed. by David Brock et al. 1999. LC 99-12839. 248p. (C). text 110.00 (*0-415-19216-1*) Routledge.

Restructuring the American Health Market - Separating Myth Reality No. 1: Health Trends Issue Brief. Sylvia Fubini. 1996. 52p. (Orig.). pap. text 110.00 (*1-887324-01-1*) Hlth Trends.

Restructuring the Professional Organisation: Accounting Healthcare & Law. David Brock et al. 1999. LC 99-12839. x, 259p. pap. 36.95 (*0-415-19217-X*) Routledge.

Results & Evaluation of New Methodology in Cardiology: Proceedings of the Cardiovascular Disease Conference, 8th, Snowmass at Aspen, Colorado, Jan. 10-14, 1977. Cardiovascular Disease Conference Staff. Ed. by J. H. Vogel. 1977. (Advances in Cardiology Ser.: Vol. 22). 117.50 (*3-8055-2748-9*) S Karger.

Results in Neuroanatomy, Motor Organization, Cerebral Circulation & Modelling: Recent Developments of Neurobiology in Hungary, Vol. 8. K. Lissak. 1979. (Recent Developments of Neurobiology in Hungary Ser.: No. 8). 242p. (C). (*963-05-1594-6*) Akade Kiado HUN. *Dist:* St Mut.

Results in Neuroanatomy, Neurochemistry, Neurophysiology & Neuropathology: Recent Developments of Neurobiology in Hungary, Vol. 9. K. Lissak. 1982. (Recent Developments of Neurobiology in Hungary Ser.: No. 9). 232p. (C). (*963-05-2947-5*) Akade Kiado HUN. *Dist:* St Mut.

Results in Neuroendocrinology, Neurochemistry & Sleep Research. K. Lissak. 1978. (Recent Developments of Neurobiology in Hungary Ser.: No. 7). 189p. (C). (*963-05-1587-3*) Akade Kiado HUN. *Dist:* Intl Spec Bk, St Mut.

Resume Writing for the Professional Nurse. Nancy Kuzmich. rev. ed. 1998. (Illus.). 110p. 39.95 (*0-916780-31-7*) CES Assocs.

Resumes & Personal Statements for Health Professionals. James W. Tysinger. 2nd ed. 1998. LC 98-20357. pap. 18.95 (*1-883620-01-5*) Galen AZ.

Resumes for Health & Medical Careers. VGM Career Horizons Staff. 1995. LC 92-48533. (VGM Professional Resumes Ser.). vii, 151p. pap. 9.95 (*0-8442-4154-7*, VGM Career Bks) McGraw-Hill Trade.

Resumes for Health & Medical Careers. VGM Career Horizons Editors. 2nd rev. ed. 1997. LC 97-35374. (VGM Professional Resumes Ser.). (Illus.). 455p. pap. 9.95 (*0-8442-4515-1*, 45151, VGM Career Bks) McGraw-Hill Trade.

Resumes for Nursing Careers. VGM Career Horizons Staff & Robert T. Teske. 1996. LC 96-25596. (VGM Professional Resumes Ser.). 462p. pap. 9.95 (*0-8442-4524-0*, 45240) NTC Contemp Pub Co.

Resumes for the Health Care Professional. Kim Marino. 1993. LC 91-44718. 208p. pap. 14.95 (*0-471-55862-1*); 2nd ed. 2000. LC 99-52757. 224p. pap. 14.95 (*0-471-38073-3*) Wiley.

***Resurgent - Emergent Infectious Diseases.** Ed. by Brian G. Spratt. 1998. (British Medical Bulletin Ser.: Vol. 54, No. 3). 243p. pap. (*1-85315-344-3*) Royal Soc of Medicine Pr Ltd GBR. *Dist:* Balogh.

***Resurrecting the Body: Feminism, Religion & Psychoanalysis.** Naomi R. Goldenberg. 2001. 255p. reprint ed. pap. text 15.00 (*0-7881-9825-4*) DIANE Pub.

Resuscitation. Lonny J. Ashworth. 1998. (CPG Mentor - Patient Cases in Respiratory Care Ser.: Unit 7). (*0-8151-2300-0*) Mosby Inc.

Resuscitation & Emergency Care. Royal Life Saving Society-Australia Staff. 1994. 96p. (C). (gr. 13). pap. text (*0-8151-7322-9*) Mosby Inc.

Resuscitation Handbook, No. 2. Peter J. F. Baskett. 1993. 136p. (C). (gr. 13). (*1-56375-620-X*) Gower-Mosby.

Resuscitation in Pregnancy: A Practical Approach. Philip Jevon & Margaret Raby. 2001. (Illus.). 128p. pap. text 25.00 (*0-7506-4457-5*) Buttrwrth-Heinemann.

Resuscitation in Primary Care. Michael Colquhoun & Philip Jevon. 2001. LC 00-66775. (Illus.). 136p. pap. text 34.00 (*0-7506-4249-1*) Buttrwrth-Heinemann.

Resuscitation of the Newborn: A Practical Approach. David Drew et al. 2000. LC 00-58502. (Illus.). 144p. pap. text 30.00 (*0-7506-4378-1*) Buttrwrth-Heinemann.

Resuscitation Rules. Ed. by Tim Hodgetts & Nick Castle. 1999. (Illus.). 116p. pap. text (*0-7279-1371-9*) BMJ Pub GBR. *Dist:* AIDC.

RET Resource Book for Practitioners. Ed. by Janet L. Wolfe & Michael E. Bernard. 1993. 275p. (Orig.). (C). pap. 39.95 (*0-917476-22-0*) A Ellis Institute.

Retard. Diane O'Reilly. Ed. by James A. Keene. 1989. LC 88-83478. 200p. 18.95 (*0-944435-05-X*) Glenbridge Pub.

Retardation in Young Children: A Developmental Study of Cognitive Deficit. Sarah H. Broman et al. 1987. 376p. text 69.95 (*0-89859-989-X*) L Erlbaum Assocs.

Retarded Australians. Clifford Judge. 1975. pap. 19.95 (*0-522-84082-5*) Intl Spec Bk.

Retention & Productivity Strategies for Nurse Managers. Carol J. Huston & Bessie L. Marquis. 1989. (Nursing Management Ser.). (Illus.). 494p. text 37.50 (*0-397-54739-0*) Lppncott W & W.

Retention & Stability in Orthodontics. Ed. by Ravindra Nanda & Charles J. Burstone. 1993. (Illus.). 176p. text 79.00 (*0-7216-4342-6*) Saunders.

Rethinking AIDS Prevention: Cultural Approaches. Ed. by Ralph Bolton & Merrill Singer. 1992. LC 92-13820. 367p. pap. text 36.00 (*2-88124-552-8*) Gordon & Breach.

Rethinking Alzheimer's Care. Sam Fazio et al. 1999. LC 99-41163. xviii, 174p. pap. 26.95 (*1-878812-62-9*) Hlth Prof Pr.

Rethinking Attention Deficit Disorders. Miriam C. Julkowski et al. 1998. LC 97-6106. 250p. (Orig.). pap. 27.95 (*1-57129-037-0*) Brookline Bks.

Rethinking Clinical Audit: Psychotherapy Services in the NHS. Rachael Davenhill & Matthew Patrick. 1998. LC 97-47788. 208p. (C). 78.95 (*0-415-16207-6*); pap. 26.95 (*0-415-16208-4*) Routledge.

Rethinking Health Care: Innovation & Change in America. Max Heirich. 1998. LC 97-42611. 464p. (C). text 91.00 (*0-8133-3454-3*) Westview.

Rethinking Health Care Policy: The New Politics of State Regulation. Robert B. Hackey. LC 97-37198. (American Governance & Public Policy Ser.). 1998. 253p. pap. 23.95 (*0-87840-669-7*); 1997. 272p. 49.95 (*0-87840-668-9*) Georgetown U Pr.

Rethinking How We Age: A New View of the Aging Mind, 28. C. G. Prado. 1986. LC 85-9862. (Contributions in Philosophy Ser.: No. 28). 185p. 55.00 (*0-313-24785-4*, PRA/, Greenwood Pr) Greenwood.

Rethinking Innateness: A Connectionist Perspective on Development. Jeffery L. Elman et al. 1996. LC 96-15522. (Neural Networks & Connectionist Modeling Ser.). (Illus.). 475p. 65.00 (*0-262-05052-8*, Bradford Bks) MIT Pr.

Rethinking Life & Death. Peter Albert David Singer. 2nd ed. 1996. LC 96-3653. 320p. pap. 14.95 (*0-312-14401-6*) St Martin.

Rethinking Methods in Psychology. Ed. by Jonathan Smith et al. 1995. LC 95-70199. (Rethinking Psychology Ser.). 224p. 74.50 (*0-8039-7732-8*, 1391); pap. 25.95 (*0-8039-7733-6*, 1392) Sage.

Rethinking Psychiatry: From Cultural Category to Personal Experience. Arthur Kleinman. 1988. 256p. text 29.95 (*0-02-917441-4*) Free Pr.

Rethinking Psychiatry from Cultural Category to Personal Experience. Arthur Kleinman. 1991. LC 80-60855. 237p. pap. 18.95 (*0-02-917442-2*) Free Pr.

Rethinking Psychology, Vol. 3. Ed. by Jonathan Smith et al. 1995. 256p. 74.50 (*0-8039-7734-4*, 1425); 3rd ed. pap. 25.95 (*0-8039-7735-2*, 1426) Sage.

Rethinking the Sociology of Mental Health. Ed. by Joan Busfield. 2001. LC 00-54682. (Sociology of Health & Illness Monographs). 224p. pap. 34.95 (*0-631-22185-9*) Blackwell Pubs.

Reticulocyte Counting by Flow Cytometry: Proposed Guideline (1993) Contrib. by John A. Koepke. 1993. 75.00 (*1-56238-207-1*, H44-P) NCCLS.

Reticuloendothelial System: A Comprehensive Treatise, Vol. 7A: Physiology. Ed. by Sherwood M. Reichard & James P. Filkens. 1984. LC 79-25933. 436p. 105.00 (*0-306-41422-8*, Plenum Trade) Perseus Pubng.

Reticuloendothelial System Vol. 3: A Comprehensive Treatise: Phylogeny & Ontogeny. Ed. by Nicholas Cohen & Michael Sigel. 1982. LC 79-25933. 790p. 135.00 (*0-306-40928-3*, Plenum Trade) Perseus Pubng.

Reticuloendothelial System Vol. 6: A Comprehensive Treatise: Immunology. Ed. by Joseph A. Bellanti & Herbert B. Herscowitz. 1984. LC 79-25933. 370p. 95.00 (*0-306-41421-X*, Plenum Trade) Perseus Pubng.

Reticuloendothelial System Vol. 7B: A Comprehensive Treatise: Physiology. Ed. by Sherwood M. Reichard & James P. Filkins. 1984. LC 79-25933. 558p. 115.00 (*0-306-41423-6*, Plenum Trade) Perseus Pubng.

Reticuloendothelial System Vol. 8: A Comprehensive Treatise: Pharmacology. Ed. by John W. Hadden & Andor Szentivanyi. 1985. LC 79-25933. 490p. 115.00 (*0-306-41792-8*, Plenum Trade) Perseus Pubng.

Reticuloendothelial System Vol. 10: A Comprehensive Treatise; Infection. M. R. Escobar & J. P. Utz. 1988. LC 79-25933. (Illus.). 376p. (C). 110.00 (*0-306-42846-6*, Kluwer Plenum) Kluwer Academic.

Retina. Bressler. 1996. text (*0-7216-6731-7*) Saunders.

Retina. Ed. by Stephen J. Ryan. 2nd ed. 1994. LC 93-40452. (Illus.). 2800p. (C). (gr. 13). text 440.00 (*0-8016-8032-8*, 08032) Mosby Inc.

Retina Stephen J. Ryan et al. 3rd ed. 1999. LC 2001-266503. (Illus.). xxix, 2601p. (C). text 499.95 (*0-323-00804-6*) Mosby Inc.

Retina: The Fundamentals. Gloria Wu. 1995. (Illus.). 256p. text 75.00 (*0-7216-6691-4*) Saunders.

Retina & Vitreous. Ed. by Rudolph M. Franklin. 1993. LC 93-12350. (Illus.). lib. bdg. (*90-6299-091-6*) Kugler NLD. *Dist:* Lib Res.

Retina & Vitreous. Gouras. 1993. (*0-397-44692-6*) Gower-Mosby.

Retina Atlas. David R. Guyer et al. 1995. LC 94-31577. (Illus.). 800p. (C). (gr. 13). text 268.00 (*0-8151-3432-0*, 24716) Mosby Inc.

Retina, Vitreous & Choroid: Clinical Procedures. Robert L. Johnston. Ed. by Chris J. Cakanac. 1995. LC 95-14051. (Clinical Procedure Ser.). (Illus.). 137p. spiral bd. 44.99 (*0-7506-9615-X*) Buttrwrth-Heinemann.

Retina-Vitreous-Macula. David R. Guyer et al. Ed. by Richard Lampert. 1998. LC 97-16250. (Illus.). 1776p. (C). text 395.00 (*0-7216-6756-2*) Saunders.

Retinal Basis of Vision. J. I. Toyoda et al. 1999. LC 00-698593. (Illus.). 300p. pap. 69.00 (*0-444-50299-8*, Excerpta Medica) Elsevier.

Retinal Degeneration: Clinical & Laboratory Applications. Ed. by Joe G. Hollyfield et al. 1993. (Illus.). 380p. (C). text 110.00 (*0-306-44570-0*, Kluwer Plenum) Kluwer Academic.

Retinal Degeneration & Regeneration: Proceedings of an International Symposium, Kanazawa, Japan, July 8-9, 1995. Ed. by Shinzi Kato et al. 1996. LC 96-1713. (*90-6299-143-2*) Kugler NLD. *Dist:* Lib Res.

Retinal Degenerations. Robert E. Anderson et al. 1991. (Illus.). 544p. lib. bdg. 116.00 (*0-8493-0178-5*, RE551, CRC Reprint) Franklin.

Retinal Degenerative Diseases & Experimental Therapy. Joe G. Hollyfield et al. 1999. LC 99-40819. (*0-306-46193-5*, Kluwer Plenum) Kluwer Academic.

Retinal Detachment see Michels's Retinal Detachment

Retinal Detachment: A Colour Manual of Diagnosis & Treatment. Jack J. Kanski & Zdenek Gregor. 2nd ed. 1995. LC 94-27820. (Colour Manuals in Opthalmology Ser.). (Illus.). 128p. text 88.00 (*0-7506-1768-3*) Buttrwrth-Heinemann.

Retinal Detachment: Diagnosis & Management. William E. Benson. 2nd ed. 1988. LC 65-10911. (Illus.). 224p. text 68.25 (*0-397-50926-X*, Lippncott) Lppncott W & W.

Retinal Detachment: Diagnosis & Management. Carl D. Regillo & William E. Benson. 3rd ed. 1998. LC 98-12131. 240p. text 135.00 (*0-7817-1646-2*) Lppncott W & W.

Retinal Detachment: Principles & Practice. George F. Hilton et al. 2nd rev. ed. 1995. LC 94-43382. (Ophthalmology Monographs: Vol. 1). (*1-56055-028-7*) Am Acad Ophthal.

Retinal Detachment: The Essentials of Management. Hector Bryson Chawla. 3rd ed. 1998. LC 98-28063. 144p. pap. text 70.00 (*0-7506-3980-6*) Buttrwrth-Heinemann.

Retinal Detachment Surgery. A. H. Chignell. 1980. (Illus.). 45.00 (*0-387-09475-X*) Spr-Verlag.

Retinal Diseases. Mark O. Tso. 1988. LC 65-8261. (Illus.). 480p. text 85.00 (*0-397-50661-9*, Lippnctt) Lppncott W & W.

Retinal Diseases: Pathogenesis, Laser Therapy, & Surgery. Jesse Sigelman. 1984. 130.00 (*0-316-79052-4*, Little Brwn Med Div) Lppncott W & W.

Retinal Diseases 2. Ed. by R. Brancato et al. 1987. LC 87-22626. (Illus.). 392p. lib. bdg. (*90-6299-037-1*) Kugler NLD. *Dist:* Lib Res.

Retinal Muller Cell: Structure & Function. Vijay Sarthy & Harris Ripps. 2001. LC 00-58749. (Perspectives in Vision Research Ser.). (Illus.). xiv, 278p. 95.00 (*0-306-46470-5*, Kluwer Plenum) Kluwer Academic.

Retinal Pigment Epithelial Transplantation. Devjani Lahiri-Munir & C. Garcia. 1995. LC 95-7452. (Medical Intelligence Unit Ser.). 133p. 79.00 (*1-57059-255-1*) Landes Bioscience.

Retinal Pigment Epithelium. Michael F. Marmor & Thomas J. Wolfensberger. 1998. LC 97-18098. (Illus.). 776p. text 198.50 (*0-19-510956-2*) OUP.

Retinal Pigment Epithelium. Ed. by M. Zingirian & F. C. Piccolino. 1990. LC 89-19878. (Illus.). 326p. lib. bdg. (*90-6299-055-X*) Kugler NLD. *Dist:* Lib Res.

Retinal Pigment Epithelium. Ed. by Keith M. Zinn & Michael F. Marmor. 1979. (Illus.). 531p. (C). 68.00 (*0-674-76684-9*) HUP.

Retinal Pigment Epithelium & Macular Diseases. European Macula Group Staff. Ed. by Gabriel Coscas. 1998. LC 98-22538. (Documenta Ophthalmologica Proceedings Ser.). 457p. (*0-7923-5144-4*) Kluwer Academic.

Retinal Proteins. Ed. by Yu A. Ovchinnikov. 1987. 590p. lib. bdg. (*90-6764-102-2*) VSP NLD. *Dist:* Coronet Bks.

Retinal Transmitters & Modulators: Models for the Brain, Vol. I. Ed. by William W. Morgan. 1985. 176p. 132.00 (*0-8493-5691-1*, QP479) CRC Pr.

Retinal Transmitters & Modulators: Models for the Brain, Vol. 2. William W. Morgan. 1984. LC 84-12068. 176p. 105.00 (*0-8493-5692-X*, QP479) Franklin.

Retine, Vieillissement et Transplantation. Ed. by Y. Christen et al. 200p. Vol. 5. 1994. 55.00 (*2-906077-42-9*); Vol. 6. 1995. 58.00 (*2-906077-60-7*) Elsevier.

Retinitis Pigmentosa: Proceedings of the 4th Congress of the International Retinitis Pigmentosa Association, Bad Nauheim 1986, FRG, Pt. 2. F. Brunsmann & R. von Gizycki. 1988. (Advances in the Biosciences Ser.: Vol. 63). 322p. 100.50 (*0-08-035725-3*, North Holland) Elsevier.

Retinoid Protocols. Ed. by Christopher Redfern. 1998. LC 97-44455. (Methods in Molecular Biology Ser.: Vol. 89). (Illus.). 456p. 110.00 (*0-89603-438-0*) Humana.

Retinoids: Biology, Chemistry, & Medicine. Ed. by Michael B. Sporn et al. 2nd ed. 1993. LC 93-3451. 704p. text 199.00 (*0-7817-0082-5*) Lppncott W & W.

Retinoids: From Basic Science to Clinical Applications. Ed. by M. A. Livrea & G. Vidali. 1994. LC 94-16145. (Molecular & Cell Biology Updates Ser.). 396p. 128.00 (*0-8176-2812-6*) Birkhauser.

Retinoids: Progress in Research & Clinical Applications. M. A. Livrea. Ed. by Lester Packer. 1993. (Basic & Clinical Dermatology Ser.: Vol. 5). (Illus.). 672p. text 250.00 (*0-8247-8758-7*) Dekker.

Retinoids: Ten Years On. Ed. by J. H. Saurat. 1991. (Illus.). x, 356p. 291.50 (*3-8055-5387-0*) S Karger.

Retinoids - Experimental & Clinical Results: Seventeenth World Congress of Dermatology, Berlin, May 1987, Journal: Dermatologica, Vol. 175, suppl. 1. Ed. by R. Stadler et al. 1987. (Illus.). iv, 204p. pap. 63.50 (*3-8055-4708-0*) S Karger.

Retinoids in Clinical Practice: The Risk-Benefit Ratio. Ed. by Gideon Koren. 1992. (Medical Toxicology Ser.: Vol. 1). (Illus.). 296p. text 155.00 (*0-8247-8778-1*) Dekker.

Retinoids in Normal Development & Teratogenesis. Ed. by Gillian Morriss-Kay. 1992. (Illus.). 320p. 95.00 (*0-19-854770-6*) OUP.

Retinoids in Oncology. European School of Oncology Staff. Ed. by L. Degos & D. R. Parkinson. 1995. LC 95-14259. (ESO Monographs). (Illus.). 128p. 104.00 (*3-540-59181-8*) Spr-Verlag.

Retinoids in Oncology. Ed. by Waun Ki. Hong & Reuben Lotan. 1993. LC 93-10155. (Basic & Clinical Oncology Ser.: Vol. 4). (Illus.). 352p. text 185.00 (*0-8247-9048-0*) Dekker.

Retinoids, Their Physiological Function & Therapeutic Potential. Ed. by E. Edward Bittar & G. V. Sherbet. 1997. (Advances in Organ Biology Ser.: Vol. 3). 312p. 90.00 (*0-7623-0285-2*) Jai Pr.

Retinopathy of Prematurity. Marilyn M. Miller & Michael J. Shapiro. 1995. (*90-6299-125-4*) Kugler NLD. *Dist:* Lib Res.

Retinopathy of Prematurity: A Clinician's Guide. Ed. by J. T. Flynn & William S. Tasman. 1992. (Illus.). 162p. 105.00 (*0-387-97635-3*) Spr-Verlag.

Retinoscopy Book: An Introductory Manual for Eye Care Professionals. John M. Corboy. 4th ed. 1995. LC 79-65451. (Illus.). 160p. pap. 40.00 (*1-55642-271-7*, 62717) SLACK Inc.

Retiree Health Benefits: Employer Obligations, Retiree Rights. William J. Danish. 1994. (Employee Benefits - Human Resource Library). 400p. (*0-471-57510-0*, Pergamon Pr) Elsevier.

Retiree Health Benefits: Field Test of the FASB Proposal. Harold Dankner et al. 1989. LC 89-84509. (Illus.). 215p. pap. 25.00 (*0-910586-74-8*, 079-89) Finan Exec.

Retiree Health Benefits: How to Cope with the Accounting, Actuarial, & Management Issues. Murray S. Akresh et al. Ed. by Claire Barth & Jennifer Strand. 1991. (Bold Step Ser.). (Illus.). 134p. (Orig.). pap. 40.00 (*0-86641-194-1*, 91256) Inst Mgmt Account.

Retiree Health Care Crisis. Ed. by James H. Ballagh. 1989. (Current Issues Ser.: No. 12). 100p. (Orig.). pap. 10.00 (*0-89215-159-5*) U Cal LA Indus Rel.

Retirement: Coping with Emotional Upheavals. Leland Bradford & Martha Bradford. 1979. LC 79-4101. text 29.95 (*0-88229-564-0*) Burnham Inc.

Retirement: The Challenge of Change. E. Michael Brady. 1988. (Orig.). pap. 8.00 (*0-939561-02-6*) Univ South ME.

Retirement Counseling: A Handbook for Gerontology Practitioners. Virginia E. Richardson. 1993. LC 92-48349. (Life Styles & Issues in Aging Ser.: Vol. 1). 224p. 31.95 (*0-8261-7020-X*) Springer Pub.

Retraining Cognition: Techniques & Applications. Rick Parente & Douglas Herrmann. 2000. LC 96-12260. 304p. 65.00 (*0-8342-0764-8*) PRO-ED.

***Retraining Cognition Techniques Applications.** Rick Parente. 2nd ed. 1996. (*0-8342-2074-1*) PRO-ED.

Retransplantation: Symposium Foundation Marcel Merieux. Ed. by Jean-Louis Touraine et al. 1998. LC 97-46901. (Transplantation & Clinical Immunology Ser.). 352p. 170.00 (*0-7923-4937-7*) Kluwer Academic.

Retreat into the Mind: Victorian Poetry & the Rise of Psychiatry. Ekbert Faas. 1991. 320p. pap. 18.95 (*0-691-01511-2*) Princeton U Pr.

Retreat of Tuberculosis, 1850-1950. F. B. Smith. 1988. 288p. lib. bdg. (*0-7099-3383-5*) C Helm GBR. *Dist:* Routldge.

Retrieval of Medicinal Chemical Information. Ed. by W. Jeffrey Howe et al. 1978. LC 78-21611. (ACS Symposium Ser.: No. 84). 29.95 (*0-8412-0465-9*) Am Chemical.

Retroactive Inhibition As Affected by Conditions of Learning. Edward C. Tolman. 1974. (Psychology Monographs General & Applied: Vol. 25). reprint ed. pap. 55.00 (*0-8115-1424-2*) Periodicals Srv.

Retroperitoneal Laparascopy for the Urologist. Durga D. Gaur. 1998. LC 97-913994. (Illus.). 280p. text 195.00 (*0-19-564143-4*) OUP.

Retroperitoneum & Intestine. Kenneth C. Suen. 2nd ed. 1994. LC 94-4776. (Guides to Clinical Aspiration Biopsy Ser.). (Illus.). 304p. 98.50 (*0-89640-256-8*) Igaku-Shoin.

***Retroviral & Related Nucleic Acid Processing Enzymes Expression & Detection: Applications on Clinical Studies of HIV & HERVs.** Raymond Awad. 2001. (Comprehensive Summaries of Uppsala Dissertations from the Faculty of Medicine Ser.: No. 1083). (Illus.). 100p. pap. (*91-554-5132-2*) Acta Univ SWE. *Dist:* Coronet Bks.

Retroviral Immunology: Immune Response & Restoration. Ed. by Giuseppe Pantaleo & Bruce D. Walker. 2001. LC 00-54274. (Infectious Disease Ser.). 337p. 135.00 (*0-89603-675-8*) Humana.

Retroviral Latency. Ed. by Mark A. Laughlin & Roger J. Pomerantz. 1994. (Medical Intelligence Unit Ser.). 115p. 99.00 (*1-57059-034-6*, LN9034) Landes Bioscience.

Retroviral Proteases. Ed. by Lawrence C. Kuo et al. 1994. (Methods in Enzymology Ser.: Vol. 241). (Illus.). 432p. text 94.00 (*0-12-182142-0*) Acad Pr.

Retroviral Reverse Transcriptases. Simon Litvak. 1996. (Molecular Biology Intelligence Unit Ser.). 205p. 99.00 (*1-57059-369-8*) Landes Bioscience.

Retroviral Testing: Essentials of Quality Control & Lab Diagnosis. Neil T. Constantine. 1992. 256p. 115.95 (*0-8493-4429-8*, RC607) CRC Pr.

Retroviridae. Ed. by J. A. Levy. (Viruses Ser.). (Illus.). (C). Vol. 1. 1992. 504p. text 110.00 (*0-306-44074-1*); Vol. 2. 1993. 458p. text 110.00 (*0-306-44369-4*); Vol. 3. 1994. 564p. text 120.00 (*0-306-44693-6*) Kluwer Academic (Kluwer Plenum).

Retrovirus Biology & Human Disease. Robert,C. Gallo & Flossie Wong-Staal. 1989. (Illus.). 432p. text 165.00 (*0-8247-7874-X*) Dekker.

Retroviruses. Ed. by John M. Coffin et al. (Illus.). (C). 1999. 843p. pap. 95.00 (*0-87969-571-4*); 1997. LC 97-32263. 900p. text 185.00 (*0-87969-497-1*) Cold Spring Harbor.

Retroviruses & Human Pathology. Ed. by Robert,C. Gallo et al. 1986. LC 85-31692. (Experimental Biology & Medicine Ser.: Vol. 11). 557p. 139.50 (*0-89603-098-9*) Humana.

Retroviruses in Human Lymphoma-Leukemia: Proceedings of the 15th International Symposium of the Princess Takamatsu Cancer Research Fund, Japan, 1984. Ed. by M. Miwa et al. 1985. 352p. lib. bdg. (*90-6764-057-3*) VSP NLD. *Dist:* Coronet Bks.

Retroviruses of Human AIDS & Related Animal Diseases. Ed. by M. Girard & B. Dodet. 1996. 384p. 61.00 (*2-906077-75-5*) Elsevier.

Rett Syndrome - Clinical & Biological Aspects: Studies on 130 Swedish Females. Bengt Hagberg. 1993. (Clinics in Developmental Medicine Ser.: No. 127). 120p. (C). text 49.95 (*0-521-41283-8*) Cambridge U Pr.

Return of Blood to the Heart. Gardner. 2nd ed. 268p. (*0-86196-387-3*) J Libbey Med GBR. *Dist:* Bks Intl VA.

Return of the French Freud. Ed. by Todd Dufresne. 1997. 252p. (C). 75.00 (*0-415-91525-2*); LC 95-53176. pap. 21.95 (*0-415-91526-0*) Routledge.

Return of w3 Fatty Acids into the Food Supply: I. Land-Based Animal Food Products & Their Health Effects. International Conference, Bethesda, Md., September 1997. Ed. by A. P. Simopoulos. 1998. LC 98-17779. (World Review of Nutrition & Dietetics Ser.: Vol. 83). (Illus.). xii, 240p. 215.00 (*3-8055-6694-8*) S Karger.

Return to Center: The Flowering of Self-Trust. Bobbie Probstein. 1985. LC 85-70723. (Illus.). 242p. (Orig.). pap. 10.95 (*0-87516-554-0*) DeVorss.

Return to Community: Building Support Systems for People with Psychiatric Disabilities. Paul J. Carling. 1994. LC 94-29724. 348p. text 42.00 (*0-89862-299-9*) Guilford Pubns.

Return to Glory Days. Dean Gelfand et al. 1997. LC 97-18379. 288p. per. 14.00 (*0-671-56323-8*, PB Trade Paper) PB.

Return to Harmony: Creating Harmony & Balance Through the Frequencies of Sound. Nicole LaVoie. Ed. by Jill Lawrence et al. 1996. LC 96-92084. (Illus.). 260p. pap. 13.00 (*0-9650387-4-2*) Snd Wave Energy.

Return to Health. Jess Kraft. Ed. by Barbara A. Kraft. 1987. LC 87-60170. 140p. (Orig.). pap. 6.95 (*0-9618099-0-6*) Red Lantern Pr.

Return to Herbal Medicine. LaDean Griffin. 1979. pap. 6.95 (*0-89036-073-1*) Liahona Pub Trust.

Return to Spirit: After the Mythic Church. Desmond Murphy. 1997. LC 97-14140. 264p. pap. 19.95 (*0-8245-1685-0*) Crossroad NY.

Return to the Joy of Health: Natural Medicine & Alternative Treatments for All Your Health Complaints. Zoltan P. Rona & Jeanne M. Martin. 1995. LC 95-910586. 425p. pap. 19.95 (*0-920470-62-9*) Alive Bks.

Return to Wholeness: Embracing Mind, Body & Spirit in the Face of Cancer. David Simon. 1998. LC 98-18402. (Illus.). 288p. 24.95 (*0-471-29577-9*) Wiley.

Return to Work after Coronary Artery Bypass Surgery. Ed. by Paul J. Walter. 1985. (Illus.). 480p. 62.00 (*0-387-13591-X*) Spr-Verlag.

Reunion in Vienna. Edith Foster. 1991. (Studies in Austrian Literature, Culture & Thought). 180p. pap. 16.00 (*0-929497-40-6*) Ariadne CA.

Reuse of Effluents - Methods of Wastewater Treatment & Health Safeguards: Proceedings of the WHO Expert Committee, Geneva, 1971. WHO Staff. 1973. (Technical Reports: No. 517). pap. text 7.00 (*92-4-120517-2*, 1100517) World Health.

Reuse of Hemodialyzer Blood Tubing. 1989. 48p. pap. 90.00 (*0-910275-83-1*, TIR6-209) Assn Adv Med Instrn.

Reuse of Hemodialyzers. 2nd ed. 1993. 26p. pap. 82.00 (*0-910275-15-7*, RD47-209) Assn Adv Med Instrn.

***Reuse of Single-Use Medical Devices: Congressional Hearing.** Ed. by Fred Upton. 2001. 184p. (C). pap. text 35.00 (*0-7567-1197-5*) DIANE Pub.

Reuse of Single-Use Medical Devices: Guidelines for Healthcare Facilities. Canadian Healthcare Association Staff & Association for the Advancement of Medical Instruments Staff. 1996. LC 97-209735. xii, 127p. (*1-57020-073-4*) Assn Adv Med Instrn.

Reve et l'existence; Traum und Existenz see Dream & Existence

Reversal of Multidrug Resistance in Cancer. Ed. by J. A. Kellen. 1993. 160p. 149.95 (*0-8493-4744-0*) CRC Pr.

Reversal Theory: Applications & Development. Ed. by M. F. Apter et al. 1985. LC 85-170010. 212p. (C). text 39.95 (*0-906449-74-X*) L Erlbaum Assocs.

Reversal Theory: Motivation, Emotion & Personality. Michael J. Apter. 1989. 224p. 45.00 (*0-415-01581-2*) Routledge.

Reversals: A Personal Account of Victory over Dyslexia. Eileen M. Simpson. 1998. 246p. pap. 13.00 (*0-374-52316-9*) FS&G.

Reverse Effect: How Vitamins & Minerals Promote Health & Cause Disease. Walter A. Heiby. 1988. (Illus.). 1216p. (Orig.). 59.50 (*0-938869-01-9*) MediSci Pubs.

Reverse Osmosis: A Practical Guide for Industrial Users. Wes Byrne. 1995. LC 95-60061. 461p. 90.00 (*0-927188-03-1*) Tall Oaks Pub.

Reverse the Aging Process Naturally: How to Build the Immune System with Antioxidants, the Supernutrients of the Nineties. Gary Null & Martin Feldman. 1993. LC 92-56703. (Gary Null's Natural Health Library). 207p. pap. 12.95 (*0-679-74509-2*) Villard Books.

Reversibility in Testicular Toxicity Assessment. Anthony R. Scialli. 1992. 192p. lib. bdg. 125.00 (*0-8493-5980-5*, RA1224) CRC Pr.

Reversible Airway Obstruction: Neurohumoral Mechanisms & Treatment. Ed. by S. Bianco et al. 1987. (Journal: Vol. 50, Suppl. 2, 1986). (Illus.). vi, 326p. pap. 102.75 (*3-8055-4524-X*) S Karger.

Reversing Diabetes. Julian M. Whitaker. rev. ed. 2001. LC 00-47230. (Illus.). 448p. pap. (*0-446-67658-6*) Warner.

Reversing Diabetes. Julian M. Whitaker. 1990. LC 86-40416. (Illus.). 389p. pap. 14.99 (*0-446-38563-8*) Warner Bks.

Reversing Fibromyalgia: How to Treat & Overcome Fibromyalgia & Other Arthritis-Related Diseases. Joe M. Elrod. 1997. 223p. pap. 12.95 (*1-58054-005-8*) Woodland UT.

Reversing Heart Disease. Julian M. Whitaker. 1988. LC 84-40089. (Illus.). 272p. pap. 14.99 (*0-446-38548-4*) Warner Bks.

***Reversing Heart Disease.** Julian Whitaker. rev. ed. 2002. 416p. pap. (*0-446-67657-8*) Warner Bks.

Reversing Human Aging. Michael Fossel. 1996. LC 95-36636. xii, 307p. 25.00 (*0-688-14324-5*, Wm Morrow) Morrow Avon.

Reversing Hypertension: A Vital New Program to Prevent, Treat & Reduce High Blood Pressure. Julian Whitaker. 2001. LC 99-39815. (Illus.). 336p. pap. (*0-446-67663-2*) Warner.

Reversing Multiple Sclerosis: 9 Effective Steps to Recover Your Health. Celeste Pepe & Lisa Hammond. 2001. LC 00-111725. xxvii, 465p. pap. 15.95 (*1-57174-226-3*) Hampton Roads Pub Co.

Reversing the Aging Process. Gene Davis. 1987. 332p. (Orig.). pap. 29.95 (*0-9618919-0-4*) Life Res Found.

Reversing the Aging Process: Twelve Steps Toward Growing Younger. Kimberly Wittman. 1997. 95p. (Orig.). mass mkt. 14.95 (*1-885351-22-4*) Cheval Intl.

Review. Husband. 1989. text 110.00 (*0-443-04179-2*) Saunders.

Review & Appraisal of the World Population Plan of Action. 1989. 53p. pap. text 5.50 (*92-1-151185-2*, E.89.XIII.11) UN.

Review & Evaluation of Smoking Cessation Methods: The U. S. & Canada, 1978-1985. Jerome L. Schwartz. 1992. (Illus.). 299p. (C). pap. text 40.00 (*1-56806-109-9*) DIANE Pub.

Review Body for Nursing Staff, Midwives, Health Visitors & Professions Allied: 16th Report. 1999. (Command Papers: No. 4240). 45p. pap. (*0-10-142402-7*, HM24027); 39p. pap. (*0-10-142412-4*, HM24124) Statnry Office GBR. *Dist:* Bernan Associates.

Review Body for Nursing Staff, Midwives, Health Visitors & Professions Allied 15th Report, 1998: Command Paper 3833. 1998. (Command Papers: No. 81011068). 39p. pap. (*0-10-138332-0*, HM83320) Statnry Office GBR. *Dist:* Bernan Associates.

Review Body on Doctors & Dentists Remuneration Reports: 28th Report, 1999. 1999. 73p. pap. (*0-10-142432-9*, HM24329) Statnry Office GBR. *Dist:* Bernan Associates.

Review Book for Invasive CV Technology Vol. III: Hemodynamics. 1998. (Cardiovascular Review Bks.). (Illus.). 305p. spiral bd. 80.00 (*0-9653568-5-X*) Cardiac Self Assessmnt.

Review Book on Ophthalmology. S. Seal. 1986. (C). (*0-7855-4668-5*) Current Dist IND. *Dist:* St Mut.

Review Course for the N. E. S. P. A. Chad Nye. l.t. ed. 1998. LC 97-41312. (Illus.). 208p. pap. 119.25 net. (*1-56593-741-4*, 1440) Thomson Learn.

***Review for NCLEX-RN.** Diane M. Billings. 7th ed. 2001. (Illus.). 864p. pap. text 32.95 (*0-7817-3069-4*) Lppncott W & W.

Review for Physician Assistants. Patrick Auth & Morris Kerstein. 2001. LC 00-46426. 512p. pap. text 40.00 (*0-7817-1927-5*) Lppncott W & W.

Review for the USMLE Step 2. Carlyle H. Chan. 3rd rev. ed. 1999. LC 99-54040. (Illus.). 361p. (C). pap. 39.95 (*0-8385-0341-1*, A-0341-6) McGraw-Hill Prof.

Review for USMILE Step 1: United States Medical Licensing Examination, Step 1. John S. Lazo et al. 5th ed. 1998. LC 98-33988. (National Medical Series for Independent Study). (Illus.). 350p. pap. text 36.95 (*0-683-30490-9*) Lppncott W & W.

Review for USMLE. Steps 2 & 3. Carlos Ayala & Brad Spellberg. 2000. LC 99-49379. (Boards & Wards Ser.). (Illus.). 352p. pap. 28.95 (*0-632-04493-4*) Blackwell Sci.

Review for USMLE: United States Medical Licensing Examination, Step 1. John S. Lazo et al. 3rd ed. 1994. LC 93-41661. (National Medical Series for Independent Study). (Illus.). 300p. 29.95 (*0-683-06265-4*) Lppncott W & W.

Review for USMLE: United States Medical Licensing Examination, Step 1. Barbara Fadem et al. 4th ed. 1996. LC 93-41661. (National Medical Series for Independent Study). 115p. pap. text 16.95 (*0-683-02940-1*) Lppncott W & W.

Review for USMLE Step 2: United States Medical Licensing Examination. National Medical School Review Staff. 2nd ed. 1998. 506p. pap. text 36.95 (*0-683-30283-3*) Lppncott W & W.

Review Guide for LPN-LVN Pre-Entrance Exam. Ed. by Mary McDonald. 1999. LC 99-42996. (Illus.). 368p. (C). pap. text 24.95 (*0-7637-1061-X*, 1061-X, N L N Bart) Jones & Bartlett.

Review Guide for RN Pre-Entrance Exam. Ed. by Mary McDonald. 1999. (Illus.). 368p. (C). pap. text 24.95 (*0-7637-1062-8*, 1062-8, N L N Bart) Jones & Bartlett.

Review Manual for Neurology in Clinical Practice. Karl E. Misulis. Ed. by Walter G. Bradley et al. 3rd ed. 2000. LC 00-35808. 368p. pap. text 49.99 (*0-7506-7192-0*) Buttrwrth-Heinemann.

Review Manual for the Emt-Intermediate: Self-Assessment Practice Tests. Donald J. Ptacnik. 3rd ed. 1993. 246p. pap. 27.00 (*0-7216-5042-2*) Saunders.

Review Manual of Health Information: Management of Strategic Resources. Mervat Abdelhak. 1996. 784p. pap. text 31.50 (*0-7216-5148-8*) Saunders.

Review of Amino Acid Transport Processes in Animal Cells & Tissues. Joseph Lerner. 1977. LC 78-55683. text 20.00 (*0-89101-036-X*) U Maine Pr.

Review of Approaches to Viral Chemotherapy. Maxwell Gordon et al. 1981. 96p. 35.00 (*0-915340-08-9*) PJD Pubns.

Review of Behavior Therapy Vol. 12: Theory & Practice. Cyril M. Franks et al. 1990. 382p. text 57.50 (*0-89862-752-4*) Guilford Pubns.

Review of Biostatistics. Paul E. Leaverton. 3rd ed. 1986. 128p. pap. 16.50 (*0-316-51853-0*, Little Brwn Med Div) Lppncott W & W.

Review of Child Development Research Ed. by Martin L. Hoffman & Lois W. Hoffman. LC 64-20472. Set. 1966. (*0-87154-383-4*); Vol. 1. 1964. 548p. 55.00 (*0-87154-384-2*); Vol. 2. 1966. 598p. 55.00 (*0-87154-385-0*) Russell Sage.

Review of Child Development Research, Vol. 3. Bettye M. Caldwell & Henry N. Ricciuti. 1976. 600p. pap. text 10.00 (*0-226-09044-2*, P680) U Ch Pr.

Review of Chiropractic Boards, & IV. Gibson & George Birnback. 1998. LC 99-177807. 288p. (C). pap. 39.95 (*0-8385-0386-1*) McGraw-Hill Prof.

Review of Clinical Anesthesia. David G. Silverman & Neil Roy Connelly. 3rd ed. 2001. LC 00-46431. 320p. pap. text 49.95 (*0-7817-2919-X*) Lppncott W & W.

Review of Critical Care Nursing: Case Studies & Applications. Sheila D. Melander. Ed. by Barbara N. Cullen. 1996. LC 95-39975. (Illus.). 426p. pap. text 32.00 (*0-7216-5537-8*) Saunders.

Review of Dental Assisting. Hazel O. Torres & Lois E. Mazzucchi. 1983. (Illus.). 350p. pap. text 37.95 (*0-7216-8883-7*) Saunders.

Review of Dental Hygiene. Caren M. Barnes. 4th ed. 1994. LC 94-20015. (Review Ser.). 304p. (C). pap. 37.80 (*0-8385-0230-X*, A0230-1) P-H.

Review of Fluoride: Benefits & Risks: Report of the Ad Hoc Subcommittee on Fluoride. 1994. (Illus.). 240p. (Orig.). (C). pap. text 50.00 (*0-7881-0729-1*) DIANE Pub.

Review of General Psychiatry. Howard H. Goldman. 5th ed. 2000. (Lange Medical Bks.). (Illus.). 704p. pap. 44.95 (*0-8385-8434-9*) McGraw-Hill Prof.

Review of Health & Social Services for Mentally Disordered Offenders (Mental Handicap) or Autism. HMSO Staff. 1994. (People with Learning Disabilities Ser.: Vol. 7). 206p. pap. (*0-11-321701-3*, HM17013) Statnry Office GBR. *Dist:* Bernan Associates.

Review of Hemodialysis for Nurses & Dialysis Patients, No. 6. C. F. Gutch et al. 6th ed. 1999. LC 99-461823. (Review of Hemodialysis for Nurses & Dialysis Patients Ser.: Vol. 6). (Illus.). 352p. (C). (gr. 13). pap. text 36.95 (*0-8151-2099-0*, 28866) Mosby Inc.

Review of Intensive Care Medicine. Nicholas A. Smyrnios et al. 2nd ed. 2000. 288p. pap. text 59.95 (*0-7817-2021-4*) Lppncott W & W.

Review of Internal Medicine. David R. Schlossberg. 2nd ed. 2000. 320p. pap. text 45.00 (*0-7817-1967-4*) Lppncott W & W.

Review of Maternal Child Nursing. Judith Green. 1978. text 17.95 (*0-07-024302-6*) McGraw.

Review of Medical Physiology. Edward G. Schneider. 1997. LC 97-18245. (Illus.). 304p. pap. text 17.95 (*0-397-58403-2*) Lppncott W & W.

Review of Medical Physiology. William F. Ganong. 20th ed. 2001. (Lange Medical Bks.). (Illus.). 870p. pap. 49.95 (*0-8385-8282-6*) McGraw-Hill Prof.

***Review of Medical Technologies.** Ciulla. 3rd ed. 2001. LC 2001-51363. 570p. pap. 42.67 (*0-8385-0340-3*) P-H.

Review of Mental Health Nursing. P. Haring. 1979. text 20.95 (*0-07-026415-5*) McGraw.

Review of Neuroradiology. Val M. Runge. 1995. 160p. pap. text 45.00 (*0-7216-5134-8*) Saunders.

Review of Neuroscience. Ben Pansky et al. 2nd ed. 1991. 576p. text 39.00 (*0-07-105304-2*) McGraw-Hill Med Pub.

Review of NiAAA's Neuroscience & Behavioral Research Portfolio. Ed. by Antonio Noronha et al. 2000. 562p. pap. text 60.00 (*0-7567-0441-3*) DIANE Pub.

Review of Nuclear Medicine Technology. Ann M. Stevens. 2nd ed. 1996. LC 96-578. 141p. pap. 42.00 (*0-932004-45-8*) Soc Nuclear Med.

Review of Nurse Anesthesiology. John J. Nagelhout. 1999. LC 99-19474. xix, 186p. pap. text 49.95 (*0-7216-7531-X*) Saunders.

Review of Obstetrics & Gynecology. Louis A. Vontver et al. 6th ed. 1999. LC 99-54037. (Illus.). 416p. pap. 39.95 (*0-8385-0323-3*) McGraw-Hill Prof.

Review of Ophthalmology. Kenneth C. Chern & Kenneth W. Wright. 1997. LC 96-20671. (Illus.). 600p. 79.00 (*0-683-18239-0*) Lppncott W & W.

Review of Ophthalmology. G. N. Seal. 1989. (C). (*0-89771-363-X*) Current Dist IND. *Dist:* St Mut.

Review of Organic Functional Groups: Introduction to Medicinal Organic Chemistry. Thomas L. Lemke. 3rd ed. 1991. LC 91-4855. (Illus.). 148p. pap. 29.00 (*0-8121-1428-0*) Lppncott W & W.

Review of Orthopaedic Trauma. Mark R. Brinker. 2001. LC 00-59544. (Illus.). 496p. pap. text 55.00 (*0-7216-8191-3*) Saunders.

Review of Orthopaedics. Mark D. Miller. Ed. by Richard Lampert. 2nd ed. 1996. LC 95-24469. (Illus.). 432p. pap. text 52.95 (*0-7216-5901-2*) Saunders.

Review of Orthopaedics. Mark R. Brinker & Mark D. Miller. 3rd ed. 2000. LC 99-16737. xv, 622p. (C). pap. text (*0-7216-8153-0*) Saunders.

Review of Pain Medicine. Roger W. Davis. 1993. 148p. pap. 24.70 (*1-884401-00-7*) Pain Review.

Review of Pathology. Ivan Damjanov & Emanuel Rubin. 2nd ed. 1998. LC 99-33310. (Illus.). 250p. pap. text 27.95 (*0-397-58408-3*); 1997. 225p. text 399.00 (*0-7817-1635-7*) Lppncott W & W.

Review of Pediatric Critical Care. Sandra Czerwinski & Patricia A. Moloney-Harmon. Ed. by Barbara N. Cullen. 1996. LC 96-15372. (Illus.). 250p. pap. text 34.00 (*0-7216-6159-9*) Saunders.

Review of Pediatric Over-the-Counter Drugs. Ed. by Peter Allen. 1989. 25p. pap. 250.00 (*0-941285-41-3*) FIND-SVP.

Review of Pediatric Psychology, Vol. 1. Ed. by William J. Burns & John V. LaVigne. 1984. 304p. text 56.00 (*0-8089-1602-5*, 790727, Grune & Strat) Harcrt Hlth Sci Grp.

Review of Pediatrics. Fredric D. Burg. 1999. LC 00-38810. xxx, 593p. pap. text 49.00 (*0-7216-1754-9*) Saunders.

Review of Pediatrics. Martin I. Lorin & Dimitri A. Sotiropoulos. 5th ed. 1993. (Review Ser.). (Illus.). 222p. (C). pap. 39.95 (*0-8385-0057-9*, A0057-8) McGraw-Hill Prof.

Review of Perioperative Nursing. Mark L. Phippen et al. Ed. by Maura Connor. 1999. LC 96-16726. 300p. pap. text 29.95 (*0-7216-3413-3*) Saunders.

Review of Personality Theories. Victor J. Drapela. 2nd ed. 1994. LC 94-36205. (Illus.). 184p. (C). pap. text 25.95 (*0-398-05957-8*); text 40.95 (*0-398-05943-8*) C C Thomas.

Review of Published Research on the Relationship of Some Personality Variables to ESP Scoring Level. Gordon L. Mangan. 1958. (Parapsychological Monographs: No. 1). pap. 5.00 (*0-912328-03-7*) Parapsych Foun.

Review of Pulmonary & Critical Care Medicine. Reuben M. Cherniack. 1996. 281p. pap. (*1-55009-027-5*) DEKR.

Review of Radiologic Physics. Walter Huda & Richard M. Sloan. 1995. LC 94-25711. (Illus.). 286p. 34.95 (*0-683-04230-0*) Lppncott W & W.

Review of Research in Nursing Education, Vol. I. Ed. by William L. Holzemer. 1986. 208p. pap. 19.95 (*0-88737-340-2*, 15-2170) Natl League Nurse.

Review of Research in Nursing Education, Vol. III. Ed. by Gloria Clayton & Pamela Baj. 1990. 192p. 9.95 (*0-88737-486-7*) Natl League Nurse.

Review of Research in Nursing Education, Vol. IV. Ed. by Pamela Baj & Gloria Clayton. 1991. 192p. pap. 9.95 (*0-88737-504-9*) Natl League Nurse.

Review of Research in Nursing Education, Vol. V. Ed. by Lois R. Allen. 1992. (C). pap. text 9.95 (*0-88737-542-1*, 15-2448) Natl League Nurse.

Review of Research in Nursing Education, Vol. VII. Ed. by Kathleen R. Stevens. 1996. 211p. pap. 34.95 (*0-88737-671-1*, 19-6711, NLN Pr) Natl League Nurse.

Review of Skeletal Radiology. Terry R. Yochum et al. 1998. LC 97-42362. 750p. pap. 42.00 (*0-683-30139-X*) Lppncott W & W.

Review of Sports Medicine & Arthroscopy. Ed. by Mark D. Miller et al. 1995. LC 94-22156. (Illus.). pap. text 56.95 (*0-7216-5281-6*) Saunders.

Review of Surgery. David C. Sabiston. Ed. by Lisette Bralow. 2nd ed. 1996. 368p. pap. text 38.95 (*0-7216-8671-0*) Saunders.

Review of the Department of Defense's Program for Breast Cancer Research. Institute of Medicine Staff. 1997. LC 97-67577. 100p. pap. 20.00 (*0-309-05780-9*) Natl Acad Pr.

Review of the Fialuridine (FIAU) Clinical Trials. Institute of Medicine Staff. 1995. LC 95-68327. 280p. pap. text 34.00 (*0-309-05279-3*) Natl Acad Pr.

Review of the Hanford Thyroid Disease Study Draft Final Report. National Academy of Sciences Staff. 2000. 228p. pap. 46.50 (*0-309-06883-5*) Natl Acad Pr.

Review of the Health & Nutritional Properties of Cocoa & Chocolate. Ian Knight. 1999. LC 99-17982. 149.95 (*0-632-05415-8*) Blackwell Sci.

Review of the Nature & Uses of Examinations in Medical Education. J. Charvat et al. 1968. (Public Health Papers: No. 36). 74p. pap. text 7.00 (*92-4-130036-1*, 1110036) World Health.

Review of the Scientific Literature as It Pertains to Gulf War Illness Vol. 4: Stress. Grant N. Marshall et al. 2000. 142p. (C). pap. 15.00 (*0-8330-2860-X*); 1999. LC 98-31679. (Illus.). 130p. pap. 15.00 (*0-8330-2679-8*, MR-1018/4-OSD) Rand Corp.

Review of the Scientific Literature As It Pertains to Gulf War Illnesses: Chemical & Biological Warfare Agents. William S. Augerson. 2000. LC 98-31679. (Gulf War Illnesses Ser.). (Illus.). 265p. pap. 30.00 (*0-8330-2680-1*) Rand Corp.

Review of the Scientific Literature As It Pertains to Gulf War Illnesses: Immunizations. Beatrice Alexandra Golomb. 2001. pap. 15.00 (*0-8330-2678-X*) Rand Corp.

Review of the Scientific Literature As It Pertains to Gulf War Illnesses: Infectious Diseases. Lee H. Hilborne & Beatrice Alexandra Golomb. 2001. LC 98-31679. (Gulf War Illnesses Ser.). (Illus.). 119p. pap. 15.00 (*0-8330-2676-3*) Rand Corp.

Review of the Scientific Literature As It Pertains to Gulf War Illnesses: Pesticides, 8. Gary Checchine et al. 2001. LC 98-31679. (Gulf War Illnesses Ser.). (Illus.). pap. 15.00 (*0-8330-2682-8*) Rand Corp.

Review of the Scientific Literature As it Pertains to Gulf War Illnesses: Volume 7: Depleted Uranium, Vol. 7. Naomi Harley et al. 1999. LC 98-31679. (Gulf War Illnesses Ser.). (Illus.). 144p. pap. 15.00 (*0-8330-2681-X*, MR-1018/7-OSD) Rand Corp.

Review of the Scientific Literature as It Pertains to Gulf War Illnesses Vol. 6: Oil Well Fires. Dalia M. Spektor. 1998. LC 98-31679. (Gulf War Illnesses Ser.). (Illus.). 93p. pap. 15.00 (*0-8330-2668-2*, MR-1018-OSD) Rand Corp.

Review of the Technological Efficacy of Some Antioxidants & Synergists. FAO-WHO Expert Committee on Food Additives. 1972. (WHO Food Additives Ser.: No. 3). 144p. pap. text 8.00 (*92-4-166003-1*, 1270003) World Health.

Review of Thoracic Imaging & Chest Disease: A Practical Approach. Richard Slone et al. 1998. LC 98-15834. (Illus.). 432p. text 89.00 (*0-07-058223-8*) McGraw-Hill Prof.

Review of Vascular Surgery. Ed. by William C. Krupski. 1994. LC 94-10941. 170p. pap. text 35.00 (*0-7216-4843-6*) Saunders.

Review Questions & Answers for Veterinary Boards: Ancillary Topics. James Pratt. 2nd ed. 1997. LC 97-39805. (Mosby's Review Questions & Answers for Veterinary Boards Ser.: Vol. 2). 312p. (C). (gr. 13). pap. text 36.95 (*0-8151-7468-3*, 28276) Mosby Inc.

Review Questions & Answers for Veterinary Boards: Basic Science. James Pratt. 2nd ed. 1997. LC 97-37952. (Mosby's Review Questions & Answers for Veterinary Boards Ser.: Vol. 2). 264p. (C). (gr. 13). pap. text 36.95 (*0-8151-7389-X*, 28272) Mosby Inc.

Review Questions & Answers for Veterinary Boards: Clinical Sciences. James Pratt. 2nd ed. 1997. LC 97-37128. (Mosby's Review Questions & Answers for Veterinary Boards Ser.: Vol. 2). (Illus.). 312p. (C). (gr. 13). pap. text 36.95 (*0-8151-7462-4*, 28273) Mosby Inc.

Review Questions & Answers for Veterinary Boards: Large Animal Medicine & Surgery, No. 2. James Pratt. 2nd ed. 1997. LC 97-39808. (Mosby's Review Questions & Answers for Veterinary Boards Ser.: Vol. 2). 288p. (C). (gr. 13). pap. text 36.95 (*0-8151-7466-7*, 28275) Mosby Inc.

Review Questions & Answers for Veterinary Boards: Series. Paul W. Pratt. 2nd ed. 1998. (Illus.). 160.00 (*0-323-00145-9*) Mosby Inc.

Review Questions & Answers for Veterinary Boards: Small Animal Medicine & Surgery, No. 2. James Pratt. 2nd ed. 1997. LC 97-34834. (Mosby's Review Questions & Answers for Veterinary Boards Ser.: Vol. 2). 288p. (C). (gr. 13). pap. text 36.95 (*0-8151-7465-9*, 28274) Mosby Inc.

Review Questions & Answers for Veterinary Technicians. Thomas P. Colville. 2nd ed. 1995. LC 95-44415. 368p. (C). (gr. 13). pap. text 34.95 (*0-8151-1850-3*, 27466) Mosby Inc.

Review Questions & Explanations in Computed Tomography. Lois E. Romans. 1996. LC 96-1773. 300p. pap. 26.95 (*0-683-07330-3*) Lppncott W & W.

Review Questions for Clinical Neurology Board Review. D. J. Coffey. 2001. (Review Questions Ser.). (Illus.). 200p. pap. 34.95 (*1-85070-054-0*, Parthenon Pbng) CRC Pr.

Review Questions for CT. Euclid Seeram. 1997. LC 97-4140. (Illus.). 128p. pap. 29.95 (*0-86542-529-9*) Blackwell Sci.

Review Questions for Gross Anatomy & Embryology. T. R. Gest et al. 1993. (Review Questions Ser.). (Illus.). 401p. (C). 24.95 (*1-85070-503-8*, Parthenon Pbng) CRC Pr.

Review Questions for Health Information Management: RRA & ART Examination Preparation. Mary R. Burns et al. 1997. LC 96-29845. (Review Questions Ser.). 138p. 21.95 (*1-85070-737-5*, B2658, Parthenon Pbng) CRC Pr.

Review Questions for Human Anatomy: A Program of Study Through Regional Self-Assessment. Patrick W. Tank. 1996. LC 96-2871. (Review Questions Ser.). 154p. 24.95 (*1-85070-795-2*, T0806, Parthenon Pbng) CRC Pr.

Review Questions for Human Embryology. T. R. Gest & J. M. Anderson. 1995. (Review Questions Ser.). (Illus.). 104p. (C). lib. bdg. 19.95 (*1-85070-591-7*, Parthenon Pbng) CRC Pr.

Review Questions for Human Histology. E. Robert Burns. 1995. LC 95-17810. (Review Questions Ser.). 216p. lib. bdg. 21.95 (*1-85070-594-1*, Parthenon Pbng) CRC Pr.

Review Questions for Human Pathology. Robin R. Jones. 1999. LC 97-47206. (Review Questions Ser.). (Illus.). 322p. 21.95 (*1-85070-599-2*, Parthenon Pbng) CRC Pr.

Review Questions for Human Physiology. James N. Pasley. 1998. (Review Questions Ser.). (Illus.). 142p. lib. bdg. 21.95 (*1-85070-601-8*, Parthenon Pbng) CRC Pr.

Review Questions for Microbiology & Immunology: A Review for the USMLE, Step 1, 2 & 3 Examinations. A. C. Reese & C. N. Nair. 2000. LC 98-35193. (Review Questions Ser.). (Illus.). 124p. lib. bdg. 27.95 (*1-85070-020-6*) CRC Pr.

Review Questions for MRI. Carolyn Kaut & William Faulkner. 1994. LC 94-24135. 192p. pap. 37.95 (*0-632-03905-1*) Blackwell Sci.

Review Questions for Neuroanatomy: Structural & Functional. William T. Mosenthal. 1996. LC 96-2843. (Review Questions Ser.). 134p. lib. bdg. 21.95 (*1-85070-653-0*, Parthenon Pbng) CRC Pr.

Review Questions for Nuclear Medicine: The Technology Registry Examination. Anna M. Gallo-Foss. 1997. LC 96-29859. (Review Questions Ser.). (Illus.). 176p. 21.95 (*1-85070-703-0*, GO883, Parthenon Pbng) CRC Pr.

Review Questions for Phlebotomy: A Subject Review & Questions for ASCP Phlebotomy Technician Examinations. S. A. Taylor. 2000. LC 99-44543. (Review Questions Ser.). 112p. 27.95 (*1-85070-755-3*, T0638, Parthenon Pbng) CRC Pr.

Review Questions for the Adult & Family Nurse Practitioner Certification Examination. Jill E. Winland-Brown & Lynne M. Dunphy. 1999. LC 99-12943. (Illus.). 352p. (C). pap. text 46.95 (*0-8036-0471-8*) Davis Co.

Review Questions for the NCLEX-RN. Sandra F. Smith. 3rd ed. 1997. LC 98-197992. 240p. (C). pap. 24.95 (*0-8385-8445-4*) Appleton & Lange.

Review Questions for the Physician Assistant Certifying Examination. David F. Irvine. 1998. LC 98-14472. (Review Questions Ser.). (Illus.). 172p. 28.95 (*1-85070-663-8*, I0125, Parthenon Pbng) CRC Pr.

Review Questions for the USMLE Step 3 Examination. Ed. by Arshad Majid. 2001. LC 00-64941. (Review Questions Ser.). (Illus.). 122p. pap. 35.95 (*1-85070-063-X*, Parthenon Pbng) CRC Pr.

Review Questions for Ultrasound: A Sonographer's Exam Guide. Joyce Miller et al. 1998. LC 97-42674. (Review Questions Ser.). (Illus.). 190p. 43.95 (*1-85070-704-9*, M1957, Parthenon Pbng) CRC Pr.

Review Questions in Intraoperative Monitoring. ASET Committee. 1999. 48p. spiral bd. 24.00 (*1-57797-036-5*) ASET.

Review Questions in Polysomnography. ASET Committee. 1999. (Illus.). 64p. spiral bd. 24.00 (*1-57797-037-3*) ASET.

Reviewed Contents of Major Diabetes Congresses. F. Belfiore. 1981. (Frontiers in Diabetes Ser.: Vol. 1). xii, 162p. 77.50 (*3-8055-3414-0*) S Karger.

Reviewing Health Manpower Development: A Method of Improving National Health Systems. M. Roemer. 1987. (Public Health Papers: No. 83). 149p. 13.00 (*92-4-130083-3*) World Health.

Reviews in Child & Adolescent Psychiatry: Reprinted from the Journal of the American Academy of Child & Adolescent Psychiatry, Volume 1. David Herzog. 1998. 146p. 25.00 (*0-683-18376-1*) Lppncott W & W.

Reviews in Environmental Health (1999) Ed. by Gary E. R. Hook & George W. Lucier. 2000. (Illus.). 224p. (C). pap. text 40.00 (*0-7881-8554-3*) DIANE Pub.

Reviews in Pediatric Hem-Oncology VI. Ed. by Carl Pochedly. 1985. LC 85-9547. 218p. 65.00 (*0-275-91306-6*, C1306, Praeger Pubs) Greenwood.

Reviews of Environmental Contamination & Toxicology. Ed. by G. W. Ware. Vol. 101. 1987. 169p. 89.95 (*0-387-96593-9*); Vol. 108. 1988. (Illus.). 184p. 89.95 (*0-387-96902-0*); Vol. 110. 1989. (Illus.). 190p. 89.95 (*0-387-97158-0*); Vol. 116. 1990. 200p. 99.00 (*0-387-97334-6*); Vol. 127. 1992. 176p. 108.00 (*0-387-97829-1*); Vol. 128. 1992. 124p. 108.00 (*0-387-97899-2*); Vol. 129. 1992. 144p. 108.00 (*0-387-97900-X*); Vol. 154. 1997. (Illus.). 148p. 64.95 (*0-387-98371-6*) Spr-Verlag.

Reviews of Physiology, Vol. 115. 1990. 90.00 (*0-387-51712-X*) Spr-Verlag.

Reviews of Physiology, Biochemistry & Pharmacology, Vol. 87. 1980. (Illus.). 232p. 71.00 (*0-387-09944-1*) Spr-Verlag.

Reviews of Physiology, Biochemistry & Pharmacology. Ed. by Richard H. Adrian. 1981. (Illus.). Vol. 88. 264p. 76.00 (*0-387-10408-9*); Vol. 89. 260p. 70.00 (*0-387-10495-X*) Spr-Verlag.

Reviews of Physiology, Biochemistry & Pharmacology. Ed. by Richard H. Adrian et al. (Illus.). Vol. 90. 1981. 300p. 76.00 (*0-387-10657-X*); Vol. 91. 1981. 227p. 67.00 (*0-387-10961-7*); Vol. 92. 1981. 223p. 67.00 (*0-387-11105-0*); Vol. 94. 1982. 207p. 76.00 (*0-387-11701-6*) Spr-Verlag.

Reviews of Physiology, Biochemistry & Pharmacology, Vol. 95. Ed. by Richard H. Adrian. 1982. (Illus.). 223p. 76.00 (*0-387-11736-9*) Spr-Verlag.

Reviews of Physiology, Biochemistry & Pharmacology. Ed. by Richard H. Adrian et al. (Illus.). Vol. 96. 1982. 194p. 72.00 (*0-387-11849-7*); Vol. 97. 1983. 176p. 67.00 (*0-387-12135-8*) Spr-Verlag.

Reviews of Physiology, Biochemistry & Pharmacology, Vol. 98. H. Blashko et al. 1983. (Illus.). 255p. 93.00 (*0-387-12817-4*) Spr-Verlag.

Reviews of Physiology, Biochemistry, & Pharmacology, Vol. 110. 1988. (Illus.). 292p. 113.00 (*0-387-18736-7*) Spr-Verlag.

Reviews of Physiology, Biochemistry & Pharmacology. Ed. by M. P. Blaustein et al. 1989. (Illus.). Vol. 113. 146p. 80.00 (*0-387-50948-8*); Vol. 114. 272p. 113.00 (*0-387-51693-X*) Spr-Verlag.

Reviews of Physiology, Biochemistry & Pharmacology, Vol. 116. D. Pette et al. Ed. by M. P. Blaustein et al. 1990. (Illus.). 176p. 98.00 (*0-387-52880-6*) Spr-Verlag.

Reviews of Physiology, Biochemistry & Pharmacology. Ed. by M. P. Blaustein et al. (Illus.). Vol. 118. 1991. 128p. 76.00 (*0-387-54211-6*); Vol. 120. 1992. 208p. 140.00 (*0-387-55364-9*); Vol. 122. 1993. 264p. 143.00 (*0-387-56380-6*); Vol. 123. 1994. 266p. 133.00 (*0-387-57536-7*); Vol. 127. 1995. 272p. 163.00 (*3-540-60135-X*); Vol. 128. 1996. 192p. 116.00 (*3-540-61343-9*) Spr-Verlag.

Reviews of Physiology, Biochemistry & Pharmacology, Vol. 132. Ed. by M. P. Blaustein. 1998. (Illus.). 131p. 79.95 (*3-540-63492-4*) Spr-Verlag.

Reviews of Physiology, Biochemistry & Pharmacology. Ed. by M. P. Blaustein et al. (Illus.). Vol. 133. 1998. 120p. 89.95 (*3-540-63945-4*); Vol. 134. 1998. 324p. 149.00 (*3-540-64753-8*); Vol. 135. 1998. 216p. 115.00 (*3-540-64779-1*); Vol. 140. 2000. 146p. 92.00 (*3-540-66603-6*) Spr-Verlag.

Reviews of Physiology, Biochemistry & Pharmacology: Special Issue on Signal Transduction, Vol. 119, Pt. I. Ed. by M. P. Blaustein et al. 1992. (Illus.). 264p. 147.00 (*0-387-55192-1*) Spr-Verlag.

Reviews of Physiology, Biochemistry & Pharmacology: Special Issue on Signal Transduction II, Vol. 121. Ed. by M. P. Blaustein et al. 1992. (Illus.). 216p. 140.00 (*0-387-55969-8*) Spr-Verlag.

Reviews of Physiology, Biochemistry & Pharmacology Vol. 138: Special Issue on the Tird Filament System. Ed. by M. P. Blaustein et al. 1999. (Illus.). 278p. 119.00 (*3-540-65484-4*) Spr-Verlag.

Revised Protocol to the European Agreement on the Exchange of Tissue-Typing Reagents. Council of Europe Staff. 1985. (Conventions & Agreements Ser.: No. 84a). (ENG & FRE.). (*92-871-0767-X*) Council of Europe FRA. *Dist:* Manhattan Pub Co.

Revised Social Service Care Plans for Nursing Homes. Marylou Hughes & Manuela Espinosa. rev. ed. 1993. 136p. (Orig.). (C). 16.50 (*1-877735-11-6*, 2114PP) Prof Prnting & Pub.

Revising the Tax Treatment of Employer-Provided Health Insurance. Glied. 1994. 50p. (Orig.). pap. 9.95 (*0-8447-7029-9*) Am Enterprise.

Revision for MRCPsych, Pt. 1. Basant K. Puri & John Sklar. 1990. 232p. pap. text (*0-443-04331-0*) Church.

Revision Hip Arthroplasty: A Practical Approach to Bone Stock Loss. Richard N. Villar & Derek McMinn. 1997. LC 96-9042. (Illus.). 136p. (*0-7506-1640-7*) E A GBR. *Dist:* OUP.

Revision in Sciences Basic to Ophthalmology. Ramen Malhotra & David Easty. 1997. LC 97-9710. (An Arnold Publication). 256p. pap. (*0-340-67678-7*) E A GBR. *Dist:* OUP.

Revision Notes on Surgical Care. P. J. Wormald & J. D. Knottenbelt. 1995. (Illus.). 384p. pap. (*0-340-61377-7*) E A GBR. *Dist:* OUP.

Revision of Failed Arthroscopic & Ligament Surgery. Bertram Zarins & Richard A. Marder. 1998. LC 97-43315. (Illus.). 172p. 105.00 (*0-86542-437-3*) Blackwell Sci.

Revision of the Fungi Formerly Classified As Nectria Subgenus Hyphonectria. Gary J. Samuels. 1976. LC 66-6394. (Memoirs Ser.: Vol. 26, No. 3). (Illus.). 126p. pap. 9.00 (*0-89327-008-3*) NY Botanical.

Revision of the Genus Synchiropus (Teleostei: Callionymidae) Ronald Fricke. 1981. (Theses Zoological Ser.: Vol. 1). (Illus.). 194p. text 34.00 (*3-7682-1306-4*) Lubrecht & Cramer.

Revision Otologic Surgery. Ed. by Vincent N. Carrasco & Harold C. Pillsbury. 1997. LC 97-1120. (Illus.). 304p. text 109.00 (*0-86577-610-5*) Thieme Med Pubs.

Revision Questions in Pediatrics: For Postgraduate Examinations. Patrick Cartlidge et al. 1999. LC 99-28871. (Illus.). ix, 280p. text (*0-443-06246-3*) Church.

Revision Spine Surgery. Joseph Y. Margulies et al. 1998. LC 98-36265. (Illus.). 887p. (C). (gr. 13). text 195.00 (*0-8151-4591-8*, 30029) Mosby Inc.

Revision Surgery in Total Hip Arthroplasty. B. B. Wroblewski. 1990. (Illus.). 236p. 158.00 (*0-387-19618-8*) Spr-Verlag.

Revision Surgery in Total Hip Arthroplasty. Boguslaw M. Wroblewski. 1990. 236p. 144.00 (*3-540-19618-8*) Spr-Verlag.

Revision Total Hip Arthroplasty. Ed. by James V. Bono et al. 1999. LC 97-42562. (Illus.). 637p. 179.00 (*0-387-98391-0*) Spr-Verlag.

Revision Total Hip Arthroplasty. Marvin E. Steinberg. 1998. LC 98-19477. 608p. text 179.00 (*0-7817-1424-9*) Lppncott W & W.

Revision Total Knee Arthroplasty. Gerard A. Engh et al. 1997. LC 96-39068. 485p. text 169.00 (*0-683-02827-8*) Lppncott W & W.

Revision Total Knee Arthroplasty. Paul A. Lotke & Jonathan P. Garino. rev. ed. 1998. LC 98-6927. 560p. text 179.00 (*0-7817-1024-3*) Lppncott W & W.

Revisional Surgery in Rheumatoid Arthritis. Ed. by F. W. Hagena. 1990. (Rheumatology, the Interdisciplinary Concept Ser.: Vol. 13). (Illus.). x, 266p. 226.25 (*3-8055-4930-X*) S Karger.

Revisioning Men's Lives: Gender, Intimacy & Power. Terry A. Kupers. 1993. LC 92-36142. 200p. pap. 18.95 (*0-89862-271-9*) Guilford Pubns.

Revisioning Phenomenology: Nursing & Health Science Research. Patricia L. Munhall. 1994. LC 94-1454. 326p. pap. 33.95 (*0-88737-597-9*) Natl League Nurse.

Revisioning Women, Health & Healing: Feminist, Cultural & Technoscience Perspectives. Ed. by Adele Clarke & Virginia L. Olesen. 1999. LC 98-9685. x, 374p. (C). pap. 25.95 (*0-415-91846-4*) Routledge.

Revitalize Your Body with Nature's Secrets. Edwin Flatto. 1981. pap. 9.95 (*0-935540-14-8*) Plymouth Pr.

Revitalize Your Life: Improve Your Health, Your Sex Life,& Your Looks after Age Fifty. Jack Lalanne. 2001. LC 93-78853. 208p. pap. 15.95 (*0-8038-9356-6*) Hastings Hse.

Revival of Interest in the Dream. Robert Fliess. 1953. 164p. 27.50 (*0-8236-5820-1*) Intl Univs Pr.

Reviving Primary Care: A U. S. - U. K. Comparison. John Fry et al. 1995. LC 95-15842. (*1-85775-001-2*) Radcliffe Med Pr GBR. *Dist:* Balogh.

Revolucion Psiquiatrica: Del Manicomio a la Comunidad. Ed. by Michael A. Woodbury. Tr. by Gallogo Mere & Lilita B. Diaz from ENG. 1987. (SPA.). 275p. (Orig.). pap. 40.00 (*0-9619117-0-0*) Veritas Ed Pub.

Revolution in Perception: The Ecological Psychology of James J. Gibson. Edward S. Reed. 1988. (C). 45.00 (*0-300-04289-2*) Yale U Pr.

Revolution in Psychiatry. Hornstein. 1997. 25.00 (*0-02-914962-2*) Free Pr.

Revolution in the Physiology of the Living Cell & Beyond. Gilbert N. Ling. 1992. LC 89-11068. 404p. lib. bdg. 64.50 (*0-89464-398-3*) Krieger.

Revolutionary Approach to Prostate Cancer. Aubrey Pilgrim & E. David Crawford. rev. ed. 2001. LC 99-64526. (Illus.). 300p. pap. 18.95 (*1-58501-015-4*) CeShore Pubg.

Revolutionary Medicine, 1700-1800. C. Keith Wilbur. 1996. LC 96-43016. (Illustrated Living History Ser.). (Illus.). 112p. (Orig.). (YA). (gr. 5-7). 19.95 (*0-7910-4532-3*, Chelsea Juniors) Chelsea Hse.

Revolutionary Medicine, 1700-1800. C. Keith Wilbur. 2nd ed. 1997. LC 97-27608. (Illustrated Living History Ser.). (Illus.). 88p. (Orig.). pap. 14.95 (*0-7627-0139-0*) Globe Pequot.

Revolutionary New Approach: Uncovering the Secret Power of Your Hidden Emotions. Samuel J. Mann. 1998. LC 98-17434. (Illus.). 256p. 24.95 (*0-471-17547-1*) Wiley.

Rewiring the Brain: A Lifeline to New Connections. Carolyn E. Dolen. 1998. 59.92 (*1-57444-192-2*) St Lucie Pr.

Rewriting Family Scripts: Improvisation & Systems Change. John Byng-Hall. 1995. LC 95-16208. (Family Therapy Ser.). 288p. text 40.00 (*0-89862-876-8*) Guilford Pubns.

Rewriting Love Stories: Brief Marital Therapy. Patricia O. Hudson & William H. O'Hanlon. 1994. LC 93-29294. 192p. pap. 11.95 (*0-393-31094-9*) Norton.

Rewriting Nursing History. Ed. by Celia Davies. 1980. 226p. 44.00 (*0-389-20153-7*, N6982) B&N Imports.

Rewriting the Soul: Multiple Personality & the Sciences of Memory. Ian Hacking. 1998. 352p. pap. 17.95 (*0-691-05908-X*) Princeton U Pr.

Rhabdomyosarcoma & Related Tumors in Children & Adolescents. Harold M. Maurer & Frederick B. Ruymann. 1991. (Illus.). 472p. 189.00 (*0-8493-6902-9*, RC281) CRC Pr.

Rhabdoviruses. R. R. Wagner. 1987. LC 87-12279. (Viruses Ser.). (Illus.). 562p. (C). text 139.50 (*0-306-42453-3*, Kluwer Plenum) Kluwer Academic.

Rhabdoviruses, Vol. I. David H. Bishop. 1979. 208p. 92.95 (*0-8493-5913-9*, QR415) CRC Pr.

Rhabdoviruses David H. Bishop. 1980. Vol. II. 256p. 141.00 (*0-8493-5914-7*, QR415); Vol. III. 272p. 148.00 (*0-8493-5915-5*) Franklin (CRC Reprint).

Rhea Complex: A Detour Around the Oedipus Complex. Akhter Ahsen. 1984. LC 84-72149. 279p. 35.00 (*0-913412-24-4*) Brandon Hse.

Rheology of Blood, Blood Vessels & Associated Tissues. D. R. Gross & N. H. Hwang. 1981. (NATO Advanced Science Institutes Ser.: No. 41). 382p. text 138.50 (*90-286-0950-4*) Kluwer Academic.

Rheology of Food, Pharmaceutical & Biological Materials with General Rheology: Proceedings of the Annual Meeting of the British Society of Rheology, University of Warwick, Coventry, U. K., 12- 15 Sept. 1989. Ed. by R. E. Carter. 1990. 342p. pap. 109.95 (*1-85166-525-0*) Elsevier.

Rherythropoietin in Cancer Supportive Treatment. Ed. by John F. Smyth et al. 1996. LC 96-13976. (Illus.). 280p. text 115.00 (*0-8247-9761-2*) Dekker.

Rhetorical Voice of Psychoanalysis: Displacement of Evidence by Theory. Donald P. Spence. 1994. LC 93-6344. 232p. 39.50 (*0-674-76874-4*) HUP.

Rhetorics of Self Making. Ed. by Debbora Battaglia. 1995. LC 94-398. text 40.00 (*0-520-08798-4*); pap. text 18.95 (*0-520-08799-2*) U CA Pr.

Rheumaderm: Current Issues in Rheumatology & Dermatology. Carmel Mallia. 1999. LC 98-31757. (Advances in Experimental Medicine & Biology Ser.). 562p. text (*0-306-46047-5*, Kluwer Plenum) Kluwer Academic.

Rheumaorthopadie. 1995. 139.00 (*3-540-60040-X*) Spr-Verlag.

Rheumatic Diseases: Immunological Mechanisms & Prospects for New Therapies. John Stanley Hill Gaston. 1999. LC 98-11713. (Illus.). 296p. (C). text 85.00 (*0-521-59327-1*) Cambridge U Pr.

Rheumatic Diseases: Report of a WHO Scientific Group. 1992. (Technical Reports: No. 816). (CHI, ENG, FRE, RUS & SPA.). vii, 59p. pap. text 10.00 (*92-4-120816-3*, 1100816) World Health.

Rheumatic Diseases & Sports. Ed. by H. W. Baenkler. 1992. (Rheumatology Ser.: Vol. 16). (Illus.). vii, 232p. 191.50 (*3-8055-5425-7*) S Karger.

Rheumatic Diseases & the Heart. J. A. Cosh & J. L. Lever. 1989. (Illus.). 250p. 121.00 (*0-387-19524-6*) Spr-Verlag.

Rheumatic Fever. Angelo Taranta & Milton Markowitz. 2nd ed. 1990. (C). text 59.00 (*0-7462-0106-0*) Kluwer Academic.

Rheumatic Fever & Rheumatic Heart Disease: Report on a WHO Study Group. WHO Staff. 1988. (Technical Report Ser.: No. 764). 58p. 8.00 (*92-4-120764-7*) World Health.

Rheumatic Fever & Streptococcal Infection: Unraveling the Mysteries of a Dread Disease. Benedict F. Massell. 1997. LC 97-205903. (Francis Countway Library of Medicine). 400p. 25.00 (*0-674-76877-9*) HUP.

Rheumatic Fever in America & Britain: A Biological, Epidemiological & Medical History. Peter C. English. 1999. LC 99-14094. 320p. 50.00 (*0-8135-2710-4*) Rutgers U Pr.

Rheumatism: Materia Medica Relating to Rheumatism. 2000. LC 99-97768. 169p. pap. 7.95 (*1-929410-07-7*) dttm.

Rheumatoid Arthritis. Ed. by Michael Fischbach. 1991. (Contemporary Management in Internal Medicine Ser.: Vol. 1, No. 6). (Illus.). 228p. text (*0-443-08827-6*) Church.

Rheumatoid Arthritis. Ed. by J. J. Goronzy & C. M. Weyand. 2001. LC 00-48164. (Current Directions in Autoimmunity Ser.: 3). (Illus.). viii, 282p. 170.50 (*3-8055-7120-8*) S Karger.

Rheumatoid Arthritis. Edward D. Harris, Jr. Ed. by Richard Zorab. 1997. LC 96-40173. (Illus.). 432p. text 131.00 (*0-7216-5249-2*) Saunders.

Rheumatoid Arthritis. Lipsky. 1997. (*0-397-51589-8*, L1216) Lppncott W & W.

Rheumatoid Arthritis: A Separate World: A Personal Account of Living with Rheumatoid Arthritis. Eileen Courtnay. Ed. by Adolph Caso. 2000. LC 00-63038. (Illus.). 140p. pap. 19.95 (*0-8283-2058-6*) Branden Bks.

Rheumatoid Arthritis: An Illustrated Guide to Pathogenesis, Diagnosis & Management. Ralph Schumacher & Eric P. Gall. 1988. LC 65-40264. (Illus.). 420p. (C). (gr. 13). text (*0-397-44653-5*, GM0068) Gower-Mosby.

Rheumatoid Arthritis: Frontiers in Pathogenesis & Treatment. Gary S. Firestein et al. 2000. LC 99-59424. (Illus.). xv, 581p. text 198.50 (*0-19-262972-7*) OUP.

Rheumatoid Arthritis: Pathogenesis, Assessment, Outcome, & Treatment. Ed. by Frederick Wolfe & Theodore Pincus. 1994. (Illus.). 544p. text 195.00 (*0-8247-8878-8*) Dekker.

Rheumatoid Arthritis: Recent Research Advances. Ed. by J. S. Smolen et al. 1992. LC 91-5068. 399p. 126.00 (*0-387-53315-X*) Spr-Verlag.

Rheumatoid Arthritis: Your Medication Explained. Mary-Claire Mason & Elaine Smith. 2001. 112p. pap. (*0-85969-836-X*) Sheldon Pr GBR. *Dist:* Intl Pubs Mktg.

Rheumatoid Arthritis & Related Diseases. Robert P. Sundel. 1998. (Illus.). 144p. pap. text 34.00 (*1-879772-10-8*) Health Studies.

Rheumatoid Arthritis Surgery of the Complex Hand & Foot. Ed. by F. W. Hagena. 1987. (Rheumatology Ser.: Vol. 11). (Illus.). xiv, 190p. 154.00 (*3-8055-4408-1*) S Karger.

Rheumatoid Arthritis Surgery of the Elbow. Ed. by M. J. Hamalainen & F. W. Hagena. 1991. (Rheumatology, the Interdisciplinary Concept Ser.: Vol. 15). (Illus.). x, 130p. 108.00 (*3-8055-5327-7*) S Karger.

Rheumatoid Arthritis Surgery of the Shoulder. Ed. by A. W. Lattin & C. Petersson. 1989. (Rheumatology, the Interdisciplinary Concept Ser.: Vol. 12). (Illus.). xiv, 138p. 121.75 (*3-8055-4804-4*) S Karger.

Rheumatoid Hand & Wrist. Ed. by J. Stanley. 1998. (Illus.). 256p. text (*0-443-04836-3*) Church.

Rheumatoid Hip. H. Thabe & Bad Kreuznach. 1990. (Illus.). 185p. 71.95 (*0-387-52884-9*) Spr-Verlag.

Rheumatologic Rehabilitation Vol. I: Assessment & Mangement. Ed. by Jeanne L. Melvin & Gail Jensen. 1997. LC 98-204415. (Illus.). 450p. text 50.00 (*1-56900-086-7*, 1201) Am Occup Therapy.

Rheumatological Physiotherapy. Carol David & Jill Lloyd. 1999. (Illus.). 208p. pap. 32.00 (*0-7234-2594-9*) Mosby Inc.

Rheumatology. Harold M. Adelman. 2001. (Questions & Answers Ser.). (Illus.). 148p. pap. text 26.95 (*1-873413-73-4*) Merit Pub Intl.

Rheumatology. Moll. 2nd ed. 1998. 158p. pap. text 16.95 (*0-443-05887-3*) Saunders.

Rheumatology. J. M. Moll. 2nd ed. 1997. LC 96-39719. (Colour Guide Ser.). (*0-443-05805-9*) Harcrt Hlth Sci Grp.

Rheumatology: Diagnosis & Therapeutics. John J. Cash et al. 1998. LC 97-42809. 472p. pap. 39.95 (*0-683-30014-8*) Lppncott W & W.

***Rheumatology & the Kidney.** Ed. by Dwomo Adu et al. 2001. (Illus.). 368p. 90.00 (*0-19-263178-0*) OUP.

Rheumatology, Arthritis & Musculoskeletal Disease Two Thousand. Panush. 2000. (Illus.). 400p. text 84.95 (*0-8151-2926-2*, 31667) Mosby Inc.

Rheumatology Examination & Injection Techniques. Michael Doherty et al. 1992. (Illus.). 143p. text (*0-7020-1442-7*) W B Saunders GBR. *Dist:* Saunders.

***Rheumatology Examination & Injection Techniques.** Michael Doherty et al. 2nd ed. 1999. (Illus.). 168p. (*0-7020-2387-6*) W B Saunders GBR. *Dist:* Saunders.

Rheumatology for the Health Care Professional. Harry Spiera & Irwin Oreskes. 1991. 480p. (Orig.). (C). pap. 42.50 (*0-87527-464-1*) Green.

Rheumatology Guidebook. R. Ferrari et al. 1996. LC 97-17007. 200p. (Orig.). pap. (*1-85996-215-7*) Bios Sci GBR. *Dist:* Bks Intl VA.

Rheumatology in Chinese Medicine. Gerard Guillaume & Mach Chieu. Tr. by David Vachon from FRE. 1996. LC 95-83689. (Illus.). 430p. 95.00 (*0-939616-26-2*) Eastland.

Rheumatology in Primary Care. Juan J. Canoso. Ed. by Ray Kersey. 1997. LC 96-40174. 432p. text 47.00 (*0-7216-6080-0*) Saunders.

Rheumatology Nursing. Hill. 1998. LC 98-9759. (C). pap. text (*0-443-05792-3*) Church.

Rheumatology Nursing: A Problem-Oriented Approach. Janice S. Pigg et al. 1989. LC 84-19551. 462p. text 39.95 (*0-8273-4333-7*) Delmar.

Rheumatology Pearls. Ed. by Richard M. Silver & Edwin A. Smith. 1997. LC 96-49763. (Pearls Ser.). (Illus.). 180p. pap. 45.00 (*1-56053-201-7*) Hanley & Belfus.

Rheumatology Secrets. Ed. by Sterling West. 1996. LC 96-32241. (Secrets Ser.). (Illus.). 575p. pap. 45.95 (*1-56053-154-1*) Hanley & Belfus.

Rhinitis. Ed. by Robert M. Naclerio & Steven R. Durham. 1998. LC 98-39370. (Lung Biology in Health & Disease Ser.). (Illus.). 558p. text 195.00 (*0-8247-0189-5*) Dekker.

Rhinitis. Ed. by Guy A. Settipane. 2nd ed. 1991. LC 90-64470. (Illus.). 300p. text 68.00 (*0-936587-04-0*) OceanSide Pubns.

Rhinitis: Immunopathology & Pharmacotherapy. D. Raeburn & Mark A. Giembycz. 1997. LC 96-37785. (Respiratory Pharmacology & Pharmacotherapy Ser.). 165.00 (*3-7643-5301-5*) Birkhauser.

Rhino-Otological Microsurgery of the Skull Base. Michael Portmann et al. 1995. LC 93-33094. (Practice of Surgery Ser.). (Illus.). 320p. text (*0-443-04539-9*) Church.

Rhinologic Diagnosis & Treatment. Thomas V. McCaffrey. 1996. (Illus.). 432p. text 79.00 (*0-86577-619-9*) Thieme Med Pubs.

Rhinology: A State of the Art: Proceedings of the XVth Congress of the European Phinologic Society & the XIIIth International Symposium on Infection & Allergy of the Nose, Copenhagen, Denmark, June 19-23, 1994. Ed. by Mirkos Tos et al. 1995. LC 95-35522. (*90-6299-119-X*) Kugler NLD. *Dist:* Lib Res.

Rhinology & Nasal Allergy Year Book, 1998, No. 2. Ed. by David W. Kennedy et al. 1998. 404p. 67.00 (*0-936587-12-1*) OceanSide Pubns.

Rhinology & Nasal Allergy Yearbook, 1996. David W. Kennedy & Paul A. Greenberger. 1996. (Illus.). 325p. 30.00 (*0-936587-08-3*) OceanSide Pubns.

Rhinology & Sinus Disease: A Problem-Oriented A . . . Steven D. Schaeffer. 1998. LC 97-50427. (Illus.). 320p. (C). (gr. 13). text 75.00 (*0-8016-7800-5*, 07800) Mosby Inc.

Rhinoplasty. Cook. 2000. 452p. 185.00 (*0-86577-763-2*, C3687) Thieme Med Pubs.

Rhinoplasty. Fernando Ortiz-Monasterio. 1994. LC 93-33891. (Illus.). 304p. text 152.00 (*0-7216-6786-4*) Saunders.

Rhinoplasty: A Practical Guide to Functional & Aesthetic Surgery of the Nose. Ed. by G. J. Nolst-Trenite. 1998. (Illus.). xi, 298p. (*90-6299-164-5*) Kugler NLD. *Dist:* Lib Res.

Rhinoplasty: An Atlas of Surgical Techniques. Rollin K. Daniel. 1999. LC 98-27807. 556p. 395.00 (*0-387-94458-3*) Spr-Verlag.

Rhinoplasty: The Art & the Science, Set. Eugene Tardy, Jr. Ed. by Larry McGrew. 1996. LC 95-41653. (Illus.). 912p. text 405.00 (*0-7216-8755-5*) Saunders.

Rhinoplasty Dissection Manual. Contrib. by Dean M. Toriumi & Daniel G. Becker. 1999. LC 99-26058. 208p. text 125.00 (*0-7817-1783-3*) Lppncott W & W.

Rhinoplasty Tetrology: Corrective, Secondary, Congenital, Reconstructive. D. Ralph Millard, Jr. 1996. LC 96-1014. 552p. text 425.00 (*0-316-57156-3*, Little Brwn Med Div) Lppncott W & W.

Rhizoctonia Species: Taxonomy, Molecular Biology, Ecology, Pathology & Disease Control. Buruch Sneh. 1996. LC 96-30327. lib. bdg. 224.00 (*0-7923-3644-5*) Kluwer Academic.

Rhode Island Health Care in Perspective 2000. Ed. by Kathleen O'Leary Morgan & Scott E. Morgan. 2000. 21p. spiral bd. 19.00 (*0-7401-0238-9*) Morgan Quitno Corp.

Rhythm Factor in Human Behavior. Salvatore J. Garzino. 1982. LC 81-81611. 15.00 (*0-87212-151-8*) Libra.

Rhythm Quizlets: Self Assessment. Henry J. Marriott. LC 87-2802. (Illus.). 1987. 189p. pap. text 29.00 (*0-8121-1110-9*); 2nd ed. 1996. 288p. pap. 39.95 (*0-683-05582-8*) Lppncott W & W.

Rhythmic Breathing Plus Olfactory Nerve Influence on Respiration (1908) Richard B. Noble. 1996. 165p. reprint ed. pap. 11.95 (*1-56459-835-7*) Kessinger Pub.

Rhythmic Breathings & Olfactory Nerve Influence on Respiration. Richard B. Noble. 1991. lib. bdg. 79.95 (*0-8490-4958-X*) Gordon Pr.

Rhythmic Integration: Finding Wholeness in the Cycle of Change. Ronald Robbins. 1990. pap. 13.95 (*0-88268-099-4*) Station Hill Pr.

Rhythmic Medicine - Music with a Purpose. Janalea Hoffman. 1995. 208p. (Orig.). pap. 14.95 (*1-886051-18-6*) Rhythmic Med.

Ribonucleic Acids. Ed. by P. R. Stewart & D. S. Letham. 2nd ed. 1977. LC 77-4899. (Illus.). 374p. 105.00 (*0-387-90281-3*) Spr-Verlag.

Ribozymes in Gene Therapy of Cancer. Kevin J. Scanlon. 1998. LC 98-28767. (Biotechnology Intelligence Unit Ser.). 231p. 99.00 (*1-57059-552-6*) Landes Bioscience.

Richard Selzer & the Rhetoric of Surgery. Charles M. Anderson. 1989. LC 88-26454. 160p. (C). 21.95 (*0-8093-1502-5*) S Ill U Pr.

Richtlinien Zur Infusiontherapie Mit Aminosaeuren. Ed. by P. Schoelmerich & H. Schoenborn. 1979. (Beitraege zur Infusionstherapie und Klinische Ernaehrung Ser.: Band 4). (Illus.). pap. 15.00 (*3-8055-3058-7*) S Karger.

Rickettsial & Chlamydial Diseases of Domestic Animals. Ed. by Zerai Woldehiwet & Miodrag Ristic. 1993. LC 92-34988. 170.00 (*0-08-040831-1*, Pergamon Pr) Elsevier.

Rickettsial Infection & Immunity. Ed. by Burt Anderson et al. 1997. LC 97-22825. (Infectious Agents & Pathogenesis Ser.). (Illus.). 264p. (C). text 79.50 (*0-306-45528-5*, Kluwer Plenum) Kluwer Academic.

Riddle of AIDS: Was AIDS Made in a Lab. 1992. lib. bdg. 75.00 (*0-8490-8708-2*) Gordon Pr.

Riddle of Freud: Jewish Influences on His Theory of Female Sexuality. Estelle Roith. 1987. 250p. (C). pap. text (*0-422-61760-1*); lib. bdg. (*0-422-61380-0*) Tavistock GBR. *Dist:* Routldge.

Riddles of Eros: Exploring, Sex, Psyche & Culture. William Manson. 1994. LC 93-38164. 128p. (C). pap. text 25.00 (*0-8191-9370-4*) U Pr of Amer.

Rift Valley Fever. Ed. by N. Goldblum et al. 1981. (Contributions to Epidemiology & Biostatistics Ser.: Vol. 3). (Illus.). xii, 196p. pap. 72.25 (*3-8055-1770-X*) S Karger.

Rift Valley Fever: An Emerging Human & Animal Problem. WHO Staff. 1982. (WHO Offset Publications: No. 63). 69p. 6.00 (*92-4-170063-7*) World Health.

Right & Left Hemispheres of the Animal Brain: Cerebral Lateralization of Function. V. L. Bianki. 1987. (Monographs in Neuroscience: Vol. 3). xvi, 423p. text 189.00 (*2-88124-197-2*) Gordon & Breach.

Right Brain - Left Brain Reflexology: A Self-Help Approach to Balancing Life Energies with Color, Sound, & Pressure-Point Techniques. Madeleine Turgeon. 1993. LC 93-6778. (Illus.). 224p. pap. text 14.95 (*0-89281-432-2*, Heal Arts VT) Inner Tradit.

Right Brain & Religion: A Discussion of Religion in the Context of the Right-&-Left-Brain Theory. C. W. Dalton. Ed. by L. D. Garland. 1990. LC 90-81587. (Illus.). pap. 11.95 (*0-916969-02-9*) Big Blue Bks.

Right Choice Vol. 1: A Guide to Missouri & Illinois Nursing Homes & Supportive Living Settings, 1989. Health Care Creative Services Staff. Ed. by Catherine L. Collins. 1988. 88p. (Orig.). pap. text 6.95 (*0-923109-00-5*) Hlth Care Creat.

Right Choices: An Insider's Guide to Selecting a Nursing Home. Lynn Smith. 1992. 100p. pap. 9.95 (*0-9633706-0-X*) L Smith Ent.

Right Fruteful Treatise for the Artificial Cure of Struma. William Clowes. 1970. LC 72-25835. (English Experience Ser.: No. 238). 68p. reprint ed. 15.00 (*90-221-0238-6*) Walter J Johnson.

Right Hand: Left-Handedness. Daniel Wilson. LC 78-72830. (Brainedness, Handedness, & Mental Abilities Ser.). reprint ed. 41.50 (*0-404-60898-1*) AMS Pr.

Right Hemisphere: Neurology & Neuropsychology. Alfredo Ardila & Peggy Ostosky-Solis. 1984. (Monographs in Neuroscience). xvi, 278p. text 235.00 (*2-88124-103-4*) Gordon & Breach.

Right Hemisphere & Verbal Communication. Yves Joanette et al. 1989. 228p. 148.00 (*0-387-97101-7*) Spr-Verlag.

Right Hemisphere Communication Disorders: Theory & Management. Connie Tompkins. 1994. (Illus.). 386p. (C). text 45.00 (*1-56593-381-8*, 0770) Singular Publishing.

Right Hemisphere Communication Disorders: Theory & Management. Connie Tompkins. 1994. (Clinical Competence Ser.). (Illus.). 386p. (C). spiral bd. 67.95 (*1-56593-176-9*, 0483) Thomson Learn.

Right Hemisphere Damage: Disorders of Communication & Cognition. Penelope S. Myers. 1998. LC 98-22184. (Illus.). 360p. text 65.95 (*1-56593-224-2*, 0584) Thomson Learn.

Right Hemisphere Stroke: A Victim Reflects on Rehabilitative Medicine. Fred K. Johnson. 1990. LC 89-70612. (William Beaumont Hospital Speech & Language Pathology Ser.). 136p. (C). text 19.95 (*0-8143-2172-0*) Wayne St U Pr.

Right in the Middle: Selective Trunk Activity in the Treatment of Adult Hemiplegia. P. M. Davies. 1996. (Illus.). 288p. 49.00 (*0-387-51242-X*) Spr-Verlag.

Right Medicine: How to Make Health Care Reform Work Today. David Cundiff & Mary Ellen McCarthy. 1994. LC 94-27992. 220p. 29.50 (*0-89603-284-1*) Humana.

Right Mind. Robert Ornstein. 1997. LC 97-21659. 200p. 22.00 (*0-15-100324-6*) Harcourt.

Right Start: Guidelines for Your Baby's Nutrition & Lifelong Health. Marcia E. Young. 1987. 224p. 17.95 (*0-8027-0968-0*); pap. 10.95 (*0-8027-7305-2*) Walker & Co.

Right Test: A Physician's Guide to Laboratory Medicine. Carl E. Speicher. Ed. by Ray Kersey. 3rd ed. 1998. LC 97-43314. (Illus.). 288p. (C). pap. text 29.95 (*0-7216-5123-2*) Saunders.

Right Test: International Edition. Speicher. 3rd ed. 1998. (C). pap. text 20.00 (*0-8089-2065-0*, Grune & Strat) Harcrt Hlth Sci Grp.

Right Thing: Ten Years of Ethics Columns from the Healthcare Forum Journal. Emily Friedman. 1996. LC 96-3295. (Health Ser.). 394p. pap. 38.00 (*0-7879-0225-X*) Jossey-Bass.

Right to Die: Decision & Decision Makers. Group for the Advancement of Psychiatry Staff. 1983. LC 84-45126. 96p. 20.00 (*0-87668-721-4*) Aronson.

Right to Health As a Human Right: Colloquim 1978 of the Hague Academy of International Law. Ed. by Rene-Jean Dupuy. 1979. 513p. lib. bdg. 129.00 (*90-286-1028-6*) Kluwer Academic.

Right to Health Care: An Advocate's Guide to the Hill-Burton Uncompensated Care & Community Services Requirements. Armin Freifeld. 1986. 326p. (Orig.). pap. 15.00 (*0-941077-16-0*, 41,900) NCLS Inc.

Right to Health Care in Several European Countries: Expert Meeting, Held in Rotterdam, The Netherlands, April 27-28, 1998. Andre den Exter & Herbert E. Hermans. 1999. LC 98-39191. (Studies in Social Policy). 208p. text 66.00 (*90-411-1087-9*) Kluwer Law Intl.

Right to Health in the Americas: A Comparative Constitutional Study. Ed. by H. L. Fuenzalida-Puelma & S. S. Connor. 1989. (PAHO Scientific Publications: No. 509). (ENG & SPA.). xvii, 716p. pap. text 60.00 (*92-75-11509-5*, 1610509) World Health.

Right to Innocence: Healing the Trauma of Childhood Sexual Abuse. Beverly Engel. 1990. 272p. mass mkt. 6.99 (*0-8041-0585-5*) Ivy Books.

Right to Live: The Right to Die. C. Everett Koop. 1981. 160p. reprint ed. pap. 4.95 (*0-919225-02-0*) Life Cycle Bks.

Right to Refuse Mental Health Treatment. Bruce J. Winick. 1996. LC 96-42913. (Law & Public Policy Ser.). 427p. text 49.95 (*1-55798-369-0*, 431-6770) Am Psychol.

Right to Treatment for Mental Patients. Ed. by Stuart Golann & William J. Fremouw. 1976. (Illus.). 320p. (C). 32.95 (*0-8290-0863-2*) Irvington.

Right Ventricle. Ed. by Marvin A. Konstam & Jeffrey M. Isner. 1988. (C). text 249.50 (*0-89838-987-9*) Kluwer Academic.

Right Ventricular Hypertrophy & Function in Chronic Lung Disease. Ed. by V. Jezek et al. 1992. LC 92-2330. (Current Topics in Rehabilitation Ser.). (Illus.). 200p. 69.95 (*0-387-19774-5*) Spr-Verlag.

Righthandedness & Lefthandedness: With Chapters Treating of the Writing Posture, the Rule of the Road, Etc. George M. Gould. LC 78-72794. reprint ed. 26.50 (*0-404-60859-0*) AMS Pr.

Rights & Responsibilities of Doctors. 1992. 226p. pap. text (*0-7279-0753-0*) BMJ Pub GBR. *Dist:* AIDC.

Rights of Patients: The Basic ACLU Guide to Patient Rights. George J. Annas. 2nd rev. ed. 1992. LC 88-29893. 328p. 39.50 (*0-89603-182-9*) Humana.

Rights of Patients: The Basic ACLU Guide to Patient Rights. George J. Annas. 2nd rev. ed. 1989. LC 88-29893. (American Civil Liberties Union Handbook Ser.). 312p. (C). pap. 10.95 (*0-8093-1527-0*) S Ill U Pr.

Rights of People Who Are HIV Positive: The Basic ACLU Guide to the Rights of People Living with HIV Disease & AIDS. William B. Rubenstein et al. 1996. LC 95-52122. 488p. (C). pap. 13.95 (*0-8093-1992-6*) S Ill U Pr.

Rights of People with Mental Disabilities: The Basic ACLU Guide to the Rights of People with Mental Illness & Mental Retardation. Robert M. Levy & Leonard S. Rubenstein. 1996. LC 95-36408. (American Civil Liberties Union Handbook Ser.). 424p. (C). pap. 13.95 (*0-8093-1990-X*) S Ill U Pr.

Rights to Health Care. Thomas J. Bole, III & William B. Bondeson. 1991. 318p. (C). lib. bdg. (*0-7923-1137-X*) Kluwer Academic NLD. *Dist:* Kluwer Academic.

Rigid Fixation of the Craniomaxillofacial Skeleton. Michael J. Yaremchuk et al. Ed. by Joseph S. Gruss. 1992. 712p. text (*0-7506-9197-2*) E A GBR. *Dist:* OUP.

Ring of the Dove: A Treatise on the Art & Practice of Arab Love. Ali ibn Ahmad Ibn-Hazm. Tr. by Arthur John Arberry. LC 78-63500. 288p. reprint ed. 34.50 (*0-404-17148-6*) AMS Pr.

Ringing Ears Vol. 1: A Tinnitus Victim's Guide. John D. Griggs. Ed. by Cynthia M. Buddy et al. 1982. (Illus.). 60p. (Orig.). pap. 10.00 (*0-9612648-1-0*) Natl Tinn Fund.

Rings of Fire: Primitive Affects & Object Relations in Group Psychotherapy. Ed. by Victor L. Schermer & Malcolm Pines. 1994. LC 93-34089. (International Library of Group Psychotherapy & Group Process). 336p. (C). 89.95 (*0-415-06681-6*); pap. 31.95 (*0-415-06682-4*) Routledge.

***Rise & Fall of American Post-Acute Health Care.** Gerbew De Young. 2001. (Illus.). 320p. 39.95 (*1-886236-31-3*) ABI Prof Pubns.

Rise & Fall of Managed Care. Linda L. Miles. Ed. by Virginia McCullough. 1997. 96p. pap. 12.95 (*0-9658409-0-5*) Link Pub VA.

Rise of a University Teaching Hospital: A Leadership Perspective: The University of Iowa Hospitals & Clinics. Samuel Levey. 1996. LC 96-36389. 618p. 24.00 (*1-56793-048-4*) Health Admin Pr.

Rise of Surgery: From Empiric Craft to Scientific Discipline. Owen H. Wangensteen & Sarah D. Wangensteen. 1978. LC 77-87933. (Illus.). xv, 785p. 50.00 (*0-8166-0829-6*) Midewiwin.

Rising Curve: Long-Term Gains in IQ & Related Measures. Ed. by Ulric Neisser. 1998. LC 97-52183. (APA Science Volumes Ser.). 415p. 39.95 (*1-55798-503-0*) Am Psychol.

Rising Tide of Suicide: A Guide to Prevention, Intervention & Postvention. L. Richard Batzler. 1988. LC 85-82029. 200p. (Orig.). pap. 10.00 (*0-935710-08-6*) Hid Valley MD.

Rising Trends in Asthma - Symposium, No. 206. CIBA Foundation Staff & Stephen T. Holgate. 1997. LC 96-40339. (CIBA Foundation Symposia Ser.: Vol. 206). 290p. 128.00 (*0-471-97012-3*) Wiley.

Risk. Ed. by Edward J. Burger. 1993. 288p. pap. text 22.95 (*0-472-08222-1*, 08222) U of Mich Pr.

Risk Adjustment for Measuring Healthcare Outcomes. Lisa I. Iezzoni. 2nd ed. 1997. LC 97-21. 70.00 (*1-56793-054-9*) Health Admin Pr.

***Risk Analysis: Foundations, Models, & Methods.** Louis A. Cox. 2001. LC 2001-54399. (International Series in Operations Research & Management Science: Vol. 45). 568p. (*0-7923-7615-3*) Kluwer Academic.

Risk Analysis: Prospects & Opportunities. C. Zervos et al. 1992. (Advances in Risk Analysis Ser.: Vol. 8). (Illus.). 780p. (C). text 185.00 (*0-306-44113-6*, Kluwer Plenum) Kluwer Academic.

Risk & Economic Consequences of Contagious Animal Disease Introduction. H. S. Horst. 1997. 145p. pap. (*90-6754-516-3*) Backhuys Pubs NLD. *Dist:* Balogh.

Risk & Prevention of Arterial Lipidoses. P. Schwandt. 1990. 194p. pap. 22.50 (*0-87527-232-0*) Green.

Risk & Progression Factors in Carcinogenesis. Ed. by H. K. Muller-Hermelink et al. 1996. LC 96-12853. (Recent Results in Cancer Research Ser.: Vol. 143). (Illus.). 392p. 157.00 (*3-540-60953-9*) Spr-Verlag.

Risk & Protective Factors in the Development of Psychopathology. Ed. by Jon Rolf et al. (Illus.). 570p. (C). 1993. pap. text 37.95 (*0-521-43972-8*); 1990. text 100.00 (*0-521-35099-9*) Cambridge U Pr.

Risk & Recovery: AIDS, HIV, & Alcohol: A Handbook for Providers. Marcia Quackenbush et al. 1995. LC 92-26635. 256p. text 16.95 (*0-89087-690-8*) Celestial Arts.

Risk & Reward: A "How-To" Guide to Choosing an MSO. David W. Hilgers et al. 1997. (Illus.). 130p. pap. 49.00 (*0-9640262-6-0*) TX Med Assn.

Risk Approach in Health Care with Special Reference to Maternal & Child Health, including Family Planning. E. M. Backett et al. 1984. (Public Health Papers: No. 76). 121p. pap. text 11.00 (*92-4-130076-0*, 1110076) World Health.

Risk Assessment & Decision Making Using Test Results: The Carcinogenicity Prediction & Battery Selection Approach. J. Pet-Edwards et al. 1989. (Illus.). 220p. (C). 85.00 (*0-306-43067-3*, Plenum Trade) Perseus Pubng.

Risk Assessment & Management Handbook: For Environmental, Health, & Safety Professionals. Robin Pitblado et al. 1995. LC 95-21284. 688p. text 99.00 (*0-07-035987-3*) McGraw-Hill Prof.

Risk Assessment for Deliberate Releases. W. Klingmuller. 1988. (Illus.). 193p. 63.95 (*0-387-18930-0*) Spr-Verlag.

Risk Assessment for Neurobehavioral Toxicity. Ed. by Bernard Weiss & Jurg Elsner. 1997. (Illus.). 418p. (Orig.). (C). pap. text 50.00 (*0-7881-4487-1*) DIANE Pub.

Risk Assessment in Chemical Carcinogenesis. Ed. by Dietrich Schmahl et al. 1991. (Sitzungsberichte der Heidelberger Akademie der Wissenschaften Ser., Mathematisch-Naturwissenschaftliche Klasse, Jahrgang 1991: Suppl. 1). (Illus.). 180p. 39.95 (*0-387-54149-7*) Spr-Verlag.

Risk Assessment in the Federal Government: Managing the Process. National Research Council Staff. 1983. 191p. (C). pap. text 27.95 (*0-309-03349-7*) Natl Acad Pr.

Risk Assessment Methods: Approaches for Assessing Health & Environmental Risks. Vincent T. Covello & Miley W. Merkhoher. 1994. (Illus.). 334p. (C). 83.00 (*0-306-44382-1*, Plenum Trade) Perseus Pubng.

Risk Assessment of Chemicals: An Introduction. C. J. Van Leeuwen. Ed. by J. L. Hermens. 1995. 392p. (C). lib. bdg. 94.00 (*0-7923-3740-9*) Kluwer Academic.

Risk Assessment of N-Nitroso Compounds for Human Health. Dietrich Schmahl. 1980. (Journal: Vol. 37, No. 4). (Illus.). 120p. pap. 53.25 (*3-8055-1137-X*) S Karger.

Risk Assessment of Prenatally-Induced Adverse Health Effects. Diether Neubert et al. 1992. LC 92-26482. 565p. 125.00 (*0-387-55890-X*) Spr-Verlag.

Risk Assessment of Ventricular Tachyarrhythmias, No. 3. Mark H. Anderson. 1995. LC 94-23609. (Clinical Approaches to Tachyarrhythmias Ser.: Vol. 3). (Illus.). 80p. 16.00 (*0-87993-612-6*) Futura Pub.

Risk at Delivery. Ed. by G. P. Mandruzzato. 1977. (Contributions to Gynecology & Obstetrics Ser.: Vol. 3). (Illus.). 42.75 (*3-8055-2421-8*) S Karger.

Risk-Based Contributions to Private Health Insurance, Vol. 12. Ed. by Mark C. Hornbrook. 1991. (Advances in Health Economics & Health Services Research Ser.). 268p. 73.25 (*1-55938-241-4*) Jai Pr.

Risk-Based Payments under Public Programs, Vol. 10. Ed. by Richard M. Scheffler et al. 1989. (Advances in Health Economics & Health Services Research Ser.). 376p. 73.25 (*0-89232-976-9*) Jai Pr.

Risk-Benefit Analysis for the Use & Approval of Thrombolytic, Antiarrhythmic, & Hypolipidemic Agents. Ed. by Joel Morganroth & E. Neil Moore. 1989. (C). text 145.00 (*0-7923-0294-X*) Kluwer Academic.

Risk Communication: A Bibliography of Risk Communication & Environmental Health Risk Literature. Daniel T. Boatright et al. 1996. 139p. (Orig.). pap. 55.00 (*0-944111-14-9*) Natl Environ Health.

Risk Contracting & Capitation Answer Book: Strategies for Managed Care. Sheryl Tatar Dacso & Clifford C. Dacso. 1999. LC 99-11154. 432p. 99.00 (*0-8342-0988-8*, 09888) Aspen Pub.

Risk Estimates for Radiation Protection. Intro. by Charles B. Meinhold. 1993. LC 93-44242. (Report Ser.: No. 115). 148p. (Orig.). pap. text 35.00 (*0-929600-34-7*) NCRP Pubns.

***Risk Factors & Adverse Pregnancy Outcomes in Small-for-Gestational-Age Births.** Britt Clausson. 2000. (Comprehensive Summaries of Uppsala Dissertations from the Faculty of Medicine Ser.: No. 973). (Illus.). 41p. pap. (*91-554-4858-5*) Uppsala Universitet SWE. *Dist:* Coronet Bks.

Risk Factors & Implant Treatment: Clinical Assessment & Rationale. Frank Renouard & Bo Rangert. 1999. LC 99-19894. text 78.00 (*0-86715-355-5*) Quint Pub Co.

Risk Factors for Adverse Drug Reactions: Epidemiological Approaches. R. Hoigne et al. 1990. (Agents & Actions Supplements Ser.: No. 29). 150p. 47.00 (*0-8176-2372-8*) Birkhauser.

Risk Factors for Cancer in the Workplace. Jack Siemiatycki. 1991. (Illus.). 176p. lib. bdg. 139.00 (*0-8493-5018-2*, RC268) CRC Pr.

Risk Factors for Cardiovascular Disease in Non-Smokers. Ed. by D. F. Weetman & D. Wood. 1993. (Illus.). x, 150p. 128.75 (*3-8055-5682-9*) S Karger.

Risk Factors for Cataract Development. Ed. by Otto Hockwin et al. 1989. (Developments in Ophthalmology Ser.: Vol. 17). (Illus.). xi, 217p. 161.00 (*3-8055-4906-7*) S Karger.

Risk Factors for Post-Traumatic Stress Disorder. Ed. by Rachel Yehuda. 1999. LC 98-43412. (Progress in Psychiatry Ser.: Vol. 17). xxi, 250p. 44.00 (*0-88048-816-6*) Am Psychiatric.

Risk Factors for Youth Suicide. Ed. by Lucy Davidson & Markku Linnoila. 1990. (Death Education, Aging & Health Care Ser.). 275p. 57.95 (*1-56032-138-5*) Hemisp Pub.

Risk Factors in Infancy. Ed. by Alice S. Honig. 1986. (Special Aspects of Education Ser.: Vol. 7). x, 176p. text 142.00 (*0-677-21420-0*); 176, xp. pap. text 35.00 (*0-677-21430-8*) Gordon & Breach.

Risk Factors in the Development of Cardiovascular Disorders: A Review of the Literature & an Empirical Cross- Sectional Study of 120 Subjects. Ping Zhuang. 1992. LC 92-49841. (European University Studies: Ser. VI, Vol. 378). (Illus.). 262p. 53.00 (*3-631-45223-3*) P Lang Pubng.

Risk Management: Health & Safety in Primary Care. N. Higson. 1996. LC 96-13133. 128p. pap. text 42.00 (*0-7506-3064-7*) Buttrwrth-Heinemann.

***Risk Management & Litigation in Obstetrics & Gynaecology.** Roger Clements. 2001. 428p. pap. (*1-85315-480-6*) Royal Soc of Medicine Pr Ltd GBR. *Dist:* Balogh.

Risk Management Basics: Protecting Profits & Product Safety in Medical Product Industries Through Risk-Based Decision-Making in Change Control, Deviation Investigations & Corrective/Preventative Action Programs. Carol DeSain & Charmaine Vercimak Sutton. 2000. LC 00-106392. (Basics Ser.). (Illus.). viii, 147p. 124.95 (*0-929870-55-7*) Advanstar Commns.

Risk Management Handbook: Protecting You & Your Practice from Legal Action. Maryann Ricardo. 1995. 250p. reprint ed. ring bd. 49.95 (*1-57066-033-6*, ME057) Practice Mgmt Info.

Risk Management in Health Care Institutions: A Strategic Approach. Florence Kavaler & Allen D. Spiegel. 1997. LC 96-39658. (Health Science Ser.). (Illus.). 400p. (C). text 54.95 (*0-7637-0257-9*, 0257-9) Jones & Bartlett.

Risk Management Pointers: Practical Advice for Busy Physicians. RiskCare Staff. 1998. 100p. pap. text 135.00 (*1-893929-00-0*) RiskCare.

Risk Management Strategies for Physicians in Managed Care. RiskCare Staff & Fay Rozovsky. 1999. 100p. pap. 135.00 (*1-893929-11-6*) RiskCare.

Risk Management Techniques in Perinatal & Neonatal Practice. Ed. by Steven M. Donn & Charles W. Fisher. 1996. LC 96-12740. (Illus.). 720p. 115.00 (*0-87993-640-1*) Futura Pub.

Risk Management with Suicidal Patients. Ed. by Bruce Bongar et al. 197p. 1999. pap. 21.00 (*1-57230-498-7*, C0498); 1997. LC 97-48981. 35.00 (*1-57230-302-6*, C0302) Guilford Pubns.

Risk Manager's Desk Reference. Barbara J. Youngberg. 2nd ed. 1998. LC 97-45703. 544p. 105.00 (*0-8342-1016-9*, 10169) Aspen Pub.

Risk Markers for Oral Diseases Vol. 1: Dental Caries: Markers of High & Low Risk Groups & Individuals. Ed. by N. W. Johnson. 1991. 525p. (C). text 150.00 (*0-521-37563-0*) Cambridge U Pr.

Risk Markers for Oral Diseases Vol. 2: Oral Cancer: Detection of Patients & Lesions at Risk. Ed. by N. W. Johnson. 1991. (Illus.). 420p. (C). text 150.00 (*0-521-37421-9*) Cambridge U Pr.

Risk Markers for Oral Diseases Vol. 3: Periodontal Diseases: Markers of Disease Susceptibility & Activity. Ed. by N. W. Johnson. 1991. (Illus.). 480p. (C). text 150.00 (*0-521-38566-0*) Cambridge U Pr.

***Risk Matters in Healthcare: Communicating, Explaining & Managing Risk.** Kay Mohanna & Ruth Chambers. 2000. 128p. pap. (*1-85775-456-5*) Radcliffe Med Pr GBR. *Dist:* Balogh.

Risk of Malnutrition in Nursing Homes: Forum Before the Special Committee on Aging, United States Senate, One Hundred Fifth Congress, First Session, Washington, DC, October 22, 1997. U. S. Government Staff. 1997. LC 98-144086. (S. Hrg. Ser.). iii, 42 p. (*0-16-056116-7*) USGPO.

Risk Prevention Skills: Communicating for Pharmacists. David M. Angaran et al. 1995. iv, 83p. pap. 39.00 (*1-930548-26-5*) Tennenhouse Prof Pubns.

Risk Prevention Skills: Communicating in Extended & Subacute Care Facilities. Holly Bratt & Dan J. Tennenhouse. 1998. iv, 80p. pap. 21.95 (*1-930548-18-4*) Tennenhouse Prof Pubns.

Risk Prevention Skills: Record Keeping for Pharmacists. David M. Angaran et al. 1995. iv, 83p. pap. 39.00 (*1-930548-27-3*) Tennenhouse Prof Pubns.

Risk Prevention Skills: Record Keeping in Extended & Subacute Care Facilities. Holly Bratt & Dan J. Tennenhouse. 1998. iv, 76p. pap. 21.95 (*1-930548-19-2*) Tennenhouse Prof Pubns.

Risk Prevention Skills for Cardiologists: Communicating & Record Keeping in Clinical Practice. Dan J. Tennenhouse et al. 1999. (Illus.). viii, 221p. pap. 79.00 (*1-930548-23-0*) Tennenhouse Prof Pubns.

Risk Prevention Skills for Gastroenterologists: Communicating & Record Keeping in Clinical Practice. Dan J. Tennenhouse & Mary P. Kasher. 1998. (Illus.). viii, 221p. pap. 79.00 (*1-930548-24-9*) Tennenhouse Prof Pubns.

Risk Prevention Skills for Nurses: Communicating & Record Keeping in Clinical Practice. Dan J. Tennenhouse et al. 2nd ed. 1988. (Illus.). viii, 198p. pap. 39.00 (*1-930548-20-6*) Tennenhouse Prof Pubns.

Risk Prevention Skills for Office & Clinic Medical Assistants: Communicating & Record Keeping in Clinical Practice. Dan J. Tennenhouse. 1990. (Illus.). iv, 136p. pap. 35.00 (*1-930548-21-4*) Tennenhouse Prof Pubns.

Risk Prevention Skills for Pediatricians. Dan J. Tennenhouse et al. 1998. (Illus.). viii, 167p. pap. 79.00 (*1-930548-25-7*) Tennenhouse Prof Pubns.

Risk Prevention Skills for Physicians: Communicating & Record Keeping in Clinical Practice. Dan J. Tennenhouse & Mary P. Kasher. 1995. (Illus.). viii, 167p. pap. 64.00 (*1-930548-22-2*) Tennenhouse Prof Pubns.

Risk Profiles in Clinical Nephrology. Ed. by G. Buccianti. 1984. (Contributions to Nephrology Ser.: Vol. 37). (Illus.). x, 202p. pap. 29.75 (*3-8055-3739-5*) S Karger.

Risk Quantitation & Regulatory Policy. Ed. by David G. Hoel et al. 1985. (Banbury Reports: No. 19). 368p. 67.00 (*0-87969-219-7*) Cold Spring Harbor.

Risk Taking: A Study in Cognition & Personality. Nathan Kogan & Michael A. Wallach. 1983. LC 83-12584. 278p. reprint ed. lib. bdg. 59.75 (*0-313-23250-4*, KORT, Greenwood Pr) Greenwood.

Risking Connection: A Training Curriculum for Working with Survivors of Childhood Abuse. Karen W. Saakvitne. 1999. LC 99-52278. lib. bdg. (*1-886968-08-X*) Sidran Pr.

Risks & Outcomes in Developmental Psychopathology. Ed. by Hans-Christoph Steinhausen & Frank C. Verhulst. 1999. LC 98-52302. (Illus.). 344p. text 57.50 (*0-19-262799-6*) OUP.

Risks from Radium & Thorotrast. Ed. by D. M. Taylor. 1990. (BIR Reports Ser.: No. 21). (Illus.). 300p. pap. text (*0-905749-22-7*) Med Physics Pub.

Risks in Labor & Delivery & Pediatrics. Meridith B. Cox. 1997. (Risk Management Ser.). (C). pap. text, wbk. ed. 20.00 (*0-912665-25-4*) BusinessWatch.

Risks in O. R. & Post-Op Care. Meridith B. Cox. 1997. (Risk Management Ser.). (Orig.). (C). pap. text, wbk. ed. 25.00 (*0-912665-26-2*) BusinessWatch.

Risks of Carcinogenesis from Urethane Exposure. Andrew G. Salmon & Lauren Zeise. 1991. (Illus.). 240p. lib. bdg. 110.00 (*0-8493-5587-7*, R) CRC Pr.

Risks of Knowing: Developmental Impediments to School Learning. K. Zelan. 1991. LC 90-29300. (Perspectives in Developmental Psychology Ser.). (Illus.). 334p. (C). 54.50 (*0-306-43759-7*, Plenum Trade) Perseus Pubng.

***Risks to Human Reproduction: NTP-Cerhr Expert Panel Reports on DI(2-Ethylhexyl) Phthalate & Other Phthalates.** Ed. by Robert Kavlock. 2001. 300p. (C). pap. text 40.00 (*0-7567-0783-8*) DIANE Pub.

Risky Sex: Gay Men & HIV Prevention. Dwayne Turner. 1997. LC 96-40290. (Between Men-Between Women: Lesbian & Gay Studies). 208p. 47.50 (*0-231-10574-6*); pap. 17.50 (*0-231-10575-4*) Col U Pr.

Risky Sexual Behaviors among African-Americans. Ernest H. Johnson. 1993. LC 92-28483. 192p. 67.00 (*0-275-94162-0*, C4162, Praeger Pubs) Greenwood.

Risky Times: How to Be AIDS-Smart & Stay Healthy. Jeanne Blake. 1999. LC 89-40728. (Illus.). 196p. (YA). (gr. 8 up). pap. 5.95 (*0-89480-656-4*, 1656) Workman Pub.

Ritalin: Theory & Patient Management. Laurence L. Greenhill & Betty B. Osman. 1991. 338p. 158.00 (*0-913113-53-0*) M Liebert.

***Ritalin Fact Book.** Breggin. 2002. 208p. pap. 12.00 (*0-7382-0450-1*) Perseus Bks Grp.

Ritalin-Free Child: Managing Hyperactivity & Attention Deficits Without Drugs. Diana Hunter. Ed. by Joseph Pappas. 1995. LC 95-47004. 160p. pap. 12.95 (*0-9628336-8-1*, Womens Pubns) Consumer Press.

Ritalin-Free Kids: Safe & Effective Homeopathic Medicine for ADHD & Other Behavioral & Learning Problems. Judyth Reichenberg-Ullman & Robert Ullman. 2nd rev. ed. 2000. LC 00-62356. (Illus.). 320p. pap. 16.95 (*0-7615-2769-9*, Prima Health) Prima Pub.

Ritalin Nation: Rapid-Fire Culture & the Transformation of Human Consciousness. Richard J. DeGrandpre. 2000. LC 2001-278262. 288p. pap. 13.95 (*0-393-32025-1*) Norton.

Rittenhouse Cookbook: A Year of Heart-Healthy Recipes. Jim Coleman et al. 1997. LC 97-15249. (Illus.). 234p. 29.95 (*0-89815-864-8*) Ten Speed Pr.

Ritual. Theodor Reik. 1976. pap. 24.95 (*0-8236-8269-2*, 025840) Intl Univs Pr.

Ritual & Pastoral Care. Elaine Ramshaw. 1987. LC 85-45487. (Theology & Pastoral Care Ser.). 128p. pap. 14.00 (*0-8006-1738-X*, 1-1738, Fortress Pr) Augsburg Fortress.

Ritual & Religion in the Making of Humanity. Roy A. Rappaport. 1999. LC 98-24494. (Studies in Social & Cultural Anthropology: No. 110). 562p. (C). pap. text 19.95 (*0-521-29690-0*) Cambridge U Pr.

Rituals for Women Coping with Breast Cancer. Rosalie Muschal-Reinhardt et al. 2000. (Illus.). 60p. pap. 12.00 (*1-890662-10-0*) Prism Coll.

Rituals in Families & Family Therapy. Ed. by Evan Imber-Black et al. 1988. 414p. 34.95 (*0-393-70064-X*) Norton.

Rituals in Psychotherapy: Transition & Continuity. Onno Van der Hart. Tr. by Angie Pleit-Kuiper from DUT. 220p. 1982. text 27.50 (*0-8290-0537-4*); 1986. (C). reprint ed. pap. text 14.95 (*0-8290-1925-1*) Irvington.

Rituals of Healing. Dossey Achterberg et al. 1994. LC 93-37375. 384p. pap. 15.95 (*0-553-37347-1*) Bantam.

River: A Journey to the Source of HIV & AIDS. Edward Hooper. 2000. LC 2001-265779. (Illus.). 1168p. pap. 24.95 (*0-316-37137-8*, Back Bay) Little.

River of Tears: The Politics of Black Women's Health. Ed. by Delores P. Aldridge & LaFrancis Rodgers-Rose. 1993. 174p. (Orig.). (C). pap. text 13.95 (*0-934185-01-8*) Traces Inst.

RN Boards Review for NCLEX, 1987. Ed. by Alice Stein & Nancy Jacobson. 1986. 650p. (Orig.). pap. 17.95 (*0-935236-49-X*) Genl Med Pub.

RN Core Competencies. Julia Fulton. 1998. 174p. spiral bd. 130.00 (*1-879575-76-0*) Acad Med Sys.

RN First Assistant. Jane C. Rothrock. 3rd ed. 1998. LC 98-20816. 496p. pap. text 45.95 (*0-7817-1501-6*) Lppncott W & W.

RN Magazine's NDR - 95. George R. Spratto & Adrienne L. Woods. 1995. 1395p. pap. 26.95 (*0-8273-6548-9*) Delmar.

RN Magazine's NDR - 94 Nurse's Drug Reference. George R. Spratto & Adrienne L. Woods. 1994. 1290p. pap. 25.95 (*0-8273-5711-7*) Delmar.

RN Magazine's NDR - 91. Adrienne L. Woods et al. 2nd ed. 1991. pap. 25.95 (*0-8273-4737-5*) Delmar.

RN Magazines NDR 1994 - Display Dump. George R. Spratto. 1994. (Professional Reference - Nursing Ser.). 259.50 (*0-8273-6202-1*) Delmar.

RN Magazine's Nurses' Drug Reference, '92. George R. Spratto & Adrienne L. Woods. 1992. pap. 25.95 (*0-8273-4844-4*) Delmar.

RNA Isolation & Characterization Protocols. Ed. by Ralph Rapley & David L. Manning. 1998. LC 98-12453. (Methods in Molecular Biology Ser.: Vol. 86). (Illus.). 280p. 109.50 (*0-89603-494-1*) Humana.

RNA Methodologies: A Laboratory Guide for Isolation & Characterization. Ed. by Robert E. Farrell, Jr. 1993. (Illus.). 319p. pap. 53.00 (*0-12-249700-7*) Acad Pr.

RNA Methodologies: A Laboratory Guide for Isolation & Characterization. Robert E. Farrell, Jr. 2nd ed. 1998. LC 98-84574. (Illus.). xx, 533 p. (C). 59.95 (*0-12-249695-7*) Acad Pr.

RNA Polymerase & Associated Factors, Pt. B. Ed. by Sankar Adhya et al. 1996. (Methods in Enzymology Ser.: Vol. 274). (Illus.). 566p. text 89.00 (*0-12-182175-7*) Acad Pr.

RNA Processing: A Practical Approach, Vol. II. Ed. by Stephen J. Higgins & B. David Hames. 1994. (Practical Approach Ser.: Vol. 136). (Illus.). 278p. pap. text 45.00 (*0-19-963470-X*) OUP.

RNA Processing Pt. B: Specific Methods. Ed. by John N. Abelson et al. 1990. (Methods in Enzymology Ser.: Vol. 181). 650p. text 136.00 (*0-12-182082-3*) Acad Pr.

***RNA-Protein Interactions in the Bacteriophage MS2.** Elin Grahn. 2001. (Comprehensive Summaries of Uppsala Dissertations from the Faculty of Science & Technology Ser.: No. 642). (Illus.). 62p. pap. (*91-554-5066-0*) Uppsala Universitet SWE. *Dist:* Coronet Bks.

RNA Tumor Viruses, Oncogenes, Human Cancer & AIDS: On Frontiers of Understanding. Ed. by Philip Furmanski et al. 1985. (Developments in Oncology Ser.). text 132.50 (*0-89838-703-5*) Kluwer Academic.

RNP Particles, Splicing & Autoimmune Diseases. Ed. by Johannes Schenkel. 1998. LC 97-34400. (Springer Lab Manuals Ser.). (Illus.). 230p. ring bd. 79.95 (*3-540-62448-1*) Spr-Verlag.

RN's Legally Speaking: How to Protect Your Patients & Your License. Sullivan. 1997. (Illus.). xiv, 331p. pap. text 25.00 (*1-56363-274-8*, PDR) Med Econ.

RN's Pocket Assessment Guide: Quick, Accurate Evaluation of Adult Acute Care Patients. 1997. (Illus.). 204p. spiral bd. 30.00 (*1-56363-273-X*, PDR) Med Econ.

Road Ahead: A Stroke Recovery Guide. Ed. by Thelma Edwards. 4th ed. 1998. 196p. reprint ed. pap. text (*0-9624876-1-9*) Natl Stroke Assn.

Road Back to Health: Coping with the Emotional Aspects of Cancer. Neil A. Fiore. rev. ed. 1995. LC 90-2160. 238p. reprint ed. pap. 14.95 (*0-89087-617-7*) Celestial Arts.

Road Blocks to Rehabilitation: Recovery from a Work-Related Injury. Barbara J. Headley. Ed. by Francis E. LaFave & Edward J. Hughes. 1988. (Illus.). 24p. pap. text 2.00 (*0-929538-03-X*) Innovat Systems.

Road Map of Head & Neck Anatomy. Rumy Hilloowala. 1996. (Illus.). 115p. (Orig.). (C). pap. text 21.95 (*0-943025-85-0*) Cummngs & Hath.

Road to Birth Game. Julie Burns & Frank Bialosiewicz. 1983. (Technical Notes Ser.: No. 24). (Illus.). 33p. (Orig.). pap. text 2.00 (*0-932288-71-5*) Ctr Intl Ed U of MA.

Road to Daulis: Psychoanalysis, Psychology & Classical Mythology. Robert Eisner. 1987. 284p. 42.50 (*0-8156-0210-3*) Syracuse U Pr.

Road to Immunity: How to Survive & Thrive in a Toxic World. Kenneth Bock & Nellie Sabin. 1997. LC 97-18169. 464p. per. 14.00 (*0-671-54507-8*, PB Trade Paper) PB.

Road to Nowhere: The Genesis of President Clinton's Plan for Health Security. Jacob S. Hacker. 1996. LC 96-8083. (Princeton Studies in American Politics). (Illus.). 239p. 49.50 (*0-691-04423-6*) Princeton U Pr.

Road to Reform: The Future of Health Care in America. Eli Ginzberg. 1994. 180p. 24.95 (*0-02-911715-1*) Free Pr.

***Road Traffic Law: Medicolegal Essentials.** Payne-James & Wall. 2003. 180p. pap. (*1-900151-94-4*) Greenwich Med GBR. *Dist:* JAMCO Dist.

Rob & Smith's Operative Surgery: Genitourinary Tract Hugh N. Whitfield et al. Ed. by David C. Carter et al. 5th ed. LC 92-22884. (Illus.). 700p. (C). (gr. 13). 1995. pap. 754.95 (*0-7506-1242-8*); Vols. 1 & 2. 1993. pap. 215.95 (*0-7506-0903-6*) Chapman & Hall.

Rob & Smith's Operative Surgery: Head & Neck, 1. Ian A. McGregor & David J. Howard. 4th ed. 1993. (Illus.). 350p. (C). (gr. 13). text 410.95 (*0-7506-0296-1*) Chapman & Hall.

Rob & Smith's Operative Surgery: Head & Neck, Set. Ian A. McGregor & David J. Howard. 4th ed. 1992. (Illus.). 700p. text 595.00 (*0-7506-0298-8*) Oxford Pr Inc.

Rob & Smith's Operative Surgery: Neurosurgery. Lindsay Symon. 4th ed. 1993. 516p. pap. 220.50 (*0-407-00668-0*) Chapman & Hall.

Rob & Smith's Operative Surgery: Neurosurgery. Symon et al. 4th ed. 1991. (C). text 99.95 (*0-8016-4418-6*) Mosby Inc.

Rob & Smith's Operative Surgery: Ophthalmic Surgery. J. C. Gottsched. 5th ed. 1999. (Illus.). 528p. text (*0-340-74091-4*) E A GBR. *Dist:* OUP.

Robbins Clinical Pathology. Laposata. 1999. text 30.00 (*0-7216-7027-X*) Harcourt.

Robbins Pathologic Basis of Disease. Ramzi S. Cotran et al. 5th ed. 1994. LC 94-2629. (Illus.). 1414p. (C). text 75.00 (*0-7216-5032-5*) Saunders.

Robbin's Pathologic Basis of Disease. Ramzi S. Cotran et al. Ed. by Bill Schmitt. 6th ed. 1998. LC 98-36022. (Illus.). xv, 1424p. (C). text 75.00 (*0-7216-7335-X*) Saunders.

Robbins Review of Pathology. Edward Klatt & Vinay Kumar. 2000. (Illus.). 285p. (C). pap. text (*0-7216-8259-6*) Saunders.

Robert Crayhon's Nutrition Made Simple: A Comprehensive Guide to the Latest Findings in Optimal Nutrition. Robert Crayhon. 1996. LC 95-43216. 320p. pap. 14.95 (*0-87131-796-6*) M Evans.

Roberts' Nutrition Work with Children. Ethel A. Martin & Virginia A. Beal. 4th ed. 1994. LC 77-13972. (Illus.). reprint ed. lib. bdg. 19.00 (*0-226-50738-6*) U Ch Pr.

Roberts' Practical Guide to Common Medical Emergencies. 1997. LC 96-40889. 302p. pap. text 59.95 (*0-397-51838-2*) Lppncott W & W.

Robots & Biological Systems: Towards a New Bionics? Ed. by P. Dario et al. 1993. (NATO ASI Ser.: Vol. 102). (Illus.). 786p. 231.00 (*0-387-56158-7*) Spr-Verlag.

Roche Lexikon Medizin. 1993. (GER.). 1,849p. (*3-541-11213-1*) Urban & S DEU. *Dist:* IBD Ltd.

Roche Lexikon Medizin. Hoffmann-La Roche. 3rd ed. 1993. (GER.). 1849p. 85.00 (*0-7859-8421-6*, 3541112131) Fr & Eur.

Roche Lexikon Medizin. 4th ed. (GER.). cd-rom (*3-541-17124-3*) Urban & Schwarz AUT. *Dist:* IBD Ltd.

Rochester Manual - Practical Patient Care: Medicine, Surgery, Pediatrics, OB-Gyn & Psychiatry. Karl A. Illig & Wendy C. Husser. Date not set. (Illus.). 690p. text (*1-886128-07-3*) Laennec Pub.

Rock-a-By Baby. Verta Taylor. 1996. LC 96-19519. 240p. (C). pap. 24.95 (*0-415-91292-X*) Routledge.

Rock-a-By Baby. Verta A. Taylor. 1996. LC 96-19519. 240p. (C). 70.00 (*0-415-91291-1*) Routledge.

Rockefeller Foundation Archives Series 1.1 (Projects) Series 600 (Asia) & Series 601 (China): Guide to the Scholarly Resources Microfilm Edition. 1994. LC 94-16888. 10.00 (*0-8420-4141-9*) Scholarly Res Inc.

Rockwood & Green's Fractures in Adults. Ed. by Charles A. Rockwood, Jr. 4th ed. 1996. Vol. 1. (*0-397-51510-3*); Vol. 2. (*0-397-51511-1*) Lppncott W & W.

Rockwood & Green's Fractures in Adults, Volumes 1 and 2. James D. Heckman & Robert W. Bucholz. 5th ed. 2001. LC 00-65515. text 375.00 (*0-7817-2508-9*) Lppncott W & W.

***Rockwood & Wilkins' Fractures in Children,** Volume 3. Charles A. Rockwood et al. 5th ed. 2001. LC 2001-29220. (Illus.). 1,264p. text 225.00 (*0-7817-2509-7*) Lppncott W & W.

***Rockwood, Green & Wilkins' Fractures,** Set. James D. Heckman et al. 5th ed. 2001. 4168p. text 550.00 incl. cd-rom (*0-7817-1935-6*) Lppncott W & W.

Rodd's Chemistry of Carbon Compounds Ed. by M. F. Ansell. Suppl. Vol. 1 C & D. 1973. 464p. 286.00 (*0-444-41072-4*); Suppl. Vol. 1 A & B. 1975. xvi,268p. 204.00 (*0-444-40972-6*); Suppl. Vol. 2, Pts. C-E. 1974. 318p. 226.00 (*0-444-41135-6*) Elsevier.

Rodd's Chemistry of Carbon Compounds Pt. K: Six Membered Heterocyclic Compounds with Two or More Hetero-Atoms, Vol. 4. S. Coffey. 1979. 552p. 357.50 (*0-444-41647-1*) Elsevier.

Rodent Tumor Models in Experimental Cancer Therapy. Ed. by Robert F. Kallman. 1987. 432p. 88.00 (*0-08-033145-9*, H220, H230, Pergamon Pr) Elsevier.

Roenigk & Roenigk's Dermatologic Surgery: Principles & Practice. Ed. by Randall K. Roenigk & Henry H. Roenigk, Jr. 2nd ed. 1996. LC 95-46848. (Illus.). 1408p. text 225.00 (*0-8247-9503-2*) Dekker.

Roentgen Diagnosis of the Urogenital System. O. Olsson. 1974. LC 73-14486. (Encyclopedia of Medical Radiology Ser.: Vol. 13, Pt. 1). (Illus.). 690p. 300.00 (*0-387-06514-8*) Spr-Verlag.

Roentgenographic Diagnosis of Renal Mass Lesions. Erich K. Lang. 1971. LC 70-125008. (Illus.). 190p. 12.50 (*0-87527-047-6*) Green.

Roentgenologist. Jack Rudman. 1994. (Career Examination Ser.: C-697). pap. 39.95 (*0-8373-0697-3*) Nat Learn.

Roentgenology of the Foot: Principles & Practice. Frank Weinstein. 1974. LC 73-11606. (Illus.). 352p. 32.50 (*0-87527-137-5*) Green.

Rogers' Scientific Art of Nursing Practice. Ed. by Mary Madrid & Elizabeth A. Manhart Barrett. 1994. LC 94-202074. 451p. 33.95 (*0-88737-608-8*, 15-2610, NLN Pr) Natl League Nurse.

Roitt's Essential Immunology. Ivan M. Roitt. 9th ed. 1997. LC 97-7044. (Illus.). 476p. pap. 48.95 (*0-86542-729-1*) Blackwell Sci.

Role & Competencies of Graduates of Diploma Programs in Nursing. NLN Council of Diploma Programs Staff. 2nd ed. 1989. 4p. 5.95 (*0-88737-474-3*, 16-1735) Natl League Nurse.

Role & Education of Nurses. 1995. (*92-871-2782-4*) Council of Europe FRA. *Dist:* Manhattan Pub Co.

Role & Training of Community Pharmacists. 1993. (*92-871-2209-1*) Council of Europe FRA. *Dist:* Manhattan Pub Co.

Role Motivation Theories. John B. Miner. 1993. LC 92-28816. (People & Organizations Ser.). (Illus.). 304p. (C). text 49.95 (*0-415-08486-5*, B0012) Routledge.

Role of Adenosine in Cerebral Metabolism & Blood Flow. Ed. by V. Stefanovich & I. Okyayuz-Baklouti. 1987. 141p. lib. bdg. (*90-6764-098-0*) VSP NLD. *Dist:* Coronet Bks.

Role of Aggression in Human Pathology. Ed. by H. Musaph & P. J. Mettrop. 1972. (Psychotherapy & Psychosomatics Ser.: Vol. 20, No. 5). (Illus.). pap. 15.75 (*3-8055-1562-6*) S Karger.

Role of Antihormones. Ed. by Anthony Howell. 1990. (Current Controversies in the Treatment of Breast Cancer Ser.: Vol. 1). (Illus.). 182p. (C). lib. bdg. 71.95 (*1-85070-295-0*, Parthenon Pbng) CRC Pr.

Role of Apoptosis in Development, Tissue Homeostasis & Malignancy: Death from Inside Out. T. M. Dexter et al. 1995. (Illus.). 112p. (C). pap. text 101.95 (*0-412-63810-X*, Chap & Hall NY) Chapman & Hall.

Role of B1-Integrins in Skeletal Muscle Differentiation & Extracellular Matrix Assembly. Lars Lohikangas. 2000. (Comprehensive Summaries of Uppsala Dissertations from the Faculty of Medicine Ser.: No. 939). 44p. pap. (*91-554-4752-X*) Uppsala Universitet SWE. *Dist:* Coronet Bks.

Role of Bacterial Antigens in Organ Specific Autoimmunity. Bernice M. Wenzel. 1990. 106p. text 123.00 (*3-7186-5081-9*, Harwood Acad Pubs) Gordon & Breach.

Role of Beta Agonist Therapy in Asthma Mortality. Richard Beasley. 1993. 288p. lib. bdg. 199.00 (*0-8493-6761-1*, QR201) CRC Pr.

Role of Brain Dopamine. Ed. by Edward Fluckiger et al. 1989. (Basic & Clinical Aspects of Neuroscience Ser.: Vol. 3). (Illus.). 55p. 27.95 (*0-387-50040-5*) Spr-Verlag.

Role of Calcium in Biological Systems, Vol. I. Ed. by Leopold J. Anghileri & Ann M. Tuffet-Anghileri. 1982. 288p. 163.00 (*0-8493-6280-6*, QP535, CRC Reprint) Franklin.

Role of Calcium Ions in Drug Action. M. Denborough. 1987. (International Encyclopedia of Pharmacology & Therapeutics Ser.: No. 124). (Illus.). 200p. 192.50 (*0-08-034193-4*, Pergamon Pr) Elsevier.

Role of Cell Surface Development, Vol. I. Salem S. Rao. 1987. 152p. 88.00 (*0-8493-4688-6*, CRC Reprint) Franklin.

Role of Cell Types in Hepatocarcinogenesis. Alphonse E. Sirica. 1992. 368p. lib. bdg. 239.00 (*0-8493-4746-7*, RC280) CRC Pr.

Role of Central Conceptual Structures in the Development of Children's Thought. Robbie Case & Yukari Okamoto. 1996. 225p. pap. text 19.50 (*0-226-09540-1*) U Ch Pr.

Role of Children's Hospices in the Provision of Respite Care. Carol Robinson. 1998. 76p. pap. (*1-900990-26-1*) Natl Childrens Bur GBR. *Dist:* Paul & Co Pubs.

Role of Chromium in Animal Nutrition. National Research Council Staff. 1997. LC 97-80669. 100p. pap. 23.00 (*0-309-06354-X*) Natl Acad Pr.

Role of Consciousness in the Physical World. R. G. Jahn. 1981. (AAAS Selected Symposium Ser.: No. 57). 136p. text 27.00 (*0-89158-955-4*) Westview.

Role of Cytokines in Cancer Treatment. Ed. by F. Takaku. 1994. (Journal: Vol. 51, No. 2, 1994). (Illus.). 96p. pap. 88.75 (*3-8055-5948-8*) S Karger.

Role of Cytokines in the Inflammatory Response. Ed. by S. L. Kunkel. 1996. (Journal: Vol. 5, No. 4, 1996). (Illus.). 54p. pap. 28.00 (*3-8055-6380-9*) S Karger.

Role of Dietary Supplements for Physically Active People: Current Bibliographies in Medicine: January 1966 Through April 1996. Kristine M. Scannell et al. 1996. 53p. (Orig.). pap. text 25.00 (*0-7881-3347-0*) DIANE Pub.

***Role of Dopamine-Metabolising Enzymes in Renal Sodium Handing: An Experimental Study in Vivo.** Cecilia Odlind. 2001. (Comprehensive Summaries of Uppsala Dissertations from the Faculty of Medicine Ser.: No. 1026). (Illus.). 47p. (*91-554-4998-0*) Uppsala Universitet SWE. *Dist:* Coronet Bks.

Role of Drugs & Electrolytes in Hormonogenesis. Ed. by K. Fotherby & S. B. Pal. 1984. LC 84-7611. (Illus.). xii, 360p. 138.50 (*3-11-008463-5*) De Gruyter.

Role of Drugs in Community Psychiatry. Ed. by Charles Shagass. 1971. (Modern Problems of Pharmacopsychiatry Ser.: Vol. 6). 30.50 (*3-8055-1200-7*) S Karger.

***Role of Duplex Scanning in the Management of Carotid Artery Disease.** Karl Logason. 2001. (Comprehensive Summaries of Uppsala Dissertations from the Faculty of Medicine Ser.: No. 1030). (Illus.). 49p. (*91-554-5004-0*) Uppsala Universitet SWE. *Dist:* Coronet Bks.

***Role of Early Detection & Complementary & Alternative Medicine in Women's Cancers: Congressional Hearing.** Dan Burton. 2001. 189p. (C). pap. text 35.00 (*0-7567-1814-7*) DIANE Pub.

Role of Endorphins & Neuropsychiatry. Ed. by H. M. Emrich. 1981. (Modern Problems of Pharmacopsychiatry Ser.: Vol. 17). (Illus.). viii, 292p. 115.75 (*3-8055-2918-X*) S Karger.

Role of Enzyme Treatment in Pancreatic Disease. Ed. by H. G. Beger et al. 1993. (Journal: Vol. 54, Suppl. 2, 1993). (Illus.). vi, 54p. pap. 26.25 (*3-8055-5861-9*) S Karger.

Role of Epidemiology in Regulatory Risk Assessment. Ed. by John D. Graham. 1995. LC 95-36824. (International Congress Ser.: Vol. 1092). 166p. 138.50 (*0-444-82201-1*) Elsevier.

Role of Exercise in Internal Medicine. Ed. by E. Jokl & D. Brunner. 1976. (Medicine & Sport Science Ser.: No. 10). 160p. 85.25 (*3-8055-2362-9*) S Karger.

Role of Fats in Human Nutrition. J. Podmore. 1985. LC 85-5491. 210p. text 65.00 (*3-527-26219-9*, Wiley-VCH) Wiley.

Role of Glia in Neurotoxicity. Ed. by Michael Aschner et al. 1996. LC 95-37895. 384p. 199.95 (*0-8493-4792-0*, 4792) CRC Pr.

Role of Gut Bacteria in Human Toxicology & Pharmacology. Ed. by M. Hill. 1995. LC 95-201332. 350p. (*0-7484-0110-5*) Tay Francis Ltd GBR. *Dist:* Taylor & Francis.

Role of Health Centres in the Development of Urban Health Systems: Report of a WHO Study Group on Primary Health Care in Urban Areas. 1992. (Technical Reports: No. 827). (ENG, FRE & SPA.). iv, 38p. pap. text 7.00 (*92-4-120827-9*, 1100827) World Health.

Role of Health Information Managers in CPR Projects: A Practical Guide. Margret Amatayakul. 1999. (Illus.). 292p. pap. text 55.00 (*1-58426-032-7*, AB102699) Am Hlth Info.

Role of Health Insurance in the Health Services Sector. Universities-National Bureau Staff & Richard N. Rosett. 1976. LC 76-8856. (Universities-National Bureau Conference Ser.: No. 27). 584p. reprint ed. 140.50 (*0-87014-272-0*) Natl Bur Econ Res.

Role of Herpesviruses in a Atherogenesis. Ed. by David P. Hajjar & Stephen M. Schwartz. 1998. (Advances in Vascular Biology Ser.: Vol. 4). 180p. text 75.00 (*90-5702-321-0*, ECU75, Harwood Acad Pubs) Gordon & Breach.

Role of High Energy Electrons in the Treatment of Cancer. Ed. by J. M. Vaeth & J. L. Meyer. 1991. (Frontiers of Radiation Therapy & Oncology Ser.: Vol. 25). (Illus.). x, 342p. 282.75 (*3-8055-5235-1*) S Karger.

Role of Hospitals in Ambulatory & Domiciliary Medical Care. 1959. (Technical Report Ser.: No. 176). 32p. pap. text 3.00 (*92-4-120176-2*) World Health.

Role of Immune Complexes in Disease: Report of a WHO Scientific Group, 1977. 1977. (Technical Report Ser.: No. 606). 58p. pap. text 8.00 (*92-4-120606-3*, 1100606) World Health.

Role of Interleukin-2 in the Treatment of Cancer Patients. Ed. by John Wagstaff. 1993. LC 93-104. 200p. (C). text 147.00 (*0-7923-2164-2*) Kluwer Academic.

Role of ISC's. Anne C. Ward & Robert L. Sandidge. 1996. pap. 27.50 (*1-57654-003-0*, Creative Core) Creat Core.

Role of Laser in Gastroenterology: Analysis of Eight Years' Experience. Lisabeth M. Mathus-Vliegen. 1989. (Developments in Gastroenterology Ser.). (C). text 191.50 (*0-7923-0425-X*) Kluwer Academic.

Role of Melatonin & Pineal Peptides in Neuroimmunomodulation. F. Fraschini & R. J. Reitner. 1991. (NATO Advanced Science Institutes Ser.: Vol. 204). (Illus.). 344p. (C). text 115.00 (*0-306-43921-2*, Kluwer Plenum) Kluwer Academic.

Role of Membranes in Lens Ageing & Cataract: Proceedings of the Spring Meeting, 1995. Ed. by G. F. Vrensen & T. Libondi. 1996. (Journal: Vol. 28, Suppl. 1, 1996). (Illus.). xii, 106p. pap. 36.50 (*3-8055-6304-3*) S Karger.

Role of Mental Health Professionals in the Prevention & Treatment of Child Abuse & Neglect. Marilyn S. Peterson. 1995. 73p. (Orig.). (C). pap. text 35.00 (*0-7881-1664-9*) DIANE Pub.

***Role of Mental Illness in Criminal Trials: Insanity & Mental Incompetence.** Ed. by Jane Moriarty. 2001. (C). lib. bdg. 125.00 (*0-8153-4062-1*) Garland.

***Role of Mental Illness in Criminal Trials: Insanity & Mental Incompetence.** Ed. by Jane Moriarty. 2001. (C). lib. bdg. 125.00 (*0-8153-4063-X*); lib. bdg. 125.00 (*0-8153-4064-8*) Garland.

Role of Micro-Organisms in Non-Infectious Disease. Ed. by R. R. De Vries et al. 1990. (Argenteuil Symposia Ser.). (Illus.). 208p. 83.00 (*0-387-19623-4*) Spr-Verlag.

Role of Microenvironment in Axonal Regeneration: Influence of Lesion-Induced Changes & Glial Implants on the Regeneration of the Postcommissural Fornix. Christine C. Stichel-Gunkel. Ed. by F. Beck et al. 1997. LC 97-10368. (Advances in Anatomy, Embryology & Cell Biology Ser.: No. 137). (Illus.). 80p. pap. 65.00 (*3-540-62787-1*) Spr-Verlag.

Role of Microglial Cells & Astrocytes in Pathology. Ed. by J. E. Merrill. 1994. (Journal: Vol. 16, No. 3-4, 1994). (Illus.). 124p. pap. 50.50 (*3-8055-6086-9*) S Karger.

Role of Multiple Intensification in Medical Oncology. Ed. by M. S. Aapro & D. Maraninchi. 1997. LC 97-40470. (ESO Monographs). (Illus.). 54p. 44.00 (*3-540-63543-2*) Spr-Verlag.

Role of Neuroplasticity in the Response to Drugs. 1993. lib. bdg. 259.95 (*0-8490-8505-5*) Gordon Pr.

Role of Neurotransmitter Systems in Anxiety Modulation. 1984. (Journal: Vol. 17, Suppl. 3, 1984). (Illus.). iv, 84p. pap. 24.50 (*3-8055-3983-5*) S Karger.

Role of Neurotransmitters in Brain Injury. M. Y. Globus & W. D. Dietrich. 1992. LC 92-49215. (Illus.). 390p. (C). text 110.00 (*0-306-44255-8*, Kluwer Plenum) Kluwer Academic.

Role of Nitric Oxide & Sepsis & ARDS. Ed. by M. P. Fink & D. Payen. 1995. LC 95-37672. (Update in Intensive Care & Emergency Medicine Ser.: No. 24). (Illus.). 416p. 147.00 (*3-540-60128-7*) Spr-Verlag.

Role of Oxygen Radicals in Cardiovascular Disease. Ed. by Antonia L'Abbate. 1988. (C). text 173.50 (*0-89838-407-9*) Kluwer Academic.

Role of Pharmacoeconomics in Outcomes Management. Ed. by Nelda E. Johnson & David B. Nash. 1996. LC 96-35331. 112p. (Orig.). pap. 35.00 (*1-55648-169-1*, 169111) AHPI.

Role of Pharmacology in Pediatric Oncology. Ed. by L. Massimo et al. 1987. (Developments in Oncology Ser.). lib. bdg. 197.00 (*0-89838-795-7*) Kluwer Academic.

Role of Phosphonates in Living Systems. Ed. by Richard L. Hilderbrand. 1983. 216p. lib. bdg. 144.00 (*0-8493-5724-1*, QP801) CRC Pr.

Role of Platelet-Activating Factor in Immune Disorders, Part 2. Ed. by Pierre Braquet. 1988. (New Trends in Lipid Mediators Research Ser.: Vol. 2). (Illus.). viii, 214p. 172.25 (*3-8055-4744-7*) S Karger.

Role of Platelets in Blood-Biomaterial Interactions. Ed. by Y. F. Missirlis & J. L. Wautier. 1993. LC 93-2728. text 148.50 (*0-7923-2162-6*) Kluwer Academic.

Role of Procoagulant Activity in Health & Disease. Gary A. Levy. 1993. 240p. 179.00 (*0-8493-5566-4*, QP93) CRC Pr.

Role of Prolactin in Human Reproduction. Ed. by M. Mizuno et al. 1988. (Illus.). x, 314p. 225.25 (*3-8055-4786-2*) S Karger.

Role of Protein Kinase C in Insulin Action, Resistance & Secretion. Robert V. Farese. 1994. LC 95-142286. (Medical Intelligence Unit Ser.). 112p. 99.00 (*1-57059-218-7*) Landes Bioscience.

Role of Proteoglycans & Glycosaminoglycans in Aging. K. Sames. 1994. (Interdisciplinary Topics in Gerontology Ser.: Vol. 28). (Illus.). xiv, 140p. 128.75 (*3-8055-5925-9*) S Karger.

Role of Psychiatry in Medical Education: An Appraisal & a Forecast. Sidney L. Werkman. 1966. LC 66-10810. (Commonwealth Fund Publications). (Illus.). 203p. 22.00 (*0-674-77730-1*) HUP.

Role of Psychoanalysis in Psychiatric Education: Past, Present, & Future. Ed. by Sidney H. Weismann & Robert Thurnblad. 1987. (Emotions & Behavior Monographs: No. 7). (C). 55.00 (*0-8236-5850-3*) Intl Univs Pr.

Role of Psychosocial Factors in the Pathogenesis of Coronary Heart Disease, 1980. Ed. by A. D. Appels & P. Falger. 1981. (Journal: Vol. 34, No. 2-3). (Illus.). iv, 160p. pap. 35.75 (*3-8055-2286-X*) S Karger.

Role of Public Health Officers & General Practitioners in Mental Health Care. 1962. (Technical Report Ser.: No 235). 54p. pap. text 3.00 (*92-4-120235-1*) World Health.

***Role of Reactive Oxygen Species in Traumatic Brain Injury: Experimental Studies in the Rat.** Niklas Marklund. 2001. (Comprehensive Summaries of Uppsala Dissertatons from the Faculty of Medicine: No. 1048). (Illus.). 73p. pap. (*91-554-5053-9*) Uppsala Universitet SWE. *Dist:* Coronet Bks.

Role of Religion & Ethics in the Prevention & Control of Aids: Health Education Through Religion, 6. 1992. pap. text 10.00 (*92-9021-153-9*) World Health.

Role of RNA & DNA in Brain Function. Ed. by Antonia Giuditta et al. 1986. text 127.50 (*0-89838-814-7*) Kluwer Academic.

Role of Serotonin in Psychiatric Disorders. Ed. by Serena-Lynn Brown & Herman M. Van Praag. 1991. LC 90-2285. (Einstein Clinical & Experimental Psychiatry Monograph Ser.: No. 4). (Illus.). 352p. text 51.95 (*0-87630-589-3*) Brunner-Routledge.

Role of Sexual Abuse in the Etiology of Borderline Personality Disorder, No. 49. Ed. by Mary C. Zanarini. 1997. LC 95-26270. (Progress in Psychiatry Ser.: No. 52). 259p. text 42.00 (*0-88048-496-9*, 8496) Am Psychiatric.

Role of Somatostatin-Analogues in Gastrointestinal Diseases. Ed. by C. Beglinger & M. W. Buchler. 1999. (Digestion Ser.: Vol. 60, Suppl. 2 (1999)). (Illus.). iv, 58p. pap. 25.25 (*3-8055-6878-9*) S Karger.

Role of Somatostatin Analogues in Oncology: European Neuroendocrine Tumour Network (E. N. E. T.), Innsbruck (Austria), February 2000. K. Oberg. 2000. (Digestion Ser.: Vol. 62). (Illus.). iv, 112p. pap. 34.00 (*3-8055-6931-9*) S Karger.

Role of Somatostatin & Octreotide in Pancreatic Disease: Proceedings of a Symposium During the EPC Meeting, Ulm, October 1992. Ed. by M. W. Buechler et al. 1993. (Journal: Vol. 55, Suppl. 1, 1994). (Illus.). vi, 52p. pap. 25.25 (*3-8055-5950-X*) S Karger.

Role of the Charge Nurse. Linda Greenberg et al. Ed. by Patricia A. Wentworth et al. unabr. ed. 1998. (Regional Conference Ser.). (Illus.). ring bd. 475.00 (*0-935890-20-3*) Emerg Nurses IL.

Role of the Community Hospital in the Care of the Dying Patient & Bereaved. Ed. by Elias Gerchick et al. 1976. 250p. 42.50 (*0-8422-7278-X*) Irvington.

Role of the Community Hospital in the Care of the Dying Patient, & the Bereaved. Elias Gerchick. 1979. 19.95 (*0-405-12506-2*) Ayer.

Role of the Family in Psychiatric Rehabilitation: A Workbook. LeRoy Spaniol et al. 2000. 224p. pap., wbk. ed. 32.95 (*1-878512-09-9*) Boston Univ Ctr Psy Rehab.

Role of the Family in TBI Rehab. Ed. by William H. Burke. 2nd rev. ed. 1996. (Professional Series on Traumatic Brain Injury: Vol. 19). 56p. pap. 9.50 (*1-882855-46-9*) HDI Pubs.

Role of the Forebrain in Sensation & Behavior: Proceedings of the Symposium, Moffett Field, CA, May 26-27, 1989. Ed. by G. Holstege. 1991. (Progress in Brain Research Ser.: No. 87). 430p. 277.25 (*0-444-81181-8*) Elsevier.

Role of the Health Sector in Food & Nutrition. 1981. (Technical Report Ser.: No. 667). 92p. pap. text 6.00 (*92-4-120667-5*) World Health.

Role of the Laser in Dermatology: An Atlas. Toshio Ohshiro. 1997. LC 96-30947. 294p. 560.00 (*0-471-96630-4*) Wiley.

Role of the Liver in Maintaining Glucose Homeostasis. Alan D. Cherrington et al. 1994. (Medical Intelligence Unit Ser.). 118p. 99.00 (*1-57059-006-0*, LN9006) Landes Bioscience.

Role of the Mental Health Nurse. Ed. by Sheila Forster. 2000. (Illus.). 224p. pap. (*0-7487-3893-2*) Nelson Thornes GBR. *Dist:* Intl Spec Bk, Trans-Atl Phila.

Role of the Minister in Caring for the Dying Patient & the Bereaved. Brian P. O'Connor et al. 19.95 (*0-405-12504-6*) Ayer.

Role of the Nurse in Clinical Medical Education. Norma A. Wylie. 1988. LC 87-63229. (Medical Humanities Ser.). (Illus.). 274p. 18.95 (*0-931369-21-5*) Southern IL Univ Sch.

Role of the Physician Executive: Cases & Commentary. Ed. by David A. Kindig & Anthony R. Kovner. 1992. LC 92-49823. 268p. (C). pap. text 18.00 (*0-910701-88-1*, 0922) Health Admin Pr.

***Role of the Plasminogen Activator - Plasmin Pathway in Bone Metabolism.** Evis Daci. 2000. (Acta Biomedica Lovanuensia Ser.: No. 223). (Illus.). 108p. pap. (*90-5867-081-3*) Leuven Univ BEL. *Dist:* Coronet Bks.

Role of the Preceptor: A Guide for Nurse Educators & Clinicians. Ed. by Jean P. Flynn. 1997. LC 96-41728. (Illus.). 160p. 32.95 (*0-8261-9460-5*) Springer Pub.

Role of the Registry in Cancer Control. Ed. by D. M. Parkin et al. 1986. (IARC Scientific Publications Ser.: No. 66). (Illus.). 150p. 20.00 (*0-19-723066-0*) OUP.

Role of the Thymus in Health & Senescence, Vol. 1: Thymus & Immunity. Ed. by Nate F. Cardarelli. 1989. LC 88-39539. 368p. 172.00 (*0-8493-6909-6*, QP188);II. 197.00 (*0-8493-6910-X*, QP188) Franklin (CRC Reprint).

Role of the Thymus in Tolerance Induction Ed. by Marion D. Kendall. 1990. (Thymus Update Ser.: Vol. 3). x, 327p. text 223.00 (*3-7186-5020-7*, Harwood Acad Pubs) Gordon & Breach.

Role of the Volunteer Director in the Care of the Terminal Patient & the Family. Harriet H. Naylor. 1981. 19.95 (*0-405-13092-9*) Ayer.

Role of the Volunteer in the Care of the Terminal Patient & the Family. Harriet H. Naylor. 1981. 18.95 (*0-405-13091-0*) Ayer.

Role of Trace Elements for Health Promotion & Disease Prevention: Proceedings of the 1996 Annual Meeting of the European Academy of Nutritional Sciences, Copenhagen, August 1996. Ed. by Paul Walter & Brittmarie Sandstrom. 1998. LC 98-9428. (Bibliotheca Nutritio et Dieta Ser.: No. 54, 1998). (Illus.). viii, 170p. 198.25 (*3-8055-6628-X*) S Karger.

Role of Traditional Medicine in Primary Health Care. Ed. by Ivan Wolffers. 1991. 75p. pap. (*90-6256-936-6*) VU Univ Pr NLD. *Dist:* Paul & Co Pubs.

Role of Trazodone in Antidepressant Therapy: Safety & Clinical Efficacy. Ed. by B. Silvestrini et al. 1984. (Journal: Vol. 17, Supp. 2). (Illus.). iv, 104p. pap. 50.50 (*3-8055-3884-7*) S Karger.

Role of Values in Psychology & Human Development. Ed. by William M. Kurtines et al. 1992. LC 91-18870. 304p. 200.00 (*0-471-53945-7*) Wiley.

Role-Play: A Practical Guide. Ed. by Elizabeth Milroy. 1982. (Illus.). 150p. text 22.00 (*0-08-025744-5*, R130); pap. text 17.90 (*0-08-025745-3*, R132) Elsevier (Pergamon Pr).

Role Theory: Expectations, Identities & Behaviors. Bruce J. Biddle. 1979. text 70.00 (*0-12-095950-X*) Acad Pr.

Role Theory & Illness. Gerald Gordon. pap. 22.95 (*0-8084-0270-6*) NCUP.

Role Viruses & the Immune System in Diabetes Mellitus. Ed. by T. Dyrberg. 1990. (Current Topics in Microbiology & Immunology Ser.: Vol. 156). (Illus.). 139p. 95.00 (*0-387-51918-1*) Spr-Verlag.

Roleplays in Health Information Management: An Instructional Resource. Susan P. Bailey & Joanne Muller. 1997. v, 153p. pap. text 44.95 (*0-9657783-2-0*) Lenox Pub Co.

Roles & Paradigms in Psychotherapy. Ed. by Marie C. Nelson et al. 1968. LC 67-28011. (Illus.). 384p. text 89.00 (*0-8089-0344-6*, 793095, Grune & Strat) Harcrt Hlth Sci Grp.

Roles & Responsibilities of the Ethics Consultant: A Retrospective Analysis of Cases. Benjamin Freedman. Ed. by Francoise Baylis. 2000. (Ethics in Clinical Medicine Ser.). 176p. (C). pap. 16.95 (*1-55572-058-7*) Univ Pub Group.

Roles & Tasks of Community Mental Health Teams. Gerald Wistow & Stephen Brown. 1990. (Avebury Studies of Care in the Community). 144p. text (*1-85628-003-9*) Avebury GBR. *Dist:* Ashgate Pub Co.

Roles of Occupational Therapists in Continuity of Care. Ed. by Florence S. Cromwell. 1985. LC 85-899. (Occupational Therapy in Health Care Ser.: Vol. 2, No. 1). 159p. text 5.95 (*0-86656-392-X*); pap. text 19.95 (*0-86656-393-8*) Haworth Pr.

Roles of Physician Assistants & Nurse Practitioners in Primary Care. Ed. by Marian Osterweis & Stephen Garfinkel. 1993. (Orig.). pap. (*1-879694-07-7*) AAH Ctrs.

Rolfing: The Integration of Human Structures. Ida P. Rolf. 1977. LC 76-52192. (Illus.). 27.50 (*0-930422-10-4*) Dennis-Landman.

Rolle der Anthrazykline in der Therapie des Mamma - und Ovarialkarzinoms: Symposium Berlin, November 1999. 2000. (Onkologie Ser.: Band 23, suppl. 2). (GER.). 32p. pap. 25.25 (*3-8055-7084-8*) S Karger.

***Roman Catholic Perspective on the Morality of Withdrawing or Withholding Food & Fluid Administered Artificially to an Individual in the Persistent Vegetative State.** David M. O'Leary. 2001. 192p. pap. 20.00 (*0-9677471-2-0*) Catholic Ctr at Tufts Univ.

Romance of American Psychology: Political Culture in the Age of Experts. Ellen Herman. 1995. LC 94-26930. 512p. text 40.00 (*0-520-08598-1*) U CA Pr.

Romance of Proctology. Charles E. Blanchard. LC 75-23684. reprint ed. 49.50 (*0-404-13237-5*) AMS Pr.

Romance of the Fungus World: An Account of Fungus Life in Its Numerous Guises, Both Real & Legendary. R. T. Rolfe & F. W. Rolfe. 1974. LC 74-81401. (Illus.). 352p. reprint ed. pap. 6.95 (*0-486-23105-4*) Dover.

Romance, Poetry & Surgical Sleep: Literature Influences Medicine, 42. E. M. Papper. 1995. LC 94-24189. (Contributions in Medical Studies Ser.: Vol. 42). 176p. 62.50 (*0-313-29405-4*, Greenwood Pr) Greenwood.

Rome II: The Functional Gastrointestinal Disorders: Diagnosis, Pathophysiology & Treatment - A Multinational Consensus. Ed. by Douglas A. Drossman et al. 2nd rev. unabr. ed. 2000. LC 99-40667. Orig. Title: The Functional Gastrointestinal Disorders. 800 p. pap. text 99.95 (*0-9656837-2-9*); (Illus.). 800p. text 79.95 (*0-9656837-1-0*) Degnon Assocs.

Ronald Ross: Malariologist & Polymath : A Biography. E. R. Nye & M. E. Gibson. 1997. LC 96-8835. (Illus.). 352p. text 59.95 (*0-312-16296-0*) St Martin.

Root Atlas of Lympho-Graphy. 1975. text 155.50 (*90-207-0479-6*) Kluwer Academic.

Root Canal Cover-Up. George E. Meinig. Ed. by Charlene Koonce & Mark Lovendale. 2nd ed. 1994. LC 93-72133. (Illus.). 257p. pap. 19.95 (*0-945196-14-8*) Bion Pub.

Root Canal Cover-Up. George E. Meinig. Ed. by Mark Lovendale & Charlene Koonce. 6th ed. 1993. LC 93-72133. (Illus.). 230p. reprint ed. pap. 19.95 (*0-945196-19-9*) Bion Pub.

Roots & Shoots see Tree of Healing: Psychological & Biblical Foundations for Counseling & Pastoral Care

Roots of Behaviourism, Set. Ed. by Robert H. Wozniak. 1993. 2488p. (C). 651.00 (*0-415-10165-4*) Routledge.

Roots of Crime: Selected Papers on Psychoanalysis, Vol. 2. Edward Glover. 1960. pap. 24.95 (*0-8236-8270-6*, 025860) Intl Univs Pr.

Roots of Delinquency: Infancy, Adolescence & Crime. Michael Wadsworth. 1979. LC 79-10065. 150p. text 44.00 (*0-06-497305-0*, N6726) B&N Imports.

Roots of Healing: The New Medicine. Michael Toms et al. 1997. LC 96-49306. 200p. (Orig.). pap. 12.95 (*1-56170-422-9*, 891) Hay House.

Roots of Modern Gerontology & Geriatrics: An Original Anthology. Ed. by Gerald J. Gruman & Robert J. Kastenbaum. 1979. LC 78-22184. (Aging & Old Age Ser.). lib. bdg. 33.95 (*0-405-11801-5*) Ayer.

Roots of Modern Social Psychology (1872-1954) Robert M. Farr. 1997. (Illus.). 208p. (C). 60.95 (*0-631-15251-2*) Blackwell Pubs.

Roots of Prosocial Behavior in Children. Nancy Eisenberg. Ed. by Paul H. Mussen. 1989. (Cambridge Studies in Social & Emotional Development). (Illus.). 208p. (C). pap. text 15.95 (*0-521-33771-2*) Cambridge U Pr.

Roots of Psychotherapy. Carl A. Whitaker & Thomas P. Malone. 1981. LC 80-24437. (Brunner Mazel Classics in Psychoanalysis & Psychotherapy: No. 9). 272p. reprint ed. text 39.95 (*0-87630-265-7*) Brunner-Routledge.

Rorschach Assessment of Children & Adolescents: A Comprehensive System, Vol. 3. John E. Exner. 2nd ed. 1994. LC 85-17870. (Personality Processes Ser.: Vol. 3). 448p. 110.00 (*0-471-55927-X*) Wiley.

Rorschach - A Comprehensive System: Assessment of Personality & Psychopathology, Vol. 2, Interpretation. John E. Exner. 2nd ed. 1991. LC 90-13160. (Personality Processes Ser.: Vol. 2). 496p. 110.00 (*0-471-85080-2*) Wiley.

Rorschach - A Comprehensive System Basic Foundations, Vol. 1. John E. Exner. 3rd ed. 1993. LC 93-9878. (Personality Processes Ser.: Vol. 1). 672p. (Orig.). pap. 110.00 (*0-471-55902-4*) Wiley.

PQR

Rorschach Assessment of Aggressive & Psychopathic Personalities. Carl B. Gacono & J. Reid Meloy. 1994. LC 94-11478. (Personality & Clinical Psychology Ser.). 432p. text 44.00 (0-8058-0980-5) L Erlbaum Assocs.

Rorschach Content Interpretation. Edward Aronow & Marvin Reznikoff. 1976. LC 76-25544. 384p. text 63.00 (0-8089-0961-4, 790200, Grune & Strat) Harcrt Hlth Sci Grp.

Rorschach Interpretation: Advanced Technique. Leslie Phillips & Joseph G. Smith. 1953. LC 53-9833. (Illus.). 400p. text 39.00 (0-8089-0361-6, 793287, Grune & Strat) Harcrt Hlth Sci Grp.

Rorschach Introduction: Content & Perceptual Approaches. Ed. by Edward Aronow & Marvin Reznikoff. 1982. 160p. text 23.95 (0-8089-1516-9, 790201, Grune & Strat) Harcrt Hlth Sci Grp.

Rorschach Location & Scoring Manual. Leonard Small. 1956. LC 55-10398. (Illus.). 224p. text 56.00 (0-8089-0432-9, 794140, Grune & Strat) Harcrt Hlth Sci Grp.

Rorschach Responses in Old Age. Louise B. Ames et al. rev. ed. 1995. LC 95-14106. (Master Work Ser.). 242p. pap. 60.00 (1-56821-490-1) Aronson.

Rorschach Study of Child Development. Nettie H. Ledwith. 1975. LC 75-26632. 336p. reprint ed. lib. bdg. 59.75 (0-8371-8365-0, LERS, Greenwood Pr) Greenwood.

Rorschach Systems. John F. Exner. 1969. LC 68-31431. 392p. text 56.00 (0-8089-0128-1, 791180, Grune & Strat) Harcrt Hlth Sci Grp.

Rorschach Technique with Children & Adolescents: Application & Norms. Eugene E. Levitt & Aare Truumaa. 1972. LC 72-7362. 160p. text 47.00 (0-8089-0785-9, 792520, Grune & Strat) Harcrt Hlth Sci Grp.

Rorschach Test: Theory & Practice. Rajendra K. Misra et al. 1996. LC 96-28316. 295p. 32.00 (0-8039-9328-5, 80595) Sage.

Rorschach Test Scoring. Alvin G. Burstein & Sandra Loucks. 1989. LC 66-56615. 300p. pap. 39.95 (0-89116-780-3) Hemisp Pub.

Rorschach Tests: Index of New Information for Reference & Research. David I. Rochman. 1997. 160p. 57.50 (0-7883-1698-2); pap. 47.50 (0-7883-1699-0) ABBE Pubs Assn.

Rorschach Workbook. Lucille H. Blum et al. rev. ed. 1975. LC 74-10227. 193p. spiral bd. 25.00 (0-8236-5901-1) Intl Univs Pr.

Rorschachiana. Ed. by Irving B. Weiner. 1993. (Yearbook of the International Rorschach Society Ser.: Vol. 18). (Illus.). 160p. text 34.00 (0-88937-114-8) Hogrefe & Huber Pubs.

Rorschachiana: Yearbook of the International Rorschach Society, Vol. 20. Ed. by Irving B. Weiner. 1995. (Illus.). 216p. text 38.00 (0-88937-141-5) Hogrefe & Huber Pubs.

Rorschachiana Vol. 23: Yearbook of the International Rorschach Society. Ed. by A. Andronikof-Sanglade. 1999. 152p. text 38.00 (0-88937-201-2) Hogrefe & Huber Pubs.

Rorschachiana Vol. 24: Yearbook of the International Rorschach Society. Ed. by A. Andronikof-Sanglade. 2000. (Illus.). 188p. 38.00 (0-88937-226-8) Hogrefe & Huber Pubs.

Rosacea Handbook: A Self-Help Guide. Ann-Marie Lindstrom. 2000. LC 00-131566. (Illus.). 178p. pap. 12.95 (1-887053-14-X) United Res CA.

Rose & Black's Clinical Patterns in Nephrology. Robert M. Black. 1995. 597p. text 139.00 (0-316-75652-0, Little Brwn Med Div) Lppncott W & W.

***Rosemary Gladstar's Family Herbal: A Guide to Living Life with Energy, Health & Vitality.** Rosemary Gladstar. 2001. LC 2001-32783. 408p. 24.95 (1-58017-425-6) Storey Bks.

Rosen's Breast Pathology. Paul P. Rosen. 2nd ed. 2001. LC 00-52058. (Illus.). 1,024p. text 299.00 (0-7817-2379-5) Lppncott W & W.

Rosen's Emergency Medicine, Concepts & Clinical Practice. John Marx et al. 5th ed. Date not set. 3165p. text (0-323-01185-3) Mosby Inc.

Rosen's Management of Labor: Physician's Judgment & Patient Care. Ralph W. Hale & Mortimer G. Rosen. 2nd ed. 1997. LC 97-3650. 224p. (0-412-13811-5) E A GBR. *Dist:* OUP.

Ross & Wilson: Anatomy & Physiology in Health & Illness. Kathleen J. Wilson. 7th ed. 1990. (Illus.). 412p. pap. text (0-443-04243-8) Church.

***Ross & Wilson - Anatomy & Physiology in Health & Illness.** Anne Waugh & Allison Grant. 9th ed. 2001. LC 2001-28776. (Illus.). pap. (0-443-06468-7) Church GBR. *Dist:* Saunders.

Ross & Wilson Anatomy & Physiology in Health & Illness. Kathleen J. Wilson et al. 8th ed. 1996. LC 96-25832. 465p. pap. text (0-443-05156-9) Church.

Ross Information Processing Assessment (RIPA-2) Complete Kit. Deborah R. Swain. 2nd ed. 1996. 44p. 106.00 (0-88120-379-3, 7640) PRO-ED.

Rossetti Infant-Toddler Language Scale: A Measure of Communication & Interaction. Louis M. Rossetti. 1990. 165p. spiral bd. 43.00 (1-55999-121-6) LinguiSystems.

Rossetti Infant-Toddler Language Scale Kit: A Measure of Communication & Interaction. Louis M. Rossetti. 1990. (J). (ps). tchr. ed., spiral bd., suppl. ed. 69.95 (1-55999-143-7, 143-7A1) LinguiSystems.

Roster of All Regimental Surgeons & Assistant Surgeons in the Late War. 1989. 304p. reprint ed. 30.00 (0-942211-75-8) Olde Soldier Bks.

Rotary Blood Pumps: New Developments & Current Applications. Ed. by H. Matsuda. 2000. (Illus.). 150p. 64.00 (4-431-70280-6) Spr-Verlag.

Rotation Manual for Clinical Laboratory Science. Lori Rice-Spearman & Hal S. Larsen. 1994. LC 94-38433. (0-683-04821-X) Lppncott W & W.

Rotator Cuff: Current Concepts & Complex Problems. Louis U. Bigliani. Ed. by Joseph P. Iannotti. 1998. LC 97-52637. (Monograph Ser.). (Illus.). 120p. pap. 38.00 (0-89203-171-9) Amer Acad Ortho Surg.

Rotator Cuff Disorders. Ed. by Wayne Z. Burkhead, Jr. 1996. LC 95-14112. (Illus.). 500p. text 159.00 (0-683-01215-0) Lppncott W & W.

Rotator Cuff Disorders: Evaluation & Treatment. Ed. by J. P. Iannotti. 1991. LC 91-33008. 88p. pap. 38.00 (0-89203-051-8) Amer Acad Ortho Surg.

Rotator Cuff Repair: A Guide for Patients. David Collins. 1997. (Ortho Ser.). 32p. pap. text 2.95 (1-885274-52-1) Health InfoNet Inc.

Rotaviruses: Methods & Protocols. Ed. by James Gray & Ulrich Desselberger. 2000. LC 99-23881. (Methods in Molecular Medicine Ser.: Vol. 34). (Illus.). 272p. 99.50 (0-89603-736-3) Humana.

Rote List 1998 (German Physician's Desk Reference) 1998. (GER.). 1380p. 295.00 (0-7859-9656-7) Fr & Eur.

Rote List 1999. annuals Ed. by French and European Staff. Tr. of German Physician's Desk Reference. (GER.). 295.00 (0-320-03687-1) Fr & Eur.

Rote List, 1996 (German Physician's Desk Reference) 1996. (GER.). 195.00 (0-7859-9764-4) Fr & Eur.

Rothman-Simeone the Spine. Harry N. Herkowitz et al. Ed. by Richard Lampert. 4th ed. 1999. LC 97-2672. (Illus.). 1535p. (C). text 295.00 (0-7216-7176-4) Saunders.

Rough Medicine: Surgeons at Sea in the Age of Sail. Joan Druett. 2000. LC 00-34474. (Illus.). x, 270p. 27.50 (0-415-92451-0) Routledge.

***Rough Medicine: Surgeons at Sea in the Age of Sail.** Joan Druett. 2001. reprint ed. pap. 16.95 (0-415-92452-9) Routledge.

Routes to Hospital: A Sociological Analysis of the Paths to Psychiatric Hospitalization. Roger Manktelow. 1994. LC 94-9576. (1-85628-492-1) Avebry GBR. *Dist:* Ashgate Pub Co.

Routine Surveillance for Radionuclides in Air & Water. 1968. (Illus.). 64p. pap. text 8.00 (92-4-156005-3, 1150136) World Health.

Routine Urinalysis & Collection, Transportation, & Preservation of Urine Specimens: Approved Guideline (1995) Contrib. by Helen M. Free. 1995. 95.00 (1-56238-282-9, GP16-A) NCCLS.

Routledge Langenscheidt German Dictionary of Medicine, Vol. 2. Fritz-Jurgen Nohring. 3rd ed. 1998. LC 97-43142. (Bilingual Specialist Dictionaries Ser.). (GER.). 904p. (C). 125.00 (0-415-17337-X) Routledge.

Routledge Langenscheidt German Dictionary of Medicine: Germanenglish, Vol. 1. Ed. by Fritz-Jurgen Nohring. 2nd ed. 1998. LC 97-43142. (Bilingual Specialist Dictionaries Ser.). (GER.). 975p. (C). 125.00 (0-415-17130-X) Routledge.

Roxburgh's Common Skin Diseases. R. M. Marks. 16th ed. 1993. (Illus.). 344p. (gr. 13). pap. (0-412-41130-X) E A GBR. *Dist:* OUP.

Roxene, Vol. 1. Wendy Stephenson. 1983. 70p. (Orig.). pap. 5.95 (0-920490-28-X) Temeron Bks.

Roy Adaptation Model: The Definitive Statement. Callista Roy. 2nd ed. 1998. LC 98-33477. 492p. (C). pap. 49.00 (0-8385-8248-6) P-H.

Roy Adaptation Model-Based Research: 25 Years of Contributions to Nursing Science. Boston Based Adaptation Research in Nursing Society. 1999. (Monographs). (Illus.). 371p. pap. text 39.95 (0-9656391-8-5, 1086) Sigma Theta Tau.

Royal College of General Practitioners: The First 25 Years. John Fry et al. 1982. (Illus.). 350p. text 29.00 (0-85200-360-9) Kluwer Academic.

Royal Marsden Hospital Handbook of Wound Management in Cancer Care. Wayne Naylor et al. 2001. LC 00-66723. (Illus.). 256p. pap. 31.95 (0-632-05751-3) Blackwell Sci.

Royal Marsden Hospital Manual of Clinical Nursing Procedures. Jane Mallett et al. 5th ed. 2000. LC 00-23642. (Illus.). pap. 49.95 (0-632-05235-X) Blackwell Sci.

Royal Marsden Hospital Manual of Multidisciplinary Standards of Care. Joanna M. Luthert & Lorraine Robinson. 1993. (Illus.). 256p. pap. 26.95 (0-632-03386-X) Blackwell Sci.

Royal Marsden NHS Trust Manual of Clinical Nursing Procedures. Jane Mallett & Christopher Bailey. 4th ed. 1996. LC 96-19076. 662p. pap. 34.95 (0-632-04068-8) Blackwell Sci.

Royal Pharmacopoeia Society of Great Britain, 1841-1991. Ed. by Holloway. 1991. (0-85369-244-0) Pharmaceutical Pr GBR. *Dist:* Rittenhouse.

Royal Vic: The Story of Montreal's Royal Victoria Hospital, 1894-1994. Neville Terry. 1994. LC 95-113778. (Illus.). 288p. (0-7735-1170-9) McG-Queens Univ Pr CAN. *Dist:* CUP Services.

Roy's Pocket Guide - Medication Drip Constants & Reference Tables. Roy G. Bridges. 1998. LC 98-92100. (Illus.). 106p. ring bd. 10.00 (0-9666974-0-5) R Bridges Enter.

RPA, NIDDK Meeting - Selected Presentations, 1995: Joint Annual Meeting of Renal Physicians Association & National Institute of Diabetes, Digestive & Kidney Diseases, Washington, May 1995. Ed. by T. A. Golper & M. J. Scherbenske. 1996. (Journal: Vol. 14, No. 4, 1996). (Illus.). 62p. pap. 44.50 (3-8055-6371-X) S Karger.

RSI & the Experts: The Construction of Medical Knowledge. Hilary Arksey. 1999. LC 98-230629. (1-85728-864-5) UCL Pr Ltd.

RSI Assorted Nutritional Therapy. Ed. by RSI Promotions Staff. 1998. pap. 14.95 (0-8092-2677-4) NTC Contemp Pub Co.

RSNA, 1992: Selected Scientific Exhibits. Radiological Society of North America-RadioGraphic. 1994. 500.00 (1-56815-024-5, 10024) Mosby Inc.

RU 486: The Pill That Could End the Abortion Wars & Why American Women Don't Have It. Lawrence Lader. 1992. pap. 9.57 (0-201-60819-7); 1991. 16.30 (0-201-57069-6) Addison-Wesley.

Rubber Dam in Clinical Practice. J. S. Reid et al. 1991. (Illus.). 108p. pap. text 34.00 (1-85097-011-4) Quint Pub Co.

Rudolf Steiner on Nutrition & Stimulants. Rudolf Steiner. Tr. by K. Castelliz & B. Saunders-Davies from GER. 1991. 238p. (C). pap. text 12.95 (0-938250-29-9) Bio-Dynamic Farm.

Rudolph Virchow: Doctor, Statesman, Anthropologist & Virchow-Bibliographie 1843-1901 Erwin H. Ackerknecht. Ed. by J. Schwalbe & I. Bernard Cohen. 1981. LC 80-2112. (Development of Science Ser.). (Illus.). reprint ed. lib. bdg. 49.95 (0-405-13832-6) Ayer.

Rudolph's Fundamentals of Pediatrics. Abraham M. Rudolph & Robert Kamei. 1994. (Illus.). 780p. (C). pap. 39.95 (0-8385-8233-8, A8233-7) McGraw-Hill Prof.

Rudolph's Fundamentals of Pediatrics. Abraham M. Rudolph et al. 2nd ed. 1998. 800p. (C). pap. text 44.95 (0-8385-8236-2, A-8236-0, Apple Lange Med) McGraw.

***Rudolph's Fundamentals of Pediatrics.** Abraham M. Rudolph et al. 3rd ed. 2002. LC 2001-54631. (Illus.). 848p. pap. 64.95 (0-8385-8450-0, Apple Lange Med) McGraw.

Rudolph's Pediatrics. Abraham Rudolph. 20th ed. 1995. (Illus.). 2337p. (C). text 150.00 (0-8385-8492-6, A8492-9) McGraw-Hill Prof.

Rudolph's Pediatrics. Rudolph. 21st ed. 1999. pap. text, stu. ed. 55.00 (0-8385-8286-9) Appleton & Lange.

Rudolph's Pediatrics. Abraham M. Rudolph. 21st ed. 2001. LC 00-68714. (C). 99.95 (0-8385-8285-0, Apple Lange Med) McGraw.

Rudolph's Pediatrics: A Study Guide. Robert Pantell. 2nd ed. 1992. 256p. pap. text 29.95 (0-8385-8489-6, A8489-5) Appleton & Lange.

Rule-Governed Behavior: Cognition, Contingencies, & Instructional Control. S. C. Hayes. 1989. LC 89-35845. (Applied Clinical Psychology Ser.). (Illus.). 412p. (C). 75.00 (0-306-43172-6, Plenum Trade) Perseus Pubng.

Rules & Representations. Noam Chomsky. 1982. LC 79-26145. (Woodbridge Lectures Ser.: No. 11). pap. text 22.00 (0-231-04827-0) Col U Pr.

Rules for Medical Terminology. Lois Mack. 2nd ed. 1996. 256p. (C). spiral bd. 42.95 (0-7872-2844-3, 41284401) Kendall-Hunt.

Rules Governing Medicinal Products in the European Union Vol. I: Pharmaceutical Legislation/Medicinal Products for Human Use. European Communities Commission, Directorate-General for Industry, Pharmaceuticals and Cosmetics. 1997. (Eudralex Collection). 294p. pap. (92-828-2032-7, CO-08-97-856ENC) Comm Europ Commun BEL. *Dist:* Bernan Associates, Balogh.

Rules Governing Medicinal Products in the European Union Vol. II: Notice to Applicants: Medicinal Products for Human Use/Presentation & Content of Dossier, Set. European Communities Commission, Directorate-General for Industry, Pharmaceuticals and Cosmetics. 1997. (Eudralex Collection). 425p. pap. (0-11-975780-X, CO-41-97-000-EN-C) Statnry Office GBR. *Dist:* Balogh, Bernan Associates.

Rules Governing Medicinal Products in the European Union Vol. III: Guidelines - Medicinal Products for Human Use. European Communities Commission, Directorate-General for Industry, Pharmaceuticals and Cosmetics. 1998. (Eudralex Collection). 1055p. pap. (92-828-2436-5, CO-54-97-000ENC) Comm Europ Commun BEL. *Dist:* Balogh, Bernan Associates.

Rules Governing Medicinal Products in the European Union Vol. IV: Good Manufacturing Practices/Medicinal Products for Human & Veterinary Use. European Communities Commission, Directorate-General for Industry, Pharmaceuticals and Cosmetics. 1997. (Eudralex Collection). 153p. pap. (92-828-2029-7, CO-08-97-977-EN) Comm Europ Commun BEL. *Dist:* Balogh, Bernan Associates.

Rules Governing Medicinal Products in the European Union Vol. V: Pharmaceutical Legislation/Veterinary Medicinal Products. European Communities Commission, Directorate-General for Industry, Pharmaceuticals and Cosmetics. 1997. (Eudralex Collection). 281p. pap. (92-828-2037-8, CO-08-97-864-EN) Comm Europ Commun BEL. *Dist:* Balogh, Bernan Associates.

Rules of Hope. James R. Averill et al. 1990. (Recent Research in Psychology Ser.). 134p. 44.95 (0-387-97219-6) Spr-Verlag.

Rules of Insanity: Moral Responsibility & the Mentally Ill. Carl Elliott. 1996. LC 95-34254. 143p. (C). pap. text 19.95 (0-7914-2952-0) State U NY Pr.

Rules of the Mind. John R. Anderson. 1993. 336p. pap. 32.50 (0-8058-1200-8); text 69.95 (0-8058-1199-0) L Erlbaum Assocs.

Rules That Babies Look By: The Organization of Newborn Visual Activity. Marshall M. Haith. 1980. LC 80-10601. (Child Psychology Ser.). (Illus.). 159p. text 29.95 (0-89859-033-7) L Erlbaum Assocs.

Rumen Microbes & Digestive Physiology in Ruminants: Satellite Symposium of the 8th Animal Science Congress, Kyoto October 1996. Ed. by Ryoji Onodera et al. 1997. LC 98-117971. (Illus.). x, 260p. text 222.75 (3-8055-6588-7) S Karger.

Ruminant Feed Evaluation & Utilisation. Ed. by D. I. Givens & J. M. Wilkinson. 1988. 110p. (Orig.). pap. text (0-948617-18-7) Chalcombe Pubns GBR. *Dist:* Scholium Intl.

Ruminant Pestivirus Infections: Virology, Pathogenesis, & Perspectives of Prophylaxis. Ed. by B. Liess et al. 1993. (Archives of Virology Ser.: Supplementum 3). (Illus.). 271p. 187.00 (0-387-82279-8) Spr-Verlag.

Runaway Learning Machine: Growing up Dyslexic. James J. Bauer. 1992. LC 92-71009. 96p. (C). pap. text 6.95 (0-932796-43-5) Ed Media Corp.

Running as Therapy: An Integrated Approach. Ed. by Michael L. Sachs & Gary W. Buffone. 1997. LC 97-16480. (Master Work Ser.). 360p. pap. text 50.00 (0-7657-0093-X) Aronson.

Running Hot: Structure & Stress in Ambulance Work. Donald L. Metz. 1984. 252p. reprint ed. lib. bdg. 23.50 (0-8191-4069-4) U Pr of Amer.

Running Injuries. Gary N. Guten. Ed. by Richard Lampert. 1997. LC 96-27149. (Illus.). 304p. text 58.00 (0-7216-6843-7) Saunders.

Running, Walking & Jumping: The Science of Locomotion. A. J. Dagg. 1977. 143p. pap. 18.00 (0-85109-530-5) Taylor & Francis.

Running Your Own Private Residential or Nursing Home. Colin M. Barron. 1990. 148p. 29.95 (1-85302-062-1) Taylor & Francis.

Ruptured Cerebral Aneurysm. Oliver D. Grin & Dorothy L. Bouwman. Ed. by Carol E. Roberts. rev. ed. 1989. (Patient Education Ser.). (Illus.). 26p. pap. text 4.00 (0-929689-36-4) Ludann Co.

Rupturierte Bauaortenaneurysma: Klinisches Expertengespraech Ueber Anaesthesie und Chirurgie, Hamburg, January 1993. Ed. by H. Imig. 1993. (Illus.). viii, 70p. pap. 33.25 (3-8055-5826-0) S Karger.

Rural Children in Selected Counties of North Carolina. U. S. Children's Bureau Staff. Ed. by Francis S. Bradley & Margaretta A. Williamson. 1969. LC 76-78778. (Illus.). 118p. reprint ed. lib. bdg. 55.00 (0-8371-1399-7, RCN&) Greenwood.

Rural Emergency Medical Services. 1990. lib. bdg. 75.00 (0-8490-4026-4) Gordon Pr.

Rural Health. N. D. Kamble. 1985. (0-8364-1327-X) Ashish Pub Hse IND. *Dist:* S Asia.

Rural Health: An Evolving System of Accessible Services. Tracey M. Orloff & Barbara Tymann. 1996. 293p. pap. 33.00 (1-55877-250-2) Natl Governor.

Rural Health & Aging Research: Theory, Methods & Practical Applications. NC Rural Aging Program Staff. Ed. by Wilbert M. Gesler et al. 1998. LC 97-28444. (Society & Aging Ser.). 248p. text 49.00 (0-89503-183-3) Baywood Pub.

Rural Health Care: Innovation in a Changing Environment. Ed. by LaVonne A. Straub & Norman L. Walzer. 1992. LC 92-11921. 240p. 55.00 (0-275-94315-1, C4315, Praeger Pubs) Greenwood.

Rural Health Challenges in the 1990s: Strategies from the Hospital-Based Rural Health Care Program. Karin Gillespie. Ed. by Victoria D. Weisfeld. 1996. 176p. (Orig.). (0-942054-10-5) R W Johnson Found.

Rural Health Nursing. Ed. by Patricia F. Winstead-Fry et al. 1991. 424p. 17.95 (0-88737-524-3) Natl League Nurse.

Rural Health Services: A Management Perspective. Ed. by Joyce E. Beaulieu & David E. Berry. 1994. LC 94-20578. 350p. pap. 20.50 (1-56793-018-2, 0948) Health Admin Pr.

***Rural Health Services Funding: A Resource Guide.** Jenny F. Harriman. rev. ed. 2001. 56p. (C). pap. text 25.00 (0-7567-1089-8) DIANE Pub.

Rural Healthcare. Ed. by Iain Mungall & Jim Cox. 1998. LC 99-187727. (Illus.). 184p. pap. (1-85775-267-8) Radcliffe Med Pr GBR. *Dist:* Balogh.

Rural Hospital: Its Structure & Organization. R. F. Bridgman. 1955. (Monographs: No. 21). (ENG & FRE., Illus.). 162p. pap. text 20.00 (92-4-140021-8, 1140021) World Health.

Rural Hospitals in Evolution: State Policy Issues & Initiatives. Stephen Phillips & John Luehrs. Ed. by Karen Glass. 1989. 40p. (Orig.). pap. text 20.00 (1-55877-067-4) Natl Governor.

Rural Psychology. Ed. by Alan W. Childs & Gary B. Melton. 1983. 458p. 75.00 (0-306-41045-1, Plenum Trade) Perseus Pubng.

Rural Rescue & Emergency Care. Ed. by Robert Worsing. 1993. (Illus.). 368p. pap. text 36.95 (0-89203-075-5, 075-5) Jones & Bartlett.

Rural Water Supplies. 1983. (Euro Reports & Studies Ser.: No. 87). 66p. pap. text 7.00 (92-890-1253-6) World Health.

Rush University Review of Surgery. Steven G. Economou et al. 2nd ed. 1993. LC 93-6622. (Illus.). 512p. pap. text 42.00 (0-7216-3780-9) Saunders.

Rush University Review of Surgery. Daniel J. Deziel et al. 3rd ed. 1999. LC 99-23140. (Illus.). 575p. (C). pap. text 47.95 (0-7216-7581-6) Saunders.

***Russ Coile's Health Care Forecast: Special Report.** Russell C. Coile, Jr. 2001. pap. (0-8342-1872-0) Aspen Pub.

Russell & Rubinstein's Pathology of Tumors of the Nervous System Ed. by Darell D. Bigner et al. 6th ed. 1998. LC 97-37688. (An Arnold Publication). (Illus.). 1424p. text (0-340-58113-1) E A GBR. *Dist:* OUP.

Russian-Arabic Medical Dictionary. G. T. Arslanian. 1983. (ARA & RUS.). 622p. 49.95 (0-8288-1158-X, M15440) Fr & Eur.

Russian Emergency Services Directory. Global Investment and Business Center, Inc. Staff. (Russian Business Library: Vol. 27). (Illus.). 350p. 2000. pap. 99.95 (0-7397-3076-2); 1999. pap. 99.00 (0-7397-0627-6) Intl Business Pubns.

Russian-English Medical Dictionary Phrase Book. V. I. Petrov. 3rd ed. 1993. 595p. 95.00 (0-7859-9075-5) Fr & Eur.

Russian-English Medical Dictionary Phrase-Book. V. I. Petrov et al. 3rd ed. 1993. 596p. (C). reprint ed. 32.95 (0-8285-5177-4) Firebird NY.

Russian-English Veterinary Dictionary. R. Mack. 1972. 104p. (Orig.). (C). (0-89771-927-1) Collets GBR. *Dist:* St Mut.

Russian Health Care Crisis: History, Evaluation, & Recommendations. David E. Powell. 1997. (Twentieth Century Fund Bk.). 120p. (C). pap. 9.95 (0-87078-373-4) Century Foundation.

Russian Industry: Medical Equipment Industry. 2nd rev. ed. 1996. (Russian & Nis Industrial Directories Ser.). (Illus.). 250p. pap. 99.00 (1-57751-120-4) Intl Business Pubns.

Russian Industry-97: Medical Equipment. Russian Information and Business Center, Inc. Staff. 3rd ed. 1997. (Russian Industrial Directories Ser.: Vol. 17). 400p. pap. 99.00 (1-57751-266-9) Intl Business Pubns.

Russian Medical Equipment Industry: Company Name, Address, Number of Employees, CEO, Phone, Fax, Main Products... And More, Set. Contrib. by Global Investment and Business Center, Inc. Staff & International Business Publications Staff. 2000. (Russian Industrial & Business Library: Vol. 46). (Illus.). 350p. pap. 99.95 (0-7397-3466-0) Intl Business Pubns.

Russian Medical Services & Recreation Facilities Directory, '96. 1996. (Russian Business Library). 300p. (Orig.). pap. 99.00 (1-57751-018-6) Intl Business Pubns.

Russian Medical Services Directory. Global Investment and Business Center, Inc. Staff. (Russian Business Library: Vol. 28). (Illus.). 350p. 2000. pap. 99.95 (0-7397-3077-0); 1999. pap. 99.00 (0-7397-0628-4) Intl Business Pubns.

Russian Medicine. William A. Gantt. 1978. LC 75-23669. (Clio Medica Ser.: 20). (Illus.). reprint ed. 40.00 (0-404-58920-0) AMS Pr.

Russian Psychology: Past, Present & Future. Ed. by Elena L. Grigorenko et al. 1996. LC 97-150898. 457p. (C). lib. bdg. 85.00 (1-56072-389-0) Nova Sci Pubs.

Russian Psychology in Transition: Interviews with Moscow Psychologists. Maureen Cote. 1998. LC 98-29055. 75.00 (1-56072-601-6) Nova Sci Pubs.

Rutgers University College of Pharmacy: A Centennial History. David L. Cowen & Roy A. Bowers. 1991. LC 90-39149. (Illus.). 175p. (C). text 35.00 (0-8135-1634-X) Rutgers U Pr.

Rx: For a Liberated Childbirth. Bev Smucha & Alice Unger. Ed. by Evie Heilbrun. 1979. LC 77-80302. 19.95 (0-87949-098-5) Ashley Bks.

RX 2000 see Our Medical Future: Breakthroughs in Health & Longevity by the Year 2000 & Beyond

RX & OTC Cough & Cold Products. Ed. by Peter Allen. 1985. 206p. pap. text 2955.00 (0-931634-51-2) FIND-SVP.

Rx Factor: Strategic Creativity in Pharmaceutical Marketing. Pavan Choudary. 1997. LC 97-18645. 26.00 (0-8039-9378-1) Sage.

***Rx Facts: Drug Interactions.** Ed. by Facts and Comparisons Staff. 2001. (Drug Interaction Facts). per. 7.95 (1-57439-101-1) Facts & Comparisons.

Rx for Living! Cofactors: The Bridge Between Medicine & Healing. Jay M. Stinson. 1998. LC 97-97228. (Illus.). 220p. (Orig.). pap. text 19.95 (0-9663067-0-8) Pollywog Pr.

Rx for the Soul: Moments from a Physician's Practice That Brings Inspiration & Encouragement. David B. Wilhelm. 1997. LC 96-40023. 228p. pap. 10.99 (0-7852-7245-3) Nelson.

RX: Prescription for the Boards: Usmle Step 2: A Student-to-Student Guide. Kate C. Feibusch & Radhika S. Breaden. 2nd ed. 1998. LC 98-25208. 496p. pap. text 32.95 (0-7817-1427-3) Lppncott W & W.

Ryan: A Mother's Story of Her Hyperactive-Tourette Syndrome Child. Susan Hughes. 1990. LC 89-83295. 160p. (Orig.). 14.95 (1-878267-25-6); pap. 9.95 (1-878267-26-4) Hope Pr CA.

Ryan's Occupational Therapy Assistant. Sally E. Ryan & Karen Sladyk. 3rd ed. 2000. 80p. pap. text (1-55642-514-7) SLACK Inc.

Rycroft on Analysis Creativity. Charles Rycroft. 1992. 192p. (C). pap. text 19.50 (0-8147-7428-8) NYU Pr.

***Rypins' Basic Sciences Review.** Harold Rypins & Edward D. Frohlich. 18th ed. 2001. LC 00-69648. (Illus.). xvi, 810p. pap. text 39.95 (0-7817-2518-6) Lppncott W & W.

S

***S-EMG Muscular Assessment Reference Manual.** Gabriel E. Sella. 2001. 25.00 (1-884325-16-5) G E Sella.

S. T. A. R. Instructor's Guide. Sheila Greeley. 1992. 65p. (Orig.). spiral bd. 15.95 (0-9622812-0-4) FAFCTPC.

S. T. A. R. Strategic Thinking & Reading. Rhonda Holt Atkinson et al. 1996. LC 96-21078. 500p. (J). mass mkt. 38.00 net. (0-314-20181-5) West Pub.

S-V Forty Viruses. Keerti V. Shah et al. 1973. (Illus.). 220p. (C). text 30.50 (0-8422-7064-7) Irvington.

Sabiston Essentials of Surgery. Ed. by David C. Sabiston, Jr. & H. Kim Lyerly. 2nd rev. ed. 1994. LC 93-33972. pap. text 43.00 (0-7216-5019-8) Saunders.

Sabiston Textbook of Surgery: The Biological Basis of Modern Surgical Practice. Courtney M. Townsend, Jr. et al. 16th ed. 2000. LC 00-30778. (Illus.). 2175p. text 125.00 (0-7216-8269-3) Saunders.

***Sabiston Textbook of Surgery: The Biological Basis of Modern Surgical Practice, Pocket Companion.** Courtney M. Townsend, Jr. 2001. (Illus.). 2175p. (0-7216-9279-6) Saunders.

Sabiston's Review of Surgery. Courtney M. Townsend, Jr. et al. 3rd ed. 2001. LC 00-46406. viii, 167p. text (0-7216-9258-3) Saunders.

Saccadic Eye Movements in Neurological & Ophthalmological Diagnosis. Otmar Meienberg. 1988. (Neurology Ser.: Vol. 29). (Illus.). xii, 115p. 94.95 (0-387-18547-X) Spr-Verlag.

Saccharin: Current Status. Ed. by L. Goldberg & D. M. Conning. 1985. (Illus.). 148p. pap. (0-08-032009-0, H221, H120) PPL GBR. *Dist:* Elsevier.

Saccharin & Its Health Risk Controversy: Index of New Information. American Health Research Institute Staff. Date not set. 160p. 57.50 (0-7883-1860-8); pap. 47.50 (0-7883-1861-6) ABBE Pubs Assn.

Sacred Leaves of Candomble: African Magic, Medicine, & Religion in Brazil. Robert A. Voeks. 1997. LC 96-51297. (Illus.). 256p. pap. 17.95 (0-292-78731-6) U of Tex Pr.

Sacred Mushroom Seeker: Tributes to R. Gordon Wasson. Terence McKenna et al. Ed. by Thomas J. Riedlinger. 1997. LC 96-54885. (Illus.). 304p. pap. 24.95 (0-89281-338-5, Heal Arts VT) Inner Tradit.

Sacred Plant Medicine: Explorations in Indigenous Herbalism. Stephen H. Buhner. 1996. LC 96-67085. (Illus.). 240p. pap. text 18.95 (1-57098-091-8) Roberts Rinehart.

***Sacred Plant Medicine: Explorations in the Practice of Indigenous Herbalism.** Stephen Buhner. 2001. 210p. pap. 18.95 (0-9708696-0-6) Raven Pr ID.

Sacred Plant Medicine: Explorations in the Practice of Indigenous Herbalism. Stephen H. Buhner. 1996. (Illus.). 240p. 30.00 (1-57098-085-3) Roberts Rinehart.

Sacred Space: Stories from a Life in Medicine. Clif Cleaveland. 1998. LC 97-36741. 210p. text 21.95 (0-943126-64-9) Amer Coll Phys.

Sadomasochism: Etiology & Treatment. Suzanne P. Schad-Somers. 1996. LC 95-52080. (Master Work Ser.). 304p. pap. 50.00 (1-56821-789-7) Aronson.

Safe Alternatives in Childbirth. David Stewart et al. 4th rev. ed. 1992. LC 76-19336. 268p. pap. 12.95 (0-934426-47-3) NAPSAC Reprods.

Safe & Good Use of Blood in Surgery (Sanguis) Use of Blood Products & Artifical Colloids in 43 European Hospitals, No. EUR 15398. Girolamo Sirchia et al. 1994. (Illus.). 235p. (92-826-4118-X, CD-NA-15-398ENC) Comm Europ Commun BEL. *Dist:* Bernan Associates.

Safe & Healthy: A Parent's Guide to Children's Illnesses & Accidents. William M. Sears. 1989. (Growing Family Ser.). 239p. (Orig.). pap. 8.95 (0-912500-22-0) La Leche.

Safe & Sound. Elena Bosque & Sheila Watson. rev. ed. 1997. LC 96-34318. (Illus.). 160p. pap. 10.95 (0-312-15204-3) St Martin.

Safe & Voluntary Surgical Contraception: Guidelines for Service Programs. AVSC International Staff. 1997. 104p. reprint ed. pap. text 8.00 (1-885063-06-7) EngenderHlth.

Safe Choices Guide: AIDS & HIV Policies & Prevention Programs for High-Risk Youth. National Network of Runaway and Youth Services Staff. 1990. 252p. ring bd. 30.00 (1-878848-01-1) Natl Res Ctr.

Safe Current Limits for Electromedical Apparatus. 3rd ed. 1993. (AAMI Technical Information Report Ser.). 14p. pap. 70.00 (1-57020-007-6, ES1-209) Assn Adv Med Instrn.

Safe Handling Cytotoxic Drugs: An Independent Study Module. Carol S. Blecher et al. Ed. by Jacqueline Welch & Joyce M. Silveria. rev. ed. 1997. (Illus.). 20p. pap. text 15.00 (1-890504-00-9) Oncology Nursing.

Safe in the Sun. Mary E. Siegel. rev. ed. 1995. LC 95-9685. 96p. pap. 8.95 (0-8027-7459-8) Walker & Co.

Safe Medical Devices Act of 1990: A Legislative History of Public Law No. 101-629, Set. Ed. by Bernard D. Reams. 1996. LC 96-75096. (Federal Health Law Ser.: Part 10). 490.00 (1-57588-093-8, 309070) W S Hein.

Safe Medical Devices Act of 1990: Implications for Healthcare Personnel. 1992. 101p. pap. 95.00 (1-57020-053-X, MDR91-209) Assn Adv Med Instrn.

Safe Passage Questioned: Medical Care & Safety for the Polar Tourist. Ed. by John M. Levinson & Errol Ger. 1998. LC 97-41984. (Illus.). 192p. pap. 24.95 (0-87033-504-9) Cornell Maritime.

Safe Place: A Journal for Women with Breast Cancer. Jennifer Pike. rev. ed. 1999. LC 98-32412. 216p. reprint ed. spiral bd. 22.95 (0-8118-2267-2) Chronicle Bks.

Safe Place: Laying the Groundwork of Psychotherapy. Leston L. Havens. 1996. 192p. pap. 12.00 (0-674-00086-2) HUP.

Safe Return Home: An Inspirational Book for Caregivers of Alzheimer's Patients. Tom Batiuk & Chuck Ayers. 1998. LC 98-3785. 112p. 12.95 (0-8362-6913-6) Andrews McMeel.

Safe Use of Pesticides. 1985. (Technical Reports: No. 720). 60p. pap. text 6.00 (92-4-120720-5, 1100720) World Health.

Safe Use of Pesticides: Proceedings of the WHO Expert Committee on Insecticides, 20th, Geneva, 1972. WHO Staff. 1973. (Technical Reports: No. 513). pap. text 6.00 (92-4-120513-X, 1100513) World Health.

Safe Use of Pesticides: Third Report of the WHO Expert Committee on Vector Biology & Control. 1979. (Technical Report Ser.: No. 634). 44p. pap. text 5.00 (92-4-120634-9, 1100634) World Health.

Safe Use of Pesticides in Public Health: Sixteenth Report of the WHO Expert Committee on Insecticides. 1967. (Technical Report Ser.: No. 356). 65p. pap. text 5.00 (92-4-120356-0, 1100356) World Health.

Safe Use of Radioactive Tracers in Industrial Processes. 1974. (Safety Ser.: No. 40). 54p. (Orig.). pap. (92-0-123074-5, ISP369) IAEA AUT. *Dist:* Bernan Associates.

Safe Use of Vitamin A. J. Christopher Bauernfeind. Ed. by G. Arroyave et al. 1980. (Illus.). 44p. (Orig.). pap. text 3.50 (0-935368-24-8) ILSI.

Safe Uses of Cortisol. William M. Jefferies. 2nd ed. 1996. (Illus.). 228p. 58.95 (0-398-06620-5); pap. 41.95 (0-398-06621-3) C C Thomas.

Safe Work in the 21st Century: Education & Training Needs for the Next Decade's Occupational Safety & Health Personnel. Institute of Medicine Staff & Board on Health Sciences Staff. 2000. LC 00-55005. (Illus.). xxi, 242p. pap. 44.00 (0-309-07026-0) Natl Acad Pr.

Safeguarding the Public Health. Stuart Galishoff. 1975. LC 75-66. (Illus.). 191p. 62.50 (0-8371-7956-4, GPH/, Greenwood Pr) Greenwood.

Safer Childbirth? A Critical History of Maternity Care. Marjorie Tew. 1990. 250p. pap. 32.50 (0-412-33740-1, A4423) Chapman & Hall.

Safer Death: Multidisciplinary Aspects of Terminal Care. Ed. by A. Gilmore & S. Gilmore. 1988. LC 88-12414. (Illus.). 228p. 75.00 (0-306-42912-8, Plenum Trade) Perseus Pubng.

Safer Prescribing: A Guide to Some Problems in the Use of Drugs. Linda Beeley. 5th ed. 1991. 128p. pap. 16.95 (0-632-03292-8) Blackwell Sci.

Safer Sex: Guidelines to Live By. David Wiemers & Paul Turner. 1995. (Illus.). 32p. (Orig.). pap. 4.95 (0-9648684-0-7) InfoPlus.

Safer Sex: How Safe Is Safe? Christina Dye. rev. ed. 2000. pap. 0.50 (0-89230-221-6) Do It Now.

Safer Sex Photobook: Photographs & Video Prints. Wieland Speck & Harry Cane. 1997. (Illus.). 62p. (C). reprint ed. pap. text 10.00 (0-7881-5072-3) DIANE Pub.

Safety & Clinical Efficacy of Implanted Neuroaugmentive Devices. Ed. by Philip L. Gildenberg. 1978. (Applied Neurophysiology Ser.: Vol. 40, Nos. 2-4). (Illus.). pap. 50.50 (3-8055-2925-2) S Karger.

Safety & Efficacy of Radiopharmaceuticals. Ed. by Knud Kristensen & Elisabeth Norbygaard. 1983. (Developments in Nuclear Medicine Ser.). text 206.50 (0-89838-609-8) Kluwer Academic.

Safety & Efficacy of Radiopharmaceuticals, 1987. Ed. by Knud Kristensen & Elisabeth Norbygaard. 1987. (Developments in Nuclear Medicine Ser.). (C). text 234.00 (0-89838-986-0) Kluwer Academic.

Safety & Environmental Training: Using Compliance to Improve Your Company. Dawn A. Baldwin. 1992. LC 92-15212. 256p. text 60.95 (0-442-01066-4, VNR) Wiley.

Safety & Equipment Risks: Do You Prevent Injuries? Meridith B. Cox. 1991. (Orig.). (C). pap. text 55.00 (0-912665-24-6) BusinessWatch.

Safety & Health in the Use of Agrochemicals: A Guide. 1991. v, 79p. (Orig.). pap. 22.50 (92-2-107281-9) Intl Labour Office.

Safety & Health of Migrant Workers: International Symposium. 1983. (Occupational Safety & Health Ser.: No. 41). 337p. 27.00 (92-2-001906-X) Intl Labour Office.

Safety & Health Program. Mark M. Moran. 1992. (OSHA Written Compliance Programs Ser.: No. 24). (Illus.). 37p. ring bd. 169.00 (1-890966-18-5) SafetyCertified.

Safety & Health Requirements Manual 1994. lib. bdg. 650.95 (0-8490-8509-8) Gordon Pr.

***Safety & Health Resource Guide for Small Business.** Barry Leonard. 2001. 51p. (C). pap. text 20.00 (0-7567-0861-3) DIANE Pub.

Safety & Infection Control. SPC Staff. 1997. LC 97-27724. (Healthcare Professional Guides: Vol. 6). (Illus.). 288p. spiral bd. 26.95 (0-87434-916-8) Springhouse Corp.

Safety & Security Administration in Health Care Facilities: Forms, Checklists & Guidelines. Aspen Reference Group Staff. Ed. by Sara N. Di Lima & Dwayne E. Eutsey. 1995. LC 94-48768. ring bd. 220.00 (0-8342-0657-9) Aspen Pub.

Safety & the Executive. James V. Findlay. LC 79-54954. (Illus.). 128p. 18.00 (0-88061-008-5) Intl Loss Cntrl.

Safety Assessment for Pharmaceuticals. Ed. by Shayne C. Gad. 512p. 1995. text 92.95 (0-442-00123-1); 1994. 125.00 (0-471-28385-1) Wiley (VNR).

Safety at Scene: Manual for Paramedics & Immediate Care Doctors. Vic Calland. 2000. LC 00-58233. (Illus.). xi, 226p. (0-7234-3199-X) Mosby Inc.

Safety Engineer. Jack Rudman. 1994. (Career Examination Ser.: C-797). pap. 34.95 (0-8373-0797-X) Nat Learn.

Safety Evaluation of Biotechnologically-Derived Pharmaceuticals: Facilitating a Scientific Approach. Ed. by Susan A. Griffiths & Cyndy E. Lumley. 1998. LC 98-196381. (Centre for Medicines Research Workshop Ser.). 200p. 95.00 (0-7923-8732-5) Kluwer Academic.

Safety Evaluation of Chemicals in Food Pt. 1: Toxicological Data Profiles for Pesticides: Carbamate & Organophosphorus Insecticides Used in Agriculture & Public Health. 1975. (Progress in Standardization: No. 3). pap. text 10.00 (92-4-068522-7, 1260003) World Health.

Safety Evaluation of Drugs & Chemicals. Ed. by W. Eugene Lloyd. 1986. LC 84-12912. (Illus.). 487p. (C). text 140.00 (0-89116-352-2) Hemisp Pub.

Safety Evaluation of Medical Devices. A. Gad. 1997. LC 96-53470. (Illus.). 400p. text 185.00 (0-8247-9827-9) Dekker.

Safety for the Forensic Identification Specialist. Nancy E. Masters. 1995. LC 95-75630. (Illus.). 258p. (C). pap. 39.95 (0-9622305-1-0) Lightning Powder.

Safety in Clinical & Biomedical Laboratories. Ed. by C. H. Collins. 1988. (Illus.). 176p. (Orig.). (C). (gr. 13). pap. 37.95 (0-412-28370-0) Chapman & Hall.

Safety in Electromedical Technology. Norbert Leitgeb. 1996. (Illus.). 184p. 119.00 (1-57491-014-0) IHS Health Grp.

Safety in Numbers: Safer Sex & Gay Men. Edward King. 1993. LC 93-5200. (Lesbian & Gay Studies). 288p. text 90.00 (0-304-32699-2) Continuum.

Safety in the Use of Asbestos: An ILO Code of Practice. 1990. xiii, 116p. pap. 18.00 (92-2-103872-6) Intl Labour Office.

Safety in the Use of Asbestos: Proceedings of the International Labour Conference, 72nd Session, 1986, Report IV. 1985. 68p. (Orig.). pap. 13.50 (92-2-105174-9) Intl Labour Office.

Safety Management for Health Care Facilities. Linda D. Lee. 1989. (Management & Compliance Ser.: Vol. 5). (Illus.). 275p. ring bd. 110.00 (0-87258-512-3, 055204) Am Hospital.

Safety Manual on Magnetic Resonance Imaging Contrast Agents. Emanuel Kanal & Frank G. Shellock. 1995. LC 95-33162. pap. (0-397-51619-3) Lppncott W & W.

Safety Measures for Use in Outbreaks of Communicable Disease. Donald J. Dunsmore. 1986. 99p. pap. text 17.00 (92-4-154206-3, 1150250) World Health.

Safety Meetings for Health Care Workers. Barbara Kelly et al. 1996. LC 98-203746. (1-55645-044-3) Busn Legal Reports.

Safety, Nutrition & Health. Robertson. 1998. (Early Childhood Education Ser.). 64p. tchr. ed. 12.00 (0-8273-7330-9) Delmar.

Safety, Nutrition and, Health In Early Education. Robertson. 1998. LC 97-41064. (Early Childhood Education Ser.). 528p. (C). pap. text 64.95 (0-8273-7329-5) Delmar.

Safety of Anaesthetic Drugs. 104p. pap. text (0-86471-045-3) Adis Intl NZL. *Dist:* Lppncott W & W.

Safety of Diagnostic Ultrasound. Ed. by Stanley B. Barnett & George Kossoff. 1997. LC 97-38076. (Progress in Obstetric & Gynecological Sonography Ser.). 158p. lib. bdg. 85.95 (1-85070-646-8, Parthenon Pbng) CRC Pr.

Safety of Irradiated Foods. J. F. Diehl. 2nd ed. 1995. LC 95-9488. (Food Science & Technology Ser.: Vol. 68). (Illus.). 464p. text 199.00 (0-8247-9344-7) Dekker.

Safety of Silicone Breast Implants. Institute of Medicine Staff. Ed. by Stuart Bondurant et al. 2000. LC 99-40812. xvi, 540p. 49.00 (0-309-06532-1) Natl Acad Pr.

S

S

Safety of the Blood Supply: Report of a Roundtable Discussion. Robert E. Stein. 1992. 24p. pap. 20.00 (*0-933067-12-7*) Roscoe Pound Inst.

Safety Performance Management. George L. Germain. (Illus.). 38p. ring bd. 57.50 (*0-88061-019-0*) Intl Loss Cntrl.

Safety Policies & Procedures for Health Care Facilities. John S. Klare. 1992. (Orig.). pap. 100.00 (*0-87258-593-X*, 055452) Am Hospital.

***Safety Standards & Infection Control for Dental Hygienists.** Ellen Dietz & Raula Badavinac. 2002. 368p. text 38.95 (*0-7668-2660-0*) Delmar.

***Safety Standards for Infection Control for Dental Assistants.** Ellen Dietz. 2001. LC 2001-53763. 352p. pap. 33.95 (*0-7668-2659-7*) Delmar.

Safety with Lasers & Other Optical Sources: A Comprehensive Handbook. D. Sliney & M. L. Wolbarsht. 1980. LC 80-16591. (Illus.). 1064p. (C). text 135.00 (*0-306-40434-6*, Kluwer Plenum) Kluwer Academic.

Saffron Scourge: A History of Yellow Fever in Louisiana, 1796-1905. Jo A. Carrigan. 1993. LC 93-73292. (Illus.). 480p. (C). 27.50 (*0-940984-86-5*) Univ LA Lafayette.

Saga of a Surgeon: The Life of Daniel Brainard, M. D. Janet Kinney. 1987. LC 87-62176. (Medical Humanities Ser.). (Illus.). 246p. (C). 17.95 (*0-931369-20-7*) Southern IL Univ Sch.

SAGES Manual: Fundamentals of Laparoscopy & GI Endoscopy. Ed. by Carol E. H. Scott-Conner. 1998. LC 98-29512. (Illus.). 622p. pap. 53.95 (*0-387-98496-8*) Spr-Verlag.

St. Anthony's Clinical Coder. Marleeta K. Jones & Connie Johnson. Ed. by Karen M. Schmidt. 1996. 210p. (C). (*1-56329-347-1*) Ingenix Inc.

St. Anthony's Color-Coded Compact ICD-9-CM Code Book for Physician Payment Ed. by Laurie Castillo & Catherine Hopkins. 1996. 1418p. 49.95 (*1-56329-356-0*) Ingenix Inc.

St. Anthony's DRG Guidebook (DRG) Ed. by Cathleen Culbertson & Karen Schmidt. 1997. 620p. pap. 79.95 (*1-56329-470-2*) Ingenix Inc.

1999 Drg Guidebook. Ed. by Cathleen Culbertson & Karen Schmidt. rev. ed. 1999. 620p. (C). pap. 79.95 (*1-56329-571-7*) Thomson Learn.

St. Anthony's DRG Optimizer (OPT) Ed. by Cay Moriarity & Julia Palmer. rev. ed. 1997. 400p. pap. 149.00 (*1-56329-497-4*) Ingenix Inc.

St. Anthony's Guide to E/M Coding & Documentation (RGEM) rev. ed. 1999. 500p. (C). pap. 129.00 (*1-56329-533-4*) Thomson Learn.

St. Anthony's Guide to Radiology Managed Care & Capitation: Radiology, Diagnostic Imaging, Radiation Therapy. Michael J. Monea. Ed. by Jay Lechtman & John F. Persinos. Date not set. 200p. (C). 349.00 (*1-56329-312-9*) Ingenix Inc.

St. Anthony's HCPCS Level II Code Book (HBIN) Ed. by Anita Hart & Laurie Castillo. 1998. 375p. pap. 49.95 (*1-56329-473-7*) Ingenix Inc.

St. Anthony's HCPCS Level II Code Book (HBK) Ed. by Anita Hart & Laurie Castillo. rev. ed. 1998. 540p. spiral bd. 85.00 (*1-56329-474-5*) Ingenix Inc.

St. Anthony's HCPCS Level II Codebook - Short Version: HBIN. Ed. by Laurie Castillo & Carol Endahl. 1997. (C). (*1-56329-390-0*) Ingenix Inc.

St. Anthony's HCPCS Level II Codebook: HBK. Ed. by Laurie Castillo & Carol Endahl. 1997. (C). 75.00 (*1-56329-389-7*) Ingenix Inc.

St. Anthony's I-9 Express, ICD-9-CM Softbound Codebook for Physician Payment (REZ) 1999. 600p. (C). pap. 99.95 (*1-56329-561-X*) Thomson Learn.

St. Anthony's ICD-9-CM Code Book Ed. by Karen Schmidt et al. 1997. 1300p. pap. 69.95 (*1-56329-432-X*) Ingenix Inc.

St. Anthony's ICD-9-CM Code Book for Home Health Services, Nursing Homes & Hospices. Ed. by Karen Schmidt & Anita Hart. 1997. 1250p. 125.00 (*1-56329-427-3*) Ingenix Inc.

St. Anthony's ICD-9-CM Code Books for Physician's Payment, Vol. 1 & 2. 1996. (*0-8273-8249-9*) Delmar.

St. Anthony's ICD-9-CM Code Books for Physician's Payment, Vol. 1 & 2. St. Anthony's. 1996. (*0-8273-8248-0*) Delmar.

St. Anthony's ICD-9-CM Code Books for Physician's Payment, Vol. 1 & 2. St. Anthony's Staff. 1996. pap. (*0-8273-8247-2*) Delmar.

St. Anthony's Illustrated ICD-9-CM Code Book (SIAS) 1999. 500p. (C). pap. 99.95 (*1-56329-596-2*) Thomson Learn.

St. Anthony's Illustrated ICD-9-CM Code Book for Physician Payment. Ed. by Laurie Castillo & Catherine Hopkins. 1997. (Illus.). 1110p. pap. 79.95 (*1-56329-424-9*) Ingenix Inc.

St. Anthony's Illustrated ICD-9-CM Code Book Ed. by Karen Schmidt & Anita Hart. 1997. (Illus.). 1630p. 195.00 (*1-56329-430-3*) Ingenix Inc.

St. Anthony's Integrated Health Care Directory. Ed. by Susan Namovicz-Peat & Mary Darby. 2nd ed. Date not set. 600p. (C). 595.00 (*1-56329-319-6*) Ingenix Inc.

St. Anthony's Medicare Billing Compliance Guide. Carol F. Endahl. Ed. by Karen M. Schmidt & Paul H. Hubbard. Date not set. 200p. 259.00 (*1-56329-323-4*) Ingenix Inc.

St. Anthony's Medicare Correct Coding & Payment Manual for Procedures & Services. Ed. by Anita Hart & Sheila R. Parvis. 1999. 450p. (C). 279.00 (*1-56329-407-9*) Ingenix Inc.

St. Anthony's Reengineering the Medical Practice: Profit Through Efficiency in a Medical Office Environment. Jon Hultman. rev. ed. 1996. (Illus.). 206p. 199.00 (*1-56329-308-0*) Ingenix Inc.

St. Anthony's Reimbursement Guide to Radiology Services, 1992. E. Lorenz. 1992. 340p. (C). ring bd. 177.00 (*1-56329-093-6*, SRA) Ingenix Inc.

St. Anthony's Softbound ICD-9-CM Code Book for Physician Payment Ed. by Laurie Castillo & Catherine Hopkins. 1996. 982p. 59.95 (*1-56329-353-6*) Ingenix Inc.

St. Anthony's Spiral ICD-9-CM Code Book for Physician Payment Ed. by Laurie Castillo & Catherine Hopkins. 1996. 982p. 59.95 (*1-56329-354-4*) Ingenix Inc.

St. Anthony's Spiral ICD-9-CM Codebook for Physician Payment (RSIS) 1999. 800p. (C). pap. 69.95 (*1-56329-556-3*) Thomson Learn.

St. Anthony's Standard ICD-9-CM Code Book Ed. by Karen Schmidt & Anita Hart. 1997. 1250p. 49.95 (*1-56329-426-5*) Ingenix Inc.

St. Anthony's Three-in-One Code Book for ENT: 1993 Edition. Ed. by Kathy Brouch. 1992. 167.00 (*1-56329-110-X*, SEN) Ingenix Inc.

St. Anthony's UB-92 Editor. Carol F. Endahl & Greg Britt. Ed. by Julia R. Palmer. Date not set. (Illus.). 600p. 199.00 (*1-56329-385-4*) Ingenix Inc.

St. Anthony's Updatable ICD-9-CM Code Book for Outpatient Services. Ed. by Karen Schmidt & Lolita Jones. 1997. 1282p. 139.00 (*1-56329-428-1*) Ingenix Inc.

St. Anthony's Updatable ICD-9-CM Code Book Ed. by Karen Schmidt et al. 1997. 1300p. 139.00 (*1-56329-433-8*) Ingenix Inc.

St. Anthony's Version 2.0 APG Guidebook, 1997. Lolita M. Jones. 1997. 410p. pap. 79.00 (*1-56329-388-9*) Ingenix Inc.

St. Elizabeth Hospital: Looking Back, Looking Forward. Margaret Finnerty. Ed. by Rodney Nelson & Amy Phillips. 1993. 110p. (C). 25.00 (*0-929690-18-4*) Herit Pubs AZ.

Saint-Frances Guide to Cardiology. Andrew Michaels et al. 2000. LC 00-56541. (Illus.). 400p. pap. text 25.95 (*0-683-30660-X*) Lppncott W & W.

Saint-Frances Guide to Outpatient Medicine. Stephen A. Benton et al. 1999. LC 99-24904. (Illus.). 550p. 19.95 (*0-683-30187-X*) Lppncott W & W.

Saint-Frances Guide to Psychiatry. Malia McCarthy et al. 2000. LC 00-45340. (Illus.). 300p. pap. text 25.95 (*0-683-30661-8*) Lppncott W & W.

St. John's Tower & Health Care Facility: An Architectural Evaluation. William F. Gartz et al. Ed. by Gary T. Moore. 1987. (Publications in Architecture & Urban Planning: No. R81-7). (Illus.). iv, 135p. reprint ed. 13.00 (*0-938744-20-8*) U of Wis Ctr Arch-Urban.

St. John's Wort: The Herbal Way to Feeling Good. Norman Rosenthal. 2000. 235p. text 24.00 (*0-7881-9143-8*) DIANE Pub.

St. John's Wort: The Miracle Medicine. Alan H. Pressman & Nancy Burke. 1998. LC 98-223315. 224p. mass mkt. 5.99 (*0-440-22605-8*) Dell.

St. Kitts Vervet. Ed. by M. T. McGuire. 1974. (Contributions to Primatology Ser.: Vol. 1). 202p. 48.75 (*3-8055-1692-4*) S Karger.

Saints, Scholars & Schizophrenics: Mental Illness in Rural Ireland. Nancy Scheper-Hughes. 1979. 259p. pap. 18.95 (*0-520-04786-9*) U CA Pr.

Salary Survey, 1992. Medical Library Association Staff. 1992. 39p. pap. 52.00 (*0-912176-33-4*) Med Lib Assn.

Sale of Body Parts by the People's Republic of China. U. S. Government Printing Office Staff. 1998. LC 98-215434. v, 184 p. (*0-16-057455-2*) USGPO.

Saline Solution Video Participant's Guide: Sharing Christ in a Busy Practice. Walter L. Larimore & William C. Peel. 2000. (Illus.). 160p. pap., wbk. ed. 9.99 (*0-9666809-4-4*) Christ Med & Dental Assns.

Saliva: Composition & Secretion. Ira L. Shannon & R. P. Suddick. Ed. by M. Myers Howard. 1974. (Monographs in Oral Science: Vol. 2). (Illus.). 135p. 42.75 (*3-8055-1455-7*) S Karger.

Salivary Gland Biogenesis & Function Vol. 842: Annals of the New York Academy of Sciences. Ed. by Maria A. Kukuruzinska & Lawrence A. Tabak. 1998. LC 98-15976. (Annals of the New York Academy of Sciences Ser.: No. 842). 232p. 110.00 (*1-57331-135-9*); pap. 110.00 (*1-57331-136-7*) NY Acad Sci.

Salivary Gland Tumours. Ed. by J. Klijanienko & P. Vielh. 2000. (Monographs in Clinical Cytology Ser.: Vol. 15). (Illus.). xii, 142p. 172.25 (*3-8055-7024-4*) S Karger.

Salivary System. Ed. by Leo M. Sreebny. 1987. LC 87-5139. 256p. 140.00 (*0-8493-6689-5*, QP188, CRC Reprint) Franklin.

Salmonella. Rufus K. Guthrie. 1991. 240p. 131.95 (*0-8493-5419-6*, QR201) CRC Pr.

Salmonella: A Practical Approach to the Organism & Its Control in Foods. Chris Bell & Alec Kyriakides. 2001. LC 00-66804. (Illus.). 200p. pap. 39.95 (*0-632-05519-7*) Blackwell Sci.

Salmonella Enterica Serovar Enteritidis in Humans & Animals: The Epidemiology, Pathogenesis & Control. Ed. by A. M. Saeed et al. 1999. LC 98-39318. (Illus.). 464p. (C). text 159.95 (*0-8138-2707-8*) Iowa U Pr.

Salmonid Ecosystems of the North Pacific. Ed. by William J. McNeil & Daniel C. Himsworth. 1980. LC 80-17800. (Illus.). 348p. pap. 26.95 (*0-87071-335-3*) Oreg St U Pr.

Salmonid Reproduction: Review Papers from an International Symposium. Ed. by Robert N. Iwamoto & Stacia Sower. 1985. LC 85-13764. (Illus.). viii, 167p. (Orig.). pap. text 10.00 (*0-934539-00-6*, WSG-WO85-2) Wash Sea Grant.

Salt & Hypertension. Ed. by R. Rettig et al. 1989. (Illus.). 363p. 118.00 (*0-387-50063-4*) Spr-Verlag.

Salt & Water. Horacio J. Adrogue & Donald E. Wesson. 1994. LC 94-18242. (Basics of Medicine Ser.). (Illus.). 320p. pap. 10.95 (*0-86542-426-8*) Blackwell Sci.

Salt, Diet & Health. G. A. MacGregor & H. E. De Wardener. 1998. LC 98-17411. (Illus.). 245p. (C). text 74.95 (*0-521-58352-7*) Cambridge U Pr.

Salud! A Latina's Guide to Total Health - Body, Mind, & Spirit. Jane L. Delgado. 1997. LC 97-19202. 400p. pap. 20.00 (*0-06-095187-7*, Perennial) HarperTrade.

***Salud! A Latina's Guide to Total Health - Body, Mind, & Spirit.** Jane L. Delgado & National Hispanic Women's Health Initiative Staff. 2002. (Illus.). 416p. pap. 23.95 (*0-06-000621-8*, Rayo) HarperCollins Gen Bks.

***Salud! Guia Integral Para la Mujer Latina.** Jane L. Delgado. 2002.Tr. of Salud: A Latina's Guide to Total Health. (SPA.). 448p. pap. 19.95 (*0-06-093740-8*) HarperCollins Pubs.

Salud: A Latina's Guide to Total Health see Salud!: Guia Integral Para la Mujer Latina

Salud en Casa (Healthwise Handbook) Guia Practica de Healthwise. Donald W. Kemper & Healthwise Staff. Ed. by Terrance Smith. 2nd rev. ed. 1998. (SPA.). 423p. pap. text 9.95 (*1-877930-47-4*) Healthwise.

Salud en el Siglo XXI, "Sobreviviran Los Medicos? see Health in the 21st Century: Will Doctors Survive?

Salud Herbal de Hoy. Louise Tenney. 1994. (Today's Herbal Health Ser.). (SPA.). 308p. pap. 14.95 (*0-913923-93-1*) Woodland UT.

Saludo en el Siglo: Sobreviviran los Medicas? Francisco Contreras. Ed. by Pamela M. Lowe. Tr. by Luisa Ruiz. 1997.Tr. of Health in the 21st Century: Will Doctors Survive?. (SPA., Illus.). 456p. (Orig.). mass mkt. 19.95 (*1-57946-001-1*) Interpacific Pr.

Salvat Encyclopedia of Health, Set. Salvat Staff. 1983. (SPA.). 1295.00 (*0-8288-8240-1*, 8471374803) Fr & Eur.

Salvat Medicina, Enciclopedia de Conocimientos Basicos, Set. 1974. (SPA.). 3000p. 1200.00 (*0-8288-6210-9*, S-50559) Fr & Eur.

Salyer & Bardach's Atlas of Craniofacial & Cleft Surgery: Cleft Lip & Palate Surgery, Vol. 2. Kenneth E. Salyer & Janusz Bardach. 1999. text 250.00 (*0-7817-2605-0*) Lppncott W & W.

Salyer & Bardach's Atlas of Craniofacial & Cleft Surgery: Craniofacial Surgery, Vol. 1. Kenneth E. Salyer & Janusz Bardach. 1999. text 250.00 (*0-7817-2604-2*) Lppncott W & W.

SAM-e Handbook: The Fast, Natural Way to Relieve the Pain of Arthritis, Alleviate the Discomfort of Fibromyalgia & Overcome Depression. Nancy Stedman. 2000. LC 00-37430. xiii, 162p. pap. 9.95 (*0-609-80654-8*, Three Riv Pr) Crown Pub Group.

SAM-e Solution: The Essential Guide to the Revolutionary Antidepression Supplement. Deborah Mitchell. 1999. LC 99-65497. xvii, 220p. pap. (*0-446-67637-3*) Warner.

SAM Model of Senescence: Proceedings of the First International Conference on Senescence, the SAM Model, Kyoto, 17-18 March, 1994. Ed. by Toshio Takeda. 1994. LC 94-20411. (International Congress Ser.: No. 1062). 474p. 227.25 (*0-444-81695-X*, Excerpta Medica) Elsevier.

Sam Woods. Stanley E. Rushworth. Ed. by Peter Greenwood. 1992. LC 92-81553. 176p. (Orig.). (C). pap. 14.95 (*0-9632574-9-8*) Talk Leaves.

Samadhi: Self Development in Zen, Swordsmanship, & Psychotherapy. Mike Sayama. 1985. LC 85-9894. (Series in Transpersonal & Humanistic Psychology). 160p. (C). text 51.50 (*0-88706-146-X*); pap. text 18.95 (*0-88706-147-8*) State U NY Pr.

Same-Day Diagnosis of Human Virus Infections. Donald M. McLean & Kathleen K. Wong. 1984. 144p. 49.50 (*0-8493-6590-2*, QR387, CRC Reprint) Franklin.

SAMe (S-Adenosylmethionine) The European Arthritis & Depression Breakthrough. Sol Grazie & Marie Costa. 1999. LC 98-34443. 256p. pap. 14.00 (*0-7615-1627-1*, Prima Health) Prima Pub.

Samman's the Nails in Disease. Peter D. Samman & David A. Fenton. 5th ed. 1995. LC 94-34926. (Illus.). 224p. text 80.00 (*0-7506-0189-2*) Buttrwrth-Heinemann.

Samoan Medical Belief & Practice. Cluny MacPherson & La'avasa MacPherson. 1990. 280p. (*1-86940-045-3*) Auckland Univ NZL. *Dist:* Paul & Co Pubs.

Sample Preparation for Biomedical & Environmental Analysis. D. Stevenson & I. D. Wilson. 1994. (Chromatographic Society Symposium Ser.). (Illus.). 256p. (C). text 85.00 (*0-306-44663-4*) Kluwer Academic.

Sample Size Determination in Health Studies: A Practical Manual. Stephen K. Lwanga & S. Lemeshow. 1991. (ENG, FRE & SPA.). viii, 80p. pap. text 16.00 (*92-4-154405-8*, 1150336) World Health.

Sample Size Tables for Clinical Studies. D. Machin et al. 2nd ed. 1997. LC 96-29177. (Illus.). 110.95 (*0-86542-870-0*) Blackwell Sci.

Sample Water for Legionella? Weighing the Benefits Against the Costs. Matthew R. Freije. 1998. LC 98-92506. 14p. pap. 14.00 (*0-9649926-5-5*, 305) HC Info Res.

Samples, Reagents & Assessment of Results, Vol. 2, Samples, Reagents, Assessment of Results. Ed. by Hans U. Bergmeyer. 3rd ed. 1983. LC 84-105641. 539p. 320.00 (*3-527-26042-0*, Wiley-VCH) Wiley.

Sampling & Identifying Allergenic Pollens & Molds: An Illustrated Identification Manual for Air Samplers. E. Grant Smith. 1990. LC 86-70134. (Illus.). 196p. (Orig.). (C). pap. text 125.00 (*0-930961-02-1*) Blewstone Pr.

Sampling Design & Statistical Methods for Environmental Biologists. Roger H. Green. 1979. LC 78-24422. 272p. 140.00 (*0-471-03901-2*) Wiley.

Sampling Inner Experience in Disturbed Affect. R. T. Hurlburt. 1993. (Emotions, Personality, & Psychotherapy Ser.). (Illus.). 264p. (C). 52.50 (*0-306-44377-5*, Plenum Trade) Perseus Pubng.

Sampling Methods in Morbidity Surveys & Public Health Investigations. 1966. (Technical Report Ser.: No. 336). 29p. pap. text 5.00 (*92-4-120336-6*) World Health.

Sampling Normal & Schizophrenic Inner Experience. R. T. Hurlburt. 1990. (Emotions, Personality, & Psychotherapy Ser.). (Illus.). 306p. (C). 52.50 (*0-306-43284-6*, Plenum Trade) Perseus Pubng.

Sam's WIT: Water Interval Training for Fabulous People of Every Kind. Sam Rettig & Drucie French. l.t. ed. 1993. (Illus.). 118p. pap. 20.00 (*0-9637470-2-9*) DFC Seminars.

Samter's Immunologic Diseases, Set. Ed. by Michael M. Frank et al. 5th rev. ed. 1995. LC 94-11310. Orig. Title: Immunological Diseases. (Illus.). 1,680p. reprint ed. text 350.00 (*0-316-29237-0*, Little Brwn Med Div) Lppncott W & W.

Samuel Johnson in the Medical World: The Doctor & the Patient. John Wiltshire. 1991. (Illus.). 303p. (C). text 85.00 (*0-521-38326-9*) Cambridge U Pr.

Samuel S. White Catalogue of Dental Instruments & Equipment. Samuel S. White. 1995. (Illus.). 408p. reprint ed. 150.00 (*0-930405-63-3*) Norman SF.

San Francisco General Hospital Handbook of HIV Management: A Guide to the Practical Management of HIV-Infected Patients. P. A. Volberding & J. A. Aberg. 1999. LC 99-34250. (Illus.). 222p. lib. bdg. 43.95 (*1-85070-938-6*, Parthenon Pbng) CRC Pr.

Sanapia: Comanche Medicine Woman. David E. Jones. 1984. 107p. (C). reprint ed. pap. text 10.95 (*0-88133-041-8*) Waveland Pr.

Sanctity of Life & Human Dignity. Ed. by Kurt Bayertz. 1996. LC 95-36283. (Philosophy & Medicine Ser.: Vol. 52). 328p. (C). text 161.50 (*0-7923-3739-5*) Kluwer Academic.

Sanctity of Social Life: Physicians' Treatment of Critically Ill Patients. Diana Crane. 1975. LC 74-15510. 186p. 30.00 (*0-87154-209-9*) Russell Sage.

Sanctity of Social Life: Physician's Treatment of Critically Ill Patients. Diana Crane. 1977. LC 74-15510. (Illus.). 286p. reprint ed. pap. text 21.95 (*0-87855-648-6*) Transaction Pubs.

Sandler Heart Failure. 1989. lib. bdg. (*0-85200-678-0*) Kluwer Academic.

Sandor Ferenczi: Reconsidering Active Intervention. Martin Stanton. 1991. LC 90-14523. 240p. 45.00 (*0-87668-569-6*) Aronson.

Sandor Ferenczi: The Psychotherapist of Tenderness & Passion. Arnold W. Rachman. 1997. LC 94-32540. 488p. 60.00 (*1-56821-100-7*) Aronson.

Sandostatin in the Treatment of Acromegaly: Consensus Round Table, Amsterdam, 1987. 1988. (Illus.). 184p. 51.95 (*0-387-19269-7*) Spr-Verlag.

Sandostatin in the Treatment of GEP Endrocine Tumors. Ed. by T. M. O'Dorisio. 1989. (Illus.). 156p. 51.95 (*0-387-50715-9*) Spr-Verlag.

Sandplay: A Psychotherapeutic Approach to the Psyche. Dora M. Kalff. Tr. by Hilde Kirsch & Wendayne Ackerman. rev. ed. 1981. LC 80-27195. (Illus.). 166p. pap. 17.95 (*0-938434-00-4*) Sigo Pr.

Sandplay: Past, Present, & Future. R. Rogers Mitchell & Harriet S. Friedman. 1994. LC 93-8079. (Illus.). 192p. (C). pap. 27.95 (*0-415-10137-9*) Routledge.

Sandplay: Silent Workshop of the Psyche. Katherine Bradway & Barbara McCoard. 1997. LC 96-16802. (Illus.). 264p. pap. 29.95 (*0-415-15075-2*); (C). 89.95 (*0-415-15074-4*) Routledge.

Sandplay Therapy with Children & Families. Lois J. Carey. 1998. LC 97-50266. xxix, 205 p. 40.00 (*0-7657-0161-8*) Aronson.

Sandra Smith's Review for NCLEX-M. Sandra F. Smith. 2000. 781p. pap. 34.95 (*0-13-089121-5*) P-H.

SANE (Sexual Assault Nurse Examiner) Development & Operation Guide. Lindra E. Ledray. 2000. (Illus.). 302p. pap. text 40.00 (*0-7567-0091-4*) DIANE Pub.

Sane Society. Erich Fromm. 1990. LC 55-8006. 384p. pap. 16.00 (*0-8050-1402-0*, Owl) H Holt & Co.

Sanford Guide to Antimicrobial Therapy, 1997. Jay P. Sanford et al. rev. ed. 1997. pap. 7.00 (*0-933775-30-X*) Antimicrob Ther.

***Sanford Guide to Antimicrobial Therapy, 1997: Medical Book System.** Sanford. 27th ed. 47.95 (*1-56712-422-4*) Franklin Elect.

Sanford Guide to Antimicrobial Therapy & HIV-AIDS Therapy, 1997. Jay P. Sanford et al. l.t. rev. ed. 1997. pap. 25.00 (*0-933775-32-6*) Antimicrob Ther.

Sanford Guide to HIV-AIDS Therapy, 1997. Merle A. Sande et al. 6th ed. 1997. pap. 7.00 *(0-933775-31-8)* Antimicrob Ther.

Sangoma: My Odyssey into the Spirit World of Africa. James A. Hall. 1995. LC 95-157. (Illus.). 272p. pap. 12.00 *(0-684-81506-0*, Fireside) S&S Trade Pap.

Sanitarians: A History of American Public Health. John Duffy. 1992. 344p. (C). pap. text 16.95 *(0-252-06276-0)* U of Ill Pr.

Sanitary Condition of Boston: The Report of a Medical Commission. Boston Medical Commission Staff. Ed. by Barbara G. Rosenkrantz. 1977. LC 76-25655. (Public Health in America Ser.). reprint ed. lib. bdg. 19.95 *(0-405-09808-1)* Ayer.

Sanitary Condition of the Laboring Population of New York, with Suggestions for Its Improvement. John H. Griscom. 1976. LC 75-125742. (American Environmental Studies). reprint ed. 16.95 *(0-405-02667-6)* Ayer.

Sanitary Lessons of the War & Other Papers. George M. Sternberg. Ed. by Barbara G. Rosenkrantz. 1977. LC 76-40647. (Public Health in America Ser.). reprint ed. lib. bdg. 19.95 *(0-405-09832-4)* Ayer.

Sanitation - Practices & Methods for Health Protection & Disease Prevention: Index of New Information. Hollis H. Bester. 1997. 160p. 57.50 *(0-7883-1708-3)*; pap. 47.50 *(0-7883-1709-1)* ABBE Pubs Assn.

Sanity Manual: The Therapeutic Uses of Writing. Alan Hunter. 1998. LC 98-35922. 18.95 *(1-56072-609-1*, Nova Kroshka Bks) Nova Sci Pubs.

Sante Naturelle - Encyclopedie Maladies, Traitements. R. Dalet. 1996. (FRE.). 200p. 49.95 *(0-320-00647-6)* Fr & Eur.

Saphenous Vein Bypass Graft Disease. Eric R. Bates & David R. Holmes. 1998. LC 98-5321. (Fundamental & Clinical Cardiology Ser.). (Illus.). 352p. text 165.00 *(0-8247-9902-X)* Dekker.

Sapira's Art & Science of Bedside Diagnosis. Contrib. by Jane M. Orient & Joseph D. Sapira. 2nd ed. 1999. LC 99-30301. (Illus.). 704p. text 79.95 *(0-683-30714-2)* Lppncott W & W.

Saponins Used in Traditional & Modern Medicine: Proceedings of the 20th National Meeting of the American Chemical Society Symposium on Saponins: Chemistry & Biological Activity Held in Chicago, Illinois, August 20-24, 1995. Ed. by George R. Waller & Kazuo Yamasaki. 1996. LC 96-2902. (Advances in Experimental Medicine & Biology Ser.: Vol. 404). (Illus.). 619p. 174.00 *(0-306-45393-2*, Kluwer Plenum) Kluwer Academic.

Sar. Eric J. Lien. 1987. (Medicinal Research Ser.: Vol. 11). (Illus.). 384p. text 199.00 *(0-8247-7686-0)* Dekker.

Sarah: A Sexual Biography. Paul R. Abramson. 1984. LC 83-17983. 142p. (C). pap. text 20.95 *(0-87395-863-2)* State U NY Pr.

***Saratov Fall Meeting '99: Optical Technologies in Biophysics & Medicine: International Workshop & Fall School for Young Scientists & Students on Optics, Laser Physics, & Biophysics: 5-8 October 1999, Saratov, Russia.** Ed. by V. V. Tuchin et al. 2000. LC 00-711277. (Illus.). xiv, 460p. *(0-8194-3626-7)* SPIE.

Sarcocystosis of Animals. J. P. Dubey et al. 1989. LC 88-15684. 224p. 130.00 *(0-8493-6364-0*, QR201, CRC Reprint) Franklin.

Sarcoidosis & Other Granulomatous Disorders. Ed. by D. Geraint James. 1994. (Lung Biology in Health & Disease Ser.: Vol. 73). (Illus.). 896p. text 250.00 *(0-8247-9126-6)* Dekker.

Sarcoidosis & Other Granulomatous Disorders. D. Geraint James & W. Jones Williams. 1985. (Problems in Internal Medicine Ser.: Vol. 24). (Illus.). 256p. text 99.00 *(0-7216-1044-7)* Saunders.

Sarcoidosis Resource Guide & Directory. Sandra Conroy. 1992. (Illus.). 304p. (Orig.). pap. 19.95 *(0-9631222-5-8)* PC Pubns.

Sarcoidosis Resource Guide & Directory for Health Care Professionals. Sandra Conroy. 1991. (Illus.). 250p. pap. *(0-9631222-6-6)* PC Pubns.

Sarcolemmal Biochemistry, Vol. 1. Abdul M. Kidwai. 1987. LC 86-26358. reprint ed. 106.00 *(0-8493-5909-0*, CRC Reprint) Franklin.

Sarngadhara Samhita: A Treatise on Ayurveda. Sarngadhara. Tr. by Srikanata K. Murthy from SAN. 1984. 335p. text 42.00 *(0-89744-056-0)* Auromere.

Sastun: One Woman's Apprenticeship with a Maya Healer & their Efforts to Save the Vanishing Tradition of Rainforest Medicine. Rosita Arvigo & Nadine Epstein. 1995. LC 93-37439. 208p. pap. 15.00 *(0-06-250259-X)* Harper SF.

Satanism: Psychiatric & Legal Views. George B. Palermo & Michele C. Del Re. 1999. LC 99-41451. (American Series in Behavioral Science & Law: Vol. 1099). xvii, 205p. text 44.95 *(0-398-07007-5)*; pap. text 31.95 *(0-398-07008-3)* C C Thomas.

Satellite Cells of the Sensory Ganglia. Ennio Pannese. 1981. (Advances in Anatomy, Embryology & Cell Biology Ser.: Vol. 65). (Illus.). 111p. 48.95 *(0-387-10219-1)* Spr-Verlag.

Satiation: From Gut to Brain. Ed. by Gerard P. Smith. 1997. LC 97-14182. (Oxford Neuroscience Ser.). (Illus.). 304p. text 65.00 *(0-19-510515-X)* OUP.

Saturated Heterocyclic Chemistry. M. F. Ansell & G. Pattenden. LC 72-83454. Vol. 2. 1974. 47.00 *(0-85186-532-1)*; Vol. 3. 1975. 43.00 *(0-85186-562-3)*; Vol. 4. 1977. 77.00 *(0-85186-592-5)*; Vol. 5. 1978. 66.00 *(0-85186-622-0)* Am Chemical.

Saudia Arabia Medical Review. IMMEL Publishing Ltd. Staff. 1995. 98p. (C). pap. *(0-907151-57-4)* IMMEL Pubng GBR. *Dist:* Trans-Atl Phila, St Mut.

Sauer's Herbal Cures: America's First Book of Botanic Healing, 1762-1778. William Woys Weaver. 2000. LC 00-56128. (Illus.). 336p. 37.50 *(0-415-92360-3)* Routledge.

Sauer's Manual of Skin Diseases. Contrib. by John C. Hall & Gordon C. Sauer. 8th ed. 1999. LC 99-26912. (Illus.). 464p. pap. text 64.95 *(0-7817-1629-2)* Lppncott W & W.

Sauna Detoxification Therapy: A Guide for the Chemically Sensitive. Marilyn G. McVicker. 1997. LC 96-51802. (Illus.). 175p. per. 29.95 *(0-7864-0359-4)* McFarland & Co.

Saunders Cardiology CD-ROM: Containing Braunwald, 5/E, Skorton et al., 2/E & Smith. Ed. by Richard Zorab. 1998. text 415.00 *(0-7216-7168-3)* Saunders.

Saunders Comprehensive Review for NCLEX-PN. Linda Anne Silvestri. 2000. LC 99-23882. (Illus.). xxvii, 1051p. (C). pap. text 31.95 *(0-7216-7794-0)* Saunders.

Saunders Comprehensive Veterinary Dictionary. Blood. 2nd ed. 1998. (Illus.). 1394p. (C). text *(0-7020-2442-2)* W B Saunders GBR. *Dist:* Saunders.

Saunders Drug Handbook for Health Professionals 2000. Robert J. Kizior & Barbara B. Hodgson. 1999. LC 00-269537. (Illus.). xxii, 1275p. pap. text 29.95 *(0-7216-8568-4)* Saunders.

Saunders Drugs for Nursing Practice. Linda Harner. 1996. LC 95-17704. 1024p. pap. text *(0-7216-5402-9)* Saunders.

Saunders First Responder. Bovia. 1999. pap. text 29.95 *(0-7216-8660-5)* Saunders.

Saunders Fundamental Nursing Assistance. Polaski. 1994. 345.00 *(0-7216-4309-4)* Harcourt.

Saunders Fundamentals for Nursing Assistants. Arlene L. Polaski & Judith P. Warner. 1994. (Illus.). pap., tchr. ed. *(0-7216-3612-8)*; 944p. pap. text 29.95 *(0-7216-3608-X)*; pap. text, stu. ed. 17.95 *(0-7216-3613-6)*;Set. 944p. pap., stu. ed. 38.95 *(0-7216-4516-X)* Saunders.

Saunders Gastroenterology. Saunders, W.B., Publishing Staff. cd-rom *(0-7216-7884-X)* Saunders.

Saunders Infection Control Reference Service. Elias Abrutyn. Ed. by Lisa Biello. 1997. LC 96-38025. 1536p. text 295.00 *(0-7216-6443-1)* Saunders.

Saunders Infection Control Reference Service: A Guide to the Guidelines. Elias Abrutyn. 2nd ed. 2000. (Illus.). 1310p. 325.00 *(0-7216-8468-8)* Harcrt Hlth Sci Grp.

Saunders Instructor's Resource Package for NCLEX-RN. Linda Anne Silvestri. Ed. by Maura Connor. 1999. (Illus.). 315p. text, tchr. ed. 850.00 *(0-7216-7797-5)* Saunders.

Saunders International Medical Word Book. 1991. 1100p. text 75.00 *(0-7216-3620-9)* Saunders.

Saunders Manual for Veterinary Technology. Peter. Date not set. text *(0-7216-4193-8)* Saunders.

Saunders Manual of Clinical Laboratory Science. Craig A. Lehmann. Ed. by Selma Kaszczuk. 1998. LC 97-27842. (Illus.). 1104p. text 69.95 *(0-7216-2185-6)* Saunders.

Saunders Manual of Medical Assisting Practice. Ed. by Karen Lane. 1992. LC 92-49703. (Illus.). 888p. text 49.95 *(0-7216-3063-4)* Saunders.

Saunders Manual of Medical Practice. Robert E. Rakel. Ed. by Darlene Pedersen. 1996. LC 95-6354. (Illus.). 1287p. text 105.00 *(0-7216-5192-5)* Saunders.

Saunders Manual of Medical Practice. Robert E. Rakel. Ed. by Ray Kersey. 2nd ed. 1999. (Illus.). 1340p. text *(0-7216-8002-X)* Saunders.

Saunders Manual of Nursing Care. Saunders. Ed. by Joan Luckmann et al. 1997. LC 95-50014. (Illus.). 1885p. text 51.00 *(0-7216-5017-1)* Saunders.

Saunders Manual of Pediatric Practice. Laurence Finberg. Ed. by Judy Fletcher. 1998. LC 97-5188. (Illus.). 976p. pap. text 75.00 *(0-7216-6537-3)* Saunders.

***Saunders Manual of Pediatric Practice.** Laurence Finberg. 2nd ed. 2001. *(0-7216-9242-7)* Saunders.

Saunders Manual of Physical Therapy Practice. Rose S. Myers. 1995. LC 94-452. (Illus.). 1072p. text 87.00 *(0-7216-3671-3)* Saunders.

Saunders Manual of Small Animal Practice. Stephen J. Birchard & Robert G. Sherding. 1993. (Illus.). 1424p. text 130.00 *(0-7216-3219-X)* Saunders.

Saunders' Manual of Small Animal Practice. Stephen J. Birchard & Robert G. Sherding. 2nd ed. 1999. LC 98-26528. (Illus.). xxii, 1636p. (C). text 110.00 *(0-7216-7078-4)* Saunders.

***Saunders' Medical Assisting Exam Review.** Deborah E. Barbier Holmes & Joanna Bligh. 2001. LC 2001-34267. *(0-7216-9566-3)* Saunders.

Saunders Medical Assisting Review. Newsome. Date not set. pap. text *(0-7216-4331-0)* Harcourt.

Saunders Nursing Drug Handbook. Barbara B. Hodgson & Robert J. Kizior. Ed. by Maura Connor. 99th ed. 1998. (Illus.). 1328p. (C). pap. text 28.95 *(0-7216-7398-8)* Saunders.

Saunders Nursing Drug Handbook 2000. Saunders, W.B., Publishing Staff. 2000. (Saunders Nursing Drug Handbooks Ser.). 1392p. pap. text 31.95 *(0-7216-7400-3)* Saunders.

Saunders Ophthalmology Word Book. Laurie Adams. 4th ed. 1991. 368p. pap. text 35.00 *(0-7216-3672-1)* Saunders.

Saunders Paramedic Care. Thomas. 2000. text *(0-7216-6274-9)* Saunders.

Saunders Pharmaceutical Word Book. Ellen Drake & Randy Drake. 2000. 720p. 32.95 *(0-7216-9331-8)*; 98th ed. 1997. pap. text 29.95 *(0-7216-7261-2)* Saunders.

Saunders Pharmaceutical XRef Book, 2000. Ellen Drake & Randy Drake. Date not set. 605p. pap. text *(0-7216-8412-2)* Saunders.

Saunder's Pocket Essentials of Clinical Medicine. Ann Ballinger & Steve Patchett. 1995. (Illus.). 547p. pap. text *(0-7020-1921-6)* W B Saunders GBR. *Dist:* Saunders.

Saunders Pocket Reference for Nurses. Kathleen Melonakos. 2nd ed. 1994. LC 94-20443. (Illus.). 733p. pap. text 24.00 *(0-7216-4459-7)* Saunders.

Saunders Q & A Review for NCLEX-RN. Linda Anne Silvestri. Ed. by Maura Connor. 1998. LC 98-3395. (Illus.). 1215p. (C). 39.25 *(0-7216-7793-2)* Saunders.

Saunders Review for NCLEX-RN. Esther Matassarin-Jacobs. 2nd ed. 1994. LC 93-22879. (Illus.). 800p. pap. text 32.00 *(0-7216-4993-9)*; 1995. pap. text 33.00 *(0-7216-6323-0)* Saunders.

Saunders Review of Dental Hygiene. Debralee McKelvey Nelson. 2000. LC 99-27192. (Illus.). xix, 666p. text 58.75 *(0-7216-7576-X)* Saunders.

Saunders Review of Family Practice. Edward T. Bope et al. Ed. by Ray Kersey. 2nd ed. 1996. LC 96-16715. (Illus.). 416p. pap. text 52.00 *(0-7216-5817-2)* Saunders.

***Saunders Review of Family Practice.** Edward T. Bope et al. 3rd ed. 2001. 360p. *(0-7216-8821-7)* Saunders.

Saunder's Review of Practical Nursing for NCLEX-PN. Esther Matassarin-Jacobs. Ed. by Maura Connor. 3rd rev. ed. 1996. (Illus.). 480p. pap. text 28.95 *(0-7216-5872-5)* Saunders.

Saunders Student Nurse Planner. Susan C. DeWit. 1995. LC 95-11490. pap. text 15.00 *(0-7216-5831-8)* Saunders.

Savage God: A Study of Suicide. A. Alvarez. 1990. pap. 11.95 *(0-393-30657-7)* Norton.

Savage Mind. Claude Levi-Strauss. 1968. LC 66-28197. (Nature of Human Society Ser.). pap. 16.95 *(0-226-47484-4*, P325) U Ch Pr.

Save Lives! Report Recommendations & Community Action Guide of the Join Together Public Policy Panel on Underage Access to Alcohol. 1994. (Illus.). 56p. (Orig.). (C). pap. text 20.00 *(0-7881-0778-X)* DIANE Pub.

Save Your Back. H. Duane Saunders & Michael S. Melnick. Ed. by Robin Saunders & Beth Solheim. 1981. (Illus.). (Orig.). pap. text 5.00 *(0-9616461-4-4)* Saunders Grp.

Save Your Knees. James Fox & Rick Mcguire. 1988. LC 88-153566. 304p. (Orig.). pap. 13.95 *(0-440-50011-7*, Dell Trade Pbks) Dell.

Save Your Sight! Natural Ways to Prevent & Reverse Macular Degeneration & Other Eye Diseases. Marc R. Rose et al. 1998. LC 97-41030. (Illus.). 304p. pap. *(0-446-67402-8)* Warner.

Saving Face: My Victory over Skin Cancer. Carolyn Shuck. 2000. LC 00-37555. 256p. 26.95 *(0-8397-7340-4)* Eriksson.

***Saving Money on Medicines: The Drugs Budget Handbook.** Penny Blanch. 2000. 280p. pap. *(1-85775-433-6)* Radcliffe Med Pr GBR. *Dist:* Balogh.

Saving Your Skin: Prevention, Early Detection & Treatment of Melanoma & Other Skin Cancers. Barney Kenet. 2nd ed. 1998. (Illus.). 224p. pap. 16.95 *(1-56858-124-6)* FWEW.

Saving Yourself from the Disease-Care Crises. Walt Stoll. 1996. (Illus.). 210p. (Orig.). pap. 9.95 *(0-9653171-0-2)* Sunrise Hlth.

Savvy Medical Consumer. Charles B. Inlander & People's Medical Society Staff. rev. ed. 1997. LC 97-8923. 128p. pap. 10.95 *(1-882606-31-0)* Peoples Med Soc.

Saw Palmetto: Nature's Prostate Healer & Other Breakthrough Herbal & Nutritional Remedies. Ray Sahelian. 1998. LC 99-173859. 160p. pap. 5.99 *(1-57566-300-7*, Knsington) Kensgtn Pub Corp.

Saw Palmetto: The Natural Choice for Prostate Health. Kate G. Udall. 1998. (Woodland Health Ser.). 32p. pap. 3.95 *(1-885670-59-1)* Woodland UT.

Saw Palmetto Story. Michael Murray. rev. ed. 1991. 14p. reprint ed. pap. 2.95 *(0-9647080-2-7)* Healing Wisdom.

Say Goodbye to Back Pain: A Successful Alternative for the Treatment of Back Pain. Richard Stuckey. 1994. (Illus.). 122p. pap. 14.95 *(0-85572-248-7)* Seven Hills Bk.

Say Goodbye to Illness. Devi S. Nambudripad. 2nd ed. 1999. (Say Goodbye Ser.). (Illus.). xxxiv, 521p. pap. 24.00 *(0-9658242-1-7)* Delta Pubng.

Say It in Spanish: A Guide for Health Care Professionals. Esperanza V. Joyce & Maria E. Villanueva. 1995. 304p. pap. text 16.95 *(0-7216-4955-6)*; 2nd ed. 2000. LC 99-51713. (Illus.). 350p. pap. text 19.95 incl. audio *(0-7216-8613-3)* Saunders.

Say No to Cancer. Barbara Waters. 1984. LC 83-90862. (Illus.). 453p. (Orig.). (C). pap. 12.00 *(0-930107-01-2)* Waters Pub.

Say That Again, Please! Insights in Dealing with a Hearing Loss. Thomas H. Bradford. 1991. LC 91-92991. (Illus.). 382p. (Orig.). pap. 16.95 *(0-9630738-5-0)* Bradford Pubns.

Saying Good-Bye to Managed Care: Building an Independent Psychotherapy Practice. Sandra Haber et al. 2000. LC 00-63527. (Illus.). xi, 217p. *(0-8261-1383-4)* Springer Pub.

***Saying Good-Bye to Managed Care: Building Your Independent Psychotherapy Practice.** Sandra Haber et al. 2000. LC 00-63527. (Illus.). xi, 217p. *(0-8261-1463-6)* Springer Pub.

Saying Goodbye: A Casebook of Termination in Child & Adolescent Analysis & Therapy. Ed. by Anita G. Schmukler. 1991. 400p. text 49.95 *(0-88163-106-X)* Analytic Pr.

Saying Goodbye in Child Psychotherapy: Planned, Unplanned, & Premature Endings in Child Psychotherapy. Donna Cangelosi. 1997. LC 96-49473. 192p. 40.00 *(1-56821-677-7)* Aronson.

Saying Goodbye to a Baby Vol. 2: A Counselor's Guide to Birthparent Loss & Grief in Adoption, Vol. 2. Patricia E. Roles. 1989. 34p. pap. 10.95 *(0-87868-393-3)* Child Welfare.

Saying Goodbye to Grandma. Moshe Spero. 1997. (Illus.). 64p. (J). (gr. k-5). 14.95 *(0-943706-46-7)* Pitspopany.

Saying "No" Its Meaning in Child Development, Psychoanalysis, Linguistics & Hegel. Wilfried Ver Eecke. 1984. LC 84-1617. 224p. text 18.50 *(0-8207-0169-6)* Duquesne.

Scabies. K. Mellanby. 1972. 87p. 20.00 *(0-7855-0673-X)* St Mut.

Scale for Measuring the Antero-Posterior Posture of Ninth Grade Boys. C. L. Brownell. LC 74-176601. (Columbia University. Teachers College. Contributions to Education Ser.: No. 325). reprint ed. 37.50 *(0-404-55325-7)* AMS Pr.

Scales for Rating Behavioral Characteristics of Superior Students. Joseph S. Renzulli et al. 1997. (gr. k-12). pap. 8.95 *(0-936386-00-2*, 662) Creative Learning.

Scalpel & the Sword: The Story of Doctor Norman Bethune. Ted Allan & Sydney Gordon. rev. ed. 1974. LC 73-8059. 336p. reprint ed. pap. 10.00 *(0-85345-302-0)* Monthly Rev.

***Scan: How It Relates to Our Health & Improves Our Functioning.** Raymond K. Brown. 2001. LC 00-193480. 25.00 *(0-7388-5788-2)*; pap. 16.00 *(0-7388-5787-4)* Xlibris Corp.

Scanning Electron Microscope Studies of the Brain Ventricular Surfaces. Ed. by Om Johari. 1978. (Illus.). reprint ed. pap. text 15.00 *(0-931288-03-7)* Scanning Microscopy.

Scanning Electron Microscopy: Atlas of Corneal Pathology. Frank M. Polack. 1983. (Illus.). 168p. (gr. 13). 74.50 *(0-89352-203-1)* Mosby Inc.

Scanning Electron Microscopy 1978: International Review of Advances in Techniques & Applications of the Scanning Electron Microscope, 1978 Ed. by Om Johari & Robert P. Becker. 1978. LC 72-626068. (Illus.). Pt. I. text 37.00 *(0-931288-01-0)*; Pt. II. text 37.00 *(0-931288-02-9)*; Set. text 65.00 *(0-931288-00-2)* Scanning Microscopy.

Scanning Electron Microscopy 1979: International Review of Advances in Techniques & Applications of the Scanning Electron Microscope, 1979 Ed. by Om Johari & Robert P. Becker. 1979. LC 72-626068. (Illus.). *(0-931288-06-1)*;Pt. II. text 37.00 *(0-931288-05-3)*;Pts. I & II. text 65.00 *(0-931288-08-8)* Scanning Microscopy.

Scanning Electron Microscopy, 1980, Pt. I. Om Johari. 1980. LC 72-626068. (Illus.). xvi, 608p. 52.00 *(0-931288-11-8)* Scanning Microscopy.

Scanning Electron Microscopy, 1980. Ed. by Om Johari & R. P. Becker. (Illus.). Pt. III. 1980. LC 72-62608. xx, 670p. 52.00 *(0-931288-13-4)*; Pt. IV. 1981. iv, 220p. 52.00 *(0-931288-14-2)* Scanning Microscopy.

Scanning Electron Microscopy, 1982, Pt. I. Ed. by Om Johari et al. 1983. LC 72-626068. (Illus.). xvi, 464p. 52.00 *(0-931288-23-1)* Scanning Microscopy.

Scanning Electron Microscopy 1982, Pt. II. Ed. by Om Johari et al. 1983. LC 72-626068. (Illus.). xvi, 432p. 52.00 *(0-931288-24-X)* Scanning Microscopy.

Scanning Electron Microscopy, 1982, Set. Ed. by Om Johari et al. 1983. LC 72-626068. (Illus.). xvi, 464p. 109.00 *(0-931288-27-4)* Scanning Microscopy.

Scanning Electron Microscopy Atlas of Normal & Malignant Leukocytes. Aaron Polliack et al. 1993. LC 92-49075. 95p. text 107.00 *(3-7186-5362-1)* Gordon & Breach.

Scanning Electron Microscopy, 1980, Pt. II. R. P. Becker & Om Johari. 1980. LC 72-626068. (Illus.). xiv, 658p. 52.00 *(0-931288-12-6)* Scanning Microscopy.

Scanning Electron Microscopy of Cells in Culture. Ed. by Paul B. Bell, Jr. 1984. (Illus.). vi, 314p. reprint ed. pap. 29.00 *(0-931288-31-2)* Scanning Microscopy.

Scanning Electron Microscopy of Vascular Casts: Methods & Applications. Ed. by P. M. Motta et al. 1992. (Electron Microscopy in Biology & Medicine Ser.). 416p. (C). text 350.50 *(0-7923-1297-X)* Kluwer Academic.

Scanning Patterns of Human Infants: Implications for Visual Learning. Gordon Bronson. 1982. LC 81-20543. (Monographs on Infancy Ser.: Vol. 2). 136p. 77.00 *(0-89391-114-3*, Ablex) Greenwood.

Scanning the Global Environment: A Framework & Methodolgy for Integrating Environmental Reporting & Assessment. National Institute of Public Health and the Environment. 68p. 20.00 *(92-807-1491-0)* UN.

Scaphoid Fractures & Complications. Ed. by James H. Herndon. 1994. 88p. pap. 38.00 (*0-89203-084-4*) Amer Acad Ortho Surg.

Scar Revision. Terence M. Davidson. 4th rev. ed. 1998. LC 98-14945. (Self-Instructional Package Ser.). (Illus.). 113p. (Orig.). pap. text 25.00 (*1-56772-063-3*, 5506035) AAO-HNS.

***Scarce Goods: Justice, Fairness & Organ Transplantation.** Tom Koch. 2001. LC 2001-32936. 256p. 65.00 (*0-275-97432-4*); pap. 25.00 (*0-275-97433-2*) Greenwood (Praeger Trade).

Scarce Medical Resources & Justice: Proceedings of 1987 Bishops' Workshop. Ed. by Donald G. McCarthy. 1987. LC 87-18302. 308p. (Orig.). pap. 17.95 (*0-935372-21-0*) NCBC.

Scared Child: Helping Kids Overcome Traumatic Events. Barbara Brooks & Paula M. Siegel. 1996. LC 96-10330. 176p. pap. 16.95 (*0-471-08284-8*) Wiley.

Scarlet Survey. Kevin Sherlock. 1997. 272p. (Orig.). pap. 19.95 (*0-9654036-1-0*, VSC497) Brennyman Bks.

Scarred Minds: The Psychological Impact of War on Sri Lankan Tamils. Daya Somasundaram. 1998. LC 98-7050. 42.95 (*0-7619-9267-7*, 83579) Sage.

Scarred Soul: Understanding & Ending Self-Inflicted Violence. Tracy Alderman. 1997. LC 97-66073. (Illus.). 224p. pap. 14.95 (*1-57224-079-2*) New Harbinger.

Scars of Venus: A History of Venereology. J. D. Oriel. 1994. LC 93-34554. 248p. (Illus.). 98.00 (*3-540-19844-X*); 98.00 (*0-387-19844-X*) Spr-Verlag.

Scattered: How Attention Deficit Disorder Originates & What You Can Do about It. Gabor Mate. 2000. LC 99-12999. (Illus.). 348p. pap. 14.95 (*0-452-27963-1*, Plume) Dutton Plume.

Scenario Development & Costing in Health Care: Methodological Accomplishments & Practical Guidelines. STG Foundation for Future Health Scenarios Staff. 2000. LC 98-148829. 96p. (Orig.). pap. (*90-6224-877-2*) Uitgeverij Arkel NLD. *Dist:* LPC InBook.

Scenes from Surgical Life. David LeVay. 1976. 200p. 22.95 (*0-8464-0813-9*) Beekman Pubs.

Scenes of Madness: A Psychiatrist at the Theatre. Derek R. Davis. 1995. LC 95-18951. 224p. (C). pap. 29.95 (*0-415-13173-1*) Routledge.

***Scent Therapy: Health & Well-being Through Fragrance.** Raje Airey. 2001. (Illus.). 64p. 9.95 (*0-7548-0821-1*, Lorenz Bks) Anness Pub.

Sceptic's Medical Dictionary. Michael O'Donnell. 1997. 209p. pap. (*0-7279-1204-6*) BMJ Pub GBR. *Dist:* AIDC.

Schalm's Veterinary Hematology. Nemi C. Jain. 4th ed. 1986. LC 84-27811. (Illus.). 1221p. text 149.00 (*0-8121-0942-2*) Lppncott W & W.

Schalm's Veterinary Hematology. Bernard F. Feldman et al. 5th ed. 2000. LC 99-89116. (Illus.). 1,376p. text 159.00 (*0-683-30692-8*) Lppncott W & W.

Schedules for Clinical Assessment in Neuropsychiatry, Version 2.0 (SCAN) Glossary. World Health Organization Staff. 1994. 237p. spiral bd. 18.95 (*0-88048-984-7*, 8984) Am Psychiatric.

Schedules for Clinical Assessment in Neuropsychiatry, Version 2.0 (SCAN) Manual. WHO Staff. 1994. 332p. spiral bd. 20.95 (*0-88048-976-6*, 8976) Am Psychiatric.

Schedules for Clinical Assessment in Neuropsychiatry, Version 2.0 (SCAN) Recording Booklets. World Health Organization Staff. 1994. LC 95-187319. 103p. pap. text 16.00 (*0-88048-985-5*, 8985) Am Psychiatric.

Scheduling Patients & Appointment Book Control: A Complete How-to Manual for the Doctor & Staff. Robert D. Westerman. 1991. (Classic Practice Ser.: Vol. 1). 290p. ring bd. 295.00 (*0-9629983-0-3*) R Westerman.

Scheimpflung Lens Documentation: New Developments & Applications. Ed. by A. Wegener. 1992. (Journal: Vol. 24, Suppl. 1, 1992). (Illus.). iv, 72p. pap. 23.50 (*3-8055-5702-7*) S Karger.

Schein's Common Sense Emergency Abdominal Surgery: A Small Book for Residents, Thinking Surgeons & Even Students. Moshe Schein. 2000. 320p. pap. 52.00 (*3-540-66654-0*) Spr-Verlag.

Schema in Clinical Psychoanalysis. Joseph Slap & Laura Slap-Shelton. 1991. 184p. 29.95 (*0-88163-089-6*) Analytic Pr.

Schemas. Beauvois. 1996. (C). pap. text, tchr. ed. 28.00 (*0-15-501702-0*); pap. text 49.00 (*0-15-501282-7*) Harcourt Coll Pubs.

Schemas in Problem Solving. Sandra P. Marshall. 1995. (Illus.). 438p. (C). text 85.00 (*0-521-43072-0*) Cambridge U Pr.

Schemata. Beverly Moser et al. 1996. LC 95-82111. (GER.). 304p. (C). pap. text 32.00 (*0-03-010104-2*) Holt R&W.

Schematic Replica of the Cardiac Cycle. Bernard M. Bane. 1981. 45p. pap. 3.00 (*0-930924-11-8*) BMB Pub Co.

Schilddruesentumoren. Ed. by K. Krisch. 1983. (Beitraege Zur Onkologie, Contributions to Oncology Ser.: Vol. 16). (Illus.). vi, 82p. pap. 35.75 (*3-8055-3695-X*) S Karger.

Schistosomes, Liver Flukes, & Helicobacter Pylori. 1994. (IARC Scientific Publications Ser.: Vol. 61). 270p. pap. text 70.00 (*92-832-1261-4*, 1720061) World Health.

Schistosomiasis. Ed. by A. Mahmoud. 1999. (Tropical Medicine Ser.). 550p. (*1-86094-146-X*) Imperial College GBR. *Dist:* World Scientific Pub.

Schistosomiasis & 200 Million World-Wide Infections: Index of New Information. Lorrie M. Gilbertson. 1998. (Illus.). 160p. 57.50 (*0-7883-1770-9*); pap. 47.50 (*0-7883-1771-7*) ABBE Pubs Assn.

Schistosomiasis Control: Proceedings of the WHO Expert Committee, Geneva, 1972. WHO Staff. 1973. (Technical Reports: No. 515). pap. text 6.00 (*92-4-120515-6*, 1100515) World Health.

Schistosomiasis in Egypt. Ed. by M. F. Abd-El-Wahab. 1982. 256p. 142.00 (*0-8493-6220-2*, RC182, CRC Reprint) Franklin.

Schistosomiasis in Twentieth Century Africa: Historical Studies on West Africa & Sudan. K. David Patterson & Gerald W. Hartwig. 1984. pap. 15.00 (*0-918456-54-1*) African Studies Assn.

Schizoid Phenomena, Object Relations & the Self. Harry Guntrip. 1969. LC 68-56426. 438p. 65.00 (*0-8236-5985-2*) Intl Univs Pr.

***Schizoid Phenomena, Object Relations & the Self.** Harry Guntrip. 2001. (Books-on-Demand Ser.). 437p. pap. text 39.95 (*0-8236-8310-9*, 25985) Intl Univs Pr.

***Schizophrenia.** Ed. by Scott Barbour. 2001. LC 2001-33015. (Contemporary Issues Companion Ser.). 191p. pap. 19.95 (*0-7377-0636-8*); lib. bdg. 31.20 (*0-7377-0637-6*) Gale (Greenhaven Pr).

Schizophrenia. Ed. by Steven Hirsch & Daniel Weinberger. 1995. LC 94-26616. (Illus.). 656p. 178.95 (*0-632-03276-6*) Blackwell Sci.

Schizophrenia. Ed. by Eckart R. Straube & Kurt Hahlweg. 1990. (Illus.). 244p. 72.00 (*0-387-50573-3*) Spr-Verlag.

Schizophrenia. John S. Strauss & William T. Carpenter. 1981. (Critical Issues in Psychiatry Ser.). (Illus.). 232p. (C). text 65.00 (*0-306-40704-3*, Kluwer Plenum) Kluwer Academic.

Schizophrenia. Sophia Frangou & Robin Murray. 2nd ed. 2000. 120p. pap. (*1-85317-920-5*) Martin Dunitz GBR. *Dist:* Blackwell Sci.

Schizophrenia: A Comprehensive Text. Marvin Herz & Stephen Marder. 2002. LC 2001-38950. 600p. text 59.95 (*0-683-30709-6*) Lppncott W & W.

***Schizophrenia: A Workbook for Healthcare Professionals.** Ed. by Peter Thompson. 3rd ed. 2000. 200p. pap., wbk. ed. (*1-85775-461-1*) Radcliffe Med Pr GBR. *Dist:* Balogh.

Schizophrenia: Breaking Down the Barriers. Stephen G. Holliday et al. 1997. LC 96-2847. 262p. 135.00 (*0-471-96703-3*) Wiley.

Schizophrenia: Current Concepts & Research. D. Siva Sankar. 1969. LC 70-95390. 49.95 (*0-9600290-0-1*) PJD Pubns.

Schizophrenia: Emperical Research & Findings. Eckart R. Straube. 1992. (Personality, Psychopathology & Psychotherapy Ser.). (Illus.). 637p. text 74.95 (*0-12-673010-5*) Acad Pr.

Schizophrenia: From Mind to Molecule. Ed. by Nancy C. Andreasen. 1994. LC 93-9585. (American Psychopathological Association Ser.). 278p. text 36.00 (*0-88048-950-2*, 8950) Am Psychiatric.

Schizophrenia: Latest Advances in Understanding & Drug Development. Ed. by Lori Dirks. 1996. (Biomedical Library). 296p. pap. 795.00 (*1-57936-016-5*) Drug & Market Dev.

Schizophrenia: Origins, Processes, Treatment, & Outcome. Ed. by Rue L. Cromwell & C. R. Snyder. 1993. LC 92-48996. (Illus.). 384p. (C). text 115.00 (*0-19-506922-6*) OUP.

Schizophrenia: Psychotic Continuum or Distinct Entities. Ed. by Ming T. Tsuang et al. 1995. LC 94-47536. (Illus.). 167p. 83.95 (*3-540-58820-5*); (*0-387-58820-5*) Spr-Verlag.

Schizophrenia: Recent Biosocial Developments. Costas N. Stefanis & Andreas D. Rabuilas. 1987. LC 86-27353. 286p. 43.95 (*0-89885-345-1*, Kluwer Acad Hman Sci) Kluwer Academic.

Schizophrenia: Science & Practice. Ed. by John C. Shershow. 1978. LC 78-6317. (Illus.). 256p. 36.50 (*0-674-79112-6*) HUP.

Schizophrenia: Selected Papers. David Shakow. 1977. LC 76-45548. (Psychological Issues Monographs: No. 38). 354p. 52.50 (*0-8236-6003-6*); 42.50 (*0-8236-6002-8*) Intl Univs Pr.

Schizophrenia: Symptoms, Causes, Treatments. Kayla F. Bernheim & Richard R. Lewine. 1979. (Illus.). (C). pap. text 13.00 (*0-393-09017-5*) Norton.

Schizophrenia: The Facts. Ming T. Tsuang & Stephen V. Farraone. 2nd ed. 1997. (Facts Ser.). 190p. pap. 19.95 (*0-19-262760-0*) OUP.

Schizophrenia: The First Ten Dean Award Lectures. Ed. by Stanley R. Dean. 1973. LC 73-6815. text 32.50 (*0-8422-7115-5*) Irvington.

Schizophrenia: The Positive Perspective. Peter K. Chadwick. 1997. LC 96-40143. 240p. (C). 89.95 (*0-415-14287-3*); pap. 27.95 (*0-415-14288-1*) Routledge.

Schizophrenia: The Sacred Symbol of Psychiatry. Thomas Szasz. 1988. LC 87-26769. (Illus.). 237p. (C). reprint ed. pap. 18.95 (*0-8156-0224-3*) Syracuse U Pr.

Schizophrenia: Towards a New Synthesis. J. Wing. 1978. 304p. text 44.00 (*0-8089-1140-6*, 794857, Grune & Strat) Harcrt Hlth Sci Grp.

Schizophrenia: Treatment, Management, & Rehabilitation. Ed. by Alan S. Bellack. 1984. 432p. text 48.00 (*0-8089-1640-8*, 790497, Grune & Strat) Harcrt Hlth Sci Grp.

Schizophrenia - The Way Out. Maria Kuman. pap. 20.00 (*1-893637-23-9*) Hlth & Hap.

Schizophrenia & Bipolar Disease: Often Misdiagnosed, Often Mistreated. Herbert Wagemaker. Ed. by Ann Bucholz. 1996. (Illus.). 155p. (Orig.). pap. 12.00 (*0-9654996-1-8*) Ponte Vedra Pub.

Schizophrenia & Comorbid Conditions: Diagnosis & Treatment. Ed. by Michael Y. Hwang & Paul C. Bermanzohn. 2001. LC 00-58661. xvii, 238p. 46.00 (*0-88048-771-2*, 8771) Am Psychiatric.

Schizophrenia & Mood Disorders: The New Drug Therapies in Clinical Practice. Ed. by Peter F. Buckley & John L. Waddington. 2001. (Illus.). 368p. (Orig.). pap. text 49.50 (*0-7506-4096-0*) OUP.

Schizophrenia & the Family. Theodore Lidz & Stephen Fleck. rev. ed. 1985. LC 65-23613. x, 494p. 72.50 (*0-8236-6001-X*, 06001) Intl Univs Pr.

Schizophrenia & the Family: A Practitioner's Guide to Psychoeducation & Management. Carol M. Anderson et al. 1986. LC 85-17218. 365p. text 41.95 (*0-89862-065-1*) Guilford Pubns.

Schizophrenia from a Neurocognitive Perspective: Probing the Impenetrable Darkness. Michael F. Green. 1997. LC 97-26855. 190p. 70.00 (*0-205-18477-4*) Allyn.

Schizophrenia Genesis: The Origins of Madness. Irving L. Gottesman. 1990. (Series of Books in Psychology). 296p. (C). pap. text 20.95 (*0-7167-2147-3*) W H Freeman.

Schizophrenia in Focus: Guidelines for Treatment & Rehabilitation. David Dawson et al. 1983. 190p. 32.95 (*0-89885-096-7*, Kluwer Acad Hman Sci) Kluwer Academic.

Schizophrenia Revealed. Michael Greene. 2001. LC 2001-18041. (Professional Book Ser.). (Illus.). 240p. 32.00 (*0-393-70334-7*) Norton.

Schizophrenia Simplified: A Field Guide to Schizophrenia for Frontline Workers, Families, & Professionals. Ed. by Mary V. Seeman & J. F. Thornton. 1995. LC 91-20806. (Illus.). 160p. reprint ed. spiral bd. 16.95 (*0-920887-17-1*) Hogrefe & Huber Pubs.

Schizophrenias: A Biological Approach to the Schizophrenia Spectrum Disorders. Mary Coleman & Christopher Gillberg. 1996. LC 95-53058. (Series on Psychiatry). (Illus.). 288p. 46.95 (*0-8261-9290-4*) Springer Pub.

Schizophrenic Disorders: Sense & Nonsense in Conceptualization, Assessment, & Treatment. L. C. Whitaker. 1992. (Perspectives on Individual Differences Ser.). (Illus.). 272p. (C). 45.00 (*0-306-44156-X*, Plenum Trade) Perseus Pubng.

Schizophrenic Disorders: Theory & Treatment from a Psychodynamic Point of View. Ping-Nie Pao. 1979. LC 77-92180. 456p. 70.00 (*0-8236-5990-9*) Intl Univs Pr.

Schizophrenic Psychology: Index of New Information with Authors, Subjects & Bibliography. Harold P. Drummond. 1993. 180p. pap. 44.50 (*1-55914-811-X*) ABBE Pubs Assn.

Schizophrenics in the Community: An Experimental Study in the Prevention of Hospitalization. Benjamin Pasamanick et al. 1967. LC 66-25455. (Illus.). 32.50 (*0-89197-390-7*) Irvington.

Schizotypal Personality. Ed. by Adrian Raine et al. 1995. (Illus.). 528p. (C). text 120.00 (*0-521-45422-0*) Cambridge U Pr.

Schizotypy: Implications for Illness & Health. Ed. by Gordon Claridge. 1997. LC 96-45523. (Illus.). 354p. text 115.00 (*0-19-852353-X*) OUP.

Schmerzbehandlung in der Rheumatologie. Ed. by G. Kaganas et al. 1989. (Fortbildungskurse fuer Rheumatologie Ser.: Vol. 8). (Illus.). xii, 248p. 55.00 (*3-8055-4901-6*) S Karger.

Schmerzmessung und Schmerzdiagnostik: Methoden, Analysen, Ergebnisse am Beispiel Rheumatischer Erkrankungen. O. B. Scholz. 1994. (Illus.). xiv, 288p. 80.00 (*3-8055-5792-2*) S Karger.

Schmidek & Sweet's Operative Neurosurgical Techniques Henry H. Schmidek & William H. Sweet. 4th ed. 2000. LC 99-38473. (Illus.). xxxii, 2473p. (*0-7216-7815-7*) Saunders.

Schmidt's Anatomy of a Successful Dental Practice. Duane A. Schmidt. 1996. LC 96-33681. 44.95 (*0-87814-585-0*) PennWell Corp.

Scholars & Personal Computers: Microcomputing in the Human & Social Sciences. George M. Kren. 1988. LC 86-27615. 209p. 35.95 (*0-89885-358-3*, Kluwer Acad Hman Sci) Kluwer Academic.

Scholarship in the Discipline of Nursing. Ed. by G. Gray & R. Pratt. 1996. 432p. pap. (*0-443-05109-7*) Church.

Scholarships & Loans for Nurse Education. NLN Research Division Staff. 2nd ed. 2002. (Illus.). (C). pap. text 26.95 (*0-7637-1440-2*, 1440-2, N L N Bart) Jones & Bartlett.

Scholarships & Loans for Nursing Education, 1997-1998. Regina Fawcett. 1997. 125p. pap. 23.95 (*0-88737-730-0*, 41-7300, NLN Pr) Natl League Nurse.

***Scholastic Tradition & Humanist Innovation: The Concept of Neutrum in Renaissance Medicine.** Timo Joutsivuo. 1999. pap. (*951-41-0863-9*) Finnish Acad FIN. *Dist:* Intl Spec Bk.

School & Community Resources for the Behaviorally Handicapped. Ed. by Thomas J. Kelly et al. 1974. 333p. text 32.50 (*0-8422-5163-4*); pap. text 12.75 (*0-8422-0392-3*) Irvington.

School-Based Affective & Social Interventions. Ed. by Susan G. Foreman. 1988. LC 87-25151. (Special Services in the Schools Ser.: Vol. 3, Nos. 3 & 4). 169p. text 39.95 (*0-86656-702-X*) Haworth Pr.

School Based Clinics That Work. Jane K. Martin. 1995. (Illus.). 73p. (Orig.). (C). pap. text 20.00 (*0-7881-1885-4*) DIANE Pub.

School-Based Prevention Programs for Children & Adolescents. Joseph A. Durlak. 1995. LC 95-12680. (Development Clinical Psychology & Psychiatry Ser.: Vol. 34). 136p. (C). pap. 34.95 (*0-8039-5632-0*, 4940) Sage.

School Consultation: A Guide to Practice & Training. Jane C. Conoley & Collie W. Conoley. 2nd ed. 1991. (Psychology Practitioner Guidebooks Ser.). 204p. (C). text (*0-08-037901-X*); pap. text (*0-08-037900-1*) PPI GBR. *Dist:* Elsevier.

School Crisis Survival Guide: Management Techniques & Materials for Counselors & Administrators. Suni Petersen & Ronald Straub. 1991. LC 91-21679. 216p. (J). (gr. k-12). pap. 29.95 (*0-87628-806-9*) Ctr Appl Res.

School Emergencies Manual. Dee K. Bauer & MESD School Health Services Staff. rev. ed. 1994. ring bd. 37.50 (*1-880118-05-X*, 245-01) MESD Pr.

School Failure. Ed. by David W. Kaplan. 1987. (Journal: Vol. 13, No. 2-3, 1986). (Illus.). 88p. pap. 51.50 (*3-8055-4550-9*) S Karger.

School Health. Warren Schaller. 5th ed. 1981. (C). text 29.95 (*0-03-057702-0*) Harcourt Coll Pubs.

School Health: Findings from Evaluated Programs. 1994. lib. bdg. 250.00 (*0-8490-8408-3*) Gordon Pr.

School Health Education to Prevent AIDS & Sexually Transmitted Diseases. WHO Staff. 1992. (WHO AIDS Ser.: Vol. 10). (CHI, FRE, RUS & SPA.). v, 79p. pap. text 18.00 (*92-4-121010-9*, 1870010) World Health.

School Health Practice. William H. Creswell & Ian M. Newman. 10th ed. 1992. (Illus.). 528p. (C). text 68.75 (*0-8016-6746-1*) McGrw-H Hghr Educ.

School Life & Organizational Psychology. American Psychological Association Staff. 1981. (Human Behavior Curriculum Project Ser.). 64p. (Orig.). tchr. ed. 9.95 (*0-8077-2618-4*); pap. text 3.95 (*0-8077-2617-6*) Tchrs Coll.

School Nurse Practitioner. Jack Rudman. 1994. (Certified Nurse Examination Ser.: CN-3). pap. 27.95 (*0-8373-6103-6*) Nat Learn.

School Nurse's Source Book of Individualized Healthcare Plans. Marykay B. Haas. 1993. LC 92-48666. pap. 39.95 (*0-9624814-1-6*) Sunrise River Pr.

School Nurse's Survival Guide: Ready-to-Use Tips, Techniques & Materials for the School Health Professional. Richard M. Adams, II. 1995. LC 95-18454. 354p. spiral bd. 34.95 (*0-13-186727-X*) P-H.

School Nursing. Lewis. 2nd ed. 2001. pap. text (*0-7216-8521-8*) Saunders.

School Nursing & Health Services: A Resource & Planning Guide. Cindy S. Erickson. 1998. LC 98-220071. (Bulletin Ser.). 325p. pap. 27.00 (*1-57337-048-7*) WI Dept Pub Instruct.

School of Natural Healing. John R. Christopher. 1996. LC 90-205323. 724p. 39.95 (*1-879436-01-9*, 99101) Christopher Pubns.

School Phobia & Its Treatment. Nigel Blagg. 1987. 240p. pap. (*0-7099-5050-0*); lib. bdg. (*0-7099-3938-8*) C Helm GBR. *Dist:* Routldge.

School Planning: A Guide for Parents of Children with Seizure Disorders. Epilepsy Foundation of America Staff. 1994. 125p. pap. 12.95 (*0-916570-14-2*) Epilepsy Foundation of America.

School Psychologist: An Introduction. Ed. by George W. Hynd. 1983. 352p. text 47.95 (*0-8156-2289-9*) Syracuse U Pr.

School Psychologist in Nontraditional Settings: Integrating Clients, Services, & Settings. Ed. by R. C. D'Amato & R. S. Dean. 1989. 240p. 49.95 (*0-89859-996-2*) L Erlbaum Assocs.

School Psychology. Jack Rudman. 1994. (National Teacher Examination Ser.: NT-40). pap. 23.95 (*0-8373-8450-8*) Nat Learn.

School Psychology: Past, Present & Future. Thomas K. Fagan & Paula Sachs Wise. 2nd ed. 2000. 537p. pap. text 67.50 (*0-932955-90-8*, N0014) Natl Assn Schl Psych.

School Psychology at a Turning Point: Ensuring a Bright Future for the Profession. Beeman N. Phillips. 1990. LC 89-27510. (Social & Behavioral Sciences Ser.). 328p. 47.00 (*1-55542-195-4*) Jossey-Bass.

School Refusal: Assessment & Treatment. Neville J. King et al. 1995. LC 94-34941. (Practitioner Guidebook Ser.). 192p. (C). 52.00 (*0-205-16071-9*, Longwood Div) Allyn.

School Stress & Anxiety. Beeman N. Phillips. 1978. LC 77-21658. 165p. 32.95 (*0-87705-324-3*, Kluwer Acad Hman Sci) Kluwer Academic.

Schools—Progress, Activities, & Trends: Index of New Information with Authors, Subjects, & References. Chester M. Lukeman. 1995. pap. 47.50 (*0-7883-0465-8*) ABBE Pubs Assn.

Schools & Drugs: A Handbook for Parents & Educators. Joyce M. Tobias. 2nd rev. ed. 1989. LC 89-48781. 48p. (Orig.). (C). 4.00 (*0-9616700-4-5*) Panda Press VA.

Schools & Health: Our Nation's Investment. Lois Nicholson et al. 1997. 350p. 59.95 (*0-309-05435-4*) Natl Acad Pr.

Schoolsearch Guide to Colleges with Programs or Services for Students with Learning Disabilities. Midge Lipkin. 1993. 928p. (Orig.). pap. text 34.95 (*0-9620326-5-4*) Schoolsearch Pr.

Schreiner Festschrift, George E. Journal: Mineral & Electrolyte Metabolism, Vol. 13, No. 6, 1987. Ed. by J. M. Letteri. 1987. (Illus.). vi, 118p. pap. 69.75 (*3-8055-4651-3*) S Karger.

Schriften Zur Psychologie: Neu Herausgegeben, Eingeleitet und Mit Einer Biographischen Einfuhrung Versehen von Helga Sprung Unter Mitarbeit von Lothar Sprung. Carl Stumpf. 1997. (Beitrage Zur Geschichte der Psychologie Ser.: Bd. 14). (GER.). 411p. 56.95 (*3-631-31367-5*) P Lang Pubng.

Schulkinder unter Stress: Theoretische Ueberlegungen zum Stressmodell. Hans R. Mueller. Ed. by G. Ritzel. 1976. (Sozialmedizinische und Paedagogische Jugendkunde Ser.: Band 12). 140p. 21.00 (*3-8055-2299-1*) S Karger.

Schweizerische Gesellschaft fuer Dermatologie und Venerologie, Genf, September 30-October 1, 1977: 59 Jahresversammlung - Journal: Dermatologica, Vol. 157, No. 5. Ed. by R. Schuppli. 1978. (Illus.). pap. 22.75 (*3-8055-2964-3*) S Karger.

Schweizerische Gesellschaft fuer Gynaekologie, Bericht ueber die Jahresversammlung Davos 1976. 1977. (Journal: Vol. 16, Suppl. 1). (Illus.). 24.50 (*3-8055-2669-5*) S Karger.

Schweizerische Gesellschaft fuer Gynaekologie, Bericht ueber die Jahresversammlung, Montreux, Juni 1979. Ed. by E. Dreher. 1980. (Journal: Vol. 19, Suppl. 2). pap. 28.75 (*3-8055-0456-X*) S Karger.

Schweizerische Gesellschaft fuer Gynaekologie Bericht ueber die Jahresversammlung, St. Gallen. J 1980. Ed. by E. Dreher. 1981. (Journal: Vol. 20, No. 1). (Illus.). iv, 144p. pap. 28.75 (*3-8055-2126-X*) S Karger.

Schweizerische Gesellschaft fuer Gynaekologie und Geburtshilfe: Societe Suisse de Gynecologie et Obstetrique , Bericht ueber die Jahresversammlung, St. Moritz, April 1984. Ed. by E. Dreher. 1985. (Journal: Vol. 24, Suppl. 1). iv, 160p. pap. 41.75 (*3-8055-3964-9*) S Karger.

Schweizerische Gesellschaft fuer Gynaekologie und Geburtshilfe: Societe Suisse de Gynecologie et Obstetrique, Bericht ueber die Jahresversammlung Lugano, Juni 1, 1985. Ed. by E. Dreher. 1986. (Journal: Vol. 25, Suppl. 2, 1985). (Illus.). ii, 92p. pap. 24.50 (*3-8055-4242-9*) S Karger.

Schweizerische Gesellschaft fuer Gynaekologie und Geburtshilfe, Bericht ueber die Jahresversammlung, Lausanne, Juni 1983. Ed. by E. Dreher. 1984. (Journal: Vol. 23, Suppl. 4). (Illus.). iv, 116p. pap. 28.75 (*3-8055-3815-4*) S Karger.

Schweizerische Gesellschaft fuer Gynaekologie und Geburtshilfe unter Mitkirkung der Schweizerischen Gesellschaft fuer Medizinische Genetik. Bericht ueber die Jahresversammlung, Zuerich, 1982. Ed. by E. Dreher. 1983. (Journal: Vol. 22, Suppl. 3). (Illus.). xiv, 104p. pap. 34.00 (*3-8055-3656-9*) S Karger.

Schweizerische Gesellschaft fuer Senologie, Kongress in Zuerich, November Nineteen Seventy-Nine. Ed. by W. E. Schreiner. 1981. (Journal: Vol. 21, Suppl. 1). (Illus.). vi, 198p. pap. 52.25 (*3-8055-2837-X*) S Karger.

Schwindel. P. Liard et al. 1994. (Illus.). x, 102p. pap. 33.25 (*3-8055-5814-7*) S Karger.

Sciatica. William Hunter. 1985. 48p. 4.00 (*0-8187-0060-2*) Harlo Press.

Sciatica Relief Handbook. Chet Cunningham. 1998. LC 97-60209. (Illus.). 261p. pap. 14.95 (*1-887053-09-3*) United Res CA.

Science & Art of Dental Ceramics, Vol. II. John McLean. 1980. (Illus.). 496p. text 160.00 (*0-931386-11-X*) Quint Pub Co.

Science & Art of Living a Longer & Healthier Life. Carl E. Bartecchi & Robert W. Schrier. 1997. LC 97-214604. (Illus.). 207p. (Orig.). pap. 14.95 (*0-929240-80-4*) EMIS.

Science & Art of Living a Longer & Healthier Life: Charting a Course for the New Millennium. Carl E. Bartecchi & Robert W. Schrier. 2nd rev. ed. 2000. LC 99-58003. (Illus.). 271p. pap. 14.95 (*0-917634-04-7*) EMIS.

Science & Art of the Pendulum: A Complete Course in Radiesthesia. Gabriele Blackburn. 1984. LC 83-83220. (Illus.). 96p. (Orig.). (C). pap. 10.00 (*0-9613054-1-X*) Idylwild Bks.

Science & Babies: Private Decisions, Public Dilemmas. Suzanne Wymelenberg & Institute of Medicine Staff. 1990. 184p. pap. 14.95 (*0-309-04136-8*) Natl Acad Pr.

Science & Behavior Quickprint. Ashcraft. 1998. pap. text 35.00 (*0-536-01781-6*) Pearson Custom.

Science & Empire: East Coast Fever in Rhodesia & the Transvaal. Paul F. Cranefield. 1991. (Cambridge History of Medicine Ser.). (Illus.). 403p. (C). text 100.00 (*0-521-39253-5*) Cambridge U Pr.

Science & Gender: A Critique of Biology & Its Theories on Women. Ruth Bleier. 1984. (Athene Ser.). (Illus.). 250p. text 45.00 (*0-08-030972-0*); pap. text 18.95 (*0-08-030971-2*) Elsevier (Pergamon Pr).

Science & Gender: A Critique of Biology & Its Theories on Women. Ruth Bleier. 1984. LC 97-7367. (Athene Ser.). 240p. (C). pap. text 18.95 (*0-8077-6200-8*) Tchrs Coll.

Science & Health Experiments & Demonstrations in Smoking Education. 1989. 11.85 (*0-917160-19-3*) Am Sch Health.

Science & Health with Key to the Scriptures. Mary Baker Eddy. 1989. 700p. reprint ed. pap. 15.95 (*0-930227-11-5*) Bookmark CA.

Science & Human Behavior. B. F. Skinner. 1965. LC 53-7045. 461p. reprint ed. pap. 17.95 (*0-02-929040-6*) Free Pr.

Science & Innovation: The U. S. Pharmaceutical Industry During the 1980s. Alfonso Gambardella. 1995. (Illus.). 215p. (C). text 64.95 (*0-521-45118-3*) Cambridge U Pr.

Science & Medicine. Ed. by Michael Cole. 1990. 246p. (*1-870773-17-9*) Spoon River.

Science & Medicine in Imperial Russia. Anatoly Bezkorovainy. 1980. (Illus.). 271p. pap., spiral bd. 12.00 (*0-9607600-0-8*) Bezkorovainy.

Science & Medicine in Islam: A Collection of Essays. Franz Rosenthal. 1991. (Collected Studies: No. 330). 250p. text (*0-86078-282-4*) Variorum GBR. *Dist:* Ashgate Pub Co.

Science & Medicine in Shakespeare's Time: A Guide to the Microfiche Collection. 1991. (Shakespeariana Ser.). 43p. (Orig.). pap. 20.00 (*0-8357-2175-2*) Univ Microfilms.

Science & Medicine in Sport. Ed. by John Bloomfield. 2nd ed. 1995. 648p. pap. 89.95 (*0-86793-321-6*) Blackwell Sci.

Science & Medicine in Twentieth-Century China: Research & Education. Ed. by John Z. Bowers et al. 1989. (Science, Medicine, & Technology in East Asia Ser.: No. 3). 283p. LC 88-36952. text 50.00 (*0-89264-077-4*); pap. text 25.00 (*0-89264-078-2*) Ctr Chinese Studies.

Science & Philosophy of the Organism, Set. Hans Adolf Eduard Driesch. LC 77-27217. (Gifford Lectures: 1907-08). reprint ed. 89.50 (*0-404-60500-1*) AMS Pr.

Science & Politics of I. Q. Leon J. Kamin. 1974. LC 74-13883. 183p. (C). text 39.95 (*0-89859-129-5*) L Erlbaum Assocs.

Science & Practice in Clinical Neurology. Ed. by Simon C. Gandevia et al. 1994. (Illus.). 471p. (C). text 74.95 (*0-521-43119-0*) Cambridge U Pr.

Science & Practice of Cognitive Behaviour Therapy. Ed. by David M. Clark & Christopher G. Fairburn. 1996. (Illus.). 452p. pap. text 51.95 (*0-19-262725-2*) OUP.

Science & Practice of Gerontology: A Multidisciplinary Guide. Ed. by Nancy J. Osgood & Ann H. Sontz. 1989. LC 88-25100. 204p. lib. bdg. 62.50 (*0-313-26161-X*, OSP/, Greenwood Pr) Greenwood.

Science & Practice of Iridology, Vol. I. Bernard Jensen. 1952. pap. 39.99 (*0-9608360-5-5*) B Jensen.

Science & Practice of Occlusion. Ed. by Charles McNeill. 1997. LC 97-18246. (Illus.). 550p. text 148.00 (*0-86715-304-0*) Quint Pub Co.

Science & Practice of Pediatric Cardiology Arthur Garson, Jr. et al. 1990. LC 90-5544. (Illus.). 2557p. text 395.00 (*0-8121-1167-2*) Lppncott W & W.

Science & Practice of Pediatric Cardiology, In Two Volumes. Arthur Garson. 2nd ed. 1997. LC 96-16213. 2,600p. text 399.00 (*0-683-03417-0*) Lppncott W & W.

Science & Psychotherapy, Vol. 1. Ed. by Raphael Stern & Louise Horowitz. 1979. (Philosophy & Science Ser.). text 50.00 (*0-930586-02-6*) Haven Pubns.

Science & Psychotherapy, Vol. 2. Raphael Stern. 1984. (Philosophy & Science Ser.). 65.00 (*0-930586-39-5*) Haven Pubns.

Science & Quiet Art: The Role of Medical Research in Health Care. David Weatherall. 1996. 384p. pap. 15.95 (*0-393-31564-9*) Norton.

Science & Service in Mental Retardation: Proceedings of the Seventh Congress of the International Association for the Scientific Study of Mental Deficiency. Ed. by Joseph M. Berg. 1986. 512p. text 47.50 (*0-416-40650-5*, 1042) Routledge.

Science & Society: Historical Essays on the Relations of Science, Technology & Medicine. A. Rupert Hall. 1994. (Collected Studies: No. CS 434). (Illus.). 350p. (*0-86078-400-2*) Variorum GBR. *Dist:* Ashgate Pub Co.

Science & the Practice of Medicine in the Nineteenth Century. W. F. Bynum. 1994. (Cambridge History of Science Ser.). (Illus.). 301p. (C). text 59.95 (*0-521-25109-5*); pap. text 21.95 (*0-521-27205-X*) Cambridge U Pr.

Science & the Primacy of Consciousness: Intimation of a 21st Century Revolution. Ed. by Richard L. Amoroso et al. 2000. LC 00-100695. (Readings in Consciousness Studies: Vol. 1). (Illus.). xiii, 360p. (C). pap. 37.95 (*0-9678687-1-8*) Noetic Pr CA.

Science, Animals & Evolution: Reflections on Some Unrealized Potentials of Biology & Medicine, 14. Catherine Roberts. 1980. LC 79-52322. (Contributions in Philosophy Ser.: No. 14). 221p. 62.50 (*0-313-21479-4*, RSA/, Greenwood Pr) Greenwood.

Science at the Bedside: Clinical Research in American Medicine, 1905-1945. A. McGehee Harvey. 1981. LC 80-28786. 576p. 54.00 (*0-8018-2562-8*) Johns Hopkins.

Science Book of Wonder Drugs. Donald G. Cooley. 1977. LC 72-99627. (Essay Index Reprint Ser.). (Illus.). 25.95 (*0-8369-1562-3*) Ayer.

Science Challenging AIDS. Ed. by G. Giraldo et al. 1991. (Illus.). xx, 300p. 191.50 (*3-8055-5485-0*) S Karger.

***Science Fictions: A Scientific Mystery, A Massive Cover-Up, & the Dark Legacy of Robert Gallo.** John Crewdson. 2002. LC 2001-34450. (Illus.). 672p. 27.95 (*0-316-13476-7*) Little.

Science Friction: Grins & Groans among the Titles of Scientific Studies. Lubertus Berrens. 1995. LC 95-4088. (Illus.). 92p. pap. 19.50 (*0-88937-146-6*) Hogrefe & Huber Pubs.

Science, Ideology & the Media: The Cyril Burt Scandal. Ronald Fletcher. 1991. LC 90-40836. 196p. (C). text 44.95 (*0-88738-376-9*) Transaction Pubs.

Science in Nursing. Cree. 3rd rev. ed. 1995. pap. text 54.00 (*0-7295-1422-6*) Saunders.

***Science in Nursing.** Laurie Cree & Sandra Rishmiller. 4th ed. 2001. 430p. (*0-7295-3260-7*) Harcourt AUS. *Dist:* Saunders.

Science in the Art of Osteopathy: Osteopathic Principles & Practice. Caroline Stone. 2000. (Illus.). 400p. pap. (*0-7487-3328-0*) Nelson Thornes GBR. *Dist:* Intl Spec Bk.

Science Medicale Occidentale Entre Deux Renaissances, Vols. XII-XV. Danielle Jacquart. 1997. LC 96-40471. (Variorum Collected Studies: Vol. 567). (FRE.). 336p. (*0-86078-621-8*) Variorum GBR. *Dist:* Ashgate Pub Co.

Science, Medicine & Cultural Imperialism. Ed. by Teresa Meade & Mark Walker. 1991. LC 90-45331. 215p. 45.00 (*0-312-04779-7*) St Martin.

Science, Medicine, & History Ed. by E. Ashworth Underwood. 1975. LC 74-26300. (History, Philosophy, & Sociology of Science Ser.). (Illus.). reprint ed. Set. 108.95 (*0-405-06624-4*); Vol. 1. 54.95 (*0-405-06640-6*); Vol. 2. 54.95 (*0-405-06641-4*) Ayer.

Science, Medicine & Technology: English Grammar & Technical Writing. Peter A. Master. 1986. (Illus.). 320p. (C). pap. text 16.00 (*0-13-795469-7*) P-H.

Science, Medicine & the State in Germany: The Case of Baden, 1815-1871. Arleen M. Tuchman. 1993. LC 92-23470. (Illus.). 216p. text 45.00 (*0-19-508047-5*) OUP.

Science, Mind & Psychology: Essays in Honor of Grover Maxwell. Ed. by Mary L. Maxwell & C. Wade Savage. 1989. LC 89-36360. 476p. (C). lib. bdg. 76.00 (*0-8191-7557-9*) U Pr of Amer.

Science Museum Book of Medicine. S. Angliss. (Illus.). mass mkt. (*0-340-71476-X*) Hodder & Stought Ltd GBR. *Dist:* Lubrecht & Cramer, Trafalgar.

Science of Advanced Behavioral Modeling. Wyatt Woodsmall. 1998. (Advanced Neuro Linguistic Programming Applications Ser.). 97p. spiral bd. 35.00 (*1-892876-05-1*) Next Step Pr.

Science of Animal Agriculture. Ray V. Herren. 1993. LC 92-21483. 335p. mass mkt. 39.75 (*0-8273-4546-1*) Delmar.

Science of Animal Agriculture: Lab Manual Answer Key. Frank Flanders & Ray V. Herren. 1994. 32p. 12.75 (*0-8273-6683-3*) Delmar.

Science of Breath. Yogi Ramacharaka. reprint ed. 11.00 (*0-911662-00-6*) Yoga.

Science of Cancer Treatment. Ed. by Michael J. Waring & B. A. Ponder. 1990. 224p. text 118.50 (*0-7923-8905-0*) Kluwer Academic.

Science of Cancerous Disease from Earliest Times to the Present. Jacob Wolff. 1990. (Resources in Medical History Ser.). 600p. 60.00 (*0-88135-085-0*, Sci Hist) Watson Pub Intl.

Science of Cancerous Disease from Earliest Times to the Present. J. G. Wolff. 1989. (C). reprint ed. 50.00 (*81-205-0092-X*) S Asia.

Science of Dentistry. Sturdevant et al. 2nd ed. 1984. (Illus.). 608p. (C). (gr. 13). text 27.50 (*0-8016-4926-9*, 04926) Mosby Inc.

Science of Emotion: Research & Tradition in the Psychology of Emotions. Randolph R. Cornelius. 1995. LC 95-37946. 260p. (C). pap. text 39.60 (*0-13-300153-9*) P-H.

Science of Food: An Introduction to Food Science, Nutrition & Microbiology. P. M. Gaman & K. B. Sherrington. 2nd ed. 1981. (Illus.). 224p. text 44.00 (*0-08-025896-4*); pap. text 21.00 (*0-08-025895-6*) Elsevier (Pergamon Pr).

Science of Food Regulation: Food Intake, Taste, Nutrient Partitioning, & Energy Expenditure. Ed. by George A. Bray & Donna H. Ryan. 1992. LC 91-29389. (Pennington Center Nutrition Ser.: Vol. 2). 440p. text 80.00 (*0-8071-1741-2*) La State U Pr.

Science of Hair Care. Ed. by Charles Zviak. 1986. (Dermatology Ser.: Vol. 7). (Illus.). 624p. text 245.00 (*0-8247-7378-0*) Dekker.

Science of Happiness: Acupuncture - How & Why It Works on Aging Pain & Inflammation. Anuthep Benja-Athon & Christopher A. L. Cox. Ed. by Sandra H. Guiducci. 2000. (Acupuncture Ser.). (Illus.). 54p. pap. 12.95 (*0-9706580-0-1*) Muscle Joint.

Science of Human Nutrition. Judith E. Brown. 1990. 619p. (C). pap. text 34.00 (*0-15-578688-1*) SCP.

Science of Human Nutrition. Judith F. Brown. 2nd ed. 1996. 640p. (C). text (*0-03-005084-7*) SCP.

Science of Low Power Laser Therapy. Ed. by Tiina Karu. 1998. 320p. text (*90-5699-108-6*) GBSP NLD. *Dist:* Gordon & Breach.

Science of Mental Illness. Ethan E. Gorenstein. 1992. (Illus.). 158p. text 34.95 (*0-12-291745-6*) Acad Pr.

Science of Mind. Ernest Holmes. 1998. LC 88-29848. 672p. reprint ed. 15.95 (*0-87477-921-9*, Tarcher Putnam) Putnam Pub Group.

Science of Nutrition of Farm Livestock. D. Cuthbertson & H. Sinclair. 1969. LC 69-14229. (International Encyclopedia of Food & Nutrition Ser.: Vol. 17, Pt. 1). (*0-08-012709-6*) Pergamon Repr GBR. *Dist:* Franklin.

Science of Opticianry, Vol. II. William A. Borover. 1982. (Illus.). 300p. per. 48.00 (*0-9606398-2-9*) Gracie Ent.

Science of Photomedicine. Ed. by James D. Regan et al. 1982. LC 82-9072. (Photobiology Ser.). 680p. 125.00 (*0-306-40924-0*, Plenum Trade) Perseus Pubng.

Science of Psychology. Raygor. Date not set. (C). text (*0-15-507244-7*); pap. text, stu. ed. (*0-15-507245-5*) Harcourt Coll Pubs.

Science of Psychotherapy. Harvey J. Fischer. 1990. 288p. 59.95 (*1-56032-122-9*) Taylor & Francis.

Science of Regeneration: Physiological, Nutritional & Blood Methods of Regeneration. Universal Research Staff. Ed. by Manuel Grace. 1995. (Illus.). 150p. (Orig.). lib. bdg. 10.95 (*0-942951-04-2*) Universal Res MA.

Science of the Mind. Owen Flanagan. 2nd exp. rev. ed. 1991. LC 90-42948. (Illus.). 128p. (Orig.). pap. 26.95 (*0-262-56056-9*, Bradford Bks) MIT Pr.

Science of the Singing Voice. Johan Sundberg. 1992. 228p. pap. 34.95 (*1-56593-583-7*, 0809) Singular Publishing.

Science of Vision. Ed. by K. N. Leibovic. 1990. (Illus.). 487p. 96.00 (*0-387-97270-6*) Spr-Verlag.

Science of Well-Being. Judith L. Powell & Wallace D. Wattles. 1993. LC 93-17454. 160p. (Orig.). pap. 8.95 (*1-56087-059-1*) Top Mtn Pub.

Science of Woman: Gynaecology & Gender in England, 1800-1929. Ornella Moscucci. 1993. (History of Medicine Ser.). (Illus.). 288p. (C). pap. text 28.95 (*0-521-44795-X*) Cambridge U Pr.

Science on Trial: The Clash of Medical Evidence & the Law in the Breast Implant Case. Marcia Angell. 1996. LC 95-50081. 288p. 27.50 (*0-393-03973-0*) Norton.

Science on Trial: The Clash of Medical Evidence & the Law in the Breast Implant Case. Marcia Angell. 1997. LC 98-113190. 256p. pap. 13.95 (*0-393-31672-6*) Norton.

Science, Philosophy & ESP. Charles McCreery. 1989. (C). 120.00 (*0-900076-03-8*) St Mut.

Science-Royal Society of Chemistry Medicinal Chemistry Symposium, 2nd, No. 50. J. C. Emmett. 1989. (Special Publications). 342p. (C). (*0-85186-935-1*) Royal Soc Chem GBR. *Dist:* Spr-Verlag.

Science, Spread & Therapy of HIV Disease: Everything You Need to Know, but Had No Idea Who to Ask. Michael Anthony DiSpezio. 1998. (Science Fundamentals Ser.). (Illus.). 142p. (Orig.). (YA). (gr. 7 up). LC 97-19710. 26.95 (*1-882360-20-6*); pap. 13.95 (*1-882360-19-2*) ATL Pr Sci.

Science, Systems & Psychoanalysis. Robert J. Langs. 1992. 288p. pap. text (*1-85575-036-8*) Karnac Bks GBR. *Dist:* Other Pr LLC.

Science, Technology, & the Art of Medicine: European-American Dialogues. Ed. by Corinna Delkeskamp-Hayes & Mary A. Cutter. Tr. by Ruth W. Moskop & S. G. Engelhardt. 1993. LC 92-18579. (Philosophy & Medicine Ser.: Vol. 44). 346p. (C). lib. bdg. (*0-7923-1869-2*) Kluwer Academic NLD. *Dist:* Kluwer Academic.

Science That Colonizes: A Critique of Fertility Studies in Africa. Agnes Riedmann. 1993. LC 92-26098. 256p. 49.95 (*1-56639-042-7*) Temple U Pr.

Science Tracer Bullets: A Reference Guide to Scientific, Technological, Health, & Environmental Information Sources, Set. Ed. by Helene Henderson. 1990. liv, 402p. lib. bdg. 180.00 (*1-55888-925-6*) Omnigraphics Inc.

Science Tracer Bullets Vol. 3: Medical & Biological Sciences. Ed. by Helene Henderson. 1990. liv, 430p. lib. bdg. 53.00 (*1-55888-262-6*) Omnigraphics Inc.

***Sciences - Research & Medicine: Using the Internet to Find a Job & Get Hired.** Princeton Review Staff. 2002. (Job Surfing Ser.). 352p. pap. 14.95 (*0-375-76237-X*) PRP NY.

Sciences Basic to Psychiatry. Basant K. Puri & Peter J. Tyrer. 2nd ed. 1998. LC 98-14946. (C). pap. text (*0-443-05514-9*) Church.

Sciences of Cognition: Theory & Research in Psychology & Artificial Intelligence. Morton Wagman. 1995. LC 94-28001. 184p. 62.50 (*0-275-94948-6*, Praeger Pubs) Greenwood.

Sciences of Fish Health Management: Master Volume. John Gratzek. (Aquariology Ser.). 34.95 (*1-56465-105-3*, 16855) Tetra Pr.

Sciences of the Flesh: Representing Body & Subject in Psychoanalysis. Dianne F. Sadoff. 1998. LC 98-16198. 372p. 55.00 (*0-8047-3084-9*) Stanford U Pr.

Scientific American Medicine Ed. by D. Dale & D. Federman. 1996. LC 77-92625. (Illus.). ring bd. 328.00 (*0-89454-000-9*) Sci Am Medicine.

Scientific American Molecular Neurology. Joseph B. Martin & Scientific American Editors. 1998. LC 98-5123. (Introduction to Molecular Medicine Ser.). 79.00 (*0-89454-030-0*) WebMD.

Scientific American Molecular Oncology. John Michael Bishop. 1996. 79.00 (*0-89454-023-8*) WebMD.

Scientific American Reader Psychology. Gray. 3rd ed. 2000. pap. text 10.60 (*0-7167-5149-6*) W H Freeman.

S

Scientific American Surgery. Set. Ed. by Douglas Wilmore et al. 1996. (Illus.). ring bd. 250.00 (*0-89454-019-X*) Sci Am Medicine.

Scientific & Clinical Applications of Magnetic Carriers: Proceedings of an International Conference Held in Rostock, Germany, September 5-7-, 1996. Ed. by Urs Hafeli et al. 1997. LC 97-23537. 644p. (C). text 149.50 (*0-306-45687-7*, Kluwer Plenum) Kluwer Academic.

Scientific & Clinical Literature for the Decade of the Brain. Ed. by Tony Stankus. 1993. LC 93-4490. (Science & Technology Libraries Ser.: Vol. 13, Nos. 3-4). 254p. lib. bdg. 7.95 (*1-56024-481-X*) Haworth Pr.

Scientific & Pastoral Perspectives on Intercessory Prayer: An Exchange Between Larry Dossey, M. D. & Health Care Chaplains. Larry Dossey. Ed. by Larry VandeCreek. 1998. LC 98-12323. 140p. 29.95 (*0-7890-0518-2*, Haworth Pastrl); pap. 14.95 (*1-56023-113-0*, Harrington Park) Haworth Pr.

Scientific Approaches to Consciousness. Ed. by Jonathan D. Cohen & Jonathan W. Schooler. 1996. (Carnegie Mellon Symposia on Cognition Ser.). 300p. text 119.00 (*0-8058-1471-X*); pap. text 45.00 (*0-8058-1472-8*) L Erlbaum Assocs.

Scientific Approaches to Health & Health Care. Ed. by B. Z. Nizetic et al. 1986. 186p. pap. text 15.00 (*92-890-1032-0*, 1340030) World Health.

Scientific Background of International Sanitary Conferences, 1851-1938. N. Howard-Jones. 1975. (History of International Public Health Ser.: No. 1). (Illus.). pap. text 12.00 (*92-4-156055-X*, 1290001) World Health.

Scientific Bases of Cancer Chemoprevention: Proceedings of the International Forum on the Scientific Bases of Cancer Chemoprevention, 31 March-2 April 1996. Cesare Maltoni et al. 1996. LC 96-36161. (International Congress Ser.). 310p. 148.00 (*0-444-82453-7*) Elsevier.

Scientific Basis for Selected Environmental Medicine Techniques. Sherry A. Rogers. 1994. LC 94-69079. 130p. reprint ed. pap. 17.95 (*0-9618821-6-6*) SandKey.

Scientific Basis for Vitamin Intake in Human Nutrition. Ed. by P. J. Walter. 1995. LC 95-24755. (Bibliotheca Nutritio et Dieta Ser.: No. 52). (Illus.). vi, 178p. 198.25 (*3-8055-6166-0*) S Karger.

Scientific Basis of Child Custody Decisions. Ed. by Robert M. Galatzer-Levy & Louis Kraus. 1999. LC 98-55271. 480p. 145.00 (*0-471-17478-5*) Wiley.

Scientific Basis of Health Services. Ed. by Michael Peckham & Richard Smith. 1996. 186p. pap. text (*0-7279-1029-9*) BMJ Pub GBR. *Dist:* AIDC.

Scientific Basis of Modern Radiotherapy. Ed. by N. J. McNally. 1989. (British Institute Radiology Report Ser.: No. 19). pap. (*0-905749-20-0*) Med Physics Pub.

Scientific Basis of Noise-Induced Hearing Loss. Ed. by Alf Axelsson et al. 1996. LC 95-45011. 472p. 99.00 (*0-86577-596-6*) Thieme Med Pubs.

Scientific Basis of Phototherapy. Leonard I. Grossweiner. 1994. 227p. lib. bdg. 149.00 (*0-8493-4980-X*) CRC Pr.

Scientific Basis of Transfusion Medicine. Kenneth C. Anderson & Paul M. Ness. Ed. by Marc Strauss. 2nd ed. 1999. LC 99-37690. (Illus.). 658p. text (*0-7216-7684-7*) Saunders.

Scientific Basis of Vegetarianism: Determining Our Natural Dietary Needs. Arthur M. Baker. 1994. 30p. (Orig.). pap. 7.95 (*1-883989-46-9*) Self Hlth Care.

Scientific Credibility of Freud's Theories & Therapy. Seymour Fisher & Roger P. Greenberg. 1985. LC 85-9722. 502p. pap. text 26.50 (*0-231-06215-X*) Col U Pr.

Scientific Dialogue: From Basic Research to Clinical Intervention. Ed. by H. G. Zapotoczky & T. Wenzel. 1990. (Annual Series of European Research in Behavior Therapy: Vol. 5). xii, 316p. (*90-265-1106-X*) Swets.

Scientific Essentials of Reproduction. Hillier. 1996. text 125.00 (*0-7020-1826-0*) Saunders.

Scientific Evidence for Dietary Targets in Europe. Ed. by J. C. Somogyi & A. Trichopoulou. 1985. (Bibliotheca Nutritio et Dieta Ser.: No. 37). (Illus.). vi, 162p. 130.50 (*3-8055-4161-9*) S Karger.

Scientific Evidence in Personal Injury Litigation. Elliott B. Oppenheim. 2000. 250p. 250.00 (*1-930263-04-X*) Terra Firma NM.

***Scientific Evidence on Condom Effectiveness for Sexually Transmitted Disease (STD) Prevention: Workshop Summary.** Ed. by Penny Hitchcock. 2001. 51p. pap. text 20.00 (*0-7567-1504-0*) DIANE Pub.

Scientific Expert in Court: Principles & Guidelines. Richard C. Froede. 1997. 92p. pap. 21.00 (*0-915274-93-0*, 202736, AACC Pr) Am Assn Clinical Chem.

Scientific Foundations & Biochemistry in Clinical Practice. Williams & Marks. 1998. 800p. pap. text (*0-7506-4221-1*) E A GBR. *Dist:* OUP.

Scientific Foundations of Biochemistry in Clinical Practice. Ed. by David L. Williams & Vincent Marks. 2nd ed. 1995. (Scientific Foundations of Clinical Biochemistry Ser.). (Illus.). 896p. 205.00 (*0-7506-0167-1*) Buttrwrth-Heinemann.

Scientific Foundations of Chronic Pain Therapy. Ed. by Rajesh Munglani. 2002. (Greenwich Medical Media Ser.). (Illus.). 350p. text 89.50 (*1-900151-83-9*) OUP.

Scientific Foundations of Cognitive Theory & Therapy of Depression. David A. Clark et al. 1999. LC 98-44674. 504p. 85.00 (*0-471-18970-7*) Wiley.

Scientific Foundations of Neurology. A. Norman Guthkelch & Karl E. Misulis. 1996. LC 96-14099. (Illus.). 512p. 135.00 (*0-86542-408-X*) Blackwell Sci.

Scientific Foundations of the Ovulation Method. Thomas W. Hilgers. 1995. LC 95-69119. (Illus.). 81p. pap. 16.00 (*0-9626485-3-1*) Pope Paul Sixth.

Scientific Foundations of Trauma. Graham Cooper et al. 1997. LC 97-199803. (Illus.). 848p. text 310.00 (*0-7506-1585-0*) Buttrwrth-Heinemann.

Scientific Guide to Peaceful Living. Betty Yulin Ho. 1973. LC 77-142457. (System of Government in the Living Body Ser.). (Illus.). 170p. pap. 25.00 (*0-9600148-2-9*) Juvenescent.

Scientific Healing Affirmations. Paramahansa Yogananda. 1981. LC 81-53040. (Illus.). 100p. pap. 3.50 (*0-87612-144-X*) Self Realization.

Scientific Hydrotherapy. William L. McKie. 1993. 134p. reprint ed. spiral bd. 16.50 (*0-7873-0599-5*) Hlth Research.

Scientific Illustration. Phyllis Wood. 2nd ed. 1994. LC 93-3317. pap. 29.95 (*0-442-01316-7*, VNR) Wiley.

***Scientific Investigations into Chinese Qi-Gong.** Richard H. Lee. 2nd rev. ed. (Illus.). 80p. reprint ed. pap. 4.95 (*1-889983-06-3*) China Hlthways.

Scientific Issues in Quantitative Cancer Risk Assessment. Suresh H. Moolgavkar. 1990. 320p. 77.95 (*0-8176-3501-7*) Birkhauser.

Scientific Meeting on Rehabilitation in Leprosy. 1961. (Technical Report Ser.: No. 221). 37p. pap. text 3.00 (*92-4-120221-1*) World Health.

Scientific Methods & Behavioral Analysis. Ed. by Perone. 1999. (C). text (*0-321-01186-4*) Addson-Wesley Educ.

Scientific Principles of Anesthesia. Debra Schwinn. 1998. LC 97-11333. (Atlas of Anesthesia Ser.). text (*0-443-07901-3*) Church.

Scientific Principles of Psychopathology. P. McGuffin et al. 1984. 780p. text 78.00 (*0-8089-1667-X*, 792837, Grune & Strat) Harcrt Hlth Sci Grp.

Scientific Proceedings American Animal Hospital Association Annual Meeting. 1986. 662p. 42.00 (*0-9616498-5-2*) Am Animal Hosp Assoc.

Scientific Proceedings of the Annual Meeting of the American Animal Hospital Association. American Animal Hospital Association Staff. 1984. 467p. 9.50 (*0-9616498-7-9*) Am Animal Hosp Assoc.

Scientific Revolution in Victorian Medicine. Youngson. 1996. (Australian National University Press Ser.). text (*0-08-032982-9*, Pergamon Pr) Elsevier.

Scientific Study of Human Nature: Tribute to Hans J. Eysenck at Eighty. Ed. by Helmuth Nyborg. 1997. LC 97-15771. 654p. 99.00 (*0-08-042787-1*, Pergamon Pr) Elsevier.

Scientific Study of Personality. Hans J. Eysenck. 1982. LC 81-20077. 320p. reprint ed. lib. bdg. 45.50 (*0-313-23241-5*, EYSS, Greenwood Pr) Greenwood.

Scientific Validation of Herbal Medicine. Daniel B. Mowrey. 1990. 336p. pap. 16.95 (*0-87983-534-6*, 35346K, Keats Pubng) McGraw-Hill Trade.

Scientific Vegetarianism. Edmond B. Szekely. 1977. (Illus.). 56p. pap. 3.50 (*0-89564-041-4*) IBS Intl.

Scientific Watergate - Dyslexia: How & Why Countless Millions Are Deprived of Breakthrough Medical Treatment. Harold N. Levinson. 1994. LC 93-87064. (Illus.). 455p. 24.95 (*0-9639303-0-3*) Stonebrdge Pubng.

***Scientific Workshop on Lesbian Health 2000: Steps for Implementing the Iom Report.** Suzanne G. Hayes. 2001. 100p. (C). pap. text 25.00 (*0-7567-1404-4*) DIANE Pub.

Scientist Practitioner: Research & Accountability in Clinical & Educational Settings. David H. Barlow et al. 1983. (General Psychology Ser.: No. 128). 360p. text 65.00 (*0-08-027217-7*); pap. text 26.50 (*0-08-027216-9*) Elsevier (Pergamon Pr).

Scientist-Practitioner Perspectives on Test Interpretation. Ed. by James W. Lichtenberg & Rodney K. Goodyear. 1998. LC 98-20688. 192p. (C). pap. text 37.00 (*0-205-17481-7*) Allyn.

Scientists of the Mind: Intellectual Founders of Modern Psychology. Clarence J. Karier. 1986. LC 85-996. (Illus.). 368p. text 29.95 (*0-252-01182-1*) U of Ill Pr.

SciLogP. Academic Press Staff. 1999. 136p. 895.00 (*0-12-606309-5*) Acad Pr.

Scintigraphy of Inflammation with Nanometer-Sized Colloidal Tracers. Marc De Schrijver. 1989. (Developments in Nuclear Medicine Ser.). (C). text 135.00 (*0-7923-0272-9*) Kluwer Academic.

Scintillation Detectors. 1983. (Advanced Health Physics Training Ser.). (Illus.). 170p. ring bd. 60.00 (*0-87683-193-5*) GP Courseware.

Sclera. C. Stephen Foster & Maria Sainz De La Maiza. 1993. LC 93-10235. (Illus.). 316p. 203.00 (*0-387-94058-8*) Spr-Verlag.

Sclera & Systemic Disorders. Peter G. Watson. 2001. (Illus.). 384p. 220.00 (*0-7506-3909-1*) Buttrwrth-Heinemann.

Scleroderma: Caring for Your Hands & Face. Jeanne L. Melvin. 1994. (Illus.). 28p. pap. text 6.00 (*1-56900-006-9*) Am Occup Therapy.

Scleroderma: The New Boston Study & the Therapy That Can Save Your Life. Henry Scammell. 1998. LC 97-61593. 192p. 19.95 (*0-87131-842-3*) M Evans.

Scleroderma Book: A Guide for Patients & Families. Maureen D. Mayes. 1999. LC 98-54669. (Illus.). 192p. 23.00 (*0-19-511507-4*) OUP.

Sclerosis: Index of New Information & Research Bible of Current Reviews. Leonard F. Selinsky. 1997. 143p. 57.50 (*0-7883-1612-5*); 1997. 143p. pap. 47.50 (*0-7883-1613-3*); 1994. 150p. pap. 47.50 (*0-7883-0039-3*) ABBE Pubs Assn.

***Sclerosis: Index of New Information & Research Bible of Current Reviews.** Leonard F. Selinsky. 2001. 151p. 57.50 (*0-7883-2521-3*) ABBE Pubs Assn.

Sclerotheraphy: Treatment of Varicose & Telangiectatic Veins. Mitchel P. Goldman & John J. Bergan. 3rd ed. LC 00-67896. 445p. text (*0-323-01468-2*) Saunders.

Sclerotherapy: Treatment of Varicose & Telangiectatic Leg Virus. Mitchel P. Goldman. 2nd ed. 1995. LC 94-44914. (Illus.). 544p. (C). (gr. 13). text 195.00 (*0-8151-4011-8*, 24425) Mosby Inc.

Sclerotherapy of Spider Veins. Victoria Vitale-Lewis. 1995. (Illus.). 142p. text (*0-7506-9459-9*) E A GBR. *Dist:* OUP.

Scoliosis: Ascending the Curve. Brooke Lyons et al. 1999. LC 99-28380. (Illus.). x, 306p. 24.95 (*0-87131-883-0*) M Evans.

Scoliosis: Collection of Published Articles. R. B. Mawhiney. 1989. (Illus.). 66p. 45.00 (*0-931764-08-4*) Roberts Pub Co.

Scoliosis: Diagnosis & Management. Rene Cailliet. 1975. LC 75-6709. (Illus.). 121p. text 22.95 (*0-8036-1640-6*) Davis Co.

Scoliosis: Identifiable Causes Detection & Correction. Vol. III. Frederick H. Barge. 2nd exp. ed. 1996. 347p. text 75.95 (*1-885048-02-5*) Barge Chiropract.

Scoliosis Care. R. B. Mawhiney. 1998. (Illus.). 100p. pap. 12.95 (*0-931764-01-7*) Roberts Pub Co.

Scoliosis Prevention. Ed. by J. O. Warner et al. 1985. LC 84-26400. (Proceedings of the Seventh Phillip Zorab Symposium). 316p. 72.50 (*0-275-91327-9*, C1327, Praeger Pubs) Greenwood.

Scoliosis Sourcebook. Michael Neuwirth & Kevin Osborn. 2001. LC 00-69643. (Illus.). 272p. pap. 16.95 (*0-7373-0321-2*, 03212W) McGraw-Hill Prof.

Scope & Standards of Advanced Clinical Practice in Rehabilitation Nursing. 2000. 30p. pap. (*1-884278-12-4*) Rehab Nursing.

Scope & Standards of Pediatric Oncology Nursing Practice. Association of Pediatric Oncology Nurses & American Nurses Association Staff. 2000. LC 00-48523. ix, 44p. pap. text (*1-55810-154-3*, SSPONP-20, Am Nurses Fnd) Am Nurses Pub.

Scope & Standards of Psychiatric-Mental Health Clinical Nursing Practice. 2000. pap. 14.95 (*1-55810-153-5*) Am Nurses Pub.

Scope of Ambulatory Monitoring in Ischemic Heart Disease: Proceedings. Conference on Ambulatory Monitoring, 3rd, 1977. Ed. by Nancy K. Jacobsen et al. 1978. 18.50 (*0-917054-15-6*) Med Communications.

Scope of Epidemiological Psychiatry: Essays in Honor of Michael Shepherd. Ed. by Paul Williams et al. 1989. 200p. 53.00 (*0-415-01814-5*) Routledge.

Scorecards for Abdominal Sonography. Jann Dolk. Ed. by Edward G. Grant. 2001. LC 00-60162. (Illus.). 762p. pap. 49.95 (*0-941022-47-1*, 11027) Davies Pubng.

Scorecards for Vascular Technology. Cindy A. Owen. Ed. by D. E. Strandness. 2001. LC 00-60161. (Illus.). 854p. pap. 49.95 (*0-941022-48-X*) Davies Pubng.

Scots Herbal. Tess Darwin. 1997. LC 98-187777. 208p. (*1-873644-60-4*) Mercat Pr Bks GBR. *Dist:* St Mut.

Scott: An Aid to Clinical Surgery. Ed. by H. A. Dudley & B. P. Waxman. 4th ed. 1988. (Illus.). 320p. pap. text (*0-443-03839-2*) Church.

Scott, an Aid to Clinical Surgery. Robin C. Williamson et al. 6th ed. 1998. LC 97-39864. (C). pap. text (*0-443-05603-X*); (*0-443-05609-9*) Church.

Scottish Medical Societies, 1731-1939: Their History & Records. Jacqueline Jenkinson. 1993. 256p. text (*0-7486-0390-5*) Edinburgh U Pr GBR. *Dist:* Col U Pr.

***Scourge: The Once & Future Threat of Smallpox.** Jonathan B. Tucker. 2001. LC 2001-22913. 291p. 26.00 (*0-87113-830-1*, Atlntc Mnthly) Grove-Atltic.

Scrapie Disease in Sheep: Historical, Clinical, Epidemiological, Pathological & Practical Aspects of the Natural Disease. Herbert B. Parry. 1984. text 104.00 (*0-12-545750-2*) Acad Pr.

Screaming Room: A Mother's Journal of Her Son's Struggle with AIDS. Barbara Peabody. 1987. 288p. mass mkt. 4.99 (*0-380-70345-9*, Avon Bks) Morrow Avon.

Screen Film Mammography: Imaging Considerations & Medical Physics Responsibilities. Ed. by Gary Barnes & G. Donald Frey. 1991. (Illus.). 242p. (C). reprint ed. pap. text 43.95 (*0-944838-12-X*) Med Physics Pub.

***Screening.** Ed. by Catherine Peckham & Carol Dezateux. 1998. (British Medical Bulletin Ser.: Vol. 54, No. 4). 259p. pap. (*1-85315-345-1*) Royal Soc of Medicine Pr Ltd GBR. *Dist:* Balogh.

Screening & Assessment for Alcohol & Other Drug Abuse among Adults in the Criminal Justice System. Ed. by Anna Marsh & Sandra Clunies. 1999. (Illus.). 129p. (C). pap. text 25.00 (*0-7881-7599-8*) DIANE Pub.

Screening & Assessment of Alcohol & Other Drug-Abusing Adolescents: A Treatment Improvement Protocol. 1994. (Illus.). 201p. (Orig.). (C). pap. text 35.00 (*0-7881-1167-1*) DIANE Pub.

Screening & Diagnostic Procedures. 1983. 1.50 (*0-939418-50-9*) Ferguson-Florissant.

Screening & Management of Potentially Treatable Genetic Metabolic Disorders. Ed. by P. F. Benson. 1984. 176p. text 164.50 (*0-85200-784-1*) Kluwer Academic.

Screening & Surveillance in General Practice. Ed. by Cyril Hart & John Bain. 1992. (Illus.). 392p. text (*0-443-04160-1*) Church.

Screening Children for Auditory Function. Ed. by Fred H. Bess & James W. Hall, III. 1992. LC 92-70246. (Illus.). 560p. (C). text 55.00 (*0-9631439-0-5*) Vanderbilt Wilkerson.

Screening, Diagnosis, Management & Counseling, Clinical Practice Guideline for Sickle Cell Disease in Newborns & Infants. 1997. lib. bdg. 250.95 (*0-8490-8139-4*) Gordon Pr.

Screening for Biological Response Modifiers: Methods & Rationale. James E. Talmadge et al. 1985. (Developments in Oncology Ser.). text 86.50 (*0-89838-712-4*) Kluwer Academic.

Screening for Brain Dysfuction in Psychiatric Patients. Cooper B. Holmes. 1998. LC 98-27914. 148p. text 38.95 (*0-398-06921-2*); pap. text 24.95 (*0-398-06907-7*) C C Thomas.

Screening for Brain Impairment: A Manual for Mental Health Practice. Richard A. Berg et al. 2nd ed. 1994. 264p. 33.95 (*0-8261-5741-6*) Springer Pub.

Screening for Cancer of the Uterine Cervix. Ed. by M. Hakama et al. 1987. (IARC Scientific Publications Ser.: No. 76). (Illus.). 320p. text 55.00 (*92-832-1176-6*) OUP.

Screening for Colorectal Carcinoma: Proceedings of International Meeting Organized by the United Kingdom Coordinating Committee on Cancer Research. Ed. by Jack D. Hardcastle. 1990. (Illus.). 110p. pap. 15.00 (*0-926592-03-3*) Normed Verlag.

Screening for Down's Syndrome. Ed. by J. Gedes Grudzinskas et al. 1995. (Illus.). 358p. (C). text 90.00 (*0-521-45271-6*) Cambridge U Pr.

Screening for Hearing Loss & Otitis Media in Children. Jackson Roush. 2001. LC 00-49254. (Illus.). 272p. pap. text 49.95 (*0-7693-0000-6*) Singular Publishing.

Screening for Inborn Errors of Metabolism: Proceedings of the WHO Scientific Group, Geneva, 1967. WHO Staff. 1968. (Technical Reports: No. 401). 57p. pap. text 5.00 (*92-4-120401-X*, 1100401) World Health.

Screening for Infectious Diseases among Substance Abusers: A Treatment Improvement Protocol. 1994. (Illus.). 160p. (Orig.). (C). pap. text 35.00 (*0-7881-1162-0*) DIANE Pub.

Screening Handbook. John Fry et al. 1990. 160p. pap. text 59.00 (*0-7923-8926-3*) Kluwer Academic.

Screening in Chronic Disease. Alan S. Morrison. 2nd ed. 1992. (Monographs in Epidemiology & Biostatistics: No. 19). (Illus.). 272p. text 49.50 (*0-19-506390-2*) OUP.

Screening in Primary Health Care: Setting Priorities with Limited Resources. P. A. Braveman & E. Tarimo. 1994. LC 96-139939. (CHI, ENG, FRE & SPA.). viii, 196p. pap. text 30.00 (*92-4-154473-2*, 1150424) World Health.

Screening the Body: Tracing Medicine's Visual Culture. Lisa Cartwright. 1995. LC 94-30340. 199p. pap. 17.95 (*0-8166-2290-6*); text 49.95 (*0-8166-2289-2*) U of Minn Pr.

Scripture & Science: A Physician's Reflections on Judaic Doctrine. Harold Speert. 1995. LC 95-18835. 10.00 (*1-57059-256-X*) Landes Bioscience.

Scrisori Din Tinerete Catre Eduard Silberstein, 1871-1881. Sigmund Freud. Ed. by Florin V. Vladescu. Tr. by Ioan Milea. 1993. (Illus.). 196p. (Orig.). pap. text 19.95 (*1-883881-01-3*) S Freud RT&PF.

Scruffy's Pawsitive Mission: A Tail of a Dog & Her Master Attacking Panic. Patricia L. Pleban. 1999. (Illus.). 149p. pap. 12.95 (*1-58446-003-2*, Legacy OH) Temple Pubg.

Scuba Diving First Aid. National Safety Council Staff. 1995. LC 94-48302. (Emergency Care Ser.). (Illus.). 64p. (C). pap. text 15.00 (*0-86720-944-5*, 944-5) Jones & Bartlett.

SE Switch: Evolution & Our Self-Esteem. Leonard A. Zimmerman. 2000. LC 00-36914. 127p. pap. 17.95 (*1-58141-021-2*) Rivercross Pub.

Sea Life. 1981. 85p. (*0-9607580-3-8*) S Stafford.

Sea of Grass: The Maritime Drug War, 1970-1990. Charles M. Fuss, Jr. 1996. LC 96-16534. (Illus.). 352p. 34.95 (*1-55750-276-5*) Naval Inst Pr.

Sea Salt's Hidden Powers. Jacques De Langre. 2nd ed. 1993. (Illus.). 101p. 8.00 (*0-916508-42-0*) Happiness Pr.

Seafood-Analysis & Research for Health & Disease: Index of New Information with Authors, Subjects & References. Marvin H. Vensko. 1997. 164p. 57.50 (*0-7883-1362-2*); pap. 47.50 (*0-7883-1363-0*) ABBE Pubs Assn.

Seafood Safety. Institute of Medicine Staff. 1991. 452p. text 49.95 (*0-309-04387-5*) Natl Acad Pr.

Seamless Connections: Refocusing Your Organization to Create a Successful Continuum of Care. Connie Evashwick. 1997. LC 96-29703. (Illus.). 168p. (Orig.). pap. 45.00 (*1-55648-183-7*, 067105) AHPI.

Search for an Abortionist. Nancy H. Lee. 1993. LC 74-75135. lib. bdg. 13.00 (*0-226-47001-6*) U Ch Pr.

Search for an AIDS Vaccine: Ethical Issues in the Development & Testing of a Preventive HIV Vaccine. Christine Grady. 1995. LC 94-35650. (Medical Ethics Ser.). 192p. text 26.50 (*0-253-32619-2*) Ind U Pr.

Search for Anti-Inflammatory Drugs: Case Histories from Concept to Clinic. Ed. by Vincent J. Merluzzi & Julian Adams. 1995. LC 95-1583. (Illus.). 314p. 96.50 (*0-8176-3685-4*) Birkhauser.

Search for Antiviral Drugs: Case Histories from Concept to Clinic. Ed. by Julian Adams & Vincent J. Merluzzi. 1993. LC 93-16405. (Illus.). xiii, 240p. 63.50 (*0-8176-3606-4*) Birkhauser.

Search for Authenticity: An Existential-Analytic Approach to Psychotheraphy. James F. Bugental. enl. ed. 477p. reprint ed. 1997. pap. text 19.95 (*0-8290-1298-2*); 1989. text 49.50 (*0-8290-0108-5*) Irvington.

Search for Connections: Studies of Regeneration in the Nervous System of the Leech. John G. Nicholls. 1987. LC 86-22061. (Magnes Memorial Lectures: Vol. 2). (Illus.). 86p. (Orig.). pap. text 21.95 (*0-87893-577-0*) Sinauer Assocs.

Search for Health: A Classic Anthology. Tom Valentine et al. 1995. (Illus.). 520p. pap. 35.00 (*0-9648325-0-X*) Valentine Commun.

Search for Man's Sanity. Trigant Burrow. Ed. by Gerald N. Grob. 1980. LC 78-22553. (Historical Issues in Mental Health Ser.). reprint ed. lib. bdg. 50.95 (*0-405-11907-0*) Ayer.

Search for Maturity: Personality, Conscience, Religion. Zdzislaw Chlewinski. 1998. (American University Studies: Vol. 198). VII, 137p. (C). text 32.95 (*0-8204-3471-X*) P Lang Pubng.

Search for New Anticancer Drugs. Ed. by Michael J. Waring & B. A. Ponder. 1992. LC 92-49744. (Cancer Biology & Medicine Ser.: Vol. 3). (C). text 177.50 (*0-7923-8959-X*) Kluwer Academic.

Search for New Vaccines: The Effects of the Vaccines for Children Program. Henry Grabowski & John Vernon. 1997. LC 97-30439. 100p. (Orig.). pap. 14.95 (*0-8447-4033-0*) Am Enterprise.

Search for Oneness. Lloyd H. Silverman et al. 1983. LC 82-4658. x, 306p. 45.00 (*0-8236-6013-3*) Intl Univs Pr.

Search for Security: An Ethno-Psychiatric Study of Rural Ghana. Margaret J. Field. 1970. (C). reprint ed. pap. 2.50 (*0-393-00508-9*) Norton.

Search for the Causes of Schizophrenia. Ed. by H. Hafner et al. 1987. (Illus.). 389p. 167.00 (*0-387-17376-5*) Spr-Verlag.

Search for the Causes of Schizophrenia. Vol. III. Ed. by H. Hafner & W. F. Gattaz. 1995. (Illus.). 352p. 108.00 (*3-540-58751 9*) Spr-Verlag.

Search for the Self: Selected Writings of Heinz Kohut. Ed. by Paul H. Ornstein. 1991. Vol. 3. 400p. 62.50 (*0-8236-6017-6*); Vol. 4. 500p. 67.50 (*0-8236-6018-4*) Intl Univs Pr.

Search for the Self: Selected Writings of Heinz Kohut 1950-1978 Ed. by Paul H. Ornstein. 1978. LC 77-90229. 1. 75.00 (*0-8236-6015-X*); 2. 67.50 (*0-8236-6016-8*) Intl Univs Pr.

Search for the Tourette Syndrome & Human Behavior Genes. David E. Comings. 1996. 34.00 (*1-878267-36-1*); pap. 29.95 (*1-878267-41-8*) Hope Pr CA.

Search Is an Emergency: Text for Managing Search Operations. Brady Games Staff et al. 1995. (Illus.). 480p. 30.00 (*0-913724-28-9*) Emerg Response Inst.

Search PsycINFO: Instructor Guide. Ed. by Carolyn G. Gosling et al. 1989. 49p. pap., tchr. ed. 15.00 (*1-55798-056-X*) Am Psychol.

Searching for Health. Robert J. Peshek. 1982. 15.95 (*0-9605902-4-2*) Color Coded Charting.

Searching for Health Information: The Cancer Information Service Model. Vicki S. Freimuth et al. 1989. LC 88-38116. (Illus.). 264p. (C). text 65.00 (*0-8122-8123-3*); pap. text 24.95 (*0-8122-1272-X*) U of Pa Pr.

Searching for Magic Bullets: Orphan Drugs, Consumer Activism, & Pharmaceutical Development. Lisa R. Basara & Michael Montagne. 1994. LC 93-35534. (Illus.). 276p. lib. bdg. 39.95 (*1-56024-858-0*); pap. 14.95 (*1-56024-859-9*) Haworth Pr.

Searching for Memory: The Brain, the Mind & the Past. Daniel L. Schacter. 1997. LC 96-19521. 398p. pap. 16.50 (*0-465-07552-5*) Basic.

Searchlights on Delinquency. Ed. by K. R. Eissler. 1967. 80.00 (*0-8236-6020-6*) Intl Univs Pr.

Sear's Anatomy & Physiology for Nurses. 6th ed. (*0-7131-4463-7*) E A GBR. *Dist:* Routldge.

Season to Taste: Low Salt - No Salt. Carol E. Goodkind & Abby L. Sproul. 1986. (Illus.). 64p. (Orig.). pap. 5.95 (*0-9610600-1-8*) Sea to Sea.

Seasonal Affective Disorder & Beyond: Light Treatment for SAD & Non-SAD Conditions. Ed. by Raymond W. Lam. 1998. LC 97-4720. 327p. text 47.00 (*0-88048-867-0*, 8867) Am Psychiatric.

Seasonal Affective Disorders & Phototherapy. Ed. by Norman E. Rosenthal & Mary C. Blehar. 1989. LC 88-24402. 386p. 60.00 (*0-89862-741-9*, 2741) Guilford Pubns.

Seasonal Food Medicine. Timothy Yeh et al. 1996. (Illus.). 300p. (Orig.). pap. text 49.95 (*0-9652967-0-9*) Yehs Ctr Nat Med.

***Seasonal Patterns of Immune Function & Disease.** Randy J. Nelson et al. 2002. 260p. text 64.95 (*0-521-59068-X*) Cambridge U Pr.

Seasonal Spermatogenesis in the Mute Swan (Cygnus Olor) H. Breucker. 1982. (Advances in Anatomy, Embryology & Cell Biology Ser.: Vol. 72). (Illus.). 94p. 39.95 (*0-387-11326-6*) Spr-Verlag.

Seasonal Variation in Health & Diseases: With Sections on Effects of Weather & Temperature; a Bibliography. T. M. Allan & A. S. Douglas. 1995. LC 94-14865. 496p. 150.00 (*0-7201-2211-2*) Continuum.

Seasonality & Human Ecology. Ed. by Stanley J. Ulijaszek & S. S. Strickland. 1993. LC 92-43449. (Society for the Study of Human Biology Symposium Ser.: Vol. 35). (Illus.). 262p. (C). text 74.95 (*0-521-43147-6*) Cambridge U Pr.

Seasoned Psychotherapist: Triumph over Adversity. Carl Goldberg. 1992. LC 92-16191. 200p. (C). 24.95 (*0-393-70146-8*) Norton.

Seasons of Grief & Grace: A Sister's Story of AIDS. Susan F. Wiltshire. LC 94-26440. (Illus.). 216p. 1994. (C). 29.95 (*0-8265-1261-5*); 1995. reprint ed. pap. 14.95 (*0-8265-1271-2*) Vanderbilt U Pr.

Seat Belts & Other Devices to Reduce Injuries from Traffic Accidents: Report on a WHO Technical Group. 1981. (Euro Reports & Studies Ser.: No. 40). 53p. pap. text 4.00 (*92-890-1206-4*) World Health.

Seating & Moving Through the Decades: A Literature Review of Seating & Mobility through 1992. Jean A. Zollars. 2nd ed. 1993. (C). pap. text 29.95 (*1-882632-03-6*) PAX Pr.

Seattle - Tacoma Health Care Choices: The Families U. S. A. Guide to Quality & Cost. Marc S. Miller. 1996. (Illus.). 240p. (Orig.). pap. 10.95 (*0-9617893-1-X*) Fam USA Found.

Seattle Psychotherapy Language Analysis Schema. Peter E. Maxim. 1986. 66p. pap., ring bd. 24.95 (*0-295-96459-6*) U of Wash Pr.

Sebaceous Glands, Acne & Related Disorders: Basic & Clinical; Research, Clinical Entities & Treatment. 4th International Dermatology Symposium, Berlin, April 1997. Ed. by Ch. C. Zouboulis. 1998. (Dermatology Ser.: Vol. 196, No. 1, 1998). (Illus.). 118p. pap. 59.25 (*3-8055-6648-4*) S Karger.

Second AAS Symposium on Physical & Biological Phenomena under Zero G Conditions, Jan. 18, 1963, Los Angeles, CA. Ed. by Elliot T. Benedikt & Robert W. Halliburton. 1963. LC 57-43769. (Advances in the Astronautical Sciences Ser.: Vol. 14). 382p. 30.00 (*0-87703-015-4*, Am Astronaut Soc) Univelt Inc.

Second Annual Nicholas E. Davies CPR Recognition Symposium Proceedings. Ed. by Elaine B. Steen. 1997. (Illus.). 123p. (Orig.). pap. 24.00 (*0-9649285-1-5*, D596-5) Comp-based Patient Rec.

Second Asian Regional Workshop on Injectable Contraceptives. Ed. by Edwin B. McDaniel. 1982. (Illus.). 93p. pap. 5.00 (*0-942716-04-3*) World Neigh.

Second Brain: A History of the Spinal Cord from Ancient Egy. Fiffer. 2001. text (*0-7167-4109-1*) W H Freeman.

Second Brain: The Scientific Basis of Gut Instinct & a Groundbreaking New Understanding of Nervous Disorders of the Stomach & Intestine. Michael Gershon. 1999. LC 98-28577. (Illus.). 336p. pap. 14.00 (*0-06-093072-1*) HarperCollins Pubs.

Second Decade of AIDS: A Mental Health Practice Handbook. Ed. by Walt Odets & Michael Shernoff. 1995. LC 94-40679. 320p. pap. 19.95 (*1-886330-01-8*) Hatherleigh.

Second Fifty Years: Promoting Health & Preventing Disability. Institute of Medicine Staff. Ed. by Robert L. Berg & J. S. Cassells. 1992. 344p. pap. 19.95 (*0-309-04681-5*) Natl Acad Pr.

Second Forty Years. Edward J. Stieglitz. Ed. by Robert J. Kastenbaum. 1979. LC 78-22218. (Aging & Old Age Ser.). (Illus.). reprint ed. lib. bdg. 30.95 (*0-405-11831-7*) Ayer.

Second Generation of Calcium Antagonists. W. G. Nayler. 1991. (Illus.). 226p. 103.00 (*0-387-54215-9*) Spr-Verlag.

Second-Hand Knowledge: An Inquiry into Cognitive Authority, 44. Patrick Wilson. 1983. LC 82-21069. (Contributions in Librarianship & Information Science Ser.: No. 44). 211p. 37.50 (*0-313-23763-8*, WWK/, Greenwood Pr) Greenwood.

Second Handbook of Psychological & Social Instruments. D. M. Pestonjee. 1990. (C). (*81-7022-193-5*) Concept IND. *Dist:* S Asia.

Second HGH Symposium, Amsterdam, June 1991. Ed. by J. Girard & J. S. Christiansen. 1991. (Journal: Vol. 36, Suppl. 1, 1991). (Illus.). iv, 84p. pap. 38.50 (*3-8055-5552-0*) S Karger.

Second International Aphasia Rehabilitation Congress: Proceedings of the Conference, Goteborg, Sweden, June 1986. Ed. by Chris Code & Dave J. Muller. 1987. (Aphasiology Special Issue Ser.: Vol. 1, No. 3, May-June 1987). 116p. pap. 25.00 (*0-85066-913-8*) Taylor & Francis.

Second International Conference on Frontal Lobe Degeneration of Non-Alzheimer Type, Lund, Sweden, September 1992. Ed. by Victoria E. Chan-Palay. 1993. (Journal: Vol. 4, No. 3-4, 1993). (Illus.). 116p. pap. 45.25 (*3-8055-5824-4*) S Karger.

Second International Congress of Neuroendocrinology Abstracts, Bordeaux, June 1990: Journal: Neuroendocrinology, Vol. 52, Suppl. 1. Ed. by J. D. Vincent & D. A. Poulain. 1990. (Illus.). iv, 178p. pap. 56.75 (*3-8055-5252-1*) S Karger.

Second Japan Conference on Endometriosis: Biology of Endometrium vs. Endometriosis: Proceedings of the 2nd Japan Conference on Endometriosis, Kanagawa, May, 1999. Ed. by H. Hoshiai et al. 1999. (Gynecologic & Obstetric Investigation Ser.: Vol. 48, Suppl. 1). (Illus.). iv, 58p. pap. 25.25 (*3-8055-6987-4*) S Karger.

Second-Line Agents in the Treatment of Arthritis. Ed. by Jonathan S. Dixon & D. E. Furst. 1991. (Infectious Disease & Therapy Ser.: Vol. 9). (Illus.). 640p. text 255.00 (*0-8247-8541-X*) Dekker.

Second Look: The Reconstruction of Personal History in Psychiatry & Psychoanalysis. Samuel Novey. Ed. by Chicago Institute for Psychoanalysis Staff. 1986. LC 85-10884. (Classics in Psychoanalysis Monograph: No. 3). xiv, 162p. reprint ed. 30.00 (*0-8236-6022-2*, 06022) Intl Univs Pr.

Second Nuclear Era: A New Start for Nuclear Power. Alvin M. Weinberg et al. 1985. LC 85-26613. 460p. 69.00 (*0-275-90183-1*, C0183, Praeger Pubs) Greenwood.

Second Opinion: A Holistic Approach to Treating Adults with A. D. D. Richard C. Bennett. 1994. 110p. pap. text 19.95 (*1-885988-00-1*) Add Resources.

Second Opinion: The Columbia-Presbyterian Guide to Surgery. Eric Rose. 2000. LC 2001-34957. (Illus.). xvii, 336p. 27.95 (*0-312-20584-8*) St Martin.

Second Opinion Elective Surgery. Eugene McCarthy et al. 1981. LC 81-3471. 206p. 60.00 (*0-86569-079-0*, Auburn Hse) Greenwood.

Second Opinions: Americans' Changing Views on Healthcare Reform. John Immerwahr & Jean Johnson. 1994. 40p. pap. 15.00 (*1-889483-26-5*) Public Agenda.

Second Part of the Popular Errors. Tr. & Anno. by Gregory D. De Rocher. 1995. LC 94-4708. 336p. text 49.95 (*0-8173-0758-3*) U of Ala Pr.

Second Part of the Secretes of Maister Alexis of Piemont. Piemontese Alessio. Tr. by W. Ward. 1977. LC 77-6843. (English Experience Ser.: No. 839). reprint ed. lib. bdg. 20.00 (*90-221-0839-2*) Walter J Johnson.

Second Plague of Europe: AIDS Prevention & Sexual Transmission among Men in Western Europe. Michael Pollak. 1994. LC 92-18354. pap. 9.95 (*1-56023-020-7*, Harrington Park); (Illus.). 104p. 39.95 (*1-56024-306-6*) Haworth Pr.

Second Sandoz Symposium on the Treatment of Parkinson's Disease, Tokyo, October 1993. Ed. by I. Goto. 1994. (Journal: Vol. 34, Suppl. 3, 1994). (Illus.). iv, 40p. pap. 19.25 (*3-8055-6058-3*) S Karger.

Second Sickness: Contradictions of Capitalist Health Care. Howard Waitzkin. 2nd ed. 1999. LC 99-46590. 288p. text 69.00 (*0-8476-9886-6*) Rowman.

Second Symposium by the Eight Winners of the Grants from Sandoz Foundation for Gerontological Research: Annual Meeting of the Japan Gerontological Society, Kochi-Japan, November 1990 - Journal: Gerontology, Vol. 37, Suppl. 1, 1991. Ed. by H. Orimo. 1991. (Illus.). iv, 64p. pap. 21.00 (*3-8055-5473-7*) S Karger.

Second Ten Years of the World Health Organization, 1958-1967. 1968. text 29.00 (*92-4-156015-0*, 1150139) World Health.

Second Trimester Abortion. Ed. by G. Berger et al. 1981. text 162.50 (*90-247-2487-2*) Kluwer Academic.

Second Year: The Emergence of Self-Awareness. Jerome Kagan. 1981. 171p. LC 81-4214. (Illus.). (C). 30.00 (*0-674-79662-4*); pap. 14.50 (*0-674-79663-2*) HUP.

Secondary & Teritiary Prevention of Stroke: Patient Outcomes Research Team (PORT) Final Report - Phase 1. David B. Matchar & Gregory P. Samsa. 2000. pap. (*1-58763-009-5*) Agency Healthcare.

Secondary Detachment of the Retina: Proceedings of the Collogue du Club Jules Gonin, 7th & the Assemblee de la Societe Suisse d'Ophthalmologie, 63rd, Lausanne, 1970. Colloque du Club Jules Gonin Staff & Assemblee de la Societe Suisse d'Ophthalmologie Staff. Ed. by R. Dufour. 1972. (Modern Problems in Ophthalmology Ser.: Vol. 10). (Illus.). 139.25 (*3-8055-1300-3*) S Karger.

Secondary Hypertension. Ed. by H. Vetter. 1985. (Journal: Vol. 72, Suppl. 1, 1985). (Illus.). iv, 196p. pap. 51.50 (*3-8055-4079-5*) S Karger.

Secondary Infections & ISR Testing. Katherine E. Anderson. 1998. 150p. pap., spiral bd. 19.95 (*1-57876-930-2*, Love Lives) Triple U Enterprises.

Secondary Metabolism & Differentiation in Fungi. J. W. Bennett & Alex Ciegler. 1983. (Mycology Ser.: Vol. 5). (Illus.). 504p. text 225.00 (*0-8247-1819-4*) Dekker.

Secondary Metabolism in Microorganisms, Plants & Animals. M. Luckner. 3rd ed. 1990. 549p. 129.00 (*0-387-50287-4*) Spr-Verlag.

Secondary Neoplasias Following Chemotherapy, Radiotherapy & Immunosuppression. Ed. by U. Ruther et al. 2000. LC 00-66398. (Contributions to Oncology Ser.: Vol. 55). (Illus.). viii, 376p. 172.25 (*3-8055-7116-X*) S Karger.

Secondary Prevention in Coronary Artery Disease & Myocardial Infarction. Ed. by P. Mathes. 1985. (Developments in Cardiovascular Medicine Ser.). lib. bdg. 223.50 (*0-89838-736-1*) Kluwer Academic.

Secondary Prevention of Colorectal Cancer. Ed. by P. Rozen & S. J. Winawer. 1986. (Frontiers of Gastrointestinal Research Ser.: Vol. 10). (Illus.). xiv, 274p. 172.50 (*3-8055-4252-6*) S Karger.

Secondary Progressions in Eidetic Analysis. Laurie Purcell. 1993. 121p. pap. 11.00 (*0-913412-69-4*) Brandon Hse.

***Secondary Rhinoplasty: Including Reconstruction of the Nose.** R. Meyer. 2nd ed. 2001. (Illus.). 560p. 279.00 (*3-540-65884-X*) Spr-Verlag.

Secondary Rhinoplasty & Nasal Reconstruction. Rod J. Rohrich et al. Ed. by James C. Grotting. 1995. (Illus.). 160p. text 125.00 (*0-942219-80-5*) Quality Med Pub.

Secondary Sources in the History of Canadian Medicine Vol. 2: A Bibliography/Bibliographie de l'Histoire de la Medicine. Charles G. Roland & Jacques Bernier. 2000. LC 99-932186. (FRE.). 264p. (C). 55.00 (*0-88920-344-X*) Wilfrid Laurier.

Secret Doctors: Ethnomedicine of African-Americans. Wonda L. Fontenot. 1994. LC 93-40560. 192p. 60.00 (*0-89789-354-9*, Bergin & Garvey) Greenwood.

Secret for Winning the Weight Control Game: The Almost-Too-Good-to-Be-True Cure for Obesity (after Which, You Can't Stay Fat) John A. Van Koevering. 1991. 100p. (Orig.). pap. 35.00 (*0-9601346-1-1*) Caballero Pr.

Secret Language of Eating Disorders: The Revolutionary New Approach to Understanding & Curing Anorexia & Bulimia. Peggy Claude-Pierre. 2000. (Illus.). 288p. (C). reprint ed. 25.00 (*0-7881-9541-7*) DIANE Pub.

Secret Language of the Mind: A Visual Inquiry into the Mysteries of Consciousness. David Cohen. 1996. LC 96-10435. (Illus.). 192p. pap. 19.95 (*0-8118-1431-9*) Chronicle Bks.

Secret Life of the Unborn Child. Verny Thomas. 1982. 256p. pap. 13.95 (*0-440-50565-8*, Dell Trade Pbks) Dell.

Secret Life of Your Cells. Robert S. Stone. 1989. LC 89-50767. 196p. pap. 12.95 (*0-914918-96-6*, Whitford) Schiffer.

Secret Malady: Venereal Disease in Eighteenth-Century Britain & France. Ed. by Linda E. Merians. 1997. LC 96-20580. 280p. pap. 18.00 (*0-8131-0888-8*); (Illus.). text 42.50 (*0-8131-1989-8*) U Pr of KY.

Secret Medicine of the Pharoahs: Ancient Egyptian Medicine. Cornelius Stetter. 1993. LC 92-48470.Tr. of Denn alles steht seit Ewigkeit geschrieben. (ENG & GER., Illus.). 182p. pap. 19.95 (*0-86715-265-6*) Quint Pub Co.

Secret of Childhood. Maria Montessori. 1982. 416p. mass mkt. 6.99 (*0-345-30583-3*) Ballantine Pub Grp.

Secret of Chinese Pulse Diagnosis. Bob Flaws. 1995. LC 95-80457. 160p. pap. 29.95 (*0-936185-67-8*) Blue Poppy Pr.

Secret of Healing. Jack E. Addington. 1979. 204p. pap. 10.95 (*0-911336-80-X*) Sci of Mind.

Secret of Instantaneous Healing. Harry D. Smith. 1986. 8.95 (*0-13-797951-7*, Reward) P-H.

Secret Plague: Venereal Disease in Canada, 1838-1939. Jay Cassel. 1987. 539p. pap. 17.95 (*0-8020-6617-8*); text 35.00 (*0-8020-2593-5*) U of Toronto Pr.

Secret Ring: Freud's Inner Circle & the Politics of Psychoanalysis. Phyllis Grosskurth. 1999. (Illus.). 245p. reprint ed. text 23.00 (*0-7881-6401-5*) DIANE Pub.

Secret Strength of Depression. Frederic F. Flach. 2nd rev. ed. 1995. LC 95-50893. 256p. pap. 14.95 (*1-886330-02-6*) Hatherleigh.

Secret Teachings of the Espiritistas: Unravelling the Enigma of Psychic Surgery. Harvey J. Martin, III. Ed. by Kathryn R. Butler & Ann K. Fisher. Tr. by Seigfreid Sepulveda from SPA. 1998. LC 99-184224. (Illus.). xviii, 267p. 24.95 (*0-9660843-8-1*) Metamind Ent.

Secret to Hunza Superior Health. Carl Classic. Ed. by Gordon F. Richiusa. 1991. 203p. (Orig.). reprint ed. pap. 7.95 (*0-9628298-7-0*) Ctr Human Natural Nrtn.

Secret World of Drawings: Healing Through Art. Gregg M. Furth. 1989. (Illus.). 150p. (Orig.). (C). 40.00 (*0-938434-47-0*); pap. 19.95 (*0-938434-46-2*) Sigo Pr.

Secretarial Dental Assistant. Douglas. 1976. (Dental Assisting Procedures Ser.). tchr. ed. 9.00 (*0-8273-0350-5*) Delmar.

Secretin, Cholecystokinin-Pancreozymin & Gastrin. Ed. by T. E. Jorpes & Viktor Mutt. 1973. (Handbook of Experimental Pharmacology Ser.: Vol. 34). (Illus.). 376p. 144.00 (*0-387-05952-0*) Spr-Verlag.

Secretion & Action of Gonadotropins. Ed. by B. Runnebaum et al. 1984. (Illus.). 105p. 47.95 (*0-387-13854-4*) Spr-Verlag.

Secrets: Therapy for Adults Molested As Children. Bobbi Hobbs. Ed. by F. Beard. 1988. 150p. 23.95 (*0-941819-16-7*) Windrose Pubs CA.

Secrets for a Healthier Longer Life. 1992. lib. bdg. 75.00 (*0-8490-8712-0*) Gordon Pr.

Secrets of a Long Life: How to Remain Healthy, Sexual, & Actively Working Beyond 100. Morton Walker. 1984. (Dr. Morton Walker Better Health Booklets Ser.). (Illus.). 56p. (Orig.). pap. 4.95 (*0-8159-6850-7*) Devin.

***Secrets of Chinese Herbal Medicine.** Penelope Ody. 2001. LC 2001-28330. (Illus.). 224p. pap. 9.95 (*0-7894-7776-9*) DK Pub Inc.

Secrets of Complete Nutrition: Maintaining Your Health & Energy Potential. Michael Sharon. 1986. LC 85-23309. (Illus.). 224p. pap. 7.95 (*0-668-06192-8*) P-H.

Secrets of Eternal Youth: Why Diet Should Be Based upon Bio-Chemical Food Analysis for Health & Long Life. Victor G. Rocine. 1991. (Longevity Ser.). lib. bdg. 79.95 (*0-8490-4103-1*) Gordon Pr.

S

Secret(s) of Good Patient Care: Thoughts on Medicine in the 21st Century. William C. Felch. 1996. LC 95-25334. 208p. 58.00 (*0-275-95448-X*, Praeger Pubs) Greenwood.

Secrets of Indian Medicine. R. S. Agarwal. 4th ed. 1996. 240p. pap. (*81-7058-068-4*) SAA Pubn Dept IND. *Dist:* Auromere, Lotus Pr, E-W Cultural Ctr, Matagiri Bks, SABDA.

Secrets of Natural Health. Shyam Singha. 1997. LC 96-48639. 288p. pap. 14.95 (*1-85230-938-5*) Element MA.

Secrets of Oriental Physicians. Paul M. Kourenoff. 1996. 146p. reprint ed. spiral bd. 17.50 (*0-7873-0512-X*) Hlth Research.

Secrets of Oriental Physicians: Two Hundred Natural Healing Formulas for Nearly Every Ailment. 1991. (Alternative Medicine Ser.). lib. bdg. 79.95 (*0-8490-4307-7*) Gordon Pr.

Secrets of the Stork: A Workbook for Expecting Mothers & Their Families. Linda R. Yerger & Susan O. Diket. Ed. by John P. Yerger. 1996. (Illus.). 110p. spiral bd., wbk. ed. 14.95 (*0-9655414-0-1*) L Y A N Pub.

Secrets of Wise Men, Chemists & Great Physicians: A Book of Rare Formulas, Recipes & Prescriptions. W. K. David. 1991. (Alternative Medicine Ser.). lib. bdg. 79.95 (*0-8490-4306-9*) Gordon Pr.

Secrets to Happiness, Inner Peace & Health: Complete Guide to Optimal Wellness of Body, Mind & Spirit. Brian K. Bailey. 1997. (Illus.). 320p. (Orig.). pap. 15.95 (*0-9654904-0-8*) Hlth Unltd.

Section Eighty-Nine Companion. Ed. by Ari Cowan & Lee T. Paterson. 1989. (Orig.). pap. 38.00 (*0-932823-01-7*) Am Somerset.

Sectional Anatomy by MRI. Georges Y. El-Khoury et al. 2nd ed. 1994. LC 94-32581. (Illus.). 776p. text (*0-443-08890-X*) Church.

Sectional Anatomy for Imaging Professionals. Lorrie L. Kelley & Connie M. Petersen. 1997. LC 97-42675. (Illus.). 160p. pap. text, stu. ed. 19.95 (*0-8151-8667-3*, 28946) Mosby Inc.

Sectional Anatomy for Imaging Professionals. Lorrie L. Kelley & Connie M. Peterson. 1997. (Illus.). 160p. pap. text, tchr. ed. (*0-8151-4933-6*, 29039) Mosby Inc.

Sectional Anatomy for Imaging Professionals. Kelley & Connie M. Petersen. 1996. (Illus.). 320p. (C). (gr. 13). text 52.00 (*0-8151-8665-7*, 28944) Mosby Inc.

***Sectional Anatomy Learning System** Edith Applegate. 2nd ed. 2001. LC 2001-40049. (Illus.). 515p. pap. (*0-7216-8443-2*) Saunders.

Sectional Anatomy Learning System: Concepts & Applications. Edith J. Applegate. 1991. (Illus.). 600p. tchr. ed. (*0-7216-3240-8*); text 61.50 (*0-7216-3269-6*) Saunders.

***Sectional Anatomy Learning System Set.** Edith Applegate. 2001. (Illus.). pap., tchr. ed. (*0-7216-8444-0*) Saunders.

Sectional Anatomy of the Head & Neck: A Detailed Atlas. John H. Lillie & Brent A. Bauer. 1994. (Illus.). 224p. text 57.95 (*0-19-504297-2*) OUP.

Sectional Fetal Anatomy in Ultrasound. Ed. by A. Staudach. 1987. (Illus.). 198p. 147.00 (*0-387-18213-6*) Spr-Verlag.

Sectional Human Anatomy: Correlated with CT & MRI. Man-Chung Han & Chu-Wan Kim. 3rd ed. 1995. (Illus.). 336p. 95.00 (*0-89640-279-7*) Igaku-Shoin.

Sectional MRI Anatomy of the Human Body: A Photographic Atlas. S. Marinkovich. 2000. (Illus.). 540p. 139.00 (*0-86577-899-X*) Thieme Med Pubs.

Secular Bioethics in Theological Perspective. Ed. by Earl E. Shelp. 1996. LC 95-20651. (Theology & Medicine Ser.: Vol. 8). 236p. (C). text 140.00 (*0-7923-3735-2*) Kluwer Academic.

Secure Base: Clinical Applications of Attachment Theory. John Bowlby. 1988. LC 99-207166. (Illus.). (*0-415-00640-6*) Routledge.

Security & Access: Guidelines for Managing Electronic Patient Information. Sandra R. Fuller. 1997. 98p. pap. text 37.00 (*1-58426-010-6*, AB101797) Am Hlth Info.

Security in the Health Care Environment. David H. Sells, Jr. 2000. LC 99-51847. 500p. 79.00 (*0-8342-1225-0*) Aspen Pub.

Security Measures - for Professionals, Patients, Hospitals & Data Protection: Index of New Information. Jeff M. Davidson. 1994. 160p. 57.50 (*0-7883-0214-0*); pap. 47.50 (*0-7883-0215-9*) ABBE Pubs Assn.

Sedation: A Guide to Patient Management. Stanley F. Malamed. 3rd ed. 1994. LC 94-32507. (Illus.). 656p. (C). (gr. 13). pap. text 54.00 (*0-8151-5736-3*, 24148) Mosby Inc.

Sedation: A Guide to Patient Management. Stanley F. Malamed. 3rd ed. 1995. (Illus.). 656p. pap. (*84-8174-136-1*) Mosby-Doyma Libros ESP. *Dist:* Mosby Inc.

Sedation Analgesia for Diagnostic & Therapeutic Procedures. Ed. by Shobha Malviya et al. 2001. (Contemporary Clinical Neuroscience Ser.). 300p. 125.00 (*0-89603-863-7*) Humana.

***Sedation & Analgesia for Beginners.** Park et al. 2002. (Illus.). 140p. pap. (*1-84110-057-9*) Greenwich Med GBR. *Dist:* JAMCO Dist.

Sedation & Analgesia in the Critically Ill. G. R. Park et al. 1995. LC 94-43108. (Illus.). 250p. 89.95 (*0-86542-905-7*) Blackwell Sci.

***Seduction, Suggestion, Psychoanalysis.** Ed. by Philippe Van Haute & Jozef Vorveleyn. 2001. (Figures of the Unconscious Ser.). 125p. (*90-5867-127-5*) Leuven Univ BEL. *Dist:* Coronet Bks.

Seductions of Psychoanalysis: Freud, Lacan & Derrida. John Forrester. 1991. (Cambridge Studies in French: No. 26). (Illus.). 436p. (C). pap. text 29.95 (*0-521-42466-6*) Cambridge U Pr.

Seductive Mirage: An Exploration of the Work of Sigmund Freud. Allen Esterson. 1993. LC 93-994. 280p. 52.95 (*0-8126-9230-6*); pap. 18.95 (*0-8126-9231-4*) Open Court.

See Again! Reversing & Preventing Macular Degeneration. Alexander Eaton. 1999. LC 99-12339. 240p. pap. 15.00 (*0-609-80334-4*) Harmony Bks.

See Us Hear Us: Voices of Breast Cancer. Ed. by Kana Riley. 1994. 128p. (Orig.). pap. 5.00 (*0-9644254-0-8*) NH Breast Cancer.

Seed & the Soil: Gender & Cosmology in Turkish Village Society. Carol L. Delaney. 1991. LC 90-28545. (Comparative Studies on Muslim Societies: No. 11). (Illus.). 393p. text 55.00 (*0-520-07314-2*); pap. text 22.50 (*0-520-07550-1*) U CA Pr.

Seed of Madness: Constitutional Environmental Fantasy Org. Psychiatric Core. Vamik D. Volkan & Salman Akhtar. 1997. LC 96-25084. 213p. 35.00 (*0-8236-6023-0*) Intl Univs Pr.

Seeds of Hope: A Physician's Personal Triumph over Prostate Cancer. Michael A. Dorso. Ed. by Doreen L. Skardarasy. 2000. LC 00-10024. (Illus.). (*0-9678801-6-5*) Acorn MI.

Seeing Both Sides: Classic Controversies in Abnormal Psychology. Scott O. Lilienfeld. 1994. LC 94-18083. (Psychology Ser.). 512p. pap. text 46.95 (*0-534-25134-X*) Brooks-Cole.

Seeing in Special Ways: Children Living with Blindness. Thomas Bergman. 2000. (Illus.). 54p. text 20.00 (*0-7881-9062-8*) DIANE Pub.

Seeing in the Dark: Reflections on Dreams & Dreaming. Bert O. States. 1997. LC 96-20997. 288p. 50.00 (*0-300-06910-3*) Yale U Pr.

Seeing is Believing: 700 Years of Scientific & Medical Illustration. Jennifer B. Lee & Miriam Mandelbaum. 1999. LC 99-46587. (*0-87104-449-8*) NY Pub Lib.

Seeing Things Differently: Activities, Exercises & Cognitive Treatment Strategies for Special Populations. James Haaven. 2000. 180p. pap. 27.95 (*1-885473-34-6*) Wood N Barnes.

Seeing Through the Visible World: Jung Gnosis & Chaos see Modern Woman in Search of Soul: A Jungian Guide to the Visible & Invisible Worlds

Seeing Well Again Without Your Glasses. Christopher Markert. (Illus.). 128p. 17.95 (*0-8464-4288-4*) Beekman Pubs.

Seeing Young Children. Warren R. Bentzen. 3rd ed. 1997. (Early Childhood Education Ser.). 10.50 (*0-8273-7666-9*) Delmar.

Seeing Young Children: A Guide for Observing & Recording Behavior. Warren R. Bentzen. 1985. LC 85-1564. 272p. (C). pap. 27.00 (*0-8273-2329-8*) Delmar.

Seeing Young Children: A Guide to Observing & Recording Behavior. Warren R. Bentzen. 2nd ed. 1991. 269p. pap., tchr. ed. 9.50 (*0-8273-4478-3*); 2nd ed. 1991. 269p. pap. 28.50 (*0-8273-4477-5*); 3rd ed. 1996. (Illus.). 384p. (C). pap. text 44.95 (*0-8273-7665-0*) Delmar.

Seeking Strategic Advantage Through Health Policy Analysis. Beaufort B. Longest, Jr. 1996. LC 96-26898. (Orig.). pap. 40.00 (*1-56793-047-6*) Health Admin Pr.

Seelenleben des Kruppels: Kruppelseelen Kundliche Erziehung und das Gesetz Betr. Hans Wurtz. Ed. by William R. Phillips & Janet Rosenberg. 1980. LC 79-6007. (Physically Handicapped in Society Ser.). (GER.). reprint ed. lib. bdg. 16.95 (*0-405-13138-0*) Ayer.

Seeley, A&P No. 2: LM. Jay M. Templin. 2nd ed. 1992. 736p. spiral bd. 29.95 (*0-8016-6653-8*) Mosby Inc.

Seeley, A&P No. 2: Study Guide. Tate. 2nd ed. 1991. 624p. pap. 25.62 (*0-8016-4803-3*) Mosby Inc.

Seems Like Yesterday: A Surgeon's Odyssey. Charles C. Kissinger. Ed. by Anna M. Nesmith. 1988. LC 88-81078. (Illus.). 254p. (Orig.). pap. 14.95 (*0-9620330-0-6*) Henderson Pr.

Segmental Idiopathic Necrosis of the Femoral Head, Vol. 5. Ed. by U. H. Weil. 1981. (Progress in Orthopedic Surgery Ser.). (Illus.). 121p. 55.95 (*0-387-10718-5*) Spr-Verlag.

Segmental Motor System. Ed. by Marc D. Binder & Lorne M. Mendell. 1989. (Illus.). 416p. text 68.00 (*0-19-505484-9*) OUP.

Seis Dias de Noviembre: El Fusilamiento de los Estudiantes de Medicina. Byron Miguel. 1990. LC 90-84963. (Coleccion Cuba y sus Jueces). (SPA., Illus.). 96p. (Orig.). pap. 9.95 (*0-89729-586-2*) Ediciones.

Seized: My Life with Epilepsy. Teresa McLean. 1996. 174p. pap. (*1-86066-013-4*) R Cohen Bks GBR. *Dist:* Trafalgar.

Seizing Control: Live with Epilepsy. Betts. Date not set. (*0-7190-3814-6*); 1998. (*0-7190-3813-8*) Manchester Univ Pr.

Seizure Disorders in the Elderly & the Mentally Handicapped in the Long-Term Care Facility. Ed. by Chris Fellner. 1995. (*1-57130-022-8*) Medicine Grp USA.

Seizure Free: From Epilepsy to Brain Surgery, I Survived & You Can, Too! English Press Staff. 2nd ed. 2000. pap. 12.95 (*0-9663819-0-4*) English Press.

Seizure Recognition & Observation: A Guide for Allied Health Professionals. Epilepsy Foundation of America Staff. 1992. 12p. pap. 2.95 (*0-916570-17-7*) Epilepsy Foundation of America.

Seizure Training: Instructor's Guide. Illus. by Bonnie Kline. 2000. 158p. pap. 39.95 (*1-928752-19-5*) Mc Gowan Pubns.

Seizures: Medical Causes & Management. Ed. by Norman Delanty. 2001. (Current Clinical Practice Ser.). 376p. 125.00 (*0-89603-827-0*) Humana.

Seizures & Epilepsy in Childhood: A Guide for Parents. John M. Freeman et al. 2nd ed. 1997. LC 96-31617. (Health Bks.). (Illus.). 352p. 45.00 (*0-8018-5497-0*) Johns Hopkins.

Seizures & Epilepsy in the Elderly. A. James Rowan. 1996. LC 96-28927. 343p. text 110.00 (*0-7506-9622-2*) Buttrwrth-Heinemann.

Seizures Training: Participant's Guide. Illus. by Bonnie Kline. 2000. 112p. pap. 19.95 (*1-928752-18-7*) Mc Gowan Pubns.

Selbstbewusstsein und Unbewusstes: Studien Zu Freud und Heidegger. Martin Bartels. 1976. (Quellen und Studien zur Philosophie: Vol. 10). (C). 92.30 (*3-11-005778-6*) De Gruyter.

Seldin, Donald W. Festschrift: Journal: Mineral & Electrolyte Metabolism, Vol. 11, No. 4, 1985. Ed. by N. A. Kurtzman. 1985. (Illus.). 76p. pap. 28.00 (*3-8055-4063-9*) S Karger.

Selected Aspects of Nursing. Searle. 1989. pap. text 30.00 (*0-409-10008-0*) Buttrwrth-Heinemann.

Selected Atlases of Bone Scintigraphy. Ed. by Douglas Van Nostrand et al. 1992. LC 92-2321. (Atlases of Clinical Nuclear Medicine Ser.). (Illus.). 140p. 136.00 (*0-387-97823-2*) Spr-Verlag.

Selected Atlases of Cardiovascular Nuclear Medicine. Ed. by Douglas Van Nostrand. 1993. LC 93-10234. (Atlases of Clinical Nuclear Medicine Ser.). (Illus.). 168p. 141.00 (*0-387-94045-6*) Spr-Verlag.

Selected Atlases of Gastrointestinal Scintigraphy. Ed. by Harvey A. Ziessman & Douglas Van Nostrand. 1991. (Atlases of Clinical Nuclear Medicine Ser.). (Illus.). 173p. 132.00 (*0-387-97618-3*) Spr-Verlag.

Selected Bibliography of Pediatric Orthopaedics. Ed. by James H. Beaty & Charles T. Price. 4th ed. 1996. 333p. pap. 35.00 (*0-89203-158-1*) Amer Acad Ortho Surg.

Selected Bibliography of the Foot & Ankle with Commentary. Ed. by Glen Pfeffer & Mark S. Mizel. 1992. 321p. pap. 25.00 (*0-89203-061-5*) Amer Acad Ortho Surg.

Selected Bibliography on Detection of Dependence-Producing Drugs in Body Fluids. T. L. Chruscie & M. Chrusciel. 1975. (Offset Publications: No. 17). pap. text 15.00 (*92-4-052004-X*, 1120017) World Health.

Selected Cases in General & Systemic Pathology. American Registry of Pathology Staff & Armed Forces Institute of Pathology Staff. 1991. (C). 250.00 incl. disk (*1-56815-000-8*) Mosby Inc.

Selected Correspondence of Dr. Karl A. Menninger, 1945-1965. Ed. by Howard J. Faulkner & Virginia D. Pruitt. 1995. LC 95-8760. (Illus.). 294p. pap. 29.95 (*0-8262-0998-X*) U of Mo Pr.

Selected Models of Anxiety, Depression & Psychosis. Ed. by P. Simon et al. 1988. (Animal Models of Psychiatric Disorders Ser.: Vol. 1). (Illus.). vi, 198p. 155.75 (*3-8055-4667-X*) S Karger.

Selected Models of Practice in Geriatric Psychiatry: A Task Force Report of the American Psychiatric Association. APA Task Force on Models of Practice in Geriatric Psychiatry. 1993. LC 92-48940. 82p. 12.95 (*0-89042-239-7*, 2239) Am Psychiatric.

Selected Mycotoxins: Ochratoxins, Trichotecenes, Ergot. 1990. (Environmental Health Criteria Ser.: No. 105). 263p. pap. text 46.00 (*92-4-157105-5*, 1160105) World Health.

Selected Options for Expanding Health Insurance Coverage. Jack Rodgers. 1994. (Illus.). 79p. (Orig.). (C). pap. text 30.00 (*0-7881-0418-7*) DIANE Pub.

Selected Papers: Psychoanalysis & Group Analysis. S. H. Foulkes. 1990. 370p. pap. text (*0-946439-56-7*) Karnac Bks GBR. *Dist:* Brunner-Routledge.

Selected Papers & Discussion from the Second Annual Meeting of the SISE June 2-3, 1989, Geneva, Switzerland. Ed. by D. J. Leaper. 1990. (Surgical Research Communications Ser.). ii, 138p. pap. text 130.00 (*3-7186-5023-1*) Gordon & Breach.

Selected Papers Fourth International Conference on Malignant Lymphoma, June 6-9, 1990, lugano. Ed. by J. E. Ultmann. 1993. (C). pap. text 88.50 (*0-7923-1116-7*) Kluwer Academic.

Selected Papers from the 1st Meeting of the SISE, Vol. 5, No. 1. Ed. by D. J. Leaper. 1989. (Surgical Research Communications Ser.). ii, 94p. pap. text 74.00 (*3-7186-4894-6*) Gordon & Breach.

Selected Papers from the International Symposium on Mast Cell, October 29, 1990, Hiroshima, Japan & the 7th Annual Symposium of the Skin Pharmacology Society on Immunopharmacology & Carcinogenesis, October 30, 1990, Hiroshima, Japan: Journal: Skin Pharmacology, Vol. 4, Suppl. 1, 1991. Ed. by S. Yamamoto. 1991. (Illus.). iv, 100p. pap. 31.50 (*3-8055-5497-4*) S Karger.

Selected Papers of Ludwig Jekels. Ludwig Jekels. 1970. reprint ed. pap. 24.95 (*0-8236-8305-2*, 26025) Intl Univs Pr.

Selected Papers of the International Migraine-Headache Symposium: Proceedings of the International Symposium, Florence, 1970. International Migraine-Headache Symposium Staff. Ed. by F. Sicuteri. 1972. (Pain & Headache Ser.: Vol. 3). 121.75 (*3-8055-1295-3*) S Karger.

Selected Papers of Wolfgang Kohler. Wolfgang Kohler. Ed. by Solomon E. Asch & Mary Henle. 1971. 465p. (C). 13.00 (*0-87140-505-9*) Liveright.

Selected Papers on Direct Psychoanalysis, Vol. 2. John N. Rosen. 1968. 172p. text 37.00 (*0-8089-0387-X*, 793622, Grune & Strat) Harcrt Hlth Sci Grp.

Selected Papers on Laser Beam Diagnostics. Robert N. Hindy & Jeffrey H. Hunt. 1996. LC 96-26559. (Milestone Ser.). 110.00 (*0-8194-2283-5*, MS126) SPIE.

Selected Papers on Laser Safety. Ed. by David H. Sliney & Brian J. Thompson. 1995. LC 95-20693. (SPIE Milestone Ser.: Vol. MS 117). 118.00 (*0-8194-2014-X*) SPIE.

Selected Papers on Optical Fibers in Medicine. Ed. by A. Katzir. 1990. (Milestone Ser.). 736p. 65.00 (*0-8194-0368-7*, VOL. MS11(H)); pap. 50.00 (*0-8194-0369-5*, VOL. MS11(S)) SPIE.

Selected Papers on Optical Tomography: Fundamentals & Applications in Medicine. Olaf Minet et al. 1998. LC 98-3470. (Milestone Ser.). 118.00 (*0-8194-2877-9*) SPIE.

Selected Papers on Optometry. Ed. by William M. Rosenblum & William J. Benjamin. 1992. LC 92-29543. (Milestone Ser.: Vol. MS 62). pap. 50.00 (*0-8194-1050-0*) SPIE.

Selected Papers on Photodynamic Therapy. Ed. by David Kessel. 1993. LC 93-5236. (Milestone Ser.: Vol. MS 82/HC). 65.00 (*0-8194-1368-2*); pap. 50.00 (*0-8194-1367-4*) SPIE.

Selected Papers on the Pathogenic Rickettsiae. Ed. by Nicholas Hahon. 1968. LC 68-17625. (Illus.). 382p. 46.50 (*0-674-79890-2*) HUP.

Selected Papers on Tissue Optics: Applications in Medical Diagnostics & Therapy. Ed. by Valery V. Turchin. 1994. LC 94-28511. (Milestone Ser.: MS. 102). 50.00 (*0-8194-1695-9*) SPIE.

Selected Practical Problems in Health & Social Research. Ed. by Thomas E. Dinero. 1996. LC 96-30652. (Journal of Health & Social Policy: Vol. 8, No. 1). 107p. (C). 29.95 (*1-56024-832-7*) Haworth Pr.

Selected Problems of Adolescence: With Emphasis on Group Formation. Helene Deutsch. 1967. LC 67-28587. (Psychoanalytic Study of the Child Monographs: No. 3). 246p. (Orig.). 27.50 (*0-8236-6040-0*) Intl Univs Pr.

Selected Proceedings from the First & Second Delft Pain Symposia: Journal: Applied Neurophysiology, Vol. 47, No. 4-6. Ed. by Janine M. Pernak et al. 1986. (Illus.). 112p. pap. 64.50 (*3-8055-4044-2*) S Karger.

Selected Proceedings from the Scientific Program - The 1998 North American Veterinary Conference: Respiratory Disease, Antimicrobial Therapy, Dermatology. Intro. by Veterinary Learning Systems Staff. 1998. (Illus.). 84p. pap. text (*1-884254-43-8*) Vet Lrn Syst.

Selected Proceedings of the Annual Meeting of the American Society of Pediatric Neurosurgeons, San Juan, Puerto Rico, January 1991. Ed. by A. E. Marlin. 1992. (Journal of Pediatric Neurosurgery: Vol. 18, Nos. 5-6, 1992). (Illus.). iv, 108p. pap. 96.75 (*3-8055-5711-6*) S Karger.

Selected References in Elective Orthopaedics. A. H. Ratliff et al. 1991. 204p. 39.00 (*0-387-19682-X*) Spr-Verlag.

Selected References in Orthopaedic Trauma. A. H. Ratliff et al. 1989. 124p. 41.95 (*0-387-19556-4*) Spr-Verlag.

Selected Synthetic Organic Fibres. Ed. by World Health Organization Staff. 1993. (Environmental Health Criteria Ser.: No. 151). (ENG, FRE & SPA.). 100p. pap. text 26.00 (*92-4-157151-9*, 1160151) World Health.

Selected Topics in Clinical Enzymology: Vol. 2, Proceedings (Selected) of the 4th International Congress on Clinical Enzymology, Washington, D.C., July 30 - August 2, 1983. Ed. by M. Werner & D. M. Goldberg. 1985. (Illus.). xxii, 667p. 200.00 (*3-11-010233-1*) De Gruyter.

Selected Topics in Clinical Oncology: An In-Depth Study of 18 Cancers Usually Neglected. J. M. Debois. 2000. LC 00-21826. (Illus.). xi, 596p. 236.00 (*0-7923-6195-4*) Kluwer Academic.

Selected Topics in Medical Artificial Intelligence. Ed. by P. L. Miller. 1988. (Computers & Medicine Ser.). (Illus.). 236p. 74.00 (*0-387-96701-X*) Spr-Verlag.

Selected Vitamins, Minerals & Functional Consequences of Maternal Malnutrition. Ed. by Artemis P. Simopoulos. 1991. (World Review of Nutrition & Dietetics Ser.: Vol. 64). (Illus.). x, 180p. 170.50 (*3-8055-5168-1*) S Karger.

Selected Writings, 1877 to 1930. D'Arcy Power. 1970. LC 78-95632. (Illus.). x, 368p. reprint ed. 45.00 (*0-678-03750-7*) Kelley.

Selected Writings from a Connectionist's Psychology. Edward Lee Thorndike. 1969. LC 76-94621. 370p. reprint ed. lib. bdg. 59.75 (*0-8371-2570-7*, THWP, Greenwood Pr) Greenwood.

Selected Writings in Medical Sociological Research. Ed. by Michael Bloor. 1997. LC 97-73458. (Cardiff Papers in Qualitative Research). 224p. text (*1-85972-676-3*) Ashgate Pub GBR. *Dist:* Ashgate Pub Co.

Selected Writings of Anna Freud. Anna Freud. 2001. 336p. pap. (*0-14-026814-6*) Pnguin Bks Ltd GBR. *Dist:* Trafalgar.

Selected Writings of Bertram D. Lewin, M. D. Ed. & Intro. by Jacob A. Arlow. 1973. LC 72-94802. (Illus.). 608p. 25.00 (*0-911194-02-9*) Psych Qtly.

Selected Writings of Rosemary Ellis: In Search of the Meaning of Nursing Science. Ed. by Joyce J. Fitzpatrick & Ida Martinson. 1996. LC 96-68450. 152p. 44.95 (*0-8261-9400-1*) Springer Pub.

Selecting a Pediatric Residency: An Employment Guide. American Academy of Pediatrics Staff. 1993. 110p. pap. 20.00 (*0-910761-47-7*) Am Acad Pediat.

Selecting Access Systems for Individuals with Physical Disabilities. Kathy S. Lee & Debra J. Thomas. 1990. 310p. pap. text 50.00 (*0-8020-6695-X*) U of Toronto Pr.

Selecting & Evaluating a Referral Laboratory: Tentative Guideline (1991) Contrib. by Robert R. Rickert. 1991. 75.00 (*1-56238-139-3*, GP9-T) NCCLS.

Selecting Effective Treatments: A Comprehensive, Systematic Guide for Treating Mental Disorders. Linda Seligman. rev. ed. 1998. LC 98-17919. (Psychology Ser.). 512p. pap. 45.00 (*0-7879-4307-X*) Jossey-Bass.

Selecting Students for Training in Health Care: A Practical Guide to Improving Selection Procedures. M. Bennet & R. Wakeford. 1983. (WHO Offset Publications: No. 74). 38p. 7.00 (*92-4-170074-2*) World Health.

Selecting Treatment Interventions: A Casebook for Clinical Practice in Child & Adolescent Managed Mental Health. John B. Mordock. 2nd ed. 1999. 172p. pap. 79.95 (*1-884937-59-4*) Manisses Communs.

Selectins: Initiators of Leukocyte Endothelial Adhesion. Ed. by Dietmar Vestweber. 1997. 240p. text (*90-5702-074-2*, ECU75) GBSP NLD. *Dist:* Gordon & Breach.

Selection & Use of Chemical Indicators for Steam Sterilization Monitoring in Health Care Facilities. 1988. 49p. pap. 90.00 (*0-910275-87-4*, TIR3-209) Assn Adv Med Instrn.

Selection of Doses in Chronic Toxicity-Carcinogenicity Studies. Ed. by Harold C. Grice. 1983. (Current Issues in Toxicology Ser.). (Illus.). 130p. 37.95 (*0-387-12845-X*) Spr-Verlag.

Selection of Primary Sources for the History of Pharmacy in the United States: Books & Trade Catalogs from the Colonial Period to 1940. Nydia M. King. 1987. 123p. (Orig.). pap. 11.00 (*0-931292-16-6*) Am Inst Hist Pharm.

Selection of Treatment for Alcoholics. Ed. by E. Mansell Pattison. 1982. LC 79-620007. (NIAAA-RUCAS Alcoholism Treatment Ser.: No. 1). pap. 22.50 (*0-911290-47-8*) Rutgers Ctr Alcohol.

Selections from Public Health in Reports & Papers: American Public Health Association (1873-1883) Ed. by Barbara G. Rosenkrantz. 1977. LC 76-4065. (Public Health in America Ser.). reprint ed. lib. bdg. 34.95 (*0-405-09838-3*) Ayer.

Selections from Public Health Reports & Papers Presented at the Meetings of the American Public Health Association (1884-1907) An Original Anthology. Ed. by Barbara G. Rosenkrantz. 1977. LC 76-40657. (Public Health in America Ser.). reprint ed. lib. bdg. 21.95 (*0-405-09883-9*) Ayer.

Selections from the Health-Education Series: An Original Anthology. Ed. by Barbara G. Rosenkrantz. 1977. LC 76-40664. (Public Health in America Ser.). reprint ed. lib. bdg. 18.95 (*0-405-09873-1*) Ayer.

Selections from the Journal of the Massachusetts Association of Boards of Health, 1891-1904: An Original Anthology. Ed. by Barbara G. Rosenkrantz. 1977. LC 76-40669. (Public Health in America Ser.). lib. bdg. 41.95 (*0-405-09878-2*) Ayer.

Selective Activation of Drugs by Redox Processes. Ed. by G. E. Adams et al. 1990. LC 90-14335. (NATO Advanced Science Institutes Ser.: Vol. 198). (Illus.). 370p. (C). text 138.00 (*0-306-43735-X*, Kluwer Plenum) Kluwer Academic.

Selective Arteriography of the Spinal Cord. John L. Doppman et al. 1969. LC 68-58106. (Illus.). 157p. 14.50 (*0-87527-006-9*) Green.

Selective Attention & the Control of Binocular Rivalry. Leon C. Lack. 1978. (Psychological Studies: No. II). pap. text (*90-279-7644-9*) Mouton.

Selective Cox-2 Inhibitors: Pharmacology, Clinical Effects & Therapeutic Potential. Ed. by John R. Vane & Jack H. Botting. 1998. LC 98-139493. 160p. 85.00 (*0-7923-8729-5*) Kluwer Academic.

***Selective Estrogen Receptor Modulators: Research & Clinical Applications.** Ed. by Andrea Manni & Michael Verderame. 2002. (Contemporary Endocrinology Ser.). 384p. 175.00 (*0-89603-912-9*) Humana.

***Selective Estrogen Receptor Modulators (SERMs)** Ed. by Marietta Anthony et al. 2001. LC 2001-51416. (Annals of the New York Academy of Sciences Ser.: Vol. 949). 450p. 140.00 (*1-57331-358-0*) NY Acad Sci.

Selective Feeding Programmes. Tim Lusty & Pat Diskett. 1984. (Practical Guide Ser.: No. 1). (Illus.). 96p. (C). pap. (*0-85598-097-4*) Oxfam Pub GBR. *Dist:* Stylus Pub VA.

Selective 5-HT Reuptake Inhibitors: Novel or Commonplace Agents? Ed. by M. Gastpar & Jennifers S. Wakelin. 1988. (Advances in Biological Psychiatry Ser.: Vol. 17). (Illus.). viii, 108p. 85.25 (*3-8055-4776-5*) S Karger.

Selective Immunosuppression: Basic Concepts & Clinical Applications. Ed. by Luciano Adorini. 1994. (Chemical Immunology Ser.: Vol. 60). (Illus.). x, 166p. 151.50 (*3-8055-6034-6*) S Karger.

Selective Inhibitors of Viral Functions. Ed. by W. A. Carter. 1973. LC 73-81479. (Uniscience Ser.). 377p. 70.50 (*0-87819-027-9*, CRC Reprint) Franklin.

Selective Mutism: Implications for Research & Treatment. Thomas R. Kratochwill. 1981. LC 80-18631. 208p. text 39.95 (*0-89859-064-7*) L Erlbaum Assocs.

Selective Mutism in Children. Tony Cline. 1994. 184p. (Orig.). (C). pap. text 45.00 (*1-56593-257-9*, 0546) Singular Publishing.

Selective Neuronal Death. CIBA Foundation Staff. 1987. LC 86-28082. (CIBA Foundation Symposia Ser.: No. 126). 292p. 128.00 (*0-471-91092-9*) Wiley.

Selective Neurotoxity. Ed. by H. Herken & F. Hucho. 1994. LC 94-7806. (Illus.). 905p. 140.00 (*0-387-57815-3*); 158.00 (*3-540-57815-3*) Spr-Verlag.

Selective Serotonin Re-Uptake Inhibitors: Advances in Basic Research & Clinical Practice. Ed. by J. P. Feighner & W. F. Boyer. 2nd ed. 1996. LC 95-39512. (Perspectives in Psychiatry Ser.: Vol. 5). 388p. 199.95 (*0-471-95600-7*) Wiley.

Selective Studies in Health & Social Services. Ed. by A. G. McDonald. 1981. (OMEGA Special Issue Ser.: Vol. 9, No. 5). 104p. pap. 35.00 (*0-08-023620-0*, Pergamon Pr) Elsevier.

Selenium. 1997. (Woodland Health Ser.). pap. 3.95 (*1-58054-000-7*) Woodland UT.

Selenium. 1987. (Environmental Health Criteria Ser.: No. 58). 276p. pap. text 38.00 (*92-4-154258-6*, 1160058) World Health.

Selenium: Index of New Information & Research Bible. Sidney K. Winnans. 1996. LC 96-12483. 49.50 (*0-7883-0800-9*); 1996. LC 96-12483. pap. 44.50 (*0-7883-0801-7*); 1994. 57.50 (*0-7883-0210-8*); 1994. pap. 47.50 (*0-7883-0211-6*) ABBE Pubs Assn.

Selenium in Biology & Human Health. Ed. by Raymond F. Burk. 1993. LC 93-4691. (Illus.). 221p. 99.00 (*0-387-94080-4*) Spr-Verlag.

Selenium in Biology & Medicine. Ed. by A. Wendel. 1989. (Illus.). 330p. 153.00 (*0-387-50755-8*) Spr-Verlag.

Self. Jonathan D. Brown. 1997. LC 97-1298. 368p. pap. 34.06 (*0-07-008306-1*) McGrw-H Hghr Educ.

Self: Interdisciplinary Approaches (Second G. Stanley Hall Symposium) Ed. by J. Strauss, II & G. R. Geothals. 1991. (Illus.). 278p. 97.00 (*0-387-97536-5*) Spr-Verlag.

Self Across Psychology: Self Recognition, Self-Awareness, & the Self Concept, Vol. 818. Ed. by Joan G. Snodgrass & Robert L. Thompson. 1997. LC 97-20571. (Annals of the New York Academy of Sciences Ser.: No. 818). 301p. 80.00 (*1-57331-034-4*) NY Acad Sci.

Self-Actuated Healing: The Alternative to Doctors & Drugs Is Within You. Lonny Brown. 1988. LC 89-9249. 176p. (Orig.). pap. 8.95 (*0-87961-185-5*) Naturegraph.

Self-Administered Patient Education Audit for Family Practices. Ed. by John H. Renner. 1990. 19p. 10.00 (*0-9626145-1-3*) Health Facts Pub.

Self-Analysis: Critical Inquiries, Personal Visions. Ed. by James W. Barron. 1993. LC 93-15733. 320p. text 45.00 (*0-88163-143-4*) Analytic Pr.

Self Analysis for Analysts. Karl Konig. 1997. LC 97-198053. 144p. pap. (*1-85302-476-7*) Jessica Kingsley GBR. *Dist:* Taylor & Francis.

Self & Identity: Fundamental Issues. Ed. by Richard D. Ashmore & Lee Jussim. 1997. LC 96-8402. (Rutgers Series on Self & Social Identity: Vol. 1). (Illus.). 256p. pap. 29.95 (*0-19-509827-7*) OUP.

Self & Identity: Perspectives Across the Lifespan. T. Honess & K. M. Yardley. 1987. (International Library of Philosophy, Psychology, & Scientific Method). 416p. lib. bdg. 67.50 (*0-7102-0829-4*, Routledge Thoemms) Routledge.

Self & Its Brain. Karl R. Popper & John C. Eccles. rev. ed. 1985. (Illus.). 597p. 86.95 (*0-387-08307-3*) Spr-Verlag.

Self & Its Pleasures: Bataille, Lacan, & the History of the Decentered Subject. Carolyn J. Dean. 1992. LC 92-52748. (Illus.). 288p. 49.95 (*0-8014-2660-X*); pap. 19.95 (*0-8014-9954-2*) Cornell U Pr.

Self & Motivational Systems: Toward a Theory of Psychoanalytic Technique. Joseph D. Lichtenberg et al. 2001. LC 92-49414. (Psychoanalytic Inquiry Ser.: Vol. 13). 272p. reprint ed. pap. 32.50 (*0-88163-154-X*) Analytic Pr.

Self & Object Constancy: Clinical & Theoretical Perspectives. Ed. by Ruth F. Lax et al. 1985. LC 85-27365. (Psychiatry Ser.). 355p. 47.00 (*0-89862-226-3*) Guilford Pubns.

Self & Others: Object Relations Theory in Practice. N. Gregory Hamilton. 1992. LC 87-19479. 352p. reprint ed. pap. 40.00 (*0-87668-544-0*) Aronson.

Self & Process: Brain States & the Conscious Present. J. W. Brown. 1991. (Illus.). xiii, 201p. 57.95 (*0-387-97514-4*) Spr-Verlag.

Self & the Ego in Psychotherapy: A New Approach to Object Relations Theory & Therapy. N. Gregory Hamilton. 1996. LC 95-39263. 200p. 40.00 (*1-56821-659-9*) Aronson.

Self As Agent. John Macmurray. 1991. LC 91-21419. 232p. (C). pap. 17.50 (*0-391-03715-3*) Brill Academic Pubs.

Self-Assembling Complexes for Gene Delivery: From Laboratory to Clinical Trial. Ed. by Alexander V. Kabanov et al. 1998. LC 97-42812. 460p. 190.00 (*0-471-97269-X*) Wiley.

Self-Assessment Atlas of Gastroenterology. Ed. by Tadataka Yamada et al. 1994. (Illus.). 200p. 49.95 (*0-397-51367-4*) Lppncott W & W.

Self-Assessment Color Review of Avian Medicine. Ed. by Robert B. Altman & Neil A. Forbes. 1998. (Sacr Ser.). (Illus.). 192p. pap. 34.95 (*0-8138-2339-0*) Iowa U Pr.

Self-Assessment Color Review of Cardiothoracic Critical Care. Ed. by Riyad C. Karmy-Jones & H. Mathilda Horst. 1997. 160p. pap. text 24.95 (*0-316-74755-6*) Lppncott W & W.

Self-Assessment Color Review of Clinical Haematology. Atul B. Mehta. 1995. pap. text 32.95 (*0-316-56557-1*, Little Brwn Med Div) Lppncott W & W.

Self-Assessment Color Review of Equine Internal Medicine. Tim S. Mair. 1997. (Illus.). 192p. pap. text 34.95 (*0-8138-2864-3*) Iowa U Pr.

Self-Assessment Color Review of Equine Orthopedics & Rheumatology. Stephen C. May et al. 1998. LC 99-169788. (Illus.). 176p. pap. text 34.95 (*0-8138-2137-1*) Iowa U Pr.

Self-Assessment Color Review of Equine Reproduction & Stud Medicine. Jonathan F. Pycock. 1997. LC 97-179510. (Illus.). 208p. pap. 34.95 (*0-8138-2303-X*) Iowa U Pr.

Self-Assessment Color Review of Renal Medicine. Timothy H. J. Goodship & Bradley J. Maroni. 1997. (Illus.). 192p. pap. text 32.95 (*0-316-83932-9*) Lppncott W & W.

Self-Assessment Color Review of Respiratory Medicine. S. G. Spiro. 1997. 192p. pap. text 27.95 (*0-316-80697-8*) Lppncott W & W.

Self-Assessment Color Review of Small Animal Emergency & Critical Care Medicine. Ed. by Rebecca Kirby. 1998. (Sacr Ser.). (Illus.). 192p. pap. 34.95 (*0-8138-2959-3*) Iowa U Pr.

Self-Assessment Color Review of Small Animal Neurology. Simon J. Wheeler. 1996. (Illus.). 152p. pap. text (*0-8138-2217-3*) Manson Pubng GBR. *Dist:* Iowa U Pr.

Self-Assessment Color Review of Small Animal Orthopedics. Ed. by Daniel Lewis et al. 1998. LC 99-174419. (Illus.). 192p. pap. text 34.95 (*0-8138-2947-X*) Iowa U Pr.

Self-Assessment Color Review of Small Animal Soft Tissue Surgery. Ed. by Stephen Gilson. 1998. LC 98-146718. (Illus.). 192p. pap. text 34.95 (*0-8138-2866-X*) Iowa U Pr.

Self-Assessment Color Review of Small Mammals. Ed. by Susan A. Brown & Karen Rosenthal. 1997. LC 97-164753. (Illus.). 192p. pap. 34.95 (*0-8138-2092-8*) Iowa U Pr.

Self-Assessment Color Review of Veterinary Dentistry. Ed. by Frank J. Verstraete. 1999. (Illus.). 224p. (C). pap. text 34.95 (*0-8138-2548-2*) Iowa U Pr.

Self Assessment for Managers of Health Care: How Can I Be a Better Manager. 1987. (Offset Publications: No. 97). 60p. pap. text 10.00 (*92-4-170097-1*, 1120097) World Health.

Self Assessment for MRCP, Pt. I. C. F. Corke. 4th ed. 1995. LC 95-32582. pap. 29.95 (*0-86542-937-5*) Blackwell Sci.

Self-Assessment for Teachers of Health Workers: How to Be a Better Teacher. A. Rotem & F. Abbatt. 1982. (WHO Offset Publications: No. 68). 59p. 8.00 (*92-4-170068-8*) World Health.

Self Assessment for the Diploma in Child Health. Wai-Ching Leung & Adrian Mindford. 1997. LC 97-20459. (An Arnold Publication). (Illus.). 208p. pap. (*0-340-67720-1*) E A GBR. *Dist:* OUP.

***Self-Assessment for the MRCP Part 2 Written Paper.** Narinder Bajaj. 2001. LC 2001-37620. (*0-632-06439-0*); (*0-632-06443-9*) Blackwell Sci.

Self-Assessment Guide to Hematology. Sona Holmes et al. 1993. (C). 30.95 (*0-8151-4626-4*, 22970) Mosby Inc.

Self-Assessment in Accident & Emergency Medicine. Ian Greaves et al. 1996. LC 96-7480. (Illus.). 232p. pap. text (*0-7506-2215-6*) E A GBR. *Dist:* OUP.

Self-Assessment in Chest Medicine. Ronald B. George et al. 1996. LC 95-35114. 196p. 49.95 (*0-683-03460-X*) Lppncott W & W.

Self-Assessment in Clinical Medicine: Preparation & Revision for the MRCP. S. Kaddoura et al. 1998. (Illus.). 116p. pap. (*0-443-05380-4*) Church.

Self-Assessment in Histology: Questions & Quiz Micrographs. Paul R. Wheater & H. George Burkitt. 1981. (Illus.). 176p. pap. text (*0-443-02109-0*) Church.

Self Assessment in Immediate Medical Care. Richard M. Hodgetts. 1990. text 19.95 (*0-7020-1510-5*) Saunders.

Self Assessment in Multidisciplinary Critical Care: A Comprehensive Review. Ed. by Phillip Dellinger & Robert Taylor. 1986. LC 86-60806. (*0-936145-25-0*) SCCM Fullerton.

Self-Assessment in Nephrology. Sanford E. Warren et al. 1987. LC 86-30559. (Illus.). 270p. (C). text 90.00 (*0-306-42342-1*, Kluwer Plenum) Kluwer Academic.

***Self-Assessment in Obstetrics & Gynaecology.** Marcus Setchell & Basky Thilaganathan. 4th ed. 2001. (Arnold Publication). 192p. (Orig.). pap. text 14.95 (*0-340-76068-0*) OUP.

Self Assessment in Pediatrics. David Milner & Stefan Herber. 1996. 28.00 (*0-7234-2920-0*) Mosby Inc.

Self-Assessment Picture Test in Veterinary Medicine: Exotic Species. J. E. Cooper. 1994. (C). (gr. 13). text 32.95 (*0-8151-1861-9*, 22825) Mosby Inc.

Self-Assessment Picture Tests. V. R. Tindall. 1996. (*0-7234-2554-X*) Wolfe Publishing GBR. *Dist:* Mosby Inc.

Self-Assessment Picture Tests: Avian Medicine. Brian H. Coles & Maria-Elizabeth Krautwald-Junghanns. 10th ed. 1999. LC 98-31100. (Illus.). 224p. pap. 39.95 (*0-7234-3008-X*) Mosby Inc.

Self Assessment Picture Tests: Clinical Cardiology. D. L. Patterson. 2nd ed. 1997. pap. (*0-7234-2591-4*) Martin Dunitz GBR. *Dist:* Mosby Inc.

Self-Assessment Picture Tests: Dermatology. G. Kavanaugh & J. J. Savin. 1998. (Illus.). 128p. text (*0-7234-2553-1*) Martin Dunitz GBR. *Dist:* Mosby Inc.

Self-Assessment Picture Tests: Gastroenterology. David Allison. 2nd ed. 1997. pap. 15.95 (*0-7234-2589-2*) Mosby Inc.

Self Assessment Picture Tests Cardiology, Vol. 2. Wajdi Turkie & Derek Rowlands. 1996. 144p. (*0-7234-2452-7*) Martin Dunitz GBR. *Dist:* Mosby Inc.

Self Assessment Picture Tests in Clinical Medicine. C. D. Forbes & William F. Jackson. 1995. pap. 15.95 (*0-7234-2118-8*) Mosby Inc.

Self Assessment Picture Tests in Dentistry. Glyn & Jones Staff. 1993. 144p. (C). (gr. 13). pap. text 32.95 (*0-8151-4023-1*, 23066) Mosby Inc.

Self Assessment Picture Tests in Dentistry. L. Shaw. 1993. (Illus.). 144p. (C). (gr. 13). pap. text 32.95 (*0-8151-7664-3*, 23065) Mosby Inc.

Self Assessment Picture Tests in Dentistry. R. Winstanley. 1994. (Illus.). 205p. (C). (gr. 13). pap. text 32.95 (*0-8151-9336-X*, 23044) Mosby Inc.

Self Assessment Picture Tests in Dentistry - Endod... R. T. Walker. 1994. (Illus.). 144p. (C). (gr. 13). 32.95 (*0-8151-9148-0*, 23002) Mosby Inc.

Self-Assessment Picture Tests in Medicine. Pierre-Marc G. Bouloux. 1996. mass mkt. (*0-7234-2467-5*) Wolfe Publishing GBR. *Dist:* Mosby Inc.

Self Assessment Picture Tests in Medicine, Set. Pierre-Marc G. Bouloux. 1997. 488p. pap. 57.00 (*0-7234-2468-3*) Mosby Inc.

Self-Assessment Picture Tests in Medicine, Vol. 2. Pierre-Marc G. Bouloux. 1997. pap. (*0-7234-2465-9*) Mosby Inc.

Self Assessment Picture Tests in Medicine: Otolaryngology, Head & Neck Surgery. M. Hawthorne et al. 1995. 144p. (*0-7234-2021-1*) Martin Dunitz GBR. *Dist:* Mosby Inc.

Self-Assessment Picture Tests in Medicine: Pediatrics. Ed. by David Milner. 1994. (Illus.). 148p. (C). (gr. 13). pap. text 15.95 (*0-8151-5916-1*, 23092) Mosby Inc.

Self-Assessment Picture Tests in Medicine, '97. Pierre-Marc G. Bouloux. 1997. Vol. 1. pap. (*0-7234-2464-0*); Vol. 3. pap. (*0-7234-2466-7*) Mosby Inc.

Self-Assessment Picture Tests in Rheumatology Medicine. Michael Doherty & Emmanuel George. 1995. (Illus.). 144p. 19.95 (*0-7234-1968-X*) Mosby Inc.

Self-Assessment Picture Tests in Small Animal Dermatology. Kummel. 1994. mass mkt. (*0-7234-1944-2*) Wolfe Publishing GBR. *Dist:* Mosby Inc.

Self-Assessment Picture Tests in Veterinary Medicine: Clinical Anatomy. Boyd. 1995. mass mkt. 32.95 (*0-7234-2142-0*) Mosby Inc.

Self-Avoiding Walk. Neal Madras & Gordon Slade. 1996. (Illus.). 448p. pap. 43.95 (*0-8176-3891-1*) Birkhauser.

Self-Awareness & Drug Abuse & Drug Control. L. Pickens. Ed. by Therese A. Zak. 1981. (Lifeworks Ser.). (Illus.). 128p. text 13.96 (*0-07-049910-1*) McGraw.

Self-Awareness in Animals & Humans: Developmental Perspectives. Ed. by Sue T. Parker et al. 1994. (Illus.). 464p. (C). text 110.00 (*0-521-44108-0*) Cambridge U Pr.

Self-Care: Lay Initiatives in Health. Lowell S. Levin et al. 1976. LC 76-29361. pap. 7.95 (*0-88202-111-7*) Watson Pub Intl.

Self-Care: Your Family Guide to Symptoms & How to Treat Them. Don R. Powell. 1996. LC 95-34190. (Illus.). 280p. 29.95 (*1-882606-24-8*) Peoples Med Soc.

Self Care Acupressure Kit. David G. Williams. 1992. 26p. pap. 15.95 incl. VHS (*0-944649-13-0*) Mtn Home Pub.

Self-Care Advisor. Health Publishing Group Editors. 1996. (Illus.). 336p. (Orig.). pap. (*0-9644119-1-1*) Time Inc Health.

Self-Care Advisor: The Essential Home Health Guide for You & Your Family. Ed. by Health Magazine Editors. 2000. LC 00-44741. (Illus.). 352p. pap. (*0-7370-1620-5*) Time-Life Bks GBR. *Dist:* AOL Time Warner.

Self-Care & Self-Help Groups for the Elderly. 1991. lib. bdg. 69.95 (*0-8490-4487-1*) Gordon Pr.

S

Self Care Deficit Nursing Theory: In Practice. Connie M. Dennis. 1996. (Illus.). 176p. (C). (gr. 13). pap. text 28.00 (*0-8151-2426-0*, 28191) Mosby Inc.

Self Care Deficit Theory of Nursing. Joan Munley. 1984. 128p. (C). pap. text (*0-910973-03-2*) Arrowhead AZ.

***Self-Care Essentials: A Simple Guide to Managing Your Health Care & Living Well.** Chad Abresch et al. Ed. by David M. Hunnicutt. 2001. (Illus.). 128p. lib. bdg. 0.00 (*0-9628334-9-5*) WELCOA.

Self-Care Guide to Holistic Medicine: Creating Optimal Health. Robert S. Ivker et al. 2000. LC 00-56366. (Illus.). 512p. pap. 15.95 (*1-58542-056-5*, Avery) Putnam Pub Group.

Self-Care Nursing in a Multicultural Context. Juliene Lipson & Nancy Steiger. 1996. LC 96-4508. 352p. 74.95 (*0-8039-7054-4*, 2789); pap. 37.95 (*0-8039-7055-2*, 2788) Sage.

Self Care Versus Medical Care. 1992. lib. bdg. 69.99 (*0-8490-8793-7*) Gordon Pr.

Self Change: Social Psychological & Clinical Perspectives. Ed. by Y. Klar et al. 1992. (Illus.). 285p. 64.95 (*0-387-97811-9*) Spr-Verlag.

Self Concept. John Hattie. 1992. 320p. text 59.95 (*0-89859-629-7*) L Erlbaum Assocs.

Self-Concept Vol. 1: A Review of Methodological Considerations & Measuring Instruments. Ruth C. Wylie. rev. ed. 1974. LC 72-97165. 433p. text 50.00 (*0-8032-0830-8*) U of Nebr Pr.

Self-Concept of the Young Child: An Anthology. Ed. by Thomas D. Yawkey. 1982. LC 80-13812. vii, 274p. (Orig.). pap. 12.95 (*0-8425-1815-0*, Friends of the Library) Brigham.

Self-Conscious Emotions: The Psychology of Shame, Guilt, Embarrassment & Pride. Ed. by June P. Tangney & Kurt W. Fischer. 1995. LC 94-31710. 542p. 60.00 (*0-89862-264-6*, 2264) Guilford Pubns.

Self-Consistency: A Theory of Personality. Prescott Lecky. 1982. LC 82-82238. 144p. pap. 6.95 (*0-87208-221-0*); 1994. LC 93-81260. 176p. (C). pap. 12.95 (*0-87208-310-1*) Shoeless Pub.

Self-Contained Breathing Apparatus. J. Steven Kidd & John Czajkowski. 1995. 30p. wbk. ed. (*0-8151-5119-5*) Mosby Inc.

Self-Control & Self-Modification of Emotional Behavior. Ed. by Kirk R. Blankstein et al. 1982. (Advances in the Study of Communication & Affect Ser.: Vol. 7). 216p. 42.50 (*0-306-40945-3*, Plenum Trade) Perseus Pubng.

Self-Defeating Behaviors: Experimental Research, Clinical Impressions, & Practical Implications. R. C. Curtis. 1989. (Social - Clinical Psychology Ser.). (Illus.). 398p. (C). 65.00 (*0-306-43129-7*, Plenum Trade) Perseus Pubng.

Self-Delight in a Harsh World: The Main Stories of Individual, Marital, & Family Psychotherapy. James P. Gustafson. 1992. LC 92-5034. 200p. (C). 22.95 (*0-393-70136-0*) Norton.

Self-Destruction in the Promised Land: A Psychocultural History. Howard I. Kushner. 1989. 280p. 24.95 (*0-8135-1377-4*) Rutgers U Pr.

Self-Directed Behavior. David L. Watson. 4th ed. 1985. (Psychology Ser.). tchr. ed. (*0-534-04777-7*) Wadsworth Pub.

Self-Directed Behavior: Self-Modification for Personal Adjustment. David L. Watson & Roland G. Tharp. 5th ed. 1988. LC 88-19920. 334p. (C). mass mkt. 29.00 (*0-534-09276-4*) Brooks-Cole.

Self-Directed Program Reorder: Protocols & Programs. Richard E. Gans. 1996. 39.95 (*1-56593-805-4*, 1576) Thomson Learn.

Self-Directed Search & Related Holland Career Materials: A Practitioner's Guide. Robert C. Reardon & Janet G. Lenz. 1997. LC 97-45675. 320p. pap. text 33.00 (*0-911907-28-9*) Psych Assess.

Self-Directedness: Causes & Effects Throughout the Life Course. Ed. by Judith Rodin et al. 1990. 280p. 59.95 (*0-8058-0562-1*) L Erlbaum Assocs.

Self-Disclosure: Theory, Research, & Therapy. Valerian J. Derlega & J. H. Berg. 1987. LC 87-18654. (Perspectives in Social Psychology Ser.). (Illus.). 380p. (C). 70.00 (*0-306-42635-8*, Plenum Trade) Perseus Pubng.

Self-Disclosure in the Therapeutic Relationship. G. Stricker & M. Fisher. 1990. LC 90-6740. (Illus.). 310p. (C). 59.50 (*0-306-43448-2*, Plenum Trade) Perseus Pubng.

Self-Envy: Therapy & the Divided Internal World. Rafael E. Lopez-Corvo. 1995. LC 94-7733. 248p. 40.00 (*1-56821-252-6*) Aronson.

Self-Esteem: Paradoxes & Innovations in Clinical Theory & Practice. Richard L. Bednar & Scott R. Peterson. 2nd ed. 1995. LC 95-16098. 433p. text 34.95 (*1-55798-305-4*); pap. text 24.95 (*1-55798-290-2*) Am Psychol.

Self-Esteem & Mental Health: Health Facts. Nora J. Krantzler & Kathleen R. Miner. 1994. LC 93-43820. 12.95 (*1-56071-181-7*, H301) ETR Assocs.

Self-Esteem Enhancement with Children & Adolescents. A. W. Pope et al. 1988. 160p. text 30.00 (*0-08-032765-6*); pap. text 15.95 (*0-08-032764-8*) Elsevier (Pergamon Pr).

Self-Esteem for Tots to Teens. Eugene Anderson et al. 1991. LC 90-92130. pap. 8.95 (*1-879276-00-3*) Parent Tching Pubns.

Self Esteem, Mood & Evolutionary Fitness: A Synthesis. Eric A. Stone. 1992. (Illus.). 12p. (C). pap. 9.95 (*0-9631937-0-8*) BioPsych Pr.

Self-Esteem Problems of Children: Psychodynamics & Psychotherapy. Richard A. Gardner. 1992. LC 92-9573. 584p. text 40.00 (*0-933812-26-4*) Creative Therapeutics.

Self-Esteem Therapy. R. A. Steffenhagen. 1990. LC 89-49159. 208p. 62.50 (*0-275-93193-5*, Praeger Pubs) Greenwood.

Self-Evaluation for BMET Certification. 1994. pap. 50.00 (*1-57020-040-8*, SG1-209) Assn Adv Med Instrn.

Self-Evaluation in Young Children. Deborah J. Stipek et al. 1992. (Child Development Research & Social Policy Ser.). (Illus.). 142p. pap. text 15.00 (*0-226-77487-2*) U Ch Pr.

Self-Experiences in Group Intersubjective & Self-Psychological Pathways to Human Understanding. Ed. by Irene Harwood & Malcolm Pines. 1998. LC 98-152024. 350p. (*1-85302-596-8*) Jessica Kingsley GBR. *Dist:* Taylor & Francis.

Self-Experiences in Group Intersubjective & Self-Psychological Pathways to Human Understanding. Ed. by Irene Harwood & Malcolm Pines. 1998. LC 98-152024. (International Library of Group Analysis: Vol. 4). 350p. pap. (*1-85302-597-6*) Jessica Kingsley GBR. *Dist:* Taylor & Francis.

Self-Funding of Health Care Benefits. Carlton Harker. Ed. by Mary E. Brennan. 4th ed. 1997. LC 97-74488. 872p. (Orig.). pap. text 90.00 (*0-89154-514-X*) Intl Found Employ.

Self-Funding Your Employee Medical Benefits: A Survival Guide & How-To-Do-It Book. Thomas R. Young. Ed. by Gulf Coast Offset, Inc. Staff. 1985. (Orig.). (C). pap. (*0-9614151-1-8*); lib. bdg. (*0-9614151-0-X*) Young.

Self-Handicapping: The Paradox That Isn't. R. L. Higgins et al. 1990. (Social-Clinical Psychology Ser.). (Illus.). 312p. (C). 49.50 (*0-306-43540-3*, Plenum Trade) Perseus Pubng.

***Self Heal with Herbs & Nutrition.** Jill Rosemary Davies. 2001. LC 2001-47253. 270p. pap. 18.95 (*1-58091-111-0*) Crossing Pr.

Self-Healing: Powerful Techniques. Ranjie N. Singh. Date not set. 252p. 24.95 (*1-896826-00-8*) APG Trade.

Self Healing: The Secret of the Ring Muscles. Paula Garbourg. 1992. 184p. pap. (*0-86689-032-7*) Balaban Intl Sci Serv.

Self-Healing by Thought Force. William W. Atkinson. 1996. 91p. reprint ed. pap. 7.95 (*1-56459-646-X*) Kessinger Pub.

Self-Healing Cookbook: A Macrobiotic Primer for Healing Body, Mind & Moods with Whole, Natural Foods. Kristina Turner. 6th rev. ed. 1998. (Illus.). 216p. (Orig.). reprint ed. pap. 16.50 (*0-945668-10-4*) Earthtones Pr.

Self-Healing Dynamics for Cancer & Other Illnesses. Jan K. Garverick. 1991. 96p. (Orig.). pap. text 7.95 (*0-9630177-0-5*) Morgana Pubns.

Self-Healing Handbook: Nutrition & the Harston Method of Deep Muscle Therapy. Anna W. Harston. 1993. LC 93-78404. (Illus.). 248p. pap. 12.95 (*0-9636998-0-6*) LHC Pubs.

Self-Healing Workbook: Your Personal Plan for Stress-Free Living. C. Norman Shealy. 1993. (Home Library of Alternative Medicine). (Illus.). 160p. pap., stu. ed. 14.95 (*1-85230-429-4*) Element MA.

Self-Health: The Perfect Health Plan. Richard D. Pinson. 1999. LC 99-96631. (Illus.). X,335p. 19.95 (*0-9671059-1-9*) Well Being.

Self-Health Handbook: Low-Cost, Easy-to-Use Therapies from Around the World. Kenneth A. Dachman & Joen P. Kinnan. 1996. LC 95-46516. 304p. 26.75 (*0-8160-3201-7*) Facts on File.

Self-Help & Mutual Aid Groups: International & Multicultural Perspectives. Ed. by Francine Lavoie et al. 1995. LC 94-44762. (Prevention in Human Services Ser.). 363p. 49.95 (*1-56024-716-9*) Haworth Pr.

***Self-Help for Hyperventilitation Syndrome: Recognizing & Correcting Your Breathing Pattern Disorder.** Dinah Bradley. 3rd ed. 2001. LC 2001-26468. (Illus.). 128p. pap. 12.95 (*0-89793-348-6*) Hunter Hse.

Self-Help for Your Anxiety: The Proven Anxiety Antidote Method. Robert Sharpe. 1997. (Illus.). 260p. pap. (*0-285-62986-7*) Souvenir Pr Ltd GBR. *Dist:* IPG Chicago.

Self-Help Groups & Voluntary Action: International Perspectives. Alfred H. Katz & David H. Smith. 250p. text (*0-8290-1274-5*) Irvington.

Self-Help Guide to Managing Depression. Barker. 1993. 78p. pap. 16.00 (*1-56593-216-1*, 0575) Singular Publishing.

Self-Help Revolution. Ed. by Alan Gartner & Frank Riessman. 1984. (Community Psychology Ser.: Vol. X). 304p. 42.95 (*0-89885-070-3*, Kluwer Acad Hman Sci) Kluwer Academic.

Self-Hypnosis. C. F. Freimuth. 1979. 12p. pap. 5.00 (*0-933992-07-6*) Coffee Break.

Self-Hypnosis: Its Theory, Technique & Application. Melvin Powers. 1975. pap. 7.00 (*0-87980-138-7*) Wilshire.

Self-Hypnosis: The Chicago Paradigm. Erika Fromm et al. 1990. LC 90-3167. (Guilford Clinical & Experimental Hypnosis Ser.). 254p. 35.00 (*0-89862-341-3*) Guilford Pubns.

Self-Hypnosis: The Complete Manual for Health & Self-Change. Brian M. Alman & Peter T. Lambrou. 2nd ed. 1991. LC 91-29007. (Illus.). 304p. pap. 22.95 (*0-87630-650-4*) Brunner-Routledge.

Self-Hypnosis & Other Mind Expanding Techniques. Charles Tebbetts. 2nd ed. 1977. 141p. (C). pap. 9.95 (*0-930298-18-7*) Westwood Pub Co.

Self-Hypnosis for Health & Personal Growth: A Practical Method to Help You Solve Your Problems & Realize Your Dreams. George Gamez. Ed. by Elizabeth Ferrant. 1999. LC 98-68339. 144p. pap. 13.95 (*0-9650590-4-9*, PG102) Peak Pubns CA.

Self-Hypnosis Step by Step: The 30 Essential Techniques. J. P. Guyonnaud & Giovanni Sciuto. 1996. (Illus.). 208p. pap. text (*0-285-63324-4*) Souvenir Pr Ltd GBR. *Dist:* IPG Chicago.

Self in Emotional Distress: Cognitive & Psychodynamic Perspectives. Ed. by Zindel V. Segal & Sidney J. Blatt. 1993. LC 92-49988. 386p. 45.00 (*0-89862-256-5*) Guilford Pubns.

Self in Infancy: Theory & Research. Ed. by Philippe Rochat. 1995. LC 95-35838. (Advances in Psychology Ser.: Vol.112). 496p. 130.50 (*0-444-81925-8*) Elsevier.

Self in Process: Toward a Post-Rationalist Cognitive Therapy. Vittorio F. Guidano. 1991. LC 90-14129. 237p. 40.00 (*0-89862-447-9*, 2447) Guilford Pubns.

Self in Social Psychology: Essential Readings. Ed. by Roy F. Baumeister. 1999. LC 99-16279. (Key Readings in Social Psychology Ser.). 492p. (C). pap. (*0-86377-573-X*) Psychol Pr GBR. *Dist:* Taylor & Francis.

Self in the Family: A Classification of Personality, Criminality & Psychopathology. Luciano L'Abate & Margaret Baggett. 1996. LC 96-19639. (Couples & Family Dynamics & Treatment Ser.). 404p. 110.00 (*0-471-12247-5*) Wiley.

Self in the System: Expanding the Limits of Family Therapy. Michael P. Nichols. 1987. LC 87-13773. 328p. text 40.95 (*0-87630-472-2*) Brunner-Routledge.

Self in Transition: Infancy to Childhood. Ed. by Dante Cicchetti & Marjorie Beeghly. 1990. LC 90-35059. (John D. & Catherine T. MacArthur Foundation Series on Mental Health & Development). (Illus.). 412p. 41.95 (*0-226-10662-4*) U Ch Pr.

Self-Injurious Behavior. Judith E. Favell. 1982. pap. 53.00 (*0-08-028824-3*) Elsevier.

Self-Injurious Behavior: A Somatosensory Treatment Approach. Haru Hirama. 1989. 38p. (C). pap. text 11.50 (*0-935273-01-8*) Chess Pub.

Self-Injurious Behavior: Analysis, Assessment & Treatment. Ed. by J. K. Luiselli et al. 1991. (Disorders of Human Learning, Behavior, & Communication Ser.). (Illus.). 393p. 97.00 (*0-387-97580-2*) Spr-Verlag.

Self-Injurious Behaviors: Assessment & Treatment. Ed. by Daphne Simeon & Eric Hollander. 2001. LC 00-61807. xii, 210p. pap. 34.00 (*0-88048-808-5*, 8808) Am Psychiatric.

Self Injurious Behaviour: A Collection of Published Papers on Prevalence, Causes, & Treatment in People with Mental Handicap or Autism. G. Murphy & B. Wilson. Ed. by BIMH Publications Staff. 1985. 500p. 90.00 (*0-906054-55-9*); pap. 80.00 (*0-906054-49-4*) St Mut.

Self-Instruction Workbook Emergency. Elling. 8th ed. 1997. pap. text 21.15 net. (*0-8359-5098-0*) P-H.

Self-Interest & Universal Health Care: Why Well-Insured Americans Should Support Coverage for Everyone. Larry Churchill. 1994. LC 94-14568. 112p. text 23.95 (*0-674-80092-3*, CHUSEL) HUP.

Self-Knower: A Hero under Control. R. A. Wicklund et al. 1992. (Social-Clinical Psychology Ser.). (Illus.). 184p. (C). 47.00 (*0-306-43988-3*, Plenum Trade) Perseus Pubng.

Self-Learning Materials & Modules for Health Workers: A Guide for Their Development, Utilization & Evaluation. 1985. (SEARO Technical Publications Ser.: No. 6). 18p. pap. text 3.00 (*92-9022-145-3*) World Health.

Self-Managed Work Teams in Health Care Organizations. Elizabeth D. Becker-Reems. 1994. LC 94-1253. 231p. pap. 52.00 (*1-55648-122-5*, 169109) AHPI.

Self-Management for Adolescents: A Skills Training Program. Thomas A. Brigham. 1988. LC 88-19031. (Treatment Manuals for Practitioners Ser.). 161p. pap. 30.00 (*0-89862-202-6*) Guilford Pubns.

Self-Management of Asthma. Harry Kotses & Andrew Harver. 1998. LC 97-49681. (Lung Biology in Health & Disease Ser.). (Illus.). 440p. text 175.00 (*0-8247-9858-9*) Dekker.

Self-Massage for Your Arthritis. Simon Wang. 1998. (Chinese Health Library Ser.: Vol. 2). 38p. pap. 4.98 (*0-9641605-5-2*) East Hlth Dev.

Self-Massage for Your Asthma. Simon Wang. 1998. (Chinese Health Library Ser.: Vol. 4). (Illus.). 40p. pap. 4.98 (*0-9641605-7-9*) East Hlth Dev.

Self-Massage for Your Eyes. Simon Wang. 1998. (Chinese Health Library Ser.: Vol. 3). (Illus.). 40p. pap. 4.98 (*0-9641605-6-0*) East Hlth Dev.

Self-Massage for Your Headache. Simon Wang. 1998. (Chinese Health Library Ser.: Vol. 5). (Illus.). 40p. pap. 4.98 (*0-9641605-8-7*) East Hlth Dev.

Self-Massage for Your Hypertension. Simon Wang. 1998. (Chinese Health Library Ser.: Vol. 6). (Illus.). 40p. pap. 4.98 (*0-9641605-9-5*) East Hlth Dev.

Self-Mastery. Swami Paramananda. 5th ed. 1961. pap. 4.95 (*0-911564-08-X*) Vedanta Ctr.

Self-Mutilation: Theory, Research & Treatment. Barent W. Walsh & Paul M. Rosen. 1988. LC 88-5154. 273p. 40.00 (*0-89862-731-1*, 2731) Guilford Pubns.

Self-Narratives: The Construction of Meaning in Psychotherapy. Hubert J. Hermans & Els Hermans-Jansen. 1995. LC 95-8249. (Practicing Professional Ser.). 306p. 40.00 (*0-89862-878-4*, C2878) Guilford Pubns.

Self-Neglect: Challenges for Helping Professionals. Ed. by James G. O'Brien. 2000. LC 00-21100. xii, 101p. pap. text 14.95 (*0-7890-0993-5*) Haworth Pr.

Self-Neglecting Elders: A Clinical Dilemma. Ed. by Eloise Rathbone-McCuan & Dorothy R. Fabian. 1992. LC 91-36343. 216p. 57.50 (*0-86569-047-2*, T047, Auburn Hse) Greenwood.

Self-Organization & Psychotherapy. Ed. by A. L. Goudsmit. 1990. (Recent Research in Psychology Ser.). 189p. 47.95 (*0-387-52161-5*) Spr-Verlag.

Self-Parenting: The Complete Guide to Your Inner Conversations. John K. Pollard, III. 1987. LC 86-83037. (Illus.). 250p. (Orig.). pap. 9.95 (*0-942055-25-X*) Generic Human Studies.

Self-Presentation. Ed. by S. L. Zelen. 1988. (Recent Research in Psychology Ser.). 178p. 63.95 (*0-387-96862-8*) Spr-Verlag.

Self-Process & Development: The Minnesota Symposia on Child Psychology, Vol. 23. Ed. by Megan R. Gunnar & L. Alan Sroufe. 1990. 280p. (C). text 69.95 (*0-8058-0695-4*) L Erlbaum Assocs.

Self-Psychology & Diagnostic Assessment: Identifying Selfobject Functions Through Psychological Testing. annuals Marshall L. Silverstein. 1999. LC 98-27593. (Personality & Clinical Psychology Ser.). 312p. (ps-3). 34.50 (*0-8058-2280-1*) L Erlbaum Assocs.

Self-Psychology in Clinical Social Work. Miriam Elson. 1988. (Professional Bks.). (C). pap. text 14.00 (*0-393-95797-7*) Norton.

Self-Regulation Theory: Applying Theory to Your Practice. Jean E. Johnson et al. 1997. (Illus.). 130p. (Orig.). pap. text, spiral bd. 29.50 (*1-890504-02-5*) Oncology Nursing.

Self-Related Cognitions in Anxiety & Motivation. Ed. by Ralf Schwarzer. 1985. 360p. (C). text 69.95 (*0-89859-513-4*) L Erlbaum Assocs.

Self-Relaxation: Comfort in Times of Tension. Harley D. Christiansen. 1981. LC 81-2595. (Illus.). 96p. pap. 15.95 (*0-915456-02-8*) P Juul Pr.

Self-Representation: Life Narrative Studies in Identity & Ideology, 18. Gary S. Gregg. 1991. LC 91-7227. (Contributions in Psychology Ser.: No. 18). 248p. 60.00 (*0-313-27862-8*, GGA/, Greenwood Pr) Greenwood.

Self, Social Identity, & Physical Health: Interdisciplinary Explorations. Ed. by Richard J. Contrada & Richard D. Ashmore. 1999. LC 98-20149. (Rutgers Series on Self & Social Identity: Vol.2). (Illus.). 296p. text 60.00 (*0-19-512730-7*); pap. text 29.95 (*0-19-512731-5*) OUP.

Self-Society Dynamic: Cognition, Emotion, & Action. Ed. by Judith A. Howard & Peter J. Callero. 1991. (Illus.). 351p. (C). text 69.95 (*0-521-38433-8*) Cambridge U Pr.

Self-Starvation: From Individual to Family Therapy in the Treatment of Anorexia Nervosa. Mara P. Selvini. 1996. LC 84-45722. 312p. pap. 50.00 (*1-56821-822-2*) Aronson.

Self-Studies: On the Psychology of Self & Identity. Karl E. Scheibe. 1995. LC 94-40037. 240p. 67.00 (*0-275-94538-3*, Praeger Pubs) Greenwood.

Self-Studies: The Psychology of Self & Identity. Karl E. Scheibe. 1998. LC 94-40037. 240p. pap. 23.95 (*0-275-96291-1*, Praeger Pubs) Greenwood.

Self-Study Course for Paraoptometric Certification. AOA Staff. Ed. by Mary Jameson. 2nd ed. 2000. LC 96-30878. (Illus.). 358p. pap. text 54.99 (*0-7506-7266-8*) Buttrwrth-Heinemann.

Self-Study Exercises in Radiography. William L. Leonard. 2nd ed. 1998. (Illus.). 260p. (C). pap. text 29.95 (*0-9644624-3-5*) JLW Pub.

Self-Study Modules on Tuberculosis. Ed. by Barry Leonard. 2000. (Illus.). 235p. reprint ed. pap. text 50.00 (*0-7567-0087-6*) DIANE Pub.

Self-System: Developmental Changes Between & Within Self-Concepts. Annerieke Oosterwegel & Louis Oppenheimer. 1993. 208p. text 39.95 (*0-8058-1216-4*) L Erlbaum Assocs.

Self-Teaching Study Guide & Workbook for "The Sensation of Being Somebody" Maurice E. Wagner. 3rd ed. 1985. 148p. 10.00 (*0-940445-00-X*) Christ Growth Pubs.

Self-Therapy for Sex Problems. Daniel Steele. 1987. LC 86-62950. 211p. pap. 20.00 (*0-9618277-0-X*) Human Rsch.

Self-Therapy for the Stutterer. Malcolm Fraser. 1985. pap. 3.00 (*0-87980-415-7*) Wilshire.

Self to the Self. Dora Wilson. 1947. (C). pap. 4.00 (*0-87574-035-9*) Pendle Hill.

Self-Treatment for AIDS: Oxygen Therapy. Betsy Russell-Manning. rev. ed. 1989. per. 16.95 (*0-930165-12-8*) Greensward Pr.

Selfish Brain: Learning from Addiction. Robert L. DuPont. 1997. LC 96-8593. 589p. 32.95 (*0-88048-686-4*, 8686) Am Psychiatric.

Selfish Gene. Richard Dawkins. 2nd ed. 1990. 366p. pap. text 12.95 (*0-19-286092-5*) OUP.

Self's Better Body Book. Self Magazine Staff. 1998. pap. (*0-609-80318-2*, Clarkson Potter) Crown Pub Group.

Sell Yourself to Science: The Complete Guide to Selling Your Organs, Body Fluids, Bodily Functions & Being a Human Guinea Pig. Jim Hogshire. 1992. LC 92-81803. (Illus.). 166p. (Orig.). pap. 16.95 (*1-55950-084-0*, 94129) Loompanics.

Selling of Contraception: The Dalkon Shield Case, Sexuality, & Women's Autonomy. Nicole J. Grant. 1993. LC 91-41227. (Women & Health Ser.). 223p. pap. 18.95 (*0-8142-0615-8*) Ohio St U Pr.

Selling of DSM III: The Rhetoric of Science in Psychiatry. Stuart A. Kirk & Herb Kutchins. 1992. (Social Problems & Social Issues Ser.). 280p. lib. bdg. 50.95 (*0-202-30431-0*) Aldine de Gruyter.

Selling of DSM-III: The Rhetoric of Science in Psychiatry. Stuart A. Kirk & Herb Kutchins. 1992. (Social Problems & Social Issues Ser.). 280p. pap. text 25.95 (*0-202-30432-9*) Aldine de Gruyter.

Semantic & Conceptual Development: An Ontological Perspective. Frank C. Keil. 1979. LC 79-10491. (Cognitive Science Ser.: Vol. 1). (Illus.). 229p. 30.00 (*0-674-80100-8*) HUP.

Semantic Theory of Evolution. Marcello Barbieri. 1985. (Models of Scientific Thought Ser.: Vol. 2). xii, 188p. text 96.00 (*3-7186-0243-1*) Gordon & Breach.

Semantics & Cognition. Ray S. Jackendoff. Ed. by Joan Bresnan et al. 1985. (Current Studies in Linguistics). (Illus.). 304p. (C). pap. 22.95 (*0-262-60013-7*) MIT Pr.

Seminaire Vol. 11: Les Quatre Concepts Fodaementaux de la Psychanalyse. Jacques Lacan. 1990. (FRE.). pap. 19.95 (*0-7859-2719-0*) Fr & Eur.

Seminal Research Papers, 11. John Dewey et al. 1977. LC 77-72191. (Contributions to the History of Psychology Ser.: No. 11, Pt. A, Orientations). 454p. reprint ed. lib. bdg. 78.50 (*0-313-26935-1*, U6935, Greenwood Pr) Greenwood.

Seminal Vesicles & Fertility. Ed. by C. G. Bollack & A. Clavert. 1984. (Progress in Reproductive Biology & Medicine Ser.: Vol. 12). (Illus.). x, 182p. 129.75 (*3-8055-3907-X*) S Karger.

Seminar at Sea: Second International Hemex Symposium on the Duromedics Bileaflet Valve. Ed. & Illus. by Silent Partners, Inc. Staff. 1986. 144p. pap. (*1-878353-06-3*) Silent Partners.

Seminar of Jacques Lacan: The Psychoses 1955-1956, Bk. 3. Jacques Lacan. Ed. by Jacques-Alain Miller. Tr. by Russell Grigg. 1993. LC 92-28360. (Seminar of Jacques Lacan Ser.: Vol. 3). 352p. 35.00 (*0-393-03467-4*) Norton.

Seminar of Jacques Lacan Bk. 2: The Ego in Freud's Theory & in the Technique of Psychoanalyis, 1954-1955. Ed. by Jacques-Alain Miller. Tr. by Sylvana Tomaselli. 1991. (Seminar of Jacques Lacan Ser.: Vol. 2). pap. 17.95 (*0-393-30709-3*) Norton.

Seminar on Ambulatory Pediatrics: Journal: Paediatrician, Vol. 5, No. 3. Ed. by George D. Maragos. 1977. (Illus.). 26.25 (*3-8055-2433-1*) S Karger.

Seminar on Bibliotherapy: Proceedings of Sessions on Bibliotherapy Madison, Wisconsin, June 21-23, 1978. Ed. by Margaret E. Monroe. 1978. 180p. pap. 6.00 (*0-936442-07-7*) U Wis Sch Lib.

Seminar on Delivery of Child Health Care. Ed. by O. P. Petersson. 1979. (Journal: Vol. 9, No. 1, 1980). 52p. pap. 28.75 (*3-8055-0800-X*) S Karger.

Seminar on Environmental Pharmacology. Ed. by Ryuta Ito. 1977. (Journal: Vol. 6, No. 1). (Illus.). 27.00 (*3-8055-2794-2*) S Karger.

Seminar on Geographical Pediatrics. Ed. by George D. Maragos. 1977. (Journal: Vol. 6, No. 2). (Illus.). 27.00 (*3-8055-2795-0*) S Karger.

Seminar on Haematology & Oncology. Ed. by H. Ekert. 1980. (Journal: Vol. 9, No. 2). (Illus.). 88p. pap. 28.75 (*3-8055-1302-X*) S Karger.

Seminar on Human Genetics. Ed. by George D. Maragos. 1978. (Journal: Vol. 6, No. 6). (Illus.). 27.00 (*3-8055-2909-0*) S Karger.

Seminar on Immunological Aspects of Kidney Diseases in Children. Ed. by George D. Maragos. 1981. (Journal: Vol. 10, No. 5-6). (Illus.). 164p. pap. 61.00 (*3-8055-3488-4*) S Karger.

Seminar on Infectious Diseases in Childhood. Ed. by George D. Maragos. 1979. (Journal: Vol. 8, No. 1-2). (Illus.). pap. 57.50 (*3-8055-3027-7*) S Karger.

Seminar on Kidney Diseases in Children. Ed. by F. Mota-Hernandez. 1979. (Journal: Vol. 8, No. 5-6, 1979). pap. 57.50 (*3-8055-0344-X*) S Karger.

Seminar on Neonatology. Ed. by George D. Maragos. 1977. (Journal: Vol. 5, No. 5). (Illus.). 26.25 (*3-8055-2702-0*) S Karger.

Seminar on Office Pediatrics, Pt. II. Ed. by George D. Maragos. 1979. (Journal: Vol. 8, No. 3). (Illus.). pap. 28.75 (*3-8055-3074-9*) S Karger.

Seminar on Pediatric Allergy. Ed. by George D. Maragos. 1977. (Journal: Vol. 5, No. 4). (Illus.). 80p. 26.25 (*3-8055-2648-2*) S Karger.

Seminar on Pediatric Cardiology. Ed. by George D. Maragos. 1978. (Journal: Vol. 7, No. 1-3). (Illus.). pap. 81.00 (*3-8055-2912-0*) S Karger.

Seminar on Pediatric Cardiology. Ed. by J. G. Shakibi. 1981. (Journal: Vol. 10, No. 1-3). (Illus.). 180p. pap. 91.50 (*3-8055-2675-X*) S Karger.

Seminar on Public Health. Ed. by George D. Maragos. 1982. (Journal: Vol. II, No. 1-2, 1982). (Illus.). Pt. I. iv, 120p. pap. 67.00 (*3-8055-3533-3*); Pt. 2. 126p. pap. 67.00 (*3-8055-3532-5*) S Karger.

Seminar on Spinal Cord Stimulation for the Control of Pain & other Neurological Disorders. Ed. by Philip L. Gildenberg & D. M. Long. 1982. (Journal: Vol. 44, No. 4). (Illus.). vi, 84p. pap. 42.75 (*3-8055-3531-7*) S Karger.

Seminar on the Role & Training of Community Pharmacists: (Proceedings of the Seminar, Strasbourg, 2-4 October, 1991) 1993. (*92-871-2296-2*) Council of Europe FRA. *Dist:* Manhattan Pub Co.

Seminar on Tubal Physiology & Biochemistry. Ed. by Carl J. Pauerstein. 1975. (Journal: Vol. 6, Nos. 3-4). iv, 160p. reprint ed. 48.75 (*3-8055-2252-5*) S Karger.

Seminars in the Psychiatry of Learning Disabilities. Ed. by Oliver Russell. 1997. LC 97-173712. 282p. pap. (*1-901242-02-1*) Royal Coll Psych GBR. *Dist:* Balogh.

Seminars of Jacques Lacan: Freud's Writings on Technique 1953-1954. Jacques Lacan. Ed. by Jacques-Alain Miller. Tr. by John Forrester & Sylvana Tomaselli from FRE. 1988. (Seminar of Jacques Lacan Ser.: Bk. 1). 314p. 24.95 (*0-393-01895-4*) Norton.

Semiotic Approaches to Human Relations. Jurgen Ruesch. 1972. (*90-279-2299-3*) Mouton.

Semiotic Approaches to Psychiatry. Harley C. Shands. 1970. (Approaches to Semiotics Ser.: No. 2). text (*90-279-0506-1*) Mouton.

Semiotic Foundations of Drug Therapy: The Placebo Problem in a New Perspective. Klaus Schonauer. 1994. LC 93-36818. (Approaches to Semiotics Ser.: Vol. 112). (Illus.). x, 258p. (C). lib. bdg. (*3-11-013532-9*) Mouton.

Semiotic Perspectives on Clinical Theory & Practice: Medicine, Neuropsychiatry & Psychoanalysis. Ed. by Bonnie E. Litowitz & Phillip S. Epstein. 1991. (Approaches to Semiotics Ser.: No. 98). (Illus.). xii, 206p. (C). lib. bdg. (*3-11-012632-X*, 140-91) Mouton.

Semiotics of Cellular Communication in the Immune System. N. Avrion Mitchison & Eli E. Sercarz. 1988. (NATO ASI Ser.: Vol. 23). (Illus.). 335p. 147.00 (*0-387-18552-6*) Spr-Verlag.

Semrad: The Heart of a Therapist. Ed. by Susan Rako & Harvey Mazer. 1983. LC 84-45091. 208p. 40.00 (*0-87668-684-6*) Aronson.

Send Us a Lady Physician: Women Doctors in America, 1835-1920. Ruth Abram. 1986. LC 85-13856. (Illus.). 255p. pap. 12.95 (*0-393-30278-4*) Norton.

Senescence & Rejuvenescence. Charles M. Child. Ed. by Robert J. Kastenbaum. 1979. LC 78-22192. (Aging & Old Age Ser.). (Illus.). reprint ed. lib. bdg. 39.95 (*0-405-11809-0*) Ayer.

Senescence, the Last Half of Life. G. Stanley Hall. 1979. LC 73-169385. (Family in America Ser.). 530p. reprint ed. 31.95 (*0-405-03860-7*) Ayer.

Senile Dementia: Policy & Services. Bernard Ineichen. 1989. 180p. 47.50 (*0-412-33790-8*) Chapman & Hall.

Senior Care Acquisition Report, 2000. annuals Irving Levin Associates, Inc. Staff. 5th ed. 2000. (Illus.). vii, 132p. per. 495.00 (*1-930625-10-3*) I Levin.

Senior Citizens' Club Leader. Jack Rudman. 1994. (Career Examination Ser.: C-2745). pap. 27.95 (*0-8373-2745-8*) Nat Learn.

Senior Citizens' Information & Referral Specialist. Jack Rudman. 1994. (Career Examination Ser.: C-2814). pap. 27.95 (*0-8373-2814-4*) Nat Learn.

Senior Citizens' Nutrition Center Manager. Jack Rudman. 1994. (Career Examination Ser.: C-3356). pap. 34.95 (*0-8373-3356-3*) Nat Learn.

Senior Citizens' Program Coordinator. Jack Rudman. 1994. (Career Examination Ser.: C-2811). pap. 34.95 (*0-8373-2811-X*) Nat Learn.

Senior Clinical Psychologist. Jack Rudman. 1994. (Career Examination Ser.: C-1906). pap. 39.95 (*0-8373-1906-4*) Nat Learn.

Senior Community Narcotic Education Representative. Jack Rudman. 1994. (Career Examination Ser.: C-1942). pap. 34.95 (*0-8373-1942-0*) Nat Learn.

Senior Dental Hygienist. Jack Rudman. 1994. (Career Examination Ser.: C-2855). pap. 34.95 (*0-8373-2855-1*) Nat Learn.

Senior Dentist. Jack Rudman. 1994. (Career Examination Ser.: C-711). pap. 54.95 (*0-8373-0711-2*) Nat Learn.

Senior Drug Abuse Educator. Jack Rudman. 1994. (Career Examination Ser.: C-2520). pap. 34.95 (*0-8373-2520-X*) Nat Learn.

Senior Drug Abuse Rehabilitation Counselor. Jack Rudman. 1994. (Career Examination Ser.: C-2928). pap. 34.95 (*0-8373-2928-0*) Nat Learn.

Senior Drug & Alcohol Counselor. Jack Rudman. 1994. (Career Examination Ser.: C-2742). pap. 34.95 (*0-8373-2742-3*) Nat Learn.

Senior Hospital Administration Consultant. Jack Rudman. 1994. (Career Examination Ser.: C-2769). pap. 44.95 (*0-8373-2769-5*) Nat Learn.

Senior Hospital Care Investigator. Jack Rudman. 1994. (Career Examination Ser.: C-715). pap. 29.95 (*0-8373-0715-5*) Nat Learn.

Senior Licensed Practical Nurse. Jack Rudman. 1994. (Career Examination Ser.: C-3500). pap. 34.95 (*0-8373-3500-0*) Nat Learn.

Senior Medicaid Claims Examiner. Jack Rudman. 1994. (Career Examination Ser.: C-2692). pap. 29.95 (*0-8373-2692-3*) Nat Learn.

Senior Medical Conduct Investigator. Jack Rudman. 1994. (Career Examination Ser.: C-2610). pap. 29.95 (*0-8373-2610-9*) Nat Learn.

Senior Medical Emergency Dispatcher. Jack Rudman. 1994. (Career Examination Ser.: C-2332). pap. 29.95 (*0-8373-2332-0*) Nat Learn.

Senior Medical Laboratory Technician. Jack Rudman. 1994. (Career Examination Ser.: C-2496). pap. 29.95 (*0-8373-2496-3*) Nat Learn.

Senior Medical Records Clerk. Jack Rudman. 1994. (Career Examination Ser.: C-2310). reprint ed. pap. 29.95 (*0-8373-2310-X*) Nat Learn.

Senior Medical Services Specialist. Jack Rudman. 1994. (Career Examination Ser.: C-2747). pap. 39.95 (*0-8373-2747-4*) Nat Learn.

Senior Medical Social Worker. Jack Rudman. 1994. (Career Examination Ser.: C-2629). pap. 34.95 (*0-8373-2629-X*) Nat Learn.

Senior Medical Stenographer. Jack Rudman. 1994. (Career Examination Ser.: C-2940). pap. 27.95 (*0-8373-2940-X*) Nat Learn.

Senior Mental Health Worker. Jack Rudman. 1994. (Career Examination Ser.: C-1925). pap. 29.95 (*0-8373-1925-0*) Nat Learn.

Senior Moments: Growing Old Is Not for Sissies. Don Core. 2000. LC 99-90399. (Illus.). 128p. pap. 10.95 (*1-879752-03-4*) SOFITS.

Senior Occupational Therapist. Jack Rudman. 1994. (Career Examination Ser.: C-2174). pap. 34.95 (*0-8373-2174-3*) Nat Learn.

Senior Pharmacist. Jack Rudman. 1994. (Career Examination Ser.: C-722). pap. 34.95 (*0-8373-0722-8*) Nat Learn.

Senior Pharmacy Inspector. Jack Rudman. 1994. (Career Examination Ser.: C-2532). pap. 39.95 (*0-8373-2532-3*) Nat Learn.

Senior Physical Therapist. Jack Rudman. 1994. (Career Examination Ser.: C-1018). pap. 34.95 (*0-8373-1018-0*) Nat Learn.

Senior Psychiatric Social Worker. Jack Rudman. 1994. (Career Examination Ser.: C-2487). pap. 34.95 (*0-8373-2487-4*) Nat Learn.

Senior Psychologist. Jack Rudman. 1994. (Career Examination Ser.: C-2173). pap. 39.95 (*0-8373-2173-5*) Nat Learn.

Senior Public Health Educator. Jack Rudman. 1994. (Career Examination Ser.: C-3475). pap. 34.95 (*0-8373-3475-6*) Nat Learn.

Senior Public Health Engineer. Jack Rudman. 1994. (Career Examination Ser.: C-3346). pap. 39.95 (*0-8373-3346-6*) Nat Learn.

Senior Public Health Nutritionist. Jack Rudman. 1994. (Career Examination Ser.: C-1592). pap. 29.95 (*0-8373-1592-1*) Nat Learn.

Senior Public Health Representative. Jack Rudman. 1994. (Career Examination Ser.: C-2385). pap. 34.95 (*0-8373-2385-1*) Nat Learn.

Senior Public Health Sanitarian. Jack Rudman. 1994. (Career Examination Ser.: C-2002). pap. 34.95 (*0-8373-2002-X*) Nat Learn.

Senior Radiologic Technologist. Jack Rudman. 1994. (Career Examination Ser.: C-1545). pap. 34.95 (*0-8373-1545-X*) Nat Learn.

Senior Security Hospital Treatment Assistant. Jack Rudman. 1994. (Career Examination Ser.: C-1617). pap. 27.95 (*0-8373-1617-0*) Nat Learn.

Senior Social Services Medical Assistance Specialist. Jack Rudman. 1994. (Career Examination Ser.: C-2432). pap. 39.95 (*0-8373-2432-7*) Nat Learn.

Senior Speech & Hearing Therapist. Jack Rudman. 1994. (Career Examination Ser.: C-2273). reprint ed. pap. 34.95 (*0-8373-2273-1*) Nat Learn.

Senior X-Ray Technician. Jack Rudman. 1994. (Career Examination Ser.: C-731). pap. 34.95 (*0-8373-0731-7*) Nat Learn.

Senior's Guide to Pain-Free Living. Doug Dollemore. Ed. by Prevention Health Books for Seniors Staff. 2000. LC 00-24809. (*1-57954-127-5*) Rodale Pr Inc.

Seniors Health Journal. Ina Yalof & Joann Lamb. 2000. LC 00-40235. 112p. pap. 17.95 (*0-312-26388-0*) St Martin.

Senna & Its Rational Use. Ed. by Elke Leng-Peschlow. 1992. (Journal: Vol. 44, Suppl. 1, 1992). (Illus.). iv, 52p. pap. 17.50 (*3-8055-5574-1*) S Karger.

Sensation & Measurement: Papers in Honor of S. S. Stevens. Ed. by H. R. Moskowitz et al. 1974. LC 74-77966. 550p. text 226.00 (*90-277-0474-0*) Kluwer Academic.

Sensation & Perception. E. Bruce Goldstein. 2nd ed. 1984. 481p. (C). pap. 41.25 (*0-534-03035-1*) Brooks-Cole.

Sensation & Perception. Margaret W. Matlin. 3rd ed. 1992. LC 91-26132. 533p. 55.00 (*0-205-13519-6*) Allyn.

Sensation & Perception. Stanley Coren et al. 4th ed. 1994. (Illus.). (C). text 83.50 (*0-15-500103-5*) Harcourt Coll Pubs.

Sensation & Perception. Stanley Coren et al. 5th ed. 1999. LC 98-72167. (Illus.). 720p. (C). text 100.50 (*0-15-508050-4*) Harcourt Coll Pubs.

Sense & Senility: The Neuropathology of the Aged Human Brain. David M. Mann. 1997. (Neuroscience Intelligence Unit Ser.). 198p. pap. 89.95 (*0-412-13431-4*) Chapman & Hall.

Sense & Senility: The Neuropathy of the Aged Human Brain. D. M. Mann. 1997. LC 96-29707. (Neuroscience Intelligence Unit Ser.). 206p. 99.00 (*1-57059-422-8*) Landes Bioscience.

Sense & Sensibility in Health Care. Ed. by Marshall Marinker. Date not set. 296p. (Orig.). (C). pap. text (*0-7279-1111-2*) BMJ Pub GBR. *Dist:* AIDC.

Sense of Asher. Richard Asher. 1984. (Illus.). 112p. pap. (*0-7279-0136-2*) BMJ Pub GBR. *Dist:* AIDC.

Sense of Coherence & Resiliency: Stress, Coping, & Health. Ed. by Hamilton I. McCubbin et al. 1994. LC 94-60612. (Resiliency & Families Ser.). 300p. (Orig.). (C). pap. (*0-9639334-0-X*) U of Wis CEFM.

Sense of Direction: Activities to Build Functional Directional Skills. Laura Sena. Ed. by Cindy Drolet. 1999. LC 98-47876. (Illus.). 221p. spiral bd. 44.00 (*1-883315-38-7*, 8491) Imaginart Intl.

Sense of Humor: Explorations of a Personality Characteristic. W. Ruch. 1998. LC 98-15494. (Humor Research Ser.). 498p. 132.00 (*3-11-016207-5*) De Gruyter.

Sense of Self: Research & Theory. Alan O. Ross. 1992. LC 91-868. 208p. (C). text 32.95 (*0-8261-7430-2*) Springer Pub.

Sense of Smell. Ed. by R. H. Wright. 1982. 248p. 141.00 (*0-8493-5232-0*, QP458, CRC Reprint) Franklin.

Sense of Vocation: A Study of Career & Life Development. Larry Cochran. 1990. LC 89-34226. 211p. (C). text 25.50 (*0-7914-0245-2*) State U NY Pr.

Senses & the Intellect, 4. Alexander Bain. 1977. LC 77-72191. (Contributions to the History of Psychology Ser.: No. 4, Pt. A, Orientations). 605p. reprint ed. lib. bdg. 95.00 (*0-313-26928-9*, U6928, Greenwood Pr) Greenwood.

Sensible Analysis of the 12-Lead ECG. Kathleen A. Handal & Kathryn Monica Lewis. 2000. LC 99-44880. (Allied Health Ser.). 275p. (C). pap. text 33.95 (*0-7668-0524-7*) Delmar.

Sensible ECG Analysis. Kathleen A. Handal & Kathryn Monica Lewis. 1999. LC 99-29634. (Allied Health Ser.). (Illus.). 250p. (C). pap. text 44.95 (*0-7668-0520-4*) Delmar.

Sensible Sex. Curtis. 9.95 (*1-56684-236-0*) Evans Bk Dist.

Sensitive Gut. Ed. by Harvard Medical School Staff. 2001. LC 2001-50153. (Illus.). 224p. pap. 13.00 (*0-7432-1504-4*, Fireside) S&S Trade Pap.

Sensitive Periods in Development: Interdisciplinary Perspectives. Ed. by Marc Bornstein. 1987. (Crosscurrents in Contemporary Psychology Ser.). 304p. text 59.95 (*0-89859-696-3*) L Erlbaum Assocs.

Sensitivity Training: Processes, Problems & Applications. Arthur Blumberg. 1971. LC 74-157409. (Notes & Essays Ser.: No. 68). pap. 2.50 (*0-87060-040-0*, NES 68) Syracuse U Cont Ed.

Sensitization in the Nervous System. Ed. by Charles Barnes & Peter W. Kaliuas. 1988. (Illus.). 300p. lib. bdg. 77.00 (*0-936923-12-1*) Telford Pr.

Sensorimotor Impairment in the Elderly: Proceedings of the NATO Advanced Research Workshop, Bad Windsheim, Germany, September 11-13, 1992. Ed. by George E. Stelmach & Volker Homberg. 1993. LC 93-5120. (NATO Advanced Science Institutes Ser.: Vol. 75). 480p. (C). text 285.50 (*0-7923-2393-9*) Kluwer Academic.

Sensorimotor Integration for Developmentally Disabled Children: A Handbook. Eileen W. Richter & Patricia C. Montgomery. 2nd ed. 1991. LC 76-62660. 100p. pap. 49.50 (*0-87424-142-1*, W-142A) Western Psych.

Sensorimotor Interactions in Space Perception & Action. Ed. by D. G. Bouwhuis et al. 1987. 352p. reprint ed. 123.00 (*0-444-70185-0*, North Holland) Elsevier.

Sensory Awareness & Music Focus. Katherine Clipp & Betty Cox. 1994. 60p. (C). pap. text 12.00 (*0-935273-08-5*) Chess Pub.

Sensory Evaluation Techniques. Morten C. Meilgaard et al. 2nd rev. ed. 1991. 376p. (C). 136.95 (*0-8493-4280-5*, TA418) CRC Pr.

Sensory Experience, Adaptation & Perception: Festschrift for Ivo Kohler. Ed. by Lothar Spillmann & Bill Wooten. 1984. 775p. (C). text 160.00 (*0-89859-218-6*) L Erlbaum Assocs.

Sensory Guidance of Movement, Vol. 218. Gregory Bock & Jamie Goode. 1998. LC 98-38056. (Novartis Foundation Symposium Ser.). 354p. 125.00 (*0-471-98262-8*) Wiley.

Sensory Hair Cells: Synaptic Transmission. G. N. Akoev & Y. N. Andrianov. 1993. LC 93-7183.Tr. of Sinapticheskaia Peredacha v Retsoptarakh Akustiko-Lateralnoi Sistemy. (Illus.). 194p. 212.00 (*0-387-56186-2*) Spr-Verlag.

Sensory Integration: Theory & Practice. Anne G. Fisher et al. 1991. LC 92-2139. (Illus.). 418p. text 41.95 (*0-8036-3565-6*) Davis Co.

Sensory Integration Vol. 40-2: Behavioral Aspects of Vision Care. 1999. (Illus.). 64p. pap. 20.00 (*0-943599-30-X*) OEPF.

Sensory Integration & Learning Disorders. A. Jean Ayres. 1973. LC 72-91446. 294p. (C). 69.50 (*0-87424-303-3*, W-303) Western Psych.

Sensory Integration & the Child. A. Jean Ayres. 1979. LC 79-66987. 191p. pap. text 23.50 (*0-87424-158-8*, W-158) Western Psych.

Sensory Integrative Approaches in Occupational Therapy. Zoe Mailloux. 1987. LC 87-2878. (Occupational Therapy in Health Care Ser.: Vol. 4, No. 2). 179p. 49.95 (*0-86656-665-1*) Haworth Pr.

Sensory Mechanisms of the Spinal Cord. W. D. Willis, Jr. 2nd ed. 1991. (Illus.). 590p. (C). text 115.00 (*0-306-43781-3*, Kluwer Plenum) Kluwer Academic.

Sensory Motor Handbook: A Guide for Implementing & Modifying Activities in the Classroom. Julie Bissell et al. 1988. LC 88-60760. (Illus.). 150p. pap. 18.00 (*1-882068-02-5*) Sensory Integration.

Sensory-Motor Integration: Implication for Neurological Disease. Ed. by A. Struppler et al. 1987. (Journal: Vol. 49, No. 5, 1987). (Illus.). 48p. pap. 38.50 (*3-8055-4633-5*) S Karger.

Sensory Motor Issues in Autism. Johanna Anderson. 1999. (Illus.). 64p. (C). pap. text 35.00 (*0-12-785073-2*) Acad Pr.

Sensory Nerves & Neuropeptides in Gastroenterology: From Basic Science to Clinical Perspectives. Ed. by M. Costa et al. 1991. (Advances in Experimental Medicine & Biology Ser.). (Illus.). 318p. (C). text 126.00 (*0-306-43911-5*, Kluwer Plenum) Kluwer Academic.

Sensory Neurons: Diversity, Development & Plasticity. Sheryl A. Scott. 1992. (Illus.). 464p. text 80.00 (*0-19-506676-6*) OUP.

Sensory Research: Multimodal Perspectives. Ed. by Ronald T. Verrillo. 1993. 328p. 69.95 (*0-8058-1342-X*) L Erlbaum Assocs.

Sensory Systems of Arthropods. Ed. by K. Wiese et al. 1993. LC 93-22173. (Advances in Life Sciences Ser.). (Illus.). 696p. 162.00 (*0-8176-2795-2*) Birkhauser.

Sensory Testing Methods. Ed. by Edgar Chambers, 4th & Mona Baker Wolf. 2nd ed. 1996. LC 96-32386. (Manual Ser.: Vol. 26). (Illus.). 120p. pap. 33.00 (*0-8031-2068-0*, MNL26) ASTM.

Sensory to Motor Transformation: Pre-Motor Mechanisms. Ed. by B. Blum et al. 1989. (Journal: Vol. 33, Nos. 2-3, 1989). (Illus.). 136p. pap. 81.75 (*3-8055-5061-8*) S Karger.

Sensual Healing: An Elemental Guide to Feeling Good. Teresa Kennedy. 1996. LC 96-8368. 224p. pap. 12.95 (*0-87131-806-7*) M Evans.

Sensual Sex: Arousing Your Senses & Deepening the Passion in Your Relationship. Beverly Engel. 1999. LC 98-52742. (Illus.). 246p. pap. 14.95 (*0-89793-245-5*) Hunter Hse.

Sensuous Heart: Guidelines for Sex after a Heart Attack or Heart Surgery. Suzanne Cambre. Ed. by Faye Hoffman & Nancy Hull. 1990. LC 90-8192. (Illus.). 20p. (Orig.). pap. text 5.75 (*0-939838-28-1*) Pritchett & Hull.

Sentinel for Health: A History of the Centers for Disease Ccontrol. Elizabeth W. Etheridge. 1991. LC 90-24679. (Illus.). 384p. text 55.00 (*0-520-07107-7*) U CA Pr.

Sentinel HIV Seroprevalence Surveys. 1995. (Illus.). 103p. (Orig.). (C). pap. text 25.00 (*0-7881-1914-1*) DIANE Pub.

Sentinel Node in Surgical Oncology. M. R. S. Keshtgar et al. 1999. LC 98-52045. (Illus.). 201p. 119.00 (*3-540-65176-4*) Spr-Verlag.

Sepa Todo Sobre Addicciones. Editorial America, S. A. Staff. Ed. by Maria E. Del Real. 1990. (SPA., Illus.). 360p. (Orig.). pap. (*0-944499-90-2*) Editorial Amer.

Separate Social Worlds of Siblings: The Impact of Nonshared Environment on Development. Ed. by E. Mavis Hetherington et al. 1993. (Advances in Family Research Ser.). 232p. text 49.95 (*0-8058-1311-X*) L Erlbaum Assocs.

Separating Together: How Divorce Transforms Families. Abigail J. Stewart et al. 1997. LC 97-8707. 293p. text 38.00 (*1-57230-235-6*, 0235) Guilford Pubns.

Separation: Anxiety & Anger. John Bowlby. 2000. LC 70-78464. (Basic Books Classics: Vol. 2). 476p. pap. 25.00 (*0-465-09716-2*) Basic.

Separation - Individuation: Theory & Application. Joyce Edward et al. 2nd ed. 1992. LC 92-31503. 385p. text 47.95 (*0-87630-697-0*) Brunner-Routledge.

Separation Anxiety & the Dread of Abandonment in Adult Males. Gwendolyn Stevens & Sheldon Gardner. 1994. LC 93-37884. 208p. 64.00 (*0-275-94609-6*, Praeger Pubs) Greenwood.

Separation Anxiety Disorder: Psychodynamics & Psychotherapy. Richard A. Gardner. 1985. LC 84-26348. ix, 180p. 22.50 (*0-933812-10-8*) Creative Therapeutics.

Separation-Individuation: Essays in Honor of Margaret S. Mahler. Ed. by John B. McDevitt & Calvin F. Settlage. 1971. LC 78-143378. 520p. 77.50 (*0-8236-6065-6*) Intl Univs Pr.

Separations Technology: Pharmaceutical & Biotechnology Applications. Ed. by Wayne P. Olson. 1995. 505p. 179.00 (*0-935184-72-4*) IHS Health Grp.

Sepsis. Ed. by K. Reinhardt & K. Eyrich. 1989. (Illus.). 391p. 123.00 (*0-387-17763-9*) Spr-Verlag.

Sepsis & Multiorgan Failure. Alan M. Fein et al. 1997. LC 96-40538. (Illus.). 675p. text 120.00 (*0-683-03097-3*) Lppncott W & W.

***Sepsis & Multiple Organ Dysfunction.** Deitch. 2001. (Illus.). 605p. (*0-7020-2165-2*) W B Saunders GBR. *Dist:* Saunders.

Sepsis & Organ Dysfunction: A Tribute to Roger Bone. Ed. by A. E. Baue et al. 1999. 200p. pap. (*88-470-0052-1*) Spr-Verlag ITA. *Dist:* Spr-Verlag.

Sepsis & Organ Dysfunction: Epidemiology & Scoring Systems, Pathophysiology & Therapy. Ed. by A. E. Baue et al. 1998. LC 98-15825. (Illus.). 200p. 89.00 (*88-470-0297-4*) Spr-Verlag.

Sepsis unter besonderer Beruecksichtigung der Ernaehrungsprobleme. Ed. by J. Eckhart. 1983. (Beitraege zur Infusionstherapie und Klinische Ernaehrung Ser.: Vol. 10). (Illus.). viii, 208p. pap. 43.50 (*3-8055-3677-1*) S Karger.

Septic Shock. Ed. by Jean Francois Dhainaut et al. 2000. (Illus.). 300p. text 120.00 (*0-7020-1773-6*) Saunders.

Septic Shock. Ed. by Richard K. Root & Merle A. Sande. 1985. (Contemporary Issues in Infectious Diseases Ser.: Vol. 4). (Illus.). 281p. text (*0-443-08397-5*) Church.

Septic Shock. Ed. by J. L. Vincent & L. G. Thijs. 1987. (Intensive Care & Emergency Medicine Ser.: Vol. 4). (Illus.). 291p. 85.95 (*0-387-17861-9*) Spr-Verlag.

Septic Shock: Methods & Protocols. Ed. by Thomas J. Evans. 2000. LC 99-29663. (Methods in Molecular Medicine Ser.: Vol. 36). (Illus.). 224p. 99.50 (*0-89603-730-4*) Humana.

Sequelae of Low Birthweight. Ed. by Henry G. Dunn. 1991. LC 65-80534. (Clinics in Developmental Medicine Ser.: No. 95-96). (Illus.). 306p. (C). text (*0-521-41215-3*) Mc Keith Pr GBR. *Dist:* Cambridge U Pr.

Sequences of Proteins of Immunological Interest, Set. Elvin A. Kabat. 5th ed. 1992. (Illus.). 2719p. (C). pap. text 175.00 (*0-941375-65-X*) DIANE Pub.

Sequential Analysis. John Gottman & Anup K. Roy. 1990. (Illus.). 287p. (C). text 80.00 (*0-521-34665-7*) Cambridge U Pr.

Sequential Traumatization in Children. Hans Keilson. 1993. 464p. (Orig.). pap. 30.00 (*965-223-806-6*) Gefen Bks.

Serca2-Type Ca (2+)-Transport ATPases in the Pig (Sus Scrofa) Isoform Diversity & Regulation by Phospholamban. Hilde Verboomen. 1995. (Acta Biomedica Lovaniensia Ser.: Vol. 106). (Illus.). 89p. (Orig.). pap. (*90-6186-666-9*) Leuven Univ BEL. *Dist:* Coronet Bks.

Serial Casts. Cusick. 1998. (C). pap. 29.95 (*0-12-784575-5*) Acad Pr.

Serial Changes in Subcutaneous Fat Thicknesses of Children & Adults. Alex F. Roche et al. 1982. (Monographs in Pediatrics: Vol. 17). (Illus.). x, 110p. pap. 68.75 (*3-8055-3496-5*) S Karger.

Serial Publications Containing Medical Classics. Lee Ash & Gertrude L. Annan. 2nd ed. 1979. 35.00 (*0-9603990-0-3*) Antiquarium.

Serial Reactions Considered As Conditioned Reactions. William M. Lepley. 1974. (Psychology Monographs General & Applied: Vol. 46). reprint ed. 55.00 (*0-8115-1445-5*) Periodicals Srv.

Series in Depression & Anxiety. S. A. Montgomery & Johan A. Den-Boer. 1998. LC 98-3702. (Perspectives in Psychiatry Ser.). 202p. 110.00 (*0-471-97877-9*) Wiley.

Series in Medicinal Chemistry Handbook Chemotherapeutic Agents, No. 2. Matthew Verderame. LC 84-24410. reprint ed. 366.00 (*0-8493-3285-0*, CRC Reprint) Franklin.

Series in Radiation Meaurement & Protection, No. 2. A. Brodsky. 1982. LC 78-10558. reprint ed. 781.00 (*0-8493-3750-X*, CRC Reprint) Franklin.

Series of Slides for the Atlas of Histopathology of the Cervix Uteri. Gisela Dallenbach-Hellweg & Hemming Poulsen. 1992. 40p. 224.00 incl. sl. (*0-387-92119-2*) Spr-Verlag.

Series on Nursing Administration, Vol. I. Alice R. Johnson & Joanne McCloskey. Ed. by Debra Hunter. 1988. 216p. (C). text 39.95 (*0-201-12778-4*) Mosby Inc.

Series on Nursing Administration, Vol. 2. Marion Johnson & Joanne C. McCloskey. 1989. 212p. text 23.96 (*0-201-12928-0*) Addison-Wesley.

Series on Nursing Administration, Vol. 3. Joyce Young Johnson & Joanne McCloskey. Ed. by Debra Hunter. 1990. (C). text (*0-201-12937-X*) Addison-Wesley.

Serine Proteases & Their Serpin Inhibitors in the Nervous System: Regulation in Development & in Degenerative & Malignant Disease. Ed. by B. W. Festoff. 1990. (NATO ASI Ser.: Vol. 191). (Illus.). 384p. 150.00 (*0-306-43584-5*, Plenum Trade) Perseus Pubng.

Serious & Unstable Condition: Financing America's Health Care. Henry J. Aaron. 1991. 158p. 32.95 (*0-8157-0051-2*) Brookings.

Serious Mental Health Problems. Brooker. 1998. pap. text 29.00 (*0-7020-2127-X*) Saunders.

Serious Mental Illness & the Family: The Practitioner's Guide. Diane T. Marsh. 1998. LC 98-9521. (Couples & Family Dynamics & Treatment Ser.). 374p. 55.00 (*0-471-18180-3*) Wiley.

Serious Symptoms, Simple Solutions: What To Do When You've Tried Everything Else. FC and A Publishing Staff. 1997. 390p. pap. 9.99 (*0-915099-99-3*) FC&A Pub.

Serious Symptoms, Simple Solutions: What to Do When You've Tried Everything Else. FC and A Publishing Staff. 1998. 367p. 27.96 (*0-915099-98-5*) FC&A Pub.

Serologic Diagnosis of Celiac Diseases. Chorzelski. 1990. 216p. 121.00 (*0-8493-5436-6*, RC862, CRC Reprint) Franklin.

Serologic Problem-Solving Strategies: A Systematic Approach. Ed. by Susan T. Johnson et al. 1996. (Illus.). 158p. pap. text 60.00 (*1-56395-066-9*, PC97-960019) Am Assn Blood.

Serological Cancer Markers. Ed. by Stewart Sell. 1992. LC 92-1428. (Contemporary Biomedicine Ser.: Vol. 11). (Illus.). 552p. 145.00 (*0-89603-209-4*) Humana.

Serological Tumour Markers: An Introduction. J. E. Roulston & R. C. Leonard. 1993. LC 92-49368. (Illus.). 192p. text (*0-443-04511-9*) Church.

Serology of Tuberculosis & BCG Vaccination. Ed. by W. Fox. 1983. (Advances in Tuberculosis Research Ser.: Vol. 21). (Illus.). viii, 192p. 143.50 (*3-8055-3855-3*) S Karger.

Serotonin. Syd Baumel. 1998. LC 98-200779. (Good Health Guides). 48p. pap. 3.95 (*0-87983-823-X*, 3823XK, Keats Pubng) McGraw-Hill Trade.

Serotonin: From Cell Biology to Pharmacology & Therapeutics. Ed. by Paul M. Vanhoutte. 1993. LC 93-20892. (Medical Science Symposia Ser.). 445p. (C). text 200.50 (*0-7923-2518-4*) Kluwer Academic.

Serotonin & Gastrointestinal Function. Ed. by Timothy S. Gaginella & James J. Galligan. 1995. LC 95-14338. (Pharmacology & Toxicology Ser.). 192p. 159.95 (*0-8493-8387-0*, 8387) CRC Pr.

Serotonin & Microcirculation. Ed. by R. S. Reneman & A. Bollinger. 1986. (Mikrozirkulation in Forschung und Klinik Ser.: Vol. 10). (Illus.). x, 92p. pap. 57.50 (*3-8055-4163-5*) S Karger.

Serotonin & Serotonin Antagonists: Journal: Clinical Physiology & Biochemistry, Vol. 8, Suppl. 3. Ed. by J. Rosenthal & Pieter A. Van Zwieten. 1991. (Illus.). iv, 128p. pap. 40.00 (*3-8055-5456-7*) S Karger.

Serotonin in Affective Disorders. Ed. by J. Menlewicz et al. 1984. (Advances in Biological Psychiatry Ser.: Vol. 14). (Illus.). vi, 90p. 47.00 (*3-8055-3898-7*) S Karger.

Serotonin in Antipsychotic Treatment. Ed. by John M. Kane et al. 1996. (Medical Psychiatry Ser.: Vol. 3). (Illus.). 408p. text 150.00 (*0-8247-9302-1*) Dekker.

Serotonin Receptor Subtypes: Pharmacological Significance & Clinical Implications. Giorgio Racagni & Julien Mendlewicz. 1992. (International Academy for Biomedical & Drug Research Ser.: Vol. 1). (Illus.). x, 146p. 117.50 (*3-8055-5550-4*) S Karger.

Serotonin Receptors. Ed. by Elaine Sanders-Bush. 1989. LC 88-26646. (Receptors Ser.). 402p. 145.00 (*0-89603-142-X*) Humana.

Serotonin Receptors & Their Ligands, Vol. 27. Ed. by Berend Olivier et al. 1997. LC 97-24994. (Pharmacochemistry Library). 378p. 248.50 (*0-444-82041-8*) Elsevier.

Serotonin, Sleep & Mental Disorder. Ed. by C. Idzikowski & P. J. Cowen. 1991. 312p. (*1-871816-06-8*) Wrightson Biomed GBR. *Dist:* Taylor & Francis.

Serotonin Solution: The Potent Substance That Can Help You Stop Bingeing, Lose Weight, & Feel Great. Judith J. Wurtman & Susan Suffes. 1999. 288p. text 24.00 (*0-7881-5949-6*) DIANE Pub.

Serotoninergic Neurons & 5-HT Receptors in the CNS. Ed. by H. G. Baumgarten et al. 1997. LC 97-23528. (Handbook of Experimental Pharmacology Ser.: No. 129). (Illus.). 656p. 399.00 (*3-540-62666-2*) Spr-Verlag.

Serum Proteins in Clinical Medicine Vol. II: Clinical Section. Date not set. (Illus.). 420p. ring bd. 125.00 (*0-9653655-2-2*) Fnd Blood Res.

Service Delivery Guidelines for Family Planning Service Programs. Ed. by Noel McIntosh & Elizabeth Oliveras. 1996. LC 96-205961. (Illus.). 110p. pap. text 15.00 (*0-929817-10-9*) JHPIEGO.

Service Delivery in Educational Settings. Goldsmith. Date not set. 40.00 (*0-7506-9573-0*) Buttrwrth-Heinemann.

Service Load of a Staff Nurse in One Official Public Health Agency. Marion Ferguson. LC 71-176768. (Columbia University. Teachers College. Contributions to Education Ser.: No. 915). reprint ed. 37.50 (*0-404-55915-8*) AMS Pr.

Service Needs of the Seriously Mentally Ill: Training Implications for Psychology. Ed. by Dale L. Johnson. 1991. LC 90-1229. 160p. pap. 19.95 (*1-55798-102-7*) Am Psychol.

Service of Curing, the Art of Caring: A History of Expanding Health Care in the Pecos Valley. Charles W. Sanford. 1995. LC 95-76625. 88p. 15.00 (*0-929690-26-5*) Herit Pubs AZ.

Service Quality Improvement: The Customer Satisfaction Strategy for Health Care. Wendy Leebov & Gail Scott. 1993. LC 93-32889. 380p. pap. 58.00 (*1-55648-110-1*, 136107) AHPI.

Service Quality Management in Hospitality, Tourism & Leisure. Ed. by Jay Kandampully et al. 2000. LC 00-27256. (Illus.). 340p. pap. text 39.95 (*0-7890-1141-7*) Haworth Pr.

Service Savvy Health Care: One Goal at a Time. Wendy Leebov et al. 1998. LC 97-50160. 276p. pap. 38.00 (*1-55648-225-6*) AHPI.

Services for Cardiovascular Emergencies: Proceedings of the WHO Expert Committee, Geneva, 1974. WHO Staff. 1975. (Technical Reports: No. 562). pap. text 10.00 (*92-4-120562-8*, 1100562) World Health.

Services for the Prevention & Treatment of Dependence on Alcohol & Other Drugs: 14th Report of the WHO Expert Committee on Mental Health. Date not set. (Technical Report Ser.: No. 363). pap. text 5.00 (*92-4-120363-3*, 1100363) World Health.

Services for the Seriously Mentally Ill in Texas: Facts & Issues. Mary A. Pisani. 1988. 39p. (Orig.). pap. 1.00 (*0-915757-11-7*) League Women Voters TX.

Services to the Aging & Aged: Public Policies & Programs. Ed. by Paul K. Kim. 11th ed. 1994. LC 94-28668. (Issues in Aging Ser.: Vol. 3). 344p. text 62.00 (*0-8153-0611-3*, SS802) Garland.

Services to the Orthopedically Handicapped. Louis Hoyer & Charles K. Hay. Ed. by William R. Phillips & Janet Rosenberg. 1980. LC 79-6906. (Physically Handicapped in Society Ser.). (Illus.). reprint ed. lib. bdg. 18.95 (*0-405-13115-1*) Ayer.

Serving African American Children. Ed. by Sandra Jackson & Sheryl Brissett-Chapman. 1998. LC 98-9773. 278p. pap. text 24.95 (*0-7658-0434-4*) Transaction Pubs.

Serving Children with HIV Infection in Child Day Care: A Guide for Center-Based & Family Day Care Providers. Child Welfare League of America Staff. 1991. 48p. pap. 11.95 (*0-87868-439-5*) Child Welfare.

Serving HIV-Infected Children, Youth & Their Families: A Guide for Residential Group Care Providers. Paul Gitelson & L. Jean Emery. 1989. pap. 9.95 (*0-87868-367-4*) Child Welfare.

***Serving Medicine: The Nevada State Medical Association & the Politics of Medicine.** Richard G. Pugh. 2001. LC 2001-23999. (Golden Age of Medicine in Nevada Ser.: Vol. 2). (*0-9649759-8-X*) Greasewood.

Serving the Seriously Mentally Ill: Public-Academic Linkages in Services, Research, & Training. Ed. by Paul Wohlford et al. 1993. 275p. pap. 19.95 (*1-55798-216-3*) Am Psychol.

Serving the Underserved: Caring for People Who Are Both Old & Mentally Retarded. Ed. by Mary C. Howell et al. 1989. 508p. pap. 29.95 (*0-930958-08-X*) Excptnl Parent.

Sesame. Betty Kamen. 1989. 30p. pap. 1.95 (*0-87983-436-6*, Keats Pubng) McGraw-Hill Trade.

Set for Life: Eat More - Weigh Less - Feel Terrific! Jane P. Merrill & Karen M. Sunderland. 2nd rev. ed. 1995. (Illus.). 326p. pap. 19.95 (*0-9621168-3-1*, 3000427) Sunrise Pubs.

Set No Limits: A Rebuttal to Daniel Callahan's Proposal to Limit Health Care for the Elderly. Ed. by Robert L. Barry & Gerard V. Bradley. 1991. LC 91-10448. 160p. text 26.95 (*0-252-01860-5*) U of Ill Pr.

Setting a Course for Health. Deborah Catesby. 1994. 236p. pap. (*1-85609-077-9*) Witherby & Co GBR. *Dist:* St Mut.

Setting Allocation Priorities & Genetic & Reproductive Technologies. Ed. by Robert H. Blank & Andrea L. Bonnicksen. 1993. (Emerging Issues in Biomedical Policy Ser.: Vol. 1). 315p. pap. 23.00 (*0-231-07411-5*) Col U Pr.

Setting Limits: Medical Goals in An Aging Society, with "A Reponse to My Critics" Daniel Callahan. 1995. LC 94-34439. 272p. pap. 16.95 (*0-87840-572-0*) Georgetown U Pr.

Setting New Priorities in Health Care. Jack A. Meyer et al. 1993. (Illus.). 60p. (Orig.). pap. text (*0-9629870-2-6*) Milbank Memorial.

Setting Priorities for Clinical Practice Guidelines. Institute of Medicine Staff. Ed. by Marilyn J. Field. 1995. LC 95-67087. 176p. pap. text 33.00 (*0-309-05247-5*) Natl Acad Pr.

Setting Priorities in Health Care. Ed. by Mo Malek. 1994. LC 94-215318. 348p. 196.50 (*0-471-94394-0*) Wiley.

Setting Rates for Hospital & Nursing Home Care. Paul L. Grimaldi. 1985. LC 84-17838. 360p. text 27.50 (*0-88331-196-8*) R B Luce.

Setting Standards for Professional Nursing: The Marker Model. Carolyn G. Smith-Marker. 1987. 39.00 (*0-932491-84-7*) Res Appl Inc.

Setting the Limit: Occupational Health Standards & the Limits of Science. Sven O. Hansson. 1998. LC 97-34725. (Illus.). 176p. (C). text 35.00 (*0-19-512160-0*) OUP.

Setting the Seen: Creative Visualization for Healing. Alan Cohen. 1982. (Illus.). 27p. (Orig.). (C). pap. 2.95 (*0-910367-33-7*) A Cohen.

Setting up Your Own Prepaid Plan: A Do-It-Yourself Guide. Dale E. Wagman. 1989. 283p. 10.00 (*0-87814-340-8*, D4272) PennWell Corp.

Setting Your Weight. 1988. (Fitness, Health & Nutrition Ser.). (Illus.). 144p. 17.27 (*0-8094-6191-9*); lib. bdg. 23.27 (*0-8094-6192-7*) Time-Life.

Settings for Health Promotion: Linking Theory & Practice. Blake D. Poland et al. 1999. LC 99-50471. viii, 373p. pap. 29.95 (*0-8039-7419-1*, 1416) Sage.

Seven Countries: A Multivariate Analysis of Death & Coronary Heart Disease. Ancel Keys. 1980. LC 79-9163. (Commonwealth Fund Publications). (Illus.). 392p. 54.00 (*0-674-80237-3*) HUP.

Seven Countries Study: A Scientific Adventure in Cardiovascular Disease Epidemiology. D. Kromhout et al. 1994. 218p. (*90-6960-048-X*) H Blackburn.

Seven Levels of Healing. Lilla Bek & Philippa Pullar. 1987. 160p. pap. (*0-7126-9473-0*) CEN3 GBR. *Dist:* Trafalgar.

Seven-Minute Rotator Cuff Solution. Jerry Robinson & Joseph Horrigan. 1990. (Illus.). 64p. (Orig.). pap. 16.95 (*0-944831-25-7*) Health Life.

7 Pillars of Health. Joseph Christiano. 2000. 288p. 19.99 (*0-88419-693-3*) Creation House.

Seven Sacred Rites of Menopause: The Spiritual Journey to the Wise-Woman Years. Kristi Meisenbach Boylan. 2000. LC 00-44542. 160p. pap. 11.95 (*1-891661-13-2*) Snta Monica.

Seven Secrets of Anti-Aging. John P. Lenhart. Ed. by Diane Marcou. 2000. pap. 24.95 (*1-930822-00-6*) Medfo.

Seven Service Strategies That Work: The Health Care Manager's Guide to Great Customer Service. Wendy Leebov et al. 1998. LC 97-51922. 291p. pap. (*1-55648-230-2*) American Host.

***Seven Steps to a Pain Free Life.** Robin A. McKenzie. 2001. (Illus.). 224p. pap. 15.00 (*0-452-28277-2*, Plume) Dutton Plume.

7 Steps to a Pain-Free Life: How to Rapidly Relieve Back & Neck Pain Using the McKenzie Method. Robin A. McKenzie & Craig Kubey. 2000. LC 00-33567. (Illus.). 256p. 23.95 (*0-525-94560-1*) Dutton Plume.

Seven Steps to HIM Compliance. Ruthann Russo. 1998. LC 98-230630. (Illus.). 146p. pap. text 97.00 (*1-57839-043-5*) Opus Communs.

7 Steps to Normal Bladder Control: Simple, Practical Tips & Techniques for Staying Dry. Elizabeth Vierck. 1998. LC 98-6574. (Health Ser.). (Illus.). 192p. pap. 16.95 (*0-936197-29-3*) Harbor Pr.

Seven Steps to Peak Performance: The Mental Training Manual for Athletes. Richard M. Suinn. 1987. LC 86-10427. 64p. spiral bd. 12.90 (*0-920887-12-0*) Hogrefe & Huber Pubs.

Seven Strategies for the Future of Nursing: Changing Roles, Responsibilities & Employment Patterns of Registered Nurses. Ed. by Edward H. O'Neil et al. 1998. LC 97-45454. 233p. 42.00 (*0-7879-4028-3*) Jossey-Bass.

Seven Styles of Parenting. Patricia Hershey Owen. 1994. LC 93-80895. 96p. pap. 10.00 (*1-882657-08-X*) Health Digest.

Seven-Week Victory Diet: Win the Food Fight. Sam Grossman. 1990. mass mkt. 4.95 (*0-312-92258-2*) St Martin.

Seven Weeks to a Settled Stomach. Ronald L. Hoffman. Ed. by Julie Rubenstein. 1991. 352p. reprint ed. mass mkt. 6.99 (*0-671-73425-3*) PB.

Seven Weeks to Sobriety. Loan M. Larson et al. rev. ed. 1997. LC 97-214438. pap. 12.95 (*0-449-00259-4*) Fawcett.

***17 Lies That Are Holding You Back & the Truth That Will Set You Free.** Steve Chandler. 2001. 240p. pap. 15.95 (*1-58063-215-7*) Renaissance.

XVIIes Journees Nationales de Neonatologie, 1987. Ed. by J. P. Relier. 1987. (Paris, Mai Ser.: Vol. 7). vi, 382p. pap. 139.25 (*3-8055-4652-1*) S Karger.

***Seventh Conference on Health Survey Research Methods.** Conference on Health Survey Research Methods Staff et al. 2001. LC 00-69532. (DHHS Publication Ser.: Nos. 01-1013). pap. (*0-8406-0567-6*) Natl Ctr Health Stats.

Seventh General Programme of Work Covering the Period, 1984-1989. 1982. text (*92-4-180008-9*) World Health.

Seventh hGH Symposium. Ed. by J. Girard & J. S. Christiansen. 1996. (Journal: Vol. 46, No. 4-5). (Illus.). 104p. pap. 88.75 (*3-8055-6432-5*) S Karger.

7th World Congress on Animal, Plant & Microbial Toxins: Proceedings of the International Symposium, 7th, Brisbane, Australia, July 11-16, 1982. International Symposium on Animal, Plant and Microbi & R. Endean. 1983. (Illus.). 544p. pap. 145.00 (*0-08-029803-6*, Pergamon Pr) Elsevier.

Seventy Birth Control Clinics: A Survey & Analysis Including the General Effects of Control on Size & Quality of Population. Caroline H. Robinson. 1972. LC 71-169398. (Family in America Ser.). 380p. reprint ed. 19.95 (*0-405-03875-5*) Ayer.

70 Essential TCM Formulas for Beginners. Bob Flaws. 1994. 265p. (Orig.). pap. 21.95 (*0-936185-59-7*) Blue Poppy Pr.

Seventy Steps Toward Wisdom. Sigmund Lowe. 2nd ed. 1981. 95p. pap. 3.50 (*0-87516-050-6*) DeVorss.

73 Practical Strategies for Medicare Compliance. Ed. by AIS Editorial Staff. 2nd rev. ed. 1998. 85p. spiral bd. 54.00 (*0-929156-74-9*) Atlantic Info Services Inc.

Severe Asthma, No. 86. Ed. by Donald Y. M. Leung & S. J. Szefler. 1995. LC 95-31819. (Lung Biology in Health & Disease Ser.: Vol. 86). (Illus.). 640p. text 225.00 (*0-8247-9511-3*) Dekker.

Severe Behavior Problems: A Functional Communication Training Approach. V. Mark Durand. 1990. LC 90-44746. (Treatment Manuals for Practitioners Ser.). 183p. pap. 22.00 (*0-89862-217-4*, 2217) Guilford Pubns.

Severe Burns: A Family Guide to Medical & Emotional Recovery. Glorya Hale. 1993. LC 93-870. (Illus.). 272p. (C). 24.95 (*0-8018-4653-6*) Johns Hopkins.

Severe Communication Disorders: Intervention Strategies. Ed. by Katharine G. Butler. 1993. LC 93-36267. 240p. pap. 44.00 (*0-8342-0589-0*) PRO-ED.

Severe Depression: A Practitioner's Guide. Philip J. Barker. 1992. LC 92-33173. 296p. 42.50 (*1-56593-051-7*, 0299) Thomson Learn.

Severe Depressive Disorders. Ed. by Leon Grunhaus & John F. Greden. 1994. LC 93-47693. (Progress in Psychiatry Ser.: No. 44). 368p. text 17.95 (*0-88048-472-1*, 8472) Am Psychiatric.

Severe Head Injuries: Pathology, Diagnosis & Treatment. B. L. Bauer & T. J. Kuhn. 1997. LC 97-16897. (Illus.). 154p. 87.00 (*3-540-62701-4*) Spr-Verlag.

Severe Learning Disabilities & Challenging Behaviors. Carol Martin et al. Ed. by Eric Emerson. 2nd ed. 1993. LC 86-5291. 192p. pap. 49.95 (*1-56593-130-0*, 0442) Singular Publishing.

Severe Personality Disorders: Psychotherapeutic Strategies. Otto F. Kernberg. 1993. 384p. (C). reprint ed. pap. 24.00 (*0-300-05349-5*) Yale U Pr.

Severe Spondylolisthesis: Pathogenetic - Diagnostic - Therapeutic Considerations. Ed. by J. Harms & H. Sturtz. 2000. 150p. (*3-7985-1253-1*) D Steinkopff DEU. *Dist:* Spr-Verlag.

Severe Stress & Mental Disturbance in Children. Ed. by Cynthia R. Pfeffer. 1996. LC 95-23086. 697p. text 72.95 (*0-88048-657-0*, 8657) Am Psychiatric.

Severed Trust: Why American Medicine Hasn't Been Fixed. George D. Lundberg & James H. Stacey. 2001. LC 00-49814. 336p. text 26.00 (*0-465-04291-0*) Basic.

***Severed Trust: Why American Medicine Hasn't Been Fixed.** George D. Lundberg & James Stacey. rev. ed. 2002. 368p. pap. text 16.00 (*0-465-04292-9*) Perseus Bks Grp.

Severely & Profoundly Handicapped: A Practical Approach to Teaching. Ed. by Edward T. Donlon & Louise F. Burton. 1976. LC 76-17293. 272p. text 52.50 (*0-8089-0952-5*, 791058, Grune & Strat) Harcrt Hlth Sci Grp.

Severely Disturbed Youngsters & the Parental Alliance. Ed. by Jacquelyn S. Sanders & Barry L. Childress. 1993. LC 92-1554. (Residential Treatment for Children & Youth Ser.). 100p. (C). 39.95 (*1-56024-319-8*) Haworth Pr.

Severely Emotionally Disturbed Youth in Texas: Financing & Coordinating Services. Pat Wong & David C. Warner. 1991. (Policy Research Project Report Ser.: Vol. 91). 430p. 13.00 (*0-89940-699-8*) LBJ Sch Pub Aff.

Severin's Veterinary Ophthalmology Notes. Glenn A. Severin. 3rd ed. 1995. (Illus.). 546p. pap. text 50.00 (*0-9646143-0-8*) Vet Ophthal Notes.

Sevilla HGH Symposium: Clinical Aspects of Growth Hormone Replacement Therapy, Proceedings, Seville, Spain, April 1990. Ed. by J. Girard & J. S. Christiansen. 1990. (Illus.). iv, 108p. pap. 48.75 (*3-8055-5290-4*) S Karger.

Sevillana Medicina, Burgos, 1545. Juan De Avinon. Ed. by Eric W. Naylor. 1987. (Medieval Spanish Medical Texts Ser.: No. 8). (SPA.). 6p. 10.00 incl. fiche (*0-940639-03-3*) Hispanic Seminary.

Seward's Bedside Diagnosis. David M. Mattingly & Charles Seward. 13th ed. 1989. (Illus.). 373p. pap. text (*0-443-04077-X*) Church.

Sewering the Cities: An Original Anthology. Ed. by Barbara G. Rosenkrantz. 1977. LC 76-40352. (Public Health in America Ser.). (Illus.). reprint ed. lib. bdg. 23.95 (*0-405-09879-0*) Ayer.

Sex: An Encyclopedia for the Bewildered. K. S. Daly. 1996. LC 97-118632. (Illus.). 256p. (*1-85410-359-8*) Aurum Press Ltd GBR. *Dist:* London Brdge.

Sex: The Relationship Between Sex & Spiritual Development. J. G. Bennett. 1981. 74p. reprint ed. pap. 7.95 (*0-87728-533-0*) Red Wheel ME.

Sex: What You Don't Know Can Kill You. Joe S. McIlhaney, Jr. & Marion McIlhaney. adapted rev. ed. 1997. LC 96-43362. 128p. (gr. 12). pap. 11.99 (*0-8010-5737-X*, Sexuality and S) Baker Bks.

Sex Vol. 3: True Homosexual Experiences from S. T. H. Writers. Ed. by Boyd McDonald. 1996. LC 82-15393. (Illus.). 192p. (Orig.). reprint ed. pap. 14.95 (*0-917342-98-4*) Gay Sunshine.

Sex, Abortion, & Unmarried Women, 133. Paul Sachdev. 1993. LC 92-33303. (Contributions in Women's Studies: No. 133). 336p. 68.50 (*0-313-24071-X*, SAU, Greenwood Pr) Greenwood.

Sex Abuse Hysteria Salem Witches Trials Revisited: Causes of the Present Child Sex Abuse Hysteria in the United States. Richard A. Gardner. 1991. LC 90-20218. (Illus.). 150p. 18.00 (*0-933812-22-1*) Creative Therapeutics.

Sex & Back Pain: Advice on Restoring Comfortable Sex Lost to Back Pain. Lauren Andrew Hebert. 1992. LC 92-70997. (Illus.). 108p. (Orig.). pap. 12.95 (*1-879864-00-2*) IMPACC USA.

Sex & Bisexuality: Index of Modern Information. Rosalie F. Zoltano. 1990. LC 88-47995. 150p. 47.50 (*1-55914-200-6*); pap. 44.50 (*1-55914-201-4*) ABBE Pubs Assn.

Sex & Character. Otto Weininger. LC 72-11295.Tr. of Geschlecht & Charakter. reprint ed. 40.00 (*0-404-57507-2*) AMS Pr.

Sex & Cognition. Doreen Kimura. 1999. LC 98-26802. (Bradford Book Ser.). (Illus.). 217p. 42.00 (*0-262-11236-1*, Bradford Bks) MIT Pr.

Sex & Dehumanization. David Holbrook. 1998. LC 97-27082. (Social Policy & Social Theory Ser.). 238p. pap. text 24.95 (*0-7658-0402-6*) Transaction Pubs.

Sex & Family Planning - How We Teach the Young: Report on a Study. B. Lewin. 1984. (Public Health in Europe Ser.: No. 23). 170p. pap. text 19.00 (*92-890-1159-9*) World Health.

Sex & Gender. John Archer & Barbara Lloyd. 1985. (Illus.). 286p. pap. text 19.95 (*0-521-31921-8*) Cambridge U Pr.

Sex & Gender. Doyle. 3rd ed. 1994. tchr. ed. 9.68 (*0-697-12736-2*) McGraw.

Sex & Human Life. Eric T. Pengelley. 2nd ed. 1978. LC 77-77720. (Life Sciences Ser.). (Illus.). pap. text (*0-201-05770-0*) Addison-Wesley.

Sex & Insanity. Melvin Anchell. 1983. LC 83-81798. 169p. pap. 12.95 (*0-89420-238-3*, 110020, Halcyon) Natl Book.

Sex & Love: Addiction, Treatment & Recovery. Eric Griffin-Shelley. LC 90-21283. 1997. pap. 24.95 (*0-275-96065-X*); 1991. 224p. 65.00 (*0-275-93794-1*, C3794) Greenwood (Praeger Pubs).

Sex & Masochism: Index of New Information. Jerry S. Hartford. 1997. 150p. 57.50 (*0-7883-0962-5*); pap. 47.50 (*0-7883-0963-3*) ABBE Pubs Assn.

Sex & Medicine: Gender, Power & Authority in the Medical Profession. Rosemary Pringle. 1998. LC 97-46532. 250p. (C). text 69.95 (*0-521-57093-X*); pap. text 24.95 (*0-521-57812-4*) Cambridge U Pr.

Sex & Pedophilia: Index of New Information Including Analysis & Results. Arlene S. Shank. 1996. LC 96-12663. 57.50 (*0-7883-0772-X*); pap. 47.50 (*0-7883-0773-8*) ABBE Pubs Assn.

Sex & Peyronie's Disease (Penile Induration-Strabismus) Index of New Information. Hector H. Blickstein. 1994. 150p. 57.50 (*0-7883-0048-2*); pap. 47.50 (*0-7883-0049-0*) ABBE Pubs Assn.

Sex & Peyronie's Disease (Penile Induration, Strabismus) Index of New Information. Hector H. Blickstein. rev. ed. 1998. 127p. 57.50 (*0-7883-1854-3*); pap. 47.50 (*0-7883-1855-1*) ABBE Pubs Assn.

Sex & Psychology of Sexual Offenses: Index of New Information with Authors, Subjects & Bibliography. Joanna J. Levitt. 1993. 180p. 47.50 (*1-55914-768-7*); 1993. 180p. pap. 44.50 (*1-55914-769-5*); 1998. 151p. 57.50 (*0-7883-1850-0*) ABBE Pubs Assn.

Sex & Psychosexual Development: Index of New Information with Authors, Subjects & Bibliography. Allison C. Ledger. 1993. 180p. 47.50 (*1-55914-824-1*); pap. 44.50 (*1-55914-825-X*) ABBE Pubs Assn.

Sex & Repression in Savage Society. Bronislaw Malinowski. 1996. LC 85-971. xii, 300p. pap. text 16.00 (*0-226-50287-2*) U Ch Pr.

Sex & Sanity: The Myths & Realities of Human Sexuality. Tom-Blaise Shepherd. 2nd rev. ed. 1996. 60p. (Orig.). pap. 7.98 (*1-888716-09-6*) Xandex Pr.

Sex & Self-Respect: The Quest for Personal Fulfillment. Philip M. Helfaer. 1998. LC 98-4945. 256p. 72.50 (*0-275-96185-0*, Praeger Pubs) Greenwood.

Sex & Status: Hierarchies in the Health Workforce. Ruth J. Simmons. Ed. by Irene Butter et al. 1985. LC 85-72881. 80p. 12.00 (*0-87553-134-2*) Am Pub Health.

Sex & Suffering: Women's Health & a Women's Hospital: The Royal Women's Hospital, Melbourne, 1856-1996. Janet McCalman. 1999. 432p. (*0-522-84837-0*) Melbourne Univ Pr AUS. *Dist:* Paul & Co Pubs.

Sex & the Biology of Coitus: Index of Modern Authors & Subjects with Guide for Rapid Research. Helen M. Markle. 1991. LC 88-47980. 153p. 47.50 (*1-55914-220-0*); pap. 44.50 (*1-55914-221-9*) ABBE Pubs Assn.

Sex & the Population Crisis. John A. Loraine. 1986. LC 85-24774. 213p. reprint ed. lib. bdg. 62.50 (*0-313-22505-2*, LOSP, Greenwood Pr) Greenwood.

Sex & Transsexualism: Index of Modern Information. Rosalie F. Zoltano. 1989. LC 88-47994. 150p. 47.50 (*1-55914-048-8*); pap. 44.50 (*1-55914-049-6*) ABBE Pubs Assn.

Sex at Risk: Lifetime Number of Partners, Frequency of Intercourse & the Low AIDS Risk of Vaginal Intercourse. Stuart Brody. 1997. LC 97-12110. 120p. 32.95 (*1-56000-309-X*) Transaction Pubs.

Sex Behavior, HIV & AIDS: Index of New Information with Authors & Subjects. Martine M. Yannock. 1992. 180p. 47.50 (*1-55914-648-6*); pap. 44.50 (*1-55914-649-4*) ABBE Pubs Assn.

Sex Book for Those Who Think They Know It All. Charles L. Pelton. Ed. by Sheryl Klinkel. 1980. (Illus.). 227p. pap. 14.95 (*0-931470-04-8*); lib. bdg. 24.95 (*0-931470-03-X*) Fam Health Media.

Sex by Prescription: The Startling Truth about Today's Sex Therapy. Thomas Szasz. 1990. 224p. reprint ed. pap. 18.95 (*0-8156-0250-2*) Syracuse U Pr.

Sex, Cells & Same-Sex Desire: The Biology of Sexual Preference. John P. Dececco. 1995. LC 95-6140. pap. text 34.95 (*1-56023-060-6*, Harrington Park) Haworth Pr.

Sex, Cells, & Same-Sex Desire: The Biology of Sexual Preference. Ed. by David A. Parker & John P. De Cecco. 1995. LC 95-6140. 49.95 (*1-56024-700-2*) Haworth Pr.

Sex Chromosomes & Sex Determination in Vertebrates. Alberto J. Solari. 1993. LC 93-7964. 336p. 220.95 (*0-8493-4571-5*, QH600) CRC Pr.

Sex Determination. G. Bacci & G. A. Kerkut. 1965. LC 65-17948. (International Series of Monographs on Pure & Applied Mathematics: Vol. 26). (*0-08-011291-9*) Pergamon Repr GBR. *Dist:* Franklin.

Sex Determination & Sexual Dimorphism in Mammals. Alfred Glucksmann & M. I. Smith. 1979. LC 78-63273. (Wykeham Science Ser.: No. 54). 174p. (C). pap. 18.00 (*0-8448-1370-2*, Crane Russak) Taylor & Francis.

Sex Determination in Mouse & Man. Ed. by M. A. Ferguson-Smith. 1989. (Illus.). 158p. reprint ed. text 99.00 (*0-85403-369-6*) Scholium Intl.

Sex, Diet & Debility in Jacksonian America: Sylvester Graham & Health Reform, 4. Stephen Nissenbaum. 1980. LC 79-8280. (Contributions in Medical History Ser.: No. 4). 198p. 49.95 (*0-313-21415-8*, NSY/, Greenwood Pr) Greenwood.

Sex Differences in Depression. Susan Nolen-Hoeksema. 1990. LC 89-27303. 270p. 56.00 (*0-8047-1640-4*) Stanford U Pr.

Sex, Disease & Society: A Comparative History of Sexually Transmitted Diseases & HIV AIDS in Asia & the Pacific, 43. Milton J. Lewis et al. 1997. LC 96-28065. (Contributions in Medical Studies Ser.). 312p. 72.50 (*0-313-29442-9*, Greenwood Pr) Greenwood.

Sex, Drugs & HIV/AIDS in Brazil. James A. Inciardi et al. 2000. LC 00-43784. (Illus.). 304p. pap. text 30.00 (*0-8133-3424-1*) Westview.

Sex, Drugs & the Continuing Spread of AIDS. Clyde B. McCoy & James A. Inciardi. 1995. LC 94-13908. (Illus.). 181p. (C). pap. text 34.95 (*0-935732-64-0*) Roxbury Pub Co.

Sex Education. Ed. by Tamara L. Roleff. 1998. LC 98-35008. (At Issue Ser.). (Illus.). 96p. (YA). (gr. 9-12). pap. 12.45 (*0-7377-0008-4*); lib. bdg. 21.20 (*0-7377-0009-2*) Gale (Greenhaven Pr).

Sex Education: Syllabus. Lester A. Kirkendall & Ruth F. Osborne. 1971. (gr. 7-12). pap. text 7.80 (*0-89420-087-9*, 216786) Natl Book.

Sex Education: Teacher's Guide & Resource Manual. Steven Bignell. Ed. by Jane Hiatt & Mary Nelson. rev. ed. 1982. 277p. 29.95 (*0-941816-08-7*) ETR Assocs.

Sex Education for the Health Professional: A Curriculum Guide. Ed. by Norman Rosenzweig & F. Paul Pearsall. 1978. (Seminars in Psychiatry Ser.). 352p. text 49.00 (*0-8089-1100-7*, 793645, Grune & Strat) Harcrt Hlth Sci Grp.

Sex Education in the Classroom. J. C. Willke. 1977. 4.95 (*0-910728-11-9*) Hayes.

Sex Education in the Eighties: The Challenge of Healthy Sexual Evolution. Ed. by Lorna Brown. 1981. LC 81-15738. (Perspectives in Sexuality Ser.). 278p. (C). 49.50 (*0-306-40762-0*, Plenum Trade) Perseus Pubng.

Sex, Gay Men, & AIDS. Ed. by Peter M. Davies et al. 1993. LC 93-16012. (Social Aspects of AIDS Ser.). x, 199p. 85.00 (*0-7507-0095-5*); pap. 27.95 (*0-7507-0096-3*) Taylor & Francis (Falmer Pr).

Sex, Gender & Pain. Ed. by Roger B. Fillingim. 2000. LC 00-33589. (Progress in Pain Research & Management Ser.: Vol. 17). (Illus.). xiv, 393p. 79.00 (*0-931092-35-3*) Intl Assn Study Pain.

***Sex Hormone Replacement Therapy.** Ed. by Henry G. Burger. 2000. LC 00-61078. (Endocrine Updates Ser.). 152p. 135.00 (*0-7923-7965-9*, Kluwer Acad) Kluwer Academic.

Sex Hormones & Antihormones in Endocrine Dependent Pathology: Proceedings of an International Symposium, Milano, 10-14 April 1994. Ed. by Marcella Motta & Mario Serio. 1994. LC 94-32151. (International Congress Ser.: Vol. 1064). 448p. 233.50 (*0-444-81879-0*) Elsevier.

Sex in Education: or A Fair Chance for the Girls. Edward Clarke. 1977. LC 74-180566. (Medicine & Society in America Ser.). 190p. reprint ed. 18.95 (*0-405-03943-3*) Ayer.

Sex in the Therapy Hour: A Case of Professional Incest. Carolyn M. Bates & Annette M. Brodsky. 1993. LC 88-19032. 236p. pap. 20.00 (*0-89862-098-8*) Guilford Pubns.

Sex Life in Marriage. Oliver M. Butterfield. (Illus.). 12.95 (*0-87523-035-0*) Emerson.

Sex Linkage of Intelligence: The X-Factor. Robert Lehrke. 1997. LC 96-53612. (Human Evolution, Behavior, & Intelligence Ser.). 208p. 60.00 (*0-275-95903-1*, Praeger Pubs) Greenwood.

Sex Murder & Sex Aggression: Phenomenology, Psychopathology, Psychodynamics & Prognosis. Eugene Revitch & Louis B. Schlesinger. 1989. (Illus.). 152p. (C). text 43.95 (*0-398-05556-4*) C C Thomas.

Sex Offender Treatment: Psychological & Medical Approaches. Ed. by Eli Coleman et al. 1996. LC 92-48795. (Journal of Offender Rehabilitation: Vol. 18, Nos. 3/4). 233p. pap. 19.95 (*0-7890-0069-5*) Haworth Pr.

Sex on the Brain: The Biological Differences Between Men & Women. Deborah Blum. 1998. LC 96-52034. 352p. pap. 13.95 (*0-14-026348-9*) Penguin Putnam.

Sex, Orgasm & the Mind of Clear Light: The Sixty-Four Acts of Gay Male Love. Jeffrey Hopkins. 1998. LC 97-43909. (Illus.). 150p. pap. 14.95 (*1-55643-274-7*) North Atlantic.

Sex Preferences: Origins & Influences. Mon Roes. 1988. 126p. (Orig.). (C). pap. 8.95 (*0-9618960-0-0*) M M Fain.

Sex Profession: What Sex Therapy Can Do. Patricia Schiller. 1980. 250p. (Orig.). 20.00 (*0-937532-00-2*); pap. 15.00 (*0-937532-01-0*) Chilmark Hse.

Sex Research - Early Literature from Statistics to Erotica: Guide to the Microfilm Collection. Ed. by Research Publications, Inc. Staff. 1983. 130p. 110.00 (*0-89235-075-X*, PSM) Gale.

Sex Role Attitudes among High School Seniors: Views about Work & Family Roles. A. Regula Herzog & Jerald G. Bachman. 1982. 272p. (Orig.). pap. 16.00 (*0-87944-275-1*) Inst Soc Res.

Sex Role Attitudes & Cultural Change. Ira Gross et al. 1982. text 112.50 (*90-277-1340-5*) Kluwer Academic.

S

Sex Role Stereotyping in Occupational Choices: A Career Counseling Manual. Claudia G. Meer et al. 1982. 62p. 6.00 (*0-941312-01-1*) Inst Mgmt & Labor.

Sex Roles & Aging: Theory & Research from a Systems Perspective. Jan D. Sinnott. 1986. (Contributions to Human Development Ser.: Vol. 15). xiv, 134p. 38.50 (*3-8055-4207-0*) S Karger.

Sex Roles & Psychopathology. Ed. by Cathy S. Widom. 1984. 390p. 60.00 (*0-306-41406-6*, Plenum Trade) Perseus Pubng.

Sex Rx. Theresa Crenshaw. 1998. 288p. pap. 12.00 (*0-06-272052-X*, Perennial) HarperTrade.

Sex Satisfaction & Happy Marriage. Alfred H. Tyrer. 1951. (Illus.). 9.95 (*0-87523-039-3*) Emerson.

Sex, Sensibility & the Gendered Body. Ed. by Janet Holland & Lisa Adkins. 1996. LC 96-491. 256p. pap. 19.95 (*0-312-16082-8*) St Martin.

Sex Steroids & Bone. Ed. by R. Ziegler et al. (Schering Foundation Workshop Ser.: Vol. 9). (Illus.). 1994. vii, 205p. 59.00 (*0-387-57374-7*); 1993. LC 93-43028. 205p. (*0-347-57374-6*) Spr-Verlag.

Sex Steroids & the Cardiovascular System. Ed. by P. Ramwell et al. 1993. LC 92-49749. (Schering Foundation Workshop Ser.: Vol. 5). (Illus.). xii, 201p. 59.00 (*3-540-55728-8*); 201p. 64.95 (*0-387-55728-8*) Spr-Verlag.

Sex Steroids & the Cardiovascular System: The Proceedings of the 1st Interdisciplinary Workshop, Tuebingen, Germany, October 1996. Lippert, T. H., Ary Workshop Staff. Ed. by T. H. Lippert et al. 1997. LC 97-7110. (Illus.). 256p. lib. bdg. 60.95 (*1-85070-956-4*, Parthenon Pbng) CRC Pr.

Sex Therapy: A Practical Guide. Keith E. Hawton. 1986. LC 86-17422. 273p. reprint ed. 22.50 (*0-87668-934-9*) Aronson.

Sex Therapy: A Practical Guide. Keith E. Hawton. 1985. (Illus.). 280p. pap. text 45.00 (*0-19-261413-4*) OUP.

Sex Therapy Handbook: A Clinical Manual for the Diagnosis & Treatment of Sexual Disorders. E. C. Krohne. 1982. LC 80-26504. (Illus.). 128p. text 19.50 (*0-88331-197-6*) R B Luce.

Sex Variants: A Study of Homosexual Patterns, Set. George W. Henry. LC 78-22292. (Gay Experience Ser.). (Illus.). reprint ed. 75.00 (*0-404-61525-2*) AMS Pr.

Sex Without Love: A Philosophical Exploration. Russell Vannoy. 1980. LC 79-57534. 234p. (C). pap. 25.00 (*0-87975-129-0*) Prometheus Bks.

***Sex, Work, & Professionalism: Working in HIV/AIDS.** Katie Deverell. 2001. LC 2001-20491. (Social Aspects of AIDS Ser.). 90.00 (*0-415-23320-8*); pap. 28.95 (*0-415-23321-6*) Routledge.

Sexaholics Anonymous. 1989. LC 89-10261. 212p. pap. 10.00 (*0-9622887-0-5*) SA Literature.

Sexing the Body: Gender Politics & the Construction of Sexuality. Anne Fausto-Sterling. LC 00-703212. (Illus.). xii, 473p. 2001. pap. 20.00 (*0-465-07714-5*); 2000. 35.00 (*0-465-07713-7*) Basic.

Sexism & Stereotypes in Modern Society: The Gender Science of Janet Taylor Spence. Ed. by William B. Swann, Jr. et al. 1998. LC 98-24925. 324p. pap. 39.95 (*1-55798-531-6*, 431-8770) Am Psychol.

Sexocize: A Female Genitourinary Program. Janan Clark. 2nd ed. 1998. (Illus.). 41p. pap. 12.95 (*0-929593-01-4*) West Pine Pub.

Sexology Encyclopedia Vol. 1: Sex & Intercourse Research: Index & Reference Books of New Information. American Health Research Institute Staff. Ed. by John C. Bartone. 1996. (Illus.). 175p. pap. 47.50 (*0-7883-0851-3*);Set. 57.50 (*0-7883-0850-5*) ABBE Pubs Assn.

Sexology Encyclopedia Vol. 4: Sex Offenses: Index & Reference Books of New Information. Harold P. Drummond. Ed. by John C. Bartone. 1996. (Illus.). 157p. pap. 47.50 (*0-7883-0857-2*) ABBE Pubs Assn.

Sexology Encyclopedia Vol. 5: Intra-Uterine Devices: Index & Reference Books of New Information. Doris E. Rockford. Ed. by John C. Bartone. 1996. (Illus.). 151p. pap. 47.50 (*0-7883-0859-9*) ABBE Pubs Assn.

Sexology Encyclopedia Vol. 5: Intra-Uterine Devices: Index & Reference Books of New Information, Set. Doris E. Rockford. Ed. by John C. Bartone. 1996. (Illus.). 170p. 57.50 (*0-7883-0858-0*) ABBE Pubs Assn.

Sexology Encyclopedia Vol. 6: Impotence: Index & Reference Books of New Information. Alexander D. Farrell. Ed. by John C. Bartone. 1996. (Illus.). 151p. pap. 47.50 (*0-7883-0861-0*);Set. 57.50 (*0-7883-0860-2*) ABBE Pubs Assn.

Sexology Encyclopedia Vol. 7: Sexually Transmitted Diseases: Index & Reference Books of New Information. Helen M. Markle & John C. Bartone. 1996. (Illus.). 159p. pap. 47.50 (*0-7883-0863-7*) ABBE Pubs Assn.

Sexology Encyclopedia Vol. 7: Sexually Transmitted Diseases: Index & Reference Books of New Information, Set. Helen M. Markle. Ed. by John C. Bartone. 1996. (Illus.). 159p. 57.50 (*0-7883-0862-9*) ABBE Pubs Assn.

Sexology Encyclopedia Vol. 8: Sex & Transsexualism: Index & Reference Books of New Information. Rosalie F. Zoltano. Ed. by John C. Bartone. 1996. (Illus.). 129p. pap. 47.50 (*0-7883-0865-3*);Set. 57.50 (*0-7883-0864-5*) ABBE Pubs Assn.

Sexology Encyclopedia Vol. 9: Incest: Index & Reference Books of New Information. Lottie F. Lydeen. Ed. by John C. Bartone. 1996. (Illus.). 163p. pap. 47.50 (*0-7883-0867-X*);Set. 57.50 (*0-7883-0866-1*) ABBE Pubs Assn.

Sexology Encyclopedia Vol. 10: Homosexuality: Index & Reference Books of New Information. Sanivar H. Clygout. Ed. by John C. Bartone. 1996. (Illus.). 155p. pap. 47.50 (*0-7883-0869-6*);Set. 57.50 (*0-7883-0868-8*) ABBE Pubs Assn.

Sexology Encyclopedia Vol. 11: Sex Disorders: Sex Disorders: Index & Reference Books of New Information. American Health Research Institute Staff. Ed. by John C. Bartone. 1996. (Illus.). 153p. pap. 47.50 (*0-7883-0871-8*);Set. 57.50 (*0-7883-0870-X*) ABBE Pubs Assn.

Sexology Encyclopedia Vol. 12: Vagina Research: Index & Reference Books of New Information. Judy J. Hallcrest. Ed. by John C. Bartone. 1996. (Illus.). 143p. pap. 47.50 (*0-7883-0873-4*);Set. 57.50 (*0-7883-0872-6*) ABBE Pubs Assn.

Sexology Encyclopedia Vol. 13: Prostate Research: Index & Reference Books of New Information. Virginia L. Jensen. Ed. by John C. Bartone. 1996. (Illus.). 163p. pap. 47.50 (*0-7883-0875-0*);Set. 57.50 (*0-7883-0874-2*) ABBE Pubs Assn.

Sexology Encyclopedia Vol. 14: Menstruation Disorders: Index & Reference Books of New Information. Bette M. Parkenham. Ed. by John C. Bartone. 1996. (Illus.). 150p. 57.50 (*0-7883-0876-9*); pap. 47.50 (*0-7883-0877-7*) ABBE Pubs Assn.

Sexology Encyclopedia Vol. 15: Sex Behavior: Index & Reference Books of New Information. American Health Research Institute Staff. Ed. by John C. Bartone. 1996. (Illus.). 153p. 57.50 (*0-7883-0878-5*); pap. 47.50 (*0-7883-0879-3*) ABBE Pubs Assn.

Sexology Encyclopedia Vol. 16: Herpes Genitalis: Index & Reference Books of New Information. Marian L. Rice. Ed. by John C. Bartone. 1996. (Illus.). 145p. 57.50 (*0-7883-0880-7*); pap. 47.50 (*0-7883-0881-5*) ABBE Pubs Assn.

Sexology Encyclopedia Vol. 17: Sex & Bisexuality: Index & Reference Books of New Information. Rosalie F. Zoltano. Ed. by John C. Bartone. 1996. (Illus.). 149p. 57.50 (*0-7883-0882-3*); pap. 47.50 (*0-7883-0883-1*) ABBE Pubs Assn.

Sexology Encyclopedia Vol. 18: Sex Research: Index & Reference Books of New Information. Rosalie F. Zoltano. Ed. by John C. Bartone. 1996. (Illus.). 167p. 57.50 (*0-7883-0884-X*); pap. 47.50 (*0-7883-0885-8*) ABBE Pubs Assn.

Sexology Encyclopedia Vol. 19: Vasectomy & Medicine: Index & Reference Books of New Information. Ed. by John C. Bartone. 1996. (Illus.). 145p. 57.50 (*0-7883-0886-6*) ABBE Pubs Assn.

Sexology Encyclopedia Vol. 19: Vasectomy & Medicine: Index & Reference Books of New Information. Benard I. Valahos. Ed. by John C. Bartone. 1996. (Illus.). 145p. pap. 47.50 (*0-7883-0887-4*) ABBE Pubs Assn.

Sexology Encyclopedia Vol. 20: Female Genital Diseases: Index & Reference Books of New Information. Patricia S. Hurley. Ed. by John C. Bartone. 1996. (Illus.). 155p. 57.50 (*0-7883-0888-2*); pap. 47.50 (*0-7883-0889-0*) ABBE Pubs Assn.

Sexology Encyclopedia Vol. 21: Sexual Harassment: Index & Reference Book of New Information. Simon H. Bonner. 1996. (Illus.). 143p. 57.50 (*0-7883-0890-4*); pap. 47.50 (*0-7883-0891-2*) ABBE Pubs Assn.

Sexology Encyclopedia Vol. 23: Premenstrual Syndromes: Index & Reference Books of New Information. Jacob L. Liehaus. 1996. (Illus.). 123p. 57.50 (*0-7883-0894-7*); pap. 47.50 (*0-7883-0895-5*) ABBE Pubs Assn.

Sexology Uncensored. Bland. 1999. LC 98-16624. 261p. pap. text 18.00 (*0-226-05669-4*); lib. bdg. 45.00 (*0-226-05668-6*) U Ch Pr.

Sexual Aberrations. Wilhelm Stekel. 1971. pap. 5.95 (*0-87140-246-7*) Liveright.

Sexual Abuse. Ed. by Levine. 1997. (Psychoanalytic Inquiry Ser.: Vol. 17, No. 3). pap. 20.00 (*0-88163-934-6*) Analytic Pr.

Sexual Abuse & Eating Disorders. Ed. by Mark F. Schwartz & Leigh Cohn. Date not set. LC 95-26500. 240p. text 27.95 (*0-87630-794-2*) Brunner-Routledge.

Sexual Abuse & the Primary Care Doctor. G. Wakely. 1991. 128p. pap. 24.95 (*0-412-41580-1*, A6372) Chapman & Hall.

Sexual Abuse of Children Ed. by W. T. O'Donohue & James H. Geer. 1992. 424p. pap. 45.00 (*0-8058-0340-8*); 544p. pap. 55.00 (*0-8058-0955-4*) L Erlbaum Assocs.

Sexual Abuse of Children: A Resource Guide & Annotated Bibliography. Benjamin Schlesinger. 1982. 212p. pap. text 11.95 (*0-8020-6481-7*) U of Toronto Pr.

Sexual Abuse of Children: Index of Modern Information. Lottie F. Lydeen. 1990. LC 89-47967. 150p. 47.50 (*1-55914-038-0*); pap. 44.50 (*1-55914-039-9*) ABBE Pubs Assn.

***Sexual Abuse of Children: Understanding, Intervention & Prevention.** Diana Riley. 1991. 96p. pap. (*1-870905-76-8*) Radcliffe Med Pr GBR. *Dist:* Balogh.

Sexual Abuse of Children in the 1980s: Issues & Annotated Bibliography, 1980-1984. Benjamin Schlesinger. 1986. 208p. pap. 16.95 (*0-8020-6622-4*) U of Toronto Pr.

Sexual Abuse Recalled: Treating Trauma in the Era of the Recovered Memory Debate. Ed. by Judith L. Alpert. 1995. LC 95-4702. 440p. 50.00 (*1-56821-363-8*) Aronson.

Sexual Addiction: An Integrated Approach. Aviel Goodman. 1998. LC 97-27415. 456p. 65.00 (*0-8236-6063-X*) Intl Univs Pr.

Sexual Adjustment: A Guide for the Spinal Cord Injured. Martha F. Gregory. Ed. by Raymond C. Cheever. 1974. 70p. pap. 4.95 (*0-915708-00-0*, #1410) Cheever Pub.

Sexual & Reproductive Neurorehabilitation. Ed. by Mindy L. Aisen. 1997. LC 97-12460. (Current Clinical Neurology Ser.). (Illus.). 256p. 145.00 (*0-89603-376-7*) Humana.

Sexual Aspects of Cardiovascular Disease, 10. Chris Papadopoulos. 1989. LC 89-3973. (Sexual Medicine Ser.: No. 10). 120p. 60.00 (*0-275-92523-4*, C2523, Praeger Pubs) Greenwood.

Sexual Aspects of Headaches. Ed. by Seymour Diamond & Michael Maliszewski. 1992. LC 91-46626. 520p. (C). 75.00 (*0-8236-6071-0*) Intl Univs Pr.

Sexual Assault: The Medical-Legal Examination. Sharon R. Crowley. 1999. LC 98-37949. (Illus.). 240p. (C). text 59.95 (*0-8385-8533-7*) McGraw-Hill Prof.

Sexual Assault of Children & Adolescents. Ann Wolbert Burgess et al. 1978. LC 77-10217. 250p. 35.00 (*0-669-01892-9*) Lxngtn Bks.

Sexual Aversion, Sexual Phobias, & Panic Disorder. Helen S. Kaplan & Donald F. Klein. 1987. LC 86-28331. 168p. text 52.95 (*0-87630-450-1*) Brunner-Routledge.

Sexual Barrier: Legal, Medical, Economic & Social Aspects of Sex Discrimination. Marija M. Hughes. 1977. LC 77-83214. 70.00 (*0-912560-04-5*) Hughes Pr.

Sexual Behavior: Problems & Management. N. McConaghy. 1993. (Applied Clinical Psychology Ser.). (Illus.). 426p. (C). 75.00 (*0-306-44177-2*, Plenum Trade) Perseus Pubng.

Sexual Behavior & AIDS in Britain. HMSO Staff. 1993. 250p. pap. (*0-11-701748-5*, HM17485) Statnry Office GBR. *Dist:* Bernan Associates.

Sexual Behavior & Preventing Pregnancy. Frances S. Sizer & Eleanor N. Whitney. 1993. LC 92-39463. mass mkt. 12.25 (*0-314-01685-6*) West Pub.

Sexual Behaviour & AIDS in India. Moni Nag. 1997. LC 96-902172. (C). (*81-259-0125-6*) Vikas IND. *Dist:* S Asia.

Sexual Concerns When Illness or Disability Strikes. Carol L. Sandowski. 1989. (Illus.). 304p. (C). text 61.95 (*0-398-05612-9*) C C Thomas.

Sexual Conduct: The Social Sources of Human Sexuality. John H. Gagnon & William Simon. 1973. 328p. (C). lib. bdg. 37.95 (*0-202-30261-X*) Aldine de Gruyter.

Sexual Counseling Skills Workshop: A Trainers' Handbook. Robert R. Wilson. 1977. pap. 2.00 (*0-89055-120-0*) Carolina Pop Ctr.

Sexual Cultures & the Construction of Adolescent Identities. Ed. by Janice M. Irvine. 1994. (Health, Society, & Policy Ser.). 336p. 69.95 (*1-56639-135-0*); LC 93-22144. pap. 22.95 (*1-56639-136-9*) Temple U Pr.

Sexual Development of Young Children. Virginia Lively & Edwin Lively. 1991. 192p. pap., tchr. ed. 8.50 (*0-8273-4199-7*); 198p. (C). mass mkt. 24.50 (*0-8273-4198-9*) Delmar.

Sexual Deviance: Theory, Assessment & Treatment. Ed. by D. Richard Laws & William O'Donohue. 1997. LC 97-25929. 514p. text 65.00 (*1-57230-241-0*, 0241) Guilford Pubns.

Sexual Deviancy & Social Proscription: The Social Context of Carnal Behavior. Clifton D. Bryant. 1982. LC 81-6216. 432p. 52.00 (*0-89885-024-X*); pap. 24.95 (*0-89885-094-0*) Kluwer Academic (Kluwer Acad Hman Sci).

Sexual Deviation. Ed. by Ismond Rosen. 3rd ed. 1996. (Illus.). 508p. (C). text 125.00 (*0-19-262516-0*) OUP.

Sexual Deviation in American Society: A Social-Psychological Study of Sexual Nonconformity. Bernard J. Oliver, Jr. 1967. pap. 18.95 (*0-8084-0277-3*) NCUP.

Sexual Difference: Masculinity & Psychoanalysis. Stephen Frosh. 1994. LC 93-5902. 192p. (C). text 62.95 (*0-415-06843-6*) Routledge.

Sexual Differentiation. A. A. Gerall et al. 1992. LC 92-4962. (Handbook of Behavioral Neurobiology Ser.: Vol. 11). (Illus.). 384p. (C). text 95.00 (*0-306-43983-2*, Kluwer Plenum) Kluwer Academic.

Sexual Dimorphism in Homo Sapiens: A Question of Size. Ed. by Robert L. Hall. 1984. LC 81-5907. 429p. 89.50 (*0-275-91365-1*, C1365, Praeger Pubs) Greenwood.

Sexual Dimorphism in Human & Mammalian Biology & Pathology. Alfred Glucksmann. 1981. LC 80-42373. 374p. text 157.00 (*0-12-286960-5*) Acad Pr.

Sexual Disorders: Treatment, Theory & Research. C. David Tollison & Henry E. Adams. 1979. LC 79-20853. text 34.95 (*0-89876-029-1*) Gardner Pr.

Sexual Dysfunction: A Guide for Assessment & Treatment. John P. Wincze & Michael P. Carey. 1991. LC 91-16339. (Treatment Manuals for Practitioners Ser.). 212p. pap. 22.00 (*0-89862-218-2*, 2218); text 49.95 (*0-89862-207-7*) Guilford Pubns.

Sexual Dysfunction in Aging Males. R. H. W. Van Lunsen. 2001. 200p. 75.00 (*1-84214-034-5*, Parthenon Pbng) CRC Pr.

Sexual Exploitation in Professional Relationships. Ed. by Glen O. Gabbard. 1989. LC 88-3280. 257p. text 34.00 (*0-88048-290-7*, 8290) Am Psychiatric.

Sexual Exploitation of Patients by Health Professionals, 4. Ed. by Ann Wolbert Burgess & Carol R. Hartman. 1986. LC 86-9318. (Sexual Medicine Ser.: Vol. 4). 207p. 68.50 (*0-275-92171-9*, C2171, Praeger Pubs) Greenwood.

Sexual Expression: A Manual for Trainers. Carl Hartman et al. 1981. LC 81-6760. (Illus.). 152p. pap. 19.95 (*0-89885-053-3*, Kluwer Acad Hman Sci) Kluwer Academic.

Sexual Feelings in Psychotherapy: Explorations for Therapists & Therapists-in-Training. Kenneth S. Pope et al. 1993. LC 93-7139. 304p. pap. text 24.95 (*1-55798-201-5*) Am Psychol.

Sexual Fitness. 1988. (Fitness, Health & Nutrition Ser.). (Illus.). 144p. 17.27 (*0-8094-6110-2*); lib. bdg. 23.27 (*0-8094-6111-0*) Time-Life.

Sexual Harassment: A Special Issue of Military Psychology. Ed. by Fritz Grasgow. 1999. 128p. pap. 20.00 (*0-8058-9786-0*) L Erlbaum Assocs.

Sexual Harassment in the Workplace & Academia: Psychiatric Issues. Ed. by Diane K. Shrier. 1996. LC 95-26269. (Clinical Practice Ser.: No. 38). 304p. text 39.50 (*0-88048-490-X*, 8490) Am Psychiatric.

Sexual Healing Journey: A Guide for Survivors of Sexual Abuse. Wendy Maltz. 1992. LC 90-55934. (Illus.). 368p. reprint ed. pap. 14.00 (*0-06-092155-2*, Perennial) HarperTrade.

Sexual Health: Foundations for Practice. Ed. by Heather A. Wilson & Sue McAndrew. 2000. 295p. pap. text (*0-7020-2269-1*) W B Saunders GBR. *Dist:* Saunders.

Sexual Health: Questions You Have... Answers You Need. Michael V. Reitano. 1999. LC 98-44625. (Illus.). 192p. pap. 12.95 (*1-882606-43-4*) Peoples Med Soc.

Sexual Health Concerns: Interviewing & History Taking for Health Practitioners. Michael W. Ross et al. 2nd ed. 1999. (Illus.). 220p. (C). pap. text 26.95 (*0-8036-0668-0*) Davis Co.

***Sexual Health Matters in Primary Care.** Gill Wakley & Ruth Chambers. 2001. 248p. pap. (*1-85775-414-X*) Radcliffe Med Pr GBR. *Dist:* Balogh.

Sexual Health Promotion in General Practice. Hilary Curtis. 1995. 144p. pap. (*1-85775-131-0*) Radcliffe Med Pr GBR. *Dist:* Balogh.

Sexual Hormones: Influence on the Electrophysiology of the Brain. Manuel Alcaraz et al. 1974. LC 74-4137. 223p. text 31.00 (*0-8422-7214-3*) Irvington.

Sexual Images of the Self: The Psychology of Erotic Sensations & Illusions. S. Fisher. 1989. 360p. 69.95 (*0-8058-0439-0*) L Erlbaum Assocs.

Sexual Impotence in the Male & Female. William A. Hammond. 1974. LC 73-20626. (Sex, Marriage & Society Ser.). 310p. reprint ed. 26.95 (*0-405-05802-0*) Ayer.

Sexual Interactions: Basic Understandings. Elizabeth R. Allgeier & Albert Richard Allgeier. 1999. LC 97-72430. (Illus.). (*0-395-84600-5*) HM.

Sexual Interactions & HIV Risk: New Conceptual Perspectives in European Research. Ed. by L. Van Campenhoudt. 1995. LC 95-17936. (Social Aspects of AIDS Ser.). pap. 29.95 (*0-7484-0346-9*) Taylor & Francis.

Sexual Intimacy Between Therapists & Patients. Kenneth S. Pope et al. LC 86-15165. (Sexual Medicine Ser.: No. 5). 1988. 196p. pap. 18.95 (*0-275-92953-1*); 5. 1986. 197p. 59.00 (*0-275-92253-7*, B2953) Greenwood (Praeger Pubs).

Sexual Inversion. Havelock Ellis & John A. Symonds. 1975. LC 75-12312. (Homosexuality: Lesbians & Gay Men in Society, History & Literature Ser.). reprint ed. 32.95 (*0-405-07363-1*) Ayer.

Sexual Involvement with Therapists: Patient Assessment, Subsequent Therapy, Forensics. Kenneth S. Pope. 1994. LC 94-11534. 249p. pap. 24.95 (*1-55798-248-1*) Am Psychol.

Sexual Life: A Clinician's Guide. S. B. Levine. 1992. (Critical Issues in Psychiatry Ser.). (Illus.). 250p. (C). 54.00 (*0-306-44287-6*, Plenum Trade) Perseus Pubng.

Sexual Life of the Child. Albert Moll. Tr. by Eden Paul from GER. LC 72-11290. reprint ed. 39.00 (*0-404-57483-1*) AMS Pr.

Sexual Medicine in Primary Care. William L. Maurice. 1998. LC 98-39997. (Illus.). xxix, 366p. (C). (gr. 13). pap. text 39.95 (*0-8151-2797-9*, 31217) Mosby Inc.

Sexual Neurasthenia, Its Hygiene, Causes, Symptoms & Treatment with a Chapter on Diet for the Nervous. George M. Beard. Ed. by A. D. Rockwell. 5th ed. 1972. LC 76-180553. (Medicine & Society in America Ser.). 312p. reprint ed. 20.95 (*0-405-03933-6*) Ayer.

Sexual Nutrition. Morton Walker & Joan Walker. 1984. 400p. mass mkt. 3.95 (*0-8217-1390-6*, Zebra Kensgtn) Kensgtn Pub Corp.

Sexual Nutrition. Morton Walker. rev. ed. 1996. 264p. 29.98 (*0-941683-34-6*) Instant Improve.

Sexual Offender Treatment: Biopsychosocial Perspective. Ed. by Eli Coleman & Michael Miner. 2000. LC 00-36965. 118p. (C). 39.90 (*0-7890-1017-8*) Haworth Pr.

Sexual Offender Treatment: Biopsychosocial Perspectives. Ed. by Eli Coleman & Michael Miner. 2000. LC 00-36965. 118p. (C). pap. 14.95 (*0-7890-1018-6*) Haworth Pr.

Sexual Offending Against Children: Assessment & Treatment of Male Abusers. Ed. by Tony Morrison et al. 1994. LC 94-1687. 240p. (C). pap. 27.95 (*0-415-05505-9*, B4373) Routledge.

Sexual Options for Paraplegics & Quadriplegics. Thomas O. Mooney et al. 1975. (Illus.). 150p. pap. 29.95 (*0-316-57937-8*, Little Brwn Med Div) Lppncott W & W.

Sexual Organism: Its Healthful Management. James C. Jackson. 1974. LC 73-20632. (Sex, Marriage & Society Ser.). 296p. reprint ed. 25.95 (*0-405-05807-1*) Ayer.

Sexual Orientation: Toward Biological Understanding. Ed. by Lee Ellis & Linda Ebertz. 1997. LC 97-8864. 304p. 70.00 (*0-275-95651-2*, Praeger Pubs) Greenwood.

Sexual Pharmacology. Ed. by Alan J. Riley et al. 1994. (Illus.). 248p. text 75.00 (*0-19-262283-8*) OUP.

Sexual Pharmacology: Drugs That Affect Sexual Function. Theresa L. Crenshaw & James P. Goldberg. 1996. LC 95-42109. 500p. (C). 75.00 (*0-393-70144-1*) Norton.

Sexual Physiology. R. T. Trall. 1974. LC 73-20640. (Sex, Marriage & Society Ser.). 310p. reprint ed. 26.95 (*0-405-05821-7*) Ayer.

Sexual Politics of Jean-Jacques Rousseau. Joel Schwartz. LC 83-18141. xii, 208p. 1996. 20.50 (*0-226-74223-7*); 1985. pap. text 9.95 (*0-226-74224-5*) U Ch Pr.

Sexual Rehabilitation of the Spinal-Cord Injured Patient. Ed. by J. F. J. Leyson. 1991. LC 90-4685. (Illus.). 572p. 135.00 (*0-89603-145-4*) Humana.

Sexual Self: How Character Shapes Sexual Experience. Avodah K. Offit. rev. ed. 1995. LC 95-22483. (Master Work Ser.). 336p. pap. 25.00 (*1-56821-548-7*) Aronson.

Sexual Strands: Understanding & Treating Sexual Anomalies in Men. R. Langevin. 1983. (Illus.). 560p. (C). text 99.95 (*0-89859-205-4*) L Erlbaum Assocs.

Sexual Strategy. Tim Halliday. 1995. LC 82-2607. (Phoenix Fiction Ser.). (Illus.). 160p. (C). pap. 14.95 (*0-226-31387-5*) U Ch Pr.

Sexual Subjects: Lesbians, Gender & Psychoanalysis. Adria E. Schwartz. LC 97-21490. 200p. (C). 1998. 90.00 (*0-415-91092-7*); 1997. pap. 24.95 (*0-415-91093-5*) Routledge.

Sexual Transmission of HIV Infection: Risk Reduction, Trauma, & Adaptation. Ed. by Lena N. Schonnesson. 1993. LC 92-49781. (Journal of Psychotherapy & the Family Ser.: Vol. 5, Nos. 1-2, 1992). (Illus.). 168p. 39.95 (*1-56024-332-5*) Haworth Pr.

Sexual Transmission of HIV Infection: Risk Reduction, Trauma & Adaptation. Ed. by Lena N. Schonnesson. 1993. LC 92-49781. (Journal of Psychotherapy & the Family Ser.: Vol. 5, Nos. 1-2, 1992). (Illus.). 168p. pap. 19.95 (*1-56023-024-X*, Harrington Park) Haworth Pr.

Sexual Trauma & Psychopathology: Clinical Intervention with Adult Survivors. Shanti Shapiro & George M. Dominiak. 1992. LC 92-25642. 192p. 30.95 (*0-669-27357-0*) Lxngtn Bks.

Sexual Unfolding: Sexual Development & Sex Therapies in Late Adolescence. Lorna J. Sarrel & Philip M. Sarrel. 1995. LC 95-22326. (Master Work Ser.). 378p. reprint ed. 50.00 (*1-56821-675-0*) Aronson.

Sexual Victimisation: Two Recent Researches into Sex Problems & Their Social Effects. Ed. by D. J. West. 1985. 194p. text (*0-566-00832-7*) Avebry GBR. *Dist:* Ashgate Pub Co.

Sexual Visions: Images of Gender in Science & Medicine Between the Eighteenth & Twentieth Centuries. Ludmilla Jordanova. 1993. LC 92-41729. (Science & Literature Ser.). (Illus.). 208p. (C). reprint ed. pap. 14.95 (*0-299-12294-8*) U of Wis Pr.

Sexualitat des Menschen: Handbuch und Atlas. Erwin J. Haeberle. 1983. (GER.). 559p. 41.55 (*3-11-008753-7*) De Gruyter.

Sexualities & Homosexualities. Jaime P. Stubrin. 1994. 176p. pap. text (*1-85575-065-1*) Karnac Bks GBR. *Dist:* Other Pr LLC.

Sexualities in Health & Social Care: A Textbook. Contrib. by Tamsin Wilton. 2000. LC 99-56511. (*0-335-20026-5*) OpUniv Pr GBR. *Dist:* Taylor & Francis.

***Sexualities Lost & Found: Psychoanalytic Perspectives on Lesbian Experience.** Ed. by Edith Gould & Sandra Kiersky. unabr. ed. 2001. LC 2001-16859. 225p. pap. text 32.95 (*0-8236-6062-1*) Intl Univs Pr.

Sexuality. Greenberg. 3rd ed. 1993. 22.50 (*0-697-17222-8*); trans. 84.68 (*0-697-10114-2*) McGraw.

Sexuality: A Developmental Approach to Problems. Betty N. Gordon & Carolyn S. Schroeder. 1995. LC 95-17305. (Clinical Child Psychology Library). (Illus.). 176p. (C). 42.00 (*0-306-45039-9*); pap. 23.00 (*0-306-45040-2*) Perseus Pubng (Plenum Trade).

Sexuality: A Nursing Perspective. Ferm Mims & Melinda Swenson. 1979. pap. text 25.95 (*0-07-042388-1*) McGraw.

Sexuality: New Perspectives, 6. Ed. by Zira DeFries et al. 1985. LC 84-28991. (Contributions in Psychology Ser.: No. 6). (Illus.). 362p. 75.00 (*0-313-24207-0*, DFS/, Greenwood Pr) Greenwood.

Sexuality Across the Life Course. Ed. by Alice S. Rossi. 1994. LC 93-41706. (John D. & Catherine T. MacArthur Foundation Series on Mental Health & Development). 435p. 34.95 (*0-226-72833-1*) U Ch Pr.

Sexuality after TBI. William H. Burke. 2nd ed. 1995. (Professional Series on Traumatic Brain Injury: Vol. 10). 68p. pap. 9.50 (*1-882855-41-8*) HDI Pubs.

Sexuality & Aging. Robert L. Solnick. rev. ed. 1978. LC 78-51932. pap. 14.00 (*0-88474-023-4*, 05752-5) Free Pr.

Sexuality & Aging: An Annotated Bibliography. George F. Wharton. 1981. LC 81-5097. 251p. 26.50 (*0-8108-1427-7*) Scarecrow.

Sexuality & Chronic Illness: A Comprehensive Approach. Leslie R. Schover & Soren B. Jensen. 1988. LC 87-23640. 357p. 49.95 (*0-89862-715-X*) Guilford Pubns.

Sexuality & Disability. Maddie Blackburn, MSc, RGN. 2002. 192p. pap. 29.99 (*0-7506-2252-0*) Buttrwrth-Heinemann.

Sexuality & Family Planning: Report of a Consultation & Research Findings. T. Langfeldt & M. Porter. 1986. 62p. pap. 8.00 (*92-890-1042-8*) World Health.

***Sexuality & Health Care.** Ed. by Hazel Heath & Isabel White. 2001. 224p. pap. 33.95 (*0-632-04804-2*) Blackwell Sci.

Sexuality & Medicine Vol. I: Conceptual Roots. Ed. by Earl E. Shelp. 5th ed. 1986. (Philosophy & Medicine Ser.: No. 22). 304p. pap. text 65.50 (*90-277-2386-9*) Kluwer Academic.

Sexuality & Medicine Vol. II: Ethical Viewpoints in Transition. Ed. by Earl E. Shelp. 5th ed. 1987. (Philosophy & Medicine Ser.: No. 23). 312p. pap. text 65.50 (*1-55608-016-6*); lib. bdg. 118.50 (*1-55608-013-1*) Kluwer Academic.

Sexuality & Patient Care: A Guide for Nurses & Teachers. Els Van Ooijen & Andrew Charnock. 1994. LC 93-39266. 42.50 (*1-56593-305-2*, 0629) Singular Publishing.

Sexuality & Serious Mental Illness. Ed. by Peter F. Buckley. 1999. (Chronic Mental Illness Ser.). 335p. text 40.00 (*90-5702-598-1*, Harwood Acad Pubs) Gordon & Breach.

Sexuality & the Devil: Symbols of Love, Power & Fear in Male Psychology. Edward J. Tejirian. 1990. 272p. (C). 60.00 (*0-415-90205-3*) Routledge.

Sexuality & the Person with Traumatic Brain Injury: A Guide for Families. Ernest R. Griffith & Sally Lemberg. 1992. LC 92-32994. (Illus.). 170p. pap. 18.95 (*0-8036-4408-6*) Davis Co.

Sexuality & the Psychology of Love. Sigmund Freud. 1993. 213p. (C). pap. 10.00 (*0-02-050986-3*) Macmillan.

Sexuality Counseling: A Training Program. Kay F. Schepp. 1986. LC 86-70572. x, 510p. 31.95 (*0-915202-47-6*) Accel Devel.

Sexuality Education in Postsecondary & Professional Training Settings. Ed. by James W. Maddock. 1997. LC 97-14977. 193p. 39.95 (*0-7890-0027-X*) Haworth Pr.

Sexuality in America: Contemporary Perspectives on Sexual Identity, Dysfunction & Treatment. Donald A. Brown & Chanda Clary. 1981. LC 81-81824. 24.50 (*0-87650-132-3*) Pierian.

Sexuality in the Second Decade. Raymond R. Willoughby. 1937. (SRCD M Ser.: Vol. 2, No. 3). pap. 25.00 (*0-527-01496-6*) Periodicals Srv.

Sexuality, Politics & AIDS in Brazil: In Another World? Richard Parker & Herbert Daniel. 1993. (Social Aspects of AIDS Ser.). 196p. 85.00 (*0-7507-0135-8*); pap. 29.95 (*0-7507-0136-6*) Taylor & Francis (Falmer Pr).

Sexuality Today. Gilbert D. Nass & Mary P. Fisher. 1988. (Illus.). 488p. (C). text 41.25 (*0-86720-408-7*, 408-7); pap. text, tchr. ed. 10.00 (*0-86720-414-1*, 414-1) Jones & Bartlett.

Sexuality, War & Schizophrenia: Collected Psychoanalytic Papers. Victor Tausk. Ed. & Intro. by Paul Roazen. 1991. 224p. (C). text 44.95 (*0-88738-365-3*) Transaction Pubs.

Sexually Adequate Female. Caprio. 1979. pap. 3.00 (*0-87980-146-8*) Wilshire.

Sexually Adequate Male. Caprio. 1979. pap. 3.00 (*0-87980-147-6*) Wilshire.

Sexually Aggressive Women: Current Perspectives & Controversies. Peter B. Anderson & Cynthia Struckman-Johnson. 1998. LC 98-2635. 244p. text 32.00 (*1-57230-165-1*, C0165) Guilford Pubns.

Sexually Disturbed: Treating Psychosexual Disorders. Averil M. Doyle. 1992. LC 91-45565. 168p. 58.00 (*0-275-94294-5*, C4294, Praeger Pubs) Greenwood.

Sexually Transmitted Diseases. Ed. by William Dudley. 1998. LC 98-38040. (At Issue Ser.). 95p. (YA). (gr. 9-12). pap. 13.70 (*0-7377-0010-6*); lib. bdg. 21.20 (*0-7377-0011-4*) Gale (Greenhaven Pr).

Sexually Transmitted Diseases. D. Goldmeier & S. Barton. 1986. 188p. 25.95 (*0-387-17056-1*) Spr-Verlag.

Sexually Transmitted Diseases. Ed. by Melanie C. Karaffa. 1992. 400p. text 49.95 (*1-878487-35-3*, ME220) Practice Mgmt Info.

Sexually Transmitted Diseases. Ed. by Gerald L. Mandell & Michael F. Rein. 1996. LC 95-32207. (Atlas of Infectious Diseases Ser.: Vol. 5). (Illus.). 294p. text (*0-443-07720-7*) Church GBR. *Dist:* Saunders.

Sexually Transmitted Diseases. A. McMillan & G. Scott. 1991. (Colour Aids Ser.). (Illus.). 112p. (Orig.). (C). pap. text (*0-443-04052-4*) Church.

Sexually Transmitted Diseases. A. McMillan. 2nd ed. 2000. 125p. (Orig.). pap. text 0.00 (*0-443-06229-3*) Saunders.

Sexually Transmitted Diseases. Tsieh Sun. 2nd ed. Date not set. (*0-938607-37-5*) Field & Wood Inc Medical.

Sexually Transmitted Diseases. Ed. by King K. Holmes et al. 3rd ed. 1998. LC 98-31523. (Illus.). 1344p. text 169.00 (*0-07-029688-X*) McGraw-Hill Prof.

Sexually Transmitted Diseases: A Guide for Clinicians. Ed. by F. Gashnait & Lawrence C. Parish. 1988. (Illus.). 388p. 121.00 (*0-387-96776-1*) Spr-Verlag.

Sexually Transmitted Diseases: A Physician Tells You What You Need to Know. Lisa Marr. 1999. LC 98-25952. (Johns Hopkins Press Health Bks.). (Illus.). 355p. 44.50 (*0-8018-6042-3*); 264p. pap. 16.95 (*0-8018-6043-1*) Johns Hopkins.

Sexually Transmitted Diseases: A Practical Guide. NIAID Staff. Ed. by Robert/J. Banis. 1997. LC 97-62235. (Illus.). 140p. pap. 16.95 (*1-888725-06-0*) Sci & Human Pr.

Sexually Transmitted Diseases: Advances in Diagnosis & Treatment. Ed. by P. Elsner & A. Eichmann. 1996. (Current Problems in Dermatology Ser.: Vol. 24, 1996). (Illus.). x, 268p. 249.75 (*3-8055-6220-9*) S Karger.

Sexually Transmitted Diseases: An Essential Slide Collection. James S. Bingham. 99p. incl. sl. (*0-397-46361-8*, GM0016) Gower-Mosby.

Sexually Transmitted Diseases: Epidemiology, Pathology, Diagnosis, & Treatment. Kenneth A. Borchardt & Michael A. Noble. 1997. LC 96-39561. 368p. 94.95 (*0-8493-9476-7*) CRC Pr.

Sexually Transmitted Diseases: Methods & Protocols. Ed. by Rosanna Peeling & P. Frederick Sparling. 1999. LC 98-18197. (Methods in Molecular Medicine Ser.: Vol. 20). (Illus.). 256p. 99.50 (*0-89603-535-2*) Humana.

Sexually Transmitted Diseases & Adverse Outcomes of Pregnancy. Ed. by Penelope J. Hitchcock et al. 1999. LC 99-11079. (Illus.). 320p. 99.95 (*1-55581-132-9*) ASM Pr.

Sexually Transmitted Diseases & AIDS. David Daniels et al. 1993. LC 92-2331. (Brainscan MCQs Ser.). 195p. 44.95 (*0-387-19762-1*) Spr-Verlag.

Sexually Transmitted Diseases & Appearance of Warts & Papillomas: Index of Modern Authors & Subjects with Guide for Rapid Research. Helen M. Markle. 1991. LC 90-56248. 190p. 47.50 (*1-55914-264-2*); pap. 44.50 (*1-55914-265-0*) ABBE Pubs Assn.

Sexually Transmitted Diseases Sourcebook: Basic Consumer Health Information about Sexually Transmitted Diseases. Ed. by Dawn D. Matthews. 2nd ed. 2001. LC 00-47878. (Health Reference Ser.). (Illus.). xiv, 538p. lib. bdg. 78.00 (*0-7808-0249-7*) Omnigraphics Inc.

Sexually Transmitted Diseases Sourcebook: Basic Information about Herpes, Chlamydia, Gonorrhea & More. Ed. by Linda M. Ross. 1997. LC 97-17036. (Health Reference Ser.: Vol. 26). 564p. 78.00 (*0-7808-0217-9*) Omnigraphics Inc.

***Sexually Transmitted Infections.** Edwards et al. 2001. (Fast Facts Ser.). (Illus.). 60p. pap. (*1-899541-04-7*) Health Pr GBR. *Dist:* JAMCO Dist.

Sexually Transmitted Infections: Nursing Care & Management. Tracy Steadman. 1998. (Illus.). 240p. pap. (*0-7487-3337-X*) Nelson Thornes GBR. *Dist:* Intl Spec Bk, Trans-Atl Phila.

Sexually Transmitted Infections & Aids in the Tropics. Ed. by O. P. Arya & C. A. Hart. 1998. LC 98-23327. (CAB International Publication). 400p. 110.00 (*0-85199-262-5*) OUP.

***SF-36 Physical & Mental Health Summary Scales: A Manual for Users of Version 1.** John E. Ware, Jr. et al. 2nd rev. ed. 2001. (Illus.). 248p. pap. text 89.95 (*1-891810-09-X*) Quality Metric.

SGNA Manual of Gastrointestinal Procedures: Publication of the Society of Gastroenterology Nurses & Associates. Marilyn Schaffner. 3rd ed. 1994. (Illus.). 210p. 59.95 (*0-683-07587-X*) Lppncott W & W.

Shackelford's Surgery of the Alimentary Tract George D. Zuidema. 4th ed. 1995. (Illus.). 3200p. text 479.00 (*0-7216-4982-3*) Saunders.

Shadow & Light: A Practical Guide to Caregiving. South Carolina Agencies on Aging Staff. 1994. (Illus.). 56p. (Orig.). pap. (*0-917069-08-0*) Univ SC Inst Pub Affairs.

Shadow & Self: Selected Papers in Analytical Psychology. Joseph L. Henderson. 1990. LC 89-36875. 564p. (Orig.). pap. 9.95 (*0-933029-33-0*) Chiron Pubns.

Shadow & the Counsellor: Working with Darker Aspects of the Person, Role & Profession. Steve Page. 1999. LC 98-45952. (Illus.). xii, 169p. 80.00 (*0-415-13144-8*); pap. 26.95 (*0-415-13145-6*) Routledge.

Shadow Culture: Psychology & Spirituality in America. Eugene Taylor. 1999. (*0-201-60880-4*) Addison-Wesley.

Shadow of the Object: Psychoanalysis of the Unthought Known. Christopher Bollas. 1989. 274p. pap. text 19.50 (*0-231-06627-9*) Col U Pr.

Shadow of the Other: Intersubjectivity & Gender in Psychoanalysis. Jessica Benjamin. 1997. LC 97-14660. 149p. (C). 80.00 (*0-415-91236-9*); 3rd ed. pap. 20.95 (*0-415-91237-7*) Routledge.

Shadow on My Soul: Overcoming Addiction to Suicide. Paula M. Quinn. 1995. 188p. (Orig.). pap. 14.95 (*1-879198-13-4*) Knwldg Ideas & Trnds.

Shadow Syndromes: The Mild Forms of Major Mental Disorders That Sabotage Us. John J. Ratey & Catherine Johnson. 1998. LC 96-33422. 400p. reprint ed. pap. 13.00 (*0-553-37959-3*) Bantam.

Shadows Linger. Glen Cook. 1984. 320p. mass mkt. 2.95 (*0-8125-3372-0*, Tor Books) T Doherty Assocs.

***Shaken Baby Syndrome: A Multidisciplinary Approach.** Ed. by Stephen Lazoritz & Vincent J. Palusci. 2001. LC 2001-51555. (*0-7890-1351-7*); pap. (*0-7890-1352-5*) Haworth Pr (Maltreatment & Trauma Pr).

***Shakespeare's Physic.** John Crawford Adams. 2000. LC 2001-347845. (Illus.). 192p. pap. (*1-85315-463-6*) Royal Soc of Medicine Pr Ltd GBR. *Dist:* Balogh.

***Shaking up Parkinson Disease: Fighting Like a Tiger, Thinking Like a Fox.** Abraham Lieberman. 2001. (Illus.). (C). pap. text 18.95 (*0-7637-1866-1*, 1866-1) Jones & Bartlett.

Shall I Study Pharmacy? AACP Staff. 7th ed. 1980. 32p. pap. 0.75 (*0-937526-08-8*) AACP Alexandria.

Shallow-Water Asteroidea & Ophiuroidea of Hawaii. Charles A. Ely. 1974. (BMB Ser.). (Illus.). reprint ed. 25.00 (*0-527-02284-5*) Periodicals Srv.

Shamanism: Activities & Index of New Information. James K. Hong. 1998. 57.50 (*0-7883-1836-5*); pap. 47.50 (*0-7883-1837-3*) ABBE Pubs Assn.

Shamanism: The Neural Ecology of Consciousness & Healing. Michael Winkelman. 2000. LC 99-40409. 336p. 65.00 (*0-89789-704-8*, Bergin & Garvey) Greenwood.

Shamanism & the Drug Propaganda: Patriarchy & the Drug War. Dan Russell. annot. unabr. ed. 1998. LC 98-91312. (Illus.). 357p. (Orig.). pap. 24.95 (*0-9650253-1-4*) Kalyx.com.

Shamans, Healers & Medicine. Holger Kalweit. 2000. (Illus.). 320p. pap. 17.95 (*1-57062-712-6*) Shambhala Pubns.

Shamans, Mystics & Doctors: A Psychological Inquiry into India & Its Healing Traditions. Sudhir Kakar. 1990. LC 90-20821. x, 320p. pap. text 16.00 (*0-226-42279-8*) U Ch Pr.

Shambaugh's Surgery of the Ear. Glasscock. 4th ed. 1990. (Illus.). 656p. text 179.00 (*0-7216-2063-9*) Saunders.

Shambhala Guide to Traditional Chinese Medicine. Daniel Reid. 1996. LC 95-23897. (Illus.). 224p. (Orig.). pap. 12.00 (*1-57062-141-1*) Shambhala Pubns.

Shame! An Other Guide for the Perplexed. John W. McGinley. 1993. LC 93-18431. 310p. (Orig.). (C). 58.00 (*0-8191-9093-4*); pap. 32.50 (*0-8191-9094-2*) U Pr of Amer.

Shame: Interpersonal Behavior, Psychopathology & Culture. Ed. by Paul Gilbert & Bernice Andrews. 1998. LC 97-44735. (Series in Affective Science). (Illus.). 304p. text 60.00 (*0-19-511479-5*) OUP.

Shame & Pride: Affect, Sex & the Birth of the Self. Donald L. Nathanson. 1994. 496p. pap. 18.95 (*0-393-31109-0*) Norton.

Shame Faced: The Road to Recovery. Kojiro Miyasaka. 1986. 28p. (Orig.). pap. 3.00 (*0-89486-358-4*, 5452B) Hazelden.

Shame, Guilt & Alcoholism: Treatment Issues in Clinical Practice. Ronald T. Potter-Efron. (Addiction Treatment Ser.: Vol. 2). 287p. 1989. LC 87-29724. text 8.95 (*0-86656-855-7*); 1988. LC 88-32058. pap. text 24.95 (*0-86656-856-5*, Harrington Park) Haworth Pr.

Shame of the States. Albert Deutsch. 1980. LC 73-2394. (Mental Illness & Social Policy; the American Experience Ser.). reprint ed. 19.95 (*0-405-05202-2*) Ayer.

Shang Han Lun: Wellspring of Chinese Medicine. Chang Chung-Ching. 1994. pap. 14.95 (*0-941942-02-3*) Orient Heal Arts.

Shang Han Lun & Other Traditional Formulas: A Clinical Reference. J. Michael Moore. 1993. LC 93-35804. (*0-941942-42-2*) Orient Heal Arts.

Shaolin Secret Formulas for the Treatment of External Injury. Monk De Qian. Tr. by Zhang Ting-liang & Bob Flaws from CHI. 2nd ed. 1995. 185p. 18.95 (*0-936185-08-2*) Blue Poppy Pr.

Shape Memory Implants. Ed. by L. Yahia. 2000. LC 00-38819. (Illus.). xxiii, 349p. 112.00 (*3-540-67229-X*) Spr-Verlag.

Shapedown: Just for Kids!, Level 3, Ages 11-12. Laurel M. Mellin. 5th ed. 1995. LC 88-70316. (Illus.). 202p. pap. 18.95 (*0-935902-23-6*) Balboa Pub.

Shaping an Integrated Delivery Network: Home Care's Role in Improving Service, Outcomes & Profitability. Connie R. Curran. 1998. LC 98-19918. 162p. 46.00 (*1-56793-085-9*) Health Admin Pr.

Shaping Effective Healthcare in Kenya: An Example for Developing Countries. Simon Kangethe. 1998. 96p. pap. 10.00 (*0-8059-4445-1*) Dorrance.

Shaping of a Profession: Physicians in Norway, Past & Present. Ivind Larsen & Bent O. Olsen. 1996. LC 96-46645. (*0-88135-168-7*) Watson Pub Intl.

Shaping of Modern Psychology. Leslie S. Hearnshaw. 1989. pap. 14.95 (*0-415-03903-7*) Routledge.

Shaping of Modern Psychology: An Historical Introduction. Leslie S. Hearnshaw. 1987. 408p. text 49.95 (*0-7102-0576-7*, 05767, Routledge Thoemms) Routledge.

Shaping of the Socio-Economic Systems. Thomas Baumgartmer et al. 1986. (Studies in Cybernetics: Vol. 11). xiv, 360p. text 106.00 (*2-88124-003-8*); pap. text 59.00 (*2-88124-027-5*) Gordon & Breach.

Shaping Psychology: How We Got Where We're Going. Timothy Gannon. 1991. (Sources in Semoitics Ser.: Vol. X). 322p. (C). 63.50 (*0-8191-7757-1*) U Pr of Amer.

Shaping the Future: Biology & Human Values. Steve Olson. 1989. 132p. 17.95 (*0-309-03947-9*) Natl Acad Pr.

Shaping the Future of Feminist Psychology: Education, Research, & Practice. Ed. by Judith Worell & Norine G. Johnson. 1997. LC 97-17947. (Psychology of Women Bks.). 266p. text 34.95 (*1-55798-448-4*, 431-6940) Am Psychol.

Share Borne by the Beneficiary of the Cost of Medical Care & of Medical Rehabilitation Supplies: (Situation at 1 July, 1988) Council of Europe Staff. 2nd ed. 1990. (*92-871-1858-2*) Council of Europe FRA. *Dist:* Manhattan Pub Co.

Share the Care: An Evaluation of a Family-Based Respite Care Service. Kirsten Stalker. 1990. 160p. 42.50 (*1-85302-038-9*) Taylor & Francis.

Share the Care: How to Organize a Group to Care For Someone Who is Seriously Ill. Cappy Capossela & Sheila Warnock. 1995. LC 95-34631. 288p. pap. 14.00 (*0-684-81136-7*, Fireside) S&S Trade Pap.

Shared Beliefs in a Society: Social Psychological Analysis. Daniel Bar-Tal. 2000. LC 00-8359. xviii, 211p. 53.95 (*0-7619-0658-4*, 53.95) Sage.

Shared Care: A Model for Clinical Management. Peter Edwards et al. 1996. LC 95-47038. 137p. pap. (*1-85775-165-5*) Radcliffe Med Pr GBR. *Dist:* Balogh.

***Shared Care for Hypertension.** Neil Poulter et al. 2001. (Shared Care Ser.). 200p. pap. (*1-899066-80-2*) Isis Med GBR. *Dist:* Bks Intl VA.

***Shared Care for Prostatic Diseases.** Fitzpatrick et al. Ed. by Roger Kirby. 2nd ed. 2001. (Illus.). 160p. pap. (*1-901865-60-6*) Isis Med GBR. *Dist:* Bks Intl VA.

***Shared Care in Mental Health.** Mynors-Wallace et al. 2001. (Shared Care Ser.). (Illus.). 224p. pap. (*1-901865-73-8*) Isis Med GBR. *Dist:* Bks Intl VA.

Shared Experience: The Psychoanalytic Dialogue. Luciana Nissim-Momigliano & Andreina Robutti. 1992. 272p. pap. text (*1-85575-034-1*) Karnac Bks GBR. *Dist:* Other Pr LLC.

Shared Governance Implementation Manual. Tim Porter-O'Grady. 1992. (Illus.). 208p. (C). (gr. 13). pap. text 36.95 (*0-8016-6317-2*, 06317) Mosby Inc.

Sharing Birth: A Father's Guide to Giving Support During Labor. Carl Jones. 1989. LC 89-6658. (Illus.). 195p. (Orig.). reprint ed. 29.95 (*0-89789-209-7*); pap. 12.95 (*0-89789-208-9*) Greenwood (Bergin & Garvey).

Sharing Care: The Integration of Family Approaches with Child Treatment. Robert G. Ziegler. 1999. LC 99-12989. 336p. pap. 39.95 (*0-87630-974-0*) Brunner-Routledge.

***Sharing Risk & Reward: Public-Private Collaboration to Eliminate Micronutrient Malnutrition.** Micronutrient Initiative Association Staff. 1996. (Micronutrient Initiative Ser.). 66p. pap. (*0-662-24368-4*) IDRC-CRDI CAN. *Dist:* Stylus Pub VA.

Sharpening Your Image: How to Get, Keep & Expand a Healthcare Business. Lisa Mosing. 1992. 238p. pap. 29.95 (*0-9633990-0-4*) Nutrition Wks.

Shattered Assumptions: Towards a New Psychology of Trauma. Ronnie Janoff-Bulman. 1992. LC 91-34496. 250p. 29.95 (*0-02-916015-4*) Free Pr.

Shattered Dreams: Healing the Hurt of Miscarriage & Stillbirths. Jacqueline Grekin. Date not set. pap. (*0-9659685-3-7*) J Grekin.

Shattered Images: The Phenomenological Language of Sexual Trauma. Dee Spring. 1993. LC 92-50849. (Illus.). 305p. pap. 29.95 (*0-9613309-2-9*) Magnolia St Pub.

Shattered Innocence: A Practical Guide for Counseling Women Survivors of Childhood Sexual Abuse. Neil Weiner & Sharon E. Robinson-Kurpius. 1995. LC 95-13954. 240p. 69.95 (*1-56032-347-7*) Taylor & Francis.

Shattered Mirrors: Our Search for Identity & Community in the AIDS Era. Monroe E. Price. 1989. LC 89-33265. 160p. text 32.00 (*0-674-80590-9*) HUP.

Shattered Self: A Psychoanalytic Study of Trauma. Richard B. Ulman & Doris Brothers. 1993. 344p. reprint ed. pap. text 29.95 (*0-88163-174-4*) Analytic Pr.

Shattered Selves: Multiple Personality in a Postmodern World. James M. Glass. 208p. 1995. pap. 15.95 (*0-8014-8256-9*); 1993. LC 92-33928. 39.95 (*0-8014-2809-2*) Cornell U Pr.

Shattering Myths & Mysteries of Alcohol: Insights & Answers to Drinking, Smoking & Drug Use. Raymond V. Haring. 1998. LC 97-94070. (Illus.). 264p. (Orig.). pap. 14.95 (*0-9643673-1-9*) Hlthspan.

She: Understanding Feminine Psychology. Robert A. Johnson. rev. ed. 1989. LC 89-45098. 96p. reprint ed. pap. 10.00 (*0-06-096397-2*, Perennial) HarperTrade.

She Never Said Goodbye: My Wife's Disappearance down a Road of No Return - Alzheimer's. George Vernon Ellison & Loy Young. Ed. by Wendy Ruiz. Tr. by Francine Dufour. 2000. LC 00-190041. (Illus.). 240p. pap. 19.95 (*1-882888-52-9*) Aquarius Hse.

She Speaks, He Listens: Women on the French Analysts' Couch. Elaine H. Baruch & Lucienne J. Serrano. 1995. 207p. (C). pap. 19.95 (*0-415-91127-3*) Routledge.

Shedding Life: Disease, Politics, & Other Human Conditions. Miroslav Holub. Tr. by David Young from CZE. 1997. LC 97-10712. 306p. 22.95 (*1-57131-217-X*) Milkweed Ed.

***Shedding Life: Disease, Politics & Other Human Conditions.** Miroslav Holub. Tr. by David Young. 2001. 279p. reprint ed. 23.00 (*0-7881-9769-X*) DIANE Pub.

Sheep Ailments: T. V. Vet Sheep Book. 6th ed. 1992. (T. V. Vet Ser.). (Illus.). 192p. (*0-85236-212-9*) Farming Pr GBR. *Dist:* Diamond Farm Bk.

Sheep & Goat Practice 2. Boden. 2nd ed. 1997. 223p. pap. text 55.00 (*0-7020-2330-2*) Saunders.

Sheep Diseases. A. Brightling. 1988. 54.95 (*0-909605-52-1*) Intl Spec Bk.

Sheffield Dawson Guide to Prognosis & Management of CAP & HAP. Lionel A. Mandell & Richard Wiederman. 1999. 90p. pap. 29.95 (*0-9668202-4-X*) S Dawson Pubs.

Sheffield Dawson Guide to Urinary Tract Infections. George A. Pankey. 2000. 70p. pap. 23.95 (*0-9668202-5-8*) S Dawson Pubs.

Shell & the Kernel: Renewals of Psychoanalysis. Nicholas Abraham & Maria Torok. Tr. by Nicholas T. Rand. 1994. LC 93-47621. (Illus.). 240p. pap. text 24.00 (*0-226-00088-5*); lib. bdg. 45.00 (*0-226-00087-7*) U Ch Pr.

Shell-Shock & Other Neuropsychiatric Problems Presented in Five Hundred & Eighty-Nine Case Histories from the War Literature, 1914-1918. Elmer E. Southard. 1973. LC 73-2416. (Mental Illness & Social Policy; the American Experience Ser.). reprint ed. 68.95 (*0-405-05226-X*) Ayer.

Shellfish & Public Health: Lead, Cadmium, Chromium, Arsenic, & Nickel in Shellfish. Michael A. Adams et al. 1994. (Illus.). 212p. (Orig.). (C). pap. text 50.00 (*0-7881-0588-4*) DIANE Pub.

Shen Nong Ben Cao Jing see Divine Farmer's Materia Medica: A Translation of the Shen Nong Ben Cao Jing

Shepard's Contemporary Health Care Issues. Ed. by James H. Cooper & Vera D. Cooper. 1994. LC 94-19056. (*0-07-172577-6*) Shepards.

Sherris Medical Microbiology. Kenneth J. Ryan. 4th ed. 1999. 74.95 (*0-8385-8529-9*, Medical Exam) Appleton & Lange.

Sherris Medical Microbiology. Kenneth J. Ryan. 3rd ed. 1999. LC 94-14526. (Illus.). 890p. (C). pap. text 69.95 (*0-8385-8541-8*, A8541-3, Apple Lange Med) McGraw.

Shiatzu Accupuncture Without a Needle. Yukiko Irwin. 1976. pap. 16.95 (*0-397-01107-5*) Lppncott W & W.

Shielding Techniques for Radiation Oncology Facilities. Patton H. McGinley. 1998. LC 97-36743. text 62.95 (*0-944838-81-2*) Med Physics Pub.

Shifting Contexts: The Generation of Effective Psychotherapy. Bill O'Hanlon & James Wilk. 1987. LC 86-26986. 289p. 38.00 (*0-89862-677-3*, 2677) Guilford Pubns.

Shifting Safety & Health Paradigms. F. David Pierce. 1996. 239p. text 75.00 (*0-86587-527-8*) Gov Insts.

Shifting Sands: Government-Group Relationships in the Health Care Sector. Joan P. Boase. 1994. LC 93-90659. (Canadian Public Administration Ser.). 240p. (*0-7735-1158-X*) McG-Queens Univ Pr CAN. *Dist:* CUP Services.

Shifting Sources of Power & Influence. Charles E. Dwyer. 1993. LC 92-74648. 80p. (Orig.). (C). pap. text 25.95 (*0-924674-12-1*) Am Coll Phys Execs.

Shiftwork in the 21st Century: Challenges for Research & Practice. Ed. by Sonia Hornberger et al. 2000. LC 00-50706. (Arbeitswissenschaft in der Betrieblichen Praxis Ser.: Vol. 17). (Illus.). 430p. (C). pap. text 52.95 (*0-8204-4364-6*) P Lang Pubng.

Shingles & PHN. Thomas C. Thomsen & Eleanor Mann. rev. ed. 1994. 168p. pap. 10.95 (*0-945288-03-4*) Cross River Pubns.

Shining Affliction: A Story of Harm & Healing in Psychotherapy. Annie G. Rogers. 1996. LC 94-45171. 336p. pap. 13.95 (*0-14-024012-8*, Penguin Bks) Penguin Putnam.

Shining Light on Constipation: Rectal Descent & Other Colon, Rectal & Anal Problems. Christopher J. Lahr. Ed. by Brian J. Lindgren. 1997. (Illus.). 112p. (Orig.). pap. 12.95 (*0-9648176-4-0*) Pink Hse.

Ship Captain's Medical Guide. Maritime and Coastguard Agency Staff. 22nd ed. 1999. (Illus.). 248p. (*0-11-551658-1*) Statnry Office GBR. *Dist:* Balogh, Bernan Associates.

***Ship of Thought.** Ed. by Duncan Barford. 2001. (*1-85575-286-7*) Karnac Bks GBR. *Dist:* Other Pr LLC.

Ship of Thought: Essays on Psychoanalysis & Learning. Ed. by Duncan Burford. 2000. (Encyclopedia of Psychoanalysis Ser.: Vol. 4). 250p. pap. (*1-900877-25-2*) Rebus Pr Ltd GBR. *Dist:* Intl Spec Bk.

Ship's Doctor. Terrence Riley. 1995. LC 95-8186. (Illus.). 312p. 34.95 (*1-55750-721-X*) Naval Inst Pr.

Ships' Medicine Chest & Medical Aid at Sea, Set. 1994. lib. bdg. 595.00 (*0-8490-5746-9*) Gordon Pr.

Shisandra Berry, Schisandra Chinensis: Analytical, Quality Control & Therapeutic Monograph. Roy Upton et al. 1999. (Illus.). 25p. 19.95 (*1-929425-05-8*) Amer Herbal.

Shock: Metabolism, Physiology & Therapeutics. Ed. by James B. Heneghan. 1990. 49.95 (*0-915340-17-8*) PJD Pubns.

Shock & Resuscitation. Ed. by Evan R. Geller. 1993. (Illus.). 592p. text 75.00 (*0-07-023500-7*) McGraw-Hill Educ Grp.

Shock & the Adult Respiratory Distress Syndrome. Ed. by W. J. Kox & D. J. Bihari. 1990. (Current Concepts in Critical Care Ser.). (Illus.). 238p. 46.95 (*0-387-17484-2*) Spr-Verlag.

Shock, from Molecular & Cellular Level to Whole Body: Proceedings of the Third International Shock Congress, Shock '95, Hamamatsu, Japan, 21-23 October 1995. Ed. by Kazuo Okada & Hiromaru Ogata. 1996. LC 96-5881. (International Congress Ser.: No. 1102). 410p. 194.50 (*0-444-82285-2*) Elsevier.

Shock, Sepsis & Organ Failure: I-Brain Damage Secondary to Hemorrhagic-Traumatic Shock: II-Brain Damage Secondary to Sepsis: III-Brain Damage Secondary to Traumatic Brain Injury. Gunther O. Schlag et al. 1997. LC 96-40408. (*0-387-62419-8*) Spr-Verlag.

Shock, Sepsis & Organ Failure: I-Brain Damage Secondary to Hemorrhagic-Traumatic Shock: II-Brain Damage Secondary to Sepsis: III-Brain Damage Secondary to Traumatic Brain Injury. Daniel L. Traber. 1997. LC 96-40408. (Illus.). 304p. 98.00 (*3-540-62419-8*) Spr-Verlag.

Shock, Sepsis, & Organ Failure: Proceedings of the 3rd Wiggers-Bernard Conference on Cytokine Networks, 1992, Styria Austria. Ed. by Gunther O. Schlag et al. 1995. LC 93-12635. (Illus.). 426p. 89.00 (*0-387-55339-8*) Spr-Verlag.

Shock, Sepsis & Organ Failure: Scavenging of Nitric Oxide & Inhibition of Its Production, Sixth Wiggers Bernard Conference 1997. Ed. by Guenther Schlag & Heinz Redl. 1999. LC 98-36986. (Illus.). 307p. 132.00 (*3-540-64544-6*) Spr-Verlag.

Shock, Sepsis & Organ Failure-Nitric Oxide. Ed. by Gunther O. Schlag & H. Redl. 1995. (Illus.). 488p. 140.00 (*3-540-58549-4*) Spr-Verlag.

Shock Wave Lithotripsy Vol. 1: State of the Art. Ed. by James E. Lingeman & D. M. Newman. 1988. (Illus.). 432p. 110.00 (*0-306-43112-2*, Plenum Trade) Perseus Pubng.

Shock Wave Lithotripsy Vol. 2: Urinary & Biliary Lithotripsy. Ed. by James E. Lingeman & D. M. Newman. 1989. LC 89-70948. (Illus.). 476p. 110.00 (*0-306-43416-4*, Plenum Trade) Perseus Pubng.

Shocks to the System: Psychotherapy of Traumatic Disability Syndromes. Laurence Miller. 1998. LC 98-14545. 256p. 40.00 (*0-393-70256-1*) Norton.

Shook over Hell: Post-Traumatic Stress, Vietnam, & the Civil War. Eric T. Dean, Jr. 1997. LC 97-9737. (Illus.). 352p. 37.95 (*0-674-80651-4*) HUP.

Shop Talk: A Prevocational Language Program for Students with Developmental Disabilities. Louise Kent-Udolf & Eileen R. Sherman. 1983. LC 83-61810. 236p. pap. text 25.95 (*0-87822-229-4*, 2294) Res Press.

***Shopping for Assisted Living: What Customers Need to Make the Best Buy: Congressional Hearing.** Ed. by Charles E. Grassley. 2001. 221p. (C). reprint ed. pap. 35.00 (*0-7567-0979-2*) DIANE Pub.

Short Account of the Malignant Fever, Lately Prevalent in Philadelphia: With a Statement of the Proceedings That Took Place on the Subject in Different Parts of the United States. Mathew Carey. 1970. LC 73-112531. (Rise of Urban America Ser.). reprint ed. 16.95 (*0-405-02441-X*) Ayer.

Short & Long Term Effects of Breast Feeding on Child Health. Ed. by Berthold Koletzko et al. 2000. LC 00-34930. (Advances in Experimental Medicine & Biology Ser.: Vol. 478). (Illus.). xiii, 447p. 105.00 (*0-306-46405-5*, Kluwer Plenum) Kluwer Academic.

Short & Profitable Treatise Touching the Cure of the Morbus Gallicus by Unctions. William Clowes. 1972. LC 75-38166. (English Experience Ser.: No. 443). 118p. reprint ed. 20.00 (*90-221-0443-5*) Walter J Johnson.

***Short Answer Questions for the FRCA,** Pt. 2. Maher Michel et al. 2001. 219p. pap. (*0-443-06409-1*) Church GBR. *Dist:* Saunders.

Short Cases for Pediatric Exams. Adam Glasser et al. 2000. LC 99-57054. (Illus.). 225p. pap. text (*0-7020-2162-8*) W B Saunders GBR. *Dist:* Saunders.

Short Cases for the MRCP. Charles R. Hind. 2nd ed. 1990. 172p. pap. text (*0-443-04190-3*) Church.

***Short Cases in General Surgery.** Ramachandran. 2001. (Illus.). 427p. pap. (*0-443-07044-X*) Church GBR. *Dist:* Saunders.

***Short Cases in Paediatrics.** Alan Cade & Donald Hodge. 2000. (Greenwich Medical Media Ser.). (Illus.). 244p. (*1-84110-009-9*) Greenwich Med GBR. *Dist:* JAMCO Dist.

Short Course in Adolescent Psychiatry. Ed. by Joseph R. Novello. 1994. LC 93-74373. (Master Work Ser.). 288p. pap. 45.00 (*1-56821-195-3*) Aronson.

Short Course in Clinical Pharmacokinetics. Dennis A. Noe. 1994. LC 93-74962. 154p. (Orig.). (C). pap. 27.00 (*0-915486-19-9*) Applied Therapeutics.

Short Course in Pathology. Nancy Standler. 1994. LC 94-3037. pap. text (*0-443-08955-8*) Church.

Short Dialysis. Ed. by Vincenzo Cambi. 1987. (Topics in Renal Medicine Ser.). (C). text 183.50 (*0-89838-858-9*) Kluwer Academic.

***Short Essay Questions for MRCOG Part 2: A Self-Assessment Guide.** Pallavi Latthe et al. 2001. (Arnold Publication). 288p. (Orig.). pap. text 29.50 (*0-340-76255-1*) OUP.

Short History of Anaesthesia: The First 150 Years. G. B. Rusham et al. 1996. LC 96-31494. 218p. pap. text 37.50 (*0-7506-3066-3*) Buttrwrth-Heinemann.

Short History of Aryan Medical Science. Bhagavat Simhaji. LC 75-23683. reprint ed. 45.00 (*0-404-13236-7*) AMS Pr.

Short History of Biology. Isaac Asimov. 1980. LC 80-15464. (American Museum Science Bks.). (Illus.). 189p. reprint ed. lib. bdg. 47.50 (*0-313-22583-4*, ASSB, Greenwood Pr) Greenwood.

Short History of Breast Cancer. Daniel De Moulin. 1983. lib. bdg. 32.50 (*90-247-2814-2*) Kluwer Academic.

Short History of British Psychology, 1840-1940. Leslie S. Hearnshaw. 1986. LC 86-22840. (Methuen's Manuals of Modern Psychology Ser.). 342p. reprint ed. lib. bdg. 92.50 (*0-313-25278-5*, HEAS, Greenwood Pr) Greenwood.

Short History of Cardiology. James B. Herrick. LC 75-23720. reprint ed. 49.50 (*0-404-13278-2*) AMS Pr.

Short History of Medical Ethics. Albert R. Jonsen. 1999. LC 99-14646. 168p. text 34.95 (*0-19-513455-9*) OUP.

Short History of Medicine. Erwin H. Ackerknecht. rev. ed. 1982. LC 81-48194. 304p. (C). reprint ed. pap. text 17.95 (*0-8018-2726-4*) Johns Hopkins.

Short History of Nautical Medicine. Louis H. Roddis. LC 75-23757. reprint ed. 39.50 (*0-404-13363-0*) AMS Pr.

Short History of Neurology. F. Clifford Rose. 1999. LC 99-10462. 282p. pap. text 50.00 (*0-7506-4165-7*) Buttrwrth-Heinemann.

Short History of Surgery. D'Arcy Power. LC 75-23751. reprint ed. 32.50 (*0-404-13357-6*) AMS Pr.

Short History of the Early American Microscopes, Vol. 12. Donald L. Padgitt. 1975. LC 74-30750. (Illus.). 30.00 (*0-904962-04-0*) Microscope Pubns.

Short History of Tuberculosis. George N. Meachen. LC 75-23738. reprint ed. 31.50 (*0-404-13295-2*) AMS Pr.

Short History Western Civilizations, Vol. 2. Joyce E. Salisbury. 8th ed. 1993. (C). pap., stu. ed. 16.88 (*0-07-026903-3*) McGraw-H Hghr Educ.

Short Practice of Spinal Surgery. Henry V. Crock. 2nd ed. 1993. (Illus.). 319p. 154.00 (*3-211-82351-4*); LC 92-48889. 344p. 169.00 (*0-387-82351-4*) Spr-Verlag.

Short-Term Approaches to Psychotheraphy. Ed. by Henry Grayson & Paul T. Olsen. 1979. LC 78-27605. (New Directions in Psychotherapy Ser.: Vol. III). 285p. 35.95 (*0-87705-345-6*, Kluwer Acad Hman Sci) Kluwer Academic.

Short-Term Counseling: A Psychoanalytic Approach. Barbara W. Tilley. 1985. LC 84-9008. xii, 358p. (C). 52.50 (*0-8236-6072-9*, BN#06072) Intl Univs Pr.

Short-Term Counseling: Guidelines Based on Recent Research. Irving L. Janis. 1983. LC 83-3488. 240p. pap. 16.00 (*0-300-03125-4*, Y-480) Yale U Pr.

Short-Term Counseling: Theory & Practice. Kathleen Black. 1982. pap. (*0-201-00073-3*, 00073, Health Sci) Addison-Wesley.

Short-Term Couple Therapy. Ed. by James M. Donovan. 1999. LC 98-32163. (Guilford Family Therapy Ser.). (Illus.). 417p. text 45.00 (*1-57230-431-6*, C0431) Guilford Pubns.

Short-Term Couples Therapy Bk. 8027: The Imago Model in Action. Wade Luquet. 1996. LC 96-1961. 224p. pap. text 47.95 (*0-87630-802-7*) Brunner-Routledge.

Short-Term Dynamic Hypnotherapy & Hypnoanalysis: Clinical Research & Treatment Strategies. Milton V. Kline. 1992. (Illus.). 334p. (C). text 65.95 (*0-398-05796-6*) C C Thomas.

Short-Term Dynamic Psychotherapy: Evaluation & Technique. Peter E. Sifneos. 2nd ed. 1987. LC 87-2346. (Topics in General Psychiatry Ser.). (Illus.). 348p. (C). text 54.00 (*0-306-42341-3*, Kluwer Plenum) Kluwer Academic.

Short-Term Family Therapy with Borderline Patients. Craig A. Everett & Sandra Volgy-Everett. 1998. 200p. (C). pap. text 29.95 (*1-884228-25-9*) Geist & Russell.

Short-Term Play Therapy for Disruptive Children. Cheryl B. McNeel et al. 1996. 129p. 37.95 (*1-882732-51-0*) Childswork.

Short-Term Psychotherapy & Brief Treatment Techniques: An Annotated Bibliography, 1920-1980. Harvey P. Mandel. 1981. LC 81-221. 704p. 95.00 (*0-306-40658-6*, Plenum Trade) Perseus Pubng.

Short-Term Psychotherapy & Emotional Crisis. Peter E. Sifneos. 1972. LC 78-172323. (Illus.). 219p. 36.95 (*0-674-80720-0*) HUP.

Short-Term Tests for Chemical Carcinogens. Ed. by H. F. Stich & R. H. San. 1981. (Topics in Environmental Physiology & Medicine Ser.). (Illus.). 518p. 227.00 (*0-387-90496-4*) Spr-Verlag.

***Short Term Therapy, Long Term Change.** Marion Solomon et al. 2001. LC 2001-30684. (Professional Book Ser.). (Illus.). 256p. 28.00 (*0-393-70333-9*) Norton.

Short-Term Therapy Techniques. Christ L. Zois & Margaret Scarpa. 1997. LC 96-26113. 352p. 50.00 (*0-7657-0026-3*) Aronson.

Short-Term Therapy with Children: A Multi-Modal Approach to Helping Children with Their Problems. Lawrence E. Shapiro. rev. ed. 1994. (Illus.). xiii, 213 p. text 34.95 (*1-882732-13-8*) Childswork.

Short-Term Treatment in Occupational Therapy. Diane Gibson & Kathy Kaplan. 1984. LC 84-9115. (Occupational Therapy in Mental Health Ser.: Vol. 4, No. 3). 114p. 39.95 (*0-86656-342-3*) Haworth Pr.

Short Text Book of Surgery, Vol. II. B. P. Chatterjee. 1989. (C). (*0-89771-365-6*); (*0-89771-364-8*) Current Dist IND. *Dist:* St Mut.

Short Textbook of Clinical Imaging. Ed. by D. Sutton & J. W. Young. 1990. (Illus.). 868p. 155.00 (*0-387-19592-0*) Spr-Verlag.

Short Textbook of Clinical Imaging. David Sutton & Jeremy W. Young. 1990. 856p. 145.00 (*3-540-19592-0*) Spr-Verlag.

Short Textbook of Medical Jurisprudence. C. C. Mallik. 1985. (*0-7855-0749-3*) Current Dist IND. *Dist:* St Mut.

Short Textbook of Otolaryngology. A. L. Mukherjee. 1985. (*0-7855-0825-2*) Current Dist IND. *Dist:* St Mut.

Short Textbook of Radiotherapy. H. Miller et al. 4th ed. 1979. (Illus.). 299p. (*0-443-01389-6*) Church.

Short Title Catalogue of Eighteenth Century Printed Books in the National Library of Medicine. John Blake. 1998. 501p. reprint ed. 75.00 (*1-57898-086-0*) Martino Pubng.

Shorter Term Treatments for Borderline Personality Disorders. John D. Preston. 1997. LC 97-66082. 184p. text 49.95 (*1-57224-092-X*) New Harbinger.

Shortest Distance: The Pursuit of Independence for Persons with Acquired Brain Injury. Ed. by Brian T. McMahon & Randall W. Evans. 1994. LC 93-87363. 156p. (C). per. 47.95 (*1-878205-68-4*) St Lucie Pr.

Shortness of Breath: A Guide to Better Living & Breathing. Andrew L. Ries. 6th ed. 2000. LC 00-40197. (Illus.). xvii, 133p. pap. 9.95 (*0-323-01064-4*) Mosby Inc.

***Shots in the Dark: The Wayward Search for an AIDS Vaccine.** Jon Cohen. 2001. 464p. reprint ed. pap. 15.95 (*0-393-32225-4*) Norton.

Shots in the Dark: The Wayward Search for the AIDS Vaccine. Jon Cohen. 2001. LC 00-61635. (Illus.). 384p. 27.95 (*0-393-05027-0*) Norton.

Should Healthy People Pay More for Health Insurance? John C. Goodman. 1992. (Illus.). 17p. pap. 5.00 (*0-943802-94-6*, BG115) Natl Ctr Pol.

Should Medical Care Be Rationed by Age? Ed. by Timothy M. Smeeding et al. 1987. 192p. 57.00 (*0-8476-7521-1*) Rowman.

Should Psychology Be a Science? Pros & Cons. Jock Abra. 1998. LC 97-21853. 272p. 72.50 (*0-275-95476-5*, Praeger Pubs) Greenwood.

Should the Baby Live? The Problem of Handicapped Infants. Helga Kuhse & Peter Albert David Singer. 1994. (Modern Revivals in Philosophy Ser.). 240p. (*0-7512-0313-0*) Gregg Revivals GBR. *Dist:* Ashgate Pub Co.

Shoulder. Ed. by Carter R. Rowe. 1987. (Illus.). 1988p. text (*0-443-08457-2*) Church.

Shoulder Charles A. Rockwood, Jr. & Frederick A. Matsen, III, 3rd. Ed. by Lew Reines. 2nd ed. 1998. (Illus.). 1472p. (C). text 225.00 (*0-7216-8134-4*) Saunders.

Shoulder: A Method of Evaluation & Assessment. David W. Altchek. 1995. 160p. 55.00 (*0-07-001284-9*) McGraw.

Shoulder: Operative Technique. Melvin Post et al. 1998. LC 97-42619. 400p. text 129.00 (*0-683-06947-0*) Lppncott W & W.

Shoulder: Periarticular Degenerative Pathology. Ed. by L. Celli. Tr. by S. Notini. 1991. (Current Concepts in Orthopedic Surgery Ser.: Vol. 1). (Illus.). 144p. 135.00 (*0-387-82219-4*) Spr-Verlag.

Shoulder: Rupture of the Supraspinatus Tension & Other Lesions in or about the Subacronial Bursa. E. A. Codman. 1984. LC 83-25154. 495p. reprint ed. 84.50 (*0-89874-731-7*) Krieger.

Shoulder & Elbow, Vols. 5 & 5a. Jules R. Kalisch & Harold Williams. 1970. (Courtroom Medicine Ser.). 417.00 (*0-8205-1246-X*, 246) Bender.

Shoulder Arthrography. Ed. by Amy B. Goldman et al. 1982. 52.50 (*0-316-31931-7*, Little Brwn Med Div) Lppncott W & W.

Shoulder Arthroplasty. Ed. by Gilles Walch & Pascal Boileau. 1998. LC 97-29884. (Illus.). 466p. 185.00 (*3-540-63349-9*) Spr-Verlag.

Shoulder Arthroscopy. Stephen J. Snyder. 1994. (Illus.). 271p. text 175.00 (*0-07-059526-7*) McGraw-Hill Educ Grp.

Shoulder in Hemiplegia. Rene Cailliet. 1980. LC 79-18598. (Illus.). 130p. text 15.95 (*0-8036-1602-3*) Davis Co.

Shoulder Injuries in Sport: Evaluation, Treatment, & Rehabilitation. Jerome V. Ciullo. 1996. LC 95-41120. (Illus.). 304p. text 62.00 (*0-87322-651-8*, BCIU0651) Human Kinetics.

Shoulder Injuries in the Athlete: Surgical Repair & Rehabilitation. Ed. by Richard J. Hawkins & Gary W. Misamore. 1995. LC 95-36792. (Illus.). 470p. text (*0-443-08947-7*) Church.

Shoulder (Master Techniques in Orthopaedic Surgery) Master Techniques in Orthopaedic Surgery. Ed. by Edward V. Craig. 1995. (Master Techniques in Orthopaedic Surgery Ser.). (Illus.). 496p. text 199.00 (*0-7817-0035-3*) Lppncott W & W.

Shoulder Pain. Rene Cailliet. 3rd ed. 1991. LC 91-9421. (Pain Ser.). (Illus.). 277p. pap. 21.95 (*0-8036-1614-7*) Davis Co.

Shoulder Pathophysiology: Rehabilitation & Treatment. Scott V. Haig. 1988. 360p. 65.00 (*0-8342-0622-6*) PRO-ED.

Shoulder Reconstruction. Neer. 1990. 624p. text 189.00 (*0-7216-2832-X*) Saunders.

Shoulder Replacement. Ed. by R. Kolbel et al. Tr. by Terry C. Telger from GER. 1987. (Illus.). 222p. 97.00 (*0-387-17129-0*) Spr-Verlag.

Shoulder Surgery. Copeland. 1996. text 102.00 (*0-7020-2063-X*) Saunders.

Shoulder Trauma. Hawkins. 1998. text (*0-443-07565-4*) Church.

Shoulders, Upper Back & Neck: Free Yourself from Pain! Rosemarie Atencio. 1995. LC 94-79485. (Illus.). 128p. (Orig.). pap. 17.95 (*0-9637360-9-4*) HWD Pub.

Shouldn't I Be Happy? Emotional Problems of Pregnant & Postpartum Women. Shaila Misri. 2000. 340p. reprint ed. text 23.00 (*0-7881-6879-7*) DIANE Pub.

Shouldn't I Be Happy? Emotional Problems of Pregnant & Postpartum Women. Shaila Misri. 1995. LC 95-2848. 368p. 23.00 (*0-02-921405-X*) Free Pr.

Show Me How: A Manual for Parents of Preschool Visually Impaired & Blind Children. Mary Brennan. 1982. 56p. pap. 12.95 (*0-89128-113-4*) Am Foun Blind.

Shrink Rap: Sixty Psychotherapists Discuss Their Work, Their Lives, & the State of Their Field. Lee D. Kassan. 1996. LC 96-18541. 600p. 50.00 (*0-7657-0017-4*) Aronson.

Shrink to Fit: Answers to Your Questions about Therapy. Dale A. Masi et al. 1998. LC 98-38164. 200p. pap. 10.95 (*1-55874-620-X*) Health Comm.

Shrink Yourself. Ted Meyer. 2001. LC 00-45835. (Illus.). x, 85p. pap. 9.95 (*0-312-27222-7*) St Martin.

Shrinks: The Analysts Analyzed. James Park. 1993. 224p. text 34.95 (*0-7475-0794-5*) Trafalgar.

Shunts & Problems in Shunts. Ed. by M. Choux. 1982. (Monographs in Neural Sciences: Vol. 8). (Illus.). x, 230p. pap. 100.00 (*3-8055-2465-X*) S Karger.

Shy Children, Phobic Adults: Nature & Treatment of Social Phobia. Deborah C. Beidel & Samuel M. Turner. 1997. LC 97-33477. 324p. 39.95 (*1-55798-461-1*) Am Psychol.

Shyness. Philip G. Zimbardo. 2000. pap. 15.00 (*0-201-55018-0*) Perseus Bks Grp.

Shyness & Embarrassment: Perspectives from Social Psychology. Ed. by W. Ray Crozier. 1990. (Illus.). 375p. (C). text 69.95 (*0-521-35529-X*) Cambridge U Pr.

Shyness & Social Anxiety Workbook: Proven Techniques for Overcoming Your Fears. Martin M. Anthony et al. 2000. LC 00-134875. 256p. pap., wbk. ed. 15.95 (*1-57224-216-7*) New Harbinger.

Si Su Hijo Tartamudea: Una Guia Para los Padres. 1990. (Publications on Stuttering: No. 15). (SPA.). 48p. pap. 1.00 (*0-933388-12-8*) Stuttering Fnd Am.

SI Units for Clinical Measurement. Ed. by Donald S. Young & Edward J. Huth. 1997. LC 96-30174. (Medical Writing & Communication Ser.). 331p. (Orig.). (C). pap. text 36.00 (*0-943126-51-7*) Amer Coll Phys.

Sialadenosis & Sialadenitis. Ed. by R. Chilla. 1981. (Advances in OtoRhinoLaryngology Ser.: Vol. 26). (Illus.). viii, 252p. 137.50 (*3-8055-1669-X*) S Karger.

Sialic Acids: Chemistry, Metabolism, & Function. Ed. by R. Schauer. 1983. (Cell Biology Monographs: Vol. 10). (Illus.). 344p. 144.95 (*0-387-81707-7*) Spr-Verlag.

Sibling Abuse Trauma: Assessment & Intervention Strategies for Children, Families & Adults. John V. Caffaro & Allison Conn-Caffaro. 1998. LC 98-8166. (Illus.). 303p. 49.95 (*0-7890-6007-8*, Maltreatment & Trauma Pr) Haworth Pr.

Sibling Abuse Trauma: Assessment & Intervention Strategies for Children, Families, & Adults. John V. Caffaro & Allison Conn-Caffaro. 1998. LC 98-8166. (Illus.). 303p. pap. 24.95 (*0-7890-0491-7*, Maltreatment & Trauma Pr) Haworth Pr.

Sibling Interaction Across Cultures. Ed. by P. G. Zukow. 1988. 207p. 71.95 (*0-387-96784-2*) Spr-Verlag.

Sibling Relationships: Their Nature & Significance Across the Lifespan. Ed. by Michael E. Lamb & Brian Sutton-Smith. 1982. 416p. 79.95 (*0-89859-189-9*) L Erlbaum Assocs.

Sibling Relationships Vol. 10: Their Causes & Consequences. Judy Dunn et al. Ed. by Gene H. Brody. 1996. (Advances in Applied Developmental Psychology Ser.). (Illus.). 263p. pap. 39.50 (*1-56750-181-8*);10. LC 96-136098. 73.25 (*1-56750-180-X*) Greenwood (Ablex).

Sibling Relationships Across the Life Span. Victor G. Cicirelli. 1995. LC 95-18584. (Illus.). 268p. (C). 45.00 (*0-306-45025-9*, Kluwer Plenum) Kluwer Academic.

Siblings: Love, Envy, & Understanding. Judy Dunn & Carol Kendrick. 1982. LC 81-7251. (Developing Child Ser.). (Illus.). 304p. 37.95 (*0-674-80735-9*) HUP.

Siblings in the Unconscious & Psychopathology: Womb Fantasies, Claustrophobias, Fear of Pregnancy, Murderous Rage, Animal Symbolism, Christmas & Easter Neuroses, & Twinnings or Identifications with Sisters & Brothers. Vamik D. Volkan & Gabriele Ast. 1997. LC 96-30832. 184p. 27.50 (*0-8236-6067-2*) Intl Univs Pr.

Siblings in Therapy: Life Span & Clinical Issues. Ed. by Michael D. Kahn & Karen G. Lewis. 1988. (Professional Bks.). (Illus.). 469p. 34.95 (*0-393-70058-5*) Norton.

Siblings of Children with Autism: A Guide for Families. Sandra L. Harris. Ed. by Michael D. Powers. 1994. LC 94-18177. (Topics in Autism Ser.). 127p. (Orig.). pap. 12.95 (*0-933149-71-9*) Woodbine House.

Sicilian Folk Medicine. Giuseppe Pitre. 1971. (Illus.). 320p. 48.50 (*0-87291-013-X*) Coronado Pr.

Sick & Tired of Being Sick & Tired: Black Women's Health Activism in America, 1890-1950. Susan L. Smith. 1995. LC 95-11310. (Studies in Health, Illness, & Caregiving). (Illus.). 288p. pap. text 16.95 (*0-8122-1449-8*) U of Pa Pr.

Sick & Tired of Feeling Sick & Tired: Living with Invisible Chronic Illness. Paul J. Donoghue & Mary E. Siegel. 2000. LC 2001-267010. xxii, 284p. pap. 14.95 (*0-393-32065-0*); 1992. LC 92-6400. 288p. 22.95 (*0-393-03408-9*) Norton.

Sick Building Syndrome: How Indoor Air Pollution Is Poisoning Your Life & What You Can Do. Nicholas Tate. 1993. 23.95 (*0-88282-085-0*); LC 93-84519. 182p. pap. 13.95 (*0-88282-082-6*) New Horizon NJ.

Sick Building Syndrome: Sources, Health Effects, Mitigation. M. C. Baechler et al. 1992. LC 91-20423. (Pollution Technology Review Ser.: No. 205). (Illus.). 328p. 98.00 (*0-8155-1289-9*) Noyes.

Sick Building Syndromes & Distressed Employees: Index of New Information. Dennis D. Patuznik. 1998. 160p. 57.50 (*0-7883-1754-7*); pap. 47.50 (*0-7883-1755-5*) ABBE Pubs Assn.

Sick Newborn Baby. Christopher J. Kelnar. 3rd ed. 1995. pap. text 30.00 (*0-7020-1647-0*) Saunders.

Sick, Not Dead: The Health of British Workingmen During the Mortality Decline. James C. Riley. 1997. LC 96-26961. 384p. 61.00 (*0-8018-5411-3*) Johns Hopkins.

Sick Not Sick: A Guide to Rapid Patient Assessment. Mike Helbock et al. 2000. LC 99-40734. (Illus.). 104p. (C). pap. text 26.95 (*0-7637-1191-8*, 1191-8) Jones & Bartlett.

Sicke Womans Private Looking Glasse Wherein Methodically Are Handled All Uterine Affects, or Diseases Arising from Ye Wombe. John Sadler. 1977. LC 77-7430. (English Experience Ser.: No. 891). reprint ed. lib. bdg. 25.00 (*90-221-0891-0*) Walter J Johnson.

Sickle Cell Anemia. Anthony Cerami & Washington. 1973. LC 72-93681. 25.95 (*0-89388-068-X*) Okpaku Communications.

Sickle Cell Anemia: A Source Guide. 1991. lib. bdg. 250.00 (*0-8490-4868-0*) Gordon Pr.

Sickle Cell Disease. Jacqueline L. Harris. 2001. LC 00-47932. (Medical Library). (Illus.). 96p. (J). 24.90 (*0-7613-1459-8*) TFC Bks NY.

Sickle Cell Disease: Basic Principles & Clinical Practice. Ed. by Stephen H. Embury et al. 1994. LC 93-50787. 928p. text 169.00 (*0-7817-0142-2*) Lppncott W & W.

Sickle Cell Disease: Pathophysiology, Diagnosis, & Management. Ed. by Vipul N. Mankad & Blaine R. Moore. 1992. LC 91-32168. 432p. 100.00 (*0-275-92503-X*, C2503, Praeger Pubs) Greenwood.

Sickle Cell Disease: Screening, Diagnosis, Management & Counseling in Newborns & Infants. 1994. lib. bdg. 250.00 (*0-8490-8401-6*) Gordon Pr.

Sickle Cell Disease: Screening, Diagnosis, Management, & Counseling in Newborns & Infants. 1995. lib. bdg. 253.99 (*0-8490-6805-3*) Gordon Pr.

Sickle Cell Disease: Screening, Diagnosis, Management, & Counseling in Newborns & Infants. Jeanne A. Smith & Thomas R. Kinney. Ed. by Mary L. Grady. 1997. (Illus.). 97p. reprint ed. pap. text 25.00 (*0-7881-4703-X*) DIANE Pub.

Sickle Cell Pain. Samir K. Ballas. 1998. LC 98-2595. (Progress in Pain Research & Management Ser.: Vol. 11). (Illus.). 389p. 87.00 (*0-931092-22-1*) Intl Assn Study Pain.

Sickled Cell: From Myths to Molecules. Stuart J. Edelstein. 1986. LC 86-2003. (Illus.). 224p. 44.50 (*0-674-80737-5*) HUP.

Sickness & Health in America: Readings in the History of Medicine & Public Health. Ed. by Judith W. Leavitt & Ronald L. Numbers. 3rd rev. ed. 1997. LC 96-44916. (Illus.). 600p. 65.00 (*0-299-15320-7*); pap. 29.95 (*0-299-15324-X*) U of Wis Pr.

Sickness & Senility Are Unnecessary. Leon De Seblo. 1996. 111p. reprint ed. spiral bd. 13.50 (*0-7873-0270-8*) Hlth Research.

Sickness & the State: Health & Illness in Colonial Malaya, 1870-1940. Lenore Manderson. 1996. LC 95-42786. (Illus.). 335p. (C). text 64.95 (*0-521-56008-X*) Cambridge U Pr.

Sickness in Small Scale Industries. K. C. Reddy. 1988. (C). (*81-7024-212-6*) Ashish Pub Hse IND. *Dist:* S Asia.

Side-Effects of Anti-Inflamatory Drugs 3. Ed. by Kim D. Rainsford & G. P. Velo. 1992. (Inflammation & Drug Therapy Ser.). (C). text 223.00 (*0-7923-8966-2*) Kluwer Academic.

Side Effects of Anti-Inflammatory Drugs IV. Ed. by K. D. Rainsford. 1997. LC 97-180927. 384p. text 234.00 (*0-7923-8713-9*) Kluwer Academic.

Side Effects of Drugs Annual, 18. Ed. by J. K. Aronson & C. J. Van Boxtel. 1995. 558p. 233.50 (*0-444-81939-8*) Elsevier.

Side Effects of Drugs Annual: A Worldwide Yearly Survey of New Data & Trends, Vol. 21. J. K. Aronson. 1998. 590p. 197.00 (*0-444-82818-4*) Elsevier.

Side Effects of Drugs Annual 15, 1991, Vol. 15. M. N. Dukes & J. K. Aronson. 1991. 586p. 216.50 (*0-444-89171-4*) Elsevier.

Side Effects of Drugs Annual 17: A Worldwide Yearly Critical Survey of New Data & Trends. Ed. by J. K. Aronson & C. J. Van Boxtel. 1994. 648p. 228.00 (*0-444-82005-1*) Elsevier.

Side Effects of Drugs Annual 16: A Yearly Critical Survey of the World's Literature on Adverse Reactions to Drugs. Ed. by M. N. Dukes & J. K. Aronson. 1993. 646p. 221.00 (*0-444-89657-0*) Elsevier.

Side Effects of Estrogen Drug Therapy. Harold E. Simmons. 1979. pap. 8.00 (*0-87312-007-8*) Psychogenic Disease.

Sideline Help. Marshall K. Steele, III. 1996. LC 95-38863. (Illus.). 152p. pap. 14.95 (*0-87322-786-7*, PSTE0786) Human Kinetics.

Sidney M. Jourard: Selected Writings. Ed. by Michael Lowman et al. 1994. (Illus.). 371p. (Orig.). (C). pap. text 23.95 (*0-917982-49-5*) Capitol Enquiry.

SIDS Survival Guide: Information & Comfort for Grieving Family & Friends & Professionals Who Seek to Help Them. Joani N. Horchler & Robin D. Morris. 1994. LC 94-66748. (Illus.). 290p. (Orig.). pap. 14.95 (*0-9641218-7-5*) SIDS Educ Srvs.

Sieben S-Immunglobulin Zur Intravenoesen Anwendung. Ed. by F. R. Seiler & R. G. Geursen. 1982. (Beitraege zur Infusionstherapie und Klinische Ernaehrung Ser.: Vol. 9). (Illus.). viii, 176p. pap. 43.50 (*3-8055-3632-1*) S Karger.

Siete Necesidades Basicas Del Nino: Seven Things Children Need. John M. Drescher. 1983. (SPA.). 128p. reprint ed. pap. 7.99 (*0-311-46085-2*) Casa Bautista.

Sigh of Relief: The First-Aid Handbook for Childhood Emergencies. Martin Green. 1995. mass mkt. 22.95 (*0-553-85064-4*) Bantam.

Sigler & Flanders' Nonprescription Drug Cards. Jeffrey D. Sigler. 1997. 106p. ring bd. 24.95 (*1-880579-27-8*) Sigler & Flanders.

Sigma Receptors. Ed. by Yossef Itzhak. 1994. (Neuroscience Perspectives Ser.). (Illus.). 360p. text 78.00 (*0-12-376350-9*) Acad Pr.

Sigmund & Freud: Critical Assessments. Ed. by Laurence Spurling. 1989. 500p. 295.00 (*0-415-02088-3*, A3445) Routledge.

Sigmund Freud. Intro. by Harold Bloom. 1985. (Modern Critical Views Ser.). 222p. 29.95 (*0-87754-600-2*) Chelsea Hse.

Sigmund Freud. Ed. by Robert Bocock. 1983. (Key Sociologists Ser.). 128p. pap. (*0-85312-580-5*, NO. 3754) Tavistock-E Horwood GBR. *Dist:* Routldge.

Sigmund Freud. Michael Jacobs. 1992. (Key Figures in Counselling & Psychotherapy Ser.). 160p. (C). pap. 25.95 (*0-8039-8465-0*, 9290) Sage.

***Sigmund Freud.** Nick Rennison. 2001. 96p. pap. (*1-903047-54-4*) Pocket Essentials GBR. *Dist:* Trafalgar.

Sigmund Freud. Richard Wollheim. 1990. 336p. pap. text 22.95 (*0-521-28385-X*) Cambridge U Pr.

Sigmund Freud: His Life & Mind. Helen W. Puner. 1992. 295p. (C). pap. text 24.95 (*1-56000-611-0*) Transaction Pubs.

Sigmund Freud: His Personality, His Teaching & His School. Fritz Wittels. Tr. by Eden Paul & Cedar Paul from GER. 1977. LC 79-161001. (Select Bibliographies Reprint Ser.). reprint ed. 25.95 (*0-8369-5869-1*) Ayer.

Sigmund Freud: Man & Father. Martin Freud. 1983. 224p. 45.00 (*0-87668-722-2*) Aronson.

Sigmund Freud - The Standard Edition: The Ego & the Id. Sigmund Freud. Ed. by James Strachey. Tr. by Joan Riviere. 1990. (Standard Edition of the Complete Psychological Works of Sigmund Freud). 86p. pap. 8.95 (*0-393-00142-3*) Norton.

Sigmund Freud As a Consultant. Edoardo Weiss. 1991. 81p. (C). text 39.95 (*0-88738-423-4*) Transaction Pubs.

Sigmund Freud Presente par Lui-Meme. Sigmund Freud. 1987. (FRE.). pap. 10.95 (*0-7859-2804-9*) Fr & Eur.

Sigmund Freud: The Standard Edition: Group Psychology & the Analysis of the Ego. Sigmund Freud. Ed. & Tr. by James Strachey. 1990. (Norton Library: Vol. N770). 85p. reprint ed. pap. 8.95 (*0-393-00770-7*) Norton.

Sigmund Freud: The Standard Edition: Inhibitions, Symptoms, & Anxiety. Sigmund Freud. Ed. by James Strachey. Tr. by Alix Strachey. 1990. (Standard Edition of the Complete Psychological Works of Sigmund Freud). 132p. pap. 8.95 (*0-393-00874-6*) Norton.

Sigmund Freud: The Standard Edition: New Introductory Lectures on Psychoanalysis. Sigmund Freud. Ed. & Tr. by James Strachey. 1990. pap. 10.95 (*0-393-00743-X*) Norton.

Sigmund Freud: The Standard Edition: On the History of the Psycho-Analytic Movement. Sigmund Freud. Ed. by James Strachey. Tr. by Joan Riviere. 1990. LC 91-114587. (Standard Edition of the Complete Psychological Works of Sigmund Freud). 99p. pap. 4.95 (*0-393-00150-4*) Norton.

Sigmund Freud: The Standard Edition: Totem & Taboo. Sigmund Freud. Tr. by James Strachey. 1990. LC 91-120509. (Standard Edition of the Complete Psychological Works of Sigmund Freud). 213p. pap. 10.95 (*0-393-00143-1*) Norton.

Sigmund Freud's Dreams. Alexander Grinstein. 1980. LC 79-2485. 486p. 72.50 (*0-8236-6074-5*) Intl Univs Pr.

Sigmund Freud's Mission: An Analysis of His Personality & Influence. Erich Fromm. 1990. 20.50 (*0-8446-4544-3*) Peter Smith.

Sigmund Freud's Writings: A Comprehensive Bibliography. Ed. by Alexander Grinstein. 1977. LC 76-46812. 181p. 30.00 (*0-8236-6076-1*) Intl Univs Pr.

Sign Communication for Everyday Use: A Multimedia Guide. Nanci A. Scheetz. 1988. LC 97-45851. 171p. spiral bd. 65.00 (*0-8342-1095-9*, 10959) PRO-ED.

Sign Communication for Health Care Professionals. Scheetz. 1993. tchr. ed. 59.00 (*0-8342-1208-0*) PRO-ED.

Sign Language: Fourth Most Used Language in the U. S. A. Louie J. Fant, Jr. 1977. LC 77-93544. (Illus.). pap. 19.95 (*0-917002-13-X*, 159) Joyce Media.

Sign Language: The Study of Deaf People & Their Language. Jim Kyle et al. 1988. (Illus.). 326p. pap. text 31.95 (*0-521-35717-9*) Cambridge U Pr.

S

Sign Language & the Deaf Community: Essays in Honor of William Stokoe. Charlotte Baker & Robbin M. Battison. 1981. (Illus.). 267p. pap. text 8.95 (*0-913072-36-2*) Natl Assn Deaf.

Sign Language & the Health Care Professional. Debbie L. Cole. 1990. LC 89-20083. 92p. (C). pap. 12.50 (*0-89464-417-3*) Krieger.

Sign Language for Everyone. California State Department of Health Staff et al. LC 75-70066. (Illus.). 14.95 (*0-917002-02-4*) Joyce Media.

Sign Language for Everyone: A Basic Course in Communication with the Deaf. Cathy Rice. 1978. LC 77-14592. 19.99 (*0-8407-9002-3*) Nelson.

Sign Language Research: Theoretical Issues. Ed. by Ceil Lucas. 1990. LC 89-28131. (Illus.). 398p. text 49.95 (*0-930323-58-0*) Gallaudet Univ Pr.

Sign Language Structure: An Outline of Visual Communication Systems of the American Deaf. William C. Stokoe. 1993. 94p. (C). reprint ed. pap. text 16.95 (*0-932130-03-8*, LP407) Linstok Pr.

Sign Languages of Deaf People & Psycholinguistics. A. Van Uden. 1986. viii, 120p. (*90-265-0701-1*) Swets.

Signal Analysis & Pattern Recognition in Biomedical Engineering. Ed. by G. F. Inbar. 1975. 324p. 3.5 hd 70.50 (*0-7065-1465-3*) Coronet Bks.

Signal Averaged Electrocardiography: Concepts, Methods, & Applications. J. Anthony Gomes. 1993. LC 93-5136. 608p. (C). text 267.50 (*0-7923-2390-4*) Kluwer Academic.

Signal Averaging: AAMI TIR23. 2000. pap. 100.00 (*1-57020-129-3*) Assn Adv Med Instrn.

Signal Detection Theory & ROC Analysis in Psychology & Diagnostics: Collected Papers. John A. Swets. 1996. (Scientific Psychology Ser.). 328p. text 69.95 (*0-8058-1834-0*) L Erlbaum Assocs.

***Signal Transduction & Human Disease.** Finkel. 2002. 320p. (*0-471-02011-7*) Wiley.

Signal Transduction by Integrins. Paola Defilippi et al. 1997. LC 97-24582. (Molecular Biology Intelligence Unit Ser.). 188p. pap. 89.95 (*0-412-13301-6*) Chapman & Hall.

Signal Transduction in Affective Disorders. Nihon Seishin Shinkei Gakkai. Ed. by H. Ozawa et al. 1997. LC 97-44757. (Illus.). 160p. 105.00 (*4-431-70210-5*) Spr-Verlag.

Signal Transduction in Chemosensitive Receptor Cells. Ed. by S. J. Fidone & B. W. Ache. rev. ed. 1999. (Biological Signals & Receptors Ser.: Vol. 8, No. 6, 1999). (Illus.). 68p. pap. 25.25 (*3-8055-6957-2*) S Karger.

Signal Transduction in Leukocytes: G Protein-Related & Other Pathways. Ed. by Pramod M. Lad et al. 1995. LC 95-16903. 400p. 189.95 (*0-8493-6694-1*, 6694) CRC Pr.

Signal Transduction in Lung Cells. Jerome S. Brody et al. Ed. by Vsevolod A. Tkacuk. 1993. (Lung Biology in Health & Disease Ser.: Vol. 65). (Illus.). 704p. text 275.00 (*0-8247-8813-3*) Dekker.

***Signal Transduction in Mast Cell Migration.** Magnus Sundstrom. 2001. (Comprehensive Summaries of Uppsala Dissertations from the Faculty of Medicine Ser.: No. 1081). (Illus.). 53p. pap. (*91-554-5130-6*) Acta Univ SWE. *Dist:* Coronet Bks.

Signal Transduction in Testicular Cells. Ed. by V. Hansson et al. 1996. (Ernst Schering Research Foundation Ser.: Suppl. 2). (Illus.). 351p. 66.95 (*3-540-60910-5*) Spr-Verlag.

Signal Transduction in Testicular Cells: Basic & Clinical Aspects. Ed. by V. Hansson et al. 1996. LC 96-10610. (Ernst Schering Research Foundation Ser.: Supplement No. 2). (*0-387-60910-5*) Spr-Verlag.

***Signal Transduction Pathways in Autoimmunity.** Vol.5. Ed. by A. Altmann & Argyrios N. Theofilopoulos. 2001. LC 2001-50451. (Current Directions in Autoimmunity Ser.: Vol. 5). (Illus.). 198p. 198.25 (*3-8055-7308-1*) S Karger.

Signaling & Gene Expression in the Immune System. 2000. (Symposia on Quantitative Biology Ser.: Vol. LXIV). (Illus.). 600p. pap. text 110.00 (*0-87969-570-6*); (C). text 258.00 (*0-87969-569-2*) Cold Spring Harbor.

Signaling Mechanisms & Gene Expression in the Ovary. Ed. by G. Gibori. 1991. (Serono Symposia Ser.). (Illus.). 487p. 157.00 (*0-387-97653-1*) Spr-Verlag.

Signaling Networks & Cell Cycle Control: The Molecular Basis of Cancer & Other Diseases. Ed. by J. Silvio Gutkind. 2000. LC 99-56127. (Cancer Drug Discovery & Development Ser.: Vol. 5). (Illus.). xiv, 578p. 165.00 (*0-89603-710-X*) Humana.

Signaling Pathways in the Control of Apoptosis by UVB or Hypericin. Zerihun Assefta Tereffe. 1999. (Illus.). 134p. (*90-5867-002-3*) Leuven Univ BEL. *Dist:* Coronet Bks.

Signalling in the Liver. Ed. by D. Haussinger. 1998. LC 99-191556. 224p. 140.00 (*0-7923-8744-9*) Kluwer Academic.

Signals & Images: Proceedings, GIRI Meeting on Signals & Images (7th/8th, 1993-1994, Montepellier, France/Israel, December) Ed. by Madeleine Bastide. 1997. LC 97-868. 300p. text 167.00 (*0-7923-4466-9*) Kluwer Academic.

Signals & Systems for Speech & Hearing. Stuart Rosen & Peter Howell. 1991. 332p. (C). pap. text 44.95 (*0-12-597231-8*) Acad Pr.

Signet-Mosby Medical Encyclopedia. Ed. by Walter D. Glanze et al. rev. ed. 1996. (Illus.). 912p. pap. 7.99 (*0-451-18409-2*, Sig) NAL.

Significance of Children's Play. Joan E. Cass. 1977. 22.95 (*0-7134-0689-5*) Trafalgar.

Significance of Infant Observational Research for Clinical Work with Children, Adolescents, & Adults. Ed. by Scott Dowling & Arnold Rothstein. 1989. (Workshop Series of the American Psychoanalytic Association: Monograph 5). 300p. 40.00 (*0-8236-6073-7*) Intl Univs Pr.

Significance of the Physical Constitution in Mental Disease: Medicine Monographs, Vol. X. F. I. Wertheimer & Florence E. Hesketh. Ed. by Gerald N. Grob. 1980. LC 78-22594. (Historical Issues in Mental Health Ser.). (Illus.). reprint ed. lib. bdg. 16.95 (*0-405-11944-5*) Ayer.

Significant Differences: Feminism in Psychology. Corinne Squire. 1989. 176p. 45.00 (*0-415-01224-4*, A2447); pap. 12.95 (*0-415-01225-2*, A3580) Routledge.

***Significant Disability: Issues Affecting People with Significant Disabilities from a Historical Policy, Leadership, & Systems Perspective.** Ed. by E. Davis Martin. 2001. LC 2001-27143. 244p. text 59.95 (*0-398-07192-6*); pap. text 34.95 (*0-398-07193-4*) C C Thomas.

Signs & Symptoms. Klippel & Liang. 1994. (C). (gr. 13). 190.00 (*0-8151-5214-0*, 24338) Mosby Inc.

Signs & Symptoms in Emergency Medicine: An Evidence-Based Manual. Mark A. Davis. 1999. (Illus.). 560p. pap. (*84-8174-450-6*) Mosby-Doyma Libros ESP. *Dist:* Mosby Inc.

Signs & Symptoms in Emergency Medicine: Literature-based Guide to Emergent Conditions. Mark A. Davis et al. 1999. LC 98-49185. pap. 25.95 (*0-323-00211-0*) Mosby Inc.

Signs & Symptoms in Pediatrics. Walter W. Tunnessen & Kenneth B. Roberts. 3rd ed. 1999. LC 98-51161. 880p. text 59.95 (*0-7817-1639-X*) Lppncott W & W.

Signs & Symptoms of Athletic Injuries. James B. Gallaspy & J. Douglas May. 1995. (Illus.). 528p. (C). pap. text 59.38 (*0-8151-4039-8*) McGrw-H Hghr Educ.

Signs of Drug Use. James Woodward. 1980. pap. text 9.95 (*0-932666-04-3*) T J Pubs.

Signs of Health: Traditional Chinese Medicine for Modern Living. Ed. by Ramona A. Moody & Lee C. Overholser. 1991. LC 91-70385. (Illus.). 182p. (Orig.). pap. 19.95 (*0-9627734-0-9*); lib. bdg. 19.95 (*0-9627734-1-7*) Empire CA.

Signs of Life: The Five Universal Shapes & How to Use Them. Angeles Arrien. 1998. LC 98-14989. (Illus.). 96p. 19.95 (*0-87477-933-2*, Tarcher Putnam) Putnam Pub Group.

Signs of Sexual Behavior. James Woodward. 1980. pap. text 9.95 (*0-932666-02-7*) T J Pubs.

Silage Fermentation. Michael F. Woolford. 1984. (Microbiology Ser.: Vol. 14). (Illus.). 368p. text 195.00 (*0-8247-7039-0*) Dekker.

Silence of the Body: Materials for the Study of Medicine. Guido Ceronetti. Tr. by Michael Moore from ITA. 1993.Tr. of Silencio del Corpo. 233p. 22.00 (*0-374-26405-8*) FS&G.

Silence of the Body: Materials for the Study of Medicine. Guido Ceronetti. Tr. by Michael Moore from ITA. 1998.Tr. of Silenzio del Corpo. 234p. text 22.00 (*0-7881-5654-3*) DIANE Pub.

Silence of the Spheres: The Deaf Experience in the History of Science. Harry G. Lang. 1994. LC 93-20838. 224p. 57.75 (*0-89789-368-9*, Bergin & Garvey) Greenwood.

***Silencing, Heterochromatin & DNA Double Strand Break Repair.** Kevin D. Mills. 2000. LC 00-61051. (Illus.). 136p. 99.95 (*0-7923-7982-9*, Kluwer Acad) Kluwer Academic.

Silencing the Self: Women & Depression. Dana C. Jack. 1991. 256p. (C). text 29.00 (*0-674-80815-0*) HUP.

Silencing the Self: Women & Depression. Dana C. Jack. 1993. LC 92-53406. 272p. pap. 13.00 (*0-06-097527-X*, Perennial) HarperTrade.

Silencio del Corpo see Silence of the Body: Materials for the Study of Medicine

Silent Alarm: On the Edge with a Deaf EMT. Steven L. Schrader. 1995. LC 95-34074. 144p. pap. text 17.95 (*1-56368-044-0*) Gallaudet Univ Pr.

***Silent Body.** Robert Murphy. 2001. 256p. reprint ed. pap. 13.95 (*0-393-32042-1*) Norton.

Silent Clots, Life's Biggest Killers: Lockstep Medicine's Conspiracy to Suppress the Test That Should Be Done in Emergency Rooms Throughout the World. James R. Privitera & Alan Stang. 1.t. unabr. ed. 1997. LC 96-72237. (Illus.). 290p. (Orig.). pap. 19.95 (*0-9656313-0-3*) Catacombs Pr.

Silent Enemies. Justina H. Hill. 1977. LC 79-134093. (Essay Index Reprint Ser.). 25.95 (*0-8369-1954-8*) Ayer.

Silent Enemies: The Story of the Diseases of War & Their Control. Justina H. Hill. 1982. (Essay Index Reprint Ser.). 275p. reprint ed. lib. bdg. 20.00 (*0-8290-0789-X*) Irvington.

Silent Grief: Living in the Wake of Suicide. Christopher Lukas & Henry M. Seiden. 1997. LC 96-37735. (Master Works). 264p. pap. 40.00 (*0-7657-0056-5*) Aronson.

Silent Knife: Cesarean Prevention & Vaginal Birth after Cesarean. Nancy W. Cohen & Lois J. Estner. 1983. LC 82-24276. (Illus.). 456p. pap. 44.95 (*0-89789-027-2*, Bergin & Garvey) Greenwood.

Silent Language. Edward T. Hall. 1980. LC 79-25399. 217p. reprint ed. lib. bdg. 67.00 (*0-313-22277-0*, HASN, Greenwood Pr) Greenwood.

Silent Language of Psychotherapy: Social Reinforcement of Unconscious Processing. Ernst G. Beier & David M. Young. 3rd rev. ed. 1998. LC 97-48669. 323p. pap. text 25.95 (*0-202-30610-0*); lib. bdg. 49.95 (*0-202-30609-7*) Aldine de Gruyter.

Silent Myocardial Ischemia: A Critical Appraisal. Ed. by J. J. Kellermann & E. Braunwald. 1990. (Advances in Cardiology Ser.: Vol. 37). (Illus.). viii, 358p. 207.00 (*3-8055-5196-7*) S Karger.

Silent Myocardial Ischemia & Angina: Prevalence, Prognostic & Therapeutic Significance. Bramah N. Singh. 1988. 320p. 48.00 (*0-08-036078-5*, Pergamon Pr) Elsevier.

Silent Myocardial Ischemia & Infarction. Pete F. Cohn. 3rd ed. 1993. LC 92-48488. (Fundamental & Clinical Cardiology Ser.: Vol. 13). (Illus.). 288p. text 115.00 (*0-8247-9054-5*) Dekker.

Silent Myocardial Ischemia & Infarction. Peter F. Cohn. 4th ed. 2000. LC 00-22916. (Fundamental & Clinical Cardiology Ser.). (Illus.). 360p. text 125.00 (*0-8247-0354-5*) Dekker.

Silent Passage. Gail Sheehy. Ed. by Julie Rubenstein. rev. ed. 1995. LC 95-69194. 336p. mass mkt. 12.00 (*0-671-51951-4*) PB.

Silent Passage: Menopause. Gail Sheehy. Ed. by Julie Rubenstein. 1993. 256p. reprint ed. mass mkt. 6.50 (*0-671-79931-2*) PB.

Silent People Dwelling in a World Without Sound: All about Deaf Mutes. J. N. Williams. 1972. 250.00 (*0-8490-1054-3*) Gordon Pr.

Silent Sorrow: Pregnancy Loss: Guidance & Support for You & Your Family. Ingrid Kohn et al. 2nd rev. ed. 2000. LC 99-25720. xx, 299p. pap. 15.95 (*0-415-92481-2*) Routledge.

Silent War: Infection Control for Emergency Responders. OnGuard Inc. Staff. 1992. (Student Textbook Ser.). 232p. pap. text, stu. ed. 13.95 (*1-56916-403-7*); 410p. tchr. ed., ring bd. 35.95 (*1-56916-402-9*) OnGuard.

Silent War: Infection Control for Law Enforcement. OnGuard Inc. Staff. Ed. by Susan Peterson. 1996. (Illus.). 144p. pap. text 7.95 (*1-56916-710-9*, 40SWP) OnGuard.

Silent War: Infection Control for Law Enforcement: Post-Incident Procedures. OnGuard Inc. Staff. 1993. (Illus.). 116p. tchr. ed., ring bd. 30.95 (*1-56916-709-5*) OnGuard.

Silent War: Infection Control for Law Enforcement: Reducing Your Risk. OnGuard Inc. Staff. 1993. (Illus.). 59p. tchr. ed., ring bd. 30.95 (*1-56916-706-0*) OnGuard.

Silent War: Infection Control for Law Enforcement: Understanding Contagious Diseases. OnGuard Inc. Staff. 1993. (Illus.). 53p. tchr. ed., ring bd. 30.95 (*1-56916-703-6*) OnGuard.

***Silent Waves, Theory & Practice of Lymph Drainage Therapy: With Applications for Lymphedema, Chronic Pain, & Inflammation.** Bruno Chikly. Ed. by George Lord, Jr. 2001. LC 00-134580. (Illus.). 440p. 65.00 (*0-9700530-5-3*) Intl Health.

Silent World of Doctor & Patient. Jay Katz. 263p. reprint ed. pap. text 15.95 (*0-8018-5780-5*) Johns Hopkins.

Silenzio del Corpo see Silence of the Body: Materials for the Study of Medicine

Silica & Silica-Induced Lung Diseases: Current Concepts. Ed. by Vincent Castranova et al. 1995. 432p. 244.95 (*0-8493-4709-2*, 4709) CRC Pr.

Silica, Silicosis & Cancer: Controversy in Occupational Medicine, 2. Ed. by David F. Goldsmith et al. 1985. LC 85-640225. (Cancer Research Monographs: Vol. 2). 560p. 80.00 (*0-275-91305-8*, C1305, Praeger Pubs) Greenwood.

Silica, the Amazing Gel: An Essential Mineral for Radiant Health, Recovery & Rejuvenation. Klaus Kaufmann. 1993. LC 93-910249. (Kaufmann Foods Ser.). (Illus.). 159p. (Orig.). pap. 9.95 (*0-920470-30-0*) Alive Bks.

Silicon & Siliceous Structures in Biological Systems. Ed. by T. L. Simpson & B. E. Volcani. 1981. (Illus.). 587p. 294.00 (*0-387-90592-8*) Spr-Verlag.

Silicone Oil in the Treatment of Complicated Retinal Detachments: Techniques, Results, & Complications. K. Lucke & H. Laqua. 1990. (Illus.). 161p. 65.00 (*0-387-53035-5*) Spr-Verlag.

Silicone Oil in Vitreoretinal Surgery. R. Zivojnovic. 1987. (Monographs in Ophthalmology). (C). text 211.50 (*0-89838-879-1*) Kluwer Academic.

Silicone Spills: Breast Implants on Trial. Mary W. Stewart. 1998. LC 97-41006. (*0-89789-515-0*, Bergin & Garvey) Greenwood.

Silicone Spills: Breast Implants on Trial. Mary White Stewart. 1998. LC 97-41006. 240p. 27.95 (*0-275-96359-4*, Praeger Pubs) Greenwood.

Silicone Survival Handbook: How to Get Well from Silicone Poisoning Caused by Breast Implants. I Am Staff. 2002. pap. 19.95 (*1-892177-51-X*, Lightning Source) HEAVEN-ON-EARTH.

Silicone Survivors: Women's Experiences with Breast Implants. Susan M. Zimmerman. 1998. LC 97-45536. 240p. (C). text 59.95 (*1-56639-611-5*); pap. text 19.95 (*1-56639-612-3*) Temple U Pr.

Silicosis: Records of International Conference, Johannesburg, August, 1930, (I. L. O. Studies & Reports) 1974. (Series F: No. 13, Vol. 31). reprint ed. 65.00 (*0-8115-3263-1*) Periodicals Srv.

Sillas Especiales. Jean A. Zollars. Ed. by Macrina C. Montano. Tr. by Alejandra Millar. 1993. (SPA., Illus.). 95p. (Orig.). pap. 20.00 (*1-882632-02-8*); pap. 19.95 (*1-882632-04-4*) PAX Pr.

Silva Mind Control Through Psychorientology. Harry F. McKnight. 5.95 (*0-913343-40-4*) Inst Psych Inc.

Silver Dental Fillings: The Toxic Timebomb. Sam Ziff. 1984. 220p. pap. 16.95 (*0-943358-24-8*) Aurora Press.

Silver Linings: The Other Side of Cancer. Ed. by Shirley Gollo & Elaine Glass. 1997. LC 97-66193. (Illus.). 260p. (Orig.). pap. 19.50 (*1-890504-01-7*) Oncology Nursing.

Silver Threads: A Personal Look at the First Twenty-Five Years of the Registry of Interpreters for the Deaf. Lou Fant. 1990. 152p. (Orig.). (C). pap. text 12.95 (*0-916883-08-6*) RID Pubns.

Silvergirls Surgery: The Breast. Harris B. Shumacker. 1991. (*0-941432-30-0*) Mosby Inc.

Simian Immuno-Deficiency Virus. Ed. by N. L. Letvin & R. C. Desrosiers. 1994. LC 15-12910. (Currents Topics in Microbiology & Immunology Ser.: Vol. 188). (Illus.). 241p. 159.00 (*0-387-57274-0*) Spr-Verlag.

Simian Virus 40 (SV40) - A Possible Human Polyomavirus: Workshop, Natcher Auditorium, National Institute of Health, Bethesda, MD, January 1997. Ed. by Fred Brown & Andrew M. Lewis. 1998. (Illus.). xii, 412p. 330.50 (*3-8055-6733-2*) S Karger.

Similarities & Differences Between Children & Adults: Implications for Risk Assessment. Ed. by P. S. Guzelian et al. 1992. LC 92-81193. 300p. pap. text 35.00 (*0-944398-07-3*) ILSI.

Similarity & Symbols in Human Thinking. Ed. by Steven A. Sloman et al. 1998. LC 98-7439. (Cognition Special Issues Ser.). (Illus.). 227p. pap. text 25.00 (*0-262-69214-7*) MIT Pr.

Similarity in Visually Perceived Forms. Erich Goldmeier. 1972. LC 72-83230. (Psychological Issues Monographs: No. 29, Vol. 8, No. 1). 135p. 27.50 (*0-8236-6077-X*) Intl Univs Pr.

Simkin Handbook of Therapeutic Monitoring. Ed. by William J. Taylor & Daniel J. Robinson. 2nd ed. 1993. LC 93-83709. v, 174p. pap. 14.00 (*0-929375-10-6*) H W Bks.

Simon Baruch: Rebel in the Ranks of Medicine, 1840-1921. Patricia S. Ward. Ed. by Lester D. Stephens. 1994. LC 93-31300. (History of American Science & Technology Ser.). (Illus.). 416p. text 49.95 (*0-8173-0589-0*) U of Ala Pr.

Simple Acts of Kindness: Volunteering in the Age of AIDS. Ed. by John Griggs. 1989. LC 89-5131. 127p. pap. 5.95 (*0-934459-56-8*) United Hosp Fund.

Simple Earth Solutions: Powerful Paths to Health & Healing Through Natural Remedies. Ronald J. Vaillancourt. 1995. LC 95-90285. 351p. (Orig.). pap. 29.95 (*0-9645645-1-3*) Abundant Hlth Pub.

Simple Eye Care for Health Care Workers. Helen Keller International Staff. 2nd ed. 1993. LC 93-1669.Tr. of Guides des Soins Oculaires Primaires pour le Personnel de Sante. pap. 5.00 (*0-915173-23-9*) Helen Keller Intl.

Simple Guide to Blood Gas Analysis. Peter Driscoll et al. 1997. (Illus.). 191p. pap. text (*0-7279-1107-4*) BMJ Pub GBR. *Dist:* AIDC.

Simple Guide to Orthopaedics. R. L. Kuckstep. 1993. 450p. (Orig.). pap. text (*0-443-04385-X*) Church.

Simple Guide to Trauma. Ronald L. Huckstep. 4th ed. 1989. (Illus.). 397p. pap. text (*0-443-03350-1*); 5th ed. 1995. LC 95-6577. pap. text (*0-443-04679-4*) Church.

Simple Guide to Using Herbal Medicine. Philip Evans. 2001. (Simple Guides to Natural Health Ser.). 112p. pap. (*1-86034-052-0*) Global Bks GBR. *Dist:* Midpt Trade.

Simple Matter of Salt: An Ethnography of Nutritional Deficiency in Spain. Renate L. Fernandez. 1990. LC 90-33972. (Comparative Studies of Health Systems & Medical Care: Vol. 25). (Illus.). 225p. text 50.00 (*0-520-06910-2*) U CA Pr.

Simple Minds. Dan Lloyd. 1989. LC 88-26808. 280p. 35.00 (*0-262-12140-9*, Bradford Bks) MIT Pr.

Simple Plants: Traditional Medicinal Herbs of Northern Illinois. Valerie Morris. 1994. 84p. pap. 9.95 (*1-888342-01-3*); 1996. 100p. pap. text 12.95 (*1-888342-02-1*) Flying Pig.

Simple Process of Getting Healthy: The Total Book for Good Health & Well-Being. Ted Landau. 1994. 66p. (Orig.). pap. 10.95 (*0-9640599-0-8*) Apollo Pub OR.

Simple Remedies for the Home. C. W. Dail & C. S. Thomas. 1991. LC 91-61468. (Illus.). 158p. (Orig.). per. 11.95 (*0-945383-30-4*, 945-5820) TEACH Servs.

Simple Screening Instruments for Outreach for Alcohol & Other Drug Abuse & Infectious Diseases. Randi Henderson et al. Ed. by Ken C. Winters. 1998. (Illus.). 74p. (C). pap. text 30.00 (*0-7881-4840-0*) DIANE Pub.

Simple Skin Surgery. Susan Burge et al. 2nd ed. 1996. LC 95-50692. (Illus.). 104p. pap. 41.95 (*0-86542-690-2*) Blackwell Sci.

Simple Steps to Health: A Self-Help Guide. Madeline Goulard. 1996. (Illus.). 250p. pap. 14.00 (*0-9642335-2-5*) Simple Life Bks.

Simple Truth: Ideas & Experiences for Humans from Less-Than-Perfect Families. Thom Rutledge. 1994. 105p. pap. 8.95 (*0-9627963-0-1*) T W Rutledge.

Simplified Approach to Electrocardiography. Richard A. Johnson & Mark Schwartz. 1986. (Illus.). 331p. pap. text 34.00 (*0-7216-1738-7*) Saunders.

Simplified Drugs & Solutions for Health Care Professionals. Norma Dison. 11th ed. 1996. (Illus.). 352p. (C). (gr. 13). pap. text 21.00 (*0-8151-2505-4*, 28190) Mosby Inc.

Simplified EKG Analysis: A Sequential Guide to Interpretation. Ed. by Charles B. Seelig. 1992. (Illus.). 120p. (Orig.). pap. text 22.00 (*1-56053-010-3*) Hanley & Belfus.

Simplified Extended, Deep & or Meditative Relaxation, Set-R. Russell E. Mason. 1975. (Train-Ascendance Ser.). pap. 23.00 incl. audio (*0-89533-004-0*, 53.GT-RM) F I Comm.

Simplified Guide to Nutritional Supplements. Sam Ziff & Michael F. Ziff. 1994. 160p. (Orig.). pap. 12.00 (*0-941011-10-0*) Bio-Probe.

Simplified Relaxation, Problem Solutions & Substitutions & Value Considerations, Set-S. Russell E. Mason. 1975. (Train-Ascendance Ser.). pap. 65.00 incl. audio (*0-89533-020-2*, 65.GT-SV) F I Comm.

Simplifying Phacoemulsification: Safe & Efficient Methods for Cataract Surgery. Paul S. Koch. 5th ed. 1997. LC 97-9765. 240p. text 65.00 (*1-55642-352-7*, 63527) SLACK Inc.

Simply Nutritious: Recipes & Recommendations to Reduce Your Risk of Cancer. Sabine M. Artaud-Wild. 1987. LC 86-71576. 182p. lib. bdg. 6.00 (*0-9617128-0-5*); spiral bd. 8.00 (*0-9617128-1-3*) Amer Cancer Soc OR.

Simpson's Forensic Medicine. Bernard Knight. 11th ed. (Illus.). 224p. pap. (*0-340-61370-X*) E A GBR. *Dist:* OUP, Routldge.

Simulating the Medical Office Software for Windows 95, Set. Jerry Belch. Ed. by Valerie Harris et al. 1999. (Illus.). 600p. tchr. ed., ring bd. 249.95 incl. disk (*0-89262-528-7*) Career Pub.

Simulating the Medical Office Software for Windows 95: Appointments Instructor's Guide. Jerry Belch. Ed. by Valerie Harris et al. 1999. (Illus.). 42p. tchr. ed., spiral bd. 49.95 incl. disk (*0-89262-540-6*) Career Pub.

Simulating the Medical Office Software for Windows 95: Business Checking Instructor's Guide. Jerry Belch. Ed. by Valerie Harris et al. 1999. (Illus.). 44p. tchr. ed., spiral bd. 49.95 incl. disk (*0-89262-541-4*) Career Pub.

Simulating the Medical Office Software for Windows 95: Insurance Claims Instructor's Guide. Jerry Belch. Ed. by Valerie Harris et al. 1999. (Illus.). 36p. tchr. ed., spiral bd. 49.95 incl. disk (*0-89262-544-9*) Career Pub.

Simulating the Medical Office Software for Windows 95: Patient Billing Instructor's Guide. Jerry Belch. Ed. by Valerie Harris et al. 1999. (Illus.). 80p. tchr. ed., spiral bd. 49.95 incl. disk (*0-89262-543-0*) Career Pub.

Simulating the Medical Office Software for Windows 95: Purchase Orders Instructor's Guide. Jerry Belch. Ed. by Valerie Harris et al. 1999. (Illus.). 32p. tchr. ed., spiral bd. 49.95 incl. disk (*0-89262-542-2*) Career Pub.

Simulating the Medical Office Software for Windows 95: Record Management Instructor's Guide. Jerry Belch. Ed. by Valerie Harris et al. 1999. (Illus.). 52p. tchr. ed., spiral bd. 49.95 incl. disk (*0-89262-538-4*) Career Pub.

Simulation & Imaging of the Cardiac System. Ed. by Samuel Sideman & Rafael Beyar. 1985. (Developments in Cardiovascular Medicine Ser.). text 256.50 (*0-89838-687-X*) Kluwer Academic.

Simulation Approach to the Study of Human Fertility. Gigi Santow. 1978. (Publications of the Netherlands Inter-University Demographic Institute & the Population & Family Study Centre: Vol. 5). pap. text 77.50 (*90-207-0765-5*) Kluwer Academic.

Simulation Fidelity in Training System Design: Bridging the Gap Between Reality & Training. R. T. Hays & M. J. Singer. 1990. (Recent Research in Psychology Ser.). (Illus.). 415p. 58.95 (*0-387-96846-6*) Spr-Verlag.

Simulation in Emergency Management & Engineering: Simulation in Health Care. Ed. by Jim D. Sullivan et al. 1991. 269p. pap. 48.00 (*0-911801-86-3*, MC91-2) Soc Computer Sim.

Simulation in Health Care Delivery Systems, 1984. Stanridge. 1984. 120p. pap. 20.00 (*0-911801-02-2*, MC84-1) Soc Computer Sim.

Simulation in Health Sciences & Services: 1993 Conference. James G. Anderson & Meyer Katzper. 1993. 116p. pap. 48.00 (*1-56555-021-8*, MC93-2) Soc Computer Sim.

Simulation in the Medical Sciences. Ed. by James G. Anderson & Meyer Katzper. 1996. 226p. pap. 80.00 (*1-56555-091-9*, HSS-96) Soc Computer Sim.

Simulation in the Medical Sciences Held in Phoenix, Arizona - January, 1997. Ed. by James G. Anderson & Meyer Katzper. 1998. 199p. pap. 80.00 (*1-56555-105-2*, HSS-97) Soc Computer Sim.

Simulation Model for the Future Analysis of Cardiovascular Disease. O. J. Frieze et al. 2000. 408p. (Orig.). pap. incl. disk (*90-6224-878-0*) Uitgeverij Arkel NLD. *Dist:* LPC InBook.

Simulators in Anesthesiology Education: Proceedings of the Second Conference Held in Rochester, New York, May 31-June 2, 1996. Ed. by Lindsey C. Henson & Andrew C. Lee. 1998. LC 97-46469. (Illus.). 132p. 65.00 (*0-306-45775-X*, Kluwer Plenum) Kluwer Academic.

Simultaneous Horizontal & Cyclovertical Strabismus Surgery. Marc H. Govin & Jos J. Bierlaagh. 1994. LC 93-18643. (Monographs in Ophthalmology: Vol. 15). 216p. (C). text 293.00 (*0-7923-2246-0*) Kluwer Academic.

Sinapticheskaia Peredacha v Retsoptarakh Akustiko-Lateralnoi Sistemy see Sensory Hair Cells: Synaptic Transmission

Sindrome de Down: Biologia, Desarrollo, Educacion. Nuevas Perspectivas. Contrib. by J. Florez et al. 1997. (SPA.). 248p. pap. (*84-458-0519-3*, 5193) Ediciones Cientificas ESP. *Dist:* P H Brookes.

Sindrome de Down: Hacia un Futuro Mejor Guia Para los Padres. Siegfried M. Pueschel. 1993. (SPA.). 286p. pap. (*84-345-2429-5*) Ediciones Cientificas ESP. *Dist:* P H Brookes.

Sindrome de Down: Problematica Biomedica. Jeanette K. Pueschel & Siegfried M. Pueschel. 1994. (SPA.). 352p. pap. (*84-458-0202-X*) Ediciones Cientificas ESP. *Dist:* P H Brookes.

Sindrome de Down y Educacion. Jesus Florez & Troncoso. 1991. (SPA.). 318p. (C). pap. (*84-458-0118-X*) Ediciones Cientificas ESP. *Dist:* P H Brookes.

Sindrome Premenstrual - Premenstrual Syndrome. Marvin Eastlund. 1995. (Serie Enfoque a la Familia - Focus on the Family Ser.). (SPA.). 55p. (*1-56063-709-9*) Editorial Unilit.

Singing on the Throne: And Other Tales of a Country Vet in the South. Clifton C. McLean. Ed. by MaryBelle Campbell. (Illus.). 160p. 1993. pap., per. 18.00 (*1-879009-12-9*); 2nd ed. 1994. pap., per. 16.95 (*1-879009-16-1*) Old Barn Entrprs.

Single Case Experimental Designs: Strategies for Studying Behavior Change. David H. Barlow & Michel Hersen. 2nd ed. 1984. (General Psychology Ser.: No. 56). 432p. text 70.00 (*0-08-030136-3*); pap. text 26.50 (*0-08-030135-5*) Elsevier (Pergamon Pr).

Single-Case Research Designs: Methods for Clinical & Applied Settings. Alan E. Kazdin. 1982. (Illus.). 384p. (C). pap. text 36.95 (*0-19-503021-4*) OUP.

Single-Dose Therapy of Urinary Tract Infections: Modern Trend in the Treatment of Lower Urinary Tract Infections. Ed. by A. Jardin & J. D. Williams. 1987. (Journal: Vol. 13, Suppl. 1, 1987). (Illus.). iv, 136p. pap. 43.50 (*3-8055-4559-2*) S Karger.

Single-Session Therapy: Maximizing the Effect of the First (& Often Only) Therapeutic Encounter. Moshe Talmon. 1990. LC 90-36407. (Social & Behavioral Science Ser.). 170p. 36.00 (*1-55542-260-8*) Jossey-Bass.

Single-Subject Research: Application in Educational & Clinical Settings. Stephen B. Richards et al. 1998. LC 98-28028. (Illus.). 308p. pap. text 50.95 (*1-56593-799-6*, 1652) Thomson Learn.

Singles Scene: A Psychoanalytic Study of the Breakdown of Intimacy. Gerald Alper. 1995. LC 93-6446. 128p. 37.95 (*1-883255-15-5*) Intl Scholars.

Singles Scene: A Psychoanalytical Study of the Breakdown of Intimacy. Gerald Alper. 1995. LC 93-6446. pap. 14.95 (*1-883255-14-7*) Intl Scholars.

Singular View: The Art of Seeing with One Eye. Frank B. Brady. 5th ed. 1994. LC 94-189866. (Illus.). 144p. reprint ed. pap. 15.00 (*0-9614639-2-9*) Frank B Brady.

Singulars Encyclopedia & Speech-Language Pathology Singh. 2001. pap. 79.25 net. (*0-7693-0104-5*); pap. 100.00 net. (*0-7693-0105-3*) Singular Publishing.

Singular's Encyclopedia of Audiology Brad A. Stach. 2001. pap. 79.25 net. (*0-7693-0151-7*) Singular Publishing.

Singular's Illustrated Dictionary of Medical Audiology. Stephen Singular. 2001. pap. 40.00 net. (*0-7693-0163-0*) Singular Publishing.

Singular's Illustrated Dictionary of Pediatric Comm Disorders. Singular Publishing Staff. 2001. pap. 40.00 net. (*0-7693-0164-9*) Singular Publishing.

Singular's Medical Dictionary of Speech-language Pathology. Stephen Singular. 2001. pap. 40.00 net. (*0-7693-0162-2*) Singular Publishing.

Sinn Als Bedeutung: Bedeutungstheoretische Untersuchungen zur Psychoanalyse Sigmund Freuds. Stephan Achim. 1989. (Quellen und Studien zur Philosophie: Vol. 24). (GER.). xvi, 174p. (C). lib. bdg. 78.25 (*3-11-011949-8*) De Gruyter.

Sintomas, Sus Causas y Curas - Symptoms, Their Causes & Cures: How to Understand & Treat 265 Health Concerns. Prevention Magazine Editors. 1996. (SPA.). 29.95 (*0-87596-366-8*) Rodale Pr Inc.

Sinus Bone Graft. Ole T. Jensen. 1998. LC 98-35893. (Illus.). 234p. text 138.00 (*0-86715-343-1*) Quint Pub Co.

Sinus Cure: 7 Simple Steps to Relieve Sinusitis & Other Ear, Nose & Throat Conditions. Debra Fulghum Bruce & Murray Grossan. 2001. LC 00-110367. (Illus.). 288p. pap. 12.95 (*0-345-43971-6*, Ballantine) Ballantine Pub Grp.

Sinus Disease: Current Therapy. Kennedy. 1997. (*0-7216-5406-1*) Saunders.

Sinus Handbook: A Self-Help Guide. Muriel K. MacFarlane. 1997. LC 96-61828. (Illus.). 312p. pap. 12.95 (*1-887053-08-5*) United Res CA.

Sinus Health: How to Prevent & Correct Sinus Problems. Mary VanderWall. unabr. ed. 1998. LC 97-46165. 30p. pap. 6.95 (*0-9617223-4-7*, 8) Hughes Henshaw.

Sinus Node: Structure, Function, & Clinical Relevance. Felix I. Bonke. 1978. text 199.50 (*90-247-2064-8*) Kluwer Academic.

Sinus Node Inhibitors: A New Concept in Angina Pectoris. Ed. by A. Hjalmarson & W. I. Remme. 1992. 72p. 29.00 (*0-387-91393-9*) Spr-Verlag.

***Sinus Source Book: Everything You Need to Know.** Deborah Rosin. 2002. (Illus.). 191p. 26.00 (*0-7567-5275-2*) DIANE Pub.

Sinus Sourcebook. Deborah F. Rosin. 1998. LC 97-50154. 208p. 25.00 (*1-56565-643-1*, 06431W) Lowell Hse.

Sinus Sourcebook. Deborah F. Rosin. rev. ed. 1999. LC 97-50154. (Illus.). 208p. pap. 15.95 (*0-7373-0083-3*, 00833W) NTC Contemp Pub Co.

Sinuses. Ed. by Paul J. Donald et al. 1994. LC 94-13768. 688p. text 239.00 (*0-7817-0041-8*) Lppncott W & W.

Sinusitis: Pathogenesis & Treatment. Ed. by Howard M. Druce. 1993. LC 93-20821. (Clinical Allergy & Immunology Ser.: Vol. 1). (Illus.). 352p. text 155.00 (*0-8247-8845-1*) Dekker.

Sinusitis Help Book: A Comprehensive Guide to a Common Problem. M. Lee Williams. 1998. 400p. pap. 17.95 (*0-471-34702-7*); LC 98-230250. (Illus.). pap. 16.95 (*1-56561-163-2*) Wiley.

Sir Alexander Fleming: Man of Penicillin. John Malkin. 1985. 92p. (*0-907526-06-3*) Alloway Pub GBR. *Dist:* St Mut.

Sir Arthur Newsholme & State Medicine, 1885-1935. John M. Eyler. 1997. (History of Medicine Ser.). (Illus.). 443p. (C). text 69.95 (*0-521-48186-4*) Cambridge U Pr.

Sir Jason Winters Story: From Deadly Cancer to Perfect Health. Benjamin Roth Smythe. rev. ed. 1997. pap. 19.95 (*1-885026-06-4*) Vinton Pubng.

Sisters on a Journey: Portraits of American Midwives. Penfield Chester. 1997. LC 97-7711. (Illus.). 288p. (C). pap. 19.95 (*0-8135-2408-3*); text 50.00 (*0-8135-2407-5*) Rutgers U Pr.

Sisyphus: The Old Stone, a New Way: A Jungian Approach to Midlife Crisis. Verena Kast. 1995. LC 76-15656. 214p. pap. 15.00 (*3-85630-527-0*) Continuum.

Sites of Drug Action in the Human Brain. Ed. by Anat Biegon & Nora D. Volkow. 1995. LC 94-25232. 192p. 199.95 (*0-8493-7653-X*, 7653) CRC Pr.

Sitosterol. David Kritchevsky & O. J. Pollak. 1981. (Monographs on Atherosclerosis: Vol. 10). (Illus.). vii, 220p. pap. 128.75 (*3-8055-0568-X*) S Karger.

Situation Analysis Approach to Assessing Family Planning & Reproductive Health Services: A Handbook. Robert Miller. 1997. LC 97-5428. (*0-87834-090-4*) Population Coun.

Situation des Menschen: German Translation. Harvey Jackins. Tr. by Dietmar Kreuer from ENG. 1984. pap. 7.00 (*0-911214-75-5*) Rational Isl.

Six Etudes de Psychologie. Jean Piaget. 1987. (FRE.). pap. 12.95 (*0-7859-2805-7*) Fr & Eur.

Six Group Therapies. S. Long. 1987. LC 87-7187. (Illus.). 358p. (C). 80.00 (*0-306-42642-0*, Plenum Trade) Perseus Pubng.

Six Hundred MCQs in Anaesthesia: Basic Sciences. Neville W. Goodman & Chris Johnson. 2nd ed. 1993. LC 93-12699. 264p. pap. text (*0-443-04831-2*) Church.

Six Hundred MCQs in Anaesthesia: Clinical Practice. P. J. Simpson & N. W. Goodman. 1987. LC 86-14728. 256p. (Orig.). pap. text (*0-443-03155-X*) Church.

600 MCQs in Anaesthesia: Clinical Practice. Neville W. Goodman & Chris Johnson. 2nd ed. 1996. LC 95-20318. pap. text (*0-443-04835-5*) Church.

630 Questions & Answers about Chinese Herbal Medicine: A Workbook & Study Guide. Bob Flaws. 1999. LC 98-94962. 159p. pap. text 29.95 (*1-891845-04-7*) Blue Poppy Pr.

Six Key Approaches to Counselling & Therapy. Richard Nelson-Jones. 2000. 256p. pap. text 21.95 (*0-8264-4969-7*) Continuum.

***6 Minutes to Superior Dental Health: How to Protect Your Family in a Dental Disease Society.** Rodney S. Katayama. LC 99-68390. pap. 19.95 (*1-58619-002-4*, Authors Pub NA) Elton-Wolf Pub.

Six Perspectives on Theory for the Practice of Occupational Therapy see Perspectives on Theory for the Practice of Occupational Therapy

Six Practical Lessons for an Easier Childbirth. Elisabeth D. Bing. 3rd rev. ed. 1994. LC 93-26507. (Illus.). 176p. pap. 11.95 (*0-553-37369-2*) Bantam.

Six Psychological Studies. Jean Piaget. Ed. by David Elkind. Tr. by Anita Tenzer. 1968. (Orig.). mass mkt. 8.80 (*0-394-70462-2*) Vin Bks.

Six Steps in the Treatment of Borderline Personality Organization. Vamik D. Volkan. 1995. LC 95-205493. (Master Work Ser.). 250p. pap. text 40.00 (*1-56821-726-9*) Aronson.

Six Steps to the Fountain of Youth Workbook, Vol. 1. Dennis Kelly. l.t. unabr. ed. 1997. (Illus.). 192p. pap. 12.95 (*1-890243-04-3*) Trineurogenics.

Six Talks on Jung's Psychology. Robert A. Clark. 1953. (Orig.). pap. 4.50 (*0-910286-07-8*) Boxwood.

Six Therapists & One Client. Ed. by Frank Dumont & Raymond Corsini. 2000. 322p. pap. (*1-85343-519-8*) Free Assoc Bks GBR. *Dist:* Intl Spec Bk.

Six Therapists & One Client. Contrib. by Frank Dumont et al. 2nd ed. 2000. LC 99-58723. (Illus.). xv, 336p. (*0-8261-1319-2*) Springer Pub.

Six Weeks to a Toxic-Free Body. Dean Kimmel. 1992. 146p. (Orig.). pap. 9.95 (*0-9621446-2-2*) Corbin Hse.

Sixteen PF Fifth Edition: Administrator's Manual. Mary T. Russell & Darcie L. Karol. 1994. 162p. (Orig.). pap. 40.00 (*0-918296-21-8*) Inst Personality & Ability.

Sixteen PF Fifth Edition: Technical Manual. Ed. by Steven R. Conn & Mark L. Rieke. 1994. 324p. (Orig.). (C). pap. 55.00 (*0-918296-22-6*) Inst Personality & Ability.

Sixteenth Century Physician & His Methods. Richard L. Sutton, Jr. 1986. LC 85-82669. (Illus.). 276p. 37.50 (*0-932845-12-6*) Lowell Pr.

6th Annual Report on Carcinogens (1991) 1994. 461p. (Orig.). (C). pap. text 65.00 (*0-7881-0423-3*) DIANE Pub.

Sixth HGH Symposium. Ed. by J. S. Christiansen & J. Girard. 1996. (Journal: Vol. 45, Nos. 1 & 2, 1996). (Illus.). 112p. pap. 88.75 (*3-8055-6280-2*) S Karger.

Sixth International Symposium on Pediatric Neuro-Oncology, Marseille, June 1993: Abstracts. Ed. by M. Choux. 1993. (Journal: Vol. 19, No. 6, 1993). (Illus.). 62p. pap. 48.00 (*3-8055-5883-X*) S Karger.

6th International Visual Field Symposium. Ed. by A. Heijl & Erik L. Greve. 1985. (Documenta Ophthalmologica Proceedings Ser.). text 366.50 (*90-6193-524-5*) Kluwer Academic.

***Sixth Report of the Joint National Committee on Prevention, Detection, Evaluation & Treatment of High Blood Pressure.** Sheldon G. Sheps. 2002. (Illus.). 70p. (C). pap. text 20.00 (*0-7567-1919-4*) DIANE Pub.

Sixth Report of the Joint National Committee on Prevention, Detection, Evaluation, & Treatment of High Blood Pressure. NIH Staff & National Heart, Lung and Blood Institute Staff. 6th ed. 1997. (Illus.). 78p. (C). pap. 8.95 (*1-883205-42-5*) Intl Med Pub.

Sixth Symposium by the 5 Winners of the Grants from Sandoz Foundation for Gerontological Research: Annual Meeting of the Japan Gerontological Society, Tokyo, Japan, September 1994. Ed. by H. Orimo. 1995. (Journal: Vol. 41, Suppl. 1, 1995). (Illus.). iv, 34p. pap. 21.75 (*3-8055-6235-7*) S Karger.

Sixth Symposium on a Long Term Clinical Care of Parkinson's Disease, Tokyo, October 1991. Ed. by T. Nakanishi. 1992. (Journal: Vol. 32, Suppl. 1, 1992). (Illus.). vi, 54p. pap. 26.25 (*3-8055-5664-0*) S Karger.

Sixty-Five-Year Index to Physical Therapy. 1987. 120p. pap. 20.00 (*0-912452-65-X*, C-11) Am Phys Therapy Assn.

Sixty-Plus & Fit Again: Exercises for Older Men & Women. Magda Rosenberg & Isadore Rossman. 1977. LC 76-49130. (Illus.). 156p. 12.95 (*0-87131-224-7*) M Evans.

60 Second EMT. Gideon Bosker et al. 2nd ed. 1995. LC 95-30731. (Illus.). 256p. (C). (gr. 13). pap. text 23.95 (*0-8016-7812-9*, 07812) Mosby Inc.

60 Second Menopause Management: The Quickest Ways to Handle Problems & Discomfort. Carol R. Schulz. 1995. LC 95-69344. 240p. pap. 20.95 (*0-88282-137-7*) New Horizon NJ.

67 Good Ways to Sleep: A People's Medical Society Book. Charles B. Inlander & Cynthia K. Moran. 1995. LC 95-6993. 96p. 14.95 (*0-8027-1306-8*); pap. 7.95 (*0-8027-7448-2*) Walker & Co.

Sixty-Seven Ways to Good Sleep. Charles B. Inlander. 1998. 6.99 (*0-517-18138-X*) Random Hse Value.

62 Natural Ways to Beat Jet Lag. Charles B. Inlander & Cynthia K. Moran. 1997. LC 97-227969. 192p. mass mkt. 5.99 (*0-312-96325-4*) St Martin.

60 Ways to Relieve Stress in 60 Seconds. Manning Rubin. 1993. LC 92-50932. (Illus.). 128p. pap. 5.95 (*1-56305-338-1*, 3338) Workman Pub.

Sixty Years in Search of Cures: An Herbalist's Success with Chinese Herbs. Fung Fung & John Fung. Date not set. LC 95-172921. 174p. pap. 15.95 (*0-9638285-1-7*) Get Well Fnd.

Size & Growth of the Nutritionally Improved Farm Market. Elizabeth Frazao & Jane E. Allshouse. 1997. (Illus.). 41p. (Orig.). (C). pap. text 25.00 (*0-7881-3699-2*) DIANE Pub.

Size Exclusion Chromatography (GPC) Ed. by Theodore J. Provder. 1980. LC 80-22015. (ACS Symposium Ser.: No. 138). 41.95 (*0-8412-0586-8*) Am Chemical.

Sjogren's Syndrome: Model for Understanding Autoimmunity. Ed. by Norman Talal. 1989. (Second International Symposium Ser.). 275p. pap. text 83.00 (*0-12-682345-6*) Acad Pr.

Sjogren's Syndrome: State of the Art. M. Homma & T. Tojo. 1994. LC 94-15740. (Illus.). xxxviii, 620p. text (*90-6299-107-6*) Kugler NLD. *Dist:* Lib Res.

Sjogren's Syndrome Handbook. Elaine K. Harris & Steven Caroons. 1988. 29.95 (*0-9621157-0-3*) Sjogrens Syndrome.

Skeletal Anatomy. Glenda J. Bryan. 3rd ed. 1996. pap. text (*0-443-05150-X*, B2220) Church.

Skeletal Growth & Development: Clinical Issues & Basic Science Advances. Ed. by Joseph A. Buckwalter et al. 1998. LC 98-26059. (Symposium Ser.). (Illus.). 668p. 105.00 (*0-89203-183-2*) Amer Acad Ortho Surg.

Skeletal Growth Factors. Ernesto Canalis. 2000. LC 99-52559. 512p. text 149.00 (*0-7817-2474-0*) Lppncott W & W.

S

Skeletal Injury in the Child. John A. Ogden. 2nd ed. 1989. 960p. text 240.00 (*0-7216-2955-5*) Saunders.

Skeletal Injury in the Child. John A. Ogden. 3rd ed. 2000. LC 98-51165. (Illus.). 1200p. 295.00 (*0-387-98510-7*) Spr-Verlag.

Skeletal Muscle. Ed. by Stuart Binder-Macleod. 1994. 133p. 30.00 (*0-912452-93-5*, P-105) Am Phys Therapy Assn.

Skeletal Muscle. H. Schalmbruch. 1985. (Handbuch der Mikroskopischen Anatomie Des Menschen Ser.: Vol. 2, Pt. 6). (Illus.). 440p. 464.00 (*0-387-15608-9*) Spr-Verlag.

Skeletal Muscle: Form & Function. Alan J. McComas. 1996. LC 95-24525. (Illus.). 416p. text 62.00 (*0-87322-780-8*, BMCC0780) Human Kinetics.

***Skeletal Muscle: Pathology, Diagnosis & Management of Disease.** Peters. Ed. by Victor R. Preedy. 2002. (Illus.). 500p. (*1-84110-029-3*) Greenwich Med GBR. *Dist:* JAMCO Dist.

Skeletal Muscle in Health & Disease: A Textbook of Muscle Physiology. Dorothy A. Jones & J. M. Round. 1990. LC 90-5631. text (*0-7190-3164-8*) Manchester Univ Pr GBR. *Dist:* St Martin.

Skeletal Muscle Metabolism in Exercise & Diabetes: Proceedings of the Copenhagen Muscle Research Center Symposium on Regulation of Skeletal Muscle Metabolism: Focus on Glucose Transport, Held in Copenhagen, Denmark, October 23-26, 1997. Ed. by Erik A. Richter & Bengt Saltin. 1998. LC 98-26175. (Advances in Experimental Medicine & Biology Ser.: Vol. 441). (Illus.). 340p. 95.00 (*0-306-45920-5*, Kluwer Plenum) Kluwer Academic.

Skeletal Muscle Microcirculation. Ed. by K. Messmer & F. Hammersen. 1984. (Mikrozirkulation in Forschung und Klinik Ser.: Vol. 5). (Illus.). vii, 148p. pap. 64.50 (*3-8055-3920-7*) S Karger.

Skeletal Muscle Pathology. Ed. by John Walton & Frank L. Mastaglia. 2nd ed. 1992. (Illus.). 803p. text (*0-443-04241-1*) Church.

Skeletal Muscle Structure & Function. Richard L. Lieber. 1994. (Illus.). 314p. 41.95 (*0-683-05026-5*) Lppncott W & W.

Skeletal Nuclear Medicine. Ed. by B. David Collier, Jr. et al. 1996. (Illus.). 512p. (C). (gr. 13). text 195.00 (*0-8151-3273-5*, 23963) Mosby Inc.

Skeletal Radiology. Martin H. Reed. 1991. (Illus.). 696p. 150.00 (*0-683-07212-9*) Lppncott W & W.

Skeletal Radiology: Atlas of the Spine & Extremities. John Taylor & Donald Resnick. 2000. LC 99-59402. (Illus.). 605p. text (*0-7216-7510-7*) Saunders.

Skeletal Reconstruction & Bioimplantation: Demineralized Bone Matrix, Non-Collagenous, Native & Recombinant Bonemorphogenetic Proteins. T. Sam Lindholm. 1998. LC 97-34263. (Medical Intelligence Unit Ser.). 225p. 99.00 (*1-57059-506-2*) Landes Bioscience.

Skeletal Tissue Mechanics. R. B. Martin et al. 1998. LC 98-2906. (Illus.). 406p. 67.95 (*0-387-98474-7*) Spr-Verlag.

Skeletal Trauma. Bruce D. Browner. 1999. text (*0-7216-5993-4*) Saunders.

***Skeletal Trauma: Fractures, Dislocations, Ligamentous Injuries**, Set. Bruce D. Browner et al. 2nd ed. 1998. (Illus.). 2540p. 510.00 incl. cd-rom (*0-7216-7614-6*) Saunders.

Skeletal Trauma: Fractures, Dislocations, Ligamentous Injuries, Set. Bruce D. Browner et al. 2nd ed. 1997. (Illus.). 2540p. text 445.00 (*0-7216-7526-3*) Saunders.

Skeletal Trauma: Fractures, Dislocations, Ligamentous Injuries, Set. Bruce D. Browner et al. Ed. by Richard Lampert. 2nd ed. 1997. LC 96-50086. (Illus.). 2400p. text 325.00 (*0-7216-6884-4*) Saunders.

Skeletal Trauma in Children, Vol. 3. Neil E. Green & Marc F. Swiontkowski. Ed. by Richard Lampert. 2nd ed. 1997. LC 96-49870. (Illus.). 626p. text 170.00 (*0-7216-6735-X*) Saunders.

Skeletal Trauma in Old Age. Ed. by David I. Rowley & Benedict Clift. 1994. LC 94-70928. (Illus.). 240p. (gr. 13). (*0-412-48750-0*) E A GBR. *Dist:* OUP.

Skeleton. Steve Parker. 1996. LC 96-7962. (Look at Your Body Ser.). (Illus.). 32p. (J). (gr. 4-6). 22.90 (*0-7613-0529-7*, Copper Beech Bks) Millbrook Pr.

Skeleton Keys: An Introduction to Human Skeletal Morphology, Development, & Analysis. Jeffrey H. Schwartz. 1995. (Illus.). 376p. text 62.95 (*0-19-505638-8*) OUP.

Skeptic's Guide to Alternative Medicine: The Holistic Approach to Well Being. Carlos A. Bonilla. Ed. by Carlos A. Bonilla & Katherine Lauderdale. 1998. LC 97-74916. (Illus.). 64p. pap. 19.95 (*1-879774-13-5*) ICA Pub Co.

Sketch of a System of the Philosophy of the Human Mind, 1. Thomas Brown. 1977. LC 77-72191. (Contributions to the History of Psychology Ser.: Pt. A, Orientations). 320p. reprint ed. lib. bdg. 69.50 (*0-313-26925-4*, U6925, Greenwood Pr) Greenwood.

SKIBO - Diseases & Disorders Affecting the Skin & Bones: A Clinical, Dermatologic & Radiologic Synopsis. Juergen Freyschmidt & Gisela Freyschmidt. 1998. LC 98-10617. (Illus.). 224p. 129.00 (*3-540-64042-8*) Spr-Verlag.

Skiing Trauma & Safety: Fifth International Symposium - STP 860. Ed. by Robert J. Johnson & C. Daniel Mote. 1985. LC 85-3897. (Illus.). 500p. text 62.00 (*0-8031-0429-4*, STP860) ASTM.

Skilful Physician. Carey Balaban et al. 1997. 266p. text 69.00 (*90-5702-531-0*); pap. text 29.95 (*90-5702-532-9*) Gordon & Breach (Harwood Acad Pubs).

Skill Acquisition & Human Performance. Robert W. Proctor & Addie Dutta. 1995. (Advanced Psychology Texts Ser.: Vol. 1). 400p. 76.95 (*0-8039-5010-1*, 4705) Sage.

Skill Acquisition Rates & Patterns. N. E. Lane. 1987. (Recent Research in Psychology Ser.). (Illus.). 143p. 56.95 (*0-387-96579-3*) Spr-Verlag.

Skill Building Activities for Alcohol & Drug Education. Carson Bates & James Wigtil. 1994. (Illus.). 100p. (C). pap. text 38.95 (*0-86720-757-4*, 757-4) Jones & Bartlett.

Skill with Illustrations of Chinese Acupuncture & Moxibustion. Yan Jie. Tr. by Yin Ganglin from CHI. 1993. (Illus.). 462p. text (*0-535-70931-5*) Akade Kiado HUN. *Dist:* Intl Spec Bk.

Skilled Consultant: A Systematic Approach to the Theory & Practice of Consultation. Richard D. Parsons. 1995. LC 95-20870. 352p. 87.00 (*0-205-16119-7*) Allyn.

Skilled Helper: A Systematic Approach to Effective Helping. Gerard Egan. 4th ed. 1990. LC 89-38002. (Psychology Ser.). 432p. (C). 38.95 (*0-534-12138-1*) Brooks-Cole.

Skilled Helper: Model Skills & Methods for Effective Helping. Gerard Egan. 3rd ed. 1985. LC 85-14956. (Psychology Ser.). 384p. (C). pap. 30.50 (*0-534-05904-X*) Brooks-Cole.

Skilled Nursing Facilities: Approval Process for Certain Services May Result in Higher Medicare Costs. Janet L. Shikles. 1999. (Illus.). 133p. reprint ed. pap. text 25.00 (*0-7881-7876-8*) DIANE Pub.

Skilled Nursing Facility Management: Cost Reporting. Michael E. Lesnick. 1995. LC 97-13983. (HFMA Healthcare Financial Management Ser.). 250p. 175.00 (*1-55738-637-4*, Irwn Prfssnl) McGraw-Hill Educ Grp.

Skilled Nursing Facility Management: Coverage Issues. Michael E. Lesnick. 1995. 200p. 175.00 (*1-55738-638-2*, Irwn Prfssnl) McGraw-Hill Educ Grp.

Skilled Nursing Facility Management: New Directions in Long Term Care. Michael E. Lesnick. 1995. 250p. 50.00 (*1-55738-639-0*, Irwn Prfssnl) McGraw-Hill Educ Grp.

Skilled Nursing Facility Management: Optimizing Reimbursement. Michael E. Lesnick. 1995. 300p. 175.00 (*1-55738-636-6*, Irwn Prfssnl) McGraw-Hill Educ Grp.

Skills Analysis Model: An Effective Curriculum for Children with Severe Learning Difficulties. J. M. Gardner et al. 1985. 130p. 40.00 (*0-906054-41-9*) St Mut.

Skills & Procedures of Emergency & General Medicine. Harvey W. Meislin & Stephen J. Dresnick. 1981. 250p. text 31.50 (*0-8359-7009-4*) P-H.

Skills Clinical Supervision: A Practical Guide for Supervisees, Clinical Supervisors & Managers. M. Bond. 1997. LC 97-15164. (Supervision in Context Ser.). pap. (*0-335-19660-8*) OpUniv Pr.

Skills for Communicating with Patients. Jonathan Silverman et al. 1998. LC 98-14385. 200p. pap. (*1-85775-189-2*) Radcliffe Med Pr GBR. *Dist:* Balogh.

Skills for Midwifery Practice. Ruth Johnson & Wendy Taylor. 2000. 335p. pap. text (*0-443-06243-9*) Saunders.

Skills for the Patient Care Technician. Susan K. Strasinger & Marjorie A. Di Lorenzo. 1999. LC 98-44093. (Illus.). 487p. pap. 39.95 (*0-8036-0355-X*) Davis Co.

Skills Manual for the EMT. Faught. pap. text (*0-7216-6386-9*) Saunders.

Skills of Argument. Deanna Kuhn. 1991. (Illus.). 334p. (C). text 26.95 (*0-521-40451-7*); pap. text 31.95 (*0-521-42349-X*) Cambridge U Pr.

Skills Practice Manual to Accompany Health Unit Coordinating. Myrna LaFleur Brooks & Elaine T. Gillingham. 4th ed. 1998. LC 97-44166. 656p. (C). pap. 27.00 (*0-7216-7613-8*) Saunders.

Skills Training for Children with Behavior Disorders: A Parent & Therapist Guidebook. Michael L. Bloomquist. 1996. LC 96-27. 272p. pap., instr.'s gde. ed. 32.00 (*1-57230-080-9*, 0080) Guilford Pubns.

Skills Training Manual for Treating Borderline Personality Disorder. Marsha M. Linehan. 1993. LC 93-15216. (Diagnosis & Treatment of Mental Disorder Ser.). (Illus.). 180p. pap., stu. ed. 30.00 (*0-89862-034-1*, C2034) Guilford Pubns.

Skin. Ed. by W. S. Symmers & D. Weedon. 3rd ed. 1992. (Systemic Pathology Ser.: Vol. 9). (Illus.). 1095p. text (*0-443-03201-7*) Church.

Skin: Drug Application & Evaluation of Environmental Hazards, Proceedings of the Oholo Biological Conference, 22nd, Ma'alot, March 1977. Oholo Biological Conference Staff. Ed. by J. W. Mali et al. 1977. (Current Problems in Dermatology Ser.: Vol. 7). (Illus.). 86.25 (*3-8055-2797-7*) S Karger.

Skin: Interface of a Living System: Perspective for Skin Care System in the Future: Proceedings of the Shiseido Science Symposium Held in Tokyo on 5 July, 1997. H. Tagami et al. 1998. LC 98-38388. (International Congress Ser.). 212p. 112.00 (*0-444-82964-4*) Elsevier.

Skin & Aging Processes. Barbara A. Gilchrest. 1984. 136p. lib. bdg. 139.00 (*0-8493-5472-2*, RL73) CRC Pr.

Skin & Its Troubles. Compiled by Health Research Staff. 1994. 88p. reprint ed. spiral bd. 11.00 (*0-7873-1119-7*) Hlth Research.

Skin & Systemic Disease. Mark G. Lebwohl. 1995. (Illus.). 251p. text (*0-443-08739-3*) Church GBR. *Dist:* Saunders.

Skin Barrier: Principles of Percutaneous Absorption. H. Schaefer & T. E. Redelmeier. 1996. LC 96-24964. (Illus.). xvi, 310p. 191.50 (*3-8055-6326-4*) S Karger.

Skin Bioengineering: Techniques & Applications in Dermatology & Cosmetology. Ed. by Peter Elsner et al. 1998. LC 97-52829. (Current Problems in Dermatology Ser.: Vol. 26, 1998). (Illus.). x, 250p. 216.50 (*3-8055-6519-4*) S Karger.

Skin Cancer. Ed. by J. A. Bishop et al. 1996. LC 96-190934. (Cancer Surveys Ser.: Vol. 26). (Illus.). 300p. (C). text 56.00 (*0-87969-483-1*) Cold Spring Harbor.

Skin Cancer. Rona M. Mackie. 1996. (*1-85317-203-0*) Martin Dunitz GBR. *Dist:* Mosby Inc.

Skin Cancer. R. A. Schwartz. 1988. (Illus.). 427p. 120.00 (*0-387-96612-9*) Spr-Verlag.

Skin Cancer. Arthur J. Sober & Frank G. Haluska. 2000. LC 2001-430140. (ACS Atlas of Clinical Oncology Ser.). (Illus.). 320p. incl. cd-rom (*1-55009-108-5*) DEKR.

Skin Cancer: Basic Science, Clinical Research, & Treatment. Ed. by C. Garbe et al. 1995. (Recent Results in Cancer Research Ser.: Vol. 139). (Illus.). 456p. 137.00 (*0-387-57630-4*) Spr-Verlag.

Skin Cancer: Mechanisms & Human Relevance. Hasan Mukhtar. 1994. 464p. 178.95 (*0-8493-7358-1*) CRC Pr.

Skin Cancer & UV-Radiation. Ed. by Peter Altmeyer et al. 1997. LC 97-10068. (Illus.). 1136p. 235.00 (*3-540-62723-5*) Spr-Verlag.

Skin Carcinogenesis in Man & in Experimental Models. Ed. by Erich Hecker et al. 1993. LC 92-48377. (Recent Results in Cancer Research Ser.: Vol. 128). 168.00 (*3-540-56321-0*); (Illus.). 364p. 152.00 (*0-387-56321-0*) Spr-Verlag.

Skin Care: Clear & Simple. Ligaya H. Buchbinder. Ed. by Erica Orloff. 1997. LC 96-93067. 192p. (Orig.). pap. 12.95 (*1-885843-05-4*) Saturn Press.

Skin Care in Health, Disease, Wounds, Cosmetics & Management Variations Including Products: Index of New Information. James K. Tullar. 1997. 150p. 57.50 (*0-7883-1360-6*); pap. 47.50 (*0-7883-1361-4*) ABBE Pubs Assn.

Skin Changes & Diseases in Pregnancy. Marwali Harahap. Ed. by Robert C. Wallach. 1996. (Basic & Clinical Dermatology Ser.: Vol. 11). (Illus.). 416p. text 175.00 (*0-8247-9401-X*) Dekker.

Skin Cleansing with Synthetic Detergents: Chemical, Ecological, & Clinical Aspects. Griesbach Conference Staff. Ed. by O. Braun-Falco & H. C. Korting. 1992. LC 92-13632. (Illus.). 264p. (*3-540-55409-2*); 71.95 (*0-387-55409-2*) Spr-Verlag.

Skin Cover in the Injured Hand. Ed. by David M. Evans. 9th ed. 1992. (Hand & Upper Limb Ser.: No. 9). (Illus.). 207p. text (*0-443-03799-X*) Church.

Skin Deep: An A-Z of Skin Disorders, Treatments & Health, Updated Edition. Carol A. Turkington & Jeffrey S. Dover. rev. ed. 1996. LC 95-10187. (Illus.). 416p. 40.00 (*0-8160-3071-5*) Facts on File.

Skin Disease: Diagnosis & Treatment. Thomas P. Habif. (Illus.). (C). 2000. 570p. (gr. 13). text 49.00 (*0-8151-3762-1*, 28122); 1998. LC 97-35557. 320p. text 99.00 (*0-8151-2886-X*, 30735) Mosby Inc.

Skin Disease in Childhood & Adolescence. Elisabeth Higgins et al. 1996. LC 95-6273. (Illus.). 256p. 170.00 (*0-86542-835-2*) Blackwell Sci.

Skin Diseases of the Cat. Sue Paterson. 2000. LC 00-708873. (Illus.). 244p. pap. text (*0-632-04805-0*) Blckwell Science GBR. *Dist:* Iowa U Pr.

Skin Diseases of the Dog. Sue Paterson. 1999. LC 98-34064. (Illus.). 310p. (C). pap. text (*0-632-04808-5*) Blckwell Science GBR. *Dist:* Iowa U Pr.

Skin Diseases of the Feet. Richard C. Gibbs. 1979. LC 96-176169. (Illus.). 238p. 32.50 (*0-87527-105-7*) Green.

Skin Disorders: Journal: Pediatrician, Vol. 18, No. 3, 1991. Ed. by David W. Kaplan. 1991. (Illus.). 72p. pap. 43.50 (*3-8055-5460-5*) S Karger.

Skin Disorders Sourcebook: Basic Information about Common Skin & Scalp Conditions. Ed. by Allan R. Cook. 1997. LC 97-6570. (Health Reference Ser.: Vol. 22). xvi, 647p. lib. bdg. 78.00 (*0-7808-0080-X*) Omnigraphics Inc.

Skin Flaps. Bennett. 1998. text (*0-7216-3414-1*) Saunders.

Skin Flaps. Ed. by William C. Grabb & M. Bert Myers. 1975. LC 74-20219. 440p. 130.00 (*0-316-32267-9*, Little Brwn Med Div) Lppncott W & W.

Skin for Thought: Interviews with Gilbert Tarrab on Psychology & Psychoanalysis. Didier Anzieu. 1990. 186p. pap. text (*0-946439-86-9*) Karnac Bks GBR. *Dist:* Other Pr LLC.

Skin Grafting. Ross Rudolph et al. 1979. 42.95 (*0-316-76109-5*, Little Brwn Med Div) Lppncott W & W.

Skin Immune System: Cutaneous Immunology & Clinical Immunodermatology. Ed. by Jan D. Bos. 2nd ed. 1997. LC 96-41754. 752p. 179.95 (*0-8493-4016-0*) CRC Pr.

Skin Immune System (SIS) Ed. by Jan D. Bos. 1990. 520p. 239.00 (*0-8493-4945-1*, RL97) CRC Pr.

Skin Langerhans (Dendritic) Cells in Virus Infections & AIDS. Ed. by Yechiel Becker. 1990. (Developments in Medical Virology Ser.). (C). text 208.00 (*0-7923-1015-2*) Kluwer Academic.

Skin Lesions: A Practical Guide to Diagnosis, Management & Minor Surgery. J. Schofield & Ronald Kneebone. 1996. (Illus.). 144p. (*0-412-63140-7*) E A GBR. *Dist:* OUP.

***Skin Lesions & Environmental Exposure: Rash Decisions.** Alan H. Hall. Ed. by Daniel J. Hogan. 2001. (Illus.). 51p. (C). reprint ed. pap. text 20.00 (*0-7567-1213-0*) DIANE Pub.

Skin Manifestations in Visceral Cancer. V. C. Andreev. 1978. (Current Problems in Dermatology Ser.: Vol. 8). (Illus.). pap. 86.25 (*3-8055-2878-7*) S Karger.

Skin Microflora & Microbial Skin Disease. Ed. by W. C. Noble. 1993. (Illus.). 402p. (C). text 100.00 (*0-521-40198-4*) Cambridge U Pr.

Skin Painting Techniques & in vivo Carcinogenesis Bioassays. Ed. by F. Homburger. 1983. (Progress in Experimental Tumor Research Ser.: Vol. 26). (Illus.). vi, 314p. 191.50 (*3-8055-3556-2*) S Karger.

Skin Penetration: Hazardous Chemicals at Work. Philippe Grandjean. 1990. 220p. (*0-85066-834-4*) Tay Francis Ltd GBR. *Dist:* Taylor & Francis.

Skin Permeability. Hans Schaefer et al. 1983. (Illus.). 360p. 115.00 (*0-387-11797-0*) Spr-Verlag.

Skin Pharmacology & Toxicology: Recent Advances. Ed. by Corraldo L. Galli et al. 1990. LC 89-26614. (NATO ASI Series A, Life Sciences: Vol. 181). (Illus.). 326p. 95.00 (*0-306-43404-0*, Plenum Trade) Perseus Pubng.

Skin Problems of the Amputee. William S. Levy. 1983. LC 78-50196. (Illus.). 324p. 49.95 (*0-87527-181-2*) Green.

Skin Reactions to Drugs. Kirsti Kauppinen & Kristiina Alanko. 1998. LC 98-22072. (CRC Series in Dermatology Ser.). 224p. lib. bdg. 139.95 (*0-8493-8376-5*) CRC Pr.

Skin Resurfacing. William P. Coleman, III & Naomi Lawrence. 1998. LC 97-48638. (Illus.). 400p. text 159.00 (*0-683-30165-9*) Lppncott W & W.

Skin Saver Remedies: Don't Hide Behind a Mask. Juta Stepanovs. 2000. (Illus.). 139p. pap. 12.95 (*0-8464-5201-4*) Beekman Pubs.

***Skin Sense: A Derrmatologist's Complete Guide to Your Family's Skin Care.** Garry Gewirtzman. 2001. 287p. reprint ed. pap. 13.00 (*0-7567-5136-5*) DIANE Pub.

Skin Signs of Systemic Disease. Irwin M. Braverman. Ed. by Judy Fletcher. 3rd ed. 1997. LC 96-6572. (Illus.). 704p. text 145.00 (*0-7216-3745-0*) Saunders.

Skin Signs of Systemic Disease: An Essential Slide Collection. Denis E. Sharvill. 1988. 96p. (gr. 13). (*0-397-46423-1*, GM0158) Gower-Mosby.

Skin, Soft Tissue, Bone & Joint Infections. Ed. by Dennis L. Stevens. 1995. (Atlas of Infectious Diseases Ser.: Vol. 2). (Illus.). 250p. text 135.00 (*1-878132-44-X*) Current Med.

Skin Sourcebook. Alan S. Boyd. 1998. LC 98-51989. (Illus.). 416p. pap. 22.95 (*0-7373-0003-5*, 00035W) NTC Contemp Pub Co.

Skin Surgery. Marwali Harahap. 1985. (Illus.). 1032p. 125.00 (*0-87527-317-3*) Green.

Skin Tumors of the Dog & Cat. Goldschmidt. 1998. 328p. pap. text 70.00 (*0-7506-4269-6*) Buttrwrth-Heinemann.

Skin Tumors of the Dog & Cat. M. H. Goldschmidt & F. Shofer. 1992. (Illus.). 232p. text 105.00 (*0-08-040823-0*, Pergamon Pr) Elsevier.

Skin Wise: A Guide to Healthy Skin for Women. Ed. by Annette Callan. 1996. (Illus.). 208p. (C). pap. 22.95 (*0-19-553745-9*) OUP.

Skinny Potatoes: Over One Hundred Delicious, New Low-Fat Recipes for the World's Most Versatile Vegetable. Barbara Grunes. 1993. (Skinny Cookbook Ser.). (Illus.). 78p. (Orig.). pap. 20.95 (*0-940625-72-5*) Surrey Bks.

Skull Vol. 1: Development. Ed. by James Hanken & Brian K. Hall. 1993. LC 92-49119. (Skull Ser.: Vol. 1). (Illus.). 608p. (C). pap. text 37.50 (*0-226-31567-3*); lib. bdg. 82.50 (*0-226-31566-5*) U Ch Pr.

Skull Vol. 2: Patterns of Structural & Systematic Diversity. Ed. by James Hanken & Brian K. Hall. 1993. LC 92-49119. (Skull Ser.: Vol. 2). (Illus.). 592p. (C). pap. text 34.95 (*0-226-31570-3*); 226th ed. lib. bdg. 82.50 (*0-226-31568-1*) U Ch Pr.

Skull Vol. 3: Functional & Evolutionary Mechanisms. Ed. by James Hanken & Brian K. Hall. 1993. LC 92-49119. (Skull Ser.: Vol. 3). (Illus.). (C). 480p. lib. bdg. 77.00 (*0-226-31571-1*); 468p. pap. text 29.95 (*0-226-31573-8*) U Ch Pr.

***Skull Base Meningioma.** Olafur Gudjonnsson. 2001. (Comprehensive Summaries of Uppsala Dissertations from the Faculty of Medicine Ser.: No. 1041). (Illus.). 59p. (*91-554-5034-2*) Uppsala Universitet SWE. *Dist:* Coronet Bks.

Skull Base Surgery: Anatomy, Biology, & Technology. Ed. by Ivo P. Janecka & Klaus Tiedemann. 1996. 432p. text 179.00 (*0-397-51716-5*) Lppncott W & W.

Skull Base Surgery: Anatomy, Diagnosis & Treatment. Ed. by Madjid Samii. 1994. (Illus.). xx, 1276p. 574.00 (*3-8055-5967-4*) S Karger.

Skull Base Surgery Update: Update I: Proceedings of the First Congress of the European Skull Base Society, Held in Riva del Garda, Italy, September 25-30, 1993. European Skull Base Society Staff. Ed. by A. Mazzoni & Mario Sanna. 1995. LC 94-46322. (Illus.). xii, 504p. pap. text (*90-6299-115-7*) Kugler NLD. *Dist:* Lib Res.

Skull, Spine & Contents Pt. 1: Procedures & Indications. Ed. by H. J. Kaufmann. 1975. (Progress in Pediatric Radiology Ser.: Vol. 5). 300p. 112.25 (*3-8055-1382-8*) S Karger.

Skull, Spine & Contents Pt. 2: Clinical Aspects. Ed. by H. J. Kaufmann. 1977. (Progress in Pediatric Radiology Ser.: Vol. 6). (Illus.). 140.00 (*3-8055-2337-8*) S Karger.

Sky Is Falling: Understanding & Coping with Phobias, Panic & Obsessive-Compulsive Disorders. Raeann Dumont. 1996. LC 95-30992. 352p. 25.00 (*0-393-03848-3*) Norton.

Slang & Jargon of Drugs & Drink. Richard A. Spears. 1986. LC 85-26277. 601p. 45.00 (*0-8108-1864-7*) Scarecrow.

Slanted Truths: Essays on Gaia, Symbiosis & Evolution. Lynn Margulis & Dorion Sagan. 1997. LC 97-2160. (Illus.). 368p. 27.00 (*0-387-94927-5*) Spr-Verlag.

SLATTER Fundamentals of Veterinary Ophthalmology. Slatter. 2nd ed. 1990. LC 89-70312. (Illus.). 576p. pap. text 69.00 (*0-7216-2463-4*) Saunders.

Slaughter of the Innocent. Hans Ruesch. 1992. 446p. reprint ed. pap. 4.95 (*0-9610016-0-7*) CIVIS-Civitas.

Slavery & Medicine: Enslavement & Medical Practices in Antebellum Louisiana. Katherine K. Bankole. 1998. LC 97-35394. (Studies in African American History & Culture). 274p. 56.00 (*0-8153-3059-6*) Garland.

Slaying the Giant: Practical Help for Understanding Preventing & Overcoming Depression. French O'Shields. 1998. 145p. (Orig.). reprint ed. pap. 9.95 (*0-9641901-0-9*) Hem Of His Garment.

Sleep. Ed. by Rosemary Cooper. 1993. LC 93-3996. (Illus.). 720p. (*0-412-39150-3*) E A GBR. *Dist:* OUP.

Sleep. J. Allan Hobson. 1989. LC 88-37027. (Scientific American Library). 213p. text 32.95 (*0-7167-5050-3*) W H Freeman.

Sleep. ASET Staff et al. 4th rev. ed. 1998. (Illus.). iv, 156p. spiral bd. 25.00 (*1-57797-015-2*) ASET.

Sleep, Aging & Related Disorders. Ed. by W. Emser et al. 1987. (Interdisciplinary Topics in Gerontology Ser.: Vol. 22). (Illus.). x, 166p. 108.75 (*3-8055-4451-0*) S Karger.

Sleep & Biological Rhythms: Basic Mechanisms & Applications to Psychiatry. Ed. by Jacques Montplaisir & Roger Godbout. 1990. (Illus.). 256p. text 49.95 (*0-19-505825-9*) OUP.

Sleep & Breathing. Ed. by Nicholas A. Saunders & Colin E. Sullivan. 2nd ed. 1993. LC 93-28482. (Lung Biology in Health & Disease Ser.: Vol. 71). (Illus.). 1002p. text 275.00 (*0-8247-8877-X*) Dekker.

***Sleep & Breathing in Children: A Developmental Approach.** Ed. by Gerald M. Loughlin et al. 2000. LC 00-708684. (Lung Biology in Health & Disease Ser.: Vol. 147). (Illus.). xxv, 867p. text 235.00 (*0-8247-0300-6*) Dekker.

Sleep & Disease & the Immune Response. Richard Brown. Date not set. 89.95 (*0-8493-7698-X*) CRC Pr.

Sleep & Dreams. Duane Michals. 1984. (Illus.). 64p. pap. 11.95 (*0-912810-46-7*) Lustrum Pr.

Sleep & Health Risk. Ed. by J. H. Peter et al. 1991. (Illus.). 573p. 138.00 (*0-387-53083-5*) Spr-Verlag.

Sleep & Its Disorders Vol. 1i: What You Should Know. Robert Hooper. rev. ed. 2000. (Illus.). 184p. pap. 14.95 (*0-9700026-4-5*) Just Peachy.

Sleep & Movement Disorders. Sudhansu Chokroverty et al. 2001. (Illus.). 540p. 135.00 (*0-7506-7200-5*) Buttrwrth-Heinemann.

Sleep Apnea: Implications in Cardiovascular & Cerebrovascular Disease. T. Douglas Bradley & John S. Floras. 2000. LC 00-29048. (Lung Biology in Health & Disease Ser.). (Illus.). 584p. text 195.00 (*0-8247-0299-9*) Dekker.

Sleep Apnea & Rhonchopathy. Ed. by K. Togawa et al. 1993. (Illus.). x, 178p. 214.00 (*3-8055-5611-X*) S Karger.

Sleep, Arousal, & Performance. Robert D. Ogilvie. Ed. by Roger J. Broughton. 1991. (Illus.). xvi, 286p. 120.50 (*0-8176-3518-1*) Birkhauser.

***Sleep-Deficiency, Deprivations, Disturbances & Disorders: Index of New Information & Guide-Book for Consumers, Reference & Research.** Jamin K. Mottolova. 2002. 180p. 47.50 (*0-7883-2494-2*); pap. 47.50 (*0-7883-2495-0*) ABBE Pubs Assn.

Sleep Demons: An Insomniac's Memoir. Bill Hayes. 2001. LC 00-68228. (Illus.). 368p. 24.95 (*0-671-02814-6*, WSP) PB.

***Sleep Disordered Breathing: Natural Evolution & Metabolism.** Ahmed Elmasry. 2000. (Comprehensive Summaries of Uppsala Dissertations from the Faculty of Medicine Ser.: No. 970). (Illus.). 66p. (Orig.). pap. (*91-554-4848-8*) Uppsala Universitet SWE. *Dist:* Coronet Bks.

***Sleep Disorders.** 2002. (Diseases & Disorders Ser.). 27.45 (*1-56006-909-0*, Lucent Books) Gale.

Sleep Disorders: America's Hidden Nightmare. Roger Fritz. Ed. by Carol Haralson. 1993. 180p. (Orig.). pap. 12.95 (*0-9635137-0-2*) Nat Sleep Alert.

Sleep Disorders: An Alternative Medicine Definitive Guide. Herbert Ross et al. 2000. LC 00-38581. (Illus.). 275p. pap. 14.95 (*1-887299-20-3*) AlternMed Bks.

Sleep Disorders: Diagnosis & Treatment. Ed. by J. Steven Poceta & Merrill M. Mitler. 1998. LC 98-16257. (Current Clinical Practice Ser.). (Illus.). 250p. 79.50 (*0-89603-527-1*) Humana.

Sleep Disorders & Insomnia in the Elderly. Ed. by J. L. Albarede et al. 1993. 232p. 39.95 (*0-8261-8171-6*) Springer Pub.

Sleep Disorders & Neurological Disease. Antonio Culebras. 1999. LC 99-40800. (Neurological Disease & Therapy Ser.). (Illus.). 464p. text 195.00 (*0-8247-7605-4*) Dekker.

Sleep Disorders in Childhood & Adolescence. Ed. by David W. Kaplan. 1990. (Journal: Vol. 17, No. 1). (Illus.). 52p. pap. text 29.75 (*3-8055-5151-7*) S Karger.

Sleep Disorders Medicine: Basic Science, Technical Considerations & Clinical Aspects. Sudhansu Chokroverty. 1993. (Illus.). 504p. text 140.00 (*0-7506-9002-X*); 2nd ed. 1998. LC 98-4115. 781p. text 150.00 (*0-7506-9954-X*) Buttrwrth-Heinemann.

Sleep Disorders of Older People. 1992. lib. bdg. 250.00 (*0-8490-5543-1*) Gordon Pr.

Sleep Disorders Sourcebook: Basic Consumer Health Information about Sleep & Its Disorders. Ed. by Jennifer Swanson. 1998. LC 98-37257. (Health Reference Ser.). (Illus.). 600p. lib. bdg. 78.00 (*0-7808-0234-9*) Omnigraphics Inc.

Sleep, Dreaming, & Sleep Disorders: An Introduction. William H. Moorcroft. 2nd ed. 1993. 508p. (Orig.). (C). 75.50 (*0-8191-9250-3*); LC 93-5259. pap. 46.00 (*0-8191-9251-1*) U Pr of Amer.

Sleep '86. Ed. by W. P. Koella et al. 1988. LC 87-36156. 466p. lib. bdg. (*0-89574-252-7*) Gustav Fischer DEU. *Dist:* Lubrecht & Cramer, Balogh.

Sleep Medicine: Normal Sleep & Its Disorders. Michael S. Aldrich. 1999. LC 98-30554. (Contemporary Neurology Ser.: Vol. 53). (Illus.). 408p. text 110.00 (*0-19-512957-1*) OUP.

Sleep, 1980: Proceedings of the European Congress on Sleep Research, 5th, Amsterdam, September 1980. European Congress on Sleep Research Staff. Ed. by W. P. Koella. 1981. (Illus.). xiv, 466p. 215.75 (*3-8055-2045-X*) S Karger.

Sleep, 1982: Proceedings of the 9th European Congress on Sleep Research, Jerusalem, September 4-9, 1988. Ed. by Jim Horne. 1990. 310p. text (*0-89574-301-9*) Gustav Fischer DEU. *Dist:* Lubrecht & Cramer, Balogh.

Sleep Nineteen Eighty-Two: Sixth European Congress on Sleep Research, Zurich, March 1982. Ed. by W. P. Koella. 1983. (Illus.). xiv, 438p. 274.00 (*3-8055-3577-5*) S Karger.

Sleep, 1978: Proceedings of the European Congress on Sleep Research, 4th, Tirgu-Mures, September 1978. European Congress on Sleep Research Staff. Ed. by L. Popoviciu et al. 1980. 171.50 (*3-8055-0778-X*) S Karger.

Sleep, 1974: Instinct, Neurophysiology, Endocrinology, Episodes, Dreams, Epilepsy & Intracranialpathology: Proceedings of the European Congress on Sleep Research, 2nd, Rome, April 8-11, 1974. European Congress on Sleep Research Staff. Ed. by W. P. Koella et al. 1975. 400p. 164.50 (*3-8055-2069-7*) S Karger.

Sleep, 1976: Proceedings of the European Congress on Sleep Research, 3rd, Montpellier, September 1976. European Congress on Sleep Research Staff. Ed. by W. P. Koella & P. Levin. 1977. 161.00 (*3-8055-2663-6*) S Karger.

Sleep Onset: Normal & Abnormal Processes. Ed. by John R. Harsh & Robert D. Ogilvie. 1994. LC 94-41375. (Illus.). 397p. text 29.95 (*1-55798-266-X*, 431-8320) Am Psychol.

Sleep Related Breathing Disorders. Ed. by Hartmut Zwick. 1992. LC 92-24922. 100p. 33.95 (*0-387-82376-X*); pap. 25.00 (*3-211-82376-X*) Spr-Verlag.

Sleep Research & Polysomnography: Index of New Information. Ruth M. DeVecchia. 1994. 150p. 57.50 (*0-7883-0044-X*); pap. 47.50 (*0-7883-0045-8*) ABBE Pubs Assn.

Sleep Research & Polysomnography: Index of New Information. Ruth M. De Vecchia. rev. ed. 1997. 180p. 57.50 (*0-7883-1596-X*); pap. 47.50 (*0-7883-1597-8*) ABBE Pubs Assn.

Sleep Secrets for Shift Workers & People with Off-Beat Schedules. David Morgan. 1996. LC 96-9961. 176p. pap. 15.95 (*1-57025-118-5*) Whole Person.

Sleep-Talking: Psychology & Psychophysiology. Arthur M. Arkin. 1982. LC 81-3300. (Illus.). 640p. text 99.95 (*0-89859-031-0*) L Erlbaum Assocs.

Sleep-Wake Disorders: Proceedings of a Japanese-German International Symposium Held in Erfurt, Germany, October 9-10, 1996. K. Meier-Evert & M. Okawa. 1998. LC 97-42703. (Illus.). 199p. 95.00 (*0-306-45771-7*, Kluwer Plenum) Kluwer Academic.

Sleeping & Sexual Symptoms, Vol. 3. W. Klunker. 1987. 434p. 112.00 (*3-7760-0561-0*) Medicina Bio.

Sleeping Through the Night: How Infants, Toddlers & Their Parents Can Get a Good Night's Sleep. Jodi A. Mindell. 1997. LC 96-39372. 304p. pap. 14.00 (*0-06-273409-1*) HarperCollins Pubs.

Sleeping Well: The Sourcebook for Sleep & Sleep Disorders. Jan Yager & Michael J. Thorpy. 2001. LC 2001-28323. 256p. pap. 16.95 (*0-8160-4090-7*, Checkmark) Facts on File.

Sleepwatcher's. William C. Dement. 1996. 234p. (Orig.). (C). pap. text 16.95 (*0-9649338-0-2*) Nychthemeron Pr.

Sleisenger & Fordtran's Gastrointestinal & Liver Disease: Pathophysiology/Diagnosis/Management, Set. Mark Feldman et al. Ed. by Richard Zorab. 6th ed. 1997. LC 96-21131. (Illus.). 1920p. text 195.00 (*0-7216-6291-9*) Saunders.

Sleisenger & Fordtran's Gastrointestinal & Liver Disease Review & Assessment. Richard A. Weisiger & Lyman E. Bilhartz. Ed. by Richard Zorab. 2nd ed. 1998. LC 98-223589. 224p. (C). pap. text 40.00 (*0-7216-7703-7*) Saunders.

Slender Me Naturally. Bernard Jensen. 1986. pap. 12.99 (*0-932615-00-7*) B Jensen.

Slender Thread: Rediscovering Hope at the Heart of Crisis. Diane Ackerman. 1998. LC 96-8721. 320p. pap. 14.00 (*0-679-77133-6*) Vin Bks.

Slicing Through Your Emotional Luggage. Jerome Hart. 4th ed. 1998. 64p. (C). per. 19.95 (*0-7872-5360-X*, 41536001) Kendall-Hunt.

Slide Atlas of Clinical Dermatology, Set. Anthony Du Vivier. 406p. incl. sl. (*0-397-46303-0*, GM0113) Gower-Mosby.

Slide Atlas of Diagnostic Oncology Unit 2: Slide Atlas of Lung Cancer & Tumors of the Heart & Mediastinum. Arthur T. Skarin. 1991. 42p. (gr. 13). (*1-56375-032-5*, GM0202) Gower-Mosby.

Slide Atlas of Diagnostic Oncology Unit 9: Slide Atlas of Skin Cancer. Michael M. Wick. 1991. 28p. (gr. 13). (*1-56375-039-2*, GM0209) Gower-Mosby.

Slide Atlas of Diagnostic Oncology Unit 11: Slide Atlas of Acute & Chronic Leukemias. Arthur T. Skarin. 1991. 40p. (gr. 13). (*1-56375-041-4*, GM0211) Gower-Mosby.

Slide Atlas of Diagnostic Oncology Unit 13: Slide Atlas of Multiple Myeloma & Plasma Cell Dyscrasias. Arthur T. Skarin. 1991. 24p. (gr. 13). (*1-56375-043-0*, GM0213) Gower-Mosby.

***Slide Atlas of Ear, Nose & Throat Disorders on CD-ROM.** A. J. Gulya & Wilson. 2001. ring bd. 74.95 (*1-84214-109-0*, Parthenon Pbng) CRC Pr.

Slide Atlas of Endovascular Surgery: Interventional Techniques in Vascular Disease. R. White & G. White. 1992. (Illus.). 176p. ring bd. 595.00 (*0-442-31556-2*) Chapman & Hall.

Slide Atlas of Gastrointestinal Endoscopy, Set. Fred E. Silverstein & Guido Tytgat. 1992. 279p. (gr. 13). (*1-56375-028-7*, GM0132) Gower-Mosby.

Slide Atlas of Gynecological Endoscopy. Alan G. Gordon & B. Victor Lewis. 180p. (*0-397-46473-8*, GM0186) Gower-Mosby.

Slide Atlas of Human Anatomy. J. A. Gosling et al. 2nd ed. 1991. 340p. (gr. 13). text (*0-397-44806-6*, GM0104) Gower-Mosby.

Slide Atlas of Infections of the Skin. Anthony Du Vivier. 1991. 208p. (gr. 13). text incl. sl. (*1-56375-502-5*, GM0238) Gower-Mosby.

Slide Atlas of Infectious Diseases, Set. W. Edmund Farrar et al. 2nd ed. 1992. 384p. (gr. 13). (*1-56375-504-1*, GM0261) Gower-Mosby.

Slide Atlas of MRI: Central Nervous System. Walter Kucharczyk. 264p. sl. (*0-397-46477-0*, GM0187) Gower-Mosby.

Slide Atlas of MRI of the Musculoskeletal System. Javier Beltran. 312p. incl. sl. (*0-397-46476-2*, GM0013) Gower-Mosby.

Slide Atlas of Neurology. George D. Perkin et al. 220p. sl. (*0-397-46309-X*, GM0116) Gower-Mosby.

Slide Atlas of Neuropathology. Haruo Okazaki & Bernd W. Scheithauer. 1988. 279p. (gr. 13). (*0-397-46403-7*, GM0141) Gower-Mosby.

Slide Atlas of Ophthalmic Surgery. Norman S. Jaffe. 1989. 345p. (gr. 13). text (*0-397-46428-2*, GM0159) Gower-Mosby.

Slide Atlas of Orthopedic Radiology. Adam Greenspan. 592p. sl. (*0-397-46405-3*, GM0143) Gower-Mosby.

Slide Atlas of Pathology of AIDS. Harry L. Ioachim. 1989. 244p. (gr. 13). text (*0-397-46437-1*, GM0168) Gower-Mosby.

Slide Atlas of Pathology of the Skin Phillip H. McKee. 1989. text (*0-397-46468-1*, GM0184) Gower-Mosby.

Slide Atlas of Pediatric Physical Diagnosis Unit 11: Slide Atlas of Pediatric Hematology & Oncology. J. Jeffrey Malatack et al. 2nd ed. 1992. 36p. (gr. 13). (*1-56375-056-2*) Gower-Mosby.

Slide Atlas of Pediatric Physical Diagnosis Unit 14: Slide Atlas of Pediatric Urologic Disorders. Mark F. Bellinger. 2nd ed. 1992. 18p. (gr. 13). (*1-56375-059-7*) Gower-Mosby.

Slide Atlas of Pediatric Physical Diagnosis Unit 20: Slide Atlas of Pediatric Oral Disorders. M. M. Nazif et al. 2nd ed. 1992. 21p. (gr. 13). (*1-56375-065-1*) Gower-Mosby.

Slide Atlas of Radiologic Imaging. E. George Kassner. 1989. 649p. (gr. 13). (*0-397-46418-5*, GM0144) Gower-Mosby.

Slide Atlas of Radiologic Imaging Unit 1: Slide Atlas of Bone & Joint Radiology. Nancy Baker. 1989. 58p. (gr. 13). (*0-397-46417-7*, GM0145) Gower-Mosby.

Slide Atlas of Radiologic Imaging Unit 5: Slide Atlas of Abdominal Sonography. Mordecai Koenigsberg & Janet Hoffman-Tretin. 1989. 60p. (gr. 13). (*0-397-46414-2*, GM0149) Gower-Mosby.

Slide Atlas of Radiologic Imaging Unit 9: Slide Atlas of Interventional Radiology. Robert J. Rosen. 1989. 32p. (gr. 13). (*0-397-46410-X*) Gower-Mosby.

Slide Atlas of Radiologic Imaging Unit 10: Slide Atlas of Imaging of Nonskeletal Trauma. Robert J. Rosen. 1989. 24p. (gr. 13). (*0-397-46409-6*) Gower-Mosby.

Slide Atlas of Radiologic Imaging Unit 11: Slide Atlas of Radiology of the Brain. George Lantos. 1989. 68p. (gr. 13). (*0-397-46408-8*, GM0155) Gower-Mosby.

Slide Atlas of Radiologic Imaging Unit 12: Slide Atlas of Diagnostic Imaging of the Head & Neck. Arnold M. Noyek. 1989. 50p. (gr. 13). (*0-397-46407-X*, GM0156) Gower-Mosby.

Slide Atlas of Radiology of the Chest, Set. Margaret E. Turner-Warwick et al. 1991. 320p. (C). (gr. 13). text (*1-56375-515-7*, GM0242) Gower-Mosby.

Slide Atlas of Rheumatology. P. A. Dieppe et al. 382p. incl. sl. (*0-397-46342-1*); 1986. (gr. 13). incl. sl. (*0-397-46343-X*, GM00127) Gower-Mosby.

Slide Atlas of Sexually Transmitted Diseases. Stephen Morse et al. 1989. 250p. (gr. 13). text (*0-397-46438-X*, GM0169) Gower-Mosby.

Slide Atlas of Sexually Transmitted Diseases: The Acquired Immune Deficiency Syndrome. Stephen Morse et al. 1989. 42p. (gr. 13). (*0-397-46450-9*, GM0177) Gower-Mosby.

Slide Atlas of Strabismus Surgery. R. Richards. 1991. (Illus.). 240p. ring bd. 895.00 (*0-442-31557-0*) Chapman & Hall.

Slide Atlas of Surgical Exposures in Orthopaedics. Stanley Hoppenfeld & Piet De Boer. 1987. 530p. (gr. 13). text (*0-397-46348-0*, GM0130) Gower-Mosby.

Slide Atlas of Surgical Exposures of the Limbs. Neil Rushton et al. 1986. 218p. (gr. 13). text (*0-397-46345-6*, GM0128) Gower-Mosby.

Slide Atlas of the Heart. J. Willis Hurst. 364p. sl. (*0-397-46401-0*, GM0140) Gower-Mosby.

Slide Interpretation. H. L. Beynon et al. 1991. (Complete MRCP Ser.). (Illus.). 232p. (Orig.). pap. text (*0-443-04309-4*) Church.

Slide Interpretation from the MRCP. Hugh J. Kennedy et al. 1987. (Illus.). 224p. (Orig.). pap. text (*0-443-03638-1*) Church.

Slide Preparation & Staining of Blood Films for the Laboratory Diagnosis of Parasitic Diseases: Tentative Guideline (1992) Contrib. by Lynne S. Garcia. 1992. 75.00 (*1-56238-161-X*, M15-T) NCCLS.

Slide Set for Biochemistry. Robert Roskoski, Jr. 1996. (STARS Ser.). (Illus.). 24p. ring bd. 625.00 incl. sl. (*0-7216-6527-6*) Saunders.

Slides in Human Arthrology. B. N. Tillman. 1985. (Illus.). 171p. 463.00 (*0-387-00350-9*) Spr-Verlag.

Slides to Sectional Anatomy Learning Section. Applegate. 1991. 520.00 (*0-7216-3239-4*) Saunders.

Slim Deception - Fat Reflection: One Woman's Struggle with Bulimia. Deborah Yelinek. 1987. 96p. pap. 2.50 (*0-919797-61-X*) Kindred Prods.

Slings & Arrows: Narcissistic Injury & Its Treatment. Jerome D. Levin. 1993. LC 93-13285. 336p. 50.00 (*0-87668-550-5*) Aronson.

Slip & Fall Handbook. Stephen I. Rosen. 2000. (Illus.). 400p. pap. 125.00 (*0-9703549-1-6*) Hanrow.

Slipping, Tripping & Falling Accidents. Ed. by P. R. Davis. 1985. (Ergonomics Ser.: Vol. 28). 168p. pap. 23.00 (*0-85066-950-2*) Taylor & Francis.

Sloane-Dorland Annotated Medical-Legal Dictionary: 1992 Supplement. Richard Sloane. 1992. LC 92-5676. pap. text 64.75 (*0-314-00807-1*) West Pub.

Slow Cures & Bad Philosophers: Essays on Wittgenstein, Medicine & Bioethics. Carl Elliott. 2001. LC 00-63661. 224p. 18.95 (*0-8223-2646-9*) Duke.

Slow Cures & Bad Philosophers: Essays on Wittgenstein, Medicine & Bioethics. Ed. by Carl Elliott. 2001. LC 00-63661. 224p. 54.95 (*0-8223-2657-4*) Duke.

Slow-Down Therapy. Linus Mundy. 1990. LC 90-81236. (Illus.). 72p. pap. 4.95 (*0-87029-229-3*) Abbey.

Slow Infections of the Central Nervous System: The Legacy of Dr. Bjorn Sigurdsson. Ed. by Johannes Bjornsson. 1994. LC 94-12040. (Annals Ser.: Vol. 724). (*0-89766-843-X*); pap. 135.00 (*0-89766-844-8*) NY Acad Sci.

Slow Motion: Changing Masculinities, Changing Men. Lynne Segal. 1990. 396p. (Orig.). (C). pap. 15.95 (*0-8135-1620-X*); text 45.00 (*0-8135-1619-6*) Rutgers U Pr.

Slow Potential Changes in the Human Brain. W. C. McCallum & S. H. Curry. 1993. LC 93-26280. (NATO Advanced Science Institutes Ser.: Vol. 254). (Illus.). 326p. (C). text 114.00 (*0-306-44596-4*, Kluwer Plenum) Kluwer Academic.

Slow-Release Delivery of Antimicrobials As Adjunct to Standard Periodontal Therapy. Betty N. Vandekerckhove. 1997. (Acta Biomedica Lovaniensia Ser.: Vol. 150). 118p. pap. (*90-6186-812-2*) Leuven Univ BEL. *Dist:* Coronet Bks.

Slow Virus Diseases. Ed. by J. Hotchin. 1974. (Progress in Medical Virology Ser.: Vol. 18). 380p. 118.50 (*3-8055-1700-9*) S Karger.

Slow Virus Infections of the Central Nervous System. Ed. by V. Ter Meulen & M. B. Katz. 1977. LC 77-1570. (Illus.). 258p. 136.00 (*0-387-90188-4*) Spr-Verlag.

SLR 87: Papers from the Fourth International Symposium on Sign Language Research. Ed. by W. H. Edmondson & F. Karlsson. 1990. LC 90-231230. (International Studies on Sign Language & Communication of the Deaf: Vol. 10). (Illus.). 288p. pap. text (*3-927731-06-4*) Signum-Verlag DEU. *Dist:* Gallaudet Univ Pr.

Slumber of Apollo: Reflections on Recent Art, Literature, Language & the Individual Consciousness. John

S

Holloway. 1984. LC 83-14279. (Illus.). 176p. text 59.95 (*0-521-24804-3*) Cambridge U Pr.

Small Animal Allergy: A Practical Guide. Edward Baker. 1990. LC 90-5615. (Illus.). 144p. pap. 42.50 (*0-8121-1240-7*) Lppncott W & W.

Small Animal Anesthesia, II. Diane McKelvey & K. Wayne Hollingshead. 1994. (Fundamentals Ser.: Vol. II). (Illus.). 352p. (C). (gr. 13). pap. text 33.00 (*0-8016-7961-3*, 07961) Mosby Inc.

Small Animal Anesthesia & Analgesia. K. Wayne Hollingshead & Diane McKelvey. 2nd ed. 1999. LC 99-25655. (Illus.). 334p. text 31.95 (*0-323-00273-0*) Mosby Inc.

Small Animal Cardiology. Keene. 1999. text (*0-7216-5497-5*) Saunders.

Small Animal Cardiology. Nelson. 2002. 256p. pap. 25.00 (*0-7506-7298-6*) Buttrwrth-Heinemann.

Small Animal Cardiology Secrets. Ed. by Jonathan A. Abbott. 2000. LC 00-23234. (Secrets Ser.). (Illus.). 350p. pap. 39.95 (*1-56053-352-8*) Hanley & Belfus.

Small Animal Cardiovascular Medicine. Mark D. Kittleson & Richard D. Kienle. 1998. LC 97-49052. (Illus.). 611p. (gr. 13). text 95.00 (*0-8151-5140-3*, 24180) Mosby Inc.

Small Animal Care. Dean Warren. 1994. LC 94-17075. (Illus.). 480p. (J). 69.95 (*0-8273-4557-7*) Delmar.

Small Animal Care & Management. Dean Warren. 2nd ed. (Agriculture Ser.). 2000. LC 00-20911. (Illus.). 560p. (C). text 69.95 (*0-7668-1424-6*); 1992. 64p. pap., tchr. ed. 12.75 (*0-8273-4558-5*) Delmar.

Small Animal Care & Management CTB. Dean Warren. 1995. (Agriculture Ser.). text 105.95 (*0-8273-7076-8*) Delmar.

Small Animal Clinical Diagnosis by Laboratory Methods. Michael D. Willard et al. 2nd ed. 1994. LC 93-31784. (Illus.). 416p. pap. text 50.00 (*0-7216-5202-6*) Saunders.

Small Animal Clinical Diagnosis by Laboratory Methods. Michael D. Willard et al. Ed. by Ray Kersey. 3rd ed. 1999. LC 98-34636. (Illus.). 415p. (C). pap. text 45.00 (*0-7216-7160-8*) Saunders.

Small Animal Clinical Nutrition. Ed. by Michael S. Hand et al. 4th rev. ed. 1999. LC 00-268836. (Illus.). xxi, 1192p. text (*0-945837-05-4*) M Morris Assocs.

Small Animal Clinical Oncology. Stephen J. Withrow & E. Gregory MacEwen. 2nd ed. 1995. LC 95-23427. (Illus.). 480p. text 94.00 (*0-7216-5592-0*) Saunders.

***Small Animal Clinical Pharmacology.** Jill E. Maddison et al. 2001. (Illus.). 507p. pap. (*0-7020-2573-9*) W B Saunders GBR. *Dist:* Saunders.

Small Animal Clinical Pharmacology & Therapeutics. Dawn Merton Booth. 1997. LC 99-87178. (Illus.). xiv, 806p. text 89.00 (*0-7216-4364-7*) Saunders.

Small Animal Dentistry. Colin E. Harvey & Peter P. Emily. 1993. (Illus.). 408p. (C). (gr. 13). text 71.00 (*0-8016-6076-9*, 06076) Mosby Inc.

Small Animal Dentistry. Harvey. 2nd ed. 2000. text (*0-323-00561-6*) Mosby Inc.

Small Animal Dermatology: A Practical Guide to Performing & Interpreting Diagnostic. Peter Barrie Hill. 2002. 256p. pap. 70.00 (*0-7506-4804-X*) Buttrwrth-Heinemann.

Small Animal Diagnosis. Ed. by Michael D. Lorenz & Larry M. Cornelius. 2nd ed. 1993. LC 92-46032. 652p. pap. text 49.50 (*0-397-51200-7*) Lppncott W & W.

Small Animal Ear Diseases: An Illustrated Guide. Louis N. Gotthelf. 2000. LC 99-40018. (Illus.). xiii, 270p. pap. text 47.00 (*0-7216-7750-9*) Saunders.

Small Animal ECGs: An Introductory Guide for Veterinary Surgeons. Mike Martin. 2000. LC 99-40470. (Illus.). 128p. pap. text (*0-632-05216-3*) Blckwell Science GBR. *Dist:* Iowa U Pr.

Small Animal Emergency Manual: First 24 Hours. Kirby. Date not set. text (*0-7216-7863-7*) Saunders.

Small Animal Endoscopy. Todd R. Tams. 2nd ed. 1998. LC 99-178834. (Illus.). 510p. (C). (gr. 13). text 119.00 (*0-8151-8743-2*, 23778) Mosby Inc.

Small Animal Internal Medicine. Darcy H. Shaw & Sherri L. Ihle. 1997. LC 97-3958. (National Veterinary Medical Series for Independent Study). 630p. pap. 35.95 (*0-683-07670-1*) Lppncott W & W.

Small Animal Internal Medicine. Richard W. Nelson & C. Guillermo Couto. 2nd ed. 1998. LC 98-221791. (Illus.). 1376p. (C). (gr. 13). text 125.00 (*0-8151-6351-7*, 26032) Mosby Inc.

Small Animal Internal Medicine. Richard W. Nelson & C. Guillermo Couto. 2nd ed. 1998. (Illus.). 1376p. (*84-8174-461-1*) Mosby-Doyma Libros ESP. *Dist:* Mosby Inc.

Small Animal Internal Medicine Case Management Test Booklet. Darcy H. Shaw & Sherri L. Ihle. 1997. LC 97-8339. (National Veterinary Medical Series for Independent Study). 150p. pap. 14.95 (*0-683-30348-1*) Lppncott W & W.

Small Animal Lameness. Schrader. Date not set. text (*0-7216-7778-9*) Saunders.

Small Animal Medical Therapeutics. Michael D. Lorenz et al. 1991. (Illus.). 656p. pap. text 49.50 (*0-397-50994-4*) Lppncott W & W.

Small Animal Nursing. Denis R. Lane et al. 1998. LC 98-53103. (Illus.). 288p. pap. text 35.00 (*0-7506-3615-7*) Buttrwrth-Heinemann.

Small Animal Nutrition. Sandie Agar. 2001. LC 2001-25326. 208p. pap. text 29.95 (*0-7506-4575-X*) Buttrwrth-Heinemann.

Small Animal Oncology. Joanna Morris & Jane M. Dobson. 2000. LC 00-58599. (Illus.). 256p. pap. 64.95 (*0-632-05282-1*) Blackwell Sci.

Small Animal Oncology: A Practitioner's Guide. Caroline Prymak. 2001. 224p. pap. 60.00 (*0-7506-4574-1*) Buttrwrth-Heinemann.

Small Animal Ophthalmic Surgery: A Practical Guide for the Practicing Veterinarian. Janice P. Gelatt. 2001. (Illus.). 408p. pap. 75.00 (*0-7506-4805-8*) Buttrwrth-Heinemann.

Small Animal Ophthalmology: A Problem Oriented Approach. Peiffer. 2nd ed. 1996. (Illus.). 205p. pap. text (*0-7020-2017-6*) W B Saunders GBR. *Dist:* Saunders.

Small Animal Opthalmology, '94. Riis. 1994. text (*0-7234-2003-3*) Wolfe Publishing GBR. *Dist:* Mosby Inc.

Small Animal Orthopedics. Robert L. Leighton. 1993. LC 92-35357. 225p. (gr. 13). (*1-56375-082-1*) Gower-Mosby.

Small Animal Orthopedics. Marvin L. Olmstead. 1995. LC 95-15902. (Illus.). 592p. (C). (gr. 13). text 80.00 (*0-8016-5874-8*, 05874) Mosby Inc.

Small Animal Paediatric Medicine & Surgery. Giselle Hosgood & Johnny D. Hoskins. 1998. LC 97-31809. 324p. text 85.00 (*0-7506-3599-1*) Buttrwrth-Heinemann.

Small Animal Physical Diagnosis & Clinical Procedures. Dennis M. McCurnin & Poffenbarger. 1990. (Illus.). 244p. text 54.00 (*0-7216-5931-4*) Saunders.

Small Animal Radiology & Ultrasonography: A Diagnostic Atlas & Text. Ronald L. Burk & Norman Ackerman. Ed. by Ray Kersey. 2nd ed. 1996. (Illus.). 560p. text 120.00 (*0-7216-5270-0*) Saunders.

Small Animal Surgery. Fossum. 1997. (Illus.). 1216p. (C). (gr. 13). text 142.00 (*0-8151-3238-7*, 24202) Mosby Inc.

Small Animal Surgery. Ed. by Joseph Harari. 1996. LC 95-35809. (National Veterinary Medical Series for Independent Study). 475p. 34.95 (*0-683-03910-5*) Lppncott W & W.

Small Animal Surgery. Saunders. 1995. text 70.00 (*0-7020-1688-8*) Saunders.

Small Animal Surgery. Fossum. 2nd ed. 2002. text (*0-323-01238-8*) Mosby Inc.

Small Animal Surgery Secrets. Ed. by Joseph Harari. 2000. LC 00-23119. (Secrets Ser.). (Illus.). xiii, 381p. pap. 39.95 (*1-56053-355-2*) Hanley & Belfus.

Small Animal Surgical Nursing. Diane L. Tracy. 3rd ed. 2000. (Illus.). 434p. text 37.00 (*1-55664-503-1*) Mosby Inc.

Small Animal Surgical Nursing, Vol. 2. Diane L. Tracy & McBride. 2nd ed. 1994. (Illus.). 384p. (C). (gr. 13). pap. text 32.00 (*0-8016-6813-1*, 06813) Mosby Inc.

Small Animal Toxicology. Michael E. Peterson. 1999. LC 00-30095. (Illus.). xix, 796p. text 59.00 (*0-7216-7826-2*) Saunders.

Small Animal Ultrasound. Ronald W. Green. 1995. 400p. 195.00 (*0-7817-1775-2*) Lppncott W & W.

Small Animal Ultrasound. Ed. by Ronald W. Green. 1995. 400p. text 84.00 (*0-397-51387-9*) Lppncott W & W.

Small Animal Veterinary Nerdbook. Sophia A. Yin. 2nd ed. 1998. LC 97-94752. (Illus.). 456p. (C). ring bd. 48.95 (*0-9641518-1-2*) CattleDog Pubng.

Small Animal Wound Management. Steven F. Swaim & Ralph A. Henderson. 1990. LC 89-12383. (Illus.). 252p. pap. text 49.50 (*0-8121-1239-3*) Lppncott W & W.

Small Animal Wound Management. Stephen F. Swaim & Ralph A. Henderson, Jr. 2nd ed. 1997. LC 96-29668. 460p. 62.00 (*0-683-30276-0*) Lppncott W & W.

Small Bowel Disorders. Ed. by Ranjit N. Ratnaike. 2000. (Arnold Publication). 545p. 195.00 (*0-340-76008-7*) OUP.

Small Bowel Enterocyte Culture & Transplantation. F. C. Campbell. 1994. (Medical Intelligence Unit Ser.). 116p. 99.00 (*1-57059-004-4*, LN9004) Landes Bioscience.

Small Bowel Radiology. G. Antes & F. Eggemann. 1988. (Illus.). 207p. 139.00 (*0-387-15263-6*) Spr-Verlag.

Small Bowel Transplantation. Ed. by David Grant & Richard F. Wood. 1994. 160p. (*0-340-57322-8*) E A GBR. *Dist:* OUP.

Small Cell Lung Cancer: Proceedings of the International Conference on Small Cell Lung Cancer, Ravenna, Italy, 27-28 March, 1987. Ed. by M. Marangolo & G. Fiorentini. 1988. (Advances in the Biosciences Ser.: Vol. 72). (Illus.). 182p. 78.00 (*0-08-036631-7*, Pergamon Pr) Elsevier.

Small French & English Lexicon of Animal Physiology & Nutrition: Petit Lexique de Physiologie et de Nutrition Animales. Alice Daifuku. 1986. (ENG & FRE.). 52p. pap. 27.95 (*0-8288-0749-3*, F25160) Fr & Eur.

Small, Good Thing: Stories of Children with HIV & Those Who Care for Them. Anne Hunsaker Hawkins. 2000. LC 00-27018. xv, 286p. 23.95 (*0-393-04944-2*) Norton.

Small Groups in Counseling & Therapy: Process & Leadership. Barbara W. Posthuma. 3rd ed. 1998. LC 98-8516. 285p. (C). pap. text 78.00 (*0-205-29126-0*) Allyn.

Small GTPases & Their Regulators Pt. C: Proteins Involved in Transport. Melvin I. Simon. Ed. by W. E. Balch et al. 1995. (Methods in Enzymology Ser.: Vol. 257). (Illus.). 360p. text 79.00 (*0-12-182158-7*) Acad Pr.

Small GTPases & Their Regulators Pt. B: Rho Family. Melvin I. Simon. Ed. by W. E. Balch et al. 1995. (Methods in Enzymology Ser.: Vol. 256). (Illus.). 401p. text 84.00 (*0-12-182157-9*) Acad Pr.

Small Intestine. Ed. by Lawrence R. Schiller. 1997. LC 97-5655. (Gastroenterology & Hepatology Ser.: Vol. 7). (Illus.). 244p. text (*0-443-07865-3*) Church GBR. *Dist:* Saunders.

***Small Intestine in Experimental Peritonitis: An Experimental Study Focusing on Intestinal Energy Metabolism, Bacterial Translocation & Mucosal Immunology.** Mikael Ljungdahl. 2000. (Comprehensive Summaries of Uppsala Dissertations from the Faculty of Medicine Ser.: No. 908). 51p. pap. (*91-554-4655-8*) Uppsala Universitet SWE. *Dist:* Coronet Bks.

Small Medical Encyclopedia (Petite Encyclopedie Medicale) J. Hamburger. 17th ed. 1987. (FRE.). 1600p. 195.00 (*0-7859-4745-0*, M15436) Fr & Eur.

Small Medical Lexicon: French/English/French. Masson Staff. 4th ed. 1998. (ENG & FRE.). 192p. 29.95 (*0-320-00160-1*) Fr & Eur.

Small Peptides: Chemistry, Biology, & Clinical Studies. A. S. Dutta. 1993. LC 93-11629. (Pharmacochemistry Library: Vol. 19). 632p. 300.00 (*0-444-88655-9*) Elsevier.

Small Pox: Epidemics Deadly Diseases Throughout History. Tom Ridgway. 2000. LC 00-9890. (Epidemics! Ser.). (Illus.). 64p. (J). (gr. 7-12). lib. bdg. 19.95 (*0-8239-3346-6*) Rosen Group.

Small Wonders: Healing Childhood Trauma with EMDR. Joan Lovett. 1999. LC 98-30742. 256p. 27.95 (*0-684-84446-X*) S&S Trade.

Smallholder's Vet Book. Andrew Coe. 1985. (Illus.). 224p. 29.95 (*0-7134-4150-X*) Trafalgar.

Smallpox: When Should Routine Vaccination Be Discontinued. J. C. Frauenthal. 1981. 55p. pap. text 12.95 (*0-8176-3042-2*) Birkhauser.

Smallpox & Its Eradication. Frank Fenner et al. 1988. (Illus.). 1500p. text 140.00 (*92-4-156110-6*, 1150277) World Health.

Smallpox & the Iroquois Wars: An Ethnohistorical Study of the Influence of Disease & Demographic Change in Iroquoian Culture History, 1630-1700. Stephen Clark. 1981. (Illus.). vi, 121p. reprint ed. pap. text 14.38 (*1-55567-027-X*) Coyote Press.

Smallpox Eradication: Proceedings of the WHO Scientific Group, Geneva, 1967. WHO Staff. 1968. (Technical Reports: No. 393). 52p. pap. text 5.00 (*92-4-120393-5*, 1100393) World Health.

Smallpox in Colonial America: An Original Anthology. Ed. by Barbara G. Rosenkrantz. 1977. LC 76-40353. (Public Health in America Ser.). (Illus.). reprint ed. lib. bdg. 23.95 (*0-405-09880-4*) Ayer.

Smallpox Vaccination: A Survey of Recent Legislation. WHO Staff. 1954. (International Digest of Health Legislation Offprints: Vol. 5, No. 3). 42p. 3.00 (*92-4-169052-6*) World Health.

Smart but Stuck: Emotional Aspects of Learning Disabilities & Imprisoned Intelligence. Ed. by Myrna Orenstein. rev. ed. 2000. LC 00-47283. xvii, 228p. (C). 34.95 (*0-7890-1466-1*); pap. text 19.95 (*0-7890-1467-X*) Haworth Pr.

Smart Choices, Small Changes: The Healthy Lifestyle Planning Kit. Judith D. Grillo. 1995. (Illus.). 125p. (Orig.). pap. text 9.95 (*0-9643606-0-8*) Cricket Commun.

Smart Drugs II - The New Generation: New Drugs & Nutrients to Improve Your Memory & Increase Your Intelligence, No. II. Ward Dean et al. 1993. LC 93-78074. 287p. pap. 14.95 (*0-9627418-7-6*) Smart Pubns CA.

Smart Fats: How Dietary Fats & Oils Affect Mental, Physical, & Emotional Intelligence. Michael Schmidt. 1997. LC 96-37578. 250p. pap. 16.95 (*1-883319-62-5*) Frog Ltd CA.

Smart Girls: A New Psychology of Girls, Women & Giftedness. Barbara A. Kerr. 3rd rev. ed. 1997. LC 97-23100. Orig. Title: Smart Girls, Gifted Women; Smart Girls Two. (Illus.). 270p. (gr. k-12). pap. 24.00 (*0-910707-26-X*) Great Potential Pr.

Smart Girls, Gifted Women; Smart Girls Two see Smart Girls: A New Psychology of Girls, Women & Giftedness

Smart Guide to Sports Medicine. Sheila Sobell. 1999. LC 99-27222. (Smart Guides Ser.). 220p. pap. 12.95 (*0-471-35647-6*) Wiley.

Smart Love: A Codependence Recovery Program Based on Relationship Addiction Support Group. Jody Hayes & Maureen Redl. 1989. LC 88-32451. 208p. 13.95 (*0-87477-472-1*, Tarcher Putnam) Putnam Pub Group.

Smart Patient, Good Medicine: Working with Your Doctor to Get the Best Medical Care. Richard L. Sribnick & Wayne B. Sribnick. 1994. 144p. pap. 8.95 (*0-8027-7414-8*) Walker & Co.

Smart Questions to Ask Your Doctor. Dorothy Leeds & Jon M. Strauss. 1992. 192p. mass mkt. 8.99 (*0-06-104086-X*, Harp PBks) HarperCollins Pubs.

Smart Tracks: Systems Management for Orthopaedic Rehabilitation. James Hoyme et al. 1996. 300p. (Orig.). text 249.95 (*0-9643582-1-2*) Learn Pubns.

Smart Ways to Stay Young & Healthy. Bradley Gascoigne & Julie Irwin. 1992. 128p. (Orig.). pap. 7.95 (*0-914171-49-6*) Ronin Pub.

Smart Women, Strong Bones. Ronda Gates & Beverly Whipple. 2000. LC 00-108287. (Illus.). ix, 160p. (*1-878319-02-7*) Lifestyles Four.

SmartMedicine: How to Cut Medical Costs & Cure Cancer. Kent Wallner. 2000. LC 99-95168. (Illus.). 242p. pap. 24.95 (*0-9648991-2-4*) SmartMedicine.

Smile, Be True to Your Teeth & They'll Never Be False to You. Robert S. Rauch. 2nd rev. ed. 1991. (Illus.). 105p. pap. 9.95 (*0-9624076-0-7*) R S Rauch.

Smiling Spleen. W. Pagel. 1984. (Illus.). x, 214p. 133.25 (*3-8055-3707-7*) S Karger.

Smith & Nephew in the Health Care Industry. James Foreman-Peck. 1995. LC 94-21252. 304p. 100.00 (*1-85898-085-2*) E Elgar.

Smith's Anesthesia for Infants & Children. Etsuro K. Motoyama. Ed. by Peter J. Davis. 6th ed. 1995. (Illus.). 1024p. (C). (gr. 13). text 139.00 (*0-8151-5937-4*, 23779) Mosby Inc.

Smith's General Urology. Jack W. McAninch. 15th ed. 2000. (Lange Medical Bks.). (Illus.). 888p. (C). pap. 54.95 (*0-8385-8607-4*) McGraw-Hill Prof.

Smith's Recognizable Patterns of Human Deformation. Graham. 2nd ed. 1988. 208p. text 59.00 (*0-7216-2338-7*) Saunders.

Smith's Recognizable Patterns of Human Malformation. Kenneth Lyons Jones. Ed. by Judy Fletcher. 5th ed. 1997. LC 96-16722. (Illus.). 875p. text 75.00 (*0-7216-6115-7*) Saunders.

Smith's Textbook of Endourology, Set. Ed. by Arthur D. Smith et al. 1996. (Illus.). 1571p. (C). text 295.00 (*0-942219-81-3*) Quality Med Pub.

Smith's the Critically Ill Child: Diagnosis & Medical Management. Joseph D. Dickerman & Jerold F. Lucey. 3rd ed. 1985. (Illus.). 352p. text 85.00 (*0-7216-8386-X*) Saunders.

Smog, Health & Disease: Index of New Information. Dennis D. Patuznik. 1998. 160p. 57.50 (*0-7883-1758-X*); pap. 47.50 (*0-7883-1759-8*) ABBE Pubs Assn.

Smoke Away: Quit Smoking Now. Jay Burchett. 1989. 31p. (Orig.). pap. 4.95 (*0-929013-04-2*) Newport Pub Hse.

Smoked: The Inside Story of the Minnesota Tobacco Trial. Deborah C. Rybak & David Phelps. Ed. by Tom Mason. 1998. (Illus.). 480p. pap. 17.95 (*0-9641908-4-2*) MSP Communs.

SmokeFree - Worksite Smoking Control, Discouragement, & Cessation. Harold H. Dawley, Jr. 1987. (Illus.). 90p. (Orig.). pap. 14.95 (*0-9617202-1-2*) Wellness Inst.

Smokeless Tobacco Control: Report of a WHO Study Group, 1988. 1988. (Technical Report Ser.: No. 773). 81p. pap. text 11.00 (*92-4-120773-6*, 1100773) World Health.

Smokeless Tobacco or Health: An International Perspective. 1995. (Illus.). 389p. (Orig.). (C). pap. text 50.00 (*0-7881-2067-0*) DIANE Pub.

Smoker's Heaven: You Don't Have to Die to Go There. Martin Ehde, Jr. 1980. LC 79-57444. (Illus.). 132p. (Orig.). pap. 4.95 (*0-936188-01-4*) Ehde Pub Co.

Smoking: Facilitator's Manual. Sabina M. Dunton & Melody S. Fanning. Ed. by Richard A. McNeely. 1982. (Well Aware About Health Risk Reduction Ser.). (Illus.). 186p. (Orig.). 29.95 (*0-943562-51-1*) Well Aware.

Smoking: Individual Differences, Psychopathology, & Emotion. David G. Gilbert. 1995. (Series in Health Psychology & Behavioral Medicine). 307p. 59.95 (*1-56032-171-7*) Taylor & Francis.

Smoking: Psychology & Pharmacology. Heather Ashton & Rod Stepney. 1982. LC 81-18829. 250p. pap. (*0-422-77710-2*, NO. 3836) Tavistock GBR. *Dist:* Routldge.

Smoking: To Be or Not to Be. Robert Horning. 1993. LC 93-85796. 144p. (Orig.). pap. 6.95 (*0-9637330-0-1*) Portage Pub.

Smoking: Workbook. Sabina M. Dunton & Melody S. Fanning. Ed. by Richard A. McNeely. 1982. (Well Aware About Health Risk Reduction Ser.). (Illus.). 109p. (Orig.). pap. 8.50 (*0-943562-52-X*) Well Aware.

Smoking & Arterial Disease. Ed. by R. M. Greenhalgh. 1981. 315p. pap. 62.95 (*0-8464-1215-2*) Beekman Pubs.

Smoking & Health in the Americas: A 1992 Report of the Surgeon General, in Collaboration with the Pan American Health Organization. 1995. 213p. (Orig.). (C). pap. text 50.00 (*0-7881-2310-6*) DIANE Pub.

Smoking & Hospitals Are a Bad Match! American Hospital Association Staff. 1988. (Illus.). 47p. 35.00 (*0-87258-517-4*, 166901) Am Hospital.

Smoking & Illicit Drug Use. Ed. by Mark S. Gold. 1998. LC 97-52072. 128p. 39.95 (*0-7890-0507-7*, Hawrth Medical) Haworth Pr.

Smoking & Reproduction: A Comprehensive Bibliography. Ernest L. Abel. 1982. LC 82-15660. 163p. lib. bdg. 59.00 (*0-313-23663-1*, ASR/, Greenwood Pr) Greenwood.

Smoking & Reproduction: An Annotated Bibliography. Ernest L. Abel. 1984. 160p. 98.00 (*0-8493-6481-7*, Z6671, CRC Reprint) Franklin.

Smoking As a Cardiovascular Risk Factor: New Strategies for Smoking Cessation. Ed. by Lars Wilhelmsen. 1991. LC 91-20878. (Illus.). 80p. text 16.00 (*0-88937-069-9*) Hogrefe & Huber Pubs.

Smoking Behavior from Pre-Adolescence to Young Adulthood. Anthony V. Swan & Michael Murray. Ed. by Linda Jarrett. 1991. 254p. text (*1-85628-033-0*) Avebry GBR. *Dist:* Ashgate Pub Co.

Smoking Cigarettes - The Unfiltered Truth: Understanding Why & How to Quit. Janet Benner. 1987. LC 87-80270. 144p. (Orig.). pap. 10.95 (*0-942723-12-0*) Joelle Pub.

Smoking in Adolescence: Images & Identities. Barbara B. Lloyd et al. 1998. LC 97-37982. (Illus.). 232p. (C). 78.95 (*0-415-17859-2*); pap. 26.95 (*0-415-17860-6*) Routledge.

Smoking, Personality & Stress: Psychosocial Factors in the Prevention of Cancer & Coronary Heart Disease. Hans J. Eysenck. 2nd ed. 1995. (Illus.). 130p. 66.95 (*0-387-97493-8*) Spr-Verlag.

Smoking-Related Behavior & Attitudes: A Report on Research Using the ONS OMNIB. Fiona Dawe & Eileen Goddard. 1997. LC 98-133888. (*0-11-620948-8*, HM094888) Statnry Office GBR. *Dist:* Bernan Associates.

Smoking Scare De-Bunked. W. T. Whitby. 1990. 118p. pap. 9.50 (*0-9595564-1-9*) Green.

Smoking, Stop: Quit for Good! Rhoderick Elin & Elin Rhoderick. 1990. 31p. pap. 39.50 incl. audio (*0-88432-287-4*, S01670) J Norton Audio-Forum.

Smooth Muscle Cells in Atherosclerosis. J. C. Geer. Ed. by M. Daria Haust et al. 1972. (Monographs on Atherosclerosis: Vol. 2). 49.75 (*3-8055-1377-1*) S Karger.

Smooth Muscle Contraction: New Regulatory Modes. Ed. by K. Saida & Kazuhiro Kohama. 1995. (Illus.). xvi, 160p. 172.25 (*3-8055-6123-7*) S Karger.

Smooth Muscle Excitation. Ed. by T. B. Bolton & Tadao Tomita. 1996. (Illus.). 560p. text 120.00 (*0-12-112360-X*) Acad Pr.

Smooth Muscle Regeneration: A Review & Experimental Study. J. McGeachie. 1975. (Monographs in Developmental Biology: Vol. 9). (Illus.). vii, 90p. 48.00 (*3-8055-2058-1*) S Karger.

Snail Hosts of Schistosomiasis & Other: A Manual. Emile A. Malek. 1985. (Scientific Publications: Vol. 478). 334p. 12.00 (*92-75-11478-1*) PAHO.

Snail Transmitted Parasitic Diseases Emile A. Malek. 1980. Vol. 1. 352p. 193.00 (*0-8493-5269-X*, RC119); Vol. 2. 344p. 188.00 (*0-8493-5270-3*) Franklin (CRC Reprint).

Snake Bites & Their Treatment. Wee Y. Chin et al. 1991. pap. 19.95 (*9971-69-151-5*) Intl Spec Bk.

Snake-Oil Syndrome: Patent Medicine Advertising. A. Walker Bingham. 1994. LC 93-72216. (Illus.). 40.00 (*0-8158-0484-9*) Chris Mass.

Snake Venom Poisoning. Findlay Russell. rev. ed. 1983. LC 83-3134. (Illus.). 576p. text 57.50 (*0-87936-015-1*) Scholium Intl.

Snakebite Assessment & Treatment in the Eastern United States: A Merging of the Methods of Top Experts into a Guidebook for Nurses & Physicians, Including Comprehensive Protocols Plus Patient Assessment & Treatment Records Designed for Photocopying. Jon E. Soskis. 1995. LC 94-80125. (Illus.). 107p. pap. 95.00 (*0-9639911-5-9*) Snakebite.

Snakebite First Aid. Thomas G. Glass, Jr. 1981. (Illus.). 41p. reprint ed. pap. 9.95 (*0-9614759-0-0*) Glass Pub Co.

Snakebite Protocols/Consultant Directory. Jon E. Soskis. 1994. 32p. spiral bd. 30.00 (*0-9639911-7-5*) Snakebite.

Snakes of Medical Importance & Snake-Bite Treatment. Indramani Jena & Akulananada Sarangi. 1993. (Illus.). xxxv, 293p. (*81-7024-577-X*) Ashish Pub Hse IND. *Dist:* Nataraj Bks.

Snellen Sel Papers Electrocard. 1977. text 135.00 (*90-6021-420-X*) Kluwer Academic.

Snoezelen: Evidence from Practice. Patricia Schofield & Roger Hutchinson. 2000. 240p. (*1-85343-490-6*) Free Assoc Bks GBR. *Dist:* Intl Spec Bk.

Snomed International: The Systematized Nomenclature of Human & Veterinary Medicine Roger A. Ccotbe & College of American Pathologists Staff. 3rd ed. 1993. LC 98-221770. (*0-930304-48-9*) Coll Am Pathol.

Snore No More: Your Complete Guide to a Quiet Night's Sleep. Jeffrey Hausfield. 1998. LC 98-28777. 256p. pap. 12.00 (*0-609-80154-6*) Crown Pub Group.

Snoring & Obstructive Sleep Apnea. Ed. by David N. Fairbanks & Shiro Fujita. 2nd ed. 1994. LC 94-2841. 272p. text 99.00 (*0-7817-0196-1*) Lppncott W & W.

Snoring & Sleep Apnea: Personal & Family Guide to Diagnosis & Treatment. Ralph A. Pascualy & Sally Warren Soest. 2nd ed. 1995. LC 95-46517. (Illus.). 256p. pap. 24.95 (*0-939957-82-5*) Demos Medical.

Snoring & Sleep Apnea: Sleep Well, Feel Better. Ralph A. Pascualy & Sally Warren Soest. 3rd rev. ed. 2000. LC 00-31445. 222p. pap. 24.95 (*1-888799-29-3*) Demos Medical.

Snoring from A to ZZZZ: Proven Cures for the Night's Worst Nuisance. Derek S. Lipman. 1998. (Illus.). 236p. pap. text 14.00 (*0-7881-5867-8*) DIANE Pub.

Snowshoe & Lancet: Memoirs of a Frontier Newfoundland Doctor, 1937-1947. Robert Skidmore Ecke. 2000. LC 00-35305. (Illus.). 240p. 24.95 (*0-914339-85-0*) P E Randall Pub.

So Hakase No Kampoh: Dr. Tsung's Chinese Medicine. Pi-Kwang Tsung. unabr. ed. 1996. (JPN.). 116p. (Orig.). pap. 14.95 (*0-9655166-0-1*) Am Inst Chinese Herbs.

So-o You Are Going to the Hospital. Carol Zimet. 1993. (Illus.). 24p. pap. (*0-9639659-0-5*) C Zimet.

So That His Death Will Have Not Been in Vain: The Sickel Cell Trait: A Serious Factor to Be Observed by the Military. Peggy D. Friend. 1994. LC 92-50578. 675p. (Orig.). (gr. 10-12). pap. 19.95 (*0-936026-77-4*) R&M Pub Co.

***So That Was Life.** P. H. Schurr. (History of Medicine Ser.). (*1-85315-305-2*) Royal Soc of Medicine Pr Ltd GBR. *Dist:* Balogh.

So That's What They're For: Breastfeeding Basics. Janet Tamaro-Natt. 2nd ed. 1998. LC 98-14249. (Illus.). 256p. pap. 10.95 (*1-58062-041-8*) Adams Media.

So, Who Do You Think You Are? Face Your Wounds, Heal Them & Change Your Life. David W. Pendlum. Ed. by Susan Chinn & Nora Macaluso. 2000. LC 99-68285. 160p. pap. 9.95 (*0-9672942-1-5*) Grnlf Ent.

So You Have High Blood Cholesterol. 1995. (Illus.). 34p. (C). pap. text 12.00 (*0-7881-2170-7*) DIANE Pub.

So You Have High Blood Cholesterol. 1990. lib. bdg. 75.00 (*0-8490-3996-7*) Gordon Pr.

So You Want to See a Psychiatrist? Ed. by Bruce L. Danto et al. 1980. LC 79-23225. 170p. lib. bdg. 19.95 (*0-405-12622-0*) Ayer.

So You're Going to Have Puppies. Mari Stein. 1973. (Illus.). pap. 3.95 (*0-918546-03-6*) Quarterdeck.

So You're on the Hospital Board! Richard J. Umbdenstock. 4th ed. 1992. LC 92-29099. 41p. pap. 18.00 (*1-55648-095-4*, 196115) AHPI.

So You're Thinking of Going to a Chiropractor. Robert Dryburgh. 1984. 160p. pap. 3.95 (*0-87983-355-6*, Keats Pubng) McGraw-Hill Trade.

Soap, Water, & Sex: A Lively Guide to the Benefits of Sexual Hygiene & to Coping with Sexually Transmitted Diseases. Jacob Lipman. 1998. LC 97-31405. 191p. pap. text 23.00 (*1-57392-193-9*) Prometheus Bks.

Sober Alcoholic: An Organizational Analysis of Alcoholics Anonymous. Irving P. Gellman. 1964. 24.95 (*0-8084-0279-X*) NCUP.

Sober Days, Golden Years: Alcoholism & the Older Person. 1982. 48p. pap. 4.95 (*0-935908-06-4*, 3263, HazeldenJohnson Inst) Hazelden.

Soccer. Ed. by Bjorn Ekblom. 2nd ed. 1995. (Handbook of Sports Medicine & Science Ser.). (Illus.). 240p. pap. 41.95 (*0-632-03328-2*, BEKB3328) Blackwell Sci.

Social Accountability Program: Continuing the Community Benefit Tradition of Not-for-Profit Homes & Services for the Aging. Catholic Health Association of the United States Staff & American Association of Homes and Services for the Aging Staff. 1993. 98p. pap. 9.95 (*0-943774-47-0*, 812) Cath Health.

Social Amnesia: A Critique of Contemporary Psychology. Intro. by Russell Jacoby. 1997. LC 96-5599. 223p. pap. text 24.95 (*1-56000-892-X*) Transaction Pubs.

Social & Behavioral Aspects of AIDS, Vol. 3. Ed. by Gary L. Albrecht & Rick Zimmerman. 1993. (Advances in Medical Sociology Ser.). 227p. 78.50 (*1-55938-439-5*) Jai Pr.

Social & Behavioral Aspects of Female Alcoholism: An Annotated Bibliography. Compiled by H. Paul Chalfant & Brent S. Roper. 1980. LC 80-1021. 145p. lib. bdg. 59.00 (*0-313-20947-2*, CAL/, Greenwood Pr) Greenwood.

Social & Behavioral Aspects of Malaria Control: A Study Among the Murut of Sabah. Kin Foong. 2000. (Borneo Research Council Occasional Papers: Vol. 1). 241p. pap. text 20.00 (*1-929900-00-7*) Borneo Res.

Social & Behavioral Aspects of Pharmaceutical Care. Ed. by Mickey C. Smith & Albert I. Wertheimer. 1996. (Illus.). 838p. lib. bdg. 89.95 (*1-56024-952-8*, Pharmctl Prods) Haworth Pr.

Social & Biological Aspects of Mental Disease. Benjamin Malzberg. Ed. by Gerald N. Grob. 1980. LC 78-22573. (Historical Issues in Mental Health Ser.). (Illus.). reprint ed. lib. bdg. 28.95 (*0-405-11926-7*) Ayer.

Social & Cognitive Aspects of Normal & Atypical Language Development. Ed. by S. Von Tetzchner et al. 1989. (Cognitive Development Ser.). (Illus.). 182p. 150.00 (*0-387-96882-2*) Spr-Verlag.

Social & Cultural Perspectives on Blindness: Barriers to Community Integration. C. Edwin Vaughan. 1998. LC 97-52371. 220p. text 46.95 (*0-398-06854-2*); pap. text 31.95 (*0-398-06855-0*) C C Thomas.

Social & Economic Factors Affecting Morality: Confluence 5. Bernard Benjamin. 1965. text (*3-11-000279-5*) Mouton.

Social & Emotional Development of Exceptional Students: Handicapped & Gifted. Carroll J. Jones. 1992. 218p. text 43.95 (*0-398-05781-8*) C C Thomas.

Social & Ethical Interpretations in Mental Development. James M. Baldwin. 2nd ed. 1977. LC 73-2960. (Classics in Psychology Ser.). reprint ed. 40.95 (*0-405-05133-6*) Ayer.

Social & Health Aspects of Sexually Transmitted Diseases Principles of Control Measures. 1977. (Public Health Papers: No. 65). 56p. pap. text 8.00 (*92-4-130065-5*, 1110065) World Health.

Social & Medical Aspects of Drug Abuse. Ed. by George Serban. 1984. 288p. text 40.00 (*0-88331-201-8*) R B Luce.

Social & Personality Development. David R. Shaffer. (Psychology Ser.). 1979. LC 78-12032. (Illus.). (C). mass mkt. 32.00 (*0-8185-0289-4*); 2nd ed. 1987. LC 87-10958. 516p. (C). mass mkt. 50.00 (*0-534-08412-5*); 3rd ed. 1993. LC 93-18915. 569p. mass mkt. 53.50 (*0-534-20760-X*) Brooks-Cole.

Social & Personality Development: An Evolutionary Synthesis. K. B. MacDonald. 1988. (Perspectives in Developmental Psychology Ser.). (Illus.). 340p. (C). 70.00 (*0-306-42891-1*, Plenum Trade) Perseus Pubng.

Social & Personality Development: Essays on the Growth of the Child. William Damon. 1983. 504p. (C). pap. text 24.50 (*0-393-95307-6*) Norton.

Social & Personality Development: From Infancy Through Adolescence. William Damon. 1983. (Illus.). 392p. (C). pap. text 26.50 (*0-393-95248-7*) Norton.

Social & Psychological Aspects of Aging. Ed. by Clark Tibbitts et al. 1980. LC 79-8691. (Growing Old Ser.). reprint ed. lib. bdg. 88.95 (*0-405-12787-1*) Ayer.

Social & Psychological Contexts of Language. Ed. by Robert N. St. Clair & Howard Giles. 1980. LC 79-28232. 352p. text 69.95 (*0-89859-021-3*) L Erlbaum Assocs.

Social Animal. Elliot Aronson. 7th ed. 1994. LC 94-27611. (Series of Books in Psychology). (Illus.). 528p. (C). (gr. 11-12). pap. text 38.95 (*0-7167-2618-1*) W H Freeman.

Social Anxiety. Mark R. Leary & Robin M. Kowalski. 1995. LC 95-32612. (Emotions & Social Behavior Ser.). 244p. 39.95 (*1-57230-007-8*) Guilford Pubns.

Social Anxiety Disorder: A Guide. John H. Greist et al. 2000. 61p. pap. 4.95 (*1-890802-23-9*) Madison Inst of Med.

Social Assumptions, Medical Categories. Barbara Hansen. 1997. LC 98-209952. (Advances in Medical Sociology Ser.: Supplement 1). 78.50 (*0-7623-0243-7*) Jai Pr.

Social Attitudes & Psychophysical Measurement. Bernd Wegener. 1982. 512p. text 99.95 (*0-89859-083-3*) L Erlbaum Assocs.

Social Basis of Health & Healing in Africa. Ed. by Steven Feierman & John M. Janzen. 1998. 487p. (C). text 30.00 (*0-7881-5432-X*) DIANE Pub.

Social Basis of Health & Healing in Africa. Ed. by Steven Feierman & John M. Janzen. 1992. LC 90-44243. (Comparative Studies of Health Systems & Medical Care: Vol. 30). (C). text 75.00 (*0-520-06680-4*); pap. text 24.95 (*0-520-06681-2*) U CA Pr.

Social Behavior As Exchange. George C. Homans. 1993. (Reprint Series in Social Sciences). (C). reprint ed. pap. text 5.00 (*0-8290-2665-7*, S-122) Irvington.

Social Behavior from Fish to Man. William Etkin. abr. ed. 1967. LC 67-28654. pap. text 2.45 (*0-226-22037-0*, P533) U Ch Pr.

Social Behavior in Autism. E. Schopler & G. B. Mesibov. 1986. (Current Issues in Autism Ser.). (Illus.). 402p. (C). 66.00 (*0-306-42163-1*, Plenum Trade) Perseus Pubng.

Social Beliefs, Cultural Practices in Health & Disease. K. L. Pokarna. 1994. (C). (*81-7033-254-0*) Rawat Pubns IND. *Dist:* S Asia.

Social Causes of Psychological Distress. John Mirowsky & Catherine E. Ross. 1989. (Social Institutions & Social Change Ser.). 224p. (C). pap. text 25.95 (*0-202-30355-1*) Aldine de Gruyter.

Social Change & Personality: Essays in Honor of Nevitt Sanford. Ed. by M. B. Freedman. 1987. (Recent Research in Psychology Ser.). 231p. 64.95 (*0-387-96485-1*) Spr-Verlag.

Social Change & Women's Reproductive Health Care: A Guide to Physicians & Their Patients, 8. Nada L. Stotland. 1988. LC 87-27591. 266p. 77.00 (*0-275-92570-6*, Praeger Pubs) Greenwood.

Social Cognition & Clinical Psychology: A Synthesis. Ed. by Lyn Y. Abramson. 1988. LC 86-18453. 372p. 47.95 (*0-89862-011-2*) Guilford Pubns.

Social Cognition & Development: Studies of the Development of Understanding. George E. Butterworth & Paul Charles Light. 1997. LC 81-24075. 282p. (C). 24.00 (*0-226-08609-7*) U Ch Pr.

Social Cognition & Individual Change: A Cognitive-Ecological Approach to Practice. Aaron M. Brower. 1993. LC 93-29475. (Sourcebooks for the Human Services: Vol. 26). 89.95 (*0-8039-3883-7*, 7513); pap. 39.95 (*0-8039-3884-5*, 7514) Sage.

Social Cognition, Inference, & Attribution. Robert S. Wyer, Jr. & D. E. Carlston. 1979. 400p. 89.95 (*0-89859-499-5*) L Erlbaum Assocs.

Social Cognitive Psychology: History & Current Domains. David F. Barone et al. 1997. LC 97-1614. (Series in Social/Clinical Psychology). 508p. (C). pap. 42.50 (*0-306-45475-0*); (Illus.). 102.00 (*0-306-45474-2*) Perseus Pubng (Plenum Trade).

Social Comparison: Contemporary Theory & Research. Ed. by T. A. Wills & Jerry Suls. 1990. 432p. (C). pap. 49.95 (*0-8058-0550-8*); text 99.95 (*0-8058-0549-4*) L Erlbaum Assocs.

Social Comparison, Social Justice, & Relative Deprivation: Theoretical, Empirical, & Policy Perspectives. Ed. by John C. Masters & William P. Smith. 1987. (Greenwald & Krauss Ser.). 320p. text 59.95 (*0-89859-632-7*) L Erlbaum Assocs.

Social Construction in Couple & Family Counseling. Ed. by John D. West et al. 1998. LC 97-49144. xx, 187p. pap. text 21.95 (*1-55620-165-6*, 72672) Am Coun Assn.

Social Construction of Context Through Play. M. Nawal Lutfiyya. 1987. 238p. pap. 27.00 (*0-8191-6135-7*) U Pr of Amer.

Social Construction of Illness: Historical, Sociological & Anthropological Perspectives. Ed. by Jens Lachmund & Gunnar Stollberg. 1992. 240p. (Orig.). pap. 68.50 (*3-515-05839-7*) Coronet Bks.

Social Context of Caring in a Mixed Economy. Open Learning Foundation Staff. 1996. 144p. pap. (*0-443-05732-X*) Church.

Social Context of Chronic Pain Sufferers. Ranjan Roy. 1992. 450p. text 50.00 (*0-8020-2860-8*) U of Toronto Pr.

Social Context of Cognitive Development. Mary Gauvain. 2000. LC 00-62259. (Guilford Series on Social & Emotional Development Ser.). (Illus.). 249p. pap. 22.00 (*1-57230-610-6*) Guilford Pubns.

Social Context of Conduct: Psychological Writings of Theodore R. Sarbin. Ed. by Vernon L. Allen & Karl E. Scheibe. 1982. LC 82-473. 273p. 68.50 (*0-275-90752-X*, C0752, Praeger Pubs) Greenwood.

Social Context of Coping. J. Eckenrode. 1991. (Stress & Coping Ser.). (Illus.). 306p. (C). 49.50 (*0-306-43783-X*, Plenum Trade) Perseus Pubng.

Social Context of Health. M. Harding. 1998. LC 98-4843. (Health Psychology Ser.). (*0-335-19864-3*); pap. (*0-335-19863-5*) OpUniv Pr.

Social Context of the Chronic Pain Sufferer. Ranjan Roy. 1992. 310p. pap. text 19.95 (*0-8020-7360-3*) U of Toronto Pr.

Social Control of Deviance. Nanette J. Davis & Clarice Stasz. 2nd ed. 1990. 384p. (C). text 47.50 (*0-07-015930-0*) McGrw-H Hghr Educ.

Social Control of the Mentally Deficient. Stanley P. Davies. 1976. LC 75-17215. (Social Problems & Social Policy Ser.). (Illus.). reprint ed. 35.95 (*0-405-07486-7*) Ayer.

Social Correlates of Infant & Reproductive Mortality in the United States: A Reference Guide. Ann Creighton-Zollar. 1993. LC 92-41215. 224p. text 41.00 (*0-8153-0221-5*, SS766) Garland.

Social Costs & Rewards of Caring. Dermot Clifford. 1990. 261p. text (*1-85628-074-8*) Avebry GBR. *Dist:* Ashgate Pub Co.

Social Desirability Variable in Personality Assessment & Research. Allen L. Edwards. 1982. LC 81-20141. 108p. reprint ed. lib. bdg. 49.75 (*0-313-23245-8*, EDSD, Greenwood Pr) Greenwood.

Social Development. Nancy Eisenberg. 1994. (Review of Personality & Social Psychology Ser.: Vol. 15). 352p. pap. 42.95 (*0-8039-5685-1*, 3964) Sage.

Social Development. J. E. Grusec & H. Lytton. 1996. (Illus.). 545p. 69.95 (*0-387-96591-2*) Spr-Verlag.

Social Deviancy & Adolescent Personality. John C. Ball. 1973. LC 72-12308. (Illus.). 119p. reprint ed. lib. bdg. 52.50 (*0-8371-6687-X*, BASD, Greenwood Pr) Greenwood.

Social Dimensions of Development. Margaret Hardiman & James Midgley. 1989. 328p. reprint ed. text (*0-566-07044-8*) Avebry GBR. *Dist:* Ashgate Pub Co.

Social Dimensions of Health: The Israeli Experience. Judith T. Shuval. 1992. LC 92-14557. 224p. 65.00 (*0-275-93495-0*, C3495, Praeger Pubs) Greenwood.

Social Dimensions of Mental Illness, Alcoholism, & Drug Dependence, 9. Don Martindale & Edith Martindale. 1971. LC 72-133499. 330p. 72.50 (*0-8371-5175-9*, MAM/, Greenwood Pr) Greenwood.

Social Dreaming at Work. W. Gordon Lawrence. 1998. 224p. pap. (*1-85575-209-3*) Karnac Bks GBR. *Dist:* Other Pr LLC.

Social Economics of Health Care. John B. Davis. 2001. LC 00-51778. (Advances in Social Economics Ser.). (*0-415-25162-1*) Routledge.

Social Economics of Health Care. John Bryan Davis. 2001. LC 00-51778. (Advances in Social Economics Ser.). lib. bdg. 110.00 (*0-415-20765-7*) Routledge.

Social Effects of Health Policy: Experiences of Health & Health Care in Contemporary Britain. John Eyles & Jenny Donovan. 1990. 142p. text (*0-566-07084-7*) Avebry GBR. *Dist:* Ashgate Pub Co.

Social Environment & Health. Stewart G. Wolf. 1981. LC 80-50868. (Jessie & John Danz Lectures). (Illus.). 112p. 20.00 (*0-295-95777-8*) U of Wash Pr.

Social Exchange: Advances in Theory & Research. Ed. by Kenneth J. Gergen et al. 1980. LC 80-18170. 324p. 55.00 (*0-306-40395-1*, Plenum Trade) Perseus Pubng.

***Social Fabric of Health: An Introduction to Medical Anthropology.** John Janzen. 2001. 336p. text 45.94 (*0-07-032831-5*) McGrw-H Hghr Educ.

Social Factors in Medical Progress. Bernhard J. Stern. LC 68-57582. (Columbia University. Studies in the Social Sciences: No. 287). reprint ed. 20.00 (*0-404-51287-9*) AMS Pr.

Social Factors in the Personality Disorders: A Biopsychosocial Approach to Etiology & Treatment. Joel Paris. 1996. (Studies in Social & Community Psychiatry). (Illus.). 244p. (C). text 69.95 (*0-521-47224-5*) Cambridge U Pr.

Social Forces & Aging: An Introduction to Social Gerontology. Robert C. Atchley. (C). 4th ed. 1984. 510p. pap. 24.75 net. (*0-534-04338-0*); 5th ed. 1987. 527p. pap. 32.00 net. (*0-534-08790-6*) Wadsworth Pub.

Social Foundations of Thought & Action: A Social Cognitive Theory. Albert Bandura. 1985. LC 85-9310. (Prentice-Hall Series in Social Learning Theory Ser.). (Illus.). 544p. 116.00 (*0-13-815614-X*) P-H.

S

Social Function in Psychiatry: The Hidden Axis of Classification Exposed. Ed. by Peter Tyrer & Patricia Casey. 1993. LC 93-28470. 176p. (*1-871816-23-8*) Wrightson Biomed GBR. *Dist:* Taylor & Francis.

Social Functioning Patterns in Families of Offspring Receiving Treatment for Drug Abuse. Sharol Cannon. 1975. LC 75-42602. 10.95 (*0-87212-040-6*) Libra.

Social Functions & Economic Aspects of Health Insurance. William A. Rushing. 1987. (S. S. Huebner International Ser.: Vol. 5). lib. bdg. 112.00 (*0-89838-219-X*) Huebner Foun Insur.

Social Gerontology: A Multidisciplinary Perspective. Nancy R. Hooyman & H. Asuman Kiyak. 2nd ed. 1991. 656p. pap. text 42.00 (*0-205-12793-2*, H27931) Allyn.

Social Gerontology: New Directions. Ed. by Silvana Di Gregorio. 1987. 300p. lib. bdg. (*0-7099-3894-2*) C Helm GBR. *Dist:* Routldge.

Social Group Work with Older People. National Association of Social Workers Staff. Ed. by Leon Stein. 1980. LC 79-8684. (Growing Old Ser.). reprint ed. lib. bdg. 19.95 (*0-405-12801-0*) Ayer.

Social Groupwork & Alcoholism. Ed. by Marjorie Altman & Ruth Crocker. LC 82-2998. (Social Work with Groups Ser.: Vol. 5, No. 1). 92p. 1985. pap. text 14.95 (*0-86656-439-X*); 1982. text 39.95 (*0-917724-94-1*) Haworth Pr.

***Social Health Insurance.** 1998. (Social Security Ser.: No. 5). vi, 100p. pap. 12.95 (*92-2-110738-8*) Intl Labour Office.

Social History of Medicine: Health Healing & Disease in England 1750-1950. Contrib. by Joan Lane. 2001. LC 00-62758. lib. bdg. 85.00 (*0-415-20037-7*) Routledge.

Social History of Medicine in England, 1750-1950. Joan Lane. 2001. LC 00-62758. (Illus.). 256p. pap. 27.95 (*0-415-20038-5*) Routledge.

Social History of the Asylum: Mental Illness & Its Treatment in the Late 19th & Early 20th Century. Thomas G. Ebert. 1999. 320p. pap. text 40.00 (*1-55605-291-X*) Wyndham Hall.

Social History of the Minor Tranquilizers: The Quest for Small Comfort in the Age of Anxiety. Ed. by Mickey C. Smith. 1991. LC 91-13143. 259p. reprint ed. pap. 19.95 (*1-56024-142-X*) Haworth Pr.

Social History of Wet Nursing in America: From Breast to Bottle. Janet Golden. 1996. (History of Medicine Ser.). (Illus.). 232p. (C). text 69.95 (*0-521-49544-X*) Cambridge U Pr.

Social Hygiene in Twentieth Century Britain. Greta Jones. 1987. (Welcome Institute Ser.). 192p. (*0-7099-1481-4*) C Helm GBR. *Dist:* Routldge.

Social Ideas of American Physicians, 1776-1976: Studies of the Humanitarian Tradition in Medicine. Eugene P. Link. 1993. LC 91-50603. (Illus.). 320p. 46.50 (*0-945636-34-2*) Susquehanna U Pr.

Social Impact of AIDS in the United States. National Research Council Staff. 1993. LC 92-38885. 336p. 39.95 (*0-309-04628-9*) Natl Acad Pr.

Social Implications of Spina Bifida. Margaret Woodburn. 1975. (Education Ser.). pap. (*0-85633-061-2*) N F E R-Nelson Pub Co.

Social Inequalities & Cancer. Ed. by Manolis Kogevinas et al. 1997. LC 98-127171. (IARC Scientific Publications Ser.: No. 138). (Illus.). 428p. pap. text 89.50 (*92-832-2138-9*) OUP.

Social Influence, Vol. 5. Ed. by Peter Herman et al. 1987. (Ontario Symposia on Personality & Social Psychology Ser.: Vol. V). 312p. (C). text 59.95 (*0-89859-678-5*) L Erlbaum Assocs.

***Social Influence: Direct & Indirect Processes.** Joseph P. Forgas & Kipling D. Williams. 2001. LC 2001-16242. (Sydney Symposium of Social Psychology Ser.: Vol. 3). (Illus.). xxi, 367p. pap. (*1-84169-039-2*) Psychol Pr GBR. *Dist:* Taylor & Francis.

Social Influence Processes & Prevention. J. Edwards et al. 1990. LC 89-23236. (Social Psychological Applications to Social Issues Ser.: Vol. 1). (Illus.). 368p. (C). 65.00 (*0-306-43293-5*, Plenum Trade) Perseus Pubng.

***Social Influences.** Ed. by Joseph P. Forgas & Kipling D. Williams. 2001. LC 2001-16242. (Sydney Symposia in Social Psychology Ser.: Vol. 3). (Illus.). xxi, 367p. (C). text (*1-84169-038-4*) Psychol Pr GBR. *Dist:* Taylor & Francis.

Social Influences Affecting the Behavior of Young Children. Ruth P. Koshuk. 1941. (SRCD M Ser.: Vol. 6, No. 2). pap. 25.00 (*0-527-01518-0*) Periodicals Srv.

Social Influences on Behavior: Student Booklet. American Psychological Association Staff. 1981. (Human Behavior Curriculum Project Ser.). 80p. (Orig.). (gr. 9-12). pap. text 3.95 (*0-8077-2619-2*) Tchrs Coll.

Social Influences on Behavior: Teachers Handbook. American Psychological Association Staff. 1981. (Human Behavior Curriculum Project Ser.). 48p. (Orig.). pap. 9.95 (*0-8077-2620-6*) Tchrs Coll.

Social Inhibition & Socioemotional Functioning in Middle Childhood. Kerstin Bengtsgard. 2000. (Comprehensive Summaries of Uppsala Dissertations from the Faculty of Social Sciences Ser.: No. 91). (Illus.). 57p. pap. (*91-554-4748-1*) Uppsala Universitet SWE. *Dist:* Coronet Bks.

Social Integration of People with Schizophrenia. Lesley Cotterill. 1994. (Studies of Care in the Community). 154p. (*1-85628-841-2*) Avebry GBR. *Dist:* Ashgate Pub Co.

Social Inter-Personal Interactions: Index of Modern Authors & Subjects with Guide for Rapid Research. Marcus R. Soviero. 1991. LC 90-56318. 165p. 47.50 (*1-55914-442-4*); pap. 44.50 (*1-55914-443-2*) ABBE Pubs Assn.

Social Interaction. Michael Argyle. 1973. pap. (*0-422-75480-3*) Tavistock GBR. *Dist:* Routldge.

Social Interaction & Cognitive Development in Children. Anne N. Perret-Clermont. 1980. (European Monographs in Social Psychology: No. 19). text 139.95 (*0-12-551950-8*) Acad Pr.

Social Interaction & Its Management. Judy Gahagan. Ed. by Peter Herriot. 1984. LC 83-15129. (New Essential Psychology Ser.). 187p. pap. 7.50 (*0-416-33780-5*, NO. 4043) Routledge.

Social Interaction & the Development of Children's Understanding. Ed. by Lucien T. Winegar. 1989. LC 89-31305. 232p. (C). 77.00 (*0-89391-533-5*, Ablex) Greenwood.

Social Learning & Imitation. Neal E. Miller & John Dollard. 1979. LC 78-23728. (Illus.). 341p. reprint ed. lib. bdg. 35.00 (*0-313-20714-3*, MISL, Greenwood Pr) Greenwood.

Social Life of Children in a Changing Society. K. M. Borman. 1982. (Illus.). 320p. (C). text 69.95 (*0-89859-187-2*) L Erlbaum Assocs.

Social Marketing: Strategies for Changing Public Behavior. Philip Kotler & Eduardo L. Roberto. 1989. LC 89-45735. (Illus.). 352p. 40.00 (*0-02-918461-4*) Free Pr.

Social Meaning of Surgery. Nicholas J. Fox. 1991. 192p. (*0-335-09943-2*); pap. (*0-335-09942-4*) OpUniv Pr.

Social Medicine in Eastern Europe: The Organization of Health Services & the Education of the Medical Personnel in Czechoslovakia, Hungary, & Poland. Richard E. Weinerman & Shirley B. Weinerman. 1960. LC 72-78525. (Commonwealth Fund Publications). (Illus.). 217p. 23.50 (*0-674-81380-4*) HUP.

Social Medicine of Old Age: Report of an Inquiry in Wolverhampton. J. H. Sheldon. 1980. LC 79-8688. (Growing Old Ser.). reprint ed. lib. bdg. 24.95 (*0-405-12804-5*) Ayer.

Social Medicine Reader. Gail E. Henderson. Ed. by Nancy M. King et al. 1997. LC 96-50376. (Illus.). 528p. 79.95 (*0-8223-1957-8*); 632p. pap. 29.95 (*0-8223-1965-9*) Duke.

Social Mobility & Controlled Fertility. H. Y. Tien. 1965. 23.95 (*0-8084-0280-3*) NCUP.

Social Nature of Mental Illness. Len Bowers. 1998. LC 97-42740. 232p. (C). 89.95 (*0-415-17002-8*) Routledge.

Social Networks & Health of the Frail Elderly. Michal E. Mor-Barak. 1991. LC 91-28275. (Studies on the Elderly in America). 192p. text 30.00 (*0-8153-0515-X*) Garland.

Social Networks, Drug Abuse, & HIV Transmission. 1997. lib. bdg. 250.99 (*0-8490-6077-X*) Gordon Pr.

Social Networks, Drug Injectors' Lives & HIV-AIDS. S. R. Friedman et al. 1999. LC 98-55920. (AIDS Prevention & Mental Health Ser.). (Illus.). 294p. (C). text 75.00 (*0-306-46079-3*, Kluwer Plenum) Kluwer Academic.

Social Order - Mental Disorder: Anglo-American Psychiatry in Historical Perspective. Andrew T. Scull. 1992. (Medicine & Society Ser.: Vol. 3). (C). pap. text 18.95 (*0-520-07889-6*) U CA Pr.

Social Order-Mental Disorder: Anglo-American Psychiatry in Historical Perspective. Andrew T. Scull. 1989. (Medicine & Society Ser.: Vol. 3). text 40.00 (*0-520-06406-2*) U CA Pr.

Social Organization of Doctor-Patient Communication. Sue Fisher & Alexandra D. Todd. 2nd ed. 1993. 320p. (C). 77.00 (*0-89391-694-3*); pap. 39.50 (*0-89391-699-4*) Greenwood (Ablex).

Social Organization of Medical Work. Anselm L. Strauss. 1997. LC 96-53073. 313p. pap. text 24.95 (*1-56000-968-3*) Transaction Pubs.

Social Organization of Medical Work. Anselm L. Strauss et al. 1995. LC 84-23995. (Illus.). 33.00 (*0-226-77707-3*) U Ch Pr.

Social Organization of Mental Illness. Lindsay Prior. 1993. LC 93-84109. (Illus.). 240p. (C). 74.50 (*0-8039-8499-5*, 9201); 2nd ed. pap. 25.95 (*0-8039-8500-2*, 9202) Sage.

Social Origins of Depression: A Study of Psychiatric Disorder in Women. George W. Brown & Tirril O. Harris. 1978. LC 78-3209. 399p. 50.00 (*0-02-904890-7*) Free Pr.

Social Origins of Mental Ability. Gary Collier. 1993. LC 93-3625. (Personality Processes Ser.). 300p. 185.00 (*0-471-30407-7*) Wiley.

Social Pediatrics. Ed. by Bengt Lindstrom & Nick Spencer. 1995. (Illus.). 628p. text 135.00 (*0-19-262179-3*) OUP.

Social Perception. Leslie Zebrowitz. Ed. by Anthony S. Manstead. 1990. (Mapping Social Psychology Ser.). 248p. (*0-335-09861-4*) OpUniv Pr.

Social Perception in Clinical & Counseling Psychology. J. H. Harvey et al. Ed. by R. P. McGlynn et al. 1984. (Interfaces in Psychology Ser.: No. 2). 185p. 29.95 (*0-89672-127-2*); pap. 17.95 (*0-89672-126-4*) Tex Tech Univ Pr.

Social Perspectives on Pregnancy & Chilbirth for Nurses & the Caring Professions. Contrib. by Julie Kent. 2000. LC 99-25146. (Social Science for Nurses & the Caring Professions Ser.). 251p. (*0-335-19911-9*) OpUniv Pr GBR. *Dist:* Taylor & Francis.

Social Phobia: A Guide. John H. Greist et al. 1997. 61p. pap. 4.50 (*1-890802-09-3*) Madison Inst of Med.

Social Phobia: Clinical & Research Perspectives. Ed. by Murray B. Stein. 1995. LC 95-2031. 384p. text 49.00 (*0-88048-653-8*, 8653) Am Psychiatric.

Social Phobia: Clinical Application of Evidence-Based Psychotherapy. Ronald M. Rapee & William C. Sanderson. 1997. LC 97-19446. (Clinical Application of Evidence-Based Psychotherapy Ser.). 184p. text 35.00 (*0-7657-0004-2*) Aronson.

Social Phobia: Diagnosis, Assessment & Treatment. Richard G. Heimberg. 1995. LC 95-34091. 435p. 50.00 (*1-57230-012-4*, 0012) Guilford Pubns.

Social Policy: Nurses & Patients. Jill Manthorpe. 1999. 224p. (C). (gr. 13). 75.00 (*0-415-16158-4*, D6313) Routledge.

Social Policy for Nurses & the Caring Professions. Louise Ackers & Pamela Abbott. 1996. LC 95-49768. (Social Science for Nurses & the Caring Professions Ser.). 192p. (C). (*0-335-19360-9*) OpUniv Pr.

Social Policy/Health Care. Gormley. 1998. (C). pap. text (*0-443-05747-8*) Church.

Social Processes in Clinical & Counseling Psychology. Ed. by J. E. Maddux et al. 1987. (Illus.). 205p. 52.95 (*0-387-96533-5*) Spr-Verlag.

Social Psychiatry: Eighteen Essays. Ed. by Ari Kiev. 1970. 32.95 (*0-8464-0855-4*) Beekman Pubs.

Social Psychiatry: Theory, Methodology, & Practice. Ed. by Paul E. Bebbington. 1991. 420p. (C). text 44.95 (*0-88738-403-X*) Transaction Pubs.

Social Psychiatry Across Cultures: Studies from North America, Asia, Europe & Africa. Ed. by Rumi K. Price et al. 1995. (Topics in Social Psychiatry Ser.). (Illus.). 244p. (C). 45.00 (*0-306-44971-4*, Plenum Trade) Perseus Pubng.

Social Psychiatry & Community Attitudes. 1959. (Technical Report Ser.: No. 177). 42p. pap. text 3.00 (*92-4-120177-0*) World Health.

Social Psychiatry & International Accord. Ed. by Jules H. Masserman & Christine M. Masserman. 1993. 221p. (C). text 19.95 (*0-89876-201-4*) Gardner Pr.

Social Psychiatry in the Late Twentieth Century: Selected Proceedings - XII World Congress of Social Psychiatry. Ed. by Eliot Sorel et al. 1993. LC 92-48296. (*1-881901-02-5*) LEG7AS.

Social Psychology. 1999. (*0-13-022215-1*) P-H.

Social Psychology Ed. by Elliot Aronson & Anthony R. Pratkanis. 1993. (International Library of Critical Writings in Business History). 1800p. (C). lib. bdg. 525.00 (*0-8147-0609-6*) NYU Pr.

Social Psychology Brehm. (C). Date not set. text, tchr. ed., suppl. ed. 61.16 (*0-395-76069-0*); 1995. pap., tchr. ed., suppl. ed. 11.96 (*0-395-74526-8*) HM.

Social Psychology. Sharon S. Brehm & Saul M. Kassin. 1989. (C). pap. text 2.76 (*0-395-52640-X*); pap. text 2.76 (*0-395-52641-8*) HM.

Social Psychology. Donelson R. Forsyth. 1986. LC 86-17102. (Psychology Ser.). 651p. (C). 48.95 (*0-534-06744-1*) Brooks-Cole.

Social Psychology. Franzoi. 1995. 101.25 (*0-697-17477-8*, WCB McGr Hill) McGrw-H Hghr Educ.

Social Psychology. Ed. by Gilovich. 1999. (C). text (*0-321-01385-9*); pap. text, stu. ed. (*0-321-01386-7*) Addson-Wesley Educ.

Social Psychology. Kenrick & Neuberg. 1997. (C). pap. text, stu. ed. 20.00 (*0-205-27426-9*) P-H.

Social Psychology. Alan Marks. 1994. 208p. pap. text, stu. ed. 20.95 (*0-87901-749-X*) Worth.

Social Psychology. Roger Brown. 2nd ed. 1985. LC 85-13114. (Illus.). 720p. (C). 35.00 (*0-02-908300-1*) Free Pr.

Social Psychology. Eliot R. Smith & Diane Mackie. 2nd ed. 2000. LC 99-42560. 673p. 49.95 (*0-86377-587-X*) L Erlbaum Assocs.

Social Psychology. James W. Vander Zanden. 2nd ed. 1980. 524p. (C). text 24.50 (*0-394-32427-7*) Random.

Social Psychology Brehm. 3rd ed. 1995. (C). pap. text, stu. ed. 19.56 (*0-395-74527-6*) HM.

Social Psychology. H. Andrew Michener. 4th ed. 1997. (C). pap. text, tchr. ed. 42.00 (*0-15-504129-0*) Harcourt.

Social Psychology. H. Andrew Michener. 3rd ed. 1994. (C). pap. text, tchr. ed., suppl. ed. 33.75 (*0-15-500764-5*) Harcourt Coll Pubs.

Social Psychology. H. Andrew Michener. 4th ed. 1998. LC 98-87316. (Illus.). 688p. (C). text 87.95 (*0-15-504128-2*) Wadsworth Pub.

Social Psychology. Kay Deaux & Lawrence S. Wrightsman. 5th ed. 1987. LC 87-15798. 650p. (C). mass mkt. 46.00 (*0-534-08226-2*) Brooks-Cole.

Social Psychology. David G. Myers. 5th ed. 1995. (C). pap., stu. ed. 25.63 (*0-07-044360-2*) McGrw-H Hghr Educ.

Social Psychology. Alfred R. Lindesmith et al. 8th ed. 1999. LC 98-58146. pap. 34.95 (*0-7619-0746-7*, 81454) Sage.

Social Psychology. 9th ed. 1999. (C). text (*0-205-29805-2*, Longwood Div) Allyn.

Social Psychology: 3/e. Elliot Aronson et al. 3rd ed. 1998. LC 98-20751. 704p. (C). 91.00 (*0-321-02435-4*, Prentice Hall) P-H.

Social Psychology: An Analysis of Human Behavior. Leonard William Doob. 1971. LC 79-136063. 583p. reprint ed. lib. bdg. 38.50 (*0-8371-5213-5*, DOSP, Greenwood Pr) Greenwood.

Social Psychology: An Introduction. Michael A. Hogg & Graham M. Vaughan. 1995. LC 94-38461. pap. 60.00 (*0-7450-1625-1*); 2nd ed. 1998. LC 97-32382. (*0-13-486770-X*) P-H.

Social Psychology: Handbook of Basic Principles. Ed. by E. Tory Higgins & Arie W. Kruglanski. 1996. LC 96-22623. 948p. 100.00 (*1-57230-100-7*) Guilford Pubns.

Social Psychology: Index of Modern Authors & Subjects with Guide for Rapid Research. Salvatore S. Pequeno. 1991. LC 90-56329. 160p. 47.50 (*1-55914-454-8*); pap. 44.50 (*1-55914-455-6*) ABBE Pubs Assn.

Social Psychology: Instructor's Manual. Eliot R. Smith & Diane M. Mackie. 1995. tchr. ed. (*0-87901-801-1*) Worth.

Social Psychology: Instructor's Resource Guide. Irwin A. Horowitz & Kenneth S. Bordens. 1994. 249p. (C). pap. text, tchr. ed. (*0-87484-977-2*, 977) Mayfield Pub.

Social Psychology: Sociological Perspectives. Ed. by Morris Rosenberg & Ralph H. Turner. 1990. 798p. (C). pap. 29.95 (*0-88738-854-X*) Transaction Pubs.

Social Psychology: Student Study Guide. Irwin A. Horowitz & Kenneth S. Bordens. 1994. 143p. (C). pap. text 20.95 (*0-87484-978-0*, 978) Mayfield Pub.

Social Psychology: Test Bank. Lord. 1997. (C). pap. text 44.50 (*0-03-019104-1*) Harcourt.

Social Psychology: Test Item File. Franzoi. 1995. 19.37 (*0-697-17476-X*) McGraw.

Social Psychology: Unraveling the Mystery. Douglas T. Kenrick et al. 1998. LC 98-51504. (Illus.). 648p. (C). 93.00 (*0-205-16521-4*) Allyn.

Social Psychology A to Z. Elliott McGinnies. 1993. 356p. pap. text 32.50 (*0-89876-210-3*) Gardner Pr.

Social Psychology & Culture. Fathali Moghaddam. 1998. tchr. ed. 24.00 (*0-7167-3231-9*) W H Freeman.

Social Psychology & Dysfunctional Behavior. Mark R. Leary & R. S. Miller. 1986. (Social Psychology Ser.). (Illus.). 262p. 59.00 (*0-387-96325-1*) Spr-Verlag.

Social Psychology & Health. Wolfgang Stroebe. 2000. LC 99-59166. (*0-335-19922-4*) Open Univ TX.

Social Psychology & Health. Wolfgang Stroebe & Margaret Stroebe. Ed. by Anthony S. Manstead. 1994. (Mapping Social Psychology Ser.). 304p. (*0-335-09858-4*); pap. (*0-335-09857-6*) OpUniv Pr.

Social Psychology & Health. Wolfgang Stroebe & Margaret S. Stroebe. 1995. LC 95-3089. (Mapping Social Psychology Ser.). 290p. mass mkt. 33.50 (*0-534-26004-7*) Brooks-Cole.

Social Psychology & Health. Wolfgang Stroebe. 2nd ed. 2000. LC 99-59166. (Mapping Social Psychology Ser.). 288p. pap. (*0-335-19921-6*) OpUniv Pr.

Social Psychology & Health: European Perspectives. D. R. Rutter & Lyn Quine. 1994. 232p. (*1-85628-562-6*) Avebry GBR. *Dist:* Ashgate Pub Co.

Social Psychology at the Crossroads: Conference on Social Psychology, University of Oklahoma, 1950. Ed. by John N. Rohrer & Muzafer Sherif. 1977. LC 73-111822. (Essay Index Reprint Ser.). 30.95 (*0-8369-1600-X*) Ayer.

Social Psychology: Conflicts & Continuities: An Introduction Textbook. Dennis Howitt et al. 1989. 208p. pap. (*0-335-09882-7*) OpUniv Pr.

Social Psychology for Nurses. 256p. pap. (*0-7131-4577-3*) E A GBR. *Dist:* Routldge.

Social Psychology in the '80s. Kay Deaux et al. 4th ed. 1984. LC 83-7379. (Psychology Ser.). 700p. (C). mass mkt. 33.50 (*0-534-02926-4*) Brooks-Cole.

Social Psychology of Adolescent Delinquency. Nicholas Emler & Stephen Reicher. 1995. (Social Psychology & Society Ser.). 240p. (C). pap. 28.95 (*0-631-16823-0*) Blackwell Pubs.

Social Psychology of Aging. Vern L. Bengtson. 1973. LC 73-4918. pap. 3.50 (*0-672-61339-5*, Bobbs) Macmillan.

Social Psychology of Education: Current Research & Theory. Ed. by Robert S. Feldman. 1986. (Illus.). 401p. text 80.00 (*0-521-30620-5*) Cambridge U Pr.

Social Psychology of Facial Appearance. R. Bull & N. Rumsey. 1988. (Social Psychology Ser.). 355p. 137.00 (*0-387-96607-2*) Spr-Verlag.

Social Psychology of Groups. John W. Thibaut & Harold H. Kelley. 1986. 334p. pap. text 29.95 (*0-88738-633-4*) Transaction Pubs.

Social Psychology of Health & Illness. Ed. by G. S. Sanders & Jerry Suls. 1989. LC 82-1465. (Environment & Health Ser.). 368p. pap. text 39.95 (*0-8058-0554-0*) L Erlbaum Assocs.

Social Psychology of HIV Infection. Ed. by John B. Pryor & Glenn Reeder. 1993. 376p. text 75.00 (*0-8058-0991-0*) L Erlbaum Assocs.

Social Psychology of Interaction. Jerold Heiss. 1981. (Biology Ser.). 400p. pap. text 20.95 (*0-13-817718-X*) P-H.

Social Psychology of Intergroup Conflict. Ed. by Wolfgang Stroebe et al. 1988. (Social Psychology Ser.). 198p. 120.00 (*0-387-17695-0*) Spr-Verlag.

Social Psychology of Leisure. Roger C. Mannell & Douglas A. Kleiber. 1997. LC 97-60787. 450p. text 37.95 (*0-910251-88-6*, PSY92) Venture Pub PA.

Social Psychology of Mental Health: Basic Mechanisms & Applications. Ed. by Diane N. Ruble & Mary Ellen Oliveri. 1992. LC 92-1540. 365p. 46.95 (*0-89862-136-4*) Guilford Pubns.

Social Psychology of Organizations. Daniel Katz & Robert L. Kahn. 2nd ed. 1978. LC 77-18764. 848p. 105.95 (*0-471-02355-8*) Wiley.

Social Psychology of Organizing. Karl E. Weick. 1979. LC 79-10015. (Topics in Social Psychology Ser.). 294p. (C). pap. 40.00 (*0-07-554808-9*) McGrw-H Hghr Educ.

Social Psychology of Self-Referent Behavior. H. B. Kaplan. 1987. (Illus.). 224p. (C). 49.50 (*0-306-42356-1*, Plenum Trade) Perseus Pubng.

Social Psychology of the Self-Concept. Ed. by Morris Rosenberg & Howard B. Kaplan. 1982. (Illus.). 576p. (C). text 32.50 (*0-88295-214-5*); pap. text 22.50 (*0-88295-215-3*) Harlan Davidson.

Social Psychology of Tourist Behaviour. P. L. Pearce. 1982. (International Series of Monographs in the Sciences: Vol. 3). 142p. (*0-08-025794-1*) Pergamon Repr GBR. *Dist:* Franklin.

Social Psychology, Past & Present: An Integrative Orientation. J. M. Jackson. 1993. 184p. pap. 22.50 (*0-8058-1572-4*) L Erlbaum Assocs.

Social Psychology Readings: A Century of Research. Amy G. Halberstadt & Steve L. Ellyson. 1989. 512p. (C). pap. 46.88 (*0-07-025543-1*) McGrw-H Hghr Educ.

Social Realities & Community Psychiatry. H. Warren Dunham. 1976. LC 74-10967. 252p. 42.95 (*0-87705-215-8*, Kluwer Acad Hman Sci) Kluwer Academic.

Social Reality of Clinical Nursing in a Rural Hospital. Alan Pearson. 1989. 35p. (C). pap. (*0-7300-0694-8*, NPR803) Deakin Univ AUS. *Dist:* St Mut.

Social Reality of Death: Death in Contemporary America. Kathleen C. Charmaz. 1980. (Sociology Ser.). text 13.50 net. (*0-201-01033-X*) Addison-Wesley.

Social Referencing & the Social Construction of Reality in Infancy. S. Feinman. 1992. LC 92-11922. (Illus.). 440p. (C). 75.00 (*0-306-43850-X*, Plenum Trade) Perseus Pubng.

Social Responsibility in Science, Technology, & Medicine. Paul T. Durbin. 1993. LC 92-72013. 232p. (C). 31.50 (*0-934223-27-0*) Lehigh Univ Pr.

Social Science & Medicine: Seventh International Conference Background Papers. Ed. by Peter J. McEwan. 1981. (Journal of Social Science & Medicine Ser.: Vol. 15A, No. 3). 100p. pap. 18.00 (*0-08-028130-3*, Pergamon Pr) Elsevier.

Social Science Perspectives on Medical Ethics. Ed. by George Weisz. 1990. 312p. (C). lib. bdg. (*0-7923-0566-3*) Kluwer Academic NLD. *Dist:* Kluwer Academic.

Social Science Perspectives on Medical Ethics. Ed. by George Weisz. 1990. LC 90-13026. 320p. (C). reprint ed. pap. text 19.95 (*0-8122-1349-1*) U of Pa Pr.

Social Scientists & the Physically Handicapped: An Original Anthology. Ed. by William R. Phillips & Janet Rosenberg. 1980. LC 79-6011. (Physically Handicapped in Society Ser.). lib. bdg. 35.95 (*0-405-13103-8*) Ayer.

Social Security & Medicare: A Policy Primer. Eric R. Kingson & Edward D. Berkowitz. 1993. LC 92-43384. 224p. pap. 21.95 (*0-86569-201-7*, R201, Auburn Hse) Greenwood.

Social Security & Medicare: Individual Versus Collective Risk & Responsibility. Ed. by Sheila Burke et al. 2000. LC 99-50627. 232p. pap. text 20.95 (*0-8157-1283-9*) Brookings.

Social Security & Medicare Answer Book. Sean K. Hornbeck & David A. Pratt. 1999. 480p. 125.00 (*1-56706-132-X*) Aspen Pub.

Social Security & Medicare with Medigap: Approved 1990 Guide to Your Benefits, What They Are - How to Get Them. Wm. J. Williams. 1990. LC 90-81879. 130p. (Orig.). 15.95 (*0-9626952-1-1*); pap. 10.95 (*0-9626952-0-3*) Gamala Pub Co.

Social Security Benefits - A Guide to Accessing Services for Persons with Traumatic Brain Injury. Ed. by Linda J. Courtney. 1994. 40p. pap. 6.50 (*1-882855-28-0*) HDI Pubs.

Social Security Disability Benefits: How to Get Them! How to Keep Them! James W. Ross. rev. ed. 1984. 104p. pap. 19.95 (*0-9615202-5-6*) Ross Pub Co.

Social Security, Medicare & Pensions: Get the Most Out of Your Retirement & Medical Benefits. Joseph L. Matthews et al. 6th l.t. ed. LC 96-38562. 1997. pap. 20.00 (*0-7838-1984-6*); 1996. 651p. lib. bdg. 25.95 (*0-7838-1983-8*) Gale (Macmillan Ref).

Social Sensibility & Neural Function. Jay Schulkin. 2000. LC 00-26950. (Illus.). xviii, 206p. (C). 35.00 (*0-262-19447-3*, Bradford Bks) MIT Pr.

Social Service & the Art of Healing. Richard C. Cabot. 1973. LC 73-84257. (NASW Classics Ser.). 192p. reprint ed. pap. text 9.95 (*0-87101-062-3*) Natl Assn Soc Wkrs.

Social Service Policies & Procedures for Long-Term Care Facilities. Marylou Hughes. 1991. 100p. (C). 29.50 (*1-877735-33-7*, 2181PP) Prof Prntng & Pub.

Social Services Medical Assistance Specialist. Jack Rudman. 1994. (Career Examination Ser.: C-2431). pap. 34.95 (*0-8373-2431-9*) Nat Learn.

Social Situations. Michael Argyle et al. 1981. (Illus.). 462p. pap. text 29.95 (*0-521-29881-4*) Cambridge U Pr.

Social Skills. Matson. 1984. (Applied Research in Mental Retardation Ser.). pap. 18.25 (*0-08-030959-3*, Pergamon Pr) Elsevier.

Social Skills Basis of Psychopathology: Alternatives to Abnormal Psychology. E. Lakin Phillips. 1978. (Current Issues in Behavioral Psychology Ser.). 304p. text 47.00 (*0-8089-1126-0*, 793285, Grune & Strat) Harcrt Hlth Sci Grp.

Social Skills for Nursing Practice. Peter French. 1983. (Illus.). 272p. pap. (*0-7099-1009-6*) C Helm GBR. *Dist:* Routldge.

Social Skills for Nursing Practice. Peter French. 2nd ed. 1993. LC 93-33906. (*0-412-94740-4*, Chap & Hall NY) Chapman & Hall.

Social Skills for Nursing Practice. Peter French. 2nd ed. 1994. LC 93-33906. 312p. pap. 44.75 (*1-56593-228-5*, 0571) Singular Publishing.

Social Skills for People with Learning Disabilities: A Social Capability Approach. M. Burton et al. 1995. 282p. pap. 44.75 (*1-56593-194-7*, 0509) Singular Publishing.

Social Skills Training for Psychiatric. Robert Paul Liberman. 1992. 272p. (C). pap. text 60.50 (*0-205-14407-1*, H4407) Allyn.

Social Skills Training for Psychiatric Patients. Robert P. Liberman et al. 1989. (Psychology Practitioner Guidebooks). 250p. text 35.00 (*0-08-034695-2*); pap. text 17.95 (*0-08-034694-4*) Elsevier (Pergamon Pr).

Social Skills Training for Schizophrenia: A Step-by-Step Guide. Alan S. Bellack et al. 1997. LC 96-52826. (Treatment Manuals for Practitioners Ser.). 288p. 35.00 (*1-57230-177-5*, 0177) Guilford Pubns.

Social Skills Training Treatment for Depression. Robert E. Becker et al. 1987. 128p. text 28.00 (*0-08-032818-0*); pap. text 14.95 (*0-08-032817-2*) Elsevier (Pergamon Pr).

Social Sources of Delinquency: An Appraisal of Analytic Models. Ruth R. Kornhauser. LC 78-3776. (Illus.). 1995. pap. text 9.00 (*0-226-45114-3*); 1994. lib. bdg. 22.00 (*0-226-45113-5*) U Ch Pr.

Social Space for Domestic Animals. Ed. by R. Zayan. 1985. (Current Topics in Veterinary Medicine & Animal Science Ser.). text 191.00 (*0-89838-773-6*) Kluwer Academic.

Social Stratification & Psychiatric Disorders. August B. Hollinghead & Frederick C. Redlich. 1993. (Reprint Series in Social Sciences). (C). reprint ed. pap. text 5.00 (*0-8290-3793-4*, S-120) Irvington.

Social Stress & the Family: Advances & Developments in Family Stress Therapy & Research. Ed. by Hamilton I. McCubbin et al. 1983. LC 83-190. (Marriage & the Family Ser.: Vol. 6, Nos. 1-2). 231p. text 49.95 (*0-86656-163-3*) Haworth Pr.

Social Stress in Domestic Animals. Ed. by R. Zayan & R. Dantzer. 1990. (Current Topics in Veterinary Medicine & Animal Science Ser.). (C). text 195.50 (*0-7923-0615-5*) Kluwer Academic.

Social Stress in the United States: Links to Regional Patterns in Crime & Illness. Arnold S. Linsky & Murray A. Straus. 1986. LC 86-14192. 186p. 60.00 (*0-86569-149-5*, Auburn Hse) Greenwood.

Social Structure & Testosterone: Explorations of the Socio-Bio-Social Chain. Theodore D. Kemper. 1990. LC 89-70040. 265p. (C). text 40.00 (*0-8135-1550-5*); pap. text 17.00 (*0-8135-1551-3*) Rutgers U Pr.

Social Suffering. Arthur Kleinman et al. 1997. LC 97-201. 425p. text 55.00 (*0-520-20993-1*); pap. text 22.00 (*0-520-20995-8*) U CA Pr.

Social Support: An International View. Barbara R. Sarason et al. 1990. LC 89-27301. (Personality Processes Ser.). 528p. 240.00 (*0-471-60624-3*) Wiley.

Social Support & Cardiovascular Disease. Ed. by S. A. Shumaker & S. M. Czajkowski. 1994. (Behavioral Psychophysiology Ser.). (Illus.). 382p. (C). text 65.00 (*0-306-43982-4*, Kluwer Plenum) Kluwer Academic.

Social Support & Patient Adherence: Experimental & Survey Findings. Robert D. Caplan et al. 1980. 283p. (Orig.). pap. 16.00 (*0-87944-260-3*) Inst Soc Res.

Social Support & Psychiatric Disorder: Research Findings & Guidelines for Clinical Practice. Ed. by T. S. Brugha. 1995. (Studies in Social & Community Psychiatry). (Illus.). 361p. (C). text 90.00 (*0-521-44238-9*) Cambridge U Pr.

Social Systems & Schizophrenia: Selected Papers. H. Warren Dunham. 1980. LC 80-14193. 316p. 72.95 (*0-275-90472-5*, C0472, Praeger Pubs) Greenwood.

Social Transformation of American Medicine: The Rise of a Sovereign Profession & the Making of a Vast Industry. Paul Starr. 1984. LC 81-68412. 528p. pap. 25.00 (*0-465-07935-0*) Basic.

Social Trust: Toward a Cosmopolitan Society. Timothy C. Earle & George T. Cvetkovich. 1995. LC 94-45265. 240p. 62.50 (*0-275-94845-5*, Praeger Pubs) Greenwood.

***Social Values & Attitudes Surrounding New Reproductive Technologies.** 505p. pap. (*0-662-21376-9*) Can7 Govern Pub CAN. *Dist:* Intl Spec Bk.

Social Welfare of Women & Children with HIV & AIDS: Legal Protections, Policy & Programs. Theodore J. Stein. 1997. LC 96-50095. (Child Welfare Ser.). (Illus.). 272p. (C). pap. text 20.95 (*0-19-510942-2*) OUP.

Social Withdrawal, Inhibition, & Shyness in Childhood. Ed. by Kenneth H. Rubin & Jens Asendorpf. 1993. 368p. pap. 39.95 (*0-8058-1220-2*); text 79.95 (*0-8058-1219-9*) L Erlbaum Assocs.

Social Work: Disabled People & Disabling Environments. Ed. by Michael Oliver. 1991. 160p. 49.50 (*1-85302-042-7*) Taylor & Francis.

Social Work: Essays on the Meeting-Ground of Doctor & Social Worker. Richard C. Cabot. 1972. LC 76-180561. (Medicine & Society in America Ser.). 224p. reprint ed. 19.95 (*0-405-03940-9*) Ayer.

Social Work Administration in Health Care. Ed. by Abraham Lurie & Gary Rosenberg. 1984. LC 84-799. 310p. pap. 49.95 (*0-86656-314-8*); text 59.95 (*0-917724-42-9*) Haworth Pr.

Social Work & Alzheimer's Disease: Practice Issues with Victims & Their Families. Ed. by Rose Dobrof. 1986. LC 85-220269. (Journal of Gerontological Social Work Ser.: Vol. 9, No. 2). 126p. text 39.95 (*0-86656-402-0*) Haworth Pr.

Social Work & Child Sexual Abuse. Ed. by Jon R. Conte & David A. Shore. 1982. LC 82-11952. (Journal of Social Work & Human Sexuality: Vol. 1, Nos. 1-2). 184p. text 39.95 (*0-917724-98-4*) Haworth Pr.

Social Work & Health Care. Ed. by Rex Taylor & Jill Ford. 1989. (Research Highlights in Social Work Ser.: Vol. 19). 144p. (*1-85302-016-8*) Jessica Kingsley GBR. *Dist:* Taylor & Francis.

Social Work & Psychoanalysis. Margaret Yelloly. 1980. pap. 30.95 (*0-442-30167-7*) Chapman & Hall.

Social Work & Terminal Care, 2. Ed. by Lee H. Suszycki et al. 1984. LC 84-11615. (Foundation of Thanatology Ser.: Vol. 2). 176p. 29.95 (*0-275-91280-9*, C1280, Praeger Pubs) Greenwood.

Social Work & Thanatology. Ed. by Ben A. Orcutt et al. 1980. LC 79-22448. 300p. lib. bdg. 27.95 (*0-405-12621-2*) Ayer.

Social Work & the Family Unit. Ed. by David J. Ludwig. 2000. LC 00-40845. (Illus.). xii, 100p. (C). 34.95 (*0-7890-1196-4*); pap. 24.95 (*0-7890-1197-2*) Haworth Pr.

Social Work & Transplantation of Human Organs. Surjit S. Dhooper. 1993. LC 93-14136. 256p. 70.00 (*0-275-94338-0*, C4338, Praeger Pubs) Greenwood.

Social Work Constructivist Research. Mary K. Rodwell. 1998. LC 98-19159. (Social Psychology Reference Ser.). (Illus.). 328p. 70.00 (*0-8153-2552-5*, SS1134) Garland.

Social Work in Ambulatory Care: New Implications for Health & Social Services. Ed. by Gary Rosenberg & Andrew Weissman. 1994. (Social Work in Health Care Ser.). (Illus.). 108p. lib. bdg. 19.95 (*1-56024-697-9*) Haworth Pr.

Social Work in Health Care: A Guide to Professional Practice. Neil F. Bracht. 1978. LC 78-7881. 346p. 49.95 (*0-917724-04-6*); pap. 7.95 (*0-917724-05-4*) Haworth Pr.

Social Work in Health Care: A Handbook for Practice. Ed. by Kay W. Davidson. 1990. LC 89-24535. 517p. (C). text 19.95 (*0-86656-846-8*); pap. text 49.95 (*0-86656-907-3*) Haworth Pr.

Social Work in Health Care: A Review of the Literature. Society for Hospital Social Work Directors Staff. 1988. 91p. (Orig.). pap. 27.00 (*0-87258-477-1*, 187902) Am Hospital.

Social Work in Health Care in the 21st Century. Surjit S. Dhooper. 1997. LC 96-45777. (Sourcebooks for the Human Serives Ser.). 416p. 89.95 (*0-8039-5932-X*, 1543); pap. 39.95 (*0-8039-5933-8*, 1454) Sage.

Social Work in Health Settings: Practice in Context. Ed. by Toba Schwaber Kerson and Associates Staff. 1989. LC 89-1684. (Social Work Practice Ser.: No. 4). 523p. text 49.95 (*0-86656-811-5*); pap. text 24.95 (*0-86656-851-4*) Haworth Pr.

Social Work in Health Settings: Practice in Context. Ed. by Toba S. Kerson. 2nd ed. 1997. LC 96-51915. (Illus.). 700p. (C). 89.95 (*0-7890-6018-3*); pap. 49.95 (*0-7890-6019-1*) Haworth Pr.

Social Work in Mental Health: Trends & Issues. Ed. by Uri Aviram. 1997. LC 97-37786. (Social Work in Health Care Ser.). 134p. 29.95 (*0-7890-0383-X*) Haworth Pr.

Social Work in Pediatrics. Ed. by Ruth B. Smith & Helen G. Clinton. 1995. 130p. 24.95 (*1-56024-765-7*) Haworth Pr.

Social Work in the Health Field: A Care Perspective. Lois A. Fort Cowles. 1999. LC 99-16078. (Illus.). 354p. (C). pap. text 29.95 (*0-7890-0913-7*); lib. bdg. 49.95 (*0-7890-6033-7*) Haworth Pr.

Social Work Licensure Examination Study Manual - Basic. Eli Fresquez & Frances Goddard. 1998. (Illus.). 160p. stu. ed., spiral bd. 230.00 (*1-892380-00-5*) Ventajas.

Social Work Practice & Medication Use. Sophia F. Dziegielewski & Ana Leon. 2001. LC 00-51574. (Social Work Ser.). xvii, 326p. (*0-8261-1394-X*) Springer Pub.

Social Work Practice in Health Care: An Ecological View. Carel B. Germain. 1984. LC 83-48757. (Fields of Practice Ser.). 336p. (C). 35.00 (*0-02-911660-0*) Free Pr.

Social Work Practice in Sexual Problems. Ed. by James Gripton & Mary Valentich. 1986. LC 85-21992. (Journal of Social Work & Human Sexuality: Vol. 4, Nos. 1-2). 139p. text 4.95 (*0-86656-485-3*); pap. text 14.95 (*0-86656-526-4*) Haworth Pr.

Social Work Practice with Groups: A Clinical Perspective. Kenneth Reid. 1996. 311p. (C). pap. 49.75 (*0-534-14820-4*) Brooks-Cole.

Social Work Services & Patient Decision Making. Patricia Hansen. 1998. LC 97-77389. (Illus.). 164p. text (*1-84014-152-2*) Ashgate Pub GBR. *Dist:* Ashgate Pub Co.

Social Work Theory & Practice with the Terminally Ill. Ed. by Joan K. Parry. LC 88-29623. 130p. 1996. pap. 14.95 (*0-7890-0084-9*); 1989. (Social Work Practice Ser.: No. 3). (Illus.). 39.95 (*0-86656-750-X*) Haworth Pr.

Social Work Treatment of Alcohol Problems. Ed. by D. Cook et al. 1983. LC 82-620033. (NIAAA-RUCAS Alcoholism Treatment Ser.: No. 5). pap. 15.00 (*0-911290-15-X*) Rutgers Ctr Alcohol.

Social Work with Groups in Health Settings. Ed. by Abraham Lurie et al. 1982. LC 82-18151. 124p. pap. 7.95 (*0-88202-137-0*) Watson Pub Intl.

Social Worker & Psychotropic Medication: Toward Effective Collaboration with Mental Health Clients, Families, & Providers. Kia J. Bentley & Joseph Walsh. 1995. LC 95-35303. 230p. 44.95 (*0-534-34004-0*) Brooks-Cole.

Social Workers in Health Care Management: The Move to Leadership. Ed. by Gary Rosenberg & Sylvia S. Clarke. LC 87-15026. (Social Work in Health Care Ser.: Vol. 12, No. 3). 159p. 1988. pap. text 14.95 (*0-86656-815-8*); 1987. 39.95 (*0-86656-672-4*) Haworth Pr.

Social Workers Speak Out on the HIV/AIDS Crisis: Voices from & to African-American Communities. Larry M. Gant & Patricia A. Stewart. 1998. LC 98-21658. 176p. 60.00 (*0-275-96093-5*, Praeger Pubs) Greenwood.

Socialism & the NHS: Fabian Essays in Health Care. Ed. by John Carrier & Ian Kendall. 1990. (Illus.). 120p. text (*0-566-07110-X*) Avebry GBR. *Dist:* Ashgate Pub Co.

Socialist Health - Capitalist Health: Is There a Difference?: A Special Issue of the Journal Medical Anthropology. Ed. by M. Singer & H. A. Baer. 1989. ii, 126p. pap. text 43.00 (*2-88124-343-6*) Gordon & Breach.

Socialization of Emotions. M. Lewis & C. Saarni. 1985. (Genesis of Behavior Ser.: Vol. 5). (Illus.). 334p. (C). 75.00 (*0-306-41851-7*, Plenum Trade) Perseus Pubng.

Socialization of Family Size Values: Youth & Family Planning in an Indian Village. Thomas Poffenberger & Kim Sebaly. 1976. LC 76-53996. (Michigan Papers on South & Southeast Asia: No. 12). (Illus.). xiv, 159p. (Orig.). pap. 3.00 (*0-89148-012-9*) Ctr S&SE Asian.

Societas Ergophthalmologica Internationalis: 5th Symposium, Bordeux 1974. 6th Symposium, Hamburg 1976. 7th Symposium, Nagoya 1978. Ed. by H. J. Merte. 1982. (Problems of Industrial Medicine in Ophthalmology Ser.: Vol. 5-7). (Illus.). xx, 760p. pap. 216.75 (*3-8055-3003-X*) S Karger.

Societe Belge de Dermatologie et de Syphiligraphie: Belgische Vereniging voor Dermatologie en Syfiligrafie - Journal: Dermatologica, Vol. 158, No. 3. Ed. by R. Schuppli. 1979. (Illus.). pap. 28.75 (*3-8055-3018-8*) S Karger.

Societe Suisse de Gynecologie, Bericht ueber die Jahresversammlung, Genf, 1981. Ed. by E. Dreher. 1981. (Gynaekologische Rundschau Journal: Vol. 21, Suppl. 3). (Illus.). iv, 88p. pap. 25.25 (*3-8055-3479-5*) S Karger.

Society & Fertility. Malcolm Potts & Peter Selman. 1979. (Illus.). 384p. 32.50 (*0-7121-1960-4*) Trans-Atl Phila.

Society & Health. Ed. by Benjamin Amick, III et al. 1995. LC 95-30314. (Illus.). 392p. text 52.50 (*0-19-508506-X*) OUP.

Society & Health in Guyana: The Sociology of Health Care in a Developing Nation. Marcel Fredericks et al. 1986. LC 84-70752. (Illus.). 189p. (Orig.). (C). pap. 12.50 (*0-89089-296-2*); lib. bdg. 29.95 (*0-89089-295-4*) Carolina Acad Pr.

Society & Identity: Toward a Sociological Psychology. Andrew J. Weigert et al. 1986. (ASA Rose Monographs). 162p. text 54.95 (*0-521-32325-8*) Cambridge U Pr.

Society & Medicine. New York Academy of Medicine Staff. Ed. by Iago Galdston. 1977. LC 74-142684. (Essay Index Reprint Ser.). 18.95 (*0-8369-2124-0*) Ayer.

Society & Personality: The Interactionist Approach to Social Psychology. Tamotsu Shibutani. 1991. 646p. pap. text 29.95 (*0-88738-688-1*) Transaction Pubs.

Society for Natural Immunity, 5th Annual Meeting: 17th International Natural Killer Cell Workshop, Warrenton, VA., October 17-21, 1998: Abstracts. Ed. by William H. Chambers & John R. Ortaldo. 1999. (Natural Immunity Ser.: Vol. 16, Nos. 2 & 3 (1998)). (Illus.). 80p. pap. 25.25 (*3-8055-6857-6*) S Karger.

Society for Vascular Surgery: A History, Nineteen Forty-Five to Nineteen Eighty-Three. Harris B. Shumacker. Ed. by James N. Rogers. 1984. LC 83-20450. (Illus.). 450p. text 15.00 (*0-9612978-0-8*) Society Vascular Surgery.

Society, Health, & Population During the Demographic Transition. Anders Brandstrom & Lars-Goran Tedebrand. 1988. (Illus.). 514p. lib. bdg. 78.50 (*91-22-01216-8*) Coronet Bks.

Society of Critical Care Medicine—Self-Assessment in Multidisciplinary Critical Care, Vol. 2: A Comprehensive Review. Ed. by R. Phillip Dellinger et al. 1989. 500p. (Orig.). pap. 47.00 (*0-936145-29-3*) SCCM Fullerton.

Society of the Spectacle. Guy Debord. Tr. by Donald Nicholson-Smith from FRE. 1995. LC 89-39940. 154p. pap. 10.95 (*0-942299-79-5*) Zone Bks.

Society's Choices: Social & Ethical Decision Making in Biomedicine. Institute of Medicine Staff. Ed. by Harvey V. Feinberg et al. 1995. LC 94-39354. 550p. (C). text 59.95 (*0-309-05132-0*) Natl Acad Pr.

Society's Mirror: Reflections on Healthcare Reform. John Gollatz. 1997. LC 97-41805. (Illus.). 250p. (Orig.). 21.95 (*1-885987-09-9*, ME084, Health Info Pr) Practice Mgmt Info.

Socio-Cultural Matrix of Alcohol & Drug Use: A Sourcebook of Patterns & Factors. Ed. by Brenda Forster & Jeffrey C. Salloway. 1990. LC 89-13794. (Interdisciplinary Studies in Alcohol & Drug Use & Abuse: Vol. 4). 587p. lib. bdg. 119.95 (*0-88946-285-2*) E Mellen.

Socio-Economic Re-Evaluation of the Torts Law of Liability for Personal Injuries. S. M. Hasan. 1962. 115p. pap. 30.00 (*0-7855-1358-2*) St Mut.

Socio-Egocentrism: Theory, Research & Practice. James S. Peters, II. 2001. LC 95-32069. 76p. pap. 69.95 (*1-57309-035-2*) Intl Scholars.

Socio-Egocentrism: Theory, Research & Practice. James S. Peters, II. 2002. LC 95-32069. 76p. pap. 49.95 (*1-57309-034-4*) Intl Scholars.

Socio-Medical Health Indicators. Ed. by Jack Elinson & Athilia E. Siegmann. 1979. LC 78-74484. 240p. pap. 29.95 (*0-89503-013-6*) Baywood Pub.

Sociobiology & Psychology: Ideas, Issues & Applications. Ed. by Charles Crawford et al. 1987. LC 87-6783. 446p. 89.95 (*0-89859-580-0*) L Erlbaum Assocs.

Sociodemographic Factors in the Epidemiology of Multiple Sclerosis: An Annotated Bibliography, 5. Compiled by George W. Lowis. 1991. LC 90-14016. (Bibliographies & Indexes in Medical Studies: No. 5). 256p. lib. bdg. 68.50 (*0-313-26838-X*, LSY/, Greenwood Pr) Greenwood.

Sociogenesis of Language & Human Conduct. Ed. by Bruce Bain. 1983. 580p. 110.00 (*0-306-41041-9*, Plenum Trade) Perseus Pubng.

Sociological & Medical Aspects of Nutrition. Ed. by Geoffrey H. Bourne. 1988. (World Review of Nutrition & Dietetics Ser.: Vol. 55). (Illus.). xii, 252p. 201.00 (*3-8055-4703-X*) S Karger.

Sociological Insight: An Introduction to Non-Obvious Sociology. Randall Collins. 2nd ed. 1992. 224p. (C). pap. text 19.95 (*0-19-507442-4*) OUP.

Sociological Perspectives on the New Genetics. Peter Conrad & Jonathan Gabe. 1999. LC 99-51435. (Sociology of Health & Illness Ser.). pap. text 32.95 (*0-631-21599-9*) Blackwell Pubs.

Sociological Studies of Children, Vol. 1. Ed. by Nancy Mandell. 1986. 303p. 73.25 (*0-89232-565-8*) Jai Pr.

Sociology & Health Care: An Introduction for the Health Care Professionals. John Bond & Senga Bond. 2nd ed. 1995. (Illus.). 280p. pap. text (*0-443-04059-1*) Church.

Sociology & Occupational Therapy: An Integrated Approach. Derek Jones. 1998. LC 98-23328. (C). pap. text (*0-443-05515-7*) Church.

Sociology & Politics of Health: A Reader. Michael Purdy & David Banks. 2001. LC 00-51818. 29.95 (*0-415-23319-4*) Routledge.

Sociology & Politics of Health: A Reader. Ed. by Michael Purdy & David Banks. 2001. LC 00-51818. 90.00 (*0-415-23318-6*) Routledge.

Sociology & the Field of Public Health. Edward A. Suchman. 1963. LC 63-21228. 182p. pap. 9.95 (*0-87154-864-X*) Russell Sage.

Sociology Applied to Nursing. Joan M. Birchenall. 1998. (C). pap. text 25.00 (*0-7020-1932-1*) Saunders.

Sociology As Applied to Medicine. Graham Scambler. 4th ed. 1997. pap. text (*0-7020-2275-6*) Bailliere Tindall.

Sociology for Nursing & Health Care. Martin Joseph. 1994. 256p. (C). pap. text 26.95 (*0-7456-0906-6*) Blackwell Pubs.

Sociology in Medicine. Mervyn W. Susser et al. 3rd ed. 1985. (Illus.). 470p. text 59.95 (*0-19-503444-9*) OUP.

Sociology, Nursing & Health. Anne Williams & Hannah Cooke. 1998. LC 98-26504. (Illus.). 256p. pap. text 35.00 (*0-7506-3619-X*) Buttrwrth-Heinemann.

Sociology of Chiropractic. Saul Rosenthal. 1986. LC 86-8532. (Studies in Health & Human Services: Vol. 6). lib. bdg. 89.95 (*0-88946-130-9*) E Mellen.

Sociology of Fertility: Determinants of Fertility Differentials in South India. Kuttan Mahadevan. 1978. 11.00 (*0-8364-0293-6*) S Asia.

Sociology of Health. Andrew C. Twaddle & Richard M. Hessler. 2nd ed. 1987. 427p. (C). text 88.00 (*0-02-421870-7*, Macmillan Coll) P-H.

Sociology of Health & Health Care: An Introduction for Nurses. Ed. by Steve Taylor & David Field. 1993. LC 93-7900. pap. 26.95 (*0-632-03402-5*) Blackwell Sci.

Sociology of Health & Health Care: An Introduction for Nurses. Steve Taylor. 2nd ed. 1997. LC 97-22077. (Illus.). 288p. pap. 38.95 (*0-632-04093-9*) Blackwell Sci.

Sociology of Health & Health Care: An Introduction for Nurses. Steve Taylor & David Field. 2nd ed. 1997. LC 97-22077. 238p. pap. 38.95 (*0-632-04147-1*) Blackwell Sci.

Sociology of Health & Illness. Kenneth Jones. 1991. (Illus.). 494p. (C). pap. text (*0-7021-2441-9*) Juta & Co ZAF. *Dist:* Intl Spec Bk.

Sociology of Health & Illness. Sarah Nettleton. 1995. 280p. (C). 64.95 (*0-7456-0893-0*); pap. 29.95 (*0-7456-0894-9*) Blackwell Pubs.

Sociology of Health & Illness, 001. Ed. by Gillian Lupton & Jake Najman. 1995. 420p. 69.95 (*0-7329-2800-1*); pap. 34.95 (*0-7329-2799-4*) Paul & Co Pubs.

Sociology of Health & Illness: Australian Readings. Ed. by Gillian Lupton. 1989. 389p. pap. (*0-333-50220-5*) Intl Spec Bk.

Sociology of Health & Medicine: A Critical Introduction. Ellen Annadale. 1998. LC 97-45218. 250p. 62.95 (*0-7456-1357-8*); pap. 28.95 (*0-7456-1358-6*) Blackwell Pubs.

Sociology of Health, Healing & Illness. Lynne E. Lonnquist & Gregory L. Weiss. 3rd ed. 1999. LC 99-26763. (Illus.). 403p. (C). 62.67 (*0-13-099928-8*) P-H.

Sociology of Health, Healing & Illness. Ed. by Prentice-Hall Staff. 3rd ed. 2000. (C). text (*0-13-021801-4*) P-H.

Sociology of Health, Illness, & Health Care: A Critical Approach. Rose Weitz. 1995. LC 95-303. 476p. (C). pap. 64.95 (*0-534-20742-1*) Wadsworth Pub.

Sociology of Health, Illness, & Health Care: A Critical Approach. Rose Weitz. 2nd ed. 2000. LC 00-42301. (Sociology - Intro Level Ser.). (Illus.). 496p. 70.95 (*0-534-24756-3*) Wadsworth Pub.

Sociology of Health Inequalities. Mel Bartley et al. 1998. (Sociology of Health & Illness Ser.). 256p. pap. 30.95 (*0-631-20929-8*) Blackwell Pubs.

***Sociology of Healthcare.** Alan Clarke. 2001. LC 2001-16391. vii, 310p. pap. (*0-582-36954-1*) Pearson Educ.

Sociology of HIV Transmission. Michael Bloor. 1995. LC 95-68522. 176p. pap. 27.95 (*0-8039-8750-1*, 9442) Sage.

Sociology of Human Fertility: An Annotated Bibliography. Ronald Freedman. 1975. LC 73-12272. (Population & Demography Ser.). 283p. 29.00 (*0-8290-2302-X*) Irvington.

Sociology of Medical Science & Technology. Ed. by Mary A. Elston. 1997. LC 98-111017. (Sociology of Health & Illness, Special Issues Ser.). 160p. pap. 26.95 (*0-631-20447-4*) Blackwell Pubs.

Sociology of Mental Disorders. William E. Eaton. 3rd ed. 2000. LC 99-55308. (Illus.). 400p. 80.00 (*0-275-96323-3*); pap. 27.50 (*0-275-96324-1*) Greenwood (Praeger Pubs).

Sociology of Mental Health & Illness. David Pilgrim & Anne Rogers. 2nd ed. 1999. LC 98-44939. (Illus.). xv, 238p. (*0-335-20348-5*) OpUniv Pr.

Sociology of Mental Illness. Howard B. Kaplan. 1972. pap. 17.95 (*0-8084-0356-7*) NCUP.

Sociology of Mental Illness. Mark Tausig et al. 1998. LC 98-42451. 240p. pap. text 40.00 (*0-13-459637-4*) P-H.

Sociology of Mental Illness. Bernard J. Gallagher, III & Corinne J. Rita. 3rd ed. 1998. LC 94-35083. 496p. 61.33 (*0-13-014408-8*) P-H.

Sociology of Physical Disability & Rehabilitation. Ed. by Gary L. Albrecht. 1982. LC 75-33544. (Contemporary Community Health Ser.). 613p. (C). reprint ed. pap. 12.95 (*0-8229-5341-2*) U of Pittsburgh Pr.

Sociology of the Caring Professions. Pamela Abbott & Claire Wallace. 1990. 200p. 65.00 (*1-85000-819-1*); pap. 34.95 (*1-85000-824-8*) Taylor & Francis (Falmer Pr).

Sociology of the Mentally Disordered Offender. Tom Mason & David Mercer. 1999. LC 98-51542. pap. text (*0-582-31741-X*) Longman.

Sociology/Health Care. Bond. 3rd ed. 1999. pap. text 29.95 (*0-443-05530-0*) Saunders.

Sociomedical Perspectives on Patient Care. Ed. by Jeffrey M. Clair & Richard M. Allman. 1993. LC 92-48516. 304p. (C). pap. text 19.00 (*0-8131-0819-5*) U Pr of KY.

Sociomedical Perspectives on Patient Care Relationships. Ed. by Jeffrey M. Clair & Richard M. Allman. 1993. LC 92-48516. 304p. (C). text 39.95 (*0-8131-1815-8*) U Pr of KY.

Sociopsychological Aspects of Sexually Transmitted Diseases. Ed. by Margaret Rodway & Marianne Wright. 1988. LC 88-638. (Journal of Social Work & Human Sexuality: Vol. 6, No. 2). (Illus.). 162p. text 49.95 (*0-86656-737-2*) Haworth Pr.

***Sod-Gliadin: The Ultimate Defense Against Disease & Aging.** Carl Germano. 2001. mass mkt. 5.99 (*1-57566-819-X*, Knsington) Kensgtn Pub Corp.

Sodium: Its Biological Significance. Solomon Papper. 1981. (CRC Uniscience Ser. on Cations of Biological Significance). 304p. 113.95 (*0-8493-5873-6*, RC632) CRC Pr.

Sodium Content of Your Food. 1984. lib. bdg. 79.95 (*0-87700-547-8*) Revisionist Pr.

Sodium Counter. Annette B. Natow & JoAnn Hesun. Ed. by Sally Peters. 1993. 576p. (Orig.). pap. text 5.99 (*0-671-69566-5*) PB.

Sodium Glutamate (MSG) Index of New Information & Medical Research Bible. Morton N. Willette. 1997. LC 96-12485. 135p. 57.50 (*0-7883-1106-9*); 1997. LC 96-12485. 135p. pap. 47.50 (*0-7883-1107-7*); 1994. 150p. 57.50 (*0-7883-0134-9*); 1994. 150p. pap. 47.50 (*0-7883-0135-7*) ABBE Pubs Assn.

Sodium in Diets, Food & Health: Index of New Information. Mattie N. Rodriguez. Date not set. 160p. 57.50 (*0-7883-1880-2*); pap. 47.50 (*0-7883-1881-0*) ABBE Pubs Assn.

Sodium Transport Inhibitors. Ed. by G. S. Stokes & J. F. Marwood. 1988. (Progress in Biochemical Pharmacology Ser.: Vol. 23). (Illus.). xiv, 162p. 129.75 (*3-8055-4707-2*) S Karger.

Soft & Hard Tissue Repair: Biological & Clinical Aspects, 2. Ed. by Thomas K. Hunt et al. 1984. LC 83-24595. (Surgical Science Ser.: Vol. II). 624p. 99.75 (*0-275-91434-8*, C1434, Praeger Pubs) Greenwood.

Soft Neurological Signs. David E. Tupper & Robert W. Johnson. 1986. 416p. text 41.00 (*0-8089-1841-9*, 794641, Grune & Strat) Harcrt Hlth Sci Grp.

Soft Tissue & Muscoskeletal System. Ed. by Ulrich Mohr. 1993. LC 93-178961. (Illus.). 72p. pap. text 30.00 (*92-832-0122-1*) OUP.

Soft Tissue Arthritis: Bursitis, Fibromyalgia, Fibromyositis, Fibrositis, Rheumatism. Anthony Di Fabio & Paul Jaconello. 1998. LC 97-71310. 104p. pap. 10.00 (*0-9615437-4-4*) Arthritis Trust.

Soft Tissue Changes in Contractures, Vol. 1. Gordon Cummings et al. 1983. (Orthopedic Physical Therapy Ser.). (Illus.). pap. 30.00 (*0-936030-02-X*) Stokesville Pub.

Soft Tissue Implant Markets: Manufacturers Address Regulations & Defend Against Litigation. Market Intelligence Staff. 1993. 221p. 1895.00 (*1-56753-454-6*) Frost & Sullivan.

Soft Tissue Injuries: Diagnosis & Treatment. Robert E. Windsor & Dennis Lox. 1997. LC 97-13858. 379p. 49.95 (*1-56053-212-2*) Hanley & Belfus.

Soft Tissue Injuries: Management & Prevention with Aromatherapy. Maureen Farrell & Leslie Thompson. 2001. (Illus.). 192p. pap. 38.00 (*0-7506-4164-9*) Buttrwrth-Heinemann.

Soft Tissue Injuries in Sports Medicine. Louis C. Almekinders. 1995. LC 95-36197. 288p. pap. 54.95 (*0-86542-382-2*) Blackwell Sci.

***Soft Tissue Injury Evaluation: Forensic Criteria: A Practical Manual.** Gabriel E. Sella. 1997. 60.00 (*1-884325-12-2*) G E Sella.

Soft-Tissue Manipulation: A Practitioner's Guide to the Diagnosis & Treatment of Soft-Tissue Dysfunction & Reflex Activity. Leon Chaitow. 1988. 272p. text 49.95 (*0-89281-276-1*, Heal Arts VT) Inner Tradit.

***Soft Tissue Massage for Pain Relief: How You Can Massage the Pain from 37 Health Conditions.** Bernard Schatz. 2001. pap. 18.95 (*1-57174-264-6*) Hampton Roads Pub Co.

Soft Tissue Pain & Disability. Rene Cailliet. 3rd ed. 1996. LC 95-39159. (Pain Ser.). (Illus.). 545p. (C). pap. text 32.95 (*0-8036-0110-7*) Davis Co.

Soft Tissue Reconstruction in the Upper Extremity. Richards. 1995. text 135.00 (*0-443-08926-4*) Harcourt.

Soft Tissue Rheumatic Pain: Recognition, Management, & Prevention. Robert P. Sheon et al. 3rd ed. 2002. (Illus.). 432p. 59.95 (*0-683-07678-7*) Lppncott W & W.

***Soft Tissue Rheumatology.** Speed et al. 2001. (Fast Facts Ser.). (Illus.). 96p. pap. (*1-899541-38-1*) Health Pr GBR. *Dist:* JAMCO Dist.

Soft Tissue Sarcomas. Ed. by Laurence H. Baker. 1983. (Cancer Treatment & Research Ser.). text 98.00 (*0-89838-584-9*) Kluwer Academic.

Soft Tissue Sarcomas. Raphael E. Pollock. 2000. (ACS Atlas of Clinical Oncology Ser.). 400p. incl. cd-rom (*1-55009-128-X*) DEKR.

Soft Tissue Sarcomas: New Developments in the Multidisciplinary Approach to Treatment. Ed. by Herbert M. Pinedo et al. 1991. (C). text 159.50 (*0-7923-1139-6*) Kluwer Academic.

Soft Tissue Sarcomas: Present Achievements & Future Prospects. J. Verweij et al. 1997. LC 97-9988. (Cancer Treatment & Research Ser.). text 269.50 (*0-7923-9913-7*) Kluwer Academic.

Soft Tissue Sarcomas in Adults, No. 138. Ed. by D. K. Hossfeld et al. 1994. LC 94-22889. (Recent Results in Cancer Research Ser.: Vol. 138). (Illus.). 176p. 127.00 (*0-387-57629-0*) Spr-Verlag.

Soft Tissue Tumors. Ed. by Dieter Harms & Dietmar Schmidt. 1994. LC 94-29977. (Current Topics in Pathology Ser.: 89). (*3-540-55150-6*) Spr-Verlag.

Soft Tissue Tumors. Sharon W. Weiss & John S. Brooks. 1996. (International Academy of Pathology Monographs Ser.: Vol. 24). (Illus.). 268p. 79.00 (*0-683-08963-3*) Lppncott W & W.

Soft Tissue Tumors. Franz M. Enzinger & Sharon W. Weiss. 3rd ed. 1994. LC 94-32118. (Illus.). 1104p. (C). (gr. 13). text 240.00 (*0-8151-3132-1*, 23703) Mosby Inc.

Soft Tissue Tumors, 89. Ed. by Dieter Harms & Dietmar Schmidt. 1994. LC 94-29977. (Current Topics in Pathology Ser.: Vol. 89). (Illus.). 398p. 199.00 (*0-387-55150-6*) Spr-Verlag.

Soft Tissue Tumours. Ed. by V. Eusebi. 1988. (Journal: Vol. 6, No. 3). (Illus.). 92p. pap. 50.50 (*3-8055-4794-3*) S Karger.

Soft Tissues: Trauma & Sports Injuries. Ed. by G. McLatchie & C. M. Lennox. 1993. 496p. pap. text 67.50 (*0-7506-3065-5*, 71307) Buttrwrth-Heinemann.

Soft Tissues of the Extremities: A Radiologic Study of Rheumatic Disease. W. J. Weston & D. G. Palmer. 1978. LC 77-7951. (Comprehensive Manuals in Radiology Ser.: Vol. 1). (Illus.). 128p. 115.00 (*0-387-90259-7*) Spr-Verlag.

Soft Workouts. 1988. (Fitness, Health & Nutrition Ser.). (Illus.). 144p. 17.27 (*0-8094-6195-1*) Time-Life.

Softdesk Civil: Using the Power of Softdesk. Phillip Zimmerman. 1997. LC 97-34724. (Illus.). 512p. (C). pap. 76.95 incl. disk (*0-8273-8440-8*) Delmar.

Software Applications for Mental Health. 1993. 40p. pap. 15.00 (*1-883066-00-X*) Natl Comm Mental.

Software Engineering in Medical Informatics. T. Timmers & B. I. Blum. 1991. 548p. 186.00 (*0-444-89013-0*, North Holland) Elsevier.

Soigner en Deux Langues (Nursing in Two Languages) French/English. Huguette Fizaine. 1995. (ENG & FRE.). 305p. pap. 62.00 (*2-87209-394-X*) IBD Ltd.

Soil Transmitted Helminths: Proceedings of the WHO Expert Committee on Helminthiasis, Rio de Janeiro, 1963. WHO Staff. 1964. (Technical Reports: No. 277). (ENG, FRE, RUS & SPA.). 70p. pap. text 5.00 (*92-4-120277-7*, 1100277) World Health.

Soins Apres Abortement: Guide Practique pour Ameliorer Qualite des Soins. Ed. by Judith Winkler et al. 1996. (FRE., Illus.). (Orig.). pap. 15.00 (*0-929817-32-X*) JHPIEGO.

Soins Infirmiers, Enfermeria see Nursing Practice: Report of a WHO Expert Committee

Sol-Gel Processes for Ceramic Fuels. International Atomic Energy Agency Staff. 1969. (Panel Proceedings Ser.). (Illus.). 179p. pap. (*92-0-141068-9*, ISP207) IAEA AUT. *Dist:* Bernan Associates.

Solace: The Missing Dimension in Psychiatry. Paul C. Horton. LC 81-2794. 184p. 1994. pap. 7.95 (*0-226-35387-7*); 1992. lib. bdg. 15.00 (*0-226-35386-9*) U Ch Pr.

Solar & Ultraviolet Radiation. WHO Staff. 1992. (IARC Scientific Publications Ser.: Vol. 55). 316p. pap. text 72.00 (*92-832-1255-X*, 1720055) World Health.

Solar Neutrinos & Neutrino Astronomy. Ed. by M. L. Cherry et al. 1984. LC 84-63143. (AIP Conference Proceedings Ser.: No. 126). 320p. (C). 44.00 (*0-88318-325-0*) Am Inst Physics.

Solar Plexus. Theron Q. Dumont. reprint ed. pap. 3.00 (*0-911662-40-5*) Yoga.

Solcoderm. Ed. by M. Weiner & P. Hafner. 1984. (Journal: Vol. 168, Suppl. 1). (Illus.). iv, 68p. pap. 28.00 (*3-8055-3890-1*) S Karger.

Soldier in Science: The Autobiography of Bailey K. Ashford, Colonel M. C., U. S. A. Bailey K. Ashford. 1998. LC 98-26039. xxxiii, 425 p. (*0-8477-0351-7*) U of PR Pr.

Soldier's Heart: Survivors' Views of Combat Trauma. Ed. by Sarah Hansel et al. 1995. LC 94-69895. (Illus.). xii, 242p. (Orig.). pap. 19.95 (*0-9629164-6-3*) Sidran Pr.

Soleil Noir: Depression et Melancholie. Julia Kristeva. 1989. (FRE.). pap. 11.95 (*0-7859-2817-0*) Fr & Eur.

Solid Organ Transplant Rejection: Mechanisms, Pathology, & Diagnosis. Ed. by Kim Solez et al. 1996. (Illus.). 656p. text 215.00 (*0-8247-9510-5*) Dekker.

Solid Organ Transplantation Pathology. Ed. by Elizabeth H. Hammond. 1994. LC 93-36143. (Major Problems in Pathology Ser.: No. 30). (Illus.). 304p. text 75.00 (*0-7216-4482-1*) Saunders.

Solid-State & Chemical Radiation Dosimetry in Medicine & Biology. International Atomic Energy Agency Staff. 1967. (Proceedings Ser.). (Illus.). 471p. pap. (*92-0-010167-4*, ISP138) IAEA AUT. *Dist:* Bernan Associates.

Solid Tumor in Childhood. Norman S. Jaffe. 1983. 176p. 103.00 (*0-8493-5732-2*, RC281, CRC Reprint) Franklin.

Solide Maligne Tumoren im Kindesalter. Ed. by E. Bern Rossi. 1974. (Paediatrische Fortbildungskurse fuer die Praxis Ser.: Vol. 39). (Illus.). 100p. 28.75 (*3-8055-1691-6*) S Karger.

Solo Sex: Advanced Techniques see Joy of Solo Sex

Solubility & Related Properties. Kenneth C. James. 1986. (Drugs & the Pharmaceutical Sciences Ser.: Vol. 28). (Illus.). 432p. text 185.00 (*0-8247-7484-1*) Dekker.

Solubility Test to Confirm the Presence of Sickling Hemoglobins. 1995. (Approved Standard Ser.: Vol. 6). 75.00 (*1-56238-274-8*, H10-A2) NCCLS.

Solubility Testing of Actinides on Breathing-Zone & Area Air Samples. 1997. lib. bdg. 250.95 (*0-8490-7722-2*) Gordon Pr.

Solution Focused Group Therapy. Linda Metcalf. 1998. LC 98-26800. (Illus.). 256p. 29.95 (*0-684-84744-2*) S&S Trade.

Solution-Focused Therapy: A Casebook. 1996. 184p. pap. 9.00 (*1-879771-14-4*) Global Pub NJ.

Solution Focused Therapy: A Handbook for Health Care Professionals. Dave Hawkes et al. 1998. LC 98-27521. 208p. pap. text 32.50 (*0-7506-1978-3*) Buttrwrth-Heinemann.

Solution-Focused Therapy: Managing Human Relationships. Ron Wilgosh et al. 1998. (Illus.). 192p. pap. 32.50 (*0-7506-2037-4*) Buttrwrth-Heinemann.

Solution of Nutritional Problems: The Contribution of Producers, Distributors & Nutritionists. Ed. by J. C. Somogyi. 1979. (Bibliotheca Nutritio et Dieta Ser.: No. 28). (Illus.). pap. 126.25 (*3-8055-3025-0*) S Karger.

Solution-Oriented Hypnosis: An Ericksonian Approach. William H. O'Hanlon & Michael Martin. 1992. LC 92-16410. 180p. (C). 25.00 (*0-393-70149-2*) Norton.

Solution-Oriented Therapy for Chronic & Severe Mental Illness. Tim Rowan & Bill O'Hanlon. 1998. LC 98-14865. 177p. 59.95 (*0-471-18362-8*) Wiley.

Solutioning: Solution-Focused Interventions for Counselors. Willy H. Webb. 1999. LC 98-41205. 328p. pap. text 29.95 (*1-56032-744-8*) Hemisp Pub.

Solutions: Practical & Effective Antidotes for Sexual & Relationship Problems. Leslie Cameron-Bandler. rev. ed. 1985. LC 85-70138. 259p. (C). pap. 11.95 (*0-932573-01-0*) Real People.

***Solutions for the "Treatment Resistant" Addicted Client: Therapeutic Techniques for Engaging Difficult Clients.** Nicholas A. Roes. 2001. LC 2001-16625. 177p. pap. 22.95 (*0-7890-1121-2*) Haworth Pr.

***Solutions for the "Treatment-Resistant" Addicted Client: Therapeutic Techniques for Engaging Difficult Clients.** Nicholas A. Roes. 2001. LC 2001-16625. (Illus.). 177p. lib. bdg. 39.95 (*0-7890-1120-4*) Haworth Pr.

Solutions, Minerals & Equilibria. Robert M. Garrels & Charles L. Christ. 1990. (Illus.). 464p. (C). text 65.95 (*0-86720-148-7*, 148-7) Jones & Bartlett.

Solutions to Selected Problems: From the Physics of Radiology. Harold E. Johns & John R. Cunningham. 4th ed. 1991. (Illus.). 148p. (C). pap. text 33.95 (*0-398-05750-8*) C C Thomas.

Solved - The Riddle of Weight Loss: Restore Healthy Body Chemistry & Lose Weight Naturally. Stephen Langer & James F. Scheer. 1989. LC 89-7572. Orig. Title: How to Win at Weight Loss. 256p. pap. 12.95 (*0-89281-296-6*, Heal Arts VT) Inner Tradit.

Solvent Abuse: A Population-Based Neuropsychological Study. O. Chadwick et al. 1991. (Recent Research in Psychology Ser.). (Illus.). 150p. 63.95 (*0-387-97607-8*) Spr-Verlag.

Solvent Neurotoxicity. Peter Arlien-Soborg. 1991. 400p. lib. bdg. 195.00 (*0-8493-6234-2*, RC347) CRC Pr.

Solving Common Sexual Problems: Toward a Problem-Free Sexual Life. Stephen B. Levine. 1997. LC 97-28092. 296p. pap. 30.00 (*0-7657-0121-9*) Aronson.

Solving Patient Problems In Internal Medicine. Steven M. Mitchell. 1998. 190p. pap. 28.95 (*1-889325-07-4*) Blackwell Sci.

Solving Patient Problems In Psychiatry. Terry A. Travis. 1998. (Clerkship Ser.). pap. 27.95 (*1-889325-10-4*) Blackwell Sci.

Solving Problems in Couples & Family Therapy: Techniques & Tactics. Robert Sherman et al. 1991. LC 91-25757. 352p. text 49.95 (*0-87630-647-4*) Brunner-Routledge.

Solving Problems with NMR Spectroscopy. Atta-ur-Rahman et al. 1995. LC 95-15392. (Illus.). 430p. pap. text 39.95 (*0-12-066320-1*) Acad Pr.

Solving Sexual Problems in the 1990's. Ben N. Ard, Jr. 1989. (American University Studies: Ser. VIII, Vol. 15). XIV, 302p. (C). text 44.95 (*0-8204-1061-6*) P Lang Pubng.

Solving the Anorexia Puzzle: A Scientific Approach. W. Frank Epling & W. D. Pierce. 1992. LC 90-4426. (Illus.). 256p. pap. text 34.95 (*0-88937-034-6*) Hogrefe & Huber Pubs.

Solving the Frontline Crisis in Long-Term Care Vol. 1: A Practical Guide to Finding & Keeping Quality Nursing Assistants. Karl A. Pillemer. Ed. by Richard Hoffman & Martin Schumacher. 1996. 124p. (Orig.). pap. 39.00 (*0-9653629-0-6*) Frontline Pub.

Solving the Mystery of Breast Discharge. Judy C. Kneece. 1996. (Illus.). 56p. pap. 7.95 (*1-886665-07-9*) EduCare Pub.

Solving the Mystery of Breast Pain. Judy C. Kneece. 1996. (Illus.). 56p. pap. 7.95 (*1-886665-06-0*) EduCare Pub.

Solving the Puzzle of Chronic Fatigue Syndrome. Murray Susser & Michael Rosenbaum. 1992. LC 91-53018. (Illus.). 190p. (Orig.). pap. 14.95 (*0-943685-11-7*) Essential Science.

Solving the Puzzles in Medical Terminology: An Interactive Study Guide to Accompany the Telecourse Medical Terminology. Vikki Wetle & Glen Longshore. 1996. (Illus.). 400p. (C). pap. text 31.95 (*0-7637-0214-5*, 0214-5) Jones & Bartlett.

Solving Your Child's Behavior Problems: An Everyday Guide for Parents. Jeffrey A. Kelly. 1983. 224p. pap. 8.95 (*0-316-48695-7*, Little Brwn Med Div) Lppncott W & W.

Solving Your Problems Together: Family Therapy for the Whole Family. Jana Annunziata & Phyllis Jacobson-Kram. 1994. LC 94-29708. (Illus.). 37p. 19.95 (*1-55798-268-6*, 4317460) Am Psychol.

Somatic & Autonomic Regulations in Sleep: Physiological & Clinical Aspects. E. Lugaresi & P. L. Parmeggiani. 1997. LC 97-28727. 140p. 55.00 (*3-540-75046-0*) Spr-Verlag.

Somatic & Endocrine Studies of Puberal & Adolescent Boys. William W. Greulich. 1942. (SRCD Ser.: Vol. 7, No. 3). pap. 25.00 (*0-527-01524-5*) Periodicals Srv.

Somatic Diversification of Immune Responses. Ed. by M. Flajnik & G. Kelsoe. 1997. (Current Topics in Microbiology & Immunology Ser.: Vol. 229). (Illus.). 221p. 139.00 (*3-540-63608-0*) Spr-Verlag.

Somatic Empathy. Leslie Korn. 2nd ed. 1996. (Illus.). 56p. pap. 15.00 (*1-893710-07-6*) Ctr for World Studies.

Somatic Gene Therapy. Ed. by Patricia L. Chang. 1994. LC 94-17728. 320p. 104.95 (*0-8493-2440-8*) CRC Pr.

Somatic Hypermutation in V-Regions. Ed. by Edward J. Steele. 1991. 200p. lib. bdg. 142.00 (*0-8493-5348-3*, QR186) CRC Pr.

Somatics: Reawakening the Mind's Control of Movement, Flexibility, & Health. Thomas Hanna. 2000. 176p. pap. 17.00 (*0-201-07979-8*) Perseus Bks Grp.

Somatisierte Angst und Depressivitaet. Ed. by W. Poeldinger. 1984. (Illus.). vi, 136p. 35.00 (*3-8055-3844-8*) S Karger.

Somatization: Bodily Experience & Mental States. Ed. by Levinson & Droga. 1997. (Psychoanalytic Inquiry Ser.: Vol. 17, No.2). pap. 20.00 (*0-88163-935-4*) Analytic Pr.

Somatization Disorder in the Medical Setting. 1994. (Illus.). 98p. (Orig.). (C). pap. text 25.00 (*0-941375-81-1*) DIANE Pub.

Somatization Disorder in the Medical Setting. G. Richard Smith, Jr. 1991. LC 91-6429. 97p. text 10.95 (*0-88048-374-1*, 8374) Am Psychiatric.

Somatizing Child. E. G. Shapiro & A. A. Rosenfeld. 1987. (Contributions to Psychology & Medicine Ser.). (Illus.). 147p. 99.00 (*0-387-96363-4*) Spr-Verlag.

SomatoEmotional Release & Beyond. John E. Upledger. 1990. (Illus.). 266p. text 40.00 (*0-9627157-0-0*) UI Pub.

***Somatoform & Factitious Disorders.** Ed. by Katherine A. Phillips. 2001. LC 00-67403. (Review of Psychiatry Ser.: Vol. 20). 208p. pap. 29.95 (*1-58562-029-7*, 62029) Amer Psych Assn.

Somatoform Disorders: A Worldwide Perspective. Y. Ono. 1999. LC 99-14495. (Keio University Symposia for Life Science & Medicine Ser.). (Illus.). 308p. 145.00 (*4-431-70248-2*) Spr-Verlag.

Somatostatin: Recent Advances in Basic Research & Clinical Applications. Ed. by Emilio Del Pozo. 1988. (Journal: Vol. 29, No. 2-3). 88p. (Orig.). pap. 102.75 (*3-8055-4809-5*) S Karger.

Somatostatin Analogues: Basic & Clinical Perspectives Meeting, Sorrento, November, 1995. Ed. by R. Arnold. 1996. (Journal: Vol. 57, Suppl. 1, 1996). (Illus.). vi, 120p. pap. 50.50 (*3-8055-6337-X*) S Karger.

Somatostatin & Its Receptors, Symposium No. 190. CIBA Foundation Staff. 1995. LC 94-43530. (CIBA Foundation Symposia Ser.: Vol. 190). 284p. 128.00 (*0-471-95382-2*) Wiley.

Somatotrophic Axis & the Reproductive Process in Health & Disease: Proceedings of the Symposium, Held October 28 to 31, 1993. Ed. by Eli Y. Adashi & Michael O. Thorner. 1995. LC 94-39174. (Illus.). 307p. 159.00 (*0-387-94419-2*) Spr-Verlag.

Some Aromatic Amines, Hydrazines & Related Substances, N-Nitroso Compounds & Miscellaneous Alkylating Agents. 1974. (IARC Scientific Publications Ser.: Vol. 4). 286p. 24.00 (*92-832-1204-5*, 1720004) World Health.

Some Aspects of Human & Veterinary Nutrition. Ed. by Geoffrey H. Bourne. 1978. (World Review of Nutrition & Dietetics Ser.: Vol. 28). 140.00 (*3-8055-2672-5*) S Karger.

Some Aspects of Human Nutrition. Ed. by H. C. Bourne. 1977. (World Review of Nutrition & Dietetics Ser.: Vol. 27). 99.25 (*3-8055-2393-9*) S Karger.

Some Aspects of Strontium Radiobiology. 1991. LC 91-25467. (Report Ser.: No. 110). 95p. pap. text 30.00 (*0-929600-19-3*) NCRP Pubns.

Some Aspects of the Effect of the Dominant American Culture Upon Children of Italian-Born Parents. Joseph W. Tait. 1972. LC 72-81351. (Illus.). ix, 74p. reprint ed. lib. bdg. 25.00 (*0-678-00919-8*) Kelley.

***Some Became Flowers: Living with Dying at Home.** Sharon Brown. 200p. pap. (*1-55017-087-2*) Harbour Pub Co.

Some British Pioneers of Social Medicine. Major Greenwood. 1977. LC 71-126320. (Biography Index Reprint Ser.). reprint ed. 18.95 (*0-8369-8026-3*) Ayer.

Some Chemicals Used in Plastics & Elastomers. 1986. (IARC Scientific Publications Ser.: Vol. 39). 403p. pap. text 83.00 (*92-832-1239-8*, 1720039) World Health.

Some Choice: Law, Medicine & the Market. George J. Annas. 1998. LC 97-48975. 320p. text 29.95 (*0-19-511832-4*) OUP.

Some Clinical Experiences of E. E. Case, M. D. Ed. by Jay Yasgur. 1992. (C). pap. text 28.50 (*1-886149-01-1*) Van Hoy Pubs.

Some Days Are Better Than Others: A Book About Breastfeeding. Diane Reukauf & Mary A. Trause. 3rd ed. 1989. pap. text 23.00 (*0-8359-7054-X*) P-H.

Some Experimental Evidence of the Perception of Dot Patterns & Two-Dimensional Shapes. Michael F. Dacey & Gerald J. Karaska. 1963. (Discussion Papers: No. 2). pap. 10.00 (*1-55869-115-4*) Regional Sci Res Inst.

Some Factors Influencing the Non-Expert. Elaine Vaughan. 1990. LC 90-13855. (Environment: Problems & Solutions Ser.: Vol. 5). 230p. text 20.00 (*0-8240-0422-1*) Garland.

Some Famous Medical Trials. Leonard A. Parry. 1976. LC 74-95631. x, 326p. reprint ed. 45.00 (*0-678-03754-X*) Kelley.

Some Flame Retardants & Textile Chemicals, & Exposures in the Textile Manufacturing Industry. 1990. (IARC Scientific Publications Ser.: Vol. 48). 345p. pap. text 72.00 (*92-832-1248-7*, 1720048) World Health.

Some Fundamental Approaches in Skin Research. Ed. by J. W. Mali. 1981. (Current Problems in Dermatology Ser.: Vol. 9). (Illus.). viii, 152p. pap. 85.25 (*3-8055-3080-3*) S Karger.

***Some Good in the World: A Life of Purpose: A Memoir.** Told to Edward J. Piszek & Jake Morgan. 2001. LC 2001-2738. (Illus.). xxviii, 235p. 29.95 (*0-87081-627-6*) Univ Pr Colo.

Some Lesser Known Herbal Drugs in Ayurveda. Gyanendra Pandey. 1996. (C). (*81-7030-512-8*) Sri Satguru Pubns IND. *Dist:* S Asia.

Some Mathematical Questions in Biology. Ed. by George F. Oster. 1980. LC 77-25086. (Lectures on Mathematics in the Life Sciences: Vol. 13). 274p. pap. 39.00 (*0-8218-1163-0*, LLSCI/13) Am Math.

Some Mathematical Questions in Biology. Ed. by Simon A. Levin. 1979. LC 77-25086. (Lectures on Mathematics in the Life Sciences: Vol. 12). 218p. reprint ed. pap. 36.00 (*0-8218-1162-2*, LLSCI/12) Am Math.

Some Mathematical Questions in Biology, Pt. I. Ed. by Murray Gerstenhaber. 1970. (Lectures on Mathematics in the Life Sciences: Vol. 2). 156p. reprint ed. pap. 27.00 (*0-8218-1152-5*, LLSCI/2) Am Math.

Some Mathematical Questions in Biology. Ed. by J. D. Cowan. 1972. (Lectures on Mathematics in the Life Sciences: Vol. 3). Pt. II. 121p. pap. 28.00 (*0-8218-1153-3*, LLSCI/3); Pt. III. 151p. pap. 31.00 (*0-8218-1154-1*, LLSCI/4) Am Math.

Some Mathematical Questions in Biology, Pt. IV. Ed. by J. D. Cowan et al. 1973. (Lectures on Mathematics in the Life Sciences: Vol. 5). 150p. pap. 40.00 (*0-8218-1155-X*, LLSCI/5) Am Math.

Some Mathematical Questions in Biology, Pt. V. Ed. by J. D. Cowan. 1974. (Lectures on Mathematics in the Life Sciences: Vol. 6). 141p. pap. 32.00 (*0-8218-1156-8*, LLSCI/6) Am Math.

Some Mathematical Questions in Biology. Ed. by Simon A. Levin. (Lectures on Mathematics in the Life Sciences: Vol. 7). Pt. VI. 1974. 232p. pap. 49.00 (*0-8218-9902-3*, LLSCI/7); Pt. IX. 1978. 244p. pap. 36.00 (*0-8218-1160-6*, LLSCI/0); Pt. X. 1979. 179p. pap. 27.00 (*0-8218-1161-4*, LLSCI/11) Am Math.

Some Mathematical Questions in Biology - Neurobiology. Ed. by Robert M. Miura. 1982. LC 82-18418. (Lectures on Mathematics in the Life Sciences: Vol. 15). 122p. pap. 32.00 (*0-8218-1165-7*, LLSCI/15) Am Math.

Some Methods for Microbiological Assay. Ed. by R. G. Board & D. W. Lovelock. 1975. text 152.00 (*0-12-108240-7*) Acad Pr.

Some Naturally Occurring Substances: Food Items & Constituents, Heterocyclic Aromatic Amines & Mycotoxins. 1993. (IARC Scientific Publications Ser.: Vol. 56). 599p. pap. text 95.00 (*92-832-1256-8*, 1720056) World Health.

Some of It Was Funny. Mary B. Hamlin. 1982. 119p. (Orig.). 10.95 (*0-9610242-1-6*); pap. 7.95 (*0-9610242-0-8*) Murrayhollow.

Some Pharmaceutical Drugs. 1996. (IARC Scientific Publications Ser.: Vol. 66). 514p. pap. 72.00 (*92-832-1266-5*, 1720066) World Health.

Some Pharmaceutical Drugs: The Evaluation of Carcinogenic Risks to Humans. 1980. (IARC Scientific Publications Ser.: No. 24). 335p. text 48.00 (*92-832-1224-X*) World Health.

Some Pitfalls & Problems in Neurosurgery. Ed. by J. C. De Villiers. 1990. (Progress in Neurological Surgery Ser.: Vol. 13). (Illus.). xii, 208p. 172.25 (*3-8055-4989-X*) S Karger.

Some Social Aspects of Dentistry. Ed. by W. R. Ayer. 1981. 100p. pap. 18.00 (*0-08-028132-X*, Pergamon Pr) Elsevier.

Some Special Aspects of Nutrition. Ed. by Geoffrey H. Bourne. 1979. (World Review of Nutrition & Dietetics Ser.: Vol. 33). (Illus.). 137.50 (*3-8055-2942-2*) S Karger.

Some Stories Are Better Than Others: Doing What Works in Brief Therapy & Managed Care. Michael F. Hoyt. 2000. LC 99-89147. (Illus.). xvii, 320p. 34.95 (*1-58391-041-7*) Brunner-Routledge.

Some Systems of Biological Communication: Journal: Biosciences Communications, Vol. 3, Nos. 5 & 6. Ed. by Stacey B. Day. 1977. (Illus.). 49.75 (*3-8055-2817-5*) S Karger.

Somebody Else's Kids. Torey L. Hayden. 1982. 336p. pap. 6.50 (*0-380-59949-X*, Avon Bks) Morrow Avon.

Someone I Know Has Multiple Personalities: A Book for Significant Others—Friends. Sandra J. Hocking. 1994. LC 94-11538. 84p. (Orig.). pap. 9.95 (*1-877872-08-3*) Launch Pr.

Somesthesis & the Neurobiology of the Somatosensory Cortex. Ed. by O. Franzen et al. 1996. LC 96-6739. 421p. 113.00 (*0-8176-5322-8*); (Illus.). 448p. 124.50 (*3-7643-5322-8*) Birkhauser.

Something about X-Rays for Everybody. Edward Trevert. 1989. (Illus.). 82p. (C). reprint ed. 16.95 (*0-944838-05-7*) Med Physics Pub.

Something to Draw On: Activities & Interventions Using an Art Therapy Approach. Carol Ross. 1996. 150p. (*1-85302-363-9*) Jessica Kingsley GBR. *Dist:* Taylor & Francis.

Sometimes My Heart Goes Numb: Love & Cargeiving in a Time of Aids. Charles Garfield et al. 1997. LC 97-10993. (Harvest Book Ser.). 352p. pap. 13.00 (*0-15-600495-X*, Harvest Bks) Harcourt.

Sometimes Words Are Not Enough. Sue P. Heiney et al. 2000. (Illus.). 30p. pap. 10.00 (*1-889863-02-5*) Palmetto Richland.

Sommeil Provoque et les Etats Anolagues. Ambroise-Auguste Liebeault. 1976. LC 75-16716. (Classics in Psychiatry Ser.). reprint ed. 28.95 (*0-405-07444-1*) Ayer.

Song of Symptoms. Patersimilias. 1980. 30.00 (*0-85032-186-7*) St Mut.

Song of the Coyote: Freeing the Imagination Through the Arts. Phyllis L. Sawyers & Frances L. Henry. 1980. (Illus.). 302p. pap. text 21.95 (*0-89641-036-6*) American Pr.

Sonographic Review of the Abdomen. Janice Hickey. 1998. LC 98-15839. 320p. pap. text 47.50 (*0-397-51691-6*) Lppncott W & W.

Sonography in Obstetrics & Gynecology: Principles & Practice. Arthur C. Fleischer et al. 6th ed. 2001. (Illus.). 1270p. (C). text 175.00 (*0-8385-8614-7*) McGraw-Hill Prof.

Sonography of the Infant Hip: An Atlas. Reinhard Graf & Peter Schuler. Tr. by Terry Telger. 1986. LC 86-13178. 276p. 170.00 (*0-89573-451-6*, Wiley-VCH) Wiley.

Sonography of the Infant Hip & Its Therapeutic Implications. Reinhard Graf et al. 1996. LC 95-25117. 127p. pap. 64.95 (*3-8261-0041-7*, Chap & Hall NY) Chapman & Hall.

Sonoma County Physician Directory, 2000. 2000. 144p. 19.95 (*0-9677244-0-6*) Sonoma County Med.

Sons, Lovers & Fathers: Understanding Male Sexuality. Didier Dumas et al. Tr. by Anne Trager from FRE. 1997. LC 96-31300. 200p. 35.00 (*0-7657-0033-6*) Aronson.

Soothing the Troubled Mind: Treatment & Prevention of Schizophrenia with Acupuncture & Moxibustion. Ed. by Nigel Wiseman. Tr. by Thomas I. DeYoung from CHI. 1999. LC 99-50641. Orig. Title: Zhen Jiu Fang Zhi Shen Fen Lie Zheng. 164p. (Orig.). pap. 17.95 (*0-912111-60-7*) Paradigm Publns.

SOPHE Heritage Collection of Health Education Monographs Society for Public Health Education Staff. 1982. LC 81-51486. 1000p. text 40.00 (*0-89914-013-0*);Sct. text 60.00 (*0-89914-008-4*) Third Party Pub.

Soranus' Gynecology. Tr. by Owsei Temkin et al from GRE. 1991. LC 91-20791. (Softshell Bks.). (Illus.). 312p. reprint ed. pap. text 22.50 (*0-8018-4320-0*) Johns Hopkins.

Sorcerer & Witch in Melanesia. Ed. by Michele Stephen. 1987. 208p. (C). text 40.00 (*0-8135-1227-1*) Rutgers U Pr.

Soren Kierkegaard's Christian Psychology: Insight for Counseling & Pastoral Care. C. Stephen Evans. 1990. 160p. mass mkt. 12.99 (*0-310-43751-2*) Zondervan.

Sorensen & Luckmann's Basic Nursing: A Psychophysiologic Approach. Verolyn B. Bolander. 3rd ed. 1994. 379p. (*0-7216-5237-9*) Saunders.

Sorensen & Luckmann's Basic Nursing: A Psychophysiologic Approach. Ed. by Verolyn R. Bolander. 3rd ed. 1994. LC 93-21589. (Illus.). 1664p. text 61.00 (*0-7216-4013-3*) Saunders.

Sorensen & Luckmann's Basic Nursing: A Psychophysiologic Approach, Study Guide/Checklist Package. Ed. by Verolyn B. Bolander. 3rd ed. 1994. (Illus.). stu. ed. 87.00 (*0-7216-5218-2*) Saunders.

Sorensen & Luckmann's Basic Nursing: Performing Checklist. Bolander. 3rd ed. 1994. wbk. ed. 17.95 (*0-7216-5216-6*) Harcourt.

Sorensen's Basic Nursing. Bolande. 3rd ed. 1994. 77.00 (*0-7216-5217-4*) Harcourt.

Sorrow Built a Bridge: Friendship & AIDS. Daniel Berrigan. 1989. 231p. (Orig.). pap. 14.95 (*1-879175-04-5*) Fortkamp.

SOS Video, No. 2. 1995. (Exploring Transcription Practices Ser.). 10p. stu. ed. 200.00 (*0-935229-25-6*) Am Assoc Med.

Sota Omoigui's Pain Drugs Handbook. Sota Omoigui. 2nd ed. 1999. LC 98-40987. (Illus.). xliv, 816p. pap. 39.95 (*0-632-04419-5*) St-of-the-Art Tech.

Sotai: Balance & Health Through Natural Movement. Keizo Hashimoto & Yoshizaki Kawakami. 1983. (Illus.). 240p. pap. 18.00 (*0-87040-534-9*) Japan Pubns USA.

Sotos Syndrome: A Handbook for Families. Rebecca R. Anderson & Bruce A. Buehler. 1992. (Illus.). 55p. (Orig.). spiral bd. 11.00 (*1-889843-01-6*) Munroe-Meyer Inst.

Soul Approach to Depression: Our Normal Transitional Emotions. Kathy Oddenino. 1995. LC 96-109469. (Illus.). 348p. (Orig.). pap. 24.95 (*0-923081-05-4*) Joy Pubns MD.

Soul-Birthing: How to Choose, Attract & Influence the Soul of Your Baby Before Conception or Birth. Linda Day-Schmal. 2000. LC 00-191549. (Illus.). 235p. pap. 14.95 (*1-929341-04-0*) SpiritPassage.

Soul in Distress: What Every Pastoral Counselor Should Know about Emotional & Mental Illness. Richard W. Roukema. 1997. LC 96-48818. 274p. 49.95 (*0-7890-0168-3*); pap. 19.95 (*0-7890-0198-5*) Haworth Pr (Haworth Pastrl).

Soul Medicine: Medical Challenges on Life's Uncertain Journey. John E. Postley. 1995. 288p. (Orig.). pap. 14.95 (*0-944634-33-8*) Love & Logic.

Soul Murder Revisited: Thoughts about Therapy, Hate, Love & Memory. Leonard Shengold. 2000. 328p. pap. 18.95 (*0-300-08699-7*); 1999. LC 98-27156. 311p. 40.00 (*0-300-07594-4*) Yale U Pr.

Soul on the Couch: Spirituality, Religion, & Morality in Contemporary Psychoanalysis. Ed. by Charles Spezzano & Gerald J. Gargiulo. 1997. LC 97-16523. (Relational Perspectives Bks.: No. 7). 272p. 45.00 (*0-88163-181-7*) Analytic Pr.

Soul Recovery & Extraction. Ai G. Waya. 1993. 74p. (Orig.). pap. 9.95 (*0-9634662-0-8*) Blue Turtle.

S

Soul's Logical Life: Towards a Rigorous Notion of Psychology. Wolfgang Giegerich. 1998. 282p. 45.95 (*3-631-33277-7*) P Lang Pubng.

Souls to Soles: A Self-Help Exploration of Reflexology. Paul Rude. 1997. LC 97-71445. (Illus.). 160p. (Orig.). pap. 12.95 (*0-914955-51-9*) Lotus Pr.

Sound Guide for Physiology. Abaco. 1995. 19.00 (*0-205-18373-5*) Allyn.

Sound Language & Awareness Psychology. Joseph M. Jones. 1985. LC 85-90320. (Illus.). 236p. (Orig.). pap. 12.50 (*0-9615111-1-7*) Sandbird Pub.

Sound Medicine: Healing with Music, Voice & Song. Laeh M. Garfield. 1995. LC 87-13223. 192p. pap. 9.95 (*0-89087-483-2*) Celestial Arts.

Sound of a Miracle. Annabel Stehli. 1992. 256p. mass mkt. 4.99 (*0-380-71739-5*, Avon Bks) Morrow Avon.

Sound Sex & the Aging Heart: Sex in the Mid & Later Years with Special Reference to Cardiac Problems. Lee Scheingold & Nathaniel N. Wagner. 1974. LC 74-662. (Illus.). 168p. 32.95 (*0-87705-155-0*, Kluwer Acad Hman Sci) Kluwer Academic.

Sounding the Silence: or Why People Sing in the Shower. Sue Parker & Rebekah Nix. 1994. LC 94-219605. (Illus.). 172p. (Orig.). pap. 12.99 (*0-9641407-0-5*) RNIX.

S

Sounds of Healing: A Physician Reveals the Therapeutic Power of Sound, Voice & Music. Mitchell L. Gaynor. 2000. 288p. pap. 13.00 (*0-7679-0266-1*) Broadway BDD.

Sounds of the Diseased Heart. Aldo A. Luisada. 1973. LC 74-176171. (Illus.). 416p. text 32.50 (*0-87527-113-8*) Green.

Sounds of the Normal Heart. Aldo A. Luisada. 1972. LC 78-176172. (Illus.). 280p. 32.50 (*0-87527-051-4*) Green.

Source Book in Animal Biology. Thomas S. Hall. 1951. LC 74-120317. (Source Books in the History of the Sciences). (Illus.). 732p. 70.00 (*0-674-82141-6*) HUP.

Source Book in Bioethics: A Documentary History. Ed. by Albert R. Jonsen et al. 1998. LC 97-41521. 510p. 95.00 (*0-87840-683-2*) Georgetown U Pr.

Source-Book of Biological Names & Terms. Edmund C. Jaeger. 3rd ed. 1977. (Illus.). 360p. 61.95 (*0-398-00916-3*) C C Thomas.

Source Book of Educational Materials for Medical Radiographers. 1986. lib. bdg. 79.95 (*0-8490-3806-5*) Gordon Pr.

Source Book of Enzymes. John Stephen White & Dorothy Chong White. 1997. LC 97-191848. 1328p. 199.95 (*0-8493-9470-8*) CRC Pr.

Source Book of Indian Medicine: An Anthology. K. H. Krishnamurthy. 1991. (C). (*81-7018-612-9*) BR Pub IND. *Dist:* S Asia.

Source Book of Medical History. Logan Clendening. 1960. 685p. (C). pap. 15.95 (*0-486-20621-1*) Dover.

Source Book of Ophthalmology. Daniel M. Albert. 1995. (Illus.). 416p. 104.95 (*0-86542-240-0*) Blackwell Sci.

Source Book of Practical Experiments in Physiology Requiring Minimal Equipment. International Union of Physiological Sciences Congress Staff. 1991. 204p. (C). text 44.00 (*981-02-0570-8*); pap. text 18.00 (*981-02-0571-6*) World Scientific Pub.

Source Book of Substance Abuse & Addiction. Lawrence Friedman et al. 1996. (Illus.). 256p. pap. 49.95 (*0-683-03364-6*) Lppncott W & W.

Sourcebook for Helping People with Spiritual Problems. Emma Bragdon. 2nd rev. ed. 1994. (Illus.). 320p. (C). reprint ed. pap. 14.95 (*0-9620960-1-6*) Lightening Up Pr.

***Sourcebook for Medical Audiology.** Enid Smith. 2002. 49.95 (*0-7693-0247-5*) Singular Publishing.

Sourcebook for Medical Speech Pathology. Lee A. Golper. 2nd ed. 1997. LC 97-24423. (Clinical Competence Ser.). 447p. spiral bd. 62.95 (*1-56593-861-5*, 1686) Thomson Learn.

Sourcebook for Speech, Language & Cognition: Stimulus Materials for Rehabilitation. Susan H. Brubaker. 1992. LC 92-13721. (William Beaumont Hospital Speech & Language Pathology Ser.: Bks. 1-2). Bk. 1. 200p. 48.00 (*0-8143-2411-8*); Bk. 2. 194p. 48.00 (*0-8143-2412-6*) Wayne St U Pr.

Sourcebook of Adult Assessment Strategies. Nicola S. Schutte & John M. Malouff. 1995. LC 95-9524. (Applied Clinical Psychology Ser.). (Illus.). 488p. (C). text 70.00 (*0-306-45029-1*, Kluwer Plenum) Kluwer Academic.

Sourcebook of Apraxia Remediation Activities. Sharon M. Nakamura et al. 1990. 160p. pap. text 32.00 (*0-930951-47-6*) Acad Comm.

Sourcebook of Medical Illustration. Ed. by P. Cull. 1989. (Illus.). 481p. 85.00 (*1-85070-255-1*, Parthenon Pbng) CRC Pr.

Sourcebook of Occupational Rehabilitation. P. M. King. 1998. LC 98-39286. (Series in Rehabilitation & Health). (Illus.). 370p. (C). 70.00 (*0-306-45842-X*, Plenum Trade) Perseus Pubng.

Sourcebook of Pediatric Psychology. Ed. by Roberta A. Olson et al. 1994. LC 93-23443. 608p. (C). 103.00 (*0-205-15182-5*, Longwood Div) Allyn.

Sourcebook of Phonological Awareness Activities Goldsworthy. 2000. 360p. pap. text 51.95 (*0-7693-0090-1*) Singular Publishing.

Sourcebook of Psychological Treatment Manuals for Adult Disorders. Ed. by Vincent B. Van Hasselt & Michel Hersen. 1995. (Illus.). 732p. (C). 100.00 (*0-306-45144-1*, Plenum Trade) Perseus Pubng.

Sourcebook of Reference Methods, Materials & Related Information for the Clinical Laboratory: Proposed Guideline (1994) Contrib. by Harry S. Hertz. 1994. 75.00 (*1-56238-222-5*, NRSC12-P) NCCLS.

Sourcebook on Asbestos Diseases: Asbestos Abatement, Vol. 5. George A. Peters & Barbara J. Peters. 1991. 800p. 85.00 (*0-88063-792-7*, MICHIE) LEXIS Pub.

Sourcebook on Asbestos Diseases: Asbestos Control & Medical Treatment, Vol. 7. George A. Peters & Barbara J. Peters. 1993. 95.00 (*0-88063-797-8*, MICHIE) LEXIS Pub.

Sourcebook on Asbestos Diseases: Asbestos Medical Research, Vol. 4. George A. Peters & Barbara J. Peters. 1989. 75.00 (*0-88063-759-5*, MICHIE) LEXIS Pub.

Sourcebook on Asbestos Diseases: International Asbestos Medical Research, Vol. 6. Ed. by George A. Peters & Barbara J. Peters. 1991. 600p. 95.00 (*0-88063-796-X*, MICHIE) LEXIS Pub.

Sourcebook on Asbestos Diseases Vol. Medical, Legal & Engineering Aspects. George A. Peters & Barbara J. Peters. Vol. 1. 1980. 75.00 (*0-88063-756-0*); Vol. 2. 1986. 75.00 (*0-88063-757-9*); Vol. 3. 1988. 75.00 (*0-88063-758-7*) LEXIS Pub (MICHIE).

Sourcebook on Asbestos Diseases Case Law Quarterly. Quarterly Journal Staff. 1989. 75.00 (*0-8240-7348-7*, 82414-10, MICHIE) LEXIS Pub.

Sourcebook on Asbestos Diseases, 1980-1993: Medical, Legal & Engineering Aspects, Set. George A. Peters & Barbara J. Peters. 1993. 7100p. 500.00 (*0-8240-7175-1*, 82410-10, MICHIE) LEXIS Pub.

Sourcebook on Postretirement Health Care Benefits. Ed. by Robert D. Paul & Diane M. Disney. 1988. LC 88-15194. 603p. 89.00 (*0-916592-76-6*) Panel Pubs.

Sourcebook on Substance Abuse: Etiology, Epidemiology, Assessment, & Treatment. Ed. by Peggy J. Ott et al. 1999. LC 98-35240. 472p. 91.00 (*0-205-19802-3*) Allyn.

Sources: Notable Selections in Psychology. Ed. by Terry F. Pettijohn. 1993. LC 93-34527. 384p. (C). text 14.95 (*1-56134-263-7*, Dshkn McG-Hill) McGrw-H Hghr Educ.

Sources: Notable Selections in Psychology. Terry F. Pettijohn. 2nd ed. 1996. LC 96-85797. 384p. (C). text 14.00 net. (*0-697-34331-6*, WCB McGr Hill) McGrw-H Hghr Educ.

Sources & Magnitude of Occupational & Public Exposures from Nuclear Medicine Procedures: Recommendations of the National Council on Radiation Protection & Measurements. Intro. by Charles B. Meinhold. 1996. LC 96-690. (NCRP Reports: Vol. 124). 77p. (Orig.). pap. 25.00 (*0-929600-51-7*) NCRP Pubns.

Sources & Traditions of Classification in Psychiatry. Ed. by Norman Sartorius et al. 1990. LC 89-24610. 254p. text 49.00 (*0-920887-74-0*) Hogrefe & Huber Pubs.

Sources for the History of Medicine in Late Medieval England. Tr. & Intro. by Carole Rawcliffe. 1995. LC 94-45554. (Documents of Practice Ser.). pap. 6.00 (*1-879288-54-0*) Medieval Inst.

Sources in the History of American Pharmacology. John Parascandola & Elizabeth Keeney. 1983. pap. 5.60 (*0-931292-12-3*) Am Inst Hist Pharm.

Sources of Medical Technology: Universities & Industry, Vol. 5. Institute of Medicine Staff. Ed. by Annetine C. Gelijns et al. 1995. LC 94-43303. (Medical Innovation at the Crossroads Ser.: Vol. 5). 280p. (Orig.). (C). pap. text 32.00 (*0-309-05189-4*) Natl Acad Pr.

Sources of Mortality Changes in Italy since Unification. Elizabeth Hoffman. Ed. by Stuart Bruchey. 1981. LC 80-2811. (Dissertations in European Economic History Ser.). (Illus.). lib. bdg. 30.95 (*0-405-13995-0*) Ayer.

South African Disease: Apartheid Health & Health Services. Cedric De Beer. 1986. LC 86-70877. 240p. 19.95 (*0-86543-038-1*); pap. 7.95 (*0-86543-039-X*) Africa World.

South Carolina Health Care in Perspective 2000. Ed. by Kathleen O'Leary Morgan & Scott E. Morgan. 2000. 21p. spiral bd. 19.00 (*0-7401-0239-7*) Morgan Quitno Corp.

South Carolina Health Care Perspective, 1998. Ed. by Kathleen O'Leary Morgan & Scott E. Morgan. 1998. 20p. pap. 19.00 (*1-56692-839-7*) Morgan Quitno Corp.

South Dakota Health Care in Perspective 2000. Ed. by Kathleen O'Leary Morgan & Scott E. Morgan. 2000. 21p. spiral bd. 19.00 (*0-7401-0240-0*) Morgan Quitno Corp.

South Dakota Health Care Perspective, 1998. Ed. by Kathleen O'Leary Morgan & Scott E. Morgan. 1998. 20p. pap. 19.00 (*1-56692-840-0*) Morgan Quitno Corp.

South Florida Rehab & Healthcare Directory, 1991. Ed. by Kester J. Nedd. 1991. 490p. 39.00 (*1-879657-00-7*, Nedmar Graphics) HealthNet Pages.

Southeast Asian Birth Customs: Three Studies in Human Reproduction. Donn V. Hart et al. 1965. LC 65-18348. (Monographs). 315p. pap. 15.00 (*0-87536-318-0*) HRAFP.

Southern Folk Medicine, 1750-1820: 1750-1820. Kay K. Moss. 1999. LC 98-40223. (Illus.). xv, 259p. 29.95 (*1-57003-289-0*) U of SC Pr.

Southwestern Medical Dictionary: Spanish-English & English-Spanish. Margarita A. Kay. 1977. LC 00-9994. (ENG & SPA.). 217p. pap. 12.50 (*0-8165-0529-2*) U of Ariz Pr.

***Southwestern Medical Dictionary: Spanish-English, English-Spanish.** Margarita Artschwager Kay. 2nd ed. 2001. LC 00-9994. (ENG & SPA., Illus.). xxi, 308p. pap. 17.95 (*0-8165-2155-7*) U of Ariz Pr.

Southwick's the Law of Healthcare Administration. J. Stuart Showalter & Arthur F. Southwick. 3rd ed. 1999. LC 98-53747. 9p. 68.00 (*1-56793-101-4*) Health Admin Pr.

Soviet & American Psychology During World War II, 34. Albert R. Gilgen et al. 1997. LC 97-8773. (Contributions in Psychology Ser.: Vol. 34). 264p. 67.00 (*0-313-28794-5*, Greenwood Pr) Greenwood.

Soviet Art of Brainwashing. Kenneth Goff. 1979. 64p. pap. 3.50 (*0-911038-27-2*, 0026, Noontide Pr) Legion Survival.

Soviet Medical Reviews Section F Oncology Reviews. N. N. Blokhin & Trapeznikov. 1987. Vol. 1. xii, 222p. text 389.00 (*3-7186-0313-6*); Vol. 2. ix, 130p. text 237.00 (*3-7186-0436-1*) Gordon & Breach.

Soviet Military Psychiatry: The Theory & Practice of Coping with Battle Stress, 53. Richard A. Gabriel. 1986. LC 85-24795. (Contributions in Military Studies Ser.: No. 53). (Illus.). 186p. 60.00 (*0-313-25225-4*, GSM/, Greenwood Pr) Greenwood.

Soviet Psycholinguistics. Jan Prucha. 1972. (Janua Linguarum, Ser. Minor: No. 143). 117p. (Orig.). pap. text (*90-279-2317-5*) Mouton.

Soviet Psychology: Philosophical, Theoretical & Experimental Issues. Levy Rahmani. 1973. LC 72-182041. 560p. 65.00 (*0-8236-6110-5*) Intl Univs Pr.

Soviet Psychotherapy. Tr. by E. Salisbury & Ann Lauterbach. 1984. (Illus.). 255p. (*0-08-024291-X*) Pergamon Repr GBR. *Dist:* Franklin.

Sowing the Body: Psychoanalysis & Ancient Representations of Women. Page DuBois. 1996. (Women in Culture & Society Ser.). (Illus.). xvi, 248p. 35.95 (*0-226-16757-7*) U Ch Pr.

Soy: Asia's Hidden Healer. Deanne Tenney. 1998. (Woodland Health Ser.). 30p. pap. 3.95 (*1-58054-018-X*) Woodland UT.

Soy Smart Health: Discover the "Super Food" That Fights Breast Cancer, Heart Disease, Osteoporosis, Menopausal Discomforts & Estrogen. Duane E. Townsend et al. 2001. LC 00-10269. 303p. pap. 14.95 (*1-58054-044-9*) Woodland UT.

Soziale Phobie: Eine Anleitung Zur Durchfuehrung Einer Exposition in Vivo. Z. Wlazlo. 1995. xii, 128p. pap. 35.00 (*3-8055-5918-6*) S Karger.

Space & Its Exploration. Ed. by J. D. Rummel et al. 1993. (Space Biology & Medicine Ser.: Vol. 1). 338p. 99.95 (*1-56347-061-6*, 61-6) AIAA.

Space & Place: Theories of Identity & Location. Ed. by Erica Carter et al. 1993. LC 94-172821. 256p. (C). pap. (*0-85315-775-8*) Lawrence & Wishart GBR. *Dist:* NYU Pr.

Space Clinical Medicine: A Prospective Look at Medical Problems from Hazards of Space Operations. D. E. Busby. 1968. 276p. text 106.00 (*90-277-0110-5*) Kluwer Academic.

Space Flight: Index of Modern Authors & Subjects with Guide for Rapid Research. Vasnil S. Sokov. rev. ed. 1994. LC 94-31237. 157p. pap. 47.50 (*0-7883-0403-8*); text 57.50 (*0-7883-0402-X*) ABBE Pubs Assn.

Space Physiology & Medicine. 1994. lib. bdg. 260.95 (*0-8490-6402-3*) Gordon Pr.

Space Physiology & Medicine. Arnauld E. Nicogossian et al. 3rd ed. 1994. (Illus.). 481p. text 95.00 (*0-8121-1595-3*) Lppncott W & W.

Spacious Body: Explorations in Somatic Ontology. Jeffrey Maitland. 1995. LC 95-8725. 250p. pap. 12.95 (*1-55643-188-0*) North Atlantic.

Spadacrene Anglica: Or, the English Spaw-Fountaine in Yorkshire. Edmund Deane. 1974. LC 74-80172. (English Experience Ser.: No. 651). 32p. reprint ed. 15.00 (*90-221-0651-9*) Walter J Johnson.

Span. see Enciclopedia de la Sexualidad

Spanisches Supplement Zu Medizinisches Woerterbuch. E. Veillon & Albert Nobel. 1971. (GER.). 48.00 (*0-7859-0834-X*, M-7623) Fr & Eur.

Spanish - English Handbook for Medical Professionals: Compendio en Ingles y Espanol Para Profesionales de la Medicine. Jesus Perez-Sabido. Ed. by Gregg Rogers. 4th ed. 1993. LC 93-37022. (ENG & SPA.). 378p. spiral bd. 29.95 (*1-878487-61-2*, ME054) Practice Mgmt Info.

Spanish - English Patient Education Collection: Women & Infants. Aspen Reference Group Staff & Sara N. Di Lima. Ed. by Sandra J. Painter. 1995. LC 95-12765. (ENG & SPA.). 672p. spiral bd. 60.00 (*0-8342-0717-6*) PRO-ED.

Spanish Course for Health Care Professionals, Level 1. Bess I. Kennedy. (Hablar el Idioma de Su Cliente). (ENG & SPA., Illus.). 1998. pap. text, stu. ed., wbk. ed. 63.95 incl. audio (*0-9660225-4-8*, SPHC1); 1997. 108p. pap. text, wbk. ed. Price not set. (*0-9660225-0-5*, SWHC1) Manzana.

Spanish Course for Health Care Professionals Level 1: Instructor's Aid. Bess I. Kennedy. 1997. (Hablar el Idioma de Su Cliente). (Illus.). 72p. tchr. ed., ring bd. 25.00 (*0-9660225-2-1*, IAHC1) Manzana.

Spanish Course for Health Care Professionals Level 1: Instructor's Manual. Bess I. Kennedy. 1997. (Hablar el Idioma de Su Cliente). (ENG & SPA., Illus.). 148p. tchr. ed. 87.50 (*0-9660225-1-3*, IMHC1) Manzana.

Spanish Course for Health Care Professionals Level I: Instructor's Packet. Bess I. Kennedy. 1998. (Hablar el Idioma de Su Cliente). (ENG & SPA., Illus.). tchr. ed., spiral bd. 175.00 incl. audio (*0-9660225-5-6*, IPHC1) Manzana.

Spanish Course for Healthcare Professional, Level I. Bess I. Kennedy. 1998. (ENG & SPA., Illus.). 82p. pap., stu. ed. 19.95 (*0-9660225-7-2*, SGHCI) Manzana.

Spanish Course for Healthcare Professionals Level 1: Tests. Bess I. Kennedy. 1998. (Hablar el Idioma de Su Cliente). (ENG & SPA.). 13p. pap., tchr. ed. 19.95 (*0-9660225-6-4*, THCI) Manzana.

Spanish-English - English-Spanish Glossary of Psychiatric Terminology. J. C. Nemiah & F. P. Gallardo. 1996. (ENG & SPA.). 504p. pap. (*84-7978-234-X*) Ediciones Diaz ESP. *Dist:* IBD Ltd.

Spanish-English Illustrated Medical Dictionary Dorlands. 27th ed. 1992. (ENG & SPA., Illus.). 250.00 (*0-7859-8835-1*) Fr & Eur.

Spanish-English/English-Spanish Medical Dictionary, Vol. 1. Onyria H. McElroy & L. L. Grabb. 2nd ed. 1996. LC 96-20619. (ENG & SPA.). 560p. pap. text 39.95 (*0-316-55448-0*, LBC448) Lppncott W & W.

***Spanish Flu Pandemic of 1918: New Perspectives.** Ed. by Howard Phillips & David Killingray. 2001. (Studies in the Social History of Medicine). 224p. (C). (gr. 13). lib. bdg. 90.00 (*0-415-23445-X*) Routledge.

Spanish for Health Care Professionals. William C. Harvey. 1994. (ENG & SPA.). 256p. pap. 13.95 (*0-8120-1730-7*, BA7307) Barron.

***Spanish for Health Care Professionals: With Optional Cassettes**, Set. William C. Harvey. 2nd ed. 2000. (Illus.). 288p. pap. 21.95 (*0-7641-7300-6*) Barron.

Spanish for Health Care Workers: Communication & Culture. Robert O. Chase et al. 1998. LC 97-34802. (Yale Language Ser.). (SPA., Illus.). 272p. 20.00 (*0-300-07077-2*) Yale U Pr.

Spanish for Health Professionals: Interactive Language Exercises: Doctors, Dentists, Nurses, Psychologists, Social Workers & Related Fields = Ingles para Profesionistas de la Salud: Ejercicios Interactivos de Lenguaje: Doctores, Dentistas, Enfermeras, Sicologos, Trabajadores Sociales Y Campos Afines. Contrib. by Dario Sanchez & Ruben Juarez. 1997. LC 99-173326. (Illus.). (*0-9658803-0-3*) Comp Res Assocs.

Spanish for Medical Personnel. Janet E. Meizel. 1999. LC 93-244744. (ENG & SPA.). 310p. per. 24.95 (*1-56930-001-1*) Delmar.

Spanish for Medical Personnel. Ana C. Jarvis & Raquel Lebredo. 5th ed. 2000. LC 97-102932. (C). pap. text 28.36 (*0-669-35459-7*) HM Trade Div.

Spanish for Nursing. Sam L. Slick. 1998. 106p. ring bd. 49.50 incl. audio (*1-888467-13-4*) Command Spanish.

Spanish for Pediatric Medicine: A Practical Communication Guide. American Academy of Pediatrics Staff & Edward Machtinger. 1997. LC 97-71403. (SPA.). 219p. spiral bd. 34.95 (*0-910761-84-1*) Am Acad Pediat.

Spanish Made Easy: Spanish for the Medical Worker. Phanis Kennedy. Ed. & Tr. by Mitchell Kennedy. Tr. by Cecilee Lindsey. 1996. 32p. pap. 4.95 (*0-9661893-0-2*) M Kennedy Enter.

Spanish/English Dictionary of Medical Sciences: Spanish - English Stedman. 25th ed. 1993. (ENG & SPA.). 1530p. 295.00 (*0-7859-9305-3*) Fr & Eur.

Spare Parts: Organ Replacement in American Society. Renee C. Fox & Judith P. Swazey. 1992. LC 91-39727. 272p. text 39.95 (*0-19-507650-8*) OUP.

Spas, Hot Tubs & Whirlpool Bathtubs: A Guide for Disease Prevention. Matthew R. Freije. 2000. 29p. pap. 25.00 (*1-930488-11-4*) HC Info Res.

Spasticity: Mechanisms & Management. Ed. by A. F. Thilmann et al. 1994. LC 93-34850. (Illus.). 463p. 103.00 (*0-387-56981-2*) Spr-Verlag.

Spasticity Management: Rehabilitation Strategies. Linda A. Preston & Jeffrey S. Hecht. 1999. LC 00-500435. (Illus.). pap. text 20.00 (*1-56900-117-0*) Am Occup Therapy.

Spatial Child. John P. Dixon. 1983. (Illus.). 248p. (C). 49.95 (*0-398-04821-5*) C C Thomas.

Spatial Cognition: The Structure & Development of Mental Representations of Spatial Relations. David R. Olson & Ellen Bialystok. 1983. 296p. text 69.95 (*0-89859-252-6*) L Erlbaum Assocs.

Spatial Hearing: The Psychophysics of Human Sound Localization. Jens Blauert. Tr. by John S. Allen from GER. rev. ed. 1996. LC 96-12637.Tr. of Raumliches Horen. (Illus.). 480p. (C). 52.95 (*0-262-02413-6*) MIT Pr.

***Spatial Neglect: A Clinical Handbook for Diagnosis & Treatment.** Ian H. Robertson & Peter W. Halligan. 2001. 192p. pap. (*0-86377-810-0*) Psychol Pr GBR. *Dist:* Taylor & Francis.

Spatial Organization of Cerebral Processes. M. N. Livanov. 1975. 178p. 3.5 hd 48.00 (*0-7065-1514-5*) Coronet Bks.

Spatial Planning of Health Services Vol. 33: Case Studies in Warsaw, Poland. Jacek Malczewski. 1990. (Progressin Planning Ser.: No. 2). (Illus.). 63p. pap. 41.50 (*0-08-040171-6*, Pergamon Pr) Elsevier.

Spatial Structure of the Medical Care Process. Jerry B. Schneider. 1967. (Discussion Papers: No. 14). pap. 10.00 (*1-55869-120-0*) Regional Sci Res Inst.

Spatially Oriented Behavior. Ed. by A. Hein & M. Jeanherod. 1983. (Illus.). 365p. 107.00 (*0-387-90789-0*) Spr-Verlag.

Spatiotemporal Environmental Health Modelling: A Tractatus Stochasticus. George Christakos & Dionissios T. Hristopulos. 1998. LC 98-24443. 400p. 130.00 (*0-7923-8211-0*) Kluwer Academic.

Speak Now or Forever Rest in Peace: The Very Real Dangers of HMOs - & What You Can Do about Them. Tom Mann. 1997. LC 99-173185. (Illus.). iv, 110 p. 7.99 (*0-9659594-0-6*) G Miller.

Speak to Me. Marcia Calhoun Forecki. 2nd rev. ed. 1985. LC 84-28740. 160p. pap. 12.95 (*0-930323-68-8*) Gallaudet Univ Pr.

Speakers: The Role of Listeners. Ed. by Carl F. Graumann. 1989. 128p. (*1-85359-059-2*) Multilingual Matters GBR. *Dist:* Taylor & Francis.

Speaking Desires Can Be Dangerous: The Poetics of the Unconscious. Elizabeth Wright. 2000. LC 99-43571. 200p. pap. 22.95 (*0-7456-1968-1*) Blackwell Pubs.

Speaking of Ayurvedic Remedies for Common Diseases. T. L. Devaraj. 1995. (C). pap. (*81-207-1611-6*) Sterling Pubs.

Speaking of Life: Horizons of Meaning for Nursing Home Residents. Jaber F. Gubrium. 1993. LC 93-28591. (Communication & Social Order Ser.). 213p. pap. text 26.95 (*0-202-30482-5*); lib. bdg. 49.95 (*0-202-30481-7*) Aldine de Gruyter.

Speaking of Man. Abraham Myerson. Ed. by Gerald N. Grob. 1980. LC 78-22577. (Historical Issues in Mental Health Ser.). reprint ed. lib. bdg. 23.95 (*0-405-11929-1*) Ayer.

Speaking of Operations. Irvin Shrewsbury Cobb. 1998. (Collected Works of Irvin S. Cobb). 64p. reprint ed. lib. bdg. 88.00 (*1-58201-610-0*) Classic Bks.

Speaking of Operations. Irvin Shrewsbury Cobb. 1928. LC 71-92422. 65p. reprint ed. 39.00 (*0-403-00556-6*) Scholarly.

Speaking of Sadness: Depression, Disconnection & the Meanings of Illness. David A. Karp. 1997. 256p. reprint ed. pap. 13.95 (*0-19-511386-1*) OUP.

Speaking Out: Partners in Advocacy - Family Action Guide. Epilepsy Foundation of America Staff. 1992. 50p. pap. 9.95 (*0-916570-07-X*) Epilepsy Foundation of America.

Speaking Out: Partners in Advocacy - Tools & Resources. Epilepsy Foundation of America Staff. 1992. 89p. pap. 10.95 (*0-916570-08-8*) Epilepsy Foundation of America.

Speaking Out: Partners in Advocacy - Understanding the Process. Epilepsy Foundation of America Staff. 1992. 20p. pap. 5.95 (*0-916570-09-6*) Epilepsy Foundation of America.

Speaking Out on Health: An Anthology. Ed. by Literacy Volunteers of New York City Staff. 1989. (New Writers' Voices Ser.). 64p. pap. text 4.75 (*0-929631-05-6*, 3105-6) New Readers.

Speaking, Relating, & Learning: A Study of Hawaiian Children at Home & at School. Stephen T. Boggs. 1986. LC 85-7388. 216p. (C). 77.00 (*0-89391-330-8*, Ablex) Greenwood.

Speaking the Language of Respiratory Care. California College for Health Sciences Staff. 1991. LC 85-4141. 48p. (C). pap. 22.95 incl. audio (*0-933195-00-1*) CA College Health Sci.

Speaking with Deaf - Blind Children. Judy Katz-Levine. 1983. (Illus.). 20p. (Orig.). (C). pap. 4.25 (*0-930707-00-1*) Free Begin Pr.

Special Applications of REBT: A Therapist's Casebook. Joseph Yankura & Windy Dryden. 1997. LC 97-23193. 32.95 (*0-8261-9801-5*) Springer Pub.

Special Aspects of the Therapy for Gastric Carcinoma. Ed. by R. Kirchner & K. Maruyama. 1995. (Journal: Vol. 11, No. 2, 1994). (Illus.). 82p. pap. 68.00 (*3-8055-6134-2*) S Karger.

Special Courses for National Staff with Higher Administrative Responsibilities in the Health Services. 1965. (Technical Report Ser.: No. 311). 31p. pap. text 3.00 (*92-4-120311-0*) World Health.

Special Delivery. Rahima Baldwin. 1995. LC 78-61611. 192p. pap. 18.95 (*0-89087-934-6*) Celestial Arts.

Special Education: Research & Practice: Synthesis of Findings. Ed. by Margaret C. Wang et al. 1990. 236p. pap. 49.95 (*0-08-040237-2*, Prgamon Press) Buttrwrth-Heinemann.

Special Education Handbook: An Introductory Reference. Phillip Williams. 1990. 320p. (*0-335-09314-0*) OpUniv Pr.

Special Focus: Surveillance for Reproductive Health. Ed. by Richard A. Goodman. 1998. (Illus.). 98p. (C). pap. text 25.00 (*0-7881-7055-4*) DIANE Pub.

Special Infant: An Interdisciplinary Approach to the Optimal Development of Infants. Ed. by Jack M. Sack. 1982. LC 81-4478. 351p. 45.95 (*0-89885-028-2*, Kluwer Acad Hman Sci) Kluwer Academic.

Special Issue on Signal Transduction III. Ed. by M. P. Blaustein et al. 1994. (Reviews of Physiology, Biochemistry & Pharmacology Ser.: Vol. 124). (Illus.). 140p. 113.00 (*0-387-57587-1*) Spr-Verlag.

Special Issues in Nutrition. Ed. by Lucille S. Hurley. 1987. 96p. (Orig.). reprint ed. pap. 17.50 (*0-943029-00-7*) Am Soc Nutr Sci.

Special Kind of Parenting: Meeting the Needs of Handicapped Children. Julia Darnell Good & Joyce Good Reis. 1985. LC 85-80903. (Illus.). 172p. pap. 6.50 (*0-912500-27-1*, 163-12) La Leche.

Special-Needs Adoption: A Study of Intact Families. James A. Rosenthal & Victor K. Groze. 1992. LC 91-30278. 264p. 68.00 (*0-275-93790-9*, C3790, Praeger Pubs) Greenwood.

Special Needs Dementia Units: Design, Development & Operations. Nancy R. Peppard. 1991. LC 91-12278. 152p. 29.95 (*0-8261-5950-8*) Springer Pub.

Special Neuroendocrine Systems: Journal: Neuroendocrinology, Vol. 53, Suppl. 1, 1991. Ed. by S. F. Pang & F. Tang. 1991. (Illus.). iv, 84p. pap. 54.00 (*3-8055-5357-9*) S Karger.

Special Observations in the Last Time of the Pestilence. 1971. LC 72-171780. (English Experience Ser.: No. 405). 28p. reprint ed. 10.00 (*90-221-0405-2*) Walter J Johnson.

***Special Physical Education: Adapted, Individualized, Developmental with PowerWeb.** John Dunn. 7th ed. 2001. pap. 77.19 (*0-07-250526-5*) McGrw-H Hghr Educ.

Special Populations in the Community: Advances in Reducing Health Disparities. Juliann G. Sebastian & Angeline Bushy. 1999. LC 99-23669. 405p. pap. 47.00 (*0-8342-1364-8*) Aspen Pub.

Special Problems in Counseling the Chemically Dependent Adolescent. Eileen S. Sweet. 1991. LC 91-20804. (Journal of Adolescent Chemical Dependency). (Illus.). 170p. pap. 39.95 (*1-56024-162-4*); lib. bdg. 14.95 (*1-56024-163-2*) Haworth Pr.

Special Problems in Managing Eating Disorders. Ed. by Joel Yager et al. 1991. LC 91-4580. (Clinical Practice Ser.: No. 20). 245p. text 14.95 (*0-88048-457-8*, 8457) Am Psychiatric.

Special Report: A Doctor's Proven New Way to Conquer Back Pain. John E. Eichenlaub. 1992. LC 92-28322. 152p. pap. text 24.95 (*0-13-827049-X*, Parker Publishing Co) P-H.

Special Report: A Doctor's Proven New Way to Conquer Rheumatism & Arthritis. James K. Vanfleet. rev. ed. 1995. LC 91-30291. 152p. (C). pap. text 31.00 (*0-13-832650-9*) P-H.

Special Report on Medical Records. Meridith B. Cox. 1999. (Risk Management Ser.). pap. 50.00 (*0-912665-29-7*) BusinessWatch.

Special Research Methods for Gerontology. Ed. by M. P. Lawton & A. R. Herzog. 1989. (Society & Aging Ser.: Vol. 2). 330p. text 46.95 (*0-89503-061-6*); 257p. pap. text 36.00 (*0-89503-053-5*) Baywood Pub.

Special Seating. Jean A. Zollars. 1993. (Illus.). 95p. (Orig.). pap. 20.00 (*1-882632-01-X*); pap. 10.00 (*1-882632-05-2*) PAX Pr.

Special Section on Termination: A Special Issue of Psychoanalytic Psychology. Ed. by Robert C. Lane & Marvin Hyman. 1997. 176p. pap. 20.00 (*0-8058-9866-2*) L Erlbaum Assocs.

Special Senses. Thomas Braem. 1994. (Organs of the Human Anatomy: Vol. 4). 92p. (C). spiral bd. 15.95 (*1-878576-29-1*) Flash Anatomy Inc.

Special Skills & Techniques. Gretchen B. Van Boemel. 1999. LC 98-54626. (Basic Bookshelf for Eyecare Professionals Ser.). (Illus.). 272p. pap. text 30.00 (*1-55642-349-7*) SLACK Inc.

Special Study of the Incidence of Retardation. L. B. Blan. LC 79-176569. (Columbia University. Teachers College. Contributions to Education Ser.: No. 40). reprint ed. 37.50 (*0-404-55040-1*) AMS Pr.

Special Techniques for the Enzymologist. Ed. by Sidney P. Colowick & Nathan O. Kaplan. 1957. (Methods in Enzymology Ser.: Vol. 4). text 209.00 (*0-12-181804-7*) Acad Pr.

Special Techniques for Working with Older Adults: Exam. Elinor Waters. 70.00 Am Coun Assn.

Special Techniques in Internal Fixation. C. F. Brunner & B. G. Waber. 1981. (Illus.). 208p. 155.00 (*0-387-11056-9*) Spr-Verlag.

Special Tests for Orthopedic Examination. Jeff Konin et al. 1997. LC 97-21469. (Illus.). 296p. 29.50 (*1-55642-351-9*, 43519) SLACK Inc.

Special Tests of Visual Function. Ed. by E. Zrenner. 1984. (Developments in Ophthalmology Ser.: Vol. 9). (Illus.). xii, 240p. 129.75 (*3-8055-3885-5*) S Karger.

Special Topics in Gynecologic Ultrasound. 1998. (Ultrasound & Women's Health Ser.: Pt. II). (*1-930047-47-9*, 98II); (*1-930047-51-7*, 98II-P) Am Inst Ultrasound.

Special Twentieth Anniversary Issue of the ASME Biomechanics Symposium. 1993. 160p. 20.00 (*0-7918-0695-2*, I00358) ASME.

Special Way to Care: A Guide for Neighbors, Friends, & Community in their Efforts to Provide Financial & Emotional Support for Terminally & Catastrophically Ill Children. Sheila Petersen. 1988. 180p. (Orig.). pap. (*0-9619785-0-3*) Friends Karen.

Special Women? The Experience of Women in the Special Hospital System. Ed. by Catherine Hemingway. 1996. LC 96-84601. 172p. (*1-85628-868-4*) Avebry GBR. *Dist:* Ashgate Pub Co.

Special Women: The Role of the Professional Labor Assistant. Paulina Perez & Cheryl Snedeker. 2nd ed. 1994. LC 94-94211. (Illus.). 157p. pap. 9.95 (*0-9641159-9-9*) Doubleday.

Special Women: The Role of the Professional Labor Assistant. Paulina Perez & Cheryl Snedeker. 1994. (Illus.). 157p. pap. 12.95 (*0-937604-10-0*, Pennypr) Intl Childbirth.

Specialist Foster Family Care: A Normalizing Experience. Ed. by Joe Hudson. 1989. LC 89-15648. (Child & Youth Services Ser.: Vol. 12, Nos. 1 & 2). (Illus.). 273p. text 49.95 (*0-86656-939-1*) Haworth Pr.

***Specialist Registrar Handbook.** John Gatrell & Tony White. 2nd ed. 2001. 336p. pap. (*1-85775-464-6*) Radcliffe Med Pr GBR. *Dist:* Balogh.

Specialization of Medicine with Particular Reference to Ophthalmology. George Rosen. 1972. LC 79-180586. (Medicine & Society in America Ser.). 106p. reprint ed. 14.95 (*0-405-03966-2*) Ayer.

Specialized Drug Delivery Systems: Manufacturing & Production Technology. Ed. by Praveen Tyle. 1989. (Drugs & the Pharmaceutical Sciences Ser.: Vol. 41). (Illus.). 496p. text 185.00 (*0-8247-8190-2*) Dekker.

Specialized Medical Education in the European Region. J. Parkhouse & J. Menu. 1989. (Euro Reports & Studies Ser.: No. 112). 266p. pap. text 18.00 (*92-890-1278-1*) World Health.

Specialized Pharmaceuticals Dictionary: Diccionario de Especialidades Farmaceuticas. Emilio S. Rosenstein. 28th ed. 1982. (SPA.). 1350p. 49.95 (*0-8288-1877-0*, S39848) Fr & Eur.

Specialized SOPs for General Surgeons. Melinda Coburn. 1998. ring bd. 50.00 incl. disk (*0-910167-58-3*) Comm Unltd CA.

Specialized SOPs for OBGYNs. Leila Chambers & Robyn Hayes. 1998. ring bd. 50.00 incl. disk (*0-910167-57-5*) Comm Unltd CA.

Specialized SOPs for Oral Surgeons. Marsha Freeman. 1998. 34p. ring bd. 35.00 incl. disk (*0-910167-50-8*, Dental Commun) Comm Unltd CA.

Specialized SOPs for Orthodontists. Marsha Freeman. 1998. 36p. ring bd. 35.00 incl. disk (*0-910167-48-6*, Dental Commun) Comm Unltd CA.

Specialized SOPs for Pediatric Dentists. Marsha Freeman. 1998. 69p. ring bd. 45.00 incl. disk (*0-910167-52-4*, Dental Commun) Comm Unltd CA.

Specialized SOPs for Pediatricians. Leila Chambers & Robyn Hayes. 1998. 52p. ring bd. 45.00 incl. disk (*0-910167-44-3*, Dental Commun) Comm Unltd CA.

Specialized SOPs for Periodontists. Marsha Freeman. 1998. 24p. ring bd. 35.00 incl. disk (*0-910167-49-4*, Dental Commun) Comm Unltd CA.

Specialized SOPs for Primary Care Physicians. Leila Chambers & Robyn Hayes. 1998. 44p. ring bd. 45.00 incl. disk (*0-910167-56-7*, Dental Commun) Comm Unltd CA.

Specialty Board Review: Neurology. Barbara S. Giesser et al. 4th ed. 1997. 252p. (C). pap. text 42.50 (*0-8385-8650-3*, A8650-2, Apple Lange Med) McGraw.

Specialty Contact Lenses: A Fitter's Guide. Carol A. Schwartz. 1995. LC 95-17561. (Illus.). 288p. pap. text 62.00 (*0-7216-4747-2*) Saunders.

Specialty Fiber Optics for Biomedical & Industrial Applications, Vol. 2977. Ed. by Abraham Katzir & James A. Harrington. 1997. 172p. 59.00 (*0-8194-2388-2*) SPIE.

Specialty Practice of Rehabilitation Nursing: A Core Curriculum. Ed. by Patricia A. Edwards. 4th ed. 2000. LC 00-190797. (Illus.). xiv, 424p. pap. (*1-884278-11-6*) Rehab Nursing.

Species & Specificity: An Interpretation of the History of Immunology. Pauline M. Mazumdar. 1995. LC 93-31219. (Illus.). 473p. (C). text 69.95 (*0-521-43172-7*) Cambridge U Pr.

***Specific Anti-Tumour Effects of 6-Diazo-5-Oxo-L-Norleucine (DON) on Carcinoid Tumour Cells.** Feng Wu. 2000. (Comprehensive Summaries of Uppsala Dissertations from the Faculty of Medicine Ser.: No. 918). (Illus.). 67p. pap. (*91-554-4690-6*) Uppsala Universitet SWE. *Dist:* Coronet Bks.

Specific Diagnosis. John M. Scudder. 1994. 387p. reprint ed. 48.00 (*1-888483-04-0*) Eclectic Med.

Specific Malformations, Vol. 2. Helen B. Taussig. 2nd ed. 1961. (Commonwealth Fund Publications). (Illus.). 1059p. 65.00 (*0-674-16151-3*) HUP.

Specific Phobias: Clinical Applications of Evidence-Based Psychotherapy. Timothy J. Bruce & William C. Sanderson. 1998. LC 97-42371. (Clinical Application of Evidence-Based Psychotherapy Ser.). (Illus.). 280p. 40.00 (*1-56821-883-4*) Aronson.

Specific Reading Disability. Dirk J. Bakker. Ed. by Paul Satz. 1970. (Modern Approaches to the Diagnosis & Instruction of Multi-Handicapped Children Ser.: Vol. 3). xii, 166p. 25.00 (*90-237-4103-X*) Taylor & Francis.

Specific Reading Disability: A View of the Spectrum. Bruce K. Shapiro et al. 1998. LC 98-9512. pap. 33.50 (*0-912752-45-9*) York Pr.

Specific Receptors of Antibodies, Antigens & Cells: Proceedings of the International Convocation on Immunology, 3rd, Buffalo, 1972. International Convocation on Immunology Staff. Ed. by N. R. Rose. 1973. 300p. 134.00 (*3-8055-1372-0*) S Karger.

Specific Speech & Language Disorders in Children. Ed. by Paul Fletcher et al. 1992. LC 92-19316. 272p. (Orig.). pap. 49.95 (*1-879105-59-4*, 0238) Thomson Learn.

Specific Techniques for the Psychotherapy of Schizophrenic Patients. Andrew Lotterman. 1996. LC 95-16237. 172p. 35.00 (*0-8236-6130-X*) Intl Univs Pr.

Specification of Gamma-Ray Brachytherapy Sources. 1974. LC 73-94306. (Report Ser.: No. 41). 24p. pap. text 20.00 (*0-913392-23-5*) NCRP Pubns.

Specifications for Immunological Testing for Infectious Diseases: Approved Guideline (1994) Contrib. by A. Myron Johnson. 1994. 75.00 (*1-56238-251-9*, I/LA18-A) NCCLS.

Specifications for Pesticides Used in Public Health: Insecticides - Molluscicides - Repellents - Methods. 6th ed. 1985. (ENG, FRE & SPA.). 384p. pap. text 48.00 (*92-4-156084-3*, 1150259) World Health.

Specifications for the Identity & Purity of Some Food Colours, Flavour Enhancers, Thickening Agents & Certain Other Food Additives. 1976. (Food Additives Ser.: No. 7). pap. text 22.00 (*92-4-166007-4*, 1270007) World Health.

Specificity, Function & Development of NK Cells: NK Cells: The Effector Arm of Innate Immunity. Ed. by K. Karre & M. Colonna. 1998. (Current Topics in Microbiology & Immunology Ser.: Vol. 230). (Illus.). 280p. 149.00 (*3-540-63941-1*) Spr-Verlag.

Specificity in Biological Interactions. Ed. by Bernard Pullman. 1984. text 270.00 (*90-277-1813-X*) Kluwer Academic.

Specificity of Serological Reactions. Karl Landsteiner. 1990. 348p. pap. 8.95 (*0-486-66203-9*) Dover.

Specimen Collection & Transport for Microbiological Investigation. K. Engbaek & M. El-Nageh. 1995. LC 96-168039. (WHO Regional Publications, Eastern Mediterranean Ser.: No. 8). pap. text 12.00 (*92-9021-196-2*) World Health.

Specimen Dissection & Photography: For the Pathologist, Anatomist & Biologist. M. Donald McGavin & Samuel W. Thompson. 1988. (Illus.). 300p. (C). text 75.95 (*0-398-05451-7*) C C Thomas.

SPECT: Single-Photon Emission Computed Tomography: A Primer. Robert J. English. 3rd ed. 1995. LC 95-40807. 223p. pap. text 42.00 (*0-932004-43-1*) Soc Nuclear Med.

Spect Imaging of the Brain. Ed. by R. Duncan. 1997. LC 96-28961. (Developments in Nuclear Medicine Ser.: No. 29). 260p. (C). text 169.00 (*0-7923-4186-4*) Kluwer Academic.

Spectacle Frame Dispensing. George Clayton. 1989. (C). (*0-900099-04-6*) Assn Brit Dispen Opticians GBR. *Dist:* St Mut.

***Spectacle Lenses: Theory & Practice.** Colin Fowler & Keziah Latham Petre. 2001. LC 00-54373. (Illus.). 160p. pap. text 40.00 (*0-7506-2370-5*) Buttrwrth-Heinemann.

Spectacular Healing Foods. Dubin. 1998. (C). pap. 13.95 (*0-13-621251-4*) P-H.

Spectral Atlas of Polycyclic Aromatic Compounds: Including Data on Occurrence & Biological Activity. Ed. by Walter Karcher et al. 1985. lib. bdg. 284.50 (*90-277-1652-8*) Kluwer Academic.

Spectral Atlas of Polycyclic Aromatic Compounds Vol. 3: Including Information on Aquatic Toxicity, Occurrence & Biological Activity. Ed. by Walter Karcher et al. 1991. 1168p. lib. bdg. 355.00 (*0-7923-1464-6*) Kluwer Academic.

Spectral Data for Steroids. 1994. LC 93-60264. text 250.00 (*1-883400-00-7*) TX A&M Thermodyn.

Spectro-Chrome Metry Encyclopedia. Dinshah P. Chadiali. 3rd ed. 1992. (Illus.). 240p. 14.00 (*0-933917-08-2*) Dinshah Hlth Soc.

Spectroscopic Membrane Probes. Ed. by Leslie M. Loew. 1988. Vol. I. 240p. 137.00 (*0-8493-4535-9*); Vol. II. 208p. 126.00 (*0-8493-4536-7*); Vol. III. 240p. 137.00 (*0-8493-4537-5*) Franklin (CRC Reprint).

Spectrum of Child Abuse: Assessment, Treatment, & Prevention. R. Kim Oates. 1996. (Basic Principles into Practice Ser.: Vol. 8). 208p. pap. text 22.95 (*0-87630-807-8*) Brunner-Routledge.

Spectrum of Factitious Disorders. Ed. by Marc D. Feldman & Stuart J. Eisendrath. 1996. (Clinical Practice Ser.: No. 40). 304p. text 38.00 (*0-88048-909-X*, 8909) Am Psychiatric.

Spectrum of Normal Aging, Mild Cognitive Impairment & Alzheimer's Disease. Ed. by Ronald C. Peterson & Mayo Foundation for Medical Education and Research. 2001. (Illus.). 300p. text 55.00 (*0-19-512342-5*) OUP.

Spectrum of Psychoanalysis: Essays in Honor of Martin S. Bergmann. Arnold D. Richards. 1994. 378p. 60.00 (*0-8236-4505-3*) Intl Univs Pr.

Speculations J. H. Hacsi. 1983. 205p. (Orig.). pap. text 9.95 (*0-9612146-0-0*) Champagne Pr.

Speculations after Freud: Psychoanalysis, Philosophy, & Culture. Ed. by Sonu Shamdasani & Michael Munchow. 1994. LC 93-26967. 208p. (C). 80.00 (*0-415-07655-2*); (gr. 13). pap. 26.95 (*0-415-07656-0*) Routledge.

Speech: A Special Code. Alvin M. Liberman. 1996. LC 95-30668. (Learning, Development, & Conceptual Change Ser.). (Illus.). 472p. 70.00 (*0-262-12192-1*, Bradford Bks) MIT Pr.

Speech Acoustics & Perception. Philip Lieberman. 1972. LC 70-183114. (Studies in Communicative Disorders). (C). (*0-672-61293-3*, Bobbs) Macmillan.

Speech after Stroke: A Manual for the Speech-Language Pathologist & the Family Member. S. Stryker. 2nd ed. 1981. (Illus.). 442p. spiral bd. 51.95 (*0-398-04122-9*) C C Thomas.

Speech & Communication Disorder in Psychiatry. Rosemary Gravell & Jenny France. (Therapy in Practice Ser.: No. 22). 29.95 (*0-412-34700-8*) Chapman & Hall.

S

Speech & Communication Problems in Psychiatry. Ed. by Rosemary Gravell & Jenny France. 1991. (Illus.). 364p. (Orig.). (C). pap. text 51.50 (*1-879105-58-6*, 0254) Thomson Learn.

Speech & Hearing in Communication. Harvey Fletcher. Ed. by J. B. Allen. 1995. LC 94-47509. 49.00 (*1-56396-393-0*) Acoustical Soc Am.

Speech & Hearing Science: Anatomy & Physiology. W. R. Zemlin. 2nd ed. 1981. (Illus.). 704p. text 42.00 (*0-13-827378-2*) P-H.

Speech & Hearing Science: Anatomy & Physiology. Willard R. Zemlin. 4th ed. 1997. LC 96-53899. 610p. 92.00 (*0-13-827437-1*) P-H.

Speech & Hearing Science: Selected Readings. Ed. by Norman J. Lass. 1974. 382p. text 52.50 (*0-8422-5154-5*); pap. text 17.50 (*0-8422-0377-X*) Irvington.

Speech & Hearing Therapist. Jack Rudman. 1994. (Career Examination Ser.: C-754). pap. 29.95 (*0-8373-0754-6*) Nat Learn.

Speech & Language: Principles & Processes of Behavior Change. C. Woodruff Starweather. 1983. (Illus.). 448p. text 48.30 (*0-13-832501-4*) P-H.

Speech & Language Evaluation in Neurology: Adult Disorders. Ed. by John Darby, Jr. 1985. 460p. text 61.00 (*0-8089-1719-6*, 790976, Grune & Strat) Harcrt Hlth Sci Grp.

Speech & Language Evaluation in Neurology: Childhood Disorders. Ed. by John Darby, Jr. 1985. 304p. text 84.00 (*0-8089-1720-X*, 790979, Grune & Strat) Harcrt Hlth Sci Grp.

Speech & Language Impairments in Children: Causes, Characteristics, Intervention & Outcome. Dorothy V. M. Bishop & Laurence B. Leonard. 2000. 352p. (*0-86377-568-3*) Psychol Pr GBR. *Dist:* Taylor & Francis.

Speech & Language Problems in Children: A Practical Guide. Dilys Treharne. Ed. by Jo Campling. 1990. (Therapy in Practice Ser.). 120p. pap. (*0-412-37650-4*, A4408) Chapman & Hall.

Speech & Reticence: Sounds & Silence. Carl Johnson. 1973. LC 73-83225. (C). pap. 4.95 (*0-88310-001-0*) Publishers Consult.

Speech & the Hearing Impaired Child: Theory & Practice. Daniel Ling. 1976. LC 76-21920. (Illus.). text 27.95 (*0-88200-074-8*, A0669) Alexander Graham.

Speech & Voice Quality: Index of New Information for Reference & Research. Lynn W. Ennes & Claire D. Basill. 1997. 160p. 57.50 (*0-7883-1780-6*); pap. 47.50 (*0-7883-1781-4*) ABBE Pubs Assn.

Speech Art Classification. T. T. Ballmer & W. Brennenstuhl. 1980. (Language & Communication Ser.: Vol. 8). (Illus.). 274p. 46.95 (*0-387-10294-9*) Spr-Verlag.

Speech Audiologist. Jack Rudman. 1994. (Career Examination Ser.: C-753). pap. 27.95 (*0-8373-0753-8*) Nat Learn.

Speech Correction: An Introduction to Speech Pathology & Audiology. Charles Van Ripper & Robert L. Erickson. 9th ed. 1995. LC 95-41718. 512p. 85.00 (*0-13-825142-8*) P-H.

Speech Evaluation in Medicine. John K. Darby, Jr. 1981. 464p. text 55.50 (*0-8089-1359-X*, 790978, Grune & Strat) Harcrt Hlth Sci Grp.

Speech Evaluation of the Patient with a Tracheostomy Tube. Nancy Conway. Ed. by Cindy Drolet. 1997. (Illus.). 124p. ring bd. 46.00 (*1-883315-23-9*, 7097) Imaginart Intl.

Speech, Language & Hearing: Normal Processes & Disorders. Paul H. Skinner & Ralph L. Shelton. 1978. LC 77-73956. (Speech Pathology & Audiology Ser.). tchr. ed. (*0-201-07462-1*); text 17.50 net. (*0-201-07461-3*) Addison-Wesley.

***Speech, Language & Hearing Programs in Schools.** O'Connell. 1990. tchr. ed. (*0-8342-1031-2*) PRO-ED.

Speech-Language Pathologist in Home Health Care. Cecil G. Betros, Jr. 1995. LC 98-48636. (Illus.). 225p. pap. 51.00 (*0-8342-0919-5*, 20919) PRO-ED.

Speech-language Pathologist's Guide to Managing the New Medicare. Susan Rigby & Peggy Kipping. 2000. LC 99-55580. (*0-89079-847-8*) PRO-ED.

***Speech-Language Pathology: A Simplified Guide to Structures, Functions, & Clinical Implications.** Carl R. Schneiderman & Robert E. Potter. 2001. LC 2001-94341. (Illus.). 250p. pap. 39.95 (*0-12-627874-1*) Acad Pr.

Speech-Language Pathology: Services in the Schools. Joyce S. Taylor. 1981. 224p. (C). text 30.00 (*0-8089-1385-9*, 794543, Grune & Strat) Harcrt Hlth Sci Grp.

Speech-Language Pathology & Audiology: Issues & Management. Robert M. McLauchlin. 1986. LC 79-2843. 464p. text 56.00 (*0-8089-1770-6*, 792843, Grune & Strat) Harcrt Hlth Sci Grp.

Speech-Language Pathology Services. Joyce S. Taylor. 2nd ed. 1991. 270p. (C). 92.00 (*0-205-13262-6*) Allyn.

Speech-Language Treatment of the Aphasias - Workbook I: Treatment Materials for Auditory Comprehension & Reading Comprehension. Anita S. Halper & Martha S. Burns. 1993. (Rehabilitation Institute of Chicago Ser.). 383p. 68.00 (*0-8342-0079-1*) PRO-ED.

Speech-Language Treatment of the Aphasias - Workbook II: Treatment Materials for Oral Expression & Written Expression. Anita S. Halper & Martha S. Burns. 1995. (Rehabilitation Institute of Chicago Ser.). 9p. 65.00 (*0-8342-0080-5*) PRO-ED.

Speech Motor Control & Stuttering: Proc. of the 2nd Internat. Conf., Held in Nijmegen, The Netherlands, June 13-16, 1990. Ed. by H. F. Peters et al. 1991. (International Congress Ser.: No. 950). 582p. 273.50 (*0-444-81408-6*, Excerpta Medica) Elsevier.

Speech Motor Dynamics in Stuttering. Ed. by H. F. Peters & W. Hulstijn. 1987. (Illus.). 420p. 89.95 (*0-387-81971-1*) Spr-Verlag.

Speech of Primates. Philip Lieberman. 1972. (Janua Linguarum, Ser. Minor: No. 148). (Illus.). 133p. (Orig.). pap. text (*90-279-2321-3*) Mouton.

Speech Pathologist. Jack Rudman. 1994. (Career Examination Ser.: C-755). pap. 29.95 (*0-8373-0755-4*) Nat Learn.

Speech Pathology: A Dynamic Neurological Treatment of Normal Speech & Speech Deviations. Lee E. Travis. LC 78-72851. (Brainedness, Handedness, & Mental Abilities Ser.). reprint ed. 42.50 (*0-404-60895-7*) AMS Pr.

Speech Pathology & Audiology. Jack Rudman. (Undergraduate Program Field Tests Ser.: Vol. 25). 43.95 (*0-8373-6075-7*); 1994. pap. 23.95 (*0-8373-6025-0*) Nat Learn.

Speech Pathology Desk Reference. Ed. by Ross J. Roeser et al. 1998. LC 97-22115. (Illus.). 448p. pap. 45.00 (*0-86577-696-2*) Thieme Med Pubs.

Speech Production - EMIC #1146: Proceedings of the 3rd International Conference on Speech Motor Control & Stuttering, Nijmegen, The Netherlands, 5-8 June 1996. Ed. by W. L. Hulstijn et al. 1997. LC 97-24975. (International Congress Ser.: No. 1146). 652p. 221.00 (*0-444-82460-X*, Excerpta Medica) Elsevier.

Speech Protocols in Audiology. Ed. by Ralph R. Rupp & Kenneth Stockdell, Sr. 1980. 436p. text 47.00 (*0-8089-1254-2*, 793680, Grune & Strat) Harcrt Hlth Sci Grp.

Speech Reticence: Sounds & Silence. Carl Johnson. 1973. LC 73-83225. (C). 8.95 (*0-88310-015-0*) Publishers Consult.

***Speech Sound Disorders Resource Guide for School-age Children.** Ann Bosma Smit. 2002. 336p. pap. text 49.95 (*0-7693-0075-8*) Singular Publishing.

Speech Teacher: A Random Narrative. Loren Reid. 1990. LC 90-63139. (Illus.). 109p. (C). pap. 7.00 (*0-944811-05-1*) Natl Comm Assn.

Speech Therapy Techniques for Cleft Palate & Related Disorders. Karen J. Golding-Kushner. 2000. 175p. pap. 40.00 net. (*0-7693-0161-X*) Singular Publishing.

Speechless: Living with Spasmodic Dysphonia. Dot Sowerby et al. 1999. (Illus.). ix, 130p. (Orig.). pap. (*0-9659941-1-2*) Natl Spasmodic Dysphonia.

Speechreading: A Way to Improve Understanding. Harriet Kaplan et al. 2nd rev. ed. 1985. LC 87-7599. (Illus.). 162p. pap. text 14.95 (*0-930323-32-7*, Clerc Bks) Gallaudet Univ Pr.

Speechreading (Lipreading) Janet Jeffers & Margaret Barley. 1980. (Illus.). 408p. 62.95 (*0-398-02185-6*) C C Thomas.

Speed Culture: Amphetamine Use & Abuse in America. Lester Grinspoon & Peter Hedblom. 1976. LC 74-27257. (Harvard Paperbacks Ser.). 368p. pap. text 13.00 (*0-674-83194-2*) HUP.

Speed Culture: Amphetamine Use & Abuse in America. Lester Grinspoon et al. 1975. LC 74-27257. (Harvard Paperbacks Ser.). 368p. 39.00 (*0-674-83192-6*) HUP.

Speed of Thought: Information Processing in the Cerebral Cortex. Martin Tovee. 1998. LC 98-11141. (Neuroscience Intelligence Unit Ser.). 183p. 129.00 (*1-57059-488-0*) Landes Bioscience.

Speedwriting Medical Dictation Course. Goodwin W. Gilson & David Werheimer. 1960. 266p. 232.92 incl. audio (*0-672-97884-9*); tchr. ed. (*0-672-96154-7*); text (*0-672-96153-9*) Macmillan.

Speedwriting Medical Dictionary. Schaefer. 2nd ed. 1988. 11.19 net. (*0-02-679731-3*) Glencoe.

Speedy Spanish for Medical Personnel. T. L. Hart. Ed. & Tr. by Babe Hart. 1980. (Speedy Language Ser.). (SPA., Illus.). 24p. (C). pap. 4.95 (*0-9602838-6-2*) Baja Bks.

Speedy Spanish for Nursing Personnel. T. L. Hart. 1988. (ENG & SPA.). (Orig.). pap. 4.95 (*0-9615829-4-4*) Baja Bks.

Spehlmann's EEG Primer. Ed. by B. J. Fisch. 2nd enl. rev. ed. 1991. 650p. pap. 95.50 (*0-444-81420-5*); 238.50 (*0-444-81242-3*) Elsevier.

Speller's Law Relating to Hospitals. John Finch. 7th ed. 1994. LC 93-74217. (Illus.). 968p. (C). (gr. 13 up). pap. 214.95 (*0-412-41000-1*, Chap & Hall NY) Chapman & Hall.

Spellright: A Medical Word Book. Jane Rice. 1991. 780p. (C). pap. 30.40 (*0-8385-6290-6*, A6290-9) Appleton & Lange.

Spencer's Pathology of the Lung. Ed. by Philip S. Hasleton. 5th ed. 1996. LC 95-19711. (Illus.). 1282p. text 199.00 (*0-07-105448-0*) McGraw-Hill Prof.

Sperm Action: Proceedings of the International Seminar on Reproductive Physiology & Sexual Endocrinology, 5th, Brussels, May, 1975. International Seminar on Reproductive Physiology &. Ed. by P. O. Hubinont. 1976. 85.25 (*3-8055-2244-4*) S Karger.

Sperm Causing Diseases: A Major Medical Breakthrough. Donald E. Tyler. 1990. LC 90-84852. 95p. pap. 25.00 (*1-884981-04-6*) Discov Bks.

Sperm Cell. Ed. by Jean Andre. 1982. text 234.00 (*90-247-2784-7*) Kluwer Academic.

Sperm Competition & Sexual Selection. Ed. by Tim R. Birkhead & Anders P. Moller. 1998. (Illus.). 650p. (C). pap. text 59.95 (*0-12-100543-7*) Morgan Kaufmann.

Sperm Competition in Birds: Evolutionary Causes & Consequences. Tim R. Birkhead & A. P. Moller. 1991. (Illus.). 282p. pap. text 53.00 (*0-12-100541-0*) Acad Pr.

Sperm Confirm: Comprehensive Morphology Atlas of Sperm. Susan A. Rothmann. 1997. (Illus.). 127p. sl. 363.00 (*0-9660540-0-8*, SC100) Fertil Solns.

Sperm Confirm: Comprehensive Morphology Atlas of Sperm. Ed. by Susan A. Rothmann. 1997. (Illus.). 127p. 375.00 (*0-9660540-1-6*, SC101) Fertil Solns.

Spermatozoa: The Probable Etiology of Gonorrhea, Nonspecific Urethritis & Other Diseases. Donald E. Tyler. 1990. LC 90-80362. 90p. pap. 25.00 (*1-884981-03-8*) Discov Bks.

Spex Success: Full Length Practice Test. Stanley Zaslau. 1995. 156p. (C). pap. text 30.00 (*1-886468-08-7*) FMSG.

Sphincter of Oddi: Proceedings of the Gastroenterological Symposium, 3rd. Gastroenterological Symposium Staff. Ed. by J. Delmont. 1977. (Illus.). 54.00 (*3-8055-2623-7*) S Karger.

Sphincters: Normal Function - Changes in Diseases. Daniel. 1992. 464p. 184.00 (*0-8493-6748-4*, QP322) CRC Pr.

Sphingolipid-Mediated Signal Transduction. Yusuf A. Hannun. 1997. LC 97-7230. (Molecular Biology Intelligence Unit Ser.). 236p. 99.00 (*1-57059-436-8*) Landes Bioscience.

Sphingolipids As Signaling Modulators in the Nervous System. Ed. by Robert W. Leeden et al. 1998. LC 98-15146. (Annals of the New York Academy of Sciences Ser.: No. 845). 435p. 140.00 (*1-57331-137-5*) NY Acad Sci.

***Spicelegia: Polychromatic Gleanings.** Farid S. Haddad & S. H. Abul-Husn. 2002. (Illus.). 278p. pap. 30.00 (*1-886465-03-7*) Shad Board.

Spices & Herbs: Their Lore & Use. Elizabeth S. Hayes. 1980. (Illus.). 256p. reprint ed. pap. 6.95 (*0-486-24026-6*) Dover.

Spices of Life: The Well Being Handbook for Older Americans. Ruth Fort. 1990. 160p. (Orig.). pap. 8.00 (*0-936758-27-9*) Ctr Responsive Law.

Spiegelungen. Ernst Renk. 1985. (GER.). 291p. text 29.50 (*0-930329-40-6*) Kabel Pubs.

Spikes: Exploring the Neural Code. Fred Rieke et al. 1996. LC 95-46161. (Computational Neuroscience Ser.). (Illus.). 413p. 49.50 (*0-262-18174-6*, Bradford Bks) MIT Pr.

Spin Choreography: Basic Steps in High Resolution NMR. Ray Freeman. 1998. (Illus.). 404p. reprint ed. text 67.95 (*0-19-850481-0*) OUP.

Spinal Afferent Processing. Ed. by Tony L. Yaksh. 1986. (Illus.). 574p. (C). text 150.00 (*0-306-42046-5*, Kluwer Plenum) Kluwer Academic.

Spinal Anatomy. Gregory D. Cramer & Susan A. Darby. 1995. (Illus.). 448p. (C). (gr. 13). text 99.95 (*0-8016-6467-5*, 06467) Mosby Inc.

Spinal & Supraspinal Mechanisms of Voluntary Motor Control & Locomotion. Ed. by J. E. Desmedt. 1980. (Progress in Clinical Neurophysiology Ser.: Vol. 8). (Illus.). x, 374p. 120.00 (*3-8055-0022-X*) S Karger.

Spinal Center: Role Play Peacegames. David W. Felder. 1996. 44p. pap. text 8.95 (*0-910959-69-2*, B&G 13E) Wellington Pr.

Spinal Cord Disease: Basic Science, Diagnosis & Management. Ed. by E. Critchley & A. Eisen. 1999. (Illus.). xiv, 610p. (C). pap. (*1-85233-121-6*) Spr-Verlag GBR. *Dist:* Spr-Verlag.

Spinal Cord Disease: Basic Science, Diagnosis & Management, Vol. XIV. Ed. by E. M. Critchley & Andrew A. Eisen. 2nd rev. ed. 1996. LC 96-24791. (Illus.). 624p. 179.00 (*3-540-19935-7*) Spr-Verlag.

Spinal Cord Diseases: Diagnosis & Treatment. Ed. by Gordon Engler & Jonathan Cole. 1998. LC 98-4261. (Neurological Disease & Therapy Ser.). (Illus.). 696p. text 215.00 (*0-8247-9489-3*) Dekker.

Spinal Cord Dysfunction: Functional Stimulation, Vol. III. Ed. by L. S. Illis. 1992. (Illus.). 376p. 115.00 (*0-19-261919-5*) OUP.

***Spinal Cord Injuries.** Elaine Landau. 2001. LC 2001-1045. (Diseases & People Ser.). (Illus.). 128p. (J). (gr. 6-12). lib. bdg. 20.95 (*0-7660-1474-6*) Enslow Pubs.

Spinal Cord Injuries: Psychological, Social, & Vocational Rehabilitation. Roberta B. Trieschmann. 2nd ed. 1988. LC 87-71320. 360p. text 54.95 (*0-939957-08-6*) Demos Medical.

Spinal Cord Injury. Ed. by N. E. Naftchi. 1982. LC 81-8573. (Illus.). 306p. text 45.00 (*0-88331-202-6*) R B Luce.

***Spinal Cord Injury.** Yasakawa. 2nd ed. 2001. 72.00 (*0-8342-1972-7*) PRO-ED.

Spinal Cord Injury: A Guide for Living. Sara Palmer et al. 2000. LC 99-52572. (Johns Hopkins Press Health Bks.). (Illus.). 288p. 44.50 (*0-8018-6352-X*); pap. 15.95 (*0-8018-6353-8*) Johns Hopkins.

Spinal Cord Injury: A Guide for Patient & Family. Lynn Phillips et al. 1987. 320p. text 18.00 (*0-88167-274-2*) Lppncott W & W.

Spinal Cord Injury: A Guide to Functional Outcomes in Occupational Therapy. Ed. by Judy P. Hill. 1984. LC 84-25852. 264p. (C). pap. 79.00 (*0-87189-604-4*) PRO-ED.

Spinal Cord Injury: A Guide to Functional Outcomes in Physical Therapy Management. Nixon. 1993. LC 84-18474. (Illus.). 251p. (C). spiral bd. 76.00 (*0-89443-552-3*) PRO-ED.

Spinal Cord Injury: An Analysis of Medical & Social Costs. Monroe Berkowitz et al. 1998. LC 98-4054. 200p. 89.95 (*1-888799-17-X*) Demos Medical.

Spinal Cord Injury: An Illustrated Guide for Health Care Professionals. Marcia Hanak & Anne Scott. 2nd ed. 1993. 188p. pap. text 29.95 (*0-8261-4172-2*) Springer Pub.

Spinal Cord Injury: Clinical Outcomes from the Model Systems. Samuel L. Stover et al. 1992. 376p. 88.00 (*0-8342-0697-8*) PRO-ED.

Spinal Cord Injury: Medical Management & Rehabilitation. Ed. by Gary M. Yarkony. 1998. LC 94-14208. (Rehabilitation Institute of Chicago Procedure Manual Ser.). 252p. 83.00 (*0-8342-0553-X*, 20553) PRO-ED.

Spinal Cord Injury Desk Reference: Guidelines for Life Care Planning & Case Management. Terry L. Blackwell et al. 2000. LC 00-65790. (Illus.). 300p. pap. text 59.95 (*1-888799-49-8*) Demos Medical.

Spinal Cord Injury Pathway. McDermott. 1998. (C). pap. text 75.00 (*0-12-785067-8*) Acad Pr.

Spinal Cord Injury Patient Education Manual. Aspen Reference Group Staff. 1997. pap. 79.00 (*0-8342-1064-9*, 21064) PRO-ED.

***Spinal Cord Injury Rehabilitation.** pap. 34.95 (*0-412-47680-0*) Chapman & Hall.

***Spinal Cord Ischemia: An Experimental Study of the Spinal Cord Blood Supply & Preoperative Ischemia Detection by a New Method of Intrathecal Monitoring.** Lennart Christiansson. 2000. (Comprehensive Summaries of Uppsala Dissertations from the Faculty of Medicine Ser.: No. 921). (Illus.). 56p. pap. (*91-554-4699-X*) Uppsala Universitet SWE. *Dist:* Coronet Bks.

Spinal Cord Monitoring: Basic Principles, Regeneration, Pathophysiology, & Clinical Aspects. Ed. by H. S. Sharma & Y. Olsson. 1998. LC 98-25818. (Illus.). 400p. 189.00 (*3-211-82923-7*) Spr-Verlag.

Spinal Cord Oxygenation During Thoracic Aortic Clamping in Pigs. Anders Hellberg. 2000. (Comprehensive Summaries of Uppsala Dissertations from the Faculty of Medicine Ser.: No. 930). (Illus.). 56p. pap. (*91-554-4722-8*) Uppsala Universitet SWE. *Dist:* Coronet Bks.

Spinal Cord (Spinal Medulla) Primatologia, Vol. 2, Pt. 2. C. R. Noback & J. K. Harting. Ed. by H. Hofer et al. 1971. (Illus.). pap. 39.25 (*3-8055-1205-8*) S Karger.

Spinal Cord Stimulation: An Innovative Method for Critical Limb Ischemia. Ed. by S. Horsch & L. Claeys. 1994. 59.95 (*0-387-91463-3*) Spr-Verlag.

Spinal Cord Trauma: Handbook of Clinical Neurology, Vol. 61. Ed. by Pierre J. Vinken et al. 1992. LC 92-48797. 586p. 260.50 (*0-444-81280-6*) Elsevier.

Spinal Discord. Spengler. 1998. pap. 10.00 (*0-8050-5553-3*, Owl) H Holt & Co.

Spinal Disorders in Growth & Aging. Ed. by H. E. Takahashi. 1995. LC 95-218845. (Illus.). 338p. 158.00 (*0-387-70141-9*) Spr-Verlag.

Spinal Fitness Class. Raymond K. Woltz. Ed. by T. Bruce Henderson. 1983. (Illus.). 92p. pap. 14.95 (*0-9613447-0-9*) R K Woltz.

Spinal Fusion: Science & Technique. J. M. Cotler & H. B. Cotler. 1990. (Illus.). 407p. 341.00 (*0-387-97054-1*) Spr-Verlag.

Spinal Injuries Handbook. Hugh Dickson et al. 2nd ed. 1992. pap. text 25.00 (*0-07-470001-4*) McGraw-Hill Med Pub.

Spinal Instability. Ed. by Robert N. Holtzman et al. 1993. LC 92-48680. (Contemporary Perspectives in Neurosurgery Ser.). (*3-540-97941-7*); (Illus.). 531p. 168.00 (*0-387-97941-7*) Spr-Verlag.

Spinal Meningiomas. A. Pansini & P. Conti. 1996. LC 96-37039. (Illus.). 215p. 298.00 (*3-540-75030-4*) Spr-Verlag.

Spinal MRI: A Teaching File Approach. John H. Bisese. 1992. (Illus.). 304p. text 45.00 (*0-07-005406-1*) McGraw-Hill Educ Grp.

Spinal Narcotics. Ed. by Narinder Rawal & Dennis W. Coombs. 1989. (Current Management of Pain Ser.). (C). text 131.50 (*0-7923-0374-1*) Kluwer Academic.

Spinal Opiate Analgesia: Experimental & Clinical Studies. Ed. by Tony L. Yaksh & H. Mueller. 1982. (Anaesthesiology & Intensive Care Medicine Ser.: Vol. 144). (Illus.). 147p. 51.00 (*0-387-11036-4*) Spr-Verlag.

Spinal Stenosis. Nixon. 1991. 416p. 150.00 (*0-7131-4525-0*) Routledge.

Spine. Michael W. Spence. 1987. LC 87-2452. (Illus.). 76p. pap. 13.95 (*0-911198-89-X*) Purdue U Pr.

Spine Contrib. by Richard H. Rothman & Frederick A. Simeone. 3rd ed. 1991. (Illus.). 2172p. text 335.00 (*0-7216-3203-3*) Saunders.

S

Spine: Basic Evaluation & Mobilization Techniques. Freddy M. Kaltenborn. 3rd ed. 1993. (Illus.). 289p. pap. text 39.95 (*82-7054-052-8*) Orthopedic Phys.

Spine Dictionary. Christopher J. Centeno. 1998. LC 98-3975. 290p. 29.95 (*1-56053-270-X*) Hanley & Belfus.

Spine Imaging: Case Review. Brian C. Bowen. 2001. LC 2001-30078. (Case Review Ser.). (Illus.). 320p. text (*0-323-00507-1*) Mosby Inc.

Spine in Sports. Robert G. Watkins. 1995. (Illus.). 688p. (C). (gr. 13). text 108.00 (*0-8016-7502-2*, 05366) Mosby Inc.

Spine Secrets. Ed. by Fred Naraghi. 2001. (Secrets Ser.). (Illus.). 350p. pap. 39.95 (*1-56053-358-7*) Hanley & Belfus.

Spine Surgery. Vaccaro. 2001. text 195.00 (*0-323-01077-6*) Mosby Inc.

Spine Surgery: A Practical Atlas. Wetzel. 1999. LC 2001-31258. (C). pap. text 150.00 (*0-8385-8617-1*) Appleton & Lange.

Spine Surgery: Complication Avoidance & Management. Benzel. 1998. LC 98-25169. (C). text (*0-443-07540-9*, B2227) Church.

Spine Trauma. Alan M. Levine. Ed. by Richard Lampert. 1998. LC 97-39760. (Illus.). 720p. text 140.00 (*0-7216-2957-1*) Saunders.

Spinning Inward: Using Guided Imagery with Children. Maureen Murdock. enl. rev. ed. 1987. LC 87-9740. (Illus.). 158p. pap. 26.95 (*0-87773-422-4*) Shambhala Pubns.

Spinning Straw into Gold: Your Emotional Recovery from Breast Cancer. Ronnie Kaye. 1991. 224p. (Orig.). pap. 12.00 (*0-671-70164-9*, Fireside) S&S Trade Pap.

Spionidae: Invertebrates of the San Francisco Bay Estuary System, Vol. 1. William J. Light. Ed. by Welton L. Lee. 1978. (Illus.). text 12.50 (*0-910286-58-2*) Boxwood.

Spiral CT: A Teaching File. Elliot K. Fishman & R. Brooke Jeffrey. 1996. LC 96-30754. 336p. text 169.00 (*0-397-51668-1*) Lppncott W & W.

Spiral CT: Principles, Techniques, & Clinical Applications. Elliot K. Fishman & R. Brooke Jeffrey. 2nd ed. 1998. LC 97-50463. 448p. text 135.00 (*0-7817-1251-3*) Lppncott W & W.

***Spiral CT of the Abdomen.** Ed. by A. L. Baert & K. Sartor. 2002. (Medical Radiology Ser.). (Illus.). 555p. pap. 89.95 (*3-540-42291-9*) Spr-Verlag.

Spiral CT of the Abdomen. Ed. by F. Terrier et al. 1999. LC 98-52822. (Medical Radiology Ser.). (Illus.). 450p. 279.00 (*3-540-63463-0*) Spr-Verlag.

Spiral Manual of Sports Medicine. Marc R. Safran et al. 1998. LC 98-4821. (*0-7817-1755-8*); 752p. spiral bd. 39.95 (*0-7817-1222-X*) Lppncott W & W (Lippncott).

Spires of Form: Glimpses of Evolution. Victor B. Scheffer. 1985. LC 84-22374. (Illus.). 178p. reprint ed. pap. 7.95 (*0-15-684744-2*, Harvest Bks) Harcourt.

Spirit & Soul: Essays in Philosophical Psychology. Edward S. Casey. 1991. LC 91-13223. xii, 314p. pap. 18.00 (*0-88214-346-8*) Spring Pubns.

Spirit-Centered Wholeness: Beyond the Psychology of Self. Ed. by H. Newton Malony. 1987. LC 87-23028. (Studies in the Psychology of Religion: Vol. 2). 256p. lib. bdg. 89.95 (*0-88946-246-1*) E Mellen.

Spirit of Counsel. Swainson. 1977. 158p. (*0-85435-103-5*) C W Daniel GBR. *Dist:* Natl Bk Netwk.

Spirit of Homeopathic Medicines: Essential Insights to 300 Remedies. Didier Grandgeorge. Tr. by Juliana Barnard from FRE. 1998. LC 97-38032.Tr. of Esprit du Remede Homeopathique. 240p. pap. 20.00 (*1-55643-261-5*) North Atlantic.

***Spirit of Sanity.** Neville Symington. 2001. 176p. pap. (*1-85575-265-4*) Karnac Bks GBR. *Dist:* Other Pr LLC.

Spirit of Swiftwater. Jeff Widmer. 1998. LC 98-40902. 1182p. text 19.95 (*0-940866-74-9*) U Scranton Pr.

Spirit vs. Scalpel: Traditional Healing & Modern Psychotherapy. Leonore L. Adler & Runi B. Mukherji. 1995. LC 94-29715. 248p. 67.00 (*0-89789-406-5*, Bergin & Garvey) Greenwood.

Spirits & Demons at Work: Alcohol & Other Drugs on the Job. Harrison M. Trice & Paul M. Roman. 2nd ed. 1979. LC 78-23804. 294p. pap. 15.95 (*0-87546-072-0*, ILR Press) Cornell U Pr.

Spirits Captured in Stone: Shamanism & Traditional Medicine among the Taman of Borneo. Jay H. Bernstein. 1996. LC 96-43233. 220p. pap. text 17.95 (*1-55587-692-7*, 876927); lib. bdg. 49.95 (*1-55587-691-9*, 876919) L Rienner.

Spiritual Art Therapy: An Alternate Path. Ellen G. Horovitz-Darby. 1994. LC 94-26380. (Illus.). 186p. (C). 46.95 (*0-398-05927-6*) C C Thomas.

Spiritual Aspects of Psychiatric Practice. Paul R. Fleischman. 1993. LC 93-91043. (Illus.). 128p. (Orig.). pap. 10.95 (*0-9638398-2-9*) Bonne Chance.

Spiritual Dimensions of Healing: From Native Shamanism to Contemporary Health Care. Stanley Krippner & Patrick Welch. 1992. LC 92-159. (Frontiers of Consciousness Ser.). (Illus.). 302p. 19.95 (*0-8290-2462-X*); text 39.95 incl. audio (*0-8290-3162-6*) Irvington.

Spiritual Dimensions of Nursing Practice. Carson. 1989. 400p. pap. text 39.50 (*0-7216-2249-6*) Saunders.

Spiritual Healing. Nelson White & Anne White. 1985. LC 85-50745. (Illus.). 65p. (Orig.). pap. text 18.00 (*0-939856-42-5*) Tech Group.

Spiritual Healing. Swami Paramananda. 4th ed. 1975. pap. 4.95 (*0-911564-10-1*) Vedanta Ctr.

Spiritual Healing: Doctors Examine Therapeutic Touch & Other Holistic Treatments. Ed. by Dora Kunz. 2nd ed. 1995. 320p. pap. 15.00 (*0-8356-0714-3*, Quest) Theos Pub Hse.

Spiritual Path: An Introduction to the Psychology of the Spiritual Traditions. Han F. De Wit. Tr. by Henry Jansen & Lucia Hofland-Jansen from DUT. 1999. LC 98-58115. 320p. 53.00 (*0-8207-0307-9*) Duquesne.

Spiritual Pilgrims: Carl Jung & Teresa of Avila. John W. Welch. 1982. LC 82-80164. 208p. pap. 16.95 (*0-8091-2454-8*) Paulist Pr.

Spiritual Properties of Herbs. Gurudas. 1988. (Illus.). 288p. (Orig.). pap. 14.95 (*0-9615875-7-1*) Cassandra Pr.

Spiritual Psychology: A Course for Renewalin Body, Mind & Spirit. Jim Morningstar. rev. ed. 1999. (Illus.). 140p. pap. 18.00 (*0-9604856-3-5*) Transform Inc.

Spiritual Resources in Family Therapy. Ed. by Froma Walsh. 1999. LC 99-38031. 302p. 36.00 (*1-57230-508-8*) Guilford Pubns.

Spiritual Science & the Art of Healing: Rudolf Steiner's Anthroposophical Medicine. Victor Bott. 1996. LC 96-4207. (Illus.). 208p. reprint ed. pap. 12.95 (*0-89281-636-8*, Heal Arts VT) Inner Tradit.

Spiritual Sex Manual. Charlene Webster. 1982. LC 82-72079. (Illus.). 176p. pap. 12.95 (*0-910315-01-9*) Pts of Light Distributing.

Spiritual Strategy for Counseling & Psychotherapy. P. Scott Richards & Allen E. Bergin. 1997. LC 97-8297. 391p. text 39.95 (*1-55798-434-4*) Am Psychol.

Spiritual Sunlight for the Weary Soul: Meditations for the Chronically Fatigued. Lynn Vanderzalm. 2000. LC 98-23003. 176p. pap. 11.99 (*0-87788-823-X*, H Shaw Pubs) Waterbrook Pr.

Spiritualism & the Foundations of C. G. Jung's Psychology. F. X. Charet. 1993. LC 91-23521. 329p. (C). text 64.50 (*0-7914-1093-5*); pap. text 22.95 (*0-7914-1094-3*) State U NY Pr.

Spirituality & Chemical Dependency: Guidelines for Treatment. Kitty Joachim. Ed. by Virginia Biegun. 1988. 29p. (Orig.). pap. text 4.00 (*0-944335-00-4*) Oxford Inst.

Spirituality & Couples Therapy: Heart & Soul in the Therapy Process. Pref. by Barbara J. Brothers. 1993. LC 93-4262. (Journal of Couples Therapy Ser.: Vol. 3, No.1). (Illus.). 158p. lib. bdg. 39.95 (*1-56024-312-0*) Haworth Pr.

Spirituality & Healthcare: Reaching Toward a Holistic Future. John Shea. 2001. 168p. pap. 12.95 (*0-945482-02-7*) Park Ridge Ctr.

Spirituality in Nursing: From Traditional to New Age. Barbara J. S. Barnum. 1996. LC 95-25630. 176p. 29.95 (*0-8261-9180-0*) Springer Pub.

Spirituality of Work: Nurses. William Droel. 1991. (Spirituality of Work Ser.). 48p. (Orig.). pap. 2.95 (*0-914070-71-1*, 130) ACTA Pubns.

Spirometry & Lung Volume Measurement. Lonny J. Ashworth. 1998. (CPG Mentor - Patient Cases in Respiratory Care Ser.: Unit 8). (*0-8151-2301-9*) Mosby Inc.

Spirulina Platensis (Arthrospira) Physiology, Cell Biology & Biotechnology. Ed. by Avigad Vonshak. 1997. LC 97-179798. 256p. (*0-7484-0674-3*) Tay Francis Ltd GBR. *Dist:* Taylor & Francis.

Spitz & Fisher's Medicolegal Investigation of Death: Guidelines for the Application of Pathology to Crime Investigation. Werner U. Spitz. 3rd ed. 1993. (Illus.). 856p. (C). text 95.95 (*0-398-05818-0*) C C Thomas.

Splanchnic Circulation: No Longer a Silent Partner, No. 23. Ed. by M. R. Pinsky et al. 1995. LC 95-37674. (Update in Intensive Care & Emergency Medicine Ser.: Vol. 23). (Illus.). 201p. 123.00 (*3-540-59198-2*) Spr-Verlag.

Spleen. Ed. by A. J. Bowdler. 1990. (Illus.). 536p. 159.95 (*0-442-31209-1*) Chapman & Hall.

Spleen & Nostalgia: A Life & Work in Psychoanalysis. John E. Gedo. 1997. LC 97-9834. 360p. text 40.00 (*0-7657-0082-4*) Aronson.

Splendor of Truth & Health Care: Proceedings of the Fourteenth Workshop for Bishops, Dallas, Texas. Ed. by Russell E. Smith. 1995. LC 95-39696. 250p. pap. 19.95 (*0-935372-39-3*) NCBC.

Splinting. Coppard. 2nd ed. 2000. (Illus.). 448p. spiral bd. 38.00 (*0-323-00934-4*) Mosby Inc.

Splitting & Projective Identification. James S. Grotstein. 2000. pap. 40.00 (*0-7657-0297-5*); 1985. LC 84-45724. 256p. 40.00 (*0-87668-756-7*) Aronson.

Spoiled: Why Our Food Is Making Us Sick & What We Can Do about It. Nicols Fox. 1998. 224p. pap. 14.95 (*0-14-027555-X*) Penguin Putnam.

Spoken Language Comprehension: An Experimental Approach to Disordered & Normal Processing. Lorraine K. Tyler. 1992. (Bradford Bks.). (Illus.). 288p. 48.00 (*0-262-20088-0*) MIT Pr.

Spoken Word Production & Its Breakdown in Aphasia. Lyndsey Nickels. 1997. LC 98-106170. (Illus.). x, 230p. (*0-86377-466-0*) Psychol Pr GBR. *Dist:* Taylor & Francis.

Spondylarthritides. Ed. by Andrei Calin & Joel D. Taurog. 1998. LC 97-25516. (Illus.). 366p. (C). text 98.50 (*0-19-262749-X*) OUP.

Spongiform Encephalopathies. Allen. 1993. text 107.00 (*0-443-04928-9*) Saunders.

Spontaneous Abortion: Diagnosis & Treatment. Ed. by Tim Chard et al. 1992. (Illus.). 231p. 174.00 (*0-387-19712-5*) Spr-Verlag.

Spontaneous Alternation Behavior. Ed. by W. N. Dember. 1989. (Illus.). 211p. 78.95 (*0-387-96963-2*) Spr-Verlag.

Spontaneous & Induced Abortion: Proceedings of the WHO Scientific Group, Geneva, 1970. WHO Staff. 1970. (Technical Reports: No. 461). 51p. pap. text 5.00 (*92-4-120461-3*, 1100461) World Health.

Spontaneous & Induced Intima Formation in Blood Vessels. Mark M. Kockx. 1995. (Medical Intelligence Unit Ser.). 107p. 69.00 (*1-57059-220-9*) Landes Bioscience.

Spontaneous Animal Models of Human Disease, Vol. 2. Ed. by Edwin J. Andrews et al. 1980. LC 78-20039. (American College of Laboratory Animal Medicine Ser.). text 104.00 (*0-12-058502-2*) Acad Pr.

Spontaneous Cognitive Processes in Handicapped Children. M. Cherkes-Julkowski & N. Gertner. 1988. (Disorders of Human Learning, Behavior, & Communication Ser.). (Illus.). 171p. 89.95 (*0-387-96801-6*) Spr-Verlag.

Spontaneous Creative Imagery: Problem-Solving & Life-Enhancing Skills. Aina O. Nucho. 1995. LC 95-20397. (Illus.). 174p. text 46.95 (*0-398-06549-7*) C C Thomas.

Spontaneous Healing see Curacion Espontanea

Spontaneous Healing: How to Discover & Enchance Your Body's Natural Ability to Maintain & Heal Itself. Andrew Weil. 1996. LC 98-96001. 320p. pap. 12.95 (*0-449-91064-4*) Fawcett.

Spontaneous Intracerebral Haematomas: Advances in Diagnosis & Therapy. Ed. by H. W. Pia et al. 1981. (Illus.). 415p. 158.00 (*0-387-10146-2*) Spr-Verlag.

Sporopollenin Dinoflagellate Cysts: Their Morphology & Interpretation. William R. Evitt. 1985. LC 84-72457. (Illus.). 349p. (C). 30.00 (*0-931871-00-X*) Am Assn Strat.

Sport & Exercise Science: Essays in the History of Sports Medicine. Ed. by Jack W. Berryman & Roberta J. Park. 1992. 392p. (C). text 18.95 (*0-252-01896-6*) U of Ill Pr.

Sport & Remedial Massage Therapy. Mel Cash. 1997. (Illus.). 288p. pap. (*0-09-180956-8*) Ebury Pr GBR. *Dist:* Trafalgar.

Sport First Aid Updated Edition. Melinda J. Flegel. rev. ed. 1996. LC 96-22584. (Illus.). 200p. pap. 21.95 (*0-88011-556-4*, PFLE0556) Human Kinetics.

Sport Medicine: Incidence & Treatment of Athletic Injuries. E. C. Percy et al. 1973. LC 73-10382. (Sport Medicine Ser.: Vol. 1). 32.00 (*0-8422-7142-2*) Irvington.

Sport Medicine: Pathology. Olof Ringertz et al. 1973. LC 73-10369. (Sport Medicine Ser.: Vol. 3). 32.00 (*0-8422-7141-4*) Irvington.

Sport Medicine: Physiology. Kenneth D. Rose et al. 1974. LC 73-11032. (Sport Medicine Ser.: Vol. 4). 202p. text 32.00 (*0-8422-7139-2*) Irvington.

Sport Medicine: Protection, Treatment & Nutrition. Russel M. Lane et al. 1974. LC 73-10420. (Sport Medicine Ser.: Vol. 2). 32.00 (*0-8422-7140-6*) Irvington.

***Sport Psychology.** 3rd ed. 2001. 612p. 67.95 (*0-534-57719-9*) Wadsworth Pub.

Sport Psychology. Richard H. Cox. 3rd ed. 1993. tchr. ed. 9.68 (*0-697-12622-6*) McGraw.

***Sport Psychology: Concepts & Applications with Powerweb.** Richard Cox. 5th ed. 2001. pap. 55.31 (*0-07-248915-4*) McGrw-H Hghr Educ.

Sport Psychology Interventions. Ed. by Shane M. Murphy. 1995. LC 94-10390. (Illus.). 400p. text 50.00 (*0-87322-659-3*, BMUR0659) Human Kinetics.

Sport Pyschology Workbook for Riders. Ann S. Reilly. 2001. (Illus.). 132p. (*0-85131-771-5*) J A Allen GBR. *Dist:* Trafalgar.

Sport Safety Training. American Red Cross Staff. 1997. (Illus.). 192p. (C). (gr. 13). spiral bd. 12.50 (*0-8151-0983-0*, 29435) Mosby Inc.

Sport Safety Training Course Text Package. American Red Cross Staff. 1997. (C). (gr. 13). pap. text 15.75 (*0-8151-0998-9*, 29483) Mosby Inc.

Sport Scientists: Research Adventures. Gary G. Brannigan. 1998. LC 98-20915. 25.31 (*0-673-98454-0*) Addison-Wesley.

Sporting Body. Mervyn Cross et al. 1994. (Illus.). 192p. text 29.00 (*0-07-452830-0*) McGraw-Hill Prof.

Sporting Injuries. Peter Dornan & Richard Dunn. 2nd ed. 1988. (Illus.). 256p. pap. text (*0-7022-2064-7*) Univ Queensland Pr AUS. *Dist:* Intl Spec Bk.

Sports - Mental Health, Psychic Stress & Emotional Reactions: Index of New Information with References. Hugo H. Bronsen. 1996. 150p. 57.50 (*0-7883-0818-1*); pap. 47.50 (*0-7883-0819-X*) ABBE Pubs Assn.

Sports - Mental Health, Stress Forms & Emotional Reactions: Index of New Information with Authors, Subjects, Research Categories & References. Hugo H. Bronsen. 1995. pap. 47.50 (*0-7883-0675-8*) ABBE Pubs Assn.

Sports - Performance & Circadian Rhythms: Index of Modern Authors & Subjects with Guide for Rapid Research. Riley N. Wiseman. 1991. 200p. 47.50 (*1-55914-278-2*); pap. 44.50 (*1-55914-279-0*) ABBE Pubs Assn.

Sports—It's Shoes & Sole: Quality, Action, Choices, Safety, Problems & Shoe Therapy: Index of New Information with References. Hugo H. Bronsen. 1999. 150p. 57.50 (*0-7883-2162-5*); pap. 47.50 (*0-7883-2163-3*) ABBE Pubs Assn.

Sports & Competitive Behavior: Index of Modern Information. Vicky W. Holibrook. 1990. LC 90-31768. 141p. 47.50 (*1-55914-226-X*); pap. 44.50 (*1-55914-227-8*) ABBE Pubs Assn.

Sports & Exercise in Midlife. Ed. by Stephan L. Gordon et al. 1994. 570p. pap. 45.00 (*0-89203-078-X*) Amer Acad Ortho Surg.

Sports & Exercise Injuries: Conventional, Homeopathic & Alternative Treatments. Steven I. Subotnick. 1991. LC 91-20892. 393p. pap. 18.95 (*1-55643-114-7*) North Atlantic.

Sports & Exercise Medicine, No. 76. Ed. by Stephen C. Wood & Robert C. Roach. 1994. (Lung Biology in Health & Disease Ser.: Vol. 76). (Illus.). 314p. text 140.00 (*0-8247-9190-8*) Dekker.

Sports & New Exercise Research: Index of Current Information. Lindy H. Price. 1997. 171p. 57.50 (*0-7883-1608-7*); pap. 47.50 (*0-7883-1609-5*) ABBE Pubs Assn.

Sports & Psychological Influences: Index of Modern Authors & Subjects with Guide for Rapid Research. Hugo H. Bronsen. rev. ed. 1994. LC 94-34382. 145p. 57.50 (*0-7883-0250-7*); pap. 47.50 (*0-7883-0251-5*) ABBE Pubs Assn.

Sports & Recreation for the Disabled. Michael J. Paciorek & Jeffery A. Jones. 1994. LC 94-16013. (Illus.). 468p. reprint ed. pap. 19.95 (*1-57028-012-6*, Mstrs Press) McGraw-Hill Trade.

Sports & Stress Therapy: Athletic Rehabilitation on Massage, Stretching & Strengthening. Eskay Shazryl & Jarrod Hanks. Ed. by Judy LeBlanc & Dave Henley. 1994. LC 93-74515. (Illus.). 144p. 19.95 (*0-9639757-8-1*) Eskay.

***Sports & What's New with Anabolic Steroids: Index of New Information for Reference & Research Including Uses, Risks & Dangers.** Ed. by Research and Development Division Staff & John C. Bartone. 2001. 180p. 47.50 (*0-7883-2558-2*); pap. 44.50 (*0-7883-2559-0*) ABBE Pubs Assn.

Sports Chiropractic. Robert D. Mootz & Kevin A. McCarthy. 1999. LC 99-31781. 200p. pap. 45.00 (*0-8342-1375-3*) Aspen Pub.

Sports, Drugs & Doping: Index of Modern Information. Hugo H. Bronsen. 1990. LC 89-77608. 175p. 47.50 (*1-55914-126-3*); pap. 44.50 (*1-55914-127-1*) ABBE Pubs Assn.

Sports Endocrinology. Ed. by Michelle P. Warren & Naama W. Constantini. 2000. (Contemporary Endocrinology Ser.: Vol. 23). (Illus.). 496p. 135.00 (*0-89603-586-7*) Humana.

Sports Fitness for Women. Elizabeth Day & Ken Day. 1986. (Illus.). 120p. 29.95 (*0-7134-4692-7*) Trafalgar.

Sports Guide: A Planning Guide for Cardiovascular Risk Reduction Projects at Sporting Events. 1996. (Illus.). 64p. (Orig.). pap. text 25.00 (*0-7881-2823-X*) DIANE Pub.

Sports Gynecology: Problems & Care of the Athletic Female. Michelle P. Warren & Mona M. Shangold. 1997. LC 96-48787. (Illus.). 265p. pap. 47.95 (*0-86542-463-2*) Blackwell Sci.

Sports Injuries. Ed. by Vivian Grisogono. 1989. (Illus.). 264p. pap. text (*0-443-03175-4*) Church.

Sports Injuries: A Self-Help Guide. Vivian Grisogono. 1989. (Illus.). 294p. pap. (*0-7195-4111-5*) John Murray GBR. *Dist:* Trafalgar.

Sports Injuries: A Unique Guide to Self-Diagnosis & Rehabilitation. Malcolm Read & Paul Wade. 2nd ed. 1997. (Illus.). 192p. pap. text (*0-7506-3112-0*) Buttrwrth-Heinemann.

Sports Injuries: Causes, Diagnosis, Treatment & Prevention. S. Bird et al. 1997. (Illus.). 320p. (Orig.). pap. 55.00 (*1-56593-196-3*, 0511) Singular Publishing.

Sports Injuries: Diagnosis & Management. Garrick & Webb. 1990. 368p. text 69.00 (*0-7216-2127-9*) Saunders.

Sports Injuries: Diagnosis & Treatment. James G. Garrick & David Ray Webb. 2nd ed. 1999. LC 98-28594. text 55.00 (*0-7216-4434-1*) Harcourt.

Sports Injuries: Mechanisms, Prevention, & Treatment. Freddie H. Fu & David A. Stone. 2nd ed. 2001. 1,264p. text 169.00 (*0-683-30477-1*) Lppncott W & W.

Sports Injuries: Their Treatment by Homeopathy & Acupressure. Leslie J. Speight. 1991. 76p. (Orig.). pap. 11.95 (*0-8464-1535-6*) Beekman Pubs.

Sports Injuries & Illnesses: Their Prevention & Treatment. Rob O'Connor et al. 1998. (Illus.). 208p. (*1-86126-107-1*) Crowood Pr GBR. *Dist:* Trafalgar.

Sports Injuries & Their Treatment. Ed. by Basil Helal et al. 1987. (Illus.). 520p. (C). (gr. 13). pap. 174.95 (*0-412-23950-7*) Chapman & Hall.

Sports Injuries of the Ankle & Foot. George J. Lian & Richard A. Marder. 1996. LC 96-7605. (Illus.). 205p. 154.00 (*0-387-94687-X*) Spr-Verlag.

Sports Injuries of the Hand & Upper Extremity. Chan. 1995. text 115.00 (*0-443-07780-0*) Harcourt.

Sports Injuries of the Shoulder: Conservative Management. Ed. by Thomas Souza. 1993. (Illus.). 640p. text (*0-443-08844-6*) Church.

Sports Injuries Sourcebook: Basic Consumer Health Information about Common Sports Injuries. Ed. by Heather E. Aldred. 1999. LC 99-29624. (Health Reference Ser.). (Illus.). xiv, 606p. lib. bdg. 78.00 (*0-7808-0218-7*) Omnigraphics Inc.

S

Sports Injury Assessment & Rehabilitation. David C. Reid. 1991. (Illus.). 1269p. text (*0-443-08662-1*) Church.

Sports Injury Assessment & Rehabilitation. D. C. Reid. 2nd ed. 1998. (*0-443-08996-5*) Church.

Sports Injury Care. Thomas E. Abdenour & Alton L. Thygerson. 1993. (Fitness & Health Ser.). (Illus.). 264p. spiral bd. 30.95 (*0-86720-282-3*, 282-3) Jones & Bartlett.

***Sports Injury Handbook: An Athlete's Guide to Causes, Prevention & Treatment.** Hans Kraus. 2001. LC 2001-271050. (Illus.). 168p. pap. 14.95 (*1-58574-317-8*, Lyons) Globe Pequot.

Sports Injury Handbook: Professional Advice for Amateur Athletes. Allan M. Levy & Mark L. Fuerst. 1993. LC 92-29435. 304p. pap. 19.95 (*0-471-54737-9*) Wiley.

Sports Injury Management. Marcia K. Anderson & Susan J. Hall. 1995. LC 94-22447. (Illus.). 844p. 49.95 (*0-683-00175-2*); 1994. 43.95 (*0-8121-1754-9*) Lppncott W & W.

Sports Massage. Hungerford. 1998. (C). pap. text 34.95 (*0-8385-8653-8*) P-H.

Sports Massage. Jari Ylinen & Mel Cash. 1989. (Illus.). 192p. pap. (*0-09-173746-X*) S Paul GBR. *Dist:* Trafalgar.

Sports Medicine. William Ray Heitzmann. (Opportunities in... Ser.). (Illus.). 160p. 1993. pap. 10.95 (*0-8442-6241-2*); 1988. 13.95 (*0-8442-6240-4*) McGraw-Hill Trade (VGM Career Bks).

Sports Medicine. Ed. by J. B. King. 1992. (Illus.). 250p. text (*0-443-04719-7*) Church.

Sports Medicine. Ed. by J. B. King. 1994. LC 93-29874. (Colour Guide Ser.). (Illus.). 112p. 17.95 (*0-443-04972-6*) Saunders.

Sports Medicine. Irvin et al. 2nd ed. 1998. LC 97-45694. 600p. 86.00 (*0-13-037466-0*) P-H.

Sports Medicine. Richard H. Strauss. 2nd ed. 1991. (Illus.). 656p. text 85.00 (*0-7216-3734-5*) Saunders.

Sports Medicine: A Practical Guide for Youth Sports Coaches & Parents. Jerald D. Hawkins. 1992. 105p. pap. text 10.95 (*0-944183-09-3*) PRC Pub.

Sports Medicine: Colour Guide. Sherry. 1997. pap. text (*0-443-05482-7*, S2138) Church.

Sports Medicine: Curriculum Guide for Family Practice Residencies. STFM Task Force on Sports Medicine Staff. 1990. 41p. (Orig.). pap. 10.00 (*0-942295-21-8*, 85) Soc Tchrs Fam Med.

Sports Medicine: Ethics & the Law. Edward Grayson & Catherine Bond. 1999. LC 00-265730. 216p. pap. text 40.00 (*0-7506-1576-1*) Buttrwrth-Heinemann.

Sports Medicine: Fitness, Training, Injuries. Otto Appenzeller. 3rd ed. 1988. LC 88-10689. 528p. pap. text (*0-683-00233-3*) Urban & S DEU. *Dist:* Williams & Wilkins.

Sports Medicine: Health Care for Young Athletes. American Academy of Pediatrics Staff. 2nd ed. 1991. 328p. pap. 42.95 (*0-910761-28-0*) Am Acad Pediat.

Sports Medicine: Practical Guidelines for General Practice. Domhnall MacAuley et al. 1998. LC 98-42535. 288p. pap. text 40.00 (*0-7506-3730-7*) Buttrwrth-Heinemann.

Sports Medicine: Primary Care & Rehabilitation. Ed. by Giles R. Scuderi & Peter D. McCann. 1996. LC 96-28208. (Illus.). 656p. (C). (gr. 13). text 89.95 (*0-8151-7771-2*, 25524) Mosby Inc.

Sports Medicine: The School Age Athlete. Bruce Reuder. Ed. by Richard Lampert. 2nd ed. 1996. LC 95-36916. (STARS Ser.). (Illus.). 704p. text 149.00 (*0-7216-5673-0*) Saunders.

Sports Medicine & Athletic Training Patient Education Manual. Ed. by Sara N. Di Lima et al. 1995. LC 98-198010. 138p. ring bd. 199.00 (*0-8342-1078-9*, S473) Aspen Pub.

Sports Medicine & Rehabilitation: A Sport-Specific Approach. Ed. by Ralph M. Buschbacher & Randall L. Braddom. 1994. 319p. 52.00 (*1-56053-133-9*) Hanley & Belfus.

Sports Medicine Bible: Prevent, Detect, & Treat Your Sports Injuries Through the Latest Medical Techn. Lyle J. Micheli & Mark Jenkins. 1995. LC 95-2316. (Illus.). 352p. pap. 23.95 (*0-06-273143-2*, Harper Ref) HarperCollins Pubs.

***Sports Medicine Bible for Young Athletes.** Lyle J. Micheli & Mark Jenkins. 2001. LC 2001-31322. (Illus.). xii, 252p. pap. 19.95 (*1-57071-710-9*) Sourcebks.

Sports Medicine for Coaches & Athletes - Soccer. Adil E. Shamoo. 1995. 120p. text 28.00 (*3-7186-0600-3*); pap. text 15.00 (*3-7186-0601-1*) Gordon & Breach (Harwood Acad Pubs).

Sports Medicine for Coaches & Trainers. Edward J. Shahady & Michael J. Petrizzi. 2nd ed. 1991. LC 91-2604. (Illus.). xvi, 192p. pap. 24.95 (*0-8078-4331-8*) U of NC Pr.

Sports Medicine for Parents & Coaches. Daniel J. Boyle. 1999. LC 99-13392. (Illus.). ix, 117p. 29.95 (*0-87840-732-4*); pap. 12.95 (*0-87840-733-2*) Georgetown U Pr.

Sports Medicine for Primary Care. John C. Richmond et al. 1995. LC 95-32073. 608p. 79.95 (*0-86542-348-2*) Blackwell Sci.

***Sports Medicine for Specific Ages & Abilities.** Ed. by Nicola Maffulli. 1991. LC 2001-17368. x, 471p. (*0-443-06128-9*) Church.

Sports Medicine for the Primary Care Physician. Ed. by Richard B. Birrer. 2nd ed. 1994. LC 93-45708. 656p. per. 83.95 (*0-8493-2741-5*) CRC Pr.

Sports Medicine for Young Athletes: A Guide for Parents, Teachers & Coaches. Institute for Athletic Medicine Staff. 1998. LC 98-16095. (Illus.). 256p. pap. 14.95 (*1-57749-066-5*) Fairview Press.

Sports Medicine in General Practice. Randell K. Wexler. 1995. (Illus.). 130p. (Orig.). pap. 22.95 (*0-9646891-1-1*) Anadem Pubng.

Sports Medicine of the Lower Extremity. Steven I. Subotnick. Ed. by Mark Strauss. 2nd ed. 1998. LC 98-21519. (Illus.). 832p. (C). text (*0-443-08999-X*) Church.

Sports Medicine Roles & Responsibilities for High School Team Physicians & Athletic Trainers. Ohio State Medical Association Staff et al. 1997. LC 96-70418. 72p. (Orig.). pap. 9.95 (*0-944183-20-4*) PRC Pub.

Sports Medicine Secrets. Morris B. Mellion. 2nd rev. ed. 1998. LC 98-43414. (Secrets Ser.). (Illus.). 500p. pap. 39.95 (*1-56053-308-0*) Hanley & Belfus.

Sports Medicine Standards Book. David L. Herbert. 1993. LC 91-68119. 50p. pap. 29.95 (*0-944183-10-7*) PRC Pub.

Sports Neurology. Ed. by Barry D. Jordan et al. 2nd ed. 1998. LC 98-23250. (Illus.). 528p. text 110.00 (*0-397-51629-0*) Lppncott W & W.

Sports Nutrition: A Guide for Professionals Working with Active People. Dan Benardot. 2nd ed. 1992. LC 92-49945. pap. 35.00 (*0-88091-110-7*) Am Dietetic Assn.

Sports Nutrition: Minerals & Electrolytes. Ed. by Constance V. Kies & Judy A. Driskell. 1995. LC 94-18438. (CRC Series on Nutrition in Exercise & Sport Ser.). 352p. 104.95 (*0-8493-7916-4*) CRC Pr.

***Sports Nutrition for Women.** Anita Bean & Peggy Wellington. 2001. LC 2001-46330. 15.95 (*0-89793-350-8*) Hunter House.

Sports Ophthalmology. Bruce M. Zagelbaum. 1996. LC 95-42108. (Illus.). 256p. 89.95 (*0-86542-365-2*) Blackwell Sci.

Sports Performance - Analysis, Skills, Conditions, Training, & Human Factors: Index to New Information with Authors & Subjects. Jerry B. Holtz. rev. ed. 1994. LC 94-34141. 155p. 57.50 (*0-7883-0497-6*); pap. 47.50 (*0-7883-0498-4*) ABBE Pubs Assn.

Sports Physical Therapy. Ed. by Donna B. Bernhardt. 1986. (Clinics in Physical Therapy Ser.: Vol. 10). (Illus.). 223p. (C). text (*0-443-08444-0*) Church.

Sports Physiology. Richard W. Bowers & Edward L. Fox. 3rd ed. 1992. 464p. (C). text 68.75 (*0-697-13008-8*, WCB McGr Hill) McGrw-H Hghr Educ.

Sports Physiotherapy: Applied Science & Practice. Joan McMeeken et al. 1995. LC 94-47028. xix, 780p. text (*0-443-04804-5*) Church.

Sports-Prevention & Control of Athletic Injuries: Index of New Information with Authors & Subjects. Hugo H. Bronsen. rev. ed. 1994. 57.50 (*0-7883-0156-X*); pap. 47.50 (*0-7883-0157-8*) ABBE Pubs Assn.

Sports, Prevention & Control of Athletic Injuries: Index of New Information with Authors & Subjects. Hugo H. Bronsen. rev. ed. 1994. LC 94-24773. 157p. 57.50 (*0-7883-0264-7*); pap. 47.50 (*0-7883-0265-5*) ABBE Pubs Assn.

Sports Psychology in Action. Richard J. Butler. 1996. (Illus.). 224p. pap. text (*0-7506-2436-1*) E A GBR. *Dist:* OUP.

Sports Related Concussion. Julian E. Bailes et al. 1998. LC 98-30556. 261p. 30.00 (*1-57626-050-X*) Quality Med Pub.

Sports Report - Tennis Elbow: Index of New Information with Authors, Subjects & References. Hugo H. Bronsen. 1994. 47.50 (*1-55914-738-5*); pap. 44.50 (*1-55914-739-3*) ABBE Pubs Assn.

Sports Therapy: A Practical Approach. Mark Hudson. 1999. (Illus.). 256p. pap. (*0-7487-3374-4*) Nelson Thornes GBR. *Dist:* Trans-Atl Phila.

Sports Varieties - Studies of Exercise Using Human Saliva As a Diagnostic Instrument: Index of New Information & Bibliography. Boris A. Mormons. 1997. 150p. 57.50 (*0-7883-0988-9*) ABBE Pubs Assn.

Sports Vision. Michael W. Stoner & Alan W. Reichow. Ed. by Timothy G. Ramage. 1993. (Introduction to Behavioral Optometry Ser.). (Illus.). 80p. lib. bdg. 18.00 (*0-943599-64-4*) OEPF.

Sports Women. Ed. by Marlene J. Adrian. 1987. (Medicine & Sport Science Ser.: Vol. 24). (Illus.). viii, 160p. 128.75 (*3-8055-4501-0*) S Karger.

Sportsmassage: A Complete Program for Increasing Performance in Fifteen Popular Exercises. Jack Meagher & Pat Boughton. rev. ed. 1990. (Illus.). 224p. pap. 16.95 (*0-88268-096-X*) Station Hill Pr.

Sportsmedicine Book. Gabe Mirkin & Marshall Hoffman. 1978. LC 78-14908. 24.95 (*0-316-57434-1*, Little Brwn Med Div) Lppncott W & W.

SportsMedicine for the Combat Arts. Joseph J. Estwanik. 1996. LC 96-83747. (Illus.). 288p. (Orig.). pap. 24.95 (*1-888926-00-7*) Boxergenics.

***Spotlight on Clinical Practice: Preparing for the Demands of Clinical Governance & Revalidation.** Sally Irvine & Hilary Haman. 2000. 232p. pap. (*1-85775-496-4*) Radcliffe Med Pr GBR. *Dist:* Balogh.

Spotlight on the Cities: Improving Urban Health in Developing Countries. I. Tabibzadeh et al. 1989. (ENG, FRE & SPA.). iv, 174p. pap. text 27.00 (*92-4-156131-9*, 1150329) World Health.

Sprache den Familientherapie-Ein Vokabular see Language of Family Therapy: A Systemic Vocabulary & Sourcebook

Sprachfuehrer fuer die Krankenpflege. Deutsche Schwestergemeinschaft Staff. 1968. 253p. pap. 19.95 (*0-8288-6662-7*, M-7627) Fr & Eur.

Spread of AIDS in the Developing World: Congressional Hearing. Ed. by Benjamin A. Gilman. 2000. 141p. (C). reprint ed. pap. text 25.00 (*0-7881-8837-2*) DIANE Pub.

Spread of AIDS in the Developing World: Hearing Before the Committee on International Relations, House of Representatives, One Hundred Fifth Congress, Second Session, September 16, 1998. Contrib. by U. S. Congress, House Committee on International Relations. 1998. LC 99-184732. (Illus.). (*0-16-057755-1*) USGPO.

Spread Sheet Application for Health Care & Business Professionals: A Self Aided Instruction. Edward Khiwa-Kiwuwa. 1994. 75p. text, stu. ed. 30.95 (*0-9643899-1-6*) E K Kiwuwa.

Spreading Depression. Ed. by R. J. Do Carmo. 1992. (Experimental Brain Research Ser.: Vol. 23). (Illus.). 120p. 82.95 (*0-387-55532-3*) Spr-Verlag.

Spreading Germs: Disease, Theories & Medical Practice in Britain, 1860-1900. Michael Worboys. 2000. LC 00-23501. (Cambridge Studies in the History of Medicine). (Illus.). 344p. text 59.95 (*0-521-77302-4*) Cambridge U Pr.

Spreadsheet Applications to Animal Nutrition & Feeding. Ronald J. Lane & Tim L. Cross. 1985. text 43.80 (*0-8359-6965-7*); pap. text 21.33 (*0-8359-6964-9*) P-H.

***Springer GroBworterbuch Medizin: Deutsch-Englisch.** Peter Reuter. 2001. LC 2001-49123.Tr. of Medical Dictionary: English-German. (ENG & GER.). (*3-540-41980-2*) Springer Pub.

Springhouse Certification Review: Critical Care Nursing. Springhouse Publishing Company Staff. 1995. LC 95-35911. 400p. pap. 32.95 (*0-87434-782-3*) Springhouse Corp.

Springhouse Certification Review: Emergency Nursing. Ed. by Springhouse Publishing Company Staff & June Norris. 1996. LC 96-31612. (Illus.). 384p. pap. 32.95 (*0-87434-846-3*) Springhouse Corp.

Springhouse Nurse's Drug Guide, '98. SPC Staff. Ed. by David Moreau. 1997. (Illus.). 1488p. 28.95 incl. disk (*0-87434-892-7*) Springhouse Corp.

Sprinkles of Love: A Parent's Guide to Infant Message. Michelle Moe. Ed. by Phyllis Woung. Date not set. (Illus.). 24p. pap. 14.95 (*0-9659509-0-5*) Kisses from Heaven.

Sprituality & Nursing Practice. Judy Harrison & Philip Burnard. 1993. 218p. (*1-85628-509-X*) Avebry GBR. *Dist:* Ashgate Pub Co.

SPSS for Psychologists: A Guide to Data Analysis Using SPSS for Windows. Richard Kemp et al. 2000. LC 00-20564. (Illus.). vii, 287p. pap. 24.95 (*0-8058-3755-8*) L Erlbaum Assocs.

Spurgeon's Color Atlas of Large Animal Anatomy: The Essentials. Thomas O. McCracken & Robert A. Kainer. 1999. LC 99-20525. 170p. pap. text 55.00 (*0-683-30673-1*) Lppncott W & W.

Spy in the Nursing Home: Inside Tips & Tactics for Choosing the Right One in 5 Days. Eileen Kraatz. 1999. 100p. pap. 14.95 (*1-885987-17-X*, ME091) Practice Mgmt Info.

Square Pegs, Round Holes: The Learning-Disabled Child in the Classroom & at Home. Harold B. Levy. 1974. LC 73-3422. (Illus.). 288p. 8.95 (*0-316-52232-5*, Little Brwn Med Div) Lppncott W & W.

Squares of the Natural Numbers in Radiation Protection. Herbert M. Parker. 1977. LC 77-81781. (Taylor Lectures: No. 1). pap. 20.00 (*0-913392-39-1*) NCRP Pubns.

Squire's Fundamentals of Radiology. Robert A. Novelline & Lucy F. Squire. 5th ed. 1997. LC 96-36574. (Illus.). 640p. 76.00 (*0-674-83339-2*) HUP.

SRS-A to Leukotrienes: The Dawning of a New Treatment. Stephen T. Holgate & Sven-Erik Dahlen. 1997. LC 97-18092. 24.95 (*0-632-04288-5*) Blackwell Sci.

St. Anthony's Illustrated ICD-9-CM Code Book Ed. by Laurie Castillo & Catherine Hopkins. 1997. (Illus.). 1110p. (*1-56329-423-0*) Ingenix Inc.

St. Anthony's Updatable ICD-9-CM Code Book for Physician Payment Ed. by Laurie Castillo & Catherine Hopkins. 982p. Date not set. 129.00 (*1-56329-420-6*); 1997. pap. 59.95 (*1-56329-421-4*); 1997. spiral bd. 59.95 (*1-56329-422-2*) Ingenix Inc.

St. John's Wort: Improve Your Moods & Immunity. Stephanie Pedersen. 2000. LC 99-43066. (Natural Cure Library). (Illus.). 64p. pap. 3.95 (*0-7894-5189-1*, D K Ink) DK Pub Inc.

St. John's Wort: Nature's Mood Booster. Michael E. Thase & Elizabeth E. Loredo. 1998. LC 98-215113. mass mkt. 5.99 (*0-380-80288-0*, Avon Bks) Morrow Avon.

Stabilitat und Wandel Im Unternehmen: Das Management Zwischen Tradition und Innovation. Wolfgang Battmann. 1997. (Wirtschaftspsychologie Ser.: Bd. 6). (GER., Illus.). VIII, 157p. 35.95 (*3-631-32430-8*) P Lang Pubng.

Stability - Indicating HPLC Methods for Drug Analysis. Quanyun A. Xu & Lawrence A. Trissel. unabr. ed. 1999. LC 99-20308. 391p. pap. text 125.00 (*0-917330-95-1*) Am Pharm Assn.

Stability & Characterization of Protein & Peptide Drugs: Case Histories. Ed. by Y. J. Wang & Rodney Pearlman. 1993. (Pharmaceutical Biotechnology Ser.: Vol. 5). (Illus.). 351p. (C). text 85.00 (*0-306-44365-1*, Kluwer Plenum) Kluwer Academic.

Stability of Drugs & Dosage Forms. Sumie Yoshioka & Valentino J. Stella. 2000. LC 00-35697. (Illus.). x, 268p. 75.00 (*0-306-46404-7*, Kluwer Plenum) Kluwer Academic.

Stability of Insulin. Jens Brange. 1995. 128p. (C). text 55.50 (*0-7923-8874-7*) Kluwer Academic.

Stability of Protein Pharmaceuticals Pt. A: Chemical & Physical Pathways of Protein Degradation. T. J. Ahern & M. C. Manning. 1992. (Pharmaceutical Biotechnology Ser.: Vol. 2). (Illus.). 462p. (C). text 105.00 (*0-306-44152-7*, Kluwer Plenum) Kluwer Academic.

Stability of Protein Pharmaceuticals Pt. B: In Vivo Pathways of Degradation & Strategies for Protein Stabilization. T. J. Ahern & M. C. Manning. 1992. (Pharmaceutical Biotechnology Ser.: Vol. 3). (Illus.). 354p. (C). text 95.00 (*0-306-44153-5*, Kluwer Plenum) Kluwer Academic.

Stabilization & Transport of the Critically Ill. Ed. by N. S. Morton et al. 1996. (Illus.). 256p. (*0-443-05176-3*) Church.

Stable Fixation of the Hand & Wrist. A. E. Freeland et al. 1986. (Illus.). 285p. 170.00 (*0-387-96300-6*) Spr-Verlag.

Stable Internal Fixation in Maxillofacial Bone Surgery. R. Texhammar & R. R. Schmoker. 1986. (Illus.). 105p. 65.00 (*0-387-13593-6*) Spr-Verlag.

Stable Isotope Pharmaceuticals for Clinical Research & Diagnosis: Drug Development & Evaluation. Peter Krumbiegel. 1992. (Illus.). 210p. (Orig.). pap. (*1-56081-327-X*) Gustav Fischer DEU. *Dist:* Lubrecht & Cramer, Balogh.

Stable Isotopes in Ecology & Environmental Science. K. Lajtha & R. Michener. 1994. LC 93-28720. (Illus.). 250p. pap. 68.95 (*0-632-03154-9*) Blackwell Sci.

Stable Isotopes in Nutrition. Judith R. Turnlund & Phyllis E. Johnson. 1984. LC 84-12430. (ACS Symposium Ser.: No. 258). 240p. 43.95 (*0-8412-0855-7*) Am Chemical.

Stable Isotopes in Pharmaceutical Research. Ed. by T. R. Browne. 1997. (Pharmacochemistry Library: Vol. 26). 482p. 259.00 (*0-444-81941-X*, North Holland) Elsevier.

Stable Veterinary Handbook. Colin J. Vogel. 1990. (Illus.). 160p. pap. (*0-7153-9448-7*) Trafalgar.

Staff & the Serpent: Pertinent & Impertinent Observations on the World of Medicine. Allen B. Weisse. 1998. LC 97-5480. 224p. 29.95 (*0-8093-2149-1*) S Ill U Pr.

Staff Development Handbook for Long-Term Care Facilities. Charlotte K. Eliopoulos & Katherine Seiler. 62nd ed. 1997. 109p. 69.95 (*1-882515-03-X*) Hlth Educ Netwk.

Staff Development Training Program for Nursing Homes & ACLF's. Alan Meyers. 1995. 150p. wbk. ed. 89.95 (*0-937119-03-2*) Meyers Pub.

Staff Manual for Adolescent Substance Abuse Intervention Workbook: Taking a First Step. Steven L. Jaffe. Date not set. 16p. pap., wbk. ed. 19.95 (*1-58562-018-1*, 62018) Am Psychiatric.

Staff Nurse. Jack Rudman. 1994. (Career Examination Ser.: C-756). pap. 27.95 (*0-8373-0756-2*) Nat Learn.

Staff Physician. Jack Rudman. 1994. (Career Examination Ser.: C-1493). pap. 44.95 (*0-8373-1493-3*) Nat Learn.

Staff Recruitment & Retention: Study Results & Intervention Strategies. Sheryl A. Larson et al. 1998. LC 98-10508. pap. 31.95 (*0-940898-56-X*) Am Assn Mental.

Staff Support in Health Care. David J. Stoter. 1997. LC 97-10863. 224p. (Orig.). pap. 41.95 (*0-632-04098-X*) Blackwell Sci.

Staffing Management & Methods: Tools & Techniques for Nursing Leaders. AONE Management Staff & Maryann F. Fralic. 2000. LC 00-131120. 256p. pap. 35.00 (*0-7879-5536-1*) Jossey-Bass.

Stage & Structure: Reopening the Debate, 1. Ed. by Iris Levin & Sidney Strauss. 1986. LC 85-15624. (Human Development Ser.: Vol. 1). 336p. 77.00 (*0-89391-224-7*, Ablex) Greenwood.

Stage II Recovery: Life Beyond Addiction. Earnie Larsen. 1984. LC 85-51017. 112p. pap. 13.00 (*0-86683-460-5*) Harper SF.

Staged Diabetes Management: A Systematic Approach to the Prevention, Detection & Treatment of Diabetes & Its Complications. R. S. Mazze & International Diabetes Center Staff. 1999. LC 99-21829. (Illus.). 342p. (*1-885115-55-5*) IDC Pubng.

Staging & Treatment of Gastric Cancer. C. Cordiano & D. De Manzoni. 1991. 330p. text (*1-57235-016-4*) Piccin Nuova.

***Staging Laparoscopy.** Ed. by K. C. P. Conlon & P. Hohenberger. 1999. (Illus.). 300p. pap. (*3-540-65632-4*) Spr-Verlag.

StairMaster Fitness Handbook: A User's Guide to Exercise Testing & Prescription. Ed. by James A. Peterson & Cedric X. Bryant. 1995. LC 95-70429. (Health, Fitness, & Wellness Ser.). (Illus.). 340p. (Orig.). pap. 19.95 (*1-57167-024-6*) Sagamore Pub.

Stalingrad: The Defeat of the German 6th Army. Paul Carell. 1992. LC 92-62188. (Illus.). 352p. 29.95 (*0-88740-469-3*) Schiffer.

Stalking the Healthful Herbs. Euell Gibbons. 1989. (Illus.). 303p. reprint ed. pap. 17.50 (*0-911469-06-0*) A C Hood.

Stand Tall! Every Woman's Guide to Preventing & Treating Osteoporosis. Morris Notelowitz et al. 2nd rev. ed. 1998. LC 97-43586. (Illus.). 240p. 24.95 (*0-937404-38-1*) Triad Pub FL.

Standard Acupuncture Nomenclature. 2nd ed. 1993. iii, 266p. pap. text 16.00 (*92-9061-105-7*, 1512001) World Health.

Standard & Transmission-Based Precautions: The New Infection Control System. Charles A. Illian. 1997. (Illus.). 87p. pap. 29.95 (*1-888343-09-5*) Hartman Pub.

Standard Biphasic-Contrast Examination of the Stomach & Duodenum: Method Results & Radiological Atlas. J. Odo Op den Orth. 1979. 182p. text 176.50 (*90-247-2159-8*) Kluwer Academic.

Standard Emergency Procedures for the Small Animal Veterinarian. Signe J. Plunkett. 1993. LC 92-39992. pap. text 33.00 (*0-7216-6781-3*) Saunders.

Standard for Medical & Dental Equipment: UL 544. 4th ed. 1998. (C). pap. text 172.00 (*0-7629-0349-X*) Underwrtrs Labs.

Standard for Real-Time Display of Thermal & Mechanical Acoustic Output Devices on Diagnostic Ultrasound Equipment: Revision 1. 1998. (Illus.). 49p. pap. 36.00 (*1-930047-20-7*, RTD 1) Am Inst Ultrasound.

Standard Haematology Practice/3. British Committee for Standards in Haematology Staff. Ed. by Keith Wood. 3rd ed. 1999. LC 99-25479. (Illus.). x, 285p. 143.95 (*0-632-05322-4*) Blackwell Sci.

Standard Haematology Practice. J. K. Wood. 2nd ed. 1994. (Illus.). 304p. 120.00 (*0-632-03739-3*) Blackwell Sci.

Standard History of the Medical Profession of Philadelphia. Burton A. Konkle. 2nd enl. ed. LC 75-17803. reprint ed. 115.00 (*0-404-13201-4*) AMS Pr.

Standard Marketing Procedures for Dentists. Gordon Burgett. 1997. (Illus.). 224p. (Orig.). pap. 149.00 incl. disk (*0-910167-36-2*, Dental Commun) Comm Unltd CA.

Standard Marketing Procedures for Dentists. Gordon Burgett & Reece Franklin. 2nd rev. ed. 1998. 188p. (Orig.). ring bd. 149.00 incl. disk (*0-910167-45-1*, Dental Commun) Comm Unltd CA.

Standard Methods for Measuring Performance of Pulse-Echo Ultrasound Imaging Equipment. 1990. (Illus.). 53p. pap. 51.00 (*1-930047-23-1*, SMP) Am Inst Ultrasound.

Standard Methods of Chemical Analysis: Instrumental Methods, Vol. IIIB. Ed. by Frank J. Welcher. 6th ed. 1975. LC 74-23465. 1060p. reprint ed. 115.00 (*0-88275-253-7*) Krieger.

Standard Methods of Chemical Analysis Vol. IIA: Vol. IIA Industrial & Natural Products & Noninstrumental Methods. Ed. by Frank J. Welcher. 6th ed. 1975. LC 74-23465. 1372p. reprint ed. 148.00 (*0-88275-340-1*) Krieger.

Standard Model Designs for Rural Water Supply. 1986. (Illus.). 235p. pap. text 60.00 (*92-890-1030-4*, 1340031) World Health.

Standard 1972. 1973. (Illus.). 664p. pap. 110.00 (*92-0-010272-7*, ISP310) Bernan Associates.

Standard of Care: The Law of American Bioethics. George J. Annas. 1997. 304p. reprint ed. pap. text 27.50 (*0-19-512006-X*) OUP.

Standard Operating Procedures for All Dentists. Marsha Freeman. 3rd ed. 1998. ring bd. 225.00 incl. disk (*0-910167-47-8*); 4th ed. 2000. 487p. ring bd. 325.00 (*0-910167-62-1*) Comm Unltd CA (Dental Commun).

Standard Operating Procedures for All Doctors. Robyn Freeman & Leila Chambers. 1998. 221p. ring bd. 195.00 incl. disk (*0-910167-53-2*, Medical Comm) Comm Unltd CA.

Standard Operating Procedures for Dentists. Marsha Freeman. 2nd rev. ed. 1997. (Illus.). 400p. (Orig.). pap. 225.00 incl. disk (*0-910167-43-5*, Dental Commun) Comm Unltd CA.

Standard Operating Procedures for Good Clinical Practice at the Investigative Site. Arna P. Shefrin & Carol A. Saunders. 1998. 162p. 695.00 (*0-9663593-1-3*) Ctr for Clin Res.

Standard Operating Procedures for Pediatric Dentists. Marsha Freeman. 2nd rev. ed. 1996. (Illus.). 304p. pap. 179.00 incl. disk (*0-910167-34-6*, Dental Commun) Comm Unltd CA.

Standard Orthopaedic Operations. John C. Adams & Clifford A. Stossel. 4th ed. 1992. (Illus.). 485p. text (*0-443-04351-5*) Church.

Standard Presentation & Labeling of Ultrasound Images: A Stage 2 Standard. 1999. (Illus.). 22p. spiral bd. 24.00 (*1-930047-19-3*, SPL) Am Inst Ultrasound.

Standard Welding Procedure Specification for Gas Tungsten Arc Welding of Carbon Steel, (M-I, Group 1), 10 Through 18 Gauge, in the As-Welded Condition, with or Without Backing (B2.1.008-90) 1990. 6p. 39.00 (*0-87171-337-3*) Am Welding.

Standardization & Control of Biologicals Produced by Recombinant DNA Technology. Ed. by F. T. Perkins & W. Hennessen. 1985. (Developments in Biological Standardization Ser.: Vol. 59). (Illus.). viii, 216p. pap. 61.00 (*3-8055-4027-2*) S Karger.

Standardization in Blood Fractionation Including Coagulation Factors: Joint IABS-CSL Symposium, Melbourne, May 1986. Ed. by P. Schiff & W. Hennessen. 1987. (Developments in Biological Standardization Ser.: Vol. 67). (Illus.). viii, 388p. pap. 61.00 (*3-8055-4607-6*) S Karger.

Standardization of Albumin, Plasa Substitutes & Plasmapheresis. Ed. by W. Hennessen. 1981. (Developments in Biological Standardization Ser.: Vol. 48). (Illus.). viii, 326p. pap. 61.00 (*3-8055-2496-X*) S Karger.

Standardization of Cell Substrates for the Production of Virus Vaccines: Proceedings of the Joint WHO-IABS, Geneva, 1976. Joint WHC-IABS Staff. Ed. by International Association of Biological Standardiz & R. H. Regamey. 1977. (Developments in Biological Standardization Ser.: Vol. 37). (Illus.). 61.00 (*3-8055-2784-5*) S Karger.

Standardization of Epidemiological Studies of Host Susceptibility. Ed. by Janice Dorman. 1995. LC 94-48569. (NATO Advanced Science Institutes Ser.: Vol. 270). (Illus.). 298p. (C). text 95.00 (*0-306-44892-0*, Kluwer Plenum) Kluwer Academic.

Standardization of Growth Hormone Measurement Evidence-Based Medicine: 3rd KIGS/KIMS Expert Meeting on Growth & Growth Disorders, Sorrento, November 1998. Ed. by M. B. Ranke & J. Dowie. 1999. (Hormone Research Ser.: Vol. 51, Suppl. 1 (1999)). (Illus.). iv, 88p. pap. 34.00 (*3-8055-6898-3*) S Karger.

Standardization of Radiation Dosimetry in the Soviet Union, France, the United Kingdom, the Federal Republic of Germany & Czechoslavakia. 1973. (Illus.). 101p. (Orig.). pap. (*92-0-117073-4*, ISTR4) IAEA AUT. *Dist:* Bernan Associates.

Standardization of the Immunopharmacology of Natural & Synthetic Immunomodulators. Ed. by F. Brown & J. P. Revillard. 1992. (Developments in Biological Standardization Ser.: Vol. 77). (Illus.). x, 254p. pap. 182.75 (*3-8055-5619-5*) S Karger.

Standards & Ethics for Counselling in Action. Tim Bond. 1993. (Counselling in Action Ser.: Vol. 17). (Illus.). 160p. (C). 57.95 (*0-8039-8645-9*, 9877) Sage.

Standards & Guidelines for the Psychotherapies. Ed. by Paul Cameron et al. 1998. LC 99-166523. (Illus.). 902p. text 70.00 (*0-8020-0804-6*); 780p. pap. text 24.95 (*0-8020-7166-X*) U of Toronto Pr.

Standards & Guidelines in Urological Oncology. Ed. by M. P. Wirth et al. 1999. (Urologia Internationalis Ser.: Vol. 63, No. 1). (Illus.). 86p. pap. 34.00 (*3-8055-7023-6*) S Karger.

Standards & Scope of Advanced Rehabilitation Nursing Practice. Association of Rehabilitation Nurses Staff. 1996. 25p. (Orig.). (C). pap. text 7.00 (*1-884278-06-X*) Rehab Nursing.

Standards for Blood Banks & Transfusion Services. Ed. by Jay E. Menitove. 17th rev. ed. 1996. 86p. pap. text 75.00 (*1-56395-086-3*, PC97-ST9617) Am Assn Blood.

Standards for Blood Banks & Transfusion Services. 20th ed. 2000. pap. text (*1-56395-132-0*) Am Assn Blood.

Standards for Emergency Nursing Practice. National Emergency Nurses' Association Staff. 2nd ed. 1993. 104p. (C). (gr. 13). pap. text 22.00 (*0-8016-8094-8*, 08094) Mosby Inc.

Standards for Health Services in Correctional Institutions. American Public Health Association Staff. Ed. by Nancy N. Dubler. 2nd ed. 1986. LC 86-14078. 160p. 15.00 (*0-87553-143-1*) Am Pub Health.

Standards for Hematopoietic Progenitor Cells. Ed. by Jay E. Menitove. 1996. 36p. pap. text 30.00 (*1-56395-071-5*, PC97-935720) Am Assn Blood.

Standards for Hospital Libraries. Compiled by Hospital Library Standards and Practices Committee. 1984. 12.00 (*0-912176-17-2*) Med Lib Assn.

Standards for Parentage Testing Laboratories. Ed. by AABB Parentage Testing Committee. 2nd rev. ed. 1994. 24p. pap. text 20.00 (*1-56395-037-5*) Am Assn Blood.

Standards for Parentage Testing Laboratories. AABB Parentage Testing Committee. 4th ed. 1999. 34p. pap. (*3-8055-7032-5*) S Karger.

Standards for Paternity Testing Laboratories. Ed. by Robert W. Allen. 3rd ed. 1998. pap. text 55.00 (*1-56395-096-0*) Am Assn Blood.

Standards for Performance of the Abdominal & Retroperitoneal Ultrasound Examination see Guias para Efectuar el Examen de Ultrasonido Abdominal y Retroperitoneal

Standards for Performance of the Abdominal & Retroperitoneal Ultrasound Examination. rev. ed. 2000. 8p. pap. 10.00 (*1-930047-79-7*) Am Inst Ultrasound.

Standards for Performance of the Antepartum Obstetrical Ultrasound see Normas para Llevar A Cabo el Examen Obstetrico Prenatal Con Ultrasonido

Standards for Performance of the Hip Ultrasound Examination for Developmental Dysplasia of the Hip. 2000. (Illus.). 20p. pap. 10.00 (*1-930047-81-9*) Am Inst Ultrasound.

Standards for Performance of the Scrotal Ultrasound Examination. rev. ed. 2000. 10p. pap. 10.00 (*1-930047-78-9*) Am Inst Ultrasound.

Standards for Performance of the Thyroid & Parathyroid Ultrasound Examination. rev. ed. 2000. 8p. pap. 10.00 (*1-930047-80-0*) Am Inst Ultrasound.

Standards for Performance of the Ultrasound Examination of the Prostate & Surrounding Tissues. rev. ed. 2000. 16p. pap. 10.00 (*1-930047-77-0*) Am Inst Ultrasound.

Standards for Performance of the Vascular/Doppler Ultrasound Examination see Normas para la Realizacion del Estudio Vascular/Doppler Por Ultrasonido

Standards for Performance of the Visceral Vascular Doppler Ultrasound Examination. rev. ed. 2000. 20p. pap. 10.00 (*1-930047-82-7*) Am Inst Ultrasound.

Standards for Suicide Prevention & Crisis Centers. Jerome A. Motto et al. 1974. LC 73-17029. 114p. 32.95 (*0-87705-105-4*, Kluwer Acad Hman Sci) Kluwer Academic.

Standards for the Performance of the Ultrasound Examination of the Female see Normas para la Realizacion del Estudio Pelvico Femenino Por Medio de Ultrasonido

Standards for the Practice of Therapeutic Recreation & Self Assessment Guide. American Training Association Staff. 1993. 32p. (Orig.). pap. text 18.75 (*1-889435-02-3*) Am Therapeutic.

Standards in Absorption Spectrometry. C. Burgess & A. Knowles. 1981. (Techniques in Visible & Ultraviolet Spectrometry Ser.). (C). text 29.95 (*0-412-22470-4*, 2230) Chapman & Hall.

Standards of Care for the Health Care Professional. Meridith B. Cox. 1984. (Legal Aspects of Medical & Health Records Ser.). (Illus.). xiii, 130p. (C). pap. 40.00 (*0-912665-05-X*) BusinessWatch.

Standards of Care in Emergency Medicine: A Practical Guide to Emergency Procedures & Legal Liability. Herbert N. Wigder & Jeffrey C. Moffat. 1998. ring bd. 159.00 (*0-8342-1106-8*, S733) Aspen Pub.

Standards of Clinical Practice for Nephrology Nursing. Ed. by Sally Burrows-Hudson. exp. rev. ed. 1999. 107p. pap. 50.00 (*0-9653379-1-X*) Am Nephrology.

Standards of Emergency Nursing Practice. Ed. by Marylou Killian et al. 4th ed. 1999. 92p. pap. (*0-935890-59-9*) Emerg Nurses IL.

Standards of Human Occlusal Development. Moyers et al. 1976. (Craniofacial Growth Ser.: Vol. 5). (Illus.). 371p. 65.00 (*0-929921-03-8*) UM CHGD.

Standards of Oncology Nursing Practice. Mary H. Brown et al. 1989. LC 86-11102. 622p. pap. text 39.95 (*0-8273-4212-8*) Delmar.

Standards, Recommended Practices, & Guidelines: An Independent Study Activity. 1998. 60p. pap. text 99.00 (*0-939583-99-2*) AORN.

Standards, Recommended Practices & Guidelines 1998: With Official AORN Statements. AORN Staff. 1998. 341p. pap. text 48.75 (*1-888460-00-8*) AORN.

Standing & Walking with Functional Electrical Stimulation (FES) for People with Paralysis. Carole Kantor. 1992. 5p. pap. text 5.00 (*1-888470-02-X*) FES Info Ctr.

Standing in the Spaces: Essays on Clinical Process, Trauma & Dissociation. Philip M. Bromberg. 2001. LC 98-29429. 376p. pap. 36.00 (*0-88163-246-5*) Analytic Pr.

Standing Room Only: The World's Exploding Population. Karl Sax. 1983. LC 83-1757. Orig. Title: The Challenge of Overpopulation, 1955 edition. 206p. (C). reprint ed. lib. bdg. 60.00 (*0-313-23968-1*, SAST, Greenwood Pr) Greenwood.

Stanford Manual of Cardiopulmonary Transplantation. Ed. by Julian A. Smith et al. 1996. (Illus.). 320p. 65.00 (*0-87993-637-1*) Futura Pub.

Stanford University Healthy Heart Cookbook & Life Plan: Over 200 Delicious Low-Fat Recipes. Helen C. Page et al. 1997. 608p. pap. 17.95 (*0-8118-1750-4*) Chronicle Bks.

Staphylococcal Disease in the Soviet Union - Epidemiology & Response to a National Epidemic. Daivd Shrayer. Ed. by Michael Oxman. 1989. (Illus.). 144p. (Orig.). pap. 75.00 (*1-55831-113-0*) Delphic Associates.

***Staphylococci in Cardio-Thoracic Surgery: Epidemiological & Clinical Studies.** Ann Tammelin-Brandemark. 2001. (Comprehensive Summaries of Uppsala Dissertations from the Faculty of Medicine Ser.: No. 1031). 43p. (*91-554-5005-9*) Uppsala Universitet SWE. *Dist:* Coronet Bks.

Staphylococci in Human Disease. Kent B. Crossley & Gordon Archer. 1996. LC 96-49803. text (*0-443-07644-8*) Church.

Star-Junior First Aid. Sheila Greeley. rev. ed. 1989. LC 89-51922. (Illus.). 76p. (Orig.). per. 8.95 (*0-936029-19-6*) Western Bk Journ.

Star Medicine: Native American Path to Emotional Healing. Wolf Moondance. 1997. LC 97-1003. (Illus.). 192p. pap. 12.95 (*0-8069-9547-5*) Sterling.

Star Profile: Social Training Achievement Record. C. Williams. 1985. 35p. tchr. ed. (*0-906054-39-7*) Brit Inst Lrning GBR. *Dist:* Taylor & Francis.

Star Profile: Social Training Achievement Record. C. Williams. 1985. 35p. lp 15.00 (*0-7855-0760-4*) St Mut.

Star Track Reading & Spelling: A Training Manual for Low Flyers. Cosette Beadle & Joan Hampshire. 1997. 250p. pap. 95.00 (*1-56593-606-X*, 1258) Singular Publishing.

StarHanger. 1997. 298p. pap. (*0-9677836-0-7*) C Lincoln.

Starlight Elixirs & Cosmic Vibrational Healing. Michael Smulkis & Fred Rubenfeld. 352p. pap. 31.95 (*0-8464-4294-9*) Beekman Pubs.

Starling's Law of the Heart Revisited. Ed. by H. E. Ter Keurs & M. I. Noble. 1988. (Developments in Cardiovascular Medicine Ser.). 168p. (C). text 160.50 (*0-89838-382-X*) Kluwer Academic.

Start Over Every Morning. Harvey Jackins. 1989. 16.00 (*0-913937-36-3*); pap. 13.00 (*0-913937-35-5*) Rational Isl.

Start to Finish: Developmentally Sequenced Fine Motor Activities for Preschool Children. Nory Marsh. Ed. by Kirsteen Anderson. 1998. LC 98-193659. (Illus.). 213p. spiral bd. 42.50 (*1-883315-29-8*, 8512) Imaginart Intl.

Starting a Chiropractic Practice: A Comprehensive Guide to Clinic Management. Gayle A. Jensen & Rudolf P. Vrugtman. 3rd ed. 1997. LC 97-18284. (Illus.). 344p. pap. 36.95 (*0-945213-25-5*) Rudi Pub.

Starting a Medical Practice: The Physician's Handbook for Successful Start-Up. American Medical Association Staff. 1996. (Practice Success Ser.). pap. 54.00 (*0-89970-786-6*, OP315296WE) AMA.

Starting a Medical Practice in Texas. Donald P. Wilcox & Christopher K. Davis. 1997. 47p. (C). pap. 29.00 (*0-9640262-7-9*) TX Med Assn.

Starting Again: Early Rehabilitation after Traumatic Brain Injury. Patricia M. Davies. 1994. LC 94-9131. (Illus.). 442p. 42.00 (*0-387-55934-5*) Spr-Verlag.

Starting & Sustaining Genetic Support Groups. Joan O. Weiss & Jayne S. Mackta. 1996. 152p. (C). pap. text 19.95 (*0-8018-5264-1*) Johns Hopkins.

Starting Out, Starting Over: Finding the Work That's Waiting for You. Linda Peterson. 1995. LC 95-4177. 394p. pap. 14.95 (*0-89106-073-1*, 7230, Davies-Black Pub) Consulting Psychol.

Starting Young: School-Based Health Centers at the Elementary Level. National Health & Education Consortium Staff. 1995. 50p. 10.00 (*0-937846-42-2*) Inst Educ Lead.

Startling New Facts about Osteoporosis: Why Calcium Alone Does Not Prevent Bone Disease. Betty Kamen. rev. ed. 1989. (Illus.). 42p. pap. 4.00 (*0-944501-02-8*) Nutrition Encounter.

Starving for Salvation: The Spiritual Dimensions of Eating Problems among American Girls & Women. Michelle Mary Lelwica. 1999. LC 98-50120. 224p. 25.00 (*0-19-512743-9*) OUP.

Starving in the Silences: An Exploration of Anorexia Nervosa. Matra Robertson. 1992. LC 92-16188. 125p. (C). pap. text 15.00 (*0-8147-7435-0*) NYU Pr.

***Starving Madness: Tales of Hunger, Hope & Healing in Psychotherapy.** Judith Ruskay Rabinor. 2001. LC 2001-53186. (*0-936077-41-7*) Gurze Bks.

Stat: Special Techniques in Assertiveness Training for Women in the Health Professions. Melodie Chenevert. 4th rev. ed. 1993. LC 93-26505. Orig. Title: STAT Special Techniques in Assertiveness Training for Women in the Health Professions. (Illus.). 168p. (C). pap. text 20.95 (*0-8016-7233-3*, 07233) Mosby Inc.

Stat: The Laboratory's Role. Kathleen Sazama & Mary G. Haugh. 1986. LC 86-17353. 89p. pap. text 28.00 (*0-89189-210-9*) Am Soc Clinical.

STAT! Medical Office Emergency Manual. Jeryll A. Tuttle-Yoder. 1996. (Medical Assisting Ser.). tchr. ed. 14.95 (*0-8273-7090-3*) Delmar.

Stat! Medical Office Emergency Manual. Jeryll A. Tuttle-Yoder et al. 1995. LC 95-14211. (Medical Assisting Ser.). 324p. (C). otabind 40.95 (*0-8273-6489-X*) Delmar.

STAT Special Techniques in Assertiveness Training for Women in the Health Professions see Stat: Special Techniques in Assertiveness Training for Women in the Health Professions

State & Federal Prohibitions on Physician Referrals: A Guide to Compliance. Robert W. McAdams, Jr. et al. 1998. LC 99-202067. 466p. ring bd. 199.00 (*0-8342-1214-5*) Aspen Pub.

State & Future Directions of Acute Myocardial Infarction. A. Raineri et al. 1988. xii, 484p. text 348.00 (*3-7186-4808-3*) Gordon & Breach.

State & Local Government Responsibilities to Provide Medical Care for Indigents. Michael Dowell. 1985. (Illus.). 384p. (Orig.). pap. 25.00 (*0-941077-02-0*, 40,275) NCLS Inc.

State & the Medical Profession: A Cross-National Comparison of the Health Policy Arena in the United Kingdom & Sweden, 1945-1985. Peter Garpenby. 1989. (Linkoping Studies in Arts & Sciences: No. 39). 252p. (Orig.). pap. 96.50 (*91-7870-455-3*) Coronet Bks.

State Antidiscrimination Laws: Protected Classes Disability Discrimination Family & Medical Leave. Ed. by Catherine T. Long. 1997. LC 98-207643. (Employment & Human Resources Professional Ser.). 2012p. pap. 125.00 (*0-8080-0201-5*) CCH INC.

State-Approved Schools of Nursing - LPN-LVN 1997. National League for Nursing Staff. 1997. 96p. pap. 32.95 (*0-88737-738-6*, 19-7386, NLN Pr) Natl League Nurse.

State-Approved Schools of Nursing - LPN-LVN 1999. NLN Research Division Staff. 1999. (Illus.). 128p. (C). pap. text 42.95 (*0-7637-1139-X*, 1139-X, N L N Bart) Jones & Bartlett.

State-Approved Schools of Nursing - LPN-LVN (Annual) 1997. 96p. 27.95 (*0-88737-556-1*) Natl League Nurse.

State-Approved Schools of Nursing - LPN/LVN Programs, 2000. NLN Research Division Staff. 2nd ed. 2002. (Illus.). 160p. (C). pap. text 41.95 (*0-7637-1420-8*, 1420-8, N L N Bart) Jones & Bartlett.

State-Approved Schools of Nursing - RN, 1997. 1997. 128p. 33.95 (*0-88737-735-1*, 19-7351, NLN Pr) Natl League Nurse.

State-Approved Schools of Nursing - RN (Annual) 1992. 128p. 23.95 (*0-88737-555-3*) Natl League Nurse.

State-Approved Schools of Nursing - RN Programs, 2000. NLN Research Division Staff. 2nd ed. 2002. (Illus.). 160p. (C). pap. text 41.95 (*0-7637-1436-4*, 1436-4, N L N Bart) Jones & Bartlett.

State Board Exam Review for Skin Care Specialist. 1980. pap. 12.95 (*0-87350-094-6*) Milady Pub.

State-by-State Health Care Collection Laws & Regulations. annuals Aspen Health and Administration Development Group. 2000. LC 2001-271740. viii, 327p. pap. 99.00 (*0-8342-1881-X*, 1881x) Aspen Pub.

***State-by-State Health Care Collection Laws & Regulations.** HADG Staff. 2001. 110p. pap. 89.00 (*0-8342-2016-4*) Aspen Pub.

State-by-state Survey of the Statutes of Limitation & Repose Applicable to Pharmaceutical & Medical Device Litigation: A Report of the Subcommittee on Pharmaceutical & Medical Devices, Products Liability Litigation Committee, Section of Litigation, American Bar Association. Barry F. McNeil. 1997. LC 98-119466. (*1-57073-470-4*) Amer Bar Assn.

State Compensation Laws & Regulations: Minimum Wage/Overtime, Prevailing Wage, Wage Payment. CCH Editorial Staff. Ed. by Sharon A. Shipley. 1997. LC 98-135805. (Employment & Human Resources Professional Ser.). 2400p. pap. 125.00 (*0-8080-0202-3*) CCH INC.

State Definitions & Reporting Requirements for Live Births, Fetal Deaths & Induced Termination of Pregnancy. National Center for Health Statistics Staff. 1997. LC 97-29256. (*0-8406-0534-X*, (PHS) 98-1119) Natl Ctr Health Stats.

State Drug Resources National Directory (1992) 1993. 130p. (Orig.). (C). pap. text 30.00 (*0-7881-0164-1*) DIANE Pub.

State Efforts to Improve the Primary Care Workforce: Scholarship/Loan Programs & Medical Evaluation Reforms. Tim M. Henderson & Wendy Fox-Grage. 1997. LC 98-120736. 70p. 35.00 (*1-55516-602-4*, 6732) Natl Conf State Legis.

State Exam Review for the Theory & Practice of Therapeutic Massage. Ed. by Barbara Jewett. 2nd ed. 1994. LC 94-220687. 94p. pap. 13.50 (*1-56253-223-5*) Milady Pub.

State Guide to Complementary Alternative Medicine Specialties. Alternative Link Staff. 2001. LC 00-65922. 1026p. pap. text 58.95 (*0-7668-2797-6*) Delmar.

State Guide to the Legal Scope of Practice for Nursing. Alternative Link Staff. 2001. LC 00-65923. 524p. pap. text 46.95 (*0-7668-2798-4*) Delmar.

State Health Care Reform under the Clinton Administration. John C. Goodman & Gerald L. Musgrave. 1992. 66p. pap. 10.00 (*0-943802-76-8*, 173) Natl Ctr Pol.

State Hospital Reform: Why Was It So Hard to Accomplish? David B. Pharis. 1999. LC 98-40711. 300p. pap. 30.00 (*0-89089-886-3*) Carolina Acad Pr.

State Hospitals in the Depression. National Committee for Mental Health. Ed. by Gerald N. Grob. 1980. LC 78-22579. (Historical Issues in Mental Health Ser.). reprint ed. lib. bdg. 18.95 (*0-405-11931-3*) Ayer.

State-Level Databook on Health Care Access & Financing. David W. Liska et al. 3rd ed. 1998. LC 98-9660. 249p. pap. 42.50 (*0-87766-677-6*) Urban Inst.

State Medical Boards & the Politics of Public Protection. Carl F. Ameringer. 1999. LC 98-21738. (Illus.). 188p. 43.95 (*0-8018-5987-5*) Johns Hopkins.

State Medical Licensure Guidelines, 1999 Edition. Hospital Association American Staff. 1999. 250p. pap. text (*1-887617-64-7*) St Bart Pr Ltd.

State Medical Licensure Guidelines, 1997: Information Manual for MD & DO Physicians in the United States of America. Jason F. Janoulis & Brenda H. Janoulis. rev. ed. 1997. 150p. reprint ed. pap. 89.00 (*1-887617-53-1*) St Bart Pr Ltd.

State Medicine Licensure Requirements & Statistics. 2000. 49.95 (*0-89970-544-8*, OP399093) AMA.

State Mental Hospitals: Problems & Potentials. Ed. by John Talbott. 1980. LC 79-21928. 219p. 35.95 (*0-87705-394-4*, Kluwer Acad Hman Sci) Kluwer Academic.

State Mental Patient & Urban Life: Moving in & Out of the Institution. Dan A. Lewis & Arthur J. Lurigio. 1994. 146p. (C). text 41.95 (*0-398-05901-2*) C C Thomas.

State Methadone Treatment Guidelines: A Treatment Improvement Protocol. 1994. (Illus.). 222p. (Orig.). (C). pap. text 50.00 (*0-7881-1166-3*) DIANE Pub.

State Nursing Boards for Practical Nurse (SNB-PN) Jack Rudman. (Admission Test Ser.: Vol. 46). 49.95 (*0-8373-5146-4*); 1994. pap. 29.95 (*0-8373-5046-8*) Nat Learn.

State Nursing Boards for Registered Nurse (SNB-RN) Jack Rudman. (Admission Test Ser.: Vol. 45). 49.95 (*0-8373-5145-6*); 1994. pap. 29.95 (*0-8373-5045-X*) Nat Learn.

State of Health Atlas. Judith MacKay et al. 1993. LC 92-27298. 128p. pap. 16.00 (*0-671-79375-6*, Touchstone) S&S Trade Pap.

State of Health in America. Michael Scigliano. 1997. (Illus.). 160p. pap. (*0-9656924-1-8*) Uptime Sprts Nutrit.

State of New York City's Municipal Hospital System, Fiscal Year 1995: Report of the City Hospital Visiting Committee. United Hospital Fund, City Hospital Visiting Committee. 1995. 56p. pap. 10.00 (*1-881277-26-7*) United Hosp Fund.

State of New York City's Municipal Hospital System, Fiscal Year 1996: Report of the City Hospital Visiting Committee. United Hospital Fund, City Hospital Visiting Committee. 1996. 48p. pap. 10.00 (*1-881277-30-5*) United Hosp Fund.

State of the Art in Digital Mammographic Image Analysis. K. W. Bowyer & S. Astley. 1994. (Series in Machine Perception & Artificial Intelligence: Vol. 9). 308p. text 109.00 (*981-02-1509-6*) World Scientific Pub.

State of the Art in Family Therapy Research: Controversies & Recommendations. Ed. by Lyman C. Wynne. 1987. text 18.00 (*0-9615519-2-5*) Family Process.

State of the Art in Family Therapy Research: Controversies & Recommendations. Intro. by Lyman C. Wynne. 1988. LC 87-951. 312p. pap. 18.00 (*0-9615519-3-3*) Family Process.

State of the Art in Quantitative Coronary Arteriography. Ed. by Johan H. Reiber & Patrick W. Serruys. 1986. (Developments in Cardiovascular Medicine Ser.). text 251.50 (*0-89838-804-X*) Kluwer Academic.

State of the Art of Surgery, Nineteen Seventy-Nine to Nineteen Eighty. Ed. by M. Allgower & F. Arder. 1980. 116p. 18.95 (*0-387-10136-5*) Spr-Verlag.

State of the Art of the IUD: Liber Amicorum Professor Thiery. Ed. by H. Van der Pas. 1990. 240p. text 146.00 (*0-7923-8922-0*) Kluwer Academic.

State of the Art Technology in Anesthesia & Intensive Care: Proceedings of the 18th International Symposium on Computing in Anesthesia & Intensive Care, Hamamatsu City, Japan, 18-21 March 1998. Ed. by Kazuyuki Ikeda et al. 1998. (International Congress Ser.). 350p. 140.50 (*0-444-50008-1*, Excerpta Medica) Elsevier.

State of the Child. Mark Testa & Fred Wulczyn. 1980. LC 80-70497. (Research Reports on Children in Illinois Ser.: Vol. 1). xiv, 111p. (Orig.). pap. text 10.00 (*0-932132-33-2*) Natl Opinion Res.

State of the Heart: The Practical Guide to Your Heart & Heart Surgery. Larry W. Stephenson & Jeffrey L. Rodengen. 2000. (Illus.). 287p. pap. 29.95 (*0-945903-63-4*, Write) Write Stuff Syndicate.

State Options for Expanding Children's Health Insurance. Shelly Gehshan. 1997. 20p. 15.00 (*1-55516-753-5*, 6733) Natl Conf State Legis.

State, Politics, & Health: Essays for Rudolf Klein. Ed. by Patricia Day et al. 1995. LC 95-36573. xii, 243p. 58.95 (*1-55786-868-9*) Blackwell Pubs.

State Programs for Providing Children's Health Insurance: A Resource Notebook. Forum for Providing Health Policy Leadership Staff. 1997. LC 98-117243. 236p. 40.00 (*1-55516-750-0*, 6734) Natl Conf State Legis.

State Resources & Services Related to Alcohol & Drug Problems for Fiscal Year 1993: An Analysis of State Alcohol & Drug Abuse Profile Data. John S. Gustafson et al. 1996. 395p. (Orig.). pap. text 45.00 (*0-7881-2799-3*) DIANE Pub.

State Sanitation: A Review of the Work of the Massachusetts State Board of Health George C. Whipple. Ed. by Barbara G. Rosenkrantz. 1977. LC 76-40652. (Public Health in America Ser.). (Illus.). reprint ed. lib. bdg. 69.95 (*0-405-09835-9*) Ayer.

State Strategies for Financing Graduate Medical Education: A Special Report. Edward S. Salsberg. 1997. LC 97-30705. (*1-881277-35-6*) United Hosp Fund.

Statement of Conditions Manual: A Comprehensive Guide to JCAHO Compliance. David M. Birk & James K. Lathrop. 1998. LC 99-212068. (Illus.). 850p. pap. text 247.00 (*1-57839-048-6*) Opus Communs.

Statement on the Scope & Standards of Advanced Practice in Oncology Nursing. Joanne Lester et al. rev. ed. 1997. LC 98-204655. 28p. pap. text 13.95 (*1-890504-05-X*) Oncology Nursing.

Statement on the Scope & Standards on Oncology Nursing Practice. American Nurses Association Staff & Oncology Nursing Society Staff. 1996. LC 96-2450. 50p. pap. 14.95 (*1-55810-121-7*, MS-23) Am Nurses Pub.

Statements of Fact in Traditional Chinese Medicine. Bob Flaws. 1994. 120p. pap. 12.95 (*0-936185-52-X*) Blue Poppy Pr.

States Manual of Spinal, Pelvic & Extravertebral Technics. C. R. Kirk et al. 2nd ed. 1986. (Illus.). 245p. (C). text 40.00 (*0-9615849-0-4*) Natl Coll Chiro.

States of Brain & Mind. Allan J. Hobson. 1988. (Readings from the Encyclopedia of Neuroscience Ser.). 144p. 38.00 (*0-8176-3409-6*) Birkhauser.

States of Consciousness. American Psychological Association Staff et al. 1981. (Human Behavior Curriculum Project Ser.). 55p. tchr. ed. 9.95 (*0-8077-2616-8*); pap. text 3.95 (*0-8077-2615-X*) Tchrs Coll.

States of Exile: Correspondences Between Art, Literature & Nursing. Jeanine Young-Mason. 1995. 24.95 (*0-88737-626-6*) Natl League Nurse.

States of Health: Health & Illness in Australia. Janet M. George & Alan Davis. 1998. LC 98-199352. (*0-582-81014-0*) Longman.

States of Mind: American & Post-Soviet Perspectives on Contemporary Issues in Psychology. Ed. by Diane F. Halpern & Alexander E. Voiskounsky. 1997. LC 96-28089. (Illus.). 448p. pap. 40.00 (*0-19-510351-3*) OUP.

States of Mind: Configurational Analysis of Individual Psychology. M. J. Horowitz. 2nd ed. 1987. LC 87-2571. (Critical Issues in Psychiatry Ser.). (Illus.). 292p. (C). 65.00 (*0-306-42449-5*, Plenum Trade) Perseus Pubng.

States of Mind: New Discoveries about How Our Brains Make Us Who We Are. Ed. by Roberta Conlan. 1999. LC 98-11719. (Illus.). 224p. 24.95 (*0-471-29963-4*) Wiley.

Statistical Analysis of Medical Data: New Developments. Ed. by Brian S. Everitt & Graham Dunn. 1998. LC 98-229709. (Arnold Publication). (Illus.). 352p. pap. 45.00 (*0-340-67775-9*) OUP.

Statistical & Methodological Advances in Psychiatric Research. Ed. by Robert D. Gibbons & Dysken. 1983. 184p. 29.95 (*0-88331-203-4*) R B Luce.

Statistical Applications for Health Information Management. Carol E. Osborn. 2000. LC 00-21793. (Illus.). 352p. pap. 59.00 (*0-8342-1243-9*) Aspen Pub.

Statistical Aspects of BSE & VCJD: Models for an Epidemic. C. A. Donelley. 1999. LC 99-35812. (Monographs on Statistics & Applied Probability Ser.: Vol. 84). 256p. 69.95 (*0-8493-0386-9*, Chap & Hall CRC) CRC Pr.

Statistical Bases of Reference Values in Laboratory Medicine. Eugene K. Harris & James C. Boyd. 1995. LC 95-9589. (Statistics: Textbooks & Monographs: Vol. 146). (Illus.). 384p. text 195.00 (*0-8247-9339-0*) Dekker.

Statistical Computerized Electrocardiogram Norm for Males & Females 26 Yrs. Old to 65 Yrs. Old. Ralph H. Kapilian. 1984. 79p. (Orig.). spiral bd. 29.95 (*0-916311-00-7*) R H Kapilian.

Statistical Concepts & Applications in Medicine. J. Aitchison & I. J. Lauder. 1993. (Monographs on Statistics & Applied Probability). (Illus.). 400p. 60.00 (*0-412-30430-9*) Chapman & Hall.

Statistical Design & Analysis of Pharmaceutical Sciences: Validation, Process Controls, & Stability, No. 143. Ed. by Shein-Chung Chow & Jen-pei Liu. 1995. LC 94-43570. (Statistics: Textbooks & Monographs: Vol. 143). (Illus.). 580p. text 75.00 (*0-8247-9336-6*) Dekker.

Statistical Epidemiology in Veterinary Science. F. B. Leech & K. C. Sellers. 1979. 30.00 (*0-85264-211-3*) Lubrecht & Cramer.

Statistical First Aid: Instructor's Guide. R. P. Hirsch & Richard K. Riegelman. 1992. (Illus.). 80p. tchr. ed. (*0-86542-192-7*) Blackwell Sci.

Statistical Ideas for Health Care Research. Nicola Crichton. 2001. (Arnold Publication). (Illus.). 224p. pap. text 24.95 (*0-340-69164-6*) OUP.

Statistical Imperative-Practical Quantitative Tools for Healthcare Managers. Eric Joseph. 2nd ed. 1994. 124p. pap. text 50.00 (*0-916499-66-9*) Care Educ Grp.

Statistical Indicators for the Planning & Evaluation of Public Health Programmes: Proceedings of the WHO Expert Committee on Health Statistics, 14th, Geneva, 1970. WHO Staff. 1971. pap. text 5.00 (*92-4-120472-9*, 1100472) World Health.

Statistical Indices of Family Health: Report. WHO Staff. 1976. (Technical Reports: No. 587). pap. text 8.00 (*92-4-120587-3*, 1100587) World Health.

Statistical Issues in Analyzing the NHANES I Epidemiologic Followup Study. 1994. LC 93-46586. (Vital & Health Statistics Ser. 2: Data Evaluation & Methods Research: No. 121). (*0-8406-0487-4*) Natl Ctr Health Stats.

Statistical Issues in Drug Research & Development. Ed. by Karl A. Peace. 1989. (Statistics: Textbooks & Monographs: Vol. 106). (Illus.). 384p. text 175.00 (*0-8247-8290-9*) Dekker.

Statistical Methodology in the Pharmaceutical Sciences. Donald A. Berry. 1989. (Statistics: Textbooks & Monographs: Vol. 104). (Illus.). 600p. text 195.00 (*0-8247-8117-1*) Dekker.

Statistical Methods for Anaesthesia & Intensive Care. Tony Gin & Paul Myles. 2000. LC 00-57925. (Illus.). 152p. pap. text 42.50 (*0-7506-4065-0*) Buttrwrth-Heinemann.

Statistical Methods for Cancer Studies. Richard G. Cornell. 1984. (Statistics: Textbooks & Monographs: Vol. 51). (Illus.). 496p. text 165.00 (*0-8247-7169-9*) Dekker.

Statistical Methods for Clinical Trials. Mark X. Norleans. 2000. LC 00-47465. (Biostatistics Ser.). (Illus.). xviii, 257p. text 99.75 (*0-8247-0467-3*) Dekker.

Statistical Methods for Health Care Research. Barbara Hazard Munro. 4th ed. 2001. LC 00-37064. 480p. pap. text 45.95 (*0-7817-2175-X*) Lppncott W & W.

Statistical Methods for Health Sciences. M. M. Shoukri & V. L. Edge. 1995. LC 95-39160. 320p. 79.95 (*0-8493-7644-0*) CRC Pr.

Statistical Methods for Health Sciences. M. M. Shoukri & C. A. Pause. 2nd ed. 1998. LC 98-40852. 400p. 94.95 (*0-8493-1095-4*) CRC Pr.

Statistical Methods for Medical Investigations. Brian S. Everitt. 2nd ed. 1994. LC 94-8091. (An Arnold Publication). 256p. pap. (*0-340-61431-5*) E A GBR. *Dist:* OUP.

Statistical Methods for Pharmaceutical Research Planning. Sten W. Bergman & John C. Gittins. 1985. (Statistics: Textbooks & Monographs). (Illus.). 272p. text 150.00 (*0-8247-7146-X*) Dekker.

Statistical Methods for Psychology. David C. Howell. 4th ed. 1996. mass mkt. 18.75 net. (*0-534-51999-7*) Brooks-Cole.

Statistical Methods for Psychology. David C. Howell. 2nd ed. 1987. (C). pap. 40.25 (*0-87150-068-X*, 36G0140) PWS Pubs.

Statistical Methods for Psychology. David C. Howell. 5th ed. 2001. LC 00-66738. (Illus.). xiv, 802p. pap. 55.00 net. (*0-534-37770-X*) Thomson Learn.

Statistical Methods for Psychology. David C. Howell. 3rd ed. 1992. 693p. text 50.50 (*0-534-92955-9*) Wadsworth Pub.

Statistical Methods for Psychology: Solutions Manual. David C. Howell. 3rd ed. Date not set. tchr. ed. (*0-534-92956-7*) Brooks-Cole.

Statistical Methods For Psychology with infotrac. Howell. 4th ed. 1998. (Statistics Ser). 61.25 incl. cd-rom (*0-534-36347-4*) Brooks-Cole.

Statistical Methods for Survival Data Analysis. Elisa T. Lee. 2nd ed. 1992. LC 91-27926. (Probability & Statistics Ser.). 496p. 105.00 (*0-471-61592-7*) Wiley.

Statistical Methods for the Analysis of Biomedical Data. Robert F. Woolson. 1987. LC 87-6069. (Probability & Statistics Ser.). 544p. 175.00 (*0-471-80615-3*) Wiley.

Statistical Methods in Cancer Research: The Design & Analysis of Cohort Studies, Vol. 2. N. E. Breslow & N. E. Day. 1994. (IARC Scientific Publications Ser.: No. 82). (Illus.). 418p. reprint ed. pap. text 49.50 (*92-832-0182-5*) OUP.

Statistical Methods in Cancer Research Vol. 1: The Analysis of Case-Control Studies, Vol. 1. N. E. Breslow & N. E. Day. 1993. (IARC Scientific Publications Ser.: No. 32). (Illus.). 352p. (C). reprint ed. pap. text 39.50 (*92-832-0132-9*, 11877) OUP.

Statistical Methods in Cancer Research Vol. 3: The Design & Analysis of Long-Term Animal Experiments, III Vol. J. J. Gart et al. 1987. (IARC Scientific Publications Ser.: No. 79). (Illus.). 230p. text 45.00 (*92-832-1179-0*) OUP.

Statistical Methods in Clinical Trials. David L. DeMets. 1997. (Texts in Statistical Science Ser.). (C). (gr. 13). pap. 54.95 (*0-412-06361-1*) Chapman & Hall.

Statistical Methods in Epidemiology. Harold A. Kahn & Christopher T. Sempos. 1989. (Monographs in Epidemiology & Biostatistics: No. 12). (Illus.). 320p. pap. text 39.95 (*0-19-505049-5*) OUP.

Statistical Methods in Laboratory Medicine. P. W. Strike. 2nd ed. 1991. (Monographs in Medical Laboratory Science). (Illus.). 541p. text 195.00 (*0-7506-1345-9*) Buttrwrth-Heinemann.

Statistical Methods in Medical Research. P. Armitage & G. Berry. 3rd ed. 1994. LC 93-22118. (Illus.). 640p. (*0-632-03695-8*) Blckwell Science.

Statistical Methods in Spatial Epidemiology. A. B. Lawson. 2001. LC 00-43389. (Probability & Statistics Ser.). (Illus.). 298p. 89.95 (*0-471-97572-9*) Wiley.

Statistical Models for the Social & Behavioral Sciences: Multiple Regression & Limited-Dependent Variable Models. William H. Crown. 1998. LC 97-5583. 200p. 68.00 (*0-275-95316-5*, Praeger Pubs) Greenwood.

Statistical Models in Behavioral Research. William K. Estes. 1991. LC 90-43392. 168p. pap. 19.95 (*0-8058-0688-1*) L Erlbaum Assocs.

Statistical Models in Epidemiology. David Clayton & Michael Hills. 1993. (Illus.). 376p. (C). text 69.95 (*0-19-852221-5*, 7713) OUP.

Statistical Models in Psychological & Educational Testing. D. N. De Gruijter & Leo J. Van der Kamp. 1984. x, 294p. pap. (*90-265-0517-5*) Swets.

Statistical Operations: Analysis of Health Research Data. R. Hirsch & Richard K. Riegelman. 1995. LC 94-33711. (Illus.). 500p. pap. 49.95 incl. disk (*0-86542-258-3*) Blackwell Sci.

Statistical Process Control for Health Care. Hart. 2001. LC 2001-43508. (Illus.). 370p. 67.95 (*0-534-37865-X*) Thomson Learn.

Statistical Reasoning in Medicine: The Intuitive P Value Primer. Lemuel A. Moye. 2000. LC 99-46511. (Illus.). 224p. pap. 39.00 (*0-387-98933-1*) Spr-Verlag.

Statistical Reasoning in Psychology & Education. Edward W. Minium. 3rd ed. 1993. 280p. pap., wbk. ed. 32.95 (*0-471-82473-9*) Wiley.

Statistical Record of Health & Medicine. Ed. by Charity Anne Dorgan. 94th ed. 1994. (Illus.). 1218p. 109.00 (*0-8103-9745-5*) Gale.

Statistical Record of Health & Medicine. Gale Research Staff. 95th ed. 1997. (Illus.). 1300p. 125.00 (*0-7876-0093-8*, GML14099-108823) Gale.

Statistical Study of Certain Aspects of the Time Factor in Intelligence. Frederick C. Walters. LC 77-177666. (Columbia University. Teachers College. Contributions to Education Ser.). reprint ed. 37.50 (*0-404-55248-X*) AMS Pr.

Statistical Techniques in Bioassay. Z. Govindarajulu. 1988. (Illus.). xiv, 166p. 60.00 (*3-8055-4630-0*) S Karger.

Statistical Tools for the Health Science. Fallon. 1993. text (*0-442-00349-8*, VNR) Wiley.

Statistics: A Guide for Therapists. John McCall. 1997. LC 96-8890. (Skills for Practice Ser.). (Illus.). 288p. pap. text 39.50 (*0-7506-2104-4*) Buttrwrth-Heinemann.

Statistics: A Guide to Biological & Health Sciences. Richard S. Pieters & Gerald R. Rising. 1977. LC 76-50856. reprint ed. pap. text 8.95 (*0-8162-8564-0*) Holden-Day.

Statistics: A Health Sciences Introduction Minitab. Biles. 1993. 160p. pap. 16.95 (*0-8016-6534-5*) Mosby Inc.

Statistics: Learning in the Presence of Variation. Robert L. Wardrop. 736p. 42.95 (*0-8016-7505-7*); 1993. 250.00 (*0-8016-5682-6*); 1993. 250.00 (*0-8016-5690-7*); 1993. 100.00 (*0-8016-5681-8*); 1993. 75.00 (*0-8016-5684-2*); 1993. 384p. pap. 16.95 (*0-8016-7506-5*) Mosby Inc.

Statistics & Experimental Design for Toxicologists. Shayne C. Gad & Carrol S. Weil. 2nd ed. 1989. (Telford Press Ser.). 400p. 89.95 (*0-936923-17-2*, RA1199); per. 59.95 (*0-936923-18-0*) CRC Pr.

Statistics at Square I. Ed. by T. D. Swinscow. 9th rev. ed. 1996. 152p. pap. text (*0-7279-0916-9*) BMJ Pub GBR. *Dist:* AIDC.

***Statistics at Square Two: Understanding Modern Statistical Applications in Medicine.** M. J. Campbell. 2001. (Illus.). 134p. pap. (*0-7279-1394-8*) BMJ Pub GBR. *Dist:* AIDC.

Statistics for Clinicians. Basant K. Puri. 1996. pap. text 28.50 (*0-7020-1876-7*) Saunders.

Statistics for Engineers. James T. McClave & Richard L. Scheaffer. 1982. 480p. (C). pap. 30.75 (*0-87872-298-X*, 6950) PWS Pubs.

Statistics for Health Professionals. Susan Shott. 1990. (Illus.). 432p. pap., tchr. ed. (*0-7216-3472-9*); text 43.00 (*0-7216-8254-5*) Saunders.

Statistics for Pharmacists. Alain W. Li et al. 1997. LC 97-20887. (Illus.). 256p. pap. 46.95 (*0-632-04881-6*) Blackwell Sci.

Statistics for Psycholgy. Arthur Aron. 2nd ed. 1998. LC 98-7802. 643p. (C). 92.00 (*0-13-914078-6*) P-H.

Statistics for the Behavioral Sciences. James Jaccard. 1983. 384p. (C). mass mkt. 40.00 (*0-534-01247-7*) Brooks-Cole.

Statistics for the Behavioral Sciences. Sharon L. Weinberg & Kenneth P. Goldberg. 1990. 635p. pap. text 39.95 (*0-521-40873-3*) Cambridge U Pr.

Statistics for the Behavioral Sciences. James Jaccard & Michael A. Becker. 2nd ed. 1990. 520p. (C). text 47.50 (*0-534-10326-X*) Brooks-Cole.

Statistics for the Behavioral Sciences. Frederick J. Gravetter & Larry B. Wallnau. Ed. by Baxter Staff. 3rd ed. 1992. 632p. (C). text 63.00 (*0-314-90876-5*) West Pub.

Statistics for the Behavioral Sciences. James Jaccard & Michael A. Becker. 3rd ed. 1996. LC 96-15744. (Psychology Ser.). 672p. (C). spiral bd. 96.95 (*0-534-17406-X*) Brooks-Cole.

Statistics for the Behavioral Sciences. B. Michael Thorne & J. Martin Giesen. 3rd ed. 1999. LC 99-33807. 416p. (C). text 66.95 (*0-7674-1064-5*) Mayfield Pub.

***Statistics for the Behavioral Sciences.** James Jaccard & Michael A. Becker. 4th ed. 2001. 672p. 99.95 (*0-534-56925-0*) Wadsworth Pub.

Statistics for the Biological Sciences. William C. Schefler. 2nd ed. 1979. LC 78-55830. (Illus.). text (*0-201-07500-8*) Addison-Wesley.

Statistics for the Health Professional. Shott. 2nd ed. 2000. pap. (*0-7216-5979-9*) Saunders.

Statistics from Scratch: An Introduction for Health Care Professionals. David Bowers. 1996. LC 95-49518. 192p. pap. 44.95 (*0-471-96325-9*) Wiley.

Statistics Further from Scratch: For Health Care Professionals. 1997. LC 96-47783. 180p. pap. 44.95 (*0-471-97136-7*) Wiley.

Statistics in Clinical Practice. Ed. by David Coggan. 1995. 120p. (Orig.). pap. text (*0-7279-0907-X*) BMJ Pub GBR. *Dist:* AIDC.

Statistics in Medical Research: Developments in Clinical Trials. E. A. Gehan & N. A. Lemak. 1994. (Illus.). 224p. (C). text 45.00 (*0-306-44863-7*, Kluwer Plenum) Kluwer Academic.

Statistics in Medicine. Theodore Colton. 1975. LC 73-1413. 372p. pap. text 45.00 (*0-316-15250-1*) Lppncott W & W.

Statistics in Public Health: Quantitative Approaches to Public Health Problems. Ed. by Donna F. Stroup & Steven M. Teutsch. 1998. LC 97-47073. (Illus.). 256p. text 39.95 (*0-19-511498-1*) OUP.

Statistics in Toxicology. Ed. by D. Krewski & C. Franklin. 1991. xiii, 677p. text 409.00 (*2-88124-340-1*) Gordon & Breach.

Statistics of Health Services & of Their Activities: Proceedings of the WHO Expert Committee on Health Statistics, 13th, Geneva, 1968. WHO Staff. 1969. (Technical Reports: No. 429). pap. text 5.00 (*92-4-120429-X*, 1100429) World Health.

Statistics on Psychotropic Substances. 1989. 196p. (Orig.). 22.00 (*92-1-048048-1*) UN.

Statistics on Psychotropic Substances for 1988. 116p. 19.00 (*92-1-048046-5*, EFS.89.XI.4) UN.

Statistics on Psychotropic Substances for 1990. 1991. 196p. 38.00 (*92-1-048051-1*, 91.XI.3) UN.

Statistics with Confidence. Ed. by Douglas A. Altman et al. 2nd ed. 2000. 240p. pap. text (*0-7279-1375-1*) BMJ Pub GBR. *Dist:* AIDC.

Stats on Psychotropic Substances, 1987. 1988. 19.00 (*92-1-048043-0*, TR88.XI.3) UN.

Status Epilepticus: Its Clinical Features & Treatment in Children & Adults. Simon D. Shorvon. 1994. LC 93-24228. (Illus.). 400p. (C). text 95.00 (*0-521-42065-2*) Cambridge U Pr.

Status of Alternative Methods in Toxicology. Anderson. 1996. 168p. (C). (*0-85404-404-3*) Royal Soc Chem GBR. *Dist:* Spr-Verlag.

Status of Common Sense in Psychology. Ed. by Jurg Siegfried. 1994. LC 92-48700. 388p. 85.00 (*0-89391-873-3*, Ablex) Greenwood.

Status of Invertebrate Paleontology, 1953, Vol. 112. Ed. by Bernhard Kummel & Stephen Jay Gould. 1980. LC 79-8351. (History of Paleontology Ser.). (Illus.). reprint ed. lib. bdg. 21.95 (*0-405-12715-4*) Ayer.

Status of Ketamine in Anesthesiology: Pros & Cons. Ed. by E. F. Domino. 1990. LC 89-92147. (Illus.). 583p. 95.00 (*0-916182-07-X*) NPP Bks.

Status One: The New Practice of High Risk Population Health Management. Samuel Forman. 1999. LC 99-18725. 251p. 47.00 (*0-7879-4154-9*) Jossey-Bass.

Stay Fit & Healthy until You're Dead. Dave Barry. Ed. by Roger B. Yepsen. 2000. LC 85-11931. (Illus.). 96p. pap. 12.95 (*0-87857-570-7*, 10-136-1) Rodale Pr Inc.

Stay Well Without Going Broke: Winning the War over Medical Bills. Pattie Vargas et al. 1993. LC 93-84015. 384p. 22.95 (*0-914984-52-7*) Starburst.

Staying Alive: The Complete Guide to Energy Renewal. Marylil K. Humphreys. 1990. LC 89-82616. (Illus.). 184p. (Orig.). pap. 12.95 (*0-9625645-0-8*) Avocet Pub.

Staying Clean: Living Without Drugs. 1989. 76p. (Orig.). pap. 8.00 (*0-89486-447-5*, 5150A) Hazelden.

Staying Dry: A Practical Guide to Bladder Control. Kathryn L. Burgio et al. 1989. LC 89-45480. (Illus.). 192p. pap. 13.95 (*0-8018-3909-2*) Johns Hopkins.

***Staying Fit after Forty: A Plan for Healthy & Active Living.** Ed. by Don S. Otis. 2001. LC 00-53186. 192p. pap. 9.99 (*0-87788-453-6*) Waterbrook Pr.

Staying Flexible. 1987. (Fitness, Health & Nutrition Ser.). (Illus.). 144p. 17.27 (*0-8094-6167-6*); lib. bdg. 23.27 (*0-8094-6168-4*) Time-Life.

Staying Healthy. Janus. 1997. (Illus.). (gr. 6-12). text Price not set. (*0-8359-3350-4*) Globe Fearon.

Staying Healthy: 10 Easy Steps for Women. Carolle Jean-Murat. 1994. (Illus.). 120p. (Orig.). pap. 14.94 (*0-9627145-7-7*) Waterside Prodns.

Staying Healthy: A Bibliography of Health Promotion Materials. 1986. lib. bdg. 79.95 (*0-8490-3807-3*) Gordon Pr.

Staying Healthy: A Bibliography of Health Promotion Materials. 1984. lib. bdg. 250.00 (*0-87700-550-8*) Revisionist Pr.

***Staying Healthy on Hajj & Umrah: Practical Approaches to Obtaining & Maintaining a Healthy State During Hajj & Umrah.** A. H. Luqman & A. M. Luqman. 2001. (Illus.). 40p. pap. 14.95 (*0-9710958-0-9*) Medsurg.

Staying Healthy with Nutrition: The Complete Guide to Diet & Nutritional Medicine. Elson M. Haas. 1995. LC 90-38517. 1200p. pap. 37.95 (*0-89087-481-6*) Celestial Arts.

Staying Human During Residency Training. Allan D. Peterkin. 2nd ed. 1998. LC 98-167109. 284p. pap. 15.00 (*0-8020-8148-7*) U of Toronto Pr.

Staying Out of Court: A Self-Assessment Guide for Nurses. Barbara E. Calfee. 4th ed. 1994. 90p. pap. text, per., ring bd. 19.95 (*0-9633540-3-5*) ARC Pub.

Staying Safe: Preventing Child Abuse. Girl Scouts of the U. S. A. Staff. 1986. (Contemporary Issues Ser.). 16p. pap. 1.50 (*0-88441-461-2*, 26-821) Girl Scouts USA.

Staying Sober: A Guide for Relapse Prevention. Terence T. Gorski & Merlene Miller. 1986. 228p. pap. 12.00 (*0-8309-0459-X*, 17-0120-7) Herald Pub Hse.

Staying Sober Recovery Education Modules. Terence T. Gorski & Marlene Miller. 1989. pap. 150.00 (*0-8309-0542-1*, 17-0166-5) Herald Pub Hse.

Staying Sober Recovery Education Modules: Exercise Manual. Terence T. Gorski & Marlene Miller. 1989. pap., stu. ed. 8.00 (*0-8309-0602-9*, 17-0188-6) Herald Pub Hse.

Staying Well. American Institute for Preventive Medicine Staff. 1993. LC 93-34773. (For Your Information Ser.). 9.50 (*1-56420-027-2*) New Readers.

Staying Well in a Toxic World: Understanding Environmental Illness, Multiple Chemical Sensitivities, Chemical Injuries, & Sick Building Syndrome. Lynn Lawson. 1996. (Orig.). LC 00-93212. 80p. pap. 15.95 (*0-9653659-1-3*); LC 96-94641. 488p. pap. 15.95 (*0-9653659-0-5*) Lynnwrd Pr.

STD: Health Facts. Lucas Stang & Kathleen R. Miner. 1996. LC 93-43843. 12.95 (*1-56071-183-3*, H303) ETR Assocs.

STD: Sexually Transmitted Diseases, Including HIV-AIDS. John T. Daugirdas. 3rd rev. ed. 1992. 14.95 (*0-9629279-1-0*) Medtext.

STD Blues: A Self-Defense Guide. Judy Ismach. rev. ed. 2000. pap. 0.50 (*0-89230-185-6*) Do It Now.

STDs & HIV: A Guide for Today's Young Adults. William L. Yarber. 1992. 103p. pap. text, tchr. ed. 17.00 (*0-88314-534-0*) AAHPERD.

Steal This Urine Test: Fighting the Drug Hysteria in America. Abbie Hoffman & Jonathan Silvers. 1987. LC 87-12093. 192p. pap. 12.95 (*0-14-010400-3*, Penguin Bks) Penguin Putnam.

Stealing the Dragon's Fire: A Personal Guide & Resource for Dealing with Breast Cancer. Clo Wilson-Hashiguchi. Ed. by Margaret D. Smith et al. 1995. LC 93-94147. (Illus.). 334p. (Orig.). pap. 19.95 (*0-9638590-0-5*) Wilson Pubng.

Stealth Health. Evelyn Tribole. 2000. (Illus.). 256p. pap. 12.95 (*0-14-028205-X*) Penguin Putnam.

Stealth Liposomes. Ed. by F. J. Martin & Danilo D. Lasic. 1995. LC 94-32683. (Pharmacology & Toxicology Ser.). 320p. 179.95 (*0-8493-8383-8*) CRC Pr.

***Steatohepatitis (nash & Ash)** U. Leuschner et al. 2001. (Falk Symposium Ser.: Vol. 121). 400p. 193.00 (*0-7923-8769-4*) Kluwer Academic.

Stedman Portuguese-English, English-Portuguese Medical Dictionary. 25th ed. 1996. (ENG & POR.). 1658p. 295.00 (*0-7859-9348-7*) Fr & Eur.

Stedman's - Bergey Bacteria Word Book. 1992. 392p. pap. 28.00 (*0-683-07945-X*) Lppncott W & W.

Stedman's Alternative Medicine Words. Williams and Wilkins Staff. 2000. (Illus.). 600p. pap. text 38.95 (*0-7817-2161-X*) Lppncott W & W.

Stedman's ATCC Fungus Names. Shung-Chang Jong et al. 1992. LC 92-22845. 272p. pap. 28.00 (*0-683-07957-3*) Lppncott W & W.

Stedman's Cardiology & Pulmonary Words. Helen E. Littrell & Thomas L. Stedman. 2nd ed. 1997. LC 96-45978. (Stedman's Word Bks.). 601p. 35.95 (*0-683-40081-9*) Lppncott W & W.

***Stedman's Cardiology & Pulmonary Words: Includes Respiratory.** 3rd ed. 2001. 800p. pap. text 38.95 (*0-7817-3056-2*) Lppncott W & W.

Stedman's Cardiology Words. Stedman. 1992. LC 92-21067. 256p. 28.00 (*0-683-07953-0*) Lppncott W & W.

Stedman's Concise Medical Dictionary. Ed. by Stedman's Medical Dictionary Staff. rev. ed. 1994. LC 93-21060. 25.00 (*0-671-87473-X*, Webs New Wrld) Hungry Minds.

Stedman's Concise Medical Dictionary Illustrated. Stedman. 2nd ed. 1994. LC 93-41724. (Illus.). 1286p. pap. 24.95 (*0-683-07917-4*) Lppncott W & W.

Stedman's Dermatology & Immunology Words. Darla Haberer. 1997. LC 96-36759. (Stedman's Word Bks.). 544p. 38.95 (*0-683-40080-0*) Lppncott W & W.

***Stedman's Dermatology & Immunology Words.** 2nd ed. 2001. LC 2001-50427. 700p. pap. text 38.95 (*0-7817-3059-7*) Lppncott W & W.

Stedman's Diccionario de Ciencas Medicas Illustrado. Stedman. 25th ed. 1993. (SPA., Illus.). 1568p. 59.95 (*0-683-07912-3*) Lppncott W & W.

Stedman's English-Japanese-English Medical Dictionary. Medical View Staff. 2nd ed. 1984. 1973p. 250.00 (*0-8288-1850-9*) Fr & Eur.

Stedman's English-Portuguese Medical Dictionary Stedman. 1979. (ENG & POR.). 195.00 (*0-7859-7528-4*, 8522602247) Fr & Eur.

***Stedman's GI & GU Words: Includes Urology.** Thomas Lathrop Stedman. 3rd ed. 2001. LC 2001-50350. 800p. pap. text 38.95 (*0-7817-3058-9*) Lppncott W & W.

Stedman's GI Words. Stedman. 1992. 360p. 28.00 (*0-683-07943-3*) Lppncott W & W.

Stedman's GI/GU Words: Including: Nephrology. Ed. by Darla Haberer. 2nd ed. 1996. 731p. pap. 38.95 (*0-683-18145-9*) Lppncott W & W.

Stedman's ICTV Virus Words. Charles H. Calisher & Claude M. Fauquet. 1992. LC 92-12319. 304p. pap. 28.00 (*0-683-07956-5*) Lppncott W & W.

Stedman's Medical Dictionary. 10th ed. 2000. 2,000p. text 99.95 (*0-683-40008-8*) Lppncott W & W.

Stedman's Medical Dictionary. Thomas Lathrop Stedman. 22nd ed. 1976. 1586p. reprint ed. 9.95 (*0-683-07919-0*) Krieger.

Stedman's Medical Dictionary. Thomas Lathrop Stedman. 10th ed. 2000. LC 99-56094. (Stedman's Medical Dictionary Ser.). 2,098p. text 49.95 (*0-683-40007-X*) Lppncott W & W.

***Stedman's Medical Dictionary.** Stedman. 26th ed. 99.95 (*1-56712-420-8*) Franklin Elect.

Stedman's Medical Dictionary. Ed. by Lippincott, Williams and Wilkins Staff. 27th ed. 2000. LC 99-56094. (Illus.). 2098p. 59.95 incl. cd-rom (*0-7817-2728-6*, Lippncttt) Lppncott W & W.

Stedman's Medical Dictionary: Deluxe Version. 25th ed. 1990. (Illus.). 1920p. 89.95 (*0-683-07925-5*) Lppncott W & W.

Stedman's Medical Eponyms. Pat Forbis et al. 1998. LC 98-17560. 524p. pap. text 34.00 (*0-683-07965-4*) Lppncott W & W.

Stedman's Medical Equipment Words. Stedman. 1993. 608p. 34.00 (*0-683-07954-9*) Lppncott W & W.

Stedman's OB-GYN Words. 1992. 272p. pap. 28.00 (*0-683-07942-5*) Lppncott W & W.

Stedman's Oncology Words. 1992. LC 92-49350. 300p. 28.00 (*0-683-07951-4*); 3rd ed. 2000. pap. text 38.95 (*0-7817-2654-9*) Lppncott W & W.

Stedman's Ophthalmology Words. Thomas L. Stedman. 2nd ed. 1999. LC 99-89436. (Community Builders Ser.). (Illus.). 592p. pap. text 38.95 (*0-683-30776-2*) Lppncott W & W.

***Stedman's Organisms & Infectious Disease Words.** Thomas Lathrop Stedman. 2001. LC 2001-50348. 800p. pap. text 38.95 (*0-7817-3351-0*) Lppncott W & W.

Stedman's Orthopaedic & Rehab Words: With Podiatry, Chiropractic, Physical Therapy & Occupational Therapy Words. Contrib. by Thomas Lathrop Stedman. 3rd ed. 1999. LC 99-16399. (Stedman's Word Book Ser.). 826p. pap. text 38.95 (*0-683-30778-9*) Lppncott W & W.

Stedman's Pathology & Lab Medicine Words. Ed. by Christa Scott. 2nd ed. 1997. LC 97-15929. 688p. 38.95 (*0-683-40191-2*) Lppncott W & W.

***Stedman's Pediatric Words: Including Neonatology.** 2001. 650p. pap. text 38.95 (*0-7817-3057-0*) Lppncott W & W.

Stedman's Plastic Surgery ENT Dentistry Words. Thomas L. Stedman. 1998. LC 98-33791. (Stedman's Word Books Ser.). 753p. pap. 38.95 (*0-683-40460-1*) Lppncott W & W.

Stedman's Podiatry Words. 1995. 350p. 28.00 (*0-683-07961-1*) Lppncott W & W.

Stedman's Psychiatry, Neurology & Neurosurgery Words. 2nd ed. 1999. (Stedman's Word Bks.). 1039p. pap. text 38.95 (*0-683-30775-4*) Lppncott W & W.

Stedman's Radiology Words. 1992. 308p. 28.00 (*0-683-07940-9*) Lppncott W & W.

Stedman's Radiology Words. Williams and Wilkins Staff. 3rd ed. 2000. pap. text 38.95 (*0-7817-2653-0*) Lppncott W & W.

Stedman's Surgery Words. Sandy Kovacs. 1997. LC 97-20704. (Stedman's Word Book Ser.). 829p. text 38.95 (*0-683-40190-4*) Lppncott W & W.

Stedman's Urology Words. Stedman. 1993. 350p. 28.00 (*0-683-07960-3*) Lppncott W & W.

Stell & Maran's Head & Neck Surgery. John Watkinson et al. 4th ed. 2000. (Illus.). 528p. (*0-7506-3366-2*) E A GBR. *Dist:* OUP.

Stella: One Woman's Victory over Cancer. Stella Andres & Brad Steiger. 1986. 160p. 14.95 (*0-86700-015-5*, Synergy Bks) P Walsh Pr.

Stem Cell Biology & Gene Therapy. Ed. by Peter J. Quesenberry et al. 1998. LC 97-48252. 566p. 120.00 (*0-471-14656-0*, Wiley-Liss) Wiley.

Stem Cell Transplantation: A Clinical Textbook. Ed. by Patricia Buchsel & Pamela M. Kapustay. 2000. LC 00-100252. (Illus.). 304p. ring bd. 52.00 (*1-890504-15-7*) Oncology Nursing.

***Stem Cell Transplantation & Tissue Engineering.** Ed. by A. Haverich & H. Graf. 2001. LC 2001-54968. (Ernst Schering Research Foundation Workshop: Vol. 35). (*3-540-41495-9*) Springer Pub.

***Stem Cell Transplantation in the Young.** Paulette Mehta. 2002. (Illus.). (C). text 134.95 (*0-7637-1855-6*, 1855-6) Jones & Bartlett.

Stem Cells. Ed. by C. S. Potten. 1996. (Illus.). 496p. text 99.95 (*0-12-563455-2*) Acad Pr.

Stem Cells & CNS Development. Ed. by Mahendra S. Rao. 2001. LC 00-58081. (Contemporary Neuroscience Ser.). (Illus.). x, 370p. 125.00 (*0-89603-886-6*) Humana.

Steno on Muscles: Introduction, Texts & Translation. Troels Kardel et al. 1994. LC 93-73911. (Transactions Ser.: Vol. 84, Pt. 1). (Illus.). 252p. (C). pap. 20.00 (*0-87169-841-2*, T841-KAT) Am Philos.

Stenosis of the Cervical Spine: Causes, Diagnosis, & Treatment. V. Denaro. 1991. (Illus.). 203p. 225.00 (*0-387-53328-1*) Spr-Verlag.

Stent-Grafts: Current Clinical Practice. Bart L. Dolmatch. 1999. LC 99-44547. (Illus.). 272p. 99.00 (*0-86577-893-0*) Thieme Med Pubs.

Step by Step: Sixteen Steps Toward Legally Sound Sexual Abuse Investigations. Jan Hindman. 1987. 44p. pap. 5.95 (*0-9611034-3-4*) AlexAndria OR.

Step-by-Step Guide to a Higher Score on the Nab Exam. Peter J. Buttaro. 1999. LC 98-32393. 144p. pap. 65.00 (*0-8342-1314-1*) Aspen Pub.

Step-by-Step Guide to Completing the MDS. Janet I. Feldman & R. W. Baker. 1999. LC 00-500768. (Aspen Publication Ser.). (Illus.). 192p. 95.00 (*0-8342-1366-4*) Aspen Pub.

Step by Step Guide to the Estimation of Child Mortality. 1989. 83p. 19.00 (*92-1-151183-6*, 89.XIII.9) UN.

Step-by-Step Learning Guide for Older Retarded Children. Vicki M. Johnson & Roberta A. Werner. 1977. (Step-By-Step Learning Guide Series; 2 Ser.). 214p. (C). pap. 16.95 (*0-8156-2181-7*) Syracuse U Pr.

Step-by-Step Learning Guide for Retarded Infants & Children. Vicki M. Johnson & Roberta A. Werner. 1975. LC 75-22172. (Illus.). 208p. (C). pap. 16.95 (*0-8156-2174-4*) Syracuse U Pr.

Step-by-Step Medical Coding. Ed. by Carol J. Buck. 1996. (Illus.). pap., tchr. ed. (*0-7216-5345-6*) Saunders.

Step-by-Step Medical Coding. Carol J. Buck. Ed. by Margaret Biblis. 2nd ed. 1998. LC 97-20508. (Illus.). 560p. (C). pap. text 36.95 (*0-7216-7536-0*) Saunders.

Step-by-Step Medical Coding. Carol J. Buck. 2nd ed. 1998. (Illus.). 555p. pap. (*0-7216-7537-9*) Saunders.

S

S

Step by Step to Peer Health Education Programs: A Planning Guide. Malcolm Goldsmith & Sherri T. Reynolds. 1996. LC 96-32280. pap. (*1-56071-517-0*) ETR Assocs.

Step Four for Young Adults. Paul E. Bjorklund. 1981. 44p. pap. 3.25 (*0-89486-118-2*, 1129B) Hazelden.

Step One: The Foundation of Recovery. William Springborn. 1977. 24p. (Orig.). pap. 2.00 (*0-89486-017-8*, 1425B) Hazelden.

Step One for Young Adults. Della Van Dyke & Jane Nakken. 1985. (Step Pamphlets for Young Adults Ser.). 24p. (Orig.). pap. 3.25 (*0-89486-304-5*, 1362B) Hazelden.

Step 1 Success: Full Length Practice Test for the USMLE. Stanley Zaslau. Ed. & Illus. by Paul McGrath. 1995. 240p. spiral bd., wbk. ed. 26.00 (*1-886468-07-9*) FMSG.

Step Ten: A Good Tenth Step. Mel B. 1982. 20p. (Orig.). pap. 2.00 (*0-89486-153-0*) Hazelden.

Step Three for Young Adults. Della Van Dyke. 1986. (Step Pamphlets for Young Adults Ser.). 20p. (Orig.). pap. 3.25 (*0-89486-352-5*, 5502B) Hazelden.

Step 3 Simulated Exam. John R. Thornborough. 1996. (Pretest Simulated Exam Ser.). (Illus.). 192p. text 32.00 (*0-07-052067-4*) McGraw-Hill Med Pub.

Step 3 Success: Full Length Practice Test. Stanley Zaslau. 1995. 202p. (C). pap. text 26.00 (*1-886468-05-2*) FMSG.

Step 2 Success: Full Length Practice Test for the USMLE. Stanley Zaslau. Ed. & Illus. by Paul L. McGrath. 1995. 228p. spiral bd., wbk. ed. 26.00 (*1-886468-06-0*) FMSG.

Stepfamilies: A Guide to Working with Stepparents & Stepchildren. Emily B. Visher & John S. Visher. 1984. LC 78-25857. 300p. text 35.95 (*0-87630-190-1*) Brunner-Routledge.

Stepfamilies: The Step by Step Model of Brief Therapy. Mala S. Burt & Roger B. Burt. 1996. LC 96-32988. 208p. 29.95 (*0-87630-832-9*) Brunner-Routledge.

***Stepping into Palliative Care: A Handbook for Community Professionals.** Ed. by Jo Cooper. 2000. 288p. pap. (*1-85775-303-8*) Radcliffe Med Pr GBR. *Dist:* Balogh.

Stepping off Life's Sad Merry-Go-Round: Metaphorically Speaking. Patricia Topp. 1998. (Illus.). xi, 283p. pap. 25.00 (*0-9667369-0-7*) P Topp.

Stepping Stones to Recovery for Women. Ed. by B. Mary. LC 89-17751. 240p. (Orig.). pap. 6.95 (*0-934125-15-5*) Hazelden.

Stepping Stones to Recovery from Cocaine-Crack Addiction. Mark R. & Mary L. LC 90-20336. 128p. pap. 7.95 (*0-934125-10-4*) Hazelden.

Stepping Toward Control: A Book for People Who Live with Diabetes. Twila Okerlund. Ed. by Susan D. Allen & Colleen A. Holloran. 2001. LC 94-11662. (Illus.). 64p. pap. text 3.75 (*0-916999-15-7*) HERC Pubng.

Steps to an Ecology of Mind. Gregory Bateson. 1988. LC 87-24133. 545p. reprint ed. 50.00 (*0-87668-950-0*) Aronson.

Steps to Better Health for Children. Ann R. Cox et al. 1985. pap. 13.95 (*0-8359-7110-4*) P-H.

Steps to Follow: A Guide for the Treatment of Adult Hemiplegia. P. M. Davies. 1996. (Illus.). 335p. 46.00 (*0-387-13436-0*) Spr-Verlag.

Steps to Follow: The Comprehensive Treatment of Patients with Hemiplegia. Patricia M. Davies. 2nd exp. rev. ed. 2000. LC 00-20621. (Illus.). 512p. pap. 54.00 (*3-540-60720-X*) Spr-Verlag.

Steps to Help Your School Set up an AIDS Education Program. rev. ed. 1995. (Illus.). 23p. pap. 4.00 (*1-880002-04-3*) Natl Coal Advocates.

Steps to Language. I. M. Schlesinger. 1982. 448p. text 79.95 (*0-89859-045-0*) L Erlbaum Assocs.

Stereo Atlas of Fluorescein & Indocyanine Green Angiograph. Patrick J. Saine et al. 1999. LC 98-45258. 147p. text 99.00 (*0-7506-7001-0*) Buttrwrth-Heinemann.

Stereo Atlas of Glaucoma. Campbell Netland. 1997. LC 97-22257. (Illus.). 272p. text 149.00 (*0-8151-1399-4*, 26953) Mosby Inc.

Stereoencephalotomy Symposium, 5th, International, 1970. Stereoencephalotomy Symposium Staff. Ed. by F. Mundinger et al. 1972. (Advances in Stereoencephalotomy Ser.: Vol. 6). pap. 70.50 (*3-8055-1358-5*) S Karger.

Stereoscopic Acuity in Ocular Pursuit of Moving Objects: Dynamic Stereoscopy & Movement Parallax: Relevance to Road Safety & Occupational Medicine. Matthias Sachsenweger & Ulrich Sachsenweger. 1992. 136p. (C). pap. text 126.50 (*0-7923-1486-7*) Kluwer Academic.

Stereotactic & Functional Neurosurgery. Ed. by Philip L. Gildenberg & Ronald R. Tasker. 1997. (Illus.). 2174p. text 399.00 (*0-07-023604-6*) McGraw-Hill Prof.

Stereotactic Radiosurgery: For Brain Tumors. 1996. (Illus.). (*0-944093-42-6*) Am Brain Tumor.

Stereotactic Techniques in Clinical Neurosurgery. D. A. Bosch. 1986. (Illus.). 290p. 119.00 (*0-387-81878-2*) Spr-Verlag.

Stereotaxic Atlas of the New Zealand Rabbit's Brain. Ivan Urban & Philippe Richard. 1972. (Illus.). 92p. 24.95 (*0-398-02431-6*) C C Thomas.

Stereotaxic Surgery in the Rat. Richard K. Cooley & C.H. Vanderwolf. 2nd ed. 1990. pap. (*0-920700-00-4*) A J Kirby.

Stereotyped Movements: Brain & Behavior Relationships. Ed. by Robert L. Sprague & Karl M. Newell. 1996. LC 95-4732. (APA Science Conference Ser.). (Illus.). 211p. 24.95 (*1-55798-301-1*) Am Psychol.

Stereotypes & Social Cognition. Jacques-Philippe Leyens et al. 1994. LC 94-67832. 256p. 74.50 (*0-8039-8583-5*, 2939) Sage.

Steric Factor in Medicinal Chemistry: Dissymmetric Probes of Pharmacological Receptors. A. F. Casy. 1994. (Illus.). 590p. (C). text 135.00 (*0-306-44289-2*, Kluwer Plenum) Kluwer Academic.

Steric Fit in Quantitative Structure-Activity Relations. Ed. by Alexandru T. Balaban et al. 1980. (Lecture Notes in Chemistry: Vol. 15). (Illus.). 178p. 27.95 (*0-387-09755-4*) Spr-Verlag.

***Sterically Stabilised Liposomes & Related Lipid Aggregates: Fundamental Studies on Aggregate Strucure & Stability.** Markus Johnsson. 2001. (Comprehensive Summaries of Uppsala Dissertations from the Faculty of Science & Technology Ser.: No. 629). (Illus.). 69p. (*91-554-5027-X*) Uppsala Universitet SWE. *Dist:* Coronet Bks.

Sterile Filtration: A Practical Approach. Maik W. Jornitz & Theodore H. Meltzer. 2000. LC 00-50926. (Illus.). xv, 623p. text 195.00 (*0-8247-0282-4*) Dekker.

Sterile-Male Technique for Eradication or Control of Harmful Insects. 1969. (Panel Proceedings Ser.). pap. (*92-0-111369-2*, ISP224) IAEA AUT. *Dist:* Bernan Associates.

Sterile Pharmaceutical Manufacturing: Applications for the 1990s. Ed. by Michael J. Groves et al. 1991. Vol. I. 244p. 86.50 (*0-935184-21-X*); Vol. II. 243p. 86.50 (*0-935184-22-8*) IHS Health Grp.

Sterile Pharmaceutical Products: Process Engineering Applications I. Ed. by Kenneth Avis. 1995. LC 95-24999. (Drug Manufacturing Technology Ser.). (Illus.). 415p. 189.00 (*0-935184-81-3*) IHS Health Grp.

Sterile Product Facility Design & Project Management. Jeffery N. Odum. 1996. (Illus.). 320p. ring bd. 194.00 (*1-57491-020-5*) IHS Health Grp.

Sterilization & Disinfection: Index of Modern Information for Medicine & Research with Bibliography. Stanley B. Gessler. rev. ed. 1994. 149p. 57.50 (*0-7883-0192-6*); pap. 47.50 (*0-7883-0193-4*) ABBE Pubs Assn.

Sterilization for Human Betterment. E. S. Gosney & Paul Popenoe. Ed. by Gerald N. Grob. 1980. LC 78-22561. (Historical Issues in Mental Health Ser.). reprint ed. lib. bdg. 19.95 (*0-405-11915-1*) Ayer.

Sterilization of Drugs & Devices: Technologies for the 21st Century. Ed. by Fred M. Nordhauser & Wayne P. Olson. 1998. LC 98-176740. (Illus.). 552p. 239.00 (*1-57491-060-4*) IHS Health Grp.

Sterilization of Health Care Products: Requirements for Validation & Routine Control - Industrial Moist Heat Sterilization. 1993. (Illus.). 19p. (Orig.). pap. 74.00 (*1-57020-017-3*, ST1134-209) Assn Adv Med Instrn.

Sterilization of Health Care Products - Biological Indicators - General Pt. 1: ANSI/AAMI ST59:1999. 2000. (Illus.). pap. 90.00 (*1-57020-122-6*) Assn Adv Med Instrn.

Sterilization of Health Care Products - Biological Indicators for Ethylene Oxide Sterilization Pt. 2: ANSI/AAMI ST21:1999. 2000. (Illus.). pap. 70.00 (*1-57020-123-4*) Assn Adv Med Instrn.

Sterilization of Health Care Products - Biological Indicators for Moist Heat Sterilization Pt. 3: ANSI/AAMI ST19:1999. 1999. (Illus.). pap. 70.00 (*1-57020-124-2*) Assn Adv Med Instrn.

Sterilization of Health Care Products - Chemical Indicators: Class 2 Indicators for Air Removal Test, ANSI/AAMI ST66:1999. 2000. (Illus.). 80.00 (*1-57020-125-0*) Assn Adv Med Instrn.

Sterilization of People with Mental Disabilities. 1995. LC 94-38499. 288p. 68.00 (*0-86569-225-4*) Greenwood.

Sterilization Technology for the Health Care Facility. Ed. by Marimargaret Reichert & Jack H. Young. 2nd ed. 1997. LC 97-8366. 336p. 109.00 (*0-8342-0838-5*, 20838) Aspen Pub.

Steroid Action on Brain & Behavior: 10th Annual Workshop, Los Angeles, California, November 1998. Ed. by J. G. Dulka. 1999. (Brain, Behavior & Evolution Ser.: Vol. 54, No. 1). (Illus.). 70p. pap. 25.25 (*3-8055-6969-6*) S Karger.

Steroid Analysis by HPLC: Recent Applications. Kautsky. 1981. (Chromatographic Science Ser.: Vol. 16). (Illus.). 424p. text 225.00 (*0-8247-1324-9*) Dekker.

Steroid Analysis in the Pharmaceutical Industry. Sandor Gorog. 1989. 560p. 94.95 (*0-470-21178-4*) P-H.

Steroid & Sterol Hormone Action. Ed. by T. C. Spelsberg & R. Kumar. 1987. (C). text 164.50 (*0-89838-894-5*) Kluwer Academic.

Steroid Contraceptives & Women's Response: Regional Variability in Side-Effects & Steroid Pharmacokinetics. R. Snow & P. Hall. 1994. (Illus.). 276p. (C). text 114.00 (*0-306-44718-5*, Kluwer Plenum) Kluwer Academic.

Steroid Converting Enzymes & Diseases. Ed. by K. Fotherby & S. B. Pal. 1984. LC 84-17034. (Illus.). ix, 261p. 138.50 (*3-11-009556-4*) De Gruyter.

Steroid Hormone Receptors: Basic & Clinical Aspects. Ed. by Virinder K. Moudgil. 1993. LC 93-33850. (Hormones in Health & Disease Ser.). xiv, 522p. 99.00 (*0-8176-3694-3*) Birkhauser.

Steroid Hormone Resistance: Mechanisms & Clinical Aspects. Ed. by George P. Chrousos et al. 1986. LC 85-23250. (Advances in Experimental Medicine & Biology Ser.: Vol. 196). 454p. 95.00 (*0-306-42229-8*, Plenum Trade) Perseus Pubng.

Steroid Hormones & the T-Cell Cytokine Profile. Ed. by G. A. Rook & Stafford L. Lightman. 1997. LC 97-15904. (Illus.). 300p. 125.00 (*3-540-76057-1*) Spr-Verlag.

Steroid Receptor Methods: Protocols & Assays. Ed. by Benjamin A. Lieberman. 2001. LC 2001-24304. (Methods in Molecular Biology Ser.: Vol. 176). (Illus.). xiv, 381p. 99.50 (*0-89603-754-1*) Humana.

Steroid Receptors & Antihormones: Proceedings. Ed. by David Henderson et al. 1995. LC 95-11022. (Annals of the New York Academy of Sciences Ser.: Vol. 761). 416p. pap. 120.00 (*0-89766-938-X*) NY Acad Sci.

Steroid Receptors & the Management of Cancer E. Brad Thompson & Marc E. Lippman. 1979. Vol. 1. 272p. 148.00 (*0-8493-5477-3*, RC271); Vol. 2. 176p. 94.00 (*0-8493-5478-1*, RC271) Franklin (CRC Reprint).

Steroids. S. Coffey. Vol. 2, Pt. D. 1970. 500p. 315.00 (*0-444-40774-X*); Vol. 2, Pt. E. 1971. 290p. 268.75 (*0-444-40775-8*) Elsevier.

Steroids & Isoprenoids. Ed. by Sidney P. Colowick & Nathan O. Kaplan. 1985. (Methods in Enzymology Ser.: Vol. 110). Pt. A. text 188.00 (*0-12-182010-6*); Pt. B. text 188.00 (*0-12-182011-4*) Acad Pr.

Steroids & Neuronal Activity - Symposium No. 153. CIBA Foundation Staff et al. 1990. LC 90-12763. (CIBA Foundation Symposia Ser.: No. 153). 294p. 128.00 (*0-471-92689-2*) Wiley.

Steroids & Terpenoids. Ed. by R. B. Clayton et al. 1969. (Methods in Enzymology Ser.: Vol. 15). text 209.00 (*0-12-181872-1*) Acad Pr.

Steroids Game. Charles E. Yesalis & Virginia S. Cowart. 1998. LC 97-45859. (Illus.). 216p. pap. 16.95 (*0-88011-494-0*, PYES0494) Human Kinetics.

Steve: Remembrances of Stephen W. Kuffler. Ed. by U. J. McMahan. 1990. LC 90-10383. (Illus.). 142p. pap. 19.95 (*0-87893-516-9*) Sinauer Assocs.

Stevens' Handbook of Experimental Psychology Ed. by Richard C. Atkinson et al. 2nd ed. 1988. 1078p. 770.00 (*0-471-61625-7*) Wiley.

Stevens' Handbook of Experimental Psychology Vol. 1: Perception & Motivation, Vol. 1, Perception and Motivation. Ed. by Richard C. Atkinson et al. 2nd ed. 1988. LC 87-31637. 905p. 385.00 (*0-471-04203-X*) Wiley.

Stevens' Handbook of Experimental Psychology Vol. 2: Learning & Cognition, Vol. 2. Ed. by Richard C. Atkinson et al. 2nd ed. 1988. 1027p. 385.00 (*0-471-04207-2*) Wiley.

Stewards of Life: Bioethics & Pastoral Care. Sondra E. Wheeler. 1996. LC 96-17677. 144p. (Orig.). pap. text 13.00 (*0-687-02087-5*) Abingdon.

Stewart's Operative Urology, Set. Andrew C. Novick et al. 2nd ed. 1989. (Illus.). 908p. 225.00 (*0-683-06589-0*) Lppncott W & W.

Stick Figure: A Personal Journey Through Anorexia & Bulimia. Christine Fontana. 1996. pap. text (*0-85572-257-6*) Hill Content Pubng AUS. *Dist:* Seven Hills Bk.

Sticking to the Point: A Rational Method for the Step by Step Formulation of Administration of an Acupuncture Treatment. Bob Flaws. 1990. 150p. (Orig.). (C). pap. text 18.95 (*0-936185-17-1*) Blue Poppy Pr.

Sticking to the Point Vol. 2: A Study of Acupuncture & Moxibution Formulas & Strategies. Bob Flaws. 1998. LC 91-168430. 276p. pap. 21.95 (*0-936185-97-X*) Blue Poppy Pr.

Sticks & Stones: Identifying & Avoiding All Forms of Abuse. Miriam Adahan. 1997. LC 97-7351. 17.95 (*0-87306-793-2*) Feldheim.

Stigma: A Social Psychological Analysis. Irwin Katz. 1981. LC 80-20765. 160p. text 39.95 (*0-89859-078-7*) L Erlbaum Assocs.

Stigma: Notes on the Management of Spoiled Identity. Irving Goffman. 1963. (Orig.). pap. 5.95 (*0-13-846626-2*, Spectrm) Hungry Minds.

Stigma & Mental Illness. Ed. by Paul J. Fink & Allan Tasman. 1992. LC 91-26135. 236p. text 37.00 (*0-88048-405-5*, 8405) Am Psychiatric.

***Stigma & Social Exclusion in Healthcare.** Ed. by Tom Mason. 2001. LC 2001-19139. pap. 27.95 (*0-415-22200-1*) Routledge.

Still Going Against the Grain: Wheat-Free Cookery. Phyllis L. Potts. 1994. LC 94-94308. (Illus.). 260p. (Orig.). pap. 14.95 (*0-9630479-1-4*) Central Pt.

Still to Be Born: A Guide for Bereaved Parents Who are Making Decisions about Their Future. Pat Schwiebert & Paul Kirk. 1993. 120p. 5.50 (*0-9615197-2-X*) Perinatal Loss.

Stillness Built of Motion: Living with Tourette's. Emma Morgan. 2nd ed. 1996. (Illus.). (Orig.). reprint ed. pap. 7.00 (*0-9650733-4-3*, ECHO-003) Echolalia Pr.

Stimulants & Narcotics: Medically, Philosophically, & Morally Considered. George M. Beard. Ed. by Gerald N. Grob. 1981. LC 80-1213. (Addiction in America Ser.). reprint ed. lib. bdg. 19.95 (*0-405-13569-6*) Ayer.

Stimulants & Narcotics: Their Mutual Relations. Francis E. Anstie. Ed. by Gerald N. Grob. 1981. LC 80-1212. (Addiction in America Ser.). reprint ed. lib. bdg. 40.95 (*0-405-13568-8*) Ayer.

Stimulated Recall: Personalized Assessment of Clinical Reasoning. Howard S. Barrows. 2000. 31p. 12.00 (*0-931369-35-5*) Southern IL Univ Sch.

Stimulation & Control of Cardiac System Samuel Sideman & R. Beyar. 1987. LC 87-9352. reprint ed. Set. 363.00 (*0-8493-6512-0*); Vol. 2. 224p. 126.00 (*0-8493-6514-7*); Vol. 3. 240p. 134.00 (*0-8493-6515-5*) Franklin (CRC Reprint).

Stimulation of Fracture Healing with Ultrasound. H. G. Knoch & W. Klug. 1991. (Illus.). 96p. 75.00 (*0-387-53674-4*) Spr-Verlag.

Stimulus Class Formation in Humans & Animals, Vol. 117. Thomas R. Zentall & Paul M. Smeets. 1996. LC 96-34862. (Advances in Psychology Ser.). 322p. 112.00 (*0-444-82401-4*) Elsevier.

Stimulus-Response Compatibility: An Integrated Perspective. Ed. by R. W. Proctor & T. G. Reeve. 1989. (Advances in Psychology Ser.: No. 65). 508p. 199.00 (*0-444-88092-5*, North Holland) Elsevier.

Stimulus Secretion Coupling in Chromaffin Cells, Set. K. Rosenheck & P. I. Lelkes. 1987. LC 87-6378. 214.00 (*0-8493-6534-1*, CRC Reprint) Franklin.

Stimulus-Secretion Coupling in Chromaffin Cells, Vol. 2. K. Rosenheck & P. I. Lelkes. 1987. LC 87-6378. 100.00 (*0-8493-6537-6*, CRC Reprint) Franklin.

Stinking Thinking. Gayle Rosellini. 1985. 24p. (Orig.). pap. 2.00 (*0-89486-326-6*, 5451B) Hazelden.

Stochastic Models for Carcinogenesis. W. Y. Tan. 1991. (Statistics: Textbooks & Monographs: Vol. 116). (Illus.). 264p. text 155.00 (*0-8247-8427-8*) Dekker.

Stochastic Models of Cancer. Suresh H. Moolgavkar. 1996. (Monographs on Statistics & Applied Probability). 54.95 (*0-412-99481-X*, Chap & Hall NY) Chapman & Hall.

Stochastic Models of Tumor Latency & Their Applications. B. Asselain et al. 1996. 250p. text 61.00 (*981-02-1831-1*) World Scientific Pub.

Stochastic Population Theories. D. Ludwig. 1978. (Lecture Notes in Biomathematics: Vol. 3). reprint ed. pap. 22.00 (*0-387-07010-9*) Spr-Verlag.

Stochastic Processes in the Neurosciences. Henry Tuckwell. 1989. LC 89-6115. (CBMS-NSF Regional Conference Series in Applied Mathematics: No. 56). v, 129p. pap. 35.50 (*0-89871-232-7*) Soc Indus-Appl Math.

Stochastic Transport Processes in Discrete Biological Systems. E. Frehland. 1982. (Lecture Notes in Biomathematics: Vol. 47). 169p. 31.95 (*0-387-11964-7*) Spr-Verlag.

Stock Diseases. Brightling. 1997. 328p. 145.00 (*0-409-30476-X*) Buttrwrth-Heinemann.

Stoking the Fire: A Surgical Memoir of London. Charles S. Roberts. 1998. LC 98-36943. (Illus.). 200p. 40.00 (*0-87993-422-0*) Futura Pub.

***Stolen Child: Aspects of Autism & Asperger Syndrome.** Ann Hewetson. 2002. LC 2001-43015. 248p. 27.95 (*0-89789-844-3*, H844, Bergin & Garvey) Greenwood.

Stoma Care Nursing. 320p. pap. (*0-340-59491-8*) E A GBR. *Dist:* Routldge.

Stomach. Ed. by W. Domschke & S. J. Konturek. 1993. (Illus.). 420p. pap. (*3-540-56613-9*); LC 93-21900. 396p. 145.00 (*0-387-56613-9*) Spr-Verlag.

Stomach. Ed. by Sven Gustavsson et al. 1991. (Illus.). 444p. text (*0-443-04417-1*) Church.

Stomach. Ed. by Leo Van der Reis. 1980. (Frontiers of Gastrointestinal Research Ser.: Vol. 6). (Illus.). xii, 188p. 80.00 (*3-8055-3071-4*) S Karger.

Stomach & Duodenum. Ed. by Mark Feldman. 1996. (Gastroenterology & Hepatology Ser.: Vol. 3). (Illus.). 233p. text (*0-443-07843-2*) Church GBR. *Dist:* Saunders.

Stomach Virus & Other Forms of Family Bonding. Kathy Peel. 1993. 236p. pap. 9.99 (*0-8499-3477-X*) W Pubng Grp.

Stomal Therapy. Bokey & Shell. 1985. 33.00 (*0-08-029865-6*); pap. 20.00 (*0-08-029862-1*, Pergamon Pr) Elsevier.

Stone Diseases. Ed. by D. Hauri & O. Schmucki. 1987. (Urologia Internationalis Ser.: Vol. 41, No. 5, 1986). 76p. pap. 67.00 (*3-8055-4523-1*) S Karger.

Stone Surgery. Michael Marberger et al. 1991. (Practice of Surgery Ser.). (Illus.). 320p. text (*0-443-03522-9*) Church.

Stools & Bottles. Gayle Rosellini. 160p. 10.00 (*0-89486-027-5*, 1040A) Hazelden.

Stop Committing Voice Suicide. Martin Cooper. 1996. LC 95-62223. 172p. pap. text 10.00 (*0-87980-437-8*) Wilshire.

Stop Drinking & Start Living. Stephen E. Schlesinger & John J. Gillick. 1985. (Illus.). 154p. 12.95 (*0-8306-1937-2*, 1937H) McGraw-Hill Educ Grp.

Stop Drinking & Start Living. Stephen E. Schlesinger. 2nd ed. 1989. pap. 7.95 (*0-8306-3227-1*) McGraw-Hill Educ Grp.

Stop Hair Loss. Paavo O. Airola. 1984. 32p. pap. 2.95 (*0-932090-06-0*) Health Plus.

Stop Heart Disease Now! Atherolysis: My Program for the Prevention & Reversal of Heart Disease. Narendra M. Pai. 1999. LC 98-92140. (Dr. Pai Publications). (Illus.). 134p. pap. 23.98 (*0-9667295-0-1*, 001, Left Front) Dr Pai Pubns.

Stop, Listen, & Look: Child's Health Surveillance in Primary Care. Barbara Robson & Lesley Lamont-Herps. 1999. 144p. pap. 35.00 (*0-8036-0402-5*) Davis Co.

Stop Managing Costs: Designing Healthcare Organizations Around Core Business Systems. James P. Mozena et al. 1999. LC 98-55718. (*0-87389-449-9*) ASQ Qual Pr.

Stop Smoking in a Nutshell. Kevin Brandt. deluxe ltd. ed. 1999. 142p. pap. 29.95 (*1-928813-01-1*) K Brandt.

Stop the Medicine! A Medical Doctor's Miraculous Recovery with Natural Healing. Cynthia A. Foster. 1999. LC 00-500201. 295p. (Orig.). pap. 15.95 (*1-891173-70-7*) Break on Through.

Stop the Nightmares of Trauma: Thought Field Therapy - The Power of Therapy for the 21st Century. Roger J. Callahan & Joanne Callahan. 2000. 334p. pap. 24.95 (*1-57087-505-7*) Prof Pr NC.

Stop the Rollercoaster: How to Take Charge of Your Blood Sugars in Diabetes. John Walsh et al. 1996. (Illus.). 230p. (Orig.). pap. 21.95 (*1-884804-82-9*) Torrey PP.

Stop the Snoring! At Last, End Your Mate's Nocturnal Noise. Ralph Schoenstein. 1997. LC 98-202436. 93p. (Orig.). mass mkt. (*0-446-60460-7*) Warner.

Stop Walking on Eggshells: Taking Your Life Back When Someone You Care about Has Borderline Personality Disorder. Paul T. Mason & Randi Kreger. 1998. LC 97-75479. 240p. pap. 14.95 (*1-57224-108-X*) New Harbinger.

***Stop Your Cravings: A Balanced Approach to Burning Fat, Increasing Energy & Reducing Stress.** Jennifer Workman. 2002. LC 2001-40893. 368p. 25.00 (*0-7432-1705-5*) S&S Trade.

Stop Your Herpes Now. Healthworks Medical Group Staff. 1981. 52p. (Orig.). pap. 4.50 (*0-938480-01-4*) Healthworks.

Stop Your Indigestion: Causes, Remedies, Recipes. Phyllis Avery. 1993. (Illus.). 228p. (Orig.). pap. 14.95 (*1-880598-36-1*) P Avery.

Stop Your Tinnitus: Causes, Preventatives, & Alternatives. Phyllis Avery. 1991. (Illus.). 192p. (Orig.). pap. 14.95 (*1-880598-22-1*) P Avery.

Stoplight Diet for Children: An Eight-Week Program for Parents & Children. Leonard H. Epstein & Sally Squires. 1988. 16.95 (*0-316-24575-5*, Little Brwn Med Div) Lppncott W & W.

Stopping Aids. Kaye Wellings. 1997. 224p. (C). pap. 34.60 (*0-582-29227-1*) Addison-Wesley.

Stopping Anxiety Medication: Panic Control Therapy for Benzodiazepine Discontinuation (PCT-BD) Michael W. Otto et al. 2000. (Illus.). 157p. pap. 32.00 (*0-12-784451-1*); 136p. pap. 26.00 (*0-12-784452-X*) Acad Pr.

Stopping Restless Legs Syndrome. L. E. Mills et al. 2000. LC 00-699667. 64p. pap. 12.95 (*1-887053-16-6*) United Res CA.

Stories for the Third Ear: Using Hypnotic Fables in Psychology. Lee Wallas. 1985. (Professional Bks.). 178p. 20.95 (*0-393-70019-4*) Norton.

Stories from the Heart: Case Studies of Emotional Abuse. Ed. by M. T. Loring. 1997. 200p. 45.00 (*3-7186-0585-6*) Gordon & Breach.

Stories of Hope & Healing: Six Women Confront Breast Cancer. Leslie E. Strong. 1993. 46p. pap. 14.95 (*1-881025-07-1*) Equinox Pr.

Stories of Hospital & Camp. C. E. McKay. 1977. LC 70-37312. (Black Heritage Library Collection). reprint ed. 25.95 (*0-8369-8949-X*) Ayer.

Stories That Heal: Reparenting Adult Children of Dysfunctional Families Using Hypnotic Stories in Psychotherapy. Lee Wallas. 1991. 220p. (C). 22.95 (*0-393-70106-9*) Norton.

Stories the Feet Can Tell Thru Reflexology. Eunice Ingham. rev. ed. 1984. (Illus.). 226p. pap. 11.50 (*0-9611804-3-9*) Ingham Pub.

Stork & the Syringe: A Political History of Reproductive Medicine. Naomi Pfeffer. 1993. LC 93-32897. (Feminist Perspectives Ser.). 244p. pap. 26.95 (*0-7456-1187-7*) Blackwell Pubs.

Storm over Biology: Essays on Science, Sentiment, & Public Policy. Bernard D. Davis. 1986. LC 85-63388. 330p. 36.00 (*0-87975-324-2*) Prometheus Bks.

Story of a Cancer Cure, Bk. I. Thomas B. Caulfield. 1983. LC 83-26160. (Story of a Cancer Cure Ser.: Vol. 1). 224p. lib. bdg. 27.95 (*0-9611788-0-9*) Ctr Adv Psychic Res.

Story of a Mental Hospital: Fulbourn 1858-1983. David H. Clark. 1996. pap. (*1-899209-03-4*) Process Pr GBR. *Dist:* Intl Spec Bk.

Story of Anna O: The Woman Who Led Freud to Psychoanalysis. Lucy Freeman. 1994. LC 94-70015. 282p. pap. 40.00 (*1-56821-226-7*) Aronson.

Story of Blindness. Gabriel Farrell. 1956. LC 56-7212. 280p. 36.50 (*0-674-83940-4*) HUP.

Story of Dentistry. Kenneth Wilson. 1986. 88p. pap. (*0-7223-1989-4*) A H S Ltd GBR. *Dist:* St Mut.

Story of Innovation: The Alexian Village Health Center, Milwaukee. Mark A. Proffitt & Chen-Jui Yang. 1995. (Illus.). xi, 75p. (C). per. 15.00 (*0-938744-86-0*, R94-5) U of Wis Ctr Arch-Urban.

Story of Intermountain Health Care. Tom Vitelli. 1995. (Illus.). 365p. LC 95-76430. 25.00 (*0-9646476-0-5*); pap. 18.00 (*0-9646476-1-3*) Intermtn Hlth Care.

Story of Medicine: Medicine Around the World & Across the Ages. Richard Walker. 2000. (Exploring History Ser.). (Illus.). 64p. (gr. 4-7). 15.00 (*0-7548-0531-X*) Anness Pub.

Story of My Childhood. Clara Barton. Ed. by Annette K. Baxter. 1980. LC 79-8773. (Signal Lives Ser.). (Illus.). reprint ed. lib. bdg. 19.95 (*0-405-12823-1*) Ayer.

Story of Psychology. Morton Hunt. 1994. 784p. pap. 21.00 (*0-385-47149-1*) Doubleday.

Story of Rebirthing. Leonard D. Orr. 1990. 5.00 (*0-945793-08-1*) Inspir Univ.

Story of Taxol: Nature & Politics in the Pursuit of an Anti-Cancer Drug. Jordan Goodman & Vivien Walsh. 2001. LC 00-34230. (Illus.). 296p. (C). text 27.95 (*0-521-56123-X*) Cambridge U Pr.

Story of the NIH Grants Program. Stephen P. Strickland. 1989. LC 88-38887. 110p. (C). 48.00 (*0-8191-7322-3*) U Pr of Amer.

Storymaking & Creative Groupwork with Elderly People. Paula Crimmens. 1997. LC 96-48680. pap. (*1-85302-440-6*) Jessica Kingsley GBR. *Dist:* Taylor & Francis.

Storymaking in Education & Therapy. Alida Gersie & Nancy King. 1990. 416p. 49.50 (*1-85302-519-4*); pap. 29.95 (*1-85302-520-8*) Taylor & Francis.

Storytelling & Conversation: Discourse in Deaf Communities. Ed. by Elizabeth Winston. 1999. LC 00-697710. (Sociolinguistics in Deaf Communities Ser.: Vol. 5). (Illus.). x, 227p. 55.00 (*1-56368-081-5*) Gallaudet Univ Pr.

Storytelling in Psychotherapy with Children. Richard Gardner. 1993. LC 93-14898. 296p. pap. 35.00 (*1-56821-032-9*) Aronson.

Storytelling, Narrative & the Thematic Apperception Test. Phebe Cramer. 1996. LC 96-5520. (Assessment of Personality & Psychopathology Ser.). 374p. text 45.00 (*1-57230-094-9*, 0094) Guilford Pubns.

Strabismus. Julio Prieto-Diaz & Carlos R. Souza-Dias. 4th ed. 1999. LC 99-23502. 554p. text 185.00 (*0-7506-7129-7*) Buttrwrth-Heinemann.

Strabismus: A Neurodevelopmental Approach. J. T. Flynn. 1990. (Nature's Experiment Ser.). (Illus.). 142p. 99.00 (*0-387-97409-1*) Spr-Verlag.

Strabismus & Amblyopia: Experimental Basis for Advances in Clinical Management. Ed. by G. Lennerstrand et al. 1988. (Wenner-Gren International Symposia Ser.: Vol. 49). (Illus.). 452p. 110.00 (*0-306-42943-8*, Plenum Trade) Perseus Pubng.

Strabismus & Amblyopia: Visual Training. Donald J. Getz. rev. ed. 1990. (Introduction to Behavioral Optometry Ser.). (Illus.). 105p. reprint ed. pap. text 18.00 (*0-943599-08-3*) OEPF.

Strabismus & Ocular Motility Disorders. Ed. by Emilio Campos. 1990. text 95.00 (*0-333-51224-3*) Intl Spec Bk.

Strabismus & the Sensorimotor Reflex. Y. Mitsui. 1986. 228p. 100.00 (*4-900392-74-X*) Elsevier.

Strabismus & Tumors of the Uvea. Ed. by H. Saraux. 1981. (Journal: Vol. 182, No. 2). (Illus.). 84p. pap. 38.50 (*3-8055-3418-3*) S Karger.

Strabismus Management. William V. Good et al. 1995. (Illus.). 379p. text 110.00 (*0-7506-9075-5*) Buttrwrth-Heinemann.

Strabismus Symposium, Amsterdam, September 3-4, 1981. A. T. Van Balen & W. A. Houtman. 1982. text 199.50 (*90-6193-728-0*) Kluwer Academic.

Straight Dope on Hormones. Delia Van Maris. Ed. by JoAnn Roberts. 24p. (Orig.). (C). pap. text 4.00 (*1-880715-11-2*) Creat Des Srvs.

Straight from the Heart. Rita Dervin et al. 1990. (Illus.). 64p. pap. text 3.15 (*0-916999-08-4*) HERC Pubng.

Straight from the Heart. Ina L. Yalof. 1996. LC 96-76487. 192p. 20.00 (*1-57566-094-6*, Knsington) Kensgtn Pub Corp.

Straight, Male, Modern: A Cultural Critique of Psychoanalysis. John Brenkman. 1993. LC 93-14035. 320p. (C). pap. 25.95 (*0-415-90218-5*, A3974) Routledge.

Straight Talk about Breast Cancer: From Diagnosis to Recovery. Suzanne Braddock et al. Ed. by Melanie M. Clark. 1994. LC 94-72529. 144p. (Orig.). pap. 12.95 (*1-886039-21-6*) Addicus Bks.

Straight Talk about Psychiatric Medications for Kids. Timothy E. Wilens. 1998. LC 98-7275. (Illus.). 280p. pap. 15.95 (*1-57230-204-6*, C0204) Guilford Pubns.

Straight Talk about Psychiatric Medications for Kids. Timothy E. Wilens & Alden Studebaker. 1998. LC 98-7275. (Illus.). 280p. 33.00 (*1-57230-404-9*) Guilford Pubns.

Straight Talk on Spondylitis. Rodney Bluestone et al. Ed. by Robert L. Swezey et al. 2nd ed. 1993. LC 92-36216. (*1-881941-01-9*) Spondylitis Assn.

Straight Talk on Stuttering: Information, Encouragement & Counsel for Stutterers, Caregivers, & Speech-Language Clinicians. Lloyd M. Hulit. 1996. 278p. 60.95 (*0-398-06591-8*); pap. 39.95 (*0-398-06592-6*) C C Thomas.

Straight Talk with Your Gynecologist: How to Get Answers That Will Save Your Life. Eddie C. Sollie. Ed. by Julie Livingston. 1993. LC 92-42738. 240p. (Orig.). pap. 12.95 (*0-941831-83-3*) Beyond Words Pub.

Straight Wire. Lawrence F. Andrews. Ed. by John Valleau & Julie T. Olfe. 1990. (Illus.). 448p. (C). text 125.00 (*0-9616256-0-0*) L A Wells.

Strains of Human Viruses. Ed. by M. Majer & S. A. Plotkin. 1972. 160p. 85.25 (*3-8055-1401-8*) S Karger.

Stramonium: With an Introduction to Analysis Using Cycles & Segments. Paul Herscu. 1996. LC 96-70061. (Illus.). 239p. (Orig.). pap. 28.00 (*0-9654004-0-9*) New Engld Schl Homeopthy.

Strange Attractors: Chaos, Complexity, & the Art of Family Therapy. Michael R. Butz et al. 1996. LC 96-1600. (Couples & Family Dynamics & Treatment Ser.). 267p. 100.00 (*0-471-07951-0*) Wiley.

Strange Case of T. L. Art by Tony Labat & Fiction by Carlo McCormick. Carlo McCormick. 1995. 56p. 15.00 (*0-9631095-4-5*) Artspace Bks.

Stranger: A Psychological Study of Adolf Hitler. David M. Moriarty. 1993. (Illus.). 302p. (Orig.). pap. text 27.50 (*0-87527-491-9*) Green.

Stranger in My Own Body: Atypical Gender Identity Development & Mental Health. Ed. by David Freedman & Domenico Di Ceglie. 1998. LC 00-500753. 360p. pap. (*1-85575-183-6*) Karnac Bks GBR. *Dist:* Other Pr LLC.

***Stranger in the Mirror: Dissociation: The Secret Epidemic of Our Time.** Marlene Steinberg. 2001. 344p. pap. 14.00 (*0-06-095487-6*, Cliff Street) HarperTrade.

Stranger in the Mirror: Dissociation: The Secret Epidemic of Our Time. Marlene Steinberg. 2000. LC 00-31705. (Illus.). 336p. 25.00 (*0-06-019564-9*, Cliff Street) HarperTrade.

Stranger in Your Bed: A Guide to Emotional Intimacy. Dean C. Dauw. 1979. LC 78-23444. 120p. text 25.95 (*0-88229-472-5*) Burnham Inc.

Stranger on the Planet: The Small Book of Laurie. Claire Burch. 1997. 175p. pap. 10.00 (*0-916147-67-3*) Regent Pr.

Stranger Than Fiction: When Our Minds Betray Us. Marc D. Feldman et al. 1998. LC 97-5481. 320p. 24.95 (*0-88048-930-8*, 8930) Am Psychiatric.

Strangers at the Bedside: A History of How Law & Bioethics Transformed Medical Decision-Making. David J. Rothman. 1992. LC 90-55598. 320p. pap. 20.00 (*0-465-08210-6*) Basic.

Strategic Alignment: Managing Integrated Health Systems. Ed. by Douglas A. Conrad & Geoffrey A. Hoare. 1993. LC 93-34353. 303p. (Orig.). (C). pap. text 20.00 (*1-56793-003-4*, 0937) Health Admin Pr.

***Strategic Application of Information Technology in Health Care Organizations.** John Glaser. 2nd ed. 2002. LC 2001-38581. (Jossey-Bass Health Ser.). 208p. 65.00 (*0-7879-5987-1*) Wiley

Strategic Approaches in Coronary Intervention. Stephen Ellis & David Holmes. 2nd ed. 1999. LC 99-33460. (Illus.). 640p. text 125.00 (*0-683-30729-0*) Lppncott W & W.

Strategic Assessment of U. S., Japanese & Canadian Healthcare. Ed. by Frost and Sullivan Staff. 1995. 413p. spiral bd. 1295.00 (*0-7889-0262-8*, 5243-59) Frost & Sullivan.

Strategic Brief Therapy. Giorgio Nardone. 2001. LC 00-56939. 30.00 (*0-7657-0280-0*) Aronson.

Strategic Choices for a Changing Health Care System. Ed. by Stuart H. Altman & Uwe E. Reinhardt. 1996. LC 96-2630. (Baxter Health Policy Review Ser.: Vol. 2). 413p. 54.00 (*1-56793-040-9*, 0975) Health Admin Pr.

Strategic Family Therapy. Cloe Madanes. 1991. LC 80-26286. (Social & Behavioral Science Ser.). 272p. pap. 28.00 (*1-55542-363-9*) Jossey-Bass.

Strategic Financial Planning for Healthcare Organizations: An Executive Guide to Capital Debt. Christopher T. Payne. 1994. 300p. (C). text 60.00 (*1-55738-615-3*, Irwn Prfssnl) McGraw-Hill Educ Grp.

Strategic Health Planning: Methods - Techniques Applied to Marketing - Management. Allen D. Spiegel & Herbert H. Hyman. Ed. by Glenn R. Caddy. 1991. (Developments in Clinical Psychology Ser.). 544p. (C). pap. 49.50 (*0-89391-892-X*, Ablex) Greenwood.

Strategic Health Planning: Methods & Techniques Applied to Marketing - Management. Allen D. Spiegel & Herbert H. Hyman. Ed. by Glenn R. Caddy. 1991. (Developments in Clinical Psychology Ser.). 544p. (C). 130.00 (*0-89391-742-7*, Ablex) Greenwood.

Strategic Issues in Health Care Management. Ed. by Mo Malek et al. 1993. 298p. 181.95 (*0-471-93964-1*) Wiley.

Strategic Leadership for Medical Groups: Navigating Your Strategic Web. John D. Blair & Myron D. Fottler. 1998. LC 97-50436. 238p. 50.00 (*0-7879-0853-3*) Jossey-Bass.

Strategic Management for Health Care Entities: Creative Frameworks for Financial & Operational Analysis. Thomas R. Prince. 1998. LC 98-9419. 543p. 100.00 (*1-55648-214-0*) AHPI.

Strategic Management of Behavioral Problems. Mary M. Kerr & Michael C. Nelson. 3rd ed. 1997. LC 97-15169. 447p. pap. text 70.00 (*0-02-363527-4*, Macmillan Coll) P-H.

Strategic Management of Health Care Organizations. W. Jack Duncan et al. 3rd ed. 1997. LC 97-12153. (Illus.). 960p. text 79.95 (*1-55786-968-5*) Blackwell Pubs.

***Strategic Management of Health Care Organizations.** Peter M. Ginter et al. 4th ed. 2002. LC 2001-37504. 960p. 89.95 (*0-631-22586-2*) Blackwell Pubs.

Strategic Management of Human Resources in Health Services Organizations. Myron D. Fottler et al. 1989. LC 87-34059. (Health Services Ser.). 454p. text 47.50 (*0-8273-4240-3*) Delmar.

Strategic Marketing: How to Achieve Independence & Prosperity in Your Mental Health Practice. Kalman M. Heller. 1997. LC 97-25932. 160p. (Orig.). pap. 26.45 (*1-56887-031-0*, SMBP, Prof Resc Pr) Pro Resource.

Strategic Plan to Combat HIV & AIDS in the U. S. 1993. (Illus.). 52p. (Orig.). (C). pap. text 20.00 (*1-56806-188-9*) DIANE Pub.

Strategic Planning in Health Care: A Guide for Board Members. Ernst and Young Staff et al. 1994. LC 94-33244. 140p. pap. 40.00 (*1-55648-127-6*, 196130) AHPI.

Strategic Planning in Healthcare: Building a Quality-Based Plan Step by Step. Bernard J. Horak. 1997. LC 96-53418. 175p. 42.50 (*0-527-76314-4*) Product Pr.

Strategic Planning Workbook. American Hospital Association Staff. 1989. (Illus.). 114p. 60.00 (*0-87258-520-4*, 184205) Am Hospital.

Strategies. Wyatt Woodsmall. 1998. (Advanced Neuro Linguistic Programming Applications Ser.). 100p. spiral bd. 35.00 (*1-892876-04-3*) Next Step Pr.

Strategies & Environments of America's Small, Rural Hospitals: A Report on a Study Funded by the Pew Charitable Trusts. John W. Seavey et al. 1992. LC 92-7079. (Illus.). 336p. (Orig.). pap. text 29.95 (*0-87258-623-5*, 184160) Am Hospital.

S

Strategies for Analyzing Neuropeptide Systems. Ed. by R. M. Dores & T. C. Stevenson. 1993. (Journal: Vol. 3, No. 3-4, 1993). (Illus.). 88p. pap. 75.75 (*3-8055-5803-1*) S Karger.

Strategies for Assessing the Safety of Foods Produced by Biotechnology: Report of a Joint FAO-WHO Consultation. 1991. (ENG, FRE & SPA.). iv, 59p. pap. text 11.00 (*92-4-156145-9*, 1150369) World Health.

Strategies for Developing Primary Care in the South Bronx. Kathryn Haslanger. 1993. 50p. pap. 10.00 (*0-934459-96-7*) United Hosp Fund.

Strategies for Immunointerventions in Dermatology. Ed. by Gunter Burg & Richard G. Dummer. 1997. LC 97-8062. (Illus.). 418p. 142.00 (*3-540-62680-8*) Spr-Verlag.

Strategies for Integrated Health Care: Emerging Practices in Information Management & Cross-Continuum Care. Ed. by Erica Drazen & Jane Metzger. 1998. LC 98-40134. (Business & Management Ser.). 256p. 52.00 (*0-7879-4159-X*) Jossey-Bass.

Strategies for Integrating Substance Abuse Treatment & the Juvenile Justice System: A Practical Guide. Laura Burney-Nissen. 2000. 239p. (C). pap. text 35.00 (*0-7567-0166-X*) DIANE Pub.

Strategies for Long-Term Care. 1988. 528p. pap. 13.50 (*0-88737-413-1*, 20-2231) Natl League Nurse.

***Strategies for Nursing Leadership.** Harriet R. Feldman. 2001. LC 00-69815. 296p. (*0-8261-1414-8*) Springer Pub.

Strategies for Organic Drug Synthesis & Design. Daniel Lednicer. 1997. LC 97-11813. 500p. 99.50 (*0-471-19657-6*) Wiley.

Strategies for Primary Health Care: Technologies Appropriate for the Control of Disease in the Developing World. Ed. by Julia A. Walsh & Kenneth S. Warren. 1986. LC 86-50118. (Studies in Infectious Disease Research). xii, 344p. lib. bdg. 42.00 (*0-226-87207-6*) U Ch Pr.

***Strategies for Public Mental Health Workforce Development.** Barry Leonard. 2001. 54p. (C). reprint ed. pap. text 20.00 (*0-7567-0610-6*) DIANE Pub.

Strategies for Resolving Individual & Family Problems. Fred W. Vondracek & Sherry Corneal. 1994. LC 94-21195. (Counseling Ser.). 512p. 91.95 (*0-534-25470-5*) Brooks-Cole.

Strategies for Selecting & Verifying Hearing Aid Fittings. Ed. by Michael Valente. 1994. LC 93-33542. 52.00 (*0-86577-500-1*) Thieme Med Pubs.

Strategies for Short-Term Testing for Mutagens-Carcinogens. Byron E. Butterworth. 1979. 160p. 87.00 (*0-8493-5661-X*, QH465, CRC Reprint) Franklin.

Strategies for Stroke Prevention: Sanofi Wintrop Symposium to the Third European Stroke Conference, Stockholm, May 1994. Ed. by J. Bogousslavsky & H. P. Adams. 1995. (Journal: Vol. 4, Suppl. 4, 1994). (Illus.). iv, 38p. pap. 21.75 (*3-8055-6073-7*) S Karger.

Strategies for Studying Suicide & Suicidal Behavior. Ed. by Irma S. Lann et al. 1989. 164p. 20.95 (*0-89862-383-9*) Guilford Pubns.

Strategies for Success in Biotechnology As Applied to the Healthcare Industry. Kewal Jain. Ed. by Susan C. DiClemente. 1997. (Illus.). 225p. spiral bd. 1195.00 (*1-57936-079-3*) Drug & Market Dev.

Strategies for Success in Coaching: A Sports Medicine Paradigm. C. Douglas Clinger et al. 1992. LC 91-36524. (*0-87949-366-6*) Ashley Bks.

Strategies for Supporting Classroom Success: Focus on Communication - an Audio Workshop. Ed. by Nickola W. Nelson & Barbara Hoskins. 1997. (School-Age Children Ser.). (Illus.). 132p. (Orig.). pap. 156.95 (*1-56593-810-0*, 1586) Singular Publishing.

Strategies for Teaching At-Risk & Handicapped Infants & Toddlers. Sharon A. Raver. 1991. LC 90-46743. 460p. (C). text 73.00 (*0-675-21202-2*, Merrill Coll) P-H.

Strategies for Teaching Nursing. Rheba De Tornyay & Martha A. Thompson. 3rd ed. 1989. LC 86-19060. 353p. (C). mass mkt. 35.50 (*0-8273-4228-4*) Delmar.

Strategies for the Chemoprevention of Prostate Cancer. Ed. by C. C. Schulman & G. J. Kelloff. 1999. LC 99-232361. (European Urology Ser.: Vol. 35, No. 5-6, 1999). (Illus.). iv, 156p. 77.50 (*3-8055-6866-5*) S Karger.

Strategies for the New Health Care Marketplace: Managing the Convergence of Consumerism & Technology. Dean C. Coddington et al. 2001. LC 00-12247. (Jossey-Bass Health Ser.). (Illus.). 448p. 50.00 (*0-7879-5593-0*) Jossey-Bass.

Strategies for the Prevention of Blindness in National Programmes: A Primary Health Care Approach. 2nd ed. 1997. (Illus.). 104p. pap. 25.20 (*92-4-154492-9*, 1152223) Am Soc Clinical.

Strategies for the Treatment of Hepatobiliary Disease. Ed. by G. Paumgartner et al. 1990. (Falk Symposium Ser.). (C). text 138.00 (*0-7923-8903-4*) Kluwer Academic.

Strategies for Theory Construction in Nursing. Lorraine W. Walker & Kay C. Avant. 3rd ed. 1994. LC 94-7951. 240p. (C). pap. 59.00 (*0-8385-8688-0*, A8688-2) P-H.

Strategies for Therapy with the Elderly: Living with Hope & Meaning. Claire M. Brody & Vicki G. Semel. 1993. LC 93-3273. 200p. 32.95 (*0-8261-8010-8*) Springer Pub.

Strategies in Genetic Counseling: The Challenge of the Future. Ed. by Susie Ball. 1988. (National Society of Genetic Counselors Ser.: Vol. 1). 216p. 35.95 (*0-89885-388-5*, Kluwer Acad Hman Sci) Kluwer Academic.

Strategies in Genetic Counseling - Tools for Professional Advancement, Vol. 2. Ed. by N. J. Zellers. 1989. (National Society of Genetic Counselors Ser.). (Illus.). 236p. 38.00 (*0-89885-450-4*, Kluwer Acad Hman Sci) Kluwer Academic.

Strategies in Gynecologic Surgery. Ed. by Herbert J. Buchsbaum & L. A. Walton. 1986. (Clinical Perspectives in Obstetrics & Gynecology Ser.). (Illus.). 231p. 135.00 (*0-387-96278-6*) Spr-Verlag.

Strategies in Primary & Secondary Prevention of Coronary Artery Disease. Ed. by T. Ischinger & H. Gohlke. 1992. (Illus.). 304p. text (*3-88603-440-2*) W Zuckschwerdt DEU. *Dist:* Scholium Intl.

Strategies in Vaccine Design. Ed. by Gordon L. Ada. 1994. LC 93-46422. (Medical Intelligence Unit Ser.). 232p. 99.00 (*1-57059-094-X*, LN9094) Landes Bioscience.

Strategies of Adjuvant Therapy. John M. Kirkwood. 2000. (Illus.). 240p. (*1-85317-317-7*) Martin Dunitz GBR. *Dist:* Blackwell Sci.

Strategies of European OTC Pharmaceuticl Markets. Ed. by Frost and Sullivan Staff. 1997. 368p. spiral bd. 3950.00 (*0-7889-0721-2*, 3205-59) Frost & Sullivan.

Strategies of Intervention with Public Offenders. Ed. by Sol Chaneles. 1982. LC 82-15383. (Journal of Offender Counseling, Services & Rehabilitation: Vol. 6, Nos. 1-2). 137p. pap. text 19.95 (*0-86656-171-4*) Haworth Pr.

Strategies of Microsurgery in Problematic Brain Areas: With Special Reference to NMR. Wolfgang Seeger. 1990. 398p. 195.00 (*3-211-82189-9*) Spr-Verlag.

Strategies of Microsurgery in Problematic Brain Areas with Special Reference to NMR. Wolfgang Seeger. 1990. (Illus.). 398p. 214.00 (*0-387-82189-9*) Spr-Verlag.

Strategies of Psychotherapy. Jay Haley. 1963. LC 63-16660. 216p. text 29.95 (*0-8089-0168-0*, 791825, Grune & Strat) Harcrt Hlth Sci Grp.

Strategies to Protect the Health of Deployed U. S. Forces: Analytical Framework for Assessing Risks. Lorenz Rhomberg. 2000. LC 00-269890. xiv, 113p. 29.75 (*0-309-06895-9*) Natl Acad Pr.

Strategies to Protect the Health of Deployed U. S. Forces: Detecting, Characterizing & Documenting Exposures. National Research Council Staff et al. 2000. LC 00-698252. (Illus.). xxviii, 242p. pap. 73.25 (*0-309-06875-4*) Natl Acad Pr.

Strategy & Architecture of Health Care Information Systems. Michael K. Bourke. 1996. LC 93-27727. (Computers in Health Care Ser.). (Illus.). 356p. 69.95 (*0-387-97982-4*) Spr-Verlag.

Strategy Book for Health Care Compliance Officers. Ed. by Nina Youngstrom & Mark J. Pastin. 1999. 370p. pap. 273.00 (*0-929156-69-2*) Atlantic Info Services Inc.

Strategy Development Workshop for Public Education on Weight & Obesity: Summary Report. 1995. 139p. (Orig.). (C). pap. text 30.00 (*0-7881-2467-6*) DIANE Pub.

Strategy for a Loss of Faith: Jung's Proposal. John P. Dourley. 1992. (Studies in Jungian Psychology by Jungian Analysts: Vol. 56). 144p. pap. (*0-919123-57-0*) Inner City Bks CAN. *Dist:* BookWorld.

Strategy for Research in Space Biology & Medicine into the Next Century. National Research Council Staff. 1998. LC 98-86544. 296p. pap. text 49.00 (*0-309-06047-8*) Natl Acad Pr.

Strategy in Head Injury Management. Richard H. Simon & James T. Sayre. 1992. 214p. (C). pap. text 65.00 (*0-8385-8682-1*, A8682-5, Apple Lange Med) McGraw.

Strategy of a Megamerger: An Insider's Account of the Baxter Travenol-American Hospital Supply Combination. Thomas G. Cody. 1992. LC 92-30382. pap. 23.95 (*0-275-94518-9*, B4518, Praeger Pubs) Greenwood.

Strategy of Preventive Medicine. Geoffrey Rose. 1994. (Illus.). 150p. reprint ed. pap. text 32.50 (*0-19-262486-5*) OUP.

Stratified Process Model for Planning & Designing in Psychoanalytic Therapy Research. Bengt J. Eriksson. 1989. (Studia Psychologica Clinica Upsaliensia: No. 1). (Illus.). 592p. (Orig.). pap. 77.50 (*91-554-2408-2*) Coronet Bks.

Stratum Corneum. Ed. by R. M. Marks & Gerd Plewig. 1983. (Illus.). 265p. 68.95 (*0-387-11704-0*) Spr-Verlag.

Strauss & Welt's Diseases of the Kidney: Roche Edition Lawrence E. Earley. 1980. 1. 8.88 (*0-316-20316-5*); 2. 8.87 (*0-316-20317-3*) Little.

Strauss's Pharmacy Law Examination Review - Florida. Steven Strauss. 5th ed. 1999. 388p. pap. text 85.00 (*0-9625324-8-7*) Strauss Pub.

Strauss's Pharmacy Law Examination Review - New Jersey. Steven Strauss. 4th ed. 1999. 339p. (C). pap. text 85.00 (*0-9625324-9-5*) Strauss Pub.

Street Addict Role: A Theory of Heroin Addiction. Richard C. Stephens. 1991. LC 90-39205. (SUNY Series, the New Inequalities). 223p. (C). text 64.50 (*0-7914-0619-9*); pap. text 22.95 (*0-7914-0620-2*) State U NY Pr.

Street Drugs: A Reference Guide to Controlled Substances. Carl L. Vidano. Ed. by Kenneth M. Goddard. 1986. (Illus.). 100p. (Orig.). pap. text 10.95 (*0-9616606-0-0*) C L Vidano Pub.

Street Drugs: The Facts Explained, the Myths Exploded. Andrew Tyler. 1996. 518p. mass mkt. (*0-340-60975-3*) Hodder & Stought Ltd GBR. *Dist:* Lubrecht & Cramer, Trafalgar.

***Street Medicine Medical Hazmat Series** EMEDIA Staff. 1996. tchr. ed. 299.00 incl. VHS (*0-8151-3553-X*) Mosby Inc.

Street Scenarios for the EMT & Paramedic. Brent Braunworth & Albert L. Howe. Ed. by Laurence W. Schlanger. 1993. LC 93-14345. 256p. pap. text 49.00 (*0-89303-976-4*) P-H.

Streetmedic's Handbook. Owen T. Traynor et al. 1995. LC 95-13932. (Illus.). 503p. (C). pap. text 26.95 (*0-8036-0012-7*) Thomson Learn.

Streetsense: Communication, Safety & Control. Kate B. Dernocoeur. 3rd rev. ed. 1996. LC 96-31540. (Illus.). 330p. pap. 22.95 (*0-938106-21-X*) Laing Res Servs.

Streetwise! Practical Risk Management for Practicing Physicians. Rosemary Gafner. 1992. 101p. stu. ed. 45.00 (*1-884269-00-1*) Med Risk Mgmt.

Streetwise Guide to Chinese Herbal Medicine. Martha Dahlen & Wong Kang Ying. 1996. (Illus.). pap. 11.95 (*962-7316-02-4*) China Bks.

Strength & Compassion in Kidney Failure: Writings of Mildred (Barry) Friedman Professional Kidney Patients. Eli A. Friedman & Belding H. Scribner. 1998. 248p. 39.00 (*0-7923-5236-X*) Kluwer Academic.

Strength Training for Preventive Medicine. Denton Smith & E. Leslie Knight. 1994. (*0-929736-16-8*) ISC Div Wellness.

***Strength Training for Strong Bones: A Step-by-Step Program to Prevent Osteoporosis & Stay Fit & Active for Life.** Susie Dinan & Joan Basset. 2001. (Illus.). 96p. pap. 21.95 (*0-06-095926-6*, HarpRes) HarpInfo.

Strengthen Your Immune System! Gun Agell. 1994. 180p. pap. (*0-9640299-0-1*) G Agell.

Strengthening Family Resilience. Froma Walsh. 1998. LC 98-8527. (Guilford Family Therapy Ser.). 338p. 37.00 (*1-57230-408-1*, C0408) Guilford Pubns.

Strengthening Geriatric Nursing Education. Ed. by Terry Fulmer & Marianne Matzo. 1995. LC 95-2116. (Illus.). 200p. 33.95 (*0-8261-8940-7*) Springer Pub.

Strengthening Health Management in Districts & Provinces. Andrew Cassels & Katja Janovsky. 1995. (FRE & SPA.). vi, 75p. (C). pap. text 20.00 (*92-4-154483-X*, 1150428) World Health.

Strengthening Maternal & Child Health Programmes Through Primary Health Care: Guidelines for Countries of the Eastern Mediterranean Region. 1991. (WHO EMRO Technical Publications: No. 18). 75p. pap. text 3.00 (*92-9021-131-8*, 1450018) World Health.

***Strengthening Medicare for Future Generations: Congressional Hearing.** William M. Thomas. 2001. 91p. (C). reprint ed. pap. text 20.00 (*0-7567-1489-3*) DIANE Pub.

Strengthening Ministries of Health for Primary Health Care: Report of a WHO Expert Committee. 1988. (Technical Report Ser.: No. 766). 110p. pap. text 12.00 (*92-4-120766-3*, 1100766) World Health.

Strengthening Research in Academic OB-GYN Departments. Institute of Medicine Staff. Ed. by Jessica Townsend. 1992. LC 92-70987. 320p. pap. text 30.00 (*0-309-04697-1*, RG648) Natl Acad Pr.

Strengthening Stepfamilies. Elizabeth A. Einstein & Linda Albert. 1986. pap., tchr. ed. 45.95 (*0-88671-218-1*, 6471) Am Guidance.

Strengths Model: Case Management with People Suffering from Severe & Persistent Mental Illness. Charles A. Rapp. 1997. LC 96-50963. (Illus.). 240p. (C). pap. 41.95 (*0-19-511444-2*) OUP.

Streptococcal & Staphylococcal Infections: Proceedings of the WHO Expert Committee, Geneva, 1967. WHO Staff. 1968. (Technical Reports: No. 394). 56p. pap. text 5.00 (*92-4-120394-3*, 1100394) World Health.

Streptococcal Infections: Clinical Aspects, Microbiology & Molecular Pathogenesis. Ed. by Dennis L. Stevens & Edward L. Kaplan. 2000. LC 98-55466. (Illus.). 474p. text 98.50 (*0-19-509921-4*) OUP.

Streptococci & the Host: Proceedings of the XIIIth Lancefield International Symposium Held in Paris, France, September 16-20, 1996. Ed. by Thea Horaud et al. 1997. LC 97-13635. (Advances in Experimental Medicine & Biology Ser.: Vol. 418). 1094p. 195.00 (*0-306-45603-6*, Kluwer Plenum) Kluwer Academic.

Streptokinase Treatment in Chronic Arterial Occlusions & Stenoses. Ed. by Michael Martin. 1982. 208p. 120.00 (*0-8493-5046-8*, RC694, CRC Reprint) Franklin.

Stress. Greg Wilkinson. 1999. LC 98-44062. (DK Medical Guides Ser.). 6.95 (*0-7894-4165-9*) DK Pub Inc.

Stress: A Nutritional Approach. Louise Tenney. 1997. (Woodland Health Ser.: No. 5). 32p. pap. 3.95 (*0-913923-32-X*) Woodland UT.

Stress: Causes & Symptoms & the Use of Herbs, Vitamins & Minerals & Diet to Fight Stress. 1991. lib. bdg. 79.95 (*0-8490-5107-X*) Gordon Pr.

Stress: Conceptual & Biological Aspects. Fredrick Toates & Milton Keynes. 1996. LC 95-10939. 352p. 215.00 (*0-471-96021-7*) Wiley.

Stress: From Synapse to Syndrome. Ed. by S. Clare Stanford et al. 1993. (Illus.). 376p. text 100.00 (*0-12-663370-3*) Acad Pr.

Stress: Handbook of Psychology & Health, Vol. 5. Ed. by Andrew Baum & Jerome E. Singer. 1987. 352p. text 79.95 (*0-89859-209-7*) L Erlbaum Assocs.

Stress: Neurobiology & Neuroendocrinology. Ed. by Marvin Brown et al. 1990. (Illus.). 720p. text 250.00 (*0-8247-8325-5*) Dekker.

Stress: Neurochemical & Humoral Mechanisms: Proceedings of the 4th Symposium on Catecholamines & Other Neurotransmitters in Stress, Czechoslovakia, June 1987, Set. Ed. by Glen R. Van Loon. 1989. liv, 1074p. text 633.00 (*2-88124-339-8*) Gordon & Breach.

Stress: Neuroendocrine & Molecular Approaches, Vols. 1 & 2. 1992. LC 91-46587. Lii, 1044p. text 330.00 (*2-88124-506-4*) Gordon & Breach.

Stress: Perspectives & Processes. Dean Bartlett. 1998. LC 98-14536. (Health Psychology Ser.). (*0-335-19928-3*); 192p. pap. (*0-335-19927-5*) OpUniv Pr.

Stress: Physiological & Psychological Aspects: A Source Guide. 1991. lib. bdg. 76.00 (*0-8490-4902-4*) Gordon Pr.

Stress: The Nature & History of Engineered Grief. Robert Kugelmann. 1992. LC 92-8381. 224p. 67.00 (*0-275-94271-6*, C4271, Praeger Pubs) Greenwood.

Stress: The Role of Catecholamines & Other Neurotransmitters, Set. Earl Usdin et al. 1984. lx, 1100p. text 585.00 (*2-88124-102-6*) Gordon & Breach.

Stress: Theory & Practice. King. 1985. text 33.95 (*0-8089-1874-5*, Grune & Strat) Harcrt Hlth Sci Grp.

Stress Vol. I: The Cause of Disease. Ingrid Naiman. 5th ed. 1997. (Astrology of Healing Ser.). (Illus.). 274p. reprint ed. pap. 35.00 (*1-882834-01-1*) Seventh Ray.

Stress - Basis Mechanisms & Clinical Implications: Proceedings of the First World Congress on Stress, Held October 2-7, 1994, Vol. 771. Ed. by George P. Chrousos et al. 1995. pap. 165.00 (*0-89766-944-4*) NY Acad Sci.

Stress A-Z: A Sourcebook for Facing Everyday Challenges. Ada P. Kahn. 1998. LC 97-51580. 400p. 40.00 (*0-8160-3295-5*, Checkmark) Facts on File.

Stress among Older Adults: Understanding & Coping. James H. Humphrey. 1992. 172p. (C). text 39.95 (*0-398-05790-7*) C C Thomas.

Stress & Adaptation in the Context of Culture: Depression in a Southern Black Community. William W. Dressler. 1991. LC 89-26307. 354p. (C). pap. text 24.95 (*0-7914-0414-5*) State U NY Pr.

Stress & Addiction. Edward Gottheil et al. 1987. LC 87-7987. (Psychosocial Stress Ser.: No. 9). 352p. 49.95 (*0-87630-463-3*) Brunner-Routledge.

Stress & Adversity over the Life Course: Trajectories & Turning Points. Ed. by Ian H. Gotlib & Blair Wheaton. 1997. (Illus.). 311p. (C). text 52.95 (*0-521-55075-0*) Cambridge U Pr.

Stress & Anxiety. Ed. by Charles D. Spielberger et al. (Clinical & Community Psychology Ser.). Vol. 9. 1985. LC 74-28292. (Illus.). 283p. text 68.95 (*0-89116-310-7*); Vol. 11. 1988. 258p. 78.95 (*0-89116-312-3*) Hemisp Pub.

Stress & Anxiety, Vol. 12. Ed. by Charles D. Spielberger & Irwin G. Sarason. 1989. (Clinical & Community Psychology Ser.). 360p. 78.95 (*0-89116-890-7*) Hemisp Pub.

Stress & Anxiety, Vol. 13. Ed. by Charles D. Spielberger et al. 1990. (Clinical & Community Psychology Ser.). 336p. 89.95 (*1-56032-139-3*) Hemisp Pub.

Stress & Anxiety, Vol. 10: A Sourcebook of Theory & Research, Vol. 10. Ed. by Charles D. Spielberger & Irwin G. Sarason. 1986. (Clinical & Community Psychology Ser.). (Illus.). 450p. pap. 36.95 (*0-89116-460-X*) Hemisp Pub.

Stress & Burnout among Providers Caring for the Terminally Ill & Their Families. Ed. & Intro. by Lenora F. Paridis. 1988. LC 87-25949. (Hospice Journal: Vol. 3, Nos. 2-3). 276p. text 39.95 (*0-86656-674-0*) Haworth Pr.

Stress & Common Gastrointestinal Disorders: A Comprehensive Approach, 3. Gerhard Dotevall. 1985. LC 85-6565. (Gastroenterology Ser.: Vol. 3). 192p. 67.00 (*0-275-91310-4*, C1310, Praeger Pubs) Greenwood.

Stress & Coping Across Development. Tiffany M. Field et al. 1988. 288p. 59.95 (*0-89859-960-1*) L Erlbaum Assocs.

Stress & Coping in Child Health. Ed. by Annette M. La Greca et al. 1991. LC 91-38224. (Advances in Pediatric Psychology Ser.). 413p. 46.95 (*0-89862-112-7*) Guilford Pubns.

Stress & Coping in Later-Life Families. Mary A. Stephens et al. 1990. (Series in Applied Psychology: Social Issues & Questions). 304p. 66.95 (*0-89116-928-8*) Hemisp Pub.

Stress & Coping in Mental Health. Carson. 1994. 221p. pap. 41.50 (*1-56593-330-3*, 0660) Singular Publishing.

***Stress & Coping in Mental Health Nursing.** Carson. 1994. pap. (*0-412-59270-3*) Chapman & Hall.

Stress & Coping in Nursing. Roy Bailey & Margaret Clarke. 1990. 352p. pap. 32.50 (*0-412-33830-0*, A4441) Chapman & Hall.

Stress & Disease Processes: Perspectives in Behavioral Medicine. Ed. by Andrew Baum et al. 1992. (Advances in Behavioral Medicine Ser.). 328p. text 69.95 (*0-8058-1161-3*) L Erlbaum Assocs.

Stress & Emotion, Vol. 14. Ed. by Charles D. Spielberger et al. 1991. (Series in Stress & Emotion: Anxiety, Anger, & Curiosity). 340p. 99.95 (*1-56032-187-3*) Hemisp Pub.

Stress & Emotional Health: Applications of Clinical Anthropology. John A. Rush. 1999. LC 99-11414. (Illus.). 232p. 72.50 (*0-86569-290-4*, T290); pap. 22.95 (*0-86569-291-2*, T290) Greenwood (Auburn Hse).

Stress & Health. Rice. 3rd ed. 1998. LC 98-7726. (Psychology Ser.). 498p. pap. text 50.95 (*0-534-26502-2*) Brooks-Cole.

Stress & Health: A Reversal Theory Perspective. Sven Svebak & Michael J. Apter. 1997. LC 96-28946. (Health Psychology & Behavioral Medicine Ser.). 215p. 69.95 (*1-56032-473-2*) Taylor & Francis.

Stress & Health: A Reversal Theory Perspective. Sven Svebek & Michael J. Apter. 1997. LC 96-28946. (Health Psychology & Behavioral Medicine Ser.). pap. 29.95 (*1-56032-474-0*) Taylor & Francis.

Stress & Health: Biological & Psychological Interactions. William R. Lovallo. 1997. (Behavioral Medicine & Health Psychology Ser.: Vol. 1). 224p. 76.95 (*0-8039-7000-5*, 2911) Sage.

Stress & Health: Principles & Practice for Coping & Wellness. Phillip L. Rice. 1987. LC 86-26875. (Psychology Ser.). 380p. (C). mass mkt. 21.25 (*0-534-07608-4*) Brooks-Cole.

Stress & Health among the Elderly. Ed. by May L. Wykle et al. 1992. LC 91-4873. 280p. 36.95 (*0-8261-7320-9*) Springer Pub.

Stress & Heart Disease. Ed. by R. E. Beamish et al. 1985. (Developments in Cardiovascular Medicine Ser.). text 146.50 (*0-89838-709-4*) Kluwer Academic.

Stress & Human Performance. Ed. by James E. Driskell & Eduardo Salas. 1996. LC 96-3785. (Applied Psychology Ser.). 360p. text 65.00 (*0-8058-1182-6*) L Erlbaum Assocs.

Stress & Hypertension. Ed. by J. Bahlmann & H. Liebau. 1982. (Contributions to Nephrology Ser.: Vol. 30). (Illus.). xiv, 206p. pap. 29.75 (*3-8055-3450-7*) S Karger.

Stress & Immunity. Nicholas P. Plotnikoff et al. 1991. (Illus.). 528p. lib. bdg. 129.00 (*0-8493-8845-7*, QP82) CRC Pr.

Stress & Its Management by Yoga. Ed. by K. N. Udupa & R. C. Prasad. 1999. 395p. pap. (*81-208-0052-4*); reprint ed. (*81-208-0000-1*) Motilal Bnarsidass IND. *Dist:* S Asia, St Mut.

Stress & Mental Health: Contemporary Issues & Prospects for the Future. Ed. by W. R. Avison & I. Gotlib. 1994. (Stress & Coping Ser.). (Illus.). 358p. (C). 52.50 (*0-306-44687-1*, Plenum Trade) Perseus Pubng.

Stress & Nervous Disorders. Jan De Vries. 1998. (By Appointment Only Ser.). 126p. pap. (*1-85158-651-2*) Mainstream Pubng GBR. *Dist:* Trafalgar.

Stress & Organizational Problems in Hospitals. Ed. by Don Wallis & Charles J. De Wolff. 1988. 256p. 49.95 (*0-7099-5255-4*) Routledge.

Stress & Performance Effectiveness Vol. 3: Stress & Performance Effectiveness. Ed. by Earl A. Alluisi & Edwin A. Fleishman. 1982. (Human Performance & Productivity Ser.). 288p. text 69.95 (*0-89859-091-4*) L Erlbaum Assocs.

Stress & Pregnancy. John J. Sullivan & Joyce C Foster. 1990. LC 86-82022. (Stress in Modern Society Ser.: No. 8). 32.50 (*0-404-63261-0*) AMS Pr.

Stress & Productivity. Ed. by Leonard W. Krinsky et al. 1984. LC 83-22606. (Problems of Industrial Psychiatric Medicine Ser.: Vol. 9). 176p. 35.95 (*0-89885-137-8*, Kluwer Acad Hman Sci) Kluwer Academic.

Stress & Recovery. Patricia Hoolihan. 1984. 24p. (Orig.). (C). pap. 2.00 (*0-89486-236-7*, 1414B) Hazelden.

Stress & Satisfaction on the Job: Work Meanings & Coping of Mid-Career Men. Patricia E. Benner. 1984. LC 84-3252. 203p. 62.50 (*0-275-91127-6*, C1127, Praeger Pubs) Greenwood.

Stress & Tension Control, Vol. 2. Ed. by Frank J. McGuigan et al. 1985. 420p. 85.00 (*0-306-41815-0*, Plenum Trade) Perseus Pubng.

Stress & Tension Control Vol. 3: Stress Management. Ed. by Frank J. McGuigan et al. 1989. (Illus.). 298p. (C). 114.00 (*0-306-43327-3*, Plenum Trade) Perseus Pubng.

Stress & the Blood System. P. D. Gorizontov et al. 1989. LC 88-13625. 250p. 35.00 (*0-8236-6162-8*) Intl Univs Pr.

Stress & the Family Vol. I: Coping with Normative Transitions. Ed. by Hamilton I. McCubbin & Charles R. Figley. 1983. LC 83-6048. (Psychosocial Stress Ser.: No. 2). 296p. text 35.95 (*0-87630-321-1*) Brunner-Routledge.

Stress & the Family Vol. II: Coping with Catastrophe, Vol. 2. Ed. by Charles R. Figley & Hamilton I. McCubbin. 1983. LC 83-6048. (Psychosocial Stress Ser.: No. 2). 272p. text 35.95 (*0-87630-332-7*) Brunner-Routledge.

Stress & the Healthy Family. Dolores Curran. 1985. 192p. 13.95 (*0-86683-863-5*) Harper SF.

***Stress & the Heart: Psychosocial Pathways to Coronary Heart Disease.** Ed. by Stephen A. Stansfield & Michael G. Marmot. 2001. 328p. pap. (*0-7279-1277-1*) BMJ Pub GBR. *Dist:* AIDC.

Stress & the Heart: Storm in a Bottle. Sander Orent. 1989. LC 87-7540. 256p. text 24.95 (*0-89876-139-5*) Gardner Pr.

Stress & the Military Family. Carol B. Richardson. 1993. (Family Forum Library). 16p. 1.95 (*1-56688-070-X*) Bur For At-Risk.

Stress & the Police Officer. Katherine W. Ellison & John L. Genz. 1983. (Illus.). 224p. 39.95 (*0-398-04829-0*) C C Thomas.

Stress & Trauma. Patricia A. Resick. 2000. LC 00-55381. (Clinical Psychology Ser.). (Illus.). ix, 205p. (*1-84169-190-9*); (*1-84169-163-1*) Psychol Pr GBR. *Dist:* Taylor & Francis.

Stress & Vision. Elliott B. Forrest. Ed. by Frances Conkey & Sally M. Corngold. 1988. (Illus.). 325p. 30.00 (*0-943599-00-8*) OEPF.

Stress & Well-Being at Work: Assessments & Interventions for Occupational Mental Health. Ed. by James C. Quick et al. 1992. 372p. pap. text 19.95 (*1-55798-175-2*) Am Psychol.

Stress & Wellness Reference Guide: A Comprehensive Index to the Chalktalks, Processes, & Activities in the Whole Person Structured Exercises Series. Ed. by Nancy L. Tubesing. 1995. LC 95-33567. (Structured Exercises Ser.). 192p. (Orig.). otabind 29.95 (*1-57025-080-4*) Whole Person.

Stress & Women Physicians. Marjorie A. Bowman & Deborah I. Allen. 2nd ed. 1990. (Illus.). 216p. 19.50 (*0-387-97319-2*) Spr-Verlag.

Stress, Anxiety, & Depression: The Natural Way of Healing. Natural et al. 1995. LC 95-157966. 304p. mass mkt. 5.99 (*0-440-21659-1*) Dell.

Stress, Appraisal, & Coping. Richard S. Lazarus & Susan Folkman. 1984. 464p. (C). pap. 46.95 (*0-8261-4191-9*) Springer Pub.

Stress, Attitudes & Decisions: Selected Papers. Irving L. Janis. 1982. LC 82-9007. 352p. 82.50 (*0-275-90826-7*, C0826, Praeger Pubs) Greenwood.

Stress Between Work & Family. J. Eckenrode & S. Gore. 1989. (Stress & Coping Ser.). (Illus.). 248p. (C). 42.50 (*0-306-43318-4*, Plen Insight) Perseus Pubng.

Stress Burnout: An Annotated Bibliography. T. F. Riggar. 1985. LC 84-5447. 319p. 21.95 (*0-8093-1186-0*) S Ill U Pr.

Stress Busters: Bust the Stress Before It Busts You. Jack Hofer. 1986. LC 85-62946. 100p. 11.95 (*0-9615743-0-5*) SunShine CO.

Stress, Catecholamines & Cardiovascular Disease. David S. Goldstein. 1995. LC 94-19852. (Illus.). 576p. text 79.50 (*0-19-506538-7*) OUP.

Stress Control. Vernon Coleman. 1979. 214p. 20.00 (*0-85117-167-2*) Transatl Arts.

Stress Control. Darrell Franken. 1986. 48p. pap. 5.95 (*0-934957-14-2*) Wellness Pubns.

Stress Control: Save Your Life from Distress the Real Disease. Jonathon D. Miller. 1999. pap. 4.98 (*0-935815-06-6*) Lifecircle.

Stress, Coping & Cardiovascular Disease. Ed. by Philip M. McCabe et al. 1999. LC 99-23561. 250p. (*0-8058-3419-2*) L Erlbaum Assocs.

Stress, Coping & Developing: An Integrative Perspective. Carolyn M. Aldwin. 1999. LC 94-18295. 331p. pap. 23.00 (*1-57230-543-6*, C0543) Guilford Pubns.

Stress, Coping & Development: A Integrative Perspective. Carolyn M. Aldwin. 1994. LC 94-18295. 331p. 40.00 (*0-89862-261-1*, 2261) Guilford Pubns.

Stress, Coping & Development in Children. Norman Garmezy & Michael Rutter. 1988. LC 87-46302. (Illus.). 382p. (C). reprint ed. pap. text 19.95 (*0-8018-3651-4*) Johns Hopkins.

Stress, Coping & Disease. Jay S. Skyler & Neil Schneiderman. 1991. 264p. 39.95 (*0-8058-0408-0*) L Erlbaum Assocs.

Stress, Coping, & Health: A Situation-Behavior Approach - Theory, Methods, Applications. Meinrad Perrez & Michael Reicherts. 1992. LC 91-35352. (Illus.). 233p. pap. text 24.00 (*0-88937-065-6*) Hogrefe & Huber Pubs.

Stress, Coping, & Health in Families: Sense of Coherence & Resiliency. Hamilton I. McCubbin et al. 1998. LC 98-9082. (Resiliency in Families Ser.). 336p. 91.95 (*0-7619-1396-3*, 82375) Sage.

Stress, Coping & Health in Families: Sense of Coherence & Resiliency. Hamilton I. McCubbin et al. 1998. LC 98-9082. (Resiliency in Families Ser.). 336p. pap. 42.95 (*0-7619-1397-1*, 82376) Sage.

Stress, Coping & Relationships in Adolescence. Inge Seiffge-Krenke. 1995. (Research Monographs in Adolescence). 296p. text 59.95 (*0-8058-1235-0*) L Erlbaum Assocs.

Stress, Coping, & Resiliency in Children & Families. Ed. by E. Mavis Hetherington & Elaine A. Blechman. 1996. LC 95-41029. (Advances in Family Research Ser.). 256p. text 55.00 (*0-8058-1710-7*) L Erlbaum Assocs.

Stress, Culture & Community: The Psychology & Philosophy of Stress. S. E. Hobfoll. 1998. LC 98-39939. (Plenum Series on Stress & Coping). (Illus.). 296p. (C). 45.00 (*0-306-45942-6*) Plenum.

Stress Disorders. Douglas M. Baker. 1977. pap. (*0-906006-11-2*) Baker Pubns GBR. *Dist:* New Leaf Dist.

Stress Disorders among Vietnam Veterans: Theory, Research, & Treatment. Ed. by Charles R. Figley. 1978. LC 77-94734. (Psychosocial Stress Ser.: No. 1). 356p. text 34.95 (*0-87630-164-2*) Brunner-Routledge.

Stress, Distress & Illness. Ian Hislop. 1991. (Illus.). 224p. pap. text 27.00 (*0-07-452809-2*) McGraw-Hill Med Pub.

Stress Doppler Echocardiography. Ed. by Steve M. Teague. 1990. (Developments in Cardiovascular Medicine Ser.). (C). text 248.50 (*0-7923-0499-3*) Kluwer Academic.

Stress Echocardiography. Eugenio Picano. 2nd ed. 1996. LC 94-29136. (Illus.). 198p. 84.95 (*0-387-58137-5*); 3rd ed. 1997. LC 97-4381. 306p. (C). 81.00 (*3-540-62620-4*) Spr-Verlag.

Stress Echocardiography: Its Role in the Diagnosis & Evaluation of Coronary Artery Disease, Vol. 149. Thomas H. Marwick. 1994. LC 93-41121. (Developments in Cardiovascular Medicine Ser.: No. 149). 192p. (C). text 123.00 (*0-7923-2579-6*) Kluwer Academic.

Stress Effects on Family Caregivers of Alzheimer's & Related Dementias: Research & Interventions. Ed. by Enid Light et al. 1994. 440p. 58.95 (*0-8261-7890-1*) Springer Pub.

Stress Encyclopedia. Frank J. McGuigan. 1998. LC 98-28926. 276p. pap. text 53.00 (*0-205-17876-6*) Allyn.

Stress-Free, Anti-Aging Diet. D. R. Morse & R. L. Pollack. 1989. (Stress in Modern Society Ser.: No. 19). 32.50 (*0-404-63270-X*) AMS Pr.

Stress-Free Living Kit. Incl. Handbook for Achieving Stress-Free Living. Lilburn S. Barksdale. unabr. ed. 1980. pap., vinyl bd. 43.95 incl. audio (*0-918588-24-3*, 207) Barksdale Foun.

Stress, Gender, & Alcohol-Seeking Behavior. Ed. by Walter A. Hunt & Sam Zakhari. 1996. (Illus.). 364p. (Orig.). (C). pap. text 45.00 (*0-7881-2675-X*) DIANE Pub.

Stress, Immunity & Aging. Edwin L. Cooper. 1984. (Immunology Ser.: Vol. 24). (Illus.). 336p. text 155.00 (*0-8247-7114-1*) Dekker.

Stress in Childhood. Ed. by James H. Humphrey. 1984. LC 83-45028. (Studies in Modern Society: Political & Social Issues: No. 17). 32.50 (*0-404-61624-0*) AMS Pr.

Stress in Children. Bettie B. Youngs. 1986. 192p. mass mkt. 4.50 (*0-380-70161-8*, Avon Bks) Morrow Avon.

Stress in College Athletics: Causes, Consequences, Coping. James H. Humphrey et al. 2000. LC 99-56493. (Illus.). xiii, 183p. (C). pap. text 24.95 (*0-7890-0935-8*) Haworth Pr.

Stress in College Athletics: Causes, Consequences, Coping. Deborah A. Yow et al. 2000. LC 99-56493. (Illus.). xiii, 183p. (C). lib. bdg. 59.95 (*0-7890-0934-X*) Haworth Pr.

Stress in Industry: Cause, Effects, & Prevention. L. Levi. 1984. (Occupational Safety & Health Ser.: No. 51). vi, 70p. (Orig.). pap. 11.25 (*92-2-103539-5*) Intl Labour Office.

Stress in Organizations: Toward a Phase Model of Burnout. Robert T. Golembiewski et al. 1985. LC 85-16744. 284p. 72.50 (*0-275-90024-X*, C0024, Praeger Pubs) Greenwood.

Stress in Psychiatric Disorders. Ed. by Robert P. Liberman & Joel Yager. 1994. LC 93-41244. 208p. 34.95 (*0-8261-8310-7*) Springer Pub.

Stress in Psychotherapists. Ed. by Ved P. Varma. 1997. LC 96-4647. 256p. (C). 89.95 (*0-415-12174-4*); pap. 27.95 (*0-415-12175-2*) Routledge.

Stress in the American Workplace: Alternatives for the Working Wounded. Donald T. De Carlo & Deborah H. Gruenfeld. 1989. LC 89-13187. 188p. (Orig.). pap. 19.95 (*0-934753-34-2*) LRP Pubns.

Stress in Young People: What's New & What to Do. Sarah MacNamara. 2000. 208p. pap. 24.95 (*0-8264-4920-4*) Continuum.

Stress-Inducible Cellular Responses. U. Feige. 1996. LC 96-22168. (Experientia Supplementum Ser.). 180.00 (*0-8176-5205-1*); 512p. 180.00 (*3-7643-5205-1*) Birkhauser.

Stress Inoculation Training. Donald Meichenbaum. 1985. (Psychology Practitioner Guidebooks). 128p. text 28.00 (*0-08-031597-6*); pap. text 14.95 (*0-08-031596-8*) Elsevier (Pergamon Pr).

Stress Management. Corbin. 2000. pap. text 11.97 net. (*0-395-97328-7*) HM.

Stress Management. James S. Gordon. 2000. LC 00-24063. (Twenty-First Century Health & Wellness Ser.). 112p. (J). (gr. 7-12). 24.95 (*0-7910-5987-1*) Chelsea Hse.

Stress Management: An Integrated Approach. Dorothy H. Cotton. 1990. LC 89-38991. (Psychosocial Stress Ser.: No. 17). 288p. text 38.95 (*0-87630-557-5*) Brunner-Routledge.

Stress Management: HP 630. California College for Health Sciences Staff. 1990. 23p. (C). stu. ed. (*0-933195-30-3*) CA College Health Sci.

Stress Management: Psychological Foundations. Stephen M. Auerbach & Sandy E. Gramling. 1997. LC 97-5294. 272p. pap. text 57.00 (*0-13-722281-5*) P-H.

Stress Management: The Quest for Zest. Aina O. Nucho. 1988. (Illus.). 194p. (C). text 38.95 (*0-398-05478-9*) C C Thomas.

Stress Management & Counselling: Theory, Practice, Research & Methodology. Ed. by Stephen Palmer & Windy Dryden. 1996. LC 96-5302. (Stress Counselling Ser.). (Illus.). 160p. text 90.00 (*0-304-33564-9*) Continuum.

Stress-Management & Relaxation Activities for Trainers. Robert Epstein. 1998. 275p. ring bd. 89.95 (*0-07-021763-7*) McGraw.

Stress-Management & Relaxation Activities for Trainers. Robert Epstein. 1998. LC 98-68035. (Illus.). 275p. pap. 34.95 (*0-07-021762-9*) McGraw-Hill Prof.

Stress Management for Cancer Patients: A Self-Help Care Manual. Morry Edwards. 2000. (Illus.). x, 159p. 22.95 (*0-9678801-1-4*) Acorn MI.

Stress Management for Chronic Disease. Ed. by Michael L. Russell. 1988. (General Psychology Ser.). 400p. 55.00 (*0-08-032807-5*, Pergamon Pr) Elsevier.

Stress Management for Educators: A Guide to Manage Our Response to Stress (Staff) Bettie B. Youngs. 1992. LC 92-52732. 112p. pap. 16.95 (*0-915190-77-X*, JP 9077-X) Jalmar Pr.

Stress Management for HIV: Clinical Validation & Intervention Manual. Michael H. Antoni et al. Ed. by Jean Kristeller. 1996. LC 97-9633. (Behavioral Medicine - from Research to Practice). 300p. pap. (*0-8058-2246-1*) L Erlbaum Assocs.

Stress Management for the Healthy Type A: A Skills-Training Program. Ethel Roskies. 1987. LC 86-31856. 224p. spiral bd. 22.95 (*0-89862-692-7*) Guilford Pubns.

Stress Management for the Healthy Type A: Theory & Practice. Ethel Roskies. 1987. LC 86-31856. 252p. 32.50 (*0-89862-689-7*) Guilford Pubns.

Stress Management for the Veterinary Practice Team. A. D. Elkins & Sandra Brackenridge. 1996. 42p. (Orig.). (C). pap. 25.00 (*0-9603534-9-6*) Vet Practice.

Stress Management Guide for Administrators. 1989. 96p. pap. 10.00 (*0-940221-02-0*) Lrng Tools.

Stress Management Guide for Educators. 1989. 92p. pap. 9.95 (*0-940221-03-9*) Lrng Tools.

Stress Management Handbook: Strategies for Health & Inner Peace. Lori A. Leyden-Rubenstein. 1998. LC 97-39243. 208p. pap. 14.95 (*0-87983-794-2*, 37942K, Keats Pubng) McGraw-Hill Trade.

Stress Management in Primary Care. Kenneth Hambly & Alice J. Muir. 1997. LC 96-40480. (Illus.). 224p. pap. text 37.50 (*0-7506-2737-9*) Buttrwrth-Heinemann.

Stress Management Skillbook. Educational Foundation of the National Restaurant Association Staff. 1993. (Management Skills Program Ser.). 28p. (Orig.). pap. 10.95 (*0-915452-40-5*) Educ Found.

Stress Management Sourcebook. J. Barton Cunningham. 2nd ed. 2000. LC 00-57187. (Illus.). 336p. pap. 17.95 (*0-7373-0508-8*, Contemporary) McGraw-Hill Trade.

Stress Management Sourcebook: Everything You Need to Know. J. Barton Cunningham. 1998. LC 97-37447. 336p. reprint ed. 27.00 (*1-56565-792-6*, 07926W, Extension Pr) Lowell Hse.

Stress Management Training: A Group Leader's Guide. Nancy Norvell & Dale Belles. 1990. LC 89-62711. 96p. pap. 17.95 (*0-943158-33-8*, SM-GBP, Prof Resc Pr) Pro Resource.

Stress Mess Solution. George S. Everly & Daniel A. Girdano. 1981. LC 79-14652. 174p. 11.50 (*0-13-852616-8*) P-H.

Stress of Life. Hans Selye. 2nd ed. 1978. LC 77-14023. (Paperbacks Ser.). 516p. (C). reprint ed. pap. 14.95 (*0-07-056212-1*) McGraw-Hill Prof.

Stress of Life: From Molecules to Man. Ed. by Peter Csermely. 1998. LC 98-6826. (Annals of the New York Academy of Sciences Ser.: Vol. 851). 547p. 140.00 (*1-57331-116-2*); pap. 140.00 (*1-57331-117-0*) NY Acad Sci.

Stress Owner's Manual: Meaning, Balance & Health in Your Life. Edmond W. Boenisch & Michele Haney. 1996. LC 96-26977. 208p. (Orig.). pap. 14.95 (*0-915166-84-4*) Impact Pubs CA.

Stress Pack. Journey Editions Staff. 1997. (Cures for Modern Times Ser.). (Illus.). 64p. 16.95 (*1-885203-45-4*) Jrny Editions.

Stress Physiology in Animals Vol. 2: Sheffield Biological Sciences. Ed. by Paul H. M. Balm. 1999. (Sheffield Biological Sciences Ser.: Vol. 2). 288p. (*1-85075-908-1*) Sheffield Acad GBR. *Dist:* CUP Services.

Stress Reduction & Prevention. D. Meichenbaum & M. Jaremko. 1983. (Illus.). 512p. (C). 52.50 (*0-306-41066-4*, Plenum Trade) Perseus Pubng.

Stress Reduction for Caregivers. Jody Olshevski. 1999. LC 98-55754. 208p. pap. text 24.95 (*0-87630-941-4*) Brunner-Routledge.

Stress Reduction for Mormons. John C. Turpin. 1983. 56p. 5.50 (*0-939506-01-7*) Turpin & Assocs.

Stress Release. Wayne W. Topping. rev. ed. 1985. (Illus.). 163p. (Orig.). pap. 13.00 (*0-935299-03-3*) Topping Inst.

Stress Response Syndromes. Mardi J. Horowitz. 2nd ed. LC 85-71507. 1986. 358p. 50.00 (*0-87668-811-3*); 1992. 384p. reprint ed. pap. 50.00 (*0-87668-298-0*) Aronson.

Stress Response Syndromes: Personality Styles & Interventions. Mardi J. Horowitz. 4th ed. 2001. LC 00-52205. 50.00 (*0-7657-0313-0*) Aronson.

Stress Response Syndromes: PTSD, Grief, & Adjustment Disorders. Mardi J. Horowitz. 3rd ed. 1997. LC 97-209669. 384p. 50.00 (*0-7657-0025-5*) Aronson.

Stress Revisited, Set, Vols. 1 & 2. Ed. by G. Jasmin & M. Cantin. 1991. (Methods & Achievements in Experimental Pathology Ser.: Vols. 14-15). (Illus.). xxviii, 400p. 347.00 (*3-8055-5404-4*) S Karger.

Stress Revisited: Neuroendocrinology of Stress. Ed. by M. Cantin & G. Jasmin. 1991. (Methods & Achievements in Experimental Pathology Ser.: Vol. 14). (Illus.). xii, 176p. 169.75 (*3-8055-5374-9*) S Karger.

Stress Revisited Vol. 2: Systemic Effects of Stress. Ed. by G. Jasmin & M. Cantin. 1991. (Methods & Achievements in Experimental Pathology Ser.: Vol. 15). (Illus.). xvi, 224p. 215.75 (*3-8055-5403-6*) S Karger.

Stress Scripting: A Guide to Stress Management. Jonathan C. Smith. 1990. LC 90-38840. 280p. 52.95 (*0-275-93639-2*, C3639, Praeger Pubs) Greenwood.

Stress, Self-Concept, & Violence. John A. Corson. Ed. by James H. Humphrey. 1989. LC 86-82026. (Stress in Modern Society Ser.: No. 11). 32.50 (*0-404-63271-8*); pap. 14.95 (*0-404-63263-7*) AMS Pr.

Stress, Stress Hormones & the Immune System. J. C. Buckingham et al. 1997. LC 97-5380. 426p. 147.95 (*0-471-95886-7*) Wiley.

Stress Test: Cartoons on Medicine. Sidney Harris. 1994. LC 93-31590. (Illus.). 150p. (Orig.). pap. 10.95 (*0-8135-2065-7*) Rutgers U Pr.

Stress Test Biofeedback Card & Booklet. Alfred A. Barrios. 1985. pap. 3.95 (*0-9601926-3-8*) Self-Prog Control.

Stress, the Aging Brain, & the Mechanisms of Neuron Death. Robert M. Sapolsky. 1992. LC 91-46530. (Illus.). 448p. 70.00 (*0-262-19320-5*, Bradford Bks) MIT Pr.

Stress Therapy. Tom McGrath. 1997. LC 96-79961. (Elf-Help Bks.). (Illus.). 96p. pap. 4.95 (*0-87029-301-X*, 20153) Abbey.

Stress Training for Life. Herbert Kindler & Marilyn Ginsburg. 1990. 160p. 14.95 (*0-89397-335-1*) Nichols Pub.

Stress Without Tears. Tom Rhodes. 1990. (Illus.). 130p. (Orig.). 22.50 (*0-9615234-1-7*) Jacobs Pub.

Stress, You Can't Live with It & You Can't Live Without It: Changing Stress into Success. James P. Cima. 1997. 150p. (Orig.). pap. 19.95 (*0-9659476-2-9*) JPC Pubng.

StressBusters: Tips to Feel Healthy, Alive & Energized. Katherine Butler. 1996. 192p. pap. 8.95 (*0-471-34706-X*) Wiley.

Stressbusters Five Minute Massage see 5 Minute Massage: Quick & Simple Exercises to Reduce Tension & Stress

Stressechocardiography Interactive: Strategies for Interpretation. Ed. by S. Beckmann & G. Haug. 1999. 160p. incl. cd-rom (*3-7985-1150-0*) D Steinkopff DEU. *Dist:* Spr-Verlag.

Stressed Heart. Ed. by Marianne J. Legato. 1987. (Developments in Cardiovascular Medicine Ser.). text 174.00 (*0-89838-849-X*) Kluwer Academic.

Stressful Life Events. Ed. by Thomas W. Miller. 1989. (Stress & Health Ser.: No. 4). 838p. 90.00 (*0-8236-6165-2*, BN#00165) Intl Univs Pr.

Stressful Life Events & Their Contexts. Ed. by Barbara Snell Dohrenwend & Bruce P. Dohrenwend. 1984. (Monographs in Psychosocial Epidemiology). 287p. pap. text 15.00 (*0-8135-1004-X*) Rutgers U Pr.

Stressors & the Adjustment Disorders. Joseph D. Noshpitz & R. Dean Coddington. 1990. LC 89-25065. (Personality Processes Ser.). 693p. 275.00 (*0-471-62186-2*) Wiley.

Stricken: Voices from the Hidden Epidemic of Chronic Fatigue Syndrome. Peggy Munson. 2000. LC 00-31930. xxv, 270p. pap. 24.90 (*0-7890-0895-5*, Hawrth Medical) Haworth Pr.

Stricken: Voices from the Hidden Epidemic of Chronic Fatigue Syndrometc. Peggy Munson. 2000. LC 00-31930. 270p. 59.90 (*0-7890-0894-7*, Hawrth Medical) Haworth Pr.

Strings: The Miracle of Life. John Robbins. 1998. 220p. 23.95 (*1-880823-17-9*) N Star Pubns.

Strip AIDS U. S. A. A Collection of Cartoon Art to Benefit People with AIDS. Trina Robbins. 1988. (Illus.). 140p. pap. text 9.95 (*0-86719-373-5*) Last Gasp.

Striving Toward Improvement. Joint Commission on Accreditation of Healthcare Organizations. 1992. 55.00 (*0-86688-255-3*) Joint Comm Hlthcare.

Stroke. (*0-340-57719-3*) E A GBR. *Dist:* Routldge.

***Stroke.** Brown & Benavente. 2002. (Fast Facts Ser.). (Illus.). pap. (*1-903734-02-9*) Health Pr GBR. *Dist:* JAMCO Dist.

***Stroke.** Ed. by Martin M. Brown. 2000. (British Medical Bulletin Ser.: Vol. 56, No. 2). 576p. pap. (*1-85315-457-1*) Royal Soc of Medicine Pr Ltd GBR. *Dist:* Balogh.

S

Stroke. Charles Warlow et al. 2nd ed. 2000. LC 00-59905. (Illus.). xi, 804p. 208.95 (*0-632-05418-2*) Blackwell Sci.

Stroke: A Clinical Approach. Louis R. Caplan. 3rd ed. 2000. LC 99-54757. (Illus.). 568p. text 99.00 (*0-7506-9953-1*) Buttrwrth-Heinemann.

Stroke: A Guide for Patients & Their Families. John E. Sarno. 1991. pap. (*0-13-853730-5*, Fireside) S&S Trade Pap.

Stroke: A Practical Guide to Management. C. P. Warlow et al. 1997. (Illus.). pap. 199.95 (*0-632-05005-5*) Blackwell Sci.

Stroke: A Practical Guide to Management. Charles P. Warlow et al. Ed. by Martin Dennis et al. 1996. LC 96-5661. (Illus.). 900p. 199.95 (*0-86542-874-3*) Blackwell Sci.

Stroke: A Self-Help Manual for Stroke Sufferers & Their Relatives. R. M. Youngson. 1992. (Take Control Ser.). 144p. (Orig.). pap. (*0-7153-8945-9*) Trafalgar.

Stroke: An Owner's Manual: The Invaluable Guide to Life after Stroke. Arthur Josephs. 1992. LC 91-77440. 160p. (Orig.). pap. 14.95 (*0-9631493-9-3*) Amadeus CA.

Stroke: Animal Models: Proceedings of an International Symposium Held at Wiesbaden, Germany, 16 November 1981. Ed. by Hoechst Stefanovich. 1982. (Illus.). 196p. 67.00 (*0-08-029799-4*, Pergamon Pr) Elsevier.

Stroke: Current & Future Trends in Disease Management. K. K. Jain. Ed. by Susan D. DiClemente. 1998. (Illus.). 458p. 4950.00 (*1-57936-112-9*, 1980) International Business.

Stroke: Diagnosis & Treatment. Ed. by Marc Fisher. 1993. LC 92-49808. 300p. (gr. 13). (*1-56375-091-0*) Gower-Mosby.

Stroke: Emergency Management & Critical Care. Thorsten Steiner et al. 1998. LC 98-4649. (Update in Intensive Care & Emergency Medicine Ser.). (Illus.). 194p. 109.00 (*3-540-61880-5*) Spr-Verlag.

Stroke: Pathophysiology, Diagnosis & Management. Barnett. 3rd ed. 1998. LC 98-3396. (C). text (*0-443-07551-4*, B1184) Church.

Stroke: Questions You Have - Answers You Need. Jennifer Hay. 1995. LC 95-21858. 192p. pap. 10.95 (*1-882606-22-1*) Peoples Med Soc.

Stroke . . . Now What? Neub Petschulat & Joyce Corinna. 1991. 240p. (Orig.). 17.95 (*0-9631426-0-7*) CAM Pub.

Stroke & Head Injury: A Guide to Functional Outcomes in Physical Therapy. Ann L. Charness. 1993. (Illus.). 330p. (C). spiral bd. 83.00 (*0-87189-226-X*) PRO-ED.

Stroke Data Banks: Challenges for Research. Ed. by M. Brainin & M. A. Foulkes. 1994. (Journal: Vol. 13, No. 6, 1994). (Illus.). iv, 104p. pap. 47.00 (*3-8055-6016-8*) S Karger.

Stroke Diagnosis & Management: Current Procedures & Equipment. William S. Fields et al. 1973. LC 72-13847. (Illus.). 298p. 18.50 (*0-87527-101-4*) Green.

Stroke Free for Life: A Breakthrough Medical Plan for Risk Assesment & Prevention. David O. Wiebers. 2001. LC 00-65688. (Illus.). 352p. 25.00 (*0-06-019823-0*) HarperCollins Pubs.

Stroke in Children & Young Adults. Ed. by Jose Biller et al. 1994. LC 93-49468. 280p. text 99.00 (*0-7506-9203-0*) Buttrwrth-Heinemann.

Stroke Manual for Families. Tampa General Rehabilitation Center Staff. 1989. 60p. (Orig.). pap. 6.50 (*1-882855-05-1*) HDI Pubs.

Stroke Prevention. Ed. by W. Dorndorf & P. Marx. 1994. LC 93-38418. (Illus.). viii, 200p. 64.50 (*3-8055-5882-1*) S Karger.

Stroke Prevention by the Practitioner. Ed. by J. Bogousslavsky. 1999. (Cerebrovascular Diseases Ser.: Vol. 9, Suppl. 4, 1999). (Illus.). vi, 70p. pap. 25.25 (*3-8055-6881-9*) S Karger.

Stroke Recovery Book: A Guide for Patients & Families. Kip Burkman. 1998. LC 98-6547. (Illus.). 172p. pap. 14.95 (*1-886039-30-5*) Addicus Bks.

Stroke Recovery Pathway. McDermott. 1998. (C). pap. text 75.00 (*0-12-785068-6*) Acad Pr.

Stroke Rehabilitation: A Function-Based Approach. Ed. by Gillen. 1997. LC 98-111015. (Illus.). 640p. (gr. 13). text 65.00 (*0-8151-3460-6*, 29193) Mosby Inc.

Stroke Rehabilitation: A Function-Based Approach. Glen Gillen & Ann Burkhardt. 1998. tchr. ed. (*0-8151-2894-0*) Mosby Inc.

Stroke Rehabilitation: Basic Concepts & Research Trends. William S. Fields & William A. Spencer. 1967. LC 67-19383. (Illus.). 184p. 18.50 (*0-87527-034-4*) Green.

Stroke Rehabilitation: Scientific & Evidence-Based Exercise & Training. Roberta B. Shepherd. 2001. 192p. pap. 63.00 (*0-7506-4712-4*) Buttrwrth-Heinemann.

Stroke Rehabilitation Patient Education Manual. Aspen Reference Group Staff. Ed. by Sara N. De Lima. 1995. LC 95-35240. 454p. ring bd. 189.00 (*0-8342-0675-7*) Aspen Pub.

***Stroke Services: Policy & Practice Across Europe.** Ed. by Charles Wolfe et al. 2001. 152p. pap. (*1-85775-455-7*) Radcliffe Med Pr GBR. *Dist:* Balogh.

Stroke Therapy: Basic, Preclinical, & Clinical Directions. Ed. by Leonard P. Miller. 1998. LC 98-22640. (Illus.). 456p. 147.00 (*0-471-18347-4*, Wiley-Liss) Wiley.

Stroke Treatment & Prevention: From Clinical Trials to Daily Practice: 51st Meeting of the Spanish Society of Neurology Barcelona, December 1998. Ed. by A. Chamarro. 1999. (Cerebrovascular Diseases Ser.: Vol. 9, Suppl. 3). (Illus.). iv, 50p. pap. 25.25 (*3-8055-6926-2*) S Karger.

Stroke: Treatment, Prevention & Rehabilitation: Perugia 1st International Stroke Meeting, Perugia, November 1999. Ed. by V. Gallai & L. Parnetti. 1999. (Cerebrovascular Diseases Ser.: 10, Suppl. 4 (2000)). iv, 52p. 25.25 (*3-8055-6973-4*) S Karger.

Stroke/Head Injury: A Guide to Functional Outcomes in Physical Therapy - Rehabilitation Institute of Chicago Procedure Manual. Ann L. Charness & RIC Staff. 2nd ed. 2001. 65.00 (*0-8342-1802-X*) Aspen Pub.

Strombeck's Small Animal Gastroenterology. W. Grant Guilford et al. 3rd rev. ed. 1996. LC 95-22527. 1072p. text 150.00 (*0-7216-3760-4*) Saunders.

Strong Enough for Two. James L. Mastrich & William J. Birnes. 1991. 256p. pap. 9.95 (*0-02-034520-8*) Macmillan.

Strong Medicine: A Century of High Desert Remedies. Robert G. Boyd & Vivian Adams. Ed. by Jack Cooper. 1998. (Western Heritage Ser.: Vol. 2). (Illus.). 40p. pap. 12.95 (*0-9663487-0-2*) High Desert Mus.

Strong Medicine: Health Politics in the 21st Century. Iliffe. 1988. (C). pap. (*0-85315-694-8*) Lawrence & Wishart GBR. *Dist:* NYU Pr.

Strong Medicine: How to Save Canada's Health-Care System. Michael Rachlis. 1994. LC 94-189706. 396p. (*0-00-255281-7*, R0122) HarpCollins.

Strong Medicine: How To Save Canada'S Health-Care System. Michael Rachlis. 1995. 448p. reprint ed. pap. (*0-00-638061-1*, R0549) HarpCollins.

Strong Medicine: The Ethical Rationing of Health Care. Paul T. Menzel. 1990. 256p. (C). text 37.95 (*0-19-505710-4*) OUP.

Strong Shadows: Scenes from an Inner City AIDS Clinic. Abigail Zuger. 1997. 264p. pap. text 11.95 (*0-7167-3100-2*); 1995. LC 95-7587. 243p. text 22.95 (*0-7167-2916-4*) W H Freeman.

Strong Women Stay Young. Miriam E. Nelson & Sarah Wernick. 1997. LC 96-41541. 288p. 24.95 (*0-553-10347-4*) Bantam.

Stronger Pump: A Guide for People with Heart Failure. Julia A. Purcell & Barbara J. Fletcher. Ed. by Nancy R. Hull. rev. ed. 1994. LC 80-10191. (Illus.). 40p. pap. text 6.50 (*0-939838-05-2*) Pritchett & Hull.

Strongyloidiasis: A Major Roundworm Infection of Man. Ed. by D.I. Grove. 1989. 220p. (*0-85066-732-1*) Tay Francis Ltd GBR. *Dist:* Taylor & Francis.

Structural Abnormalities & Reproductive Failure: An Evidence Based Approach to Diagnosis & Management. Gerard S. Letterie. 1997. LC 96-47749. pap. 135.00 (*0-86542-434-9*) Blackwell Sci.

Structural & Contractile Proteins Pt. D: Extracellular Matrix. Ed. by Leon W. Cunningham. 1987. (Methods in Enzymology Ser.: Vol. 144). 521p. text 157.00 (*0-12-182044-0*) Acad Pr.

Structural & Contractile Proteins Pt. A: Extracellular Matrix. Ed. by Sidney P. Colowick & Leon W. Cunningham. 1982. (Methods in Enzymology Ser.: Vol. 82). text 188.00 (*0-12-181982-5*) Acad Pr.

Structural & Functional Abnormalities in Subclinical Diabetic Angiopathy. Ed. by B. Weber et al. 1992. (Pediatric & Adolescent Endocrinology Ser.: Vol. 22). (Illus.). x, 242p. 213.25 (*3-8055-5606-3*) S Karger.

Structural & Functional Organization of the Neocortex: Proceedings of a Symposium in the Memory of Otto D. Creutzfeldt, May 1993. Ed. by B. Albowitz et al. 1994. LC 94-16023. 135.00 (*0-387-57205-8*) Spr-Verlag.

Structural & Functional Organization of the Placenta. Ed. by P. Kaufmann & B. F. King. 1982. (Bibliotheca Anatomica Ser.: No. 22). (Illus.). viii, 164p. 133.25 (*3-8055-3520-1*) S Karger.

***Structural & Functional Studies of the Density Enhanced Receptor-Like Protein Tyrosine Phosphatase DEP-1.** Maria Sorby. 2001. 42p. pap. (*91-554-5063-6*) Uppsala Universitet SWE. *Dist:* Coronet Bks.

Structural Basis of Behavior. J. Anthony Deutsch. 1995. LC 60-12466. lib. bdg. 19.50 (*0-226-14345-7*) U Ch Pr.

Structural Basis of Muscular Contraction. John M. Squire. 1981. LC 81-2321. 716p. 120.00 (*0-306-40582-2*, Plenum Trade) Perseus Pubng.

Structural Biomaterials. Julian F. Vincent. rev. ed. 1990. (Illus.). 256p. pap. 32.50 (*0-691-02513-4*) Princeton U Pr.

Structural Carbohydrates in the Liver: Falk Symposium, No 34. Ed. by Werner Reutter et al. 1983. 600p. text 272.50 (*0-85200-711-6*) Kluwer Academic.

Structural Fat Grafting. Sydney R. Coleman. 2000. (Illus.). 400p. text 250.00 (*1-57626-133-6*) Quality Med Pub.

Structural Fetal Abnormalities: The Total Picture. Ed. by Roger C. Sanders et al. 1995. LC 95-23082. (Illus.). 296p. (C). (gr. 13). pap. text 64.95 (*0-8151-7838-7*, 24633) Mosby Inc.

Structural Modified Food Fats: Synthesis, Biochemistry & Use. Ed. by Armond Christophe. 1998. LC 98-17717. (Illus.). 256p. lib. bdg. 90.00 (*0-935315-93-4*, PC114) Am Oil Chemists.

Structural-Process Models of Complex Human Behavior, No. 26. M. N. Scandura. 1978. (NATO Advanced Science Institutes Ser.). 620p. lib. bdg. 162.50 (*90-286-0578-9*) Kluwer Academic.

Structural Shielding Design & Evaluation for Medical Use of X-Rays & Gamma-Rays of Energies up to Ten MeV. 1976. LC 76-22969. (Report Ser.: No. 49). 134p. pap. text 40.00 (*0-913392-31-6*) NCRP Pubns.

***Structural Studies on Cytochrome BC(1) Complex from Bovine Heart Mitochondria.** Momi Iwata. 2001. (Comprehensive Summaries of Uppsala Dissertations from the Faculty of Science & Technology Ser.: No. 643). (Illus.). 81p. pap. (*91-554-5069-5*) Uppsala Universitet SWE. *Dist:* Coronet Bks.

Structural Theory of the Emotions. Joseph De Rivera. 1977. LC 76-53916. (Psychological Issues Monographs: No. 40). 178p. 32.50 (*0-8236-6171-7*); pap. 27.50 (*0-8236-6170-9*) Intl Univs Pr.

Structuralist Program in Psychology: Foundations & Applications. Ed. by Hans Westmeyer. 1992. LC 92-48722. (Illus.). 290p. text 35.90 (*0-88937-100-8*) Hogrefe & Huber Pubs.

Structure Activity Correlation as a Predictive Tool in Toxicology: Fundamentals, Methods & Applications. Ed. by Leon Golberg. 1983. LC 82-3007. (Chemical Industry Institute of Toxicology Ser.). (Illus.). 330p. 145.00 (*0-89116-276-3*) Hemisp Pub.

Structure & Activity of Anti-Tumour Agents. D. N. Reinhoudt. 1982. text 155.50 (*90-247-2783-9*) Kluwer Academic.

Structure & Dynamics of Health Research & Public Funding: An International Institution Comparison. Dietmar Braun. Tr. by Neil Solomon. 1994. LC 94-7725. 216p. (C). lib. bdg. 127.50 (*0-7923-2777-2*) Kluwer Academic.

Structure & Dynamics of Nucleic Acids & Proteins. Ed. by Enrico Clementi et al. 1983. (Illus.). 500p. (C). lib. bdg. 80.00 (*0-940030-04-7*) Adenine Pr.

Structure & Fiber Connections of the Hippocampus. Walter K. Schwerdtfeger. 1984. (Advances in Anatomy, Embryology & Cell Biology Ser.: Vol. 83). (Illus.). 743p. 41.95 (*0-387-13092-6*) Spr-Verlag.

Structure & Function - Special Edition. Gary A. Thibodeau & Kevin T. Patton. 9th ed. 1991. (Illus.). 496p. (C). (gr. 13). text 30.95 (*0-8016-6403-9*, 06403) Mosby Inc.

Structure & Function in Normal & Abnormal Hips: How to Rescue Mechanically Jeopardized Hips. Renato Bombelli. 3rd enl. rev. ed. 1993. (Illus.). LC 93-18576. 211p. 310.00 (*0-387-56266-4*); 235p. (*3-540-56266-4*) Spr-Verlag.

Structure & Function of Alzheimer's Amyloid Beta Proteins. David Schubert. 1994. (Molecular Biology Intelligence Unit Ser.). 100p. 99.00 (*1-57059-216-0*) Landes Bioscience.

Structure & Function of Domestic Animals. Bruce W. Currie. 1992. 464p. 79.95 (*0-8493-8766-3*) CRC Pr.

Structure & Function of Endothelial Cells. F. Hammersen. Ed. by K. Messmer. 1983. (Mikrozirkulation in Forschung und Klinik Ser.: Vol. 1). (Illus.). x, 138p. pap. 40.00 (*3-8055-3635-6*) S Karger.

Structure & Function of Invertebrate Oxygen Carriers. Ed. by S. N. Vinogradov & O. H. Kapp. 1991. (Illus.). 352p. 89.95 (*0-387-97585-3*) Spr-Verlag.

Structure & Function of Invertebrate Respiratory Proteins. Ed. by E. J. Wood. 1983. (Life Chemistry Reports). xvi, 416p. text 220.00 (*3-7186-0155-9*) Gordon & Breach.

Structure & Function of the Bladder Neck. W. Dorschner et al. 2001. LC 00-51602. (Advances in Anatomy, Embryology & Cell Biology Ser.: Vol. 159). (Illus.). 122p. pap. 85.00 incl. cd-rom (*3-540-67998-7*) Spr-Verlag.

Structure & Function of the Body. Linda Swisher. 10th ed. 1997. (Illus.). 304p. pap. text, stu. ed. 15.95 (*0-8151-8716-5*) Mosby Inc.

Structure & Function of the Body. Gary A. Thibodeau & Kevin T. Patton. 10th ed. 1997. LC 96-17642. (C). text 35.95 (*0-8151-8714-9*, 28293) Mosby Inc.

Structure & Function of the Body. Gary Thibodeau & Kevin T. Patton. 10th ed. 1997. (Illus.). 512p. pap., tchr. ed. (*0-8151-8717-3*) Mosby Inc.

Structure & Function of the Body. Gary A. Thibodeau & Kevin T. Patton. 11th ed. 2000. LC 99-59495. (Illus.). 582p. 37.95 incl. cd-rom (*0-323-01082-2*); pap. 34.95 incl. cd-rom (*0-323-01081-4*) Mosby Inc.

***Structure & Function of the Body: Electronic Image Collection.** Gary A. Thibodeau & Kevin T. Patton. 2000. 582p. 300.00 incl. cd-rom (*0-323-01170-5*) Mosby Inc.

***Structure & Function of the Body: Instructor's Resource Manual.** Gary A. Thibodeau & Kevin T. Patton. 2000. 250.00 incl. cd-rom (*0-323-01079-2*) Mosby Inc.

Structure & Function of the Circulation, Vol. 3. Ed. by Colin J. Schwartz et al. 1981. 564p. 95.00 (*0-306-40751-5*, Plenum Trade) Perseus Pubng.

Structure & Function of the Human Auditory System. Champlin. 2002. pap. 44.00 net. (*0-7693-0170-3*) Singular Publishing.

Structure & Function of the Kidney. Ed. by R. K. Kinne. 1989. (Comparative Physiology Ser.: Vol. 1). viii, 198p. 143.50 (*3-8055-4886-9*) S Karger.

Structure & Function of the Musculoskeletal System. James Watkins. 1998. LC 98-27930. (Illus.). 376p. text 52.00 (*0-88011-686-2*, BWAT0686) Human Kinetics.

***Structure & Function of the Stratum Corneum as Border Organ.** Ed. by J. Lademann & W. Sterry. 2001. (Skin Pharmacology & Applied Skin Physiology Ser.: Vol. 14, Suppl. 1). (Illus.). iv, 104p. pap. 34.00 (*3-8055-7292-1*) S Karger.

Structure & Functions of Amine Oxidases. Ed. by Bruno Mondovi. 1986. 304p. 167.00 (*0-8493-5869-8*, QP603, CRC Reprint) Franklin.

Structure & Gestalt: Philosophy & Literature in Austria-Hungary & Her Successor States. Ed. by Barry Smith. 1981. (Linguistic & Literary Studies in Eastern Europe: Vol. 7). x, 349p. 86.00 (*90-272-1510-3*) J Benjamins Pubng Co.

Structure & Insight. Pierree M. Van Hiele. 1985. (Developmental Psychology Ser.). pap. text 55.00 (*0-12-714161-8*) Acad Pr.

Structure-Based Drug Design. Ed. by Veerapandian. 1997. LC 97-20396. (Illus.). 664p. text 195.00 (*0-8247-9869-4*) Dekker.

Structure-Based Drug Design: Experimental & Computational Approaches. Penelope W. Codding. 1998. LC 98-28192. (NATO Advanced Science Institutes Ser.). vii, 289p. 129.00 (*0-7923-5201-7*) Kluwer Academic.

Structure-Based Drug Design: Thermodynamics, Modeling & Strategy. John E. Ladbury & Pat R. Connelly. 1997. LC 97-21929. (Biotechnology Intelligence Unit Ser.). 183p. 109.00 (*1-57059-469-4*) Landes Bioscience.

Structure-Based Drug Design: Thermodynamics, Modeling & Strategy. Ed. by John E. Ladbury & Pat R. Connelly. 1997. LC 97-21929. (Biotechnology Intelligence Unit Ser.). (Illus.). 187p. 117.00 (*3-540-63250-6*) Spr-Verlag.

Structure, Cellular Synthesis, & Assembly of Biopolymers. Ed. by Steven T. Case. 1992. LC 92-36490. (Results & Problems in Cell Differentiation Ser.: Vol. 19). (Illus.). 350p. 239.00 (*0-387-55549-8*) Spr-Verlag.

Structure, Development, & Phykogeny of Cranial Nerves. Ed. by R. L. Boord. 1993. (Journal: Vol. 148, Nos. 2-3, 1993). (Illus.). 104p. pap. 214.00 (*3-8055-5909-7*) S Karger.

Structure du Comportement. Maurice Merleau-Ponty. 1990. (FRE.). pap. 21.95 (*0-7859-3015-9*) Fr & Eur.

Structure, Dynamics, & Biogenesis of Biomembranes. Ed. by Ryo Sato & Shun-Ichi Ohnishi. 1982. LC 83-51051. 188p. 65.00 (*0-306-41283-7*, Plenum Trade) Perseus Pubng.

Structure for Population Education: Goals, Generalizations, & Behavioral Objectives. Mary T. Lane & Ralph E. Wileman. 2nd ed. 1978. LC 74-77985. pap. 4.00 (*0-89055-128-6*) Carolina Pop Ctr.

Structure, Function & Genetics of Ribosomes. Ed. by G. W. Kramer & B. Hardesty. 1986. (Molecular Biology, Biochemistry & Biophysics Ser.). (Illus.). 810p. 288.00 (*0-387-96233-6*) Spr-Verlag.

Structure, Function & Modulation of Striated Muscle Calcium Channels. David J. Pelzer. 1994. (Molecular Biology Intelligence Unit Ser.). 115p. 89.95 (*1-57059-057-5*) CRC Pr.

Structure, Function, & Regulation of Molecules Involved in Leukocyte Adhesion: Proceedings of the Second International Conferences on "Structure & Function of Molecules Involved in Leukocyte Adhesion II" Held in Titisee, Germany, October 2-6, 1991. Ed. by Peter E. Lipsky et al. 1992. LC 92-2337. (Illus.). 396p. 150.00 (*0-387-97870-4*) Spr-Verlag.

Structure of Antigens, Vol. 3. Ed. by Mare H. Van Regenmortel. 1995. (Structure of Antigens Ser.: Vol. 3). 432p. 224.95 (*0-8493-9225-X*, 9225) CRC Pr.

Structure of Freudian Thought: The Problem of Immutability & Discontinuity in Developmental Theory. Melvin Feffer. 1981. LC 81-23610. 298p. 45.00 (*0-8236-6185-7*) Intl Univs Pr.

Structure of Human Abilities. Philip E. Vernon. 2nd ed. 1979. LC 79-9751. 208p. reprint ed. lib. bdg. 35.00 (*0-313-20804-2*, VEST, Greenwood Pr) Greenwood.

Structure of Individual Psychotherapy. Bernard D. Beitman. 1990. LC 86-3160. 330p. reprint ed. pap. 24.00 (*0-89862-461-4*, 2461) Guilford Pubns.

Structure of Mind in History: Five Major Figures in Psychohistory. Philip Pomper. 1985. LC 84-22988. 192p. text 40.50 (*0-231-06064-5*) Col U Pr.

Structure of Psychiatry in the U. S. S. R. Edward A. Babayan. 1986. LC 85-18100. 350p. 55.00 (*0-8236-6169-5*) Intl Univs Pr.

Structure of Psychoanalytic Theory: A Systematizing Attempt. David Rapaport. 1967. (Psychological Issues Monographs: No. 6, Vol. 2, No. 2). 158p. (Orig.). 27.50 (*0-8236-6180-6*) Intl Univs Pr.

Structure of Psychological Well-Being. Norman M. Bradburn. 1969. LC 67-27388. (Monographs in Social Research: No. 15). (Illus.). 15.00 (*0-202-25029-6*) Natl Opinion Res.

Structure of the Human Brain: A Photographic Atlas. Stephen J. DeArmond et al. 3rd ed. 1989. (Illus.). 208p. spiral bd. 29.50 (*0-19-504357-X*) OUP.

Structure-Property Correlations in Drug Research. Ed. by Han Van de Waterbeemd. 1996. LC 96-3247. (Biotechnology Intelligence Unit Ser.). 210p. text 79.00 (*0-12-711650-8*) Landes Bioscience.

Structured Clinical Interview. Spitzer. 1990. 45.95 (*0-88048-411-X*) Am Psychiatric.

Structured Clinical Interview for DSM-IV Axis I Disorders (SCID-I), Clinical Version: Set of Administration Booklet & Packet of 5 Scoresheets. Michael B. First et al. 1997. pap. text 43.50 (*0-88048-934-0*, 8934) Am Psychiatric.

Structured Clinical Interview for DSM-IV Axis II Personality Disorders (SCID-II) Set of User's Guide, Interview & Questionnaire. Michael B. First et al. 1997. pap. text 47.00 (*0-88048-812-3*, 8812) Am Psychiatric.

Structured Clinical Interview for DSM-IV Axis I Disorders (SCID-I), Clinician Version: Administration Booklet. Michael B. First et al. 1997. 96p. tchr. ed., spiral bd. 26.00 (*0-88048-932-4*, 8932) Am Psychiatric.

Structured Clinical Interview for DSM-IV Axis I Disorders (SCID-I), Clinician Version: Score Sheets. Michael B. First et al. 1997. 64p. pap. text, tchr. ed. 22.95 (*0-88048-933-2*, 8933) Am Psychiatric.

Structured Clinical Interview for DSM-IV Axis I Disorders (SCID-I), Clinician Version: Set of User's Guide, Administration Booklet, & Package of 5 Scoresheets. Michael B. First et al. 1997. pap. text 67.00 (*0-88048-935-9*, 8935) Am Psychiatric.

Structured Clinical Interview for DSM-IV Axis I Disorders (SCID-I), Clinician Version: User's Guide. Michael B. First et al. 1997. 160p. pap. text, stu. ed. 28.50 (*0-88048-931-6*, 8931) Am Psychiatric.

Structured Clinical Interview for DSM-IV Axis II Personality Disorders (SCID-II) User's Guide. Michael B. First et al. 1997. 80p. pap. text 31.95 (*0-88048-810-7*, 8810) Am Psychiatric.

Structured Clinical Interview for DSM-IV Dissociative Disorders (SCID-D) Marlene Stein. rev. ed. 1994. 86p. pap. text 22.95 (*0-88048-860-3*, 8860) Am Psychiatric.

Structured Clinical Interview for DSM-IV Personality Disorders (SCID-II) Interview & Questionnaire. Michael B. First et al. 1997. 64p. pap. text 22.95 (*0-88048-811-5*, 8811) Am Psychiatric.

Structured Exercises for Promoting Family & Group Strengths: A Handbook for Group Leaders, Trainers, Educators, Counselors, & Therapists. Ed. by Ron McManus & Glen H. Jennings. LC 95-4829. 303p. (C). 1997. pap. 19.95 (*0-7890-0224-8*); 1996. (Illus.). 39.95 (*1-56024-978-1*) Haworth Pr.

Structured Exercises in Healing for Adult Survivors of Childhood Sexual Abuse: A 12-Session Program. Bonnie J. Collins & Kathryn Marsh. 1998. LC 98-8937. 24.95 (*1-57025-165-7*) Whole Person.

Structured Exercises in Stress Management. Ed. by Nancy L. Tubesing & Donald A. Tubesing. 1994. (Stress Management Handbook Ser.). 192p. Vol. 2. pap. text 29.95 (*1-57025-015-4*); Vol. 4. pap. text 29.95 (*1-57025-017-0*) Whole Person.

Structured Exercises in Stress Management, Vol. 5. Ed. by Nancy L. Tubesing & Sandy S. Christian. 1995. LC 83-61073. (Stress Management Handbook Ser.). 192p. otabind 29.95 (*1-57025-016-2*) Whole Person.

Structured Exercises in Wellness Promotion. Ed. by Nancy L. Tubesing & Donald A. Tubesing. 1994. (Wellness Promotion Handbook Ser.). 192p. Vol. 1. pap. text 29.95 (*1-57025-018-9*); Vol. 2. pap. text 29.95 (*1-57025-019-7*) Whole Person.

Structured Exercises in Wellness Promotion: Loose-Leaf Edition, Vol. 4. Ed. by Nancy L. Tubesing & Donald A. Tubesing. 1994. (Wellness Promotion Handbook Ser.). 192p. (Orig.). ring bd. 54.95 (*0-938586-41-6*) Whole Person.

Structured Group Psychotherapy for Bipolar Disorder: The Life Goals Program. Mark S. Bauer & Linda McBride. 1996. LC 96-3140. (Illus.). 280p. (Orig.). 43.95 (*0-8261-9300-5*) Springer Pub.

Structured Interview for DSM-IV Personality (SIDP-IV) Bruce Pfohl et al. 1997. 48p. pap. text 22.95 (*0-88048-937-5*, 8937) Am Psychiatric.

***Structured Sensory Intervention for Traumatized Children, Adolescents & Parents: Strategies to Alleviate Trauma.** William Steele & Melvyn Raider. 2002. LC 2001-42765. (Mellen Studies in Social Work: Vol. 1). 256p. 89.95 (*0-7734-7347-5*) E Mellen.

Structured Specifying: Techniques & Applications. Ali Mili. 1990. (Information Technology Ser.). 143p. 39.95 (*0-470-21527-5*) P-H.

Structures & Function of Low Affinity FC Receptors. Ed. by W. H. Fridman. 1989. (Chemical Immunology Ser.: Vol. 47). (Illus.). xii, 260p. 187.00 (*3-8055-4959-8*) S Karger.

Structures & Procedures of Implicit Knowledge. Arthur C. Graesser & Leslie F. Clark. 1985. LC 85-7336. (Advances in Discourse Processes Ser.: Vol. 17). 336p. pap. 42.50 (*0-89391-362-6*);17. 85.00 (*0-89391-192-5*) Greenwood (Ablex).

Structures of Antigens, Vol. I. Ed. by M. H. V. Van Regenmortel. 1992. 432p. 169.00 (*0-8493-8865-1*, QR186) CRC Pr.

Structures of Knowing. Katherine Arens. 1989. 440p. (C). lib. bdg. (*0-7923-0009-2*) Kluwer Academic NLD. *Dist:* Kluwer Academic.

Structures of Subjectivity: Explorations in Psychoanalytic Phenomenology. George E. Atwood & Robert D. Stolorow. 1993. (Psychoanalytic Inquiry Bk.: Vol. 4). 144p. (C). reprint ed. pap. 22.50 (*0-88163-166-3*) Analytic Pr.

Structuring Change: Effective Practice for Common Client Problems. Ed. by Kevin J. Corcoran. 1992. LC 91-43836. 340p. (C). pap. text 39.95 (*0-925065-14-5*) Lyceum IL.

Structuring the Therapeutic Process: Compromise with Chaos - a Therapist's Response to the Individual & the Group. Murray Cox. 1978. pap. 27.00 (*1-85302-028-1*) Taylor & Francis.

Struggle for Control: A Study of Law, Disputes, & Deviance. Pat Lauderdale & Michael Cruit. 1993. LC 91-47942. (SUNY Series in Deviance & Social Control). 256p. (C). pap. text 22.95 (*0-7914-1312-8*) State U NY Pr.

Struggle for Workers' Health. Ed. by Ray H. Elling. 1986. 500p. (C). text 47.95 (*0-89503-047-0*) Baywood Pub.

Struktur des Verhaltens. Maurice Merleau-Ponty. 1976. (Phaenomenologisch-Psychologische Forschungen Ser.: Vol. 13). xxvi, 278p. (C). text 75.40 (*3-11-004469-2*) De Gruyter.

Struktur, Spleissprozesse und Funktionen Mitochondrialer Introne: Das "Mobile" Intron des Ascomyceten Podospora Anserina. Udo Schmidt. 1989. (Bibliotheca Mycologica: Vol. 127). (GER., Illus.). 124p. (*3-443-59028-4*) Gebruder Borntraeger DEU. *Dist:* Balogh.

Struktur und Funktion Endothelialer Zellen. Ed. by K. Messmer & F. Hammersen. 1983. (Illus.). x, 150p. pap. 42.75 (*3-8055-3712-3*) S Karger.

Struktur und Funktionen Mitochondrialer Dna Bei Pilzen. H. U. Kueck. 1981. (Bibliotheca Mycologica Ser.: No. 84). (GER., Illus.). 148p. pap. text 24.00 (*3-7682-1323-4*) Lubrecht & Cramer.

Stuart & Sundeen's Pocket Guide to Psychiatric Nursing. Gail W. Stuart & Michele T. Laraia. 4th ed. 1997. LC 98-115972. (Mosby's Pocket Guide Ser.). (Illus.). 480p. (C). (gr. 13). pap. text 22.95 (*0-8151-2602-6*, 31072) Mosby Inc.

Stuart & Sundeen's Principles & Practice of Psychiatric Nursing. Gail W. Stuart & Michele T. Laraia. 6th ed. 1997. LC 97-36169. (Illus.). 936p. (C). (gr. 13). text 53.00 (*0-8151-2603-4*, 31073) Mosby Inc.

Stuart & Sundeen's Principles & Practice of Psychiatric Nursing: Includes Testbank. Gail W. Stuart & Michele T. Laraia. 6th ed. 1998. (Illus.). 936p. tchr. ed. (*1-55664-439-6*) Mosby Inc.

Student-Directed Learning: Teaching Self-Determination Skills. Martin Agran. 1996. LC 96-34861. (Special Education Ser.). (Illus.). 288p. pap. text 67.95 (*0-534-15942-7*) Brooks-Cole.

***Student Education Evaluation Disk for Nursing Assistant.** Sheila A. Sorrentino. 1996. pap. 17.95 incl. disk (*0-8151-8554-5*) Mosby Inc.

Student-Faculty Relations in Medical School: A Study of Professional Socialization. David Caplovitz. Ed. by Harriet Zuckerman & Robert K. Merton. 1980. LC 79-8980. (Dissertations on Sociology Ser.). lib. bdg. 29.95 (*0-405-12956-4*) Ayer.

Student Guide Health Occupation Clinical Experience. Thomson. 1996. (Health Occupations Ser.). tchr. ed. 12.00 (*0-8273-6291-9*) Delmar.

Student Guide to the Registered Nurse (R.N.) Examination. Maryanne C. Glynn. Ed. by David M. Tarlow. 1981. (Illus.). pap. 12.95 (*0-931572-03-7*) Datar Pub.

Student Guide to the World's Medical Schools Where the Language of Instruction Is in English. David M. Tarlow. 1993. pap. 12.95 (*0-931572-02-9*) Datar Pub.

Student Health Problems: An Educator's Reference. Wilma W. Tompkins & Theodore P. Shannon. 1993. LC 92-35114. 261p. (C). mass mkt. 29.25 (*0-8273-4989-0*) Delmar.

Student Manual to Accompany the Administrative Medical Assistant. Mary E. Kinn. 4th ed. 2000. 482p. (C). pap., stu. ed. 12.00 (*0-7216-7296-5*) Saunders.

Student Mastery & Competency Package for the Medical Assistant: Administrative & Clinical. Mary E. Kinn et al. Ed. by Adrianne Williams. 8th ed. 2000. (Illus.). 540p. pap., stu. ed. (*0-7216-7302-3*) Saunders.

Student Nurse Handbook: Difficult Concepts Made Easy. B. Gayle Twiname et al. 1998. LC 98-37951. 400p. (C). pap., stu. ed. 17.95 (*0-8385-8681-3*) P-H.

Student Nurses in Clinical Practice: Studies on Independence, Assessment & Performance. Anna Lofmark. 2000. (Comprehensive Summaries of Uppsala Dissertations from the Faculty of Social Sciences Ser.: No. 92). (Illus.). 59p. pap. (*91-554-4749-X*) Uppsala Universitet SWE. *Dist:* Coronet Bks.

Student Psychiatry Today: A Comprehensive Textbook. Robert I. Cohen & Jerome J. Hart. 2nd ed. 1995. LC 95-4192. 448p. pap. text 44.95 (*0-7506-1586-9*) E A GBR. *Dist:* OUP.

Student Recruitment in Psychosocial Occupational Therapy: Intergenerational Approaches. Susan Haiman. 1990. LC 90-4541. (Occupational Therapy in Mental Health Ser.: Vol. 10, No. 1). 84p. text 3.95 (*0-86656-993-6*) Haworth Pr.

Student Review for Clinical Medicine. Woods. 1993. (C). pap. text, stu. ed. 17.95 (*0-7216-5238-7*) Harcourt.

Student Stress: A Classroom Management System. Kevin J. Swick. 1987. 96p. pap. 9.95 (*0-8106-1696-3*) NEA.

Student Study Guide for Biology: Concepts & Connections. Richard M. Liebaert. 2nd ed. 1996. 480p. (C). pap. text 25.00 (*0-8053-2023-7*) Addison-Wesley.

Student Study Guide for Sorensen & Luckmann's Basic Nursing: A Psychophysiologic Approach. Verolyn B. Bolander. 3rd ed. 1994. (Illus.). 380p. pap. text 19.00 (*0-7216-4327-2*) Saunders.

Student Suicide: A Guide for Intervention. John A. Vidal. 1989. 56p. pap. 7.95 (*0-8106-0244-X*) NEA.

Student Syllabus: The SUM Program Beginning Medical Transcription Course. Susan M. Turley & Linda C. Campbell. 1992. pap. 5.00 (*0-934385-52-1*) Hlth Prof Inst.

Student to Student Guide to Medical School. William R. Betcher. 1985. 278p. pap. 19.95 (*0-316-09246-0*, Little Brwn Med Div) Lppncott W & W.

Student Workbook for Comprehensive Maternity Nursing: Nursing Process & the Childbearing Family. A. & Mehlmeister. 2nd ed. 1990. 272p. text 15.95 (*0-397-54754-4*) Lppncott W & W.

Student Workbook for Essentials of Anatomy & Physiology. Valerie C. Scanlon. 2nd ed. 1994. 417p. pap., wbk. ed. 18.95 (*0-8036-7736-7*) Davis Co.

Student Workbook for Essentials of Anatomy & Physiology. Valerie C. Scanlon & Tina Sanders. 3rd ed. 1998. (Illus.). 440p. pap., stu. ed. 19.95 (*0-8036-0408-4*) Davis Co.

Student Workbook for Health Careers Today. Judith A. Gerdin. 1990. (Illus.). 368p. (C). (gr. 13). pap. text 14.95 (*0-8016-2470-3*, 02470) Mosby Inc.

Student Workbook for Understanding Human Structure & Function. Valerie C. Scanlon & Tina Sanders. 1997. (Illus.). 356p. pap., stu. ed. 17.95 (*0-8036-0242-1*) Davis Co.

Student Workbook to Accompany Clinical Pharmacology & Nursing Management. Laurel Eisenhauer et al. 5th ed. 1997. 368p. pap. text, wbk. ed. 17.95 (*0-397-55332-3*) Lppncott W & W.

Students & Dyslexia: Growing up with a Specific Disability. Barbara Riddick et al. 1997. 180p. 39.95 (*1-56593-886-0*, 1736) Singular Publishing.

Student's Atlas of Nueroanatomy. Walter J. Hendelman. 1994. LC 93-41702. pap. text 34.00 (*0-7216-5428-2*) Saunders.

Students Dictionary of Psychological Terms. Reinhard O. Schmidt. 2000. 96p. pap. text 16.00 (*1-55605-314-2*) Wyndham Hall.

Student's Dictionary of Psychology. Peter Stratton & Nicky Hayes. 1989. 224p. (*0-7131-6500-6*); 1989. 224p. pap. (*0-7131-6501-4*); 2nd ed. 1995. LC 92-30214. (Illus.). 240p. pap. text (*0-340-56926-3*) E A GBR. *Dist:* Routldge, OUP.

Student's Dictionary of Psychology. Peter Stratton & Nicky Hayes. 3rd ed. 1998. LC 98-25917. (Arnold Publication). (Illus.). 336p. pap. text 16.95 (*0-340-70583-3*) OUP.

***Student's Guide to Studying Psychology.** Thomas Heffernan. 2000. (*0-86377-870-4*) Psychol Pr.

Student's Manual for Balancing Body Chemistry with Nutrition. Robert J. Peshek. 1977. 20.00 (*0-9605902-1-8*) Color Coded Charting.

Student's Pocket Medical Lexicon. Elias Longley. 2000. 303p. pap. 25.00 (*0-7884-1545-X*, 1545) Heritage Bk.

Student's Rorschach Manual: An Introduction to Administering, Scoring & Interpreting Researcher's Psychodiagnostic Inkblot Test. Robert M. Allen. rev. ed. 1978. LC 77-14710. xii, 361p. 52.50 (*0-8236-6201-2*) Intl Univs Pr.

Students Speak: A Survey of Health Interests & Concerns: Kindergarten Through Twelfth Grade. Lucille Trucano. 1984. 208p. (Orig.). pap. 6.50 (*0-935529-02-0*) Comprehen Health Educ.

Student's Textbook of Surgery. William M. Rambo. 1995. (Illus.). 400p. pap. 22.95 (*0-86542-485-3*) Blackwell Sci.

Students with Autism: Characteristics & Instruction Programming. Jack Scott et al. 1999. LC 99-27449. (Illus.). 435p. pap. text 69.95 (*1-56593-630-2*, 1306) Thomson Learn.

Students with Mild Disabilities. Tom E. Smith et al. 1993. LC 92-70786. (Illus.). 450p. (C). text 76.00 (*0-03-047519-8*) Harcourt Coll Pubs.

Students with Seizures: A Manual for School Nurses. Nancy Santilli et al. 1991. LC 91-72641. (Illus.). (Orig.). spiral bd. (*0-941932-25-7*) HealthScan.

Studies & Essays on International Humanitarian Law & Red Cross Principles. Ed. by Christophe Swinarski. 1984. lib. bdg. 50.00 (*90-247-3078-3*) Kluwer Academic.

Studies Concerning Organisms Occurring in Water Supplies. L. B. Walton. 1930. (Bulletin Ser.: No. 24). pap. text 2.00 (*0-86727-023-3*) Ohio Bio Survey.

***Studies in Alternative Therapy**, Vol. 3. 1996. pap. 32.00 (*87-7838-206-8*) Intl Spec Bk.

Studies in Analytical Psychology. Gerhard Adler. 1967. LC 67-10652. (Illus.). 10.00 (*0-913430-14-5*) C G Jung Foun.

Studies in Child Guidance. Jean W. Macfarlane. 1938. (SRCD M Ser.: Vol. 3, No. 6). 25.00 (*0-527-01506-7*) Periodicals Srv.

Studies in Childhood, 3. James Sully. 1977. LC 77-72191. (Contributions to the History of Psychology Ser.: Psychometrics & Educational Psychology). 527p. reprint ed. lib. bdg. 92.50 (*0-313-26938-6*, U6938, Greenwood Pr) Greenwood.

Studies in Clinical Psychodiagnostics & Psychotherapy. L. Kardos et al. 1987. 191p. (C). pap. (*963-05-4068-1*) Akade Kiado HUN. *Dist:* Intl Spec Bk, St Mut.

Studies in Clinical Psychology, Vol. 3. Ed. by Lee E. Travis. 1974. (Psychology Monographs General & Applied: Vol. 49). reprint ed. 55.00 (*0-8115-1448-X*) Periodicals Srv.

Studies in Crime: Introduction to Forensic Archaeology. John Hunter. 1996. (Illus.). 160p. pap. 50.00 (*0-7134-7901-9*) Trafalgar.

Studies in Crisis Behavior. Ed. by Michael Brecher. 1979. 384p. (C). text 44.95 (*0-87855-292-8*) Transaction Pubs.

Studies in Drug Utilization: Methods & Applications. U. Bergman et al. 1979. (WHO Regional Publications, European Ser.: No. 8). 185p. 20.00 (*92-9020-108-8*, 1310008) World Health.

Studies in Economic Appraisal in Health Care Michael F. Drummond. 1. 1981. 224p. text 39.95 (*0-19-261274-3*); 2. 1986. 304p. text 49.00 (*0-19-261398-7*) OUP.

Studies in Inherited Metabolic Disease: Lipoproteins; Ethical Issues. Ed. by R. J. Pollitt et al. 1988. (C). text 185.00 (*0-7462-0101-X*) Kluwer Academic.

Studies in Inherited Metabolic Diseases: Prenatal & Perinatal Diagnosis. Ed. by G. M. Addison et al. 1989. (C). text 226.50 (*0-7923-8916-6*) Kluwer Academic.

Studies in Learning & Memory: Selected Papers. Benton J. Underwood. Ed. by Charles D. Spielberger. 1982. LC 81-22694. (Centennial Psychology Ser.). 331p. 72.50 (*0-275-90917-4*, C0917, Praeger Pubs) Greenwood.

Studies in Mental Health Policy. Ed. by Kenneth Whittemore. 1994. 152p. (Orig.). pap. 15.00 (*0-944285-39-2*) Pol Studies.

Studies in Natural Products Chemistry: Stereoselective Synthesis, Pt. E. A. Rahman. 1991. (Studies in Natural Products Chemistry: Vol. 8). 500p. 240.50 (*0-444-88967-1*) Elsevier.

Studies in Neotropical Ornithology Honoring Ted Parker. Ed. by J. V. Remsen, Jr. 1997. (Ornithological Monographs: Vol. 48). (Illus.). 918p. 49.95 (*0-935868-93-3*) Am Ornithologists.

Studies in Neuropsychology: Selected Papers of Arthur Benton. Arthur L. Benton. Ed. by Otfried Spreen & Louis Costa. 1985. (Illus.). 320p. text 47.50 (*0-19-503636-0*) OUP.

Studies in Non-Determining Psychology. Ed. by Gerald N. Epstein. 1992. 294p. pap. 18.00 (*1-883148-02-2*) ACMI Pr.

Studies in Osteoarthrosis: Pathogensis, Intervention, Assessment. Ed. by D. J. Lott et al. 1987. LC 86-23428. 136p. 525.00 (*0-471-91336-7*) Wiley.

Studies in Pessimism. Arthur Schopenhauer. 1970. reprint ed. 49.00 (*0-403-00044-0*) Scholarly.

Studies in Pharmaceutical Economics. Ed. by Mickey C. Smith. 1996. LC 96-4736. (Illus.). 682p. lib. bdg. 79.95 (*0-7890-0062-8*, Pharmctl Prods) Haworth Pr.

Studies in Psychology. William Reich. 2nd ed. 1991. (C). pap. text 32.20 (*0-536-58075-8*) Pearson Custom.

Studies in Psychology of Reading, No. 4— William C. Morse et al. 1968. LC 68-54427. (Michigan University Monographs in Education: No. 4). 188p. reprint ed. lib. bdg. 35.00 (*0-8371-0176-X*, MOPR, Greenwood Pr) Greenwood.

Studies in Psychopathology: The Descriptive Psychology Approach. Ed. by Raymond M. Bergner. 1993. 256p. (C). pap. 19.95 (*0-9625661-3-6*) Descriptive Psych Pr.

Studies in Radiotherapeutics. Joseph S. Mitchell. 1960. LC 60-3368. (Illus.). 281p. 23.95 (*0-674-84930-2*) HUP.

Studies in Reflecting Abstraction. Jean Piaget. Ed. & Tr. by Robert L. Campbell. 2000. LC 00-44553. 336p. (*1-84169-157-7*) Psychol Pr GBR. *Dist:* Taylor & Francis.

Studies in Remembering: The Reproduction of Connected & Extended Verbal Material. I. H. Paul. 1959. (Psychological Issues Monographs: No. 2, Vol. 1, No. 2). 152p. (Orig.). 27.50 (*0-8236-6240-3*) Intl Univs Pr.

Studies in Social Identity. Theodore R. Sarbin & Karl E. Scheibe. 1983. LC 82-16580. 400p. 75.00 (*0-275-91073-3*, C1073, Praeger Pubs) Greenwood.

Studies in Stomatology & Craniofacial Biology. Ed. by M. Cohen & B. Baum. 1997. LC 96-77470. 633p. 125.00 (*90-5199-283-1*, 283-1) IOS Press.

Studies in the Acquisition of Anaphora. Ed. by Barbara Lust. 1986. pap. text 62.50 (*90-277-2122-X*) Kluwer Academic.

Studies in the Acquisition of Anaphoria. Ed. by Barbara Lust. 1986. lib. bdg. 154.50 (*90-277-2121-1*) Kluwer Academic.

Studies in the Medicine of Ancient India, Pt. 1: Osteology, or the Bones of the Human Body, Pt. 1. August F. Hoernle. LC 75-23723. reprint ed. 45.00 (*0-404-13281-2*) AMS Pr.

Studies in the Paleopathology of Egypt. Marc A. Ruffer. Ed. by Roy L. Moodie. LC 75-23758. reprint ed. 135.00 (*0-404-13364-9*) AMS Pr.

Studies in the Pathology of Radiation Disease. N. Krayevskii & A. Lieberman. 1965. LC 64-21692. 429p. (*0-08-010772-9*) Pergamon Repr GBR. *Dist:* Franklin.

Studies in the Psychology of Intemperance. G. E. Partridge. Ed. by Gerald N. Grob. 1981. LC 80-1244. (Addiction in America Ser.). reprint ed. lib. bdg. 29.95 (*0-405-13614-5*) Ayer.

Studies in Tibetan Medicine. Elisabeth Finckh. 1989. LC 88-39158. (Illus.). 95p. pap. 9.95 (*0-937938-61-0*) Snow Lion Pubns.

Studies in Viable Cell Immobilization. Ed. by Colin Webb & George A. Dervakos. 1996. (Molecular Biology Intelligence Unit Ser.). 118p. 99.00 (*1-57059-018-4*, LN9018) Landes Bioscience.

Studies of Aging: Protocols. Ed. by Hal Sternberg & Paola S. Timiras. 1999. LC 99-20522. (Lab Manual Ser.). (Illus.). 256p. 82.00 (3-540-64600-0) Spr-Verlag.

Studies of Brain Metabolism in Psychiatric Patients: Can Standards Be Drawn? Ed. by H. Agren et al. 1992. (Journals of Neural Transmission: Suppl. 37). (Illus.). 100p. 63.95 (0-387-82346-8) Spr-Verlag.

Studies of Illnesses of Children Followed from Birth to Eighteen Years. Isabelle Valadian et al. 1961. (SRCD M Ser.: Vol. 26, No. 3). 25.00 (0-527-01590-3) Periodicals Srv.

Studies of Mind & Brain. Stephen Grossberg. 1982. 660p. pap. text 79.50 (90-277-1360-X); lib. bdg. 165.00 (90-277-1359-6) Kluwer Academic.

Studies of Narcosis. Charles E. Overton. Ed. by Robert L. Lipnick. 1990. xi, 203p. (C). text 65.00 (0-412-35240-0) Chapman & Hall.

***Studies of Neuropeptides in Pancreatic Beta Cell Function with Special Emphasis on Islet Amyloid Polypeptide (IAPP)** Ella Karlsson. 2000. (Comprehensive Summaries of Uppsala Disertations from the Faculty of Medicine: No. 980). (Illus.). 68p. (Orig.). pap. (91-554-4890-9) Uppsala Universitet SWE. *Dist:* Coronet Bks.

Studies of Reading & Arithmetic in Mentally Retarded Boys. L. Dunn & R. J. Capobianco. 1954. (SRCD M Ser.: Vol. 19, No. 1). pap. 25.00 (0-527-01560-1) Periodicals Srv.

Studies of the Normal & Abnormal Development of the Nervous System. Ed. by W. Lierse & F. Beck. 1980. (Bibliotheca Anatomica Ser.: No. 19). (Illus.). pap. 162.75 (3-8055-1039-X) S Karger.

Studies of the Yoruba Therapeutic System in Nigeria. Ed. by D. Michael Warren et al. 1997. (Studies in Technology & Social Change: No. 28). (Illus.). 230p. (C). pap. 20.00 (0-945271-44-1) ISU-CIKARD.

Studies on Child Language & Aphasia. Roman Jakobson. 1971. (Janua Linguarum, Ser. Minor: No. 114). (Orig.). pap. text (90-279-1640-3) Mouton.

***Studies on Cytotoxic & Neutrophil Challenging Polypeptides & Cardiac Glycosides of Plant Origin.** Senia Johansson. 2001. (Comprehensive Summaries of Uppsala Dissertations from the Faculty of Pharmacy Ser.: No. 255). (Illus.). 74p. pap. (91-554-5092-X) Uppsala Universitet SWE. *Dist:* Coronet Bks.

Studies on Dextropropoxyphene: With Special Reference to Dependence among Chronic Pain Patients, Classification of the Manner of Death in Fatal Poisoning & Characteristics of the Fatal Poisoning Victims. Birgitta Jonasson. 2000. (Comprehensive Summaries of Uppsala Dissertations from the Faculty of Medicine Ser.: No. 933). (Illus.). 60p. pap. (91-554-4729-5) Uppsala Universitet SWE. *Dist:* Coronet Bks.

Studies on Effects of Antioxidants on Arterial Thrombosis & Endothelial Cell Injury: With Special Reference to Tocopherols & ApoA1 Milano. Dayuan Li. 2000. (Comprehensive Summaries of Uppsala Dissertations from the Faculty of Medicine Ser.: No. 936). (Illus.). 47p. pap. (91-554-4740-6) Uppsala Universitet SWE. *Dist:* Coronet Bks.

Studies on Excitation & Inhibition in the Retina. Ed. by Floyd Ratliff. 1974. LC 73-89539. (Illus.). 688p. 17.50 (0-87470-019-1) Rockefeller.

Studies on Hysteria. Josef Breuer & Sigmund Freud. 1982. LC 57-12310. (Basic Books Classics). 320p. pap. 22.00 (0-465-08276-9) Basic.

Studies on Indian Medical History: Papers Presented at the International Workshop on the Study of Indian Medicine Held at the Wellcome Institute for the History of Medicine, Sept. 2-4, 1985. Ed. by G. Jan Meulenbeld & Dominik Wujastyk. 1987. (Groningen Oriental Studies: Vol. II). 247p. (Orig.). (C). pap. (90-6980-015-2) Egbert Forsten NLD. *Dist:* Hodlder & Stoughton.

Studies on Neuromuscular Diseases: Proceedings of the Quantitative Methods of Investigations in the Clinics of Neuromuscular Diseases International Symposium, Giessen, April 1974. Quantitative Methods of Investigations in the Clinics of Neuromuscular Diseases Staff. Ed. by K. Kunze & J. E. Desmedt. 1975. 250p. 132.25 (3-8055-1749-1) S Karger.

Studies on Normal Pressure Glaucoma. H. Caroline Geijssen. 1991. (Illus.). 240p. lib. bdg. (90-6299-068-1) Kugler NLD. *Dist:* Lib Res.

***Studies on Rotavirus Replication.** Alexis Fuentes. 2000. (Comprehensive Summaries of Uppsala Dissertations from the Faculty of Medicine Ser.: No. 919). (Illus.). 53p. pap. (91-554-4693-0) Uppsala Universitet SWE. *Dist:* Coronet Bks.

***Studies on the Bcl-2 Family of Apoptosis Regulators in the Nervous System.** Susanne Hamner. 2000. (Comprehensive Summaries of Uppsala Disertations from the Faculty of Medicine: No. 977). (Illus.). 66p. (Orig.). pap. (91-554-4870-4) Uppsala Universitet SWE. *Dist:* Coronet Bks.

Studies on the Biology & Pathology of the Skin. Ed. by L. Robert. 1977. (Frontiers of Matrix Biology Ser.: Vol. 4). (Illus.). 220p. 118.50 (3-8055-2666-0) S Karger.

Studies on the Development of Consciousness. Yves Chesni. Tr. by Joseph Zenk. 1994. 153p. text 37.50 (0-931095-02-6) Live Oak.

***Studies on the Differential Specificity of Protein Kinases & Its Applications.** Mart Loog. 2001. (Comprehensive Summaries of Uppsala Dissertations from the Faculty of Medicine Ser.: No. 1073). (Illus.). 47p. pap. (91-554-5116-0) Acta Univ SWE. *Dist:* Coronet Bks.

Studies on the Piriform Lobe. Facundo Valverde-Garcia. 1965. LC 65-16689. (Illus.). 138p. 18.00 (0-674-85200-1) HUP.

Studies on the Self & Social Cognition. M. F. Pichevin et al. 1993. 344p. text 109.00 (981-02-1237-2) World Scientific Pub.

Studies on Tick-Borne Encephalitis. D. Blaskovic et al. 1967. (Bulletin of WHO Ser.: Suppl. No. 1 to Vol. 36). 94p. pap. 9.00 (92-4-068361-5, 1033601) World Health.

Studies on Trophoblastic Disease in China. Hongzhao Song & Baozhen Wu. 1989. (International Academic Publishers Ser.). (Illus.). 300p. 105.00 (0-08-036144-7, Pergamon Pr) Elsevier.

Studies on William Harvey. Ed. by I. Bernard Cohen. 1981. LC 80-2101. (Development of Science Ser.). (Illus.). lib. bdg. 71.95 (0-405-13866-0) Ayer.

Studies to Enhance the Evaluation of Family Planning Programs, No. 87. 1998. 246p. 25.00 (92-1-151106-2, E.84.XIII.9) UN.

Study & Analysis of the Conditional Reflex. Ignatius A. Hamel. 1974. (Psychology Monographs General & Applied: Vol. 27). reprint ed. pap. 55.00 (0-8115-1426-9) Periodicals Srv.

Study & Review for EMT Prehospital Care. Mark C. Henry & Edward R. Stapleton. 2nd rev. ed. 1997. LC 99-161759. (Illus.). 765p. pap. text, stu. ed. 16.95 (0-7216-6102-5) Saunders.

Study Course in Homeopathy. Phyllis Speight. 1979. 145p. (C). pap. 27.95 (0-8464-1052-4) Beekman Pubs.

Study Course in Homeopathy. Phyllis Speight. 1980. 30.00 (0-85032-164-6) St Mut.

Study Guide. C. A. Mutzebaugh. 9th ed. 1999. 32p. 99.50 (0-88937-223-3) Hogrefe & Huber Pubs.

Study Guide & Computerized Learning Resources T-A Nursing Research: Methods, Critical Appraisal & Utilization. Kathleen Rose-Grippa & Mary Jo Gorney-Moreno. 4th ed. 1998. 240p. stu. ed. (0-8151-2810-X) Mosby Inc.

Study Guide & Exam Review for Comprehensive Dent. Finkbeiner. 1993. text (0-397-54924-5) Lppncott W & W.

Study Guide & Learning Activities for Training Manual for IV Admixture Personnel. Vicente J. Tormo & Max L. Hunt. 1997. 96p. pap. 19.95 (0-944496-57-1) Precept Pr.

Study Guide & Manual for the National Certification Examinations for Nurse Practitioners & Other Primary Health Care Providers. Patricia Martinell et al. 1989. 125p. pap. text 19.95 (0-8290-1279-6) Irvington.

Study Guide & Practice Tests to Accompany Zimbardo's Psychology & Life. Philip G. Zimbardo. 13th ed. 1992. (C). pap. text 21.00 (0-673-46628-0) Addson-Wesley Educ.

Study Guide & Review Manual of Human Embryology: Review Manual. Keith L. Moore & T. V. Persaud. Ed. by William Schmitt. 5th ed. 1998. LC 97-33990. (Illus.). 176p. (C). pap. text, stu. ed. 22.95 (0-7216-7378-3) Saunders.

Study Guide & Self-Examination Review for Kaplan & Sadock's Synopsis of Psychiatry. Harold I. Kaplan & Benjamin J. Sadock. 1998. Orig. Title: Study Guide & Self-Examination Review for Synopsis of Psychiatry & Comprehensive Textbook of Psychiatry. 5th ed. (Illus.). 544p. (0-683-23141-3); 6th ed. LC 98-14746. 500p. 59.95 (0-683-30591-3) Lppncott W & W.

Study Guide & Self-Examination Review for Synopsis of Psychiatry & Comprehensive Textbook of Psychiatry see Study Guide & Self-Examination Review for Kaplan & Sadock's Synopsis of Psychiatry

Study Guide & Self-Examination Review for Understanding Human Behavior in Health & Illness. Richard C. Simons. 3rd ed. 348p. (0-683-04571-7) Lppncott W & W.

Study Guide for Biological Psychology. James W. Kalat. 5th ed. 1994. (Psychology Ser.). mass mkt., stu. ed. 18.75 (0-534-21110-0) Brooks-Cole.

Study Guide for Children in a Changing World. Edward F. Zigler. 2nd ed. 1992. (Psychology Ser.). mass mkt., stu. ed. 18.00 (0-534-14240-0) Brooks-Cole.

Study Guide for Comprehending Behavioral Statistics. Russell T. Hurlburt. 1993. LC 93-24308. 561p. mass mkt. 54.75 (0-534-17418-3) Brooks-Cole.

Study Guide for Emergency Care in the Streets. Nancy L. Caroline. 5th ed. 1995. (Illus.). 592p. pap. text, stu. ed. 26.95 (0-316-12893-7) Lppncott W & W.

Study Guide for Fundamentals of Contemporary Nursing. Carol Lindeman. Date not set. (Illus.). 350p. stu. ed. (0-7216-8308-8) Saunders.

Study Guide for Health, Safety & Nutrition for the Young Child. Lynn R. Marotz et al. 3rd ed. 1993. (Illus.). 169p. stu. ed. 14.95 (0-8273-6060-6) Delmar.

Study Guide for Motor Learning & Performance: A Problem Based Learning Approach. Craig N. Wrisberg. 2000. LC 99-58645. (Illus.). 184p. pap. text 18.00 (0-7360-0000-3, BWRI0000) Human Kinetics.

Study Guide for National Certification in Therapeutic Recreation. Gerald O'Morrow & Ron Reynolds. 1990. LC 90-71335. 89p. 11.95 (0-910251-38-X) Venture Pub PA.

Study Guide for Obstetrics & Gynecology. Ling. 2001. 280p. pap. 55.00 (0-8385-8683-X, Apple Lange Med) McGraw.

Study Guide for Pharmacology: A Nursing Process Approach. Joyce L. Kee & Evelyn Hayes. 3rd ed. 2000. (Illus.). 300p. pap., stu. ed. (0-7216-8565-X) Saunders.

Study Guide for Physical Agents. Michelle H. Cameron. Ed. by Andrew Allen. 1999. 105p. stu. ed. (0-7216-6246-3) Saunders.

Study Guide for Practice of Nursing Research: Conduct, Critique & Utilization. Nancy Burns & Susan K. Grove. 3rd ed. 1997. (Illus.). 715p. pap. text, stu. ed. 22.95 (0-7216-2587-8) Saunders.

Study Guide for Preventive Medicine Certification: A Manual for Specialists in Occupational Medicine, Aerospace Medicine & Public Health & General Preventive Medicine. Nick A. Vlachos et al. 9th ed. 1997. 296p. pap. text, stu. ed. 80.00 (1-883595-17-7, OEM Pr) OEM Health.

Study Guide for Radiation Oncology Physics Board Exams. Brian Berman & Bruce Thomadsen. 2000. (Illus.). 75p. pap. text 29.95 (0-944838-94-4) Med Physics Pub.

Study Guide for the Discovering Psychology Telecourse, Myers, Psychology. Richard O. Straub. 4th ed. 1995. 468p. pap. text 16.95 (0-87901-777-5) Worth.

Study Guide for the Nata Board of Certification, Inc. Entry-Level Athletic Trainer Certification Examination. NATA Board of Certification Staff. 2nd ed. 1999. (Illus.). 146p. (C). pap. text, stu. ed. 35.95 (0-8036-6501-6) Davis Co.

Study Guide for the Textbook of Gynecology. Larry J. Copeland. 1993. 304p. pap. text, stu. ed. 39.95 (0-7216-3383-8) Saunders.

Study Guide for the Therapeutic Recreation Certification Examination. Norma Stumbo & Jean Folkerth. 2nd ed. 1997. pap. 21.95 (1-57167-034-3) Sagamore Pub.

Study Guide for Understanding Medical-Surgical Nursing. Paula D. Hopper & Linda S. Williams. 1999. (Illus.). 349p. pap., stu. ed. 17.95 (0-8036-0332-0) Davis Co.

Study Guide for Understanding Nursing Research. Nancy Burns & Susan K. Grove. 2nd ed. 255p. pap. text (0-7216-8108-5) Saunders.

Study Guide of Clinical Hematology: Theory & Practice. Janice Hudson & Robert F. Bunting, Jr. 1994. LC 93-41166. (Illus.). 259p. (C). pap. text 25.95 (0-8036-4604-6) Davis Co.

Study Guide T/A the Dissectable Human CD-ROM & Mosby's System Atlas. Lindsay. 1997. 144p. stu. ed. incl. cd-rom (0-8151-4541-1) Mosby Inc.

Study Guide to Accompany Anthony Textbook. Kathleen S. Prezbindowski. 11th ed. 1983. 370p. pap. text 13.95 (0-8016-4011-3) Mosby Inc.

Study Guide to Accompany Brunner & Suddarth's Textbook of Medical Surgical Nursing. Mary Jo Boyer. 9th ed. 1999. 400p. pap. text 19.95 (0-7817-2305-1) Lppncott W & W.

Study Guide to Accompany Clinical Drug Therapy. Anne Collins Abrams. 6th ed. pap. text (0-7817-1813-9) Lppncott W & W.

Study Guide to Accompany Computed Tomography. Euclid Seeram. Ed. by Lisa Biello. 1996. LC 96-41148. 416p. pap. text, stu. ed. 37.00 (0-7216-6103-3) Saunders.

Study Guide to Accompany Essentials of Nursing Research: Methods, Appraisal, & Utilization. Denise F. Polit & Bernadette P. Hungler. 5th ed. 2000. 272p. pap. text 19.95 (0-7817-2558-5) Lppncott W & W.

Study Guide to Accompany Fundamental Skills & Concepts in Patient Care. Barbara Kuhn Timby. 7th ed. 2000. 368p. pap. text 19.95 (0-7817-2317-5) Lppncott W & W.

Study Guide to Accompany Fundamentals of Nursing: The Art & Science of Nursing Care. Carol Taylor et al. 4th ed. 2000. 384p. pap. text 19.95 (0-7817-2285-3) Lppncott W & W.

Study Guide to Accompany Human Anatomy & Physiology. Elaine Nicpon Marieb. 3rd ed. 1995. LC 94-39756. (C). pap. text 27.19 (0-8053-4283-4) Benjamin-Cummings.

Study Guide to Accompany Introductory Clinical Pharmacology. Sally S. Roach. 6th ed. 1999. 256p. pap. text 19.95 (0-7817-1751-5) Lppncott W & W.

Study Guide to Accompany Jacob & Francone's Elements of Anatomy & Physiology. Terry Bristol. 2nd ed. 1992. (Illus.). 183p. pap. text 17.95 (0-7216-3644-6) Saunders.

Study Guide to Accompany Lippincott's Textbook for Medical Assistants. Herschfelt & Brill. 1997. 400p. pap. text, stu. ed. 22.95 (0-397-55107-X) Lppncott W & W.

Study Guide to Accompany Maternity Nursing: An Introductory Text. Arlene Burroughs. 6th ed. 1992. (Illus.). 224p. pap. text, stu. ed. 19.95 (0-7216-3314-5) Saunders.

Study Guide to Accompany Nursing Pharmacology & Clinical Management. Venable. 1998. 368p. pap. text 19.95 (0-397-55245-9) Lppncott W & W.

Study Guide to Accompany Psychiatric Mental Health Nursing. Mary Ann Boyd & Mary Ann Nihart. 1998. 224p. pap. text 18.95 (0-397-55179-7) Lppncott W & W.

Study Guide to Accompany Psychopathology & Psychotherapy: Diagnosis & Treatment. Jon Carlson et al. 1998. LC 97-43842. 9.95 (1-56032-554-2) Hemisp Pub.

Study Guide to Core Curriculum for Critical Care Nursing. Maurene A. Harvey. Ed. by Thomas Eoyang. 3rd ed. 1999. (Illus.). 380p. (C). pap. text 35.00 (0-7216-8344-4) Saunders.

Study Guide to DSM-IV. Michael A. Fauman. 1994. LC 94-7366. 420p. pap. text 34.50 (0-88048-696-1, 8696) Am Psychiatric.

Study Guide to Epidemiology & Biostatistics. J. Richard Hebel et al. 5th ed. 2000. LC 00-38571. 224p. pap. 37.00 (0-8342-1758-9, 17589) Aspen Pub.

Study Guide to Essentials of Clinical Psychiatry: Based on the American Psychiatric Press Textbook of Psychiatry. Ed. by Donald M. Hilty et al. 3rd ed. 1999. pap. text, stu. ed. 32.00 (0-88048-842-5, 8842) Am Psychiatric.

Study Guide to Pharmacology Essentials. Jody A. Eckler et al. Ed. by Ilze Rader. 1996. 176p. pap. text, stu. ed. 17.95 (0-7216-6487-3) Saunders.

Study Guide to the American Psychiatric Press Textbook of Consultation-Liaison Psychiatry. Judith Berman et al. 1999. LC 98-53143. 226p. pap. 25.00 (0-88048-805-0) Am Psychiatric.

Study Guide to the American Psychiatric Press Textbook of Geriatric Psychiatry. F. M. Baker. 2001. 192p. pap. 29.50 (0-88048-697-X, 8697) Am Psychiatric.

Study Guide to the American Psychiatric Press Textbook of Neuropsychiatry. Jude Berman et al. 3rd ed. 1997. 256p. pap. text, stu. ed. 26.00 (0-88048-804-2, 8804) Am Psychiatric.

Study Guide to Treatments of Psychiatric Disorders. Sarah D. Atkinson & Glen O. Gabbard. 2nd ed. 1996. 525p. pap. text, stu. ed. 39.95 (0-88048-858-1, 8858) Am Psychiatric.

Study Guide to Understanding Pharmacology. Turley. 2nd ed. 1999. 112p. pap. text, stu. ed. 18.40 (0-13-081090-8) P-H.

Study Guide to Understanding Radiography. Stephen S. Hiss. 3rd ed. 1993. LC 93-8612. (Illus.). 206p. (C). text 39.95 (0-398-05880-6) C C Thomas.

Study in Disguised Intelligence Tests: Interview Form. Donald S. Snedden. LC 71-177765. (Columbia University. Teachers College. Contributions to Education Ser.: No. 291). reprint ed. 37.50 (0-404-55291-9) AMS Pr.

Study in Reaction Time & Movement. T. V. Moore. 1974. (Psychology Monographs General & Applied: Vol. 6). reprint ed. pap. 55.00 (0-8115-1405-6) Periodicals Srv.

Study of Abortion in Primitive Societies. George Devereux. rev. ed. 1976. LC 75-10572. 390p. 57.50 (0-8236-6245-4); pap. 24.95 (0-8236-8311-7, 26245) Intl Univs Pr.

Study of Biology. Jeffrey J. Baker & Garland A. Allen. 4th ed. 1982. LC 81-17550. (Illus.). 1040p. text (0-201-10180-7); stu. ed. (0-201-10182-3) Addison-Wesley.

Study of Brief Psychotherapy. D. H. Malan. 1976. LC 75-30916. 326p. pap. 27.50 (0-306-20019-8, Plenum Trade) Perseus Pubng.

Study of Chinese Alchemy. Obed S. Johnson. 1974. LC 74-352. (Gold Ser.: Vol. 12). 156p. reprint ed. 20.95 (0-405-05914-0) Ayer.

Study of Cranial & Skeletal Material Excavated at Nippur. D. R. Swindler. 1956. (University Museum Monographs: No. 12). (Illus.). v, 40p. pap. 10.00 (0-934718-04-0) U Museum Pubns.

Study of Daoist Acupuncture & Moxibustion. Liu Zheng-cai. 1999. LC 98-74995. (Illus.). viii, 223p. pap. 29.95 (1-891845-08-X) Blue Poppy Pr.

Study of Delaware Indian Medicine Practice & Folk Beliefs. Gladys Tantaquidgeon. LC 76-43864. (Pennsylvania Historical & Musuem Commission Anthropological Ser.). reprint ed. 35.50 (0-404-15724-6) AMS Pr.

Study of Deviates in Versatility & Sociability of Play Interest. Paul A. Witty. LC 73-177630. (Columbia University. Teachers College. Contributions to Education Ser.: No. 470). reprint ed. 37.50 (0-404-55470-9) AMS Pr.

Study of Handedness. Wallace F. Jones. LC 78-72804. (Brainedness, Handedness, & Mental Abilities Ser.). reprint ed. 32.50 (0-404-60867-1) AMS Pr.

Study of Human Abilities. Shao Liu. 1937. (American Oriental Ser.: Vol. 11). 25.00 (0-527-02685-9) Periodicals Srv.

Study of Institutional Children with Particular Reference to the Caloric Value As Well As Other Factors of the Dietary. Pauline B. Mack & C. Urbach. 1948. (SRCD M Ser.: Vol. 13, No. 1). pap. 25.00 (0-527-01543-1) Periodicals Srv.

Study of Intelligence Test Elements. Elizabeth L. Vincent. (Columbia University. Teachers College. Contributions to Education Ser.: No. 152). reprint ed. 37.50 (0-404-55152-1) AMS Pr.

Study of Introvert-Extrovert Responses to Certain Test Situations. Raymond A. Schwegler. LC 76-177805. (Columbia University. Teachers College. Contributions to Education Ser.: No. 361). reprint ed. 37.50 (*0-404-55361-3*) AMS Pr.

Study of Learning & Retention in Young Children. Lois H. Stolz. LC 71-177067. (Columbia University. Teachers College. Contributions to Education Ser.: No. 164). reprint ed. 37.50 (*0-404-55164-5*) AMS Pr.

Study of Man & the Way to Health. J. D. Buck. 1994. 260p. reprint ed. pap. 17.95 (*1-56459-421-1*) Kessinger Pub.

Study of Medical Sciences (Theodor Billroth & Abraham Flexner) An Analysis from Past to Present. Karel B. Absolon. 1986. (Illus.). 170p. pap. 49.50 (*0-930329-10-4*) Kabel Pubs.

Study of Neurosis. John S. Duryee. 1984. LC 84-18699. 300p. (C). text 29.95 (*0-940524-02-3*); pap. text 19.95 (*0-940524-03-1*) G Handwerk.

Study of Ovulation & Early Pregnancy, Vol. 2. Ed. by Y. Boutaleb & A. Gzouli. 1991. (Recent Developments in Fertility & Sterility Ser.). (Illus.). 158p. (C). ring bd. (*1-85070-285-3*, Parthenon Pbng) CRC Pr.

Study of Sensory Control in the Rat. Florence Richardson. 1974. (Psychology Monographs General & Applied: Vol. 12). reprint ed. pap. 55.00 (*0-8115-1411-0*) Periodicals Srv.

Study of Shamanism & Alternate Modes of Healing: The Proceedings of the Fifth International. Ruth-Inge Heinze. 1992. pap. 18.95 (*0-8290-2471-9*) Irvington.

Study of Surgery. Glenn W. Geelhoed. 1995. 392p. pap. 40.00 (*0-8036-0719-9*) Davis Co.

Study of Surgery. Glenn W. Geelhoed. 1994. LC 94-79793. (Illus.). 392p. pap. 40.00 (*0-9632873-6-2*) J & S Pub VA.

Study of the Evolution, Effectiveness & Financing of Public & Private Drug Treatment Services. 1994. lib. bdg. 250.95 (*0-8490-6424-4*) Gordon Pr.

Study of the Knowledge & Use of Hospice by Health Care Professionals in Omaha. Carole M. Davis et al. 1984. 48p. (Orig.). pap. 3.50 (*1-55719-093-3*) U NE CPAR.

***Study of the Myenteric Plexus in Neuropathy: Correlation of Plexus Myentericus Changes & Motility Disturbances in Rats. Implications for Human Pathology.** Ingrid Demedts. 2001. (Acta Biomedica Lovaniensia Ser.: No. 243). (Illus.). 108p. pap. (*90-5867-153-4*) Leuven Univ BEL. *Dist:* Coronet Bks.

Study of the Nature, Incidence & Consequences of Elementary School Playground Related Injuries: Final Report. 1996. (Illus.). 100p. (Orig.). (C). pap. text 30.00 (*0-7881-2700-4*) DIANE Pub.

Study of Two Levels of Bread Enrichment in Children's Diets. Pauline B. Mack et al. 1953. (SRCD M Ser.: Vol. 18, No. 2). pap. 25.00 (*0-527-01558-X*) Periodicals Srv.

Study Outlines in Physics: Construction & Experimental Evaluation. Jessie Clemensen. LC 71-176654. (Columbia University. Teachers College. Contributions to Education Ser.: No. 553). reprint ed. 37.50 (*0-404-55553-5*) AMS Pr.

Study Skills for Nurses. Jayne Taylor. 1992. LC 92-49336. 17.95 (*0-412-44070-9*) Chapman & Hall.

Study Skills for Nurses. Jayne Taylor. 1992. LC 92-49336. 112p. pap. 28.75 (*1-56593-066-5*, 0380) Singular Publishing.

Study Skills for Nursing: A Practical Guide. Joan W. Parnell & Kevin D. Kendrick. 1994. LC 94-26096. pap. text (*0-443-04686-7*) Church.

Study Toxicology Through Questions. John A. Timbrell. 1997. LC 97-201773. 134p. pap. (*0-7484-0695-6*) Tay Francis Ltd GBR. *Dist:* Taylor & Francis.

Studying a Study & Testing a Test: How to Read the Health Science Literature. Richard K. Riegelman. 4th ed. 1999. LC 99-56118. (Illus.). 356p. pap. text 39.95 (*0-7817-1860-0*) Lppncott W & W.

Studying a Study & Testing a Test: How to Read the Medical Literature. Richard K. Riegelman. 1981. pap. 19.50 (*0-316-74518-9*, Little Brwn Med Div) Lppncott W & W.

Studying for Psychology. Donna L. Mealey & William D. McIntosh. Ed. by Brenda D. Smith. 1997. LC 94-12577. (Studying for Ser.). (Illus.). 208p. (C). pap. 23.20 (*0-06-500648-8*) Addson-Wesley Educ.

Studying Health & Disease. Ed. by Kevin McConway. 1994. LC 93-43194. (Health & Disease Ser.: Bk. 2). 132p. pap. (*0-335-19252-1*) OpUniv Pr.

***Studying Health & Disease.** Ed. by Kevin McConway & Basiro Davey. 2001. (Health & Disease Ser.). 208p. pap. (*0-335-20835-5*) OpUniv Pr GBR. *Dist:* Taylor & Francis.

Studying Hygiene Behaviour: Methods, Issues, & Experiences. Ed. by Sandy Cairncross & Vijay Kochar. 1994. LC 93-44528. (Illus.). 334p. 36.00 (*0-8039-9159-2*, 8771) Sage.

***Studying Judgement: Models & Methods.** Nigel Harvey. 2001. 120p. (C). pap. (*1-84169-904-7*) Psychol Pr GBR. *Dist:* Taylor & Francis.

***Studying Organization & Delivery of Health Services: Research Methods.** Ed. by Naomi Fulop et al. 2002. LC 2001-19651. (Social Aspects of AIDS Ser.). (Illus.). 224p. (C). pap. 27.95 (*0-415-25763-8*); lib. bdg. 80.00 (*0-415-25762-X*) Routledge.

Studying Personality: Student Booklet. American Psychological Association Staff. 1981. (Human Behavior Curriculum Project Ser.). 75p. (Orig.). (gr. 9-12). pap. text 3.95 (*0-8077-2627-3*) Tchrs Coll.

Studying Personality: Teachers Manual & Duplication Masters. American Psychological Association Staff. 1981. (Human Behavior Curriculum Project Ser.). 64p. (Orig.). pap. 9.95 (*0-8077-2628-1*) Tchrs Coll.

Studying the Clinician: Judgment Research & Psychological Assessment. Howard N. Garb. 1998. LC 97-47679. 333p. 39.95 (*1-55798-483-2*) Am Psychol.

Studying the Novice Programmer. E. Soloway & James C. Spohrer. 1988. (Interacting with Computers Ser.). 504p. 99.95 (*0-8058-0002-6*); pap. 55.00 (*0-8058-0003-4*) L Erlbaum Assocs.

Studying the Social Worlds of Children. Frances C. Waksler. 1991. 282p. 75.00 (*1-85000-910-4*); pap. 27.95 (*1-85000-911-2*) Taylor & Francis (Falmer Pr).

Stuettgen, G., Festschrift: Journal: Skin Pharmacology, Vol. 4, No. 3, 1991. Ed. by H. Schaefer. 1991. (Illus.). 112p. pap. 41.75 (*3-8055-5465-6*) S Karger.

Stuff We're Made Of: The Positive Approach to Health Through Nutrition. Jorian Jenks. 1959. 5.00 (*0-8159-6829-9*) Devin.

Stunned Myocardium: Properties, Mechanisms, & Clinical Manifestations. Ed. by Robert A. Kloner & Karin Przyklenk. 1992. LC 92-49722. (Fundamental & Clinical Cardiology Ser.: Vol. 11). (Illus.). 488p. text 135.00 (*0-8247-8722-6*) Dekker.

Stunning, Hibernation, & Calcium in Myocardial Ischemia & Reperfusion. Ed. by Lionel H. Opie. 1992. LC 92-17257. (C). pap. text 132.50 (*0-7923-1793-9*) Kluwer Academic.

Stunted Lives, Stagnant Economies: Poverty, Disease, & Underdevelopment. Eileen Stillwaggon. 1998. LC 97-22317. (Illus.). 384p. 50.00 (*0-8135-2493-8*) Rutgers U Pr.

Stunted Lives, Stagnant Economies: Poverty, Disease & Underdevelopment. Eileen Stillwaggon. 1998. LC 97-22317. xv, 342p. pap. 23.00 (*0-8135-2494-6*) Rutgers U Pr.

Sturge-Weber Syndrome. E. S. Roach et al. 1999. (Illus.). 175p. (*0-9670484-0-0*) Sturge Weber.

Stuttering. Ed. by H. H. Gregory. 1995. (Journal: Vol. 46, No. 5, 1994). (Illus.). 56p. pap. 33.25 (*3-8055-6132-6*) S Karger.

Stuttering. Edward G. Conture. 2nd ed. 1989. 320p. (C). 89.00 (*0-13-853631-7*) P-H.

Stuttering: A Psychoanalytic Study. I. Peter Glauber. Ed. by Helen M. Glauber. 1982. LC 82-8125. 208p. 35.95 (*0-89885-154-8*, Kluwer Acad Hman Sci) Kluwer Academic.

Stuttering: A Short History of a Curious Disorder. Marcel E. Wingate. 1997. LC 97-10408. 272p. 62.95 (*0-89789-530-4*, Bergin & Garvey) Greenwood.

Stuttering: An Integrated Approach to Its Nature & Treatment. Theodore J. Peters & Barry Guitar. 1991. (Illus.). 392p. 42.00 (*0-683-06870-9*) Lppncott W & W.

Stuttering: An Integration of Contemporary Therapies, No. 16. Theodore J. Peters & Barry Guitar. 1980. LC 80-51679. pap. 2.00 (*0-933388-15-2*) Stuttering Fnd Am.

Stuttering: Differential Evaluation & Therapy. Hugo H. Gregory. 1973. LC 73-4549. (Studies in Communicative Disorders). (C). pap. text (*0-672-61291-7*, Bobbs) Macmillan.

Stuttering: Differential Evaluation & Therapy. Hugo H. Gregory. Ed. by Harvey Halpern. 1986. LC 86-490. (PRO-ED Studies in Communicative Disorders). (Illus.). 64p. pap. text 9.00 (*0-89079-093-0*, 1383) PRO-ED.

Stuttering: From Theory to Practice. Margaret Fawcus. 1995. 164p. pap. text 49.95 (*1-56593-497-0*, 1152) Singular Publishing.

Stuttering & Other Fluency Disorders: An Overview for Beginning Clinicians. Franklin H. Silverman. 2nd ed. 1995. LC 95-24637. 368p. 88.00 (*0-205-17514-7*) Allyn.

Stuttering & Related Disorders of Fluency. Curlee. 2nd rev. ed. 1998. (Illus.). 320p. 45.00 (*0-86577-764-0*) Thieme Med Pubs.

Stuttering & Science. William H. Perkins. 1995. 156p. pap. 35.00 (*1-56593-284-6*, 1244) Thomson Learn.

Stuttering & Your Child: Questions & Answers, No. 22. Ed. by Jane Fraser & Edward G. Conture. 1993. 64p. pap. 1.00 (*0-933388-28-4*) Stuttering Fnd Am.

Stuttering Intervention: A Collaborative Journey to Fluency Freedom. David A. Shapiro. 1998. LC 97-31307. 600p. 42.00 (*0-89079-740-4*, 8509) PRO-ED.

Stuttering Prevented: A Guide for Parents. William H. Perkins. 1991. (Illus.). 204p. (Orig.). (C). pap. text 39.95 (*1-879105-50-0*, 0235) Thomson Learn.

Stuttering Self-Help for Adults. Morris V. Jones. 1989. 144p. (C). pap. text 38.95 (*0-398-05568-8*) C C Thomas.

Stuttering Therapy: An Integrated Approach to Theory & Practice. Richard Culatta & Stanley Goldberg. 1994. LC 94-33140. (Illus.). 442p. pap. 88.00 (*0-02-326311-3*) P-H.

Stuttering Therapy: Prevention & Intervention with Children, No. 20. Ed. by Gregory H. Hugo & Hugo H. Gregory. 1985. LC 85-189819. 152p. pap. 2.00 (*0-933388-22-5*) Stuttering Fnd Am.

Stuttering Therapy, Transfer & Maintenance, No. 19. Jane Fraser. 1985. LC 83-240657. 112p. pap. 2.00 (*0-933388-19-5*) Stuttering Fnd Am.

Stuttering Words. 1997. LC 86-82260. (Publications on Stuttering: No. 2). 64p. pap. 1.00 (*0-933388-25-X*) Stuttering Fnd Am.

Su Hijo: Momentos Claves en su Desarrollo Desde el Periodo Prenatal Hasta los Seis Anos. T. Berry Brazelton. 2001. LC 94-29561. (SPA., Illus.). 560p. reprint ed. pap. 20.00 (*0-201-40919-4*) Perseus Bks Grp.

Sub-Acute Spongiform Encephalopathies: Proceedings of a Seminar in the CEC Agricultural Research Programme, Held in Brussels, November 12-14, 1990. Ed. by Raymond S. Bradley et al. 1991. (Current Topics in Veterinary Medicine & Animal Science Ser.). 304p. text 180.50 (*0-7923-1458-1*) Kluwer Academic.

Subacute Care Operations: A Management Guide for the Free-Standing or Hospital-Based Unit. Laura Z. Hyatt. 1995. 250p. (C). text 75.00 (*1-55738-630-7*, Irwn Prfssnl) McGraw-Hill Educ Grp.

Subacute Care Services: The Evolving Opportunities & Challenges. Marshall W. Kelly. 1995. LC 95-24869. 200p. (C). text 55.00 (*1-55738-621-8*, Irwn Prfssnl) McGraw-Hill Educ Grp.

Subarachnoid Hemorrhage. R. P. Sengupta & V. L. McAllister. 1986. (Illus.). 378p. 317.00 (*0-387-15534-1*) Spr-Verlag.

Subarachnoid Hemorrhage. M. Vermeulen et al. 1992. (Major Problems in Neurology Ser.: Vol. 25). (Illus.). 140p. text (*0-7020-1486-9*) W B Saunders GBR. *Dist:* Saunders.

Subarachnoid Hemorrhage: Causes & Cures. Bryce Weir. 1998. (Contemporary Neurology Ser.: 52). (Illus.). 324p. text 120.00 (*0-19-512875-3*) OUP.

Subcelluar Taxonomy: An Ultrastructural Classification System with Diagnostic Applications. Ed. by A. L. McLay & Peter G. Toner. 1985. LC 83-10856. (Ultrastructural Pathology Publication). 86p. 78.95 (*0-89116-293-3*) Hemisp Pub.

Subcellular Basis of Contractile Failure. Ed. by Borivoj Korecky & Naranjan S. Dhalla. 1990. (Developments in Cardiovascular Medicine Ser.). (C). text 157.00 (*0-7923-0890-5*) Kluwer Academic.

Subcellular Biochemistry Vol. 18: Intracellular Parasites. J. L. Avila & J. R. Harris. 1992. (Illus.). 450p. (C). text 150.00 (*0-306-44065-2*, Kluwer Plenum) Kluwer Academic.

Subcommissural Organ: An Ependymal Brain Gland. Ed. by A. Oksche et al. 1993. LC 93-9609. (Illus.). 333p. 180.00 (*0-387-56336-9*) Spr-Verlag.

Subcortical Functions in Language & Memory. Bruce Crosson. 1992. LC 91-42906. 374p. 50.00 (*0-89862-790-7*, 2790) Guilford Pubns.

***Subcortical Stroke.** Ed. by G. A. Donnan. 2nd ed. 2001. LC 2001-50040. (Oxford Medical Publications). (*0-19-263157-8*) OUP.

Subcortical Visual Systems. Ed. by David J. Ingle & G. E. Schneider. 1971. (Journal: Vol. 3, No. 1-4). reprint ed. pap. 80.00 (*3-8055-1149-3*) S Karger.

Subfertility Handbook: A Clinician's Guide. Ed. by Gab Kovacs. 1997. LC 97-9495. (Illus.). 285p. (C). text 69.95 (*0-521-56016-0*) Cambridge U Pr.

Subject & Agency in Psychoanalysis: Which Is to Be Master? Frances M. Moran. 1993. LC 92-48288. (Psychoanalytic Crosscurrents Ser.). 208p. (C). text 45.00 (*0-8147-5482-1*) NYU Pr.

Subject & Author Index to Physical Therapy, 1986-1997. rev. ed. 1997. 123p. pap. 37.00 (*1-887759-14-X*, C-13) Am Phys Therapy Assn.

Subject Catalog of the Library of the New York Academy of Medicine. New York Academy of Medicine Library Staff. 1970. 3695.00 (*0-8161-1460-9*); Supplement 1. 1980. suppl. ed. 625.00 (*0-8161-1273-8*) Gale (Macmillan Ref).

Subject Directory of Special Libraries Vol. 3: Health Science Libraries. 26th ed. 2001. 375.00 net. (*0-7876-3525-1*) Gale.

Subject Dose in Radiological Imaging. Ed. by Kwan-Hoong Ng et al. 1998. LC 99-206988. 318p. 129.50 (*0-444-82989-X*) Elsevier.

Subject Matter in Health Education: An Analysis & Evaluation of the Contents of Some Courses of Study & Textbooks Dealing with Health & Suggestions for Using Such an Analysis. Ruth M. Strang. LC 70-177814. (Columbia University. Teachers College. Contributions to Education Ser.: No. 222). reprint ed. 37.50 (*0-404-55222-6*) AMS Pr.

Subject of Semiotics. Kaja Silverman. 1984. 316p. pap. text 24.95 (*0-19-503178-4*) OUP.

Subject Relations: Unconscious Experience & Relational Psychoanalysis. Naomi Rucker & Karen Lombardi. 1997. LC 97-16984. (C). 256p. 75.00 (*0-415-91422-1*); 224p. pap. 23.99 (*0-415-91423-X*) Routledge.

Subject to Ourselves: Social Theory, Psychoanalysis & Postmodernity. Anthony Elliott. 1996. 175p. (*0-7456-1422-1*); pap. (*0-7456-1423-X*) Polity Pr GBR. *Dist:* Blackwell Pubs.

Subjected to Science: Human Experimentation in America Before the Second World War. Susan E. Lederer. 1997. (Henry E. Sigerist Series in the History of Medicine). 216p. pap. text 17.95 (*0-8018-5709-0*) Johns Hopkins.

Subjection & Subjectivity: Psychoanalytic Feminism & Moral Philosophy. Diana T. Meyers. 1994. LC 94-20584. (Thinking Gender Ser.). 256p. (C). 80.00 (*0-415-90471-4*, A6579); pap. 22.95 (*0-415-90508-7*, A6583) Routledge.

Subjective Experience in Social Cognition & Behavior. Herbert Bless. 1999. LC 99-51588. 352p. 54.95 (*0-86377-690-6*) L Erlbaum Assocs.

Subjective Well-Being. R. Nagpal & H. Sell. 1985. (SEARO Regional Health Papers: No. 7). 161p. pap. text 10.00 (*92-9022-176-3*, 1580007) World Health.

Subjective Well-Being: An Interdisciplinary Perspective. Ed. by F. Strack et al. 1991. (International Series in Experimental Social Psychology: Vol. 21). (Illus.). 300p. text 96.00 (*0-08-037264-3*, CRC Reprint) Franklin.

Subjectivity & Method in Psychology: Gender, Meaning & Science. Wendy Hollway. 1989. (Gender & Psychology Ser.). 160p. (C). 74.50 (*0-8039-8207-0*) Sage.

Subjectivity, Information, Systems: Introduction to a Theory of Relativistic Cybernetics. Guy M. Jumarie. 1986. (Studies in Cybernetics: Vol. 12). xviii, 356p. text 195.00 (*2-88124-011-9*) Gordon & Breach.

Subjects of Analysis. Thomas H. Ogden. 240p. 1996. pap. text 40.00 (*1-56821-803-6*); 1994. LC 93-43113. 40.00 (*1-56821-185-6*) Aronson.

Sublime Surrender: Male Masochism at the Fin-de-Siecle. Suzanne R. Stewart. 1998. LC 98-15731. (Cornell Studies in the History of Psychiatry). (Illus.). 240p. 45.00 (*0-8014-3434-3*); pap. 17.95 (*0-8014-8450-2*) Cornell U Pr.

Subliminal Treatment Procedures: A Clinician's Guide. Paul G. Swingle. 1991. 300p. (C). 45.00 (*0-8058-0894-9*); pap. 22.50 (*0-8058-0895-7*) L Erlbaum Assocs.

Subliminal Treatment Procedures: A Clinician's Guide. Paul G. Swingle. 1992. LC 90-3857. 192p. pap. 24.45 (*0-943158-77-X*, STPBP, Prof Resc Pr) Pro Resource.

Subrarachnoid Hemmorage: Medical & Surgical Management. Ed. by Takehiko Yanagihara et al. 1997. LC 97-36798. (Illus.). 584p. text 195.00 (*0-8247-9519-9*) Dekker.

Subspecialty Care. Ed. by Stanley Muravchick. 1998. LC 97-47123. (Atlas of Anesthesia Ser.: no. 5). (C). text (*0-443-07904-8*) Church.

Substance Abuse: A Comprehensive Textbook. Joyce H. Lowinson et al. 2nd ed. 1992. (Illus.). 1136p. text 142.00 (*0-683-05211-X*) Lppncott W & W.

Substance Abuse: A Multidimensional Assessment & Treatment Approach. Penelope A. Moyers. 1992. LC 88-43456. (Illus.). 216p. (C). pap. 24.00 (*1-55642-084-6*) SLACK Inc.

Substance Abuse: A Self Teaching Guide for Health Professionals. American Academy of Pediatrics Staff. 1988. 193p. pap. 44.95 (*0-910761-20-5*) Am Acad Pediat.

Substance Abuse: Drugs. Ed. by Joan Cochran et al. 2nd rev. ed. 1994. 132p. (Orig.). pap. text 37.00 (*1-879772-03-5*) Health Studies.

Substance Abuse: The Nation's Number One Health Problem. Brandeis University, Institute for Health Policy Staff. 1993. (Key Indicators for Policy Ser.). (Illus.). 68p. (Orig.). pap. (*0-942054-08-3*) R W Johnson Found.

***Substance Abuse: The Nation's Number One Health Problem.** Constance Horgan. Ed. by Jane J. Stein. rev. ed. 2001. (Illus.). 128p. (C). pap. text 35.00 (*0-7567-1119-3*) DIANE Pub.

Substance Abuse Accounts Auditor. Jack Rudman. 1994. (Career Examination Ser.: C-3478). pap. 29.95 (*0-8373-3478-0*) Nat Learn.

Substance Abuse among Women & Parents. James Colliver et al. 1996. (Illus.). 62p. (Orig.). (C). pap. text 20.00 (*0-7881-2746-2*) DIANE Pub.

Substance Abuse & Family Therapy. Edward Kaufman. 1985. 256p. text 30.00 (*0-8089-1679-3*, 792254, Grune & Strat) Harcrt Hlth Sci Grp.

Substance Abuse & Mental Health Statistics Sourcebook. Ed. by Beatrice A. Rouse. 1996. (Illus.). 193p. pap. text 35.00 (*0-7881-2985-6*) DIANE Pub.

Substance Abuse & Misuse: In the Older Adult. Sharon Edwards. 1997. (Illus.). 88p. pap. 29.95 (*1-888343-06-0*) Hartman Pub.

Substance Abuse & Physical Disability. Ed. by Allen W. Heinemann. 1993. LC 92-1443. (Illus.). 270p. lib. bdg. 49.95 (*1-56024-289-2*) Haworth Pr.

Substance Abuse & the New Road to Recovery: A Practioner's Guide. Glenn D. Walters. 1996. LC 97-6610. 217p. 54.95 (*1-56032-427-9*); pap. 24.95 (*1-56032-428-7*) Hemisp Pub.

Substance Abuse as Symptom: A Psychoanalytic Critique of Treatment Approaches & the Cultural Beliefs That Sustain Them. Louis S. Berger. 1991. 272p. text 45.00 (*0-88163-102-7*) Analytic Pr.

Substance Abuse Counseling: An Individualized Approach. Judith A. Lewis et al. 1987. LC 87-24618. 281p. (C). pap. 34.50 (*0-534-08448-6*); 2nd ed. 1993. LC 93-8054. 243p. mass mkt. 46.75 (*0-534-20053-2*) Brooks-Cole.

Substance Abuse Curriculum Development in Family Medicine: An Instructor's Manual in Two Parts. 1994. 111p. (Orig.). (C). pap. text 30.00 (*0-7881-0273-7*) DIANE Pub.

Substance Abuse Disorders in Clinical Practice. Edward C. Senay. 2nd ed. 1989. (*0-8151-7712-7*) Mosby Inc.

Substance Abuse Disorders in Clinical Practice. Edward C. Senay. 2nd ed. 1999. LC 98-21154. 272p. 37.00 (*0-393-70291-X*) Norton.

S

Substance Abuse During Pregnancy & Childhood. Ed. by Ronald R. Watson. 1995. LC 94-44482. (Drug & Alcohol Abuse Reviews Ser.: Vol. 8). 144p. 89.50 (*0-89603-295-7*) Humana.

Substance Abuse Education for Nursing: A Model Curriculum. Ed. by Madeline Naegle. 1992. Vol. I. 602p. pap. 34.95 (*0-88737-523-5*); Vol. II. 660p. pap. 34.95 (*0-88737-545-6*); Vol. III. 402p. pap. 34.95 (*0-88737-546-4*) Natl League Nurse.

Substance Abuse in Adolescents & Young Adults: A Guide to Treatment. Joseph K. Nowinski. 1990. 246p. (C). 29.95 (*0-393-70097-6*) Norton.

Substance Abuse in Children & Adolescents: Intervention & Evaluation. Steven P. Schinke et al. 1991. (Developmental Clinical Psychology & Psychiatry Ser.: Vol. 22). (Illus.). 112p. 74.95 (*0-8039-3748-2*, 7563); pap. 34.95 (*0-8039-3749-0*, 7564) Sage.

Substance Abuse in the Workplace: An Employer Perspective. 1987. 69p. pap. 7.00 (*0-939900-30-0*, PB43) Soc Human Resc Mgmt.

Substance Abuse Issues among Families in Diverse Populations. Ed. by Jorge Delva. 2000. LC 00-31968. (Journal of Family Social Work Ser.: Vol. 4, No. 4). 97p. (C). 39.90 (*0-7890-1194-8*) Haworth Pr.

Substance Abuse I: Drug Abuse: A Bibliography. Ed. by Joan Nordquist. 1989. (Contemporary Social Issues: A Bibliographic Ser.: No. 16). 64p. (C). pap. 20.00 (*0-937855-31-6*) Ref Rsch Serv.

Substance Abuse Prevention: A Multicultural Perspective. Ed. by Snehendu B. Kar. 1999. LC 98-47889. 336p. text 42.00 (*0-89503-194-9*) Baywood Pub.

Substance Abuse Prevention Activities for Secondary Students: Ready-to-Use Lessons, Fact Sheets & Resources for Grades 7-12. Patricia Gerne & Timothy A. Gerne. 1991. LC 91-19746. 336p. (YA). (gr. 7-12). pap. text 27.95 (*0-13-876707-6*, 710704) P-H.

Substance Abuse Prevention in Multicultural Communities. Ed. by Jeanette M. Valentine et al. 1998. LC 97-36612. 171p. 39.95 (*0-7890-0343-0*) Haworth Pr.

Substance Abuse Problems. Sidney Cohen. 1981. LC 80-21280. 392p. text 6.95 (*0-917724-18-6*); pap. text 24.95 (*0-917724-22-4*) Haworth Pr.

Substance Abuse Problems Vol. 2: New Issues for the 1980s, Vol. 2. Sidney Cohen. 1985. LC 80-21280. (Substance Abuse Problems Ser.: Vol. 2). 323p. text 6.95 (*0-86656-368-7*); pap. text 24.95 (*0-86656-369-5*) Haworth Pr.

Substance Abuse Problems & Programs in Newark: A Needs Assessment for Newark's Fighting Back Initiative. Patricia A. Ebener et al. 1993. LC 93-21520. pap. text 13.00 (*0-8330-1420-X*, MR-282-BGC/DPRC) Rand Corp.

Substance Abuse Program Specialist. Jack Rudman. 1994. (Career Examination Ser.: C-3336). pap. 29.95 (*0-8373-3336-9*) Nat Learn.

Substance Abuse Treatment: A Family Systems Perspective. Edith M. Freeman. 1993. (Sourcebooks for the Human Services: Vol. 25). (Illus.). 330p. (C). 89.95 (*0-8039-4889-1*, 4333); LC 93-9209. pap. 39.95 (*0-8039-4890-5*, 4334) Sage.

Substance Abuse Treatment for Persons with Child Abuse & Neglect Issues. Ed. by Judy Howard. 2000. 181p. pap. text 35.00 (*0-7567-0081-7*) DIANE Pub.

***Substance Abuse Treatment Parity: A Viable Solution to the Nation's Epidemic of Addiction?: Congressional Hearing.** Ed. by John L. Mica. 2001. 112p. (C). pap. text 25.00 (*0-7567-1804-X*) DIANE Pub.

Substance Abuse Treatment Program Assistant. Jack Rudman. 1994. (Career Examination Ser.: C-3479). pap. 27.95 (*0-8373-3479-9*) Nat Learn.

Substance Abuse II: Alcohol Abuse: A Bibliography. Ed. by Joan Nordquist. 1990. (Contemporary Social Issues: A Bibliographic Ser.: No. 17). 60p. (Orig.). pap. 20.00 (*0-937855-32-4*) Ref Rsch Serv.

Substance-Abusing High Achievers: Addiction As an Equal Opportunity Destroyer. Abraham Twerski. 1998. LC 97-23008. (Library of Substance Abuse & Addiction Treatment). 232p. 30.00 (*0-7657-0110-3*) Aronson.

Substance & Shadow: Women & Addiction in the United States. Stephen R. Kandall. 1999. (Illus.). 367p. pap. text 16.95 (*0-674-85361-X*) HUP.

Substance Called Food: How to Understand, Control, & Recover from Addictive Eating. Gloria Arenson. 2nd ed. 1989. 256p. pap. 11.95 (*0-8306-3430-4*) McGraw-Hill Educ Grp.

Substance Called Food: How to Understand, Control & Recover from Addictive Eating. Gloria Arenson. 2nd ed. 1989. 294p. pap. 12.95 (*0-07-156827-1*) McGraw.

Substance Use among Children & Adolescents: Its Nature, Extent & Effects from Conception to Adulthood. Ann M. Pagliaro & Louis A. Pagliaro. 1996. LC 95-25496. 416p. 110.00 (*0-471-58042-2*) Wiley.

Substance Use & Misuse: Nature, Context, & Clinical Interventions. G. Hussein Rassool. 1998. LC 98-2838. 282p. pap. 49.95 (*0-632-04884-0*) Blackwell Sci.

Substances & Naturally Occurring Goitrogens. P. Langer & M. A. Greer. 1978. (Illus.). 67.00 (*3-8055-2659-8*) S Karger.

***Succeeding As a Hospital Doctor: The Experts Share Their Secrets.** Kirby & Mundy. 2001. (Illus.). 178p. pap. (*1-899541-68-3*) Health Pr GBR. *Dist:* JAMCO Dist.

Succeeding As Homemaker - Home-Health Aide. Lane. 1994. (Home Care Aide Ser.). wbk. ed. 13.95 (*0-8273-5365-0*) Delmar.

Succeeding As Homemaker - Home Health Aide Guide. Lane. 1994. (Home Care Aide Ser.). 12.95 (*0-8273-5530-0*) Delmar.

Success & Crisis in National Health Systems: A Comparative Approach. Ed. by Mark G. Field. 1989. (Contemporary Issues in Health, Medicine, & Social Policy Ser.). 320p. 45.00 (*0-415-01289-9*); pap. 18.95 (*0-415-01290-2*) Routledge.

Success & Understanding. Jean Piaget. 1978. LC 78-16435. (Illus.). 248p. 28.00 (*0-674-85387-3*) HUP.

Success in Practical Nursing: Personal & Vocational Issues. Ed. by Signe S. Hill & Helen A. Howlett. 2nd ed. 1993. (Illus.). pap., tchr. ed. (*0-7216-6466-0*) Saunders.

Success in Practical Nursing: Personal & Vocational Issues. Signe S. Hill & Helen A. Howlett. 3rd ed. 1997. (Illus.). pap., tchr. ed. (*0-7216-6878-X*) Saunders.

Success in Practical Nursing: Personal & Vocational Issues. Signe S. Hill & Helen A. Howlett. Ed. by Ilze Rader. 3rd ed. 1997. LC 96-35766. (Illus.). 448p. pap. text 23.00 (*0-7216-6877-1*) Saunders.

***Success in Practical/Vocational Nursing: From Student to Leader.** Signe S. Hill & Helen Stephens Howlett. 2001. pap., tchr. ed. 250.00 (*0-7216-9084-X*) Saunders.

Success or Failure? Family Planning Programs in the Third World, 4. Donald J. Hernandez. 1985. LC 84-6653. (Studies in Population & Urban Demography: No. 4). (Illus.). 161p. 55.00 (*0-313-24401-4*, HSU/, Greenwood Pr) Greenwood.

Success over Stress. Joseph L. Palotta. 1990. 184p. pap. 6.95 (*0-9604852-3-6*) Revelation Hse.

Success with Heart Failure: Help & Hope for Those with Congestive Heart Failure. Marc A. Silver. 1998. LC 98-12364. (Illus.). 272p. (C). pap. 19.95 (*0-306-45985-X*) Da Capo.

Successful Administration in Senior Housing: Working with Elderly Residents. Nancy W. Sheehan. 1992. LC 92-18609. (Illus.). 240p. (C). 59.95 (*0-8039-4524-8*, 4757); pap. 31.95 (*0-8039-4525-6*, 4758) Sage.

Successful Aging: Perspectives from the Behavioral Sciences. Ed. by Paul B. Baltes & Margaret M. Baltes. 1993. (European Network on Longitudinal Studies on Individual Development). (Illus.). 413p. (C). pap. text 35.95 (*0-521-43582-X*) Cambridge U Pr.

Successful Aging: The MacArthur Foundation Study Shows How the Lifestyle Choices You Make Now—More Than Heredity—Determine Your Health & Vitality. John W. Rowe & Robert L. Kahn. l.t. ed. 1999. 288p. pap. 12.95 (*0-440-50863-0*) Dell.

Successful Aging: The MacArthur Foundation Study Shows How the Lifestyle Choices You Make Now—More Than Heredity—Determine Your Health & Vitality. John W. Rowe & Robert L. Kahn. 1998. LC 97-36900. 288p. 26.50 (*0-375-40045-1*) Pantheon.

Successful Assertiveness. Dena Michelli. 1997. LC 96-32472. pap. 6.95 (*0-7641-0071-8*) Barron.

Successful Breastfeeding. Royal College of Midwives Staff. 2nd ed. 1991. (Illus.). 88p. pap. text (*0-443-04460-0*) Church.

Successful Breastfeeding. Royal College of Midwives Staff. 2nd ed. 2000. LC 2001-28188. (Illus.). 110p. 15.95 (*0-443-05967-5*) Harcrt Hlth Sci Grp.

Successful Cardiac Rehabilitation: The Complete Guide for Building Cardiac Rehab Programs. Peggy Pashkow et al. 1988. 39.95 (*0-9619796-0-7*) HeartWatchers Pr.

Successful Case Management in Long-Term Care. Joan Quinn. 1993. LC 92-49033. (Illus.). 176p. 32.95 (*0-8261-7750-6*) Springer Pub.

Successful Communication with Alzheimer's Disease Patients: An In-Service Training Manual. Elizabeth E. Ostuni et al. 1997. LC 96-54719. 288p. text 44.99 (*0-7506-9564-1*) Buttrwrth-Heinemann.

Successful Dental Practice in Good Times & Bad. Morton M. Ehudin. 1991. 10.00 (*0-87814-361-0*, D4296) PennWell Corp.

Successful Enrollment Management: A Workbook for Nursing Education Recruitment Professionals. American Association of Colleges of Nursing Staff. Ed. by Barbara K. Redman. 1989. 250p. (Orig.). stu. ed. 35.00 (*0-922148-01-5*) AACN.

Successful Faculty in Academic Medicine: Essential Skills & How to Acquire Them. Ed. by Carole J. Bland et al. 1989. LC 89-21921. (Medical Education Ser.: Vol. 12). 336p. 44.95 (*0-8261-6730-6*) Springer Pub.

Successful Financial Management for the Veterinary Practice. Robert E. Froehlich. 1987. 92p. (Orig.). pap. text 24.95 (*0-941451-01-1*) Am Animal Hosp Assoc.

Successful Grant Writing: Strategies for Health & Human Service Professionals. Laura N. Gitlin & Kevin J. Lyons. 1996. LC 95-46547. (Illus.). 235p. pap. 34.95 (*0-8261-9260-2*) Springer Pub.

Successful Home Birth & Midwifery: The Dutch Obstetric Model. Ed. by Eva Abraham-Van de Mark. 1993. LC 92-42901. 248p. 72.50 (*0-89789-295-X*, H295, Bergin & Garvey) Greenwood.

Successful Medical Student. John R. Thornborough. 1995. 14.95 (*1-882531-03-5*) ILOC.

Successful Models of Community Long Term Care Services for the Elderly. Ed. by Eloise H. Killeffer. 1990. LC 89-29378. (Physical & Occupational Therapy in Geriatrics Ser.: Vol. 8, Nos. 1 & 2). (Illus.). 178p. text 39.95 (*0-86656-987-1*) Haworth Pr.

Successful Movement Challenges: Movement Activities for the Developing Child. Jack Capon. Ed. by Frank Alexander & Diane Alexander. 1981. (Illus.). 129p. (Orig.). pap. 14.00 (*0-915256-07-X*) Front Row.

Successful Operations in the Treatment Outcomes Driven World of Managed Care. Roberta A. Kreb & Kenneth E. Wolf. 1997. (Clinical Ser.: No. 13). 90p. pap. text 12.00 (*0-910329-84-2*, 0310226) Am Speech Lang Hearing.

Successful Partnerships for the Future: The Administrator - Physician Dynamic. Mary A. Krill. 1994. 98p. (Orig.). pap. 25.00 (*1-56829-048-9*, 4819) M G M A.

Successful Physician: A Productivity Handbook for Practitioners. Marshall O. Zaslove. 1998. LC 98-4368. 336p. pap. 36.00 (*0-8342-1098-3*, 10983) Aspen Pub.

Successful Physician Negotiator: How to Get What You Deserve. James Mangraviti, Jr. & Steven J. Babitsky. 1998. 284p. 59.95 (*0-9652197-7-1*) SEAK.

Successful Private Practice in the 1990s: A New Guide for the Mental Health Professional. Joan K. Beigel & Ralph H. Earle. 1990. LC 90-2053. 224p. pap. text 25.95 (*0-87630-586-9*, 5869) Brunner-Routledge.

Successful Problem Solving & Test Taking for the NCLEX-PN. Patricia A. Hoefler. 2nd rev. ed. 1998. 166p. (C). pap. text 29.95 (*1-56533-029-3*) M E D S Inc.

Successful Problem Solving & Test Taking for the Nursing Assistant's Exam. Patricia A. Hoefler. 3rd ed. 1998. (C). pap. text 29.95 (*1-56533-030-7*) M E D S Inc.

Successful Psychiatric Practice: Current Dilemmas, Choices, & Solutions. Ed. by Edward K. Silberman. 1995. (Clinical Practice Ser.: No. 33). 272p. text 16.95 (*0-88048-486-1*, 8486) Am Psychiatric.

Successful Psychotherapy: A Caring, Loving Relationship. C. H. Patterson & Suzanne C. Hidore. 1997. LC 95-52030. 280p. 40.00 (*1-56821-795-1*) Aronson.

Successful Scientific Writing: A Step-by-Step Guide for the Biological & Medical Sciences. Janice R. Matthews et al. (Illus.). 1996. 195p. (C). pap. text 21.95 (*0-521-55948-0*); 2nd ed. 2000. LC 00-36043. 252p. pap. text 24.95 (*0-521-78962-1*) Cambridge U Pr.

Successful Stuttering Management Program. Dorvan H. Breitenfeldt & Delores R. Lorenz. 1989. 164p. stu. ed. 47.50 (*0-910055-10-6*) East Wash Univ.

Successful Surgery: A Doctor's Mind & Body Guide to Help You Through Surgery. Robert Baker. 1996. LC 95-49049. 288p. pap. 12.00 (*0-671-51900-X*, PB Trade Paper) PB.

Successful Test Taking: Learning Strategies for Nursing Students. Marian B. Sides & Nancy Korchek. 3rd ed. 1998. LC 97-42752. 448p. pap. text 29.95 (*0-7817-9202-9*) Lppncott W & W.

SuccessTypes for Medical Students: A Program for Improving Academic Performance. John W. Pellev & Bernell K. Dalley. unabr. ed. 1997. (SuccessTypes Ser.: Vol. 1). (Illus.). 242p. pap. 23.95 (*0-9665049-0-9*) Extend Studies.

Such Agreeable Friends. Gay L. Balliet. 1987. 266p. (Orig.). pap. (*0-910119-33-3*) SOCO Pubns.

Such Stuff as Dreams Are Made On: The Autobiography & Journals of Helen M. Luke. Helen M. Luke. 2001. LC 00-62120. (Illus.). 288p. pap. 14.95 (*0-609-80589-4*) Harmony Bks.

Such Stuff as Dreams Are Made On: The Autobiography & Journals of Helen M. Luke. Helen M. Luke. Ed. by Barbara A. Mowat. 2000. LC 99-51411. (Illus.). 267p. 29.95 (*0-930407-47-4*) Parabola Bks.

Sucralfate: From Basic Science to the Bedside. Ed. by D. Hollander & Guido N. Tytgat. 1995. LC 94-45587. (Illus.). 392p. (C). text 75.00 (*0-306-44740-1*, Kluwer Plenum) Kluwer Academic.

Sudden Cardiac Death. 1985. (Technical Reports: No. 726). 25p. pap. text 4.00 (*92-4-120726-4*, 1100726) World Health.

Sudden Cardiac Death. Ed. by A. Bayes De Luna et al. 1990. (C). lib. bdg. 196.50 (*0-7923-0716-X*) Kluwer Academic.

Sudden Cardiac Death. Sidney Goldstein. 1994. LC 94-9562. (Illus.). 346p. 75.00 (*0-87993-589-8*) Futura Pub.

Sudden Cardiac Death. Ed. by Robert J. Myerburg. 1987. (Journal: Vol. 74, Suppl. 2, 1987). (Illus.). iv, 72p. pap. 23.50 (*3-8055-4629-7*) S Karger.

Sudden Cardiac Death: Past, Present, & Future. Ed. by Sandra B. Dunbar et al. 1997. LC 96-47804. (American Heart Association Monograph Ser.). (Illus.). 440p. 78.00 (*0-87993-666-5*) Futura Pub.

Sudden Cardiac Death & Congestive Heart Failure. Joel Morganroth & E. Neil Moore. 1983. text 158.50 (*0-89838-580-6*) Kluwer Academic.

***Sudden Cardiac Death in Swedish Orienteers.** Lars Wesslen. 2001. (Comprehensive Summaries of Uppsala Dissertations from the Faculty of Medicine Ser.: No. 1017). (Illus.). 44p. (*91-554-4986-7*) Uppsala Universitet SWE. *Dist:* Coronet Bks.

Sudden Cardiac Death in the Athlete. Ed. by Paul J. Wang et al. 1998. LC 97-52288. (Illus.). 600p. 89.00 (*0-87993-691-6*) Futura Pub.

Sudden Cardiac Death in the Community. Ed. by Mickey S. Eisenberg et al. 1984. LC 83-21156. 163p. 50.00 (*0-275-91428-3*, C1428, Praeger Pubs) Greenwood.

Sudden Coronary Death: Proceedings of the Paavo Nurmi Symposium, 4th, Helsinki, September 15-17, 1977. Paavo Nurmi Symposium Staff. Ed. by V. Manninen. 1978. (Advances in Cardiology Ser.: Vol. 25). (Illus.). 102.75 (*3-8055-2881-7*) S Karger.

Sudden Deafness: A Controversial Issue. Ed. by Jean-Philippe Guyot. 2000. (Oto-Rhino-Laryngologia Nova Ser.: Vol. 9, No. 5). (Illus.). 60p. pap. 25.25 (*3-8055-7091-0*) S Karger.

Sudden Death. Ed. by Henri E. Kulbertus & Hein J. Wellens. 1980. (Developments in Cardiovascular Medicine Ser.: Vol. 4). (Illus.). xiv, 406p. text 199.50 (*90-247-2290-X*) Kluwer Academic.

Sudden Death: Cardiac & Other Causes. Donald B. Hackel & Keith A. Reimer. 1993. LC 93-70292. (Illus.). 168p. (Orig.). 75.00 (*0-89089-546-5*) Carolina Acad Pr.

Sudden Death: Intervention Skills for the Caring Professions. Bob Wright. 1990. (Illus.). 180p. pap. text (*0-443-04133-4*) Church.

Sudden Death & the Myth of CPR. Stefan Timmermans. 1999. LC 99-17282. (Illus.). 272p. 59.50 (*1-56639-715-4*); pap. 22.95 (*1-56639-716-2*) Temple U Pr.

Sudden Death Due to Acute Myocardial Infarction. L. Szekeres. 1986. LC 85-29941. 296p. 169.00 (*0-8493-6545-7*, CRC Reprint) Franklin.

Sudden Death in Infancy, Childhood & Adolescence. Roger W. Byard & Stephen D. Cohle. 1994. LC 93-43607. (Illus.). 561p. (C). text 120.00 (*0-521-42031-8*) Cambridge U Pr.

***Sudden Death in Ischemic Heart Disease: An Altnerative View on the Significance of Morphologic Findings.** Giorgio Baroldi & Malcolm D. Silver. 1996. LC 95-22875. (Medical Intelligence Unit Ser.). (Illus.). 200p. (C). 125.00 (*3-540-59499-X*) Spr-Verlag.

Sudden Hearing Loss. Charles P. Kimmelman & Lyon L. Gleich. 1993. (Self-Instructional Package Ser.). (Illus.). 43p. (Orig.). pap. text 25.00 (*1-56772-001-3*) AAO-HNS.

Sudden Infant Death Syndrome: Journal: Pediatrician, Vol. 15, No. 4, 1988. Ed. by David W. Kaplan. 1988. (Illus.). 80p. pap. 41.00 (*3-8055-4892-3*) S Karger.

Sudden Infant Death Syndrome: Who Can Help & How. Ed. by Charles Corr et al. 1991. 272p. 36.95 (*0-8261-6720-9*) Springer Pub.

Sudden Loss of Cochlear & Vestibular Function. Ed. by M. Hoke. 1981. (Advances in OtoRhinoLaryngology Ser.: Vol. 27). (Illus.). x, 198p. 128.75 (*3-8055-2630-X*) S Karger.

Sudden Menopause: Restoring Health & Emotional Well-Being. Debbie DeAngelo. 2000. LC 00-143905. (Illus.). 256p. pap. 15.95 (*0-89793-325-7*) Hunter Hse.

Suddenly Successful: How Behavioral Optometry Helps You Overcome Learning Health & Behavior Problems. Ellis S. Edelman et al. Ed. by Sally M. Corngold & Marcia Castaneda. 1991. (Illus.). 306p. 22.95 (*0-943599-14-8*) OEPF.

Sue, Settle or Be Silent? A. Anthony Piazza. 1994. pap. 18.95 (*0-9635237-0-8*) P M C & B.

Suffer the Children: A Pediatrician's Reflections on Abuse. Rosamond L. Murdock & Mariette Hartley. 1992. LC 91-35371. 220p. 19.95 (*0-929173-09-0*) Health Press.

Suffering. Betty Ferrell. 1996. LC 95-544. (Nursing Ser.). (Illus.). 192p. (C). text 53.95 (*0-86720-723-X*, 723-X) Jones & Bartlett.

Suffering: Psychological & Social Aspects in Loss, Grief, & Care. Ed. by Robert DeBellis et al. 1986. LC 85-31744. (Loss, Grief & Care Ser.: Vol. 1, Nos. 1 & 2). 196p. text 49.95 (*0-86656-558-2*) Haworth Pr.

Suffering from Illusion: The Secret Victory of Self-Defeat. Sayers R. Brenner. 1994. LC 94-65657. (Illus.). 341p. reprint ed. pap. 16.95 (*0-9640827-0-5*) Paradox Bks.

Suffering Presence: Theological Reflections on Medicine, the Mentally Handicapped & the Church. Stanley M. Hauerwas. 1986. LC 85-40603. 224p. (Orig.). pap. text 14.00 (*0-268-01722-0*) U of Notre Dame Pr.

Sugar Blues. William Dufty. 1986. 255p. reprint ed. mass mkt. 6.99 (*0-446-34312-9*) Warner Bks.

Sugar Control Bible & Cookbook: The Complete Nutrition Guide to Revitalizing Your Health. Jacqueline L. Paltis. 1998. 220p. (Orig.). pap. 29.95 (*1-892241-02-1*) New Energy.

Sugar Free . . . Microwavery. Judith S. Majors. LC 80-67167. pap. 6.95 (*0-9602238-3-5*) Apple Pr.

Sugar Free . . . That's Me. Judith S. Majors. 1978. LC 78-74029. (Illus.). pap. 6.95 (*0-9602238-0-0*) Apple Pr.

Sugarcane Pathology Vol. 1: Fungal Diseases. Ed. by G. P. Rao et al. 2000. (Illus.). 320p. 86.00 (*1-57808-046-0*) Science Pubs.

Sugars That Heal: The New Healing Science of Glyconutrients. Emil I. Mondoa & Mindy Kitei. 2001. LC 2001-35219. 288p. 22.00 (*0-345-44106-0*, Ballantine) Ballantine Pub Grp.

Suggested Guidelines for Nutrition & Metabolic Management of Adult Patients Receiving Nutrition Support. Ed. by Marion F. Winkler et al. 1993. LC 93-851. (Illus.). spiral bd. (*0-88091-113-1*) Am Dietetic Assn.

Suggestion in the Cure of Diseases & the Correction of Vices. George C. Pitzer. 1991. lib. bdg. 79.95 (*0-8490-4493-6*) Gordon Pr.

Suggestive Inquiry into the Hermetic Mystery: With a Dissertation on the More Celebrated of the Alchemical Philosophers Being an Attempt Towards the Recovery of the Ancient Experiment of Nature (1918) Mary Anne Atwood. 1999. 692p. reprint ed. pap. 29.95 (*0-7661-0811-2*) Kessinger Pub.

Suggestive Therapeutics. Hippolyte Bernheim. 440p. 100.00 (*1-85506-673-4*) Thoemmes Pr.

Suggestopedic Methods & Applications. Ludiger Schiffler. Tr. by Kay U. Herr from GER. 1992. LC 92-27764. 196p. text 85.00 (*2-88124-522-6*); pap. text 36.00 (*2-88124-571-4*) Gordon & Breach.

Suicidal Adolescent. Ed. by Moses Laufer. 1996. 162p. 28.50 (*0-8236-6697-2*, BN 06697) Intl Univs Pr.

Suicidal Adolescent. Ed. by Moses Laufer. 1995. 168p. pap. text (*1-85575-121-6*) Karnac Bks GBR. *Dist:* Other Pr LLC.

Suicidal Behavior in the Asia-Pacific Region. Ed. by Kok L. Peng & Wen-Shing Tseng. 1992. 267p. (*9971-69-165-5*) Sngapore Univ Pr SGP. *Dist:* Coronet Bks.

Suicidal Behaviors: Diagnosis & Management. Ed. by H. L. Resnik. 1995. LC 94-32435. 568p. pap. text 50.00 (*1-56821-263-1*) Aronson.

Suicidal Behaviour in Europe. Crepet. 328p. (*0-86196-356-3*) J Libbey Med GBR. *Dist:* Bks Intl VA.

Suicidal Child. Cynthia R. Pfeffer. 1986. LC 85-31710. 318p. 39.95 (*0-89862-664-1*) Guilford Pubns.

Suicidal Mind. Edwin S. Shneidman. 1998. (Illus.). 208p. reprint ed. pap. 13.95 (*0-19-511801-4*) OUP.

Suicidal Patient: Clinical & Legal Standards of Care. Bruce Bongar. 1991. LC 91-4568. 311p. 39.95 (*1-55798-109-4*) Am Psychol.

Suicidal Women: Their Thinking & Feeling Patterns. Charles Neuringer & Dan J. Lettieri. 1982. LC 81-6294. 250p. text 26.95 (*0-89876-023-2*) Gardner Pr.

Suicide. R. V. Clarke. 1989. (Illus.). 130p. 81.95 (*0-387-97004-5*) Spr-Verlag.

Suicide. Emile Durkheim. 1966. pap. 16.95 (*0-02-908660-4*) Free Pr.

Suicide: A Social & Historical Study. Henry R. Fedden. 1980. LC 72-80703. (Illus.). 351p. reprint ed. (*0-405-08498-6*) Blom Pubns GBR. *Dist:* Ayer.

Suicide: An Essay on Comparative Moral Statistics. Henry Morse. 1975. LC 74-25770. (European Sociology Ser.). 402p. reprint ed. 29.95 (*0-405-06524-8*) Ayer.

Suicide: Biopsychosocial Approaches. Alexander Botsis et al. 1997. LC 97-46414. (International Congress Ser.: 1145). (Illus.). 284p. 152.50 (*0-444-82755-2*) Elsevier.

Suicide: Clinical & Epidemiological Studies. Brian Barraclough. 1987. 200p. lib. bdg. (*0-7099-5009-8*) C Helm GBR. *Dist:* Routldge.

Suicide: Prevention, Intervention, Postvention. Earl A. Grollman. 2nd rev. ed. 1988. LC 87-47880. 188p. pap. 15.00 (*0-8070-2707-3*) Beacon Pr.

Suicide: The Tragedy of Hopelessness. David Aldridge. 1998. LC 98-152420. 300p. pap. (*1-85302-444-9*) Jessica Kingsley GBR. *Dist:* Taylor & Francis.

Suicide: The Ultimate Rejection; a Psycho-Social Study. Colin Pritchard. 1995. LC 94-43417. 209p. pap. (*0-335-19032-4*) OpUniv Pr.

Suicide: The Will to Live vs the Will to Die. Norman Linzer. 1984. 240p. 35.95 (*0-89885-156-4*); pap. 20.95 (*0-89885-190-4*) Kluwer Academic (Kluwer Acad Hman Sci).

Suicide: Understanding & Responding. Ed. by Douglas G. Jacobs & Herbert N. Brown. 1989. 510p. 72.50 (*0-8236-6695-6*) Intl Univs Pr.

***Suicide - Violence - Aggression.** Pamela Marcus. 16.95 (*0-8151-7291-5*) Mosby Inc.

Suicide Across the Life Span: Premature Exits. Judith M. Stillion & Eugene E. McDowell. 1996. (Series in Death Education, Aging, & Health Care). 325p. 89.95 (*1-56032-303-5*); 2nd ed. pap. 34.95 (*1-56032-304-3*) Hemisp Pub.

Suicide after Sixty: The Final Alternative. Marv Miller. 1979. LC 79-4246. (Death & Suicide Ser.: Vol. 2). 128p. pap. 21.95 (*0-8261-2781-9*) Springer Pub.

Suicide among the Elderly in Long-Term Care Facilities, 19. Nancy J. Osgood et al. 1990. LC 90-36738. (Contributions to the Study of Aging Ser.: No. 19). 216p. 62.50 (*0-313-26522-4*, ODD, Greenwood Pr) Greenwood.

Suicide & Attempted Suicide. Ed. by E. M. Brooke. 1974. (Public Health Papers: No. 58). pap. text 8.00 (*92-4-130058-2*, 1110058) World Health.

Suicide & Attempted Suicide: Methods & Consequences. Geo Stone & Brian W. Aldiss. 1999. LC 97-22792. 480p. 27.95 (*0-7867-0492-6*) Carroll & Graf.

Suicide & Clinical Practice. Ed. by Douglas G. Jacobs. 1992. LC 91-17193. (Clinical Practice Ser.: No. 21). 189p. text 11.95 (*0-88048-455-1*, 8455) Am Psychiatric.

Suicide & Depression in Late Life: Critical Issues in Treatment, Research & Public Policy. Gary J. Kennedy. 1996. LC 95-37313. (Publication Series of the Einstein-Monte: Vol. 13). 192p. 110.00 (*0-471-12913-5*) Wiley.

***Suicide & Euthanasia in Older Adults: A Transcultural Journey.** Diego De Leo. 2001. (Illus.). 224p. 24.50 (*0-88937-251-9*) Hogrefe & Huber Pubs.

Suicide & Homicide: Some Economic, Sociological & Psychological Aspects of Aggression. Andrew F. Henry & James F. Short, Jr. Ed. by Robert J. Kastenbaum. 1977. LC 76-19575. (Death & Dying Ser.). (Illus.). reprint ed. lib. bdg. 23.95 (*0-405-09573-2*) Ayer.

Suicide & Its Psychological Influences: Index of Authors & Subjects with Guide for Rapid Research. Sidney J. Hopkins. rev. ed. 1994. LC 94-34384. 171p. 57.50 (*0-7883-0246-9*); pap. 47.50 (*0-7883-0247-7*) ABBE Pubs Assn.

Suicide & the Elderly: An Annotated Bibliography & Review, 3. Compiled by Nancy J. Osgood & John L. McIntosh. 1986. LC 86-14935. (Bibliographies & Indexes in Gerontology Ser.: No. 3). 206p. lib. bdg. 72.95 (*0-313-24786-2*, OSE/, Greenwood Pr) Greenwood.

Suicide & the Inner Voice: Risk Assessment, Treatment & Case Management. Robert W. Firestone. 1997. LC 96-51212. 352p. 81.95 (*0-7619-0554-5*, 80533); pap. 39.95 (*0-7619-0555-3*, 80534) Sage.

Suicide & the Soul. James Hillman. 1997. (Dunquin Ser.: ol. 8). 330p. pap. 18.00 (*0-88214-227-5*) Spring Pubns.

Suicide by Lifestyle. Courtney Hafela. l.t. ed. 1997. 205p. 24.95 (*0-9660181-2-5*) Two Blond Gdes.

Suicide in Adolescence. Ed. by Rene F. Diekstra & Keith E. Hawton. 1987. text 111.00 (*0-89838-780-9*) Kluwer Academic.

Suicide in Alcoholism. George E. Murphy. 1992. (Monographs in Psychiatry: No. 1). (Illus.). 336p. text 49.95 (*0-19-507153-0*) OUP.

Suicide in Later Life: Recognizing the Warning Signs. Nancy J. Osgood. 1992. 168p. 23.95 (*0-669-21214-8*) Free Pr.

Suicide Intervention in the Schools. Scott Poland. 1989. LC 88-36988. (Guilford School Practitioner Ser.). 214p. pap. 24.00 (*0-89862-232-8*, 2232); text 49.95 (*0-89862-353-7*) Guilford Pubns.

Suicide Notes: Predictive Clues & Patterns. Antoon A. Leenaars. 1988. 272p. 42.95 (*0-89885-399-0*, Kluwer Acad Hman Sci) Kluwer Academic.

Suicide over the Life Cycle: Risk Factors, Assessment, & Treatment of Suicidal Patients. Ed. by Susan J. Blumenthal & David J. Kupfer. 1990. LC 89-18368. 799p. text 85.50 (*0-88048-307-5*, 8307) Am Psychiatric.

Suicide Prevention: Case Consultations. Ed. by Alan L. Berman. 1990. LC 89-26342. (Death & Suicide Ser.: Vol. 10). 176p. 29.95 (*0-8261-7120-6*) Springer Pub.

Suicide Prevention: The Global Context: Proceedings of the XIXth Congress of the International Association for Suicide Prevention Held in Adelaide, Australia, March 23-27, 1997. Ed. by Robert J. Kosky et al. 1998. LC 98-9502. (Illus.). 424p. 115.00 (*0-306-45815-2*, Kluwer Plenum) Kluwer Academic.

Suicide Prevention in Schools. Antoon A. Leenaars & Susanne Wenkstern. 1990. 89.95 (*0-89116-954-7*); pap. 39.95 (*1-56032-081-8*) Hemisp Pub.

Suicide Risk: Assessment & Response Guidelines. William J. Fremouw et al. 1990. (Psychology Practitioner Guidebooks Ser.). 160p. text (*0-08-036445-4*); pap. text (*0-08-036444-6*) PPI GBR. *Dist:* Elsevier.

Suicide with Assistance: Index of New Information. Shirley S. Taube. 1994. 150p. 57.50 (*0-7883-0030-X*); pap. 47.50 (*0-7883-0031-8*) ABBE Pubs Assn.

Suicidology: Contemporary Developments. Ed. by Edwin S. Shneidman. 1976. LC 76-7031. (Seminars in Psychiatry Ser.). 592p. text 89.00 (*0-8089-0930-4*, 794030, Grune & Strat) Harcrt Hlth Sci Grp.

Suing for Medical Malpractice. Frank A. Sloan et al. 1993. LC 92-48268. (Illus.). 272p. (C). 39.95 (*0-226-76279-3*) U Ch Pr.

Sujet Freudien see Freudian Subject

Suki & Massry's Therapy of Renal Diseases & Related Disorders. Wadi N. Suki & Shaul G. Massry. 3rd ed. 1997. LC 96-49630. 1320p. lib. bdg. 475.00 (*0-7923-4368-9*) Kluwer Academic.

Sulfatases of Microbial Origin. Ed. by K. S. Dodgeson et al. 1982. Vol. 1. 216p. 122.00 (*0-8493-6035-8*, QP609); Vol. 2. 208p. 122.00 (*0-8493-6036-6*) Franklin (CRC Reprint).

Sulfation of Drugs & Related Compounds. Gerald J. Mulder. 1981. 248p. 142.00 (*0-8493-5920-1*, RM301, CRC Reprint) Franklin.

Sulfur & Sulfur Amino Acids, Vol. 143. Ed. by William B. Jakoby & Owen W. Griffith. 1987. (Methods in Enzymology Ser.). 504p. text 149.00 (*0-12-182043-2*) Acad Pr.

Sulfur Bacteria - STP 650. Ed. by E. Fjerdingstad. 1985. 129p. pap. 15.00 (*0-8031-0582-7*, STP650) ASTM.

Sulfur in Pesticide Action & Metabolism. Ed. by Joseph D. Rosen et al. 1981. LC 81-7916. (ACS Symposium Ser.: No. 158). 38.95 (*0-8412-0635-X*) Am Chemical.

Sulfur in Proteins. Yu. M. Torchinsky. 1981. (Illus.). 304p. (*0-08-023778-9*) Pergamon Repr GBR. *Dist:* Franklin.

Sulfur Oxides & Suspended Particulate Matter. 1979. (Environmental Health Criteria Ser.: No. 8). 107p. pap. text 16.00 (*92-4-154068-0*, 1160008) World Health.

Sulphur-Containing Drugs & Related Organic Compounds: Chemistry, Biochemistry & Toxicology: Metabolism & Pharmacokinetics of Sulpher-Containing Drugs, Vol. 3, Pt. B. Ed. by L. A. Damani. 1989. (Adolescent Medicine Ser.). 280p. 74.95 (*0-470-21514-3*) P-H.

Sulphur-Containing Drugs & Related Organic Compounds Vol. 2, Pt. A: Chemistry, Biochemistry & Toxicology: Analytical, Biochemical & Toxicological Aspects of Sulphur Xenobiochemistry, Vol. 2. Ed. by L. A. Damani. 1989. (Adolescent Medicine Ser.). 163p. 74.95 (*0-470-21500-3*) P-H.

Sulphur-Containing Drugs & Related Organic Compounds Vol. 2, Pt. B: Chemistry, Biochemistry & Toxicology: Analytical, Biochemical & Toxicological Aspects of Sulphur Xenobiochemistry, Vol. 2. Ed. by L. A. Damani. 1989. (Adolescent Medicine Ser.). 175p. 74.95 (*0-470-21501-1*) P-H.

Sulphur-Containing Drugs & Related Organic Compounds Vol. 3, Pt. A: Chemistry, Biochemistry & Toxicology: Metabolism & Pharmacokinetics of Sulphur Containing Drugs, Vol. 3. Ed. by L. A. Damani. 1989. (Adolescent Medicine Ser.). 204p. 74.95 (*0-470-21513-5*) P-H.

SUM Program Beginning Medical Transcription. Linda Campbell et al. 1994. 300p. pap. text 840.00 incl. audio (*0-934385-60-2*) Hlth Prof Inst.

SUM Program Pathology Transcription Unit. 2nd rev. ed. 1992. 72p. pap. text 280.00 incl. audio (*0-934385-65-3*) Hlth Prof Inst.

SUM Program Radiology Transcription Unit. 2nd rev. ed. 1990. 72p. pap. text 210.00 incl. audio (*0-934385-64-5*) Hlth Prof Inst.

Sumario de la Medicina, Francisco Lopez de Villalobos, I-1169: Biblioteca Nacional de Madrid. Maria Nieves-Sanchez. 1987. (Medieval Spanish Medical Texts Ser.: No. 13). (SPA.). 8p. 10.00 incl. fiche (*0-940639-09-2*) Hispanic Seminary.

Sumatripian - From Molecule to Man: An Official Session at the 8th Migraine Trust Symposium - Journal: European Neurology, Vol. 31, No. 5, 1991. Ed. by J. Lance & V. Pfaffenrath. 1991. (Illus.). 72p. pap. 31.50 (*3-8055-5437-0*) S Karger.

Summaries of State Laws Relating to the Insane. John Koren. Ed. by Gerald N. Grob. 1980. LC 78-22570. (Historical Issues in Mental Health Ser.). reprint ed. lib. bdg. 20.95 (*0-405-11923-2*) Ayer.

Summary of Contraindications to Oral Contraceptives, Vol. 2. S. C. M. Knijff & E. M. Goorissen. 2000. LC 99-27096. (Summary of Oral Contraceptive Data Ser.: Vol. 2). (Illus.). 602p. lib. bdg. 85.95 (*1-85070-691-3*, Parthenon Pbng) CRC Pr.

Summary of Drug Interactions with Oral Contraceptives. T. B. Geurts et al. Ed. by J. M. Sitsen. 1993. (Summary of Oral Contraceptive Data Ser.). (Illus.). 130p. (C). lib. bdg. 42.95 (*1-85070-518-6*, Parthenon Pbng) CRC Pr.

Summary of Evaluations Performed by the Joint FAO-WHO Expert Committee on Food Additives (JECFA) 1956-1993 (First Through Forty-First Meetings) United Nations Food and Agriculture Organization Staff & World Health Organization Staff. 1994. LC 96-144817. iii, 284p. pap. text 99.00 (*92-4-156172-6*, 1930059) World Health.

Summary Report on the Evaluation of Short-Term Tests for Carcinogens: Collaborative Study on in Vitro Tests. WHO Staff. 1985. (Environmental Health Criteria Ser.: No. 47). 77p. 15.00 (*92-4-154187-3*) World Health.

Summary Report on the Evaluation of Short-Term Tests for Carcinogens: Collaborative Study on in Vivo Tests. 1990. (Environmental Health Criteria Ser.: No. 109). 96p. pap. text 18.90 (*92-4-157109-8*, 1160109) World Health.

Summer of the Pestilence: A History of the Ravages of the Yellow Fever in Norfolk, Virginia A. D. 1855. George D. Armstrong. 3rd ed. 1995. LC 94-67855. 76p. pap. 10.00 (*1-57000-037-9*) W S Dawson.

Summer Plague: Polio & Its Survivors. Tony Gould. 1995. LC 94-47253. 366p. 45.00 (*0-300-06292-3*) Yale U Pr.

Summon up the Blood: In Dogged Pursuit of the Blood Cell Regulators. Donald Metcalf. 2000. (Illus.). 214p. 49.95 (*1-880854-27-9*); pap. 29.95 (*1-880854-28-7*) AlphaMed Pr.

Sun, Air & Light Baths: How They Cure Disease. 1991. (Alternative Medicine Ser.). lib. bdg. 79.95 (*0-8490-4546-0*) Gordon Pr.

Sun Can Shine Again: A Journey Through Heartache. Orrie Snyder. 1997. LC 97-60122. 352p. pap. 12.99 (*1-57921-006-6*) WinePress Pub.

Sun Is Feminine: A Study on Language & Acquisition in Bilingual Children. T. Taeschner. 1983. (Language & Communication Ser.: Vol. 13). (Illus.). 246p. 92.00 (*0-387-12238-9*) Spr-Verlag.

Sun Sense: A Complete Guide to the Prevention, Early Detection, & Treatment of Skin Cancer. Perry Robins. 1990. (Illus.). 272p. pap. 109.95 (*0-9627688-0-4*) Skin Cancer Fndtn.

Sun, the Rain & the Insulin: Growing up with Diabetes. Joan MacCracken. Ed. by Donna Hoel & Greg Hoel. 1996. LC 96-90047. (Illus.). 250p. (Orig.). pap. 12.95 (*0-9646018-5-0*) Tiffin Pr ME.

Sundt's Occlusive Cerebrovascular Disease. Ed. by Fredric B. Meyer. 2nd rev. ed. 1994. LC 94-18063. text 175.00 (*0-7216-4911-4*) Saunders.

Sunlight & Health: Lowering Cholesterol, Blood Pressure & Blood Sugar Through the Positive Effects of the Sun. 1992. lib. bdg. 88.00 (*0-8490-8815-1*) Gordon Pr.

Sunlight Could Save Your Life. Zane R. Kime. 1980. LC 80-51038. 312p. 15.95 (*0-9604268-0-9*); pap. 11.95 (*0-9604268-1-7*) Wrld Hlth Pubns.

Sunscreen Photobiology: Molecular, Cellular & Physiological Aspects. Francis P. Gasparro. 1997. LC 97-21826. (Biotechnology Intelligence Unit Ser.). 182p. 109.00 (*1-57059-468-6*) Landes Bioscience.

SUNY Downstate Medical Center. Jack E. Termine. 2000. LC 99-69492. (College History Ser.). (Illus.). 128p. pap. 19.99 (*0-7385-0069-0*) Arcadia Publng.

Super Anti-Oxidants: Why They Will Change the Face of Healthcare in the 21st Century. James F. Balch. 1999. LC 99-232631. 320p. pap. 21.95 (*0-87131-851-2*) M Evans.

Super Aspirin Cure for Arthritis: What You Need to Know About the Breakthrough Drugs That Stop Pain & Reverse Arthritis Symptoms Without Side Effects. Harris H. McIlwain et al. 1999. LC 99-200327. 208p. mass mkt. 5.99 (*0-553-58107-4*) Bantam.

Super Brain Breathing for Super Health & High Energy see Super Power Breathing: For Super Energy, High Health & Longevity

Super Calcium Miracle: The Calcium Citrate Malate Breakthrough. Mark Andon. 1998. LC 98-25969. 240p. pap. 15.00 (*0-7615-1456-2*, Prima Health) Prima Pub.

Super Healing Foods. 1994. 192p. (Orig.). pap. 14.95 (*1-57327-012-1*, M Pr CA) Busn Concepts.

Super Health Through Super Foods: How to Eat High in the Rating Chart. 1992. lib. bdg. 88.75 (*0-8490-8792-9*) Gordon Pr.

Super Nutrients Handbook: The Hidden Power in Plant Foods That Benefit Body & Mind. Lyndel Costain. 2001. LC 00-53107. (Healing Handbooks Ser.). (Illus.). 128p. pap. 12.95 (*0-7894-7179-5*) DK Pub Inc.

Super Nutrition for Men: And the Women Who Love Them. Ann L. Gittleman. 2nd ed. 1997. 224p. reprint ed. pap. 14.95 (*0-87131-834-2*) M Evans.

Super Nutrition for Menopause. Anne L. Gittleman. 1993. 256p. (Orig.). mass mkt. 5.99 (*0-671-78100-6*) PB.

Super Potency at Any Age. Edwin Flatto. 1991. LC 91-73635. 288p. 29.98 (*0-941683-09-5*) Instant Improve.

Super Potency at Any Age. Edwin Flatto. 8th rev. ed. 1998. (FRE, GER, IND & POL., Illus.). 235p. lib. bdg. 24.95 (*0-935540-18-0*) Plymouth Pr.

Super Power Breathing: For Super Energy, High Health & Longevity. Paul C. Bragg & Patricia Bragg. 21st rev. ed. 1999. Orig. Title: Super Brain Breathing for Super Health & High Energy. (Illus.). 160p. pap. 7.95 (*0-87790-020-5*) Hlth Sci.

Super Searchers on Health & Medicine: The Online Secrets of Top Health & Medical Researchers. Susan Detwiler. Ed. by Reva Basch. 2000. LC 00-43006. (Super Searchers Ser.: Vol. 5). (Illus.). 260p. pap. 24.95 (*0-910965-44-7*, CyberAge Bks) Info Today Inc.

Super Shrink II. Joseph Lowman. 1990. 119p. (C). pap. text 51.50 (*0-15-584764-3*) Harcourt Coll Pubs.

Super Shrink II: Jennifer. Lowman. 1990. (C). pap. text, tchr. ed. 7.00 (*0-15-584765-1*) Harcourt Coll Pubs.

Super "T" The Complete Guide to Creating an Effective, Safe & Natural Testosterone Supplement Program for Men & Women. Karlis Ullis et al. 1999. LC 99-14572. (Illus.). 272p. pap. 12.00 (*0-684-86335-9*, Fireside) S&S Trade Pap.

Superbiomin: The "Superbiomin" with Its 26 Mineral Elements for Human Beings, Animals & Nature. Robert Schindele. 1995. 88p. pap. (*3-85068-285-4*) Ennsthaler AUT. *Dist:* Am Educ Systs.

Superbugs: Microorganisms in Extreme Environments. Ed. by Koki Horikoshi & W. D. Grant. 1991. (Illus.). 299p. 108.00 (*0-387-52825-3*) Spr-Verlag.

***Superficial Esophageal Neoplasm: Pathology, Diagnosis, & Therapy.** Masayuki Imamura. 2001. LC 2001-49711. (*4-431-70317-9*) Springer Pub.

***Superficial Fungal Infections.** Richardson & Boni E. Elewski. 2000. (Fast Facts Ser.). (Illus.). 56p. pap. (*1-899541-76-4*) Health Pr GBR. *Dist:* JAMCO Dist.

Superficial Fungal Infections. Ed. by Julian L. Verbov. 1986. (New Clinical Applications in Dermatology Ser.). lib. bdg. 82.00 (*0-85200-943-7*) Kluwer Academic.

Superficial Keratitis. Ed. by P. C. Maudgal & L. Missotten. 1981. text 141.50 (*90-6193-801-5*) Kluwer Academic.

Superficial Liposculpture: Manual of Technique. Carson M. Lewis et al. 1996. LC 92-49210. (Illus.). 137p. 198.00 (*0-387-97917-4*) Spr-Verlag.

Superior Nutrition. 1994. pap. 8.95 (*0-9606948-1-1*) Willow Pub.

SuperLab LT: Experimental Software for Psychology Students. Hisham Abboud & Christopher Chase. 1997. (Illus.). 50p. (Orig.). (C). pap. text 30.00 (*0-9661842-0-3*) Cedrus Corp.

Superoxide Dismutase. Ed. by Larry W. Oberley. 1982. Vol. I. 168p. 97.00 (*0-8493-6240-7*, QP603); Vol. II. 192p. 110.00 (*0-8493-6241-5*) Franklin (CRC Reprint).

Superoxide Ion: Chemistry & Biological Implications, Vol. I. Igor B. Afanas'Ev. 1989. 296p. 219.00 (*0-8493-5451-X*, QP535) CRC Pr.

Supershrink II: 5.25" Joseph Lowman. 1990. 119p. (C). pap. text 51.50 (*0-15-584763-5*) Harcourt.

Supervising Addiction Specialist. Jack Rudman. 1994. (Career Examination Ser.: C-1501). pap. 34.95 (*0-8373-1501-8*) Nat Learn.

Supervising Air Pollution Inspector. Jack Rudman. 1994. (Career Examination Ser.: C-1502). pap. 34.95 (*0-8373-1502-6*) Nat Learn.

Supervising Audiologist. Jack Rudman. 1994. (Career Examination Ser.: C-2237). pap. 34.95 (*0-8373-2237-5*) Nat Learn.

Supervising Drug & Alcohol Community Coordinator. Jack Rudman. 1994. (Career Examination Ser.: C-2777). pap. 39.95 (*0-8373-2777-6*) Nat Learn.

Supervising Emergency Medical Service Specialist. Jack Rudman. 1994. (Career Examination Ser.: C-3480). pap. 34.95 (*0-8373-3480-2*) Nat Learn.

Supervising Hospital Care Investigator. Jack Rudman. 1994. (Career Examination Ser.: C-779). pap. 29.95 (*0-8373-0779-1*) Nat Learn.

Supervising Medicaid Claims Examiner. Jack Rudman. 1994. (Career Examination Ser.: C-2693). pap. 34.95 (*0-8373-2693-1*) Nat Learn.

Supervising Medical Services Specialist. Jack Rudman. 1994. (Career Examination Ser.: C-3616). pap. 39.95 (*0-8373-3616-3*) Nat Learn.

Supervising Medical Social Worker. Jack Rudman. 1994. (Career Examination Ser.: C-2630). pap. 34.95 (*0-8373-2630-3*) Nat Learn.

Supervising Nurse. Jack Rudman. 1994. (Career Examination Ser.: C-1883). pap. 34.95 (*0-8373-1883-1*) Nat Learn.

Supervising Physical Therapist. Jack Rudman. 1994. (Career Examination Ser.: C-2904). pap. 34.95 (*0-8373-2904-3*) Nat Learn.

Supervising Physician & Surgeon. Jack Rudman. 1994. (Career Examination Ser.: C-2195). pap. 49.95 (*0-8373-2195-6*) Nat Learn.

Supervising Professional Development in Health Care Practice. Jenny Spouse & Liz Redfern. 1999. LC 99-38176. pap. 47.95 (*0-632-05159-0*) Blackwell Sci.

Supervising Public Health Nurse. Jack Rudman. 1994. (Career Examination Ser.: C-1748). (Orig.). reprint ed. pap. 34.95 (*0-8373-1748-7*) Nat Learn.

Supervising Public Health Sanitarian. Jack Rudman. 1994. (Career Examination Ser.: C-2275). reprint ed. pap. 34.95 (*0-8373-2275-8*) Nat Learn.

Supervising the Counsellor: A Cyclical Model. Steve Page & Val Wosket. 1994. LC 94-8492. (Illus.). 256p. (C). 84.95 (*0-415-10213-8*, B4078) Routledge.

Supervising Therapist. Jack Rudman. 1994. (Career Examination Ser.: C-2253). pap. 34.95 (*0-8373-2253-7*) Nat Learn.

***Supervision: A Pharmacy Perspective.** Jeannette Y. Wick. 2002. 200p. pap. text 30.00 (*1-58212-013-7*) Am Pharm Assn.

Supervision & Related Issues: A Handbook for Professionals. Cathy A. Malchiodi & Shirley Riley. 1996. 250p. pap. 28.95 (*0-9613309-7-X*) Magnolia St Pub.

Supervision & Training: Models, Dilemmas, & Challenges. Ed. by Florence W. Kaslow. 1986. LC 85-27037. (Clinical Supervisor Ser.: Vol. 4, Nos. 1 & 2). 259p. text 49.95 (*0-86656-528-0*); pap. text 19.95 (*0-86656-529-9*) Haworth Pr.

Supervision & Treatment of Sex Offenders. I. Glen Kercher. rev. ed. 1998. LC 98-215941. 304p. pap. 29.95 (*1-55691-129-7*) Learning Pubns.

Supervision for Midwives. Ed. by Mavis Kirkham. 1997. LC 97-144815. 227p. pap. text 32.50 (*1-898507-14-7*) Buttrwrth-Heinemann.

Supervision in Healthcare Facilities. Winborn Davis. 1999. (Illus.). 138p. (C). pap. 32.50 (*0-929442-54-7*) Prof Prnting & Pub.

Supervision in the Health Care Organizations. Richard I. Lyles & Carl Joiner. 1989. LC 85-17799. 245p. text 33.50 (*0-8273-4294-2*) Delmar.

Supervision of Health Personnel at District Level. D. Flahault & M. Piot. 1988. 100p. 18.00 (*92-4-154229-2*) World Health.

Supervision of Psychologist & Counsellor. G. Shipton. 1997. LC 96-33218. 159p. (*0-335-19513-X*); pap. (*0-335-19512-1*) OpUniv Pr.

Supervisor (Medical & Psychiatric Social Work) Jack Rudman. 1994. (Career Examination Ser.: C-1052). pap. 34.95 (*0-8373-1052-0*) Nat Learn.

Supervisor of Vocational Rehabilitation Unit. Jack Rudman. 1994. (Career Examination Ser.: C-1742). pap. 34.95 (*0-8373-1742-8*) Nat Learn.

Supervisor's Guide to On-the-Job Alcoholism & Drug Problems. Business and Legal Reports Staff. 1986. pap. 9.95 (*1-55645-432-5*) Busn Legal Reports.

Supervisor's Role in Early Recovery. Brenda R. Blair. 1991. 24p. pap. 3.25 (*1-56246-014-5*, 3285, HazeldenJohnson Inst) Hazelden.

Supervisory Couple in Broad-Spectrum Psychotherapy. Wyn Bramley. 1997. 180p. (C). LC 97-189700. (*1-85343-353-5*); pap. (*1-85343-354-3*) Free Assoc Bks GBR. *Dist:* Intl Spec Bk, NYU Pr.

Supervisory Management for Health Care Organizations. Theo Haimann. 4th ed. 1990. 448p. (C). per. 48.50 net. (*0-697-14126-8*) Brown & Benchmark.

Supplement B, Suppl. B. 51st ed. 1997. 200p. (Orig.). pap. text, suppl. ed. Not sold separately (*1-56363-223-3*) Med Econ.

Supplement Shopper: An Alternative Medicine Definitive Guide. Gregory Pouls et al. 1999. LC 99-12466. (Illus.). 500p. pap. 14.95 (*1-887299-17-3*) AlternMed Bks.

Supplement to a Programmed Manual for Nursing Home Administrator Examinees. Edmond Boudreaux. 11th ed. 1995. 20p. (C). pap. text 5.00 (*1-878199-06-4*) Pro Exam Review.

Supplement to Glossary of Indian Medicinal Plants. R. N. Chopra. 1988. (C). (*0-7855-2288-3*) Scientific GBR. *Dist:* St Mut.

Supplement to Handbook on Injectable Drugs. Lawrence A. Trissel. (Orig.). 8th ed. 1995. 96p. pap. text (*1-879907-54-2*); 9th rev. ed. 1997. LC 97-176916. 112p. pap. text 31.00 (*1-879907-72-0*, P470S); 10th ed. 1999. 96p. pap. (*1-879907-95-X*) Am Soc Hlth-Syst.

Supplement to Reports on AIDS in the African Press: An Annotated Bibliography. Nancy J. Schmidt. 1990. 72p. pap. 3.00 (*0-941934-61-6*) Indiana Africa.

Supplement to the Eleventh Mental Measurements Yearbook. Ed. by Jane C. Conoley & James C. Impara. 1994. LC 39-3422. (Mental Measurements Yearbook Ser.). 323p. pap. 55.00 (*0-910674-34-5*) Buros Inst Mental.

Supplement to the Ninth Mental Measurements Yearbook. Ed. by Jane C. Conoley et al. 1988. (Mental Measurements Yearbook Ser.). xiii, 279p. (Orig.). pap. 65.00 (*0-910674-30-2*) Buros Inst Mental.

Supplement to the Residential Alternatives Series: Leisure Volunteer's Guide. C. E. Gathercole. 1985. 8p. (*0-906054-54-0*) Brit Inst Lrning GBR. *Dist:* Taylor & Francis.

Supplement to Twists & Turns, a Mother's Caring Journey: Two Children with Schizophrenia. Ruth C. Ackerman. 1997. (Illus.). 6p. pap. 3.00 (*0-9637493-1-5*) Paths of Life.

Supplemental Health Insurance. Ed. by Jane J. Stein. 1999. LC 98-177773. (Insurance Education Ser.). 283p. pap. 30.00 (*1-879143-42-9*) Health Ins Assn Am.

Supplemental Health Insurance Study Manual. HIAA Staff. 1998. 56p. pap., stu. ed. 10.00 (*1-879143-43-7*) Health Ins Assn Am.

Supplements for Bodybuilding. Woodland Publishing Staff. 1999. pap. text 3.95 (*1-58054-049-X*) Woodland UT.

Supply-Demand Model of Health Care Financing with an Application to Zaire. Ricardo A. Bitran. 1994. LC 93-20079. (EDI Technical Materials Ser.). 92p. pap. 24.00 (*0-8213-2342-3*, 12342) World Bank.

Support Groups - The Human Face of the HIV-AIDS Epidemic: A Handbook for Health Care Professionals, People with AIDS, Their Loved Ones, & the Community-at-Large. Gail Barouh. 1992. LC 92-81221. x, 94p. pap. 10.00 (*1-881305-00-7*) LIAAC.

Support Groups for Children. Kathleen O'Rourke & John C. Worzbyt. 1996. 425p. pap. 39.95 (*1-56032-395-7*) Hemisp Pub.

Support of the Acutely Failing Liver. Achilles A. Demetriou. 2nd ed. 2000. (Tissue Engineering Intelligence Unit Ser.). 156p. 89.00 (*1-57059-585-2*) Landes Bioscience.

Support of the Acutely Failing Liver. Ed. by Achilles A. Demetriou & Frederick D. Watanabe. 2nd ed. 2000. (Tissue Engineering Intelligence Unit Ser.). 156p. 99.00 (*1-58706-001-9*) Eurekah.

Supported Cancer Care: The Complete Guide for Patients & Their Families. Ernest H. Rosenbaum. 2001. LC 00-66170. 496p. pap. 24.95 (*1-57071-696-X*) Sourcebks.

Supported Complex & High Risk Coronary Angioplasty. Ed. by Fayez A. Shawl. 1991. (Interventional Cardiology Ser.). (C). text 159.50 (*0-7923-1121-3*) Kluwer Academic.

Supported Employment & TBI. Ed. by William H. Burke. 2nd ed. 1995. (Professional Series on Traumatic Brain Injury: Vol. 18). 64p. (Orig.). pap. 9.50 (*1-882855-38-8*) HDI Pubs.

Supporting Emotional Needs of Family Members: A Module for Training Personnel Serving Families of Deaf & Hard of Hearing Infants & Young Children. Ed. by Valerie Schuyler. 1993. (Early Intervention Ser.). 39p. (C). 89.00 incl. VHS (*0-9618297-4-5*) Hearing & Speech.

Supporting Language Learning in Everyday Life. Judith F. Duchan. 1994. LC 94-29227. (School-Age Children Ser.). 224p. (Orig.). (C). pap. text 44.95 (*1-56593-221-8*, 0581) Thomson Learn.

Supporting Sick Children. Penny Cook. 1999. 269p. (C). pap. text (*0-7020-2207-1*) W B Saunders GBR. *Dist:* Saunders.

Supporting the Pediatric Transfusion Recipient. Ed. by Linda A. Chambers & Linda A. Issitt. 1994. LC 94-32346. (Illus.). 161p. (C). 50.00 (*1-56395-032-4*) Am Assn Blood.

Supportive & Active Psychotherapies: A Dynamic Approach. Paul A. Dewald. 1997. LC 93-74969. 354p. pap. 50.00 (*1-56821-221-6*) Aronson.

***Supportive Cancer Care: A Comprehensive Guide for Patients & Their Families.** Ernest H. Rosenbaum & Isadora R. Rosenbaum. 2001. LC 00-66170. 496p. pap. 19.95 (*1-57071-787-7*) Sourcebks.

***Supportive Care & Midwifery.** Rosemary Mander. 2001. LC 2001-25254. ix, 190p. (*0-632-05425-5*) Blackwell Sci.

Supportive Care in Cancer: A Handbook for Oncologists. Jean Klastersky et al. 2nd exp. rev. ed. 1999. LC 99-32709. (Basic & Clinical Oncology Ser.). (Illus.). 824p. text 195.00 (*0-8247-1998-0*) Dekker.

Supportive Care in Cancer Patients. Ed. by H. J. Senn & L. Schmid. 1988. (Recent Results in Cancer Research Ser.: Vol. 108). (Illus.). 342p. 137.00 (*0-387-17150-9*) Spr-Verlag.

Supportive Care in Cancer Patients: Recent Developments. Ed. by M. Karthaus & Arnold Ganser. 2000. (Antibiotics & Chemotherapy Ser.: Vol. 50). (Illus.). viii, 196p. 137.50 (*3-8055-6910-6*) S Karger.

Supportive Care in Cancer Therapy. Ed. by Donald J. Higby. 1983. (Cancer Treatment & Research Ser.). text 213.50 (*0-89838-569-5*) Kluwer Academic.

Supportive Care of Children with Cancer: Current Therapy & Guidelines from the Children's Cancer Group. Arthur R. Ablin. 2nd ed. 1997. LC 97-26952. (Series in Hematology/Oncology). 352p. pap. text 32.95 (*0-8018-5727-9*) Johns Hopkins.

Supportive Care of the Cancer Patient. Ed. by Chris Williams & John W. Sweetenham. 1998. LC 98-121489. (An Arnold Publication). (Illus.). 336p. (*0-340-56171-8*) E A GBR. *Dist:* OUP.

Supportive Therapy: A Psychodynamic Approach. Lawrence H. Rockland. 1989. LC 89-42801. 320p. (C). pap. 45.00 (*0-465-08337-4*) Basic.

Supportive Therapy for Borderline Patients: A Psychodynamic Approach. Lawrence H. Rockland. 1992. LC 92-1538. (Diagnosis & Treatment of Mental Disorders Ser.). 308p. 40.00 (*0-89862-182-8*, 2182) Guilford Pubns.

Supportive Therapy in Haematology. Ed. by P. C. Das et al. 1985. LC 85-4977. text 213.00 (*0-89838-700-0*) Kluwer Academic.

Suppressed Madness of Sane Men: Forty-Four Years of Exploring Psycho-Analysis. Marion Milner. 1987. (Illus.). 250p. (C). pap. (*0-422-61690-7*); lib. bdg. (*0-422-61020-8*) Tavistock GBR. *Dist:* Routldge.

Suppressor B Lymphocytes, Vol. 1. R. V. Petrov et al. Tr. by V. E. Tatarchenko from RUS. 1988. (Soviet Medical Reviews, Immunology Series Supplement: Vol. 1). xii, 208p. text 348.00 (*3-7186-4800-8*) Gordon & Breach.

Suppressor Cells & Their Factors. Ed. by Randall S. Krakauer & John D. Clough. 1981. 184p. 109.00 (*0-8493-6185-0*, QR185, CRC Reprint) Franklin.

Suprachiasmatic Nucleus: The Mind's Clock. R. Moore & S. Reppert. Ed. by Donald F. Klein et al. 1991. (Illus.). 488p. text 88.00 (*0-19-506250-7*) OUP.

Supreme Green Medicine. Harald W. Tietze. 2000. (Illus.). 105p. pap. 12.95 (*0-8464-5202-2*) Beekman Pubs.

Suprofen. Ed. by M. E. Rosenthale. 1983. (Journal: Vol. 27, Suppl. 1). (Illus.). viii, 96p. pap. 33.25 (*3-8055-3789-1*) S Karger.

Sur le Reve. Sigmund Freud. 1990. (FRE.). pap. 10.95 (*0-7859-2821-9*) Fr & Eur.

Surface Anatomy. Backhouse. 1991. (*0-8151-0372-7*) Mosby Inc.

Surface Anatomy: The Anatomical Basis of Clinical Examination. John S. Lumley. 2nd ed. 1996. LC 96-10352. (Illus.). pap. text (*0-443-05302-2*) Church.

Surface Anatomy & Palpation Skills for Chiropractors. Stuart Kinsinger. 2002. (Illus.). 256p. pap. 42.50 (*0-7506-4484-2*) Buttrwrth-Heinemann.

Surface Anatomy for Clinical Needle Electromyography. Hang J. Lee & Joel A. Delisa. 1999. (Illus.). 240p. pap. text 44.95 (*1-888799-41-2*) Demos Medical.

Surface & Dermal Monitoring for Toxic Exposures. Shirley A. Ness. 1994. (Industrial Health & Safety Ser.). 576p. 125.00 (*0-471-28564-1*, VNR) Wiley.

Surface Modification of Polymeric Biomaterials: Proceedings of the American Chemical Society Division of Polymer Chemistry International Symposium Held in Anaheim, California, April 2-6, 1995. Ed. by Buddy D. Ratner & David G. Castner. 1997. LC 96-40102. (Illus.). 214p. (C). text 85.00 (*0-306-45512-9*, Kluwer Plenum) Kluwer Academic.

Surfactant in Lung Injury & Lung Transplantation. James F. Lewis & Richard J. Novick. 1997. (Medical Intelligence Unit Ser.). 218p. 99.00 (*1-57059-432-5*) Landes Bioscience.

Surfactant System of the Lung: Prevention & Treatment of Neonatal & Adult Respiratory Distress Syndrome. Ed. by Ermelando V. Cosmi et al. 1991. text (*0-333-55856-1*) Intl Spec Bk.

Surfactantsystem der Lunge. Konrad Morgenroth & M. Newhouse. 1986. viii, 110p. (C). lib. bdg. 79.25 (*3-11-011015-6*) De Gruyter.

SurfLess Find More! World's Leading Medicine Internet Sites Quickly & Easily. 2000. spiral bd. 14.95 (*1-893957-09-8*) SurfLess.

Surgeon. Jack Rudman. 1994. (Career Examination Ser.: C-790). pap. 49.95 (*0-8373-0790-2*) Nat Learn.

Surgeon & the Hospital in the Civil War. Albert G. Hart. 1987. pap. 10.00 (*0-942211-54-5*) Olde Soldier Bks.

Surgeon General's Report on. Pruitt. 1994. (C). pap. text 22.50 (*0-03-010248-0*) Harcourt Coll Pubs.

Surgeon General's Report on Nutrition & Health. U. S. Department of Health & Human Services Staff. 1989. 128p. mass mkt. 6.95 (*0-446-39061-5*) Warner Bks.

Surgeon General's Report on Nutrition & Health. U. S. Department of Health and Human Resources Staff. 1989. 768p. pap. 18.95 (*0-914629-96-4*) Prima Pub.

Surgeon General's Report on Nutrition & Health: Summary & Recommendations. C. Everett Koop. 1994. 78p. (Orig.). (C). pap. text 25.00 (*0-7881-0744-5*) DIANE Pub.

Surgeon Major Parke's African Journey, 1887-1889. J. B. Lyons. 1994. LC 94-158925. 282p. 39.95 (*1-874675-20-1*) Dufour.

Surgeons at War: Medical Arrangements for the Treatment of the Sick & Wounded in the British Army During the Late 18th & 19th Centuries, 205. Matthew H. Kaufman. 2000. LC 00-34079. (Contributions in Military Studies Ser.: Vol. 205). (Illus.). 240p. 68.00 (*0-313-31665-1*, GM1665, Greenwood Pr) Greenwood.

Surgeon's Fight to Rebuild Men. Fred Albee. 1995. (American Autobiography Ser.). 270p. reprint ed. lib. bdg. 79.00 (*0-7812-8441-4*) Rprt Serv.

Surgeon's Guide to Endoscopic & Laparoscopic Ultrasonography of the Colon, Rectum, & Anus. Ed. by W. Douglas Wong et al. 1997. LC 96-52546. (Illus.). text (*0-89640-338-6*) Igaku-Shoin.

Surgeon's Guide to Staging, Grading & Classifications. Lisa R. David & Andrew M. Schneider. 2001. LC 00-38807. (Illus.). xx, 216p. text 41.50 (*0-7216-8807-1*) Saunders.

Surgeon's Little Instruction Book. Daniel J. Waters. 1998. LC 98-233813. 183p. pap. 10.00 (*1-57626-082-8*, QMP) Quality Med Pub.

Surgeons, Smallpox & the Poor: A History of Medicine & Social Conditions in Nova Scotia, 1749-1799. Allan E. Marble. (Illus.). 376p. 1997. pap. (*0-7735-1639-5*); 1993. (*0-7735-0988-7*) McG-Queens Univ Pr CAN. *Dist:* CUP Services.

Surgeon's Surgeon see Belle Epoque of Surgery: The Life & Times of Theodor Billroth

Surgeon's Surgeon Vol. 1: Theodor Billroth (1829-1894), Vol. 1. Karel B. Absolon. 1979. (Illus.). 25.00 (*0-87291-129-2*) Coronado Pr.

Surgeon's Surgeon Vol. 3: Theodor Billroth (1829-1894) Karel B. Absolon. 1987. (Illus.). 280p. 30.00 (*0-87291-163-2*) Coronado Pr.

Surgery. John D. Corson & Robin C. N. Williamson. 2000. (Illus.). 1660p. text 150.00 (*0-7234-3069-1*) Mosby Inc.

Surgery. Nikos M. Linardakis. 1999. (Digging Up the Bones Ser.). (Illus.). 130p. pap. text 18.95 (*0-07-038367-7*) McGraw-Hill Med Pub.

Surgery. Molly Shapiro. 1998. LC 98-26910. (Vital Information Ser.). 160p. pap. 11.95 (*0-89594-898-2*) Crossing Pr.

Surgery. Taylor. 1999. pap. text (*0-7216-7642-1*) Saunders.

Surgery. L. Skrbic. 1991. (Illus.). 127p. (Orig.). (C). reprint ed. (*0-9626486-1-2*) Postgraduate Med Rev Ed.

Surgery. Bruce E. Jarrell & R. Anthony Carabasi, III. 2nd ed. 1990. (National Medical Ser.). (Illus.). 570p. 27.00 (*0-683-06270-0*) Lppncott W & W.

Surgery: A Clinical Approach. Bongard. 1996. LC 96-41027. pap. text 49.00 (*0-443-08994-9*) Saunders.

Surgery: A Clinical Approach. Michael J. Stamos & Edward Passaro. 1996. LC 96-41027. (*0-443-08995-7*) Church.

Surgery: A Core Text with Self-Assessment Covering Orthopaedics, Ear, Nose & Throat, Vol. 2. John A. Dent. 1997. pap. text (*0-443-05171-2*) Church.

Surgery: A Patient's Guide from Diagnosis to Recovery. Claire Mailhot et al. 1999. 254p. pap. 20.00 (*0-943671-19-1*) UCSF Schl Nursing.

Surgery: An Illustrated History. Ira M. Rutkow. 1993. LC 93-9820. (Illus.). 560p. (C). (gr. 13). text 135.00 (*0-8016-6078-5*, 06078) Mosby Inc.

Surgery: Basic Science & Clinical Evidence. Ed. by Jeffrey A. Norton et al. 2000. LC 00-40049. (Illus.). 2170p. 119.00 (*0-387-98447-X*) Spr-Verlag.

Surgery: Diagnosis & Therapy. Richard M. Stillman. 1989. (Illus.). 663p. (C). pap. 31.95 (*0-8385-1283-6*, A1283-9, Apple Lange Med) McGraw.

Surgery: Foot & Ankle. Michael J. Coughlin & Roger A. Mann. 7th ed. 1999. LC 99-20312. 1605p. text 295.00 (*0-323-00327-3*) Mosby Inc.

Surgery: PreTest Self-Assessment & Review. Peter L. Geller. 9th ed. 2000. (Pretest Clinical Science Ser.). (Illus.). 328p. pap. 24.95 (*0-07-135954-0*) McGraw-Hill Prof.

Surgery: Review for New National Boards. Glenn W. Geelhoed. 1995. (Illus.). 246p. pap. 25.00 (*0-8036-0718-0*) Davis Co.

Surgery: Review for New National Boards. Glenn W. Geelhoed. 1994. LC 94-79792. (Illus.). 246p. pap. 25.00 (*0-9632873-5-4*) J & S Pub VA.

Surgery & Arthroscopy of the Knee. Ed. by W. E. Muller & W. Hackenbruch. 1988. (Illus.). 730p. 199.00 (*0-387-17982-8*) Spr-Verlag.

Surgery & Pathology of the Middle Ear. Ed. by Jean F. Marquet. 1985. text 281.50 (*0-89838-707-8*) Kluwer Academic.

Surgery & Support of the Premature Infant. Ed. by P. Puri. 1985. (Modern Problems in Pediatrics Ser.: Vol. 23). (Illus.). x, 210p. 141.75 (*3-8055-4073-6*) S Karger.

Surgery, Anesthesia & Experimental Techniques in Swine. M. Michael Swindle. 1998. LC 98-24474. (Illus.). 320p. (C). text 99.95 (*0-8138-1829-X*) Iowa U Pr.

Surgery Annual 1983, Vol. 15. Lloyd M. Nyhus. 1983. (Illus.). 416p. (C). pap. text 95.00 (*0-8385-8721-6*, A8721-1, Apple Lange Med) McGraw.

Surgery Annual 1982, Vol. 14. Lloyd M. Nyhus. 1982. (Illus.). (C). pap. text 95.00 (*0-8385-8719-4*, A8719-5, Apple Lange Med) McGraw.

Surgery Annual, 1993, Vol. 25, Pt. 1. Lloyd M. Nyhus. 1992. (Illus.). 272p. (C). text 90.00 (*0-8385-8798-4*, A8798-9) Appleton & Lange.

Surgery Annual 1992, Vol. 24, Pt. 1. Ed. by Lloyd M. Nythus. 1991. 258p. (C). pap. text 95.00 (*0-8385-8745-3*, A8745-0, Apple Lange Med) McGraw.

Surgery Annual 1992, Vol. 24, Pt. 2. Lloyd M. Nyhus. 1992. (Illus.). 272p. (C). pap. text 95.00 (*0-8385-8748-8*, A8748-4, Apple Lange Med) McGraw.

Surgery at a Glance. P. A. Grace & N. R. Borley. 1999. LC 98-42494. (At a Glance Ser.). (Illus.). 168p. pap. 26.95 (*0-632-04958-8*) Blackwell Sci.

Surgery at the District Hospital: Obstetrics, Gynaecology, Orthopaedics, & Traumatology. Ed. by J. Cook et al. 1991. (ENG, FRE, RUS & SPA.). 207p. pap. text 22.50 (*92-4-154413-9*, 1150351) World Health.

Surgery Book. Robert M. Youngson. 1997. LC 96-31915. (Illus.). 448p. pap. 17.95 (*0-312-15218-3*) St Martin.

Surgery Book: An Illustrated Guide to 73 of the Most Common Operations. Robert M. Youngson. 1998. (Illus.). 448p. pap. text 18.00 (*0-7881-5927-5*) DIANE Pub.

***Surgery, Ethics & the Law.** Brendan J. Dooley. 2001. pap. 39.00 (*0-86793-021-7*) Blackwell Sci.

Surgery for Anaesthetists. Richard Zorab. 1989. 193.00 (*0-632-01371-0*) CRC Pr.

Surgery for Bone & Soft-Tissue Tumors. Ed. by Michael Simon & Dempsey Springfield. 1997. (Illus.). 784p. text 259.00 (*0-397-51396-8*) Lppncott W & W.

Surgery for Cancer of the Larynx & Related Structures. Carl E. Silver. Ed. by Larry McGrew. 2nd ed. 1996. LC 95-17699. (Illus.). 288p. text 145.00 (*0-7216-5266-2*) Saunders.

Surgery for Cerebrovascular Disease. Ed. by Wesley S. Moore. 2nd ed. 1996. (Illus.). 736p. text 230.00 (*0-7216-3624-1*) Saunders.

Surgery for Endocrinological Diseases & Malformations in Childhood. Ed. by M. W. Gauderer & T. A. Angerpointner. 1991. (Progress in Pediatric Surgery Ser.: Vol. 26). (Illus.). 144p. 137.00 (*0-387-52524-6*) Spr-Verlag.

Surgery for Finals. Andrew Goldberg & Gerard Stansby. 1997. 200p. (*1-86094-077-3*) Imperial College GBR. *Dist:* World Scientific Pub.

Surgery for Gastrointestinal Cancer: A Multidisciplinary Approach. Ed. by Harold J. Wanebo et al. 1996. LC 96-14257. 900p. text 199.00 (*0-397-51518-9*) Lppncott W & W.

Surgery for Hyperopia & Presbyopia. Neal A. Sher. 1997. LC 96-24160. (*4-260-14340-9*) Igaku-Shoin.

Surgery for Hyperopia & Presbyopia. Ed. by Neal A. Sher. 1997. LC 96-24160. (Illus.). text (*0-89640-340-8*) Igaku-Shoin.

Surgery for Mechanical Complications of Myocardial Infarction. Ed. by Tirone E. David. 1993. LC 93-23998. (Illus.). 252p. 156.00 (*1-879702-67-3*, R) CRC Pr.

Surgery for Morbid Obesity. John H. Linner. 1984. (Illus.). 208p. 138.00 (*0-387-90888-9*) Spr-Verlag.

Surgery for Movement Disorders. Joachim K. Krauss et al. 2001. text 159.00 (*0-7817-2244-6*) Lppncott W & W.

Surgery for Retinal & Vitreous Disease. John D. Scott. 1998. LC 97-27013. (Illus.). 385p. text 285.00 (*0-7506-3824-9*) Buttrwrth-Heinemann.

Surgery for Retinal & Vitreous Disease. John D. Scott. 1998. (Illus.). 524p. (C). text (*0-443-04983-1*) Church.

Surgery for Rheumatoid Arthritis: A Comprehensive Team Approach. Mack L. Clayton & Charley J. Smyth. 1992. (Illus.). 414p. text (*0-443-08217-0*) Church.

Surgery Handbook: A Guide for Patients & Families. Paul Ruggieri. 1999. LC 99-50492. (Illus.). vii, 149p. pap. 14.95 (*1-886039-38-0*) Addicus Bks.

Surgery in AIDS. Forse. 1999. text (*0-7216-5139-9*) Saunders.

Surgery in America: From the Colonial Era to the Twentieth Century. A. S. Earle. 2nd ed. 1983. LC 83-17808. (Illus.). 407p. 110.00 (*0-275-91389-9*, C1389, Praeger Pubs) Greenwood.

Surgery in & Around the Brain Stem & Third Ventricle. Ed. by Madjid Samii. 1986. (Illus.). 599p. 333.00 (*0-387-16581-9*) Spr-Verlag.

Surgery in Gynecological Oncology. A. P. Heintz. Ed. by C. Thomas Griffiths. 1983. (Developments in Oncology Ser.). text 191.50 (*0-89838-604-7*) Kluwer Academic.

Surgery in Rheumatoid Arthritis. Ed. by Ian F. Goldie. 1981. (Reconstruction Surgery & Traumatology Ser.: Vol. 18). (Illus.). vi, 214p. 95.75 (*3-8055-1445-X*) S Karger.

Surgery in Solitary Kidney & Corrections of Urinary Transport Disturbances. Ed. by T. A. Angerpointner et al. 1989. (Process in Pediatric Surgery Ser.: Vol. 23). (Illus.). 205p. 133.00 (*0-387-50485-0*) Spr-Verlag.

***Surgery in the Surgery.** Sidha Sambandan. 1999. 280p. pap., wbk. ed. (*1-85775-284-8*) Radcliffe Med Pr GBR. *Dist:* Balogh.

Surgery in World War II 2 vols., Set. 1995. lib. bdg. 599.99 (*0-8490-6582-8*) Gordon Pr.

Surgery Nutrition Handbook. Mary Marian et al. 1995. LC 95-16240. (Nutrition Handbks.: Vol. 4). 85p. pap. 21.00 (*0-412-07521-0*) Aspen Pub.

Surgery of Basal Cell Carcinoma. Daniel Marchac. 1987. (Illus.). 113p. 150.00 (*0-387-18034-6*) Spr-Verlag.

Surgery of Childhood Tumors. Robert Carachi. 1999. (Arnold Publication). (Illus.). 273p. text 250.00 (*0-340-69269-3*) OUP.

Surgery of Congenital Heart Disease: The Pediatric Cardiac Care Consortium 1984-1995. Ed. by James H. Moller. 1997. (Perspectives in Pediatric Cardiology Ser.: No. 6). (Illus.). 412p. pap. 97.00 (*0-87993-678-9*) Futura Pub.

Surgery of Cranial Base Tumors. Laligam N. Sekhar & Ivo P. Janecka. 896p. 1993. sl. 359.00 (*0-7817-0052-3*); 1992. text 289.00 (*0-88167-877-5*, 2378) Lppncott W & W.

Surgery of Facial Bone Fractures. Ed. by Craig A. Foster & John E. Sherman. 1986. (Illus.). 273p. text (*0-443-08436-X*) Church.

Surgery of Female Incontinence. Ed. by S. L. Stanton & Emil A. Tanagho. 2nd rev. ed. 1986. (Illus.). 285p. 218.00 (*0-387-15821-9*) Spr-Verlag.

Surgery of Hand-Unit in Adults & Children. Hosein A. Motamed. 2001. LC 77-78228. (Illus.). reprint ed. Vol. I. Not sold separately (*0-910161-03-8*); Vol. II. Not sold separately (*0-910161-04-6*) Motamed Med Pub.

Surgery of Infants & Children: Scientific Principles & Practice. Keith T. Oldham. 1996. LC 96-43070. 1,880p. text 279.00 (*0-397-51417-4*) Lppncott W & W.

Surgery of Inflammatory Bowel Disorders Vol. 14: CSI. E. Lee & Nolan. 1987. (Illus.). pap. (*0-443-03439-7*) Church.

Surgery of Male Infertility. Ed. by Marc Goldstein. 1994. LC 94-7749. (Illus.). 336p. 89.00 (*0-7216-6693-0*) Saunders.

Surgery of Occlusive Cerebrovascular Disease. R. S. Lord. 1998. (Illus.). 300p. (*0-443-04951-3*) Church.

Surgery of Peripheral Nerves. G. Morello & F. Pluchino. 1988. (Surgical Technique Ser.: Vol. XIV). 392p. text (*1-57235-043-1*) Piccin Nuova.

Surgery of Skull Base Meningiomas: With a Chapter on Pathology by G. F. Walter. Madjid Samii & M. Ammirati. 1993. (Illus.). 146p. 175.00 (*0-387-54016-4*) Spr-Verlag.

Surgery of Skull Base Tumors. Ed. by C. Gary Jackson. 1990. (Illus.). 291p. text (*0-443-08596-X*) Church.

Surgery of Spinal Trauma. Cotler. 1999. 416p. text 169.00 (*0-683-18108-4*) Lppncott W & W.

Surgery of the Alimentary Tract. George Zuidema & Charles Yeo. 5th ed. 2001. LC 00-30058. (Illus.). 2895p. text 495.00 (*0-7216-8203-0*) Saunders.

Surgery of the Alimentary Tract: Mesentary Vasculature, Hernias, Small Intestine, Peritoneum, Omentum, Mesentary & Retroperitoneum, Surgical Nutrition, Set. Richard T. Shackelford & George D. Zuidema. 2nd ed. 1986. (Illus.). 600p. 490.00 (*0-7216-8087-9*) Saunders.

Surgery of the Aorta & Its Branches. Bruce L. Gewertz. 2000. LC 99-23552. (Illus.). 479p. text (*0-7216-7751-7*) Saunders.

Surgery of the Arteria Profunda Femuralis. Ed. by Marco P. Merlini. 1994. LC 94-12558. (Illus.). 182p. 140.00 (*0-387-58067-0*) Spr-Verlag.

Surgery of the Arteries to the Head. Ramon Berguer & Edouard Kieffer. 1992. (Illus.). 236p. 231.00 (*0-387-97748-1*) Spr-Verlag.

Surgery of the Biliary Tract. Ed. by James Toouli. 1993. LC 92-49459. (Illus.). 408p. text (*0-443-04361-2*) Church.

Surgery of the Breast: Principles & Art. Scott L. Spear & John W. Little. 1998. LC 98-9429. 1,008p. text 299.00 (*0-397-51584-7*) Lppncott W & W.

Surgery of the Cervical Spine. Howard S. An. 1994. (Illus.). 350p. 150.00 (*0-683-00128-0*) Lppncott W & W.

Surgery of the Cervical Spine. Emery. 1999. LC 2001-49785. text (*0-7216-5780-X*) Saunders.

Surgery of the Chest, Set. David C. Sabiston, Jr. & Frank C. Spencer. 6th ed. 1995. LC 94-22780. (Illus.). 2272p. text 310.00 (*0-7216-5271-9*) Saunders.

Surgery of the Colon & Rectum. Nicholls. 1999. text (*0-443-05962-4*) Church.

Surgery of the Colon & Rectum. Nicholls. 1997. text 235.00 (*0-443-05565-3*) Saunders.

Surgery of the Colon, Rectum & Anus. Patrick W. Mazier et al. 1994. LC 93-40034. (Illus.). 992p. text 250.00 (*0-7216-4689-1*) Saunders.

Surgery of the Colon, Rectum & Anus. Ed. by L. P. Fielding & S. M. Goldberg. 5th ed. 1993. (Rob & Smith's Operative Surgery Ser.). (Illus.). 940p. (C). pap. 496.95 (*0-7506-1255-X*, Chap & Hall NY) Chapman & Hall.

Surgery of the Craniovertebral Junction. Curtis A. Dickman et al. 1997. LC 97-25003. (*3-13-107181-8*) G Thieme DEU. *Dist:* Thieme Med Pubs.

Surgery of the Craniovertebral Junction. Curtis Dickman et al. 1998. LC 97-25003. (Illus.). 784p. 299.00 (*0-86577-681-4*) Thieme Med Pubs.

Surgery of the Ear & Temporal Bone. Ed. by Joseph B. Nadol, Jr. & Harold F. Schuknecht. 1992. (Illus.). 494p. text 219.00 (*0-88167-803-1*, 2287) Lppncott W & W.

Surgery of the Elbow: Practical & Scientific Aspects. Ed. by David Stanley & Neville R. Kay. 1998. (Arnold Publication). (Illus.). 422p. 175.00 (*0-340-59805-0*) OUP.

Surgery of the Esophagus, Stomach, & Small Intestine. Ed. by Christopher Wastell et al. 5th ed. 1995. LC 94-21059. 1,040p. text 225.00 (*0-316-92442-3*, Little Brwn Med Div) Lppncott W & W.

Surgery of the Eye Stephen R. Waltman et al. 1987. (Illus.). 1157p. text (*0-443-08354-1*) Church.

Surgery of the Eyelid, Orbit, & Lacrimal System. Ed. by William B. Stewart. 1993. LC 93-19768. (Ophthalmology Monographs). (*1-56055-069-4*) Am Acad Ophthal.

Surgery of the Eyelids & Orbit: An Anatomical Approach. Bradley N. Lemke & Robert C. Della Rocca. 1992. (Illus.). 322p. (C). pap. text 199.00 (*0-8385-7500-5*, A7500-0, Apple Lange Med) McGraw.

Surgery of the Foot & Ankle. Basil Helal. 1995. 800p. text 199.00 (*0-397-51423-9*) Lppncott W & W.

Surgery of the Foot & Ankle. Kenneth A. Johnson. 1989. (Illus.). 320p. text 175.00 (*0-88167-398-6*) Lppncott W & W.

Surgery of the Foot & Ankle. Coughlin. 7th ed. 1999. (C). text 295.00 (*0-323-00899-2*) Mosby Inc.

Surgery of the Foot & Ankle Cd-ROM. Michael J. Coughlin & Roger A. Mann. 7th ed. 1999. 395.00 incl. cd-rom (*0-323-00900-X*) Mosby Inc.

Surgery of the Gallbladder & Bile Ducts. Lawrence M. Way & Carlos A. Pellegrini. 1987. (Illus.). 726p. text 155.00 (*0-7216-9139-0*) Saunders.

Surgery of the Hand & Upper Extremity. Clayton A. Peimer. 1. (*0-07-049388-X*); 2. (*0-07-049389-8*) McGraw.

Surgery of the Hand & Upper Extremity, Set. Ed. by Clayton A. Peimer. 1996. LC 95-32395. 2468p. text 189.00 (*0-07-049293-X*) McGraw-Hill Prof.

Surgery of the Heart & Aorta. Cooley. pap. text (*0-7216-4371-X*) Saunders.

Surgery of the Hip Joint. Ed. by Raymond G. Tronzo. 2nd ed. (Illus.). Vol. 1. 1984. 428p. 186.00 (*0-387-90922-2*); Vol. 2. 1987. 442p. 296.00 (*0-387-96275-1*) Spr-Verlag.

Surgery of the Intracranial Venous System: Embryology, Anatomy, Pathophysiology, Neuroradiology, Diagnosis, & Treatments. Ed. by A. Hakuba. 1996. (Illus.). 619p. 280.00 (*4-431-70167-2*) Spr-Verlag.

Surgery of the Iris & the Ciliary Body: Proceedings of the Ophthalmic Microsurgery Study Group, 4th, Lund, Sweden, July 4-7, 1972. Ophthalmic Microsurgery Study Group Staff. Ed. by E. Palm & G. Mackensen. 1975. (Advances in Ophthalmology Ser.: Vol. 30). 300p. 172.25 (*3-8055-1844-7*) S Karger.

Surgery of the Knee. Ed. by John N. Insall. 2nd ed. 1993. (Illus.). 1344p. text (*0-443-08734-2*) Church.

Surgery of the Knee John N. Insall & W. Norman Scott. 3rd ed. 2000. LC 00-24855. (Illus.). 1310p. text 395.00 (*0-443-06545-4*) Saunders.

Surgery of the Larynx. Byron J. Bailey & Hugh F. Biller. 1985. (Illus.). 471p. text 142.00 (*0-7216-1472-8*) Saunders.

Surgery of the Leg & Foot. August Rutt. 1980. (Hackenbroch Ser.). text 142.00 (*0-7216-4446-5*) Saunders.

Surgery of the Liver & Biliary Tract. Ed. by Leslie H. Blumgart & Y. Fong. 1998. (Illus.). incl. cd-rom (*0-443-05996-9*) Church.

Surgery of the Liver & Biliary Tract Ed. by Leslie H. Blumgart. 2nd ed. 1994. LC 94-5894. (Illus.). text (*0-443-04500-3*) Church.

Surgery of the Liver & Biliary Tract. Ed. by L.H. Blumgart. 3rd ed. 2000. 2075p. text (*0-7020-2501-1*) W B Saunders GBR. *Dist:* Saunders.

Surgery of the Liver & Intrahepatic Bile Ducts. I. Fagarasanu. Ed. by Henry J. Heimlich. 1972. LC 77-86984. (Illus.). 490p. 32.50 (*0-87527-007-7*) Green.

Surgery of the Lumbar Spine. Sanford J. Larson & Dennis Maiman. 1999. LC 99-22441. (Illus.). 336p. 149.00 (*0-86577-758-6*) Thieme Med Pubs.

Surgery of the Lung, Pleura & Chest: The Requisites. 2000. 512p. text 75.00 (*0-8151-2613-1*, 31644) Mosby Inc.

Surgery of the Male Reproductive Tract. Ed. by Larry I. Lipshultz et al. 1980. (Clinics in Andrology Ser.: No. 2). (Illus.). 275p. text 211.50 (*90-247-2315-9*) Kluwer Academic.

Surgery of the Middle Ear, Vol. 2. Robert Vincent et al. 1998. pap. text 310.00 (*0-7506-3062-0*) Buttrwrth-Heinemann.

Surgery of the Musculoskeletal System Ed. by C. McCollister Evarts. 2nd ed. 1989. (Illus.). 5214p. text (*0-443-08516-1*) Church.

Surgery of the Neck. P. G. Cevese et al. 1988. (Surgical Technique Ser.: Vol. XII). 422p. text (*1-57235-037-7*) Piccin Nuova.

Surgery of the Neurogenic Bladder. P. Magasi. 1982. 148p. (C). (*963-05-2892-4*) Akade Kiado HUN. *Dist:* St Mut.

Surgery of the Newborn. Neill V. Freeman et al. 1995. text (*0-443-04346-9*) Church.

Surgery of the Oesophagus. Ed. by Glyn G. Jamieson. 1988. (Illus.). 960p. text (*0-443-03409-5*) Church.

Surgery of the Pancreas. John R. Brooks. 1983. (Illus.). 528p. text 142.00 (*0-7216-2082-5*) Saunders.

Surgery of the Pancreas. M. Trede & David C. Carter. 2nd ed. 1998. LC 97-7856. text (*0-443-05522-X*) Church.

Surgery of the Paranasal Sinuses. Andrew Blitzer et al. 2nd ed. 1991. (Illus.). 480p. text 175.00 (*0-7216-3583-0*) Saunders.

Surgery of the Peripheral Nerve. Susan E. Mackinnon. 1988. (Illus.). 662p. 199.00 (*0-86577-283-5*) Thieme Med Pubs.

Surgery of the Prostate. Martin I. Resnick & Ian M. Thompson. 1997. LC 97-23368. (*0-04-435576-9*) Church.

Surgery of the Sellar Region & Paranasal Sinuses. Ed. by Madjid Samii. 1991. (Illus.). 583p. 325.00 (*0-387-53697-3*) Spr-Verlag.

Surgery of the Shoulder: Proceedings of the Sixth International Congress on Surgery of the Shoulder, Held in Helsinki, 27 June-1 July 1995 & Stockholm, 2-4 July 1995. Ed. by Martti Vastamaki & Pekka Jalovaara. 1995. LC 95-11221. (International Congress Ser.: Vol. 1085). 536p. 275.50 (*0-444-81913-4*, Excerpta Medica) Elsevier.

Surgery of the Skull Base. Madjid Samii. 1989. (Illus.). 525p. 373.00 (*0-387-18448-1*) Spr-Verlag.

Surgery of the Skull Base: An Interdisciplinary Approach. Madjid Samii & Wolfgang Draf. 1989. 525p. 342.00 (*3-540-18448-1*) Spr-Verlag.

Surgery of the Spinal Cord. August Livshitz. Tr. by V. E. Tatarchenko from RUS. 1991. LC 90-4997. 440p. 72.50 (*0-8236-6257-8*) Intl Univs Pr.

Surgery of the Spinal Cord: Potential for Regeneration & Recovery. Ed. by Robert N. Holtzman & B. M. Stein. 1991. (Contemporary Perspectives in Neurosurgery Ser.). (Illus.). 359p. 163.00 (*0-387-97625-6*) Spr-Verlag.

Surgery of the Spine: Surgical Anatomy & Operative Approaches. R. Louis. 1983. (Illus.). 328p. 288.00 (*0-387-11412-2*) Spr-Verlag.

Surgery of the Stomach. Ed. by H. D. Becker et al. 1988. (Illus.). 374p. 284.00 (*0-387-17116-9*) Spr-Verlag.

***Surgery of the Temporomandibular Joint.** Norma James & Ellis. 2000. (Illus.). 379p. (*0-7020-2548-8*) W B Saunders GBR. *Dist:* Saunders.

Surgery of the Third Ventricle. Michael L. J. Apuzzo. 2nd ed. 1997. LC 96-29699. 1,284p. text 269.00 (*0-683-00249-X*) Lppncott W & W.

Surgery of the Thymus. Ed. by J. C. Givel. 1990. (Illus.). 360p. 238.00 (*0-387-16315-8*) Spr-Verlag.

***Surgery of the Upper Gastrointestinal Tract.** Ed. by Tom R. DeMeester & J. R. Siewert. 2001. (Surgery Atlas Ser.). (Illus.). 450p. incl. cd-rom (*3-540-41100-3*) Spr-Verlag.

Surgery of the Upper Gastrointestinal Tract. G. G. Jamieson & H. T. Debas. 5th ed. 1994. (Rob & Smith's Operative Surgery Ser.). (Illus.). 640p. (*0-412-53550-5*) E A GBR. *Dist:* OUP.

Surgery of the Upper Respiratory System. William W. Montgomery. (Illus.). Vol. 1. 3rd ed. 1997. LC 96-5668. 704p. text 169.00 (*0-683-06121-6*); Vol. 2. 2nd ed. 1988. LC 78-9004. 760p. text 110.00 (*0-8121-1142-7*) Lppncott W & W.

Surgery of Vertebrobasilar Aneurysms: London, Ontario, Experience on 1,767 Patients. C. G. Drake et al. 1996. LC 97-10380. (Illus.). 400p. 205.00 (*3-211-82696-3*) Spr-Verlag.

Surgery Office Manual. David E. Eisenbud. 1995. (Office Manual Ser.). 222p. 145.00 (*1-890018-08-2*) Anadem Pubng.

Surgery on Call. Lefor Gomella. 3rd ed. 2001. (Illus.). 544p. (C). pap. 29.95 (*0-8385-8817-4*) McGraw-Hill Prof.

Surgery 101 Basic Science Review Vol. 2: The Blue Manual. Raffy Leon Karamanoukian. 1999. 178p. ring bd. 39.00 (*0-9663292-3-6*) Magalhaes Sci Pr.

Surgery 101 Basic Science Review Vol. 3: The Blue Manual. Raffy Leon Karamanoukian. 2000. 169p. ring bd. 39.00 (*0-9663292-4-4*) Magalhaes Sci Pr.

Surgery Reconstruction of the Upper Extremity. James Herndon. 1999. LC 98-41104. 992p. (C). text 225.00 (*0-8385-9304-6*) McGraw-Hill Prof.

Surgery Review: A Self-Assessment Study Manual. Ed. by M. D. Ram. 1987. LC 87-14466. 225p. pap. 32.50 (*0-941022-09-9*) Davies Pubng.

Surgery Study Cards. Gott. 1989. pap. text 75.00 (*0-7216-2804-4*) Saunders.

Surgery Survival Guide: A Manual for Interns & Medical Students. Michael S. Godin. 3rd ed. 1993. (Illus.). 128p. pap. 16.95 (*0-9621594-2-5*) Bluebelle Med Co.

Surgery Two Thousand. Edward Copeland. 2000. (Illus.). 624p. text 74.00 (*0-8151-1502-4*, 29695) Mosby Inc.

Surgery Upper GI Tract. Jamison. 5th ed. Date not set. (Operative Surgery Ser.). (*0-7506-0317-8*) Chapman & Hall.

Surgical Abortion. Eugene Glick. unabr. ed. 1998. (Illus.). 90p. pap. text 10.00 (*0-9662827-0-1*) WEWMG.

Surgical Adhesives & Sealants: Current Technology & Applications. Ed. by David Sierra & Renato Saltz. 1998. LC 95-61620. 247p. 79.95 (*1-56676-327-4*) CRC Pr.

Surgical Anatomy & Technique: A Pocket Manual. John E. Skandalakis et al. 2nd ed. 1999. LC 98-54986. (Pocket Manual Ser.). (Illus.). 720p. pap. 39.00 (*0-387-98752-5*) Spr-Verlag.

Surgical Anatomy for Neurosurgeons Vol. 2: Anatomy Review & Dissection Manual. Ghassan K. Bejjani & Donald Wright. 2002. (Illus.). 448p. 129.00 (*0-86577-879-5*) Thieme Med Pubs.

Surgical Anatomy of Head & Neck. J. Krmpotic-Nenanic et al. 1988. (Illus.). 331p. 454.00 (*0-387-17414-1*) Spr-Verlag.

Surgical Anatomy of the Head & Neck. Parviz Janfaza et al. 2000. LC 00-38466. 928p. text 349.00 (*0-683-06302-2*) Lppncott W & W.

Surgical Anatomy of the Nose. M. Eugene Tardy, Jr. 1990. (Illus.). 128p. text 139.00 (*0-88167-636-5*, 2098) Lppncott W & W.

Surgical Anatomy of the Orbit. Barry M. Zide & Glenn W. Jelks. 1985. (Illus.). 88p. text 129.00 (*0-88167-054-5*);Set. sl. 205.00 (*0-88167-203-3*) Lppncott W & W.

Surgical & Dental Instruments: Snowden & Brother (1860) & John Weiss & Son (1863) James M. Edmonson & Snowden and Brother Staff. 1997. LC 97-13781. (Illus.). 340p. reprint ed. 150.00 (*0-930405-72-2*, NP33942) Norman SF.

Surgical & Interventional Cardiovascular Pathology: Basic Principles & Clinical Correlations. Schoen. 1989. 320p. 120.00 (*0-7216-2457-X*) Saunders.

Surgical & Prosthetic Voice Restoration after Total & Subtotal Laryngectomy: Proceedings of the 6th International Congress, San Sebastian, 29 September-1 October 1995. Ed. by J. Algaba. 1996. (International Congress Ser.: No. 1112). 432p. 162.50 (*0-444-82345-X*, Excerpta Medica) Elsevier.

Surgical Applications of Energy, Vol. 3249. Ed. by Thomas P. Ryan. 1998. LC 98-171723. 288p. 69.00 (*0-8194-2688-1*) SPIE.

Surgical Approach to Head & Neck Anatomy. Dolwick. 1993. (*0-397-50970-7*) Lppncott W & W.

Surgical Approaches for Internal Fixation. T. Ruedi et al. 1983. (Illus.). 187p. 165.00 (*0-387-12809-3*) Spr-Verlag.

Surgical Approaches in Otorhinolaryngology. Walter F. Thumfart. 1999. LC 98-50616. (Illus.). 439p. 179.00 (*0-86577-834-5*) Thieme Med Pubs.

Surgical Approaches to Cutaneous Melanoma. Ed. by C. M. Balch. 1985. (Pigment Cell Ser.: Vol. 7). (Illus.). viii, 212p. 148.00 (*3-8055-4055-8*) S Karger.

Surgical Approaches to the Facial Skeleton. Ed. by Edward Ellis, III & Michael F. Zide. 1995. LC 94-27364. (Illus.). 304p. text 199.00 (*0-683-02794-8*) Lppncott W & W.

Surgical Approaches to the Foot & Ankle. George B. Holmes, Jr. 1994. LC 93-46581. 255p. text 99.00 (*0-07-030029-1*) McGraw-Hill Educ Grp.

Surgical Approaches to the Spine. Todd A. Albert et al. 1997. LC 96-29395. (Illus.). 272p. text 125.00 (*0-7216-4554-2*) Saunders.

Surgical-Assist Systems. Ed. by Marilyn S. Bogner et al. 1998. LC 98-227294. (Proceedings of SPIE Ser.: Vol. 3262). 316p. 99.00 (*0-8194-2701-2*) SPIE.

Surgical Atlas of External Rhinoplasty: Decortication Approach. Slobodan B. Jugo. 1995. LC 95-8380. (Illus.). text (*0-443-04690-5*) Church.

Surgical Atlas of Gynecologic Oncology. Ed. by Donald D. Gallup & O. Eduardo Talledo. 1994. LC 93-32871. text 92.00 (*0-7216-3980-1*) Saunders.

Surgical Atlas of Sports Medicine. Miller. 1999. text (*0-7216-7307-4*) Saunders.

Surgical Attending Rounds. F. Lee & C. Dyke. 1992. 393p. pap. 29.50 (*0-8121-1470-1*) Lppncott W & W.

Surgical Attending Rounds. K. Francis Lee & Cornelius M. Dyke. 1999. LC 98-45984. 494p. pap. text 45.00 (*0-683-30585-9*) Lppncott W & W.

Surgical Care for the Elderly. R. Benton Adkins, Jr. & H. William Scott, Jr. 2nd ed. 1997. LC 97-23283. 560p. text 149.00 (*0-7817-1450-8*) Lppncott W & W.

Surgical Care of Voice Disorders. W. J. Gould & V. L. Lawrence. 1984. (Disorders of Human Communication Ser.: Vol. 7). (Illus.). 116p. 54.95 (*0-387-81777-8*) Spr-Verlag.

***Surgical Case-Histories from the Past.** Harold Ellis. 1994. (History of Medicine Ser.). 235p. (*1-85315-222-6*) Royal Soc of Medicine Pr Ltd GBR. *Dist:* Balogh.

Surgical Complications: A Self-Instructional Guide, Bk. 4. Dale S. Bloomquist et al. Ed. by James R. Hooley & James R. Whitacre. 3rd rev. ed. 1983. (Illus.). 64p. pap. 7.95 (*0-89939-041-2*) Stoma Pr.

Surgical Complications & Wound Healing in the Small Animal Practice. Joseph Harari. 1993. LC 92-20695. (Illus.). 432p. pap. text 65.00 (*0-7216-3984-4*) Saunders.

Surgical Consultations: Update 2. Oliver Beahrs et al. 1994. 512p. 75.00 (*0-8151-0553-3*) Mosby Inc.

Surgical Consultations: Update 3. Oliver Beahrs et al. 1995. 512p. 75.00 (*0-8151-0554-1*) Mosby Inc.

Surgical Consultations: Update 4. Oliver Beahrs et al. 1996. 75.00 (*0-8151-0555-X*) Mosby Inc.

Surgical Correction of Dentofacial Deformities William H. Bell et al. 1980. LC 76-27050. 1. text 235.00 (*0-7216-1675-5*); 2. text 235.00 (*0-7216-1707-7*) Saunders.

Surgical Correction of Dentofacial Deformities, 3. Ed. by William H. Bell et al. 1985. LC 76-27050. (Illus.). 2565p. 680.00 (*0-7216-1740-9*) Saunders.

***Surgical Critical Care.** Robert U. Ashford & T. Neal Evans. 2001. (Illus.). 248p. pap. (*1-84110-066-8*) Greenwich Med GBR. *Dist:* JAMCO Dist.

Surgical Critical Care. Howard Corwin. Date not set. (*0-393-71031-9*) Norton.

Surgical Critical Care. Frank R. Lewis, Jr. & John A. Weigelt. 1995. LC 94-44206. (Illus.). 416p. text 105.00 (*0-7216-3368-4*) Saunders.

***Surgical Cross Coder 2001.** Ingenix, Inc. Staff. pap. 139.95 (*1-56337-365-3*) Ingenix Inc.

Surgical Decision Making. Lawrence Norton et al. 3rd ed. 1992. (Illus.). 368p. text 95.00 (*0-7216-6598-5*) Saunders.

Surgical Decision Making. Karen E. Monks. 4th ed. 1999. LC 00-38804. (Illus.). xviii, 357p. text 79.00 (*0-7216-7985-4*) Saunders.

Surgical Dermatology. David J. Eedy et al. 1996. LC 95-52144. (Illus.). 288p. 147.95 (*0-632-03425-4*) Blackwell Sci.

Surgical Dermatology: Advances in Current. Henry H. Roenigk. 1993. 567p. (C). (gr. 13). text 139.00 (*0-8151-7414-4*, 23486) Mosby Inc.

Surgical Dermatopathology. Ed. by Mary E. Maloney et al. 1999. LC 98-33478. (Illus.). xi, 506p. 168.95 (*0-86542-299-0*) Blackwell Sci.

Surgical Diagnosis & Management: A Guide to General Surgical Care. David C. Dunn & Nigel Rawlinson. 3rd ed. 1999. LC 98-14103. (Illus.). 736p. pap. 52.95 (*0-86542-718-6*) Blackwell Sci.

Surgical Diagnosis & Methods of Examination. B. P. Chatterjee. 1989. (C). (*0-89771-366-4*) Current Dist IND. *Dist:* St Mut.

Surgical Diseases in Pregnancy. Ed. by Luis A. Cibils. 1990. (Clinical Perspectives in Obstetrics & Gynecology Ser.). (Illus.). 208p. 105.00 (*0-387-97203-X*) Spr-Verlag.

Surgical Diseases of the Pancreas. John M. Howard et al. 3rd ed. 1998. LC 97-22075. 868p. text 189.00 (*0-683-18019-3*) Lppncott W & W.

Surgical Diseases of the Pleura & Chest Wall. R. Maurice Hood. 1986. (Illus.). 269p. text 85.00 (*0-7216-1401-9*) Saunders.

Surgical Diseases of the Spleen. J. R. Hiatt et al. 1996. LC 96-41244. (Illus.). 344p. 149.00 (*3-540-61781-7*) Spr-Verlag.

Surgical Disorders of the Fourth Ventricle. Alan R. Cohen. 1995. 512p. 235.00 (*0-86542-360-1*) Blackwell Sci.

Surgical Disorders of the Peripheral Nerves. R. Birch et al. 1998. (Illus.). 450p. (*0-443-04443-0*) Church.

Surgical Disorders of the Shoulder. Ed. by Michael S. Watson. 1991. (Illus.). 662p. text (*0-443-03889-9*) Church.

Surgical Emergencies. John R. Monson et al. 1999. LC 98-17789. (Illus.). 406p. 131.95 (*0-632-05047-0*) Blackwell Sci.

Surgical Emergencies in Children: A Practical Guide. Ed. by Peter A. Raine et al. 1994. LC 94-27819. (Illus.). 416p. text 150.00 (*0-7506-1389-0*) Buttrwrth-Heinemann.

Surgical Endocrinology. John Lynn & Stephen Bloom. 1993. (Illus.). 592p. 265.00 (*0-7506-1390-4*) Buttrwrth-Heinemann.

Surgical Endocrinology: A Clinical Syndromes Approach. Gerard M. Doherty & Britt Skogseid. 2000. LC 00-56577. 640p. text 179.00 (*0-7817-1922-4*) Lppncott W & W.

Surgical Endodontics: A Colour Manual. Ian E. Barnes et al. 2nd ed. 1991. (Illus.). 128p. text 95.00 (*0-7236-1571-3*) Buttrwrth-Heinemann.

Surgical Ethics. Ed. by Laurence B. McCullough et al. 1998. LC 97-29008. 416p. text 52.50 (*0-19-510347-5*) OUP.

Surgical Exposures in Orthopaedic Surgery: The Anatomic Approach. Stanley Hoppenfeld & Piet DeBoer. 1984. (Illus.). 640p. text 165.00 (*0-397-50597-3*, 65-07628, Lippnctt) Lppncott W & W.

Surgical Exposures in Orthopaedics. Stanley Hoppenfeld. 2nd ed. 1994. 624p. (C). text 199.00 (*0-397-51044-6*) Lppncott W & W.

Surgical Geriatric Gynecology. V. Jaluvka. 1980. (Contributions to Gynecology & Obstetrics Ser.: Vol. 7). (Illus.). x, 174p. pap. 71.50 (*3-8055-3070-6*) S Karger.

Surgical Gynecologic Oncology. Ed. by E. Burghardt et al. 1993. LC 92-49606. 249.00 (*0-86577-473-0*) Thieme Med Pubs.

Surgical Gynecologic Techniques. F. Novak. 1978. 422p. text (*1-57235-025-3*) Piccin Nuova.

Surgical Hemotherapy. Ed. by P. Lundsgaard-Hansen. 1980. (Bibliotheca Haematologica Ser.: No. 46). (Illus.). viii, 252p. pap. 78.50 (*3-8055-0361-X*) S Karger.

Surgical Infections. E. H. Farthman et al. 1998. (Illus.). 500p. (*0-683-18049-5*) Lppncott W & W.

Surgical Infections: Diagnosis & Treatment. Ed. by Jonathan L. Meakins. 1993. LC 93-29195. (Illus.). 500p. (C). text 89.00 (*0-89454-016-5*) Sci Am Medicine.

Surgical Instruments: A Pocket Guide. MaryAnn Papanier Wells & Mary Bradley. Ed. by Maura Connor. 2nd ed. 1998. LC 98-5488. (Illus.). 480p. (C). pap. text 32.00 (*0-7216-7801-7*) Saunders.

Surgical Instruments in Greek & Roman Times. J. G. Milne. 1991. (Illus.). 201p. 25.00 (*0-89005-127-5*) Ares.

Surgical Instruments of the Hindus Girindranath Mukhopadhyaya. LC 75-23714. reprint ed. 65.00 (*0-404-13340-1*) AMS Pr.

Surgical Intern Pocket Survival Guide. Ronald Chamberlain. 1993. 78p. pap. text 7.50 (*0-9634063-5-3*) Intl Med Pub.

Surgical Intuition: What It Is & How to Get It. Ed. by Robert M. Hamm & Charles M. Abernathy. 1995. LC 93-77760. (Illus.). 436p. 45.00 (*1-56053-059-6*) Hanley & Belfus.

Surgical Judgement Using Decision Sciences, 3. John R. Clarke. 1984. LC 83-24594. (Surgical Science Ser.: Vol. III). 106p. 52.50 (*0-275-91425-9*, C1425, Praeger Pubs) Greenwood.

Surgical Knots & Suturing Techniques: A Handbook for Students of Surgery. F. D. Giddings. 1997. LC 97-93710. Orig. Title: The Handbook of Surgical Knot Tying. (Illus.). 38p. spiral bd. 15.00 (*1-889326-00-3*) Giddings Studio Pub.

Surgical Laparoscopy. Karl A. Zucker. 2nd ed. 2000. 864p. text 275.00 (*0-683-30670-7*) Lppncott W & W.

Surgical Laparoscopy Update. Ed. by Karl A. Zucker. 1993. LC 92-49363. (Illus.). 493p. 145.00 (*0-942219-26-0*) Quality Med Pub.

Surgical Management. Geoffrey D. Chisholm et al. Ed. by R. C. Williamson. 2nd rev. ed. 1991. 848p. pap. text 150.00 (*0-7506-0025-X*) Buttrwrth-Heinemann.

Surgical Management of Cerebrovascular Disease. Ed. by R. Eugene Zierler. 1994. LC 94-20311. 416p. text 80.00 (*0-07-072792-9*) McGraw-Hill Med Pub.

Surgical Management of Coexisting Glaucoma & Cataract. Ed. by E. L. Greve. 1987. (Illus.). 108p. lib. bdg. (*90-6299-028-2*) Kugler NLD. *Dist:* Lib Res.

Surgical Management of Crohn's Disease & Ulcerative Colitis. Devinder Kumar & John Alexander-Williams. 1993. LC 93-4186. (Illus.). 244p. 195.00 (*0-387-19730-3*) Spr-Verlag.

Surgical Management of Crohn's Disease & Ulcerative Joints. Devinder Kumar & John Alexander-Williams. 1993. (Illus.). 260p. (*3-540-19730-3*) Spr-Verlag.

Surgical Management of Cutaneous Ulcers & Pressure Sores. Bok Y. Lee & Burton L. Herz. 1997. LC 96-8950. 272p. (*0-412-99421-6*) E A GBR. *Dist:* OUP.

Surgical Management of Deformities in Leprosy & Other Peripheral Neuropathies. Noshir H. Antia et al. 1993. LC 92-911926. (Illus.). 172p. text 45.00 (*0-19-563058-0*) OUP.

Surgical Management of Epilepsy. Ed. by Allen R. Wyler & Bruce P. Hermann. 1993. (Illus.). 277p. text 105.00 (*0-7506-9416-5*) Buttrwrth-Heinemann.

Surgical Management of External Diseases of the Eye. Susan M. Stenson. 1995. LC 94-32668. (Illus.). 344p. 145.00 (*0-89640-274-6*) Igaku-Shoin.

Surgical Management of Soft Tissue Sarcomas. Myron Arlen & Ralph C. Marcove. 1987. (Illus.). 344p. text 142.00 (*0-7216-1399-3*) Saunders.

Surgical Management of Sterility. E. Cittadini et al. 1976. 150p. text (*1-57235-057-1*) Piccin Nuova.

Surgical Management of Tumors of the Oropharynx. Steven M. Zeitels & Arnold Komisar. 1997. LC 97-16822. (Self-Instructional Package Ser.). (Illus.). 72p. pap. text 25.00 (*1-56772-056-0*, 5506310) AAO-HNS.

Surgical Management of Vascular Disease. Ed. by Peter R. Bell et al. 1992. (Illus.). 1436p. text (*0-7020-1514-8*) W B Saunders GBR. *Dist:* Saunders.

Surgical Management of Venous Disease. Seshardi Raju & L. Leonel Villavicencio. 1997. LC 96-31993. (Illus.). 567p. 125.00 (*0-683-07111-4*) Lppncott W & W.

Surgical MCQS. Craven. 3rd ed. 1993. pap. 26.95 (*0-443-04702-2*) Saunders.

Surgical Neonate: Anaesthesia & Intensive Care. David Hatch et al. 3rd ed. 1996. 320p. (*0-340-55305-7*) E A GBR. *Dist:* OUP.

Surgical Neuroangiography Pierre L. Lasjaunias et al. 2nd rev. ed. 2001. LC 00-49688. (Illus.). 850p. 350.00 (*3-540-41204-2*) Spr-Verlag.

Surgical Neuroangiography. Pierre L. Lasjaunias & A. Berenstein. (Functional Anatomy of Craniofacial Arteries Ser.). (Illus.). Vol. 1. 1994. 426p. 230.00 (*0-387-16534-7*); Vol. 2. 1996. 450p. 199.00 (*0-387-16535-5*) Spr-Verlag.

Surgical Neuroangiography, Vol. 3. A. Berenstein & P. Lasjaunias. 1997. (Illus.). 337p. 240.00 (*0-387-17501-6*) Spr-Verlag.

Surgical Neuroangiography Vol. 4: Endocascular Treatment of Cerebral Problems, Vol. 4. A. Berenstein & P. Lasjaunias. 1993. (Illus.). 344p. 230.00 (*0-387-17500-8*) Spr-Verlag.

Surgical Neuroangiography Vol. 5: Endocascular Treatment of Spine & Spinal Cord. A. Berenstein & P. Lasjaunias. 1994. (Illus.). 250p. 240.00 (*0-387-55043-7*) Spr-Verlag.

Surgical Nursing. Ed. by K. Manley & L. Bellman. 1998. (Illus.). 544p. pap. (*0-443-05421-5*) Church.

Surgical Nursing of Children. Margaret Chambers. 2002. (Illus.). 256p. pap. 40.50 (*0-7506-4807-4*) Buttrwrth-Heinemann.

Surgical Nutrition. 1996. (Illus.). 215p. 120.00 (*3-540-59291-1*) Spr-Verlag.

Surgical Oncology. T. G. Allen-Mersh. 1995. (Illus.). 480p. (*0-412-48940-6*) E A GBR. *Dist:* OUP.

Surgical Oncology. David N. Krag. 2001. LC 00-61999. (Vademecum Ser.). (Illus.). spiral bd. (*1-57059-633-6*) Landes Bioscience.

Surgical Oncology. Raphael E. Pollock. 1997. LC 97-5016. (Cancer Treatment & Research Ser.). text 384.00 (*0-7923-9900-5*) Kluwer Academic.

Surgical Oncology. Ed. by U. Veronesi et al. 1989. (Illus.). 999p. 304.00 (*0-387-17770-1*) Spr-Verlag.

Surgical Oncology: Contemporary Principles & Practice. Bland et al. 2001. (Illus.). 1223p. text 185.00 (*0-8385-8736-4*) McGraw-Hill Prof.

***Surgical Oncology: Multidisciplinary Approach to Difficult Problems.** Howard Silberman & Allan W. Silberman. 2001. (Arnold Publication). 600p. 198.50 (*0-340-76242-X*) OUP.

Surgical Oncology: The Requisites. 2000. (Illus.). 544p. pap. text 65.00 (*0-8151-4385-0*, 31679) Mosby Inc.

Surgical Ophthalmology One. Frederic C. Blodi et al. 1991. (Illus.). 598p. 350.00 (*0-387-52105-4*) Spr-Verlag.

Surgical Ophthalmology Two. Ed. by Frederic C. Blodi et al. 1992. (Illus.). 716p. 298.00 (*0-387-52107-0*) Spr-Verlag.

Surgical Orthodontics No. 2: Techniques & Instrumentation. D. B. Tuinzing et al. 1994. (Illus.). 140p. (*90-5383-231-9*) VU Univ Pr NLD. *Dist:* Paul & Co Pubs.

Surgical Outcomes in Patients with AIDS. David R. Flum & Marc K. Wallack. 1999. LC 98-44094. 356p. text 59.95 (*0-683-30219-1*) Lppncott W & W.

Surgical Pathological Anatomy of Head & Neck Specimens: A Manual Forthe Dissection of Surgical Specimens from the Upper Aerodigestive Tract. Pieter Johannes Slooteweg & J. A. M. de Goot. 1999. LC 98-43506. (Illus.). 132p. 189.00 (*1-85233-077-5*) Spr-Verlag.

Surgical Pathology. Alberto M. Marchevsky. 1990. (Lung Biology in Health & Disease Ser.: Vol. 44). (Illus.). 704p. text 230.00 (*0-8247-8106-6*) Dekker.

Surgical Pathology Walter F. Coulson. 2nd ed. 1988. LC 65-7743. (Illus.). 1824p. text 245.00 (*0-397-50609-0*, Lippnctt) Lppncott W & W.

Surgical Pathology Dissection. R. H. Hruban & William H. Westra. 1996. 50p. suppl. ed. 110.00 (*0-387-94715-9*) Spr-Verlag.

Surgical Pathology Dissection: An Illustrated Guide. William H. Westra et al. 1996. LC 95-24467. (Illus.). 232p. 61.95 (*0-387-94567-9*) Spr-Verlag.

Surgical Pathology of Laryngeal Neoplasms. Ed. by A. Ferlito. 1995. (Illus.). 504p. 303.95 (*0-412-58010-1*, Chap & Hall NY) Chapman & Hall.

Surgical Pathology of Prostate & Seminal Vesicles. Joseph Kovi. 1988. 336p. lib. bdg. 195.00 (*0-8493-4804-8*, RC899) CRC Pr.

***Surgical Pathology of Skin & Mucocutaneous.** Grace Kao. 2001. (Major Problems in Pathology Ser.). (Illus.). 399p. (*0-7216-6160-2*) Saunders.

Surgical Pathology of the Breast. Weidner. 2000. text (*0-7216-1755-7*) Harcrt Hlth Sci Grp.

Surgical Pathology of the Head & Neck. John G. Batsakis & Dale H. Rice. 1999. LC 99-35712. 208p. text 169.00 (*0-7817-2354-X*) Lppncott W & W.

Surgical Pathology of the Head & Neck, Pt. B. Barnes. 1985. (Illus.). 1896p. text 510.00 (*0-8247-7269-5*) Dekker.

Surgical Pathology of the Head & Neck, Set, Pt. A. Leon Barnes. 1985. (Illus.). 896p. text 510.00 (*0-8247-7216-4*) Dekker.

Surgical Pathology of the Head & Neck. Ed. by Leon Barnes. 2nd exp. rev. ed. (Illus.). Vol. 1. 2000. 1221p. text 575.00 (*0-8247-0109-7*, 0109-7); Vol. 2. Date not set. 736p. text 575.00 (*0-8247-0110-0*, 0110-0) Dekker.

Surgical Pathology of the Lymph Nodes & Related Organs. Ed. by Elaine S. Jaffe. 2nd ed. 1994. LC 94-13094. (Major Problems in Pathology Ser.: Vol. 16). text 82.00 (*0-7216-5136-4*) Saunders.

Surgical Pathology of the Mouth & Jaws. R. A. Cawson et al. 2000. LC 00-266878. (Illus.). ix, 326p. pap. text (*0-7236-1083-5*) John Wright GBR. *Dist:* Buttrwrth-Heinemann.

Surgical Pathology of the Nervous System & Its Coverings. Peter C. Burger et al. 3rd ed. 1990. (Illus.). 737p. text (*0-443-08687-7*) Church.

Surgical Pathology of the Ovaries. Peter Russell & Patricia Bannatyne. 1989. (Illus.). 539p. text (*0-443-03535-0*) Church.

Surgical Pathology of the Ovaries. Peter Russell & Annabelle Farnsworth. 2nd ed. 1997. LC 97-9201. text (*0-443-05384-7*) Church.

Surgical Pathology of the Pituitary Gland. Ricardo V. Lloyd. 1992. (Illus.). 271p. text 70.00 (*0-7216-6459-8*) Saunders.

Surgical Pathology of the Prostate Gland. Ro. 1999. (C). text (*0-7216-6010-X*) Saunders.

Surgical Pathology of the Salivary Glands, Vol. 25. Albert Ellis & Auclair. 1991. (Illus.). 608p. text 91.00 (*0-7216-3224-6*) Saunders.

Surgical Pathophysiology. Ed. by A. Aasen. 1990. xiii, 452p. text 176.00 (*3-7186-5038-X*, Harwood Acad Pubs) Gordon & Breach.

Surgical Pearls. Robert A. Kozol et al. 1999. LC 99-22366. (Illus.). 341p. (C). pap. text 23.95 (*0-8036-0388-6*, K2362) Davis Co.

Surgical Pediatric Otolaryngology: Head & Neck Surgery. Steven D. Handler et al. 1996. (Illus.). 400p. text 99.00 (*0-86577-153-7*) Thieme Med Pubs.

Surgical Principles. Ed. by Irving Taylor & Stephen Karran. 1996. LC 96-4700. (An Arnold Publication). 224p. pap. (*0-340-61379-3*) E A GBR. *Dist:* OUP, Routldge.

Surgical Problems in the AIDS Patient. Samuel E. Wilson & Russell A. Williams. 1994. LC 94-7074. (Illus.). 312p. 75.00 (*0-89640-247-9*) Igaku-Shoin.

Surgical Product Comparison System, 1992 Ed. by Garry Hayner. 1993. 525.00 (*0-941417-04-2*) ECRI.

Surgical Radiology: A Complement in Radiology & Imaging to the Sabiston-Davis-Christopher Textbook of Surgery J. George Teplick & Marvin E. Haskin.

1981. (Illus.). 1152p. 1. text 170.00 (*0-7216-8781-4*); 2. text 180.00 (*0-7216-8782-2*); 3. text 180.00 (*0-7216-8791-1*); Set. text 485.00 (*0-7216-8783-0*) Saunders.

Surgical Recall. Lorne Blackbourne. 1994. (Illus.). 352p. pap. 26.00 (*0-683-00835-8*) Lppncott W & W.

Surgical Recall. Lorne H. Blackbourne. 2nd ed. 1997. LC 97-25166. (Recall Ser.). 768p. pap. text 29.95 (*0-683-30102-0*) Lppncott W & W.

***Surgical Recall PDA.** Lorne Blackbourne. 2002. 29.95 (*0-7817-3299-9*) Lppncott W & W.

Surgical Reconstruction of the Face: Nose, Midface & Anterior Skull Base. Anthony J. Maniglia et al. Ed. by Stephanie Donley et al. 1999. LC 98-25699. (Illus.). 335p. text (*0-7216-6993-X*) Saunders.

Surgical Reflections: Images in Paint & Prose. Seymour I. Schwartz. 1992. LC 92-49796. (Illus.). 183p. text 79.00 (*0-942219-48-1*) Quality Med Pub.

Surgical Rehabilitation. Ed. by Jeanne Melvin & Victoria Gall. 1999. LC 00-698137. (Rheumatologic Rehabilitation Ser.: Vol. 5). (Illus.). x, 214p. pap. 52.00 (*1-56900-114-6*, 1205) Am Occup Therapy.

Surgical Rejuvenation of the Face. Thomas J. Baker & Howard L. Gordon. 2nd ed. 1995. (Illus.). 640p. (C). (gr. 13). text 272.00 (*0-8016-0153-3*, 00153) Mosby Inc.

Surgical Repair & Reconstruction in Rheumatoid Disease. A. Benjamin et al. 2nd rev. ed. 1993. (Illus.). 254p. reprint ed. 247.00 (*0-387-19727-3*) Spr-Verlag.

Surgical Research: Basic Principles & Clinical Practice. Ed. by Hans Troidl et al. 3rd ed. 1997. LC 97-13782. (Illus.). 728p. 107.00 (*0-387-94699-3*) Spr-Verlag.

Surgical Restoration of the Aging Face. Ed. by Robert W. Bernard. 1996. (Illus.). 333p. text (*0-7506-9438-6*) E A GBR. *Dist:* OUP.

Surgical Review. Larry R. Kaiser et al. 2000. LC 00-55876. 560p. pap. text 49.95 (*0-7817-2801-0*) Lppncott W & W.

Surgical Scripts: Master Surgeons Think Aloud about 43 Common Surgical Problems. Charles M. Abernathy & Robert M. Hamm. 1994. LC 93-39297. 200p. 25.00 (*1-56053-119-3*) Hanley & Belfus.

Surgical Secrets. Charles M. Abernathy. 1986. 22.95 (*0-8016-0070-7*) Mosby Inc.

Surgical Signs. Bruce Campbell & Martin Cooper. 1994. LC 93-3750. (Colour Guide Ser.). pap. text 16.95 (*0-443-04005-2*) Harcrt Hlth Sci Grp.

Surgical Signs. Bruce Campbell & M. J. Cooper. 2nd ed. 2000. LC 99-27852. (Colour Guide Ser.). (Illus.). 146p. (*0-443-06145-9*) Harcrt Hlth Sci Grp.

Surgical Teaching: Practice Makes Perfect. Neal A. Whitman & Peter Lawrence. 1991. 136p. text 30.00 (*0-940193-08-6*) Univ UT Sch Med.

Surgical Technician Operating Room Fundamentals. Baker. 1994. (Medical Lab Technician Ser.). tchr. ed. 10.00 (*0-8273-6318-4*) Delmar.

Surgical Techniques: Tools of the Trade & Rules of the Road. Edwin A. Deitch. 1997. LC 97-5053. (Illus.). 368p. pap. text 46.95 (*0-397-51393-3*) Lppncott W & W.

Surgical Techniques in Total Knee Arthroplasty. Ed. by Giles R. Scuderi & A. J. Tria. 1999. LC 98-22362. (Illus.). 608p. 125.00 (*0-387-98389-9*) Spr-Verlag.

Surgical Techniques of the Temporal Bone & Skull Base. Herbert Silverstein & Seth Rosenberg. 1992. (Illus.). 225p. text 98.50 (*0-8121-1530-9*) Lppncott W & W.

Surgical Technologist Certifying Exam Study Guide. Ed. by Association of Surgical Technologists. 1995. 158p. (Orig.). pap. text 29.95 (*0-926805-07-X*) Assn Surgical.

Surgical Technology: Principles & Practice. Joanna R. Fuller. 3rd ed. 1993. LC 92-49085. (Illus.). 752p. text 59.95 (*0-7216-4064-8*) Saunders.

Surgical Technology International Vol. III: International Developments in Surgery & Surgical Research. Ed. by Morris D. Kerstein et al. 1994. (Illus.). 604p. text 115.00 (*0-9643425-1-0*); pap. text 95.00 (*0-9643425-0-2*) Univ Med Pr.

Surgical Technology International Vol. V: International Developments in Surgery & Research. Ed. by Zoltan Szabo et al. 1996. (Illus.). 500p. text 95.00 (*0-9643425-4-5*) Univ Med Pr.

Surgical Technology International IV: International Developments in Surgery & Surgical Research. Ed. by Zoltan Szabo et al. 1995. (Illus.). 465p. text 115.00 (*0-9643425-3-7*) Univ Med Pr.

Surgical Technology International VII: International Developments in Surgery & Surgical Research. Ed. by Zoltan Szabo et al. 7th unabr. ed. 1998. (Illus.). 400p. pap. text 95.00 (*1-890131-00-8*) Univ Med Pr.

Surgical Technology International VI: International Development in Surgery & Surgical Research. Ed. by Zoltan Szabo et al. 1996. (Illus.). 500p. text 115.00 (*0-9643425-7-X*); text 95.00 (*0-9643425-6-1*) Univ Med Pr.

Surgical Technology International VIII: International Developments in Surgery & Surgical Research. Ed. by Zoltan Szabo et al. unabr. ed. 1999. (Illus.). 400p. pap. text 95.00 (*1-890131-03-2*) Univ Med Pr.

Surgical Technology Review Book. Emily H. Boegli. 1999. LC 94-6785. 320p. pap. 53.00 (*0-13-034703-5*) P-H.

Surgical Thoracoscopy. D. Gossot et al. 1993. (Illus.). 124p. 95.00 (*0-387-59577-5*) Spr-Verlag.

Surgical Thoracoscopy. Rolf Inderbitzi. 1994. LC 93-28475. (Illus.). 159p. 118.00 (*0-387-56894-8*) Spr-Verlag.

Surgical Transcription in Obstetrics & Gynecology. John E. Turrentine. 1994. (Illus.). 166p. 38.95 (*1-85070-512-7*, Parthenon Pbng) CRC Pr.

Surgical Treatment for Parkinson's Disease & Other Movement Disorders. Ed. by Daniel Tarsy et al. 2001. 400p. 145.00 (*0-89603-921-8*) Humana.

Surgical Treatment of Anal Incontinence. Charles V. Mann & Richard Glass. 2nd ed. 1996. LC 96-36555. 216p. 167.00 (*3-540-76061-X*) Spr-Verlag.

Surgical Treatment of Aortic Dissection. Hans G. Borst et al. 1995. LC 95-37913. 357p. text (*0-443-07531-X*) Church.

Surgical Treatment of Bronchial Carcinoma. J. Hasse. 1986. (Illus.). 158p. 103.00 (*0-387-16230-5*) Spr-Verlag.

***Surgical Treatment of Haemorrhoids.** Charles V. Mann. 2002. LC 2001-34455. (*1-85233-496-7*) Springer Pub.

Surgical Treatment of Hepatic Metastases of Colorectal Diseases: Report of the 94th French Congress of Surgery. Ed. by B. Nordlinger & D. Jaeck. 1993. (Monographs of the French Surgical Association). 140p. 100.00 (*0-387-55142-5*) Spr-Verlag.

Surgical Treatment of Middle Ear Cholesteatoma. M. Wayoff et al. 1987. (Advances in OtoRhinoLaryngology Ser.: Vol.36). (Illus.). x, 238p. 169.75 (*3-8055-4441-3*) S Karger.

Surgical Treatment of Mitral Stenosis. Ed. by A. N. Bakulev. 1961. 304p. 3.5 hd 84.50 (*0-7065-0099-7*) Coronet Bks.

Surgical Treatment of the Epilepsies. Ed. by Jerome Engel, Jr. 2nd ed. 1993. LC 92-49518. 816p. text 169.00 (*0-88167-988-7*) Lppncott W & W.

Surgical Word Book. Claudia J. Tessier. 2nd ed. 1991. pap. text 41.00 (*0-7216-2128-7*) Saunders.

Surgvision: The First Video Atlas of General Surgery. Ed. by Nelson Gurll. 1990. 300p. (C). 595.00 (*0-944903-06-1*) Adams Pub Group.

Surplus Powerlessness: The Psychodynamics of Everyday Life & the Psychology of Individual & Social Transformation. Michael Lerner. 1991. LC 91-7279. 424p. (C). pap. 18.50 (*0-391-03706-4*) Brill Academic Pubs.

***Surprising Blessings in Cancer.** Sallie Burdine. 2001. 125p. 14.95 (*0-9705464-2-4*) SABA Bks.

Surprising Truth about Panic, Phobia & Anxiety Disorders. Herbert Wagemaker. Date not set. (Illus.). 175p. pap. 12.00 (*0-9654996-3-4*) Ponte Vedra Pub.

Surrender. 1986. (Pocket Power Ser.). 16p. pap. 1.25 (*0-89486-325-8*, 5449B) Hazelden.

Surrogacy & the Moral Economy. Derek Morgan. 1994. (Medico-Legal Issues Ser.). (*1-85521-034-7*) Dartmth Pub GBR. *Dist:* Ashgate Pub Co.

Surrogate Markers to Assess Efficacy of Treatment in Chronic Liver Diseases: Proceedings of the International Falk Workshop Held in Basel, Switzerland, October 23-24, 1995. Ed. by J. Reichen & R. E. Poupon. 1996. LC 96-17380. xii, 213p. text 110.50 (*0-7923-8705-8*) Kluwer Academic.

Surrogate Parenting: An Annotated Review of the Literature. Sara Robbins. 1984. LC 84-1824. (CompuBibs Ser.: No. 3). 40p. pap. 10.00 (*0-914791-04-4*) Vantage Info.

Surveillance for the Prevention & Control of Health Hazards Due to Antibiotic-Resistant Enterobacteria: Report of a WHO Meeting, 1978. 1978. (Technical Report Ser.: No. 624). 54p. pap. text 6.00 (*92-4-120624-1*, 1100624) World Health.

***Surveillance for Waterborne-Disease Outbreaks: United States, 1997-1998.** Ed. by John W. Ward. 2001. (Illus.). 51p. (C). pap. text 20.00 (*0-7567-1342-0*) DIANE Pub.

Surveillance of Acute Viral Respiratory Infections in Europe: Report on a WHO Symposium. 1981. (Euro Reports & Studies Ser.: No. 47). 65p. pap. text 5.00 (*92-890-1213-7*) World Health.

Surveillance of Morbidity & Mortality Module 4: Facilitator's Guide. Martine Hilton. 1993. (Primary Health Care Management Advancement Programme Modules Ser.). 58p. pap. text (*1-882839-18-8*) Aga Khan Fnd.

Surveillance of Morbidity & Mortality Module 4: User's Guide. Pierre Claquin et al. 1993. (Primary Health Care Management Advancement Programme Modules Ser.). 126p. pap. text (*1-882839-15-3*) Aga Khan Fnd.

Survey Methods in Community Medicine: Epidemiological Studies, Programme Evaluation, Clinical Trials. J. H. Abramson. 4th ed. 1990. (Illus.). 339p. pap. text (*0-443-04196-2*) Church.

Survey of Adult Aphasia & Related. G. Albyn Davis. 2nd ed. 1992. LC 92-49840. 384p. (C). 99.00 (*0-13-878018-8*) P-H.

Survey of Blood Transfusion Services of Central & Eastern European Countries & Their Co-Operaiton with Western Transfusion Services. 1993. (*92-871-2400-0*) Council of Europe FRA. *Dist:* Manhattan Pub Co.

Survey of Compounds Which Have Been Tested for Carcinogenic Activity 1997. lib. bdg. 650.95 (*0-8490-8143-2*) Gordon Pr.

Survey of Cripples in New York City: Under the Auspices of a Special Committee on Survey of Cripples. Henry C. Wright. Ed. by William R. Phillips & Janet Rosenberg. 1980. LC 79-6014. (Physically Handicapped in Society Ser.). reprint ed. lib. bdg. 16.95 (*0-405-13137-2*) Ayer.

Survey of Early Childhood Abilities. Karen G. Codding. 1987. pap., tchr. ed. 15.00 (*0-931421-10-1*); stu. ed. 14.00 (*0-931421-23-3*); 8.00 (*0-931421-21-7*); 26.00 (*0-931421-24-1*); lp 22.00 (*0-931421-22-5*) Psychol Educ Pubns.

Survey of Functional Neuroanatomy. Bill Garoutte. 1982. LC 80-84809. (Illus.). 217p. (C). pap. text 9.75 (*0-930010-04-3*) Jones Med.

Survey of Functional Neuroanatomy. Bill Garoutte. 3rd ed. 1994. (Illus.). 224p. (C). pap. text 15.00 (*0-9643644-0-9*) Mill Valley Med.

Survey of Health Care Reform: Fifty States & Washington, D.C. Dolores A. Sands. 1994. 200p. (Orig.). (C). pap. text 40.00 (*0-7881-0750-X*) DIANE Pub.

Survey of Health Reform in Central Asia. Jeni G. Klugman & George Schieber. 1997. LC 96-38680. (Technical Papers: No. 344). 68p. pap. 22.00 (*0-8213-3804-8*, 13804) World Bank.

Survey of Lubbock's Growth As a Medical Center, 1909-1954. William R. Dunnagan. 1980. 65p. 5.00 (*0-911618-05-8*) Mus Texas.

Survey of Medical Neuroscience. Robert M. Beckstead. 1996. LC 95-11272. (Illus.). 437p. pap. 42.00 (*0-387-94488-5*) Spr-Verlag.

Survey of Models for Tumor-Immune System Dynamics. Ed. by J. A. Adam & N. Bellomo. 1996. LC 96-38754. 332p. 90.00 (*0-8176-3901-2*) Birkhauser.

Survey of Objective Studies of Psychoanalytic Concepts. Robert R. Sears. 1979. LC 79-4476. 156p. reprint ed. lib. bdg. 68.00 (*0-313-21249-X*, SESO, Greenwood Pr) Greenwood.

Survey of Salary, Benefits & Staffing Patterns of Community Mental Health Providers, 1991. 1991. 106p. pap. 34.50 (*1-883066-05-0*) Natl Comm Mental.

Survey of Social Science: Psychology Ed. by Frank N. Magill. 1993. LC 93-34708. 2923p. lib. bdg. 425.00 (*0-89356-732-9*) Salem Pr.

Survey of Traditional Chinese Medicine. Claude Larre et al. Tr. by Sarah E. Stang. 1986. (FRE., Illus.). 231p. (Orig.). pap. 24.00 (*0-912381-00-0*) Trad Acupuncture.

Surveying Memory Processes: A Special Issue of "Memory" Ed. by Daniel B. Wright & George D. Gaskell. 1998. LC 99-175227. 478p. 39.95 (*0-86377-989-1*) L Erlbaum Assocs.

Surveys of Australian Psychology. Ed. by N. T. Feather. 1985. 280p. text 25.95 (*0-86861-607-9*) Routledge.

Surveys of Drinking & Abstaining: Urban, Suburban & National Studies. 1972. (Journal of Studies on Alcohol: Suppl. No. 6). 9.00 (*0-911290-01-X*) Rutgers Ctr Alcohol.

Surveys on Surgery Theory Vol. 1: Papers Dedicated to C. T. C. Wall. Sylvain Cappell. 1999. LC 99-68088. (Annals of Mathematics Studies: Vol. 145). 448p. 89.50 (*0-691-04937-8*) Princeton U Pr.

Survival Acre - Fifty Nationwide Wild Foods & Medicines. Linda Runyon. 1985. (Illus.). 43p. (Orig.). pap. 10.00 (*0-918517-03-6*) Wild Foods Co.

Survival Analysis. John P. Klein & Melvin L. Moeschberger. 1997. LC 96-9006. (Statistics for Biology & Health Ser.). (Illus.). 502p. 76.95 (*0-387-94829-5*) Spr-Verlag.

Survival as a Response Criterion for Small-Cell Lung Cancer. Ed. by P. Drings. 2000. (Onkologie Ser.: Vol. 23, Suppl. 3, 2000). (Illus.). iv, 20p. pap. 28.75 (*3-8055-7088-0*) S Karger.

Survival Bible for Women in Medicine. Kathryn K. Ko. 1998. LC 97-15485. (Illus.). 96p. 17.95 (*1-85070-752-9*, Parthenon Pbng) CRC Pr.

Survival Guide for HMO Patients. Emerita T. Gueson. Ed. by Laurie McBrinn & Frank A. Gerolamo. abr. ed. 1997. LC 96-90337. (Do HMO's Cut Costs . . . & Lives Ser.: No. 2). pap. 14.95 (*0-9653861-1-2*) Theresevision.

Survival Guide for the Beginning Speech-Language Clinician. Susan Moon Meyer. 1996. LC 98-27314. 245p. pap. 43.00 (*0-8342-1116-5*) PRO-ED.

Survival Guide to Acute Medicine. Ed. by Lee Kang Hoe et al. 1998. (Illus.). 226p. pap. (*9971-69-220-1*) Sngapore Univ Pr SGP. *Dist:* Coronet Bks.

Survival Guide to PPS: Productivity in Home Care. Sandra L. Spoelstra. 1999. 240p. pap. 49.00 (*0-8342-1187-4*, 11874) Aspen Pub.

Survival into the Twenty-First Century. Viktoras Kulvinskas. Ed. by Hermine Hurlbut & Joan Newman. 1975. (Illus.). pap. 21.95 (*0-933278-04-7*) Twen Fir Cent.

Survival Medical Guide. George Settar. 1979. 200p. Vol. 2. (SPA.). 49.95 (*0-8288-6896-4*); Vol. 3. (GER.). 49.95 (*0-8288-6897-2*); Vol. 4. (RUM.). 49.95 (*0-8288-6898-0*); Vol. 7. (JPN.). 49.95 (*0-8288-6900-6*); Vol. 8. (CHI.). 49.95 (*0-8288-6901-4*); Vol. 10. (RUS.). 49.95 (*0-8288-6903-0*); Vol. 11. (DUT.). 49.95 (*0-8288-6904-9*); Vol. 12. (GRE.). 49.95 (*0-8288-6905-7*); Vol. 13. (SWE.). 49.95 (*0-8288-6906-5*) Fr & Eur.

Survival Medical Guide - Medicine. George Settar. 1979. 200p. Vol. 6. (ITA.). 49.95 (*0-8288-6899-9*); Vol. 9. (POR.). 49.95 (*0-8288-6902-2*) Fr & Eur.

Survival of Cancer Patients in Europe: The EUROCARE Study. M. Sant et al. 1995. (IARC Scientific Publications Ser.: No. 132). (Illus.). 488p. pap. text 98.00 (*92-832-2132-X*) OUP.

Survival of the Sanest: Order & Disorder in a Pretrial Psychiatric Clinic. Robert J. Menzies. 1989. 310p. pap. 18.95 (*0-8020-6737-9*); text 40.00 (*0-8020-5827-2*) U of Toronto Pr.

Survival Psychology. John Leach. 1994. LC 94-16099. 232p. (C). text 45.00 (*0-8147-5090-7*) NYU Pr.

***Survival Skills for GPs.** Ruth Chambers. 1999. 176p. pap. (*1-85775-334-8*) Radcliffe Med Pr GBR. *Dist:* Balogh.

***Survival Skills for Nurses: Includes Tutor's Guide.** Ruth Chambers. 1999. 184p. pap. (*1-85775-339-9*) Radcliffe Med Pr GBR. *Dist:* Balogh.

Survival Spanish: A Pocket Guide for the Medical Professional. Theodore P. Skaarup. 1991. 150p. (Orig.). spiral bd. 14.95 (*1-879671-01-8*) Key-Logic.

Survivalist's Medicine Chest. Ragnar Benson. 1982. (Illus.). 80p. pap. 14.00 (*0-87364-256-2*) Paladin Pr.

Survive & Thrive Guide to Computer Validation. Teri Stokes. 1998. LC 98-18089. (Illus.). 316p. 237.00 (*1-57491-067-1*) IHS Health Grp.

Surviving: Coping with a Life Crisis. Bob Montgomery & Laurel Morris. 1995. 210p. pap. (*0-85091-370-5*) Lothian Pub AUS. *Dist:* Seven Hills Bk.

Surviving a Competitive Healthcare Market: Strategies for the 21st Century. Jana B. Knol. 1995. 175p. (Orig.). pap. text 44.95 (*0-07-600781-2*, ME116) Practice Mgmt Info.

Surviving Alzheimer's: A Guide for Families. Florian Raymond. 1994. (Caregivers Ser.). 89p. 10.95 (*0-943873-00-2*) Elder Bks.

Surviving Alzheimer's: Caregiver's Home Management of Alzheimer's Disease. Robert H. Rogge. 2nd rev. ed. 1997. (Illus.). 73p. pap. 9.95 (*0-9657319-1-X*) Longleaf Pr NC.

Surviving & Prospering in the Managed Mental Health Care Marketplace. Tracy Todd. Ed. by Bruce D. Forman. 1994. LC 94-17985. (Practice Management Ser.). 106p. pap. 18.95 (*1-56887-004-3*, SPMBP, Prof Resc Pr) Pro Resource.

Surviving Cancer. Kay D. Quain. 1988. LC 88-62065. 126p. pap. 7.95 (*1-55612-156-3*) Sheed & Ward WI.

***Surviving Cancer.** Dee Simmons. 2001. 244p. 18.99 (*1-57794-391-0*) Harrison Hse.

Surviving Cancer: One Woman's Story & Her Inspiring Program for Anyone Facing a Cancer Diagnosis. Margie Levine. 2001. LC 2001-25165. 256p. pap. 12.95 (*0-7679-0715-9*) Broadway BDD.

Surviving Childhood Cancer: A Guide for Families. Margot J. Fromer. 1995. LC 94-32635. 240p. text 22.95 (*0-88048-668-6*, 8668) Am Psychiatric.

Surviving Childhood Cancer: A Guide for Families. Margot J. Fromer. 1998. LC 97-75471. 232p. pap. 12.95 (*1-57224-102-0*) New Harbinger.

Surviving Childhood Sexual Abuse: Practical Self-Help for Adults Who Were Sexually Abused as Children. Carolyn Ainscough & Kay Toon. rev. ed. 2000. LC 00-35431. 304p. pap. 16.00 (*1-55561-225-3*) Fisher Bks.

Surviving Disaster Stress: What to Do Before, During & after Any Crisis to Prevent Pos-Traumatic Stress Disorders. Donald E. Dossey. 1997. (Illus.). 256p. pap. 14.95 (*0-925640-08-5*) Outcomes Unltd.

Surviving Health Care Reform: A Patient's Guide. G. C. Somich. 1997. LC 97-75086. x, 110 p. (*0-9660267-0-5*) Greenaire Pr.

Surviving Hypoxia: Mechanisms of Control & Adaptation. Lutz. 1993. 592p. 166.95 (*0-8493-4226-0*, RB150) CRC Pr.

Surviving in Healthcare. Dieter R. Enzmann. 1997. LC 97-11563. (Illus.). 512p. (C). (gr. 13). pap. text 42.00 (*0-8151-2447-3*, 30821) Mosby Inc.

***Surviving Leukemia... One Man's Cord Blood Miracle.** Stephen R. Sprague. Ed. by Jessica Roe. 2001. 96p. pap. 9.95 (*0-9713426-0-1*) S R Sprague.

Surviving Lyme Disease Using Alternative Medicine. David A. Jernigan. 1999. 120p. pap. 10.95 (*0-9674623-0-4*) Somerleyton Pr.

***Surviving Manic Depression Pb.** Torrey. 2001. 416p. pap. text 15.00 (*0-465-08664-0*) Basic.

Surviving Medical School. Robert H. Coombs. 1998. LC 97-33951. 197p. pap. 36.95 (*0-7619-0529-4*, 80538) Sage.

Surviving Mental Illness: Stress, Coping & Adaptation. Agnes B. Hatfield & Harriet P. Lefley. 1993. LC 93-20492. 206p. 42.00 (*0-89862-124-0*); pap. 23.00 (*0-89862-022-8*, 2022) Guilford Pubns.

Surviving Modern Medicine: How to Get the Best from Doctors, Family, & Friends. Peter Clarke & Susan H. Evans. 1998. LC 98-6812. (Illus.). 288p. (C). 38.00 (*0-8135-2555-1*); pap. 17.00 (*0-8135-2556-X*) Rutgers U Pr.

Surviving Nursing: A Coping Manual. Emily E. Smythe. 1984. 300p. pap. (*0-201-16418-3*, Health Sci) Addison-Wesley.

Surviving Paedophilia: Traumatic Stress after Organized & Network Child Abuse. Kate Cairns. 2000. 190p. pap. 22.50 (*1-85856-136-1*, Trentham Bks) Stylus Pub VA.

Surviving Popular Psychology: Debriefing the Me Degeneration. Clint Weyand. 1980. 148p. (Orig.). pap. 8.95 (*0-938292-13-7*) Being Bks.

Surviving Pregnancy Loss. Rochelle Friedman & Bonnie Gradstein. 1982. 16.95 (*0-316-29349-0*); pap. 10.95 (*0-316-29348-2*) Lppncott W & W (Little Brwn Med Div).

Surviving Schizophrenia: A Manual for Families, Consumers & Providers. E. Fuller Torrey. 3rd ed. 1995. LC 94-10533. (Illus.). 432p. pap. 16.00 (*0-06-095076-5*) HarperTrade.

Surviving Secrets: The Experience of Abuse for the Child, the Adult, & the Helper. Moira Walker. 1992. LC 92-9376. 224p. (*0-335-09764-2*); pap. (*0-335-09763-4*) OpUniv Pr.

Surviving the AIDS Plague. Taki N. Anagnoston. Ed. by Carla Hewitt. 1991. (Illus.). 340p. (Orig.). (C). pap. text 14.95 (*0-922356-44-0*) Amer West Pubs.

Surviving the Crisis of Depression & Bipolar (Manic-Depression) Illness: Layperson's Guide to Coping with Mental Illness Beyond the Time of Crisis & Outside the Hospital. Mark A. Halebsky. 1997. LC 97-68020. 116p. pap. 18.95 (*1-880793-01-6*) Pers & Prof Growth.

Surviving the Dalkon Shield IUD: Women vs. the Pharmaceutical Industry. Karen M. Hicks. 1993. (Athene Ser.). (C). 300p. pap. 16.95 (*0-8077-6270-9*); 208p. text 37.00 (*0-8077-6271-7*) Tchrs Coll.

Surviving the Demise of Solo Practice: Mental Health Practitioners Prospering in the Era of Managed Care. Ed. by Nicholas A. Cummings et al. 1996. LC 96-14756. 356p. 52.50 (*1-887841-03-2*, Psychosocial) Intl Univs Pr.

Surviving the Toxic Crisis: Todays Ultimate Solutions to Chronic Illness. William R. Kellas & Andrea S. Dworkin. 1996. (Toxic Twins Ser.). (Illus.). 523p. pap. 29.95 (*0-9636491-2-4*) Comprehensive Hlth.

Surviving Your Health Care. Michael M. Warren. 1995. LC 93-91539. 300p. (Orig.). pap. 16.95 (*0-9627775-3-6*) Ledero Pr.

Surviving Your Role As a Lawyer. David H. Barber. 2nd rev. ed. 1987. (Illus.). 166p. pap. text 17.95 (*0-915667-07-X*) Spectra Pub Co.

Survivor: Taking Control of Your Fight Against Cancer. Laura Landro. 1998. LC 98-27002. 224p. 18.00 (*0-684-84335-8*) S&S Trade.

Survivor: Taking Control of Your Fight Against Cancer. Laura Landro. 2000. 240p. pap. 12.00 (*0-684-85678-6*, Touchstone) S&S Trade Pap.

Survivor Psychology: The Darkside of a Mental Health Mission. Susan Smith. 1995. 234p. (C). pap. 14.95 (*0-89777-138-9*, Upton Bks) SIRS Pubng.

Survivor's Guide to Breast Cancer: A Chronic Illness Specialist Tells You What to Expect & Shares the Inspiring Account of Her Own Experience As a Patient. Alice Chang et al. 2000. LC 99-75281. (Illus.). vi, 173p. pap. 13.95 (*1-57224-185-3*) New Harbinger.

Survivor's Guide to Breast Cancer: A Couple's Story of Faith, Hope & Love. Robert C. Fore & Rorie E. Fore. 1998. LC 97-48563. 144p. pap. 17.00 (*1-57312-170-3*) Smyth & Helwys.

***Survivors Recovering from Sexual Abuse, Addictions & Compulsive Behaviors: "Numb" Survivors.** Sandra Knauer. 2001. LC 2001-17010. (Illus.). 279p. pap. 34.95 (*0-7890-1458-0*, HSWPP) Haworth Pr.

***Survivors Recovering from Sexual Abuse, Addictions & Compulsive Behaviors: "Numb" Survivors.** Sandy Knauer. 2001. LC 2001-17010. (Illus.). 279p. lib. bdg. 49.95 (*0-7890-1457-2*, HSWPP) Haworth Pr.

Susceptibility to Inhaled Pollutants. Ed. by Mark J. Utell & Robert Frank. 1989. LC 89-32217. (Special Technical Publications: No. STP 1024). (Illus.). 245p. text 55.00 (*0-8031-1262-9*, STP1024) ASTM.

Suspicious Death Scene Investigation. Ed. by Peter Vanezis. 1996. (Arnold Publication). (Illus.). 208p. 65.00 (*0-340-55863-6*) OUP.

Sustainability Analysis Module 9: Facilitator's Guide. Mary Millar. 1993. (Primary Health Care Management Advancement Programme Modules Ser.). 55p. pap. text (*1-882839-16-1*) Aga Khan Fnd.

Sustainability Analysis Module 9: User's Guide. Jack Reynolds & Wayne Stinson. 1993. (Primary Health Care Management Advancement Programme Modules Ser.). 105p. pap. text (*1-882839-07-2*) Aga Khan Fnd.

Sustainable Health Care Financing in Southern Africa: Papers from an EDI Health Policy Seminar Held in Johannesburg, South Africa, June 1996. Ed. by Allison Beattie et al. 1998. LC 97-44593. (EDI Learning Resources Ser.). 192p. pap. 22.00 (*0-8213-4145-6*, 14145) World Bank.

Sustaining Safe Sex: Gay Communities Respond to AIDS. Susan Kippax et al. 1993. LC 93-24359. 228p. 85.00 (*0-7507-0133-1*); pap. 29.95 (*0-7507-0134-X*) Taylor & Francis (Falmer Pr).

Suzuki GS850-1100 Shaft Drive, 1979-1984: Service, Repair, Maintenance. 3rd ed. Date not set. (Illus.). 264p. reprint ed. pap. 28.95 (*0-89287-305-1*, M376) Primedia Bus Mag Med.

SV40 Replicon Model for Analysis of Anticancer Drugs. Robert M. Snapka. 1996. (Molecular Biology Intelligence Unit Ser.). 192p. 79.00 (*0-412-10521-7*) Landes Bioscience.

SV40 Replicon Model for Analysis of Anticancer Drugs. Robert M. Snapka. 1996. (Biotechnology Intelligence Unit Ser.). 192p. text 69.95 (*0-12-653630-9*) Acad Pr.

Swallow Right - Or Else! Daniel Garliner. 1979. LC 78-75294. 108p. 9.00 (*0-87527-195-2*) Green.

Swallowing & Pharyngology. McConnel. 2001. 65.00 (*1-56593-742-2*, M3256) Thomson Learn.

Swallowing Disorders Treatment Manual. Edward Hardy & Natalie M. Robinson. Ed. by Cindy Drolet & C. Gilles-Brown. 2nd ed. 1999. (Illus.). 227p. spiral bd. 47.00 (*1-883315-48-4*, 7201) Imaginart Intl.

Swallowing Intervention in Oncology. Ed. by Arthur M. Guilford et al. 2nd ed. 1998. LC 98-29426. (Dysphagia Ser.). (Illus.). 375p. pap. 79.95 (*1-56593-751-1*, 1460) Thomson Learn.

Swanson's Family Practice Review. John Noble. 4th rev. ed. 2000. LC 00-33875. (Illus.). xxiii, 686p. text 65.00 (*0-323-00914-X*) Mosby Inc.

Sweat Testing: Sample Collection & Quantitative Analysis; Approved Guideline (1994) Contrib. by Vicky LeGrys. 1994. 75.00 (*1-56238-188-1*, C34-A) NCCLS.

Swedish-English - English-Swedish Medical & Pharmaceutical Dictionary. Clive K. Cressy. 3rd ed. 1992. (ENG & SWE.). 682p. 248.00 (*0-7859-8923-4*) Fr & Eur.

Swedish-English, English-Swedish Medical Dictionary. Clive K. Cressy. 2nd ed. 1988. (ENG & SWE.). 547p. lib. bdg. 195.00 (*0-8288-3312-5*, F136120) Fr & Eur.

Sweeping It under the Drug: A Complete Book about Recreational Drugs & How to Create a Great Life Without Them. Dennis Marcellino. 1988. LC 88-2083. 192p. pap. 9.95 (*0-945272-04-9*) Lighthouse.

Sweet Blood & Fury. Mary Connors. 2000. 300p. pap. 15.00 (*0-9702600-6-7*) M F Connors.

Sweet Dreams: A Pediatrician's Secret for Baby's Good Night's Sleep. Paul M. Fleiss. 2000. LC 00-64149. xv, 168p. pap. 17.95 (*0-7373-0494-4*) Lowell Hse.

Sweet Invisible Body: Reflections on a Life with Diabetes. Lisa Roney. 1999. LC 98-51819. 288p. 23.95 (*0-8050-5625-4*) H Holt & Co.

Sweet Smell of Psychosis. Will Self. 1999. (Illus.). 89p. reprint ed. text 20.00 (*0-7881-6736-7*) DIANE Pub.

Sweeteners Bulletin. 1989. 46p. 1000.00 (*0-89336-687-0*, CB-001) BCC.

Sweetness & Sweeteners. Ed. by Gordon G. Birch et al. 1971. (Illus.). 176p. 47.00 (*0-85334-503-1*) Elsevier.

Swenson's Pediatric Surgery. John Raffensperger. 5th ed. 1992. (Illus.). 994p. (C). pap. text 199.00 (*0-8385-8757-7*, A8757-5, Apple Lange Med) McGraw.

Swimmer Manuscript: Cherokee Sacred Formulas & Medicinal Prescriptions. James Mooney. 1995. (Bureau of American Ethnology Ser.). 319p. lib. bdg. 99.00 (*0-7812-4099-9*) Rprt Serv.

Swimming Upstream: Teaching & Learning Psychotherapy in a Biological Era. Jerry M. Lewis. 1991. LC 90-2671. 208p. text 31.95 (*0-87630-612-1*) Brunner-Routledge.

Swine As Models in Biomedical Research. Ed. by Michael Swindle et al. 1992. LC 91-35337. (Illus.). 328p. text 69.95 (*0-8138-1472-3*) Iowa U Pr.

Swine in Biomedical Research. Ed. by M. E. Tumbleson. 1986. Vol. 1. 684p. 135.00 (*0-306-42414-2*); Vol. 2. 690p. 135.00 (*0-306-42415-0*); Vol. 3. 750p. 135.00 (*0-306-42416-9*) Perseus Pubng (Plenum Trade).

Swine in Cardiovascular Research. H. Stanton & H. Mersmann. 1986. LC 85-30734. 200p. 116.00 (*0-8493-6565-1*, CRC Reprint) Franklin.

Swine Medicine. Wolf. 1996. (C). text (*0-7216-5841-5*) Saunders.

Swine Nutrition. Austin J. Lewis & Lincoln L. Southern. 2nd ed. 2000. LC 00-49395. (Illus.). 1032p. 139.95 (*0-8493-0696-5*) CRC Pr.

Swingbeds: Assessing Flexible Health Care in Rural Communities. Ed. by Joshua M. Wiener. 1987. LC 86-73150. (Dialogues on Public Policy Ser.). 140p. pap. 11.95 (*0-8157-9283-2*) Brookings.

Swiss Ball: Theory, Basic Exercises & Clinical Application. Beate Carriere & Renate Tanzberger. 1997. LC 97-36012. (Illus.). 409p. pap. 44.00 (*3-540-61144-4*); (*0-387-61144-4*) Spr-Verlag.

Swiss Ball Applications for Orthopedic & Sports Medicine: A Guide for Home Exercise Programs Utilizing the Swiss Ball. Joanne Posner-Mayer. Ed. by Joanne Posner-Mayer et al. 1995. (Illus.). 250p. (C). pap. text 29.95 (*0-9645341-4-2*) Ball Dynam.

Swiss Nature Doctor's Guide to a Healthier Heart & Circulatory System. A. Vogel. 1990. 16p. (Orig.). pap. 2.95 (*0-87983-519-2*, Keats Pubng) McGraw-Hill Trade.

Switched-On Living: Easy Ways to Use the Mind-Body Connection to Energize Your Life. Jerry V. Teplitz & Norma Eckroate. 1994. LC 95-131058. (Illus.). 120p. pap. 10.95 (*1-878901-93-1*) Hampton Roads Pub Co.

Syllabus - European Seminars on Diagnostic & Interventional Radiology (ESDIR), Rome, Italy: Functional MRI. P. Pavone & Plinio Rossi. 1996. LC 96-26790. 160p. pap. 79.50 (*3-540-75025-8*) Spr-Verlag.

Syllabus. 5th Radiological Refresher Course: Chest, Musculoskeleton, G.I. & Abdomen, Urinary Tract. L. Dalla Palma. 1996. 200p. pap. 79.50 (*3-540-75019-3*) Spr-Verlag.

Syllabus for the Surgeon's Secretary. Jeannette A. Szulec & Z. Szulec. 4th rev. ed. 1991. (Illus.). 1144p. 95.00 (*0-913092-03-7*) Medical Arts.

Sylvia Porter's Guide to Your Health Care: How You Can Have the Best Health Care for Less. Sylvia Porter. 1990. 304p. pap. 9.95 (*0-380-89758-X*, Avon Bks) Morrow Avon.

***Sylvius 2.0: Fundamentals of Human Neural Structure.** S. Mark Williams. 2nd ed. 2000. LC 00-59496. (Illus.). xviii, 681p. cd-rom 29.95 (*0-87893-917-2*) Sinauer Assocs.

Symbiosis & Ambiguity: The Psychoanalysis of Very Early Experience. Jose Bleger. 2000. pap. (*1-899209-11-5*) Process Pr GBR. *Dist:* Intl Spec Bk.

Symbiosis & Separation: Towards a Psychology of Culture. Richard A. Koenigsberg. 1989. LC 88-93056. 89p. (Orig.). pap. 20.00 (*0-915042-20-7*) Lib Soc Sci.

Symbol & Neurosis: Selected Papers of Lawrence S. Kubie. Ed. by Herbert J. Schlesinger & Eugene B. Brody. 1978. LC 77-92177. (Psychological Issues Monographs: No. 44, Vol. 11, No. 4). 280p. 42.50 (*0-8236-6291-8*); pap. 37.50 (*0-8236-6290-X*) Intl Univs Pr.

Symbol Formation. Ed. by Heinz Werner & Bernard Kaplan. 1984. 530p. (C). pap. text 39.95 (*0-89859-370-0*) L Erlbaum Assocs.

Symbol, Story, & Ceremony: Using Metaphor in Individual & Family Therapy. Gene Combs & Jill Freedman. 1990. 279p. (C). 29.95 (*0-393-70092-5*) Norton.

Symbolic Functioning in Childhood. Ed. by Nancy R. Smith & Margery B. Franklin. 1979. 256p. 49.95 (*0-89859-491-X*) L Erlbaum Assocs.

Symbolic Images in Art As Therapy. R. M. Simon. 1997. LC 95-39590. (Illus.). 224p. (C). 89.95 (*0-415-12227-9*) Routledge.

***Symbolic Impetus: How Creative Fantasy Motivates Development.** Charles Stewart. 2001. 256p. (*1-85343-536-8*) Free Assoc Bks GBR. *Dist:* Intl Spec Bk.

Symbolic Regression Psychology. Paul D. Fairweather & Donovan Johnson. 1982. 231p. (C). text 22.50 (*0-8290-0420-3*) Irvington.

Symbolic Self Completion. R. A. Wicklund & P. M. Gollwitzer. 1982. 256p. (C). text 49.95 (*0-89859-213-5*) L Erlbaum Assocs.

Symbolization: Proposing a Developmental Paradigm for a New Psychoanalytic Theory of Mind. Anna Aragno. 1997. LC 97-15905. 432p. 65.00 (*0-8236-6294-2*) Intl Univs Pr.

Symbolization & Creativity. Susan K. Deri. 1984. LC 83-26482. xii, 364p. 55.00 (*0-8236-6292-6*) Intl Univs Pr.

Symbols of Power Self-Healing System. Richard Lewis. 1998. (Illus.). pap. 49.95 (*0-9664069-0-7*, Symbols Power) Lewis Pub CA.

Sympathetic Understanding of the Child: Birth to Sixteen. David Elkind. 3rd ed. 1994. LC 93-43166. 250p. pap. text 38.00 (*0-205-15018-7*) Allyn.

Sympathetic Vibrations: A Guide for Private Music Teachers. Amber Esping. 2000. LC 00-39211. (Illus.). xi, 181p. spiral bd. 32.95 (*0-398-07073-3*) C C Thomas.

Sympathomimetic Enantiomers in the Treatment of Asthma: The Proceedings of a Meeting Held by the Section of Respiratory Medicine, the Royal Society of Medicine, London, October 1995. Ed. by J. F. Costello. 1997. LC 96-44595. (Illus.). 138p. lib. bdg. 52.95 (*1-85070-776-6*, Parthenon Pbng) CRC Pr.

Symposium in Immunology. Ed. by M. M. Eibl et al. 1993. LC 93-7837. 79.95 (*0-387-56478-0*) Spr-Verlag.

Symposium in Immunology. Ed. by M. M. Eibl & C. Huber. 1994. (Humoral Immunodeficiencies Ser.: 3). (Illus.). 232p. pap. 85.00 (*0-387-57126-4*) Spr-Verlag.

Symposium in Immunology V Vol. 5: Antiviral Immunity. Ed. by M. M. Eibl et al. 1996. (Illus.). 132p. pap. 117.00 (*3-540-60061-2*) Spr-Verlag.

Symposium in Immunology VII: Vaccination. Ed. by M. M. Eibl et al. 1998. LC 97-41390. (Illus.). 160p. pap. 99.00 (*3-540-63360-X*) Spr-Verlag.

Symposium of the International Society for Research in Stereoencephalotomy, 7th, Sao Paulo, June 24, 1977. Ed. by Philip L. Gildenberg. 1978. (Advances in Stereoencephalotomy Ser.: Vol. 8). (Illus.). pap. 85.25 (*3-8055-2946-5*) S Karger.

Symposium on Building Partnerships for Women's Health: Implications for Managed Care. Leslie R. Wolfe & Karen Schneider. 1997. 24p. (Orig.). pap. 10.00 (*1-877966-41-X*) Ctr Women Policy.

Symposium on Byzantine Medicine. Ed. by John Scarborough. 1985. LC 85-25967. (Dumbarton Oaks Papers: No. 38). (Illus.). 298p. 40.00 (*0-88402-139-4*) Dumbarton Oaks.

Symposium on Incremental Motion Control Systems & Devices: 23rd Annual Proceedings. Ed. by Benjamin C. Kuo. 1994. (Illus.). 90.00 (*0-931538-17-3*) Incremental Motion.

Symposium on Lucunar Infarcts: Clinical Aspects & Diagnostic Examinations: Ravenna, April 1989. Ed. by G. G. Rebucci et al. 1989. (Journal: Vol. 29, Suppl. 2, 1989). 50p. (C). pap. 54.50 (*3-8055-5124-X*) S Karger.

Symposium on Medical Therapy in Glaucoma. Ed. by Erik L. Greve. 1977. (Documenta Ophthalmologica Proceedings Ser.: Vol. 12). text 85.50 (*90-6193-152-5*) Kluwer Academic.

Symposium on Nucleic Acid Metabolism of Placenta & Fetus. Ed. by T. Hayashi. 1977. (Journal: Vol. 8, No. 3). (Illus.). 26.25 (*3-8055-2771-3*) S Karger.

Symposium on Trazodone. Ed. by C. L. Cazzullo et al. 1986. (Journal: Vol. 15, Suppl. 1, 1986). (Illus.). iv, 52p. pap. 24.50 (*3-8055-4338-7*) S Karger.

Symposium sur les Tumeurs Cutanees des Enfants: Gent. November, 1978. Ed. by J. De Bersaques. 1981. (Journal: Vol. 161, Suppl. 1, 1980). (Illus.). iv, 160p. pap. 15.75 (*3-8055-2238-X*) S Karger.

Symptom Analysis: A Method of Brief Therapy. M. Gerald Edelstein. 1990. 173p. (C). 21.95 (*0-393-70094-1*) Norton.

Symptom Analysis & Physical Diagnosis. Ed. by A. Davis et al. 2nd ed. 1985. 328p. text 42.00 (*0-08-029870-2*); pap. text 25.95 (*0-08-029869-9*) Elsevier.

Symptom-Context Method: Symptoms As Opportunities in Psychotherapy. Lester Luborsky. 1996. LC 96-4876. 422p. text 29.95 (*1-55798-354-2*, 431-6730) Am Psychol.

Symptom-Focused Psychiatric Drug Therapy for Managed Care: With 100 Clinical Cases. Sonny Joseph. 1997. LC 96-26946. 510p. pap. 39.95 (*0-7890-0194-2*); (Illus.). (C). 89.95 (*0-7890-0133-0*, Hawrth Medical) Haworth Pr.

Symptom Management Algorithms for Palliative Care. Linda D. Seaman. 1996. 104p. pap. 11.50 (*1-888411-00-7*) Intellicard.

Symptom Management in Advanced Cancer. Robert G. Twycross. 1995. LC 95-34888. (*1-85775-058-6*) Radcliffe Med Pr GBR. *Dist:* Balogh.

Symptom Management in Advanced Cancer. Robert A. Twycross. 2nd ed. 1997. LC 97-30469. (*1-85775-282-1*) Radcliffe Med Pr GBR. *Dist:* Balogh.

***Symptom Management in Advanced Cancer.** Robert Twycross. 3rd ed. 2001. 432p. pap. (*1-85775-510-3*) Radcliffe Med Pr GBR. *Dist:* Balogh.

Symptom Management in Multiple Sclerosis. Randall T. Schapiro. 3rd ed. 1998. LC 98-40033. (Illus.). 204p. pap. 19.95 (*1-888799-22-6*) Demos Medical.

Symptom Management Proceedings. Ed. by Patricia J. Larson. 1995. (C). pap. 25.00 (*0-943671-13-2*) UCSF Schl Nursing.

Symptom of Beauty. Francette Pacteau. 1994. LC 93-38507. (Essays in Art & Culture Ser.). 192p. 42.50 (*0-674-85987-1*) HUP.

Symptom-Oriented Guide to Adverse Drug Reactions. Mark L. Braunstein & John D. James. 560p. pap. (*0-07-032252-X*) McGraw.

Symptom Reduction Through Clinical Biofeedback. Ivan Wentworth-Rohr. 1984. 273p. (C). 45.95 (*0-89885-135-1*); pap. 20.95 (*0-89885-366-4*) Kluwer Academic (Kluwer Acad Hman Sci).

Symptom Solver: Understanding-&-Treating-the Most Common Male Health Concerns. Alisa Bauman & Brian Kaufman. Ed. by Men's Health Books Staff. 1996. LC 96-22076. (Men's Health Life Improvement Guides: Vol. 1). (Illus.). 176p. pap. 14.95 (*0-87596-357-9*) Rodale Pr Inc.

Symptom Sorter. Keith Hopcroft & Vincent Forte. 1999. LC 99-206266. 408p. pap. (*1-85775-395-X*) Radcliffe Med Pr GBR. *Dist:* Balogh.

Symptomatology & Differential Diagnosis: A Conspectus of Clinical Semeiographies. R. C. Schafer. 1986. LC 85-71673. (Illus.). 1088p. text 90.00 (*0-9606618-1-6*, K-18) Am Chiro Assn.

Symptoms: Their Causes & Cures - How to Understand & Treat 265 Health Concerns. Ed. by Prevention Magazine Editors et al. 1994. LC 93-23014. 660p. 29.95 (*0-87596-179-7*) Rodale Pr Inc.

Symptoms & Treatment of a Child's Learning Disorders & Academic Disorders: Handbook for Parents. Morrison F. Gardner. 1990. pap. 1.95 (*0-931421-62-4*) Psychol Educ Pubns.

Symptoms in the Mind. Sims. 2nd ed. 1995. pap. text 52.50 (*0-7020-1788-4*) Saunders.

Symptoms in the Pharmacy: A Guide to the Management of Common Illness. Alison Blenkinsopp & Paul Paxton. 3rd ed. 1998. LC 98-135290. (Illus.). 304p. pap. 50.95 (*0-632-04941-3*) Blackwell Sci.

Symptoms in the Pharmacy: A Guide to the Management of Common Symptoms. Alison Blenkinsopp & Paul Paxton. 2nd ed. 1994. LC 94-11238. 256p. pap. (*0-632-03609-5*) Blckwell Science.

Symptoms of Depression. Charles G. Costello. 1993. LC 92-18109. (Personality Processes Ser.). 336p. 170.00 (*0-471-54304-7*) Wiley.

Symptoms of Disease in Childhood. T. J. David. 1995. LC 95-7187. 281p. pap. 57.95 (*0-632-03635-4*); (*0-86542-970-7*) Blackwell Sci.

Symptoms of Schizophrenia. Charles G. Castello. 1993. LC 93-16759. (Personality Processes Ser.). 336p. 170.00 (*0-471-54875-8*) Wiley.

Synaesthesia: Classic & Contemporary Readings. Simon Baron-Cohen. 1996. LC 96-5888. (Illus.). 256p. 60.95 (*0-631-19763-X*); pap. 26.95 (*0-631-19764-8*) Blackwell Pubs.

Synaptic Connections: Neuroscience Memory Cards. S. Parker Haberly & Kenneth E. Kratz. 1996. 1000p. 45.00 (*1-56593-639-6*, 1324) Thomson Learn.

Synaptic Modification, Neuron Selectivity & Nervous System Organization. Ed. by William Levy et al. 1985. 280p. (C). text 59.95 (*0-89859-344-1*) L Erlbaum Assocs.

Synaptic Modifications & Memory: An Electrophysiological Analysis. Leon L. Voronin. 1993. LC 93-6851. (Studies of Brain Function: Vol. 19). (Illus.). 303p. 220.00 (*0-387-56325-3*) Spr-Verlag.

Synaptic Organization of the Brain. Ed. by Gordon M. Shepherd. 4th ed. 1997. LC 97-2176. (Illus.). 656p. pap. text 47.50 (*0-19-511824-3*) OUP.

Synaptic Plasticity: Molecular, Cellular, & Functional Aspects. Ed. by Michel Baudry et al. 1993. LC 93-19699. (Illus.). 50.00 (*0-262-02359-8*, Bradford Bks) MIT Pr.

Synaptic Transmission: Cellular & Molecular Basis. Herbert Zimmerman. 1994. LC 93-37754. (Science Briefings Ser.). (Illus.). 160p. (C). text 66.00 (*0-19-521065-4*); pap. text 36.00 (*0-19-521073-5*) OUP.

Synchronicity: C. G. Jung, Psychoanalysis & Religion. M. D. Faber. 1998. LC 98-23555. 160p. 60.00 (*0-275-96374-8*, Praeger Pubs) Greenwood.

Synchrotron Radiation Research. Ed. by Herman Winick & Seb Doniach. 1980. LC 80-14378. (Illus.). 776p. 145.00 (*0-306-40363-3*, Plenum Trade) Perseus Pubng.

Syncope. R. T. Ross. 1989. (Major Problems in Neurology Ser.: Vol. 18). (Illus.). 176p. text (*0-7020-1326-9*) W B Saunders GBR. *Dist:* Saunders.

Syncope: Mechanisms & Management. Ed. by Blair P. Grubb & Brian Olshansky. 1997. LC 97-24424. (Illus.). 432p. 89.00 (*0-87993-683-5*) Futura Pub.

Syncope & Related Disorders. W. A. McCrea & L. J. Findley. Date not set. (Neurological Disease & Therapy Ser.). (*0-8247-9497-4*) Dekker.

Syncope in the Older Patient. R. A. Kenny. 1995. 360p. (gr. 13). 169.95 (*0-412-56810-1*) Chapman & Hall.

Syndrome of D-Glyceric Acidemia with Hyperglycinemia. Steen Kolvraa. 1988. 71p. (*87-7288-186-0*) Aarhus Univ Pr DNK. *Dist:* David Brown.

Syndrome of Nonverbal Learning Disabilities: Neurodevelopmental Manifestations. Byron P. Rourke. 1995. LC 95-3981. 518p. 55.00 (*0-89862-155-0*, 2155) Guilford Pubns.

Syndrome X: Managing Insulin Resistance. Deborah S. Romaine & Jennifer B. Marks. 2000. 224p. mass mkt. 5.99 (*0-380-81444-7*, Torch) HarperCollins Pubs.

Syndrome X: Overcoming the Silent Killer That Can Give You a Heart Attack. Gerald M. Reaven et al. 2000. LC 99-52592. (Illus.). 288p. 25.00 (*0-684-86862-8*) S&S Trade.

Syndrome X: The Complete Nutritional Program to Prevent & Reverse Insulin Resistance. Burt Berkson et al. 1999. LC 99-49639. (Illus.). 288p. 24.95 (*0-471-35835-5*) Wiley.

Syndrome X: The Complete Program to Prevent & Reverse Thgis New Epidemic. Burt Berkson et al. 2000. 288p. pap. 15.95 (*0-471-39858-6*) Wiley.

Syndrome X, the Silent Killer: The New Heart Disease Risk. Gerald M. Reaven et al. 2001. 288p. pap. 13.00 (*0-684-86863-6*, Fireside) S&S Trade Pap.

Syndromes of the Head & Neck. Robert J. Gorlin et al. 4th ed. 2001. (Oxford Monographs on Medical Genetics: No. 42). (Illus.). 1344p. text 220.00 (*0-19-511861-8*) OUP.

Synergetics of the Brain. Ed. by H. Haken et al. 1983. (Synergetics Ser.: Vol. 23). (Illus.). 390p. 89.95 (*0-387-12960-X*) Spr-Verlag.

Synergistic Approach Stuttering Therapy. Charleen Bloom & Donna K. Cooperman. 1999. LC 98-50995. 288p. text 44.99 (*0-7506-9527-7*) Buttrwrth-Heinemann.

Synergy Session: Holistic Counseling Toward the New Age. Lynn M. Buess. 1980. LC 80-67932. (Illus.). 113p. (Orig.). pap. 4.95 (*0-87516-427-7*) DeVorss.

Synesthesia. R. E. Cytowic. 1989. (Neuropsychology Ser.). (Illus.). 354p. 112.00 (*0-387-96807-5*) Spr-Verlag.

Synopses in Urology. J. K. Mellon & A. C. Thorpe. 1998. LC 97-42814. 155p. pap. 41.95 (*0-632-05072-1*) Blackwell Sci.

Synopsis Methodica Animalium Quadrupedum et Serpentini Generis. John Ray. Ed. by Keir B. Sterling. 1978. LC 77-81111. (Biologists & Their World Ser.). (LAT.). reprint ed. lib. bdg. 33.95 (*0-405-10694-7*) Ayer.

***Synopsis of Cardiac Physical Diagnosis.** Jonathan Abrams. 2nd ed. 2001. LC 00-66797. 304p. pap. text 37.50 (*0-7506-7338-9*) Buttrwrth-Heinemann.

Synopsis of Critical Care. William J. Sibbald. 3rd ed. 1988. 352p. pap. 42.00 (*0-683-07709-0*) Lppncott W & W.

Synopsis of Diseases of the Chest. J. A. Pare & Robert G. Fraser. 2nd rev. ed. 1993. LC 93-25873. (Illus.). 732p. reprint ed. text 105.00 (*0-7216-3669-1*) Saunders.

Synopsis of Eugen Bleuler's Dementia Praecox or the Group of Schizophrenias. Ed. by Nathan S. Kline. 1966. (Monograph Series on Schizophrenia). 57p. 27.50 (*0-8236-6320-5*) Intl Univs Pr.

Synopsis of Fevers & Their Treatment. J. H. Lawson. 12th ed. 1977. pap. 15.95 (*0-8151-5335-X*) Mosby Inc.

Synopsis of General Pathology for Surgeons. Dennis W. Cotton. 1997. LC 97-938. 174p. pap. text (*0-7506-3592-4*) E A GBR. *Dist:* OUP.

Synopsis of Gynecologic Oncology. C. P. Morrow. Ed. by William Schmitt. 5th ed. 1998. LC 98-21396. 736p. text 120.00 (*0-443-07509-3*) Saunders.

Synopsis of Human Anatomy & Physiology. Kent M. Van De Graaff et al. 1996. LC 95-83328. 672p. (C). text 90.63 (*0-697-04296-0*) McGrw-H Hghr Educ.

Synopsis of Intensive Care Medicine. Gary B. Smith. 2001. 512p. pap. 49.50 (*0-7506-4754-X*) Buttrwrth-Heinemann.

Synopsis of Intensive Care Medicine. L. I. Worthley. 1994. LC 93-17403. text (*0-443-04638-7*) Church.

Synopsis of Intensive Care Treatment & Technology. B. Venkatesh. 2001. (Illus.). 320p. pap. 75.00 (*0-7506-4122-3*) Buttrwrth-Heinemann.

Synopsis of Lectures on Medical Science. Alva Curtis. 1996. 27p. reprint ed. spiral bd. 8.00 (*0-7873-0232-5*) Hlth Research.

Synopsis of Minor Oral Surgery. George Dimitroulis. 1997. LC 96-23371. (*0-7236-1094-0*) John Wright GBR. *Dist:* Buttrwrth-Heinemann, Macmillan.

Synopsis of Neuropsychiatry. Barry S. Fogel & Stephen M. Rao. 1999. LC 99-28397. (Illus.). xv, 528p. pap. text 49.95 (*0-683-30699-5*) Lppncott W & W.

Synopsis of Neuropsychiatry. Ed. by Stuart C. Yudofsky & Robert E. Hales. 1994. LC 93-44844. 660p. pap. text 47.00 (*0-88048-691-0*, 8691) Am Psychiatric.

Synopsis of Ophthalmology. Jack J. Kanski. 6th ed. 1990. 237p. pap. text (*0-7236-0937-3*) John Wright GBR. *Dist:* Buttrwrth-Heinemann.

Synopsis of Orthopedics. Howard An. 1992. (Illus.). 480p. text 69.00 (*0-86577-383-1*) Thieme Med Pubs.

Synopsis of Otolaryngology. Roger F. Gray & Maurice R. Hawthorne. 5th ed. 1992. (Illus.). 624p. (*0-7506-1358-0*) E A GBR. *Dist:* OUP.

Synopsis of Pediatric Emergency Medicine. Ed. by Gary R. Fleisher & Stephen Ludwig. 1995. LC 94-39410. (Illus.). 992p. 54.95 (*0-683-03261-5*) Lppncott W & W.

Synopsis of Systemic Pathology for Surgeons. Spence et al. 2000. 272p. pap. text 30.00 (*0-7506-4731-0*) Buttrwrth-Heinemann.

Synoptic Food Composition Tables. P. Cok et al. 1987. 444p. pap. text (*1-57235-046-6*) Piccin Nuova.

Synorgon Diet: How to Achieve Healthy Weight in a World of Excess. Randy L. Wysong. 1993. (Illus.). 271p. pap. 12.95 (*0-918112-06-0*) Inquiry Pr.

Syntactic Factors in Memory? Samuel Fillenbaum. 1973. (Janua Linguarum, Series Minor: No. 168). pap. text (*90-279-2421-X*) Mouton.

Syntactic-Semantic Tagging of Medical Texts: The Multitale Project. Ed. by W. Ceusters et al. 1997. LC 97-77952. (Studies in Health Technology & Informatics: Vol. 47). 200p. (YA). (gr. 12 up). 75.00 (*90-5199-384-6*) IOS Press.

***Synthesis & Structure Activity Relationships of Competitive NMDA Antagonists with Analgesic Activity.** Britt-Marie Swahn. 1999. (Comprehensive Summaries of Uppsala Dissertations from the Faculty of Pharmacy Ser.: No. 199). (Illus.). 53p. pap. (*91-554-4396-6*) Uppsala Universitet SWE. *Dist:* Coronet Bks.

Synthesis of Self Vol. 1: The I of Consciousness: Development from Birth to Maturity R. M. Mendelsohn. 1987. LC 87-25798. (Illus.). 370p. (C). text 70.00 (*0-306-42711-7*, Kluwer Plenum) Kluwer Academic.

Synthesis of Self Vol. 2: It All Depends on How You Look at It: The Development of Pathology in the Cohesive Disorders R. M. Mendelsohn. 1987. LC 87-25798. (Illus.). 272p. (C). text 70.00 (*0-306-42712-5*, Kluwer Plenum) Kluwer Academic.

Synthesis of Self Vol. 3: Believing Is Seeing: The Pathology of Development in the Noncohesive Disorders R. M. Mendelsohn. 1987. LC 87-25798. (Illus.). 392p. (C). text 70.00 (*0-306-42713-3*, Kluwer Plenum) Kluwer Academic.

Synthesis of Self Vol. 4: The Principles That Guide the Ideal Therapist R. M. Mendelsohn. 1987. LC 87-25798. (Illus.). 266p. (C). text 70.00 (*0-306-42714-1*, Kluwer Plenum) Kluwer Academic.

Synthesis Report: Medical Prescription of Narcotics Research Programme - Final Report of the Principal Investigators. Ambros Uchtenhagen. 1998. LC 98-43240. (Medical Prescription of Narcotics Ser.: Vol. 1, 1999). (Illus.). vi, 100p. 50.50 (*3-8055-6791-X*) S Karger.

Synthesis, Storage & Secretion of Adrenal Catecholamines: Proceedings of a Satellite Symposium to the 8th International Congress of Pharmacology, 19-24 July 1981, Tokyo, Japan. Ed. by F. Izumi et al. 1982. (Illus.). 302p. 69.50 (*0-08-028012-9*, Pergamon Pr) Elsevier.

Synthetic Analgesics Pt. 2A: Morphinans. J. Hellerbach & O. Schnider. 1966. LC 59-13814. (International Series of Monographs in the Sciences: Vol. 8). (*0-08-010895-4*) Pergamon Repr GBR. *Dist:* Franklin.

Synthetic Biodegradable Polymer Scaffolds. Ed. by A. Atala et al. 1997. LC 96-45700. (Tissue Engineering Ser.). 348p. 105.00 (*0-8176-3919-5*) Birkhauser.

Synthetic Peptides As Antigens. CIBA Foundation Staff. 1986. (CIBA Foundation Symposia Ser.: No. 119). 318p. pap. 128.00 (*0-471-91203-4*) Wiley.

Synthetic Polypeptides As Antigens. Ed. by M. H. Van Regenmortel et al. 1988. (Laboratory Techniques in Biochemistry & Molecular Biology Ser.: No. 19). 228p. pap. 46.50 (*0-444-80974-0*) Elsevier.

Synthetic Reagents: Chloramine-T; Hydrogen Peroxide; Polyphosphoric Acid, Vol. 6. J. S. Pizey. 1985. (Synthetic Reagents Ser.). 160p. 111.00 (*0-470-20152-5*) P-H.

Synthetic Repertory, Set. 4th ed. 1992. (ENG, FRE & GER.). pap. text (*3-7760-1342-7*) K F Haug Pubs DEU. *Dist:* Medicina Bio.

Synthetic Substrates & Synthetic Inhibitors: The Use of Chromogenic Substrates in Studies of the Haemostatic Mechanism. Ed. by M. Blomback & P. Brakman. 1978. (Haemostasis Ser.: Vol. 7, Nos. 2-3). (Illus.). pap. 33.25 (*3-8055-2907-4*) S Karger.

Synthetic Substrates in Clinical Blood Coagulation Assays. Ed. by H. R. Lijnen et al. 1980. (Developments in Hematology & Immunology Ser.: No. 1). 142p. text 73.50 (*90-247-2409-0*) Kluwer Academic.

Synthetic Vaccines. Ed. by Bruce Nicholson. 1994. LC 93-29366. 544p. 165.00 (*0-632-03014-3*) Blackwell Sci.

Synthetic Vaccines. Ruth Arnon. 1987. Vol. I. 168p. 101.00 (*0-8493-4659-2*); Vol. II. 176p. 103.00 (*0-8493-4660-6*) Franklin (CRC Reprint).

Syphilis in Shakespeare's England. Johannes Fabricius. 1994. 380p. pap. 37.50 (*1-85302-270-5*) Taylor & Francis.

Syphilis Today & among the Ancients Frederic Buret. LC 72-9627. reprint ed. 81.50 (*0-404-57422-X*) AMS Pr.

Syrian Hamster in Toxicology & Carcinogenesis: Proceedings - Symposium on the Syrian Hamster in Toxicology & Carcinogenesis Research, Boston, November 30-December 2, 1977. Ed. by F. Homburger. 1979. (Progress in Experimental Tumor Research Ser.: Vol. 24). (Illus.). 141.75 (*3-8055-2890-6*) S Karger.

Syringobulbia: A Contribution to the Pathophysiology of the Brainstem. N. Jonesco-Sisesti. Ed. & Tr. by R. T. Ross. 1986. LC 86-9489. 328p. 88.00 (*0-275-92123-9*, C2123, Praeger Pubs) Greenwood.

Syringomyelia MPN. Barnett. 1998. text 57.00 (*0-7020-2237-3*) Saunders.

System Disorders & Atrophies Ed. by Pierre J. Vinken & George W. Bruyn. 1975. Pt. 1. 249.75 (*0-444-10845-9*); Pt. 2. 232.00 (*0-444-10861-0*) Elsevier.

System for Ophthalmic Dispensing. Clifford W. Brooks et al. 2nd ed. 1996. LC 96-9212. (Illus.). 583p. text 95.00 (*0-7506-9481-5*) Buttrwrth-Heinemann.

System of Case Taking in Medicine. S. Sarkar. 1989. (C). (*0-89771-360-5*) Current Dist IND. *Dist:* St Mut.

System of Government in the Living Body Series: A Collective Title for All 11 Books Betty Yulin Ho. Ed. by Betty Elkan. 1994. LC 92-26675. (Illus.). 1015p. pap. 130.00 (*0-9600148-8-8*) Juvenescent.

System of Orthopaedic Medicine. Ombregt. 1995. text 136.50 (*0-7020-1595-4*) Saunders.

System of Physical Examination. D. P. Kingsford & D. T. Liley. 1991. 36p. pap. text 15.00 (*0-07-452808-4*) McGraw-Hill Med Pub.

System of Scientific Medicine. Howard Berliner. 1985. 180p. (*0-422-79520-8*, 9822); pap. (*0-422-79530-5*, 9829) Tavistock GBR. *Dist:* Routldge.

System und Phylogenie der Lebewesen Vol. 1: Physikalische, Chemische und Biologische Evolution. Edwin Moehn. 1984. (Illus.). 884p. lib. bdg. (*3-510-65117-0*) E Schweizerbartsche DEU. *Dist:* Lubrecht & Cramer, Balogh.

Systema Helminthum: Acanthocephala, Vol. 5. Satyu Yamaguti. 1985. 423p. pap. (*0-7855-0399-4*) Intl Bks & Periodicals IND. *Dist:* St Mut.

Systema Helminthum: Manogenea & Aspidoeotylea, Vol. 4. Satyu Yamaguti. 1985. 699p. pap. (*0-7855-0398-6*) Intl Bks & Periodicals IND. *Dist:* St Mut.

Systema Helminthum: The Cestodes of Vertebrates, Vol. 2. Satyu Yamaguti. 1985. 860p. pap. (*0-7855-0396-X*) Intl Bks & Periodicals IND. *Dist:* St Mut.

Systema Helminthum: The Digenetic Trematodes of Vertebrates & the Digenetic Trematodes of Vertebrates, Vol. 1, Pts. 1-2. Satyu Yamaguti. 1985. 1575p. pap. (*0-7855-0395-1*) Intl Bks & Periodicals IND. *Dist:* St Mut.

Systema Helminthum: The Nematodes of Vertebrates, Vol. 3, Pts. 1-2. Satyu Yamaguti. 1985. 1261p. pap. (*0-7855-0397-8*) Intl Bks & Periodicals IND. *Dist:* St Mut.

Systematic Approach to Strabismus. Virginia C. Hansen. 1998. LC 97-42381. (Basic Bookshelf for Eyecare Professionals Ser.). 128p. 27.00 (*1-55642-326-8*) SLACK Inc.

Systematic Approach to Tsetse & TrypanOsomiasis Control. FAO Staff. 1995. LC 95-237531. (Animal Production & Health Papers: No. 121). 200p. pap. (*92-5-003554-3*, F35543) FAO ITA. *Dist:* Bernan Associates.

Systematic Aspects of Biocompatibility, Vol. 2. Ed. by D. F. Williams. 1981. 240p. 135.00 (*0-8493-6622-4*, RA1231) CRC Pr.

Systematic Classic of Acupuncture, MoxiBustion. Hung-Fu Mi. 1994. LC 91-72854. 800p. 89.95 (*0-936185-29-5*) Blue Poppy Pr.

Systematic Intervention with Disturbed Children. Ed. by Marvin I. Fine. 1984. LC 83-21519. 275p. text 37.00 (*0-88331-204-2*) R B Luce.

Systematic Medication Profile Review. Quentin M. Srnka & Timothy H. Self. 3rd ed. 1991. 151p. (Orig.). (C). pap. 15.00 (*0-910769-26-5*) Am Coll Apothecaries.

Systematic Musculoskeletal Examination: Including Manual Diagnostic Techniques. Herbert Frisch. Tr. by Terry C. Telger. 1994. LC 93-30002. (Illus.). 462p. 150.00 (*0-387-51782-0*) Spr-Verlag.

Systematic Musculoskeletal Examination: Including Manual Medicine Diagnostic Techniques. Herbert Frisch. Tr. by Terry C. Telger from GER. 1993. (Illus.). 505p. (*3-540-51782-0*) Spr-Verlag.

***Systematic Pathology: A Clinically Oriented Core Text with Self Assessment.** Susan Burroughs et al. 2001. (Illus.). 220p. pap. (*0-443-07007-5*) Church GBR. *Dist:* Saunders.

Systematic Quality Management. Gary B. Clark. 1996. 65.00 (*0-89189-312-1*) Am Soc Clinical.

Systematic Reviews: Synthesis of Best Evidence for Health Care Decisions. Ed. by Cynthia D. Mulrow & Deborah Cook. 1998. LC 97-34983. 128p. pap. text 27.00 (*0-943126-66-5*) Amer Coll Phys.

***Systematic Reviews in Health Care: A Practical Guide.** Paul Glasziou. 2001. LC 00-65170. 186p. pap. text 29.95 (*0-521-79962-7*) Cambridge U Pr.

Systematic Screening for Behavior Disorders (SSBD) Program Kit, Set. Hill M. Walker & Herbert H. Severson. 2nd ed. 1992. 368p. tchr. ed., ring bd. 95.00 incl. audio, VHS (*0-944584-73-X*, 19KIT) Sopris.

Systematic Training for Effective Parenting of Teens - Step-Teen: Leader's Guide. Don C. Dinkmeyer, Jr. et al. rev. ed. 1990. (Systematic Training for Effective Parenting of Teens Ser.). 135p. pap. text 38.95 (*0-88671-403-6*, 5752) Am Guidance.

Systematic Training in the Skills of Virginia Satir. Sharon Loeschen. 1997. LC 97-10297. (Counseling Ser.). 118p. pap. text 28.95 (*0-534-23172-1*) Brooks-Cole.

Systematics & Evolutionary Relationships of Spiny Pocket Mice, Genus Liomys. Hugh H. Genoways. 1973. (Special Publications: No. 5). (Illus.). 368p. (Orig.). pap. 10.00 (*0-89672-030-6*) Tex Tech Univ Pr.

Systematik der Individualien Keramischen Farbgestaltung see Custom Ceramic Color: A Practical System

Systematik der Neurosen see Psychology & Cognitive Therapy of the Neuroses

Systematisierung von Infusionsloesungen und Grundlagen der Infusionstherapie. I. W. Hahnefeld. 1980. (Beitraege zur Infusionstherapie und Klinische Ernaehrung Ser.: Band 5). (Illus.). 112p. pap. 78.50 (*3-8055-1395-X*) S Karger.

Systematization of Radiotherapy & the Techniques of Irradiating Cancer Patients, Vol. 3. M. Sh. Weinberg. 1989. (Soviet Medical Reviews Ser.: Vol. 3, No. 1). 68, ivp. pap. text 56.00 (*3-7186-4915-2*) Gordon & Breach.

Systematized Prevention of Oral Disease: Theory & Practice. Lars Granath & William D. McHugh. 1986. 288p. 142.00 (*0-8493-5163-4*, RK60, CRC Reprint) Franklin.

Systemic Autoimmunity. Ed. by Pierluigi E. Bigazzi & Seymour Reichlin. 1991. (Immunology Ser.: Vol. 54). (Illus.). 320p. text 195.00 (*0-8247-8550-9*) Dekker.

Systemic Disease & the Nasal Airway. Ed. by Thomas V. McCaffrey. 1993. LC 92-49198. (Rhinology & Sinusology Ser.). 65.00 (*0-86577-466-8*) Thieme Med Pubs.

Systemic Diseases, Pt. I. Ed. by Pierre J. Vinken et al. 1993. LC 93-20095. 686p. 251.50 (*0-444-81282-2*) Elsevier.

***Systemic Diseases & the Eye.** Jack J. Kanski. 2001. (Illus.). 291p. pap. (*0-7234-3216-3*) Mosby Inc.

Systemic Diseases & the Kidney Ed. by Robert W. Schrier & Saulo Klahr. 1998. LC 98-29127. (Atlas of Diseases of the Kidney Ser.: Vol. 4). (Illus.). 131.95 (*0-632-04437-3*) Blackwell Sci.

Systemic Drugs for Skin Diseases. Wolverton & Wilkin. 1991. 400p. pap. text 70.00 (*0-7216-2987-3*) Saunders.

Systemic Family Therapy: An Integrative Approach. William C. Nichols & Craig A. Everett. 1986. LC 85-17235. (Family Therapy Ser.). 442p. text 44.00 (*0-89862-066-X*) Guilford Pubns.

***Systemic Fungal Infections.** Richardson et al. 2002. (Fast Facts Ser.). (Illus.). pap. (*1-903734-03-7*) Health Pr GBR. *Dist:* JAMCO Dist.

Systemic Harpoon into Family Games: Preventive Interventions in Therapy. Giuliana Prata. 1990. LC 90-2157. 192p. text 32.95 (*0-87630-591-5*) Brunner-Routledge.

Systemic Hormones, Neurotransmitters & Brain Development. Ed. by G. Doerner & S. M. McCann. 1986. (Monographs in Neural Sciences: Vol. 12). (Illus.). x, 222p. 172.25 (*3-8055-4287-9*) S Karger.

Systemic Lupus Erythematosus. Ed. by Peter A. Miescher. 1995. LC 95-1128. 240p. 92.00 (*0-387-59039-0*) Spr-Verlag.

Systemic Lupus Erythematosus. Ed. by Robert G. Lahita. 3rd ed. 1998. LC 98-35859. (Illus.). 1051p. (C). 189.95 (*0-12-433900-X*) Acad Pr.

Systemic Lupus Erythematosus. Robert G. Lahita. 2nd ed. 1992. (Illus.). 1002p. text (*0-443-08785-7*) Church.

Systemic Lupus Erythematosus: Clinical & Theoretical Aspects. Julian L. Verbov et al. 1973. (Illus.). 220p. (C). text 29.00 (*0-8422-7104-X*) Irvington.

Systemic Lupus Erythematosus: Renal Vasculitis. Ed. by Adalberto Sessa et al. 1992. LC 92-23672. (Contributions to Nephrology Ser.: Vol. 99). (Illus.). viii, 152p. 49.75 (*3-8055-5603-9*) S Karger.

Systemic Manifestations of IBD: The Pending Challenge for Subtle Diagnosis & Treatment. Ed. by B. Lembcke et al. 1998. LC 98-133583. (Falk Symposium Ser.). 416p. 175.00 (*0-7923-8734-1*) Kluwer Academic.

Systemic Pathology: The Breast. Elston. 3rd ed. 1998. (C). text (*0-443-03723-X*) Church.

Systemic Pathology Vol. 1: Nose, Throat & Ears. Ed. by I. Friedmann. 3rd ed. 1986. (Illus.). 416p. text (*0-443-03097-9*) Church.

Systemic Pathology Vol. 2: Blood & Bone Marrow. Ed. by S. N. Wickramasinghe. 3rd ed. 1986. (Illus.). 490p. text (*0-443-03099-5*) Church.

Systemic Pathology of HIV Infections & AIDS in Children. Moran & Mullick. Date not set. 328p. pap. text 62.00 (*1-881041-40-9*) Am Registry Path.

Systemic Psychotherapy with Families, Couples & Individuals. Guido L. Burbatti et al. 1993. LC 92-9280. 224p. 45.00 (*0-87668-390-1*) Aronson.

Systemic Radiotherapy with Monoclonal Antibodies: Options & Problems. Ed. by H. Bihl & M. Wannenmacher. 1996. (Recent Results in Cancer Research Ser.: Vol. 141). (Illus.). 197p. 135.00 (*3-540-60209-7*) Spr-Verlag.

Systemic Therapist, Vol. I. Ed. by Bradford P. Keeney et al. 1990. 137p. (Orig.). pap. text 18.00 (*0-9626461-1-3*) Systemic Therapy.

Systemic Therapist, Vol. II. Ed. by Bradford P. Keeney. 1991. (Orig.). pap. text 18.00 (*0-9626461-2-1*) Systemic Therapy.

Systemic Therapy with Individuals. Luigi Boscolo & Bertrando Boscolo. 1996. 320p. pap. (*1-85575-094-5*) Karnac Bks GBR. *Dist:* Other Pr LLC.

Systemic Treatment of Incest: A Therapeutic Handbook. Terry S. Trepper & Mary J. Barrett. 1989. LC 89-9739. (Psychosocial Stress Ser.: No. 15). 304p. text 39.95 (*0-87630-560-5*) Brunner-Routledge.

Systemic Treatment Selection: Toward Targeted Therapeutic Interventions. Larry E. Beutler & John F. Clarkin. 1990. LC 89-71203. (Brunner/Mazel Integrative Psychotherapy Ser.: No. 3). 384p. text 49.95 (*0-87630-576-1*) Brunner-Routledge.

Systemic Vasculitides. Jacob Churg. Ed. by Andrew M. Churg. 1991. LC 90-15649. (Illus.). 408p. 192.50 (*0-89640-195-2*) Igaku-Shoin.

Systems Analysis in Health Care. Ed. by Vijay Mahajan & C. Carl Pegels. 1979. LC 78-19461. 504p. 83.50 (*0-275-90384-2*, C0384, Praeger Pubs) Greenwood.

Systems & Development: The Minnesota Symposia on Child Psychology, Vol. 22. Ed. by Megan R. Gunnar & Esther Thelen. 1989. (Minnesota Symposium on Child Psychology Ser.). 264p. 55.00 (*0-8058-0409-9*) L Erlbaum Assocs.

Systems & Structures Bk. I: The World's Best Anatomical Charts Collection. Anatomical Chart Company Staff. 2000. 35p. pap. 15.95 (*1-889241-07-5*, SYS-35) Anatomical Chart.

Systems & Technologies for Clinical Diagnostics & Drug Discovery, Vol. 3259. Ed. by Gerald E. Cohn. 1998. 254p. 69.00 (*0-8194-2698-9*) SPIE.

Systems & Technologies for Clinical Diagnostics & Drug Discovery II. Ed. by Gerald E. Cohn & Jack C. Owicki. 1999. LC 00-500818. (Progress in Biomedical Optics Ser.). (Illus.). ix, 326p. 84.00 (*0-8194-3073-0*) SPIE.

Systems & Theories in Psychology. Melvin H. Marx & W. A. Cronan-Hillix. 4th ed. (McGraw-Hill Psychology Ser.). 576p. (C). 1987. pap. text, tchr. ed. 21.56 (*0-07-040681-2*); 1986. text 59.74 net. (*0-07-040680-4*) McGraw.

Systems Approach to Education & Program Planning for Health Professionals. Mary Watson. 1999. text 21.59 (*1-56870-302-3*) RonJon Pub.

Systems Atlas of Male Human Anatomy. Engineering Animation Incorporated Staff. Ed. by Ron Worthington. 1996. LC 96-24276. 128p. (C). (gr. 13). spiral bd. 20.95 (*0-8151-8654-1*, 28923) Mosby Inc.

Systems-Centered Therapy for Groups. Yvonne M. Agazarian. 1997. LC 97-3418. 328p. text 42.00 (*1-57230-195-3*, 0195) Guilford Pubns.

Systems Challenge: Getting the Clinical Information Support You Need to Improve Patient Care. Ed. by Nancy A. Kreider & Becky J. Haselton. 1997. LC 97-9523. 232p. pap. 45.00 (*1-55648-199-3*, 040100) AHPI.

Systems Consultation: A New Perspective for Family Therapy. Ed. by Lyman C. Wynne et al. 1986. LC 86-4778. (Guilford Family Therapy Ser.). 487p. pap. 26.95 (*0-89862-908-X*) Guilford Pubns.

Systems Nurse: Designing Health Care Systems for Quality Care Delivery to All People. T. J. Terry. 1994. 96p. pap. 46.00 (*1-887258-01-9*); 2nd rev. ed. 1996. 102p. 46.00 (*1-887258-22-1*) T J Terry.

Systems of Accountability: Implementing Children's Health Insurance Programs. National Research Council Staff & Institute of Medicine Staff. Ed. by Molly Joel Coye & Margaret Edmunds. 1998. LC 99-188101. 40p. pap. text 10.00 (*0-309-06149-0*) Natl Acad Pr.

Systems of Continuing Education: Priority to District Health Personnel. 1990. (Technical Reports: No. 803). (ENG, FRE & SPA.). 50p. pap. text 8.00 (*92-4-120803-1*, 1100803) World Health.

Systems of Family Therapy: An Adlerian Integration. Robert Sherman & Don C. Dinkmeyer, Jr. 1987. LC 86-29897. 322p. text 39.95 (*0-87630-457-9*) Brunner-Routledge.

Systems of Psychotherapy: A Transtheoretical Analysis. James O. Prochaska. 2nd ed. 1984. 442p. (C). pap. 47.25 (*0-534-10708-7*) Brooks-Cole.

Systems of Psychotherapy: A Transtheoretical Analysis. James O. Prochaska & John C. Norcross. 3rd ed. 1996. LC 93-41023. 540p. pap. 51.00 (*0-534-22290-0*); 1994. mass mkt., tchr. ed. (*0-534-22291-9*) Brooks-Cole.

Systems of Psychotherapy: A Transtheoretical Analysis. Prochaska & Norcross. 4th ed. 1998. LC 98-28468. (Counseling Ser.). 560p. spiral bd. 73.95 (*0-534-35704-0*) Brooks-Cole.

Systems Psychology in the Schools. Jeanne M. Plas. 1986. (General Psychology Ser.: No. 141). 19209p. 35.00 (*0-08-033144-0*, J115); pap. 19.95 (*0-08-033143-2*) Elsevier (Pergamon Pr).

Systems Science in Health Care: Proceedings of the International Conference on Systems in Health Care, July 1980, Montreal, Quebec, Canada. C. Tilquin. 1981. LC 81-94784. 1888p. 829.00 (*0-08-025370-9*, Pergamon Pr) Elsevier.

Systems Theory & Family Therapy: A Primer. Raphael J. Becvar & Dorothy S. Becvar. 1982. LC 81-43721. 104p. (Orig.). (C). pap. text 16.50 (*0-8191-2444-3*); lib. bdg. 54.50 (*0-8191-2443-5*) U Pr of Amer.

Systems Theory in Immunology. Ed. by C. Bruni. 1980. (Lecture Notes in Biomathematics: Vol. 32). (Illus.). 508p. 36.95 (*0-387-09728-7*) Spr-Verlag.

Systolic & Diastolic Function of the Heart: Proceedings of the 11th International Conference of the Cardiovascular Dynamics Society, San Francisco, California, Nov 17-20, 1994. Ed. by Neil B. Ingels, Jr. et al. 1996. LC 94-7376. (Studies in Health Technology & Informatics: Vol. 21). 445p. 99.00 (*90-5199-211-4*) IOS Press.

Szycher's Dictionary of Biomaterials & Medical Devices. Michael Szycher. 1992. LC 91-67901. 272p. 94.95 (*0-87762-882-3*) CRC Pr.

T

T. A. P. P. Sources: A National Directory of Teenage Pregnancy Prevention Programs. Dominique Treboux. 1989. 565p. 50.00 (*0-8108-2277-6*) Scarecrow.

T. A. T., C. A. T., & S. A. T. in Clinical Use. Leopold Bellak. 4th ed. 1986. 408p. text 39.00 (*0-8089-1815-X*, 790516, Grune & Strat) Harcrt Hlth Sci Grp.

T. B. of Obstetrics & Neonatology. D. Dawn. 12th ed. 1990. (C). (*0-7855-4658-8*) Current Dist IND. *Dist:* St Mut.

T-Cell Autoimmunity & Multiple Sclerosis. Marco Londei. 1998. LC 99-27041. (Neuroscience Intelligence Unit Ser.: Vol. 5). (Illus.). 150p. 99.00 (*1-57059-567-4*) Landes Bioscience.

T-Cell-Directed Immunointervention. Ed. by Jean-Francois Bach. 1993. LC 92-49921. (Frontiers in Pharmacology & Therapeutics Ser.). (Illus.). 336p. 145.00 (*0-632-03105-0*) Blackwell Sci.

T Cell Hybridomas. M. J. Taussig. 1985. 296p. 167.00 (*0-8493-5202-9*, QR185, CRC Reprint) Franklin.

T-Cell Paradigms in Parasitic & Bacterial Infections. Ed. by S. H. Kaufmann. 1990. (Current Topics in Microbiology & Immunology Ser.: Vol. 155). (Illus.). 162p. 89.00 (*0-387-51515-1*) Spr-Verlag.

T-Cell Primer. Mark M. Davis. Date not set. (Illus.). 208p. (C). text 34.95 (*0-19-509337-2*) OUP.

T-Cell Subsets & Cytokines Interplay in Infectious Diseases. Ed. by A. S. Mustafa et al. 1996. LC 95-9615. (Illus.). 222p. 248.00 (*3-8055-6122-9*) S Karger.

T Cell Subsets in Infectious & Autoimmune Diseases. Nicholas A. Mitchison. 1996. (CIBA Foundation Symposia Ser.: Vol. 195). 272p. 128.00 (*0-471-95720-8*) Wiley.

T-Cell Vaccination & Autoimmune Disease. Jingwu Zhang & Jef Raus. 1995. LC 95-1239. (Medical Intelligence Unit Ser.). 174p. 79.00 (*1-57059-254-3*) Landes Bioscience.

T Cells in Arthritis. Ed. by Pierre P. Miossec et al. 1998. LC 98-19065. (Progress in Inflammation Research Ser.). 248p. 133.00 (*3-7643-5853-X*) Spr-Verlag.

T Cells in Arthritis. Pierre Miossec et al. 1998. LC 98-19065. (PIR - Progress in Inflammation Research Ser.). xii, 236p. 133.00 (*0-8176-5853-X*) Birkhauser.

T-Factor Fat Gram Counter. Ed. by Jamie Pope-Cordle & Martin Katahn. 1989. LC 00-501725. (Illus.). 103p. pap. 3.99 (*0-393-30655-0*) Norton.

T-Lymphocyte & Inflammatory Cell Research in Asthma. Ed. by Georges Jolles et al. 1993. (Illus.). 392p. text 94.00 (*0-12-388170-6*) Acad Pr.

T Lymphocyte Differentiation in the Human Thymus, Vol. 2. Ed. by Marion D. Kendall & M. A. Ritter. 1989. xii, 324p. text 231.00 (*3-7186-4932-2*) Gordon & Breach.

T Lymphocyte Subpopulations in Immunotoxicology. Ian Kimber & Mary J. Selgrade. 1998. LC 97-44163. 312p. 149.95 (*0-471-97194-4*) Wiley.

T Lymphocytes: Structure, Function & Choices. F. Celada & B. Pernis. 1992. LC 92-49284. (NATO Advanced Science Institutes Ser.: Vol. 233). (Illus.). 268p. (C). text 95.00 (*0-306-44258-2*, Kluwer Plenum) Kluwer Academic.

T-Lymphocytes & Their Receptors in Immunologic Recognition. B. D. Brondz. 1988. xxiv, 496p. text 910.00 (*3-7186-4801-6*) Gordon & Breach.

T. V. Vet Book for Stock Farmers No. 2: Calving the Cow & Care of the Calf. Ed Straiton. 1994. (T.V. Vet Ser.). (Illus.). 312p. (*0-85236-184-X*) Farming Pr GBR. *Dist:* Diamond Farm Bk.

Tabbner's Nursing Care: Theory & Practice. Ed. by J. O. Chandler. 3rd ed. 1998. (Illus.). 782p. pap. (*0-443-05434-7*) Church.

Taber's Cyclopedic Medical Dictionary. Clayton L. Thomas. 18th ed. 1998. (Illus.). 2439p. (C). text 59.95 incl. cd-rom (*0-8036-0337-1*) Davis Co.

Taber's Cyclopedic Medical Dictionary. Ed. by Clayton L. Thomas. 18th ed. 1997. LC 62-8364. (Taber's Cyclopedic Medical Dictionary Ser.). (Illus.). 2439p. (C). 31.95 (*0-8036-0194-8*) Davis Co.

Taber's Cyclopedic Medical Dictionary. Ed. & Intro. by Clayton L. Thomas. 18th ed. 1997. LC 62-8364. (Illus.). 2439p. (C). 34.95 (*0-8036-0193-X*) Davis Co.

Taber's Cyclopedic Medical Dictionary. Ed. by Clayton L. Thomas. 18th deluxe ed. 1997. (Illus.). 2439p. (C). text 69.00 (*0-8036-0195-6*) Davis Co.

Taber's Cyclopedic Medical Dictionary: Deluxe. Donald Venes & Clayton L. Thomas. 19th deluxe ed. 2001. LC 00-64688. (Illus.). 2804p. 79.00 (*0-8036-0656-7*) Davis Co.

Taber's Cyclopedic Medical Dictionary: Indexed. Doanld Venes & Clayton L. Thomas. 19th ed. 2001. LC 00-64688. (Taber's Cyclopedic Medical Dictionary Ser.: Vol. 19). (Illus.). 2804p. 35.95 (*0-8036-0654-0*) Davis Co.

Taber's Cyclopedic Medical Dictionary: Plain. Donald Venes & Clayton L. Thomas. 19th ed. 2001. LC 00-64688. (Taber's Cyclopedic Medical Dictionary Ser.). (Illus.). 2804p. 32.95 (*0-8036-0655-9*) Davis Co.

Taber's Medical Word Book with Pronunciations. Ed. by Clayton L. Thomas. 1990. LC 90-2948. 876p. (C). pap. text 19.95 incl. cd-rom (*0-8036-8265-4*) Davis Co.

Tablet Machine Instrumentation in Pharmaceutics. Watt. 1988. (Pharmaceutical Technology Ser.). 416p. 73.95 (*0-470-21088-5*) P-H.

Tableting Specification Manual. American Pharmaceutical Association Staff. Ed. by Linda Young. 4th ed. 1995. LC 95-179739. (Illus.). 128p. spiral bd. 125.00 (*0-917330-67-6*) Am Pharm Assn.

Tableting Specification Manual. TSM Steering Committee. 5th ed. 2001. LC 99-52558. (Illus.). xiii, 119p. spiral bd. 135.00 (*1-58212-005-6*) Am Pharm Assn.

Tabooed Jung: Marginalization & Influence. Christine Gallant. 1996. LC 95-51264. 192p. (C). text 37.50 (*0-8147-3087-6*) NYU Pr.

Tachycardias. Ed. by Borys Surawicz et al. 1984. (Developments in Cardiovascular Medicine Ser.). text 307.50 (*0-89838-588-1*) Kluwer Academic.

Tachycardias: Mechanisms & Management. Ed. by Mark E. Josephson & Hein J. Wellens. 2nd ed. 1993. LC 92-48867. (Bakken Research Center Ser.). (Illus.). 512p. 97.00 (*0-87993-549-9*) Futura Pub.

Tachykinin Antagonists. Ed. by R. Hakanson & F. Sundler. 1986. (Fernstrom Foundation Ser.: No. 6). 442p. 238.00 (*0-444-80735-7*) Elsevier.

Tachykinin Receptors. Ed. by Stephen H. Buck. 1994. LC 94-13436. (Receptors Ser.). 640p. 155.00 (*0-89603-266-3*) Humana.

Tachyon Energy: A New Paradigm in Holistic Healing. Gabriel Cousens & David Wagner. 1999. LC 00-271751. (Illus.). 147p. pap. 12.95 (*1-55643-310-7*) North Atlantic.

Tackling Alcohol Together. Society for the Study of Addiction Staff. 1999. 369p. pap. (*1-85343-458-2*) Free Assoc Bks GBR. *Dist:* Intl Spec Bk.

***Tackling Teenage Pregnancy: Sex, Culture & Needs.** Ruth Chambers et al. 2000. 240p. pap. (*1-85775-497-2*) Radcliffe Med Pr GBR. *Dist:* Balogh.

Tactical Decisions in a Personal Injury Case. Paul L. Stritmatter. 1988. (ATLA Monograph Ser.). 36p. (Orig.). pap. (*0-941916-48-0*) West Group.

Tactical Emergency Care: Military & Operational Out-of-Hospital Medicine. Robert A. De Lorenzo et al. 1999. LC 98-52453. 400p. pap. text 55.00 (*0-8359-5325-4*) P-H.

Tactical Psychotherapy of the Personality Disorders: A MCMI-III-Based Approach. Ed. by Paul D. Retzlaff. 1995. LC 94-44325. 288p. (C). 56.00 (*0-205-15932-X*, Longwood Div) Allyn.

Tactics & Techniques in Psychoanalytic Therapy, Vol. 1. Ed. by Peter L. Giovacchini. 1993. LC 72-144143. (Tactics & Techniques in Psychoanalytic Therapy Ser.: Vol. 1). 768p. pap. 60.00 (*1-56821-110-4*) Aronson.

Tactics & Techniques in Psychoanalytic Therapy Vol. III: Implications of Winnicott's Contributions. Ed. by Peter L. Giovacchini. 1990. LC 72-144143. 296p. 55.00 (*0-87668-789-3*) Aronson.

Tactics of Change: Doing Therapy Briefly. Richard Fisch et al. 1982. LC 81-48665. (Social & Behavioral Science Ser.). 328p. 38.00 (*0-87589-521-2*) Jossey-Bass.

Tactics of Psychotherapy: An Application of Psychoanalytic Theory to Psychotherapy. William F. Murphy. 1965. LC 65-19462. 72.50 (*0-8236-6360-4*) Intl Univs Pr.

Tactics of Scientific Research: Evaluating Experimental Data in Psychology. Murray Sidman. 1988. LC 60-13278. (Illus.). 428p. (C). reprint ed. pap. 24.95 (*0-9623311-0-4*) Authors Coop.

Tactile Aids for the Hearing Impaired. Summers. 1992. 270p. pap. 87.75 (*1-56593-582-9*, 0233) Singular Publishing.

Tactual Perception: A Sourcebook. Ed. by William Schiff & Emerson Foulke. 1982. LC 81-10172. (Illus.). 512p. text 110.00 (*0-521-24095-6*) Cambridge U Pr.

Taft Strategic Atlas: U. S. Health Care Reform. Frederick I. Taft. 1993. 686p. (Orig.). pap. 39.00 (*0-9635808-0-9*) Pub Strategy.

Tagebuch der Medicinischen Literatur der Jahre, 1745-1774. Albrecht V. Haller. 1997. (GER.). reprint ed. 458.00 (*3-487-05095-1*) G Olms Pubs.

Taheebo. Rita Elkins. 1997. (Woodland Health Ser.). 32p. pap. text 3.95 (*1-885670-40-0*) Woodland UT.

T'ai Chi Fundamentals: For Health Care Professionals & Instructors. Tricia Yu & Jill Johnson. 1999. (Illus.). 126p. pap. 29.95 (*1-877950-20-3*) Uncharted Ctry Pub.

Taigman's Advanced Cardiology: In Plain English. Syd Canan et al. 1995. LC 94-48021. 256p. pap. text 60.00 (*0-89303-999-3*) P-H.

Tailored Polymeric Materials for Controlled Delivery Systems. Ed. by Iain McCulloch & Shalaby W. Shalaby. 1998. LC 98-25962. (ACS Symposium Ser.: No. 709). (Illus.). 336p. text 120.00 (*0-8412-3585-6*) OUP.

Take Action Against Drug Abuse: How to Start a Volunteer Anti-Drug Program in Your Community. 1994. (Illus.). 53p. (Orig.). (C). pap. text 25.00 (*0-7881-0383-0*) DIANE Pub.

Take Care of the Heart You Have. Nancy Gibson et al. Ed. by Susan D. Allen & Colleen A. Holloran. (Illus.). 56p. pap. text 3.75 (*0-916999-14-9*) HERC Pubng.

Take Care of Yourself. Donald M. Vickery. 3rd ed. 1988. (SPA.). pap. (*0-201-69458-1*) Addison-Wesley.

Take Care of Yourself. Pantell. 4th ed. 1994. pap. (*0-201-40782-5*) Addison-Wesley.

Take Care of Yourself. Donald M. Vickery. 5th ed. 1995. pap. (*0-201-40710-8*) Addison-Wesley.

Take Care of Yourself. Donald M. Vickery. 6th ed. 2000. LC 95-49545. 448p. pap. 18.00 (*0-201-48989-9*) Perseus Bks Grp.

Take Care of Yourself: A Health Care Workbook for Beginning ESL Students. Marianne Brems et al. 1993. LC 93-7377. 256p. pap. text 20.93 (*0-13-882317-0*) Prentice ESL.

Take Care of Yourself: Deseret Mutual Health Version. Donald M. Vickery. 1992. pap. (*0-201-62282-3*) Addison-Wesley.

Take Care of Yourself: Franciscan Skemp Healthcare. Donald M. Vickery. 6th ed. 1996. pap. (*0-201-69459-X*) Addison-Wesley.

Take Care of Yourself: Health Track. Donald M. Vickery. 5th ed. 1995. pap. (*0-201-48990-2*) Addison-Wesley.

Take Care of Yourself: Healthplus Version. Donald M. Vickery. 1990. pap. (*0-201-62284-X*) Addison-Wesley.

Take Care of Yourself: Newport Naval Hospital. Donald M. Vickery. 6th ed. 1996. pap. (*0-201-15452-8*) Addison-Wesley.

Take Care of Yourself: Sanus Special Edition. Donald M. Vickery. 4th ed. 1992. pap. (*0-201-62260-2*) Addison-Wesley.

Take Care of Yourself: The Consumer's Guide to Medical Care. Donald M. Vickery. 1986. pap. 14.95 (*0-201-08091-5*) Addison-Wesley.

Take Care of Yourself: Wisconsin Educational Association Insurance. Donald M. Vickery. 5th ed. 1995. pap. (*0-201-48977-5*) Addison-Wesley.

Take Care of Yourself: Your Personal Guide to Self-Care & Preventing Illness. Donald M. Vickery & James F. Fries. 5th ed. 1993. LC 92-48678. pap. 17.95 (*0-201-63292-6*) Addison-Wesley.

Take Care of Yourself Guide to Treating Your Family. Donald M. Vickery. 6th ed. 1998. pap. (*0-201-33995-1*) Addison-Wesley.

Take-Charge Guide to Type I Diabetes. Betty Page Brackenridge & Richard Rubin. 1996. LC 94-17538. (Illus.). 288p. pap. 16.95 (*0-945448-35-X*, 00359Q) Am Diabetes.

Take Charge of Your Diabetes: A Guide for Patients. 1993. (Illus.). 72p. (Orig.). (C). pap. text 15.00 (*0-7881-0113-7*) DIANE Pub.

Take Charge of Your Health: Professional Secrets You Need to Know to Obtain the Best Medical Care. Stephen Astor. 1991. LC 91-90283. 216p. (Orig.). pap. 12.95 (*0-915001-07-1*) Two As Pub.

Take Charge of Your Life: What to Do When Someone in Your Family Has a Drinking or Other Drug Problem. Martin Fleming. 1993. 32p. pap. 5.95 (*1-56246-070-6*, 3113, HazeldenJohnson Inst) Hazelden.

Take Charge of Your Medical Practice... Before Someone Else Does It for You: Practical Practice Managment for the Managed Care Market. Neil Baum & Elaine Zablocki. 1996. LC 96-6738. 448p. 82.00 (*0-8342-0799-0*, 20799) Aspen Pub.

Take Control: Weight Reduction. Judd Biasiotto. 1986. (Illus.). 134p. (Orig.). pap. 8.00 (*0-933079-05-2*) World Class Enterprises.

***Take Control Diet: A Life Plan for Thinking People.** Ian Smith. 2002. LC 2001-48337. 272p. 24.95 (*0-375-50730-2*) Random.

Take Financial Control with Medicaid: How to Defend Your Money During Extended Care. Fred L. Sargent. 1997. (Illus.). vii, 66p. pap. 13.95 (*0-9659478-0-7*) Freemor.

Take Heart: The Life of Dr. Paul Dudley White. Oglesby Paul. 1986. LC 86-3170. (Francis A. Countway Library of Medicine). (Illus.). 336p. 19.95 (*0-674-86745-9*) HUP.

Take It Off & Keep It Off: Based on the Successful Methods of Overeaters Anonymous. R. Helene & Helen Lerner. 1989. LC 89-33024. 176p. pap. 8.95 (*0-8092-4493-4*, 449340, Contemporary) McGraw-Hill Trade.

Take It to Heart: CNAs' Solutions to the Staffing Crisis. Bethany Knight. 2000. 112p. pap. 12.95 (*1-888343-36-2*) Hartman Pub.

Take It to Heart: Your Complete Guide to Preventing & Treating Heart Disease. Robert Myers. 1997. (Illus.). 160p. pap. (*1-55022-339-9*) ECW CAN. *Dist:* General Distrib Services.

Take This Book & Call Me in the Morning! Mary McBride & Veronica McBride. Ed. by Helen Duffy. 1993. (Illus.). 104p. (Orig.). pap. 5.95 (*0-9627601-5-3*) Bros Grinn.

Take This Book to the Dentist with You. Charles B. Inlander et al. 1998. LC 98-2958. 244p. pap. text 14.95 (*1-882606-27-2*) Peoples Med Soc.

Take This Book to the Hospital with You: A Consumer Guide to Surviving Your Hospital Stay. Charles B. Inlander & Ed Weiner. rev. ed. 1997. LC 96-44013. (Illus.). 272p. pap. 14.95 (*1-882606-70-1*) Peoples Med Soc.

Take This Book to the Obstetrician with You. Charles B. Inlander & Karla Morales. rev. ed. 1998. LC 95-31205. (Take This Book to the Obstetrician with You Ser.: Vol. 1). 288p. pap. 5.99 (*0-312-96505-2*, Tor Books) T Doherty Assocs.

Take This Book to the Pediatrician with You: People's Medical Society Book. Charles B. Inlander & Lynne Dodson. rev. ed. 1998. LC 98-115809. 288p. mass mkt. 5.99 (*0-312-96414-5*) St Martin.

Take This Book to the Pediatrician with You: The Guide to Your Child's Health. Charles B. Inlander. 1992. (Illus.). 256p. pap. 14.95 (*0-9627334-6-6*) Peoples Med Soc.

Take Time to Talk: A Resource for Apraxia Therapy, Esophageal Speech Training, Aphasia Therapy & Articulation Therapy. Patricia F. White. 2nd ed. 1996. LC 96-14174. 185p. spiral bd. 34.99 (*0-7506-9783-0*) Buttrwrth-Heinemann.

Take Two Aspirin & See Yourself in the Morning. Robert A. Norman. 2nd ed. 1997. 218p. (Orig.). pap. 16.95 (*0-9637802-8-X*) North Shore Pr.

Take Two Crackers & Call Me in the Morning! A Real Life Guide for Surviving Morning Sickness. Miriam Erick. Ed. by Tim Champion. 1995. LC 95-80416. (Illus.). 72p. (Orig.). pap. 9.00 (*0-9613063-5-1*) Grinnen-Barrett Pub Co.

Take up Thy Bed & Walk. David Hinshaw. Ed. by William R. Phillips & Janet Rosenberg. 1980. LC 79-6905. (Physically Handicapped in Society Ser.). (Illus.). reprint ed. lib. bdg. 28.95 (*0-405-13114-3*) Ayer.

Taking a Stand: Child Psychiatrists in Custody, Access & Disputed Adoption Cases. British Agencies for Adoption and Fostering Editors Staff. 1989. (C). (*0-903534-55-X*) Brit Ag for Adopt & Fost GBR. *Dist:* St Mut.

Taking a Stand on Health Care. Helen P. Rogers. 1991. LC 91-75100. 64p. (Orig.). pap. 6.95 (*0-915915-08-1*) Wellington Pubns.

***Taking a Toxic Exposure History.** Arthur L. Frank. Ed. by Sophie J. Balk. 2001. (Illus.). 80p. (C). pap. text 20.00 (*0-7567-1824-4*) DIANE Pub.

Taking Action to Reduce Tobacco Use. National Research Council Staff & Institute of Medicine Staff. 1998. LC 98-195008. 42p. pap. text 10.00 (*0-309-06038-9*) Natl Acad Pr.

***Taking Advance Directives Seriously: Prospective Autonomy & Decisions near the End of Life.** Robert S. Olick. 2001. LC 2001-23260. 240p. 64.95 (*0-87840-868-1*) Georgetown U Pr.

Taking Asthma to School. Kim Gosselin. Ed. by Barbara Mitchell. 2nd rev. ed. 1998. LC 97-76662. (Special Kids in School Ser.: Vol. 2). (Illus.). 24p. (J). (gr. k-5). pap. 11.95 (*1-891383-01-9*) JayJo Bks.

Taking Care: Self-Care for 100 Common Symptoms & 25 Long-Term Ailments. Random House Staff. 1997. LC 96-41153. 224p. pap. 12.00 (*0-679-77794-6*) Random.

Taking Care: The Legacy of Soma Weiss, Eugene Stead & Paul Beeson. William Hollingsworth. 1994. (Illus.). 331p. pap. 16.00 (*1-57087-038-1*) Prof Pr NC.

Taking Care after 50: A Self-Care Guide for Seniors. Harvey Jay Cohen. 2000. LC 00-60731. (Illus.). 384p. pap. 17.00 (*0-8129-3174-2*, Three Riv Pr) Crown Pub Group.

Taking Care of Caregivers: For Families & Others Who Care for People with Alzheimer's Disease & Other Forms of Dementia. D. Jeanne Roberts. 1991. (Illus.). 200p. (Orig.). pap. 14.95 (*0-923521-09-7*) Bull Pub.

Taking Care of Your Child: A Parent's Guide to Complete Medical Care. Robert H. Pantell et al. 4th ed. 1993. (Illus.). 608p. pap. 17.95 (*0-201-63293-4*) Addison-Wesley.

***Taking Care of Your Child: A Parent's Guide to Complete Medical Care.** Robert Pantell & James Fries. 6th ed. 2002. (Illus.). 544p. pap. text 19.95 (*0-7382-0601-6*) Perseus Bks Grp.

Taking Chances: Derrida, Psychoanalysis, & Literature. Ed. by Joseph H. Smith & William Kerrigan. 1988. LC 83-49198. (Psychiatry & the Humanities Ser.: No. 7). 216p. reprint ed. pap. text 16.95 (*0-8018-3749-9*) Johns Hopkins.

Taking Charge: Nursing, Suffrage, & Feminism in America, 1873-1920. Sandra B. Lewenson. 1993. LC 93-11137. (Development of American Feminism Ser.: Vol. 1). 368p. text 20.00 (*0-8240-6897-1*) Garland.

Taking Charge: Nursing, Suffrage & Feminism in America, 1873-1920. Sandra Beth Lewenson. 1996. 273p. pap. 28.95 (*0-88737-684-3*) Natl League Nurse.

Taking Charge: Survival Skills for the Take Charge Nurse. Biggers & Vivian. 1997. 32p. (gr. 13). pap. text 129.95 (*0-8151-1297-1*) Mosby Inc.

Taking Charge of ADHD: The Complete, Authoritative Guide for Parents. Russell A. Barkley. rev. ed. 2000. LC 00-34130. 321p. 38.00 (*1-57230-600-9*, C0600); (Illus.). pap. 18.95 (*1-57230-560-6*, C0560) Guilford Pubns.

Taking Charge of Asthma: A Lifetime Strategy. Betty B. Wray. 1998. LC 97-48749. (Illus.). 240p. pap. 14.95 (*0-471-24704-9*) Wiley.

Taking Charge of Fibromyalgia Julie Kelly. 4th ed. 1998. pap. text 18.95 (*0-9665774-0-X*) Fibromyalgia Educ.

Taking Charge of Infertility. Patricia Irwin Johnston. LC 93-44146. 272p. 1995. pap. 14.00 (*0-944934-08-0*); 1994. 21.95 (*0-944934-07-2*) Perspect Indiana.

Taking Charge of Menopause Workbook. Robert M. Dosh et al. 1997. 195p. pap. 17.95 (*1-57224-060-1*) New Harbinger.

Taking Charge of Your Child's Allergies: The Informed Parent's Comprehensive Guide. M. Eric Gershwin & Edwin L. Klingelhofer. 2nd ed. 1998. LC 98-5850. (Illus.). 256p. 27.50 (*0-89603-455-0*) Humana.

Taking Charge of Your Fertility: The Definitive Guide to Natural Birth Control, Pregnancy Achievement, & Reproductive Health. Toni Weschler. 1995. LC 95-13496. (Illus.). 400p. pap. 22.00 (*0-06-095053-6*) HarperCollins Pubs.

Taking Charge of Your Smoking. Joyce D. Nash. 1981. 124p. (Orig.). stu. ed. 14.95 (*0-915950-50-2*) Bull Pub.

Taking Control. Lance Dodes. 2002. LC 2001-26477. 272p. 24.95 (*0-06-019811-7*) HarperCollins Pubs.

Taking Control: Living with the Mitral Valve Prolapse Syndrome. Kristine A. Scordo. 1993. 198p. (Orig.). pap. 19.95 (*0-938100-99-8*) Camden Hse.

Taking Control: Living with the Mitral Valve Prolapse Syndrome. Kristine A. Scordo. 2nd rev. ed. 1996. (Illus.). 190p. (Orig.). pap. 20.00 (*0-9650689-0-0*) Kardinal Pubng.

Taking Control of Your Headaches: How to Get the Treatment You Need. Paul N. Duckro et al. 1999. 180p. pap. 14.95 (*1-57230-471-5*) Guilford Pubns.

Taking Liberties: AIDS & Cultural Politics. Ed. by Erica Carter & Simon Watney. 1991. 240p. pap. 14.95 (*1-85242-147-9*) Serpents Tail.

***Taking Out the Violence: Shedding Light on the Science & Soul of Human Behaviour.** Ursula Anderson. 2001. 119p. pap. 17.95 (*0-9655435-7-9*) She-Bear Pubs.

Taking Responsibility: Health & Wellbeing. Barwise. LC 94-33850. (Environmental Agenda Ser.). 80p. (C). pap. text (*0-7453-0929-1*) Pluto GBR GBR. *Dist:* Stylus Pub VA.

Taking Sides: Clashing Views on Controversial Issues in Health & Society. Eileen L. Daniel. 2nd ed. 1997. (C). text 4.94 net. (*0-697-39269-4*, WCB McGr Hill) McGrw-H Hghr Educ.

Taking Sides: Clashing Views on Controversial Psychological Issues. Ed. by Joseph Rubinstein & Brent D. Slife. 8th rev. ed. 1994. LC 93-48692. (Illus.). 408p. (C). text 13.95 (*1-56134-294-7*, Dshkn McG-Hill) McGrw-H Hghr Educ.

Taking the American Medical Boards Beyond the No. 2 Pencil. Zafar Y. Ibrahim. Ed. by Debra D. Richards. 1990. 51p. lib. bdg. 12.95 (*0-9626615-0-3*) Overseas Pub.

Taking the Fear Out of Changing. Dennis E. O'Grady. 1994. LC 94-28764. 384p. pap. 14.95 (*1-55850-408-7*) Adams Media.

Taking the Fear Out of Eating: A Nutritionists' Guide to Sensible Food Choices. Charlette Gallagher & John Allred. 1992. (Illus.). 311p. (C). text 59.95 (*0-521-43124-7*); pap. text 21.95 (*0-521-43728-8*) Cambridge U Pr.

Taking the Group Seriously: Towards a Post-Foulkesian Group Analytic Theory. Farhad Dalal. 1998. LC 98-215220. (International Library of Group Analysis). 239p. (*1-85302-642-5*) Jessica Kingsley.

Taking the Lead with PACT: Peer Education in Sexuality & Health. 1989. (Illus.). 96p. (Orig.). pap. 25.00 (*1-878263-00-5*) YWCA.

Taking the "Ouch" out of Headaches. Joan Miller. 1983. (Taking the "Ouch" out of Headaches Ser.). 24.95 incl. audio (*0-9613786-0-3*) J Miller.

Taking the Pulse of a Community: Results of the Torquay Community Health Survey Research Paper. Deanne Gaskill. 1991. (Research Monographs: No. 1). (C). pap. (*0-7300-1458-4*) Deakin Univ AUS. *Dist:* St Mut.

Taking the Stress Out of Teaching. Michael E. Bernard. 19.95 (*0-85924-918-2*, B114) Inst Rational-Emotive.

Taking Time: Support for People with Cancer & the People Who Care about Them. 1992. (Illus.). 68p. (Orig.). (C). pap. text 20.00 (*1-56806-103-X*) DIANE Pub.

Taking Your Back to the Future. W. Michael Gazdar. 1997. 284p. pap. 12.95 (*0-9645301-1-2*) J Muir Chirop.

Taking Your Back to the Future: How to Get a Pain-Free Back & Total Health with Chiropractic Care. W. Michael Gazdar. Ed. by Larry Wyner & Linda Wyner. rev. ed. 1995. (Illus.). 280p. (Orig.). (C). pap. 12.95 (*0-9645301-0-4*) J Muir Chirop.

Taking Your Medications Safely. Springhouse Publishing Company Staff. 1995. LC 95-6698. (Nurseadviser Bks.). (Illus.). 512p. pap. 19.95 (*0-87434-824-2*) Springhouse Corp.

Taking Your Medicine: Drug Regulation in the United States. Peter Temin. 1980. LC 80-16680. (Illus.). 281p. 39.95 (*0-674-86725-4*) HUP.

***Tale of Healer Miguel Perdomo Neira: Medicine, Ideologies, & Power in the Nineteenth-Century Andes.** David Sowell. 2001. LC 00-67984. (Latin American Silhouettes Ser.). (Illus.). xix, 171p. 75.00 (*0-8420-2826-9*, SR Bks) Scholarly Res Inc.

Talent in Context: Historical & Social Perspectives on Giftedness. Ed. by Reva C. Friedman & Karen B. Rogers. 1998. LC 97-47678. (Illus.). 218p. 34.95 (*1-55798-493-X*) Am Psychol.

Tales & Transformation: Stories in Families & Family Therapy. Janine Roberts. 1994. LC 94-13506. 220p. (C). 27.00 (*0-393-70174-3*) Norton.

Tales for Jung Folk: Original Fairytales for Persons of All Ages Dramatizing C. G. Jung's Archetypes of the Collective Unconscious. Richard Roberts. 1983. (Illus.). 120p. pap. 8.95 (*0-942380-01-0*); 107p. lib. bdg. 15.95 (*0-942380-02-9*) Vernal Equinox.

Tales from a Traveling Couch: A Psychotherapist Revisits His Most Memorable Patients. Robert U. Akeret. 1998. 235p. text 22.00 (*0-7881-5941-0*) DIANE Pub.

Tales from Family Therapy: Life-Changing Clinical Experiences. Ed. by Frank N. Thomas. 1997. LC 97-28202. 304p. 49.95 (*0-7890-0065-2*); pap. 24.95 (*0-7890-0450-X*) Haworth Pr.

Tales from Inside the Iron Lung (And How I Got Out of It) Regina Woods. 1994. LC 93-47694. (Illus.). 160p. (Orig.). pap. 13.95 (*0-8122-1506-0*) U of Pa Pr.

Tales from My Little Black Bag. John Ibberson. 1994. 160p. pap. 18.95 (*1-55059-093-6*) Temeron Bks.

Tales in Pursuit of High-Quality Health Care. Ed. by Frederick Gale. 1994. LC 94-71700. 114p. (Orig.). pap. text 25.00 (*0-924674-29-6*) Am Coll Phys Execs.

Tales of a Country Doctor: One Hundred Years of Health Care in Lewis County. Brandt A. Bede. 1993. LC 92-85175. 124p. (C). pap. 13.50 (*1-880222-12-4*) Red Apple Pub.

Tales of a Shaman's Apprentice: An Ethnobotanist Searches for New Medicines in the Amazonian Rain Forest. Mark J. Plotkin. 1994. (Illus.). 352p. pap. 13.95 (*0-14-012991-X*, Penguin Bks) Penguin Putnam.

Tales of an Unorthodox Veterinarian. Gideon Sorokin. 1992. (Illus.). 204p. (Orig.). pap. 13.95 (*0-943376-57-2*) Magnes Mus.

Tales of Enchantment: Goal-Oriented Metaphors for Adults & Children in Therapy. Stephen R. Lankton & Carol H. Lankton. 1989. LC 89-720. 432p. text 43.95 (*0-87630-504-4*) Brunner-Routledge.

Talk & Toddle: A Commonsense Guide for the First Three Years. Anne M. Mueser & Lynne Liptay. 1983. 160p. pap. 7.95 (*0-312-78430-9*) St Martin.

Talk Medicine - The Ultimate Survival Strategy. Harvey L. Kugel. unabr. ed. 1998. LC 97-75914. (Orig.). pap. 29.95 (*1-891676-00-8*) Mantra Pr.

Talk Medicine - Your Personal Medical Diary. Harvey L. Kugel. unabr. ed. 1998. LC 97-75915. pap. 15.00 (*1-891676-01-6*) Mantra Pr.

Talk with Me: Communication with the Multi-Handicapped Deaf. California State Department of Health Staff et al. LC 75-70066. 35.00 (*0-917002-05-9*) Joyce Media.

Talk with Teens about Self & Stress: 50 Guided Discussions for School & Counseling Groups. Jean S. Peterson. Ed. by Pamela Espeland. 1993. LC 93-21514. 192p. (Orig.). (YA). (gr. 7-12). pap. 21.95 (*0-915793-55-5*, FS172) Free Spirit Pub.

Talking about Aphasia: Living with Loss of Language after Stroke. Susie Parr et al. 1997. LC 97-15402. (*0-335-19937-2*); 192p. pap. (*0-335-19936-4*) OpUniv Pr.

Talking about Dreams: Dream Reports As Personal Narratives. Roger Elbourne. 320p. (C). text (*0-8290-1582-5*) Irvington.

Talking about Health & Wellness with Patients: Integrating Health Promotion & Disease Prevention into Your Practice. Steven Jonas. 2000. LC 99-87585. xv, 144p. pap. text 29.95 (*0-8261-1338-9*) Springer Pub.

Talking about Health is Academic: Six Workshop Modules for Promoting a Coordinated Approach to School Health Programs. Education Development Center Staff. 2000. 802p. pap. text 24.95 (*0-8077-3991-X*) Tchrs Coll.

Talking about Treatment: Recommendations for Breast Cancer Adjuvant Treatment. Felicia Roberts. 1999. (Oxford Studies in Sociolinguistics). 144p. text 35.00 (*0-19-512191-0*) OUP.

Talking AIDS, a Guide for Community Work. Illus. by Petra Rohr-Rouendal. 1989. 110p. (Orig.). pap. 9.95 (*0-333-49781-3*) Scholium Intl.

Talking Back to Prozac. Peter Breggin. 1995. mass mkt. 6.99 (*0-312-95606-1*, Tor Books) T Doherty Assocs.

Talking Back to Ritalin: What Doctors Aren't Telling You about Stimulants for Children. Peter R. Breggin. LC 00-64521. rev. ed. 1998. 265p. 24.95 (*1-56751-129-5*); 2nd rev. ed. 2000. 450p. pap. 18.95 (*1-56751-128-7*) Common Courage.

Talking Cure: A Descriptive Guide to Psychoanalysis. Joseph D. Lichtenberg. 1994. 168p. (C). reprint ed. pap. 24.95 (*0-88163-192-2*) Analytic Pr.

Talking Cure: The Science Behind Psychotherapy. Susan C. Vaughan. 2000. 208p. reprint ed. 25.00 (*0-7881-9568-9*) DIANE Pub.

Talking Cure: The Science Behind Psychotherapy. Susan C. Vaughan. 1997. LC 96-45237. (Illus.). 224p. 24.95 (*0-399-14229-0*, Grosset-Putnam) Penguin Putnam.

Talking Cures: The Psychoanalyses & the Psychotherapies. Robert S. Wallerstein. 1995. LC 95-1448. 608p. 70.00 (*0-300-06107-2*) Yale U Pr.

Talking Head: The Novelist & Gullain-Barre. Jimmie R. Rankin. 1994. (Literature of a Patient Response Ser.). 770p. pap. 14.95 (*1-883938-14-7*) Dry Bones Pr.

Talking Health with Dr. Brian McDonough. Ed. by Brian P. McDonough. 1994. LC 94-6020. (Health, Society, & Policy Ser.). 288p. (C). 39.95 (*1-56639-207-1*) Temple U Pr.

Talking Points in Dermatology I. Ed. by Julian L. Verbov. 1986. (New Clinical Applications in Dermatology Ser.). lib. bdg. 82.00 (*0-85200-939-9*) Kluwer Academic.

Talking Points in Dermatology III. Ed. by Julian L. Verbov. 1989. (New Clinical Applications in Dermatology Ser.). (C). text 107.00 (*0-7462-0098-6*) Kluwer Academic.

Talking Points in Dermatology II. Ed. by Julian L. Verbov. 1987. (New Clinical Applications in Dermatology Ser.). 112p. (C). lib. bdg. 82.00 (*0-85200-689-6*) Kluwer Academic.

Talking Trauma: Paramedics & Their Stories. Timothy R. Tangherlini. 1998. LC 97-41468. 280p. pap. 18.00 (*1-57806-043-5*); text 45.00 (*1-57806-042-7*) U Pr of Miss.

Talking with Clients about Family Planning: A Guide for Health Care Providers. AVSC International Staff. 1995. 102p. pap. text 10.00 (*1-885063-11-3*) EngenderHlth.

Talking with Kids about AIDS: Resource Manual. Jennifer Tiffany et al. 1991. (Talking with Kids about AIDS: a Program for Parents & Other Adults Who Care Ser.). (Illus.). 86p. (Orig.). pap. 6.00 (*0-9629938-0-8*) Parent AIDS.

Talking with Kids about AIDS: Resource Manual & Teaching Guide, Set. Jennifer Tiffany et al. 1991. (Talking with Kids about AIDS: a Program for Parents & Other Adults Who Care Ser.). (Illus.). 178p. (Orig.). 9.50 (*0-9629938-2-4*) Parent AIDS.

Talking with Kids about AIDS: Teaching Guide. Jennifer Tiffany et al. 1991. (Talking with Kids about AIDS: a Program for Parents & Other Adults Who Care Ser.). (Illus.). 92p. (Orig.). pap., tchr. ed. 6.00 (*0-9629938-1-6*) Parent AIDS.

Talking with Patients: A Self Psychological View of Creative Intuition & Analytic Discipline. Sanford Shapiro. 1995. LC 95-14483. 224p. 40.00 (*1-56821-598-3*) Aronson.

Talking with Patients: Keys to Good Communication. Philip R. Myerscough & Michael J. Ford. 3rd ed. 1996. (Oxford Medical Publications). (Illus.). 258p. (C). pap. text 39.50 (*0-19-262570-5*) OUP.

Talking with Patients Vol. 1: The Theory of Doctor-Patient Communication. Eric J. Cassell. 1985. LC 84-26120. (Mit Press Series on the Humanistic & Social Dimensions of Medicine Ser.). (Illus.). 240p. pap. 17.95 (*0-262-53055-4*) MIT Pr.

Talking with Patients Vol. 2: Clinical Technique. Eric J. Cassell. 1985. 215p. pap. 17.95 (*0-262-53056-2*) MIT Pr.

Talking with Your Child about AIDS. Barbara Prince. 1993. LC 92-42452. (Growing Together Ser.). pap. 2.25 (*0-8298-0865-5*) Pilgrim OH.

Talks to Teachers on Psychology: And to Students on Some of Life's Ideals. William James. Ed. by Frederick Burkhardt et al. 1983. (Works of William James: No. 10). (Illus.). 368p. 44.50 (*0-674-86785-8*) HUP.

Taming Asthma & Allergy by Controlling Your Environment: A Guide for Patients. Robert A. Wood. 1995. LC 94-79901. (Illus.). 164p. (Orig.). 14.95 (*0-9643272-0-1*) A & AFOA.

Taming of Solitude: Separation Anxiety in Psychoanalysis. Jean-Michel Quinodoz. 1993. LC 93-9866. (New Library of Psychoanalysis : Vol. 20). 208p. (C). 85.00 (*0-415-09153-5*); pap. 29.99 (*0-415-09154-3*) Routledge.

Taming of the Chew: A Holistic Guide to Stopping Compulsive Eating. Denise C. Lamothe. Ed. by Laurie Blakeney. 2nd ed. 1998. (Illus.). 185p. (Orig.). pap. 14.95 (*0-9663653-0-5*) Questover Bks.

Taming Wild Thoughts. Wilfred R. Bion. 1997. 72p. pap. (*1-85575-168-2*) Karnac Bks GBR. *Dist:* Other Pr LLC.

Tamoxifen: A Guide for Clinicians & Patients. Ed. by V. Craig Jordan. 1996. 200p. (*0-9641823-4-3*) PRR.

Tamoxifen: Beyond the Antiestrogen. Ed. by John A. Kellen. 1996. 392p. 94.50 (*0-8176-3842-3*); (*3-7643-3842-3*) Birkhauser.

Tamoxifen: Index of New Information Involving Health Dangers, Risks, Adverse Reactions & Body Damage Treatments with Authors, Subjects & References. Jackson J. Tiller. 1996. 150p. 57.50 (*0-7883-1232-4*); pap. 47.50 (*0-7883-1233-2*) ABBE Pubs Assn.

Tamoxifen: Index of New Information with Authors, Subjects, Research Categories & References. Jackson J. Tiller. 1996. 150p. 57.50 (*0-7883-1230-8*); pap. 47.50 (*0-7883-1231-6*) ABBE Pubs Assn.

Tamoxifen: New Hope in the Fight Against Breast Cancer. John F. Kessler & Greg A. Annussek. 1999. LC 98-91011. 224p. mass mkt. 5.99 (*0-380-81028-X*, Avon Bks) Morrow Avon.

Tamoxifen & Breast Cancer. Michael W. DeGregorio & Valerie J. Wiebe. 1994. LC 93-43148. (Illus.). 136p. (C). 30.00 (*0-300-05907-8*) Yale U Pr.

Tamoxifen & Breast Cancer. Michael W. DeGregorio. 2nd ed. 1999. LC 99-35322. ix, 118p. pap. text 13.95 (*0-300-07951-6*) Yale U Pr.

Tamoxifen & Breast Cancer: Congressional Hearing. Ed. by Arlen Specter. 2000. 51p. (C). reprint ed. pap. text 20.00 (*0-7567-0261-5*) DIANE Pub.

Tamoxifen & Breast Cancer: Hearing before a Subcommittee of the Committee on Appropriations, United States Senate, One Hundred Fifth Congress, Second Session, Special Hearing. Contrib. by U. S. Congress, House Committee on Appropriations, Subcommittee on the Departments of Labor, Health and Human Services, Education and Related Agencies. 1998. LC 98-217010. (*0-16-057288-6*) USGPO.

Tamoxifen for the Treatment & Prevention of Breast Cancer: A Clinicians' Guide. V. Craig Jordan. 1998. LC 98-68150. (Illus.). 260p. 49.95 (*1-891483-00-5*) PRR.

Tamoxifen for the Treatment & Prevention of Breast Cancer: A Patient's Guide. Ed. by V. Craig Jordan. 1999. (Illus.). 260p. 49.95 (*1-891483-02-1*) PRR.

Tamoxifen, Molecular Basis of Use in Cancer Treatment & Prevention. Helen Wiseman. 1994. LC 94-18163. 216p. 159.95 (*0-471-94316-9*) Wiley.

Tangled Minds: Understanding Alzheimer's Disease & Other Dementias. Muriel R. Gillick. 1998. LC 97-34928. 224p. 25.95 (*0-525-94145-2*) Dutton Plume.

Taniguchi Symposia on Brain Sciences No. 18: Emotion, Memory & Behavior: Studies on Human & Nonhuman Primates. Ed. by Teruo Nakajima & Taketoshi Ono. 1995. (Taniguchi Symposia on Brain Sciences Ser.: No. 18). 99.95 (*0-8493-7777-3*, JS7777) CRC Pr.

Tao & Dharma: Chinese Medicine & Ayurveda. Robert Svoboda & Arnie Lade. 1995. LC 95-80859. 155p. (Orig.). pap. 12.95 (*0-914955-21-7*) Lotus Pr.

Tao of Chaos: DNA & the I Ching Unlocking the Code of the Universe. Katya Walter. 1996. LC 93-80811. 288p. pap. 15.95 (*1-85230-806-0*) Element MA.

Tao of Ch'i: Healing with the Unseen Life Force. Mark D. Mincolla. 1995. (Illus.). 52p. (Orig.). pap. 14.95 (*0-963281-1-9*) Pennyroyal Pr.

Tao of Health & Longevity. Liu Da. 1997. (Illus.). 224p. pap. text 10.95 (*1-56924-718-8*) Marlowe & Co.

Tao of Health, Sex & Longevity: A Modern Practical Guide to the Ancient Way. Daniel P. Reid. 1989. 416p. pap. 15.00 (*0-671-64811-X*, Fireside) S&S Trade Pap.

***Tao of Immunology: A Revolutionary New Understanding of Our Body's Defenses.** Lappe. 2001. 332p. pap. text 22.50 (*0-7382-0628-8*) Perseus Bks Grp.

Tao of Psychology: Synchronicity & the Self. Jean S. Bolen. 1982. LC 79-1778. 128p. pap. 13.00 (*0-06-250081-3*) Harper SF.

Tao Shiatsu: Life Medicine for the Twenty-First Century. Ryokyu Endo. 1994. (Illus.). 192p. pap. 19.00 (*0-87040-940-9*) Japan Pubns USA.

Tap Water & the Dynamics of Good Health. Robert A. Gegan. 1986. 84p. (Orig.). pap. text 3.95 (*0-940062-03-8*) Consumer Info Pubns.

Tapestry of Cultural Issues in Art Therapy. Ed. by Anna R. Hiscox & Abby C. Calisch. 1998. LC 98-159181. 250p. pap. (*1-85302-576-3*) Jessica Kingsley GBR. *Dist:* Taylor & Francis.

Tapestry of Service No. 1: The Evolution of Nursing in Australia. Bartz Schultz. 1991. (Illus.). 440p. text (*0-443-02719-6*) Church.

Tapetum: Cytology, Function, Biochemistry & Evolution. Ed. by M. Hesse et al. 1993. (Illus.). 159p. 150.00 (*0-387-82486-3*) Spr-Verlag.

Taping Techniques: Principles & Practice. Ed. by Rose MacDonald. 1994. (Illus.). 263p. pap. text 50.00 (*0-7506-0577-4*) Buttrwrth-Heinemann.

Taping Techniques: Principles & Practice. Rose MacDonald. 2nd ed. 2001. (Illus.). 208p. pap. 47.50 (*0-7506-4150-9*) Buttrwrth-Heinemann.

Tappan's Handbook of Healing Massage Techniques: Classic, Holistic & Emerging Methods. Frances M. Tappan & Patricia J. Benjamin. 3rd ed. 1997. LC 97-30651. (Illus.). 448p. (C). pap. 34.95 (*0-8385-3676-X*, A-3676-2) P-H.

Taproots: Underlying Principles of Milton Erickson's Therapy & Hypnosis. William H. O'Hanlon. 1987. (Professional Bks.). 180p. text 22.95 (*0-393-70031-3*) Norton.

TAPS Test of Auditory-Perceptual Skills. Morrison F. Gardner. 1985. 75p. (Orig.). pap., tchr. ed. 16.95 (*0-931421-06-3*); tchr. ed. 54.50 (*0-931421-07-1*) Psychol Educ Pubns.

Taranta Rheumatic Fever. 2nd ed. 1989. pap. text (*0-7462-0104-4*) Kluwer Academic.

Tarascon Adult Emergency Pocketbook. Steven G. Rothrock. rev. ed. 1998. 128p. pap. 9.95 (*1-882742-10-9*) Tarascon Pub.

***Tarascon Adult Emergency Pocketbook.** Steven G. Rothrock. 2nd rev. ed. 2001. 192p. pap. text 11.95 (*1-882742-23-0*) Tarascon Pub.

Tarascon Pediatric Emergency Pocketbook 3rd ed. Steven G. Rothrock. 3rd rev. ed. 1998. 128p. pap. 9.95 (*1-882742-11-7*) Tarascon Pub.

***Tarascon Pocket Orthopaedica.** Damian M. Rispoli. 2001. 192p. pap. text 11.95 (*1-882742-24-9*) Tarascon Pub.

***Tarascon Pocket Pharmacopoeia 2002 Deluxe Lab-coat pocket Edition.** Steven M. Green MD. 3rd rev. ed. 2001. 256p. pap. text 17.95 (*1-882742-22-2*) Tarascon Pub.

***Tarascon Pocket Pharmacopoeia 2002 Classic Shirt-pocket Edition.** 16th ed. 2001. 128p. pap. text 8.95 (*1-882742-21-4*) Tarascon Pub.

Tardive Dyskinesia. Ed. by H. Haag et al. 1992. LC 91-35360. (WHO Expert Series on Neuroscience: Vol. 1). (Illus.). 136p. text 29.00 (*0-88937-086-9*) Hogrefe & Huber Pubs.

Target: Techniques for Aphasia Rehabilitation - Generating Effective Treatment. Robert Goldfarb & Mary J. Santo Pietro. 1994. 400p. text 45.00 (*0-937857-50-5*, 1434) Speech Bin.

Target: The Antimicrobial Reference Guide to Effective Treatment. David Aucoin. 1994. (Illus.). (Orig.). 161p. pap. 85.00 (*1-889750-04-2*); disk 35.00 (*1-889750-05-0*) Nrth Amer Compendiums.

Target of Health in Ethiopia: A Holistic Reader in Applied Anthropology. Ed. by Simon D. Messing. 1973. 285p. text 37.50 (*0-8422-5074-3*); pap. text 16.95 (*0-8422-0261-7*) Irvington.

Target of Penicillin: The Murein Sacculus of Bacterial Cell Walls, Architecture & Growth. Ed. by R. Hakenbeck et al. 1983. LC 83-15215. xxviii, 664p. 173.10 (*3-11-009705-2*) De Gruyter.

Target Organ & the Toxic Process. Ed. by P. L. Chambers et al. 1988. (Archives of Toxicology Ser.: Suppl. 12). (Illus.). 462p. 182.00 (*0-387-18512-7*) Spr-Verlag.

Target Organ Toxicity Gerald M. Cohen. 1986. 339.90 (*0-8493-5769-1*, RA1211);Vol. I. 272p. lib. bdg. 206.00 (*0-8493-5775-6*);Vol. 2. 288p. lib. bdg. 206.00 (*0-8493-5776-4*) CRC Pr.

Target Receptors for Anxiolytics & Hypnotics: From Molecular Pharmacology to Therapeutics. Ed. by J. Mendlewicz & Giorgio Racagni. 1992. (International Academy for Biomedical & Drug Research Ser.: Vol. 3). (Illus.). vi, 162p. 152.25 (*3-8055-5602-0*) S Karger.

Targeted Drug Delivery. Ed. by R. I. Juliano et al. 1991. (Handbook of Experimental Pharmacology Ser.: Vol. 100). (Illus.). 364p. 284.00 (*0-387-52843-1*) Spr-Verlag.

Targeted Molecular Imaging in Oncology. Ed. by E. Edmund Kim & David J. Yang. 2000. LC 00-55719. (Illus.). 312p. 169.00 (*0-387-95028-1*) Spr-Verlag.

Targeted Therapeutic Systems. Praveen Tyle. Ed. by Bhanu Ram. 1989. (Targeted Diagnosis & Therapy Ser.: Vol. 3). (Illus.). 416p. text 210.00 (*0-8247-8181-3*) Dekker.

Targeting Autism: What We Know, Don't Know & Can Do to Help Young Children with Autism. Shirley Cohen. 1998. LC 97-28090. 217p. pap. text 14.95 (*0-520-21309-2*) U CA Pr.

Targeting Autism: What We Know, Don't Know, & Can Do to Help Young Children with Autism & Related Disorders. Shirley Cohen. 1998. LC 97-28090. 217p. text 40.00 (*0-520-21011-5*) U CA Pr.

Targeting Intelligible Speech: A Phonological Approach to Remediation. Barbara W. Hodson. 2nd ed. 1990. pap. 21.00 (*0-316-36801-6*, Little Brwn Med Div) Lppncott W & W.

Targeting Intelligible Speech: A Phonological Approach to Remediation. Barbara W. Hodson & Elaine P. Paden. 2nd ed. 1991. LC 90-5424. (Illus.). 190p. (C). pap. text 27.00 (*0-89079-405-7*, 1582) PRO-ED.

Targeting of Drugs: Advances in System Constructs, Vol. 4. G. Gregoriadis et al. 1995. LC 94-41747. (NATO Advanced Science Institutes Ser.: Vol. 273). (Illus.). 216p. (C). text 85.00 (*0-306-44910-2*, Kluwer Plenum) Kluwer Academic.

Targeting of Drugs 5 Vol. 5: Strategies for Oligonucleotide & Gene Delivery in Therapy; Proceedings of a NATO ASI Held in Cape Sounion, Greece, June 24-July 5, 1995, Vol. 214. Ed. by Gregory Gregoriadis & Brenda McCormack. 1997. LC 96-37079. (NATO ASI Ser.: Vol. 290). 206p. 85.00 (*0-306-45504-8*) Plenum.

Targeting of Drugs 1: Anatomical & Physiological Considerations. Ed. by George H. Poste & Gregory Gregoriadis. 1988. LC 88-28892. (Illus.). 230p. 79.50 (*0-306-43023-1*, Plenum Trade) Perseus Pubng.

Targeting of Drugs 6: Strategies for Stealth Therapeutic Systems: Proceedings of a NATO ASI Held in Cape Sounion Beach, Greece, June 24-July 5, 1997. Ed. by Gregory Gregoriadis & Brenda McCormack. 1998. LC 98-29831. (NATO ASI Series A: Vol. 300). (Illus.). 312p. (C). text 105.00 (*0-306-45937-X*) Plenum.

Targeting of Drugs 3 Vol. 3: The Challenge of Peptides & Proteins. G. Gregoriadis et al. 1993. (NATO ASI Series A, Life Sciences: Vol. 238). (Illus.). 138p. (C). text 79.50 (*0-306-44400-3*) Plenum.

Targeting of Drugs 2: Optimization Strategies. Ed. by Gregory Gregoriadis et al. 1990. LC 90-14327. (NATO Advanced Science Institutes Ser.: Vol. 199). (Illus.). 194p. (C). text 102.00 (*0-306-43739-2*, Kluwer Plenum) Kluwer Academic.

***Targets for Cancer Chemotherapy: Transcription Factors & Other Nuclear Proteins.** Ed. by Nicholas B. La & Jennifer Schussler. 2002. LC 2001-51561. (Cancer Drug Discovery & Development Ser.). 425p. 165.00 (*0-89603-938-2*) Humana.

Targets for Health for All Two Thousand: Targets in Support of the European Regional Strategy for Health for All. 1985. 201p. pap. text 18.00 (*92-890-1034-7*) World Health.

Tartan Weavers' Guide. James Scarlett. 1985. 16.95 (*0-85683-078-X*) Robin & Russ.

Taschenatlas der Genetik see Color Atlas of Genetics

Task Analysis: An Occupational Performance Approach. Diane Watson. 1997. (Illus.). 454p. (Orig.). (C). pap. text 37.00 (*1-56900-065-4*) Am Occup Therapy.

Task Force Report on Clinician Safety, No. 33. American Psychiatric Association Staff. 1993. LC 93-10489. 35p. pap. text 3.00 (*0-89042-244-3*, 2244) Am Psychiatric.

Task Talk & Text in the Operating Room - A Study in Medical Discourse, 33. Catherine J. Pettinari. Ed. by Roy O. Freedle. 1988. LC 88-10396. (Advances in Discourse Processes Ser.: Vol. 33). 192p. 85.00 (*0-89391-459-2*, Ablex) Greenwood.

Tasks of Emotional Development. Haskel Cohen & Geraldine R. Weil. LC 75-42572. 359p. reprint ed. 35.00 (*0-916598-02-0*) T E D Assocs.

Tasks of Medicine: An Ideology of Care. Ed. by Peter Baume. 1999. 324p. pap. 55.00 (*0-8036-0429-7*) Davis Co.

Taste & Smell Disorders. Allen M. Seiden. 1996. LC 96-23875. (Rhinology & Sinusology Ser.). 75.00 (*0-86577-533-8*) Thieme Med Pubs.

Taste of Home's Down-Home Diabetic Cookbook. Reiman Publications Staff. Ed. by Julie Schnittka. 1996. LC 95-71713. 320p. 17.95 (*0-89821-153-0*, 20287) Reiman Pubns.

Taste of the Good Life: A Cookbook for an Interstitial Cystitis Diet. Beverley Laumann. 1998. LC 98-73062. (Illus.). x, 240p. pap. 24.00 (*0-9665706-0-X*) Freeman Family.

Taste, Olfaction & the Central Nervous System: A Festschrift in Honor of Carl Pfaffmann. Ed. by Donald W. Pfaff. 1985. LC 84-43054. 346p. 29.95 (*0-87470-039-6*) Rockefeller.

Tasting & Smelling. Ed. by Edward C. Carterette et al. 2nd ed. 1997. LC 97-22352. (Handbook of Perception & Cognition Ser.). (Illus.). 231p. text 75.00 (*0-12-161958-3*) Morgan Kaufmann.

Taurine & the Heart. Ed. by H. Iwata et al. 1988. (Developments in Cardiovascular Medicine Ser.). 192p. text 140.50 (*0-89838-396-X*) Kluwer Academic.

Taurine 4: Taurine & Excitable Tissues. Laura Della Corte et al. 2000. (Advances in Experimental Medicine & Biology Ser.: Vol. 483). 664p. 125.00 (*0-306-46447-0*, Kluwer Plenum) Kluwer Academic.

Taurine in Health & Disease, Vol. 359. R. J. Huxtable & D. Michalk. 1994. (Illus.). 470p. (C). text 135.00 (*0-306-44812-2*, Kluwer Plenum) Kluwer Academic.

Taurine 3: Cellular & Regulatory Mechanisms, Vol. 442. Ed. by Steven Schaffer et al. 1998. LC 98-7494. (Advances in Experimental Medicine & Biology Ser.: No. 442). (Illus.). 550p. (C). text 139.50 (*0-306-45914-0*, Kluwer Plenum) Kluwer Academic.

Taurine 2: Basic & Clinical Aspects. International Society for Neurochemistry Staff. Ed. by Ryan J. Huxtable et al. 1996. LC 96-32064. (Advances in Experimental Medicine & Biology Ser.: Vol. 403). (Illus.). 671p. (C). text 167.00 (*0-306-45385-1*, Kluwer Plenum) Kluwer Academic.

Tax-Exempt Financing for Health Care Organizations. Steven B. Kite. 1996. (Health Law & Business Ser.: No. 1100). 125.00 (*1-55871-341-7*) BNA.

Tax-Exempt Status of Health Care Organizations. Bernadette M. Broccolo & Kathleen M. Niles. 1996. (Health Law & Business Ser.: No. 1900). 125.00 (*1-55871-340-9*) BNA.

Tax Treatment of Employment-Based Health Insurance. Leonard Burman. 1994. (Illus.). 59p. (Orig.). (C). pap. text 30.00 (*0-7881-1090-X*) DIANE Pub.

Taxane Anticancer Agents Vol. 583: Basic Science & Current Status. Ed. by Gunda I. Georg et al. 1995. LC 94-37226. (ACS Symposium Ser.: No. 583). (Illus.). 460p. 120.00 (*0-8412-3073-0*) Am Chemical.

Taxicokinetics & New Drug Development. Avraham Yacobi et al. 1989. (Illus.). 264p. 50.00 (*0-08-036084-X*, Pergamon Pr) Elsevier.

Taxol: Science & Applications. Ed. by Matthew Suffness. 1995. (Pharmacology & Toxicology Ser.). 448p. 179.95 (*0-8493-8382-X*, 8382) CRC Pr.

Taxonomy of Behavioral Objectives & Social Readiness Program. Ron Talarico & Francella Hewitt. 2nd rev. ed. 1993. (Illus.). 700p. 89.95 (*0-9635238-0-5*) Prtlnd Habilitat.

Taylor's Family Medicine Review. Ed. by Robert B. Taylor et al. 1998. LC 98-21884. (Illus.). 307p. pap. 46.95 (*0-387-98569-7*) Spr-Verlag.

TB- Human Biology. Daniel D. Chiras & Jay M. Templin. 3rd ed. 1999. (Illus.). 416p. (C). pap. text, tchr. ed. 15.50 (*0-7637-0959-X*, 0959-X) Jones & Bartlett.

TBI Annual Research Index. Charles-Maria V. Arokiasamy et al. 1993. 400p. pap. 29.95 (*1-878205-01-3*) St Lucie Pr.

TBI Annual Research Index, Vol. 1. Debra B. McMorrow & Gregory R. Moss. Ed. by Charles-Maria V. Arokiasamy. 1990. 280p. per. 41.95 (*1-878205-39-0*) St Lucie Pr.

TBI Tool Kit. Linda J. Courtney. Ed. by Pamela G. Burns. 1994. 224p. (Orig.). pap. 24.95 (*1-882855-07-8*) HDI Pubs.

TCM: A Woman's Guide to Healing from Breast Cancer. Nan Lu & Ellen Schaplowsky. 1999. LC 99-94877. (Traditional Chinese Medicine Ser.). (Illus.). xxiv, 358p. pap. 14.00 (*0-380-80902-8*, Avon Bks) Morrow Avon.

TCN Guide to Professional Practice in Clinical Neuropsychology. Ed. by Kenneth Adams & Byron P. Rourke. 1992. vi, 234p. (*90-265-1242-2*); pap. (*90-265-1243-0*) Swets.

Te Linde's Operative Gynecology. Ed. by John A. Rock & John D. Thompson. 8th ed. 1996. LC 96-4875. 1,696p. text 149.00 (*0-397-51399-2*) Lppncott W & W.

Tea: Bioactivity & Therapeutic Potential. Yong-su Zhen. 2000. (Medicinal & Aromatic Plants - Industrial Profiles Ser.: Vol. 17). 160p. 95.00 (*90-5823-033-3*, Harwood Acad Pubs) Gordon & Breach.

Tea Fungus Kombucha: The Natural Remedy & Its Significance in Cases of Cancer & Other Metabolic Diseases. Rosina Fasching. 1995. (Illus.). 56p. pap. (*3-85068-231-5*) Ennsthaler AUT. *Dist:* Am Educ Systs.

Tea Tree Oil. Woodland Publishing Staff. 1999. (Woodland Health Ser.). 32p. pap. text 3.95 (*1-885670-30-3*) Woodland UT.

Teach & Reach Students with Attention Deficit Disorders. Nancy L. Eisenberg & Pamela H. Esser. rev. ed. 1994. (Educator's Handbook & Resource Guide Ser.). (Illus.). 200p. tchr. ed. 19.95 (*0-9630847-0-4*) Multigrowth.

Teach Me Language: A Language Manual for Children with Autism, Asperger's Syndrome & Related Developmental Disorders. Sabrina Freeman & Lorelei Dake. 1997. LC 98-186056. (Illus.). 410p. 59.95 (*0-9657565-0-5*, TML-1) SKF Bks.

Teach Yourself Applied Psychology. Nicky Hayes. 1999. (Illus.). 192p. pap. 10.95 (*0-8442-3938-0*, Contemporary) McGraw-Hill Trade.

***Teach Yourself Herbal Medicine.** Nina Nissen. 2001. 192p. pap. 10.95 (*0-658-01621-0*) McGraw-Hill Prof.

Teach Yourself Human Anatomy & Physiology. David Le Vay. 1995. (Illus.). 384p. pap. 12.95 (*0-8442-3924-0*, Tch Yourself) McGraw-Hill Trade.

Teach Yourself Lip Reading. Olive M. Wyatt. 1974. (Illus.). 172p. 37.95 (*0-398-02128-7*) C C Thomas.

Teach Yourself to Read Modern Medical Chinese: A Step-by-Step Workbook & Guide. Bob Flaws. 1998. LC 98-71172. (CHI & ENG., Illus.). ix, 240p. spiral bd., wbk. ed. 39.95 (*0-936185-99-6*) Blue Poppy Pr.

Teacher-Clinician Planbook & Guide to the Development of Speech Skills. Daniel Ling. 1978. LC 77-93949. pap. text 12.50 (*0-88200-116-7*, A2092) Alexander Graham.

Teacher Preparation for Health Education. 1960. (Technical Report Ser.: No. 193). 19p. pap. text 5.00 (*92-4-120193-2*) World Health.

Teachers As Curriculm Planners: Narratives of Experience. F. Michael Connelly & Jean D. Clandinin. 1988. 240p. (C). text 32.95 (*0-8077-2907-8*); pap. text 18.95 (*0-8077-2906-X*) Tchrs Coll.

Teacher's Guide to Behavioral Interventions: Intervention Strategies for Behavior Problems in the Educational Environment. Kathy K. Wunderlich. 1988. 291p. pap. 28.00 (*1-878372-13-0*) Hawthorne Educ Servs.

Teacher's Guide to Beyond O. K. Win Wenger. 1985. (Psychegenic Library of Experiential Protocols). 36p. (Orig.). pap. 2.00 (*0-931865-05-0*) Proj Renaissance.

Teacher's Guide to the Psychology of Learning. Michael J. Howe. 1984. 254p. pap. 29.95 (*0-631-13578-2*) Blackwell Pubs.

Teacher's Handbook for a Functional Behavior-Based Curriculum: Communicable Models & Guides for Classroom Use. Sidney J. Drumheller. 1972. LC 72-933. 138p. pap. 24.95 (*0-87778-036-6*) Educ Tech Pubns.

Teachers Managing Stress & Preventing Burnout: The Professional Health Solution. Yvonne Gold & Robert A. Roth. 1993. LC 92-39817. 220p. 85.00 (*0-7507-0158-7*); pap. 27.95 (*0-7507-0159-5*) Taylor & Francis (Falmer Pr).

Teacher's Manual: The SUM Program Curriculum in Medical Transcription. Linda C. Campbell & Susan M. Turley. 2nd rev. ed. 1992. 177p. pap. 95.00 (*0-934385-53-X*) Hlth Prof Inst.

Teacher's Window into the Child's Mind: And Papers from the Institute for Neuro-Physiological Psychology. Sally Goddard. 1996. (Illus.). 144p. (C). pap. 19.95 (*0-9615332-5-0*) Fern Ridge Pr.

Teaching—Actions, Methods, Views, Progress, Stress & Burn-Out: Index of New Information with Authors, Subjects, & References. Mickey K. Zaharis. 1996. LC 96-12662. 57.50 (*0-7883-1018-6*); pap. 47.50 (*0-7883-1019-4*) ABBE Pubs Assn.

Teaching a Psychology of People: Resources for Gender & Sociocultural Awareness. Ed. by Phyllis Bronstein & Kathryn Quina. 1988. LC 88-16715. 220p. pap. 29.95 (*1-55798-039-X*) Am Psychol.

Teaching about AIDS: Lesson Plans for Elementary & High School. Eileen P. Flynn. 1988. LC 87-63005. (Illus.). 96p. pap., tchr. ed. 8.95 (*1-55612-113-X*) Sheed & Ward WI.

Teaching about Job Hazards: A Guide for Workers & Their Health Providers. Nina Wallerstein & Harriet Rubenstein. 1993. 141p. pap. 20.00 (*0-87553-209-8*, 008) Am Pub Health.

Teaching about Substance Abuse: A Resource Manual for Faculty Development. 1992. lib. bdg. 79.95 (*0-8490-8825-9*) Gordon Pr.

Teaching about Substance Abuse: A Resource Manual for Faculty Development. Stephen P. Flynn et al. rev. ed. 1995. 46p. (C). pap. text 20.00 (*0-7881-2580-X*) DIANE Pub.

Teaching AIDS. Douglas Tonks. 1995. LC 95-30105. 224p. (C). pap. 22.95 (*0-415-90875-2*) Routledge.

Teaching AIDS. Marcia Quackenbush & Pamela Sargent. rev. ed. 1988. 164p. pap. text 19.95 (*0-941816-41-9*); pap. text 21.95 (*1-56071-029-2*) ETR Assocs.

Teaching Aids for Home Care Nurses. Springhouse Publishing Company Staff. 1995. LC 95-36793. (Illus.). 320p. ring bd. 44.95 (*0-87434-831-5*) Springhouse Corp.

Teaching & Assessing Nurses: A Handbook for Preceptors. Robert Oliver & Colin Endersby. 1995. (Illus.). 166p. pap. text (*0-7020-1720-5*) W B Saunders GBR. *Dist:* Saunders.

Teaching & Learning Communication Skills in Medicine. Suzanne M. Kurtz et al. 1998. LC 98-14387. 272p. (*1-85775-273-2*) Radcliffe Med Pr GBR. *Dist:* Balogh.

Teaching & Learning in Medical Practice. J. W. R. Peyton. 1998. 256p. text 55.00 (*1-900887-00-2*, Manticore Europe) Manticore Pubs.

Teaching & Learning in Schools of Nursing. H. Heidgerken. 1991. 705p. (C). (*81-7002-031-X*) Himalayan Bks IND. *Dist:* St Mut.

Teaching & Learning of Psychotherapy. Rudolf Ekstein & Robert S. Wallerstein. 2nd rev. ed. 1972. LC 70-184442. 277p. 52.50 (*0-8236-6363-9*) Intl Univs Pr.

Teaching & Learning Psychiatry & Behavioral Science. Ed. by Joel Yager. 1982. 560p. text 63.00 (*0-8089-1457-X*, 794943, Grune & Strat) Harcrt Hlth Sci Grp.

Teaching & Learning Strategies in Pharmacy Ethics. Ed. by Amy M. Haddad. 2nd ed. 1997. LC 97-31729. (Journal of Pharmacy Teaching Ser.: Vol. 6, Nos. 1/2). 159p. 24.95 (*0-7890-0378-3*, Pharmctl Prods) Haworth Pr.

Teaching & the Unconscious Mind. J. C. Hill. 1971. LC 78-141661. 176p. 30.00 (*0-8236-6365-5*) Intl Univs Pr.

Teaching & Training Techniques for Hospital Doctors. Ed. by Trevor Bayley & Michael Drury. 1998. LC 99-170979. 136p. pap. (*1-85775-173-6*) Radcliffe Med Pr GBR. *Dist:* Balogh.

Teaching Art to the Deaf. Linda K. Kingsley. 1974. lib. bdg. 250.00 (*0-8490-1179-5*) Gordon Pr.

Teaching Aspects of Health Care. V. Ehlers. 1998. 142p. pap. (*0-7021-4212-3*) Juta & Co ZAF. *Dist:* Intl Spec Bk.

Teaching, Assessing & Evaluation for Clinical Competence. M. Neary. 2000. (Illus.). 224p. pap. (*0-7487-4417-7*) Nelson Thornes GBR. *Dist:* Intl Spec Bk, Trans-Atl Phila.

Teaching Atlas of Brain Imaging. Nancy J. Fischbein et al. 1999. LC 98-32391. (Illus.). 1009p. 129.00 (*0-86577-862-0*) Thieme Med Pubs.

Teaching Atlas of Breast Ultrasound. Wolfgang Leucht & Dagmar Leucht. 2nd ed. 1995. LC 95-39577. (Illus.). 250p. text 99.00 (*0-86577-572-9*) Thieme Med Pubs.

Teaching Atlas of Hand Radiology: A Self-Assessment Text. S. Gilani & B. K. Wignall. 1995. (Illus.). 213p. text (*0-7020-1731-0*) W B Saunders GBR. *Dist:* Saunders.

Teaching Atlas of Head & Neck Imaging. Ed. by Robert Lufkin et al. 1999. 470p. 99.00 (*0-86577-691-1*) Thieme Med Pubs.

Teaching Atlas of Interventional Radiology: Diagnostic & Therapeutic Angiography. Saadoon Kadir. 1999. LC 98-34890. (Illus.). 480p. 99.00 (*0-86577-777-2*) Thieme Med Pubs.

Teaching Atlas of Mammography. Laszlo Tabar & P. B. Dean. 2000. LC 00-61525. (Illus.). 230p. 119.00 (*0-86577-962-7*) Thieme Med Pubs.

Teaching Atlas of Mammography. Lazzlo Tabar & Peter B. Dean. 2nd rev. ed. 1985. (Illus.). 328p. 149.00 (*0-86577-198-7*) Thieme Med Pubs.

Teaching Atlas of Nuclear Medicine. Ed. by Kevin J. Donohoe & Annick Van den Abbeele. 2000. LC 99-40822. (Illus.). 544p. 99.00 (*0-86577-775-6*) Thieme Med Pubs.

Teaching Atlas of Spine Imaging. Ruth G. Ramsey. 1998. LC 98-27857. 149.00 (*3-13-115791-7*) Thieme Med Pubs.

Teaching Atlas of Spine Imaging. Ruth G. Ramsey. 1998. (Illus.). 912p. 149.00 (*0-86577-778-0*) Thieme Med Pubs.

Teaching Atlas of Thoracic Radiology. Sebastian Lange & Paul Stark. 1993. LC 92-49323. 109.00 (*0-86577-467-6*) Thieme Med Pubs.

Teaching Atlas of Urologic Radiology. Sebastian Lange. 1994. LC 94-35149.Tr. of Lehratlanten der Radiologischen Diagnostik. (Illus.). 300p. 109.00 (*0-86577-540-0*) Thieme Med Pubs.

Teaching Basic Behavioural Principles: A Manual for Course Tutors Using "Helping the Retarded" A. C. M. Capie et al. 1985. 88p. tchr. ed. 25.00 (*0-906054-20-6*) St Mut.

Teaching Cases from Annals of Oncology. R. L. Souhami. 1997. LC 96-21996. 196p. lib. bdg. 99.00 (*0-7923-4373-5*) Kluwer Academic.

Teaching Cases from Annals of Oncology. Robert L. Souhami. 1997. LC 96-21996. vi, 196p. pap. text 47.00 (*0-7923-4117-1*) Kluwer Academic.

Teaching Clinical Decison Making: A Handbook for Instructors. Ed. by Randall D. Cebul & Lawrence H. Beck. 1985. LC 85-3532. 192p. 37.50 (*0-275-91333-3*, C1333, Praeger Pubs) Greenwood.

Teaching Clinical Nursing. Ed. by Susan J. Hinchliff. 2nd ed. 1986. LC 85-32550. (Illus.). 296p. (Orig.). (C). pap. (*0-443-02845-1*) Church.

Teaching Comprehensive Medical Care: A Psychological Study of a Change in Medical Education. Kenneth Hammond. 1959. (Commonwealth Fund Publications). 664p. (C). 60.95 (*0-674-86910-9*) HUP.

Teaching Creatively with Video: A Guide for Health Professionals. Jane Westberg & Hilliard Jason. 1994. LC 93-43777. (Medical Education Ser.: Vol. 18). 256p. 36.95 (*0-8261-8360-3*) Springer Pub.

Teaching Developmentally Disabled Children: The Me Book. O. Ivar Lovaas. 1981. LC 80-26047. 250p. pap. 34.00 (*0-936104-78-3*, 1213) PRO-ED.

Teaching During Rounds: A Handbook for Attending Physicians & Residents. Janine C. Edwards. 1992. LC 91-35340. 144p. (Orig.). pap. text 17.95 (*0-8018-4351-0*) Johns Hopkins.

Teaching Elementary Health Science. Walter D. Sorochan & Stephen J. Bender. 2nd ed. 1979. LC 78-62551. (Health Education Ser.). (Illus.). text 28.00 net. (*0-201-07492-3*) Addison-Wesley.

Teaching Elementary School Health. Stephen J. Bender & Walter D. Sorochan. 3rd ed. 1989. (Illus.). 576p. (C). text 45.00 (*0-86720-411-7*, 411-7) Jones & Bartlett.

Teaching Family Medicine in Medical School: A Companion to Predoctoral Education in Family Medicine. David E. Swee. Ed. by STFM and AAFP Staff. 1991. 271p. 25.00 (*0-942295-23-4*) Soc Tchrs Fam Med.

Teaching Family Therapy. Ross Draper et al. 1992. (Systemic Thinking & Practice Ser.). 265p. pap. text (*1-85575-021-X*) Karnac Bks GBR. *Dist:* Other Pr LLC.

Teaching for Better Learning: A Guide for Teachers of Primary Health Care Staff. F. R. Abbatt. 2nd ed. 1992. (ENG, FRE & SPA.). vii, 190p. pap. text 41.00 (*92-4-154442-2*, 1150377) World Health.

Teaching for Health. Lyn Coutts & Leslie K. Hardy. 2nd ed. 1995. (*0-443-04126-1*) Church.

Teaching for Health: The Nurse As Health Educator. Lyn C. Coutts & Leslie K. Hardy. 1989. LC 84-11365. (Illus.). 225p. pap. text (*0-443-02751-X*) Church.

Teaching Function Nursing Practition. Margaret L. Pohl. 4th ed. 1981. 176p. (C). text 23.50 net. (*0-697-05546-9*, WCB McGr Hill) McGrw-H Hghr Educ.

Teaching Gerontology. Ed. by Verle Waters. 1991. 192p. 21.95 (*0-88737-527-8*) Natl League Nurse.

Teaching Group Dynamics: Process & Practices. Nina W. Brown. 1992. LC 92-16144. 176p. 58.00 (*0-275-94380-1*, C4380, Praeger Pubs) Greenwood.

Teaching Health & Science from a Feminist Perspective: A Practical Guide. Sue V. Rosser. 1986. (Athene Ser.). (Illus.). 200p. 36.50 (*0-08-033135-1*); pap. 19.95 (*0-08-033997-2*) Elsevier (Pergamon Pr).

Teaching Health Science. James Neutens & McGuire. 4th ed. 1997. (Health Science Ser.). (Illus.). 152p. (C). pap. text, tchr. ed. 13.95 (*0-7637-0617-5*, 0617-5) Jones & Bartlett.

Teaching Health Statistics: Twenty Lesson & Seminar Outlines. Ed. by Stephen K. Lwanga & Cho-Yook Tye. 1986. (ARA, FRE & SPA.). 230p. pap. text 39.00 (*92-4-156090-8*, 1150261) World Health.

Teaching Hospitals & the Urban Poor. Eli Ginzberg. 2000. LC 00-28294. x, 129p. 20.00 (*0-300-08232-0*) Yale U Pr.

Teaching in Nursing: A Guide to Curriculum, Teaching & Evaluation. Diane M. Billings & Judith Halstead. Ed. by Thomas Eoyang. 1998. LC 97-44011. (Illus.). 640p. text 49.00 (*0-7216-3037-5*) Saunders.

Teaching in the Community: Preparing Nurses for the 21st Century. M. Elaine Tagliareni & Barbara Marckx. 1997. LC 97-11195. 30.95 (*0-88737-726-2*) Natl League Nurse.

Teaching in the Health Related Professions. Steven B. Dowd. 1996. LC 96-14014. 292p. per. 29.95 (*0-89089-732-8*) Carolina Acad Pr.

Teaching in Your Office: A Guide to Teaching Medical Students & Residents. Patrick Alguire et al. 2000. (Illus.). 120p. (C). pap. text 25.00 (*1-930513-07-0*) Amer Coll Phys.

Teaching Interactive Skills in Health Care. Ann Faulkner. 1993. LC 93-36308. 128p. pap. 31.75 (*1-56593-227-7*, 0573) Singular Publishing.

Teaching Interpersonal Skills: A Handbook of Experiential Learning for Health Professionals. Philip Burnard. Ed. by Jo Campling. 1990. (Therapy in Practice Ser.: No. 10). 204p. pap. 23.00 (*0-412-34590-0*, A4190) Chapman & Hall.

Teaching Introductory Psychology: Survival Tips from the Experts. Ed. by Robert J. Sternberg. 1997. LC 97-3870. (Illus.). 193p. pap. text 24.95 (*1-55798-417-4*, 4316860) Am Psychol.

Teaching Job Seeking Skills. Ed. by William H. Burke. 1988. (Professional Series on Traumatic Brain Injury: Vol. 16). 100p. (Orig.). pap. 9.50 (*1-882855-23-X*) HDI Pubs.

Teaching Language-Disabled Children: A Communication Games Intervention. Susan Conant et al. 1983. LC 83-27303. 188p. pap. 17.95 (*0-914797-38-7*) Brookline Bks.

Teaching Literature & Medicine. Anne Hunsaker Hawkins & Marilyn C. McEntyre. 2000. LC 99-43455. (Options for Teaching Ser.). viii, 406p. pap. 22.00 (*0-87352-357-1*) Modern Lang.

***Teaching Made Easy: A Manual for Health Professionals.** Ruth Chambers & David Wall. 1999. 216p. pap. (*1-85775-373-9*) Radcliffe Med Pr GBR. *Dist:* Balogh.

Teaching Medical Transcription: Meeting the Challenges of the '90s! 1993. 52p. pap. 195.00 incl. VHS (*0-934385-58-0*) Hlth Prof Inst.

Teaching Medicine in the Community: A Guide for Undergraduate Education. Ed. by C. Whitehouse et al. 1997. LC 96-30191. (Oxford General Practice Ser.: No. 38). (Illus.). 238p. pap. text 69.50 (*0-19-262653-1*) OUP.

Teaching Method for Brain-Injured & Hyperactive Children: A Demonstration-Pilot Study. William M. Cruickshank. 1981. LC 81-6255. (Syracuse University Special Education & Rehabilitation Monographs: No. 6). (Illus.). 576p. reprint ed. lib. bdg. 97.50 (*0-313-23071-4*, CRTC) Greenwood.

Teaching More Than Medicine: Psychosocial Considerations in Pediatric Oncology. J. Van Eys & D. R. Copeland. 1993. 228p. pap. 24.95 (*1-85070-515-1*, Parthenon Pbng) CRC Pr.

Teaching Nursing. Sandra DeYoung. Ed. by Debra Hunter. 1999. 258p. (C). pap. text 45.00 (*0-201-09265-4*) Addison-Wesley.

Teaching Nursing in the Neighborhoods: The Northeastern University Model. Ed. by Peggy Matteson. 1995. (Teaching of Nursing Ser.). (Illus.). 256p. 34.95 (*0-8261-9100-2*) Springer Pub.

Teaching Nutrition. Joanne P. Nestor & Judith A. Glotzer. 1981. 302p. pap. text 20.00 (*0-89011-559-1*) Abt Bks.

Teaching Nutrition: A Review of Programs & Research. Ed. by Joanne P. Nestor & Judith A. Glotzer. 1984. 302p. reprint ed. pap. text 32.00 (*0-8191-4115-1*) U Pr of Amer.

Teaching Nutrition & Food Science. Margaret Knight. 1976. pap. 20.95 (*0-7134-3099-0*) Trafalgar.

Teaching of Dynamic Psychiatry: A Reappraisal of the Goals & Techniques in the Teaching of Psychoanalytic Psychiatry. Ed. by Grete L. Bibring. 1968. LC 67-27426. 277p. 40.00 (*0-8236-6380-9*) Intl Univs Pr.

Teaching of Genetics in the Undergraduate Medical Curriculum & in Postgraduate Training. 1962. (Technical Report Ser.: No. 238). 19p. pap. text 3.00 (*92-4-120238-6*) World Health.

Teaching of Human Sexuality in Schools for Health Professionals. J. Burton et al. 1974. (Public Health Papers: No. 57). pap. text 5.00 (*92-4-130057-4*, 1110057) World Health.

Teaching of Immunology in the Medical Curriculum: Report of a WHO Expert Committee, 1967. 1967. (Technical Report Ser.: No. 358). 46p. pap. text 5.00 (*92-4-120358-7*, 1100358) World Health.

Teaching of Psychosomatic Medicine & Consultation-Liaison Psychiatry. Ed. by Adam J. Krakowski & C. P. Kimball. 1979. (Bibliotheca Psychiatrica Ser.: No. 159). pap. 72.25 (*3-8055-2955-4*) S Karger.

Teaching of Public Health in Europe. J. D. Cottrell et al. 1969. (Monographs: No. 58). 246p. pap. text 36.00 (*92-4-140058-7*, 1140058) World Health.

Teaching Orthopedically Handicapped. Jack Rudman. (National Teacher Examination Ser.: NT-25). pap. 23.95 (*0-8373-8435-4*) Nat Learn.

Teaching Patient Education Skills: A Curriculum for Residents. Marion F. Fass et al. 1983. 200p. 5.00 (*0-942295-14-5*) Soc Tchrs Fam Med.

Teaching Patients with Low Literacy Skills. Cecilia C. Doak et al. 2nd ed. 1995. LC 95-11640. 224p. pap. text 30.95 (*0-397-55161-4*) Lppncott W & W.

Teaching Persons with a Brain Injury: What to Expect. Tampa General Rehabilitation Center Staff. 2nd rev. ed. 1996. (Coping Ser.: Vol. 5). 64p. pap. 9.50 (*1-882855-51-5*) HDI Pubs.

Teaching Philosophy to Gifted Students: A Secondary Level Course of Study for Teachers & Administrators. James LoGiudice. 1985. 12.00 (*0-910609-09-8*) Gifted Educ Pr.

***Teaching Physical Education for Learning with Powerweb: Health & Human Performance.** Judith Rink. 3rd ed. 2001. text 59.38 (*0-07-250617-2*) McGrw-H Hghr Educ.

Teaching Reading to Deaf Children. Beatrice O. Hart. 1978. LC 78-50668. pap. text 16.95 (*0-88200-117-5*, C1119) Alexander Graham.

Teaching Research Curriculum for Moderately & Severely Handicapped: Gross & Fine Motor. H.D. Fredericks et al. 1980. (Illus.). 264p. pap. 41.95 (*0-398-04035-4*) C C Thomas.

Teaching Research Curriculum for Moderately & Severely Handicapped: Self-Help & Cognitive. H.D. Fredericks et al. 1980. (Illus.). 280p. pap. 42.95 (*0-398-04034-6*) C C Thomas.

Teaching Slides for Respiratory Disease Slide Set: Principles of Patient Care. Robert L. Wilkins & James R. Dexter. 2nd ed. 1997. 35.00 (*0-8036-0264-2*) Davis Co.

Teaching Social Skills to Hearing-Impaired Students. Maureen A. Smith & Patrick J. Schloss. 1990. (Centennial Celebration Ser.). 203p. (Orig.). pap. text 23.95 (*0-88200-169-8*) Alexander Graham.

Teaching Sports Medicine & Recreation to Family Practice Residents. Ed. by Society for Teachers of Family Medicine, Task Forc. 1981. 122p. 5.00 (*0-942295-15-3*) Soc Tchrs Fam Med.

Teaching Strategies for Language Development. Jane Rieke et al. 1977. 119p. pap. text 24.00 (*0-8089-0996-7*, 793540, Grune & Strat) Harcrt Hlth Sci Grp.

Teaching Stress Management & Relaxation Skills: An Instructor's Guide. John D. Curtis et al. 1985. (Illus.). 280p. text 26.50 (*0-9611456-2-5*, Coulee Press) Adastra Pub.

Teaching Stress Management Skills: A Manual for Beginning & Experienced Teachers. Frances K. Wiggins & Suni Petersen. 1986. (Illus.). 167p. (Orig.). (C). pap. text 16.95 (*0-942937-01-5*) Rivijon Pr.

Teaching Students Geriatric Research. Ed. by Margaret A. Perkinson et al. 2000. LC 00-23164. (Illus.). xviii, 85p. 39.95 (*0-7890-0996-X*); pap. text 24.95 (*0-7890-0997-8*) Haworth Pr.

Teaching Students in Clinical Settings. Stengelhofen. 1992. 244p. pap. 44.75 (*1-56593-119-X*, 0422) Singular Publishing.

Teaching Students with Learning Disabilities: Strategies for Success. Ed. by Karen A. Waldron. 1992. (Illus.). 174p. (Orig.). (C). pap. 24.95 (*1-879105-40-3*, 0275) Thomson Learn.

Teaching Students with Mild & Moderate Learning Problems. John J. Langone. 1990. 472p. pap. text 44.00 (*0-205-12362-7*, H23625) Allyn.

Teaching Students with Severe Disabilities in Inclusive Settings. Maryann Demchak & American Association on Mental Retardation Staff. 1997. LC 97-36030. (Innovations Ser.). 21.95 (*0-940898-49-7*) Am Assn Mental.

Teaching Students with Severe Emotional & Learning Impairments. Ellen Browning. 1983. 331p. text 37.95 (*0-205-07677-7*, H76771) Allyn.

Teaching Teens with ADD & ADHD: A Quick Reference Guide for Teachers & Parents. Chris A. Zeigler Dendy. 2000. LC 00-63433. (Illus.). xix, 352p. pap. 18.95 (*1-890627-20-8*) Woodbine House.

Teaching the Dyslexic Child. Anita Griffiths. 1978. LC 78-12875. pap. 12.00 (*0-87879-205-8*) Acad Therapy.

Teaching the Educable Mentally Retarded. Robert A. Sedlak & Denise M. Sedlak. 1985. LC 84-16344. (SUNY Series in Special Education). (Illus.). 334p. (C). text 22.50 (*0-88706-055-2*) State U NY Pr.

Teaching the Moderately & Severely Handicapped, Vol. III. Michael Bender et al. 1976. LC 79-46596. 272p. pap. text 29.00 (*0-936104-54-6*, 1111) PRO-ED.

Teaching the Practice of Nursing. Brink & J. M. Mellish. 3rd ed. 1991. pap. text 45.00 (*0-409-11154-6*) Buttrwrth-Heinemann.

Teaching the Student with Spina Bifida. Ed. by Fern L. Rowley-Kelly & Donald H. Reigel. 1992. 496p. (Orig.). (C). pap. 40.00 (*1-55766-064-6*) P H Brookes.

Teaching the Tiger: A Handbook for Individuals Involved in the Education of Students with Attention Deficit Disorders, Tourette Syndrome or Obsessive-Compulsive Disorders. Marilyn P. Dornbush & Sheryl K. Pruitt. 1995. LC 95-2018. (Illus.). 200p. pap. 35.00 (*1-878267-34-5*) Hope Pr CA.

Teaching Transcultural Care: A Guide for Teachers of Nursing & Health Care. Paula McGee. 1992. LC 92-22885. 38.25 (*1-56593-065-7*, 0379) Singular Publishing.

Teachings from the Heart. Tarthang Tulku. 1998. LC 97-42543. (Nyingma Psychology Ser.). 400p. pap. 16.95 (*0-89800-279-6*) Dharma Pub.

Team Approach to Audiologic Assessment: A Module for Training Personnel Serving Families of Deaf & Hard of Hearing Infants & Young Children. Ed. by Valerie Schuyler. 1993. (Early Intervention Ser.). 48p. (C). ring bd. 89.00 incl. VHS (*0-9618297-9-6*) Hearing & Speech.

Team Approach to the Aquatic Continuum of Care. Charlotte O. Norton & Lynette J. Jamison. 2000. (Illus.). 200p. pap. text 29.99 (*0-7506-7168-8*) Buttrwrth-Heinemann.

Team-Based Health Care Organizations: Blueprint for Success. Jo Manion et al. 1996. LC 96-19770. 375p. 64.00 (*0-8342-0782-6*) Aspen Pub.

***Team Guide to Communication.** John Middleton. 2000. 224p. pap. (*1-85775-411-5*) Radcliffe Med Pr GBR. *Dist:* Balogh.

***Team Performance in Health Care: Assessment & Development.** Ed. by Gloria D. Heinemann & Antonette M. Zeiss. 2002. LC 2001-38934. (Issues in the Practice of Psychology Ser.). (*0-306-46707-0*, Kluwer Plenum) Kluwer Academic.

Team Physician's Handbook. Ed. by Morris B. Mellion et al. 2nd rev. ed. 1996. LC 96-45304. (Illus.). 910p. pap. 64.95 (*1-56053-174-6*) Hanley & Belfus.

Team Surgery - A Medical Information Management System: Your Guide to Successful Surgery Preparation & Recovery. Barbara Riley & Douglas Stewart. 2000. 10.00 (*0-9666043-1-8*) Team Surgery.

Teamwork for Primary & Shared Care. Peter Pritchard & James Pritchard. 2nd ed. 1994. (Practical Guides for General Practice Ser.). (Illus.). 158p. pap. text 29.95 (*0-19-262527-6*) OUP.

Tear Film: Structure, Function & Clinical Examination. Donald Korb. 2002. (Illus.). 160p. 94.50 (*0-7506-4196-7*) Buttrwrth-Heinemann.

Tears & Rage: The Nursing Crisis in America. Jane Schweitzer. 1996. LC 95-80226. (Illus.). 244p. (Orig.). pap. 18.95 (*1-883422-05-1*) Adams-Blake.

Technetium Ninety-Nine-M: Generators, Chemistry, & Preparation of Radiopharmaceuticals. William C. Eckelman. 1983. (Illus.). 168p. pap. 28.00 (*0-08-029144-9*, Pergamon Pr) Elsevier.

Technical Advances in AIDS Research in the Human Nervous System: Proceedings of a NIH Workshop Held in Washington, D. C., October 4-5, 1993. Ed. by Eugene O. Major et al. 1995. (Illus.). 352p. (C). text 110.00 (*0-306-45000-3*, Kluwer Plenum) Kluwer Academic.

Technical Advances in Biomedical Physics. Ed. by Philip P. Dendy. 1984. text 236.00 (*90-247-2934-3*) Kluwer Academic.

Technical & Biological Components of Marrow Transplantation. Ed. by C. Dean Buckner. 1995. LC 95-1584. (Cancer Treatment & Research Ser.: Vol. 76). 400p. (C). text 260.00 (*0-7923-3394-2*) Kluwer Academic.

Technical & Economic Study on Reduction, Based on Best Available Technology. European Communities Staff. 1994. 244p. pap. (*92-826-7131-3*, CR-81-43-599ENC) Comm Europ Commun BEL. *Dist:* Bernan Associates.

***Technical & Ethical Guidelines for Workers' Health Surveillance.** 1999. (Occupational Safety & Health Ser.: Vol. 72). (ENG, FRE & SPA.). x, 64p. pap. 7.95 (*92-2-110828-7*) Intl Labour Office.

Technical & Managerial Guidelines for Vasectomy Services. WHO Staff. 1988. 135p. 22.00 (*92-4-154218-7*) World Health.

Technical & Physical Parameters for Quality Assurance in Med Diag Rad. B M. Moores. 1989. (British Institute Radiology Report Ser.: No. 18). pap. (*0-905749-18-9*) Med Physics Pub.

Technical Bulletin: Color Duplex Imaging for Graft Surveillance of the Autologous Vein Graft. 1998. pap. (*1-930047-36-3*, TECH3) Am Inst Ultrasound.

Technical Bulletin: How to Interpret the Ultrasound Output Display Standard for Higher Acoustic Output Diagnostic Ultrasound Devices. 1998. (Illus.). pap. (*1-930047-38-X*, TECH1) Am Inst Ultrasound.

Technical Bulletin: Performance of the Basic Fetal Cardiac Ultrasound Examination. 1998. (Illus.). pap. (*1-930047-37-1*, TECH2) Am Inst Ultrasound.

Technical Bulletin: Transducer Manipulation. 1999. (Illus.). pap. (*1-930047-35-5*, TECH4) Am Inst Ultrasound.

Technical Knowledge in American Culture: Science, Technology, & Medicine since the Early 1800s. Ed. by Hamilton Cravens et al. 1996. LC 95-19084. (History of American Science & Technology Ser.). (FRE & GER.). 280p. (Orig.). (C). pap. text 24.95 (*0-8173-0793-1*) U of Ala Pr.

Technical Magnetic Resonance Imaging. Michael G. Aquilia et al. 1996. 287p. (C). pap. 37.50 (*0-8385-8836-0*, A8836-7) McGraw-Hill Prof.

Technical Manual. Ed. by Virginia Vengelen-Tyler. 12th rev. ed. 1996. (Illus.). 752p. 94.00 (*1-56395-062-6*, PC97-TM9612) Am Assn Blood.

Technical Manual/Standards. 3rd ed. 2000. cd-rom (*1-56395-135-5*) Am Assn Blood.

Technical, Medical, & Educational Problems of Acute Care: Proceedings of the International Symposium on Acute Care, 4th, November, 1975. International Symposium on Acute Care Staff. Ed. by B. M. Tavares. 1977. (Current Topics in Critical Care Medicine Ser.: Vol. 2). (Illus.). 200p. 42.75 (*3-8055-2374-2*) S Karger.

Technical Principles, Design, & Safety of Joint Implants. Ed. by Gottfried H. Buchhorn & Hans-Georg Willert. 1994. LC 92-1425. (Illus.). 432p. 159.00 (*0-88937-090-7*) Hogrefe & Huber Pubs.

Technical Tips for Hand Surgery. Ed. by Morton L. Kasdan et al. 1994. LC 92-55066. 328p. 71.00 (*1-56053-020-0*) Hanley & Belfus.

Technical Veterinary Dictionary. Wolfgang Lindeke. 1972. (ENG, GER, RUS & SLV.). 185p. 95.00 (*0-8288-6421-7*, M-9894) Fr & Eur.

Technicians ECG Analyzer. Burdick Corporation Staff. 1973. 1p. pap. 7.51 (*0-13-898610-X*) P-H.

Technician's Manual Veteran Dentistry. Steven E. Holmstrom. 1999. LC 99-39640. (Illus.). 355p. (C). pap. text 35.00 (*0-7216-8187-5*) Saunders.

Technicians of the Finite: The Rise & Decline of the Schizophrenic in American Thought, 1840-1960, 9. S. P. Fullinwider. 1982. LC 81-23771. (Contributions in Medical History Ser.: No. 9). 253p. 63.00 (*0-313-23021-8*, FFI/) Greenwood.

Technique & Practice Vol. 3: The Greenson Seminars on the Psychoanalytic Technique & Practice of Assessment from the Initial Contact to the Treatment Recommendation. Lee D. Jaffe. unabr. ed. 2001. 100p. pap. 26.50 (*0-8236-6423-6*, 06423) Intl Univs Pr.

Technique & Practice of Intensive Psychotherapy. Richard D. Chessick. 1983. LC 84-45011. 392p. 60.00 (*0-87668-657-9*) Aronson.

Technique & Practice of Listening in Intensive Psychotherapy. Richard D. Chessick. LC 89-104. 296p. 1989. 50.00 (*0-87668-862-8*); 1992. (Criminal Personality Ser.: Vol. 2). reprint ed. pap. 50.00 (*0-87668-300-6*) Aronson.

Technique & Practice of Psychoanalysis, Vol. 1. Ralph R. Greenson. 1967. LC 67-15417. 452p. 67.50 (*0-8236-6420-1*) Intl Univs Pr.

***Technique & Practice of Psychoanalysis**, Vol. 1. Ralph R. Greenson. 2001. xv, 452p. reprint ed. pap. text 39.95 (*0-8236-8321-4*, 26420) Intl Univs Pr.

***Technique & Practice of Psychoanalysis: A Memorial Volume to Ralph R. Greenson**, Vol. 2. Ed. by Alan Sugarman et al. 2001. xxxviii, 500p. reprint ed. pap. text 39.95 (*0-8236-8322-2*, 26421) Intl Univs Pr.

Technique & Practice of Psychoanalysis Vol. 2: A Memorial Volume to Ralph R. Greenson. Ed. by Alan Sugarman et al. 1992. LC 91-35393. (Monograph Series of the Ralph R. Greenson Memorial Library of the San Diego Psychoanalytic Institute & Society). 520p. (C). 70.00 (*0-8236-6421-X*) Intl Univs Pr.

Technique in Jungian Analysis. Ed. by M. Fordham. 1989. 336p. pap. (*0-946439-64-8*) Karnac Bks GBR. *Dist:* Other Pr LLC.

Technique in Transition. Ed. by Robert J. Langs. 1978. LC 78-65121. (Classical Psychoanalysis & Its Applications Ser.). 744p. 75.00 (*0-87668-349-9*) Aronson.

Technique of Analytical Psychotherapy. Wilhelm Stekel. 1950. (C). 7.50 (*0-87140-836-8*) Liveright.

Technique of Child Psychoanalysis: Discussions with Anna Freud. Joseph Sandler et al. 1980. 287p. pap. 18.00 (*0-674-87101-4*) HUP.

Technique of Psychiatric Self Help. Gordon R. Forrer. 1975. LC 75-42601. 12.95 (*0-87212-039-2*) Libra.

Technique of Psychoanalysis. Edward Glover. rev. ed. 1968. 404p. 60.00 (*0-8236-6400-7*) Intl Univs Pr.

Technique of Psychoanalytic Psychotherapy Vol. 1: The Initial Contact, Theoretical Framework, Understanding the Patient's Communications, the Therapist's Interventions. Robert J. Langs. 1973. LC 72-96542. 672p. 70.00 (*0-87668-104-6*) Aronson.

Technique of Psychoanalytic Psychotherapy Vol. 2: The Patient's Responses to Intervention, the Patient-Therapist Relationship, the Phases of Psychotherapy. Robert J. Langs. 1974. LC 72-96542. 544p. 60.00 (*0-87668-105-4*) Aronson.

Technique of Psychotherapy, Pt. 1. (*1-56821-496-0*) Aronson.

Technique of Psychotherapy, Set. Lewis R. Wolberg. 4th rev. ed. 1995. LC 94-74284. 1568p. 150.00 (*1-56821-498-7*) Aronson.

Technique of the Neurologic Examination: A Programmed Text. William DeMeyer. 4th ed. 1993. LC 93-25996. (Illus.). 553p. pap. 55.00 (*0-07-016353-7*) McGraw-Hill Prof.

Techniques & Issues in Abuse-Focused Therapy: Addressing the Internal Trauma. Sandra Wieland. 1998. LC 98-25306. (Interpersonal Violence Ser.). 238p. 79.95 (*0-7619-0481-6*, 80103); pap. 38.95 (*0-7619-0482-4*, 80104) Sage.

Techniques for Ablation of Benign & Malignant Prostate Tissue. Ed. by Joseph A. Smith, Jr. & Douglas F. Milam. 1996. LC 95-47709. (Topics in Clinical Urology Ser.). (Illus.). 256p. 87.95 (*0-89640-305-X*) Igaku-Shoin.

Techniques for Minimally Invasive Direct Coronary Artery Bypass Surgery. Robert W. Emery. 1997. LC 97-7042. 185p. 42.00 (*1-56053-218-1*) Hanley & Belfus.

Techniques for Nurses: A Comprehensive Clinical Approach. Barbara Kozier & Glenora L. Erb. 1982. text 33.95 (*0-201-03911-7*) Addison-Wesley.

Techniques for Observing Normal Child Behavior. Nancy T. Carbonara. 1961. LC 61-9991. 32p. (gr. 11-12). pap. 3.95 (*0-8229-5043-X*) U of Pittsburgh Pr.

Techniques for Semen Evaluation, Semen Storage, & Fertility Determination. M. R. Bakst & H. C. Cecil. 1997. (Illus.). 98p. (Orig.). pap. text, lab manual ed. 12.00 (*0-9649811-1-4*) Poultry Sci.

Techniques for the Analysis of Complex Genomes. Ed. by Rakesh Anand. 1992. (Illus.). 256p. 58.00 (*0-12-057620-1*) Acad Pr.

Techniques for the Genetic Analysis of Brain & Behavior. D. Goldowitz et al. 1992. (Techniques in the Behavioral & Neural Sciences Ser.: Vol. 8). 530p. pap. 157.00 (*0-444-89682-1*) Elsevier.

Techniques in Adlerian Psychology. Jon Carlson & Steven Slavik. 1997. LC 97-8530. 500p. pap. 41.95 (*1-56032-555-0*) Hemisp Pub.

Techniques in Biocompatibility Testing David F. Williams. 1986. 359.00 (*0-8493-6627-5*, R857) CRC Pr.

Techniques in Clinical Capillary Microscopy. Ed. by F. Mahler et al. 1986. (Mikrozirkulation in Forschung und Klinik Ser.: Vol. 11). (Illus.). xii, 152p. pap. 68.78 (*3-8055-4327-1*) S Karger.

Techniques in Clinical Electrophysiology of Vision. G. Niemeyer & Charles H. Huber. 1982. text 332.00 (*90-6193-727-2*) Kluwer Academic.

Techniques in Clinical Nursing. Barbara Kozier. 4th ed. 1992. 1038p. (C). pap. text 76.67 (*0-8053-5950-8*) Benjamin-Cummings.

Techniques in Clinical Nursing: A Nursing Process Approach. Barbara Kozier & Glenora L. Erb. 2nd ed. 1986. (Illus.). 1000p. stu. ed. (*0-201-11759-2*); pap. text 37.75 (*0-201-11755-X*) Addison-Wesley (Health Sci).

Techniques in Diagnostic Imaging. Ed. by G. H. Whitehouse & B. S. Worthington. 3rd ed. 1996. LC 95-8217. 175.00 (*0-86542-808-5*) Blackwell Sci.

Techniques in Diagnostic Pathology Vol. 2: ELISA Techniques - New Developments & Practical Applications in a Broad Field. Ed. by Gillian R. Bullock et al. 1991. (Illus.). 176p. text 83.00 (*0-12-681912-2*) Acad Pr.

Techniques in Extracoporeal Circulation. Philip Kay. 4th ed. 2001. (Illus.). 256p. 150.00 (*0-7506-4595-4*) Buttrwrth-Heinemann.

Techniques in Extracorporeal Circulation. Ed. by Philip H. Kay. 3rd ed. 1992. (Illus.). 380p. text (*0-7506-1391-2*) E A GBR. *Dist:* OUP.

Techniques in Fracture Surgery. Tornetta. 2000. (Illus.). 1250p. (C). text 199.00 (*0-8151-3666-8*, 31336) Mosby Inc.

Techniques in General Thoracic Surgery. R. Maurice Hood. 2nd ed. 1993. (Illus.). 302p. pap. text 58.00 (*0-8121-1546-5*) Lppncott W & W.

Techniques in General Thoracic Surgery. R. Maurice Hood. 1985. (Illus.). 378p. text 99.00 (*0-7216-1137-0*) Saunders.

Techniques in Glycobiology. Ed. by R. Reid Townsend & Arland T. Hotchkiss. 1997. LC 97-1913. (Illus.). 648p. text 85.00 (*0-8247-9822-8*) Dekker.

Techniques in Hand Surgery. Ed. by William F. Blair & Curtis M. Steyers. 1996. LC 95-7309. (Illus.). 1,216p. text 259.00 (*0-683-00842-0*) Lppncott W & W.

Techniques in Immunocytochemistry, Vol. 3. Gillian R. Bullock & Peter Petrusz. 1985. text 104.00 (*0-12-140403-X*) Acad Pr.

Techniques in Immunocytochemistry, Vol. 4. Gillian R. Bullock. Ed. by Peter Petrusz. 1989. 400p. text 104.00 (*0-12-140407-2*) Acad Pr.

Techniques in Insect Immunology. Ed. by A. Wiesner et al. 1998. LC 97-62347. (Illus.). 304p. (Orig.). pap. text, lab manual ed. 80.00 (*1-887052-05-4*) SOS Pubns NJ.

Techniques in Large Animal Surgery. A. Simon Turner & C. Wayne McIlwraith. 2nd ed. 1989. LC 88-13377. (Illus.). 381p. text 79.00 (*0-8121-1177-X*) Lppncott W & W.

Techniques in Marriage & Family Counseling. Ed. by Richard E. Watts. 2000. LC 99-32975. (Family Psychology & Counseling Ser.). 135p. pap. text 21.95 (*1-55620-211-3*, 72667) Am Coun Assn.

Techniques in Microbial Ecology. Ed. by Robert S. Burlage et al. 1998. LC 96-49666. (Illus.). 480p. (Orig.). spiral bd. 65.00 (*0-19-509223-6*) OUP.

Techniques in Molecular Medicine. F. Hildebrandt. 1999. (Illus.). 270p. 82.00 (*0-387-57129-9*) Spr-Verlag.

Techniques in Molecular Medicine. Ed. by Friedhelm Hildebrandt & Peter Igarashi. 1999. LC 99-31852. (Springer Lab Manuals Ser.). (Illus.). xii, 387p. ring bd. 82.00 (*3-540-57129-9*) Spr-Verlag.

Techniques in Orthopaedic Surgery. D. Evans. 1993. (Illus.). 480p. 235.00 (*0-632-02511-5*) Blackwell Sci.

Techniques in Rheological Measurement. Ed. by A. A. Collyer. 1993. 350p. 152.00 (*1-85166-885-3*) Elsevier.

Techniques in Somatic Cell Genetics. Ed. by Jerry W. Shay. 1982. LC 82-9848. (Illus.). 568p. 85.00 (*0-306-41040-0*, Plenum Trade) Perseus Pubng.

Techniques in Spinal Fusion & Stabilization. Ed. by Setti S. Rengachary et al. 1995. (Illus.). 408p. 139.00 (*0-86577-523-0*) Thieme Med Pubs.

Techniques in the Management of Gallstone Disease. A. Darzi et al. 1995. 272p. 150.00 (*0-632-03675-3*) Blackwell Sci.

Techniques in Therapeutic Arthroscopy. J. Serge Parisien. 1993. 392p. text 169.00 (*0-7817-0054-X*) Lppncott W & W.

Techniques in Therapeutic Endoscopy. Jerome D. Waye et al. 1987. (Illus.). 160p. text 142.00 (*0-03-012793-9*) Saunders.

Techniques in Therapeutic Endoscopy. J. E. Geenan et al. 2nd ed. 1992. (Illus.). 304p. (C). (gr. 13). text (*1-56375-018-X*) Gower-Mosby.

Techniques in Transactional Analysis: For Psychotherapists & Counselors. Muriel James. 1977. LC 76-9325. 558p. (C). text (*0-394-35061-8*) Random.

Techniques of Abdominal Vascular Sonography. Marsha M. Neumyer & Brian L. Thiele. Date not set. text (*0-941022-27-7*) Davies Pubng.

***Techniques of Biomedical Imaging in Neuroscience Research.** Nick Van Bruggen. 2001. (Methods & New Frontiers in Neuroscience Ser.). 356p. 89.95 (*0-8493-0122-X*, 0335) CRC Pr.

Techniques of Cerebrovascular Sonography. Jean Primozich & D. E. Strandness. Date not set. text (*0-941022-30-7*); VHS (*0-941022-33-1*) Davies Pubng.

Techniques of Chemistry - Physical Methods of Chemistry Vol. 1, Pt. 03D: X-Ray, Nuclear, Male. Ed. by Arnold Weissberger et al. 1972. LC 45-8533. 720p. 74.00 (*0-471-92733-3*) Krieger.

Techniques of Child Therapy: Psychodynamic Strategies. Morton Chethik. 1989. LC 88-24384. 276p. text 33.95 (*0-89862-745-1*); 2nd ed. 2000. LC 00-34730. (Illus.). 307p. 36.00 (*1-57230-528-2*, 8R0528) Guilford Pubns.

Techniques of Family Therapy. David S. Freeman. 1981. LC 80-69669. 368p. 60.00 (*0-87668-431-2*) Aronson.

Techniques of Lymphography & Principles of Interpretation. Hans Kuisk. 1971. LC 74-96986. (Illus.). 342p. 25.00 (*0-87527-046-8*) Green.

Techniques of Medical Litigation: A Professional's Handbook for Plaintiffs, Defendants, & Medical Consultants. Randine A. Lewis. 1997. LC 96-32508. 320p. 75.00 (*1-56720-088-5*, Quorum Bks) Greenwood.

Techniques of Peripheral Arterial Sonography. Ruth Cato & Jonathan B. Towne. Date not set. text (*0-941022-31-5*) Davies Pubng.

Techniques of Regional Anesthesia. D. Bruce Scott. 1996. (Illus.). 224p. (C). pap. text 125.00 (*0-8385-8844-1*, A8844-1, Apple Lange Med) McGraw.

Techniques of Treating Addiction: Cognitive, Emotive & Treating Addiction. F. Michler Bishop. 2001. LC 00-20329. 60.00 (*0-7657-0267-3*) Aronson.

Techniques of Venous Imaging. Steven R. Talbot & Mark A. Oliver. 1992. LC 91-31486. (Illus.). 220p. text 79.00 (*0-941022-22-6*) Davies Pubng.

Techniques of Veterinary Radiography. Ed. by Joe P. Morgan. 5th ed. 1993. LC 92-41342. (Venture Series in Veterinary Medicine). (Illus.). 496p. (C). pap. text 74.95 (*0-8138-1727-7*) Iowa U Pr.

Technological Advances in Health Sciences & the Moral & Theological Implications. Ed. by R. Borghgraef & R. Schotsmans. 1993. 90p. (Orig.). pap. (*90-6186-579-4*) Leuven Univ BEL. *Dist:* Coronet Bks.

Technological Change in the Workplace: Health Impacts for Workers. Ed. by Marianne P. Brown & John Froines. 1993. 18.50 (*0-89215-180-3*) U Cal LA Indus Rel.

Technological Developments & Trends in Pediatric Radiology. Ed. by H. J. Kaufmann. 1979. (Progress in Pediatric Radiology Ser.: Vol. 7). (Illus.). 144.50 (*3-8055-2953-8*) S Karger.

Technological Developments in Drugs & Pharmaceutical Industry in India. Husain Ahmad. 1988. (C). (*81-7013-004-2*) Navarang IND. *Dist:* S Asia.

Technological Diffusion in the Hospital Sector. Louise B. Russell & Carol S. Burke. 1976. LC 75-37308. 240p. 8.00 (*0-89068-007-8*) Natl Planning.

Technologies for Detection of DNA Damage & Mutations. Ed. by Gerd P. Pfeifer. 1996. LC 96-22324. (Illus.). 436p. (C). text 114.00 (*0-306-45237-5*, Kluwer Plenum) Kluwer Academic.

Technologies for Understanding & Preventing Substance Abuse & Addiction. 1996. (Illus.). 250p. (Orig.). pap. text 40.00 (*0-7881-2786-1*) DIANE Pub.

Technologies in Vascular Surgery. James S. Yao. 1991. text 180.00 (*0-7216-4429-5*) Saunders.

Technologies of Procreation: Kinship in the Age of Assisted Conception. Jeanette Edwards. 2nd ed. 1999. LC 98-35025. 11p. 90.00 (*0-415-17055-9*) Routledge.

Technology & Health Care in an Era of Limits. Institute of Medicine Staff. Ed. by Annetine C. Gelijns. 1992. LC 92-22704. (Medical Innovation at the Crossroads Ser.: Vol. 3). 296p. (Orig.). (C). pap. text 36.00 (*0-309-04695-5*) Natl Acad Pr.

Technology & Infertility: Clinical Psychosocial, Legal, & Ethical Aspects. Ed. by J. Bernstein et al. 1993. LC 92-2180. (Illus.). 446p. 108.00 (*0-387-97793-7*) Spr-Verlag.

Technology & Methodology in Behavioral Medicine. Ed. by David S. Krantz & Andrew S. Baum. 1998. LC 97-48632. (Perspectives on Behavioral Medicine Ser.). 240p. (*0-8058-2922-9*) L Erlbaum Assocs.

Technology & the Welfare State: The Development of Health Care in Britain & America. Stephen Uttley. 192p. (C). 1992. text 64.00 (*0-04-445840-1*, A8149); 1991. pap. text 19.95 (*0-04-445841-X*, A8150) Routledge.

Technology Assessments: Index of New Information with Authors, Subjects, & Bibliography. American Health Research Institute Staff. 1994. LC 94-30989. pap. 47.50 (*0-7883-0413-5*) ABBE Pubs Assn.

Technology Assessments in Health Sciences. American Health Research Institute Staff. 1990. 150p. 47.50 (*1-55914-110-7*); pap. 44.50 (*1-55914-111-5*) ABBE Pubs Assn.

Technology, Bureaucracy, & Healing in America: A Postmodern Paradigm. Roger J. Bulger. 1988. LC 88-20597. 141p. text 19.95 (*0-87745-219-9*) U of Iowa Pr.

Technology Explosion in Medical Science: Implications for the Health Care Industry & the Public (1981-2001) Ed. by James Gay & Barbara S. Jacobs. 1983. (Health Care Administration Ser.: Vol. 2). 176p. text 14.95 (*0-88331-205-0*) R B Luce.

Technology in a Hemodynamic Monitor. Daily. 5th ed. 1999. (C). text (*0-323-01151-9*) Mosby Inc.

Technology in Early Intervention. Ed. by James A. Blackman. 1998. LC 94-39482. (Infants & Young Children Ser.). 240p. pap. 41.00 (*0-8342-0649-8*) Aspen Pub.

Technology in Hospitals: Medical Advances & Their Diffusion. Louise B. Russell. 1979. LC 79-10737. (Studies in Social Economics). 180p. text 34.95 (*0-8157-7630-6*); pap. text 14.95 (*0-8157-7629-2*) Brookings.

Technology of Diabetes Care: Converging Medical & Psychosocial Perspectives. C. Bradley. 1991. x, 224p. text 116.00 (*3-7186-5084-3*, Harwood Acad Pubs) Gordon & Breach.

Technology Solutions Source Book for Behavioral Health Practice. Chris E. Stout. 1998. pap. 99.00 (*1-887986-05-7*) Strafford Pubns.

Technology 2000: Clinical Applications For Speech-language Pathology. American Speech, Language and Hearing Foundation Staff. 1997. LC 98-161891. 93p. (*1-58041-002-2*) Am Speech Lang Hearing.

Tecnologia Farmaceutica Industrial. Rodolfo S. Escabi. 1977. LC 76-46412. (SPA.). 356p. (Orig.). pap. 8.00 (*0-8477-2321-6*) U of PR Pr.

Teen Pregnancy & Parenting. Annette U. Rickel. 1989. 225p. 48.95 (*0-89116-808-7*); pap. 29.95 (*0-89116-908-3*) Hemisp Pub.

Teen Pregnancy & Parenting Handbook: Discussion Guide. Patricia G. Mathes & Beverly J. Irby. 1993. LC 92-85263. (Illus.). 64p. (gr. 7-12). stu. ed., spiral bd. 6.95 (*0-87822-334-7*, 4661) Res Press.

Teen Suicide: Opposing Viewpoints. Tamara L. Roleff. 2000. LC 99-55610. (Literary Companion to British Literature Ser.). (Illus.). 108p. 21.81 (*0-7377-0327-X*, Greenhaven Pr) Gale.

Teenage Addicts Can Recover: Treating the Addict, Not the Age. Shelly Marshall. 1992. 176p. pap. 12.95 (*1-880197-02-2*) Gylantic Pub.

Teenage Health Care. Gail B. Slap & Martha M. Jablow. Ed. by Paul McCarthy. 1994. LC 94-10427. 560p. (Orig.). per. 14.00 (*0-671-75412-2*) PB.

Teenage Nervous Breakdown: Music & Politics in the Post-Elvis Age. David Walley. 1998. LC 98-15095. (Illus.). 240p. (C). 24.95 (*0-306-45862-4*) Perseus Bks Grp.

Teenage Pregnancy: Developing Strategies for Change in the Twenty-First Century. Ed. by Dionne J. Jones. 1999. 175p. pap. text 21.95 (*0-88738-818-3*) Transaction Pubs.

Teenage World: Adolescents' Self-Image in Ten Countries. D. Offer et al. 1988. LC 88-4127. (Illus.). 288p. (C). 57.50 (*0-306-42747-8*, Kluwer Plenum) Kluwer Academic.

Teenagers & AIDS in America. Ed. by J. Stango. 1994. 227p. text 95.00 (*1-56072-178-2*) Nova Sci Pubs.

Teenagers Guide to A. D. D. Understanding & Treating Attention Disorders Through the Teenage Years. Antony Amen et al. 1996. 208p. pap. text 29.95 (*1-886554-05-6*) MindWrks.

Teenagers with ADD: A Parents' Guide. Chris A. Zeigler Dendy. 1995. LC 95-524. (Special Needs Collection). (Illus.). 370p. (Orig.). pap. 18.95 (*0-933149-69-7*) Woodbine House.

Teens Can Make It Happen: Nine Steps for Success. Stedman Graham. 2000. LC 00-41271. (Illus.). 256p. (J). (gr. 7-12). pap. 14.00 (*0-684-87082-7*, Fireside) S&S Trade Pap.

Teeth. Ed. by A. Oksche & L. Vollrath. 1988. (Handbook of Microscopic Anatomy Ser.: Vol. V/6). (Illus.). 560p. 464.00 (*0-387-19331-6*) Spr-Verlag.

Teeth: Form, Function & Evolution. Ed. by Bjorn Kurten. 1982. LC 81-10210. 456p. text 102.50 (*0-231-05202-2*) Col U Pr.

Tegafur-Ftorafur. Ed. by N. I. Perevodchikova et al. 1983. (Beitraege Zur Onkologie, Contributions to Oncology Ser.: Vol. 14). (Illus.). viii, 146p. pap. 40.00 (*3-8055-3653-4*) S Karger.

Telangiectasia: Procedure to Remove Dilated Blood Vessels Using the Blend Method. Michael Bono. 1996. (Illus.). 100p. pap. text 40.00 (*0-9642682-1-3*) Tortoise Press.

Tele-nurse: Telephone Triage Protocols. Baird & Lafferty. 2001. 320p. spiral bd. 62.95 (*0-7668-2047-5*) Delmar.

Telecommunications in Health Care. H. U. Brown. 1982. 112p. 69.00 (*0-8493-5588-5*, R118, CRC Reprint) Franklin.

Telecourse: Living with Health. Dallas County Community College Staff. 1994. (C). pap. text, stu. ed. 21.10 net. (*0-07-015187-3*) McGraw.

***Telehealth: A Cutting Edge Medical Tool for the 21st Century - Congressional Hearing.** Ed. by Michael Bilirakis. 2001. 87p. pap. text 20.00 (*0-7567-1768-X*) DIANE Pub.

Telematics for Health: The Role of Telehealth & Telemedicine in Homes & Communities. Eroc Verbprgj. 1995. LC 94-38840. pap. (*1-85775-023-3*) Radcliffe Med Pr GBR. *Dist:* Balogh.

Telematics in Primary Care in Europe. Ed. by J. DeMaeseneer & L. Beolchi. 1995. LC 94-7342. (Studies in Health Technology & Informatics: Vol. 20). 181p. 70.00 (*90-5199-209-2*) IOS Press.

Telemedicine: A State-by-State Analysis, 1997-98. Richard T. Hezel. 1997. 150p. (Orig.). pap. 150.00 (*1-889794-01-5*) Hezel Assocs.

Telemedicine: Federal Strategy Is Needed to Guide Investments. Sharon A. Cekala. 1999. (Illus.). 103p. (C). pap. text 30.00 (*0-7881-4372-7*) DIANE Pub.

Telemedicine: Past, Present, Future: Bibliography. January 1966 Through March 1995. 1995. 123p. (Orig.). (C). pap. text 30.00 (*0-7881-2019-0*) DIANE Pub.

Telemedicine & Telehealth: Principles, Policies, Performance & Pitfalls. Adam William Darkins & Margaret Ann Carly. 2000. 300p. pap. (*1-85343-518-X*) Free Assoc Bks GBR. *Dist:* Intl Spec Bk.

Telemedicine & Telehealth: Principles, Policies, Performance & Pitfalls. Adam William Darkins & Margaret Ann Cary. 2000. LC 99-50386. (Illus.). 320p. text 42.95 (*0-8261-1302-8*) Springer Pub.

Telemedicine & the Prospective Payment System. annuals Baker. Date not set. 200p. pap. 89.00 (*0-8342-1822-4*) Aspen Pub.

Telemedicine in Hospitals: Issues in Implementation. Sherry Emery. rev. ed. 1998. LC 98-29436. (Health Care Policy in the United States Ser.). (Illus.). 155p. 48.00 (*0-8153-3223-8*) Garland.

Telemedicine Opportunities for Medical & Electronic Providers. Ben Grimley. 1998. LC 00-550814. 241p. 3150.00 (*1-56965-394-1*, B-122) BCC.

Telemedicine Primer: Understanding the Issues. Jim Reid. 1996. LC 96-94441. xi, 294p. spiral bd. 75.00 (*0-9653045-0-7*) Innvtve Med.

Telemedicine Sourcebook, 1988. Ed. by Gwendolyn Segre. 1997. 496p. (Orig.). pap. text 265.00 (*1-57987-002-3*) Faulkner & Gray.

Telenursing: Nursing Practice in Cyberspace. Charles C. Sharpe. 2000. LC 00-38047. 280p. 67.50 (*0-86569-304-8*, T304, Auburn Hse) Greenwood.

Telepathy & the Etheric Vehicle. Alice A. Bailey. 1971. LC 50-11465. pap. 11.00 (*0-85330-116-6*) Lucis.

Telephone Health Assessment: Documentation Tablet. Sandra M. Simonsen. 1995. 1p. (C). (gr. 13). text 4.95 (*0-8151-8532-4*, 28686) Mosby Inc.

Telephone Health Assessment: Guidelines for Practice. Sandra M. Simonsen. 1997. LC 95-9442. 56p. (C). text (*0-8151-8024-1*, 27056) Mosby Inc.

Telephone Health Assessment: Guidelines for Practice. Sandra M. Simonsen. 2nd ed. 2000. 80p. 34.95 (*0-323-01164-0*) Saunders.

Telephone Medicine. Ed. by Anna Reisman & David Stevens. 2001. LC 00-69979. (Illus.). 200p. pap. 35.00 (*0-943126-87-8*, 330301000) Amer Coll Phys.

Telephone Medicine: Triage & Training - A Handbook for Primary Care Health Professionals. P. Harvey Katz. 2nd ed. 2001. LC 2001-17225. (Illus.). xviii, 279p. (C). spiral bd. 35.00 (*0-8036-0435-1*) Davis Co.

Telephone Triage: Products, Services & Successful U. S. Systems. Feedback Research Services Staff. 1997. (Illus.). 175p. spiral bd. 350.00 (*1-889713-12-0*) Feedback Rsch.

Telephone Triage: Theory, Practice, & Protocol Development. Sheila Q. Wheeler & Judith H. Windt. 1993. LC 92-18437. 336p. (C). mass mkt. 33.00 (*0-8273-4991-2*) Delmar.

Telephone Triage: Training 1996. wbk. ed. incl. VHS (*0-8151-3936-5*); wbk. ed. incl. VHS (*0-8151-4643-4*) Mosby Inc.

Telephone Triage: Training. Sandra M. Simonsen. 1997. (Illus.). pap. text, wbk. ed. 16.95 (*0-8151-3915-2*); pap. text, wbk. ed. 16.95 (*0-8151-3930-6*) Mosby Inc.

Telephone Triage: Training, Tape 2. 1996. wbk. ed. incl. VHS (*0-8151-3914-4*) Mosby Inc.

Telephone Triage & Management: A Nursing Process Approach. Reba McGear & Jo P. Simms. 1988. (Illus.). 174p. pap. text 52.00 (*0-7216-2406-5*) Saunders.

Telephone Triage Card Deck. Shea. 1994. (C). pap. text, tchr. ed. 14.00 (*0-8273-7171-3*) Delmar.

Telephone Triage Card Deck. Donna L. Shea & Carter-Ward. 1994. (Medical Assisting Ser.). 150p. 27.50 (*0-8273-6719-8*) Delmar.

Telephone Triage for Home Care. Mary Curry Narayan et al. 1997. LC 97-37808. 350p. ring bd. 149.00 (*0-8342-0978-0*, S478) Aspen Pub.

***Telephone Triage for the Obstetric Patient: A Nursing Guide.** Contrib. by W. B. Saunders. 2001. 148p. pap. 34.95 (*0-7216-9224-9*) Saunders.

Telephone Triage of the Obstetric Patient: A Nursing Guide. Deborah E. Swenson. 1998. (Illus.). 284p. pap. text 42.95 (*0-9666728-0-1*) Nthwest Shline Pub.

Telephone Triage Protocols for Adults: 18 Years & Older. Sheila Q. Wheeler. 1997. LC 97-25103. (Telephone Triage Protocols for Pediatric & Adult Populations Ser.). ring bd. 199.00 (*0-8342-0980-2*) Aspen Pub.

Telephone Triage Protocols for Ambulatory Care. Dale Woodke. rev. ed. 1997. (Quality Ambulatory Care Ser.). 1024p. pap. 135.00 (*1-884742-05-X*) Clarian Hlth.

Telephone Triage Protocols for Infants & Children: Birth to 6 Years. Sheila Q. Wheeler. 1997. LC 97-4387. (Telephone Triage Protocols for Pediatric & Adult Populations Ser.). ring bd. 199.00 (*0-8342-0982-9*) Aspen Pub.

Telephone Triage Protocols for Nurses. Julie Briggs. 1997. LC 96-39097. 448p. spiral bd. 42.50 (*0-397-55410-9*, Lippnctt) Lppncott W & W.

***Telephone Triage Protocols for Nurses.** Ed. by Julie K. Briggs. 2nd ed. 2001. LC 2001-29062. 576p. spiral bd. 42.95 (*0-7817-2786-3*, Lippnctt) Lppncott W & W.

Telephone Triage Protocols for Primary Care Centers. Dale Woodke. Ed. by Jane A. Miller. 2nd ed. 1994. (Quality Primary Care Ser.). pap. text 96.00 (*1-884742-02-5*) Clarian Hlth.

Telephone Triage Protocols for School-Age Children: 6-18 Years. Sheila Q. Wheeler. 1997. LC 97-25102. (Telephone Triage Protocols for Pediatric & Adult Populations Ser.). ring bd. 199.00 (*0-8342-0981-0*) Aspen Pub.

Telescreen & Radiographic Examination of the Urinary Transport. Endre Hajos. 1978. 116p. (C). (*963-05-1507-5*) Akade Kiado HUN. *Dist:* St Mut.

Televised Medicine Advertising & Children. Thomas S. Robertson et al. 1979. LC 79-4280. 175p. 55.50 (*0-275-90413-X*, C0413, Praeger Pubs) Greenwood.

Television: A Challenge to the Psychoanalytic Establishment. Jacques Lacan. 1990. 24.95 (*0-393-02496-2*) Norton.

Television, AIDS & Risk: A Cultural Studies Approach to Health Communication. John Tulloch & Deborah Lupton. 1997. LC 97-148062. 256p. pap. (*1-86448-224-9*) Allen & Unwin Pty AUS. *Dist:* Paul & Co Pubs.

Television Viewing Related to Aggressive & Prosocial Behaviour. O. Wiegman et al. 1986. (Selecta Reeks Ser.: Vol. 36). xii, 192p. 20.00 (*90-6472-095-9*) Taylor & Francis.

Tell Me Doctor: About Prenatal Care. American Bookworks Corporation Staff. 1991. pap. 4.95 (*0-9622813-0-1*) Amer Bookworks.

***Tell Me What to Eat If I Have Acid Reflux: Nutrition You Can Live With.** Elaine Magee. 2001. LC 2001-44809. (Tell Me What to Eat Ser.). 160p. pap. 10.99 (*1-56414-574-3*, New Page Bks) Career Pr Inc.

Tell Me What to Eat If I Have Irritable Bowel Syndrome: Nutrition You Can Live With. Elaine Magee. 2000. LC 00-31214. (Tell Me What to Eat Ser.). 160p. pap. 10.99 (*1-56414-444-5*, New Page Bks) Career Pr Inc.

Tell Me What to Eat to Help Prevent Breast Cancer: Nutrition You Can Live With. Elaine Magee. 2000. LC 00-20749. 159p. pap. 10.99 (*1-56414-447-X*, New Page Bks) Career Pr Inc.

Tell Me What to Eat to Help Prevent Colon Cancer: Nutrition You Can Live With. Elaine Magee. 2001. LC 00-46539. (Tell Me What to Eat Ser.). 159p. pap. 10.99 (*1-56414-514-X*, New Page Bks) Career Pr Inc.

Telling the Healthy Start Story: A Report on the Impact of the 22 Demonstration Projects. Mary F. Griffin et al. 1999. LC 99-70491. (Illus.). 164p. pap. (*1-57285-057-4*) Nat Ctr Educ.

Telling Without Talking: Art As a Window into the World of Multiple Personality. Barry M. Cohen & Carol T. Cox. 1995. LC 95-3602. (Illus.). 350p. (C). 45.00 (*0-393-70196-4*) Norton.

Telomeres & Telomerase: Methods & Protocols. Ed. by John A. Double & Michael J. Thompson. 2002. (Methods in Molecular Medicine Ser.: Vol. 191). (Illus.). 240p. 84.50 (*0-89603-657-X*) Humana.

Temperament: Theory & Practice. Stella Chess & Alexander Thomas. 1996. LC 96-28525. (Basic Principles into Practice Ser.: Vol. 12). 224p. pap. 24.95 (*0-87630-835-3*) Brunner-Routledge.

Temperament & Character Inventory: A Guide to Its Development & Use. D. M. Svrakic & R. D. Wetzel. 1994. LC 94-67965. 184p. text (*0-9642917-0-3*) Wash U Ctr Psychobiol.

Temperament & Character Inventory: A Guide to Its Development & Use. D. M. Svrakic et al. 1994. LC 94-67965. 184p. pap. text (*0-9642917-1-1*) Wash U Ctr Psychobiol.

Temperament & Child Psychopathology. William T. Garrison & Felton J. Earls. 1987. (Developmental Clinical Psychology & Psychiatry Ser.: Vol. 12). 160p. pap. 34.95 (*0-8039-2297-3*, 558233) Sage.

Temperament, Character & Personality: Biobehavioral Concepts in Science, Art, & Social Psychology. P. V. Simonov & P. M. Ershov. 1991. (Monographs Psychobiology Ser.). iv, 166p. text 143.00 (*2-88124-443-2*) Gordon & Breach.

Temperament in Clinical Practice. Stella Chess & Alexander Thomas. 1995. LC 85-17733. 315p. pap. 24.00 (*0-89862-813-X*, 2813) Guilford Pubns.

Temperature & Environmental Effects on the Testis. Ed. by A. W. Zorgniotti. 1991. LC 90-14362. (Advances in Experimental Medicine & Biology Ser.: Vol. 286). (Illus.). 346p. (C). text 132.00 (*0-306-43834-8*, Kluwer Plenum) Kluwer Academic.

Temperature & Life. H. Precht et al. 1973. LC 73-13495. (Illus.). 779p. 98.00 (*0-387-06441-9*) Spr-Verlag.

Temperature Calibration of Water Baths, Instruments & Temperature Sensors. 2nd ed. 1990. (Approved Standard Ser.). 75.00 (*1-56238-075-3*, I2-A2) NCCLS.

Temperature Regulation: Recent Physiological & Pharmacological Advances. Ed. by A. S. Milton. 1994. LC 93-50550. (Advances in Pharmacological Sciences Ser.). xii, 376p. 131.50 (*0-8176-2992-0*) Birkhauser.

Temperature Regulation & Drug Action: Proceedings of the Pharmacology of Thermoregulation Symposium, 2nd, Paris, 1974. Pharmacology of Thermoregulation symposium Staff. Ed. by Edward Schonbaum & P. Lommax. 1974. 450p. 129.75 (*3-8055-1756-4*) S Karger.

***Temperomandibular Joint Dysfunction: A Practitioner's Guide.** Ralph R. Isberg. 2001. (Illus.). 256p. (*1-901865-44-4*) Isis Med GBR. *Dist:* Bks Intl VA.

Temple: Concerning Diseases of the Brain & Nerves. Andrew J. Davis. 1996. 487p. reprint ed. spiral bd. 24.50 (*0-7873-0250-3*) Hlth Research.

Tempomandibular Joint Problems. 1996. lib. bdg. 250.96 (*0-8490-5881-3*) Gordon Pr.

Temporal Bone Malignancy: Anatomy, Pathology, & Treatment. John Rutka et al. 1994. LC 94-23526. (Self-Instructional Package Ser.). (Illus.). 73p. pap. text 25.00 (*1-56772-016-1*) AAO-HNS.

***Temporal Bone Malignancy: Anatomy, Pathology & Treatment.** Sukhminderjit Hehar et al. 2nd rev. ed. 2001. (Self-Instructional Package Ser.). (Illus.). 85p. pap. text 30.00 (*1-56772-037-4*, 5506270) AAO-HNS.

Temporal Codes for Memories: Issues & Problems. B. J. Underwood. 1977. 176p. 29.95 (*0-89859-142-2*) L Erlbaum Assocs.

Temporal Coding in the Brain. Ed. by G. Buzsaki et al. 1994. LC 94-12945. (Research & Perspectives in Neurosciences Ser.). (Illus.). 303p. 99.00 (*0-387-58074-3*) Spr-Verlag.

Temporal Disorder in Human Oscillatory Systems. Ed. by L. Rensing & M. C. Mackey. 1987. (Synergetics Ser.: Vol. 36). (Illus.). 259p. 79.95 (*0-387-17765-5*) Spr-Verlag.

Temporal Information Processing in the Nervous System: Special Reference to Dyslexia & Dysphasia. Ed. by Paula Tallal et al. 1993. LC 93-17625. (Annals Ser.: Vol. 682). 125.00 (*0-89766-786-7*) NY Acad Sci.

Temporal Lobe & Limbic System. Pierre Gloor. 1997. (Illus.). 888p. text 135.00 (*0-19-509272-4*) OUP.

Temporal Lobe Epilepsy, Mania & Schizophrenia & the Limbic System. Ed. by W. P. Koella & M. R. Trimble. 1982. (Advances in Biological Psychiatry Ser.: Vol. 8). (Illus.). x, 166p. pap. 68.75 (*3-8055-3494-9*) S Karger.

Temporal Lobe Epilepsy, 1948 to 1986. Christopher Ounsted et al. 1991. (Clinics in Developmental Medicine Ser.: No. 103). 129p. text 52.95 (*0-521-41220-X*) Cambridge U Pr.

Temporal Lobes & the Limbic System. Ed. by Michael R. Trimble & Tom G. Bolwig. 1992. 300p. (*1-871816-14-9*) Wrightson Biomed GBR. *Dist:* Taylor & Francis.

Temporal Order. Ed. by L. Rensing & N. I. Jaeger. 1985. (Synergetics Ser.: Vol. 29). (Illus.). 325p. 79.95 (*0-387-15274-1*) Spr-Verlag.

Temporal Variations of the Cardiovascular Systems. Ed. by T. F. Schmidt & B. T. Engel. 1992. (Illus.). 432p. 163.00 (*0-387-54776-2*) Spr-Verlag.

Temporary Cardiac Assist with an Axial Pump System. Ed. by W. Flameng. 1992. 88p. pap. 39.00 (*0-387-91413-7*) Spr-Verlag.

Temporary Dentistry. Michael Segerdal. 2nd ed. 1998. (Illus.). 122p. lab manual ed. (*1-883558-05-0*) PIBL.

Temporomandibular Disorders. Ed. by Steven L. Kraus. 2nd ed. 1994. LC 94-5632. (Clinics in Physical Therapy Ser.). 486p. text (*0-443-08924-8*) Church.

Temporomandibular Disorders & Related Pain Conditions. Ed. by Barry J. Sessle et al. 1995. LC 95-3084. (Progress in Pain Research & Management Ser.: Vol. 4). (Illus.). 506p. 23.00 (*0-931092-09-4*, PPRM4) Intl Assn Study Pain.

Temporomandibular Joint: A Biological Basis for Clinical Practice. Sarnet & Laskin. 4th ed. 1991. (Illus.). 576p. text 135.00 (*0-7216-7928-5*) Saunders.

Temporomandibular Joint & Masticatory Muscle Disorders. George A. Zarb. 1995. (Illus.). 624p. (C). (gr. 13). text 146.00 (*0-8151-9861-2*, 26651) Mosby Inc.

Tempos in Science & Nature: Structures, Relations & Complexity. C. Rossi. 1999. LC 99-28222. (Annals of the New York Academy of Sciences Ser.: Vol. 879). (Illus.). x, 450p. (*1-57331-197-9*) NY Acad Sci.

10-Minute Diagnosis Manual: How to Evaluate Symptoms & Signs in the Time-Limited Encounter. Robert B. Taylor. 2000. LC 00-20705. 416p. spiral bd. 39.95 (*0-7817-2094-X*) Lppncott W & W.

10 Best Tools to Boost Your Immune System. Elinor Levy & Tom Monte. 1997. LC 96-34239. 256p. pap. 14.00 (*0-395-69460-4*) HM.

Ten Critical Success Factors for Integrated Delivery Systems. Peter R. Kongstvedt. 1996. 39.00 (*0-8342-0858-X*, 20858) Aspen Pub.

Ten Days to Self-Esteem! David D. Burns. 1993. LC 92-38209. 240p. pap. 25.00 (*0-688-12708-8*, Wm Morrow) Morrow Avon.

Ten Essential Herbs: Everyone's Handbook to Health. Lalitha Thomas. 2nd rev. ed. 1996. LC 92-54953. (Illus.). 396p. (Orig.). pap. 16.95 (*0-934252-48-3*) Hohm Pr.

Ten Eyecare Practices: Benchmark for Success. John Brigham Pinto & Allan Walker. 1998. 98p. pap. (*1-929196-06-7*) Am Opthlmc Admin.

***Ten Golden Rules for Good Health.** Jan De Vries. 2001. 192p. pap. (*1-84018-431-0*) Mainstream Pubng GBR. *Dist:* Trafalgar.

***Ten Lectures: On the Use of Chinese Medicinals from the Personal Experience of Jiao Shu-De.** Jiao Shu-De. Ed. by Nigel Wiseman & Andrew Ellis. Tr. by Craig Mitchell. 2001. 288p. pap. 19.95 (*0-912111-62-3*) Paradigm Publns.

Ten Major Causes of Death & Disease in America: How to Beat Them. Dorie A. Erickson. exp. ed. 1998. 73p. spiral bd. 15.95 (*0-937242-15-2*) Scandia Pubs.

Ten Minute Cure for the Common Cold: A Natural Approach. James F. Dorobiala. Ed. by Kerry A. Martinez. 1988. LC 87-18114. (Illus.). 160p. (Orig.). 24.95 (*0-944346-01-4*); pap. 9.95 (*0-944346-02-2*) Sun Eagle Pub.

Ten Natural Remedies That Can Save Your Life. James F. Balch. 2000. LC 99-87660. 272p. pap. 11.95 (*0-385-49350-9*) Doubleday.

Ten Thousand Medical Words, Spelled & Divided for Quick Reference. Edward E. Byers. 1972. LC 72-2487. 128p. (gr. 9-12). text 10.24 (*0-07-009503-5*) McGraw.

Ten Years of Radiofrequency Catheter Ablation. Ed. by Jeronimo Farre & Concepcion Moro. 1998. LC 97-26375. (Illus.). 373p. 145.00 (*0-87993-684-3*) Futura Pub.

10 Years of Research on Porcine Derived Lung Surfactant. C. P. Speer & H. Walti. 1995. (Journal: Vol. 67, Suppl. 1, 1995). (Illus.). iv, 92p. pap. 29.75 (*3-8055-6196-2*) S Karger.

Tenascin: An Extracellular Matrix Protein in Differentiation, Adhesion & Cancer. Prashanta Shrestha. Ed. by Masahiko Mori. 1997. LC 97-26129. (Molecular Biology Intelligence Unit Ser.). 176p. 99.00 (*1-57059-474-0*) Landes Bioscience.

Tender Bud: A Physician's Journey Through Breast Cancer. Madeleine Meldin. 1993. LC 92-49967. 232p. 29.95 (*0-88163-157-4*) Analytic Pr.

Tender Touch: Biogenic Fulfillment. Edmond B. Szekely. 1977. (Illus.). 120p. text 5.50 (*0-89564-020-1*) IBS Intl.

Tender Touch: Massaging Your Baby to Health & Happiness. Paul Staerker. 2000. LC 00-20472. (Illus.). 128p. pap. 14.95 (*0-8431-7625-3*, Price Stern) Penguin Putnam.

Tending Inner Gardens: The Healing Art of Feminist Psychotherapy. Lesley I. Shore. 1994. LC 93-36036. 201p. (C). 39.95 (*1-56024-885-8*); pap. 14.95 (*1-56023-856-9*) Haworth Pr.

Tendon & Nerve Injuries of the Hand: Surgery & Rehabilitation. James Hunter & Schneider. 1997. LC 96-36163. (Illus.). 720p. (C). (gr. 13). text 165.00 (*0-8151-4740-6*, 28000) Mosby Inc.

Tendon Transfers of the Hand & Forearm. Richard J. Smith. 1987. (Illus.). 320p. 102.00 (*0-316-80174-7*, Little Brwn Med Div) Lppncott W & W.

***Tengo Diabetes.** Ed. by Barry Leonard. 2001. (SPA., Illus.). 123p. (C). reprint ed. pap. text 30.00 (*0-7567-0726-9*) DIANE Pub.

Tennessee Health Care in Perspective 2000. Ed. by Kathleen O'Leary Morgan & Scott E. Morgan. 2000. 21p. spiral bd. 19.00 (*0-7401-0241-9*) Morgan Quitno Corp.

Tennessee Health Care Perspective, 1998. Ed. by Kathleen O'Leary Morgan & Scott E. Morgan. 1998. 20p. pap. 19.00 (*1-56692-841-9*) Morgan Quitno Corp.

Tennis Injury Handbook: Professional Advice for Amateur Athletes. Allan M. Levy & Mark L. Fuerst. 1999. LC 98-33165. (Illus.). 192p. pap. 14.95 (*0-471-24854-1*) Wiley.

Tennis Partner: A Doctor's Story of Friendship & Loss. Abraham Verghese. 1999. LC 98-6749. 352p. pap. 14.00 (*0-06-093113-2*) HarperCollins Pubs.

Tens: Clinical Applications & Related Theory. Deirdre M. Walsh & Eric T. McAdams. 1997. LC 96-40892. text (*0-443-05323-5*) Church.

Tense Past: Cultural Essays in Trauma & Memory. Ed. by Paul Antze & Michael Lambek. 1996. LC 95-26249. 272p. (C). 90.00 (*0-415-91562-7*); pap. 27.95 (*0-415-91563-5*) Routledge.

Tensor Analysis for Physicists. J. A. Schouten. 1989. 289p. reprint ed. pap. text 10.95 (*0-486-65582-2*) Dover.

Tentative Pregnancy: How Amniocentesis Changes the Experience of Motherhood. Barbara Katz Rothman. 1993. LC 93-205351. 288p. pap. 9.95 (*0-393-30998-3*) Norton.

Tenth Anniversary of the Regional Advisory Committee on Medical Research for South-East Asia: Proceedings of the Special Session. 1986. (WHO Regional Publications, South-East Ser.: No. 15). 76p. pap. text 20.00 (*92-9022-115-1*, 1560015) World Health.

10th Global Warming International Conference & Expo (GW10), May 5-8, 1999, Mt. Fuji, Japan: Abstracts. Sinyan Shen. 1999. (Illus.). 150p. pap. 85.00 (*1-884736-10-6*) Supcon Intl.

Tenth HGH Symposium: 10th Symposium, Seville, April 1999. Ed. by J. S. Christiansen & M. B. Ranke. 1999. (Hormone Research Ser.: Vol. 51, Suppl. 3). (Illus.). iv, 180p. pap. 45.25 (*3-8055-7013-9*) S Karger.

Tenth International Symposium on Endocrinology & Development, Venice, Italy, October 1992: Growth & Metabolism: Obesity, Insulin Action & Use of Anthropometry. Ed. by A. Attanasio. 1993. (Journal: Vol. 39, Suppl. 3, 1993). (Illus.). vi, 118p. pap. 54.00 (*3-8055-5884-8*) S Karger.

Tenth Mental Measurements Yearbook. Ed. by Jane C. Conoley & Jack J. Kramer. 1989. 1000p. 135.00 (*0-910674-31-0*) Buros Inst Mental.

Tenth National ACCP Pulmonary Board Review Course Syllabus Prakash et al. Ed. by American College of Chest Physicians Staff. 1994. (Illus.). 350p. pap. text 65.00 (*0-916609-04-9*) Am Chest Phys.

Teratogens: Chemicals Which Cause Birth Defects. Ed. by Vera M. Kolb. 2nd rev. ed. 1993. LC 93-25703. 243.75 (*0-444-81482-5*) Elsevier.

Teratogens: Directory of New Medical & Scientific Reviews with Subject Index. Science and Life Consultants Association Staff. 1995. 160p. 49.50 (*0-7883-0568-9*); 1995. 160p. pap. 44.50 (*0-7883-0569-7*); 1998. 127p. 57.50 (*0-7883-1942-6*); 1998. 127p. pap. 47.50 (*0-7883-1943-4*) ABBE Pubs Assn.

Teratologies: A Cultural Study of Cancer. Jackie Stacey. 1997. LC 96-37055. (International Library of Sociology). (Illus.). 304p. pap. 26.95 (*0-415-14960-6*); (C). 80.00 (*0-415-14959-2*) Routledge.

Teratology: Principles & Techniques. Ed. by James G. Wilson & Josef Warkany. 1993. LC 65-14432. lib. bdg. 15.00 (*0-226-90049-5*) U Ch Pr.

Tercera Edad. Editorial America, S. A. Staff. Ed. by Maria E. Del Real. 1990. (SPA., Illus.). 296p. (Orig.). pap. (*0-944499-92-9*) Editorial Amer.

Terminal Care: A Source Guide. 1991. lib. bdg. 76.00 (*0-8490-4840-0*) Gordon Pr.

Terminal Care for People with AIDS. Sims. 1992. 128p. pap. 45.00 (*1-56593-547-0*, 0517) Singular Publishing.

Terminal Consent: Technology Implications for Clinical Practice. Michael Freeny. 1998. (Illus.). 20p. pap. 59.95 (*0-9663686-7-3*) W Austin Pr.

Terminal Illness: A Guide to Nursing Care. Charles Kemp. 2nd ed. 1999. LC 98-43501. 368p. pap. text 40.95 (*0-7817-1772-8*) Lppncott W & W.

Terminal Renal Failure: Therapeutic Problems, Possibilities & Potentials. Ed. by H. Klinkmann. 1990. (Contributions to Nephrology Ser.: Vol. 78). (Illus.). x, 252p. 29.75 (*3-8055-5086-3*) S Karger.

Termination: The Closing at Baker Plant. Alfred Slote. 1977. LC 69-13100. 360p. reprint ed. 12.00 (*0-87944-219-0*) Inst Soc Res.

Termination in Psychoanalysis. Stephen K. Firestein. 1978. LC 76-46811. 261p. 40.00 (*0-8236-6450-3*) Intl Univs Pr.

Terminologia Anatomica: International Anatomical Terminology. FCAT Staff. 1999. 280p. 59.00 incl. cd-rom (*0-86577-809-4*); 1998. 320p. 35.00 (*0-86577-808-6*) Thieme Med Pubs.

Terminologia, Definiciones y Criterios Diagnostieos en Endoscopia Digestiva. Z. Maratica. 3rd rev. ed. 1994. (SPA.). 124p. ring bd. 35.00 (*0-926592-13-0*) Normed Verlag.

Terminological Dictionary of the Medical Sciences see Diccionario Terminologico de Ciencias Medicas

Terminologie et Lexicographie Medicales. 1967. (FRE.). 60p. pap. 29.95 (*0-8288-6693-7*, M-6530) Fr & Eur.

Terminologie Fondamentale en Odonto-Stomatologie et Lexique: Francais-Anglais, Anglais-Francais. Roucoules. 1977. (ENG & FRE.). 259p. 35.95 (*0-8288-5524-2*, M6492) Fr & Eur.

Terminology & Communication Skills in the Health Sciences. J. Lea. 1975. pap. text 24.50 (*0-87909-821-X*) P-H.

Terminology for Allied Health Professionals. Carolee Sormunen. 3rd ed. (Medical Terminology Ser.). 1995. pap. 37.95 (*0-538-71148-5*); 1994. (C). mass mkt. 36.75 (*0-538-71151-5*) S-W Thomson.

Terminology for Allied Health Professionals. Carolee Sormunen & Marie A. Moisio. 3rd ed. 1995. 576p. pap., tchr. ed. (*0-538-71152-3*) S-W Thomson.

Terminology for Allied Health Professionals. Sormunen. 4th ed. 1998. 288p. text, tchr. ed. 26.95 (*0-7668-0241-8*) Delmar.

Terminology for Allied Health Professionals. Carolee Sormunen. 4th ed. 1998. LC 98-26137. (Allied Health Ser.). 624p. (C). pap. text 57.95 (*0-7668-0240-X*) Delmar.

Terminology for Allied Health Professionals: Tape-Text Package. Sormunen. 4th ed. 1998. text 56.95 incl. disk (*0-7668-0243-4*) Delmar.

***Terminology for Medical Administrators.** Mari Robbins & Janet Wetherfield. 1994. 129p. pap. (*1-870905-33-4*) Radcliffe Med Pr GBR. *Dist:* Balogh.

Terminology of Communication Disorders: Speech, Language & Hearing. Lucille Nicolosi et al. 4th ed. 1996. (Illus.). 384p. 42.00 (*0-683-06505-X*) Lppncott W & W.

Terminology of Health & Medicine: A Programmed Approach. Jane Rice. 1997. 350p. (C). pap. 47.00 (*0-8385-6260-4*, A-6260-2) P-H.

Terminology of Health & Medicine: Instructor's Manual. Rice. 1997. 112p. (C). pap. text, tchr. ed. 27.80 (*0-8385-8858-1*, A-8858-1) Appleton & Lange.

Terminus Brain: The Environmental Threats to Human Intelligence. Christopher Williams. 1997. LC 96-29928. (Global Issues Ser.). 288p. pap. 24.95 (*0-304-33857-5*) Continuum.

Terrains & Pathology in Acupuncture, Vol. 2. Yves Requena. Ed. by Robert L. Felt. Tr. by Allan Ducharne. 2nd ed. 1996. (Terrains & Pathology in Acupuncture Ser.: Vol. 2). (FRE., Illus.). 448p. text 30.00 (*0-912111-49-6*) Paradigm Publns.

***Terrorism & Health Science Affairs: Index of New Information & Guide-Book for Consumers, Reference & Research.** John C. Bartone. 2001. (Illus.). 200p. 57.50 (*0-7883-2548-5*); pap. 50.50 (*0-7883-2549-3*) ABBE Pubs Assn.

Test Anxiety: Theory, Assessment & Treatment. Ed. by Charles D. Spielberger & Peter R. Vagg. 1995. (Clinical & Community Psychology Ser.). 288p. (C). 52.95 (*0-89116-212-7*) Hemisp Pub.

Test Critiques. Ed. by Daniel J. Keyser & Richard C. Sweetland. LC 84-26895. (Illus.). Vol. I. 1984. 800p. text 89.00 (*0-9611286-6-6*, 1901); Vol. II. 1985. 872p. text 89.00 (*0-9611286-7-4*, 1902); Vol. III. 1985. 784p. text 89.00 (*0-9611286-8-2*, 1903); Vol. IV. 1986. 768p. text 89.00 (*0-933701-02-0*, 1904) PRO-ED.

Test Manual for Fundamentals of Contemporary Nursing Practice. Carol Lindeman. Date not set. 175p. (*0-7216-8237-5*) Saunders.

Test Manual for Introductory Nursing Care of Adults. Nancy K. Maebius & Adrianne D. Linton. 2nd ed. 2000. 155p. (*0-7216-8073-9*) Saunders.

Test Manual for Medical-Surgical Nursing Across the Health Care Continuum. Donna D. Ignatavicius et al. Ed. by Robin Carter. 1999. 315p. (*0-7216-6983-2*) Saunders.

Test of Auditory Analysis Skills (TAAS) Jerome Rosner. 1988. (gr. k-3). tchr. ed. 14.00 (*0-87879-630-4*) Acad Therapy.

Test of Auditory-Perceptual Skills: Upper Level. Morrison F. Gardner. 1994. LC 95-115070. pap. 16.95 (*0-931421-84-5*); pap. 54.50 (*0-931421-90-X*) Psychol Educ Pubns.

Test of Auditory Reasoning & Processing Skills. Morrison F. Gardner. 1992. pap., tchr. ed. 14.95 (*0-931421-79-9*) Psychol Educ Pubns.

Test of Visual - Motor Skills - Upper Level (Adolescent & Adult) Morrison F. Gardner. 1992. pap., tchr. ed. 16.95 (*0-931421-72-1*); tchr. ed. 43.95 (*0-931421-73-X*) Psychol Educ Pubns.

Test of Visual-Perceptual Skills (Non-Motor) Morrison F. Gardner. 1988. tchr. ed. 55.95 (*0-931421-41-1*); lp 9.95 (*0-931421-42-X*); (J). pap., tchr. ed., stu. ed. 18.50 (*0-931421-40-3*) Psychol Educ Pubns.

Test of Visual-Perceptual Skills (Non-Motor) Upper Level. Morrison F. Gardner. 1992. tchr. ed. 46.95 (*0-931421-77-2*) Psychol Educ Pubns.

Test Preparation for Medical Assisting. Tom Dembofsky. 1995. (C). 24.00 (*0-13-034729-9*, Macmillan Coll) P-H.

Test Procedures for the Blood Compatibility of Biomaterials. Ed. by Steen Dawids. 1993. LC 92-41726. text 255.50 (*0-7923-2107-3*) Kluwer Academic.

Test Scores & What They Mean. Howard B. Lyman. 4th ed. 1986. (Illus.). 204p. (C). pap. text 20.50 (*0-13-903832-9*) P-H.

Test-Tube Conception: A Blend of Love & Science. E. Peter Volpe. 1987. LC 87-22061. 160p. (C). 2.00 (*0-86554-287-2*, H257); pap. 14.95 (*0-86554-291-0*, MUP/P050) Mercer Univ Pr.

Test Validity. Howard Wainer & Henry Braun. 1988. 272p. (C). text 55.00 (*0-89859-997-0*) L Erlbaum Assocs.

Test Your Child: Birth to 6. Judy K. Sargent & Jeanmarie P. Scarr. 1995. LC 95-14755. (Illus.). 188p. (Orig.). pap. 14.95 (*0-940159-28-7*) Camino Bks.

Test Yourself for Maximum Health. Charles B. Inlander. 1994. LC 94-11880. 256p. pap. 14.95 (*1-882606-11-6*) Peoples Med Soc.

Test Yourself in Clinical Pharmacology for Nurses. John R. Trounce & Dinah Gould. 1999. LC 96-54720. vi, 222p. pap. text (*0-443-05783-4*) Church.

Testbank to Accompany Nursing Care of the Childbearing Family. Karen Morin. 2nd ed. 1995. (C). tchr. ed. (*0-8385-7089-5*, A7089-4) Appleton & Lange.

Tested Positive. John D. Collins. 1994. 116p. pap. 15.00 (*0-938245-13-9*) Inverted-A.

Tested Studies for Laboratory Teaching Vol. 20: Proceedings of the 20th Workshop/Conference of the Association for Biology Laboratory Education (ABLE) Ed. by Susan J. Karcher. 1999. (Illus.). 399p. pap. text 15.00 (*1-890444-02-2*) ABLE GA.

Testicular & Penile Cancer. Marc S. Ernstoff. 1998. LC 98-194786. (Illus.). viii, 173 p. 95.00 (*0-632-04319-9*) Blackwell Sci.

Testicular Cancer: Diagnosis, Surgical & Medical Therapy, Heinrich Warner Stiftung, 4th Symposium, Hamburg, November 1992. Ed. by H. Huland & U. Helmchen. 1993. (Journal: Vol. 23, Suppl. 2, 1993). (Illus.). vi, 78p. pap. 44.50 (*3-8055-5789-2*) S Karger.

Testicular Cancer: Investigation & Management. Ed. by Alan Horwich. 2nd ed. 1996. (An Arnold Publication). (Illus.). 448p. (*0-412-61210-0*) E A GBR. *Dist:* OUP.

Testicular Tumors. Robert H. Young & Robert E. Scully. 1990. (Illus.). 240p. 30.00 (*0-89189-295-8*) Am Soc Clinical.

Testifying in Court. Jack E. Horsley. 4th ed. 1992. 150p. 49.95 (*1-878487-47-7*, ME050) Practice Mgmt Info.

Testifying in Criminal Court: Emotional Effects of Criminal Court Testimony on Child Sexual Assault Victims. Gail S. Goodman et al. 1992. (Monographs of the Society for Research in Child Development: No. 229, Vol. 57, No. 5). 169p. (C). pap. text 15.00 (*0-226-30323-3*) U Ch Pr.

Testimony of Teeth: Forensic Aspects of Human Dentition. Spencer L. Rogers. 1988. (Illus.). 126p. (C). text 39.95 (*0-398-05450-9*) C C Thomas.

Testing & Assessment. Charles Desforges. Ed. by C. E. Wragg. 1989. (Education Matters Ser.). 128p. pap. text 18.95 (*0-304-31711-X*) Continuum.

Testing & Remediating Auditory Processing TRAP. Lynn V. Berk. 1997. (Illus.). 112p. 35.00 (*0-937857-76-9*, 1233) Speech Bin.

Testing & Reporting Performance Results of Ventricular Arrhythmia Detection Algorithms. 1987. 16p. pap. 70.00 (*0-910275-72-6*, ECAR-238) Assn Adv Med Instrn.

Testing CAHPS Health Plan Performance Reports in the Florida Medicaid Program. Donna O. Farley et al. 2000. 131p. (C). pap. 15.00 (*0-8330-2904-5*) Rand Corp.

Testing Drugs for the Aging Brain. 1983. (Journal: Vol. 28, Suppl. 2). (Illus.). xiv, 58p. pap. 48.00 (*3-8055-3659-3*) S Karger.

Testing for Abuse Liability of Drugs in Humans. 1990. lib. bdg. 75.00 (*0-8490-4024-8*) Gordon Pr.

Testing for HIV: What Your Lab Results Mean. Ed. by N. L. Gifford. 1995. 22p. (Orig.). (C). pap. 5.00 (*1-881818-07-1*) TBL.

Testing in Counseling, Uses & Misuses. Harley D. Christiansen. 1981. LC 81-3715. (Illus.). 96p. (Orig.). (C). pap. text 15.95 (*0-915456-03-6*) P Juul Pr.

Testing Positive: Sexually Transmitted Disease & the Public Health Response. Patricia A. Donovan. 1993. 47p. pap. 5.00 (*0-939253-28-3*) Guttmacher Inst.

Testing Programs for Behavior Toxicology Test Guides: Methodology & Interpretation of Data. Phyllis Mullinex. 1989. 58.00 (*0-911131-21-3*) Specialist Journals.

Testing the Limits of Teams: How to Implement Self-Management in Health Care. Elizabeth D. Becker-Reems & Daniel G. Garrett. 1994. LC 97-53189. (Illus.). 384p. pap. 54.00 (*1-55648-215-9*) AHPI.

Testing the Theories of Aging. Ed. by Richard C. Adelman & George S. Roth. 1982. 304p. 304.00 (*0-8493-5829-9*, QP86, CRC Reprint) Franklin.

Testing Young Children: A Reference Guide for Developmental, Psycho-Educational, & Psychosocial Assessments. Ed. by Jan L. Culbertson & Diane J. Willis. 1993. LC 92-11515. 496p. text 41.00 (*0-89079-550-9*, 1924) PRO-ED.

Testis: From Stem Cell to Sperm Function. Ed. by Erwin Goldberg. 2000. LC 00-23804. (Serono Symposia Ser.). (Illus.). 288p. 149.00 (*0-387-95024-9*) Spr-Verlag.

Testis, Epididymis & Technologies in the Year 2000 Suppl. 6: 11th European Workshop on Molecular & Cellular Endocrinology of the Testis. European Workshop on Molecular and Cellular Endocrinology of the Testis Staff et al. 2000. LC 00-39484. (Illus.). xiv, 265p. suppl. ed. 72.00 (*3-540-67345-8*) Spr-Verlag.

Testosterone: Action, Deficiency, Substitution. Ed. by E. Nieschlag & H. M. Behre. 2nd ed. 1998. LC 98-13005. (Illus.). 604p. 109.00 (*3-540-64283-8*) Spr-Verlag.

Testosterone: Action, Deficiency, Substitution. E. Nieschlag & H. M. Behre. 2nd ed. 1998. LC 98-13005. 109.00 (*0-387-64283-8*) Spr-Verlag.

Testosterone Deficiency. A. Vermeulen. 2001. 200p. 75.00 (*1-84214-043-4*, Parthenon Pbng) CRC Pr.

Testosterone Replacement Therapy. Fred C. Wu. 1996. (Illus.). 55p. pap. text 16.95 (*1-898099-12-X*) Blackwell Sci.

Testosterone Solution: Increase Your Energy & Vigor With Male Hormone Therapy. Aubrey Hill. 1997. LC 97-13864. 256p. pap. 14.00 (*0-7615-1022-2*) Prima Pub.

Testosterone Syndrome: The Critical Factor for Energy, Health & Sexuality; Reversing the Male Menopause. Eugene Shippen & William Fryer. 1998. LC 97-43349. 230p. pap. 21.95 (*0-87131-829-6*) M Evans.

Tests & Measurements for Behavioral Optometrists. Harold A. Solan & Irwin B. Suchoff. Ed. by Sally M. Corngold. 1991. LC 91-32164. (Illus.). 70p. (C). lib. bdg. 18.00 (*0-943599-21-0*) OEPF.

Tests & Measurements in Speech-Language Pathology. Dennis M. Ruscello. 2000. LC 00-46751. (Illus.). 216p. pap. text 44.99 (*0-7506-7003-7*) Buttrwrth-Heinemann.

Tests of Neuropsychological Malingering Version 2.0. 1997. 34p. 204.95 incl. cd-rom (*1-57444-122-1*) CRC Pr.

Testwell Decision Health. Bruess & Richardson. 4th ed. 1995. wbk. ed. 39.00 net. (*0-697-25961-7*, WCB McGr Hill) McGrw-H Hghr Educ.

Tetanus: Important New Concepts. Veronesi. 1981. (Symposia Foundation Merieux Ser.: Vol. 5). 284p. 100.00 (*0-444-90203-1*, Excerpta Medica) Elsevier.

Tetrabromobisphenol A & Derivatives. 1995. (Environmental Health Criteria Ser.: Vol. 172). 139p. (C). pap. 29.00 (*92-4-157172-1*, 1160172) World Health.

Tetradifon. 1986. (Environmental Health Criteria Ser.: No. 67). 47p. pap. text 11.00 (*92-4-154267-5*, 1160067) World Health.

Tetramethrin. 1990. (Environmental Health Criteria Ser.: No. 98). 69p. pap. text 19.00 (*92-4-154298-5*, 1160098) World Health.

Tetraplegia & Paraplegia: A Guide for Physiotherapists. Ida Bromley. 5th ed. 1998. LC 97-41290. (C). text (*0-443-05872-5*) Church.

Texas Atlas of Nail Disorders: Diagnosis & Treatment. Robert Baran. 1996. 224p. (*1-85317-201-4*) Martin Dunitz GBR. *Dist:* Mosby Inc.

Texas Folk Medicine, Vol. 5. Ed. by John Q. Anderson. 1970. (Texas Folklore Society Paisano Books Ser.). 15.00 (*0-88426-013-5*) Encino Pr.

Texas Health Care in Perspective 2000. Ed. by Kathleen O'Leary Morgan & Scott E. Morgan. 2000. 21p. spiral bd. 19.00 (*0-7401-0242-7*) Morgan Quitno Corp.

Texas Health Care Perspective, 1998. Ed. by Kathleen O'Leary Morgan & Scott E. Morgan. 1998. 20p. pap. 19.00 (*1-56692-842-7*) Morgan Quitno Corp.

Texas HIV-AIDS Community Resource Directory. 9th ed. 1996. 141p. (Orig.). pap. text 25.00 (*0-7881-2841-8*) DIANE Pub.

Texas Hospital Law, Issue 6. Richard L. Griffith & Dewey W. Johnston. 2nd ed. 1997. 300p. ring bd. 170.00 (*0-409-25657-9*, 82559-10, MICHIE) LEXIS Pub.

Texas Medicaid Program. Dawn Jahn & Thomas Ortiz. 1992. (Working Papers Ser.: No. 65). 63p. pap. 5.50 (*0-89940-547-9*) LBJ Sch Pub Aff.

Texas Policies & Procedures. Mattie Locke. 6th ed. 1993. 383p. (C). 65.00 (*1-877735-01-9*, 2102PP) Prof Prnting & Pub.

Text - Workbook Nursing Assistant Package. Sheila A. Sorrentino. 3rd ed. 1991. (gr. 13). text 34.95 (*0-8016-6436-5*, 06436) Mosby Inc.

Text & Atlas of Arterial Imaging: Modern & Developing Technology. Ed. by Douglas M. Cavaye & Rodney A. White. 1993. LC 92-49001. (Medical Atlas Ser.: Vol. 11). 160p. (gr. 13). pap. 209.95 (*0-412-46150-1*) Chapman & Hall.

Text & Atlas of Endoscopic Retrograde Cholangiopancreatography. Ed. by Stephen E. Silvis et al. 1995. LC 94-11089. (Illus.). 496p. 155.00 (*0-89640-265-7*) Igaku-Shoin.

Text & Atlas of Infertility Surgery. Ed. by Robert B. Hunt. 3rd ed. 1999. LC 99-22445. (Illus.). 544p. text 149.00 (*0-8151-4738-4*, 29440) Mosby Inc.

Text & Atlas of Liver Ultrasound. H. Bismuth et al. 1991. (Medical Atlas Ser.: No. 6). (Illus.). 249p. (gr. 13). pap. 171.95 (*0-412-36790-4*) Chapman & Hall.

Text & Atlas of Paediatric Orofacial Medicine & Pathology. R. K. Hall. 1993. LC 92-49028. (Medical Atlas Ser.: Vol. 13). (Illus.). 432p. (gr. 13). pap. 563.95 (*0-412-34860-8*) Chapman & Hall.

Text & Concordance of Biblioteca Nacional Manuscript 4987: Tratado Juridico. Ed. by Michelle A. Fuerch. 1986. (Spanish Aljamiado Texts Ser.: No. 1). (SPA.). 10p. 10.00 incl. fiche (*0-942260-82-1*) Hispanic Seminary.

Text & Concordance of Biblioteca Nacional, MS2147: Compendio de Cirugia. Ed. by Enrica J. Ardemagni. 1988. (Medieval Spanish Medical Texts Ser.: No. 24). (SPA.). 10p. 10.00 incl. fiche (*0-940639-23-8*) Hispanic Seminary.

Text & Concordance of Biblioteca Nacional, MS2165: Arte Complida de Cirugia. Guido Lanfranc De Milan. Ed. by Cynthia M. Wasick & Enrica J. Ardemagni. 1988. (Medieval Spanish Medical Texts Ser.: No. 26). (SPA.). 10p. 10.00 incl. fiche (*0-940639-25-4*) Hispanic Seminary.

Text & Concordance of Biblioteca Universitaria, Salamanca, MS2262: Doctor Gomez de Salamanca, Propiedades del Romero. Ed. by Marcela Lopez. 1987. (Medieval Spanish Medical Texts Ser.: No. 21). (SPA.). 6p. 10.00 incl. fiche (*0-940639-17-3*) Hispanic Seminary.

Text & Concordance of MS1-17: Biblioteca Colombina, Tesoro de los Remedios. Ed. by Maria Purificacion Zabia. 1987. (Medieval Spanish Medical Texts Ser.: No. 22). (SPA.). 6p. 10.00 incl. fiche (*0-940639-20-3*) Hispanic Seminary.

Text & Concordance of the Biblioteca del Palacio Real, MS3063: El Libro de Recetas de Gilberto. Ed. by Isabel Zurron. 1988. (Medieval Spanish Medical Texts Ser.: No. 23). (SPA.). 6p. 10.00 incl. fiche (*0-940639-22-X*) Hispanic Seminary.

Text & Concordances of Escorial Manuscript M.I.28: Tratado de las Fiebres. Isaac Israeli & Ruth M. Richards. 2nd ed. 1984. (Medieval Spanish Medical Texts Ser.: No. 1). 13p. 10.00 incl. fiche (*0-942260-44-9*) Hispanic Seminary.

Text & Text Processing. G. Denhiere & J. P. Rossi. 1991. (Advances in Psychology Ser.: Vol. 79). 414p. 169.50 (*0-444-88484-X*, North Holland) Elsevier.

Text & Transmission: Studies in Ancient Medicine & Its Transmission: Presented to Jutta Kollesch. Klau-Dietrich Fischer et al. 1998. LC 98-17523. (Studies in Ancient Medicine). xii, 342p. 137.00 (*90-04-11052-6*) Brill Academic Pubs.

Text-Atlas of Histology. C. Roland Leeson et al. 1988. (Illus.). 768p. text 78.00 (*0-7216-2386-7*) Saunders.

Text-Atlas of Histology Slide Set. C. Roland Leeson et al. 1989. 410.00 (*0-7216-2824-9*) Saunders.

Text Atlas of Lymphomas. James O. Armitage et al. 1999. 207p. (*1-85317-705-9*) Martin Dunitz.

Text Atlas of the Retina. Hamilton. 1997. (Illus.). 300p. text 110.00 (*0-7506-9786-5*) Buttrwrth-Heinemann.

Text Book of Diagonostic Microbiology. Mahon. 1995. 575.00 (*0-7216-4216-0*) Harcourt.

Text Book of Gynecology. D. C. Dutta. 1989. (C). (*0-89771-375-3*) Current Dist IND. *Dist:* St Mut.

Text Book of Medical Entomology. W. S. Patton & F. W. Cragg. 1984. 764p. pap. (*0-7855-0400-1*) Intl Bks & Periodicals IND. *Dist:* St Mut.

Text Book of Medicine. G. C. Mookherjee. 1989. (C). (*0-89771-371-0*) Current Dist IND. *Dist:* St Mut.

Text Book of Obstetrics. D. C. Dutta. 1989. (C). (*0-89771-374-5*) Current Dist IND. *Dist:* St Mut.

Text with Decision for Health. Bruess-Richardson. 4th ed. 1995. 48.25 net. (*0-697-25964-1*, WCB McGr Hill) McGrw-H Hghr Educ.

Textbook & Atlas of Diagnostic Microbiology. Elmer W. Koneman. 5th ed. 1997. LC 96-37818. 1,488p. text 72.95 (*0-397-51529-4*) Lppncott W & W.

Textbook & Color Atlas of the Temporomandibular Joint: Diseases, Disorders, Surgery. Ed. by John E. De Burgh Norman & Paul Bramley. 1990. (Illus.). 260p. (C). (gr. 13). 179.00 (*0-8151-6429-7*, 20272) Mosby Inc.

Textbook & Color Atlas of Tooth Impactions. Jens O. Andreasen et al. 1998. (C). text 198.00 (*0-323-00146-7*) Mosby Inc.

Textbook & Colour Atlas of the Cardiovascular System. C. Thomas et al. 1992. (Illus.). 162p. (gr. 13). pap. 55.95 (*0-412-43520-9*) Chapman & Hall.

Textbook for Dental Nurses. H. Levison. 8th ed. 1997. LC 97-1020. pap. 34.95 (*0-632-04031-9*) Blackwell Sci.

Textbook for Mental Health Narrative Approach. 2nd rev. ed. 2000. 500p. (C). 66.00 (*0-536-61369-9*) Pearson Custom.

Textbook for the Clinical Application of Therapeutic Drug Monitoring. Ed. by William J. Taylor & Mary H. Diers-Caviness. LC 85-71233. (Illus.). 500p. (C). text 85.00 (*0-9614903-0-6*, 9520-55) Abbott Laboratories.

Textbook in Analytic Group Psychotherapy. S. R. Slavson. 1964. LC 64-15375. 563p. 72.50 (*0-8236-6460-0*) Intl Univs Pr.

Textbook in Psychiatric Epidemiology. Ed. by Ming T. Tsuang et al. 1995. LC 94-47953. 496p. 99.95 (*0-471-59375-3*) Wiley.

Textbook of Abdominal Ultrasound. Ed. by Barry B. Goldberg. 1993. LC 92-49049. (Illus.). 552p. 135.00 (*0-683-03624-6*) Lppncott W & W.

Textbook of Accident & Emergency Medicine. Yates. 1997. 200p. (C). (gr. 13). pap. 156.95 (*0-412-45760-1*) Chapman & Hall.

Textbook of Acupuncture. Felix Mann. 1987. (Illus.). 640p. text 105.00 (*0-7506-1895-7*) Buttrwrth-Heinemann.

Textbook of Acute Pain Management. Paris. 1999. (Illus.). 800p. pap. text (*0-7216-6644-2*) Saunders.

Textbook of Administrative Psychiatry. Ed. by John A. Talbott et al. 1992. LC 92-2579. 610p. 61.95 (*0-88048-400-4*, 8400) Am Psychiatric.

Textbook of Adolescent Medicine. Elizabeth R. McAnarney et al. 1992. (Illus.). 1269p. text 152.00 (*0-7216-3077-4*) Saunders.

Textbook of Adult Emergency Medicine. Peter Cameron. 2000. LC 99-23408. text (*0-443-06280-3*) Church.

Textbook of Advanced Cardiac Life Support. Ed. by Richard O. Cummins. 1994. LC 98-203719. (Illus.). 348p. pap. text (*0-87493-626-8*) Am Heart.

Textbook of AIDS Medicine. Ed. by Thomas C. Merigan, Jr. et al. 2nd ed. 1998. LC 97-42697. 1,064p. text 169.00 (*0-683-30216-7*) Lppncott W & W.

***Textbook of Anaesthesia.** Alan Aitkenhead et al. 4th ed. 2001. (Illus.). 750p. pap. text (*0-443-06381-8*) Church GBR. *Dist:* Saunders.

Textbook of Anatomy. A. W. Rogers. 1992. (Illus.). 779p. (Orig.). pap. text (*0-443-02672-6*) Church.

Textbook of Anatomy & Physiology: High School Edition. Gary A. Thibodeau & Catherine P. Anthony. 13th ed. 1989. (Illus.). 840p. (C). (gr. 13). text 42.95 (*0-8016-6079-3*, 06079) Mosby Inc.

Textbook of Anesthesia. G. Smith & A. R. Aitkenhead. 2nd ed. 1990. (Illus.). 640p. (Orig.). pap. text (*0-443-03957-7*) Church.

Textbook of Anesthesia. Alan R. Aitkenhead. 3rd ed. 1996. 788p. pap. text (*0-443-05056-2*) Church.

Textbook of Angiology. Ed. by John B. Chang et al. 1999. LC 98-17068. (Illus.). 1376p. 250.00 (*0-387-98449-6*) Spr-Verlag.

***Textbook of Anxiety Disorders.** Ed. by Dan J. Stein & Eric Hollander. 2001. 417p. 77.00 (*0-88048-829-8*, 8829) Am Psychiatric.

Textbook of Aviation Physiology. J. Gillies. 1965. LC 65-15380. (*0-08-018999-7*) Pergamon Repr GBR. *Dist:* Franklin.

Textbook of Basic Life Support for Healthcare Providers. Retold by Pleasant DeSpain. 1997. LC 98-203738. (Illus.). 116p. pap. text (*0-87493-615-2*) Am Heart.

Textbook of Behavioral Managed Care: From Concept Through Management to Treatment. William Poynter. 1997. LC 97-33474. 153p. 37.95 (*0-87630-862-0*) Brunner-Routledge.

***Textbook of Benign Prostatic Hyperplasia.** Ed. by Roger S. Kirby et al. 2nd ed. 2001. 650p. (*1-901865-55-X*) Isis Med.

Textbook of Biological Feedback. Mariella Fischer-Williams et al. 1981. LC 80-15235. 511p. 54.95 (*0-89885-014-2*); pap. 29.95 (*0-89885-261-7*) Kluwer Academic (Kluwer Acad Hman Sci).

Textbook of Blood Banking & Transfusion Medicine. Ed. by Sally V. Rudmann. 1994. LC 93-49788. text 49.95 (*0-7216-3453-2*) Saunders.

Textbook of Bone Mestastases. Jasmin. 2001. 704p. 285.00 (*0-471-87742-5*) Wiley.

Textbook of Bronchoscopy. Steven H. Feinsilver & Alan Fein. 1995. (Illus.). 539p. 125.00 (*0-683-03107-4*) Lppncott W & W.

Textbook of Bunion Surgery. Ed. by Joshua Gerbert. 3rd ed. 1999. LC 00-49241. (Illus.). xii, 499p. text 95.00 (*0-7216-7784-3*) Saunders.

Textbook of Canine & Feline Cardiology: Principles & Clinical Practice. Philip R. Fox et al. 2nd ed. 1999. LC 96-22328. (Illus.). 830p. (C). text (*0-7216-4044-3*) Saunders.

***Textbook of Cardiothoracic Anesthesiology.** Daniel M. Thys. 2001. 1180p. text 195.00 (*0-07-079188-0*) McGraw-Hill Prof.

Textbook of Cardiovascular Medicine. Eric J. Topol. 1997. 2,760p. 224.00 (*0-7817-2552-6*); 2760p. 224.95 (*0-7817-1863-5*); LC 97-34262. (Illus.). 2,760p. text 125.00 (*0-397-51592-8*) Lppncott W & W.

Textbook of Child & Adolescent Psychiatry. Ed. by Jerry M. Wiener. 2nd ed. 1997. LC 96-20065. 1040p. text 145.00 (*1-882103-03-3*, 0303) Am Psychiatric.

Textbook of Child Behavior & Development. B. Kuppuswamy. 3rd rev. ed. 1992. pap. (*81-220-0162-9*); 1990. 300p. text (*81-220-0163-7*) Konark Pubs Pvt Ltd IND. *Dist:* Advent Bks Div.

Textbook of Children's Nursing. Tina Moules & Joan Ramsay. 1998. (Illus.). 544p. pap. (*0-7487-3340-X*) Nelson Thornes GBR. *Dist:* Intl Spec Bk, Trans-Atl Phila.

Textbook of Chiropractic. 1991. lib. bdg. 75.00 (*0-8490-5039-1*) Gordon Pr.

Textbook of Clinical Chiropractic. Ed. by Gregory Plaugher. 1993. LC 92-5613. (Illus.). 526p. 89.00 (*0-683-06897-0*) Lppncott W & W.

Textbook of Clinical Echocardiography. Catherine M. Otto & Alan S. Pearlman. (Illus.). 1994. LC 94-6846. 416p. text 110.00 (*0-7216-6634-5*); 2nd ed. 1999. LC 99-23054. 460p. (C). text 105.00 (*0-7216-7669-3*) Saunders.

Textbook of Clinical Electrocardiography. A. Bayes De Luna. 1987. pap. text 155.50 (*0-89838-835-X*); lib. bdg. 253.50 (*0-89838-826-0*) Kluwer Academic.

Textbook of Clinical (Medical) Biochemistry & Immunology. S. Ramakrishnan & Rajiswami. 1995. LC 97-111501. pap. 49.99 (*81-85427-34-8*) Intl Spec Bk.

Textbook of Clinical Medicine for Southeast Asia. Ed. by Joseph J. Sung et al. Date not set. 1000p. (C). (*962-201-773-8*) Chinese Univ HKG. *Dist:* U of Mich Pr.

Textbook of Clinical Neurology. Christopher G. Goetz & Eric J. Pappert. Ed. by Bill Schmitt. 1998. LC 97-28808. (Illus.). 1210p. (C). text 75.00 (*0-7216-6423-7*) Saunders.

***Textbook of Clinical Neuropsychiatry.** David P. Moore. 2001. (Arnold Publication). (Illus.). 720p. text 99.00 (*0-340-80624-9*) OUP.

Textbook of Clinical Occupational & Environmental Medicine. Linda Rosenstock & Mark R. Cullen. 1994. LC 93-8640. (Illus.). 944p. text 145.00 (*0-7216-3482-6*) Saunders.

Textbook of Clinical Ophthalmology. Ronald P. Crick & Peng Khaw. 2nd ed. 1997. 500p. text 99.00 (*981-02-2262-9*); pap. text 48.00 (*981-02-2373-0*) World Scientific Pub.

Textbook of Clinical Pharmacology. James M. Ritter et al. 3rd ed. 1995. 736p. pap. (*0-340-55864-4*) E A GBR. *Dist:* OUP.

Textbook of Community Children's Nursing. Julia Muir & Anna Sidey. 2000. LC 99-52566. (Illus.). xviii, 332p. text (*0-443-06368-0*) Harcrt Hlth Sci Grp.

***Textbook of Community Children's Nursing.** Julia Muir & Anna Sidey. 2000. (Illus.). 352p. pap. (*0-7020-2622-0*) W B Saunders GBR. *Dist:* Saunders.

***Textbook of Complementary & Alternative Medicine.** Jonas. 2003. 1000p. 65.00 (*0-683-04437-0*) Lppncott W & W.

Textbook of Complete Dentures. Arthur Rahn & Charles M. Heartwell, Jr. 5th ed. 1993. (Illus.). 541p. text 69.00 (*0-8121-1523-6*) Lppncott W & W.

Textbook of Contact Dermatitis. Richard J. Rycroft & Torkil Menne. 1992. LC 92-2195. (Illus.). 839p. 243.00 (*0-387-54562-X*) Spr-Verlag.

Textbook of Contact Dermatitis. Ed. by Torkil Menne et al. 2nd enl. rev. ed. 1994. LC 94-34409. (Illus.). 866p. 246.00 (*0-387-57943-5*) Spr-Verlag.

Textbook of Contact Dermatitis. Torkil Menne et al. 2nd enl. rev. ed. 1994. LC 94-34409. (Illus.). 840p. 165.00 (*3-540-57943-5*) Spr-Verlag.

Textbook of Coronary Thrombosis & Thrombolysis. Ed. by Richard C. Becker. 1998. LC 97-16368. (Developments in Cardiovascular Medicine Ser.). 704p. 398.00 (*0-7923-9923-4*) Kluwer Academic.

Textbook of Critical Care. William C. Shoemaker et al. 3rd ed. 1995. LC 94-27360. (Illus.). 1584p. text 125.00 (*0-7216-5422-3*) Saunders.

Textbook of Critical Care. William C. Shoemaker. 4th ed. 1999. LC 98-28550. text (*0-7216-7246-9*) Saunders.

Textbook of Dental Assisting. Humphrey. 1999. text (*0-7216-6136-X*); pap. text, stu. ed. (*0-7216-6138-6*) Saunders.

Textbook of Dental Homeopathy: For Dental Surgeons, Homeopathists & General Medicine Practitioners. Colin Lessell. 1995. 111p. pap. (*0-85207-281-3*) C W Daniel GBR. *Dist:* Natl Bk Netwk.

Textbook of Dental Pharmacology & Therapeutics. J. G. Walton et al. 2nd ed. 1994. (Illus.). 296p. pap. text 57.50 (*0-19-262506-3*) OUP.

Textbook of Dermatologic Surgery. Ed. by John L. Ratz et al. 1997. LC 97-41386. (Illus.). 672p. text 225.00 (*0-397-51495-6*) Lppncott W & W.

Textbook of Dermatology Ed. by Robert H. Champion et al. 5th ed. 1992. (Illus.). 3160p. cd-rom 295.00 (*0-86542-234-6*) Blackwell Sci.

Textbook of Dermatology R. H. Champion et al. 6th ed. 1998. LC 97-51464. (Illus.). 3160p. 699.00 (*0-632-03796-2*) Blackwell Sci.

Textbook of Dermatology, Set. Robert H. Champion et al. 5th ed. 1991. (Illus.). 3452p. 595.00 (*0-632-02396-1*) Blackwell Sci.

Textbook of Dermatopathology. Raymond L. Barnhill. 1998. LC 97-24101. (Illus.). 928p. text 210.00 (*0-07-005726-5*) McGraw-Hill Prof.

Textbook of Developmental Pediatrics. M. I. Gottlieb & J. E. Williams. 1987. LC 83-30411. (Illus.). 568p. (C). text 85.00 (*0-306-42334-0*, Kluwer Plenum) Kluwer Academic.

Textbook of Diabetes. John C. Pickup & Gareth Williams. 2nd ed. 1997. LC 96-25940. (Illus.). 1600p. 313.95 (*0-632-03802-0*) Blackwell Sci.

Textbook of Diabetes Slide Atlas. J. C. Pickup & G. Williams. 1993. (Illus.). 20p. 99.95 (*0-632-03569-2*) Blackwell Sci.

Textbook of Diagnostic Imaging Charles E. Putman & Carl E. Ravin. 2nd ed. 1994. LC 94-4061. (Illus.). 2368p. text 310.00 (*0-7216-3697-7*) Saunders.

***Textbook of Diagnostic Imaging in the Elderly.** Ed. by Mario Impallomeni et al. 2001. (Illus.). 650p. (*1-899066-88-8*) Isis Med.

Textbook of Diagnostic Microbiology. Ed. by Connie Mahon et al. 1995. LC 94-21550. (Illus.). 1152p. text 68.00 (*0-7216-4028-1*) Saunders.

Textbook of Diagnostic Microbiology. Connie Mahon & George Manuselis. 2nd ed. Date not set. LC 99-462321. (Illus.). 895p. text (*0-7216-7917-X*) Saunders.

Textbook of Diagnostic Ultrasonography. Sandra L. Hagen-Ansert. 4th ed. 1995. LC 94-22472. (Illus.). text 180.00 (*0-8016-7948-6*, 07948) Mosby Inc.

Textbook of Diseases of Nose, Throat & Ear. Ed. by P. B. Rao. 1990. 340p. (C). (*0-7855-6744-5*) Interprint IND. *Dist:* St Mut.

Textbook of Disorders & Injuries of Musculoskeletal Structure. Robert B. Salter. 2nd ed. 1983. (Illus.). 578p. text 56.00 (*0-683-07500-4*) Lppncott W & W.

Textbook of Disorders & Injuries of the Musculoskeletal System. Robert B. Salter. 3rd ed. 1998. LC 97-42747. (Illus.). 687p. text 58.95 (*0-683-07499-7*) Lppncott W & W.

Textbook of Dr. Voder's Manual Lymph Drainage Vol. 1: Basic Course. Hildegard Wittlinger & Gunther Wittlinger. 6th ed. 1998. (Illus.). 124p. pap. text 19.00 (*3-7760-1732-5*) Medicina Bio.

Textbook of Drug Design & Development. Ed. by Povl Krogsgaard-Larsen et al. 2nd ed. 1996. 560p. text 165.00 (*3-7186-5866-6*); pap. text 45.00 (*3-7186-5867-4*) Gordon & Breach (Harwood Acad Pubs).

Textbook of Echocardiography. Natasa Pandian & Stephen P. Sanders. 1994. 750p. (*0-683-06744-3*) Lppncott W & W.

Textbook of Echocardiography & Doppler in Adults & Children. Ed. by Martin G. St. John Sutton et al. 2nd ed. 1996. 1008p. 225.00 (*0-86542-287-7*) Blackwell Sci.

Textbook of Endocrine Physiology. Contrib. by James E. Griffin & Sergio R. Ojeda. 4th ed. 2000. LC 99-57918. (Illus.). 496p. text 65.00 (*0-19-513540-7*) OUP.

Textbook of Endocrine Surgery. Orlo H. Clark & Quan-Yang Duh. Ed. by Larry McGrew. 1997. (Illus.). 560p. text 155.00 (*0-7216-5882-2*) Saunders.

Textbook of Endourology. R. Ernest Sosa et al. Ed. by Sandra Valhoff. 1996. LC 95-41654. (Illus.). 784p. text 205.00 (*0-7216-5316-2*) Saunders.

Textbook of Endovascular Procedures. John F. Dyet et al. 2000. LC 99-40814. (Illus.). 795p. text (*0-443-06541-1*) Saunders.

Textbook of Epilepsy. Ed. by David W. Chadwick et al. 4th ed. 1992. LC 92-12309. 768p. text (*0-443-04473-2*) Church.

Textbook of Ethics in Pediatric Research. Ed. by Gideon Koren. 1993. 346p. (C). 39.50 (*0-89464-559-5*) Krieger.

Textbook of Family Medicine. John W. Saultz. 1999. LC 00-265697. (Illus.). 830p. text 95.00 (*0-07-057958-X*) McGraw-Hill Prof.

Textbook of Family Medicine. John W. Saultz. 2000. (Illus.). 655p. pap. 39.95 (*0-07-057977-6*) McGraw-Hill Prof.

Textbook of Family Medicine. Ian R. McWhinney. 2nd ed. 1997. (Illus.). 464p. text 60.00 (*0-19-511517-1*); LC 96-35096. pap. text 39.50 (*0-19-511518-X*) OUP.

Textbook of Family Practice. Dwight Robertson & E. Harvey Estes. 1991. (*0-8151-7407-1*) Mosby Inc.

Textbook of Family Practice. Robert E. Rakel. 5th ed. 1995. LC 95-6537. (Illus.). 1772p. text 125.00 (*0-7216-4053-2*) Saunders.

***Textbook of Female Urology & Urogynecology**, Set. Cardozo & D. R. Staskin. 2001. (Illus.). 800p. (*1-901865-05-3*) Isis Med GBR. *Dist:* Bks Intl VA.

Textbook of Fetal Abnormalities. Ed. by P. Twining et al. 1999. (Illus.). 668p. text (*0-443-05329-4*) Church.

Textbook of Fetal & Perinatal Pathology Jonathan S. Wigglesworth & Don B. Singer. 2nd ed. 1998. LC 97-21930. (Illus.). 1205p. 314.95 (*0-86542-396-2*) Blackwell Sci.

***Textbook of Fetal Cardiology.** Ed. by Lindsey D. Allan et al. 2000. (Greenwich Medical Media Ser.). (Illus.). 596p. text (*1-900151-63-4*) Greenwich Med GBR. *Dist:* JAMCO Dist.

Textbook of Fetal Physiology. Ed. by Geoffrey D. Thorburn & Richard Harding. 1994. (Illus.). 494p. text 98.50 (*0-19-857748-6*) OUP.

Textbook of Fetal Ultrasound. Ed. by R. Jaffe & T. H. Bui. 1999. LC 98-15514. (Illus.). 350p. 102.95 (*1-85070-017-6*) CRC Pr.

***Textbook of Forensic Addiction, Medicine & Psychiatry.** Lawrence B. Erlich. 2001. LC 2001-17414. (American Series in Behavioral Science & Law). 246p. pap. text 36.95 (*0-398-07185-3*); text 56.95 (*0-398-07184-5*) C C Thomas.

Textbook of Forensic Pharmacy. M. Mithal. 8th ed. 1988. (C). (*0-7855-4676-6*) Current Dist IND. *Dist:* St Mut.

Textbook of Gastroenterology. Tadataka Yamada. 3rd ed. 1998. LC 98-40963. 3,504p. text 279.00 (*0-397-58735-X*) Lppncott W & W.

Textbook of Gastroenterology. Tadataka Yamada et al. 3rd ed. 1999. 3,504p. 479.00 (*0-7817-2126-1*); 649.00 (*0-7817-2366-3*) Lppncott W & W.

Textbook Of Gastroenterology. Tadataka Yamada et al. 3rd ed. 1999. 3,504p. 429.00 (*0-7817-2127-X*) Lppncott W & W.

Textbook of Gastroenterology, Vol. 2. Ed. by Tadataka Yamada et al. 1995. LC 94-23213. (Illus.). (*0-397-51492-1*) Lppncott W & W.

Textbook of Gastrointestinal Radiology. Richard M. Gore & Marc S. Levine. Ed. by Lisette Bralow. 2nd ed. 1999. (Illus.). 2335p. text (*0-7216-7836-X*) Saunders.

Textbook of Gastrointestinal Radiology Ed. by Richard M. Gore et al. 1993. LC 93-24075. (Illus.). 2240p. 1. (*0-7216-3978-X*); 2. (*0-7216-3979-8*); Set. text 340.00 (*0-7216-3977-1*) Saunders.

Textbook of Gene Therapy. K. K. Jain. 1998. LC 98-14255. (Illus.). 450p. text 69.00 (*0-88937-190-3*) Hogrefe & Huber Pubs.

Textbook of General & Oral Medicine. David Wray. 1999. LC 99-10508. 359p. (*0-443-05189-5*) Saunders.

Textbook of General Practice. Ed. by Anne Stephenson. 1998. LC 97-36979. (Arnold Publication). (Illus.). 256p. pap. 24.95 (*0-340-67664-7*) OUP.

Textbook of Genito-Urinary Surgery Ed. by H. N. Whitfield & W. F. Hendry. 1985. (Illus.). 1437p. text (*0-443-02657-2*) Church.

Textbook of Genito-Urinary Surgery Hugh Whitfield et al. 2nd ed. 1998. LC 96-27776. (Illus.). 1664p. text 599.95 (*0-632-03774-1*) Blackwell Sci.

Textbook of Geriatric Medicine. Ed. by P. De V. Meiring. 1990. (Illus.). 433p. (C). pap. text (*0-7021-2387-0*) Juta & Co ZAF. *Dist:* Intl Spec Bk.

Textbook of Gerontologic Nursing. Annette Lueckenotte. 1995. (Illus.). 1024p. (C). (gr. 13). text 57.00 (*0-8016-7414-X*, 07414) Mosby Inc.

Textbook of Glaucoma. M. Bruce Shields. 3rd ed. 1991. (Illus.). 696p. 105.00 (*0-683-07695-7*); 4th ed. 1997. LC 97-983. 588p. text 149.00 (*0-683-07693-0*) Lppncott W & W.

Textbook of Gynecologic Oncology. Ed. by G. R. Blackledge et al. 1991. (Illus.). 512p. text (*0-7020-1410-9*) W B Saunders GBR. *Dist:* Saunders.

Textbook of Gynecology. Ed. by Larry J. Copeland. 1993. (Illus.). 1216p. text 120.00 (*0-7216-3401-X*) Saunders.

Textbook of Gynecology. D. Datta. 1989. (C). (*0-7855-4670-7*) Current Dist IND. *Dist:* St Mut.

Textbook of Gynecology. A. K. Ghosh. 1982. (C). (*0-89771-349-4*) Current Dist IND. *Dist:* St Mut.

Textbook of Gynecology. Larry D. Copeland. 2nd ed. 1999. text (*0-7216-5526-2*) Saunders.

Textbook of Gynecology. Contrib. by Larry J. Copeland & John F. Jarrell. 2nd ed. 2000. LC 99-26169. (Illus.). xxvi, 1539p. text (*0-7216-5552-1*) Saunders.

Textbook of Gynecology: An Evidence Based Approach. F. Sanfillipo. 2001. 800p. 130.00 (*1-84214-040-X*, Parthenon Pbng) CRC Pr.

Textbook of Head & Neck Anatomy. James L. Hiatt & Leslie P. Gartner. 3rd ed. 2000. LC 00-42121. 368p. text 50.00 (*0-7817-2166-0*) Lppncott W & W.

Textbook of Head Injury. Donald P. Becker et al. 1989. (Illus.). 576p. text 220.00 (*0-7216-1614-3*) Saunders.

Textbook of Healthcare Ethics. E. H. Loewy. 1996. LC 96-20314. (Illus.). 326p. (C). text 59.00 (*0-306-45240-5*, Kluwer Plenum) Kluwer Academic.

Textbook of Hematology. Shirlyn B. McKenzie. (Illus.). 1988. LC 87-3834. 507p. text 48.50 (*0-8121-1096-X*); 2nd ed. 1996. 768p. 58.95 (*0-683-18016-9*) Lppncott W & W.

Textbook of Holistic Aromatherapy: The Use of Essential Oils Treatments. W. E. Arnould-Taylor. 2nd ed. 1992. 104p. pap. (*0-7487-1551-7*) Nelson Thornes GBR. *Dist:* Trans-Atl Phila.

Textbook of Homosexuality & Mental Health. Ed. by Robert P. Cabaj & Terry S. Stein. 1996. LC 95-47271. 1022p. text 92.95 (*0-88048-716-X*, 8716) Am Psychiatric.

Textbook of Horseshoeing for Horseshoers & Veterinarians. Anton Lungwitz. Tr. by John W. Adams. 1995. LC 66-28443. (Illus.). 216p. reprint ed. pap. 21.95 (*0-87071-026-5*) Oreg St U Pr.

Textbook of Hypertension. Ed. by J. D. Swales. 1994. LC 93-42098. (Illus.). 1344p. 299.00 (*0-632-03527-7*) Blackwell Sci.

Textbook of Immunology. Constantin A. Bona. 2nd ed. 1996. LC 99-461715. 300p. text 80.00 (*3-7186-0596-1*); pap. text 29.50 (*3-7186-0597-X*) Gordon & Breach (Harwood Acad Pubs).

Textbook of Immunology: International Edition. James T. Barrett. 5th ed. 1987. (Illus.). 496p. (C). (gr. 13). text 23.00 (*0-8016-0406-0*, 00406) Mosby Inc.

Textbook of Immunopharmacology. Ed. by M. Maureen Dale et al. 3rd ed. 1994. LC 93-19411. (Illus.). 384p. pap. (*0-632-03025-9*) Blckwell Science.

Textbook of in Vitro Fertilization & Assisted Reproduction: The Bourn Hall Guide to Clinical & Laboratory Practice. Ed. by P. R. Brinsden. 2nd ed. 1999. LC 99-14782. (Illus.). 576p. 121.95 (*1-85070-000-1*) CRC Pr.

Textbook of Influenza. Karl G. Nicholson. 1998. (Illus.). 578p. 156.95 (*0-632-04803-4*) Blackwell Sci.

Textbook of Intensive Care. Ed. by David R. Goldhill & P. Stuart Withington. 1997. (Illus.). 912p. LC 96-84365. pap. (*0-412-60130-3*); text (*0-412-81400-5*) E A GBR. *Dist:* OUP.

Textbook of International Health. Paul F. Basch. 2nd ed. 1999. LC 98-50118. (Illus.). 576p. text 59.50 (*0-19-513204-1*) OUP.

Textbook of Interventional Cardiology. Ed. by Eric J. Topol. 2nd ed. 1993. (Illus.). 1384p. (C). text 220.00 (*0-7216-6722-8*) Saunders.

Textbook of Interventional Cardiology. Eric J. Topol. Ed. by Richard Zorab. 3rd ed. 1998. LC 98-13363. (Illus.). xv, 967p. (C). text 155.00 (*0-7216-7676-6*) Saunders.

Textbook of Intravenous Anesthesia. Paul F. White. LC 96-15025. 1996. (*0-683-02125-7*); 3rd ed. 1997. (Illus.). 617p. text 110.00 (*0-683-09000-3*) Lppncott W & W.

Textbook of Laparoscopy. Jaroslav F. Hulka & Harry Reich. Ed. by William Schmitt. 3rd ed. 1997. LC 96-29953. (Illus.). 624p. text 150.00 (*0-7216-6805-4*) Saunders.

Textbook of Mammography. Ed. by Audrey K. Tucker. 1993. LC 92-49320. 288p. text (*0-443-04208-X*) Church.

*__Textbook of Mammography.__ Audrey K. Tucker & Yin Y. Ng. 2nd ed. 2001. 334p. text (*0-443-06340-0*) Church GBR. *Dist:* Saunders.

Textbook of Materia Medica & Therapeutics of Rare Homeopathic Remedies. Oscar Hansen. 1991. lib. bdg. 75.00 (*0-87700-938-4*) Revisionist Pr.

Textbook of Materia Medica & Therapeutics of Rare Homeopathic Remedies. Oscar Hansen. 1993. 121p. reprint ed. spiral bd. 13.50 (*0-7873-0370-4*) Hlth Research.

Textbook of Medical Entomology. Edman. Date not set. (Biology Ser.). text 65.00 (*0-412-07421-4*) Chapman & Hall.

*__Textbook of Medical Imaging.__ Ronald G. Grainger et al. 2001. (Illus.). 3000p. text (*0-443-06432-6*) Church GBR. *Dist:* Saunders.

Textbook of Medical Physiology. Guyton. 9th ed. (C). text (*0-8089-2126-6*, Grune & Strat) Harcrt Hlth Sci Grp.

Textbook of Medical Physiology. Arthur C. Guyton & John E. Hall. 10th ed. 2000. LC 00-29716. (Illus.). xxxii, 1064p. text 67.95 (*0-7216-8677-X*) Saunders.

Textbook of Medical Treatment. Ed. by Ronald H. Girdwood & J. C. Petrie. 15th ed. 1987. LC 87-10282. (Illus.). 605p. (C). pap. text (*0-443-03211-4*) Church.

Textbook of Medicine. P. C. Das. 1989. (C). (*0-89771-343-5*) Current Dist IND. *Dist:* St Mut.

Textbook of Medicine. Ed. by J. Moxham & Robert L. Souhami. 1990. (Illus.). 1198p. pap. text (*0-443-03434-6*); 2nd ed. 1994. LC 93-21174. text (*0-443-04664-6*) Church.

Textbook of Medicine. R. J. Harrison. 2nd ed. 1982. (Illus.). 445p. reprint ed. pap. text 12.95 (*0-340-25165-4*, 5566-9) Appleton & Lange.

Textbook of Medicine. Souhami. 3rd ed. 1997. pap. text 62.00 (*0-443-05592-0*) Saunders.

*__Textbook of Medicine.__ Robert L. Souhami & John Moxham. 4th ed. 2001. (Illus.). 1403p. pap. (*0-443-06464-4*) Church GBR. *Dist:* Saunders.

Textbook of Medicine MCQs. Ed. by J. Moxham & Robert L. Souhami. 1992. LC 92-12584. 216p. pap. (*0-443-04663-8*) Church.

Textbook of Medicine MCQS. Souhami. 2nd ed. 1998. (C). pap. text (*0-443-06030-4*) Church.

Textbook of Men's Health. B. Lunenfeld. 2001. LC 2001-52034. (Illus.). 600p. 114.95 (*1-84214-011-6*, Parthenon Pbng) CRC Pr.

Textbook of Microscopic Anatomy. Kurt E. Johnson. 1988. (*0-471-88247-X*) Church.

Textbook of Modern Toxicology. Ernest Hodgson. 2nd rev. ed. 1997. LC 97-78. 496p. (C). pap. text 59.95 (*0-8385-8887-5*, A-8887-0) McGraw.

Textbook of Natural Medicine Joseph E. Pizzorno et al. rev. ed. 1993. (Illus.). (C). Set, Vols. 1-2. 1230p. ring bd. 295.00 (*0-9618764-0-9*, K03V2); Vol. 1. 750p. (*0-9618764-1-7*); Vol. 2. 400p. (*0-9618764-2-5*) John Bastyr.

Textbook of Neonatal Medicine: A Chinese Perspective. Tr. by Victor Y. Yu et al. 1997. LC 97-144304. 936p. (*962-209-428-7*) HK Univ Pr HKG. *Dist:* Coronet Bks.

Textbook of Neonatal Medicine: A Chinese Perspective. Ed. by Victor Y. Yu et al. 1996. LC 97-144304. (Illus.). 912p. pap. (*962-209-417-1*) HK Univ Pr HKG. *Dist:* Intl Spec Bk, Coronet Bks.

Textbook of Neonatal Resuscitation. American Academy of Pediatrics Staff & American Heart Association Staff. 2nd ed. 1994. 376p. spiral bd. 30.00 (*0-910761-61-2*) Am Acad Pediat.

Textbook of Neonatal Resuscitation. Jeanette Zaichkin. Ed. by Dana Braner & Susan Denson. 4th ed. 2000. LC 00-131686. (Illus.). 375p. pap. 39.95 (*1-58110-056-6*) Am Acad Pediat.

Textbook of Neonatal Ultrasound. Ed. by Jack O. Haller. 1998. LC 97-47603. (Illus.). 178p. 93.95 (*1-85070-902-5*, Parthenon Pbng) CRC Pr.

Textbook of Neonatology. Dharmapuri Vidyasagar. 1990. 462p. (C). (*81-85017-38-7*) Interprint IND. *Dist:* St Mut.

Textbook of Neonatology. Ed. by N. R. Roberton. 2nd ed. 1992. (Illus.). 1329p. text (*0-443-04088-5*) Church.

Textbook of Neonatology. Ed. by Janet M. Rennie & N. R. C. Roberton. 3rd ed. 1998. LC 98-48318. (C). text (*0-443-05541-6*) Church.

*__Textbook of Neuroanaesthesia & Critical Care.__ Basil Matta. 2000. (Illus.). 450p. text (*1-900151-73-1*) Greenwich Med GBR. *Dist:* JAMCO Dist.

Textbook of Neuroanatomy: With an Atlas & Dissection Guide. William T. Mosenthal. 1995. (Illus.). 528p. (C). lib. bdg. 36.95 (*1-85070-587-9*, Parthenon Pbng) CRC Pr.

Textbook of Neuroanesthesia: With Neurosurgical & Neuroscience Perspectives. Ed. by Maurice S. Albin. 1996. LC 96-24790. (Illus.). 1433p. text, tchr. ed. 195.00 (*0-07-000966-X*) McGraw-Hill Prof.

Textbook of Neurology. Julien Bogousslavsky & Marc Fisher. 1998. LC 98-21166. 896p. text 84.99 (*0-7506-9918-3*) Buttrwrth-Heinemann.

Textbook of Neurology. Ed. by Robert K. Jackler & Derald E. Brackmann. 1994. LC 93-34012. (Illus.). 1504p. (C). (gr. 13). text 210.00 (*0-8016-6383-0*, 06383) Mosby Inc.

Textbook of Neuropathology. Richard Davis & David Robertson. 2nd ed. 1990. (Illus.). 1176p. 180.00 (*0-683-02344-6*) Lppncott W & W.

Textbook of Neuropathology. Ed. by Richard L. Davis & David M. Robertson. 3rd ed. 1996. LC 96-15265. (Illus.). 1,409p. text 199.00 (*0-683-02355-1*) Lppncott W & W.

Textbook of Nuclear Medicine. Ed. by Michael A. Wilson. 1997. LC 97-34815. (Illus.). 656p. text 129.00 (*0-7817-0303-4*) Lppncott W & W.

Textbook of Nutritional Medicine. Melvyn R. Werbach & Jeffrey Moss. 1999. LC 99-73820. 740p. 74.95 (*0-9618550-9-6*) Third Line Pr.

Textbook of Obstetric Anaesthesia. Ed. by John Urquhart et al. 2002. (Medical Media Ser.). (Illus.). 400p. text (*1-900151-77-4*) Greenwich Med GBR. *Dist:* JAMCO Dist.

Textbook of Occlusion. Norman Mohl. Ed. by George A. Zarb et al. 1988. (Illus.). 413p. text 56.00 (*0-86715-167-6*, 1676) Quint Pub Co.

Textbook of Occupational Medicine Practice. J. Jeyaratnam & D. Koh. 1996. LC 97-109569. 500p. text 84.00 (*981-02-2322-6*); pap. text 42.00 (*981-02-2415-X*) World Scientific Pub.

Textbook of Ocular Pharmacology. Ed. by Thom J. Zimmerman et al. 1997. LC 97-1434. (Illus.). 928p. text 199.00 (*0-7817-0306-9*) Lppncott W & W.

Textbook of Operative Dentistry. Lloyd Baum et al. 3rd ed. 1994. LC 94-8371. (Illus.). 688p. text 72.00 (*0-7216-3484-2*) Saunders.

Textbook of Operative Urology. Fray F. Marshall. Ed. by Sandra Valkhoff et al. 1996. LC 95-17717. 992p. text 195.00 (*0-7216-5510-6*) Saunders.

Textbook of Ophthalmology. Ed. by Kenneth W. Wright. 1997. LC 96-24216. (Illus.). 950p. text 149.00 (*0-683-09292-8*, RE46) Lppncott W & W.

Textbook of Orthodontics. Ed. by T. D. Foster. 3rd ed. 1990. (Illus.). 356p. (gr. 13). 69.95 (*0-632-02654-5*) Blackwell Sci.

Textbook of Orthopaedic Medicine. James Cyriax. 8th ed. 1983. text 89.00 (*0-7216-0777-2*); Vol. 2. 11th ed. 1984. text 63.00 (*0-7216-0960-0*) Saunders.

Textbook of Orthopaedic Medicine: Diagnosis of Soft Tissue Lesions, Vol. 1. James Cyriax. 8th ed. 1982. (Illus.). text (*0-7020-0935-0*) Bailliere Tindall.

Textbook of Orthopaedic Medicine: Treatment by Manipulation, Massage & Injection, Vol. 2. James Cyriax & Margaret Coldham. 11th ed. 1984. (Illus.). 288p. text (*0-7020-1037-5*) Bailliere Tindall.

Textbook of Orthopaedic Surgery. Edward V. Craig. 1998. LC 98-15922. (Illus.). 1,070p. text 159.00 (*0-683-02180-X*) Lppncott W & W.

Textbook of Orthopaedics & Fractures. Sean P. Hughes & Richard W. Porter. 1997. LC 97-639. (An Arnold Publication). (Illus.). 248p. pap. text (*0-340-61381-5*) E A GBR. *Dist:* OUP.

Textbook of Osteopathy. American College of Mechano Therapy Staff. 1996. 96p. reprint ed. pap. 12.00 (*0-7873-1155-3*) Hlth Research.

Textbook of Osteoporosis. John A. Kanis. 1996. LC 93-43053. (Illus.). 432p. 209.95 (*0-632-03426-2*) Blackwell Sci.

Textbook of Paediatric Anaesthetic Practice. Edward Sumner & David Hatch. 1989. (Illus.). 616p. text (*0-7020-1336-6*) W B Saunders GBR. *Dist:* Saunders.

Textbook of Paediatric Dermatology. John Harper et al. 2000. LC 99-38325. (Illus.). 2064p. 519.95 (*0-86542-939-1*) Blackwell Sci.

Textbook of Pain. Ed. by Patrick D. Wall & Ronald Melzack. 3rd ed. 1993. (Illus.). text (*0-443-04757-X*) Church.

*__Textbook of Pain.__ Patrick D. Wall & Ronald Melzack. 4th ed. 2000. (Illus.). 1588p. text (*0-443-06252-8*) Church GBR. *Dist:* Saunders.

Textbook of Palliative Nursing. Betty R. Ferrell. 2000. LC 00-55060. (Illus.). 880p. text 75.00 (*0-19-513574-1*) OUP.

Textbook of Pathology. N. C. Dey. 1988. (C). (*0-7855-4661-8*) Current Dist IND. *Dist:* St Mut.

Textbook of Pediatric Advanced Life Support. (Illus.). 148p. pap. text (*0-87493-635-7*) Am Heart.

Textbook of Pediatric Basic Life Support. American Academy of Pediatrics Staff & American Heart Association Staff. 1997. LC 99-179982. (Illus.). 120p. pap. text (*0-87493-620-9*) Am Heart.

Textbook of Pediatric Critical Care. Peter R. Holbrook. 1992. (Illus.). 1256p. text 177.00 (*0-7216-2352-2*) Saunders.

Textbook of Pediatric Dermatology. Ed. by Lawrence C. Parish et al. 1989. (Illus.). 880p. text 255.00 (*0-8089-1863-X*, 793249, Grune & Strat) Harcrt Hlth Sci Grp.

Textbook of Pediatric Emergency & Critical Care Procedures. Dieckman & Steven M. Selbst. 1996. LC 96-46924. (Illus.). 864p. (C). (gr. 13). text 150.00 (*0-8016-8102-2*, 08102) Mosby Inc.

Textbook of Pediatric Emergency Procedures. Fred M. Henretig et al. 1997. LC 96-661. (Illus.). 928p. text 199.00 (*0-683-03971-7*) Lppncott W & W.

Textbook of Pediatric Infectious Diseases Ralph D. Feigin & James D. Cherry. Ed. by Judy Fletcher. 4th ed. 1997. LC 96-26904. (Illus.). 3136p. text 315.00 (*0-7216-6448-2*) Saunders.

Textbook of Pediatric Intensive Care. Ed. by Mark C. Rogers & David G. Nichols. 3rd ed. 1996. LC 96-14624. (Illus.). 1,852p. text 235.00 (*0-683-18034-7*) Lppncott W & W.

Textbook of Pediatric Intensive Care, Vol. 2. Mark C. Rogers. 2nd ed. 1992. (Illus.). 1792p. text 195.00 (*0-683-07319-2*) Lppncott W & W.

Textbook of Pediatric Neurology. G. J. Golden. 1987. LC 86-30432. (Topics in Pediatrics Ser.). (Illus.). 346p. (C). text 75.00 (*0-306-42359-6*, Kluwer Plenum) Kluwer Academic.

Textbook of Pediatric Neuropsychiatry. C. Edward Coffey & Roger A. Brumback. 1998. LC 97-15724. 1566p. 179.00 (*0-88048-766-6*, 8766) Am Psychiatric.

Textbook of Pediatric Nursing. Harjit Singh. 1996. pap. (*81-85017-80-8*) Interprint IND. *Dist:* St Mut.

Textbook of Pediatric Otohinolaryngology-Head & Neck Surgery, Vols. I & II. Chris De Souza et al. 1998. (Illus.). 767p. 434.95 (*1-56593-958-1*, 1894) Thomson Learn.

Textbook of Pediatric Respiratory Medicine. Lynn Taussig & L. Landau. 1999. LC 97-46466. (Illus.). 1320p. (C). (gr. 13). text 175.00 (*0-8016-7406-9*, 07406) Mosby Inc.

Textbook of Pediatric Rheumatology. James T. Cassidy & Ross E. Petty. 3rd ed. 1994. LC 94-33337. (Illus.). 622p. text 145.00 (*0-7216-5244-1*) Saunders.

Textbook of Pediatric Rheumatology. James T. Cassidy & Rose F. Petty. 4th ed. 2001. LC 2001-20286. (Illus.). xv, 819p. (*0-7216-8171-9*) Saunders.

Textbook of Pediatrics. Tom Lissauer & Graham Clayden. 1996. (Illus.). 330p. pap. 42.95 (*0-7234-1657-5*) Mosby Inc.

Textbook of Perinatal Medicine Ed. by A. Kurjak. 1998. LC 98-19168. (Illus.). 2042p. lib. bdg. 274.95 (*1-85070-930-0*, Parthenon Pbng) CRC Pr.

Textbook of Peritoneal Dialysis. Ed. by Ram Gokal & Karl D. Nolph. 1994. LC 93-40474. 800p. (C). lib. bdg. 247.00 (*0-7923-2661-X*) Kluwer Academic.

Textbook of Pharmaceutical Analysis. Kenneth A. Connors. 3rd ed. 1982. LC 81-19742. 680p. 160.00 (*0-471-09034-4*) Wiley.

*__Textbook of Pharmaceutical Information.__ Andrew Robson. 2001. (Illus.). 203p. pap. text (*0-443-06401-6*) Church GBR. *Dist:* Saunders.

Textbook of Pharmacotherapy for Child & Adolescent Psychiatric Disorders. Ed. by David Rosenberg et al. 1994. LC 94-6401. 576p. text 67.95 (*0-87630-740-3*) Brunner-Routledge.

Textbook of Physical Diagnosis: History & Examination. Mark H. Swartz. Ed. by William Schmitt. 3rd ed. 1997. LC 97-12945. (Illus.). 848p. text 54.95 (*0-7216-7514-X*) Saunders.

Textbook of Plastic, Maxillofacial, & Reconstructive Surgery, Set. Gregory S. Georgiade et al. 2nd ed. 1992. (Illus.). 1520p. 250.00 (*0-683-03454-5*) Lppncott W & W.

Textbook of Prematurity: Antecedents, Treatment, & Outcome. Ed. by Frank R. Witter & Louis G. Keith. 1993. LC 92-48895. (Illus.). 335p. 95.00 (*0-316-94917-5*, Little Brwn Med Div) Lppncott W & W.

Textbook of Primary Care Medicine. John Noble. (Illus.). 2nd ed. 1995. 2050p. (C). (gr. 13). text 99.95 (*0-8016-7841-2*, 07841); 3rd ed. 2001. 2048p. text 110.00 (*0-323-00828-3*) Mosby Inc.

Textbook of Prostate Cancer: Pathology, Diagnosis & Treatment. Ed. by Amir V. Kaisary. 1999. 367p. (*1-85317-422-X*) Martin Dunitz.

Textbook of Psoriasis. Ed. by Paul D. Mier & Peter C. Van de Kerkhof. 1986. LC 85-16669. (Illus.). 292p. text (*0-443-03210-6*) Church.

Textbook of Psoriasis. Petrus C. Maria Van de Kerkhof & Peter C. Van de Kerkhof. 1999. LC 99-20850. (Illus.). xii, 292p. 136.95 (*0-632-05166-3*) Blackwell Sci.

Textbook of Psychiatry. J. Graham Beaumont. 1989. 530p. (C). (gr. 13). 54.95 (*0-86793-049-7*) Mosby Inc.

Textbook of Psychiatry. Ed. by Linford Rees et al. 1996. LC 97-206881. (Illus.). 256p. pap. (*0-340-57195-0*) E A GBR. *Dist:* OUP.

Textbook of Psychiatry. Eugen Bleuler. 1977. LC 75-16685. (Classics in Psychiatry Ser.). (Illus.). reprint ed. 54.95 (*0-405-07417-4*) Ayer.

Textbook of Psychoanalysis. Ed. by Edward Nersessian & Richard G. Kopff, Jr. 1995. LC 95-8218. 768p. text 115.00 (*0-88048-507-8*, 8507) Am Psychiatric.

Textbook of Psychology. Edward B. Titchener. 1981. LC 80-14831. (History of Psychology Ser.). 608p. reprint ed. 75.00 (*0-8201-1354-9*) Schol Facsimiles.

Textbook of Pulmonary Diseases. Ed. by Gerald L. Baum. 3rd ed. 1983. 99.00 (*0-316-08386-0*, Little Brwn Med Div) Lppncott W & W.

Textbook of Pulmonary Diseases Ed. by Gerald L. Baum & Emanuel Wolinsky. 6th ed. 1997. LC 97-27989. (Illus.). 1,586p. text 299.00 (*0-316-08434-4*) Lppncott W & W.

Textbook of Rabbit Medicine. Frances Harcourt-Brown. 2001. (Illus.). 396p. 70.00 (*0-7506-4002-2*) Buttrwrth-Heinemann.

Textbook of Radiation Oncology: Principles. Steven A. Leibel & Theodore I. Phillips. 1998. LC 96-4867. 1376p. (C). text 225.00 (*0-7216-5336-7*) Saunders.

Textbook of Radiographic Positioning & Related Anatomy. Bontrager. 4th ed. 1996. LC 97-147908. (Illus.). 784p. (gr. 13). text 110.00 (*0-8151-0947-4*, 28893) Mosby Inc.

*__Textbook of Radiographic Positioning & Related Anatomy__, Set. Kenneth L. Bontrager. 5th ed. 2001. tchr. ed. (*0-323-01221-3*) Mosby Inc.

*__Textbook of Radiographic Positioning & Related Anatomy: Computerized Testbank.__ Kenneth L. Bontrager. 5th ed. 2001. (Illus.). 832p. (*0-323-01220-5*) Mosby Inc.

Textbook of Radiology & Imaging Sutton. 6th ed. 1997. LC 97-42688. (Illus.). 284p. text 349.00 (*0-443-05368-5*) Saunders.

Textbook of Radiology & Imaging. David Sutton & Richard W. Whitehouse. 6th ed. 1998. LC 97-42688. (*0-443-05562-9*) Church.

Textbook of Radiopharmacy: Theory & Practice. Ed. by Charles B. Sampson. 3rd ed. 1999. 548p. text (*90-5699-154-X*, ECU132) GBSP NLD. *Dist:* Gordon & Breach.

Textbook of Radiopharmacy: Theory & Practice. Ed. by Charles B. Sampson. 2nd ed. 1994. LC 94-7006. (Nuclear Medicine Ser.: Vol. 3). 150.00 (*2-88124-951-5*); 360p. pap. text 92.00 (*2-88124-973-6*) Gordon & Breach.

*__Textbook of Regional Anesthesia.__ Raj Prithvi. 2001. (Illus.). 1295p. text (*0-443-06569-1*) Church GBR. *Dist:* Saunders.

Textbook of Relaxation Skills: Training for Stress Relief & Pain Control. Carol Horrigan. 1997. LC 97-158522. 176p. pap. text 37.50 (*0-7506-2439-6*) Buttrwrth-Heinemann.

Textbook of Renal Disease. Ed. by Judith A. Whitworth & J. R. Lawrence. 2nd ed. 1994. (Illus.). 505p. text (*0-443-04786-3*) Church.

Textbook of Reproductive Medicine. Bruce R. Carr & Richard E. Blackwell. 2nd ed. 1998. LC 97-37910. 790p. (C). text 129.00 (*0-8385-8893-X*) McGraw-Hill Prof.

Textbook of Respiratory Care. Dean R. Hess. 2000. LC 2001-42921. (Illus.). xx, 1289p. text (*0-7216-8077-1*) Saunders.

*__Textbook of Respiratory Medicine.__ Ed. by John F. Murray & Jay A. Nadel. 2000. (Illus.). incl. cd-rom (*0-7216-9253-2*) Saunders.

Textbook of Respiratory Medicine Ed. by John F. Murray & Jay A. Nadel. 2nd ed. 1994. LC 92-48497. (Illus.). 2816p. text 305.00 (*0-7216-3890-2*) Saunders.

Textbook of Respiratory Medicine. Murray. 3rd ed. 2000. (C). text (*0-7216-7711-8*) Saunders.

Textbook of Running Medicine. Francis O'Connor et al. 2001. (Illus.). 696p. text 85.00 (*0-07-135977-X*) McGraw-Hill Prof.

Textbook of Science for the Health Professions. Barry Hinwood. 1992. LC 92-49020. 512p. pap. 57.50 (*1-56593-027-4*, 0271) Singular Publishing.

Textbook of Small Animal Medicine. Ed. by John Dunn. 1998. (Illus.). 1100p. (C). text (*0-7020-1582-2*) W B Saunders GBR. *Dist:* Saunders.

Textbook of Small Animal Surgery, Set. Ed. by Douglas H. Slatter. 2nd ed. 1993. LC 92-21883. (Illus.). 2496p. text 199.00 (*0-7216-8330-4*) Saunders.

Textbook of SPECT in Neurology & Psychiatry. De Deyn. 1997. 564p. text 166.00 (*0-86196-542-6*) Buttrwrth-Heinemann.

Textbook of Spinal Disorders. Stephen I. Esses. 1994. (Illus.). 368p. text 129.00 (*0-397-51346-1*) Lppncott W & W.

Textbook of Spinal Surgery Ed. by Keith H. Bridwell et al. 2nd ed. 1996. LC 96-7784. Set. 2,576p. text 399.00 (*0-397-51384-4*); Vol. 1. 8p. (*0-395-75179-9*); Vol. 2. (*0-397-51800-5*) Lppncott W & W.

Textbook of Surgery. Gordon J. A. Clunie et al. 1997. 600p. 95.00 (*0-86793-353-4*) Blackwell Sci.

Textbook of Surgery. I. Ahsan. 2nd ed. 1997. 410p. text 75.00 (*90-5702-139-0*); pap. text 38.00 (*90-5702-140-4*) Gordon & Breach (Harwood Acad Pubs).

Textbook of Surgery: The Biological Basis of Modern Surgical Practice. David C. Sabiston. 14th ed. 1991. (Illus.). 2272p. (*0-7216-3490-7*) Saunders.

Textbook of Surgery: The Biological Basis of Modern Surgical Practice. David C. Sabiston. Ed. by Lisette Bralow. 15th ed. 1996. (Illus.). 2304p. text 115.00 (*0-7216-5887-3*) Saunders.

Textbook of Surgery Pocket Companion. Sabiston. 2nd ed. 1998. (C). pap. text 4.75 (*0-8089-2107-X*) Harcourt.

Textbook of Surgical Technology. Keegan. 2002. text (*0-7216-8657-5*) Harcourt.

Textbook of Temporomandibular Disorders. Joel A. Kaplan. 1991. (Illus.). 848p. text 215.00 (*0-7216-5286-7*) Saunders.

Textbook of the Autoimmune Diseases. Robert G. Lahita et al. 2000. LC 99-54064. 912p. text 210.00 (*0-7817-1505-9*) Lppncott W & W.

Textbook of Therapeutics: Drug & Disease Management. Eric Toby Herfindal & Dick R. Gourley. 7th ed. 2000. 2,208p. 145.00 (*0-7817-2416-3*); text 125.00 (*0-7817-2414-7*) Lppncott W & W.

Textbook of Total Quality in Healthcare. A. F. Al-Assaf & June Schmele. 1993. LC 93-31083. (Illus.). 312p. 64.95 (*0-9634030-4-4*) St Lucie Pr.

Textbook of Transpersonal Psychiatry & Psychology. Ed. by Bruce Scotton et al. 1996. LC 95-43397. 443p. 60.00 (*0-465-09530-5*) Basic.

Textbook of Trauma Anesthesia & Critical Care. Christopher M. Grande et al. 1992. LC 92-49406. text 165.00 (*0-8016-2153-4*) Mosby Inc.

Textbook of Traumatic Injuries of the Teeth. J. O. Andreasen. 3rd ed. 1993. 500p. (*87-16-10637-7*) Black Mksgaard DNK. *Dist:* Iowa U Pr.

Textbook of Treatment Algorithms in Psychopharmacology. Jan Fawcett et al. 1999. LC 98-50140. 216p. 145.00 (*0-471-98109-5*) Wiley.

Textbook of Tuberculosis. Michael D. Iseman. 2000. LC 99-40515. (Illus.). 480p. pap. text 75.00 (*0-7817-1749-3*) Lppncott W & W.

Textbook of Uncommon Cancer. D. Raghavan. 2nd ed. 1999. LC 98-40588. 776p. (C). 395.00 (*0-471-92921-2*) Wiley.

Textbook of Urinalysis & Body Fluids: A Clinical Approach. Landy J. McBride. 1997. LC 97-38213. (Illus.). 304p. text 41.95 (*0-397-55231-9*) Lppncott W & W.

Textbook of Uroradiology. N. Reed Dunnick et al. 1990. (Illus.). 505p. 125.00 (*0-683-02696-8*) Lppncott W & W.

Textbook of Uroradiology. N. Reed Dunnick. 3rd ed. 2001. LC 00-56540. (Illus.). x, 532p. text 139.00 (*0-7817-2389-2*) Lppncott W & W.

Textbook of Vascular Medicine. John Tooke & Gordon D. O. Lowe. 1996. 674p. (*0-340-55791-5*) E A GBR. *Dist:* OUP.

Textbook of Veterinary Anatomy. K. M. Dyce et al. 2nd ed. 1995. LC 95-10076. (Illus.). 992p. text 89.00 (*0-7216-4961-0*) Saunders.

Textbook of Veterinary Diagnostic Radiology. Charles A. Thrall. Ed. by Ray Kersey. 3rd ed. 1997. LC 97-6593. (Illus.). 656p. text 85.00 (*0-7216-5092-9*) Saunders.

Textbook of Veterinary Histology. Horst-Dieter Dellmann. 4th ed. 1992. (Illus.). 351p. text 55.00 (*0-8121-1553-8*) Lppncott W & W.

Textbook of Veterinary Histology. Horst-Dieter Dellmann & Jo Ann C. Eurell. 5th ed. 1998. LC 98-4762. 356p. 62.00 (*0-683-30168-3*) Lppncott W & W.

Textbook of Veterinary Internal Medicine Stephen J. Ettinger & Edward C. Feldman. (Illus.). 4th ed. 1994. LC 93-31785. 2656p. text 199.00 (*0-7216-6795-3*); Set. 5th exp. ed. 2000. LC 98-34212. 2050p. text 195.00 (*0-7216-7256-6*); Vol. 1. 4th ed. 1994. LC 93-31785. 2656p. text (*0-7216-6796-1*); Vol. 2. 4th ed. 1994. LC 93-31785. 2656p. text (*0-7216-6797-X*) Saunders.

Textbook of Veterinary Internal Medicine: Diseases of the Dog & Cat. Ed. by Stephen J. Ettinger & Edward C. Feldman. 2000. LC 98-34212. (*0-7216-7257-4*); (*0-7216-7258-2*) Saunders.

Textbook of Veterinary Internal Medicine: Diseases of the Dog & Cat Stephen J. Ettinger. 3rd ed. 1989. 2464p. 1. text (*0-7216-1942-8*); 2. text (*0-7216-1943-6*) Saunders.

Textbook of Veterinary Ophthalmology. Kirk N. Gelatt. 3rd ed. 1991. (Illus.). 765p. text 129.00 (*0-8121-1365-9*) Lppncott W & W.

Textbook of Veterinary Physiology. James G. Cunningham. Ed. by Ray Kersey. 2nd ed. 1997. LC 96-29043. (Illus.). 688p. text 82.50 (*0-7216-6424-5*) Saunders.

Textbook of Videoscopic Surgery. Ed. by Douglas Olsen et al. 1997. 384p. text 150.00 (*90-5702-230-3*, Harwood Acad Pubs) Gordon & Breach.

Textbook of Women's Health. Lila A. Wallis et al. 1997. LC 97-37729. (Illus.). 1,088p. text 110.00 (*0-316-91991-8*) Lppncott W & W.

Textbook on Alcoholism & Drug Abuse in the Soviet Union. Edward A. Babayan & M. W. Gonopolsky. Tr. by V. Bobrov from RUS. 1985. LC 85-18086. (Illus.). vii, 353p. 52.50 (*0-8236-6470-8*) Intl Univs Pr.

Textbook on Chiropractic & Pregnancy. Joan M. Fallon. Ed. by Molly Rangnath. 1994. LC 94-79060. (Illus.). 222p. (C). text 56.00 (*1-886190-00-3*) Intl Chiropractors Assn.

*__Textbook on EDTA Chelation Therapy.__ Elmer M. Cranton. 2nd ed. 2001. LC 00-111726. (Illus.). 432p. 75.00 (*1-57174-253-0*) Hampton Roads Pub Co.

Textbook on Gerontological Nursing. Wade. 1996. 358p. (C). pap. (*0-7020-1603-9*) W B Saunders.

Textbook on Medical Law. Michael Davies. 2nd ed. 1998. LC 99-168472. 416p. pap. (*1-85431-842-X*) Blackstone Pr GBR. *Dist:* Gaunt, Intl Spec Bk.

Textes pour une Psycholinguistique. Ed. by Jacques A. Mehler & Georges Noizet. Tr. by Yvonne Noizet. 1974. (Textes de Sciences Sociales Ser.: No. 10). pap. (*90-279-7285-0*) Mouton.

Texto de Reanimacion Neonatal. American Academy of Pediatrics Staff & American Heart Association Staff. 1997. (SPA.). 376p. pap. 30.00 (*0-910761-88-4*) Am Acad Pediat.

Texto Educativo de Medicamentos Pediatricos see Pediatric Medication Education Text

Texto Ilustrado de Pediatria. Lissauer. 1998. (C). text 32.58 (*84-8174-288-0*) Mosby Inc.

Texto y Concordancia del Compendio de los Boticarios, Saladino de Ascoli, Valladolid, 1515. Ed. by Thomas M. Capuano. 1990. (Medieval Spanish Medical Texts Ser.: No. 30). (SPA.). 36p. 10.00 incl. fiche (*0-940639-60-2*) Hispanic Seminary.

Texto y Concordancias de las Melecinas, MS1743: Salamanca, Universitaria. Ed. by Sylvia Fernandez. 1989. (Medieval Spanish Medical Texts Ser.: No. 27). (SPA.). 8p. 10.00 incl. fiche (*0-940639-29-7*) Hispanic Seminary.

Textos y Concordancias del Libro de los Olios, MS2262: Salamanca, Universitaria. Ed. by M. Lopez Hernandez. 1989. (Medieval Spanish Medical Texts Ser.: No. 28). (SPA.). 8p. 10.00 incl. fiche (*0-940639-38-6*) Hispanic Seminary.

Textos y Concordancias del Libro de Medecina Llamado Macer: Andres de Burgos, Granada 1518 y 1519. Ed. by Thomas M. Capuano. 1991. (Medieval Spanish Medical Texts Ser.: No. 32). (SPA.). 20p. 10.00 incl. fiche (*0-940639-66-1*) Hispanic Seminary.

Texts & Concordances of Escorial Manuscript b.IV.34: Menor Dano de Medicina. Alfonso Chirino et al. Ed. by Enrica J. Ardemagni. 1984. (Medieval Spanish Medical Texts Ser.: No. 2). 11p. 10.00 incl. fiche (*0-942260-41-4*) Hispanic Seminary.

Textuality & Tectonics: Troubling Social & Psychological Science. Beryl Curt. 1994. 192p. (*0-335-19064-2*) OpUniv Pr.

Texture of the Nervous System of Man & the Vertebrates, Vol. I. Santiago R. y Cajal. Ed. & Tr. by Pedro Pasik & Tauba Pasik from SPA. annot. ed. 1999. LC 99-12316. (Illus.). 750p. 189.00 (*3-211-83057-X*) Spr-Verlag.

Texture of the Nervous System of Man & the Vertebrates, Vol. II. S. R. Cajal. Ed. & Tr. by P. Pasik & T. Pasik from FRE. annot. ed. 2000. (Illus.). 680p. 150.00 (*3-211-83201-7*) Spr-Verlag.

*__TGF-b & Related Cytokines in Inflammation.__ S. N. Breit & S. M. Wahl. 2001. (PIR Ser.). (Illus.). 250p. 129.00 (*3-7643-6009-7*) Spr-Verlag.

Thai Yoga Massage: A Dynamic Therapy for Physical Well-Being & Spiritual Energy. Kam Thye Chow. 2001. LC 2001-51947. (Illus.). 160p. 29.95 (*0-89281-937-5*, Heal Arts VT) Inner Tradit.

Thaianic Oscillations & Signaling. Mircea Steriade et al. 1990. LC 89-14822. 431p. 337.00 (*0-471-51508-6*) Wiley.

Thalamic Networks for Relay & Modulation. Ed. by Diego Minciacchi et al. 1993. LC 93-21166. (Studies in Neurosciences). 462p. 207.00 (*0-08-042274-8*, Pergamon Pr) Elsevier.

Thalamus. Ed. by E. G. Jones et al. 1997. LC 97-42887. 1700p. 450.00 (*0-08-042507-0*, Pergamon Pr) Elsevier.

Thalassa: A Theory of Genitality. Sandor Ferenczi. 1989. 110p. reprint ed. pap. text (*0-946439-61-3*) Karnac Bks GBR. *Dist:* Other Pr LLC.

Thalassemia: An Interdisciplinary Approach. Ed. by John T. Chirban. 1986. (Illus.). 106p. (C). text 41.50 (*0-8191-5675-2*) U Pr of Amer.

Thalidomide: Index of New Information for Research, Reference & Therapy. Max C. Dobber. 1998. 160p. 57.50 (*0-7883-1878-0*); pap. 47.50 (*0-7883-1879-9*) ABBE Pubs Assn.

Thallium & Tha-lium Compounds Health & Safety Guide. 1997. (Health & Safety Guides Ser.: Vol. 102). 35p. pap. 4.50 (*92-4-151102-8*, 1860102) Am Soc Clinical.

Thallium Myocardial Perfusion Tomography in Clinical Cardiology. D. C. Costa et al. 1994. (Illus.). 240p. 250.00 (*0-387-19675-7*) Spr-Verlag.

Thallium-201 & Technetium-99m-Pyrophosphate Nyocardial Imaging in the Coronary Care Unit. Ed. by Frans J. Wackers. 1980. (Developments in Cardiovascular Medicine Ser.: No. 9). (Illus.). 255p. text 126.50 (*90-247-2396-5*) Kluwer Academic.

Thanatologic Aspects of Aging. Ed. by Margot Tallmer et al. 1980. LC 78-70537. (Thanatology Service Ser.). 190p. pap. 9.95 (*0-930194-25-X*) Ctr Thanatology.

Thanatology Abstracts, 1977. Otto S. Margolis & Daniel J. Cherico. 1980. 19.95 (*0-405-12503-8*) Ayer.

Thanatology Abstracts, 1979. Otto S. Margolis & Daniel J. Cherico. 1981. 19.95 (*0-405-14222-6*, 19702) Ayer.

Thanatology Community & the Needs of the Movement. Ed. by Elizabeth J. Clark & Austin H. Kutscher. 1992. LC 92-10750. (Loss, Grief & Care Ser.: Vol. 6, No. 1). 125p. text 39.95 (*1-56024-218-3*) Haworth Pr.

Thanatology Course Outlines, Vol. 2. Daniel J. Cherico & Otto S. Margolis. 1979. 19.95 (*0-405-12514-3*) Ayer.

Thanatology Curriculum-Medicine. Ed. by Robert De Bellis et al. 1988. LC 88-2934. (Loss, Grief & Care Ser.: Vol. 2, Nos. 1 & 2). (Illus.). 132p. text 4.95 (*0-86656-738-0*) Haworth Pr.

Thanatology Thesaurus. Ed. by Roberta Halporn. 2000. (Thanatology Service Ser.). 50p. ring bd. 15.95 (*0-930194-17-9*) Ctr Thanatology.

Thanatos to Eros: Thirty-Five Years of Psychedelic Exploration Ethnomedicine & the Study of Consciousness. Myron J. Stolaroff. 1994. 192p. (*3-86135-453-5*) VWB DEU. *Dist:* Thaneros Pr.

That First Bite - Chance or Choice? A Working Guide Empowering Choice for Those with Eating Disorders. Rosemarie Durphy & Mary Sullivan. 1992. 128p. (Orig.). pap. 7.95 (*0-9631517-6-2*) Jeremiah Pr.

That Why Child: Problems in Psychotherapy & Counselling. Carol Jeffrey. 1996. 180p. (C). (*1-85343-338-1*); pap. (*1-85343-339-X*) Free Assoc Bks GBR. *Dist:* Intl Spec Bk, NYU Pr.

Theaters of the Body: A Psychoanalytic View of Psychosomatic Illness. Joyce McDougall. 1989. 183p. (C). 22.95 (*0-393-70082-8*) Norton.

Theaters of the Mind: Illusion & Truth on the Psychoanalytic Stage. Joyce McDougall. 1991. LC 91-20628. 320p. pap. text 28.95 (*0-87630-648-2*) Brunner-Routledge.

Theatre of the Planetary Houres for All the Days of the Yeare. George Simotta. Tr. by G. Baker from GRE. 1971. LC 73-171791. (English Experience Ser.: No. 414). 40p. reprint ed. 15.00 (*90-221-0414-1*) Walter J Johnson.

Theatre, Ritual & Transformation: The Senoi Temiar. Sue Jennings. 1995. LC 94-21644. (Illus.). 224p. (C). pap. 27.95 (*0-415-11990-1*, C0473) Routledge.

Theilheimer's Synthetic Methods of Organic Chemistry, Vol. 57. A. F. Finch. 2000. xxiv, 304p. pap. 474.00 (*3-8055-7077-5*) S Karger.

*__Theilheimer's Synthetic Methods of Organic Chemistry__, Vol. 59. Ed. by A. F. Finch. 2001. xxiv, 318p. 520.00 (*3-8055-7265-4*) S Karger.

Thematic Journal: A Diary for Self-Observation & Self-Revelation. Alan K. White. 1984. 100p. (Orig.). pap. 7.00 (*0-914865-00-5*) Mstque Pubns.

Thematic Methods & Strategies in Learning Disabilities: A Textbook for Practitioners. M. E. Lewis. 1993. LC 92-42082. (Illus.). 212p. (Orig.). (C). pap. 34.95 (*1-879105-95-0*, 0353) Thomson Learn.

Themes in Cultural Psychiatry: An Annotated Bibliography, 1975-1980. Armando R. Favazza & Ahmed D. Faheem. 1982. LC 82-2738. 208p. 32.50 (*0-8262-0377-9*) U of Mo Pr.

Themes in Medical Geography: Environment & Health. Ed. by Rais Akhtar. 1991. (*81-7024-332-7*) Ashish Pub Hse IND. *Dist:* S Asia.

Theodor Billroth, 1829-1894. Karel B. Absolon. Tr. by Ubaldo Brancato. 1995. (ITA., Illus.). 350p. (C). text 39.50 (*0-930329-76-7*) Kabel Pubs.

*__Theodoros Stamos: Allegeries of Nature: Organic Abstractions 1945-1949.__ Barbara Cavaliere. Ed. by Halley K. Harrisburg. 2001. (Illus.). 36p. pap. 15.00 (*1-930416-14-8*) M Rosenfeld.

Theological Analyses of the Clinical Encounter. Jonathan R. Sande. Ed. by Gerald P. Mckenney. 1994. LC 93-17958. (Theology & Medicine Ser.: Vol. 3). 256p. lib. bdg. (*0-7923-2362-9*) Kluwer Academic NLD. *Dist:* Kluwer Academic.

Theologies of the Body: Humanist & Christian. Benedict Ashley. 1995. LC 84-15031. (Illus.). 770p. (Orig.). reprint ed. pap. 25.95 (*0-935372-15-6*) NCBC.

Theology after Freud: An Interpretive Inquiry. Peter Homans. 1970. LC 76-84162. 29.50 (*0-672-51245-9*); pap. text 16.95 (*0-8290-1399-7*) Irvington.

Theology & Bioethics: Exploring the Foundation & Frontiers. Earl E. Shelp. 1985. 338p. text 178.50 (*90-277-1857-1*) Kluwer Academic.

*__Theology for Pastoral Psychotherapy: God's Play in Sacred Spaces.__ Brian W. Grant. 2001. LC 00-69716. 238p. 29.95 (*0-7890-1200-6*); (C). pap. text 19.95 (*0-7890-1201-4*) Haworth Pr (Haworth Pastrl).

Theology of Health Care Ministry: Faith-Filled Response to Human Suffering. Cornelius Van der Poel. 1998. LC 97-48828. 150p. pap. 12.95 (*1-55612-979-3*, LL1979) Sheed & Ward WI.

Theology of Medicine: The Political-Philosophical Foundations of Medical Ethics. Thomas Szasz. 2nd ed. 1988. LC 87-26769. 170p. (C). reprint ed. pap. 17.95 (*0-8156-0225-1*) Syracuse U Pr.

Theophrastus Bombastus von Hohenheim Called Paracelsus. John M. Stillman. LC 79-8625. (Illus.). viii, 184p. reprint ed. 34.50 (*0-404-18491-X*) AMS Pr.

Theoretical Advances in Behavior Genetics, No. 2. Ed. by Joseph R. Royce & Leendert P. Mos. 1981. (NATO Advanced Study Institutes Ser.). 722p. lib. bdg. 211.50 (*90-286-0569-X*) Kluwer Academic.

Theoretical & Clinical Aspects of Allergic Diseases. Ed. by H. Bostrom & N. Ljungstedt. 1983. (Illus.). 302p. text 49.50 (*91-22-00595-1*) Coronet Bks.

Theoretical & Conceptual Issues in Hispanic Mental Health. Ed. by Robert G. Malgady & Orlando Rodriguez. 1994. LC 93-38655. 274p. 39.50 (*0-89464-839-X*) Krieger.

Theoretical & Empirical Advances in Community Mental Health. Ed. by Edward M. Bennett & Bruce Tefft. 1985. LC 85-21371. (Studies in Health & Human Services: Vol. 5). 280p. lib. bdg. 89.95 (*0-88946-131-7*) E Mellen.

Theoretical & Practical Aspects of Allergic Disorders: Proceedings of the Collegium Internationale Allergologicum, 9th, London, Sept. 1972. Collegium Internationale Allergologicum Staff. Ed. by D. Parker et al. 1973. (International Archives of Allergy & Immunology Ser.: Vol. 45, Nos. 1-2). (Illus.). reprint ed. pap. 68.00 (*3-8055-1605-3*) S Karger.

Theoretical Approaches to Obsessive-Compulsive Disorder. Ian Jakes. 1996. (Problems in the Behavioral Sciences Ser.: No. 14). (Illus.). 215p. (C). text 64.95 (*0-521-46058-1*) Cambridge U Pr.

Theoretical Approaches to Quantitative Pharmacophore Modeling - Biological Activity Relationships. Ed. by P. G. De Benditti. 1999. (Theoretical & Computational Chemistry Ser.: Vol. 7). (*0-444-82675-0*) Elsevier.

Theoretical Basis of the Living System. Jorge Macedo. 1979. LC 75-17399. (Illus.). 84p. 10.50 (*0-87527-158-8*) Green.

Theoretical Evolutions in Person-Centered - Experiential Therapy: Applications to Schizophrenic & Retarded Psychoses. Garry Prouty. 1994. LC 93-42143. 144p. 60.00 (*0-275-94543-X*, Praeger Pubs) Greenwood.

Theoretical Foundation of Dendritic Function: Selected Papers of Wilfrid Rall. Ed. by Idam Segev et al. 1994. (Computional Neuroscience Ser.). 468p. 70.00 (*0-262-19356-6*, Bradford Bks) MIT Pr.

Theoretical Foundations & Biological Bases of Development in Adolescence. Ed. by Richard M. Lerner. 1999. LC 99-33732. (Adolescence Ser.: Vol. 1). (Illus.). 360p. reprint ed. 80.00 (*0-8153-3290-4*) Garland.

Theoretical Foundations of Behavior Therapy. Hans J. Eysenck & I. Martin. 1987. LC 87-17168. (Perspectives on Individual Differences Ser.). (Illus.). 494p. (C). 95.00 (*0-306-42634-X*, Plenum Trade) Perseus Pubng.

Theoretical Foundations of Cardiovascular Processes. Ed. by Dhanjoo N. Ghista et al. 1978. (Advances in Cardiovascular Physics Ser.: Vol. 1). (Illus.). 85.25 (*3-8055-2850-7*) S Karger.

Theoretical Issues in Language Acquisition: Continuity & Discontinuity in Development. Ed. by Juergen Weissenborn et al. 1991. 328p. pap. 32.50 (*0-8058-0380-7*); text 69.95 (*0-8058-0379-3*) L Erlbaum Assocs.

Theoretical Issues in Sign Language Research, Vol. 1: Linguistics. Ed. by Susan D. Fischer & Patricia A. Siple. 1990. LC 90-10997. (Theoretical Issues in Sign Language Research Ser.: Vol. 1). (Illus.). 352p. lib. bdg. 66.00 (*0-226-25149-7*); pap. text 36.00 (*0-226-25150-0*) U Ch Pr.

Theoretical Issues in Sign Language Research, Vol. 2: Psychology. Ed. by Patricia A. Siple & Susan D. Fischer. 1991. LC 90-10997. (Illus.). 324p. (Theoretical Issues in Sign Language Research Ser.: Vol. 2). lib. bdg. 84.00 (*0-226-25151-9*); pap. text 36.00 (*0-226-25152-7*) U Ch Pr.

Theoretical Issues in Stimulus-Response Compatibility. Bernhard Hommel & Wolfgang Prinz. 1996. LC 96-49378. (Advances in Psychology Ser.: Vol. 118). 430p. 119.50 (*0-444-82304-2*) Elsevier.

Theoretical Models & Personality Theory. Ed. by David Krech & George S. Klein. 1968. LC 68-29744. (Illus.). 142p. reprint ed. lib. bdg. 57.50 (*0-8371-0134-4*, KRTM, Greenwood Pr) Greenwood.

Theoretical Models of Human Development, Vol. 1, Theoretical Models of Human Development. Ed. by William Damon & Richard Lerner. 5th ed. 1997. LC 96-49157. (Handbook of Child Psychology Ser.: Vol. 1). 1296p. 285.00 (*0-471-05527-1*) Wiley.

Theoretical Models of Human Development/Cognition, Perception, & Language/Social, Emotional..., Set. 5th ed. Ed. by William Damon. Incl. Handbook of Child Psychology Vol. 2: Cognition, Perception & Language. Ed. by Deanna Kuhn & Robert S. Siegler. 1030p. 285.00 (*0-471-05730-4*); Handbook of Child Psychology Vol. 3: Social, Emotional, & Personality Development. Ed. by Nancy Eisenberg. 1232p. 285.00 (*0-471-07668-6*); Handbook of Child Psychology Vol. 4. Ed. by Irving E. Sigel & K. Ann Renninger. 1188p. 285.00 (*0-471-07663-5*); Vol. 1, Theoretical Models of Human Development. Theoretical Models of Human Development. Ed. by Richard Lerner. LC 96-49157. 1296p. 285.00 (*0-471-05527-1*); LC 96-49157. 3008p. 1997. 1140.00 (*0-471-17893-4*) Wiley.

Theoretical Nursing: Development & Progress. Afaf I. Meleis. 3rd ed. 1997. LC 96-36612. 688p. text 46.95 (*0-397-55259-9*) Lppncott W & W.

Theoretical Perspectives on Autobiographical Memory: Proceedings of the NATO Advanced Research Workshop, Grange-over-Sands, U. K. 4-12 July, 1991. Ed. by Martin A. Conway. 1992. (NATO Advanced Science Institutes Ser.). 516p. (C). lib. bdg. 251.00 (*0-7923-1646-0*) Kluwer Academic.

Theoretical Perspectives on Language Deficits. Yosef Grodzinsky. 1990. LC 89-39398. (Issues in the Biology of Language & Cognition Ser.). 212p. 37.95 (*0-262-07123-1*, Bradford Bks) MIT Pr.

Theoretical Population Genetics. Jeff S. Gale. 1989. 320p. (C). text 90.00 (*0-04-575026-2*) Routledge.

Theoretical Population Genetics. Jeff S. Gale. 1989. 320p. (C). pap. 54.95 (*0-04-575027-0*) Thomson Learn.

Theoretical Principles of Psychosomatic Medicine. I. I. Kurstin. 1975. 332p. 3.5 hd 83.00 (*0-7065-1510-2*) Coronet Bks.

Theoretical Psychology: The Meeting of East & West. Anand C. Paranjpe. 1984. (PATH in Pathology Ser.). 344p. 75.00 (*0-306-41400-7*, Plenum Trade) Perseus Pubng.

Theories & Methods for Practice of Clinical Psychology. Malcolm H. Robertson & Robert H. Woody. 1997. LC 96-25085. 300p. 45.00 (*0-8236-6518-6*, BN06518) Intl Univs Pr.

Theories & Methods of an Integrative Transactional Analysis: A Volume of Selected Articles. Richard G. Erskine. 1998. LC 98-209721. (Illus.). 256p. pap. 25.00 (*0-89489-004-2*) Intl Transactional.

Theories & Principles of Occupational Therapy. Mary Young & Evie Quinn. 1992. (Illus.). 224p. (Orig.). pap. text (*0-443-04060-5*) Church.

Theories & Strategies in Counseling & Psychotherapy. Burl E. Gilliland. 4th ed. 1997. 80p. (C). (*0-205-27971-6*, Macmillan Coll) P-H.

Theories & Strategies in Counseling & Psychotherapy. Burl E. Gilliland & Richard K. James. 4th ed. 1997. LC 97-20362. 436p. 77.00 (*0-205-26832-3*) Allyn.

Theories of Animal Memory: Animal Cognition. Ed. by Donald F. Kendrick et al. 1986. (Comparative Cognition & Neuroscience Bever-Alton Roeblatt Ser.). 224p. (C). pap. 29.95 (*0-89859-697-1*) L Erlbaum Assocs.

Theories of Autism. Cheryl D. Seifert. 1990. 106p. (C). pap. text 14.00 (*0-8191-7719-9*); text 37.50 (*0-8191-7718-0*) U Pr of Amer.

Theories of Behavior Therapy: Exploring Behavior Change. Ed. by William O'Donohue & Leonard Krasner. 1995. 753p. pap. 29.95 (*1-55798-488-3*); LC 94-48476. text 39.95 (*1-55798-265-1*) Am Psychol.

Theories of Child Abuse & Neglect: Differential Perspectives, Summaries, & Evaluations. Oliver C. Tzeng et al. 1991. LC 90-46516. 392p. 75.00 (*0-275-93832-8*, C3832, Praeger Pubs) Greenwood.

Theories of Consciousness: An Introduction. William Seager. 1998. LC 98-34492. (Philosophical Issues in Science Ser.). (Illus.). 296p. (C). 80.00 (*0-415-18393-6*, D6336); pap. 27.95 (*0-415-18394-4*, D6340) Routledge.

Theories of Development Psychology. Patricia H. Miller. 3rd ed. 1998. LC 92-37252. 498p. (C). pap. text 39.95 (*0-7167-2309-3*) W H Freeman.

Theories of Group Behavior. Ed. by B. Mullen & G. R. Geothals. 1986. (Social Psychology Ser.). (Illus.). 243p. 86.95 (*0-387-96351-0*) Spr-Verlag.

Theories of Human Development. Neil J. Salkind. 2nd ed. 1985. LC 84-19680. 288p. pap. 51.95 (*0-471-80575-0*) Wiley.

Theories of Human Nature: Classical & Contemporary Readings. Donald C. Abel. 1991. 432p. (C). pap. 26.25 (*0-07-000050-6*) McGrw-H Hghr Educ.

Theories of Hypnosis: Current Models & Perspectives. Ed. by Steven J. Lynn & Judith W. Rhue. 1991. LC 91-28531. (Clinical & Experimental Hypnosis Ser.). 634p. 68.00 (*0-89862-343-X*, 2343) Guilford Pubns.

Theories of Immune Networks. Ed. by H. Atlan & I. R. Cohen. 1989. (Synergetics Ser.: Vol. 46). (Illus.). 117p. 69.95 (*0-387-51678-6*) Spr-Verlag.

Theories of Love Development, Maintenance, & Dissolution: Octagonal Cycle & Differential Perspectives. Ed. by Oliver C. Tzeng. 1992. LC 91-41777. 336p. 82.50 (*0-275-94234-1*, C4234, Praeger Pubs) Greenwood.

Theories of Object Relations: Bridges to Self Psychology. Howard A. Bacal & Kenneth Newman. 1990. LC 89-28101. (Personality, Psychopathology, & Psychotherapy Ser.). 312p. text 47.50 (*0-231-06102-1*) Col U Pr.

Theories of Personality. David Lester. 1995. 200p. 69.95 (*1-56032-350-7*); pap. 34.95 (*1-56032-351-5*) Taylor & Francis.

Theories of Personality. Richard M. Ryckman. (Psychology Ser.). (C). 3rd ed. 1985. LC 84-23287. 544p. mass mkt. 34.50 (*0-534-04914-1*); 4th ed. 1988. 550p. mass mkt. 45.50 (*0-534-09996-3*); 6th ed. 1996. LC 96-5593. 635p. mass mkt. 42.50 (*0-534-33976-X*) Brooks-Cole.

Theories of Personality. Duane P. Schultz. 6th ed. 1997. (Psychology Ser.). pap. 16.75 (*0-534-35015-1*); LC 97-15794. 530p. mass mkt. 74.95 (*0-534-34119-5*) Brooks-Cole.

Theories of Personality. Richard M. Ryckman. 7th ed. 1999. LC 99-24491. (Psychology Ser.). 720p. spiral bd. 78.95 (*0-534-34898-X*) Brooks-Cole.

Theories of Populations in Biological Communities. F. B. Christiansen & T. M. Fenchel. 1977. LC 76-49871. (Ecological Studies: Vol. 20). 39.00 (*3-540-08010-4*) Spr-Verlag.

Theories of Psychotherapy. C. H. Patterson & C. Edward Watkins, Jr. 5th ed. 1997. LC 95-17191. 608p. (C). pap. text 88.00 (*0-673-99103-2*) Addson-Wesley Educ.

Theories of Psychotherapy: Origins & Evolution. Ed. by Paul L. Wachtel & Stanley B. Messer. 1997. LC 97-20793. 310p. pap. 29.95 (*1-55798-435-2*, 431-6920) Am Psychol.

Theories of Psychotherapy & Counseling: Concepts & Cases. Richard S. Sharf. 1995. LC 95-23582. 720p. mass mkt. 62.95 (*0-534-21618-8*) Brooks-Cole.

Theories of Psychotherapy & Counseling: Concepts & Cases. Richard S. Sharf. 2nd ed. 1999. LC 99-37970. (Counseling Ser.). 750p. spiral bd. 88.95 (*0-534-36485-3*) Wadsworth Pub.

Theories of Rape: Recent Inquiries into the Causes of Sexual Aggression. Ed. by Lee Ellis. 1989. 175p. 47.95 (*0-89116-172-4*) Hemisp Pub.

Theories of the Evolution of Knowing. Ed. by Gary Greenberg & Ethel Tobach. 1990. (T. C. Schneirla Conference Ser.: Vol. 4). 176p. text 65.00 (*0-8058-0755-1*) L Erlbaum Assocs.

Theories of Visual Perception. Ian E. Gordon. 1997. LC 96-3081. 312p. pap. 70.00 (*0-471-96825-0*) Wiley.

Theories on Drug Abuse: Selected Contemporary Perspectives. 1986. LC 67-11961. lib. bdg. 79.95 (*0-8490-3515-5*) Gordon Pr.

Theory & Assessment of Stressful Life Events, No. 6. Ed. by Thomas W. Miller. 1996. LC 95-40591. (Stress & Health Ser.: Monograph 6). 224p. 55.00 (*0-8236-6521-6*) Intl Univs Pr.

Theory & Measurement of Social Interest. James E. Crandall. 1981. LC 81-9973. 224p. text 56.00 (*0-231-05256-1*) Col U Pr.

Theory & Methods of Economic Evaluation of Health Care. Magnus Johannesson. 1996. (Developments in Health Economics & Public Policy Ser.: Vol. 4). 260p. (C). lib. bdg. 139.00 (*0-7923-4037-X*) Kluwer Academic.

Theory & Nursing: Integrated Knowledge Development. Peggy L. Chinn & Maeona K. Kramer. 5th ed. 1998. LC 98-31652. (Illus.). 256p. pap. text 39.00 (*0-323-00317-6*) Mosby Inc.

Theory & Practice of Brief Therapy. Simon H. Budman & Alan S. Gurman. 1988. LC 87-24847. 402p. 48.00 (*0-89862-716-8*, 2716) Guilford Pubns.

Theory & Practice of Counseling & Psychotherapy. Ed. by Gerald Corey. 4th ed. 1991. LC 90-33124. (Counseling Ser.). 512p. (C). pap., stu. ed. 13.50 (*0-534-13316-9*); text 43.25 (*0-534-13314-2*) Brooks-Cole.

Theory & Practice of Counseling & Psychotherapy. Gerald Corey. 5th ed. 1995. LC 95-15145. (Counseling Ser.). 526p. pap. 71.95 (*0-534-33856-9*) Brooks-Cole.

Theory & Practice of Counseling & Psychotherapy: HP 611. California College for Health Sciences Staff. 1991. 22p. (C). spiral bd. (*0-933195-35-4*) CA College Health Sci.

***Theory & Practice of Cultural-Historical Psychology.** Ed. by Seth Chaiklin. 2000. (Social Science Series: No. 22). 400p. pap. (*87-7288-838-5*) Aarhus Univ Pr DNK. *Dist:* David Brown.

Theory & Practice of Group Counseling. Gerald Corey. 2nd ed. 1984. LC 84-5026. (Psychology-Counseling Ser.). 600p. (C). pap. 32.75 (*0-534-03223-0*) Brooks-Cole.

Theory & Practice of Group Psychotherapy. Irvin D. Yalom. 4th ed. 1995. LC 94-33555. 608p. pap. 55.00 (*0-465-08448-6*) Basic.

Theory & Practice of Histological Techniques. Ed. by John D. Bancroft & Alan Stevens. 3rd ed. 1990. (Illus.). 726p. text (*0-443-03559-8*) Church.

Theory & Practice of Histological Techniques. Bancroft. 4th ed. 1995. text (*0-443-04760-X*, B0971) Church.

Theory & Practice of Histotechnology. Dezna C. Sheehan & Barbara B. Hrapchak. 2nd ed. 1987. LC 87-17446. 493p. (C). text 65.00 (*0-935470-39-5*) Battelle.

Theory & Practice of HIV Counselling: A Systemic Approach. Robert Bor et al. 1993. LC 92-48338. 208p. pap. text 23.95 (*0-87630-717-9*) Brunner-Routledge.

Theory & Practice of Industrial Pharmacy. Ed. by Leon Lachman et al. 3rd ed. 1986. LC 84-27806. (Illus.). 902p. text 105.00 (*0-8121-0977-5*) Lppncott W & W.

Theory & Practice of Intra-Aortic Balloon Pump Therapy. Ed. by Gerald A. Maccioli. 1996. LC 96-14625. 224p. 49.95 (*0-683-05302-7*) Lppncott W & W.

***Theory & Practice of Nursing: An Integrated Approach to Patient Care.** 1995. (Illus.). pap. (*1-873732-10-4*) Nelson Thornes GBR. *Dist:* Intl Spec Bk.

Theory & Practice of Oncology: Historical Evolution & Present Principles. Ronald W. Raven. 1990. (History of Medicine Ser.). (Illus.). 366p. lib. bdg. 104.95 (*1-85070-179-2*, Parthenon Pbng) CRC Pr.

Theory & Practice of Psychiatric Care. (*0-340-26564-7*) E A GBR. *Dist:* Routldge.

Theory & Practice of Self-Psychology. Marjorie T. White & Marcella B. Weiner. 1987. LC 86-919. 240p. text 32.95 (*0-87630-425-0*) Brunner-Routledge.

Theory & Practice of Therapeutic Touch. Jean Sayre-Adams & Stephen G. Wright. 1995. LC 95-7244. (Illus.). pap. text (*0-443-05227-1*) Church.

***Theory & Practice of Therapeutic Touch.** Jean Sayre-Adams & S. G. Wright. 2nd ed. 2001. LC 2001-17492. (Illus.). xi, 158p. (*0-443-07082-2*) Church.

Theory & Practice of 3D PET. Bernard Bendriem & David W. Townsend. 1998. LC 98-23005. (Developments in Nuclear Medicine Ser.). 167p. 78.00 (*0-7923-5108-8*) Kluwer Academic.

Theory & Problems of Child Development. David P. Ausubel et al. 3rd ed. 1980. LC 79-93284. 688p. text 47.00 (*0-8089-1183-X*, 790280, Grune & Strat) Harcrt Hlth Sci Grp.

Theory & Reality of Value-Based Medical Purchasing: Lessons from the Pioneers. Ed. by Irene Fraser. 1999. 55p. (C). reprint ed. pap. text 20.00 (*0-7881-8237-4*) DIANE Pub.

Theory & Research in Behavioral Pediatrics. Ed. by Hiram E. Fitzgerald et al. Vol. 1. 1982. 308p. 65.00 (*0-306-40851-1*); Vol. 2. 1984. 266p. 75.00 (*0-306-41566-6*); Vol. 3. 1986. (Illus.). 254p. (C). 102.00 (*0-306-42328-6*) Perseus Pubng (Plenum Trade).

Theory & Research in Behavioral Pediatrics. H. E. Fitzgerald et al. (Illus.). (C). Vol. 4. 1988. LC 82-646646. 282p. 85.00 (*0-306-42882-2*); Vol. 5. 1991. 248p. 85.00 (*0-306-43855-0*) Perseus Pubng (Plenum Trade).

Theory & Therapy in Dynamic Psychiatry. Jules H. Masserman. 1995. LC 72-96926. (Master Work Ser.). 240p. pap. 50.00 (*1-56821-511-8*) Aronson.

Theory & Treatment of Anorexia Nervosa & Bulimia: Biomedical, Sociocultural, & Psychological Perspectives. Ed. by Steven W. Emmett. 1985. LC 84-29267. 352p. text 49.95 (*0-87630-384-X*) Brunner-Routledge.

Theory Construction & Testing. Ed. by Margaret T. Beard. 1996. LC 95-60045. 328p. (C). pap. 45.95 (*0-923950-12-5*) Tucker IL.

Theory Development: What, Why, How? Jacqueline Fawcett et al. 1978. 86p. 6.00 (*0-88737-219-8*, 15-1708) Natl League Nurse.

Theory-Directed Nursing Practice. Ed. by Shirley M. Ziegler. 1993. LC 92-2379. 280p. 37.95 (*0-8261-7630-5*) Springer Pub.

Theory for Nursing: Systems, Concepts & Process. Imogene M. King. 1989. LC 81-1996. 181p. (C). mass mkt. 39.00 (*0-8273-4267-5*) Delmar.

Theory of Cognitive Dissonance. Leon Festinger. 1957. xi, 291p. 51.00 (*0-8047-0131-8*) Stanford U Pr.

Theory of Coping Systems: Change in Supportive Health Organizations. Francis D. Powell. 1975. 244p. text 34.95 (*0-87073-029-0*) Transaction Pubs.

Theory of Heat: Biomechanics, Biophysics, & Nonlinear Dynamics of Cardiac Function. Ed. by L. Glass et al. 1991. (Institute for Nonlinear Science Ser.). (Illus.). 611p. 87.95 (*0-387-97483-0*) Spr-Verlag.

Theory of Mental Tests. Harold Gulliksen. 1987. 512p. (C). reprint ed. text 89.95 (*0-8058-0024-7*) L Erlbaum Assocs.

Theory of Personality Development. Luciano L'Abate. Ed. by Charles H. Bryson. 1993. LC 93-12795. (Personality Processes Ser.). 313p. 140.00 (*0-471-30303-8*) Wiley.

Theory of Predicates. Farrell Ackerman & Gert Webelhuth. 1998. LC 97-28186. (Lecture Notes). 500p. (C). 69.95 (*1-57586-087-2*); pap. text 27.95 (*1-57586-086-4*) CSLI.

Theory of Probability for Clinical Diagnostic Testing. D. Maxwell & Eiki Satake. 1993. 123p. (C). stu. ed. 19.78 (*1-56870-062-8*) RonJon Pub.

Theory of Reasoned Action: Its Application to AIDS-Preventive Behavior. Ed. by Deborah J. Terry et al. 1998. LC 93-34087. (Social Psychology Ser.: No. 28). 362p. lib. bdg. 68.95 (*0-08-041932-1*) Routledge.

Theory of Suicide. Maurice L. Farber. Ed. by Robert J. Kastenbaum. 1979. LC 76-19568. (Death & Dying Ser.). reprint ed. lib. bdg. 19.95 (*0-405-09564-3*) Ayer.

Theory of the Striatum. Ed. by J. Wickens. 1993. LC 93-34358. (Studies in Neurosciences). 194p. 180.00 (*0-08-042278-0*, Pergamon Pr) Elsevier.

Therapeutic Action: A Guide to Psychoanalytic Therapy. Enrico E. Jones. 2000. LC 99-44464. (Illus.). xxiii, 381p. 60.00 (*0-7657-0243-6*) Aronson.

Therapeutic Activities Specialist. Jack Rudman. 1994. (Career Examination Ser.: C-889). pap. 29.95 (*0-8373-0889-5*) Nat Learn.

Therapeutic Activities with the Impaired Elderly. Phyllis M. Foster. 1986. LC 86-9945. (Activities, Adaptation & Aging Ser.: Vol. 8, Nos. 3 & 4). 204p. text 39.95 (*0-86656-566-3*) Haworth Pr.

Therapeutic Alliance. Ed. by Steven T. Levy. 2000. LC 99-22442. (Workshop Series of the American Psychoanalytic Association). 137p. 27.50 (*0-8236-6471-6*) Intl Univs Pr.

Therapeutic Alliance. William W. Meissner. 1996. LC 96-13037. 100p. 47.00 (*0-300-06684-8*) Yale U Pr.

Therapeutic Alliance in Brief Psychotherapy. Ed. by Jeremy D. Safran & J. Christopher Muran. 1998. LC 98-16497. 238p. pap. 39.95 (*1-55798-508-1*, 431-713A) Am Psychol.

Therapeutic & Everyday Discourse As Behavior Change: Towards a Microanalysis in Psychotherapy Process Research. John Kaye et al. Ed. by Jurg Siegfried. 1995. LC 93-48581. 544p. 130.00 (*0-89391-919-5*, Ablex) Greenwood.

Therapeutic & Surgical Equipment Markets: New Technologies Flourish Despite Slow FDA Approval & Reimbursement Issues. Market Intelligence Staff. 1993. 251p. 1895.00 (*1-56753-427-9*) Frost & Sullivan.

Therapeutic Angiogenesis. Ed. by G. M. Rubanyi et al. 1999. LC 99-34989. (Ernst Schering Research Foundation Ser.: Vol. 28). (Illus.). 224p. 79.00 (*3-540-65693-6*) Spr-Verlag.

Therapeutic Angiography. Ed. by C. A. Athanasoulis et al. 1981. (Illus.). 128p. 41.00 (*0-387-10526-3*) Spr-Verlag.

Therapeutic Antibodies. Ed. by J. Landon & T. Chard. 1994. LC 94-38225. (Illus.). 231p. 126.00 (*0-387-19722-2*) Spr-Verlag.

Therapeutic Applications of Cytokines: Control of Inflammation, Growth & Differentiation. Ed. by Johanna Schlegel. 1996. (Biomedical Library). 360p. pap. 795.00 (*1-57936-012-2*) Drug & Market Dev.

Therapeutic Applications of Interleukin-2. Michael B. Atkins & James W. Mier. 1993. (Basic & Clinical Oncology Ser.: Vol. 2). (Illus.). 520p. text 230.00 (*0-8247-8809-5*) Dekker.

Therapeutic Applications of NSAIDs: Subpopulations & New Formulations, No. 10. Ed. by J. P. Famaey &

Harold E. Paulus. 1992. LC 92-17090. (Infectious Disease & Therapy Ser.: Vol. 10). (Illus.). 528p. text 199.00 (*0-8247-8631-9*) Dekker.

Therapeutic Applications of Prostaglandins. (*0-340-56022-3*) E A GBR. *Dist:* Routldge.

Therapeutic Applications of Ribozymes. Kevin J. Scanlon. 1998. LC 98-21526. (Methods in Molecular Medicine Ser.: Vol. 11). (Illus.). 476p. 120.00 (*0-89603-477-1*) Humana.

Therapeutic Approaches in Mental Health - Psychiatric Nursing. David S. Bailey & Deborah R. Bailey. 4th ed. 1997. LC 96-40370. (Illus.). 481p. (C). pap. text 29.95 (*0-8036-0213-8*) Davis Co.

Therapeutic Approaches to the Treatment of Obesity. Cynthia Arbeeny. Ed. by Susan C. DiClemente. 1997. LC 98-227256. (Illus.). 300p. spiral bd. (*1-57936-062-9*, 963) Drug & Market Dev.

Therapeutic Associates Rehabilitation Guidelines. Ed. by Carol Schunk & Kelly Reed. 1996. (C). pap. text, stu. ed. 125.00 (*1-888629-04-5*) Theraputic Assoc.

Therapeutic Associates Rehabilitation Guidelines Vol. 1: Lower Extremity. Ed. by Carol Schunk & Kelly Reed. 1995. 180p. text (*1-888629-01-0*) Theraputic Assoc.

Therapeutic Associates Rehabilitation Guidelines Vol. 2: Spine & TMJ. Ed. by Carol Schunk & Kelly Reed. 1996. 150p. text (*1-888629-02-9*) Theraputic Assoc.

Therapeutic Associates Rehabilitation Guidelines Vol. 3: Upper Extremity. Ed. by Carol Schunk & Kelly Reed. 1996. text (*1-888629-03-7*) Theraputic Assoc.

Therapeutic Caregiving: A Practical Guide for Caregivers of Persons with Alzheimer's & Other Dementia Causing Diseases. Barbara J. Bridges. rev. ed. 1996. LC 95-94060. (Illus.). 256p. (Orig.). reprint ed. pap. 19.95 (*0-9645178-0-9*) BJB Pub.

Therapeutic Change: An Object Relations Perspective. Sidney J. Blatt & R. Q. Ford. 1994. (Applied Clinical Psychology Ser.). (Illus.). 336p. (C). 49.50 (*0-306-44601-4*, Plenum Trade) Perseus Pubng.

Therapeutic Claims in Multiple Sclerosis: A Guide to Treatments. William A. Sibley. 4th rev. ed. 1996. (Illus.). 213p. (Orig.). pap. 24.95 (*1-888799-08-0*) Demos Medical.

Therapeutic Communication: A Guide to Effective Interpersonal Skills for Health Care Professionals. Tova Navarra et al. 1990. LC 88-43159. 158p. pap. 23.00 (*1-55642-075-7*) SLACK Inc.

Therapeutic Communication: Knowing What to Say When. Paul L. Wachtel. LC 92-49431. 308p. 1998. (Illus.). pap. 22.00 (*1-57230-416-2*, C0416); 1993. text 37.95 (*0-89862-260-3*) Guilford Pubns.

Therapeutic Communication with Children: The Mutual Storytelling Technique in Child Psychotherapy. Richard A. Gardner. 2nd ed. 1986. LC 71-155063. 970p. 70.00 (*0-87668-856-3*) Aronson.

Therapeutic Communications for Allied Health Professions. Carol D. Tamparo & Wilburta Q. Lindh. 1993. 253p. (C). mass mkt. 31.00 (*0-8273-4999-8*) Delmar.

Therapeutic Communications for Health Professionals. Carol D. Tamparo & Wilburta Q. Lindh. 2nd ed. 1999. LC 99-33170. (Medical Assisting Ser.). 320p. (C). pap. text 38.95 (*0-7668-0921-8*) Delmar.

Therapeutic Communities: Past, Present & Future. Rex Haigh & Penelope Campling. 1998. LC 98-41230. (Therapeutic Communities Ser.). (*1-85302-614-X*) Jessica Kingsley.

Therapeutic Communities for Addictions: Readings in Theory, Research & Practice. George DeLeon & James T. Ziegenfuss, Jr. 1986. (Illus.). 282p. (C). 54.95 (*0-398-05206-9*) C C Thomas.

Therapeutic Communities for Offenders. Eric Cullen et al. 1997. LC 96-30405. (Offender Rehabilitation Ser.). 296p. pap. 75.00 (*0-471-96980-X*) Wiley.

Therapeutic Community: A Successful Approach for Treating Substance Abusers. Lewis Yablonsky. 1989. LC 87-19625. 27.95 (*0-89876-145-X*) Gardner Pr.

Therapeutic Community: Theory, Model & Method. George De Leon. 2000. LC 99-89660. (Illus.). xviii, 450p. text 41.95 (*0-8261-1349-4*) Springer Pub.

Therapeutic Community Movement: Charisma & Routinisation. Nick P. Manning. 1989. (Therapeutic Communities Section, International Library of Group Psychotherapy & Group Processes). 256p. 49.50 (*0-415-02913-9*) Routledge.

Therapeutic Community with Chronic Mental Patients. J. Maller. 1971. (Bibliotheca Psychiatrica Ser.: No. 146). pap. 38.50 (*3-8055-1157-4*) S Karger.

Therapeutic Considerations for the Elderly. Ed. by Osa L. Jackson. 1987. (Clinics in Physical Therapy Ser.: Vol. 14). (Illus.). 316p. text (*0-443-08389-4*) Church.

Therapeutic Conversations. Ed. by Stephen G. Gilligan & Reese E. Price. 1993. LC 92-31745. 250p. (C). 34.95 (*0-393-70145-X*) Norton.

Therapeutic Crafts: A Practical Approach. Cynthia Johnson et al. 1996. LC 96-2755. (Illus.). 256p. (Orig.). pap. 26.00 (*1-55642-279-2*, 32792) SLACK Inc.

Therapeutic Dialogue: A Guide to Humane & Egalitarian Psychotherapy. Sohan L. Sharma. 1995. LC 95-9602. 376p. 50.00 (*1-56821-656-4*) Aronson.

Therapeutic Dilemmas for the MRCGP. Roger Charlton & J. C. Mucklow. 1998. LC 97-45691. 176p. pap. text 35.00 (*0-7506-2918-5*) Buttrwrth-Heinemann.

Therapeutic Drug Monitoring. Gerald E. Schumacher. 1995. LC 94-40831. 660p. (C). text 70.00 (*0-8385-8946-4*, A8946-7) McGraw-Hill Prof.

Therapeutic Drug Monitoring: A Guide to Clinical Application. Ed. by Mary H. Caviness et al. 1987. LC 85-71233. (Illus.). 438p. spiral bd. 35.00 (*0-9614903-1-4*, 9520-56) Abbott Laboratories.

Therapeutic Drug Monitoring & Toxicology by Liquid Chromatography. Steven H. Y. Wong. 1985. (Chromatographic Science Ser.: Vol. 32). (Illus.). 512p. text 225.00 (*0-8247-7246-6*) Dekker.

Therapeutic Drugs. Ed. by Colin Dollery. 1991. (Illus.). 3000p. text (*0-443-02846-X*) Church.

Therapeutic Drugs Colin T. Dollery. 2nd ed. 1999. LC 98-40969. (C). text (*0-443-05148-8*) Church.

Therapeutic Drugs, Supplement 1. Ed. by Colin Dollery. 2nd ed. 1993. (Illus.). 272p. text (*0-443-04676-X*) Church.

Therapeutic Drugs & the Quality of Life. Ed. by Ivan K. Goldberg et al. 1998. LC 96-84685. (Current Thanatology Ser.). 120p. (Orig.). pap. 18.95 (*0-930194-83-7*) Ctr Thanatology.

Therapeutic Effectiveness of Methadone Maintenance Programs in the U. S. A. S. S. Wilmarth & A. Avram. 1974. (Offset Publications: No. 3). pap. text 17.00 (*92-4-170003-3*, 1120003) World Health.

Therapeutic Effects in Ocular Lesions Obtained by Systemic & Topical Administration of an Activator of the Oxygen Metabolism. Ed. by F. Menna. 1980. (Journal: Vol. 180, Suppl. 1). (Illus.). vi, 92p. 28.75 (*3-8055-1686-X*) S Karger.

Therapeutic Endoscopy: Color Atlas of Operative Techniques for the Gastrointestinal Tract. Nib Soehendra et al. 1997. LC 97-28201. (*3-13-108261-5*) G Thieme DEU. *Dist:* Thieme Med Pubs.

Therapeutic Endoscopy: Color Atlas of Operative Techniques for the GI Tract. N. Soehendra et al. 1997. LC 97-28201. (Illus.). 264p. 165.00 (*0-86577-638-5*) Thieme Med Pubs.

Therapeutic Environment. Robert J. Langs. 1979. LC 79-64458. 592p. 60.00 (*0-87668-385-5*) Aronson.

Therapeutic Exercise. Hall et al. 1998. LC 98-28903. (Illus.). 784p. text 65.50 (*0-397-55260-2*) Lppncott W & W.

Therapeutic Exercise. John V. Basmajian & Steven Wolf. 5th ed. 1990. (Illus.). 460p. 49.00 (*0-683-00433-6*) Lppncott W & W.

Therapeutic Exercise for Body Alignment & Function. Lucille Daniels & Catherine Worthingham. 2nd ed. 1977. LC 76-27058. (Illus.). pap. text 35.95 (*0-7216-2873-7*) Saunders.

Therapeutic Exercise in Developmental Disabilities. Ed. by Patricia C. Montgomery & Barbara Connolly. 2nd ed. 1993. (Illus.). 244p. (Orig.). (C). pap. text 34.95 (*1-879971-01-1*) Chattanga Grp.

Therapeutic Exercises: Foundations & Techniques. Carolyn Kisner & Lynn A. Colby. 3rd ed. 1996. (Illus.). 761p. (C). spiral bd. 51.95 (*0-8036-0038-0*) Davis Co.

***Therapeutic Exercises for Spinal Segmental Stabilization in Low Back Pain: Scientific Basis & Clinical Approach.** Carolyn Richardson. 1999. (Illus.). 202p. text (*0-443-05802-4*) Church GBR. *Dist:* Saunders.

Therapeutic Exercises for Victimized & Neglected Girls: Applications for Individual, Family, & Group Psychotherapy. Pearl S. Berman. 1994. LC 94-15881. 178p. otabind 29.45 (*1-56887-003-5*, TEVBP, Prof Resc Pr) Pro Resource.

Therapeutic Exercises in Functional Kinetics: Analysis & Instruction of Individually Adaptable Exercise. Susanne Klein-Vogelbach. Tr. by L. Sloan-Ecker from GER. 1991. (Illus.). 375p. 59.00 (*0-387-52731-1*) Spr-Verlag.

Therapeutic Experience & Its Setting: A Clinical Dialogue. Leo Stone & Robert J. Langs. 1980. LC 80-667. (Therapeutic Experience & Settin C Ser.). 382p. 50.00 (*0-87668-405-3*) Aronson.

Therapeutic Foster Care: Critical Issues. Ed. by Robert P. Hawkins & James Breiling. 1989. (Trilogy Ser.: Bk. 1). pap. 13.50 (*0-87868-355-0*, 3550) Child Welfare.

Therapeutic Gastrointestinal Endoscopy. Rosson & Bloom. 1991. (*0-8151-7399-7*) Mosby Inc.

***Therapeutic Gastrointestinal Endoscopy.** Westaby & Lombard. 2001. (Illus.). 294p. (*1-899066-95-0*) Isis Med GBR. *Dist:* Bks Intl VA.

Therapeutic Gastrointestinal Endoscopy. Stephen E. Silvis. 2nd ed. 1990. LC 89-15541. (Illus.). 400p. 115.00 (*0-89640-167-7*) Igaku-Shoin.

Therapeutic Group Analysis. Siegmund H. Foulkes. 1965. 328p. 47.50 (*0-8236-6480-5*) Intl Univs Pr.

Therapeutic Heat & Cold. Justus F. Lehmann. 4th ed. 1990. (Rehabilitation Medicine Library). (Illus.). 752p. lib. bdg. 76.00 (*0-683-04908-9*) Lppncott W & W.

Therapeutic Hemapheresis, Vol. 1. James L. MacPherson & Duke O. Kasprisin. 1985. LC 84-17637. 224p. 132.00 (*0-8493-6148-6*, RB173) Franklin.

Therapeutic Hemapheresis, Vol. 2. Ed. by Duke O. Kasprisin & James L. MacPherson. 1985. 208p. 117.00 (*0-8493-6149-4*) Franklin.

Therapeutic Hemapheresis in the 1990s. Ed. by U. E. Nydegger. 1990. (Current Studies in Hematology & Blood Transfusion: No. 57). (Illus.). viii, 282p. 232.25 (*3-8055-5166-5*) S Karger.

Therapeutic Hemorheology. A. M. Ehrly. 1991. (Illus.). 320p. 135.00 (*0-387-52263-8*) Spr-Verlag.

Therapeutic Humor with the Elderly. Ed. by Francis A. McGuire et al. 1993. LC 92-43465. (Activities, Adaptation & Aging Ser.: No. 17(1)). (Illus.). 116p. lib. bdg. 39.95 (*1-56024-310-4*) Haworth Pr.

Therapeutic Immunology. Ed. by K. Frank Austen et al. 1996. (Illus.). 650p. 215.00 (*0-86542-375-X*) Blackwell Sci.

Therapeutic Immunology. K. F. Austen et al. 2nd rev. ed. 2000. LC 00-44408. (Illus.). 672p. 209.95 (*0-632-04359-8*) Blackwell Sci.

Therapeutic Implications & Mechanisms of Angiogenesis: Inhibitors & Stimulators. Ed. by Wendy Hori. 1996. (Biomedical Library). pap. 795.00 (*1-57936-018-1*) Drug & Market Dev.

Therapeutic Intervention: Healing Strategies for Human Systems. Ed. by Uri Rueveni et al. 1982. LC 81-13501. 285p. 35.95 (*0-89885-086-X*, Kluwer Acad Hman Sci) Kluwer Academic.

***Therapeutic Interventions for Patients with Spinal Cord Injuries.** Erica Druin & Kim Planten. 2001. text (*0-323-00699-X*) Mosby Inc.

Therapeutic Interventions for the Person with Dementia. Ed. by Ellen D. Taira. 1986. LC 86-3123. (Physical & Occupational Therapy in Geriatrics Ser.: Vol. 4, No. 3). 143p. text 39.95 (*0-86656-556-6*) Haworth Pr.

Therapeutic Interventions in Alzheimer's Disease: A Program of Functional Skills for Activities of Daily Living & Communication. Joan K. Glickstein. 2nd ed. 1998. LC 96-45156. 69.00 (*0-8342-0930-6*) PRO-ED.

Therapeutic Interventions in the Complement System. Ed. by John D. Lambris & V. Michael Holers. 2000. LC 99-57866. (Contemporary Immunology Ser.). 259p. 119.50 (*0-89603-587-5*) Humana.

Therapeutic Interventions with Ethnic Elders: Health & Social Issues. Ed. by Sara Aleman et al. 2000. LC 99-45998. (Illus.). x, 219p. lib. bdg. 39.95 (*0-7890-0272-8*) Haworth Pr.

Therapeutic Laser Endoscopy in Gastrointestinal Disease. Ed. by David Fleischer et al. 1983. text 141.50 (*0-89838-577-6*) Kluwer Academic.

Therapeutic Lasers: Theory & Practice. G. David Baxter & Costas Diamantopolous. 1995. LC 93-14226. (Illus.). 192p. text (*0-443-04393-0*) Church.

Therapeutic Management of the Complicated Patient with Reflux Disease. Ed. by Chris Fellner. 1996. (*1-57130-021-X*) Medicine Grp USA.

Therapeutic Massage. Holey. 1997. 220p. pap. text (*0-7020-1923-2*) Bailliere Tindall.

Therapeutic Mastery: Becoming a More Creative & Effective Psychotherapist. Charles H. Kramer. 2000. LC 00-24659. xx, 277p. pap. text 25.95 (*1-891944-42-8*) Zeig Tucker Theisen.

Therapeutic Materials—Index of New Information & Medical Research Bible. David D. Zabarine. 1994. 150p. 47.50 (*0-7883-0092-X*); pap. 44.50 (*0-7883-0093-8*) ABBE Pubs Assn.

Therapeutic Medical Devices: Application & Design. Ed. by Albert M. Cook & John G. Webster. 1982. (Illus.). 656p. text 72.00 (*0-13-914796-9*) P-H.

Therapeutic Medications in Sports Medicine. Malissa Martin & William N. Yates, Jr. 1997. LC 97-45783. 313p. spiral bd. 29.95 (*0-683-30223-X*) Lppncott W & W.

Therapeutic Metaphors. David Gordon. 1978. LC 78-58574. pap. 21.95 (*0-916990-04-4*) META Pubns.

Therapeutic Metaphors for Children & the Child Within. Joyce C. Mills & Richard J. Crowley. 1986. LC 86-9700. 288p. text 29.95 (*0-87630-429-3*) Brunner-Routledge.

Therapeutic Modalities for Allied-Health Professionals. William E. Prentice et al. 96th ed. 1998. LC 97-48335. (Illus.). 500p. text 52.95 (*0-07-050771-6*) McGraw-Hill Educ Grp.

Therapeutic Modalities in Sports Medicine. William E. Prentice. 4th ed. 1998. LC 98-10430. 416p. text 72.81 (*0-07-092066-4*) McGrw-H Hghr Educ.

Therapeutic Nursery School. Ed. by Robert A. Furman & Anny Katan. 1969. LC 78-75187. 329p. 50.00 (*0-8236-6500-3*) Intl Univs Pr.

Therapeutic Nutrition: A Practical Guide. C. R. Pennington. 1991. (Illus.). 288p. (Orig.). (C). (gr. 13). pap. text 43.50 (*0-412-29230-0*) Chapman & Hall.

Therapeutic Opportunities in Alzheimer's Disease: Advances in Diagnostics & Drug Development. Ed. by Katherine Emory. 1996. (Biomedical Library). pap. 795.00 (*1-57936-017-3*) Drug & Market Dev.

Therapeutic Paradox. Ed. by L. Michael Ascher. 1989. LC 89-11999. 385p. text 46.50 (*0-89862-393-6*) Guilford Pubns.

Therapeutic Partnership: Ethical Concerns in Psychotherapy. Carl Goldberg. 1994. LC 94-72279. (Master Work Ser.). 290p. pap. 50.00 (*1-56821-325-5*) Aronson.

Therapeutic Peptides & Proteins: Assessing the New Technologies. Ed. by Daniel R. Marshak & Darrell T. Liu. 1988. (Banbury Reports: No. 29). (Illus.). 288p. text 77.00 (*0-87969-229-4*) Cold Spring Harbor.

Therapeutic Peptides & Proteins: Formulation, Delivery & Targeting. Ed. by Daniel R. Marshak & Darrell T. Liu. 1989. (Current Communications in Molecular Biology Ser.). (Illus.). (Orig.). pap. text 24.00 (*0-87969-328-2*) Cold Spring Harbor.

Therapeutic Perspective: Medical Practice, Knowledge & Identity in America, 1820-1885. John H. Warner. 1986. LC 85-30235. (Illus.). 376p. 45.00 (*0-674-88330-6*) HUP.

Therapeutic Perspective: Medical Practice, Knowledge & Identity in America, 1820-1885. John H. Warner. 1997. LC 97-31326. 380p. pap. 21.95 (*0-691-01209-1*) Princeton U Pr.

Therapeutic Photomedicine. Ed. by H. Hoenigsmann & G. Stingl. 1986. (Current Problems in Dermatology Ser.: Vol. 15). (Illus.). viii, 308p. 200.00 (*3-8055-4151-1*) S Karger.

Therapeutic Potential of Melatonin: 2nd Locarno Meeting on Neuroendocrinoimmunology, Locarno, May 1996. Ed. by Russell J. Reiter et al. 1997. LC 97-5492. (Frontiers of Hormone Research Ser.: Vol. 23, 1997). (Illus.). 178p. 172.25 (*3-8055-6439-2*) S Karger.

Therapeutic Presence: Bridging Expression & Form. Ed. by Arthur Robbins. 1997. LC 97-223546. 275p. pap. (*1-85302-559-3*) Jessica Kingsley GBR. *Dist:* Taylor & Francis.

Therapeutic Principles in Social Work Practice: A Primer for Clinicians. Herbert S. Strean. 1993. LC 93-31571. (Master Work Ser.). 152p. pap. 25.00 (*1-56821-137-6*) Aronson.

Therapeutic Process: Essays & Lectures. Karen Horney & Bernard J. Paris. 1999. LC 98-11729. 256p. 35.00 (*0-300-07527-8*) Yale U Pr.

Therapeutic Process, the Self, & Female Psychology: Collected Psychoanalytic Papers. Helene Deutsch. Ed. by Paul Roazen. 1991. LC 91-6761. 376p. (C). text 44.95 (*0-88738-429-3*) Transaction Pubs.

Therapeutic Program for the Patient with Arthritis. Kenneth R. Wilske et al. 3rd ed. 1980. 54p. pap. 5.00 (*0-9601944-3-6*) V Mason Clinic.

Therapeutic Progress in Ovarian Cancer, Testicular Cancer & Sarcomas. Ed. by A. T. Van Oosterom et al. 1980. (Boerhaave Series for Postgraduate Medical Education: No. 16). (Illus.). 516p. text 184.00 (*90-6021-452-8*) Kluwer Academic.

Therapeutic Protein & Peptide Formulation & Delivery, Vol. 675. Ed. by Z. Shahrokh et al. 1997. LC 97-22244. (ACS Symposium Ser.: No. 675). 230p. text 105.00 (*0-8412-3528-7*) Am Chemical.

***Therapeutic Proteins: Selected Case Studies.** Ed. by Klaus Dembowsky & Peter Stadler. 2001. 384p. 99.95 (*3-527-30270-0*) Wiley.

Therapeutic Radiology. William Mansfield. 3rd ed. 1999. pap. text 97.00 (*0-8385-8949-9*, Medical Exam) Appleton & Lange.

Therapeutic Recreation: A Helping Profession. Gerald S. O'Morrow. 2nd ed. 1980. (Illus.). 336p. text 24.00 (*0-8359-7659-9*) P-H.

Therapeutic Recreation: A Practical Approach. Marcia J. Carter et al. 2nd rev. ed. 1995. (Illus.). 593p. (C). text 46.95 (*0-88133-822-2*) Waveland Pr.

Therapeutic Recreation: Cases & Exercises. Barbara C. Wilhite & M. Jean Keller. 1992. LC 91-68519. (Illus.). 263p. (C). pap. text 22.95 (*0-910251-50-9*) Venture Pub PA.

Therapeutic Recreation - The First Steps to Reimbursement: An Overview. Linda Hutchinson-Troyer & Ann Gillespie. 1991. 26p. ring bd. 24.95 (*1-889435-00-7*) Am Therapeutic.

Therapeutic Recreation Activity Assessment. M. A. Hoss. Ed. by Joan Burlingame. 1993. 27p. ring bd. 240.00 incl. VHS (*1-882883-15-2*) Idyll Arbor.

Therapeutic Recreation for Exceptional Children: Let Me in, I Want to Play. Aubrey H. Fine & Nya M. Fine. 2nd ed. 1996. LC 96-8263. (Illus.). 422p. text 76.95 (*0-398-06661-2*); pap. text 55.95 (*0-398-06662-0*) C C Thomas.

Therapeutic Recreation for Long-Term Care Facilities. Fred S. Greenblatt. 1988. LC 86-27697. 198p. 34.95 (*0-89885-356-7*, Kluwer Acad Hman Sci) Kluwer Academic.

Therapeutic Recreation in the Nursing Home. Linda Buettner & Shelley Martin. 1995. LC 95-60609. (Illus.). 211p. (C). pap. text 29.95 (*0-910251-76-2*, TRN78) Venture Pub PA.

Therapeutic Recreation Protocol for Treatment of Substance Addictions. Rozanne W. Faulkner. 1991. LC 90-71920. (Illus.). 259p. (C). 29.95 (*0-910251-37-1*) Venture Pub PA.

Therapeutic Relationship & Its Impact. Carl Ransom Rogers. 1976. LC 76-14790. 625p. reprint ed. lib. bdg. 62.50 (*0-8371-8358-8*, ROTR, Greenwood Pr) Greenwood.

Therapeutic Relationship in Complementary Health Care. Annie Mitchell & Margaret A. Cormack. 1998. LC 97-51522. (C). pap. text 19.95 (*0-443-05319-7*) Churchill Ctr.

Therapeutic Relevance of Drug Assays. Ed. by Frederick A. DeWolff et al. 1979. (Boerhaave Series for Postgraduate Medical Education: No. 14). text 112.50 (*90-6021-443-9*) Kluwer Academic.

Therapeutic Stances: The Art of Using & Losing Control. Richard G. Whiteside. 1997. LC 97-25088. 230p. 25.95 (*0-87630-863-9*) Brunner-Routledge.

Therapeutic State: Psychiatry in the Mirror of Current Events. Thomas Szasz. 1984. LC 83-63057. 360p. pap. 26.00 (*0-87975-242-4*) Prometheus Bks.

T
U
V

Therapeutic Strategies for Treating Addiction: From Slavery to Freedom. Jerome D. Levin. 2001. LC 00-38967. 50.00 (*0-7657-0287-8*) Aronson.

Therapeutic Strategies of Modulating the Inflammatory Diseases. Inflammation Research Association Staff. Ed. by B. M. Weichman et al. 1997. LC 97-42748. (Agents & Actions Supplements Ser.: Vol. 49). 125p. text 60.00 (*3-7643-5690-1*) Birkhauser.

Therapeutic Studies. Kenneth L. Artiss. 1986. (C). text 22.50 (*0-9615865-0-8*) Psych Bks.

Therapeutic Superhighway. Kathleen M. Douglas. 1999. (Illus.). 120p. pap. 9.95 (*1-891929-09-7*) Four Seasons.

Therapeutic Surgical & Electronic Device Markets: A Detailed Database on a 13 Billion Dollar Market. Market Intelligence Staff. 1992. 280p. 995.00 (*1-56753-081-8*) Frost & Sullivan.

Therapeutic Touch: A Practical Guide. Janet Macrae. 1988. LC 87-45444. (Illus.). 112p. pap. 10.00 (*0-394-75588-X*) Knopf.

Therapeutic Trances: The Cooperation Principle in Ericksonian Hypnotherapy. Stephen G. Gilligan. 1986. LC 86-20706. 384p. text 41.95 (*0-87630-442-0*) Brunner-Routledge.

Therapeutic Use of Child's Play. Charles E. Schaefer. 1990. LC 75-9556. 688p. reprint ed. 70.00 (*0-87668-209-3*) Aronson.

Therapeutic Use of Stories: Handbook for Professionals. Kedar N. Dwivedi. 1997. LC 97-8846. (Illus.). 256p. (C). 84.95 (*0-415-15070-1*); pap. 27.95 (*0-415-15071-X*) Routledge.

Therapeutic Uses of Antioxidants for Health Improvements: Index of New Information with Authors, Subjects, & Bibliography. American Health Research Institute Staff. 1995. LC 95-16388. 57.50 (*0-7883-0468-2*) ABBE Pubs Assn.

Therapeutic Uses of Cannabis. British Medical Association Staff. 1998. 144p. text 36.00 (*90-5702-317-2*); pap. text 18.00 (*90-5702-318-0*) Gordon & Breach (Harwood Acad Pubs).

Therapeutic Uses of Music with Older Adults. Alicia A. Clair. 1996. LC 96-16282. (Illus.). 336p. (Orig.). pap. text 30.95 (*1-878812-32-7*) Hlth Prof Pr.

Therapeutic Uses of Trace Elements: Proceedings of the Fifth International Congress Held in Meribel, France, February 4-7, 1996. Ed. by Jean Neve et al. 1997. LC 96-41996. 446p. (C). text 129.50 (*0-306-45485-8*, Kluwer Plenum) Kluwer Academic.

Therapeutic Uses of Writing. Allan Hunter. 1996. 191p. lib. bdg. 65.00 (*1-56072-379-3*) Nova Sci Pubs.

Therapeutic Value of Music. Manly P. Hall. pap. 4.95 (*0-89314-815-6*) Philos Res.

Therapeutic Ways with Words. Kathleen W. Ferrara. 1994. (Oxford Studies in Sociolinguistics). (Illus.). 216p. (C). text 70.00 (*0-19-508337-7*) OUP.

Therapeutic Work with Children & Young People. Beta Copley & Barbara Forryan. 2nd ed. 1997. LC 97-179492. (Cassell Education Ser.). 256p. pap. 35.00 (*0-304-70011-8*) Continuum.

Therapeutics for Aggression: Psychological - Physical Crisis Intervention. Intro. by Michael Thackrey. 1986. 227p. 35.95 (*0-89885-305-2*, Kluwer Acad Hman Sci) Kluwer Academic.

Therapeutics in Cardiology. Ed. by A. J. De Luna. 1988. (Developments in Cardiovascular Medicine Ser.). 700p. (C). text 325.00 (*0-89838-981-X*) Kluwer Academic.

Therapeutics in Geriatric Neuropsychiatry. R. J. Ancill et al. 1998. LC 97-29971. 170p. 99.95 (*0-471-97947-3*) Wiley.

***Therapeutics in Pregnancy & Lactation.** Ed. by Anne Lee et al. 2000. 264p. pap. (*1-85775-269-4*) Radcliffe Med Pr GBR. *Dist:* Balogh.

Therapeutics in Respiratory Diseases. Peter J. Barnes et al. 1994. (*0-443-04234-9*); LC 93-3749. 180p. text (*0-443-04134-2*) Church.

Therapeutics in Terminal Cancer. Twycross. 3rd ed. 1998. text (*0-443-05294-8*) Saunders.

Therapeutics in Terminal Cancer Care. Robert G. Twycross & Sylvia A. Lack. 2nd ed. 1990. (Illus.). 237p. pap. text (*0-443-04118-0*) Church.

Therapie der Leukamien und Lymphome - Schwerpunkt Zytokine. Ed. by Juergen Fleischer et al. 1998. (Beitraege Zur Onkologie, Contributions to Oncology Ser.: Vol. 53, 1998). (Illus.). x, 272p. 143.50 (*3-8055-6571-2*) S Karger.

Therapie Urologischer Tumoren see Therapy of Urological Cancer

Therapie Urologischer Tumoren. R. Ackermann. 1991. (Illus.). 84p. pap. 35.00 (*3-8055-5294-7*) S Karger.

***Therapieoptimierungspruefung Band 23, Suppl. 9: Onkologie.** Deutsche Krebsgesellschaft Staff. 2001. (GER.). iv, 40p. 27.00 (*3-8055-7178-X*) S Karger.

Therapies for Psychosomatic Disorders in Children. Charles E. Schaefer et al. 1995. LC 94-30957. (Master Work Ser.). 380p. pap. 50.00 (*1-56821-375-1*) Aronson.

Therapist As Supervisor & Coach. Gary A. Morse. 1998. LC 98-23837. 311p. pap. text 39.99 (*0-7506-7095-9*) Buttrwrth-Heinemann.

Therapist Driven Protocols. Des Jardins & Burton. 1996. (Illus.). 272p. (gr. 13). pap. text, wbk. ed. 24.95 (*0-8151-1366-8*, 25780) Mosby Inc.

Therapist Driven Protocols Course: RCP 302 Course. Volpe & Cronin. 1994. 206p. (C). spiral bd. (*0-933195-78-8*) CA College Health Sci.

Therapist Guide to the MMPI & MMPI-2: Providing Feedback & Treatment. G. Nelson et al. 1990. LC 89-81012. xii, 364p. 31.95 (*1-55959-006-8*) Accel Devel.

Therapist Is the Therapy. Louis B. Fierman. 1997. LC 96-43253. 248p. 45.00 (*0-7657-0047-6*) Aronson.

Therapists' Dilemmas. Ed. by Wendy Dryden. 1988. 192p. 49.95 (*0-89116-775-7*) Hemisp Pub.

Therapist's Guide to Art Therapy Assessments: Tools of the Trade. Stephanie L. Brooke. 1996. LC 96-11642. (Illus.). 164p. 36.95 (*0-398-06618-3*); pap. 25.95 (*0-398-06619-1*) C C Thomas.

Therapist's Guide to Clinical Intervention: The 1-2-3s of Treatment Planning. Ed. by Sharon L. Johnson. 1997. LC 97-2832. (Illus.). 387p. pap. text 44.95 (*0-12-386585-9*) Morgan Kaufmann.

Therapist's Guide to Growing Free: A Manual for Survivors of Domestic Violence. Ed. by Wendy Susan Deaton & Michael Hertica. 2001. LC 00-47211. 105p. (C). 29.95 (*0-7890-1468-8*); pap. text 17.95 (*0-7890-1469-6*) Haworth Pr.

Therapists in the Community: Changing the Conditions That Produce Psychopathology. Matthew Dumont. 1994. LC 94-37986. (Master Work Ser.). 200p. reprint ed. pap. text 40.00 (*1-56821-405-7*) Aronson.

Therapist's Internet Handbook: More Than 1300 Web Sites & Resources for Mental Health Professionals. Robert F. Stamps & Peter M. Barach. 2001. LC 00-66213. (Professional Book Ser.). (Illus.). 258p. pap. 32.00 (*0-393-70342-8*) Norton.

Therapist's Manual for Cognitive Behavior Therapy in Groups. Lawrence I. Sank & Carolyn S. Shaffer. 1984. (Illus.). 284p. (C). 78.00 (*0-306-41229-2*, Plenum Trade) Perseus Pubng.

Therapist's Notebook: Homework, Handouts, & Activities for Use in Psychotherapy. Lorna L. Hecker et al. 1998. LC 97-26361. (Illus.). 433p. (C). pap. 49.95 (*0-7890-0400-3*) Haworth Pr.

Therapists on the Front Line: Psychotherapy with Gay Men in the Age of AIDS. Ed. by Stephen A. Cadwell et al. 1994. LC 93-46269. 608p. text 24.95 (*0-88048-558-2*, 8558) Am Psychiatric.

Therapists on Therapy. Ed. by Bob Mullan. 1996. 275p. (C). pap. (*1-85343-331-4*); pap. (*1-85343-329-2*) Free Assoc Bks GBR. *Dist:* Intl Spec Bk, NYU Pr, NYU Pr, Intl Spec Bk.

Therapist's Own Family: Toward the Differentiation of Self. Peter Titelman. 1995. 368p. pap. 50.00 (*1-56821-564-9*) Aronson.

Therapist's View of Personal Goals. Carl Ransom Rogers. 1960. LC 60-11607. (Orig.). pap. 4.00 (*0-87574-108-8*) Pendle Hill.

Therapists Who Have Sex with Their Patients: Treatment & Recovery. Herbert S. Strean. 1993. LC 93-17864. 208p. pap. 21.95 (*0-87630-724-1*) Brunner-Routledge.

Therapy: A Message of Love about a Survivor. Anne-Marie Chloe. 1996. (Illus.). xxv, 15p. (Orig.). pap. text 9.98 (*0-9655557-9-8*) Anne-Maries Peaceful Connect.

Therapy & Pathophysiology of End-Stage Renal Failure. Ed. by J. M. Scherbenske et al. 1995. (Journal: Vol. 13, No. 3-4, 1995). (Illus.). 122p. pap. 95.75 (*3-8055-6130-X*) S Karger.

Therapy & Prevention of Infections in Cancer Patients: Proceedings, Lausanne, 1978. European Organization for Research and Treatment of Cancer Staff & International Antimicrobial Therapy Group Staff. Ed. by M. Glauser & Jean Klastersky. 1979. (Illus.). pap. 41.00 (*0-08-024434-3*, Pergamon Pr) Elsevier.

Therapy for Adults Molested As Children: Beyond Survival. John Briere. 2nd exp. rev. ed. 1996. LC 96-8221. (Illus.). 272p. 36.95 (*0-8261-5641-X*) Springer Pub.

Therapy for Diabetes Mellitus & Related Disorders. American Diabetes Association. 2nd ed. 1994. 384p. pap. 34.50 (*0-945448-38-4*, PMTDRD2) Am Diabetes.

Therapy for Diabetes Mellitus & Related Disorders. Ed. by Harold E. Lebovitz. 3rd rev. ed. 1998. LC 98-4106. (Clinical Education Ser.). (Illus.). 487p. pap. 49.95 (*0-945448-94-5*) Am Diabetes.

Therapy for Genetic Disease. Ed. by Theodore Friedmann. 1991. (Molecular Medicine Ser.). (Illus.). 138p. pap. text 29.95 (*0-19-261971-3*) OUP.

Therapy for Genitourinary Cancer. Ed. by Herbert Lepor & Russell K. Lawson. 1992. (Cancer Treatment & Research Ser.). 176p. (C). text 148.50 (*0-7923-1412-3*) Kluwer Academic.

Therapy for Stutterers, No. 10. Ed. by C. Woodruff Starkweather & Malcolm Fraser. 1974. LC 74-17097. 120p. pap. 2.00 (*0-933388-08-X*) Stuttering Fnd Am.

Therapy for the Burn Patient. Ed. by Leveridge. 1991. 182p. pap. 43.25 (*1-56593-013-4*, 0255) Thomson Learn.

Therapy Guide for Language & Speech Disorders Vol. 1: A Selection of Stimulus Materials. Kathryn Kilpatrick et al. 1977. Orig. Title: Therapy Guide for the Adult with Language & Speech Disorders, Vol. 1. (Illus.). 429p. stu. ed. 37.00 (*1-880504-00-6*) Visit Nurse.

Therapy Guide for Language & Speech Disorders Vol. 2: Advanced Stimulus Materials. Kathryn Kilpatrick. rev. ed. 1987. Orig. Title: Therapy Guide for the Adult with Language & Speech Disorders, Vol. 2. 254p. stu. ed. 30.00 (*1-880504-02-2*) Visit Nurse.

Therapy Guide for Language & Speech Disorders Vol. 5: Reading Comprehension Materials. Kathryn Kilpatrick. 1987. 351p. stu. ed. 40.00 (*1-880504-05-7*) Visit Nurse.

Therapy Guide for the Adult with Language & Speech Disorders, Vol. 1 see Therapy Guide for Language & Speech Disorders, Vol. 1, A Selection of Stimulus Materials

Therapy Guide for the Adult with Language & Speech Disorders, Vol. 2 see Therapy Guide for Language & Speech Disorders, Vol. 2, Advanced Stimulus Materials

Therapy in a Nutshell: 10 Simple Lessons That Will Change Your Life. Patricia L. Bay. 1998. LC 98-175855. (Illus.). 236p. pap. 14.95 (*1-883952-07-7*) Hse of Steno.

Therapy in Motion. Ed. by Maureen N. Costonis. 1977. LC 77-9077. 298p. text 29.95 (*0-252-00586-4*) U of Ill Pr.

Therapy in Nephrology & Hypertension: A Companion to Brenner & Rector's the Kidney. Hugh R. Brady & Christopher S. Wilcox. Ed. by Richard Zorab. 1999. LC 98-21787. (Illus.). xxvii, 717p. (C). text 95.00 (*0-7216-7149-7*) Saunders.

Therapy Kit for Language Disorders. Kathryn Kilpatrick. 1994. (Illus.). 230p. 70.00 (*1-880504-09-X*) Visit Nurse.

Therapy Made Easy with Computer Assistance: Index of New Information with Authors & Subjects. American Health Research Institute Staff. rev. ed. 1994. 149p. 57.50 (*0-7883-0398-8*); pap. 47.50 (*0-7883-0399-6*) ABBE Pubs Assn.

Therapy of Advanced Melanoma. Ed. by P. Ruemke. 1990. (Pigment Cell Ser.: Vol. 10). (Illus.). viii, 230p. 172.25 (*3-8055-5032-4*) S Karger.

Therapy of Autoimmune Diseases. Ed. by J. M. Cruse & R. E. Lewis, Jr. 1989. (Concepts in Immunopathology Ser.: Vol. 7). (Illus.). viii, 216p. 167.00 (*3-8055-4931-8*) S Karger.

Therapy of Digestive Disorders: A Companion to Sleisenger & Fordtran's Gastrointestinal & Liver. M. Michael Wolfe. Ed. by Richard Zorab. 1999. LC 98-37279. (Illus.). 295p. text (*0-7216-7340-6*) Saunders.

Therapy of Hematopoietic Neoplasia. Ed. by Emil Freireich & Hagop Kantarjian. 1991. (Hematology Ser.: No. 14). (Illus.). 456p. text 230.00 (*0-8247-8455-3*) Dekker.

Therapy of Infectious Diseases. Trenholme. Date not set. (C). text (*0-7216-8145-X*) Saunders.

Therapy of Lung Metastases. Ed. by P. Drings & I. Vogt-Moykopf. 1988. (Contributions to Oncology Ser.: Vol. 30). (Illus.). viii, 222p. 58.50 (*3-8055-4749-8*) S Karger.

Therapy of Malignant Brain Tumors. K. Jellinger. 1987. (Illus.). 500p. 190.00 (*0-387-81946-0*) Spr-Verlag.

Therapy of Parkinson's Disease. Ed. by George Paulson & William C. Koller. 2nd exp. rev. ed. 1994. (Neurological Disease & Therapy Ser.: No. 34). (Illus.). 632p. text 195.00 (*0-8247-9226-2*) Dekker.

Therapy of Poetry. Molly Harrower. 1995. LC 95-33578. 132p. pap. 27.50 (*1-56821-755-2*) Aronson.

Therapy of Prostatis. Ed. by H. Weidner et al. 1986. (Clinical & Experimental Urology Ser.). (Illus.). 251p. text (*3-88603-171-3*) W Zuckschwerdt DEU. *Dist:* Scholium Intl.

Therapy of Renal Diseases & Related Disorders. Ed. by Wadi N. Suki & Shaul G. Massry. 1984. text 319.50 (*0-89838-652-7*); 2nd ed. 1991. (C). text 490.00 (*0-7923-0676-7*) Kluwer Academic.

Therapy of Systemic Rheumatic Disorders. Ed. by Van De Putte et al. 1997. LC 97-36795. (Illus.). 728p. text 225.00 (*0-8247-9516-4*) Dekker.

Therapy of the Difficult Divorce: Managing Crises, Reorienting Warring Couples, Working with the Children... Marla Beth Isaacs et al. 2000. LC 99-57414. (Master Work Ser.). 320p. 40.00 (*0-7657-0212-6*) Aronson.

Therapy of the Substance Abuse Syndromes. Henry J. Richards. 1994. LC 92-48826. 496p. 70.00 (*0-87668-539-4*) Aronson.

Therapy of Urological Cancer. R. Ackermann et al. 1991.Tr. of Therapie Urologischer Tumoren. (Illus.). viii, 178p. pap. 35.00 (*3-8055-5369-2*) S Karger.

Therapy Outcome Measures: Speech & Language Therapy. Pamela M. Enderby. 1997. 10p. (Orig.). pap. 55.00 (*1-56593-807-0*, 1578) Singular Publishing.

Therapy Outcome Measures Manual: Physiotherapy, Occupational Therapy, Rehabilitation Nursing. Pamela M. Enderby et al. 1998. LC 98-17801. pap. 55.00 (*1-56593-995-6*) Thomson Learn.

Therapy Research Processes & Practicalities. Jane Seale & Sue Barnard. 1998. LC 98-27542. 256p. pap. text 35.00 (*0-7506-3435-9*) Buttrwrth-Heinemann.

Therapy-Resistant Depressions: Proceedings of the World Congress of Psychiatry, 6th, Honolulu, Hawaii, August-September, 1977. World Congress of Psychiatry Staff. Ed. by Cesar P. De Francisco. 1979. (Journal: Vol. 14, No. 2). (Illus.). pap. 21.00 (*3-8055-3055-2*) S Karger.

Therapy Services: Organisation, Management & Autonomy. John Ovretveit. 1992. 222p. text 74.00 (*3-7186-5245-5*); pap. text 38.00 (*3-7186-5246-3*) Gordon & Breach (Harwood Acad Pubs).

Therapy Sourcebook. Francine M. Roberts. 1998. LC 97-45880. 352p. pap. 17.00 (*0-7373-0011-6*, 00116W) NTC Contemp Pub Co.

Therapy Through Drama: The Fictional Family. Muriel Gold. 2000. LC 00-41766. (Illus.). xxviii, 188p. text 44.95 (*0-398-07094-6*) C C Thomas.

Therapy Through Hypnosis. Ed. by Raphael H. Rhoades. 1976. pap. 5.00 (*0-87980-162-X*) Wilshire.

Therapy with Botulinum Toxin. Ed. by Joseph Jankovic & Mark Hallett. 1994. (Neurological Disease & Therapy Ser.: Vol. 25). (Illus.). 640p. text 240.00 (*0-8247-8824-9*) Dekker.

Therapy with Stepfamilies. Emily B. Visher & John S. Visher. 1996. LC 96-1116. (Basic Principles into Practice Ser.: Vol. 6). 208p. pap. text 23.95 (*0-87630-799-3*) Brunner-Routledge.

Therapy with Treatment Resistant Families: A Consultation-Crisis Intervention Model. William G. McCown et al. 1993. LC 93-35618. 328p. 59.95 (*1-56024-244-2*); pap. 19.95 (*1-56024-245-0*) Haworth Pr.

Therapy with Troubled Teenagers: Rewriting Young Lives in Progress. Bob Bertolino. 1998. LC 98-9520. 256p. 60.00 (*0-471-24996-3*) Wiley.

***Therascribe 4.0 User Manual.** Arthur E. Jongsma. 2001. (Practice Planners Ser.). 128p. pap. (*0-471-43644-5*) Wiley.

There Are No Incurable Diseases: Dr. Schulze's 30-Day Cleansing & Detoxification Program. Richard Schulze. 1999. LC 99-93974. 112p. pap. 12.00 (*0-9671567-3-4*) Natural Healing Pubns.

There Is a Cure for Arthritis. Paavo O. Airola. 1988. 228p. (C). pap. text 10.95 (*0-13-914698-9*) P-H.

There Is Hope: Learning to Live with HIV. Janice Ferri & Jill Schwendeman. 3rd ed. 1997. LC 97-14113. pap. 15.00 (*0-9639390-2-5*) HIV Coalition.

There Is No Gene for Good Teaching: A Handbook on Lecture Skills for Medical Teachers. Neal A. Whitman. 3rd ed. 1986. 24p. reprint ed. pap. text 10.00 (*0-940193-00-0*) Univ UT Sch Med.

There Is No Such Thing As a Therapist. Carol Holmes. 1998. 200p. pap. (*1-85575-066-X*) Karnac Bks GBR. *Dist:* Other Pr LLC.

There Is Nothing Wrong with You: Going Beyond Self-Hate. Cheri Huber. 1993. (Illus.). 234p. (Orig.). pap. 12.00 (*0-9636255-0-0*, 2097280859) Keep it Simple.

There's More to Life Than Pumpkins, Drugs & Other False Gods. Kenneth G. Reiners. 1980. LC 80-50424. 64p. (Orig.). pap. 5.95 (*0-934104-03-4*) Woodland.

There's Nothing Like a Breast: A Breast Cancer Survivor's Story of the Emotional & Sexual Effects of Reconstructive Surgery. Diane Craig Chechik. Ed. by Laurie Rosin. 2000. LC 99-90873. 133p. pap. 12.95 (*0-9620549-1-7*) Catalyst FL.

There's Nothing Like a Breast & Journey to Justice Incl. Journey to Justice: A Woman's True Story of Breast Cancer & Medical Malpractice. 2nd ed. Diane C. Chechik. Ed. by Eleanor S. Anderson. LC 88-71206. (Illus.). 168p. (C). pap. 12.95 (*0-9620549-0-9*); There's Nothing Like a Breast: A Breast Cancer Survivor's Story of the Emotional & Sexual Effects of Reconstructive Surgery. Diane Craig Chechik. Ed. by Laurie Rosin. LC 99-90873. 133p. pap. 12.95 (*0-9620549-1-7*); 2000. Set pap. 22.50 (*0-9620549-2-5*) Catalyst FL.

There's Still a Person in There: The Complete Guide to Treating & Coping with Alzheimer's. Michael Castleman et al. 2000. LC 99-34745. 384p. pap. 14.95 (*0-399-52635-8*, Perigee Bks) Berkley Pub.

Theriac. George Bartisch. Tr. by Donald Blanchard from GER. 2000.Tr. of Warhafftige. (Illus.). 44p. pap. 25.00 (*0-9700529-0-1*) Blanchards Bks.

Thermal Agents in Rehabilitation, No. 6. Ed. by Susan L. Michlovitz et al. 3rd ed. 1996. LC 95-39679. (Contemporary Perspectives in Rehabilitation Ser.). (Illus.). 405p. (C). 43.95 (*0-8036-0044-5*) Davis Co.

Thermal Balance in Health & Disease. Eduard Schonbaum et al. 1994. (Advances in Pharmacological Sciences Ser.). 540p. 160.50 (*0-8176-5054-7*) Birkhauser.

Thermal Balance in Health & Disease: Recent Basic Research & Clinical Progress. Edward Schonbaum & E. Zeisberger. Ed. by Edward Schonbaum et al. 1995. LC 94-19416. 84.00 (*0-8176-5047-4*) Birkhauser.

Thermal Processing of Bio-Materials. T Kudra & C. Strumillo. 1998. (Topics in Chemical Engineering Ser.). 654p. text (*90-5699-105-1*) GBSP NLD. *Dist:* Gordon & Breach.

Thermal Surgical Lasers: A Technical Monograph. Terry A. Fuller. 1993. (Illus.). 55p. (Orig.). pap. 50.00 (*1-883765-00-5*) Surgical Laser.

Thermal Therapy, Laser Welding & Tissue Interaction. Ed. by Stephen G. Bown et al. 1999. LC 99-192234. (Europto Ser.: Vol. 3565). 69.00 (*0-8194-3027-7*) SPIE.

Thermal Tissue Ablation. Ed. by M. Marberger. 1993. (Journal: Vol. 23, Suppl. 1, 1993). (Illus.). iv, 72p. pap. 40.00 (*3-8055-5799-X*) S Karger.

Thermobacteriology in Food Processing. C. R. Stumbo. 2nd ed. 1973. (Food Science & Technology Ser.). text 146.00 (*0-12-675352-0*) Acad Pr.

Thermographic Evidence of Soft Tissue Injury. 1987. 562p. text 95.00 (*0-07-172008-1*) Shepards.

Thermographic Investigations into the Physiological Basis of Regional Anaesthesia. G. Sprotte. 1984. (Anaesthesiology & Intensive Care Medicine Ser.: Vol. 159). (Illus.). 65p. 56.95 (*0-387-12638-4*) Spr-Verlag.

Thermography: Proceedings of the European Congress on Thermography, 1st, Amsterdam, June 1974. European Congress on Thermography Staff. Ed. by N. J. Aarts. 1975. (Bibliotheca Radiologica Ser.: Vol. 6). (Illus.). xiv, 262p. pap. 85.25 (*3-8055-2134-0*) S Karger.

Thermometry. James F. Schooley. 1986. LC 86-6142. 336p. 147.00 (*0-8493-5833-7*, QC271, CRC Reprint) Franklin.

Thermomicroscopy in the Analysis of Pharmaceuticals. M. Kuhnert-Brandstatter. 1971. 424p. (*0-08-006990-8*) Pergamon Repr GBR. *Dist:* Franklin.

Thermoradiotherapy & Thermochemotherapy Vol. 1: Biology, Physiology & Physics. Ed. by M. H. Seegenschmiedt et al. 1995. LC 95-11653. (Medical Radiology Ser.). (*3-540-57229-5*) Spr-Verlag.

Thermoradiotherapy & Thermochemotherapy Vol. 1: Biology, Physiology & Physics. Ed. by Michael H. Seegenscmiedt et al. 1995. (Medical Radiology Ser.). (Illus.). 495p. 235.00 (*0-387-57229-5*) Spr-Verlag.

Thermoradiotherapy & Thermochemotherapy Vol. 2: Clinical Applications. Ed. by M. H. Seegenschmiedt et al. 1996. (Medical Radiology Ser.). (Illus.). 420p. 212.00 (*0-387-57230-9*) Spr-Verlag.

Thermoradiotherapy & Thermochemotherapy Vol. 2: Clinical Applications. M. H. Seegenschmiedt et al. 1996. LC 95-11653. (Medical Radiology Ser.). (Illus.). 420p. 189.00 (*3-540-57230-9*) Spr-Verlag.

Thermoreception & Temperature Regulation. Ed. by J. Bligh & K. Voigt. 1990. (Illus.). 306p. 98.00 (*0-387-51711-1*) Spr-Verlag.

Thermoregulation: Pathology, Pharmacology & Therapy. P. Lomax & Edward Schonbaum. 1991. (International Encyclopedia of Pharmacology & Therapeutics Ser.). (Illus.). 692p. 230.50 (*0-08-036853-0*, Pergamon Pr) Elsevier.

Thermoregulation: Research & Clinical Applications: International Symposium on the Pharmacology of Thermoregulation, 7th, Odense, August, 1988. Ed. by Edward Schonbaum & P. Lomax. 1989. xiv, 250p. 138.50 (*3-8055-4921-0*) S Karger.

Thermoregulation: The Pathophysiological Basis of Clinical Disorders: Eighth International Symposium on the Pharmacology of Thermoregulation, Kananaskis, Alberta, August 1991. Ed. by P. Lomax & E. Schoenbaum. 1992. (Illus.). xiv, 200p. 135.75 (*3-8055-5513-X*) S Karger.

Thermoregulation Vol. 813: 10th International Symposium on the Pharmacology of Thermoregulation. Ed. by Clark M. Blatteis. 1997. LC 97-329. xvi, 878 p. pap. 170.00 (*1-57331-089-1*) NY Acad Sci.

Thermoregulation of Sick & Low Birth Weight Neonates: Temperature Control, Temperature Monitoring, Thermal Environment. Ed. by Albert A. Okken & Jochim J. Koch. 1995. (Illus.). 256p. 110.00 (*3-540-60169-4*) Spr-Verlag.

Thermoregulatory Mechanisms & Their Therapeutic Implications: Symposium, 4th, Oxford, July-August, 1979. Ed. by B. Cox et al. 1979. (Illus.). 56.75 (*3-8055-0277-X*) S Karger.

Thermosense XIX: An International Conference on Thermal Sensing & Imaging Diagnostic Applications. Ed. by Richard N. Winzbach & Douglas D. Burleigh. 1997. 80.00 (*0-8194-2471-4*) SPIE.

Thermostatic Incubator: Raising Chickens by Hand. E. S. Renwick. 98p. pap. 15.00 (*0-87556-360-0*); 1996. pap. 25.00 (*0-87556-756-8*) Saifer.

Thermotherapy & BPH. Ed. by C. C. Schulman. 1993. (Journal: Vol. 23, No. 2, 1993). (Illus.). 80p. pap. 69.75 (*3-8055-5781-7*) S Karger.

Thermotolerance. Kurt J. Henle. 1987. 192p. 112.00 (*0-8493-6459-0*, CRC Reprint) Franklin.

Thesaurus Biomedical Francais-Anglais Inserm-International Symposium Staff. 1986. (ENG & FRE.). 884p. 555.00 (*0-8288-0563-6*, M1750) Fr & Eur.

Thesaurus of Medical Informatics Terminology. Ed. by M. C. Sievert et al. 1998. 82p. pap. 39.00 (*90-5199-408-7*) IOS Press.

Thesaurus of Psychological Index Terms. Ed. by Alvin J. Walker, Jr. 8th ed. 1997. LC 97-3383. 343p. 60.00 (*1-55798-402-6*) Am Psychol.

They Bury Their Mistakes: How to Survive Your Hospitalization. Colleen O'Connor. 1994. 100p. (Orig.). pap. 10.95 (*0-9641088-3-6*) Valverde Pubns.

They Can't Talk, but Never Lie: The Making of a Zoo Vet. Theodore Zimmerman. Ed. by Elaine Zimmerman. 1996. (Illus.). 350p. 19.95 (*0-9643084-0-1*) Action Arts Pr.

They Conquered AIDS: Case Histories of People Who Have Dealt Successfully with AIDS Without Drugs & Doctors. 1992. lib. bdg. 88.95 (*0-8490-8798-8*) Gordon Pr.

They Conquered AIDS! True Life Adventures. Scott J. Gregory & Bianca Leonardo. unabr. ed. 1989. (Illus.). 360p. 24.95 (*0-930852-03-6*) Tree Life Pubns.

They Could Not Talk & So They Drew: Children's Styles of Coping & Thinking. Myra F. Levick. 1983. (Illus.). 240p. text 59.95 (*0-398-04800-2*) C C Thomas.

They Grow in Silence: Understanding Deaf Children & Adults. Ed. by Eugene D. Mindel & McCay Vernon. 1987. LC 90-21666. (Illus.). 204p. (C). reprint ed. pap. text 29.00 (*0-89079-325-5*, 1744) PRO-ED.

They Never Came Back: How to Lose Patients. Melvin A. Noonan. 1998. LC 98-96363. (Illus.). 96p. 12.95 (*0-9665934-0-5*) Timbritom.

They Say You're Crazy: How the World's Most Powerful Psychiatrists Decide Who's Normal. Paula J. Caplan. 2000. 384p. pap. 14.00 (*0-201-48832-9*) Perseus Bks Grp.

They Shall Not Hurt: Human Suffering & Human Caring. Ed. by Rodney L. Taylor & M. Jean Watson. 1989. LC 89-904. 140p. (C). text 29.95 (*0-87081-201-7*) Univ Pr Colo.

Thibodeau, Health & Disease SG. Swisher. 1992. (Illus.). 335p. (gr. 11-12). pap. text, stu. ed. 15.95 (*0-8016-6409-8*, 06409) Mosby Inc.

Thibodeau, Structure & Function. Swisher. 8th ed. 1988. (Illus.). 272p. pap. text 11.95 (*0-8016-2870-9*) Mosby Inc.

Thibodeau, Structure & Function: Study Guide. Swisher. 9th ed. 1991. (Illus.). 288p. (gr. 11-12). pap. text, stu. ed. 14.95 (*0-8016-6407-1*, 06407) Mosby Inc.

Thieme Leximed Compact English-German: Medical Dictionary. P. Reuter. 1997. 49.00 (*0-86577-734-9*); 49.00 (*0-86577-735-7*) Thieme Med Pubs.

Thieme LexiMed Pocket Medical Dictionary: English-German - German-English. Peter Reuter. 1998. (ENG & GER.). 1024p. pap. 39.00 (*0-86577-788-8*) Thieme Med Pubs.

Thin Book: Hypnotherapy Trance Scripts for Weight Mangement. Hal Brickman. 2000. 108p. pap. 24.95 (*1-891944-09-6*) Zeig Tucker Theisen.

Thin Needle Aspiration Biopsy. William J. Frable. 1983. (Major Problems in Pathology Ser.: Vol. 14). (Illus.). 384p. text 120.00 (*0-7216-3835-X*) Saunders.

Thin Woman: Feminism, Post-Structuralism & the Social Psychology of Anorexia Nervosa. 1997. LC 96-39930. (Women & Psychology Ser.). 256p. (C). 73.95 (*0-415-16332-3*) Routledge.

Thin Woman: Feminism, Post-Structuralism & the Social Psychology of Anorexia Nervosa. Helen Malson. 1997. LC 96-39930. (Women & Psychology Ser.). 256p. (C). pap. 23.95 (*0-415-16333-1*) Routledge.

Thing Apart: Love & Reality in the Therapeutic Relationship. Irving Steingart. 1995. LC 94-41351. (Critical Issues in Psychoanalysis Ser.: Vol. 2). 318p. 55.00 (*1-56821-304-2*) Aronson.

Think Fast! The ADD Experience. Ed. by Thom Hartmann & Janie Bowman. 1996. 256p. (Orig.). pap. 12.95 (*1-887424-08-3*) Underwood Bks.

Think Health. Elizabeth Blackburn. 1991. 46p. spiral bd. 7.95 (*0-87516-633-4*) DeVorss.

Think Visually! Handbook: Using Simple Shapes for Thinking, Planning & Problem Solving. Yvonne M. Hansen. 1990. (Illus.). 156p. pap. 15.00 (*0-9625347-2-2*) Gemin-Ideas Pr.

Think Yourself Slim. Bransby Clarke. 1995. 96p. (Orig.). pap. (*0-572-01471-6*) Foulsham UK GBR. *Dist:* Assoc Pubs Grp.

Thinkers & Feelers Mini Seminar Kit. William D. Murray & Rosalie R. Murray. rev. ed. 1995. (Type & Temperament Seminar Kits Ser.). 83p. ring bd. 99.95 (*1-878287-13-3*) Type & Temperament.

Thinker's Guide to Ultrasonic Imaging. Raymond L. Powis & Wendy J. Powis. 1984. LC 83-21704. (Illus.). 430p. 55.00 (*0-683-06961-6*) Lppncott W & W.

Thinking: Studies of Covert Language Processes. Ed. by Frank J. McGuigan. 1966. LC 66-15745. (Century Psychology Ser.). (Illus.). pap. text 19.95 (*0-89197-450-4*) Irvington.

Thinking about Infants & Young Children. Morag Harris. 1975. 89p. pap. (*0-902965-05-0*) Clunie Pr GBR. *Dist:* Other Pr LLC.

Thinking Across Cultures: The Third International Conference on Thinking. Ed. by Donald M. Topping et al. 1989. 512p. text 110.00 (*0-89859-913-X*) L Erlbaum Assocs.

Thinking & Problem Solving. Ed. by Robert J. Sternberg. 2nd ed. 1998. (Handbook of Perception & Cognition Ser.). (Illus.). 461p. reprint ed. pap. text 39.95 (*0-12-667260-1*) Acad Pr.

Thinking Clearly about Psychology Ed. by Dante Cicchetti & William M. Grove. 1991. 864p. text 59.95 (*0-8166-1918-2*) U of Minn Pr.

Thinking Clearly about Psychology: Essays on Matters of Public Interest, Vol. 1. Ed. by William M. Grove & Dante Cicchetti. 1991. 320p. text 39.95 (*0-8166-1891-7*) U of Minn Pr.

Thinking Clearly about Psychology Vol. 1: Essays on Matters of Public Interest, Vol. 2. Dante Cicchetti & William M. Grove. 1991. 320p. text 44.95 (*0-8166-1892-5*) U of Minn Pr.

Thinking Fragments: Psychoanalysis, Feminism, & Postmodernism in the Contemporary West. Jane Flax. 1991. 287p. pap. 18.95 (*0-520-07305-3*) U CA Pr.

Thinking in Sound: The Cognitive Psychology of Human Audition. Ed. by Stephen McAdams & Emmanuel Bigand. 1993. LC 92-26340. (Illus.). 368p. pap. text 29.95 (*0-19-852257-6*) OUP.

Thinking Like a Doctor. David Rothman. 1996. (*0-316-75781-0*) Little.

Thinking Person's Guide to Perfect Health: The Transformation of Medicine. Ron Kennedy. 1996. (Orig.). pap. 30.00 (*0-932654-13-4*) Context Pubns.

Thinking, Problem Solving, Cognition. Richard E. Mayer. 2nd ed. 1991. (C). text 41.95 (*0-7167-2214-3*); 560p. pap. text 40.95 (*0-7167-2215-1*) W H Freeman.

Thinking Styles. Robert J. Sternberg. 1997. 192p. (C). text 49.95 (*0-521-55316-4*) Cambridge U Pr.

Thinking the Difference: For a Peaceful Revolution. Luce Irigaray. Tr. by Karin Montin. 1994. LC 93-40519. 132p. (C). (gr. 13). pap. 18.95 (*0-415-90815-9*) Routledge.

Thinking Through Cultures: Expeditions in Cultural Psychology. Richard A. Shweder. 1991. LC 90-4796. (Illus.). 416p. 50.50 (*0-674-88415-9*, SHWTHI); pap. 22.50 (*0-674-88416-7*, SHWTHX) HUP.

Thinward Bound: Medical Management & Weight Loss. Mary J. Madden. Ed. by Donna Hoel. 1982. LC 82-17679. (Illus.). 112p. pap. text 11.50 (*0-89303-228-X*) P-H.

Third Component of Complement. Ed. by J. D. Lambris. 1989. (Current Topics in Microbiology & Immunology Ser.: Vol. 153). (Illus.). 251p. 123.00 (*0-387-51513-5*) Spr-Verlag.

Third HGH Symposium Sorrento, May, 1992. Ed. by J. Girard & J. S. Christiansen. 1992. (Hormone Research Ser.: Vol. 38, Suppl. 1, 1992). (Illus.). vi, 118p. pap. 54.00 (*3-8055-5742-6*) S Karger.

Third International Congress of Neuroendocrinology, Budapest, July 1994: Abstracts. Ed. by I. Gerendai & B. Halasz. 1994. (Journal: Vol. 60, Suppl. 1, 1994). iv, 104p. pap. 47.00 (*3-8055-6012-5*) S Karger.

Third International Congress on Tissue Integration in Oral & Maxillofacial Reconstruction. Minoru Ueda. 2000. (Illus.). 128p. (*4-87417-618-6*) QPC JPN. *Dist:* Quint Pub Co.

Third Joint Meeting of the European Society for Pediatric Endocrinology (ESPE) & the Lawson Wilkins Pediatric Endocrine Society (LWPES) Proceedings of the Plenary Lectures & Symposia, Jerusalem, October - November 1989. Ed. by Z. Laron. 1990. (Journal: Vol. 33, No. 2-4, 1990). (Illus.). 116p. pap. 118.50 (*3-8055-5289-0*) S Karger.

Third Opinion: An International Directory to Alternative Therapy Centers for the Treatment & Prevention of Cancer & Other Degenerative Diseases. John M. Fink. 3rd ed. 1988. 384p. pap. 16.95 (*0-89529-770-1*, Avery) Penguin Putnam.

Third Party Rape: The Conspiracy to Rob You of Health Care. C. Norman Shealy. 1993. LC 93-7684. (Illus.). 240p. (Orig.). pap. 12.95 (*1-880090-07-4*) Galde Pr.

Third SCI-RSC Medical Chemistry Symposium. Ed. by R. W. Lambert. 1986. (Special Publications: No. 55). (Illus.). 396p. (C). (*0-85186-616-6*) Royal Soc Chem GBR. *Dist:* Spr-Verlag.

Third Spring Meeting, New Insights in Haematology, Cini Foundation-Venice. Ed. by T. Chisesi. 1997. 130p. pap. text 170.00 (*90-5702-252-4*, Harwood Acad Pubs) Gordon & Breach.

Third Symposium by the Seven Winners of the Grants from Sandoz Foundation for Gerontological Research, Annual Meeting of the Japan Gerontological Society, Yokohama, November 1991. Ed. by H. Orimo. 1992. (Journal: Vol. 38, Suppl. 1, 1992). (Illus.). vi, 50p. pap. 17.50 (*3-8055-5661-6*) S Karger.

***Third Third: A Physician's Guide to a Healthy, Happy, Longer Life.** Tom Connally. 2001. LC 2001-37841. (Illus.). 288p. 24.95 (*0-9704729-2-7*) Bright Sky.

Third Wave of Asbestos Disease Vol. 643: Exposure to Asbestos in Place. Ed. by Philip J. Landrigan & Homayoun Kazemi. 1992. 628p. 190.00 (*0-89766-677-1*) NY Acad Sci.

Third Wave of Asbestos Disease, Exposure to Asbestos in Place: Public Health Control. Ed. by Philip J. Landrigan & Homayoun Kazemi. 1992. LC 92-6138. (Annals Ser.: Vol. 643). 628p. pap. 190.00 (*0-89766-678-X*, Q11) NY Acad Sci.

Thirteenth International Complement Workshop, San Diego, Calif., September 1989 Abstracts. Ed. by N. R. Cooper. 1990. (Journal: Vol. 6, No. 5). 128p. pap. 36.75 (*3-8055-5089-8*) S Karger.

Thirteenth International Congress on Thrombosis, Bilbao, Spain, June 1994 Abstracts. Ed. by J. A. Iriarte et al. 1994. (Journal: Vol. 24, Suppl. 1, 1994). viii, 410p. pap. 127.00 (*3-8055-6020-6*) S Karger.

Thirty & Terminal: Cancer Survival. John R. Wagner. 1997. LC 96-78123. 160p. (Orig.). pap. 12.95 (*0-9651590-0-0*) Infnty Pub.

35th International Symposium on Neuromedical Chemistry. Povl Krogsgaard-Larsen. 1992. 160p. pap. text 362.00 (*3-7186-5367-2*, Harwood Acad Pubs) Gordon & Breach.

Thirty-First Annual Meeting of the European Society for Paediatric Endocrinology (ESPE) Abstracts, Zaragoza, September, 1992. Ed. by A. Ferrandez Longas. 1992. (Journal: Vol. 37, Suppl. 4, 1992). viii, 76p. pap. 36.75 (*3-8055-5666-7*) S Karger.

Thirty-Five Practical Ways to Improve Your Health: A Common Sense Approach for Wholesome Living. Reid E. Lassonde. 1992. LC 91-68336. (Illus.). 142p. (Orig.). pap. 9.95 (*0-9631846-7-9*) Real-Life Pubns.

30 Low-Fat Meals in 30 Minutes. Faye Levy. 1995. LC 94-30636. 208p. (Orig.). pap. (*0-446-67059-6*) Warner.

Thirty Percent Solution: The Diet Doctor's Plan for Life Long Weight Control. Robert Stark. 1990. LC 90-80607. 112p. (Orig.). pap. 14.95 (*0-9618415-5-9*) AZ Bariatric Phy.

Thirty Plants That Can Save Your Life. Douglas Schar. 1993. LC 92-38634. 134p. (Orig.). pap. 12.95 (*1-880216-09-4*, Elliott Clark) River City Pub.

Thirty Poisonous Plants of North America. V. K. Chestnut. 1998. (Illus.). 33p. reprint ed. pap. 10.00 (*0-8466-6051-2*, S-51) Shoreys Bkstore.

36-Hour Day: A Family Guide to Caring for Persons with Alzheimer's Disease, Related Dementing Illnesses & Memory Loss in Later Life. Nancy L. Mace & Peter V. Rabins. 2001. 512p. mass mkt. (*0-446-61041-0*) Warner.

36-Hour Day: A Family Guide to Caring for Persons with Alzheimer's Disease, Related Dementing Illnesses, & Memory Loss in Later Life. Nancy L. Mace & Peter V. Rabins. 3rd ed. (Johns Hopkins Press Health Bks.). 1999. LC 98-43608. 352p. 44.00 (*0-8018-6148-9*); 1999. LC 98-43608. 352p. pap. 13.95 (*0-8018-6149-7*); 2001. LC 00-42416. (Illus.). 496p. pap. 19.95 (*0-8018-6521-2*) Johns Hopkins.

Thirty-Third Annual Meeting of the European Society for Paediatric Endocrinology (ESPE), Maastricht, June 1994, Abstracts: Hormone Research. Ed. by J. L. Van den Brande & M. Jansen. 1994. (Journal: Vol. 41, No. 2-4, 1994). viii, 104p. pap. 48.75 (*3-8055-6011-7*) S Karger.

Thirty Years in Hell: or The Confessions of a Drug Fiend. D. F. Macmartin. Ed. by Gerald N. Grob. 1981. LC 80-1256. (Addiction in America Ser.). reprint ed. lib. bdg. 29.95 (*0-405-13606-4*) Ayer.

This Book Doesn't Make Sense: Living & Learning with Dyslexia. Jean Augur. 1995. 130p. pap. 34.95 (*1-56593-605-1*, 1256) Singular Publishing.

This Book Doesn't Make Sense: Living & Learning with Dyslexia. Jean Augur. rev. ed. 1995. (*1-897635-13-3*) Whurr Pub GBR. *Dist:* Singular Publishing.

This Is My Life. Agnes Hunt. Ed. by William R. Phillips & Janet Rosenberg. 1980. LC 79-6013. (Physically Handicapped in Society Ser.). reprint ed. lib. bdg. 24.95 (*0-405-13116-X*) Ayer.

***This is Not Brain Surgery! A Mental Health Companion for the Gastric Bypass Patient.** Teri Kai Holtzclaw. 2001. 150p. pap. (*0-9712601-0-9*) T Holtzclaw.

This Is Our Work: The Legacy of Sir William Osler. Ted Grant. 1994. 220p. 75.00 (*0-9698568-0-6*) Amer Coll Phys.

This Is What We Have to Do - Are You Okay? (DINROO) Nurses Speech with Elderly Nursing Home Residents. Heather Gibb. 1991. (Research Monographs: No. 1). (C). pap. (*0-7300-1444-4*) Deakin Univ AUS. *Dist:* St Mut.

This Other Kind of Doctors: Traditional Medical Systems in Black Neighborhoods in Austin, Texas. Suzanne J. Terrell. 1990. LC 88-35024. (Immigrant Communities & Ethnic Minorities in the U. S. & Canada Ser.: No. 50). 34.50 (*0-404-19460-5*) AMS Pr.

This Sex Which Is Not One. Luce Irigaray. Tr. by Catherine Porter & Carolyn Burke from FRE. 1985. LC 84-23013. 208p. (C). 39.95 (*0-8014-1546-2*); pap. 16.95 (*0-8014-9331-5*) Cornell U Pr.

***This Side of Nirvana: Memoirs of a Spiritually Challenged Buddhist.** Sara Jenkins. 2001. 272p. 22.95 (*1-931412-73-1*) Fair Winds Pr.

This Won't Hurt (And Other Lies My Doctor Tells Me) Charles B. Inlander. 1998. LC 98-13883. 224p. pap. 14.95 (*1-882606-39-6*); 1993. LC 96-39297. (Illus.). 176p. 19.95 (*0-9627334-8-2*) Peoples Med Soc.

This World, Other Worlds: Sickness, Suicide, Death, & the Afterlife among the Vaqueiros De Alzada of Spain. Maria Catedra. Tr. by William A. Christian, Jr. 1992. (Illus.). 402p. pap. text 22.00 (*0-226-09716-1*) U Ch Pr.

Thomas Beddoes, M. D., 1760-1808: Chemist, Physician, Democrat. Dorothy A. Stansfield. 1984. (Chemists & Chemistry Ser.: Vol. 3). text 179.50 (*90-277-1686-2*) Kluwer Academic.

Thomas Cantimpratensis: Liber de Natura Rerum, Editio Princeps Secundum Codices Manuscriptos, Pt. 1. 1973. (C). 173.10 (*3-11-003789-0*) De Gruyter.

Thomas Concept. J. W. Thomas & T. J. Thomas. 1995. LC 91-143775. (Illus.). 335p. reprint ed. 25.00 (*0-9637450-0-X*) Inpsyte.

Thomas David Duane, MD: Wills Eye Hospital & Thomas Jefferson Medical College. Thomas D. Duane. 1989. (Ophthalmology Oral History Ser.). (Illus.). 178p. 35.00 (*0-926866-03-6*) FAAO.

Thomas Hodgkin: Morbid Anatomist & Social Activist. Louis Rosenfeld. 1992. LC 92-28528. (Illus.). 356p. 24.95 (*0-8191-8633-3*) Madison Bks UPA.

Thomas Jefferson Treats Himself: Herbs, Physicke, & Nutrition in Early America. John M. Holmes. Ed. by Ann A. Hunter. 1997. (Illus.). 136p. 24.95 (*0-9630797-3-5*) Loft Pr.

Thomas Jefferson University: Tradition & Heritage. Frederick B. Wagner. 1989. LC 88-8338. (Illus.). 1120p. text 120.00 (*0-8121-1210-5*) Lppncott W & W.

Thomas Spry, Lawyer & Physician: The First Attorney Admitted to Practice under English Law in the Delaware River Settlements Now Included in the States of Pennsylvania, New Jersey & Delaware. John F. Lewis. 1996. LC 96-75356. 140p. reprint ed. 45.00 (*1-56169-209-3*) Gaunt.

Thomas Szasz: Primary Values & Major Contentions. Ed. by Richard E. Vatz & Lee S. Weinberg. 1983. LC 82-62083. 253p. 41.00 (*0-87975-187-8*); pap. 26.00 (*0-87975-188-6*) Prometheus Bks.

Thomas W. Salmon: Psychiatrist. Earl D. Bond & Paul O. Komora. Ed. by Gerald N. Grob. 1980. LC 78-22550. (Historical Issues in Mental Health Ser.). (Illus.). reprint ed. lib. bdg. 19.95 (*0-405-11904-6*) Ayer.

Thomas Wharton's Adenographia. Thomas Wharton. Tr. by Stephen Freer from LAT. 1996. (Illus.). 406p. (C). text 149.50 (*0-19-854788-9*, Clarendon Pr) OUP.

***Thomas Willis 1621-1675: His Life & Work.** Trevor Hughes. 1991. (Eponymists in Medicine Ser.). 151p. (*1-85315-162-9*) Royal Soc of Medicine Pr Ltd GBR. *Dist:* Balogh.

Thompson & Thompson Genetics in Medicine. Margaret Thompson et al. 5th ed. 1991. (Illus.). 368p. pap. text 43.95 (*0-7216-2817-6*) Saunders.

Thompson & Thompson Genetics in Medicine. Robert L. Nussbaum et al. 6th ed. 1999. 444p. pap. text (*0-7216-6902-6*) Saunders.

Thompson's Introduction to Maternity & Pediatric Nursing. Hank Carbeck. Ed. by Terri Wood. 3rd ed. 1998. LC 98-38331. (Illus.). 1008p. (C). text 44.95 (*0-7216-7557-3*) Saunders.

***Thompson's Introduction to Maternity & Pediatric Nursing.** Gloria Leifer. 3rd ed. 1999. (Illus.). tchr. ed. 75.00 (*0-7216-7558-1*) Saunders.

Thompson's Pediatric Nursing: An Introductory Text. Elizabeth Schulte et al. Ed. by Ilze Rader. 7th ed. 1997. (Illus.). 512p. pap. text 31.50 (*0-7216-4239-X*) Saunders.

Thompson's Pediatric Nursing: An Introductory Text. Elizabeth Schulte et al. 7th ed. 1997. (Illus.). tchr. ed. (*0-7216-4258-6*) Saunders.

***Thompson's Pediatric Nursing: An Introductory Text.** Elizabeth Schulte et al. 8th ed. 2001. (Illus.). 464p. pap., tchr. ed. 250.00 (*0-7216-9049-1*) Saunders.

***Thompson's Pediatric Nursing: An Introductory Text - ExaMaster.** Elizabeth Schulte et al. 2001. 500.00 (*0-7216-9050-5*) Saunders.

Thompson's Resource Guide for Aging see Caregiver Sourcebook: National

Thomson's Special Veterinary Pathology. William W. Carlton et al. 3rd ed. 2000. LC 00-56224. (Illus.). xi, 755p. text 99.00 (*0-323-00560-8*) Mosby Inc.

Thomson's Special Veterinary Pathology, Vol. 2. William W. Carlton & M. Donald McGavin. 2nd ed. 1995. (Illus.). 672p. (C). (gr. 13). text 102.00 (*0-8016-7968-0*, 07968) Mosby Inc.

Th1-Th2 Paradigm & Transplantation Tolerance: Exploring the Microcosm of Transplantation-Of What Is Past, Passing & to Come. Robin P. Lowry & Takumi Takeuchi. 1994. (Medical Intelligence Unit Ser.). 118p. 99.00 (*1-57059-108-3*, LN9108) Landes Bioscience.

Thoracic Anaesthesia: Principles & Practice. Sunit Ghosh & Ray Latimer. 1999. LC 99-35760. (Illus.). 335p. text 85.00 (*0-7506-4062-6*) Buttrwrth-Heinemann.

Thoracic Anesthesia. Ed. by Joel A. Kaplan. 2nd ed. 1991. (Illus.). 769p. text (*0-443-08712-1*) Church.

Thoracic Lumbar Spine & Spinal Cord Injuries. Ed. by P. Harris. 1987. (Advances in Neurotraumatology Ser.: Vol. 2). (Illus.). 230p. 96.00 (*0-387-81928-2*) Spr-Verlag.

Thoracic Oncology. Jack Roth et al. 2nd ed. 1995. LC 94-26869. (Illus.). 608p. text 145.00 (*0-7216-4769-3*) Saunders.

Thoracic Organ Transplantation - Routine As a Challenge: Proceedings of the Third International Symposium Held in Bad Oeynhausen, 9-11 September, 1993. Ed. by Michael M. Korner et al. 1994. LC 94-3686. 350p. 201.25 (*0-444-81687-9*) Elsevier.

Thoracic Outlet Syndrome: Diagnosis & Treatment. Erich W. Pollak. 1986. (Illus.). 248p. 39.50 (*0-87993-246-5*) Fairleigh Dickinson.

Thoracic Radiology - The Requisites. Theresa C. McLoud. 1998. LC 98-18593. (Illus.). 557p. (C). (gr. 13). text 89.00 (*0-8016-6354-7*, 06354) Mosby Inc.

Thoracic Spine. Ed. by Edward C. Benzel & Charles B. Stillerman. 1998. LC 98-30127. (Illus.). 654p. 165.00 (*0-942219-75-9*) Quality Med Pub.

Thoracic Spine & Rib Cage. Timothy W. Flynn. 1996. (Illus.). 336p. text 54.99 (*0-7506-9517-X*) Buttrwrth-Heinemann.

Thoracic Surgery. A. G. Casson & M. R. Johnston. 1997. (Key Topics Ser.). 304p. pap. (*1-85996-155-X*) Bios Sci GBR. *Dist:* Coronet Bks.

Thoracic Surgery. Ed. by F. Griffith Pearson et al. 1995. LC 94-42025. text (*0-443-08798-9*) Church.

Thoracic Surgery. Ed. by H. Pichelmaier & F. W. Schildberg. 1989. (Illus.). 460p. 477.00 (*0-387-18464-3*) Spr-Verlag.

Thoracic Surgery. Pearson. 2nd ed. Date not set. (C). text (*0-443-07595-6*) Church.

Thoracic Surgical Oncology. Edward J. Beattie et al. 1992. (Illus.). 405p. text (*0-443-08589-7*) Church.

Thoracic Transplantation. R. Sibly et al. 1995. LC 94-46787. 512p. 165.00 (*0-86542-285-0*) Blackwell Sci.

Thoracic Trauma. R. Maurice Hood & A. W. Boyd. 1989. 448p. text 155.00 (*0-7216-2353-0*) Saunders.

Thoracoscopic Spine Surgery. Ed. by Curtis A. Dickman et al. 1999. LC 99-19799. (Illus.). 360p. 199.00 (*0-86577-785-3*) Thieme Med Pubs.

Thoracoscopic Spine Surgery. Curtis A. Dickman et al. 1999. LC 99-19799. (*3-13-107931-2*) Icon Lrning Systs.

Thoracoscopic Surgery. Ed. by Larry R. Kaiser & Thomas M. Daniel. 1993. LC 93-16239. (Illus.). 192p. 195.00 (*0-316-48218-8*, Little Brwn Med Div) Lppncott W & W.

Thoracoscopic Surgery. Doug Wood & Thomas Marchioro. 1995. text 150.00 (*0-07-071638-2*) McGraw.

Thoracoscopy for Surgeons: Diagnostic & Therapeutic. Ed. by Raymond A. Dieter, Jr. 1995. LC 94-29082. (Illus.). 288p. 98.50 (*0-89640-269-X*) Igaku-Shoin.

Thorax. Jean-Pierre Barral. 1991. LC 90-85570. (Illus.). 186p. (C). text 44.00 (*0-939616-12-2*) Eastland.

Thorax. Roussos. 2nd exp. rev. ed. 1995. (Lung Biology in Health & Disease Ser.: Vol. 85, Pt. C). (Illus.). Pt. C. 2892p. text 495.00 (*0-8247-9601-2*); Pt. A. LC 97-6745. 1080p. text 495.00 (*0-8247-9504-0*); Pt. B. text 495.00 (*0-8247-9600-4*) Dekker.

Thorax, Abdomen, Blood, Endocrine & Metabolic Disorders, Vol. 5. Arnold J. Rudolph. 1997. (Atlas of the Newborn Ser.: Vol. 5). (Illus.). text incl. cd-rom (*1-55009-035-6*) DEKR.

Thornton's Medical Books, Libraries & Collectors. Ed. by Alain Besson. 1990. (Illus.). 450p. text (*0-566-05481-7*) Gower GBR. *Dist:* Ashgate Pub Co.

Thorson's Introductory Guide to Kinesiology: Touch for Health. Maggie La Tourelle & Anthea Courtenay. 1993. pap. (*0-7225-2699-7*) Thorsons.

Thorson's Introductory Guide to Reflexology: A Patient's Guide. Nicola M. Hall. 1992. (Illus.). 128p. pap. (*0-7225-2528-1*) Thorsons.

Thought & Emotion: Developmental Perspectives. Ed. by David J. Bearison & Herbert Zimiles. 1985. (Jean Piaget Symposia Ser.). 256p. (C). text 49.95 (*0-89859-530-4*) L Erlbaum Assocs.

Thought & the Brain. Henri Pieron. 1980. LC 73-2981. (Classics in Psychology Ser.). reprint ed. 25.95 (*0-405-05153-0*) Ayer.

Thought, Consciousness, & Reality: Psychiatry & the Humanities, Vol. 2. Ed. by Joseph H. Smith. 1977. LC 77-77350. (Thought, Consciousness, & Reality Ser.: Vol. 2). 47.50 (*0-300-02138-0*) Yale U Pr.

Thought in the Young Child. Ed. by William Kessen & Clementina Kuhlmann. 1962. (SRCD M Ser.: Vol. 27, No. 2). 25.00 (*0-527-01593-8*) Periodicals Srv.

Thoughts on Some Questions Relating to Women, 1860-1908. Emily Davies. LC 73-14557. reprint ed. 34.50 (*0-404-56741-X*) AMS Pr.

Thoughts on the Run: Glimpses of Wholistic Spirituality. Thomas E. Legere. 1983. 144p. pap. 7.95 (*0-86683-698-5*) Harper SF.

Thoughts Without a Thinker: Psychotherapy from a Buddhist Perspective. Mark Epstein. 1996. LC 94-38063. 256p. pap. 16.00 (*0-465-08585-7*) Basic.

Thousand Marriages: A Medical Study of Sex Adjustment. Robert L. Dickinson & Lura Beam. 1970. LC 76-95093. reprint ed. lib. bdg. 85.00 (*0-8371-3085-9*, DIMA, Greenwood Pr) Greenwood.

Thousand Plateaus: Capitalism & Schizophrenia. Gilles Deleuze & Felix Guattari. 1987. LC 87-18623. 629p. pap. 19.95 (*0-8166-1402-4*); text 49.95 (*0-8166-1401-6*) U of Minn Pr.

Threatened Children: Rhetoric & Concern about Child-Victims. Joel Best. 1994. LC 89-48508. (Illus.). 256p. 29.95 (*0-226-04425-4*) U Ch Pr.

3 a.m. Handbook: The Most Commonly Asked Questions about Your Child's Health. Ed. by William Feldmen. 1998. LC 97-52235. 224p. pap. 17.95 (*0-8160-3802-3*) Facts on File.

Three Case Histories: The Wolf Man, the Rat Man, & the Psychotic Doctor Schreber. Sigmund Freud. 1993. 282p. (C). pap. 12.00 (*0-02-050988-X*) Macmillan.

Three Case Histories: The Wolf Man, the Rat Man, & the Psychotic Doctor Schreber. Sigmund Freud. 1996. LC 63-14965. 282p. per. 14.00 (*0-684-82945-2*) S&S Trade.

3-D Atlas of the Ear: Pathology of External & Middle Ear, Vol. 1. Vincent. 1997. pap. text 260.00 (*0-7506-3021-3*) Buttrwrth-Heinemann.

***3D Imaging Handbook.** Leon Shirman & Yakov Kamen. 2001. 608p. text 99.95 (*0-8493-0742-2*) CRC Pr.

3-D Imaging in Medicine. Ayaram Udupa & Gabor T. Herman. 1991. (Illus.). 576p. 149.00 (*0-8493-4294-5*, L4294BK, CRC Reprint) Franklin.

3-D Modeling Technology in Oral & Maxillofacial Surgery. J. Thomas Lambrecht. 1995. LC 94-48366. (Illus.). 160p. text 140.00 (*0-86715-287-7*, B2877) Quint Pub Co.

3-D Photon Beam Treatment Planning. Ed. by Alfred R. Smith & James A. Purdy. 1991. (Illus.). 256p. 70.50 (*0-08-041180-0*, Pergamon Pr) Elsevier.

3D Qsar in Drug Design. Hugo Kubinyi et al. 1997. LC 97-37816. (Quantitative Structure Activity Relationships Ser.). lib. bdg. 151.00 (*0-7923-4790-0*); lib. bdg. 228.00 (*0-7923-4792-7*) Kluwer Academic.

Three Determinants of Attention-Seeking in Young Children. Jacob L. Gewirtz. 1954. (Society for Research in Child Development Monographs: Vol. 19, No. 2). pap. 25.00 (*0-527-01561-X*) Periodicals Srv.

Three Dimensional Analysis of Spinal Deformities. Ed. by M. D'Amico et al. 1995. LC 94-7752. (Studies in Health Technology & Informatics: Vol. 15). 454p. 130.00 (*90-5199-181-9*) IOS Press.

Three-Dimensional & Multidimensional Microscopy: Image Acquisition & Processing V. Ed. by Carol J. Cogswell et al. 1998. LC 98-233145. (Proceedings of SPIE Ser.: Vol. 3261). 346p. 89.00 (*0-8194-2700-4*) SPIE.

Three-Dimensional Biomedical Imaging. Robert A. Robb. 1985. Vol. I. 184p. 85.00 (*0-8493-5264-9*, RC78); Vol. II, incl. poster. 160p. 85.00 (*0-8493-5265-7*) Franklin (CRC Reprint).

Three Dimensional Biomedical Imaging: Principles & Practice. Richard A. Robb. 1994. LC 94-38015. 145.00 (*1-56081-570-1*, Wiley-VCH) Wiley.

Three-Dimensional Image Reconstruction in Radiology & Nuclear Medicine. Pierre Grangeat & Jean-Louis Amans. 1996. LC 96-25828. (Computational Imaging & Vision Ser.). 315p. text 161.50 (*0-7923-4129-5*) Kluwer Academic.

Three-Dimensional Magnetic Resonance Imaging: An Integrated Clinical Update of 3D-Imaging & 3D-Postprocessing: Proceedings of a Joint Meeting in Obergurgl, Austria, 23-27 March 1992. Ed. by F. Aichner et al. 1994. LC 94-20996. 300p. 125.00 (*0-86542-800-X*) Blackwell Sci.

Three-Dimensional Microscopy Vol. 2984: Image Acquisition & Processing IV. Ed. by Carol J. Cogswell et al. 1997. LC 97-175344. 284p. 69.00 (*0-8194-2395-5*) SPIE.

Three-Dimensional Power Doppler in Obstetrics & Gynecology. Ed. by Asim Kurjak. 2000. LC 99-54491. (Illus.). 150p. lib. bdg. 118.95 (*1-85070-645-X*, Parthenon Pbng) CRC Pr.

Three-Dimensional Radiation Treatment: Technological Innovations & Clinical Results Symposium on 3-D Radiation Treatment: Technological Innovations & Clinical Results, Munich, March 1999. Ed. by H. J. Feldmann et al. 2000. LC 00-43595. (Frontiers of Radiation Therapy & Oncology Ser.: Vol. 34). (Illus.). x, 192p. 158.25 (*3-8055-6947-5*) S Karger.

Three-Dimensional Ultrasound. Thomas Nelson. 1999. LC 98-32024. (Illus.). 272p. text 95.00 (*0-7817-1997-6*) Lppncott W & W.

Three-Dimensional Ultrasound in Obstetrics & Gynecology. Ed. by K. Baba & D. Jurkovic. 1997. LC 96-51892. (Progress in Obstetric & Gynecological Sonography Ser.). (Illus.). 120p. lib. bdg. 85.95 (*1-85070-619-0*, Parthenon Pbng) CRC Pr.

Three-Edged Sword: Being Ill in America. Maureen A. Potts. 1992. 128p. (C). 43.00 (*0-8191-8669-4*) U Pr of Amer.

Three Faces of Being: Toward an Existential Clinical Psychology. Ernest Keen. 1970. LC 78-128900. (Century Psychology Ser.). (Orig.). (C). 42.50 (*0-89197-452-0*); pap. text 19.95 (*0-89197-453-9*) Irvington.

Three Hundred & Fifty Secondary Diseases-Disorders to Alcoholism. 1985. LC 85-73319. 45p. pap. 3.99 (*0-88270-610-1*) Bridge-Logos.

300 MCQS in Anatomy & Physiology for VNS. College of Animal Welfare Staff. 2000. (Veterinary Nursing Ser.: Vol. 300). (Illus.). 81p. pap. text 19.99 (*0-7506-4695-0*) Buttrwrth-Heinemann.

300 MCQS in Exotics & Wildlife for VNS. Ed. by College of Animal Welfare Staff. 2000. 82p. pap. text 19.99 (*0-7506-4696-9*) Buttrwrth-Heinemann.

300 MCQS in Medical & General Nursing for VNS. Ed. by College of Animal Welfare Staff. 2005. 128p. pap. 18.00 (*0-7506-4697-7*) Buttrwrth-Heinemann.

300 Questions & Answers in Diagnostic Aids for Veterinary Nurses. College of Animal Welfare Staff. 2000. 96p. pap. text 19.99 (*0-7506-4795-7*) Buttrwrth-Heinemann.

300 Questions & Answers in Surgical Nursing & Anaesthesia for Veterinary Nurses. Ed. by College of Animal Welfare Staff. 2000. (Veterinary Nursing Ser.: Vol. 300). 96p. pap. text 19.99 (*0-7506-4698-5*) Buttrwrth-Heinemann.

365 Days. Ronald J. Glasser. 1980. LC 77-156599. 292p. pap. 14.95 (*0-8076-0995-1*) Braziller.

Three Hundred Sixty-Five Good Health Hints. David J. Pine. 1994. LC 94-16934. 192p. (Orig.). pap. 5.95 (*1-56170-099-1*, 162) Hay House.

***365 Health & Fitness Tips.** 2001. 352p. (*3-7701-7044-X*) DuMont Buchverlag GmbH & Co DEU. *Dist:* Advanced Global.

Three Hundred Sixty-Five Ways to Manage the Business Called Private Practice. James Davis. 1990. 140p. 24.95 (*1-878487-10-8*, 9105) Practice Mgmt Info.

Three Hundred Years of Psychiatry, 1535-1860. Richard Hunter & Ida Macalpine. 1982. LC 82-73004. xxvi, 1107p. reprint ed. 135.00 (*0-910177-00-7*) Carlisle Pub.

Three in a Bed. Deborah Jackson. 1992. pap. 9.00 (*0-380-76579-9*, Avon Bks) Morrow Avon.

Three Inner Voices: Uncovering the Spiritual Roots of Addiction & Recovery. Richard G. Hartnett. 1994. LC 94-92282. (Illus.). 128p. (Orig.). pap. 10.95 (*1-885909-20-9*) Serenity NY.

Three Jewish Physicians of the Renaissance: The Marriage of Science & Ethics. Aaron Feingold. 1996. LC 96-85973. (Illus.). 63p. 18.00 (*0-9653735-0-9*) Amer Frnds.

3 Minute Consultations with America's Greatest Psychotherapists. Ed. by Jason Aronson. 2000. LC 00-46446. (Illus.). xii, 217p. pap. 8.95 (*0-7657-0305-X*) Aronson.

Three Psychologies: Perspectives from Freud, Skinner & Rogers. Robert D. Nye. (Orig.). (C). 2nd ed. 1981. LC 80-25716. 170p. mass mkt. 13.25 (*0-8185-0438-2*); 3rd ed. 1986. LC 86-9663. 162p. pap. 16.00 (*0-534-06528-7*) Brooks-Cole.

Three Psychologies: Perspectives from Freud, Skinner, & Rogers. Robert D. Nye. 5th ed. 1995. LC 94-42256. (Psychology Ser.). 192p. mass mkt. 14.00 (*0-534-26616-9*) Brooks-Cole.

Three Quarters, Two Dimes & a Nickel: A Memoir of Becoming Whole. Steve Fiffer. 1999. LC 98-47403. (Illus.). 288p. 24.00 (*0-684-85418-X*) Free Pr.

Three Realms of Managed Care: Societal, Institutional, Individual (Resources for Group Reflection & Action) Ed. by John W. Glaser & Ron P. Hamel. 1997. LC 97-33534. 288p. pap. 29.95 (*1-55612-959-9*, LL1959) Sheed & Ward WI.

Three Seductive Ideas. Jerome Kagan. 1998. LC 98-8169. 288p. 27.50 (*0-674-89033-7*) HUP.

Three Technical Papers on a Research & Demonstration Waiver for Medicare Coverage in Mexico. Policy Research Project Staff. 1999. (U. S. - Mexican Occasional Paper Ser.: Vol. 7). 79p. pap. 15.00 (*0-89940-579-7*) LBJ Sch Pub Aff.

Three Worlds of Medicine: Stories of Hope & Courage. Herbert Chasis. Ed. by Roger E. Egan, Sr. 1994. (Illus.). 160p. (Orig.). pap. 21.95 (*0-9632687-4-0*) PenRose Pub.

3D Imaging in Medicine. Jayaram K. Udupa & Gabor T. Herman. 2nd ed. 1999. LC 99-48308. 384p. 129.95 (*0-8493-3179-X*, 3179) CRC Pr.

Threefold Method for Understanding the Seven Rays & Other Essays in Esoteric Psychology. Kurt B. Abraham. 1984. LC 84-81567. 120p. (Orig.). pap. 8.50 (*0-9609002-1-7*) Lampus Pr.

Threshold. Zofia Pytowska. 1982. LC 81-21348. 176p. 18.95 (*0-87073-518-7*); pap. 14.95 (*0-87073-519-5*) Schenkman Bks Inc.

Thrills & Regressions. Michael Balint. 1959. 148p. (Orig.). 27.50 (*0-8236-6540-2*) Intl Univs Pr.

Thrinaxodon: Digital Atlas of the Skull. William Carlson et al. 1995. (Illus.). 35.00 (*0-292-77072-3*) U of Tex Pr.

36-Hour Day: A Family Guide to Caring for Persons with Alzheimer's Disease, Related Dementing Illness & Memory Loss in Later Life. Nancy L. Mace & Peter V. Rabins. rev. ed. 1992. 448p. mass mkt. 6.99 (*0-446-36104-6*) Warner Bks.

Thrival! - a Guide to Soaring with Your Spirit: Six Essential Steps to Thriving. Paul O. Radde. 21.95 (*0-9625872-1-4*) Thriving Pubns.

Thriving: The Complete Mind/Body Guide for Optimal Health & Fitness for Men. Robert Ivker & Edward Zorensky. 2000. (Illus.). 354p. text 26.00 (*0-7881-6984-X*) DIANE Pub.

Thriving in a Toxic World: Today's Ultimate Solutions to Chronic Illness. William R. Kallas & Andrea S. Dworkin. 1996. (Toxic Twins Ser.). (Illus.). 520p. pap. 29.95 (*0-9636491-1-6*) Comprehensive Hlth.

Thriving in an Age of Change: Practical Strategies for Health Care Leaders. Donald N. Lombardi. 1996. LC 96-6417. (Management Ser.). (Illus.). 44.00 (*1-56793-043-3*, 0978) Health Admin Pr.

Thriving in Capitation: A Practical Guide for the Medical Leader. Ed. by Howard Kirz. 1999. LC 97-78157. (Illus.). vi, 363p. pap. 50.00 (*0-924674-60-1*) Am Coll Phys Execs.

Thriving in Transition: Effective Living in Times of Change. Marcia Perkins-Reed. 1996. LC 95-25479. (Illus.). 272p. pap. 12.00 (*0-684-81189-8*, Touchstone) S&S Trade Pap.

Thriving on Reform: Meeting Tomorrow's Healthcare Challenges Today. E. Preston Gee. 1994. 200p. text 27.50 (*1-55738-618-8*, Irwn Prfssnl) McGraw-Hill Educ Grp.

Thriving with Your Autoimmune Disorder: A Woman's Mind-Body Guide. Simone Ravicz. 2000. LC 99-75284. (Illus.). iv, 370p. pap. 16.95 (*1-57224-189-6*) New Harbinger.

Thrombin Ed. by Raymund Machovich. 1984. Vol. I. 176p. 104.00 (*0-8493-6186-9*, QP93); Vol. II. 128p. 76.00 (*0-8493-6187-7*, QP93) Franklin (CRC Reprint).

Thrombin: Structure & Function. L. J. Berliner. 1992. (Illus.). 354p. (C). text 115.00 (*0-306-43991-3*, Kluwer Plenum) Kluwer Academic.

Thromboembolic Complications During Infancy & Childhood. Maureen Andrew. 1999. LC 00-421469. (Illus.). ix, 429p. (*1-55009-036-4*) DEKR.

Thromboembolic Diseases - Mechanisms, Prophylaxis & Treatment: 5th International Symposium, Cannes, June 1998. Ed. by V. V. Kakkar & M. M. Samama. 1998. (Haemostasis Ser.: Vol. 28, Supp. 3). (Illus.). vi, 152p. pap. 48.75 (*3-8055-6815-0*) S Karger.

Thromboembolism: New Achievements & Challenges: 6th International Symposium on Thromboembolic Diseases, Lisbon, June 1999: Proceedings. Ed. by S. Haas et al. 1999. (Haemostasis Ser.: Vol. 29, Suppl. 1). (Illus.). vi, 132p. 39.25 (*3-8055-7041-4*) S Karger.

***Thromboembolism: New Insights & Future Prospects: 7th International Symposium on Thromboembolic Diseases, Palma de Mallorca, June 2000: Proceedings.** S. Haas et al. 2001. (Supplement Issue Ser.: Vol. 30, Suppl. 2). (Illus.). viii, 178p. 45.25 (*3-8055-7177-1*) S Karger.

Thrombolysis: The Dawn of a New Era? Ed. by P. Sleight & D. A. Chamberlain. 1990. 168p. (C). (*1-85271-098-5*) IBC Tech Srvs GBR. *Dist:* St Mut.

Thrombolysis & Adjunctive Therapy for Acute Myocardial Infarction. Ed. by Eric R. Bates. 1992. LC 92-49831. (Fundamental & Clinical Cardiology Ser.: Vol. 10). (Illus.). 528p. text 140.00 (*0-8247-8664-5*) Dekker.

Thrombolytic Therapy for Stroke. Ed. by Patrick D. Lyden. 2001. LC 00-44910. (Illus.). 424p. 125.00 (*0-89603-746-0*) Humana.

Thrombolytic Therapy in Acute Ischemic Stroke III. Ed. by T. Yamaguchi et al. 1996. (Illus.). 376p. 115.00 (*0-387-70139-7*) Spr-Verlag.

Thrombolytic Therapy in Vascular Disease. Ed. by Anthony J. Comerota. 1994. (Illus.). 576p. text 89.50 (*0-397-51343-7*) Lppncott W & W.

Thrombomodulin, Thrombin, & the Control of Hemostasis. Ed. by John C. Giddings. 1994. (Medical Intelligence Unit Ser.). 113p. 99.00 (*1-57059-117-2*, LN9117) Landes Bioscience.

Thromboplastin Calibration & Oral Anticoagulant Control. Ed. by A. Van den Besselaar et al. 1984. (Developments in Hematology & Immunology Ser.). text 147.50 (*0-89838-637-3*) Kluwer Academic.

Thrombopoiesis & Thrombopoietins: Molecular, Cellular, Preclinical & Clinical Biology. Ed. by David Kuter et al. 1996. LC 96-44461. (Illus.). 456p. 170.00 (*0-89603-379-1*) Humana.

Thrombopoietin Vol. 16, Supplement 2: From Molecule to Medicine. M. J. Murphy, Jr. & D. J. Kuter. 1998. 259p. text 69.00 (*1-880854-26-0*); pap. text 49.00 (*1-880854-24-4*) AlphaMed Pr.

Thrombosis. Meade. 1995. text 105.00 (*0-443-05154-2*) Saunders.

Thrombosis & Coronary Heart Disease: Proceedings of the Paavo Nurmi Symposium, 1st, Finland, 1969. Paavo Nurmi Symposium Staff. Ed. by P. I. Halonen & A. Louhija. 1970. (Advances in Cardiology Ser.: Vol. 4). 78.50 (*3-8055-0727-5*) S Karger.

Thrombosis & Hemorrage. Joseph Loscalzo & Andrew I. Schafer. 2nd ed. 1998. LC 97-48547. (Illus.). 1,400p. text 229.00 (*0-683-30114-4*) Lppncott W & W.

Thrombosis & Hemorrhage. J. Loscalzo & A. Schafer. 1993. (Illus.). 1360p. 265.00 (*0-86542-263-X*) Blackwell Sci.

Thrombosis & Its Management. Ed. by Leon Poller & Jean M. Thomson. 1993. (Illus.). 272p. (Orig.). pap. text (*0-443-04797-9*) Church.

Thrombosis & Thrombolysis. Ed. by Eugene I. Chazov & V. N. Smirnov. 1986. LC 86-20472. (Illus.). 444p. (C). text 150.00 (*0-306-10989-1*, Kluwer Plenum) Kluwer Academic.

***Thrombotic Diseases: Current & Future Therapeutic Approaches & Market Opportunities.** George B. Zavoico. Ed. by Susan C. DiClemente. 1998. (Illus.). 481p. spiral bd. 4950.00 (*1-57936-124-2*, 912, D&MD Reports) International Business.

Through Divided Minds. Robert S. Mayer. 1992. 304p. mass mkt. 4.99 (*0-380-71920-7*, Avon Bks) Morrow Avon.

Through Divided Minds: Probing the Mysteries of Multiple Personalites - A Doctor's First-Person Story. Robert S. Mayer. 1990. 304p. pap. 8.95 (*0-380-70905-8*, Avon Bks) Morrow Avon.

Through Pediatrics to Psychoanalysis: Collected Papers. Donald Woods Winnicott. 1992. LC 92-26889. 350p. reprint ed. pap. text 37.95 (*0-87630-703-9*) Brunner-Routledge.

Through Tara's Eyes: Helping Children Cope with Alzheimer's Disease. Kathy Baumann & Erin Conners. 1995. (Illus.). 36p. pap. 5.00 (*1-930181-01-9*) A H A F.

Through the Fire & Through the Water: My Triumph over Cancer. Betty Price. 2000. 112p. pap. 7.99 (*1-883798-33-7*) Faith One.

Through the Leper-Squint. Anthony Weymouth. LC 75-23769. (Illus.). reprint ed. 37.50 (*0-404-13395-9*) AMS Pr.

Through the Looking-Glass: Personality in Culture. Ed. by Yueh-Ting Lee et al. 1998. LC 98-16383. 265p. 79.95 (*0-8058-2813-3*) L Erlbaum Assocs.

Through the Patient's Eyes: Understanding & Promoting Patient-Centered Care. Thomas L. Delbanco. Ed. by Margaret Gerteis et al. 1993. LC 93-51. (Health Management Ser.). 352p. 42.00 (*1-55542-544-5*) Jossey-Bass.

Through the Storm: A Polio Story. Robert F. Hall. 1990. LC 90-36783. 160p. pap. 9.95 (*0-87839-059-6*) North Star.

Through This Window: Views on Traumatic Brain Injury. Ed. by Patricia I. Felton. 1992. (Illus.). 278p. (Orig.). pap. text 19.50 (*0-9634461-0-X*) EBTS.

Throw Away Your Glasses. Harper West. 1994. (Illus.). 96p. pap. 7.95 (*0-9641719-0-2*) Avalanche Pub.

Thrust Plate Hip Prosthesis. Arnold H. Huggler & Hilaire A. Jacob. 1996. LC 96-34374. (Illus.). 168p. 105.00 (*3-540-61506-7*) Spr-Verlag.

Thueson's Guide to Over-the-Counter Drugs: A Symptom-by-Symptom Handbook of the Best Nonprescription Drugs. David O. Thueson. 1995. LC 94-73922. 242p. (Orig.). pap. 13.95 (*1-57224-005-9*) New Harbinger.

Thumb: The Hand & Upper Limb. Ed. by James W. Strickland. 1994. (Illus.). 240p. text (*0-443-03337-4*) Church.

Thus Speaks the Body: Attempts Toward a Personology from the Point of View of Respiration & Postures. Bjorn Christiansen. 1980. LC 72-342. (Body Movement Perspectives in Research Ser.). 246p. reprint ed. 26.95 (*0-405-03141-6*) Ayer.

Thuykdides und die Hippokratische Medizin. Georg Rechenauer. 1991. (Spudasmata Ser.: Bd. XLVII). (GER.). xii, 396p. (*3-487-09226-3*) G Olms Pubs.

Thwarting Anger: A View of Anger. Jim Cole. 1985. pap. 5.50 (*0-9601200-5-X*) Growing Images.

Thymic Tumors. Ed. by R. Sarrazin et al. 1989. (Illus.). viii, 172p. 147.00 (*3-8055-4800-1*) S Karger.

Thymopentin in Experimental & Clinical Medicine. Ed. by E. Sundal. 1985. (Journal: Vol. 4, Suppl. 1, 1985). (Illus.). iv, 156p. pap. 41.75 (*3-8055-4153-8*) S Karger.

Thymus: Diagnostic Imaging, Functions, & Pathologic Anatomy. Ed. by E. Willich et al. 1992. (Medical Radiology Ser.). (Illus.). 224p. 280.00 (*0-387-52547-5*) Spr-Verlag.

Thymus in Immunotoxicology Ed. by Marion D. Kendall. 1991. (Thymus Update Ser.: Vol. 4). xii, 360p. text 214.00 (*3-7186-5113-0*, Harwood Acad Pubs) Gordon & Breach.

Thymus Involvement in Immunity & Disease. W. D. Biggar et al. 1973. LC 72-13558. (Illus.). 220p. (C). text 32.50 (*0-8422-7068-X*) Irvington.

Thymus, Lymph Nodes, Spleen & Lymphatics. Ed. by K. Henry & W. S. Symmers. 3rd ed. 1992. (Systemic Pathology Ser.). (Illus.). 1042p. text (*0-443-03429-X*) Church.

Thymus Update Series, Vol. 4. Ed. by Marion D. Kendall. 1994. 1317p. text 314.00 (*3-7186-5073-8*) Gordon & Breach.

Thyrde & Last Parte of the Secretes of Maister Alexis of Piemont. Allesio Piemontese. Tr. by W. Warde. 1977. LC 77-6844. (English Experience Ser.: No. 840). reprint ed. lib. bdg. 20.00 (*90-221-0840-6*) Walter J Johnson.

Thyroid. Sudha R. Kini. 2nd ed. 1996. LC 95-25633. (Guides to Clinical Aspiration Biopsy Ser.). (Illus.). 536p. 98.50 (*0-89640-303-3*) Igaku-Shoin.

Thyroid & Its Diseases. Leslie J. DeGroot et al. 5th ed. 1984. LC 83-27411. 907p. (C). (*0-471-88688-2*) Church.

Thyroid & Its Diseases. Leslie J. DeGroot et al. 6th rev. ed. 1995. LC 95-36116. 793p. text (*0-443-08895-0*) Church.

Thyroid Autoimmunity. A. Pinchera et al. 1987. LC 87-29258. (Illus.). 654p. 120.00 (*0-306-42762-1*, Plenum Trade) Perseus Pubng.

***Thyroid Autoimmunity.** Ed. by David C.. Rayner & Brian R. Champion. 1996. LC 96-3286. (Medical Intelligence Unit Ser.). (Illus.). 236p. (C). 125.00 (*3-540-60351-4*) Spr-Verlag.

Thyroid Axis & Psychiatric Illness. Ed. by Russell T. Joffe & Anthony J. Levitt. 1993. 339p. text 51.95 (*0-88048-364-4*, 8364) Am Psychiatric.

Thyroid Cancer. Ed. by James A. Fagin. 1998. LC 98-45706. (Endocrine Updates Ser.). 9p. 189.00 (*0-7923-8326-5*) Kluwer Academic.

Thyroid Cancer: A Comprehensive Guide to Clinical Management. Ed. by Leonard Wartofsky. 2000. LC 99-21826. (Illus.). 528p. 175.00 (*0-89603-429-1*) Humana.

Thyroid Disease: Endocrinology, Surgery, Nuclear Medicine, & Radiotherapy. Stephen A. Falk. 2nd ed. 1997. LC 96-47104. (Illus.). 784p. text 185.00 (*0-397-51705-X*) Lppncott W & W.

Thyroid Disease: The Facts. R. I. Bayliss & W. M. Tunbridge. 3rd ed. 1998. LC 98-3834. (Facts Ser.). (Illus.). 206p. pap. 19.95 (*0-19-262946-8*) OUP.

Thyroid Disease in Clinical Practice. I. Ross McDougall. 1992. (Illus.). 344p. text 88.50 (*0-19-520936-2*) OUP.

Thyroid Diseases. Ed. by C. Beckers. 1983. 236p. 62.50 (*0-08-027094-8*, Pergamon Pr) Elsevier.

Thyroid Diseases. Ed. by Stanley G. Korenman & Martin I. Surks. 1999. LC 98-35631. (Atlas of Clinical Endocrinology Ser.: Vol. 1). (Illus.). 201p. 125.00 (*0-632-04397-0*) Blackwell Sci.

Thyroid Diseases: Clinical Fundamentals & Therapy. Fabrizio Monaco. 1993. 688p. lib. bdg. 265.00 (*0-8493-4821-8*, RC655) CRC Pr.

Thyroid Diseases: Clinical Fundamentals & Therapy. Luigi Troncone. 1993. 416p. lib. bdg. 265.00 (*0-8493-4820-X*, RC655) CRC Pr.

Thyroid Diseases of Infancy & Childhood: Effects on Behavior & Intellectual Development. Ed. by Peter Hauser & Joanne Rovet. 1998. LC 98-26778. (Progress in Psychiatry Ser.: Vol. 57). 352p. text 51.95 (*0-88048-767-4*, 8767) Am Psychiatric.

Thyroid Eye Disease. Devron H. Char. 3rd ed. 1997. LC 96-50467. (Illus.). 293p. text 110.00 (*0-7506-9893-4*) Buttrwrth-Heinemann.

Thyroid Function & Disease. Burrow et al. 1989. (Illus.). 352p. text 105.00 (*0-7216-2190-2*) Saunders.

***Thyroid Function & Iodine Nutrition in Women During Pregnancy & in Their Neonates: Studies among Sudanese Subjects.** Aboud Babiker Ali Eltom. 2000. (Comprehensive Summaries of Uppsala Dissertations from the Faculty of Medicine Ser.: No. 969). 89p. (Orig.). pap. (*91-554-4840-2*) Uppsala Universitet SWE. *Dist:* Coronet Bks.

Thyroid Hormone Metabolism: Molecular Biology & Alternate Pathways. Ed. by Sing-Yung Wu & Theo J. Visser. 1994. LC 94-15571. 266p. lib. bdg. 159.00 (*0-8493-4774-2*) CRC Pr.

***Thyroid Hormone Receptors: Methods & Protocols.** Ed. by Aria Baniahmad. 2002. (Methods in Molecular Biology Ser.: No. 202). 272p. 115.00 (*0-89603-995-1*) Humana.

Thyroid Pathology. Kurt W. Schmid & W. Bocker. 1996. LC 96-38761. (Current Topics in Pathology Ser.: Vol. 91). (Illus.). 166p. 187.00 (*3-540-61623-3*) Spr-Verlag.

Thyroid Problems: A Guide to Symptoms & Treatments. Patsy Westcott. 1999. (Illus.). 160p. pap. (*0-7225-3164-8*) Thorsons GBR. *Dist:* Natl Bk Netwk.

Thyroid Solution: A Mind-Body Program for Beating Depression & Regaining Your Emotional & Physical Health. Ridha Arem. 2000. 400p. pap. 16.00 (*0-345-42920-6*, Ballantine) Ballantine Pub Grp.

Thyroid Sourcebook. M Sara Rosenthal. 4th ed. 2000. LC 2001-53692. (Illus.). 288p. pap. 16.95 (*0-7373-0495-2*, Contemporary) McGraw-Hill Trade.

Thyroid Sourcebook: Everything You Need to Know. M Sara Rosenthal. 1996. 272p. pap. 16.00 (*1-56565-482-X*) Lowell Hse.

Thyroid Sourcebook: Everything You Need to Know. M Sara Rosenthal. 3rd ed. 1998. LC 93-10425. (Illus.). 288p. pap. 16.00 (*0-7373-0014-0*, 00140W) NTC Contemp Pub Co.

Thyroid Sourcebook for Women. M Sara Rosenthal. 3rd ed. 1999. LC 99-39865. (Illus.). 336p. pap. 17.95 (*0-7373-0264-X*, 0264XW) NTC Contemp Pub Co.

Thyroid Tumors. Ed. by O. Clark & H. D. Roeher. 1988. (Progress in Surgery Ser.: Vol. 19). (Illus.). viii, 228p. 165.25 (*3-8055-4713-7*) S Karger.

Thyroid Tumours. D. Wynford-Thomas & E. D. Williams. 1989. (Illus.). 176p. text (*0-443-03568-7*) Church.

Thyroiditis. Virginia A. Livolsi & Paul Logerfo. 1981. 224p. 126.00 (*0-8493-5705-5*, RC657, CRC Reprint) Franklin.

Thyrotropin: Ultrasensitive TSH Measurement in Clinical Research & Diagnostics. A. Passath & H. Hoefler. Ed. by G. Leb et al. 1987. (Illus.). x, 361p. (C). 113.85 (*0-89925-209-5*) De Gruyter.

Tibetan Ayurveda: Health Secrets from the Roof of the World. Robert Sachs. 2001. LC 00-50577. (Illus.). 255p. pap. 14.95 (*0-89281-936-7*) Inner Tradit.

Tibetan Buddhist Medicine & Psychiatry: The Diamond Healing. Terry Clifford. 1990. LC 82-61872. (Illus.). 288p. pap. 12.95 (*0-87728-710-4*) Red Wheel ME.

Tibetan Healing: The Modern Legacy of Medicine Buddha. Peter Fenton. 1999. LC 99-16623. (Illus.). 272p. pap. 22.95 (*0-8356-0776-3*, Quest) Theos Pub Hse.

***Tibetan Medicine.** Gerti Samel. 2001. 160p. pap. (*0-316-85845-5*) Little GBR. *Dist:* Trafalgar.

Tibetan Medicine: The Buddhist Way of Healing. Dolkar Khangkar. 2000. (Illus.). 84p. 16.95 (*0-89346-919-X*) Heian Intl.

Tibetan Medicine: Theory & Practice. Vaidya B. Dash. 1997. (C). (*81-7030-519-5*) Sri Satguru Pubns IND. *Dist:* S Asia.

Tibetan Medicine & Healing. Namgyal Qusar & Jean Sergen. Date not set. 320p. pap. 15.00 (*0-465-08481-8*) Basic.

Tibia & Fibula. Ed. by Charles Court-Brown & Dietmar Pennig. 1997. (Musculoskeletal Trauma Ser.). (Illus.). 288p. text 130.00 (*0-7506-0529-4*) Buttrwrth-Heinemann.

Tibial Nonunion: Diagnosis & Treatment. Ed. by John F. Connolly. 1991. LC 91-4558. 71p. pap. 38.00 (*0-89203-048-8*) Amer Acad Ortho Surg.

Tibial Plateau Fractures. H. Mason Hohl. Ed. by Richard Lampert. 1997. LC 96-9599. 224p. text 135.00 (*0-7216-7015-6*) Saunders.

Tick-Borne Encephalitis & Haemorrhagic Fever with Renal Syndrome in Europe. 1986. (EURO Reports & Studies: No. 104). 79p. pap. text 8.00 (*92-890-1270-6*, 1330104) World Health.

Tick Vector Biology: Medical & Veterinarian Aspects. Ed. by B. Fifaz et al. 1993. (Illus.). 193p. (C). 120.00 (*0-387-54045-8*) Spr-Verlag.

Ticks & Tick-Borne Diseases. R. W. Sutherst. 1986. 160p. pap. 96.00 (*0-949511-27-7*) St Mut.

Ticlopidine, Platelets, & Vascular Disease. Ed. by William K. Hass & J. Donald Easton. 1994. LC 92-48386. 162p. 104.00 (*0-387-94009-X*); (*3-540-94009-X*) Spr-Verlag.

Tidbits for Young Doctors & Their Patients: Journal of a Country Doctor, Pt. II. Donald L. Martin. 1993. pap. 9.95 (*1-55673-528-6*, Fairway Pr) CSS OH.

Tidy's Physiotherapy. Ann M. Thompson et al. 12th ed. 1991. (Illus.). 448p. pap. (*0-7506-1346-7*) John Wright GBR. *Dist:* Buttrwrth-Heinemann.

Tierischer Magnetismus—Entlarvt see Animal Magnetism—Unmasked

Ties That Bind: Men's & Women's Social Networks. Ed. by Laura Lein & Marvin B. Sussman. 1983. LC 82-23230. (Marriage & the Family Ser.: Vol. 5, No. 4). 111p. text 39.95 (*0-86656-161-7*) Haworth Pr.

Tietz Fundamentals of Clinical Chemistry. Carl A. Burtis & Edward R. Ashwood. 4th rev. ed. 1995. LC 95-5400. (Illus.). 880p. text 66.00 (*0-7216-3763-9*) Saunders.

Tietz Textbook of Clinical Chemistry. Carl A. Burtis et al. Ed. by Adrianne Williams. 3rd ed. 1998. LC 97-31212. (Illus.). 2000p. (C). text 195.00 (*0-7216-5610-2*) Saunders.

Til Death Do Us Part: A Basic Education in Total Health: How to Keep Body & Soul Happily Together. Martin P. Cornelius, III. 1981. 256p. (Orig.). (C). pap. 15.00 (*0-9607142-0-0*) Health Ed & Life Exp Res.

Till Break of Day: Meeting the Challenge of HIV & AIDS at London Lighthouse. Marina Cantacuzino. 1994. 278p. pap. 17.95 (*0-434-10806-5*) Trafalgar.

***Till the Break of Day: A History of Mental Health Services in Singapore, 1841-1993.** Ng Beng Yeong. 2001. (Illus.). 312p. pap. (*9971-69-245-7*) Sngapore Univ Pr SGP. *Dist:* Coronet Bks.

Tilt: Teaching Individuals to Live Together. Kalman J. Kaplan. 1998. LC 98-25595. 264p. 74.95 (*0-87630-927-9*); pap. 29.95 (*0-87630-928-7*) Brunner-Routledge.

Time Codes. Wyatt Woodsmall. 1998. (Advanced Neuro Linguistic Programming Applications Ser.). 23p. spiral bd. 15.00 (*1-892876-08-6*) Next Step Pr.

Time-Conscious Psychological Therapy: A Life Stage to Go Through. Jenifer E. Wilson. 1996. LC 95-9188. 208p. (C). 85.00 (*0-415-11457-8*); pap. 29.95 (*0-415-11458-6*) Routledge.

Time-Dependent Structure & Control of Arterial Blood Pressure. Ed. by Francesco Portaluppi & Michael H. Smolensky. 1996. LC 96-7856. (Annals of the New York Academy of Sciences Ser.: Vol. 783). pap. 100.00 (*1-57331-009-3*) NY Acad Sci.

Time Distortion in Hypnosis: An Experimental & Clinical Investigation. Linn F. Cooper & Milton H. Erickson. 2nd ed. 1982. LC 82-663. (Illus.). 206p. reprint ed. text 29.50 (*0-8290-0702-4*) Irvington.

Time, Dose & Fractionation in the Radiation Therapy of Cancer: A Frontier Revisited. Ed. by J. M. Vaeth & J. Meyer. 1988. (Frontiers of Radiation Therapy & Oncology Ser.: Vol. 22). (Illus.). x, 194p. 155.75 (*3-8055-4654-8*) S Karger.

Time Enough? States Respond to Term Limits. Frwd. by Daniel M. Fox & William Pound. 1997. LC 97-199199. 40p. (Orig.). pap. (*1-887748-12-1*) Milbank Memorial.

Time for Alzheimers. Florence Baurys. 1998. LC 98-19749. 196p. pap. 16.95 (*1-885373-13-9*) Emerald Ink.

Time for Dying. Barney G. Glaser & Anselm L. Strauss. 1968. LC 67-17601. 285p. lib. bdg. 35.95 (*0-202-30027-7*) Aldinc de Gruyter.

Time, Health & Medicine. Ronald Frankenberg. 1992. LC 91-51133. 176p. (C). 47.00 (*0-8039-8678-5*, 9377) Sage.

Time, Internal Clocks & Movement. Ed. by Maria A. Pastor & Julio Artieda. 1996. LC 96-18161. (Advances in Psychology Ser.: Vol. 115). 324p. 115.00 (*0-444-82114-7*, North Holland) Elsevier.

Time-Limited Day Treatment for Personality Disorders: Integration of Research & Practice in a Group Program. William E. Piper et al. 1996. LC 96-20928. 360p. 29.95 (*1-55798-370-4*) Am Psychol.

Time-Limited Dynamic Psychotherapy: A Guide to Clinical Practice. Hanna Levenson. 1995. LC 95-13934. 256p. 48.00 (*0-465-08651-9*) Basic.

Time-Limited, Intermittent Therapy with Children & Families. Thomas Kreilkamp. 1989. LC 88-30229. 264p. text 32.95 (*0-87630-532-X*) Brunner-Routledge.

Time-Limited Psychotherapy. James Mann. 1973. LC 72-96631. (Commonwealth Fund Publications). 212p. pap. 20.50 (*0-674-89191-0*) HUP.

***Time-Limited Psychotherapy in Practice.** Gaby Shefler. 2001. 320p. (C). pap. 29.95 (*1-58391-140-5*); text 64.95 (*1-58391-139-1*) Brunner-Routledge.

Time-Limited Therapy in a General Practice Setting: How to Help Within Six Sessions. Glyn Hudson-Allez. 1997. LC 97-68970. 208p. 57.95 (*0-7619-5656-5*, 81577); pap. 25.95 (*0-7619-5657-3*, 81578) Sage.

Time Line Therapy. 1988. LC 87-63197. pap. 24.95 (*0-916990-21-4*) META Pubns.

Time-Managed Group Psychotherapy: Effective Clinical Applications. K. Roy MacKenzie. 1997. LC 96-21267. 466p. text 69.50 (*0-88048-863-8*, 8863) Am Psychiatric.

Time, Mind & Behavior. J. A. Michon & J. L. Jackson. 1985. (Illus.). 313p. 105.00 (*0-387-15444-2*) Spr-Verlag.

Time of Her Life: Menopause, Health & Well Being. Myra Hunter & Jean Coope. 1995. (Illus.). 192p. pap. (*0-563-36759-8*) BBC GBR. *Dist:* Parkwest Pubns.

Time of Personal Regeneration. Richard J. Aschwanden & Maria Aschwanden. Ed. by Charles R. Aschwanden. 1984. 60p. pap. 3.40 (*0-913071-00-5*, TX1-202-40) Rama Pub Co.

Time on Fire: My Comedy of Terrors. Evan Handler. 1997. LC 97-1750. 288p. pap. 12.95 (*0-8050-5067-1*) H Holt & Co.

Time, Roles & Self in Old Age. Ed. by Jaber F. Gubrium. 1976. LC 74-12131. 363p. 45.95 (*0-87705-230-1*); pap. 24.95 (*0-87705-350-2*) Kluwer Academic (Kluwer Acad Hman Sci).

Time Series in Psychology. Robert A. Gregson. 1983. 456p. (C). text 89.95 (*0-89859-250-X*) L Erlbaum Assocs.

Time to be Born & a Time to Die: The Ethics of Choice. Ed. by Barry S. Kogan. 1991. 277p. pap. text 28.95 (*0-202-30389-6*); lib. bdg. 51.95 (*0-202-30388-8*) Aldine de Gruyter.

Time to Begin. Valentine Dmitriev. 1983. 248p. (Orig.). (C). pap. 20.00 (*0-911163-01-8*) Caring.

Time to Die: The Place for Physician Assistance. Charles F. McKhann. 2000. 282p. pap. 17.00 (*0-300-08698-9*) Yale U Pr.

Time to Heal: American Medical Education from the Turn of the Century to the Era of Managed Care. Kenneth M. Ludmerer. 1999. LC 98-55496. (Illus.). xxvi, 514p. text 29.95 (*0-19-511837-5*) OUP.

Time to Hear, a Time to Help: Listening to People with Cancer. Daniel Rosenblum. 1993. 250p. text 27.95 (*0-02-927105-3*) Free Pr.

Time to Say Good-Bye: Moving Beyond Loss. Mary M. Goulding. 1996. LC 95-26563. 168p. (Orig.). pap. 14.00 (*0-918949-74-2*) Elder Bks.

Time Trends in Cancer Incidence & Mortality. P. Damiecki. Ed. by M. Coleman et al. 1993. (IARC Scientific Publications Ser.: No. 121). (Illus.). 814p. text 195.00 (*92-832-2121-4*) OUP.

Timebomb: The Coming Epidemic of Multi-Drug Resistant Tuberculosis. Lee Reichman & Janice Hopkins. 2001. LC 2001-34523. (Illus.). 304p. text 24.95 (*0-07-135924-9*) McGraw-Hill Prof.

Timeless Healing: The Power & Biology of Belief. Herbert Benson. 1996. LC 96-3311. 352p. 24.00 (*0-684-81441-2*) S&S Trade.

Timeless Healing: The Power & Biology of Belief. Herbert Benson & Marg Stark. l.t. ed. 1996. LC 96-2763. 24.95 (*1-56895-366-6*, Compass) Wheeler Pub.

Timetables: Structuring the Passage of Time in Hospital Treatment & Other Careers. Julius A. Roth. 1963. (Orig.). pap. 4.95 (*0-672-60851-0*, Bobbs) Macmillan.

Timing of Behavior: Neural, Psychological, & Computational Perspectives. Ed. by David A. Rosenbaum & Charles E. Collyer. 1998. LC 97-37189. (Bradford Book Ser.). (Illus.). 396p. 55.00 (*0-262-18188-6*, Bradford Bks) MIT Pr.

Timing of Toxicological Studies to Support Clinical Trials: Proceedings: C. M. R. Discussion Meeting on the Timing of Toxicological Studies (1994: Nutfield, U. K.) Ed. by Christopher Parkinson. 1995. LC 95-129065. 150p. text 92.50 (*0-7923-8872-0*) Kluwer Academic.

Timolol Ophthalmic Solution in the Treatment of Glaucoma. D. Dausch & H. Honegger. 1978. LC 78-72505. 3.00 (*0-911910-95-6*) Merck-Sharp-Dohme.

Tin & Organotin Compounds: A Preliminary Review. 1980. (Environmental Health Criteria Ser.: No. 5). 109p. pap. text 12.00 (*92-4-154075-3*, 1160015) World Health.

Tin As a Vital Nutrient: Implications in Cancer Prophylaxis & Other Physiological Processes. Ed. by Nate F. Cardarelli. 1986. 336p. 138.00 (*0-8493-6579-1*, RC271, CRC Reprint) Franklin.

Tin-Based Antitumour Drugs. Ed. by Marcel Gielen. 1990. (NATO ASI Ser.: Vol. 37). (Illus.). 226p. 95.00 (*0-387-50417-6*) Spr-Verlag.

Tincture of Tears & Laughter. Marcos Krausz. Ed. by Bernadette Garzarelli. 1995. LC 95-75678. (Illus.). 90p. (Orig.). pap. 15.00 (*0-9639838-1-4*) Little Treasure.

Tincture of Time: The Story of 150 Years of Medicine in Atlanta. Martin Moran. 1995. 140p. 45.00 (*0-9647461-0-7*) Med Assn Atlanta.

Tinnitus. Masaaki Kitahara. 1988. LC 99-12777. (Illus.). 140p. 66.00 (*0-89640-174-X*) Igaku-Shoin.

Tinnitus: Diagnosis & Treatment. Shulman. 2nd ed. 2001. pap. 74.75 net. (*0-7693-0022-7*) Singular Publishing.

Tinnitus: Diagnosis-Treatment. Abraham Shulman et al. 1991. LC 90-5759. (Illus.). 571p. text 99.50 (*0-8121-1121-4*) Lppncott W & W.

Tinnitus: Facts, Theories, & Treatments. National Research Council Staff. 1982. 150p. (C). pap. text 14.95 (*0-309-03328-4*) Natl Acad Pr.

Tinnitus: Treatment & Relief. Jack A. Vernon. 1997. LC 97-19661. (Illus.). 234p. (C). 34.00 (*0-205-18269-0*) Allyn.

Tinnitus - New Hope for a Cure. Paul Van Valkenburgh. 1995. (Illus.). 128p. (Orig.). (C). pap. 14.95 (*0-9617425-2-6*) Van Valkenburgh.

Tinnitus - Turning the Volume Down: Proven Strategies for Quieting the Noise in Your Head. Kevin Hogan. unabr. ed. 1998. (Illus.). 240p. pap. 19.95 (*0-9635085-9-8*) Network Three Thous.

Tinnitus Handbook. Ed. by Richard S. Tyler. 2000. LC 99-57052. (Audiology Textbks.). 493p. pap. 48.75 net. (*1-56593-922-0*) Singular Publishing.

Tinnitus Handbook: A Self-Help Guide. Bill Habets. 1997. (Illus.). 240p. (Orig.). pap. 14.95 (*1-887053-06-9*) United Res CA.

Tinnitus-Hilfe: Ein Arbeitsbuch Fuer Patienten und Ihre Aerztlichen und Nichtaerztlichen Helfer. Bernhard Kellerhals & Regula Zogg. 2nd rev. ed. 1997. (Illus.). xii, 90p. pap. 28.00 (*3-8055-6527-5*) S Karger.

Tinnitus, 1991: Proceedings of the Fourth International Tinnitus Seminar, Bordeaux, France, August 27-30, 1991. Ed. by J. M. Aran & R. Dauman. 1992. LC 92-49982. (Illus.). 575p. lib. bdg. (*90-6299-087-8*) Kugler NLD. *Dist:* Lib Res.

Tinnitus Rehabilitation by Retraining: A Workbook for Sufferers, Their Doctors & Other Health Care Professionals. B. Kellerhals & R. Zogg. 1999. LC 99-16567. (Illus.). xii, 84p. pap., wbk. ed. 24.50 (*3-8055-6930-0*) S Karger.

Tipping the Balance Towards Primary Health Care: A Pan-European Analysis. Ed. by Tom Rathwell et al. 1995. 200p. (*1-85628-941-9*) Avebry GBR. *Dist:* Ashgate Pub Co.

Tips & Techniques, Secrets from a Lifetime in Dentistry, 1. Tr. by Jerald L. Weitzel. 1987. (Illus.). 51p. (C). pap. 39.95 (*0-944375-00-6*) United Prof Pubns.

Tips & Techniques, Secrets from a Lifetime in Dentistry, Set 1. Tr. by Jerald L. Weitzel. 1987. (Illus.). 51p. (C). (*0-944375-01-4*) United Prof Pubns.

Tips & Timesavers for Home Health Nurses. SPC Staff. Ed. by David Moreau. 1997. LC 97-65380. (Springhouse Home Care Ser.). (Illus.). 192p. (Orig.). pap. 22.95 (*0-87434-917-6*) Springhouse Corp.

Tips for Growing Your Practice. Anne Barber et al. 1999. 88p. pap. 20.00 (*0-943599-32-6*) OEPF.

Tired or Toxic? Sherry A. Rogers. 1990. 438p. pap. 17.95 (*0-9618821-2-3*) SandKey.

Tissot: Physician of the Enlightenment. Antoinette S. Emch-Deriaz. 1992. LC 91-46129. (American University Studies: Ser. IX, Vol. 126). 339p. (C). text 49.95 (*0-8204-1819-6*) P Lang Pubng.

Tissue Adhesives in Wound Care. James V. Quinn. 1998. 88p. text incl. cd-rom (*1-55009-067-4*) DEKR.

Tissue & Organ Regeneration in Adults: Synthesis of Skin & Peripheral Nerves. Ioannis V. Yannas. 2001. LC 00-53199. (Illus.). 520p. 89.95 (*0-387-95214-4*) Spr-Verlag.

Tissue Augmentation in Clinical Practice: Procedures & Techniques. Arnold W. Klein. 1998. LC 98-15510. (Basic & Clinical Dermatology Ser.). (Illus.). 416p. text 150.00 (*0-8247-0124-0*) Dekker.

Tissue Characterization with Ultrasound. Ed. by James F. Greenleaf. 1986. Vol. I: Methods. 272p. 136.00 (*0-8493-6221-0*, RC78); Vol. II: Results & Applications. 304p. 155.00 (*0-8493-6222-9*) Franklin (CRC Reprint).

Tissue Cleansing Through Bowel Management. Bernard Jensen. 1981. 175p. pap. 12.99 (*0-9608360-7-1*) B Jensen.

Tissue Culture As a Plant Production System for Horticultural Crops. Ed. by Richard H. Zimmerman et al. 1986. (Current Plant Science & Biotechnology in Agriculture Ser.). text 169.50 (*90-247-3378-2*) Kluwer Academic.

Tissue Culture Investigations. Ed. by Universities Federation for Animal Welfare Staff. 1982. 20.00 (*0-7855-1108-3*) St Mut.

Tissue Culture Techniques. Luccio Nuzzolo & Augusto Vellucci. 1983. LC 67-26015. (Illus.). 258p. 37.50 (*0-87527-117-0*) Green.

Tissue Culture Techniques: An Introduction. Bernice M. Martin. LC 94-6357. xi, 247p. 1997. (Illus.). 49.95 (*0-8176-3643-9*); 1994. 99.00 (*0-8176-3718-4*) Birkhauser.

Tissue Donations in Health, Disease & Post-Mortem Gifts: Index of Authors & Subjects. American Health Research Institute Staff. 1993. 180p. 47.50 (*1-55914-932-9*); pap. 44.50 (*1-55914-933-7*) ABBE Pubs Assn.

Tissue Engineering. E. Bell. 1993. LC 93-28004. 241p. 82.50 (*0-8176-3687-0*) Birkhauser.

Tissue Engineering. Jeffrey R. Morgan & Martin L. Yarmush. 1998. LC 98-11174. (Methods in Molecular Medicine Ser.: Vol. 18). (Illus.). 648p. 115.00 (*0-89603-516-6*) Humana.

Tissue Engineering: Dental Applications & Future Directions. Ed. by Samuel E. Lynch et al. 1999. LC 98-35196. (Illus.). 297p. text 98.00 (*0-86715-346-6*) Quint Pub Co.

Tissue Engineering for Therapeutic Use: Organ Regeneration: Proceedings of the First International Symposium of Tissue Engineering for Therapeutic Use, Kyoto, 27-28 March, 1997. Yoshito Y. Ikada & Yoshio Yamaoka. 1998. LC 98-35191. 188p. 112.00 (*0-444-82993-8*) Elsevier.

Tissue Engineering of Prosthetic Vascular Grafts. P. P. Zilla & Howard P. Greisler. 1999. LC 98-24890. (Tissue Engineering Intelligence Unit Ser.). (Illus.). 621p. 200.00 (*1-57059-549-6*) Landes Bioscience.

Tissue Expansion. Rolf E. Nordstrom. 1996. LC 96-6179. (Illus.). 288p. text (*0-7506-9711-3*) E A GBR. *Dist:* OUP.

Tissue Expansion in Reconstructive Surgery. Gordon H. Sasaki. 1998. LC 98-9639. (Illus.). 384p. (C). (gr. 13). text 165.00 (*0-8016-4320-1*, 04320) Mosby Inc.

Tissue Growth Factors. Ed. by Renato Baserga. 1981. (Handbook of Experimental Pharmacology Ser.: Vol. 57). (Illus.). 630p. 272.00 (*0-387-10623-5*) Spr-Verlag.

Tissue Inhibitors of Metalloproteinase in Development & Disease (TIMPs '96) Proceedings of the Inhibitors of Metalloproteinases Conference Held at Banff, Alberta, Canada, September 25-29, 1996. Ed. by Susan P. Hawkes et al. 2000. 264p. 95.00 (*90-5702-599-X*, Harwood Acad Pubs) Gordon & Breach.

Tissue-Integrated Prostheses. Per-Ingvar Branemark et al. 1985. (Illus.). 352p. text 96.00 (*0-86715-129-3*) Quint Pub Co.

Tissue Integration in Oral, Orthopedic, & Maxillofacial Reconstruction. Ed. by William R. Laney & Dan E. Tolman. 1992. (Illus.). 396p. pap. text 72.00 (*0-86715-251-6*) Quint Pub Co.

Tissue Optics: Light Scattering Methods & Instruments for Medical Diagnosis. Contrib. by V. Tuchin. 2000. LC 99-53491. (Tutorial Texts in Optical Engineering Ser.: Vol. 38). (Illus.). xxv, 352p. pap. 50.00 (*0-8194-3459-0*) SPIE.

Tissue Oxygen Deprivation. Ed. by Gabriel G. Haddad & George Lister. 1996. LC 96-19881. (Lung Biology in Health & Disease Ser.: Vol. 95). (Illus.). 1120p. text 265.00 (*0-8247-9493-1*) Dekker.

Tissue Oxygenation in Acute Medicine. Ed. by W. J. Sibbald et al. 1998. LC 98-30787. (Update in Intensive Care & Emergency Medicine Ser.: Vol. 33). (Illus.). 392p. 129.00 (*3-540-64086-X*) Spr-Verlag.

Tissue Perfusion & Organ Function. T. Kamada et al. 1995. 276p. 206.50 (*0-444-81967-3*) Elsevier.

Tissue Renin-Angiotensin System: Physiologic & Pharmacologic Implications. Ed. by Victor J. Dzau. 1988. LC 73-3001. (Circulation Monographs: No. 12). 78p. 9.60 (*0-87493-261-0*) Am Heart.

Tissue Renin-Angiotensin Systems: Current Concepts of Local Regulators in Reproductive & Endocrine Organs. Ed. by Amal K. Mukhopadhyay & Mohan K. Raizada. 1995. (Advances in Experimental Medicine & Biology Ser.: Vol. 377). (Illus.). 470p. (C). text 130.00 (*0-306-45077-1*, Kluwer Plenum) Kluwer Academic.

Tissue Repair & Fibrosis: The Role of the Myofibroblast. Ed. by Alexis Desmouliere et al. 1999. LC 99-19995. (Current Topics in Pathology Ser.: Vol. 93). (Illus.). 242p. 179.00 (*3-540-65244-2*) Spr-Verlag.

Tissue-Specific Metabolic Alterations in Diabetes. Ed. by F. Belfiore & S. Gregorio. 1990. (Frontiers in Diabetes Ser.: Vol. 10). viii, 192p. 168.00 (*3-8055-5171-1*) S Karger.

Tissue Specific Toxicity: Biochemical Mechanisms. Ed. by Wolfgang Dekant & H. G. Neumann. 1992. (Illus.). 263p. text 110.00 (*0-12-208860-3*) Acad Pr.

Tissue Substitutes, Phantoms & Computational Modelling in Medical Ultrasound. 1998. LC 98-28850. (ICRU Report Ser.: Vol. 61). 65.00 (*0-913394-60-2*) Intl Comm Rad Meas.

Tissue-Type Plasminogen Activator (t-PA) Physiological & Clinical Aspects, Vol. II. Cornelis Kluft. 1988. 192p. 111.00 (*0-8493-4609-6*, QP93, CRC Reprint) Franklin.

Titanium Alloys in Surgical Implants - STP 796. Ed. by Hugh A. Luckey & Fred Kubli, Jr. 1983. LC 84-72888. 295p. text 37.50 (*0-8031-0241-0*, STP796) ASTM.

***Titanium in Medicine: Material Science, Surface Science, Engineering, Biological Responses & Medical Applications.** Ed. by D. M. Brunette et al. 2001. LC 2001-269649. (Engineering Materials Ser.). (Illus.). xiii, 1019p. 199.00 (*3-540-66936-1*) Spr-Verlag.

Title Catalog, Pt. 7. Marine Biological Laboratory Staff & Woods Hole Oceanographic Institution Staff. 1971. 1215.00 (*0-8161-0937-0*, Macmillan Ref) Gale.

Tm & Cult Mania. Michael A. Persinger et al. 1980. 208p. 12.95 (*0-8158-0392-3*) Chris Mass.

TMJ: Clinical & Practice Managememt. Errol Lader. 116p. ring bd. 85.00 (*0-9610782-0-0*) Vadare.

TMJ: Its Many Faces. Wesley E. Shankland, 2nd. 2nd ed. 1998. (Illus.). 232p. pap. 19.50 (*1-890018-23-6*) Anadem Pubng.

TMJ: Systems Manual of Insurance & Practice Management. Errol Lader. 97p. spiral bd. 65.00 (*0-9610782-1-9*) Vadare.

TMJ: The Self Help Program. John J. Taddey et al. rev. ed. 1991. LC 90-90095. (Illus.). 240p. 21.95 (*0-9625540-9-X*); pap. 13.95 (*0-9625540-3-0*) Surrey Park Pr.

TMJ - The Jaw Connection, the Overlooked Diagnosis: A Self-Care Guide to Diagnosing & Managing this Hidden Ailment. Greg Goddard. 1991. LC 91-75870. (Illus.). 200p. (Orig.). pap. 12.50 (*0-943358-35-3*) Aurora Press.

TMJ Disorders: Management of the Craniomandibular Complex. Ed. by Steven L. Kraus. 1987. (Clinics in Physical Therapy Ser.: Vol. 18). (Illus.). 422p. pap. (*0-443-08484-X*) Church.

TMJ Iatroepidemic: Unintentional Confessions of a Profession. Webby & Chang. Ed. by Sabra Broock & Tim Dixon. 1997. LC 97-72277. 443p. (Orig.). pap., per. 29.95 (*0-9657526-0-7*) BrierNet.

TMJ Pain Control: A Self-Help Program. Sharon L. Carr & Terry L. Daugherty. 1989. (Illus.). 40p. 29.95 incl. audio (*0-924728-00-0*, TMJ Stress Ctr) MyoData.

TMJ Therapy Balances Body Chemistry. Robert J. Peshef. 1983. 65.00 (*0-9605902-6-9*) Color Coded Charting.

TMRL: Management of Coronary Artery Diseases. Ed. by M. Klien et al. 1998. LC 98-2506. (Illus.). 290p. 129.00 (*3-540-64064-9*) Spr-Verlag.

TNM Atlas. Ed. by M. Graf et al. 4th ed. 1997. (Illus.). 393p. pap. 32.00 (*3-540-62704-9*) Spr-Verlag.

TNM Atlas: Illustrated Guide to the TNM-PTNM Classification of Malignant Tumours. Ed. by G. Wagner et al. 3rd ed. 1995. (UICC International Union Against Cancer Ser.). (Illus.). xix, 343p. reprint ed. 29.00 (*0-387-17721-3*) Spr-Verlag.

TNM Classification of Malignant Tumours. P. Hermanek & L. H. Sobin. 4th rev. ed. 1996. 197p. 31.95 (*3-540-17366-8*) Spr-Verlag.

TNM Classification of Malignant Tumours. Ed. by UICC Staff et al. 4th rev. ed. 1996. (International Union Against Cancer Ser.). (Illus.). 170p. 29.00 (*0-387-17366-8*) Spr-Verlag.

TNM Classification of Malignant Tumours. Leslie H. Sobin & Christian Wittekind. 5th ed. 1997. LC 97-9162. 256p. pap. 39.50 (*0-471-18486-1*) Wiley.

***TNM Classification of Malignant Tumours.** Ed. by Leslie H. Sobin & Christian Wittekind. 6th ed. 2002. (UICC Ser.). pap. (*0-471-22288-7*) Wiley.

TNM Interactive: An Illustrated Resource for the Classification & Staging of Malignant Tumors. Ed. by L. H. Sobin. 5th ed. 1998. 173.50 incl. cd-rom (*0-471-29696-1*) Wiley.

TNM Supplement, 1993: A Commentary on Uniform Use. Ed. by E. Hermanek et al. 1994. LC 93-10973. (Illus.). 141p. suppl. ed. 45.00 (*0-387-56556-6*) Spr-Verlag.

TNM Supplement 2000: A Commentary on Uniform Use. Ch Wittekind et al. 2nd ed. 2001. LC 2001-33257. 168p. pap. 45.00 (*0-471-37939-5*) Wiley.

TNP Handbook of Drug-Herb & Drug-Nutrient Interactions: A Guide for Health Professionals. Richard Harkness et al. 2002. LC 00-52409. (Natural Pharmacist Ser.). (Illus.). 208p. 39.99 (*0-7615-2753-2*) Prima Pub.

TNP Handbook of Herbs, Supplements & Conditions: A Guide for Health Professionals. Andrea M. Girman & Steven Bratman. 2002. LC 00-53052. (Natural Pharmacist Ser.). (Illus.). 800p. pap. 39.99 (*0-7615-2773-7*, Prima Health) Prima Pub.

To a Patient Named Nick: A Different Kind of Story of a Nurse & an AIDS Patient. Eva L. Altarejos-Espinosa. 1998. LC 95-71609. 152p. 14.95 (*0-9648529-0-X*) Carelife Pubng.

To Air Is Human: A Manual for People with Chronic Lung Disease. Madeline H. Barrow. l.t. ed. 1999. (Illus.). 72p. pap. 7.95 (*0-939838-51-6*) Pritchett & Hull.

To America's Health: A Proposal to Reform the Food & Drug Administration. Henry Miller. 2000. LC 00-31937. (Publication Ser.: Vol. P482). 112p. pap. 14.95 (*0-8179-9902-7*) Hoover Inst Pr.

To Be a Man: In Search of the Deep Masculine. Ed. by Keith Thompson. 1991. (New Consciousness Reader Ser.). 320p. (Orig.). 13.95 (*0-87477-637-6*, Tarcher Putnam) Putnam Pub Group.

To Be a Nurse. Linda Strangio et al. Ed. by Lisa Ruggerio & Carolyn S. Zagury. 1995. LC 94-61761. 216p. pap. 12.95 (*1-880254-22-0*) Vista.

To Be a Nurse: Personal-Vocational Relations for the LPN/LVN. Mary Ann Anderson. 2000. LC 99-58026. (Illus.). 360p. pap. text 24.95 (*0-8036-0573-0*) Davis Co.

To Be a Nurse & Nursing Leadership, Management & Professional Practice for the LPN/LVN, Set. Mary Ann Anderson. 2nd ed. 2001. LC 00-47411. pap. 44.95 (*0-8036-0854-3*) Davis Co.

To Be a Woman: The Birth of the Conscious Feminine. Ed. by Connie Zweig. 1990. (New Consciousness Reader Ser.). 288p. (Orig.). pap. 14.95 (*0-87477-561-2*, Tarcher Putnam) Putnam Pub Group.

To Be or Not to Be: Reflections on Modern Bioethical Choices. Donald V. Paone. 1999. 116p. pap. 9.95 (*0-9667222-0-5*) Blue Skies.

To Breathe Freely: Risk, Consent, & Air. Ed. by Mary Gibson. 1985. LC 84-22278. (Maryland Studies in Public Philosophy). 312p. (C). 56.50 (*0-8476-7416-9*) Rowman.

To Buy or Not to Buy: A Profile of California's Non-Poor Uninsured. Jill M. Yegian et al. 1999. (Illus.). 25p. pap. (*1-929008-20-1*) CA HlthCare Fnd.

To Comfort the Dying: Pain Control in Advanced Cancer. Charles O. O'Shaughnessy. Ed. by John R. Kirschner. 1996. (Illus.). 250p. (Orig.). pap. 21.95 (*0-9654910-0-5*) Lovejoy Hospice.

To Die or Not to Die. Nathan Breslau. 1982. (Orig.). pap. 2.95 (*0-9610716-0-5*) N Breslau.

To Die Or Not to Die? Cross-disciplinary, Cultural & Legal Perspectives on the Right to Choose Death. Ed. by Arthur S. Berger & Joyce Berger. 1990. LC 90-34370. 208p. 62.50 (*0-275-93585-X*, C3585, Praeger Pubs) Greenwood.

To Do No Harm: A Journey Through Medical School. Philip R. Reilly. 1987. LC 86-26576. 309p. 49.95 (*0-86569-162-2*); pap. 16.95 (*0-86569-163-0*) Greenwood (Auburn Hse).

To Do No Harm: Learning to Care for the Seriously Ill. Alan C. Mermann. 1998. 128p. 45.00 (*0-391-04084-7*); pap. 15.00 (*0-391-04085-5*) Brill Academic Pubs.

To Do No Harm: Learning to Care for the Seriously Ill. Alan C. Mermann. 1999. LC 99-10115. 128p. pap. 17.00 (*1-57392-666-3*, Humanity Bks) Prometheus Bks.

To Dream the Perfect Organization. Joel Fort & Lothar Salin. 1981. LC 80-53829. (Illus.). 144p. (C). pap. text 9.95 (*0-89914-005-X*) Third Party Pub.

To Ensure Individual & Family Security Through Health Care Coverage for All Americans, Set. 1994. lib. bdg. 2555.95 (*0-8490-5818-X*) Gordon Pr.

To Err Is Human: Building a Safer Health System. Linda T. Kohn et al. 2000. LC 99-88993. (Illus.). 300p. 34.95 (*0-309-06837-1*) Natl Acad Pr.

To Have & to Hold: Marriage, the First Baby, & Preparing Couples for Parenthood. C. F. Clulow. 1982. 168p. text 21.00 (*0-08-028470-1*, Pergamon Pr) Elsevier.

To Heal Again: Toward Serenity & the Resolution of Grief. Rusty Berkus. 1996. (Illus.). 64p. (Orig.). pap. 19.95 (*0-9609888-2-3*) Red Rose Pr.

To Heal the Heart of a Child: Helen Taussig, M.D. Joyce Baldwin. 1992. LC 91-41058. 128p. (J). (gr. 7 up). lib. bdg. 15.85 (*0-8027-8167-5*) Walker & Co.

To Improve Health & Health Care, 1997: The Robert Wood Johnson Anthology. Stephen L. Isaacs. 1997. LC 97-16892. (Robert Wood Johnson Foundation Anthology Ser.). 268p. pap. 21.00 (*0-7879-0909-2*) Jossey-Bass.

To Improve Health & Health Care, 2001. Stephen L. Isaacs & James R. Knickman. 2000. LC 00-10983. (Robert Wood Johnson Foundation Anthology Ser.). (Illus.). 288p. pap. 21.00 (*0-7879-5276-1*) Jossey-Bass.

To Improve Health & Health Care, 2000: The Robert Wood Johnson Foundation Anthology. Stephen L. Isaacs. 1999. LC 99-38570. (Robert Wood Johnson Foundation Anthology Ser.). (Illus.). 292p. pap. 21.00 (*0-7879-4976-0*) Jossey-Bass.

To Mock Doctor's Rules: A History of Education in Public Health. Elizabeth Fee & Roy M. Acheson. 1991. (Illus.). 360p. 49.95 (*0-19-261757-5*) OUP.

To Pace or Not to Pace, Controversial Subjects on Cardiac Pacing: Proceedings of the European Pacemaker Colloquium, 2nd, Brussels, April 1977. European Pacemaker Colloquium Staff. Ed. by Hilbert J. Thalen & J. Warren Hawthorne. 1978. text 199.50 (*90-247-2070-2*) Kluwer Academic.

To Redeem One Person Is to Redeem the World: The Life of Frieda Fromm-Reichmann. Gail A. Hornstein. 2000. LC 00-57316. (Illus.). 512p. 35.00 (*0-684-82792-1*) Free Pr.

To Relieve the Human Condition: Bioethics, Technology, & the Body. Gerald P. McKenny. 1997. LC 96-45998. 279p. (C). text 60.50 (*0-7914-3473-7*); pap. text 20.95 (*0-7914-3474-5*) State U NY Pr.

To Serve the Greatest Number: A History of Group Health Cooperative of Puget Sound. Walt Crowley & Group Health Cooperative of Puget Sound Staff. 1997. LC 96-38972. (Illus.). 312p. 19.95 (*0-295-97587-3*) U of Wash Pr.

To Speak Again: My Victory over Throat Cancer. Raymond A. Berte. 1988. 192p. 24.95 (*0-8159-6923-6*) Devin.

To Stretch a Plank: A Survey of Psychokinesis. Diana M. Robinson. 1981. LC 80-12335. 282p. 32.95 (*0-88229-404-0*) Burnham Inc.

To the Ends of the Earth: Women's Search for Education in Medicine. Thomas N. Bonner. 1992. (Illus.). 264p. (C). 45.95 (*0-674-89303-4*) HUP.

To the Point. 1989. (*0-9627652-0-1*, TXU 380-459) A A Wenger.

To the Point: Effective Communications for the Medical Staff. Steve Rivkin et al. 1996. LC 97-159307. (Medical Staff Reengineering Ser.). vi, 28 p. 32.00 (*1-885829-25-6*) Opus Communs.

To the Stutterer, No. 9. Intro. by Malcolm Fraser. 1972. LC 76-376781. 116p. pap. 2.00 (*0-933388-07-1*) Stuttering Fnd Am.

To Thine Own Self Be Good. Slightly Off Center Writers Group Staff. 1995. (Orig.). pap. 9.95 (*1-56721-125-9*) Twnty-Fifth Cent Pr.

To Treat or Not to Treat: Bioethics & the Handicapped Newborn. Richard Sparks. 1988. 352p. pap. 9.95 (*0-8091-2993-0*) Paulist Pr.

To Understand & to Help: The Life Work of Susan Isaacs (1885-1948) Lydia A. Smith. 1985. LC 83-48187. (Illus.). 352p. 45.00 (*0-8386-3211-4*) Fairleigh Dickinson.

To Understand Your Child. Kay Kuzma. rev. ed. 1985. 128p. pap. 5.95 (*0-910529-00-0*) Family Mtrs.

To Wake in Tears: Understanding Intersitial Cystitis. Catherine M. Simone. 1998. LC 98-74050. 225p. pap. 19.95 (*0-9667750-0-7*) IC Hope.

To Your Good Health. David L. Vastola. 2000. LC 97-48255. 64p. pap. 9.95 (*1-56825-040-1*) Rainbow Books.

Tobacco. Mark S. Gold. 1995. (Drugs of Abuse: Vol. 4). (Illus.). 224p. 45.00 (*0-306-44933-1*) Kluwer Academic.

Tobacco: A Major International Health Hazard. Ed. by D. Zaridze & Richard Peto. 1987. (IARC Scientific Publications Ser.: No. 74). (Illus.). 200p. text 46.00 (*92-832-1174-X*) OUP.

Tobacco: Biology & Politics. Stanton A. Glantz. 1994. 3.95 (*1-56796-071-5*) WRS Group.

Tobacco: Health Facts. Nora J. Krantzler & Kathleen R. Miner. 1995. LC 94-42445. 12.95 (*1-56071-477-8*, H414) ETR Assocs.

Tobacco: Index of Modern Information with Bibliography. Scott T. Dowling. 1990. LC 90-32063. 160p. 47.50 (*1-55914-154-9*); pap. 44.50 (*1-55914-155-7*) ABBE Pubs Assn.

***Tobacco - Control Activities in the United States 1992-1993: Biennial Report to Congress.** Pref. by Donna E. Shalala. 2001. (Illus.). 72p. (C). reprint ed. pap. text 20.00 (*0-7567-0606-8*) DIANE Pub.

Tobacco, Alcohol & Cancer Prevention. Ernest H. Rosenbaum et al. Ed. by Sheila Mahoney & Nancy Wiltsek. 1984. (Illus.). 29p. pap. 2.50 (*0-933161-02-6*) Better H Prog.

***Tobacco & Health.** R. Doll & J. Crofton. 1996. (British Medical Bulletin Ser.: Vol. 52, No. 1). 228p. pap. (*1-85315-272-2*) Royal Soc of Medicine Pr Ltd GBR. *Dist:* Balogh.

Tobacco & Health: Proceedings of the 9th World Conference Held in Paris, France, October 10-14, 1994. Ed. by Karen Slama. 1995. (Illus.). 1072p. 185.00 (*0-306-45111-5*, Plenum Trade) Perseus Pubng.

Tobacco & Marijuana. Ochsner et al. 1976. per. 16.00 (*0-88252-048-2*) Paladin Hse.

Tobacco & the Clinician: Interventions for Medical & Dental Practice. 1994. (Illus.). 389p. (Orig.). (C). pap. text 50.00 (*0-7881-1142-6*) DIANE Pub.

Tobacco & Your Oral Health. Arden Christen & Jennifer Klein. 1997. LC 97-25101. (Illus.). 36p. pap. 22.00 (*0-86715-326-1*) Quint Pub Co.

***Tobacco (CEOs) Congressional Hearing.** Ed. by John McCain. 2001. 96p. (C). pap. text 25.00 (*0-7567-0947-4*) DIANE Pub.

Tobacco Control Laws: Implementation & Enforcement. Peter D. Jacobson & Jeffrey Wasserman. 1997. LC 97-5328. 180p. pap. 15.00 (*0-8330-2486-8*, MR-841-RWJ) Rand Corp.

Tobacco Effects in the Mouth. R. E. Mecklenburg et al. 1995. (Illus.). 28p. (Orig.). (C). pap. text 25.00 (*0-7881-2182-0*) DIANE Pub.

Tobacco Epidemic. Ed. by C. T. Bolliger & K. O. Fagerstrom. 1997. LC 97-29285. (Progress in Respiratory Research Ser.: No. 28). (Illus.). x, 266p. 82.75 (*3-8055-6531-3*) S Karger.

Tobacco Habits Other Than Smoking: Betel-Quid & Areca-Nut Chewing; & Some Related Nitrosamines. 1985. (IARC Scientific Publications Ser.: Vol. 37). 291p. pap. text 77.00 (*92-832-1537-0*, 1720037) World Health.

Tobacco or Health: Status in the Americas: A Report of the Pan American Health Organization. 1992. (PAHO Scientific Publications: No. 536). (ENG & SPA.). xiv, 387p. pap. text 40.00 (*92-75-11536-2*, 1610536) World Health.

Tobacco Smoke in Active & Passive Pollution: Reports of Harmful Conditions & Effects: Index of Authors & Subjects. Wayne W. Weiss. 1994. LC 94-31240. 57.50 (*0-7883-0362-7*); pap. 47.50 (*0-7883-0363-5*) ABBE Pubs Assn.

Tobacco Smoking & Atherosclerosis: Pathogenesis & Cellular Mechanisms. Ed. by J. N. Diana. 1990. LC 90-7922. (Advances in Experimental Medicine & Biology Ser.: Vol. 273). (Illus.). 404p. (C). text 156.00 (*0-306-43668-X*, Kluwer Plenum) Kluwer Academic.

Tobacco Smoking & Nicotine: A Neurobiological Approach. Ed. by W. R. Martin et al. 1987. LC 87-18513. (Advances in Behavioral Biology Ser.: Vol. 31). (Illus.). 534p. 120.00 (*0-306-42611-0*, Plenum Trade) Perseus Pubng.

Tobacco Smoking & Nutrition: Influence of Nutrition on Tobacco-Associated Health Risks. Ed. by John N. Diana & William A. Pryor. 1993. LC 93-10409. (Annals Ser.: Vol. 686). 366p. pap. 90.00 (*0-89766-808-1*) NY Acad Sci.

Today & Tommorrow's Woman - Menopause: Before & After (Girls of 16 to Women of 99) Virginia L. Millonig. 1996. LC 95-48849. 300p. (Orig.). pap. text 10.00 (*1-878028-23-5*) Hlth Lead Assoc.

Today, I Have Cancer: A Daily Journal of Life with Cancer. Debi Estabrook. 1995. 376p. (Orig.). pap. 9.95 (*1-56383-049-3*, 9250) G & R Pub.

Today's Art of Peritoneal Dialysis: Proceedings of the International Symposium, 1st Chapala, Jalisco, Mexico, June 25-28, 1978. International Symposium on Peritoneal Dialysis Staff. Ed. by A. T. Becerra & F. S. Boen. 1979. (Contributions to Nephrology Ser.: Vol. 17). (Illus.). 29.75 (*3-8055-3006-4*) S Karger.

Today's Health Alternative. Raquel Martin. 1992. (Illus.). 456p. (Orig.). (C). pap. text 16.95 (*0-922356-45-9*) Amer West Pubs.

Todays Healthy Eating. Louise Tenney. 1993. 249p. pap. 12.95 (*0-913923-09-5*) Woodland UT.

Today's Herbal Health: The Essential Guide to Understanding Herbs Used for Medicinal Purposes. Louise Tenney. 1997. pap. text 16.95 (*1-885670-76-1*) Woodland UT.

Today's Herbal Health for Women. Louise Tenney. 1996. 256p. pap. text 12.95 (*1-885670-35-4*) Woodland UT.

Today's Management Methods: A Guide for the Health Care Executive. Ed. by Robert G. Gift & Catherine F. Kinney. 1996. LC 96-5097. (Illus.). 313p. (Orig.). pap. 69.00 (*1-55648-153-5*, 001117) AHPI.

Today's Woman: Prenatal Care & Beyond. Paula Baran. Ed. by Carolyn S. Zagury & Margaret C. Ciocco. 1998. LC 97-62502. 128p. pap. 12.95 (*1-880254-53-0*) Vista.

Toddlers & Their Mothers: A Study in Early Personality Development. Erna Furman. 1992. LC 91-35415. 420p. (C). 60.00 (*0-8236-6555-0*) Intl Univs Pr.

Toddlers & Their Mothers: Abridged Version for Parents & Educators. Erna Furman. 1993. LC 93-1871. 243p. pap. 24.95 (*0-8236-8318-4*, 26555) Intl Univs Pr.

Toddler's Behavior with Agemates: Issues of Interaction, Cognition & Affect. Wanda C. Bronson. 1981. LC 81-12896. (Monographs on Infancy Ser.: Vol. 1). 128p. (C). 77.00 (*0-89391-080-5*, Ablex) Greenwood.

Toga Therapy: Safe, Natural Methods to Promote Healing & Restore Health & Well-Being. Stella Weller. 1995. (Illus.). 154p. pap. (*0-7225-2998-8*) Thorsons GBR. *Dist:* Natl Bk Netwk.

Togaviridae & Flaviviridae. S. Schlesinger & M. Schlesinger. 1986. LC 86-4914. (Viruses Ser.). (Illus.). 470p. (C). text 120.00 (*0-306-42176-3*, Kluwer Plenum) Kluwer Academic.

Toil & Toxics: Workplace Struggles & Political Strategies for Occupational Health. James C. Robinson. 1991. LC 90-20986. 253p. text 40.00 (*0-520-07164-6*); pap. text 14.95 (*0-520-08448-9*) U CA Pr.

Toilet Learning: The Picture Book Technique for Children & Parents. Alison Mack. 1983. LC 77-24305. 109p. pap. 12.95 (*0-316-54237-7*) Little.

Toilet Training to Independence for the Handicapped: A Manual for Trainers. Sue Bettison. 1982. (Illus.). 144p. (C). pap. 30.95 (*0-398-04678-6*) C C Thomas.

Tom Brown's Guide to Wild Edible & Medicinal Plants. Tom Brown, Jr. 1986. LC 86-109262. 288p. pap. 12.95 (*0-425-10063-4*) Berkley Pub.

Tomographic Methods in Nuclear Medicine: Physical Principles, Instruments, & Clinical Applications. Ed. by Bhagwat D. Ahluwalia. 1989. 288p. lib. bdg. 195.00 (*0-8493-6198-2*, RC78) CRC Pr.

Tomorrow I'll Be Different. Beauchamp Colclough. 1995. 240p. pap. 11.95 (*0-87951-629-1*) Overlook Pr.

Tomorrow's Hospital: A Look to the Twenty-First Century. Eli Ginzberg. 176p. 1998. pap. 14.00 (*0-300-07270-8*); 1996. LC 95-39952. 35.00 (*0-300-06574-4*) Yale U Pr.

Tomorrow's Medicine. Richard Grossman. 1998. (*0-201-62689-6*) Addison-Wesley.

Tongan Herbal Medicine. W. Arthur Whistler. 1992. (Illus.). 122p. pap. 12.95 (*0-8248-1527-0*) Isle Botanica.

Tongue Diagnosis in Chinese Medicine. Giovanni Maciocia. 2nd rev. ed. 1995. LC 94-61961. (Illus.). 210p. (C). text 45.00 (*0-939616-19-X*) Eastland.

Tonsils: A Clinical-Oriented Update. Ed. by G. B. Galioto. 1992. LC 92-49677. (Advances in OtoRhinoLaryngology Ser.: Vol. 47). (Illus.). x, 350p. 195.75 (*3-8055-5604-7*) S Karger.

Tonsils & Adenoids: A Guide for Parents. Jack Paradise. Ed. by Frank A. Oski. 1995. (Pediatrics Ser.). (Illus.). 16p. pap. 2.95 (*1-885274-11-4*) Health InfoNet Inc.

Too Ill to Talk? User Involvement & Palliative Care. Neil Small & Penny J. Rhodes. 2000. LC 00-55815. pap. 25.95 (*0-415-23317-8*) Routledge.

Too Ill to Talk? User Involvement & Palliative Care. Contrib. by Neil Small & Penny J. Rhodes. 2000. LC 00-55815. lib. bdg. 85.00 (*0-415-23316-X*) Routledge.

Too Much of a Good Thing? Why Health Care Spending Won't Make U. S. Sick. Charles R. Morris. 2000. 80p. pap. 9.95 (*0-87078-441-2*) Century Foundation.

Too Old to Cry, Too Hurt to Laugh: Abused Teens in Today's America. Robert J. Ackerman & Lee M. Joiner. 1989. 140p. pap. 9.95 (*0-8306-3407-X*) McGraw-Hill Educ Grp.

Too Poor to Be Sick: Access to Medical Care for the Uninsured. Patricia A. Butler. 1988. 128p. 17.50 (*0-87553-151-2*) Am Pub Health.

Too Scared to Cry: Psychic Trauma in Childhood. Lenore Terr. 1992. LC 89-46121. 372p. reprint ed. pap. 17.00 (*0-465-08644-6*) Basic.

Toohey's Medicine: A Textbook for Students in the Health Care Professions. Ed. by Stephen R. Bloom. 15th ed. 1994. 377p. pap. text (*0-443-04704-9*) Church.

Toohey's Medicine for Nurses. Arnold Bloom & Stephen Bloom. 14th ed. 1986. (Illus.). 335p. text (*0-443-03076-6*) Church.

Toolbook for Health Care Redesign. Ruth I. Hansten & Marilynn J. Washburn. 1997. LC 97-21698. 296p. spiral bd. 68.00 (*0-8342-0907-1*, 20907) Aspen Pub.

***Toolbox for Portfolio Development: A Practical Guide for the Primary Health Care Team.** Roger Pietroni. 2001. 208p. pap. (*1-85775-444-1*) Radcliffe Med Pr GBR. *Dist:* Balogh.

Tools for Evaluating Health Technologies. 1997. lib. bdg. 250.95 (*0-8490-6232-2*); 1996. lib. bdg. 250.99 (*0-8490-6892-4*) Gordon Pr.

Tools for Evaluating Health Technologies: Five Background Papers. 1995. (Illus.). 149p. (Orig.). (C). pap. text 40.00 (*0-7881-1832-3*) DIANE Pub.

Tools for Healing: Working Toward Harmony & Balance. Kathy Mengle. 1985. LC 84-72359. (Illus.). 160p. (Orig.). pap. 10.95 (*0-87516-548-6*) DeVorss.

Tools of Biochemistry. Terrance C. Cooper. 1977. 448p. 125.00 (*0-471-17116-6*) Wiley.

Tools of the Trade. Gordon Stokes & Daniel Whiteside. (Illus.). 101p. (Orig.). pap. 16.50 (*0-918993-25-3*) Thoth NV.

Tooth Development & Caries F. C. Driessens & J. H. Woltgens. 1986. 239.95 (*0-8493-6500-7*, RK331) CRC Pr.

Tooth Development & Caries. F. Driessens & J. H. Woltgens. 1986. LC 85-27002. Vol. 1. 108p. 132.00 (*0-8493-6503-1*); Vol. 2. 208p. 158.00 (*0-8493-6504-X*) Franklin (CRC Reprint).

Tooth Enamel Microstructure. Ed. by W. Von Koenigswald & P. M. Sander. 1997. (Illus.). 288p. (C). text (*90-5410-667-0*) A A Balkema NLD. *Dist:* Ashgate Pub Co.

Tooth Extraction - A Practical Guide. Paul Robinson. 2000. (Illus.). 144p. pap. text 30.00 (*0-7236-1071-1*) Buttrwrth-Heinemann.

Tooth Fairy's Guide, Photo Album & Scorecard. Elaine F. Keenan. 1997. 16p. (J). (ps-8). 29.95 (*0-9663273-0-6*) Heirloom Memories.

Top Docs: Managing the Search for Physician Leaders. George F. Longshore. 2nd ed. 1999. LC 99-62337. 125p. pap. 42.00 (*0-924674-71-7*) Am Coll Phys Execs.

***Top Doctors: New York Metro Area.** 6th ed. 2001. pap. 24.95 (*1-883769-28-0*) Castle Connolly Med.

Top 50 Spinal Pain Syndromes. Lynton Giles. 2004. (Illus.). 160p. pap. 55.00 (*0-7506-4008-1*) Buttrwrth-Heinemann.

Top 100 Drug Interactions: A Guide to Patient Management. Philip D. Hansten & John R. Horn. 1999. (Illus.). 160p. pap. 10.00 (*0-9674718-0-X*) H & H Pub WA.

***Top Tips for GPs: A Beginner's Guide to General Practice.** Knut Schroeder. 2000. 160p. pap. (*1-85775-440-9*) Radcliffe Med Pr GBR. *Dist:* Balogh.

Top Tips in Gastrointestinal Surgery. Ciaran J. Walsh et al. 1999. LC 98-38634. (Illus.). xix, 148p. pap. 44.95 (*0-632-04253-2*) Blackwell Sci.

Top Tips in Primary Care Management. Derek Gallen & Glynis Buckle. 1997. LC 97-3775. (Illus.). 208p. pap. 29.95 (*0-86542-976-6*) Blackwell Sci.

Top Tips in Urology. Ed. by J. McLoughlin et al. 1995. LC 95-11624. (Illus.). 117p. pap. 14.95 (*0-86542-610-4*) Blackwell Sci.

Top Twenty Medical Staff Policies & Procedures. Hugh Greeley & Herman Williams. 1998. LC 99-189151. (Illus.). 144p. pap. text 147.00 (*1-57839-030-3*) Opus Communs.

Top 200 "Meds" for the Surgical Patient. Robert L. McEntyre. 1991. 263p. pap. 19.95 (*0-942219-23-6*) Quality Med Pub.

Topical Application of Antibiotics: Recent Advances in Ophthalmology. Ed. by Yoshihito Honda & Wolfgang Behrens-Baumann. 1997. (Opthalmologica Ser.: Vol. 211, Suppl. 1, 1997). (Illus.). vi, 82p. pap. 38.25 (*3-8055-6479-1*) S Karger.

Topical Child Development. James Cantrell. 1994. 186p. stu. ed. 25.50 (*0-8273-6092-4*) Delmar.

Topical Corticosteroids. Ed. by Howard I. Maibach & C. Surber. 1991. (Illus.). viii, 518p. 275.75 (*3-8055-5332-3*) S Karger.

Topical Diagnosis in Neurology: Anatomy, Physiology, Sight, Symptoms. Peter Daus. 3rd ed. 1997. LC 97-3148. (Illus.). 348p. pap. 35.00 (*0-86577-711-X*) Thieme Med Pubs.

Topical Drug Bioavailability, Bioequivalence & Penetration. V. P. Shah & H. I. Maibach. 1994. (Illus.). 476p. (C). text 144.00 (*0-306-44367-8*, Kluwer Plenum) Kluwer Academic.

Topical Drug Delivery Formulations. David W. Osborne & Anton H. Amann. 1989. (Drugs & the Pharmaceutical Sciences Ser.: Vol. 42). (Illus.). 352p. text 225.00 (*0-8247-8183-X*) Dekker.

Topical Glucocorticoids with Increased Benefit - Risk Ratio. Ed. by H. C. Korting & Howard I. Maibach. 1993. (Current Problems in Dermatology Ser.: Vol. 21). (Illus.). viii, 208p. 182.75 (*3-8055-5712-4*) S Karger.

Topical Minoxidil: Experimental & Clinical Results. Ed. by J. J. Voorhees. 1987. (Journal: Vol. 175, Suppl. 2, 1987). (Illus.). iv, 60p. pap. 20.00 (*3-8055-4723-4*) S Karger.

Topical Reviews in Accident Surgery, Vol. 1. N. Tubbs & P. S. London. 1980. (Topical Reviews Ser.). (Illus.). 240p. pap. text (*0-7236-0534-3*) John Wright.

Topics in Behavioral Medicine: Annual Series of European Research in Behavior Therapy, Vol. 1. Ed. by J. Vinck. 1986. vii, 348p. pap. (*90-265-0762-3*) Swets.

Topics in Carbon-13 NMR Spectroscopy, Vol. 4. Ed. by George C. Levy. 1984. (Topics in Carbon-13 NMR Spectroscopy Ser.: 1-683). 282p. 220.00 (*0-471-09857-4*) Wiley.

Topics in Child Neurology, Vol. 2. Ed. by G. Wise et al. 1983. (Illus.). 280p. text 42.50 (*0-88331-207-7*) R B Luce.

Topics in Clinical Cardiology: Indications for Diagnostic Procedures. Albert E. Raizner. 1996. LC 96-30883. (Topics in Clinical Cardiology Ser.). (*4-260-14318-2*) Igaku-Shoin.

Topics in Clinical Cardiology: Indications for Diagnostic Procedures. Ed. by Albert E. Raizner. 1996. LC 96-30883. (Topics in Clinical Cardiology Ser.). (Illus.). 176p. 69.50 (*0-89640-318-1*) Igaku-Shoin.

Topics in Clinical Pharmacology & Therapeutics. Ed. by R. F. Maronde. 1986. (Illus.). 518p. 138.00 (*0-387-96196-8*) Spr-Verlag.

Topics in Environmental Epidemiology. Ed. by Kyle Steenland & David A. Savitz. 1997. LC 96-29398. (Illus.). 376p. text 49.50 (*0-19-509564-2*) OUP.

Topics in Enzyme & Fermentation Biotechnology. Alan Wiseman. Vol. 5. 1981. LC 80-41326. 359p. 143.00 (*0-470-27089-6*); Vol. 6. 1982. 232p. 99.95 (*0-470-27304-6*); Vol. 9. 1984. 192p. 65.95 (*0-470-20031-6*) P-H.

Topics in Gerontology: Selected Annotated Bibliographies, 22. Ed. by Thomas O. Blank. 1993. LC 93-9311. (Bibliographies & Indexes in Gerontology Ser.: No. 22). 256p. lib. bdg. 72.95 (*0-313-28337-0*, BTY/, Greenwood Pr) Greenwood.

Topics in Imaging Processing Techniques in Cardiac Dynamics: Special Issue Journal Automedica, Vol. 10, No. 1. Ed. by Michiyoshi Kuwahara & Barry W. Hyndman. 1988. 92p. text 291.00 (*0-677-25710-4*) Gordon & Breach.

Topics in Medicinal Chemistry, No. 65. Ed. by P. R. Leeming. 1988. (Special Publications). 362p. (C). (*0-85186-726-X*) Royal Soc Chem GBR. *Dist:* Spr-Verlag.

TUV

Topics in Medicinal Chemistry: 4th SCI-RSC Medicinal Chemistry Symposium Special Publication. Ed. by P. R. Leeming. 1988. (Cambridge Biennial Ser.: No. 65). (Illus.). 360p. pap. text 99.00 (*0-85186-706-5*) Scholium Intl.

***Topics in Neuroanaesthesia & Intensive Care: Experimental & Clinical Studies on Cerebral Circulation, Metabolism & Intracranial Pressure.** G. E. Cold & B. L. Dahl. 2001. xv, 410p. 149.00 (*3-540-41871-7*) Spr-Verlag.

Topics in Neuroscience: From Basic Immunology to Immune-Mediated Demyelination. G. Martino & Luciano Adorini. 1999. LC 99-17459. 329p. (C). (*88-470-0054-8*) Spr-Verlag ITA. *Dist:* Spr-Verlag.

Topics in Ophthalmology. Jack J. Kanski. 1985. (*0-7020-1103-7*) Saunders.

Topics in Pallative Care, Vol. 3. Ed. by Russell K. Portenoy & Eduardo Bruera. 1998. (Illus.). 328p. text 55.00 (*0-19-510246-0*) OUP.

Topics in Palliative Care, Vol. 1. Ed. by Russell K. Portenoy & Eduardo Bruera. 1997. LC 96-22250. (Illus.). 328p. text 55.00 (*0-19-510244-4*) OUP.

Topics in Palliative Care, Vol. 2. Ed. by Eduardo Bruera & Russell K. Portenoy. 1998. (Topics in Palliative Care Ser.). (Illus.). 368p. text 55.00 (*0-19-510245-2*) OUP.

Topics in Palliative Care, Vol. 5. Ed. by Russell Portenoy & Eduardo Bruera. 2000. (Illus.). 344p. text 49.95 (*0-19-513220-3*) OUP.

Topics in Pathology for Hong Kong. P. C. Wu. 1995. 176p. (Orig.). pap. (*962-209-336-1*) HK Univ Pr HKG. *Dist:* Intl Spec Bk, Coronet Bks.

Topics in Pathophysiology of Hypertension. Ed. by Herman Villarreal & Mohinder P. Sambhi. 1983. text 340.00 (*0-89838-595-4*) Kluwer Academic.

Topics in Pediatric Gastroenterology. Ed. by J. A. Dodge. 1976. (Illus.). pap. 40.00 (*0-8464-0931-3*) Beekman Pubs.

Topics in Pediatrics: A Festschrift for Lewis A. Barness. Ed. by H. H. Pomerance & Barry B. Bercu. 1990. (Illus.). 307p. 169.00 (*0-387-96964-0*) Spr-Verlag.

Topics in Preventive Psychiatry. Ed. by G. N. Christodoulou & V. Kontaxakis. 1994. (Bibliotheca Psychiatrica Ser.: No. 165). (Illus.). viii, 152p. 121.75 (*3-8055-5877-5*) S Karger.

Topics in the History of Psychology, Vol. I. Ed. by Gregory A. Kimble & Kurt Schlesinger. 1985. 424p. (C). text 49.95 (*0-89859-311-5*) L Erlbaum Assocs.

Topics in the History of Psychology, Vol. II. Gregory A. Kimble & Kurt Schlesinger. 1985. 448p. (C). 49.95 (*0-89859-312-3*) L Erlbaum Assocs.

Topics in Therapeutics. Royal College of Physicians Staff. Ed. by A. M. Breckenridge. 1974. pap. text 45.00 (*0-7855-7134-5*) St Mut.

Topics in Therapeutics. Ed. by D. W. Vere. 1978. 224p. pap. 35.00 (*0-8464-1144-X*) Beekman Pubs.

Topics in Therapeutics, 1976. Royal College of Physicians Staff. Ed. by R. G. Shanks. 1976. pap. text 65.00 (*0-7855-7135-3*) St Mut.

Topics in Urology: New Diagnostic Tests. Ed. by Martin I. Resnick & J. Patrick Spirnak. 1995. LC 95-32007. (Topics in Clinical Urology Ser.). (Illus.). 216p. 69.50 (*0-89640-290-8*) Igaku-Shoin.

Topics in Vaccine Adjuvant Research. Dale R. Spriggs & Koff. 1990. 168p. 139.00 (*0-8493-5719-5*, RC919) CRC Pr.

Topics of Psychosomatic Research: Proceedings of the European Conference on Psychomatic Research, 9th, Vienna, April 1972. European Conference on Psychosomatic Research Staff. Ed. by H. Freyberger. 1973. (Journal: Vol. 22, Nos. 2-6). 305p. reprint ed. 78.50 (*3-8055-1616-9*) S Karger.

Topics on Biomedical Physics: Proceedings of the 6th National Congress of the Italian Association of Medical Physicians. L. Andreucci & A. Schenone. 1992. 700p. text 121.00 (*981-02-1037-X*) World Scientific Pub.

Topley & Wilson's Microbiology & Microbial Infections Ed. by Leslie Collier et al. 9th ed. 1998. (Arnold Publication). (Illus.). text 1250.00 incl. cd-rom (*0-340-70069-6*) OUP.

Topley & Wilson's Microbiology & Microbial Infections Ed. by Leslie Collier et al. 9th ed. 1998. LC 98-137864. (An Arnold Publication). 4500p. (*0-340-61470-6*) E A GBR. *Dist:* OUP.

Topley & Wilson's Microbiology & Microbial Infections: Parasitology, Vol. 5. F. Cox. 9th ed. 1998. (Illus.). 750p. text (*0-340-66320-0*) E A GBR. *Dist:* OUP.

Topley & Wilson's Microbiology & Microbial Infections: Volume 4: Medical Mycology. L. Ajello. 9th ed. 1998. (Illus.). 750p. text (*0-340-66319-7*) E A GBR. *Dist:* OUP.

Topley & Wilson's Microbiology & Microbial Infections Vol. 1: Virology. Leslie Collier. 9th ed. 1998. (Illus.). 750p. text (*0-340-66316-2*) E A GBR. *Dist:* OUP.

Topley & Wilson's Microbiology & Microbial Infections Vol. 2: Systematic Bacteriology. Albert Balows. 9th ed. 1998. (Illus.). 750p. text (*0-340-66317-0*) E A GBR. *Dist:* OUP.

Topley & Wilson's Microbiology & Microbial Infections: Volume 3: Bacterial Infections Vol. 3: Bacterial Infections. Ed. by Leslie Collier et al. 9th ed. 1998. 750p. (*0-340-66318-9*) E A GBR. *Dist:* OUP.

Topley & Wilson's Principles of Bacteriology, Virology & Immunity. 8th ed. 124p. text (*0-7131-4593-5*) E A GBR. *Dist:* Routldge.

Topley & Wilson's Principles of Bacteriology, Virology & Immunity. Leslie H. Collier. 8th ed. 736p. text (*0-7131-4592-7*) E A GBR. *Dist:* Routldge.

Topley & Wilson's Principles of Bacteriology, Virology & Immunity. Alan H. Linton. 8th ed. 484p. text (*0-7131-4589-7*) E A GBR. *Dist:* Routldge.

Topley & Wilson's Principles of Bacteriology, Virology & Immunity. Tom Parker. 8th ed. 724p. text (*0-7131-4590-0*) E A GBR. *Dist:* Routldge.

Topley & Wilson's Principles of Bacteriology, Virology & Immunity. Geoffrey R. Smith. 8th ed. text (*0-7131-4591-9*) E A GBR. *Dist:* Routldge.

Topley & Wilson's Principles of Bacteriology, Virology & Immunity, Set. M. T. Parker. 8th ed. 2742p. text (*0-7131-4594-3*) E A GBR. *Dist:* Routldge.

Topographic Positions of the Measurement Points in Electro-Acupuncture Vol. 3: Textual & Illustrated, Vol. III. Reinhold Voll. Tr. by Hartwig Schuldt from GER. 1978. (Electro-Acupuncture According to Voll Ser.). (Illus.). 152p. text (*3-88136-060-3*) ML-Verlag DEU. *Dist:* Medicina Bio.

Topographical & Motion Palpation of the Appendicular Skeleton. Kent L. Boyer. 1995. LC 95-9283. (Illus.). 184p. pap. text 29.95 (*0-7734-9919-9*) E Mellen.

Topographical & Motion Palpation of the Axial Skeleton. Kent L. Boyer. 1991. LC 91-19648. (Illus.). 128p. pap. 39.95 (*0-7734-9904-0*) E Mellen.

Topography & Systems in Psychoanalytic Theory. Merton M. Gill. 1963. LC 59-9821. (Psychological Issues Monographs: No. 10, Vol. 3, No. 2). 179p. (Orig.). 27.50 (*0-8236-6560-7*); pap. 22.50 (*0-8236-6580-1*) Intl Univs Pr.

Topology for Physicists. Albert S. Schwarz. Tr. by Silvio Levy. 1996. LC 96-15840. (Grundlehren der Mathematischen Wissenschaften Ser.: Vol. 308). (*3-540-54754-1*) Spr-Verlag.

Torah, Light & Healing: Mystical Insights into Healing Based on the Hebrew Language. Matityahu Glazerson. 1996. LC 95-50733. 232p. pap. 30.00 (*1-56821-934-2*) Aronson.

Torasemide - Clinical Pharmacology & Therapeutic Applications: Proceedings of the International Symposium on Torasemide, Munich, October 21-23, 1988. Ed. by F. Kruck et al. 1991. (Progress in Pharmacology & Clinical Pharmacology Ser.: Vol. 8, No. 1). 273p. (Orig.). pap. text (*0-89574-321-3*) Gustav Fischer DEU. *Dist:* Lubrecht & Cramer, Balogh.

Torch Syndrome: Infections of the Human Fetus. Gilles R. Monif. 1993. (Illus.). 172p. text 14.95 (*1-880906-02-3*) IDI Pub.

Torn Between Two Systems: Improving Chronic Care in Medicare & Medicaid. Ed. by Charles E. Grassley. 1998. (Illus.). 175p. (C). pap. text 30.00 (*0-7881-7252-2*) DIANE Pub.

Torres & Ehrlich Modern Dental Assisting. Doni Bird & Debbie S. Robinson. Ed. by Shirley Kuhn. 6th ed. 1999. LC 98-40582. (Illus.). 765p. (C). text 47.00 (*0-7216-7627-8*) Saunders.

Torrey's Morphogenesis of the Vertebrates. Alan Feduccia & Edward McCrady. 5th ed. 1991. LC 90-24801. 528p. text 84.95 (*0-471-62314-8*) Wiley.

Torticollis: Differential Diagnosis, Assessment & Treatment, Surgical Management & Bracing. Ed. by Karen Karmel-Ross. 1997. LC 97-10982. (Physical & Occupational Therapy in Pediatrics Ser.: Vol. 17, No. 2). 124p. 39.95 (*0-7890-0316-3*) Haworth Pr.

Tortipelvis: The Slipped Disc Syndrome, Its Cause & Correction. Frederick H. Barge. 4th ed. 1994. LC 94-72716. 164p. text 38.95 (*1-885048-00-9*) Barge Chiropract.

Torture: Human Rights, Medical Ethics & the Case of Israel. Ed. by Neve Gordon & Ruchama Marton. 1995. LC 95-13688. (C). (*1-85649-313-X*) Zed Books GBR. *Dist:* St Martin.

Tortured Mind: The Many Faces of Manic Depression. Ann Holmes & Dan Harmon. Ed. by Carol C. Nadelson. 1998. LC 97-44058. (Encyclopedia of Psychological Disorders Ser.). (Illus.). 144p. 24.95 (*0-7910-4900-0*) Chelsea Hse.

Total Abolition of Personal Restraint in the Treatment of the Insane. Robert G. Hill. 1976. LC 75-16725. (Classics in Psychiatry Ser.). reprint ed. 22.95 (*0-405-07433-6*) Ayer.

Total Breast Health. Robin Keuneke. LC 97-74361. 1998. 240p. 23.00 (*1-57566-269-8*); 2000. 512p. pap. 16.00 (*1-57566-459-3*) Kensgtn Pub Corp (Knsington).

Total Burn Care. Herndon. 1995. text 157.00 (*0-7020-1827-9*) Saunders.

Total Communication: Structure & Strategy. Lionel Evans. 1982. LC 81-85672. (Illus.). 176p. 13.95 (*0-913580-75-9*) Gallaudet Univ Pr.

Total Concentration: How to Understand Attention Deficit Disorder, Maximize Your Mental Energy & Reach Your Full Potential. Harold N. Levinson. 2000. LC 90-48943. 200p. pap. 15.95 (*0-87131-708-7*) M Evans.

Total-Condylar Knee Arthroplasty. Ed. by C. S. Ranawat. 1985. (Illus.). 282p. 191.00 (*0-387-96043-0*) Spr-Verlag.

Total Customer Satisfaction: A Comprehensive Approach for Health Care Providers. Stephanie G. Sherman & V. Clayton Sherman. 1998. LC 98-38362. (Health & Psychology Ser.). 376p. pap. 58.00 (*0-7879-4392-4*) Jossey-Bass.

Total Exposure & Assessment Methodology (TEAM) Toxic Substances & Chemicals, an International Symposium, Pt. I. Ed. by Steve Colome et al. 1991. (Journal of Exposure Analysis & Environmental Epidemiology Ser.: Vol. 1, No. 1). (Illus.). pap. text 60.00 (*0-911131-30-2*) Specialist Journals.

Total Exposure & Assessment Methodology (TEAM) Toxic Substances & Chemicals, an International Symposium, Pt. II. Ed. by Michael J. Dellarco et al. 1991. (Journal of Exposure Analysis & Environmental Epidemiology Ser.: Vol. 1, No. 2). (Illus.). pap. text 60.00 (*0-911131-73-6*) Specialist Journals.

Total Fitness in Thirty Minutes. Laurence E. Morehouse. 1990. pap. 5.99 (*0-671-72993-4*) S&S Trade.

Total Guide to a Healthy Heart: Integrative Strategies for Preventing & Reversing Heart Disease. Seth J. Baum. 1999. LC 98-75687. 304p. 25.00 (*1-57566-448-8*, Knsington) Kensgtn Pub Corp.

Total Health & Food Power: Famous Recipes & a Plan for Health. Rose B. Ludlow. 1986. LC 85-29594. (Illus.). 240p. pap. 7.95 (*0-88007-158-3*) Woodbridge Pr.

Total Health at the Computer: A How-to Guide to Saving Your Eyes & Body at the VDT Screen in 3 Minutes a Day. Martin A. Sussman et al. 1993. LC 93-1721. 176p. pap. 13.95 (*0-88268-162-1*) Station Hill Pr.

Total Health for Men: How to Prevent & Treat the Health Problems That Trouble Men Most. Ed. by Neil Wertheimer. 1995. LC 95-15909. 600p. 31.95 (*0-87596-312-9*) Rodale Pr Inc.

Total Health for Women: From Allergies & Back Pain to Overweight & PMS, the Best Preventive & Curative Advice for Over 110 Women's Health Problems. Ellen Michaud et al. 1995. LC 95-9810. 31.95 (*0-87596-311-0*) Rodale Pr Inc.

Total Health for Women: From Allergies & Back Pain to Overweight & PMS, the Best Preventive & Curative Advice for over 110 Women's Health Problems. Ellen Michaud et al. 1997. LC 97-8823. 608p. pap. 15.95 (*0-87596-463-X*) Rodale Pr Inc.

Total Hip Arthroplasty. Robert E. Booth et al. 1988. (Illus.). 336p. text 135.00 (*0-03-013328-9*) Saunders.

Total Hip Arthroplasty Outcomes. Gerald A. Finerman et al. 1997. LC 97-36174. (Illus.). 250p. pap. text (*0-443-07657-X*) Church.

Total Hip Prostheses. Ed. by M. E. Muller & R. Ganz. 1976. 79p. 280.00 (*0-387-92103-6*) Spr-Verlag.

Total Hip Replacement. E. Eggers. 1994. (Orthopedic Ser.). 32p. pap. text 3.95 (*1-885274-02-5*) Health InfoNet Inc.

Total Hip Replacement (THR) Surgery & You Vol. 1: Absolute Must Reading for Those Involved in THR Surgery. Paul B. Malone, III. 1998. (Illus.). 176p. pap. 14.95 (*0-9616548-3-X*) Synergy Pr.

Total Institutions. Ed. by Samuel E. Wallace. 1971. 198p. reprint ed. text 32.95 (*0-87855-057-7*); pap. text 18.95 (*0-87855-550-1*) Transaction Pubs.

Total Intravenous Anaesthesia. Nicholas L. Padfield. 2000. LC 00-57145. (Illus.). 304p. text 75.00 (*0-7506-4171-1*) Buttrwrth-Heinemann.

Total Intravenous Anaesthesia. Ed. by Jan Smith & Paul F. White. 1998. (Illus.). 168p. pap. (*0-7279-1191-0*) BMJ Pub GBR. *Dist:* AIDC.

Total Joint Replacement. Petty. 1991. (Illus.). 896p. text 187.00 (*0-7216-3367-6*) Saunders.

Total Knee Arthroplasty. Ed. by James A. Rand. 1992. LC 92-12132. 480p. text 159.00 (*0-88167-930-5*) Lppncott W & W.

Total Knee Replacement. 1988. (Illus.). 256p. 107.00 (*0-387-70031-5*) Spr-Verlag.

Total Knee Replacement. Ed. by R. S. Laskin. 1991. (Illus.). 268p. 192.00 (*0-387-19644-7*) Spr-Verlag.

Total Knee Replacement: A Guide for Patients. David S. Hungerford. Ed. by David Seligson. 1995. (Orthopedic Ser.). (Illus.). 32p. (Orig.). pap. 3.95 (*1-885274-06-8*) Health InfoNet Inc.

Total Parenteral Nutrition. Josef E. Fischer. 1976. LC 75-30283. 45.00 (*0-316-28370-3*, Little Brwn Med Div); 2nd ed. 1991. 95.00 (*0-316-28379-7*) Lppncott W & W.

Total Parenteral Nutrition in the Hospital & at Home. Ed. by K. N. Jeejeebhoy. 1983. 255p. 152.00 (*0-8493-6120-6*, RM224, CRC Reprint) Franklin.

Total Project Management: Strategies & Tactics for the Healthcare Industries. Roger Dabbah. 1993. (Illus.). 340p. 98.00 (*0-935184-45-7*) IHS Health Grp.

Total Purchasing: A Model for Locality Commissioning. Ed. by Rod Smith et al. 1996. (*1-85775-146-9*) Radcliffe Med Pr GBR. *Dist:* Balogh.

Total Quality Management: The Health Care Pioneers. Mara M. Melum & Marie K. Sinioris. 1992. LC 92-11056. 404p. pap. 69.00 (*1-55648-089-X*, 169410) AHPI.

Total Quality Management for Home Care. Elaine R. Davis. 1994. 368p. pap. 91.00 (*0-8342-0332-4*, 20332) Aspen Pub.

Total Quality Management for Hospital Nutrition Services. M. Rosita Schiller et al. 1994. LC 93-39360. 400p. pap. 77.00 (*0-8342-0551-3*) Aspen Pub.

Total Quality Management in Geriatric Care. Douglas K. Miller et al. 1995. LC 94-48380. 176p. 31.95 (*0-8261-8840-0*) Springer Pub.

Total Quality Management in Healthcare: From Theory to Execution. Dean H. Stamatis. 1996. LC 96-1634. 336p. text 45.00 (*0-7863-0980-6*, Irwn McGrw-H) McGrw-H Hghr Educ.

Total Relaxation: Healing Practice for Body, Mind & Spirit. John Harvey. 1998. LC 97-32360. (Illus.). 192p. pap. 20.00 (*1-56836-224-2*) Kodansha.

Total Service Medical Practice: 17 Steps to Satisfying Your Internal & External Customers. Vicky Bradford. 1996. (C). text 45.00 (*0-7863-1244-0*, Irwn McGrw-H) McGrw-H Hghr Educ.

Total Synthesis II. 2nd ed. 1998. (Illus.). 291p. pap. 35.00 (*0-9658291-2-X*) Panda Ink.

Total Wellness Program for Women over 30: Comprehensive Manual with Medical Guidelines for Health Care Professionals. Barbara Kass-Annese. Ed. by Jerry Byrd. 1997. LC 97-70430. 350p. spiral bd. 35.95 (*0-9655715-0-5*) Health Choice.

Totally Awesome Health Teacher Resource Binder: Grade 6. Linda Brower Meeks & Philip Heit. Ed. by Julie DeVillers. 1997. (Illus.). 650p. tchr. ed., ring bd. 205.00 (*1-886693-19-6*) Everyday Learn.

Totem & Taboo: Resemblances Between the Psychic Lives of Savages & Neurotics. Sigmund Freud. 1976. 27.95 (*0-8488-1331-6*) Amereon Ltd.

Totem & Taboo: Resemblances Between the Psychic Lives of Savages & Neurotics. Sigmund Freud. unabr. ed. 1998. LC 98-27922. (Thrift Editions Ser.). 176p. pap. 2.00 (*0-486-40434-X*) Dover.

Totem et Tabou: Interpretation par la Psychanalyse de la Vie Sociale. Sigmund Freud. 1989. (FRE.). pap. 19.95 (*0-7859-3038-8*) Fr & Eur.

Tot's 'n Tension. Rita T. Liberman & Hal Liberman. 1985. 100p. (Orig.). pap. 5.95 (*0-9614923-0-9*) Tranquil Pr.

Touch: The Foundation of Experience. Ed. by Kathryn E. Barnard & T. Berry Brazelton. 1990. (Clinical Infant Reports: No. 4). 610p. 75.00 (*0-8236-6605-0*, BN 06605) Intl Univs Pr.

Touch & Emotion in Manual Therapy. Bevis Nathan. 1999. LC 99-37127. 222p. 25.95 (*0-443-05657-9*) Saunders.

Touch for Health: A New Approach to Restoring Our Natural Energies. John F. Thie. 1996. LC 73-86019. (Illus.). 132p. reprint ed. pap. 27.95 (*0-87516-180-4*) DeVorss.

Touch in Early Development. Ed. by Tiffany M. Field. 1995. 136p. text 34.50 (*0-8058-1890-1*) L Erlbaum Assocs.

Touch in Psychotherapy: Theory, Research & Practice. Ed. by Edward W. Smith et al. 1997. LC 97-41416. 248p. text 36.00 (*1-57230-269-0*, C0269) Guilford Pubns.

Touch of Diabetes: A Straightforward Guide for People Who Have Type 2 Diabetes. Lois Jovanovic-Peterson et al. rev. ed. 1998. 192p. pap. 13.95 (*1-56561-169-1*) Wiley.

Touch of Diabetes: A Straightforward Guide for People Who Have Type II Diabetes. Lois Jovanovic-Peterson et al. 1998. 176p. pap. 13.95 (*0-471-34754-X*) Wiley.

Touch of Healing: Energizing the Body, Mind & Spirit with the Art of Jin Shin Jyutsu. Alice Burmeister & Tom Monte. 1997. LC 96-36960. (Illus.). 208p. pap. 15.95 (*0-553-37784-1*) Bantam.

Touch of Hope: A Hands-on Healer Shares the Miraculous Power of Touch. Dean Kraft & Rochelle Kraft. 1999. LC 99-462618. 306p. reprint ed. pap. 12.95 (*0-425-16868-9*) Berkley Pub.

Touch of Magic at Brentwood: The History of an Osteopathic Hospital. Tabac and Associates, Inc. Staff. 2000. (Illus.). 62p. pap. (*0-9678781-0-1*) Brentwood Fndt.

Touch, Temperature, & Pain in Health & Disease: Mechanisms & Assessments. Ed. by Jorgen Boivie et al. 1994. LC 94-36236. (Progress in Pain Research & Management Ser.: 3). (Illus.). 548p. 27.00 (*0-931092-08-6*, PPRM3) Intl Assn Study Pain.

Touch Therapy. Helen Colton. 1988. Orig. Title: The Gift of Touch. 320p. mass mkt. 4.95 (*0-8217-2361-8*, Zebra Kensgtn) Kensgtn Pub Corp.

Touch Therapy. Helen Colton. 1989. Orig. Title: The Gift of Touch. pap. 4.95 (*0-8217-2774-5*) NAL.

Touch Therapy. Tiffany M. Field. 2000. LC 99-35908. (*0-443-05791-5*) Church.

Touched with Fire: Manic-Depressive Illness & the Artistic Temperament. Kay Redfield Jamison. 1996. LC 96-21444. (Illus.). 384p. pap. 15.00 (*0-684-83183-X*) Free Pr.

Touching: The Human Significance of the Skin. Ashley Montagu. 1971. LC 75-151290. (Illus.). text 52.50 (*0-231-03488-1*) Col U Pr.

Touching: The Human Significance of the Skin. Ashley Montagu. 3rd ed. 1986. LC 85-45216. 512p. pap. 16.00 (*0-06-096028-0*, Perennial) HarperTrade.

Touching Horses. Marion Kaselle & Pamela Hannay. 1994. 232p. (*0-85131-579-8*) J A Allen GBR. *Dist:* Trafalgar.

Touching the Future: The Foundation for Physical Therapy. Victoria Stuart. Ed. by Holtzman, Robert, and Assoc., Inc. Staff. 1997. (Illus.). 70p. (Orig.). pap. (*0-9628807-2-8*) FPT VA.

Touching the Mountain: The Self Breema Handbook: Ancient Exercises for the Modern World. Jon Schreiber. 1989. LC 89-85099. (Illus.). 189p. (Orig.). pap. 24.95 (*0-9623581-2-6*) CA Health Pubns.

Touching Thomas. Thomas Crain. 1996. 130p. (Orig.). pap. 8.99 (*0-9627099-6-4*) Zephyr Pub Corp.

Tough Choices: In Vitro Fertilization & the Reproductive Technologies. Ed. by Patricia Stephenson & Marsden G. Wagner. 1993. LC 92-48989. (Health, Society, & Policy Ser.). 192p. (C). 69.95 (*1-56639-060-5*) Temple U Pr.

Tough Choices: Living & Dying in the 21st Century. Maureen A. McTeer. 1999. xii, 212p. pap. (*1-55221-040-5*) Irwin Law CAN. *Dist:* Gaunt.

Tough Love: How Parents Can Deal with Drug Abuse. Pauline Neff. 1984. 160p. reprint ed. pap. 10.95 (*0-687-42407-0*) Abingdon.

Tough Questions, Great Answers: Responding to Patient Concerns about Today's Dentistry. Robin Wright. 1997. LC 97-19573. (Illus.). 152p. pap. text 26.00 (*0-86715-320-2*) Quint Pub Co.

Toughing Out Tourette's & ADHD-ADD. Intro. by Joan E. Murphy. 1989. 240p. (Orig.). pap. text 12.00 (*0-9625194-0-5*) Baton Rouge Tourette Grp.

Tourette Syndrome & Human Behavior. David E. Comings. 1990. LC 89-83294. 828p. pap. 39.95 (*1-878267-28-0*) Hope Pr CA.

Tourette's & Attention Deficit Hyperactivity Disorder: Toughing It Out at Home & at School. Ed. & Intro. by Joan E. Murphy. 1995. 218p. (Orig.). pap. 18.00 (*0-9625194-1-3*) Baton Rouge Tourette Grp.

***Tourette's Syndrome: Finding Answers & Getting Help.** Mitzi Waltz. Ed. by Nancy Keene. 2001. LC 2001-18507. (Patient-Centered Guides Ser.). xv, 400p. 24.95 (*0-596-50007-6*) OReilly & Assocs.

Tourette's Syndrome: Index of Modern Authors & Subjects with Guide for Rapid Research. Jesse S. Winograd. rev. ed. 1992. LC 92-27855. 180p. 47.50 (*1-55914-752-0*); pap. 44.50 (*1-55914-753-9*) ABBE Pubs Assn.

Tourette's Syndrome: The Facts. Mary M. Robertson & Simon Baron-Cohen. 2nd ed. 1998. (Facts Ser.). (Illus.). 122p. pap. 19.95 (*0-19-852398-X*) OUP.

***Tourette's Syndrome — Tics, Obsessions, Compulsions: Developmental Psychopathology & Clinical Care.** James F. Leckman. 2001. 600p. pap. 55.00 (*0-471-11375-1*) Wiley.

Tourette's Syndrome - Tics, Obsessions, Compulsions: Developmental Psychopathology & Clinical Care. Ed. by James F. Leckman & Donald J. Cohen. 2nd ed. 1998. LC 98-9988. 600p. 165.00 (*0-471-16037-7*) Wiley.

Tourism & Health: Risks, Research & Responses. Stephen Clift & Peter Grabowski. 1997. LC 96-39581. (Cutting Edge of Tourism Ser.). (Illus.). 256p. text (*1-85567-474-2*) P P Pubs GBR. *Dist:* Continuum.

Toward a Caring Curriculum: A New Pedagogy for Nursing. Em Oliva Bevis & Jean Watson. 1989. 416p. pap. 34.95 (*0-88737-440-9*) Natl League Nurse.

Toward a General Theory of the Paranormal. Lawrence LeShan. 3rd ed. 1969. LC 73-80027. (Parapsychological Monographs: No. 9). pap. 7.00 (*0-912328-13-4*) Parapsych Foun.

Toward a Genetics of Language. Ed. by Mabel L. Rice. 1996. 432p. text 89.95 (*0-8058-1677-1*); pap. 49.95 (*0-8058-1678-X*) L Erlbaum Assocs.

Toward a Holistic Developmental Psychology. Ed. by Seymour Wapner & Bernard Clark. 1983. 272p. (C). text 59.95 (*0-89859-262-3*) L Erlbaum Assocs.

Toward A Molecular Basis of Alcohol Use & Abuse. Ed. by B. Jansson. 1994. LC 94-10167. (EXS Ser.: Vol. 7). x, 407p. 103.00 (*0-8176-2940-8*); 118.00 (*3-7643-2940-8*) Birkhauser.

Toward a National Health Care Survey: A Data System for the 21st Century. National Research Council Staff & Institute of Medicine Staff. Ed. by Gooloo S. Wonderlich. 1992. 204p. (C). pap. text 27.00 (*0-309-04692-0*) Natl Acad Pr.

Toward a National Policy on Drug & AIDS Testing. Ed. by Mathea Falco & Warren I. Cikins. 1989. (Brookings Dialogues on Public Policy Ser.). 80p. pap. text 10.95 (*0-8157-2733-X*) Brookings.

Toward a New Brain: Evolution & the Human Mind. Stuart Litvak & A. Wayne Senzee. 1985. 250p. 17.95 (*0-13-926056-0*) P-H.

Toward a New Philosophical Basis for Parapsychological Phenomena. Hornell Hart. 1965. LC 65-15951. (Parapsychological Monographs: No. 6). pap. 5.00 (*0-912328-09-6*) Parapsych Foun.

Toward a New Psychology of Gender: A Reader. Ed. by Mary M. Gergen & Sara N. Davis. 640p. (C). 1997. 90.00 (*0-415-91307-1*); 1996. LC 95-52893. pap. 29.95 (*0-415-91308-X*) Routledge.

Toward a New Psychology of Women. Jean B. Miller. 2nd ed. 1987. LC 86-47553. 192p. reprint ed. pap. 14.00 (*0-8070-2909-2*) Beacon Pr.

Toward a Philosophy of the Science of Chiropractic. Joseph C. Keating. 1993. (Illus.). 451p. text 59.95 (*0-9614296-9-0*) Wrld-Wide Bks.

***Toward a Psychology of Awakening: Buddhism, Psychotherapy & the Path of Personal & Spiritual Transformation.** John Welwood. 2002. 352p. pap. 16.95 (*1-57062-823-8*) Shambhala Pubns.

Toward a Psychology of Being. Abraham H. Maslow. 2nd ed. 1968. 256p. pap. 38.95 (*0-442-03805-4*); 3rd ed. 1998. LC 98-3766. 320p. 40.00 (*0-471-29309-1*) Wiley (VNR).

Toward a Psychology of Situations: An Interactional Perspective. Ed. by David Magnusson. 1981. 480p. text 89.95 (*0-89859-061-2*) L Erlbaum Assocs.

Toward a Renewed Mind. Richard F. Gottier. 1990. (Illus.). 276p. 19.95 (*0-9625671-0-8*) R F Gottier.

Toward a Sound Philosophy of Nursing. Ed. by June F. Kikuchi & Helen Simmons. 1994. LC 93-34604. (C). pap. 31.95 (*0-8039-5423-9*, 4820) Sage.

Toward a Theory of Psychosomatic Disorders: Proceedings of the European Conference on Psychosomatic Research, 11th, Heidelberg, September 14-17, 1976. European Conference on Psychosomatic Research Staff. Ed. by Walter Brautigam & Michael Von Rad. 1977. (Journal: Vol. 28, Nos. 1-4). 85.25 (*3-8055-2747-0*) S Karger.

Toward a Typology of Juvenile Offenders: Implications for Therapy & Prevention. Sheldon Glueck & Eleanor T. Glueck. 1970. LC 71-115014. 200p. text 56.00 (*0-8089-0648-8*, 791600, Grune & Strat) Harcrt Hlth Sci Grp.

Toward a Typology of Opiate Users. William Bates & Betty Crowther. 1974. 160p. pap. text 13.95 (*0-87073-960-3*) Schenkman Bks Inc.

Toward a Unified Psychology: Incommensurability, Hermeneutics & Morality. Stephen Yanchar & Brent D. Slife. 2000. (Special Issue of the Journal of Mind & Behavior Ser.). 102p. pap. text 19.00 (*0-930195-09-4*) Inst Mind Behavior.

Toward a Virtuous Circle: A Nutrition Review of the Middle East & North Africa. Atsuko Aoyama. 1999. LC 99-35061. (Health, Nutrition, & Population Ser.). 124p. pap. 25.00 (*0-8213-4557-5*, 14557) World Bank.

Toward a Visible Constituency for Health: A Guide to Citizen Action on Health Legislation. United Hospital Fund Staff. 1980. 64p. 5.00 (*0-934459-28-2*) United Hosp Fund.

Toward an Ecology of the Brain. R. Walsh. 1981. (Illus.). 285p. text 29.95 (*0-88331-208-5*) R B Luce.

Toward an Electronic Health Record Europe, 2000: Conference on the Creation of a European Electronic Health Record. 2000. 297p. pap. 60.00 (*1-893378-04-7*) Medical Recs.

Toward an Electronic Health Record Europe '98: Conference on the Creation of a European Health Record. 1998. 400p. pap. 153.00 (*1-893378-00-4*) Medical Recs.

Toward an Electronic Patient Record '95: Eleventh International Symposium on the Creation of Electronic Health Records & Global Conference on Patient Cards, Set. Ed. by C. Peter Waegemann. 1995. (Illus.). 1040p. (Orig.). pap. 89.95 (*0-9640667-5-0*) Medical Recs.

Toward an Electronic Patient Record '99: Proceedings Manual. 1999. pap. 150.00 (*1-893378-01-2*) Medical Recs.

Toward an Electronic Patient Record '96: International Symposium on the Creation of Electronic Health Records & Global Conference on Patient Cards. Ed. by C. Peter Waegemann. 1996. (Illus.). (Orig.). pap. text (*0-9640667-7-7*) Medical Recs.

Toward an Integrated Medicine: Classics from Psychosomatic Medicine 1959 - 1979. American Psychosomatic Society Staff. 1995. 358p. text 16.50 (*0-88048-727-5*, 8727) Am Psychiatric.

Toward an Optimal Health Program. 1994. lib. bdg. 250.95 (*0-8490-5670-5*) Gordon Pr.

Toward Anti-Adhesion Therapy for Microbial Diseases: Proceedings of the Bat-Sheva Seminar Held in Zichron Yaakov, Israel, February 25-March 1, 1996. Ed. by Itzhak Kahane & Itzhak Ofek. 1996. LC 96-31493. (Advances in Experimental Medicine & Biology Ser.: Vol. 408). (Illus.). 297p. 107.00 (*0-306-45397-5*, Kluwer Plenum) Kluwer Academic.

Toward Better Blood Pressure. Linda Pietz et al. 1992. 48p. stu. ed. (*1-884153-06-2*) Prk Nicollet.

Toward Chronopharmacology: Proceedings of Satellite Symposium to the 8th International Congress of Pharmacology, Nagasaki, Japan, 27-28 July, 1981. International Congress of Pharmacology Staff. Ed. by R. Takahashi & Franz Halberg. 1982. (Illus.). 456p. 69.50 (*0-08-027977-5*, Pergamon Pr) Elsevier.

Toward Comprehensive Theory for Alzheimer's Disease. Ed. by Zaven S. Khachaturian & M. Marcel Mesulam. 2000. 220p. 85.00 (*1-57331-297-5*) NY Acad Sci.

Toward Consilience: The Bioneurological Basis of Behavior, Thoughts, Experience & Language. Gerald A. Cory, Jr. 2000. LC 00-42337. xii, 420p. 95.00 (*0-306-46436-5*, Kluwer Plenum) Kluwer Academic.

Toward Equality of Well-Being: Strategies for Improving Minority Health. 1994. lib. bdg. 250.00 (*0-8490-8527-6*) Gordon Pr.

Toward Ethnic Diversification in Psychology Education & Training. Ed. by George Stricker et al. 1990. 251p. pap. 19.95 (*1-55798-088-8*) Am Psychol.

Toward Fitness: Guided Exercise for Those with Health Problems. Robert Cantu. 1980. LC 79-27686. 258p. 32.95 (*0-87705-496-7*, Kluwer Acad Hman Sci) Kluwer Academic.

Toward Healthy Aging. Priscilla Ebersole. 5th ed. 1997. LC 97-29887. (Illus.). 1128p. (C). (gr. 13). text 57.00 (*0-8151-2879-7*, 31040) Mosby Inc.

Toward Healthy Aging: Includes Testbank. Priscilla Ebersole & Patricia Hess. 5th ed. 1998. (Illus.). 1128p. tchr. ed. (*1-55664-424-8*) Mosby Inc.

Toward Painless Writing: A Guide for Health Professionals. Tova Navarra. 1998. LC 98-12762. 128p. pap. text 19.95 (*1-55642-293-8*, 42938) SLACK Inc.

Toward Self & Sanity: On the Genetic Origins of the Human Character. A. M. Benis. 1985. LC 84-26313. 528p. 39.95 (*0-88437-074-7*) Psych Dimensions.

Toward the Conquest of Beriberi. Robert R. Williams. 1961. LC 61-7397. (Illus.). 360p. 39.00 (*0-674-89790-0*) HUP.

Toward the 21st Century: Incorporating Genetics into Primary Health Care. Nancy Touchette. 1997. LC 97-19247. 29.00 (*0-87969-499-8*) Cold Spring Harbor.

Toward the Validation of Dynamic Psychotherapy: A Replication. D. H. Malan. 1976. LC 76-10182. 308p. 59.50 (*0-306-30896-7*, Plenum Trade) Perseus Pubng.

Towards a Comprehensive Therapy of Schizophrenia. Ed. by H. D. Brenner et al. rev. ed. 1997. LC 96-931627. (Illus.). 288p. text 49.00 (*0-88937-175-X*) Hogrefe & Huber Pubs.

Towards a Discipline of Nursing. Ed. by Genevieve Gray & Rosalie Pratt. 1992. (Illus.). 400p. (Orig.). pap. text (*0-443-04438-4*) Church.

Towards a Healthy Baby: Congenital Disorders & the New Genetics in Primary Health Care. Bernadette Modell & Michael Modell. 1992. (Illus.). 432p. 95.00 (*0-19-262234-X*) OUP.

Towards a Healthy District: Organizing & Managing District Health Systems Based on Primary Health Care. E. Tarimo. 1990. (CHI, ENG, FRE & SPA.). v, 105p. pap. text 19.00 (*92-4-154412-0*, 1150353) World Health.

Towards a National Nutrition Policy: Guidelines for Countries of the Eastern Mediterranean Region. Ed. by K. Bagchi. 1990. 65p. pap. text 2.00 (*92-9021-118-0*, 1450017) World Health.

Towards a New Alchemy Vol. 1: The Millennium Science. Nick Begich. Ed. by Thomas Begich. 1996. LC 96-96347. (Illus.). 180p. (Orig.). pap. 14.95 (*0-9648812-2-5*) Earthpulse Pr.

Towards a New Pharmacotherapy of Pain. Ed. by A. I. Basbaum & Jean-Marie Besson. 1991. LC 90-42921. (Dahlem Workshop Reports). 468p. 350.00 (*0-471-92854-2*) Wiley.

Towards a New Science of Health. Ed. by Robert Lafaille & Stephen Fulder. 1993. LC 93-3282. 208p. (C). 90.00 (*0-415-08171-8*) Routledge.

Towards a Science of Healing Vol. II: Advanced Human Ecology & Energy Balancing Sciences. Steven Rochlitz. deluxe ed. 1991. (Illus.). 100p. (C). spiral bd. 59.95 (*0-945262-40-X*) HEBS.

Towards a Sociology of Schizophrenia: Humanistic Reflections. Keith Doubt. 1996. LC 96-167200. 220p. pap. 13.95 (*0-8020-7830-3*); 350p. text 30.00 (*0-8020-0845-3*) U of Toronto Pr.

Towards Advanced Nursing Practice. Schober. 296p. pap. (*0-340-59358-X*) E A GBR. *Dist:* Routldge.

Towards Advanced Practice: Key Concepts for Care. Jane E. Schober & Susan M. Hinchliff. 1995. 320p. pap. 45.00 (*1-56593-592-6*, 1230) Singular Publishing.

Towards an Mphil or Phd in Health & Social Care. Immy Holloway & Jan Walker. 1999. LC 99-35390. pap. 38.95 (*0-632-05057-8*) Blackwell Sci.

Towards an Understanding of Integrative Brain Functions; Analyses at Multiple Levels: Proceedings of the Nobel Symposium 103. Ed. by K. Fuxe et al. 1998. LC 00-273706. 316p. 90.00 (*0-444-50097-9*) Elsevier.

Towards Coordination of Cancer Research in Europe: Results of the 4th EC Biomedical & Health Research Program. Ed. by A. J. M. Vermorken & F. A. J. M. Schermer. 1994. LC 94-7542. (Biomedical & Health Research Ser.: Vol. 5). 189p. 93.00 (*90-5199-157-6*) IOS Press.

Towards Earlier Diagnosis: A Guide to Primary Care. Keith Hodgkin. 5th ed. 1985. LC 84-7103. (Illus.). 784p. pap. text (*0-443-03131-2*) Church.

Towards Human Work: Solutions to Problems in Occupational Health & Safety. Ed. by M. Kumashiro & E. D. Megaw. 1991. 438p. (*0-7484-0039-7*) Tay Francis Ltd GBR. *Dist:* Taylor & Francis.

Towards Migraine 2000. F. Clifford Rose. 1996. LC 96-38504. (Developments in Neurology Ser.: 12). (Illus.). 328p. 218.50 (*0-444-82494-4*) Elsevier.

Towards Minimally Invasive Neurosurgery. Ed. by P. K. Pillay et al. 1995. (Journal: Vol. 64, No. 2, 1995). (Illus.). 44p. pap. 21.75 (*3-8055-6269-1*) S Karger.

Towards Natural Medicine Research in the 21st Century: Proceedings of the International Symposium on Natural Medicines, Kyoto, Japan, 28-30 October 1997. Ed. by Hiroyuki Ageta et al. 1998. LC 99-187096. (International Congress Ser.). 596p. 198.00 (*0-444-82898-2*, Excerpta Medica) Elsevier.

Towards Reproductive Certainty: Fertility & Genetics Beyond 1999: The Plenary Proceedings of the 11th World Congress on In Vitro Fertilization & Human Reproductive Genetics. Ed. by R. Jansen & D. Mortimer. 1999. LC 99-26998. (Illus.). 534p. lib. bdg. 141.95 (*1-85070-084-2*) CRC Pr.

Towards Resident-Oriented Environments. Ed. by Stella Dixon. 1989. (C). (*0-86242-098-9*) Age Concern Eng GBR. *Dist:* St Mut.

Towards Security in Medical Telematics: Legal & Technical Aspects. Ed. by B. Barber et al. 1996. (Studies in Health Technology & Informatics: Vol. 27). 262p. 98.00 (*90-5199-246-7*, 246-7) IOS Press.

Towards Teaching Communication Skills: A Model for Use with the Profoundly & Severely Mentally Handicapped. C. Williams. 1985. 62p. 45.00 (*0-906054-23-0*) St Mut.

Towards the Neurobiology of Chronic Pain. G. Carli & M. Zimmermann. 1996. LC 96-40280. (Progress in Brain Research Ser.: 110). 290p. 183.00 (*0-444-82149-X*) Elsevier.

Towards Understanding Relationships. Robert A. Hinde. 1980. LC 79-40921. (European Monographs in Social Psychology: No. 18). text 65.00 (*0-12-349250-5*) Acad Pr.

Toxemia Explained: The True Interpretation of the Cause of Disease (1926) J. H. Tilden. 1996. 137p. reprint ed. pap. 14.95 (*1-56459-869-1*) Kessinger Pub.

Toxic & Carcinogenic Effects of Solid Particles in the Respiratory Tract. Ed. by Ulrich Mohr et al. 1994. LC 94-75676. (Illus.). 652p. 95.00 (*0-944398-14-6*) ILSI.

Toxic Circles: Environmental Hazards from the Workplace into the Community. Ed. by Helen E. Sheehan & Richard P. Weeden. 1993. LC 92-48258. (Illus.). 290p. (C). text 45.00 (*0-8135-1990-X*) Rutgers U Pr.

Toxic Food: What You Need to Know to Feed Your Family Safely. Carl Lowe & Philip Lief Group Inc. Staff. 1990. 128p. mass mkt. 3.95 (*0-380-76001-0*, Avon Bks) Morrow Avon.

Toxic Immune Syndrome Cookbook: Yeast-Free Hypoallergenic Recipes to Support Your Immune System. William R. Kellas. rev. ed. 1995. (Illus.). 192p. pap. 16.95 (*0-9636491-0-8*) Comprehensive Hlth.

Toxic Nephropathies: Proceedings. Congress on Toxic Nephropathies Staff. Ed. by Geoffrey Merton Berlyne et al. 1978. (Contributions to Nephrology Ser.: Vol. 10). (Illus.). 29.75 (*3-8055-2832-9*) S Karger.

Toxic Oil Syndrome: Current Knowledge & Future Perspectives. 1992. (WHO Regional Publications, European Ser.: No. 42). (ENG & SPA.). xvii, 163p. pap. text 31.00 (*92-890-1305-2*, 1310042) World Health.

Toxic Oil Syndrome Mass Food Poisoning in Spain. 1984. pap. text 12.00 (*92-890-1021-5*) World Health.

Toxic Shock Syndrome. Merlin S. Bergdoll & P. Joan Chesney. 1990. (Illus.). 248p. 139.00 (*0-8493-6671-2*, R) CRC Pr.

Toxic Substances & Mental Retardation: Neurobehavioral Toxicology & Teratology. Ed. by S. Schroeder. 1987. LC 87-1776. (Monographs of the American Association on Mental Retardation: No. 8). 188p. (C). pap. 8.00 (*0-940898-15-2*) Am Assn Mental.

Toxic Substances in the Environment. Bettina M. Francis. 1994. LC 92-26896. (Environmental Science & Technology Ser.). 384p. 74.95 (*0-471-50781-4*) Wiley.

Toxic Terror: The Truth Behind the Cancer Scares. Elizabeth M. Whelan. 1993. LC 92-34154. (Consumer Health Ser.). 476p. (C). 34.00 (*0-87975-788-4*) Prometheus Bks.

Toxic Torts: Litigation of Hazardous Substance Cases. Gary Z. Nothstein. 1984. LC 83-27128. (Trial Practice Ser.). 776p. text 95.00 (*0-07-047454-0*) Shepards.

***Toxic Treatment: Surviving the Cancer Wars.** Penny Williams. 2001. 304p. pap. (*1-55263-360-8*) Key Porter CAN. *Dist:* Firefly Bks Limited.

Toxicants f Plant Origin Proteins & Amino Acids, Vol. III. Peter R. Cheeke. 1989. 288p. 229.00 (*0-8493-6992-4*) CRC Pr.

Toxicants of Plant Origin Peter R. Cheeke. 1989. 288p. 239.00 (*0-8493-6991-6*, SF757);Vol. I. 352p. 249.00 (*0-8493-6990-8*, SF757);Vol. IV. 240p. 210.00 (*0-8493-6993-2*, SF757) CRC Pr.

***Toxicity Caused by Benzene, Toluene, Ethlene/Propylene Glycol, Gasoline, Jet Fuel & Stoddard Solvent.** James E. Conel. 2001. 138p. (C). reprint ed. pap. text 30.00 (*0-7567-1831-7*) DIANE Pub.

***Toxicity Caused by Lead Vinyl Chloride, Chromium, Arsenic, Cadmium, Cyanide, Nitrate/Nitrite, Mercury, Carbon Tetrachloride & Methanol; & Reproductive & Developmental Hazards.** Sarae Royce. 2002. 273p. reprint ed. pap. text 45.00 (*0-7567-1832-5*) DIANE Pub.

Toxicity of Anticancer Drugs: A Study in Human Toxicity. Ed. by Garth Powis & M. Hackar. 1991. 256p. text (*0-07-105305-0*) PPI GBR. *Dist:* McGraw.

Toxicity of Hormones in Perinatal Life. Ed. by Takao Mori & Hiroshi Nagasawa. 1988. 208p. 114.00 (*0-8493-6862-6*, RG627, CRC Reprint) Franklin.

Toxicity of Pesticides to Fish, Vol. II. Ed. by A. S. Murty. 1986. 192p. 92.00 (*0-8493-6059-5*, SH174, CRC Reprint) Franklin.

Toxicity Screening Procedures Using Bacterial Systems. Dickson Liu & Dutka. 1984. (Drug & Chemical Toxicology Ser.: Vol. 1). (Illus.). 496p. text 199.00 (*0-8247-7171-0*) Dekker.

Toxicity Testing: Strategies to Determine Needs & Priorities. National Research Council Staff. 1984. 382p. pap. text 34.95 (*0-309-03433-7*) Natl Acad Pr.

Toxicity Testing of Dental Materials. Ed. by Harold R. Stanley. 1985. 176p. 104.00 (*0-8493-5916-3*, RA1270, CRC Reprint) Franklin.

Toxicity Testing Using Microorganisms. Bernard J. Dutka & Gabriel Bitton. 1986. Vol. I. 168p. 103.00 (*0-8493-5256-8*, RA1199); Vol. II. 240p. 123.00 (*0-8493-5257-6*, RA1199) Franklin (CRC Reprint).

T
U
V

Toxicologic Assessment of the Army's Zinc Cadmium Sulfide Dispersion Tests. 1997. 350p. pap. 49.00 (*0-309-05783-3*) Natl Acad Pr.

Toxicologic, Pharmacodynamic & Kinetic Studies Following Spinal Administration of U Opioid, GabaB & A2 Adrenergic Agonists. Marc Sabbe. 1997. (Acta Biomedica Lovaniensia Ser.: Vol. 142). (Illus.). 141p. pap. (*90-6186-787-8*) Leuven Univ BEL. *Dist:* Coronet Bks.

Toxicological Appraisal of Halogenated Aromatic Compounds Following Groundwater Pollution: Report on a WHO Working Group. 1980. (EURO Nonserial Publication Ser.). 58p. 8.00 (*92-9020-196-7*, 1340001) World Health.

Toxicological Evaluation of Certain Food Additives & Contaminants. Contrib. by FAO-WHO Expert Committee on Food Additives. 1993. (WHO Food Additives Ser.: No. 32). vii, 301p. pap. text 45.00 (*92-4-166032-5*, 1270032) World Health.

Toxicological Evaluation of Certain Food Additives & Contaminants, 22. FAO-WHO Expert Committee on Food Additives. 1988. (Illus.). 192p. pap. text 21.95 (*0-521-36928-2*) Cambridge U Pr.

Toxicological Evaluation of Certain Food Additives & Naturally Occurring Toxicants. Contrib. by FAO-WHO Expert Committee on Food Additives. 1993. (WHO Food Additives Ser.: No. 30). vii, 399p. pap. text 45.00 (*92-4-166030-9*, 1270030) World Health.

Toxicological Evaluation of Certain Veterinary Drug Residues in Food. Contrib. by FAO-WHO Expert Committee on Food Additives. (WHO Food Additives Ser.: No. 33). 1994. vi, 152p. pap. text 40.00 (*92-4-166033-3*, 1270033); 1993. vii, 216p. pap. text 40.00 (*92-4-166031-7*, 1270031); 1992. vii, 237p. pap. text 40.00 (*92-4-166029-5*, 1270029); 1991. vii, 227p. pap. text 25.00 (*92-4-166027-9*, 1270027) World Health.

Toxicological Evaluation of Certain Veterinary Drug Residues in Food. Contrib. by Forty-Third Meeting of Joint FAO-WHO Expert Commit. 1995. (WHO Food Additives Ser.: No. 34). vi, 173p. pap. text 45.00 (*92-4-166034-1*, 1270034) World Health.

Toxicological Evaluation of Certain Veterinary Drug Residues in Food: 34th Meeting of the Joint FAO/WHO Expert Committee on Food Additives. WHO Staff. 1990. (WHO Food Additives Ser.: No. 25). 175p. 22.00 (*92-4-166025-2*) World Health.

Toxicological Evaluation of Certain Veterinary Drug Residues in Food: 45th Meeting of the Joint FAO-WHO Expert Committee on Food Additives (JECFA) 1996. (Food Additives Ser.: Vol. 36). 157p. pap. 45.00 (*92-4-166036-8*, 1270036) World Health.

Toxicological Evaluation of Certain Veterinary Drug Residues in Food: 47th Meeting of the Joint FAO/WHO Expert Committee on Food Additives (JECFA) 1996. (WHO Food Additives Ser.: Vol. 38). 194p. pap. 45.00 (*92-4-166038-4*, 1270038) Am Soc Clinical.

Toxicological Evaluation of Certain Veterinary Drug Residues in Food: Meeting of the Joint FAO/WHO Expert Committee on Food Additives (JECFA) WHO Staff. 1997. (WHO Food Additives Ser.: No. 39). 45.00 (*92-4-166039-2*) World Health.

Toxicological Evaluation of Some Enzymes, Modified Starches & Certain Other Substances. FAO-WHO Expert Committee on Food Additives. 1972. (WHO Food Additives Ser.: Vol. 1). 109p. pap. text 5.40 (*92-4-166001-5*, 1270001) World Health.

Toxicological Evaluation of Some Food Colours, Enzymes, Flavour Enhancers, Thickening Agents & Certain Other Food Additives. 1975. (Food Additives Ser.: No. 6). pap. text 13.00 (*92-4-166006-6*, 1270006) World Health.

Toxicological Evaluation of Some Food Colours, Thickening Agents & Certain Other Substances. 1975. (Food Additives Ser.: No. 8). pap. text 12.00 (*92-4-166008-2*, 1270008) World Health.

Toxicological Evaluations Vol. 2: Potential Health Hazards of Existing Chemicals. Ed. by B. G. Chemie. 1991. LC 90-10020. (Illus.). 224p. 69.95 (*0-387-53435-0*) Spr-Verlag.

Toxicological Evaluations Vol. 3: Potential Health Hazards of Existing Chemicals. Ed. by B. G. Chemie. 1991. LC 90-10020. (Illus.). 192p. 59.95 (*0-387-54331-7*) Spr-Verlag.

Toxicological Evaluations Vol. 4: Potential Health Hazards of Existing Chemicals. BG Chemie Staff. 1992. (Illus.). 309p. 67.95 (*0-387-54984-6*) Spr-Verlag.

Toxicological Evaluations Vol. 6: Potential Health Hazards of Existing Chemicals. 1993. 237p. 67.95 (*0-387-56980-4*) Spr-Verlag.

Toxicological Evaluations Vol. 8: Potential Health Hazards of Existing Chemicals. Ed. by B. G. Chemie & Heidelberg. 1994. 277p. 67.95 (*0-387-58287-8*) Spr-Verlag.

Toxicological Evaluations Vol. 11: Potential Health Hazards of Existing Chemicals, Vol. 11. Ed. by Berufsgenossenschaft der Chemischen Industrie Staff. 1997. (Illus.). 241p. 56.95 (*3-540-61391-9*) Spr-Verlag.

Toxicological Evaluations Vol. 14: Potential Health Hazards of Existing Chemicals. Berufsgenossenschaft der Chemischen Industry Staff. 1998. LC 90-10020. 371p. 64.95 (*3-540-63084-8*) Spr-Verlag.

***Toxicological Profile for Asbestos.** Prod. by Jeffrey P. Koplan. rev. ed. 2001. (Illus.). 208p. reprint ed. pap. text 50.00 (*0-7567-0748-X*) DIANE Pub.

***Toxicological Profile for Benzidine.** Gangadhar Choudhary & Susan Gold Haber. rev. ed. 2001. 181p. (C). reprint ed. pap. text 50.00 (*0-7567-0776-5*) DIANE Pub.

***Toxicological Profile for Carbon Tetrachloride.** Frwd. by Jeffrey P. Koplan. rev. ed. 2001. (Illus.). 240p. (C). reprint ed. pap. text 50.00 (*0-7567-0747-1*) DIANE Pub.

***Toxicological Profile for Chlorophenols.** H. Edward Murray & Diane Wong. rev. ed. 2001. (Illus.). 239p. (C). reprint ed. pap. text 50.00 (*0-7567-0775-7*) DIANE Pub.

***Toxicological Profile for Fluorides, Hydrogen Fluoride & Fluorine (F)** Frwd. by Jeffrey P. Koplan. 2001. 257p. (C). reprint ed. pap. text 50.00 (*0-7567-0749-8*) DIANE Pub.

***Toxicological Profile for Formaldehyde.** Prod. by Jeffrey P. Koplan. 2001. 450p. (C). reprint ed. pap. text 50.00 (*0-7567-0752-8*) DIANE Pub.

***Toxicological Profile for Lead.** Jeffrey P. Koplan. rev. ed. 2001. 622p. (C). reprint ed. pap. text 75.00 (*0-7567-0750-1*) DIANE Pub.

Toxicological Risk Assessment: Biological & Statistical Criteria, Vol. I. D. Krewski & D. B. Clayson. Ed. by I. C. Munro et al. 1985. 244p. 138.00 (*0-8493-5976-7*, RA1199, CRC Reprint) Franklin.

Toxicological Risk Assessment: Biological & Statistical Criteria, Vol. II. Ed. by I. C. Munro et al. 1985. LC 84-12679. 276p. 156.00 (*0-8493-5977-5*, RA1199, CRC Reprint) Franklin.

Toxicologist As Expert Witness: A Hint Book for Courtroom Procedure. Arthur Furst. 1996. LC 96-21820. 150p. 74.95 (*1-56032-531-3*) Taylor & Francis.

Toxicologist's Pocket Handbook. Michael J. Derelanko. 2000. 256p. per. 39.95 (*0-8493-0009-6*) CRC Pr.

Toxicology. 1994. 160.00 (*1-56238-204-7*, SC13-L) NCCLS.

Toxicology. Ed. by Thomas J. Haley & William O. Berndt. 1988. 697p. pap. 74.95 (*0-89116-810-9*) Hemisp Pub.

Toxicology. Gary D. Osweiler. 1996. LC 94-49123. (National Veterinary Medical Series for Independent Study). 400p. 29.95 (*0-683-06664-1*) Lppncott W & W.

Toxicology: Principles & Applications. Ed. by John De Vries et al. 1996. LC 95-23711. 1312p. (C). 199.95 (*0-8493-9232-2*, 9232) CRC Pr.

Toxicology: Stories. Steve Aylett. 1999. LC 99-33899. 208p. pap. 12.95 (*1-56858-131-9*) FWEW.

Toxicology - from Cells to Man: Proceedings of the 1995 EUROTOX Congress Meeting Held in Prague, Czech Republic, August 27-30, 1995. Ed. by J. P. Seiler et al. 1996. LC 95-47133. (Archives of Toxicology Ser.: Supplement No. 18). (*0-387-60673-4*); (Illus.). 441p. 157.00 (*3-540-60673-4*) Spr-Verlag.

Toxicology & Clinical Pharmacology of Herbal Products. Melanie Johns Cupp. 2000. LC 99-46505. (Forensic Science & Medicine Ser.). 344p. 89.50 (*0-89603-791-6*) Humana.

Toxicology Desk Reference: The Toxic Exposure & Medical Monitoring Index Ed. by Robert P. Ryan & Claude E. Terry. 4th ed. 1997. 2200p. pap. 450.00 (*1-56032-615-8*) Hemisp Pub.

Toxicology Desk Reference: The Toxic Exposure & Medical Monitoring Index. Robert P. Ryan. 5th ed. 1999. 1024p. 550.00 (*1-56032-855-X*); 450.00 (*1-56032-795-2*) Taylor & Francis.

Toxicology for Non-Toxicologists. Mark E. Stelljes. 1999. LC 99-51974. 168p. pap. 85.00 (*0-86587-611-8*, 611) Gov Insts.

Toxicology in the Use, Misuse, & Abuse of Food, Drugs & Chemicals. Ed. by P. L. Chambers et al. 1983. (Archives of Toxicology Ser.: Suppl. 6). (Illus.). 380p. 85.00 (*0-387-12392-X*) Spr-Verlag.

Toxicology Laboratory Design & Management for the 80's & Beyond. Ed. by A. S. Tegeris. 1984. (Concepts in Toxicology Ser.: Vol. 1). (Illus.). xii, 320p. 129.75 (*3-8055-3797-2*) S Karger.

Toxicology of Aflatoxins: Human Health, Veterinary & Agricultural Significance. Ed. by David L. Eaton & John D. Groopman. 1993. LC 93-13269. (Illus.). 544p. text 73.00 (*0-12-228255-8*) Acad Pr.

Toxicology of Botanical Medicines. Francis Brinker. 3rd ed. 2000. LC 99-85790. 296p. (C). pap. 35.00 (*1-888483-09-1*, 1-888483-09-1) Eclectic Med.

Toxicology of Chemical Mixtures: Case Studies, Mechanisms & Novel Approaches. Ed. by Raymond S. Yang. 1994. LC 93-39555. (Illus.). 720p. text 125.00 (*0-12-768350-X*) Acad Pr.

Toxicology of Contact Dermatitis: Allergy, Irritancy & Urticaria. David Basketter. 1999. LC 98-48821. (Current Toxicology Ser.). (Illus.). 188p. 135.00 (*0-471-97201-0*) Wiley.

Toxicology of Contact Hypersensitivity. Ed. by Ian Kimber & Thomas Maurer. 1996. 130p. 89.95 (*0-7484-0349-3*) Taylor & Francis.

Toxicology of Insecticides. Fumio Matusmura. 2nd ed. 1985. LC 85-12371. 618p. 75.00 (*0-306-41979-3*, Plenum Trade) Perseus Pubng.

Toxicology of Metals, Vol. 1. Ed. by Louis W. Chang et al. 1996. LC 95-42586. (Toxicology of Metals Ser.: Vol. 1). 1232p. lib. bdg. 139.00 (*0-87371-803-8*, L803) Lewis Pubs.

Toxicology of Pesticides in Animals. T. S. S. Dikshith. 1990. 264p. lib. bdg. 210.00 (*0-8493-6907-X*, RA1270) CRC Pr.

Toxicology of Recombinant Proteins. Johnson. 1994. (*0-8493-8874-0*) CRC Pr.

Toxicology of the Eye: Effects on the Eyes & Visual System from Chemicals, Drugs, Metals & Minerals, Plants, Toxins & Venoms; Also, Systemic Side Effects from Eye Medications W. Morton Grant & Joel S. Schuman. 4th ed. 1993. LC 93-12521. 1626p. (C). 276.95 (*0-398-05860-1*) C C Thomas.

Toxicology of the Immune System: A Human Approach. Robert Burrell et al. 1992. 322p. 199.00 (*0-471-29069-6*, VNR) Wiley.

Toxicology of the Liver. Gabriel L. Plaa & William R. Hewitt. 2nd ed. 1997. LC 97-22577. 456p. 135.00 (*1-56032-719-7*) Hemisp Pub.

Toxicology of the Liver. Gabriel L. Plaa & William R. Hewitt. 2nd ed. 1993. (Target Organ Toxicology Ser.). text 121.00 (*0-88167-886-4*) Lppncott W & W.

Toxicology of the Lung. Donald E. Gardner. 3rd rev. ed. 1999. LC 99-34751. 500p. 135.00 (*1-56032-801-0*) Taylor & Francis.

Toxicology of the Male & Female Reproductive System. Ed. by Peter K. Working. 1989. (Chemical Industry Institute of Toxicology Ser.). 384p. 130.00 (*0-89116-583-5*) Hemisp Pub.

Toxicology Risk Assessment. Hong Y. Fan. Ed. by Louis W. Chang. 1995. (Illus.). 888p. text 235.00 (*0-8247-9490-7*) Dekker.

Toxics A to Z: A Guide to Everyday Pollution Hazards. John Harte et al. 1991. LC 90-25860. (Illus.). 576p. pap. 27.50 (*0-520-07224-3*); text 75.00 (*0-520-07223-5*) U CA Pr.

Toxics Crisis: What the States Should Do. Jeffrey Tryens. 1983. 100p. 8.95 (*0-89788-072-2*) CPA Washington.

Toxin-Induced Models of Neurological Disorders. M. L. Woodruff & A. J. Nonneman. 1994. (Illus.). 366p. (C). text 85.00 (*0-306-44614-6*, Kluwer Plenum) Kluwer Academic.

Toxins As Tools in Neurochemistry. Ed. by F. Hucho & Y. A. Ovchinnikov. 1983. xiv, 368p. 138.50 (*3-11-009593-9*) De Gruyter.

Toxins of Animal & Plant Origin, Vol. 3. Ed. by A. DeVries & E. Kochva. 1973. LC 71-130967. (Illus.). 1088p. text 849.00 (*0-677-14710-4*) Gordon & Breach.

***Toxoplasmosis.** D. H. M. Joynson & T. G. Wreghitt. 2001. 280p. text 100.00 (*0-521-44328-8*) Cambridge U Pr.

Toxoplasmosis. Ed. by Judith E. Smith. 1994. LC 93-35674. (NATO ASI Ser.: Vol. 78). (Illus.). 258p. 165.00 (*0-387-57305-4*) Spr-Verlag.

Toxoplasmosis: Proceedings of the WHO Expert Committee of Investigators, Geneva, 1968. WHO Staff. 1969. (Technical Reports: No. 431). pap. text 5.00 (*92-4-120431-1*, 1100431) World Health.

Toxoplasmosis of Animals & Man. J. P. Dubey & C. P. Beattie. 1988. 232p. 214.95 (*0-8493-4618-5*, SF809) CRC Pr.

Toy Boy & the Burgundy Car. Andrew Levy. 1999. LC 99-21518. (Video Casebook Ser.: Vol. I). (Illus.). ix, 160p. pap. 38.95 incl. cd-rom (*0-632-05122-1*) Blackwell Sci.

Trace Amines: Comparative & Clinical Neurobiology. Ed. by Alan A. Boulton et al. 1988. LC 88-6847. (Experimental & Clinical Neuroscience Ser.). (Illus.). 496p. 145.00 (*0-89603-144-6*) Humana.

Trace Element Analysis in Biological Specimens. Ed. by R. F. Herber & M. Stoeppler. 1994. LC 94-11681. (Techniques & Instrumentation in Analytical Chemistry Ser.: Vol. 15). 590p. 276.50 (*0-444-89867-0*) Elsevier.

Trace Element Analytical Chemistry in Medicine & Biology, Vol. 2. Ed. by Peter Braetter & Peter Schramel. 1983. 1189p. 253.85 (*3-11-008681-6*) De Gruyter.

Trace Element Analytical Chemistry in Medicine & Biology Vol. 3: Proceedings of the 3rd International Workshop. Ed. by P. Braetter & Peter Schramel. 1984. LC 80-26803. (Illus.). xvi, 763p. 219.25 (*3-11-009821-0*) De Gruyter.

Trace Element Medicine & Chelation Therapy. David M. Taylor & David R. Williams. 1995. (RSC Paperback Ser.). 134p. (C). pap. (*0-85404-503-1*) Royal Soc Chem GBR. *Dist:* Spr-Verlag.

Trace Elements & Free Radicals in Oxidative Diseases. Ed. by Alain Favier et al. 1994. LC 94-10023. (Illus.). 288p. lib. bdg. 75.00 (*0-935315-53-5*, PC073) Am Oil Chemists.

Trace Elements & Man. Henry A. Schroeder. 1973. LC 72-85731. (Illus.). 192p. pap. 7.95 (*0-8159-6907-4*) Devin.

Trace Elements in Clinical Medicine: Proceedings of the Second Meeting of the International Society for Trace Element Research in Humans (ISTERH), August 28-September 1, 1989, Tokyo. Ed. by H. Tomita. 1990. (Illus.). 522p. 99.00 (*0-387-70060-9*) Spr-Verlag.

Trace Elements in Health & Disease. Antero Aito & J. Jarvisalo. 1991. 244p. (C). (*0-85186-976-9*) Royal Soc Chem GBR. *Dist:* Spr-Verlag.

Trace Elements in Health & Disease. Ed. by H. Bostrom & N. Ljungstedt. 1985. (Illus.). 285p. text 86.00 (*91-22-00733-4*) Coronet Bks.

Trace Elements in Human & Animal Nutrition, Vol. 1. Walter Mertz. 5th ed. 1987. 480p. text 104.00 (*0-12-491251-6*) Acad Pr.

Trace Elements in Human Nutrition: Proceedings of the WHO Expert Committee, Geneva, 1973. WHO Staff. 1973. (Technical Reports: No. 532). pap. text 7.00 (*92-4-120532-6*, 1100532) World Health.

Trace Elements in Human Nutrition & Health. 1996. LC 96-211990. (FRE.). 343p. (Orig.). (C). pap. 85.00 (*92-4-156173-4*, 1150431) World Health.

Trace Elements in Human Plasma or Serum. Ed. by Jacques Versieck. 1988. 224p. 135.00 (*0-8493-6810-3*, QP99, CRC Reprint) Franklin.

Trace Elements in Man & Animals 6. Ed. by Lucille S. Hurley et al. 6th ed. 1988. (Illus.). 676p. 135.00 (*0-306-43004-5*, Plenum Trade) Perseus Pubng.

Trace Elements in Man & Animals 10. Ed. by Ann-Marie Roussel et al. 2000. LC 00-27446. (Illus.). xii, 1172p. 199.00 (*0-306-46378-4*, Kluwer Plenum) Kluwer Academic.

Trace Elements in Relation to Cardiovascular Diseases: Status of the Joint WHO-IAEA Research Programme. Ed. by R. Masironi. 1974. (Offset Publications: No. 5). pap. text 7.00 (*92-4-170005-X*, 1120005) World Health.

Trace Elements in Renal Insufficiency. Ed. by E. Quellhorst et al. 1984. (Contributions to Nephrology Ser.: Vol. 38). (Illus.). x, 206p. 29.75 (*3-8055-3676-3*) S Karger.

Trace Elements, Micronutrients & Free Radicals. Ed. by Ivor E. Dreosti. 1991. LC 91-13721. (Contemporary Issues in Biomedicine, Ethics & Society Ser.). (Illus.). 239p. 119.50 (*0-89603-188-8*) Humana.

Trace Minerals in Foods. Kenneth T. Smith. 1988. (Food Science & Technology Ser.: Vol. 28). (Illus.). 675p. text 225.00 (*0-8247-7835-9*) Dekker.

Tracheal Intubation. Cros. 1992. 70.00 (*0-683-08584-0*) Lppncott W & W.

Tracheal Reconstruction in Infancy. Thom E. Lobe. 1991. text 115.00 (*0-7216-5779-6*) Saunders.

Tracheostomy & Ventilator Dependency: Management of Breathing, Speaking & Swallowing. Donna C. Tippett. 2000. LC 99-10470. (Illus.). 320p. 69.00 (*0-86577-774-8*) Thieme Med Pubs.

Tracheostomy Care. Springhouse Publishing Company Staff. 1992. (Procedures Video Ser.). 36.95 incl. VHS (*0-87434-468-9*) Springhouse Corp.

Tracheotomy. Ed. by Eugene N. Myers et al. 1985. (Illus.). 318p. text (*0-443-08381-9*) Church.

Tracheotomy. Johannes J. Fagan et al. 3rd rev. ed. 1997. LC 96-52775. (SIPac - Self-Instructional Package Ser.). (Illus.). 60p. pap. text 25.00 (*1-56772-053-6*) AAO-HNS.

Tracing Neural Connections with Horseradish Peroxidase. M. Marsel Mesulam. 1982. (IBRO Handbook Ser.). 268p. pap. 289.95 (*0-471-10029-3*, Wiley-Interscience) Wiley.

Tracking down Hidden Food Allergy. William G. Crook. 2nd ed. 1980. (Illus.). 104p. (Orig.). pap. 6.95 (*0-933478-05-4*) Prof Bks Future Health.

Tracking Mental Health Outcomes: A Therapist's Guide to Measuring Client Progress, Analyzing Data, & Improving Your Practice. Donald E. Wiger & Kenneth B. Solberg. 2001. LC 00-63350. (Illus.). 304p. pap. 49.95 (*0-471-38875-0*) Wiley.

Tracking State Oversight of Managed Care. Frwd. by John M. Colmers & Daniel M. Fox. 1999. LC 00-501909. (Illus.). x, 33p. pap. (*1-887748-32-6*) Milbank Memorial.

Tracking the Elusive Human Vol. 1: A Practical Guide to C. G. Jung's Psychological Types, W. H. Sheldon's Body & Temperament Types, & Their Integration. Tyra Arraj & James Arraj. 1988. LC 87-30213. (Illus.). 184p. (Orig.). pap. 12.00 (*0-914073-16-8*) Inner Growth Bks.

Tracking the Elusive Human Vol. 2: An Advanced Guide to the Typological Worlds of C. G. Jung, W. H. Sheldon, Their Integration & the Biochemical Typology of the Future. James Arraj. 1990. LC 87-30213. (Illus.). 336p. (Orig.). pap. 14.00 (*0-914073-36-2*) Inner Growth Bks.

Trade, Jobs & Wages. Hian Teck Hoon. 2000. LC 00-29413. (Illus.). 224p. 90.00 (*1-85898-712-1*) E Elgar.

Tradition & Change in Psychoanalysis. Roy Schafer. 1997. LC 96-46630. 272p. 42.50 (*0-8236-6632-8*, BN06632) Intl Univs Pr.

Tradition & Innovation in Psychoanalytic Education: Clark Conference on Psychoanalytic Training for Psychologists. E. R. Shapiro & Murray Meisels. 1989. 312p. 59.95 (*0-8058-0386-6*) L Erlbaum Assocs.

Tradition & Reality. McCoppin. 1994. 34.00 (*0-443-04217-9*) Harcourt.

Traditional Acupuncture: The Law of Five Elements. Dianne M. Connelly. 1994. pap. 16.00 (*0-912381-03-5*) Trad Acupuncture.

Traditional Acupuncture: The Law of Five Elements. Diane M. Connelly. 3rd ed. (Illus.). 157p. pap. 12.00 (*0-912379-01-4*) Ctr Traditional Acupuncture.

Traditional & Modern Medical Systems. Ed. by Ray H. Elling. 1981. (Illus.). 100p. pap. 18.00 (*0-08-028097-8*, Pergamon Pr) Elsevier.

Traditional Birth Attendant in Seven Countries: The Case Studies in Utilization & Training. A. Mangay-Maglacas & H. Pizurki. 1981. (Public Health Papers: No. 75). 211p. pap. text 15.00 (*92-4-130075-2*, 1110075) World Health.

Traditional Birth Attendants: A Joint WHO-UNFPA-UNICEF Statement. 1992. (ENG, FRE & SPA.). 18p. pap. text 9.00 (*92-4-156150-5*, 1150388) World Health.

Traditional Chinese Acupuncture: Meridians & Points. J. R. Worsley. 2nd rev. ed. 2000. (Illus.). 327p. 50.00 (*0-7881-9452-6*) DIANE Pub.

***Traditional Chinese Health Secrets: The Essential Guide to Harmonious Living.** Xu Xiangcai. 2001. 144p. pap. 16.95 (*1-886969-89-2*) YMAA Pubn.

Traditional Chinese Medicine. Richard Craze & Jen T. Fou. 1998. (Teach Yourself Ser.). (Illus.). 190p. pap. 9.95 (*0-8442-0019-0*, 00190, Tch Yourself) McGraw-Hill Trade.

Traditional Chinese Medicine. Sheila McNamara. 1995. LC 95-45945. 320p. pap. 14.00 (*0-465-00629-9*) Basic.

Traditional Chinese Medicine: A Woman's Guide to Trouble-Free Menopause. Nan Lu & Ellen Schaplowsky. 2000. LC 00-42518. (Illus.). xxxii, 352p. pap. 14.00 (*0-380-80904-4*) Morrow Avon.

Traditional Chinese Medicine: Ancient Wisdom for a Modern World. Heidi Nye. 1998. (Good Health Guides). 48p. pap. 3.95 (*0-87983-898-1*, 38981K, Keats Pubng) McGraw-Hill Trade.

Traditional Chinese Medicine Formula. Qiao Yi & Al Stone. Ed. by Peter Holmes & Laurel Redmon. 1999. 365p. pap., stu. ed. 40.00 (*1-890029-40-8*) Snow Lotus.

Traditional Chinese Therapeutic Exercises - Standing Pole. 1994. (Illus.). 89p. pap. (*7-119-00696-7*) Beijing Foreign Lang CHN. *Dist:* China Bks.

Traditional Flower Remedies of Edward Bach. Leslie J. Kaslof. 1988. (Good Health Guides). 32p. pap. 2.95 (*0-87983-624-5*, 36245K, Keats Pubng) McGraw-Hill Trade.

Traditional Foods Are Your Best Medicine: Improving Health & Longevity with Native Nutrition. Ronald F. Schmid. 1997. LC 97-1070. (Illus.). 288p. 14.95 (*0-89281-735-6*, Heal Arts VT) Inner Tradit.

Traditional Healers & Childhood in Zimbabwe. Pamela Reynolds. 1995. LC 94-47391. (Illus.). 208p. (C). text 39.95 (*0-8214-1121-7*); pap. text 17.95 (*0-8214-1122-5*) Ohio U Pr.

Traditional Health Systems & Public Policy: Proceedings of the International Workshop on Traditional Health Systems & Public Policy, Ottawa, Canada, 1994. Ed. by Anwar Islam & Rosina Wiltshire. 1995. LC 95-136507. 184p. pap. (*0-88936-751-5*) IDRC-CRDI.

Traditional Home & Herbal Remedies. Jan De Vries. 1988. (By Appointment Only Ser.). 158p. pap. (*1-85158-012-3*) Mainstream Pubng GBR. *Dist:* Trafalgar.

Traditional Home Remedies: Time-Tested Methods for Staying Well the Natural Way. Martha White & Old Farmers' Almanac Editors. rev. ed. 1997. LC 96-52374. (Old Farmer's Almanac Home Library). (Illus.). 160p. pap. 12.95 (*0-7835-4868-0*) Time Life.

Traditional Medical Systems in East Asia. Seung-Pyo Hong. 1988. (Bibliographies in Technology & Social Change Ser.: No. 3). 44p. (Orig.). (C). pap. 6.00 (*0-945271-06-9*) ISU-CIKARD.

Traditional Medicine. Ed. by Bharati Mukherjee. 1993. 420p. (C). text 45.00 (*1-881570-32-0*) Science Pubs.

Traditional Medicine in Contemporary China. Nathan Sivin. 1987. LC 86-31730. (Science, Medicine, & Technology in East Asia Ser.: No. 2). 549p. text 60.00 (*0-89264-073-1*); reprint ed. pap. text 35.00 (*0-89264-074-X*) Ctr Chinese Studies.

Traditional Native American Healing & Child Sexual Abuse. Ed. by David W. Lloyd. 1994. 62p. (Orig.). (C). pap. text 30.00 (*0-7881-1306-2*) DIANE Pub.

Traditional Reiki for Our Times: Practical Methods for Personal & Planetary Healing. Amy Z. Rowland. 1998. LC 98-10603. (Illus.). 256p. pap. 19.95 (*0-89281-777-1*, Heal Arts VT) Inner Tradit.

Traditional Wisdom for Heart Care. H. S. Wasir. 1995. (C). (*0-7069-9739-5*) Vikas IND. *Dist:* S Asia.

Trafficking of Bacterial Toxins. Ed. by Catharine Saelinger. 1989. 184p. lib. bdg. 153.00 (*0-8493-4787-4*, QP632) CRC Pr.

Tragedy-Contradiction & Repression. Richard Kuhns. 1991. LC 90-20279. 190p. 31.95 (*0-226-45826-1*) U Ch Pr.

Tragedy of Black Lung: Federal Compensation for Occupational Disease. Peter S. Barth. 1987. LC 87-8332. 292p. pap. 19.00 (*0-88099-044-9*) W E Upjohn.

Tragedy of the Self: Individual & Social Disintegration Viewed Through the Self Psychology of Heinz Kohut. Gary F. Greif. 2000. LC 99-86744. 152p. 37.50 (*0-7618-1623-2*) U Pr of Amer.

Tragic Vision Vol. 1: The Confrontation of Extremity. Murray Krieger. 1973. (Tragic Vision Ser.: Vol. 1). 295p. pap. text 17.95 (*0-8018-1550-9*) Johns Hopkins.

Trail Guide to the Body: How to Locate Muscles, Bones & More! Andrew R. Biel. 1997. LC 97-93767. (Illus.). 302p. reprint ed. pap. text 42.95 (*0-9658534-0-3*) Bks of Discov.

***Trail Guide to the Body: How to Locate Muscles, Bones & More!** Andrew R. Biel. 2nd rev. ed. 2001. 340p. (C). per. 49.95 (*0-9658534-1-1*) Bks of Discov.

Trained Mind. 1988. (Fitness, Health & Nutrition Ser.). (Illus.). 144p. 17.27 (*0-8094-6118-8*); lib. bdg. 23.27 (*0-8094-6119-6*) Time-Life.

Trainee Handbook: A Guide for Counseling & Psychotherapy Trainees. Robert Bor & Mary Watts. 1998. LC 98-61584. 290 p. pap. 29.95 (*0-7619-5852-5*, 85014) Sage.

Trainee's Companion to General Practice. Ed. by Joe Rosenthal et al. 1993. LC 93-3406. 320p. text (*0-443-04703-0*) Church.

Trainer's Handbook: What Infant-Family Specialists Need to Know & How to Teach It. Ed. by Nancy Rushmer & Valerie Schuyler. 1993. (Early Intervention Ser.). 90p. (C). 45.00 (*1-883204-00-3*) Hearing & Speech.

Training & Continuing Education: A Handbook for Health Care Institutions. 1970. 261p. 17.50 (*0-87914-006-2*) Hosp Res & Educ.

Training & Continuing Education in Early Intervention. Ed. by James A. Blackman. 1995. LC 94-24185. (Infants & Young Children Ser.). 240p. pap. 41.00 (*0-8342-0650-1*) Aspen Pub.

Training & Preparation of Teachers for Medical Schools with Special Regard to the Needs of Developing Countries. 1966. (Technical Report Ser.: No. 337). 26p. pap. text 3.00 (*92-4-120337-4*) World Health.

Training & Preparation of Teachers for Schools of Medicine & of Allied Health Sciences: Proceedings of the WHO Scientific Group, Geneva, 1972. WHO Staff. 1973. (Technical Reports: No. 521). pap. text 4.00 (*92-4-120521-0*, 1100521) World Health.

Training & Supervision for Counselling in Action. Windy Dryden & Brian Thorne. 1991. (Counselling in Action Ser.: Vol. 14). 192p. (C). pap. 24.95 (*0-8039-8336-0*, 9306) Sage.

Training & Teaching the Mental Health Professional: An In-Depth Approach. Jed A. Yalof. 1996. LC 95-21425. 320p. pap. 50.00 (*1-56821-710-2*) Aronson.

Training & Use of Dental Auxiliary Personnel. H. Alfred. 1977. (Public Health in Europe Ser.: No. 7). 70p. 9.00 (*92-9020-126-6*, 1320007) World Health.

Training & Utilization of Auxiliary Personnel for Rural Health Teams in Developing Countries: Report of a WHO Expert Committee. 1979. (Technical Report Ser.: No. 633). 35p. pap. text 5.00 (*92-4-120633-0*, 1100633) World Health.

Training & Utilization of Feldshers in the U. S. S. R. 1974. (Public Health Papers: No. 56). pap. text 5.00 (*92-4-130056-6*, 1110056) World Health.

Training Behavioral Healthcare Professionals: Higher Learning in an Era of Managed Care. James M. Schuster et al. 1997. LC 96-41553. (Managed Behavioral Healthcare Library). 180p. 43.00 (*0-7879-0795-2*) Jossey-Bass.

Training for a Rapidly Changing Workplace: Applications of Psychological Research. Ed. by Miguel A. Quinones & Addie Ehrenstein. 1996. LC 96-29550. 345p. pap. 29.95 (*1-55798-386-0*) Am Psychol.

Training for Sports & Fitness. Brent S. Ruchall & Frank S. Pyke. 1991. (*0-7329-0190-1*); pap. (*0-7329-0189-8*) Intl Spec Bk.

Training for the Healthcare Manufacturing Industries: Tools & Techniques to Improve Performance. James L. Vesper. 1993. (Illus.). 413p. 98.75 (*0-935184-43-0*) IHS Health Grp.

Training Health Workers to Recognize, Treat, Refer & Educate. Paul Courtright & Susan Lewallen. 1993. 60p. pap. text 23.00 (*981-02-1329-8*) World Scientific Pub.

Training in Medical Psychotherapy: Cross-Cultural Diversity. Ed. by H. Costa & P. Herrmann. 1990. (Psychotherapy & Psychosomatics Ser.: Vol. 53, No. 1-4, 1990). (Illus.). 208p. pap. 150.50 (*3-8055-5321-8*) S Karger.

Training in Neurosurgery. Ed. by H. J. Reulen et al. 1997. (Acta Neurochirurgica Ser.: Suppl. 69). (Illus.). 220p. 84.00 (*3-211-83002-2*) Spr-Verlag.

Training in Radiological Protection for Nuclear Programs. 1975. (Technical Reports: No. 166). 116p. pap. (*92-0-125075-4*, IDC166) IAEA AUT. *Dist:* Bernan Associates.

Training Manual & Video for Dementia Care Specialists. Jean M. Stehman et al. 1996. LC 95-44411. (Illus.). 232p. (C). 115.00 (*0-8018-5268-4*) Johns Hopkins.

Training Manual for Central Service Technicians. American Society for Healthcare Education and Training Staff. 1986. LC 86-3332. (Illus.). 278p. pap. text 70.00 (*0-87258-442-9*, 031802) Am Hospital.

Training Manual for Central Service Technicians: Instructor's Manual. American Society for Healthcare Education and Training Staff. 1991. (Illus.). 94p. (Orig.). pap. text 35.00 (*0-87258-615-4*, 031084) Am Hospital.

Training Manual for Central Service Technicians: Workbook. American Society for Healthcare Education and Training Staff. 1994. (Illus.). 173p. (C). 35.00 (*0-87258-678-2*, 031803) Am Hospital.

Training Manual for Enteral Feeding. Richard E. Dean. 1990. LC 90-62727. 88p. pap. 22.95 (*0-944496-17-2*) Precept Pr.

Training Manual for Human Service Workers in Major Disasters. Ed. by Norman L. Faberow. 1999. 45p. (C). reprint ed. pap. text 20.00 (*0-7881-7653-6*) DIANE Pub.

Training Manual for Intravenous Admixture Personnel. Max L. Hunt, Jr. Ed. by Vicente J. Tormo. 5th rev. ed. 1995. 153p. pap. 29.95 (*0-944496-44-X*) Precept Pr.

Training Manual for SENG Guided Discussion Groups see Gifted Parent Groups: The SENG Model

Training Manual for Total Parenteral Nutrition. Richard E. Dean. 1990. LC 90-62754. 140p. pap. 22.95 (*0-944496-18-0*) Precept Pr.

Training Manual in Applied Medical Anthropology. Ed. by Carole E. Hill. 1991. pap. 20.00 (*0-913167-46-0*) Am Anthro Assn.

Training Nurse Practitioners & Physician Assistants: How Important Is State Financing? Tim M. Henderson et al. 1997. LC 98-211852. iv, 30 p. 20.00 (*1-55516-817-5*) Natl Conf State Legis.

Training of Good Physicians: Critical Factors in Career Choices. Fremont J. Lyden et al. 1968. LC 68-21977. (Commonwealth Fund Publications). (Illus.). 262p. 37.95 (*0-674-90285-8*) HUP.

Training of Health Laboratory Personnel (Technical Staff) Fourth Report of the WHO Expert Committee on Health Laboratory Services, 1966. 1966. (Technical Report Ser.). 31p. pap. text 3.00 (*92-4-120345-5*, 1100345) World Health.

Training of Medical Assistants & Similar Personnel: Seventeenth Report of the WHO Expert Committee on Professional & Technical Education of Medical & Auxiliary Personnel. 1968. (Technical Report Ser.: No. 385). 26p. pap. text 3.00 (*92-4-120385-4*, 1100385) World Health.

Training of Occupational Health Personnel: Report on a Consultation. 1982. (Euro Reports & Studies Ser.: No. 58). 22p. pap. text 4.00 (*92-890-1224-2*) World Health.

Training of Primary Physicians. Ed. by Stephen J. Kunitz et al. 1986. LC 85-22745. (Illus.). 428p. (Orig.). text 75.50 (*0-8191-5030-4*); pap. text 40.00 (*0-8191-5031-2*) U Pr of Amer.

Training of Psychiatrists. 1963. (Technical Report Ser.: No. 252). 39p. pap. text 3.00 (*92-4-120252-1*) World Health.

Training of Research Workers in the Medical Sciences: Proceedings of the CIOMS Round Table conference, Geneva, 1970. CIOMS Round Table Conference Staff. 1972. 186p. pap. text 24.00 (*92-4-156040-1*, 1830005) World Health.

Training of Staff, Other Than Health Care Staff, Concerned with Rehabilitation. Council of Europe Staff. 1992. (*92-871-1966-X*) Council of Europe FRA. *Dist:* Manhattan Pub Co.

Training of the Physician for Family Practice. 1963. (Technical Report Ser.: No. 257). 39p. pap. text 3.00 (*92-4-120257-2*) World Health.

Training of Trainers for Health Systems Research. I. Pathmanathan & N. I. Nik-Safiah. 1992. 282p. pap. (*0-88936-589-X*) IDRC-CRDI CAN. *Dist:* Stylus Pub VA.

Training on AIDS for Personnel in Drug Treatment Centres. 1988. (ENG & GER.). v, 27p. pap. text 8.00 (*92-890-1056-8*, 1340039) World Health.

Training Program for Operation of Emergency Vehicles 1992. lib. bdg. 375.00 (*0-8490-8864-X*) Gordon Pr.

Training Programs in Assistive Technology: 1992 Guide. Lynn R. Bryant. 1992. 87p. pap. 15.00 (*0-9635859-1-6*) RehabTech.

Training Strategies for Health Information Systems. 1996. (*92-871-2946-0*) Council of Europe FRA. *Dist:* Manhattan Pub Co.

Training Teachers of the Gifted & Talented. Margaret Lindsey. Ed. by Abraham J. Tannenbaum. 1980. LC 80-11867. (Perspectives on Gifted & Talented Education Ser.). 60p. (Orig.). pap. text 8.95 (*0-8077-2590-0*) Tchrs Coll.

Training Techniques in Cardiac Rehabilitation. Paul Fardy et al. 1997. LC 97-16033. (Current Issues in Cardiac Rehabilitation Ser.). (Illus.). 152p. pap. text 25.00 (*0-87322-536-8*, BFAR0536) Human Kinetics.

Training the Food Service Worker. 1967. 155p. tchr. ed. 9.95 Hosp Res & Educ.

Training the Housekeeping Aide. 1967. 271p. tchr. ed. 9.95 Hosp Res & Educ.

Training the Physical Therapist. Thut. 1998. (C). text 44.00 (*0-12-784588-7*) Acad Pr.

Training Therapy: Prophylaxis & Rehabilitation. Gustavsen Rolf & Renate Streeck. Tr. & Adapted by Wolfgang G. Gilliar. 2nd rev. ed. 1993. LC 92-48359. (Flexibook Ser.). (Illus.). 240p. pap. text 29.90 (*0-86577-483-8*) Thieme Med Pubs.

Training Verification for Laboratory Personnel: Approved Guideline (1995) Contrib. by David E. Nevalainen. 1995. 85.00 (*1-56238-286-1*, GP21-A) NCCLS.

Traite de Gastro-Enterologie J. J. Bernier et al. 1984. (FRE., Illus.). 1600p. 295.00 (*2-257-10431-5*) S M P F Inc.

Traite de Mycologie Medicale see Medical Mycology

Traite Des Degenerescences Physiques, Intellectuelles et Morales De L'espece Humaine Benedict A. Morel. 1976. LC 75-16721. (Classics in Psychiatry Ser.). (FRE., Illus.). reprint ed. 62.95 (*0-405-07446-8*) Ayer.

Traite des Maladies du Cerveau et de Ses Membranes: Maladies Mentales. Antoine L. Bayle. 1976. LC 75-16682. (Classics in Psychiatry Ser.). (FRE.). reprint ed. 51.95 (*0-405-07414-X*) Ayer.

Traite Medico-Philosophique sur l'Alienation Mentale. Philippe Pinel. 2nd ed. 1976. LC 75-16727. (Classics in Psychiatry Ser.). (FRE.). reprint ed. 48.95 (*0-405-07450-6*) Ayer.

Traits As Dispositions for Psychopathology: Congress, Dresden, September 1998. Ed. by Petra Netter & Burkhard Brocke. 2000. (Neuropsychobiology Ser.: Vol. 41, No. 1). (Illus.). 54p. pap. 25.25 (*3-8055-6911-4*) S Karger.

Trance & Treatment: Clinical Uses of Hypnosis. Herbert Spiegel et al. 1987. LC 86-20627. (Illus.). 382p. pap. 26.00 (*0-88048-264-8*, 8264) Am Psychiatric.

Trance on Trial. Alan W. Scheflin & Jerrold L. Shapiro. 1989. LC 88-1674. (Clinical & Experimental Hypnosis Ser.). 338p. pap. 25.00 (*0-89862-340-5*, 2340) Guilford Pubns.

Trancework: An Introduction to the Practice of Clinical Hypnosis. Michael D. Yapko. 2nd enl. rev. ed. 1990. LC 89-22173. 464p. text 44.95 (*0-87630-568-0*) Brunner-Routledge.

Tranquilizer Use & Well-Being: A Longitudinal Study of Social & Psychological Effects. Robert D. Caplan et al. 1984. (ISR Research Report Ser.). 442p. (Orig.). pap. text 25.00 (*0-87944-296-4*) Inst Soc Res.

Tranquillisation. James G. Speight. 1990. 111p. pap. (*0-85207-228-7*) C W Daniel GBR. *Dist:* Natl Bk Netwk.

Tranquillisers: Social, Psychological & Clinical Perspectives. Jonathan Gabe & Paul Williams. 1986. 350p. (*0-422-79930-0*, 1025) Tavistock GBR. *Dist:* Routldge.

Trans Cultural Society Health & Disease. Ed. by Eugene B. Gallagher & Janardan Subedi. 1995. LC 94-35679. 345p. pap. text 48.00 (*0-13-669094-7*) P-H.

Trans Kit Fund Nursing. Barbara Kozier et al. Ed. by Debra Hunter. 3rd ed. 1989. 954p. (C). trans. 175.00 (*0-201-11777-0*) Addison-Wesley.

Trans Matnl Newborn Nrsg. Sally B. Olds. Ed. by Patti Cleary. 4th ed. 1994. 1328p. (C). pap. text 211.73 (*0-8053-5583-9*) Addison-Wesley.

Transactional Analysis at Work. Keith Carby & Manab Thakur. 1976. 98p. (C). 80.00 (*0-85292-133-0*) St Mut.

Transactional Analysis in Health Care. Jean Elder. 1978. LC 78-57376. pap. text (*0-201-01512-9*, Health Sci) Addison-Wesley.

Transactions: 1984 Reports of Mortality, Morbidity & Other Experience. 1988. text 75.00 (*0-938959-11-5*) Soc Actuaries.

Transactions: Proceedings of the American Association for the Study & Prevention of Infant Mortality Meeting, 1st, New Haven, 1909. American Association for the Study and Prevention of Infant Mortality. 1974. LC 74-1663. (Children & Youth Ser.). 356p. reprint ed. 31.95 (*0-405-05944-2*) Ayer.

Transactions: The Interplay Between Individual, Family, & Society. John Spiegel. 1983. LC 84-45129. 480p. 65.00 (*0-87668-699-4*) Aronson.

Transactions 23rd Meeting European Strabismological Association. Ed. by Micheline Spiritus. 1996. (Transactions Meetings European Strabismological Association Ser.). (Illus.). 554p. (*90-70430-23-1*) Swets.

Transblepharoplasty Subperiosteal Forehead & Midface Lift. Malcolm Paul. 1998. LC 98-4297. (Illus.). 32p. pap. 189.00 (*0-387-98482-8*) Spr-Verlag.

Transcendence in Relationships: Existentialism & Psychotherapy. Robert Willis. 1994. (Frontiers in Psychotherapy Ser.). 240p. pap. 39.50 (*1-56750-074-9*); LC 94-28155. (Illus.). 77.00 (*1-56750-073-0*) Greenwood (Ablex).

Transcendence of Loss over the Life-Span. Patricia Weenolsen. 1988. LC 66-56391. (Death Education, Aging & Health Care Ser.). 500p. 125.00 (*0-89116-736-6*); pap. text 49.95 (*0-89116-582-7*) Hemisp Pub.

Transcending Addiction & Other Afflictions: Lifehealing. Angela Browne-Miller. 1993. LC 93-2901. (Frontiers in Psychotherapy Ser.). 77.00 (*0-89391-900-4*); pap. 39.50 (*0-89391-903-9*) Greenwood (Ablex).

Transcending the Psychoneurotic Disturbances: New Approaches in Psychospirituality & Personality Development. Edward B. Bynum. 1994. LC 92-1577. (Illus.). 414p. lib. bdg. 49.95 (*1-56024-338-4*) Haworth Pr.

Transcending the Self: An Object Relations Model of Psychoanalytic Therapy. Frank L. Summers. 1999. LC 98-42974. 280p. 45.00 (*0-88163-231-7*) Analytic Pr.

Transcending Turmoil: Survivors of Dysfunctional Families. Donna F. LaMar. Ed. by Bonnie Tilson. Date not set. 328p. (Orig.). pap. 13.95 (*1-884570-39-9*) Research Triangle.

Transcortical Aphasias. Marcelo L. Berthier. 1999. LC 00-501116. (Brain Damage, Behaviour & Cognition Ser.). 272p. 54.95 (*0-86377-840-2*) L Erlbaum Assocs.

Transcranial Doppler. David W. Newell & Rune Aaslid. 1991. 288p. text 199.00 (*0-88167-836-8*) Lppncott W & W.

Transcranial Doppler Imaging: Techniques & Interpretation. Ed. by Mira L. Katz & Anthony J. Comerota. 1999. (Illus.). 250p. 99.00 (*1-56757-062-3*) Appleton Comms.

Transcranial Doppler Sonography. Ed. by Rune Aaslid. 1992. (Illus.). 190p. 55.92 (*0-387-81935-5*) Spr-Verlag.

Transcranial Doppler-Sonography. Ulrich Bogdahn. 1998. (Illus.). 209.95 (*0-632-04856-5*) Blackwell Sci.

Transcranial Doppler Ultrasonography. Viken L. Babikian et al. 2nd ed. 1999. LC 99-12513. 512p. text 155.00 (*0-7506-9969-8*) Buttrwrth-Heinemann.

Transcranial Magnetic Stimulation. Ed. by W. Paulus. 1999. LC 99-36369. (Supplements to Electroencephalography & Clinical Neurophysiology Ser.: Vol. 50). 386p. 180.50 (*0-444-50070-7*) Elsevier.

Transcription Factors. Joseph Locker. 2000. (Human Molecular Genetics Ser.). 300p. 115.00 (*0-12-454345-6*) Acad Pr.

T U V

Transcription Factors: A Practical Approach. Ed. by David S. Latchman. 2nd ed. 1999. LC 98-40981. (Practical Approach Ser.: No. 201). (Illus.). 325p. text 120.00 (*0-19-963697-4*); pap. text 60.00 (*0-19-963696-6*) OUP.

Transcription Factors & Cell Aging. Ed. by A. Y. Liu et al. 1996. (Journal: Vol. 5, No. 3, 1996). (Illus.). 70p. pap. 28.00 (*3-8055-6366-3*) S Karger.

Transcription Factors & DNA Replication. David S. Pederson & Nicholas H. Heintz. 1994. LC 94-33851. (Molecular Biology Intelligence Unit Ser.). 125p. 99.00 (*1-57059-069-9*, LN9069) Landes Bioscience.

Transcription Factors & Human Disease. Gregg L. Semenza. 1998. LC 97-47791. (Oxford Monographs on Medical Genetics: No. 37). (Illus.). 384p. text 49.95 (*0-19-511239-3*) OUP.

Transcription for Medical Office Assistant. Baker. 1998. 99.95 incl. audio (*0-8273-7907-2*); (C). tchr. ed. 16.00 (*0-8273-7906-4*) Delmar.

Transcriptional Regulation. Ed. by Steven L. McKnight & Keith R. Yamamoto. 1993. LC 92-31461. (Monographs: Vol. 22). 1335p. 120.00 (*0-87969-410-6*); pap. 71.00 (*0-87969-425-4*) Cold Spring Harbor.

Transcultural Aspects of Psychiatric Art: Proceedings of the International Congress of Psychopathology of Expression, 7th, Boston, Mass., Oct., 1973. International Congress of Psychopathology of Expre. Ed. by Irene Jakab. 1975. (Journal: Vol. 4). 111.50 (*3-8055-2138-3*) S Karger.

Transcultural Child Development: A Context for Psychological Assessment & Treatment. Ed. by Gloria Johnson-Powell et al. 1997. LC 97-8358. 400p. 110.00 (*0-471-17479-3*) Wiley.

Transcultural Communication in Health Care. Joan Luckmann & Sylvia Tindell Nobles. 1999. LC 99-40689. (Allied Health Ser.). 256p. (C). pap. text 24.95 (*0-7668-0593-X*) Delmar.

Transcultural Communication in Nursing. Joan Luckmann. 1998. LC 98-50682. 400p. pap. text 28.95 (*0-7668-0256-6*) Delmar.

Transcultural Concepts in Nursing. Margaret M. Andrews & Joyceen Boyle. 3rd ed. 1998. LC 98-3026. 592p. pap. text 34.95 (*0-7817-1038-3*) Lppncott W & W.

Transcultural Counselling in Action. Patricia D'Ardennes & Aruna Mahtani. 1989. (Counselling in Action Ser.: Vol. 6). 144p. (C). text 49.95 (*0-8039-8110-4*); pap. 19.95 (*0-8039-8111-2*, 7003) Sage.

Transcultural Dimensions in Medical Ethics. Ed. by Edmund D. Pellegrino et al. 1992. 225p. 35.00 (*1-55572-015-3*) Univ Pub Group.

Transcultural Health Care. George Henderson & Martha Primeaux. 1981. 24.50 (*0-201-03237-6*); pap. (*0-201-03452-2*) Addison-Wesley (Health Sci).

Transcultural Health Care: A Culturally Competent Approach. Ed. by Larry D. Purnell & Betty J. Paulanka. 1997. LC 97-5282. (Illus.). 511p. (C). pap. text 34.95 (*0-8036-0208-1*) Davis Co.

Transcultural Medicine: Principles & Practice. B. Qureshi. 1989. (C). text 84.00 (*0-85200-938-0*) Kluwer Academic.

Transcultural Nursing: Assessment & Intervention. Joyce N. Giger. 2nd ed. 1995. (Illus.). 640p. (C). (gr. 13). pap. text 37.00 (*0-8016-7411-5*, 07411) Mosby Inc.

Transcultural Nursing: Assessment & Intervention. Giger. 3rd ed. 1999. (Illus.). 672p. text 31.00 (*0-323-00287-0*) Mosby Inc.

Transcultural Nursing for Advanced Practice. Ed. by Jane L. Echols et al. 1999. (Illus.). 448p. pap. text 38.95 (*0-07-105486-3*) McGraw-Hill Med Pub.

Transcutaneous Electrical Nerve Stimulators. 1986. 10p. pap. 70.00 (*0-910275-60-2*, NS4-209) Assn Adv Med Instrn.

Transcutaneous Monitoring of Oxygen. 1978. (Illus.). pap. 28.75 (*3-8055-2883-3*) S Karger.

Transdermal Controlled Systemic Medications. Yie W. Chien. 1987. (Drugs & the Pharmaceutical Sciences Ser.: Vol. 31). (Illus.). 464p. text 199.00 (*0-8247-7760-3*) Dekker.

Transdermal Delivery of Drugs Agis F. Kydonieus. Ed. by Bret Berner. 1987. 300p. 499.85 (*0-8493-6483-3*, RS201) CRC Pr.

Transdermal Delivery of Drugs. Agis F. Kydonieus & B. Berner. 1986. LC 86-2585. 216p. 125.00 (*0-8493-6484-1*, CRC Reprint) Franklin.

Transdermal Delivery of Drugs, Vol. II. Agis F. Kydonieus. 1987. 168p. 191.00 (*0-8493-6485-X*) CRC Pr.

Transdermal Delivery of Drugs, Vol. 3. Agis F. Kydonieus & B. Berner. 1987. LC 86-2585. 101.00 (*0-8493-6486-8*, CRC Reprint) Franklin.

Transdermal Drug Delivery: Developmental Issues & Research Initiatives. Jonathan Hadgraft & Richard A. Guy. 1988. (Drugs & the Pharmaceutical Sciences Ser.: Vol. 35). (Illus.). 336p. text 175.00 (*0-8247-7991-6*) Dekker.

Transdermal Fentanyl. Ed. by K. A. Lehmann & D. Zech. 1991. (Illus.). 192p. 69.95 (*0-387-54440-2*) Spr-Verlag.

Transdisciplinary Play-Based Assessment & Intervention: Child & Program Summary Forms. Toni W. Linder. 1993. 58p. 27.00 (*1-55766-163-4*) P H Brookes.

Transducing the Genome: Information, Anarchy & Revolution in the Biomedical Sciences. Gary Zweiger. 2001. LC 00-49628. (Illus.). 269p. text 24.95 (*0-07-136980-5*) McGraw-Hill Prof.

Transesophageal Echocardiography. De Bruijn. 1991. 133.00 (*0-316-17816-0*, Little Brwn Med Div) Lppncott W & W.

Transesophageal Echocardiography. Ed. by R. Erbel et al. 1991. (Illus.). 360p. 211.00 (*0-387-50507-5*) Spr-Verlag.

Transesophageal Echocardiography. Ed. by William K. Freeman et al. 1994. LC 93-5357. 624p. text 275.00 (*0-316-29293-1*) Lppncott W & W.

Transesophageal Echocardiography. C. Carl Jaffe & Patrick J. Lynch. 1992. (C). 500.00 incl. disk (*1-56815-014-8*) Mosby Inc.

Transesophageal Echocardiography: A New Monitoring Technique. N. Kolev et al. 1996. LC 94-42060. 200p. 91.00 (*3-211-82650-5*) Spr-Verlag.

Transesophageal Echocardiography: Clinical & Intraoperative Applications. Ed. by Jose C. Missri. 1992. LC 92-23799. (Illus.). 248p. text (*0-443-08852-7*) Church.

Transesophageal Echocardiography in Anesthesea. Uriel A. Yodfat. 2001. (Illus.). 300p. 145.00 (*0-7506-7104-1*) Buttrwrth-Heinemann.

Transesophageal Echocardiography in Congenital Heart Disease. Ed. by Oliver Stumper & George R. Sutherland. 1994. (Illus.). 296p. text (*0-340-55653-6*) E A GBR. *Dist:* OUP.

Transfatty Acids in Human Nutrition. Ed. by Jean L. Sebedio & William W. Christie. unabr. ed. 1998. (Oily Press Lipid Library). (Illus.). 320p. (C). (*0-9514171-8-5*) Oily Pr GBR. *Dist:* Matreya.

Transfer of Care: Psychiatric Deinstitutionalization & Its Aftermath. Phil Brown. 1988. 292p. (C). pap. text 13.95 (*0-415-00188-9*) Routledge.

Transference & Countertransference. Heinrich Racker. 1968. 216p. 33.00 (*0-8236-6640-9*) Intl Univs Pr.

Transference & Empathy in Asian American Psychotherapy: Cultural Values & Treatment Needs. Jean L. Chin et al. 1993. LC 92-48757. 168p. 60.00 (*0-275-94493-X*, C4493, Praeger Pubs) Greenwood.

Transference & Its Context: Selected Papers on Psychoanalysis. Leo Stone. 1984. LC 83-25807. 470p. 60.00 (*0-87668-655-2*) Aronson.

Transference & Transcendence: Ernest Becker's Contribution to Psychotherapy. Daniel Liechty. 1995. LC 94-39365. 224p. 45.00 (*1-56821-434-0*) Aronson.

Transference in Psychotherapy: Clinical Management. Ed. by Evelyne A. Schwaber. 1986. LC 84-12958. 181p. (C). 30.00 (*0-8236-6625-5*, 06625) Intl Univs Pr.

Transference Neurosis & Psychoanalytic Experience: Perspectives on Contemporary Clinical Practice. Gail S. Reed. 1994. LC 94-1406. 240p. 45.00 (*0-300-05957-4*) Yale U Pr.

Transference Neurosis & Transference Psychosis. Margaret I. Little. LC 80-66925. 1993. 352p. pap. 50.00 (*1-56821-074-4*); 1980. 350p. 40.00 (*0-87668-421-5*) Aronson.

Transference/Countertransference. Ed. by Nathan Schwartz-Salant & Murray Stein. 1992. LC 91-40546. (Chiron Clinical Ser.: Vol. 1984). (Illus.). 200p. (Orig.). pap. 24.95 (*0-933029-63-2*) Chiron Pubns.

Transferrin: The Iron Carrier. Alan J. Welch. 1992. 304p. lib. bdg. 169.00 (*0-8493-6793-X*, QP552) CRC Pr.

Transferring to a United States Medical School. Stanley Zaslau. 2nd rev. ed. 1996. 125p. (C). pap. text 18.00 (*1-886468-11-7*) FMSG.

Transfigure System. Health for Life Staff. 1989. (Illus.). 127p. pap. 19.95 (*0-944831-21-4*) Health Life.

Transform Your Emotional DNA: Understanding the Blueprint of Your Life. Theresa Dale. 2nd rev. ed. 1997. LC 96-90408. (Illus.). 103p. mass mkt. 19.95 (*0-9652947-6-5*) Wellness Ctr.

Transformation: Emergence of the Self. Murray Stein. 1998. LC 97-41052. (Carolyn & Ernest Fay Series in Analytical Psychology). (Illus.). 208p. 22.95 (*0-89096-780-6*) Tex A&M Univ Pr.

Transformation & Recovery: A Guide for the Design & Development of Acupuncture-Based Chemical Dependency Treatment Programs. Alex Brumbaugh. 1994. 650p. pap. 39.00 (*0-9639791-0-8*) Stillpoint Pr.

Transformation Assay of Established Cell Lines: Mechanisms & Application. Ed. by T. Kakunaga & H. Yamasaki. 1986. (IARC Scientific Publications Ser.: No. 67). (Illus.). 200p. 40.00 (*0-19-723067-9*) OUP.

Transformation in Clinical & Developmental Psychology. Ed. by D. A. Kramer & M. J. Bopp. 1989. (Illus.). 263p. 140.00 (*0-387-96901-2*) Spr-Verlag.

Transformation of Consciousness in Myth: Integrating the Thought of Jung & Campbell. John W. Tigue. 1994. LC 93-12339. (Reshaping of Psychoanalysis Ser.: Vol. 4). 162p. (C). text 39.95 (*0-8204-2130-8*) P Lang Pubng.

Transformation of German Academic Medicine, 1750-1820. Thomas H. Broman. 1996. (Cambridge History of Medicine Ser.). 222p. (C). text 59.95 (*0-521-55231-1*) Cambridge U Pr.

Transformation of Human Diploid Fibroblasts. Ed. by George E. Milo. 1990. 304p. 202.00 (*0-8493-4956-7*, RC268) CRC Pr.

Transformation of Human Epithelial Cells. George E. Milo. 1992. 336p. 206.00 (*0-8493-6382-9*, RC280) CRC Pr.

Transformation of Meaning in Psychological Therapies: Integrating Theory & Practice. Michael J. Power & Chris R. Brewin. 1997. LC 96-48034. 228p. pap. 55.00 (*0-471-97005-0*) Wiley.

Transformation of Meaning in the Psychological Therapies: Integrating Theory & Practice. Mick Power & Chris R. Brewin. 1997. LC 96-48034. (Clinical Psychology & Personality Ser.). 228p. 150.00 (*0-471-95826-3*) Wiley.

Transformation Through Bodywork: Using Touch Therapy to Find Inner Peace. Dan Menkin. 1996. (Illus.). 248p. pap. 16.00 (*1-879181-34-7*) Bear & Co.

Transformation Through Menopause. Marian Van Eyck McCain. 1991. 200p. pap. 19.95 (*0-89789-269-0*); LC 91-12685. 60.00 (*0-89789-268-2*, H268) Greenwood (Bergin & Garvey).

Transformation Workbook: Colour Healing & Yoga. Pauline Wills & Theodore Gimbel. 1992. (Illus.). 224p. (Orig.). pap. (*0-572-01599-2*) W Foulsham GBR. *Dist:* Trans-Atl Phila.

Transformational Leadership: Renewing Fundamental Values & Achieving New Relationships in Health Care. Barbara A. Donaho et al. Ed. by Eric B. Linne. 1995. LC 95-35494. 305p. pap. 40.00 (*1-55648-144-6*, 001116) AHPI.

Transformational Nursing Leadership: A Vision for the Future. Anne M. Barker. 1992. 256p. (C). reprint ed. pap. text 34.95 (*0-88737-551-0*, 15-2473) Natl League Nurse.

Transformational Reiki: Trans-Reiki. Karyn Mitchell. 1997. 250p. (Orig.). pap. 19.96 (*0-9640822-6-8*) Mind Rivers.

Transformations: Countertranference During the Psychoanalytic Treatment of Incest, Real & Imagined. Elaine V. Siegel. 1996. LC 96-12828. 208p. 36.00 (*0-88163-117-5*) Analytic Pr.

Transformations of Consciousness: Conventional & Contemplative Perspectives on Development. Ken Wilber et al. 1986. LC 85-2486. 325p. pap. 40.00 (*0-394-74202-8*) Shambhala Pubns.

Transformations of Gender & Race: Family & Developmental Perspectives. Ed. by Rhea V. Almeida. 1999. LC 98-48952. 155p. 34.95 (*0-7890-0655-3*) Haworth Pr.

Transformations of Gender & Race: Family & Developmental Perspectives. Rhea V. Almeida. 1998. LC 98-48952. xiii, 135p. (*0-7890-0673-1*) Haworth Pr.

Transformations of the Animal World: Being the Authorized Translation of "Les Transformations Du Monde Animal. Charles Deperet. Ed. by Stephen Jay Gould. 1980. LC 79-8330. (History of Paleontology Ser.). reprint ed. lib. bdg. 35.95 (*0-405-12711-1*) Ayer.

Transformed Cell: Unlocking the Mysteries of Cancer. Steven A. Rosenberg & John M. Barry. 2000. 353p. 26.00 (*0-7881-9396-1*) DIANE Pub.

Transformed Cell: Unlocking the Mysteries of Cancer. Steven Rosenberg & John M. Barry. 1993. viii, 376p. reprint ed. pap. 12.50 (*0-380-72115-5*, Avon Bks) Morrow Avon.

Transforming Aggression: Psychotherapy with the Difficult-to-Treat Patient. Frank Lachmann. 2001. LC 00-38963. xiii, 264p. 45.00 (*0-7657-0293-2*) Aronson.

Transforming Growth Factor-B in the Kidney & Renal Diseases. Ed. by Raimund Hirschberg. 1998. (Mineral & Electrolyte Metabolism Ser.: Vol. 24, Nos. 2-3). (Illus.). 100p. pap. 77.50 (*3-8055-6651-4*) S Karger.

Transforming Hate to Love: An Outcome Study of the Peper Harow Adolescent Treatment Process. Melvyn Rose. 1997. LC 96-46581. 168p. (C). 84.95 (*0-415-13831-0*); pap. 26.95 (*0-415-13832-9*) Routledge.

Transforming Health Care: Action Strategies for Health Care Leaders. Daniel J. Anderson et al. 1998. LC 98-12341. 125p. 40.00 (*1-55648-232-9*) AHPI.

Transforming Health Care Through Information: Case Studies. Ed. by Nancy M. Lorenzi et al. 1995. LC 95-17731. (Computers in Health Care Ser.). (Illus.). 431p. 69.00 (*0-387-94455-9*) Spr-Verlag.

Transforming Healthcare Organizations: How to Achieve & Sustain Organizational Excellence. Ellen Marszalek-Gaucher & Richard J. Coffey. 1990. LC 90-4777. (Health Management Ser.). 288p. 48.00 (*1-55542-250-0*) Jossey-Bass.

Transforming Home Care: Quality, Cost, & Data Management. Donna Ambler Peters & Tad McKeon. 1998. LC 98-15281. 450p. 72.00 (*0-8342-1072-X*, 1072X) Aspen Pub.

Transforming Medicaid. League of Women Voters Education Fund Staff. 1996. 19p. 3.99 (*0-89959-399-2*, 1047) LWVUS.

Transforming Nurses Anger & Pain: Steps Toward Healing. Sandra P. Thomas. 1998. 296p. 40.95 (*0-8261-1209-9*) Springer Pub.

Transforming Nursing Through Reflective Practice. Christopher Johns & Dawn Freshwater. 1998. LC 97-31578. (Illus.). 288p. pap. 41.95 (*0-632-04784-4*) Blackwell Sci.

Transforming Proteins of DNA Tumor Viruses. Ed. by R. Knippers & A. J. Levine. 1989. (Current Topics in Microbiology & Immunology Ser.: Vol. 144). (Illus.). 284p. 135.00 (*0-387-50909-7*) Spr-Verlag.

Transforming RN Education: Dialogue & Debate. Ed. by Nancy L. Dickelmann & Marsha L. Rather. 1993. (Illus.). 366p. (C). pap. text 35.95 (*0-88737-573-1*, 14-2511) Natl League Nurse.

Transforming State Health Agencies to Meet Current & Future Challenges. Marie Maralit et al. 1997. 86p. pap. 22.00 (*1-55877-279-0*) Natl Governor.

Transforming Supervision in Health Care. Don Mason. 1999. 160p. pap. 19.95 (*0-304-70463-6*) Continuum.

Transforming the Delivery of Health Care. Timothy Carse & Jeffrey Slater. 1995. text 95.00 (*0-07-413100-1*, Irwn McGrw-H) McGrw-H Hghr Educ.

Transforming the Pain: A Workbook on Vicarious Traumatization. Karen W. Saakvitne et al. 1996. LC 96-21879. 159p. pap. 17.00 (*0-393-70233-2*) Norton.

Transforming Therapy: A New Approach to Hypnotherapy. Gil Boyne. 2nd ed. 1989. 400p. 37.50 (*0-930298-13-6*) Westwood Pub Co.

Transforming Trauma: A Guide to Understanding & Treating Adult Survivors of Child Sexual Abuse. Anna C. Salter. 1995. LC 95-7710. (Illus.). 353p. 74.95 (*0-8039-5508-1*, 3857); 360p. pap. 39.95 (*0-8039-5509-X*, 3858) Sage.

Transforming Trauma - EDMR: The Revolutionary New Therapy for Freeing the Mind, Clearing the Body, & Opening the Mind. Laurel Parnell. 1997. LC 96-44478. 208p. (C). 21.00 (*0-393-04053-4*) Norton.

Transfusion & Hemaopoietic Stem Cells: Proceedings of the 6th Hokkaido Symposium on Transfusional Medicine, July 22-23, Sapporo, Japan, 1994. Sadayoski Sekiguchi. 1996. LC 96-13647. (Illus.). 256p. 125.00 (*0-86542-911-1*) Blackwell Sci.

Transfusion-Associated AIDS. Robert K. Jenner. 1995. LC 95-9195. 364p. kivar 30.00 (*0-913875-14-7*, 1078-R) Lawyers & Judges.

Transfusion Immunology & Medicine: Proceedings of the Twelfth International Convocation on Immunology. Ed. by Carel J. Van Oss. 1995. LC 94-23955. (Illus.). 480p. text 195.00 (*0-8247-9640-3*) Dekker.

Transfusion Medicine: A Practical Guide. Jeffrey McCullough. 1997. LC 97-29682. (Illus.). 528p. pap. 49.95 (*0-07-045113-3*) McGraw-Hill Prof.

Transfusion Medicine - Fact & Fiction: Proceedings of the 16th Annual Symposium on Blood Transfusion, Groningen, 1991, Organized by the Red Cross Blood Bank Groningen-Drenthe. Ed. by C. T. Sibinga et al. 1992. LC 92-12547. (Developments in Hematology & Immunology Ser.: Vol. 27). 240p. (C). text 94.00 (*0-7923-1732-7*) Kluwer Academic.

Transfusion Practice in Cardiac Surgery. Michael L. Baldwin & Sanford R. Kurtz. 1991. LC 91-4865. (Illus.). 58p. (C). text 9.00 (*1-56395-005-7*) Am Assn Blood.

Transfusion Reactions. Ed. by Mark A. Popovsky. 1996. (Illus.). 404p. 99.00 (*1-56395-055-3*, PC97-PR9602) Am Assn Blood.

Transfusion Science. J. Overfield et al. 1999. LC 99-33335. (Biomedical Sciences Explained Ser.). 216p. pap. (*0-7506-3415-4*) E A GBR. *Dist:* OUP.

Transfusion Service Manual of SOPs, Training Guides, & Competence Assessment Tools. 1996. (Orig.). pap. text 50.00 (*1-56395-070-7*, PC97-OP9602) Am Assn Blood.

Transfusion Therapy. Ed. by P. D. Mintz. 1999. (Illus.). xviii, 482p. (*3-8055-6900-9*) S Karger.

Transfusion Therapy: Clinical Principles & Practice. Ed. by Paul D. Mintz. 1998. LC 98-42095. (*1-56395-099-5*) Am Assn Blood.

Transfusion Therapy: From Donor to Patient. Ed. by Christina A. Kasprisin & Linda A. Chambers. 1992. LC 92-49978. 67p. 9.00 (*1-56395-014-6*) Am Assn Blood.

Transfusion Therapy: Guidelines for Practice. Ed. by Stephanie H. Summers. 1990. LC 90-955. 180p. (C). text 9.00 (*0-915355-85-X*) Am Assn Blood.

Transfusion Transmitted Infections. Dennis M. Smith et al. 1991. LC 91-4561. 330p. 65.00 (*0-89189-289-3*) Am Soc Clinical.

Transfusionsmedizin 1986 - Infektionen, Autotransfusion, Lymphokine. Ed. by V. Kretschmer & W. Stangel. 1987. (Beitraege zur Infusionstherapie und Klinische Ernaehrung Ser.: Vol. 18). (Illus.). xii, 412p. 87.00 (*3-8055-4696-3*) S Karger.

Transfusionsmedizin 1987 - Notfall - und Massivtransfusion, Autoimmunhaemolysen, Infektionen, Stammzelluebertragung. Ed. by V. Kretschmer et al. 1988. (Contributions to Infusion Therapy Ser.: Vol. 21). (Illus.). xiv, 360p. 73.25 (*3-8055-4840-0*) S Karger.

Transfusionsmedizin 1996/97: 29.Kongress der Deutschen Gesellschaft fur Transfusionsmedizin und Immunhamatologie (DGTI), Essen, September 1996. Ed. by Walter Sibrowski et al. 1997. (Beitraege Zur Infusionstherapie und Transfusionsmedizin/Contributions to Infusion Therapy & Transfusion Medicine Ser.: No. 34, 1997). (Illus.). xii, 282p. 156.50 (*3-8055-6562-3*) S Karger.

Transfusionsmedizin Aktuell: Infektionen, Thrombozyten, Granulozyten. Ed. by V. Kretschmer & W. Stangel. 1986. (Beitraege zur Infusionstherapie und Klinische Ernaehrung Ser.: Vol. 15). (Illus.). viii, 294p. 58.50 (*3-8055-4340-9*) S Karger.

Transfusionsmedizin, 1988: Infektionen, Plasmaprodukte, Transplantationen, Antikoerper. Ed. by V. Kretschmer et al. 1989. (Beitraege zur Infusionstherapie und Klinische Ernaehrung Ser.: Vol. 24). (Illus.). viii, 242p. 68.75 (*3-8055-5055-3*) S Karger.

Transfusionsmedizin, 1989-1990. Ed. by V. Kretschmer et al. 1990. (Beitraege zur Infusionstherapie und Klinische Ernaehrung Ser.: Vol. 26). (Illus.). viii, 454p. 105.25 (*3-8055-5251-3*) S Karger.

Transfusionsmedizin, 1990-1991. Ed. by V. Kretschmer et al. 1991. (Beitraege zur Infusionstherapie und Klinische Ernaehrung Ser.: Vol. 28). (Illus.). xii, 378p. 105.25 (*3-8055-5478-8*) S Karger.

Transfusionsmedizin, 1991-1992. Ed. by V. Kretschmer et al. 1993. (Beitraege zur Infusionstherapie und Klinische Ernaehrung Ser.: Vol. 30). (Illus.). xiv, 482p. 105.25 (*3-8055-5687-X*) S Karger.

Transfusionsmedizin, 1993-1994. Ed. by W. Sibrowski et al. 1994. (Beitraege Zur Infusinstherapie und Transfusionsmedizin. Band 32 Contributions to Infusion Therapy & Transfusion Medicine Ser.). (Illus.). xii, 536p. 143.50 (*3-8055-6025-7*) S Karger.

Transfusionsmedizin, 1992-1993. Ed. by V. Kretschmer et al. 1993. (Beitraege zur Infusionstherapie und Klinische Ernaehrung Ser.: Vol. 31). (Illus.). x, 230p. 81.75 (*3-8055-5841-4*) S Karger.

Transfusionsmedizin und Schock. H. Reissigl & D. Schoenitzer. 1986. (Handbuch der Infusionstherapie und Klinischen Ernaehrung Ser.: Band 3). xii, 256p. 108.75 (*3-8055-3744-1*) S Karger.

Transgender & HIV: Risks, Prevention & Care. Ed. by Walter O. Bockting & Sheila Kirk. 2001. LC 00-63367. 182p. pap. 24.95 (*0-7890-1268-5*); (C). 49.95 (*0-7890-1267-7*) Haworth Pr.

Transgender Care: Recommended Guidelines, Practical Information, & Personal Accounts. Gianna E. Israel & Donald E. Tarver, II. 2001. 304p. LC 97-17280. lib. bdg. 59.50 (*1-56639-571-2*); reprint ed. pap. text 22.95 (*1-56639-852-5*) Temple U Pr.

Transgenerational Family Therapies. Laura G. Roberto. 1992. LC 92-1530. (Family Therapy Ser.). 219p. 30.00 (*0-89862-107-0*) Guilford Pubns.

Transgenic Animals As Model Systems for Human Diseases. Ed. by Erwin Wagner & Franz Theuring. 1995. LC 93-18847. (Schering Foundation Workshop Ser.: Vol. 6). (Illus.). 163p. 82.95 (*0-387-56281-8*) Spr-Verlag.

Transgenic Mouse Model for Alzheimer's Disease. Dieder Moechars. 1996. (Acta Biomedica Lovaniensia Ser.: No. 122). (Illus.). 113p. (Orig.). pap. (*90-6186-727-4*) Leuven Univ BEL. *Dist:* Coronet Bks.

Transgenic Organisms: Biological & Social Implications. Ed. by J. Tomiuk et al. 1996. LC 96-6480. (Advances in Life Sciences Ser.). 263p. 83.95 (*3-7643-5262-0*) Birkhauser.

Transgenics in Endocrinology. Ed. by Martin Matzuk et al. 2001. LC 00-67291. (Contemporary Endocrinology Ser.). (Illus.). 550p. 149.50 (*0-89603-764-9*) Humana.

Transglutaminase. Ed. by Victor A. Najjar & Laszlo Lorand. 1984. (Developments in Molecular & Cellular Biochemistry Ser.). text 141.00 (*0-89838-593-8*) Kluwer Academic.

Transient Amnesia: Clinical & Neuropsychological Aspects. John R. Hodges. 1991. (Major Problems in Neurology Ser.: Vol. 24). (Illus.). 171p. text (*0-7020-1553-9*) W B Saunders GBR. *Dist:* Saunders.

Transient Enzyme Kinetics. Bagshaw. 1999. (Illus.). 200p. (Orig.). pap. 46.00 (*0-412-60310-1*, Chap & Hall NY) Chapman & Hall.

Transient Global Amnesia & Related Disorders. Ed. by Hans J. Markowitsch. 1990. LC 90-4811. (Illus.). 260p. text 58.00 (*0-920887-70-8*) Hogrefe & Huber Pubs.

Transient Ischaemic Attacks of the Brain & Eye. Graeme J. Hankey & Charles P. Warlow. 1994. (Major Problems in Neurology Ser.: Vol. 27). (Illus.). 422p. text (*0-7020-1590-3*) W B Saunders GBR. *Dist:* Saunders.

Transition from School to Adult Services in Prader-Willi Syndrome: What Parents Need to Know. Julie A. Seguin & Robert M. Hodapp. 1998. (Prader-Willi Syndrome Information Ser.: Vol. 6). 65p. pap. 10.00 (*0-9646533-1-1*) P-W Perspect.

Transition Metal Complexes As Drugs & Chemotherapeutic Agents. Nicholas Farrell. 1989. (C). text 191.50 (*90-277-2828-3*) Kluwer Academic.

***Transitional Approach to Change.** Gilles Amado. 2001. 250p. pap. (*1-85575-226-3*) Karnac Bks GBR. *Dist:* Other Pr LLC.

Transitional Care: The Problem of Alternate Level of Care in New York City. Dana G. Safran & Elizabeth A. Eastwood. 1989. (Papers: No. 13). 48p. 5.00 (*0-934459-60-6*) United Hosp Fund.

Transitional Man: The Anatomy of a Miracle. Franklin Earnest, III. 1981. LC 81-68047. 76p. pap. 7.00 (*0-914480-06-5*) Far West Edns.

Transitional Space in Mental Breakdown & Creative Integration. Peter L. Giovacchini. 1996. LC 95-53722. (Master Work Ser.). 385p. 50.00 (*1-56821-776-5*) Aronson.

Transitioning from Individual to Family Counseling. Ed. by Charles H. Huber. 1994. LC 93-37731. (Family Ser.: No. 2). 143p. pap. text 17.95 (*1-55620-132-X*, 72563) Am Coun Assn.

Transitions: Handbook of Managed Care for Inpatient to Outpatient Treatment. Ed. by Douglas H. Ruben & Chris E. Stout. 1993. LC 92-45144. 184p. 62.95 (*0-275-94064-0*, C4064, Praeger Pubs) Greenwood.

Transitions for Persons with Deaf-Blindness & Other Profound Handicaps: State of the Art. Ed. by Angela Covert & H.D. Fredericks. 1987. 180p. (Orig.). 10.00 (*0-944232-00-0*) Teaching Res.

Transitions in a Woman's Life: Major Life Events in Developmental Context. Ramona T. Mercer et al. 1989. (Focus on Women Ser.). 224p. 32.95 (*0-8261-6560-5*) Springer Pub.

Transjugular Intrahepatic Portal-Systemic Shunts. Ed. by Harold O. Conn et al. 1996. LC 95-48166. (Illus.). 400p. 108.00 (*0-89640-300-9*) Igaku-Shoin.

Translabyrinthine Acoustic Neuroma Surgery: A Surgical Manual. Mirko Tos & J. Thomsen. 1991. (Illus.). 79p. 45.00 (*0-86577-397-1*) Thieme Med Pubs.

Translocations in Solid Tumors. Colin S. Cooper & Jonathan A. Fletcher. 2001. (Medical Intelligence Unit Ser.). 262p. 99.00 (*1-58706-033-7*) Eurekah.

Transmembrane Signaling & Sensation. Ed. by Fumio Oosawa et al. 1984. (Taniguchi Symposia on Brain Sciences Ser.: No. 7). 278p. lib. bdg. (*90-6764-041-7*) VSP NLD. *Dist:* Coronet Bks.

Transmembrane Signaling Protocols. Ed. by Dafna Bar-Sagi. 1998. LC 97-45056. (Methods in Molecular Biology Ser.: Vol. 84). (Illus.). 320p. 120.00 (*0-89603-488-7*); spiral bd. 94.50 (*0-89603-432-1*) Humana.

Transmissible Spongiform Enecephalopathies: Impact on Animal & Human Health. Ed. by F. Brown. 1993. (Developments in Biological Standardization Ser.: Vol. 80). (Illus.). x, 234p. pap. 191.50 (*3-8055-5831-7*) S Karger.

Transmissible Subacute Spongiform Encephalopathies: Prion Diseases. Ed. by L. Court & B. Bodet. 1996. 508p. pap. 99.00 (*2-906077-91-7*) Elsevier.

Transmission of Depression in Families & Children: Assessment & Intervention. Ed. by Pirooz G. Sholevar. 1994. LC 93-24688. 368p. 50.00 (*1-56821-088-4*) Aronson.

Transmission of Epidemic Influenza. R. E. Hope-Simpson. 1991. (Illus.). 272p. (C). text 54.50 (*0-306-44073-3*, Kluwer Plenum) Kluwer Academic.

Transmural Plasma Flow in Atherogenesis. H. Jellinek et al. 1983. 190p. (C). (*963-05-3205-0*) Akade Kiado HUN. *Dist:* St Mut.

Transnational Evaluation of the E.C.HO Project. Ed. by Chantal van Audenhove et al. 1997. LC 98-179453. (*90-5350-690-X*) Garant Uitgevers BEL. *Dist:* Gaunt.

Transoesophageal Echocardiography in Anaesthesia. Ed. by Jan Poelaert & Karl Skarvan. 2000. (Illus.). 256p. (*0-7279-1278-X*) BMJ Pub GBR. *Dist:* AIDC.

Transorbital Intracranial Penetrating Injury. Martin T. Van Duinen. 1999. LC 99-40694. (*0-7923-5915-1*) Kluwer Academic.

Transosseous Osteosynthesis: Theoretical & Clinical Aspects of the Regeneration & Growth of Tissue. G. A. Ilizarov. 1991. (Illus.). 800p. 325.00 (*0-387-53534-9*) Spr-Verlag.

Transparencies for the Human Body in Health & Illness. Barbara Herlihy & Nancy K. Maebius. trans. (*0-7216-6113-0*) Saunders.

Transparencies to Accompany Sorensen & Luckmann's Basic Nursing: A Psychophysiologic Approach. Verolyn B. Bolander. 3rd ed. 1994. 160p. incl. trans. (*0-7216-4745-6*) Saunders.

Transparency & Refraction of the Cornea. Feher Janos. 1996. LC 97-132372. (Pathophysiology of the Eye Ser.: No. 3). 230p. pap. (*963-05-6996-5*) Akade Kiado HUN. *Dist:* Intl Spec Bk, St Mut.

Transparenzkriterien fur Pflanzliche, Homoopathische und Anthroposophische Arzneimittel. Ed. by Theodor Dingermann. 2000. (GER.). 76p. pap. 35.00 (*3-8055-7045-7*) S Karger.

Transpersonal: Psychotherapy & Counselling. John Rowan. 1993. LC 92-15268. (Illus.). 304p. (C). (gr. 13). pap. 27.95 (*0-415-05362-5*, A7787) Routledge.

Transpersonal Development: The Development Beyond Psychosynthesis. Robert Assagioli. 1991. pap. (*1-85274-062-0*) Aqrn Pr GBR. *Dist:* Harper SF.

Transpersonal Development: The Development Beyond Psychosynthesis. Roberto Assagioli. rev. ed. 1993. (*1-85538-291-1*) Thorsons GBR. *Dist:* Natl Bk Netwk.

Transpersonal Knowing: Exploring the Horizon of Consciousness. Ed. by Tobin Hart et al. 2000. LC 99-49022. (Suny Series, Transpersonal & Humanistic Psychology Ser.). x, 341p. pap. text 21.95 (*0-7914-4616-6*); (C). text 63.50 (*0-7914-4615-8*) State U NY Pr.

Transpersonal Psychology in Psychoanalytic Perspective. Michael Washburn. 1994. LC 93-38025. 367p. (C). text 26.50 (*0-7914-1953-3*); pap. text 25.95 (*0-7914-1954-1*) State U NY Pr.

Transpersonal Psychotherapy: Theory & Practice. Ed. by Elizabeth Wilde McCormick & Nigel Wellings. 2000. 224p. 74.95 (*0-8264-4845-3*); pap. 28.95 (*0-304-70678-7*) Continuum.

Transpersonal Research Methods in the Social Sciences: Honoring Human Experience. Rosemarie Anderson & William Braud. 1998. LC 98-8870. (Qualitative Ser.). 62.00 (*0-7619-1012-3*, 81383); pap. 31.00 (*0-7619-1013-1*, 81384) Sage.

Transpetalation: Beyond Quantitative & Qualitative Research, Applied to Multiple Sclerosis. Eleanor Treece. 1999. 264p. pap. 17.00 (*0-8059-4599-7*) Dorrance.

Transplant Coronary Artery Disease: The Nemesis of Heart Transplantation. Johan Van Cleemput. 2000. LC 00-691689. (Acta Biomedica Lovaniensia Ser.: No. 219). 141p. pap. (*90-5867-044-9*) Leuven Univ BEL. *Dist:* Coronet Bks.

Transplant Infections. Ed. by Raleigh A. Bowden et al. 1998. LC 98-17228. 448p. text 179.00 (*0-397-58776-7*) Lppncott W & W.

Transplant International: Proceedings of the 6th ESOT Congress, Rodos, October 25-28, 1993. Ed. by C. Hammer Munich et al. 1994. (Official Journal of the European Society for Organ Transplantation). 705p. 168.00 (*0-387-57835-8*) Spr-Verlag.

Transplant International: Proceedings of the Fifth Congress of the European Society for Organ Transplantation Maastricht, October 7-10, 1991. Ed. by G. Kootstra et al. 1992. (Official Journal of the European Society for Organ Transplantation: Vol. 5, Suppl. 1, 1992). (Illus.). 729p. 176.00 (*0-387-55342-8*) Spr-Verlag.

Transplant International, Official Journal of the European Society for Organ Transplantation Suppl. 1, Vol. 13: Proceedings of the 9th Congress of the European Society for Organ Transplantation, Osio, June 20-24, 1999. Ed. by P. F. Pfeffer. 2000. (Illus.). xviii, 622p. pap. (*3-540-67571-X*) Spr-Verlag.

Transplant Pathology: Clinical & Anatomic Principles. Ed. by Peter C. Kolbeck et al. 1994. LC 93-1867. 327p. 50.00 (*0-89189-364-4*) Am Soc Clinical.

Transplant Patient: Biological, Psychiatric & Ethical Issues in Organ Transplantation. Ed. by Paula Trzepacz & Andrea DiMartini. 2000. LC 99-25872. (Psychiatry & Medicine Ser.). (Illus.). 324p. text 64.95 (*0-521-55354-7*) Cambridge U Pr.

Transplant Production Systems: Proceedings of the International Symposium on Transplant Production Systems, Yokohama, Japan, 21-26 July 1992. Ed. by Toyoki Kozai & K. Kurata. 1992. LC 92-15554. 344p. (C). text 185.00 (*0-7923-1797-1*) Kluwer Academic.

Transplant Protocols. Ed. by Alexander M. Walker. 1990. LC 90-3166. 328p. (Orig.). 45.00 (*0-917227-05-0*) Epidemiology.

Transplant Success Stories, 1993. Ed. by Jane Schoenberg & Paul I. Terasaki. 1993. 5.00 (*1-880318-00-8*) UCLA Tissue.

Transplant Surgery. Ed. by John Forsythe. 1997. (Companion Guide to Specialist Surgical Practice Ser.: Vol. 7). (Illus.). 280p. text (*0-7020-2146-6*) W B Saunders GBR. *Dist:* Saunders.

Transplant Vascular Sclerosis. Charles Orosz. 1996. (Medicine Ser.). 251p. pap. 89.95 (*0-412-10121-1*) Chapman & Hall.

Transplant Vascular Sclerosis. Charles Orosz. 1996. LC 95-31248. (Medical Intelligence Unit Ser.). 222p. 99.00 (*1-57059-287-X*) Landes Bioscience.

Transplantation. Ed. by Graeme R. Catto. 1989. (New Clinical Applications in Nephrology Ser.). (C). text 121.50 (*0-7462-0116-8*) Kluwer Academic.

Transplantation. Leo C. Ginns et al. 1999. LC 98-37281. (Illus.). 968p. 295.00 (*0-86542-520-5*) Blackwell Sci.

Transplantation. Ed. by M. Gumpel. 1992. (Journal: Vol. 14, No. 2, 1992). (Illus.). 112p. pap. 41.75 (*3-8055-5658-6*) S Karger.

Transplantation: Anaesthesia & Critical Care Procedures at the University of Pittsburgh. Leonard Firestone. 1995. 656p. pap. 45.00 (*0-7506-9565-X*) Buttrwrth-Heinemann.

Transplantation: In Focus. J. Fabre. 2001. (In Focus Ser.). (Illus.). 86p. (C). pap. text 13.95 (*0-19-963193-X*) OUP.

Transplantation & Clinical Immunology: Proceedings of the 16th International Course, Lyon, France, 28-30 May; 1984 Symposia Fondation Merieux, 10, Vol. XVI. Ed. by J. L. Touraine et al. 1985. 302p. 192.00 (*0-444-80682-2*, Excerpta Medica) Elsevier.

Transplantation & Clinical Immunology, Vol. XVII—the Hyperimmunized Patient: Proceedings of the Seventeenth International Course, Lyon, France, 20-22 May 1985. Ed. by J. L. Touraine et al. 1986. (Symposia Foundation Merieux Ser.: Vol. 11). 264p. 150.00 (*0-444-80760-8*) Elsevier.

Transplantation & Developmental Biology of the Liver. Ed. by H. S. Rosenberg. 1991. (Perspectives in Pediatric Pathology Ser.: Vol. 14). xii, 220p. 240.00 (*3-8055-5156-8*) S Karger.

Transplantation & Replacement of Thoracic Organs: The Present Status of Biological & Mechanical Replacement. Ed. by David K. Cooper & Dimitry Novitzky. 1990. (C). text 398.00 (*0-7923-8909-3*) Kluwer Academic.

Transplantation & Replacement of Thoracic Organs: The Present Status of Biological & Mechanical Replacement of the Heart & Lungs. Ed. by D. K. Cooper et al. 2nd ed. 1997. LC 97-136519. 830p. text 350.00 (*0-7923-8898-4*) Kluwer Academic.

Transplantation Biology: Cellular & Molecular Aspects. Nicholas L. Tilney. 1996. 778p. text 189.00 (*0-397-51683-5*) Lppncott W & W.

Transplantation Biology: Cellular & Molecular Aspects. Ed. by Nicholas L. Tilney et al. 1996. (*0-516-83503-3*) Lppncott W & W.

Transplantation Drug Manual. John D. Pirsch. Ed. by William Simmons & Hans Sollinger. 3rd ed. 1999. LC 99-28833. (Vademecum Ser.). 15p. 45.00 (*1-57059-593-3*) Landes Bioscience.

Transplantation Ethics. Robert M. Veatch. 2000. LC 00-26843. (Illus.). xvii, 427p. text 65.00 (*0-87840-811-8*) Georgetown U Pr.

***Transplantation Ethics.** Robert M. Veatch. 2002. 448p. pap. text 29.95 (*0-87840-812-6*) Georgetown U Pr.

Transplantation Immunology. Ed. by Fritz H. Bach & Hugh Auchincloss. 1995. LC 94-49601. (Illus.). 424p. 165.00 (*0-471-30448-4*) Wiley.

Transplantation in Primates. Ed. by Gerald P. Murphy. 1972. (Primates in Medicine Ser.: Vol. 7). 51.50 (*3-8055-1408-5*) S Karger.

Transplantation in the 1980s: Recent Advances. Ed. by Rex Jamison. 1984. LC 84-6783. 128p. 55.00 (*0-275-91436-4*, C1436, Praeger Pubs) Greenwood.

Transplantation Nursing. Ed. by Marie T. Nolan & Sharon M. Agustine. 1995. LC 94-31323. 425p. (C). text 59.95 (*0-8385-8989-8*, A8989-4) McGraw-Hill Educ Grp.

Transplantation of Muscles in Animals. A. N. Studitsky. 1988. (C). (*81-7087-023-2*) Oxford IBH IND. *Dist:* S Asia.

Transplantation of Neural Tissue into the Spinal Cord. Gerta Vrbova et al. 1994. (Neuroscience Intelligence Unit Ser.). 128p. 99.00 (*1-57059-169-5*, LN9037) Landes Bioscience.

Transplantation of Organs & Cells: Contribution of Clinical Biochemistry to Clinical Success. Knut Kleesiek. 1997. 147.95 (*3-89412-306-0*) Blackwell Sci.

Transplantation of Ovarian & Testicular Tissues. Robert G. Gosden. 1996. (Medical Intelligence Unit Ser.). 158p. 99.00 (*1-57059-336-1*) Landes Bioscience.

Transplantation of Ovarian & Testicular Tissues. Lennart Sjolin et al. 1996. (Molecular Biology Intelligence Unit Ser.). 144p. pap. 89.95 (*0-412-10531-4*) Landes Bioscience.

Transplantation of the Liver. Ronald W. Busutil & Goran B. Klintmalm. Ed. by Lisette Bralow. 1996. (Illus.). 784p. text 275.00 (*0-7216-4942-4*) Saunders.

Transplantation of the Liver. Willis C. Maddrey. 3rd ed. 2000. LC 00-45341. (Illus.). ix, 506p. text 169.00 (*0-7817-2039-7*) Lppncott W & W.

Transplantation Pathology: A Guide for Practicing Pathologists. Ed. by Colin L. Berry & J. Pratt. 1998. (Current Topics in Pathology Ser.: Vol. 92). (Illus.). 231p. 155.00 (*3-540-64096-7*) Spr-Verlag.

Transplantation Reviews, Vol. 3. Morris & Tilney. 1989. (Illus.). 240p. text 92.00 (*0-7216-3288-2*) Saunders.

***Transplantation Surgery.** N. Hakim & G. Danovitch. 2001. LC 00-37332. (Specialist Surgery Ser.). (Illus.). xiv, 450p. 125.00 (*1-85233-286-7*) Spr-Verlag.

***Transplantation Surgery: A Companion to Specialist Surgical Practice.** John L. R. Forsythe. 2nd ed. 2001. (Illus.). 349p. (*0-7020-2588-7*) W B Saunders GBR. *Dist:* Saunders.

Transplantation Techniques & Use of Cryopreserved Allograft Cardiac Valves & Vascular Tissue. Ed. by David R. Clarke. 1989. (Illus.). 237p. (C). pap. 345.00 (*0-944903-03-7*) Adams Pub Group.

Transplantation Therapeutics. Ed. by A. P. Monaco. 1987. (Journal: Vol. 46, Suppl. 1, 1987). (Illus.). iv, 60p. pap. 20.00 (*3-8055-4642-4*) S Karger.

Transplantation Tolerance Induction. J. Wesley Alexander. 1996. (Medical Intelligence Unit Ser.). 275p. 99.00 (*1-57059-282-9*) Landes Bioscience.

Transplantation Tolerance Induction. J. Wesley Alexander & Robert A. Good. 1996. (Medical Intelligence Unit Ser.). 280p. pap. 89.95 (*0-412-10161-0*, VNR) Wiley.

Transplanting Your Head: And Other Feats of the Future. Scientific American Editors. Ed. by Peter Jedicke. 2nd ed. 2001. LC 2001-42405. (Extreme Science Ser.). 256p. pap. 14.95 (*0-312-26819-X*, St Martin Griffin) St Martin.

Transplants & Implants in Otology. Ed. by G. Babighian et al. 1988. LC 88-12784. (Illus.). 402p. text (*90-6299-047-9*) Kugler NLD. *Dist:* Lib Res.

Transplants & Implants in Otology II. Ed. by N. Yanagihara et al. 1992. LC 92-10385. (Illus.). 413p. lib. bdg. (*90-6299-084-3*) Kugler NLD. *Dist:* Lib Res.

Transplants & Implants in Otology III: Proceedings of the Third International Symposium on Transplants & Implants in Otology, Bordeaux, France, June 10-14, 1995. Ed. by M. Portmann et al. 1996. LC 96-4640. (*90-6299-142-4*) Kugler NLD. *Dist:* Lib Res.

Transport & Bioenergetics In Biomembranes. Ed. by Ryo Sato & Yasuo Kagawa. 1982. 262p. 65.00 (*0-306-41282-9*, Plenum Trade) Perseus Pubng.

Transport & Inherited Disease. Ed. by N. R. Belton & C. Toothill. 1982. text 183.00 (*0-85200-391-9*) Kluwer Academic.

Transport in the Liver: Proceedings of the 74th Falk Symposium Held in Heidelberg, Germany, January 27-18, 1994. Ed. by D. Keppler & K. Jungermann. 1994. LC 94-17600. xii, 258p. text 115.00 (*0-7923-8858-5*) Kluwer Academic.

Transport of Neurotransmitters. Ed. by D. M. Paton. 1980. (Journal: Vol. 21, No. 2). (Illus.). 74p. pap. 21.00 (*3-8055-1316-X*) S Karger.

Transport Processes in Pharmaceutical Systems. Ed. by Gordon L. Amidon. 1999. LC 99-51470. (Drugs & the Pharmaceutical Sciences Ser.: Vol. 102). (Illus.). ix, 727p. text 225.00 (*0-8247-6610-5*) Dekker.

Transport Processes in Pharmaceutical Systems. Gordon Amidon & Ping I. Lee. Date not set. (Drugs & the Pharmaceutical Sciences Ser.). (*0-8247-9374-9*) Dekker.

T U V

Transportation & Behavior. Ed. by Irwin Altman et al. 1982. LC 76-382942. (Human Behavior & Environment Ser.: Vol. 5). 304p. (C). 65.00 (*0-306-40773-6*, Plenum Trade) Perseus Pubng.

Transportation Physical Exam & Health Assessment. Jarvis. 2nd ed. 1996. 160.00 (*0-7216-6539-X*) Saunders.

Transportation Systems, Medical Ergonomics & Training. Ed. by Don Harris. 1999. (Engineering Psychology & Cognitive Ergonomics Ser.: Vol. 3). 482p. text (*1-84014-546-3*) Ashgate Pub GBR. *Dist:* Ashgate Pub Co.

Transpupillary Thermotherapy. J. G. Journee-de Korver. 1998. (Illus.). iv, 108p. (*90-6299-161-0*) Kugler NLD. *Dist:* Kugler Pubns.

Transracial Adoption: A Bibliography. Kathleen K. Harris. 1989. (C). (*0-903534-59-2*) Brit Ag for Adopt & Fost GBR. *Dist:* St Mut.

Transsexuals: Candid Answers to Private Questions. Gerald Ramsey. 1996. (Illus.). 192p. (Orig.). 24.95 (*0-89594-790-0*) Crossing Pr.

Transsexuals: Life from Both Sides. Lynn Hubschman. 2000. (Illus.). 277p. pap. text 20.00 (*0-7881-8749-X*) DIANE Pub.

Transtemporal Surgery of the Internal Auditory Canal: Proceedings. International Otoneurological Symposium Staff. Ed. by C. R. Pfaltz & Ugo Fisch. 1970. (Advances in OtoRhinoLaryngology Ser.: Vol. 17). 72.25 (*3-8055-0237-0*) S Karger.

Transthoracic Echocardiography. C. Carl Jaffe & Patrick J. Lynch. 1992. (C). 500.00 incl. disk (*1-56815-015-6*) Mosby Inc.

Transurethral Surgery. W. Mauermayer. 1982. (Illus.). 473p. 535.00 (*0-387-11869-1*) Spr-Verlag.

Transvaginal Colour Doppler: The Scientific Basis & Practical Application of Colour Doppler in Gynaecology. Ed. by Tom H. Bourne et al. 1995. LC 95-2189. (Illus.). 206p. 154.00 (*3-540-58432-3*) Spr-Verlag.

Transvaginal Sonography. I. E. Timor-Trishsch & Shraga Rottem. 2nd ed. 1991. (Arnold Publication). (Illus.). 554p. text 97.95 (*0-412-04651-2*) OUP.

Transvaginal Sonography. Ilan E. Timor-Tritsch. 3rd ed. 1998. pap. 85.00 (*0-412-98231-5*, T5303) Chapman & Hall.

Transvaginal Sonography: A Clinical Atlas. Arthur C. Fleischer & Donna M. Kepple. 2nd ed. 1995. LC 95-7919. 448p. text 115.00 (*0-397-51513-8*) Lppncott W & W.

Transvaginal Sonography in Infertility. Bill Yee. 1995. LC 95-17693. (Illus.). 224p. text 99.00 (*0-7817-0305-0*) Lppncott W & W.

Transvaginal Sonography of the Normal & Abnormal Fetus. I. E. Timor-Tritsch. Ed. by M. Bronshtein & E. Z. Zimmer. 2001. LC 00-40673. (Illus.). xii, 268p. 114.95 (*1-85070-693-X*, Parthenon Pbng) CRC Pr.

Transvaginal Ultrasound. Melvin G. Dodson. 2nd ed. 1994. LC 94-36305. (Illus.). 352p. text (*0-443-08953-1*) Church.

Transverse Paraphysics: The New Science of Space, Time & Gravity Control. J. G. Gallimore. 1982. LC 82-50823. (Illus.). 359p. (Orig.). pap. text 35.00 (*0-9603536-4-X*) Tesla Bk Co.

Transvestism: A Handbook for Psychologists, Psychiatrists & Counsellors. Harry Brierley. 1979. (Illus.). 160p. (*0-08-022268-4*) Pergamon Repr GBR. *Dist:* Franklin.

Transvestite & the Transexual: A Case Study of Public Categories & Private Indentities. Dave King. 1993. 229p. text (*1-85628-134-5*) Avebry GBR. *Dist:* Ashgate Pub Co.

Transvestites & Transsexuals: Toward a Theory of Cross-Gender Behavior. R. F. Docter. 1988. LC 88-19586. (Perspectives in Sexuality Ser.). (Illus.). 266p. (C). 45.00 (*0-306-42878-4*, Plenum Trade) Perseus Pubng.

Tranx: Minor Tranquilizers, Major Problems. Jim Parker. rev. ed. 2000. (Illus.). pap. 3.50 (*0-89230-180-5*) Do It Now.

Trastorno por Deficit de Atencion e Hiperactividad: Un Manual de Trabajo Clinico. Russell A. Barkley et al. Tr. by Maribel Matos et al. 2nd ed. 1998. (SPA.). 174p. pap. text 32.00 (*1-57230-388-3*, 0388) Guilford Pubns.

Trastornos Digestivos (Digestive System Problems) Como Controlarlos. Frank Calderon. 1998. (SPA.). 192p. pap. 5.95 (*0-939193-22-1*) Edit Concepts.

Tratado de Enfermeria Medico Quirurgica. Lillian S. Brunner. 6th ed. 1989. text 79.95 (*0-07-104007-2*) McGraw.

Tratado de Enfermeria Practica. Beverly W. Dugas. 4th ed. 1986. pap. text 39.95 (*0-07-104008-0*) McGraw.

Tratado de la Epidemia e de la Pestilenc: Biblioteca Nacional de Madrid, I-51. Vasco De Taranto. Ed. by Maria Purificacion Zabia. 1987. (Medieval Spanish Medical Texts Ser.: No. 16). (SPA.). 6p. 10.00 incl. fiche (*0-940639-12-2*) Hispanic Seminary.

Tratado de la Phisonomia: Biblioteca Nacional, Madrid, I-51. Vernon Hicks. Ed. by Maria Nieves-Sanchez & Tim Dennison. 1987. (Medieval Spanish Medical Texts Ser.: No. 14). (SPA., Illus.). 8p. 10.00 incl. fiche (*0-940639-10-6*) Hispanic Seminary.

Tratado Nuevo: Alvarez Chanca, Biblioteca Nacional, Madrid, I-51. Ed. by Maria Purificacion Zabia. 1987. (Medieval Spanish Medical Texts Ser.: No. 19). (SPA.). 6p. 10.00 incl. fiche (*0-940639-15-7*) Hispanic Seminary.

Tratado Util, Licenciado Fores: Biblioteca Nacional de Madrid, I-51. Ed. by Maria Purificacion Zabia. 1987. (Medieval Spanish Medical Texts Ser.: No. 17). (SPA.). 6p. 10.00 incl. fiche (*0-940639-13-0*) Hispanic Seminary.

Tratameinto Medico Emergencia para Adultos. Stephen Vogel & David H. Manhoff. 1991. (SPA.). pap. 7.95 (*0-916363-09-0*) Beechwood Hlthbks.

Tratamiento de las Fracturas en Atencion Primaria (Fracture Management for Primary Care. M. Patrice Eiff et al. 1998. (ENG & SPA., Illus.). 293p. (*84-8174-431-X*) Mosby-Doyma Libros ESP. *Dist:* Mosby Inc, Saunders.

Tratamiento Endodoncico. Franklin S. Weine. 5th ed. 1997. (C). text 120.96 (*84-8174-189-2*) Mosby Inc.

Tratamiento Medico de Emergencia para Infantes. Stephen Vogel & David H. Manhoff. 1990. pap. 7.95 (*0-916363-03-1*) Beechwood Hlthbks.

Tratamiento Medico de Emergencia para Ninos. Stephen Vogel & David H. Manhoff. 1990. pap. 7.95 (*0-916363-02-3*) Beechwood Hlthbks.

Trauma. Ed. by Ian Greaves et al. 1998. LC 97-36978. (An Arnold Publication). (Illus.). 448p. pap. text (*0-340-69201-4*) E A GBR. *Dist:* OUP.

Trauma M. Houts. 1959. 1787.00 (*0-8205-1740-2*) Bender.

Trauma. Frederick A. Jakobiec. 1995. 39.00 (*0-316-06076-3*, Little Brwn Med Div) Lppncott W & W.

Trauma. Skinner. 1999. (Companion Series to Bailey & Love's Short Practice of Surgery). (Illus.). 512p. (C). pap. 36.95 (*0-412-61950-4*); pap. 110.00 (*0-412-61940-7*) Chapman & Hall (Chap & Hall NY).

Trauma. D. V. Skinner. 1999. (Illus.). 380p. 98.50 (*0-340-74101-5*) OUP.

Trauma. Ernest E. Moore et al. 3rd ed. 1998. (Illus.). (C). pap. text 165.00 (*0-8385-9010-1*, A9010-8, Apple Lange Med) McGraw.

Trauma. Ed. by Kenneth L. Mattox et al. 4th ed. 1999. LC 99-12957. (Illus.). 1514p. pap. 199.00 (*0-8385-9012-8*) McGraw-Hill Prof.

Trauma: A Genealogy. Ruth Leys. 1999. LC 99-52681. (Illus.). x, 318p. pap. text 19.00 (*0-226-47766-5*) U Ch Pr.

***Trauma: A Practitioner's Guide to Counselling.** Ed. by Thom Spiers. 2001. LC 2001-37525. (*0-415-18694-3*); pap. (*0-415-18695-1*) Brunner-Routledge.

Trauma: A Scientific Basis for Care. Ed. by Emin Kaya Alpar & Peter Gosling. 1999. (An Arnold Publication). (Illus.). 400p. text (*0-340-70093-9*) E A GBR. *Dist:* OUP.

Trauma: An Osteopathic Approach. Jean-Pierre Barral & Alain Croibier. 2000. LC 99-72891. (Illus.). vii, 329p. (C). 60.00 (*0-939616-32-7*) Eastland.

Trauma: Explorations in Memory. Cathy Caruth. 1995. LC 94-46167. 288p. pap. text 18.95 (*0-8018-5007-X*) Johns Hopkins.

***Trauma: Practical Application of Recent Advances.** Ed. by David W. Yates. 1999. (British Medical Bulletin Ser.: Vol. 55, No. 4). 237p. pap. (*1-85315-440-7*) Royal Soc of Medicine Pr Ltd GBR. *Dist:* Balogh.

Trauma & Adolescence. Ed. by Max Sugar. 1999. LC 98-52743. (Monograph Series of the International Society for Adolescent Psychiatry Ser.: Vol. 1). 322p. 49.95 (*0-8236-6626-3*, 06626) Intl Univs Pr.

Trauma & Fulfillment Therapy: A Wholistic Framework. Paul Valent. 1998. LC 98-30412. (Series in Trauma & Loss). 62.95 (*0-87630-938-4*); pap. 26.95 (*0-87630-939-2*) Brunner-Routledge.

Trauma & Its Metabolic Problems. Ed. by R. N. Barton. 1985. (British Medical Bulletin Ser.: Vol. 41, No. 3). (Illus.). 104p. (*0-443-03250-5*) Church.

Trauma & Its Wake Vol. 1: The Study & Treatment of Post-Traumatic Stress Disorder. Ed. by Charles R. Figley. 1985. LC 84-29344. (Psychosocial Stress Ser.: No. 4). 484p. text 50.95 (*0-87630-385-8*) Brunner-Routledge.

Trauma & Its Wake Vol. 2: Traumatic Stress Theory, Research, & Intervention. Ed. by Charles R. Figley. 1986. LC 84-29344. (Psychosocial Stress Ser.: No. 8). 368p. text 49.95 (*0-87630-431-5*) Brunner-Routledge.

Trauma & Memory. Linda M. Williams & Victoria L. Banyard. 1998. LC 98-25342. 384p. 97.95 (*0-7619-0771-8*, 80873); pap. 46.95 (*0-7619-0772-6*, 80874) Sage.

Trauma & Memory: Clinical & Legal Controversies. Ed. by Paul S. Applebaum et al. 1997. (Illus.). 568p. text 59.50 (*0-19-510065-4*) OUP.

Trauma & Mobile Radiography. Michael W. Drafke. 2nd ed. 2000. (Illus.). 392p. 26.95 (*0-8036-0694-X*) Davis Co.

Trauma & Recovery: The Aftermath of Violence, from Domestic Abuse to Political Terror. Judith Herman. 1997. LC 97-12136. 288p. pap. 16.00 (*0-465-08730-2*) Basic.

Trauma & Self. Charles B. Strozier & Michael Flynn. 1996. LC 96-1354. 280p. 58.50 (*0-8476-8228-5*); pap. 22.95 (*0-8476-8229-3*) Rowman.

Trauma & the Vietnam War Generation: Report of Findings from the National Vietnam Veterans Readjustment Study. Intro. by Richard A. Kulka et al. 1990. LC 89-71185. (Brunner-Mazel Psychosocial Stress Ser.: No. 18). (Illus.). 352p. 34.95 (*0-87630-573-7*) Brunner-Routledge.

Trauma & Transformation: Growing in the Aftermath of Suffering. Richard G. Tedeschi & Lawrence G. Calhoun. 1995. LC 95-11803. 163p. (C). 86.95 (*0-8039-5256-2*, 4453) Sage.

Trauma Assessments: A Clinician's Guide. Eve B. Carlson. 1997. LC 97-17254. 307p. text 30.00 (*1-57230-251-8*, 0231) Guilford Pubns.

Trauma Care Beyond the Resuscitation Room: Beyond Resuscitation Room. Ed. by Peter A. Driscoll & David V. Skinner. 1998. 312p. text (*0-7279-0933-9*) BMJ Pub GBR. *Dist:* AIDC.

Trauma Care Manual. Ed. by Ian Greaves et al. 2001. (An Arnold Publication). 339p. (Orig.). pap. text (*0-340-75979-8*) E A GBR. *Dist:* OUP.

Trauma Care Systems: Clinical, Financial, & Political Considerations. Ed. by John G. West et al. 1983. LC 83-11223. 182p. 59.95 (*0-275-91418-6*, C1418, Praeger Pubs) Greenwood.

Trauma Code: On the Scene with Fire & Rescue. Sonny Shepherd. 1996. (Illus.). 130p. (Orig.). pap. 24.95 (*0-9655450-6-7*) Raven Ent.

Trauma, Dissociation, & Impulse Dyscontrol in Eating Disorders. Johan Vanderlinden & Walter Vandereycken. 1997. LC 97-9766. 228p. 29.95 (*0-87630-843-4*) Brunner-Routledge.

Trauma, Growth, & Personality. Phyllis Greenacre. 1969. LC 71-75188. reprint ed. 50.00 (*0-8236-6645-X*) Intl Univs Pr.

Trauma Handbook. Ernest Moore. 1999. (C). pap. text 35.00 (*0-8385-9011-X*) Appleton & Lange.

Trauma in the Lives of Children: Crisis & Stress Management Techniques for Counselors, Teachers, & Other Professionals. Kendall Johnson. 2nd ed. 1998. LC 97-31056. (gr. k-12). 256p. 29.95 (*0-89793-233-1*); (Illus.). 352p. pap. 19.95 (*0-89793-232-3*) Hunter Hse.

Trauma Informatics. Ed. by Kimball I. Maull & Jeffrey S. Augenstein. 1998. LC 97-8491. (Computers in Health Care Ser.). (Illus.). 282p. 64.95 (*0-387-94359-5*) Spr-Verlag.

Trauma Management. David J. Kreis & Geraldo Gomez. 1989. 600p. 120.00 (*0-316-50371-1*, Little Brwn Med Div) Lppncott W & W.

Trauma Management: An Emergency Medicine Approach. Peter C. Ferrera et al. 1999. (Illus.). 730p. text 95.00 (*0-323-00210-2*) Mosby Inc.

Trauma Manual. Andrew Peitzman et al. 1997. LC 97-29878. (Illus.). 624p. spiral bd. 39.95 (*0-316-69834-2*, Little Brwn Med Div) Lppncott W & W.

Trauma, Memory, & Dissociation. Ed. by J. Douglas Bremner & Charles R. Marmar. 1998. LC 97-3211. (Progress in Psychiatry Ser.: Vol. 54). 439p. text 56.00 (*0-88048-753-4*, 8753) Am Psychiatric.

Trauma Nursing: Comprehensive Curriculum. Elizabeth W. Bayley & Turcke. 1992. (Illus.). (C). text 54.95 (*0-86720-628-4*, 628-4) Jones & Bartlett.

Trauma Nursing: From Resuscitation Through Rehabilitation. Virginia D. Cardona et al. 2nd ed. 1993. LC 92-49094. (Illus.). 944p. text 104.00 (*0-7216-4333-7*) Saunders.

***Trauma Nursing: From Resuscitation Through Rehabilitation.** Karen A. McQuillan et al. 3rd ed. 2001. LC 2001-42916. (Illus.). 955p. (*0-7216-8441-6*) Saunders.

Trauma Nursing: Principles & Practice. Barbara A. Knezevich Brown. 2nd ed. 1992. (Illus.). 638p. (C). text 54.95 (*0-8385-9006-3*, A9006-6) McGraw-Hill Educ Grp.

Trauma Nursing: The Art & Science. Janet A. Neff & Pamela S. Kidd. 1992. LC 92-16291. (Illus.). 808p. (C). (gr. 13). text 57.95 (*0-8016-6655-4*, 06655) Mosby Inc.

Trauma of Birth. Otto Rank. 1994. LC 93-21385. (Illus.). 256p. reprint ed. pap. 7.95 (*0-486-27974-X*) Dover.

Trauma of the Foot & Ankle. Bruce Sangeorzan. 1996. text (*0-7817-0300-X*) Lppncott W & W.

Trauma of the Middle Ear. Michael Strohm. 1986. (Advances in OtoRhinoLaryngology Ser.: Vol. 35). (Illus.). x, 254p. 151.50 (*3-8055-4087-6*) S Karger.

Trauma of the Nose & Paranasal Sinuses. Robert H. Mathog et al. Ed. by Howard Levine. 1994. LC 94-26571. (Rhinology & Sinusology Ser.). (Illus.). 184p. 79.00 (*0-86577-526-5*) Thieme Med Pubs.

Trauma of the Spine. B. Wimmer et al. 1990. (Radiology of the Spine Ser.). (Illus.). 90p. 118.00 (*0-387-50977-1*) Spr-Verlag.

Trauma of War: Stress & Recovery in Vietnam Veterans. Ed. by Stephen M. Sonnenberg et al. 1985. LC 85-6094. 454p. text 25.95 (*0-88048-048-3*, 8048) Am Psychiatric.

Trauma-Organized Systems: Physical & Sexual Abuse in Families. Arnon Bentovim. rev. ed. 1992. 148p. pap. text (*1-85575-012-0*) Karnac Bks GBR. *Dist:* Other Pr LLC.

Trauma Radiography Papoose Table: Trauma Radiography Made Easier by This Invention. Ricardo Scott. 1999. (Ricardo Re-Invents Radiography Beyond 2000 Ser.). (Illus.). 75p. pap. (*1-58470-016-5*, RAS1949) Crnerstone GA.

Trauma Radiology Companion: Methods, Guidelines & Imaging Fundamentals. Eric J. Stern. 1997. LC 97-4092. (Illus.). 416p. pap. text 79.95 (*0-397-51733-5*) Lppncott W & W.

Trauma Ready Reference. Susan B. Sheehy. 1994. (Illus.). 44p. (C). (gr. 13). spiral bd. 15.00 (*0-8151-7823-9*, 24839) Mosby Inc.

Trauma Recovery & Empowerment: A Clinician's Guide for Working with Women in Groups. Maxine Harris. 1998. LC 98-23590. (Illus.). 432p. 32.95 (*0-684-84323-4*) Free Pr.

Trauma, Repetition & Affect Regulation: The Work of Paul Russell. Ed. by Judith Guss Teicholz & Daniel Kreigman. 1999. LC 98-36921. 154p. pap. 22.00 (*1-892746-00-X*) Other Pr LLC.

Trauma Research Methodology. Ed. by Eve B. Carlson. 1996. LC 95-26829. viii, 291p. (Orig.). pap. text 18.95 (*0-9629164-8-X*, CATR) Sidran Pr.

Trauma Response: Treatment for Emotional Injury. Diane S. Everstine & Louis Everstine. 1993. LC 92-49171. 240p. (C). 27.95 (*0-393-70123-9*) Norton.

Trauma Secrets. Ed. by Gideon P. Naude et al. 1998. LC 98-27476. (Secrets Ser.). (Illus.). 300p. pap. 39.95 (*1-56053-256-4*) Hanley & Belfus.

Trauma, Sepsis, & Shock: The Physiological Basis of Therapy. George H. A. Clowes, Jr. 1988. (Science & Practice of Surgery Ser.: Vol. 15). (Illus.). 616p. text 190.00 (*0-8247-7502-3*) Dekker.

Trauma Surgery. Donald D. Trunkey et al. 4th ed. 1993. (Rob & Smith's Operative Surgery Ser.). (Illus.). 482p. (C). text 275.00 (*0-407-00677-X*, Chap & Hall NY) Chapman & Hall.

Trauma Surgery & Surgical Critical Care: The Requisitese. Hiatt et al. 2000. (Illus.). 544p. (C). (gr. 13). text 65.00 (*0-8151-2624-7*, 31643) Mosby Inc.

Trauma to the Genito-Urinary Tract: A Practical Guide to Management. Nicholas Cetti & Roger S. Kirby. 1997. LC 96-39334. 96p. pap. text 63.00 (*0-7506-1587-7*) Buttrwrth-Heinemann.

Trauma to the Middle & Inner Ear. Michael D. Dilea et al. 1997. LC 96-50974. (Self-Instructional Package Ser.). (Illus.). 60p. (Orig.). pap. text 25.00 (*1-56772-054-4*, 5506300) AAO-HNS.

Trauma, Transformation, & Healing: An Integrative Approach to Theory, Research, & Post-Traumatic Therapy. John P. Wilson. 1989. LC 89-639. (Psychosocial Stress Ser.: No. 14). 368p. text 47.95 (*0-87630-540-0*) Brunner-Routledge.

Trauma Victim: Practical Suggestions. Hyer, Lee, and Associates Staff. 1994. 768p. (C). 45.95 (*1-55959-047-5*) Accel Devel.

Traumatic Abuse & Neglect of Children. Gertrude Williams & John Money. abr. ed. 1982. LC 79-3684. 400p. pap. text 20.95 (*0-8018-2926-7*) Johns Hopkins.

Traumatic & Reconstructive Urology. Jack W. McAninch. Ed. by Richard Zorab. 1996. LC 95-10055. 640p. text 163.00 (*0-7216-3886-4*) Saunders.

Traumatic Aphasia: Its Syndromes, Psychology & Treatment. A. R. Luria. Tr. by Douglas M. Bowden. 1970. LC 68-17903. (Janua Linguarum, Ser. Major: No. 5). text (*90-279-0717-X*) Mouton.

Traumatic Bond Between the Psychotherapist & Managed Care. Ed. by Karen Weisgerber. 1998. LC 98-23700. xvi, 264p. 40.00 (*0-7657-0180-4*) Aronson.

Traumatic Brain Edema. Ed. by F. Cohadon et al. 1987. (FIDIA Research Ser.). 186p. 90.00 (*0-387-96507-6*) Spr-Verlag.

Traumatic Brain Injury. Donald W. Marion. 1998. LC 98-17720. (Illus.). 320p. 99.00 (*0-86577-727-6*) Thieme Med Pubs.

Traumatic Brain Injury. Bruce E. Murdoch & Deborah G. Theodoros. 2001. LC 00-52371. 416p. pap. text 57.95 (*0-7693-0017-0*) Thomson Learn.

Traumatic Brain Injury: Evaluation & Litigation. Richard W. Petrocelli et al. 1994. 643p. 95.00 (*1-55834-172-2*, 65861-10, MICHIE) LEXIS Pub.

Traumatic Brain Injury: Mechanisms of Damage, Assessment, Intervention, & Outcome. Ed. by Erin D. Bigler. 1990. LC 90-3855. 458p. text 41.00 (*0-89079-201-1*, 1484) PRO-ED.

Traumatic Brain Injury: Pathophysiology & Neuropsychological Evaluation, Vol. 1. Ralph M. Reitan & Deborah Wolfson. 1986. LC 86-60951. (Illus.). 425p. text 59.95 (*0-934515-06-9*) Neuropsych Pr.

Traumatic Brain Injury: Recovery & Rehabilitation, Vol. 2. Ralph M. Reitan & Deborah Wolfson. 1987. LC 86-60952. (Illus.). 400p. text 59.95 (*0-934515-07-7*) Neuropsych Pr.

Traumatic Brain Injury Activities: Back into Life. Andrew K. Gruen & Lynn S. Gruen. 1994. LC 93-46707. pap. 42.00 (*0-930599-95-0*) Thinking Pubns.

Traumatic Brain Injury & Neuropsychological Impairment. R. S. Parker. 1990. (Illus.). 452p. 126.00 (*0-387-97239-0*) Spr-Verlag.

Traumatic Brain Injury in Children & Adolescents: A Sourcebook for Teachers & Other School Personnel. Mary P. Mira et al. 1992. LC 92-3454. 152p. (Orig.). pap. text 21.00 (*0-89079-531-2*, 4037) PRO-ED.

Traumatic Brain Injury in Children & Adolescents: A Sourcebook for Teachers & Other School Personnel. Janet S. Tyler & Mary P. Mira. 2nd ed. 1999. LC 98-30833. (*0-89079-805-2*) PRO-ED.

***Traumatic Brain Injury in Children & Adolescents: Assessment & Intervention.** Margaret Semrud-Clikeman. 2001. LC 2001-23143. (Guilford School Practitioner Ser.). (Illus.). xii, 211p. (*1-57230-686-6*) Guilford Pubns.

Traumatic Brain Injury Rehabilitation. Ed. by Mark J. Ashley & David K. Krych. 1995. LC 95-7284. 448p. 139.95 (*0-8493-9463-5*, 9463) CRC Pr.

*Traumatic Brain Injury Rehabilitation.** Chamberlain. 1995. pap. 35.95 (*0-412-48970-8*) Chapman & Hall.

Traumatic Brain Injury Rehabilitation: A Guide for Speech-Language Pathologists. Rita J. Gillis. 1996. 342p. text 49.99 (*0-7506-9650-8*) Buttrwrth-Heinemann.

Traumatic Brain Injury Rehabilitation: Children & Adolescents. Mark Ylvisaker. 2nd ed. 1997. LC 97-26005. 476p. text 64.99 (*0-7506-9972-8*) Buttrwrth-Heinemann.

Traumatic Brain Injury Rehabilitation: Services, Treatments & Outcomes. Ed. by M. Anne Chamberlain et al. 1995. LC 95-69154. 286p. pap. 45.00 (*1-56593-307-9*, 0631) Singular Publishing.

Traumatic Disorders of the Ankle. Ed. by W. C. Hamilton. 1984. (Illus.). 293p. 200.00 (*0-387-90831-5*) Spr-Verlag.

Traumatic Disorders of the Knee. Ed. by John M. Siliski. 1994. LC 93-46007. (Illus.). 431p. 196.00 (*0-387-94171-1*) Spr-Verlag.

Traumatic Events & Mental Health. L. Stephen O'Brien. 1998. LC 97-22865. (Psychiatry & Medicine Ser.). (Illus.). 312p. (C). text 110.00 (*0-521-57027-1*); pap. text 46.95 (*0-521-57886-8*) Cambridge U Pr.

Traumatic Events Treatment Planner. Tammi Kolski et al. 2001. LC 00-43922. 272p. pap. 175.00 incl. disk (*0-471-39588-9*) Wiley.

Traumatic Experiences of Nurses: When Your Profession Becomes a Nightmare. Huub Buyssen. 1996. LC 96-164781. 112p. pap. (*1-85302-377-9*) Jessica Kingsley GBR. *Dist:* Taylor & Francis.

Traumatic Hip Dislocation in Childhood. A. Barquet. 1987. (Illus.). 146p. 94.00 (*0-387-17009-X*) Spr-Verlag.

Traumatic Incident Reduction (TIR) Gerald D. French & Chrys Harris. 1998. LC 98-3810. (Innovations in Psychology Ser.). 216p. 49.95 (*1-57444-215-5*, SL2155) St Lucie Pr.

Traumatic Stress: From Theory to Practice. Ed. by John R. Freedy & Stevan E. Hobfoll. 1995. (Series on Stress & Coping). (Illus.). 420p. (C). 62.50 (*0-306-45020-8*, Plenum Trade) Perseus Pubng.

Traumatic Stress: The Effects of Overwhelming Experience on Mind, Body & Society. Ed. by Bessel A. Van der Kolk et al. 1996. LC 96-10818. 596p. 62.00 (*1-57230-088-4*, 0088) Guilford Pubns.

Traumatic Stress in Critical Occupations: Recognition, Consequences & Treatment. Douglas Paton & John M. Violanti. 1996. LC 95-47069. (Illus.). 260p. 65.95 (*0-398-06577-2*); pap. 43.95 (*0-398-06578-0*) C C Thomas.

Traumatic Subarachnoid Haemorrhage. A. Kakarieka. 1996. LC 96-3359. (Illus.). 109p. pap. 32.95 (*3-540-60771-4*) Spr-Verlag.

Traumatized Hand & Wrist: Radiographic & Anatomic Correlation. Gelula. 1991. (Illus.). 288p. text 91.00 (*0-7216-1217-2*) Saunders.

Traumatologie und Rehabilitation No. 2: Organverletzungen. Ed. by U. Laffer et al. 1992. (Basler Beitraege zur Chirurgie Ser.: Vol. 4). (Illus.). vi, 118p. 77.50 (*3-8055-5459-1*) S Karger.

Traumatology of the Skull Base: Anatomy, Clinical & Radiological Diagnosis, Operative Treatment. Ed. by Madjid Samii & J. Brihaye. 1983. (Illus.). 240p. 79.95 (*0-387-12528-0*) Spr-Verlag.

Travel & Tropical Medicine Manual. Elaine C. Jong & Russell McMullen. 2nd ed. 1995. (Illus.). 448p. pap. text 52.00 (*0-7216-4214-4*) Saunders.

Travel & Tropical Medicine Manual. Jong. 3rd ed. 1999. (C). text (*0-7216-7678-2*) Saunders.

Travel for the Disabled: A Handbook of Travel Resources & 500 Worldwide Access Guides. Helen Hecker. l.t. ed. LC 85-16471. (Illus.). 192p. 19.95 (*0-933261-00-4*) Twin Peaks Pr.

Travel Health Clinic Pocket Guide to Healthy Travel. Lawrence Bryson. 1994. 175p. (Orig.). pap. 13.95 (*0-9624945-4-2*) Silvercat Pubns.

*Travel Medicine.** Pollard & Murdoch. 2001. (Fast Facts Ser.). (Illus.). 152p. pap. (*1-899541-59-4*) Health Pr GBR. *Dist:* JAMCO Dist.

Travel Medicine. Ed. by R. Steffen et al. 1989. (Illus.). 596p. 127.00 (*0-387-19356-1*) Spr-Verlag.

*Travel Medicine: Color Guide.** Eric Walker et al. 2001. (Illus.). 147p. pap. (*0-443-06164-5*) Church GBR. *Dist:* Saunders.

Traveler's Diarrhea: Recent Advances. Ed. by C. Scarpignato & P. Rampal. 1995. (Journal: Vol. 41, Suppl. 1, 1995). (Illus.). iv, 82p. pap. 24.50 (*3-8055-6125-3*) S Karger.

Travelers Guide to International Drugs: European, Vol. 1. G. John DiGregorio et al. 2000. (Travelers Guide To International Drugs: 1). 150p. pap. 8.95 (*0-942447-33-6*) Med Surveill.

*Travelers Guide to International Drugs: European 2001.** G. John DiGregorio et al. rev. ed. 2000. 155p. pap. 14.00 (*0-942447-39-5*) Med Surveill.

Travelers Guide to International Drugs: European Volume II, Vol. 1. G. John DiGregorio et al. 2000. (Travelers Guide To International Drugs). 150p. pap. 8.95 (*0-942447-34-4*) Med Surveill.

*Travelers Guide to International Drugs: Middle East.** G. John DiGregorio et al. 116p. pap. 14.00 (*0-942447-32-8*) Med Surveill.

*Travelers Guide to International Drugs: Western Hemisphere 2001** G. John DiGregorio et al. rev. ed. 2000. (Travelers Guide to International Drugs Ser.). 129p. pap. 14.00 (*0-942447-40-9*) Med Surveill.

Travelers' Guide to U. S. Certified Doctors Abroad. 1976. LC 76-10128. 9.95 (*0-672-50833-8*, Bobbs) Macmillan.

Traveler's Health Sourcebook: Basic Consumer Health Information for Travelers. Ed. by Joyce Brennfleck Shannon. 2000. LC 00-36311. (Health Reference Ser.). (Illus.). xv, 635p. lib. bdg. 78.00 (*0-7808-0384-1*) Omnigraphics Inc.

Traveling . . . Like Everybody Else: A Practical Guide for Disabled Travelers. Jacqueline Freedman & Susan Gersten. 1987. 224p. pap. 11.95 (*0-915361-77-9*) Lambda Pubs.

Travell & Simons' Myofascial Pain & Dysfunction Vol. 1: The Trigger Point Manual, Upper Half of Body, Volume 1: The Upper Extremities. David G. Simons et al. 2nd ed. 1998. LC 98-36642. 970p. 102.00 (*0-683-08363-5*) Lppncott W & W.

Travell & Simons' Trigger Point Flip Charts. Janet G. Travell & David G. Simons. 1996. (Illus.). 24p. 61.00 (*0-683-18008-8*) Lppncott W & W.

Traveller's Guide to Homeopathy. Phyllis Speight. 1990. 64p. (Orig.). pap. 12.95 (*0-8464-1337-X*) Beekman Pubs.

Travellers Guide to Homoeopathy. Phyllis Speight. 1989. 111p. pap. (*0-85207-212-0*) C W Daniel GBR. *Dist:* Natl Bk Netwk.

Travellers Medical Services Directory: 1993 Edition. Ed. by Milan Korcok. 1992. 144p. pap. 7.95 (*0-9635675-0-0*) Intl Med Srvs.

Travels with a Stethoscope: A Physician Looks at the 20th Century. Ronald H. Girdwood. 1989. 250p. (C). text (*0-85976-334-X*) J Donald GBR. *Dist:* St Mut.

Trazodone, New Avenues in Psycho-Pharmaco-Therapy: Proceedings of the International Symposium, Montreal, October, 1973. Ed. by T. Ban & B. Silvestrini. 1974. (Modern Problems of Pharmacopsychiatry Ser.: Vol. 9). 250p. 65.25 (*3-8055-1718-1*) S Karger.

Treadmill Walking: A Motivational Resource for Treadmill Training. R. Sweetgall & Robert Neeves. 1989. 96p. pap. 9.95 (*0-939041-08-1*) Creative Walking.

Trease & Evans' Pharmacognosy. Evans. 14th ed. 1996. pap. text 78.95 (*0-7020-1899-6*) Saunders.

Treasure of Euonymus: Conteyninge the Hid Secretes of Nature. Conrad Gesner. Tr. by P. Morwyng. 1969. LC 63-6477. (English Experience Ser.: No. 97). 408p. reprint ed. 45.00 (*90-221-0097-9*) Walter J Johnson.

Treasury of Medical Humor. Ed. by James E. Myers. 1992. LC 92-71388. 350p. (Orig.). pap. 10.95 (*0-942936-21-3*) Lincoln-Herndon Pr.

Treasury of Natural First Aid Remedies from A-Z. James Kusick. 1994. LC 94-30472. 368p. (C). pap. text 11.95 (*0-13-063181-7*) P-H.

Treasury of Veterinary Humor. Ed. by Seymour Glasofer. 1997. LC 97-74590. 200p. pap. 12.95 (*0-942936-33-7*) Lincoln-Herndon Pr.

Treat Me Right! Understanding the Ethical Dilemmas Facing Doctors & Patients. Bruce Hatfield. 2nd ed. 1996. 192p. pap. (*1-55145-085-2*) NStone Publ.

Treat Your Back Without Surgery: The Best Non-Surgical Alternatives to Eliminating Back & Neck Pain. Stephen H. Hochschuler & Bob Reznik. 1998. LC 98-4613. (Illus.). 224p. 24.95 (*0-89793-235-8*); pap. 14.95 (*0-89793-234-X*) Hunter Hse.

Treat Your Child the Natural Way. Amanda Cochrane. 2001. pap. (*0-00-711073-1*) Thorsons GBR. *Dist:* Natl Bk Netwk.

Treat Your Own Neck. Robin A. McKenzie. 3rd ed. 1997. (Illus.). 63p. reprint ed. pap. text (*0-473-00209-4*) Spinal Pubns Ltd NZL. *Dist:* Orthopedic Phys.

Treating Abused Adolescents. Eliana Gil. 1996. LC 96-12550. 228p. pap. 22.00 (*1-57230-115-5*, 0115); text 42.00 (*1-57230-114-7*) Guilford Pubns.

Treating Abused Adolescents: A Program for Providing Individual & Group Therapy. Darlene A. Merchant. 1990. (gr. 8-12). pap. text 14.95 (*1-55691-017-7*, 177) Learning Pubns.

Treating Acromegaly: 100 Years On. Ed. by J. A. Wass. 1994. 221p. pap. 29.95 (*1-898099-05-7*) Blackwell Sci.

Treating Addiction as a Human Process. Edward J. Khantzian. 1999. LC 98-36955. 712p. 70.00 (*0-7657-0186-3*) Aronson.

Treating Addictive Behaviors. Ed. by William R. Miller & Nick Heather. 2nd ed. 1998. LC 98-27475. (Applied Clinical Psychology Ser.). (Illus.). 372p. (C). text 54.50 (*0-306-45852-7*, Kluwer Plenum) Kluwer Academic.

Treating Addictive Behaviors: Processes of Change. W. R. Miller & N. H. Heather. 1986. (Applied Clinical Psychology Ser.). 484p. 75.00 (*0-306-42248-4*, Plenum Trade) Perseus Pubng.

Treating Adolescents. Ed. by Hans Steiner et al. 1996. LC 95-44176. (Library of Current Clinical Technique). 448p. pap. 33.00 (*0-7879-0206-3*, E343-Y2T) Jossey-Bass.

Treating Adolescents by Family Therapy: A Developmental & Narrative Approach. Anne K. Fishel. 1999. LC 98-51012. xxi, 290p. 40.00 (*0-7657-0192-8*) Aronson.

Treating Adult Survivors of Childhood Sexual Abuse. William C. Nichols. 1992. LC 91-50913. (Practitioner's Resource Ser.). 80p. pap. 15.95 (*0-943158-68-0*, TASBP, Prof Resc Pr) Pro Resource.

Treating AIDS with Chinese Medicine. Mary K. Ryan & Arthur Shattuck. 1993. LC 93-85212. 384p. pap. 29.95 (*1-881896-07-2*) Pacific View Pr.

Treating Alcohol & Drug Users in the Community. T. A. Waller. 2nd ed. 2002. 256p. pap. 38.95 (*0-632-03575-7*) Blackwell Sci.

Treating Alcohol Dependence: A Coping Skills Training Guide. Peter M. Monti et al. 1989. LC 88-36838. (Treatment Manuals for Practitioners Ser.). 240p. pap. 24.00 (*0-89862-215-8*, 2215) Guilford Pubns.

Treating Alcohol Problems: Marital & Family Interventions. Ed. by Timothy J. O'Farrell. 1993. LC 93-3061. (Substance Abuse Ser.). 446p. 50.00 (*0-89862-195-X*, 2195) Guilford Pubns.

Treating Alcoholism & Drug Abuse among Homeless Men & Women: Nine Community Demonstration Grants. Milton Argerion & Dennis McCarty. 1990. LC 90-4301. (Alcoholism Treatment Quarterly Ser.: Vol. 7, No. 1). (Illus.). 164p. text 39.95 (*0-86656-992-8*) Haworth Pr.

Treating Alzheimer's & Other Dementias: Recent Research Advances. Ed. by Manfred Bergener & Sanford I. Finkel. 1995. LC 94-45399. 61.95 (*0-8261-8930-X*) Springer Pub.

Treating & Managing Sleep Disorders: A Primer. Max Hirshkowitz et al. 2000. 320p. 45.00 (*0-471-36175-5*) Wiley.

Treating & Overcoming Anorexia Nervosa. Steven Levenkron. 1988. 240p. mass mkt. 5.99 (*0-446-34416-8*) Warner Bks.

Treating Anger, Anxiety, & Depression in Children & Adolescents: A Cognitive-Behavioral Perspective. Jerry Wilde. 1995. LC 95-36561. 187p. 39.95 (*1-56032-481-3*); pap. 19.95 (*1-56032-482-1*) Accel Devel.

Treating Anxiety Disorders. Walton T. Roth & Irvin D. Yalom. 1996. LC 96-28708. (Library of Current Clinical Technique). 288p. pap. 35.00 (*0-7879-0316-7*) Jossey-Bass.

Treating Anxious Children & Adolescents: An Evidence-Based Approach. Ronald M. Rapee et al. 2000. LC 99-75287. (Illus.). 195p. 49.95 (*1-57224-192-6*) New Harbinger.

Treating Attachment Abuse: A Compassionate Approach. Steven Stosny. 1995. LC 95-7295. (Illus.). 304p. 39.95 (*0-8261-8960-1*) Springer Pub.

Treating Bulimia: A Psychoeducational Approach. Sharlene A. Wolchik et al. 1985. (Psychology Practitioner Guidebooks). 144p. text 28.00 (*0-08-032400-2*); pap. text 14.95 (*0-08-032399-5*) Elsevier (Pergamon Pr).

Treating Cancer with Chinese Herbs. Hong-yen Hsu. 1993. 346p. pap. 12.95 (*0-941942-04-X*) Orient Heal Arts.

Treating Cardiovascular Diseases in the Elderly. 168p. pap. text (*0-86471-069-0*) Adis Intl NZL. *Dist:* Lppncott W & W.

Treating Cerebral Palsy: For Clinicians by Clinicians. Ed. by Eugene T. McDonald. 1987. LC 86-22568. (For Clinicians by Clinicians Ser.). (Illus.). 312p. pap. text 31.00 (*0-89079-141-4*, 1412) PRO-ED.

Treating Chemically Dependent Families: A Practical Systems Approach for Professionals. John T. Edwards. 1991. 200p. pap. 17.95 (*0-935908-56-0*, 3275, HazeldenJohnson Inst) Hazelden.

Treating Child Abuse & Family Violence in Hospitals: A Program for Training & Services. Kathleen M. White et al. 1989. 186p. 37.00 (*0-669-20822-1*) Lxngtn Bks.

Treating Childhood & Adolescent Obesity. Ed. by Daniel S. Kirschenbaum et al. 1987. (Psychology Practitioner Guidebooks). 160p. 30.00 (*0-08-032414-2*); pap. 15.95 (*0-08-032413-4*) Elsevier (Pergamon Pr).

Treating Children & Adolescents in Residential & Inpatient Settings. Robert D. Lyman & Nancy R. Campbell. 1996. LC 96-10054. (Developmental Clinical Psychology & Psychiatry Ser.: Vol. 36). 160p. 74.95 (*0-8039-7046-3*, 2771) Sage.

Treating Children in Out-of-Home Placements. Marvin Rosen. 1998. LC 97-45116. 216p. lib. bdg. 39.95 (*0-7890-0163-2*, Hawrth Medical) Haworth Pr.

Treating Children with Sexually Abusive Behavior Problems: Guidelines for Child & Parent Intervention. Jan E. Burton & Lucinda A. Rasmussen. 1998. LC 98-6095. (Illus.). 279p. pap. 29.95 (*0-7890-0473-9*); lib. bdg. 49.95 (*0-7890-0472-0*) Haworth Pr (Maltreatment & Trauma Pr).

Treating Children's Fears & Phobias. Thomas R. Kratochwill & Richard J. Morris. 2nd ed. 1998. (C). 37.95 (*0-205-16827-2*, Macmillan Coll) P-H.

Treating Children's Fears & Phobias: A Behavioral Approach. Richard J. Morris & Thomas R. Kratochwill. 1983. LC 82-10186. (General Psychology Ser.: No. 114). (Illus.). 375p. text 65.00 (*0-08-025999-5*, J115); pap. text 24.50 (*0-08-025998-7*) Elsevier (Pergamon Pr).

Treating Coexisting Psychiatric & Addictive Disorders: A Practical Guide. Ed. by Norman S. Miller. 1994. LC 94-4696. 24.95 (*0-89486-972-8*, 1499) Hazelden.

Treating Complex Cases: The Cognitive Behavioural Therapy Approach. Adrian Wells et al. 2000. LC 98-25593. (Clinical Psychology & Personality Ser.). 456p. pap. 44.95 (*0-471-97839-6*) Wiley.

Treating Conduct & Oppositional Defiant Disorders in Children. Arthur M. Horne & Thomas V. Sayger. 1990. (Psychology Practitioner Guidebooks Ser.). 200p. text (*0-08-036438-1*); pap. text (*0-08-036437-3*) PPI GBR. *Dist:* Elsevier.

Treating Couples. Ed. by Hilda Kessler. 1996. LC 95-42119. (Library of Current Clinical Technique). 304p. pap. 33.00 (*0-7879-0205-5*) Jossey-Bass.

Treating Couples: The Intersystem Model of the Marriage Council of Philadelphia. Ed. by Gerald R. Weeks. 1989. LC 88-24231. 368p. text 52.95 (*0-87630-534-6*) Brunner-Routledge.

Treating Depression in Children & Adolescents. J. L. Matson. 1989. (Psychology Practitioner Guidebooks). 144p. text 28.00 (*0-08-035874-8*); pap. text 14.95 (*0-08-035875-6*) Elsevier (Pergamon Pr).

Treating Depression in Primary Care: A Manual for Primary Care & Mental Health Providers. Patricia Robinson et al. 1996. (Illus.). 265p. (Orig.). (C). pap. 42.95 (*1-878978-26-8*) Context Pr.

Treating Depression in the Elderly. Stephen Curran et al. 2000. 256p. pap. text (*0-7506-4379-X*) E A GBR. *Dist:* OUP.

Treating Difficult Personality Disorders. Michael Rosenbluth & Irvin D. Yalom. 1996. LC 96-8761. (Jossey-Bass Library of Current Clinical Technique). 288p. pap. 35.00 (*0-7879-0315-9*) Jossey-Bass.

Treating Disordered Speech Motor Control: For Clinicians by Clinicians. Ed. by Deanie Vogel & Michael P. Cannito. 1991. LC 90-9167. (For Clinicians by Clinicians Ser.). 410p. pap. text 36.00 (*0-89079-299-2*, 1943) PRO-ED.

Treating Dissociative Identity Disorder. James L. Spira. 1996. (Jossey Bass Library Of Current Clinical). 416p. pap. 28.00 (*0-7879-0329-9*) Jossey-Bass.

Treating Dissociative Identity Disorder: The Power of the Collective Heart. Sarah Y. Krakauer. 2001. LC 00-65184. xxv, 246p. 34.95 (*0-87630-975-9*) Brunner-Routledge.

Treating Drug Abusers: New Directions. Gerald A. Bennett. 1989. 200p. 49.50 (*0-415-02039-5*, A3461); pap. 15.95 (*0-415-05837-6*, A5206) Routledge.

Treating Drug Abusers Effectively. Ed. by Daniel M. Fox et al. 1997. LC 96-27367. (Illus.). 448p. (C). text 66.95 (*1-57718-041-0*) Blackwell Pubs.

Treating Drug Problems, Vol. 1. Institute of Medicine Staff. Ed. by Dean R. Gerstein & Henrick J. Harwood. 1990. 356p. text 29.95 (*0-309-04285-2*) Natl Acad Pr.

Treating Eating Disorders. Walter Vandereycken & Pierre J. Beumont. 1998. LC 98-4523. 304p. text 55.00 (*0-8147-8753-3*); 286p. pap. text 19.50 (*0-8147-8754-1*) NYU Pr.

Treating Eating Disorders. Joellen Werne. 1996. (Jossey-Bass Library of Current Clinical Technique). 377p. pap. 35.00 (*0-7879-0330-2*) Jossey-Bass.

Treating Epilepsy Naturally: A Guide to Alternative & Adjunct Therapies. Patricia A. Murphy. 2001. LC 2001-29778. 288p. pap. 16.95 (*0-658-01379-3*) McGraw-Hill Trade.

Treating Families of Brain Injury Survivors. Paul R. Sachs. 1991. LC 91-4612. (Series on Rehabilitation: Vol. 9). 232p. 33.95 (*0-8261-6920-1*) Springer Pub.

Treating Family of Origin Problems: A Cognitive Approach. Richard C. Bedrosian & George D. Bozicas. 1994. LC 93-33386. 384p. 40.00 (*0-89862-178-X*) Guilford Pubns.

Treating Fearful Dental Patients: A Patient Management Handbook. Philip Weinstein et al. 2nd ed. 1995. (Illus.). 359p. (C). pap. 37.50 (*1-880291-01-0*) Cont Dental Educ.

Treating Food Allergy, My Way! see Food Allergy Book: The Foods That Cause You Pain & Discomfort & How to Eliminate Them from Your Diet

*Treating Huckleberry Finn: A New Narrative Approach to Working with Kids Diagnosed ADD/ADHD.** David Nylund. 2002. pap. 25.00 (*0-7879-6120-5*) Jossey-Bass.

Treating Huckleberry Finn: A New Narrative Approach to Working with Kids Diagnosed ADD/ADHD. David Nylund. 2000. LC 00-8176. 256p. 39.95 (*0-7879-5229-X*) Jossey-Bass.

Treating Lesbians & Bisexual Women: Challenges & Strategies for Health Professionals. Elisabeth Page Gruskin. 1999. LC 98-25343. 73.95 (*0-7619-0044-6*, 1653); pap. 36.95 (*0-7619-0045-4*, 1654) Sage.

Treating Malpractice: Report of the Twentieth Century Fund Task Force on Medical Malpractice Insurance. 1986. 70p. (Orig.). (C). pap. text 7.50 (*0-87078-173-1*) Century Foundation.

Treating Mental Illness & Behavior Disorders in Children & Adults with Mental Retardation. Ed. by Anton Dosen & Kenneth Day. 2001. LC 00-32793. xv, 561p. 79.00 (*0-88048-850-6*, 8850) Am Psychiatric.

Treating Mind & Body: Essays in the History of Science, Professions, & Society under Extreme Conditions. Geoffrey Cocks. 1997. LC 97-20184. 283p. text 34.95 (*1-56000-310-3*) Transaction Pubs.

Treating Obsessive-Compulsive. Samuel M. Turner. 1992. (Practitioner Guidebook Ser.). 140p. (C). pap. text 47.00 (*0-205-14488-8*, H4488, Longwood Div) Allyn.

Treating Obsessive-Compulsive Disorder. Samuel M. Turner & Deborah C. Beidel. 1988. 140p. text 28.00 (*0-08-034232-9*); pap. text 14.95 (*0-08-034231-0*) Elsevier (Pergamon Pr).

T U V

Treating Panic Disorder & Agoraphobia: A Step-by-Step Clinical Guide. Elke Zuercher-White. 1997. LC 97-66078. 296p. text 49.95 (*1-57224-084-9*) New Harbinger.

Treating Patients with Alcohol & Other Drug Problems: An Integrated Approach. Robert D. Margolis & Joan E. Zweben. 1998. LC 97-42378. (Psychologists in Independent Practice Bks.). (Illus.). 358p. pap. 29.95 (*1-55798-518-9*) Am Psychol.

Treating Patients with Memories of Abuse: Legal Risk Management. Samuel J. Knapp & Leon VandeCreek. 1997. LC 97-15987. (Psychologists in Independent Practice Bks.). 197p. 24.95 (*1-55798-441-7*) Am Psychol.

Treating People in Families: An Integrative Framework. William C. Nichols. 1995. LC 95-25437. (Guilford Family Therapy Ser.). (Illus.). 331p. 36.00 (*1-57230-036-1*, 0036) Guilford Pubns.

***Treating People with Anxiety & Stress: A Practical Guide for Primary Care.** Ed. by Greg Wilkinson et al. 2000. LC 00-344698. (Illus.). 288p. pap. (*1-85775-139-6*) Radcliffe Med Pr GBR. *Dist:* Balogh.

Treating People with Chronic Disease: A Psychological Guide. Carol D. Goodheart & Martha H. Lansing. 1996. LC 96-30817. (Psychologists in Independent Practice Ser.). 229p. pap. text 24.95 (*1-55798-387-9*, 431-7750) Am Psychol.

Treating People with Depression: A Practical Guide for Primary Care. Ed. by Greg Wilkinson et al. 1999. LC 99-206277. (Illus.). 168p. pap. (*1-85775-391-7*) Radcliffe Med Pr GBR. *Dist:* Balogh.

Treating Post-Natal Depression: A Psychological Approach for Health Care Practitioners. Paul R. Martin et al. 2000. LC 99-45635. (Illus.). 292p. pap. 45.00 (*0-471-98645-3*) Wiley.

Treating Preschool Children. Hans Steiner & Irvin D. Yalom. 1997. LC 97-20811. (Volume in the Jossey-Bass Library of Current Clinical Technique). 256p. pap. 33.00 (*0-7879-0877-0*) Jossey-Bass.

Treating PTSD: Cognitive-Behavioral Strategies. Ed. by David W. Foy. 1992. LC 92-1463. (Treatment Manuals for Practitioners Ser.). 172p. pap. 21.00 (*0-89862-220-4*, 2220) Guilford Pubns.

Treating Schizophrenia. Ed. by Sophia Vinogradov. 1995. LC 94-44052. (Social & Behavioral Sciences-Health Ser.). 372p. 39.00 (*0-7879-0079-6*) Jossey-Bass.

Treating School-Age Children. Ed. by Hans Steiner & Irvin D. Yalom. 1997. LC 97-5198. (Library of Current Clinical Technique). 298p. pap. 35.00 (*0-7879-0878-9*) Jossey-Bass.

Treating Sex Offenders in Correctional Institutions & Outpatient Clinics: A Guide to Clinical Practice. William E. Prendergast. 1991. 220p. 49.95 (*1-56024-206-X*) Haworth Pr.

Treating Sexual Disorders. Randolph S. Charlton. 1996. LC 96-8762. (Jossey-Bass Library of Current Clinical Technique). 384p. pap. 28.00 (*0-7879-0311-6*) Jossey-Bass.

Treating Sexual Shame: A New Map for Overcoming Dysfunction, Abuse, & Addiction. Anne S. Hastings. 1997. LC 97-15765. 344p. 40.00 (*0-7657-0103-0*) Aronson.

Treating Sexually Abused Boys: A Practical Guide for Therapists & Counselors. Lisa Camino. 1999. LC 99-16647. 288p. pap. 37.00 (*0-7879-4793-8*) Jossey-Bass.

Treating Sinus, Migraine, & Cluster Headaches, My Way! Vol. II: An Allergist's Approach to Headache Treatment. William E. Walsh. 1993. LC 93-90632. (Food Allergy Book Ser.). 269p. (Orig.). pap. 12.95 (*0-9631544-5-1*) ACA Pubns.

Treating Stress in Families. Ed. by Charles R. Figley. 1989. LC 88-8554. (Psychosocial Stress Ser.: No. 13). 300p. text 45.95 (*0-87630-530-3*) Brunner-Routledge.

Treating Substance Abuse: Theory & Technique. Ed. by Frederick Rotgers et al. 1995. LC 95-25144. (Substance Abuse Ser.). 328p. text 36.00 (*1-57230-025-6*, 0025) Guilford Pubns.

Treating Suicidelike Behavior in a Preschooler. Paul V. Trad. 1990. LC 89-36105. 490p. 70.00 (*0-8236-6649-2*, BN 06649) Intl Univs Pr.

Treating Survivors of Satanist Abuse. Ed. by Valerie Sinason. 1994. LC 93-41461. 332p. (C). pap. 29.99 (*0-415-10543-9*) Routledge.

Treating Survivors of Satanist Abuse: An Invisible Trauma. Ed. by Valerie Sinason. 1994. 320p. (C). pap. 18.95 (*0-415-10607-9*) Routledge.

Treating Teenage Drug Abuse in a Day Care Setting. William Feigelman. 1990. LC 89-26538. 160p. 52.95 (*0-275-93379-2*, C3379, Greenwood Pr) Greenwood.

Treating the Adult Survivor of Childhood Sexual Abuse: A Psychoanalytic Perspective. Jody M. Davies & Mary G. Frawley. 1994. LC 93-34377. 304p. pap. 50.00 (*0-465-06633-X*) Basic.

Treating the Aftermath of Sexual Abuse: A Handbook for Working with Children in Care. Margaret Osmond et al. 1998. LC 97-52025. 176p. pap. 18.95 (*0-87868-693-2*, 6932) Child Welfare.

Treating the Alcoholic: A Social Work Challange: A Special Issue of Social Casework. 1989. 72p. pap. 8.95 (*0-87304-234-4*) Manticore Pubs.

Treating the Changing Family: Handling Normative & Unusual Events. Michele Harway. 1995. LC 95-11794. (Couples & Family Dynamics & Treatment Ser.). 374p. 95.00 (*0-471-07905-7*) Wiley.

Treating the Chemically Dependent & Their Families. Dennis C. Daley & Miriam S. Raskin. 1991. (Sourcebooks for the Human Services: Vol. 16). (Illus.). 244p. (C). pap. 39.95 (*0-8039-3298-7*, 6289) Sage.

Treating the Elderly. Ed. by Javaid I. Sheikh & Irvin D. Yalom. 1996. LC 95-26782. (Jossey-Bass Library of Current Clinical Technique Ser.). 288p. pap. 33.00 (*0-7879-0219-5*) Jossey-Bass.

Treating the Homeless Mentally Ill: A Task Force Report of the American Psychiatric Association. Ed. by H. Richard Lamb et al. 1992. LC 92-10470. 315p. text 11.95 (*0-89042-236-2*, 2236) Am Psychiatric.

Treating the Mentally Disabled. Ed. by Gary E. McCuen. 1988. (Ideas in Conflict Ser.). (Illus.). 140p. (YA). (gr. 7-12). lib. bdg. 15.95 (*0-86596-066-6*) G E M.

Treating the Neurotic Patient in Brief Psychotherapy. Ed. by Althea J. Horner. 1994. LC 93-74779. (Master Work Ser.). 256p. pap. 40.00 (*1-56821-212-7*) Aronson.

Treating the Oedipal Patient in Brief Psychotherapy. Ed. by Althea J. Horner. 1985. LC 84-24300. 256p. 45.00 (*0-87668-759-1*) Aronson.

Treating the Poor: A Personal Sojourn Through the Rise & Fall of Community Mental Health. Matthew P. Dumont. Ed. by Judy Kaplan. 2nd ed. 1994. LC 92-97289. 149p. (Orig.). 26.95 (*0-9634975-1-0*); pap. 15.95 (*0-9634975-0-2*) Dymphna Pr.

Treating the Psychological Consequences of HIV. Michael F. O'Connor & Irvin D. Yalom. 1996. LC 96-31519. (Library of Current Clinical Technique). 464p. pap. 35.00 (*0-7879-0314-0*) Jossey-Bass.

Treating the Remarried Family. Clifford J. Sager et al. 1986. LC 82-17811. 406p. text 47.95 (*0-87630-323-8*) Brunner-Routledge.

Treating the School Age Stutterer: A Guide for Clinicians, No. 14. Carl W. Dell, Jr. 1997. LC 79-67284. 110p. (Orig.). pap. 2.00 (*0-933388-11-X*) Stuttering Fnd Am.

Treating the Sexual Offender. Barry M. Maletzky. 1991. 320p. (C). pap. 32.95 (*0-8039-3663-X*, 32003) Sage.

Treating the Trauma of Rape: Cognitive-Behavioral Therapy for PTSD. Edna B. Foa & Barbara O. Rothbaum. 1997. LC 97-30807. (Treatment Manuals for Practitioners Ser.). 286p. 32.00 (*1-57230-178-3*, C0178) Guilford Pubns.

Treating the Treatment Failures: The Challenge of Chronic Schizophrenia. Arnold M. Ludwig. 1971. LC 75-155998. 236p. text 78.00 (*0-8089-0707-7*, 792595, Grune & Strat) Harcrt Hlth Sci Grp.

Treating the Troubled Family. Nathan W. Ackerman. 1994. LC 94-71150. (Master Work Ser.). 320p. pap. 40.00 (*1-56821-268-2*) Aronson.

Treating the Whole Patient: BPH & Beyond. Ed. by J. E. Altwein & R. S. Kirby. 1996. (Journal: Vol. 29, Suppl. 1, 1996). (Illus.). iv, 52p. pap. 21.75 (*3-8055-6295-0*) S Karger.

Treating Tobacco Use & Dependence: Clinical Practice Guideline. Michael C. Fiore et al. 2000. 126p. (*1-58763-007-9*) Agency Healthcare.

Treating Traumatized Children: New Insights & Creative Interventions. Beverly James. 1989. 320p. 36.95 (*0-669-20994-5*) Free Pr.

Treating Troubled Adolescents: A Family Therapy Approach. H. Charles Fishman. 1988. LC 87-47838. 336p. pap. 42.00 (*0-465-08742-6*) Basic.

Treating Women Molested in Childhood. Catherine Classen. 1995. LC 94-39886. (Jossey-Bass Library of Current Clinical Technique). 242p. 39.00 (*0-7879-0078-8*) Jossey-Bass.

Treating Women's Fear of Failure. Ed. by Esther D. Rothblum & Ellen Cole. 1988. LC 87-25134. (Women & Therapy Ser.: Vol. 6, No. 3). 105p. text 29.95 (*0-86656-676-7*) Haworth Pr.

Treating Youth Who Sexually Abuse: An Integrated Multi-Component Approach. Paul Stephen Lundrigan. 2001. LC 00-33532. 306p. 59.95 (*0-7890-0936-6*) Haworth Pr.

Treatise Concerning the Medicinal Philosophic Stone. Philippus Aureolus Paracelsus. 1989. pap. 3.95 (*1-55818-161-X*) Holmes Pub.

Treatise of Health & Long Life with the Future Means of Attaining It. Leonard Lessius & Luigi Cornaro. Ed. by Robert J. Kastenbaum. Tr. by Timothy Smith. 1979. LC 78-22206. (Aging & Old Age Ser.). reprint ed. lib. bdg. 18.95 (*0-405-11821-X*) Ayer.

Treatise of 113 Diseases of the Eyes. Richard Banister. 1971. LC 79-37135. (English Experience Ser.: No. 297). 480p. reprint ed. 35.00 (*90-221-0297-1*) Walter J Johnson.

Treatise of the Hypochondriack & Hysterick Diseases. Bernard Mandeville. 1976. LC 76-45623. 432p. reprint ed. 60.00 (*0-8201-1277-1*) Schol Facsimiles.

Treatise of the Hypochondriack & Hysterick Passions. Bernard De Mandeville. 1976. LC 75-16717. (Classics in Psychiatry Ser.). reprint ed. 27.95 (*0-405-07445-X*) Ayer.

Treatise of the Organ of Hearing. Guichard J. Duverney. LC 77-147969. reprint ed. 41.50 (*0-404-08221-1*) AMS Pr.

Treatise of the Plague: Containing the Nature, Signes & Accidents of the Same. Thomas Lodge. 1979. LC 79-84119. (English Experience Ser.: No. 938). 92p. reprint ed. lib. bdg. 20.00 (*90-221-0938-0*) Walter J Johnson.

Treatise on Analytical Chemistry: Theory & Practice, Vol. 8, Pt. 1. Ed. by Philip J. Elving et al. 2nd ed. 1986. (Treatise on Analytical Chemistry Ser.). 767p. (*0-471-07995-2*) Interscience GBR. *Dist:* Wiley.

Treatise on Aphasia & Other Speech Defects. Henry C. Bastian. LC 78-72786. (Brainedness, Handedness, & Mental Abilities Ser.). reprint ed. 49.50 (*0-404-60851-5*) AMS Pr.

Treatise on Children's Disease. T. Datta. 1984. (C). (*0-7855-4653-7*) Current Dist IND. *Dist:* St Mut.

Treatise on Controlled Drug Delivery: Fundamentals - Optimization - Applications. Ed. by Agis F. Kydonieus. 1991. (Illus.). 568p. text 75.00 (*0-8247-8519-3*) Dekker.

Treatise on Glaucoma. Robert H. Elliot. 2nd ed. 1979. LC 78-20807. (Classics in Ophthalmology Ser.). (Illus.). 680p. reprint ed. lib. bdg. 54.00 (*0-88275-842-X*) Krieger.

Treatise on Hygiene. William Hammond. 1991. (American Civil War Medical Ser.: No. 5). (Illus.). 604p. reprint ed. 60.00 (*0-930405-38-2*) Norman SF.

Treatise on Hygiene & Public Health Albert H. Buck. Ed. by Barbara G. Rosenkrantz. 1977. LC 76-25654. (Public Health in America Ser.). reprint ed. lib. bdg. 116.95 (*0-405-09810-3*);Vol. 1. lib. bdg. 58.95 (*0-405-09811-1*);Vol. 1. lib. bdg. 58.95 (*0-405-09812-X*) Ayer.

Treatise on Insanity & Other Disorders Affecting the Mind. James C. Prichard. 1973. LC 73-2412. (Mental Illness & Social Policy; the American Experience Ser.). reprint ed. 26.95 (*0-405-05222-7*) Ayer.

Treatise on Insanity in Its Medical Relations. William A. Hammond. 1973. LC 73-2402. (Mental Illness & Social Policy; the American Experience Ser.). reprint ed. 50.95 (*0-405-05208-1*) Ayer.

Treatise on Man & the Development of His Faculties, 1842. Lambert A. Quetelet. 1969. LC 77-81364. (History of Psychology Ser.). (Illus.). 150p. 50.00 (*0-8201-1061-2*) Schol Facsimiles.

Treatise on Mental Diseases. Henry J. Berkley. Ed. by Gerald N. Grob. 1980. LC 78-22549. (Historical Issues in Mental Health Ser.). (Illus.). reprint ed. lib. bdg. 50.95 (*0-405-11903-8*) Ayer.

Treatise on Poisons in Relation to Medical Jurisprudence, Physiology & the Practice of Physic. Robert Christison. LC 79-156011. reprint ed. 67.50 (*0-404-09111-3*) AMS Pr.

Treatise on the Canon of Medicine of Avicenna. Avicenna. LC 73-12409. reprint ed. 145.00 (*0-404-11231-5*) AMS Pr.

Treatise on the Management of Pregnant & Lying-In Women. Charles White. 1988. LC 86-6600. 15.00 (*0-88135-081-8*) Watson Pub Intl.

Treatise on the Medical Jurisprudence of Insanity. Isaac Ray. 5th ed. 1977. LC 75-16732. (Classics in Psychiatry Ser.). reprint ed. 54.95 (*0-405-07453-0*) Ayer.

Treatise on the Nature, Symptoms, Causes & Treatment of Insanity. William C. Ellis. 1976. LC 75-16700. (Classics in Psychiatry Ser.). reprint ed. 32.95 (*0-405-07427-1*) Ayer.

Treatise on the Spleen & Stomach: A Translation of the Pi Wei Lun. Li Dong-Yuan. Ed. by Bob Flaws. Tr. by Yang Shou-Zhong & Li Jian-Yong from CHI. 1993. LC 92-75135. 275p. pap. 22.95 (*0-936185-41-4*) Blue Poppy Pr.

Treatise on the Teeth. John A. Skinner. 1967. (Illus.). reprint ed. 15.00 (*0-87266-027-3*) Argosy.

Treatise Wherein Is Declared the Sufficiencie of English Medicines, for Cure of All Diseases, Cured with Medicine. Timothy Bright. 1977. LC 77-6860. (English Experience Ser.: No. 854). reprint ed. lib. bdg. 15.00 (*90-221-0854-6*) Walter J Johnson.

Treatment: What It Is & How to Do It. Raymond C. Barker. 16p. pap. 3.50 (*0-87516-504-4*) DeVorss.

Treatment & Care in Old Age Psychiatry. Ed. by Raymond Levy et al. 1993. LC 93-3405. 256p. pap. (*1-871816-17-3*) Wrightson Biomed GBR. *Dist:* Taylor & Francis.

Treatment & Disposal of Wastes: Report of a WHO Scientific Group, 1967. 1967. (Technical Report Ser.: No. 367). 30p. pap. text 3.00 (*92-4-120367-6*, 1100367) World Health.

Treatment & Prevention of Alcohol Problems. W. Miles Cox. 1986. (Personality, Psychopathology & Psychotherapy Ser.). text 53.00 (*0-12-194470-0*) Acad Pr.

Treatment & Prevention of Childhood Sexual Abuse. Ed. by Sandra A. Burkhardt & Anthony F. Rotatori. 1995. LC 95-7942. 220p. 34.95 (*1-56032-320-5*) Taylor & Francis.

Treatment & Rehabilitation of Fractures. Stanley Hoppenfeld. 1999. LC 99-16183. (Illus.). xviii, 606p. pap. text 69.95 (*0-7817-2197-0*, Lippnctt) Lppncott W & W.

Treatment & Security Needs of Special Hospital Patients. Tony Maden et al. 1995. 150p. pap. text 150.00 (*1-56593-501-2*, 1160) Singular Publishing.

Treatment Approaches with Suicidal Adolescents, No. 11. Ed. by James K. Zimmerman & Gregory M. Asnis. 1995. LC 94-30990. (Einstein Psychiatry Publication Ser.: Vol. 11). 320p. 140.00 (*0-471-10236-9*) Wiley.

Treatment Aspects of Drug Dependence. Ed. by Arnold J. Schecter. 1978. (Uniscience Ser.). 148.00 (*0-8493-5476-5*, RC566, CRC Reprint) Franklin.

Treatment by Neuropathy & the Encyclopedia of Physical & Manipulative Therapeutics. Thomas T. Lake. 1996. 684p. reprint ed. spiral bd. 38.50 (*0-7873-0519-7*) Hlth Research.

Treatment Costs for Very Low Birthweight Infants: The California Medicaid Experience. Jeannette A. Rogowski & Ellen R. Harrison. 1995. 66p. (Orig.). pap. text 13.00 (*0-8330-2345-4*, MR-451-AHCPR) Rand Corp.

Treatment Drug Courts: Integrating Substance Abuse Treatment with Legal Case Processing. Ed. by Sandra Clunies. 1999. 65p. (C). pap. text 20.00 (*0-7881-7593-9*) DIANE Pub.

Treatment Efficacy for Stuttering: A Search for Empirical Bases. Anne K. Cordes & Roger J. Ingham. 1998. LC 98-5956. xiv, 323p. (*1-56543-904-X*) Mt SA Coll Philos.

Treatment Efficacy for Stuttering: A Search for Empirical Buses. Anne K. Cordes & Roger J. Ingham. 1998. (Illus.). 304p. pap. 65.00 (*1-56593-904-2*, 1790) Thomson Learn.

Treatment for Adolescent Substance Abusers. 1992. lib. bdg. 250.00 (*0-8490-5495-8*); 1991. lib. bdg. 250.00 (*0-8490-5046-4*) Gordon Pr.

Treatment for Chronic Depression: Cognitive Behavioral Analysis System of Psychotherapy (CBASP) James P. McCullough, Jr. 1999. 326p. text 37.00 (*1-57230-527-4*, 8R0527) Guilford Pubns.

Treatment for Developmentally Disabled Persons with Sexual Behavior Problems: Community-Based Treatment, Management & Supervision of Sexual Behavior Problems among Developmentally Disabled Persons/Accompianied by programs book. Gerry D. Blasingame. 2001. 180p. pap. 42.95 (*1-885473-45-1*) Wood N Barnes.

Treatment for Stimulant Use Disorders. Ed. by Richard A. Rawson & Rose M. Urban. 2000. 226p. (C). pap. text 40.00 (*0-7881-8902-6*) DIANE Pub.

Treatment Guidelines for Medicine & Primary Care, 2002. Paul D. Chan & Margaret T. Johnson. 2000. 268p. 19.95 (*1-929622-00-7*) Current Clin Strat.

Treatment in Crisis Situations. Naomi Golan. 1978. LC 77-85350. (Treatment Approaches in the Human Services Ser.). 35.00 (*0-02-912060-8*) Free Pr.

Treatment in Dermatology. Ed. by Julian L. Verbov. 1987. (New Clinical Applications in Dermatology Ser.). lib. bdg. 82.00 (*0-85200-955-0*) Kluwer Academic.

Treatment in Dermatology. Barbara Leppard & Richard Ashton. Ed. by Joshua Wieder & Nicholas J. Lowe. rev. ed. 1995. LC 94-40427. (*1-85775-135-3*); text (*1-85775-130-2*) Radcliffe Med Pr GBR. *Dist:* Balogh.

Treatment Interventions In Human Sexuality. Ed. by Carol C. Nadelson & David B. Marcotte. 1983. LC 83-4078. (Critical Issues in Psychiatry Ser.). 502p. 89.50 (*0-306-41082-6*, Plenum Trade) Perseus Pubng.

Treatment Issues & Innovations in Mental Retardation. Ed. by Johnny L. Matson & Frank Andrasik. 1983. (Applied Clinical Psychology Ser.). 666p. 95.00 (*0-306-40935-6*, Plenum Trade) Perseus Pubng.

Treatment Manual for Adolescents with Anorexia Nervosa: A Family-Based Approach. James E. Lock et al. 2000. LC 00-61757. 270p. text 35.00 (*1-57230-607-6*, C0607) Guilford Pubns.

Treatment Modalities in Lung Cancer. Ed. by R. Arriagada & T. Le Chevalier. 1988. (Antibiotics & Chemotherapy Ser.: Vol. 41). (Illus.). xii, 248p. 172.25 (*3-8055-4775-7*) S Karger.

Treatment Monitoring & Reporting Systems, No. 4. Ed. by R. Simon. 1999. (European Addiction Research Ser.: Vol. 5). (Illus.). 54p. pap. 25.25 (*3-8055-7025-2*) S Karger.

Treatment of Abuse & Addiction: A Holistic Approach. Arthur P. Ciaramicoli. 1997. LC 97-11439. 264p. 50.00 (*0-7657-0087-5*) Aronson.

Treatment of Acute Leukemias: New Directions for Clinical Research. Ed. by Ching-Hon Pui. 2001. (Current Clinical Oncology Ser.). 550p. 125.00 (*0-89603-834-3*) Humana.

Treatment of Addiction: Current Issues for Arts Therapies. Diane Waller & Jacqueline Mahony. 1999. LC 98-17017. (Illus.). 224p. (C). 80.00 (*0-415-16996-8*); pap. 27.95 (*0-415-16997-6*) Routledge.

Treatment of Adult Survivors of Childhood Abuse. Eliana Gil. 1988. LC 88-80275. 250p. (Orig.). (C). pap. 18.95 (*0-9613205-6-7*, 0007) Launch Pr.

Treatment of Adult Survivors of Incest. Ed. by Patricia L. Paddison. 1993. LC 92-17653. (Clinical Practice Ser.: No. 27). 148p. text 12.95 (*0-88048-469-1*, 8469) Am Psychiatric.

Treatment of Age-Related Cognitive Dysfunction: Pharmacological & Clinical Evaluation. Ed. by Giorgio Racagni et al. 1992. (International Academy for Biomedical & Drug Research Ser.: Vol. 2). (Illus.). vi, 154p. 121.00 (*3-8055-5551-2*) S Karger.

Treatment of Alcoholism & Other Addictions: A Self-Psychology Approach. Jerome D. Levin. 1987. LC 87-19563. 433p. 60.00 (*0-87668-947-0*) Aronson.

Treatment of Anxiety Disorders: Clinician's Guide & Treatment Manuals. Gavin Andrews et al. 1995. (Illus.). 438p. (C). pap. text 47.95 (*0-521-46927-9*) Cambridge U Pr.

Treatment of Aphasia: From Theory to Practice. Ed. by Chris Code & Dave J. Muller. 1995. 250p. (Orig.). (C). pap. text 49.95 (*1-56593-255-2*, 0430) Singular Publishing.

Treatment of Asthma: The Long-Acting Beta-2-Agonists. Ed. by Friedrich Kummer. 1998. LC 98-19197. (Illus.). 200p. pap. 36.00 (*3-211-83124-X*) Spr-Verlag.

Treatment of Benign Prostatic Hyperplasia. Ed. by Ken Koshiba et al. 2000. LC 00-30777. (Recent Advances in Endourology Ser.: 2). (Illus.). 208p. 99.00 (*4-431-70284-9*) Spr-Verlag.

Treatment of Black Alcoholics. Ed. by Frances L. Brisbane & Maxine Womble. 1985. LC 85-13975. (Alcoholism Treatment Quarterly Ser.: Vol. 2, No. 3-4). 270p. text 49.95 (*0-86656-403-9*) Haworth Pr.

Treatment of Bleeding Disorders with Blood Components. Ed. by Eberhard F. Mammen et al. 1980. (Reviews of Hematology: Vol. I). 49.95 (*0-915340-01-1*) PJD Pubns.

Treatment of Blood Diseases with Chinese Medicine see Handbook of Chinese Hematology

Treatment of Burns: Principles & Practice. William W. Monafo & Carlos Pappalardo. 1971. LC 71-138827. (Illus.). 286p. 22.50 (*0-87527-055-7*) Green.

Treatment of Cancer. Ed. by Karol Sikora & K. Halnan. 2nd ed. 1990. (Illus.). 936p. pap. 251.95 (*0-412-29400-1*) Chapman & Hall.

Treatment of Cancer. P. Price. 3rd ed. 1995. 1160p. (gr. 13). 249.95 (*0-412-56010-0*) Chapman & Hall.

Treatment of Cardiovascular Disease. James T. Willerson. 1992. (gr. 13). text (*0-397-44695-0*) Gower-Mosby.

Treatment of Cats by Homeopathy. K. Sheppard. 1979. pap. 10.00 (*0-85032-120-4*) Formur Intl.

Treatment of Cattle by Homeopathy. Macleod. 1981. 129p. pap. (*0-85207-247-3*) C W Daniel GBR. *Dist:* Natl Bk Netwk.

Treatment of Cattle by Homeopathy. MacLeod. 1997. pap. 26.95 (*0-8464-1210-1*) Beekman Pubs.

Treatment of Cattle by Homeopathy. George MacLeod. 160p. (Orig.). pap. 26.95 (*0-8464-4303-1*) Beekman Pubs.

Treatment of Cerebral Infarction. J. Suzuki. 1987. (Illus.). 400p. 120.00 (*0-387-81933-9*) Spr-Verlag.

Treatment of Cerebral Palsy in Motor Disorders. Sophie Levitt. 3rd ed. 1995. LC 94-16798. (Illus.). 312p. pap. 52.95 (*0 632 03873 X*) Blackwell Sci.

Treatment of Chemical Agent Casualties & Conventional Military Chemical Injuries. 1991. lib. bdg. 79.95 (*0-8490-4087-6*) Gordon Pr.

Treatment of Childhood Disorders. Ed. by Eric J. Mash & Russell A. Barkley. 2nd ed. 1998. LC 98-24806. 771p. 69.95 (*1-57230-276-3*, C0276) Guilford Pubns.

Treatment of Children & Adolescents in Residential & Inpatient Settings, No. 36. Robert D. Lyman & Nancy R. Campbell. 1996. LC 96-10054. (Developmental Clinical Psychology & Psychiatry Ser.: Vol. 36). 160p. pap. 34.95 (*0-8039-7047-1*, 2770) Sage.

***Treatment of Chronic Fatigue Snydrome in the Antiviral Revolution Era.** Ed. by Roberto Patarca-Montero. 2001. 115p. pap. text 19.95 (*0-7890-1254-5*, Hawrth Medical) Haworth Pr.

***Treatment of Chronic Fatigue Syndrome in the Antiviral Revolution Era.** Ed. by Roberto Patarca-Montero. 2001. 115p. 34.95 (*0-7890-1253-7*, Hawrth Medical) Haworth Pr.

Treatment of Chronic Pain. Ed. by Mark Mumenthaler. 1990. 337p. text 176.00 (*3-7186-5026-6*); pap. text 114.00 (*3-7186-5027-4*) Gordon & Breach (Harwood Acad Pubs).

Treatment of Cocaine Abuse: An Annotated Bibliography, 9. John J. Miletich. 1992. LC 91-35403. (Bibliographies & Indexes in Medical Studies: No. 9). 256p. lib. bdg. 62.95 (*0-313-27839-3*, MTQ/, Greenwood Pr) Greenwood.

Treatment of Communication Disorders in Culturally & Linguistically Diverse Populations. Orlando Taylor. 1986. LC 82-22431. 209p. (Orig.). (C). text 37.50 (*0-89079-365-4*, 1558) Buttrwrth-Heinemann.

Treatment of Complicated Epilepsies in Adults. Ed. by P. Berner & L. W. Diehl. 1978. (Bibliotheca Psychiatrica Ser.: No. 158). (Illus.). 50.50 (*3-8055-2814-0*) S Karger.

Treatment of Convulsive Status Epilepticus. Working Group on Status Epilepticus Staff. 1995. 32p. (Orig.). pap. (*0-916570-21-5*) Epilepsy Foundation of America.

Treatment of Dementias: A New Generation of Progress. E. M. Meyer et al. 1992. (Advances in Behavioral Biology Ser.: Vol. 40). (Illus.). 448p. (C). text 130.00 (*0-306-44228-0*, Kluwer Plenum) Kluwer Academic.

Treatment of Depression. Ian H. Gotlib. 1987. (Practitioner Guidebook Ser.). 208p. (C). pap. text 54.95 (*0-205-14358-X*, H4358, Longwood Div) Allyn.

Treatment of Depression: A Holistic Approach. David McMillin. 1997. LC 97-8533. (Edgar Cayce Health Ser.). 352p. (Orig.). pap. 16.95 (*0-87604-386-4*, 498) ARE Pr.

Treatment of Depression: An Interpersonal Systems Approach. Ian H. Gotlib & Catherine A. Colby. 1987. (Psychology Practitioner Guidebooks: No. 5). 180p. text 30.00 (*0-08-033634-5*); pap. text 15.95 (*0-08-033633-7*) Elsevier (Pergamon Pr).

Treatment of Depression: Bridging the 21st Century. Ed. by Myrna M. Weissman. 2001. LC 00-55838. (Illus.). xx, 357p. 64.00 (*0-88048-397-0*, 8397) Am Psychiatric.

Treatment of Depression - Newer Pharmacotherapies: Evidence Report - Technology Assessment. Ed. by Cynthia D. Mulrow. 2000. (Illus.). 365p. (C). pap. text 40.00 (*0-7881-8540-3*) DIANE Pub.

Treatment of Depression in Managed Care. Mark Mays & James W. Croake. Ed. by S. Richard Sauber. 1997. LC 96-36748. (Mental Health Practice under Managed Health Care Ser.: Vol. 7). 256p. 27.95 (*0-87630-829-9*) Brunner-Routledge.

Treatment of Disease in TCM Vol. 1: Diseases of the Head & Face Including Mental/Emotional Disorders. Philippe Sionneau & Lu Gang. Ed. by Bob Flaws. 1996. LC 95-83249. 260p. pap. text 21.95 (*0-936185-69-4*) Blue Poppy Pr.

Treatment of Disease in TCM Vol. III: Disease of the Mouth, Lips, Tongue, Teeth & Gums. Philippe Sionneau & Lii Gang. Ed. by Bob Flaws. 1997. LC 95-83249. 242p. (Orig.). pap. 21.95 (*0-936185-79-1*) Blue Poppy Pr.

Treatment of Disease in TCM Vol. 5: Diseases of the Chest, Abdomen, & Ribside. Philippe Sionneau & Lii Gang. 1998. LC 95-83249. 390p. pap. text 29.95 (*1-891845-02-0*) Blue Poppy Pr.

Treatment of Disease in TMC Vol. 7: General Symptoms. Philippe Sionneau & Lu Gang. 2000. LC 95-83249. 7p. pap. text 24.95 (*1-891845-14-4*) Blue Poppy Pr.

Treatment of Disease with Acupuncture: Complete Course in Acupuncture, Vol. II. James Tin Yao So. Ed. by Richard Feit. 1993. (Treatment of Disease with Acupuncture Ser.: Vol. II). 379p. (C). text 37.00 (*0-912111-08-9*) Paradigm Publns.

Treatment of Dogs by Homoeopathy. K. Sheppard. 1981. pap. 10.00 (*0-85032-079-8*) Formur Intl.

Treatment of Drinking Problems: A Guide for Helping Professions. Griffith Edwards et al. 1997. LC 96-53577. (Illus.). 380p. (C). text 110.00 (*0-521-49696-9*); pap. text 41.95 (*0-521-49793-0*) Cambridge U Pr.

Treatment of Drug Dependent Individuals with Comorbid Mental Disorders. Ed. by Lisa S. Onken et al. 1998. (Illus.). 170p. (C). pap. text 35.00 (*0-7881-2782-9*) DIANE Pub.

Treatment of Early Stage Breast Cancer. 1994. lib. bdg. 250.00 (*0-8490-8523-3*) Gordon Pr.

Treatment of Emotional Disorders. Seymour L. Halleck. 1978. LC 77-18374. (Treatment of Emotional Disorder CL Ser.). 544p. 45.00 (*0 87668 263 8*) Aronson.

Treatment of End-Stage Coronary Artery Disease. P. J. Walter. 1988. (Advances in Cardiology Ser.: Vol. 36). (Illus.). x, 306p. 164.50 (*3-8055-4717-X*) S Karger.

Treatment of Endometriosis & Other Disorders & Infections, Vol. 4. Ed. by Y. Boutaleb & A. Gzouli. 1991. (Recent Developments in Fertility & Sterility Ser.). (Illus.). 196p. (C). ring bd. (*1-85070-287-X*, Parthenon Pbng) CRC Pr.

Treatment of Epilepsy. Ed. by Simon D. Shorvon et al. 1996. LC 95-36763. (Illus.). 900p. 225.00 (*0-632-03782-2*) Blackwell Sci.

Treatment of Epilepsy: Principles & Practice. Elaine Wyllie. 1992. LC 92-49990. (Illus.). 1100p. text 105.00 (*0-8121-1504-X*) Lppncott W & W.

***Treatment of Epilepsy: Principles & Practice.** Elaine Wyllie. 3rd ed. 2001. LC 00-54583. (Illus.). 1,328p. text 199.00 (*0-7817-2374-4*) Lppncott W & W.

Treatment of Families in Conflict: The Clinical Study of Family Process. Group for the Advancement of Psychiatry Staff. 1983. LC 84-45131. 352p. 55.00 (*0-87668-724-9*) Aronson.

Treatment of Families in Crisis. Donald G. Langsley & David M. Kaplan. 1968. LC 68-29400. 208p. text 47.00 (*0-8089-0251-2*, 792440, Grune & Strat) Harcrt Hlth Sci Grp.

Treatment of Fractures in Children & Adolescents. Ed. by B. G. Weber. 1979. LC 79-16985. (Illus.). 408p. 271.00 (*0-387-09313-3*) Spr-Verlag.

Treatment of Fractures in the Elderly. Ed. by Kenneth J. Koval et al. 1997. LC 97-14316. (Illus.). 295p. text 139.00 (*0-397-51825-0*) Lppncott W & W.

Treatment of Functional Somatic Symptoms. Ed. by Richard Mayou et al. 1995. (Illus.). 466p. (C). text 89.50 (*0-19-262499-7*) OUP.

Treatment of Genetic Diseases. Ed. by Robert J. Desnick. 1991. (Illus.). 350p. text (*0-443-08773-3*) Church.

Treatment of Haemoglobinopathies & Allied Disorders: Proceedings of the WHO Scientific Group, Geneva, 1971. WHO Staff. 1972. (Technical Reports: No. 509). pap. text 5.00 (*92-4-120509-1*, 1100509) World Health.

Treatment of Homosexuals with Mental Health Disorders. Ed. by Michael Ross & John P. DeCecco. 1988. LC 87-30826. (Journal of Homosexuality Ser.: No. 15, No. 1-2). (Illus.). 222p. pap. 17.95 (*0-918393-47-7*, Harrington Park) Haworth Pr.

Treatment of Horses by Acupuncture. Erwin Westermayer. 2nd ed. 1985. (Illus.). 40p. pap. 37.95 (*0-8464-4304-X*) Beekman Pubs.

Treatment of Horses by Acupuncture. Erwin Westermayer. 1979. 130p. (*0-85032-161-1*) C W Daniel GBR. *Dist:* Natl Bk Netwk.

Treatment of Horses by Homeopathy. George MacLeod. 1977. 130p. pap. (*0-85207-249-X*) C W Daniel GBR. *Dist:* Natl Bk Netwk.

Treatment of Horses by Homeopathy. G. MacLeod. rev. ed. 1993. 182p. pap. 26.95 (*0-8464-1284-5*) Beekman Pubs.

Treatment of Horses by Homoeopathy. G. Macleod. 1980. 40.00 (*0-85032-155-7*) St Mut.

Treatment of Hospitalized Cystic Fibrosis Patient. Ed. by David M. Orentsein & Robert C. Stern. 1997. LC 97-31070. (Lung Biology in Health & Disease Ser.). (Illus.). 472p. text 195.00 (*0-8247-9500-8*) Dekker.

Treatment of Infantile Hydrocephalus Concezio Di Rocco. 1987. LC 86-24451. 205.00 (*0-8493-5720-9*, RJ469);Vol. 1. 96.00 (*0-8493-5721-7*, RJ496);Vol. 2. 184p. reprint ed. 109.00 (*0-8493-5722-5*) Franklin (CRC Reprint).

Treatment of Infants, Child & Adolescents. Fredric D. Burg. 1990. 432p. pap. text 37.00 (*0-7216-2139-2*) Saunders.

Treatment of Infertility, Vol. 1. Ed. by Y. Boutaleb & A. Gzouli. 1991. (Recent Developments in Fertility & Sterility Ser.). (Illus.). 258p. (C). ring bd. (*1-85070-284-5*, Parthenon Pbng) CRC Pr.

***Treatment of Infertility: Assisted Reproductive Technologies.** 669p. pap. (*0-662-21383-1*) Can7 Govern Pub CAN. *Dist:* Intl Spec Bk.

Treatment of Insanity. John M. Galt. 1973. LC 73-2397. (Mental Illness & Social Policy; the American Experience Ser.). reprint ed. 35.95 (*0-405-05205-7*) Ayer.

Treatment of Late-Life Insomnia. Kenneth L. Lichstein & Charles M. Morin. 2000. LC 99-50603. (Illus.). 354p. pap. 33.95 (*0-7619-1507-9*, 82554) Sage.

Treatment of Mandibular Fractures. Jonas T. Johnson et al. 2nd ed. 1995. LC 95-8250. (Self-Instructional Package Ser.). (Illus.). 112p. pap. text 25.00 (*1-56772-018-8*) AAO-HNS.

Treatment of Mental Disorders. Ed. by John H. Greist et al. 1982. 584p. (C). pap. text 32.50 (*0-19-503107-5*) OUP.

Treatment of Mental Disorders: A Review of Effectiveness. Ed. by Norman Sartorius et al. 1993. LC 93-2989. text 30.95 (*0-88048-975-8*, 8975) Am Psychiatric.

Treatment of Migraine: Pharmacological & Biofeedback Considerations. Ed. by Roy J. Mathew. 1981. (Illus.). 170p. text 27.50 (*0-88331-209-3*) R B Luce.

Treatment of Mild Cognitive & Emotional Sequelae of Neurologic Dysfunction. Sarah Raskin & Catherine Mateer. 1999. LC 99-13808. (Illus.). 312p. text 49.95 (*0-19-508527-2*) OUP.

***Treatment of Modern Western Diseases with Chinese Medicine: A Textbook & Clinical Manual.** Bob Flaws & Philippe Sionneau. 2001. LC 2001-35418. (*1-891845-20-9*) Blue Poppy Pr.

Treatment of Multiple Sclerosis: Trial Design, Results & Future Perspectives. Ed. by R. A. Rudick et al. 1992. (Clinical Medicine & the Nervous System Ser.). (Illus.). 313p. 150.00 (*0-387-19683-8*) Spr-Verlag.

Treatment of Multiple Sclerosis: Trial Design, Results, & Future Perspectives. Richard A. Rudick & Donald E. Goodkin. 1991. (Clinical Medicine & the Nervous System Ser.). 290p. 145.00 (*3-540-19683-8*) Spr-Verlag.

Treatment of Neurosis in the Young: A Psychoanalytic Perspective. Ed. by M. Hossein Etezady. 1993. LC 93-231. 320p. 55.00 (*0-87668-500-9*) Aronson.

Treatment of Obsessive & Compulsive Behaviors. Leon Salzman. 1995. LC 94-38376. (Master Work Ser.). 274p. reprint ed. pap. text 50.00 (*1-56821-422-7*) Aronson.

Treatment of Obsessive Compulsive Disorder. Lata K. McGinn & William C. Sanderson. 1999. LC 98-54404. (Clinical Application of Evidence-Based Psychotherapy Ser.). xiv, 296p. 40.00 (*0-7657-0211-8*) Aronson.

Treatment of Obsessive Compulsive Disorder. Gail S. Steketee. 1996. LC 93-15832. (Treatment Manuals for Practitioners Ser.). 224p. pap. 23.00 (*0-89862-911-X*, 2911) Guilford Pubns.

Treatment of Offenders with Mental Disorders. Robert M. Wettstein. 1998. LC 97-42397. 438p. text 45.00 (*1-57230-271-2*, C0271) Guilford Pubns.

Treatment of Opiate Addiction Using Methadone: A Counselor's Manual. Michael J. McCann et al. 1995. 335p. (Orig.). (C). pap. text 55.00 (*0-7881-2534-6*) DIANE Pub.

Treatment of Pain. Ed. by Harold J. Wain & Dionisios P. Devaris. 1982. LC 81-65783. 208p. 40.00 (*0-87668-607-2*) Aronson.

Treatment of Panic Disorder: A Consensus Development Conference. Ed. by Barry E. Wolfe & Jack D. Maser. 1994. LC 93-17653. 377p. text 19.95 (*0-88048-685-6*, 8685) Am Psychiatric.

Treatment of Parkinson's Disease: 4th Sandoz Symposium, Tokyo, October 1995. Ed. by Hisayuki Kowa. 1997. (European Neurology Ser.: Vol. 38, Suppl. 1 (1997)). (Illus.). iv, 58p. pap. 26.25 (*3-8055-6565-8*) S Karger.

Treatment of Parkinson's Disease: 5th Sandoz Symposium, Tokyo, November 1997. Ed. by Ichiro Kanazawa. 1997. (European Neurology Ser.: Vol. 38, Suppl. 2, 1997). (Illus.). iv, 70p. pap. 30.50 (*3-8055-6611-5*) S Karger.

Treatment of Patients in the Borderline Spectrum. William W. Meissner. 1995. LC 88-10526. 648p. pap. 60.00 (*1-56821-495-2*) Aronson.

Treatment of Personality Disorders. Ed. by Jan Derksen et al. 1999. LC 99-47601. 312p. 149.50 (*0-306-46215-X*, Kluwer Plenum) Kluwer Academic.

Treatment of Persons with Severe Mental Disorders. Ed. by Jeffrey R. Bedell. 1993. 239p. 39.95 (*1-56032-292-6*) Taylor & Francis.

Treatment of Precancerous Lesions & Early Breast Cancer: Diagnosis & Management. Irving M. Ariel & Anthony C. Cahan. 1993. 416p. 89.00 (*0-683-00255-4*) Lppncott W & W.

Treatment of Pressure Ulcers: Clinical Prctice Guideline. Nancy Bergstrom. 1997. (Illus.). 154p. (C). reprint ed. pap. text 40.00 (*0-7881-2418-8*) DIANE Pub.

Treatment of Primitive Mental States. Peter L. Giovacchini. 536p. 1996. LC 96-152696. pap. 65.00 (*1-56821-808-7*); 1978. LC 78-74990. 60.00 (*0-87668-347-2*) Aronson.

Treatment of Psychiatric Disorders: Revised for DSM-4. William H. Reid et al. 3rd rev. ed. 1997. LC 96-7478. 514p. 69.95 (*0-87630-765-9*) Brunner-Routledge.

Treatment of Psychiatric Disorders: Revised for the DSM-III-R. William H. Reid. 2nd enl. rev. ed. 1989. LC 88-19468. 438p. text 43.95 (*0-87630-536-2*) Brunner-Routledge.

Treatment of Radiation Injuries. Ed. by D. Browne et al. 1990. LC 90-14216. (Illus.). 260p. 79.50 (*0-306-43729-5*, Plenum Trade) Perseus Pubng.

Treatment of Rape Victims: Facilitating Psychosocial Adjustment. K. S. Calhoun & B. M. Atkeson. 1991. (Psychology Practitioner Guidebooks Ser.). 160p. text (*0-08-031576-3*); pap. text (*0-08-031575-5*) PPI GBR. *Dist:* Elsevier.

***Treatment of Recurrent Depression.** Ed. by John F. Greden. 2001. LC 00-69520. (Review of Psychiatry Ser.: Vol. 20). 208p. pap. 29.95 (*1-58562-025-4*, 62025) Am Psychiatric.

Treatment of Renal Anemia: Mini-Symposium on Recombinant Human Erythropoietin - Journal: Blood Purification, Vol. 8, No. 5, 1990. Ed. by B. Canaud & K. M. Koch. 1991. (Illus.). 76p. pap. 40.00 (*3-8055-5344-7*) S Karger.

Treatment of Renal Anemia with Recombinant Human Erythropoietin. Ed. by K. M. Koch. 1988. (Contributions to Nephrology Ser.: Vol. 66). (Illus.). viii, 212p. 29.75 (*3-8055-4764-1*) S Karger.

Treatment of Schizophrenia. Leland E. Hinsie. Ed. by Gerald N. Grob. 1980. LC 78-22565. (Historical Issues in Mental Health Ser.). reprint ed. lib. bdg. 19.95 (*0-405-11919-4*) Ayer.

Treatment of Schizophrenia: A Holistic Approach Based on the Readings of Edgar Cayce. David McMillin. 1997. LC 97-8463. (Edgar Cayce Health Ser.). 521p. (Orig.). pap. 16.95 (*0-87604-384-8*, 493) ARE Pr.

Treatment of Schizophrenia: Progress & Prospects. L. J. West & D. E. Flinn. 1976. LC 76-47510. (Illus.). 320p. text 71.00 (*0-8089-0970-3*, 794805, Grune & Strat) Harcrt Hlth Sci Grp.

Treatment of Schizophrenia: Status & Emerging Trends. Ed. by Hans Dieter Brenner et al. rev. ed. 2000. LC 00-39544. (Illus.). xii, 259p. text 39.00 (*0-88937-195-4*) Hogrefe & Huber Pubs.

Treatment of Serious Infections in the 1990s. Ed. by Merle A. Sande & Richard K. Root. 1991. (Contemporary Issues in Infectious Diseases Ser.: Vol. 9). (Illus.). 243p. text (*0-443-08799-7*) Church.

Treatment of Severe Dyslipoproteinemia in the Prevention of Coronary Heart Disease. Ed. by A. M. Gotto, Jr. et al. 1992. (Illus.). x, 366p. 105.25 (*3-8055-5539-3*) S Karger.

Treatment of Severe Dyslipoproteinemia in the Prevention of Coronary Heart Disease: Fourth International Symposium, Munich, October 1992. Ed. by A. M. Gotto, Jr. et al. 1993. (Illus.). x, 242p. 216.75 (*3-8055-5843-0*) S Karger.

Treatment of Severe Hypercholesterolemia in the Prevention of Coronary Heart Disease. Ed. by A. M. Grotto et al. 1988. (Contributions to Infusion Therapy Ser.: Vol. 23). (Illus.). viii, 198p. 55.00 (*3-8055-4905-9*) S Karger.

Treatment of Severe Hypercholesterolemia in the Prevention of Coronary Heart Disease - 2. M. Mancini et al. Ed. by A. M. Gotto, Jr. et al. 1990. viii, 274p. 68.75 (*3-8055-5085-5*) S Karger.

Treatment of Sexual Dysfunction: A Bio-Psycho-Social Approach. William E. Hartman & Marilyn A. Fithian. 1972. LC 72-93106. (Illus.). 282p. 14.95 (*0-9600626-1-0*) Ctr Marital Sexual.

Treatment of Small Bowel Diseases: Proceedings of the Hepato-Gastroenterology Symposium, University Hospital Center of Nice, 1st, August 1972. Hepato-Gastroenterology Symposium Staff. Ed. by J. Delmont. 1973. (Illus.). 200p. 38.50 (*3-8055-1490-5*) S Karger.

Treatment of Soft Tissue Sarcomas. Ed. by Herbert M. Pinedo & Jaap Verweij. 1988. (Cancer Treatment & Research Ser.). (C). text 114.00 (*0-89838-391-9*) Kluwer Academic.

Treatment of Substance Abuse: Psychosocial Occupational Therapy Approaches. Ed. by Diane Gibson. 1989. LC 88-21309. (Occupational Therapy in Mental Health Ser.: Vol. 8, No. 2). (Illus.). 80p. text 29.95 (*0-86656-838-7*) Haworth Pr.

Treatment of Suicidal Patients in Managed Care. Ed. by James M. Ellison. 2001. LC 00-56946. xvi, 218p. pap. 39.00 (*0-88048-828-X*, 8828) Am Psychiatric.

Treatment of the Addictions: Applications of Outcome Research for Clinical Management. Ed. & Intro. by Norman S. Miller. 1994. LC 94-22157. (Alcoholism Treatment Quarterly Ser.: Vol. 12, No. 2). (Illus.). 135p. lib. bdg. 39.95 (1-56024-686-3) Haworth Pr.

Treatment of the Addictions: Applications of Outcome Research for Clinical Management. Intro. by Norman S. Miller. 1994. LC 94-22157. (Alcoholism Treatment Quarterly Ser.: Vol. 12, No. 2). (Illus.). 135p. pap. 14.95 (1-56023-064-9, Harrington Park) Haworth Pr.

Treatment of the Alcohol-Abusing Offender. Robert R. Ross & Lynn O. Lightfoot. 1985. 164p. (C). 33.95 (0-398-05090-2) C C Thomas.

Treatment of the Borderline Adolescent: A Developmental Approach. James F. Masterson. 5th ed. 1985. LC 85-4236. 305p. reprint ed. text 38.95 (0-87630-394-7) Brunner-Routledge.

***Treatment of the Borderline Patient: Applying Fairbairn's Object Relations Theory in the Clinical Setting.** David P. Celani. 2001. (Books-on-Demand Ser.). xxi, 210p. reprint ed. pap. text 25.95 (0-8236-8324-9, 26644) Intl Univs Pr.

Treatment of the Chronic Schizophrenic Patient. Ed. by Diane Gibson. 1986. LC 86-18451. (Occupational Therapy in Mental Health Ser.: Vol. 6, No. 2). 87p. text 39.95 (0-86656-578-7) Haworth Pr.

Treatment of the Edentulous Patient. Victor O. Lucia. 1986. LC 85-30060. (Illus.). 248p. text 148.00 (0-86715-122-6, 1226) Quint Pub Co.

Treatment of the Insane Without Mechanical Restraints. John Conolly. 1973. LC 73-2392. (Mental Illness & Social Policy; the American Experience Ser.). reprint ed. 28.95 (0-405-05200-6) Ayer.

Treatment of the Masochistic Personality: An Interactional-Object Relations Approach to Psychotherapy. Cheryl G. Hughes & Marolyn Wells. 1995. LC 94-34953. 288p. text 40.00 (1-56821-384-0) Aronson.

Treatment of the Narcissistic Neuroses. Hyman Spotnitz & Phyllis W. Meadow. rev. ed. 1995. LC 94-36858. 304p. pap. text 50.00 (1-56821-416-2) Aronson.

Treatment of the Postmenopausal Woman: Basic & Clinical Aspects. Contrib. by Rogerio A. Lobo. 2nd ed. 1999. LC 99-34504. (Illus.). 704p. text 129.00 (0-7817-1559-8) Lppncott W & W.

Treatment of the Pregnant Addict. Janice Pringle et al. 1994. 135p. pap. 49.97 (1-884937-16-0) Manisses Communs.

Treatment of the Rheumatic Diseases: A Companion to Kelley's Textbook of Rheumatology. Michael H. Weisman et al. 2nd ed. 2000. LC 99-51710. (Illus.). 495p. text 125.00 (0-7216-8464-5) Saunders.

Treatment of the Rheumatic Diseases: Companion to the Textbook of Rheumatology. Ed. by Michael H. Weisman & Michael E. Weinblatt. 1994. LC 94-28994. Orig. Title: Drug Therapy of the Rheumatic Diseases. (Illus.). 384p. text 58.00 (0-7216-5382-0) Saunders.

Treatment of the Seriously Obese Patient. Ed. by Thomas A. Wadden & Theodore B. VanItallie. 1992. LC 92-1459. 524p. 60.00 (0-89862-879-2) Guilford Pubns.

Treatment of the Severely Disturbed Adolescent. Donald B. Rinsley. LC 80-66922. 1994. 364p. pap. 45.00 (1-56821-222-4); 1983. 368p. 45.00 (0-87668-415-0) Aronson.

Treatment of the Uncomplicated Aural Cholesteatoma. Andrew J. Miller et al. 2nd rev. ed. 1999. LC 99-38642. (Self-Instructional Ser.). (Illus.). 60p. pap. text 25.00 (1-56772-025-0) AAO-HNS.

Treatment of Tuberculosis: Guidelines for National Programmes. 1993. (ENG, FRE & SPA.). vii, 43p. pap. text 9.00 (92-4-154451-1, 1150397) World Health.

Treatment of War Wounds in Graeco-Roman Antiquity. Christine F. Salazar. 1999. LC 99-89213. (Studies in Ancient Medicine: Vol. 21). (Illus.). xxvii, 299p. (90-04-11479-3) Brill Academic Pubs.

Treatment of Water, Electrolyte, & Acid-Base Disorders in the Surgical Patient. L. Beaty Pemberton & Deloras Pemberton. 1994. LC 93-28458. 416p. pap. 32.00 (0-07-049363-4) McGraw-Hill Educ Grp.

Treatment Options for Meniere's Disease: Endolymphatic Sac Surgery. I. Kaufman Arenberg & Malcolm D. Graham. 1998. LC 98-12943. (Illus.). 188p. 155.95 (1-56593-734-1, 1428) Thomson Learn.

Treatment Options in Early Intervention. Ed. by James A. Blackman. 1994. LC 94-38449. (Infants & Young Children Ser.). 260p. pap. 41.00 (0-8342-0645-5) PRO-ED.

Treatment Outcomes in Psychotherapy & Psychiatric Interventions. Len Sperry et al. 1996. LC 96-26029. (Mental Health Practice under Managed Care Ser.: Vol. 6). 256p. pap. 27.95 (0-87630-826-4) Brunner-Routledge.

Treatment Perspectives in Urologic Oncology. Richard D. Williams. Ed. by Peter R. Carroll. 1990. (Illus.). 256p. (0-08-040298-4) PPI GBR. *Dist:* McGraw.

Treatment Planning - A Clinician's Desk Reference. Victoria J. Ficklin & Maria H. Miyares-Piper. unabr. ed. 1997. 79p. wbk. ed. 19.95 (0-9661796-0-9) Santee Pub.

Treatment Planning & Dose Calculation & Treatment Planning in Radiation Oncology. Gunilla C. Bentel et al. 1982. (Illus.). 265p. text 54.00 (0-08-027176-6, H230); pap. text 24.00 (0-08-027175-8) Elsevier (Pergamon Pr).

Treatment Planning & Dose Calculation in Radiation Oncology. Gunilla C. Bentel et al. 4th ed. 1991. 352p. text 42.00 (0-07-105246-1) McGraw-Hill Med Pub.

Treatment Planning & Dose Calculation in Radiation Oncology. Thomas K. Noell et al. 4th ed. 1989. 368p. text 43.00 (0-08-034328-7); pap. text 25.00 (0-08-034327-9) Elsevier (Pergamon Pr).

Treatment Planning for Pedodontic Patients. Anthony S. Blinkhorn. 1992. (Illus.). 152p. text 62.00 (1-85097-014-9) Quint Pub Co.

Treatment Planning for Psychotherapists. Richard B. Makover. 1996. LC 95-47205. 256p. text 37.00 (0-88048-743-7, 8743) Am Psychiatric.

Treatment Planning for Traumatized Teeth. Mitsuhiro Tsukiboshi. 2000. LC 99-56647. (Illus.). 120p. text 72.00 (0-86715-374-1) Quint Pub Co.

Treatment Planning in Radiation Oncology. Faiz M. Khan & Roger A. Potish. 1997. LC 97-6377. (Illus.). 608p. 129.00 (0-683-04607-1) Lppncott W & W.

Treatment Planning in the Radiation Therapy of Cancer. Ed. by J. M. Vaeth & J. Meyer. 1987. (Frontiers of Radiation Therapy & Oncology Ser.: Vol. 21). (Illus.). x, 342p. 282.75 (3-8055-4377-8) S Karger.

Treatment Plans & Interventions for Depression & Anxiety Disorders. Robert L. Leahy & Stephen J. Holland. 2000. LC 99-59385. (Clinician's Toolbox Ser.). 332p. pap. 55.00 incl. cd-rom (1-57230-514-2, 8R0514) Guilford Pubns.

Treatment Procedures in Communicative Disorders. M. N. Hegde. 3rd rev. ed. 1998. LC 97-26808. 508p. text 39.00 (0-89079-729-3, 8494) PRO-ED.

Treatment Protocols in Communicative Disorders: Targets & Strategies. M. N. Hegde. rev. ed. 1998. LC 97-23918. 413p. spiral bd. 44.00 (0-89079-730-7, 8493) PRO-ED.

Treatment Resistance: A Guide for Practitioners. Salvatore Cullari. 1996. LC 95-43196. 288p. (C). 60.00 (0-205-15572-3) Allyn.

Treatment Services for Adolescent Substance Abusers. 1986. lib. bdg. 79.95 (0-8490-3496-5) Gordon Pr.

Treatment Stimulators. 1989. (British Institute Radiology Supplement Ser.: No. 23). pap. (0-905749-19-7) Med Physics Pub.

Treatment Strategies for Chronic Renal Failure: Limitations of Resources & Priorities, the Dilemma of the Nineties. Ed. by C. Zoccali. 1994. (Contributions to Nephrology Ser.: Vol. 109). (Illus.). x, 120p. 49.75 (3-8055-5868-6) S Karger.

Treatment Strategies for Patients with Psychiatric Comorbidity. Ed. by Scott Wetzler & William C. Sanderson. 1997. LC 96-34774. (Publication Series of the Department of Psychiatry Albert Einstein College of Medicine of Yeshiva University). 368p. 140.00 (0-471-11773-0) Wiley.

Treatment Strategies in Child & Adolescent Psychiatry. Ed. by J. G. Simeon & H. B. Ferguson. 1990. LC 90-7429. (Illus.). 250p. (C). 47.50 (0-306-43466-0, Plenum Trade) Perseus Pubng.

Treatment Techniques for Common Mental Disorders. Joan Atwood & Robert Chester. 1987. LC 87-17471. 352p. 50.00 (0-87668-962-4) Aronson.

Treatment Unit Clerk. Jack Rudman. 1994. (Career Examination Ser.: C-319). pap. 23.95 (0-8373-0319-2) Nat Learn.

Treatment with GnRH Analogs: Controversies & Perspectives. Ed. by Marco Filicori & Carlo Flamigni. 1996. LC 96-33672. (Illus.). 276p. lib. bdg. 74.95 (1-85070-690-5, Parthenon Pbng) CRC Pr.

Treatment Without Consent: Law, Psychiatry & the Treatment of Mentally Disordered People since 1845. Phil Fennell. 1995. LC 95-21254. (Social Ethics & Policy Ser.). 368p. (C). 89.95 (0-415-07787-7) Routledge.

Treatment Works for Major Depressive Disorder: A Patient & Family Guide. American Psychiatric Association Staff. 2000. 12p. pap. 19.95 (0-89042-288-5, 2288) Am Psychiatric.

Treatments of Psychiatric Disorders Ed. by Glen O. Gabbard. 3rd ed. 2001. 3088p. 279.00 (0-88048-910-3, 8910); Vol. II. (0-88048-911-1) Am Psychiatric.

Treatments of Psychiatric Disorders for DSM-IV, Set. Ed. by Glen O. Gabbard. 2nd ed. 1995. LC 95-5770. 2800p. 258.00 (0-88048-700-3, 8700) Am Psychiatric.

Tree of Healing: Psychological & Biblical Foundations for Counseling & Pastoral Care. Roger F. Hurding. 1988. Orig. Title: Roots & Shoots. 464p. reprint ed. 18.95 (0-310-25140-0, 11022) Zondervan.

Tree of Knowledge: The Biological Roots of Human Understanding. Humberto R. Maturano & Francisco J. Varela. rev. ed. 1998. LC 91-50781. (Illus.). 264p. pap. 29.95 (0-87773-642-1) Shambhala Pubns.

Tree of Life: Paths in Jungian Individuation. J. Marvin Spiegelman. 1993. LC 74-81034. 368p. (Orig.). pap. 14.95 (1-56184-062-9) New Falcon Pubns.

Trembling Mountain: A Personal Account of Kuru, Cannibals, & Mad Cow Disease. Robert Klitzman. 1998. LC 98-14386. (Illus.). 235p. (C). 27.95 (0-306-45792-X) Perseus Bks Grp.

Tremor the Most Common Complaints. Plotkin. 2001. 208p. pap. 24.99 (0-7506-7284-6) Buttrwrth-Heinemann.

Trends & Changes in Drug Research & Development. Ed. by S. R. Walker & B. C. Walker. 1989. 120p. (C). text 111.00 (0-85200-839-2) Kluwer Academic.

Trends & Future Perspectives in Peptide & Protein Drug Delivery. Ed. by V. Lee. 1995. (Drug Targeting & Delivery Ser.). 340p. text 132.00 (3-7186-5641-8, Harwood Acad Pubs) Gordon & Breach.

Trends & Issues in Nursing. Marilyn H. Oermann. 1993. (0-397-54919-9) Lppncott W & W.

Trends & Issues in Professional Nursing. Lois J. Rew. 1998. (Nursing Education Ser.). (C). 31.95 (0-8273-7879-3) Delmar.

Trends & Issues in Theoretical Psychology. Ed. by Ian Lubek et al. 1995. LC 96-102095. 412p. pap. 69.95 (0-8261-8810-9) Springer Pub.

Trends & Regional Variations in Amphetamine-Related Emergency Admissions Vol. 1: California, 1984-1993. James K. Cunningham & Margaret A. Thielemeir. 1995. (Illus.). 98p. (Orig.). reprint ed. pap. 16.00 (0-9651259-3-9) Public Statistics.

Trends & Variations in Fertility in the United States. Clyde V. Kiser et al. 1968. LC 68-25613. (Vital & Health Statistics Monographs, Am). (Illus.). 368p. 39.50 (0-674-90780-9) HUP.

Trends in Cancer Incidence & Mortality. Ed. by R. Doll et al. 1994. (Cancer Surveys Ser.: Vol. 19/20). (Illus.). 583p. (C). 108.00 (0-87969-391-6) Cold Spring Harbor.

Trends in Cancer Research. 1966. (ENG, FRE & RUS.). 84p. pap. text 5.40 (92-4-156000-2, 1150151) World Health.

Trends in Cognitive & Behavioural Therapies. Paul M. Salkovskis. 1996. LC 95-31227. 174p. 175.00 (0-471-96172-8); pap. 47.00 (0-471-95788-7) Wiley.

Trends in Contrast Media. Ed. by Henrik S. Thomsen et al. 1999. LC 98-28592. (Medical Radiology Ser.). (Illus.). 480p. 249.00 (3-540-60924-5) Spr-Verlag.

Trends in Drug Research II: Proceedings of the 11th Noordwijkerhout-Camerino Symposium, 11-15 May, 1997, Noordwijkerhout. H. Van der Goot. 1998. LC 97-43576. (Pharmacochemistry Library). 258p. 187.00 (0-444-82633-5) Elsevier.

***Trends in Gastroenterology & Hepatology: Millennium 2000.** Ed. by H. Asakura & S. Nakzawa. 2001. (Illus.). xviii, 370p. 139.00 (4-431-70302-0) Spr-Verlag.

Trends in Haemostasis, 1995. Losonczy Hajna & David Marianna. 1995. LC 96-133465. 204p. pap. (963-05-6844-6) Akade Kiado HUN. *Dist:* Intl Spec Bk, St Mut.

Trends in Health Benefits. 1994. lib. bdg. 300.00 (0-8490-9049-0) Gordon Pr.

Trends in Health Care Provider Liability II: An Analysis of Jury Verdicts. Brian Shenker. 1992. LC 92-36273. 49.50 (0-934753-81-4) LRP Pubns.

Trends in Health Spending: An Update. 1993. (Illus.). 80p. (Orig.). (C). pap. text 40.00 (1-56806-549-3) DIANE Pub.

Trends in Health Spending: An Update. 1994. (Orig.). lib. bdg. 250.00 (0-8490-5745-0) Gordon Pr.

Trends in Health Status, Services, & Finance: The Transition in Central & Eastern Europe. Ellen Goldstein et al. 1996. LC 96-40968. (Technical Papers: No. 341). 56p. pap. 22.00 (0-8213-3751-3, 13751) World Bank.

Trends in Health Status, Services, & Finance: The Transition in Central & Eastern Europe, Statistical Annex, Vol. II. Gnanaraj Chellaraj et al. 1997. LC 96-40968. (Technical Papers: No. 348). 152p. pap. 22.00 (0-8213-3828-5, 13828) World Bank.

Trends in Hospital Utilization: United States, 1988-92. Brenda Gillum et al. 1996. LC 96-8988. (Vital & Health Statistics Ser.: Series 13, No. 124). (0-8406-0516-1) Natl Ctr Health Stats.

Trends in Hospital Utilization: United States, 1988-92. Brenda Gilum. 1997. (Illus.). 71p. (C). pap. text 25.00 (0-7881-4534-7) DIANE Pub.

Trends in Infant Mortality by Cause of Death & Other Characteristics. 1994. lib. bdg. 250.00 (0-8490-5744-2) Gordon Pr.

Trends in Inflammation Research Two. R. Hirschelmann. Ed. by H. Bekemeier. 1982. (Agents & Actions Supplements Ser.: Vol. 10). 315p. 87.50 (0-8176-1344-7) Birkhauser.

Trends in Inflammatory Bowel Disease Therapy. Ed. by C. N. Williams. 1991. (Falk Symposium Ser.). 480p. text 229.00 (0-7923-8952-2) Kluwer Academic.

Trends in Inflammatory Bowel Disease Therapy, 1992. Ed. by C. N. Williams. 1993. LC 93-234830. (Falk Symposium Ser.). 384p. (C). text 174.50 (0-7923-8827-5) Kluwer Academic.

Trends in Inflammatory Bowel Disease Therapy, 1996. Ed. by R. S. McLeod et al. 1997. LC 98-172294. 320p. text 151.00 (0-7923-8718-X) Kluwer Academic.

Trends in Inflammatory Bowel Disease Therapy 1999. Ed. by C. Noel Williams. 2000. 288p. 145.00 (0-7923-8762-7) Kluwer Academic.

Trends in Medicinal Chemistry. Shalom Sarel. 1992. 132.00 (0-632-03364-9) CRC Pr.

Trends in Memory Development Research. Ed. by M. T. Chi. 1983. (Contributions to Human Development Ser.: Vol. 9). (Illus.). xii, 128p. pap. 42.75 (3-8055-3661-5) S Karger.

Trends in Neuroimmunology. Ed. by M. G. Marrosu et al. 1990. LC 90-6764. (Illus.). 178p. 55.00 (0-306-43510-1, Plenum Trade) Perseus Pubng.

Trends in Oral Contraception. Ed. by R. F. Harrison et al. 1983. 70p. text 59.00 (0-85200-771-X) Kluwer Academic.

Trends in Organ Transplantation. Ed. by Barbara A. Williams & Doris M. Sandiford-Guttenbiel. 1996. LC 95-24993. (Illus.). 272p. 49.95 (0-8261-9150-9) Springer Pub.

Trends in Pregnancies & Pregnancy Rates by Outcome: Estimates for the United States, 1976-96. National Center for Health Statistics Staff. 1999. LC 99-88898. (Vital & Health Statistics Ser.). pap. (0-8406-0561-7) Natl Ctr Health Stats.

Trends in Radiation Dosimetry. Ed. by W. L. McLaughlin. 1983. (Illus.). 320p. pap. 28.00 (0-08-029143-0, Pergamon Pr) Elsevier.

Trends in Research & Treatment of Joint Diseases. Ed. by Kazushi Hirohata et al. 1992. (Illus.). 192p. 123.00 (0-387-70095-1) Spr-Verlag.

Trends in Specialization: Tomorrow's Medicine. Ed. by Donald G. Langsley & James H. Darragh. 1985. LC 85-73107. (Illus.). 128p. lib. bdg. 29.95 (0-934277-06-0) Am Bd Med Spec.

Trends in the Health of Older Americans: U. S., 1994. Ed. by R. A. Cohen et al. 1995. LC 94-44483. (Vital & Health Statistics, Series 3, Analytical & Epidemiological Studies: No. 30). 328p. 21.00 (0-8406-0504-8) Natl Ctr Health Stats.

Trends in the Health of Older Americans: U. S., 1994. R. A. Cohen & J. F. Van Nostrand. 1996. (Illus.). 326p. pap. text 45.00 (0-7881-2796-9) DIANE Pub.

Trends in the Management of Systemic Fungal Infections. Ed. by D. W. Denning. 1992. (Journal: Vol. 38, Suppl. 1, 1992). (Illus.). iv, 96p. pap. 30.50 (3-8055-5627-6) S Karger.

Trends in the Study of Morbidity & Mortality. D. Curiel et al. 1965. (Public Health Papers: No. 27). (ENG, FRE, RUS & SPA.). 196p. pap. text 8.00 (92-4-130027-2, 1110027) World Health.

Trends of Mental Disease. American Psychopathological Association Staff. Ed. by Gerald N. Grob. 1980. LC 78-22547. (Historical Issues in Mental Health Ser.). (Illus.). reprint ed. lib. bdg. 18.95 (0-405-11901-1) Ayer.

Trepanations-Metapher: Ueber den Literarischen Umgang Mit Einem Medizinischen Thema. Roman Fischer. 1997. (GER., Illus.). 80p. pap. 28.00 (3-8055-6493-7) S Karger.

Treponema Pallidum: A Bibliographical Review of the Morphology, Culture & Survival of T. Pallidum & Associated Organisms. 1966. (WHO Bulletin Supplement Ser.: Vol. 35). pap. text 12.00 (92-4-068351-8, 1033501) World Health.

Treponemal Infections. 1982. (Technical Report Ser.: No. 674). 75p. pap. text 6.00 (92-4-120674-8) World Health.

Treponematoses Research: Proceedings of the WHO Scientific Group, Geneva, 1969. WHO Staff. 1970. (Technical Reports: No. 455). 91p. pap. text 7.00 (92-4-120455-9, 1100455) World Health.

Tretinoin - Actions, Harmful Reactions, & Variations in Therapy: Index of New Information with Authors, Subjects, & References. American Health Research Institute Staff. rev. ed. 1996. LC 96-3122. 151p. 57.50 (0-7883-1046-1); pap. 47.50 (0-7883-1047-X) ABBE Pubs Assn.

Treves: A Mystery Unravelled. Stephen Trombley. 1989. 224p. 47.50 (0-415-03423-X) Routledge.

Tri-Color Diet: A Miracle Breakthrough in Diet & Nutrition for a Longer, Healthier Life. Martin Katahn. 2000. 270p. reprint ed. text 23.00 (0-7881-6881-9) DIANE Pub.

Tri-Color Diet: A Miracle Breakthrough in Diet & Nutrition for a Longer, Healthier Life. Martin Katahn. 1996. LC 95-26434. (Illus.). 240p. 23.00 (0-393-03920-X) Norton.

Tri-n-Butyl Phosphate. 1990. (Environmental Health Criteria Ser.: No. 112). (ENG, FRE & SPA.). 80p. pap. text 19.00 (92-4-157112-8, 1160112) World Health.

Triage: Meeting the Challenge. 2nd rev. ed. 1997. (Orig.). 43.00 (0-935890-13-0) Emerg Nurses IL.

Triage in Emergency Practice. Gail Handysides. 1996. LC 95-10713. (Illus.). 400p. (C). (gr. 13). text 36.95 (0-8016-7892-7, 07892) Mosby Inc.

Triage Spanish: Basic Conversation for Health Professionals. Irwin Stern. 1994. LC 93-86874. (SPA.). x, 149p. pap. 19.95 incl. audio (0-9638926-0-6) Span-Text Bks.

Trial. Charles E. Harman. 1995. (Illus.). 721p. (Orig.). pap. 29.50 (0-9649391-0-X) Old Ct Pr.

Trial of John W. Hinckley Jr. A Case Study in the Insanity Defense. Peter W. Low et al. 1986. (University Casebook Ser.). 137p. pap. text 10.50 (0-88277-333-X) Foundation Pr.

Trial of the Assassin Guiteau: Psychiatry & the Law in the Gilded Age. Charles E. Rosenberg. 1976. LC 68-16713. pap. 14.95 (0-226-72717-3, P682) U Ch Pr.

Trial of the Templars in Cyprus: A Complete English Edition. Ed. & Tr. by Anne Gilmour-Bryson from LAT. 1998. LC 98-12850. (Medieval Mediterranean Ser.). xviii, 502p. 168.00 (90-04-10080-6) Brill Academic Pubs.

Trial Psychology: Communication & Persuasion in the Courtroom. Margaret C. Roberts. 1987. 490p. 95.00 (0-409-25105-4, 82475-10, MICHIE) LEXIS Pub.

Trials for Acute Stroke Therapy. Ed. by J. Bogousslavsky et al. 1995. (Journal: Vol. 5, Suppl. 1, 1995). (Illus.). iv, 34p. pap. 15.75 (3-8055-6228-4) S Karger.

Trials of an Expert Witness: Tales of Clinical Neurology & the Law. Harold L. Klawans. 1998. 280p. 19.95 (*1-888799-19-6*) Demos Medical.

Trials of an Ordinary Doctor: Joannes Groenevelt in Seventeenth-Century London. Harold J. Cook. 1994. LC 93-39733. (Illus.). 328p. 50.95 (*0-8018-4778-8*) Johns Hopkins.

Trials of Labour: The Re-Emergence of Midwifery. Brian Burtch. 1994. LC 93-49582. (Critical Perspectives on Public Affairs Ser.). 288p. (*0-7735-1141-5*); pap. (*0-7735-1143-1*) McG-Queens Univ Pr CAN. *Dist:* CUP Services.

Trials of Prophylactic Agents for the Control of Communicable Diseases: A Guide to Their Organization & Evaluation. T. M. Pollock. 1966. (Monographs: No. 52). (ENG, FRE, RUS & SPA.). 92p. pap. text 7.00 (*92-4-140052-8*, 1140052) World Health.

Trial(s) of Psychoanalysis. Francoise Meltzer. 1988. LC 87-34687. 296p. pap. text 17.00 (*0-226-51970-8*); 306p. lib. bdg. 34.00 (*0-226-51969-4*) U Ch Pr.

Trials of the Visionary Mind: Spiritual Emergency & the Renewal Process. John W. Perry. 1998. LC 98-23483. (Series in Transpersonal & Humanistic Psychology). 200p. (C). text 59.50 (*0-7914-3987-9*) State U NY Pr.

Trials of Thinking, Feeling & Willing. Carl Unger. 1980. pap. 2.50 (*0-916786-47-1*, Saint George Pubns) R Steiner Col.

Tribal Ecosystem & Malnutrition in India. Ed. by P. D. Tiwari & A. N. Sharma. 1989. (*81-85119-74-0*) Northern Bk Centre IND. *Dist:* S Asia.

Tribal Ethnomedicine: Continuity & Change. Jose K. Boban. 1998. LC 98-909143. (*81-7648-027-4*) Ashish Pub Hse IND. *Dist:* S Asia.

Tributyltin Compounds. 1990. (Environmental Health Criteria Ser.: No. 116). (ENG, FRE & SPA.). 273p. pap. text 46.00 (*92-4-157116-0*, 1160116) World Health.

Trichinella & Trichinosis. Ed. by William C. Campbell. 1983. LC 82-2390. 606p. 125.00 (*0-306-41140-7*, Plenum Trade) Perseus Pubng.

Trichlorfon. 1992. (Environmental Health Criteria Ser.: No. 132). (ENG, FRE & SPA.). 162p. pap. text 36.00 (*92-4-157132-2*, 1160132) World Health.

Trichomoniasis. Ed. by H. Ruettgers. 1983. (Journal: Vol. 23, Suppl. 2, 1983). (Illus.). iv, 92p. pap. 24.50 (*3-8055-3751-4*); viii, 92p. pap. 24.50 (*3-8055-3646-1*) S Karger.

Trichothecene Mycotoxicosis: Pathophysiologic Effects Ed. by Val R. Beasley. 1989. Vol. I. 208p. 109.00 (*0-8493-5088-3*, RA1242); Vol. II. 224p. 121.00 (*0-8493-5089-1*, RA1242) Franklin (CRC Reprint).

Trichotillomania: A Guide. Jeffrey L. Anders & James W. Jefferson. rev. ed. 1998. 49p. pap. 4.95 (*1-890802-14-X*) Madison Inst of Med.

Trichotillomania: New Developments. Ed. by Dan Stein et al. 1999. LC 98-29254. 344p. 47.00 (*0-88048-759-3*, 8759) Am Psychiatric.

Tricontinental Symposium on Autoimmune Skin Diseases, Proceedings, Kyodai Kaikan, Kyoto - Japan, November 1, 1993. Ed. by T. Nishikawa et al. 1994. (Journal: Vol. 189, Suppl. 1, 1994). (Illus.). xii, 138p. pap. 62.75 (*3-8055-5993-3*) S Karger.

Tricresyl Phosphate. 1990. (Environmental Health Criteria Ser.: No. 110). (ENG, FRE & SPA.). 122p. pap. text 24.00 (*92-4-157110-1*, 1160110) World Health.

Trigeminal Neuralgia. Zakrzewska. 1995. text 76.00 (*0-7020-1696-9*) Saunders.

Trigeminal Neuralgia: Current Concepts Regarding Pathogenesis & Treatment. Gerhard H. Fromm & Barry J. Sessle. 1990. (Illus.). 256p. text 75.00 (*0-409-90126-1*) Buttrwrth-Heinemann.

Trigeminal System in Man. Kamen G. Usunoff et al. Ed. by F. Beck et al. 1997. LC 97-11159. (Advances in Anatomy, Embryology & Cell Biology Ser.: No. 136). (Illus.). 96p. pap. 69.00 (*3-540-62786-3*) Spr-Verlag.

Trigger Points: Understanding Myofascial Pain & Discomfort. Anatomical Chart Company Staff. 1994. (Illus.). 9p. pap. 29.95 (*0-9603730-6-3*, TPCB2) Anatomical Chart.

Triggering of Acute Coronary Syndromes: Implications for Prevention. Ed. by Stefan N. Willich & James E. Muller. 1995. LC 95-21135. (Developments in Cardiovascular Medicine Ser.: Vol. 170). 424p. (C). text 213.50 (*0-7923-3605-4*) Kluwer Academic.

Triggering of Ovulation in Stimulated Cycles: HCG or LH? The Proceedings of an International Symposium Held under the Auspices of the French Endocrinology Society. Ed. by J. C. Emperaire. 1994. LC 93-46967. (Studies in Profertility: Vol. 1). 288p. lib. bdg. 71.95 (*1-85070-539-9*, Parthenon Pbng) CRC Pr.

Triglyceride, High Density Lipoprotein & Coronary Heart Disease. 1994. lib. bdg. 255.75 (*0-8490-5630-6*) Gordon Pr.

Trimipramin - Schlafentzug - Licht: Neurobiologische & Psychopathologische Verlaufsmessungen bei Depressionstherapie. Edith Holsboer-Trachsler. 1994. (Bibliotheca Psychiatrica Ser.: No. 166). (Illus.). xii, 138p. 129.75 (*3-8055-5920-8*) S Karger.

Trinucleotide Diseases & Instability. Ed. by B. A. Oostra. 1998. LC 97-51981. (Results & Problems in Cell Differentiation Ser.: Vol. 21). (Illus.). 178p. 109.00 (*3-540-63993-4*) Spr-Verlag.

Trip to the Hospital. Janet Tubbs. 2000. (Illus.). 16p. (J). (ps-4). pap. 19.95 (*1-881185-24-9*) Arcadia AZ.

Triphenyl Phosphate. 1991. (Environmental Health Criteria Ser.: No. 111). (ENG, FRE & SPA.). 80p. pap. text 19.00 (*92-4-157111-X*, 1160111) World Health.

Triple Threat: Defending Against Alcohol Abuse, Sexual Promiscuity & Gambling. Elliot Johnson. 2000. (Illus.). 28p. pap. 3.95 (*1-929478-09-7*) Cross Trng.

Trissel's Stability of Compounded Formulations. Lawrence A. Trissel. 1995. LC 95-80392. 296p. 60.00 (*0-917330-74-9*); 2nd ed. 2000. 475p. 88.00 (*1-58212-007-2*) Am Pharm Assn.

Tritium & Other Radionuclide Labeled Organic Compounds Incorporated in Genetic Material. 1979. LC 79-84486. (Report Ser.: No. 63). 147p. pap. text 35.00 (*0-913392-47-2*) NCRP Pubns.

Triumph: Improving the Management of Lower Urinary Tract Symptoms in Real Life Practice. Ed. by C. R. Chapple. 2001. (European Urology Ser.: Vol. 39, Suppl. 3, 2001). iv, 48p. 25.25 (*3-8055-7206-9*) S Karger.

Triumph over Cancer - Up Close & Personal. Stanley Millman. 2000. 53p. (*0-9679053-0-3*) Hands Across Sea.

Trocars & Pneumoperitoneum Needles in Minimally Invasive Surgery: Litigation, Legal, Marketing & Design. George Cristino. 1996. 465.00 (*1-886974-14-4*) Inst Knowledge.

***Tropenchirurgie III (Tropical Surgery III)** Ed. by W. Strecker & L. Kinzl. 1999. (Hefte zur Zeitschrift "Der Unfallchirurg" Ser.: Heft 274). (GER., Illus.). xviii, 441p. pap. 154.00 (*3-540-66038-0*) Spr-Verlag.

Trophoblast Research Vol. 4: Trophoblast Invasion & Endometerial Receptivity, Novel Aspects of the Cell Biology of Embryo Implantation. Ed. by H. W. Denker & J. D. Aplin. 1990. LC 90-7197. (Illus.). 463p. (C). text 180.00 (*0-306-43520-9*, Kluwer Plenum) Kluwer Academic.

Tropic Regulation of the Basal Ganglia: Focus on Dopamine Neurons. L. F. Agnati et al. Ed. by K. Fuxe et al. 1994. LC 93-34086. (Wenner-Gren International Ser.: 62). 628p. 219.50 (*0-08-042276-4*) Elsevier.

Tropical & Geographical Medicine: Companion Handbook. Ed. by Adel A. F. Mahmoud. 2nd ed. 1993. (Companion Handbook Ser.). (Illus.). 464p. 32.00 (*0-07-039625-6*) McGraw-Hill Med Pub.

Tropical Animal Health. Horst S. Seifert. 2nd ed. 1996. LC 95-40167. 548p. (C). text 199.00 (*0-7923-3821-9*) Kluwer Academic.

Tropical Dermatology. Roberto Arenas & Roberto Estrada. 2000. LC 99-10905. (Vademecum Ser.). (Illus.). 358p. spiral bd. 45.00 (*1-57059-493-7*) Landes Bioscience.

Tropical Disease. Ricardo V. Cohen & Frederico Aun. 1997. LC 96-27741. (On Call In...Ser.). 362p. (*1-57059-356-6*) Landes Bioscience.

Tropical Disease Research: Progress, 1975-94; Highlights, 1993-1994. Ed. by R. Walgate. 1995. LC 96-161788. (FRE.). v, 167p. (C). pap. text 26.00 (*92-4-156179-3*, 1150427) World Health.

Tropical Disease Research: Progress, 1991-1992, 11th Report. 1993. (FRE.). 140p. (C). pap. text 26.00 (*92-4-156158-0*, 1150400) World Health.

Tropical Disease Research: Seventh Programme Report, January 1, 1983 - December 31, 1984. 1985. 267p. pap. 45.00 (*92-4-156085-1*, 1150234) World Health.

Tropical Diseases: Control & Prevention in the Context of the New World Order. Ed. by James House et al. 2000. LC 00-56629. (Annals of the New York Academy of Sciences Ser.: Vol. 916). (Illus.). xv, 698p. 160.00 (*1-57331-281-9*) NY Acad Sci.

Tropical Diseases: From 50,000 BC to 2500 AD. Robert S. Desowitz. 2000. 256p. reprint ed. text 30.00 (*0-7881-9032-6*) DIANE Pub.

Tropical Diseases Research: A Global Partnership Eight Programme Report, the First Ten Years, with Highlights of the 1985-86 Biennium. 1987. 202p. pap. text 45.00 (*92-4-156106-8*, 1150267) World Health.

***Tropical Infectious Diseases: Epidemiology, Investigation, Diagnosis & Management.** Ranjan L. Fernando et al. 2001. (Greenwich Medical Media Ser.). (Illus.). 332p. pap. (*1-900151-39-1*) Greenwich Med GBR. *Dist:* JAMCO Dist.

Tropical Infectious Diseases: Principles, Pathogens, & Practice Richard L. Guerrant et al. Ed. by Marc Strauss. 1999. LC 99-20414. (Illus.). 1790p. (C). text (*0-443-07908-0*) Church.

Tropical Legumes in Animal Nutrition. Ed. by J. P. D'Mello & C. Devendra. 1995. (Illus.). 352p. (C). text 120.00 (*0-85198-926-8*) OUP.

***Tropical Medicine: Achievements & Prospects.** Ed. by David A. Warrell. 1998. (British Medical Bulletin Ser.: Vol. 54, No. 2). 254p. (*1-85315-343-5*) Royal Soc of Medicine Pr Ltd GBR. *Dist:* Balogh.

***Tropical Medicine & Parasitology.** Wallace Peters & Geoffrey Pasvol. 5th expurg. ed. 2001. (Illus.). 267p. pap. (*0-7234-3191-4*) Mosby Inc.

Tropical Medicine in the Twentieth Century: A History of the Liverpool School of Tropical Medicine. Helen L. Power. 1998. LC 97-48878. (Illus.). 200p. (*0-7103-0604-0*) Kegan Paul Intl GBR. *Dist:* Col U Pr.

Tropical Molecular Medicine. Madhav G. Deo. 1999. LC 99-937586. (Illus.). 208p. text 36.50 (*0-19-564630-4*) OUP.

Tropical Neurology. Shakir. 1995. text 82.95 (*0-7020-1922-4*) Saunders.

Tropical Pathology. Ed. by W. Doerr & Gerhard Seifert. 2nd ed. (Illus.). 1996. 1104p. 698.00 (*3-540-59391-8*); 1995. (Spezielle Pathologische Anatomie Ser.: Vol. 8). 1424p. 767.00 (*0-387-57673-8*) Spr-Verlag.

Tropical Surgery. Ed. by Ricardo Cohen et al. 1997. LC 96-27741. (Vademecum Ser.). (Illus.). xx, 338p. 98.00 (*3-8055-6497-X*) S Karger.

***Tropical Veterinary Diseases: Control & Prevention in the Context of the New World Order.** Ed. by James A. House et al. 2000. LC 00-56629. (Annals of the New York Academy of Sciences Ser.: Vol. 916). (Illus.). xv, 698p. (*1-57331-282-7*) NY Acad Sci.

Tropospheric Ozone: Human Health & Agricultural Impacts. David J. McKee. 1993. 352p. lib. bdg. 99.95 (*0-87371-475-X*, L475) Lewis Pubs.

Trouble-Free Menopause: Every Woman's Guide to Living a Fit & Healthy Life. Linda Konner & Judy E. Marshel. 1995. (Orig.). pap. 5.50 (*0-380-77732-0*, Avon Bks) Morrow Avon.

Trouble in the Prostate? The New Short Guide to Intelligent Choices. 1996. (Illus.). 90p. (Orig.). pap. 10.95 (*0-9653110-0-7*) T H Coleman.

Trouble in the Prostate? The New Short Guide to Intelligent Decisions. 2nd rev. ed. 1996. (Illus.). 82p. (Orig.). pap. 11.95 (*0-9653110-1-5*) T H Coleman.

Troubled Adolescent. Joseph L. White. 1989. (General Psychology Ser.). 400p. text 45.00 (*0-08-036820-4*); pap. text 19.50 (*0-08-036819-0*) Elsevier (Pergamon Pr).

Troubled Adolescent: As He Emerges on Psychological Tests. Ernest A. Hirsch. 1970. LC 72-110262. 645p. 95.00 (*0-8236-6650-6*) Intl Univs Pr.

Troubled Bodies: Critical Perspectives on Postmodernism, Medical Ethics & the Body. Ed. by Paul A. Komesaroff. 1995. LC 95-16274. 296p. pap. 17.95 (*0-8223-1688-9*); text 49.95 (*0-8223-1676-5*) Duke.

Troubled Bodies: Medical Ethics in the Postmodern Era. Ed. by Paul A. Komesaroff. 1996. 224p. pap. (*0-522-84684-X*) Melbourne Univ Pr AUS. *Dist:* Paul & Co Pubs.

Troubled Children - Troubled Systems. Ed. by Steven J. Apter. rev. ed. 1982. (General Psychology Ser.: No. 104). 285p. text 60.00 (*0-08-027167-7*); pap. text 25.00 (*0-08-027166-9*) Elsevier (Pergamon Pr).

Troubled Children in a Troubled World. Edith Buxbaum. 1970. LC 79-128623. 341p. (Orig.). 50.00 (*0-8236-6653-0*) Intl Univs Pr.

Troubled Dream of Life: In Search of a Peaceful Death. Daniel Callahan. 2000. LC 00-26365. 256p. reprint ed. pap. 15.95 (*0-87840-815-0*) Georgetown U Pr.

Troubled Families - Problem Children: Working with Parents: A Collaborative Process. Carolyn Webster-Stratton & Martin Herbert. 1994. LC 93-47493. 368p. pap. 85.00 (*0-471-94448-3*); 245.00 (*0-471-94251-0*) Wiley.

Troubled Helix: Social & Psychological Implications of the New Human Genetics. Ed. by Theresa Marteau & Martin Richards. 1996. (Illus.). 377p. (C). text 90.00 (*0-521-46288-6*) Cambridge U Pr.

Troubled Journey: Coming to Terms with the Mental Illness of a Sibling or Parent. Diane T. Marsh & Rex M. Dickens. 1997. LC 96-6815. 288p. 24.95 (*0-87477-875-1*, Tarcher Putnam) Putnam Pub Group.

Troubled Voices: Stories of Ethics & Illness. Richard M. Zaner. 1993. LC 93-3823. 192p. 19.95 (*0-8298-0964-3*) Pilgrim OH.

Troubled Youth in Treatment Homes: A Handbook of Therapeutic Foster Care. Ed. by Pamela Meadowcroft & Barbara A. Trout. 1990. (Trilogy Ser.: Bk. 2). pap. 11.50 (*0-87868-354-2*) Child Welfare.

Troubles of Children & Adolescents. Ed. by Ved Varma. 1997. LC 97-197653. 250p. pap. (*1-85302-323-X*) Jessica Kingsley GBR. *Dist:* Taylor & Francis.

Troubleshooting Histology Stains. R. W. Horobin & J. D. Bancroft. 1998. (Illus.). 256p. text (*0-443-05312-X*) Church.

Troublesome Disguises. Dinesh Bhugra et al. 1997. LC 97-4247. (Illus.). 352p. 81.95 (*0-86542-674-0*) Blackwell Sci.

Troubling the Angels: Women Living with HIV/AIDS. Patricia A. Lather. 1997. LC 97-3989. 288p. (C). pap. text 23.00 (*0-8133-9016-8*) Westview.

Truants from Life: The Rehabilitation of Emotionally Disturbed Children. Bruno Bettelheim. 1964. LC 55-7331. (Illus.). 516p. pap. 16.95 (*0-02-903450-7*) Free Pr.

Truck Company Operations. J. Steven Kidd & John Czajkowski. 1995. pap. text, wbk. ed. (*0-8151-5100-4*) Mosby Inc.

Trudging the Road: A Work-Study Journey Through the Twelve Steps of Alcoholics Anonymous. Chris F. Gladding. 1991. 170p. stu. ed. 16.00 (*0-9629091-0-6*) Glad Pubn.

True & False Allegations of Child Sexual Abuse: Assessment & Case Management. Ed. by Tara Ney. 1995. LC 94-47941. 400p. text 45.95 (*0-87630-758-6*) Brunner-Routledge.

True & False Experience: The Human Element in Psychotherapy. Peter Lomas. 1994. 170p. (C). pap. text 24.95 (*1-56000-733-8*) Transaction Pubs.

True Healing Art or Hygienic vs. Drug Medication (1880) R. T. Trall. 1996. 109p. reprint ed. pap. 11.95 (*1-56459-808-X*) Kessinger Pub.

Trust after Trauma: A Guide to Relationships for Survivors & Those Who Love Them. Aphrodite Matsakis. 1998. LC 97-75470. 344p. pap. 15.95 (*1-57224-101-2*) New Harbinger.

Trust & Betrayal in the Treatment of Child Abuse. Laurie K. MacKinnon. 1998. LC 97-43972. 260p. text 35.00 (*1-57230-298-4*) Guilford Pubns.

Trust Building with Children Who Hurt: A One-to-One Support Program for Children Ages 5-14. Ruth P. Arent. 1991. 224p. (J). (gr. k-9). text 29.95 (*0-87628-191-9*) Ctr Appl Res.

Trust Matters: New Directions in Health Care Leadership. Michael H. Annison & Dan S. Wilford. 1998. LC 98-18743. (Business & Management Ser.). 160p. 35.00 (*0-7879-4389-4*) Jossey-Bass.

"Trust Me, I'm a Doctor" Understanding & Surviving Modern Health Care. Thomas L. Minogue. 1996. xiv, 326p. (Orig.). (YA). (gr. 7 up). pap. 16.95 (*0-9654891-0-8*) TLM Cnslting.

Trust Your Body! Trust Your Baby! Childbirth Wisdom & Cesarean Prevention. Ed. by Andrea F. Henkart. 1995. LC 94-30915. 200p. pap. 15.75 (*0-89789-294-1*, Bergin & Garvey) Greenwood.

Trustee Handbook for Health Care Governance. James E. Orlikoff et al. 1998. LC 97-31677. (Trustee Ser.). 152p. 60.00 (*1-55648-220-5*) AHPI.

Trustee's Guide to Board Duties, Responsibilities & Liabilities. Charles F. MacKelvie & Marcia S. Handler. 1993. LC 92-48301. 92p. per. 24.95 (*1-882198-15-8*) Hlthcare Fin Mgmt.

Trustee's Guide to Compensation for Healthcare Executives. Michael F. Doody. 1993. LC 93-257. (Hospital Trustee Guide Ser.). 96p. per. 24.95 (*1-882198-16-6*) Hlthcare Fin Mgmt.

Trustee's Guide to Understanding Healthcare Antitrust Law Issues. Jonathan P. Tomes. 1992. 76p. 24.95 (*0-930228-89-8*) Hlthcare Fin Mgmt.

Trustee's Guide to Understanding Healthcare Environmental Law. Jonathan P. Tomes. 1992. 75p. per. 24.95 (*0-930228-88-X*) Hlthcare Fin Mgmt.

Trustee's Guide to Understanding Hospital Business Fundamentals. James J. Unland. 1992. 92p. per. 24.95 (*0-930228-81-2*) Hlthcare Fin Mgmt.

Trustee's Guide to Understanding Medical Staff Privileges. Jonathan P. Tomes. 1992. 85p. per. 24.95 (*0-930228-90-1*) Hlthcare Fin Mgmt.

Trusting Ourselves: The Complete Guide to Emotional Well-Being for Women. Karen Johnson. 1991. LC 89-38637. 496p. pap. 19.95 (*0-87113-447-0*, Atlntc Mnthly) Grove-Atltic.

Truth about Addiction & Recovery. Stanton Peele et al. 1992. 432p. pap. 14.00 (*0-671-75530-7*, Fireside) S&S Trade Pap.

Truth about Breast Cancer. Hay. 1996. LC 97-137478. 288p. pap. text (*0-7737-5794-5*) Stoddart Publ.

Truth about Breast Cancer: A 7-Step Prevention Plan. Joseph Keon. 1998. LC 94-12045. (Illus.). 304p. (Orig.). pap. 18.00 (*0-9648974-7-4*) Parissound.

Truth about Breast Cancer Risk Assessment. Alan Hollingsworth. 2000. LC 00-101498. 110p. 24.00 (*0-88100-115-5*) Natl Writ Pr.

Truth about Breast Implants. Randolph H. Guthrie. 1994. 145p. pap. 14.95 (*0-471-59418-0*) Wiley.

Truth about Chiropractic. Debra Levinson. 1993. (Illus.). 39.95 (*0-9633577-0-0*) Max Pubns.

Truth about Freud's Technique: The Encounter with the Real. M. Guy Thompson. 1994. LC 94-2933. (Psychoanalytic Crosscurrents Ser.). 296p. (C). text 45.00 (*0-8147-8206-X*) NYU Pr.

Truth about Herpes. Stephen L. Sacks. 3rd ed. 1988. (Illus.). 216p. pap. 14.95 (*0-919574-58-0*) Gordon Soules Bk.

Truth & Consequences of Sexually Transmitted Diseases. Carole Marsh. 1994. (Smart Sex Stuff Ser.). (Orig.). pap. 29.95 (*1-55609-212-1*) Gallopade Intl.

***Truth Behind Growth Hormone: Its Promise & Its Peril.** D. Gary Young. 1999. (Illus.). 46p. pap. text 3.95 (*0-943685-24-9*) Essential Science.

Truth Games: Lies, Money & Psychoanalysis. John Forrester. 1997. LC 97-17559. 224p. 24.95 (*0-674-53962-1*) HUP.

Truth, Trust & Medicine. Ed. by Jennifer Jackson. 2001. LC 00-56027. 192p. 65.00 (*0-415-18547-5*) Routledge.

Truth, Trust, & Relationships: Healing Interventions in Contextual Therapy. Barbara R. Krasner & Austin J. Joyce. 1995. LC 95-8927. 256p. text 31.95 (*0-87630-755-1*) Brunner-Routledge.

Try Being Healthy. Alec Forbes. 1976. 188p. pap. 11.95 (*0-8464-4305-8*) Beekman Pubs.

Try Being Healthy. Alec Forbes. 1980. 50.00 (*0-85032-140-9*) St Mut.

Try to Feel it My Way: New Help for Touch Dominant People & Those Who Care about Them. Suzette Haden Elgin. 1996. LC 96-15553. 176p. 40.00 (*0-471-00669-6*); 178p. pap. 14.95 (*0-471-00670-X*) Wiley.

Trying Again: A Guide to Pregnancy after Miscarriage, Stillbirth, & Infant Loss. Ann Douglas & John R. Sussman. 2000. LC 00-44683. xii, 311p. pap. 16.95 (*0-87833-182-4*) Taylor Pub.

Trying to Give Ease Vol. 1: Tommie Bass & the Story of Herbal Medicine. John K. Crellin & Jane Philpott. 1997. LC 97-15490. 335p. pap. 16.95 (*0-8223-2017-7*) Duke.

Tryptophan, Serotonin & Melatonin. Ed. by Gerald Huether. 1999. LC 99-42731. (Advances in Experimental Medicine & Biology Ser.). 852p. (0-306-46204-4, Kluwer Plenum) Kluwer Academic.

TSHR Universal Spinal Implementation. C. E. Johnston, II et al. 1993. 200p. text (0-9635430-1-6) Hundley & Assocs.

Tsubo: Vital Points of Oriental Therapy. Katsusuke Serizawa. 1998. LC 77-352739. (Illus.). 256p. pap. 25.00 (0-87040-900-X) Japan Pubns USA.

Tsutsugamushi Disease: An Overview. Ed. by Akiyoshi Kawamura, Jr. 1996. LC 97-140816. 361p. 120.00 (0-86008-512-0) Col U Pr.

Tubal Infertility. Ivo A. Brosens & Alan G. Gordon. 1989. (Illus.). 130p. (gr. 13). text (0-397-44572-5, GM0020) Gower-Mosby.

Tuberculosis. Ed. by William N. Rom & Stuart M. Garay. 1995. LC 95-10766. 1,002p. text 225.00 (0-316-75574-5, Little Brwn Med Div) Lppncott W & W.

Tuberculosis. Ed. by Milton D. Rossman & Rob R. MacGregor. 1994. 426p. text 69.00 (0-07-053950-2) McGraw-Hill Educ Grp.

Tuberculosis. William H. Hay et al. 1996. 37p. reprint ed. spiral bd. 11.00 (0-7873-1020-4) Hlth Research.

Tuberculosis. Ed. by David L. Schlossberg. 2nd ed. 1987. (Clinical Topics in Infectious Disease Ser.). (Illus.). 227p. 106.00 (0-387-96552-1) Spr-Verlag.

Tuberculosis: A Clinical Handbook. Ed. by Larry I. Lutwick. 1994. (Illus.). 392p. pap. (0-412-60740-9) E A GBR. *Dist:* OUP.

Tuberculosis: A Comprehensive International Approach. Ed. by Lee Reichman & Earl Hershfield. 1993. LC 93-20307. (Lung Biology in Health & Disease Ser.: Vol. 66). (Illus.). 784p. text 240.00 (0-8247-8852-4) Dekker.

Tuberculosis: A Half-Century of Study & Conquest. Jay A. Myers. 1970. LC 75-96989. (Illus.). 378p. 17.50 (0-87527-059-X) Green.

Tuberculosis: A Sourcebook for Nursing Practice. Ed. by Felissa Cohen & Jerry Durham. 1995. LC 94-35452. (Illus.). 312p. 49.95 (0-8261-8720-X) Springer Pub.

Tuberculosis: A State-of-the-Art Series. 1999. (Respiration Ser.: Vol. 65 (1998)). (Illus.). iv, 68p. pap. 30.50 (3-8055-7000-7) S Karger.

Tuberculosis: An International Perspective. Ed. by John D. Porter & John M. Grange. 1999. LC 98-43593. (Illus.). xvii, 509p. (1-86094-143-5) Imperial College GBR. *Dist:* World Scientific Pub.

Tuberculosis: And Non Tuberculous Myobacterial Infections. David L. Schlossberg. Ed. by Richard Zorab. 4th ed. 1999. LC 98-33386. (Illus.). 415p. (C). text 95.00 (0-7216-7308-2) Saunders.

Tuberculosis: Costly & Preventable Cases Continue in Five Cities. 1995. (Illus.). 55p. (Orig.). (C). pap. text 25.00 (0-7881-2048-4) DIANE Pub.

Tuberculosis: Current Concepts & Treatment. Lloyd N. Friedman. 2nd ed. 2000. LC 00-25394. (Illus.). 536p. 99.95 (0-8493-1565-4) CRC Pr.

Tuberculosis: Epidemics Deadly Diseases Throughout History. Fred Ramen. 2000. LC 00-9965. (Epidemics! Ser.). (Illus.). 64p. (J). (gr. 7-12). lib. bdg. 19.95 (0-8239-3349-0) Rosen Group.

Tuberculosis: Pathogenesis, Protection & Control. Ed. by Barry R. Bloom. 1994. LC 94-2932. (Illus.). 500p. 119.95 (1-55581-072-1) ASM Pr.

Tuberculosis among Certain Indian Tribes of the United States. Ales Hrdlicka. (Bureau of American Ethnology Ser.). 1995. 99p. lib. bdg. 69.00 (0-7812-4042-5); 1988. reprint ed. lib. bdg. 49.00 (0-7812-0016-4) Rprt Serv.

Tuberculosis among Certain Indian Tribes of the United States. Ales Hrdlicka. 1980. 96p. reprint ed. 49.00 (0-403-02467-6) Scholarly.

Tuberculosis & AIDS: The Relationship Between Mycrobacteria TB & the HIV Type 1. Lawrence L. Scharer & John M. McAdam. 1995. (Illus.). 160p. 33.95 (0-8261-9000-6) Springer Pub.

Tuberculosis & Its Prevention. Stefan Grzybowski. 1983. (Illus.). 124p. 19.75 (0-87527-198-7) Green.

Tuberculosis & Veterans' Medical Centers. 1994. (Illus.). 69p. (Orig.). (C). pap. text 20.00 (0-7881-0659-7) DIANE Pub.

Tuberculosis As a Disease of the Masses & How to Combat It. S. Adolphus Knopf. Ed. by Barbara G. Rosenkrantz. 1977. LC 76-40633. (Public Health in America Ser.). reprint ed. lib. bdg. 19.95 (0-405-09824-3) Ayer.

Tuberculosis Bacteriology: Organization & Practice. C. H. Collins et al. 2nd ed. 1997. LC 97-3038. 152p. (0-7506-2458-2) E A GBR. *Dist:* OUP.

Tuberculosis Control. 1982. (Technical Report Ser.: No. 671). 26p. pap. text 3.00 (92-4-120671-3) World Health.

Tuberculosis Current Concepts & Treatment: A Comprehensive Update. Lloyd N. Friedman. 1994. 384p. 115.95 (0-8493-4825-0) CRC Pr.

***Tuberculosis in the Workplace.** Ed. by Marilyn J. Field. 2001. LC 2001-30369. (Illus.). xiv, 340p. pap. 49.00 (0-309-07330-8) Natl Acad Pr.

Tuberculosis Movement: A Public Health Campaign in the Progressive Era, 22. 1988. LC 87-29432. (Contributions in Medical Studies Ser.: No. 22). 195p. 60.00 (0-313-25748-5, TCD/, Greenwood Pr) Greenwood.

Tuberculosis of the Bones & Joints. Ed. by M. Martini. 1988. (Illus.). 219p. 118.00 (0-387-18166-0) Spr-Verlag.

Tuberculosis Pearls. Ed. by Neil Schluger. 1995. (Pearls Ser.). 210p. (Orig.). pap. 45.00 (1-56053-156-8) Hanley & Belfus.

Tuberculosis Resource Guide. P. Heinsohn. 1996. 143p. (Orig.). pap. text 35.00 (0-7881-3337-3) DIANE Pub.

Tuberculosis Resurgent. Ed. by Richard Westlund et al. 2nd rev. ed. 1995. 95p. (Orig.). pap. text 22.00 (1-879772-02-7) Health Studies.

Tuberculosis Revival: Individual Rights & Societal Obligations in a Time of AIDS. 1992. LC 92-40474. (Special Reports). 10.00 (1-881277-12-7) United Hosp Fund.

Tuberculosis Statistics in the U. S. 1994. lib. bdg. 250.00 (0-8490-8409-1) Gordon Pr.

Tuberculosis Training & Education Resource Guide. Ed. by Barry Leonard. 2000. 61p. (C). pap. text 20.00 (0-7567-0190-2) DIANE Pub.

Tuberous Sclerosis Complex. Manuel R. Gomez. 3rd ed. 1999. LC 98-4111. (Illus.). 368p. text 79.95 (0-19-512210-0) OUP.

Tubular Disease. Michael Michelis. Date not set. (0-938607-33-2) Field & Wood Inc Medical.

Tubulointerstitial & Cystic Disease of the Kidney. Ed. by S. M. Dodd et al. 1995. LC 95-3278. (Current Topics in Pathology Ser.: Vol. 88). (Illus.). 304p. 143.00 (3-540-58842-6) Spr-Verlag.

Tubulo-Interstitial Nephropathies. Ed. by Alberto Ameria et al. 1991. (Developments in Nephrology Ser.). (C). text 163.50 (0-7923-1200-7) Kluwer Academic.

Tufts University Guide to Total Nutrition: Second Edition. Stanley Gershoff et al. 2nd rev. ed. 1996. LC 95-6386. (Illus.). 368p. (Orig.). pap. 16.00 (0-06-273316-8, Harper Ref) HarperCollins Pubs.

Tuftsin: Biochemistry, Immunology & Clinical Prospects. Nishioka. 1995. 177.95 (0-8493-6701-8) CRC Pr.

Tulapai to Tokay: A Bibliography of Alcohol Use & Abuse Among Native Americans of North America. Patricia D. Mail & David R. McDonald. 1981. LC 80-81243. (Bibliographies Ser.). 372p. 20.00 (0-87536-253-2) HRAFP.

Tumescent Technique. Gerald H. Pitman. 1995. (Illus.). 19p. pap. 85.00 (0-942219-95-3) Quality Med Pub.

Tumescent Technique: Local Anesthesia, Liposuction & Dermatologic Plastic Surgery. Jeffrey A. Klein. 2000. (Illus.). 300p. (C). (gr. 13). text 185.00 (0-8151-5205-1, 26543) Mosby Inc.

Tummy: An Owner's Manual. Judson P. Cone. 1974. 63p. (Orig.). pap. 1.95 (0-89074-008-9) Charing Cross.

Tumor & Non-Tumor Aspects of Angiogenesis. Jacqueline B. Weiss & Barry McLaughlin. 1994. (Medical Intelligence Unit Ser.). 118p. 89.95 (1-57059-038-9, LN9038) CRC Pr.

Tumor Aneuploidy. Ed. by T. Buchner et al. 1985. LC 85-9897. (Illus.). 141p. 42.95 (0-387-15376-4) Spr-Verlag.

Tumor Biology: Regulation of Cell Growth, Differentiation & Genetics in Cancer. NATO Scientific Affairs Organization Staff. Ed. by Asterios S. Tsiftoglou. 1996. LC 96-32244. (NATO ASI Ser.). 331p. 149.50 (3-540-61492-3) Spr-Verlag.

Tumor Blood Circulation: Angiogenesis, Vascular Morphology & Blood Flow of Experimental & Human Tumors. Hans-Inge Peterson. 1979. 240p. 138.00 (0-8493-5695-4, RC255, CRC Reprint) Franklin.

Tumor Blood Supply & Metabolic Microenvironment: Characterization & Implications for Therapy. Rakesh K. Jain & Peter W. Vaupel. 1991. (Illus.). 340p. (Orig.). pap. 78.00 (1-56081-328-8) Balogh.

Tumor Board: Cancer Diagnosis & Treatment. David Winchester et al. 1996. LC 96-23252. (Illus.). 788p. text 110.00 (0-397-51340-2) Lppncott W & W.

Tumor Bone Diseases & Osteoporosis in Cancer Patients. Jean J. Body. 1999. LC 99-39513. (Illus.). 584p. text 195.00 (0-8247-6399-8) Dekker.

Tumor Cell Differentiation: Biology & Pharmacology. Ed. by Jarle Aarbakke et al. 1987. LC 87-17012. (Experimental Biology & Medicine Ser.: Vol. 17). (Illus.). 360p. (C). 150.00 (0-89603-134-9) Humana.

Tumor Diagnosis by Electron Microscope, Vol. 3. Jose Russo. 1989. 75.00 (0-938607-22-7) Field & Wood Inc Medical.

Tumor Immunology. Ed. by A. G. Dalgleish & M. J. Browning. 1996. (Cancer: Clinical Science in Practice Ser.). (Illus.). 369p. (C). text 90.00 (0-521-47237-7) Cambridge U Pr.

Tumor Immunology: Symposium in Immunology IV. Ed. by Martha Eibl & C. Huber. 1997. LC 96-35941. (Illus.). 172p. pap. 110.00 (3-540-61755-8) Spr-Verlag.

Tumor Immunology & Cancer Therapy. Ed. by Ronald H. Goldfarb & Theresa L. Whiteside. 1993. LC 93-39772. (Immunology Ser.: Vol. 61). (Illus.). 344p. text 175.00 (0-8247-9179-7) Dekker.

Tumor Invasion & Metastasis. Lance A. Liotta & I. R. Hurt. 1982. text 366.50 (90-247-2611-5) Kluwer Academic.

Tumor Marker Protocols. Ed. by Margaret Hanausek & Zbigniew Walaszek. 1998. LC 97-51263. (Methods in Molecular Medicine Ser.: Vol. 14). (Illus.). 512p. 129.50 (0-89603-380-5) Humana.

Tumor Markers. S. Eissa. 1999. LC 99-203423. (Illus.). 416p. text (0-412-81720-9) E A GBR. *Dist:* OUP.

Tumor Markers: Biology & Clinical Applications, 4. Ed. by Nasser Javadpour. 1987. LC 85-30014. (Cancer Research Monographs: Vol. 4). 304p. 99.75 (0-275-92145-X, C2145, Praeger Pubs) Greenwood.

Tumor Matrix Biology. Ed. by Roza Adany. 1995. LC 94-44953. 272p. lib. bdg. 205.00 (0-8493-4882-X, 4882) CRC Pr.

Tumor Metastasis, Vol. 1. Ed. by Bruce R. Zetter. Date not set. 128.50 (0-7623-0400-6) Jai Pr.

Tumor Models in Cancer Research. Ed. by Beverly A. Teicher. 2001. (Cancer Drug Discovery & Development Ser.). 500p. 145.00 (0-89603-887-4) Humana.

Tumor Necrosis Factor: Molecular & Celullar Biology & Clinical Relevance. International Conference on Tumor Necrosis Factor. Ed. by Walter Fiers & Wim A. Buurman. 1993. LC 92-48509. (Illus.). x, 256p. 281.00 (3-8055-5676-4) S Karger.

Tumor Necrosis Factor: Structure Function Relationship & Clinical Application. Ed. by T. Osawa & B. Bonavida. 1992. (Illus.). x, 292p. 242.75 (3-8055-5458-3) S Karger.

Tumor Necrosis Factor: Structure, Mechanism of Action, Role in Disease & Therapy. Ed. by B. Bonavida et al. 1990. (Illus.). x, 254p. 172.25 (3-8055-4966-0) S Karger.

Tumor Necrosis Factor & Related Cytotoxins. CIBA Foundation Staff. 1987. LC 87-18975. (CIBA Foundation Symposia Ser.: No. 131). 252p. 128.00 (0-471-91097-X) Wiley.

Tumor Necrosis Factor-Cachectin & Related Cytokines. Ed. by B. Bonavida et al. 1988. (Illus.). viii, 276p. 172.25 (3-8055-4755-2) S Karger.

Tumor Response Monitoring & Treatment Planning. Ed. by A. Breit. 1992. (Illus.). 740p. 185.00 (0-387-54783-5) Spr-Verlag.

Tumor Stereotaxis. Kelly. 1990. (Illus.). 442p. text 179.00 (0-7216-5360-X) Saunders.

Tumor Suppressor Genes in Human Cancer. Ed. by David E. Fisher. 2001. LC 00-27593. (Cancer Drug Discovery & Development Ser.). (Illus.). xii, 386p. 135.00 (0-89603-807-6) Humana.

Tumor Surgery of the Head & Neck. R. S. Pollack. 1975. (Illus.). x, 206p. 63.50 (3-8055-2092-1) S Karger.

Tumor Therapy with Tumor Cells & Neuraminidase: Cell Physiological, Immunological, & Oncological Aspects. H. H. Sedlacek. 1987. (Beitraege Zur Onkologie, Contributions to Oncology Ser.: Vol. 27). (Illus.). viii, 96p. 43.50 (3-8055-4549-5) S Karger.

Tumorbiologie. J. G. Birkmayer. 1984. (Illus.). viii, 230p. 49.75 (3-8055-3892-8) S Karger.

Tumorchirurgie und Lebensqualitaet. Ed. by M. Duerig & U. Laffer. 1989. (Basler Beitraege zur Chirurgie Ser.: Vol. 2). (Illus.). x, 168p. 65.25 (3-8055-5070-7) S Karger.

Tumorimmunologie & Tumortherapie. H. H. Sedlacek. 1986. (Beitraege Zur Onkologie, Contributions to Oncology Ser.: Vol. 25). (Illus.). x, 186p. 55.00 (3-8055-4447-2) S Karger.

Tumors: Structure & Diagnosis. R. C. Curran & E. L. Jones. 1991. (Harvey Miller Publications). (Illus.). 812p. text 275.00 (0-19-261840-7) OUP.

Tumors & Related Lesions of the Female Genital Tract: Proceedings of the Fifty Sixth Annual Anatomic Pathology Slide Seminar of the ASCP. Ed. by William R. Hart et al. 1991. 136p. 35.00 (0-89189-337-7) Am Soc Clinical.

Tumors & Tumor-Like Conditions of the Kidneys & Ureters. Ed. by John N. Eble. 1990. (Contemporary Issues in Surgical Pathology Ser.: Vol. 16). (Illus.). 268p. text (0-443-08674-5) Church.

Tumors & Tumor-Like Lesions of Bone & Joints. Fritz Schajowicz. 1981. (Illus.). 581p. 280.00 (0-387-90492-1) Spr-Verlag.

Tumors & Tumor-Like Lesions of Soft Tissues. Ed. by Vito Ninfo & E. B. Chung. 1991. (Contemporary Issues in Surgical Pathology Ser.: Vol. 18). (Illus.). 295p. text (0-443-08672-9) Church.

Tumors & Tumor-Like Lesions of the Lung. Darryl Carter & Arthur S. Patchefsky. 1998. LC 97-23526. (Major Problems in Pathology Ser.). (Illus.). 448p. (C). text 85.00 (0-7216-3312-9) Saunders.

Tumors & Tumor-Like Lesions of the Uterine Corpus & Cervix. Philip B. Clement & Robert H. Young. 1993. (Contemporary Issues in Surgical Pathology Ser.). (Illus.). 504p. text (0-443-08801-2) Church.

Tumors & Tumorlike Lesions of Bone: Pathology, Radiology, & Treatment. Fritz Schajowicz. 2nd ed. 1993. LC 92-49404. (3-540-55366-5); 1995. (Illus.). 752p. 348.00 (0-387-55366-5) Spr-Verlag.

Tumors in Aquatic Animals. Ed. by F. Homburger. 1976. (Progress in Experimental Tumor Research Ser.: Vol. 20). 400p. 134.00 (3-8055-2254-1) S Karger.

Tumors in Urology. D. E. Neal. 1995. LC 94-14579. (Illus.). 298p. 136.00 (3-540-19867-9) Spr-Verlag.

Tumors in Urology: Biology & Clinical Management. Ed. by David E. Neal. 1994. LC 94-14579. (Illus.). 298p. 159.00 (0-387-19867-9) Spr-Verlag.

Tumors of Skin Appendages. Ken Hashimoto et al. 1987. (Illus.). 208p. pap. text (0-409-95159-5) E A GBR. *Dist:* OUP.

Tumors of Soft Tissues. Tapas K. Das Gupta & Prabir K. Chaudhuri. 2nd ed. 1998. LC 97-40497. 636p. (C). text 179.00 (0-8385-9044-6, A-9044-7, Apple Lange Med) McGraw.

Tumors of the Brain & Skull Ed. by Pierre J. Vinken & George W. Bruyn. 1975. Pt. 1. 292.00 (0-444-10495-X); Pt. 2. 292.00 (0-444-10573-5); Pt. 3. 232.00 (0-444-10842-4) Elsevier.

Tumors of the Cardiovascular System. 1995. lib. bdg. 257.95 (0-8490-6722-7) Gordon Pr.

Tumors of the Central Nervous System. Burger & Scheithauer. 1994. (AFIP Atlas of Tumor Pathology Ser.: Vol. 10). (Illus.). 452p. pap. text 60.00 (1-881041-10-7) Am Registry Path.

Tumors of the Central Nervous System, Set. 1995. lib. bdg. 600.99 (0-8490-6726-X) Gordon Pr.

Tumors of the Epidermis. Ken Hashimoto & Amir H. Mehregoan. 1990. (Illus.). 288p. text (0-409-90163-6) E A GBR. *Dist:* OUP.

Tumors of the Esophagus & Stomach 1991. lib. bdg. 600.95 (0-8490-4334-4) Gordon Pr.

Tumors of the Exocrine Pancreas. 1995. lib. bdg. 251.99 (0-8490-6715-4) Gordon Pr.

Tumors of the Eye. Ed. by N. Bornfeld et al. 1991. LC 91-35368. (Illus.). 700p. lib. bdg. (90-6299-082-7) Kugler NLD. *Dist:* Lib Res.

Tumors of the Eye & Ocular Adnexa. McLean et al. 1995. (AFIP Atlas of Tumor Pathology Ser.: Vol. 12). (Illus.). 322p. pap. text 56.00 (1-881041-11-5) Am Registry Path.

Tumors of the Fetus & Newborn. Hart Issacs. 1997. LC 96-38016. (C). text 105.00 (0-7216-3813-9) Harcourt.

Tumors of the Head & Neck in Children. Robert O. Greer et al. 1983. LC 82-19114. 416p. 105.00 (0-275-91391-0, C1391, Praeger Pubs) Greenwood.

Tumors of the Heart & Great Vessels. Allen Burke & Renu Virmani. 1996. (AFIP Atlas of Tumor Pathology Ser.: Vol. 16). (Illus.). 231p. pap. text 58.00 (1-881041-20-4) Am Registry Path.

Tumors of the Intestines, Set. 1995. lib. bdg. 605.75 (0-8490-7565-3) Gordon Pr.

Tumors of the Kidney. Michele Pavone-Macaluso & Jean B. DeKernion. 1986. (Surgery Ser.). (Illus.). 340p. 86.75 (0-683-02426-4) Lppncott W & W.

Tumors of the Kidney & Urinary Tract. Steen Olsen. 1985. (Illus.). 291p. text 142.00 (0-7216-1588-0) Saunders.

Tumors of the Liver & Extrahepatic Bile Ducts. 1995. lib. bdg. 252.99 (0-8490-6718-9) Gordon Pr.

Tumors of the Lower Respiratory Tract. Colby et al. 1995. (AFIP Atlas of Tumor Pathology Ser.: Vol. 13). (Illus.). 554p. pap. text 69.00 (1-881041-17-4) Am Registry Path.

Tumors of the Lung, Vol. 24. Bruce MacKay et al. 1990. (Illus.). 432p. text 92.00 (0-7216-5807-5) Saunders.

Tumors of the Lung: Contemporary Issues. B. Corrin. 1997. LC 97-7855. text (0-443-05367-7) Church.

Tumors of the Lymph Nodes & Spleen. Warnke et al. 1995. (AFIP Atlas of Tumor Pathology Ser.: Vol. 14). (Illus.). 544p. pap. text 69.00 (1-881041-18-2) Am Registry Path.

Tumors of the Male Genital System. 1995. lib. bdg. 257.99 (0-8490-6720-0) Gordon Pr.

Tumors of the Mediastinum. Shimosato & Mukai. 1997. (AFIP Atlas of Tumor Pathology Ser.: Vol. 21). (Illus.). 278p. pap. text 60.00 (1-881041-30-1) Am Registry Path.

Tumors of the Mediastinum. J. M. Verley & K. H. Hollmann. 1992. LC 91-35327. (Current Histopathology Ser.). 136p. (C). text 251.00 (0-7923-8986-7) Kluwer Academic.

Tumors of the Pediatric Nervous System. Robert Keating. 2001. LC 00-53279. 400p. 189.00 (0-86577-848-5) Thieme Med Pubs.

Tumors of the Salivary Glands. Ellis & Auclair. 1996. (AFIP Atlas of Tumor Pathology Ser.: Vol. 17). (Illus.). 468p. pap. text 69.00 (1-881041-26-3) Am Registry Path.

Tumors of the Serosal Membranes. Battifora & McCaughey. 1995. (AFIP Atlas of Tumor Pathology Ser.: Vol. 15). (Illus.). 128p. pap. text 45.00 (1-881041-19-0) Am Registry Path.

Tumors of the Soft Tissues. 1995. lib. bdg. 275.95 (0-8490-6725-1) Gordon Pr.

Tumors of the Spine: Diagnosis & Clinical Management. Sundaresan et al. 1990. (Illus.). 576p. text 335.00 (0-7216-2896-6) Saunders.

Tumors of the Spine & Spinal Cord Ed. by Pierre J. Vinken & George W. Bruyn. 1976. Pt. 1. 156.50 (0-444-10783-5); Pt. 2. 311.00 (0-444-10929-3) Elsevier.

Tumors of the Upper Respiratory Tract & Ear. 1995. lib. bdg. 278.95 (0-8490-6723-5) Gordon Pr.

Tumors of the Urinary Bladder. 1995. lib. bdg. 263.95 (0-8490-6716-2) Gordon Pr.

Tumors of the Urinary Bladder & Related Urinary Structures: Tumors of the Kidney, Bladder & Related Urinary Structures. William M. Murphy et al. Ed. by George M. Farrow. 1994. (AFIP Atlas of Tumor Pathology Ser.: Vol. 11). (Illus.). 362p. pap. text 55.00 (1-881041-15-8) Am Registry Path.

Tumors of the Uterine Corpus & Gestational Trophoblastic Disease. Silverbery & Robert J. Kurman. 1992. (AFIP Atlas of Tumor Pathology Ser.: Vol. 3). (Illus.). 290p. pap. text 45.00 (1-881041-01-8) Am Registry Path.

Tumour Angiogenesis. Ed. by Roy Bicknell et al. 1997. LC 96-52106. (Illus.). 396p. text 195.00 (0-19-854937-7) OUP.

Tumour Localization with Radioactive Agents. International Atomic Energy Agency Staff. 1976. LC 76-7616. (Panel Proceedings Ser.). (Illus.). 142p. pap. (*92-0-111276-9*, ISP451) IAEA AUT. *Dist:* Bernan Associates.

Tumours, Lymphomas & Selected Paraproteinaemias. Ed. by Julian L. Verbov. 1988. (New Clinical Applications in Dermatology Ser.). (C). text 99.50 (*0-7462-0082-X*) Kluwer Academic.

Tumours of the Brain & Skull, Pt. III. Pierre J. Vinken & George W. Bruyn. 1975. (Handbooks of Clinical Neurology: Vol. 18). 582p. 349.00 (*0-7204-7218-0*) Elsevier.

Tumours of the Epidermis & Ache. Marks. 1997. (Illus.). 208p. (C). pap. 119.95 (*0-412-63530-5*, Chap & Hall NY) Chapman & Hall.

Tumours of the Larynx. A. Burkhardt & E. Meyer-Breiting. 1988. (Illus.). 221p. 224.00 (*0-387-16342-5*) Spr-Verlag.

Tumours of the Nervous System. Ironside. 2001. (C). text 248.00 (*0-443-04558-5*) Saunders.

Tumours of the Spine & Spinal Cord, Pt. I. Pierre J. Vinken & George W. Bruyn. 1975. (Handbooks of Clinical Neurology: Vol. 19). 394p. 235.50 (*0-7204-7219-9*) Elsevier.

Tumours of the Upper Jaw. Ed. by Donald Harrison & Valerie J. Lund. 1993. LC 92-49458. 360p. text (*0-443-04017-6*) Church.

Tungara Frog: A Study in Sexual Selection & Communication. Michael J. Ryan. LC 84-24110. (Illus.). xvi, 230p. 1994. lib. bdg. 33.00 (*0-226-73228-2*); 1992. pap. text 14.95 (*0-226-73229-0*) U Ch Pr.

Tuning the Therapeutic Instrument: Affective Learning of Psychotherapy. David E. Scharff & Jill Savege Scharff. 2000. LC 99-48775. 440p. 60.00 (*0-7657-0245-2*) Aronson.

Tunnel of Hope. Sheri J. Vitolo. Ed. by Gwen Costa. 1990. LC 90-22321. 165p. 13.95 (*0-87949-348-8*) Ashley Bks.

Tunnel Syndromes: Peripheral Nerve Compression Syndromes. Marko M. Pecina et al. 2nd ed. 1996. LC 96-21241. 304p. 104.95 (*0-8493-2629-X*) CRC Pr.

Turek's Orthopaedics, Principles & Their Application. Ed. by Stuart L. Weinstein & Joseph A. Buckwalter. 5th ed. 1994. LC 93-39198. 736p. text 139.00 (*0-397-50692-9*) Lppncott W & W.

Turn off the Fat Genes! The Revoluntionary Guide to Taking Charge of the Genes That Control Your Weight. Neal Barnard & Jennifer Raymond. 2001. LC 00-33466. (Illus.). 368p. 23.95 (*0-609-60631-X*) Harmony Bks.

***Turn off the Fat Genes: The Revolutionary Guide to Losing Weight.** Neal Barnard. 2001. 368p. pap. 14.00 (*0-609-80904-0*, Three Riv Pr) Harmony Bks.

Turnaround Imperative: A Leader's Guide for Survival in a Turbulent Health Care Environment. Victor A. Cocowitch & Kevin M. Fickenscher. 1996. LC 95-79896. 117p. (Orig.). (C). pap. text 44.00 (*0-924674-37-7*) Am Coll Phys Execs.

***Turnbull's Obstetrics.** Geoffrey Chamberlain & Philip Steer. 3rd ed. 2001. (Illus.). 940p. (*0-443-06365-6*) Church GBR. *Dist:* Saunders.

Turner Syndrome in a Life Span Perspective: Research & Clinical Aspects : Proceedings of the 4th International Symposium, Gothenburg, 12-21 May, 1995. Ed. by K. Albertsson-Wikland & M. B. Ranke. 1995. (International Congress Ser.: Vol. 1089). 340p. 185.00 (*0-444-82188-0*) Elsevier.

Turning a "Little Light" on Multiple Sclerosis: I'm Not Crazy, I'm Not Drunk, Well Maybe a Little Nuts. Kathy D. Kvaale. Ed. by Fern Erdahl et al. 1997. (Orig.). pap. 5.00 (*0-9643922-2-4*) K Kvaale.

Turning Awareness into Action: What Your Community Can Do about Drug Use in America. rev. ed. 1993. (ENG & SPA.). 148p. (C). pap. text 20.00 (*0-7881-0208-7*) DIANE Pub.

Turning Back the Aging Clock: Dr. Lee-Benners' Scientifically Designed & Medically Based Longevity Program. Lee-Benner. 1991. (Illus.). 230p. (Orig.). pap. 25.00 (*0-944213-05-7*) World Hlth Found.

Turning Every Stone: Autism with Love - Reality Therapy. Phyllis H. Lambert. 1990. (Illus.). 96p. pap., per. 18.00 (*0-9624737-4-X*) Old Barn Entrprs.

Turning Point: How Men of Conscience Brought about Major Change in the Care of America's Mentally Ill. Alex Sareyan. 1993. LC 93-9227. (Illus.). 314p. text 18.95 (*0-88048-560-4*, 8560) Am Psychiatric.

Turning Point: How Persons of Conscience Brought about Major Change in the Care of America's Mentally Ill. Alex Sareyan. 1994. LC 94-26396. 314p. pap. 17.99 (*0-8361-3596-2*) Herald Press.

Turning Point: The Other Side of Menopause. C. Sue Hudson-Ferman. 1995. LC 94-16479. 224p. 25.00 (*0-19-508773-9*) OUP.

Turning Points: Treating Families in Transition & Crisis. Frank S. Pittman, III. 1987. (Professional Bks.). 370p. 34.95 (*0-393-70040-2*) Norton.

Turning Points in Analytic Therapy: From Winnicott to Kernberg. Gerald Schoenewolf. 1990. LC 89-17949. 256p. 50.00 (*0-87668-809-1*) Aronson.

Turning Points in Analytic Therapy: The Classic Cases. Gerald Schoenewolf. 1990. LC 89-17949. 256p. 50.00 (*0-87668-819-9*) Aronson.

Turning Points in Cataract Formation, Syndromes & Retinoblastoma. Ed. by W. Straub. 1982. (Developments in Ophthalmology Ser.: Vol. 7). (Illus.). viii, 100p. 81.75 (*3-8055-3564-3*) S Karger.

Turning Points in Retinal Surgery: Proceedings of the Jules Gorin Club Meeting, Lausanne, June 1976. Gorin, Jules, Club Staff. Ed. by E. W. Norton et al. 1977. (Modern Problems in Ophthalmology Ser.: Vol. 18). (Illus.). 213.25 (*3-8055-2425-0*) S Karger.

Tuskegee's Truths: Rethinking the Tuskegee Syphilis Study. Ed. by Susan M. Reverby. 2000. LC 99-56379. (Studies in Social Medicine). (Illus.). xviii, 630p. pap. 27.50 (*0-8078-4852-2*); lib. bdg. 69.95 (*0-8078-2539-5*) U of NC Pr.

Tutorial Essays in Psychology, Vol. 1. Ed. by Norman S. Sutherland. 1977. 182p. 36.00 (*0-89859-148-1*) L Erlbaum Assocs.

Tutorial Essays in Psychology, Vol. 2. Ed. by N. S. Sutherland. 1979. 160p. 36.00 (*0-89859-199-6*) L Erlbaum Assocs.

Tutorials for Junior Students of Surgery. Graham D. Hill & Andrew G. Hill. 1990. 124p. pap. text (*0-443-04449-X*) Church.

Tutorials for the Biomedical Sciences: Animations, Simulations & Calculations. C. Pidgeon. 1996. 328p. pap. 110.00 (*0-471-18637-6*, Wiley-VCH) Wiley.

Tutorials for the Biomedical Sciences: Animations, Simulations, & Calculations Using Mathematica. Ed. by Charles Pidgeon. 1996. LC 95-25624. (Illus.). xxviii, 300p. pap. 79.95 incl. disk (*1-56081-928-6*, Wiley-VCH) Wiley.

Tutorials in Clinical Surgery in General. F. G. Smiddy. 1991. 256p. (Orig.). pap. text (*0-443-04577-1*) Church.

Tutorials in Clinical Surgery in General - Two. F. G. Smiddy. 2nd ed. 1992. 292p. (Orig.). pap. text (*0-443-04796-0*) Church.

***Tutorials in Differential Diagnosis.** Robert L. Souhami et al. 2001. (Illus.). 267p. pap. (*0-443-06157-2*) Church GBR. *Dist:* Saunders.

Tutorials in Differential Diagnosis. Eric R. Beck et al. 3rd ed. 1992. (Illus.). 236p. (Orig.). pap. text (*0-443-04472-4*) Church.

Tutorials in General Practice. Michael Mead & Henry Patterson. 2nd ed. 1992. (Illus.). 206p. pap. text (*0-443-04332-9*) Church.

Tutorials in Motor Behavior. George E. Stelmach & Jean Requin. 1987. (Advances in Psychology Ser.: Vol. 1). 680p. 183.00 (*0-444-85466-5*, North Holland) Elsevier.

Tutorials in Motor Behavior II. Jean Requin & G. E. Stelmach. 1992. (Advances in Psychology Ser.: Vol. 87). 960p. 198.50 (*0-444-88801-2*, North Holland) Elsevier.

Tutorials in Motor Neuroscience: Proceedings of the NATO Advanced Study Institute. Jean Requin & George E. Stelmach. 1991. 696p. (C). text 326.00 (*0-7923-1385-2*) Kluwer Academic.

Tutorials in Surgery. F. G. Smiddy. 1977. pap. 39.00 (*0-8464-0938-0*) Beekman Pubs.

Tutorials in Surgery, Vol. 2. F. G. Smiddy. 2nd ed. 1986. LC 83-19302. (Illus.). 319p. (C). pap. (*0-443-03603-9*) Church.

Twelfth I. S. C. E. R. G. Symposium. 1976. (Documenta Ophthalmologica Proceedings Ser.: Vol. 10). pap. text 226.00 (*90-6193-150-9*) Kluwer Academic.

Twelve Counseling Programs for Children at Risk. Susan T. Dennison. 1989. (Illus.). 430p. (C). text 83.95 (*0-398-05626-9*) C C Thomas.

Twelve Health Center Districts in Need: A Birth Atlas. Constance T. Gager et al. 1988. LC 89-170901. 161p. 13.00 (*0-88156-065-0*) Comm Serv Soc NY.

Twelve Hundred MCQ's in Medicine. Michael J. Ford. 2nd ed. 1991. (Illus.). 196p. pap. text (*0-443-04252-7*) Church.

Twelve-Lead ECG. Springhouse Publishing Company Staff. 1992. (Procedures Video Ser.). 36.95 incl. VHS (*0-87434-375-5*) Springhouse Corp.

12 Lead ECG: The Art of Interpretation. Tomas B. Garcia & Neil E. Holtz. 2000. LC 00-55359. (Illus.). 552p. pap. text 46.95 (*0-7637-1284-1*, 1284-1) Jones & Bartlett.

Twelve Lead ECG Interpretation: A Self-Teaching Manual. Ann E. Norman. 1992. (Illus.). 299p. pap. 29.00 (*0-07-105396-4*) McGraw-Hill Prof.

12-Lead ECG in Acute Myocardial Infarction. Tim Phalen. 1995. LC 95-45315. (Illus.). 252p. (C). (gr. 13). pap. text 29.00 (*0-8151-6752-0*, 25863) Mosby Inc.

12-Lead ECGS: A "Pocket Brain" for Easy Interpretation. Ken Grauer. 1998. (Illus.). iv, 60p. pap. text 10.00 (*0-9663389-0-1*) KG-EKG.

Twelve Lead Egg Interpretation: The Self-Assessment Approach. Zainul Abedin & Robert P. Conner. 1989. 336p. pap. text 35.00 (*0-7216-2846-X*) Saunders.

Twelve Lead EKG. Carolyn G. Smith-Marker. rev. ed. 1984. 53p. pap. text 7.00 (*0-932491-01-4*); VHS 297.00 (*0-932491-14-6*) Res Appl Inc.

Twelve-Lead Electrocardiography for ACLS Providers. Bruce Foster. 1995. (Illus.). 174p. pap. text 22.00 (*0-7216-5873-3*) Saunders.

12-Lead Workbook for the Medical Practitioner. Vernon R. Stanley. 1996. (Illus.). 93p. (Orig.). pap. 15.00 (*0-9651073-1-0*) Kopy Xpress.

Twelve-Month Pregnancy: What You Need to Know Before You Conceive to Ensure a Healthy Beginning for You & Your Baby. Barry Herman & Susan K. Perry. 240p. 1992. LC 91-46748. pap. 12.95 (*0-929923-51-0*); 2nd ed. 1996. pap. 16.00 (*1-56565-480-3*, 04803W) Lowell Hse.

Twelve Problems in Health Care Ethics. Thomas A. Shannon. 1984. LC 84-22654. (Studies in Health & Human Services: Vol. 2). 320p. lib. bdg. 99.95 (*0-88946-127-9*) E Mellen.

Twelve Stages of Healing: A Network Approach to Wholeness. Donald M. Epstein & Nathaniel Altman. 1994. LC 94-21081. (Illus.). 256p. pap. 14.00 (*1-878424-08-4*) Amber-Allen Pub.

12 Step Approach to Healing in Nursing. Mikiuscak. 2002. (Professional Reference - Nursing Ser.). pap. 20.95 (*0-8273-6604-3*) Delmar.

Twelve Step Facilitation Therapy Manual. 1994. (Illus.). 134p. pap. text 35.00 (*1-57979-139-5*) DIANE Pub.

12 Step Prayer Book: A Collection of Favorite 12 Step Prayers & Inspirational Readings. Bill Pittman. 128p. (Orig.). pap. 5.95 (*0-934125-11-2*) Hazelden.

Twelve-Step Workbook of Overeaters Anonymous. Overeaters Anonymous, Inc. Staff. 1993. LC 93-83640. pap. 8.35 (*0-9609898-5-4*) Overeaters Anym.

Twelve Steps & Twelve Traditions. 1989. (RUS.). 213p. 2.75 (*0-916856-26-7*); 1953. LC 53-5454. 192p. 2.70 (*0-916856-01-1*) AAWS.

Twelve Steps & Twelve Traditions. Alcoholics Anonymous World Services, Inc., Staff. 1953. (LIT.). 192p. pap. 5.25 (*0-916856-48-8*) AAWS.

Twelve Steps & Twelve Traditions of Overeaters Anonymous. Overeaters Anonymous, Inc. Staff. 1993. LC 93-85052. pap. 10.99 (*0-9609898-6-2*) Overeaters Anym.

Twelve Steps for Tobacco Users: For Recovering People Addicted to Nicotine. Jeanne F. 1984. 25p. (Orig.). pap. 2.50 (*0-89486-229-4*, 1419) Hazelden.

Twelve Steps of Phobics Anonymous. Contrib. by Marilyn Gellis & Rosemary Muat. 1989. 156p. (Orig.). pap. 9.95 (*0-9627373-0-5*) Inst Phobic Awareness.

Twelve Steps to Self Parenting for Adult Children. Patricia O'Gormand et al. 1988. 135p. pap. 7.95 (*0-932194-68-0*) Health Comm.

12 Things You Should Know about Your Diabetes - Right Now! Irl B. Hirsch. 2001. LC 00-32272. (Illus.). ix, 180p. 14.95 (*1-58040-061-2*) Am Diabetes.

Twelve Tissue Remedies of Schuessler. William Boericke & Willis Dewey. 10.95 (*0-89378-065-0*) Formur Intl.

Twelve Weeks to a Successful Data Dictionary. Maida R. Herbst. 1997. LC 97-170659. (Illus.). 125p. (Orig.). pap. text 77.00 (*1-57839-000-1*) Opus Communs.

Twentieth Anniversary Symposium—PCMR: Maximizing the Quality of Life for Individuals with Mental Retardation & Other Developmental Disabilities. 1988. 194p. (*1-55672-008-4*) US HHS.

Twentieth Annual Northeast Bioengineering Conference, 1994. IEEE, Engineering in Medicine and Biology Staff. Ed. by Institute of Electrical and Electronics Engineers, Inc. Staff. 1994. LC 88-646567. 110p. pap. text (*0-7803-1930-3*); lib. bdg. (*0-7803-1931-1*, 94CH3439-7); fiche (*0-7803-1932-X*) Inst Electrical.

Twentieth-Century Doctor: House Calls to Space Medicine. Mavis P. Kelsey, Sr. 1999. LC 98-44065. (Sara & John Lindsey Series in the Arts & Humanities: Vol. 4). (Illus.). 416p. 29.95 (*0-89096-866-7*) Tex A&M Univ Pr.

Twentieth Century Neurology: The British Contribution. F. Clifford Rose. 2000. 250p. (*1-86094-245-8*) Imperial College GBR. *Dist:* World Scientific Pub.

Twentieth Century Psychiatry: Its Contribution to Man's Knowledge of Himself. William A. White. 1973. LC 73-2428. (Mental Illness & Social Policy; the American Experience Ser.). reprint ed. 19.95 (*0-405-05236-7*) Ayer.

Twentieth Century Psychology: Recent Developments. Ed. by Philip Harriman et al. 1977. LC 75-128255. (Essay Index Reprint Ser.). 43.95 (*0-8369-1948-3*) Ayer.

Twentieth-Century Surgeon: My Life in the Massachusetts General Hospital. Claude E. Welch. (Illus.). 1992. xx, 392p. 24.95 (*0-88135-181-4*); 1993. xviii, 394p. 24.95 (*0-88135-182-2*) Watson Pub Intl.

20 Common Behavioral Problems in Primary Care. Frank V. DeGruy. 2002. (Illus.). 382p. pap. 49.95 (*0-07-016438-X*) McGraw-Hill Prof.

20 Common Ethical Problems in Primary Care. Jeremy Sugarman. 2000. LC 00-268934. (Illus.). xvi, 279p. pap. text 45.00 (*0-07-063369-X*) McGraw-Hill Educ Grp.

20 Common Problems in Geriatrics. Alan M. Adelman. 2000. LC 00-20707. (Twenty Common Problems Ser.). (Illus.). 432p. pap. 45.00 (*0-07-000518-4*) McGraw-Hill Prof.

Urology: 20 Common Problems. Joel Teichman. 2000. LC 00-33236. (Illus.). 335p. pap. 45.00 (*0-07-063413-0*) McGraw-Hill Prof.

20 Common Problems in Clinical Laboratory Management. Judith A. O'Brien. 1999. LC 99-13820. (Clinical Laboratory Science Ser.). (Illus.). 557p. pap. 45.00 (*0-07-048265-9*) McGraw-Hill Prof.

***20 Common Problems in Gastroenterology.** Steven Edmundowicz. 2001. LC 2001-30900. (Illus.). 317p. pap. 45.00 (*0-07-022055-7*) McGraw-Hill Prof.

20 Common Problems in Pediatrics. Abraham B. Bergman. 2000. LC 00-20236. (Illus.). 355p. pap. 45.00 (*0-07-134901-4*) McGraw-Hill Prof.

20 Common Problems in Preventive Health Care. Doug Campos-Outcalt. 2000. LC 99-89081. (Twenty Common Problems Ser.). 510p. pap. 45.00 (*0-07-012044-7*) McGraw-Hill Prof.

20 Common Problems in Primary Care. Barry Weiss. 1998. LC 98-29864. (Twenty Common Problems Ser.). (Illus.). 592p. pap. 45.00 (*0-07-069609-8*) McGraw-Hill Prof.

20 Common Procedures in Primary Care. Dana Lynge & Barry Weiss. 2001. LC 00-32922. (Twenty Common Problems Ser.). (Illus.). 457p. pap. 45.00 (*0-07-136002-6*) McGraw-Hill Prof.

28-Day Antioxidant Diet Program. Steven Masley. Ed. by Claire Gervs. 1997. (Illus.). xii, 308p. pap. 13.75 (*0-9659977-6-6*) Vitality Bks.

XXVes Journees Nationales de Neonatologie, 1995. Ed. by J. P. Relier. 1995. (Progres en Neonatologie Ser.: Vol. 15). (Illus.). vi, 332p. pap. 170.50 (*3-8055-6208-X*) S Karger.

21st Century Health Care Leader. Ed. by Roderick W. Gilkey. 1999. LC 98-39561. (Business & Management Ser.). (Illus.). 432p. 44.00 (*0-7879-4157-3*) Jossey-Bass.

21st Century Miracle Medicine: RoboSurgery, Wonder Cures, & the Quest for Immortality. Alexandra Wyke. 1997. LC 96-45680. (Illus.). 366p. (C). 26.95 (*0-306-45565-X*) Perseus Bks Grp.

Twenty-First Century Obstetrics Now! David Stewart & Lee Stewart. 2nd ed. 1978. LC 77-72854. (Illus.). pap. 14.95 (*0-917314-09-3*);1. pap. 7.95 (*0-917314-07-7*);2. pap. 7.95 (*0-917314-08-5*) NAPSAC.

XXIes Journees Nationales de Neonatologie, 1990. Ed. by J. P. Relier. 1990. (Progres en Neonatologie Ser.: Vol. 10). (Illus.). vi, 312p. pap. 137.50 (*3-8055-5249-1*) S Karger.

Twenty-First Journees Nationales de Neonatologie, 1991. Ed. by J. P. Relier. 1991. (Progres en Neonatologie Ser.: Vol. 11). (Illus.). vi, 370p. pap. 161.00 (*3-8055-5446-X*) S Karger.

25 Most Difficult Nursing Situations. Sutton. 1998. (Nursing Education Ser.). pap. 20.95 (*0-8273-5680-3*) Delmar.

25 Natural Ways to Control Irritable Bowel Syndrome: A Mind-Body Approach to Health & Well-Being. James Scala. 2000. LC 00-63036. 160p. pap. 12.95 (*0-658-00701-7*) McGraw-Hill Trade.

25 Natural Ways to Lower Blood Pressure: A Mind-Body Approach to Health & Well-Being. James Scala. 2001. LC 2001-29857. 160p. pap. 14.95 (*0-658-00702-5*, Keats Pubng) McGraw-Hill Trade.

***25 Natural Ways to Relieve Allergies & Asthma.** Romy Fox. 2001. LC 2001-38132. (25 Natural Ways ... Ser.). 160p. pap. 14.95 (*0-658-01374-2*) McGraw-Hill Prof.

***25 Natural Ways to Relieve PMS.** Nadine Taylor. 2002. LC 2001-50251. (25 Natural Ways ... Ser.). 160p. pap. 14.95 (*0-658-01376-9*, Contemporary) McGraw-Hill Trade.

Twenty-Five Objections to Divine Healing & the Bible Answers. Gordon Lindsay. 1971. 1.95 (*0-89985-030-8*) Christ for the Nations.

Twenty-Five Years of Building the Future: Doctors Hospital, Pinole, CA. Margaret Finnerty. Ed. by John Myers & Robert Gryder. 1992. 100p. (C). 15.00 (*0-929690-15-X*) Herit Pubs AZ.

25 Years of Innovation: The Story of Pfizer Central Research. Ogden Tanner. 1996. LC 95-82399. (Illus.). 216p. (*0-944641-17-2*) Greenwich Pub Group.

Twenty-Five Years of Peptic Ulcer Research in Hungary: From Basic Sciences to Clinical Practice, 1971-1995. Contrib. by G. Y. Mozsik et al. 1997. 448p. (*963-05-7436-5*) Akade Kiado HUN. *Dist:* Intl Spec Bk, St Mut.

Twenty-Four Hour ACE Inhibition: Current & Future Perspectives: Journal: Cardiology, Vol. 79, Suppl. 1, 1991. Ed. by C. Johnston. 1991. (Illus.). 84p. pap. 52.25 (*3-8055-5461-3*) S Karger.

Twenty-Four Hour Drink Book. Ralph Maloney. 1962. (Illus.). 12.95 (*0-8392-1121-X*) Astor-Honor.

***24th Annual FIGO Report.** Pecorelli. 2001. (Illus.). 170p. (*1-901865-39-8*) Isis Med GBR. *Dist:* Bks Intl VA.

XXIVemes Journees Nationales de Neonatologies, 1994, No. 14. Ed. by J. P. Relier. 1994. (Progres en Neonatologie Ser.: Vol. 14). (Illus.). iv, 256p. pap. 170.50 (*3-8055-6015-X*) S Karger.

Twenty Myths about National Health Insurance. John C. Goodman & Gerald L. Musgrove. 1991. (Illus.). 87p. (C). pap. 10.00 (*0-943802-69-5*, 166) Natl Ctr Pol.

Twenty-Ninth Congress of the European Society for Surgical Research (ESSR), Abstracts, Montpellier, France, May 1994. Ed. by L. Teot. 1994. (Journal: Vol. 26, Suppl. 1, 1994). xii, 118p. pap. 36.75 (*3-8055-6002-8*) S Karger.

21 Words for Nurses. Jeanine Young-Mason. 1995. 50p. 12.95 (*0-912083-85-9*); LC 95-30678. pap. 5.95 (*0-912083-88-3*) Diamond Communications.

XXIIes Journees Nationales De Neonatologie Paris, May 1992. Ed. by J. P. Relier. 1992. (Progres en Neonatologie Ser.: Vol. 12). (Illus.). vi, 326p. pap. 169.75 (*3-8055-5636-5*) S Karger.

XXIIIes Journees Nationales de Neonatologie, 1993, Paris, May 1993. 1993. (Progres en Neonatologie Ser.: Vol. 13). (Illus.). vi, 292p. pap. 169.75 (*3-8055-5828-7*) S Karger.

Twenty Thousand Medical Words. Robert W. Prichard & Robert E. Robinson. 1972. 288p. (gr. 13). pap. text 11.95 (*0-07-050874-7*) Mosby Inc.

2020 Vision: Health in the 21st Century. Institute of Medicine Staff. 1996. 134p. (Orig.). pap. text 32.00 (*0-309-05488-5*) Natl Acad Pr.

Twenty-Two Years: Causes & Consequences of Mental Retardation. Stephen A. Richardson & Helene Koller. 1996. LC 96-28834. (Illus.). 416p. 48.95 (*0-674-21297-5*) HUP.

Twenty Years of Community Medicine: A Hunterdon Medical Center Symposium. Henderson et al. 1974. LC 74-80237. (Illus.). 192p. 15.00 (*0-914366-01-7*) Columbia Pub.

Twenty Years of Psychoanalysis. Ed. by Franz Gabriel Alexander & Helen Ross. 1977. LC 77-93312. (Essay Index Reprint Ser.). 30.95 (*0-8369-1541-0*) Ayer.

Twenty Years of Toxicology. Conning. 1982. (Food & Chemical Toxicology Ser.). pap. 48.00 (*0-08-028856-1*, Pergamon Pr) Elsevier.

Twin Block Funct Therapy. Clark. 1995. text (*0-7234-2120-X*) Wolfe Publishing GBR. *Dist:* Mosby Inc.

***Twin Block Functional Therapy: Applications in Dentofacial Orthopaedics.** William Clark. 2nd ed. 2001. (Illus.). (*0-7234-3170-1*) Mosby Inc.

Twin-Block Functional Therapy: Applications in Dentofacial Orthopedics. William J. Clark. 1995. (Illus.). 240p. (*84-8174-310-0*) Mosby-Doyma Libros ESP. *Dist:* Mosby Inc.

Twins As a Tool of Behavior Genetics: Report of the Dahlem Worshop on What Are the Mechanisms Mediating the Genetic & Environmental Determinants of Behavior? Ed. by Thomas J. Bouchard, Jr. & Peter Propping. 1993. LC 93-8773. (Dahlem Workshop Reports: Vol. 53). 326p. 245.95 (*0-471-94174-3*) Wiley.

Twins, Triplets, & More: From Pre-Birth Through High School - What Every Parent Needs to Know When Raising Two or More. Elizabeth Bryan. 1992. LC 92-1095. 160p. 19.95 (*0-312-07876-5*) St Martin.

Twists & Turns, a Mother's Caring Journey - Two Children with Schizophrenia. Ruth C. Ackerman. 1993. LC 93-94015. (Illus.). 149p. (Orig.). pap. 12.00 (*0-9637493-0-7*) Paths of Life.

***Two at a Time: Having Twins: The Journey Through Pregnancy & Birth.** Jane Seymour. 2002. 224p. pap. 14.00 (*0-671-03678-5*) PB.

Two at a Time: Having Twins: The Journey Through Pregnancy & Birth. Jane Seymour & Pamela Patrick Novotny. 2001. (Illus.). 224p. 24.95 (*0-671-03677-7*, PB Hardcover) PB.

Two Butterflies on My Head: Psychoanalysis in the Interdisciplinary Scientific Dialogue. Ed. by M. Leuzinger-Bohleber et al. 1992. (Illus.). 280p. 41.00 (*0-387-53899-2*) Spr-Verlag.

Two Choose to Continue. Bobbie G. Custer. 2nd rev. ed. 1991. 106p. reprint ed. pap. text 9.95 (*0-9620061-0-6*) BGC Pub Co.

Two-Dimensional Echocardiographic Atlas: Congenital Heart Disease, Vol. 1. James B. Seward et al. 1987. (Illus.). 598p. 374.00 (*0-387-96473-8*) Spr-Verlag.

Two-Dimensional Echocardiography: Clinical Pathological Correlations in Adult & Congenital Heart Disease. Arthur D. Hagan et al. 1983. text 82.50 (*0-316-33781-1*, Little Brwn Med Div) Lppncott W & W.

Two-Dimensional Echocardiography in Infants & Children. J. P. Lintermans. 1986. text 281.00 (*0-89838-778-7*) Kluwer Academic.

Two-Dimensional Electrophoresis & Immunological Techniques. Bonnie S. Dunbar. 1988. LC 86-30393. (Illus.). 388p. (C). spiral bd. 44.50 (*0-306-42839-3*, Kluwer Plenum) Kluwer Academic.

Two-Dimensional Electrophoresis & Immunological Techniques. Bonnie S. Dunbar. 1988. LC 86-30393. (Illus.). 388p. (C). 85.00 (*0-306-42439-8*, Plenum Trade) Perseus Pubng.

Two-Dimensional Real-Time Ultrasonic Imaging of the Heart. Ed. by Emilio R. Giuliana. 1985. text 247.50 (*0-89838-671-3*) Kluwer Academic.

Two Discourses Concerning the Soul of Brutes, Which Is That of the Sensations of Man. Thomas Willis. Tr. by S. Pordage from LAT. 1971. LC 72-161936. (History of Psychology Ser.). 264p. 50.00 (*0-8201-1096-5*) Schol Facsimiles.

Two-Edged Sword: A Study of the Paranoid Personality in Action. William H. Hampton & Virginia S. Burnham. Ed. by James C. Smith, Jr. 1990. LC 90-37097. (Illus.). 160p. (Orig.). pap. 14.95 (*0-86534-147-8*) Sunstone Pr.

Two Faces of Swedish Psychology Vol. 1: An Evaluation of Swedish Research in Cognitive Psychology. Ed. by Arne Ohman & Bo Ohngren. 1991. 168p. (Orig.). pap. 38.50 (*91-86362-16-X*) Coronet Bks.

Two Faces of Swedish Psychology Vol. 2: An Evaluation of Swedish Research in Biological Psychology. Barry Everitt et al. 1992. 209p. (Orig.). pap. 44.00 (*91-86362-19-4*) Coronet Bks.

Two-Generation Programs for Families in Poverty: A New Intervention Strategy. Ed. by Sheila Smith & Foundation for Child Development Staff. 1995. (Advances in Applied Developmental Psychology Ser.: Vol. 9). (Illus.). 300p. pap. 39.50 (*1-56750-100-1*, Ablex) Greenwood.

Two Headed Dragon: Exploring the Gifts of AIDS. Sean M. Hoag. 2000. 140p. pap. 13.95 (*1-892038-04-8*) Ravenwood Pub.

Two Hearts, One Fire: A Glimpse Behind the Mask of Leprosy. Howard E. Crouch & Sister Mary Augustine. 1989. LC 89-50271. 240p. pap. 12.00 (*0-9606330-1-4*) Damien-Dutton Soc.

250 Short Cases in Clinical Medicine. Baliga. 2nd ed. 1997. 645p. pap. text (*0-7020-2205-5*) Bailliere Tindall.

***250 Short Cases in Clinical Medicine.** Baliga. 3rd ed. 2001. 656p. pap. (*0-7020-2624-7*) W B Saunders GBR. *Dist:* Saunders.

250 Tips for Making Life with Arthritis Easier. Arthritis Foundation Staff. 1997. LC 96-79812. 128p. (Orig.). pap. 9.95 (*1-56352-381-7*) Longstreet.

200 Kid-Tested Ways to Lower the Fat in Your Child's Favorite Foods: How to Make the Brand-Name & Homemade Foods Your Kids Love More Healthful - & Delicious. Elaine Moquette-Magee. 1994. 297p. pap. 12.95 (*1-56561-034-2*, 004231) Wiley.

260 Essential Chinese Medicinals. Bob Flaws. 1999. LC 98-74794. 288p. pap. 32.95 (*1-891845-03-9*) Blue Poppy Pr.

200 Tips for Passing the Oral Psychiatry Exam. Ed. by Donald R. Hall. 1997. LC 96-33251. 110p. 14.95 (*1-56053-202-5*) Hanley & Belfus.

2000 Year Book of Medicine. Roger M. Barkin. 2000. (Illus.). 629p. text 82.00 (*0-8151-2903-3*, 31814) Mosby Inc.

Two Lions of Lyons: The Tale of Two Surgeons - Alexis Carrel & Rene Leriche. Angelo M. May & Alice G. May. rev. ed. 1994. (Illus.). 319p. (C). 49.50 (*0-930329-45-7*) Kabel Pubs.

Two Lives to Lead: Bisexuality in Men & Women. Ed. by Fritz Klein & Timothy J. Wolf. 1985. LC 85-5868. (Journal of Homosexuality Ser.: Vol. 11, Nos. 1 & 2). 255p. reprint ed. pap. 14.95 (*0-918393-22-1*, Harrington Park) Haworth Pr.

2-Methoxyethanol, 2-Ethoxyethanol, & Their Acetates. 1990. (Environmental Health Criteria Ser.: No. 115). 126p. pap. text 24.00 (*92-4-157115-2*, 1160115) World Health.

Two Million-Year-Old Self. Anthony Stevens. 1993. LC 92-48861. (Carolyn & Ernest Fay Series in Analytical Psychology: No. 3). (Illus.). 162p. 24.50 (*0-89096-536-6*) Tex A&M Univ Pr.

2-Nitropropane. 1992. (Environmental Health Criteria Ser.: No. 138). (ENG, FRE & SPA.). 108p. pap. text 26.00 (*92-4-157138-1*, 1160138) World Health.

2-Propanol. 1990. (Environmental Health Criteria Ser.: No. 103). 132p. pap. text 26.00 (*92-4-157103-9*, 1160103) World Health.

Two Sciences of Mind: Readings in Cognitive Science & Consciousness. Ed. by Sean O'Nuallain et al. 1997. LC 96-52164. (Advances in Consciousness Research Ser.: Vol. 9). xii, 490p. pap. 79.95 (*1-55619-189-8*) J Benjamins Pubng Co.

Two Sexes: Growing up Apart, Coming Together. Eleanor E. MacCoby. 1999. LC 97-30594. (Family & Public Policy Ser.). 384p. text 39.95 (*0-674-91481-3*, Belknap) HUP.

Two Social Psychologies: An Integrative Approach. Cookie W. Stephan & Walter G. Stephan. 1985. 435p. (C). pap. 28.75 net. (*0-534-10849-0*) Wadsworth Pub.

2002 Year Book of Dermatology. Mosby Medical Library Staff. 2002. text 81.00 (*0-323-00449-0*) Mosby Inc.

***2000 Annual Report of the Scientific Registry & the OPTN.** Ed. by Carol M. Smith et al. 2001. (Illus.). 589p. pap. 15.00 (*1-886651-41-8*) United Network.

2000 Coding for Optimal Reimbursement. Robert D. Keene. 2000. 250p. pap. 75.00 (*1-58383-056-1*); pap. 245.00 incl. audio (*1-58383-102-9*) Robert D Keene.

2000 Computers in Cardiology. IEEE, Engineering in Medicine and Biology Staff. 2000. LC 80-641097. 850p. pap. (*0-7803-6557-7*, 00CH37163) IEEE Standards.

2000 National Directory of Fire Chiefs & EMS Administrators. 2000. 1158p. lib. bdg. 99.00 (*1-880245-23-X*) SPAN Pub.

2000 Dorland's Medical Directory, Northern Florida. Contrib. by Russell Perkins. 1999. 424p. pap. 49.95 (*1-880874-59-8*) Dorland Hlthcare.

2000 Dorland's Medical Directory, Southern Florida. Contrib. by Russell Perkins. 1999. 431p. pap. 49.95 (*1-880874-60-1*) Dorland Hlthcare.

2000 Dorland's Medical Directory, Eastern Pennsylvania. Contrib. by Russell Perkins. 2000. 1000p. pap. 79.95 (*1-880874-61-X*) Dorland Hlthcare.

2000 Evaluation & Management Chart Auditing. Robert D. Keene. Ed. by Tony Mistretta. 2000. 240p. pap. 165.00 incl. cd-rom (*1-58383-110-X*) Robert D Keene.

2000 Evaluation & Management Toolbox. Robert D. Keene. 2000. 200p. pap. 225.00 incl. disk (*1-58383-097-9*) Robert D Keene.

2000 Fee Schedule & Payment Policies for Physician's Medicare Services. 500p. pap. text 40.00 (*0-8080-0440-9*) CCH INC.

2000 1st IEEE EMBS Special Topics Conference on Microtechnology in Meicine & Biology. IEEE, Engineering in Medicine and Biology Staff. 2000. LC 00-108164. 700p. pap. (*0-7803-6603-4*, 00EX451) IEEE Standards.

2000 HCPCS: Level II Codes. Robert D. Keene. 1999. 230p. pap. 65.00 (*1-58383-064-2*) Robert D Keene.

***2001 IEEE Engineering in Medicine & Biology 23rd Annual Conference.** IEEE Engineering in Medicine and Biology Society Staff. 2001. 6000p. pap. (*0-7803-7211-5*, 01CH37272) IEEE Standards.

2000 Making the Best Medical Records & Documentation. Robert D. Keene. 2000. 145p. pap. 45.00 (*1-58383-096-0*) Robert D Keene.

2000 Medical Office Policy Manual. Robert D. Keene. 2000. pap. 142.00 incl. cd-rom (*1-58383-067-7*, MOPDSK0) Robert D Keene.

2000 Medicare & Coding for Allergy. Robert D. Keene. 2000. 240p. pap. 145.00 (*1-58383-071-5*) Robert D Keene.

2000 Medicare & Coding for Anesthesia. Robert D. Keene. 2000. 240p. pap. 145.00 (*1-58383-072-3*) Robert D Keene.

2000 Medicare & Coding for Cardiology. Robert D. Keene. 2000. 250p. pap. 145.00 (*1-58383-073-1*) Robert D Keene.

2000 Medicare & Coding for Dermatology. Robert D. Keene. 2000. 235p. pap. 145.00 (*1-58383-074-X*) Robert D Keene.

2000 Medicare & Coding for Emergency Medicine. Robert D. Keene. 2000. 240p. pap. 145.00 (*1-58383-075-8*) Robert D Keene.

2000 Medicare & Coding for Endocrinology. Robert D. Keene. 2000. 230p. pap. 145.00 (*1-58383-076-6*) Robert D Keene.

2000 Medicare & Coding for Family Practice. Robert D. Keene. 2000. 248p. pap. 145.00 (*1-58383-077-4*) Robert D Keene.

2000 Medicare & Coding for Gastroenterology. Robert D. Keene. 2000. 245p. pap. 145.00 (*1-58383-078-2*) Robert D Keene.

2000 Medicare & Coding for General Surgery. Robert D. Keene. 2000. 240p. pap. 145.00 (*1-58383-079-0*) Robert D Keene.

2000 Medicare & Coding for Internal Medicine. Robert D. Keene. 2000. 240p. pap. 145.00 (*1-58383-080-4*) Robert D Keene.

2000 Medicare & Coding for Neurology. Robert D. Keene. 2000. 240p. pap. 145.00 (*1-58383-081-2*) Robert D Keene.

2000 Medicare & Coding for OB/GYN. Robert D. Keene. 2000. 245p. pap. 145.00 (*1-58383-082-0*) Robert D Keene.

2000 Medicare & Coding for Oncology. Robert D. Keene. 2000. 240p. pap. 145.00 (*1-58383-083-9*) Robert D Keene.

2000 Medicare & Coding for Orthopedics. Robert D. Keene. 2000. 248p. pap. 145.00 (*1-58383-085-5*) Robert D Keene.

2000 Medicare & Coding for Otolaryngology. Robert D. Keene. 2000. 240p. pap. 145.00 (*1-58383-086-3*) Robert D Keene.

2000 Medicare & Coding for Pediatrics. Robert D. Keene. 2000. 240p. pap. 145.00 (*1-58383-087-1*) Robert D Keene.

2000 Medicare & Coding for Physical Therapy. Robert D. Keene. 2000. 230p. pap. 145.00 (*1-58383-088-X*) Robert D Keene.

2000 Medicare & Coding for Psychiatry & Mental Health. Robert D. Keene. 2000. 250p. pap. 145.00 (*1-58383-089-8*) Robert D Keene.

2000 Medicare & Coding for Pulmonology. Robert D. Keene. 2000. 240p. pap. 145.00 (*1-58383-090-1*) Robert D Keene.

2000 Medicare & Coding for Rheumatology. Robert D. Keene. 2000. 235p. pap. 145.00 (*1-58383-092-8*) Robert D Keene.

2000 Medicare & Coding for Urology. Robert D. Keene. 2000. 240p. pap. 145.00 (*1-58383-093-6*) Robert D Keene.

2000 Medicare & Medicaid Benefits. CCH Editorial Staff. pap. 10.00 (*0-8080-0443-3*) CCH INC.

2000 Medicare Coding & Compliance Regulations. Robert D. Keene. unabr. ed. 2000. pap. 245.00 incl. audio (*1-58383-100-2*) Robert D Keene.

2000 Medicare Covered & Noncovered Services. Robert D. Keene. 2000. 350p. 228.00 (*1-58383-060-X*) Robert D Keene.

2000 Medicare Explained. CCH Editorial Staff. pap. 30.00 (*0-8080-0444-1*) CCH INC.

2000 Medicare Rules & Regulations. Robert D. Keene. 2000. 245p. pap. 75.00 (*1-58383-066-9*); pap. 245.00 incl. audio (*1-58383-104-5*) Robert D Keene.

2000 Mosby's Genrx: Book. Mosby Staff. 10th ed. 1999. (Mosby's Physicians GenRx Ser.). (Illus.). 1504p. text 49.95 (*0-323-00627-2*) Mosby Inc.

2000 National Correct Coding Manual. Robert D. Keene. 2000. 250p. pap. 250.00 (*1-58383-109-6*) Robert D Keene.

2000 Nursing Drug Reference. Paul Skidmore. 1999. (Illus.). 1220p. text 29.95 (*0-323-00306-0*) Mosby Inc.

2000 Nursing Licensure Guidelines: State Information Manual for Nurses. Brenda H. Janoulis & Jason F. Janoulis. 2000. 145p. pap. 69.00 (*1-887617-77-9*) St Bart Pr Ltd.

***2001 Bell's Palsy (TM) Cause, Treatment & Prevention.** Anuthep Benja-Athon & Theda Benja-Athon. 2001. (Illus.). 57p. pap. 65.95 (*0-9706580-8-7*) Muscle Joint.

2001 Business of Medicine. 11th ed. 2001. 350p. 328.00 (*1-58383-121-5*, BOMED1) Robert D Keene.

***2001 California Master Medicaid Guide.** Teresa Zak et al. 2001. 500p. pap. 199.00 (*0-8080-0625-8*) CCH INC.

2001 Coding & Medicare for Ophthalmology. 11th ed. 2001. 240p. pap. text 145.00 (*1-58383-146-0*, MEDOPT1) Robert D Keene.

2001 Coding & Medicare for Orthopedics. 11th ed. 2001. 250p. pap. text 145.00 (*1-58383-147-9*, MEDORTHO1) Robert D Keene.

2001 Coding & Medicare for Otolaryngology. 11th ed. 2001. 250p. pap. text 145.00 (*1-58383-148-7*, MEDOTO1) Robert D Keene.

2001 Coding & Medicare for Pediatrics. 11th ed. 2001. 250p. pap. text 145.00 (*1-58383-149-5*, MEDPED1) Robert D Keene.

2001 Coding & Medicare for Psychiatry. 11th ed. 2001. 250p. pap. text 145.00 (*1-58383-150-9*, MEDPSY1) Robert D Keene.

2001 Coding & Medicare for Physical Therapy. 11th ed. 2001. 225p. pap. text 145.00 (*1-58383-151-7*, MEDPT1) Robert D Keene.

2001 Coding & Medicare for Pulmonology. 11th ed. 2001. 250p. pap. text 145.00 (*1-58383-152-5*, MEDPUL1) Robert D Keene.

2001 Coding & Medicare for Radiology. 11th ed. 2001. 250p. pap. text 145.00 (*1-58383-153-3*, MEDRAD1) Robert D Keene.

2001 Coding & Medicare for General Surgery. 11th ed. 2001. 250p. pap. text 145.00 (*1-58383-154-1*, MEDSUR1) Robert D Keene.

2001 Coding & Medicare for Urology. 11th ed. 2001. 250p. pap. text 145.00 (*1-58383-163-0*, MEDURO1) Robert D Keene.

2001 Coding & Medicare for Allergy. 11th ed. 2001. 250p. pap. text 145.00 (*1-58383-133-9*, MEDALL1) Robert D Keene.

2001 Coding & Medicare for Anesthesiology. 11th ed. 2001. 250p. pap. text 145.00 (*1-58383-134-7*, MEDANEST1) Robert D Keene.

2001 Coding & Medicare for Cardiology. 11th ed. 2001. 250p. pap. text 145.00 (*1-58383-135-5*, MEDCARD1) Robert D Keene.

2001 Coding & Medicare for Emergency Medicine. 11th ed. 2001. 250p. pap. text 145.00 (*1-58383-136-3*, MEDEMR1) Robert D Keene.

2001 Coding & Medicare for Endocrinology. 11th ed. 2001. 250p. pap. text 145.00 (*1-58383-137-1*, MEDENDO1) Robert D Keene.

2001 Coding & Medicare for Dermatology. 11th ed. 2001. 250p. pap. text 145.00 (*1-58383-138-X*, MEDDERM1) Robert D Keene.

2001 Coding & Medicare for Family Practice. 11th ed. 2001. 250p. pap. text 145.00 (*1-58383-139-8*, MEDFAM1) Robert D Keene.

2001 Coding & Medicare for Gastroenterology. 11th ed. 2001. 250p. pap. text 145.00 (*1-58383-140-1*, MEDGAS1) Robert D Keene.

2001 Coding & Medicare for Internal Medicine. 11th ed. 2001. 250p. pap. text 145.00 (*1-58383-142-8*, MEDINT1) Robert D Keene.

2001 Coding & Medicare for Neurology. 11th ed. 2001. 250p. pap. text 145.00 (*1-58383-143-6*, MEDNEURO1) Robert D Keene.

2001 Coding & Medicare for OB/GYN. 11th ed. 2001. 250p. pap. text 145.00 (*1-58383-144-4*, MEDOB1) Robert D Keene.

2001 Coding & Medicare for Oncology. 11th ed. 2001. 250p. pap. text 145.00 (*1-58383-145-2*, MEDONC1) Robert D Keene.

2001 Coding & Medicare for Rheumatology. 11th ed. 2001. 250p. pap. text 145.00 (*1-58383-162-2*, MEDRHEUM1) Robert D Keene.

2001 Coding for Optimal Reimbursement. 11th ed. 2001. 250p. pap. text 75.00 (*1-58383-122-3*, CODOPT1) Robert D Keene.

***2001 Coding Workbook for the Physician's Office.** Covell. 4th ed. 2001. pap. text 27.95 (*0-7668-4008-5*) Delmar.

2001 Collections & Insurance. 11th ed. 2001. 200p. pap. text 65.00 (*1-58383-123-1*, COLINS1) Robert D Keene.

2001 Complete Guide to Prescription & Nonprescription Drugs 2001. H. Winter Griffith. 2000. (Complete Guide to Prescription & Non-Prescription Drugs Ser.). 1104p. pap. 16.95 (*0-399-52634-X*, Perigee Bks) Berkley Pub.

2001 Draft Compliance Program Guidance for Individual & Small Group Physician Practices. 11th ed. 2001. 110p. pap. text 45.00 (*1-58383-118-5*, PHYCOMP1) Robert D Keene.

2001 Evaluation & Management Percentages & Policies. 11th ed. 2001. 150p. pap. text 79.00 (*1-58383-119-3*, EMPAP1) Robert D Keene.

2001 Financial Planning for a Medical Practice. 11th ed. 2001. 200p. pap. text 45.00 (*1-58383-125-8*, FIPLAN1) Robert D Keene.

2001 HCFA Common Procedure Coding System. 11th ed. 2001. 250p. pap. text 65.00 (*1-58383-128-2*, HCPCS1) Robert D Keene.

2001 Marketing Your Practice in an Era of Medical Reform. 11th ed. 2001. 200p. pap. text 45.00 (*1-58383-131-2*, MARKET1) Robert D Keene.

2001 Medical Office Policy Manual. 11th ed. 2001. 350p. pap. 142.00 (*1-58383-155-X*, MOPDSK1) Robert D Keene.

2001 Medicare Covered & Noncovered Services. 11th ed. 2001. 350p. 228.00 (*1-58383-124-X*, COVER1) Robert D Keene.

2001 Medicare Rules & Regulations. 11th ed. 2001. 250p. pap. text 75.00 (*1-58383-141-X*, MEDICR1) Robert D Keene.

2001 Negotiating Managed Care Contracts. 11th ed. 2001. 200p. pap. text 75.00 (*1-58383-130-4*, MANCRE1) Robert D Keene.

2001 PDR for Ophthalmic Medicines. Medical Economics Staff. 29th rev. ed. 2000. (Physicians' Desk Reference for Ophthalmology Ser.: Vol. 29). (Illus.). 250p. 59.00 (*1-56363-366-3*, PDR) Med Econ.

2001 PDR Nurse's Drug Handbook. George R. Spratto. 2000. (Physicians' Desk Reference Nurse's Handbook Ser.). 1392p. pap. text 32.95 (*0-7668-2136-6*) Delmar.

2001 Pfizer Medical School Manual: A Practical Guide to Admission to American Medical Schools. Mike Magee. 4th ed. 2001. 100p. (Orig.). (C). pap. 9.95 (*1-889793-06-X*) Spencer Bks.

2001 Physician's Pricing Guide. 11th ed. 2001. 30p. pap. text 279.00 (*1-58383-164-9*, PRICE1) Robert D Keene.

2001 Residency Directory. Accreditation Services Division Staff. rev. ed. 2000. Vol. 2. 244p. pap. text 20.95 (*1-58528-021-6*); Vols. 1 & 2. 484p. pap. text 32.95 (*1-58528-020-8*) Am Soc Hlth-Syst.

***2001 Update to Competence Assessment Tools for Health-System Pharmacies.** Lee B. Murdaugh. 2001. 75p. ring bd. (*1-58528-025-9*) Am Soc Hlth-Syst.

2001 Year Book of Dermatology. Mosby Medical Library Staff. 2001. text 81.00 (*0-323-00448-2*) Mosby Inc.

2001 Year Book of Cardiology. Ed. by Robert C. Schlant. 2001. (Illus.). 475p. (*0-323-01542-5*) Mosby Inc.

2001 Year Book of Critical Care. Ed. by Joseph E. Parrillo. 2001. (Illus.). 380p. (*0-323-01517-4*) Mosby Inc.

2001 Year Book of Dentistry. Ed. by Kenneth Zakariasen. 2001. (Illus.). 500p. (*0-323-01543-3*) Mosby Inc.

2001 Year Book of Endocrinology. Ed. by Ernest L. Mazzaferri. 2001. (Illus.). 450p. (*0-323-01513-1*) Mosby Inc.

2001 Year Book of Hand Surgery. Ed. by Amy Ladd & Richard Berger. 2001. 345p. (*0-323-01544-1*) Mosby Inc.

2001 Year Book of Neonatal & Perinatal Medicine. Ed. by Avroy A. Fanaroff. 2001. (Illus.). 450p. (*0-323-01546-8*) Mosby Inc.

2001 Year Book of Nephrology, Hypertension & Mineral Metabolism. Ed. by Steve J. Schwab. 2001. (Illus.). 300p. (*0-323-01511-5*) Mosby Inc.

2001 Year Book of Neurology & Neurosurgery. Gibbs Bradley. 2001. (Illus.). 512p. text 78.00 (*0-8151-0930-X*, 30638) Mosby Inc.

2001 Year Book of Oncology. Ed. by Patrick Loehrer, Sr. 2001. (Illus.). 420p. (*0-323-01509-3*) Mosby Inc.

2001 Year Book of Pulmonary Disease. Ed. by James Jett. 2001. (Illus.). 424p. (*0-323-01515-8*) Mosby Inc.

2001 Year Book of Rheumatology, Arthritis & Musculoskeletal Disease. Ed. by Richard S. Panush. 2001. (Illus.). 385p. (*0-323-01519-0*) Mosby Inc.

2001 Year Book of Sports Medicine. Shephard. 2001. text 88.00 (*0-323-00731-7*) Mosby Inc.

2000 Personnel Management of a Medical Practice. Robert D. Keene. 2000. 220p. pap. 65.00 (*1-58383-094-4*) Robert D Keene.

2000 Resource Based Relative Value System, Vols. 1 & 2. Robert D. Keene. 1999. 400p. pap. 65.00 (*1-58383-062-6*) Robert D Keene.

2000 State Medical Licensure Guidelines: Information Manual for MD & DO Physicians. Brenda H. Janoulis & Jason F. Janoulis. rev. ed. 2000. 81p. pap. 89.00 (*1-887617-76-0*) St Bart Pr Ltd.

***2003 Year Book of Critical Care.** Ed. by Joseph E. Parrillo. 2003. (Illus.). 380p. (*0-323-01525-5*) Mosby Inc.

2003 Year Book of Family Practice. Ed. by Marjorie A. Bowman. Date not set. 550p. (*0-323-01524-7*) Mosby Inc.

2003 Year Book of Rheumatology, Arthritis & Musculoskeletal Disease. Ed. by Richard S. Panush. 2003. (Illus.). 385p. (*0-323-01521-2*) Mosby Inc.

2000-2001 Medical & Healthcare Marketplace Guide 16th ed. 2000. 680p. pap. 690.00 (*1-880874-71-7*) Dorland Hlthcare.

2000-2001 NABCO Breast Cancer Resource List. 2000. 84p. pap. text (*0-9703468-0-8*) National Alliance.

***2002 Oncology Nursing Drug Handbook.** Gail M. Wilkes et al. 2001. (C). pap. 53.95 (*0-7637-1990-0*, 1990-0, N L N Bart) Jones & Bartlett.

2002 Year Book of Critical Care. Ed. by Joseph E. Parrillo. 2002. (Illus.). 380p. (*0-323-01518-2*) Mosby Inc.

2002 Year Book of Endocrinology. Ed. by Ernest L. Mazzaferri. 2002. (Illus.). 450p. (*0-323-01514-X*) Mosby Inc.

2002 Year Book of Family Practice. Berg. 2002. (*0-8151-2037-0*, 31733) Mosby Inc.

***2002 Year Book of Gastroenterology.** Ed. by Gary R. Lichtenstein. 2002. (Illus.). 360p. (*0-323-01533-6*) Mosby Inc.

2002 Year Book of Nephrology, Hypertension & Mineral Metabolism. Ed. by Steve J. Schwab. 2002. (Illus.). 300p. (*0-323-01512-3*) Mosby Inc.

2002 Year Book of Neurology & Neurosurgery. Ed. by Bradley Gibbs. 2002. (Illus.). 512p. text (*0-8151-1998-4*, 30639) Mosby Inc.

2002 Year Book of Nuclear Medicine. Ed. by Alexander Gottschalk. 2002. vinyl bd. (*0-323-01551-4*) Mosby Inc.

2002 Year Book of Obstetrics & Gynecology. Mishell. 2002. (*0-8151-2207-1*, 31736) Mosby Inc.

2002 Year Book of Oncology. Ed. by Patrick Loehrer, Sr. 2002. (Illus.). 420p. (*0-323-01510-7*) Mosby Inc.

2002 Year Book of Pulmonary Disease. Ed. by James Jett. 2002. (Illus.). 424p. (*0-323-01516-6*) Mosby Inc.

2002 Year Book of Rheumatology, Arthritis & Musculoskeletal Disease. Ed. by Richard S. Panush. 2002. (Illus.). 385p. (*0-323-01520-4*) Mosby Inc.

2002 Year Book of Surgery. Ed. by Edward M. Copeland, III. 2002. vinyl bd. (*0-323-01552-2*) Mosby Inc.

2000 Update to Competence Assessment Tools for Health-System Pharmacists. Lee B. Murdaugh. 2000. 50p. (*1-58528-014-3*) Am Soc Hlth-Syst.

2000 Year Book of Allergy, Asthma & Clinical Immunology. 2000. (Volume in the Year Books Ser.). (*1-55664-516-3*) Mosby Inc.

2000 Year Book of Anesthesiology & Pain Management. John H. Tinker. 2000. (*0-323-00704-X*) Mosby Inc.

2000 Year Book of Cardiology. Schlant. 2000. text 90.30 (*0-323-00513-6*) Mosby Inc.

2000 Year Book of Chiropractic. 1999. (Illus.). 350p. text 73.00 (*0-8151-2859-2*, 31805) Mosby Inc.

2000 Year Book of Critical Care Medicine. Ed. by Joseph Parrillo. 2000. (Illus.). 400p. 84.00 (*0-323-01500-X*) Mosby Inc.

2000 Year Book of Dentistry. Kenneth Zakariasen. 2000. (Illus.). 500p. 79.00 (*0-323-01501-8*) Mosby Inc.

2000 Year Book of Emergency Medicine. Ed. by William Burdick. 2000. (Illus.). 400p. 88.00 (*0-323-01508-5*) Mosby Inc.

2000 Year Book of Endocrinology. Ed. by Ernest L. Mazzaferri. 2000. (Illus.). 432p. 85.00 (*0-323-01502-6*) Mosby Inc.

2000 Year Book of Gastroenterology. Ed. by Gary R. Lichtenstein. 2000. (Illus.). 350p. 81.00 (*0-323-01503-4*) Mosby Inc.

2000 Year Book of Hand Surgery. Peter C. Amadio. 2000. (Illus.). 350p. text 80.00 (*0-8151-0165-1*, 25766) Mosby Inc.

2000 Year Book of Nephrology, Hypertension & Mineral Metabolism. Ed. by Steve J. Schwab. 2000. (Illus.). 89.00 (*0-323-01507-7*) Mosby Inc.

2000 Year Book of Neurology & Neurosurgery. Gibbs Bradley. 2000. (Illus.). 512p. text 78.00 (*0-8151-0322-0*, 30637) Mosby Inc.

2000 Year Book of Nuclear Medicine. Ed. by Alexander Gottschalk. 2000. (Illus.). 496p. 93.00 (*0-323-01504-2*) Mosby Inc.

2000 Year Book of Oncology. Ed. by Patrick Loehrer, Sr. 2000. (Illus.). 395p. 89.00 (*0-323-01505-0*) Mosby Inc.

2000 Year Book of Sports Medicine. Shephard. 2000. text 84.00 (*0-323-00730-9*) Mosby Inc.

2000 Year Book of Dermatology. Mosby Medical Library Staff. 2000. text 81.00 (*0-323-00447-4*) Mosby Inc.

Two Treatises Concerning the Perservation of Eye-Sight. Walter Bailey. 1975. LC 74-28827. (English Experience Ser.: No. 709). reprint ed. 20.00 (*90-221-0709-4*) Walter J Johnson.

Two-Valued Iterative Systems of Mathematical Logic. Emil L. Post. 1941. (Annals of Mathematics Studies). pap. 25.00 (*0-527-02721-9*) Periodicals Srv.

Two Views of Mind: Abhidharma & Brain Science. Christopher Decharms. 1997. LC 97-41162. 229p. pap. text 14.95 (*1-55939-081-6*) Snow Lion Pubns.

Two Weeks with the Psychic Surgeons. Marti Sladek. 1977. LC 76-45732. (Illus.). 273p. 17.95 (*0-917816-01-3*) DOMA Pr.

Two Years' Service on the Reorganized State Board of Insanity in Massachusetts, August, 1914 to August, 1916. Lloyd V. Briggs. Ed. by Gerald N. Grob. 1980. LC 78-22551. (Historical Issues in Mental Health Ser.). (Illus.). reprint ed. lib. bdg. 50.95 (*0-405-11905-4*) Ayer.

***TxMxM1: The Anatomy & Clinics of Metastatic Cancer.** J. M. Debois. 2001. LC 2001-50384. 768p. (*0-7923-6793-6*) Kluwer Academic NLD. *Dist:* Kluwer Academic.

Tyler's Guide: The Healthcare Executive's Job Search. Larry J. Tyler. 2nd ed. 1998. LC 97-49119. xi, 233p. pap. 42.00 (*1-56793-075-1*) Health Admin Pr.

Tyler's Herbs of Choice: The Therapeutic Use of Phytomedicinals. James E. Robbers & Varro E. Tyler. 2nd ed. 1999. LC 98-28809. 287p. pap. 19.95 (*0-7890-0160-8*); (Illus.). 49.95 (*0-7890-0159-4*) Haworth Pr.

Tyler's Honest Herbal: A Sensible Guide to the Use of Herbs & Related Remedies. Steven Foster & Varro E. Tyler. 4th ed. 1999. LC 98-43234. 442p. 49.95 (*0-7890-0705-3*) Haworth Pr.

Tympano-Ossicular, Allograft Tympanoplasty: A Manual of Techniques. Bernard Ars & Nicole Ars-Piret. 1993. (Illus.). 55p. pap. text (*90-6299-093-2*) Kugler NLD. *Dist:* Lib Res.

Tympanoplasty: Repair of the Tympanic Membrane. Peter S. Roland. 1999. LC 99-14321. (Self-Instructional Package Ser.). (Illus.). 89p. 25.00 (*1-56772-071-4*, 5506340) AAO-HNS.

Tympanoplasty, Mastoidectomy & Stapes Surgery. Ugo Fisch. 1994. (Illus.). 304p. 125.00 (*0-86577-559-1*) Thieme Med Pubs.

Type A Behavior: Its Diagnosis & Treatment. Meyer Friedman. 1996. LC 96-44150. (Prevention in Practice Library). (Illus.). 164p. (C). pap. text 23.00 (*0-306-45357-6*, Kluwer Plenum) Kluwer Academic.

Type A Behavior: Its Diagnosis & Treatment. Meyer Friedman. 1996. LC 96-44150. (Prevention in Practice Library). (Illus.). 164p. (C). 45.00 (*0-306-45356-8*, Plenum Trade) Perseus Pubng.

Type A Personality: Index of Authors & Subjects with Guide for Rapid Research. D. J. Randall. rev. ed. 1994. 57.50 (*0-7883-0182-9*); pap. 47.50 (*0-7883-0183-7*) ABBE Pubs Assn.

Type & Team Development Seminar Kit: Using Type to Unleash the Power of Your Team. William D. Murray & Peter Walsh. rev. ed. 1996. (Type & Temperament Seminar Kits Ser.). 160p. ring bd. 159.95 (*1-878287-14-1*) Type & Temperament.

Type I Diabetes: Molecular, Cellular & Clinical Immunology. Ed. by George S. Eisenbarth & Kevin J. Lafferty. 1996. (Illus.). 320p. text 69.50 (*0-19-509126-4*) OUP.

Type I Diabetes in Clinical Practice: Etiology & Treatment. Ed. by Mark A. Sperling. 2002. (Contemporary Endocrinology Ser.). 500p. 135.00 (*0-89603-931-5*) Humana.

***Type 2 Diabetes: An Essential Guide for the Newly Diagnosed.** Gretchen Becker. 2001. LC 2001-41043. (First Year Ser.). (Illus.). 336p. pap. 14.95 (*1-56924-546-0*) Marlowe & Co.

Type 2 Diabetes: Prediction & Prevention. Graham Hitman. 1999. LC 98-48819. (Practical Diabetes Ser.). 412p. 190.00 (*0-471-98595-3*) Wiley.

Type 2 Diabetes: Questions & Answers. Gerald M. Reaven. 2001. (Questions & Answers Ser.). (Illus.). 168p. pap. text 29.95 (*1-873413-17-3*) Merit Pub Intl.

Type 2 Diabetes: Your Healthy Living Guide. American Diabetes Association. 1996. LC 92-17906. (Illus.). 248p. pap. 24.95 (*0-945448-27-9*); 2nd ed. 2000. LC 00-64288. vii, 176p. 16.95 (*1-58040-060-4*); 2nd ed. 1997. LC 96-54838. 280p. pap. 16.95 (*0-945448-79-1*, 00791Q) Am Diabetes.

Type II Diabetes & Your Health. Helen V. Fisher. 2000. LC 00-32165. 240p. pap. 14.95 (*1-55561-280-6*) Fisher Bks.

Type 2 Diabetes Basics. Patti Rickheim et al. 2000. LC 00-266800. (Illus.). iii, 107p. (*1-885115-54-7*) IDC Pubng.

Type II Diabetes Diet Book. Cal Ezrin & Rubert E. Kowalski. 2nd rev. ed. 1997. 304p. pap. 16.00 (*1-56565-807-8*, Anodyne) Lowell Hse.

Type 2 Diabetes Diet Book. Calvin Ezrin & Robert E. Kowalski. 3rd rev. ed. 1999. LC 99-16753. 336p. pap. 16.95 (*0-7373-0103-1*, 01031W) NTC Contemp Pub Co.

Type II Diabetes Diet Book: The Insulin Control Diet. Calvin Ezrin & Robert E. Kowalski. 1995. 304p. pap. 16.00 (*1-56565-334-3*) Lowell Hse.

***Type 2 Diabetes in Practice.** Andrew J. Krentz & Cliff Bailey. 2001. 150p. pap. (*1-85315-482-2*) Royal Soc of Medicine Pr Ltd GBR. *Dist:* Balogh.

Type II Diabetes Sourcebook. David Drum & Terry Zierenberg. 1998. LC 97-651. 334p. pap. 18.00 (*1-56565-862-0*, 08620W) Lowell Hse.

***Type-2 Diabetic Nephropathy in Japan: From Bench to Bedside.** Ed. by Y. Tomino. 2001. (Contributions to Nephrology Ser.: Vol. 134). (Illus.). viii, 140p. 172.25 (*3-8055-7274-3*) S Karger.

Type 2 Diabetic Woman. M Sara Rosenthal. 1999. LC 99-13013. 358p. pap. 17.95 (*0-7373-0078-7*, 00787W) NTC Contemp Pub Co.

Types, Levels-Irregularities of Response to a Nursery School Situation of 40 Children Observed with Special Reference to the Home Environment. E. C. Slater. 1939. (SRCD M Ser.: Vol. 4, No. 2). 25.00 (*0-527-01509-1*) Periodicals Srv.

Typhoid & the Politics of Public Health in Nineteenth Century Philadelphia. Michael P. McCarthy. 1988. LC 86-72881. (Memoirs Ser.: Vol. 179). (Illus.). 150p. (Orig.). (C). pap. 10.00 (*0-87169-179-5*, M179-MCM) Am Philos.

Typhoid Fever: Its Nature, Mode of Spreading & Prevention. William Budd. Ed. by Barbara G. Rosenkrantz. 1977. LC 76-25656. (Public Health in America Ser.). (Illus.). reprint ed. lib. bdg. 21.95 (*0-405-09809-X*) Ayer.

Typhoid Fever: Strategies for the '90s. T. Pang. 1992. 300p. text 95.00 (*981-02-0953-3*) World Scientific Pub.

Typhus & Doughboys: The American Polish Typhus Relief Expedition, Nineteen Nineteen to Nineteen Twenty-One. Alfred E. Cornebise. 1983. LC 81-70530. (Illus.). 240p. 29.50 (*0-87413-216-9*) U Delaware Pr.

Tyranny of Health: Doctors & the Regulation of Lifestyle. Michael Fitzpatrick. 2000. LC 00-42470. 192p. 16.95 (*0-415-23572-3*) Routledge.

Tyranny of the Normal: Essays on Bioethics, Theology, & Myth. Leslie A. Fiedler. 1996. LC 95-34579. 176p. 22.95 (*1-56792-003-9*) Godine.

Tyranny of the Spirit: Domination & Submission in Adolescent Relationships. David K. Curran. 1996. LC 96-11820. 344p. 50.00 (*1-56821-833-8*) Aronson.

Tyrosine Kinases & Neoplastic Transformation. S. Kellie. 1994. (Molecular Biology Intelligence Unit Ser.). 100p. 99.00 (*1-57059-075-3*) Landes Bioscience.

U

U. K. Health Markets. 1987. 100p. 180.00 (*0-7855-7256-2*) St Mut.

U. S. A. Medical Directories: Dallas - Fort Worth, 1995-96 Issue. American Medical Sales School, Inc. Staff. Ed. & Intro. by Diane Huggins. rev. ed. 1995. (Illus.). 410p. 42.50 (*1-882328-03-5*) Am Med Sales.

U. S. Allergy & Asthma Markets. Market Intelligence Staff. 1994. LC 97-212932. 300p. 3295.00 (*0-7889-0158-3*) Frost & Sullivan.

U. S. Allergy & Asthma Therapeutics Markets. Ed. by Frost and Sullivan Staff. 1997. 546p. spiral bd. 3495.00 (*0-7889-0692-5*, 5492-45) Frost & Sullivan.

U. S. Analytical Laboratory Instrumentation Markets: Industry Markets & Software Enhancements Reshape Competitive Strategies. 1995. 414p. spiral bd. 2395.00 (*0-7889-0376-4*, 0907-30) Frost & Sullivan.

U. S. & Canadian Medical Schools 1999. Peterson's Guides Staff. 2nd ed. 1998. (Peterson's Guides Ser.). 254p. pap. text 24.95 (*0-7689-0150-2*) Petersons.

U. S. Anesthesia & Gas Monitoring Equipment Markets Continuing Development of Integrated & Compact Products. Market Intelligence Staff. 1994. 210p. 1995.00 (*0-7889-0027-7*) Frost & Sullivan.

U. S. Antifungal Markets: High Growth Era for Systemic & OTC Products. Market Intelligence Staff. 1994. 340p. (Orig.). 2495.00 (*1-56753-899-1*) Frost & Sullivan.

U. S. Army Special Forces Medical Handbook. Glen K. Craig. 1988. (Illus.). 608p. pap. 27.00 (*0-87364-454-9*) Paladin Pr.

U. S. Autoimmune Disease Markets. Market Intelligence Staff. 1994. LC 97-213049. 370p. 2395.00 (*0-7889-0138-9*) Frost & Sullivan.

U. S. Autoimmune Disease Therapeutic Markets: Betaseron & Other New Compounds Advance Through Clinical Trials. Market Intelligence Staff. 1993. 450p. 1995.00 (*1-56753-545-3*) Frost & Sullivan.

U. S. Biotechnology & Pharmaceutical Instrument Markets. Frost and Sullivan Staff. 1996. 506p. spiral bd. 2495.00 (*0-7889-0415-9*, 5310-55) Frost & Sullivan.

U. S. Breast Cancer Diagnostics, Therapeutics & Prosthetics Markets. Frost and Sullivan Staff. 1996. 255p. spiral bd. 1995.00 (*0-7889-0499-X*, 5345-50) Frost & Sullivan.

U. S. Complex Carbohydrate Therapeutics Markets. Market Intelligence Staff. 1994. 2195.00 (*0-7889-0135-4*) Frost & Sullivan.

U. S. Critical Care Drug Markets. Ed. by Frost and Sullivan Staff. 1997. 240p. spiral bd. 2895.00 (*0-7889-0687-9*, 5488-44) Frost & Sullivan.

U. S. Dental Esthetics, Therapeutics & Hygiene Product Markets. Ed. by Frost and Sullivan Staff. 1995. 323p. spiral bd. 5199.50 (*0-7889-0229-6*, 0958-54) Frost & Sullivan.

U. S. Dental Laboratories Industry. Marketdata Enterprises, Inc. Staff. 1998. 19p. 59.00 (*1-891084-20-8*) Mktdata Ent.

U. S. Disposable Medical Gloves & Condom Markets: Gloves & Condoms. Frost Sullivan Staff. 1996. 364p. spiral bd. 1895.00 (*0-7889-0498-1*, 5480-51) Frost & Sullivan.

U. S. Dual-Use Exports to Iraq & Their Impact on the Health of the Persian Gulf War Veterans. 1997. (Illus.). 551p. reprint ed. pap. text 50.00 (*0-7881-3825-1*) DIANE Pub.

U. S. Emergency & Trauma Care Device Markets: New Technologies Focus on Safety & Ease of Use. Market Intelligence Staff. 1995. 342p. (Orig.). spiral bd. 1895.00 (*0-7889-0119-2*, 5078-54) Frost & Sullivan.

U. S. Endoscope Markets: Intracranial & Spinal Markets Emerge. Frost and Sullivan Staff. 1995. 363p. spiral bd. 2295.00 (*0-7889-0400-0*, 5231-57) Frost & Sullivan.

U. S. Ethical Nutrition Markets: Manufacturers Target Home Healthcare for Growth. Market Intelligence Staff. 1994. 1895.00 (*0-7889-0061-7*) Frost & Sullivan.

U. S. Experiment in Social Medicine: The Community Health Center Program, 1965-1986. Alice Sardell. 1988. LC 87-35847. (Series in Policy & Institutional Studies). (Illus.). 288p. (Orig.). (C). pap. 19.95 (*0-8229-5803-1*) U of Pittsburgh Pr.

U. S. Fluid & Drug Delivery System Markets. Market Intelligence Staff. 1994. (Orig.). 2295.00 (*0-7889-0097-8*) Frost & Sullivan.

U. S. Health Care Crisis: The Fight over Access, Quality, & Cost. Victoria Sherrow. 1994. LC 93-51508. (Issue & Debate Ser.). 128p. (gr. 7-11). lib. bdg. 23.90 (*1-56294-364-2*) Millbrook Pr.

U. S. Health Care Workforce: Realigning to Meet the Future: Congressional Hearing. Ed. by Bill Frist. 2000. 118p. reprint ed. pap. text 25.00 (*0-7567-0055-8*) DIANE Pub.

U. S. Health Law & Policy, 1999: A Guide to the Current Literature. Donald H. Caldwell. 1998. LC 98-18221. 450p. 110.00 (*1-55648-236-1*) AHPI.

U. S. Health Policy Groups: Institutional Profiles. Ed. by Craig Ramsay. 1995. LC 94-27942. 488p. lib. bdg. 90.00 (*0-313-28618-3*) Greenwood.

U. S. Health Politics: Public Policy & Political Theory. C. R. Paton. 1990. 240p. text (*0-566-07101-0*) Avebry GBR. *Dist:* Ashgate Pub Co.

U. S. Health System: Origins & Function. Marshal W. Raffel & Norma K. Raffel. 3rd ed. 1989. pap. text 41.95 (*0-8273-4336-1*) Delmar.

U. S. Health System: Origins & Functions. Marshall W. Raffel & Norma K. Raffel. 4th ed. 1993. LC 93-11931. 302p. (C). mass mkt. 42.25 (*0-8273-5408-8*) Delmar.

U. S. Health System Origins & Functions. Marshall W. Raffel & Camille K. Barsukiewicz. 5th ed. 2001. LC 2001-28360. (Illus.). viii, 211p. (C). text 64.95 (*0-7668-0714-2*) Delmar.

U. S. Health Workforce: Power, Politics & Policy. Marian Osterweis et al. 1996. 300p. pap. 25.00 (*1-879694-11-5*) AAH Ctrs.

U. S. Healthcare Compendium Vol. I: A Demographic & Statistical Analysis. Market Intelligence Staff. 1994. 221p. (Orig.). 795.00 (*0-7889-0127-3*) Frost & Sullivan.

U. S. Healthcare Delivery System in the Year 2000: Opportunities for Suppliers, Goods & Services. 1993. 120p. 2450.00 (*0-89336-965-9*, B-101) BCC.

U. S. Home Care Monitoring & Telemedicine Markets: Issues, Market Forecasts, & Trends. Feedback Research Services Staff. 1997. (Illus.). 205p. spiral bd. 595.00 (*1-889713-11-2*) Feedback Rsch.

U. S. Home Diagnostic & Monitoring Product Markets: An Evolution in Self-Help Spawns a Revolution in Preventive Care. Frost and Sullivan Staff. 1996. 333p. spiral bd. 2295.00 (*0-7889-0460-4*, 5315-54) Frost & Sullivan.

U. S. Home Diagnostic & Monitoring Product Markets: Cost Containment Pressures Motivate Self-Testing. Market Intelligence Staff. 1994. 289p. 1995.00 (*0-7889-0018-8*) Frost & Sullivan.

U. S. Home Healthcare Market Overview. Ed. by Frost and Sullivan Staff. 1997. 270p. spiral bd. 2295.00 (*0-7889-0777-8*, 5614-59) Frost & Sullivan.

U. S. Hospital Infection Control Equipment & Supply Markets: New Sterilization Systems Lead Industry Growth. Frost and Sullivan Staff. 1995. LC 98-168748. 389p. spiral bd. 2295.00 (*0-7889-0267-9*, 5302-54) Frost & Sullivan.

U. S. Hospital Information System Markets. Ed. by Frost and Sullivan Staff. 1995. 509p. spiral bd. 2295.00 (*0-7889-0232-6*, 5226-74) Frost & Sullivan.

U. S. Hospital Information Systems Market. Market Intelligence Staff. 1992. 388p. 2600.00 (*1-56753-683-2*, A2546) Frost & Sullivan.

U. S. Hospital Kit & Tray Markets: Manufacturers Meet User Demands with Customization & Safety Features. Market Intelligence Staff. 1994. 358p. 1895.00 (*0-7889-0107-9*) Frost & Sullivan.

U. S. Immunotherapeutic Markets. 1996. 530p. spiral bd. 3295.00 (*0-7889-0558-9*, 5481-43) Frost & Sullivan.

U. S. Implantable & Interventional Cardiovascular Device Markets. Market Intelligence Staff. 1995. 328p. (Orig.). spiral bd. 2295.00 (*0-7889-0130-3*, 5084-54) Frost & Sullivan.

U. S. Implantable Cardiovascular Device Markets. Frost & Sullivan. 1996. 305p. spiral bd. 2895.00 (*0-7889-0617-8*, 5348-54) Frost & Sullivan.

U. S. Implementation of Telemedicine: Survey-Based Progress Updates & Market Forecasts. Feedback Research Services Staff. 1997. (Illus.). 388p. spiral bd. 1495.00 (*1-889713-17-1*) Feedback Rsch.

U. S. Incontinence & Ostomy Product Markets. Ed. by Frost and Sullivan Staff. 1995. 371p. spiral bd. 1895.00 (*0-7889-0261-X*, 5238-51) Frost & Sullivan.

U. S. Information Systems for Physician Markets: From the Doctor's Office to the Clinics Without Walls. Frost and Sullivan Staff. 1996. spiral bd. 2295.00 (*0-7889-0424-8*, 5334-74) Frost & Sullivan.

U. S. Intravenous Equipment & Supply Markets Vol. 1: Intravenous Solutions. Market Intelligence Staff. 1993. 101p. 1295.00 (*1-56753-532-1*) Frost & Sullivan.

U. S. Intravenous Equipment & Supply Markets Vol. 2: Vascular Access Devices. Market Intelligence Staff. 1993. 182p. 1295.00 (*1-56753-533-X*) Frost & Sullivan.

U. S. Intravenous Equipment & Supply Markets Vol. 3: Infusion Devices. Market Intelligence Staff. 1993. 155p. 1295.00 (*1-56753-534-8*) Frost & Sullivan.

U. S. IV Vein Access Markets: Mini-Series. 1995. spiral bd. 1495.00 (*0-7889-0377-2*, 5304-54) Frost & Sullivan.

U. S. Livestock Market for Veterinary Medical Services & Products. Center for Info. Management Staff. 2nd ed. 1995. Orig. Title: The U. S. Market for Food Animal Veterinary Medical Services. (Illus.). 103p. (Orig.). pap. 74.50 (*1-882691-08-3*) Am Veterinary Med Assn.

U. S. Market for Food Animal Veterinary Medical Services see U. S. Livestock Market for Veterinary Medical Services & Products

U. S. Medical & Dental Suction & Irrigation Equipment Markets: Manufacturer's Focus on Portability & Product Integration. 1995. LC 98-168752. spiral bd. 1895.00 (*0-7889-0382-9*, 5307-54) Frost & Sullivan.

U. S. Medical & Pharmaceutical Packaging Markets: Blister Packaging & Roll Stock Lead Industry Growth. Frost and Sullivan Staff. 1996. LC 98-168944. 334p. spiral bd. 1895.00 (*0-7889-0410-8*, 5076-37) Frost & Sullivan.

U. S. Medical & Pharmaceutical Packaging Markets: Manufacturers Focus on Cost Containment & Waste Reduction. Market Intelligence Staff. 1993. 300p. (Orig.). 1695.00 (*1-56753-628-X*) Frost & Sullivan.

U. S. Medical Disposable Product Markets Vol. 3: Needles, Syringes & Related Products. Market Intelligence Staff. 1994. 370p. (Orig.). 1895.00 (*1-56753-924-6*) Frost & Sullivan.

U. S. Medical Glove End-User Study. 1996. 138p. spiral bd. 1495.00 (*0-7889-0563-5*, 5525-51) Frost & Sullivan.

U. S. Medical License Examination Jack Rudman. 1994. (Admission Test Ser.: ATS-104). pap. 89.95 (*0-8373-5804-3*) Nat Learn.

U. S. Medical License Examination Step I: Basic Medical Sciences. Jack Rudman. 1994. (Admission Test Ser.: ATS-104A). pap. 49.95 (*0-8373-6967-3*) Nat Learn.

U. S. Medical License Examination Step II: Clinical Sciences. Jack Rudman. 1994. (Admission Test Ser.: ATS-104B). pap. 49.95 (*0-8373-6968-1*) Nat Learn.

U. S. Medical Licensing Exam (USMLE) Step I: Basic Medical Sciences. Jack Rudman. (Admission Test Ser.: Vol. 104A). 69.95 (*0-8373-6992-4*) Nat Learn.

U. S. Medical Licensing Exam (USMLE) Step II: Clinical Sciences. Jack Rudman. (Admission Test Ser.: Vol. 104B). 69.95 (*0-8373-6993-2*) Nat Learn.

U. S. Medical Licensing Examination Step III: Patient Management. Jack Rudman. 1996. (Admission Test Ser.: ATS-104C). pap. 49.95 (*0-8373-6969-X*) Nat Learn.

U. S. Medical Licensing Examination (USMLE) Jack Rudman. (Admission Test Ser.: Vol. 104). 109.95 (*0-8373-5854-X*) Nat Learn.

U. S. Medical Waste Management & Disposal Markets: Huge Impact on Alternate Cites Due to Stringent Regulation Enforcement. Market Intelligence Staff. 1994. 560p. 1995.00 (*0-7889-0012-9*) Frost & Sullivan.

U. S. Mental Health Telemedicine: Survey-Based Overview of Usage & Successful Systems. Feedback Research Services Staff. 1997. (Illus.). 79p. spiral bd. 100.00 (*1-889713-15-5*) Feedback Rsch.

U. S. National Health Policy: An Analysis of the Federal Role. Jennie J. Kronenfeld & Marcia L. Whicker. 1984. LC 84-2169. 274p. 77.00 (*0-275-91207-8*, C1207, Praeger Pubs) Greenwood.

U. S. Neurodiagnostic & Neurosurgical Product Markets. Market Intelligence Staff. 1995. LC 98-168738. 344p. 1995.00 (*0-7889-0151-6*, 5197-54) Frost & Sullivan.

U. S. Neurotherapeutic Pharmaceuticals Markets by Disease. Ed. by Frost and Sullivan Staff. 1995. 309p. spiral bd. 2295.00 (*0-7889-0199-0*, 5203-45) Frost & Sullivan.

U. S. Obsterics & Gynecology Pharmaceutical Markets. Ed. by Frost and Sulllivan Staff. 1995. 301p. spiral bd. 2295.00 (*0-7889-0260-1*, 5202-44) Frost & Sullivan.

U. S. Ophthalmic Diagnostic Equipment Markets: Manufacturers Visualize High Growth from Emerging Technologies. Market Intelligence Staff. 1994. 320p. 1895.00 (*0-7889-0050-1*) Frost & Sullivan.

U. S. Ophthalmic Surgical Device Markets. Market Intelligence Staff. 1994. 288p. (Orig.). 1895.00 (*0-7889-0103-6*) Frost & Sullivan.

U. S. Organ Transplant & Artificial Organ Product Markets. Market Intelligence Staff. 1995. LC 98-167119. 309p. spiral bd. 1995.00 (*0-7889-0165-6*, 5081-54) Frost & Sullivan.

U. S. Osteoporosis Diagnostics & Therapeutics Market. Ed. by Frost and Sullivan Staff. 1997. 323p. spiral bd. 2995.00 (*0-7889-0685-2*, 5527-44) Frost & Sullivan.

U. S. Osteoporosis Markets. Market Intelligence Staff. 1994. LC 98-167130. 412p. 2295.00 (*0-7889-0122-2*) Frost & Sullivan.

U. S. Pain Management Pharamaceutical Markets. Ed. by Frost and Sullivan Staff. 1997. 274p. spiral bd. 2295.00 (*0-7889-0664-X*) Frost & Sullivan.

U. S. Patient & Mobility Aid Markets. Market Intelligence Staff. 1994. 345p. 1895.00 (*0-7889-0155-9*) Frost & Sullivan.

U. S. Patient & Mobility Aid Markets: Niche Markets on the Move. Market Intelligence Staff. 1994. (Orig.). 1895.00 (*0-7889-0123-0*) Frost & Sullivan.

U. S. Patient Monitoring Markets. Market Intelligence Staff. 1995. 308p. spiral bd. 2195.00 (*0-7889-0161-3*, 5196-56) Frost & Sullivan.

U. S. Prescription Anti-Imflammatory Pharmaceutical Markets: Aggressive R&D Enhances New Compounds & Treatments. 1995. LC 98-168538. spiral bd. 2495.00 (*0-7889-0395-0*, 5027-44) Frost & Sullivan.

U. S. Prescription Gastrointestinal Pharmaceutical Markets in a Period of Transition. Market Intelligence Staff. 1994. 2495.00 (*0-7889-0064-1*) Frost & Sullivan.

U. S. Prescription Generic Pharmaceutical Markets. Market Intelligence Staff. 1993. (Quarterly Business Planning Ser.). 260p. 3295.00 (*0-7889-0099-4*) Frost & Sullivan.

U. S. Prescription Generic Pharmaceutical Markets: Quarterly. Frost and Sullivan Staff. 1996. LC 98-168561. 507p. spiral bd. 4295.00 (*0-7889-0422-1*, 5353-44) Frost & Sullivan.

U. S. Prescription Neurological - Psychotherapeutic Pharmaceuticals: R & D Efforts Paying Off. Market Intelligence Staff. 1993. 300p. 2295.00 (*1-56753-617-4*) Frost & Sullivan.

U. S. Prescription Respiratory Pharmaceutical Markets: New Asthma Treatment Guidelines Breathe Life into Industry. Market Intelligence Staff. 1994. 300p. 2295.00 (*1-56753-962-9*) Frost & Sullivan.

U. S. Prosthetic Joint Implants Market. 1996. 279p. spiral bd. 2995.00 (*0-7889-0559-7*, 5229-58) Frost & Sullivan.

U. S. Psychotherapeutics Pharmaceuticals Markets by Disease. Ed. by Frost and Sullivan Staff. 1995. 343p. spiral bd. 2295.00 (*0-7889-0194-X*, 5242-45) Frost & Sullivan.

U. S. Rehabilitation Product Markets. Market Intelligence Staff. 1994. 300p. 1895.00 (*0-7889-0048-X*) Frost & Sullivan.

U. S. Rural Health Telemedicine: Overview of Usage & Successful Systems. Feedback Research Services Staff. 1997. 80p. spiral bd. 100.00 (*1-889713-16-3*) Feedback Rsch.

U. S. Sexually Transmitted Disease, Diagnostic & Therapeutic Markets. Market Intelligence Staff. 1994. (Orig.). 2295.00 (*0-7889-0136-2*) Frost & Sullivan.

U. S. Soft Tissue Implant Markets. Ed. by Frost and Sullivan Staff. 1997. 347p. spiral bd. 2695.00 (*0-7889-0704-2*, 5487-54) Frost & Sullivan.

U. S. Specialty Biocide Markets: EPA Regulations Redefine Industry Focus. Market Intelligence Staff. 1994. 510p. 1995.00 (*1-56753-997-1*) Frost & Sullivan.

U. S. Spinal Implants & Surgical Product Markets: Implant Market Rebounds. Frost and Sullivan Staff. 1995. LC 98-168623. 338p. spiral bd. 2495.00 (*0-7889-0401-9*, 5347-58) Frost & Sullivan.

U. S. Telemedicine Market: Issues, Forecasts, & Trends, 1995-2000. Feedback Research Services Staff. 1996. (Illus.). 207p. spiral bd. 495.00 (*1-889713-01-5*) Feedback Rsch.

U. S. Thrombosis Markets: Anticoagulants, Antithrombotics & Thrombolytics: New Drugs, New Indications Expand Market. Market Intelligence Staff. 1994. LC 97-203018. 290p. 2495.00 (*1-56753-957-2*) Frost & Sullivan.

U. S. Urology Product Markets: Infection Control in an Aging Population Stimulates Growth. Market Intelligence Staff. 1993. 250p. 1995.00 (*1-56753-619-0*) Frost & Sullivan.

U. S. Wound Management Markets: The Quest for Less Damaging, More Active Products. Market Intelligence Staff. 1994. 300p. (Orig.). 2295.00 (*1-56753-887-8*) Frost & Sullivan.

U. S. Wound Management Product Markets: Newest Dressings Setting the Pace. Frost and Sullivan Staff. 1996. spiral bd. 2495.00 (*0-7889-0432-9*, 5344-51) Frost & Sullivan.

UC Berkeley Wellness Self-Care Handbook: The Everyday Guide to Home Remedies. John E. Swartzberg & Sheldon Margen. 1998. LC 97-52213. 34.95 (*0-929661-42-7*) Rebus.

UCH Handbook of Psychiatry. Ed. by R. Tredgold & H. Wolff. 1984. 240p. pap. 18.95 (*0-7156-0937-8*) Focus Pub-R Pullins.

UCH Textbook of Psychiatry: An Integrated Approach. D. Wolff. 1989. pap. 37.95 (*0-7156-2289-7*) Focus Pub-R Pullins.

UCLA Geriatric Curriculum Guide for Residency Training. UCLA, Division of Geriatrics Staff. 1998. 14p. (C). pap. 50.00 (*0-9661178-0-8*) Regents U CA.

UCLA International Conference on Imaging Detectors in High Energy, Astroparticle & Medical Physics. 1996. 200p. lib. bdg. 33.00 (*981-02-2895-3*) World Scientific Pub.

UCSD Healthy Diet for Diabetes: A Comprehensive Nutritional Guide & Cookbook. University of California, San Diego, School of Med et al. 1991. 352p. pap. 18.00 (*0-395-57225-8*) HM.

Ueber die Beeinflussbarkeit Psychiatrischer Krankheitsverlaeufe, 1980, Vol. 13, No. 3-4. Ed. by E. Gabriel. 1981. (Illus.). iv, 136p. pap. 28.75 (*3-8055-2336-X*) S Karger.

Ueber die Wirksamkeit der Daseinanalytischen Therapie Bei Psychosomatischen Stoerungen. B. Weber. 1994. (Journal: Vol. 11, No. 1, 1994). (Illus.). 98p. pap. 26.25 (*3-8055-5952-6*) S Karger.

Ueberlebenszeiten Beim Mammakarzinom. H. E. Wander. 1991. (Illus.). viii, 24p. pap. 42.75 (*3-8055-5248-3*) S Karger.

UFAW Handbook on the Care & Management of Laboratory Animals. Universities Federation for Animal Welfare Staff. Ed. by T. B. Poole. 6th ed. 1989. (Illus.). 933p. text (*0-582-40911-X*) Univs Fed Animal Welfare GBR. *Dist:* St Mut.

Ulcer & Non-Ulcer Dyspepsias. Ed. by M. J. Smith. 1987. (Practical Clinical Medicine Ser.). lib. bdg. 101.50 (*0-85200-970-4*) Kluwer Academic.

Ulcer Disease: New Aspects of Pathogenesis & Pharmacology. Ed. by Sandor Szabo & Carl J. Pfeiffer. 1989. 448p. lib. bdg. 248.00 (*0-8493-6216-4*, RC822) CRC Pr.

Ulcer Story: The Authoritative Guide to Ulcers, Dyspepsia, & Heartburn. W. Grant Thompson. 1996. (Illus.). 386p. (C). 29.95 (*0-306-45275-8*) Da Capo.

Ulcerative Colitis. Calm A. O'Morain. 1991. 208p. 129.00 (*0-8493-5498-6*, RC862) CRC Pr.

Ulcerative Lesions of the Oral Cavity. Nicole Murray et al. 2000. LC 00-59400. (Self-Instructional Package Ser.). (Illus.). 51p. pap. text 30.00 (*1-56772-030-7*, 5506365) AAO-HNS.

Ulla-Maija Grace's Aromatherapy for Practitioners. 1996. 17.95 (*0-8464-4572-7*) Beekman Pubs.

Ullstein Lexikon der Medizin. 1970. (GER.). 49.95 (*0-8288-6557-4*, M-7674) Fr & Eur.

Ulrich Wolf Dedication Volume. Ed. by M. Schmidt & H. P. Klinger. 2001. (Cytogenetics & Cell Genetics Ser.: Vol. 91, No. 1-4). (Illus.). iv, 310p. 80.00 (*3-8055-7176-3*) S Karger.

Ultimate Back Book: Understand, Manage & Conquer Your Back Pain. Judylaine Fine. 1997. LC 99-181172. (Illus.). 368p. pap. (*0-7737-5863-1*) Stoddart Publ.

***Ultimate Book of Women's Health.** Nan Kathryn Fuchs. Ed. by Steven E. Kroening. 2001. 450p. pap. 19.95 (*1-885385-01-3*) Soundview Pubns.

Ultimate Breastfeeding Book of Answers: The Most Comprehensive Problem-Solution Guide to Breastfeeding. Jack Newman. 2000. LC 00-57435. (Illus.). 464p. pap. 19.95 (*0-7615-2996-9*) Prima Pub.

Ultimate Colonisation. R. Klein. 1993. (C). 45.00 (*1-85594-032-9*) St Mut.

Ultimate Consumer's Guide to Diets & Nutrition. James Marti. 1997. LC 96-53266. 480p. pap. 16.00 (*0-395-72860-6*) HM.

Ultimate Diet Tool Kit: Ohio Distinctive Software Guide to Diet & Nutrition. Stanford Apseloff & Glen Apseloff. 1994. 250p. (Orig.). pap. 8.95 (*0-9647934-0-7*) OH Distinct Pub.

Ultimate Guide for Pharmaceutical Reps. Andy Farah. 2000. (Illus.). 158p. pap. 24.00 (*0-9678437-1-5*) Farah Consult.

Ultimate Guide to Pregnancy for Lesbians: Tips & Techniques from Conception Through Birth - How to Stay Sane & Care for Yourself. Rachel Pepper. 1999. LC 99-22669. (Illus.). xii, 211p. pap. 14.95 (*1-57344-080-9*) Cleis Pr.

Ultimate HMO Handbook: How to Make the Most of the Revolution in Managed Care. Rhys W. Jones. 1994. 140p. (Orig.). pap. 7.95 (*0-9635819-1-0*) TTM Pub.

Ultimate Patient Satisfaction: Designing & Implementing an Effective Patient Satisfaction Program. John F. O'Malley. 1997. LC 97-26913. (HFMA Healthcare Financial Management Ser.). 336p. 55.00 (*0-7863-1219-X*, Irwn Prfssnl) McGraw-Hill Educ Grp.

Ultimate Rape: What Every Woman Should Know about Hysterectomies & Ovarian Removal. Elizabeth L. Plourde & M. T. Plourde. 1998. LC 97-92836. (Informed Health Care Ser.). 288p. 19.95 (*0-9661735-0-3*) New Voice.

Ultimate Recipe for Fitness. Sheila Cluff & Eleanor Brown. 1990. (Illus.). 192p. pap. 14.95 (*0-9618805-3-8*) Fitness Ojai.

Ultimate Sports Nutrition. Frederick C. Hatfield. 1987. (Illus.). 192p. (Orig.). pap. 16.95 (*0-8092-4887-5*, 488750, Contemporary) McGraw-Hill Trade.

Ultimate Sports Nutrition Handbook. Ellen Coleman & Suzanne Nelson Steen. 1996. (Illus.). 240p. pap. 14.95 (*0-923521-34-8*) Bull Pub.

Ultimate Stranger: The Autistic Child. Carl H. Delacato. rev. ed. 1984. 240p. reprint ed. pap. 15.00 (*0-87879-446-8*, 446-8) Acad Therapy.

Ultimate Training: Gary's Null's Complete Guide to Eating Right, Exercising & Living Longer. Gary Null. 1993. LC 92-44033. 224p. pap. 12.95 (*0-312-08796-9*) St Martin.

Ultimate Transformation. R. P. Kaushik. 2nd ed. 1977. LC 77-85215. pap. 8.95 (*0-918038-04-9*) Journey Pubns.

Ultra High Dilution: Physiology & Physics. Ed. by P. C. Endler & J. Schulte. 1994. LC 93-48594. 280p. (C). text 156.00 (*0-7923-2676-8*) Kluwer Academic.

Ultra-High Molecular Weight Polyethylene as a Biomaterial in Orthopedic Surgery. Ed. by H. Willert et al. 1991. LC 89-24609. (Illus.). 350p. text 94.00 (*0-920887-60-0*) Hogrefe & Huber Pubs.

Ultra Low Doses. Ed. by Christian Doutremepuich. 1991. LC 92-107886. 180p. (*0-7484-0021-4*) Tay Francis Ltd GBR. *Dist:* Taylor & Francis.

Ultra-Solutions: How to Fail Most Successfully. Paul Watzlawick. 1987. 110p. 12.95 (*0-393-02514-4*) Norton.

Ultrafit Older Cat. Claire Bessant & Bradley Viner. 1997. LC 96-43186. 10.95 (*0-8120-9856-0*) Barron.

Ultrasensitive Biochemical Diagnostics II, Vol. 2985. Ed. by Gerald E. Cohn & Steven A. Spoer. 1997. LC 97-193041. 306p. 80.00 (*0-8194-2396-3*) SPIE.

Ultrasonic Diagnosis of Cerebrovascular Disease. Ed. by Merrill P. Spencer. 1987. (Developments in Cardiovascular Medicine Ser.). text 206.50 (*0-89838-836-8*) Kluwer Academic.

Ultrasonic Diagnosis of Digestive Diseases. Francis S. Weill et al. 4th rev. ed. 1996. LC 95-39184. 743p. 212.00 (*3-540-60412-X*) Spr-Verlag.

Ultrasonic Imaging & Animal Reproduction. O. J. Ginther. 1995. Bk. 1, Fundamentals. (Illus.). 225p. (C). 45.00 (*0-9640072-3-1*); Bk. 2, Horses. 375p. 75.00 (*0-9640072-4-X*) Equisrvs Pubng.

Ultrasonic Physics & Instrumentation. Beth Anderhub & O'Brien Anderhub. 1988. (Illus.). 304p. pap. text (*0-316-03918-7*, Little Brwn Med Div) Lppncott W & W.

Ultrasonic Surgical Techniques for the Pelvic Surgeon. Ed. by Janet S. Rader & Neil B. Rosenhein. 1994. LC 94-21216. (Illus.). 112p. 97.00 (*0-387-94244-0*) Spr-Verlag.

Ultrasonic Tissue Characterization. Ed. by F. Dunn et al. 1996. (Illus.). 250p. 149.00 (*4-431-70162-1*) Spr-Verlag.

Ultrasonic Tissue Characterization. Ed. by J. M. Thijssen & D. Nicholas. 1982. text 112.50 (*90-247-2757-X*) Kluwer Academic.

Ultrasonic Tomography in Obstetrics & Gynecology. E. G. Loch. 1973. (Advances in Obstetrics & Gynaecology Ser.: Vol. 51). (Illus.). 35.00 (*3-8055-1585-5*) S Karger.

Ultrasonics in Early Pregnancy: Diagnostic Scanning & Fetal Motor Activity. E. Reinold. Ed. by P. J. Keller. 1976. (Contributions to Gynecology & Obstetrics Ser.: Vol. 1). 51.50 (*3-8055-2332-7*) S Karger.

Ultrasonography: An Introduction to Normal Structure & Functional Anatomy. Ed. by Reva A. Curry & Betty B. Tempkin. 1995. (Illus.). 492p. tchr. ed. (*0-7216-4748-0*); LC 93-26475. 800p. text 71.00 (*0-7216-4585-2*) Saunders.

Ultrasonography for Surgeons. Meyers. 1999. text (*0-7216-7236-1*) Saunders.

Ultrasonography in Infants & Children. Teele & Share. 1991. (Illus.). 528p. text 142.00 (*0-7216-8775-X*) Saunders.

Ultrasonography in Obstetrics & Gynecology. Ed. by Peter W. Callen. 3rd ed. 1993. LC 93-6621. (Illus.). 736p. text 89.95 (*0-7216-6712-0*) Saunders.

Ultrasonography in Obstetrics & Gynecology. Peter W. Callen. 4th ed. 2000. LC 99-45309. (Illus.). 925p. (C). text (*0-7216-8132-8*) Saunders.

Ultrasonography in Ophthalmology. Ed. by J. M. Thijssen & A. M. Verbeek. 1981. text 332.00 (*90-6193-724-8*) Kluwer Academic.

Ultrasonography in Ophthalmology 14: Proceedings of the 14th SIDUO Congress, Tokyo, Japan 1992. Ed. by J. M. Thijssen et al. 1995. LC 95-14247. (Documenta Ophthalmologica Proceedings Ser.: Vol. 58). 324p. (C). text 146.50 (*0-7923-3475-2*) Kluwer Academic.

Ultrasonography in Ophthalmology 15. G. Cennamo. 1997. LC 97-231. (Documenta Ophthalmologica Proceedings Ser.). 624p. text 314.50 (*0-7923-4464-2*) Kluwer Academic.

Ultrasonography in Ophthalmology II: Proceedings of the 11th SIDUO Congress, Capri 1986. Ed. by J. M. Thijssen et al. 1988. (Documenta Ophthalmologica Proceedings Ser.). (C). text 237.50 (*0-89838-378-1*) Kluwer Academic.

Ultrasonography in the Assessment of Ovarian & Tamoxifen-Associated Endometrial Pathology. Dirk Timmerman. 1998. (Acta Biomedica Lovaniensia Ser.: Vol. 163). (Illus.). 139p. pap. (*90-6186-857-2*) Leuven Univ BEL. *Dist:* Coronet Bks.

Ultrasonography of the Placenta: A Review. Lewis H. Nelson, III. 1994. (Illus.). 49p. pap. 57.00 (*1-930047-17-7*, UP) Am Inst Ultrasound.

Ultrasonography of the Spleen. J. N. Bruneton et al. 1988. (Illus.). 89p. 86.95 (*0-387-18595-X*) Spr-Verlag.

Ultrasonography on Ophthalmology, Siduo 5: Proceedings of the International Society for Ultrasonic Diagnosis in Ophthalmology, Ghent, May, 1973. International Society for Ultrasonic Diagnosis in Ophthalmology. Ed. by J. Francois & F. Goes. 1975. (Bibliotheca Ophthalmologica Ser.: Vol. 83). (Illus.). 450p. 153.25 (*3-8055-1777-7*) S Karger.

Ultrasound. Edward I. Bluth. 1999. (Illus.). 768p. 159.00 (*0-86577-861-2*) Thieme Med Pubs.

Ultrasound. Alfred B. Kurtz & William D. Middleton. 1995. LC 95-11324. (Requisites Ser.). text 89.00 (*0-8016-8096-4*) Taylor & Francis.

Ultrasound: Its Chemical, Physical, & Biological Effects. Kenneth S. Suslick. 1988. LC 87-28050. 336p. 75.00 (*0-89573-328-5*, Wiley-VCH) Wiley.

Ultrasound: Medical Applications, Biological Effects, & Hazard Potential. Ed. by M. H. Repacholi et al. 1987. 386p. 89.50 (*0-306-42411-8*, Plenum Trade) Perseus Pubng.

Ultrasound & Ballistocardiography in Cardiovascular Research: Proceedings of the Ballistocardiography & Cardiovascular Dynamics Congress, 3rd World, 9th European, Sofia, 1973. Ballistocardiograph Research Society Staff. Ed. by Jan Baan. 1974. (Bibliotheca Cardiologica Ser.: No. 34). (Illus.). 120p. 47.00 (*3-8055-1763-7*) S Karger.

Ultrasound & Early Pregnancy. Ed. by D. Jurkovic & E. Juaniaux. 1995. LC 95-33638. (POGSS Ser.). (Illus.). 164p. lib. bdg. 85.95 (*1-85070-615-8*, Parthenon Pbng) CRC Pr.

Ultrasound & Fetal Growth. J. M. Carrera & G. P. Mandruzzato. 2001. LC 99-16520. (Progress in Obstetric & Gynecological Sonography Ser.). (Illus.). xi, 117p. 77.95 (*1-85070-618-2*, Parthenon Pbng) CRC Pr.

Ultrasound & Fetal Therapy. Ed. by Mark I. Evans & C. H. Rodeck. 2000. LC 99-34251. (Progress in Obstetric & Gynecological Sonography Ser.). (Illus.). 166p. lib. bdg. 85.95 (*1-85070-671-9*, Parthenon Pbng) CRC Pr.

Ultrasound & Infertility. Ed. by S. Kupesic & D. De Ziegler. 1999. LC 99-49905. (Illus.). 312p. lib. bdg. 85.95 (*1-85070-620-4*, Parthenon Pbng) CRC Pr.

Ultrasound & Multifetal Pregnancy. Ana Monteagudo & Ilan E. Timor-Tritsch. 1997. LC 97-39909. (Progress in Obstetric & Gynecological Sonography Ser.). 228p. lib. bdg. 85.95 (*1-85070-986-6*, Parthenon Pbng) CRC Pr.

Ultrasound & the Endometrium. S. Granberg. Ed. by A. C. Fleischer & Asim Kurjak. 1997. LC 97-2669. (Progress in Obstetric & Gynecological Sonography Ser.). (Illus.). 160p. 85.95 (*1-85070-906-8*, F1073, Parthenon Pbng) CRC Pr.

Ultrasound & the Fallopian Tube. Ed. by Ilan E. Timor-Tritsch & Asim Kurjak. 1996. (Progress in Obstetric & Gynecological Sonography Ser.). (Illus.). 132p. lib. bdg. 85.95 (*1-85070-616-6*, Parthenon Pbng) CRC Pr.

Ultrasound & the Fetal Brain. Ed. by Frank A. Chervenak et al. 1995. LC 95-23988. (Progress in Obstetric & Gynecological Sonography Ser.). (Illus.). 254p. lib. bdg. 85.95 (*1-85070-612-3*, Parthenon Pbng) CRC Pr.

Ultrasound & the Fetal Heart. Ed. by Juri W. Wladimiroff & G. Pilu. 1996. LC 96-3059. (Progress in Obstetric & Gynecological Sonography Ser.). (Illus.). 138p. lib. bdg. 85.95 (*1-85070-617-4*, Parthenon Pbng) CRC Pr.

Ultrasound & the Ovary. Ed. by Asim Kurjak. 1994. LC 94-2029. (Progress in Obstetric & Gynecological Sonography Ser.: Vol. 1). 280p. lib. bdg. 85.95 (*1-85070-508-9*, Parthenon Pbng) CRC Pr.

Ultrasound & the Umbilical Cord. Ed. by W. Sepulveda & E. Jauniaux. 2001. (Progress in Obstetric & Gynecological Sonography Ser.). (Illus.). 200p. 88.00 (*1-85070-662-X*, Parthenon Pbng) CRC Pr.

Ultrasound & the Uterus. R. Osmers & Asim Kurjak. 1995. (Progress in Obstetric & Gynecological Sonography Ser.). (Illus.). 138p. (C). lib. bdg. 85.95 (*1-85070-613-1*, Parthenon Pbng) CRC Pr.

Ultrasound & Women's Health. 1998. (*1-930047-45-2*);Set. (Illus.). pap. (*1-930047-44-4*, 98UWH2) Am Inst Ultrasound.

Ultrasound & Women's Health: March 1998 Syllabus. Beryl R. Benacerraf et al. 2nd ed. 1998. (Illus.). 110p. pap. 68.00 (*1-930047-16-9*, UWH2) Am Inst Ultrasound.

Ultrasound Angioplasty. Ed. by Robert J. Siegel. 1996. (Developments in Cardiovascular Medicine Ser.: Vol. 178). 304p. text 248.00 (*0-7923-3722-0*) Kluwer Academic.

Ultrasound-Assisted Liposuction. Rod J. Rohrich et al. 1998. LC 98-24569. (Illus.). 412p. 225.00 (*1-57626-081-X*, QMP) Quality Med Pub.

Ultrasound Atlas of Disease Processes. Carol A. Krebs. 1997. (Illus.). 432p. (C). pap. text 189.00 (*0-8385-9245-7*, A9245-0, Apple Lange Med) McGraw.

Ultrasound Biomicroscopy of the Eye. Charles J. Pavlin & F. Stuart Foster. 1994. LC 93-40948. (Illus.). 214p. 147.00 (*0-387-94206-8*) Spr-Verlag.

Ultrasound Board Review: Questions & Answers for Self-Assessment. Michael M. Abiri. 1998. LC 98-41914. (Illus.). 192p. pap. 24.95 (*0-86577-815-9*) Thieme Med Pubs.

Ultrasound Companion. Philip W. Ralls & Nabil A. Yassa. 2003. 352p. pap. text 59.95 (*0-7817-2623-9*) Lppncott W & W.

Ultrasound Contrast Agents. Barry B. Goldberg. 1997. 216p. (*1-85317-283-9*) Martin Dunitz GBR. *Dist:* Mosby Inc.

Ultrasound Diagnosis in Obstetrics & Gynecology. Manfred Hansmann et al. Ed. by B. K. Wittman. Tr. by Terry C. Telger from GER. 1986. (Illus.). 495p. 352.00 (*0-387-15348-9*) Spr-Verlag.

Ultrasound Diagnosis of Breast Disease. Eriko Tohno et al. 1994. (Illus.). 160p. text (*0-443-04387-6*) Church.

Ultrasound Diagnosis of Cerebrovascular Disease: Doppler Sonography of the Extra- & Intracranial Arteries Duplex Scanning. Gerhard-Michael Von Reutern & Hans J. Von Budingen. Tr. by T. C. Telger. 1993. LC 93-28853. 397p. 169.00 (*0-86577-457-9*) Thieme Med Pubs.

Ultrasound Eighty-Two. Lerski & Morley. 1983. (Ultrasound in Medicine & Biology Ser.). pap. 8.65 (*0-08-030769-8*, Pergamon Pr) Elsevier.

Ultrasound Examination Review: Sonographer's Self-Assessment. Marveen Craig et al. 2nd ed. 1994. LC 93-41354. (Illus.). 304p. pap. text 40.00 (*0-397-55021-9*) Lppncott W & W.

Ultrasound for Surgeons. Ed. by Junji Machi & Bernard Sigel. 1997. LC 96-9300. (Illus.). 368p. 110.00 (*0-89640-321-1*) Igaku-Shoin.

Ultrasound for the Surgeon. Ed. by Edgar D. Staren & Maurice E. Arregui. 1996. 304p. text 139.00 (*0-397-51587-1*) Lppncott W & W.

Ultrasound Handbook: Clinical, Etiologic & Pathologic Implications of Sonographic Findings. Rebecca Hall. 3rd ed. 1999. LC 98-40629. 264p. spiral bd. 29.95 (*0-7817-1711-6*) Lppncott W & W.

Ultrasound in Ambulatory Medicine. Eric R. Snoey. Ed. by Barry C. Simon. 1996. (Illus.). 304p. (C). (gr. 13). text 64.95 (*0-8151-8519-7*, 28609) Mosby Inc.

Ultrasound in Cardiology. Kurt Schmailzl & Oliver Ormerod. 1994. LC 95-169809. (Illus.). 450p. 241.95 (*0-86542-802-6*) Blackwell Sci.

Ultrasound in Coronary Artery Disease. Ed. by Sabino Iliceto et al. 1990. (Developments in Cardiovascular Medicine Ser.). (C). text 268.50 (*0-7923-0784-4*) Kluwer Academic.

Ultrasound in Dermatology. Ed. by P. Altmeyer et al. 1992. (Illus.). 449p. 285.00 (*0-387-53750-3*) Spr-Verlag.

Ultrasound in Emergency Medicine. Michael Heller. 1995. LC 94-13906. (Illus.). 240p. text 58.00 (*0-7216-4506-2*) Saunders.

Ultrasound in Fetal Syndrome. Benacerraf. 1998. LC 98-5489. text (*0-443-07968-4*) Church.

Ultrasound in Gastroenterology. Paul A. Dubbins & A. E. Joseph. 1994. LC 94-16246. (Clinics in Diagnostic Ultrasound Ser.: Vol. 29). text (*0-443-08905-1*) Church.

Ultrasound in Gastroenterology & Hepatology. M. Gebel. 2000. (Illus.). 270p. pap. 133.95 (*0-632-05528-6*) Blackwell Sci.

Ultrasound in Gynecology. Steven R. Goldstein & Ilan E. Timor-Tritsch. 1995. LC 95-4803. 321p. text (*0-443-08957-4*) Church.

Ultrasound in Gynecology & Oabstetrics: Textbook & Atlas. E. Merz. 1991. (Illus.). 343p. text 159.00 (*0-86577-376-9*) Thieme Med Pubs.

Ultrasound in Infertility. A. Kurjak. 1989. 224p. lib. bdg. 159.00 (*0-8493-4766-1*, RC889) CRC Pr.

Ultrasound in Medicine & Biology: EUROSON '87—Proceedings of the Sixth Congress, Helsinki. S. Bondestam et al. 1987. 413p. pap. 67.50 (*951-99835-2-X*) Coronet Bks.

Ultrasound in Orthopedics. 1988. 209.00 (*0-387-91327-0*) Spr-Verlag.

Ultrasound in Othopedics. 1988. 209.00 (*0-387-91328-9*) Spr-Verlag.

Ultrasound in Surgical Practice: Principles & Clinical Applications. Jay K. Harness. 2001. LC 98-32455. (Illus.). 552p. 149.00 (*0-471-24538-0*) Wiley.

Ultrasound in Urology: Journal: Urologia Internationalis, Vol. 45, No. 4, 1990. Ed. by D. Hauri. 1990. (Illus.). 76p. pap. 55.00 (*3-8055-5226-2*) S Karger.

Ultrasound Mammography: Methods, Results, Diagnostic Strategies. B. J. Hackeloer et al. 1988. (Illus.). 144p. 170.00 (*0-387-96494-0*) Spr-Verlag.

Ultrasound Markers for Fetal Chromosomal Defects. Ed. by R. J. Snijders & K. H. Nicolaides. 1995. (Frontiers in Fetal Medicine Ser.). (Illus.). 200p. lib. bdg. 71.95 (*1-85070-610-7*, Parthenon Pbng) CRC Pr.

Ultrasound of Fetal Anomalies. David A. Nyberg. 1995. text 710.00 (*1-56815-017-2*, 10027) Mosby Inc.

Ultrasound of Human Diseases. Jones Staff. 1998. text (*0-7216-4929-7*) Saunders.

Ultrasound of Superficial Structures: High Frequencies, Doppler, & Interventional Procedures. Ed. by Luigi Salbiati et al. 1995. 416p. text (*0-443-05131-3*) Church.

Ultrasound of the Breast. 1998. (Ultrasound & Women's Health Ser.: Vol. 3). (*1-930047-48-7*, 98III); (Illus.). (*1-930047-52-5*, 98III-P) Am Inst Ultrasound.

Ultrasound of the Breast. Fornage. 1998. (C). text (*0-443-07658-8*) Church.

***Ultrasound of the Breast: An Atlas of Diagnostic & Interventional Procedures.** Bruno D. Fornage. 2001. (Illus.). 310p. (*0-443-06472-5*) Church GBR. *Dist:* Saunders.

Ultrasound of the Head & Neck. Ed. by C. D. Verwoerd. 1993. (Journal: Vol. 55, No. 5, 1993). (Illus.). 68p. pap. 58.50 (*3-8055-5836-8*) S Karger.

Ultrasound of the Infant Brain. Malcolm I. Levene et al. 1991. (Clinics in Developmental Medicine Ser.: No. 92). (Illus.). 148p. (C). text (*0-521-41212-9*) Mc Keith Pr GBR. *Dist:* Cambridge U Pr.

Ultrasound of the Prostate. Bruno D. Fornage. 2nd ed. 1997. 352p. 145.00 (*0-471-14969-1*, F1049) Wiley.

Ultrasound of the Prostate. Matthew D. Rifkin. 2nd ed. 1996. LC 96-23896. 480p. text 175.00 (*0-397-51769-6*) Lppncott W & W.

Ultrasound Physics & Instrumentation. Wayne R. Hendrick & David L. Hykes. 3rd ed. 1994. LC 94-21585. (Illus.). 432p. (C). (gr. 13). text 49.00 (*0-8151-4246-3*, 24085) Mosby Inc.

Ultrasound Physics Review. Cindy A. Owen. 2000. LC 00-60160. (Illus.). 175p. pap. 55.00 (*0-941022-52-8*, 11029) Davies Pubng.

Ultrasound Renal Stone Surgery. 1982. 545.00 (*0-387-91211-8*) Spr-Verlag.

Ultrasound Review of Obstetrics & Gynecology. Janice Hickey & Franklin Goldberg. 1996. 192p. pap. text 47.50 (*0-397-51654-1*) Lppncott W & W.

Ultrasound Scanning: Principles & Protocols. Betty B. Tempkin. 1992. (Illus.). 347p. (C). pap. text 61.00 (*0-7216-3706-X*) Saunders.

Ultrasound Scanning: Principles & Protocols. Betty B. Tempkin. Ed. by Andrew Allen. 2nd ed. 1998. LC 97-44164. (Illus.). 668p. (C). text 69.00 (*0-7216-6879-8*) Saunders.

Ultrasound Scanning Guide. Lisa Bachan. 1996. (Orig.). pap. (*0-9651644-0-3*) Chrlston Ultrasnd.

Ultrasound Screening for Fetal Anomalies: Is It Worth It? Ed. by Salvator Levi & Frank A. Chervenak. 1998. LC 98-17556. (Annals of the New York Academy of Sciences Ser.). 350p. 140.00 (*1-57331-123-5*); pap. 140.00 (*1-57331-124-3*) NY Acad Sci.

Ultrasound Teaching Manual. Daphne M. Cohen & M. Hofer. 1999. (Illus.). 80p. pap. 16.95 (*0-86577-725-X*) Thieme Med Pubs.

Ultrasounography in Obstetrics & Gynecology: A Practical Approach. Carol B. Benson. 2000. LC 99-54407. 59.00 (*0-86577-895-7*) Thieme Med Pubs.

Ultrastructural Appearances of Tumours. Douglas W. Henderson et al. 2nd ed. 1986. (Illus.). 456p. text (*0-443-03111-8*) Church.

Ultrastructural Effects of Radiation on Tissues & Cells. Ed. by K. E. Carr & T. M. Seed. 1983. (Illus.). 172p. (Orig.). pap. text 18.00 (*0-931288-29-0*) Scanning Microscopy.

Ultrastructural Kidney Pathology. Ed. by V. Marinozzi. 1985. (Journal: Vol. 2, No. 4, 1984). (Illus.). 52p. pap. 41.75 (*3-8055-4251-8*) S Karger.

Ultrastructural Pathology: An Introduction to Interpretation. Norman F. Cheville. 1994. LC 93-37657. (Illus.). 954p. (C). text 199.95 (*0-8138-2398-6*) Iowa U Pr.

Ultrastructural Pathology of the Cell & Matrix: 2 Volume Set Feroze N. Ghadially. 4th ed. 1996. LC 96-18218. 1322p. (*0-7506-9635-4*) E A GBR. *Dist:* OUP.

Ultrastructural Pathology of the Kidney. Ed. by C. L. Pirani. 1987. (Journal: Vol. 5, No. 2, 1987). (Illus.). 68p. pap. 39.25 (*3-8055-4634-3*) S Karger.

Ultrastructure, Macromolecules, & Evolution. Lawrence S. Dillon. 1981. LC 80-20550. 716p. 120.00 (*0-306-40528-8*, Plenum Trade) Perseus Pubng.

Ultrastructure, Membrane & Cell Interactions. Horst Robenek. Ed. by Nicholas J. Severs. 1992. 336p. lib. bdg. 229.00 (*0-8493-5505-2*, RC692) CRC Pr.

Ultrastructure of Brain Tumors & Biopsies: A Diagnostic Atlas, 5. C. L. Dolman. 1984. LC 84-3469. (Methods in Laboratory Medicine Ser.: Vol. 5). 266p. 62.95 (*0-275-91426-7*, C1426, Praeger Pubs) Greenwood.

Ultrastructure of Endocrine Cells & Tissues: Electron Microscopy in Biology & Medicine. Ed. by P. M. Motta. 1983. text 240.00 (*0-89838-568-7*) Kluwer Academic.

Ultrastructure of Human Gametogenesis & Early Embryogenesis. Ed. by Jonathan Van Blerkom & Pietro M. Motta. 1989. (Electron Microscopy in Biology & Medicine Ser.). (C). text 159.50 (*0-89838-383-8*) Kluwer Academic.

Ultrastructure of Male Urogenital Glands: Prostrate, Semial Vesicles, Urethral, & Bulbourethral Glands. Ed. by Alessandro Riva et al. 1994. LC 94-11636. (Electron Microscopy in Biology & Medicine Ser.: EMBM 11). 224p. (C). text 247.00 (*0-7923-2800-0*) Kluwer Academic.

Ultrastructure of Reproduction Gametogenesis, Fertilization & Embryogenesis. Ed. by Jonathan Van Blerkom & Pietro M. Motta. 1983. (Electron Microscopy in Biology & Medicine Ser.). text 197.50 (*0-89838-572-5*) Kluwer Academic.

Ultrastructure of Skeletal Tissue. Ed. by E. Bonucci & P. M. Motta. 1990. (Electron Microscopy in Biology & Medicine Ser.). (C). text 320.00 (*0-7923-0373-3*) Kluwer Academic.

Ultrastructure of the Animal Cell. L. T. Threadgold. Ed. by G. A. Kerkut. 2nd ed. 1976. 472p. (*0-08-018958-X*) Pergamon Repr GBR. *Dist:* Franklin.

Ultrastructure of the Conjunctival Epithelium. K. P. Steuhl. 1989. (Developments in Ophthalmology Ser.: Vol. 19). (Illus.). x, 106p. 83.50 (*3-8055-4943-1*) S Karger.

Ultrastructure of the Digestive Tract. Ed. by P. M. Motta & Hisao Fujita. 1988. (Electron Microscopy in Biology & Medicine Ser.). (C). text 197.00 (*0-89838-893-7*) Kluwer Academic.

Ultrastructure of the Extraparietal Glands of the Digestive Tract. Ed. by Alessandro Riva & Pietro M. Motta. 1989. (Electron Microscopy in Biology & Medicine Ser.). (C). text 246.50 (*0-7923-0303-2*) Kluwer Academic.

Ultrastructure of the Small Intestinal Mucosa: Normal & Disease-Related Appearances. Margot Shiner. 1983. (Illus.). 163p. 170.00 (*0-387-11732-6*) Spr-Verlag.

Ultraviolet Radiation. 1979. (Environmental Health Criteria Ser.: No. 14). 110p. pap. text 16.00 (*92-4-154074-5*, 1160014) World Health.

Ultraviolet Radiation: An Authoritative Scientific Review of Environmental & Health Effects of Ultraviolet Radiation, with Reference to Global Ozone Layer Depletion. 1994. (Environmental Health Criteria Ser.: No. 160). 352p. pap. text 67.00 (*92-4-157160-8*, 1160160) World Health.

***Ultraviolet Radiation & Squamous Cell Carcinoma in Human Skin.** Cecilia Wassberg. 2001. (Comprehensive Summaries of Uppsala Dissertations from the Faculty of Medicine Ser.: No. 1079). (Illus.). 53p. pap. (*91-554-5126-8*) Acta Univ SWE. *Dist:* Coronet Bks.

Ultraviolet Radiation in Antarctica: Measurements & Biological Effects. Ed. by C. Susan Weiler & Polly A. Penhale. 1994. LC 94-1422. (Antarctic Research Ser.: Vol. 62). 257p. 70.00 (*0-87590-841-1*) Am Geophysical.

Umfangreiches Agyptisches Traum-Deutungs Buch by Nostradamus see Nostradamus's Dream Interpretations

Umgang mit Schwierigen Kindern und Jugendlichen. H. J. Von Schumann. 1973. (Psychologische Praxis Ser.: No. 48). 80p. 17.00 (*3-8055-1561-8*) S Karger.

Unarius Publications Catalogue. Unarius Educational Foundation Staff. 1995. (Illus.). 36p. pap. 2.00 (*0-935097-01-5*) Unarius Acad Sci.

Unassisted Childbirth. Laura K. Shanley. 1993. LC 93-5268. 176p. 57.75 (*0-89789-370-0*); pap. 19.95 (*0-89789-377-8*) Greenwood (Bergin & Garvey).

Unbiased Stereology: A Practical Guide. M. Reed & V. Howard. 1998. LC 97-45235. (Microscopy Handbooks). (Illus.). 144p. pap. 32.95 (*0-387-91516-8*) Spr-Verlag.

T U V

Unborn Baby Book. Jack H. McCubbin & Marjorie V. Fuqua. 1985. (Illus.). 128p. (Orig.). pap. 7.95 (*0-9615085-7-4*) Tex Med Pr.

Unborn Baby Book. Jack H. McCubbin & Marjorie F. McCubbin. 2nd ed. 1986. LC 85-51698. (Illus.). 144p. (Orig.). pap. 7.95 (*0-9615085-8-2*) Tex Med Pr.

Unborn Patient: Prenatal Diagnosis & Treatment. Harrison & Roy A. Filly. 2nd ed. 1990. (Illus.). 674p. text 210.00 (*0-7216-4538-0*) Saunders.

Unborn Patient: Prenatal Diagnosis & Treatment. Michael R. Harrison. 3rd ed. 2000. LC 00-58853. 688p. text 220.00 (*0-7216-8446-7*) Saunders.

Unbound: A Book of Aids. Aaron Shurin. 1997. 96p. 19.95 (*1-55713-112-0*) Sun & Moon CA.

Uncertain Lives, Untimely Deaths: Experiences & Psychological Needs of the Young Adult with Serious Chronic Illness. Suzanne Quin. 1996. (Developments in Nursing & Health Care Ser.). 176p. text (*1-85972-497-3*) Avebry GBR. *Dist:* Ashgate Pub Co.

Uncertainties in Fatal Cancer Risk Estimates Used in Radiation Protection. 1997. LC 97-41391. (NCRP Reports: No. 126). 165p. pap. 25.00 (*0-929600-57-6*) NCRP Pubns.

***Uncertainties in Radiation Dosimetry & Their Impact on Dose-Response Analyses.** Ed. by Elaine Ron & F. Owen Hoffman. 2001. (Illus.). 317p. pap. 40.00 (*0-7567-1304-8*) DIANE Pub.

Uncertainty: Behavioral & Social Dimensions. Ed. by Seymour Fiddle. 1980. LC 80-82073. 401p. 75.00 (*0-275-90480-6*, C0480, Praeger Pubs) Greenwood.

Uncertainty in Environmental Health Risk Assessment. Kenneth T. Bogen. 1990. LC 90-3766. (Environment: Problems & Solutions Ser.). 219p. text 15.00 (*0-8240-0407-8*) Garland.

Uncertainty in the Risk Assessment of Environmental & Occupational Hazards: An International Workshop. Contrib. by A. John Bailer. 1999. LC 99-52620. (Annals of the New York Academy of Sciences Ser.: Vol. 895). (Illus.). xii, 377p. (*1-57331-236-3*) NY Acad Sci.

TUV

Uncharted Seas. Fuller Albright & Read Ellsworth. deluxe ed. 1990. 124p. ring bd. 59.95 (*0-945892-02-0*) JBK Pub.

Uncheese Cookbook. Joanne Stepaniak. 1994. LC 93-42489. 192p. pap. 12.95 (*0-913990-42-6*) Book Pub Co.

Uncommon Care for Common Animals: 1995 IWRC Conference Proceedings. Ed. by Mary D. Reynolds. 1996. (Illus.). 223p. (Orig.). pap. 18.00 (*1-884196-05-5*) IWRC.

Uncommon Causes of Stroke. Ed. by Julien Bogousslavsky & Louis Caplan. 2nd ed. 2001. LC 00-64231. (Illus.). 410p. (C). text 240.00 (*0-521-77145-5*) Cambridge U Pr.

Uncommon Child. Ed. by Michael Lewis & Leonard A. Rosenblum. 1981. LC 80-20601. (Genesis of Behavior Ser.: Vol. 3). 354p. 65.00 (*0-306-40499-0*, Plenum Trade) Perseus Pubng.

Uncommon Infections & Special Topics. Ed. by Louis G. Keith. 1985. text 248.00 (*0-85200-861-9*) Kluwer Academic.

Uncommon Men of Medicine: From Rabelais to Maugham. B. Mahendra. 1991. 305p. (C). 60.00 (*0-86332-604-8*) St Mut.

Uncommon Plant Drugs of Ayurveda. Gyanendra Pandey. 1995. LC 94-904592. (C). (*81-7030-404-0*) Sri Satguru Pubns IND. *Dist:* S Asia.

Uncommon Problems in Intensive Care. J. F. Cade. 1998. (Illus.). 600p. (*0-443-05104-6*) Church.

Uncommon Psychiatric Syndromes. M. David Enoch & Ball. 4th ed. 2000. 288p. pap. text (*0-7506-4314-5*) E A GBR. *Dist:* OUP.

Uncommon Voyage: Parenting a Special Needs Child in the World of Alternative Medicine. Laura S. Kramer. 1997. 224p. pap. 14.95 (*0-571-19928-3*) Faber & Faber.

Uncommon Voyage: Parenting a Special Needs Child in the World of Alternative Medicine. Laura Shapiro Kramer. 2nd ed. 2001. LC 2001-16264. 240p. pap. 14.95 (*1-55643-370-0*) North Atlantic.

Uncomplicated Guide to Diabetes Complications. Michael A. Pfeiffer. Ed. by Marvin E. Levin. 1998. LC 98-7166. (Illus.). 374p. pap. 18.95 (*0-945448-87-2*, 00872Q) Am Diabetes.

Unconditional Demand for Health Care in Cote D'Ivoire: Does Selection on Health Status Matter? William H. Dow. 1996. LC 96-34971. (Living Standards Measurement Study Working Papers: No. 127). 62p. pap. 22.00 (*0-8213-3757-2*, 13757) World Bank.

Unconscious: The Fundamentals of Human Personality Normal & Abnormal. Morton Prince. 2nd ed. 1973. LC 73-2411. (Mental Illness & Social Policy; the American Experience Ser.). reprint ed. 44.95 (*0-405-05221-9*) Ayer.

Unconscious, a Symposium. Charles M. Child et al. 1977. LC 67-22125. (Essay Index Reprint Ser.). 19.95 (*0-8369-0957-7*) Ayer.

Unconscious & the Theory of Psychoneuroses. Zvi Giora. 1992. LC 94-150166. (Psychoanalytic Crosscurrents Ser.). 256p. (C). pap. text 18.50 (*963-7977-06-6*) NYU Pr.

Unconscious as Infinite Sets. Ignacio Matte-Blanco. 1998. LC 98-209638. 504p. reprint ed. pap. (*1-85575-202-6*) Karnac Bks GBR. *Dist:* Other Pr LLC.

Unconscious Beethoven: An Essay in Musical Psychology. Ernest Newman. 1990. 154p. reprint ed. lib. bdg. 59.00 (*0-7812-9045-7*) Rprt Serv.

Unconscious Communication in Everyday Life. Robert J. Langs. 1993. LC 82-1669. 224p. pap. 40.00 (*1-56821-106-6*) Aronson.

Unconscious Communication in Practice. E. Mary Sullivan. 1998. LC 98-16395. (*0-335-20199-7*) OpUniv Pr.

Unconscious Contracts: A Psychoanalytic Theory of Society. Michael Allingham. 1988. 176p. text 45.00 (*0-7102-0996-7*, Routledge Thoemms) Routledge.

Unconscious Fantasy in Psychotherapy: Its Meaning & Mastery in Psychotherapy. Kenneth Levin. 1994. LC 92-49153. 320p. 50.00 (*0-87668-260-3*) Aronson.

Unconscious for Sale: Advertising, Psychoanalysis, & the Public. Doris-Louise Haineault & Jean-Yves Roy. Tr. by Kimball Lockhart & Barbara Kerslake. 1993. LC 92-32340. (Theory & History of Literature Ser.: Vol. 86). (Illus.). 240p. (C). pap. 19.95 (*0-8166-2186-1*); text 49.95 (*0-8166-2185-3*) U of Minn Pr.

Unconscious Logic: An Introduction to Matte Blanco's Bi-Logic & Its Uses. Eric Rayner. 1995. LC 94-45146. (New Library of Psychoanalysis). 176p. (C). pap. 29.95 (*0-415-12726-2*, C0566) Routledge.

Unconscious Today: Essays in Honor of Max Schur. Ed. by Mark Kanzer. 1971. LC 74-14337. 544p. 80.00 (*0-8236-6680-8*) Intl Univs Pr.

Uncontrollable Kids: From Heartbreak to Hope. Foster W. Cline. 1995. 338p. per. 14.95 (*0-944634-19-2*) Love & Logic.

Unconventional Agents & Unclassified Viruses: Recent Advances in Biology & Epidemiology. Ed. by Wolfgang Eichhorn et al. 1996. 340p. pap. 185.00 (*0-387-82480-4*) Spr-Verlag.

Unconventional Cancer Treatments. 1991. lib. bdg. 250.00 (*0-8490-4956-3*) Gordon Pr.

Unconventional Sources of Dietary Fiber. Ed. by Ivan Furda. 1983. LC 83-2691. (ACS Symposium Ser.: No. 214). 315p. lib. bdg. 64.95 (*0-8412-0768-2*) Am Chemical.

Uncovering Shame: An Approach Integrating Individuals & Their Family Systems. James M. Harper & Margaret H. Hoopes. 1990. 350p. 34.95 (*0-393-70100-X*) Norton.

Undaunted Psychologist: Adventures in Research. Ed. by Gary G. Brannigan & Matthew R. Merrens. 1992. LC 92-16793. 320p. (C). 59.95 (*1-56639-015-X*) Temple U Pr.

Undaunted Spirits: Portraits of Recovery from Trauma. Mary Baures. 1994. LC 93-37931. 232p. pap. 16.95 (*0-914783-71-8*) Charles.

Undead Mother: Psychoanalytic Explorations of Masculinity, Feminity & Matricide. Christina Wieland. 2000. 244p. pap. (*1-900877-23-6*) Rebus Pr Ltd GBR. *Dist:* Intl Spec Bk, Other Pr LLC.

Under My Skin: A Kid's Guide to Atopic Dermatitis. Karen Crowe. 2000. (Illus.). 48p. (J). (gr. 3-8). pap. 5.95 (*0-9702446-2-2*) Fujisawa Health.

Under the Fig Leaf: A Comprehensive Guide to the Care & Maintenance of the Penis, Prostate & Related Organs. Angelo S. Paola. 1998. LC 98-39340. (Illus.). 320p. pap. 14.95 (*1-885987-15-3*, ME090) Practice Mgmt Info.

Under the Influence: A Guide to the Myths & Realities of Alcoholism. James R. Milam & Katherine Ketcham. 1984. 256p. mass mkt. 7.50 (*0-553-27487-2*) Bantam.

Under the Influence? Drugs & the American Workforce. National Research Council, Institute of Medicine. Ed. by Jacques Normand et al. 1993. LC 93-44292. 336p. (C). text 39.95 (*0-309-04885-0*) Natl Acad Pr.

Under the Influence of Modern Medicine. Terry A. Rondberg. 1998. 156p. lib. bdg. 12.95 (*0-9647168-3-6*) Chiropractic Jrnl.

Under the Mask: A Guide to Feeling Secure & Comfortable During Anesthesia & Surgery. James E. Cottrell & Stephanie Golden. 2001. LC 00-34202. (Illus.). viii, 280p. 39.00 (*0-8135-2877-1*); pap. 20.00 (*0-8135-2878-X*) Rutgers U Pr.

Under the Medical Gaze: Facts & Fictions of Chronic Pain. Susan Greenhalgh. 2001. LC 00-48890. (Illus.). xii, 371p. pap. 18.95 (*0-520-22398-5*); text 48.00 (*0-520-22397-7*) U CA Pr.

Undercurrents: A Therapist's Reckoning with Depression. Martha Manning. 1995. LC 94-33043. 208p. pap. 14.00 (*0-06-251184-X*) Harper SF.

Undercurrents: A Therapist's Reckoning with Her Own Depression. Martha Manning. 1998. 197p. text 20.00 (*0-7881-5241-6*) DIANE Pub.

Undercurrents of Anxiety: The Revolutionary Approach to Dealing with & Recovering from . . . Elizabeth Trego & Judith Trego. 1998. LC 98-90827. 200p. pap. (*1-57502-963-4*, PO2641) Morris Pubng.

Underdevelopment & Health Care in Africa: The Ghanaian Experience. Randolph Quaye. 1996. LC 95-687. 188p. text 79.95 (*0-7734-2254-4*) E Mellen.

Undergraduate Education in Cancer in the European Region: Report on a UICC/WHO Meeting. 1981. (Euro Reports & Studies Ser.: No. 49). 30p. pap. text 4.00 (*92-890-1215-3*) World Health.

Undergraduate Obstetrics & Gynecology. Michael Hull et al. 3rd ed. 1997. LC 96-24741. 480p. pap. text 55.00 (*0-7506-1351-3*) Buttrwrth-Heinemann.

Underground Cancer Book: A New Cancer Theory. Jack R. Ferber. 1998. LC 97-76170. 400p. pap. 49.95 (*0-9662282-0-0*) Jalsa Pubs.

Underlying Molecular, Cellular & Immunological Factors in Cancer & Aging. S. S. Yang. 1993. (Advances in Experimental Medicine & Biology Ser.: Vol. 330). (Illus.). 350p. (C). text 110.00 (*0-306-44411-9*, Kluwer Plenum) Kluwer Academic.

Underpinning & Retention. Ed. by S. Thorburn & G. S. Littlejohn. 1992. (Illus.). 416p. lib. bdg. (*0-7514-0094-7*) B Acad & Prof GBR. *Dist:* Routldge.

Underpinnings of Medical Ethics. Edmond A. Murphy et al. 1997. LC 97-1405. (Illus.). 496p. 53.95 (*0-8018-5568-3*) Johns Hopkins.

Underprivileged Areas & Health Care. Brian Jarman & Madhavi Bajekal. 1997. 200p. pap. 26.00 (*1-86094-014-5*) World Scientific Pub.

Understand & Control Your Asthma. Helene Boutin & Louis-Philippe Boulet. 1995. (Illus.). 120p. (*0-7735-1210-1*); LC 95-182066. pap. (*0-7735-1263-2*) McG-Queens Univ Pr CAN. *Dist:* CUP Services.

Understand & Treat Alcoholism. Paul Berenson. Date not set. 19.95 (*0-465-08875-9*) Basic.

Understand Your Backache: A Guide to Prevention, Treatment, & Relief. Rene Cailliet. 1984. LC 83-24071. (Illus.). 194p. pap. 13.95 (*0-8036-1647-3*) Davis Co.

Understandable Jung: The Personal Side of Jungian Psychology. Harry A. Wilmer. 1994. LC 93-10581. (Illus.). 642p. (Orig.). pap. 19.95 (*0-933029-69-1*) Chiron Pubns.

Understanding: Eliminating Stress & Finding Serenity in Life & Relationships. Jane Nelsen. 1986. LC 85-63353. 141p. pap. 8.95 (*0-9606896-2-1*) Empowering People.

Understanding Abnormal Behavior David Sue et al. (C). 3rd ed. 1990. 249.96 (*0-395-53264-7*); 3rd ed. 1989. pap. text, tchr. ed. 3.96 (*0-395-53262-0*); 3rd ed. 1989. pap. text, tchr. ed. 3.96 (*0-395-53263-9*); 5th ed. 1996. text, stu. ed. 20.36 (*0-395-78827-7*); 5th ed. 1996. 570p. text 70.36 (*0-395-78826-9*) HM.

Understanding Abnormal Behavior: Description, Explanation, Management. Leonard D. Goodstein & James F. Calhoun. 1982. LC 81-17669. (Illus.). (C). text (*0-394-34768-4*); stu. ed. 5.75 (*0-394-34769-2*) Random.

Understanding Abnormal Psychology. Neil Frude. 1997. LC 97-16962. (Basic Psychology Ser.). (C). 366p. text 68.95 (*0-631-16194-5*); 400p. pap. text 36.95 (*0-631-16195-3*) Blackwell Pubs.

Understanding Abortion. Mary Pipes. pap. (*0-7043-4480-7*) Womens Press GBR. *Dist:* Trafalgar.

Understanding Acid-Base. Benjamin Abelow. 1997. LC 97-3514. (Illus.). 320p. pap. 26.95 (*0-683-18272-2*) Lppncott W & W.

Understanding Acupuncture. Robert L. Felt & Stephen Birch. 1999. LC 98-36985. xv, 335p. pap. text (*0-443-06179-3*) Church.

Understanding Addictive Disease: A Tool for Preventing Relapse. Terrence Gorski & Merlene Miller. 1991. 30p. pap. 4.00 (*0-8309-0608-8*) Herald Pub Hse.

Understanding ADHD. Christopher Green. 1998. LC 98-96349. 320p. pap. 12.95 (*0-449-00152-0*) Fawcett.

Understanding ADHD: Attention Deficit Hyperactivity Disorder & the Feeling Brain. Sandra K. Woods & Willis H. Ploof. 1997. LC 97-4853. 208p. 74.95 (*0-8039-7422-1*, 1413); pap. 37.95 (*0-8039-7423-X*, 1414) Sage.

Understanding Adolescence: Issues & Implications for Effective Schools. Barbara Z. Presseisen. 1990. 60p. reprint ed. pap. 16.95 (*1-56602-002-6*) Research Better.

Understanding Advanced Statistics: A Guide for Nurses & Health Care Researchers. Denis Anthony. 1999. LC 98-3310. (*0-443-05933-0*) Saunders.

Understanding Aggressive Behavior in Children. Craig F. Ferris & Thomas Grisso. 1996. LC 96-34935. (Annals of the New York Academy of Sciences Ser.). pap. 125.00 (*1-57331-013-1*) NY Acad Sci.

Understanding Aging: Images, Attitudes & Professional Practice. Simon J. Biggs. 1993. LC 92-46227. pap. (*0-335-15724-6*) OpUniv Pr.

Understanding AIDS: Advances in Research & Treatment. Seth C. Kalichman. 2nd ed. 1998. LC 98-7455. 509p. 39.95 (*1-55798-529-4*); pap. 29.95 (*1-55798-530-8*) Am Psychol.

Understanding Alcoholism: A Starting Point for Families. Ted Lawson. 1991. LC 90-64269. 64p. pap. 3.95 (*0-89243-341-8*) Liguori Pubns.

Understanding Allergy, Sensitivity, & Immunity: A Comprehensive Guide. Janice Vickerstaff Joneja & Leonard Bielory. 1990. (Illus.). 350p. (C). pap. 16.95 (*0-8135-1521-1*) Rutgers U Pr.

Understanding Allergy, Sensitivity, & Immunity: A Comprehensive Guide. Janice Vickerstaff Joneja et al. 1990. LC 96-6476. (Illus.). 350p. (C). text 45.00 (*0-8135-1520-3*) Rutgers U Pr.

Understanding Alternative Medicine: New Health Paths in America. Lawrence Tyler. 2000. LC 99-37570. xii, 112p. 49.95 (*0-7890-0741-X*); pap. 19.95 (*0-7890-0902-1*) Haworth Pr (Haworth Herbal Pr).

Understanding Alzheimer's Disease. Neal R. Cutler & John J. Sramek. 1996. LC 96-20284. (Understanding Health & Sickness Ser.). 151p. pap. 12.00 (*0-87805-911-3*); text 28.00 (*0-87805-910-5*) U Pr of Miss.

Understanding Alzheimer's Disease: What It Is, How to Cope with It, Future Directions. Ed. by Miriam K. Aronson. 1998. (Illus.). 380p. reprint ed. text 17.00 (*0-7881-5582-2*) DIANE Pub.

Understanding Anaesthesia. Len E. S. Carrie et al. 3rd ed. 1996. LC 95-25188. 544p. pap. text 47.50 (*0-7506-2079-X*) Buttrwrth-Heinemann.

***Understanding Anaesthesia.** Peter J. Simpson & Mansukh Popat. 4th rev. ed. 2001. (Illus.). 480p. pap. 49.99 (*0-7506-4853-8*) Buttrwrth-Heinemann.

Understanding & Applying Medical Anthropology. Peter J. Brown. 1998. LC 97-31050. xii, 451p. pap. text 43.95 (*1-55934-723-6*, 1726) Mayfield Pub.

Understanding & Caring for Human Diseases. Marcia Borgstadt. rev. ed. 1995. LC 95-13518. (Health Occupations Ser.). 352p. (C). 39.95 (*0-8273-6605-1*) Delmar.

Understanding & Caring for Human Diseases. Borgstadt. 2nd ed. 1996. (Health Occupations Ser.). 56p. pap. text, tchr. ed. 12.50 (*0-8273-7431-3*) Delmar.

Understanding & Changing Health Behaviour: From Health Beliefs to Self-Regulation. Ed. by Paul Norman et al. 2000. 410p. pap. 23.00 (*90-5823-074-0*, Harwood Acad Pubs) Gordon & Breach.

Understanding & Diagnosing Pediatric Heart Disease. David W. Sapire. 1992. LC 90-14476. (Illus.). 197p. (C). pap. text 44.95 (*0-8385-9254-6*, A9254-2, Apple Lange Med) McGraw.

Understanding & Evaluating Commonly Requested Laboratory Tests. Gail Vaughn. 1999. LC 98-31573. 480p. (C). pap. 41.00 (*0-8385-9273-2*) P-H.

Understanding & Helping the Schizophrenic: A Guide for Family & Friends. Silvano Arieti. 1995. LC 94-77917. 252p. pap. text 28.50 (*1-56821-269-0*) Aronson.

Understanding & Living with People Who Are Mentally Ill: Techniques to Deal with Mental Illness in the Family. James E. Soukup. 1994. 192p. (C). LC 94-3543. pap. 30.95 (*0-398-05949-7*); LC 94-35453. text 46.95 (*0-398-05940-3*) C C Thomas.

Understanding & Management of Nausea & Vomiting. Jan Hawthorn. 1994. LC 94-31283. (Illus.). 224p. pap. 41.95 (*0-632-03819-5*) Blackwell Sci.

Understanding & Management of Pain. Jan Hawthorn et al. 1996. LC 98-25009. 250p. (Orig.). pap. 41.95 (*0-632-04033-5*) Blackwell Sci.

Understanding & Managing Child Sexual Abuse. Ed. by R. Kim Oates. 1990. (Illus.). 422p. text (*0-7295-0322-4*) Bailliere Tindall.

Understanding & Managing Children's Classroom Behavior. Sam Goldstein. 1994. LC 94-9332. (Personality Processes Ser.). 528p. 99.95 (*0-471-57946-7*, J328-Y3H) Wiley.

Understanding & Managing Endometriosis: Advances in Research & Practice. Ed. by A. Lemay & R. Maheux. 1999. LC 99-30330. (Illus.). 288p. lib. bdg. 107.95 (*1-85070-070-2*, Parthenon Pbng) CRC Pr.

Understanding & Managing Vision Defects: A Guide for Occupational Therapists. Mitchell Scheiman. 1996. LC 96-30414. 432p. pap. 32.00 (*1-55642-283-0*, 32830) SLACK Inc.

Understanding & Managing Vision Deficits: A Guide for Occupational Therapists. Mitchell Scheiman. 2nd ed. 2001. 500p. pap. text 35.00 (*1-55642-528-7*) SLACK Inc.

Understanding & Preventing HIV Risk Behavior. Stuart Oskamp & Suzanne Thompson. 1996. LC 96-10121. (Claremont Symposium on Applied Social Science Ser.: Vol. 9). 248p. 81.95 (*0-8039-7424-8*, 80287);No. 9. (Illus.). pap. 37.95 (*0-8039-7425-6*, 80288) Sage.

Understanding & Responding. Lynette Long & Penny Prophit. 2nd ed. 1991. (Nursing Ser.). (Illus.). (C). pap. text 42.95 (*0-86720-433-8*, 433-8) Jones & Bartlett.

Understanding & Supporting Young People. Jenny Sazama. Tr. by Mako Ameniya et al. 1999. (JPN.). pap. 2.00 (*1-58429-066-8*) Rational Isl.

Understanding & Teaching Emotionally Disturbed Children & Adolescents. Phyllis L. Newcomer. 2nd rev. ed. 1993. LC 92-33990. 620p. (C). text 41.00 (*0-89079-575-4*, 6575) PRO-ED.

Understanding & Treating ADD. Kirby et al. 1986. (Practitioner Guidebook Ser.). 52p. (C). pap. text 48.00 (*0-205-14391-1*, H4391, Longwood Div) Allyn.

Understanding & Treating Adolescent Substance Abuse. Philip P. Muisener. 1994. LC 93-32463. (Sage Sourcebooks for the Human Services Ser.: Vol. 27). (Illus.). 252p. (C). pap. 39.95 (*0-8039-4276-1*, 7524) Sage.

Understanding & Treating Alcoholism J. Littrell. 1991. (C). text 99.95 (*0-8058-0872-8*);Vol. I. 408p. text 75.00 (*0-8058-0870-1*);Vol. II. 296p. text 49.95 (*0-8058-0871-X*) L Erlbaum Assocs.

Understanding & Treating Aspiration. David E. Eibling et al. 1993. (Self-Instructional Package Ser.). (Illus.). 69p. pap. text 25.00 (*1-56772-002-1*) AAO-HNS.

Understanding & Treating Attention Deficit Disorder. Edward A. Kirby & Liam K. Grimley. 1986. (Psychology Practitioner Guidebooks). 152p. text 28.00 (*0-08-033134-3*, J115); pap. text 14.95 (*0-08-033133-5*) Elsevier (Pergamon Pr).

Understanding & Treating Depressed Adolescents & Their Families. Gerald D. Oster & Janice E. Caro. 1990. LC 89-37665. (Personality Processes Ser.). 228p. 160.00 (*0-471-60897-1*) Wiley.

Understanding & Treating Glaucoma. Contrib. by Tim Peters and Company, Inc. 1997. LC 97-220971. (Illus.). (*1-879874-66-0*) T Peters & Co.

Understanding & Treating Mental Illness: The Strength & Limits of Modern Psychiatry. J. M. Cleghorn & B. L. Lee. 1991. LC 90-4429. 250p. pap. text 16.95 (*0-920887-73-2*) Hogrefe & Huber Pubs.

Understanding & Treating Violent Psychiatric Patients. Ed. by Martha L. Crowner. 2000. LC 99-49869. (Progress in Psychiatry Ser.: Vol. 60). xii, 192p. 34.50 (*0-88048-752-6*, 8752) Am Psychiatric.

Understanding & Using Groups. Brenda Vernelle. 1994. LC 95-118430. 212p. (*1-871177-60-X*); pap. (*1-871177-61-8*) Whiting & Birch GBR. *Dist:* Paul & Co Pubs.

Understanding Anemia. Ed Uthman. 1998. LC 97-29076. (Understanding Health & Sickness Ser.). 160p. text 28.00 (*1-57806-038-9*); (Illus.). pap. 12.00 (*1-57806-039-7*) U Pr of Miss.

Understanding Anesthesia Equipment. Jerry A. Dorsch & Susan E. Dorsch. 4th ed. 1998. 1,012p. 129.00 (*0-683-30487-9*) Lppncott W & W.

Understanding Animal Breeding. Richard M. Bourdon. 2nd ed. 1999. LC 99-34849. (Illus.). 538p. (C). 96.00 (*0-13-096449-2*) P-H.

Understanding Anorexia Nervosa. Felicia F. Romeo. 1986. 116p. (C). 32.95 (*0-398-05191-7*) C C Thomas.

Understanding Anorexia Nervosa. Debbie Stanley. 1999. LC 99-15943. (Teen Eating Disorder Prevention Book Ser.). 104p. (YA). (gr. 7-12). lib. bdg. 17.95 (*0-8239-2877-2*, E2ANNE) Rosen Group.

Understanding Aphasia. Harold Goodglass. 1993. LC 93-1533. (Foundations of Neuropsychology Ser.). (Illus.). 297p. text 59.95 (*0-12-290040-5*) Acad Pr.

Understanding Arthritis. Myron G. Rosenbaum. 1975. LC 73-9498. (Illus.). 112p. 10.00 (*0-87527-121-9*) Green.

Understanding Arthritis. Ann F. Irving et al. l.t. ed. 1997. LC 96-48727. (Spec-Hall Ser.). 309p. lib. bdg. 24.95 (*0-7838-8043-X*, Macmillan Ref) Gale.

Understanding Arthritis: The Way Forward. William Fox & David Freed. 1990. text 54.00 (*0-333-44440-X*) Intl Spec Bk.

Understanding Arthritis: What It Is, How to Treat It, How to Cope with It. Arthritis Foundation Staff. 1986. (Illus.). 290p. pap. 12.00 (*0-684-18736-1*) S&S Trade.

Understanding Asthma. Phil Lieberman. 1999. LC 99-13753. (Understanding Health & Sickness Ser.). (Illus.). x, 124p. pap. 12.00 (*1-57806-142-3*); 28.00 (*1-57806-141-5*) U Pr of Miss.

Understanding Basic Pharmacology: Practical Approaches for Effective Application. Barbara MacDermott & Judith H. Deglin. 1994. LC 93-23657. 546p. (C). pap. text 29.95 (*0-8036-5714-5*) Davis Co.

Understanding Behavior: What Primate Studies Tell Us about Human Behavior. Ed. by James Loy & Calvin B. Peters. 1991. (Illus.). 280p. (C). text 55.00 (*0-19-506020-2*) OUP.

Understanding Biopharmaceuticals: Manufacturing & Regulatory Issues. June N. Grindley & Jill E. Ogden. 1999. LC 99-43041. (Illus.). xv, 325p. 209.00 (*1-57491-083-3*) IHS Health Grp.

Understanding Black Adolescent Male Violence: Its Remediation & Prevention. Amos N. Wilson. 1992. 92p. (Orig.). pap. 7.95 (*1-879164-03-5*) Afrikan World.

Understanding Blindness: An Integrative Approach. Mark Hollins. 1989. 200p. 39.95 (*0-89859-952-0*) L Erlbaum Assocs.

Understanding Breast Cancer. Peter A. Dervan. 2001. LC 00-54808. (Illus.). 197p. per. 29.50 (*0-7864-1004-3*) McFarland & Co.

Understanding Breast Cancer Risk. Patricia T. Kelly. 1991. (Health, Society, & Policy Ser.). 195p. 49.95 (*0-87722-812-4*); pap. 22.95 (*0-87722-813-2*) Temple U Pr.

Understanding Caffeine: A Biobehavioral Analysis. Jack E. James. 1997. LC 96-45893. (Behavioral Medicine & Health Psychology Ser.: Vol. 2). 238p. (C). 76.95 (*0-8039-7182-6*, 71826); pap. 37.95 (*0-8039-7183-4*, 71834) Sage.

Understanding Cancer. Mark Renneker. 3rd ed. 1991. pap. 39.95 (*0-923521-29-1*) Bull Pub.

Understanding Cancer: A Patient's Guide to Diagnosis, Prognosis & Treatment. Norman C. Coleman. 1999. LC 98-18732. 192p. 39.95 (*0-8018-6019-9*); pap. 14.95 (*0-8018-6020-2*) Johns Hopkins.

Understanding Cancer: A Scientific & Clinical Guide for the Lay Person. Peter A. Dervan & John L. DiGaetani. 1999. LC 99-14626. (Illus.). 208p. per. 29.50 (*0-7864-0628-3*) McFarland & Co.

Understanding Cancer: From Basic Science to Clinical Practice. Malcolm Alison & Catherine Sarraf. 1997. (Postgraduate Medical Science Ser.). (Illus.). (C). 276p. text 95.00 (*0-521-56154-X*); 277p. pap. text 34.95 (*0-521-56751-3*) Cambridge U Pr.

Understanding Candida: Treatment & Recipes. Peter De Ruyter. 1989. 160p. (Orig.). pap. (*1-85327-035-0*) Prism Pr GBR. *Dist:* Assoc Pubs Grp.

Understanding Cardiac Pacing: A Guide for Nurses. Kevan Metcalfe. 1992. (Illus.). 197p. (C). pap. text 36.95 (*0-8385-9258-9*, A9258-3, Apple Lange Med) McGraw.

Understanding Challenging Behavior: A Step-by-Step Behavior Analysis Guide. Gerald Groden et al. 1993. 125p. ring bd. 89.00 (*1-884937-03-9*) Manisses Communs.

Understanding Chest Radiographers. Joseph L. Rau. 1985. 23.95 (*0-8016-4026-1*) Mosby Inc.

Understanding Child Abuse & Neglect. Cynthia C. Tower. 1989. 496p. pap. text 23.00 (*0-205-11767-8*, H17676) Allyn.

Understanding Child Behavior Disorder. Gelfand. 2nd ed. 1988. (C). pap. text, tchr. ed. 66.50 (*0-03-016619-5*) Harcourt Coll Pubs.

Understanding Child Behavior Disorders. Donna M. Glefand et al. 3rd ed. 1997. LC 96-77605. 496p. (C). text 95.50 (*0-15-501701-2*) Harcourt Coll Pubs.

Understanding Child Development. Spencer A. Rathus. 1988. (C). tchr. ed. 409.50 (*0-03-001843-9*); pap. text, stu. ed. 28.50 (*0-03-001839-0*) Harcourt Coll Pubs.

Understanding Child Development. Spencer A. Rathus & Peter Favaro. 1988. (Illus.). 688p. (C). text 69.50 (*0-03-001837-4*) Harcourt Coll Pubs.

Understanding Child Development. Rosalind Charlesworth. 3rd ed. 1992. 640p. (Orig.). pap. 40.00 (*0-8273-4891-6*) Delmar.

Understanding Child Development. Phyllis M. Click. 3rd ed. 1992. 640p. pap., stu. ed. 15.95 (*0-8273-4893-2*) Delmar.

Understanding Child Development. Charlesworth. 4th ed. 1996. (Early Childhood Education Ser.). 96p. (C). tchr. ed. 18.95 (*0-8273-7334-1*) Delmar.

Understanding Child Development. Delmar Publishing Staff. 4th ed. 1996. (Early Childhood Education Ser.). 15.00 (*0-8273-7335-X*) Delmar.

Understanding Child Development. Charles Worth. 4th ed. 1996. (C). pap. text, stu. ed. 20.95 (*0-8273-7333-3*) Delmar.

Understanding Child Development. Rosalind Charlesworth. 5th ed. 1999. LC 99-49326. (Early Childhood Education Ser.). (Illus.). 608p. (Orig.). (C). pap. text 70.95 (*0-7668-0338-4*) Delmar.

Understanding Child Sexual Maltreatment. Kathleen C. Faller. 1990. (Sourcebooks for the Human Services: Vol. 12). (Illus.). 256p. (C). pap. 39.95 (*0-8039-3842-X*, 7510) Sage.

Understanding Childhood Obesity. J. Clinton Smith. 1999. LC 98-44680. (Understanding Health & Sickness Ser.). (Illus.). 120p. pap. 12.00 (*1-57806-134-2*); text 28.00 (*1-57806-133-4*) U Pr of Miss.

Understanding Children. Jeannette Harrison. 1990. (C). (*0-86431-087-0*) Aust Council Educ Res AUS. *Dist:* St Mut.

Understanding Children. Richard A. Gardner. 1992. LC 84-45133. 256p. reprint ed. 40.00 (*0-87668-726-5*) Aronson.

Understanding Children & Adolescents. Judith A. Schickendanz. 3rd ed. 1999. 77.25 (*0-205-29960-1*) Allyn.

Understanding Children & Adolescents: Examination Copy. Judith A. Schickedanz et al. 3rd annot. ed. 1997. (C). text, tchr. ed. (*0-205-27341-6*, T7341-5) Allyn.

Understanding Chronic Fatigue Syndrome: An Empirical Guide to Assessment & Treatment. Fred Friedberg & Leonard A. Jason. 1998. LC 98-21293. 266p. 39.95 (*1-55798-511-1*, 431-715A) Am Psychol.

Understanding Chronic Fatigue Syndrome: Better Ways of Managing Your Lifestyle. Alastair Jackson. 2000. 208p. pap. (*1-86508-407-7*) Allen & Unwin Pty AUS. *Dist:* IPG Chicago.

Understanding Chronic Illness: The Medical & Psychosocial Dimensions of Nine Diseases. Toba S. Kerson & Lawrence A. Kerson. 1985. LC 84-28622. 368p. (C). 35.00 (*0-02-918200-X*) Free Pr.

Understanding Clergy Misconduct in Religious Systems: Scapegoating, Family Secrets & the Abuse of Power. Candace R. Benyei. 1998. LC 97-37001. 197p. pap. 19.95 (*0-7890-0452-6*) Haworth Pr.

Understanding Clinical Disease Processes for ICD-9-CM Coding. Launa L. Graham. rev. ed. 1999. (Illus.). 160p. pap. text 70.00 (*1-58426-016-5*, AC200799) Am Hlth Info.

Understanding Clinical Investigations. Skinner. 1995. pap. text 42.00 (*0-7020-1821-X*) Saunders.

Understanding Clinical Nutrition. Corinne B. Cataldo et al. Ed. by Marshall. 1992. 382p. (C). pap. text 52.00 (*0-314-20865-8*) West Pub.

Understanding Clinical Nutrition. Eleanor Noss Whitney & Corinne Balog Cataldo. 2nd ed. 1997. LC 97-41849. (Health Sciences Ser.). 600p. (C). pap. text 72.95 (*0-534-53341-8*) Wadsworth Pub.

Understanding Co-Dependency. Sharon Wegscheider-Cruse & Joseph R. Cruse. 1990. 150p. pap. 7.95 (*1-55874-077-5*, 0775) Health Comm.

Understanding Cognitive Science. Michael R. Dawson. 1998. LC 98-13849. (Illus.). 320p. 59.95 (*0-631-20894-1*); pap. 29.95 (*0-631-20895-X*) Blackwell Pubs.

Understanding Creativity: The Interplay of Biological, Psychological & Social Factors. John S. Dacey & Kathleen H. Lennon. 1998. LC 98-19770. (Health & Psychology Ser.). 320p. 43.00 (*0-7879-4032-1*) Jossey-Bass.

Understanding Cultural Identity in Intervention & Assessment. Richard Dana. 1998. LC 97-45247. (Multicultural Aspects of Counseling Ser.). pap. 34.95 (*0-7619-0364-X*, 2550) Sage.

Understanding Cultural Identity in Intervention & Assessment. Richard Henry Dana, Jr. 1998. LC 97-45247. (Multicultural Aspects of Counseling Ser.). 89.95 (*0-7619-0363-1*, 2549) Sage.

Understanding Cystic Fibrosis. Karen Hopkin. 1998. LC 97-38646. (Understanding Health & Sickness Ser.). 128p. pap. 12.00 (*0-87805-967-9*); text 28.00 (*0-87805-966-0*) U Pr of Miss.

Understanding Dementia. Alan Jacques & Graham A. Jackson. 3rd ed. 2000. 408p. (Orig.). (C). pap. text 37.95 (*0-443-05512-2*) Saunders.

Understanding Dental Caries, Vols. 1 & 2. Ed. by G. Nikiforuk. 1985. (Illus.). xxviii, 596p. 101.00 (*3-8055-3906-1*) S Karger.

Understanding Dental Caries Vol. 1: Etiology & Mechanisms. Ed. by G. Nikiforuk. 1985. (Illus.). xiv, 306p. 50.50 (*3-8055-3864-2*) S Karger.

Understanding Dental Health. Francis G. Serio. 1998. LC 97-15276. (Understanding Health & Sickness Ser.). (Illus.). 128p. text 28.00 (*1-57806-009-5*) U Pr of Miss.

Understanding Depression. Paul R. Robbins. 1993. LC 92-56685. (Illus.). 200p. lib. bdg. 28.50 (*0-89950-878-2*) McFarland & Co.

Understanding Depression: A Complete Guide to Its Diagnosis & Treatment. Donald F. Klein & Paul H. Wender. 1994. 192p. (C). reprint ed. pap. 10.95 (*0-19-508669-4*, 6287) OUP.

*__Understanding Diabetes.__ Sydney's St. Vincents Hospital Staff. 2001. (Illus.). 128p. pap. 13.00 (*0-7432-1818-3*) S&S Trade.

Understanding, Diagnosing & Treating ADHD in Children & Adolescents: An Integrative Approach. James A. Incorvaia et al. 1999. LC 98-36494. (Illus.). 544p. 55.00 (*0-7657-0184-7*) Aronson.

Understanding Diagnostic Tests in the Childbearing Year: A Holistic Guide to Evaluating the Health of Mother & Baby. Anne Frye. 6th rev. unabr. ed. 1997. LC 97-94295. (Illus.). 981p. pap. 43.00 (*1-891145-50-9*) Labrys Pr.

Understanding Digitally Programmable Hearing Aids. Ed. by Robert E. Sandlin. 1993. LC 93-14194. 416p. (C). 111.00 (*0-205-14845-X*) Allyn.

Understanding Disease. John Ball. 1990. 111p. pap. (*0-85207-229-5*) C W Daniel GBR. *Dist:* Natl Bk Netwk.

Understanding Disease: A Health Practitioner's Handbook. John Ball. (Illus.). 264p. (Orig.). pap. 29.95 (*0-8464-4307-4*) Beekman Pubs.

Understanding Disease: Pathology & Prevention. S. Mera. 1997. 856p. pap. (*0-7487-3178-4*) Nelson Thornes GBR. *Dist:* Intl Spec Bk, Trans-Atl Phila.

Understanding Disease: Pathology & Prevention. S. Mera. 1997. (Illus.). 600p. (C). pap. text 55.00 (*1-56593-428-8*, 1095) Singular Publishing.

Understanding Diverse Families: What Practitioners Need to Know. Barbara F. Okun. 1998. 376p. pap. 24.00 (*1-57230-417-0*, C0417) Guilford Pubns.

Understanding Down Syndrome: An Introduction for Parents. Cliff Cunningham. 1998. LC 95-25997. 244p. pap. 14.95 (*1-57129-009-5*) Brookline Bks.

Understanding Drug Therapies. Skinner. 1999. LC 98-36988. pap. text 29.95 (*0-7020-2024-9*) Saunders.

Understanding Drugs of Abuse: The Processes of Addiction, Treatment & Recovery. Mim J. Landry. 1993. LC 93-26208. 363p. 22.95 (*0-88048-533-7*, 8533) Am Psychiatric.

Understanding Dying, Death & Bereavement. Leming. 3rd ed. 1994. (C). pap. text, tchr. ed. 8.50 (*0-15-501311-4*) Harcourt Coll Pubs.

Understanding Ear Infections. Peter Allen. 1993. (Illus.). 28p. (C). reprint ed. pap. 24.95 (*0-9622326-1-0*) The Davis Ctr.

Understanding Eating Disorders: Anorexia Nervosa, Bulimia Nervosa, & Obesity. LeeAnn Alexander-Mott & Barry D. Lumsden. LC 94-8719. pap. 29.50 (*1-56032-295-0*) Taylor & Francis.

Understanding Eating Disorders: Anorexia Nervosa, Bulimia Nervosa, & Obesity. Ed. by LeeAnn Alexander-Mott & D. Barry. 1994. 275p. (*1-56032-249-7*) Taylor & Francis.

Understanding ECGs in Infants & Children. L. C. Harris & Ellen Feinstein. 2nd ed. 1979. text 19.50 (*0-316-34826-0*, Little Brwn Med Div) Lppncott W & W.

Understanding EKGs: A Practical Approach. Brenda M. Beasley. 1999. LC 99-14784. 192p. pap. 41.00 (*0-8359-8571-7*) P-H.

Understanding Electrocardiography. Mary B. Conover. 7th ed. 1995. LC 95-32204. (Illus.). 560p. (C). (gr. 13). pap. text 37.95 (*0-8151-1927-5*, 27202) Mosby Inc.

Understanding Emptiness: The Think - Feel Conflict. Robert A. Moss. 1993. 128p. pap. 9.95 (*0-9638848-0-8*) R A Moss.

Understanding Epidemiology. Mary E. Torrence. 1997. LC 96-39467. (Biomedical Science Ser.). (Illus.). 192p. (C). (gr. 13). pap. text 23.00 (*0-8151-8887-0*, 28668) Mosby Inc.

Understanding EPM: Your Guide to Horse Health Care & Management. David E. Granstrom. 1997. (Horse Health Care Library). (Illus.). 96p. (Orig.). pap. 14.95 (*0-939049-93-7*) Blood-Horse.

*__Understanding Equine Acupuncture.__ Rhonda Rathgeber. 2001. pap. 16.95 (*1-58150-068-8*) Blood-Horse.

Understanding Equine Lameness: Your Guide to Horse Health Care & Management. Les Sellnow. 1998. (Horse Health Care Library). (Illus.). 124p. pap. 14.95 (*0-939049-94-5*) Blood-Horse.

*__Understanding Equine Medications.__ Barbara D. Forney. 2002. pap. 16.95 (*1-58150-069-6*) Blood-Horse.

*__Understanding Equine Neurological Disorders.__ Bradford G. Bentz. 2001. (Illus.). 120p. pap. 14.95 (*1-58150-062-9*) Blood-Horse.

Understanding Estimates of National Health Expenditures under Health Reform. 1994. (Illus.). 216p. (Orig.). (C). pap. text 50.00 (*0-7881-1041-1*) DIANE Pub.

Understanding Evolution. Earl D. Hanson. 1981. (Illus.). 556p. (C). text 35.95 (*0-19-502784-1*) OUP.

Understanding Executive Stress. Cary L. Cooper & Judi Marshall. 1978. LC 77-16077. text 17.50 (*0-89433-059-4*) Petrocelli.

Understanding First Class Dental Care: A Human Interest Story. David Vine. 2001. (Illus.). 166p. pap. 49.00 (*0-9703471-0-3*) D Vine.

Understanding Food Science & Technology. Murano. 2001. (Health Sciences Ser.). pap. 48.00 (*0-534-54486-X*) Wadsworth Pub.

Understanding Freud: The Man & His Ideas. Ed. by Emanuel E. Garcia. 1992. LC 92-4146. 200p. (C). text 45.00 (*0-8147-3045-0*) NYU Pr.

Understanding Gene Therapy. N. R. Lemoine. 1999. LC 99-40701. (Medical Perspectives Ser.). 192p. pap. 35.95 (*0-387-91512-5*) Spr-Verlag.

Understanding Genital Herpes: To Conquer a Dragon. Gilles R. G. Monif. 2nd ed. 1994. (Women's Health Care Ser.). (Illus.). 80p. pap. 6.95 (*1-880906-38-4*) IDI Pub.

Understanding Genital Warts: A Guide for Women. Patricia A. Cooper. 1997. (Women's Health Care Ser.). (Illus.). 103p. (Orig.). pap. 6.95 (*1-880906-29-5*) IDI Pub.

Understanding Gestational Diabetes. 1994. (Illus.). 46p. (Orig.). pap. text 15.00 (*0-7881-1057-8*) DIANE Pub.

Understanding Girls with AD/HD. Kathleen Nadeau et al. 1999. LC 99-22182. (Illus.). xii, 291p. pap. 19.95 (*0-9660366-5-4*) Advantage Books.

Understanding Glaucoma. 1995. (Illus.). 23p. pap. 3.00 (*1-930181-10-8*) A H A F.

Understanding GMP. Martyn Becker. Date not set. (Illus.). 69.50 (*1-930114-22-2*) Davis Horwood Intl.

Understanding Good Clinical Practice. Lisa Forsman & Brooke Lucas. 2000. (Illus.). 100p. 69.50 (*1-930114-01-X*) Davis Horwood Intl.

Understanding Group Behavior Vol. 1: Consensual Action by Small Groups. Ed. by Erich H. Witte & James H. Davis. 1996. LC 96-12707. 320p. pap. 34.50 (*0-8058-1640-2*); 375p. text 69.95 (*0-8058-1639-9*) L Erlbaum Assocs.

Understanding Group Behavior Vol. 2: Small Group Processes & Interpersonal Relations. Ed. by Erich H. Witte & James H. Davis. 1996. LC 96-12707. pap. 34.50 (*0-8058-1642-9*); 328p. text 69.95 (*0-8058-1641-0*) L Erlbaum Assocs.

Understanding Health Care Budgeting: An Introduction. Allen G. Herkimer, Jr. 1988. 238p. (C). 84.00 (*0-87189-772-5*) Aspen Pub.

Understanding Health Care Financial Management: Text, Cases, & Models. Louis C. Gapenski. 2nd ed. 1996. 872p. text 75.00 (*1-56793-041-7*) Health Admin Pr.

Understanding Health Care Outcomes Research. Robert L. Kane. 1997. LC 97-6839. 278p. 58.00 (*0-8342-0959-4*) Aspen Pub.

Understanding Health Care Reform. Theodore R. Marmor. 1994. LC 94-15886. 288p. 50.00 (*0-300-05878-0*); pap. 19.00 (*0-300-05879-9*) Yale U Pr.

Understanding Health Insurance: A Guide to Professional Billing. Rowell. 5th ed. 1999. (Allied Health Ser.). 12.00 net. (*0-7668-1309-6*) Delmar.

Understanding Health Insurance: A Guide to Professional Billing. Jo Ann Rowell. 5th ed. 1999. LC 99-42099. (Allied Health Ser.). 576p. pap. text 64.95 (*0-7668-1308-8*) Delmar.

Understanding Health Insurance - IML. Rowell. 4th ed. 1998. 176p. tchr. ed. 18.95 (*0-8273-8409-2*) Delmar.

Understanding Health Policy: A Clinical Approach. Thomas S. Bodenheimer. 2nd ed. 1998. (Illus.). 322p. (C). pap. 39.95 (*0-8385-9075-6*) McGraw-Hill Prof.

*__Understanding Health Policy: A Clinical Approach.__ Thomas S. Bodenheimer & Kevin Grumbach. 3rd ed. 2001. (Illus.). 222p. pap. 34.95 (*0-07-137815-4*) McGraw-Hill Prof.

Understanding Health Wellness. Shappell. 1998. 17.50 net. (*0-07-234380-X*) McGraw.

Understanding Healthcare Compliance. James Georgoulakis & Bolko Zimmer. unabr. ed. 1998. (Illus.). 30p. 195.00 (*1-892923-00-9*) Med-Natl Consult.

Understanding Healthcare Financial Management. Louis C. Gapenski & Association of University Programs in Health Administration Staff. 3rd ed. 2000. LC 00-61341. (*1-56793-144-8*) Health Admin Pr.

Understanding Hearing Loss. Kenneth Lysons. rev. ed. 1995. 150p. pap. (*1-85302-214-4*) Jessica Kingsley GBR. *Dist:* Taylor & Francis.

Understanding Heart Disease. Arthur Selzer. 1991. LC 92-4854. (Illus.). 325p. text 40.00 (*0-520-06560-3*) U CA Pr.

*__Understanding Heart Sounds & Murmurs: With an Introduction to Lung Sounds.__ Ara G. Tilkian & Mary Boudreau Conover. 2001. (Illus.). 321p. pap. (*0-7216-7643-X*) Saunders.

Understanding Heart Sounds & Murmurs: With an Introduction to Lung Sounds. Ara G. Tilkian & Mary B. Conover. 3rd ed. 1993. (Illus.). 298p. pap. 39.50 (*0-7216-6784-8*) Saunders.

Understanding Helical Scanning. Cheryl A. Blanck. 1998. LC 97-48630. 80p. 24.95 (*0-683-30304-X*) Lppncott W & W.

Understanding Herpes. Lawrence R. Stanberry. 1998. LC 97-39627. (Understanding Health & Sickness Ser.). 120p. pap. 12.00 (*1-57806-041-9*); (Illus.). text 28.00 (*1-57806-040-0*) U Pr of Miss.

Understanding Hospital Financial Management. Allen G. Herkimer, Jr. 2nd ed. 1986. 456p. (C). 85.00 (*0-87189-392-4*) Aspen Pub.

Understanding Human Anatomy & Physiology. Eldra P. Solomon & Gloria A. Phillips. 1987. LC 86-17759. (Illus.). 400p. pap. text 33.00 (*0-7216-1994-0*) Saunders.

Understanding Human Anatomy & Physiology. Sylvia S. Mader. (C). 2nd ed. 1994. 464p. text, stu. ed. 24.37 (*0-697-13673-6*); 3rd ed. 1996. LC 95-83238. 480p. text 34.00 net. (*0-697-25170-5*) McGrw-H Hghr Educ (WCB McGr Hill).

Understanding Human Anatomy & Physiology. Sylvia S. Mader & Jay M. Templin. 3rd ed. 1996. (C). pap., stu. ed. 27.81 (*0-697-25173-X*) McGrw-H Hghr Educ.

Understanding Human Behavior. Clifford R. Mynatt & Michael E. Doherty. 1998. LC 98-7068. 448p. (*0-205-29082-5*); 430p. (C). pap. text 54.00 (*0-205-14000-9*) Allyn.

Understanding Human Behavior. Philipchal. 8th ed. 1994. (C). pap. text, tchr. ed. 35.00 (*0-15-501419-6*); pap. text, stu. ed. 30.50 (*0-15-501420-X*) Harcourt Coll Pubs.

Understanding Human Behavior. Ronald P. Philipchalk & James V. McConnell. 8th ed. 1994. (Illus.). 704p. (C). text 92.00 (*0-15-500991-5*) Harcourt Coll Pubs.

Understanding Human Behavior: A Guide for Health Care Providers. Mary E. Milliken. 4th ed. 1987. LC 86-16758. (Illus.). 304p. (C). (gr. 9-12). tchr. ed. 12.00 (*0-8273-2799-4*); 4th ed. 1987. LC 86-16758. 304p. (C). pap. 28.95 (*0-8273-2797-8*); 4th ed. 1987. LC 86-16758. (Illus.). 304p. (C). (gr. 9-12). text 28.50 (*0-8273-2798-6*); 5th ed. 1993. LC 92-14880. 78p. pap., tchr. ed., stu. ed. 14.00 (*0-8273-5475-4*); 5th ed. 1993. LC 92-14880. 78p. pap. 29.95 (*0-8273-5473-8*) Delmar.

Understanding Human Behavior: A Guide For Health Care Providers. Mary E. Milliken. 6th ed. 1997. LC 97-13707. 448p. (C). pap. text 48.95 (*0-8273-8221-9*) Delmar.

Understanding Human Behavior: Test Bank. Philipchal. 8th ed. 1994. (C). pap. text 44.50 (*0-15-501421-8*) Harcourt Coll Pubs.

Understanding Human Behavior for Effective Police Work. Harold E. Russell & Allan Beigel. 3rd ed. 1990. LC 90-80676. 464p. pap. 45.00 (*0-465-08859-7*) Basic.

Understanding Human Behavior in Health & Illness. Richard C. Simons. 3rd ed. 1985. (Illus.). 822p. (C). text 35.00 (*0-683-07741-4*) Lppncott W & W.

Understanding Human Nature. Alfred Adler. Tr. by Colin Brett. 1998. LC 97-49425. 250p. reprint ed. pap. 13.95 (*1-56838-195-6*) Hazelden.

Understanding Human Sexuality. Janet S. Hyde. 5th ed. 1993. LC 93-24355. (C). text 57.00 net. (*0-07-031615-5*) McGraw.

Understanding Human Structure & Function. Valerie C. Scanlon & Tina Sanders. 1997. LC 96-37146. (Illus.). 454p. pap. 31.95 (*0-8036-0236-7*) Davis Co.

Understanding (in 30 Minutes) & Eliminating (in 30 Days) Pain. Daniel A. Twogood. 1996. 42p. (Orig.). pap. 7.95 (*0-9631125-3-8*) Wilhelmina.

Understanding Insulin Action: Principles & Molecular Mechanisms. Splittstoesser. 1989. (Ellis Horwood Series in Biomedical Sciences). 300p. (C). (gr. 13). pap. 71.95 (*0-412-02261-3*) Chapman & Hall.

Understanding Intelligence. Ken Richardson. 1990. 192p. pap. (*0-335-09397-3*) OpUniv Pr.

Understanding Kidney Transplantation. Edith T. Oberley & Neal R. Glass. 1987. (Illus.). 160p. (C). 37.95 (*0-398-05277-8*) C C Thomas.

Understanding Laboratory & Diagnostic Tests. Marie A. Moisio & Elmer W. Moisio. 1997. LC 97-13352. (Health Information Management Ser.). 432p. (C). pap. text 49.95 (*0-8273-7854-8*) Delmar.

Understanding Laboratory Investigations: A Text for Nurses & Other Health Care Professionals. Christopher Higgins. 2000. LC 00-44463. (Illus.). 320p. pap. 31.95 (*0-632-04245-1*) Blackwell Sci.

Understanding Laminitis: Your Guide to Horse Health Care & Management. Ric Redden. Ed. by Jacqueline Duke. 1998. (Horse Health Care Library). (Illus.). 144p. pap. 14.95 (*0-939049-98-8*) Blood-Horse.

Understanding Language Disorders: The Impact on Learning. Vivienne L. Ratner & Laura R. Harris. 1994. LC 93-23636. 55.00 (*0-930599-90-X*) Thinking Pubns.

Understanding Lens Surfacing. Clifford W. Brooks. 1991. (Illus.). 416p. text 95.00 (*0-7506-9177-8*) Buttrwrth-Heinemann.

Understanding Lens Surfacing Laboratory Exercises: A Laboratory Manual in Lens Surfacing. Clifford W. Brooks. 1995. (Illus.). 128p. pap. text, lab manual ed. 34.99 (*0-7506-9617-6*) Buttrwrth-Heinemann.

Understanding Leukaemia & Related Cancers. Tariq I. Mughal & John M. Goldman. 1999. LC 00-500436. (Illus.). xvi, 107p. pap. 34.95 (*0-632-05346-1*) Blackwell Sci.

Understanding Life. Alfred Adler & Colin Brett. 1998. LC 97-49424. 180p. reprint ed. pap. 13.95 (*1-56838-196-4*) Hazelden.

Understanding Life-Style: The Psycho-Clarity Process. Robert L. Powers & Jane Griffith. 1987. LC 87-13146. 336p. text 42.50 (*0-918287-02-2*); pap. text 32.50 (*0-918287-03-0*) APA.

Understanding Low Vision. Randall T. Jose. 1983. LC 83-21446. 560p. text 53.00 (*0-89128-119-3*) Am Foun Blind.

Understanding Lung Sounds. Steven Lehrer. 2nd ed. 1993. (Illus.). 160p. pap. text 46.00 (*0-7216-4902-5*) Saunders.

Understanding Major Mental Disorder: The Contribution of Family Interaction Research. Ed. by Kurt Hahlweg & Michael J. Goldstein. 1987. 30.00 (*0-9615519-4-1*) Family Process.

Understanding Managed Care: An Introduction for Health Care Professionals. A. U. Rickel & T. N. Wise. 1999. LC 99-42843. (Illus.). x, 122p. pap. 35.00 (*3-8055-6960-2*) S Karger.

Understanding Managed Care: Challenges & Opportunities for Nurses. Barbara Youngberg. Tr. by Kathy Johnson. 1998. (Illus.). 120p. pap. 59.95 (*1-57801-025-X*) Western Schls.

Understanding Managed Care Contracts: A Practical Guide for Dental Professionals. David H. Lees & Mark D. Steisel. 1999. LC 99-44719. (Illus.). xvii, 271p. pap. 64.95 (*0-87814-772-1*) PennWell Corp.

Understanding Managed Health Care: A Guide for Seniors. William J. Pokluda. 1997. LC 96-35275. (Patient Information Ser.). 63p. 6.50 (*1-57626-021-6*) Quality Med Pub.

Understanding Masculinities: Social Relations & Cultural Arenas. Mairtin Mac An Ghaill. 1996. 224p. pap. (*0-335-19460-5*) OpUniv Pr.

Understanding Medical Coding: A Comprehensive Guide. Sandra L. Johnson. 1999. LC 98-53981. (Allied Health Ser.). 832p. (C). pap. text 58.95 (*0-7668-0104-7*) Delmar.

Understanding Medical Immunology. Evelyne M. Kirkwood & Catriona J. Lewis. 2nd ed. 1991. LC 87-31747. 192p. pap. 74.95 (*0-471-91577-7*) Wiley.

Understanding Medical Information: A User's Guide to Informatics & Decision-Making. Theresa Jordan. 2001. (Illus.). 300p. (C). pap. 29.95 (*0-8385-9272-4*, A-9272-4, Apple Lange Med) McGraw.

Understanding Medical Insurance. JoAnn C. Rowell. (Medical Assisting Ser.). 1989. pap. 29.95 (*0-8273-3352-8*); 1989. pap., tchr. ed. 14.00 (*0-8273-3353-6*); 2nd ed. 1995. (C). pap. text, suppl. ed. 12.95 (*0-8273-6085-1*); 3rd ed. 1996. LC 95-19490. 384p. text 35.95 (*0-8273-7268-X*); 3rd ed. 1996. tchr. ed. 16.00 (*0-8273-7269-8*) Delmar.

Understanding Medical Insurance: A Step-by-Step Guide. Joann C. Rowell. 2nd ed. 1994. LC 93-2680. 336p. pap. 29.95 (*0-8273-4966-1*) Delmar.

Understanding Medical Research: A Practitioner's Guide. Jane L. Garb. 1996. LC 96-17216. 173p. pap. text 39.95 (*0-316-29169-2*) Lppncott W & W.

Understanding Medical-Surgical Nursing. Linda S. Williams & Paula D. Hopper. 1999. (Illus.). 1296p. 51.95 (*0-8036-0331-2*) Davis Co.

Understanding Medical-Surgical Nursing, Taber's Cyclopedic Medical Dictionary. Linda S. Williams. 18th ed. 2000. (Illus.). 81.90 (*0-8036-0537-4*) Davis Co.

Understanding Medical Terminology. Rose M. Mahoney. 8th ed. 1990. 640p. (C). text 37.00 net. (*0-697-14056-3*, WCB McGr Hill) McGrw-H Hghr Educ.

Understanding Medical Terminology. Agnes C. Frenay & Rose M. Mahoney. 9th ed. 1992. 640p. (C). text 36.50 net. (*0-697-14058-X*) Brown & Benchmark.

Understanding Medical Terminology. Agnes C. Frenay & Rose M. Mahoney. 10th ed. 1997. LC 96-86396. 592p. (C). pap. 58.13 (*0-697-21943-7*, WCB McGr Hill) McGrw-H Hghr Educ.

Understanding Medical Terms. Walter F. Stanaszek & Mary J. Stanaszek. 2nd ed. 1998. 412p. 41.95 (*1-56676-595-1*) CRC Pr.

Understanding Medical Terms: A Guide for Pharmacy Practice. Walter F. Stanaszek et al. 1992. LC 91-66131. 320p. (Orig.). 39.95 (*0-87762-885-8*) CRC Pr.

Understanding Medicare. T. J. Steskal. 1980. 93p. (Orig.). pap. 9.95 (*0-937978-00-0*, MC-1) Info Prods.

Understanding Medicare Managed Care: How Competing Choices Meet the Economic, Strategic & Policy Challenges Facing Our Health Care System. Louis F. Rossiter. 2000. LC 00-58207. (Illus.). xviii, 373p. pap. (*1-56793-143-X*) Health Admin Pr.

Understanding Medications: What the Label Doesn't Tell You. Alfred Burger. 1995. LC 95-17498. 220p. 45.00 (*0-8412-3210-5*); pap. 24.95 (*0-8412-3246-6*) Am Chemical.

Understanding Melanoma: What You Need to Know. Perry Robins & Maritza Perez. 1996. (Illus.). 80p. (Orig.). mass mkt. 10.00 (*0-9627688-2-0*) Skin Cancer Fndtn.

Understanding Mental Disorders Due to Medical Conditions or Substance Abuse: What Every Therapist Should Know, No. 3. Ghazi Asaad. 1995. LC 94-11620. (Basic Principles into Practice Ser.: Vol. 3). (Illus.). 172p. pap. text 22.95 (*0-87630-751-9*) Brunner-Routledge.

Understanding Mental Illness & Its Nursing. Trick. 2nd ed. 1976. pap. 30.00 (*0-8464-0947-X*) Beekman Pubs.

Understanding Mental Objects. Meir Perlow. 1995. LC 94-45147. (New Library of Psychoanalysis). 224p. (C). pap. 29.95 (*0-415-12179-5*, C0225) Routledge.

Understanding Mental Retardation. Edward F. Zigler & Robert M. Hodapp. 1986. (Illus.). 306p. pap. text 21.95 (*0-521-31878-5*) Cambridge U Pr.

Understanding Mentally Retarded Children. Harriet E. Blodgett & Grace J. Warfield. 1959. LC 59-12295. (Illus.). (Orig.). pap. text 8.95 (*0-89197-457-1*) Irvington.

Understanding Misbehavior: Using Misbehavior As a Guide to Children's & Adolescent's Needs. John F. Taylor. 1993. LC 93-79229. (Counselor Survival Ser.: Vol. 6). 48p. 10.95 (*1-884063-01-2*) Mar Co Prods.

Understanding MRI. Jeffrey H. Newhouse. 1991. 54.95 (*0-316-60474-7*, Little Brwn Med Div) Lppncott W & W.

Understanding Narrative Therapy: A Guidebook for the Social Worker. Paul Abelson & Sonia L. Abels. 2001. LC 00-53828. (Series on Social Work). xiii, 217p. (*0-8261-1382-6*) Springer Pub.

Understanding Neuroscience. William R. Klemm. 1995. LC 95-36633. (Mosby's Biomedical Science Ser.). (Illus.). 304p. (gr. 13). pap. text 24.00 (*0-8151-5223-X*, 26579) Mosby Inc.

Understanding Normal & Clinical Nutrition. Eleanor N. Whitney et al. Ed. by Marshall. 3rd ed. 1991. 954p. (C). text 65.25 (*0-314-87426-7*) West Pub.

Understanding Normal & Clinical Nutrition Student Study Guide. Whitney. 4th ed. 1994. 17.25 net. (*0-314-04934-7*) Thomson Learn.

Understanding Nursing. Leslie D. Atkinson. 6th ed. 2000. (*0-07-135079-9*) McGraw.

Understanding Nursing Care. Ed. by Anne M. Chilman & Margaret Thomas. 3rd ed. 1987. LC 85-24653. (Illus.). 681p. (Orig.). pap. text (*0-443-03040-5*) Church.

Understanding Nursing Care. Ed. by Stanley Walker & Patricia I. Peattie. 4th ed. 1995. pap. text (*0-443-04636-0*) Church.

Understanding Nursing Research. Nancy Burns. 1995. (C). pap. text, stu. ed. 18.95 (*0-7216-4437-6*) Harcourt.

Understanding Nursing Research. Nancy Burns & Susan K. Grove. 1995. (Illus.). 560p. pap. text 32.00 (*0-7216-4436-8*); 1994. 208p. tchr. ed. (*0-7216-4439-2*); 2nd ed. 1999. LC 98-43924. (Illus.). 555p. (C). pap. (*0-7216-8106-9*) Saunders.

Understanding Nutrition. Eleanor N. Whitney & Sharon R. Rolfes. Ed. by Marshall. 6th ed. 1993. 603p. (C). text 55.25 (*0-314-01239-7*) West Pub.

Understanding Nutrition. Eleanor N. Whitney & Sharon R. Rolfes. 7th ed. 1995. 750p. (C). 56.95 (*0-314-06385-4*) West Pub.

*__Understanding Nutrition.__ Eleanor Noss Whitney & Sharon Rady Rolfes. 9th ed. 2001. 882p. pap. 76.95 (*0-534-59005-5*) Duxbury.

*__Understanding Nutrition.__ Eleanor Noss Whitney & Sharon Rady Rolfes. 9th ed. 2001. LC 2001-23758. (Illus.). (*0-534-59004-7*) Wadsworth Pub.

Understanding Obesity: The Five Medical Causes. Lance Levy. 2000. (Your Personal Health Ser.). (Illus.). 208p. pap. 14.95 (*1-55209-479-0*) Firefly Bks Limited.

Understanding Obsessive-Compulsive Behavior. Ed. by Michael A. Jenike & M. Asberg. 1991. (Illus.). 60p. text 16.00 (*0-88937-046-X*) Hogrefe & Huber Pubs.

Understanding Obstetric Ultrasound: Its Use & Interpretation. Jean Proud. 2nd ed. 1997. LC 97-200254. 104p. pap. text 29.99 (*1-898507-60-0*, RG527) Buttrwrth-Heinemann.

Understanding Osteoporosis & It's Treatment: A Guide for Physicians & their Patients. G. T. Birdwood. 1995. (Illus.). 192p. lib. bdg. 60.95 (*1-85070-409-0*, Parthenon Pbng) CRC Pr.

Understanding Other Minds: Perspectives from Developmental Cognitive Neuroscience. Ed. by Simon Baron-Cohen et al. 2nd ed. 2000. LC 99-37353. (Illus.). 560p. text 100.00 (*0-19-852446-3*) OUP.

Understanding Pacemakers. David Sonnenburg et al. 1988. LC 80-22912. (Illus.). 175p. 24.95 (*0-935576-04-5*); pap. 16.95 (*0-935576-05-3*) Kesend Pub Ltd.

Understanding Pain: Interpretation & Philosophy. Mitchell T. Smolkin. 1989. LC 88-23590. 102p. (Orig.). 14.00 (*0-89464-308-8*) Krieger.

Understanding Pain & Its Relief in Labour. Susan Moore. 1996. (Illus.). 184p. pap. (*0-443-05026-0*) Church.

Understanding Panic & Other Anxiety Disorders. Benjamin Root. 2000. LC 00-21977. (Understanding Health & Sickness Ser.). (Illus.). x, 109p. pap. 12.00 (*1-57806-245-4*); text 28.00 (*1-57806-244-6*) U Pr of Miss.

Understanding Parkinson's Disease: A Self-Help Guide. David L. Cram. 1999. LC 99-17981. (Illus.). 184p. pap. 14.95 (*1-886039-40-2*) Addicus Bks.

Understanding Pathology. Huether. 2nd ed. 1999. (C). text 300.00 (*0-323-01002-4*) Harcourt Coll Pubs.

Understanding Pathology. Ed. by Sue E. Huether & Kathryn L. McCance. 2nd ed. 1999. 1195p. text 63.00 (*0-323-00791-0*) Mosby Inc.

Understanding Pathophysiology. Sue E. Heuther & Kathryn L. McCance. 1996. tchr. ed., suppl. ed. (*0-8151-4731-7*) Mosby Inc.

Understanding Pathophysiology. Sue E. Huether & Kathryn L. McCance. 1995. (Illus.). 1248p. (C). (gr. 13). text 63.00 (*0-8151-4081-9*, 24416) Mosby Inc.

Understanding Pathophysiology. Clayton Parkinson. 1996. 368p. (C). (gr. 13). pap. text, stu. ed. (*0-8151-7299-0*, 28196) Mosby Inc.

Understanding Pathophysiology. Parkinson et al. 2nd ed. 1999. (Illus.). stu. ed. (*0-323-00792-9*) Mosby Inc.

Understanding Pathophysiology: Includes Testbank. Sue E. Huether. 2nd ed. 1999. tchr. ed. (*0-323-00793-7*) Mosby Inc.

Understanding Payment for Advanced Practice Nursing Services Vol. 1: Medicare Reimbursement. Sheila Abood & David Keepnews. 2000. 214p. pap. 34.95 (*1-55810-148-9*) Am Nurses Pub.

Understanding Pediatric Heart Sounds. Steven Lehrer. 1991. (Illus.). 248p. pap. 51.00 incl. audio (*0-7216-2387-5*) Saunders.

Understanding Periodontal Diseases. Joel M. Berns. rev. ed. 1993. LC 92-37495. (Illus.). 74p. pap. 26.00 (*0-86715-239-7*) Quint Pub Co.

Understanding Pharmacology for the Health Professions. Susan M. Turley. 2nd ed. 1998. LC 98-2930. 432p. pap. 50.67 (*0-13-675729-4*) P-H.

Understanding Physical, Sensory & Health Impairments: Characteristics & Educational Implications. Kathryn W. Heller et al. 1995. LC 95-9010. 464p. 96.95 (*0-534-33913-1*) Brooks-Cole.

Understanding Post-Traumatic Fibromyalgia: A Helpful Guide to Post-Traumatic Fibromyalgia. Mark J. Pellegrino. 1996. LC 97-205619. (Illus.). 130p. pap. 16.25 (*0-9646891-8-9*) Anadem Pubng.

Understanding Post-Traumatic Stress: A Psychosocial Perspective on PTSD & Treatment. Stephen Joseph et al. 1997. LC 96-41655. 200p. pap. 70.00 (*0-471-96801-3*) Wiley.

Understanding Practice: Perspectives on Activity & Context. Ed. by Seth Chaiklin & Jean Lave. 1996. (Learning in Doing). (Illus.). 426p. (C). pap. text 22.95 (*0-521-55851-4*) Cambridge U Pr.

Understanding Pregnancy & Childbirth. Sheldon H. Cherry. 3rd rev. ed. 1992. LC 91-37781. (Illus.). 288p. pap. 11.95 (*0-02-030981-3*) Hungry Minds.

Understanding Pregnancy & Childbirth. Sheldon H. Cherry. 1973. LC 72-89700. 8.95 (*0-672-51614-4*, Bobbs); 1983. LC 82-17800. 272p. (*0-672-52758-8*) Macmillan.

Understanding Prostate Disease. Charles B. Inlander & Janet Worsley Norwood. 1999. LC 98-50713. (Understanding Ser.). 256p. pap. 14.95 (*0-02-862436-X*) Hungry Minds.

Understanding Psychiatric Medications in the Treatment of Chemical Dependency & Dual Diagnoses. John D. Preston et al. 1995. (Illus.). 134p. (C). text 41.95 (*0-398-05963-2*); pap. text 28.95 (*0-398-05964-0*) C C Thomas.

Understanding Psychiatric Treatment: Therapy for Serious Mental Disorder in Adults. Ed. by Gerald O'Mahony & James V. Lucey. 1998. LC 97-43723. 172p. pap. 70.00 (*0-471-97570-2*) Wiley.

Understanding Psychological Assessment. William I. Dorfman & Michel Hersen. 2001. LC 00-33114. (Perspectives on Individual Differences Ser.). (Illus.). 382p. 54.50 (*0-306-46268-0*, Kluwer Plenum) Kluwer Academic.

Understanding Psychological Research. Miriam Lewin. 1987. LC 87-3507. 464p. (C). reprint ed. lib. bdg. 49.50 (*0-89464-230-8*) Krieger.

Understanding Psychological Science. Janet L. Jones. 1997. LC 94-8456. 512p. (C). pap. 100.00 (*0-06-501459-6*) Addson-Wesley Educ.

Understanding Psychological Testing in Children: A Guide for Health Professionals. S. Gabel et al. 1986. LC 86-15104. (Illus.). 194p. (C). 45.00 (*0-306-42244-1*, Kluwer Plenum) Kluwer Academic.

Understanding Psychology. Ken Richardson. 1989. 160p. (*0-335-09843-6*); pap. (*0-335-09842-8*) OpUniv Pr.

Understanding Psychology. Bishop. 3rd ed. 1996. pap. text, stu. ed. 20.00 (*0-13-443508-7*) P-H.

Understanding Psychology. Communications Research Machines, Inc. Staff. 4th ed. 1983. LC 79-19647. 498p. (C). pap. text, stu. ed. (*0-394-33823-5*) Random.

Understanding Psychology. Robert S. Feldman. 4th ed. 1995. LC 95-7190. 754p. (C). text 53.00 net. (*0-07-021249-X*); 5th ed. 1998. LC 97-46348. 53.00 net. (*0-07-289146-7*) McGraw.

Understanding Psychology. Robert S. Feldman. 4th ed. 1995. (C). pap., stu. ed. 24.69 (*0-07-021281-3*) McGrw-H Hghr Educ.

Understanding Psychology. Charles G. Morris & Albert A. Maisto. 5th ed. 2000. LC 00-37495. (Illus.). 640p. pap. 65.00 (*0-13-018934-0*) P-H.

Understanding Psychology. James W. Vander Zanden et al. 5th ed. 1987. 608p. text 32.52 (*0-07-555247-7*) McGraw.

Understanding Psychology Student Handbook: A Review Guide, Activities Manual & Reader. Martin Schulman. 2nd ed. 1977. (*0-394-32205-3*) Random.

Understanding Psychology Without Mind Matters. Charles G. Morris & Albert A. Maisto. 5th ed. 2000. 608p. pap. 52.00 (*0-13-029073-4*) P-H.

Understanding Psychotherapy: The Science Behind the Art. Michael F. Basch. 1990. LC 88-47763. (Illus.). 352p. pap. 17.50 (*0-465-08860-0*) Basic.

Understanding Radiography. Stephen S. Hiss. 3rd ed. 1993. (Illus.). 574p. (C). 68.95 (*0-398-05827-X*) C C Thomas.

Understanding Reality Therapy: A Metaphorical Approach. Robert E. Wubbolding. 1991. LC 90-55519. 160p. (Orig.). pap. 11.50 (*0-06-096572-X*, Perennial) HarperTrade.

Understanding Recovery from Eating Disorders. Toni L. Rocha. 1999. LC 99-26582. (Teen Eating Disorder Prevention Book Ser.). 136p. (YA). (gr. 7-12). lib. bdg. 18.95 (*0-8239-2884-5*, E2UNRE) Rosen Group.

Understanding Research in Nursing. Shirley Chater. 1975. (Offset Publications: No. 14). pap. text 3.60 (*92-4-170014-9*, 1120014) World Health.

Understanding-Responding: A Communication Manual for Nurses. Lynette Long & Penny Prophit. 1981. LC 80-17977. (Illus.). (C). pap. text 30.00 (*0-87872-284-X*, 284-X) Jones & Bartlett.

Understanding Rett Syndrome: A Practical Guide for Parents, Teachers & Therapists. Barbro Lindberg. 1997. LC 90-34409. (Illus.). 184p. text 26.00 (*0-88937-033-8*) Hogrefe & Huber Pubs.

Understanding Rheumatoid Arthritis. Stanton Newman et al. 1995. LC 95-16023. 256p. (C). 90.00 (*0-415-10540-4*); pap. 26.95 (*0-415-10541-2*) Routledge.

Understanding Schizophrenia: A Guide to the New Research on Causes & Treatment. Richard S. Keefe & Philip D. Harvey. 1994. LC 94-8270. 286p. 25.95 (*0-02-917247-0*) Free Pr.

Understanding "Senility" A Layperson's Guide. Virginia Fraser & Susan M. Thornton. 1987. LC 86-30662. (Golden Age Bks.). 103p. pap. 19.00 (*0-87975-392-7*) Prometheus Bks.

Understanding Sex & Relationships. Rosemary Stones. 2001. (Overcoming Common Problems Ser.). 128p. (J). (gr. 7-12). pap. (*0-85969-767-3*) Sheldon Pr GBR. *Dist:* Intl Pubs Mktg.

Understanding Sexual Medicine. Ivor Felstein. 1986. pap. text 73.50 (*0-85200-982-8*) Kluwer Academic.

Understanding Sickle Cell Disease. Miriam Bloom. 1995. LC 94-44275. (Understanding Health & Sickness Ser.). 128p. pap. 11.95 (*0-87805-745-5*) U Pr of Miss.

Understanding Sjogren's Syndrome. Sue Dauphin. enl. ed. 1993. LC 93-85164. (Illus.). 245p. (Orig.). pap. 16.95 (*0-9620354-2-4*) Pixel Pr.

Understanding Sleep: The Evaluation & Treatment of Sleep Disorders. Ed. by Mark R. Pressman & William C. Orr. 1997. LC 97-1393. (Application & Practice in Health Psychology Ser.: Vol. 4). 566p. 49.95 (*1-55798-419-0*, 4317870) Am Psychol.

Understanding Social Psychology. Stephen Worchel et al. 5th ed. 1991. LC 90-47466. 688p. (C). mass mkt. 53.50 (*0-534-13626-5*) Brooks-Cole.

Understanding Social Psychology: Study Guide. Stephen Worchel & Joel Cooper. 5th ed. 1991. (Psychology Ser.). mass mkt., stu. ed. 17.00 (*0-534-13627-3*) Brooks-Cole.

Understanding Sports Massage. Patricia Benjamin & Scott P. Lamp. 1996. LC 95-49158. (Illus.). 136p. (Orig.). pap. text 26.00 (*0-87322-976-2*, BBEN0976) Human Kinetics.

Understanding Statistics in the Behavioral Sciences. Robert R. Pagano. Ed. by Clyde Perlee. 4th ed. 1994. LC 93-41157. 550p. (C). mass mkt. 52.50 (*0-314-02691-6*) West Pub.

Understanding Stepfamilies: Implications for Assessment & Treatment. Debra K. Huntley. 1995. LC 94-34581. (Family Ser.). 155p. pap. text 21.95 (*1-55620-142-7*, 72590) Am Coun Assn.

Understanding Stress: A Psychological Perspective for Health Professionals. Cary L. Cooper & Valerie Sutherland. 1990. 250p. 19.95 (*0-412-33930-7*, A4406) Chapman & Hall.

Understanding Stress in Doctors' Families. Usha R. Rout & Jaya K. Rout. 2000. LC 00-132819. 144p. 59.95 (*1-85972-591-0*) Ashgate Pub Co.

Understanding Stress Using Pointed Illustrations. Ivor L. Livingston & Shaffiran Livingston. 1994. (Illus.). 143p. pap. (*0-9631535-0-1*) I L Livingston.

***Understanding Stroke: Information about Stroke & Recovery.** 2001. (Illus.). 72p. 14.95 (*1-931876-04-5*) Allina Health Pr.

Understanding Substance Abuse Prevention Toward the 21st Century: A Primer on Effective Programs. Paul J. Brounstein & Janine M. Zweig. 2000. (Illus.). 80p. (C). pap. text 20.00 (*0-7567-0164-3*) DIANE Pub.

***Understanding Surgery: A Comprehensive Guide for Every Family.** Joel A. Berman. Ed. by Adolph Caso. 2001. LC 2001-18500. (Illus.). 500p. pap. 19.95 (*0-8283-2061-6*) Branden Bks.

Understanding Surgical Disease: The Miami Manual of Surgery. University of Miami Staff et al. Ed. by Mark G. McKenney et al. 1997. LC 97-33685. 464p. pap. text 59.95 (*0-316-56001-4*, Little Brwn Med Div) Lppncott W & W.

Understanding the ABCs of Alzheimer's Disease: A Guide for Caregivers. Frances Oakley. 1993. (Illus.). 20p. (Orig.). pap. text 6.00 (*0-910317-94-1*) Am Occup Therapy.

Understanding the Alcoholic's Mind: The Nature of Craving & How to Control It. Arnold M. Ludwig. 1989. (Illus.). 208p. reprint ed. pap. 13.95 (*0-19-505918-2*) OUP.

Understanding the Autopsy. Samuel B. Burgess. 1993. LC 92-74142. (Illus.). 224p. (Orig.). pap. 22.50 (*0-923687-26-2*) Celo Valley Bks.

Understanding the Biochemistry of Respiration. David James & Guy Matthews. 1991. (Illus.). 96p. (C). pap. text 17.95 (*0-521-39993-9*) Cambridge U Pr.

Understanding the Borderline Mother (A1) Helping Her Childrens Transcend the Intense, Unpredictable & Volatile Relationship. Christine Lawson. 2000. LC 00-38966. xvii, 330p. 40.00 (*0-7657-0288-6*) Aronson.

Understanding the Brain & Its Development: A Chemical Approach. Harun K. Yusuf. 1992. 400p. (C). pap. 37.00 (*981-02-0492-2*); text 114.00 (*9971-5-0756-0*) World Scientific Pub.

Understanding the Brain Through the Hippocampus: The Hippocampal Region As a Model for Studying Brain Structure & Function. Jon Storm-Mathisen et al. Ed. by J. Zimmer & Ole P. Ottersen. 1990. (Progress in Brain Research Ser.: No. 83). 488p. 290.75 (*0-444-81149-4*) Elsevier.

Understanding the Concept of Empathy & Its Foundations in Psychoanalysis. Renuka M. Sharma. 1993. LC 93-34149. 132p. text 69.95 (*0-7734-9375-1*) E Mellen.

Understanding the Control of Metabolism. D. Fell. Ed. by Keith Snell. 1996. (Frontiers in Metabolism Ser.: No. 2). (Illus.). 300p. (Orig.). (C). pap. (*1-85578-047-X*) Portland Pr Ltd GBR. *Dist:* Ashgate Pub Co.

Understanding the Drug-Exposed Child: Approaches to Behavior & Learning. Ira J. Chasnoff et al. 1998. LC 98-70479. 216p. (Orig.). pap. 29.95 (*1-879176-29-7*) Imprint Pubns.

Understanding the Emotionally Depleted Woman. Anne Bowie & P. S. Bowie. 1996. LC 95-77815. 221p. pap. 12.95 (*0-9646913-0-2*) Gldn Quill NV.

Understanding the Equine Foot: Your Guide to Horse Health Care & Management. Fran Jurga. 1998. (Horse Health Care Library). (Illus.). 108p. pap. 14.95 (*0-939049-96-1*) Blood-Horse.

Understanding the Gifted Adolescent. Ed. by Marlene Bireley & Judy L. Genshaft. 1991. (Education & Psychology of the Gifted Ser.: No. 5). 296p. (C). pap. text 22.95 (*0-8077-3072-6*) Tchrs Coll.

Understanding the Horse's Back. Sara Wyche. 1998. (Illus.). 160p. (*1-86126-114-4*) Crowood Pr GBR. *Dist:* Trafalgar.

Understanding the Human Being: The Importance of the First Three Years of Life. Silvana Q. Montanaro. 1991. (Illus.). 166p. (Orig.). (C). pap. text 14.95 (*1-879341-00-X*) N Montessori.

Understanding the Human Body. Philip Tate. 1994. (C). text 55.94 (*0-8151-8805-6*) McGrw-H Hghr Educ.

Understanding the Human Body. Philip Tate et al. 1993. (Illus.). 336p. (C). pap., stu. ed. 26.25 (*0-8016-7198-1*) McGrw-H Hghr Educ.

Understanding the Immune System: The Immune System in the Human Body & How It Works. 1984. lib. bdg. 250.00 (*0-87700-620-2*) Revisionist Pr.

Understanding the Legislative & Regulatory Process. Ed. by Barbara Cordell et al. unabr. ed. Date not set. (Regional Conference Ser.). ring bd. 475.00 (*0-935890-29-7*) Emerg Nurses IL.

Understanding the Liver: A History, 14. Thomas S. Chen & Peter S. Chen. 1984. LC 83-22631. (Contributions in Medical History Ser.: No. 14). (Illus.). 293p. 82.50 (*0-313-23472-8*, CLV/, Greenwood Pr) Greenwood.

Understanding the Male Hustler. Samuel M. Steward. 1991. 150p. pap. 4.95 (*1-56024-111-X*) Haworth Pr.

Understanding the Nature of Autism: A Practical Guide. Janice E. Janzen. 1998. 454p. pap. text 54.00 (*0-12-784559-3*) Acad Pr.

Understanding the Nervous System: An Engineering Perspective. Sid Deutsch & Alice Deutsch. 1993. LC 92-49854. (Illus.). 306p. (C). pap. 43.95 (*0-87942-296-3*, PP0291-5, Wiley-IEEE) Wiley.

Understanding the Neurotransmitters: Key to the Workings of the Brain. W. Birkmayer & P. Riederer. 1989. (Illus.). 160p. 35.95 (*0-387-82100-7*) Spr-Verlag.

Understanding the NHS Reforms: The Creation of Incentives? Peter West. 1997. LC 97-3914. (State of Health Ser.). 208p. pap. (*0-335-19243-2*) OpUniv Pr.

Understanding the Nursing Process: Fundamentals of Care Planning. Leslie D. Atkinson & Mary E. Murray. 4th ed. 1990. (Illus.). 319p. pap. text (*0-08-040299-2*) PPI GBR. *Dist:* McGraw.

Understanding the Nursing Process in a Changing Care Environment. Leslie D. Atkinson & Mary Ellen Murray. 6th ed. 2000. (Illus.). 243p. pap. 32.95 (*0-07-135078-0*) McGraw-Hill Prof.

Understanding the Pill: A Consumer's Guide to Oral Contraceptives. Greg Juhn. 1994. LC 93-38903. (Illus.). 105p. pap. 9.95 (*1-56024-908-0*); lib. bdg. 39.95 (*1-56024-851-3*) Haworth Pr.

Understanding the Self-Help Organization: Frameworks & Findings. Ed. by Thomas J. Powell. 1994. LC 94-3376. 345p. 67.95 (*0-8039-5487-5*, 3659); 336p. pap. 36.95 (*0-8039-5488-3*, 3660) Sage.

Understanding the Tin Man: Why So Many Men Avoid Intimacy. William July, II. 2001. LC 00-46746. 240p. reprint ed. pap. 12.95 (*0-7679-0566-0*) Broadway BDD.

Understanding the Twelve Steps: A Guide for Counselors, Therapists, & Recovering People. Terence T. Gorski. 1989. pap. 8.95 (*0-8309-0559-6*, 17-0187-8) Herald Pub Hse.

Understanding the U. S. Health Services System. Phoebe L. Barton. 1998. LC 98-3742. 473p. 65.00 (*1-56793-081-6*) Health Admin Pr.

Understanding Therapeutic Action: Psychodynamic Concepts of Cure. Ed. by Lawrence Lifson. 1996. LC 95-35827. (Psychoanalytic Inquiry Ser.: No. 15). 280p. text 45.00 (*0-88163-205-8*) Analytic Pr.

Understanding Tourette Syndrome, Obsessive-Compulsive Disorder & Related Problems: A Developmental & Catastrophe Theory Perspective. John M. Berecz. 1991. LC 91-4824. (Illus.). 366p. 44.95 (*0-8261-7390-X*) Springer Pub.

Understanding Toxicology: Chemicals, Their Benefits & Risks. Brono H. Schiefer et al. 1997. LC 96-41143. 160p. 34.95 (*0-8493-2686-9*) CRC Pr.

Understanding Transference: The Core Conflictual Relationship Theme Method. Lester Luborsky & Paul Crits-Christoph. 2nd rev. ed. 1997. LC 97-26192. 379p. text 39.95 (*1-55798-453-0*) Am Psychol.

Understanding Trauma: A Psychoanalytical Approach. Caroline Garland. 1998. LC 98-21050. (Tavistock Clinic Ser.). 224p. (C). 90.00 (*0-415-92187-2*); pap. 24.95 (*0-415-92188-0*) Routledge.

Understanding Troubled Minds: A Guide to Mental Illness & Its Treatment. Sidney Bloch & Bruce Singh. 1997. LC 98-170613. 320p. pap. (*0-522-84642-4*) Melbourne Univ Pr AUS. *Dist:* Paul & Co Pubs.

Understanding 12 Lead EKGs: A Practical Approach. Brenda M. Beasley & Michael C. West. 2000. LC 00-58902. (Illus.). 352p. pap. 43.00 (*0-13-027281-7*, Prentice Hall) P-H.

Understanding Ultrasound Physics: Fundamentals & Exam Review. Sidney K. Edelman. 2nd ed. 1994. (Illus.). 385p. (C). text 46.00 (*0-9626444-3-9*) ESP TX.

Understanding Urology. S. N. Rous. 1973. (Perspectives in Medicine Ser.: No. 5). (Illus.). 16.75 (*3-8055-0000-9*) S Karger.

Understanding Violence: An Introduction to Research on Aggressive Individuals, Families, & Groups. Elizabeth Kandel-Englander. 1997. LC 96-34117. 200p. 45.00 (*0-8058-1939-8*); pap. 19.98 (*0-8058-1940-1*) L Erlbaum Assocs.

Understanding Vision. Roger Watt. 1991. (Illus.). 301p. (C). text 99.95 (*0-12-738500-2*); pap. text 55.00 (*0-12-738501-0*) Acad Pr.

Understanding Voice Problems. Raymond Colton et al. 1989. (Illus.). 376p. pap. 43.00 (*0-683-02058-7*) Lppncott W & W.

Understanding Voice Problems: A Physiological Perspective for Diagnosis & Treatment. Raymond H. Colton & Janina K. Casper. 2nd ed. 1996. LC 95-33492. (Illus.). 400p. 54.95 (*0-683-02059-5*) Lppncott W & W.

Understanding Woman's Behaviour. Parveen Kumar. 1990. LC 89-50185. 134p. (Orig.). pap. 7.00 (*0-916383-90-3*) Aegina Pr.

Understanding Women in Distress. Ed. by Pamela Ashurst & Zaida Hall. 1989. 272p. 49.95 (*0-415-01832-3*) Routledge.

Understanding Women's Recovery from Illness & Trauma. Margaret H. Kearney. 1999. LC 99-6104. (Women's Mental Health & Development Ser.: Vol. 4). xii, 186p. 79.95 (*0-7619-0558-8*, 81049) Sage.

Understanding Wound Healing & Principles of Wound Management. Janet Stoia-Davis & Marcia Gay-Bales. 1999. (Illus.). 139p. pap. (*1-57801-029-2*) Western Schls.

Understanding Your Digestive System. Michael F. Elmore. 1991. (Illus.). 20p. (Orig.). pap. (*0-9631030-0-8*) Creat Ideas.

Understanding Your Health. James F. Mckenzie. 4th ed. 1994. 288p. (C). text, stu. ed. 20.62 (*0-8151-5777-0*, WCB McGr Hill) McGrw-H Hghr Educ.

Understanding Your Health. Payne. 4th ed. 1995. tchr. ed. (*0-8151-6803-9*) Mosby Inc.

Understanding Your Health. Wayne A. Payne. 4th ed. 1994. tchr. ed. (*0-8151-6807-1*) Mosby Inc.

Understanding Your Health Study Guide. McKenzie et al. 1991. 288p. pap. 14.95 (*0-8016-6654-6*) Mosby Inc.

***Understanding Your Health with HealthQuest 2.0, Healthnet, Online Learning Center Passcard & E-Text.** Wayne A. Payne & Dale B. Hahn. 6th ed. 2000. (C). 58.13 (*0-07-242088-X*) McGrw-H Hghr Educ.

Understanding Your Horse's Lameness. Diane Morgan. 1992. LC 92-13128. (Illus.). 152p. 19.95 (*0-939481-26-X*) Half Halt Pr.

Understanding Your Immune System. Eve Potts & Marion Morra. 1986. 224p. pap. 3.95 (*0-380-89728-8*, Avon Bks) Morrow Avon.

Understanding Your New Life with Dialysis: A Patient Guide for Physical & Psychological Adjustment. Edith T. Oberley & Terry D. Oberley. 4th ed. 1992. (Illus.). 194p. (C). pap. text 35.95 (*0-398-05774-5*) C C Thomas.

Understanding Yourself & Others: An Introduction to Temperament. Linda V. Berens. 2000. (Understanding Yourself & Others Ser.). 44p. 5.95 (*0-9664624-4-0*) Telos Pubns.

Undertaking Midwifery Research: A Basic Guide to Design & Analysis. Carolyn M. Hicks. 1996. pap. text (*0-443-05230-1*) Church.

Undiscovered Mind: How the Human Brain Defies Replication, Medication & Explanation. John Horgan. 2000. 336p. pap. 14.00 (*0-684-86578-5*, Touchstone) S&S Trade Pap.

Undiscovered Mind: How the Human Brain Defies Replication, Medication & Explanation. John Horgan. 1999. LC 99-31051. 336p. 25.00 (*0-684-85075-3*) Free Pr.

Undiscovered Self. Carl Gustav Jung. 1976. 126p. 17.95 (*0-8488-0547-X*) Amereon Ltd.

Undiscovered Self: With Symbols & the Interpretation of Dreams. Carl Gustav Jung. Tr. & Rev. by R. F. C. Hull. rev. ed. 1990. LC 89-38499. (Bollingen Ser.: Vol. 20). 166p. pap. 10.95 (*0-691-01894-4*) Princeton U Pr.

Undoing Depression: What Therapy Doesn't Teach You & Drugs Can't Give You. Richard O'Connor. 1997. LC 96-50214. 416p. 23.95 (*0-316-62643-0*) Little.

UNDP/UNFPA/WHO/World Bank Special Programme of Research, Development & Research Training in Human Reproduction: Biennial Report, 1994-1995. UNDP/UNFPA/WHO. 1996. 111p. (Orig.). pap. 23.40 (*92-4-156183-1*, 1150443) World Health.

Undue Risk: Secret State Experiments on Humans. Jonathan D. Moreno. 2000. LC 00-59140. 368p. reprint ed. pap. 18.95 (*0-415-92835-4*) Routledge.

Uneasy Endings: Daily Life in an American Nursing Home. Renee R. Shield. 1988. LC 88-47743. (Anthropology of Contemporary Issues Ser.). 304p. 42.50 (*0-8014-2159-4*); pap. 18.95 (*0-8014-9490-7*) Cornell U Pr.

Uneasy Equilibrium: Private & Public Financing of Health Services in the United States, 1875-1965. Odin W. Anderson. 1968. pap. 9.95 (*0-8084-0305-2*) NCUP.

Uneasy Sensations: Smollett & the Body. Aileen Douglas. 1995. LC 95-1786. 232p. 29.95 (*0-226-16051-3*) U Ch Pr.

Unequal Burden of Cancer: An Assessment of NIH Research & Programs for Ethnic Minorities & the Medically Underserved. Institute of Medicine Staff. Ed. by M. Alfred Haynes & Brian D. Smedley. 1999. LC 99-6105. 352p. text 47.95 (*0-309-07154-2*) Natl Acad Pr.

Unequal Treatment. Eileen Nechas. 1994. LC 93-47632. 272p. 22.00 (*0-671-79186-9*) S&S Trade.

Unexplained Fever. Benedict Isaac & Serge Kernbaum. 1990. 560p. lib. bdg. 254.95 (*0-8493-4556-1*, RB129) CRC Pr.

Unexplained Infertility. Patrick J. Taylor & John A. Collins. 1993. LC 92-23032. (Illus.). 294p. text 42.50 (*0-19-262290-0*) OUP.

Unfavorable Result in Plastic Surgery Robert M. Goldwyn. 2nd ed. 1984. 1134p. 285.00 (*0-316-31975-9*, Little Brwn Med Div) Lppncott W & W.

***Unfavorable Result in Plastic Surgery: Avoidance & Treatment.** Ed. by Robert M. Goldwyn & Mimis Cohen. 3rd ed. 2001. LC 2001-23445. text 239.00 (*0-7817-1819-8*) Lppncott W & W.

Unfinished Health Agenda: Lessons from Hawai'i. Ed. by Bob Grossman & Jim Shon. 1994. 256p. (Orig.). (C). pap. text 19.00 (*0-8248-1690-0*) HI St Primary.

Unfinished Revolution: Women & Health Care in America. Emily Friedman. 1994. LC 94-5940. 304p. pap. 20.00 (*1-881277-17-8*) United Hosp Fund.

Unfolding Case Studies: Experiencing the Realities of Clinical Nursing Practice. Kellie J. Glendon & Deborah L. Ulrich. 2000. 262p. pap. 32.60 (*0-13-089279-3*) P-H.

Unfolding Self: Psychosynthesis & Counseling. Molly Y. Brown. 1983. LC 83-61449. (Illus.). 181p. (C). reprint ed. pap. 20.00 (*0-9611444-0-8*) Psychosynth Pr.

Unformulated Experience: From Dissociation to Imagination in Psychoanalysis. Donnel B. Stern. 1997. LC 97-25923. (Relational Perspectives Bks.: Vol. 8). 312p. 45.00 (*0-88163-141-8*) Analytic Pr.

***Unfortunate Folk: Essays on Mental Health Treatment, 1863-1992.** Ed. by Barbara Brookes & Jane Thomson. 2001. 296p. pap. (*1-877276-09-X*) Univ Otago Pr NZL. *Dist:* Intl Spec Bk.

Unhealthy Decade: A Sociological Study of the State of Public Health in Russia 1990-1999. Per Carlson. 2000. (Acta Universitatis Stockholmiensis Ser.: No. 10). (Illus.). 164p. pap. (*91-22-01870-0*) Almqvist & Wiksell SWE. *Dist:* Coronet Bks.

Unhealthy Societies: From Inequality to Well-Being. Richard G. Wilkinson. 1996. LC 96-21560. 272p. (C). 85.00 (*0-415-09234-5*); pap. 28.95 (*0-415-09235-3*) Routledge.

Unholy Hungers: Encountering the Vampire in Ourselves & Others. Barbara E. Hort. Ed. by David O'Neal. 1996. LC 95-25783. 272p. (Orig.). pap. 16.00 (*1-57062-181-0*) Shambhala Pubns.

Unholy Madness: The Church's Surrender to Psychiatry. Seth Farber. 1999. LC 99-21613. 162p. pap. 12.99 (*0-8308-1939-8*) InterVarsity.

UNIDO Guides to Information Sources: Pharmaceutical Industry, No. 20. pap. 4.00 (*92-1-106150-4*, ID/162) UN.

Unification Through Division: Histories of the Divisions of the American Psychological Association, Vol. 2. Ed. by Donald A. Dewsbury. 1997. LC 96-41480. (Histories of the Divisions of the American Psychological Association Ser.: Vol. 2). 325p. pap. text 24.95 (*1-55798-430-1*) Am Psychol.

Unification Through Division Vol. 1: Histories of the Divisions of the American Psychological Association. Ed. by Donald A. Dewsbury. 1996. LC 96-41480.

TUV

(Histories of the Divisions of the American Psychological Association Ser.: Vol. 1). 317p. pap. 24.95 (1-55798-379-8) Am Psychol.

Unified Fitness: A 35-Day Exercise Program for Sustainable Health. John Alton. 2002. pap. 22.95 (1-57174-224-7) Hampton Roads Pub Co.

Unified Medical Dictionary: English, Arabic, French. 1983. text (88-7674-000-7) World Health.

Unified Medical Language System: Current Bibliographies in Medicine (Jan. '86-Dec. '96) Catherine R. Selden & Betsy L. Humphreys. 1997. 54p. (Orig.). (C). pap. text 25.00 (0-7881-4481-2) DIANE Pub.

Unified Theories of Cognition. Allen Newell. (Illus.). 1994. 576p. pap. 24.95 (0-674-92101-1); 1990. 544p. 57.00 (0-674-92099-6) HUP.

Uniform Drug Code. Peter D. Hays. 2nd rev. ed. 1994. 10p. (Orig.). pap. 3.00 (1-885554-02-8) P D Hays.

Uniform Pharmaceutical Pricing: An Economic Analysis. Berndt. 1994. 50p. (Orig.). pap. 9.95 (0-8447-7028-0) Am Enterprise.

Uniformity of Claims for In Vitro Diagnostic Tests: Proposed Guideline (1996) 1996. 25.00 (1-56238-303-5, EP11-P) NCCLS.

Unifying Concepts of Leukemia: Proceedings of the International Symposium on Comparative Leukemia Research, 5th, Padova, Venice, 1971. International Symposium on Comparative Leukemia Research Staff. Ed. by R. M. Dutcher. 1973. (Bibliotheca Haemotologica Ser.: No. 39). 196.75 (3-8055-1383-6) S Karger.

Unilateral Renal Function Studies: Proceedings of the International Symposium, 1st, Monecatini Terme, May, 1977. International Symposium on Unilateral Renal Functions Studies Staff. Ed. by C. P. Bianchi et al. 1978. (Contributions to Nephrology Ser.: Vol. 11). (Illus.). 29.75 (3-8055-2858-2) S Karger.

Uninformed Consent: The Hidden Dangers in Dental Care. Hal A. Huggins & Thomas E. Levy. 1998. LC 98-71590. (Illus.). 280p. pap. 14.95 (1-57174-117-8) Hampton Roads Pub Co.

Uninvited Guest: Emerging from Narcissism Towards Marriage in Psychoanalytic Therapy with Couples. James Fisher. 1999. 336p. pap. (1-85575-196-8) Karnac Bks GBR. Dist: Other Pr LLC.

Unipac 5: Communication & the Interdisciplinary Team Approach. Porter Storey & Carol F. Knight. 1997. (Hospice & Palliative Care Training for Physicians Ser.: Vol. 5). 80p. (Orig.). pap. 20.00 (1-889296-05-8) Am Acad Hospice.

Unipac Five: Communication & the Physician's Role on the Interdisc. Porter Storey. 1998. LC 99-191374. 160p. spiral bd. 20.00 (0-7872-5144-5) Kendall-Hunt.

Unipac 4: Management of Selected Nonpain Symptoms in the Terminally Ill. Porter Storey & Carol F. Knight. 1996. (Hospice & Palliative Care Training for Physicians Ser.: Vol. 4). 80p. (Orig.). pap. text 20.00 (1-889296-04-X) Am Acad Hospice.

Unipac 1: The Hospice/Palliative Approach to Caring for the Terminally Ill. Porter Storey & Carol F. Knight. 1997. 80p. (Orig.). pap. 20.00 (1-889296-01-5) Am Acad Hospice.

Unipac One: The Hospice/Palliative Medicine Medicine Approach to. Porter Storey. 1998. LC 99-191374. 160p. spiral bd. 20.00 (0-7872-5081-3) Kendall-Hunt.

Unipac 6: Ethical & Legal Decision Making When Caring for the Terminally Ill. Porter Storey & Carol F. Knight. 1996. (Hospice & Palliative Care Training for Physicians Ser.: Vol. 6). 112p. (Orig.). pap. text 20.00 (1-889296-06-6) Am Acad Hospice.

Unipac 3: Assessment & Treatment of Pain in the Terminally Ill. Porter Storey & Carol F. Knight. 1996. (Hospice & Palliative Care Training for Physicians Ser.: Vol. 3). 86p. (Orig.). pap. text 20.00 (1-889296-03-1) Am Acad Hospice.

Unipac 2: Psychological, Spiritual, & Physiological Aspects of Dying & Bereavement. Porter Storey & Carol F. Knight. 1997. (Hospice & Palliative Care Training for Physicians Ser.: Vol. 2). 80p. (Orig.). pap. 20.00 (1-889296-02-3) Am Acad Hospice.

Unique Physician Identification Number for All States. Set. 1994. lib. bdg. 495.00 (0-8490-8402-4) Gordon Pr.

Unique Properties of Melanocytes: Proceedings of the International Pigment Cell Conference, Houston, Texas, Jan., 1975. International Pigment Cell Conference Staff. Ed. by V. Riley. 1977. (Pigment Cell Ser.: Vol. 3). (Illus.). 133.25 (3-8055-2371-8) S Karger.

Uniquely Human: The Evolution of Speech, Thought, & Selfless Behavior. Philip Lieberman. 1993. (Illus.). 224p. (C). pap. 17.00 (0-674-92183-6) HUP.

Uniqueness: The Human Pursuit of Difference. C. R. Snyder & H. L. Fromkin. 1980. LC 79-18764. (Perspectives in Social Psychology Ser.). (Illus.). 250p. (C). 42.50 (0-306-40376-5, Plenum Trade) Perseus Pubng.

Unit-Based Nursing Staff Development: A Handbook for Clinical Nurses. Joan S. Lockhart. 2000. 300p. pap. 39.00 (0-8342-0887-3, 20887) Aspen Pub.

Unit 731 Testimony: Testimony: Japan's Wartime Human Experimentation Program. Hal Gold. 1995. LC 95-60907. (Illus.). 256p. pap. text (4-900737-39-9) Yen Bks JPN. Dist: Tuttle Pubng.

Unit 2000: A Nursing Unit Design Symposium Addressing Patient Beds for the Future. Ed. by Kirkham R. Hamilton. 1993. 391p. 35.00 (0-9636950-0-2) W C H Architects.

Unitas: Building Healing Communities for Children. Edward P. Eismann. 2nd ed. 1996. LC 96-16790. xvi, 214p. pap. 25.00 (0-8232-1686-1) Fordham.

Unitas: Hispanic & Black Children in a Healing Community. Anne Farber & Lloyd H. Rogler. 1982. 128p. 18.95 (0-87073-505-5); pap. 11.95 (0-87073-506-3) Schenkman Bks Inc.

United States Health Care Laws & Rules. Ed. by Peter A. Pavarini. 1995. 1700p. 75.00 (0-314-06827-9) Am Hlth Lawyers.

United Way's Donor Option Program: Background Paper on the Reasons for Problems with DOPs & Suggestions for a Model Donor Option Program. Jennifer Henry & Steven Paprocki. 1989. 30p. pap. 15.00 (1-891465-04-X) Natl Comm Philan.

Uniting Psychology & Biology: Integrative Perspectives on Human Development. Ed. by Nancy L. Segal et al. 1997. LC 97-10903. 568p. 39.95 (1-55798-428-X) Am Psychol.

***Units, Symbols, Abbreviations: A Guide for Medical & Scientific.** Ed. by D. N. Baron. 5th ed. 1994. 64p. pap. (0-905958-78-0) Royal Soc of Medicine Pr Ltd GBR. Dist: Balogh.

Unity & Diversity of Membrane Function. Ed. by Gerhard H. Giebisch & J. F. Hoffman. 1994. (Journal: Vol. 17, No. 3-4, 1994). (Illus.). 110p. pap. 38.50 (3-8055-5980-1) S Karger.

Unity of Mistakes: A Phenomenological Interpretation of Medical Work. Marianne A. Paget. 1988. LC 87-26716. 224p. (C). 34.95 (0-87722-533-8) Temple U Pr.

Unity of Self. Stephen L. White. 1991. LC 90-29869. (Representation & Mind Ser.). (Illus.). 464p. 65.00 (0-262-23162-X) MIT Pr.

Univers de la Psychologie, 1: Champ, Histoire et Methodes de la Psychologie. Ed. by Yves Pelicier. 1977. (FRE.). 512p. 150.00 (0-8288-5525-0, M6537) Fr & Eur.

Univers de la Psychologie, 3: Le Development Psychologique Normale, Lavie Psychologie Pathologique. Ed. by Yves Pelicier. 1977. (FRE.). 523p. 150.00 (0-8288-5527-7, M6539) Fr & Eur.

Univers de la Psychologie, 2: La Vie Psychologique Normale. Ed. by Yves Pelicier. 1977. (FRE.). 509p. 150.00 (0-8288-5526-9, M6538) Fr & Eur.

Universal Childbirth Picture Book see Libro Universal de Ilustraciones del Parto

Universal Drug Infusion Ruler. Sota Omoigui. 1995. (Illus.). 4p. spiral bd. 29.00 (0-9650767-0-9) St-of-the-Art Tech.

Universal Experience of Adolescence. Norman Kiell. 1964. LC 63-22359. 942p. 80.00 (0-8236-6720-0) Intl Univs Pr.

Universal Grammar & Second Language Acquisition. Lydia White. 1989. LC 89-48055. (Language Acquisition & Language Disorders Ser.: Vol. 1). xii, 198p. 62.00 (1-55619-092-1); pap. 24.95 (1-55619-093-X) J Benjamins Pubng Co.

Universal Health Care: What the United States Can Learn from the Canadian Experience. Pat Armstrong et al. LC 97-41011. 192p. 1998. text 24.00 (1-56584-410-6); 1999. (Illus.). reprint ed. pap. text 14.95 (1-56584-515-3) New Press NY.

Universal Health Insurance Coverage Using Medicare's Payment Rates. 1992. (Illus.). 61p. (Orig.). (C). pap. text 20.00 (1-56806-125-0) DIANE Pub.

Universal Healthcare Almanac. Ed. by Linda L. Cherner. 1988. 450p. (C). 140.00 (0-933311-02-8) R-C Pubns.

Universal Healthcare Almanac: Quarterly Updates. Linda L. Cherner. 1989. 480p. ring bd. 195.00 (0-9645024-0-2) Silver Cherner.

Universal Medical Device Nomenclature System. ECRI Staff. 1994. (ENG & SPA.). 300p. pap. 99.00 (0-941417-30-1) ECRI.

Universal Multiplication of Intelligence. Glenn Doman & J. Michael Armentrout. 1980. LC 80-66236. (Gentle Revolution Ser.). 223p. 12.50 (0-936676-02-7) Inst Achieve Human Pot.

Universal Newborn Hearing Screening: A Practical Guide. Lynn Spivak. 1997. LC 97-22870. (Illus.). 256p. 49.00 (0-86577-699-7) Thieme Med Pubs.

Universal Standard Benefits Set, Enrollee Cost Sharing & Affordability Report. 1995. (Illus.). 99p. (Orig.). (C). pap. text 30.00 (0-7881-2365-3) DIANE Pub.

Universals of Psychoanalysis: In the Treatment of Psychotic & Borderline States. Henri Rey. Ed. by Jeanne Magagna. 1994. 319p. (C). pap. (1-85343-370-5) Free Assoc Bks GBR. Dist: Intl Spec Bk.

Universe of Consciousness: How Matter Becomes Imagination. Colin McGin et al. 2000. LC 00-271748. (Illus.). 288p. 27.50 (0-465-01376-7) Basic.

Universitaets-Klinik und Poliklinik fuer Hals -, Nasen- und Ohren-Krankheiten Basel 1876-1976. 1976. 16.75 (3-8055-2405-6) S Karger.

University Chemical Dependency Project. Steven Ungerleider & Steven A. Bloch. 1987. 113p. (Orig.). (0-943277-00-0) Integrated Res Servs.

University Health Services. 1966. (Technical Report Ser.: No. 320). 21p. pap. text 3.00 (92-4-120320-X) World Health.

University Hospitals & School Managers Guide to Environment: A Guide for University, Hospital, & School Managers. James T. O'Reilly et al. 1996. LC 95-38757. (Industrial Health & Safety Ser.). 368p. text 78.95 (0-442-02123-2, VNR) Wiley.

University in the Urban Community: Responsibilities for Public Health. Ed. by John R. Hogness et al. 1995. LC 95-5244. 250p. pap. (1-879694-09-3) AAH Ctrs.

University of California, Davis Book of Horses: Complete Medical Reference for Horses & Foals, A. Mordecai Siegal. 1996. LC 96-10907. (Animal & Pet Care Ser.). (Illus.). 528p. 32.00 (0-06-270139-8, Harper Ref) HarperCollins Pubs.

University of Iowa Family Practice. Mark A. Graber et al. Ed. by Robert L. Herting. 3rd ed. 1997. LC 97-2674. (Illus.). 864p. (C). (gr. 13). pap. text 36.95 (0-8151-2395-7, 30999) Mosby Inc.

University of Iowa Family Practice Handbook. Mark Graber. 4th ed. 2001. LC 2001-30389. (Illus.). xxviii, 849p. text (0-323-01209-4) Mosby Inc.

University of Kansas Medical Center: A Pictorial History. Lawrence H. Larsen & Nancy J. Hulston. 1992. LC 91-44669. (Illus.). x, 222p. 35.00 (0-7006-0539-8) U Pr of KS.

University of Kentucky Elder Care Handbook: Resources & Guidance for University Employees Helping Older Family Members. Ronald L. Burdon. 1995. 88p. pap. (0-9647559-0-4) Am Wellness.

University of Melborune - Nucleus Multi-Electrode Cochlear Implant. G. M. Clark et al. 1987. (Advances in OtoRhinoLaryngology Ser.: Vol. 38). (Illus.). x, 190p. 116.75 (3-8055-4575-4) S Karger.

University of Oklahoma College of Medicine & Health Sciences Center, 1964-1996. Mark Allen Everett. 2000. LC 70-177333. (Medical Education in Oklahoma Ser.: Vol. 3). 192p. 35.00 (0-8061-3268-X) U of Okla Pr.

Unjust Punishments: Mandatory HIV Testing of Women Sex Workers & Pregnant Women. Lisa Bowleg. 1992. (Women & AIDS Ser.). (C). pap. 8.00 (1-877966-13-4) Ctr Women Policy.

Unkonventionelle Rheumatherapie. Ed. by W. Muller et al. 1985. (Fortbildungskurse fuer Rheumatologie Ser.: Vol. 7). (GER., Illus.). viii, 192p. pap. 65.25 (3-8055-4005-1) S Karger.

Unleashing Our Unknown Selves: An Inquiry into the Future of Feminity & Masculinity. France Morrow. 1990. LC 90-39262. 288p. 72.50 (0-275-93587-6, C3587); pap. 22.95 (0-275-93837-9, B3837) Greenwood (Praeger Pubs).

Unlikely Entrepreneurs: A Complete Guide to Business Start-Ups for Individuals with Disabilities & Chronic Health Conditions. RoseAnne Herzog. 1998. LC 98-91687. 250p. pap. 21.95 (0-9664862-0-X) Northpeak Pubng.

Unlimited Sex: Beck's Three-Step Method for Achieving Unlimited Male Potency Forever. Francine Beck. 1996. pap. text 14.95 (0-935016-37-6) Arrowood Pr.

Unlock Your Mind & Be Free! A Practical Approach to Hypnotherapy. Edgar Barnett. 1984. 153p. reprint ed. pap. 9.95 (0-930298-49-7) Westwood Pub Co.

Unlocking the Doctor's Little Black Bag. Charles W. Snook. 1999. LC 99-31701. 184p. 18.95 (1-882897-35-8) Lost Coast.

Unlocking the Healing Powers in Your Hands: The 18 Mudra System of Qigong. A. S. Umar Sharif. Ed. & Illus. by Alexis A. Thielke. unabr. ed. 2000. 115p. pap. 22.00 (0-9637036-3-3) Sharif Ent.

Unlocking the Mysteries of Sensory Dysfunction. Elizabeth Anderson & Pauline Emmons. 1996. 91p. (Orig.). pap. 19.95 (1-885477-25-2) Fut Horizons.

Unmarried Mother: A Study of 500 Cases. Percy G. Kammerer. 1969. LC 69-14935. (Criminology, Law Enforcement, & Social Problems Ser.: No. 58). reprint ed. 24.00 (0-87585-058-8) Patterson Smith.

Unmasking PMS. Joseph Martorano et al. 1993. LC 93-72. 240p. 21.95 (0-87131-692-7) M Evans.

Unmedical Book. Elizabeth Baker & Elton Baker. 1987. 263p. (Orig.). pap. 11.95 (0-918880-14-9) Intl Promotions.

Unmedical Miracle - Oxygen. Elizabeth Baker. rev. ed. 1994. 150p. pap. 11.95 (0-937766-12-7) Drelwood Comns.

Unmotivated Child. Natalie Rathvon. 1996. LC 96-30263. 240p. per. 13.00 (0-684-80306-2) S&S Trade.

Unnatural Causes: The Three Leading Killer Diseases in America. Ed. by Russell C. Maulitz. 1989. 210p. text 37.00 (0-8135-1405-3); pap. text 18.00 (0-8135-1406-1) Rutgers U Pr.

Unnatural Death: Confessions of a Medical Examiner. Michael M. Baden & Judith A. Hennesee. 1990. 240p. mass mkt. 5.99 (0-8041-0599-5) Ivy Books.

Unnecessary Cesarean Sections: Curing a National Epidemic. Mary Gabay & Sidney M. Wolfe. enl. ed. 1994. 589p. (C). pap. text 60.00 (0-937188-55-7) Pub Citizen.

Unnecessary Cesareans: Ways to Avoid Them. Diony Young & Charles Mahan. 1980. 27p. 1.50 (0-934024-00-6) Intl Childbirth.

Unnecessary Losses: Costs to Americans of the Lack of Family & Medical Leave. Roberta M. Spalter-Roth & Heidi Hartmann. 1990. LC 89-82427. 73p. pap. 15.00 (1-878428-00-4) Inst Womens Policy Rsch.

Unnoticed Majority in Psychiatric Inpatient Care. C. A. Kiesler & C. G. Simpkins. 1993. (Stress & Coping Ser.). (Illus.). 270p. (C). 45.00 (0-306-44363-5, Plenum Trade) Perseus Pubng.

Unofficial Guide to Alternative Medicine. Macmillan Publishing Company Staff et al. 1998. LC 00-500405. (Unofficial Guides Ser.). (Illus.). 528p. pap. 15.95 (0-02-862526-9, Unoffic Guide) Hungry Minds.

Unofficial Guide to Living with Diabetes. Maria Thomas & Loren W. Greene. 1999. (Unofficial Guides Ser.). (Illus.). 592p. pap. 15.95 (0-02-862919-1, Unoffic Guide) Hungry Minds.

Unofficial Guide to Menopause. Unofficial Panel of Experts Staff et al. 1999. (Unofficial Guides). (Illus.). 448p. pap. 15.95 (0-02-862694-X, Unoffic Guide) Hungry Minds.

Unofficial Guide to Women's Health. Carol Turkington. 2000. LC 00-699301. (Unofficial Guides Ser.). 400p. pap. 15.95 (0-02-863666-X) Hungry Minds.

Unquiet Mind: A Memoir of Moods & Madness. Kay R. Jamison. 1995. LC 95-14273. 240p. 26.95 (0-679-44374-6) Random.

Unquiet Mind: A Memoir of Moods & Madness. Kay R. Jamison. 1997. LC 95-14273. 224p. pap. 12.00 (0-679-76330-9) Vin Bks.

Unraveling DNA. Maxim D. Frank-Kamenetskii. 1993. 216p. 64.95 (0-471-18852-2, Wiley-VCH) Wiley.

***Unraveling the ADD-ADHD Fiasco: Successful Parenting Without Drugs.** David B. Stein. 2001. LC 2001-22654. (Illus.). 256p. pap. 14.95 (0-7407-1859-2) Andrews McMeel.

Unrelated Business Income Tax Issues in Health Care. Brian D. Lepard & Frederick J. Gerhart. 1996. (Health Law & Business Ser.: No. 2000). 125.00 (1-55871-342-5) BNA.

Unresolved Grief: A Practical, Multicultural Approach for Health Professionals. John C. Gunzburg. 1993. 416p. pap. 54.25 (1-56593-198-X, 0513) Singular Publishing.

Unresolved Questions in the Freud-Jung Debate: On Psychosis, Sexual Identity & Religion. P. Vandermeersch. 1991. (Louvain Philosophical Studies: No. 4). 304p. (Orig.). pap. (90-6186-436-4) Leuven Univ BEL. Dist: Coronet Bks.

Unrolithiasis Research. Nath and Thind, S. K. Staff. 1989. (C). (81-7024-244-4) Ashish Pub Hse IND. Dist: S Asia.

Unsafe in Their Own Homes: State Programs Fail to Protect Elderly from Indignity, Abuse & Neglect. 1993. 27p. (Orig.). (C). pap. text 20.00 (1-56806-373-3) DIANE Pub.

Unsaturated Fatty Acids in Foods: The Report of the British Nutrition Foundation's Task Force. British Nutrition Foundation Staff. 1992. 300p. 89.95 (0-442-31621-6) Chapman & Hall.

Unscientific Psychology: A Cultural-Performatory Approach to Understanding Human Life. Fred Newman & Lois Holzman. 1996. LC 96-2801. 232p. 59.95 (0-275-95412-9, Praeger Pubs) Greenwood.

Unshielded: The Human Cost of the Dalkon Shield IUD. Mary Hawkins. 1997. LC 98-106169. 258p. pap. text 17.95 (0-8020-7861-3) U of Toronto Pr.

Unspoken Art: Profiles of Veterinary Life. Lee Gutkind. 1998. LC 98-17749. 256p. pap. 15.00 (0-8050-5811-7, Owl) H Holt & Co.

Unstable Angina. 1995. lib. bdg. 251.95 (0-8490-6848-7) Gordon Pr.

Unstable Angina. Ed. by John D. Rutherford. 1991. (Fundamental & Clinical Cardiology Ser.: Vol. 4). (Illus.). 328p. text 145.00 (0-8247-8618-1) Dekker.

Unstable Angina: Diagnosis & Management - Clinical Practice Guideline. Eugene Braunwald. 1997. (Illus.). 154p. (C). pap. text 30.00 (0-7881-4607-6) DIANE Pub.

Unstable Angina: Diagnosis & Management: Commentary on the Agency for Health Care Policy & Research Clinical Practice Guidelines. Michael H. Crawford. 1997. LC 96-26865. 190p. pap. (0-412-09771-0) E A GBR. Dist: OUP.

Unstable Angina Order. Adelman. 1981. lib. bdg. (90-247-2486-4) M Nijhoff NLD. Dist: Kluwer Academic.

Unstable Coronary Artery Syndromes: Pathophysiology, Diagnosis & Treatment. Robert L. Wilensky. 1998. LC 98-21789. (Developments in Cardiovascular Medicine Ser.). (0-7923-8201-3) Kluwer Academic.

Unstable Frontiers: Technomedicine & the Cultural Politics of "Curing" AIDS. John N. Erni. 1994. LC 94-773. text 39.95 (0-8166-2380-5) U of Minn Pr.

Unstable Ideas: Temperament, Cognition, & Self. Jerome Kagan. (Illus.). 1992. 328p. pap. 18.50 (0-674-93039-8); 1989. LC 88-28376. 352p. 39.95 (0-674-93038-X) HUP.

Unstable Shoulder. Ed. by Louis U. Bigliani. 1996. LC 96-2510. (American Academy of Orthopaedic Surgeons Monograph Ser.). 90p. pap. 38.00 (0-89203-120-4) Amer Acad Ortho Surg.

Unstable Shoulder. Russell F. Warren. 1998. LC 98-22298. 512p. text 189.00 (0-397-51677-0) Lppncott W & W.

Unsupervised Learning & Map Formation: Foundations of Neural Computation. Terrence J. Ejnowski. Ed. by Geoffrey E. Hinton. 1999. LC 98-14784. (Computational Neuroscience Ser.). (Illus.). 397p. pap. text 30.00 (0-262-58168-X) MIT Pr.

Unsupported Middle: Future Developments in a Primary Care-LED NHS. Geoff Meads. 1997. LC 97-5138. (1-85775-109-4) Radcliffe Med Pr GBR. Dist: Balogh.

Untapped Options: Building Links Between Marketing & Human Resources to Achieve Organizational Goals

in Health Care. Bea Northcott & Janette Helm. 2000. 240p. 52.00 (*0-7879-5537-X*) Jossey-Bass.

Untapped Resource: Working with Volunteers Who Are Mentally Ill. John D. Weaver. 1993. (C). pap. 12.50 (*0-945795-10-6*) MBA Pub.

Untersuchungen uber die Grundfragen des Sprachlebens, Vol. 5. Philipp Wegener. Ed. by E. F. K. Koerner. 1991. LC 90-357. (Classics in Psycholinguistics Ser.: Vol. 5). (GER.). lii, viii 214p. reprint ed. 65.00 (*90-272-1894-3*) J Benjamins Pubng Co.

Untersuchungen Zum Abbau der Buchenblattstreu Durch Pilze. Martina Kloidt. 1989. (Dissertationes Botanicae Ser.: Band 130). (GER., Illus.). 182p. pap. (*3-443-64042-7*) Gebruder Borntraeger DEU. *Dist:* Balogh.

Until the Cure: Caring for Women with HIV. Ed. by Ann Kurth. 1993. LC 93-5550. (Yale FastBack Ser.). 336p. 42.50 (*0-300-05806-3*) Yale U Pr.

Unto the Least of These: Special Education in the Church. Andrew H. Wood. 1984. LC 84-16077. 143p. reprint ed. pap. 5.99 (*0-87227-099-8*, RBP5127) Reg Baptist.

Untold Lives: The First Generation of American Women Psychologists. Elizabeth Ann Scarborough & Laurel Furumoto. 1989. LC 86-20715. (King's Crown Paperback Ser.). 236p. pap. text 19.50 (*0-231-05155-7*) Col U Pr.

Untold Truth about Fatness. Dean Kimmel. 1988. 42p. (Orig.). pap. 2.95 (*0-9621446-0-6*) Corbin Hse.

Untouched Key: Tracing Childhood Trauma in Creativity & Destructiveness. Alice Miller. 1991. LC 91-219126. 192p. pap. 13.95 (*0-385-26764-9*) Doubleday.

Unusual Occurrences of Cancer As a Clue of Cancer Etiology: Proceedings of the 18th International Symposium of the Princess Takamatsu Cancer Research Fund, November 1987, Tokyo. Joseph F. Fraumeni, Jr. et al. 1989. 350p. 143.00 (*0-85066-459-4*) Taylor & Francis.

Unvividness Paradox: Dynamics of Imagery Formation. Akhter Ahsen. 1990. LC 89-62540. 250p. pap. text 24.95 (*0-913412-46-5*) Brandon Hse.

Unwanted Effects of Cosmetics & Drugs Used in Dermatology. Ed. by A. C. De Groot et al. 3rd rev. ed. 1993. 782p. 272.50 (*0-444-89775-5*) Elsevier.

Unwelcome Intruder: Freud's Struggle with Cancer. Sharon Romm. 1983. LC 83-13649. (Illus.). 164p. 60.00 (*0-275-91409-7*, C1409, Praeger Pubs) Greenwood.

Unwind: Turkeys Do Fly. Merrie Farrell. 1994. LC 94-29892. 15.95 (*1-885275-59-5*) C J Howie.

Unwomanly Conduct: The Challenges of Intentional Childlessness. Carolyn M. Morell. 1994. LC 93-45984. 240p. (C). pap. 20.95 (*0-415-90678-4*) Routledge.

Up from Scapegoating: Awakening Consciousness in Groups. Arthur D. Colman. 1995. LC 95-14098. 160p. (Orig.). pap. 19.95 (*0-933029-95-0*) Chiron Pubns.

Up from the Ashes: There Is Life after a Stroke. James A. Young. Ed. by BookWorld Staff. 1996. (Illus.). 160p. (Orig.). pap. 14.95 (*0-9651506-0-7*) Inner Path.

Up-Front Sleeper: The Federal Witness "Protection" Programs: A "Letter" to Janet Reno Corrupt Jurisprudence Unchecked. Martin Porozynski. 3rd rev. ed. 2000. 198p. spiral bd. 14.95 (*0-9644416-2-4*) Doublenight Pr.

Update for the MRCP. Thomasin C. Andrews. 1996. LC 96-30950. pap. text (*0-443-05589-0*) Church.

Update in Critical Care Medicine: Management of the Critical Care Patient. Pierre Casthely et al. 1989. LC 89-91693. (Illus.). 200p. (Orig.). 59.00 (*0-9623083-0-7*) P A Castheley.

Update in Intensive Care & Emergency Medicine. Ed. by J. L. Vincent. 1985. (Anaesthesiology & Intensive Care Medicine Ser.: Vol. 178). (Illus.). xiv, 304p. 71.95 (*0-387-15261-X*) Spr-Verlag.

Update in Intensive Care & Emergency Medicine, 1986. J. L. Vincent. 1986. (Illus.). 561p. 79.95 (*0-387-16508-8*) Spr-Verlag.

Update in Ob/Gyn Ultrasound, Vol. II. Beryl R. Benacerraf et al. 1997. (Illus.). 116p. pap. 57.00 (*1-930047-18-5*, UOG2) Am Inst Ultrasound.

Update in Stroke Prevention: Problems of the Stroke Recurrence: Sanofi Winthrop Symposium to the 3rd World Stroke Congress & the 5th European Stroke Conference, Munich, September 1996. Ed. by J. Bogousslavsky & J. D. Easton. 1997. (Journal: Vol. 7, Supplement 1, 1997). (Illus.). iv, 28p. pap. 21.75 (*3-8055-6462-7*) S Karger.

Update, 1991. Ed. by J. L. Vincent. 1991. (Update in Intensive Care & Emergency Medicine Ser.: Vol. 14). (Illus.). 608p. 130.00 (*0-387-53672-8*) Spr-Verlag.

Update on Adolescent Gynecology & Endocrinology: Basic & Clinical Aspects. Ed. by George Creatsas et al. 1997. LC 97-13702. (Annals of the New York Academy of Sciences Ser.: Vol. 816). pap. 140.00 (*1-57331-039-5*);Vol. 816. 140.00 (*1-57331-038-7*) NY Acad Sci.

Update on Childhood Asthma. Ed. by M. H. Schoni & R. Kraemer. 1993. LC 93-12413. 221p. 90.00 (*0-8176-2867-3*) Spr-Verlag.

Update on Hemostasis. David H. Boldt. 1990. (Contemporary Management in Internal Medicine Ser.: Vol. 1, No. 2). (Illus.). 240p. text (*0-443-08823-3*) Church.

Update on Hepatobiliary Diseases, 1996. Ed. by S. K. Lam. 1997. (Falk Symposium Ser.). 336p. (C). text 157.50 (*0-7923-8715-5*) Kluwer Academic.

Update on Hormonal Treatment in the Menopause. Ed. by M. L'Hermite. 1989. (Progress in Reproductive Biology & Medicine Ser.: Vol. 13). (Illus.). viii, 108p. 85.25 (*3-8055-4904-0*) S Karger.

Update on Neonatal Respiratory Disorders & Surfactant: 14th International Workshop on Surfactant Replacement, Skagen, June 1999: Proceedings. Ed. by H. Verder et al. 1999. (Biology of the Neonate Ser.: Vol. 76, Suppl. 1 (1999)). (Illus.). iv, 52p. pap. 25.25 (*3-8055-6897-5*) S Karger.

Update on Non-Narcotic Analgesic Research: Fiuggi, Italy, October 2-3, 1992. Ed. by Giuseppe Nappi & W. D. Gerber. 1993. LC 93-11312. (*0-8176-2917-3*) Birkhauser.

Update on Strabismus & Pediatric Ophthalmology: Proceedings of the June, 1994 Joint ISA & AAPO&S Meeting, Vancouver, Canada. Ed. by Gunnar Lennerstrand & American Association for Strabismus and Pediatric Ophthalmology Staff. 1995. LC 94-46587. 752p. 244.95 (*0-8493-8961-5*, 8961) CRC Pr.

Update to Glaucoma, Ocular Blood Flow & Drug Treatment. Ed. by Stephen M. Drance. 1995. LC 95-17698. (Illus.). 144p. text (*90-6299-124-6*) Kugler NLD. *Dist:* Lib Res.

Update to Joint Commission Hospital Accreditation Standards: Supplement to the Elements of Quality in Pharmaceutical Care. Charles P. Coe. 1994. LC 94-218227. (Orig.). pap. text 35.00 (*1-879907-45-3*) Am Soc Hlth-Syst.

Updated ENT. G. G. Browning. 3rd ed. 1999. (Illus.). 184p. pap. text (*0-7506-1921-X*) E A GBR. *Dist:* OUP.

Updates in Advances in Lung Cancer. Ed. by J.H. Schiller. 1997. LC 97-34804. (Progress in Respiratory Research Ser.: No. 29). (Illus.). x, 192p. 160.00 (*3-8055-6557-7*) S Karger.

Updates in Colo-Proctology. Ed. by J. C. Givel et al. 1993. LC 92-49863. (Illus.). 210p. 158.00 (*0-387-55327-4*) Spr-Verlag.

Updates on Human Immuno-Deficiency Virus Which Causes the A.I.D.S. Disease & the Third World. Michael Akpan & Juliana Akpan. 1993. 88p. (Orig.). pap. 8.95 (*1-56411-048-6*) Khalifahs Booksellers.

Updates to Critical Care Pharmocotherapy: Focus on Sedation & Analgesia. Bart Chernow & Joseph F. Dasta. 1996. 16p. pap. (*0-683-18054-1*) Lppncott W & W.

Updating the Core Psychology Course: Integrating Gender into the Curriculum. Toby R. Silverman-Dresner. 1989. (American University Studies: Ser. VIII, Vol. 16). 115p. (C). text 24.95 (*0-8204-1098-5*) P Lang Pubng.

Upper Cervical Syndrome: Chiropractic Diagnosis & Treatment. Howard Vernon. 1988. (Illus.). 272p. 62.00 (*0-683-08591-3*) Lppncott W & W.

Upper Digestive Surgery. Taylor. 1999. (C). text 295.00 (*0-7020-1434-6*) Harcourt.

Upper Extremities Orthotics. Miles H. Anderson. fac. ed. 1979. (Illus.). 476p. 73.95 (*0-398-00044-1*) C C Thomas.

Upper Extremity: Traumatic Injuries & Conditions. Sharon G. Childs et al. 1999. vi, 114p. pap. 55.00 (*1-892665-02-6*) Natl Assn Ortho Nurse.

Upper Extremity Casting. Kelly. 1998. (C). pap. text 47.50 (*0-12-784577-1*) Acad Pr.

Upper Extremity Disorders: Frequency, Impact & Cost. Jennifer L. Kelsey. 1997. LC 96-53383. (*0-443-07912-9*) Church.

Upper Extremity in Sports Injuries. Frank W. Jobe. Ed. by Marilyn M. Pink. 1995. (Illus.). 752p. (C). (gr. 13). text 210.00 (*0-8016-7207-4*, 07207) Mosby Inc.

Upper Extremity Injuries in the Athlete. Ed. by Arthur M. Pappas et al. 1994. LC 94-33757. (Illus.). 514p. text (*0-443-08836-5*) Church.

Upper Extremity Neuroanatomy & Clinical Examination: A Programmed Text. David P. Nichols. 1997. 56p. spiral bd. 24.00 (*90-5702-530-2*, Harwood Acad Pubs) Gordon & Breach.

Upper Gastrointestinal Cancer: Esophagus & Stomach. Mitchell C. Posner et al. 2000. (ACS Atlas of Clinical Oncology Ser.). 350p. incl. cd-rom (*1-55009-101-8*) DEKR.

Upper Gastrointestinal Surgery. Ed. by Michael Griffin & Stephen Raimes. 1997. (Companion Guide to Specialist Surgical Practice Ser.: Vol. 2). (Illus.). 380p. text (*0-7020-2141-5*) W B Saunders GBR. *Dist:* Saunders.

***Upper Gastrointestinal Surgery: A Companion to Specialist Surgical Practice.** Michael Griffin & Simon A. Raimes. 2nd ed. 2001. 300p. (*0-7020-2587-9*) W B Saunders GBR. *Dist:* Saunders.

Upper Limb, Vol. 6. 1972. (*0-443-00878-7*) Church.

Upper Limb & Hand. Nicholas Barton & Patrick J. Mulligan. 1998. 256p. (C). text 57.00 (*0-7020-2236-5*) Saunders.

Upper Limb Deficiencies in Children. Douglas W. Lamb & Hamish Law. 1987. 152p. 100.00 (*0-316-51269-9*, Little Brwn Med Div) Lppncott W & W.

Upper Limb Orthotics. Wilton. 1997. pap. text (*0-7020-2214-4*) Bailliere Tindall.

Upper Motor Neurons Functions & Dysfunctions. John C. Eccles. 1985. (Recent Achievements in Restorative Neurology Ser.: Vol. 1). (Illus.). xvii, 346p. 242.75 (*3-8055-4020-5*) S Karger.

Upper Respiratory & Head & Neck Infections. Ed. by Gerald L. Mandell & Itzhak Brook. 1995. LC 95-1977. (Atlas of Infectious Diseases Ser.: Vol. 4). (Illus.). 215p. text (*0-443-07710-X*) Church GBR. *Dist:* Saunders.

Uppers, Downers, All Arounders. Darryl S. Inaba et al. 3rd ed. 1997. LC 96-71688. (Illus.). 496p. pap. text 38.00 (*0-926544-25-X*) CNS.

Upset Workbook: Health Care Edition. Pennie Myers & Don W. Nance. 1989. 118p. 59.00 (*0-9620723-2-X*) MAS.

Upset Workbook: Patient Representative Edition. Pennie Myers & Don W. Nance. 1990. 130p. 59.00 (*0-9620723-3-8*) MAS.

Upside-down Kids: Helping Dyslexic Children Understand Themselves & Overcome Their Disorder. Harold N. Levinson & Addie Sanders. 1991. LC 91-4420. 168p. (ps up). 17.95 (*0-87131-625-0*) M Evans.

Upward Journey: The Story of Internal Medicine at Georgetown: 1851-1981. John F. Stapleton. 1996. LC 96-76436. (Illus.). 304p. (C). (*0-9652807-0-5*) Georgetown U Med.

Ur-ine Trouble: Think You Would Pass a Drug Test? Don't Be So Sure! Kent Holtorf & Stephanie Cartozian. 1997. (Illus.). 165p. (Orig.). 24.95 (*0-9657467-3-9*) Vandalay Pubs.

Urban African American Health Care. Eric J. Bailey. 1991. 206p. (C). text 57.50 (*0-8191-8276-1*); pap. text 27.50 (*0-8191-8277-X*) U Pr of Amer.

Urban Air Pollution: Proceedings of the WHO Expert Committee with Particular Reference to Motor Vehicles, Geneva, 1968. WHO Staff. 1969. (Technical Reports: No. 410). 53p. pap. text 5.00 (*92-4-120410-9*, 1100410) World Health.

Urban Districts & Drug Scenes: Prevention of Drug Dependence. 1996. LC 97-105702. 288p. pap. (*92-827-7759-6*, CE91-95-576-ENC) Comm Europ Commun BEL. *Dist:* Bernan Associates.

Urban Ecology & Health in the Third World. Ed. by Lawrence M. Schell et al. 1993. (Society for the Study of Human Biology Symposium Ser.: No. 32). (Illus.). 301p. (C). text 85.00 (*0-521-41159-9*) Cambridge U Pr.

Urban Environmental Health & Hygiene in Sub-Saharan Africa. Erik Nordberg & Uno Winblad. 1994. LC 95-200662. (Current African Issues Ser.: No. 18). 26p. (*91-7106-364-1*) Nordic Africa SWE. *Dist:* Transaction Pubs.

Urban Family & Family Planning in India. A. R. Desai. 1980. 224p. reprint ed. 22.95 (*0-940500-70-1*) Asia Bk Corp.

Urban Family Medicine. Ed. by R. Birrer. 1986. (Illus.). 287p. 176.00 (*0-387-96301-4*) Spr-Verlag.

Urban Health Crisis: Strategies for Health for All in the Face of Rapid Urbanization. 1993. xvi, 80p. pap. text 20.00 (*92-4-156159-9*, 1150402) World Health.

Urban Health in Developed Countries. Ed. by Trudy Harpham & Marcel Tanner. 1995. LC 95-228399. 228p. text 55.00 (*0-312-15831-9*) St Martin.

Urban Health Services. 1963. (Technical Report Ser.: No. 250). 35p. pap. text 4.00 (*92-4-120250-5*) World Health.

Urban Hospital Location. Leslie Mayhew. 1985. LC 85-15820. (London Research Series in Geography: No. 4). (Illus.). 176p. text 60.00 (*0-04-362054-X*) Routledge.

Urbanization & Environmental Quality. Isao Orishimo. 1982. (Studies in Applied Regional Science). 192p. lib. bdg. 111.00 (*0-89838-080-4*) Kluwer Academic.

Urbanization & Its Implications for Child Health Potential for Action. WHO Staff. 1988. 86p. 16.00 (*92-4-156123-8*) World Health.

***Urea & Non-Protein Nitrogen Metabolism in Infants: With Special Reference to the Sudden Infant Death Syndrome (SIDS)** Mary George. 2001. (Comprehensive Summaries of Uppsala Dissertations from the Faculty of Medicine Ser.: No. 1087). 43p. pap. (*91-554-5141-1*) Uppsala Universitet SWE. *Dist:* Coronet Bks.

Urea-Formaldehyde Resins. Beat Meyer. 1979. (Illus.). text (*0-201-04558-3*) Addison-Wesley.

Uremic Toxins. Ed. by S. Ringoir et al. 1987. LC 87-25936. (Illus.). 308p. 85.00 (*0-306-42771-0*, Plenum Trade) Perseus Pubng.

Ureter. Ed. by H. Bergman. 2nd ed. 1981. (Illus.). 780p. 250.00 (*0-387-90561-8*) Spr-Verlag.

Ureteroscopy. Jeffry Huffman et al. 1987. (Illus.). 200p. pap. text 69.00 (*0-7216-2148-1*) Saunders.

Urgent & Emergency Admissions to Hospital: The Report of a CSAG Committee. 1995. 96p. pap. (*0-11-321835-4*, HM18354) Statnry Office GBR. *Dist:* Bernan Associates.

Urgent Care in the Dental Office: An Essential Handbook. G. T. Terezhalmy & Levente G. Batizy. 1998. LC 97-36190. 264p. ring bd. 68.00 (*0-86715-323-7*) Quint Pub Co.

Urgent Care Medicine. Tanise Edwards & Thom Mayer. 2002. LC 2001-31616. (Illus.). 504p. pap. 79.00 (*0-07-022068-9*) McGraw-Hill Prof.

Urgent Endoscopy of Digestive & Abdominal Diseases: New Fields of Gastrointestinal Endoscopy. 1972. (Illus.). 260p. 108.00 (*3-8055-1349-6*) S Karger.

Urinalysis: Methods, Diagnostics, Influence of Sexually Transmitted Diseases & Abuse-Injury Implications. Shelly S. Scarre. 1995. LC 95-15409. 57.50 (*0-7883-0720-7*); pap. 47.50 (*0-7883-0721-5*) ABBE Pubs Assn.

Urinalysis & Body Fluids. Mobley. 1996. (Medical Lab Technician Ser.). pap., lab manual ed. 32.95 (*0-8273-5951-9*) Delmar.

Urinalysis & Body Fluids. Susan K. Strasinger. 3rd rev. ed. 1994. LC 94-18792. (Illus.). 233p. pap. 37.95 (*0-8036-8103-8*) Davis Co.

Urinalysis & Body Fluids: A Color Text & Atlas. Karen M. Ringsrud & Jean Jorgenson Linne. 1994. (Illus.). 272p. (gr. 13). pap. text 43.00 (*0-8016-7043-8*, 07043) Mosby Inc.

Urinary & Fecal Incontinence: Nursing Management. Ed. by Dorothy Beckley Doughty. 2nd ed. 2000. LC 99-40801. (Illus.). 456p. (C). text 41.95 (*0-8151-2912-2*, 31812) Mosby Inc.

Urinary & Fecal Incontinence: Nursing Management (IAET) Doughty. 1991. (Illus.). 296p. (C). (gr. 13). text 45.00 (*0-8016-1444-9*, 01444) Mosby Inc.

Urinary Calculi: Recent Advances in Aetiology, Stone Structure & Treatment, Proceedings of the Renal Stone Research Symposium, Madrid, Sept. 1972. Renal Stone Research Symposium Staff. Ed. by L. Cifuentes Delatte et al. 1974. (Illus.). 113.25 (*3-8055-1618-5*) S Karger.

Urinary Calculus: Proceedings of the International Urinary Stone Conference, Australia, 1979. International Urinary Stone Conference Staff et al. 1989. 518p. 59.50 (*0-88416-294-X*) Mosby Inc.

***Urinary Continence.** Shah & Leach. 2nd ed. 2000. (Fast Facts Ser.). (Illus.). 88p. pap. (*1-899541-64-0*) Health Pr GBR. *Dist:* JAMCO Dist.

Urinary Continence: Assessment & Promotion. Mary Palmer. 1996. 256p. pap. 48.00 (*0-8342-0747-8*, 20747) Aspen Pub.

Urinary Cytology: Manual & Atlas. P. Rathert et al. Tr. by Terry C. Telger from GER. 2nd rev. ed. 1992. LC 92-49568. (Illus.). 224p. 158.00 (*0-387-53312-5*) Spr-Verlag.

Urinary Cytology: Phase-Contrast Microscopy & Analysis of Stained Smears. H. J. De Voogt et al. 1977. (Illus.). 194p. 114.00 (*0-387-08042-2*) Spr-Verlag.

Urinary Cytopathology. William M. Murphy. 2000. (Illus.). 96p. 60.00 (*0-89189-445-4*) Am Soc Clinical.

Urinary Diversion. Ed. by M. H. Ashken. 1982. (Clinical Practice in Urology Ser.). (Illus.). 143p. 114.00 (*0-387-11273 1*) Spr-Verlag.

Urinary Enzymes in Clinical & Experimental Medicine. Ed. by K. Jung et al. 1992. (Illus.). 326p. 136.00 (*0-387-53188-2*) Spr-Verlag.

Urinary Incontinence. Ed. by James G. Malone-Lee & Adrian Wagg. 2000. (Illus.). 256p. pap. text (*1-900151-16-2*) Greenwich Med GBR. *Dist:* OUP.

Urinary Incontinence. Pat D. O'Donnell. 1997. LC 98-132082. (Illus.). 496p. (C). (gr. 13). text 84.95 (*0-8151-6517-X*, 26546) Mosby Inc.

Urinary Incontinence. Ed. by Adolphe Steg. 1993. (International Society of Urology Reports). (Illus.). 304p. text (*0-443-04643-3*) Church.

Urinary Incontinence & How to Overcome It. 1991. lib. bdg. 250.00 (*0-8490-5123-1*) Gordon Pr.

Urinary Incontinence in Adults. 1995. lib. bdg. 251.95 (*0-8490-6803-7*) Gordon Pr.

Urinary Incontinence in Adults: Clinical Practice Guideline. Ananias Diokno & Kathleen A. McCormick. 1997. (Illus.). 125p. (C). reprint ed. pap. text 30.00 (*0-7881-4612-2*) DIANE Pub.

Urinary Incontinence in Adults No. 2: Acute & Chronic. USPHS Staff. 1996. pap. 7.50 (*1-883205-26-3*) Intl Med Pub.

Urinary Incontinence in the Elderly: Pharmacotherapy Treatment. Ed. by James W. Cooper. 1997. LC 97-16252. (Journal of Geriatric Drug Therapy Ser.). 72p. 24.95 (*0-7890-0327-9*) Haworth Pr.

Urinary Incontinence in Women: A Guide for Women. Joseph Khoury. Ed. by G. D. Webster. 1997. (Urology Ser.). (Illus.). 32p. (Orig.). pap. text 2.95 (*1-885274-41-6*) Health InfoNet Inc.

Urinary Incontinence Sourcebook. Diane Newman & Mary K. Dzurinko. 1997. LC 97-6722. 368p. 32.00 (*1-56565-648-2*, 06482W) Lowell Hse.

Urinary Incontinence Sourcebook. Diane Kaschak Newman. rev. ed. 1999. LC 99-6722. (Illus.). 368p. pap. 19.95 (*0-7373-0261-5*, 02615W) NTC Contemp Pub Co.

Urinary Proteins. Ed. by L. Migone. 1981. (Contributions to Nephrology Ser.: Vol. 26). (Illus.). viii, 124p. pap. 29.75 (*3-8055-1848-X*) S Karger.

Urinary Sediment. Patrick C. Ward. 1992. (C). 410.00 incl. disk (*1-56815-009-1*) Mosby Inc.

Urinary Sediment: A Textbook Atlas. Meryl H. Haber. 1981. LC 81-4413. (Illus.). 126p. pap. 80.00 (*0-89189-103-X*); 158p. sl. 180.00 (*0-89189-106-4*) Am Soc Clinical.

Urinary Sediment: An Integrated View. G. B. Fogazzi et al. 1994. (Illus.). 160p. (*0-412-59300-9*) E A GBR. *Dist:* OUP.

***Urinary Sphincter.** Corcos & Schick. 2001. 225.00 (*0-8247-0477-0*) Dekker.

***Urinary Stones.** Tolley & Segura. 2002. (Fast Facts Ser.). (Illus.). 80p. pap. (*1-899541-09-8*) Health Pr GBR. *Dist:* JAMCO Dist.

Urinary System. Ed. by Ulrich Mohr et al. 1993. (Illus.). 56p. pap. text 30.00 (*92-832-0123-X*) OUP.

Urinary System. Ed. by Thomas C. Jones et al. 2nd ed. 1997. LC 97-25783. (Monographs in Pathology of Laboratory Animals). (Illus.). 483p. 284.00 (*3-540-61847-3*) Spr-Verlag.

Urinary System. Thomas C. Jones et al. 2nd ed. 1997. LC 97-25783. (Monographs on Pathology of Laboratory Animals). (*0-944398-76-6*) ILSI.

Urinary Tract Cancer: State of the Art: EORTC Data Center, Brussels, November 1995. Ed. by Louis Denis. 1997. (Journal: Vol. 31, Supplement 1, 1997). (Illus.). vi, 82p. pap. 69.75 (*3-8055-6466-X*) S Karger.

Urinary Tract Infection in Clinical & Laboratory Practice. Rosalind Maskell. 1988. (Illus.). 284p. (C). text (*0-683-13061-7*) E A GBR. *Dist:* Williams & Wilkins.

Urinary Tract Infections. Ed. by Tom Bergan. 1997. LC 97-2774. (Infectiology Ser.: Vol. 1, 1997). (Illus.). 142p. 97.50 (*3-8055-6440-6*) S Karger.

Urinary Tract Infections. Ed. by David Brooks. 1987. LC 87-4115. (Practical Clinical Medicine Ser.). (C). pap. text 73.50 (*0-85200-695-0*) Kluwer Academic.

Urinary Tract Infections. Ed. by Graeme R. Catto. 1989. (New Clinical Applications in Nephrology Ser.). (C). text 111.00 (*0-7462-0115-X*) Kluwer Academic.

***Urinary Tract Infections.** Hannan et al. 2002. (Fast Facts Ser.). (Illus.). 60p. pap. (*1-899541-26-8*) Health Pr GBR. *Dist:* JAMCO Dist.

Urinary Tract Infections. Ed. by F. Nordbring & L. G. Burman. 1981. (Illus.). 151p. (Orig.). pap. text 34.00 (*91-22-00455-6*) Coronet Bks.

Urinary Tract Infections: Detection, Prevention, & Management. Calvin M. Kunin. 5th ed. 1996. LC 96-26585. (Illus.). 400p. pap. 45.00 (*0-683-18102-5*) Lppncott W & W.

Urinary Tract Infections: Molecular Pathogenesis & Clinical Management. Ed. by Harry L. Mobley & John W. Warren. 1995. LC 95-24719. 99.95 (*1-55581-093-4*) ASM Pr.

Urinary Tract Infections & Infections of the Female Pelvis. Ed. by Gerald L. Mandell & Jack D. Sobel. 1997. LC 96-24706. (Atlas of Infectious Diseases Ser.: Vol. 9). (Illus.). 205p. text (*0-443-07770-3*) Church GBR. *Dist:* Saunders.

Urine - Therapy - It May Save Your Life. Beatrice Bartnett. 1992. 52p. (Orig.). pap. 5.90 (*0-9622182-3-5*) Lifestyle Inst.

Urine & Polymedicine: Guidebook with Bibiliography. Gwen V. Hassig. rev. ed. 1991. LC 87-47634. 160p. 44.50 (*1-55914-216-2*); pap. 39.50 (*1-55914-217-0*) ABBE Pubs Assn.

Urine Studies in Labs & Practice: Index of Modern Authors & Subjects with Guide for Rapid Research. Jerry C. Ewald. 1991. LC 90-56292. 160p. 47.50 (*1-55914-378-9*); pap. 44.50 (*1-55914-379-7*) ABBE Pubs Assn.

Urine-Therapy: It May Save Your Life. Beatrice Barnett. 7th rev. ed. 1992. 56p. pap. 9.95 (*0-9622182-5-1*) Lifestyle Inst.

Urine Therapy for AIDS & Cancer. 1991. lib. bdg. 250.00 (*0-8490-5032-4*) Gordon Pr.

Urinzytologie. 1995. 194.00 (*3-540-59248-2*) Spr-Verlag.

Urodynamic & Reconstructive Surgery: The Practice of Surgery. A. R. Mundy. 1993. (Illus.). 348p. text (*0-443-03348-X*) Church.

Urodynamics. Paul Abrams. 2nd ed. 1997. LC 96-51999. (Illus.). 356p. 105.00 (*3-540-19678-1*) Spr-Verlag.

Urodynamics: Principles, Practice & Application. Ed. by A. R. Mundy et al. 2nd ed. 1994. (Illus.). 542p. text (*0-443-04081-8*) Church.

Urodynamics & the Evaluation of Female Incontinence: A Practical Guide. Peter K. Sand & Donald R. Ostergard. 1995. LC 94-24640. 89.00 (*0-387-19904-7*) Spr-Verlag.

Urodynamics Made Easy. Christopher R. Chapple & Timothy J. Christmas. 1991. (Illus.). 92p. pap. text (*0-443-04356-6*) Church.

Urogenital Ageing. Ed. by B. Von Schoultz. 1994. (Illus.). 84p. 27.95 (*1-85070-537-2*, Parthenon Pbng) CRC Pr.

Urogenital Infections. Ed. by A. Bondi et al. 1988. LC 87-14209. (Advances in Experimental Medicine & Biology Ser.: Vol. 224). (Illus.). 146p. 65.00 (*0-306-42799-0*, Plenum Trade) Perseus Pubng.

Urogenital Manipulation. Jean-Pierre Barral. 1993. LC 93-72643. (Illus.). 249p. (C). text 48.00 (*0-939616-18-1*) Eastland.

Urogenital System. Thomas Braem. 1994. (Organs of the Human Anatomy: Vol. 9). 24p. (C). spiral bd. 12.95 (*1-878576-33-X*) Flash Anatomy Inc.

Urogynecologic Surgery. W. Glenn Hurt. 2nd ed. 2000. LC 99-86184. 224p. text 99.00 (*0-7817-1963-1*) Lppncott W & W.

Urogynecology. Cardozo. 1997. text (*0-443-05058-9*, C0827) Church.

Urogynecology: Diagnosis & Treatment of Female Incontinence. Ed. by Gretchen M. Lentz. 1997. LC 97-6755. 300p. pap. 85.00 (*0-412-06691-2*) Chapman & Hall.

Urogynecology & Reconstructive Pelvic Surgery. Ed. by Morton A. Stenchever & J. Thomas Benson. 2000. LC 99-33745. (Atlas of Clinical Gynecology Ser.: Vol. 5). (Illus.). 280p. text 185.00 (*0-8385-0320-9*) McGraw-Hill Prof.

Urogynecology & Urodynamics. Donald R. Ostergard & Alfred E. Bent. 3rd ed. 1991. (Illus.). 692p. 98.00 (*0-683-06647-1*) Lppncott W & W.

Urogynecology & Urodynamics: Theory & Practice. Ed. by Donald R. Ostergard & Alfred E. Bent. 4th ed. 1996. LC 95-47708. (Illus.). 726p. text 125.00 (*0-683-06648-X*) Lppncott W & W.

Urolithiasis. Donald Resnick & Charles Y. Pak. 1990. (Illus.). 352p. text 115.00 (*0-7216-2439-1*) Saunders.

Urolithiasis. Ed. by R. A. Sutton. 1987. (Journal: Vol. 13, No. 4, 1987). 96p. pap. 97.50 (*3-8055-4567-3*) S Karger.

Urolithiasis. Ed. by V. R. Walker et al. 1989. (Illus.). 1102p. 165.00 (*0-306-43249-8*, Plenum Trade) Perseus Pubng.

Urolithiasis 2: Proceedings of the International Symposium on Urolithiasis, 7th, Cairns, Australia, Held August 1992. R. Ryall et al. 1994. (Illus.). 726p. 165.00 (*0-306-44727-4*, Kluwer Plenum) Kluwer Academic.

Urologic Cancer. Marc S. Ernstoff. 1996. LC 96-34918. 215.00 (*0-86542-497-7*) Blackwell Sci.

Urologic Cancer. Ed. by Richard E. Peschel et al. 1995. 500p. (C). (*0-393-71029-7*, Norton Medical Bks) Norton.

Urologic Cancer: Chemotherapeutic Principles & Management. Ed. by F. M. Torti. 1983. (Recent Results in Cancer Research Ser.: Vol. 85). (Illus.). 151p. 76.00 (*0-387-12163-3*) Spr-Verlag.

Urologic Disorders. Jonathan I. Epstein. 1992. LC 91-35399. (Differential Diagnosis in Pathology Ser.). (Illus.). 208p. 89.00 (*0-89640-222-3*) Igaku-Shoin.

Urologic Endocrinology. Jacob Rajfer. 1986. (Illus.). 448p. text 115.00 (*0-7216-7426-7*) Saunders.

Urologic Endoscopy: A Manual & Atlas. Demetrius H. Bagley et al. 1985. 336p. 165.00 (*0-316-07518-3*, Little Brwn Med Div) Lppncott W & W.

Urologic Malignancies. Hamdy. 2001. (Illus.). 384p. (C). text 125.00 (*0-443-05478-9*) Harcrt Hlth Sci Grp.

Urologic Malignancies: Quality of Life Issues. Ed. by Emil A. Tanagho & P. R. Carroll. 1991. (Urologia Internationalis Ser.: Vol. 46, No. 3, 1991). (Illus.). 68p. pap. 69.75 (*3-8055-5399-4*) S Karger.

Urologic Oncology. Ed. by William J. Catalona & T. Ratliff. 1984. (Cancer Treatment & Research Ser.). text 187.00 (*0-89838-628-4*) Kluwer Academic.

Urologic Oncology. Ed. by Herbert Lepor & William L. McGuire. 1989. (Cancer Treatment & Research Ser.). (C). text 174.00 (*0-7923-0161-7*) Kluwer Academic.

Urologic Oncology. Joseph E. Oesterling & Jerome Richie. Ed. by Richard Zorab. 1997. LC 96-41702. 864p. text 165.00 (*0-7216-6347-8*) Saunders.

Urologic Prostheses: The Complete Practical Guide to Devices, Their Implantation & Patient Followup. Ed. by Culley C. Carson, III. 2001. LC 2001-24826. (Current Clinical Urology Ser.). 328p. 125.00 (*0-89603-894-7*) Humana.

Urologic Surgery. James F. Glenn. 5th ed. 1998. LC 98-5457. 1,184p. text 225.00 (*0-397-58737-6*) Lppncott W & W.

Urologic Surgery in Infants & Children. Lowell R. King. Ed. by Stephanie Donley. 1997. LC 97-4118. (Illus.). 320p. text 130.00 (*0-7216-6857-7*) Saunders.

Urologic Surgery in Neonates & Young Infants. Lowell King. 1989. (Illus.). 432p. text 125.00 (*0-7216-2370-0*) Saunders.

Urologic Surgical Pathology. Young. Ed. by David G. Bostwick & John N. Eble. 1996. (Illus.). 800p. (C). (gr. 13). text 250.00 (*0-8016-7503-0*, 05572) Mosby Inc.

Urological Complications in Gynecological Surgery & Radiotherapy. J. Kunz. 1984. (Contributions to Gynecology & Obstetrics Ser.: Vol. 11). (Illus.). viii, 220p. 117.50 (*3-8055-3759-X*) S Karger.

Urological Disease in the Fetus & Infant: Diagnosis & Management. D. F. Thomas. 1997. LC 97-26049. 352p. text (*0-7506-0768-8*) E A GBR. *Dist:* OUP.

Urological Nursing. Fillingham. 2nd ed. 1997. pap. text (*0-7020-2303-5*) Bailliere Tindall.

Urological Pathology. William M. Murphy. Ed. by Leslie Day. 2nd ed. 1997. LC 96-46546. 656p. text 195.00 (*0-7216-6029-0*) Saunders.

Urological Pathology: Based on the Proceedings of the Sixtieth Annual Anatomic Pathology Slide Seminar of the American Society of Clinical Pathologists: October 27 & 28, 1994, Washington, DC. Contrib. by William M. Murphy et al. 1995. 112p. 40.00 (*0-89189-393-8*) Am Soc Clinical.

Urological Prostheses, Appliances & Catheters. Ed. by J. P. Pryor & Geoffrey D. Chisholm. 1992. (Clinical Practice in Urology Ser.). (Illus.). 288p. 196.00 (*0-387-17490-7*) Spr-Verlag.

Urological Radiology: Radiological Diagnosis of Urological Diseases: Plain Film, Sonography, Angiography, CT, & MRI. Ed. by Eberhard Lohr & Klaus Sievers. 1995. LC 94-34633. (Illus.). 256p. text 89.00 (*0-88937-131-8*) Hogrefe & Huber Pubs.

Urology: A Core Textbook. Stephen N. Rous. 2nd ed. 1996. LC 95-39429. (Illus.). 365p. pap. 54.95 (*0-86542-493-4*) Blackwell Sci.

Urology: Core Textbook. Stephen N. Rous. Date not set. pap. (*0-393-71033-5*) Norton.

Urology: From Antiquity to the 20th Century. Leonard P. Wershub. 1970. LC 71-78017. (Illus.). 320p. 18.70 (*0-87527-086-7*) Green.

Urology: Illustrated Case Histories. Helen Parkhouse & Krishna Sethia. 1995. 92p. (gr. 13). (*0-7234-2234-6*) Wolfe Publishing GBR. *Dist:* Mosby Inc.

Urology & Nephrology: An Internet Resource Guide. Ed. by Dan Goldenson. 2001. pap. 24.95 (*0-9700525-3-7*) eMedguides.

Urology & Oncology. Waxman. 1992. 100.00 (*0-340-54926-2*) Trafalgar.

Urology & Reproduction. Elizabeth K. White. 3rd ed. 1993. LC 92-48863. (Regents - Prentice-Hall Medical Assistant Kit Ser.). pap. 23.09 (*0-13-035676-X*) P-H.

Urology & the Male Reproductive System. 2nd ed. 1984. (Medical Ser.). (Illus.). (C). 12.95 (*0-935920-17-X*, Ntl Pubs Blck) P-H.

Urology Annual, 1991, Vol. 5. Stephen N. Rous. 1990. (Illus.). 288p. (C). pap. text 95.00 (*0-8385-9323-2*, A9323-5, Apple Lange Med) McGraw.

Urology Annual, 1997, Vol. 11. Ed. by Stephen N. Rous. 1997. (Illus.). 321p. 125.00 (*0-86542-567-1*) Blackwell Sci.

Urology Annual 1996, Vol. 10. Stephen N. Rous. 1996. 368p. 95.00 (*0-86542-488-8*) Blackwell Sci.

Urology Annual 1996, Vol. 10. Stephen N. Rous. Date not set. (*0-393-71034-3*) Norton.

Urology for Primary Care Physicians. Unyime Nseyo et al. Ed. by Stephanie Donley. 1999. LC 98-40584. (Illus.). 365p. (C). text (*0-7216-7148-9*) Saunders.

Urology for the House Officer. Michael Macfarlane. 1988. (House Officer Ser.). (Illus.). 300p. (Orig.). (C). pap. 20.00 (*0-683-05324-8*) Lppncott W & W.

***Urology Highlights 2000-2001.** Shah. 2001. (Fast Facts Ser.). (Illus.). 92p. pap. (*1-899541-79-9*) Health Pr GBR. *Dist:* JAMCO Dist.

Urology in Childhood, Vol. 15. Ed. by C. E. Alken et al. 1958. (Illus.). 353p. 144.00 (*0-387-02303-8*) Spr-Verlag.

Urology in Childhood, Vol. 15, Supplement. D. I. Williams et al. Ed. by C. E. Alken et al. 1974. (Illus.). 458p. 118.00 (*0-387-06406-0*) Spr-Verlag.

Urology Office Manual. Neil H. Baum. 1994. (Office Manual Ser.). 200p. 145.00 (*1-890018-04-X*) Anadem Pubng.

Urology Pearls. Ed. by Martin I. Resnick & Anthony Schaeffer. 1999. LC 99-32134. (Pearls Ser.). (Illus.). 250p. pap. 45.00 (*1-56053-351-X*) Hanley & Belfus.

Urology Secrets. Ed. by Martin I. Resnick & Andrew Novick. 2nd ed. 1999. LC 99-24451. (Secrets Ser.). (Illus.). 300p. pap. 39.95 (*1-56053-320-X*) Hanley & Belfus.

Uropathology Ed. by Gary S. Hill. 1989. (Illus.). 1427p. text (*0-443-08194-8*) Church.

Urticaria: Clinical, Diagnostic & Therapeutic Aspects. Ed. by B. M. Henz et al. 1997. LC 97-20558. (Illus.). 210p. 70.00 (*3-540-62973-4*) Spr-Verlag.

U.S. & Canadian Medical Schools: A Comprehensive Guide to All 159 Accredited Medical Schools. Peterson's Guides Staff. 4th ed. 1999. 254p. pap. text 24.95 (*0-7689-0285-1*) Petersons.

Us Four: A Senator, His Family, Their Brain-injured Child. Marion Menning. 1986. (Illus.). 160p. pap. (*0-9615632-0-6*) Alpha Pub MN.

***U. S. Health Law & Policy, 2001: A Guide to the Current Literature.** Donald H. Caldwell. 2nd ed. 2001. LC 00-54593. (Jossey-Bass Health Ser.). 624p. 100.00 (*0-7879-5504-3*) Jossey-Bass.

Usage Prudent de la Vitamine A. J. Christopher Bauernfeind. Ed. by G. Arroyave et al. Tr. by Marc Vincent. 1984. (FRE., Illus.). 77p. (Orig.). pap. text 3.50 (*0-935368-39-6*) ILSI.

Use & Abuse of Biology: An Anthropological Critique of Sociobiology. Marshall D. Sahlins. 1976. 136p. pap. text 15.95 (*0-472-76600-7*, 76600) U of Mich Pr.

Use & Abuse of Medicine. Marten DeVries et al. 1982. LC 82-7563. 296p. 78.75 (*0-275-91362-7*, C1362, Praeger Pubs) Greenwood.

Use & Approval of Antihypertensive Agents & Surrogate Endpoints for the Approval of Drugs Affecting Antiarrhythmic Heart Failure & Hypolipidemia: Proceedings of the Tenth Annual Symposium on New Drugs & Devices, Oct. 31-Nov. 1, 1989. Ed. by Joel Morganroth & E. Neil Moore. 1990. (C). text 133.50 (*0-7923-0756-9*) Kluwer Academic.

Use & Impact of Computers in Clinical Medicine. Ed. by J. G. Anderson & S. J. Jay. 1986. (Computers & Medicine Ser.). (Illus.). 362p. 63.95 (*0-387-96362-6*) Spr-Verlag.

Use & Standardization of Chemically Defined Antigens. Ed. by W. Hennessen & Girish N. Vyas. 1986. (Developments in Biological Standardization Ser.: Vol. 63). (Illus.). viii, 176p. pap. 61.00 (*3-8055-4280-1*) S Karger.

Use & Standardization of Combined Vaccines. Ed. by A. L. Van Wezel & W. Hennessen. 1987. (Developments in Biological Standardization Ser.: Vol. 65). (Illus.). viii, 288p. 61.00 (*3-8055-4461-8*) S Karger.

Use & Usefulness of the ICIDH for Health Professions (Nursing, Physical Therapy, Speech Therapy, Occupational Therapy, Chiropody & Orthoptics) 1996. (*92-871-3004-3*) Council of Europe FRA. *Dist:* Manhattan Pub Co.

Use of ACE Inhibitors in General Practice. George Strube & Gillian Strube. 1992. 128p. text 45.50 (*0-7923-8963-8*) Kluwer Academic.

Use of Animal Models for Research in Human Nutrition. Ed. by Anton C. Beynen & C. E. West. 1989. (Comparative Animal Nutrition Ser.: Vol. 6). (Illus.). v, 190p. 146.25 (*3-8055-4802-8*) S Karger.

Use of Antibiotics: A Clinical Review of Antibacterial, Antifungal & Antiviral Drugs. A Kucers et al. 5th ed. 1997. LC 97-21384. (Illus.). 1968p. (*0-7506-0155-8*) E A GBR. *Dist:* OUP.

Use of Anticonvulsants in Psychiatry: Recent Advances. Post et al. Ed. by Pope. 1988. LC 88-60779. 192p. 22.50 (*0-945986-00-9*) Health Care NJ.

Use of Applicable Biotechnological Methods for Diagnosing Haemoparasites. Ed. by G. Uilenberg & A. Permin. 1994. 188p. pap. (*92-5-103503-2*, F35032) FAO ITA. *Dist:* Bernan Associates.

Use of Calcium Antagonists in Cardiology: Proceedings of the 1st International Symposium on Tiapamil, Lausanne, April 1981. B. N. Singh. 1982. (Journal: Vol. 69, Suppl. 1, 1982). (Illus.). xii, 242p. pap. 65.25 (*3-8055-3588-0*) S Karger.

Use of Cannabis: Proceedings of the WHO Scientific Group, Geneva, 1970. WHO Staff. 1971. (Technical Reports: No. 478). pap. text 5.00 (*92-4-120478-8*, 1100478) World Health.

Use of Ceramics in Surgical Implants. S. F. Hulbert & F. A. Young, Jr. 1978. LC 73-99078. viii, 270p. text 262.00 (*0-677-13870-9*) Gordon & Breach.

Use of Ciprofloxacin in the Treatment of Chronic Otitis & Sinusitis & Malignant External Otitis. Ed. by F. Legent. 1994. (Journal: Vol. 40, Suppl. 1, 1994). (Illus.). iv, 42p. pap. 14.00 (*3-8055-6071-0*) S Karger.

Use of Computers & Statistics in Toxicology, Vol. 10. Ed. by M. J. Ord et al. 1985. 102p. 32.00 (*0-85066-977-4*) Taylor & Francis.

Use of Computers in General Practice. John F. Preece. 2nd ed. 1989. (Illus.). 256p. pap. text (*0-443-04258-6*) Church.

Use of Computers in General Practice. Preece. 3rd ed. 1994. pap. text 38.00 (*0-443-04938-6*) Saunders.

Use of Computers in Radiation Therapy: XIIIth International Conference, Heidelberg, Germany May 22-25, 2000. Ed. by Wolfgang Schlegel & Thomas Bortfeld. 2000. 500p. pap. 99.00 (*3-540-67176-5*) Spr-Verlag.

Use of Epidemiology in Local Health Planning: A Training Manual. Axel Kroeger et al. LC 96-36126. 192p. 1997. (*1-85649-481-0*); 1996. pap. (*1-85649-482-9*) Zed Books GBR. *Dist:* St Martin.

Use of Essential Drugs: Model List of Essential Drugs (Eighth List) Sixth Report of the WHO Expert Committee. 1995. (Technical Reports: No. 850). (FRE & SPA.). iv, 138p. (C). pap. text 21.00 (*92-4-120850-3*, 1100850) World Health.

Use of Essential Drugs: Model List of Essential Drugs Fourth Report of the WHO Expert Committee. 1990. (Technical Reports: No. 796). 57p. pap. text 8.00 (*92-4-120796-5*, 1100796) World Health.

Use of Essential Drugs Model List of Essential Drugs (9th List) Seventh Report of the WHO Expert Committee. WHO Staff. 1997. (Technical Report Ser.: No. 867). 80p. 13.50 (*92-4-120867-8*) World Health.

Use of Essential Drugs (The) Model List of Essential Drugs (Fifth List) Third Report of the WHO Expert Committee. WHO Staff. 1988. (Technical Report Ser.: No. 770). 63p. 8.00 (*92-4-120770-1*) World Health.

Use of Factory Statistics in the Investigation of Industrial Fatigue. Philip S. Florence. LC 76-76627. (Columbia University. Studies in the Social Sciences: No. 190). reprint ed. 39.50 (*0-404-51190-2*) AMS Pr.

Use of Fungi As Food & in Food Processing, Pt. 2. William D. Gray. 1973. (Monotopic Reprint Ser.). 22.00 (*0-8493-0118-1*, CRC Reprint) Franklin.

Use of Group Services in Permanency Planning for Children. Ed. by Sylvia Morris. 1983. LC 82-23389. (Social Work with Groups Ser.: Vol. 5, No. 4). 109p. text 32.95 (*0-86656-199-4*) Haworth Pr.

Use of Growth Factors in Cancer Therapy. 1995. lib. bdg. 250.99 (*0-8490-7582-3*); 1994. lib. bdg. 258.95 (*0-8490-8525-X*) Gordon Pr.

Use of Health Service Facilities in Medical Education: Sixteenth Report of the WHO Expert Committee on Professional & Technical Education of Medical & Auxiliary Personnel. 1967. (Technical Report Ser.: No. 355). 65p. pap. text 5.00 (*92-4-120355-2*, 1100355) World Health.

Use of Herbal Remedies in Two Haitian Communities & Implications for Health-Care Providers Worldwide. Richbe C. Zamor. 2001. LC 00-53718. (Studies in Health & Human Services: Vol. 40). (Illus.). 204p. 89.95 (*0-7734-7488-9*) E Mellen.

Use of Heteroploid & Other Cell Substrates for the Production of Biologicals. Ed. by W. Hennessen. 1982. (Developments in Biological Standardization Ser.: Vol. 50). (Illus.). x, 402p. pap. 61.00 (*3-8055-3472-8*) S Karger.

Use of Human Immunoglobulin. 1966. (Technical Report Ser.: No. 327). 29p. pap. text 3.00 (*92-4-120327-7*) World Health.

Use of Human Tissues & Organs for Therapeutic Purposes: A Survey of Existing Legislation. 1969. (International Digest of Health Legislation Offprints: Vol. 20, No. 1). pap. text 5.00 (*92-4-169201-4*, 1956901) World Health.

Use of Humor in Psychotherapy. Herbert S. Strean. 1994. LC 93-25547. 248p. pap. 35.00 (*1-56821-084-1*) Aronson.

Use of Hypnosis in Surgery & Anesthesiology: Psychological Preparation of the Surgical Patient. Lillian E. Fredericks. 2000. LC 00-60769. (Illus.). xxv, 240p. 58.95 (*0-398-07128-4*) C C Thomas.

Use of Hypnosis in Surgery & Anesthesiology: Psychological Preparation of the Surgical Patient. Lillian E. Fredericks & Frederick J. Evans. 2000. LC 00-60769. xxv, 240p. pap. 38.95 (*0-398-07129-2*) C C Thomas.

Use of Interpretation in Treatment: Technique & Art. Ed. by Emanuel F. Hammer. 1993. LC 93-30193. 392p. pap. 50.00 (*1-56821-111-2*) Aronson.

Use of Language in Clinical Practice Guidelines. 1995. (Medical Ser.). lib. bdg. 253.99 (*0-8490-6840-1*) Gordon Pr.

Use of Longer-Acting Agents in Cardiac Therapy: Recent Advances. Abrams et al. Ed. by Stanley B. Garbus. 1989. 25.00 (*0-945986-11-4*) Health Care NJ.

Use of Medical Evidence: Low-Back Permanent Partial Disability Claims in Maryland. Leslie I. Boden. 1986. 60p. (Orig.). pap. 35.00 (*0-935149-02-3*, SP-86-1) Workers Comp Res Inst.

Use of Medical Evidence: Low-Back Permanent Partial Disability Claims in New Jersey. Leslie I. Boden. 1987. LC 87-31628. 35.00 (*0-935149-07-4*, WC-87-2) Workers Comp Res Inst.

Use of Mercury & Alternative Compounds As Seed Dressings: Report of the FAO-WHO Meeting, Geneva, 1974. FAO-WHO Meeting Staff. 1974. (Technical Reports: No. 555). pap. text 5.00 (*92-4-120555-5*, 1100555) World Health.

Use of Microphysiological Recordings During Stereotactic Neurosurgery Journal: Stereotactic & Functional Neurosurgery, 1989, Vol. 52, No. 2-4. Ed. by P. L. Gildenberg et al. 1989. (Illus.). 200p. pap. 91.50 (*3-8055-5039-1*) S Karger.

Use of Multi-State Life Tables in Estimating Places for Biomedical & Behavioral Scientists: A Technical Paper. National Research Council Staff. 1997. LC 98-102273. 42p. (C). pap. text 10.00 (*0-309-05794-9*) Natl Acad Pr.

Use of Neuroleptics in Children. Ed. by Mary A. Richardson & Gary Haugland. 1995. (Clinical Practice Ser.: No. 37). 256p. text 36.00 (*0-88048-475-6*, 8475) Am Psychiatric.

Use of Physicians' Services by Low-Income Children. Margo L. Rosenbach. 1993. LC 92-48901. (Children of Poverty Ser.). 200p. text 15.00 (*0-8153-1113-3*) Garland.

Use of Projective Techniques with Persons with Mental Retardation: A Guide for Assessment Instrument Selection. Paul E. Panek. 1997. LC 96-53508. (Illus.). 188p. text 47.95 (*0-398-06756-2*); pap. text 35.95 (*0-398-06757-0*) C C Thomas.

Use of Psychological Testing for Treatment Planning & Outcome Assessment. Ed. by Mark E. Maruish. 2nd ed. 1999. LC 98-34838. (Illus.). xvi, 1507p. 250.00 (*0-8058-2761-7*) L Erlbaum Assocs.

Use of Psychotropic Drugs in the Medically Ill. Ed. by G. A. Fava & H. Freyberger. 1988. (Journal: Vol. 49, No. 2, 1988). (Illus.). 80p. pap. 48.75 (*3-8055-4927-X*) S Karger.

Use of Public Attitude Assessment in the Development of Emergency Service Policy for the City of Austin, Texas. William E. Coll et al. 1989. (Special Project Reports: Vol. SP-UP). 218p. pap. 10.00 (*0-89940-865-6*) LBJ Sch Pub Aff.

Use of Quinolones in Travel Medicine: Second Conference on International Travel Medicine. Ed. by H. L. DuPont. 1992. (Illus.). 56p. 21.95 (*0-387-54778-9*) Spr-Verlag.

Use of Resealed Erthrocytes As Carriers & Bioreactors. M. Magnani & J. R. DeLoach. 1993. (Advances in Experimental Medicine & Biology Ser.: Vol. 326). (Illus.). 357p. (C). text 110.00 (*0-306-44345-7*, Kluwer Plenum) Kluwer Academic.

Use of Restricted Significance Tests in Clinical Trials. D. Salsburg & Stephen E. Fienberg. Ed. by J. O. Berger et al. 1992. (Series in Statistics in the Health Sciences). (Illus.). 173p. 74.95 (*0-387-97798-8*) Spr-Verlag.

Use of Science & Technology in Service to Children in Courts. Contrib. by Michael Edmond Donnelly. Date not set. LC 97-38842. (*0-8204-1385-2*) P Lang Pubng.

***Use of Seclusion & Restraints in Mental Hospitals: Hearing Before the Committee on Finance, U. S. Senate.** Ed. by William V. Roth, Jr. 2001. (Illus.). 156p. (C). reprint ed. pap. text 30.00 (*0-7567-1625-X*) DIANE Pub.

Use of Self in Therapy. Virginia M. Satir & Michele Baldwin. 1987. LC 87-90. (Journal of Psychotherapy & the Family Ser.: Vol. 3, No. 1). 155p. (Orig.). text 39.95 (*0-86656-544-2*); pap. text 19.95 (*0-86656-545-0*) Haworth Pr.

Use of Self in Therapy. Ed. by Michele Baldwin. 2nd abr. ed. 2000. LC 99-36719. xxv, 293p. 49.95 (*0-7890-0744-4*); pap. 24.95 (*0-7890-0745-2*) Haworth Pr.

Use of Synthetic Antigens for Diagnosis of Infectious Diseases: Report of a WHO Scientific Group, 1987. 1989. (Technical Report Ser.: No. 784). 74p. pap. text 9.00 (*92-4-120784-1*, 1100784) World Health.

Use of Technology in the Care of the Elderly & the Disabled. Ed. by Jean Bray & Sheila Wright. 1980. LC 80-17847. 267p. 68.00 (*0-313-22616-4*, BTC/, Greenwood Pr) Greenwood.

Use of the Body in Relation to the Mind. George Moore. LC 78-72812. reprint ed. 32.50 (*0-404-60882-5*) AMS Pr.

Use of the Eyes in Movement. Jack Heggie. 1985. 54p. (Orig.). pap. 9.95 (*0-939866-03-X*) Woodstone Bks.

Use of the International Classification of Impairments, Disabilities & Handicaps (ICIDH) in Mental Health. Council of Europe Staff. 1991. (*92-871-1939-2*) Council of Europe FRA. *Dist:* Manhattan Pub Co.

Use of the International Classification of Impairments, Disabilities & Handicaps (ICIDH) in Rehabilitation. Council of Europe Staff. 1989. (*92-871-1767-5*) Council of Europe FRA. *Dist:* Manhattan Pub Co.

Use of the International Classification of Impairments, Disabilities & Handicaps (ICIDH) in the Assessment of Technical Aids. Council of Europe Staff. 1992. (*92-871-2137-0*) Council of Europe FRA. *Dist:* Manhattan Pub Co.

Use of the Physical & Social Environment of the General Hospital for Therapeutic Purposes, Pt. 1. Esther L. Brown. 1961. 160p. pap. 16.50 (*0-87154-183-1*) Russell Sage.

Use of the Self: Countertransference & Communication in the Analytic Situation. Theodore Jacobs. 1991. LC 90-4926. 224p. 35.00 (*0-8236-6710-3*) Intl Univs Pr.

Use of the Telephone in Psychotherapy. Joyce K. Aronson. 2000. LC 00-41618. xxxvi, 468p. 45.00 (*0-7657-0268-1*) Aronson.

Use of Time & Resources by Provisioned Troops of Monkeys: Social Behaviour, Time & Energy in the Barbary Macaque (Macaca Sylanus L.) at Gibraltar. John E. Fa. 1986. (Contributions to Primatology Ser.: Vol. 23). (Illus.). xii, 380p. 150.50 (*3-8055-4263-1*) S Karger.

Use of Viruses for the Control of Insect Pests & Disease Vectors: Report of the FAO-WHO Meeting on Insect Viruses, Geneva, 1972. FAO-WHO Meeting on Insect Viruses Staff. 1973. (Technical Reports: No. 531). pap. text 4.00 (*92-4-120531-8*, 1100531) World Health.

Use of X-Ray Diffraction in the Study of Protein & Nucleic Acid Structure. K. C. Holmes & D. M. Blow. Ed. by David Glick. rev. ed. 1979. LC 79-20293. 132p. lib. bdg. 15.00 (*0-89874-046-0*) Krieger.

Useful & Harmful Interactions of Antibiotics. M. Neuman. 1985. LC 84-1607. 288p. 164.00 (*0-8493-6061-7*, CRC Reprint) Franklin.

Useful Information on Alzheimer's Disease: Diagnosis, Causes, Treatment & Research. 1991. lib. bdg. 65.00 (*0-8490-4336-0*) Gordon Pr.

Useful Servants: Psychodynamic Theories from a Clinical Perspective. Susan Levine. 1996. LC 96-12695. 320p. 40.00 (*1-56821-844-3*) Aronson.

Useful Spanish for Medical & Hospital Personnel. Francesco Cordasco. 1977. 146p. pap. 14.95 (*1-879170-62-0*) St Aedans Pr & Bk.

User Acceptance of Health Telematics Applications: Looking for Convincing Cases. Ed. by I. Iakovidis et al. 1998. LC 98-73205. (Studies in Health Technology & Informatics: Vol. 56). 189p. 79.00 (*90-5199-415-X*) IOS Press.

User Education in Health Sciences Libraries: A Reader. Ed. by M. Sandra Wood. 1995. LC 95-30629. (Illus.). 298p. (C). pap. text 14.95 (*1-56024-995-1*); lib. bdg. 39.95 (*1-56024-964-1*) Haworth Pr.

User Precision Performance of Clinical Chemistry Devices: Tentative Guideline, Vol. 4. National Committee for Clinical Laboratory Standards. 2nd ed. 1992. 85.00 (*1-56238-145-8*, EP5-T2) NCCLS.

Users & Abusers of Psychiatry: A Critical Look at Traditional Psychiatric Practice. Lucy Johnstone. 1989. 288p. 45.00 (*0-415-02839-6*) Routledge.

User's Guide to a Better Bod: "Wisdom for Facing the Trials of Creating a Healthier, Happier You" Jo Elder & M. I. Wiser. 1993. LC 92-21172. (Illus.). 160p. pap. 6.50 (*0-941361-96-9*) One More Pr.

User's Guide to Bypass Surgery. Ted Klein. 1996. LC 95-48908. (Illus.). 170p. (Orig.). pap. 14.95 (*0-8214-1143-8*) Ohio U Pr.

User's Guide to Community Entry for the Severely Handicapped. Ed. by Ernest Pancsofar & Robert Blackwell. 1985. LC 84-24139. (SUNY Series in Special Education). 182p. (C). pap. text 21.95 (*0-88706-035-8*) State U NY Pr.

User's Guide to Deleuze & Guattari's Capitalism & Schizophrenia. Brian Massumi. 1992. LC 91-30392. 236p. 26.95 (*0-262-13282-6*); pap. text 13.95 (*0-262-63143-1*) MIT Pr.

***Users' Guides to the Medical Literature: Essentials of Evidence-Based Clinical Practice.** 2001. 512p. 34.95 incl. cd-rom (*1-57947-191-9*, OP740001BKG) AMA.

User's Manual for Conducting Child Nutrition Surveys in Developing Countries. CFNPP Staff & Victoria Quinn. 1992. (Working Papers). (C). pap. text 7.00 (*1-56401-121-6*) Cornell Food.

User's Resource to Accompany Management in Healthcare. Marreel-McLellan. 1999. 96p. tchr. ed. 17.95 (*0-7668-1256-1*) Delmar.

Uses & Abuses of Air: Showing Its Influence in Sustaining Life & Producing Disease. John H. Griscom. 1972. LC 79-125743. (American Environmental Studies). reprint ed. 19.95 (*0-405-02668-4*) Ayer.

Uses & Actions of 1,25 Dihyroxyvitamin D3 in Uremia. Ed. by Shaul G. Massry & J. W. Coburn. 1980. (Contributions to Nephrology Ser.: Vol. 18). (Illus.). x, 218p. 29.75 (*3-8055-3064-1*) S Karger.

Uses of Elemental Diets in Clinical Situations. Ed. by Gustavo Bounous. 1992. LC 87-24283. 352p. 235.00 (*0-8493-6680-1*, RM229, CRC Reprint) Franklin.

Uses of Epidemiology in Housing Programmes & in Planning Human Settlements: Proceedings of the WHO Expert Committee on Housing & Health, Geneva, 1972. WHO Staff. 1974. (Technical Reports: No. 544). pap. text 6.00 (*92-4-120544-X*, 1100544) World Health.

Uses of Epidemiology in the Study of the Elderly. 1984. (Technical Report Ser.: No. 706). 84p. pap. text 10.00 (*92-4-120706-X*) World Health.

Uses of Health Systems Research. C. Taylor. 1984. (Public Health Papers: No. 78). 49p. pap. text 9.00 (*92-4-130078-7*, 1110078) World Health.

Uses of Psychiatry in the Law: A Clinical View of Forensic Psychiatry. Walter Bromberg. 1979. LC 78-22724. (Illus.). 442p. 75.00 (*0-89930-000-6*, BRP/, Quorum Bks) Greenwood.

Uses of Water in Health & Disease: A Practical Treatise on the Bath, Its History & Uses. J. H. Kellogg. 1998. LC 97-60504. 154 p. 7.95 (*1-57258-085-2*) TEACH Servs.

Uses of Writing in Psychotherapy. Ed. by Patricia Kelley. 1990. LC 89-26938. (Journal of Independent Social Work: Vol. 4, No. 2). 160p. (C). text 39.95 (*0-86656-967-7*) Haworth Pr.

Usher's Syndrome: What It Is, How to Cope, & How to Help. Earlene Duncan et al. 1988. (Illus.). 106p. (C). text 36.95 (*0-398-05481-9*) C C Thomas.

Using & Conducting Nursing Research in the Clinical Setting. Magdalena A. Mateo & Karin T. Kirchhoff. Ed. by Thomas Eoyang. 2nd ed. 1999. LC 98-4260. (Illus.). 392p. (C). text 44.00 (*0-7216-7165-9*) Saunders.

Using & Understanding Medical Statistics. D. E. Matthews & Vernon T. Farewell. 3rd rev. ed. 1996. LC 96-1017. (Illus.). xiv, 246p. pap. 35.00 (*3-8055-6276-4*) S Karger.

Using Antibodies: A Laboratory Manual. Ed Harlow & David Lane. 1998. LC 98-42802. (Illus.). 512p. (C). text 230.00 (*0-87969-543-9*); pap. text 135.00 (*0-87969-544-7*) Cold Spring Harbor.

Using Books in Clinical Social Work Practice: A Guide to Bibliotherapy. John T. Pardeck. 1997. LC 97-30713. 157p. (C). 29.95 (*0-7890-0120-9*); pap. 19.95 (*0-7890-0430-5*) Haworth Pr.

Using Clinical Practice Guidelines to Evaluate Quality of Care: Issues & Methods, Set. 1995. (Illus.). 166p. (Orig.). (C). pap. text 40.00 (*0-7881-2474-9*) DIANE Pub.

Using Cognitive Approaches with the Seriously Mentally Ill: Dialogue Across the Barrier. Barbara A. Olevitch. 1995. LC 95-6348. 184p. 62.50 (*0-275-95244-4*, Praeger Pubs) Greenwood.

Using Computers in Clinical Practice: Psychotherapy & Mental Health Applications. Ed. by Marc D. Schwartz. 1984. LC 83-18648. 510p. text 15.95 (*0-86656-208-7*) Haworth Pr.

Using CPT for Cardiothoracic Reimbursement: A Manual for Surgeons & Insurance Billing Specialists. Ed. by Sidney Levitsky & Jeanne T. Fitzgerald. 1990. 105p. (Orig.). 25.00 (*0-9626174-0-7*) Soc Thor Surgeons.

Using Designed Experiments to Shrink Healthcare Costs. M. Daniel Sloan. 1997. LC 96-17217. (Illus.). 215p. pap. 40.00 (*0-87389-367-0*, H0931) ASQ Qual Pr.

Using Drawings in Assessment & Therapy: A Guide for Mental Health Professionals. Gerald D. Oster & Patricia Gould. 1987. LC 86-30958. (Illus.). 208p. pap. text 31.95 (*0-87630-478-1*) Brunner-Routledge.

Using DSM-IV: A Clinician's Guide to Psychiatric Diagnosis. Anthony L. LaBruzza. 1996. LC 97-117198. 472p. pap. 45.00 (*0-7657-0053-0*) Aronson.

Using DSM-IV: A Clinician's Guide to Psychiatric Diagnosis. Anthony L. Labruzza & Jose M. Mendez-Villarrubia. 1995. LC 94-28534. (Illus.). 459p. 60.00 (*1-56821-333-6*) Aronson.

Using Groups to Help People. Dorothy Stock Whitaker. 1987. (International Library of Philosophy, Psychology, & Scientific Method). 448p. (C). pap. 31.95 (*0-415-04283-6*) Routledge.

Using Herbs: Choose the Best Manufactured Products, Understand Herb Supplement Labels, Design Your Own Herbal Program. annuals Logan V. Chamberlain. 1998. LC 98-8457. (Illus.). 96p. pap. 9.95 (*1-883010-49-7*) Interweave.

Using Imagery to Develop Memory. Michael T. Bagley. 1987. 118p. pap. 9.99 (*0-89824-040-9*) Trillium Pr.

Using MDS Quality Indicators to Improve Outcomes. Marilyn J. Rantz & Lori L. Popejoy. 1998. LC 97-32677. 200p. spiral bd. 62.00 (*0-8342-1047-9*, 10479) Aspen Pub.

Using Metaphors in Psychotherapy. Philip Barker. 1992. LC 85-15171. 236p. pap. text 28.95 (*0-87630-716-0*) Brunner-Routledge.

Using Nursing Case Management to Improve Health Outcomes: Recasting Theory, Tools & Care Delivery. Michael Newell. 1995. 304p. 79.00 (*0-8342-0623-4*, 20623) Aspen Pub.

Using Nursing Research: Process, Critical Evaluation & Utilization. Patricia Ann Dempsey & Arthur D. Dempsey. 5th ed. 1999. LC 99-16519. 384p. pap. text 34.95 (*0-7817-1790-6*) Lppncott W & W.

Using Outplacement Services Effectively. Marilyn M. Kennedy. Ed. by Wesley Curry. 1991. LC 91-75795. 20p. (Orig.). (C). pap. text 5.95 (*0-924674-11-3*) Am Coll Phys Execs.

Using Performance Measurement to Improve Outcomes in Ambulatory Care. Joint Commission on Accreditation of Healthcare Organizations. 1999. (Illus.). 171p. pap. 49.00 (*0-86688-603-6*, ACPM-50) Joint Comm Hlthcare.

Using Performance Measurement to Improve Outcomes in Home Care & Hospice Settings. Joint Commission on Accreditation of Healthcare Organizations. 1999. (Illus.). 172p. pap. 50.00 (*0-86688-573-0*, HCPM-50) Joint Comm Hlthcare.

Using Projective Techniques with Children: A Guide to Clinical Assessment. Louis A. Chandler & Virginia J. Johnson. 1991. (Illus.). 140p. (C). text 36.95 (*0-398-05726-5*) C C Thomas.

Using Psychosocial Counselling Techniques in Primary Health Care. Ellen Jespersen & P. F. Pegg. 1988. 230p. text 72.95 (*0-566-05463-9*) Ashgate Pub Co.

Using Qualitative Methods in Psychology. Mary Kopala & Lisa A. Suzuki. 1999. LC 98-25463. 54.95 (*0-7619-1036-0*, 81481); pap. 27.95 (*0-7619-1037-9*, 81482) Sage.

Using Qualitative Research: A Practical Introduction for Occupational & Physical Therapists. Karen Whalley Hammell et al. 2000. LC 99-38187. viii, 125p. (*0-443-06232-3*) Church.

Using Race & Culture in Counseling & Psychotherapy: Theory & Process. Janet E. Helms & Donelda A. Cook. 1998. LC 98-36029. 374p. (C). 75.00 (*0-205-28565-1*) Allyn.

Using Rational-Emotive Therapy Effectively: A Practitioner's Guide. M. E. Bernard. 1991. (Illus.). 366p. (C). 102.00 (*0-306-43754-6*); pap. 42.50 (*0-306-43755-4*) Perseus Pubng (Plenum Trade).

Using REBT with Common Psychological Problems: A Therapist's Casebook. Ed. by Joseph Yankura & Windy Dryden. 1997. LC 97-14148. (Illus.). 264p. pap. 33.95 (*0-8261-9800-7*) Springer Pub.

Using Research for Effective Health Promotion. Sandy Oliver & Greet Peersman. 2001. LC 00-65245. 176p. (*0-335-20870-3*) OpUniv Pr GBR. *Dist:* Taylor & Francis.

Using Self Psychology in Psychotherapy. Ed. by Helene Jackson. 1994. LC 90-1236. 296p. pap. 40.00 (*1-56821-044-2*) Aronson.

***Using Statistics in Psychological Research.** Kathryn M. LaFontana. 3rd ed. 2000. 246p. pap. 33.44 (*0-07-245283-8*) McGrw-H Primis Cstm.

Using Strategic & Tactical Planning to Make Your Veterinary Practice More Profitable. Brian M. Hayden. 1999. LC 99-59473. 108p. pap. (*1-58326-019-6*) Am Animal Hosp Assoc.

Using the Appropriateness Method in Clinical Practice Guideline Development. Paul G. Shekelle & David L. Schriger. 1995. 85p. (Orig.). pap. text 13.00 (*0-8330-1458-7*, MR-233-AHCPR) Rand Corp.

Using the Arts & Humanities to Teach Nursing: A Creative Approach. Theresa M. Valiga & Elizabeth R. Bruderle. 1997. LC 96-26797. (Teaching of Nursing Ser.). (Illus.). 320p. 41.95 (*0-8261-9420-6*) Springer Pub.

Using the Bodies of the Dead: Legal, Ethical & Organisational Dimensions of Organ Transplantation. Nora Machado. 1998. LC 98-19209. 264p. 74.95 (*1-85521-973-5*) Ashgate Pub Co.

***Using the Civil Society Index - Assessing the Health of Civil Society: A Handbook for Using the Civicus Index on Civil Society as a Self-Assessment Tool.** Richard Holloway. 2001. 80p. pap. 5.00 (*1-929842-08-2*) CIVICUS.

Using the Creative Arts in Therapy: A Practical Introduction. Ed. by Bernie Warren. 2nd ed. 1993. LC 92-48527. (Illus.). 208p. (C). pap. 27.95 (*0-415-08814-3*, B0886) Routledge.

Using the ECG to Detect MI: CE Booklet. Julia Ann Purcell. 2000. 28p. pap. text 39.95 (*0-7817-1899-6*) Lppncott W & W.

Using the Library to Find Out about Parapsychology. Rhea A. White. 1989. 40p. (Orig.). pap. 5.00 (*0-944446-16-7*) EHE Network.

Using Your Medicines Wisely: A Passport to Good Health Care. 1990. lib. bdg. 75.00 (*0-8490-3999-1*) Gordon Pr.

USMLE Behavioral Science Made Ridiculously Simple. Frederick S. Sierles. 1998. (Illus.). 171p. (Orig.). pap. text 16.95 (*0-940780-34-8*) MedMaster.

USMLE Board Certification Review: Steps 2 & 3. D. Kanjilal. 1999. LC 99-26612. 149.00 (*1-58141-035-2*) Rivercross Pub.

USMLE Pharmacology Review Book. Hobart Walling. Ed. by Mauricio Waintrub. 1999. (USMLE Ser.). (Illus.). 260p. lib. bdg. 18.00 (*1-884083-86-2*) Maval Pub.

USMLE Step 1: The Study Guide. Joel S. Goldberg. 1996. LC 95-41811. (USMLE Step 1 Review Ser.). (Illus.). 473p. pap., stu. ed. 39.95 (*0-8039-7284-9*, 8388) Sage.

USMLE Step 1: United States Medical Licensing Examination. Jonathan Cargan et al. 1998. LC 97-67179. 1200p. pap. 39.95 (*0-87891-074-3*) Res & Educ.

USMLE Step 1 Basic Sciences Simulated Test 1, Vol. 1. Hobart Walling et al. Ed. & Illus. by Maria Luder. 1999. (USMLE Ser.). 120p. (C). pap. text 18.00 (*1-884083-18-8*) Maval Pub.

USMLE Step 1 Basic Sciences Simulated Test 2, Vol. 2. Valentin A. Waintrub & Mauricio L. Waintrub. Ed. by Maria Luder. 1999. (USMLE Ser.). (Illus.). 180p. (C). lib. bdg. 18.00 (*1-884083-19-6*) Maval Pub.

USMLE Step 1 Quickie. 1998. pap. 19.95 (*0-9654687-4-7*) Emrani Publns.

USMLE Step 1 Recall: Buzzwords for the Boards. Brent A. Reinheimer. 1999. 304p. pap. text 29.95 (*0-683-30639-1*); 2nd ed. LC 98-55690. 136p. pap. text 17.95 (*0-683-30713-4*) Lppncott W & W.

***USMLE Step 1 Recall PDA.** Brent A. Reinheimer. 2002. 29.00 (*0-7817-3343-X*) Lppncott W & W.

USMLE Step 3: United States Medical Licensing Examination. Rose S. Fife et al. 1999. LC 98-66567. 1008p. pap. 39.95 (*0-87891-076-X*) Res & Educ.

USMLE Step 2: United States Medical Licensing Examination. Rose S. Fife et al. 1998. LC 98-66565. 1200p. pap. 39.95 (*0-87891-075-1*) Res & Educ.

USMLE Step 2 Starter Kit. Kaplan Educational Consultants Staff. 1999. (Illus.). 208p. (C). pap. 29.95 (*0-8385-8666-X*, A-8666-8) Appleton & Lange.

USMLE Success. FMSG, Inc. Staff & Stanley Zaslau. 4th rev. ed. 1999. (Illus.). 280p. (C). pap. text, wbk. ed. 20.00 (*1-886468-30-3*) FMSG.

USP Vol. I: Drug Information for the Healthcare Professional. Medical Economics Staff & U. S. Pharmacopeia Staff. Ed. by T. A. Hutchinson. 20th rev. ed. 2000. (Usp Di Ser.: Vol. 1). (Illus.). 3548p. 135.00 (*1-56363-331-0*) Med Econ.

USP DI Vol. 2: Advice of the Patient. Medical Economics Staff & U. S. Pharmacopeia Staff. Ed. by T. A. Hutchinson. 20th rev. ed. 2000. (Illus.). 1666p. 75.00 (*1-56363-332-9*) Med Econ.

USP DI Vol. 3: Approved Drug Products & Legal Requirements. Medical Economics Staff & U. S. Pharmacopeia Staff. Ed. by T. A. Hutchinson. 20th rev. ed. 2000. (Usp Di Ser.: Vol. 3). 1480p. 120.00 (*1-56363-333-7*) Med Econ.

***USP DI Desktop Series 2002.** Medical Economics Co. Staff & Micromedex Staff. 2002. cd-rom 199.00 (*1-56363-408-2*) Med Econ.

***USP DI 2002: Approved Drug Produces & Legal Requirements.** Medical Economics Co. Staff. rev. ed. 2002. (Illus.). 145.00 (*1-56363-407-4*) Med Econ.

***USP DI 2002: Drug Information for the Helthcare Professional.** Medical Economics Co. Staff. 2002. (Illus.). reprint ed. 164.00 (*1-56363-405-8*) Med Econ.

***USP DI 2002 Vol. II: Advice for the Patient. Drug Information in Lay Language.** Medical Economics Co. Staff. rev. ed. 2002. (Illus.). 88.00 (*1-56363-406-6*) Med Econ.

USP Guide to Heart Medicines: U. S. Pharmacopeia. U. S. Pharmacopeia Staff. 1996. (Illus.). (Orig.). pap. 6.99 (*0-380-78094-1*, Avon Bks) Morrow Avon.

USP Guide to Medicines. U. S. Pharmacopeia Staff. 1996. LC 95-94723. pap. 6.99 (*0-380-78092-5*, Avon Bks) Morrow Avon.

USP Guide to Vitamins & Minerals. Contrib. by U. S. Pharmacopeia Staff. 1996. LC 95-94914. pap. 6.99 (*0-380-78093-3*, Avon Bks) Morrow Avon.

USP Pill Book of Prescription Drugs, Bk. 1. U. S. Pharmacopeia Staff. 1994. (Orig.). pap. (*0-446-60032-6*) Warner Bks.

USSF Sports Medicine Book of Soccer. Ed. by William E. Garrett, Jr. et al. 1996. LC 96-1088. (Illus.). 512p. 55.00 (*0-683-18249-8*) Lppncott W & W.

Utah Guide to Alternative Health Care. Lisa Kingsbury & Cam Williams. Ed. by Connie Adler & Mary Kingsbury. 1996. 300p. pap. 14.95 (*0-9653267-0-5*) S L C Pubns.

Utah Health Care in Perspective 2000. Ed. by Kathleen O'Leary Morgan & Scott E. Morgan. 2000. 21p. spiral bd. 19.00 (*0-7401-0243-5*) Morgan Quitno Corp.

Utah Health Care Perspective, 1998. Ed. by Kathleen O'Leary Morgan & Scott E. Morgan. 1998. 20p. pap. 19.00 (*1-56692-843-5*) Morgan Quitno Corp.

Uterine & Embryonic Factors in Early Pregnancy. Ed. by Jerome F. Strauss, III & C. R. Lyttle. 1991. (Reproductive Biology Ser.). (Illus.). 312p. (C). text 114.00 (*0-306-44042-3*, Kluwer Plenum) Kluwer Academic.

Uterine Artery Embolization: A Systematic Review of the Literature & Proposal for Research. Michael S. Broder et al. 2000. 58p. (C). pap. 6.00 (*0-8330-2808-1*, MR-1158-CIRREF) Rand Corp.

Uterine Contractility: Mechanisms of Control. Ed. by Robert E. Garfield. 1990. (Serono Symposia, U. S. A. Ser.). (Illus.). 400p. (C). text 70.00 (*1-878601-05-9*) Serono Symposia USA.

Uterine Fibroids: What Every Woman Needs to Know. Nelson H. Stringer. 1996. LC 96-69941. (Illus.). 130p. (Orig.). pap. 17.95 (*0-924428-10-4*) Phys Sci Pub.

Uterine Function: Molecular & Cellular Aspects. M. E. Carsten & J. D. Miller. 1990. LC 90-6882. (Illus.). 628p. (C). text 169.50 (*0-306-43446-6*, Kluwer Plenum) Kluwer Academic.

Uterine Natural Killer Cells. Ed. by Anne Croy. 1997. (Journal: Vol. 15, No. 1, 1996-97). (Illus.). 70p. pap. 26.25 (*3-8055-6395-7*) S Karger.

Uterus. Ed. by T. Chard & J. Gedes Grudzinskas. 1995. (Cambridge Reviews in Human Reproduction Ser.). (Illus.). 399p. (C). pap. text 34.95 (*0-521-42453-4*) Cambridge U Pr.

Uterus: Endometrium & Myometrium. Ed. by Carlo Bulletti et al. 1997. LC 97-18287. (Annals of the New York Academy of Sciences Ser.). pap. 110.00 (*1-57331-105-7*); 368p. 110.00 (*1-57331-104-9*) NY Acad Sci.

Uterus: Pathology, Diagnosis & Management. Ed. by A. Altcheck et al. 1991. (Clinical Perspectives in Obstetrics & Gynecology Ser.). (Illus.). 446p. 161.00 (*0-387-97422-9*) Spr-Verlag.

Utilization Case Management. Olga Cotera. 1997. 121p. spiral bd. 110.00 (*1-879575-77-9*) Acad Med Sys.

Utilization Management: A Handbook for Psychiatrists. APA Committee on Managed Care. 1992. LC 91-47117. 65p. pap. text 9.95 (*0-89042-235-4*, 2235) Am Psychiatric.

Utilization Management & Capitation Strategies. Margaret D. Bischel. 1998. (Illus.). 413p. ring bd. 225.00 (*1-893826-07-4*) Apollo Managed.

Utilization of Classroom Peers As Behavior Change Agents. Ed. by Phillip S. Strain. 1981. (Applied Clinical Psychology Ser.). 376p. 65.00 (*0-306-40618-7*, Plenum Trade) Perseus Pubng.

UV-B Radiation & Immunosuppression. Frances P. Noonan. 1996. (Medical Intelligence Unit Ser.). 250p. 89.95 (*0-412-11611-1*) Chapman & Hall.

UV Curing: Science & Technology. Ed. by S. Peter Pappas. 1978. LC 78-56293. (Illus.). per. 95.00 (*0-936840-04-8*) Tech Marketing.

Uvea. N. A. Rao et al. 1992. (Textbook of Ophthalmology Ser.). 256p. (gr. 13). text (*1-56375-084-8*) Gower-Mosby.

Uveitis. Ed. by Susan Lightman & Hamish Towler. 1998. 176p. text (*0-7279-1202-X*) BMJ Pub GBR. *Dist:* AIDC.

Uveitis: A Clinical Approach to Diagnosis & Management. Ronald E. Smith & Robert A. Nozik. 2nd ed. 1988. (Illus.). 288p. 87.00 (*0-683-07769-4*) Lppncott W & W.

Uveitis: A Clinical Manual for Ocular Inflammation. E. Mitchel Opremack. 1994. LC 94-13826. (Illus.). 278p. 181.00 (*0-387-94247-5*) Spr-Verlag.

***Uveitis: An Illustrated Manual.** Nicholas P. Jones. 2001. (Illus.). 376p. pap. 69.95 (*0-7506-5463-5*) Buttrwrth-Heinemann.

Uveitis: An Illustrated Manual. Nicholas P. Jones. 1998. LC 98-28349. 392p. text 100.00 (*0-7506-3230-5*) Buttrwrth-Heinemann.

Uveitis: Fundamentals & Clinical Practice. Robert B. Nussenblatt et al. 2nd ed. 1995. (Illus.). 432p. (C). (gr. 13). text 118.00 (*0-8151-6446-7*, 23708) Mosby Inc.

***Uveitis in the Third Millennium: Proceedings of the Fifth International Symposium on Uveitis Held in Buenos Aires on 26-29 March 2000.** Ed. by Emilio M. Dodds & Cristobal A. Couto. 2000. LC 2001-23271. (International Congress Ser.: Vol. 1204). 338p. 129.50 (*0-444-50521-0*, Excerpta Medica) Elsevier.

Uveitis Scoring System. R. B. Nussenblatt et al. 1991. (Illus.). 20p. 20.00 (*0-387-54957-9*) Spr-Verlag.

Uveitis Today: Proceedings of the Fourth International Symposium on Uveitis, Held in Yokohama, Japan, 10-14 October, 1997. Shigeaki Ohno. 1998. LC 98-18044. 346p. 138.50 (*0-444-82983-0*) Elsevier.

Uveitis Update. Ed. by D. BenEzra. 1999. LC 99-40686. (Developments in Ophthalmology Ser.: Vol. 31). (Illus.). viii, 190p. 165.25 (*3-8055-6891-6*) S Karger.

V

V. A. Innovations in Ambulatory Care. Ed. by Ronald Goldman. 1998. 235p. (C). pap. text 40.00 (*0-7881-4670-X*) DIANE Pub.

V. M. Bekhterev's Collective Reflexology. Ed. by L. H. Strickland & E. Lockwood. 1993. 257p. lib. bdg. 125.00 (*1-56072-142-1*) Nova Sci Pubs.

VA & Defense Health Care: Evolving Health Care Systems Require Rethinking of Resource Sharing Strategies. Ed. by Ann Calvaresi-Barr & Karyn Papineau. 2000. (Illus.). 56p. (C). pap. text 20.00 (*0-7567-0301-8*) DIANE Pub.

VA Health Care: Albuquerque Medical Center Not Recovering Full Costs of Lithotripsy Services. 1995. (Illus.). 50p. (Orig.). (C). pap. text 30.00 (*0-7881-2240-1*) DIANE Pub.

VA Health Care: Effects of Facility Realignment on Construction Needs Are Unknown. 1996. (Illus.). 43p. (Orig.). (C). pap. text 25.00 (*0-7881-3229-6*) DIANE Pub.

VA Health Care: Issues Affecting Eligibility Reform Efforts. 1996. (Illus.). 148p. (Orig.). (C). pap. text 35.00 (*0-7881-3591-0*) DIANE Pub.

VA Health Care: Need for Brevard Hospital Not Justified. 1996. (Illus.). 60p. reprint ed. pap. text 20.00 (*0-7881-3206-7*) DIANE Pub.

VA Health Care: Opportunities for Service Delivery Efficiencies Within Existing Resources. 1996. (Illus.). 64p. (Orig.). (C). pap. text 25.00 (*0-7881-3459-0*) DIANE Pub.

VA Health Care: Retargeting Needed to Better Meet Veterans' Changing Needs. 1995. (Illus.). 72p. (Orig.). (C). pap. text 25.00 (*0-7881-1816-1*) DIANE Pub.

VA Healthcare: More Veterans Are Being Served, But Better Oversight Is Needed. Bruce D. Layton & James C. Musselwhite. 2000. (Illus.). 58p. (C). reprint ed. pap. text 20.00 (*0-7881-8716-3*) DIANE Pub.

***VA Research: Protections for Human Subjects Need to Be Strengthened.** Cynthia A. Bascetta. 2001. 56p. (C). pap. text 20.00 (*0-7567-1321-8*) DIANE Pub.

VA (Veterans Administration) Health Care: Comparison of VA Benefits with Other Public & Private Programs. 1994. (Illus.). 89p. (Orig.). (C). pap. text 30.00 (*0-7881-0197-8*) DIANE Pub.

VA (Veterans Administration) Health Care: Variabilities in Outpatient Care, Eligibility & Rationing Decisions. 1994. (Illus.). 56p. (Orig.). (C). pap. text 30.00 (*0-7881-0216-8*) DIANE Pub.

Vaccination: A Natural Approach. Ed. by Christine Murphy. 2001. 96p. pap. 20.00 (*1-930051-10-7*) Lantern Books.

Vaccination Against Smallpox. Edward Jenner. 1996. LC 96-7788. (Great Minds Ser.). 91p. pap. text 7.00 (*1-57392-064-9*) Prometheus Bks.

Vaccination Against Tuberculosis. 1980. (Technical Report Ser.: No. 651). 21p. pap. text 2.00 (*92-4-120651-9*) World Health.

Vaccination & Control of Aujeszky's Disease. Ed. by J. T. Van Oirschot. 1989. (Current Topics in Veterinary Medicine & Animal Science Ser.). (C). text 160.00 (*0-7923-0184-6*) Kluwer Academic.

Vaccination & Immunisation: Dangers, Delusions & Alternatives (What Every Parent Should Know) Leon Chaitow. 5th ed. 192p. pap. 20.95 (*0-8464-4308-2*) Beekman Pubs.

Vaccination, Social Violence & Criminality: The Medical Assault on the American Brain. Harris L. Coulter. 1990. LC 90-7991. 300p. (Orig.). 25.00 (*1-55643-103-1*); pap. 14.95 (*1-55643-084-1*) Ctr Emp Med.

Vaccination Strategies of Tropical Diseases. Ed. by F. Y. Liew. 1989. 320p. 206.00 (*0-8493-6189-3*, RC119) CRC Pr.

Vaccinations: A Thoughtful Parent's Guide - How to Make Safe, Sensible Decisions about the Risks, Benefits, & Alternatives. Aviva Jill Romm. 2001. LC 2001-24673. (Illus.). 288p. pap. 16.95 (*0-89281-931-6*, Heal Arts VT) Inner Tradit.

Vaccinations & Immune Malfunction. Harold E. Buttram & John C. Hoffman. 3rd ed. 1987. 75p. (Orig.). pap. 4.00 (*0-916285-36-7*) Humanitarian.

Vaccine Adjuvants: Immunological & Clinical Principles. Charles Hackett & Donald A. Harn, Jr. Date not set. (Infectious Disease Ser.). 500p. (*0-89603-892-0*) Humana.

Vaccine Adjuvants: Preparation Methods & Research Protocols. Ed. by Derek T. O'Hagan. 2000. LC 99-88373. (Methods in Molecular Medicine Ser.: Vol. 42). 352p. 99.50 (*0-89603-735-5*) Humana.

Vaccine & Serum Evils. Herbert M. Shelton. 1996. 46p. reprint ed. spiral bd. 9.00 (*0-7873-0784-X*) Hlth Research.

Vaccine Design: The Role of Cytokine Networks. Ed. by Gregory Gregoriadis et al. 1998. LC 98-12983. (NATO Advanced Science Institutes Ser.: No. 293). (Illus.). 220p. (C). text 107.00 (*0-306-45818-7*, Kluwer Plenum) Kluwer Academic.

Vaccine Design: The Subunit & Adjuvant Approach. Ed. by Michael F. Powell & Mark J. Newman. 1995. LC 95-16401. (Pharmaceutical Biotechnology Ser.: Vol. 6). (Illus.). 994p. (C). text 165.00 (*0-306-44867-X*, Kluwer Plenum) Kluwer Academic.

Vaccine Guide: Making an Informed Choice. Randall Neustaedter. 2nd ed. 1996. LC 95-48308. Orig. Title: The Immunization Decision. (Illus.). 250p. (Orig.). pap. 16.95 (*1-55643-215-1*) North Atlantic.

Vaccine Manual. Noel Mowat & Mark Rweyemamu. 1997. LC 98-224049. (Animal Production & Health Ser.: No. 35). 434p. pap. (*92-5-103774-4*, F37744) FAO ITA. *Dist:* Bernan Associates.

Vaccine Research & Development, Vol. 1. Ed. by Wayne C. Koff & Howard R. Six. 1992. (Illus.). 264p. text 175.00 (*0-8247-8619-X*) Dekker.

Vaccine Supply & Innovation. Institute of Medicine Staff. 1985. 210p. pap. text 21.00 (*0-309-03544-9*) Natl Acad Pr.

Vaccines. Stanley A. Plotkin & Edward A. Mortimer, Jr. 2nd ed. 1994. LC 93-10761. (Illus.). 1024p. reprint ed. text 185.00 (*0-7216-6584-5*) Saunders.

Vaccines. Stanley A. Plotkin & Walter A. Orenstein. Ed. by Richard Zorab. 3rd ed. 1999. LC 98-31650. 1055p. (C). text 287.25 (*0-7216-7443-7*) Saunders.

Vaccines: Are They Really Safe & Effective? Neil Z. Miller. 10th rev. ed. 2001. LC 92-81105. (Illus.). 80p. pap. 8.95 (*1-881217-10-8*) New Atlantean.

Vaccines: New Advances in Technologies & Applications. Ed. by Rebecca Ostriker. 1996. (Biomedical Library). 356p. pap. 795.00 (*1-57936-013-0*) Drug & Market Dev.

Vaccines: New Generation Immunological Adjuvants: Proceedings of a NATO ASI Held in Cape Sounion, Greece, June 24-July 5, 1994. Ed. by Gregory Gregoriadis et al. 1996. (NATO ASI Ser.: Vol. 282). (Illus.). 200p. 85.00 (*0-306-45283-9*) Plenum.

Vaccines: Recent Trends & Progress. Ed. by Gregory Gregoriadis et al. 1991. (NATO Advanced Science Institutes Ser.: Vol. 215). (Illus.). 168p. (C). text 102.00 (*0-306-44044-X*, Kluwer Plenum) Kluwer Academic.

Vaccines Vol. II: New Advances in Technologies & Applications. 1997. (Biomedical Library). pap. (*1-57936-033-5*) Drug & Market Dev.

***Vaccines - Finding the Balance Between Public Safety & Personal Choice: Congressional Hearing.** Ed. by Dan Burton. 2001. 313p. reprint ed. pap. text 45.00 (*0-7567-1813-9*) DIANE Pub.

Vaccines Against Virally Induced Cancers: Symposium No. 187. CIBA Foundation Staff. 1995. LC 94-33207. (CIBA Foundation Symposia Ser.: Vol. 187). 292p. 128.00 (*0-471-95026-2*) Wiley.

Vaccines & Immunotherapy. Ed. by S. J. Cryz. 1991. 496p. text 94.50 (*0-07-105380-8*) McGraw-Hill Med Pub.

Vaccines & Immunotherapy. S. J. Cryz. 1991. (Illus.). 448p. (*0-08-036083-1*) PPI GBR. *Dist:* McGraw.

Vaccines & World Health: Science, Policy & Practice. Paul F. Basch. 1994. LC 93-23283. (Illus.). 288p. text 49.95 (*0-19-508532-9*) OUP.

Vaccines Are Dangerous: A Warning to the Black Community. Curtis Cost. 1992. 160p. pap. text 9.95 (*1-881316-08-4*) A&B Bks.

Vaccines 88, New Chemical & Genetic Approaches to Vaccination: Prevention of Aids & Other Viral, Bacterial & Parasitic Diseases. Ed. by Robert Chanock et al. 1987. LC 87-13175. (Vaccines Ser.). (Illus.). 460p. pap. text 95.00 (*0-87969-310-X*) Cold Spring Harbor.

Vaccines, '85: Molecular & Chemical Basis of Resistance to Parasitic, Bacterial & Viral Diseases. Ed. by Richard A. Lerner et al. 1985. LC 84-29372. 407p. (Orig.). pap. 75.00 (*0-87969-181-6*) Cold Spring Harbor.

Vaccines, '89: Modern Approaches to New Vaccines Including the Prevention of AIDS. Ed. by Richard A. Lerner et al. 1989. (Illus.). 425p. pap. 100.00 (*0-87969-323-1*) Cold Spring Harbor.

Vaccines, '86: New Approaches to Immunization—Developing Vaccines Against Parasitic, Bacterial & Viral Diseases. Ed. by Fred Brown et al. 1986. LC 86-2589. 418p. (Orig.). pap. 75.00 (*0-87969-190-5*) Cold Spring Harbor.

Vaccines for Children Program: A Critique. Robert Goldberg. 1995. LC 96-177554. 50p. (Orig.). pap. 9.95 (*0-8447-7052-3*) Am Enterprise.

Vaccines for the 21st Century: A Tool for Decision-Making. Division of Health Promotion and Disease Prevention & Institute of Medicine Staff. Ed. by Kathleen R. Stratton et al. 2001. LC 00-25528. (Illus.). xi, 460p. (C). 49.95 (*0-309-05646-2*) Natl Acad Pr.

Vaccines for Vet Applications. Ed. by A. R. Peters. 1993. (Illus.). 304p. 115.00 (*0-7506-1126-X*) Buttrwrth-Heinemann.

Vaccines, from Concept to Clinic: A Guide to the Development & Clinical Testing of Vaccines for Human Use. Lawrence C. Paoletti & Pamela M. McInnes. 1998. LC 98-21739. 224p. 109.95 (*0-8493-1168-3*) CRC Pr.

Vaccines, 1992: Modern Approaches to New Vaccines Including Prevention of AIDS. Ed. by Fred Brown et al. 1992. (Illus.). 400p. (C). text 100.00 (*0-87969-405-X*) Cold Spring Harbor.

Vaccines, '90: Modern Approaches to New Vaccines Including Prevention of AIDS. Ed. by Fred Brown et al. 1990. (Illus.). 528p. pap. 100.00 (*0-87969-341-X*) Cold Spring Harbor.

Vaccines, '91: Modern Approaches to New Vaccines Including Prevention of AIDS. Ed. by Robert M. Chanock et al. 1991. (Illus.). 425p. pap. text 85.00 (*0-87969-367-3*) Cold Spring Harbor.

Vaccines, '97: Molecular Approaches to the Control of Infectious Diseases. Ed. by Fred Brown et al. 1997. (Illus.). 367p. (C). pap. text 100.00 (*0-87969-516-1*) Cold Spring Harbor.

Vaccinia, Vaccination, Vaccinology: Jenner, Pasteur & Their Successors. Ed. by S. A. Plotkin & B. Fantini. 1996. 380p. pap. 76.00 (*2-906077-83-6*) Elsevier.

Vacuum Extraction. Vacca. 1992. 35.00 (*0-340-54849-5*) Trafalgar.

Vacuum Extraction in Modern Obstetric Practice: Instruments, Operations, Risks & Benefits. J. P. O'Grady et al. 1995. LC 94-49184. (Illus.). 154p. lib. bdg. 30.95 (*1-85070-665-4*, Parthenon Pbng) CRC Pr.

Vademecum Clinique du Medecin Praticien. Vittorio Fattorusso. 14th ed. 1995. (FRE.). 1760p. 185.00 (*0-7859-9766-0*) Fr & Eur.

Vademecum de la Patologia Infecciosa de las Aves Domesticas. Pastor E. Zarzuelo. 1982. 356p. 55.00 (*0-8288-2392-8*, S39832) Fr & Eur.

Vademecum du Veterinaire: Therapeutique, Pharmacologie et Hygiene. A. Brion. 14th ed. 1984. 816p. 39.95 (*0-8288-1793-6*) Fr & Eur.

Vademecum Encyclopedique du Medecin Praticien: Encyclopedic Vademecum of Medical Practice. H. Dousset. 9th ed. 1980. 1266p. 110.00 (*0-8288-1801-0*, M15580) Fr & Eur.

Vademecum fuer Pilzfreunde: Taschenbuch Zur Bequemen Bestimmung Aller in Mittel-Europa Vorkommenden Ansehnlichen Pilzkoerper. A. Ricken. 1969. reprint ed. 24.00 (*3-7682-0603-3*) Lubrecht & Cramer.

Vademecum International, 1997: Especialidades Farmaceutica. 1997. 1700p. 295.00 (*0-7859-9486-6*) Fr & Eur.

Vademecum of Antibiotics: Vadecum de los Antibioticos. Newman. 1981. (SPA.). pap. 19.95 (*0-8288-4681-2*, S34979) Fr & Eur.

Vademecum of Pharmacology: Vademecum de Pharmacie. Paul Schiltz & Colette Schlitz. 17th ed. 1985. (FRE.). 882p. 42.50 (*0-8288-1827-4*, M6820) Fr & Eur.

Vademekum Fuer Den Pharmazeuten. Rudolf Schmidt-Wetter. 39.95 (*0-8288-7982-6*, M7138); 10th ed. (GER.). 39.95 (*3-7948-0066-4*, M-7138) Fr & Eur.

Vagal Control of the Heart Vol. 7: Experimental Basis & Clinical Implications, No. 7. Ed. by Peter J. Schwartz & Matthew N. Levy. 1993. LC 93-23821. (Bakken Research Center Ser.). (Illus.). 644p. 115.00 (*0-87993-561-8*) Futura Pub.

Vagina: An Owner's Manual. Judson P. Cone. 1974. 87p. (Orig.). pap. 1.95 (*0-89074-007-0*) Charing Cross.

Vaginal Birth after Cesarean: The Smart Women's Guide to VBAC. Elizabeth Kaufmann. 1996. LC 96-16960. (Illus.). 224p. (Orig.). pap. 12.95 (*0-89793-202-1*) Hunter Hse.

Vaginal Birth after Cesarean (VBAC) Experience: Birth Stories by Parents & Professionals. Lynn B. Richards et al. 1987. LC 87-15107. (Illus.). 304p. pap. 22.95 (*0-89789-120-1*, Bergin & Garvey) Greenwood.

***Vaginal Hysterectomy.** Sheth & Studd. 2001. (Illus.). 336p. (*1-901865-43-6*) Isis Med GBR. *Dist:* Bks Intl VA.

Vaginal Surgery. David H. Nichols & Clyde L. Randall. 3rd ed. 1989. (Illus.). 480p. 89.00 (*0-683-06494-0*) Lppncott W & W.

Vaginal Surgery. David H. Nicholas & Clyde L. Randall. 4th ed. 1996. LC 95-17805. (Illus.). 520p. 129.00 (*0-683-06491-6*) Lppncott W & W.

Vaginal Therapeutics Education Course. Competence Assurance Systems Staff. 1984. (Illus.). pap. text 55.00 (*0-89147-110-3*) CAS.

Vaginale Hysterektomie und Inkontinenz-Operationen. Ed. by H. A. Hirsch. 1979. (Gynaekologische Rundschau Journal: Supplement 1, Vol. 19). (Illus.). 36.75 (*3-8055-3072-2*) S Karger.

Vaginalmykose und Perinatale Pilzinfektion. J. D. Schnell. 1982. (Illus.). x, 142p. 57.50 (*3-8055-2854-X*) S Karger.

Valerian: The Relaxing & Sleep Herb. Christopher Hobbs. Ed. by Michael Miour. 1993. (Illus.). 53p. pap. 5.95 (*0-9618470-9-3*) Botanica CA.

Validate Your Pain! Exposing the Chronic Pain Cover-Up. Allan F. Chino & Corinne D. Davis. 2000. LC 97-65268. 391p. pap. 19.95 (*0-9673439-2-5*) InSync Commn.

Validation Breakthrough: Simple Techniques for Communicating with People with "Alzheimer's-Type Dementia" Naomi Feil. 1993. LC 93-4077. 356p. (Orig.). (C). pap. 22.95 (*1-878812-11-4*) Hlth Prof Pr.

Validation for Medical Device & Diagnostic Manufacturers. Carol DeSain & Charmaine V. Sutton. 2nd ed. 1997. LC 97-31031. 192.00 (*1-57491-063-9*) IHS Health Grp.

Validation Fundamentals: How to, What to, When to Validate. William Gibson & Keith Powell-Evans. 1998. LC 98-12065. (Illus.). 170p. 139.00 (*1-57491-070-1*) IHS Health Grp.

Validation in Blood Establishments & Transfusion Services. Ed. by Sallie M. Holliman. 1996. (Illus.). 166p. (Orig.). pap. text 89.00 (*1-56395-056-1*, PC97-960080) Am Assn Blood.

Validation in the Clinical Theory of Psychoanalysis: A Study in the Philosophy of Psychoanalysis. Adolf Grunbaum. 1993. LC 92-48956. (Psychological Issues Monographs: No. 61). 450p. 57.50 (*0-8236-6722-7*, BN#06722) Intl Univs Pr.

Validation Instruments for Community Pharmacy: Pharmaceutical Care for the Third Millennium. Lilian M. Azzopardi. 2000. LC 00-20476. (Illus.). xiv, 281p. 89.95 (*0-7890-0900-5*); 282p. pap. 39.95 (*0-7890-1109-3*) Haworth Pr (Pharmctl Prods).

Validation of Biopharmaceutical Manufacturing Processes. Ed. by Brian D. Kelley & R. Andrew Ramelmeier. LC 98-18617. (ACS Symposium Ser.: No. 698). (Illus.). 208p. text 110.00 (*0-8412-3567-8*) Am Chemical.

Validation of Pharmaceutical Processes. F. J. Carleton & J. P. Agalloco. 2nd exp. rev. ed. 1998. LC 98-44757. (Illus.). 856p. text 195.00 (*0-8247-9384-6*, 9384-6) Dekker.

Valium & Other Tranquilizers. Gail Winger. 1992. (Encyclopedia of Psychoactive Drugs Ser.: No. 1). (Illus.). 124p. (YA). (gr. 7 up). lib. bdg. 19.95 (*0-87754-759-9*) Chelsea Hse.

Valium, Librium & the Benzodiazepine Blues. Jim Parker. rev. ed. 2000. pap. 0.50 (*0-89230-163-5*) Do It Now.

Valkyries: The Women Around Jung. Maggy Anthony. 1993. 144p. pap. 14.95 (*1-85230-187-2*) Element MA.

Valproate. Wolfgang Lhoscher. 1999. LC 99-18269. (Milestones in Drug Therapy Ser.). (*0-8176-5836-X*) Birkhauser.

Valuation of Hospitals & Medical Centers. James J. Unland. 1989. 355p. (Orig.). 45.00 (*1-882198-11-5*) Hlthcare Fin Mgmt.

Valuation of Hospitals & Medical Centers. James J. Unland. 1993. (Orig.). text 60.00 (*0-7602-0118-8*, Irwn Prfssnl) McGraw-Hill Educ Grp.

Valuation of Medical Practice. Reed Tinsley et al. 1999. LC 99-10467. (Illus.). 278p. 105.00 (*0-471-29965-0*) Wiley.

Valuation of Physician Practices & Clinics. Bruce G. Krider. 1997. LC 97-23180. 200p. 153.00 (*0-8342-0962-4*, 20962) Aspen Pub.

***Valuation of Psychictric Services.** David Schultz & Crystell Penderson. 2001. (Illus.). 160p. pap. 25.00 (*0-9710235-0-6*) Amer Psych Soc Inc.

Value Areas & Their Development. H. J. Hermans. 1976. 306p. (*90-265-0225-7*) Swets.

Value-Based Cost Management for Healthcare: Linking Costs to Quality & Delivery. Kicab Castaneda-Mendez. 1996. 189p. 32.95 (*0-527-76304-7*) Product Pr.

Value for Value Psychotherapy: The Economic & Therapeutic Barter. Paul S. Rappoport. 1983. LC 82-16573. 195p. 55.50 (*0-275-91724-X*, C1724, Praeger Pubs) Greenwood.

Value of Life: An Introduction to Medical Ethics. John Harris. 1985. 320p. pap. 13.95 (*0-7102-0437-X*, Routledge Thoemms) Routledge.

Value of New Serological Probes for the Study of Putative Periodontal Pathogens: A Survey after Five Years of Application. Rudolf Gmur. 1995. LC 95-31863. pap. text 38.00 (*0-86715-316-4*) Quint Pub Co.

Value of Psychiatric Treatment: Its Efficacy in Severe Mental Disorders. Ed. by Samuel J. Keith & Susan M. Matthews. 1996. (Illus.). 112p. (C). reprint ed. pap. text 35.00 (*0-7881-3094-3*) DIANE Pub.

Value of Psychological Treatment: Collected Papers of Nicholas A. Cummings. Nicholas A. Cummings et al. 2000. LC 98-50582. 446p. 48.95 (*1-891944-12-6*) Zeig Tucker Theisen.

Value Orientations in Counseling & Psychotherapy: The Meanings of Mental Health. C. Marshall Lowe. 2nd ed. 1976. LC 76-25957. 320p. pap. text 19.50 (*0-910328-09-9*) Sulzburger & Graham Pub.

Value Presuppositions in Theories of Human Development. Leonard Cirillo & Seymour Wapner. 1986. 184p. text 39.95 (*0-89859-753-6*) L Erlbaum Assocs.

***Value Rx: It's Time to Manage & Measure What Matters in Healthcare.** Edward J. Giniat & Barry D. Libert. 2001. (Illus.). 256p. 32.00 (*0-06-662095-3*) HarperCollins Pubs.

***Values & Ethics in the Practice of Psychotherapy & Counselling.** Ed. by Fiona Barnes Palmer & Lesley Murdin. 2001. 224p. pap. (*0-335-20475-9*); LC 00-50504. text (*0-335-20476-7*) OpUniv Pr GBR. *Dist:* Taylor & Francis.

Values & Work: A Special Issue of the Journal Applied Psychology. Robert A. Roe. 1999. 104p. pap. 24.95 (*0-86377-994-8*) L Erlbaum Assocs.

Values in Conflict: Christian Nursing in a Changing Profession. Judith A. Shelly & Arlene B. Miller. 1991. LC 91-20901. 215p. pap. 14.99 (*0-8308-1330-6*, 1330) InterVarsity.

Values in Conflict: Christianity, Marxism, Psychoanalysis & Existentialism. Ed. by Victor Comerchero. 1970. LC 74-111099. 986p. (Orig.). (C). pap. text 22.95 (*0-89197-463-6*) Irvington.

Values in Conflict: Resolving Ethical Issues in Health Care. American Hospital Association Staff. 2nd ed. 1994. 120p. (Orig.). pap. 29.00 (*0-87258-668-5*, 025002) Am Hospital.

Values in Medical Practice: A Statement of Philosophy for Physicians & Model for Teaching a Healing Science. Rudolph J. Napodano. 1986. LC 85-19742. 144p. 32.95 (*0-89885-268-4*, Kluwer Acad Hman Sci) Kluwer Academic.

Values of Psychotherapy. Jeremy Holmes & Richard Lindley. 1989. (Studies in Bioethics). 272p. 33.95 (*0-19-217759-1*) OUP.

Values, Self, & Society: Toward a Humanist Social Psychology. M. Brewster Smith. 1991. 278p. (C). text 39.95 (*0-88738-373-4*) Transaction Pubs.

Valuing Health Care: Costs, Benefits, & Effectiveness of Pharmaceuticals & Other Medical Technologies. Frank A. Sloan. 1996. (Illus.). 287p. pap. text 24.95 (*0-521-57646-6*) Cambridge U Pr.

Valuing Health Care: Costs, Benefits, & Effectiveness of Pharmaceuticals & Other Medical Technologies. Ed. by Frank A. Sloan. 1995. LC 94-9554. (Illus.). 287p. (C). text 69.95 (*0-521-47020-X*) Cambridge U Pr.

Valuing Health for Policy: An Economic Approach. Ed. by George Tolley et al. 1994. LC 94-9537. 436p. 55.00 (*0-226-80713-4*) U Ch Pr.

Valuing the Global Environment: Actions & Investments for a 21st Century. Global Environment Facility Staff. 1998. (Illus.). 120p. pap. text (*1-884122-28-0*) Global Environ.

Valva & Treatment of the Patient with Diarrhea. Paul F. Miskovitz & Arnold Rochwarger. 1992. (Illus.). 179p. text 84.99 (*1-56372-059-0*) Buttrwrth-Heinemann.

Valve Morphology in the Genus Cymbella: C. A. Agardh. Kurt Krammer. Ed. by Kurt Krammer & J. G. Helmcke. 1982. (Micromorphology of Datom Valves Ser.: No. XI). (Illus.). 300p. (Orig.). 99.00 (*3-7682-1333-1*) Lubrecht & Cramer.

Valvular Heart Disease. Ed. by Muayed Al-Zaibag & Carlos Duran. 1994. LC 93-46486. (Fundamental & Clinical Cardiology Ser.: Vol. 20). (Illus.). 760p. text 250.00 (*0-8247-8861-3*) Dekker.

Valvular Heart Disease. James E. Dalen & Joseph S. Alpert. 1986. 125.00 (*0-316-17171-9*, Little Brwn Med Div) Lppncott W & W.

Valvular Heart Disease. Catherine M. Otto. Ed. by Richard Zorab. 1999. LC 98-47450. (Illus.). 575p. text (*0-7216-7139-X*) Saunders.

Valvular Heart Disease. Joseph S. Alpert et al. 3rd ed. 1999. LC 99-16809. (Illus.). xv, 478p. text 149.00 (*0-7817-2310-8*) Lppncott W & W.

Vampire, Dracula & Incest: The Vampire Myth, Stoker's Dracula, & Psychotherapy of Vampiric Sexual Abuse. Daniel Lapin. 1995. LC 95-75221. 252p. (Orig.). pap. 14.95 (*0-9644983-0-8*) Gargoyle Pub.

Vanadium: Trace Mineral for Health. 1996. lib. bdg. 250.99 (*0-8490-5914-3*) Gordon Pr.

Vanadium Compounds: Biochemical & Therapeutic Applications. Ed. by Ashok K. Srivastava & Jean-Louis Chiasson. 1996. (Developments in Molecular & Cellular Biochemistry Ser.: Vol. 16). 256p. (C). text 254.00 (*0-7923-3762-X*) Kluwer Academic.

Vanadium in Biological Systems: Physiology & Biochemistry. Ed. by N. Dennis Chasteen. 1990. (C). text 166.50 (*0-7923-0733-X*) Kluwer Academic.

Vandalized Lovemaps: Paraphilic Outcome of Seven Cases in Pediatric Sexology. John Money & Margaret Lamacz. 1989. LC 89-4037. 224p. 38.00 (*0-87975-513-X*) Prometheus Bks.

Vandals at the Gates of Medicine: Historic Perspectives on the Battle over Health Care Reform. Miguel Faria, Jr. 1995. (Illus.). 403p. 41.95 (*0-9641077-0-8*) Hacienda Pub.

Vanishing Bile Duct Syndrome - Pathophysiology & Treatment. Ed. by D. Alvaro. 1997. (Falk Symposium Ser.). 272p. (C). text 127.00 (*0-7923-8721-X*) Kluwer Academic.

Vanishing Mind: A Practical Guide to Alzheimer's Disease & Other Dementias. Leonard L. Heston & June A. White. 3rd ed. 1991. (Illus.). 191p. (C). text 26.95 (*0-7167-2131-7*); pap. text 16.95 (*0-7167-2192-9*) W H Freeman.

Vapor-Liquid Equilibrium Data Collection Tables & Diagrams of Data for Binary & Multicomponent Mixtures up to Moderate Pressures; Constants of Correlation Equations for Computer Use: Part 2b: Organic Hydroxy Compounds: Alcohols & Phenols. Ed. by J. Gmehling et al. 1978. LC 79-670289. (Dechema Chemistry Data Ser.: Vol. 1). text (*3-926959-18-5*) Dechema DEU. *Dist:* Scholium Intl.

Variability in Human Drug Response. Ed. by G. T. Tucker. 1999. LC 00-702809. (International Congress Ser.: Vol. 1178). 316p. 125.00 (*0-444-82958-X*, Excerpta Medica) Elsevier.

Variability in Human Fertility. Ed. by L. Rosetta & C. G. Mascie-Taylor. 1996. (Studies in Biological Anthropology: Vol. 19). (Illus.). 235p. (C). text 69.95 (*0-521-49569-5*) Cambridge U Pr.

Variability in Response to Anti-Rheumatic Drugs. Ed. by Peter M. Brooks et al. 1993. LC 93-2005. (Agents & Actions Supplements Ser.: Vol. 44). xi, 227p. 90.00 (*0-8176-2869-X*) Birkhauser.

Variable Force Technique. Peter Leighton. 1988. LC 87-63607. (Illus.). 199p. ring bd. 39.95 (*0-945817-01-0*) Origin Bks.

Variants & Pitfalls in Body Imaging. Ali Shirkhoda. 1999. LC 99-35193. 768p. text 199.00 (*0-683-30058-X*) Lppncott W & W.

Variation & Adaptive Expression of Antibodies. George P. Smith. 1973. LC 72-95186. 192p. 29.00 (*0-674-93205-6*) HUP.

Variation in the Human Genome. CIBA Foundation Staff et al. 1996. LC 95-54159. (CIBA Foundation Symposia Ser.: Vol. 197). 340p. 128.00 (*0-471-96152-3*) Wiley.

Variation of Basidiospores in the Hymenomycetes & Its Significance to Their Taxonomy. Erast Parmasto & Ilmi Parmasto. 1987. (Bibliotheca Mycologica: Vol. 115). (GER., Illus.). 168p. (*3-443-59016-0*) Gebruder Borntraeger DEU. *Dist:* Balogh.

Variations in Human Physiology. Ed. by R. M. Case. 1988. LC 84-11301. (Integrative Studies in Human Physiology). 241p. text (*0-7190-1086-1*) Manchester Univ Pr GBR. *Dist:* St Martin.

Variations in the Use of Cesarean Sections: Literature Synthesis. Joanna Z. Heilbrunn & Rolla E. Park. 1995. LC 95-35760. 80p. pap. text 9.00 (*0-8330-2306-3*, MR-330-AHCPR) Rand Corp.

Variations on a Theme: Diversity & the Psychology of Women. Ed. by Joan C. Chrisler & Alyce H. Hemstreet. 1995. LC 94-26207. (SUNY Series in the Psychology of Women). 238p. (C). text 21.50 (*0-7914-2435-9*) State U NY Pr.

Variations on Teaching & Supervising Group Therapy. Intro. by Karen G. Lewis. 1989. LC 89-19970. (Journal of Independent Social Work: Vol. 3, No. 4). (Illus.). 151p. text 29.95 (*0-86656-921-9*) Haworth Pr.

Varicose Veins: A Guide for Patients. Bandyk. Ed. by Ellis & Larry Carey. 1995. (Surgery Ser.). (Illus.). 24p. (Orig.). pap. 2.95 (*1-885274-22-X*) Health InfoNet Inc.

Varicose Veins: A Guide to Prevention & Treatment. Howard C. Baron & Barbara A. Ross. 1995. LC 95-12535. (Illus.). 160p. 24.95 (*0-8160-2986-5*) Facts on File.

Varicose Veins, Venous Disorders, & Lymphatics Problems in the Lower Limbs. David Tibbs et al. 1998. LC 96-39274. (Illus.). 264p. (C). text 139.50 (*0-19-262762-7*) OUP.

Varieties of Affect. Claire Armon-Jones. 1992. LC 92-137326. (Studies in Philosophy). 410p. text 50.00 (*0-8020-2823-3*) U of Toronto Pr.

Varieties of Juvenile Delinquency. C. Frankenstein. 1970. xii, 252p. text 174.00 (*0-677-02820-2*) Gordon & Breach.

Varieties of Memory & Consciousness: Essays in Honour of Endel Tulving. Ed. by H. L. Roediger, III & F. I. Craik. 1989. 464p. 89.95 (*0-89859-935-0*); pap. 45.00 (*0-8058-0546-X*) L Erlbaum Assocs.

Varieties of Moral Personality: Ethics & Psychological Realism. Owen Flanagan. 1991. (Illus.). pap. 22.50 (*0-674-93219-6*) HUP.

Varieties of Religious Experience. William James. 1958. 408p. pap. 6.99 (*0-451-62743-1*, ME2069, Ment) NAL.

Varney's Midwife. Dixie Rasmussen. 2000. (Illus.). 256p. (C). pap. text, stu. ed. 37.50 (*0-7637-1082-2*) Jones & Bartlett.

Varney's Midwifery. Helen Varney. 3rd ed. 1996. LC 96-38376. (Nursery Ser.). (Illus.). 944p. (C). text 95.95 (*0-86720-748-5*, 748-5) Jones & Bartlett.

***Varney's Midwifery.** Helen Varney-Burst et al. 4th ed. 2002. (Illus.). (C). text 109.95 (*0-7637-1856-4*, 1856-4) Jones & Bartlett.

Varney's Midwifery: Pocket Notebook. Helen Varney et al. 3rd ed. 1998. LC 97-42676. (Nursing Ser.). (Illus.). 352p. (C). pap. text 37.95 (*0-7637-0546-2*, 0546-2) Jones & Bartlett.

Vascular Access. Ingemar Davidson. 1996. (On Call In Ser.). 450p. pap. 39.95 (*0-412-13551-5*) Chapman & Hall.

Vascular Access: Principles & Practice. Ed. by Samuel E. Wilson. 3rd rev. ed. 1995. (Illus.). 336p. (C). (gr. 13). text 86.95 (*0-8151-9226-6*, 24313) Mosby Inc.

***Vascular Access: Principles & Practice.** Samuel E. Wilson. 4th ed. 2001. (Illus.). 350p. (*0-323-01188-8*) Mosby Inc.

***Vascular Access Devices: A Clinician's Guide.** Suzanne F. Herbst & Robert O. Hickman. 2001. (Illus.). (C). text 54.95 (*0-7637-1689-8*, 1689-8) Jones & Bartlett.

Vascular Access Surgery. Rowe. 1999. (C). pap. text 60.00 (*0-8385-9353-4*) P-H.

Vascular Anatomy & Physiology: An Introductory Text. Ann C. Belanger. 1990. LC 90-925. 200p. pap. 39.95 (*0-941022-11-0*) Davies Pubng.

Vascular Anatomy of the Spinal Cord. A. K. Thron. 1988. (Illus.). 114p. 79.95 (*0-387-82015-9*) Spr-Verlag.

***Vascular & Endovascular Opportunities.** R. M. Greenhalgh. 2000. 672p. text (*0-7020-2610-7*) W B Saunders GBR. *Dist:* Saunders.

Vascular & Endovascular Surgery. Ed. by Jonathon Beard & Peter Gaines. 1997. (Companion Guide to Specialist Surgical Practice Ser.: Vol. 6). (Illus.). 380p. text (*0-7020-2144-X*) W B Saunders GBR. *Dist:* Saunders.

***Vascular & Endovascular Surgery.** Ed. by Jonathan D. Beard & Peter A. Gaines. 2nd ed. 2001. (Illus.). 408p. pap. (*0-7020-2591-7*) W B Saunders GBR. *Dist:* Saunders.

Vascular & Endovascular Surgical Techniques: An Atlas. Ed. by Roger M. Greenhalgh. 3rd ed. 1994. (Illus.). 544p. text (*0-7020-1901-1*) W B Saunders GBR. *Dist:* Saunders.

***Vascular & Interventional Imaging Case Review.** Steven B. Oglevie. 2001. (Illus.). 190p. (*0-323-01352-X*) Mosby Inc.

Vascular & Interventional Radiology. Yukiyoshi Kimura Fujikami. 1999. pap. text 80.00 (*0-7817-1661-6*) Lppncott W & W.

Vascular & Interventional Radiology. Karim Valji. Ed. by Lisette Bralow. 1999. LC 98-36266. (Illus.). 509p. text 145.00 (*0-7216-7003-2*) Saunders.

Vascular & Interventional Radiology: Principles & Practices. Curtis W. Bakal et al. 2001. (Illus.). 608p. 139.00 (*0-86577-678-4*) Thieme Med Pubs.

Vascular & Interventional Radiology: The Requistes. 2000. (Illus.). 512p. text 75.00 (*0-8151-4369-9*, 31224) Mosby Inc.

Vascular & Neurologic Complications of Diabetes Mellitus. Ed. by F. Belfiore et al. 1987. (Frontiers in Diabetes Ser.: Vol. 8). (Illus.). xii, 256p. 172.25 (*3-8055-4452-9*) S Karger.

Vascular & Peritoneal Access for Dialysis. Ed. by Vittorio E. Andreucci. 1989. (Topics in Renal Medicine Ser.). (C). text 246.50 (*0-7923-0119-6*) Kluwer Academic.

Vascular Andrology: Erectile Dysfunction/Priapism Varicocele. Ed. by A. Ledda. 1996. (Illus.). 149p. pap. 53.95 (*3-540-59472-8*) Spr-Verlag.

Vascular Anesthesia: A Practical Handbook. Lawrence Caldicott et al. 1998. 288p. text 52.00 (*0-7506-3468-5*) Buttrwrth-Heinemann.

Vascular Aphasia. Joseph M. Tonkongy. 1986. (Illus.). 248p. 32.50 (*0-262-20054-6*, Bradford Bks) MIT Pr.

Vascular Brachytherapy. Ed. by Ron Waksman. 2nd ed. 1998. LC 98-28924. (Illus.). 656p. 149.00 (*0-87993-413-1*, Futura Media) Futura Pub.

T U V

*__Vascular Brachytherapy.__ Ed. by Ron Waksman. 3rd ed. 2001. (Illus.). 800p. 175.00 (*0-87993-489-1*) Futura Pub.

Vascular Brain Disease in Old Age. Ed. by W. Meier-Ruge. 1989. (Teaching & Training in Geriatric Medicine Ser.: Vol. 2). viii, 188p. pap. 24.50 (*3-8055-4477-4*) S Karger.

Vascular Brain Stem Diseases. Ed. by B. Hofferberth et al. 1990. (Illus.). viii, 282p. 69.75 (*3-8055-5031-6*) S Karger.

*__Vascular Complications of Diabetes: Current Issues in Pathogenesis & Treatment.__ Ed. by Richard Donnelly & Jost Jonas. 2001. LC 2001-52645. pap. (*0-632-06513-3*) Blackwell Sci.

Vascular Control of Hemostasis. Ed. by Victor W. Van Hinsbergh. 1996. (Advances in Vascular Biology Ser.). 320p. text 110.00 (*3-7186-5796-1*) Gordon & Breach.

Vascular Dementia. Ed. by John Stirling Meyer et al. 2000. LC 00-39355. (Illus.). x, 310p. 88.00 (*0-87993-425-5*) Futura Pub.

Vascular Dementia: A Review of Concepts & Ideas. Ed. by I. Prohovnik et al. 1996. LC 95-45454. 362p. 234.95 (*0-471-95294-X*) Wiley.

Vascular Dementia: Etiological, Pathogenetic, Clinical & Treatment Aspects. Ed. by L. A. Carlson et al. 1994. (Journal: Vol. 5, Nos. 3-4, 1994). (Illus.). iv, 86p. pap. 97.50 (*3-8055-5984-4*) S Karger.

Vascular Diagnosis. Ed. by Eugene F. Bernstein. 4th ed. 1993. LC 93-4086. (Illus.). 1058p. (C). (gr. 13). text 258.00 (*0-8016-6557-4*, 06557) Mosby Inc.

Vascular Diagnosis with Ultrasound: Clinical Reference with Case Studies. Michael Hennerici & Doris Neuerburg-Heusler. Tr. by Christopher Kronen. 1998. LC 97-34733. (Illus.). 464p. text 159.00 (*0-86577-603-2*) Thieme Med Pubs.

Vascular Diagnostics: Noninvasive & Invasive Techniques-Periinterventional Evaluations. Ed. by Peter Lanzer & Josef Roesch. 1994. LC 94-28254. (Illus.). 528p. 166.00 (*0-387-57939-7*) Spr-Verlag.

Vascular Diagnostics: Principles & Technology. Martin J. Lipton & Peter Lanzer. 1996. LC 96-41507. (Illus.). 362p. 175.00 (*3-540-61541-5*); (*0-387-61541-5*) Spr-Verlag.

Vascular Disease, Vol. VII. Ed. by Mark Creager. 1996. LC 95-24438. (Atlas of Heart Diseases Ser.: Vol. 7). (Illus.). 232p. 134.00 (*1-878132-26-1*) Current Med.

Vascular Disease: A Multi-Specialty Approach to Diagnosis & Management. Eton. 1997. (On Call In Ser.). 200p. pap. 49.95 (*0-412-11761-4*, E0551) Chapman & Hall.

Vascular Disease: A Multi-Specialty Approach to Diagnosis & Management. Darwin Eton & Fred A. Weaver. 2nd ed. 1999. LC 99-36129. (Vademecum Ser.). (Illus.). 685p. spiral bd. 45.00 (*1-57059-561-5*) Landes Bioscience.

Vascular Disease: Molecular Biology & Gene Transfer Protocols. Ed. by Andrew H. Baker. 1999. LC 98-55168. (Methods in Molecular Medicine Ser.: Vol. 30). (Illus.). xiv, 441p. 125.00 (*0-89603-731-2*) Humana.

Vascular Disease & Injury: Preclinical Research. Ed. by Daniel I. Simon & Campbell Rogers. 2000. LC 00-39603. (Contemporary Cardiology Ser.). (Illus.). 368p. 135.00 (*0-89603-753-3*) Humana.

Vascular Disease in the Elderly. Edward A. Stemmer. Ed. by Wilbert S. Aronow et al. 1997. LC 96-50375. (Illus.). 600p. 120.00 (*0-87993-646-0*) Futura Pub.

Vascular Disease in the Older Person. Ed. by E. G. Lakatta. 1997. LC 97-41937. (Novartis Foundation for Gerontological Research Ser.). 166p. lib. bdg. 52.95 (*1-85070-010-9*) CRC Pr.

Vascular Diseases, Pt. I. Ed. by Pierre J. Vinken et al. 1989. 600p. 265.00 (*0-444-90503-0*); 498p. 219.00 (*0-444-90482-4*); 498p. 110.50 Elsevier.

Vascular Diseases: Surgical & Interventional Therapy Ed. by D. Eugene Strandness, Jr. & Arina Van Breda. 1993. (Illus.). 1472p. text (*0-443-08841-1*) Church.

Vascular Diseases in Neonates, Infants & Children: Interventional Neuroradiology Management: P. Lasjaunias. Pierre L. Lasjaunias. LC 96-29097. 1997. (Illus.). 707p. 260.00 (*3-540-60845-1*); 1996. (*0-387-60845-1*) Spr-Verlag.

Vascular Diseases of the Nervous System Ed. by Pierre J. Vinken & George W. Bruyn. 1972. Pt. 1. 281.75 (*0-444-10060-1*); Pt. 2. 272.50 (*0-444-10061-X*) Elsevier.

Vascular Disorders of the Upper Extremity. Ed. by Herbert I. Machleder. 3rd ed. 1998. LC 98-21934. (Illus.). 515p. 98.00 (*0-87993-409-3*, Futura Media) Futura Pub.

Vascular Dynamics: Physiological Perspectives. Ed. by N. Westerhoff & D. R. Gross. 1989. (NATO ASI Series A, Life Sciences: Vol. 166). (Illus.). 334p. 89.50 (*0-306-43210-2*, Plenum Trade) Perseus Pubng.

*__Vascular Endothelial Growth Factor Receptors in Angiogenesis.__ Kui Huang. 2001. (Comprehensive Summaries of Uppsala Dissertations from the Faculty of Medicine Ser.: No. 986). (Illus.). 60p. pap. (*91-554-4909-3*) Uppsala Universitet SWE. *Dist:* Coronet Bks.

Vascular Endothelium: Physiological Basis of Clinical Problems. Ed. by J. D. Catravas et al. 1991. (NATO Advanced Science Institutes Ser.: Vol. 208). (Illus.). 318p. (C). text 126.00 (*0-306-44012-1*, Kluwer Plenum) Kluwer Academic.

Vascular Endothelium: Responses to Injury. Ed. by J. D. Catravas et al. 1996. (NATO Advanced Science Institutes Ser.: Vol. 281). (Illus.). 364p. 115.00 (*0-306-45282-0*, Kluwer Plenum) Kluwer Academic.

Vascular Endothelium Vol. 2: Physiological Basis of Clinical Problems. J. D. Catravas et al. 1993. (NATO Advanced Science Institutes Ser.: Vol. 257). (Illus.). 240p. (C). text 95.00 (*0-306-44633-2*, Kluwer Plenum) Kluwer Academic.

Vascular Endothelium Vol. 4: Pharmacologic & Genetic Manipulations. J. D. Catravas et al. 1998. LC 98-9865. (NATO Advanced Science Institutes Ser.: No. 294). (Illus.). 308p. (C). text 110.00 (*0-306-45819-5*, Kluwer Plenum) Kluwer Academic.

Vascular Endothelium & Basement Membranes. Ed. by B. M. Altura. 1979. (Advances in Microcirculation Ser.: Vol. 9). (Illus.). 53.25 (*3-8055-3054-4*) S Karger.

Vascular Endothelium in Health & Disease. Ed. by Shu Chien. 1988. LC 88-26583. (Advances in Experimental Medicine & Biology Ser.: Vol. 242). (Illus.). 246p. 75.00 (*0-306-43034-7*, Plenum Trade) Perseus Pubng.

*__Vascular Factors in Alzheimer's Disease.__ Ed. by Raj N. Kalaria & Paul Ince. 2001. 555p. pap. 42.00 (*0-8018-6695-2*) NY Acad Sci.

Vascular Factors in Alzheimer's Disease. Ed. by Raj N. Kalaria & Paul Ince. 2000. 555p. 180.00 (*1-57331-251-7*) NY Acad Sci.

Vascular Graft Infections. Ed. by T. J. Bunt. 1994. (Illus.). 420p. 69.00 (*0-87993-576-6*) Futura Pub.

Vascular Graft Update: Safety & Performance. Helen E. Kambic et al. 1986. LC 86-14077. (Special Technical Publications: No. 898). (Illus.). 360p. text 54.00 (*0-8031-0462-6*, STP898) ASTM.

Vascular Growth Factors & Angiogenesis. Ed. by Lena Claesson-Welsh et al. 1998. (Current Topics in Microbiology & Immunology Ser.: Vol. 237). (Illus.). 197p. 129.00 (*3-540-64731-7*) Spr-Verlag.

Vascular Imaging: Principles & Techniques. Ed. by Bonnie L. Johnson & Thomas J. Fogarty. Date not set. (Illus.). 400p. 89.00 (*1-56757-063-1*) Appleton Comms.

Vascular Imaging by Color Doppler & Magnetic Resonance. Ed. by A. P. Yoganathan & Peter Lanzer. 1991. (Illus.). 338p. 253.00 (*0-387-53320-6*) Spr-Verlag.

Vascular Imaging for Surgeons. Greenhalgh. 1995. text 175.00 (*0-7020-2015-X*) Saunders.

Vascular Injuries & Diseases of the Upper Limb. E. Shaw Wilgis. 1983. 183p. 51.50 (*0-316-94066-6*, Little Brwn Med Div) Lppncott W & W.

Vascular Injuries in Surgical Practice. Fred Bongard et al. 1991. (Illus.). 339p. (C). text 85.00 (*0-8385-9383-6*, A9383-9, Apple Lange Med) McGraw.

Vascular Intervention: A Clinical Approach. Ed. by Bruce A. Perler & Gary J. Becker. 1997. LC 97-30187. (Illus.). 608p. 139.00 (*0-86577-694-6*) Thieme Med Pubs.

Vascular Laboratory Operations Manual: A Guide to Survival. Ed. by Claudia B. Rumwell. 2nd rev. ed. 1997. LC 92-48990. (Illus.). 350p. ring bd. 295.00 (*0-941022-24-2*) Davies Pubng.

Vascular Laboratory Physician's Manual: Indications, Interpretation, & Clinical Decision Making. Marsha M. Neumyer et al. Date not set. (*0-941022-29-3*) Davies Pubng.

Vascular Laboratory Policies & Procedures Manual-Windows 95, 98, NT. Ed. by Claudia Rumwell & Michalene McPharlin. 1998. ring bd. 795.00 incl. disk (*0-941022-49-8*) Davies Pubng.

Vascular Laboratory Policies & Procedures Manual-MSR 1.1. Ed. by Claudia B. Rumwell & Michalene McPharlin. 1995. ring bd. 795.00 incl. disk (*0-941022-41-2*) Davies Pubng.

Vascular Laboratory Policies & Procedures Manual-Windows 2.1.1. Ed. by Claudia B. Rumwell & Michalene McPharlin. 1995. ring bd. 795.00 incl. disk (*0-941022-42-0*) Davies Pubng.

Vascular Laboratory Quality Assurance Manual. Terence Needham. Date not set. (*0-941022-26-9*) Davies Pubng.

Vascular Malformations of the Central Nervous System. Ed. by Jafar J. Jafar et al. 1999. LC 99-23053. (Illus.). xvii, 540p. text 179.00 (*0-7817-1472-9*) Lppncott W & W.

Vascular Medicine. Pearce & Yao. 1999. (C). pap. text 145.00 (*0-8385-9378-X*) P-H.

Vascular Medicine: A Textbook of Vascular Biology & Diseases. Ed. by Joseph Loscalzo et al. 2nd ed. 1996. LC 95-39262. 1,328p. text 229.00 (*0-316-53400-5*, Little Brwn Med Div) Lppncott W & W.

Vascular Medicine from Endothelium to Myocardium. Ed. by Ernst E. Van der Wall et al. 1997. LC 97-28767. (Developments in Cardiovascular Medicine Ser.: No. 197). 240p. text 99.00 (*0-7923-4740-4*) Kluwer Academic.

Vascular Morphogenesis: In Vivo, In Vitro, In Mente. Charles D. Little et al. 1997. LC 97-37689. (Molecular Biology of Cardiovascular Development Ser.). xiv, 265p. (*3-7643-3920-9*) Birkhauser.

Vascular Morphogenesis in the Female Reproductive System. Hellmut Augustin. 2001. LC 00-65098. (Cardiovascular Molecular Morphogenesis Ser.). (Illus.). xii, 333p. 159.00 (*0-8176-4221-8*) Birkhauser.

Vascular Morphogenesis in Vivo, in Vitro, in Mente: In Vivo, In Vitro, In Mente. C. Little et al. 1998. LC 97-37689. (Illus.). 325p. 90.00 (*0-8176-3920-9*) Birkhauser.

Vascular Neuroeffector Mechanisms: Proceedings of the Symposium, 2nd International, Odense, July-August, 1955. Vascular Neuroeffector Mechanism Symposium Staff. 1976. (Illus.). 300p. 109.75 (*3-8055-2325-4*) S Karger.

Vascular Neuroeffector Systems, Physiology & Pharmacology: Proceedings of the Symposium, Interlaken, 1969. Physiology and Pharmacology of Vascular Neuroeffecto. Ed. by J. A. Bevan et al. 1971. (Illus.). viii, 350p. 62.75 (*3-8055-1184-1*) S Karger.

Vascular Neuroeffectors Mechanisms Journal: Blood Vessels, Vol. 28, No. 103, 1991. Ed. by J. A. Bevan et al. 1991. (Illus.). 268p. pap. 187.00 (*3-8055-5380-3*) S Karger.

Vascular Nursing. Ed. by Victoria A. Fahey. 2nd ed. 1993. LC 93-11267. (Illus.). 626p. text 93.50 (*0-7216-6589-6*) Saunders.

Vascular Nursing. Victoria A. Fahey. Ed. by Robin Carter. 3rd ed. 1999. LC 98-37280. (Illus.). 495p. text (*0-7216-7657-X*) Saunders.

Vascular Pathology. Ed. by William E. Stehbens & J. T. Lie. 1994. LC 94-69665. (Illus.). 816p. (*0-412-48640-7*) E A GBR. *Dist:* OUP.

Vascular Perfusion in Cancer Therapy. Ed. by K. Schwemmle & K. Aigner. 1983. (Recent Results in Cancer Research Ser.: Vol. 86). (Illus.). 295p. 99.00 (*0-387-12346-6*) Spr-Verlag.

Vascular Physics Review. Ed. & Intro. by Barton A. Bean et al. 1995. (Illus.). 180p. pap. text 55.00 (*0-941022-36-6*) Davies Pubng.

Vascular Pole of the Renal Glomerulus of Rats. M. Elger et al. 1997. LC 97-22646. (Advances in Anatomy, Embryology & Cell Biology Ser.: Vol. 139). (Illus.). 98p. pap. 96.00 (*3-540-63241-7*) Spr-Verlag.

Vascular Reconstruction: Anatomy, Exposure & Techniques. Jamal J. Hoballah. 2000. LC 99-29750. (Illus.). xiii, 393p. wbk. ed. 95.00 (*0-387-98500-X*) Spr-Verlag.

Vascular Risk Factors & Neuroprotection in Glaucoma: Update, 1996. Stephen M. Drance. 1997. LC 97-17662. (*90-6299-137-8*) Kugler NLD. *Dist:* Lib Res.

Vascular Smooth Muscle in Culture Ed. by Julie H. Campbell & Gordon R. Campbell. 1987. 212.00 (*0-8493-4325-9*, QP110);I. 168p. 98.00 (*0-8493-4327-5*) Franklin (CRC Reprint).

Vascular Smooth Muscle in Culture, Vol. I. Julie H. Campbell. 1987. 200p. 114.00 (*0-8493-4326-7*, CRC Reprint) Franklin.

Vascular Surgery. Beard. 1998. (Illus.). 380p. (C). text 90.00 (*0-7020-2145-8*) Saunders.

Vascular Surgery. Ed. by G. Herberer & R. J. Van Dongen. 1989. (Illus.). 811p. 477.00 (*0-387-18280-2*) Spr-Verlag.

Vascular Surgery. Crawford W. Jamieson & James S. Yao. 1993. (Rob & Smith's Operative Surgery Ser.). (Illus.). 700p. 435.00 (*0-7506-0588-X*) Chapman & Hall.

Vascular Surgery. Peter M. Lamont et al. 1999. LC 98-37284. (Illus.). 224p. text 145.00 (*0-19-262523-3*) OUP.

Vascular Surgery. MacVittie. 1997. (Perioperative Nursing Ser.). (Illus.). 272p. (C). (gr. 13). text 54.95 (*0-8151-7031-9*, 27475) Mosby Inc.

*__Vascular Surgery.__ Robert B. Rutherford. 2000. 1110p. (*0-7216-8100-X*); 1999. 1156p. (*0-7216-8101-8*) Saunders.

Vascular Surgery. R. E. Norton. 1982. (Illus.). 1177p. reprint ed. pap. text 11.50 (*0-340-22496-7*, 5567-7) Appleton & Lange.

Vascular Surgery Ed. by Robert B. Rutherford. 4th ed. 1995. LC 93-40051. (Illus.). 2033p. 260.00 (*0-7216-3837-6*) Saunders.

Vascular Surgery. C. W. Jamieson & J. S. T. Yao. 5th ed. 1993. (Rob & Smith's Operative Surgery Ser.). (Illus.). 696p. (*0-412-58630-4*) E A GBR. *Dist:* OUP.

Vascular Surgery, Set. Robert B. Rutherford. 5th ed. 2000. LC 98-52324. (Illus.). 2266p. (C). text (*0-7216-8078-X*) Saunders.

Vascular Surgery: A Comprehensive Review. Wesley S. Moore. Ed. by Lisette Bralow. 5th ed. 1997. LC 96-35522. (Illus.). 832p. text 195.00 (*0-7216-6962-X*) Saunders.

Vascular Surgery: Guide & Handbook. G. Pratt. 1976. LC 75-27628. (Illus.). 416p. 32.50 (*0-87527-138-3*) Green.

Vascular Surgery: Principles & Practice. Ed. by Frank J. Veith et al. 2nd ed. 1994. (Illus.). 1250p. text 179.00 (*0-07-070813-4*) McGraw-Hill Educ Grp.

Vascular Surgery: The Requisites. 2000. 544p. text 65.00 (*0-8151-2911-4*, 31821) Mosby Inc.

Vascular Surgery: Theory & Practice. Allan Callow & Calvin B. Ernst. 1996. 1776p. (C). text 235.00 (*0-8385-9384-4*, A9384-7) McGraw-Hill Educ Grp.

*__Vascular Surgery Highlights 2000-2001.__ Davies. 2001. (Fast Facts Ser.). (Illus.). 96p. pap. (*1-899541-84-5*) Health Pr GBR. *Dist:* JAMCO Dist.

Vascular Surgery Review. Roy L. Tawes, Jr. 1999. 144p. pap. 28.95 (*1-56757-060-7*) Appleton Comms.

Vascular Surgery, 2000. John M. Porter. 2000. 86.00 (*0-8151-2736-7*, 31319) Mosby Inc.

Vascular Surgery, 2002. John M. Porter. 2002. 86.00 (*0-8151-2738-3*, 31321) Mosby Inc.

Vascular Surgical Approaches. Ed. by Alain Branchereau & Ramon Berguer. 1999. LC 98-43503. (Illus.). 344p. 115.00 (*0-87993-664-9*) Futura Pub.

Vascular Technology: An Illustrated Review. Claudia Rumwell & Michalene McPharlin. 2nd ed. 2000. LC 99-86818. (Illus.). xiii, 322p. pap. text 64.95 (*0-941022-45-5*, 11026) Davies Pubng.

Vascular Technology: An Illustrated Review for the Registry Exam. Claudia B. Rumwell & Michalene McPharlin. 1995. (Illus.). 267p. pap. text 59.95 (*0-941022-43-9*) Davies Pubng.

Vascular Technology Review. Ed. by Barton A. Bean. 3rd ed. 1989. LC 88-34404. pap. text 55.00 (*0-941022-15-3*) Davies Pubng.

Vascular Technology Review. Ed. by Donald P. Ridgway & D.E. Strandness, Jr. 4th ed. 2001. LC 2001-47133. pap. text 55.00 (*0-941022-19-6*) Davies Pubng.

Vascular Trauma. Rich. 2nd ed. 2000. (C). text (*0-7216-4071-0*) Saunders.

Vascular Tumors & Malfunctions of the Ocular Fundus. J. D. Delaey & M. Hanssens. 1990. (Monographs in Ophthalmology). (C). text 201.00 (*0-7923-0750-X*) Kluwer Academic.

Vasculature of the Brain & Cranial Base: Variations in Clinical Anatomy. Walter Grand & L. N. Hopkins. 1998. LC 98-26777. (Illus.). 248p. 149.00 (*0-86577-784-5*); 149.00 (*3-13-111221-2*) Thieme Med Pubs.

*__Vasculitis.__ Ed. by Eugene Ball & S. Louis Bridges, Jr. 2001. (Illus.). 512p. text 168.95 (*0-19-263053-9*) OUP.

Vasculitis, Rheumatic Disease, & the Nervous System. Peter Berlit. Ed. by Patricia Moore. 1992. LC 92-48500. 35.00 (*0-387-54853-X*) Spr-Verlag.

Vasectomy: The Decision-Making Process. S. D. Mumford. 1978. (Illus.). pap. 10.00 (*0-911302-33-6*) San Francisco Pr.

Vasectomy Counseling. S. D. Mumford. 1977. (Illus.). 15.00 (*0-911302-31-X*) San Francisco Pr.

Vaskulaere Hirnerkrankung im Alter. Ed. by W. Meier-Ruge. 1989. (Geriatrie fuer die Taegliche Praxis Ser.: Vol. 2). viii, 188p. pap. 21.00 (*3-8055-4508-8*) S Karger.

Vasoactive Renal Hormones. Ed. by G. M. Eisenbach & J. Brod. 1978. (Contributions to Nephrology Ser.: Vol. 12). (Illus.). pap. 29.75 (*3-8055-2839-6*) S Karger.

Vasodilator Mechanisms. Ed. by P. M. Vanhoutte & St. F. Vatner. 1985. (Bibliotheca Cardiologica Ser.: No. 38). (Illus.). viii, 284p. 120.00 (*3-8055-3903-7*) S Karger.

Vasomotion & Flow Modulation in the Microcirculation. Ed. by Marcos Intaglietta. 1989. (Progress in Applied Microcirculation Ser.: Vol. 15). (Illus.). viii, 104p. 68.00 (*3-8055-5014-6*) S Karger.

Vasomotion & Quantitative Kapillaroskopie. Ed. by K. Messmer & F. Hammersen. 1984. (Progress in Applied Microcirculation Ser.: Vol. 3). (Illus.). viii, 152p. pap. 71.50 (*3-8055-3809-X*) S Karger.

Vasopressin: Disturbed Secretion & Its Effects. L. Kovacs. 1990. (Developments in Nephrology Ser.). (C). text 160.00 (*0-7923-0249-4*) Kluwer Academic.

Vasopressin: Principles & Properties. D. M. Gash & G. J. Boer. 1987. (Illus.). 654p. (C). text 135.00 (*0-306-42515-7*, Kluwer Plenum) Kluwer Academic.

Vasopressin & Oxytocin: Molecular, Cellular & Clinical Advances. Hans H. Zingg et al. 1998. LC 98-40029. (Advances in Experimental Medicine & Biology Ser.). (C). text (*0-306-45928-0*, Kluwer Plenum) Kluwer Academic.

Vast Sea of Misery: A History & Guide to the Union & Confederate Field Hospitals at Gettysburg, July 1-November 20, 1863. Gregory A. Coco. 1988. (Illus.). 224p. (C). pap. text 21.95 (*0-939631-88-1*) Thomas Publications.

VAT: Veterinary Aptitude Test Practice Examination. David M. Tarlow. 1992. (Practice Examination Ser.: No. 3). 40p. pap. 16.95 (*0-931572-56-8*);No. 2. pap. 16.95 (*0-931572-54-1*) Datar Pub.

VAT (Veterinary Aptitude Test) David M. Tarlow. 1992. (Practice Examination Ser.: No. 4). 40p. pap. text 16.95 (*0-931572-55-X*) Datar Pub.

VAT (Veterinary Aptitude Test) Practice Examination. David M. Tarlow. 1992. (Practice Examination Ser.). 40p. (C). No. 1. pap. 16.95 (*0-931572-27-4*); No. 5. pap. text 16.95 (*0-931572-28-2*) Datar Pub.

VBAC Companion: The Expectant Mother's Guide to Vaginal Birth after Cesarean. Diane Korte. 1997. LC 97-31338. (Illus.). 256p. 21.95 (*1-55832-128-4*) Harvard Common Pr.

VCAT - Veterinary College Admission Test: Comprehensive Manual for Self Study. David M. Tarlow. 2nd rev. ed. 1999. (Illus.). 150p. (C). pap. text 19.95 (*1-57732-122-7*) Datar Pub.

VCAT - Veterinary College Admission Test No. 1: Practice Exam Annotated Answers. David M. Tarlow. rev. ed. 1999. 20p. (C). pap. text 5.95 (*1-57732-124-3*) Datar Pub.

VCAT - Veterinary College Admission Test No. 1: Practice Examination. David M. Tarlow. 1999. 40p. (C). pap. text 18.95 (*1-57732-123-5*) Datar Pub.

VCAT - Veterinary College Admission Test No. 2: Practice Exam Annotated Answers. David M. Tarlow. 2nd rev. ed. 1999. 20p. (C). pap. text 6.95 (*1-57732-126-X*) Datar Pub.

VCAT - Veterinary College Admission Test No. 2: Practice Examination. David M. Tarlow. 2nd rev. ed. 1999. 40p. (C). pap. text 18.95 (*1-57732-125-1*) Datar Pub.

TUV

VCAT - Veterinary College Admission Test No. 3: Practice Exam Annotated Answers. David M. Tarlow. 3rd rev. ed. 1999. 20p. (C). pap. text 6.95 (*1-57732-128-6*) Datar Pub.

VCAT - Veterinary College Admission Test No. 3: Practice Examination. David M. Tarlow. 2nd rev. ed. 1999. 40p. (C). pap. text 18.95 (*1-57732-127-8*) Datar Pub.

VCAT - Veterinary College Admission Test No. 4: Practice Exam Annotated Answers. David M. Tarlow. 2nd rev. ed. 1999. 20p. (C). pap. text 6.95 (*1-57732-130-8*) Datar Pub.

VCAT - Veterinary College Admission Test No. 4: Practice Examination. David M. Tarlow. 2nd rev. ed. 1999. 40p. (C). pap. text 18.95 (*1-57732-129-4*) Datar Pub.

VCAT - Veterinary College Admission Test No. 5: Practice Exam Annotated Answers. David M. Tarlow. 2nd rev. ed. 1999. 20p. (C). pap. text 6.95 (*1-57732-132-4*) Datar Pub.

VCAT - Veterinary College Admission Test No. 5: Practice Examination. David M. Tarlow. 2nd rev. ed. 1999. 40p. (C). pap. text 18.95 (*1-57732-131-6*) Datar Pub.

VCAT - Veterinary College Admission Test - Core Content. David M. Tarlow. 2nd rev. ed. 1999. (Illus.). 400p. pap. 49.95 (*1-57774-009-2*) Educ Tsting Cnslts.

VCAT Exam No. 5 Annotated Answers (Veterinary College Admissions Test) David M. Tarlow. 1996. pap. 5.95 (*1-57732-054-9*) Datar Pub.

VCAT Exam No. 5 (Veterinary College Admission Test) David M. Tarlow. 7th ed. 1996. pap. 19.95 (*1-57732-045-X*) Datar Pub.

VCAT Exam No. 4 Annotated Answers (Veterinary College Admissions Test) David M. Tarlow. 7th ed. 1996. pap. 5.95 (*1-57732-053-0*) Datar Pub.

VCAT Exam No. 4 (Veterinary College Admission Test) David M. Tarlow. 1996. pap. 19.95 (*1-57732-049-2*) Datar Pub.

VCAT Exam No. 1 Annotated Answers (Veterinary College Admission Test) David M. Tarlow. 7th ed. 1996. (Orig.). pap. 5.95 (*1-57732-050-6*) Datar Pub.

VCAT Exam No. 1 (Veterinary College Admission Test) David M. Tarlow. 7th ed. 1996. (Illus.). (Orig.). pap. 19.95 (*1-57732-046-8*) Datar Pub.

VCAT Exam No. 3 Annotated Answers (Veterinary College Admissions Test) David M. Tarlow. 7th ed. 1996. pap. 5.95 (*1-57732-052-2*) Datar Pub.

VCAT Exam No. 3 (Veterinary College Admission Test) David M. Tarlow. 1996. (Orig.). pap. 19.95 (*1-57732-048-4*) Datar Pub.

VCAT Exam No. 2 Annotated Answers (Veterinary College Admission Test) David M. Tarlow. 7th ed. 1996. (Orig.). pap. 5.95 (*1-57732-051-4*) Datar Pub.

VCAT Exam No. 2 (Veterinary College Admission Test) David M. Tarlow. 7th ed. 1996. (Orig.). pap. 19.95 (*1-57732-047-6*) Datar Pub.

VCAT (Veterinary College Admission Test) For Comprehensive Review. David M. Tarlow. 7th ed. 1996. (Illus.). (Orig.). pap., stu. ed. 19.95 (*1-57732-044-1*) Datar Pub.

VD: The Love Epidemic. Mari Stein. rev. ed. 1977. (Illus.). reprint ed. pap. 3.95 (*0-918546-00-1*) Quarterdeck.

VD Book: For People Who Care about Themselves & Others. Joseph A. Chiappa & Joseph J. Forish. 1977. LC 76-17596. (Illus.). 145p. pap. 6.95 (*0-8290-0287-1*) Irvington.

VDU-Manual: A Practical Guide to Solving VDU-Related Eye Problems. David Thomson. 2001. 256p. pap. 45.00 (*0-7506-3785-4*) Buttrwrth-Heinemann.

Vector-Borne Pathogens: International Trade & Tropical Animal Diseases. Emmanuel Camus et al. 1996. LC 96-31285. (Annals of the New York Academy of Sciences Ser.). (*0-89766-955-X*); pap. 130.00 (*0-89766-956-8*) NY Acad Sci.

Vector-Borne Pathogens: International Trade & Tropical Animal Diseases. James A. House. 1999. 504p. pap. text 24.95 (*0-8018-6305-8*) Johns Hopkins.

Vector Control. 1963. (WHO Bulletin Supplement Ser.: Vol. 29). pap. text 12.00 (*92-4-068291-0*, 1032901) World Health.

Vector Control for Malaria & Other Mosquito-Borne Diseases: Report of a WHO Study Group. 1995. (Technical Reports: Vol. 857). (FRE & SPA.). 91p. (C). pap. 15.00 (*92-4-120857-0*, 1100857) World Health.

Vector Control in International Health. 1972. 144p. pap. text 32.00 (*92-4-154016-8*, 1150160) World Health.

Vector Control in Primary Health Care: Report of a WHO Scientific Group, 1987. WHO Staff. 1987. (Technical Report Ser.: No. 755). 61p. 9.00 (*92-4-120755-8*) World Health.

Vector Ecology: Proceedings of the WHO Scientific Group, Geneva, 1972. WHO Staff. 1972. (Technical Reports: No. 501). pap. text 4.00 (*92-4-120501-6*, 1100501) World Health.

Vectors: Cloning Applications. P. Gacesa & D. Ramji. 1998. LC 97-32758. (Essential Techniques Ser.). 172p. pap. 48.95 (*0-471-96266-X*) Wiley.

Vectors of Disease Agents: Interactions with Plants, Animals, & Men. Ed. by John J. McKelvey, Jr. et al. 1980. LC 80-18676. 229p. 75.00 (*0-275-90521-7*, C0521, Praeger Pubs) Greenwood.

Vectors of Diseases of Natural Foci. Ed. by P. A. Petrishcheva. 1965. 336p. 3.5 hd 82.00 (*0-7065-0566-2*) Coronet Bks.

Vedic Medicine. Rita Singh. 1998. (*81-7488-836-5*) Anmol IND. *Dist:* S Asia.

Vegetable Materia Medica of India & Ceylon. E. Roberts. 1984. 437p. (C). (*0-7855-3298-6*) Scientific GBR. *Dist:* St Mut.

Vegetables & Health Sciences: Index of Modern Information. Victor K. Elwood. rev. ed. 1992. LC 92-31218. 144p. 47.50 (*1-55914-750-4*); pap. 44.50 (*1-55914-751-2*) ABBE Pubs Assn.

Vegetarian Baby: A Sensible Guide for Parents. Sharon K. Yntema. LC 79-24623. (Illus.). 224p. 1991. pap. 11.95 (*0-935526-02-1*); 1980. lib. bdg. 14.95 (*0-935526-01-3*) McBooks Pr.

Vegetarian Journal Reports. Ed. by Charles Stahler et al. 1990. (Illus.). 112p. (Orig.). pap. 10.00 (*0-931411-07-6*) Vegetarian Resc.

Vegetarian Medicines. Clarence Meyer. Ed. by David C. Meyer. 1981. (Illus.). 96p. (Orig.). pap. 5.95 (*0-916638-06-5*) Meyerbooks.

Vegetarian Pregnancy: The Definitive Nutritional Guide to Having a Healthy Baby. Sharon K. Yntema. 1994. LC 94-8073. (Illus.). 336p. pap. 15.95 (*0-935526-21-8*) McBooks Pr.

Vegetarianism & the Jewish Tradition. Louis A. Berman. 1982. LC 81-11729. 120p. 19.95 (*0-87068-756-5*) Ktav.

***Vegetative State.** Bryan Jennett. 2001. LC 2001-37373. 200p. pap. text 42.95 (*0-521-44158-7*) Cambridge U Pr.

Vehicle Extrication: A Training Manual. Steven Kidd & John D. Czajkowski. 1991. LC 89-84561. 253p. 40.95 (*0-87814-915-5*); 260p. stu. ed. 5.00 (*0-87814-929-5*) Fire Eng.

Vehicle Extrication & Rescue. Ronald E. Moore. 1997. (C). (gr. 13). tchr. ed. 65.00 (*0-8151-2274-8*, 31739) Mosby Inc.

Vehicle Rescue. James B. Gargan. 2nd ed. 1996. LC 96-1797. 352p. pap. text 59.00 (*0-8359-8374-9*) P-H.

Vehicles: Experiments in Synthetic Psychology. Valentino Braitenberg. 1986. 168p. (C). pap. 16.95 (*0-262-52112-1*, Bradford Bks) MIT Pr.

Vein Diagnosis & Treatment: A Comprehensive Approach. Robert A. Weiss et al. 2000. LC 00-32912. (Illus.). 304p. text 149.00 (*0-07-069201-7*) McGraw-Hill Prof.

Veins: Their Functional Role in the Circulation. Hirakawa et al. 1994. LC 93-36742. (Illus.). 153p. 126.00 (*0-387-70126-5*) Spr-Verlag.

Venereal Disease Bibliography for 1966-1970. Stephen H. Goode. 1972. LC 71-189843. 400p. 22.50 (*0-87875-023-1*) Whitston Pub.

Venereal Disease Bibliography for 1973. Stephen H. Goode. 1975. LC 71-189843. xxiii, 276p. 11.00 (*0-87875-058-4*) Whitston Pub.

Venereal Disease Bibliography for 1974. Compiled by Judith Kramer-Greene. 1976. LC 71-189843. 15.00 (*0-87875-080-0*) Whitston Pub.

Venereal Disease Bibliography for 1975. Compiled by Judith Kramer-Greene. 1977. LC 71-189843. 25.00 (*0-87875-097-5*) Whitston Pub.

Venereal Disease Control: A Survey of Recent Legislation. 1975. (International Digest of Health Legislation Offprints: Vol. 26, No. 1). pap. text 8.00 (*92-4-169261-8*, 1957501) World Health.

Venereal Diseases: A Survey of Existing Legislation. WHO Staff. 1956. (International Digest of Health Legislation Offprints: Vol. 7, No. 2). 44p. 3.00 (*92-4-169072-0*) World Health.

Venipuncture Technique for Contrast Media Administration. Robert J. Parelli. 1998. (Illus.). 136p. 80.00 (*1-880359-16-2*) Par Rad.

Venom Phospholipase A2 Enzymes: Structure, Function & Mechanism. R. M. Kini. 1997. LC 96-27171. 528p. 200.00 (*0-471-96189-2*) Wiley.

Venomous Animals & Their Toxins. G. Habermehl. 1981. (Illus.). 195p. 37.95 (*0-387-10780-0*) Spr-Verlag.

Venomous Snakes: Ecology, Evolution, & Snakebite. Ed. by Roger S. Thorpe et al. 1996. (Symposia of the Zoological Society of London Ser.: No. 70). (Illus.). 296p. text 150.00 (*0-19-854986-5*) OUP.

Venous Access Management. McCowan. 1998. (C). text (*0-443-07786-X*) Church.

Venous & Arterial Thrombosis: Pathophysiological & Clinical Aspects, Selected Plenary Lectures: 15th International Congress on Thrombosis, Antalya, October 1998. Ed. by S. Levy-Toledano & H. C. Hemker. 1999. (Haemostasis Ser.: Vol. 29, Nos. 2 & 3). (Illus.). 116p. pap. 34.00 (*3-8055-6958-0*) S Karger.

Venous Catheters: A Practical Manual. Philip C. Pieters et al. 2001. (Illus.). 304p. pap. 39.00 (*0-86577-921-X*) Thieme Med Pubs.

Venous Disorders. John J. Bergan. 2000. (Vademecum Ser.). spiral bd. 45.00 (*1-57059-528-3*) Landes Bioscience.

Venous Disorders of the Legs: Principles & Practice. L. L. Tretbar. 1998. LC 98-6341. (Illus.). 150p. disk 159.00 (*1-85233-007-4*) Spr-Verlag.

Venous Leakage: Journal: Urologia Internationalis, Vol. 49, No. 1, 1992. Ed. by W. Weidner & G. Ludwig. 1992. (Illus.). 68p. pap. 74.00 (*3-8055-5643-8*) S Karger.

Venous Surgery in the Lower Extremity. Kenneth G. Swan. 1976. LC 74-2564. (Illus.). 442p. 37.50 (*0-87527-135-9*) Green.

Venous Thromboembolism: An Evidence-Based Atlas. Ed. by Russell D. Hull et al. 1996. LC 95-39036. (Illus.). 464p. 149.00 (*0-87993-633-9*) Futura Pub.

Venous Thromboembolism: Natural History, Diagnosis, & Management. R. D. Hull. Ed. by Jack Hirsh. 1987. LC 87-8043. 192p. 100.00 (*0-8493-4761-0*, RC697, CRC Reprint) Franklin.

Venous Thrombosis: From Genes to Clinical Medicine. Ed. by D. N. Cooper & M. Krawczak. 1997. (Human Molecular Genetics Ser.). (Illus.). 352p. (*1-872748-94-5*) Bios Sci GBR. *Dist:* Bks Intl VA.

Venous Thrombosis & Pulmonary Embolism. Michael Hume et al. 1970. LC 70-122215. (Commonwealth Fund Publications). (Illus.). 472p. 45.00 (*0-674-93320-6*) HUP.

Venous Valves. R. Gottlob & R. May. 1986. (Illus.). 227p. 118.00 (*0-387-81898-7*) Spr-Verlag.

Ventilation. J. Steven Kidd & John Czajkowski. 1995. pap. text, wbk. ed. (*0-8151-5073-3*) Mosby Inc.

Ventilator-Assisted Child. Driver. 1997. 59.00 (*0-7616-1533-4*) Commun Skill.

Ventilators & Muscular Dystrophy. Nancy C. Schock & Agatha P. Colbert. 1987. 40p. 6.00 (*0-931301-03-3*) Gazette Intl.

Ventilatory Failure. Ed. by J. L. Vincent et al. 1991. (Update in Intensive Care & Emergency Medicine Ser.: Vol. 15). (Illus.). 456p. 114.95 (*0-387-54297-3*) Spr-Verlag.

Ventral Mainstem Mechanisms & Control of Respiration & Blood Pressure. Ed. by C. Ovid Trouth. 1995. LC 95-10040. (Lung Biology in Health & Disease Ser.: Vol. 82). (Illus.). 1000p. text 250.00 (*0-8247-9514-8*) Dekker.

Ventricle: Basic & Clinical Aspects. Ed. by Herbert J. Levine & William H. Gaasch. 1985. LC 85-4976. text 247.50 (*0-89838-721-3*) Kluwer Academic.

Ventricular Arrhythmias of Ischemia & Infarction: Electrophysiological Mechanisms. Andrew L. Wit & Michiel J. Janse. 1992. (Illus.). 672p. 150.00 (*0-87993-376-3*) Futura Pub.

Ventricular Fibrillation: A Pediatric Problem. Ed. by Linda Quan & Wayne H. Franklin. 2000. (American Heart Association Monograph Ser.). (Illus.). 302p. 95.00 (*0-87993-452-2*) Futura Pub.

Ventricular Septum of the Heart. Ed. by Arnold C. Wenink et al. 1981. text 162.50 (*90-6021-486-2*) Kluwer Academic.

Ventricular Support with Miniature Rotary Blood Pumps: An Experimental Study. Bart Meyns. 1997. (Acta Biomedica Lovaniensia Ser.: Vol. 145). (Illus.). 119p. pap. (*90-6186-804-1*) Leuven Univ BEL. *Dist:* Coronet Bks.

Ventricular Tachyarrhythmias in the Normal Heart. Ed. by John P. Bourke et al. 1998. LC 98-4645. (Clinical Approaches to Tachyarrhythmias Ser.: Vol. 8). (Illus.). 107p. 19.00 (*0-87993-400-X*) Futura Pub.

Ventricular Tachycardias. Ed. by Etienne Aliot & Ralph Lazzara. 1987. (Developments in Cardiovascular Medicine Ser.). lib. bdg. 230.50 (*0-89838-881-3*) Kluwer Academic.

Ventricular Vascular Coupling. Ed. by F. C. Yin. 1986. (Illus.). 406p. 129.00 (*0-387-96279-4*) Spr-Verlag.

Verbal Abuse Survivors Speak Out on Relationship & Recovery. Patricia Evans. 1993. 252p. (Orig.). pap. 10.95 (*1-55850-304-8*) Adams Media.

Verbal Processes in Children: Progress in Cognitive Developmental Research. Ed. by Charles J. Brainerd & M. Pressley. 1982. (Cognitive Development Ser.). (Illus.). 289p. 83.95 (*0-387-90648-7*) Spr-Verlag.

Verborgene Heilkuenste: Geschichte der Frauenmedzin im Spaetmittelalter. Britta-Juliane Kruse. 1995. (Quellen und Forschungen zur Literatur und Kulturgeschichte: Band 5 (239)). (GER.). xii, 498p. (C). lib. bdg. 147.70 (*3-11-014704-1*) De Gruyter.

Verbroken Verbindigen see Broken Connections: Alzheimer's Disease

Verhaltensauffaellige Schueler. B. Meile. 1982. (Sozialmedizinische und Paedagogische Jugendkunde Ser.: Band 16). xii, 84p. pap. 20.00 (*3-8055-3552-X*) S Karger.

Verhaltenstherapie Bei Kindern und Jugendlichen. Ed. by S. Schneider. 2000. (Verhaltenstherapie Ser.: Band 9, No. 4). (GER.). 60p. pap. 35.00 (*3-8055-7087-2*) S Karger.

Verify & Comply: A Quick Reference Guide to the JCAHO & NCQA Standards for Credentialing. Carol Cairns. Ed. by Steve Dorman. 2000. (Illus.). 176p. pap. text (*1-57839-075-3*) Opus Communs.

Vermont Health Care in Perspective 2000. Ed. by Kathleen O'Leary Morgan & Scott E. Morgan. 2000. 21p. spiral bd. 19.00 (*0-7401-0244-3*) Morgan Quitno Corp.

Vermont Health Care Perspective, 1998. Ed. by Kathleen O'Leary Morgan & Scott E. Morgan. 1998. 20p. pap. 19.00 (*1-56692-844-3*) Morgan Quitno Corp.

Vermont Holistic Health Directory. Alternative Medicine Research Staff. 1996. 35p. (C). pap. 20.00 (*1-893553-00-0*) AMRITA Pr.

Vermont Holistic Health Directory. Ed. by Laura Brown. 2nd rev. ed. 1998. LC 98-74454. 53p. pap. 20.00 (*1-893553-01-9*) AMRITA Pr.

Versuch. Alexander Von Humboldt. 1994. (GER.). 1100p. (C). text 89.50 (*0-930329-75-9*) Kabel Pubs.

Vertebral Artery: Surgery & Pathology. B. George & C. Laurian. 1987. (Illus.). 258p. 158.00 (*0-387-81968-1*) Spr-Verlag.

Vertebral Fracture in Osteoporosis. Ed. by Harry K. Genant et al. 1995. (Illus.). 300p. 135.00 (*0-9646199-5-4*) Radiol Res & Educ Found.

Vertebral Musculoskeletal Disorders. Alfred Brian Corrigan & Geoffrey Douglas Maitland. 1998. LC 98-20593. 288p. pap. text 95.00 (*0-7506-2965-7*) Buttrwrth-Heinemann.

Vertebrata of the Tertiary Formations of the West Edward D. Cope. Ed. by Keir B. Sterling. 1978. LC 77-81093. (Biologists & Their World Ser.). (Illus.). reprint ed. lib. bdg. 95.95 (*0-405-10672-6*);1. lib. bdg. 47.95 (*0-405-10673-4*);Vol. 2. 50.95 (*0-405-10674-2*) Ayer.

Vertebrate Cell Culture I. 1987. (Advances in Biochemical Engineering Ser.: Vol. 34). (Illus.). 175p. 109.00 (*0-387-17626-8*) Spr-Verlag.

Vertebrate Endocrinology. Ed. by David O. Norris. 3rd ed. 1996. LC 96-33146. (Illus.). 634p. (C). text 69.95 (*0-12-521670-X*) Acad Pr.

Vertebrate Gas Transport Cascade: Adaptations to Environment & Mode of Life, Proceedings of a Meeting Held in Sao Sebastiao, Sao Paulo, Brazil, September 10-15, 1991. Ed. by J. Eduardo & P. W. Bicudo. 1992. LC 92-39925. 400p. 189.00 (*0-8493-4976-1*, QP121) CRC Pr.

Vertebrate Hard Tissues. L. B. Halstead. 1974. (Wykeham Science Ser.: No. 30). 192p. pap. 18.00 (*0-85109-430-9*) Taylor & Francis.

Vertebrate Hard Tissues. L. B. Halstead & R. Hill. 1974. (Wykeham Science Ser.: No. 30). 192p. (C). 18.00 (*0-8448-1157-2*, Crane Russak) Taylor & Francis.

Vertebrate Inner Ear. Ed. by Edwin R. Lewis et al. 1985. 256p. 148.00 (*0-8493-6465-5*, QP461, CRC Reprint) Franklin.

Vertebrate Olfactory System Chemical Neuroanatomy, Function & Development: Chemical Neuroanatomy, Function & Development. Nobert Halasz. 1990. (Chemical Neuroanatomy, Function & Development Ser.). (Illus.). 280p. (C). (*963-05-5634-0*) Akade Kiado HUN. *Dist:* Intl Spec Bk, St Mut.

Vertebrate Visual System. Stephen Polyak. Ed. by Heinrich Kluver. 1957. LC 55-5153. (Illus.). lib. bdg. 100.00 (*0-226-67494-0*) U Ch Pr.

Vertebrates: Comparative Anatomy, Function, Evolution. Kenneth V. Kardong. 1990. (Illus.). 720p. 41.95 (*0-8016-2666-8*) Mosby Inc.

Vertebrobasilar Arterial Disease. Ramon Berguer & Louis R. Caplan. 1992. (Illus.). 299p. 75.00 (*0-942219-22-8*) Quality Med Pub.

Vertical Mammaplasty & Liposuction. Madeleine Lejour. 1994. (Illus.). VHS 75.00 (*1-57626-042-9*) Quality Med Pub.

Vertically Transmitted Diseases. Stavros N. Busenberg & Kenneth Cooke. 1993. LC 92-49541. (Biomathematics Ser.: Vol. 23). (*3-540-52004-X*); 248p. 136.00 (*0-387-52004-X*) Spr-Verlag.

Vertige. P. Liard et al. 1993. (Illus.). xii, 96p. pap. 33.25 (*3-8055-5822-8*) S Karger.

Vertigo: Its Multisensory Syndromes. Thomas Brandt. 2nd ed. 1999. LC 98-26294. (Clinical Medicine & the Nervous System Ser.). (Illus.). 536p. 249.00 (*3-540-19934-9*) Spr-Verlag.

Vertigo & Dizziness Rehabilitation: The MCS Method. Antonio Cesarani & Dario Alpini. 1999. LC 98-40800. (Illus.). 253p. pap. 49.00 (*3-540-64084-3*) Spr-Verlag.

Vertigo, Nausea, Tinnitus & Hearing Loss in Central & Peripheral Vestibular Diseases: Proceedings of the XXIInd Annual Meeting of the International Neurootologic & Equilibriometric Society, Hakone, Japan, 6-9 April 1995. Ed. by Claus-Frenz Claussen et al. 1995. LC 95-23632. (International Congress Ser.: No. 1087). 414p. 219.50 (*0-444-82193-7*, Excerpta Medica) Elsevier.

Vessels. 1987. (Journal: Vol. 4, No. 4, 1986). (Illus.). iv, 88p. pap. 50.50 (*3-8055-4583-5*) S Karger.

Vest Pocket Fat Counter. Susan K. Podell. 1992. LC 91-33022. 56p. pap. 2.99 (*0-385-42294-6*) Doubleday.

Vestibular & Brain Stem Control of Eye, Head & Body Movements. Ed. by Yoshikazu Shinoda & H. Shimazu. 1992. (Illus.). xii, 466p. 287.00 (*3-8055-5548-2*) S Karger.

Vestibular & Neural Front: Proceedings of the 12th International Symposium on Posture & Gait, Matsumoto, 3-7 October 1994. Ed. by Kiichiro Taguchi et al. 1994. LC 94-34759. (International Congress Ser.: 1070). 640p. 272.25 (*0-444-81933-9*) Elsevier.

Vestibular & Visual Control on Posture & Locomotor Equilibrium. M. Igarashi & O. F. Black. 1985. (Illus.). x, 366p. 164.50 (*3-8055-3951-7*) S Karger.

Vestibular Autonomic Regulation. Bill J. Yates & Alan D. Miller. 1996. LC 95-40474. 266p. 189.95 (*0-8493-7668-8*) CRC Pr.

Vestibular Dysfunction & Its Therapy. Ed. by Ulrich Buttner. 1998. LC 98-42013. (Advances in OtoRhinoLaryngology Ser.: Vol. 55). (Illus.). viii, 248p. 216.50 (*3-8055-6702-2*) S Karger.

***Vestibular Labyrinth in Health & Disease.** Ed. by Joel A. Goebel & Stephen M. Highstein. 2001. LC 2001-45569. (Annals of the New York Academy of Sciences Ser.: Vol. 942). (*1-57331-289-4*); (*1-57331-290-8*) NY Acad Sci.

Vestibular Neurotology. Ed. by P. Molina-Negro. 1982. (Advances in OtoRhinoLaryngology Ser.: Vol. 28). (Illus.). viii, 148p. 100.00 (*3-8055-3490-6*) S Karger.

Vestibular Organs: S. E. M. Atlas of the Inner Ear. Yasuo Harada. 1988. LC 87-36673. (Illus.). 216p. lib. bdg. (*90-6299-043-6*) Kugler NLD. *Dist:* Lib Res.

TUV

Vestibular Processing Dysfunction in Children. Ed. by Kenneth J. Ottenbacher & Margaret A. Short. 1985. LC 85-8636. (Physical & Occupational Therapy in Pediatrics Ser.: Vol. 5, Nos. 2 & 3). 152p. pap. text 14.95 (*0-86656-432-2*); text 49.95 (*0-86656-431-4*) Haworth Pr.

*__Vestibular Rehab for Treatment for Vertigo & Imbalance.__ Cronin. 1995. 55.00 (*0-8342-1944-1*) PRO-ED.

Vestibular Rehabilitation. Susan J. Herdman. 2nd ed. 1999. LC 99-39686. (Contemporary Perspectives in Rehabilitation Ser.). (Illus.). 597p. 75.00 (*0-8036-0444-0*) Davis Co.

Vestibular Rehabilitation: Protocols & Programs. Richard E. Gans. 1996. (Orig.). 39.95 (*1-56593-806-2*, 1574); LC 96-6911. (Illus.). 128p. pap. 150.00 (*1-56593-625-6*, 1296) Thomson Learn.

Vestibular System: Function & Morphology. Ed. by T. Gualtierotti. 1981. (Illus.). 548p. 195.00 (*0-387-90559-6*) Spr-Verlag.

Vestibular System: Fundamental & Clinical Observations. Ed. by Jan Stahle. 1984. (Illus.). 296p. text 93.50 (*91-22-00676-1*) Coronet Bks.

Vet Acupuncture 2. Ed. by Allen M. Schoen. 2nd ed. 2000. LC 00-42157. (Illus.). xviii, 628p. text 99.00 (*0-323-00945-X*) Mosby Inc.

Vet in the Vestry. Alexander Cameron. 1992. mass mkt. 4.99 (*0-312-92692-8*) St Martin.

Vet on Call: Home Remedies for Common Complaints. Ed. by Matthew Hoffman. 1998. LC 98-31657. (Dog Lovers Care Guides Ser.). 15.95 (*1-57954-048-1*) Rodale Pr Inc.

Vet on Call: Home Remedies for Common Concerns: Behavior, Grooming, Sickness, Aging. Ed. by Matthew Hoffman. 1999. LC 98-31657. (Dog Lovers Care Guides Ser.). (Illus.). 176p. pap. 14.95 (*1-57954-181-X*) Rodale Pr Inc.

Veterans & Agent Orange: Update, 1996. Institute of Medicine Staff. rev. ed. 1996. LC 96-68761. 384p. (Orig.). text 49.00 (*0-309-05487-7*) Natl Acad Pr.

Veterans & Agent Orange: Update 1998. Institute of Medicine Staff. 2nd ed. 2000. LC 00-266314. xi, 611p. pap. 79.00 (*0-309-06326-4*) Natl Acad Pr.

Veterans at Risk: The Health Effects of Mustard Gas & Lewisite. Institute of Medicine Staff. Ed. by Constance M. Pechura & David P. Rall. 1993. LC 92-40735. 448p. (Orig.). (C). pap. text 39.95 (*0-309-04832-X*) Natl Acad Pr.

Veterans' Health Care: Implications of Other Countries' Reforms for the U. S. 1995. (Illus.). 56p. (Orig.). (C). pap. text 20.00 (*0-7881-2081-6*) DIANE Pub.

Veteran's Health Care: Veteran's Perceptions of V. A. Services & V. A.'s Role in Health Care Reform. 1995. (Illus.). 40p. (Orig.). (C). pap. text 25.00 (*0-7881-1767-X*) DIANE Pub.

Veterens' Health Care: Facilities Resource Allocations Could Be More Equitable. 1996. (Illus.). 72p. (Orig.). pap. text 30.00 (*0-7881-2894-9*) DIANE Pub.

Veterinarian. Jack Rudman. 1994. (Career Examination Ser.: C-870). pap. 49.95 (*0-8373-0870-4*) Nat Learn.

Veterinarian Trainee. Jack Rudman. 1994. (Career Examination Ser.: C-1529). pap. 39.95 (*0-8373-1529-8*) Nat Learn.

Veterinarian's Anatomy & Physiology. Molgaard. 1998. (Agriculture Ser.). tchr. ed. 12.00 (*0-8273-7872-6*); tchr. ed., lab manual ed. 12.00 (*0-8273-7874-2*) Delmar.

Veterinarian's Anatomy & Physiology Lab Manual. Molgaard. 1998. (Agriculture Ser.). lab manual ed. 21.00 (*0-8273-7873-4*) Delmar.

Veterinarian's Companion for Common Dental Procedures. Heidi B. Lobprise & Robert B. Wiggs. 1999. LC 99-59463. (Illus.). 189p. pap. (*1-58326-006-4*, AAHA Pr) Am Animal Hosp Assoc.

Veterinarian's Encyclopedia of Animal Behavior. Bonnie V. Beaver. 1994. LC 94-27257. (Illus.). 320p. text 34.95 (*0-8138-2114-2*) Iowa U Pr.

Veterinarians' Guide to Natural Remedies for Cats: Safe & Effective Alternative Treatments & Healing Techniques from the Nation's Top Holistic Veterinarians. Martin Zucker. 2000. LC 99-23724. xxiii, 296p. pap. 14.95 (*0-609-80373-5*, Crown) Crown Pub Group.

Veterinarians' Guide to Natural Remedies for Dogs: Safe & Effective Alternative Treatments & Healing Techniques from the Nation's Top Holistic Veterinarians. Martin Zucker. 2000. LC 99-23709. xx, 284p. pap. 14.95 (*0-609-80372-7*, Three Riv Pr) Crown Pub Group.

Veterinarian's Guide to Your Cat's Symptoms. Michael S. Garvey et al. 1999. LC 98-39149. (Illus.). xv, 175p. (Orig.). pap. 17.95 (*0-375-75227-7*) Villard Books.

Veterinarian's Guide to Your Dog's Symptoms. Michael S. Garvey et al. 1999. LC 98-39150. (Illus.). xv, 222p. (Orig.). pap. 17.95 (*0-375-75226-9*) Villard Books.

Veterinarians' New Research Bible: Index of New Information. Max W. Denton. 1995. LC 95-19209. 57.50 (*0-7883-0494-1*); pap. 47.50 (*0-7883-0495-X*) ABBE Pubs Assn.

Veterinarian's Practical Reference Guide to Equine Nutrition. Date not set. 345p. text 45.00 (*0-9659590-0-7*) Am Equine Pract.

Veterinary Acupuncture. Alan M. Klide & Shiu H. Kung. 1977. LC 76-53193. (Illus.). 314p. 67.95 (*0-8122-7721-X*) U of Pa Pr.

Veterinary Acupuncture: Ancient Art to Modern Medicine. Ed. by Allen M. Schoen. 1994. LC 93-74075. 500p. text 94.95 (*0-939674-51-3*) Am Vet Pubns.

Veterinary Anaesthesia. Leslie Wilfred Hall et al. 10th ed. 2000. (Illus.). 470p. text (*0-7020-2035-4*) W B Saunders GBR. *Dist:* Saunders.

Veterinary Anatomy Vol. 2: The Horse. Raymond R. Ashdown & Stan Done. 1986. LC 65-73315. (Illus.). 350p. text (*0-397-58304-4*, GM0003) Gower-Mosby.

Veterinary Anatomy Vol. 3: Dog & Cat, Vol. 3. Stanley H. Done. 1995. (C). (gr. 13). (*0-397-44721-3*) Gower-Mosby.

Veterinary Anesthesia. Janyce L. Cornick-Seahorn. 2000. LC 00-44452. (Practical Veterinarian Ser.). (Illus.). 250p. pap. text 24.99 (*0-7506-7227-7*) Buttrwrth-Heinemann.

Veterinary Anesthesia. Sawyer. text (*0-7216-7942-0*) Saunders.

*__Veterinary Anesthesia & Pain Management Secrets.__ Ed. by Stephen A. Greene. 2001. LC 2001-39966. (Secrets Ser.). (Illus.). 350p. pap. text 39.95 (*1-56053-442-7*) Lppncott W & W.

Veterinary Annual. Ed. by C. S. Grunsell et al. 26th ed. 1986. (Illus.). 389p. 62.95 (*0-85608-041-1*) Buttrwrth-Heinemann.

Veterinary Annual, No. 32. Ed. by Mary-Elizabeth Raw & T. J. Parkinson. 1992. (Illus.). 320p. (C). pap. 178.95 (*0-8464-4163-2*) Beekman Pubs.

Veterinary Annual, No. 32. Mary-Elizabeth Raw & T. J. Parkinson. 32nd ed. 1992. (Illus.). 320p. 96.95 (*0-632-03406-8*) Blackwell Sci.

Veterinary Annual, No. 34. Ed. by Mary-Elizabeth Raw & T. J. Parkinson. 1994. (Illus.). 256p. 135.00 (*0-86542-809-3*) Blackwell Sci.

Veterinary Annual, No. 35. Mary-Elizabeth Raw. 1995. 364p. 113.95 (*0-632-03982-5*) Blackwell Sci.

Veterinary Annual, Vol. 31. Ed. by C. S. Grunsell et al. 31st ed. 1991. (Illus.). 232p. text 95.00 (*0-632-03264-2*) Blackwell Sci.

Veterinary Annual, 1989. F. Hill et al. 29th ed. 1989. 330p. 95.00 (*0-407-01767-4*) Blackwell Sci.

Veterinary Annual, 1996, No. 36. Ed. by Mary-Elizabeth Raw & T. J. Parkinson. 1996. (Illus.). 400p. 120.00 (*0-632-04049-1*) Blackwell Sci.

Veterinary Annual, 1993, Vol. 33. C. S. Grunsell & Mary-Elizabeth Raw. 1993. (Illus.). 288p. 104.95 (*0-632-03564-1*) Blackwell Sci.

Veterinary Aptitude Test (VAT) Student Guide. David M. Tarlow. rev. ed. 1993. (Illus.). 120p. (C). pap. 16.95 (*0-931572-06-1*) Datar Pub.

Veterinary Aromatherapy. Nelly Grosjean. 1994. 130p. pap. (*0-85207-274-0*) C W Daniel GBR. *Dist:* Natl Bk Netwk.

Veterinary Assisting. Marian Mobley. Date not set. (C). 39.93 (*0-89303-977-2*) Appleton & Lange.

Veterinary Book for Dairy Farmers. R. W. Blowey. 2nd ed. 1988. (Illus.). 496p. (*0-85236-179-3*) Farming Pr GBR. *Dist:* Diamond Farm Bk.

Veterinary Book for Sheep Farmers. Dave Brown & Sam Meadowcroft. 1990. (Illus.). 240p. (*0-85236-189-0*) Farming Pr GBR. *Dist:* Diamond Farm Bk.

Veterinary Cancer Therapy Handbook: Animal Cancer Care. All Care Animal Referral Center & AAHA Press. 2nd ed. 1999. LC 99-58917. (*1-58326-008-0*, Creat Educ) Creative Co.

Veterinary Care of the Horse. Sue Devereux & Liz Morrison. 1990. 245p. (*0-85131-543-7*) J A Allen GBR. *Dist:* Trafalgar, St Mut.

Veterinary Clinical Diagnosis. W. H. Kelly. 3rd ed. 1984. (Illus.). 430p. text (*0-7216-0947-3*) Bailliere Tindall.

Veterinary Clinical Epidemiology: A Problem-Oriented Approach. Ronald D. Smith. 1992. lib. bdg. 49.00 (*0-7506-9182-4*, R); 1992. LC 93-45328. 248p. lib. bdg. 49.95 (*0-8493-8765-5*); 2nd ed. 1995. LC 94-36939. 304p. 84.95 (*0-8493-2445-9*, 2445) CRC Pr.

Veterinary Clinical Exam & Diagnosis. Ed. by O. M. Radostits et al. 2000. 800p. text (*0-7020-2476-7*) W B Saunders GBR. *Dist:* Saunders.

Veterinary Clinical Laboratory Procedures. Ed. by Margi Sirois. 1994. LC 94-30737. (Fundamentals of Veterinary Technology Ser.). (Illus.). 256p. (C). (gr. 13). pap. text 30.00 (*0-8016-8065-4*, 08065) Mosby Inc.

Veterinary Clinical Parasitology. Margaret W. Sloss et al. 6th ed. 1994. LC 93-33959. (Illus.). 208p. pap. text 42.95 (*0-8138-1733-1*) Iowa U Pr.

Veterinary Clinical Pathology. Embert H. Coles. 4th ed. 1986. (Illus.). 486p. text 67.00 (*0-7216-1828-6*) Saunders.

Veterinary College Admission Test (College) (VCAT) Jack Rudman. 1994. (Admission Test Ser.: ATS-29). pap. 27.95 (*0-8373-5029-8*) Nat Learn.

Veterinary College Admission Test (VCAT) - Core Content. David M. Tarlow. 1996. (Medical Examinations Ser.). (Illus.). 572p. (Orig.). (C). pap. 49.95 (*1-57774-004-1*) Educ Tsting Cnslts.

Veterinary Contact Reflex Analysis: Applications in Clinical Veterinary Practice. Ron Carsten. 1996. (Illus.). 82p. (Orig.). pap. text 85.00 (*0-9649593-1-3*) Gran Farnum.

Veterinary Contribution to Public Health Practice: Report of the FAO-WHO Expert Committee on Veterinary Public Health, Geneva, 1974. FAO-WHO Expert Committee on Veterinary Public Heal. 1975. (Technical Reports: No. 573). pap. text 8.00 (*92-4-120573-3*, 1100573) World Health.

Veterinary Conversations with Mid-Twentieth Century Leaders. Ole H. Stalheim. 1996. LC 95-38586. (Illus.). 328p. text 39.95 (*0-8138-2995-X*) Iowa U Pr.

Veterinary Demographic Annual Reports, Set. 5th ed. Center for Info. Management Staff. Incl. Pt. 1: National Distribution of U. S. Veterinarians. 31p. pap. 25.00 (*1-882691-04-0*); Pt. 2: Distribution of U. S. Veterinarians by Primary Employment. 55p. pap. 25.00 (*1-882691-05-9*); Pt. 4: Distribution of U. S. Veterinarians by State. 107p. pap. 125.00 (*1-882691-07-5*); (Illus.). 1996. 295.00 (*1-882691-03-2*) Am Veterinary Med Assn.

Veterinary Demographic Data Resource, Chap. 4 see , Pt. 2, Distribution of U. S. Veterinarians by Primary Employment

Veterinary Demographic Data Resource, Chap. 6 see , Pt. 4, Distribution of U. S. Veterinarians by State

Veterinary Demographic Data Resource, Chaps. 2 & 3 see , Pt. 1, National Distribution of U. S. Veterinarians

Veterinary Dental Techniques: For the Small Animal Practitioner. Steven E. Holmstrom et al. 2nd ed. 1998. LC 98-2782. (Illus.). 464p. (C). text 79.00 (*0-7216-5839-3*) Saunders.

Veterinary Dentistry for the Small Animal Technician. M. Lynne Kesel. 2000. LC 00-24450. (Illus.). xi, 267p. pap. 34.95 (*0-8138-2037-5*) Iowa U Pr.

Veterinary Dermatology. Moriello. 2001. 256p. pap. 25.00 (*0-7506-7299-4*) Buttrwrth-Heinemann.

Veterinary Diagnostic Ultrasound. Thomas G. Nyland & John S. Mattoon. 1995. LC 94-43396. (Illus.). 512p. text 88.00 (*0-7216-2745-5*) Saunders.

Veterinary Dictionary. D. C. Blood. 2nd ed. 1998. 1394p. (C). pap. text 39.95 (*0-7020-2034-6*) Saunders.

Veterinary Dictionary: Russian-English. Roy Mack. 1972. (ENG & RUS.). 104p. pap. 35.00 (*0-8288-6425-X*, M-9710) Fr & Eur.

Veterinary Disaster Team Resource Development Guide. Patty Boge. 2nd ed. 1999. 110p. 21.95 (*0-8138-2066-9*) Iowa U Pr.

Veterinary Drug Handbook. Donald C. Plumb. 3rd rev. ed. 1999. LC 98-53001. pap. 89.95 incl. cd-rom (*0-8138-1528-2*) Iowa U Pr.

Veterinary Drug Handbook. Donald C. Plumb. 1991. LC 90-91729. 688p. pap. 39.95 (*0-9626619-0-2*) Pharmavet Pub.

Veterinary Drug Handbook: Desk Edition. Donald C. Plumb. 3rd ed. 1999. LC 98-53001. 750p. pap. text 49.95 (*0-8138-2444-3*) Iowa U Pr.

Veterinary Drug Handbook: Desk Edition & Companion. Donald C. Plumb. 3rd rev. ed. 1999. pap. 69.95 (*0-8138-0234-2*) Iowa U Pr.

Veterinary Drug Handbook: Desk Edition, CD-ROM & Companion. Donald C. Plumb. 3rd abr. rev. ed. 1999. pap. 109.95 incl. cd-rom (*0-8138-1957-1*) Iowa U Pr.

Veterinary Drug Handbook: Pocket Edition. Donald C. Plumb. 3rd ed. 1999. LC 98-53001. 750p. pap. text 49.95 (*0-8138-2353-6*) Iowa U Pr.

Veterinary Drug Handbook: Pocket Edition & CD-ROM. Donald C. Plumb. 3rd rev. ed. 1999. pap. 89.95 incl. cd-rom (*0-8138-1588-6*) Iowa U Pr.

Veterinary Drug Handbook: Pocket Edition & Companion. Donald C. Plumb. 3rd rev. ed. 1999. pap. 69.95 (*0-8138-0235-0*) Iowa U Pr.

Veterinary Drug Handbook: Pocket Edition, CD-ROM & Companion. Donald C. Plumb. 3rd abr. rev. ed. 1999. pap. 109.95 incl. cd-rom (*0-8138-1968-7*) Iowa U Pr.

Veterinary Drug Residues: Food Safety, Vol. 636. Ed. by William A. Moats & Marjorie B. Medina. 1996. LC 96-26216. (ACS Symposium Ser.: No. 636). (Illus.). 200p. text 90.00 (*0-8412-3419-1*) Am Chemical.

Veterinary Emergency & Critical Care. Douglas MacIntire. 1999. 560p. pap. text 59.95 (*0-397-58463-6*) Lppncott W & W.

Veterinary Endoscopy: Small Animal. Jones Staff. 1995. (C). text (*0-7216-3653-5*) Saunders.

Veterinary Endosurgery. Freeman. 1998. LC 98-25971. (Illus.). 295p. (gr. 13). text 99.00 (*0-8151-3321-9*, 29106) Mosby Inc.

Veterinary Entomology. Richard Wall & David Shearer. 1997. LC 96-71695. (Illus.). 456p. (Orig.). pap. (*0-412-61510-X*) Kluwer Academic.

Veterinary Epidemiology. Michael Thrusfield. 2nd ed. 1996. (Illus.). 500p. 89.95 (*0-632-04036-X*) Blackwell Sci.

Veterinary Epidemiology. Michael Thrusfield. 2nd ed. 1997. (Illus.). 496p. pap. text 52.95 (*0-632-04851-4*) Iowa U Pr.

Veterinary Epidemiology: Principles & Methods. S. Wayne Martin et al. 1987. LC 87-3169. 356p. text 49.95 (*0-8138-1856-7*) Iowa U Pr.

Veterinary Epidemiology a Clinical Evidence Based Approach. Slater. 2002. 240p. pap. 32.50 (*0-7506-7311-7*) Buttrwrth-Heinemann.

Veterinary Ethics: An Introduction. Ed. by Giles Legood. 2000. 192p. pap. 23.95 (*0-8264-4784-8*) Continuum.

Veterinary Ethics: Animal Welfare, Client Relations, Competition & Collegiality. Jerold Tannenbaum. 2nd ed. 1995. LC 95-10433. (Illus.). 650p. (C). (gr. 13). pap. text 45.00 (*0-8151-8840-4*, 23784) Mosby Inc.

Veterinary Eye Surgery. S. W. Petrick. 1983. (Illus.). text 55.00 (*0-409-11265-8*) Buttrwrth-Heinemann.

*__Veterinary Formulary.__ Bishop. 5th rev. ed. 2000. (Illus.). 712p. (*0-85369-451-6*) Pharmaceutical Pr GBR. *Dist:* Rittenhouse.

Veterinary Guide for Animal Owners. C. E. Spaulding. 1976. LC 76-10641. (Illus.). 432p. 17.95 (*0-87857-118-3*, 13-486-0) Rodale Pr Inc.

Veterinary Guide for Animal Owners: Cattle, Goats, Sheep, Horses, Pigs, Poultry, Rabbits, Dogs, Cats. C. E. Spaulding & Jackie S. Clay. 2nd ed. 1998. LC 97-33808. 432p. 22.95 (*0-87596-967-4*) Rodale Pr Inc.

Veterinary Guide to the Parasites of Reptiles: Protozoa, Vol. 1. Susan M. Barnard & Steve J. Upton. 1994. LC 93-20082. 164p. lib. bdg. 26.50 (*0-89464-832-2*) Krieger.

Veterinary Guide to the Parasites of Reptiles Vol. 2: Arthropods (Excluding Mites) Susan M. Barnard & Lance A. Durden. 2000. 298p. lib. bdg. 46.50 (*0-89464-908-6*) Krieger.

Veterinary Healthcare Services: Options in Delivery. Thomas E. Catanzaro et al. 2000. LC 99-59177. (Illus.). xiv, 166p. pap. 34.95 (*0-8138-0929-0*) Iowa U Pr.

Veterinary Helmenthology & Entomology. Moning. 1987. (*81-7089-041-1*) Intl Bk Distr IND. *Dist:* St Mut.

Veterinary Helminthology. Kassai. 1998. 296p. pap. text 60.00 (*0-7506-3563-0*) Buttrwrth-Heinemann.

Veterinary Helminthology. R. K. Reineke. 1983. (Illus.). 52.95 (*0-409-11262-3*) Buttrwrth-Heinemann.

Veterinary Hematology: Atlas of Common Domestic Species. William J. Reagan et al. 1997. LC 97-7678. (Illus.). 39.95 (*0-8138-2664-0*) Iowa U Pr.

*__Veterinary Hematology & Clinical Chemistry.__ Mary Anna Thrall. 1996. (Illus.). 544p. text 89.00 (*0-683-30415-1*) Lppncott W & W.

Veterinary Immunology. Peter M. Outteridge. 1986. 280p. pap. text 52.00 (*0-12-531131-1*) Acad Pr.

Veterinary Immunology: An Introduction. Ian R. Tizard. Ed. by Ray Kersey. 5th ed. 1996. LC 96-16337. 624p. pap. text 51.50 (*0-7216-5772-9*) Saunders.

Veterinary Information Management. D. C. Blood. 1989. text 66.00 (*0-7020-1328-5*) Saunders.

*__Veterinary Laboratory Medicine: Clinical Biochemistry & Haematology.__ Morag G. Kerr. 2nd ed. 2001. LC 2001-37683. (*0-632-04023-8*) Blackwell Sci.

Veterinary Laboratory Medicine: Clinical Pathology. J. Robert Duncan et al. 3rd ed. 1994. LC 94-1554. (Illus.). 308p. text 42.95 (*0-8138-1917-2*) Iowa U Pr.

Veterinary Laboratory Medicine: Interpretation & Diagnosis. Dennie J. Meyer & John W. Harvey. Ed. by Ray Kersey. 2nd ed. 1997. LC 97-7725. (Illus.). 352p. pap. text 39.00 (*0-7216-6222-6*) Saunders.

Veterinary Management in Transition: Preparing for the Twenty-first Century. Thomas E. Catanzaro. 2000. LC 99-58668. (Illus.). xxxi, 234p. 49.95 (*0-8138-2626-8*) Iowa U Pr.

Veterinary Manual for the Performance Horse. Nancy S. Loring & A. M. Johnston. 1995. LC 95-658. 85.00 (*0-632-03914-0*) Blackwell Sci.

Veterinary Manual for the Performance Horse. Nancy S. Loving. Ed. by Don M. Wagoner. 1993. (Illus.). 608p. (C). text 75.00 (*0-935842-06-3*) Equine Res.

Veterinary Materia Medica & Clinical Repertory. G. MacLeod. 1983. 165p. pap. (*0-85207-257-0*) C W Daniel GBR. *Dist:* Natl Bk Netwk.

Veterinary Materia Medica Repertory. A. Hora. 1986. (C). (*0-7855-2261-1*) Scientific GBR. *Dist:* St Mut.

Veterinary Material Medical & Clincial Repertory. George MacLeod. 208p. (Orig.). pap. 26.95 (*0-8464-4309-0*) Beekman Pubs.

Veterinary Medical Officer. Jack Rudman. 1994. (Career Examination Ser.: C-875). pap. 49.95 (*0-8373-0875-5*) Nat Learn.

Veterinary Medical School Admission Requirements: 2000 Edition for 2001 Matriculation. Compiled by Association of American Veterinary Medicine Staff. 2000. 176p. pap. 16.50 (*1-55753-219-2*) Purdue U Pr.

Veterinary Medical School Admissions Requirements. Jane Diehl Crawford. 12th ed. 1997. pap. text 14.95 (*0-683-30099-7*) Lppncott W & W.

Veterinary Medical Terminology. Dawn E. Christenson. Ed. by Selma Kaszczuk. 1996. LC 96-14266. 320p. pap. text 29.00 (*0-7216-4859-2*) Saunders.

Veterinary Medicine. O. M. Radostits. 9th ed. 1999. 1881p. (C). text 139.00 (*0-7020-2409-0*) Harcourt Coll Pubs.

Veterinary Medicine: A Textbook of the Diseases of Cattle, Sheep, Pigs, Goats & Horses. Ed. by O. M. Radostits et al. 8th ed. 1994. (Illus.). 1787p. text (*0-7020-1592-X*) W B Saunders GBR. *Dist:* Saunders.

*__Veterinary Medicine: Index of New Information for Reference & Research.__ Ed. by Research and Development Division Staff & John C. Bartone. 2001. 180p. 47.50 (*0-7883-2530-2*); pap. 44.50 (*0-7883-2531-0*) ABBE Pubs Assn.

Veterinary Medicine: Pocket Companion. D. C. Blood. 1994. (Illus.). 743p. pap. text (*0-7020-1695-0*) W B Saunders GBR. *Dist:* Saunders.

Veterinary Medicine in Economic Transition. Malcolm Getz. 1997. LC 96-47012. (Illus.). 288p. (C). text 44.95 (*0-8138-1814-1*) Iowa U Pr.

Veterinary Medicine in the West. Ed. by Ole H. Stalheim. 1988. (Illus.). 84p. pap. text 15.00 (*0-89745-109-0*) Sunflower U Pr.

Veterinary Microbiology. Dwight C. Hirsh & Yuan Chung Zee. 1998. LC 98-30284. (Illus.). 479p. pap. 69.95 *(0-86542-543-4)* Blackwell Sci.

Veterinary Microbiology. Ed. by R. Pandey. 1985. (Progress in Veterinary Microbiology & Immunology Ser.: Vol. 2). (Illus.). x, 222p. 128.75 *(3-8055-4067-1)* S Karger.

Veterinary Mycology Laboratory Manual. Laura Hungerford et al. 1998. LC 98-12051. (Illus.). 120p. pap. text 19.95 *(0-8138-2849-X)* Iowa U Pr.

Veterinary Neuroanatomy & Clinical Neurology. Alexander DeLahunta. 2nd ed. 1983. LC 76-4246. (Illus.). (C). text 75.00 *(0-7216-3029-4)* Saunders.

Veterinary Neurology. Shawn P. Messonnier. 1999. LC 99-44150. (Practical Veterinarian Ser.). (Illus.). 224p. pap. text 24.99 *(0-7506-7203-X)* Buttrwrth-Heinemann.

Veterinary Neuropathology. Brian A. Summers et al. 1994. (Illus.). 527p. (C). (gr. 13). text 145.00 *(0-8016-5063-1, 05063)* Mosby Inc.

Veterinary Notes for Dog Breeders. Annette M. Carricato. 1992. (Illus.). 256p. 25.95 *(0-87605-805-5*, Howell) Hungry Minds.

Veterinary Notes for Horse Owners: An Illustrated Manual of Horse Medicine & Surgery. M. Horace Hayes. 1988. 688p. 35.00 *(0-671-76561-2)* S&S Trade.

Veterinary Nursing D. R. Lane. 1996. 836p. pap. text 70.00 *(0-7506-3417-0)* Buttrwrth-Heinemann.

Veterinary Nursing Ed. by B. Cooper & D. R. Lane. 2nd ed. 1994. pap. text 65.00 *(0-08-042289-6*, Pergamon Pr) Elsevier.

Veterinary Nursing. D. R. Lane & B. Cooper. 2nd ed. 1999. LC 99-18294. 720p. pap. text 77.50 *(0-7506-3999-7)* Buttrwrth-Heinemann.

Veterinary Nursing Ed. by D. R. Lane & B. Cooper. 2nd ed. 1994. text 130.00 *(0-08-042288-8)* Elsevier.

Veterinary Nursing: A Guide to Surgical Instruments. College of Animal Welfare, U. K. Staff et al. 1997. LC 98-173413. 128p. pap. text 22.50 *(0-7506-3613-0)* Buttrwrth-Heinemann.

Veterinary Nursing: Self-Assessment Questions & Answers, Vol. 2. Julie E. Ouston. 1997. 148p. pap. text 22.50 *(0-7506-3732-3)* Buttrwrth-Heinemann.

Veterinary Nursing Vol. 1: Self-Assessment Questions & Answers. Julie E. Ouston. 1997. 128p. pap. text 22.50 *(0-7506-3731-5)* Buttrwrth-Heinemann.

Veterinary Nursing Self-Assessment Questions & Answers. Julie Elizabeth Ouston. 2nd ed. 2000. 241p. pap. text 29.99 *(0-7506-4803-1)* Buttrwrth-Heinemann.

Veterinary Nursing 300 Questions & Answers in Radiography & Fluid Therapy. College of Animal Welfare Staff. 2000. (Veterinary Nursing Ser.: Vol. 300). (Illus.). 81p. pap. text 19.99 *(0-7506-4794-9)* Buttrwrth-Heinemann.

Veterinary Oncology. Kevin A. Hahn. 2001. LC 2001-43874. (Practical Veterinarian Ser.). 256p. pap. 24.99 *(0-7506-7296-X)* Buttrwrth-Heinemann.

Veterinary Ophthalmology. Barnett. 1996. (Illus.). 184p. text *(0-7234-2956-1)* Wolfe Publishing GBR. *Dist:* Mosby Inc.

Veterinary Ophthalmology. Kirk N. Gelatt. 3rd ed. 1998. LC 98-25124. (Illus.). 1,568p. text 198.00 *(0-683-30076-8)* Lppncott W & W.

Veterinary Parasitology. Omar Barriga. 1995. (Illus.). 316p. (C). pap. text 16.00 *(1-57074-242-1)* Greyden Pr.

Veterinary Parasitology. G. M. Urquhart et al. 1989. LC 85-19789. (Illus.). 352p. text *(0-582-40906-3)* Church.

Veterinary Parasitology. G. M. Urquhart et al. 2nd rev. ed. 1996. LC 95-54099. (Illus.). 350p. (C). pap. text 62.95 *(0-632-04051-3)* Iowa U Pr.

Veterinary Parasitology Reference Manual. William J. Foreyt. 4th ed. 1999. (Illus.). 196p. pap. 34.95 *(0-8138-2377-3)* Iowa U Pr.

Veterinary Pathology. Thomas C. Jones et al. 6th ed. 1997. LC 96-32932. 1392p. 99.95 *(0-683-04481-8)* Lppncott W & W.

Veterinary Pharmaceuticals & Biological, 2001/2002. Medical Economics Staff. 12th rev. ed. 2000. 1660p. 89.95 *(0-935078-83-5)* Veterinary Hlthcare.

Veterinary Pharmacology & Therapeutics. Ed. by H. Richard Adams. (Illus.). 7th ed. 1995. LC 95-15276. 1056p. (C). text 139.95 *(0-8138-1741-2)*; 8th ed. 2001. LC 00-53953. x, 1201p. 139.95 *(0-8138-1743-9)* Iowa U Pr.

Veterinary Pharmacy Handbook: An Easy-to-Use Guide to Expanding & Improving Your Community Pharmacy Practice. D. S. Chan. 1997. 195p. (C). pap. text 32.99 *(0-9663353-0-9)* Gratefuldeb.

Veterinary Practice Management. John Bower et al. 2nd ed. 1997. LC 96-48694. (Illus.). 288p. 42.95 *(0-632-04129-3)* Blackwell Sci.

Veterinary Practice Management: Building Profit & Value. Jerry L. Simmons. 1996. LC 96-7178. (Illus.). 224p. (C). (gr. 13). text 39.95 *(0-8151-7555-8*, 23971) Mosby Inc.

Veterinary Protozoan & Hemoparasite Vaccines. Ed. by I. G. Wright. 1989. 248p. 225.00 *(0-8493-4757-2*, QR189) CRC Pr.

Veterinary Protozoology. Norman D. Levine. 1985. LC 84-27867. (Illus.). 414p. text 64.95 *(0-8138-1861-3)* Iowa U Pr.

Veterinary Receptionist's Handbook. M. T. McClister & Amy Midgley. 2nd ed. 1995. LC 95-61831. 264p. pap. 39.95 *(0-935078-56-8)* Veterinary Hlthcare.

Veterinary Reproduction & Obstetrics. David E. Noakes. 7th ed. 1995. text 82.95 *(0-7020-1785-X)* Saunders.

Veterinary Reproduction Ultrasonography, '94. Kahn. 1994. text *(0-7234-2008-4)* Wolfe Publishing GBR. *Dist:* Mosby Inc.

Veterinary Science Officer. Jack Rudman. 1994. (Career Examination Ser.: C-871). pap. 49.95 *(0-8373-0871-2)* Nat Learn.

Veterinary Technician's Guide to Medical Terminology. Barbara Handy-Marchello. 1984. (C). pap. text 12.67 *(0-8359-8313-7)* P-H.

Veterinary Treatments & Medications for Horsemen. Equine Research, Inc. Research Staff. Ed. by Don M. Wagoner. 1977. (Illus.). 628p. (C). text 75.00 *(0-935842-01-2)* Equine Res.

Veterinary Ultrasonography. Ed. by P. J. Goddard. 1995. (Illus.). 346p. text 150.00 *(0-85198-923-3)* OUP.

Veterinary Vaccines. Ed. by R. Pandey et al. 1992. (Progress in Vaccinology Ser.: Vol. 4). (Illus.). 342p. 240.00 *(0-387-97819-4)* Spr-Verlag.

Veterinary Vaccinology. Ed. by Paul-Pierre Pastoret et al. 1999. LC 97-11156. 882p. 163.50 *(0-444-81968-1)* Elsevier.

Veterinary Values: The Clinical Companion to the VPB. Robert Green et al. 5th rev. ed. 1997. 850p. pap. 29.95 *(0-935078-66-5)* Veterinary Hlthcare.

Veterinary Virology. Frederick A. Murphy et al. 3rd ed. 1999. LC 99-60582. (Illus.). 600p. (C). text 89.95 *(0-12-511340-4)* Acad Pr.

Veternarians' New Research Bible & Index of New Information. Max W. Denton. 1994. 150p. 57.50 *(0-7883-0060-1)*; pap. 47.50 *(0-7883-0061-X)* ABBE Pubs Assn.

VGM's Handbook of Health Care Careers. Ed. by VGM Career Horizons Staff. 2nd rev. ed. 1997. LC 97-34920. (VGM's Handbook Ser.). (Illus.). 112p. pap. 12.95 *(0-8442-4539-9*, 45399, VGM Career Bks) McGraw-Hill Trade.

VHS Vocal Cord Vibrations. Hirano. 65.00 incl. VHS *(1-56593-481-4*, 1046) Singular Publishing.

Viagra: A Guide to the Phenomenal Drug. annuals Susan C. Vaughan. 1998. (ps-1). mass mkt. 5.99 *(0-671-02733-6)* PB.

Viagra: How the Miracle Drug Happened & What It Can Do for You. Jonathan Jarow et al. 2000. (Illus.). 160p. pap. 14.95 *(0-87131-923-3)* M Evans.

Viagra: The Virility Breakthrough. Othniel Seiden. 1998. LC 98-19473. 224p. pap. 15.00 *(0-7615-1733-2*, Prima Health) Prima Pub.

Viagra: The Potency Pill: What You Need to Know. Consumer Guide Editors. 1998. 128p. pap. 5.99 *(0-451-19792-5)* NAL.

Viagra, What You Must Know. Mark Francis. 1998. 110p. pap. 9.95 *(1-57002-080-9)* Univ Publng Hse.

Vibrational Healing: Revealing the Essence of Nature Through Aromatherapy. Deborah Edison. 2000. LC 00-37652. (Illus.). xiii, 241p. (C). pap. 18.95 *(1-58394-031-6)* Frog Ltd CA.

Vibrational Medicine Cards: The Sacred Geometry of the Self. Rowena P. Kryder. 1997. (Illus.). 192p. (Orig.). pap. 44.00 *(0-9624716-5-8)* Golden Point Prod.

Vibrio Cholerae & Cholera: A New Perspective on a Resurgent Disease. Ed. by I. Kaye Wachsmuth et al. 1994. LC 93-39024. (Illus.). 400p. text 72.00 *(1-55581-067-5)* ASM Pr.

Vicious Circle Phenomenon: Our Battle for Self-Control - How to Win the War. Phyllis D. Brister & David M. Brister. 1987. LC 87-15434. (Illus.). 304p. (C). 19.95 *(0-939977-69-9)* Diadem Pub.

Victim of Love? How You Can Break the Cycle of Bad Relationships. Randy Petersen & Thomas Whiteman. 1998. LC 98-12182. 224p. pap. 13.00 *(1-57683-053-5)* Pinon Press.

Victim of Rape: Institutional Reactions. Lynda L. Holmstrom & Ann Wolbert Burgess. 1983. LC 83-678. 320p. pap. text 21.95 *(0-87855-932-9)* Transaction Pubs.

Victimized Daughters: Incest & the Development of the Female Self. Janet L. Jacobs. 1994. LC 93-39239. 256p. (C). 55.00 *(0-415-90626-1)* Routledge.

Victims No Longer: Men Recovering from Incest & Other Childhood Sexual Abuse. Mike Lew. 1990. LC 89-45839. 352p. reprint ed. pap. 20.00 *(0-06-097300-5*, Perennial) HarperTrade.

Victims of Abuse: The Emotional Impact of Child & Adult Trauma. Ed. by Alan Sugarman. 1993. LC 93-49082. (Ralph R. Greenson Memorial Library of the San Diego Psychoanalytic Society & Institute: Monograph 3). 250p. 35.00 *(0-8236-6730-8)* Intl Univs Pr.

Victims of Cruelty: The Body in Treatment of Post-Traumatic Stress Disorder. Marianna Eckberg. 2000. LC 00-30525. (Illus.). xix, 247p. (C). pap. 18.95 *(1-55643-353-0)* North Atlantic.

Victims of Dementia: Services, Support, & Care. William M. Clemmer. 1993. LC 91-36172. 161p. pap. 19.95 *(1-56024-265-5)*; (Illus.). 155p. lib. bdg. 39.95 *(1-56024-264-7)* Haworth Pr.

Victor Bonney: The Gynaecological Surgeon of the Twentieth Century. G. Chamberlain. 2000. LC 00-56683. (Illus.). 152p. 32.95 *(1-85070-712-X*, Parthenon Pbng) CRC Pr.

Victorian Lunacy: Richard M. Bucke & the Practice of Late 19th-Century Psychiatry. Samuel E. Shortt. 1986. (History of Medicine Ser.). (Illus.). 232p. text 44.95 *(0-521-30999-9)* Cambridge U Pr.

Victorian Lunatics: A Social Epidemiology of Mental Illness in Mid-Nineteenth-Century England. Marlene A. Arieno. 1989. LC 88-43163. (Illus.). 144p. 32.50 *(0-945636-03-2)* Susquehanna U Pr.

***Victoria's Secret Catalog Never Stops Coming.** Jennie Nash. ltd. ed. 2001. 160p. 20.00 *(0-7432-2933-9)* Scribner.

***Victoria's Secret Catalog Never Stops Coming: And Other Lessons I Learned from Breast Cancer.** Jennie Nash. 2001. LC 2001-34173. 160p. 20.00 *(0-7432-1979-1)* Scribner.

Victory: An Alcohol Drug Recovery Text. James R. Whitmer. 1989. LC 89-90683. (Illus.). 272p. pap. 16.00 *(0-9622252-0-7)* Comfort Hse Pubs.

Victory for Progress in Mental Medicine. Lloyd V. Briggs. Ed. by Gerald N. Grob. 1980. LC 78-22552. (Historical Issues in Mental Health Ser.). (Illus.). reprint ed. lib. bdg. 25.95 *(0-405-11906-2)* Ayer.

Victory over Sickness & Pain. Chuck Schiappacasse. 1997. 145p. pap. 7.95 *(0-9635913-3-9)* C Schiappacasse.

Victory Principle: An Essential Strategic Guide for the Health Care Provider. Noel K. Harper. 2000. LC 99-6682. 370p. pap. 47.50 *(0-9675782-0-5)* M L Wave.

Vidal (French Physician Desk Reference) Vidal Staff. 1999. (FRE.). 75p. 350.00 *(0-320-00691-3)* Fr & Eur.

***Video-Assisted Thoracic Surgery (VATS)** Todd L. Demmy. 2001. 181p. 45.00 *(1-57059-632-8)* Eurekah.

Video Display Terminals: Safety & Health (Excerpts from Microwave News) Louis Slesin & Martha Zybko. 1983. 84p. (Orig.). pap. 8.50 *(0-9610580-0-5)* Microwave.

Video Display Terminals & Vision. Howard D. Kahn & Sally M. Corngold. 1989. (Illus.). 60p. pap. text 18.00 *(0-943599-11-3)* OEPF.

Video-Endoscopy. Ed. by Harubumi Kato. Tr. by J. Patrick Barron. 1993. LC 92-1698. vii, 152p. text 105.00 *(3-7186-5299-4)* Gordon & Breach.

Video Seminars on Transesphageal Echocardiography: NTSC format. Terence Rafferty. 2nd ed. 1999. (Illus.). 132p. 542.00 incl. VHS *(1-893508-00-5)* Echocardio.

Video Seminars on Transesphageal Echocardiography: PAL format. Terence Rafferty. 2nd ed. 1999. (Illus.). 542.00 incl. VHS *(1-893508-01-3)* Echocardio.

Video Vein Harvesting. William Jordan. 2000. (Vademecum Ser.). spiral bd. 45.00 *(1-57059-570-4)* Landes Bioscience.

Videoendoscopy: From Velopharynx to Larynx. Michael P. Karnell. 1994. LC 94-12297. (Clinical Competence Ser.). (Illus.). 190p. (Orig.). (C). pap. text 49.95 *(1-879105-97-7*, 0352) Thomson Learn.

Videofluoroscopio Studies of Speech in Patients with Cleft Palate. M. Leon Skolnick & E. R. Cohn. 1989. (Illus.). 186p. 187.00 *(0-387-96958-6)* Spr-Verlag.

Videostroboscopic Examination of the Larynx. Minoru Hirano & Diane M. Bless. 1993. LC 93-9421. (Illus.). 260p. (Orig.). (C). pap. 65.00 *(1-879105-52-7*, 0232) Thomson Learn.

Vietnam: A Casebook. Ed. by Jacob D. Lindy et al. 1987. LC 87-15062. (Psychosocial Stress Ser.: No. 10). 384p. 53.95 *(0-87630-471-4)* Brunner-Routledge.

Vietnam Wives: Facing the Challenges of Life with Veterans Suffering Post-Traumatic Stress. Aphrodite Matsakis. 2nd rev. ed. 1996. LC 96-67798. viii, 440p. (Orig.). pap. 24.95 *(1-886968-00-4*, MAVW) Sidran Pr.

View from the Divide: The Creative Nonfiction of Health & Science. Ed. by Lee Gutkind. 1999. 192p. pap. 17.95 *(0-8229-5685-3)* U of Pittsburgh Pr.

View of the Nervous Temperament. Thomas Trotter. 1976. LC 75-16735. (Classics in Psychiatry Ser.). reprint ed. 28.95 *(0-405-07456-5)* Ayer.

Viewing Psychology As a Whole: The Integrative Science of William N. Dember. Ed. by Robert R. Hoffman et al. 1998. LC 97-47680. 704p. 49.95 *(1-55798-474-3)* Am Psychol.

Viewing the Optic Disc: A Practical Guide. Digre & Corbett. 2001. 208p. 99.00 incl. cd-rom *(0-7506-7289-7)* Buttrwrth-Heinemann.

Views on Ericksonian Brief Therapy, Process & Action. Ed. by Stephen R. Lankton et al. 1991. LC 91-16001. (Ericksonian Monographs: No. 8). 128p. text 28.95 *(0-87630-646-6)* Brunner-Routledge.

Vigilancia Epidemiologica y Ordenadores. A. Aguirre Jaime. 1996. (SPA.). 231p. pap. *(84-7978-266-8)* Ediciones Diaz ESP. *Dist:* IBD Ltd.

Vigilante Virus. R. Leland Waldrip. 1999. 333p. mass mkt. 9.95 *(1-892105-01-2)* Rappahannock Bks.

Village Health Care Manual: An Approach to Patient Care in Places with Limited Medical Resources. Trevor J. Craig. 1997. 130p. pap. text 9.99 *(0-9661484-1-X)* Stony Pt Christian.

Vindication of the Rights of Brutes. Thomas Taylor. 1966. LC 66-10010. 104p. reprint ed. 50.00 *(0-8201-1045-0)* Schol Facsimiles.

Vine of the Soul: Medicine Men, Their Plants & Rituals in the Colombian Amazon. Richard E. Schultes & Robert F. Raffauf. 1992. (Illus.). 125p. 22.95 *(0-907791-24-7)* Synerg CA.

Vinylidene Chloride. 1990. (Environmental Health Criteria Ser.: No. 100). 187p. pap. text 32.00 *(92-4-154300-0*, 1160100) World Health.

Violence: A Public Health Menace & a Public Health Approach. Ed. by Sandra Bloom. 2001. 128p. pap. *(1-85575-192-5)* Karnac Bks GBR. *Dist:* Other Pr LLC.

Violence: Basic & Clinical Science. Chris Thompson & Philip Cowen. 1993. LC 92-48198. (Mental Health Foundation Ser.). (Illus.). 272p. pap. text 97.50 *(0-7506-0926-5)* Buttrwrth-Heinemann.

Violence: From Biology to Society: Proceedings of the International Meeting on Biology & Sociology of Violence, Valencia, Spain, 16-18 September, 1996. Grisolia, James International Meeting on Biology &. 1997. LC 97-10365. (International Congress Ser.). 294p. 148.00 *(0-444-82572-X)* Elsevier.

Violence Against Children: Physical Child Abuse in the United States. David G. Gil. 1973. LC 77-130809. (Commonwealth Fund Publications). (Illus.). 230p. pap. text 8.95 *(0-674-93942-5)* HUP.

***Violence & Health Care Professions.** Wykes. 1994. pap. 34.95 *(0-412-46170-6)* Chapman & Hall.

Violence & Mental Disorder: Developments in Risk Assessment. Ed. by John Monahan & Henry J. Steadman. 1996. LC 93-1670. (John D. & Catherine T. MacArthur Foundation Series on Mental Health & Development). (Illus.). 344p. 38.50 *(0-226-53405-7)* U Ch Pr.

Violence & Mental Disorder: Developments in Risk Assessment. John Monahan & Henry J. Steadman. 1996. (John D. & Catherine T. MacArthur Foundation Series on Mental Health & Development). (Illus.). 324p. reprint ed. pap. text 17.00 *(0-226-53406-5)* U Ch Pr.

Violence & Psychosis. Taylor. 2000. 256p. text *(0-7506-4117-7)* E A GBR. *Dist:* OUP.

Violence & Suicidality: Perspectives in Clinical & Psychobiological Research. Ed. by Herman M. Van Praag et al. 1990. LC 90-1309. (Einstein Clinical & Experimental Psychiatry Monograph Ser.: No. 3). (Illus.). 332p. text 49.95 *(0-87630-551-6)* Brunner-Routledge.

Violence & the Violent Individual. Ed. by J. Ray Hays et al. 1981. LC 80-24. (Illus.). 544p. text 40.00 *(0-88331-210-7)* R B Luce.

Violence & Unintentional Injury Prevention: Abstracts of Active Projects, FY, 1993. 1994. 90p. (Orig.). (C). pap. text 30.00 *(0-7881-0612-0)* DIANE Pub.

Violence in Health Care: A Practical Guide for Coping with Violence & Caring for Victims. Ed. by Jonathan Shepherd. 1994. LC 93-43592. 208p. 48.75 *(0-19-262513-6)* OUP.

Violence in the Workplace. Raymond B. Flannery, Jr. 1995. LC 94-48654. 240p. 24.95 *(0-8245-1488-2)* Crossroad NY.

Violence Intervention & Prevention Institute Proceedings. Ed. by AAHE Staff. 1997. 92p. pap. 15.95 *(0-88314-608-8)* AAHPERD.

Violence Issues for Health Care Educators & Providers. Kevin L. Hamberger. 1998. LC 97-35184. 49.95 *(0-7890-0360-0)* Haworth Pr.

Violence Issues for Health Care Educators & Providers. Ed. by L. Kevin Hamberger et al. 1997. LC 97-35184. 333p. pap. 24.95 *(0-7890-0381-3*, Maltreatment & Trauma Pr) Haworth Pr.

Violence of Men: New Techniques for Working with Abusive Families. Cloe Madanes et al. 1995. LC 95-12239. (Psychology Ser.). 272p. 35.00 *(0-7879-0117-2)* Jossey-Bass.

Violence Through a Forensic Lens. Ann Wolbert Burgess. 2000. 335p. pap. 29.95 *(1-930745-00-1)* Nursing Spect.

Violent Aspects of Deviant Behavior. 3rd ed. 1998. 368p. (C). 66.00 *(0-536-01015-3)* Pearson Custom.

Violent Deaths in Childhood & Adolescence. Ed. by David W. Kaplan. 1985. (Journal: Vol.12, No. 1). (Illus.). 80p. pap. 43.50 *(3-8055-4231-3)* S Karger.

Violent Men: An Inquiry into the Psychology of Violence. Hans Toch. rev. ed. 1992. LC 92-10715. 286p. reprint ed. pap. 19.95 *(1-55798-172-8)* Am Psychol.

Violent Offenders: Appraising & Managing Risk. Vernon L. Quinsey et al. 1998. LC 98-4013. (Law & Public Policy: Psychology & the Social Sciences Ser.). 356p. text 39.95 *(1-55798-495-6*, 431-604A) Am Psychol.

Violent Social World of Black Men. William Oliver. 1998. LC 98-7266. (Psychology Ser.). 256p. reprint ed. pap. 25.00 *(0-7879-4305-3)* Jossey-Bass.

Violent Society. Stuart Palmer. 1972. pap. 21.95 *(0-8084-0353-2)* NCUP.

Violent Victimization see Assessing & Treating Victims of Violence

Vip, Pacap & Related Regulatory Peptides. G. Rosselini. 1994. 648p. text 137.00 *(981-02-1788-9)* World Scientific Pub.

VIP, PACAP, Glucagon & Related Peptides. Ed. by Jan Fahrenkrug & Sami Said. 2000. LC 00-48983. (Annals of the New York Academy of Sciences Ser.: Vol. 921). (Illus.). xiii, 482p. 160.00 *(1-57331-273-8)* NY Acad Sci.

VIP, PACAP, Glucagon & Related Peptides: Fourth International Symposium. International Symposium on VIP, PACAP Staff et al. 2000. LC 00-48983. (Annals of the New York Academy of Sciences Ser.: Vol. 921). (Illus.). xiii, 482p. *(1-57331-274-6)* NY Acad Sci.

Viral & Autoimmune Hepatitis: Morphologic & Pathogenetic Aspects of Cell Damage in Hepatitis with Potential Chronicity. Hans P. Dienes. 1989. LC

88-38640. (Progress in Pathology Ser.: Vol. 132). 107p. pap. text (*0-89574-280-2*) Gustav Fischer DEU. *Dist:* Lubrecht & Cramer, Balogh.

Viral & Other Infections of the Human Respiratory System. S. Myint. 1995. 504p. (C). (gr. 13). pap. text 215.95 (*0-412-60070-6*) Chapman & Hall.

Viral Chemotherapy. David Shugar. 1984. (International Encyclopedia of Pharmacology & Therapeutics Ser.). 120.00 (*0-08-030792-2*, Pergamon Pr) Elsevier.

Viral Cytopathology. H. H. Malherbe. 1980. 112p. 98.95 (*0-8493-5567-2*, RC114) CRC Pr.

Viral Diarrhea of Man & Animals. Linda J. Saif & Kenneth W. Thiel. 1989. 360p. 225.00 (*0-8493-6640-2*, QR201) CRC Pr.

Viral Disease. Ed. by Pierre J. Vinken et al. 1989. 716p. 309.50 (*0-444-90479-4*) Elsevier.

Viral Diseases in Pregnancy. Ed. by Bernard Gonik. 1994. LC 93-38947. (Clinical Perspectives in Obstetrics & Gynecology Ser.). (Illus.). 267p. 121.00 (*0-387-94207-6*) Spr-Verlag.

Viral Diseases International Nomenclature of Diseases Vol. II: Infectious Diseases, 2. 1983. (International Nomenclature of Diseases Ser.: No. 3). pap. text 20.00 (*92-9036-011-9*) World Health.

Viral Diseases of Cattle. Robert F. Kahrs. 2nd ed. 2001. LC 00-53961. (Illus.). 424p. 54.95 (*0-8138-2591-1*) Iowa U Pr.

Viral Diseases of the Fetus & Newborn. James B. Hanshaw et al. 2nd ed. 1985. (Major Problems in Clinical Pediatrics Ser.). (Illus.). 308p. text 82.00 (*0-7216-4501-1*) Saunders.

Viral DNA-Vaccines. Ed. by K. Molling. 2001. (Intervirology Ser.: Vol. 43, No. 4-6). 158p. 39.25 (*3-8055-7173-9*) S Karger.

Viral Etiology of Cervical Cancer. Ed. by Richard Peto & Harald Z. Hausen. 1986. LC 86-2227. (Banbury Reports: No. 21). 362p. text 68.00 (*0-87969-221-9*) Cold Spring Harbor.

Viral Gastroenteritis. Shunzo Chiba. 1997. LC 96-29701. (Archives of Virology Ser.). (*3-211-82875-3*) Spr-Verlag.

Viral Gastroenteritis, Vol. VII. Ed. by Shunzo Chiba et al. 1997. LC 96-29701. (Archives of Virology Ser.: Supplement 12, 1996). (Illus.). 320p. 205.00 (*3-211-82947-4*) Spr-Verlag.

Viral Genome Methods. Ed. by Kenneth W. Adolph. 1996. LC 96-11626. 320p. spiral bd. 104.95 (*0-8493-4412-3*) CRC Pr.

Viral Hemorrhagic Fever: Current Bibliographies in Medicine (January 1990-June 1996) Cynthia B. Love & Peter B. Jahrling. 1996. 65p. (Orig.). (C). pap. text 30.00 (*0-7881-3508-2*) DIANE Pub.

Viral Hemorrhagic Fevers. 1985. (Technical Reports: No. 721). 126p. pap. text 10.00 (*92-4-120721-3*, 1100721) World Health.

Viral Hepatitis. Arie J. Zuckerman. 2nd ed. 1998. (C). text 195.00 (*0-443-05797-4*) Saunders.

Viral Hepatitis: A Handbook for Clinicians & Scientists. Elizabeth A. Fagan & Tim J. Harrison. 2000. LC 00-23805. (Illus.). 303p. pap. 49.95 (*0-387-91620-2*) Spr-Verlag.

Viral Hepatitis: Clinical & Scientific Perspectives. E. A. Fagan & T. J. Harrison. 1999. 160p. pap. (*1-85996-025-1*) Bios Sci GBR. *Dist:* Bks Intl VA.

Viral Hepatitis: Current Status & Issues. Eduard Kurstak. 1992. (Illus.). 216p. 105.00 (*0-387-82387-5*) Spr-Verlag.

Viral Hepatitis: Diagnosis, Therapy & Prevention. Ed. by Steven Specter. 1999. LC 98-36841. (Illus.). 416p. 110.00 (*0-89603-424-0*) Humana.

Viral Hepatitis: Diagnosis-Treatment-Prevention. Ed. by Richard A. Wilson. 1997. LC 96-39907. (Gastroenterology Ser.: Vol. 4). (Illus.). 552p. text 195.00 (*0-8247-9416-8*) Dekker.

Viral Hepatitis: Practical Evaluation & Treatment. Teddy F. Bader. 3rd rev. ed. 2000. LC 99-67484. (Illus.). 284p. 39.00 (*0-88937-232-2*) Hogrefe & Huber Pubs.

Viral Hepatitis: Proceedings of the WHO Expert Committee, Geneva, 1974. WHO Staff. 1975. (Technical Reports: No. 570). pap. text 7.00 (*92-4-120570-9*, 1100570) World Health.

Viral Hepatitis: Standardization in Immunoprophylaxis of Infections by Hepatitis Viruses. Ed. by G. Papaevangelou & W. Hennessen. 1983. (Developments in Biological Standardization Ser.: Vol. 54). (Illus.). xviii, 590p. pap. 61.00 (*3-8055-3826-X*) S Karger.

Viral Hepatitis & Hepatocellular Carcinoma. J. Sung & D. Chen. 1990. (Current Clinical Practice Ser.: Vol. 57). 728p. 327.00 (*90-219-1780-7*, CLP 57) Elsevier.

Viral Hepatitis & Liver Disease. K. Nishioka et al. 1994. 824p. 280.00 (*0-387-70132-X*) Spr-Verlag.

Viral Hepatitis B Infection: Vaccine & Control. Ed. by C. L. Lai et al. 1984. 304p. 85.00 (*9971-950-80-4*) World Scientific Pub.

Viral Hepatitis in China: Problems & Control Strategies. Ed. by Joseph L. Melnick et al. 1991. (Monographs in Virology: Vol. 19). (Illus.). xii, 160p. 155.75 (*3-8055-5364-1*) S Karger.

Viral Hepatitis Update. Ed. by S. Iino & O. Hino. 1999. (Intervirology Ser.: Vol. 42, Nos. 2 & 3). (Illus.). 156p. pap. 39.25 (*3-8055-6962-9*) S Karger.

Viral Infections. Richard K. Root & Merle A. Sande. 1992. (Contemporary Issues in Infectious Diseases Ser.: Vol. 10). (Illus.). 218p. text (*0-443-08859-4*) Church.

Viral Infections in Obstetrics & Gynecology. Ed. by D. Jeffries & C. N. Hudson. 1999. LC 99-222953. (Illus.). 360p. (*0-340-74095-7*) E A GBR. *Dist:* OUP.

Viral Infections of Humans: Epidemiology & Control. Ed. by Alfred S. Evans & Richard A. Kaslow. 4th ed. 1997. LC 97-17146. (Illus.). (C). 1116p. text 132.00 (*0-306-44855-6*); 1051p. pap. text 59.50 (*0-306-44856-4*) Kluwer Academic (Kluwer Plenum).

Viral Infections of the Gastrointestinal Tract. Albert Z. Kapikian. 2nd ed. 1994. LC 93-46950. (Infectious Disease & Therapy Ser.: Vol. 10). (Illus.). 816p. text 250.00 (*0-8247-8860-5*) Dekker.

Viral Infections of the Heart. J. E. Banatvala. 1993. 272p. (*0-340-55737-0*) E A GBR. *Dist:* OUP.

Viral Infections of the Nervous System. Richard T. Johnson. 2nd ed. 1998. LC 97-52761. 528p. text 110.00 (*0-7817-1440-0*) Lppncott W & W.

Viral Infections of the Respiratory Tract. Raphael Dolin & Peter F. Wright. 1999. LC 98-55495. (Lung Biology in Health & Disease Ser.). (Illus.). 464p. text 195.00 (*0-8247-0195-X*) Dekker.

Viral Messenger RNA. Ed. by Yechiel Becker. 1985. (Developments in Molecular Virology Ser.). text 167.00 (*0-89838-706-X*) Kluwer Academic.

Viral Pathogenesis. Neal M. Nathanson. 1996. LC 96-23106. 960p. text 199.00 (*0-7817-0297-6*) Lppncott W & W.

Viral Pathogenesis & Immunology. Cedric A. Mims & David O. White. 1984. (Illus.). 408p. pap. 46.95 (*0-632-01193-9*) Blackwell Sci.

Viral Pollution of the Environment. Ed. by Gerald Berg. 1983. 248p. 144.00 (*0-8493-6245-8*, TD427, CRC Reprint) Franklin.

Viral Proteinases As Targets for Chemotherapy. Ed. by Hans-Georg Kraeusslich et al. 1989. (Current Communications in Molecular Biology Ser.). (Illus.). 287p. (C). pap. text 24.00 (*0-87969-335-5*) Cold Spring Harbor.

Viral Regulatory Structures. Gerald Myers. 2000. LC 98-11770. (Santa Fe Institute Studies in the Sciences of Complexity, Proceedings: Vol. 28). (Illus.). 246p. pap. 35.00 (*0-201-32822-4*) Perseus Bks Grp.

Viral Respiratory Diseases: Report of a Scientific Group. 1980. (Technical Report Ser.: No. 642). 63p. pap. text 4.00 (*92-4-120642-X*, 1100642) World Health.

Viral Safety & Evaluation of Viral Clearance from Biopharmaceutical Products: National Institute of Health, Bethesda, Md., June 1995. Ed. by Fred Brown & Anthony S. Lubiniecki. 1996. (Developments in Biological Standardization Ser.: Vol. 88, 1996). (Illus.). x, 350p. pap. 274.00 (*3-8055-6391-4*) S Karger.

Viral Safety of Plasma-Derived Replacement Factors for Hemophilia: How Safe Is Safe? Ed. by P. M. Mannucci et al. 1994. (Vox Sanguinis: Vol. 67, Supplement 4, 1994). (Illus.). iv, 28p. pap. 14.00 (*3-8055-6066-4*) S Karger.

Viral Superantigens. Ed. by Kyuhei Tomonari. 1997. LC 96-39363. 276p. 149.95 (*0-8493-7688-2*) CRC Pr.

Viral Vaccines & Antiviral Drugs. 1983. (Technical Report Ser.: No. 693). 72p. pap. text 6.00 (*92-4-120693-4*) World Health.

Viral Vectors: Tools for Study & Genetic Manipulation of the Nervous System. Ed. by Michael G. Kaplitt. 1995. LC 94-49185. (Illus.). 486p. text 99.95 (*0-12-397570-0*); pap. text 49.95 (*0-12-397571-9*) Acad Pr.

Viral Warts: Biology & Treatment. Mary H. Bunney et al. 2nd ed. 1992. (Illus.). 192p. text 85.00 (*0-19-262062-2*) OUP.

Viral Zoonoses & Food of Animal Origin: A Re-evaluation of Possible Hazards for Human Health. Ed. by O. R. Kaaden et al. 1997. 240p. 169.00 (*3-211-82927-X*) Spr-Verlag.

Viral Zoonoses & Food of Animal Origin: A Re-Evaluation of Possible Hazards for Human Health. O. R. Kaaden et al. 1997. LC 97-43178. (Archives of Virology Ser.). (Illus.). 240p. 125.00 (*3-211-83014-6*) Spr-Verlag.

Vireo-Retinal & Uveitis Update. Ed. by John B. Saer. 1998. (Illus.). x, 317p. (*90-6299-168-8*) Kugler NLD. *Dist:* Lib Res.

Virginia Health Care in Perspective 2000. Ed. by Kathleen O'Leary Morgan & Scott E. Morgan. 2000. 21p. spiral bd. 19.00 (*0-7401-0245-1*) Morgan Quitno Corp.

Virginia Health Care Perspective, 1998. Ed. by Kathleen O'Leary Morgan & Scott E. Morgan. 1998. 20p. pap. 19.00 (*1-56692-845-1*) Morgan Quitno Corp.

Virginia Henderson Reader: Excellence in Nursing. Ed. by Edward J. Halloran. 1995. LC 94-42141. 416p. 52.95 (*0-8261-8830-3*) Springer Pub.

Virginia Satir: Foundational Ideas. Barbara J. Brothers. 1991. LC 90-26287. (Journal of Couples Therapy Ser.). (Illus.). 204p. text 39.95 (*1-56024-104-7*) Haworth Pr.

Virility Factor: Masculinity Through Testosterone, the Male Hormone. Robert Bahr. 2nd rev. ed. 1993. 213p. pap. 12.95 (*0-9626531-1-X*) Factor Pr.

Virility Solution: Everything You Need to Know About Viagra, the Potency Pill That Can Restore & Enhance Male Sexuality. Steven Lamm. 1998. LC 98-5837. 224p. (YA). 23.00 (*0-684-84780-9*) S&S Trade.

*__Viroceptors, Virokines & Related Immune Modulators Encoded by DNA Viruses.__ Ed. by Grant McFadden. 1996. LC 95-19301. (Molecular Biology Intelligence Unit Ser.). (Illus.). 218p. (C). 117.00 (*3-540-58901-5*) Spr-Verlag.

Viroids. T. O. Diener. 1987. LC 87-13017. (Viruses Ser.). (Illus.). 366p. (C). text 110.00 (*0-306-42523-8*, Kluwer Plenum) Kluwer Academic.

Virological Safety Aspects of Plasma Derivatives. Ed. by F. Brown. 1994. (Developments in Biological Standardization Ser.: Vol. 81). (Illus.). x, 310p. pap. 235.00 (*3-8055-5879-1*) S Karger.

Virologie in Deutschland: Die Entwicklung Eines Fachgebietes. K. Munk. 1994. (Illus.). x, 170p. 43.50 (*3-8055-6004-4*) S Karger.

Virologie Medicale. Jacques Maurin. 1985. (Collection Traites). (FRE., Illus.). 930p. 150.00 (*2-257-10435-8*) S M P F Inc.

Virologist. Jack Rudman. (Career Examination Ser.: C-3759). pap. 27.95 (*0-8373-3759-3*) Nat Learn.

Virology. Scott. 2002. (Biology Ser.). pap. 49.95 (*0-534-23580-8*) Wadsworth Pub.

Virology. Renato Dulbecco & Harold S. Ginsberg. 2nd ed. 1988. LC 65-10705. (Illus.). 425p. text 41.95 (*0-397-50905-7*, Lippncott) Lppncott W & W.

*__Virology__ David M. Knipe et al. 4th ed. 2001. (Illus.). 3200p. text 339.00 incl. cd-rom (*0-7817-1832-5*) Lppncott W & W.

Virology Labfax. Ed. by D. Harper. 1993. (Labfax Ser.). (Illus.). 272p. 63.00 (*0-12-326320-4*) Acad Pr.

Virology Reviews. Ed. by V. M. Zhdanov. 1987. (Soviet Medical Reviews Ser.: Vol. 2). vi, 378p. (C). reprint ed. text 531.00 (*3-7186-0402-7*);Vol. 1. xii, 332p. text 500.00 (*3-7186-0314-4*) Gordon & Breach.

Virology Reviews: Influenza, Vol. 3. A. V. Frolov et al. Ed. by Dmitri K. Lvov. 1990. (Soviet Medical Reviews Ser.: Vol. 3, Pt. 3). vi, 178p. pap. text 161.00 (*3-7186-4942-X*) Gordon & Breach.

Virology Reviews: Interferon & Its Inducers, Vol. 3. I. G. Balandin et al. Ed. by Dmitri K. Lvov. 1989. (Soviet Medical Reviews Ser.: Vol. 3, Pt. 2). vi, 168p. pap. text 150.00 (*3-7186-4921-7*) Gordon & Breach.

Virology Reviews Vol. 4, Pt. 1: Chemoprophylaxis & Chemotherapy of Viral Infections, Vol. 4. E. F. Barinsky. 1991. (Soviet Medical Reviews Ser.: Section E). ii, 152p. pap. text 160.00 (*3-7186-5150-5*, Harwood Acad Pubs) Gordon & Breach.

Virology Reviews Vol. 4, Pt. 2: Viral Hepatitides A & E Part A, Vol. 4. Yu Kusov. 1992. (Soviet Medical Reviews Ser.: Section E). 88p. pap. text 88.00 (*3-7186-5259-5*, Harwood Acad Pubs) Gordon & Breach.

Virology Reviews Vol. 4, Pt. 3: Viral Hepatitides A & E Part B, Vol. 4. E. N. Peletskaya. 1992. (Soviet Medical Reviews Ser.: Section E). 83p. pap. text 84.00 (*3-7186-5260-9*, Harwood Acad Pubs) Gordon & Breach.

Virology Reviews Vol. 4, Pt. 4: Chemoprophylaxis & Chemotherapy of Viral Infections, Vol. 4. M. Balayan. 1992. (Soviet Medical Reviews Ser.: Section E). 78p. pap. text 104.00 (*3-7186-5284-6*, Harwood Acad Pubs) Gordon & Breach.

Virology Reviews Vol. 5, Pt. 1: Viral Hepatitis, Vol. 5. A. Bluger. 1992. (Soviet Medical Reviews Ser.: Section E). 148p. pap. text 235.00 (*3-7186-5356-7*, Harwood Acad Pubs) Gordon & Breach.

Virology Two: Proceedings of the International Congress for Virology, 2nd, Budapest, 1971. International Congress for Virology Staff. Ed. by Joseph L. Melnick. 1972. 82.25 (*3-8055-1290-2*) S Karger.

Viropause: The Male Menopause - Emotional & Physical Changes Midlife Men Experience. Aubrey Hill. 1993. 23.95 (*0-88282-084-2*) New Horizon NJ.

Virtual Endoscopy. D. Buthiau & D. Khayat. 2000. 220p. 95.00 (*2-287-59658-5*) Spr-Verlag.

Virtual Endoscopy & Related 3D Techniques. Ed. by Patrik Rogalla et al. 2000. LC 99-51749. (Medical Radiology Ser.). (Illus.). 200p. 112.00 (*3-540-65157-8*) Spr-Verlag.

Virtual Environments for Health Care. Judi Moline. 1997. (Illus.). 53p. (C). reprint ed. pap. text 20.00 (*0-7881-4280-1*) DIANE Pub.

Virtual Immunology. Golub. 1999. 74.95 (*0-12-298160-X*) Acad Pr.

Virtual Medicine: A New Dimension in Energy Healing. Keith Scott-mumby. 1999. (Illus.). 288p. pap. (*0-7225-3823-5*) Thorsons GBR. *Dist:* Natl Bk Netwk.

Virtual Microscope: General & Special Histology. NeoCortex Foundation Staff. 1998. 59.00 (*0-88937-205-5*) Hogrefe & Huber Pubs.

Virtual Reality for Medical Simulation & Education, Vol. 1. Metin Akay & Andy Marsh. 2001. LC 00-42259. (Illus.). 252p. 64.95 (*0-471-38863-7*) Wiley.

Virtual Reality in Neuro-Psycho-Physiology: Cognitive, Clinical & Methodological Issues in Assessment & Treatment. Ed. by G. Riva. 1997. LC 97-76731. (Studies in Health Technology & Informatics: Vol. 44). 209p. 78.00 (*90-5199-364-1*, 364-1) IOS Press.

Virtue & Medicine: Explorations in the Character of Medicine. Ed. by Earl E. Shelp. 1985. (Philosophy & Medicine Ser.: No. 17). 383p. text 167.00 (*90-277-1808-3*) Kluwer Academic.

Virtues in Medical Practice. Edmund D. Pellegrino & David C. Thomasma. 1993. LC 92-49073. 224p. text 42.50 (*0-19-508289-3*) OUP.

Virtuous Transcendence: Holistic Self-Cultivation & Self-Healing in Elderly Korean Immigrants. Keum Young Chung Pang. 2000. LC 99-55442. (Haworth Aging, Psychology, & Mental Health Ser.). xviii, 229p. pap. text 29.95 (*0-7890-0929-3*); (C). 49.95 (*0-7890-0928-5*) Haworth Pr.

Virus: The Co-Discoverer of HIV Tracks Its Rampage & Charts the Future. Luc Montagnier. 1999. LC 99-19650. (Illus.). 256p. 24.95 (*0-393-03923-4*) Norton.

Virus & the Vaccine. Debbie Bookchin. 2002. (*0-312-27872-1*) St Martin.

Virus Chemotherapy. Ed. by F. E. Hahn. 1980. (Antibiotics & Chemotherapy Ser.: Vol. 27). (Illus.). vi, 310p. 165.25 (*3-8055-0263-X*) S Karger.

Virus Diseases in Laboratory & Captive Animals. Ed. by Gholamreza Darai. 1987. (Developments in Veterinary Virology Ser.). (C). text 293.50 (*0-89838-988-7*) Kluwer Academic.

Virus Ground Zero: Stalking the Killer Viruses with the Centers for Disease Control. Ed Regis. 1996. LC 96-34299. 256p. 23.00 (*0-671-55361-5*, PB Hardcover) PB.

Virus Hepatitis & Kidney. Ed. by V. A. Mioli. 1992. (Journal: Vol. 61, No. 3, 1992). (Illus.). 128p. pap. 56.75 (*3-8055-5621-7*) S Karger.

Virus Hunter: Thirty Years of Battling Hot Viruses Around the World. C. J. Peters & Mark Olshaker. 1998. LC 97-977. (Illus.). 352p. pap. 14.95 (*0-385-48558-1*) Doubleday.

Virus Inactivation in Plasma Products. Ed. by J. J. Morgenthaler. 1988. (Current Studies in Hematology & Blood Transfusion: No. 56). (Illus.). x, 158p. 123.50 (*3-8055-4836-2*) S Karger.

Virus-Induced Immunosuppression. S. Specter & M. Bendinelli. 1989. LC 88-31629. (Infectious Agents & Pathogenesis Ser.). (Illus.). 500p. (C). text 125.00 (*0-306-43040-1*, Kluwer Plenum) Kluwer Academic.

Virus Infection & the Cell Surface. Ed. by George H. Poste & G. Nicholson. 1980. (Cell Surface Reviews Ser.: Vol. 2). 342p. 239.50 (*0-7204-0598-X*) Elsevier.

Virus Infection & the Developing Nervous System. Ed. by G. Lyon. 1988. (C). text 132.50 (*0-7462-0053-6*) Kluwer Academic.

Virus Infections & Diabetes Mellitus. Ed. by Yechiel Becker. 1987. (Developments in Medical Virology Ser.). (C). text 159.00 (*0-89838-970-4*) Kluwer Academic.

Virus Infections in Bats. S. E. Sulkin. Ed. by Rae Allen. 1974. (Monographs in Virology: Vol. 8). 100p. 60.00 (*3-8055-1696-7*) S Karger.

Virus Infections in Pregnancy. Ed. by U. G. Liebert. 1999. (Intervirology Ser.: Vol. 41, Nos. 4-5 (1998)). (Illus.). 90p. pap. 34.00 (*3-8055-6872-X*) S Karger.

Virus Infections of Birds. Ed. by J. B. McFerran & M. S. McNulty. 1993. (Virus Infections of Vertebrates Ser.: Vol. 4). 640p. 257.00 (*0-444-89899-9*) Elsevier.

Virus Infections of Equines. Ed. by Michael J. Studdert. 1996. (Virus Infections of Vertebrates Ser.: Vol. 6). 380p. 225.00 (*0-444-82527-4*) Elsevier.

Virus Infections of Equines. Michael J. Studdert. 1996. LC 96-33479. (Virus Infections of Vertebrates Ser.). (*0-04-448257-4*) Elsevier.

Virus Infections of Porcines. Ed. by M. B. Pensaert & M. C. Horzink. 1989. (Virus Infections of Vertebrates Ser.: Vol. 2). 284p. 229.50 (*0-444-42909-3*) Elsevier.

Virus Infections of Rodents & Lagomorphs. Ed. by A. D. Osterhaus. 1994. LC 94-21040. (Virus Infections of Vertebrates Ser.: Vol. 5). 432p. 228.50 (*0-444-81909-6*) Elsevier.

Virus Infections of Ruminants. Ed. by Z. Dinter & B. Morein. 1990. (Virus Infections of Vertebrates Ser.: No. 3). 592p. 266.00 (*0-444-87312-0*) Elsevier.

Virus Infections of the Nervous System. Ed. by Thomas Weber. 1997. (Intervirology Ser.: Vol. 40, No. 2-3, 1997). (Illus.). 160p. pap. 55.75 (*3-8055-6634-4*) S Karger.

Virus Invaders. Alan E. Nourse. Ed. by V. Mathews. 1992. LC 91-36650. (Venture Bks.). (Illus.). 112p. (YA). (gr. 7-12). lib. bdg. 24.00 (*0-531-12511-4*) F Watts.

Virus of the Mind: The New Science of the Meme. Richard Brodie. 1996. LC 95-79421. (Illus.). 22.00 (*0-9636001-1-7*) Integral Pr.

Virus-Resistant Transgenic Plants: Potential Ecological Impact. Ed. by Mark Tepfer & Ervin Balazs. 1997. LC 97-35755. (Illus.). 126p. 69.95 (*3-540-63257-3*) Spr-Verlag.

Virus Separation & Purification Methods. Ed. by Alfred Polson. 1993. LC 93-22933. (Illus.). 312p. text 135.00 (*0-8247-9149-5*) Dekker.

Virus Taxonomy: Classification & Nomenclature of Viruses: Sixth Report of the International Committee on Taxonomy of Viruses. International Committee on Taxonomy of Viruses & Frederick A. Murphy. 1995. LC 95-10557. (Archives of Virology Ser.: Vol. 10). (Illus.). 595p. 116.00 (*3-211-82594-0*) Spr-Verlag.

Virus Taxonomy: Seventh Report of the International Committee on Taxonomy of Viruses. Van Regengmortal et al. 1999. LC 99-65267. (Illus.). xii, 1162p. 125.00 (*0-12-370200-3*) Acad Pr.

Virus Within: A Coming Epidemic: How Medical Detectives Are Tracking a Terrifying Virus That Hides in Almost All of Us. Nicholas Regush. 2001. LC 99-58326. 272p. pap. 14.00 (*0-452-28222-5*, Plume) Dutton Plume.

Virus-X: Tracking the New Killer Plagues Out of the Present & into the Future. Frank Ryan. 1997. LC 96-30495. (Illus.). 448p. (gr. 8). 24.95 (*0-316-76383-7*) Little.

Viruses: Catalogue, Characterization & Classification. H. Fraenkel-Conrat. 1985. LC 84-1984. (Illus.). 276p. 95.00 (*0-306-41766-9*, Plenum Trade) Perseus Pubng.

Viruses Affecting Man & Animals. Murray Sanders & Morris Schaeffer. 1971. LC 75-117612. (Illus.). 478p. 27.50 (*0-87527-070-0*) Green.

Viruses, Allergies & the Immune System. Jan De Vries. 1988. (By Appointment Only Ser.). 128p. pap. (*1-85158-176-6*) Mainstream Pubng GBR. *Dist:* Trafalgar.

Viruses & Bone Marrow: Basic Research & Clinical Practice. Ed. by Neal S. Young. 1993. (Hematology Ser.: Vol. 16). (Illus.). 416p. text 210.00 (*0-8247-8833-8*) Dekker.

Viruses & Cancer: Fifty-First Symposium for the Society for General Microbiology, Held at the University of Cambridge, March 1994. Ed. by A. C. Minson et al. 1994. LC 93-46636. (Society for General Microbiology Symposia Ser.: No. 51). (Illus.). 321p. (C). text 120.00 (*0-521-45472-7*) Cambridge U Pr.

Viruses & Cancer: Proceedings of the WHO Scientific Group, Geneva, 1964. WHO Staff. 1965. (Technical Reports: No. 295). (ENG, FRE, RUS & SPA.). 60p. pap. text 5.00 (*92-4-120295-5*, 1100295) World Health.

Viruses & Human Cancer. Ed. by J. R. Arrand & D. R. Harper. 1998. (Illus.). 256p. (Orig.). pap. (*1-872748-44-9*) Bios Sci GBR. *Dist:* Bks Intl VA.

Viruses & Human Cancer. Ed. by Yohei Ito. 1977. (Progress in Experimental Tumor Research Ser.: Vol. 21). (Illus.). 97.50 (*3-8055-2701-2*) S Karger.

***Viruses & Human Disease.** James Strauss. 2001. 551p. pap. 69.95 (*0-12-673050-4*) Acad Pr.

Viruses & Reproduction: A Bibliography, 2. Compiled by Ernest L. Abel. 1988. LC 88-16575. 329p. lib. bdg. 79.00 (*0-313-26439-2*, AVR/, Greenwood Pr) Greenwood.

Viruses & the Cellular Immune Response. Ed. by D. Brain Thomas. 1993. (Illus.). 544p. text 240.00 (*0-8247-9053-7*) Dekker.

Viruses & Virus-Like Agents in Disease: A Karger Symposium, Basel, March, 1993. Ed. by R. M. Zinkernagel & W. Stauffacher. 1993. (Journal: Vol. 35, Nos. 1-4). (Illus.). 220p. reprint ed. 155.75 (*3-8055-5785-X*) S Karger.

Viruses Causing Common Respiratory Diseases in Man. George G. Jackson & Robert L. Muldoon. 1996. LC 74-8430. (Studies in Infectious Diseases Research). viii, 256p. lib. bdg. 22.00 (*0-226-38940-5*) U Ch Pr.

Viruses, Immunity, & Immunodeficiency. Ed. by Andor Szentivanyi & Herman Friedman. 1986. LC 86-3263. (University of South Florida International Biomedical Symposia Ser.). 380p. 75.00 (*0-306-42235-2*, Plenum Trade) Perseus Pubng.

Viruses, Immunity & Mental Disorders. E. Kurstak et al. 1987. (Illus.). 470p. (C). text 125.00 (*0-306-42337-5*, Kluwer Plenum) Kluwer Academic.

Viruses in Human Gene Therapy. Ed. by Jean-Michel H. Vos. 1995. LC 93-73564. (Illus.). 216p. (C). lib. bdg. 65.00 (*0-89089-559-7*) Carolina Acad Pr.

Viruses in Human Tumors. P. H. Hofschneider. Ed. by K. Munk. 1987. (Beitraege Zur Onkologie, Contributions to Oncology Ser.: Vol. 24). (Illus.). viii, 216p. 58.50 (*3-8055-4354-9*) S Karger.

Viruses in Water Systems: Detection & Identification. J. C. Block. 1989. 136p. 105.00 (*0-471-18681-3*, Wiley-VCH) Wiley.

Viruses of Legumes. John R. Edwardson & Richard G. Christie. 1991. 680p. 375.00 (*0-8493-4729-7*, SB608) CRC Pr.

Viruses of Prokaryotes Ed. by Hans-Wolfgang Ackermann & Michael S. Dubow. 1987. 268.00 (*0-8493-6054-4*, QR342, CRC Reprint) Franklin.

Viruses of Prokaryotes: General Properties of Bacteriophages, Vol. 2. Hans-Wolfgang Ackermann & M. Dubow. 1987. LC 87-9407. 256p. reprint ed. 145.00 (*0-8493-6057-9*, CRC Reprint) Franklin.

Viruses, Oncogenes & Cancer. Ed. by Joseph L. Melnick. 1985. (Progress in Medical Virology Ser.: Vol. 32). (Illus.). viii, 224p. 146.25 (*3-8055-3976-2*) S Karger.

Viruses, Plagues & History. Michael B. Oldstone. 1998. LC 97-9545. (Illus.). 224p. 25.00 (*0-19-511723-9*) OUP.

Viscera of the Domestic Mammals. R. Nickel. 1977. LC 72-95370. (Illus.). 54.95 (*0-387-91107-3*) Spr-Verlag.

Visceral Anatomy (Cardiovascular, Lymphatic, Digestive, Respiratory & Urogenital Systems), Vol. 2. Johannes Sobotta. Ed. by Frank H. Figge & Walter J. Hild. 1978. 255p. text 39.50 (*0-8067-1729-7*) Lppncott W & W.

Visceral Manipulation, Vol. 1. Jean-Pierre Barral & Pierre Mercier. 1988. LC 87-82743.Tr. of Manipulations Viscerales. (Illus.). 278p. text 50.00 (*0-939616-06-8*) Eastland.

Visceral Manipulation, Vol. 2. Jean-Pierre Barral. 1989. LC 87-82743.Tr. of Manipulations Viscerales. (Illus.). 264p. (C). text 48.00 (*0-939616-09-2*) Eastland.

Visceral Pain. Ed. by Gerald F. Gebhart. 1995. LC 95-7922. (Progress in Pain Research & Management Ser.: Vol. 5). (Illus.). 528p. 30.00 (*0-931092-10-8*, PPRM5) Intl Assn Study Pain.

Visceral Perception: Understanding Internal Cognition. G. Adam. 1998. LC 98-19005. (Plenum Series in Behavioral Psychophysiology & Medicine). (Illus.). 200p. (C). text 49.50 (*0-306-45755-5*, Kluwer Plenum) Kluwer Academic.

Viscoelastics in Ophthalmic Surgery. Lucio Buratto et al. 1999. (Illus.). 500p. 145.00 (*1-55642-448-5*) SLACK Inc.

Viscoelastics in Ophthalmic Surgery. H. B. Dick & O. Schwenn. 2000. LC 00-39482. (Illus.). 160p. 69.00 (*3-540-67330-X*) Spr-Verlag.

Visejesicki Medicinski Recnik Vol. 1: English, Latin, Serbocroatian. Aleksandar Kostic. 1987. (ENG, LAT & SER.). 1029p. 95.00 (*0-8288-0583-0*, M2040) Fr & Eur.

Visejesicki Medicinski Recnik Vol. 2: German, French, Italian, Russian. Aleksandar Kostic. 1987. (FRE, GER, ITA & RUS.). 975p. 95.00 (*0-8288-0582-2*, M2041) Fr & Eur.

Visible & Invisible Group. Yvonne Agazarian & Richard Peters. 1995. 302p. reprint ed. pap. text (*1-85575-119-4*) Karnac Bks GBR. *Dist:* Other Pr LLC.

Visible & Invisible Group: Two Perspectives on Group Psychotherapy & Group Process. Yvonne Agazarian & Richard Peters. 1989. 304p. pap. 17.95 (*0-415-03770-0*) Routledge.

Visible & Near Infrared Absorption Spectra of Human & Animal Haemoglobin: Determination & Application. W. G. Zijlistra et al. 2000. 382p. (*90-6764-317-3*) VSP NLD. *Dist:* Coronet Bks.

Visible Human Body: An Atlas of Sectional Anatomy. Gunther VonHagens et al. 1991. LC 89-13836. (Illus.). 151p. text 55.00 (*0-8121-1269-5*) Lppncott W & W.

Visible Speech the Science of Universal Alphabetics. Alexander M. Bell. 1976. reprint ed. 69.00 (*0-403-06591-7*, Regency) Scholarly.

Visible Wound: A Healing Journey Through Breast Cancer. Julie Friedeberger. 1996. LC 96-1803. 176p. pap. 12.95 (*1-85230-808-7*) Element MA.

Visibly Different: Coping with Disfigurement. Ed. by Richard Lansdown et al. 1997. LC 97-23638. (An Arnold Publication). 272p. pap. (*0-7506-3424-3*) E A GBR. *Dist:* OUP.

Vision. Pierre Buser & Michel Imbert. Tr. by Roy H. Kay from FRE. 1992. LC 91-32473. (Illus.). 576p. 60.00 (*0-262-02336-9*, Bradford Bks) MIT Pr.

Vision: A Holistic Guide to Healing the Eyesight. Joanna Rotte & Koji Yamamoto. 1986. LC 84-80538. 152p. (Orig.). pap. 18.00 (*0-87040-622-1*) Japan Pubns USA.

Vision & Aging. Ed. by Alfred J. Rosenbloom & Meredith W. Morgan. 2nd ed. 1993. (Illus.). 463p. text 89.99 (*0-7506-9311-8*) Buttrwrth-Heinemann.

Vision & Aging: Crossroads for Service Delivery. Ed. by Alberta L. Orr. 1992. LC 92-5088. 392p. pap. 47.95 (*0-89128-216-5*) Am Foun Blind.

Vision & Aging: Issues in Social Work Practice. Ed. by Nancy D. Weber. 1992. LC 91-24842. (Journal of Gerontological Social Work Ser.). (Illus.). 207p. lib. bdg. 39.95 (*1-56024-199-3*) Haworth Pr.

Vision & Mind: Modeling Mental Functions. Vadim D. Glezer. 1995. 288p. text 59.95 (*0-8058-1668-2*) L Erlbaum Assocs.

Vision & Motor Control. L. Proteau & D. Elliott. 1992. (Advances in Psychology Ser.: Vol. 85). 478p. 136.00 (*0-444-88816-0*, North Holland) Elsevier.

Vision & Reading. Ed. by Ralph P. Garzia. 1995. LC 95-24996. (Mosby's Optometric Problem Solving Ser.). (Illus.). 320p. (C). (gr. 13). pap. text 39.95 (*0-8151-3438-X*, 24263) Mosby Inc.

Vision & School Success. G. B. Spache et al. Ed. by Sally M. Corngold. 1992. (Illus.). 57p. lib. bdg. 11.00 (*0-929780-04-3*) VisionExtension.

Vision & Separation: Between Mother & Baby. Kenneth Wright. 1991. LC 90-14553. 392p. 60.00 (*0-87668-559-9*) Aronson.

Vision & Visual Dysfunction, Set. J. Cronly-Dillon. 1991. 2125.00 (*0-8493-7500-2*) CRC Pr.

Vision, Brain & Cooperative Computation. Allen R. Hanson. Ed. by Michael A. Arbib. (Computational Models of Cognition & Perception Ser.). 1987. 512p. 80.00 (*0-262-01094-1*); 1990. 744p. reprint ed. pap. 40.00 (*0-262-51049-9*, Bradford Bks) MIT Pr.

Vision Care Assistant: An Introductory Handbook. Pamela Miller. Ed. by Sally M. Corngold. 3rd ed. 1999. 144p. lib. bdg. 22.00 (*0-929780-01-9*) VisionExtension.

Vision for the Future: Jules Stein Eye Institute, 1966-1991. Compiled by Twenty-fifth Anniversary Book Committee Staff. 1992. LC 91-66445. (Illus.). 200p. (*0-9630545-1-1*) J S Eye Inst.

Vision for the Future: Meeting the Challenge of Sight Loss. Maria Conyers. 1992. 34.00 (*1-85302-110-5*) Taylor & Francis.

Vision in Context: Historical & Contemporary Perspectives on Sight. Teresa Brennan. 1996. LC 95-42441. 245p. (C). pap. 22.95 (*0-415-91475-2*) Routledge.

Vision in Vehicles II. A. G. Gale et al. 1988. 428p. 166.00 (*0-444-70423-X*, North Holland) Elsevier.

Vision in Vertebrates. M. A. Ali & M. A. Klyne. 1985. LC 85-12191. 282p. 79.50 (*0-306-42065-1*, Plenum Trade) Perseus Pubng.

Vision of the Brain. Semir Zeki. 1993. LC 92-48866. (Illus.). 380p. pap. 58.95 (*0-632-03054-2*) Blackwell Sci.

Vision, Perception, & Cognition: A Manual for the Evaluation & Treatment of the Neurologically Impaired Adult. Barbara B. Zoltan. 3rd ed. 1996. 232p. pap. 30.00 (*1-55642-265-2*, 32652) SLACK Inc.

Vision Research: A Practical Guide to Laboratory Methods. Ed. by Roger Carpenter & John Robson. 1999. LC 98-19461. (Illus.). 352p. text, lab manual ed. 55.00 (*0-19-852319-X*) OUP.

Vision Research Protocols. Ed. by Piroska Elizabeth Rakoczy. 2000. LC 00-33502. (Methods in Molecular Medicine Ser.: Vol. 47). (Illus.). x, 320p. 99.50 (*0-89603-837-8*) Humana.

Vision Therapist Vol. 34-3: Amblyopia. Anne Barber et al. 1992. (Illus.). 120p. (Orig.). pap. text 18.00 (*0-943599-52-0*) OEPF.

Vision Therapist Vol. 34-4: Infant & Toddler Vision. Carol L. Scott et al. 1992. (Illus.). 65p. (Orig.). pap. text 18.00 (*0-943599-54-7*) OEPF.

Vision Therapist Vol. 35-1: Working with the Brain Injured. 1993. (Illus.). 100p. (Orig.). pap. text 18.00 (*0-943599-60-1*) OEPF.

Vision Therapist Vol. 35-2: Communicating Effectively. Robert Williams et al. 1993. (Illus.). 122p. (Orig.). pap. text 18.00 (*0-943599-61-X*) OEPF.

Vision Therapist Vol. 35-3: Hot Topics. Diann Geisert et al. 1993. (Illus.). 101p. (Orig.). pap. text 18.00 (*0-943599-62-8*) OEPF.

Vision Therapist Vol. 35-4: Focusing on Accommodation. Cathe Kennedy et al. 1994. (Illus.). 89p. (Orig.). pap. text 18.00 (*0-943599-63-6*) OEPF.

Vision Therapist Vol. 36-2: Vision Screenings. Bobby Mansfield et al. 1994. (Illus.). 90p. (Orig.). pap. text 18.00 (*0-943599-69-5*) OEPF.

Vision Therapist Vol. 38-2: Visual Perception. 1996. (Illus.). 102p. pap. 20.00 (*0-943599-84-9*) OEPF.

Vision Therapist Vol. 38-3: Visual Thinking for Problem Solving. 1997. (Illus.). 92p. pap. 20.00 (*0-943599-85-7*) OEPF.

Vision Therapy Vol. 37-1: Training Laterality & Directionality. Anne Barber et al. 1994. (Illus.). 87p. (Orig.). pap. text 18.00 (*0-943599-75-X*) OEPF.

Vision Therapy Vol. 37-4: Tools of Behavioral Vision Care: Prisms. Paul Harris et al. 1996. (Illus.). 127p. (Orig.). pap. text 18.00 (*0-943599-78-4*) OEPF.

Vision Therapy Vol. 38-1: Tools of Behavioral Vision Care: Lenses Occluders & Filters. Homer Hendrickson et al. 1996. (Illus.). 89p. (Orig.). pap. text 20.00 (*0-943599-83-0*) OEPF.

Vision Therapy in a Primary Care Practice. Jerome Rosner et al. 1988. (Illus.). 256p. text 79.99 (*0-87873-077-X*) Buttrwrth-Heinemann.

Visions: Notes of the Seminar Given in 1930-1934. Carl Gustav Jung. Ed. by Claire Douglas. 1997. LC 96-25402. (Bollingen XLV Ser.: Vol. 99). (Illus.). 1500p. 150.00 (*0-691-09971-5*) Princeton U Pr.

Visions & Metaphysical Experiences. Manly P. Hall. pap. 4.95 (*0-89314-378-2*) Philos Res.

***Visions from the Soul: From Personality to Spirit.** Maurie D. Pressman. 2001. 261p. pap. 14.95 (*0-9658158-2-X*) Inkwell Prods.

Visions of Addiction: Major Contemporary Perspectives on Addiction & Alcoholism. Stanton Peele. 1987. LC 86-45054. 244p. 37.00 (*0-669-13092-3*) Lxngtn Bks.

Visions of Rogers's Science-Based Nursing. Ed. by Elizabeth A. Barrett. 1990. 432p. 30.95 (*0-88737-447-6*) Natl League Nurse.

Visions of Sunsets. Thea M. Kellogg. rev. ed. 1996. LC 95-90025. 192p. pap. 12.00 (*0-9645035-3-0*) WynnHart Pr.

Visions of Women. Ed. by Linda A. Bell. 1983. LC 82-4866. (Contemporary Issues in Biomedicine, Ethics, & Society Ser.). 508p. 59.50 (*0-89603-044-X*); pap. 29.95 (*0-89603-054-7*) Humana.

Visitation. Michele Roberts. 1984. pap. 8.95 (*0-7043-3909-9*) Interlink Pub.

Visiting the Sick: The Mitzvah of Bikur Cholim. Sharon Selib Epstein. 1999. LC 98-51751. xviii, 183p. 25.00 (*0-7657-6075-4*) Aronson.

Vistas in Applied Mathematics: Numerical Analysis, Atmospheric Sciences, Immunology. Ed. by A. V. Balakrishnan et al. 1986. LC 86-8340. (Translations Series in Mathematics & Engineering). 396p. text 98.00 (*0-911575-38-3*) Optimization Soft.

Visual Agnosia: Disorders of Object Recognition & What They Tell Us about Normal Vision. Martha J. Farah. 1990. (Bradford Issues in the Biology of Language Ser.). 150p. 32.50 (*0-262-06135-X*) MIT Pr.

Visual Agnosia: Disorders of Object Recognition & What They Tell Us About Normal Vision. Martha J. Farah. 1995. (Issues in the Biology of Language & Cognition Ser.). 208p. pap. text 17.50 (*0-262-56082-8*, Bradford Bks) MIT Pr.

Visual Aids to the MRCP Examination. N. K. Chakravorty. 1996. LC 94-40907. lib. bdg. 19.95 (*0-7923-8873-9*) Kluwer Academic.

Visual & Auditory Perception. Gerald M. Murch. 1973. LC 74-172349. (Illus.). (C). pap. (*0-672-60779-4*, Bobbs) Macmillan.

***Visual & Vestibular Consequences of Acquired Brain Injury.** Ed. by Irwin B. Suchoff et al. 2001. LC 2001-55181. 250p. pap. 35.00 (*0-943599-42-3*) OEPF.

Visual Attention, Vol. 8. Ed. by Richard D. Wright. 1998. LC 98-28395. (Vancouver Studies in Cognitive Science). (Illus.). 488p. pap. text 35.00 (*0-19-512693-9*) OUP.

Visual Attention & Cognition. Ed. by W. H. Zangemeister et al. 1996. LC 96-27978. (Advances in Psychology Ser.: Vol. 116). 412p. 149.50 (*0-444-82291-7*, North Holland) Elsevier.

Visual Aural Digit Span Test: VADS Test. Elizabeth M. Koppitz. 1977. 202p. text 31.00 (*0-8089-1032-9*, 792360, Grune & Strat) Harcrt Hlth Sci Grp.

Visual Awareness & Design: An Introductory Program in Perceptual Sensitivity, Conceptual Awareness, & Basic Design Skills. Philip Thiel. 1981. LC 80-51079. (Illus.). 288p. pap. 19.50 (*0-295-95786-7*) U of Wash Pr.

Visual Behavior. Beverly Jones. 1995. LC 95-75986. 228p. (Orig.). pap. 17.95 (*0-9627939-1-4*) Lockwood Pr.

Visual Coding & Adaptability. Ed. by Charles S. Harris. 1980. LC 79-26604. (Illus.). 400p. text 79.95 (*0-89859-016-7*) L Erlbaum Assocs.

Visual Development. Nigel W. Daw. 1995. (Perspectives in Vision Research Ser.). (Illus.). 242p. (C). text 54.00 (*0-306-45023-2*, Kluwer Plenum) Kluwer Academic.

Visual Diagnosis of Child Physical Abuse. American Academy of Pediatrics Staff & Kempe, C. Henry, National Center on Child Abuse. 1994. stu. ed., ring bd. 149.95 (*0-910761-46-9*) Am Acad Pediat.

Visual Diagnosis of Child Sexual Abuse from the American Academy of Pediatrics. Contrib. by Carole Jenny & Deborah Lowen. 1998. LC 98-71821. 59p. (*1-58110-011-6*) Am Acad Pediat.

Visual Diagnosis Self-Tests on Eye Diseases. Victor Chong. 2001. (Visual Diagnosis Self-Tests Ser.). (Illus.). 108p. pap. text 23.95 (*1-873413-32-7*) Merit Pub Intl.

Visual Diagnosis Self-Tests on HIV Medicine. Marc Lipman & Paul Thomas. 1997. (Visual Diagnosis Self-Tests Ser.). (Illus.). 86p. pap. 12.95 (*1-873413-41-6*) Merit Pub Intl.

Visual Diagnosis Self-Tests on Respiratory Tract Infections. Paul Thomas. 2nd rev. ed. 1997. (Visual Diagnosis Self-Tests Ser.). (Illus.). 88p. pap. 12.95 (*1-873413-31-9*) Merit Pub Intl.

Visual Diagnosis Self-Tests on Rheumatology. Paul Emery. 2nd ed. 1996. (Visual Diagnosis Self-Tests Ser.). (Illus.). 100p. pap. 23.95 (*1-873413-06-8*) Merit Pub Intl.

Visual Diagnosis Self-Tests on STDS (Sexually Transmitted Diseases) Loay M. David. 2001. (Visual Diagnosis Self-Tests Ser.). (Illus.). 100p. pap. text 23.95 (*1-873413-97-1*) Merit Pub Intl.

Visual Diagnosis Self-Tests on the Menopause & HRT: Spanish Edition. Goran Samsioe. 1996. (Visual Diagnosis Self-Tests Ser.). (SPA., Illus.). 96p. (Orig.). pap. text 12.95 (*1-873413-65-3*) Merit Pub Intl.

Visual Education Medical Terminology. Alan Cohen. 1991. pap. 10.95 (*1-55637-020-2*) Visual Educ.

Visual Electrodiagnosis in Systematic Diseases. Ed. by E. Schmoger & J. H. Kelsey. 1980. (Documenta Ophthalmologica Proceedings Ser.: No. 23). 290p. text 184.00 (*90-6193-163-0*) Kluwer Academic.

Visual Encyclopedia of Natural Healing: A Step-by-Step Pictorial Guide to Solving 100 Everyday Health Problems. 1991. LC 90-45937. 432p. 27.95 (*0-87857-928-1*, 05-998-0) Rodale Pr Inc.

***Visual Encyclopedia of Ovarian Histopathology.** V. Bychkov. 2002. 95.95 (*1-84214-179-1*, Parthenon Pbng) CRC Pr.

Visual Field in Glaucoma: Cellular Proliferation. Ed. by W. Straub. 1985. (Developments in Ophthalmology Ser.: Vol. 12). (Illus.). vi, 134p. 81.00 (*3-8055-4022-1*) S Karger.

Visual Field Symposium: 5th International, Documenta Ophthalmologica Proceedings. Ed. by Erik L. Greve & A. Heijl. 1983. text 306.00 (*90-6193-731-0*) Kluwer Academic.

Visual Fields. Neil T. Choplin & Russell P. Edwards. 1998. LC 97-48545. (Basic Bookshelf for Eyecare Professionals Ser.). 272p. pap. 33.00 (*1-55642-363-2*) SLACK Inc.

Visual Fields. David B. Henson. 2nd ed. 2000. LC 00-31206. (Illus.). 158p. pap. text 49.50 (*0-7506-4173-8*) Buttrwrth-Heinemann.

Visual Fields. David B. Henson. 1993. LC 92-49925. (Oxford Medical Publications). (C). 38.50 (*0-19-261887-3*) OUP.

Visual Fields: Clinical Case Presentations. John R. Griffin et al. 1991. (Illus.). 512p. text 100.00 (*0-409-90159-8*) Buttrwrth-Heinemann.

Visual Fields: Examination & Interpretation. Thomas J. Walsh. 2nd ed. 1996. LC 96-20818. (Ophthalmology Monographs Ser.). (*1-56055-035-X*) Am Acad Ophthal.

Visual Illusions: Their Causes, Characteristics & Applications. M. Luckiesh. 1990. (Illus.). 21.25 (*0-8446-0780-0*) Peter Smith.

Visual Illusions: Their Causes, Characteristics & Applications. Matthew Luckiesh. 1998. (Illus.). 252p. pap. 6.95 (*0-486-21530-X*) Dover.

Visual Impairment: An Overview. Ian L. Bailey & Amanda Hall. 1990. LC 90-1099. 56p. pap. 19.95 (*0-89128-174-6*) Am Foun Blind.

Visual Instrumentation Handbook: Principles of Optical Design. Pantazis Mouroulis. 1999. LC 98-49404. (Illus.). 430p. text 89.95 (*0-07-043561-8*) McGraw-Hill Prof.

Visual Intelligence: How We Create What We See. David Hoffman. 1998. LC 98-6181. (Illus.). 288p. 29.95 (*0-393-04669-9*) Norton.

Visual Intelligence: Perception, Image, & Manipulation in Visual Communication. Anne M. Barry. 1997. LC 96-42465. 425p. (C). pap. text 21.95 (*0-7914-3436-2*) State U NY Pr.

Visual Motion & Its Role in the Stabilization of Gaze. Ed. by F. A. Miles & J. Wallman. 1992. LC 92-32805.

(Reviews of Oculomotor Research Ser.: Vol. 5). 418p. 263.50 (*0-444-81195-8*) Elsevier.

Visual-Motor Development Remedial Activities. Karen G. Codding & Morrison F. Gardner. 1988. pap. 7.95 (*0-931421-16-0*); 8.95 (*0-931421-12-8*); 8.95 (*0-931421-17-9*); 8.95 (*0-931421-25-X*); 8.95 (*0-931421-26-8*); 8.95 (*0-931421-28-4*) Psychol Educ Pubns.

Visual-Motor Upper Level Remedial Activities. Morrison F. Gardner. 1993. pap. 9.95 (*0-931421-43-8*) Psychol Educ Pubns.

Visual Pathways. Ed. by H. Spekreijse & P. A. Apkarian. 1981. (Documenta Ophthalmologica Proceedings Ser.: No. 27). 472p. text 278.00 (*90-6193-723-X*) Kluwer Academic.

Visual Pattern Analyzers. Norma V. Graham. 1989. (Oxford University South Asian Studies: No. 16). (Illus.). 670p. text 80.00 (*0-19-505154-8*) OUP.

Visual Perception: A Clinical Orientation. Steven H. Schwartz. 1994. LC 93-47537. (Illus.). 368p. (C). pap. text 59.95 (*0-8385-9473-5*, A9473-8) Appleton & Lange.

***Visual Perception: An Introduction.** Nicholas Wade & Michael Swanston. 2nd ed. 2001. LC 2001-16093. pap. (*1-84169-204-2*) Psychol Pr GBR. *Dist:* Taylor & Francis.

Visual Perception: The Neurophysiological Foundations. Ed. by Lothar Spillman & John S. Werner. 1989. 531p. text 62.00 (*0-12-657675-0*) Acad Pr.

Visual-Perceptual Upper Level Remedial Activities. Karen G. Codding & Morrison F. Gardner. 1993. pap. 9.95 (*0-931421-81-0*) Psychol Educ Pubns.

Visual Processes in Reading & Reading Disabilities. Ed. by Dale M. Willows et al. 1993. LC 93-26065. 504p. pap. 55.00 (*0-8058-1332-2*); text 99.95 (*0-8058-0900-7*) L Erlbaum Assocs.

Visual Sampling Scanning Processes. John W. Senders. 1983. 160p. (C). pap. text 24.95 (*0-89859-516-9*) L Erlbaum Assocs.

Visual Space Perception: A Primer. Maurice Hershenson. 1998. LC 98-4970. (Illus.). 256p. 40.00 (*0-262-08270-5*, Bradford Bks) MIT Pr.

Visual System from Genesis to Maturity. Ed. by Roberto Lent. 1992. LC 92-21738. xii, 285p. 119.00 (*0-8176-3598-X*) Birkhauser.

Visual System in Evolution in Vertebrates. A. Hughes. 1977. LC 77-4371. (Handbook of Sensory Physiology Ser.: Vol. 7, Pt. 5). (Illus.). 813p. 299.00 (*0-387-07908-4*) Spr-Verlag.

Visual Thalamocortical System & Its Modulation by the Brain Stem Core. Mircea Steriade et al. 1990. (Progress in Sensory Physiology Ser.: Vol. 10). (Illus.). 124p. 100.00 (*0-387-51380-9*) Spr-Verlag.

Visual World of the Child. Eliane Vurpillot. 1976. LC 75-790. 372p. 55.00 (*0-8236-6749-9*) Intl Univs Pr.

Visualization & Guided Imagery in Complementary Medicine. R. D. Longacre. 2nd ed. 1998. LC 98-66043. 216p. per. 8.46 (*0-7872-4907-6*) Kendall-Hunt.

Visualization for Allergies & Asthma. Patrick Fanning. 1992. (Visualization Ser.). pap. 11.95 incl. audio (*1-879237-15-6*) New Harbinger.

Visualization in Biomedical Computing: 4th International Conference, VBC 96, Hamburg, Germany, September 1996: Proceedings. K. H. Hohne & Ron Kikinis. 1996. LC 96-35786. (Lecture Notes in Computer Science: Vol. 1131). 610p. 106.00 (*3-540-61649-7*) Spr-Verlag.

Visualization of Information Processing in the Human Brain: Recent Advances in MEG & Functional MRI. I. Hashimoto et al. 1996. LC 96-35299. (Electroencephalography & Clinical Neurophysiology Ser.). 478p. 219.50 (*0-444-82361-1*) Elsevier.

Visualizing Muscles: A New Ecorche Approach to Surface Anatomy. John Cody. 1991. LC 90-50112. (Illus.). xiv, 242p. pap. 25.00 (*0-7006-0426-X*) U Pr of KS.

Visually Limited Child. R. Bonner et al. 1970. pap. text 12.95 (*0-8422-0061-4*) Irvington.

Visually Responsive Neuron: From Basic Neurophysiology to Behavior. Ed. by T. P. Hicks et al. 1993. LC 92-48461. (Progress in Brain Research Ser.: Vol. 95). 488p. 296.50 (*0-444-89492-6*) Elsevier.

Visuals of the Clinical Histocompatibility Workshop: Jamaica Invitational, 2000: Montego Bay, Jamaica, March 1-5, 2000. Paul I. Terasaki. 2000. LC 99-70732. (Illus.). 160p. (*0-945756-10-0*) One Lambda.

Visuals of the Clinical Histocompatibility Workshop: Palm Springs Invitational. Compiled by Paul I. Terasaki. 1988. LC 88-60350. (Illus.). 173p. (Orig.). pap. 10.00 (*0-945756-00-3*, VIS88) One Lambda.

Visuals of the Clinical Histocompatibility Workshop: Palm Springs Invitational, February 1989. Compiled by Paul I. Terasaki. 1989. (Illus.). 200p. (Orig.). pap. 10.00 (*0-945756-01-1*, VIS89) One Lambda.

Vital & Health Statistics: Proceedings of the International Collaborative Effort on Automating Mortality Statistics. National Center for Health Statistics Staff. 1998. LC 98-25577. (DHHS Publications). (*0-8406-0548-X*) Natl Ctr Health Stats.

Vital & Health Statistics of the U. S. Natality & Mortality, Set. 1994. lib. bdg. 1795.95 (*0-8490-5817-1*) Gordon Pr.

Vital & Health Statistics Series: An Annotated Checklist & Index to the Publications of the "Rainbow Series", 7. Jim Walsh & A. James Bothmer. 1991. LC 91-18077. (Bibliographies & Indexes in Medical Studies: No. 7). 408p. lib. bdg. 89.50 (*0-313-27260-3*, WVH, Greenwood Pr) Greenwood.

Vital Balance: The Life Process in Mental Health & Illness. Karl Augustus Menninger. 1983. 30.25 (*0-8446-6125-2*) Peter Smith.

Vital Energy: The 7 Keys to Invigorate Mind, Body & Soul. David Simon. 1999. LC 99-28661. 261p. (C). 24.95 (*0-471-33226-7*) Wiley.

Vital Energy Easy Oriental Exercises for Health & Wellbeing. J. Young. 1991. (Illus.). 128p. text (*0-340-54549-6*) Hodder & Stought Ltd GBR. *Dist:* Lubrecht & Cramer.

Vital Health Facts & Composition of Foods. Patricia Krimmel & Edward A. Krimmel. 1994. (Illus.). 96p. (Orig.). pap. 4.50 (*0-916503-06-2*) Franklin Pubs.

Vital Link Vol. 2: With CEH Packet, Vol. 2. American College of Emergency Physicians Staff. 1994. suppl. ed. 65.00 (*0-07-000212-6*) McGraw.

Vital Meridian. Bensoussan. 1996. text 33.95 (*0-443-04255-1*) Saunders.

Vital Signs: Working Doctors Tell the Real Story Behind Medical School & Practice. Deborah Bernal et al. 1994. LC 94-28687. 219p. pap. 12.95 (*1-56079-376-7*) Petersons.

Vital Statistics for the Public Health Educator. Mark J. Kittleson. 1995. LC 94-7915. (Illus.). 184p. (C). pap. 15.95 (*0-8093-1950-0*) S Ill U Pr.

Vital Tooth Bleaching: Putting It All Together. Thomas E. Huntzinger. 1992. LC 92-24901. 152p. 29.95 (*1-881350-00-2*) Moontree Pub.

Vitalism: The History of Herbalism, Homeopathy & Flower Essences. Matthew Wood. 2nd ed. 2000. LC 00-24604. (Illus.). 160p. pap. 16.95 (*1-55643-340-9*) North Atlantic.

Vitamin A: Everything You Need to Know. Janet Benton. 1998. LC 98-36550. 128p. pap. 10.95 (*1-882606-44-2*) Peoples Med Soc.

Vitamin A & Retinoids: An Update of Biological Aspects & Clinical Applications. Contrib. by Maria A. Livrea. 1999. LC 99-36144. (Molecular & Cell Biology Updates Ser.). (Illus.). x, 300p. (*0-8176-5882-3*) Birkhauser.

Vitamin A & the Immune Function: A Symposium. Ed. by Chris Kjohhede & William R. Beisel. 1996. LC 95-45330. (Journal of Nutritional Immunology Ser.: Vol. 4, Nos. 1/2). 177p. 29.95 (*1-56024-757-6*, Hawrth Medical) Haworth Pr.

Vitamin a Deficiency: Health, Survival & Vision. Alfred Sommer & Keith P. West. 1996. (Illus.). 464p. (C). text 75.00 (*0-19-508824-7*) OUP.

Vitamin A Deficiency & Its Consequences: A Field Guide to Detection & Control. A. Sommer. 3rd ed. 1995. (FRE & SPA., Illus.). vii, 69p. (C). pap. text 17.00 (*92-4-154478-3*, 1153050) World Health.

Vitamin A Deficiency & Xerophthalmia: Report of a Joint WHO/USAID Meeting, 1976. 1976. (Technical Report Ser.: No. 590). 88p. pap. text 10.00 (*92-4-120590-3*, 1100590) World Health.

Vitamin A in Health & Disease. Rune Blomhoff. 1994. (Antioxidants in Health & Disease Ser.: Vol. 1). (Illus.). 704p. text 235.00 (*0-8247-9120-7*) Dekker.

***Vitamin A Intake, Status & Improvement Using the Dietary Approach: Studies of Vulnerable Groups in Three Asian Countries.** Viveka Persson. 2001. (Comprehensive Summaries of Uppsala Dissertations from the Faculty of Medicine Ser.: No. 1069). (Illus.). 99p. pap. (*91-554-5106-3*) Acta Univ SWE. *Dist:* Coronet Bks.

Vitamin A Supplements: A Guide to Their Use in the Treatment & Prevention of Vitamin A Deficiency & Xerophthalmia: Prepared by a WHO/UNICEF/IVACG Task Force. WHO Staff. 1988. 24p. 8.00 (*92-4-154236-5*) World Health.

Vitamin A Training Activities for Community Health & Development. Helen Keller International Staff. 1993. LC 93-395669. (Illus.). 72p. (Orig.). pap. 10.00 (*0-915173-26-3*) Helen Keller Intl.

Vitamin & Carrier Functions of Polyprenoids. Ed. by Geoffrey H. Bourne & H. R. Cama. 1978. (World Review of Nutrition & Dietetics Ser.: Vol. 31). (Illus.). 120.00 (*3-8055-2801-9*) S Karger.

Vitamin & Health Encyclopedia. Jack Ritchason. rev. ed. 1986. 129p. pap. 7.95 (*0-913923-92-3*) Woodland UT.

Vitamin & Herb Guide. Global Health Research Staff. 1997. (Illus.). 94p. pap. (*0-921202-00-8*) Gloh CAN. *Dist:* BookWorld.

Vitamin B-6 Catalysis. Ed. by T. Korpela & P. Christen. 1987. (Congress Reports: No. 1). 500p. 117.50 (*0-8176-1942-9*) Birkhauser.

Vitamin B-6 Metabolism in Pregnancy, Lactation & Infancy. Ed. by Daniel J. Raiten. 1995. LC 94-32693. 212p. 199.95 (*0-8493-4594-4*) CRC Pr.

Vitamin B1 for Dentistry! Medicine! Research! Sam Ziff & Michael F. Ziff. 1996. 120p. (Orig.). pap. 19.95 (*0-941011-15-1*) Bio-Probe.

Vitamin Book. Consumer Guide Editors. 1979. pap. 5.95 (*0-671-24819-7*, Fireside) S&S Trade Pap.

Vitamin Book. Harold M. Silverman et al. rev. ed. 1999. LC 99-461791. 512p. mass mkt. 6.50 (*0-553-57957-6*) Bantam.

Vitamin B6: Metabolism & Role in Growth. George P. Tryfiates. 1980. 377p. 71.00 (*0-917678-10-9*) Food & Nut Pr.

Vitamin C C. Alan Clemetson. 1989. Vol. 1. 336p. 169.00 (*0-8493-4841-2*, RC627); Vol. 2. 248p. 169.00 (*0-8493-4842-0*, RC627); Vol. 3. 280p. 169.00 (*0-8493-4843-9*, RC627) CRC Pr.

Vitamin C: Everything You Need to Know. Jennifer Hay. 1998. LC 98-10811. (Everything You Need to Know Ser.). (Illus.). 128p. pap. 10.95 (*1-882606-36-1*) Peoples Med Soc.

Vitamin C: Its Chemistry & Biochemistry. Davies & Austin. 1991. 164p. (C). (*0-85186-333-7*) Royal Soc Chem GBR. *Dist:* Spr-Verlag.

Vitamin C: The Future Is Now. Jeffrey S. Bland. Ed. by Don R. Bensen. 1995. (Good Health Guides). 48p. pap. 3.95 (*0-87983-685-7*, 36857K, Keats Pubng) McGraw-Hill Trade.

Vitamin C: The Pros & Cons. Stephen Sheffrey. 1991. LC 91-90308. 176p. pap. 9.95 (*0-9629372-0-7*) Service Press.

Vitamin C Controversy: Questions & Answers. Emanuel Cheraskin. 1988. LC 87-71003. (Illus.). 221p. (Orig.). pap. 12.95 (*0-942333-01-2*) Bio-Comns Pr.

Vitamin C in Health & Disease. Ed. by Lester Packer & Jurgen Fuchs. 1997. LC 97-7703. (Antioxidants in Health & Disease Ser.: Vol. 5). (Illus.). 560p. text 180.00 (*0-8247-9313-7*) Dekker.

Vitamin Contents of Arterial Tissue. J. E. Kirk. 1973. (Monographs on Atherosclerosis: Vol. 3). 43.50 (*3-8055-1466-2*) S Karger.

Vitamin D. Ed. by David Feldman et al. 1997. LC 97-23438. (Illus.). xxii, 1285 p. text 175.00 (*0-12-252685-6*) Morgan Kaufmann.

Vitamin D: Basic & Clinical Aspects. Rajiv Kumar. 1984. text 253.50 (*0-89838-620-9*) Kluwer Academic.

Vitamin D: Chemical, Biochemical & Clinical Endocrinology of Calcium Metabolism. Ed. by A. W. Norman et al. 1982. (Illus.). 1288p. text 257.70 (*3-11-008864-9*) De Gruyter.

Vitamin D: Gene Regulation, Structure-Function Analysis & Clinical Application Proceedings of the 8th Workshop on Vitamin D, Paris, France, July 5-10, 1991. Ed. by A. W. Norman et al. 1991. (Illus.). xxxviii, 995p. (C). lib. bdg. 300.00 (*3-11-012638-9*, 261-91) De Gruyter.

Vitamin D: Physiology, Molecular Biology & Clinical Applications. Ed. by Michael F. Holick. 1999. LC 98-45813. (Nutrition & Health Ser.). (Illus.). xii, 458p. 175.00 (*0-89603-467-4*) Humana.

Vitamin D - A Pluripotent Steroid Hormone: Structional Studies, Molecular Endocrinology & Clinical Applications: Proceedings of the Ninth Workshop on Vitamin D, Orlando, Florida (U. S. A.), May 28-June 2, 1994. Anthony W. Norman. 1994. LC 94-35262. 1007p. (C). lib. bdg. 361.55 (*3-11-014157-4*) De Gruyter.

Vitamin D - Chemical, Biochemical & Clinical Update: Proceedings of the 6th Workshop on Vitamin D, Italy, March 1985. Ed. by A. W. Norman et al. 1985. (Illus.). xxxxiii, 1249p. 307.70 (*0-89925-066-1*) De Gruyter.

Vitamin D - Molecular, Cellular, & Clinical Endocrinology: Proceedings of the Seventh Workshop on Vitamin D, Rancho Mirage, CA, U. S. A., April 1988. Ed. by A. W. Norman et al. 1988. xl, 1072p. (C). lib. bdg. 300.00 (*3-11-011477-1*) De Gruyter.

Vitamin D & Calcium Metabolism in the Renal Diseases. Ed. by K. Maeda et al. 1980. (Contributions to Nephrology Ser.: Vol. 22). (Illus.). vi, 122p. 29.75 (*3-8055-0389-X*) S Karger.

Vitamin D Endocrine System: Structural, Biological, Genetic & Clinical Aspects. Ed. by Anthony W. Norman & June Bishop. 2000. LC 00-107310. (Vitamin D Ser.). (Illus.). xliv, 1014p. (C). (*1-891168-04-5*) U CA Riverside.

Vitamin D in Dermatology. Ed. by Knud Kragballe. 2000. LC 99-89437. (Illus.). 408p. text 165.00 (*0-8247-7704-2*) Dekker.

Vitamin Deficiencies: Symptoms. 1996. lib. bdg. 251.75 (*0-8490-5915-1*) Gordon Pr.

Vitamin E: Everything You Need to Know. Jennifer Hay. 1998. LC 98-10812. (Everything You Need to Know Ser.). (Illus.). 128p. pap. 10.95 (*1-882606-37-X*) Peoples Med Soc.

Vitamin E: Its Usefulness in Health & in Curing Diseases. Ed. by M. Mino et al. 1993. (Illus.). xiv, 368p. 215.75 (*3-8055-5753-1*) S Karger.

Vitamin E & Disease Prevention Including Cancer: Index of New Information with Authors, Subjects & References. Gus J. Torelli. 1997. (Illus.). 150p. 57.50 (*0-7883-1342-8*); pap. 47.50 (*0-7883-1343-6*) ABBE Pubs Assn.

Vitamin E & Its Uses. 1996. lib. bdg. 250.75 (*0-8490-5913-5*) Gordon Pr.

Vitamin E Updated. Leonard Mervyn. Ed. by Richard A. Passwater & Earl R. Mindell. 1983. (Good Health Guides). 32p. (Orig.). pap. 3.95 (*0-87983-274-6*, 32746K, Keats Pubng) McGraw-Hill Trade.

***Vitamin G - Riboflavin: Index of New Information & Guide-Book for Consumers, Reference & Research.** Adolph A. Smithson. 2002. 180p. 57.50 (*0-7883-2486-1*); pap. 47.50 (*0-7883-2487-X*) ABBE Pubs Assn.

Vitamin Intake & Health: A Scientific Review. Suzanne K. Gaby et al. 1990. (Illus.). 232p. text 145.00 (*0-8247-8382-4*) Dekker.

Vitamin K & Vitamin K-Dependent Proteins. Shearer. 1993. 368p. 225.00 (*0-8493-6423-X*) CRC Pr.

Vitamin K-Dependent Biological Processes. Ed. by Maria B. Donati. 1986. (Journal: Vol. 16, No. 2, 1986). (Illus.). 132p. pap. 72.25 (*3-8055-4270-4*) S Karger.

Vitamin-Lexikon: Fur Artze, Apotheker und Ernahrungswissenschaftler. Karl-Heinz Bassler. 1992. (GER.). 432p. 105.00 (*0-7859-8360-0*, 3437006606) Fr & Eur.

***Vitamin M - Folic Acid: Index of New Information & Guide-Book for Consumers, Reference & Research.** Adolph A. Smithson. 2002. 180p. 57.50 (*0-7883-2506-X*); pap. 47.50 (*0-7883-2507-8*) ABBE Pubs Assn.

Vitamin P Complex (Bioflavanoids) Index of New Information. Wally V. Ullman. 1995. 155p. 57.50 (*0-7883-0628-6*); pap. 47.50 (*0-7883-0629-4*) ABBE Pubs Assn.

Vitamin Politics. John J. Fried. 1984. LC 83-62187. 238p. pap. 23.00 (*0-87975-222-X*) Prometheus Bks.

Vitamin Receptors: Vitamins As Ligands in Cell Communication-Metabolic Indicators. Ed. by Krishnamurti Dakshinamurti. 1994. (Intercellular & Intracellular Communications Ser.: No. 6). (Illus.). 277p. (C). text 80.00 (*0-521-39280-2*) Cambridge U Pr.

Vitamin Revolution in Health Care. Michael Janson. 1996. LC 95-81032. 236p. pap. 12.95 (*0-9649236-9-6*) Arcadia Pr NH.

Vitamin Robbers. Earl R. Mindell. Ed. by Richard A. Passwater. 1983. (Good Health Guides). (Illus.). 31p. (C). pap. 3.95 (*0-87983-275-4*, 32754K, Keats Pubng) McGraw-Hill Trade.

Vitamin Sourcebook. Tonia Reinhard. 1998. LC 98-34410. 320p. pap. 17.00 (*1-56565-878-7*, 08787W) Lowell Hse.

Vitamin Strategy: A Personalized Plan. Art Ulene & Val Ulene. 1997. 286p. (Orig.). 29.98 (*0-941683-37-0*) Instant Improve.

Vitamins. Wihelm Friedrich. 1988. 1060p. (C). lib. bdg. 307.70 (*3-11-010244-7*) De Gruyter.

Vitamins: Their Use & Abuse. Joseph V. Levy & Paul Bach-Y-Rita. 1976. 155p. 8.95 (*0-87140-616-0*) Liveright.

Vitamins & Cancer: Human Cancer Prevention by Vitamins & Micronutrients. Ed. by Frank L. Meyskens, Jr. & Kedar N. Prasad. 1986. LC 85-27134. (Experimental Biology & Medicine Ser.: Vol. 10). 481p. 139.50 (*0-89603-094-6*) Humana.

Vitamins & Cancer Prevention. Ed. by George A. Bray & Donna H. Ryan. 1992. LC 92-19677. (Pennington Center Nutrition Ser.: Vol. 3). (Illus.). 456p. (C). text 80.00 (*0-8071-1789-7*) La State U Pr.

Vitamins & Cancer Prevention Contemporary Issues in Clinical Nutrition, Vol. 14. Toni A. Laidlaw. 1991. LC 90-44657. (Contemporary Issues in Clinical Nutrition Ser.: Vol. 14). 145p. 170.00 (*0-471-56066-9*) Wiley.

Vitamins & Coenzymes, Pt. I. Ed. by John N. Abelson et al. 1997. (Methods in Enzymology Ser.: Vol. 279). (Illus.). 502p. text 99.00 (*0-12-182180-3*) Morgan Kaufmann.

Vitamins & Coenzymes, Pt. C. Ed. by Donald B. McCormick & Lemuel D. Wright. 1971. (Methods in Enzymology Ser.: Vol. 18). (C). text 209.00 (*0-12-181882-9*) Acad Pr.

Vitamins & Coenzymes, Pt. D. Ed. by Donald B. McCormick & Lemuel D. Wright. 1979. (Methods in Enzymology Ser.: Vol. 62). 616p. text 121.00 (*0-12-181962-0*) Acad Pr.

Vitamins & Coenzymes. Ed. by Donald B. McCormick & Lemuel D. Wright. (Methods in Enzymology Ser.: Vol. 18). (C). Pt. A. 1970. text 209.00 (*0-12-181879-9*); Pt. B. 1971. text 209.00 (*0-12-181880-2*) Acad Pr.

Vitamins & Coenzymes. Ed. by Donald B. McCormick & Lemuel D. Wright. 1980. (Methods in Enzymology Ser.: Vol. 66). Pt. E. LC 54-9110. 755p. text 121.00 (*0-12-181966-3*); Pt. F. 579p. text 121.00 (*0-12-181967-1*) Acad Pr.

Vitamins & Coenzymes, Pt. G. Nathan O. Kaplan. Ed. by Sidney P. Colowick. 1986. (Methods in Enzymology Ser.: Vol. 122). text 178.00 (*0-12-182022-X*) Acad Pr.

Vitamins & Coenzymes, Pt. H. Sidney P. Colowick & Nathan O. Kaplan. 1986. (Methods in Enzymology Ser.: Vol. 123). text 178.00 (*0-12-182023-8*) Acad Pr.

Vitamins & Coenzymes. Ed. by John N. Abelson et al. 1997. (Methods in Enzymology Ser.: Vol. 280). (Illus.). Pt. J. 496p. text 99.00 (*0-12-182181-1*); Pt. K. 469p. text 99.00 (*0-12-182182-X*) Morgan Kaufmann.

***Vitamins & Hormones.** Ed. by Gerald Litwack. 2000. (Vitamins & Hormones Ser.: Vol. 61). 364p. 119.95 (*0-12-709861-5*) Acad Pr.

Vitamins & Hormones, Vol. 38. Ed. by Paul L. Munson et al. 1981. (Serial Publication Ser.). text 167.00 (*0-12-709838-0*) Acad Pr.

Vitamins & Hormones, Vol. 39. 1982. text 167.00 (*0-12-709839-9*) Acad Pr.

Vitamins & Hormones, Vol. 40. Ed. by Donald D. McCormick. 1983. (Serial Publication Ser.). text 167.00 (*0-12-709840-2*) Acad Pr.

Vitamins & Hormones, Vol. 41. Ed. by Robert S. Harris & Kenneth V. Thimann. 1984. text 167.00 (*0-12-709841-0*) Acad Pr.

Vitamins & Hormones, Vol. 42. Ed. by Donald B. McCormick. 1985. 372p. text 167.00 (*0-12-709842-9*) Acad Pr.

Vitamins & Hormones, Vol. 45. Ed. by Gerald D. Aurbach & Donald B. McCormick. 1989. 375p. text 136.00 (*0-12-709845-3*) Acad Pr.

Vitamins & Hormones. Ed. by Gerald Litwack. (Illus.). Vol. 48. 1994. 306p. text 104.00 (*0-12-709848-8*); Vol. 51. 1995. 468p. text 90.00 (*0-12-709851-8*) Acad Pr.

Vitamins & Hormones: Advances in Research & Applications, Vol. 43. Ed. by Gerald D. Aurbach & Donald M. McCormick. 1986. 316p. text 136.00 (*0-12-709843-7*) Acad Pr.

Vitamins & Hormones Vol. 49: Steroids. Ed. by Gerald Litwack. 1994. (Illus.). 512p. text 94.00 (*0-12-709849-6*) Acad Pr.

Vitamins & Hormones Vol. 53: Cell Death Proteins, Vol. 53. Gerald Litwack. 1997. (Illus.). 198p. text 89.95 (*0-12-709853-4*) Morgan Kaufmann.

Vitamins & Hormones Vol. 54: Advances in Research & Applications, Vol. 54. Ed. by Gerald Litwack. 1998. (Illus.). 234p. text 84.95 (*0-12-709854-2*) Acad Pr.

Vitamins & Hormones Vol. 56, Nos. 30-55: Cumulative Subject Index. Ed. by Gerald Litwack. 1999. (Vitamins & Hormones Ser.: Vol. 56). (Illus.). 240p. (C). text 89.95 (*0-12-709856-9*) Acad Pr.

Vitamins & Minerals: An Illustrated Guide. Karen Sullivan. 1999. LC 98-20361. (Illustrated Guides Ser.). (Illus.). 144p. pap. 19.95 (*1-86204-295-0*) Element MA.

Vitamins & Minerals: Hazardous to Your Health? Mark J. Sweet & Stanley H. Freeman. 1992. 162p. pap. 8.95 (*0-930753-15-1*) Spect Ln Pr.

Vitamins & Minerals: Questions You Have - Answers You Need. Ellen Moyer. 1993. LC 93-30754. 224p. pap. 10.95 (*1-882606-05-1*) Peoples Med Soc.

Vitamins & Minerals from A to Z with Ethno-Consciousness. Jewel Pookrum. 1993. (Illus.). pap. 25.00 (*1-883104-00-9*) Jewel Pubns.

Vitamins & Minerals Handbook. Amanda Ursell. 2001. LC 00-45194. (Healing Handbooks Ser.). (Illus.). 128p. pap. 12.95 (*0-7894-7180-9*) DK Pub Inc.

Vitamins & Minerals in Health & Nutrition. Matti Tolonen. 1990. (Ellis Horwood Series in Food Science & Technology). (Illus.). 256p. (Orig.). (C). pap. text 46.50 (*0-7476-0068-6*, VNR) Wiley.

Vitamins & Minerals in the Prevention & Treatment of Cancer. Maryce M. Jacobs. 1991. 312p. 150.00 (*0-8493-4259-7*, RC271) CRC Pr.

Vitamins in Animal & Human Nutrition. Lee R. McDowell. 2nd ed. 2000. LC 00-27082. (Illus.). xvi, 793p. 99.95 (*0-8138-2630-6*) Iowa U Pr.

Vitamins in Animal Nutrition: Comparative Aspects to Human Nutrition. Lee R. McDowell. Ed. by Tony J. Cunha. 1989. (Animal Feeding & Nutrition Ser.). 486p. text 100.00 (*0-12-483372-1*) Acad Pr.

Vitamins in Human Biology & Medicine. M. H. Briggs. 1981. 272p. 152.00 (*0-8493-5673-3*, QP771, CRC Reprint) Franklin.

Vitamins, Minerals, & Dietary Supplements: A Definitive Guide to Healthy Eating. Hasnain Walji. 1995. 144p. pap. (*0-340-61905-8*) Hodder & Stought Ltd GBR. *Dist:* Lubrecht & Cramer, Trafalgar.

Vitamins, Minerals, & Food Supplements Nutrition. American Dietetic Association Staff. 1996. (Nutrition Now Ser.). 160p. pap. text 5.95 (*1-56561-092-X*) Wiley.

Vitamins, Minerals, & Protein-Amino Acids Used for Animal Health. 1993. (Illus.). 112p. 1500.00 (*0-89336-986-1*, GA-080B) BCC.

Vitamins, Minerals, & Protein-Amino Acids Used for Human Health. 1993. 176p. 1500.00 (*0-89336-985-3*, GA-080A) BCC.

Vitamins, Nutrition & Cancer. Ed. by K. N. Prasad. 1984. (Illus.). xii, 320p. 172.25 (*3-8055-3846-4*) S Karger.

Vitiligo: A Comprehensive Monograph on Basic & Clinical Science. Seung-Kyung Hann & James J. Nordlund. 2000. LC 99-46475. (Illus.). xiv, 306p. 146.95 (*0-632-05071-3*) Blackwell Sci.

***Vitiligo & Piebaldism: Treatment of Leucoderma by Transplantation of Autologous Melanocytes.** Mats J. Olsson. 2001. (Comprehensive Summaries of Uppsala Dissertations from the Faculty of Medicine Ser.: No. 1061). (Illus.). 77p. pap. (*91-554-5080-6*) Acta Univ SWE. *Dist:* Coronet Bks.

Vitreoretinal Disease: The Essentials. Carl D. Regillo et al. 1998. LC 98-24807. (Illus.). 720p. 149.00 (*0-86577-761-6*) Thieme Med Pubs.

Vitreoretinal Surgery. Zivojnovic. 1997. lib. bdg. 98.00 (*0-7923-3311-X*); lib. bdg. 98.00 (*0-7923-3312-8*); lib. bdg. 98.00 (*0-7923-3313-6*); lib. bdg. 98.00 (*0-7923-3314-4*); lib. bdg. 98.00 (*0-7923-4331-X*); lib. bdg. 98.00 (*0-7923-4332-8*) Kluwer Academic.

Vitreoretinal Surgery of the Injured Eye. D. Virgil Alfaro & Peter Liggett. 1998. LC 98-22167. 384p. text 145.00 (*0-397-58428-8*) Lppncott W & W.

Vitreous & Retinal Laser Investigation, 001. Marie-Jose Tassignon. 1994. (Illus.). 187p. pap. (*90-70289-76-8*) VUB Univ Pr BEL. *Dist:* Paul & Co Pubs.

Viviendo Sobrio. 1981.Tr. of Living Sober. (SPA.). 126p. pap. 1.50 (*0-916856-08-9*) AAWS.

Vivir despues de la Perdida. Bob Deits. 1994. LC 94-30395. (SPA.). 240p. pap. 12.95 (*1-55561-062-5*) Fisher Bks.

VNR Dictionary of Environmental Health & Safety. Frank S. Lisella. 1993. 356p. 120.00 (*0-471-28410-6*, VNR) Wiley.

Vocabulaire de la Psychanalyse. Jean-Baptiste Pontalis. Ed. by Jean Laplanche. 5th ed. 1976. (FRE.). 85.00 (*0-8288-5759-8*, M6558) Fr & Eur.

Vocabulaire de la Psychologie. Henri Pieron. 8th ed. 1990. (FRE.). 608p. 115.00 (*0-7859-4835-X*) Fr & Eur.

Vocabulaire de Medecine et des Sciences Connexes: Francais-Anglais, Anglais-Francais. W. J. Gladstone. 1971. (ENG & FRE.). 298p. 75.00 (*0-7859-5542-9*) Fr & Eur.

Vocabulaire de Psychopedagogie et de Psychiatrie de L'Enfant: Vocabulary of Child Psychiatry & Educational Psychology. Robert Lafon. 3rd ed. 1973. (FRE.). 868p. 95.00 (*0-8288-6335-0*, F-19440) Fr & Eur.

Vocabulaire Medical de Base, Set. Marie Bonvalot. 1989. (FRE.). 447p. pap. 59.95 (*0-7859-4808-2*) Fr & Eur.

Vocabulaire Psychologique et Psychiatrique. Michel Godfryd. 1993. (FRE.). 128p. pap. 16.50 (*0-7859-0977-X*, 2130452450) Fr & Eur.

Vocabulario Medico Portugues - Ingles, Ingles - Portugues. R. da Graca Veiga. 1979. (ENG & POR.). pap. 39.95 (*0-7859-0907-9*, F99490) Fr & Eur.

Vocabulary Arranged for the Instruction of the Deaf & Dumb. Wm. Vaughan. 1973. 69.95 (*0-8490-1265-1*) Gordon Pr.

***Vocabulary of Medical Signs & Symptoms.** Andre Lussier et al. 426p. pap. (*0-660-55811-4*) Can7 Govern Pub CAN. *Dist:* Intl Spec Bk.

Vocabulary of Psychoanalysis (Vocabulaire de la Psychanalyse) Jean-Baptiste Pontalis & Jean Laplanche. 10th ed. 1990. (FRE.). 544p. 105.00 (*0-7859-4741-8*, M14530) Fr & Eur.

Vocal Arts Medicine: The Care & Prevention of Professional Voice Disorders. Ed. by Michael Benninger et al. 1994. LC 93-5013. (Illus.). 374p. text 79.00 (*0-86577-439-0*) Thieme Med Pubs.

Vocal Exercise Physiology. Keith G. Saxon & Carole M. Schneider. 1995. (Illus.). 166p. (C). 45.00 (*1-56593-159-9*, 0467) Thomson Learn.

Vocal Fold Physiology: Acoustic, Perceptual, & Physiological Aspects of Voice Mechanisms. Ed. by Jan Gauffin & Britta Hammarberg. 1991. (Vocal Fold Physiology Ser.). (Illus.). 304p. (Orig.). (C). pap. 65.00 (*1-879105-51-9*, 0219) Thomson Learn.

Vocal Fold Physiology: Controlling Complexity & Chaos. Pamela J. Davis & Neville H. Fletcher. 1996. (Vocal Fold Physiology Ser.). (Illus.). 454p. (Orig.). pap. 65.00 (*1-56593-714-7*, 1404) Thomson Learn.

Vocal Fold Physiology: Voice Production, Mechanisms & Functions. Ed. by Osamu Fujimura. 1988. (Vocal Fold Physiology Ser.: Vol. 2). (Illus.). 508p. (C). 65.00 (*1-56593-456-3*, 1130) Singular Publishing.

Vocal Health & Pedagogy. Robert T. Sataloff. 1998. LC 97-42658. 488p. pap. text 61.95 (*1-56593-963-8*, 1906) Thomson Learn.

Vocal Pathologies: Diagnosis, Treatment & Case Studies. James P. Dworkin & Robert J. Meleca. 1996. LC 96-24941. 346p. pap. text, stu. ed. 65.95 (*1-56593-623-X*, 1292) Thomson Learn.

Vocal Rehabilitation: A Practice Book for Voice Improvement. Virginia Agnello & Cindy Garcia. 3rd ed. 1990. spiral bd. 24.00 (*0-89079-233-X*, 3652) PRO-ED.

Vocal Rehabilitation: Let's Talk Voice. Virginia L. Agnello. 3rd ed. 1993. LC 93-5981. (Illus.). 516p. spiral bd. 14.00 (*0-89079-591-6*, 3659) PRO-ED.

Vocational & Personal Adjustments in Practical Nursing. Betty G. Becker & Dolores T. Fender. 7th ed. 1994. (Illus.). 194p. tchr. ed. (*0-8151-4419-9*) Mosby Inc.

Vocational & Personal Adjustments in Practical Nursing. Betty G. Becker & Dolores T. Fendler. 7th ed. 1993. LC 93-8185. (Illus.). 194p. (C). (gr. 13). pap. text 24.95 (*0-8016-6839-5*, 06839) Mosby Inc.

Vocational Evaluation & Traumatic Brain Injury: A Procedural Manual. Stephen W. Thomas. 1991. 61p. (Orig.). (C). pap. 14.75 (*0-916671-94-1*) TRR.

Vocational Impact of Psychiatric Disorders: A Guide for Rehabilitation Professionals. Gary L. Fischler. 1999. LC 99-30253. 256p. 56.00 (*0-8342-1251-X*) PRO-ED.

Vocational Integration Index. Wendy S. Parent et al. 1992. 112p. pap. text 48.00 (*0-9626521-9-9*) Buttrwrth-Heinemann.

Vocational Interests: Meaning, Measurement & Counseling Use. Ed. by Mark L. Savickas & Arnold R. Spokane. 1999. LC 98-51047. (Illus.). 440p. 49.95 (*0-89106-126-6*, 7812, Davies-Black Pub) Consulting Psychol.

Vocational Rehabilitation & Employment of the Disabled: A Glossary. 1989. 182p. pap. 13.50 (*92-2-002571-X*) Intl Labour Office.

Vocational Rehabilitation for Persons with Traumatic Brain Injury. Paul Wehman & Jeffrey Kreutzer. 1995. 372p. 74.00 (*0-8342-0135-6*) PRO-ED.

Vocational Rehabilitation in Florida Workers' Compensation: Rehabilitants, Services, Costs, & Outcomes. John A. Gardner. 1988. LC 87-37119. 35.00 (*0-935149-11-2*, WC-88-1) Workers Comp Res Inst.

Vocational Rehabilitation in Workers' Compensation: Issues & Evidence. John A. Gardner. 1985. 35.00 (*0-935149-05-8*, S-85-1) Workers Comp Res Inst.

Vocational Rehabilitation Outcomes: Evidence from New York. John A. Gardner. 1986. LC 86-28144. 120p. 35.00 (*0-935149-03-1*, WC-86-1) Workers Comp Res Inst.

Voice: A Dramatic New Concept. Denton Rossell. Ed. by Delorez Westman. 1984. (Illus.). 227p. 28.50 (*0-913145-00-9*) Clark & Westman-Magnolia.

Voice: Psyche & Soma. Cornelius L. Reid. 1975. LC 74-30987. (Orig.). pap. 6.95 (*0-915282-00-3*) J Patelson Mus.

Voice & Self: A Handbook of Personal Voice Development Therapy. Ingeburg Stengel & Theo Strauch. 2000. LC 00-711421. (Illus.). xii, 201p. pap. (*1-85343-500-7*) Free Assoc Bks GBR. *Dist:* Intl Spec Bk.

Voice & Voice Therapy. Daniel R. Boone. 6th ed. 1999. LC 99-22921. (Illus.). 308p. text 77.00 incl. audio compact disk (*0-205-30843-0*, Prentice Hall) P-H.

Voice Care in the Medical Setting. Danna L. Koschkee & Linda A. Rammage. 1997. LC 97-11209. (Illus.). 224p. pap. 55.00 (*1-56593-111-4*, 0414) Thomson Learn.

Voice Clinic Handbook. Tom Harris et al. 1998. 300p. 65.00 (*1-56593-915-8*, 1812) Singular Publishing.

Voice Diagnostic Protocol: A Practical Guide to Diagnosis of Voice Disorders. Shaheen N. Awan. 1995. LC 00-45095. (Illus.). ix, 202p. pap. text 55.00 incl. disk (*0-8342-1717-1*, 17171) PRO-ED.

Voice Disorders & Their Management. Ed. by Margaret Fawcus. 2nd ed. 1991. 368p. (Orig.). pap. (*0-412-36480-8*, A4421) Chapman & Hall.

Voice Disorders & Their Management. Ed. by Margaret Fawcus. 1991. (Illus.). 400p. (Orig.). (C). pap. 54.95 (*1-879105-57-8*, 0256) Singular Publishing.

Voice from the Dumb: A Memoir of John William Lashford. W. Sleight. 1972. 59.95 (*0-8490-1266-X*) Gordon Pr.

Voice of My Own: A Verbal Box of Chocolates. Sue Chance. 1993. LC 93-91044. 260p. 19.95 (*0-9638398-0-2*) Bonne Chance.

Voice of Neurosis. Paul J. Moses. 1954. LC 54-8213. (Illus.). 140p. text 56.00 (*0-8089-0334-9*, 792985, Grune & Strat) Harcrt Hlth Sci Grp.

Voice of Shame: Silence & Connection in Psychotherapy. Ed. by Robert G. Lee & Gordon Wheeler. 1996. (Gestalt Institute of Cleveland Book Ser.). 416p. 38.95 (*0-88163-282-1*) Analytic Pr.

Voice Speech & Gesture. Hugh Campbell et al. 1977. LC 72-5589. (Granger Index Reprint Ser.). reprint ed. 57.95 (*0-8369-6381-4*) Ayer.

Voice, Speech, & Language in the Child: Development & Disorder. J. A. Martin. 1981. (Disorders of Human Communication Ser.: Vol. 4). (Illus.). 210p. 56.95 (*0-387-81629-1*) Spr-Verlag.

Voice Surgery. Ed. by Robert T. Sataloff & Wilbur J. Gould. 1992. LC 92-49947. (*0-8016-1988-2*) Mosby Inc.

Voice Technology. Ed Teja & Gary Gonnella. 1983. (C). text 39.00 (*0-8359-8417-6*) P-H.

Voice Therapy: Clinical Studies. Joseph C. Stemple. 1993. LC 92-49999. 186p. (gr. 13). text (*0-8016-4763-0*, 04763) Mosby Inc.

Voice Therapy for Adolescents. Moya L. Andrews & Anne C. Sommers. 1991. (Illus.). 220p. (Orig.). (C). reprint ed. pap. 34.95 (*1-879105-21-7*, A001) Thomson Learn.

Voice Therapy for Children. Moya L. Andrews. 1991. (Illus.). 336p. (C). reprint ed. pap. 39.95 (*1-879105-48-9*, 0231) Thomson Learn.

Voice Treatment for Children & Adolescents. Moya L. Andrews. 2001. LC 00-53778. 637p. pap. text 57.95 (*0-7693-0107-X*) Singular Publishing.

Voice Treatment for Parkinson Disease & Other Neurological Disorders. Lorraine O. Ramig et al. 2nd ed. 2000. 250p. pap. 45.00 (*1-56593-906-9*, 1794) Thomson Learn.

Voice Treatment for Parkinson's Disease & Other Neurological Disorders. Lorraine O. Ramig. 1998. 65.00 incl. audio, VHS (*1-58041-019-7*, 0112096) Am Speech Lang Hearing.

Voice Update: Proceedings of the 1st World Congress, Oporto, Portugal, April 9-13, 1995, Vol. 109. M. Pais Clemente. 1996. LC 96-29317. (International Congress Ser.). 428p. 206.25 (*0-444-82230-5*) Elsevier.

Voices of Feminist Therapy. Ed. by Elizabeth F. Williams. 1995. LC 00-501904. 190p. text 39.00 (*3-7186-0603-8*); 140p. pap. text 21.00 (*3-7186-0604-6*) Gordon & Breach (Harwood Acad Pubs).

Voices of QI: An Introductory Guide to Traditional Chinese Medicine. Alex Holland. 1997. LC 97-92547. viii, 96 p. (*0-9622665-3-1*) A Holland.

Voices of Robby Wilde. Elizabeth Kytle. 1995. LC 94-33591. 344p. pap. 14.95 (*0-8203-1715-2*) U of Ga Pr.

Voices of Strength & Hope for a Friend with AIDS. Joseph Gallagher. 1987. LC 87-61464. (Illus.). 62p. (Orig.). pap. 3.95 (*1-55612-073-7*) Sheed & Ward WI.

Voices That Care: Stories & Encouragements for People with AIDS/HIV & Those That Love Them. Neal Hitchens. 1994. LC 94-1463. 288p. pap. 11.00 (*0-671-88230-9*, Fireside) S&S Trade Pap.

Voices: The Art & Science of Psychotherapy see Carl Jung & Soul Psychology

Voiding Dysfunction: Diagnosis & Treatment. Ed. by Rodney A. Appell. 2000. LC 00-27599. (Current Clinical Urology Ser.). 336p. 125.00 (*0-89603-659-6*) Humana.

Vokabular der Psychoanalyse: The Vocabulary of Psychoanalysis Jean Laplanche. 1973. (GER.). pap. 49.95 (*0-8288-6340-7*, M-7680) Fr & Eur.

Doctors & Home Remedies. Sid Kirchheimer. 1996. mass mkt. 8.99 (*0-553-85106-3*) Bantam.

Vol. I Behavioral Medicine - Behavior Modification. Ed. by David Levinson. 1981. (Theoretical Information Control Guides Ser.). 525p. (Orig.). pap. 45.00 (*0-87536-736-4*) HRAFP.

Vol. III, Alcoholics Anonymous & Counseling. Ed. by David Levinson. 1984. (Theoretical Information Control Guides Ser.). 553p. (Orig.). pap. 45.00 (*0-87536-740-2*) HRAFP.

Volatilization Technologies for Removing Organics from Water. J. L. Fleming. 1989. LC 88-37154. (Pollution Technology Review Ser.: No. 164). (Illus.). 120p. 39.00 (*0-8155-1189-2*) Noyes.

Voles, Mice & Lemmings. Charles I. Elton. 1971. reprint ed. 70.00 (*3-7682-0275-5*) Lubrecht & Cramer.

Voltammetry in the Neurosciences: Principles, Methods & Applications. Ed. by Joseph B. Justice, Jr. 1987. LC 86-20105. (Contemporary Neuroscience Ser.). 400p. 145.00 (*0-89603-103-9*) Humana.

Volterra-Hamilton Models in the Ecology & Evolution of Colonial Organisms. P. L. Antonelli & R. H. Bradbury. 1996. 250p. text 38.00 (*981-02-2450-8*, BMBae-B2922) World Scientific Pub.

Volume & Kinetics in Tumor Control & Normal Tissue Complications No. 10: AAPM Proceedings of the 5th International Conference on Dose, Time, & Fractionation in Radiation Oncology. Ed. by Bhudatt Paliwal & Donald Herbert. 1998. LC 98-66138. 500p. pap. (*1-888340-11-8*) AAPM.

Volume Replacement. Ed. by J. F. Baron & J. Treib. 1998. LC 98-18046. (Illus.). x, 143p. pap. 65.00 (*3-540-64187-4*) Spr-Verlag.

Volume Therapy. Ed. by Johannes Treib. 1999. LC 99-42741. (Illus.). 160p. 59.95 (*3-540-65749-5*) Spr-Verlag.

Voluntary Food Intake & Diet Selection in Farm Animals. J. M. Forbes. 1995. LC 97-181254. (Illus.). 544p. text 120.00 (*0-85198-908-X*) OUP.

Voluntary HIV Counseling & Testing: Facts, Issues & Answers. 1993. (Illus.). 33p. (Orig.). pap. text 15.00 (*0-7881-0180-3*) DIANE Pub.

Volunteer in Long-Term Care. 1968. LC 68-3723. 60p. pap. 8.75 (*0-87258-043-1*, 202155) ASHAM.

Volunteer Leader: Essays on the Role of Trustees of Nonprofit Facilities & Services for the Aging. Ed. by Deborah A. Cloud. 1985. LC 84-73168. 146p. pap. text 15.00 (*0-943774-24-1*) Am Assn Homes.

Volunteer Services Department in a Health Care Institution. 1973. LC 73-77522. 72p. pap. 10.00 (*0-87258-124-1*, 202165) ASHAM.

Volunteer Services Department in a Health Care Institution. American Hospital Association Staff. 2nd rev. ed. 1988. LC 88-37456. 56p. pap. 14.00 (*0-87258-493-3*, 202166) Am Hospital.

Volunteering with Your Pet: How to Get Involved in Animal-Assisted Therapy with Any Kind of Pet. Mary R. Burch. 1996. LC 95-38944. (Illus.). 224p. pap. 19.95 (*0-87605-791-1*, Howell) Hungry Minds.

Volunteerism Marketing: New Vistas for Non-Profit & Public Sector Management. Ed. by Donald R. Self & Walter W. Wymer, Jr. 1999. LC 99-56467. (Journal of Nonprofit & Public Sector Marketing Ser.: Vol. 6, Nos. 2-3). xviii, 174p. (C). pap. text 39.95 (*0-7890-0985-4*) Haworth Pr.

Volunteers for Mental Health. Ed. by Philip Ash. 1973. LC 73-10368. 31.00 (*0-8422-5121-9*) Irvington.

Volunteers in Research & Testing. Ed. by Raid Ayesh & Anthony Hubbard. 1996. LC 97-147630. 208p. 99.95 (*0-7484-0397-3*) Taylor & Francis.

Vom Symptom zur Diagnose. Ed. by N. Zoellner & W. Hadorn. 8th ed. 1986. (Illus.). x, 682p. 108.00 (*3-8055-4030-2*) S Karger.

***Vomiting & Medicine: Subject, Reference & Research Guidebook.** Roxanne Z. Marcus. 2002. 139p. 57.50 (*0-7883-2514-0*); pap. 47.50 (*0-7883-2515-9*) ABBE Pubs Assn.

Von Normalen zum Gesunden see From Normal to Healthy: Paths to the Liberation of Consciousness

Von Willebrand Factor & the Mechanisms of Platelet Function. Zaverio M. Ruggerl. 1997. (Medical Intelligence Unit Ser.). 250p. 89.95 (*0-412-11571-9*) Chapman & Hall.

Vowel Perception & Production. B. S. Rosner & J. B. Pickering. 1994. LC 93-47078. (Psychology Ser.: No. 23). (Illus.). 444p. (C). text 120.00 (*0-19-852138-3*) OUP.

Voxel-Man Pt. 1: Brain & Skull, Version 1.1. K. H. Hohne. 2nd ed. 1997. 64p. pap. 1050.00 incl. cd-rom (*3-540-14584-2*) Spr-Verlag.

Voyage: Visions in Color & Form. Claude Sieber. 1994. LC 94-33059. 143p. text 148.00 (*0-86715-296-6*) Quint Pub Co.

Voyages Internationaux et Sante 1996 see International Travel & Health: Vaccination Requirements & Health Advice - 1996

Vrksayurveda of Parasara: A Treatise on Plant Science. Ed. by N. N. Sircar & Roma Sarkar. 1996. LC 96-901178. (C). (*81-7030-441-5*) Sri Satguru Pubns IND. *Dist:* S Asia.

Vroman Effect. Ed. by C. H. Bamford et al. 1992. 208p. 73.50 (*90-6764-139-1*) Coronet Bks.

Vulnerability & Stress in Late-Onset Psychiatric Disorders. David Gutmann. Date not set. 19.95 (*0-465-09056-7*) Basic.

Vulnerability to Drug Abuse. Ed. by Meyer Glantz & Roy Pickens. 1992. LC 91-35242. 533p. pap. text 19.95 (*1-55798-412-3*) Am Psychol.

Vulnerability to Psychopathology: A Biosocial Model. Marvin Zuckerman. 1999. LC 98-33296. 552p. 49.95 (*1-55798-566-9*) Am Psychol.

Vulnerability to Psychopathology: Risk Across the Lifespan. Ed. by Rick E. Ingram & Joseph M. Price. 2000. LC 00-59265. 476p. 55.00 (*1-57230-603-3*, C0603) Guilford Pubns.

Vulnerable Atherosclerotic Plaque: Understanding, Identification & Modification. Ed. by Valentin Fuster. 1998. LC 98-17362. (American Heart Association Monograph Ser.). (Illus.). 500p. 115.00 (*0-87993-406-9*, Futura Media) Futura Pub.

Vulnerable Brain & Environmental Risks Vol. 1: Malnutrition & Hazard Assessment. R. L. Isaacson & K. F. Jensen. 1992. (Illus.). 290p. (C). text 85.00 (*0-306-44148-9*, Kluwer Plenum) Kluwer Academic.

Vulnerable Brain & Environmental Risks Vol. 2: Toxins in Food. R. L. Isaacson & K. F. Jensen. 1992. (Illus.). 356p. (C). text 89.50 (*0-306-44165-9*, Kluwer Plenum) Kluwer Academic.

Vulnerable Brain & Environmental Risks Vol. 3: Toxins in Air & Water. Ed. by R. L. Isaacson & K. F. Jensen. 1994. (Illus.). 384p. (C). text 107.00 (*0-306-44611-1*, Kluwer Plenum) Kluwer Academic.

Vulnerable Child. Ed. by Theodore B. Cohen et al. Vol. 1. 1993. (Vulnerable Child Monographs). 300p. 45.00 (*0-8236-6755-3*); Vol. 2. 1995. (Vulnerable Child Monographs). 231p. 37.50 (*0-8236-6756-1*); Vol. III. 1998. LC 93-33421. (Vulnerable Child Ser.: Vol. 3). 354p. 52.50 (*0-8236-6757-X*, BN06757) Intl Univs Pr.

Vulnerable Populations: Evaluation & Treatment of Sexually Abused Children & Adult Survivors, Vol. 1. Suzanne M. Sgroi. 1988. LC 87-45325. 336p. 44.95 (*0-669-16336-8*) Free Pr.

Vulnerable Populations: Sexual Abuse Treatment for Children, Adult Survivors, Offenders & Persons with Mental Retardation, Vol. 2. Ed. by Suzanne M. Sgroi. 1989. 448p. 44.95 (*0-669-20942-2*); pap. 27.95 (*0-669-20943-0*) Free Pr.

Vulnerable Therapist: Practicing Psychotherapy in an Age of Anxiety. Helen W. Coale. 1998. LC 97-37272. 272p. 49.95 (*0-7890-0179-9*); pap. 24.95 (*0-7890-0480-1*) Haworth Pr.

Vulva. C. Marjorie Ridley & Sarah M. Neill. 2nd ed. 1999. LC 98-23209. (Illus.). 416p. 313.95 (*0-632-04768-2*) Blackwell Sci.

Vulvar Disease. Allison C. Ledger. 1995. (C). text (*0-7216-5317-0*) Saunders.

Vulvovaginitis. Ed. by Peter Elsner & Joachim Martius. 1993. (Illus.). 440p. text 215.00 (*0-8247-9040-5*) Dekker.

Vygotsky & Cognitive Science: Language & the Unification of the Social & Computational Mind. William Frawley. 1997. LC 96-30021. (Illus.). 384p. 43.00 (*0-674-94347-3*) HUP.

Vygotsky & the Social Formation of Mind. James V. Wertsch. 1985. 288p. reprint ed. pap. 19.95 (*0-674-94351-1*) HUP.

Vygotsky Today: On the Verge of Non-Classical Psychology. A. Asmolov. 1998. LC 98-39083. 59.00 (*1-56072-616-4*) Nova Sci Pubs.

Vygotsky's Psychology: A Biography of Ideas. Alex Kozulin. 1991. LC 90-39118. (Illus.). 294p. 41.50 (*0-674-94365-1*, KOZVYG) HUP.

W

***W. B. Saunders Fundamentals of Medical Assisting.** Sue A. Hunt & Jon Zonderman. 2001. LC 2001-49214. (*0-7216-8564-1*) Saunders.

W. R. Bion: Between Past & Future. Ed. by Parthenope Bion Talamo et al. 2000. 296p. pap. (*1-85575-187-9*) Karnac Bks GBR. *Dist:* Other Pr LLC.

Wachstum. Ed. by H. P. Schwarz. 1987. (Paediatrische Fortbildungskurse fuer die Praxis Ser.: Vol. 61). (Illus.). x, 82p. 42.75 (*3-8055-4594-0*) S Karger.

Wages of Seeking Help: Sexual Exploitation by Professionals. Contrib. by Carol Bohmer. 2000. LC 99-45991. 224p. 62.50 (*0-275-96793-X*) Greenwood.

Wages of Sickness: The Politics of Health Insurance in Progressive America. Beatrix Hoffman. 2001. LC 00-44735. (Studies in Social Medicine). (Illus.). xii, 261p. pap. 17.95 (*0-8078-4902-2*); lib. bdg. 39.95 (*0-8078-2588-3*) U of NC Pr.

Wages of Sin: Sex & Disease, Past & Present. Peter Lewis Allen. 2000. LC 99-48603. (Illus.). xxiii, 202p. 25.00 (*0-226-01460-6*) U Ch Pr.

Waianae Book on Hawaiian Health. Terry Shintani & Claire Hughes. 1990. 119p. pap. text 9.95 (*0-9646023-0-X*) Waianae Coast CHC.

Waist-High in the World: A Life among the Nondisabled. Nancy Mairs. 1998. LC 96-21819. 224p. pap. 12.00 (*0-8070-7087-4*) Beacon Pr.

Waist-High in the World: A Life among the Nondisabled. Nancy Mairs. 1999. 212p. text 20.00 (*0-7881-5998-4*) DIANE Pub.

Waiting: A Diary of Loss & Hope in Pregnancy. Ellen J. Reich. 1992. LC 91-8720. 132p. lib. bdg. 3.95 (*1-56024-087-3*); pap. 11.95 (*0-918393-88-4*) Haworth Pr.

Waiting at the Gate: Creativity & Hope in the Nursing Home. Susan L. Sandel & David R. Johnson. Ed. by Phyllis Foster. 1987. LC 87-8713. (Activities, Adaptation & Aging Ser.: Vol. 9, No. 3). 185p. 32.95 (*0-86656-631-7*) Haworth Pr.

***Waiting for a Transplant.** NKF Transaction Council Members. 2001. 64p. pap. (*1-931472-08-4*, 0656) Natl Kidney.

Waiting for Elective Surgery in Australian Public Hospitals, 1995. Lynelle Moon. 1996. LC 97-144170. viii, 55 p. (*0-642-24701-3*) Aust Inst Criminology.

Waiting to Clear: Brain Injury: Early Stages of Recovery. Mary M. Castiglione & Cynthia C. Johnson. 1994. LC 93-37557. (Illus.). 48 + 40p. pap. text 9.50 (*0-939838-35-4*) Pritchett & Hull.

Waiting to Inhale: The Politics of Medical Marijuana. Alan Bock. 2000. LC 00-48487. 224p. pap. 17.95 (*0-929765-82-6*) Seven Locks Pr.

Wake Up, a Sensory Stimulation Program. Pamela Sander. 1987. (Illus.). 89p. (C). 17.00 (*1-877735-14-0*, 2121PP) Prof Prnting & Pub.

Wake up, Rhonda: How a Courageous Family Rescued Their "Sleeping Beauty" from Severe Brain-Damage. Jo Knott. 1989. LC 89-83589. (Illus.). 242p. (Orig.). 13.95 (*0-9622992-1-9*); pap. 7.95 (*0-9622992-0-0*) Star Orange Park.

Waking Dream Therapy: Discover Your Inner Self Through Dreams & Imagination. Gerald N. Epstein. 2000. 237p. pap. 16.95 (*1-883148-03-0*) ACMI Pr.

Waking the Tiger - Healing Trauma: The Innate Capacity to Transform Overwhelming Experiences. Peter A. Levine & Ann Frederick. 1997. LC 97-3918. (Illus.). 256p. (Orig.). pap. 16.95 (*1-55643-233-X*) North Atlantic.

Waking up Well. Linda F. Fleming. Ed. by Mary Abrams. 1990. 100p. (Orig.). pap. (*1-877631-03-5*) LF Pub VA.

Walden II. Peter Ruppert. 1976. 3.50 (*0-671-00973-7*, Arc) Hungry Minds.

Waldorf Parenting Handbook: Useful Information on Child Development & Education from Anthroposophical Sources. Lois Cusick. 2nd rev. ed. 1988. pap. 17.95 (*0-916786-75-7*, Saint George Pubns) R Steiner Col.

Wales & Medicine. Ed. by John Cule. 1975. 249p. (C). pap. (*0-85088-260-5*) Gomer Pr GBR. *Dist:* St Mut.

Walk Don't Run. Elvira Monroe. 1979. LC 79-63351. pap. 3.95 (*0-933174-04-7*) Wide World-Tetra.

Walk, Don't Run: The Doctor's Book of Walking. Fred A. Stutman. 1979. LC 79-84815. 97p. pap. 6.95 (*0-934232-00-8*) Med Manor Bks.

Walk the Walk & Talk the Talk: An Ethnography of a Drug Abuse Treatment Facility. Geoffrey R. Skoll. 1992. LC 91-34771. 250p. (C). 44.95 (*0-87722-917-1*) Temple U Pr.

Walk to Win: Easy Four-Day Diet & Fitness Plan. Fred A. Stutman. 1990. LC 85-63311. (Illus.). 256p. pap. 10.95 (*0-934232-07-5*) Med Manor Bks.

Walk to Win: The Easy Four-Day Diet & Fitness Plan. Fred A. Stutman. 1990. LC 85-63311. (Illus.). 286p. 19.95 (*0-934232-08-3*) Med Manor Bks.

Walk, Wiggle, & Write: Movement Experiences Throughout Your Curriculum. Margery A. Kranyik. Ed. by Martha A. Hayes. 1991. (Illus.). 48p. pap. 6.95 (*1-878727-08-7*) First Teacher.

Walk Yourself Thin. David Rives. rev. ed. 1998. 19.95 (*1-878143-00-X*); pap. 12.95 (*1-878143-01-8*) Moon River.

Walking Cure. Bernarr Adolphus Macfadden. 1984. (Illus.). 179p. reprint ed. pap. text 15.00 (*0-87556-391-0*) Saifer.

Walking for Health. 1991. lib. bdg. 75.00 (*0-8490-5140-1*) Gordon Pr.

Walking for Health. Lon H. Seiger & James Hesson. 1990. 176p. text (*0-697-11014-1*) Brown & Benchmark.

Walking into Darkness: How to Care for the Alzheimer Patient. James J. Joyce. 8p. (Orig.). (*0-9642138-0-X*) Joyce Homecare.

Walking off Weight: A 14-Step, 14-Day Walking-Weight Loss Program That Lasts for Life. R. Sweetgall et al. 1989. 96p. pap. 8.95 (*0-939041-10-3*) Creative Walking.

Walking on the Edge Vol. 500: A Journey Through the Psychic Pain of Mental Illness. 1997. LC 98-111416. 46p. pap. 7.95 (*0-9661288-0-X*) B Starnes.

Walking Out on the Boys. Frances K. Conley. 1999. 256p. pap. 13.00 (*0-374-52595-1*) FS&G.

Walking Through the Valley: Understanding & Emerging from Clergy Depression. Robert L. Randall. 1998. LC 97-42421. 144p. pap. text 15.00 (*0-687-01463-8*) Abingdon.

Walking Through the Waters: Biblical Reflections for Families of Cancer Patients. Nancy Regensburger. Ed. by Jeannie Crawford-Lee. 2001. LC 00-43493. 108p. pap. 10.00 (*0-8358-0934-X*) Upper Room Bks.

Walking Wellness Teacher's Guide. Robert Sweetgall. Ed. by Robert Neeves. 1988. (Illus.). 144p. 13.00 (*0-939041-05-7*) Creative Walking.

Walking Wounded: Men's Lives During & since the Vietnam War. Steve Trimm. Ed. by Edward Tick. 1993. (Frontiers in Psychotherapy Ser.). 192p. (C). 77.00 (*0-89391-806-7*); pap. 39.50 (*0-89391-807-5*) Greenwood (Ablex).

Wallace St. Wold. 1998. 49.90 (*0-323-00869-0*) Mosby Inc.

Walls: Physical & Psychological. Robert E. Reuman. 1966. LC 66-24444. (Orig.). pap. 4.00 (*0-87574-147-9*) Pendle Hill.

Walrus on My Table: A Tale of Animal Healing & Human Bonding. Anthony Gugliemo & Cari Lynn. 2000. LC 00-31819. (Illus.). xiv, 192p. 22.95 (*0-312-26267-1*) St Martin.

Walsh & Hoyt's Clinical Neuro-Ophthalmology, Vol. 1. Neil R. Miller. 4th ed. 1982. (Illus.). 382p. lib. bdg. 115.00 (*0-683-06020-1*) Lppncott W & W.

Walsh & Hoyt's Clinical Neuro-Ophthalmology, Vol. 2. Neil R. Miller. 4th ed. 1984. (Illus.). 750p. 135.00 (*0-683-06021-X*) Lppncott W & W.

Walsh & Hoyt's Clinical Neuro-Ophthalmology, Vol. 3. Ed. by Neil R. Miller. 4th ed. 1987. 734p. 140.00 (*0-683-06022-8*) Lppncott W & W.

Walsh & Hoyt's Clinical Neuro-Ophthalmology. Neil R. Miller et al. 5th ed. LC 96-50372. Volume 1. 1997. 1,836p. text 199.00 (*0-683-30230-2*); Volume 2. 1997. 1,116p. text 199.00 (*0-683-30231-0*); Volume 3. 1998. 1,106p. text 199.00 (*0-683-30232-9*); Volume 4. 1998. 1022p. text 199.00 (*0-683-30233-7*); Volume 5. 1998. 7,200p. text 199.00 (*0-683-30234-5*) Lppncott W & W.

Walsh & Hoyt's Clinical Neuro-Ophthalmology: Infections & Inflammation of the Central Nervous System & Non-organic (Functional) Neuro-Opthalmologic Disease, Vol. 5, Pts. 1 & 2. Neil R. Miller. 4th ed. 1994. (Illus.). 2693p. 225.00 (*0-683-06024-4*) Lppncott W & W.

Walsh & Hoyt's Clinical Neuro-Ophthalmology Vol. 4: Vascular Disease, Vol. 4. Neil R. Miller. 4th ed. 1991. (Illus.). 947p. 170.00 (*0-683-06023-6*) Lppncott W & W.

Walter & Miller's Textbook of Radiotherapy: Radiation Physics, Therapy & Oncology. C. K. Bomford et al. 5th ed. 1993. LC 92-48182. 624p. pap. text (*0-443-02873-7*) Church.

Walter, Hamilton & Israel's Principles of Pathology for Dental Students. J. B. Walter & Margaret C. Grundy. 5th ed. 1992. (Dental Ser.). (Illus.). 496p. (Orig.). pap. text (*0-443-04124-5*) Church.

Waltham Book of Clinical Nutrition. Ed. by Josephien Wills & Kenny Simpson. 1993. LC 93-27493. 492p. 64.99 (*0-08-040839-7*) Elsevier.

Walther & Houston's Orthodontic Notes. Malcolm L. Jones & Richard G. Oliver. 6th ed. 2000. LC 00-25385. (Illus.). 252p. pap. text 31.00 (*0-7236-1065-7*) Buttrwrth-Heinemann.

Wanderjahr: The Education of a Surgeon. Edward D. Churchill. Ed. by J. Gordon Scannell. 1991. (Illus.). xi, 213p. 18.95 (*0-88135-067-2*) F A Countway.

War Against Children of Color: Psychiatry Targets Inner City Youth. Peter Breggin & Ginger R. Breggin. 1998. LC 97-13741. 400p. lib. bdg. 29.95 (*1-56751-127-9*) Common Courage.

War Against Children of Color: Psychiatry Targets Inner City Youth. Peter R. Breggin & Ginger Ross Breggin. 1999. LC 97-13741. 255p. pap. 18.95 (*1-56751-126-0*) Common Courage.

War & Children. Anna Freud & Dorothy T. Burlingham. Ed. by Philip R. Lehrman. 1973. LC 73-7699. 191p. reprint ed. lib. bdg. 41.50 (*0-8371-6942-9*, FRWC, Greenwood Pr) Greenwood.

War & Healing: Stanhope Bayne-Jones & the Maturing of American Medicine. Albert E. Cowdrey. Ed. by William J. Cooper, Jr. 1992. LC 91-32513. (Southern Biography Ser.). (Illus.). 264p. (C). text 45.00 (*0-8071-1717-X*) La State U Pr.

War Between Mentalism & Behaviorism: On the Accessibility of Mental Processes. William R. Uttal. 1999. LC 99-29247. (Scientific Psychology Ser.). 216p. 49.95 (*0-8058-3361-7*) L Erlbaum Assocs.

War Crimes in the Balkans: Medicine under Siege in the Former Yugoslavia 1991-1995. Physicians for Human Rights Staff. 1996. LC 96-67670. 100p. pap. text 10.00 (*1-879707-20-9*) Phy Human Rights.

War Dance. Eric G. Howe. 1971. LC 70-153642. (Studies in Philosophy: No. 40). reprint ed. lib. bdg. 75.00 (*0-8383-1243-8*) M S G Haskell Hse.

War Injuries of the Upper Extremity. Ed. by J. Engel & I. Kessler. 1979. (Progress in Surgery Ser.: Vol. 16). (Illus.). pap. 85.25 (*3-8055-2900-7*) S Karger.

War Is Good for Babies & Other Young Children. Deborah Dwork. 1987. 300p. (*0-422-60660-X*, 1200) Tavistock GBR. *Dist:* Routldge.

War, Medicine & Modernity. Roger Cooter. 2000. 256p. 81.00 (*0-7509-1801-2*) Sutton Publng.

War on Pain: How Breakthroughs in the New Field of Pain Medicine are Turning the Tide AgainstSuffering. Scott Fishman. 1999. LC 99-42965. 320p. 26.00 (*0-06-019297-6*) HarperCollins Pubs.

War on Pain: How Breakthroughs in the New Field of Pain Medicine are Turning the Tide AgainstSuffering. Scott Fishman. 2001. 320p. pap. 14.00 (*0-06-093078-0*, Quil) HarperTrade.

***War on Pain: How Breakthroughs in the New Field of Pain Medicine are Turning the Tide AgainstSuffering.** Scott Fishman & Lisa Berger. 2001. 301p. 26.00 (*0-7567-5134-9*) DIANE Pub.

War Syndromes of the Persian Gulf Battles: Index of New Information with References. John C. Bartone. 1997. 165p. 57.50 (*0-7883-1528-5*) ABBE Pubs Assn.

War Without a Front: The Memoirs of a French Army Nurse in Vietnam, 1950-1953. Elisabeth Sevier & Robert W. Sevier. 1999. (Illus.). 190p. pap. 14.95 (*0-9652703-1-9*) Wesley Pub Co.

Ward Attending: The Forty Day Month. Lucy M. Osborn & Neal A. Whitman. 1991. 194p. text 30.00 (*0-940193-09-4*) Univ UT Sch Med.

Ward Management & Teaching. Jean Barrett. 1989. 423p. (C). (*81-7002-032-8*) Himalayan Bks IND. *Dist:* St Mut.

Ward Management in Practice. Jennifer MacKenzie. 1998. LC 97-51523. (C). pap. text (*0-443-05702-8*) Church.

Ward Rounds for Medical Students: Clinical Medicine. G. Sandler. 1989. (Illus.). 288p. (Orig.). (C). (gr. 13). pap. text 38.00 (*0-412-30960-2*) Chapman & Hall.

Wards: An Introduction to Clinical Clerkships. Paul L. Fine. 1994. LC 94-11844. 216p. pap. text 25.95 (*0-316-28322-3*, Little Brwn Med Div) Lppncott W & W.

Ward's Anaesthetic Equipment. Andrew Davey & John T. Moyle. 4th ed. 1997. (Illus.). 399p. text (*0-7020-2169-5*) W B Saunders GBR. *Dist:* Saunders.

Ward's Natural Sign Language Thesaurus of Useful Signs 'n Synonyms. Jill Ward. Ed. by John Joyce. 1978. LC 77-93547. (Illus.). 49.00 (*0-917002-18-0*, 446) Joyce Media.

Warfarin. 1995. (Health & Safety Guides Ser.: No. 96). 24p. (C). pap. text 4.50 (*92-4-151096-X*, 1860096) Am Soc Clinical.

Warhafftige see Theriac

Warm Disease Theory. Garry Seifert. 2000. LC 00-10622. xi, 280p. 55.00 (*0-912111-61-5*) Paradigm Publns.

Warm Heart Surgery. Ed. by Tomas A. Salerno. 1995. 240p. (*0-340-61023-9*) E A GBR. *Dist:* OUP.

Warning: Inadequate Low-Income Subsidy Design Can Cause Problems for Health Care Reform. Robert Greenstein et al. 1994. 108p. (Orig.). pap. 12.00 (*1-57291-000-3*) Ctr on Budget.

Warren Cole, M. D., & the Ascent of Scientific Surgery. Dennis Connaughton. 1991. 272p. text 24.95 (*0-252-01884-2*) U of Ill Pr.

Warren Cole, M. D., & the Ascent of Scientific Surgery. Dennis Connaughton. 1991. (Illus.). 272p. 24.95 (*0-9628799-0-8*) W & C Cole Found.

Warrior Marks: Female Genital Mutilation & the Sexual Blinding of Women. Alice Walker & Pratibha Parmar. (Harvest Book Ser.). (Illus.). 1996. LC 95-25721. xxiii, 374p. pap. 15.00 (*0-15-600214-0*, Harvest Bks); 1993. LC 93-242654. 373p. 24.95 (*0-15-100061-1*) Harcourt.

Warriors & Wildmen: Men, Masculinity, & Gender. Stephen Wicks. 1996. LC 96-3623. 176p. 55.00 (*0-89789-454-5*, Bergin & Garvey) Greenwood.

Warrior's Journey Home: Healing Men, Healing the Planet. Jed Diamond. 1994. LC 93-86801. 268p. pap. 13.95 (*1-879237-60-1*) New Harbinger.

***Wartime Nurse.** Eric Taylor. 2001. (*0-7090-6777-1*) R Hale Ltd GBR. *Dist:* Trafalgar.

Warts. Michael P. Kinch. 2000. LC 98-53646. (My Heath Ser.). (Illus.). 48p. (J). (gr. 3-5). lib. bdg. 23.00 (*0-531-11625-5*) F Watts.

Warum Kennen Tiere Keinen Herzinfarkt: Aber Wir Menschen. Matthias Rath. 1997. 255p. pap. 19.80 (*0-9638768-4-8*) Health Now.

Was C. G. Jung a Mystic? And Other Essays. Aniell Jaffe. 1995. 214p. pap. 12.95 (*3-85630-508-4*) Continuum.

***Was It Something You Ate? Food Intolerance: What Causes It & How to Avoid It.** John Emsley & Peter Fell. 2002. 192p. pap. 13.95 (*0-19-850966-9*) OUP.

Was the AIDS Epidemic Unnecessary? How the Bureaucracy Has Spread the Disease. 1992. lib. bdg. 79.95 (*0-8490-5358-7*) Gordon Pr.

Washing Away of Wrongs: Forensic Medicine in Thirteenth-Century China. Sung Tz'u. Tr. by Brian E. McKnight from CHI. 1981. LC 81-6195. (Science, Medicine, & Technology in East Asia Ser.: No. 1). (Illus.). 181p. pap. text 25.00 (*0-89264-800-7*) Ctr Chinese Studies.

Washington Health Care Perspective, 1998. Ed. by Kathleen O'Leary Morgan & Scott E. Morgan. 1998. 20p. pap. 19.00 (*1-56692-846-X*) Morgan Quitno Corp.

Washington Heights-Inwood Neighborhood: Assessment of Health Care Needs. North Manhattan Health Action Group Report Staff & CCS Center for Health and Human Services Staff. 1984. 129p. (Orig.). pap. text 12.00 (*0-88156-054-5*) Comm Serv Soc NY.

Washington Heights-Inwood Neighborhoods: Assessment of Health Care Needs-Appendices. North Manhattan Health Action Group and CSS & Center for Health and Human Services. 1984. 175p. (Orig.). pap. text 15.00 (*0-88156-055-3*) Comm Serv Soc NY.

***Washington Manual Internship Survival Guide PDA.** Tammy L. Lin et al. 2001. pap. 29.95 (*0-7817-3487-8*) Lppncott W & W.

Washington Manual of Surgery. Gerard M. Doherty & Washington University Dept. of Surgery Staff. 2nd ed. 1999. LC 98-49850. (Illus.). xx, 698p. spiral bd. 39.95 (*0-7817-1640-3*) Lppncott W & W.

Wasser und Elektrolythaushalt: Physiologie und Pathophysiologie. H. Reissigl et al. 1984. (Handbuch der Infusionstherapie und Klinischen Ernaehrung Ser.: Band 1). viii, 160p. 68.75 (*3-8055-3745-X*) S Karger.

Waste Incineration & Public Health. National Research Council Staff et al. 2000. LC 00-9914. (Illus.). xvii, 335p. 49.95 (*0-309-06371-X*) Natl Acad Pr.

Waste Management for Health Care Facilities. Linda D. Lee. rev. ed. 1992. (Management & Compliance Ser.: Vol. 1). (Illus.). 300p. ring bd. 110.00 (*0-87258-585-9*, 055401) Am Hospital.

Wasted: A Memoir of Anorexia & Bulimia. Marya Hornbacher. 1997. LC 97-21375. 304p. 23.00 (*0-06-018739-5*, HarperFlamingo) HarperCollins Pubs.

Wasted Lives: A Study of Children in Mental Hospitals & Their Families. Lillian C. Kovar. 1979. LC 78-23248. text 29.95 (*0-89876-051-8*) Gardner Pr.

Wastewater Stabilization Ponds Principles of Planning & Practice. 1987. (WHO/EMRO Technical Publication Ser.: No. 10). pap. text 25.00 (*92-9021-001-X*) World Health.

Wasting Away: The Crisis of Malnutrition in India. Anthony R. Measham & Meera Chatterjee. 1999. LC 99-28089. (Directions in Development Ser.). 88p. pap. 22.00 (*0-8213-4435-8*, 14435) World Bank.

Watched Pot: How We Experience Time. Michael G. Flaherty. 1999. LC 98-25523. 190p. text 30.00 (*0-8147-2687-9*) NYU Pr.

Watching Bradley Grow: A Story about Premature Birth. Elizabeth Murphy-Melas. 1995. LC 95-62127. (Illus.). (J). (ps-3). pap. 8.95 (*1-56352-282-9*) Longstreet.

Water Analysis: A Practical Treastise on the Examination of Potable Water. J. Alfred Wanklyn & Ernest T. Chapman. Ed. by Barbara G. Rosenkrantz. 1977. LC 76-40651. (Public Health in America Ser.). (Illus.). reprint ed. lib. bdg. 19.95 (*0-405-09834-0*) Ayer.

Water & Electrolytes in Pediatrics. Laurence Finberg et al. 2nd ed. 1993. LC 92-24338. (Illus.). 288p. text 60.00 (*0-7216-3468-0*) Saunders.

Water & Sanitation in Islam: The Right Path to Health, Health Education Through Religion, 2. 1996. pap. text 9.00 (*92-9021-169-5*) World Health.

Water Balance in Schizophrenia. Ed. by David B. Schnur & Darrell G. Kirch. 1996. LC 95-46598. (Progress in Psychiatry Ser.: No. 48). 302p. text 39.50 (*0-88048-485-3*, 8485) Am Psychiatric.

Water Birth: A Midwife's Perspective. Susanna Napierala. 1994. LC 93-49703. (Illus.). 256p. pap. 19.95 (*0-89789-285-2*, Bergin & Garvey) Greenwood.

Water Borne Disease: Epidemiology & Ecology. Paul Hunter. 1997. LC 97-17109. 384p. 159.95 (*0-471-96646-0*) Wiley.

Water Contamination & Health Integration of Exposure Assessment, Toxicology, & Risk Assessment. Rhoda Wang. 1994. LC 93 48586. (Environmental Science & Pollution Ser.: Vol. 9). (Illus.). 544p. text 215.00 (*0-8247-8922-9*) Dekker.

Water, Electricity & Health: Protecting Yourself from Electrostress at Home & Work. Alan Hall. 1998. (Illus.). 192p. pap. (*1-869890-94-9*) Hawthorn Press GBR. *Dist:* Anthroposophic.

Water Fitness During Your Pregnancy. Jane Katz. 1994. LC 94-17659. 248p. pap. 17.95 (*0-87322-495-7*, PKAT0495) Human Kinetics.

Water Medicine. Harald W. Tietze. 2000. 106p. pap. 12.95 (*0-8464-5203-0*) Beekman Pubs.

Water Mite Genera & Subgenera. David Cook. 1974. (Memoir Ser.: No. 21). (Illus.). 860p. 75.00 (*1-56665-019-4*) Assoc Pubs FL.

Water of Life. John W. Armstrong. 1971. 136p. (C). pap. 19.95 (*0-8464-1060-5*) Beekman Pubs.

Water of Life. John W. Armstrong. 1980. (*0-85032-194-8*) C W Daniel GBR. *Dist:* Natl Bk Netwk.

Water Pollution Control in Developing Countries: Proceedings of the WHO Expert Committee, Geneva, 1972. WHO Staff. 1968. (Technical Reports: No. 404). pap. text 5.00 (*92-4-120404-4*, 1100404) World Health.

***Water Quality & Optical Properties of Swedish Lakes & Coastal Waters in Relation to Remote Sensing.** Niklas Strombeck. 2001. (Comprehensive Summaries of Uppsala Dissertations from the Faculty of Science & Technology Ser.: No. 633). (Illus.). 27p. (*91-554-5037-7*) Uppsala Universitet SWE. *Dist:* Coronet Bks.

Water Quality for Dialysis: Current Concepts in Hemodialyzer Reprocessing. AAMI Staff. 2nd ed. 1993. (Illus.). 59p. (Orig.). pap. 90.00 (*1-57020-003-3*, WQD-209) Assn Adv Med Instrn.

Water Rescue: Basic Skills for Emergency Responders. David Smith & Sara J. Smith. 1993. LC 93-30283. (Illus.). 368p. (C). (gr. 13). pap. text 26.95 (*0-8016-6343-1*, 06343) Mosby Inc.

Water-Soluble Vitamin Assays in Human Nutrition. Ball. 1994. (Illus.). 432p. 239.95 (*0-412-58370-4*) Chapman & Hall.

Water Virology: Water Science & Technology, Vol. 15, No. 5. Ed. by W. O. Grabow. 1983. (Illus.). 166p. pap. 44.00 (*0-08-030440-0*, Pergamon Pr) Elsevier.

***Waterbirth.** Dianne Garland. 2001. 165p. pap. text 24.99 (*0-7506-5202-0*) Buttrwrth-Heinemann.

Waterbirth Unplugged: International Perspectives on Waterbirth. Beech. 1997. 160p. pap. text 34.99 (*1-898507-53-8*) Buttrwrth-Heinemann.

Watsons Clinical Nursing. Walsh. 5th ed. 1997. pap. text (*0-7020-2025-7*) Bailliere Tindall.

Watsu: Freeing the Body in Water. Harold Dull. 2nd rev. ed. 1997. LC 93-77503. v, 160p. pap. 20.00 (*0-944202-11-X*) Harbin Springs.

Watts Hospital of Durham, North Carolina, 1895-1976: Keeping the Doors Open. P. Preston Reynolds. 1992. LC 91-77158. (Illus.). 133p. pap. 15.95 (*0-9631387-0-7*) Fund Adv Sci.

Wave Theory of Difference & Similarity. Ed. by S. W. Link. 1992. (Scientific Psychology Ser.). 384p. (C). text 79.95 (*0-8058-0926-0*) L Erlbaum Assocs.

Wave Therapy: Your Power to Heal. Samuel J. Winters. Ed. by Cynthia Snider. 1998. LC 97-97124. (Illus.). xvi, 220 p. pap. 20.00 (*0-9661900-0-9*) Winters KS.

Waves That Heal: The New Science of Radiobiology. 1991. (Alternative Energy & Medicine Ser.). lib. bdg. 69.95 (*0-8490-4311-5*) Gordon Pr.

Wax-Up for Functional Occlusion. Niklaus P. Lang et al. 1989. (Illus.). 28p. ring bd. 24.00 (*0-86715-217-6*) Quint Pub Co.

Way It Was: Sex, Surgery, Treasure, & Travel, 1907-1987. George Crile, Jr. 1992. LC 92-2971. (Illus.). 432p. 35.00 (*0-87338-465-2*) Kent St U Pr.

Way of Chinese Herbs. Michael Tierra. 1998. LC 98-15715. 496p. per. 17.00 (*0-671-89869-8*, Pocket Books) PB.

Way of Doctoring. Ainslie Meares. 1994. 180p. (Orig.). pap. (*0-85572-150-2*) Hill Content Pubng AUS. *Dist:* Seven Hills Bk.

Way of Hope: Michio Kushi's Anti-AIDS Program. Tom Monte. 1990. pap. 12.95 (*0-446-39174-3*) Warner Bks.

Way of Life. William Osler. 1937. text 11.95 (*0-06-141860-9*) Lppncott W & W.

Way of the Eagle. Jerry Fankhauser. 1987. 133p. (Orig.). pap. 10.00 (*0-9617006-4-5*) J Fankhauser.

Way of the Skeptical Nutrition. Weiner. 1981. 12.95 (*0-02-625620-7*) Macmillan.

Way of Thinking: A Primer on the Art of Being a Doctor. Eugene A. Stead, Jr. Ed. by Barton F. Haynes. 1995. LC 95-68700. (Illus.). 180p. pap. 24.95 (*0-89089-753-0*) Carolina Acad Pr.

***Way of Transition: Embracing Life's Most Difficult Moments.** William Bridges. 2001. 256p. pap. text 13.00 (*0-7382-0529-X*) Perseus Bks Grp.

Way to Health. Robert R. Leichtman & Carl Japikse. 1995. 128p. pap. 9.95 (*0-89804-805-2*, Enthea Pr) Ariel GA.

Way to Inner Freedom: A Practical Guide to Personal Development. Erik Blumenthal. 1998. LC 98-28982. 160p. reprint ed. pap. 12.95 (*1-56838-227-8*) Hazelden.

Way to Peace. 11.95 (*0-87418-037-6*) Coleman Pub.

Ways of Assessing Children & Curriculum: Stories of Early Childhood Practice, Vol. 37. Ed. by Celia Genishi. 1992. LC 92-13805. (Early Childhood Education Ser.). 232p. (C). text 17.95 (*0-8077-3186-2*) Tchrs Coll.

Ways of Knowing & Caring for Older Adults. Ed. by Mary Burke & Susan Sherman. 1993. LC 93-38938. 136p. pap. 32.95 (*0-88737-593-6*) Natl League Nurse.

Ways of Living: Self-Care Strategies for Special Needs. Ed. by Charles Christiansen. 1994. 600p. (C). text 65.00 (*1-56900-008-5*) Am Occup Therapy.

Ways of Living: Self-Care Strategies for Special Needs. Ed. by Charles H. Christiansen. 2nd ed. 2000. LC 00-267052. (Illus.). pap. (*1-56900-141-3*) Am Occup Therapy.

Ways of Studying Children: An Observation Manual for Early Childhood Teachers. Millie C. Almy & Celia Genishi. 2nd ed. 1979. LC 79-13881. 215p. pap. 17.95 (*0-8077-2551-X*) Tchrs Coll.

Ways to Better Breathing. Carola H. Speads. 1986. LC 85-90511. Orig. Title: Breathing the ABC's. (Illus.). 144p. reprint ed. pap. 8.95 (*0-9615659-1-8*) F Morrow.

Ways to Better Breathing. Carola H. Speads. 1992. Orig. Title: Breathing the ABC's. (Illus.). 144p. pap. 12.95 (*0-89281-397-0*, Heal Arts VT) Inner Tradit.

Ways Toward Wellness. Paul Terry et al. 1990. 96p. stu. ed. (*1-884153-04-6*) Prk Nicollet.

We Are Accountable. Leonard Edelestein. 1945. (C). pap. 4.00 (*0-87574-024-3*) Pendle Hill.

We Are All Water Babies. Jessica Johnson & Michel Odent. 1995. LC 95-6376. (Illus.). 128p. pap. 24.95 (*0-89087-758-0*) Celestial Arts.

We Are Not Alone: Learning to Live with Chronic Illness. Sefra Pitzele. 1985. LC 84-16378. (Illus.). 320p. pap. 14.95 (*0-918351-01-4*) Thompson Co Inc.

We Are Not Alone: Learning to Live with Chronic Illness. Sefra K. Pitzele. 1986. LC 86-40200. (Illus.). 336p. pap. 10.95 (*0-89480-139-2*, 1139) Workman Pub.

We Can Speak for Ourselves: Self-Advocacy by Mentally Handicapped People. Paul Williams & Bonnie Shoultz. 1988. 245p. (C). reprint ed. pap. text 10.00 (*0-253-36365-9*) Brookline Bks.

We Heard the Angels of Madness: A Family Guide to Coping with Manic Depression. Diane Berger. 1992. 312p. pap. 11.95 (*0-688-11615-9*, Quil) HarperTrade.

We Laughed, We Cried: Life with Fibromyalgia. Ed. by Kit Gardiser & Kathleen Kerry. 1995. (Illus.). 126p. (Orig.). pap. 12.00 (*0-9630002-1-7*) KMK Assocs.

We Need Doctors. Lola M. Schaefer. Ed. by Gail Saunders-Smith. 1999. LC 99-19423. (Helpers in Our Community Ser.). (Illus.). 24p. (J). (gr. k-1). lib. bdg. 14.60 (*0-7368-0389-0*, Pebble Bks) Capstone Pr.

We Need Each Other. Keith Hunt & Gladys Hunt. 1985. (Orig.). mass mkt. 9.99 (*0-310-26401-4*, 9965P) Zondervan.

We Never Said Goodbye: The Tragedy of Alzheimer's Disease. Isobelle Gidley & Richard Shears. 1985. 191p. 14.95 (*0-86861-551-X*) Routledge.

We Offer Ourselves As Evidence: Toward Workers' Control of Occupational Health, 19. Bennett M. Judkins. 1986. LC 85-24775. (Contributions in Labor Studies Ser.: No. 61). 261p. 68.00 (*0-313-24898-2*, JWO/, Greenwood Pr) Greenwood.

We, the Divided Self. John G. Watkins & Rhonda J. Johnson. 1982. 140p. pap. 12.00 (*0-8290-1412-8*); text 18.95 (*0-8290-1011-4*) Irvington.

We Want to Live, Set. Aajonus Vonderplanitz. 1997. LC 96-34036. 310p. 29.95 (*1-889356-77-8*, 41747) Carnelian Bay.

Wealth of Indian Alchemy & Its Medicinal Uses, Set. Rasajalanidhi. Ed. & Intro. by B. C. Mukherji. 1998. LC 98-907257. (*81-7030-582-9*) Sri Satguru Pubns IND. *Dist:* S Asia.

Weaning & Human Development. Gordon R. Forrer. 1969. LC 72-79731. 12.95 (*0-87212-020-1*) Libra.

Weaning Ways: A Mothers' Collection of Nursing & Weaning Experiences. Siena Klein-Owen. 1989. LC 89-91701. 100p. pap. 11.00 (*0-9624133-0-5*) Shared Experiences.

Weapons of Mass Destruction: Emergency Care. Robert A. De Lorenzo & Robert S. Porter. 1999. 176p. pap. 25.00 (*0-13-013923-8*) P-H.

Weapons of Our Warfare: Help for Troubled Minds. James A. Laine. 1987. (Illus.). 144p. pap. 3.95 (*0-936369-06-X*) Son-Rise Pubns.

Weapons under Fire. Lauren Holland. 1997. LC 97-21805. (Social-Psychology Reference Ser.). 335p. text 55.00 (*0-8153-2067-1*) Garland.

Wear & Tear: or Hints for the Overworked. Silas W. Mitchell. 5th ed. 1973. LC 73-2407. (Mental Illness & Social Policy; the American Experience Ser.). reprint ed. 17.95 (*0-405-05217-0*) Ayer.

Weariness, the Fever & the Fret: The Campaign Against Tuberculosis in Canada, 1900-1950. Katherine McCuaig. 1999. LC 00-341131. (Hannah Institute Studies in the History of Medicine, Health & Society: Vol. 8). (Illus.). xx, 384p. (*0-7735-1833-9*); pap. (*0-7735-1875-4*) McG-Queens Univ Pr.

Weary Sons of Freud. Catherine Clement. Tr. by Nicole Ball. 1987. 115p. (C). pap. 17.00 (*0-86091-888-2*, A0639) Verso.

Weather Matrix & Human Behavior. Michael A. Persinger. 1980. LC 80-18422. 327p. 68.50 (*0-275-90536-5*, C0536, Praeger Pubs) Greenwood.

***Weathering the Storms: Psychotherapy for Psychosis.** Murray Jackson. 2001. 360p. pap. (*1-85575-267-0*) Karnac Bks GBR. *Dist:* Other Pr LLC.

Weaving Woman: Musings & Meditations on the Feminine Mythos. Barbara Black Koltuv. rev. ed. 1995. LC 90-6736. (Illus.). 143p. pap. 9.95 (*0-89254-019-2*) Nicolas-Hays.

Web Design for Health Professionals. R. Pat Little. 1999. (Informatics Ser.: No. 2). (Illus.). pap. 15.00 (*1-893549-12-7*) Biomed Genl.

Web Doctor: Finding the Best Health Care Online. Richard M. Sharp & Vicki F. Sharp. 1998. LC 98-8657. 528p. pap. 29.95 (*0-312-19536-2*) St Martin.

Web of Inclusion: Faculty Helping Faculty. Ed. by Patricia Bayles & Jodi Parks-Doyle. 1995. 153p. pap. 31.95 (*0-88737-642-8*) Natl League Nurse.

Web Sites for Health Professionals. Mark J. Kittleson. 1997. LC 97-179628. (Health Science Ser.). (Illus.). 112p. (C). pap. text 21.95 (*0-7637-0511-X*, 0511-X) Jones & Bartlett.

Web That Has No Weaver: Understanding Chinese Medicine. Ted J. Kaptchuk. exp. rev. ed. 2000. LC 98-53193. (Illus.). xxvi, 500p. pap. 18.95 (*0-8092-2840-8*, 284080, Contemporary) McGraw-Hill Trade.

WebDoctor: Your Online Guide to Health Care & Wellness. Richard W. Sharp & Vicki F. Sharp. 1998. LC 98-12062. (Illus.). xiv, 557 p. pap. 28.00 incl. cd-rom (*1-57626-052-6*, QMP) Quality Med Pub.

Webster's American Sign Language Medical Dictionary. Elaine Costello. 2000. LC 00-59172. (Illus.). 384p. pap. 24.95 (*0-375-70927-4*) Random Ref & Info.

Webster's New Explorer Medical Dictionary. Merriam-Webster, Inc. Staff. 1999. LC 99-62652. (Webster's New Explorer Ser.). Orig. Title: Merriam Webster's Medical Dictionary. 27p. 8.98 (*1-892859-07-6*) Federal St Pr.

Wechselbeziehungen zwischen Psychiatrie, Psychologie und Philosophie, Vol. 2. Gerhard Bengesser. 1982. (European University Studies: Ser. 6, Vol. 94). (GER.). 178p. 26.00 (*3-261-05019-5*) P Lang Pubng.

Wednesday's Child Is Full of Woe: Research into Women's Experience of Neglect & Abuse in Childhood & Adult Depression. Antonia Bifulco & Patricia Moran. 1998. LC 97-26564. 224p. (C). 84.95 (*0-415-16526-1*); pap. 26.95 (*0-415-16527-X*) Routledge.

Weeds Used in Medicine. Alice Henkel. 1996. 45p. reprint ed. spiral bd. 8.00 (*0-7873-0406-9*) Hlth Research.

Week by Week: Plans for Observing & Recording Young Children. Barbara Nilsen. 1997. LC 96-12008. (Early Childhood Education Ser.). 416p. (C). pap. text 59.95 (*0-8273-7646-4*) Delmar.

Week by Week to a Strong Heart. Marvin Moser & Brenda L. Becker. 1994. 336p. mass mkt. 5.50 (*0-380-72089-2*, Avon Bks) Morrow Avon.

Weigh of Life. Beverly Slay. 1993. (Illus.). pap. 14.95 (*0-9639799-0-6*) Weigh of Life.

Weigh Out: A Medically Supervised Weight Loss Program Used for Twenty Years by a Group of California Physicians. Sandra Stoddard & Wendy Keown. 2nd ed. 1993. 200p. (Orig.). pap. 14.95 (*0-9637877-0-5*) Phys Weight.

Weighing the Options: Criteria for Evaluating Weight-Management Programs. Institute of Medicine Staff. Ed. by Paul R. Thomas. 1995. LC 94-44625. (Illus.). 296p. (Orig.). (C). pap. 24.95 (*0-309-05131-2*) Natl Acad Pr.

Weight Control, Stress & Amino Acid Therapy. 1996. lib. bdg. 251.95 (*0-8490-5895-3*) Gordon Pr.

Weight Loss & Fitness Facts: Diet - Exercise - Disease Prevention Cindy Bracken. 1994. (Illus.). 36p. (Orig.). pap. 480.00 incl. VHS (*0-9638588-0-7*) Weight Loss.

***Weight Loss for Life.** Francesca Corso. 2001. LC 00-111974. 400p. 32.95 (*1-56167-657-8*) Am Literary Pr.

Weight Loss Made Easy: Hundreds of Tips for a Weight Loss Life-Style. Cecelia Phillips. 1993. LC 88-91234. 150p. (Orig.). (*0-9618870-3-6*); pap. 14.95 (*0-9618870-2-8*) L C Ellsworth.

Weight Loss to Super Wellness. Ted L. Edwards, Jr. & Barbara Lau. 1982. (Illus.). 176p. (Orig.). pap. text 12.95 (*0-938934-07-4*) Hills Med.

Weight Loss Workbook: The Essential Companion for Any Weight Loss Program. June Rodriguez. 1998. 144p. spiral bd. 14.00 (*1-56836-201-3*) Kodansha.

Weight Management & Eating Disorders: HP 625. Rita Jones. 1993. 226p. (C). stu. ed., spiral bd. (*0-933915-48-9*) CA College Health Sci.

Weight Management for Type II Diabetes: An Action Plan. Jackie Labat. 1997. 224p. (Orig.). pap. 15.95 (*0-471-34750-7*) Wiley.

Weight Management for Type II Diabetes: An Action Plan. Jackie Labat & Annette Maggi. 1997. LC 98-231263. 224p. (Orig.). pap. 12.95 (*1-56561-114-4*) Wiley.

Weight Management the Fitness Way. Dorothy E. Dusek. 1989. (Illus.). 336p. (C). pap. text 39.95 (*0-86720-416-8*, 416-8) Jones & Bartlett.

Weight No More: A Weight-Loss Program That Can Work. Anne E. Hunt. Ed. by Eric A. Mein. 1990. (Natural Remedies for Common Ailments & Conditions Ser.). 76p. (Orig.). pap. 4.95 (*0-87604-260-4*, 351) ARE Pr.

***Weill-Cornell Illustrated Encyclopedia of Health.** Cornell University Staff. 2001. (Illus.). 1280p. 45.00 (*0-7370-1630-2*) T-L Custom Pub.

***Weir's Guide to Medical Museums.** Sue Weir. 1996. 241p. pap. (*1-85315-304-4*) Royal Soc of Medicine Pr Ltd GBR. *Dist:* Balogh.

Weir's Handbook of Experimental Immunology, Vol. 1. Donald M. Weir. 5th ed. 1996. LC 96-35330. 195.00 (*0-86542-569-8*) Blackwell Sci.

Weir's Handbook of Experimental Immunology, Vol. 1-4. Lenore Herzenberg et al. 5th ed. 1996. (Illus.). 2752p. text 595.00 (*0-86542-421-7*) Blackwell Sci.

Weir's Handbook of Experimental Immunology. Donald M. Weir. 5th ed. 1996. LC 96-35330. Vol. 2. 125.00 (*0-86542-570-1*); Vol. 4. 250.00 (*0-86542-572-8*) Blackwell Sci.

Welcome Baby: A Guide to the First Six Weeks. George E. Verrilli & Anne M. Mueser. 1981. LC 81-16696. (Illus.). 96p. pap. 6.95 (*0-312-86121-4*) St Martin.

Welcome Back to Nursing. Wendy Green. 1993. LC 92-49296. 144p. pap. 19.95 (*0-632-03556-0*) Blackwell Sci.

Welcome for Every Child: How France Protects Maternal & Child Health - A New Frame of Reference for the United States. Gail Richardson. 1994. LC 94-74638. 62p. (Orig.). pap. text 10.00 (*1-57285-011-6*) Nat Ctr Educ.

Welcome, Silence: My Triumph over Schizophrenia. Carol S. North. 1989. 240p. reprint ed. mass mkt. 4.99 (*0-380-70627-X*, Avon Bks) Morrow Avon.

Welcome to My World: Psychology 101. Nield. 1998. 116p. (C). pap. text 23.60 (*0-536-01174-5*) Pearson Custom.

Welcome to the Board! An Orientation for the New Health Care Trustee. Health Research and Educational Trust of New Jersey Staff. 1999. LC 98-52682. 153p. pap. 75.00 (*1-55648-249-3*) AHPI.

Welding Health & Safety Resource Manual. American Industrial Hygiene Association Staff. 1984. 40p. 22.00 (*0-932627-17-X*) Am Indus Hygiene.

Welfare, Choice & Solidarity in Transition: Reforming the Health Section in Eastern Europe. Janos Kornai & Karen Eggleston. 2001. LC 00-45500. (Federico Caffe Lectures). (Illus.). 380p. text 59.95 (*0-521-79036-0*) Cambridge U Pr.

Welfare Medical Care: An Experiment. Charles H. Goodrich et al. 1970. LC 77-85075. (Illus.). 361p. 34.50 (*0-674-94895-5*) HUP.

Welfare of Pigs: Current Topics in Veterinary Medicine & Animal Science, No. 11. Ed. by Watse Sybesma. 1981. x, 334p. text 184.00 (*90-247-2521-6*) Kluwer Academic.

Well Adjusted Cat: Feline Chiropractic Methods You Can Do. Daniel R. Kamen. 1997. (Illus.). 166p. pap. 13.95 (*1-57129-044-3*) Brookline Bks.

Well Adjusted Horse: Equine Chiropractic Methods You Can Do. Daniel Kamen. 1999. pap. 14.95 (*1-57129-063-X*, Lumen Eds) Brookline Bks.

W
X
Y
Z

Well & Good: Case Studies in Biomedical Ethics. John E. Thomas & Wilfrid J. Waluchow. 2nd rev. ed. 1990. 240p. pap. text (*0-921149-64-6*) Broadview.

Well Baby Book: A Comprehensive Manual of Baby Care, from Conception to Age Four. Mike Samuels & Nancy H. Samuels. enl. rev. ed. 1991. LC 90-26702. (Illus.). 464p. pap. 19.95 (*0-671-73412-1*) Summit Bks.

***Well-Being for All Beyond Generations: A Reproductive Health Review of the Middle East & North Africa Region.** Atsuko Aoyama. 2001. LC 2001-17740. (Health, Nutrition, & Population Ser.). (Illus.). 170p. 22.00 (*0-8213-4920-1*) Wrld Bank.

Well-Being for Women: A Confident Approach to Living a Joyful, Healthy & Productive Life. Stella Weller. 2000. (Illus.). 128p. pap. 14.95 (*0-8069-9330-8*, HEA024000) Sterling.

Well-Being of Video Display Terminal Users: An Exploratory Study. Steven L. Sauter et al. 1999. (Illus.). 245p. (C). reprint ed. pap. text 35.00 (*0-7881-7618-8*) DIANE Pub.

Well Cat Book: The Classic Comprehensive Handbook of Cat Care. Terri McGinnis. 1996. LC 95-25789. (Illus.). 336p. pap. 16.95 (*0-679-77000-3*) Random.

***Well Woman.** Vashti M. McKenzie. 2002. 224p. 22.00 (*0-670-88484-7*) Viking Penguin.

Well Woman. Miriam Stoppard. 1998. LC 97-43771. (DK Healthcare Ser.). (Illus.). 96p. pap. 7.95 (*0-7894-3091-6*) DK Pub Inc.

Well Women: Healing the Female Body Through Traditional Chinese Medicine. Marie E. Cargill. 1998. LC 97-16135. 144p. pap. 13.50 (*0-89789-543-6*, Bergin & Garvey) Greenwood.

Wellbeing of the Elderly: Approaches to Multidimensional Assessment. G. Fillenbaum. 1984. (WHO Offset Publications: No. 84). 99p. 11.00 (*92-4-170084-X*) World Health.

Wellness: AIDS, STD & Other Communicable Diseases. James Jackson. 1991. 184p. (C). text 13.50 (*0-87967-868-2*, Dshkn McG-Hill) McGrw-H Hghr Educ.

Wellness: Choices for Health & Fitness. Rebecca J. Donatelle. 1995. (Health Sciences Ser.). mass mkt. 28.00 (*0-534-33951-4*) Brooks-Cole.

Wellness: Choices for Health & Fitness. Rebecca J. Donatelle et al. 2nd ed. 1998. LC 98-26394. (Health Sciences Ser.). 496p. pap. text 43.95 (*0-534-34836-X*) Brooks-Cole.

Wellness: Creating a Life of Health & Fitness. Jerrold S. Greenberg et al. 1997. (C). pap., tchr. ed. (*0-205-26631-2*, T6631-0) Allyn.

***Wellness: Fundamental Concepts & Applications with HealthQuest 2.0.** David J. Anspaugh et al. 2000. (C). 22.50 (*0-07-242717-5*) McGrw-H Hghr Educ.

Wellness: Major Chronic Diseases. Paula F. Ciesielski. 1991. 176p. (C). pap. 20.00 (*0-87967-873-9*, Dshkn McG-Hill) McGrw-H Hghr Educ.

Wellness: Pregnancy, Childbirth & Parenting. Robert Kime. 1991. 160p. (C). text 13.50 (*0-87967-876-3*, Dshkn McG-Hill) McGrw-H Hghr Educ.

Wellness: Safety & Accident Prevention. David C. Lawson. 1991. 160p. (C). pap. 20.00 (*0-87967-864-X*, Dshkn McG-Hill) McGrw-H Hghr Educ.

Wellness: Stress Management. Randall Cottrell. 1991. 160p. (C). text 13.50 (*0-87967-872-0*, Dshkn McG-Hill) McGrw-H Hghr Educ.

Wellness: The Informed Health Consumer. Robert E. Kime. 1991. 160p. (C). pap. 20.00 (*0-87967-865-8*, Dshkn McG-Hill) McGrw-H Hghr Educ.

Wellness: Tobacco & Health. Richard G. Schlaadt. 1991. 160p. (C). pap. 20.00 (*0-87967-877-1*, WCB McGr Hill) McGrw-H Hghr Educ.

Wellness: Weight Control. Randall Cottrell. 1991. 176p. (C). text 13.50 (*0-87967-878-X*, Dshkn McG-Hill) McGrw-H Hghr Educ.

Wellness Against All Odds. Sherry A. Rogers. 1994. LC 94-65045. 384p. pap. 17.95 (*0-9618821-5-8*) SandKey.

Wellness & Lifestyle Renewal: A Manual for Personal Change. Mark S. Rosenfeld. 1993. (Orig.). pap. text 28.00 (*0-910317-92-5*) Am Occup Therapy.

Wellness & Prevention Sourcebook: New Approaches to Achieving Healthier Populations. Faulkner and Gray Inc. Staff. 1997. LC 98-142464. xii, 498 p. (*1-57987-016-3*) Faulkner & Gray.

Wellness Book. John R. Price. 1998. LC 97-47697. 112p. pap. 7.00 (*1-56170-500-4*, 864) Hay House.

Wellness Book: The Comprehensive Guide to Maintaining Health & Treating Stress-Related Illness. New England Deaconess Hospital and Harvard Medical S et al. 1993. LC 92-39899. (Illus.). 512p. per. 16.00 (*0-671-79750-6*) S&S Trade.

Wellness Book of I. B. S. How to Achieve Relief from Irritable Bowel Syndrome & Live a Symptom-Free Life. Deralee Scanlon & Barbara C. Becnel. 1991. 192p. pap. 11.95 (*0-312-85226-6*) St Martin.

Wellness Community Guide to Fighting for Recovery from Cancer. Harold H. Benjamin. exp. rev. ed. 1995. LC 95-11417. Orig. Title: From Victim to Victor. 256p. 15.95 (*0-87477-794-1*, Tarcher Putnam) Putnam Pub Group.

Wellness Concepts & Applications. David J. Anspaugh. 3rd ed. 1996. 403.75 (*0-8151-0973-3*) Mosby Inc.

Wellness Encyclopedia of Food & Nutrition: How to Buy, Store & Prepare Every Fresh Food. Univ. of California at Berkeley Wellness Letter Ed & Sheldon Margen. 1992. LC 92-13017. (Illus.). 512p. 29.95 (*0-929661-03-6*) Random.

Wellness for Helping Professionals: Creating Compassionate Cultures. John W. Travis & Meryn G. Callander. 1990. (Illus.). 416p. pap. 31.00 (*0-9625882-1-0*) Wellness Assocs.

***Wellness in Menopause: A Guide to Holistic Healing.** Marylyn Meek. 2001. 228p. pap. (*1-85860-064-2*) Hushion Hse.

Wellness in the Workplace: How to Plan, Implement & Evaluate a Wellness Program. Merlene T. Sherman. Ed. by Anne Knight. 1990. LC 89-81245. (Fifty-Minute Ser.). 93p. (Orig.). pap. 12.95 (*1-56052-020-5*) Crisp Pubns.

Wellness Inventory. John W. Travis. 3rd ed. 1988. (Illus.). 12p. pap. 2.95 (*0-9625882-0-2*) Wellness Assocs.

Wellness Lowfat Cookbook: Hundreds of Delicious Recipes & a Revolutionary New Eating Plan That Can Help Prevent Heart Disease. Ed. by Wellness Cooking School Staff. 1994. (Illus.). 256p. 24.95 (*0-929661-11-7*) Random.

Wellness Medicine. Robert A. Anderson. 1987. LC 87-70316. (Illus.). 520p. lib. bdg. 34.95 (*0-942767-00-4*) Amer Health Pr.

Wellness Nursing Diagnosis for Health Promotion. Karen M. Stolte. 1995. LC 95-38990. 336p. spiral bd. 25.95 (*0-397-55082-0*) Lppncott W & W.

Wellness Nutrition Counter: The Essential Guide to Complete Nutritional Information on over 6,000 Foods & Products. Sheldon Margen. 1998. LC 97-17959. 34.95 (*0-929661-38-9*) Rebus.

Wellness Practitioner: Concepts, Research, & Strategies. Carolyn C. Clark. 2nd exp. rev. ed. 1996. LC 95-47784. (Illus.). 368p. 46.95 (*0-8261-5151-5*) Springer Pub.

Wellness Program Management Yearbook. Beth-Ann Kerber. 1999. 292p. spiral bd. 195.00 (*1-882364-39-2*, Amer Busn Pub) Hlth Res Pub.

***Wellness Program Management Yearbook.** Jennifer L. Defalco. 2nd ed. 2001. 280p. pap. 159.00 (*1-882364-59-7*, Amer Busn Pub) Hlth Res Pub.

Wellness Testwell Conn For Hea. Robbins Mullen. 1996. 22.00 net. (*0-697-35774-0*, WCB McGr Hill) McGrw-H Hghr Educ.

Wellness vs. Neurotic Styles: Holistic or Monomanic Use of the Four Functions. Terence Duniho. 1991. pap. 5.95 (*1-878287-31-1*) Type & Temperament.

Wellness Way of Life. Gwen Robbins. 2nd ed. 1993. tchr. ed. 45.93 (*0-697-12660-9*) McGraw.

Wellness Way of Life. Gwen Robbins et al. 2nd ed. 1993. 496p. (C). (gr. 10-12). text 19.00 net. (*0-697-12659-5*) Brown & Benchmark.

Wellness Way of Life. Gwen Robbins. 4th ed. 1998. LC 98-5963. pap. text 15.50 (*0-697-29578-8*) McGraw.

Wellness Way of Life: With Healthquest CD-ROM. Gwen Robbins et al. 4th ed. 2000. (C). 27.50 incl. cd-rom (*0-07-242319-6*) McGrw-H Hghr Educ.

Wellness Workbook. John W. Travis & Regina S. Ryan. 2nd rev. ed. 1988. LC 86-6052. (Illus.). 568p. pap. 19.95 (*0-89815-179-1*) Ten Speed Pr.

Wells' Supportive Therapies in Health Care. Ed. by Richard Wells & Verena Tschudin. 1994. (Illus.). 299p. pap. text (*0-7020-1591-1*) W B Saunders GBR. *Dist:* Saunders.

Weltenwuerfe: Ludwig Binswangers Phaenomenologische Psychologie. Max Herzog. 1994. (Phaenomenologisch-Psychologische Forschungen Ser.: No. 17). (GER.). xxxii, 315p. (C). lib. bdg. 129.25 (*3-11-014213-9*) De Gruyter.

Werbach's Nutritional Influences on Illness. Melvyn R. Werbach. 1998. cd-rom 99.00 (*1-891710-01-X*) Third Line Pr.

We're All in This Together: Families Facing Breast Cancer. Irene Virag. 1995. (Illus.). 96p. pap. 14.95 (*0-8362-7050-9*) Andrews McMeel.

Werner & Ingbar's the Thyroid: A Fundamental & Clinical Text. Lewis E. Braverman & Robert D. Utiger. 8th ed. 2000. 1,104p. text 235.00 (*0-7817-2193-8*) Lppncott W & W.

West from Singapore. Louis L'Amour. 1987. 176p. mass mkt. 4.50 (*0-553-26353-6*) Bantam.

***West Nile Virus: A Reemerging Global Pathogen.** Peter Drotman. 2001. (Illus.). 155p. (C). pap. text 35.00 (*0-7567-1602-0*) DIANE Pub.

***West Nile Virus: Detection, Surveillance, & Control.** Ed. by Dennis J. White & Dale L. Morse. 2001. LC 2001-51398. (Annals of the New York Academy of Sciences Ser.: Vol. 951). 400p. 145.00 (*1-57331-374-2*) NY Acad Sci.

***West Nile Virus Outbreak: Lessons for Public Health Preparedness.** Janet Heinrich. 2001. (Illus.). 68p. (C). pap. text 25.00 (*0-7567-0901-6*) DIANE Pub.

West Virginia Health - Administrative Code Annotated. Ed. by C. Page Hamrick, III. 1985. 550p. ring bd. 295.00 (*0-937683-03-5*) WV Busn Pub.

West Virginia Health Care in Perspective 2000. Ed. by Kathleen O'Leary Morgan & Scott E. Morgan. 2000. 21p. spiral bd. 19.00 (*0-7401-0247-8*) Morgan Quitno Corp.

West Virginia Health Care Perspective, 1998. Ed. by Kathleen O'Leary Morgan & Scott E. Morgan. 1998. 20p. pap. 19.00 (*1-56692-847-8*) Morgan Quitno Corp.

Western Astrology & Chinese Medicine. Jonathan C. Willmott. 1985. 192p. reprint ed. pap. 9.95 (*0-89281-109-9*) Inner Tradit.

Western Attitudes Toward Death: From the Middle Ages to the Present. Philippe Aries. Tr. by Patricia M. Ranum from FRE. 1975. LC 73-19340. (Symposia in Comparative History Ser.). (Illus.). 122p. pap. text 15.95 (*0-8018-1762-5*) Johns Hopkins.

Western Diseases: Their Emergence & Prevention. Ed. by H. C. Trowell & Denis P. Burkitt. 1981. LC 80-28917. (Illus.). 474p. (C). 65.00 (*0-674-95020-8*) HUP.

Western Medical Pioneers in Feudal Japan. John Z. Bowers. 1970. LC 73-86098. (Josiah Macy Foundation Ser.). 256p. 45.00 (*0-8018-1081-7*) Johns Hopkins.

Western Medical Thought from Antiquity to the Middle Ages. Ed. by Mirko D. Grmek. Tr. by Antony Shugaar. 1999. LC 98-8462. (Illus.). 544p. text 52.00 (*0-674-40355-X*) HUP.

Western Medical Tradition: 800 B. C.-1800 A. D. Lawrence Conrad et al. 1995. (Illus.). 570p. (C). text 110.00 (*0-521-38135-5*); pap. text 39.95 (*0-521-47564-3*) Cambridge U Pr.

***Western Medicine: An Illustrated History.** Ed. by Irvine Loudon. 2001. (Illus.). 368p. pap. 27.50 (*0-19-924813-3*) OUP.

Western Medicine: An Illustrated History. Ed. by Irvine Loudon. 1997. LC 97-218848. (Illus.). 364p. (C). 49.95 (*0-19-820509-0*) OUP.

Western Rajputana States: A Medico-Topographical & General Account of Marwar, Sirohi, Jaisalmir. 1990. (C). reprint ed. (*81-85326-36-3*) Vintage IND. *Dist:* S Asia.

Westmead Pocket Anaesthetic Manual. Anthony P. Padley. 2000. (Illus.). 304p. 39.95 (*0-07-470861-9*) McGraw-Hill Educ Grp.

Wet Mind: The New Cognitive Neuroscience. Stephen M.Kosslyn et al. 1995. LC 96-149263. (Illus.). 624p. pap. 19.95 (*0-02-874085-8*) Free Pr.

Whaley & Wong's Essentials of Pediatric Nursing. Angela C. Murphy. 5th ed. 1996. 328p. (C). (gr. 13). pap. text, stu. ed. 19.95 (*0-8151-7470-5*, 28277) Mosby Inc.

Whaley & Wong's Essentials of Pediatric Nursing. Donna L. Wong. 5th ed. 1997. (Illus.). suppl. ed. (*0-8151-2522-4*); suppl. ed. (*0-8151-2523-2*) Mosby Inc.

Whaley & Wong's Essentials of Pediatric Nursing. Donna L. Wong. 5th ed. 1997. (Illus.). 1312p. (*84-8086-141-X*) Mosby-Doyma Libros ESP. *Dist:* Mosby Inc.

Whaley & Wong's Essentials of Pediatric Nursing: Includes Testbank. Donna L. Wong. 5th ed. 1997. (Illus.). tchr. ed. (*0-8151-2845-2*) Mosby Inc.

Whaley & Wong's Essentials of Pediatric Nursing: Text/Clinical Manual Package. Donna L. Wong. 5th ed. 1997. (Illus.). (*0-323-00530-6*) Mosby Inc.

Whaley & Wong's Nursing Care of Infants & Children. Donna L. Wong et al. 6th ed. 1998. 352p. (C). text, stu. ed. (*0-323-00104-1*); LC 98-41415. (Illus.). xxxvii, 2119p. (C). text 69.00 (*0-323-00150-5*);Includes Testbank. (Illus.). tchr. ed. (*0-323-00468-7*) Mosby Inc.

Whaley & Wong's Nursing Care of Infants & Children: With Dynamic Human CD-ROM for Windows. Wong Engineering Animation, Inc. Staff. 1996. (C). (gr. 13). text 81.00 incl. cd-rom (*0-8151-4627-2*, 30503) Mosby Inc.

Wharton's Cardio-Fitness Book: The Step-by-Step Program for High Energy & Endurance. Jim Wharton et al. 2001. LC 00-37725. (Illus.). 288p. pap. 16.00 (*0-8129-3161-0*) Crown Pub Group.

What a Blessing She Had Chloroform: The Medical & Social Response to the Pain of Childbirth from 1800 to the Present. Donald Caton. 1999. LC 98-36869. (Illus.). xvi, 288p. 35.00 (*0-300-07597-9*) Yale U Pr.

What a Woman Should Know about Protease Inhibitors. Leslie R. Wolfe et al. 1998. 20p. pap. 5.00 (*1-877966-55-X*) Ctr Women Policy.

What about Immunizations: Exposing the Vaccine Philosophy. Cynthia Cournoyer. 1995. 200p. (Orig.). pap. 12.95 (*0-9612188-5-1*) Nelsons Bks.

What about Me? Growing Up with a Developmentally Disabled Sibling. B. Siegel & S. C. Silverstein. 1994. LC 94-99. (Illus.). 316p. (C). 24.95 (*0-306-44650-2*) Da Capo.

What Am I Allergic To? J. J. Van Gasse. 1995. LC 95-71337. 124p. (C). 9.95 (*1-882792-17-3*) Proctor Pubns.

What an Abnormal Pap Smear Means. Margaret Wilson. 1995. (Living for Tomorrow Ser.). 137p. (Orig.). pap. (*0-85572-243-6*) Hill Content Pubng AUS. *Dist:* Seven Hills Bk.

***What Are You Feeling Doctor? Identifying & Avoiding Defensive Patterns in the Consultation.** John Salinsky & Paul Sackin. 2000. 192p. pap. (*1-85775-407-7*) Radcliffe Med Pr GBR. *Dist:* Balogh.

What Can I Do? - My Husband Has Prostate Cancer. Bev Farmer. 1995. LC 95-94781. 100p. pap. 9.95 (*0-9647936-0-1*) Pathfinder WA.

What Can I Give You? Mary Mahony. Ed. by Susan Pasternack. 1997. LC 97-91901. (Illus.). 180p. (Orig.). per. 12.95 (*0-9658879-0-1*) Redding Pr.

What Causes Men's Violence Against Women? Michele Harway & James M. O'Neil. 1999. LC 99-6400. 296p. 76.95 (*0-7619-0618-5*, 81039) Sage.

What Children Can Tell Us: Eliciting, Interpreting & Evaluating Critical Information from Children. Erikson Institute Faculty et al. 1992. LC 92-1771. (Social & Behavioral Science Ser.). 408p. reprint ed. pap. 23.00 (*1-55542-465-1*, C546-E2F) Jossey-Bass.

What Color Are You? The Way to Health Through Color. Annie Wilson & Lilla Bek. 1989. (Illus.). 160p. (Orig.). pap. (*0-85030-616-7*) Aqrn Pr GBR. *Dist:* HarperCollins Pubs.

What Constitutes the Patient in Psychotherapy? Alternative Approaches to Understanding Humans. Richard D. Chessick. 1993. LC 91-41341. 248p. 45.00 (*0-87668-549-1*) Aronson.

What Do I Do? How to Care for, Comfort, & Commune with Your Nursing Home. Katherine L. Karr. 1985. LC 85-7649. (Activities, Adaptation & Aging Ser.: Vol. 7, No. 1). (Illus.). 130p. text 19.95 (*0-86656-398-9*) Haworth Pr.

What Do I Do? Who Do I Call? Resources for Health Care Professionals Seeking Information Related to the Legal Profession. Barbara E. Calfee & David A. Calfee. 1995. 115p. (Orig.). pap. text 10.00 (*0-9633540-4-3*) ARC Pub.

What Do Psychoanalysts Want? The Problem of Aims in Psychoanalysts. Joseph Sandler & Anna U. Dreher. 1996. LC 95-9186. (New Library of Psychoanalysis : Vol. 24). 160p. (C). 84.95 (*0-415-13514-1*); pap. 29.95 (*0-415-13515-X*) Routledge.

What Do You Do with a Child Like This? Creating Change in the Lives of Troubled Children. L. Tobin. 1991. LC 91-65948. 192p. (Orig.). pap. 15.95 (*0-938586-44-0*) Whole Person.

What Do You Know about Bacteriology? Jack Rudman. 1994. (Test Your Knowledge Ser.: No. Q-13). pap. 29.95 (*0-8373-7013-2*) Nat Learn.

What Do You Know about Dental Anatomy? Jack Rudman. 1994. (Test Your Knowledge Ser.: No. Q-39). pap. 29.95 (*0-8373-7039-6*) Nat Learn.

What Do You Know about Dental Pharmacology? Jack Rudman. 1994. (Test Your Knowledge Ser.: No. Q-40). pap. 29.95 (*0-8373-7040-X*) Nat Learn.

What Do You Know about Electrocardiography? Jack Rudman. 1994. (Test Your Knowledge Ser.: No. Q-52). pap. 39.95 (*0-8373-7052-3*) Nat Learn.

What Do You Know about Endodontics/Periodontics? Jack Rudman. 1994. (Test Your Knowledge Ser.: No. Q-54). pap. 29.95 (*0-8373-7054-X*) Nat Learn.

What Do You Know about First Aid? Jack Rudman. 1994. (Test Your Knowledge Ser.: No. Q-56). pap. 23.95 (*0-8373-7056-6*) Nat Learn.

What Do You Know about Fundamentals of Nursing? Jack Rudman. 1994. (Test Your Knowledge Ser.: No. Q-59). pap. 29.95 (*0-8373-7059-0*) Nat Learn.

What Do You Know about Hematology? Jack Rudman. 1994. (Test Your Knowledge Ser.: No. Q-68). pap. 27.95 (*0-8373-7068-X*) Nat Learn.

What Do You Know about Immunohematology & Blood Banking? Jack Rudman. 1994. (Test Your Knowledge Ser.: No. Q-72). pap. 29.95 (*0-8373-7072-8*) Nat Learn.

What Do You Know about Operative Dentistry? Jack Rudman. 1994. (Test Your Knowledge Ser.: No. Q-89). pap. 29.95 (*0-8373-7089-2*) Nat Learn.

What Do You Know about Oral Pathology/Radiography? Jack Rudman. 1994. (Test Your Knowledge Ser.: No. Q-90). pap. 29.95 (*0-8373-7090-6*) Nat Learn.

What Do You Know about Oral Surgery & Anaesthesia? Jack Rudman. 1994. (Test Your Knowledge Ser.: No. Q-91). pap. 29.95 (*0-8373-7091-4*) Nat Learn.

What Do You Know about Orthodontics/Pedodontics? Jack Rudman. 1994. (Test Your Knowledge Ser.: No. Q-93). pap. 29.95 (*0-8373-7093-0*) Nat Learn.

What Do You Know about Pharmacology? Jack Rudman. 1994. (Test Your Knowledge Ser.: No. Q-95). pap. 29.95 (*0-8373-7095-7*) Nat Learn.

What Do You Know about Prosthodontics? Jack Rudman. 1994. (Test Your Knowledge Ser.: No. Q-104). pap. 29.95 (*0-8373-7104-X*) Nat Learn.

What Do You Know about Psychology? Jack Rudman. 1994. (Test Your Knowledge Ser.: No. Q-105). pap. 27.95 (*0-8373-7105-8*) Nat Learn.

What Do You See? Phenomenology of Therapeutic Art Expression. Mala G. Betensky. 1995. LC 95-5939. pap. 29.95 (*1-85302-261-6*) Taylor & Francis.

What Doctors Don't Tell You: The Truth about the Dangers of Modern Medicine. Lynne McTaggart. 1999. 416p. mass mkt. 6.99 (*0-380-80761-0*); 1998. LC 98-92431. 400p. pap. 12.50 (*0-380-79607-4*) Morrow Avon (Avon Bks).

What Doctor's, Hospitals & HMO's Don't Want You to Know: Blind Faith in the Medical System Can Kill You, You Can Take Control. L. Neely. 285p. pap. 34.95 (*0-9675896-6-5*) Gale Pubng.

What Doctors Never Have Time to Tell. Walter Julia. 2000. 64p. pap. 8.00 (*0-8059-4999-2*) Dorrance.

What Does a Woman Want? Serge Andre. 1999. LC 98-50494. (Lacanian Clinical Field Ser.). 360p. pap. 19.95 (*1-892746-28-X*, 4628X) Other Pr LLC.

What Does Everybody Know That I Don't? Social Skills Help for Adults with Attentions Deficit/Hyperactivity Disorder (AD/HD) Michele Novotni & Randy Petersen. 1999. LC 99-45492. (Illus.). 314p. pap. 14.95 (*1-886941-34-3*) Spec Pr FL.

W X Y Z

What Every Home Health Nurse Needs to Know: A Book of Readings. Ed. by Marjorie McHann. 1994. 200p. pap. 40.00 (*0-9640767-0-5*) Cnslts in Care.

What Every Home Health Nurse Needs to Know 2: A Book of Readings. Ed. & Intro. by Marjorie McHann. 1998. 200p. pap. 40.00 (*0-9640767-2-1*) Cnslts in Care.

What Every Man Should Know about Seeding. Donald F. Kaltenbach. 1996. (Illus.). 40p. (Orig.). pap. 5.00 (*0-9651827-2-X*) Proste Cancer.

What Every Parent Should Know about Childhood Immunization. Jamie Murphy. Ed. by Carol White. 1993. 192p. (Orig.). pap. 13.95 (*0-9630373-0-7*) Earth Healing.

What Every Patient, Family, Friend, & Caregiver Needs to Know about Psychiatry. Richard W. Roukema. 1998. LC 97-31951. 408p. 25.95 (*0-88048-806-9*, 8806) Am Psychiatric.

What Every Therapist Should Know about AIDS. Samuel Knapp & Leon VandeCreek. Ed. by Harold H. Smith, Jr. 1990. LC 90-52652. (Practitioner's Resource Ser.). 80p. pap. 15.95 (*0-943158-58-3*, AIDSBP, Prof Resc Pr) Pro Resource.

What Every Woman Must Know about Heart Disease: A No-Nonsense Approach to Diagnosing, Treating & Preventing the #1 Killer of Women. Siegfried J. Kra. 1997. 228p. (Orig.). pap. (*0-446-39532-3*) Warner.

What Everybody Ought to Know about Chronic Pain, Chronic Diseases & Cancer. Maria Kuman. 1996. (Illus.). pap. 20.00 (*1-893637-04-2*) Hlth & Hap.

What Good Is Free Speech in a Closet? A Story of Cover-up in Planning for Our Grandchildren's Drinking Water. Joseph L. Miller, Jr. 1985. (Illus.). 68p. pap. 4.75 (*0-9614887-0-0*) DRC Graphics Serv.

What Happened to Human Nature? Robert M. Young. 2000. pap. (*1-899209-10-7*) Process Pr GBR. *Dist:* Intl Spec Bk.

What I Heard in the Silence: Role Reversal, Trauma & Creativity in the Lives of Women. Maria V. Bergmann. 2000. LC 00-39572. xiii, 238p. pap. 29.95 (*0-8236-6842-8*) Intl Univs Pr.

What If Any Should Government's Role Be in Health Care: Selected Essays from the 1992 Harry Singer Foundation Essay Contest. Ed. by Margaret Bohannon-Kaplan. 1992. 128p. pap. 8.00 (*0-915915-22-7*) Wellington Pubns.

What Infants Know: The New Cognitive Science of Early Development. Jacques A. Mehler & Emmanuel Dupoux. Tr. by Patsy Southgate. 1994. LC 93-10147. 240p. pap. 25.95 (*1-55786-370-9*) Blackwell Pubs.

What Is A. A.? 1980. 6p. pap. 0.25 (*0-89486-109-3*, 1445) Hazelden.

What Is a Group? A New Look at Theory in Practice. Chris Oakley. 1999. LC 99-44128. pap. (*1-892746-41-7*) Other Pr LLC.

What Is a Life Worth? Ethical Considerations in Healthcare Delivery. J. Hall. rev. ed. 1995. 212p. (C). 53.95 (*0-933915-54-3*) CA College Health Sci.

What Is a Person? The Concept & the Implications for Ethics. Kevin Doran. 1989. LC 89-33546. (Studies in Health & Human Services: Vol. 14). 192p. lib. bdg. 79.95 (*0-88946-140-6*) E Mellen.

What Is Acupuncture? How Does It Work? Eric H. Stiefvater. 1980. (*0-85032-170-0*) C W Daniel GBR. *Dist:* Natl Bk Netwk.

What Is AIDS? Anna Forbes. 1996. LC 96-5879. (AIDS Awareness Library). (Illus.). 24p. (J). (gr. k-4). lib. bdg. 15.93 (*0-8239-2368-1*, PowerKids Pr) Rosen Group.

What Is an Emotion? Classic Readings in Philosophical Psychology. Ed. by Cheshire Calhoun & Robert C. Solomon. 1984. 368p. pap. text 23.95 (*0-19-503304-3*) OUP.

What Is Death? A Scientist Looks at the Cycle of Life. Tyler Volk. 2001. LC 00-59431. 256p. 27.95 (*0-471-37544-6*) Wiley.

What Is Dementia? Mary Jo Santo Pietro. 1999. 24p. pap. 4.95 (*0-937857-81-5*, 1522) Speech Bin.

What Is Diabetes? P. P. Foa. 1988. 104p. pap. (*1-57235-075-X*) Piccin Nuova.

What Is Disease? Ed. by James M. Humber & Robert F. Almeder. 1997. LC 84-640015. (Biomedical Ethics Reviews Ser.). 372p. 59.50 (*0-89603-352-X*) Humana.

What Is Effective in Psychoanalytic Therapy? The Move from Interpretation to Relation. William W. Meissner. 1991. LC 90-14509. 216p. 40.00 (*0-87668-572-6*) Aronson.

What Is Iridology? Bernard Jensen. 1984. pap. 9.99 (*0-932615-22-8*) B Jensen.

What Is Psychoanalysis? Isador H. Coriat. 1973. LC 73-2393. (Mental Illness & Social Policy; the American Experience Ser.). reprint ed. 15.95 (*0-405-05201-4*) Ayer.

What Is Psychoanalysis? Ernest Jones. 1973. LC 72-11478. 126p. reprint ed. lib. bdg. 58.00 (*0-8371-6670-5*, JOWP, Greenwood Pr) Greenwood.

What Is Psychology? Pastorino. 2001. (C). pap. text, stu. ed. (*0-15-507336-2*) Harcourt Coll Pubs.

What Is Psychology? The Inside Story. Andrew M. Colman. 2nd ed. 1989. 196p. pap. 14.95 (*0-09-172989-0*) Routledge.

What Is Psychotherapy? Proceedings of the International Congress of Psychotherapy, 9th, Oslo, June, 1973 International Congress of Psychotherapy Staff. Ed. by T. E. Mogstad & F. Magnussen. 1975. (Journal: Vol. 24, Nos. 4-6). 600p. reprint ed. 128.75 (*3-8055-2057-3*) S Karger.

What Is Qigong? Self-Healing in Chinese Medicine. 1992. (Alternative Medicine Ser.). lib. bdg. 90.00 (*0-8490-5392-7*) Gordon Pr.

What Is Self? A Study of the Spiritual Journey in Terms of Consciousness. Bernadette Roberts. 2nd ed. 1996. LC 89-91249. 216p. (Orig.). reprint ed. pap. 19.00 (*0-9623993-0-2*) M Goens Pub.

What Is Sex Education All About? A Guide for Parents. Sidney S. Ross. 1979. LC 78-64612. pap. 7.95 (*0-9602028-0-3*) Sidney Scott Ross.

What Is the Future for a Primary Care-Led NHS? Robert Boyd. 1997. LC 96-53158. (National Primary Care Research & Development Centre Ser.). (*1-85775-265-1*) Radcliffe Med Pr GBR. *Dist:* Balogh.

***What Is the U. S. Role in Combating the Global: HIV/AIDS Epidemic?: Congressional Hearing.** Ed. by John L. Mica. 2001. (Illus.). 279p. (C). reprint ed. pap. text 35.00 (*0-7567-1799-X*) DIANE Pub.

What Is Toxemia? J. H. Tilden. 1996. 50p. reprint ed. pap. 7.95 (*1-56459-870-5*) Kessinger Pub.

What Is Toxemia & Tumors? J. H. Tilden. 1996. 29p. reprint ed. spiral bd. 9.50 (*0-7873-0875-7*) Hlth Research.

What Is Wrong with Jung? Don McGowan. 1994. LC 93-38952. 219p. 35.00 (*0-87975-859-7*) Prometheus Bks.

What Kind of Life? The Limits of Medical Progress. Daniel Callahan. 1995. LC 94-34440. 320p. pap. 15.95 (*0-87840-573-9*) Georgetown U Pr.

What Language Does Your Patient Hurt In? A Practical Guide to Culturally Competent Patient Care. Suzanne Salimbeng. 2000. pap. 30.00 (*1-883998-24-7*) Amherst Educ.

What Legislators Need to Know about Children's Mental Health. 1990. 50p. 15.00 (*1-55516-688-1*, 6627) Natl Conf State Legis.

What Life Could Mean to You. Alfred Adler. 1998. LC 98-21894. 250p. reprint ed. pap. 12.95 (*1-56838-228-6*) Hazelden.

What Makes Ryan Tick? A Family's Triumph over Tourette Syndrome & Attention Deficit Disorder. Susan Hughes. 1996. LC 96-17637. pap. 15.95 (*1-878267-35-3*) Hope Pr CA.

What Makes Women Sick: Gender & the Political Economy of Health. Lesley Doyal. 1995. LC 94-47498. 320p. text 50.00 (*0-8135-2206-4*); pap. text 15.95 (*0-8135-2207-2*) Rutgers U Pr.

What Managed Care Is Doing to Outpatient Mental Health: A Look Behind the Veil of Secrecy. Ivan J. Miller. 1994. 49p. pap. 6.00 (*0-9645263-0-1*) Boulder Psychother.

What Medication Should Be Taken in America: A Guide to American Drug Products & Similar Drugs Used in Russia & CIS. Anatoliy Kleyner et al. 1997. (RUS., Illus.). 352p. pap. 10.00 (*0-9658114-0-9*) Mir Collection.

What Men Are Like. John A. Sanford & George Lough. 1988. LC 88-15271. 320p. pap. 12.95 (*0-8091-2996-5*) Paulist Pr.

What Never to Say to a Pregnant Woman: The #1 Guide to Pregnancy Etiquette. Barbara S. Glazier et al. 1996. LC 97-162464. (Illus.). 96p. pap. 7.95 (*0-930753-18-6*) Spect Ln Pr.

What People Call Pessimism: Sigmund Freud, Arthur Schnitzler & Nineteenth-Century Controversy at the University of Vienna Medical School. Mark Luprecht. 1990. (Studies in Austrian Literature, Culture & Thought). 172p. pap. 23.00 (*0-929497-28-7*) Ariadne CA.

What People Say. Kathryn A. Ordman & Mary P. Ralli. 5th ed. 1976. LC 76-6143. pap. text 11.95 (*0-88200-073-X*, B0990) Alexander Graham.

What Predicts Divorce? The Relationship Between Marital Processes & Marital Outcomes. John M. Gottman. 1993. 536p. LC 93-12547. pap. 49.95 (*0-8058-1402-7*); text 99.95 (*0-8058-1285-7*) L Erlbaum Assocs.

What Price Vaccination? Simone Delarue. 1995. pap. 15.00 (*0-916508-22-6*) Happiness Pr.

What Radiology Professionals Won't Tell You: X-Ray - The Dark Side of the Revolving Door. Ricardo A. Scott. 1995. (Techwise Ser.). (Illus.). 70p. pap. 25.95 (*1-883427-30-4*) Crnerstone GA.

What Risk? Ed. by Roger Bate. 1997. LC 97-24157. 320p. text 59.95 (*0-7506-3810-9*) Buttrwrth-Heinemann.

What the Doctors Ordered: 150 Years of Dietary Advice in Australia. Barbara Santich. 1995. (Illus.). 192p. pap. 24.95 (*1-875657-44-4*) Intl Spec Bk.

What the Face Reveals: Basic & Applied Studies of Spontaneous Expression Using the Facial Action Coding System (FACS) Ed. by Paul Ekman & Erika L. Rosenberg. 1998. LC 96-36655. (Series in Affective Science). (Illus.). 512p. text 70.00 (*0-19-510446-3*); pap. text 39.95 (*0-19-510447-1*) OUP.

What the Hands Reveal about the Brain. Howard Poizner et al. 1990. (Studies in the Biology of Language & Cog). 256p. reprint ed. pap. text 22.95 (*0-262-66066-0*) MIT Pr.

What Therapists Learn about Themselves & How They Learn It: Autognosis. Ed. by Edward Messner et al. 1994. LC 93-74196. (Master Work Ser.). 166p. pap. 40.00 (*1-56821-188-0*) Aronson.

What to Do about Your Brain-Injured Child. Glenn Doman. 1990. 19.95 (*0-944349-24-2*) Inst Achieve Human Pot.

What to Do for a Pain in the Neck: The Complete Program for Neck Pain Relief. Jerome Schofferman. 2001. LC 2001-20713. (Illus.). 304p. pap. 14.00 (*0-684-87394-X*, Fireside) S&S Trade Pap.

What to Do for Senior Health. Albert Barnett et al. 2000. (Illus.). pap. 14.95 (*0-9701245-4-6*) IHA.

What to Do for Teen Health. Gloria G. Mayer & Ann Kuklierus. 2000. (Illus.). pap. 14.95 (*0-9701245-2-X*) IHA.

What to Do If You Get Colon Cancer: A Specialist Helps You Take Charge & Make Informed Choices. Paul F. Miskovitz & Marian Betancourt. 1997. LC 97-10074. 240p. pap. 15.95 (*0-471-15984-0*) Wiley.

What to Do in a General Practice Emergency. Melanie Darwert et al. 1997. (Illus.). 98p. (*0-7279-1183-X*) BMJ Pub GBR. *Dist:* AIDC.

What to Do in an Emergency: Action Guide. Reader's Digest Editorial Staff. 1988. LC 88-18537. (Illus.). 354p. 24.95 (*0-89577-319-8*) RD Assn.

What to Do When Someone You Love is Depressed. Mitch Golant. 1998. LC 97-43348. 208p. pap. 14.00 (*0-8050-5829-X*, Owl) H Holt & Co.

What to Do When Your Baby Is Premature: A Parent's Handbook for Coping with & Preventing Premature Birth. Joseph A. Garcia-Pratts & Sharon S. Hornfischer. 2000. LC 99-86497. (Illus.). xxi, 361p. pap. 16.00 (*0-8129-3109-2*, Crown) Crown Pub Group.

What to Do When Your Child Gets Sick. Gloria G. Mayer & Ann Kuklierus. 2000. (Illus.). 181p. pap. 14.95 (*0-9701245-0-3*) IHA.

What to Do Where There Is No Doctor or Dentist, Set. 1991. lib. bdg. 129.95 (*0-8490-4679-3*) Gordon Pr.

What to Eat If You Have Cancer. Maureen B. Keane & Daniella B. Chace. 1996. LC 96-14016. (Illus.). 288p. pap. 16.95 (*0-8092-3261-8*, 326180, Contemporary) McGraw-Hill Trade.

What to Eat if You Have Cancer Cookbook. Maureen Keane & Daniella Chace. 1997. LC 96-33483. 176p. pap. 14.95 (*0-8092-3129-8*, 312980, Contemporary) McGraw-Hill Trade.

What to Eat Now: The Cancer Lifeline Cookbook. Rachel Keim & Ginny Smith. 1996. 160p. (Orig.). pap. 14.95 (*1-57061-073-8*) Sasquatch Bks.

What to Eat When Your Doctor Says It's Diabetes. Carolyn Leontos. 1998. 224p. pap. 14.95 (*0-945448-98-8*) Am Diabetes.

What to Eat When You're Expecting. Arlene Eisenberg et al. 1986. LC 85-40903. (Illus.). 349p. pap. 8.95 (*0-89480-015-9*, 1015) Workman Pub.

What to Expect When You're Expecting. Arlene Eisenberg & Heidi E. Murkoff. 2nd ed. 1996. LC 90-50951. (Illus.). 479p. 20.00 (*1-56305-875-8*, 3875) Workman Pub.

What to Expect When You're Expecting. Arlene Eisenberg et al. 2nd rev. ed. 1996. LC 90-50951. (Illus.). 504p. pap. 12.95 (*0-89480-829-X*, 1829) Workman Pub.

***What to Expect When You're Expecting.** Arlene Eisenberg et al. 3rd rev. ed. 2001. LC 2001-43523. (Illus.). 560p. 24.95 (*0-7611-2549-3*, 12549); pap. 14.95 (*0-7611-2132-3*, 12132) Workman Pub.

What to Expect When You're Expecting Pregnancy Organizer. Arlene Eisenberg et al. 1995. (Illus.). 239p. pap. 12.95 (*1-56305-872-3*) Workman Pub.

What to Order When: Pocket Guide to Diagnostic Imaging. Ronald L. Eisenberg & Alexander R. Margulis. 2nd ed. 1999. LC 99-51664. 544p. pap. text 45.00 (*0-7817-2194-6*) Lppncott W & W.

What We Know about Suicidal Behavior & How to Treat It. Ed. by Stanley Lesse. LC 88-19324. 1995. 486p. pap. 50.00 (*1-56821-063-9*); 1988. 466p. 60.00 (*0-87668-878-4*) Aronson.

What Women Need to Know: From Headaches to Heart Disease & Everything in Between. Marianne J. Legato & Carol Colman. 239p. pap. (*1-58754-100-9*) Olmstead Pr.

What Women Need to Know about Breast Self-Examination. Karen Berger & John Bostwick, III. 1995. (Illus.). 8p. pap. 1.95 (*0-942219-99-6*) Quality Med Pub.

What Women Want—What Men Want: Why the Sexes STill See Love & Commitment So Differently. John M. Townsend. 1998. LC 97-43547. 304p. 25.00 (*0-19-511488-4*) OUP.

What Women Want to Know about Breast Implants. Karen Berger & John Bostwick, III. 2nd ed. 1998. (Illus.). 57p. pap. 6.00 (*1-57626-105-0*) Quality Med Pub.

What Works? Synthesizing Effective Bio-Medical & Psychosocial Strategies for Healthy Families in the 21st Century. Ed. by Lorraine C. Blackman. 1994. (Illus.). 172p. (Orig.). (C). pap. text 29.95 (*0-9643817-0-2*) IN U Schl Soc Wrk.

What Works for Whom? A Critical Review of Psychotherapy Research. Anthony Roth & Peter Fonagy. 1998. 484p. pap. 28.00 (*1-57230-355-7*, C0355) Guilford Pubns.

What Works for Whom? A Critical Review of Psychotherapy Research. Anthony Roth et al. 1996. LC 96-22624. 484p. 50.00 (*1-57230-125-2*, 0125) Guilford Pubns.

What Works in Children's Mental Health Services? Uncovering Answers to Critical Questions. Krista Kutash & Vestena R. Rivera. 1996. LC 96-12812. (Systems of Care for Children's Mental Health Ser.: Vol. 3). 208p. (Orig.). pap. 30.00 (*1-55766-254-1*) P H Brookes.

What Works in Drug Abuse Epidemiology. Ed. by Blanche Frank & Ronald Simeone. 1992. LC 91-23375. (Journal of Addictive Diseases Ser.: Vol. 11, No. 1). (Illus.). 150p. 39.95 (*1-56024-185-3*) Haworth Pr.

***What Works with Children & Adolescents? Critical Review of Psychological Interventions with Children, Adolescents & Their Families.** Ed. by Alan Carr. 2001. (Illus.). 384p. (Orig.). (C). (gr. 13). pap. 34.95 (*0-415-23350-X*) Routledge.

What You Can Do about Diabetes. Nora Tannenhaus. 1991. (Medical Library). 144p. mass mkt. 5.99 (*0-440-20640-5*) Dell.

What You Can Do to Prevent Diabetes: Simple Changes to Improve Your Life. Annette Maggi & Jackie Boucher. 2000. LC 99-52765. 146p. pap. 12.95 (*0-471-34796-5*) Wiley.

What You Didn't Think to Ask Your Obstetrician: Revised & Expanded. Raymond I. Poliakin. exp. rev. ed. 1994. LC 94-22529. 320p. pap. 14.95 (*0-8092-3658-3*, 365830, Contemporary) McGraw-Hill Trade.

What You Don't Know about Having Babies: The Pregnancy Question & Answer Book. Joyce Armor. 1997. LC 97-20567. (*0-88166-292-5*) Meadowbrook.

What You Don't Know about Health Insurance Will Cost You. Heidi H. Hale. 1991. 67p. (Orig.). pap. 12.95 (*0-9631623-0-6*, 3160337) MediPro Mgmt.

What You Don't Know about Prescription Drugs Can Hurt You! Viviloria Frazier. 2000. 240p. pap. text 9.95 (*1-889668-17-6*) S & D.

What You Don't Know Can Heal You: The Missing Link of Wholistic Medicine. David Waldman. Ed. by Bob Owen. 1994. LC 94-76251. (Illus.). 232p. (Orig.). pap. text 12.95 (*1-882657-09-8*) Health Digest.

What You Don't Know Can Hurt You: A Guide to the Medical Literature. A. J. Longley. 1981. (Orig.). (C). pap. 3.00 (*0-937038-00-8*) Star Pr.

What You Need to Know about Breast Cancer. Pat Kelly & Mark Levine. 1999. LC 99-217325. (Illus.). ix, 110p. pap. (*1-55009-065-8*) DEKR CAN. *Dist:* Blackwell Sci.

What You Need to Know about Cancer: A Scientific American Special Issue. Weinberg & Ruosla. 1997. LC 97-3663. (Illus.). 160p. pap. text 16.95 (*0-7167-3102-9*) W H Freeman.

What You Need to Know about Psychiatric Drugs. Stuart C. Yudofsky et al. 1992. LC 91-58327. 672p. pap. 14.00 (*0-345-37334-0*) Ballantine Pub Grp.

What You Need to Know to Live with Chemicals. Ralph I. Freudenthal & Susan L. Freudenthal. 1989. LC 89-85145. (Illus.). 192p. (Orig.). pap. 12.95 (*0-9623813-0-6*) Aribet Bks.

What You Really Need to Know about Cancer: A Comprehensive Guide for Patients & Their Families. Robert Buckman. 1997. LC 97-5203. (Illus.). 384p. 44.50 (*0-8018-5594-2*); pap. 22.95 (*0-8018-5593-4*) Johns Hopkins.

What You Really Need to Know about Cancer: A Comprehensive Guide for Patients & Their Families. Robert Buckman. 1996. 485p. (*0-333-61866-1*) Macmillan GBR. *Dist:* Trans-Atl Phila.

What You Really Need to Know about Moles & Melanoma. Jill R. Schofield & William A. Robinson. 2000. LC 00-8003. (Johns Hopkins Press Health Bks.). (Illus.). 232p. 45.00 (*0-8018-6393-7*); pap. 14.95 (*0-8018-6394-5*) Johns Hopkins.

What You Should Know about Arthritic Disorders, Set. Brian Kotzin. 1992. 24p. (*1-56375-109-7*) Gower-Mosby.

What You Should Know about Herbs for Your Health. Earl L. Mindell & Virginia L. Hopkins. 1996. LC 96-4298. 120p. pap. 4.95 (*0-87983-749-7*, 37497K, Keats Pubng) McGraw-Hill Trade.

What You Should Know About Radiation. Toby J. Armellini. Ed. by Sylvia Armellini & Eve Dobkins. 2000. 112p. (C). pap. 9.95 (*0-9675953-0-4*) Armellini.

What You Should Know about Trace Minerals. Virginia L. Hopkins & Earl L. Mindell. 1996. LC 96-38359. 88p. pap. 4.95 (*0-87983-748-9*, 37489K, Keats Pubng) McGraw-Hill Trade.

What You Should Know Before Buying a Wheelchair Lift: Tips for the Prospective Buyer. Mark Hittson & Carol Hirsch. 1995. 16p. (Orig.). pap. 4.95 (*1-888349-02-6*) Katydid.

What Your Cat Is Trying to Tell You: A Head-to-Tail-Guide to Your Cat's Symptoms - & Their Solutions. John M. Simon & Stephanie Pedersen. 2000. 256p. mass mkt. 5.99 (*0-312-97288-1*, St Martins Paperbacks) St Martin.

What Your Dentist Does to Keep the Dental Office Safe. Michael Glick & Brian C. Muzyka. 1996. LC 95-45830. (Illus.). 32p. pap. 20.00 (*0-86715-314-8*) Quint Pub Co.

What Your Doctor Didn't Learn in Medical School . . . & What You Can Do About It! Stuart M. Berger. 1989. 352p. reprint ed. mass mkt. 4.95 (*0-380-70319-X*, Avon Bks) Morrow Avon.

What Your Doctor Doesn't Know Can Kill You: Advice on Health & Long Life from the Top Medical Scientists of the World. William A. Kent. 1997. 24.95 (*0-9654622-1-8*) C A Inc.

***What Your Doctor May Not Tell You about Breast Cancer: How Hormone Balance Can Save Your Life.** John R. Lee et al. 2002. LC 2001-45468. 432p. 25.95 (*0-446-52686-X*) Warner Bks.

***What Your Doctor May Not Tell You about Children's Vaccinations.** Stephanie Cave & Deborah Mitchell. 2001. LC 2001-26068. 336p. reprint ed. pap. (*0-446-67707-8*) Warner.

What Your Doctor May Not Tell You about HPV & Abnormal Pap Smears. Joel Palefsky & Jody Handley. 2002. LC 2001-56775. 400p. pap. (*0-446-67787-6*) Warner.

***What Your Doctor May Not Tell You about Knee Pain & Surgery: Learn the Truth about MRIs & Common Misdiagnoses - And Avoid Unnecessary Surgery.** Ronald P. Grelsamer. 2002. (Illus.). 400p. pap. (*0-446-67819-8*) Warner.

What Your Doctor Should Do for You: A Symptom-by-Symptom Guide to Getting Proper Treatment from Your Physician & Your Health Plan. Joel Goldberg. 1996. LC 95-50687. 368p. pap. 18.95 (*0-89733-430-2*) Academy Chi Pubs.

What Your Doctor Won't Tell You. Jane Heimlich. 1990. LC 89-46097. 288p. pap. 10.95 (*0-00-002911-4*, Perennial) HarperTrade.

What Your Doctor Won't Tell You: Today's Alternative Medical Treatments Explained to Help You Find the. Jane Heimlich. 1990. LC 89-46097. 320p. pap. 15.00 (*0-06-096539-8*, Perennial) HarperTrade.

What Your Dog Is Trying to Tell You: A Head-to-Tail Guide to Your Dog's Symptoms & Their Solutions. John M. Simon. 1998. LC 97-40592. 208p. pap. 16.95 (*0-312-18214-7*) St Martin.

What Your Unborn Baby Wants You to Know: A Complete Guide to a Healthy Pregnancy. Boris M. Petrikovsky et al. 2001. LC 00-50127. (Illus.). xvii, 296p. pap. 14.95 (*0-399-52682-X*, Perigee Bks) Berkley Pub.

Whatever Happened to General Practitioners? R. Cantafio. 1997. 268p. lib. bdg. 75.00 (*1-56072-382-3*) Nova Sci Pubs.

What's Behind the Research? Discovering Hidden Assumptions in the Behavioral Sciences. Brent D. Slife & Richard N. Williams. 1995. 264p. (C). pap. 29.95 (*0-8039-5863-3*, 7892) Sage.

What's Behind the Symptom? On Psychiatric Observation & Anthropological Understanding. Angel Martinez-Hernaez. 2000. 240p. 54.00 (*90-5702-612-0*, Harwood Acad Pubs) Gordon & Breach.

What's Going on in There? How the Brain & Mind Develop in the First Five Years of Life. Lise Eliot. 544p. 2000. pap. 16.95 (*0-553-37825-2*); 1999. LC 99-35423. 26.95 (*0-553-10274-5*) Bantam.

What's in Our Food? Fact & Fiction about Fat & Fiber, Vitamins & Minerals, Nutrients & Contaminants. Mia Parsonnet. 1996. LC 95-51724. 145p. pap. 14.95 (*1-56833-049-9*) Madison Bks UPA.

***What's in the Air: The Complete Guide to Airborne Allergies.** Gillian Shepherd & Marion Betancourt. 2002. 320p. mass mkt. 6.99 (*0-7434-4217-2*) PB.

What's New in Allergy & Asthma: New Developments & How They Help You to Overcome Allergy & Asthma. Stephen Astor. 4th rev. ed. 1996. LC 96-90200. (Illus.). 288p. (Orig.). pap. 14.95 (*0-915001-12-8*) Two As Pub.

What's New in Anesthesiology. Ed. by Theodore H. Stanley. 1988. (Developments in Critical Care, Medicine, & Anesthesiology Ser.). (C). text 147.00 (*0-89838-367-6*) Kluwer Academic.

What's New in Cardiac Imaging? SPECT, PET & MRI. Ed. by Ernst E. Van der Wall. 1992. (Developments in Cardiovascular Medicine Ser.). 580p. (C). text 332.00 (*0-7923-1615-0*) Kluwer Academic.

What's New in Cardiovascular Imaging? J. H. Reiber & E. Vander Wall. 1998. LC 98-22461. (Developments in Cardiovascular Medicine Ser.). 441p. 159.00 (*0-7923-5121-5*) Kluwer Academic.

What's New in Electrocardiography. Ed. by Hein J. Wellens & Henri E. Kulbertus. 1981. pap. text 121.50 (*90-247-2452-X*) Kluwer Academic.

What's Normal? An Anthology: Narratives of Mental & Emotional Disorders. Carol C. Donley & Sheryl Buckley. 2000. LC 99-48190. (Literature & Medicine Ser.: Vol. 3). xv, 355p. pap. 26.00 (*0-87338-653-1*) Kent St U Pr.

What's Social about Social Cognition? Social Cognition Research in Small Groups. Judith L. Nye & Aaron M. Brower. 1996. LC 96-4479. 428p. (C). pap. 39.95 (*0-8039-7205-9*, 1050) Sage.

What's the Best Way to Deal with Hyperactivity? New Update on the Attention Deficit Disorders. C. Thomas Wild. 1983. LC 83-71951. (Illus.). 52p. (Orig.). pap. 3.95 (*0-9606990-1-5*) Attent Span Advan.

What's the Diagnosis? Race Foster & Marty Smith. 1995. LC 95-21877. (Illus.). 272p. pap. 19.95 (*0-87605-788-1*, Howell) Hungry Minds.

***What's the Patient's Code Status?** Ferdinando L. Mirarchi. Ed. by James B. Caputo. 2001. LC 00-93133. (Illus.). 51p. pap. 12.95 (*1-889014-58-3*) Patient Adv Educ Res.

What's Wrong with Sex Education? Preteen & Teenage Sexual Development & Environmental Influences. Melvin Anchell. Ed. by Bobbie H. Ames. 1993. (Illus.). 108p. (Orig.). pap. 7.00 (*0-9626257-4-4*) CBCCU Amer.

What's Wrong with the Mental Health System. 1995. pap. 3.00 (*1-885357-20-6*); 1991. pap. 3.00 (*0-913937-53-3*) Rational Isl.

What's Wrong with the Mental Health System: Spanish Translation. 1994. pap. 3.00 (*1-885357-01-X*) Rational Isl.

What's Wrong with the Mental Health System & What Can Be Done About It see Ce Qui ne va Pas Dans le Systeme de la Sante Mentale et Comment y Remedier

What's Wrong with the Mental Health System & What Can Be Done About It. Tr. by Hidetoshi Mizoguchi from ENG. 1999. (JPN.). pap. 3.00 (*1-58429-047-1*) Rational Isl.

***Wheater's Basic Histopathology: A Color Atlas & Text.** Barbara Young et al. 4th ed. 2001. (Illus.). 315p. pap. (*0-443-07001-6*) Church GBR. *Dist:* Saunders.

Wheater's Basic Histopathology: A Colour Atlas & Text. Paul R. Wheater & H. George Burkitt. 3rd ed. 1996. LC 96-26701. pap. text (*0-443-05088-0*) Church.

Wheater's Functional Histology: A Text & Colour Atlas. H. George Burkitt et al. 3rd ed. 1993. LC 93-7323. (Illus.). 416p. pap. text (*0-443-04691-3*) Church.

Wheelchair Evaluation: A Practical Guide. Mitch Batavia. 1998. LC 98-2710. 360p. pap. text 19.99 (*0-7506-7037-1*) Buttrwrth-Heinemann.

Wheelchair Selection & Configuration. Rory A. Cooper. 1998. LC 98-22858. (Illus.). 424p. 34.95 (*1-888799-18-8*) Demos Medical.

Wheelchair Users & Postural Seating: A Clinical Approach. R. Ham et al. 1998. LC 97-17576. (C). pap. (*0-443-05472-X*) Church.

Wheelchair Vagabond. John G. Nelson. 14.95 (*0-933261-10-1*); 1975. pap. 9.95 (*0-933261-07-1*) Twin Peaks Pr.

Wheelchairs: A Prescription Guide. A. Bennett Wilson, Jr. 2nd ed. 1992. (Illus.). 96p. pap. 24.95 (*0-939957-39-6*) Demos Medical.

Wheeler's Atlas of Tooth Form. Major M. Ash, Jr. 5th ed. 1984. (Illus.). 158p. text 51.00 (*0-7216-1277-6*) Saunders.

Wheeler's Dental Anatomy, Physiology & Occlusion. Major M. Ash, Jr. 7th ed. 1992. (Illus.). 490p. text 54.00 (*0-7216-4374-4*) Saunders.

When a Baby Dies: A Handbook for Healing & Helping. Rana K. Limbo & Sara R. Wheeler. 1986. 168p. pap. 8.95 (*0-9612310-3-3*) Harsand Pr.

When a Child Has Diabetes. Denis Daneman et al. 1999. (Your Personal Health Ser.). (Illus.). 218p. pap. 14.95 (*1-55209-331-X*) Firefly Bks Limited.

When a Community Weeps: Case Studies in Group Survivorship. Ellen Zinner & Mary B. Williams. 1998. LC 98-25989. (Series in Trauma & Loss). 261p. 39.95 (*0-87630-953-8*) Brunner-Routledge.

When a Doctor Hates a Patient: Chapters from a Young Physician's Life. Richard E. Peschel & Enid R. Peschel. 1986. (C). pap. 13.95 (*0-520-06343-0*) U CA Pr.

When a Parent Has Cancer: A Guide to Caring for Your Children. Wendy S. Harpham. 1997. LC 96-32529. (Illus.). 208p. 26.00 (*0-06-018709-3*) HarperCollins Pubs.

When Abortion Was a Crime: Women, Medicine & Law in the United States, 1867-1973. Leslie J. Reagan. 1997. LC 96-22568. (Illus.). 400p. (C). text 45.00 (*0-520-08848-4*) U CA Pr.

When Age Grows Young. Clare H. Kirk. Ed. by Robert J. Kastenbaum. 1979. LC 78-22204. (Aging & Old Age Ser.). reprint ed. lib. bdg. 25.95 (*0-405-11819-8*) Ayer.

When AIDS Comes Home see Cuando el SIDA Llega Al Hogar

When AIDS Comes to the Church. William E. Amos, Jr. 1988. LC 87-30875. 132p. pap. 14.95 (*0-664-25009-2*) Westminster John Knox.

When AIDS Strikes. Peter A. Mozeleski. Ed. by Paul M. Mozeleski & Rosie Dominguez. 1991. (Illus.). 8p. (Orig.). (YA). (gr. 6-12). pap. 2.50 (*1-880058-85-5*) Rubbers Bros Comics.

When AIDS Strikes, Vol. 1, Nos. 1 & 2. Peter A. Mozeleski. Ed. by Paul M. Mozeleski. Ed. & Tr. by Rosie Dominguez. 1991. (Illus.). 8p. (Orig.). (YA). (gr. 6-12). pap. 2.50 (*1-880058-84-7*) Rubbers Bros Comics.

When All the Friends Have Gone: A Guide for Aftercare Providers. Ed. by O. Duane Weeks & Catherine Johnson. 2000. LC 99-462163. (Death, Value & Meaning Ser.). vii, 264p. text 44.00 (*0-89503-215-5*) Baywood Pub.

When Alzheimer's Disease Strikes. Stephen Sapp. 1996. 64p. pap. 5.95 (*0-914733-12-5*) Desert Min.

When Alzheimer's Hits Home. Jo Danna. Ed. by Carl Danna. 1995. LC 94-65719. (Illus.). 208p. (Orig.). pap. 14.95 (*0-9610036-4-2*) Palomino Pr.

When an Employee Has AIDS. Victor Schachter & Susan Von Seeburg. 1989. pap. 19.95 (*1-55840-168-7*) Exec Ent Pubns.

When Anger Hurts. Matthew McKay et al. 1993. 6.98 (*1-56731-028-1*, MJF Bks) Fine Comms.

When Anger Hurts: Quieting the Storm Within. Matthew McKay et al. 1989. 325p. pap. 15.95 (*0-934986-76-2*) New Harbinger.

When Antibiotics Fail: Restoring the Ecology of the Body. Marc Lappe. rev. ed. 1987. 288p. (Orig.). reprint ed. pap. 14.95 (*0-938190-74-1*) North Atlantic.

When Autism Strikes: Families Cope with Childhood Disintegrative Disorder. Ed. by Robert A. Catalano. 1998. LC 98-12011. (Illus.). 244p. (C). 19.95 (*0-306-45789-X*) Perseus Bks Grp.

When Baby Makes Two. Helen C. Keen. Date not set. LC 86-83412. (Illus.). 260p. (Orig.). pap. 12.95 (*0-89896-341-9*) Larksdale.

When Being a Good Parent or Teacher Is Not Enough: A Guide to Recognizing, Understanding & Supporting Difficult or Disturbed Adolescents, Vol. II. Anne E. Yarnevich & Barbara N. Buchanan. 2000. 254p. ring bd. 39.95 (*1-891330-04-7*) Health Ed Consults.

When Cancer Returns: Meeting the Challenge Again. 1995. 30p. pap. text 10.00 (*0-7881-2115-4*) DIANE Pub.

When Cancer Strikes. Nabil G. Hagag. 1998. LC 98-11744. 272p. 18.95 (*1-56072-540-0*, Nova Kroshka Bks) Nova Sci Pubs.

When Caring Isn't Enough: Meeting the Need for Long-Term Care with Long-Term Care Insurance. Samuel Larry Feldman & National LTC Network Staff. 2000. (Illus.). 344p. pap. 24.95 (*1-891042-11-4*) Million Dollar.

When Catholic & Non-Catholic Hospitals Merge: Reproductive Health Compromised. Liz Bucar. 1998. LC 98-157893. 68p. 10.00 (*0-915365-33-2*) Cath Free Choice.

When Death Is Sought: Assisted Suicide & Euthanasia in the Medical Context. NYS Task Force on Life and the Law Staff. 1994. 234p. pap. 9.00 (*1-881268-01-2*) NYS Task Force.

When Diabetes Complicates Your Life: Controlling Diabetes & Related Complications. Joseph Juliano. 2nd ed. 1998. 144p. pap. 12.95 (*0-471-34751-5*) Wiley.

When Diabetes Hits Home. Wendy Satin Rapaport. 1998. LC 98-17224. 289p. pap. 19.95 (*0-945448-88-0*, 00880Q) Am Diabetes.

When Doctors Get Sick. Ed. by Harvey Mandell & Howard Spiro. 1987. LC 87-14104. (Illus.). 484p. 35.00 (*0-306-42653-6*, Kluwer Plenum) Kluwer Academic.

When Doctors Join Unions. Gladys Budrys. 1996. LC 96-32596. (IRL Press Book). (Illus.). 224p. 39.95 (*0-8014-3277-4*) Cornell U Pr.

When Doctors Say No: The Battleground of Medical Futility. Susan B. Rubin. 1998. LC 98-6798. (Medical Ethics Ser.). 240p. 24.95 (*0-253-33463-2*) Ind U Pr.

When Every Moment Counts, Count on Provision. Leon Revien. 1987. 16p. pap. text 4.95 (*0-940429-02-0*) M B Glass Assocs.

When Families Fail: Psychological Disorders Caused by Parent-Child Relational Problems. Ann E. Holmes. Ed. by Carol C. Nadelson & Claire E. Reinburg. 1999. LC 99-13291. (Encyclopedia of Psychological Disorders Ser.). (Illus.). 93p. lib. bdg. 24.95 (*0-7910-4956-6*) Chelsea Hse.

When Father Kills Mother: Helping Children Move from Trauma to Grief. Dora Black et al. 1993. LC 92-48528. 240p. (C). text 69.95 (*0-415-07662-5*, B0869) Routledge.

When Girls Feel Fat: Helping Girls Through Adolescence. Sandra Susan Friedman. 1999. 240p. pap. 15.00 (*0-00-638561-3*) HarperCollins Pubs.

When Growing up Hurts Too Much: A Parent's Guide to Knowing When & How to Choose a Therapist for Your Teenager. Scott O. Harris & Edward N. Reynolds. 1988. 141p. pap. 10.95 (*0-02-914055-2*) Lxngtn Bks.

When Health Care Is Not Enough: Support Services for Pregnant Women & Infants. Jennifer Laman. 1994. (State Legislative Report Ser.: Vol. 19, No. 8). 9p. 15.00 (*1-55516-226-6*, 7302-1908) Natl Conf State Legis.

When Hello Means Goodbye: A Guide for Parents Whose Child Dies before Birth, at Birth or Shortly after Birth. Pat Schwiebert & Paul Kirk. Ed. by Perinatal Loss Project Staff. 2nd rev. ed. 1993. 48p. pap. 2.50 (*0-9615197-0-3*); (SPA.). pap. 2.50 (*0-9615197-1-1*) Perinatal Loss.

When Husbands Come Out of the Closet. Ed. by Jean S. Gochros. 1989. (Haworth Series on Women: No. 1). 267p. LC 88-36884. pap. text 14.95 (*0-918393-61-2*, Harrington Park); LC 88-36883. text 39.95 (*0-86656-868-9*) Haworth Pr.

When I Grow Too Old to Dream: Coping with Alzheimer's Disease. Gerry Naughtin & Terry Laidler. 1992. 13.00 (*1-86371-075-2*) Harper SF.

When Is a Dose Not a Dose? Victor Bond. 1991. LC 91-46381. (Taylor Lectures: No. 15). 41p. (Orig.). pap. text 25.00 (*0-929600-21-5*) NCRP Pubns.

When It Hurts Too Much to Quit: Smoking & Depression. Gerald S. Mayer. 1997. (Quit Smart Smoking Cessation Ser.). 12p. pap. 2.95 (*0-9642504-1-1*) Desert City Pr.

When Life Becomes Precious: A Guide for Loved Ones & Friends of Cancer Patients. Elise N. Babcock. 1997. LC 96-30256. 304p. pap. 14.95 (*0-553-37869-4*) Bantam.

When Living Hurts: Directives for Treating Depression. Michael D. Yapko. LC 87-22437. 240p. 1994. pap. 13.95 (*0-87630-757-8*); 1988. text 37.95 (*0-87630-485-4*) Brunner-Routledge.

When Love Is Not Enough: A Guide to Parenting Children with RAD Reactive Attachment. Nancy L. Thomas. 1997. (Illus.). 100p. pap. 12.00 (*0-9703525-0-6*) Fam By Design.

When Love Is Not Enough: The Management of Covert Dynamics in Organizations That Treat Children & Adolescents. Ed. by Donna P. Piazza. LC 95-44786. (Residential Treatment for Children & Youth Ser.: Vol. 13, No. 1). 105p. (C). 1997. pap. 14.95 (*0-7890-0223-X*); 1996. 29.95 (*1-56024-778-9*) Haworth Pr.

When Madness Comes Home: Help & Hope for Families of the Mentally Ill. Victoria Seconda. 1998. LC 96-28612. 362p. (J). reprint ed. pap. 15.95 (*0-7868-8326-X*) Hyperion.

When Medicare is the Secondary Payer. 1995. 200p. pap. text 45.00 (*1-58383-156-8*, SECOND1) Robert D Keene.

When Medicine Failed. Janet Leih. 1998. 181p. pap. 15.00 (*1-877649-32-5*) Tesseract SD.

When Medicine Went Mad: Bioethics & the Holocaust. Ed. by Arthur L. Caplan. 1992. LC 92-11687. (Contemporary Issues in Biomedicine, Ethics & Society Ser.). 359p. 49.50 (*0-89603-235-3*) Humana.

When Minds Go Wrong. John M. Grimes. 1954. 6.95 (*0-8159-7206-7*) Devin.

When More Is Less: The Paradox of American Health Care & How to Resolve It. Arnold S. Relman. 1993. 224p. 19.95 (*0-393-03579-4*) Norton.

When Muscle Pain Won't Go Away: The Relief Handbook for Fibromyalgia & Chronic Muscle Pain. Gayle Backstrom. 1992. LC 92-3289. 168p. pap. 12.95 (*0-87833-794-6*) Taylor Pub.

When Nothing Else Works: Innovative Interventions with Intractable Individuals. Herbert S. Strean. 1997. LC 97-5663. pap. text 40.00 (*0-7657-0074-3*) Aronson.

When One Partner Is Willing & the Other Is Not. Ed. by Barbara J. Brothers. 1997. LC 96-51966. 106p. pap. 9.95 (*0-7890-0342-2*) Haworth Pr.

When Organs Fail: The Awesome Science of Transplants. Anna Rovid Spickler. 2000. LC 00-102894. (Illus.). 249p. pap. 19.95 (*1-880319-23-3*) Biotech.

When Parents Die: Learning to Live with the Loss of a Parent. Rebecca Abrams. 2nd ed. 1999. LC 98-45977. xvi, 197p. 75.00 (*0-415-20065-2*); 224p. pap. 29.95 (*0-415-20066-0*) Routledge.

When Parkinson's Strikes Early: Voices, Choices, Resources & Treatment. Barbara Blake-Krebs & Linda Herman. 2001. LC 2001-16619. (Illus.). 288p. pap. 15.95 (*0-89793-340-0*) Hunter Hse.

***When Parkinson's Strikes Early: Voices, Choices, Resources & Treatment.** Barbara Blake-Krebs & Linda Herman. 2001. (Illus.). 288p. 25.95 (*0-89793-341-9*) Hunter Hse.

When Pregnancy Isn't Perfect: A Layperson's Guide to Complications in Pregnancy. Laurie A. Rich. 3rd ed. 1996. 349p. reprint ed. pap. 18.95 (*0-9654985-0-6*) Larata Pr.

When Psychological Problems Mask Medical Disorders: A Guide for Psychotherapists. James Morrison. 221p. 1999. pap. 20.00 (*1-57230-539-8*, C0539); 1997. LC 97-17253. text 35.00 (*1-57230-180-5*, C0180) Guilford Pubns.

When Someone Dies: A Practical Guide to Holistic Care for the Terminally Ill. Hannah Cooke. 2000. LC 99-58768. 182p. pap. text 35.00 (*0-7506-4094-4*) Buttrwrth-Heinemann.

When Someone in Your Family Has Cancer. rev. ed. 1996. (Illus.). 27p. pap. text 10.00 (*0-7881-3004-8*) DIANE Pub.

When Someone You Know Has AIDS. Anna Forbes. 1996. LC 96-1507. (AIDS Awareness Library). (Illus.). 24p. (J). (gr. k-4). lib. bdg. 15.93 (*0-8239-2369-X*, PowerKids Pr) Rosen Group.

When Someone You Love Has a Mental Illness: A Handbook for Family, Friends & Caregivers. Rebecca Woolis. 1992. LC 92-7069. 256p. 13.95 (*0-87477-695-3*, Tarcher Putnam) Putnam Pub Group.

When Someone You Love Has a Stroke. Lynn Sonberg. 1995. (Caregiving Guides). 272p. mass mkt. 5.99 (*0-440-21666-4*) Dell.

When Someone You Love Has Alzheimer's: The Caregiver's Journey. Earl A. Grollman & Kenneth S. Kosik. l.t. ed. LC 96-15884. 192p. 1997. pap. 12.00 (*0-8070-2721-9*); 1996. 22.00 (*0-8070-2720-0*) Beacon Pr.

When Someone You Love Has Cancer. Lynn Sonberg. 1995. mass mkt. 4.99 (*0-440-77889-1*) Dell.

When Someone You Love Is Depressed. Laura E. Rosen & Xavier F. Amador. 1997. 256p. per. 12.00 (*0-684-83407-3*, Fireside) S&S Trade Pap.

When Someone You Love Is Dying: A Handbook for Counselors & Those Who Care. Ruth Kopp & Stephen W. Sorenson. 2nd ed. 1985. 240p. mass mkt. 9.95 (*0-310-41601-9*, 11165P) Zondervan.

When the Air Hits Your Brain. Frank T. Vertosick. 1997. LC 96-91010. 272p. mass mkt. 5.99 (*0-449-22713-8*, Crest) Fawcett.

When the Air Hits Your Brain: Tales of Neurosurgery. Frank T. Vertosick, Jr. 1996. LC 95-9790. 288p. 23.00 (*0-393-03894-7*) Norton.

When the Bough Breaks: Pregnancy & the Legacy of Addiction. Kira Corser & Frances P. Adler. 1993. LC 93-5611. 112p. 39.95 (*0-939165-20-1*); pap. 22.95 (*0-939165-19-8*) NewSage Press.

When the Doctor Drops the Bomb. Christopher Brookes. 1997. 104p. (Orig.). pap. 9.95 (*0-9655207-0-6*) Cutters Rig Bks.

When the Doctor Says "It's Cancer" see Cuando el Medico Dice: Es Cancer

When the Man You Love Won't Take Care of His Health. Ken Goldberg. 2000. 304p. pap. 13.95 (*0-312-25471-7*) St Martin.

When the Mind Fails: A Guide to Dealing with Incompetency. Michel Silberfeld & Arthur Fish. 1994. LC 93-94593. 310p. (C). pap. 14.95 (*0-8020-6780-8*) U of Toronto Pr.

When the Nursing Home Is the Choice. Donna Du Bois. 1991. 76p. 9.50 (*1-877735-17-5*, 2130pp) Prof Prnting & Pub.

When "The Other Woman" Is His Mother: Book I: Boys & Incest Victims, & Male Multiple Personality Disorder. Faithe Brodie. 1992. LC 90-70218. 181p. pap. 13.95 (*0-9626009-0-3*) Winged Eagle Pr.

When the Tulips Bloom. Susan E. Miller. Ed. by Jerena Burdge-Rezvan. 1993. LC 93-60937. (Illus.). 152p. pap. 12.95 (*1-880254-08-5*) Vista.

When the Unthinkable Happens: A Father's Journey Through Grief. Thomas G. Crouthamel. 1995. LC 94-24127. 19.95 (*0-940701-44-8*) Keystone Pr.

When Things Get Worse: The Problem of Negative Effects in Psychotherapy. Hans H. Strupp et al. 1994. LC 94-33810. (Master Work Ser.). 366p. pap. text 50.00 (*1-56821-372-7*) Aronson.

When to Call the Surgeon: Decision Making for Primary Care Providers. Robert A. Kozol et al. 1998. LC 98-21038. (Illus.). 275p. (C). pap. text 39.00 (*0-8036-0336-3*) Davis Co.

When to Refer: The Gatekeeper's Manual. Ed. by Susan Galandiuk et al. 2000. 200p. pap. text 28.00 (*1-57626-016-X*) Quality Med Pub.

When to Refuse Treatment: A Practical Guide for Dying in Peace. Joseph F. Bentivegna. 1992. (Illus.). 190p. (Orig.). (C). 13.95 (*0-9626001-1-3*) Michelle Pub.

When We Don't Remember: A Book about Discovering Incest. Lyda W. Hersloff. 1994. LC 93-34351. 112p. pap. 9.95 (*0-942963-42-3*) Distinctive Pub.

When Words Are Not Enough: The Women's Prescription for Depression & Anxiety. Valerie D. Raskin. 1997. LC 96-38081. (Illus.). 336p. pap. 16.00 (*0-553-06713-3*) Broadway BDD.

When You Are Facing Surgery. Ron DelBene et al. 1991. (Times of Change, Times of Challenge Ser.). 31p. pap. 3.00 (*0-8358-0639-1*) Upper Room Bks.

When You Don't Know Who to Call: A Consumer's Guide to Selecting Mental Health Care. Nancy L. Schaufele & Donna B. Kennedy. Ed. by Andrea Maffetone & Euan Barr. 1998. 144p. pap. 15.00 (*1-884444-48-2*, WP060) Safer Soc.

When You Go Back to Work. Robert I. Ward. 1984. 14p. (Orig.). pap. 1.25 (*0-89486-235-9*, 1417B) Hazelden.

When You Know You're Dying: 12 Thoughts to Guide You Through the Days Ahead. James E. Miller. 1997. LC 97-60133. (Illus.). 64p. (Orig.). pap. text 6.95 (*1-885933-24-X*) Willowgreen Pubng.

***When Young Children Are Injured: Families as Caregivers in Hospitals & at Home.** Marilyn Lash et al. 1994. 49p. pap. (*0-930958-10-1*, EP085ML) Excptnl Parent.

***When Your Body Gets the Blues.** Marie-Annette Brown & Jo Robinson. 2002. LC 2001-6285. 208p. 22.95 (*1-57954-486-X*) Rodale Pr Inc.

When Your Child Is Chemically Dependent. Dennis C. Daley & Judy Miller. 1995. 16p. pap. 4.95 (*1-56246-026-9*, 3176, HazeldenJohnson Inst) Hazelden.

When Your Child Is Deaf: A Guide for Parents. David M. Luterman & Mark Ross. 1991. LC 91-3239. (Illus.). 182p. pap. text 20.25 (*0-912752-27-0*) York Pr.

When Your Child Is Ready to Return to School. 1994. (*0-944093-32-9*); 1992. (*0-944093-21-3*); 1989. (*0-944093-13-2*) Am Brain Tumor.

***When Your Child Is Seriously Injured: The Emotional Impact on Families.** Marilyn Lash. 1990. (Illus.). 39p. reprint ed. pap. (*0-930958-11-X*, EP005ML) Excptnl Parent.

When Your Child Struggles: The Myths of 20/20. David L. Cook. 4th ed. 1991. (Illus.). 173p. (Orig.). reprint ed. pap. text 22.00 (*0-9632657-0-9*) Cook Vision.

When Your Friend Gets Cancer: How You Can Help. Amy Harwell & Kristine Tomasik. 2000. LC 87-9547. 128p. (Orig.). pap. 8.99 (*0-87788-934-1*, H Shaw Pubs) Waterbrook Pr.

When You're Ill or Incapacitated/When You're the Caregiver: 12 Things to Remember in Times of Sickness, Injury or Disability/12 Things to Do if Someone You Care For is Ill or Incapacitated. James E. Miller. 1995. LC 95-90163. (Illus.). 64p. reprint ed. pap. 6.95 (*1-885933-21-5*) Willowgreen Pubng.

When You're Ready: A Woman's Healing from Childhood Physical & Sexual Abuse by Her Mother. Kathy Evert. 1987. LC 87-82076. 194p. pap. 9.95 (*0-9613205-4-0*) Launch Pr.

Where Analysis Meets the Arts: The Integration of the Arts Therapies with Psychoanalytic Theory. Ed. by Yvonne Searle & Isabelle Sterng. 2001. 220p. pap. (*1-85575-184-4*) Karnac Bks GBR. *Dist:* Other Pr LLC.

Where Coverage Ends: Catastrophic Illness & Long-Term Health Care. Ed. by Employee Benefit Research Institute Staff. 1988. LC 88-16237. (Orig.). (C). pap. text 10.25 (*0-8191-7364-9*) U Pr of Amer.

Where Coverage Ends: Catastrophic Illness & Long-Term Health Care Costs. 1988. LC 88-16237. pap. 19.95 (*0-86643-061-X*) Empl Benefit Res Inst.

Where Did Mary Go? A Loving Husband's Struggle with Alzheimers. Frank A. Wall. 1996. LC 96-16700. (Golden Age Bks.). (Illus.). 148p. 24.00 (*1-57392-070-3*) Prometheus Bks.

Where Does It Hurt? The Story of a New England Country Doctor. Aubrey V. Gould. (Orig.). 1987. (Illus.). 86p. pap. 7.95 (*0-9619628-0-1*); 2nd rev. ed. 1996. LC 90-82594. 123p. (*0-9619628-5-2*) Fieldside Pub.

***Where Id Was: Challenging Normalization in Psychoanalysis.** Ed. by Anthony Molino & Christine Ware. 2001. LC 2001-45370. (Disseminations: Psychoanalysis in Contexts Ser.). 240p. pap. 24.95 (*0-8195-6481-8*); lib. bdg. 60.00 (*0-8195-6480-X*) U Pr of New Eng (Wesleyan Univ Pr).

Where Medicine Fails. Ed. by Anselm L. Strauss. 4th ed. 1984. 400p. pap. text 24.95 (*0-87855-951-5*) Transaction Pubs.

Where Medicine Fails. Ed. by Carolyn Wiener & Anselm L. Strauss. 5th ed. 1996. LC 96-13279. 407p. pap. text 24.95 (*1-56000-869-5*) Transaction Pubs.

Where Mystery Dwells: A Psychiatrist Studies Psychical Phenomena. B. J. Laubscher. 1972. 272p. (*0-227-67801-X*) J Clarke Co Ltd GBR. *Dist:* Parkwest Pubns.

Where Remedies Lie. O. Victor Miller & James A. Hotz. Ed. by Louis Emond. 1997. LC 98-125966. (Illus.). x, 320p. 29.95 (*0-9658029-0-6*) Caduceus Pr.

Where the Roots Reach for Water: A Personal & Natural History of Melancholia. Jeffery Smith. 304p. 2001. pap. 13.00 (*0-86547-592-X*); 1999. LC 98-50420. 24.00 (*0-86547-542-3*) N Point Pr.

Where There Is No Dentist. Murray Dickson. Ed. by Michael Blake. 1983. LC 82-84067. (Illus.). 192p. pap. 12.00 (*0-942364-05-8*) Hesperian Found.

Where There Is No Doctor: A Village Health Care Handbook. David B. Werner et al. rev. ed. 1992. LC 92-1539.Tr. of Donde No Hay Doctor. (Illus.). 504p. reprint ed. pap. 17.00 (*0-942364-15-5*) Hesperian Found.

Where to Go When You're Hurting: A Healing Resource Guide. Elizabeth Rosenthal. 1998. 216p. pap. 19.95 (*0-9660472-0-6*) EMPR.

Where to Start & What to Ask: The Assessment Handbook. Susan Lukas. 1993. LC 92-49934. 220p. (C). pap. 15.95 (*0-393-70152-2*) Norton.

Where Women Have No Doctor: A Health Guide for Women. A. August Burns et al. Ed. by Sandy Niemann. 1997. LC 97-19421. pap. 20.00 (*0-942364-25-2*) Hesperian Found.

Where's the Evidence? Convtroversies in Modern Medicine. William A. Silverman. 1999. 278p. pap. text 32.50 (*0-19-263088-1*) OUP.

Which Babies Shall Live? Humanistic Dimensions of the Care of Imperiled Newborns. Ed. by Thomas H. Murray & Arthur L. Caplan. 1985. LC 85-18058. (Contemporary Issues in Biomedicine, Ethics, & Society Ser.). 238p. 49.50 (*0-89603-086-5*) Humana.

Which Doctor? David G. Green. 1985. (Research Monographs: No. 40). 84p. (Orig.). (C). pap. text (*0-255-36183-1*) Transatl Arts.

Which Tests for My Unborn Baby? Ultrasound & Other Prenatal Tests. Lachlan De Crespigny & Rhonda Dredge. 2nd ed. 1997. LC 97-180922. (Illus.). 196p. pap. 21.95 (*0-19-553954-0*) OUP.

While Dragons Sleep: How to Solve a Chemical Dependence Problem. Tom Kwasnik. 1991. LC 90-83989. (Illus.). 272p. (Orig.). pap. 12.95 (*0-9627555-0-8*) Able Pr.

Whining. Tamara Eberlein. 1997. (Child's Magazine Guide to Ser.). 208p. per. 5.99 (*0-671-88042-X*) PB.

Whiplash: Mechanisms & Management. Larry S. Nordhoff. 1992. LC 92-49445. 608p. 64.95 (*0-8016-6821-2*) Mosby Inc.

Whiplash & Related Headaches. Bernard Swerdlow. 1998. LC 98-41106. 1104p. 99.95 (*1-57444-232-5*) CRC Pr.

Whiplash & the Jaw Joint: TMJ Injury. Dale M. Foreman & Donald Rolfs. 2nd rev. ed. 1991. (Illus.). 85.00 (*0-939737-01-9*) Bk Pub Co WA.

Whiplash Encyclopedia: The Facts & Myths of Whiplash. Robert Ferrari. 1995. LC 99-21053. 920p. 132.00 (*0-8342-1661-2*) Aspen Pub.

Whiplash Handbook. Monique B. Harriton. 1989. (Illus.). 108p. 33.95 (*0-398-05598-X*); pap. 19.95 (*0-398-06380-X*) C C Thomas.

Whiplash Injuries: Current Concepts in Prevention, Diagnosis & Treatment of the Cervical Whiplash Syndrome. Marek Szpalski. 1997. LC 97-30023. 368p. text 129.00 (*0-397-51856-0*) Lppncott W & W.

Whiplash Injuries: The Cervical Acceleration/ Deceleration Syndrome. Stephen Foreman & Arthur C. Croft. 2nd ed. 1995. (Illus.). 512p. 99.00 (*0-683-03315-8*) Lppncott W & W.

Whiplash Injuries & Disequilibrium: Diagnosis & Treatment. D. Alpini & N. Cesarini. 1997. (Illus.). 260p. 130.00 (*3-540-75015-0*) Spr-Verlag.

Whipping Hidden Allergies. Harris Hosen. 1994. pap. text 17.75 (*0-9622762-2-7*) Non-Fictitious.

Whips & Kisses: Parting the Leather Curtain. Mistress Jacqueline. 1991. LC 90-27046. (Illus.). 236p. (C). 30.00 (*0-87975-656-X*) Prometheus Bks.

Whisper of Espionage: Wolfgang Kohler & the Apes of Tenerife. Ronald Ley. 1997. (Illus.). 264p. reprint ed. text 20.00 (*0-7881-5134-7*) DIANE Pub.

Whispers: The Voices of Paranoia. Ronald K. Siegel. 1996. 320p. per. 14.00 (*0-684-80285-6*, Touchstone) S&S Trade Pap.

Whispers from the East: Applying the Principles of Eastern Healing to Psychotherapy. Frances E. Steinberg & Richard G. Whiteside. 1998. LC 98-38991. (Illus.). 178p. 34.95 (*1-891944-04-5*) Zeig Tucker Theisen.

Whistleblowing in the Health Service: Accountability, Law & Professional Practice. Ed. by Geoffrey Hunt. 1994. 192p. pap. text 32.95 (*1-56593-502-0*, 1162) Singular Publishing.

Whistleblowing in the Health Service: Accountability, Law & Professional Practice. Ed. by Geoffrey Hunt. 1995. 170p. pap. (*0-340-59234-6*) E A GBR. *Dist:* Routldge.

White Blood Cells. U. Bagge & G. V. Born. 1982. text 112.50 (*90-247-2681-6*) Kluwer Academic.

White Cell. Martin J. Cline. 1975. LC 74-25998. (Commonwealth Fund Publications). (Illus.). 616p. 50.00 (*0-674-95142-5*) HUP.

White Cell Manual. Alan Winkelstein et al. 5th ed. 1998. LC 97-50157. (Illus.). 143p. (C). pap. text 22.95 (*0-8036-0305-3*) Davis Co.

White Cell Rheology & Inflammation. Ed. by K. Messmer & F. Hammersen. 1985. (Mikrozirkulation in Forschung und Klinik Ser.: Vol. 7). (Illus.). x, 124p. pap. 61.75 (*3-8055-4040-X*) S Karger.

White Chocolate. Michael D. Helzner. 1999. LC 97-66996. 176p. pap. 14.50 (*0-88739-160-5*) Creat Arts Bk.

White Coat: Becoming a Doctor at Harvard Medical School. Ellen L. Rothman. 1999. LC 98-38202. 352p. 25.00 (*0-688-15313-5*, Wm Morrow) Morrow Avon.

White Death: A History of Tuberculosis. Thomas Dormandy. 1998. LC 98-38008. (*1-85285-169-4*) Hambledon Press.

White House Doctor. T. Burton Smith & Carter Henderson. 1992. LC 92-31506. 224p. 24.95 (*0-8191-8625-2*) Madison Bks UPA.

White Knuckles & Wishful Thinking: Learning from the Moment of Relapse in Alcoholism & Other Addictions. George Manter Du Wors & Everett Washington. 2nd exp. rev. ed. 2000. LC 99-45881. (Illus.). xviii, 393p. pap. text 17.50 (*0-88937-224-1*) Hogrefe & Huber Pubs.

White Man's Medicine: Government Doctors & the Navajo, 1863-1955. Curtus et al. 1998. LC 97-36481. 290p. 39.95 (*0-8263-1839-8*) Univ of New Mexico Schl.

White Sapt Dental Technology. White. 1996. mass mkt. (*0-7234-2334-2*) Wolfe Publishing GBR. *Dist:* Mosby Inc.

White Spirit (Stoddard Solvent) 1996. (Environmental Health Criteria Ser.: No. 187). 186p. pap. 36.00 (*92-4-157187-X*, 1160187) Am Soc Clinical.

Whitman & the Romance of Medicine. Robert L. Davis. 1997. LC 96-39258. 205p. text 40.00 (*0-520-20760-2*) U CA Pr.

***WHO - Classification of Lymphomas.** H. Stein. 2002. (Illus.). 2002p. (*3-540-67709-7*) Springer Pub.

Who? What? Where? Resources for Women's Health & Aging. 1993. 82p. (Orig.). (C). pap. text 25.00 (*1-56806-943-X*) DIANE Pub.

Who Am I? Identity, Adoption & Human Fertilisation. C. Walby & B. Symons. 1989. (C). (*0-903534-87-8*) Brit Ag for Adopt & Fost GBR. *Dist:* St Mut.

Who Calls the Tune? A Psychodramtic Approach to Child Therapy. Bernadette Hoey. 1997. LC 96-6387. 168p. (C). 68.95 (*0-415-14572-4*); pap. 24.95 (*0-415-14573-2*) Routledge.

Who Cares? Institutional Barriers to Health Care for Lesbian, Gay & Bisexual Persons. Michele Eliason. 1996. LC 96-17319. 220p. pap. 29.95 (*0-88737-676-2*) Natl League Nurse.

Who Cares? True Stories of the NHS Reforms. Peter Bruggen. 1998. LC 98-175073. 720p. pap. (*1-897766-32-7*) Jon Carpenter GBR. *Dist:* Paul & Co Pubs.

Who Cares about Health? Caleb Gattegno. 1979. 166p. pap. text 14.95 (*0-87825-149-9*) Ed Solutions.

Who Cares for the Caregiver? Learning to Take Care of Yourself While Caring for Others. Sunny Bat-or. 1995. (In Service Sourcebook Ser.). 64p. pap. text 29.95 (*1-888343-03-6*) Hartman Pub.

Who Cares for Them? Workers in the Home Care Industry, 16. Penny H. Feldman et al. 1990. LC 89-17234. (Contributions to the Study of Aging Ser.: No. 16). 256p. 65.00 (*0-313-26837-1*, FWH/, Greenwood Pr) Greenwood.

Who Controls the Local Hospital? Mary Gabay & Sidney M. Wolfe. 1996. 39p. (Orig.). pap. 15.00 (*0-937188-11-5*) Pub Citizen.

Who Decides? Conflicts of Rights in Health Care. Ed. by Nora K. Bell. 1982. LC 81-83908. (Contemporary Issues in Biomedicine, Ethics & Society Ser.). 218p. 44.50 (*0-89603-034-2*) Humana.

Who Decides? Making Decisions on Behalf of Mentally Incapacitated Adults, Command Paper 3803. 1998. (Command Papers: No. 81011068). (*0-10-138032-1*, HM80321) Statnry Office GBR. *Dist:* Bernan Associates.

WHO Expert Committee on Addiction-Producing Drugs. 1964. (Technical Report Ser.: No. 273). 20p. pap. text 3.00 (*92-4-120273-4*) World Health.

WHO Expert Committee on Bilharziasis. 1965. (Technical Report Ser.: No. 299). 56p. pap. text 5.00 (*92-4-120299-8*) World Health.

WHO Expert Committee on Biological Standardization. (Technical Report Ser.: No. 700). 1984. 75p. pap. text 7.00 (*92-4-120700-0*); 1983. 184p. pap. text 13.00 (*92-4-120687-X*); 1982. 180p. pap. text 13.00 (*92-4-120673-X*); 1981. 325p. pap. text 21.00 (*92-4-120658-6*) World Health.

WHO Expert Committee on Biological Standardization: 35th Report. 1985. (Technical Reports: No. 725). 140p. pap. text 11.00 (*92-4-120725-6*, 1100725) World Health.

WHO Expert Committee on Biological Standardization: 45th Report. 1995. (Technical Report Ser.: Vol. 858). (FRE & SPA.). 102p. (C). pap. 17.00 (*92-4-120858-9*, 1100858) World Health.

WHO Expert Committee on Biological Standardization: Proceedings of the WHO Expert Committee, 26th, Geneva, 1974. WHO Staff. 1975. (Technical Reports: No. 565). pap. text 7.00 (*92-4-120565-2*, 1100565) World Health.

WHO Expert Committee on Biological Standardization: Twenty-Eighth Report of the WHO Expert Committee. 1977. (Technical Report Ser.: No. 610). 133p. pap. text 11.00 (*92-4-120610-1*, 1100610) World Health.

WHO Expert Committee on Biological Standardization Thirty Sixth Report. 1987. (Technical Reports: No. 745). 149p. pap. text 20.00 (*92-4-120745-0*, 1100745) World Health.

WHO Expert Committee on Cholera: Second Report of a WHO Expert Committee. 1967. (Technical Report Ser.). 28p. pap. text 3.00 (*92-4-120352-8*, 1100352) World Health.

WHO Expert Committee on Dependence-Producing Drugs. 1965. (Technical Report Ser.: No. 312). 16p. pap. text 3.00 (*92-4-120312-9*) World Health.

WHO Expert Committee on Dependence-Producing Drugs: Fifteenth Report of the WHO Expert Committee. 1966. (Technical Report Ser.: No. 343). 18p. pap. text 3.00 (*92-4-120343-9*, 1100343) World Health.

WHO Expert Committee on Diabetes Mellitus: Second Report of the WHO Expert Committee. 1980. (Technical Report Ser.: No. 646). 79p. pap. text 5.00 (*92-4-120646-2*, 1100646) World Health.

WHO Expert Committee on Drug Dependence: 22nd Report. 1985. (Technical Reports: No. 729). 31p. pap. text 4.00 (*92-4-120729-9*, 1100729) World Health.

WHO Expert Committee on Drug Dependence: 23rd Report. 1987. (Technical Reports: No. 741). 64p. pap. text 9.00 (*92-4-120741-8*, 1100741) World Health.

WHO Expert Committee on Drug Dependence: 27th Report. 1991. (Technical Reports: No. 808). (ENG, FRE & SPA.). 17p. pap. text 6.00 (*92-4-120808-2*, 1100808) World Health.

WHO Expert Committee on Drug Dependence: 28th Report. 1993. (Technical Reports: No. 836). (ENG, FRE & SPA.). vi, 44p. pap. text 10.00 (*92-4-120836-8*, 1101836) World Health.

WHO Expert Committee on Drug Dependence: 29th Report. 1995. (Technical Reports: No. 856). (FRE & SPA.). iv, 17p. (C). pap. text 6.00 (*92-4-120856-2*, 1100856) World Health.

WHO Expert Committee on Drug Dependence: Proceedings of the WHO Expert Committee, 17th, Geneva, 1969. WHO Staff. 1970. (Technical Reports: No. 437). pap. text 5.00 (*92-4-120437-0*, 1100437) World Health.

WHO Expert Committee on Drug Dependence: Proceedings of the WHO Expert Committee, 19th, Geneva, 1972. WHO Staff. 1973. (Technical Reports: No. 526). pap. text 4.00 (*92-4-120526-1*, 1100526) World Health.

WHO Expert Committee on Drug Dependence: Twenty-First Report of the WHO Expert Committee. 1978. (Technical Report Ser.: No. 618). 49p. pap. text 6.00 (*92-4-120618-7*, 1100618) World Health.

WHO Expert Committee on Filariasis: Proceedings of the WHO Expert Committee, 3rd, Athens, 1973. WHO Staff. 1974. (Technical Reports: No. 542). pap. text 5.00 (*92-4-120542-3*, 1100542) World Health.

WHO Expert Committee on Filariasis (Wuchereria & Brugia Infections)- Second Report of the WHO Expert Committee. 1967. (Technical Report Ser.: No. 359). 47p. pap. text 5.00 (*92-4-120359-5*, 1100359) World Health.

WHO Expert Committee on Hepatitis. 1964. (Technical Report Ser.: No. 285). 25p. pap. text 3.00 (*92-4-120285-8*) World Health.

WHO Expert Committee on Leprosy: 6th Report. WHO Staff. 1988. (Technical Report Ser.: No. 768). 51p. 8.00 (*92-4-120768-X*) World Health.

WHO Expert Committee on Leprosy: Fifth Report of the WHO Expert Committee. 1977. (Technical Report Ser.: No. 607). 48p. pap. text 6.00 (*92-4-120607-1*, 1100607) World Health.

WHO Expert Committee on Leprosy: Proceedings of the WHO Expert Committee, 4th, Geneva, 1970. WHO Staff. 1970. (Technical Reports: No. 459). pap. text 5.00 (*92-4-120459-1*, 1100459) World Health.

WHO Expert Committee on Malaria. 1964. (Technical Report Ser.: No. 291). 46p. pap. text 5.00 (*92-4-120291-2*) World Health.

WHO Expert Committee on Malaria: 18th Report. 1986. (Technical Reports: No. 735). 104p. pap. text 14.00 (*92-4-120735-3*, 1100735) World Health.

WHO Expert Committee on Malaria: Seventeenth Report of the WHO Expert Committee. 1979. (Technical Report Ser.: No. 640). 71p. pap. text 5.00 (*92-4-120640-3*, 1100640) World Health.

WHO Expert Committee on Medical Rehabilitation: Proceedings of the WHO Expert Committee, 2nd, Geneva, 1968. WHO Staff. 1969. (Technical Reports: No. 419). pap. text 3.00 (*92-4-120419-2*, 1100419) World Health.

WHO Expert Committee on Nursing: Fifth Report of the WHO Expert Committee. 1966. (Technical Report Ser.). 32p. pap. text 3.00 (*92-4-120347-1*, 1100347) World Health.

WHO Expert Committee on Onchocerciasis Third Report. 1987. (Technical Reports: No. 752). 167p. pap. text 21.60 (*92-4-120752-3*, 1100752) World Health.

WHO Expert Committee on Plague: Proceedings of the WHO Expert Committee, 4th, Geneva, 1969. WHO Staff. 1970. (Technical Reports: No. 447). pap. text 3.00 (*92-4-120447-8*, 1100447) World Health.

WHO Expert Committee on Rabies. 1966. (Technical Report Ser.: No. 321). 38p. pap. text 5.00 (*92-4-120321-8*) World Health.

WHO Expert Committee on Rabies: 8th Report. 1992. (Technical Reports: No. 824). (ENG, FRE & SPA.). vii, 84p. pap. text 12.00 (*92-4-120824-4*, 1100824) World Health.

WHO Expert Committee on Rabies: Proceedings of the WHO Expert Committee, 6th, Geneva, 1972. WHO Staff. 1973. (Technical Reports: No. 523). pap. text 4.00 (*92-4-120523-7*, 1100523) World Health.

WHO Expert Committee on Smallpox. 1964. (Technical Report Ser.: No. 283). 37p. pap. text 5.00 (*92-4-120283-1*) World Health.

WHO Expert Committee on Specifications for Pharmaceutical Preparations. (Technical Report Ser.: No. 681). 1982. 33p. pap. text 4.00 (*92-4-120681-0*); 1965. 31p. pap. text 3.00 (*92-4-120307-2*) World Health.

WHO Expert Committee on Specifications for Pharmaceutical Preparations: 32nd Report. 1992. (Technical Reports: No. 823). (ENG, FRE & SPA.). vi, 134p. pap. text 17.00 (*92-4-120823-6*, 1100823) World Health.

WHO Expert Committee on Specifications for Pharmaceutical Preparations: 33rd Report. 1993. (Technical Reports: No. 834). (ENG, FRE & SPA.). v, 30p. pap. text 7.00 (*92-4-120834-1*, 1100834) World Health.

WHO Expert Committee on Specifications for Pharmaceutical Preparations: 34th Report of a WHO Expert Committee. 1996. (WHO Technical Reports: Vol. 863). 194p. pap. 31.50 (*92-4-120863-5*, 1100863) World Health.

WHO Expert Committee on Specifications for Pharmaceutical Preparations: Proceedings of the WHO Expert Committee, 22nd, Geneva, 1968. WHO Staff. 1969. (Technical Reports: No. 418). pap. text 5.00 (*92-4-120418-4*, 1100418) World Health.

WHO Expert Committee on Specifications for Pharmaceutical Preparations: Twenty-Sixth Report of the WHO Expert Committee. 1977. (Technical Report Ser.: No. 614). 53p. pap. text 7.00 (*92-4-120614-4*, 1100614) World Health.

WHO Expert Committee on Specifications for Pharmaceutical Preparations Thirtieth Report. 1987. (Technical Reports: No. 748). 50p. pap. text 9.00 (*92-4-120748-5*, 1100748) World Health.

WHO Expert Committee on Venereal Diseases & Treponematoses: 6th Report. 1986. (Technical Reports: No. 736). 141p. pap. text 18.00 (*92-4-120736-1*, 1100736) World Health.

Who Gave Pinta to Santa Maria? Robert S. Desowitz. 1998. LC 98-15031. (Illus.). 256p. (C). pap. 13.00 (*0-15-600585-9*, Harvest Bks) Harcourt.

Who Gave Pinta to the Santa Maria? Tropical Diseases in a Temperate Climate. Robert S. Desowitz. 1997. LC 96-44741. 256p. 25.00 (*0-393-04084-4*) Norton.

Who Gets Health Care? An Arena for Nursing Action. Ed. by Barbara Kos-Munson. 1992. LC 92-48981. 80p. 22.95 (*0-8261-8240-2*) Springer Pub.

WHO Global Programme on AIDS: 1991 Progress Report. 1992. ix, 136p. pap. text 26.00 (*92-4-156156-4*, 1150391) World Health.

Who Goes First? The Story of Self-Experimentation in Medicine. Lawrence K. Altman. 1998. LC 97-42122. 454p. pap. 22.50 (*0-520-21281-9*) U CA Pr.

***Who Guide to Mental Health in Primary Care.** David Goldberg et al. 2000. 195p. pap. (*1-85315-451-2*) Royal Soc of Medicine Pr Ltd GBR. *Dist:* Balogh.

WHO Handbook for Reporting Results of Cancer Treatment. WHO Staff. 1979. (WHO Offset Publications: No. 48). 45p. 6.00 (*92-4-170048-3*) World Health.

WHO Handbook for Standardized Cancer Registries. 1976. (Offset Publications: No. 25). pap. text 9.00 (*92-4-170025-4*, 1120025) World Health.

Who Has Seen a Blood Sugar? Reflections on Medical Education. Frank Davidoff et al. 1996. LC 96-2019. 232p. 25.00 (*0-943126-47-9*) Amer Coll Phys.

WHO-Histological Typing of Tumours of the Eye & Its Adnexa. R. J. Campbell & L. E. Zimmerman. 2nd rev. ed. 1998. LC 98-26176. (International Histological Classification of Tumors Ser.). (Illus.). 123p. pap. 75.00 (*3-540-64131-9*) Spr-Verlag.

WHO in Europe: Meeting the Challenges. WHO Regional Office for Europe Staff. 1995. (WHO Regional Publications, European Ser.: No. 57). (Illus.). 17p. pap. 10.80 (*92-890-1321-4*, 1310057) World Health.

WHO in Europe, 1991. 1991. (WHO Regional Publications, European Ser.: No. 41). 17p. pap. text 12.00 (*92-890-1304-4*) World Health.

Who Is Insane? Stephen Smith. Ed. by Gerald N. Grob. 1980. LC 78-22590. (Historical Issues in Mental Health Ser.). reprint ed. lib. bdg. 23.95 (*0-405-11941-0*) Ayer.

Who Kids Turn to When They're in Trouble: Will Kids Choose You? 1992. 32p. pap. 5.50 (*1-56246-060-9*, 3205, HazeldenJohnson Inst) Hazelden.

WHO Laboratory Manual for the Examination of Human Semen & Sperm-Cervical Mucus Interaction. World Health Organization Staff. 3rd ed. 1993. (Illus.). 115p. (C). pap. text 37.95 (*0-521-42168-3*) Cambridge U Pr.

WHO Laboratory Manual for the Examination of Human Semen & Sperm-Cervical Mucus Interaction. 4th ed. 1999. LC 98-46890. (Illus.). 138p. (C). pap. text, lab manual ed. 41.95 (*0-521-64599-9*) Cambridge U Pr.

Who Lives Happily Ever After? For Families Whose Child Has Died Violently. Sharon Turnbull. Ed. by Joy Johnson. 1990. (Illus.). 24p. pap. 3.50 (*1-56123-000-6*) Centering Corp.

WHO Manual for the Standardized Investigation & Diagnosis of the Infertile Couple. Patrick J. Rowe et al. 1993. (Illus.). 91p. (C). pap. text 42.95 (*0-521-43136-0*) Cambridge U Pr.

WHO Manual for the Standardized Investigation, Diagnosis & Management of the Infertile Male. P. J. Rowe et al. 2000. LC 2001-278080. (Illus.). 102p. (C). pap. text 39.95 (*0-521-77474-8*) Cambridge U Pr.

WHO Model Prescribing Information: Drugs Used in Anaesthesia. 1989. (ENG & FRE.). 53p. pap. text 11.00 (*92-4-140101-X*, 1150333) World Health.

WHO Model Prescribing Information: Drugs Used in Mycobacterial Diseases. 1991. (ENG, FRE & SPA.). 40p. pap. text 9.00 (*92-4-140103-6*, 1150363) World Health.

Who Model Prescribing Information: Drugs Used in Parasitic Diseases. 2nd ed. 1995. (WHO Model Prescribing Information Ser.). (FRE & SPA.). 146p. (C). pap. 35.00 (*92-4-140104-4*, 1152343) World Health.

WHO Model Prescribing Information: Drugs Used in Sexually Transmitted Diseases & HIV Infection. 1995. LC 96-174708. (FRE & SPA.). 97p. (C). pap. 25.00 (*92-4-140105-2*, 1150429) World Health.

Who Needs Hair: The Flip Side of Chemotherapy. Sallie Burdine. 2001. (Illus.). 100p. pap. 16.95 (*0-9705464-8-3*) SABA Bks.

Who Needs Headaches? Why Suffer if You Don't Have To? Cass Igram. 1991. LC 91-90550. pap. 13.95 (*0-911119-32-9*) Knowledge Hse.

Who Needs Headaches? Why Suffer If You Don't Have To? Cass Igram. 1991. 18.95 (*0-911119-36-1*) Knowledge Hse.

Who Owns Our Bodies? Making Moral Choices in Health Care. John Spiers & Institute of Health Services Management Staff. 1997. LC 96-30000. 112p. pap. (*1-85775-210-4*) Radcliffe Med Pr GBR. *Dist:* Balogh.

Who Plays? Who Pays? Who Cares? A Case Study in Applied Sociology, Political Economy, & the Community Mental Health Centers Movement. Sylvia Kenig. 1992. (Critical Approaches in the Health Social Sciences Ser.). 235p. text 42.00 (*0-89503-093-4*); pap. text 31.50 (*0-89503-092-6*) Baywood Pub.

Who Pocket Guide to Classification of Mental & Behavioural Disorders: With Glossary & Diagnostic Criteria for Research. Compiled by J. E. Cooper. 1994. LC 94-26148. 422p. pap. text 27.95 (*0-88048-983-9*, 8983) Am Psychiatric.

Who Should Decide? Paternalism in Health Care. James F. Childress. 1985. 264p. pap. text 19.95 (*0-19-503976-9*) OUP.

Who Should Run the Health Service? Realignment & Reconstruction. Olusola O. Oni. 1996. LC 96-33577. (*1-85775-169-8*) Radcliffe Med Pr GBR. *Dist:* Balogh.

Who Should We Treat? Law, Patients, & Resources in the NHS. Christopher Newdick. 1995. LC 95-9156. 368p. pap. text 28.00 (*0-19-825925-5*) OUP.

Who Survives Cancer? Howard P. Greenwald. 1992. LC 91-36909. 280p. text 35.00 (*0-520-07725-3*) U CA Pr.

Who Was Zwingli? A Journal of Archetype & Culture, No. 56. Ed. by James Hillman et al. 1994. (Journal Ser.: Vol. 56). 176p. (Orig.). pap. 17.50 (*1-882670-04-3*) Spring Jrnl.

Whole Body Computed Tomography. Michael Galanski & Mathias Prokop. 2001. (Illus.). 544p. 129.00 (*0-86577-870-1*) Thieme Med Pubs.

Whole-Body Computed Tomography. Otto H. Wegener. Tr. by Suzyon O. Wandrey from GER. 2nd enl. rev. ed. 1992. LC 92-35853.Tr. of Ganzk Orper-Computertomographie. 632p. 199.95 (*0-86542-223-0*) Blackwell Sci.

Whole Body Computed Tomography CD-ROM. Otto H. Wegener. 1994. cd-rom 209.95 (*0-86542-947-2*) Blackwell Sci.

Whole Body Dentistry: Discover the Missing Piece to Better Health. Mark A. Breiner. 1999. LC 99-70461. (Illus.). 240p. pap. 19.95 (*0-9678443-0-4*) Quantum Hlth Pr.

Whole Body Hyperthermia: Biological & Clinical Aspects. Ed. by Michael Gautherie. 1992. (Clinical Thermology Ser.). (Illus.). 85p. 103.00 (*0-387-54560-3*) Spr-Verlag.

Whole-Body Irradiation. 1997. lib. bdg. 250.95 (*0-8490-7707-9*) Gordon Pr.

Whole Child Pediatrician. Mark Nesselson. 2000. 26.00 (*0-8129-3223-4*) Random.

Whole Emergency Department Catalog. Michael S. Jastremski et al. 1985. (Illus.). 416p. text 65.00 (*0-7216-1175-3*) Saunders.

Whole Health: The Guide to Wellness of Body & Mind. Joseph Keon. 1997. LC 95-70987. (Illus.). 465p. (Orig.). pap. 24.00 (*0-9648974-8-2*) Parissound.

Whole Health Shiatsu: Health & Vitality for Everyone. Shizuko Yamamoto & Patrick McCarty. 1992. (Illus.). 288p. (Orig.). pap. 25.00 (*0-87040-874-7*) Japan Pubns USA.

Whole Memory Recovery. Beverly Sheridan. 1993. 154p. pap. text 11.95 (*0-913412-68-6*) Brandon Hse.

Whole Mind: The Definitive Guide to Complementary Treatments for Mind, Mood, & Emotion. Ed. by Lynette Bassman. 1998. LC 97-31585. 574p. pap. 22.95 (*1-57731-050-0*) New Wrld Lib.

Whole Organ Approaches to Cellular Metabolism: Permeation, Cellular Uptake & Product Formation. Carl A. Goresky et al. 1998. LC 98-12963. (Illus.). 596p. 129.00 (*0-387-94975-5*) Spr-Verlag.

Whole Parent - Whole Child: A Parents Guide to Raising the Child with a Chronic Illness. Broatch Haig & Patricia M. Moynihan. 1989. LC 88-30988. (Orig.). pap. 9.95 (*0-937721-53-0*) Wiley.

Whole Surgery Handbook. David Mclanahan. 1999. text 23.95 (*0-525-93798-6*) Viking Penguin.

***Whole Surgery Handbook: How You Can Help Yourself Have Successful Surgery or Avoid It.** David McLanahan. 1999. pap. (*0-452-27188-6*) Dutton Plume.

Whole-Systems Shared Governance: Architecture for Integration. Timothy Porter-O'Grady et al. 1997. LC 97-10153. 323p. 59.00 (*0-8342-0951-9*, 20951) Aspen Pub.

Whole Tooth. Marvin Schissel. 1997. LC 96-27462. (Illus.). 320p. 23.95 (*0-312-15229-9*) St Martin.

Whole Truth about Contraception: A Guide to Safe & Effective Choices. Beverly Winikoff & Suzanne Wymelenberg. 1997. LC 97-26488. (Illus.). 242p. (Orig.). pap. 16.95 (*0-309-05494-X*, Joseph Henry Pr) Natl Acad Pr.

Whole Woman Homeopathy: The Comprehensive Guide to Treating PMS, Menopause, Cystitis & Other Problems. Judyth Reichenberg-Ullman. 4th ed. 2000. LC 00-35648. (Illus.). 368p. pap. 18.00 (*0-7615-2411-8*, Prima Health) Prima Pub.

Wholesomeness of Irradiated Food. 1981. (Technical Report Ser.: No. 659). 34p. pap. text 3.00 (*92-4-120659-4*) World Health.

Wholism & Wholistic Health: The Individual in a Personal Context - Ecology - Our Home & Heritage Held in Trust. Richard L. Crews. 1988. 40p. (C). pap. text (*0-945864-09-4*) Columbia Pacific U Pr.

Wholism & Wholistic Health: The Individual in a Personal Context - Health & Healing - Ultimate Perspectives & Practicalities. Richard L. Crews. 1988. 45p. (C). pap. text (*0-945864-10-8*) Columbia Pacific U Pr.

Wholism & Wholistic Health: The Individual in a Personal Context - Wholism - The Concept, Its Origins & Implications. Richard L. Crews. 1988. 29p. (C). pap. text (*0-945864-08-6*) Columbia Pacific U Pr.

Wholistic Healing: How to Harmonize Your Body, Mind & Spirit with Life, for Freedom, Joy, Health, Beauty, Love, Money & Psychic Powers. Elan Z. Neev. rev. ed. 1977. LC 77-71152. (Illus.). pap. 10.95 (*0-918482-00-3*) Ageless Bks.

Who's Afraid? The Phobic's Handbook. Barbara Fried. rev. ed. 1985. LC 84-28671. (Illus.). 100p. reprint ed. 16.95 (*0-89876-104-2*) Gardner Pr.

***Who's Afraid of Genetics in Medicine: Understanding the Basics of the Biogenetic Process.** Debbie Dean. 2001. 25.00 (*0-7388-6681-4*); pap. 16.00 (*0-7388-6680-6*) Xlibris Corp.

Who's Boss? Training Your Pre-Schooler in Self-Management. Francis H. Wise. Ed. & Intro. by Joyce M. Wise. 1982. LC 82-91074. (Illus.). 220p. (Orig.). (C). pap. 8.00 (*0-915766-58-2*) Wise Pub.

Who's in Charge Here? The Patient As Primary Caregiver. Jimmie R. Rankin. 1993. (Literature of Patient Response Ser.: Vol. II). 70p. pap. 12.95 (*1-883938-05-8*) Dry Bones Pr.

Who's in Charge Here? For LTC Charge Nurses: A Guidebook for the Long Term Care Charge Nurse. Sharon Baker. 1998. 132p. (C). 18.00 (*1-877735-26-4*, 2157PP) Prof Prnting & Pub.

Who's That Girl? Who's That Boy? Clinical Practice Meets Postmodern Gender Theory. Lynne Layton. LC 97-40089. 288p. 1999. pap. text 30.00 (*0-7657-0182-0*); 1998. 40.00 (*0-7657-0140-5*) Aronson.

Who's Who in American Nursing, 1996-1997. Ed. by Marquis Who's Who Staff. 6th ed. 1995. 806p. 149.95 (*0-8379-1004-8*) Marquis.

Who's Who in Managed Health Care: 1999 Edition. Brad Bangerter & Healthquest Editors. 5th rev. ed. 1999. 287p. pap. 119.00 (*0-9639238-7-0*) HlthQuest Pubs.

Who's Who in Managed Healthcare: Profiles of Key Decision Makers in Today's Leading Health Care Organizations. Brad Bangerter. Ed. by Laura Bangerter. 5th rev. ed. 1999. 287p. pap. 119.00 (*0-9639238-6-2*) HlthQuest Pubs.

Who's Who in Medicine & Healthcare. Ed. by Marquis Who's Who Staff. 985p. 2nd ed. 1998. 249.95 (*0-8379-0002-6*); 3rd ed. 2000. 249.00 (*0-8379-0004-2*) Marquis.

Who's Who in Medicine & Healthcare, 1997-1998. Ed. by Marquis Who's Who Staff. 1996. 1230p. 249.95 (*0-8379-0000-X*) Marquis.

Who's Who in Science in Europe: A Biograhical Guide in Science, Technology, Agriculture & Medicine. 9th ed. 1995. 2752p. 950.00 (*1-56159-132-7*) Groves Dictionaries.

***Whose Body Is It Anyway? Smart Alternative & Traditional Health Choices for Your Total Well-Being.** Joan Kenley & John C. Arpels. 2001. (Illus.). pap. 16.95 (*1-55704-500-3*) Newmarket.

Whose Freud? The Place of Psychoanalysis in Contemporary Culture. Ed. by Peter Brooks & Alex Woloch. 2000. LC 00-27261. (Illus.). 352p. pap. 19.95 (*0-300-08745-4*) Yale U Pr.

Whose Standards: Consumer & Professional Standards in Health Care. Charlotte Williamson. 1992. LC 92-13012. pap. (*0-335-09720-0*) OpUniv Pr.

Whose Standards: Consumer & Professional Standards in Health Care. Charlotte Williamson. 1992. LC 92-13012. (*0-335-09721-9*) OpUniv Pr GBR. *Dist:* Raincoast Bk.

Why Am I So Tired? Is Your Thyroid Making You Ill? Martin L. Budd. 2000. pap. (*0-7225-3942-8*) Thorsons GBR. *Dist:* Natl Bk Netwk.

Why Am I Up, Why Am I Down? Understanding Bipolar Disorder. Roger Granet & Elizabeth Ferber. 1999. LC 00-501567. (Laurel-Leaf Bks.). 256p. mass mkt. 5.99 (*0-440-23465-4*) Dell.

Why & How: Some Problems & Methods in Historical Biology. George G. Simpson. 1980. LC 79-42774. (Illus.). 263p. pap. 51.50 (*0-08-025784-4*, Pergamon Pr) Elsevier.

Why Animal Experimentation Matters: The Use of Animals in Medical Research. Ellen Frankel Paul et al. 2000. LC 99-47844. (New Studies in Social Policy: Vol. 2). ix, 224p. pap. text 24.95 (*0-7658-0685-1*) Transaction Pubs.

Why Animals Don't Get Heart Attacks, but People Do. Matthias Rath. rev. ed. 1997. pap. 12.95 (*0-9638768-5-6*) Health Now.

Why Be Quantitative about Radiation Risk Estimates? Edward E. Pochin. 1978. LC 78-61402. (Taylor Lectures: No. 2). 20.00 (*0-913392-42-1*) NCRP Pubns.

Why Calories Don't Count. Scott Knickelbine & Paul A. Stitt. rev. ed. 1983. (Illus.). (Orig.). pap. text 7.00 (*0-939956-05-5*) Natural Pr.

Why Did Freud Reject God? A Psychoanalytic Interpretation. Ana-Maria Rizzuto. 1998. LC 97-49877. (Illus.). 256p. 40.00 (*0-300-07525-1*) Yale U Pr.

Why Did My Baby Die? The Phenomenon of Sudden Infant Death Syndrome & How to Cope with It. Abraham Bergman & Judith Choate. 1975. LC 73-92794. 20.00 (*0-89388-146-5*) Okpaku Communications.

Why Do I Drink More Than I Want? Five Came Back; Three Did Not. Juanita M. Ferrey. 1987. LC 88-72476. 200p. (Orig.). pap. 13.00 (*0-939339-03-X*, 662-4685) AFCOM Pub.

Why Do I Eat More Than I Want Diet Book. Juanita M. Ferrey. 1987. LC 88-72476. (Illus.). 214p. (Orig.). pap. 13.00 (*0-939339-02-1*, 662-4685) AFCOM Pub.

Why Do I Wheeze? A Guide to the Effective Management of Asthma. Robert Sorensen. 2000. (Illus.). 70p. (Orig.). (J). pap. 14.95 (*0-9678835-0-4*) N Shore Asthma.

Why Do People Get Sick: The New Science of Psychoneuroimmunlogy & What It Can Do for You. 1992. lib. bdg. 88.00 (*0-8490-5402-8*) Gordon Pr.

Why Do We Fall Ill? The Story Hiding in the Body. Luis A. Chiozza. 1999. LC 98-26756. 125p. 27.50 (*1-887841-18-0*, No. 66879, Psychosocial) Intl Univs Pr.

***Why Doctors Lie.** Mel Schecter. 2001. 304p. 26.00 (*0-7867-0911-1*) Carroll & Graf.

Why Does Everything Have to Be Perfect? Understanding Obsessive-Compulsive Disorder. Lynn Schackman & Shelagh Ryan. 1999. LC 00-500744. (Laurel-Leaf Bks.). 224p. mass mkt. 5.99 (*0-440-23463-8*) Dell.

W X Y Z

Why Healing Happens. O. T. Bonnett. 1996. 209p. (Orig.). pap. 14.95 (*1-878448-70-6*) MacMurray & Beck.

Why I Am an Abortion Doctor. Suzanne T. Poppema & Mike Henderson. 1996. LC 96-2445. 266p. 31.00 (*1-57392-045-2*) Prometheus Bks.

Why I Became a Psychotherapist. Joseph Reppen. 1998. LC 98-4116. 50.00 (*0-7657-0170-7*) Aronson.

Why I Left Orthodox Medicine: Healing for the 21st Century. Derrick Lonsdale. 1994. LC 94-214685. 256p. pap. 10.95 (*1-878901-98-2*) Hampton Roads Pub Co.

Why Is Cancer Killing Our Pets? How You Can Protect & Treat Your Animal Companion. Deborah Straw. 2000. LC 00-59786. xi, 244p. pap. 14.95 (*0-89281-926-X*, Heal Arts VT) Inner Tradit.

Why Kids Kill Parents: Child Abuse & Adolescent Homicide. Kathleen M. Heide. 1992. LC 91-32556. 197p. text 37.50 (*0-8142-0563-1*) Ohio St U Pr.

Why Kill Yourself? My Heart Attack & How to Prevent Yours. Bernard Falk & Roger Blackwood. 1988. (Illus.). 192p. (*0-575-04006-8*) V Gollancz GBR. *Dist:* Trafalgar.

Why Me? How to Heal What's Hurting You. Arleen Lorrance. 1982. LC 77-88151. 186p. 11.95 (*0-916192-19-9*) L P Pubns.

Why Not Me? The Story of Gladys Milton, Midwife. Gladys Milton. 1993. LC 92-38694. (Illus.). 128p. 9.95 (*0-913990-97-3*) Book Pub Co.

Why Our Children Are Killing Themselves. Mauri Saalakhan. 2nd ed. 1993. LC 92-85134. 132p. pap. 10.00 (*0-9627854-4-X*) Writers Inc.

Why People Don't Heal & How They Can. Caroline Myss. LC 97-22798. 1998. 288p. pap. 14.00 (*0-609-80224-0*); 1997. 25.00 (*0-609-60090-7*) Harmony Bks.

Why Psychiatry Is a Branch of Medicine. Samuel B. Guze. 1992. LC 92-6001. 160p. text 26.50 (*0-19-507420-3*) OUP.

Why Psychology? Adrian Furnham & David Oakley. 1995. 128p. pap. text 17.95 (*1-85728-298-1*) Taylor & Francis.

Why Psychotherapists Fail. Richard D. Chessick. 1983. LC 84-45108. 203p. 40.00 (*0-87668-700-1*) Aronson.

Why Root Canal Therapy? Joel M. Berns. 2nd ed. 1993. LC 93-36688. (Illus.). 61p. (Orig.). pap. 28.00 (*0-86715-284-2*) Quint Pub Co.

Why Should I Nurse My Baby? Pamela K. Wiggins. 2nd rev. ed. 1996. (Illus.). 64p. pap. 4.95 (*0-9623529-1-8*, 001) Lactation Assocs Pub.

Why Some Children Succeed Despite the Odds. Ed. by Warren A. Rhodes & Waln K. Brown. 1991. LC 90-49203. 208p. 55.00 (*0-275-93705-4*, C3705, Praeger Pubs) Greenwood.

Why Some Therapies Don't Work: The Dangers of Transpersonal Psychology. Albert Ellis & Raymond Yeager. 1989. LC 88-31809. (Psychology Ser.). 189p. 31.00 (*0-87975-471-0*) Prometheus Bks.

Why the United States Does Not Have a National Health Program. Ed. by Vicente Navarro. 1992. (Policy, Politics, Health & Medicine Ser.). 266p. pap. 33.00 (*0-89503-105-1*) Baywood Pub.

Why the United States Lacks a National Health Insurance Program. Nicholas Laham. 1993. 216p. pap. 24.95 (*0-275-94779-3*, Praeger Pubs);331. LC 93-3167. (Contributions in Political Science Ser.: No. 331). 59.95 (*0-313-28745-7*, GM8745) Greenwood.

Why We Age: What Science Is Discovering about the Body's Journey Through Life. Steven N. Austad. 1997. LC 97-5542. 256p. 24.95 (*0-471-14803-2*) Wiley.

Why We Eat What We Eat: The Psychology of Eating. Ed. by Elizabeth P. Capaldi. 1996. LC 96-33870. (Illus.). 339p. 49.95 (*1-55798-366-6*, 4318500) Am Psychol.

Why We Feel: The Science of Human Emotions. Victor S. Johnston. 1999. LC 98-89426. 224p. 26.00 (*0-7382-0109-X*) Perseus Pubng.

Why We Spend Too Much on Health Care. Joseph L. Bast et al. 1992. 10p. pap. 8.95 (*0-9632027-0-7*) Heartland Inst.

Why We Spend Too Much on Health Care...& What We Can Do about It. Joseph L. Bast et al. 1993. (Illus.). 176p. (C). pap. text 8.95 (*0-9632027-2-3*) Heartland Inst.

Why Weight? A Guide to Ending Compulsive Eating. Geneen Roth. 1989. (Illus.). 224p. pap. 12.95 (*0-452-26254-2*, Plume) Dutton Plume.

Why Women? Gender Issues & Eating Disorders. Ed. by Bridget Dolan & Inez Gitzinger. 1994. LC 94-3801. 120p. (C). pap. (*0-485-12106-9*) Athlone Pr GBR. *Dist:* Transaction Pubs, Humanities.

Why You Are Being Referred to a Periodontist? Richard T. Kao. Ed. by Russell McCallion. 1998. (Illus.). 35p. (*0-914833-05-7*) Kapala Corp.

Why Zebras Don't Get Ulcers: An Updated Guide to Stress, Stress-Related Diseases & Coping. Robert M. Sapolsky. 1998. LC 98-5578. (Illus.). 434p. pap. text 16.00 (*0-7167-3210-6*) W H Freeman.

WIC Nutrition Risk Criteria: A Scientific Assessment. Contrib. by National Academy Press Staff. 1996. 377p. (Orig.). pap. text 39.00 (*0-309-05385-4*) Natl Acad Pr.

Wide Awake, Clear Headed & Refreshed: Medical Hypnoanalysis in Action. Ryan Elliott. Ed. by Gene Owens. 1991. (Illus.). 300p. (Orig.). pap. 12.95 (*0-9615140-0-0*) Relaxed Bks.

Wide Neighborhoods: A Story of the Frontier Nursing Service. Mary Breckinridge. 1981. LC 81-50181. (Illus.). 400p. reprint ed. 36.00 (*0-8131-1453-5*); pap. 18.00 (*0-8131-0149-2*) U Pr of KY.

Widening Circle: A Lyme Disease Pioneer Tells Her Story. Polly Murray. 1996. LC 95-47395. 336p. 23.95 (*0-312-14068-1*) St Martin.

Widening Scope of Self Psychology. Ed. by Arnold Goldberg. 1993. (Progress in Self Psychology Ser.: Vol. 9). 304p. text 45.00 (*0-88163-163-9*) Analytic Pr.

Widening the Scope of Cognitive Therapy: The Therapeutic Relationship, Emotion, & the Process of Change. Jeremy Safran. 1998. LC 97-37557. (Illus.). 368p. 50.00 (*0-7657-0138-3*) Aronson.

Wider Circle. Roger Hutson & Patsy Hutson. 1985. 112p. pap. 3.95 (*0-310-29421-5*, 6895P) Zondervan.

Widmann's Clinical Interpretation of Laboratory Tests. Ronald A. Sacher et al. 11th ed. 2000. LC 99-59044. (Illus.). 1104p. pap. 58.95 (*0-8036-0270-7*) Davis Co.

Widower: When Men Are Left Alone. Scott Campbell & Phyllis R. Silverman. 1996. (Death, Value & Meaning Ser.). 246p. 39.95 (*0-89503-140-X*) Baywood Pub.

Wie Sage Ichs Den Patienten: German, Turkish, Italian, Spanish, Serbocroatian. Pia M. Guardiola. 1986. 71p. lib. bdg. 45.00 (*0-8288-3591-8*, F105160) Fr & Eur.

Wild Animal Care & Rehabilitation Manual. Vicki Johnson et al. Ed. by Monica Evans. 4th ed. 1991. (Illus.). 137p. (C). pap. text 24.95 (*0-939294-16-8*) Beech Leaf.

Wild Boy of Aveyron. Jean Marc Gaspard Itard. Tr. by George Humphrey & Muriel Humphrey. 1962. pap. text 19.20 (*0-13-959494-9*) P-H.

Wild Child: How You Can Help Your Child with Attention Deficit Disorder (ADD) & Other Behavioral Disorders. Don Mordasini. 2000. LC 00-40735. 260p. 59.95 (*0-7890-1101-8*) Haworth Pr.

Wild Child: How You Can Help Your Child with Attention Deficit Disorder & Other Behavioral Disorders. Ed. by Don Mordasini. 2000. LC 00-40735. xvii, 236p. pap. 18.95 (*0-7890-1102-6*) Haworth Pr.

***Wild Genie: The Healing Power of Menstruation.** Alexandra Pope. 2001. 288p. pap. (*1-86351-279-9*) Sally Milner AUS. *Dist:* Sterling.

Wild Plant Companion: A Fresh Understanding of Herbal Food & Medicine. Kathryn G. March & Andrew L. March. 1986. (Illus.). 200p. (Orig.). pap. 11.95 (*0-940206-03-X*) Meridian Hill.

Wild Plants of Utah: Learn to Identify & Use for Emergency Food & Survival. LeArta Moulton. 2001. 89p. pap. 12.95 (*0-935596-07-0*) LM Pubns.

Wild Science: Reading Feminism, Medicine & the Media. Ed. by Janine Marchessault & Kim Sawchuk. 2000. LC 99-55545. (Writing Corporealities Ser.). (Illus.). xiii, 259p. (C). text 85.00 (*0-415-20430-5*) Routledge.

Wild Yam: Birth Control Without Fear. Willa Shaffer. 1994. (Woodland Health Ser.). 8p. pap. 2.95 (*0-913923-10-9*) Woodland UT.

Wild Yam - Nature's Source of Phytohormones. Michael Bennett. 1997. LC 97-92632. (Illus.). xii, 76p. pap. text 9.95 (*1-891410-00-8*) Optimal HealthSpan.

Wilderness EMT. Buck Tilton. 1995. (C). (*0-89303-954-3*) Appleton & Lange.

***Wilderness First Aid: A Pocket Guide.** Paul Gill. 2001. 144p. pap. 10.95 (*0-07-137962-2*) McGraw-Hill Prof.

Wilderness First Aid: Emergency Care for Remote Locations. National Safety Council Staff & Wilderness Medical Society Staff. 1997. LC 97-31077. (Illus.). 360p. (C). pap. text 19.95 (*0-7637-0407-5*, 0407-5) Jones & Bartlett.

Wilderness First Aid: When You Can't Call 911. Gilbert Preston. 1997. LC 97-11567. (Falcon's How-To Ser.). (Illus.). pap. 6.95 (*1-56044-579-3*) Falcon Pub Inc.

Wilderness First Responder: The Cutting Edge of Medical Training for Environmental Rescue Personnel. Buck Tilton. 1998. LC 98-8549. (Illus.). 288p. reprint ed. pap. 34.95 (*0-7627-0392-X*) Globe Pequot.

Wilderness Medical Associates Field Guide. Jim Morrissey. 3rd ed. 2000. (Illus.). 99p. 19.95 (*0-9704646-0-6*) Wilderness Med.

Wilderness Medicine. Paul S. Auerbach. 4th ed. 2001. LC 00-61612. (Illus.). xxiii, 1910p. 199.00 (*0-323-00950-6*) Mosby Inc.

Wilderness Medicine: Management of Wilderness & Environment Emergencies. Ed. by Paul S. Auerbach. 3rd ed. 1994. (Illus.). 1536p. (C). (gr. 13). text 179.00 (*0-8016-7044-6*, 07044) Mosby Inc.

Wilderness 911: A Step-by-Step Guide for Medical Emergencies & Improvised Care in the Backcountry. Eric A. Weiss. 1999. LC 98-39861. (Illus.). 240p. pap. 16.95 (*0-89886-597-2*) Mountaineers.

Wildlife Biotelemetry. Ed. by H. P. Kimmich. 1981. (Journal: Vol. 7, No. 3-4). (Illus.). 116p. pap. 28.75 (*3-8055-2093-X*) S Karger.

Wiley's English-Spanish, Spanish-English Dictionary of Psychology & Psychiatry. Steven M. Kaplan. LC 95-1653. 1997. (SPA.). 608p. pap. 39.95 (*0-471-19284-8*); 1995. (ENG & SPA.). 594p. 130.00 (*0-471-01460-5*) Wiley.

Wilhelm Conrad Rontgen & the Early History of the Roentgen Rays. Otto Glasser. 1993. (Illus.). 494p. reprint ed. 125.00 (*0-930405-22-6*) Norman SF.

Wilhelm Reich: The Man Who Dreamed of Tomorrow. W. Edward Mann & Edward Hoffman. 1991. (Orig.). (*1-85274-087-6*) Aqm Pr GBR. *Dist:* Harper SF.

Wilkins the Diagnosis & Treatment of Endocrine Disorders in Childhood & Adolescence. Ed. by Michael S. Kappy et al. 4th ed. 1994. LC 93-20671. (Illus.). 1270p. (C). text 164.95 (*0-398-05879-2*) C C Thomas.

Will & a Way: What the United States Can Learn from Canada about Caring for the Elderly. Robert L. Kane & Rosalie S. Kane. 1988. LC 85-16616. (Studies of Social Gerontology & Aging). 275p. pap. text 20.50 (*0-231-06137-4*) Col U Pr.

Will the Best of Intentions Be Enough; Assessing the Volunteerism Paradigm; Voluntary Health Sector Best Practices. 1996. 15.00 (*1-58534-019-7*) Points of Light.

Will They Do It Again? Risk Assessment & Management in Criminal Justice & Psychiatry. Herschel A. Prins. 1999. LC 99-21513. 176p. (C). text 85.00 (*0-415-16017-0*); xiv, 171p. pap. (*0-415-16018-9*) Routledge.

Will to Live: The Battle of a Young Boy Against Muscular Dystrophy. A. J. Mills. 1992. 100p. pap. 7.95 (*0-9633921-0-7*) Humor Bks.

Willard & Spackman's Occupational Therapy. Maureen E. Neistadt & Elizabeth Blesedell Crepeau. 9th ed. 1997. LC 97-15395. 960p. text 62.95 (*0-397-55192-4*) Lppncott W & W.

Willem Einthoven (1860-1927) Father of Electrocardiography: Life & Work, Ancestors & Contemporaries. H. A. Snellen. 1995. LC 94-43112. 144p. (C). pap. text 51.00 (*0-7923-3274-1*) Kluwer Academic.

William Alanson White: The Autobiography of a Purpose. William A. White. Ed. by Gerald N. Grob. 1980. LC 78-22596. (Historical Issues in Mental Health Ser.). reprint ed. lib. bdg. 25.95 (*0-405-11946-1*) Ayer.

William Beaumont-Frontier Doctor. Virginia Law Burns. 2nd rev. ed. 1989. LC 78-72566. (Illus.). 166p. reprint ed. lib. bdg. 17.50 (*0-9604726-4-9*) Enterprise Pr.

William Cullen & the 18th Century Medical World. Ed. by Reginald Passmore et al. 1993. LC 93-231978. (Illus.). 256p. text (*0-7486-0302-6*) Edinburgh U Pr GBR. *Dist:* Col U Pr.

William Harvey & the Use of Purpose in the Scientific Revolution: Cosmos by Chance or Universe by Design? Emerson T. McMullen. 1997. LC 97-31966. (C). 280p. 60.00 (*0-7618-0957-0*); 252p. pap. 39.00 (*0-7618-0958-9*) U Pr of Amer.

William Harvey's Natural Philosophy. Roger French. 1994. LC 93-36181. (Illus.). 405p. (C). text 80.00 (*0-521-45535-9*) Cambridge U Pr.

***William Heberden: Physician of the Age of Reason.** Ernest Heberden. 1989. (Eponymists in Medicine Ser.). 246p. (*1-85315-117-3*) Royal Soc of Medicine Pr Ltd GBR. *Dist:* Balogh.

William Henry Welch & the Heroic Age of American Medicine. Simon Flexner & James T. Flexner. 1993. LC 92-13529. (Illus.). 568p. reprint ed. 51.50 (*0-8018-4501-7*) Johns Hopkins.

William James & Henri Bergson: A Study in Contrasting Theories of Life. Horace M. Kallen. LC 75-3213. (Philosophy in America Ser.). reprint ed. 42.50 (*0-404-59209-0*) AMS Pr.

William Withering & the Foxglove. R. D. Mann et al. 1986. text 330.00 (*0-85200-950-X*) Kluwer Academic.

Williams & Lissner's Biomechanics of Human Motion. Barney F. LeVeau. 3rd ed. 1991. (Illus.). 340p. pap. text 47.00 (*0-7216-5743-5*) Saunders.

Williams & Wilkins' Dental Hygiene Handbook. Kathleen H. Alvarez. 1998. LC 97-41381. 627p. pap. 30.95 (*0-683-30089-X*) Lppncott W & W.

Williams Hematology. Ed. by Ernest Beutler et al. 5th ed. 1994. (Illus.). 1920p. text 169.00 (*0-07-070386-8*) McGraw-Hill Educ Grp.

Williams Hematology. Ernest Beutler et al. 6th ed. 2000. LC 00-58746. (Illus.). 1941p. text 169.00 (*0-07-070397-3*) McGraw-Hill Prof.

Williams Hematology: Companion Handbook. Ed. by William J. Williams. 5th ed. 1995. LC 95-4630. (Illus.). 452p. pap. 39.95 (*0-07-070394-9*) McGraw-Hill Prof.

***Williams Obstetrics.** Susan Cox et al. 21st ed. 2001. 288p. pap., stu. ed. 55.00 (*0-8385-8675-9*) McGraw-Hill Prof.

Williams Obstetrics. F. Gary Cunningham et al. 21st ed. 2001. (Illus.). 1668p. (C). text 135.00 (*0-8385-9647-9*) McGraw-Hill Prof.

***Williams Obstetrics Textbook & Study Guide.** F. Cunningham et al. 21st ed. 2001. (Illus.). text 169.00 (*0-07-138893-1*) McGraw-Hill Prof.

Williams Textbook of Endocrinology. Wilson. 1998. (C). text 35.00 (*0-8089-2112-6*, Grune & Strat) Harcrt Hlth Sci Grp.

Williams Textbook of Endocrinology. Jean D. Wilson et al. Ed. by Richard Zorab. 9th ed. 1998. LC 96-41440. (Illus.). 1552p. (C). text 150.00 (*0-7216-6152-1*) Saunders.

Williams Textbook of Endocrinology. Contrib. by Saunders, W.B., Publishing Staff. 10th ed. 2001. 210.00 incl. cd-rom (*0-7216-9268-0*) Saunders.

Willpower Is Not Enough: Understanding & Overcoming Addiction & Compulsion. Arnold M. Washton & Donna Boundy. 1990. LC 88-45069. 288p. reprint ed. pap. 13.00 (*0-06-091969-8*, Perennial) HarperTrade.

Wills Eye Hospital Atlas of Clinical Ophthalmology. Ed. by William S. Tasman & Edward A. Jaeger. 1995. 456p. text 175.00 (*0-397-51350-X*) Lppncott W & W.

***Wills Eye Hospital Atlas of Clinical Ophthalmology.** Ed. by William Tasman & Edward A. Jaeger. 2nd ed. 2001. LC 2001-20374. (Illus.). text 229.00 (*0-7817-2774-X*) Lppncott W & W.

Wilms' Tumor (Nephroblastoma) & Related Renal Neoplasms of Childhood. Ed. by Frank Gonzalez-Crussi. 1983. 304p. 171.00 (*0-8493-5670-9*, RC280, CRC Reprint) Franklin.

Wilner's Radiology of Bone Tumors. Daniel Wilner. 2nd ed. 1997. text (*0-7216-5274-3*) Saunders.

Wilson & Gisvold's Textbook of Organic Medicinal & Pharmaceutical Chemistry. Jaime N. Delgado & William A. Remers. 10th ed. 1998. LC 98-22502. 992p. text 69.50 (*0-397-51583-9*) Lppncott W & W.

Wilson's Disease. Tjaard U. Hoogenraad. 1996. (Major Problems in Neurology Ser.: Vol. 30). (Illus.). 219p. text (*0-7020-1842-2*) W B Saunders GBR. *Dist:* Saunders.

Wilson's Syndrome: The Miracle of Feeling Well. E. Denis Wilson. 1991. 346p. pap. 21.95 (*0-9629875-0-6*) Cornerstn FL.

Wilson's Topley Principles of Bacteriology, Virology & Immunity, Vol. 2. 7th ed. 1984. 576p. lib. bdg. 98.00 (*0-683-09065-8*) Lppncott W & W.

Wind & the Book: Memoirs of a Country Doctor. David D. Browne. 1976. 27.50 (*0-522-84099-X*) Intl Spec Bk.

Wind in Africa: A Story of Modern Medicine in Mali. Pascal J. Imperato. 1975. LC 73-24001. (Illus.). 363p. 10.60 (*0-87527-139-1*) Green.

Windigo Psychosis: American Ethnological Society Proceedings, 1960. Morton I. Teicher. Ed. by Verne F. Ray. 1988. LC 84-45547. reprint ed. pap. 45.00 (*0-404-62654-8*) AMS Pr.

Window of Opportunity: Interviewing by the Perinatal Nurse. Mary L. Moore & Susan R. Givens. Ed. by Karla Damus & Margaret C. Freda. 1994. LC 94-39542. (*0-86525-063-4*) March of Dimes.

Windows into the A. D. D. Mind: Understanding & Treating Attention Deficit Disorders, Childhood Through Adulthood. Daniel G. Amen. 1996. 238p. 39.95 (*1-886554-00-5*) MindWrks.

Windows Mammography. Smathers. 1995. cd-rom 325.00 (*0-7817-0320-4*) Lppncott W & W.

Windows Programming, under the Hood of MFC: A Quick Tour of Visual C++ Tools. Laura Draxler. 1997. LC 97-40627. 640p. (C). pap. text 44.95 (*0-13-488975-4*) P-H.

Windows to Cancer Rehabilitation: An Occupational Therapy Treatment Guide. Karen Kumiega. 1997. LC 98-144219. (Illus.). 153p. spiral bd. 37.00 (*1-883315-24-1*, 7108) Imaginart Intl.

Windows to Our Children: A Gestalt Therapy Approach to Children & Adolescents. Violet Oaklander. 1989. (Illus.). 352p. reprint ed. pap. 25.00 (*0-939266-06-7*) Gestalt Journal.

Winged Victory: Altered Images; Transcending Breast Cancer. Art Myers. 1996. LC 96-68207. (Illus.). 56p. (Orig.). pap. 24.95 (*1-889169-00-5*) Photo Gallery.

Wings of Gauze: Women of Color & the Experience of Health & Illness. Ed. by Barbara Bair & Susan E. Cayleff. 1993. LC 92-46308. 394p. pap. text 21.95 (*0-8143-2302-2*) Wayne St U Pr.

WinMDR/Print MDR Combination Pack annuals Medical Economics Staff. rev. ed. 1999. 499.00 (*1-56363-351-5*, PDR) Med Econ.

Winnicott. Adam Phillips. 1989. LC 88-28390. 176p. reprint ed. 31.95 (*0-674-95360-6*); pap. 16.50 (*0-674-95361-4*) HUP.

Winnicott Studies, No. 2. Ed. by Squiggle Foundation Staff. 1988. 100p. reprint ed. pap. text (*0-9510174-1-1*) Karnac Bks GBR. *Dist:* Other Pr LLC.

Winnicott Studies. Squiggle Foundation Staff. 96p. No. 6. 1992. pap. text (*1-85575-024-4*); No. 7. 1993. pap. text (*1-85575-048-1*) Karnac Bks GBR. *Dist:* Other Pr LLC.

Winnicott Studies. Ed. by Laurence Spurling. No. 8. 1993. 96p. pap. (*1-85575-067-8*); No. 10. 1996. 64p. pap. text (*1-85575-109-7*) Karnac Bks GBR. *Dist:* Other Pr LLC.

Winnicott Studies: The Journal of the Squiggle Foundation. Ed. by Squiggle Foundation Staff. reprint ed. Vol. 4, 1989. 1990. 108p. pap. text (*0-9510175-3-5*); Vol. 5, 1990. 1991. 100p. pap. text (*0-946439-99-0*) Karnac Bks GBR. *Dist:* Brunner-Routledge.

Winnicott Studies No. 3: A Celebration of the Life & Work of Marion Milner. Ed. by Squiggle Foundation Staff. 1989. 68p. reprint ed. pap. text (*0-9510174-2-X*) Karnac Bks GBR. *Dist:* Other Pr LLC.

Winning Against Relapse: A Workbook of Action Plans for Recurring Health & Emotional Problems. Mary E. Copeland. 1999. LC 98-68745. 208p. pap., wbk. ed. 14.95 (*1-57224-130-6*) New Harbinger.

Winning Medical Negligence Cases: A Guide for the Plaintiffs' Lawyer. William A. Trine & Paul N. Luvera. 1993. LC 93-2351. 45.00 (*0-941916-53-7*) West Group.

Winning of Animal Health: 100 Years of Veterinary Medicine. Ole H. Stalheim. 1994. LC 94-1629. (Illus.). 268p. text 44.95 (*0-8138-2429-X*) Iowa U Pr.

Winning Strategies for Nursing Managers. Joan O'Leary et al. 1986. (Illus.). 165p. text 16.95 (*0-397-54541-X*, Lippnctt) Lppncott W & W.

Winning the Battle: Developing Support for Sexuality & HIV/AIDS Education. Irving R. Dickman. 1991. LC 82-61000. 58p. (Orig.). pap. 12.95 (*0-9609212-0-6*) SIECUS.

Winning the Chemo Battle. Joyce S. Mitchell. 1991. pap. 11.00 (*0-393-30713-1*) Norton.

Winning the War Against Asthma & Allergies: A Drug Free Alternative Treatment Plan for Asthma Sufferers & Their Families. Ellen W. Cutler. 1997. LC 97-9404. (Instructor Material TV Ser.). 256p. pap. text 17.95 (*0-8273-8622-2*) Delmar.

Winning the War Against Immune Disorders & Allergies: A Drug Free Cure for Allergies. Ellen W. Cutler. 1998. LC 98-23746. 608p. pap. text 21.95 (*0-7668-0059-8*) Delmar.

Winning the War Against Life-Threatening Diseases. Steven Pradell. 1994. LC 94-66759. 256p. pap. 13.95 (*0-88282-125-3*) New Horizon NJ.

Winning War Against Headaches & Allergies. Ellen W. Cutler et al. 2003. 256p. pap. 16.95 (*0-7668-0058-X*) Delmar.

Winning Websites for Medical Personnel & Patients. Jennifer C. Logan. 1998. (Illus.). 111p. pap. 18.00 (*0-9664575-0-1*) La Vida Bks.

Winning with Arthritis. Harris H. McIlwain et al. LC 90-28903. 228p. 1997. pap. 5.99 (*0-471-17691-5*); 1991. pap. 15.95 (*0-471-52847-1*) Wiley.

Winning with Back Pain. Harris H. McIlwain et al. 1994. LC 93-8379. 202p. pap. 12.95 (*0-471-30328-3*) Wiley.

Winning with Back Pain: How to Beat Back Pain & Take Control of Your Life. Harris H. McIlwain. 1996. LC 93-8379. 224p. pap. 5.99 (*0-471-17694-X*) Wiley.

Winning with Chronic Pain: A Complete Program for Health & Well-Being. Harris H. McIlwain et al. 1994. LC 94-2443. (Illus.). 222p. (C). 35.00 (*0-87975-900-3*); pap. 21.00 (*0-87975-878-3*) Prometheus Bks.

Winning with Heart Attack: A Complete Program for Health & Well-Being. Debra F. Bruce et al. 1994. LC 94-25409. (Illus.). 189p. (C). 36.00 (*0-87975-914-3*) Prometheus Bks.

Winning with Osteoporosis. Harris H. McIlwain et al. 2nd ed. 1993. LC 93-7530. (Illus.). 160p. pap. 15.95 (*0-471-30489-1*) Wiley.

Winter. Auburn University Staff. 1996. (Nursing Texts Ser.). (C). (gr. 13). text 165.95 (*0-8151-4499-7*, 30629) Mosby Inc.

Wintrobe's Clinical Hematology G. Richard Lee et al. (Illus.). 10th ed. 1998. LC 96-52799. 2,680p. text 199.00 (*0-683-18242-0*); Set. 9th ed. 1992. LC 90-6194. 2320p. 175.00 (*0-8121-1188-5*) Lppncott W & W.

Wireless Phones & Health: Scientific Progress. George L. Carlo. 1998. LC 98-46064. viii, 413p. (*0-7923-8347-8*) Kluwer Academic.

Wirkung der Dosierten Distraktion auf das Ellenbogengelenk des Kaninchens. M. H. Hackenbroch. 1977. (Journal: Vol. 96, Suppl. 63-1). (Illus.). 35.75 (*3-8055-2643-1*) S Karger.

Wirkung und Nebenwirkungen Von Bleomycin. Ed. by D. K. Hossfeld & P. Engel. 1982. (Beitraege Zur Onkologie, Contributions to Oncology Ser.: Vol. 12). x, 220p. pap. 47.00 (*3-8055-3504-X*) S Karger.

WISC-III & WPPSI-R Supplement to Assessment of Children. Jerome M. Sattler. abr. ed. 1992. 200p. (C). pap. 16.00 (*0-9618209-3-4*) J M Sattler.

WISC III Clinical Use & Interpretation: Scientist-Practitioner Perspectives. Ed. by Auerelio Prifitera & Don Saklofske. 1997. LC 97-80798. (Practical Resources for the Mental Health Professional Ser.). (Illus.). 336p. text 49.95 (*0-12-564930-4*) Acad Pr.

Wisconsin & the Mentally Ill. Dale W. Robison. Ed. by Gerald N. Grob. 1980. LC 78-22588. (Historical Issues in Mental Health Ser.). lib. bdg. 28.95 (*0-405-11939-9*) Ayer.

Wisconsin Health Care in Perspective 2000. Ed. by Kathleen O'Leary Morgan & Scott E. Morgan. 2000. 21p. spiral bd. 19.00 (*0-7401-0248-6*) Morgan Quitno Corp.

Wisconsin Health Care Perspective, 1998. Ed. by Kathleen O'Leary Morgan & Scott E. Morgan. 1998. 20p. pap. 19.00 (*1-56692-848-6*) Morgan Quitno Corp.

Wisconsin Medicine: Historical Perspectives. Ronald L. Numbers & Judith W. Leavitt. 1981. LC 80-52297. (Illus.). 224p. 19.95 (*0-299-08430-2*) U of Wis Pr.

Wisconsin's Early Home Remedies. Lora Di Megilo et al. 1991. (Illus.). 172p. pap. text 9.95 (*1-878488-55-4*) Quixote Pr IA.

Wisdom: Explorations in Adult Competence. St. G. Holliday. Ed. by M. J. Chandler. 1986. (Contributions to Human Development Ser.: Vol. 17). (Illus.). x, 102p. 45.25 (*3-8055-4283-6*) S Karger.

Wisdom, Jesus & Psychotherapy. David Klimek. 1991. (Illus.). 200p. (Orig.). pap. 13.95 (*0-9630213-0-3*) Winsted Pubns.

Wisdom, Madness & Folly. R. D. Laing. 1999. pap. (*0-86241-831-3*) Canongate Books GBR. *Dist:* Grove-Atltic.

Wisdom of Amish Folk Medicine. Quillin. 1996. per. (*0-671-52812-2*) S&S Trade.

Wisdom of Healing: A Natural Mind Body Program for Optimal Wellness. David Simon. 1998. 384p. pap. 15.00 (*0-609-80214-3*, Crown) Crown Pub Group.

Wisdom of Healing: A Natural Mind Body Program for Optimal Wellness. David Simon. 2000. (Illus.). 352p. reprint ed. 27.00 (*0-7881-9312-0*) DIANE Pub.

***Wisdom of Menopause.** Christiane Northrup. 2002. 608p. pap. 18.95 (*0-553-38080-X*) Bantam Dell.

Wisdom of Menopause: Creating Physical & Emotional Health & Healing During the Change. Christiane Northrup. 2001. LC 00-51892. (Illus.). 608p. 27.95 (*0-553-80121-X*) Bantam.

Wisdom of Milton H. Erickson Vol. 1: Hypnosis & Hypnotherapy. Milton H. Erickson. Ed. by Ronald A. Havens. 1989. LC 88-31440. 297p. reprint ed. pap. 17.95 (*0-8290-2413-1*) Irvington.

Wisdom of the Body. Michael Kern. 2001. (*0-7225-3708-5*) Thorsons GBR. *Dist:* Natl Bk Netwk.

Wisdom of the Eye. David Miller. 2000. LC 00-100272. (Illus.). xi, 169p. 49.95 (*0-12-496860-0*) Acad Pr.

Wise Guide to Drugs. A. Naik. 1997. mass mkt. (*0-340-69973-6*) Hodder & Stought Ltd GBR. *Dist:* Lubrecht & Cramer, Trafalgar.

***Wise Therapy.** Tim Le Bon. 2001. 208p. 75.00 (*0-8264-5782-7*); pap. 24.95 (*0-8264-5207-8*) Continuum.

Wise Woman Herbal for the Childbearing Year. Susun S. Weed. 1986. LC 85-71064. (Wise Woman Herbal Ser.: No. 1). (Illus.). 196p. (Orig.). (C). pap. 9.95 (*0-9614620-0-0*) Ash Tree.

Wit & Wisdom in Dynamic Psychotherapy. Ed. by Gregory P. Bauer. 1990. LC 90-40191. 320p. 50.00 (*0-87668-768-0*) Aronson.

Witch & the Clown: Two Archetypes of Human Sexuality. Barry Ulanov & Ann Belford Ulanov. 1987. LC 86-21628. 337p. pap. 19.95 (*0-933029-07-1*) Chiron Pubns.

Witch Doctor's Dance. J. B. Wofford. 1999. LC 98-26405. 224p. 25.00 (*0-914875-32-9*) Bright Mtn Bks.

Witchdoctors & Psychiatrists: The Common Roots of Psychotherapy & Its Future. E. Fuller Torrey. 1987. LC 87-70297. Orig. Title: Mind Game. 320p. 30.00 (*0-87668-971-3*) Aronson.

Witchery of Sleep: An Anthology. Willard Moyer et al. 1977. lib. bdg. 59.95 (*0-8490-2828-0*) Gordon Pr.

Witches, Devils, & Doctors in the Renaissance: Johann Weyer, "De Praestigiis Daemonum" Ed. by George Mora et al. Tr. by John Shea. 1991. (Medieval & Renaissance Texts & Studies: Vol. 73). 896p. reprint ed. 55.00 (*0-86698-083-0*, MR73) MRTS.

Witches, Midwives, & Nurses: A History of Women Healers. Barbara Ehrenreich & Deirdre English. 2nd ed. 1973. LC 80-13400. (Illus.). 48p. (gr. 9-12). pap. 5.95 (*0-912670-13-4*) Feminist Pr.

With Child. Illus. by Bernie Kida et al. 1995. LC 95-41110. (*1-56796-135-5*) Childbirth Graphics.

With Child: Wisdom & Traditions for Pregnancy, Birth & Motherhood. Deborah Jackson. 1999. LC 98-46533. (Illus.). 144p. pap. 19.95 (*0-8118-2400-4*) Chronicle Bks.

With Child in Mind: Studies of the Personal Encounter with Infertility. Margarete Sandelowski. 1993. LC 92-48536. (Studies in Health, Illness, & Caregiving). 328p. (Orig.). (C). text 44.95 (*0-8122-3197-X*); pap. text 16.95 (*0-8122-1415-3*) U of Pa Pr.

With Compassion Toward Some: Homosexuality & Social Work in America. Ed. by Robert Schoenberg et al. 1985. LC 85-5838. (Journal of Social Work & Human Sexuality: Vol. 2, Nos. 2 & 3). 156p. reprint ed. pap. 14.95 (*0-918393-14-0*, Harrington Park) Haworth Pr.

With Dignity: The Search for Medicare & Medicaid, 132. Sheri I. David. 1985. LC 84-27941. (Contributions in Political Science Ser.: No. 12). 194p. 58.00 (*0-313-24720-X*, DWD/, Greenwood Pr) Greenwood.

With Stethoscope & Scapular. Joseph C. Evers. 1996. LC 96-67917. 96p. (Orig.). pap. 7.95 (*1-882972-70-8*, 3511) Queenship Pub.

With Stethoscope in Asia: Korea. Sherwood Hall. 1981. LC 77-81765. reprint ed. 19.95 (*0-930696-01-8*) MCL Assocs.

With the Armies of the Tsar: A Nurse at the Russian Front, 1914-1918. Florence Farmborough. 2000. LC 00-58998. (Illus.). 422p. reprint ed. pap. 19.95 (*0-8154-1090-5*) Cooper Sq.

With the Best of Intentions: The Child Sexual Abuse Prevention Movement. Jill D. Berrick & Neil Gilbert. 1991. LC 91-24680. 211p. 30.00 (*0-89862-564-5*) Guilford Pubns.

With the Five Year Olds. Joan Gallagher. 1969. 44p. pap. 1.95 (*0-87825-253-3*) Ed Solutions.

With the Passage of Time: The Baltimore Longitudinal Study of Aging. 1996. (Illus.). 55p. reprint ed. pap. text 25.00 (*0-7881-2840-X*) DIANE Pub.

Withdrawal of Human Projection: A Study of Culture & Internalized Objects. M. D. Faber. 1989. LC 89-80571. 99p. (Orig.). pap. 20.00 (*0-915042-21-5*) Lib Soc Sci.

***Withholding & Withdrawing Life-Prolonging Medical Treatment: Guidance for Decision Making.** Contrib. by British Mechanical Associations Staff. 2nd ed. 2001. 112p. pap. (*0-7279-1615-7*) BMJ Pub GBR. *Dist:* AIDC.

Within Hospital Walls. Kathryn Kornegay. Ed. by Carolyn S. Zagury. 1995. LC 95-61473. 150p. pap. 14.95 (*1-880254-31-X*) Vista.

Within the Hearts & Minds of Prisoners: An In-Depth View of Prisoners in Therapy. Edward M. Scott. 1998. LC 98-18638. (Illus.). 190p. 44.95 (*0-398-06876-3*); pap. 31.95 (*0-398-06877-1*) C C Thomas.

***Within Time & Beyond Time.** Ed. by Riccardo Steiner & Jennifer Johnson. 2001. 304p. pap. (*1-85575-270-0*) Karnac Bks GBR. *Dist:* Other Pr LLC.

Without Child: Experiencing & Resolving Infertility. Ellen S. Glazer & Susan L. Cooper. 1988. 226p. pap. 11.95 (*0-669-21363-2*) Jossey-Bass.

Without Conscience: The Disturbing World of the Psychopaths among Us. Robert D. Hare. 1999. LC 98-51786. 236p. pap. 16.95 (*1-57230-451-0*) Guilford Pubns.

Without Miracles: Universal Selection Theory & the Second Darwinian Revolution. Gary Cziko. 1997. LC 95-943. (Illus.). 400p. reprint ed. pap. 25.00 (*0-262-53147-X*, Bradford Bks) MIT Pr.

Without Moral Limits: Women, Reproduction & Medical Technology. Debra Evans. rev. ed. 2000. LC 00-10334. 253p. pap. 14.99 (*1-58134-201-2*) Crossway Bks.

Without Ritalin: A Natural Approach to ADD. Samuel E. Berne. 2001. LC 2001-29548. 288p. pap. 15.95 (*0-658-01215-0*) McGraw-Hill Prof.

Without Words: An Introduction to Nonverbal Communication. M. Van Schaack. 1977. 750.00 (*0-13-961417-6*) P-H.

Witness Psychology. R. Buckhout & M. Greenwald. 1981. (Monographs: No. CR-1). 4.00 (*1-55524-000-3*) Ctr Respon Psych.

Witness to Illness: Strategies for Caregiving & Coping. Karen Horowitz & Douglas M. Lanes. 1992. (Illus.). 550p. (*0-201-63229-2*) Addison-Wesley.

Witnessing, Nurturing, Protecting: Therapeutic Responses to Sexual Abuse. Alan Corbett et al. 1996. LC 96-219391. 160p. pap. (*1-85346-338-8*) David Fulton GBR. *Dist:* Taylor & Francis.

Witnessing Psychoanalysis: From Vienna Back to Vienna via Buchenwald & the U. S. A. Ernst Federn. 1990. 308p. reprint ed. pap. text (*0-946439-57-5*) Karnac Bks GBR. *Dist:* Other Pr LLC.

Wittgenstein Reads Freud: The Myth of the Unconscious. Jacques Bouveresse. Tr. by Carol Cosman from FRE. 1995. LC 94-40607. (New French Thought Ser.). (ENG & FRE.). 176p. 35.00 (*0-691-03425-7*) Princeton U Pr.

Wives & Midwives: Childbirth & Nutrition in Rural Malaysia. Carol Laderman. 1984. LC 83-47664. (Comparative Studies of Health Systems & Medical Care: Vol. 7). (Illus.). 267p. (C). pap. text 19.95 (*0-520-06036-9*) U CA Pr.

Wizard Within. A. M. Krasner. Ed. by Caroline Miller. 1990. (Illus.). (Orig.). (C). (*0-9624829-1-9*) Amer Bd Hypnotherapy.

Woerterbuch der Bildgebenden Verfahren (Dictionary of Medical Imaging) Deutsch - Englisch (English - German) H. Pucher. 2000. LC 00-44677. (ENG & GER.). vi, 901p. 40.00 (*3-540-64821-6*) Spr-Verlag.

Woerterbuch der Biochemie: Biochemistry Dictionary. K. Thielmann. 1978. (ENG, FRE, GER, RUS & SPA.). 724p. 150.00 (*0-8288-5286-3*, M7041) Fr & Eur.

Woerterbuch der Biologie. Werner Jacobs. 1976. (GER.). pap. 24.95 (*0-8288-5770-9*, M7039) Fr & Eur.

Woerterbuch der Epilepsie. H. Gastaut. 1975. (GER.). pap. 75.00 (*0-8288-5962-0*, M7013) Fr & Eur.

Woerterbuch der Medizin. Koch, Neff Oetinger Staff. 1993. (GER.). 872p. 39.95 (*0-7859-8677-4*, 342303355x) Fr & Eur.

Woerterbuch der Medizin. Margaret Minker. 1991. (GER.). 399p. 59.95 (*0-7859-8495-X*, 3806845352) Fr & Eur.

Woerterbuch der Medizin. Maxim Zetkin. 15th ed. 1992. (GER.). 2377p. 75.00 (*0-7859-8518-2*, 3861260700) Fr & Eur.

Woerterbuch der Medizinischer Fachausdrucke. Josef Hammerschmid-Gollwitzer. 1993. (GER.). 680p. 59.95 (*0-7859-8363-5*, 3442305926) Fr & Eur.

Woerterbuch der Medizinisches Informatik. H. J. Seelos. 1990. (GER.). 550p. 225.00 (*0-7859-8269-8*, 3110112248) Fr & Eur.

Woerterbuch der Pharmazie Vol. 1: Biologie, Chemie, Technologie. Harry Von Auterhoff. 1981. (GER.). 532p. 105.00 (*0-7859-8486-0*, 3804706568) Fr & Eur.

Woerterbuch der Pharmazie Vol. 2: Pharmakologie. Ernst Mutschler. 1985. (GER.). 536p. 75.00 (*0-7859-8487-9*, 3804706673) Fr & Eur.

Woerterbuch der Pharmazie Vol. 3: Arzneimittelrecht und Apothekenrecht. Karl Feiden. 1985. (GER.). 253p. 75.00 (*3-8047-0670-3*, 3804706703) Fr & Eur.

Woerterbuch der Pharmazie Vol. 3: Arzneimitttelrecht & Apothekenrecht. Karl Feiden. 1985. (GER.). 253p. pap. 75.00 (*0-7859-8488-7*) Fr & Eur.

Woerterbuch der Pharmazie Vol. 4: Geschichte der Pharmazie. Wolfgang Schneider. 1985. (GER.). 302p. 75.00 (*0-7859-8489-5*, 3804706886) Fr & Eur.

Woerterbuch der Physikalisch-Technischen Begriffe der Medizinischen Radiologie: German, French-English-Deutsch. IEC Staff. 1986. (GER.). 143p. 95.00 (*0-7859-8346-5*, 3410123334) Fr & Eur.

Woerterbuch der Psychologie. Guenther Van Clauss. 1976. (GER.). 35.00 (*0-8288-5779-2*, M6963) Fr & Eur.

Woerterbuch der Psychologie: Dictionary of Psychology. Wilhelm Hehlmann. 11th ed. 1974. (GER.). pap. 59.95 (*0-8288-6225-7*, M-6964) Fr & Eur.

Woerterbuch der Religionspsychologie. Siegfried R. Dunde. 1993. (GER.). 368p. 125.00 (*0-7859-8445-3*, 3579002864) Fr & Eur.

Woerterbuch der Veterinarmedizin Ekkehard Wiesner. 3rd ed. 1991. (GER.). 1662p. 225.00 (*0-7859-8314-7*, 3334003884) Fr & Eur.

Woerterbuch Klinisches Medizin German-English. Dressler. 1991. (ENG & GER.). 878p. 195.00 (*0-7859-7548-9*, 3527154647) Fr & Eur.

Woerterbuch Medizinischer Fachausdruecke. Fachredaktion. 2nd ed. 1973. (GER.). 59.95 (*0-8288-6348-2*, M-6913) Fr & Eur.

Woerterbuch Zur Medizinischen Soziologie. Paul Luth. 1980. (GER.). 408p. 79.95 (*0-8288-2362-6*, M15305) Fr & Eur.

Wolf Boy of Agra & Feral Children & Autistic Children. William F. Ogburn & Bruno Bettelheim. 1993. (Reprint Series in Social Sciences). (C). reprint ed. pap. text 1.90 (*0-8290-2709-2*, S-608) Irvington.

Wolf-Heidegger's Atlas of Human Anatomy, Set. 5th rev. ed. Ed. by Petra Kopf-Maier. Tr. by Arthur W. English from LAT. Incl. Wolf-Heidegger's Atlas of Human Anatomy Vol. 1: Systemic Anatomy, Body Wall, Upper & Lower Limbs. xxii, 326p. 1999. 78.25 (*3-8055-6852-5*); Wolf-Heidegger's Atlas of Human Anatomy Vol. 2: Head & Neck, Thorax, Abdomen, Pelvis, CNS, Eye, Ear. xxiv, 456p. 2000. 78.25 (*3-8055-6853-3*); LC 99-33383. (Illus.). 2000. 130.50 (*3-8055-6854-1*) S Karger.

Wolf-Heidegger's Atlas of Human Anatomy: Wolf-Heideggers Atlas der HumanAnatomie, Vols. I-III. Ed. by H. F. Frick et al. 4th rev. ed. 1990. (Illus.). 600p. 130.50 (*3-8055-4289-5*) S Karger.

Wolf-Heidegger's Atlas of Human Anatomy Vol. 1: Systemic Anatomy, Body Wall, Upper & Lower Limbs Ed. by Petra Kopf-Maier. Tr. by Arthur W. English from LAT. 5th rev. ed. 1999. LC 99-33383. (Illus.). xxii, 326p. 78.25 (*3-8055-6852-5*) S Karger.

Wolf-Heidegger's Atlas of Human Anatomy Vol. 2: Head & Neck, Thorax, Abdomen, Pelvis, CNS, Eye, Ear Ed. by Petra Kopf-Maier. Tr. by Arthur W. English from LAT. 5th rev. ed. 2000. LC 99-33383. (Illus.). xxiv, 456p. 78.25 (*3-8055-6853-3*) S Karger.

Wolf-Hirschhorn Syndrome: A Guidebook for Families. G. Bradley Schaefer et al. 1996. (Illus.). 48p. (Orig.). spiral bd. 11.00 (*1-889843-03-2*) Munroe-Meyer Inst.

Wolf Man. Ed. by Muriel Gardiner. 1991. 390p. pap. 15.00 (*0-374-52313-4*) FS&G.

Wolff-Parkinson-White Syndrome. Carlos A. Morillo et al. 1996. LC 96-36747. (Clinical Approaches to Tachyarrhythmias Ser.: Vol. 6). (Illus.). 58p. 24.00 (*0-87993-660-6*) Futura Pub.

Wolff's Anatomy of the Eye & Orbit: Including the Central Connections, Development and... Anthony J. Bron & Rama C. Tripathi. 8th ed. 1997. 752p. (C). (gr. 13). (*0-412-41010-9*) E A GBR. *Dist:* OUP.

Wolff's Law & Connective Tissue Regulation: Modern Interdisciplinary Comments on Wolff's Law of Connective Tissue Regulation & Rational Understanding of Common Clinical Problems. Ed. by Gunter Regling. 1993. LC 93-20493. 121.55 (*3-11-013909-X*) De Gruyter.

Woman: A Treatise on the Normal & Pathological Emotions of Feminine Love. Bernard S. Talmey. 7th enl. rev. ed. LC 72-9684. (Illus.). reprint ed. 34.00 (*0-404-57504-8*) AMS Pr.

Woman: Your Body, Your Health. Josleen Wilson. 1990. LC 88-21067. (Harvest Book Ser.). (Illus.). 160p. pap. 19.95 (*0-15-698150-5*, Harvest Bks) Harcourt.

Woman Beneath the Skin: A Doctor's Patients in Eighteenth-Century Germany. Barbara Duden. Tr. by Thomas J. Dunlap from GER. 1991. LC 91-4673. 248p. (C). 35.50 (*0-674-95403-3*) HUP.

Woman Beneath the Skin: A Doctor's Patients in Eighteenth-Century Germany. Barbara Duden. 1998. 256p. pap. text 16.50 (*0-674-95404-1*) HUP.

Woman Doctor's Civil War: Esther Hill Hawks' Diary. Ed. by Gerald Schwartz. 1989. LC 84-11998. (Illus.). 289p. (Orig.). pap. 14.95 (*0-87249-622-8*) U of SC Pr.

Woman Doctor's Diet for Women. 1994. 4.99 (*0-345-90195-9*) Ballantine Pub Grp.

Woman Doctor's Guide to Hormone Therapy: How to Choose What's Right for You. Nananda F. Col. 1997. LC 97-60743. 175p. 24.95 (*1-886284-03-2*, Tatnuck) Chandler Hse.

Woman for All Ages: Dr. Hallie Earle, 1880-1963. Jessie L. Janes. 1988. 61p. (Orig.). pap. 10.00 (*1-879667-14-2*) Dove Pr TX.

Woman Heal Thyself: An Ancient Healing System for Contemporary Women. Jeanne E. Blum. (Illus.). 1995. LC 94-46764. 192p. 24.95 (*0-8048-3045-2*); 1996. LC 96-8886. 328p. pap. text 18.95 (*0-8048-3101-7*) Tuttle Pubng.

Woman in Medicine. Maria Steward. 1977. lib. bdg. 59.95 (*0-8490-2832-9*) Gordon Pr.

Woman in the Mirror: Analytical Psychology & the Feminine. Claire Douglas. 1989. LC 89-21599. 260p. (Orig.). (C). 34.95 (*0-938434-58-6*); pap. 17.95 (*0-938434-57-8*) Sigo Pr.

Woman in the Surgeon's Body. Joan Cassell. 1998. LC 97-47091. 267p. 37.00 (*0-674-95467-X*) HUP.

Woman of Valor: Clara Barton & the Civil War. Stephen B. Oates. 1994. LC 93-38830. x, 527p. 27.95 (*0-02-923405-0*) Free Pr.

Woman Patient Vol. 1: Sexual & Reproductive Aspects of Women's Health Care. Ed. by Malkah T. Notman & Carol C. Nadelson. 1978. (Women in Context Ser.). (Illus.). 376p. 47.50 (*0-306-31151-8*, Plenum Trade) Perseus Pubng.

Woman Patient Vol. 2: Concepts of Femininity & the Life Cycle. Ed. by Carol C. Nadelson et al. 1982. LC 82-5326. (Women in Context Ser.). 216p. 45.00 (*0-306-40846-5*, Plenum Trade) Perseus Pubng.

Woman Patient Vol. 3: Aggressions, Adaptations, & Psychotherapy. Ed. by Malkah T. Notman & Carol C. Nadelson. 1982. LC 82-5325. (Women in Context Ser.). 326p. 45.00 (*0-306-40859-7*, Plenum Trade) Perseus Pubng.

Woman to Woman. Yvonne S. Thornton & Jo Coudert. 1998. LC 97-23547. (Illus.). 336p. pap. 13.95 (*0-452-27986-0*, Plume) Dutton Plume.

Woman Wanders Through Life & Science. Irena Koprowska. 1998. LC 96-18625. (SUNY Series in the Voices of Immigrant Women). 306p. (C). pap. text 20.95 (*0-7914-3178-9*) State U NY Pr.

Woman Who Knew Too Much: Alice Stewart & the Secrets of Radiation. Gayle Greene. 2001. (Illus.). 360p. pap. 18.95 (*0-472-08783-5*, 08783) U of Mich Pr.

Womancare: A Gynecological Guide to Your Body. Lynda Madaras & Jane Patterson. 1983. 960p. pap. 15.00 (*0-380-87643-4*, Avon Bks) Morrow Avon.

Womanly Art of Breastfeeding. La Leche League International Staff. 1991. pap. 9.95 (*0-452-26726-9*, Plume) Dutton Plume.

Woman's Best Medicine: Health, Happiness, & Long Life Through Ayur-Veda. Nancy Lonsdorf et al. 1995. LC 94-8619. 384p. 15.95 (*0-87477-785-2*, Tarcher Putnam) Putnam Pub Group.

Woman's Body: A Manual for Life. Ed. by Miriam Stoppard. 1998. LC 94-6290. (Illus.). 224p. 29.95 (*1-56458-617-0*) DK Pub Inc.

Woman's Book of Choices: Abortion, Menstrual Extraction, RU-486. Rebecca Chalker & Carol Downer. 1992. LC 92-13956. (Illus.). 192p. (Orig.). pap. 13.95 (*1-888363-28-2*) Seven Stories.

Woman's Book of Healing Herbs: Secrets from 90 Top Herbal Healers. Sari Harrar & Sara Altshul O'Donnell. 2000. (Illus.). 480p. pap. 18.95 (*1-57954-214-X*) Rodale Pr Inc.

Woman's Book of Life: Biology, Psychology & Spirituality of the Feminine Life Cycle. Joan Borysenko. 1996. LC 96-38374. 304p. 24.95 (*1-57322-043-4*, Riverhead Books) Putnam Pub Group.

Woman's Comfort Book: A Self-Nurturing Guide for Restoring Balance in Your Life. Jennifer Louden. 1992. LC 91-55316. 224p. pap. 18.00 (*0-06-250531-9*) Harper SF.

Woman's Decision: Breast Care, Treatment & Reconstruction. Karen Berger & John Bostwick, III. 3rd ed. 1998. LC 98-41310. 592p. pap. 18.95 (*0-312-18229-5*, Tor Books) T Doherty Assocs.

Woman's Decision: Breast Care, Treatment & Reconstruction. Karen Berger et al. 3rd ed. 1998. LC 98-38011. (Illus.). 680p. pap. 18.50 (*1-57626-080-1*, QMP) Quality Med Pub.

Woman's Encyclopedia of Natural Healing: The New Healing Techniques of over 100 Leading Alternative Practitioners. Gary Null. 1996. LC 96-28291. 416p. (Orig.). pap. 19.95 (*1-888363-35-5*) Seven Stories.

Woman's Guide to Making Therapy Work. Joan Shapiro & Margaret Grant. 1998. 206p. text 20.00 (*0-7881-5771-X*) DIANE Pub.

Woman's Guide to Menopause & Hormone Replacement Theory. Lorraine Dennerstein et al. 1998. LC 98-10653. 160p. 22.95 (*0-88048-782-8*, 8782) Am Psychiatric.

Woman's Guide to Overcoming Sexual Fear & Pain. Aurelie J. Goodwin & Marc E. Agronin. 1997. LC 97-66081. (Illus.). 288p. pap. 19.95 (*1-57224-089-X*) New Harbinger.

Woman's Guide to Sexual Health. Sue DeCotiis. 1989. 304p. (Orig.). mass mkt. 5.50 (*0-671-66011-X*) PB.

Woman's Guide to the Breast. Barry N. Haicken. 2nd rev. ed. 1993. (Illus.). 104p. spiral bd. 19.95 (*0-9667388-0-2*) Bay Dr Pubns.

Woman's Guide to Vitamins & Minerals. Thomas J. Sultenfuss & Sherry W. Sultenfuss. 1995. LC 94-47604. 288p. 16.95 (*0-8092-3509-9*) NTC Contemp Pub Co.

Woman's Guide to Vitamins, Minerals & Alternative Healing. Sultenfuss and Sultenfuss Staff. 2000. 288p. 7.98 (*1-56731-407-4*, MJF Bks) Fine Comms.

Woman's Guide to Yeast Infections. Naomi Bumslag & Dia L. Michaels. Ed. by Claire Zion. 1992. 288p. (Orig.). mass mkt. 5.99 (*0-671-74699-5*) PB.

Woman's Health Diary. Shelagh Wallace. 2000. (Illus.). 144p. 14.95 (*1-55209-547-9*) Firefly Bks Limited.

Woman's Health Journal. Joann L. Lamb. 2000. 112p. pap. 17.95 (*1-58238-046-5*, Whitman Coin) St Martin.

Woman's HIV Sourcebook: A Guide to Better Health & Well-Being. Patricia Kloser & Jan M. Craig. 1994. 140p. 19.95 (*0-87833-863-2*) Taylor Pub.

Woman's HIV Sourcebook: A Guide to Better Health & Well-Being. Patricia Kloser & Jane M. Craig. 1994. 176p. pap. 12.95 (*0-87833-867-5*) Taylor Pub.

Woman's Identity. Ruth T. Barnhouse. 1994. LC 93-91042. Orig. Title: Identity. 150p. reprint ed. pap. 13.95 (*0-9638398-3-7*) Bonne Chance.

Woman's Nature: Rationalizations of Inequality. Marian Lowe & Ruth Hubbard. 1983. (Athene Ser.). 140p. text 50.00 (*0-08-030143-6*); pap. text 19.95 (*0-08-030142-8*) Elsevier (Pergamon Pr).

Woman's Orgasm: A Guide to Sexual Satisfaction. Georgia Kline-Graber et al. 1988. 240p. mass mkt. 6.99 (*0-446-31503-6*) Warner Bks.

Woman's Own Guide to Pregnancy & Childbirth. Teresa Barker. 1989. 64p. (Orig.). pap. 6.95 (*0-9626223-0-3*) Womens Hlthcare Pr.

Woman's Own Remedy Box: Natural Remedies for Self-Healing. Amy Conway. 1996. (Illus.). 84p. 24.95 (*0-8048-3067-3*) Tuttle Pubng.

Woman's Quest: The Life of Marie E. Zakrzewska, M. D. Ed. by Agnes C. Vietor. 1974. LC 72-2630. (American Women Ser.: Images & Realities). (Illus.). 522p. reprint ed. 35.95 (*0-405-04486-0*) Ayer.

Woman's Right to Know: The Breast Cancer Prevention Report. Daniel A. Herman & David Zava. 1998. (Illus.). 272p. pap. text 18.99 (*0-9644403-0-X*) Advances.

Woman's Self-Esteem: Struggles & Triumphs in the Search for Identity. Nathaniel Branden. 1998. LC 98-9010. (Health & Psychology Ser.). 176p. 18.00 (*0-7879-4371-1*) Jossey-Bass.

Womb with a View. University of Wisconsin - Madison Staff. 1995. 160p. spiral bd. 14.95 (*0-7872-0552-4*) Kendall-Hunt.

Women After Treatment: A Study of Former Mental Patients & Their Normal Neighbors. Shirley S. Angrist et al. 1968. LC 68-20043. (C). 31.00 (*0-89197-471-7*) Irvington.

Women, AIDS, & Activism. ACT-UP - New York Women and AIDS Book Group Staff & New York Women's Handbook Group Staff. 1990. 294p. 25.00 (*0-89608-394-2*) South End Pr.

Women, AIDS & Communities: A Guide for Action. Gerry Pearlberg. 1991. LC 91-17428. (Illus.). 141p. 29.00 (*0-8108-2470-1*); pap. 20.50 (*0-8108-2450-7*) Scarecrow.

Women Alone: Creating a Joyous & Fulfilling Life. Julie Keene & Ione Jenson. 1995. 224p. (Orig.). pap. 12.00 (*1-56170-119-X*, 167) Hay House.

Women & Aging: An Anthology by Women. Ed. by Calyx Editorial Collective Staff et al. 1986. (Illus.). 262p. (C). 28.95 (*0-934971-07-2*); LC 90-210910. pap. 15.95 (*0-934971-00-5*) Calyx Bks.

Women & AIDS. Diane Richardson. 1987. 160p. 29.95 (*0-415-90175-8*, A0762); pap. 11.95 (*0-416-01751-7*, A0766) Routledge.

Women & AIDS: A Bibliography. Ed. by Joan Nordquist. 1993. (Contemporary Social Issues: A Bibliographic Ser.: No. 29). 64p. (Orig.). pap. 20.00 (*0-937855-56-1*) Ref Rsch Serv.

Women & AIDS: Coping & Care. Ed. by Ann O'Leary & Loretta S. Jemmott. 1996. LC 96-3254. (AIDS Prevention & Mental Health Ser.). (Illus.). 263p. 54.00 (*0-306-45258-8*, Kluwer Plenum) Kluwer Academic.

Women & AIDS: Negotiating Safer Practices, Care, & Representation. Ed. by Nancy L. Roth & Linda K. Fuller. 1997. LC 97-16980. (Haworth Innovations in Feminist Studies). 330p. 39.95 (*0-7890-6014-0*); pap. 19.95 (*1-56023-882-8*, Harrington Park) Haworth Pr.

Women & AIDS: Psychological Perspectives. Corinne Squire. 1993. (Gender & Psychology Ser.). (Illus.). 208p. pap. 27.95 (*0-8039-8588-6*, 9960) Sage.

Women & Alcohol Abuse: Prevention Resource Guide. 1993. 32p. (Orig.). (C). pap. text 25.00 (*0-7881-0167-6*) DIANE Pub.

Women & Anger. Ed. by Sandra P. Thomas et al. 1993. LC 92-44878. (Focus on Women Ser.: Vol. 15). 332p. 37.95 (*0-8261-8100-7*) Springer Pub.

Women & Anxiety: A Step-by-Step Program for Managing Anxiety & Depression. Helen A. Derosis. rev. ed. 1998. LC 97-41355. (Self-Help Classic Ser.). 296p. pap. 14.95 (*1-886330-99-9*) Hatherleigh.

Women & Borderline Personality Disorder: Symptoms & Stories. Janet Wirth Cauchon. 2001. LC 00-39037. x, 235p. 52.00 (*0-8135-2890-9*); pap. 22.00 (*0-8135-2891-7*) Rutgers U Pr.

Women & Cancer. Ed. by Steven D. Stellman. 1987. (Women & Health Ser.: Vol. 11, Nos. 3-4). 277p. LC 86-26942. text 8.95 (*0-86656-613-9*); LC 86-26943. reprint ed. pap. text 19.95 (*0-918393-31-0*, Harrington Park) Haworth Pr.

Women & Cancer: Gynecology Oncology Nursing Perspective. Giselle Moore. 1996. (Nursing Ser.). (Illus.). 624p. (C). text 68.95 (*0-86720-714-0*, 714-0) Jones & Bartlett.

Women & Children in Healthcare: An Unequal Majority. Mahowald. 1996. (Illus.). 304p. (C). pap. text 19.95 (*0-19-510870-1*) OUP.

Women & Depression: A Lifespan Perspective. Ed. by Ruth Formanek & Anita Gurian. 1987. (Focus on Women Ser.). 328p. 36.95 (*0-8261-5140-X*) Springer Pub.

Women & Diabetes. Laurinda M. Poirier & Katharine M. Coburn. 1997. LC 97-3159. (Illus.). 240p. pap. 14.95 (*0-945448-77-5*, 00775Q) Am Diabetes.

Women & Disability. Esther R. Boylan. 1991. LC 91-12443. (Women & World Development Ser.). (Illus.). (C). 111p. pap. (*0-86232-987-6*); 160p. text (*0-86232-986-8*) Zed Books GBR. *Dist:* St Martin.

Women & Drug Abuse Treatment: Needs & Services. 1986. lib. bdg. 79.95 (*0-8490-3506-6*) Gordon Pr.

Women & Drugs. 1986. lib. bdg. 79.95 (*0-8490-3507-4*) Gordon Pr.

Women & Epilepsy. Ed. by Michael R. Trimble. 1991. LC 91-84600. 294p. 256.95 (*0-471-92998-0*, Wiley-Liss) Wiley.

Women & Exercise: Physiology & Sports Medicine. Ed. by Mona M. Shangold & Gabe Mirkin. 2nd ed. 1994. (Illus.). 352p. (C). 52.00 (*0-8036-7817-7*) OUP.

Women & Fatigue. Holly Atkinson. 1989. mass mkt. 6.50 (*0-671-69216-X*) PB.

Women & Gender: Transforming Psychology. Janice Yoder. 1998. LC 98-8124. (Illus.). 450p. pap. text 60.00 (*0-13-644600-0*) P-H.

Women & Group Psychotherapy: Theory & Practice. Betsy DeChant. 1996. LC 96-20155. 618p. text 55.00 (*1-57230-098-1*, 0098) Guilford Pubns.

Women & Health. Saltman. 1992. pap. text 34.00 (*0-7295-0285-6*) Saunders.

Women & Health. Ed. by Patricia Smyke. 1991. LC 91-29612. (Women & World Development Ser.). (C). pap. 22.50 (*0-86232-983-3*) St Martin.

Women & Health: An Annotated Bibliography. Frances R. Belmonte. 1997. LC 97-22482. (Magill Bibliographies Ser.). 208p. 35.00 (*0-8108-3385-9*) Scarecrow.

Women & Health: Cross-Cultural Perspectives. Patricia Whelehan. 1988. 240p. 62.95 (*0-89789-138-4*, H138); pap. 24.95 (*0-89789-139-2*, G139) Greenwood (Bergin & Garvey).

Women & Health: Feminist Perspectives. Ed. by Sue Wilkinson & Celia Kitzinger. 1994. LC 94-24353. (Gender & Society Ser.). 208p. 85.00 (*0-7484-0148-2*) Taylor & Francis.

Women & Health in Africa. Ed. by Meredeth Turshen. 1990. LC 90-81473. 325p. (C). 49.95 (*0-86543-180-9*); pap. 16.95 (*0-86543-181-7*) Africa World.

Women & Health in America: Historical Readings. Judith W. Leavitt. 2nd ed. 1999. LC 98-14446. 65.00 (*0-299-15960-4*); 560p. pap. 29.95 (*0-299-15964-7*) U of Wis Pr.

Women & Health Psychology Cheryl B. Travis. 1988. (Environment & Health Ser.). 288p. text 45.00 (*0-8058-0253-3*); 320p. text 45.00 (*0-89859-974-1*);Set. text 70.00 (*0-8058-0292-4*) L Erlbaum Assocs.

Women & Health Research Vol. 1: Ethical & Legal Issues of Including Women in Clinical Studies. Institute of Medicine Staff. Ed. by Anne C. Mastroianni et al. 1994. LC 93-50549. 288p. (C). 34.95 (*0-309-04992-X*) Natl Acad Pr.

Women & Health Research Vol. 2: Ethical & Legal Issues of Including Women in Clinical Studies: Workshop & Commissioned Papers. Committee on the Ethical and Legal Issues Relating t. Ed. by Anna C. Mastroianni et al. 1994. LC 93-50549. (Women & Health Research; Ethical & Legal Issues of Including Women in Clinical Studies: Vol. 2). 264p. (Orig.). (C). pap. text 29.00 (*0-309-05040-5*) Natl Acad Pr.

Women & Health Services: An Agenda for Change. Lesley Doyal. 1998. LC 98-4891. xiv, 258p. (*0-335-20137-7*); pap. (*0-335-20136-9*) OpUniv Pr.

Women & Heart Disease. Desmond G. Julian & Nanette K. Wenger. 1997. 464p. (*1-85317-287-1*) Martin Dunitz GBR. *Dist:* Mosby Inc.

Women & Heart Disease. Ed. by Susan Wilansky & James T. Willerson. 2000. LC 2001-17366. (Illus.). 495p. (J). text (*0-443-07900-5*) Church.

***Women & Heart Disease: An Atlas of Racial & Ethnic Disparities in Mortality.** Ed. by Michele L. Casper. 2001. (Illus.). 239p. (C). reprint ed. pap. text 50.00 (*0-7567-0815-X*) DIANE Pub.

Women & HIV Disease: Falling Through the Cracks. 1993. (Illus.). 247p. (Orig.). (C). pap. text 40.00 (*1-56806-430-6*) DIANE Pub.

Women & HIV/AIDS (Las Mujeres y el VIH/SIDA) Issues & Perspectives (Realidades y Perspectivas) Margarita Rodriguez-Kelly. 2000. (ENG & SPA., Illus.). 300p. (*0-9664774-1-3*) Genmark DC.

Women & Hormones: An Essential Guide to Being Female. Alice T. MacMahon. Ed. by James R. MacMahon. 1990. LC 90-81214. (Illus.). 208p. (Orig.). pap. 9.95 (*0-931128-03-X*) Family Pubns.

Women & Leadership in Health Care: The Journey to Authenticity & Power. Catherine Robinson-Walker. 1999. LC 98-58078. 227p. 42.00 (*0-7879-0933-5*) Jossey-Bass.

Women & Madness. Phyllis Chesler. 3rd ed. 1997. LC 97-41573. (Illus.). 416p. reprint ed. pap. 15.00 (*1-56858-096-7*) FWEW.

Women & Madness. Phyllis Chesler. 1989. (Illus.). 400p. pap. 12.00 (*0-15-698295-1*) Harcourt.

***Women & Medicare Reform.** Marilyn Moon. 2001. 160p. pap. text 13.95 (*0-87078-471-4*) Century Foundation.

Women & Men: Gender in the Church. Ed. by Carol Penner. 1998. LC 98-72959. 152p. pap. 11.99 (*0-8361-9079-3*) Herald Press.

Women & Men: New Perspectives on Gender Differences. Ed. by Malkah T. Notman & Carol C. Nadelson. 1991. LC 90-548. (Issues in Psychiatry Ser.). 144p. pap. text 12.95 (*0-88048-136-6*, 8136) Am Psychiatric.

Women & Mental Health. Ed. by Jeri A. Sechzer et al. 1998. (Illus.). 226p. pap. text 27.00 (*0-8018-6089-X*) Johns Hopkins.

Women & Mental Health. Jeri A. Sechzer. 1996. LC 96-18877. (Annals of the New York Academy of Sciences Ser.). 215p. pap. 100.00 (*1-57331-033-6*) NY Acad Sci.

Women & Mental Health: New Directions for Change. Ed. by Carol T. Mowbray et al. 1985. LC 84-19228. (Women & Therapy Ser.: Vol. 3, Nos. 3-4). 202p. text 6.95 (*0-86656-331-8*); pap. text 19.95 (*0-86656-437-3*) Haworth Pr.

Women & Mental Health: New Directions for Change. Ed. by Carol T Mowbray et al. 1985. LC 84-22454. (Women & Therapy Ser.: Vol. 3, Nos. 3 & 4). 202p. pap. text 19.95 (*0-918393-13-2*, Harrington Park) Haworth Pr.

Women & New Reproductive Technologies: Medical, Psychosocial, Legal & Ethical Dilemmas. Ed. by A. Collins & Judith Rodin. 1991. 176p. (C). text 36.00 (*0-8058-0919-8*) L Erlbaum Assocs.

Women & Nutrition in Third World Countries. Deborah Spicer et al. 1984. LC 83-25690. 160p. 30.95 (*0-275-91185-3*, C1185, Praeger Pubs) Greenwood.

Women & Occupational Health Risks: Report on a WHO Meeting. 1983. (Euro Reports & Studies Ser.: No. 76). 41p. pap. text 4.00 (*92-890-1242-0*) World Health.

Women & Pelvic Inflammatory Diseases: Index of Modern Information. Adela I. Dione. 1991. LC 88-47953. 150p. 47.50 (*1-55914-492-0*); pap. 44.50 (*1-55914-493-9*) ABBE Pubs Assn.

Women & Population Growth: Choice Beyond Childbearing. Kathleen Newland. 1977. LC 77-91827. (Worldwatch Papers). pap. 5.00 (*0-916468-15-1*) Worldwatch Inst.

Women & Prenatal Testing: Facing the Challenges of Genetic Technology. Ed. by Karen H. Rothenberg & Elizabeth J. Thomson. 1994. LC 94-6363. (Women & Health Ser.). 305p. text 60.00 (*0-8142-0640-9*); pap. text 18.95 (*0-8142-0641-7*) Ohio St U Pr.

Women & Psychotherapy: An Assessment of Research & Practice. Ed. by Annette M. Brodsky & Rachel T. Hare-Mustin. 1986. LC 80-14842. 428p. pap. 30.00 (*0-89862-909-8*, 2909) Guilford Pubns.

Women & Relapse. Suzanne B. Cusack. 1984. 36p. (Orig.). pap. 3.00 (*0-89486-237-5*, 1379B) Hazelden.

Women & Sacrifice: Male Narcissism & the Psychology of Religion. William Beers. 1992. LC 92-13007. 214p. (C). 28.95 (*0-8143-2377-4*) Wayne St U Pr.

Women & Self-Harm: Understanding, Coping & Healing from Self-Mutilation. Gerrilyn Smith. 1999. LC 98-50423. 166p. pap. text 16.99 (*0-415-92410-3*) Routledge.

Women & Self-Harm: Understanding, Coping & Healing from Self-Mutilation. Gerrilyn Smith et al. 1999. LC 98-50423. 166p. pap. 16.95 (*0-415-92411-1*) Routledge.

Women & Sex Roles: Social Psychological Perspective. Irene H. Frieze et al. 1978. (Illus.). 444p. (C). pap. text 19.50 (*0-393-09063-9*) Norton.

Women & Substance Abuse. Ed. by Edith S. Gomberg & Ted D. Nirenberg. 1993. LC 93-23065. 400p. 85.00 (*1-56750-065-X*); pap. 42.50 (*1-56750-066-8*) Greenwood (Ablex).

Women & Substance Abuse: Gender Transparency. Ed. by Sally J. Stevens & Harry K. Wexler. 1998. LC 98-16153. 277p. pap. 24.95 (*0-7890-0389-9*) Haworth Pr.

Women & Suicidal Behavior. Ed. by Silvia S. Canetto & David Lester. 1995. LC 94-31918. (Focus on Women Ser.). (Illus.). 320p. 38.95 (*0-8261-8630-0*) Springer Pub.

Women & Tampons: Index of New Information with Authors & Subjects. Valerie J. Gibson. rev. ed. 1994. LC 94-35173. 147p. 57.50 (*0-7883-0376-7*); pap. 47.50 (*0-7883-0377-5*) ABBE Pubs Assn.

Women & the Health Care Industry: An Unhealthy Relationship? Peggy Foster. 1995. LC 94-42684. 224p. (*0-335-09473-2*); pap. (*0-335-09472-4*) OpUniv Pr.

Women & the Menopause: A Book for & about Women & the Climacteric. Brenda Millette & Joellen Hawkins. 1983. (C). pap. text 19.95 (*0-8359-8772-8*) P-H.

Women & the New Reproductive Technologies in Ireland. Fintan O'Toole. 1994. LC 95-178445. (Undercurrents Ser.). pap. (*1-85918-030-2*) Cork Univ IRL. *Dist:* Intl Spec Bk.

Women & the Ownership of PMS: The Structuring of a Psychiatric Disorder. Anne Figert. 1996. (Social Problems & Social Issues Ser.). 211p. pap. text 23.95 (*0-202-30551-1*); lib. bdg. 45.95 (*0-202-30550-3*) Aldine de Gruyter.

Women & Their Life-Styles: Index of New Information. Paul K. Vogel. 1994. 150p. 57.50 (*0-7883-0056-3*); pap. 47.50 (*0-7883-0057-1*) ABBE Pubs Assn.

Women & Tobacco. C. Chollat-Traquet et al. 1994. (Illus.). 128p. (Orig.). (C). pap. text 35.00 (*0-7881-1342-9*) DIANE Pub.

Women & Tobacco. C. Chollat-Traquet et al. 1992. (CHI, ENG, FRE, RUS & SPA.). xi, 128p. (Orig.). pap. text 26.00 (*92-4-156147-5*, 1150373) World Health.

Women & Well-Being. Ed. by Vanaja Dhruvarajan. 1990. (ENG & FRE.). 260p. (C). (*0-7735-0734-5*); pap. (*0-7735-0762-0*) McG-Queens Univ Pr CAN. *Dist:* CUP Services.

Women & Women's Cancer see Reclaiming Our Lives after Breast & Gynecologic Cancer

Women, Anger & Depression: Strategies for Self-Empowerment. Lois P. Frankel. 1991. 112p. (Orig.). pap. 8.95 (*1-55874-161-5*) Health Comm.

***Women Are Not Small Men: Live-Saving Strategies for Preventing & Healing Heart Disease in Women.** Nieca Goldberg. 2002. LC 2001-49943. 384p. 24.00 (*0-345-44098-6*, Ballantine) Ballantine Pub Grp.

Women As Healers: Cross-Cultural Perspectives. Ed. by Carol S. McClain. 1989. LC 88-16896. 272p. (C). pap. text 17.00 (*0-8135-1370-7*) Rutgers U Pr.

Women As Therapists: A Multi-Theoretical Casebook. Ed. by Dorothy W. Cantor. 1990. LC 90-35520. 272p. 33.95 (*0-8261-6910-4*) Springer Pub.

Women as Therapists: A Multi-Theoretical Casebook. Ed. by Dorothy W. Cantor. 1992. LC 92-21975. 264p. pap. 45.00 (*0-87668-313-8*) Aronson.

Women as Wombs: Reproductive Technology & the Battle over Women's Freedom. Janice G. Raymond. 1998. 288p. pap. (1-875559-41-8) Spinifex Pr AUS. *Dist:* LPC InBook, LPC InBook, Stackpole.

Women at High Risk to Breast Cancer. Ed. by Basil A. Stoll. 1989. (Developments in Oncology Ser.). (C). text 101.50 (0-89838-416-8) Kluwer Academic.

Women at Risk. David Hager & Don Joy. 1993. 159p. pap. 9.95 (0-917851-62-5) Bristol Hse.

Women at the Change: The Intelligent Woman's Guide to Menopause. Madonna S. Compton. 1999. LC 98-13884. 288p. pap. text 14.95 (1-56718-171-6) Llewellyn Pubns.

Women at War: The Story of Fifty Military Nurses Who Served in Vietnam. Elizabeth Norman. 1990. LC 90-34487. (Studies in Health, Illness, & Caregiving). (Illus.). 238p. (Orig.). (C). pap. 16.95 (0-8122-1317-3) U of Pa Pr.

Women, Babies, & Drugs: Family-Centered Treatment Options. 1990. 33p. 15.00 (1-55516-640-7, 6119) Natl Conf State Legis.

Women Beyond Freud: New Concepts of Feminine Psychology. Ed. by Milton M. Berger. 1993. 224p. text 34.95 (0-87630-709-8) Brunner-Routledge.

Women Changing Therapy: New Assessments, Values & Strategies in Feminist Therapy. Ed. by Joan H. Robbins & Rachel J. Siegel. 240p. 1985. LC 84-19276. pap. text 14.95 (0-918393-07-8, Harrington Park); 1983. LC 83-12643. (Women & Therapy Ser.: Vol. 2, Nos. 2-3). text 39.95 (0-86656-239-7); 1983. LC 83-12643. (Women & Therapy Ser.: Vol. 2, Nos. 2-3). pap. text 14.95 (0-86656-240-0) Haworth Pr.

Women, Children, & HIV - AIDS. Ed. by Felissa L. Cohen & Jerry D. Durham. 1993. LC 92-48971. 328p. 39.95 (0-8261-7880-4) Springer Pub.

Women Confront Cancer: Twenty-One Leaders Making Medical History by Choosing Alternative & Complementary Therapies. Margaret J. Wooddell & David J. Hess. 1998. LC 98-19752. 272p. pap. 15.95 (0-8147-3587-8); text 50.00 (0-8147-3586-X) NYU Pr.

Women, Crime, & Criminology: A Feminist Critique. Carol Smart. 1978. reprint ed. pap. 14.95 (0-7100-8833-7, Routledge Thoemms) Routledge.

Women, Drinking & Pregnancy. Moira Plant. 1985. 208p. (0-422-78610-1, 9483) Tavistock GBR. *Dist:* Routldge.

Women, Drug Use, & HIV Infection. Ed. by Sally J. Stevens et al. 1998. LC 98-17207. (Women & Health Ser.: Vol. 27, Nos. 1-2). 237p. 49.95 (0-7890-0351-1); pap. 19.95 (0-7890-0527-1) Haworth Pr (Hawrth Medical).

Women Drug Users: An Ethnography of a Female Injecting Community. Avril Taylor. 1993. LC 93-213810. 192p. text 39.95 (0-19-825796-1) OUP.

Women, Feminism & Family Therapy. Ed. by Lois Braverman. 1988. LC 87-63475. (Journal of Psychotherapy & the Family Ser.: Vol. 3, No. 4). 192p. text 39.95 (0-86656-696-1) Haworth Pr.

Women, Gender & Social Psychology. Ed. by Virginia O'Leary et al. 1985. 400p. (C). text 79.95 (0-89859-447-2) L Erlbaum Assocs.

Women, Girls, & Psychotherapy: Reframing Resistance. Ed. by Annie G. Rogers et al. 1991. LC 91-20845. (Women & Therapy Ser.). 243p. lib. bdg. 39.95 (1-56024-196-9) Haworth Pr.

Women Giving Birth. Saskiavan Rees et al. 1995. (Illus.). 160p. (Orig.). pap. 18.95 (0-89087-668-1) Celestial Arts.

Women Growing Older: Theoretical Perspectives in the Psychology of Aging. Ed. by Barbara F. Turner & Lillian E. Troll. 1993. LC 93-35574. (Illus.). 282p. (C). pap. 34.95 (0-8039-3987-6, 3128) Sage.

Women Healers: Portraits of Herbalists, Physicians & Midwives. Elisabeth Brooke. 1995. LC 95-23433. 176p. pap. 12.95 (0-89281-548-5, Heal Arts VT) Inner Tradit.

Women Healers in Medieval Life & Literature. Muriel J. Hughes. 1977. LC 68-57322. (Essay Index Reprint Ser.). 26.95 (0-8369-0552-0) Ayer.

Women, Health & Development: A Report by the Director-General. 1985. (WHO Offset Publications: No. 90). 41p. pap. text 7.00 (92-4-170090-4, 1120090) World Health.

Women, Health, & Development in the South-East Asia Region. 1992. (SEARO Regional Health Papers: No. 22). ix, 90p. pap. text 7.00 (92-9022-191-7, 1580022) World Health.

Women, Health & Medicine. Agnes Miles. 1991. 224p. pap. (0-335-09905-X) OpUniv Pr.

Women, Health & Medicine in America: A Historical Handbook. Ed. by Rima D. Apple. 1990. LC 90-2719. 600p. text 20.00 (0-8240-8447-0, 483) Garland.

Women, Health, & Medicine in America: A Historical Handbook. Ed. by Rima D. Apple. 1992. LC 91-20496. (Illus.). 580p. (Orig.). reprint ed. pap. text 18.95 (0-8135-1766-4) Rutgers U Pr.

Women, Health, & Poverty. Cesar A. Perales & Lauren S. Young. Ed. by Cesar A. Perales. 1989. LC 87-26274. (Women & Health Ser.: Vol. 12, Nos. 3-4). 259p. text 49.95 (0-86656-684-8) Haworth Pr.

Women, Hormones & the Menstrual Cycle: Herbal & Medical Solutions from Adolescence to Menopause. Ruth Trickey. 1998. (Illus.). 520p. pap. 24.95 (1-86448-525-6) IPG Chicago.

Women in Context: Toward a Feminist Reconstruction of Psychotherapy. Ed. by Marsha Pravder Mirkin. 1994. LC 94-5534. 502p. 55.00 (0-89862-095-3, C2095) Guilford Pubns.

Women in Families: A Framework for Family Therapy. Monica McGoldrick. 1991. pap. 20.95 (0-393-30776-X) Norton.

Women in Industry: Their Health & Efficiency. Anna M. Baetjer. Ed. by Leon Stein. 1977. LC 77-70480. (Work Ser.). (Illus.). reprint ed. lib. bdg. 35.95 (0-405-10154-6) Ayer.

Women in Medical Education: An Anthology of Experience. Ed. by Delese Wear. 1996. LC 95-49902. 183p. (C). text 21.50 (0-7914-3087-1); pap. text 21.95 (0-7914-3088-X) State U NY Pr.

Women in Medicine. Jacqueline C. Kent. 1998. LC 97-30235. (Profiles Ser.). (Illus.). 160p. (YA). (gr. 5-12). lib. bdg. 19.95 (1-881508-46-3) Oliver Pr MN.

Women in Medicine. Carol Lopate. 1968. LC 68-19526. (Josiah Macy Foundation Ser.). (Illus.). 204p. 36.00 (0-8018-0391-8) Johns Hopkins.

Women in Medicine: Getting In, Growing, & Advancing. Janet W. Bickel. 2000. LC 99-50605. 54.00 (0-7619-1818-3) Sage.

Women in Medicine & Management: A Mentoring Guide. Ed. by Deborah M. Shlian. 1995. LC 95-77323. 119p. (C). pap. text 38.00 (0-924674-35-0) Am Coll Phys Execs.

Women in Psychology: A Bio-Bibliographic Sourcebook. Ed. by Agnes N. O'Connell & Nancy F. Russo. 1990. LC 89-25787. 456p. lib. bdg. 80.00 (0-313-26091-5, OWP/, Greenwood Pr) Greenwood.

Women in Sports - Olympic Encyclopedia of Sports Medicine. Barbara L. Drinkwater. 2000. LC 99-57719. (Encyclopedia of Sports Medicine Ser.: Vol. 8). (Illus.). 608p. 129.00 (0-632-05084-5) Blackwell Sci.

Women in the Middle: Facing Midlife Challenges with Faith. Margot Hover. 1995. LC 94-60480. 88p. (Orig.). pap. 7.95 (0-89622-612-3) Twenty-Third.

Women in Therapy. Harriet G. Lerner. 1992. LC 87-19326. 320p. reprint ed. 60.00 (0-87668-978-0) Aronson.

Women in Therapy. Harriet G. Lerner. 1994. LC 88-45938. 320p. reprint ed. pap. 13.50 (0-06-097228-9, PL 7228, Perennial) HarperTrade.

Women in Therapy & Counseling. M. Walker. 1990. 208p. (0-335-09376-0); pap. (0-335-09375-2) OpUniv Pr.

Women in Veterinary Medicine: Profiles of Success. Sue Drum & H. Ellen Whitely. 1991. LC 91-7050. (Illus.). 286p. pap. 24.95 (0-8138-0667-4) Iowa U Pr.

***Women Living with Fibromyalgia: Refusing to Suffer in Silence.** Barbara Keddy. 2001. LC 2001-26469. pap. 14.95 (0-89793-342-7) Hunter Hse.

Women Living with Multiple Sclerosis. Judith Lynn Nichols et al. 1999. LC 98-35659. 256p. pap. 13.95 (0-89793-218-8) Hunter Hse.

Women, Madness, & Medicine. Denise Russell. 1995. LC 94-38395. 58.95 (0-7456-1260-1) Blackwell Pubs.

Women, Medicine & Science, 1500-1700: Mothers & Sisters of the Royal Society. Ed. by Lynette Hunter & Sarah Hutton. 1997. LC 98-100834. (Illus.). 224p. (0-7509-1334-7) Sutton Pub Ltd GBR. *Dist:* Intl Pubs Mktg.

Women, Medicine & Science, 1500-1700: Mothers & Sisters of the Royal Society. Ed. by Lynette Hunter & Sarah Hutton. 1997. (Illus.). 224p. pap. 22.95 (0-7509-1343-6) Sutton Publng.

Women, Men & Gender: Ongoing Debates. Ed. by Mary R. Walsh. 1996. LC 96-16540. 448p. pap. 26.00 (0-300-06938-3) Yale U Pr.

Women of Color: Integrating Ethnic & Gender Identities in Psychotherapy. Ed. by Lillian Comas-Diaz & Beverly Greene. 1994. LC 94-10840. 518p. 55.00 (0-89862-371-5, C2371) Guilford Pubns.

Women of Psychology: Pioneers & Innovators. Gwendolyn Stevens & Sheldon Gardner. 1982. 273p. I. text 22.95 (0-87073-443-1); I. LC 81-14394. pap. text 18.95 (0-87073-444-X); II. LC 81-14394. text 22.95 (0-87073-445-8); Set. pap. text 18.95 (0-87073-446-6) Schenkman Bks Inc.

Women of Silence: The Emotional Healing of Breast Cancer. Grace Gawler. 1995. 164p. (Orig.). pap. (0-85572-254-1) Hill Content Pubng AUS. *Dist:* Seven Hills Bk.

Women on Menopause: A Change for the Better. Anne Dickson & Nikki Henriques. 1989. 120p. pap. 9.95 (0-89281-237-0, Heal Arts VT) Inner Tradit.

Women Physicians: A Study in Roles & Role-Conflict. Nigar F. Abidi. 1993. (Illus.). xvi, 244p. (81-85445-20-6) Manak Pubns Pvt Ltd IND. *Dist:* Nataraj Bks.

Women Physicians: Careers, Status & Power. Judith Lorber. 1985. 250p. 25.00 (0-422-79040-0, NO. 9071); pap. 12.95 (0-422-79050-8, NO. 9103) Routledge.

Women Pioneers in Texas Medicine. Elizabeth Silverthorne & Geneva Fulgham. 1997. LC 97-18885. (Centennial Series of the Association of Former Students: Vol. 70). (Illus.). 304p. 24.95 (0-89096-789-X) Tex A&M Univ Pr.

Women, Poverty & AIDS: Sex, Drugs & Structural Violence. Paul Farmer et al. 1996. LC 96-27349. 350p. pap. 19.95 (1-56751-074-4) Common Courage.

Women, Power & Therapy: Issues for Women. Ed. by Marjorie Braude. 1988. LC 87-14873. (Women & Therapy Ser.: Vol. 6, Nos. 1-2). 340p. text 49.95 (0-86656-653-8) Haworth Pr.

Women, Pregnancy & Substance Abuse. Dorothy Roberts. 1991. (Law & Pregnancy Ser.). 21p. (C). pap. 8.00 (1-877966-09-6) Ctr Women Policy.

Women Resisting AIDS: Feminist Strategies of Empowerment. Ed. by Beth E. Schneider & Nancy Stoller. 1995. LC 94-31407. (Health, Society, & Policy Ser.). (Illus.). 368p. (Orig.). (C). pap. text 24.95 (1-56639-269-1) Temple U Pr.

Women, Sex, & Addiction: A Search for Love & Power. Charlotte D. Kasl. 1990. LC 89-46229. 416p. reprint ed. pap. 15.00 (0-06-097321-8, Perennial) HarperTrade.

Women Smokers Can Quit: A Different Approach. Sue F. Delaney. 1989. 64p. (Orig.). pap. 6.95 (0-9626223-1-1) Womens Hlthcare Pr.

Women, Stress, & Heart Disease. Ed. by Kristina Orth-Gomer et al. 1996. LC 97-44966. 400p. 69.95 (0-8058-2124-4) L Erlbaum Assocs.

Women Survivors of Childhood Sexual Abuse: Healing Through Group Work - Beyond Survival. Judy Chew. 1997. LC 97-7517. (Haworth Marriage & the Family Ser.). (Illus.). 160p. 39.95 (0-7890-0110-1); pap. 14.95 (0-7890-0284-1) Haworth Pr.

Women Therapists Working with Women: New Theory & Process of Feminist Therapy. Ed. by Claire Brody. 1984. (Focus on Women Ser.: Vol. 7). 192p. 42.95 (0-8261-4550-7) Springer Pub.

Women Treating Women: Case Material from Women Treated by Female Psychoanalysts. Anne E. Bernstein & Gloria M. Warner. 1985. LC 84-8996. xv, 310p. (C). 45.00 (0-8236-6863-0, 06863) Intl Univs Pr.

Women under the Knife. Herbert H. Keyser. 1986. 176p. mass mkt. 3.95 (0-446-32911-8) Warner Bks.

Women, Volunteering, & Health Policy. United Hospital Fund Staff. 1982. 81p. 5.00 (0-934459-27-4) United Hosp Fund.

Women with AIDS & Their Children. Sharon E. Walker. rev. ed. 1998. LC 97-31032. (Children of Poverty Ser.). (Illus.). 160p. text 41.00 (0-8153-3008-1) Garland.

Women with Attention Deficit Disorder: Embracing Disorganization at Home & in the Workplace. Sari Solden. 1995. LC 96-111204. (Illus.). 288p. (Orig.). pap. 11.95 (1-887424-05-9) Underwood Bks.

Women with Cancer. Ed. by B. L. Andersen. 1986. (Contributions to Psychology & Medicine Ser.). (Illus.). 330p. 159.00 (0-387-96360-X) Spr-Verlag.

Women with Disabilities: Found Voices. Ed. by Mary E. Willmuth & Lillian Holcomb. 1994. LC 93-30402. (Women & Therapy Ser.: Vol. 14, Nos. 3-4). (Illus.). 209p. lib. bdg. 39.95 (1-56024-477-1) Haworth Pr.

***Women with Epilepsy.** Ed. by Martha J. Morrell. 2002. LC 2001-52571. 192p. text 74.95 (0-521-65224-3) Cambridge U Pr.

Women, Work & Health: Stress & Opportunities. M. Frankenhaeuser et al. 1991. (Stress & Coping Ser.). (Illus.). 291p. (C). text 49.50 (0-306-43780-5, Kluwer Plenum) Kluwer Academic.

Women's Bibliography of Concerns, Care & Conditions: Index of Modern Information. Zena Y. Webster. 1990. LC 89-18646. 150p. pap. 44.50 (1-55914-125-5) ABBE Pubs Assn.

Women's Bodies: A Social History of Women's Encounter with Health, Ill-Health & Medicine. Edward Shorter. 1990. 424p. (C). pap. text 24.95 (0-88738-848-5) Transaction Pubs.

Women's Bodies, Women's Wisdom: Creating Physical & Emotional Health & Healing. Christiane Northrup. rev. ed. 1998. 944p. LC 98-72168. 35.95 (0-553-11033-0); (Illus.). pap. 18.95 (0-553-37953-4) Bantam.

Women's Bodybuilding for Beginners. Debarra Mayo. 1984. pap. 2.95 (0-02-499890-7, Macmillan Coll) P-H.

Women's Cancers: How to Prevent Them, How to Treat Them, How to Beat Them. Kerry A. McGinn. 2nd ed. 1998. LC 97-20482. (Illus.). 512p. pap. 19.95 (0-89793-223-4) Hunter Hse.

Women's Cancers: How to Prevent Them, How to Treat Them, How to Beat Them. Kerry A. McGinn & P. J. Haylock. 2nd ed. 1998. LC 97-20482. (Illus.). 512p. 29.95 (0-89793-224-2) Hunter Hse.

Women's Concise Guide to a Healthier Heart. Karen J. Carlson et al. 1997. LC 97-17310. (Illus.). 144p. 24.95 (0-674-95483-1); pap. 12.95 (0-674-95484-X) HUP.

Women's Conflicts about Eating & Sexuality: The Relationship Between Food & Sex. Rosalyn M. Meadow. 1992. LC 91-19205. 184p. pap. 10.95 (0-918393-98-1, Harrington Park) Haworth Pr.

Women's Dermatology: From Infancy to Maturity. Ed. by Lawrence Charles Parish et al. 2001. LC 00-38518. (Illus.). 640p. 97.95 (1-85070-086-9, Parthenon Pbng) CRC Pr.

Women's Education & Fertility Behaviour: A Case-Study of Rural Maharashtra, India. 41p. pap. 10.00 (92-1-151257-3, E.93.XIII.12) UN.

Women's Encyclopedia of Natural Medicine. Tori Hudson. 1997. LC 99-17382. 384p. pap. 24.95 (0-87983-788-8, 37888K, Keats Pubng) McGraw-Hill Trade.

Women's Experience of Breastfeeding. Heather MacLean. 1990. 208p. pap. 13.95 (0-8020-6756-5) U of Toronto Pr.

Women's Experience of Feminist Therapy & Counseling. Eileen McLeod. 1994. LC 93-40802. 176p. pap. (0-335-19221-1) OpUniv Pr.

Women's Experiences: A Psychological Perspective. Frances E. Donelson. 1998. LC 97-45772. xxvi, 747p. pap. 42.95 (0-7674-0043-7, 0043-7) Mayfield Pub.

Women's Experiences with HIV/AIDS: An International Perspective. Lynellen D. Long. Ed. by E. Maxine Ankrah. 1997. LC 96-31322. 352p. pap. 18.50 (0-231-10605-X) Col U Pr.

Women's Guide to Herbal Medicine. Carol Rogers. 1997. 240p. pap. (0-241-13349-1) H Hamilton GBR. *Dist:* Trafalgar.

Women's Gymnastics. Wiley Staff. 1980. (Orig.). pap. 7.95 (0-02-499910-5, Macmillan Coll) P-H.

Women's Health. 1997. LC 96-50012. (For Your Information Ser.). pap. 9.50 (1-56853-034-X) New Readers.

Women's Health. Chrisler. 2000. 53.00 (0-07-012000-5) McGraw.

Womens Health. Sample. 2000. pap. text 11.97 net. (0-395-97331-7) HM.

Womens Health. Sapsford. 1997. pap. text (0-7020-2209-8) Bailliere Tindall.

Women's Health. Ed. by Ann McPherson & Deborah Waller. 4th ed. 1997. LC 97-790. (Oxford General Practice Ser.). (Illus.). 664p. pap. text 62.50 (0-19-262750-3) OUP.

Women's Health: A Primary Care Clinical Guide. Ellis Quinn Youngkin. 2nd ed. 1998. pap. text 52.95 (0-8385-8640-6) P-H.

Women's Health: A Primary Care Clinical Guide. Ed. by Ellis Quinn Youngkin & Marcia Szmania Davis. 2nd ed. 1997. LC 97-42654. 864p. (C). pap. 60.75 (0-8385-9640-1, A-9640-2) P-H.

Women's Health: A Primary Health Care Approach. Ed. by Cath Rogers-Clark & Angie Smith. 1999. 304p. pap. 48.00 (0-8036-0423-8) Davis Co.

Women's Health: A Relational Perspective Across the Life Cycle. Judith A. Lewis & Judith Bernstein. 1996. (Nursing Ser.). (Illus.). 352p. (C). pap. text 52.95 (0-86720-485-0, 485-0) Jones & Bartlett.

Women's Health: Across Age & Frontier. 1992. (ENG & FRE.). vi, 107p. pap. text 20.00 (92-4-156152-1, 1150379) World Health.

***Women's Health: An Alternative Medicine Definitive Guide** Burton Goldberg & Alternative Medicine Editors. 2001. (Illus.). 560p. pap. 19.95 (1-887299-41-6) AlternMed Bks.

Women's Health: An Essential Guide for the Modern Woman. Karen Evennett. 1997. (Illus.). 224p. pap. (0-7063-7459-2) WrLock GBR. *Dist:* Sterling.

Women's Health: Complexities & Differences. Sheryl B. Ruzek et al. 1997. LC 96-34047. (Women & Health Ser.). 689p. text 55.00 (0-8142-0704-9); pap. text 21.95 (0-8142-0705-7) Ohio St U Pr.

***Women's Health: Expanding the Women's Health Research.** Ed. by Linda F. Wolf. 2001. (Illus.). 74p. pap. text 25.00 (0-7567-1710-8) DIANE Pub.

Women's Health: Hormones, Emotions & Behavior. Ed. by Regina C. Casper. 1997. LC 97-3022. (Psychiatry & Medicine Ser.). (Illus.). 345p. (C). text 90.00 (0-521-56341-0) Cambridge U Pr.

Women's Health: Prevention Is the Best Medicine. Ed. by George A. Bray & Donna H. Ryan. 2000. (Pennington Center Nutrition Ser.: Vol. 11). 302p. 100.00 (0-8071-2654-3) La State U Pr.

Women's Health: Quick Reference Guides for Family Physicians. Carolyn Thiedke & Joann Rosenfeld. 2000. LC 00-25887. (Academy Collection). (Illus.). 176p. pap. text 29.95 (0-7817-2447-3) Lppncott W & W.

Women's Health: The Commonwealth Fund Survey. Ed. by Marilyn M. Falik & Karen S. Collins. 1996. LC 95-46435. 408p. (C). pap. text 20.95 (0-8018-5354-0) Johns Hopkins.

Women's Health: Your Guide to a Healthier & Happier Life. David Newman et al. 1998. LC 97-77581. (Illus.). 479p. per. 19.95 (0-9661346-5-6) Better Hlth.

Women's Health - Missing from U. S. Medicine. Sue V. Rosser. 1994. LC 94-9745. (Race, Gender & Science Ser.). 224p. 31.50 (0-253-34991-5) Ind U Pr.

Women's Health Advisor. Alice Feinstein. 1995. LC 94-23193. 338p. pap. 14.95 (0-87596-230-0) Rodale Pr Inc.

Women's Health & Aging Study: Health & Social Characteristics of Older Women with Disability. 1997. lib. bdg. 253.95 (0-8490-8204-8) Gordon Pr.

Women's Health & Aging Study: Health & Social Characteristics of Older Women with Disability. Ed. by Jack M. Guralnik et al. 1996. 400p. (Orig.). pap. text 45.00 (0-7881-3122-2) DIANE Pub.

Women's Health & Development: A Global Challenge. Ed. by Beverly J. McElmurry et al. 1993. LC 93-5428. (Illus.). 400p. (C). text 57.95 (0-86720-799-X, 799-X) Jones & Bartlett.

Women's Health & Human Rights: The Promotion & Protection of Women's Health Through International Human Rights Law. R. J. Cook. 1994. LC 94-234143. (ENG, FRE & SPA.). vii, 62p. pap. text 14.00 (92-4-156166-1, 1150412) World Health.

***Women's Health & Human Rights in Afghanistn: A Population Based Assessment.** Physicians For Human Rights Staff. 2001. 200p. pap. text 10.00 (1-879707-35-7) Phy Human Rights.

Women's Health & Menopause: Risk Reduction Strategies—Improved Quality of Health. Ed. by Rodolfo Paoletti. 1999. LC 99-40693. (Medical Science Symposia Ser.: Vol. 13). (Illus.). xxiii, 289p. text 150.00 (0-7923-5906-2) Kluwer Academic.

Women's Health & Nutrition: Making a Difference. Anne Tinker. 1994. LC 94-28769. (World Bank Discussion Papers: Vol. 256). 138p. pap. 22.00 (*0-8213-2991-X*, 12991) World Bank.

Women's Health & Social Work: Feminist Perspectives. Ed. by Miriam M. Olson. 1994. LC 94-3951. (Social Work in Health Care Ser.: Vol. 19, Nos. 3-4). 175p. 39.95 (*1-56024-683-9*) Haworth Pr.

Women's Health Book. Loretta H. Kurban. 2nd ed. 1990. LC 86-91266. 90p. (Orig.). pap. 8.00 (*0-938863-24-X*) HCI Pr.

Women's Health Care: A Comprehensive Handbook. Ed. by Catherine I. Fogel & Nancy F. Woods. 1995. LC 94-36836. 900p. 123.95 (*0-8039-7022-6*, 2857); pap. 79.95 (*0-8039-7023-4*, 2856) Sage.

Women's Health Care: Movements & Models for Change. Carol S. Weisman. 1998. LC 97-34492. 320p. 49.00 (*0-8018-5825-9*); pap. text 27.95 (*0-8018-5826-7*) Johns Hopkins.

Women's Health Care Administration: Forms, Checklists, & Guidelines. Ed. by Sara N. Di Lima et al. 1996. ring bd. 199.00 (*0-8342-0773-7*) Aspen Pub.

Women's Health Care Handbook. Ed. by Cynda Johnson et al. 2nd ed. 1999. LC 99-42849. (Illus.). 740p. pap. 59.95 (*1-56053-356-0*) Hanley & Belfus.

Women's Health Care Nurse Practitioner - Nurse Midwifery Certification Review Guide. Ed. by Beth Kelsey. 2nd ed. 2001. 1100p. (C). pap. text 69.95 (*1-878028-18-9*) Hlth Lead Assoc.

Women's Health Care Nurse Practitioner Certification Review Guide. Ed. by Susan Moskosky. 1995. LC 95-33625. 500p. (C). pap. text 26.00 (*1-878028-13-8*) Hlth Lead Assoc.

Women's Health Diary: The Essential Health Record for Every Woman Aged 35 to 55. Mary F. Raver. 1995. 52p. (Orig.). pap. 4.95 (*1-886245-00-2*) Adelante CA.

Women's Health Discourses, Set. Jack Tips. 1996. 60p. 19.95 (*0-929167-18-X*) Apple-a-Day.

***Women's Health During the Childbearing Years: A Community-Based Approach, Computerized Testbank.** Peggy S. Matteson. 2001. (*0-323-00919-0*) Mosby Inc.

Women's Health Guide: A Natural Approach to Breast Cancer, Heart Disease, Fibroids, PMS, Balimia, Childbirth, Menopause, & Osteoporosis. Gale Jack & Wendy Esko. 1997. LC 97-174625. 96p. (Orig.). pap. 10.95 (*1-882984-25-0*) One Peaceful World.

Women's Health in India: Risk & Vulnerability. Ed. by Lincoln C. Chen et al. 1996. (Illus.). 332p. text 24.95 (*0-19-563620-1*) OUP.

Women's Health in Menopause: Behaviour, Cancer, Cardiovascular Disease, Vol. 7. Ed. by P. G. Crosignani. 1994. 272p. (C). text 123.00 (*0-7923-3068-4*) Kluwer Academic.

Women's Health in Menopause: Risk reduction Strategies. Ed. by R. Paoletti et al. 1997. LC 97-23945. (Medical Science Symposia Ser.: No. 11). 356p. text 115.00 (*0-7923-4697-1*) Kluwer Academic.

Women's Health in Primary Care. Ed. by Jo A. Rosenfeld et al. 1997. LC 96-13729. (Illus.). 752p. 69.95 (*0-683-07366-4*) Lppncott W & W.

Women's Health Issues: Hearings Before a Subcommittee of the Committee on Appropriations, United States Senate, One Hundred Fourth Congress, Second Session, Special Hearings, May 6, 1996—Philadelphia, PA, May 29, 1996—Beverly Hills, CA, November 15, 1996—Pittsburch, PA. U. S. Congress, Senate Committee on Appropriations, Subcommittee on Departments of Labor, Health and Human Services, Education and Related Agencies. 1997. LC 97-163616. (*0-16-054074-7*) USGPO.

Women's Health Issues: HP 570 Course Study Guide. Charlene Allert. 1992. 180p. (C). (*0-933195-21-4*) CA College Health Sci.

Women's Health Needs in Patient Education. Barbara K. Redman. 1999. LC 99-27854. (Focus on Women Ser.). (Illus.). xv, 171p. text 32.95 (*0-8261-1264-1*) Springer Pub.

Women's Health, 1999-2000. Maureen Edwards & Nora L. Howley. 2nd ed. 1999. (Annual Editions Ser.). 240p. (C). pap., stu. ed. 18.44 (*0-07-035009-4*) McGrw-H Hghr Educ.

Women's Health, 98-99. Maureen Edwards & Nora Howley. 1998. (Illus.). 256p. pap. text 12.25 (*0-07-012568-6*, Dshkn McG-Hill) McGrw-H Hghr Educ.

Women's Health Nurse Practitioner Certification Exam Review. Rebecca Donohue et al. 1998. LC 98-17718. (Nurse Practitioner Certification Review Ser.). 320p. (C). pap. 40.00 (*0-8385-9819-6*, A-9819-2) P-H.

Women's Health Nurse Practitioner Certification Review. JoAnn Zerwekh & Jo C. Clayborn. Ed. by Robin Carter. 1999. LC 98-34770. 255p. (C). pap. text 32.00 (*0-7216-7740-1*) Saunders.

Women's Health Nurse Pratitioner Certification Study Question. M. Chromecek. 1999. LC 99-22640. 300p. pap. text 35.00 (*1-878028-22-7*) Hlth Lead Assoc.

Women's Health Nursing. Sylvia K. Fields. 1992. (Nursing Examination Review Ser.: Vol. 2). (C). pap. text 21.95 (*0-8385-9818-8*, A9818-4, Apple Lange Med) McGraw.

Women's Health on the Internet. Ed. by M. Sandra Wood & Janet M. Coggan. 2000. LC 00-58213. 174p. pap. text 19.95 (*0-7890-1301-0*); 39.95 (*0-7890-1300-2*) Haworth Pr.

Women's Health over 40. Caroline Bohme et al. 2000. LC 00-699793. (What You Should Know Ser.). (Illus.). viii, 184p. pap. 6.99 (*1-55870-555-4*, Betrwy Bks) F & W Pubns Inc.

***Women's Health over 40.** Caroline J. Bohme et al. 2nd ed. 2001. (What You Should Know Ser.). (Illus.). 136p. pap. 8.99 (*0-632-04537-X*) Blackwell Sci.

Women's Health Patient Education Resource Manual. Ed. by Kenneth E. Lawrence & Sandra J. Painter. 1994. LC 93-33562. spiral bd. 209.00 (*0-8342-0547-5*) Aspen Pub.

Women's Health, Politics, & Power: Essays on Sex, Gender, Medicine, & Public Health. Ed. by Elizabeth Fee & Nancy Krieger. 1994. LC 94-42. (Policy, Politics, Health & Medicine Ser.). 382p. text 42.00 (*0-89503-120-5*) Baywood Pub.

Women's Health Products Handbook: Smart Buys for Healthy Bodies. Carol A. Rinzler. 2nd rev. ed. 1996. LC 96-27095. 288p. pap. 15.95 (*0-89793-209-9*) Hunter Hse.

Women's Health, Raising Awareness of Cervical Cancer: Hearing Before the Subcommittee on Health & Environment of the Committee on Commerce, House of Representatives, One Hundred Sixth Congress, First Session, March 16, 1999. Contrib. by U. S. Congress, House Committee on Commerce, Subcommittee on Health and the Environment. 1999. LC 99-489365. (Illus.). (*0-16-058407-8*) USGPO.

Women's Health Research: A Medical & Policy Primer. Society for the Advancement of Women's Health Research Staff. Ed. by Florence Haseltine & Beverly Jacobson. 1997. LC 96-43828. 386p. text 44.50 (*0-88048-791-7*, 8791) Am Psychiatric.

Womens Health Secrets. Date not set. pap. (*1-884350-68-2*) Alpha Pubng.

Women's Health Services: Index of New Information with Authors & Subjects. American Health Research Institute Staff. 1992. LC 92-54209. 150p. 47.50 (*1-55914-570-6*); pap. 44.50 (*1-55914-571-4*) ABBE Pubs Assn.

Women's Health Today: Perspectives on Current Research & Clinical Practice. Popkin. 1994. LC 94-22810. (Illus.). 418p. (C). lib. bdg. 82.95 (*1-85070-568-2*, Parthenon Pbng) CRC Pr.

***Women's Health under 40.** Caroline J. Bohme & Rona B. Wharton. 2nd ed. 2001. (What You Should Know Ser.). (Illus.). 136p. pap. 8.99 (*0-632-04535-3*) Blackwell Sci.

Women's Health Update. 1994. 192p. (Orig.). pap. 14.95 (*1-57327-013-X*, M Pr CA) Busn Concepts.

Women's Herbs, Women's Health. Christopher Hobbs & Kathi Keville. 1998. LC 98-4412. 220p. pap. 16.95 (*1-883010-47-0*) Interweave.

Women's Home Remedy Health Guide. Consumer Guide Editors. 1994. (Illus.). 400p. 19.98 (*0-7853-0185-2*, 3212100) Pubns Intl Ltd.

Women's Home Remedy Kit: Simple Recipes for Treating Common Health Conditions. Maribeth Riggs. 1998. 146p. (Orig.). pap. text 12.00 (*0-7881-5870-8*) DIANE Pub.

Women's Imaging. Pellerito. 1998. text 150.00 (*0-443-07611-1*) Saunders.

Women's Issues. Contrib. by APTA Staff. 1999. (Resource Guide Ser.). 190p. pap. 17.00 (*1-887759-46-8*, P-119) Am Phys Therapy Assn.

Women's Medicine. Richard E. Blackwell. 1995. LC 95-36198. 644p. 99.95 (*0-86542-373-3*) Blackwell Sci.

Women's Medicine: A Cross-Cultural Study of Indigenous Fertility Regulation. Lucile F. Newman. 1995. 203p. (Orig.). (C). pap. text 16.00 (*0-8135-2257-9*) Rutgers U Pr.

Women's Mental Health: A New Zealand Perspective. Sarah Romans. 1998. LC 99-193547. 280p. pap. (*1-877133-49-3*) Univ Otago Pr NZL. *Dist:* Intl Spec Bk.

Women's Mental Health Agenda. American Psychological Association Staff & Organizations for Professional Women Staff. Ed. by Nancy F. Russo. 1985. LC 85-72729. 99p. (Orig.). pap. 10.00 (*0-912704-44-6*) Am Psychol.

Women's Mental Health in Africa. Ed. by Esther D. Rothblum & Ellen Cole. 1990. (Women & Therapy Ser.). (Illus.). 98p. text 3.95 (*1-56024-043-1*); pap. text 9.95 (*0-918393-86-8*) Haworth Pr.

Women's Mental Health in Primary Care. Kathryn J. Zerbe. Ed. by Ray Kersey. 1999. LC 98-7959. 335p. (C). pap. text 39.00 (*0-7216-7239-6*) Saunders.

Women's Mental Health Services: A Public Health Perspective. Bruce Lubotsky Levin et al. 1998. LC 97-45341. 496p. 81.95 (*0-7619-0508-1*, 80527); pap. 39.95 (*0-7619-0509-X*, 80528) Sage.

Women's Migraine Survival Guide: The Complete, Up-to-Date Resource on the Causes of Your Migraine Pain & Treatments for Real Relief. Christina Peterson. 1999. LC 99-27288. (Illus.). 240p. pap. 12.95 (*0-06-095319-5*) HarperCollins Pubs.

Women's Moods: What Every Woman Must Know about Hormones, the Brain & Emotional Health. Deborah Sichel. 2000. 368p. pap. 14.00 (*0-380-72852-4*, Avon Bks) Morrow Avon.

Women's Nutrition Patient Education Resource Manual. Simon B. Weavers & Aspen Reference Group Staff. 2000. LC 00-36353. 478p. ring bd. 199.00 (*0-8342-1735-X*) Aspen Pub.

Women's Pharmacy: An Essential Guide to What Women Should Know about Prescription Drugs. Julie Catalano. 2000. LC 00-708758. 480p. mass mkt. 6.99 (*0-440-23537-5*, Dell Trade Pbks) Dell.

***Women's Postpartun Concerns & Midwives' Reflections on Postpartum Care: Studies in Dar es Salaam, Tanzania.** Helen Igobeko Lugina. 2001. (Illus.). 77p. pap. (*91-554-5067-9*) Uppsala Universitet SWE. *Dist:* Coronet Bks.

Women's Primary Health Care. Knuppel. 1998. pap. text 60.00 (*0-443-07914-5*) Saunders.

Women's Primary Health Care: Office Practice & Procedures. Ed. by Vicki L. Seltzer & Warren H. Pearse. 1995. LC 94-30309. (Illus.). 825p. 68.00 (*0-07-056225-3*) McGraw-Hill Med Pub.

Women's Primary Health Care: Office Practice & Procedures. Vicki L. Seltzer & Warren H. Pearse. 2nd ed. 1999. LC 00-266658. (Illus.). 1216p. text 89.00 (*0-07-058044-8*) McGraw-Hill Prof.

Women's Primary Health Care: Protocols for Practice. Ed. by Winifred L. Star et al. 1995. LC 93-39629. 62.50 (*1-55810-094-6*, MS-20) Am Nurses Pub.

Women's Problems in General Practice. Ed. by Ann McPherson. 3rd ed. 1993. LC 92-48910. (Oxford General Practice Ser.: No. 22). 512p. pap. 39.50 (*0-19-262065-7*) OUP.

Women's Reproductive Health: The Silent Emergency. Jodi L. Jacobson. 1991. 70p. (Orig.). pap. 5.00 (*1-878071-03-3*) Worldwatch Inst.

Women's Secrets: A Translation of Pseudo-Albertus Magnus' De Secretis Mulierum with Commentaries. Helen R. Lemay. 1992. LC 91-30690. (SUNY Series in Medieval Studies). 200p. (C). pap. text 22.95 (*0-7914-1144-3*) State U NY Pr.

Women's Sexual Health. Andrews. 1996. pap. text 47.00 (*0-7020-1898-8*) Saunders.

***Women's Sexual Health.** Gilly Andrews. 2001. (Illus.). 575p. pap. (*0-7020-2598-4*) W B Saunders GBR. *Dist:* Saunders.

Women's Sexuality after Childhood Incest. Elaine Westerlund. 1992. LC 92-5320. 200p. (C). 27.95 (*0-393-70141-7*) Norton.

Women's Sports Medicine & Rehabilitation: Comprehensive Understanding & Management. Nadya Gabriele Swedan. 1999. LC 00-50428. (Illus.). xlix, 398p. 79.00 (*0-8342-1731-7*, 17317) PRO-ED.

Women's Status & Fertility in Pakistan: Recent Evidence. 29p. pap. 10.00 (*92-1-151264-6*, E.94.XIII.6) UN.

Women's Symptoms: A Comprehensive Guide to Common Symptoms & Diseases: Their Causes, & Treatments. Ivan K. Strausz. 1996. LC 95-44873. 544p. pap. 14.95 (*0-440-50642-5*, Dell Trade Pbks) Dell.

Women's Therapy Groups: Paradigms of Feminist Treatment. Claire Brody. 1987. (Women's Ser.). 288p. 35.95 (*0-8261-5570-7*) Springer Pub.

***Women's Trouble: Natural & Medical Solutions.** Ruth Trickey & Kaz Cooke. rev. ed. 2001. (Illus.). 384p. pap. (*1-86508-312-7*) Allen & Unwin Pty AUS. *Dist:* IPG Chicago.

Womens Waterworks: Curing Incontinence. Pauline E. Chiarelli. 1995. (Health Bks.). 64p. pap. 8.95 (*0-9640719-0-8*) Khera Pubns.

Women's World: A Holistic Approach to Dealing with Stress. 1987. (Stress in Modern Society Ser.: No. 16). 32.50 (*0-404-63267-X*) AMS Pr.

Wonder of Being Human: Our Brain & Our Mind. John C. Eccles & Daniel N. Robinson. 1984. LC 83-49044. 192p. (C). 16.30 (*0-02-908860-7*) Free Pr.

Wonderful Art of the Eye. Benvenutus Grassus. Ed. by L. M. Eldredge. 1996. LC 95-69179. (Medieval Texts & Studies: No. 19). 120p. 24.95 (*0-87013-459-0*) Mich St U Pr.

Wonderful World Within You: Your Inner Nutritional Environment. Roger J. Williams. rev. ed. 1987. (Illus.). 278p. pap. 14.95 (*0-942333-00-4*) Bio-Comns Pr.

Wonders in Weeds. William Smith, Jr. 1977. 187p. (C). pap. 17.95 (*0-8464-1062-1*) Beekman Pubs.

Wonders in Weeds. William Smith, Jr. 1977. 111p. pap. (*0-85032-151-4*) C W Daniel GBR. *Dist:* Natl Bk Netwk.

***Wondrous Healing: Shamanism, Human Evolution & the Origin of Religion.** James M. McClenon. 2001. (Illus.). 248p. pap. 19.95 (*0-87580-590-6*) N Ill U Pr.

Wong & Whaley's Clinical Manual of Pediatric Nursing. Donna L. Wong. 4th ed. 1995. (Illus.). 704p. (C). (gr. 13). spiral bd. 35.95 (*0-8151-9442-0*, 23639) Mosby Inc.

Wong & Whaley's Clinical Manual of Pediatric Nursing. Donna L. Wong & Caryn Stoermer Hess. 5th ed. 1999. LC 99-48128. 750p. text 35.95 (*0-323-00979-4*) Mosby Inc.

Wong, Dalton College Custom Pub. Donna L. Wong. 1996. (C). (gr. 13). text 81.95 (*0-8151-2709-X*, 31344) Mosby Inc.

Wong's Essentials of Pediatric Nursing. Donna Wong. 6th ed. 2000. LC 00-58400. (Illus.). xxxii, 1350p. 66.00 (*0-323-00989-1*) Mosby Inc.

***Wong's Essentials of Pediatric Nursing: Computerized Test Bank.** Donna L. Wong et al. 6th ed. 2001. 500.00 (*0-323-01249-3*) Mosby Inc.

***Wong's Essentials of Pediatric Nursing: Electronic Image Collection.** Donna L. Wong et al. 6th ed. 2001. 300.00 (*0-323-01251-5*) Mosby Inc.

***Wong's Essentials of Pediatric Nursing: Instructor's Resource Kit.** 2001. 250.00 (*0-323-01252-3*) Mosby Inc.

Wood Becomes Water: An Introduction to Chinese Medicine & the Five Element Cycle. Gail Reichstein. 1998. LC 97-31947. (Illus.). 240p. 20.00 (*1-56836-209-9*) Kodansha.

Wood Dust & Formaldehyde. 1995. (IARC Scientific Publications Ser.: Vol. 62). viii, 405p. (C). pap. text 80.00 (*92-832-1262-2*, 1720062) World Health.

Wood Houses: Form in Rural Architecture. Werner Blaser. 2nd ed. 1985. (ENG, FRE & GER., Illus.). 216p. pap. (*0-89192-300-4*) Wepf & Co CHE. *Dist:* H B Fenn Co.

Woodcock-Johnson Psycho-Educational Battery: Recommendations & Reports. Nancy Mather & Lynne Jaffe. rev. ed. 1996. LC 96-20245. 400p. pap. 70.00 (*0-471-16210-8*) Wiley.

Woodcock-Johnson Psycho-Educational Battery: Recommendations & Reports. Nancy Mather & Lynne E. Jaffe. rev. ed. 1992. LC 91-75518. 396p. pap. text 39.50 (*0-88422-115-6*) Clinical Psych.

Woods Injurious to Human Health. Bjorn M. Hausen. 1981. (Illus.). 189p. 53.10 (*3-11-008485-6*) De Gruyter.

Woodward's Postgastrectomy Syndrome. Hocking. 2nd ed. 1991. (Illus.). 240p. text 74.00 (*0-7216-2209-7*) Saunders.

Wopert & Barnes' Pediatric Neuroradiology: Imaging of the Developing Brain. Barnes. 2000. (Illus.). 576p. text 139.00 (*0-8151-9355-6*, 28697) Mosby Inc.

Word Book in Pathology & Laboratory Medicine. Sheila B. Sloane & John L. Dusseau. 2nd ed. 1995. LC 94-30881. 960p. pap. text 41.00 (*0-7216-4040-0*) Saunders.

Word Book in Radiology: With Illustrated Anatomy. Sheila B. Sloane. 1988. LC 87-23335. (Illus.). 544p. pap. text 41.00 (*0-7216-2100-7*) Saunders.

Word Diagnostic Imaging Equipment Markets: A Comprehensive Snapshot on Medical Imaging Modalities & Related Products. Market Intelligence Staff. 1994. 570p. 2895.00 (*1-56753-987-4*) Frost & Sullivan.

Word from the Soul: Time, East-West Spirituality, & Psychotherapeutic Narrative. Stuart Sovatsky. 1998. LC 97-47049. (Series in Transpersonal & Humanistic Psychology). 256p. (C). text 60.50 (*0-7914-3949-6*); pap. text 20.95 (*0-7914-3950-X*) State U NY Pr.

Word of God & the Languages of Man: Interpreting Nature in Early Modern Science & Medicine. James J. Bono. 1995. LC 95-15652. (Science & Literature Ser.). (Illus.). 332p. 50.00 (*0-299-14790-8*); pap. 22.95 (*0-299-14794-0*) U of Wis Pr.

Word Rounds. Barton J. Gershen. 2000. LC 99-58919. 150p. 24.95 (*1-886388-16-4*) Flower Valley Pr.

Word Search: Having Fun with Medical Terminology. Cathy A. Bragg. Ed. by Carolyn S. Zagury. 1997. LC 96-62089. 280p. pap. 10.95 (*1-880254-42-5*) Vista.

Word Wizard: Medical Term Software Programming, Vol. 1. Johnson. 1993. (RT-Medical Terminolgy Ser.). (C). text 49.95 (*0-8273-5906-3*) Delmar.

Wordfinding: A Language Rehabilitation Manual for Aphasic Adults. Daniel F. Carlson. Ed. by Cindy Drolet. rev. ed. 1987. LC 87-82069. 155p. spiral bd. 65.00 (*0-9609464-4-6*, 8500) Imaginart Intl.

Words Against the Shifting Seasons: Women Speak of Breast Cancer. Illus. by Hollis Sigler. 1994. 125p. (*0-932026-34-6*) Columbia College Chi.

Words from Those Who Care: Further Case Studies of ABA with People with Autism. Ed. by Bobby Newman et al. 2000. 195p. mass mkt. 18.00 (*0-9668528-2-6*) Dove & Orca.

Words Made Flesh: Scripture, Psychology & Human Communication. Fran Ferder. 1986. LC 85-73255. 184p. pap. 10.95 (*0-87793-331-6*) Ave Maria.

Words on Aging: A Bibliography of Selected Annotated References Compiled for the Administration on Aging by the Department Library. Ed. by U. S. Department of Health, Education and Welfare Staff. 1981. LC 81-2471. 190p. reprint ed. lib. bdg. 59.50 (*0-313-22860-4*, USWA) Greenwood.

Words That Heal Today. Ernest Holmes. pap. 9.95 (*0-917849-19-1*) Sci of Mind.

Words to Say It. Marie Cardinal. Ed. & Tr. by Pat Goodheart from FRE. 9th ed. 1994.Tr. of Mots Pour le Dire. (ENG.). 308p. (Orig.). (C). pap. 22.95 (*0-941324-09-5*) Van Vactor & Goodheart.

Words Were Originally Magic. Steve De Shazer. 1994. LC 94-2713. 320p. (C). 32.00 (*0-393-70170-0*) Norton.

Wordsworth Guide to Poisons & Antidotes: A First-Aid Guide to Acids & Arsenic, Valium & Vipers. Carol Turkington. 2000. 366p. pap. text 17.00 (*0-7881-9156-X*) DIANE Pub.

Work Accidents & the Law. Crystal Eastman. 1974. LC 70-89757. (American Labor, from Conspiracy to Collective Bargaining Ser., No. 1). 361p. reprint ed. 28.95 (*0-405-02118-6*) Ayer.

Work Accidents to Miners in Illinois, Vol. 7. Earl E. Klein. 1974. LC 74-1689. (Children & Youth Ser.). 275p. reprint ed. 27.95 (*0-405-05966-3*) Ayer.

Work Alienation: An Integrative Approach. Rabindra N. Kanungo. 1982. LC 81-20959. 200p. 62.50 (*0-275-90832-1*, C0832, Praeger Pubs) Greenwood.

Work & Health: Its Your Life, an Action Guide to Job Hazards. Phillip L. Polakoff. 1984. LC 84-61087. (Orig.). pap. 7.95 (*0-918763-00-2*) Pr Assocs.

W X Y Z

Work & Illness: The Cancer Patient. Ed. by Ivan Barofsky. 1989. LC 88-25544. 195p. 62.50 (*0-275-92390-8*, C2390, Praeger Pubs) Greenwood.

Work & Its Inhibitions: Psychoanalytic Essays. Ed. by Charles W. Socarides & Selma Kramer. 1996. LC 96-9688. 280p. 42.50 (*0-8236-6866-5*, BN 06866) Intl Univs Pr.

Work & Madness: The Rise of Community Psychiatry. Diana Ralph. 1983. 425p. text (*0-919619-07-X*); 170p. pap. text (*0-919619-04-5*) Black Rose CAN. *Dist:* Consort Bk Sales.

Work & Organizational Psychology. Ed. by A. M. Koopman-Iwema & R. A. Roe. 1984. vi, 294p. pap. (*90-265-0593-0*) Swets.

Work & Play of Winnicott. Simon A. Grolnick. 1990. LC 89-18572. 232p. 40.00 (*0-87668-802-4*) Aronson.

Work & Role Redesign: Tools & Techniques for the Health Care Setting. Ruth B. Hanson & Betty Sayers. 1995. LC 95-1287. 197p. pap. 54.00 (*1-55648-135-7*) AHPI.

Work & the Eye. Rachel V. North. 1993. 288p. pap. text 50.00 (*0-7506-4045-6*); 2nd ed. 2001. LC 00-68889. (Illus.). 208p. pap. text 55.00 (*0-7506-4172-X*) Buttrwrth-Heinemann.

Work & the Health of Women. Vilma R. Hunt. 1979. 248p. 141.00 (*0-8493-5301-7*, RC963, CRC Reprint) Franklin.

Work Behavior Analysis of Professional Counselors. National Board for Certified Counselors Staff et al. 1993. LC 93-27915. 168p. 26.95 (*1-55959-053-X*) Accel Devel.

Work Book of Group-Analytic Interventions. David Kennard et al. 1993. LC 92-48526. (International Library of Philosophy, Psychology, & Scientific Method). 128p. (C). text 74.95 (*0-415-08783-X*, B0887) Routledge.

Work Environment: Healthcare, Laboratories & Biosafety, Vol. 2. Ed. by Doan J. Hansen. 1992. (Illus.). 368p. 119.95 (*0-87371-392-3*, L392) Lewis Pubs.

Work Environment: Indoor Health Hazards, Vol. 3. Ed. by Doan J. Hansen. 1993. (Illus.). 304p. 119.95 (*0-87371-393-1*, L393) Lewis Pubs.

Work Family Sex Roles Language. Ed. by Mario Barrera. 1980. LC 80-53691. pap. 6.00 (*0-89229-007-2*) TQS Pubns.

Work, Health, & Productivity. Ed. by Gareth M. Green & Frank Baker. 1991. (Illus.). 328p. text 47.50 (*0-19-505778-3*) OUP.

Work in Progress: Occupational Therapy in Work Programs. Ed. by Sarah Herfelder & Carol H. Gwin. 1989. (Illus.). 291p. (Orig.). (C). pap. text 40.00 (*0-910317-54-2*) Am Occup Therapy.

Work, Love, Play: Self Repair in the Psychoanalytic Dialogue. Joel Shor. 1992. LC 91-36576. 224p. (Orig.). text 31.95 (*0-87630-658-X*) Brunner-Routledge.

Work, Love, Play: Self Repair in the Psychoanalytic Dialogue. Joel Shor. 1990. LC 89-82165. 222p. (Orig.). lib. bdg. 20.00 (*0-930578-01-5*) Double Helix.

Work of Culture: Symbolic Transformation in Psychoanalysis & Anthropology. Gananath Obeyesekere. 1990. LC 90-10904. (Lewis Henry Morgan Lectures: Vol. 1982). 380p. lib. bdg. 60.00 (*0-226-61598-7*); pap. text 19.95 (*0-226-61599-5*) U Ch Pr.

Work of Hanna Segal: A Kleinian Approach to Clinical Practice. Hanna Segal. 1990. LC 81-7877. (Classical Psychoanalysis & Its Applications Ser.). 256p. reprint ed. 50.00 (*0-87668-422-3*) Aronson.

Work of Hans Loewald: An Introduction & Commentary. Ed. by Gerald Fogel. 1991. LC 90-22005. 296p. 50.00 (*0-87668-615-3*) Aronson.

Work of Mara Selvini Palazzoli. Ed. by Matteo Selvini. Tr. by Arnold J. Pomerans from ITA. 1988. LC 87-12438. 437p. 60.00 (*0-87668-949-7*) Aronson.

Work of WHO in the European Region, 1987: Annual Report of the Regional Director. 1988. pap. text 12.00 (*92-890-1055-X*) World Health.

Work of WHO, 1984-1985: Biennial Report of the Director-General to the World Health Assembly & to the United Nations. 1986. 284p. pap. text 45.00 (*92-4-156092-4*, 1248485) World Health.

Work of WHO Virus Reference Centres & the Services They Provide. 1968. (ENG, FRE & RUS.). 120p. pap. text 12.00 (*92-4-156035-5*, 1150161) World Health.

Work Practice: International Perspectives. Joanne Pratt & Karen Jacobs. 1997. LC 97-5624. 328p. pap. text 65.00 (*0-7506-2260-1*) Buttrwrth-Heinemann.

Work Practices Guide for Manual Lifting. 1995. lib. bdg. 251.99 (*0-8490-7525-4*) Gordon Pr.

Work Preparation for the Handicapped. David Hutchinson. 1982. (Illus.). 128p. (C). pap. (*0-7099-0283-2*) C Helm GBR. *Dist:* Routldge.

Work Related Lung Disease. 1995. lib. bdg. 254.95 (*0-8490-7524-6*) Gordon Pr.

Work-Related Lung Disease Surveillance Report (1994) Rochelle B. Althouse. 1997. (Illus.). 149p. (C). reprint ed. pap. text 40.00 (*0-7881-3336-5*) DIANE Pub.

Work-Related Lung Disease Surveillance Report (1996) Ed. by Rochelle B. Althouse. 4th ed. 1997. (Illus.). 482p. (C). pap. text 50.00 (*0-7881-3742-5*) DIANE Pub.

Work-Related Musculoskeletal Disorders: A Review of the Evidence. National Research Council Staff. 1998. 42p. pap. text 10.00 (*0-309-06327-2*) Natl Acad Pr.

Work-Related Musculoskeletal Disorders (WMSDs) A Reference for Prevention. R. Wells et al. 1994. 314p. 110.00 (*0-7484-0131-8*); LC 94-43622. 421p. pap. 44.95 (*0-7484-0132-6*) Taylor & Francis.

Work-Related Programs in Occupational Therapy. Ed. by Florence S. Cromwell. 1985. LC 85-17690. (Occupational Therapy in Health Care Ser.: Vol. 2, No. 4). 125p. 3.95 (*0-86656-487-X*); pap. text 14.95 (*0-86656-519-1*) Haworth Pr.

Work-Related Upper Limb Disorders: Recognition & Management. Michael A. Hutson. 2000. 159p. pap. (*0-7506-4548-2*) E A GBR. *Dist:* OUP.

Work Stress. Alan A. McLean. 1979. pap. 13.95 (*0-201-04592-3*) Addison-Wesley.

Work Stress: Health Care Systems in the Workplace. Ed. by James C. Quick et al. 1987. LC 86-30636. 346p. 72.50 (*0-275-92329-0*, C2329, Praeger Pubs) Greenwood.

Work with Display Units, '94: Selected Papers of the 4th International Scientific Conference on Work with Display Units, Milan, Italy, 2-5 October, 1994. International Scientific Conference on Work with Display Units Staff. Ed. by Antonio Grieco et al. 1995. LC 95-32593. 530p. 133.00 (*0-444-82145-7*) Elsevier.

Work with Display Units, '92: Selected Proceedings of the 3rd International Scientific Conference on Work with Display Units, Berlin, Germany, September 1-4, 1992. Ed. by Holger Luczak et al. 1993. LC 93-19702. 566p. 159.25 (*0-444-89759-3*, North Holland) Elsevier.

Work Worth Doing: Advances in Brain Injury Rehabilitation. Ed. by Brian T. McMahon & Linda R. Shaw. 1991. LC 91-71166. (Illus.). 432p. 57.95 (*1-878205-19-6*) St Lucie Pr.

Workbook: A Self-Study Guide for Job-Seekers with Epilepsy. Epilepsy Foundation of America Staff. 1991. 64p. pap. 9.95 (*0-916570-00-2*) Epilepsy Foundation of America.

Workbook: An Introduction to the Meridians & Points of Acupuncture. Alex Holland & James Blair. 1988. (Illus.). 202p. (Orig.). (C). 20.00 (*0-9622665-1-5*) A Holland.

Workbook Crisis Intervention: Prehospital Emergency Care. 6th ed. 1999. 368p. text 33.40 (*0-8359-5332-7*) Globe Fearon.

Workbook Dyslexia. Spafford & Grosser. 1998. 176p. (C). pap. 29.00 (*0-205-27551-6*) P-H.

Workbook for Cardiopulmonary Anatomy & Physiology: Essentials for Respiratory Care. DesJardins. 3rd ed. 1997. 224p. (C). pap., wbk. ed. 16.95 (*0-8273-8258-8*) Delmar.

Workbook for Clinical Procedures for Medical Assisting. Anne L. Lilly & Mary A. Frew. 1990. LC 90-2929. (Illus.). 269p. pap., stu. ed. 13.95 (*0-8036-3852-3*) Davis Co.

Workbook for Clinical Skills & Assisting Techniques. Sharron M. Zakus. 3rd ed. 1994. 188p. pap. text, wbk. ed. 16.95 (*0-8016-7183-3*) Mosby Inc.

Workbook for Emergency Care. Al Weigel & Robert Nixon. 2nd ed. 1983. pap. text 20.00 (*0-8359-1677-4*) P-H.

Workbook for Emergency Care in the Streets. James C. McClintock & Nancy L. Caroline. 3rd ed. 1987. 17.50 (*0-316-55437-5*, Little Brwn Med Div) Lppncott W & W.

Workbook for Medical Office Administrative Procedures. Anne L. Lilly & Mary A. Frew. 2nd ed. 1989. LC 88-31065. (Illus.). 251p. (C). pap., tchr. ed. 12.95 (*0-8036-3863-9*) Davis Co.

Workbook for MRI & CT of the Head & Neck. Anthony A. Mancuso. 2nd ed. 1988. (Illus.). 236p. 60.00 (*0-683-05478-3*) Lppncott W & W.

Workbook for Practical Nurses. Audrey L. Sutton. 3rd ed. 1969. pap. text 24.00 (*0-7216-8682-6*) Saunders.

Workbook for Providing Home Care: A Textbook for Home Care Aides. Ed. by Hartman Publishing, Inc. Staff. 1999. (Illus.). 319p. pap. text, wbk. ed. 12.50 (*1-888343-20-6*) Hartman Pub.

Workbook for Psychological Assessment with the MMPI. Alan Friedman et al. 1989. 240p. pap. 29.95 (*0-8058-0311-4*) L Erlbaum Assocs.

Workbook for Respiratory Disease: A Case Study Approach to Patient Care. David W. Chang & Fred Corn. 2nd ed. 1997. (Illus.). 233p. (C). pap. text, wbk. ed. 21.95 (*0-8036-0156-5*) Davis Co.

Workbook for the Medical Assistant. Fremgen. 1998. pap. text 22.80 net. (*0-8359-5136-7*) P-H.

Workbook for the Medical Assistant. Cooper et al. 6th ed. 1993. 320p. pap. text 19.95 (*0-8016-1011-7*) Mosby Inc.

Workbook for Today's Nursing Asstistant. Blasband. 1998. pap. text, wbk. ed. 24.80 (*0-8359-4986-9*) P-H.

Workbook in Nonlinear Phonology for Clinical Application. Barbara H. Bernhardt & Joseph P. Stemberger. 1999. LC 98-50043. 35.00 (*0-89079-810-9*) PRO-ED.

Workbook in Practical Neonatology. Ed. by Richard A. Polin et al. 2nd ed. 1993. (Illus.). 496p. pap. text, wbk. ed. 55.00 (*0-7216-4292-6*) Saunders.

Workbook in Practical Neonatology. Richard A. Polin et al. 3rd ed. 2000. (Illus.). 475p. pap. text, wbk. ed. 55.00 (*0-7216-7986-2*) Saunders.

Workbook of Clinical Chemistry: Case Presentation & Data Interpretation. Philip Mayne & Andrew P. Day. 1994. 224p. pap. text, stu. ed., wbk. ed. (*0-340-57646-4*) E A GBR. *Dist:* OUP.

Workbook on Being a Long Term Nurse. Will-Black. 4th ed. 1997. pap. text 19.80 (*0-8359-5264-9*) P-H.

Workbook on Community Accountability in Integrated Delivery. Catholic Health Association of the United States Staff. 1995. 133p. pap. 55.00 (*0-87125-230-9*) Cath Health.

Workbook on Intermediate Emergencies. Porter. 2nd ed. 1998. 128p. pap. text 30.80 (*0-8359-5263-0*) P-H.

Workbook on Redesigning Care: Becoming the Values-Driven, Low-Cost Provider. Catholic Health Association of the United States Staff. 1995. 140p. pap. 55.00 (*0-87125-229-5*) Cath Health.

Workbook to Accompany Cardiopulmonary Anatomy & Physiology Essentials for Respiratory Care. Terry R. Des Jardins. 2nd ed. 1993. 203p. (C). pap., wbk. ed. 14.95 (*0-8273-5006-6*) Delmar.

Workbook to Accompany Mosby's Paramedic Textbook. Mick J. Sanders. 1994. 416p. reprint ed. pap. text, wbk. ed. 19.95 (*0-8016-4314-7*) Mosby Inc.

Workbooks for Psychotherapists: Intervening & Validating, Vol. 3. Robert J. Langs. 1985. LC 84-62354. (Workbooks for Psychotherapists Ser.). 302p. pap. text 33.50 (*0-931231-03-5*) Newconcept Pr.

Workbooks for Psychotherapists: Listening & Formulating, Vol. 2. Robert J. Langs. 1985. LC 84-62354. (Workbooks for Psychotherapists Ser.). 304p. pap. text 36.00 (*0-931231-02-7*) Newconcept Pr.

Workbooks for Psychotherapists: Understanding Unconscious Communication, Vol. 1. Robert J. Langs. 1985. LC 84-62354. (Workbooks for Psychotherapists Ser.). 144p. pap. text 20.00 (*0-931231-01-9*) Newconcept Pr.

Workbooks in Immunology One: Antigens & Antibodies. Jules M. Elias. 1987. (Illus.). 134p. (Orig.). (C). stu. ed. 14.95 (*0-936735-00-7*) Grove Educ Tech.

Workbooks in Immunology Two: Immunoglobulins, Complement, & the Immune Response. Jules M Elias. 1987. (Illus.). 160p. (Orig.). (C). stu. ed. 15.95 (*0-936735-01-5*) Grove Educ Tech.

Worked Problems in Ophthalmic Lenses. David Jenney & Alan Tunnacliffe. 1989. (C). (*0-900099-17-8*) Assn Brit Dispen Opticians GBR. *Dist:* St Mut.

Worked Problems in Optics. Alan Tunnacliffe. 1989. (C). (*0-900099-16-X*) Assn Brit Dispen Opticians GBR. *Dist:* St Mut.

Worker Exposure to Agrochemicals: Methods for Monitoring & Assessment. Richard C. Honeycutt. 2000. LC 00-57369. (Illus.). 169p. 69.95 (*1-56670-455-3*) Lewis Pubs.

Workers' Comp Management from A to Z: A "How To" Guide with Forms. Nancy N. Menzel. 2nd ed. 1998. 224p. spiral bd. 80.00 (*1-883595-01-0*, 23025, OEM Pr) OEM Health.

Workers' Compensation & Workplace Safety: Some Lessons from Economic Theory. Richard A. Victor et al. 1982. LC 83-3145. pap. 7.50 (*0-8330-0487-5*, R-2918-1CJ) Rand Corp.

Workers' Compensation Employee Medical Guide: How to Receive Appropriate Treatment under Any Workers' Compensation System in the United States. David F. Scaccia. 2000. (Illus.). 152p. pap. 13.95 (*0-9677909-0-5*) MedPoint Pr.

Workers' Compensation Health Care Cost Containment. Ed. by Judith Greenwood & Alfred Taricco. 1992. LC 92-17565. 370p. 59.50 (*0-934753-66-0*) LRP Pubns.

Workers' Compensation Managed Care Directory & Reference Guide. Gwen, B. Lareau. Ed. by Phyllis Harris & Beth Kerber. 1999. 252p. pap. text 185.00 (*1-882364-38-4*, Amer Busn Pub) Hlth Res Pub.

Worker's Compensation Medical Care: Effective Measurement of Outcomes. Ed. by Kate Kimpan. 1996. LC 96-41336. 50.00 (*0-935149-61-9*, WC-96-7) Workers Comp Res Inst.

Workers' Emotions in Shop & Home: Study of Individual Workers from the Psychological & Physiological Standpoint. Rexford B. Hersey. Ed. by Leon Stein. 1977. LC 77-70503. (Illus.). reprint ed. lib. bdg. 41.95 (*0-405-10175-9*) Ayer.

Working Across Cultures: A Study of Expatriate Nurses Working in Developing Countries in Primary Health Care. Barbara A. Parfitt. 1998. (Developments in Nursing & Health Care Ser.). (Illus.). 212p. text (*1-85972-251-2*) Ashgate Pub GBR. *Dist:* Ashgate Pub Co.

Working after Brain Injury: What Can I Do? Dana S. DeBoskey. 1995. (Illus.). 128p. (Orig.). pap. 12.50 (*1-882855-35-3*) HDI Pubs.

Working as a Nurse: How to Make Your Career in a Fulfilling Profession. Esther Bartlett & Marion Field. 2000. (Illus.). 144p. pap. (*1-85703-443-0*) How To Bks GBR. *Dist:* Trans-Atl Phila, Midpt Trade.

Working Bibliography on Behavioral & Emotional Disorders & Assessment Instruments in Mental Retardation. Michael G. Aman. 1996. 40p. (Orig.). (C). pap. text 20.00 (*0-7881-2739-X*) DIANE Pub.

Working Brain. Aleksandr R. Luria. Tr. by B. Haigh. 1976. LC 72-95540. 408p. pap. 27.00 (*0-465-09208-X*) Basic.

Working for Equality in Health. Ed. by Paul Bywaters & Eileen McLeod. 1996. LC 95-25987. (State of Welfare Ser.). (Illus.). 240p. (C). 90.00 (*0-415-12465-4*); pap. 27.95 (*0-415-12466-2*) Routledge.

Working for Health: The History of COHSE. Carpenter. 1988. (C). pap. (*0-85315-682-4*) Lawrence & Wishart GBR. *Dist:* NYU Pr.

Working from Within: Integrating Rural Health Care. Hospital Research and Educational Trust of the AHA S. 1993. 150p. (Orig.). pap. 35.00 (*0-87258-636-7*, 184151) Am Hospital.

Working Group Report on Primary Prevention of Hypertension: National High Blood Pressure Education Program. Edward J. Roccella. 1998. (Illus.). 49p. reprint ed. pap. text 20.00 (*0-7881-4226-7*) DIANE Pub.

Working in Depth: A Clinician's Guide to Framework & Flexibility in the Analytic Relationship. Elliot Adler & Janet Lee Bachant. 1998. LC 98-4564. 60.00 (*0-7657-0160-X*) Aronson.

Working in Health Care: What You Need to Know to Succeed. Michael W. Drafke. 1994. LC 94-13881. (Illus.). 213p. pap. 23.95 (*0-8036-2808-0*) Davis Co.

Working in Orbit & Beyond: The Challenges for Space Medicine, Jul 20-21, 1987, Washington, D. C. Ed. by David Lorr & Victoria Garshnek. 1989. LC 57-43769. (Science & Technology Ser.: Vol. 72). (Illus.). 188p. 45.00 (*0-87703-295-5*); pap. 35.00 (*0-87703-296-3*) Univelt Inc (Am Astronaut Soc).

Working in the Operating Department. Bakul Kumar. 2nd ed. 1997. LC 97-25789. 317p. pap. text (*0-443-05573-4*) Church.

Working Intersubjectively: Contextualism in Psychoanalytic Practice. Donna M. Orange et al. 2001. (Psychoanalytic Inquiry Book Ser.: Vol. 17). 120p. pap. 24.95 (*0-88163-360-7*) Analytic Pr.

Working It Out: Using Exercise in Psychotherapy. Kate F. Hays. 1999. LC 99-18204. 281p. text 39.95 (*1-55798-592-8*, 431-622A) Am Psychol.

Working Man's Model Family Botanic Guide: Every Man His Own Doctor. William Fox. 1963. 310p. reprint ed. spiral bd. 16.00 (*0-7873-0331-3*) Hlth Research.

Working Memory & Human Cognition. John T. Richardson et al. 1996. LC 95-23830. (Counterpoints Ser.). (Illus.). 176p. (C). pap. text 19.95 (*0-19-510100-6*) OUP.

Working Memory & Thinking. Robert H. Logie. 1998. LC 98-153248. (Current Issues in Thinking & Reasoning Ser.). 166p. (*0-86377-514-4*) Psychol Pr GBR. *Dist:* Taylor & Francis.

Working Mind: An Introduction to Psychology. J. P. Das. 1998. LC 98-19164. 39.95 (*0-7619-9261-8*, 83503) Sage.

Working Partnership: A Collaborative Approach to Care. HMSO Staff. 1994. 74p. pap. (*0-11-321716-1*, HM17161) Statnry Office GBR. *Dist:* Bernan Associates.

Working People's Guide to Stress Management. C. Samuel Verghese. 1989. (Illus.). 219p. (Orig.). 29.95 (*0-9622041-0-2*) Pain Stress & Sleep.

Working Safely: Body Mechanics in Healthcare. Ed. by Hartman Pub. Inc., Staff. 1999. (Illus.). 90p. pap. 34.95 (*1-888343-15-X*) Hartman Pub.

Working the Countertranference. Lawrence E. Hedges. 1995. 50.00 (*0-87668-509-2*) Aronson.

Working the Organizing Experience: Transforming Psychotic, Schizoid, & Autistic States. Lawrence E. Hedges. 1995. LC 94-7821. 336p. 60.00 (*1-56821-255-0*) Aronson.

Working the Range: Essays on the History of Western Land Management & the Environment, 61. Ed. by John R. Wunder. 1985. LC 84-15693. (Contributions in Economics & Economic History Ser.: No. 61). 241p. 64.00 (*0-313-24591-6*, WUW/) Greenwood.

Working the Soul: Reflections on Jungian Psychology. Charles Ponce. 1987. LC 88-166680. (Illus.). 189p. pap. 12.95 (*1-55643-033-7*) North Atlantic.

***Working the Web: A Guide for Nurses.** Sandra DeYoung & Julie B. Bliss. 2001. 90p. pap. 12.00 (*0-13-061788-1*, Prentice Hall) P-H.

Working Together: Building Integrated Healthcare Organizations Through Improved Executive-Physician Collaboration. Seth Allcorn. 1995. 225p. text 45.00 (*1-55738-614-5*, Irwn Prfssnl) McGraw-Hill Educ Grp.

Working Together for a Healthier Scotland: A Consultation Document, Command Paper 3854. 1998. (Command Papers). (*0-10-138542-0*) Statnry Office GBR. *Dist:* Bernan Associates.

Working with Adult Incest Survivors: The Healing Journey, No. 6. Sam Kirschner et al. 1993. LC 92-33066. (Frontiers in Couples & Family Therapy Ser.: Vol. 6). 240p. text 30.95 (*0-87630-691-1*) Brunner-Routledge.

Working with Adult Survivors of Child Sexual Abuse. Elsa Jones. 1992. 112p. pap. text (*1-85575-017-1*) Karnac Bks GBR. *Dist:* Other Pr LLC.

Working with African American Males: A Guide to Practice. Larry E. Davis. 1999. LC 98-40277. 391p. 79.95 (*0-7619-0471-9*, 80031) Sage.

Working with AIDS Bereavment: A Comprehensive Approach for Mental Health Providers. Peter Goldblum & Sarah Erickson. 1999. LC 99-47163. (UCSF AIDS Health Project Monograph Ser.: No. 3). xii, 100p. pap. 10.95 (*1-879168-03-0*) AIDS Hlth Project.

Working with Behavior Disorder. Ashley. 1998. (C). pap. text 41.00 (*0-12-784586-0*) Acad Pr.

Working with Bilingual Language Disability. Ed. by Dierdre M. Duncan. 1989. (Therapy in Practice Ser.). 230p. pap. 19.95 (*0-412-33940-4*) Chapman & Hall.

Working with Child Sexual Abuse: A Post-Cleveland Guide to Effective Principles & Practice. Kieran O'Hagan. 1989. 192p. pap. (*0-335-15597-9*) OpUniv Pr.

***Working with Children.** Maureen O'Hagan. 2001. (Illus.). 251p. pap. (*0-7020-2608-5*) W B Saunders GBR. *Dist:* Saunders.

Working with Culture: Psychotherapeutic Interventions with Ethnic Minority Children & Adolescents. Ed. by Luis A. Vargas & Joan D. Koss-Chioino. 1992. LC 92-15281. (Social & Behavioral Science Ser.). 416p. 43.00 (*1-55542-469-4*, C585-E2F) Jossey-Bass.

Working with Dr. Schweitzer. Louise Jilek-Aall. 1990. 240p. (Orig.). 16.95 (*0-88839-209-5*) Hancock House.

Working with Dreams in Psychotherapy. Clara E. Hill. 1996. LC 96-14095. (Practicing Professional Ser.). 262p. text 35.00 (*1-57230-092-2*, 0092) Guilford Pubns.

Working with Drug Family Support Groups. Paul Lockley. 1996. LC 97-187552. 312p. (C). (*1-85343-336-5*); pap. (*1-85343-337-3*) Free Assoc Bks GBR. *Dist:* NYU Pr, Intl Spec Bk, NYU Pr.

Working with Drug Users. Ronno Griffiths & Brian Pearson. 1988. (Community Care Practice Handbook Ser.: Vol. 25). 117p. pap. text (*0-7045-0582-7*) Gower GBR. *Dist:* Ashgate Pub Co.

Working with Elderly People: Communication Workshops. Sue Stevens & Kate Swinburn. 2nd ed. 1995. (Illus.). ring bd. 190.00 (*1-56593-499-7*, 1156) Singular Publishing.

Working with Emotions in Psychotherapy. Leslie S. Greenberg & Sandra C. Paivio. 1997. LC 97-13521. (Practicing Professional Ser.). 303p. text 37.00 (*1-57230-243-7*, 0243) Guilford Pubns.

Working with Families of the Mentally Ill. Kayla F. Bernheim & Anthony Lehman. 1985. LC 85-18754. 244p. 22.95 (*0-393-70009-7*) Norton.

Working with Families of the Poor. Patricia Minuchin et al. 1998. LC 98-3805. (Guilford Family Therapy Ser.). 248p. 42.00 (*1-57230-406-5*, C406) Guilford Pubns.

Working with Gay Men & Lesbians in Private Psychotherapy Practice. Ed. by Christopher J. Alexander. 1998. LC 98-48951. 107p. 29.95 (*0-7890-0693-6*) Haworth Pr.

Working with Groups to Explore Food & Body Connections. Ed. by Sandy S. Christian. 1996. LC 95-49465. (Structured Exercises in Healing Ser.). pap. 24.95 (*1-57025-105-3*) Whole Person.

Working with Images: Theoretical Base of Archetypal Psychology. James Hillman et al. Ed. by Benjamin Sells. 2000. LC 00-36549. (Primary Papers in Archetypal Psychology: Vol. 1). (Illus.). 207p. pap. 18.50 (*0-88214-376-X*) Spring Pubns.

Working with Insurance & Managed Care Plans. Maxine Lewis & Jan Davison. 2nd ed. 1999. LC 99-10591. (Illus.). viii, 444p. pap. 49.95 (*1-57066-131-6*, ME125) Practice Mgmt Info.

Working with Insurance & Managed Care Plans: A Guide for Getting Paid. Jan Davison & Maxine Lewis. 1995. (Illus.). 470p. reprint ed. pap. text 44.95 (*1-57066-081-6*, Me117) Practice Mgmt Info.

Working with Involuntary Clients: A Guide to Practice. Chris Trotter. 1999. LC 99-201983. 25.95 (*0-7619-6333-2*) Sage.

Working with Men's Groups: Dancing with the Hearts & Souls of Men. Craig S. Washington. 1998. LC 98-8936. pap. 24.95 (*1-57025-123-1*) Whole Person.

Working with Older Adults: Group Process. Irene Burnside & Mary G. Schmidt. 3rd ed. 1994. (Nursing-Health Science Ser.). (Illus.). 544p. (C). pap. text 48.95 (*0-86720-679-9*, 679-9) Jones & Bartlett.

Working with Older Clients. York. 2000. (Allied Health Ser.). (C). pap. 24.00 net. (*0-7668-0538-7*) Delmar.

Working with Older People. U. S. Department of Health, Education and Welfare Staff. Ed. by Leon Stein. 1980. LC 79-8669. (Growing Old Ser.). reprint ed. lib. bdg. 18.95 (*0-405-12784-7*) Ayer.

Working with Older Persons: Cognitive & Phenomenological Methods. Edmund Sherman. 1984. LC 84-5746. lib. bdg. 91.00 (*0-89838-144-4*) Kluwer Academic.

Working with Parents: Establishing the Essential Alliance in Child Psychotherapy & Consultation. Diana Siskind. 1997. LC 96-40017. 272p. 50.00 (*0-7657-0060-3*) Aronson.

Working with Parents of Young Children with Disabilities. Elizabeth J. Webster & Louise M. Ward. 1992. LC 92-49909. (Early Childhood Intervention Ser.). (Illus.). 136p. (Orig.). (C). pap. 29.95 (*1-879105-46-2*, 0359) Thomson Learn.

Working with People Called Patients. Milton M. Berger. 1984. LC 76-46483. 176p. pap. 23.95 (*0-87630-126-X*) Brunner-Routledge.

Working with Phrases on Your Own. Kathryn Kilpatrick & Roberta DePompei. 1986. 50p. stu. ed. 8.00 (*1-880504-07-3*); 54p. stu. ed. 8.00 (*1-880504-08-1*) Visit Nurse.

Working with Pregnant & Parenting Teenage Clients. Ed. by Neil Cervera & Lynn Videka-Sherman. 1990. 256p. pap. 18.95 (*0-87304-248-4*) Manticore Pubns.

Working with Psychology: A Concise Introduction. Terry F. Pettijohn. 2nd ed. 1989. (C). per. (*0-87967-769-4*) Brown & Benchmark.

Working with Relationship Triangles: The One-Two-Three of Psychotherapy. Philip J. Guerin, Jr. et al. 1996. LC 96-33339. (Guilford Family Therapy Ser.). 251p. text 32.00 (*1-57230-143-0*, 0143) Guilford Pubns.

Working with Religious Issues in Therapy. Robert J. Lovinger. 1984. LC 84-6198. 328p. 50.00 (*0-87668-727-3*) Aronson.

Working with Schizophrenia: A Needs Based Approach. Gwen Howe. 1994. LC 94-239132. 200p. pap. 19.95 (*1-85302-242-X*) Taylor & Francis.

Working with Self-Help. Ed. by Thomas J. Powell. 1990. LC 89-14031. 355p. 28.95 (*0-87101-174-3*) Natl Assn Soc Wkrs.

Working with Seniors Vol. 39-1: Behavioral Aspects of Vision Care. 1998. (Illus.). 138p. pap. 20.00 (*0-943599-99-7*) OEPF.

Working with the Core Relationship Problem in Psychotherapy: A Handbook for Clinicians. Althea J. Horner. 1998. LC 97-52693. (Psychology Ser.). 185p. 45.00 (*0-7879-4301-0*) Jossey-Bass.

Working with the Dying & Bereaved: Systemic Approaches to Therapeutic Work. Pauline Sutcliffe et al. 1998. LC 97-24236. 232p. (C). 90.00 (*0-415-91993-2*); pap. 22.95 (*0-415-91994-0*) Routledge.

Working with the Elderly. Eunice Mortimer. Ed. by Martin Davies. 1982. (Community Care Practice Handbook Ser.: No. 9). vi, 91p. (Orig.). (C). pap. text 16.95 (*0-566-05171-0*) Ashgate Pub Co.

Working with the Elderly: An Introduction. Ed. by Elizabeth Deichman et al. 1989. LC 89-10856. (Golden Age Bks.). 299p. pap. 25.00 (*0-87975-534-2*) Prometheus Bks.

Working with the Elderly: An Introduction. Ed. by Elizabeth Deichman & Regina Kociecki. 1989. LC 89-10856. (Golden Age Bks.). 299p. 40.00 (*0-87975-520-2*) Prometheus Bks.

Working with the Family in Primary Care: A Systems Approach to Health & Illness. Janet Christie-Seely. 1984. LC 83-17772. 584p. 85.00 (*0-275-91424-0*, C1424, Praeger Pubs) Greenwood.

Working with the Family in Primary Care: A Systems Approach to Health & Illness. Ed. by Janet Christie-Seely. 1984. 584p. 49.95 (*0-03-063899-2*) Soc Tchrs Fam Med.

Working with the Mentally Disordered Offender in the Community. P. Vaughan & D. Badger. 1995. (Illus.). 288p. pap. text 51.00 (*1-56593-326-5*, 0656) Singular Publishing.

Working with the Person with Schizophrenia: The Treatment Alliance. Michael A. Selzer et al. 1989. 432p. (C). text 45.00 (*0-8147-7891-7*) NYU Pr.

Working with the Problem Drinker: A Solution-Focused Approach. Insoo K. Berg & Scott D. Miller. 1992. LC 92-12746. 240p. (C). 27.00 (*0-393-70134-4*) Norton.

Working with Traits: Psychotherapy of Personality Disorders. Joel Paris. 1998. LC 97-18482. 272p. text 50.00 (*0-7657-0096-4*) Aronson.

Working with Traumatized Children: A Handbook for Healing. Kathryn Brohl. 1996. LC 96-24093. 105p. pap. 19.95 (*0-87868-633-9*) Child Welfare.

Working with Troubled Adolescents. John Coleman. 1987. text 70.00 (*0-12-179720-1*) Acad Pr.

Working with Women & AIDS: Medical, Counselling & Social Issues. Ed. by Judy Bury et al. 1992. LC 92-9967. (Illus.). 176p. (C). 90.00 (*0-415-07658-7*, A9601); pap. 27.99 (*0-415-07659-5*, A9605) Routledge.

Working with Words, Vol. 3. Kathryn Kilpatrick. 1987. (Illus.). 289p. stu. ed. 30.00 (*1-880504-03-0*) Visit Nurse.

Working with Words on Your Own. Kathryn Kilpatrick & Roberta DePompei. 1986. 50p. stu. ed. 8.00 (*1-880504-06-5*) Visit Nurse.

Working Without a Net: Memoirs of a Small Town Surgeon. Richard Fox. 1996. LC 94-71272. (Illus.). 344p. 24.95 (*0-9641246-0-2*) Agincourt-Galen.

Working Woman's Guide to Managing Stress. J. Robin Powell & Holly George-Warren. 1994. LC 94-11400. pap. 14.95 (*0-13-969212-6*) P-H.

Working Woman's Pregnancy. Hilary Boyd. 2001. LC 00-51184. 160p. pap. 14.95 (*0-7370-0100-3*) Time-Life Educ.

Working Wounded: The Politics of Musculoskeletal Injuries. Penney Kome. 1998. LC 98-229705. 408p. pap. text 19.95 (*0-8020-7795-1*) U of Toronto Pr.

Workings of the Brain: Development, Memory & Perception. Rodolfo R. Llinas. 1989. LC 89-17196. 171p. (C). pap. 14.95 (*0-7167-2071-X*) W H Freeman.

Workplace Drug Abuse & AIDS: A Guide to Human Resource Management Policy & Practice. Donald E. Klingner & Nancy G. O'Neill. 1991. LC 90-46719. 216p. 62.95 (*0-89930-624-1*, KDR/, Quorum Bks) Greenwood.

Workplace Health Protection. Robert G. Confer. 1994. 560p. lib. bdg. 104.95 (*0-87371-387-7*, L387) Lewis Pubs.

Workplace Readiness: Health Occupations. Colbert. 1998. (Health Occupations Ser.). tchr. ed. 13.95 (*0-8273-7783-5*); 55.00 (*0-8273-7782-7*); 19.95 (*0-8273-7784-3*) Delmar.

Workplace Roulette: Gambling with Cancer. Matthew Firth et al. 1997. 280p. pap. text (*1-896357-09-1*) Betwn Lines CAN. *Dist:* U of Toronto Pr.

Workplace Wellness: The Key to Higher Productivity & Lower Health Costs. Carol B. Grant & Robert E. Brisbin. 1992. 155p. text 44.95 (*0-442-00699-3*, VNR) Wiley.

Workplace Wellness: The Key to Higher Productivity & Lower Health Costs. Carol B. Grant et al. 1992. 176p. pap. 59.95 (*0-471-28422-X*, VNR) Wiley.

Workplace Within: Psychodynamics of Organizational Life. Larry Hirschhorn. 1990. (Organization Studies). 280p. reprint ed. pap. 21.95 (*0-262-58101-9*) MIT Pr.

Works Charles Robert Darwin. LC 73-147085. reprint ed. 1485.00 (*0-404-08400-1*) AMS Pr.

Works of Robert Whytt, 1. Robert Whytt. 1978. LC 77-72191. (Contributions to the History of Psychology Ser.: Vol. I, Pt. E, Physiological Psychology). 480p. reprint ed. lib. bdg. 83.50 (*0-313-26949-1*, U6949, Greenwood Pr) Greenwood.

Works on Vision. George Berkeley. Ed. by Colin M. Turbayne. 1963. LC 62-11787. (Orig.). 6.60 (*0-672-51033-2*); pap. 4.35 (*0-672-60267-9*, LLA83) Macmillan (Bobbs).

Workshop on Drug Effects in Animals. Ed. by F. N. Krijzer & W. H. Herrmann. 1993. (Journal: Vol. 28, No. 3, 1993). (Illus.). 64p. pap. 58.50 (*3-8055-5857-0*) S Karger.

Workshop on Prevention & Treatment of Childhood Obesity: Research Directions. 1996. (Illus.). 70p. reprint ed. pap. text 30.00 (*0-7881-3302-0*) DIANE Pub.

Workshop Report on EPA Guidelines for Carcinogen Risk Assessment: Use of Human Evidence. 1994. (Illus.). 98p. (Orig.). (C). pap. text 25.00 (*0-7881-0627-9*) DIANE Pub.

Workshops in Bile Acid Research: Serum Bile Acids in Health & Disease-Pathophysiology of the Enterohepatic Circulation. E. Roda et al. 1983. 144p. text 122.00 (*0-85200-749-3*) Kluwer Academic.

Workshops in Cognitive Processes. A. Bennett et al. 2nd ed. 1982. 136p. pap. 10.95 (*0-7100-0932-1*, Routledge Thoemms) Routledge.

Workshops in Fluid & Electrolyte Disorders. Ed. by Harold M. Szerlip & Stanley Goldfarb. 1996. (Illus.). 203p. (Orig.). pap. text (*0-443-08791-1*) Church.

Worksite Health Promotion. David H. Chenoweth. 1998. LC 97-39341. (Illus.). 200p. 35.00 (*0-88011-542-4*, BCHE0542) Human Kinetics.

Worksite Nutrition: A Guide to Planning, Implementation, & Evaluation. American Dietetic Association Staff & Office of Disease Prevention and Health Promotion St. 2nd ed. 1993. LC 93-6120. 12.00 (*0-88091-126-3*) Am Dietetic Assn.

World 3-D Diagnostic Imaging System Markets. Ed. by Frost and Sullivan Staff. 1997. 306p. spiral bd. 2895.00 (*0-7889-0731-X*, 5535-50) Frost & Sullivan.

World Arthritis Treatment Products: Rx, OTC & Prosthetics: OTC Changes Dynamics of Rx Markets. Market Intelligence Staff. 1993. 280p. 2295.00 (*1-56753-496-1*) Frost & Sullivan.

World Audiology Product Markets: Competitors Keep Their Ears to the Ground for Hints of Improving Sales. Market Intelligence Staff. 1994. 310p. 1695.00 (*0-7889-0106-0*) Frost & Sullivan.

World Audiology Product Markets: Consumer Advertising Overcoming the Stigma. Market Intelligence Staff. 1992. 349p. 1495.00 (*1-56753-390-6*) Frost & Sullivan.

World Bank HIV/AIDS Interventions: Ex-Ante & Ex-Post Evaluation. Julia Dayton. 1998. LC 98-23816. (Discussion Paper Ser.: No. 389). 44p. pap. 22.00 (*0-8213-4251-7*, 14251) World Bank.

World Biomedical Sensor Markets. Market Intelligence Staff. 1994. 250p. 1895.00 (*0-7889-0036-6*) Frost & Sullivan.

World Biomedical Sensor Markets: Cross Contamination & Ease of Use Reshape the Industry. Market Intelligence Staff. 1992. 341p. 1695.00 (*1-56753-422-8*) Frost & Sullivan.

World Book Health & Medical Annual, 1999. Ed. by World Book, Inc. Staff. 1999. (Illus.). 352p. (*0-7166-1199-6*) World Bk.

World Book of Sport Psychology. John H. Salmela. 1981. text 22.95 (*0-932392-08-3*) Mouvement Pubns.

World Cancer Diagnostic Imaging & Therapeutic Equipment Markets. Ed. by Frost and Sullivan Staff. 1997. 453p. spiral bd. 2895.00 (*0-7889-0678-X*, 5521-50) Frost & Sullivan.

World Cancer Therapeutic Markets: Strategic Alliances Globalize the Marketplace. Market Intelligence Staff. 1993. 295p. 2495.00 (*1-56753-524-0*) Frost & Sullivan.

World Cancer Therapeutic Markets by Disease Cite: Accelerated R & D Intensifies Race for Cure. Market Intelligence Staff. 1994. 400p. (Orig.). 2895.00 (*1-56753-886-X*) Frost & Sullivan.

World Cancer Therapeutic Pharmaceuticals Market: Biotech Becomes Big Business. Market Intelligence Staff. 1992. 258p. (Orig.). 2295.00 (*1-56753-063-X*) Frost & Sullivan.

World Cardiac Diagnostic Equipment & Telemetry Monitoring Markets. Ed. by Frost and Sullivan Staff. 1995. 346p. spiral bd. 2295.00 (*0-7889-0228-8*, 5241-56) Frost & Sullivan.

World Cardiac Diagnostic Imaging Markets. Frost and Sullivan Staff. 1996. 346p. spiral bd. 2495.00 (*0-7889-0406-X*, 0969-50) Frost & Sullivan.

World Cardiovascular Diagnostic & Therapeutic Equipment Markets: Multi-Billion Dollar Battle, Technology Advances vs Cost Constraints. Market Intelligence Staff. 1992. 313p. (Orig.). 1995.00 (*1-56753-043-5*) Frost & Sullivan.

World Cardiovascular Drug Markets: Primary Prevention Creates Opportunities. Market Intelligence Staff. 1994. 430p. (Orig.). 2695.00 (*1-56753-925-4*) Frost & Sullivan.

World Cell Therapy Markets. Ed. by Frost and Sullivan Staff. 1997. 421p. spiral bd. 3495.00 (*0-7889-0693-3*, 5413-43) Frost & Sullivan.

World Clinical Lab Analytical Instrument Markets. Ed. by Frost and Sullivan Staff. 1995. 517p. spiral bd. 2995.00 (*0-7889-0348-9*, 5346-55) Frost & Sullivan.

World Clinical Laboratory Instrument Markets: Cost Containment...Consolidation...Point of Care; Report #909-56. Market Intelligence Staff. 1994. 306p. 2195.00 (*1-56753-702-2*) Frost & Sullivan.

World Congress for Microcirculation: Abstracts. Ed. by K. Messmer & W. M. Kuebler. 1996. (International Journal of Microcirculation Ser.: Vol. 16, Supplement 1, 1996). (Illus.). x, 308p. pap. 77.50 (*3-8055-6388-4*) S Karger.

World Congress of Psychiatry. Allan Beigel et al. 1994. LC 95-166269. 1548p. text 202.00 (*981-02-1500-2*) World Scientific Pub.

World Congresses of Gastroenterology: Congress, Vienna, September 1998: Abstracts, No. 59. Ed. by Peter Ferenci. 1998. (Digestion Ser.). ii, 820p. pap. 55.75 (*3-8055-6767-7*) S Karger.

World Congresses of Gastroenterology: Congress, Vienna, September 1998: Quadrennial. Ed. by G. J. Krejs et al. 1998. (Digestion Ser.: Vol. 59, No. 5 (1998)). (Illus.). 196p. pap. 76.50 (*3-8055-6756-1*) S Karger.

World Contrast Media Markets: New Dynamics in an Evolving Market. Market Intelligence Staff. 1994. (Orig.). 2295.00 (*0-7889-0121-4*) Frost & Sullivan.

World Databases in Medicine. 1993. 1650p. (*0-86291-613-5*) Bowker.

World Dental Products Markets: European Prosthetic Markets Triple North American Growth. 1992. 353p. 1895.00 (*1-56753-016-8*) Frost & Sullivan.

World Development Report 1993: Investing in Health. 1993. (GER.). 404p. pap. 26.00 (*0-8213-2362-8*, 12362); (SPA.). 344p. pap. 26.00 (*0-8213-2361-X*, 12361); (FRE.). 352p. pap. 26.00 (*0-8213-2360-1*, 12360) World Bank.

World Diagnostic Imaging Company Profiles. Market Intelligence Staff. 1994. 478p. (Orig.). 1595.00 (*0-7889-0131-1*) Frost & Sullivan.

World Directory of Medical Schools. WHO Staff. 6th ed. 1988. 320p. 40.50 (*92-4-150009-3*) World Health.

World Directory of Post-Basic & Post-Graduate Schools of Nursing. 1965. (ENG, FRE & RUS.). 223p. pap. text 18.00 (*92-4-150000-X*, 1150166) World Health.

World Directory of Schools for Animal Health Assistants. 1974. pap. text 24.00 (*92-4-150005-0*, 1150164) World Health.

World Directory of Schools for Dental Auxiliaries: Bilingual English/French. 1973. 379p. text 42.00 (*92-4-050003-0*) World Health.

World Directory of Schools for Medical Assistants, 1973: Bilingual English/French. 1976. 112p. pap. text 24.00 (*92-4-050002-2*) World Health.

World Directory of Veterinary Schools, 1971. 1973. pap. text 36.00 (*92-4-150004-2*, 1150169) World Health.

World Drug Situation. WHO Staff. 1988. 129p. 20.00 (*92-4-156114-9*) World Health.

World Fetal, Neonatal & Infant Monitor Markets: Manufacturers Push Hi-Tech Products Through One-Stop Shopping. Market Intelligence Staff. 1992. 433p. (Orig.). 1995.00 (*1-56753-033-8*) Frost & Sullivan.

World Gastrointestinal Drug Markets: Generic Competition Intensified As Block Buster Drugs Lose Patent Protection. Market Intelligence Staff. 1992. 537p. (Orig.). 2295.00 (*1-56753-400-7*) Frost & Sullivan.

World Geography of Human Diseases. Ed. by G. Melvyn Howe. 1978. text 272.00 (*0-12-357150-2*) Acad Pr.

World Growing Old: The Coming Health Care Challenges. Ed. by Daniel Callahan et al. 1996. LC 95-6447. (Hastings Center Studies in Ethics). 190p. pap. 16.95 (*0-87840-632-8*) Georgetown U Pr.

World Growth Factor Markets: Tissue Applications Poised for Commercialization. Market Intelligence Staff. 1993. 300p. (Orig.). 2495.00 (*1-56753-620-4*) Frost & Sullivan.

***World Health & Disease.** Alastair Gray & Philip Payne. 2001. (Health & Disease Ser.). 320p. pap. (*0-335-20838-X*) OpUniv Pr GBR. *Dist:* Taylor & Francis.

World Health & Disease. Alistair Gray & Philip Payne. Ed. by Alistair Gray. 1993. LC 92-42625. (Health & Disease Ser.: Book 3). pap. (*0-335-19078-2*) OpUniv Pr.

World Health Report, 1995: Bridging the Gaps. 1995. (ENG & FRE.). 120p. (C). pap. text 22.00 (*92-4-156178-5*, 1241995) World Health.

***World Health Report, 2000: Health Systems - Improving Performance.** Philip Musgrove. Ed. by Julio Frenk. 2001. (Illus.). 215p. (C). pap. 40.00 (*0-7567-0828-1*) DIANE Pub.

W X Y Z

*World Health Report 2001: Mental Health: New Understanding, New Hope. World Health Organisation Staff. 2001. 150p. 16.50 (92-4-156201-3) World Health.

World Health Statistics Annual, 1985: Global Overview, Vital Statistics & Life Tables, Environmental Health, Causes of Death. 1985. 531p. pap. text 76.50 (92-4-067851-4, 0178500) World Health.

World Health Statistics Annual, 1987: Global Review, Evaluation of the Global Strategy for Health for All Vital Statistics & Life Tables, Causes of Death. 1986. 472p. pap. text 81.00 (92-4-067861-1, 0178700) World Health.

World Health Statistics Annual, 1991. WHO Staff. 1992. xxii, 349p. pap. text 100.00 (92-4-067910-3, 0179100) World Health.

World Health Statistics Annual, 1994. 1995. (FRE.). 600p. (C). pap. text 100.00 (92-4-067940-5, 0179400) World Health.

World Health Statistics Annual, 1995. 1995. (Illus.). 835p. pap. 135.00 (92-4-067950-2, 0179500) World Health.

World Human Vaccine Markets. Ed. by Frost and Sullivan Staff. 1995. 482p. spiral bd. 3495.00 (0-7889-0210-5, 5227-43) Frost & Sullivan.

World Human Vaccine Markets: Over 60 Productions: Which Competitors Are Attacking Viruses? Market Intelligence Staff. 1993. 478p. 2295.00 (1-56753-460-0) Frost & Sullivan.

World Is Sound - Nada Brahma: Music & the Landscape of Consciousness. Joachim-Ernst Berendt. 1991. 240p. reprint ed. pap. 16.95 (0-89281-318-0, Destiny Bks) Inner Tradit.

World Market for Telemedicine: Products & Services: Issues, Market Forecasts, & Trends. Feedback Research Services Staff. 1997. (Illus.). 300p. spiral bd. 595.00 (1-889713-13-9) Feedback Rsch.

World Markets for Single-Use Medical Products: Industry Responds Strongly to Infection Control, AIDS Concerns. 1992. 264p. 1495.00 (1-56753-018-4) Frost & Sullivan.

World Medical Diagnostic Ultrasound Imaging Equipment Markets at the Forefront of Diagnostic. Market Intelligence Staff. 1995. 363p. spiral bd. 2495.00 (0-7889-0247-4, 5230-50) Frost & Sullivan.

World Medical Image Management. Frost & Sullivan. 1997. 356p. spiral bd. 2995.00 (0-7889-0623-2, 5355-50) Frost & Sullivan.

World Medical Imaging & Therapeutic Immunoconjugate Markets: Competitors Refocusing R&D & Marketing Strategies. Market Intelligence Staff. 1994. 351p. 2695.00 (1-56753-954-8) Frost & Sullivan.

World Medicine: East West Guide to Healing Your Body. EastWest Natural Health Editors & Tom Monte. 1993. LC 92-43052. 352p. 16.95 (0-87477-733-X, Tarcher Putnam) Putnam Pub Group.

World Meetings: Medicine, Vol. 21. Macmillan Publishing Company Staff. 1998. pap. 43.75 (0-02-865003-4); 2nd ed. per. 43.75 (0-02-865004-2); 3rd ed. per. 43.75 (0-02-865005-0); 4th ed. per. 43.75 (0-02-865006-9) Macmillan.

World Meetings: Medicine 1998, Vol. 21. Macmillan Publishing Company Staff. 1997. per. 175.00 (0-02-865002-6) Macmillan.

World Meetings Vol. 19: Medicine, 1996 Macmillan Publishing Company Staff. 1995. per. 175.00 (0-02-864646-0) Macmillan.

World Meetings Vol. 19 No. 1: Medicine. Macmillan Publishing Company Staff. 1996. per. 43.75 (0-02-864647-9) Macmillan.

World Meetings Vol. 19 No. 2: Medicine. Macmillan Publishing Company Staff. 1996. per. 43.75 (0-02-864648-7) Macmillan.

World Meetings Vol. 19 No. 3: Medicine. Macmillan Publishing Company Staff. 1996. per. 43.75 (0-02-864649-5) Macmillan.

World Meetings Vol. 19 No. 4: Medicine. Macmillan Publishing Company Staff. 1996. per. 43.75 (0-02-864650-9) Macmillan.

World Meetings Medicine. Contrib. by Gale Group Staff. 24th ed. 2001. 175.00 net. (0-02-865661-X, Macmillan Ref) Gale.

World Nuclear Medical Imaging, NMI, Market: Radiopharmaceutical Applications Drive Double-Digit Growth Despite Cost-Benefit Concerns. Market Intelligence Staff. 1992. 323p. (Orig.). 2295.00 (1-56753-074-5) Frost & Sullivan.

World Nutritional Determinants. Ed. by Geoffrey H. Bourne. 1984. (World Review of Nutrition & Dietetics Ser.: Vol. 45). (Illus.). x, 226p. 172.25 (3-8055-3948-7) S Karger.

World of Aromatherapy. Ed. by Jeanne Rose & Susan Earle. 1996. LC 95-48253. (Illus.). 350p. pap. 18.95 (1-883319-49-8) Frog Ltd CA.

World of Child Development. George S. Morrison. 1990. (Early Childhood Education Ser.). 590p. pap., stu. ed. 16.00 (0-8273-3118-5) Delmar.

World of Children's Sleep: Parent's Guide to Understanding Children & Their Sleep Problems. Alexander Z. Golbin. 1995. (Illus.). 307p. (Orig.). pap. 22.95 (1-884084-09-5) Michaelis Med.

World of Emotions: Clinical Studies of Affects & Their Expression. Ed. by Charles W. Socarides. 1977. LC 77-12735. 638p. 65.00 (0-8236-6867-3) Intl Univs Pr.

World of Francis Cooper: Nineteenth-Century Pennsylvania Photographer. Jay Ruby. 1998. LC 98-6993. (Illus.). 1200p. text 66.00 (0-271-01762-7) Pa St U Pr.

World of Microorganisms. Robert Snedden. 2000. LC 99-46864. (Microlife Ser.). (Illus.). 48p. (J). lib. bdg. 22.79 (1-57572-241-0) Heinemann Lib.

World of Natural Sciences & Its Phenomenology. H. Kuhlenbeck. Ed. by J. Gerlach. 2nd ed. 1981. (Human Brain & Its Universe Ser.: Vol. 1). (Illus.). xiv, 282p. 143.50 (3-8055-1817-X) S Karger.

World of Pastoralism: Herding Systems in Comparative Perspective. Ed. by John G. Galaty & Douglas L. Johnson. 1990. 436p. text 52.50 (0-89862-785-0) Guilford Pubns.

World of Psychology. Samuel E. Wood. 3rd ed. 1999. LC 98-21459. 77.25 (0-205-29329-8) P-H.

World of Psychology: Evaluating Psychological Information. Samuel E. Wood & Ellen R. Wood. 3rd ed. 1998. LC 98-21459. 726p. 88.00 (0-205-27467-6) Allyn.

World of Rosaphrenia: The Sexual Psychology of the Female. Major J. Baisden, Jr. 1971. LC 72-178852. 224p. 6.95 (0-912984-01-5) Allied Res Soc.

World of the Counselor: An Introduction to the Counseling Profession. Ed Neukrug. 1998. LC 98-15140. 688p. spiral bd. 76.95 (0-534-35828-4) Brooks-Cole.

World of Vocabulary, Red Level. Chester A. Halterman. annot. ed. 1985. pap., tchr. ed. 17.95 (0-8359-1308-2) Globe Fearon.

World Ophthalmic Pharmaceutical Markets. Market Intelligence Staff. 1994. 470p. (Orig.). 2395.00 (1-56753-923-8) Frost & Sullivan.

World Orthopedic & Prosthetic Product Markets: Impact of Lifestyles, Demographics & Biomaterials. Market Intelligence Staff. 1992. 627p. 1995.00 (1-56753-386-8) Frost & Sullivan.

World Pharmaceutical Industry. James Taggart. 1993. LC 92-24220. (Bus Press-Previous Routledge). 368p. (C). pap. 110.95 (0-415-02500-1, A7638) Thomson Learn.

World Pharmaceuticals Database. Ed. by Frost and Sullivan Staff. 1997. 995.00 (0-7889-0713-1, 5666-45) Frost & Sullivan.

World Population Profile, 1994: With a Special Chapter Focusing on HIV-AIDS. Ellen Jamison & Frank B. Hobbs. 1994. (Illus.). 135p. (Orig.). (C). pap. text 40.00 (0-7881-1417-4) DIANE Pub.

World Prescription Dermatology Markets. Market Intelligence Staff. 1994. 380p. 2695.00 (0-7889-0043-9) Frost & Sullivan.

World Psychology. Wood. 2nd ed. 1996. 784p. pap. text 42.00 (0-205-26718-1) P-H.

World Renal & Hemodialysis Equipment & Supply Markets: Cost Containment Pressures Influence World Markets. Market Intelligence Staff. 1994. 347p. 1995.00 (0-7889-0015-3) Frost & Sullivan.

World Renal & Hemodialysis Equipment & Supply Markets: U. S. Struggles with Cost Constraints While Europe & Japan Expand. Market Intelligence Staff. 1992. 309p. 1895.00 (1-56753-383-3) Frost & Sullivan.

World Renal Replacement Therapies Equipment & Supply Markets. Ed. by Frost and Sullivan Staff. 1997. 410p. spiral bd. 3295.00 (0-7889-0726-3) Frost & Sullivan.

World Respiratory Therapy Equipment Market: Strongest Growth Centered in Europe. 1992. 289p. 1995.00 (1-56753-027-3) Frost & Sullivan.

World Review of Nutrition & Dietetics. Ed. by Geoffrey H. Bourne. Vol. 12. 1970. 167.00 (3-8055-0663-5); Vol. 13. 1971. 85.25 (3-8055-1180-9); Vol. 14. 1972. 116.75 (3-8055-1282-1); Vol. 15. 1972. (Illus.). 300p. 99.25 (3-8055-1397-6); Vol. 17. 1973. (Illus.). 300p. 125.25 (3-8055-1336-4); Vol. 18. 1973. 143.50 (3-8055-1458-1); Vol. 19. 1974. (Illus.). 319p. 143.50 (3-8055-1589-8); Vol. 20. 1975. (Illus.). 350p. 151.25 (3-8055-1841-2); Vol. 21. 1975. (Illus.). x, 327p. 164.50 (3-8055-2133-2); Vol. 22. 1975. (Illus.). 172.25 (3-8055-2135-9); Vol. 23. 1975. (Illus.). xii, 315p. 155.00 (3-8055-2243-6); Vol. 24. 1976. (Illus.). 250p. 132.25 (3-8055-2344-0); Vol. 25. 1976. (Illus.). 300p. 149.75 (3-8055-2363-7) S Karger.

World Society for Stereotactic & Functional Neurosurery: XIIth Meeting, Lyon, July 1997: Abstracts of Poster Presentations. Ed. by M. Sindou et al. 1997. (Stereotactic & Functional Neurosurgery Ser.: Vol. 67, Nos. 1-2, 96-97). 152p. pap. 60.00 (3-8055-6556-9) S Karger.

World Society for Stereotactic & Functional Neurosurgery. Ed. by R. R. Tasker et al. 1986. (Advances in Stereoencephalotomy Ser.: Vol. 10). (Illus.). xii, 500p. pap. 172.25 (3-8055-4401-4) S Karger.

World Society for Stereotactic & Functional Neurosurgery: Proceedings of 12th Meeting, Lyon, July 1997. Ed. by M. P. Sindou et al. 1998. (Stereotactic & Functional Neurosurgery Ser.: Vol. 68, Pt. 1). (Illus.). viii, 278p. pap. 169.75 (3-8055-6688-3); viii, 318p. pap. 198.25 (3-8055-6689-1) S Karger.

World Society for Stereotactic & Functional Neurosurgery, 8th Meeting, & the European Society for Stereotactic & Functional Neurosurgery, 5th Meeting, Zurich, July 1981. World Society for Stereotactic and Functional Neuros & European Society for Stereotactic and Functional Neu. Ed. by Philip L. Gildenberg et al. 1982. (Advances in Stereoencephalotomy Ser.: Vol. 9). (Illus.). viii, 548p. pap. 135.00 (3-8055-3501-5) S Karger.

World Society for Stereotactic & Functional Neurosurgy, 10th Meeting, Maebashi, Japan, 1989: Journal: Stereotactic & Functional Neurosurgery, Vols. 54 & 55, 1990. Ed. by O. Chihiro et al. 1990. (Illus.). xiv, 564p. pap. 327.00 (3-8055-5337-4) S Karger.

World Society of Stereotactic & Functional Neurosurgery, 8th Meeting, Technical Advances. Ed. by J. M. Gybels et al. 1981. (Journal: Vol. 45, No. 4-5). (Illus.). iv, 208p. pap. 68.00 (3-8055-3499-X) S Karger.

World Stroke Congress & European Stroke Conference: 3rd Congress & 5th Conference, Munich, September 1996 - Abstracts. Ed. by J. Bogousslavsky et al. 1996. (Journal: Vol. 6, Suppl. 2, 1996). (Illus.). ii, 192p. pap. 59.25 (3-8055-6370-1) S Karger.

World Surgical Laser Markets. Ed. by Frost and Sullivan Staff. 1995. 344p. spiral bd. 2195.00 (0-7889-0244-X, 5234-57) Frost & Sullivan.

World Therapeutics Database. Ed. by Frost and Sullivan Staff. 1997. spiral bd. 995.00 (0-7889-0727-1, 5667-57) Frost & Sullivan.

World 3-D Diagnostic Medical Imaging Equipment & Software Markets: Dramatic Global Expansion Led by Clinical Applications & Ultrasound Technology. Market Intelligence Staff. 1992. 250p. 1995.00 (1-56753-413-9) Frost & Sullivan.

World Through Their Eyes: A Manual for Nursing Home Staff. Ruth Fangmeier. 1994. (Illus.). 56p. (Orig.). pap. 10.00 (0-9603444-7-0) Lighthouse NYC.

World Travel Health Guide, 1997. Ed. by Michael Hart. 1997. (Illus.). 244p. 69.95 (0-946393-71-0) SF Comns.

World Traveller's Manual of Homoeopathy. Colin Lesell. pap. 33.95 (0-8464-4497-6) Beekman Pubs.

World Travellers' Manual of Homoeopathy. Colin B. Lessell. 2nd ed. 2000. pap. (0-85207-330-5) C W Daniel GBR. *Dist:* Natl Bk Netwk.

World Ultrasound Imaging Markets: Manufacturers Focus on Developing Niche Applications. Market Intelligence Staff. 1993. 365p. 2295.00 (1-56753-618-2) Frost & Sullivan.

World-Wide Problems of Nutrition Research & Nutrition Education. J. C. Somogyi. 1982. (Bibliotheca Nutritio et Dieta Ser.: No. 32). (Illus.). xvi, 76p. pap. 65.25 (3-8055-3586-4) S Karger.

World Without Cancer: The Story of Vitamin B17. G. Edward Griffin. 2nd rev. ed. 1997. LC 96-84094. (Illus.). 368p. pap. 17.50 (0-912986-19-0) Am Media.

World Without the Rinderpest. Food and Agriculture Organization of the United Nations Staff. 1997. (Animal Production & Health Papers: No. 129). 173p. pap. (92-5-103900-3, F39003) FAO ITA. *Dist:* Bernan Associates.

World Without Words: Social Construction of Children Born Deaf & Blind. David Goode. 1994. LC 93-51038. (Health, Society, & Policy Ser.). 272p. (C). pap. text 22.95 (1-56639-216-0) Temple U Pr.

World Workshop in Clinical Periodontics - Proceedings. American Academy of Periodontology Staff. 1989. 260p. 65.00 (0-9624699-1-2) Amer Acad Periodontology.

World Wound Closure Product Markets: Developing Nations Contribute to Markets Rebound. Frost and Sullivan Staff. 1995. LC 98-168913. 343p. spiral bd. 1995.00 (0-7889-0269-5, 5090-51) Frost & Sullivan.

World Wound Closure Products: Staplers Invade Suture Markets. Market Intelligence Staff. 1992. 345p. 1695.00 (1-56753-387-6) Frost & Sullivan.

World X-Ray & Computed Tomography Equipment Markets. 1996. 358p. spiral bd. 2495.00 (0-7889-0569-4, 5391-50) Frost & Sullivan.

Worlds Apart? Long-Term Care in Australia & the United States. Ed. by Sandra J. Newman. 1988. LC 87-29770. (Home Health Care Services Quarterly Ser.: Vol. 8, No. 3). (Illus.). 113p. text 32.95 (0-86656-703-8) Haworth Pr.

World's Best Anatomical Charts. Anatomical Chart Company Staff. 2nd ed. 1993. (Illus.). 72p. pap. 15.95 (0-9603730-5-5, ACC35) Anatomical Chart.

World's Best Doctor Jokes. Raja Korale. 1998. 96p. pap. (0-00-638075-1) HarpC GBR. *Dist:* Trafalgar.

World's Easiest Guide to Using the APA. Carol J. Amato. Ed. by Claudia Suzanne. 1995. 368p. (Illus.). lib. bdg. 19.95 (0-9643853-5-X);College ed. (C). spiral bd. 19.95 (0-9643853-4-1) Stargazer.

World's Easiest Guide to Using the APA: A User-Friendly Manual for Formatting Research Papers According to the American Psychological Association Style Guide. Carol J. Amato. Ed. by Claudia Suzanne. 2nd rev. ed. 1998. LC 98-87767. 368p. (C). pap. 19.95 (0-9643853-1-7); per. 19.95 (0-9643853-2-5) Stargazer.

World's Greatest Hypnotists. John C. Hughes & Andrew E. Rothovius. 1996. LC 96-33340. 296p. text 58.00 (0-7618-0503-6); pap. text 36.00 (0-7618-0504-4) U Pr of Amer.

Worlds of Common Sense: Equality, Identity & Two Modes of Impulse Management, 26. Pauline N. Pepinsky. 1994. LC 94-7432. (Contributions in Psychology Ser.: No. 26). 232p. 68.00 (0-313-28991-3, Greenwood Pr) Greenwood.

Worlds of Hurt: Reading the Literatures of Trauma. Kali Tal. 1995. LC 96-112813. (Studies in American Literature & Culture: No. 95). 320p. (C). text 59.95 (0-521-44504-3) Cambridge U Pr.

Worlds of Illness: Biographical & Cultural Perspectives on Health & Disease. Ed. by Alan Radley. 1995. 224p. (C). pap. 29.95 (0-415-13152-9) Routledge.

Worlds of the Mentally Ill: How Deinstitutionalization Works in the City. Dan A. Lewis et al. 1990. LC 89-18058. 208p. (C). text 31.95 (0-8093-1477-0) S Ill U Pr.

World's Oldest Health Plan: Health, Nutrition & Healing from the Bible. Kathleen O'Bannon Baldinger. 1994. LC 93-85138. 352p. pap. 14.95 (0-914984-57-8) Starburst.

World's Pharmaceutical Industries: An International Perspective on Innovation, Competition & Policy. Robert Ballance et al. 1992. 288p. 100.00 (1-85278-646-9) E Elgar.

Worldwide Health Sourcebook: Basic Information about Global Health Issues. Ed. by Joyce Brennfleck Shannon. 2001. LC 00-52463. (Health Reference Ser.). xiii, 614p. lib. bdg. 78.00 (0-7808-0330-2) Omnigraphics Inc.

Worldwide Healthcare Directory. 1994. 500p. (0-86338-467-6) Euromonitor PLC GBR. *Dist:* Gale.

Worldwide Hypnotherapist's Book of Scripts & Inductions. Ed. by Katherine Zimmerman. 1999. 141p. pap. 29.00 (1-929957-03-3) TranceTime.

Worldwide Secrets for Staying Young. Paavo O. Airola. 1984. 208p. pap. 6.95 (0-932090-12-5) Health Plus.

Worldwide Variation in Human Growth. Phyllis B. Eveleth & James M. Tanner. 2nd ed. 1991. (Illus.). 409p. (C). text 100.00 (0-521-35024-7); pap. text 35.95 (0-521-35916-3) Cambridge U Pr.

*Worms & Human Disease. R. Muller. 2nd ed. 2001. LC 2001-25591. (CABI Publishing Ser.). 300p. (Orig.). pap. text 55.00 (0-85199-516-0) OUP.

Worried Sick: Our Troubled Quest for Wellness. Arthur J. Barsky, III. 1988. LC 87-32508. 17.95 (0-316-08255-4, Little Brwn Med Div) Lppncott W & W.

Worrying: Perspectives on Theory, Assessment & Treatment. Ed. by Graham C. L. Davey & Frank Tallis. 1994. LC 93-21368. (Clinical Psychology & Personality Ser.). 328p. 175.50 (0-471-94114-X) Wiley.

Worse Than the Disease: Pitfalls of Medical Progress. Diana B. Dutton. 1992. 544p. (C). pap. text 27.95 (0-521-39557-7) Cambridge U Pr.

Worst Days: A Journal from a Young Cancer Patient for Health-Care Professionals. Leonaye Bulger & Judy Dierkheising. 1996. LC 96-41962. 4.95 (1-56123-098-7) Centering Corp.

Worst Fear: One Woman's Story of Brain Surgery & Survival. Toni Ferrucci & Christopher Gilson. 1997. 194p. 19.95 (1-888770-03-1) Rising Star Publns.

Worst Pills, Best Pills: A Consumer's Guide to Preventing Drug-Induced Death or Illness. Public Citizen Health Group Staff et al. 1999. LC 00-266415. xxvi, 772p. per. 17.95 (0-671-01918-X, PB Trade Paper) PB.

Worterbuch der Ernahrungswissenschaft. C. Leitzmann. 1988. (ENG, FRE, GER, ITA & SPA.). 298p. lib. bdg. 115.00 (0-8288-3592-6, F113450) Fr & Eur.

Worterbuch der Psychologie & Psychiatrie. R. Haas. (ENG & GER.). 1988. 438p. lib. bdg. 225.00 (0-8288-3411-3, F140130); 1980. 453p. lib. bdg. 175.00 (0-8288-3410-5, F79922) Fr & Eur.

*Worterbuch Immunologie und Onkologie (Dictionary of Immunology & Oncology) Deutsch-Englisch (English-German) Peter Reuter & Christine Reuter. 2000. (ENG & GER.). xix, 806p. (3-540-66489-0) Spr-Verlag.

Worterbuch Medizin, French to German. F. Nohring. 1994. (FRE & GER.). 800p. 295.00 (0-320-00587-9) Fr & Eur.

Wound Ballistics. K. G. Selleir & B. P. Kneubuehl. 1994. (Illus.). 502p. 150.00 (0-444-81511-2) Elsevier.

Wound Ballistics in World War II & Korea, Set. 1995. lib. bdg. 599.95 (0-8490-6583-6) Gordon Pr.

Wound Care. Clark. 2000. text (0-7216-7104-7) Harcrt Hlth Sci Grp.

Wound Care. Carrie Sussman & Barbara Bates-Jensen. 2nd ed. 1996. LC 2001-33335. (Illus.). 608p. 89.00 (0-8342-1973-5) PRO-ED.

Wound Care Nursing: A Patient-Centered Approach. Sue Bale & Vanessa Jones. 1996. (Illus.). 255p. pap. text (0-7020-1870-8) W B Saunders GBR. *Dist:* Saunders.

Wound Care Patient Education Resource Manual. Ed. by Carrie Sussman. 1999. LC 99-43529. (Illus.). ring bd. 229.00 (0-8342-1673-6) Aspen Pub.

Wound Closure Biomaterials & Devices. Ed. by Chih-Chang Chu et al. 1996. LC 96-8975. 416p. 149.95 (0-8493-4964-8) CRC Pr.

Wound Healing. Ed. by J. Ian Robertson & Herwig Janssen. 1991. 232p. (1-871816-10-6) Wrightson Biomed GBR. *Dist:* Taylor & Francis.

Wound Healing: Alternatives in Management. Ed. by Joseph M. McCulloch et al. 2nd ed. 1994. LC 94-1175. (Contemporary Perspectives in Rehabilitation Ser.). (Illus.). 442p. 39.95 (0-8036-5966-0) Davis Co.

Wound Healing: Directory of Authors of New Medical & Scientific Reviews with Subject Index. Science and Life Consultants Association Staff. 1995. 160p. 57.50 (0-7883-0618-9); pap. 47.50 (0-7883-0619-7) ABBE Pubs Assn.

W X Y Z

Wound Healing & Skin Physiology. P. Altmeyer et al. 1995. LC 94-29175. (Illus.). 732p. 178.00 (*0-387-56124-2*) Spr-Verlag.

Wound Healing in Glaucoma Filtering Surgery. Franz Fankhauser. 1992. LC 92-49572. 96p. (*90-6299-088-6*) Kugler NLD. *Dist:* Lib Res.

Wound Management. Madeleine Flanagan. 1997. LC 97-16014. (Access to Clinical Education Ser.). text (*0-443-05531-9*) Church.

Wound Management & Dressings. Thomas. 1991. (*0-85369-215-7*) Pharmaceutical Pr GBR. *Dist:* Rittenhouse.

Wound Management Products in Europe. Market Intelligence Staff. 1993. 300p. 3900.00 (*1-56753-500-3*) Frost & Sullivan.

Wound Repair. Earle E. Peacock. 3rd ed. 1984. (Illus.). 544p. text 168.00 (*0-7216-7145-4*) Saunders.

***Wound Repair, Regeneration & Artificial Tissues.** Stocum. 1996. (Molecular Biology Intelligence Unit Ser.). 225p. (C). 117.00 (*3-540-58903-1*) Spr-Verlag.

Wounded Boys, Heroic Men: A Man's Guide to Recovering from Child Abuse. Daniel J. Sonkin. 1998. LC 97-47497. 256p. pap. 12.95 (*1-58062-010-8*) Adams Media.

Wounded Healer. John Gagnon. 1994. LC 93-44570. (Frontiers in Psychotherapy Ser.). 184p. 77.00 (*0-89391-973-X*); pap. 39.50 (*1-56750-063-3*) Greenwood (Ablex).

Wounded Healer: Addiction-Sensitive Therapy for the Sexually Exploitative Professional. Richard Irons & Jennifer Schneider. 1998. LC 98-21444. xvi, 252p. 35.00 (*1-56821-763-3*) Aronson.

Wounded Healer: Countertransference from a Jungian Perspective. David Sedgwick. 1994. LC 93-40465. 176p. (C). pap. 27.95 (*0-415-10620-6*, B3211) Routledge.

Wounded Healers: Creative Illness in the Pioneers of Depth Psychology. Marvin Goldwert. 1992. 164p. (Orig.). (C). 55.00 (*0-8191-8776-3*); pap. 28.00 (*0-8191-8777-1*) U Pr of Amer.

Wounded Healers: Mental Health Workers' Experiences of Depression. Ed. by Vicky Rippere & Ruth Williams. 1987. LC 84-29118. 208p. pap. 125.00 (*0-471-90592-5*) Wiley.

Wounded Woman: Healing the Father-Daughter Relationship. Linda S. Leonard. 1998. LC 83-42801. 179p. reprint ed. pap. 14.95 (*1-57062-411-9*) Shambhala Pubns.

Wounds: Biology & Management. D. J. Leaper & K. G. Harding. 1998. (Illus.). 210p. text 149.50 (*0-19-262332-X*) OUP.

Wounds & Lacerations: Emergency Care & Closure. Alexander T. Trott. 2nd ed. 1997. LC 97-22239. (Illus.). 400p. (C). (gr. 13). text 54.95 (*0-8151-8853-6*, 24725) Mosby Inc.

Wow! Resumes for Health Careers: How to Put Together a Winning Resume. Leslie Hamilton. 1998. LC 98-27257. (Career Guides). 208p. pap. 10.95 (*0-07-026028-1*, Schaums Outline) McGraw-Hill Trade.

Wrath of Angels: The American Abortion War. Jim Risen & Judy Thomas. 1997. LC 97-45936. (Illus.). 416p. 25.00 (*0-465-09272-1*) Basic.

Wright Diet - Food for Humans - The First Lesson in Medicine for Everyone. Patrick Wright. 2nd unabr. ed. 1997. Orig. Title: Grains & Greens. (Illus.). 368p. pap. 18.90 (*0-9628681-2-4*) IRFD.

Wright's Liver & Biliary Disease: Pathophysiology, Diagnosis & Management Ed. by G. H. Millward-Sadler et al. 3rd ed. 1992. (Illus.). 1667p. text (*0-7020-1392-7*) W B Saunders GBR. *Dist:* Saunders.

Wrist. Ed. by Richard H. Gelberman. 1994. LC 93-26040. (Master Techniques in Orthopaedic Surgery Ser.). (Illus.). 448p. text 199.00 (*0-7817-0037-X*) Lppncott W & W.

Wrist. R. L. Linscheid et al. Ed. by William Patrick Cooney. 1997. LC 97-14867. (Illus.). 1424p. (C). (gr. 13). text 275.00 (*0-8016-6644-9*, 06644) Mosby Inc.

Wrist. Julio Taleisnik. 1985. LC 85-13264. (Illus.). 442p. text (*0-443-08134-4*) Church.

Wrist. H. Kirk Watson & Jeffrey Weinzweig. 2000. 1,008p. text 369.00 (*0-397-51726-2*) Lppncott W & W.

Wrist & Its Disorders. David M. Lichtman. 2nd ed. 1997. LC 96-7415. text 195.00 (*0-7216-4774-X*); (*0-7216-6758-9*) Saunders.

Wrist Arthroscopy. Stanley. import ed. 1994. text 72.00 (*0-7216-5310-3*) Saunders.

Wrist Disorders: Current Concepts & Challenges. Ed. by R. Nakamura et al. 1993. LC 92-29763. 346p. 221.00 (*0-387-70102-8*) Spr-Verlag.

Wrist Imaging. G. Brunelli & P. Saffar. 1993. (Illus.). 220p. 286.00 (*0-387-59561-9*) Spr-Verlag.

Wrist in Rheumatoid Arthritis. Ed. by B. R. Simmen & N. Gschwend. 1992. (Rheumatology, the Interdisciplinary Concept Ser.: Vol. 17). (Illus.). xii, 220p. 211.50 (*3-8055-5514-8*) S Karger.

Writer & Psychoanalysis. Edmund Bergler. 2nd ed. 1992. 320p. (C). reprint ed. pap. 24.95 (*0-8236-8330-3*) Intl Univs Pr.

Writer's Guide to Nursing & Allied Health Journals. Ed. by Pamela S. Bradigan et al. 1998. 200p. pap. 48.95 (*1-55810-143-8*) Am Nurses Pub.

Writer's Workbook. Shirley Fondiller. 1992. 200p. (C). pap. text, wbk. ed. 20.95 (*0-88737-548-0*, 14-2470) Natl League Nurse.

Writing: A Guide for Therapists. Sally French & Julius Sim. 1993. (Illus.). 160p. pap. text 35.00 (*0-7506-0580-4*) Buttrwrth-Heinemann.

Writing & Madness: (Literature Philosophy Psychoanalysis) Shoshana Felman. Tr. by Martha N. Evans & Brian Massumi from FRE. LC 84-19845. 256p. (C). 1986. pap. 17.95 (*0-8014-9394-3*); 1985. 42.50 (*0-8014-1285-4*) Cornell U Pr.

Writing & Personality: Finding Your Voice, Your Style, Your Way. John K. DiTiberio & George H. Jensen. 1995. LC 94-24284. 378p. pap. 17.95 (*0-89106-071-5*, 7192, Davies-Black Pub) Consulting Psychol.

Writing & Publishing in Medicine. Edward J. Huth. 3rd ed. 1998. LC 98-35984. ix, 348p. 34.95 (*0-683-40447-4*) Lppncott W & W.

Writing & Reading in a Balanced Curriculum. Ed. by Malcolm P. Douglass. 1982. (Claremont Reading Conference Yearbook Ser.). 222p. (Orig.). pap. 5.00 (*0-941742-00-8*) Claremont Grad.

Writing Case Reports: A How-To Manual for Clinicians. 1996. 168p. pap. 65.00 (*1-887759-09-3*, C-12) Am Phys Therapy Assn.

***Writing for Health Professionals.** 1996. pap. 27.50 (*0-412-71980-0*) Chapman & Hall.

Writing for Money in Mental Health. Douglas H. Ruben. 1997. LC 96-51806. (Illus.). 290p. 49.95 (*0-7890-0101-2*); pap. 24.95 (*0-7890-0240-X*) Haworth Pr.

Writing Health Care Plans, a Handbook for Dietary Managers: A Handbook for Dietary Managers. Karen Walton. 3rd rev. ed. 1995. 162p. (C). 19.50 (*1-877735-07-8*, 2108PP) Prof Prnting & Pub.

Writing in Psychoanalysis: A Clinical Synthesis. Ed. by Emma Piccioli et al. 1996. 144p. pap. 24.95 (*0-88163-239-2*) Analytic Pr.

Writing on the Wall: Women's Autobiography & the Asylum. Mary E. Wood. 1994. LC 93-38401. 192p. pap. text 16.95 (*0-252-06389-9*) U of Ill Pr.

Writing Papers in Psychology. Ralph Rosnow & Mimi Rosnow. 4th ed. 1997. LC 97-3844. (Psychology Ser.). 143p. mass mkt. 17.95 (*0-534-34826-2*) Brooks-Cole.

Writing Papers in Psychology: A Student Guide. Ralph L. Rosnow & Mimi Rosnow. 1986. 68p. (C). mass mkt. 10.50 (*0-534-06780-8*); 3rd ed. 1995. LC 94-9163. 122p. pap. 13.95 (*0-534-24378-9*) Brooks-Cole.

Writing Psychological Reports: A Guide for Clinicians. Greg J. Wolber & William F. Carne. 1993. LC 93-26909. 128p. pap. 20.45 (*0-943158-93-1*, WPRBP, Prof Resc Pr) Pro Resource.

***Writing, Speaking & Communication Skills for Health Professionals.** Health Care Communication Group Staff. 2001. (Illus.). 352p. 40.00 (*0-300-08861-2*); pap. 17.95 (*0-300-08862-0*) Yale U Pr.

Writing Your Way Through Cancer. Chia Martin. 2000. LC 00-25175. xv, 165p. pap. 14.95 (*1-890772-00-3*) Hohm Pr.

Writings, 1878-1899: Psychology: Briefer Course; The Will to Believe; Talks to Teachers; Essays. William James. Ed. by Gerald E. Myers. 1992. LC 91-58225. (Library of America: Vol. 58). 1212p. 35.00 (*0-940450-72-0*) Library of America.

Writings of Melanie Klein Melanie Klein. 1984. 1712p. (C). 160.00 (*0-02-918460-6*) Free Pr.

Writings of Melanie Klein, I Love, Guilt & Reparation & Other Works, 1921-1945 see Iubire, Vinovatie Si Alte Lucrari, 1921-1945

Written Communication in Family Medicine. Ed. by Robert B. Taylor & K. A. Munning. 1984. (Illus.). 256p. 99.00 (*0-387-90979-6*) Spr-Verlag.

Written Expression Disorders. Noel Gregg. 1995. LC 95-1441. (Neuropsychology & Cognition Ser.: Vol. 10). xii, 145p. text 110.50 (*0-7923-3355-1*) Kluwer Academic.

Written Language Disorders. Ed. by R. Malatesha Joshi. 1991. (C). lib. bdg. 160.50 (*0-7923-0902-2*) Kluwer Academic.

Written Language Disorders: Theory into Practice. Laura L. Bailet & Louisa C. Moats. Ed. by Ann M. Bain et al. 1991. LC 89-13839. (Illus.). 209p. pap. text 27.00 (*0-89079-417-0*, 1580) PRO-ED.

Wrongful Death: A Medical Tragedy. Sandra M. Gilbert. 1995. LC 94-26732. (Illus.). 352p. 22.50 (*0-393-03721-5*) Norton.

Wrongful Death: A Memoir. Sandra M. Gilbert. 1997. LC 96-52868. 368p. pap. 13.00 (*0-393-31516-9*) Norton.

Wryneck Vol. IX: The Neck Has Gone Awry - Torticollis. Frederick H. Barge. 1998. (Illus.). 315p. (C). text 59.95 (*1-885048-11-4*); pap. text 34.95 (*1-885048-12-2*) Barge Chiropract.

Wu Wei, Negativity & Depression: The Principle of Non-Trying in the Practice of Pastoral Care. Siroj Sorajjakool. 2001. LC 00-50550. (Illus.). 211p. pap. 17.95 (*0-7890-1094-1*, Haworth Pastrl) Haworth Pr.

Wu Wei, Negativity & Depression: The Principle of Non-Trying in the Practice of Pastoral Care. Ed. by Siroj Sorajjakool. 2001. LC 00-50550. (Illus.). 184p. lib. bdg. 49.95 (*0-7890-1093-3*, Haworth Pastrl) Haworth Pr.

WWWsite Fremgen Medical Terms. Fremgen Staff. 1997. text (*0-8359-5150-2*) Brady Pub.

Wyatt vs. Stickney: Retrospect & Prospect. Ed. by L. R. Jones & R. Parlour. 1981. 245p. text 37.00 (*0-8089-1422-7*, 792209, Grune & Strat) Harcrt Hlth Sci Grp.

Wyeth Critical Care Nursing. Jonelle E. Wright & Brenda K. Shelton. 1994. (Illus.). (C). text 41.95 (*0-86720-711-6*, 711-6) Jones & Bartlett.

Wylie & Churchill-Davidson's Practice of Anaesthesia: A Practice of Anaesthesia. Ed. by Thomas E. J. Healy & Peter J. Cohen. 6th ed. 1995. (Illus.). 1560p. text (*0-340-55309-X*) E A GBR. *Dist:* OUP.

Wylie's Atlas of Vascular Surgery, In Six Volumes. Ronald J. Stoney & David J. Effeney. 1992. (Illus.). 1500p. text 550.00 (*0-397-51145-0*) Lppncott W & W.

Wyoming Health Care in Perspective 2000. Ed. by Kathleen O'Leary Morgan & Scott E. Morgan. 2000. 21p. spiral bd. 19.00 (*0-7401-0249-4*) Morgan Quitno Corp.

Wyoming Health Care Perspective, 1998. Ed. by Kathleen O'Leary Morgan & Scott E. Morgan. 1998. 20p. pap. 19.00 (*1-56692-849-4*) Morgan Quitno Corp.

X

X Factor: What It Is & How to Find It, the Relationship Between Inherited Heart Size & Racing Performance. Marianna Haun. 1997. LC 96-41931. (Illus.). 208p. pap. text 30.00 (*0-929346-46-7*) R Meerdink Co Ltd.

X-Ray Anatomy of the Vascular System. G. Luzsa. 1975. 388p. (C). (*963-05-0060-4*) Akade Kiado HUN. *Dist:* St Mut.

X-Ray & Image Analysis in Electron Microscopy. John J. Friel. 1994. LC 94-67188. 112p. pap. text 19.00 (*0-9641455-0-2*) Prncton Gamma-Tech.

X-Ray & Neutron Dynamical Diffraction, Theory & Applications: Proceedings of a NATO ASI Held in Erice, Italy, April 9-21, 1996. Ed. by Andre Authier et al. 1997. (NATO ASI Series B: Vol. 357). 430p. (C). text 125.00 (*0-306-45501-3*) Plenum.

X-Ray Assessment for Nurses. Patricia A. Dettenmeier. 1994. LC 94-242460. (Illus.). 256p. (C). (gr. 13). pap. text 35.95 (*0-8016-7245-7*, 07245) Mosby Inc.

X-Ray Coordinator. Jack Rudman. 1994. (Career Examination Ser.: C-1536). pap. 34.95 (*0-8373-1536-0*) Nat Learn.

X-Ray Diagnosis: A Physician's Approach. S. F. Lam et al. 1998. LC 97-13226. (Illus.). 210p. (C). pap. (*981-3083-24-7*) Spr-Verlag SGP. *Dist:* Spr-Verlag.

X-Ray Diagnosis in Neonates. Gy. Koteles. 1982. 174p. (C). (*963-05-3061-9*) Akade Kiado HUN. *Dist:* St Mut.

X-Ray Differential Diagnosis in Small Bowel Disease: A Practical Approach. J. L. Sellink. 1988. (Series in Radiology). (C). text 206.50 (*0-89838-351-X*) Kluwer Academic.

X-Ray Diffraction at Elevated Temperatures: A Method for in Situ Process Analysis. D. D. Chung et al. 1993. LC 92-21803. 95.00 (*0-89573-745-0*, Wiley-VCH) Wiley.

X-Ray Fluorescent Scanning of the Thyroid. Ed. by M. H. Jonckheer & F. Deconinck. 1983. text 126.50 (*0-89838-561-X*) Kluwer Academic.

X-Ray Imaging Equipment: An Introduction. Euclid Seeram. 1985. (Illus.). 610p. (C). 74.95 (*0-398-05078-3*) C C Thomas.

X-Ray Interpretation for MRCP. R. K. Hind. 2nd ed. 1992. (Illus.). 200p. (Orig.). pap. text (*0-443-04551-8*) Church.

X-Ray Interpretation for the MRCP. P. S. Parfrey & B. C. Cramer. 1983. (Illus.). 240p. pap. (*0-443-02594-0*) Church.

X-Ray Microscopy in Biology & Medicine. Ed. by K. Shinohara & K. Yada. 1990. (Illus.). 339p. 101.00 (*0-387-50702-7*) Spr-Verlag.

X-Ray Optics: Applications to Solids. Ed. by H. J. Queisser. 1977. (Topics in Applied Physics Ser.: Vol. 22). (Illus.). 227p. 61.95 (*0-387-08462-2*) Spr-Verlag.

X-Ray Physics for Radiologic Technologists. Richard H. Schmidt. 1973. LC 72-75592. (Illus.). 160p. pap. 12.50 (*0-87527-131-6*) Green.

X-Ray Repair: A Comprehensive Guide to the Installation & Servicing of Radiographic Equipment. Joseph J. Panichello. 1998. LC 97-28600. (Illus.). 284p. text 62.95 (*0-398-06815-1*) C C Thomas.

X-Ray Symposium, 1981. Ed. by A. G. Davis Philip. 1981. 76p. pap. 12.00 (*0-9607902-0-9*) L Davis Pr.

X-Ray Technician. Jack Rudman. 1994. (Career Examination Ser.: C-910). pap. 29.95 (*0-8373-0910-7*) Nat Learn.

X-Ray Technician I. Jack Rudman. 1994. (Career Examination Ser.: C-1840). pap. 29.95 (*0-8373-1840-8*) Nat Learn.

X-Ray Technician III. Jack Rudman. 1994. (Career Examination Ser.: C-1842). pap. 34.95 (*0-8373-1842-4*) Nat Learn.

X-Ray Technician II. Jack Rudman. 1994. (Career Examination Ser.: C-1841). pap. 34.95 (*0-8373-1841-6*) Nat Learn.

X-Ray Technologist Risk Management: Medico-Legal Risk Management. Ricardo A. Scott. 1994. 100p. 25.95 (*1-883427-16-9*) Crnerstone GA.

X-Rayed Without Consent: Computer Health Hazards. Bert Dumpe. Ed. by Stephen Kepple. 1989. (Illus.). 388p. (Orig.). 19.75 (*0-9622907-0-X*) Ergotec Assn.

X-Rays: Health Effects of Common Exams. John W. Gofman & Egan O'Connor. 1985. LC 84-23527. (Illus.). 440p. 25.00 (*0-87156-838-1*) Sierra.

X Y, de l'Identite Masculine see XY: On Masculine Identity

Xanthines & Cancer: An Experimental Study of Tumour Inhibition. W. J. Neish. 1988. 192p. (C). pap. (*0-08-036399-7*) Aberdeen U Pr GBR. *Dist:* Macmillan.

Xanthomonas. Ed. by J. G. Swings & E. L. Civerolo. 1994. LC 92-43468. 416p. (C). (gr. 13). pap. text 227.95 (*0-412-43420-2*) Chapman & Hall.

Xenobiotic Metabolism: In Vitro Studies. Ed. by Gaylord D. Paulson et al. 1979. LC 79-789. (ACS Symposium Ser.: No. 97). 37.95 (*0-8412-0486-1*) Am Chemical.

Xenobiotic Metabolism & Disposition: The Design of Studies on Novel Compounds. Ed. by H. P. Illing. 1989. 232p. 225.00 (*0-8493-6163-X*, QP529) CRC Pr.

Xenobiotics & Cancer: Implications for Chemical Carcinogenesis & Cancer Chemotherapy. Ed. by Lars Ernster et al. 1991. (Princess Takamatsu Symposia Ser.: No. 21). 410p. (*0-7484-0037-0*) Tay Francis Ltd GBR. *Dist:* Taylor & Francis.

Xenobiotics & Inflammation: Roles of Cytokines & Growth Factors. Ed. by Debra L. Laskin & Lawrence B. Schook. 1994. LC 93-48067. (Illus.). 361p. text 104.00 (*0-12-628930-1*) Acad Pr.

Xenotransplantation: Basic Research & Clinical Applications. Ed. by Jeffrey L. Platt. 2002. LC 2001-51652. 325p. 150.00 (*0-89603-674-X*) Humana.

Xenotransplantation: Science, Ethics, & Public Policy. Committee on Xenograft Transplantation Institute o. 1996. LC 96-69850. 136p. (Orig.). (C). pap. text 29.00 (*0-309-05549-0*) Natl Acad Pr.

Xenotransplantation: The Transplantation of Organs & Tissues Between Species. Ed. by D. Cooper & E. Kemp. 2nd ed. 1997. LC 96-39074. (Illus.). 856p. 355.00 (*3-540-61777-9*) Spr-Verlag.

Xenotransplantation from Basic Research to Clinical Application. Jeffrey L. Platt. 2000. 139.00 (*0-8493-4892-7*) CRC Pr.

XH-1 Therapy. Lai-Yin Yan. 1998. LC 99-217329. (Illus.). 168p. pap. 17.00 (*0-8059-4088-X*) Dorrance.

XXVIes Journees Nationales de Neonatologie Paris, Mai, 1996. 1996. (Progres en Neonatologie Ser.: Vol. 16, 1996). (Illus.). vi, 298p. pap. 170.50 (*3-8055-6355-8*) S Karger.

XXVII Es Journees Nationales de Neonatologie 1997: XXVII Es Journees Nationales de Neonatologies, Paris, Mai 1997. 1997. (Progres en Neonatologie Ser.: Vol. 17, 1997). (Illus.). vi, 278p. pap. 170.50 (*3-8055-6545-3*) S Karger.

XY: On Masculine Identity. Elisabeth Badinter. 1995. LC 94-41016. (European Perspectives; A Series in Social Thought & Culturall Criticism Ser.).Tr. of X Y, de l'Identite Masculine. 224p. 42.00 (*0-231-08434-X*) Col U Pr.

XYZ of Psychoanalysis: Epilogue to a Great Beginning. Harold Feldman. 1991. LC 87-21749. 192p. 62.50 (*0-275-93957-X*, C3957, Praeger Pubs) Greenwood.

W X Y Z

Y

Ya No Seas Codependiente. Melody Beattie. 1994. (Promexa/Autoayuda Ser.).Tr. of Codependent No More. (SPA.). 312p. pap. 15.00 (*968-39-0473-4*) Hazelden.

YAG Laser Bronchoscopy. Jean-Francois Dumon et al. 1985. LC 84-26310. 128p. 50.00 (*0-275-91311-2*, C1311, Praeger Pubs) Greenwood.

Yajurveda. Devi Chand. 1994. (C). (*81-215-0294-2*) M Manoharial IND. *Dist:* Coronet Bks.

Yale Guide to Children's Nutrition. Ed. by William V. Tamborlane. 1997. LC 96-44774. (Illus.). 464p. pap. 19.95 (*0-300-07169-8*) Yale U Pr.

Yale Guide to Children's Nutrition. William V. Tamborlane & Janet Z. Weiswasser. 1997. LC 96-44774. 464p. 50.00 (*0-300-06965-0*) Yale U Pr.

Yale Management Guide for Physicians. Stephen Rimar. 2001. LC 00-65288. (Illus.). 288p. 65.00 (*0-471-38458-5*) Wiley.

Yalom Reader: On Writing, Living & Practicing Psychotherapy. Irvin D. Yalom. 1998. LC 97-21790. 256p. pap. 22.00 (*0-465-03610-4*) Basic.

Yankee Surgeon: The Life & Times of Usher Parsons. Seebert J. Goldowsky. 1988. 405p. 24.50 (*0-88135-088-5*) Watson Pub Intl.

Yasgur's Homeopathic Dictionary & Holistic Health Reference. Jay Yasgur. 4th ed. 1997. LC 97-60094. Orig. Title: A Dictionary of Homeopathic Medical Terminology. 420p. (Orig.). pap. text 23.95 (*1-886149-04-6*) Van Hoy Pubs.

Year after Childbirth. Sheila Kitzinger. 1996. (Illus.). 320p. per. 13.00 (*0-684-82520-1*) S&S Trade.

Year Book of Allergy & Clinical Immunology, 1998. Lanny J. Rosenwasser. 5th ed. 1998. (Illus.). 408p. (C). (gr. 13). text 74.95 (*0-8151-7279-6*, 23108) Mosby Inc.

Year Book of Chiropractic, 1996. Phillips & Adams. 1996. (Illus.). 464p. (gr. 13). text 69.95 (*0-8151-6736-9*, 21966) Mosby Inc.

Year Book of Clinical Microbiology, 1993. James W. Snyder. 1993. 272p. 102.00 (*0-8493-3313-X*, QA) CRC Pr.

Year Book of Dermatologic Surgery. Neal A. Swanson. 2000th ed. 2000. 84.95 (*0-8151-8750-5*, 29136) Mosby Inc.

Year Book of Gastroenterology, 2001. Ed. by Gary R. Lichtenstein. 2001. (Illus.). 360p. (*0-323-01532-8*) Mosby Inc.

*__Year Book of Gastroenterology, 2003.__ Ed. by Gary R. Lichtenstein. 2003. (Illus.). 360p. (*0-323-01541-7*) Mosby Inc.

Year Book of Health Care Management, 1996. Robert Heyssel. 1996. 245p. 64.95 (*0-8151-4299-4*) Mosby Inc.

Year Book of Health Care Management, 1995. Robert Heyssel. 1995. 245p. 64.95 (*0-8151-4298-6*) Mosby Inc.

Year Book of Oncology Nursing, 1994. Christine Miaskowski et al. 1994. 320p. 39.95 (*0-8151-6140-9*) Mosby Inc.

Year Book of Oncology Nursing, 1995. Christine Miaskowski et al. 1995. 320p. 39.95 (*0-8151-6141-7*) Mosby Inc.

Year Book of Oncology Nursing, 1996. Christine Miaskowski et al. 1996. 320p. 39.95 (*0-8151-6142-5*) Mosby Inc.

Year Book of Rheumatology, Arthritis & Musculoskeletal Disease, 2005. Ed. by Richard S. Panush. Date not set. (Illus.). 385p. (*0-323-01523-9*) Harcrt Hlth Sci Grp.

Year Book of Thoracic & Cardiovascular Surgery, 1998. Andrew S. Wechsler. 5th ed. 1998. (Illus.). 440p. (C). (gr. 13). text 83.00 (*0-8151-9172-3*, 23103) Mosby Inc.

Year Book of Toxicology, 1989. Ed. by Irving Sunshine. 1989. 272p. 121.00 (*0-8493-3301-6*, RA, CRC Reprint) Franklin.

Year in Complement. Ed. by J. M. Cruse. 1993. (Journal: Vol. 12, No. 3, 1993). (Illus.). 108p. pap. 35.00 (*3-8055-5880-5*) S Karger.

Year in Immunology, Vol. 2, 1985-1986. Ed. by J. M. Cruse & R. E. Lewis, Jr. 1986. (Illus.). vi, 386p. 256.75 (*3-8055-4342-5*) S Karger.

Year in Immunology, 1988, Vol. 4 & 5. Ed. by J. M. Cruse & R. E. Lewis, Jr. 1989. (Illus.). xvi, 536p. 346.25 (*3-8055-5044-8*) S Karger.

Year in Immunology, 1988: Cellular, Molecular & Clinical Aspects. Ed. by J. M. Cruse & R. E. Lewis, Jr. 1989. (Year in Immunology Ser.: Vol. 4). (Illus.). vii, 312p. 221.75 (*3-8055-4808-7*) S Karger.

Year in Immunology, 1988: Immunoregulatory Cytokines & Cell Growth. Ed. by J. M. Cruse & R. E. Lewis, Jr. 1989. (Year in Immunology Ser.: Vol. 5). (Illus.). viii, 224p. 172.25 (*3-8055-4895-8*) S Karger.

Year in Immunology, 1984-1985. Ed. by J. M. Cruse & R. E. Lewis, Jr. 1985. (Illus.). vi, 234p. 137.50 (*3-8055-4025-6*) S Karger.

Year in Immunology, 1989-1990: Molecules & Cells of Immunity. Ed. by J. M. Cruse & R. E. Lewis, Jr. 1990. (Illus.). vi, 284p. 258.50 (*3-8055-5084-7*) S Karger.

Year in Immunology, 1986-1987. Ed. by J. M. Cruse & R. E. Lewis, Jr. 1988. (Year in Immunology Ser.: Vol. 3). (Illus.). 350p. 224.50 (*3-8055-4616-5*) S Karger.

Year in Immunology, 1983. Ed. by J. M. Cruse & L. M. Schwartz. 1984. (Journal: Vol. 3, No. 2-3). (Illus.). 156p. pap. 69.75 (*3-8055-3881-2*) S Karger.

Year in Immunology, 1982. Ed. by Lazar M. Schwartz. 1983. (Journal: Vol. 2, No. 3). (Illus.). 132p. pap. 62.75 (*3-8055-3760-3*) S Karger.

Year in Immunopathology. Ed. by J. M. Cruse & R. E. Lewis. 1987. (Journal: Vol. 5, No. 3-5, 1986). (Illus.). 248p. pap. 76.75 (*3-8055-4576-2*) S Karger.

Year of Health Hints: Three Hundred Sixty-Five Practical Ways to Feel Better & Live Longer. Don R. Powell. rev. ed. 2000. 374p. (C). reprint ed. 23.95 (*0-9635612-1-9*) Am Inst Prevent.

Year of Holidays: A Planning & Idea Book for Holiday Activities in Nursing Homes. Vicki Parsons. 1993. (Illus.). 177p. 21.50 (*1-877735-41-8*, 2225PP) Prof Prnting & Pub.

Year of Miracles: A Healing Journey from Cancer to Wholeness. Susan W. Sternberg. 1996. LC 96-92246. (Illus.). 256p. (Orig.). pap. 13.95 (*0-9653755-0-1*, YOMP) Star Mtn Pr.

Year of the Zebra. Karen Kelroy. 1997. LC 98-119157. (Illus.). pap. 10.00 (*0-9661509-0-2*) K Kelroy.

Year 2000 & Beyond: Concepts for Nurses in Reproductive Medicine. 2000. (Studies in Profertility). 50.00 (*1-84214-000-0*, Parthenon Pbng) CRC Pr.

Year 2000 Computing Crisis: Biomedical Equipment Items. Helen Lew. 1999. 117p. pap. text 30.00 (*0-7881-7640-4*) DIANE Pub.

Critical Care Medicine, Year 2000 Edition: Current Clinical Strategies. Matthew Brenner. rev. ed. 1999. (Current Clinical Strategies Ser.). 100p. pap. 16.95 (*1-881528-77-4*) Current Clin Strat.

Year 2000 Health Care Survival Guide: Strategies & Solutions for Executives. Audie G. Lewis. 1998. LC 98-36700. 104p. pap. 40.00 (*1-55648-254-X*) AHPI.

Yearbook of Cell & Tissue Transplantation, 1996-1997. Ed. by Robert P. Lanza & William L. Chick. 1996. 294p. text 184.00 (*0-7923-3844-8*) Kluwer Academic.

Yearbook of Drug Abuse, Vol. I. Ed. by Leon Brill & Ernest Harms. 1973. LC 70-174271. (Illus.). 386p. 52.00 (*0-87705-060-0*, Kluwer Acad Hman Sci) Kluwer Academic.

*__Yearbook of Intensive Care & Emergency Medicine: Jahrgang 1999.__ 1999. (Illus.). xxii, 716p. pap. 125.00 (*3-540-65288-4*) Spr-Verlag.

*__Yearbook of Intensive Care & Emergency Medicine: Jahrgang 2000.__ 2000. (Illus.). xxvi, 858p. pap. 105.00 (*3-540-66830-6*) Spr-Verlag.

Yearbook of Intensive Care & Emergency Medicine, 1993. Ed. by J. L. Vincent. 1993. (Illus.). xviii, 691p. pap. 98.00 (*0-387-56463-2*) Spr-Verlag.

Yearbook of Intensive Care Medicine, 1996. Ed. by J. L. Vincent. 1996. (Illus.). 800p. pap. 109.00 (*3-540-60552-5*) Spr-Verlag.

Yearbook of Law & Medicine, 1992. Daniel J. Sullivan. 1991. 300p. 74.95 (*0-9631342-0-5*) Phys Law Rev.

Yearbook of Morphology. Ed. by Geert Booij & Jaap Van Marle. 1988. viii, 328p. (Orig.). (C). pap. (*90-6765-376-4*) Mouton.

Yearbook of Morphology. Ed. by Geert Booy & Jaap Van Marle. 1988. viii, 328p. (Orig.). (C). (*90-6765-375-6*) Mouton.

Yearbook of Morphology, 1989. Geert Booij & Jaap Van Marle. 300p. (*90-6765-444-2*); pap. (*90-6765-445-0*) Mouton.

Yearbook of Morphology, 1993. Ed. by Geert Booij. 1994. 288p. (C). text 205.50 (*0-7923-2494-3*) Kluwer Academic.

Yearbook of Morphology, 1996. Ed. by Geert Booij & Jaap Van Marle. 1997. text 125.50 (*0-7923-4563-0*) Kluwer Academic.

Yearbook of Nephrology, 1991. Fredric L. Coe. 1991. (*0-8151-5015-6*) Mosby Inc.

Yearbook of Pharmacology. Ed. by Mannfred A. Hollinger. 1990. lib. bdg. 67.95 (*0-8493-3302-4*, RM, CRC Reprint) Franklin.

Yearbook of Pharmacology, 1991. Ed. by Mannfred A. Hollinger. 1991. 432p. lib. bdg. 73.00 (*0-8493-3306-7*, RM, CRC Reprint) Franklin.

Yearbook of Psychoanalysis & Psychotherapy, Vol. 2. Robert J. Langs. 1987. LC 86-641022. 356p. text 45.00 (*0-89876-141-7*) Gardner Pr.

Yearbook of Psychoanalysis & Psychotherapy, Vol. 1-1985. Robert J. Langs. 1985. 432p. text 49.95 (*0-931231-04-3*) Newconcept Pr.

Yearbook of Substance Use & Abuse, Vol. II. Leon Brill & Charles Winick. 1980. LC 70-174271. 360p. 52.00 (*0-87705-487-8*, Kluwer Acad Hman Sci) Kluwer Academic.

Yearbook of Substance Use & Abuse, Vol. III. Ed. by Leon Brill & Charles Winick. 1985. 351p. 52.00 (*0-89885-216-1*, Kluwer Acad Hman Sci) Kluwer Academic.

Yearbook of the Royal College of Obstetricians & Gynaecologists, 1996. Ed. by J. W. Studd. 1996. (Illus.). 400p. lib. bdg. 64.95 (*0-902331-91-4*, Parthenon Pbng) CRC Pr.

Yearbook of the Royal College of Obstetricians & Gynaecologists, 1995. Ed. by John W. Studd. 1995. (Illus.). 308p. lib. bdg. 60.95 (*0-902331-77-9*, Parthenon Pbng) CRC Pr.

Yearbook of Toxicology, 1990. Irving Sunshine. 1990. 360p. lib. bdg. 73.00 (*0-8493-3305-9*, R, CRC Reprint) Franklin.

Yearbook of Toxicology, 1991. Irving Sunshine. 1991. 408p. 225.00 (*0-8493-3309-1*, R, CRC Reprint) Franklin.

Years after Fifty. Wingate M. Johnson. 18.95 (*0-405-18502-2*) Ayer.

Yeast Connection: A Medical Breakthrough. William G. Crook. 1985. LC 83-62508. (Illus.). 304p. 15.95 (*0-933478-10-0*) Prof Bks Future Health.

Yeast Connection: A Medical Breakthrough. William G. Crook. 3rd ed. 1986. LC 86-40140. (Illus.). 434p. pap. 16.00 (*0-394-74700-3*) Vin Bks.

Yeast Connection & the Woman. William G. Crook. 1995. (Illus.). 768p. (Orig.). (C). pap. 17.95 (*0-933478-22-4*) Prof Bks Future Health.

Yeast Syndrome. John P. Trowbridge. 1986. 448p. mass mkt. 7.50 (*0-553-27751-0*) Bantam.

"Yeeks!" Getting Safely Through Perimenopause, Menopause & Beyond. Helen Greco & Jane Babin Stern. 1999. LC 99-95146. (Illus.). 110p. pap. 8.99 (*0-9674422-0-6*) Stern-Greco.

Yellow Emperor's Classic of Internal Medicine. Tr. by Ilza Veith. 1966. pap. 18.95 (*0-520-02158-4*) U CA Pr.

Yellow Emperor's Classic of Medicine: A New Translation of the Neijing Suwen with Commentary. Maoshing Ni. 1995. LC 94-44058. 316p. pap. 19.95 (*1-57062-080-6*) Shambhala Pubns.

Yellow Emperor's Medicine Classic: Treastice on Health & Long Life. Zhou Chuncai. 1996. (Illus.). 232p. pap. 14.95 (*981-3068-28-0*) China Bks.

Yellow Feaver Booklet. Absalom Jones & Richard Allen. 1993. pap. 1.75 (*0-915992-58-2*) Eastern National.

Yellow Fever & Public Health in the New South. John H. Ellis. 1992. LC 91-35692. (Illus.). 248p. text 29.95 (*0-8131-1781-X*) U Pr of KY.

Yellow Fever & the South. Margaret Humphreys. 1992. LC 91-41138. (Health & Medicine in American Society Ser.). 235p. (C). text 45.00 (*0-8135-1820-2*) Rutgers U Pr.

Yellow Fever in the North: The Methods of Early Epidemiology. William Coleman. 1987. LC 86-40456. (Wisconsin Publications in the History of Science & Medicine: No. 6). 224p. text 34.95 (*0-299-11110-5*) U of Wis Pr.

Yellow Fever Studies: An Original Anthology. Ed. by Barbara G. Rosenkrantz. 1977. LC 76-40355. (Public Health in America Ser.). reprint ed. lib. bdg. 26.95 (*0-405-09882-0*) Ayer.

Yellow-Fever Vaccinating Centres for International Travel. 1985. 68p. pap. text 11.00 (*92-4-058011-5*) World Health.

Yellow Fever Vaccinating Centres for International Travel: Situation As on 1 January 1991. 1991. 82p. pap. text 14.00 (*92-4-058012-3*, 0150357) World Health.

Yerbas Buenas. Anthony DeStefano. 2001.Tr. of Good Herbs(Latino Folk Medicine). pap. 14.95 (*0-609-81104-5*) Liv Lang.

Yersinia Enterocolitica. Ed. by Edward J. Bottone. 1981. 240p. 135.00 (*0-8493-5545-1*, QK201, CRC Reprint) Franklin.

Yersinia Enterocolitica: Proceedings of the International Symposium on Yersinia, 3rd, Montreal, September, 1977. International Symposium on Yersinia Staff. Ed. by Philip B. Carter et al. 1979. (Contributions to Microbiology & Immunology Ser.: Vol. 5). (Illus.). 135.00 (*3-8055-2927-9*) S Karger.

Yersiniosis: Present & Future. Ed. by G. Ravagnan & C. Chiesa. 1996. (Contributions to Microbiology & Immunology Ser.: Vol. 13). (Illus.). xii, 340p. 299.25 (*3-8055-6138-5*) S Karger.

YES: Shapedown Youth Evaluation Scale. Laurel M. Mellin. 2nd rev. ed. 1986. LC 86-71116. (Illus.). 269p. (*0-935902-10-4*) Balboa Pub.

Yes, You Can: A Guide to Empowerment Groups. Charlotte D. Kasl. Ed. by Charlotte D. Kasl. 1995. (Orig.). pap. 14.00 (*0-9644520-0-6*) Castle Consult.

Yes, You Can! A Guide to Self-Care for Persons with Spinal Cord Injury. Ed. by Marget C. Hammond et al. Tr. by Jorge Garcia. 2nd ed. 1993. LC 89-62035. (ENG & SPA., Illus.). 174p. pap. 9.50 (*0-929819-01-2*) Paralyzed Vets.

Yesterday, Today & Tomorrow: Take the High Road to Health with Rod Burreson. Rod Burreson et al. 2001. LC 00-11476. (Illus.). 440p. 24.95 (*1-890766-13-5*) B L Pubns.

Yesterday's Addicts: American Society & Drug Abuse, 1865-1920. H. Wayne Morgan. 1974. LC 73-7421. 220p. pap. 13.95 (*0-8061-1636-6*) U of Okla Pr.

Yesterdaze Kures. Mat Bohannon. 1993. LC 91-67745. (Illus.). 64p. pap. 9.00 (*1-56002-146-2*, Univ Edtns) Aegina Pr.

Yin Deficiency & Yin-Yang: Index of New Information & Research Guide. Helena R. Rathman. 1994. 150p. 57.50 (*0-7883-0106-3*); pap. 47.50 (*0-7883-0107-1*) ABBE Pubs Assn.

YMCA Exercise Instructor Manual. YMCA of the U. S. A. Staff. 1995. LC 94-45137. (Illus.). 216p. spiral bd. 28.00 (*0-87322-884-7*, Y5280, YMCA USA) Human Kinetics.

YMCA Prenatal Exercise Instructor Guide. YMCA of the U. S. A. Staff. 1995. LC 94-44689. (Illus.). 112p. ring bd. 36.00 (*0-87322-825-1*, Y5270, YMCA USA) Human Kinetics.

Yoga: A Gem for Women. Geeta Iyengar. 1995. LC 90-43112. (Illus.). 424p. pap. 21.95 (*0-931454-20-4*) Timeless Bks.

Yoga: An Introductory Guide to Optimum Health for Mind, Body & Spirit. Howard Kent. 2000. (New Perspectives Ser.). (Illus.). 128p. pap. (*1-86204-759-6*) Oneworld.

Yoga & Depth Psychology. I. P. Sachdeva. 1978. (*0-89684-049-2*) Motilal Bnarsidass IND. *Dist:* S Asia.

Yoga & Psychotherapy: The Evolution of Consciousness. Swami Rama et al. 1976. LC 76-356228. (Illus.). 332p. pap. 15.95 (*0-89389-036-7*) Himalayan Inst.

Yoga During Pregnancy. Vibeke Berg. 1983. 6.95 (*0-671-45987-2*, Fireside) S&S Trade Pap.

Yoga for Health. Richard Hittleman. 1985. LC 82-90825. 224p. pap. 14.95 (*0-345-32798-5*) Ballantine Pub Grp.

Yoga for Wellness: Healing with the Timeless Teachings of Viniyoga. Gary Kraftsow. 1999. pap. 19.95 (*0-14-025806-X*) Viking Penguin.

Yoga in Pregnancy. Vibeke Berg. 1983. 135p. (*0-940500-24-8*) D B Taraporevala IND. *Dist:* Asia Bk Corp.

Yoga of Nutrition. Omraam M. Aivanhov. 2nd ed. 1991. LC 91-70254. (Izvor Collection: No. 204). 139p. pap. 7.95 (*0-911857-10-9*) Prosveta USA.

Yoga Psychology: A Practical Guide to Meditation. Swami Ajaya. rev. ed. 1976. LC 76-374539. 115p. pap. 12.95 (*0-89389-052-9*) Himalayan Inst.

Yohimbe. Ita Elkins. 1997. (Woodland Health Ser.). 32p. pap. 3.95 (*1-885670-70-2*) Woodland UT.

Yokibics . . . A Mindbody Workbook for Everyday Living. Gail Chiarella. Ed. by Leah Aron. 1992. (Illus.). 120p. stu. ed. 19.95 (*0-9635553-1-2*) Yokibics.

Yoruba Medicine. Anthony D. Buckley. 2nd unabr. ed. 1997. (Illus.). 280p. reprint ed. mass mkt. 24.95 (*1-890157-01-5*) Athelia-Henrietta.

You Ain't Lived Til You Grow Old. Lenore Glassman & Yvette Jackson. 1980. (Illus.). 104p. (Orig.). pap. 4.95 (*0-918464-44-7*) LYCO Pub.

You & Leukemia. Baker. rev. ed. 1988. 205p. pap. 26.00 (*0-7216-1495-7*) Saunders.

You & Your Deaf Child: A Self-Help Guide for Parents of Deaf & Hard of Hearing Children. John W. Adams. 2nd rev. ed. 1997. LC 97-18820. Orig. Title: You & Your Hearing Impaired Child. (Illus.). 240p. 19.95 (*1-56368-060-2*, Clerc Bks) Gallaudet Univ Pr.

*__You & Your Doctor - The Essential Guide to Examinations, Tests & Investigations.__ Apple. 1997. pap. (*1-900151-80-4*) Greenwich Med GBR. *Dist:* JAMCO Dist.

You & Your Emotions see Guia Ilustrada del Medico para el Auto-Tratamiento Emocional

You & Your Hearing Impaired Child see You & Your Deaf Child: A Self-Help Guide for Parents of Deaf & Hard of Hearing Children

You & Your Hormones. Max D. Rubenstein. 1960. 15.95 (*0-8084-0387-7*) NCUP.

You & Your Pregnancy: The Most Commonly Asked Questions Before, During, & After. James P. Guerrieri & Gregory R. Moore. 1996. LC 95-49813. 133p. 9.95 (*0-915253-48-8*) Hlth Edu Lit.

You & Your Retarded Child: A Manual for Parents of Retarded Children. Samuel A. Kirk et al. 2nd ed. 1968. LC 67-20824. (Paperbounds Ser.: No. PB-2). x, 164p. (Orig.). pap. 4.95 (*0-87015-161-4*) Pacific Bks.

You Are Barbara Jordan: An In-Basket Exercise on Nursing Service Administration. 1970. (C). 7.50 (*0-87914-015-1*, 654630); tchr. ed. 7.50 (*0-87914-016-X*, 654631) Hosp Res & Educ.

You Are Not Alone. Sabra Albritton et al. Ed. by Devyani S. Raval et al. 1998. (Illus.). 216p. pap. 19.95 (*0-9666425-0-3*, 98022) Childs Med Ventures.

You Are Not Alone: Compulsive Hair Pulling, the Enemy Within. Cheryn Salazar. 1995. (Illus.). 262p. (Orig.). (YA). pap. 19.95 (*0-9650670-0-9*) Rophe Pr.

You Are Not Alone: Understanding & Dealing with Mental Illness. Clara C. Park & Leon N. Shapiro. 1979. 17.50 (*0-316-69073-2*, Little Brwn Med Div) Lppncott W & W.

You Are Not Alone: Words of Experience & Hope for the Journey Through Depression. Julia Thorne & Larry Rothstein. 1993. LC 92-56255. 192p. (Orig.). pap. 12.50 (*0-06-096977-6*, Perennial) HarperTrade.

You Are Not Your Illness: Seven Principles for Meeting the Challenge of Illness. Hal Z. Bennett & Linda N. Topf. 1995. LC 94-39618. 256p. per. 12.00 (*0-684-80124-8*, Fireside) S&S Trade Pap.

You Are What You Ate. Sherry A. Rogers. 3rd rev. ed. 1997. 308p. (Orig.). pap. 12.95 (*0-9618821-8-2*) SandKey.

You Are Your Body's Keeper: Don't Become a Medical Mistake. A. H. Felman. l.t. ed. 2000. 136p. pap. 10.00 (*0-9669018-2-7*, 2000-1) Ally.

You Bring Out the Music in Me: Music in Nursing Homes. Ed. by Beckie Karras. 1988. LC 87-22931. (Activities, Adaptation & Aging Ser.: Vol. 10, Nos. 1 & 2). (Illus.). 135p. 24.95 (*0-86656-699-6*) Haworth Pr.

You Can Be Fit! A Simple Guide to Understanding Fitness & Nutrition. Steven M. Horwitz. 1993. (Illus.). 77p. (Orig.). 10.95 (*0-9631715-3-4*) Fnd Chiro Educ Res.

You Can Beat Heart Disease: Prevention & Treatment. Lester R. Sauvage. 2nd ed. 2000. (Illus.). 336p. pap. 15.95 (*0-9663788-2-2*) Better Life Pr.

You Can Conquer Your Headaches. Frank R. Di Fiore. 1980. (Illus.). 66p. (Orig.). pap. 10.00 (*0-932896-03-0*) Westcliff Pubns.

You Can Control Diabetes: A Personal Guide to Self Empowerment. Abdul Ghani & Gary Scheiner. 1997. (Illus.). 344p. pap. 24.95 (*0-9656880-0-3*) Midtown Pub.

You Can Control Your Feelings! 24 Guides to Emotional Well-Being. Bill Borcherdt. 1993. LC 92-46866. 270p. pap. 22.45 (*0-943158-73-7*, YCCBP, Prof Resc Pr) Pro Resource.

You Can Find a Way. Patrick F. Mahony. 1985. 20.00 (*0-941694-10-0*) Inst Study Man.

You Can Get into Medical School: Letters from Premeds. Sanford J. Brown. 1986. LC 85-61493. (Illus.). 144p. (Orig.). pap. 7.95 (*0-9615167-0-4*) Mendocino Found Health.

You Can Give First Aid. 1993. 7.50 (*0-88336-550-2*); tchr. ed. 6.25 (*0-88336-551-0*) New Readers.

You Can Heal Your Life. Louise L. Hay. gif. ed. 1999. LC 98-51365. (Illus.). 304p. pap. 12.95 (*1-56170-628-0*, L446); 1987. LC 88-200391. 240p. reprint ed. pap. 12.95 (*0-937611-01-8*, 101) Hay House.

You Can Help with Your Healing: A Guide for Recovering Wholeness in Body, Mind, & Spirit. Vernon J. Bittner. rev. ed. 1992. LC 92-34279. 160p. pap. 14.99 (*0-8066-2656-9*, 9-2656) Augsburg Fortress.

You Can Kick the Habit! Walter E. Kloss. 1976. (Better Living Ser.). pap. 0.89 (*0-8127-0128-3*) Review & Herald.

You Can Lose Weight. Alan Dolit. 1980. 130p. 7.95 (*0-8290-1571-X*) Irvington.

You Can Prevent Breast Cancer. Harvey Diamond. 1995. (Illus.). 273p. (Orig.). pap. 12.95 (*1-57901-011-3*) Intl Promotions.

You Can Prevent Cancer. Ernest H. Rosenbaum. Ed. by Sheila Mahoney & Nancy Wiltsek. 1984. (Illus.). 29p. pap. 2.50 (*0-933161-00-X*) Better H Prog.

You Can Prevent or Correct Learning Disorders: The Complete Handbook of Children's Reading Disorders. Hilde Mosse. 1989. 732p. (C). reprint ed. pap. text 34.95 (*0-8077-2983-3*) Tchrs Coll.

You Can't Count on Dying. Natalie H. Cabot. Ed. by Leon Stein. 1980. LC 79-8662. (Growing Old Ser.). reprint ed. lib. bdg. 28.95 (*0-405-12779-0*) Ayer.

You Can't Quit Until You Know What's Eating You: Overcoming Compulsive Eating. Donna LeBlanc. 1990. 144p. pap. 7.95 (*1-55874-103-8*) Health Comm.

You Can't Say That to Me: Stopping the Pain of Verbal Abuse: An Eight-Step Program. Suzette Haden Elgin. 1995. LC 94-36128. 224p. 40.00 (*0-471-00395-6*); pap. 17.95 (*0-471-00399-9*) Wiley.

You Chi: The Healing Spirit. Don Boone & Laura Boone. 1993. 80p. (Orig.). pap. 9.95 (*1-56664-048-2*) WorldComm.

You Don't Have to Die from Cancer: Taking Active Charge. Abraham Khazam. 1996. pap. text (*0-85572-266-5*) Hill Content Pubng AUS. *Dist:* Seven Hills Bk.

You Don't Have to Live with Cystitis. Larrian Gillespie. rev. ed. 1996. LC 96-22962. pap. 12.00 (*0-380-78779-2*, Avon Bks) Morrow Avon.

You Don't Have to Live with Cystitis! How to Avoid It - What to Do about It. Larrian Gillespie. 1988. pap. 10.00 (*0-380-70486-2*, Avon Bks) Morrow Avon.

You Don't Have to Suffer: A Complete Guide to Relieving Cancer Pain for Patients & Their Families. Susan S. Lang & Richard B. Patt. 1995. (Illus.). 384p. pap. 12.95 (*0-19-508419-5*) OUP.

You Don't Need a Hysterectomy: New & Effective Ways of Avoiding Surgery. Ivan K. Strausz. 1993. LC 92-30268. (Illus.). xxiv, 294p. 24.95 (*0-201-60827-8*) Addison-Wesley.

You Have a Pacemaker. Barbara J. Fletcher & Julia A. Purcell. Ed. by Nancy R. Hull. rev. ed. 1996. LC 81-23461. 32p. pap. text 5.95 (*0-939838-12-5*) Pritchett & Hull.

You Have a Visitor: Observations on Pet Visitation & Therapy. Renee Lamm Esordi. 2000. LC 99-90589. (Illus.). 131p. pap. 29.95 (*0-9672532-0-9*) Blue Lamm.

You Have Choices: Recovering from Anxiety, Panic & Phobia. William N. Penzer & Bonnie Goodman. Ed. by Myra Gross. 1991. Orig. Title: Overcoming Anxiety, Panic, Phobias Through a Support Group. (Illus.). 256p. (Orig.). pap. 11.95 (*0-9622658-1-0*) William Penzer.

You Just Don't Understand: Women & Men in Conversation. Deborah Tannen. 1991. LC 90-93519. 336p. pap. 14.00 (*0-345-37205-0*) Ballantine Pub Grp.

You Know You're Pregnant When . . . Jeff Justice & Diane Pfeifer. Ed. by Diane Pfeifer. 1995. LC 94-68529. (Illus.). 96p. (Orig.). pap. 5.95 (*0-9618306-4-6*) Strawberry GA.

You Mean I Don't Have to Feel This Way? New Help for Depression, Anxiety, & Addiction. Colette Dowling. 1992. 384p. text 19.95 (*0-684-19257-8*) S&S Trade.

You Mean I Don't Have to Feel This Way? New Help for Depression, Anxiety & Addiction. Colette Dowling. 1993. LC 92-46657. 320p. reprint ed. pap. 14.95 (*0-553-37169-X*) Bantam.

You Mean I'm Not Lazy, Stupid, or Crazy?! A Self-Help Book for Adults with Attention Deficit Disorder. Kate Kelly & Peggy Ramundo. 1993. (Illus.). 350p. 19.95 (*1-882522-00-1*) Tyrell & Jerem.

You Mean I'm Not Lazy, Stupid or Crazy?! A Self-Help Book for Adults with Attention Deficit Disorder. Kate Kelly & Peggy Ramundo. 1995. LC 94-40538. (Illus.). 464p. 23.00 (*0-684-80116-7*) S&S Trade.

You Were Designed to Live for One Hundred & Forty Years. Arnold Perrin. 1979. pap. 1.00 (*0-939736-06-3*) Wings ME.

You'll Never Walk Alone: Hospital Survival Techniques. Debbie A. Weissenberg. 1998. LC 96-61584. (Illus.). 100p. pap. 9.95 (*0-9639519-8-X*) Whitewing Pr.

Youmans Neurological Surgery. H. Richard Winn. 5th ed. 2001. (Illus.). 4415p. text 795.00 (*0-7216-8291-X*) Saunders.

Young Adolescent. Peter Blos. 1974. LC 73-125597. 252p. pap. 16.50 (*0-02-904300-X*) Free Pr.

Young Adolescent Development & School Practices: Promoting Harmony. David Strahan & John Van Hoose. 1988. 48p. 8.00 (*1-56090-037-7*) Natl Middle Schl.

Young Carl Jung. Robert W. Brockway. 1997. LC 96-25223. (Illus.). 180p. pap. 17.95 (*1-888602-01-5*, 015) Chiron Pubns.

Young Child with Down Syndrome. Siegfried M. Pueschel. 1984. 371p. 45.95 (*0-89885-120-3*, Kluwer Acad Hman Sci) Kluwer Academic.

Young Children's Behavior: Implementing Your Goals. Illus. by Susan Fritts. 1978. LC 78-56624. 78p. pap. text 12.95 (*0-89334-015-4*) Humanics Pub Grp.

Young Children's Close Relationships: Beyond Attachment. Judy Dunn. 1993. (Individual Differences & Development Ser.: Vol. 4). (Illus.). 152p. (C). pap. 31.95 (*0-8039-4491-8*, 3988) Sage.

Young Deaf Adults & the Transition from High School to Postsecondary Careers. Thomas E. Allen. 1995. (Illus.). 70p. (Orig.). (C). pap. text 20.00 (*0-7881-2362-9*) DIANE Pub.

Young First Offenders: Their Criminal Careers. G. L. Webb. 1979. LC 78-72958. 9.95 (*0-933012-03-9*) Coker Pub.

Young Girl's Diary. Sigmund Freud. 1972. 300.00 (*0-87968-040-7*) Gordon Pr.

Young Hyperactive Child: Answers to Questions about Diagnosis, Prognosis & Treatment. Ed. by Jan Loney. 1987. LC 87-178. (Journal of Children in Contemporary Society: Vol. 19, Nos. 1-2). 178p. (Orig.). text 49.95 (*0-86656-670-8*) Haworth Pr.

Young Patient with Degenerative Hip Disease. Ed. by John Sevastik & Ian F. Goldie. 1986. (Illus.). 322p. (Orig.). pap. text 117.50 (*91-22-00784-9*) Coronet Bks.

Young People & Alcohol, Drugs & Tobacco. K. Anderson. 1995. (WHO Regional Publications, European Ser.: No. 66). 87p. pap. text 20.00 (*92-890-1330-3*) World Health.

Young People & Chronic Illness: True Stories, Help & Hope. Kelly Huegel. Ed. by Gretchen Bratvold & Elizabeth Verdick. 1998. LC 98-10439. (Illus.). 208p. (YA). (gr. 5-9). pap. 14.95 (*1-57542-041-4*) Free Spirit Pub.

Young People & Physical Activity. Neil Armstrong & Joanne Wellsman. 1996. LC 96-26617. (Illus.). 384p. pap. text 59.50 (*0-19-262659-0*) OUP.

Young People, Health, & Family Life. Julia Brannen et al. 1994. LC 93-22709. 229p. pap. (*0-335-19097-9*) OpUniv Pr.

Young People with Cancer: A Handbook for Parents. 1992. (Illus.). 86p. (Orig.). (C). pap. text 20.00 (*1-56806-101-3*) DIANE Pub.

Young People's Health: A Challenge for Society. 1986. (Technical Reports: No. 731). 117p. pap. text 14.40 (*92-4-120731-0*, 1100731) World Health.

Young, Sober & Free. Ed. by Shelly Marshall. 1978. 137p. 10.00 (*0-89486-055-0*, 1116A) Hazelden.

Young Surgeon Goes to War: An Autobiography. John Dziob. 1999. 96p. pap. 10.00 (*0-8059-4727-2*) Dorrance.

Young Teenagers & Alcohol, 1996. 1997. (Scotland - Education: All Publicatons Ser.: Vol. 2). (*0-11-620950-X*, HM0950X) Statnry Office GBR. *Dist:* Bernan Associates.

***Young Woman at the Rise of the 21st Century: Gynecologic & Reproductive Issues in Health & Disease.** Ed. by George Creatsas et al. 2001. 430p. pap. 32.50 (*0-8018-6694-4*) NY Acad Sci.

Young Woman at the Rise of the 21st Century Vol. 900: Gynecologic & Reproductive Issues in Health & Disease. Ed. by George Creatsas et al. 2000. LC 00-23979. (Annals of the New York Academy of Sciences Ser.: Vol. 900). (Illus.). xv, 446p. 160.00 (*1-57331-226-6*) NY Acad Sci.

Younger at Last. Steven Lamm & Gerald S. Couzens. 1997. LC 97-13557. 253p. 22.50 (*0-684-83438-3*) S&S Trade.

Younger at Last: Discover the Age-Defying Powers of Vitality Medicine. Steven Lamm. 1998. per. 6.99 (*0-671-02291-1*, Pocket Star Bks) PB.

Younger People with Dementia: Planning, Practice & Development. Sylvia Cox. 1998. LC 99-171530. 328p. pap. 29.95 (*1-85302-588-7*) Taylor & Francis.

Youniverse: Gestalt Therapy, Non-Western Religions & the Present Age. Jesse J. Thomas. 1990. LC 77-89164. (Illus.). (C). 12.95 (*0-930626-01-X*); 2nd ed. pap., stu. ed. 5.95 (*0-930626-00-1*) Psych & Consul Assocs.

Your Aching Back: A Doctor's Guide to Relief. Augustus A. White. rev. ed. 1990. 336p. per. 14.00 (*0-671-71000-1*) S&S Trade.

Your Are in Charge: The IM Method Total Fitness for the Fit & Not So Fit. Ina Marx. 1990. 148p. (Orig.). pap. text 19.95 (*0-9626194-0-X*) Esperanza Pubns.

Your Attitude Is Showing: A Primer of Human Relations. Elwood N. Chapman & Sharon L. O'Neil. 9th ed. 1998. LC 98-7522. (Illus.). 237p. (C). pap. text 34.60 (*0-13-954793-2*) P-H.

Your Baby's Development. Joan Miller. 1995. 128p. pap. (*0-572-01657-3*) Foulsham UK GBR. *Dist:* Assoc Pubs Grp.

Your Baby's Mind: Features over 200 Learning Games & Activities to Help Babies Develop to Their Full Potential During the Critical First Two Years. S. H. Jacob. rev. ed. 1992. LC 93-177109. 288p. pap. 6.95 (*1-55850-137-1*) Adams Media.

Your Baby's Secret World: Four Phases for Effective Parenting (A Professional & Practical Guide) Larry V. Cheldelin. Ed. by J. Brown. 1983. (Illus.). pap. 11.95 (*0-8283-1850-6*) Branden Bks.

Your Best Way to Health: A Primer for Better Health. 2000. 192p. pap. 19.95 (*0-9679-8916-0-4*) BEST WAY.

Your Body Can Talk: How to Use Simple Muscle Testing to Learn What Your Body Knows & Needs. Susan L. Levy, D.C. & Carol Lehr, M.A. 1996. LC 96-14124. (Illus.). 390p. (Orig.). pap. 19.95 (*0-934252-68-8*) Hohm Pr.

Your Body Doesn't Lie. John Diamond. 1989. 208p. mass mkt. 5.99 (*0-446-35847-9*) Warner Bks.

Your Body Speaks Its Mind. Stanley Keleman. 1981. LC 79-91527. 188p. reprint ed. 10.95 (*0-934320-03-9*); pap. 12.95 (*0-934320-01-2*) Center Pr.

Your Body's Many Cries for Water: You Are Not Sick, You Are Thirsty: Don't Treat Thirst with Medications. Fereydoon Batmanghelidj. 2nd ed. 1995. (Illus.). 186p. pap. 14.95 (*0-9629942-3-5*) Global Hlth.

Your Body's Most Powerful Healers: How to Stay Out of the Hospital. Edward M. Wagner & Sylvia Goldfarb. 1996. 404p. 29.98 (*0-941683-28-1*) Instant Improve.

Your Body's Red Light Warning Signals: Medical Tips That May Save Your Life. Neil Shulman et al. 1999. LC 99-218936. 416p. (Orig.). mass mkt. 5.99 (*0-440-23461-1*) Dell.

Your Body's Response. Edgar Brown & Kaye Behrens. 1985. LC 82-90165. (Illus.). 192p. (Orig.). 22.95 (*0-9613697-1-X*); pap. 16.95 (*0-9613697-0-1*) Madison Ave Pub.

Your Brain: How You Got It & How It Works. Tabitha M. Powledge. 1994. LC 94-14273. (Illus.). 224p. (J). (gr. 6-8). mass mkt. 14.95 (*0-684-19659-X*) S&S Trade.

Your Breast & You: What Every Woman Needs to Know about Breast Diseases, Breast Cancer & Cosmetic Breast Surgery Before She Has a Breast Problem. D. S. Halbert. Ed. by Delno Roberts. 1986. LC 84-72983. (Illus.). 238p. 14.95 (*0-931609-00-3*) Askon Pub.

Your Breast Cancer Treatment Handbook: Your Guide to Understanding the Disease, Treatments, Emotions & Recovery from Breast Cancer. Judy C. Kneece. Ed. by Tricia Brown. 3rd rev. ed. 1998. (Illus.). 210p. pap. text 21.95 (*1-886665-10-9*) EduCare Pub.

Your Career in Administrative Services: Teacher's Resource Package. Roberta C. Weiss. Ed. by Lisa Biello. 1996. 128p. pap. text, tchr. ed. 135.00 (*0-7216-6078-9*) Saunders.

Your Career in Cardiovascular Technology. Roberta C. Weiss. 1996. LC 95-17718. xv, 338p. text 38.00 (*0-7216-6074-6*) Saunders.

Your Career in Cardiovascular Technology: Teacher's Resource Package. Roberta C. Weiss. Ed. by Lisa Biello. 1996. 128p. pap. text, tchr. ed. 175.00 (*0-7216-6075-4*) Saunders.

Your Career in Health Care. Robert Wilson. 1996. LC 96-1229. 304p. 12.95 (*0-8120-9599-5*) Barron.

Your Career in Physical Medicine. Roberta C. Weiss. 1997. LC 97-10170. 475p. text 42.00 (*0-7216-6453-9*) Saunders.

Your Career in Physical Medicine: Teacher's Resource Package. Robert C. Weiss. Ed. by Lisa Beillo. 1997. 240p. text, tchr. ed. 175.00 (*0-7216-6454-7*) Saunders.

Your Child: A Medical Guide. Consumer Guide Editors & Ira J. Chasnoff. 1993. (Illus.). 576p. 9.98 (*0-88176-391-8*, 3200700) Pubns Intl Ltd.

Your Child & Epilepsy. Robert J. Gumnit. 1995. 256p. pap. 27.50 (*0-939957-76-0*) Demos Medical.

Your Child & X-Rays: A Parent's Guide to Radiation, X-Rays & Other Imaging Procedures. Avice M. O'Connell & Norma L. Leone. 1989. LC 87-37854. (Illus.). 104p. (Orig.). pap. 4.00 (*0-936635-05-3*) Lion Pr & Vid.

Your Child Doesn't Have to Die! How You Can Help Your Child Overcome Cancer Using Nutritional Therapy. Usa C. Ragsdale. 1996. (Orig.). pap. 12.00 (*0-9654714-0-3*) Abundant Living.

Your Child in the Hospital: A Practical Guide for Parents. Nancy Keene & Rachel Prentice. Ed. by Linda Lamb. 2nd ed. 1999. LC 99-19134. (Patient-Centered Guides Ser.). (Illus.). 172p. pap. 11.95 (*1-56592-573-4*) OReilly & Assocs.

Your Child Makes Sense: A Guidebook for Parents. Edith Buxbaum. 1961. 204p. (Orig.). pap. 24.95 (*0-8236-8350-8*, 027040) Intl Univs Pr.

Your Child Needs a Champion: Mastering the A. D. D. Challenge by Making the Right Choices. Jane F. Miller. 1997. LC 97-93086. (Illus.). 224p. pap. 16.95 (*0-9658190-0-0*) JMA Pubns.

Your Child's Doctor Visits. Marta Brandes-Miesner & Joseph M. Miesner, Sr. rev. ed. 1998. 162p. pap. 12.95 (*0-9666367-0-8*) Sun Bear.

Your Child's Food Allergies: Detecting & Treating Hyperactivity, Congestion, Irritability & Other Symptoms Caused by Common Food Allergies. Jane McNicol. 1992. LC 91-34661. 176p. pap. 9.95 (*0-471-55801-X*) Wiley.

Your Child's Health: The Parent's Guide to Symptoms, Emergencies, Common Illnesses, Behavior & School Problems. Barton D. Schmitt. rev. ed. 1991. LC 87-47687. 704p. pap. 19.95 (*0-553-35339-X*) Bantam.

Your Child's Health Abroad: A Manual for Travelling Parents. Jane Wilson-Howarth & Matthew Ellis. 1998. LC 97-42073. (Illus.). 208p. pap. (*1-898323-63-1*) Bradt Pubns GBR. *Dist:* Globe Pequot.

Your Child's Medical Journal. Sharon Larsen. 1999. 16.00 (*0-609-60434-1*) Random Hse Value.

Your Child's Speech & Language: Guidelines for Parents. Mary Brooks & Deedra Engmann-Hartung. 1978. 52p. pap. text 14.00 (*0-89079-039-6*, 1070) PRO-ED.

Your Chiropractor & You: Everything You Need to Know about Chiropractic. J. Kandel & D. Sudderth. 1999. (Illus.). 224p. pap. 14.95 (*0-7615-1712-X*) Prima Pub.

***Your Cleft-Affected Child: The Complete Book of Information, Resources & Hope.** Carrie T. Gruman-Trinkner. 2001. LC 2001-26471. (Illus.). 288p. pap. 15.95 (*0-89793-185-8*) Hunter Hse.

Your Complete Medical Record. People's Medical Society Staff. 1993. 208p. pap. 12.95 (*1-882606-00-0*) Peoples Med Soc.

Your Cure for Cancer: The Science, the Spirit & the Understanding. Robert E. Smith et al. 1998. (Illus.). 270p. pap. 19.95 (*1-57901-030-X*) Intl Promotions.

Your Drug May Be Your Problem: How & Why to Stop Taking Psychiatric Medications. Peter R. Breggin & David Cohen. 1999. LC 99-63300. ix, 272p. pap. 24.00 (*0-7382-0184-7*) Perseus Pubng.

Your Drug May Be Your Problem: How & Why to Stop Taking Psychiatric Medications. Peter R. Breggin & David Cohen. 2000. 288p. pap. text 17.00 (*0-7382-0348-3*) Perseus Bks Grp.

Your Erroneous Zones: Step-by-Step Advice for Escaping the Trap of Negative Thinking & Taking Control of Your Life. Wayne W. Dyer. 2001. LC 91-2718. 288p. reprint ed. pap. 13.00 (*0-06-091976-0*, Perennial) HarperTrade.

Your Eyes: A Book for Paramedical Personnel & the Lay Reader. Thomas Chalkley. 4th ed. 2000. LC 99-58325. (Illus.). 140p. 24.95 (*0-398-07048-2*) C C Thomas.

Your Eyes! A Comprehensive Look at the Understanding & Treatment of Vision Problems. Thomas L. D'Alonzo. rev. ed. 1991. LC 91-71193. (Illus.). 251p. (C). pap. 14.95 (*0-9629063-5-2*) Avanti.

Your Eyes: An Owner's Manual. James F. Collins. 1989. (Illus.). 224p. (Orig.). pap. (*0-9621975-0-5*) Infinity NY.

Your Eyes: Questions You Have . . . Answers You Need. Sandra Salmans. 1996. pap. 12.95 (*1-882606-59-0*) Peoples Med Soc.

***Your Eyesight & How to Take Care of It: A Collection of Patient Education Handouts Used by Leading Eye Doctors.** Lawrence Winograd & Melvin L. Rubin. 2001. 288p. pap. 24.95 (*0-937404-22-5*) Triad Pub FL.

Your Fabulous Volunteers: A History of the Washington Emergency Squad & Emergency Services in Warren County. Richard E. Harpster. Ed. by Larry K. Smith. rev. ed. 1985. (Illus.). 365p. 14.95 (*0-9604020-1-2*) Wash Emerg Squad.

Your Feet: Questions You Have . . . Answers You Need. Sandra Salmans. 1998. LC 98-3354. (Questions You Have...Answers You Need Ser.). (Illus.). 196p. pap. 12.95 (*1-882606-40-X*) Peoples Med Soc.

Your Feet Dont Have to Hurt. Suzanne Levine & Susan Jacoby. 2000. LC 00-24609. (Illus.). xxiii, 279p. 24.95 (*0-312-26276-0*) St Martin.

Your Fertility Signals: Using Them to Achieve or Avoid Pregnancy, Naturally. Merryl Winstein. 1998. LC 87-92011. (Illus.). 160p. (Orig.). pap. 13.95 (*0-9619401-0-7*) Smooth Stone Pr.

Your First Year as a Nurse: Making the Transition from Total Novice to Successful Professional. Donna Cardillo. 2001. LC 2001-21661. 288p. pap. 19.95 (*0-7615-3333-8*) Prima Pub.

Your Four Great Emotions. David Seabury. 1969. 108p. pap. 5.95 (*0-911336-22-2*) Sci of Mind.

Your Future Health Care: The Challenge & the Promise Through Better Education. Tinsley R. Harrison. 1974. LC 73-13222. 164p. 10.50 (*0-87527-132-4*) Green.

***Your Genetic Destiny: Know Your Genes & Save Your Life.** Milunsky. 2002. 432p. pap. text 18.00 (*0-7382-0684-9*) Perseus Bks Grp.

Your Good Health: A Womans A-Z. Anne McDeritt. 1994. 144p. (Orig.). pap. (*1-85594-094-9*) Attic Press.

Your Good Health: How to Stay Well, & What to Do When You're Not. Ed. by William I. Bennett et al. 1987. LC 87-19671. (Illus.). 520p. text 39.00 (*0-674-96631-7*) HUP.

Your Good Health: How to Stay Well, & What to Do When You're Not. William I. Bennett et al. Ed. by Timothy Johnson & Stephen E. Goldfinger. 1989. (Illus.). 520p. pap. text 16.50 (*0-674-96632-5*) HUP.

Your Good Health - Thank God. Yvon Morris. 1996. 51p. pap. 9.98 (*1-888139-01-3*) Y Morris Carib.

Your Good Health Garden: Food Plants That Protect Your Health. Pauline James. 1996. LC 95-11904. (Illus.). 128p. pap. 9.95 (*0-88007-208-3*) Woodbridge Pr.

Your Guide to Choosing Quality Health Care. Ed. by Donna Shalala. 2000. (Illus.). 54p. reprint ed. pap. text 20.00 (*0-7881-8370-2*) DIANE Pub.

***Your Guide to Diabetes: Type 1 & Type 2.** Ed. by Barry Leonard. 2002. (Illus.). 62p. (C). pap. text 20.00 (*0-7567-1904-6*) DIANE Pub.

***Your Guide to E-Health: Third Millennium Medicine on the Internet.** Peter Yellowlees. 2001. 204p. pap. (*0-7022-3220-3*) Univ Queensland Pr AUS. *Dist:* Intl Spec Bk.

Your Guide to Good Nutrition. Fredrick J. Stare et al. 1991. LC 91-27297. 223p. pap. 23.00 (*0-87975-692-6*) Prometheus Bks.

Your Guide to Medical Hypnosis. Lynn Phelps. 1993. LC 93-9545. (Focus on Health Ser.). (Illus.). 108p. (Orig.). pap. 7.95 (*0-944838-28-6*) Med Physics Pub.

Your Guide to Medical Schools & Residency Programs: The Information You Need to Know, You Should Know, You Must Know. Robert M. Maloney. Ed. by Richard A. DeVito. 1996. (Illus.). 250p. (Orig.). pap. 189.95 (*0-932834-25-6*) Prime Natl Pub.

Your Guide to Non-Prescription Drugs. American Pharmaceutical Association Staff. (Illus.). 500p. (*0-8290-1580-9*) Irvington.

Your Guide to Women's Health: An FDA Consumer Special Report. Ed. by Judith L. Willis. 3rd ed. 1998. (Illus.). 122p. pap. text 25.00 (*0-7881-7236-0*) DIANE Pub.

Your Gut Feelings: A Complete Guide to Living Better with Intestinal Problems. Henry D. Janowitz. 2nd rev. ed. 1994. LC 94-1717. (Illus.). 224p. pap. 13.95 (*0-19-508936-7*) OUP.

Your Handbook for Healing. Craig Carter. 1981. 64p. pap. 7.95 (*0-911336-86-9*) Sci of Mind.

Your Healing Is Within You. Canon J. Glennon. 1980. LC 80-82616. 189p. pap. 8.99 (*0-88270-457-5*) Bridge-Logos.

Your Healing Mind. Reed C. Moskowitz. 1993. 304p. reprint ed. pap. 10.00 (*0-380-71470-1*, Avon Bks) Morrow Avon.

W X Y Z

Your Health. Dianne R. Hales. 1991. 525p. pap. text 29.25 (*0-8053-2770-3*) Benjamin-Cummings.

Your Health: A Corrective System of Exercising that Revolutionizes the Entire Field of Physical Education. Joseph H. Pilates. Ed. by Judd Robbins. 1998. LC 98-223207. 63p. pap. 19.95 (*0-9614937-8-X*) Present Dynam.

Your Health & Safety at Work: A Collection of Modules. 1996. LC 97-198757. pap. 34.95 (*92-2-108014-5*) Intl Labour Office.

Your Healthy Cat: Homeopathic Medicines for Common Feline Ailments. H. G. Wolff. 1991. LC 91-163035. 131p. pap. 11.95 (*1-55643-113-9*) North Atlantic.

Your Healthy Child: A Guide to Natural Health Care. Alice L. Duncan. 2nd rev. ed. 1995. LC 95-68425. (Illus.). 272p. pap. 14.95 (*1-887020-35-7*, Sanicula Pr) Rainlight Bk.

Your Heart. James C. Thomson. Ed. by C. Leslie Thomson. 1974. 80p. pap. 6.95 (*0-8464-1058-3*) Beekman Pubs.

Your Heart: American Heart Association's Complete Guide to Heart Health. American Heart Association Staff. 1996. 432p. mass mkt. 6.99 (*0-671-53081-X*) PB.

Your Heart: In Sickness & in Health. James E. Crockett. 1984. (Illus.). 176p. (Orig.). pap. 10.00 (*0-9611980-0-1*) Eucalyptus Pr.

Your Heart: Questions You Have—Answers You Need. People's Medical Society Staff. 4th rev. ed. 1996. LC 95-49182. 222p. 13.95 (*1-882606-60-4*) Peoples Med Soc.

Your Home, Your Health & Well Being. David Rousseau et al. 1988. LC 87-7080. (Illus.). 300p. pap. 14.95 (*0-89815-223-2*) Ten Speed Pr.

Your Hormoneous Life: Learn the Secrets of Progesterone. Calvin Ross. 1996. (Illus.). 180p. (Orig.). pap. 12.95 (*1-57901-013-X*) Intl Promotions.

Your Hospital Care Guide: What You Need to Know & Questions to Ask. Sonya N. Washington. 1995. 160p. (Orig.). pap. 9.95 (*1-886583-05-6*) SeaStar Pub.

Your Hospital Care Guide Pt. 2: What You Need to Know in These Times of Health Care Changes. Sonya N. Washington. 1998. (InfoMed Book Ser.). 100p. pap. (*1-886583-06-4*) SeaStar Pub.

Your Hyperactive Child: A Parents Guide to Coping with Attention Deficit Disorder. Barbara D. Ingersoll. 1988. LC 87-36535. 240p. pap. 11.95 (*0-385-24070-8*) Doubleday.

Your Ideal Supplement Plan in 3 Easy Steps: The Essential Guide to Choosing the Herbs, Vitamins & Minerals That Are Right for You. Deborah Mitchell. 2000. LC 00-268748. (Illus.). 256p. mass mkt. 5.99 (*0-440-23554-5*) Dell.

Your Injury: A Common Sense Guide to Sports Injuries. Merrill A. Ritter & Marjorie J. Albohm. 2nd rev. ed. 2000. LC 00-103069. (Illus.). x, 188p. pap. 20.00 (*1-884125-79-4*) Cooper Pubng.

Your Inner Physician & You: Craniosacral Therapy & Somatoemotional Release. John E. Upledger. 2nd rev. ed. 1997. LC 96-37576. 163p. pap. 14.95 (*1-55643-246-1*) North Atlantic.

Your Life in Your Hands: Understanding, Preventing & Overcoming Breast Cancer. Jane Plant. 2001. LC 00-47495. 272p. 23.95 (*0-312-27561-7*, Thomas Dunne) St Martin.

Your Liver...Your Lifeline. Jack Tips. 1995. 150p. pap. 12.95 (*0-929167-06-6*) Apple-a-Day.

Your Medical Rights: How to Become an Empowered Consumer. Charles B. Inlander & Eugene I. Pavalon. 2nd ed. 1994. LC 94-1578. 416p. pap. 14.95 (*1-882606-09-4*) Peoples Med Soc.

Your Medicare Handbook. 1984. text 250.00 (*0-87700-541-9*) Revisionist Pr.

Your Medicare Handbook, 1996. Health Care Financing Administration Staff & Health and Human Services Dept. Staff. rev. ed. 1996. (Illus.). 30p. pap. 2.25 (*0-16-048594-0*, 017-060-00586-6) USGPO.

***Your Mental Health: A Layman's Guide to the Psychiatrist's Bible.** Norman Sparnon. 2001. 447p. reprint ed. 27.00 (*0-7567-5109-8*) DIANE Pub.

Your Miracle Brain: Maximize Your Brain Power, Boost Your Memory, Lift Your Mood, Improve Your IQ & Creativity, Prevent & Reverse Mental Aging. Jean Carper. 2001. 400p. reprint ed. pap. 14.00 (*0-06-098440-6*, Quil) HarperTrade.

Your Name Is Hughes Hannibal Shanks: A Caregiver's Guide to Alzheimer's. Lela K. Shanks. 1996. LC 96-3691. (Agendas for Aging Ser.). (Illus.). 197p. text 30.00 (*0-8032-4245-X*) U of Nebr Pr.

Your Natural Health Makeover. Lauri M. Aesoph. 1998. LC 97-36541. 288p. (C). text 24.95 (*0-13-628652-6*) P-H.

Your Offshore Doctor: A Manual of Medical Self-Sufficiency at Sea. Michael H. Beilan. 2nd ed. 1996. LC 96-43183. (Illus.). 184p. pap. 17.50 (*1-57409-013-5*) Sheridan.

Your Opportunities As a Dental Assistant. Margie Sherman. 1994. (Illus.). 8p. pap. 2.50 (*1-884241-03-4*, OS106) Energeia Pub.

Your Opportunities As a Massage Therapist. Laurie Bean. 1994. (Illus.). 8p. pap. 2.50 (*1-884241-11-5*, OS115) Energeia Pub.

Your Opportunities As a Physical Therapist. 1997. (Illus.). 8p. (Orig.). pap. 2.50 (*1-884241-86-7*, OS130) Energeia Pub.

Your Opportunities As an Emergency Medical Technician. 1997. 8p. (Orig.). pap. 2.50 (*1-884241-85-9*, OS127) Energeia Pub.

Your Opportunities in Medical Support. Margie Sherman. 1994. (Illus.). 8p. pap. 2.50 (*1-884241-10-7*, OS114) Energeia Pub.

Your Opportunities in Nursing. Margie Sherman. 1994. (Illus.). 8p. pap. 2.50 (*1-884241-12-3*, OS116) Energeia Pub.

Your Own Perfect Medicine. Martha M. Christy. 1994. LC 94-71171. (Illus.). 221p. (Orig.). pap. 19.95 (*0-9632091-1-6*) Wishland Inc.

Your Pain Is Real. Emile Hiesiger. 2002. 272p. pap. 13.95 (*0-06-098828-2*, ReganBooks) HarperCollins Pubs.

Your Pain Is Real: Free Yourself from Chronic Pain with Breakthrough Medical Discoveries. Emile Hiesiger. 2001. LC 00-47017. (Illus.). 272p. 25.00 (*0-06-039324-6*, ReganBooks) HarperCollins Pubs.

Your Past Lives & the Healing Process: A Psychiatrist Looks at Reincarnation & Spiritual Healing. Adrian Finkelstein. exp. ed. 1996. 187p. 15.95 (*0-9647831-1-8*) Fifty Gates.

Your Personal Guide to Immunization Exemptions. Grace Girdwain. 1992. 48p. pap. 10.95 (*0-8059-3319-0*) Dorrance.

Your Personal Guide to Living Well with Fibromyalgia. Arthritis Foundation Staff. 1997. LC 96-79811. (Illus.). 160p. (Orig.). pap. 14.95 (*1-56352-382-5*) Longstreet.

Your Personal Health Guide: The Secret to Gaining & Maintaining Health. H.L. Sam Queen. Ed. by Betty Queen. 1997. 119p. pap. 14.95 (*0-9620479-4-5*) Inst for Health Real.

Your Personality Prescription. Roberta Schwartz Wennik. 1999. LC 98-67475. 400p. pap. 14.00 (*1-57566-401-1*, Knsington) Kensgtn Pub Corp.

Your Pregnancy after Thirty. Glade B. Curtis. 1996. LC 96-22165. (Your Pregnancy Ser.). (Illus.). 384p. pap. 12.95 (*1-55561-088-9*) Fisher Bks.

Your Pregnancy Companion. Janis Graham. Ed. by Sally Peters. 1991. 256p. (Orig.). pap. 14.00 (*0-671-68557-0*) PB.

Your Pregnancy Month by Month: A Comprehensive Guide & Personal Diary from Conception to Birth. Clark Gillespie. 4th rev. ed. 1992. LC 91-58473. (Illus.). 304p. pap. 13.00 (*0-06-096533-9*) HarperTrade.

Your Pregnancy Questions & Answers. Glade B. Curtis. 1997. LC 95-24480. (Your Pregnancy Ser.). (Illus.). 416p. pap. 12.95 (*1-55561-150-8*) Fisher Bks.

Your Pregnancy Week by Week. Glade Curtis & Judith Schuler. 4th rev. ed. 2000. LC 00-34817. (Illus.). 432p. 19.95 (*1-55561-256-3*); pap. 14.95 (*1-55561-260-1*) Fisher Bks.

Your Premature Baby: Everything You Need to Know about the Childbirth Treatment & Parenting of Premature Infants. Frank P. Manginello & Theresa Foy DiGeronimo. 1991. LC 91-10572. 304p. pap. 16.95 (*0-471-53587-7*) Wiley.

Your Premature Baby: Everything You Need to know about the Childbirth, Treatment, & Parenting of Premature Infants. Frank P. Manginello. 2nd rev. ed. 1998. LC 97-31835. 336p. pap. 17.95 (*0-471-23996-8*) Wiley.

Your Premature Baby & Child: Helpful Answers & Advice for Parents. Amy Tracy et al. 1999. LC 00-265090. (Illus.). 400p. pap. 14.95 (*0-425-16506-X*) Berkley Pub.

Your Press-Away Pain Guide to Headache Relief. T. Louis Emmons. Ed. by Harmony Bentosino. 1994. (Illus.). 64p. (Orig.). pap. text 4.95 (*0-9643151-8-1*) T L Emmons.

Your Prostate: What Every Man over Forty Needs to Know, Now! Chet Cunningham. 1994. LC 90-71251. (Illus.). 192p. (Orig.). pap. 12.95 (*0-9614924-6-5*) United Res CA.

Your Psyche, the Cigarette & the Pill: The Psychogenic Theory of Disease. Harold E. Simmons. 1969. pap. 10.00 (*0-87312-003-5*) Gen Welfare Pubns.

Your Remarkable Anatomy: An Overview for Health Professionals, Students, & the General Public. Don L. Fisher. 1997. (Illus.). 128p. (gr. 7-12). pap. text 25.00 (*1-889743-01-1*) R Dean Pr.

Your Road Map to Lifelong Happiness: A Guide to the Life You Want. Ken Keyes, Jr. 1995. LC 94-45849. (Illus.). 300p. 19.95 (*0-915972-22-0*) Love Line Bks.

Your Second Pregnancy: What to Expect This Time. Katie Tamony. rev. ed. 1995. LC 94-47662. 244p. pap. 12.95 (*1-55652-234-7*) Chicago Review.

Your Sexual Health: What Every Teen Should Know about Sex. Jenny McCloskey. 1993. LC 92-35228. (Illus.). 318p. (YA). (gr. 8-12). pap. 15.95 (*1-879904-08-X*) Halo Bks.

Your Skin: An Owner's Guide. Joseph Bark. 1995. LC 95-16749. 284p. (C). pap. 12.95 (*0-13-199663-0*) PH Pr.

Your Skin Is Showing. A. Bernard Ackerman. 1979. (Illus.). 32p. text 12.00 (*0-8121-1212-1*) Lppncott W & W.

Your Special Baby: REAL Lamaze Prepared Childbirth. Stacy McCullough. exp. ed. 1995. LC 95-94033. (Illus.). 80p. pap. 11.95 (*0-9643837-0-5*, YSB95) Luckenbooth.

Your Spontaneous Healing: Your Body's Natural Ability to Maintain & Heal Itself. Andrew Weil. 1995. LC 94-48897. 309p. 28.00 (*0-679-43607-3*) Knopf.

Your Successful Massage - Bodywork Practice: Professional Edition. Jefferson Saunders & Deborah Nucci. rev. ed. 1997. (Orig.). (C). pap. text (*1-877738-03-4*) Nucci-Saunders Pubns.

Your Thyroid. Lawrence D. Wood. 1996. LC 96-96650. (Illus.). 256p. pap. 12.00 (*0-345-41006-8*) Ballantine Pub Grp.

Your Thyroid: A Home Reference. Lawrence C. Wood et al. rev. ed. 1995. (Illus.). 256p. mass mkt. 5.99 (*0-345-39170-5*) Ballantine Pub Grp.

Your Top Health Concerns. Andrew Weil. 1997. LC 97-93711. mass mkt. 2.99 (*0-8041-1677-6*) Ivy Books.

Your Total Health Handbook - Body - Soul - Spirit. Marilyn Hickey. 1993. pap. 9.95 (*1-56441-024-2*) M Hickey Min.

Your Touch Can Heal: A Guide to Healing Touch & How to Use It. Malcolm Miner. 1992. 143p. pap. 6.95 (*0-9633796-0-7*) Faith Ridge.

Your Valves: Channels to a Healthy Heart: For Valve Disease & Valve Surgery Patients. Susan D. Allen et al. 1991. (Illus.). 64p. pap. text 3.25 (*0-916999-10-6*) HERC Pubng.

You're Beautiful: Quick Reference Self Help Program for All Situations. Al G. Manning & Rachel L. Manning. 1987. LC 87-62127. pap. 7.95 (*0-941698-16-5*) Pan Ishtar.

You're in Charge: A Guide to Becoming Your Own Therapist. Janette Rainwater. 1985. LC 82-9104. 221p. reprint ed. pap. 11.00 (*0-87516-552-4*) DeVorss.

You're Not Alone: With the Personal Stories of 38 Amputees. John Sabolich. Ed. by Carol Sorrels & Linda Adlof. 1993. (Illus.). 358p. (Orig.). 14.95 (*0-9637331-2-5*) Sabolich Pros & Res.

You're Not Alone: With the Personal Stories of 38 Amputees. John Sabolich. Ed. by Carol Yandell & Linda Adlof. 1993. (Illus.). 358p. (Orig.). pap. 9.95 (*0-9637331-1-7*); lib. bdg. 6.50 (*0-9637331-0-9*) Sabolich Pros & Res.

You're OK, It's Just a Bruise: A Doctor's Sideline Secrets about Pro Football's Most... Rob Huizenga. 1995. LC 95-22962. 336p. pap. 14.95 (*0-312-13627-7*) St Martin.

Yours for Health: The Life & Times of Herbert M. Shelton. Jean A. Oswald. 1989. (Illus.). 168p. (Orig.). pap. 9.95 (*0-9620490-0-X*) Franklin Bks.

Youth, AIDS, & Sexually Transmitted Diseases. Anne Mitchell et al. 1996. LC 96-11013. (Adolescence & Society Ser.). 192p. (C). 84.95 (*0-415-10632-X*); pap. 26.95 (*0-415-10633-8*) Routledge.

Youth, Alcohol, & Social Policy. Ed. by Howard T. Blane & M. E. Chafetz. 1979. LC 79-9094. (Illus.). 450p. 65.00 (*0-306-40253-X*, Plenum Trade) Perseus Pubng.

Youth & Drugs: Proceedings of the WHO Scientific Group, Geneva, 1971. WHO Staff. 1973. (Technical Reports: No. 516). pap. text 6.00 (*92-4-120516-4*, 1100516) World Health.

Youth & Exploitation: A Process Leading to Running Away, Violence, Substance Abuse & Suicide. Alan W. McEvoy & Edsel L. Erickson. 1990. (gr. 7-12). pap. 12.95 (*1-55691-042-8*, 428) Learning Pubns.

Youth & Sex: Pleasure & Responsibility. Gordon D. Jensen. 2nd ed. 1979. LC 72-77121. (Illus.). text 29.95 (*0-911012-99-0*) Burnham Inc.

Youth Suicide. Michael Peck et al. 1986. (Death & Suicide Ser.: Vol. 6). 224p. pap. 33.95 (*0-8261-4481-0*) Springer Pub.

Youth Suicide: Issues, Assessment & Intervention. Crisis Intervention Staff. Ed. by Peter Cimbolic & David A. Jobes. 1990. 138p. (C). text 35.95 (*0-398-05706-0*) C C Thomas.

Youth Violence: Prevention, Intervention, & Social Policy. Ed. by Daniel J. Flannery & C. Ronald Huff. 1998. LC 98-22464. (Clinical Practice Ser.). 336p. text 49.50 (*0-88048-809-3*, 8809) Am Psychiatric.

You've Got a Friend: New Life After Breast Cancer. Yvonne Manley. 2001. (Illus.). 184p. pap. 14.95 (*1-57826-056-6*) Hatherleigh.

Ypsilanti-Carnegie Infant Education Project: Longitudinal Follow-Up. Ann S. Epstein & David P. Weikart. 1980. LC 80-10939. (Monographs of the High/Scope Educational Research Foundation: No. 6). 80p. (Orig.). pap. 12.95 (*0-931114-06-3*, R1026) High-Scope.

Yr Prsnl Vitamin Pfl. Michael Colgan. 1982. LC 82-12560. 304p. pap. 10.00 (*0-688-01506-9*, Quil) HarperTrade.

Y2K & You & Yours. Cherokee Chas. 1999. 50p. 9.95 (*0-9670685-0-9*) H & H Ltd.

Y2K Compliance Manual for the Medical Office. Frank J. Cohen. 1999. LC 99-25759. (*1-57066-145-6*) Practice Mgmt Info.

Z

Zab: Brevet Major Zabdiel Boylston Adams, 1829-1902, Physician. Charles N. Peabody. 1984. 255p. 17.50 (*0-8139-1066-8*) F A Countway.

Zackback Sitting: The Revolutionary Solution for Relieving Your Pain & Improving Your Posture! Dennis Zacharkow. 1998. LC 97-61826. (Illus.). 123p. pap. 13.95 (*0-9660169-3-9*, Z-49) Zackback.

Zahn - Mund - Kiefer: Rezepte und Therapien. E. Lautenbach. 1990. (Illus.). vi, 1266p. 141.75 (*3-8055-5098-7*) S Karger.

Zang Fu: The Organ Systems of Traditional Chinese Medicine. Jeremy Ross. 2nd ed. 1989. (Illus.). 200p. (C). text (*0-443-03482-6*) Church.

Zap! How Your Computer Can Hurt You & What You Can Do About It. Don Sellers. 1995. (Illus.). 160p. (C). pap. text 12.95 (*1-56609-021-0*) Peachpit Pr.

Zapp! Empowerment in Health Care. William C. Byham. 1993. LC 93-90240. 309p. pap. 11.00 (*0-449-90885-2*) Fawcett.

Zapp! How to Improve Quality, Productivity, & Employee Satisfaction. William C. Byham. rev. ed. 1997. LC 97-97003. (Illus.). 208p. pap. 12.00 (*0-449-00282-9*) Fawcett.

Zebra Cards: An Aid to Obscure Diagnosis. John G. Sotos. 1989. 92p. pap. 23.00 (*0-943126-13-4*, ZEC89) Amer Coll Phys.

Zen & the Heart of Psychotherapy. Robert Rosenbaum. 1998. LC 98-22924. 320p. 49.95 (*0-87630-891-4*) Brunner-Routledge.

Zen in the Art of Child Maintenance. Michael Pastore & Larry Pastor. 1993. LC 92-82027. 120p. pap. 14.95 (*0-927379-28-7*, ZP 99) Zorba Pr.

Zen of Eating: Ancient Answers to Modern Weight Problems. Ronna Kabatznick. 1998. LC 97-23778. 208p. pap. 13.00 (*0-399-52382-0*) Berkley Pub.

Zen-Touch & the Art of Shiatsu: Fundamental Applications in Acupressure Massage. Seymour A. Koblin. rev. ed. (Illus.). 147p. reprint ed. pap. 15.95 (*0-9625000-2-X*) Soulstar Creations.

Zerebrale Bewegungsstoerungen. Ed. by E. Koeng. 1981. (Paediatrische Fortbildungskurse fuer die Praxis Ser.: Vol. 53). (Illus.). viii, 200p. pap. 71.50 (*3-8055-3413-2*) S Karger.

Zerebrale Bewegungsstoerungen Beim Kind. Ed. by E. G. Koenig. 1974. (Paediatrische Fortbildungskurse fuer die Praxis Ser.: Vol. 40). (Illus.). 212p. 42.75 (*3-8055-1781-5*) S Karger.

Zerebrale Mikrozirkulation. Ed. by F. Hammersen & K. Messmer. 1990. (Illus.). x, 112p. pap. 71.50 (*3-8055-5208-4*) S Karger.

Zero Balancing: Touching the Energy of Bone. John Hamwee. 2000. (Illus.). 144p. pap. 17.50 (*1-55643-335-2*) North Atlantic.

Zero-Base Hospital: Survival & Success in America's Evolving Healthcare System. Matthew M. Person, III. 1997. LC 96-36383. 248p. 44.00 (*1-56793-049-2*) Health Admin Pr.

Zero Population Growth—For Whom? Differential Fertility & Minority Group Survival, 30. Ed. by Milton Himmelfarb & Victor Baras. 1978. LC 77-87966. (Contributions in Sociology Ser.: No. 30). (Illus.). 213p. 65.00 (*0-313-20041-6*, AJC/, Greenwood Pr) Greenwood.

Zhen Jiu Fang Zhi Shen Fen Lie Zheng see Soothing the Troubled Mind: Treatment & Prevention of Schizophrenia with Acupuncture & Moxibustion

Zhong Yi Fuke Shou Ce see Handbook of Traditional Chinese Gynecology

Zinc: Clinical & Biochemical Significance. Stephen C. Cunnane. 1988. 224p. 126.00 (*0-8493-6735-2*, QP535, CRC Reprint) Franklin.

Zinc & Diseases of the Digestive Tract. Ed. by J. D. Kruse-Jarres & J. Scholmerich. 1997. LC 97-188077. 144p. text 93.50 (*0-7923-8724-4*) Kluwer Academic.

Zinc & Eating Disorders. Alexander G. Schauss. 1993. 32p. pap. 2.50 (*0-87983-507-9*, Keats Pubng) McGraw-Hill Trade.

Zinc in Human Nutrition. A. Prasad. 1979. LC 79-15272. 96p. 61.00 (*0-8493-0145-9*, CRC Reprint) Franklin.

Zinc Metalloproteases in Health & Disease. N. M. Hooper. 1996. 350p. 132.00 (*0-7484-0442-2*) Taylor & Francis.

Zinssers Microbiology. Wolfgang K. Joklik. 20th ed. 1995. LC 91-41219. (Illus.). 1294p. (C). pap. text 99.00 (*0-8385-9983-4*, A9983-6, Apple Lange Med) McGraw.

Zizek Reader. Ed. by Elizabeth Wright & Edmund Wright. 1999. LC 98-8551. (Blackwell Readers Ser.). xii, 332p. 70.95 (*0-631-21200-0*); pap. 26.95 (*0-631-21201-9*) Blackwell Pubs.

ZN Superoxide Dismutase Gene in Belgian Patients with Familial or Sporadic Amyotrophic Lateral Sclerosis. Tania Aguirre. 1998. (Acta Biomedica Lovaniensia Ser.). (Illus.). 95p. pap. (*90-6186-885-8*) Leuven Univ BEL. *Dist:* Coronet Bks.

Zoloft, Paxil, Luvox & Prozac: All New Information to Help You Choose the Right Antidepressant. Donald L. Sullivan. 1999. LC 98-91016. 224p. mass mkt. 5.99 (*0-380-79518-3*, Avon Bks) Morrow Avon.

Zonal Liver Cell Heterogeneity. Ed. by K. Jungermann. 1992. (Enzyme Ser.: Vol. 46, Nos. 1-3, 1992). (Illus.). 168p. pap. 46.25 (*3-8055-5718-3*) S Karger.

Zone: A Dietary Road Map to Lose Weight Permanently, Reset Your Genetic Code, Prevent Disease. Barry Sears & Bill Lawren. 2000. 336p. mass mkt. 6.99 (*0-06-101000-6*); 1995. LC 95-17096. 352p. 25.00 (*0-06-039150-2*, ReganBooks) HarperCollins Pubs.

Zone Therapy: Using Foot Massage. Astrid I. Goosmann-Legger. 3rd ed. (Illus.). 128p. pap. 14.95 (*0-8464-4315-5*) Beekman Pubs.

Zone Therapy Using Foot Massage. Astrid Goosemann-Legger. 1986. 112p. pap. (*0-85207-170-1*) C W Daniel GBR. *Dist:* Natl Bk Netwk.

Zoo & Wild Animal Medicine. Murray E. Fowler. (Illus.). 2nd ed. 1986. 1127p. text 150.00 (*0-7216-1013-7*); 3rd ed. 1993. 864p. text 110.00 (*0-7216-3667-5*) Saunders.

Zoo & Wild Animal Medicine: Current Therapy 4. Murray E. Fowler & R. Eric Miller. Ed. by Stephanie Donley. 4th ed. 1998. LC 97-47281. (Illus.). xxiii, 747p. (C). text 89.00 (*0-7216-8664-8*) Saunders.

Zoology. Robert Dorit et al. 1991. LC 90-50861. 1136p. (C). text 129.00 (*0-03-030504-7*) SCP.

Zoonomia: or The Laws of Organic Life Erasmus Darwin. LC 79-147964. reprint ed. (*0-404-08215-7*) AMS Pr.

Zoonoses: Animal Diseases & Man. Louw W. Van den Heever & Jan H. Du Preez. 1999. (Illus.). 136p. pap. 19.95 (*0-409-11380-8*) Buttrwrth-Heinemann.

Zoonoses: Biology, Clinical Practice & Public Health Control. Ed. by Stephen R. Palmer et al. 1998. LC 97-30387. (Illus.). 968p. text 198.50 (*0-19-262380-X*) OUP.

Zoonoses: Recognition, Control & Prevention. Martin E. Hugh-Jones et al. 2000. LC 00-26919. (Illus.). 369p. pap. 39.95 (*0-8138-2542-3*) Iowa U Pr.

Zoonoses: Report of the FAO-WHO Expert Committee on Zoonoses, 3rd, Geneva, 1966. FAO-WHO Expert Committee on Zoonoses. 1967. (Technical Reports: No. 378). (ENG, FRE, RUS & SPA.). 127p. pap. text 7.00 (*92-4-120378-1*, 1100378) World Health.

Zoonoses & Communicable Diseases Common to Man & Animals. 2nd ed. 1987. (Paho Scientific Publication Ser.: No. 503). 983p. text 60.00 (*92-75-11503-6*) World Health.

Zoonotic Diseases: Special Reference Briefs Bibliography (1988-1994) Ed. by Michael D. Kreger. 2000. 84p. (C). pap. text 20.00 (*0-7881-8576-4*) DIANE Pub.

Zootoxins & Animal Envenomation. Murray E. Fowler. 1992. 272p. lib. bdg. 110.00 (*0-8493-6791-3*, SF757) CRC Pr.

Zopiclone: A Third Generation of Hypnotics. Ed. by A. Schlosberg et al. 1984. (Journal: Vol. 27, Suppl. 2). (Illus.). iv, 252p. pap. 64.50 (*3-8055-3788-3*) S Karger.

Zum Problem der Begabung und Intelligenz. Hans Werder. 1980. (Psychologische Praxis Ser.: Vol. 55). vi, 194p. pap. 24.50 (*3-8055-1123-X*) S Karger.

Zur Genese des Selbstbewusstseins: Eine Studie ueber den Beitrag des phaenomenologischen Denkens zur Frage der Entwicklung des Selbstbewusstseins. Ursula Rohr-Dietschi. 1975. LC 72-81567. (Phaenomenologisch-Psychologische Forschungen Ser.: Vol. 14). 197p. (C). 79.25 (*3-11-004048-4*) De Gruyter.

Zur Sozio-Genese des Chronischen Alkoholismus. P. Wuethrich. 1974. (Sozialmedizinische und Paedagogische Jugendkunde Ser.: Band 10). (Illus.). 200p. 35.00 (*3-8055-1695-9*) S Karger.

Zwang und Schizophrenie. H. Feer. 1973. (Bibliotheca Psychiatrica Ser.: No. 150). 108p. 39.25 (*3-8055-1546-4*) S Karger.

Zwei Hundert-Jahr-Feier der I. Universitaets-Frauenklinik Wien: Universitaets-Frauenklinik Wien. Ed. by Eduard Gitsch. 1990. (Journal: Vol. 29, Suppl. 3, 1989). (Illus.). iv, 60p. pap. 20.00 (*3-8055-5107-X*) S Karger.

Zweymuller Total Hip Prosthesis: 15 Years' Experience. Ed. by Karl Zweymuller. 1997. (Illus.). 230p. pap. text 59.00 (*0-88937-191-1*) Hogrefe & Huber Pubs.

Zwischen Leben und Tod: Aspekte der Judischen Medizinethik. Yves Nordmann. 1999. 121p. 30.95 (*3-906760-94-4*) P Lang Pubng.

PUBLISHER SYMBOL INDEX

A & AFOA, *(Asthma & Allergy Foundation of America, Maryland Chapter, Inc.; 0-9643272),* Chester Bldg., Suite 321, 8600 LaSalle Rd., Towson, MD 21286-2002 Tel 410-321-4710; Fax: 410-321-0137; Toll Free: 800-727-9333 Do not confuse with Asthma & Allergy Foundation of America, Washington, DC
E-mail: aafamd@bepl.net
Web site: http://www.aafa-md.org.

A & C Blk (GBR) *(0-245; 0-333; 0-510; 0-7136; 0-85177; 0-85314; 0-212; 0-85146; 0-85147; 0-85317; 0-86019; 0-946716; 0-9507160; 1-85691) Dist. by* **Lubrecht & Cramer.**

A A Balkema (NLD) *(0-86961; 90-5410; 90-6191; 90-5809) Dist. by* **Ashgate Pub Co.**

A A D U P A Y Publng, *(AADUPAY Publishing; 1-931386),* Div. of Hollis Enterprises, Inc., P.O. Box 20162, Beaumont, TX 77720 Tel 409-796-1711; Fax: 409-796-1406.

A A Farmar (IRL) *(1-899047) Dist. by* **Irish Bks Media.**

A A Grapevine, *(AA Grapevine, Inc.; 0-933685),* Orders Addr.: P.O. Box 1980, New York, NY 10163-1980 (SAN 662-7773); Edit Addr.: 475 Riverside Dr., No. 1040, New York, NY 10115-0122 (SAN 692-5162) Tel 212-870-3400; Fax: 212-870-3301
Web site: http://www. aagrapevine.org.

A A Wenger, *(Wenger, Allan A.; 0-9627652),* 8710 Arran Rd., Richmond, VA 23235 Tel 804-272-0037.

A Arnold, *See* **Transform WA**

A Aronowitz, *(Aronowitz, Abby; 0-9703713),* 40 Underhill Blvd., Suite LC, Syosset, NY 11791 Tel 516-682-5920.

A B Anup, *(Anup, A. B.; 0-9657083),* 15 Lucia Ct., Matawan, NJ 07747-1372 Fax: 732-441-7474.

A C Hood, *(Hood, Alan C. & Co., Inc.; 0-911469),* P.O. Box 775, Chambersburg, PA 17201 (SAN 270-8221) Tel 717-267-0867; Fax: 717-267-0572.

A Cohen, *(Cohen, Alan Pubns.; 0-910367),* 430 Kukuna, Haiku, HI 96708 (SAN 239-4227) Tel 808-572-0001; Fax: 808-572-1023
E-mail: acpubs@aloha.net; acpubs.@maui.net
Web site: htp://www.alancohen.com/
Dist(s): **Bookpeople** *(Bookpeople)*
New Leaf Dist *(New Leaf Distributing Co., Inc.).*

A E Jones Sci, *(Jones, A.E. Scientific Publishing Co., Inc.; 1-883883),* 149 Peyton Pl., SW, No. 1, Atlanta, GA 30311-1612 Tel 404-505-9706.

A Ellis Institute, *(Albert Ellis Institute; 0-917476),* 45 E. 65th St., New York, NY 10021 (SAN 210-3079) Tel 212-535-0822; Fax: 212-249-3582; Toll Free: 800-323-4738
E-mail: info@rebt.org
Web site: http://www.rebt.org.

A Finkelstein, *See* **Fifty Gates**

A Friedlander, *(Friedlander, Abraham; 0-9643008),* 1157 51st St., Brooklyn, NY 11219 Tel 718-436-1089.

A Granite Pubs, *(A Granite Pubs.; 0-935669),* 4712 Beau Lac Ln., Metairie, LA 70002-1455.

A H A F, *(American Health Assistance Foundation; 1-930181),* 15825 Shady Grove Rd., Suite 140, Rockville, MD 20850 Tel 301-948-3244; Fax: 301-258-9454; Toll Free: 800-437-2423
E-mail: aphillips@ahaf.org
Web site: http://www.ahaf.org.

A H S Ltd (GBR) *(0-7223) Dist. by* **St Mut.**

A Holland, *(Holland, Alex; 0-9622665),* 210 Polk St., No. 3, Port Townsend, WA 98368 Tel 360-385-4383.

A J Linenthal, *(Linenthal, Arthur J.; 0-9626606),* 411 Del Pond Dr., Canton, MA 02021-2756 Tel 617-828-8486.

A Kron, *(Kron, Audrey; 0-9633877),* Affil. of Center for Coping with Chronic Illness, 7466 Pebble Ln., West Bloomfield, MI 48322 Tel 248-626-6960; Fax: 248-626-1379
E-mail: shrinka@aol.com
Web site: http://www.chronicillness.com.

A M Pubng Ltd, *(AM Publishing, Ltd.; 0-9717064),* 18 Waterford Ln., Beachwood, OH 44122-7591 Do not confuse with A M Publishing in Wheatridge, CO
E-mail: cxd5@po.cwru.edu.

A Natural Path, *(A Natural Path; 0-9619435),* P.O. Box 70, Lewis, CO 81327 (SAN 244-8998) Tel 970-882-8888
E-mail: cheyannewest@frontier.net
Web site: http://www.cheyannewest.com.

A P P L E Fam, *(APPLE Family Ctr.; 0-9630874),* 70 Skyview Terr., San Rafael, CA 94903 Tel 415-492-0720.

A Paolino, *See* **Adele Roberts**

A Peters Consult, *(Peters, Andrew Consulting; 0-9702725),* 206 Royal Ct., No. 3, Appleton, WI 54915-1646 Tel 920-991-9210
E-mail: arpeters@juno.com
Web site: http://www.geocites.com/andrewpetersdc.

A R Biel, *See* **Bks of Discov**

A R Harding Pub, *(Harding, A.R. Publishing Co.; 0-936622),* 2878 E. Main St., Columbus, OH 43209 (SAN 206-4936) Tel 614-231-9585.

A S Assn, *See* **Spondylitis Assn**

A Schweitzer, *(Schweitzer, Albert Institute-Quinnipiac College Pr.; 1-885007),* P.O. Box 550, Wallingford, CT 06492-0550.

A Sharp, *(Sharp, Anne; 0-9625382),* 914 Lincoln Blvd., Apt. 308, Santa Monica, CA 90403-2827.

A Spangler, *(Spangler, Amy; 0-9627450),* P.O. Box 501046, Atlanta, GA 31150-1046 Tel 770-913-9332; Fax: 770-913-0822
E-mail: akspangler@aol.com
Dist(s): **Baker & Taylor** *(Baker & Taylor Bks.)*
Bookpeople *(Bookpeople)*
Koen Bk Distributors *(Koen Bk. Distributors)*
Quality Bks IL *(Quality Bks., Inc.).*

Aa Zz Pub, *(Aa to Zz Publishing Co.; 0-9628734),* 506 Valley Dr., E., Chittenango, NY 13037 Tel 315-687-9631.

AAAHCR, *(American Assn. for Advances in Health Care Research; 0-945769),* c/o Univ. of Rhode Island, Marketing Dept., Kingston, RI 02881.

AAAI Pr, *(AAAI Pr.; 0-262; 0-929280; 1-57735),* Div. MIT Pr., 445 Burgess Dr., Menlo Park, CA 94025 (SAN 679-1905) Tel 650-328-3123; Fax: 650-321-4457
E-mail: orders@aaai.org; press@aaai.org
Web site: http://www.aaai.org/Press/
Dist(s): **MIT Pr** *(MIT Pr.).*

AAAS, *(AAAS, The American Assn. for the Advancement of Science; 0-87168),* Orders Addr.: P.O. Box 521, Annapolis Junction, MD 20702 Tel 301-490-0056; Fax: 301-843-0159; Toll Free: 800-222-7809; Edit Addr.: 1200 New York Ave., NW, Washington, DC 20005 (SAN 201-193X) Tel 202-326-6400
E-mail: webmaster@aaas.org; jkegg@aaas.org
Web site: http://www.aaas.org.

AAASPD, *(American Assn. for the Advancement of Science, Pacific Div.; 0-934394),* Orders Addr.: Univ. of Montana, Div. of Biological Sciences, Missoula, MT 59812-1002 (SAN 204-3661) Tel 406-243-4012
E-mail: aaaspd@selway.umt.edu
Web site: http://.biology.umt.edu/aaas.

AABB Pr Imprint of Am Assn Blood

AACC Pr Imprint of Am Assn Clinical Chem

AACN, *(American Assn. of Colleges of Nursing; 0-922148),* 1 Dupont Cir., NW, Suite 530, Washington, DC 20036 (SAN 266-4496) Tel 202-463-6930; Fax: 202-785-8320.

AACP Alexandria, *(American Assn. of Colleges of Pharmacy; 0-937526),* 1426 Prince St., Alexandria, VA 22314 (SAN 202-4292) Tel 703-739-2330
Web site: http://www.aacp.org.

AAH Ctrs, *(Association of Academic Health Ctrs.; 1-879694),* 1400 16th St. NW, Suite 720, Washington, DC 20036 Tel 202-265-9600; Fax: 202-265-7514
E-mail: ahc@acadhlthctrs.org
Web site: http://www.ahcnet.org.

AAHA Pr Imprint of Am Animal Hosp Assoc

Aah-ha Bks, *(Aah-ha! Bks.; 1-889853),* 12 Virginia Ct., Amityville, NY 11701 Tel 516-598-8842; Fax: 516-691-1357; Toll Free: 888-238-1548
E-mail: book@starwater.com
Web site: http://www.starwater.com.

AAHPERD, *(American Alliance for Health, Physical Education, Recreation & Dance; 0-88314),* Orders Addr.: P.O. Box 385, Oxon Hill, MD 20750-0385 (SAN 202-3237) Tel 301-839-9808; Fax: 301-567-9553; Toll Free: 800-321-0789; Edit Addr.: 1900 Association Dr., Reston, VA 22091 Toll Free: 800-213-7193
Web site: http://www.aahperd.org.

AAL QualityLife, *(AAL QualityLife Resources; 0-9701509; 1-931380),* Div. of Aid Association for Lutherans, 4321 N. Ballard Rd., Appleton, WI 54919-0001 Tel 920-734-5721; Fax: 920-730-4725; Toll Free: 800-225-5225
E-mail: aalmail@aal.org
Web site: http://www.aal.org
Dist(s): **IPG Chicago** *(Independent Pubs. Group).*

AAO-HNS, *(American Academy of Otolaryngology-Head & Neck Surgery Foundation, Inc.; 1-56772),* Orders Addr.: 1 Prince St., Alexandria, VA 22314-3357 Tel 703-836-4444; Fax: 703-519-1570; Toll Free Fax: 888-292-2703
Web site: http://www.entnet.org.

AAPB, *(Association for Applied Psychophysiology & Biofeedback; 1-887114),* 10200 W. 44th Ave. Suite 304, Wheat Ridge, CO 80033-2840 Tel 303-422-8436; Fax: 303-422-8894
E-mail: aapb@resourcenter.com
Web site: http://www.aapb.org.

AAPM, *(American Assn. of Physicists in Medicine (AAPM); 1-888340),* One Physics Ellipse, College Park, MD 20740-3846 Tel 301-209-3350; Fax: 301-209-0862.

Aarhus Univ Pr (DNK) *(87-7288; 87-87600; 88-8145; 87-7934) Dist. by* **David Brown.**

AAWS, *(Alcoholics Anonymous World Services, Inc.; 0-916856; 1-893007),* Orders Addr.: P.O. Box 459, New York, NY 10163 (SAN 215-0441); Edit Addr.: 475 Riverside Dr., 11th Flr., New York, NY 10115 (SAN 210-7678) Tel 212-870-3400; Fax: 212-870-3137
Dist(s): **Hazelden** *(Hazelden Information & Educational Services).*

Publisher Symbol Index

A&B Bks, *(A&B Bks.; 1-881316; 1-886433),* Div. of A&B Distributors, 1000 Atlantic Ave., Brooklyn, NY 11238 (SAN 630-9216) Tel 718-783-7808; Fax: 718-783-7267; 146 Lawrence St., Brooklyn, NY 11201 (SAN 631-385X)
E-mail: maxtay@webspan.net
Dist(s): **D&J Bk Dist** *(D&J Bk. Distributors)*
Red Sea Pr *(Red Sea Pr.).*

ABA Antitrust Imprint of Amer Bar Assn

Abacus Imprint of Gordon & Breach

Abaris Bks, *(Abaris Bks.; 0-89835; 0-913870),* 70 New Canaan Ave., Norwalk, CT 06850-2600 (SAN 206-4588) Tel 203-849-1655; Fax: 203-849-9181
E-mail: abaris@abarisbooks.com; abarisbooks@worldnet.att.net
Web site: http://www.abarisbooks.com.

†**ABBE Pubs Assn,** *(ABBE Pubs. Assn. of Washington, D.C.; 0-7883; 0-88164; 0-941864; 1-55914),* Orders Addr.: 4111 Gallows Rd., Virginia Div., Annandale, VA 22003 (SAN 239-1430) Fax: 703-642-5966; Edit Addr.: Georgetown 3724, 1215 31st St., NW, Washington, DC 20007 (SAN 668-9450)
Dist(s): **Academic Bk Ctr Inc** *(Academic Bk. Ctr., Inc.)*
Am Overseas Bk Co *(American Overseas Bk. Co., Inc.)*
Baker & Taylor *(Baker & Taylor Bks.)*
Barnes & Noble Inc *(Barnes & Noble, Inc.); CIP.*

Abbey, *(Abbey Pr.; 0-87029),* 1 Hill Dr., Saint Meinrad, IN 47577-0128 (SAN 201-2057) Tel 812-357-8215; Fax: 812-357-8388; Toll Free: 800-325-2511
E-mail: customerservice@abbeypress.com
Web site: http://www.abbeypress.com/.

Abbeygate Pr, *(Abbeygate Pr.; 1-885762),* P.O. Box 117223, Burlingame, CA 94011-7223 Tel 650-343-4994
E-mail: DAAE@juno.com.

Abbott Laboratories, *(Abbott Laboratories, Diagnostics Div.; 0-9614903),* Orders Addr.: P.O. Box 152020, Irving, TX 75016 (SAN 665-8830) Tel 847-937-2845.

†**ABC-CLIO,** *(ABC-CLIO, Inc.; 0-87436; 0-903450; 1-57607; 1-85109),* Orders Addr.: P.O. Box 1911, Santa Barbara, CA 93116-1911 Tel 805-968-1911; Fax: 805-685-9685; Toll Free: 800-368-6868; Edit Addr.: 130 Cremona Dr., Santa Barbara, CA 93117 (SAN 301-5467)
E-mail: sales@abc-clio.com
Web site: http://www.abc-clio.com
Dist(s): **Baker & Taylor** *(Baker & Taylor Bks.)*
Bookhouse *(Bookhouse, The)*
netLibrary CO *(netLibrary, Inc.); CIP.*

ABCs, *(ABCs, (Applied Behaviorology Consultants); 1-882508),* 9 Farmer St., Canton, NY 13617-1120 Tel 315-386-2684
E-mail: sledoux@twcny.rr.com.

Aberdeen U Pr (GBR) *(0-08; 0-900015; 1-85752) Dist. by* **Macmillan.**

Abhinav (IND) *Dist. by* **S Asia.**

ABI Prof Pubns, *(ABI Professional Publications; 1-886236),* Orders Addr.: P.O. Box 5243, Arlington, VA 22205 Tel 703-538-5750; Fax: 703-536-9644; Toll Free: 800-551-7776; Edit Addr.: 433 N. Maple Ave., Falls Church, VA 22046.

Abiding Health, *(Abiding Health; 0-9661036),* P.O. Box 3828, Salinas, CA 93912 Tel 408-633-1607
E-mail: mmgoulding@worldnet.att.net.

Ability Workshop Pr, *(Ability Workshop Pr.; 0-929551),* 1601 Old Bayshore Hwy., Suite 260B, Burlingame, CA 94010 (SAN 249-3934) Tel 650-692-8993; Fax: 650-692-8997; Toll Free: 800-897-9001
E-mail: EldonB123@aol.com
Dist(s): **Baker & Taylor** *(Baker & Taylor Bks.).*

†**Abingdon,** *(Abingdon Pr.; 0-687),* Div. of United Methodist Publishing Hse., Orders Addr.: P.O. Box 801, Nashville, TN 37202-3919 (SAN 201-0054) Tel 615-749-6409; Fax: 615-749-6056; Toll Free Fax: 800-836-7802; Toll Free: 800-251-3320; Edit Addr.: 201 Eighth Ave., S., Nashville, TN 37202 (SAN 699-9956)
E-mail: info@abingdon.org
Web site: http://www.abingdon.org; *CIP.*

ABLE GA, *(Association for Biology Laboratory Education, Inc.-ABLE; 0-9626182; 1-890444),* c/o Susan Karcher, Dept. of Biological Science, Purdue University, West Lafayette, IN 47907 Tel 765-494-8083; Fax: 765-494-0876
E-mail: suek@bilbo.bio.purdue.edu
Web site: http://www.zoo.utoronto.ca/able; http://www.zoo.utoronto.ca/able/proc/contents.html.volume.

Able Pr, *(Able Pr.; 0-9627555),* Div. of Able Systems, Orders Addr.: P.O. Box 101, Canandaigua, NY 14424 (SAN 297-3146); Edit Addr.: 5133 Silvernail Dr., Suite E, Canandaigua, NY 14424 Tel 716-394-8926
Dist(s): **Baker & Taylor** *(Baker & Taylor Bks.).*

Ablex Imprint of Greenwood

Ablin Pr, *(Ablin Pr. Distributors; 0-9621429),* 700 John Ringling Blvd., No. 1603, Sarasota, FL 34236 (SAN 250-2216) Tel 941-361-7521; Fax: 941-363-9505.

ABPMR, *(American Board of Physical Medicine & Rehabilitation; 0-9657664),* 21 First St., Suite 674, NW., Rochester, MN 55902-3009 Tel 507-282-1776; Fax: 507-282-9242.

Abrahamson Pub, *(Abrahamson Publishing Co.; 0-9617195),* Subs. of MC Corp. of Stillwater, 10164 Norell Ave., Stillwater, MN 55082 (SAN 663-2440) Tel 612-439-2680.

Abrams, *(Abrams, Harry N. Inc.; 0-8109),* 100 Fifth Ave., New York, NY 10011 (SAN 200-2434) Tel 212-206-7715; Fax: 212-645-8437
E-mail: webmaster@abramsbooks.com
Web site: http://www.abramsbooks.com
Dist(s): **AOL Time Warner** *(AOL Time Warner Bk. Group)*
Art Inst Chi *(Art Institute of Chicago)*
Continental Bk *(Continental Bk. Co., Inc.)*
Many Feathers Bks & Maps *(Many Feathers Bks. & Maps)*
Shens Bks *(Shen's Bks.).*

Abt Bks, *(Abt Bks., Inc.; 0-89011),* 19 Follen St., Cambridge, MA 02138-3502 (SAN 207-9402) Tel 617-876-2835; Fax: 617-661-1300.

Abundant Hlth Pub, *(Abundant Health Publishers; 0-9645645),* P.O. Box 1647, Lake Panasoffkee, FL 33538 (SAN 169-1449) Tel 352-793-4571 (phone/fax)
E-mail: dvailla520@aol.com
Dist(s): **New Leaf Dist** *(New Leaf Distributing Co., Inc.).*

Abundant Living, *(Abundant Living; 0-9654714),* 346 E. State St., Saint Croix Falls, WI 54024 Tel 715-483-1430 (phone/fax); Toll Free: 888-548-4680
E-mail: woodlands@abundantlivinginc.com
Web site: http://www.abundantlivinginc.com.

Aburn Hse Paperback Imprint of Greenwood

ACA Pr, *See* **ACA Pubns**

ACA Pubns, *(ACA Pubns., Inc.; 0-9631544),* 1690 Univ. Ave. W., No. 450, Saint Paul, MN 55104 Tel 612-917-4285; Fax: 612-649-3509; Toll Free: 800-649-3523
Dist(s): **Baker & Taylor** *(Baker & Taylor Bks.)*
Bookmen Inc *(Bookmen, Inc.)*
Quality Bks IL *(Quality Bks., Inc.).*

Acad Comm, *(Academic Communication Assocs.; 0-930951; 1-57503),* Orders Addr.: P.O. Box 4279, Oceanside, CA 92052-4279 (SAN 678-8726) Tel 760-758-9593; Fax: 760-758-1604.

Acad Educ Dev, *(Academy for Educational Development, Inc.; 0-89492),* 1875 Connecticut Ave., NW, Washington, DC 20009-5721 (SAN 210-0185) Tel 202-884-8000; Fax: 202-884-8400
E-mail: admindc@aed.org
Web site: http://www.aed.org.

Acad Hospice, *See* **Am Acad Hospice**

Acad Info Systs, *(Academic Information Systems; 0-9663422),* 3205 Woodvalley Way, Columbia, MO 65203 Tel 573-882-1209; Fax: 573-884-4612
E-mail: aiscolmd@aol.com; pathdix@showme.missouri.edu
Dist(s): **Demos Medical** *(Demos Medical Publishing, Inc.).*

Acad Med Sys, *(Academy Medical Systems, Inc.; 1-879575; 1-930450),* 4000 Palos Verdes Dr. N., No 108, Rolling HIlls Estates, CA 90274 Tel 310-544-3500; Fax: 310-544-0380
Web site: http://www.academymedical.com.

†**Acad Pr,** *(Academic Pr., Inc.; 0-12),* Subs. of Harcourt, Orders Addr.: 6277 Sea Harbor Dr., Orlando, FL 32887 (SAN 206-8990) Toll Free Fax: 800-874-6418; Toll Free: 800-321-5068; Edit Addr.: 525 B St., Suite 1900, San Diego, CA 92101-4495 (SAN 241-5984) Tel 619-231-6616; Fax: 619-699-6380; Toll Free Fax: 800-336-7377
E-mail: apbcs@harcourtbrace.com; ap@acad.com
Web site: http://www.academicpress.com; *CIP.*

Acad Rsch Assocs, *(Academic Research Assocs., Inc.; 0-9629180),* 15 Cole Rd., Armonk, NY 10504 Tel 212-628-6914; Fax: 212-746-8447.

Acad Therapy, *(Academic Therapy Pubns., Inc.; 0-87879; 1-57128),* 20 Commercial Blvd., Novato, CA 94949-6191 (SAN 201-2111) Tel 415-883-3314; Fax: 415-883-3720; Toll Free: 800-422-7249 ;
Imprints: Ann Arbor Div (Ann Arbor Division)
E-mail: sales@academictherapy.com; customerservice@academictherapy.com
Web site: http://www.academictherapy.com
Dist(s): **PCI Educ Pubg** *(PCI Educational Publishing)*
PRO-ED *(PRO-ED, Inc.)*
Saddleback Pubns *(Saddleback Publishing, Inc.)*
Sopris *(Sopris West).*

†**Academy Chi Pubs,** *(Academy Chicago Pubs., Ltd.; 0-89733; 0-915864),* 363 W. Erie St., Chicago, IL 60610-3125 (SAN 213-2001) Tel 312-751-7300; Fax: 312-751-7306; Toll Free: 800-248-7323 (Orders, outside Illinois)
E-mail: academy363@aol.com
Web site: http://www.academychicago.com
Dist(s): **Baker & Taylor** *(Baker & Taylor Bks.)*
Brodart *(Brodart Co.); CIP.*

Academy Prof Inform, *(Academy Professional Information Services, Inc.; 0-934205),* 116 W. 32nd St., 16th Flr., New York, NY 10001 (SAN 693-0085) Tel 212-736-6688; Fax: 212-564-1763
E-mail: amarekl@aol.com.

Academy Pubns, *(Academy Pubns.; 0-931560),* P.O. Box 5224, Sherman Oaks, CA 91413 (SAN 212-1778) Tel 818-788-6662; Fax: 818-788-1580.

†**Accel Devel,** *(Accelerated Development; 0-915202; 1-55959),* Member of Taylor & Francis Group, 1900 Frost Rd., Suite 101, Bristol, PA 19007-1598 (SAN 210-3346); *CIP.*

Accordia Pr Imprint of FastMark

ACEBO, *(ACEBO; 1-880594),* Orders Addr.: P.O. Box 7485, Spreckels, CA 93962 Tel 408-455-1507; Fax: 408-455-1541
E-mail: orders@acebo.com; acebo@acebo.com
Web site: http://www.acebo.com
Dist(s): **Continental Bk** *(Continental Bk. Co., Inc.).*

†**ACEI,** *(Association for Childhood Education International; 0-87173),* 17904 Georgia Ave., Suite 215, Olney, MD 20832-2277 (SAN 201-2200) Tel 301-570-2111; Fax: 301-570-2212; Toll Free: 800-423-3563
E-mail: aceihq@aol.com; aceied@ad.com
Web site: http://www.udel.edu/bateman/acei; *CIP.*

Achievement Pr, *(Achievement Pr.; 0-932707),* Orders Addr.: P.O. Box 608, Sheridan, WY 82801 (SAN 687-8571); Edit Addr.: 1501 Ft. MacKenzie Rd., Sheridan, WY 82801 (SAN 665-8687) Tel 307-672-8475.

Achilles Pub, *(Achilles Pub., Inc.; 0-9647741),* 19250 Bagley Rd., No. 107, Middleburg Heights, OH 44130 Tel 440-243-9191; Fax: 440-243-9971.

Achivmnt USA, *(Achievement U.S.A. Corp.; 0-9624825),* Orders Addr.: P.O. Box 9328, Washington, DC 20005 Tel 202-319-9057; Toll Free: 800-891-3296; Edit Addr.: 1313 Q St., NW, Washington, DC 20009.

ACMI Pr, *(ACMI Pr.; 1-883148),* 351 E. 84th St., No. 10D, New York, NY 10028 Tel 212-988-7750; Fax: 212-988-7764
Dist(s): **Midpt Trade** *(Midpoint Trade Bks., Inc.).*

ACOM, *(ACOM, Inc.; 0-9658744),* P.O. Box 2186, Kensington, MD 20891 Tel 301-881-7867.

Acoma Bks, *(Acoma Bks.; 0-916552),* P.O. Box 4, Ramona, CA 92065 (SAN 207-7221).

Acorn Books, *(Acorn Bks.; 0-9648957),* P.O. Box 7348, Springfield, IL 62791-7348 Tel 217-525-8202; Fax: 217-525-8212 Do not confuse with Acorn Bks., Kansas City, MO
E-mail: amy@afterabortion.org
Web site: http://www.afterabortion.org
Dist(s): **FaithWorks NBN** *(FaithWorks/NBN)*
Lightn Source *(Lightning Source, Inc.).*

Acorn MI, *(Acorn Publishing; 0-9678801; 0-9710988),* 186 N. 23rd St., Battle Creek, MI 49015-1711 Tel 616-962-8184 (phone/fax) Do not confuse with companies with the same or similar name in Broomfield, CO, Midvale, UT, Montpelier, VT, Sisters, OR, Suffern, NY, Salt Lake City, UT, Portland, OR
E-mail: editor@acornpublishing.com
Web site: http://www.acornpublishing.com.

Acorn NC, *(Acorn Pr., The; 0-89386),* 1010 Wyldewood Rd., P.O. Box 3279, Durham, NC 27715-3279 (SAN 216-4833) Tel 919-471-3842; Fax: 919-477-2622 Do not confuse with companies with the same name in Manchester-by-the-Sea, MA, San Jose, CA, Paris, IL
E-mail: info@theacornpress.com.

Acorn Pub, *(Acorn Publishing; 0-937921),* Div. of Vitesse Pr., PMB 367, 45 State St., Montpelier, VT 05602 (SAN 659-4840) Tel 802-229-4243; Fax: 802-229-6939 Do not confuse with companies with the same or similar name in Midvale, UT, Broomfield, CO, Battle Creek, MI, Sisters, OR, Suffern, NY,Saltlake City, UT, Portland, OR
E-mail: dick@vitessepress.com
Web site: http://www.vitessepress.com
Dist(s): **A C Hood** *(Hood, Alan C. & Co., Inc.).*

Acosep Corp, *(Acosep Corp.; 0-9616402),* 401 N. Plum St., Springfield, OH 45504 (SAN 658-9677) Tel 513-322-0111; Toll Free: 800-433-1177 (in Ohio).

Acoustical Soc Am, *(Acoustical Society of America),* 1N01, 2 Huntington Quadrangle, Melville, NY 11747-4502 (SAN 226-0026) Tel 516-576-2360; Fax: 516-576-2377
E-mail: asa@aip.org
Web site: http://.asa.aip.org.

Acrpls Bks GA, *(Acropolis Bks., Inc.; 1-889051),* 8601 Dunwoody Pl., Suite 303, Atlanta, GA 30350-2509 (SAN 299-1497) Toll Free: 800-773-9923 ; *Imprints:* I Lvl (I-Level)
E-mail: acropolisbooks@mindspring.com
Web site: http://www.acropolisbooks.com.

ACTA Pr, *(ACTA Pr.; 0-88986),* 2600 Nutwood Ave., Suite 200, Fullerton, CA 92814 (SAN 671-4633)
E-mail: journals@iasted.com
Web site: http://www.iasted.com.

ACTA Pubns, *(ACTA Pubns.; 0-87946; 0-914070; 0-915388),* 4848 N. Clark St., Chicago, IL 60640-4711 (SAN 204-7489) Tel 773-271-1030; Fax: 773-271-7399; Toll Free Fax: 800-397-0079; Toll Free: 800-397-2282
E-mail: acta@one.org.

Acta Univ (SWE) *(91-554) Dist. by* **Coronet Bks.**

Action Arts Pr, *(Action Arts Pr.; 0-9643084),* P.O. Box 3192, Lake Worth, Lantana Branch, FL 33465-3192 Tel 407-588-6337; Fax: 407-588-6970.

Action Health, *(Action Health Care Services, Inc.; 0-9649636),* P.O. Box 1494, Longmont, CO 80502-1494 Fax: 303-604-1448.

Aculeus Pr, *(Aculeus Pr., Inc.; 0-9630242),* Orders Addr.: P.O. Box 142, Lexington, VA 24450 Tel 540-464-4554 (phone/fax); Edit Addr.: 1103 Bunker Hill Mill Rd., Lexington, VA 24450
E-mail: aculeus@cfw.com
Dist(s): **Baker & Taylor** *(Baker & Taylor Bks.).*

Acupinch, *(Acupinch Outreach Ctr.; 0-9607456),* 2989 McCully Dr., NE, Atlanta, GA 30345 (SAN 238-2113) Tel 404-939-1678.

Ad Center, *See* **Leathers Pub**

ADA Publng, *(ADA Publishing Co., Inc.; 1-891748),* Subs. of American Dental Assn., 211 E. Chicago Ave., Chicago, IL 60611 Tel 812-440-4671; Fax: 312-440-3538; Toll Free: 800-621-8099
E-mail: rizzoj@ADA.org
Web site: http://www.ADA.org.

Adams Bannister Cox, *(Adams, Bannister, Cox Pubs.; 0-937431),* 460 Riverside Dr., Suite 52, New York, NY 10027 (SAN 658-9707) Tel 212-222-7585.

†Adams Media, *(Adams Media Corp.; 0-937860; 1-55850; 1-58062),* 57 Littlefield St., Avon, MA 02322 (SAN 215-2886) Tel 508-427-7100; Fax: 508-427-6790; Toll Free Fax: 800-872-5628; Toll Free: 800-872-5627
E-mail: books@adamsmedia.com
Web site: http://www.adamsmedia.com
Dist(s): **IPG Chicago** *(Independent Pubs. Group); CIP.*

Adams Pub Group, *(Adams Publishing Group, Ltd.; 0-944903),* P.O. Box 263, Boston, MA 02199 (SAN 245-4971) Tel 617-965-8448.

Adams Pubng, *See* **Adams Media**

Adams-Blake, *(Adams-Blake Publishing; 1-883422),* 8041 Sierra St., Fair Oaks, CA 95628 Tel 916-962-9296; Toll Free: 800-368-2326 (credit card orders)
E-mail: abpub@nf.net
Dist(s): **Baker & Taylor** *(Baker & Taylor Bks.)*
Quality Bks IL *(Quality Bks., Inc.)*
Unique Bks Inc *(Unique Bks., Inc.).*

Adapt Bks, *(Adapt Bks.; 1-887624),* Div. of Allergy Adapt, Inc., 1877 Polk Ave., Louisville, CO 80027 Tel 303-666-8253 (phone/fax)
E-mail: foodallergy@food-allergy.org
Web site: http://www.food-allergy.org
Dist(s): **Midpt Trade** *(Midpoint Trade Bks., Inc.).*

Adastra Pub, *(Adastra Publishing; 0-9611546),* P.O. Box 5247, Madison, WI 53705 Tel 608-233-5803 ; *Imprints:* Coulee Press (Coulee Press).

Add Resources, *(Add Resources; 1-885988),* 154 Curtis, Valparaiso, IN 46383-9111 Tel 219-462-5141.

Addax Pubng, *(Addax Publishing Group, Inc.; 1-886110; 1-58497),* 8643 Hauser Dr. Suite 235, Lenexa, KS 66215-4543 Tel 913-438-5333; Fax: 913-438-2079; Toll Free: 800-598-5550
E-mail: addax1@addaxpublishing.com
Dist(s): **Baker & Taylor** *(Baker & Taylor Bks.)*
Booksource *(Booksource, The)*
Midpt Trade *(Midpoint Trade Bks., Inc.).*

Addiction Therap, *(Addiction Therapeutics Pr.; 0-9638389),* 6 Coe Dr., Durham, NH 03824 Tel 603-868-7190.

†Addicus Bks, *(Addicus Bks.; 1-886039),* Orders Addr.: P.O. Box 45327, Omaha, NE 68145 Tel 402-330-7493; Fax: 402 330-1707; Toll Free: 800-352-2873
E-mail: info@addicusbooks.com
Web site: http://www.AddicusBooks.com
Dist(s): **LPC Group** *(LPC Group)*
Quality Bks IL *(Quality Bks., Inc.)*
Unique Bks Inc *(Unique Bks., Inc.); CIP.*

†Addison-Wesley, *(Addison-Wesley Longman, Inc.; 0-201; 0-321; 0-582; 0-8053; 0-9654123),* Div. of Pearson Education Corp. Commun., Orders Addr.: 200 Old Tappan Rd., Old Tappan, NJ 07675 (SAN 299-4739) Toll Free: 800-922-0579; Edit Addr.: 75 Arlington St., Boston, MA 02116 (SAN 200-2000) Tel 617-848-6000; Toll Free: 800-447-2226 ; *Imprints:* Health Sci (Addison-Wesley Publishing Company, Incorporated, Health Sciences Division)
E-mail: pearsoned@eds.com; orderdeptnj@pearsoned.com
Web site: http://www.awl.com
Dist(s): **Continental Bk** *(Continental Bk. Co., Inc.)*
Trans-Atl Phila *(Trans-Atlantic Pubns., Inc.); CIP.*

Addison-Wesley (GBR) *(0-582) Dist. by* **Longman.**

Addison-Wesley (GBR) *(0-582) Dist. by* **Trans-Atl Phila.**

Addson-Wesley Educ, *(Addison-Wesley Educational Pubs., Inc.; 0-321; 0-328; 0-673),* Div. of Addison Wesley Longman, Inc., One Jacob Way, Reading, MA 01867 Tel 781-944-3700; Fax: 781-942-1117; Toll Free: 800-447-2226
Web site: http://www.awl.com
Dist(s): **Shens Bks** *(Shen's Bks.).*

Adebara & Honeycomb, *(Adebara & Honeycomb, Inc.; 0-942307),* 244 Fifth Ave., No. A280, New York, NY 10001 (SAN 666-9719) ; *Imprints:* Newbreed (Newbreed Books)
E-mail: adebara@netzero.net
Web site: http://www.newbreedbooks.com.

Adelaide Pr, *(Adelaide Pr.; 0-9647666),* Div. of Leora Myers & Co., 3145 Geary Blvd., No. 513, San Francisco, CA 94118-3316 Tel 415-452-0549.

Adelante CA, *(Adelante Publishing; 1-886245),* Orders Addr.: P.O. Box 501584, San Diego, CA 92150-1584 Tel 760-749-6172 (phone/fax); Edit Addr.: 8525 Circle R Course Ln., Escondido, CA 92025 Do not confuse with companies with the same or similar name in Everett, WA, Surfside, CA
E-mail: mfraver@ra.ventures.com
Dist(s): **New Leaf Dist** *(New Leaf Distributing Co., Inc.).*

Adele Roberts, *(Roberts, Adele; 0-9611448),* 4341 SR 646, Bloomingdale, OH 43910 Tel 740-765-4520.

Adell Pr, *(Adell Pr.; 0-9660078),* 900 West End Ave., Suite 14A, New York, NY 10025 (SAN 299-4194) Tel 212-865-5765; Fax: 212-678-5287
E-mail: sales@adellpress.com
Web site: http://www.adellpress.com.

†Adenine Pr, *(Adenine Pr., Inc.; 0-940030),* Orders Addr.: P.O. Box 340, Guilderland, NY 12084 (SAN 281-2428) Tel 518-456-0784; Fax: 518-452-4955; Edit Addr.: 2066 Central Ave., Schenectady, NY 12304 (SAN 281-241X) Tel 518-456-0784; Fax: 518-452-4955
E-mail: stone@adeninepress.com
Web site: http://wwwadeninepress.com; *CIP.*

Adi Gaia Esalen, *(Adi, Gaia, Esalen Pubns., Inc.; 1-886508),* 1623 Military Rd., PMB 203, Niagara Falls, NY 14304-1745 (SAN 298-4520) Toll Free Fax: 800-931-1778; Toll Free: 800-652-8574 (editorial); 888-545-0053 (orders) ; *Imprints:* Ages Pubns (Ages Publications)
E-mail: ages@800line.com
Web site: http://www.agespublications.com
Dist(s): **Baker & Taylor** *(Baker & Taylor Bks.)*
Bookpeople *(Bookpeople)*
Brodart *(Brodart Co.)*
Coutts Library Service Inc *(Coutts Library Service, Inc.)*
General Distrib Services *(General Distribution Services, Inc.)*
New Leaf Dist *(New Leaf Distributing Co., Inc.)*
Nutri-Books Corp *(Nutri-Bks. Corp.)*
Quality Bks IL *(Quality Bks., Inc.)*
Royal Pubns Inc *(Royal Pubns., Inc.)*
Unique Bks Inc *(Unique Bks., Inc.).*

Adis Intl (NZL) *(0-86471) Dist. by* **Lppncott W & W.**

Adis Pr Intl, *(Adis Pr. International, Inc.; 0-941741),* F10-940 Town Centre Dr., Langhorne, PA 19047 (SAN 666-2846) Tel 215-741-5200.

Adler Sch Prof Psy, *(Adler School of Professional Psychology; 0-918560),* 65 E. Wacker Pl., Suite 2100, Chicago, IL 60601 (SAN 201-1956) Tel 312-201-5900; Fax: 312-201-5917
E-mail: info@alder.edu; bookstore@adler.edu
Web site: http://www.adler.edu.

Adlers Foreign Bks, *(Adler's Foreign Bks., Inc.; 0-8417),* 915 Foster St., Evanston, IL 60201 (SAN 111-3089) Tel 847-864-0664; Fax: 847-864-0804; Toll Free: 800-235-3771
E-mail: info@afb-adlers.com
Web site: http://www.afb-adlers.com
Dist(s): **Distribks Inc** *(Distribooks, Inc.).*

Adonis Pr, *(Adonis Pr.; 0-932776),* 320 Rte. 21C, Ghent, NY 12075 (SAN 661-9320) Tel 518-672-4736 (phone/fax)
E-mail: adonis@taconic.net
Dist(s): **Anthroposophic** *(Anthroposophic Pr., Inc.).*

Ads-Co, *(Ads-Co, Inc.; 0-9624469),* 4213 Wiley Post Rd., Dallas, TX 75244 Tel 972-387-4733; Toll Free: 800-527-0156.

Adv Hlth Inst, *(Advanced Health Institute, Inc.; 1-888266),* 850 Sixth Ave., N., No. 2, Naples, FL 34102-5511 Tel 941-261-4335; Fax: 941-261-6713; Toll Free: 800-508-2582.

Adv Rehab Therapy, *(Advanced Rehabilitation Therapy, Inc.; 1-888131),* 7641 SW 126th St., Miami, FL 33156 (SAN 253-8164) Tel 305-378-0855; Fax: 305-378-4107; Toll Free: 800-610-4278
E-mail: info@advancedrehabtherapy.com
Web site: http://www.advancedrehabtherapy.com.

Advan Mktg Servs, *See* **Advantage Pubs**

Advanced Dev Sys, *(Advanced Development Systems, Inc.; 0-931975),* 6319 Chauncy St., Tampa, FL 33647-1106 (SAN 686-0613) Tel 813-988-0623.

Advanced Global, *(Advanced Global Distribution Services),* 5880 Oberlin Dr., San Diego, CA 32121 Toll Free Fax: 800-499-3822; Toll Free: 800-284-3580.

Advanced Research Pr, *(Advanced Research Pr., Inc.; 1-889462),* Orders Addr.: 2120 Smithtown Ave., Ronkonkoma, NY 11779 (SAN 200-4860) Tel 631-467-3140 ext. 8103; Fax: 631-630-3472; Toll Free: 888-841-8007; Edit Addr.: 150 Motor Pkwy., Suite 210, Hauppauge, NY 11788
Web site: http://www.advancedresearchpress.com
Dist(s): **Midpt Trade** *(Midpoint Trade Bks., Inc.).*

Advanced Trnging, *(Advanced Training Assocs.; 0-9655392),* 5077 E. Shore Dr., Memphis, TN 38109 Tel 901-785-8278; Fax: 901-785-7592
E-mail: ewibooks@aol.com.

Advances, *(Advances I; 0-9644403),* 1827 Kirkham St., San Francisco, CA 94122 Tel 415-661-4222; Fax: 415-665-9266; Toll Free: 800-423-8688.

Advanstar Commns, *(Advanstar Communications; 0-929870; 0-943330; 0-9630895),* 7500 Old Oak Blvd., Cleveland, OH 44130 (SAN 250-7781) Tel 440-891-2650; Fax: 440-891-2740; Toll Free: 800-598-6008
E-mail: info@advanstar.com
Web site: http://www.advanstar.com
Dist(s): **IPG Chicago** *(Independent Pubs. Group).*

Advantage Books, *(Advantage Bks., LLC; 0-9660366; 0-9714609),* 1001 Spring St., No. 206, Silver Spring, MD 20910 (SAN 253-8237) Tel 301-495-2307; Fax: 301-562-8449; Toll Free: 888-238-8588
E-mail: advantagebooks@aol.com
Web site: http://www.addvance.com.

Advantage Pubs, *(Advantage Pubs. Group; 0-934429; 1-57145),* 5880 Oberlin Dr., San Diego, CA 92121-4794 (SAN 630-8090) Tel 858-812-6492; 858-450-3562; 858-450-2347 (customer service/orders); 858-457-2500 (parent company); Fax: 619-457-2500; 858-812-6476 (customer service/orders); Toll Free Fax: 800-499-3822; Toll Free: 800-284-3580 ; *Imprints:* Laurel Glen Pub (Laurel Glen Publishing)
E-mail: apgcuserv@advmkt.com
Web site: http://www.advmket.com; http://www.advantagebooksonline.com
Dist(s): **Advanced Global** *(Advanced Global Distribution Services).*

Advocacy Pr, *(Advocacy Pr.; 0-911655),* Div. of Girls Inc. of Greater Santa Barbara, P.O. Box 236, Santa Barbara, CA 93102 (SAN 263-9114) Tel 805-962-2728; Fax: 805-963-3580; Toll Free: 800-676-1480
E-mail: advpress@impulse.net
Web site: http://www.advocacypress.com
Dist(s): **Baker & Taylor** *(Baker & Taylor Bks.)*
Bookpeople *(Bookpeople)*
Wieser Educational *(Wieser Educational, Inc.).*

Aegean Park Pr, *(Aegean Park Pr.; 0-89412),* P.O. Box 2837, Laguna Hills, CA 92654-2837 (SAN 210-0231) Tel 949-586-8811; Fax: 949-586-8269; Toll Free: 800-736-3587
E-mail: books@aegeanparkpress.com
Web site: http://www.aegeanparkpress.com
Dist(s): **Baker & Taylor** *(Baker & Taylor Bks.).*

Aegina Pr, *(Aegina Pr., Inc.; 0-916383; 1-56002),* 1905 Madison Ave., Huntington, WV 25704 (SAN 665-469X) Fax: 304-429-7234 ; *Imprints:* Univ Edtns (University Editions)
E-mail: tommcat28@aol.com.

AEI Pr Imprint of Am Enterprise

Aeolus Press (NLD) *(90-70430) Dist. by* **Swets & Zeitlinger.**

Aerial Pr, *(Aerial Pr., Inc.; 0-942344),* P.O. Box 1360, Santa Cruz, CA 95061 (SAN 239-7056) Tel 831-427-2880; Fax: 831-425-8612; Toll Free: 877-336-6400
E-mail: office@aerialpress.com
Web site: http://www.aerialpress.com
Dist(s): **Dakota Bks** *(Dakota Bks.).*

Aero Pr, *(Aero Pr. Pubs.; 0-936450),* P.O. Box 2091, Fall River, MA 02722 (SAN 207-0650) Tel 508-644-2058.

Aesthetic Realism, *(Aesthetic Realism Foundation; 0-911492),* 141 Greene St., New York, NY 10012 (SAN 205-423X) Tel 212-777-4490; Fax: 212-777-4426
Web site: http://www.aestheticrealism.org.

AF NeuroVid, *(AF NeuroVideo, Inc.; 0-9651986),* Div. of Bloch Medical Illustration, 303 Thompson Dr., Pittsburgh, PA 15229 Tel 412-359-6200.

AFCOM Pub, *(AFCOM Publishing; 0-939339),* Orders Addr.: P.O. Box H, Harbor City, CA 90710-0330 (SAN 662-4685) Tel 310-541-5304.

Affordable Adven, *(Affordable Adventures, Inc.; 0-935201; 1-56017),* 3355 Parkside Dr., Brookfield, WI 53005 (SAN 630-2998); 5686 S. 27th St., Milwaukee, WI 53213 (SAN 665-8946)
Dist(s): **ARA Services Inc** *(ARA Services, Magazine & Bk. Div.)*
Baker & Taylor *(Baker & Taylor Bks.).*

†AFH & MP, *(Air Force History & Museums Program; 0-912799),* 500 Duncan Ave., Box 94, Bolling Air Force Base, Washington, DC 20332-1111 (SAN 218-8821) Tel 202-404-2224; Fax: 202-404-2271
E-mail: mossd@pentagon.af.mil
Dist(s): **USGPO** *(U.S. Government Printing Office); CIP.*

AFH Softech, *(AFH Softech; 1-884142),* Orders Addr.: P.O. Box 620094, Cleveland, OH 44102 Fax: 216-261-8650
E-mail: info@us-medical-review.com; support@us-medical-review.com; editor@us-medical-review.com
Web site: http://www.us-medical-review.com.

Africa World, *(Africa World Pr.; 0-86543),* 11 Princess Rd., Suites D, E & F, Lawrenceville, NJ 08648 (SAN 692-3925) Tel 609-844-9583; Fax: 609-844-0198
E-mail: africawpress@nyo.com
Web site: http://www.africanworld.com.

African Am Imag, *(African American Images; 0-913543),* 1909 W. 95th St., Chicago, IL 60643 (SAN 201-2332) Tel 773-445-0322; Fax: 773-445-9844; Toll Free: 800-552-1991
E-mail: aai@africanamericanimages.com
Web site: http://www.AfricanAmericanImages.com
Dist(s): **IPG Chicago** *(Independent Pubs. Group).*

African Islam Miss Pubns, *(African Islamic Mission Pubns.; 0-916157; 1-56505),* Subs. of A.I.M. Graphics, Orders Addr.: 1390 Bedford Ave., Brooklyn, NY 11216 (SAN 294-6645); Edit Addr.: P.O. Box 4143, Brooklyn, NY 11247 Tel 718-789-0245
E-mail: aimsbooks@aol.com
Web site: http://www.afrislam.com.

†African Studies Assn, *(African Studies Assn.; 0-918456),* 132 George St., New Brunswick, NJ 08901-1400 (SAN 212-260X) Tel 732-932-8173; Fax: 732-932-3394 ; *Imprints:* Crossroads (Crossroads Press)
E-mail: callasa@rci.rutgers.edu
Web site: http://www.africanstudies.org; *CIP.*

Africana Res, *(Africana Research Pubns.; 0-933524),* 454 W. 142nd St., New York, NY 10031 (SAN 212-470X) Tel 212-281-8507.

Afrikan World, *(Afrikan World InfoSystems; 1-879164),* Div. of Harlem Graphic Arts Ctr., Inc., 743 Rogers Ave., Suite 6, Brooklyn, NY 11226 (SAN 298-1394) Tel 718-462-1830
E-mail: afrikanworld@aol.com.

Afro Res Inc, *(Afro Resources, Inc.; 0-915549),* P.O. Box 192, Temple Hills, MD 20748 (SAN 291-0659) Tel 301-894-3855.

A&G Pubg, *(A&G Publishing; 0-9665353),* 2907 Palmer Dr., Gulfport, MS 39507 Tel 228-896-9334
E-mail: GBENNETT1533@worldnet.att.net.

Aga Khan Fnd, *(Aga Khan Foundation U.S.A.; 1-882839),* 1901 L St. NW, Suite 700, Washington, DC 20036 Tel 202-293-2537; Fax: 202-785-1752.

Age Concern Eng (GBR) *(0-86242) Dist. by* **St Mut.**

Age Enlight Pr, *(Age of Enlightenment Pr.; 0-89186),* 1000 N. Fourth St., Fairfield, IA 52557 (SAN 215-2894).

Ageless Bks, *(Ageless Bks.; 0-918482),* Orders Addr.: P.O. Box 6300, Beverly Hills, CA 90212 (SAN 210-0215); Edit Addr.: 1927 W. View St., Los Angeles, CA 90016 (SAN 247-0187).

Ageless Pub, *(Ageless Publishing; 0-9623941),* 111 E. 85th St., Suite 9B, New York, NY 10028 Tel 212-348-1771.

Agency Healthcare, *(Agency for Healthcare Research & Quality; 1-58763),* Div. of Print & Electronic Publishing, 2101 E. Jefferson St., Suite 501, Rockville, MD 20852 Tel 301-594-6131; Fax: 301-594-2283
E-mail: info@ahrq.gov
Web site: http://www.ahrq.gov.

Ages Pubns Imprint of Adi Gaia Esalen

Age-Trott, *See* **Cameltrotters**

Agincourt-Galen, *(Agincourt-Galen Publishing; 0-9641246),* 12053 Foxcroft Rd., West Frankfort, IL 62896 Tel 618-932-6514; Fax: 618-932-3797.

Aglow Communs, *(Aglow Communications; 0-930756; 0-932305; 1-56616),* Div. of Aglow International, Orders Addr.: P.O. Box 1749, Edmonds, WA 98020 Toll Free Fax: 800-860-3109; Toll Free: 800-793-8126; Edit Addr.: 152 Third Ave., S., Suite 103, Edmond, WA 98020-1749 (SAN 211-8297) Tel 425-775-7282
E-mail: informationsystems@aglow.org; aglow@aglow.org
Web site: http://www.aglow.org/
Dist(s): **Riverside-World** *(Riverside World)*
Spring Arbor Dist *(Spring Arbor Distributors Inc.).*

Aglow Pubns, *See* **Aglow Communs**

Agora Financl, *(Agora Financial Publishing; 1-893479),* 1217 Saint Paul St., Baltimore, MD 21202 Tel 410-223-2592; Fax: 410-223-2548; Toll Free: 800-201-5508
E-mail: 110526.1143@compuserve.com; mgardner@agora-inc.com
Web site: http://www.taipanonline.com.

AGPS Pr (AUS) *(0-644) Dist. by* **Intl Spec Bk.**

Agriculture & Natural Res, *See* **ANR Pubns CA**

Agro-Bio Systs, *See* **S & J Unltd**

AHAB Press, *(AHAB Pr., Inc.; 1-887515),* 2 Gannett Dr., Suite 200, White Plains, NY 10604-3404 Tel 914-696-0708; Fax: 914-694-6856; Toll Free: 800-696-7090
E-mail: ahab4@aol.com
Web site: http://www.ahabpress.com.

AHD & Ref Imprint of HM

†AHPI, *(American Hospital Publishing, Inc.; 0-939450; 1-55648),* Subs. of American Hospital Assn., Orders Addr.: P.O. Box 92683, Chicago, IL 60675-2683 (SAN 661-9363) Fax: 312-422-4505; Toll Free: 800-242-2626; Edit Addr.: 1 N. Franklin St., 27th Flr., Chicago, IL 60606-3421 (SAN 216-5872) Tel 312-440-6800; Fax: 312-951-8491
Web site: http://www.amhpi.com
Dist(s): **Jossey-Bass** *(Jossey-Bass, Inc. Pubs.); CIP.*

AIA DC, *(American Institute of Architects; 1-57165; 1-879304),* 1735 New York Ave., NW, Washington, DC 20006-5292 Tel 202-626-7572; Fax: 202-626-7425; Toll Free: 800-365-2724
E-mail: kwood@aia.org
Web site: http://www.aiaonline.com.

AIA Press, *(American Institute of Architects Pr.; 0-913962; 1-55835),* Div. of American Institute of Architects, Orders Addr.: P.O. Box 60, Williston, VT 05495-0060 (SAN 661-9371) Tel 802-862-0095; Toll Free: 800-365-2724 (orders only); 800-835-2878 (customer service); Edit Addr.: 1735 New York Ave., Washington, DC 20006 (SAN 277-9536) Tel 202-626-7575; Fax: 802-864-7626.

†AIAA, *(American Institute of Aeronautics & Astronautics; 0-915928; 0-930403; 1-56347),* Orders Addr.: 9 Jay Gould Ct., P.O. Box 753, Waldorf, MD 20604 Tel 301-645-3651; Fax: 301-843-0159; Toll Free: 800-682-2422; Edit Addr.: 1801 Alexander Bell Dr., Suite 500, Reston, VA 02191-4344 (SAN 204-529X)
E-mail: custserv@aiaa.org
Web site: http://www.aiaa.org; *CIP.*

AIAS, *See* **APA**

AIDC, *(AIDC),* 50 Winter Sport Ln., Williston, VT 05495 Tel 802-862-0095; Fax: 802-864-4672-; Toll Free: 800-488-2665.

AIDS Hlth Project, *(AIDS Health Project; 1-879168),* Orders Addr.: P.O. Box 0884, San Francisco, CA 94143-0884 Fax: 415-476-7996; Edit Addr.: 1855 Folsom St., No. 506, San Francisco, CA 94103 Tel 415-476-6430
Dist(s): **Celestial Arts** *(Celestial Arts Publishing Co.).*

AIDS Hse WA, *(AIDS Housing of Washington; 0-9636595),* 2025 First Ave., Suite 420, Seattle, WA 98121-2100 Tel 206-448-5242; Fax: 206-441-9485
E-mail: info@aidshousing.org.

AIDS Ministry, *(AIDS Ministry Program of the Archdiocese of St. Paul & Minneapolis; 1-879035),* Riverside Medical Ctr., Riverside at 25th Ave., S., Minneapolis, MN 55454 Tel 612-337-4345.

AIMED, *(AIMED; 0-9641185),* 14205 Valley Vista Blvd., Sherman Oaks, CA 91423-4025 Tel 818-789-1029; Fax: 818-789-9857; Toll Free: 800-348-8441.

AIP Pr Imprint of Spr-Verlag

AJ Pub Co, *(A.J. Publishing Co.; 0-9612332),* 4200 Peach Way, Boulder, CO 80301 (SAN 289-095X) Tel 303-444-7748.

Ajanta (IND) *Dist. by* **S Asia.**

AJFP, *(American Journal of Forensic Psychiatry; 0-935645),* Div. of American College of Forensic Psychiatry, P.O. Box 5870, Balboa Island, CA 92662 (SAN 696-0774) Tel 949-673-7773; Fax: 949-673-7710.

Ajna Media, *(Ajna Media; 0-9651534),* P.O. Box 70133, Eugene, OR 97401-0107 Fax: 541-744-2243; Toll Free: 888-255-2562
E-mail: contact@ajnamedia.com
Web site: http://www.ajnamedia.com
Dist(s): **New Leaf Dist** *(New Leaf Distributing Co., Inc.).*

AK Peters, *(AK Peters, Ltd.; 1-56881),* 63 South Ave., Natick, MA 01760 (SAN 299-1810) Tel 508-655-9933 All inquiries; Fax: 508-655-5847
E-mail: service@akpeters.com
Web site: http://www.akpeters.com.

AK Sea Grant CP, *(Alaska Sea Grant College Program; 1-56612),* Div. of Univ. of Alaska, Univ. of Alaska, P.O. Box 755040, Fairbanks, AK 99775-5040 Tel 907-474-6707; Fax: 907-474-6285; Toll Free: 888-789-0090
E-mail: fypubs@uaf.edu
Web site: http://www.uaf.edu/seagrant
Dist(s): **Todd Commns** *(Todd Communications).*

Akade Kiado (HUN) *(963-05) Dist. by* **Intl Spec Bk.**

Akade Kiado (HUN) *(963-05) Dist. by* **St Mut.**

Akadem izdatelstvo (BGR) *(954-430; 954-90623) Dist. by* **Coronet Bks.**

Akadem izdatelstvo (BGR) *(954-430; 954-90623) Dist. by* **Intl Scholars.**

Akademie Verlag (DEU) *(3-05) Dist. by* **Wiley.**

Akademische Druck-und (AUT) *(3-201; 3-900144) Dist. by* **Balogh.**

Al Mai Dah, *See* **Dawud Ujamma**

Alaken, *(Alaken, Inc.; 1-880293),* 305 Magnolia St., Suite 196, Fort Collins, CO 80521 Tel 970-223-5348.

Alamitos Hlth Pubns, *(Alamitos Health Pubns.; 0-9617497),* 3801 Katella Ave., No. 230, Los Alamitos, CA 90720 (SAN 664-2098) Tel 213-598-9426.

Alana Pr, *(Alana Pr.; 0-9702258),* Orders Addr.: P.O. Box 5431, Sun City Center, FL 33571-5431 Tel 813-633-8574; Fax: 813-634-9207; Edit Addr.: 2412 Oxford Down Ct., Sun City Center, FL 33573-7046
E-mail: EN1practDrew@aol.com.

Al-Anon, *(Al-Anon Family Group Headquarters, Inc.; 0-910034),* 1600 Corporate Landing Pkwy., Virginia Beach, VA 23454-5617 (SAN 201-2391) Tel 757-563-1600; Fax: 757-563-1655
E-mail: wso@al-anon.org
Web site: http://www.al-anon.alateen.org
Dist(s): **Baker & Taylor** *(Baker & Taylor Bks.)*
Hazelden *(Hazelden Information & Educational Services).*

Alaren Pr, *(Alaren Pr.; 0-9631489),* 12500 Fair Lake Cir., Suite 145, Fairfax, VA 22033-3804
Dist(s): **IHS Health Grp** *(IHS Health Group).*

Alaska NW Bks Imprint of Gr Arts Ctr Pub

†**Alba,** *(Alba Hse.; 0-8189),* Div. of Society of St. Paul, 2187 Victory Blvd., Staten Island, NY 10314-6603 (SAN 201-2405) Tel 718-761-0047; Fax: 718-761-0057; 718-698-8390; Toll Free: 800-343-2522
E-mail: albabooks@aol.com
Web site: http://www.albahouse.org; *CIP.*

Alba Pub, *(Alba Publishing; 0-9660057),* 1133 Arthur Ave., Orlando, FL 32804-2828
E-mail: Welshreg@iag.net.

Albert Schweitzer, *(Schweitzer, Albert Fellowship; 1-881815),* 330 Brookline Ave., Boston, MA 02215-5491 (SAN 225-3968) Tel 617-667-5111; Fax: 617-667-7989
E-mail: info@schweitzerfellowship.org
Web site: http://www.schweitzerfellowship.org.

Albury Pr, *See* **Albury Pub**

Albury Pub, *(Albury Publishing; 1-57778; 1-880089; 1-59066),* Orders Addr.: P.O. Box 470406, Tulsa, OK 74147-0406 (SAN 200-920X) Tel 918-523-5650; Fax: 918-523-5855; Toll Free: 800-304-5327; Edit Addr.: 2448 E. 81st St., Suite 5600, Tulsa, OK 74137-4231
E-mail: info@alburypublishing.com
Web site: http://www.alburypublishing.com
Dist(s): **Anchor Distributors** *(Anchor Distributors)*
Appalach Bk Dist *(Appalachian Bk. Distributors)*
Harrison Hse *(Harrison Hse., Inc.)*
Spring Arbor Dist *(Spring Arbor Distributors Inc.).*

Alcena Med Comms, *(Alcena Medical Communications, Inc.; 0-9633365),* 37 Davis Ave., White Plains, NY 10605 Tel 914-682-8020; Fax: 914-682-8066.

Alcohol Con Serv, *See* **G Stone Servs**

Aldine de Gruyter, *(Aldine de Gruyter; 0-202),* Div. of Walter de Gruyter, Inc., 200 Saw Mill River Rd., Hawthorne, NY 10532 (SAN 212-4726) Tel 914-747-0110; Fax: 914-747-1326
E-mail: CS@deGruyterNY.com; aldine@degruyterny.com
Web site: http://www.deGruyter.com
Dist(s): **De Gruyter** *(De Gruyter, Walter Inc.).*

Alef Bet Comns, *(Alef Bet Communications/Wahli Printing & Media; 0-9616488; 1-883517),* 13539 US Hwy. 24 E., New Haven, IN 46774 (SAN 659-2740) Tel 219-749-2288; Fax: 219-749-0182
Web site: http://www.alefbet-wahli.com.

Alef Design, *(Alef Design Group; 1-881283),* 4423 Fruitland Ave., Los Angeles, CA 90058 Tel 323-582-1200; Fax: 323-585-0327; Toll Free: 800-845-0662
E-mail: jane@torahaura.com
Web site: http://www.torahaura.com.

Alegra Hse Pubs, *(Alegra Hse. Pubs.; 0-933879),* Orders Addr.: P.O. Box 1443A, Warren, OH 44482 (SAN 692-7858) Tel 330-443-1706; Fax: 330-399-1619; Toll Free: 800-227-2591 (orders only)
E-mail: mineral9@theworks.com
Dist(s): **Baker & Taylor** *(Baker & Taylor Bks.)*
Brodart *(Brodart Co.)*
Paperbacks for Educators *(Paperbacks for Educators)*
Soc Studies Schl *(Social Studies Schl. Service).*

Alemany Pr, *(Alemany Pr., Inc.; 0-88084),* Div. of Pearson Education Corporate Communications, 240 Frisch Ct., Paramus, NJ 07652-5240 (SAN 240-1312) Toll Free: 800-227-2375.

Alert & Oriented, *(Alert & Oriented Publishing; 0-9640124),* 319 N. West St., Apt. 318, Indianapolis, IN 46202-3261.

Aletheia CA, *(Aletheia Publishing; 0-9638662),* 936 N. Lincoln St., Redlands, CA 92374 Tel 909-794-8941 Do not confuse with Aletheia Publishing, Anacortes, WA
E-mail: elgin@aletheia.com
Web site: http://www.aletheia.com.

Aletheia Pr, *(Aletheia Pr.; 0-9623718; 1-880831),* 103 West St., Northampton, MA 01060-3712.

Alexander Graham, *(Bell, Alexander Graham Assn. for the Deaf; 0-88200),* 3417 Volta Pl., NW, Washington, DC 20007 (SAN 203-6924) Tel 202-337-5220; Fax: 202-337-8270
Web site: http://wwww.agbell.org.

AlexAndria OR, *(AlexAndria Assocs.; 0-9611034),* P.O. Box 1187, Ontario, OR 97914 (SAN 282-8804) Tel 541-889-8938; Fax: 541-889-7566.

Alin Found Pr, *(Alin Foundation Pr.; 0-9606924),* Affil. of Alin Foundation, 2107 Dwight Way, 1 Alin Plaza, Berkeley, CA 94704 (SAN 212-0682) Tel 510-644-3366
Dist(s): **Baker & Taylor** *(Baker & Taylor Bks.).*

Alive Bks, *(Alive Bks.; 0-920470),* Div. of Canadian Health Reform Products, Ltd., 8110-357 250 H St., Blaine, WA 98230 Tel 604-435-1919; Fax: 604-435-4888; Toll Free: 800-663-6513
E-mail: orders@lalivebooks.com
Dist(s): **Baker & Taylor** *(Baker & Taylor Bks.)*
Bookmen Inc *(Bookmen, Inc.)*
Distributors *(Distributors, The)*
New Leaf Dist *(New Leaf Distributing Co., Inc.)*
Nutri-Books Corp *(Nutri-Bks. Corp.).*

Alive Prodns, *(Alive Productions, Ltd.; 0-9618860),* 9 The Bridge, Port Washington, NY 11050-1405 (SAN 242-2638) Tel 516-767-9235.

All Amer Pr, *(All American Pr.; 0-940879),* 128 Eastwood Dr., Birmingham, AL 35209-6604 (SAN 664-8797) Tel 205-822-8263; 1448 Shades Crest Rd., Birmingham, AL 35226 (SAN 664-8800).

All Stars Project, *(All Stars Project, Inc.; 0-9628621),* 500 Greenwich St., Suite 201, New York, NY 10013 Tel 212-941-9400; Fax: 212-941-8340; Toll Free: 800-435-7453
Web site: http://www.allstars.org.

Allegheny Health, *(Allegheny Health, Education & Research Foundation; 0-9628790),* 320 E. North Ave., Pittsburgh, PA 15212 Tel 412-359-3074; Fax: 412-359-5123.

Allegro Pub, *(Allegro Publishing Co.; 0-9601042),* P.O. Box 29687, Los Angeles, CA 90029 (SAN 201-2464) Tel 323-665-6783 (phone/fax)
E-mail: allegropublishing@pacbell.net.

Allen & Unwin Pty (AUS) *(0-04; 0-86861; 1-86373; 1-86448; 1-86508) Dist. by* **IPG Chicago.**

Allen & Unwin Pty (AUS) *(0-04; 0-86861; 1-86373; 1-86448; 1-86508) Dist. by* **Paul & Co Pubs.**

Allergy & Asthma, *(Allergy & Asthma Network-Mothers of Asthmatic, Inc.; 1-885543),* 2751 Prosperity Ave., Suite 150, Fairfax, VA 22031-4397 Tel 703-641-9595; Fax: 703-573-7794; Toll Free: 800-878-4403
E-mail: aanma@aol.com.

Allian Pubng, *(Alliance Publishing, Inc.; 0-9641509; 1-887110),* Orders Addr.: P.O. Box 080377, Brooklyn, NY 11208-0002 Tel 718-272-3964; Fax: 718-649-6859; Edit Addr.: 595 Berriman St., Brooklyn, NY 11208
Web site: http://www.alliancepublishing.com.

Alliance Pr, *(Alliance Pr.; 0-9619913),* 3230 Chicago St., San Diego, CA 92117-6115 (SAN 247-1760) Do not confuse with companie with same name in Colorado Springs, CO, Carrollton, TX.

Alliance Schl Health, *(Alliance for Schl. Health; 0-9616270),* 1748 Park Place Dr., Carmichael, CA 95608 (SAN 658-5434) Tel 916-961-0749.

Allied Hlth Pubns, *See* **CA College Health Sci**

Allied Pubs (IND) *(81-7023) Dist. by* **S Asia.**

Allied Res Soc, *(Allied Research Society, Inc.; 0-912984),* 11057 New River Cir., Rancho Cordova, CA 95670 (SAN 201-2480) Tel 916-635-7728.

Allina Health Pr, *(Allina Health System Pr.; 1-931876),* 710 E. 24th St., Suite 400, Rte. 43400, Minneapolis, MN 55404 Tel 612-775-9615; Fax: 612-775-9625; Toll Free: 800-775-9625
E-mail: education@allina.com.

Allnce Hse, *(Alliance Hse., Inc.; 0-9665234),* 220 Ferris Ave., Suite 201, White Plains, NY 10603 Tel 914-328-5456; Fax: 914-946-1929
E-mail: alliancehs@aol.com.

Allocca Biotech, *(Allocca Biotechnology, Inc.; 0-9659987),* 19 Lorraine Ct., Northport, NY 11768 Tel 631-757-3919; Fax: 631-757-3918
E-mail: john@allocca.com
Web site: http://www.allocca.com.

Allocca Tech, *See* **Allocca Biotech**

Alloway Pub (GBR) *Dist. by* **St Mut.**

Ally, *(ALLYN; 0-9669018),* Orders Addr.: P.O. Box 4235, Brandon, FL 33509 Tel 813-681-1576; Edit Addr.: 3510 Hollow Oak Pl., Brandon, FL 33511
E-mail: felmanmd@aol.com.

†**Allyn,** *(Allyn & Bacon, Inc.; 0-205; 0-321),* Div. of Pearson Education Corp. Commun, Orders Addr.: 200 Old Tappan Rd., Old Tappan, NJ 07675 (SAN 200-2442) Toll Free Fax: 800-445-6991; Toll Free: 800-666-9433 (ordering); 800-922-0579 (customer service); 111 Tenth St., Des Moines, IA 50309 Tel 515-284-6751; Fax: 515-284-2607; Toll Free: 800-278-3525; Edit Addr.: 75 Arlington St., Suite 300, Boston, MA 02116 (SAN 201-2510) Tel 781-848-6000 ; *Imprints:* Longwood Div (Longwood Division)
E-mail: ab_webmaster@abacon.com
Web site: http://www.abacon.com; *CIP.*

ALM Pubs, *(ALM Pubs.; 0-9619041),* P.O. Box 250, Young, AZ 85554 (SAN 242-8709).

ALMA Pub, *(ALMA Publishing Co.; 0-9663299),* P.O. Box 28268, Gladstone, MO 64188 (SAN 299-5719) Tel 816-459-9644; Fax: 816-459-4837; Toll Free: 800-997-4476
Dist(s): **Quality Bks IL** *(Quality Bks., Inc.).*

Almaas Pubns, *See* **Diamond Bks CA**

Almqvist & Wiksell (SWE) *(91-22; 91-554; 91-7106; 91-21; 91-512; 91-7282; 91-7942; 91-85026; 91-20; 0-85132; 91-7265; 91-628) Dist. by* **Coronet Bks.**

Almqvist & Wiksell (SWE) *(91-22; 91-554; 91-7106; 91-21; 91-512; 91-7282; 91-7942; 91-85026; 91-20; 0-85132; 91-7265; 91-628) Dist. by* **Coronet Bks.**

Alpenglo Graphics, *(Alpenglo Graphics, Inc.; 0-9625728),* 1130 Alpine, Boulder, CO 80304 Tel 303-447-1361; Fax: 303-447-0020; Toll Free: 800-535-1287.

Alpenglow WY, *See* **Spirit Dance**

Alpert, *(Alpert, Burt; 0-9600642),* P.O. Box 1235, Kapaau, HI 96755-1235 (SAN 201-1204).

Alpha Inst, *(Alpha Institute; 0-9632360),* Orders Addr.: P.O. Box 2463, Alameda, CA 94501; Edit Addr.: 1525 Broadway, Suite 2, Alameda, CA 94501 Tel 510-521-1916.

Alpha Pub MN, *(Alpha Pubs.; 0-9615632),* 712 Fairway Dr., Rock Valley, IA 51247 (SAN 696-0618) Tel 612-721-7856.

Alpha Pubng, *(Alpha Publishing, Inc.; 1-884350),* 13751 Benson Ave., Chino, CA 91710 Tel 909-464-0500; Fax: 909-464-0502 Do not confuse with companies with same or similar names in Mamaroneck, NY, Annapolis, MD, Louisville, KY, Chino, CA, Mont Clair, CA, Pheonix, AZ, Lafayette, LA
Web site: http://www.booksale.com.

AlphaMed Pr, *(AlphaMed Pr.; 1-880854),* One Prestige Pl., Suite 290, Miamisburg, OH 45342-3758 Tel 937-291-2355; Fax: 937-291-4229; Toll Free: 800-206-9850
E-mail: AlphaMedPress@AlphaMedpress.com
Web site: htttp://www.AlphaMedPress.com.

Alpine Guild, *(Alpine Guild, Inc.; 0-931712),* P.O. Box 4848, Dillon, CO 80435 (SAN 281-255X) Tel 970-262-6505; Fax: 970-262-9378; Toll Free: 800-869-9559
E-mail: alpgld@sni.net; information@alpineguild.com
Web site: http://www.alpineguild.com
Dist(s): **Hinshaw Music** *(Hinshaw Music Textbook Div.).*

Alpine Pr, *(Alpine Pr.; 0-9615114),* P.O. Box 1930, Mills, WY 82644 (SAN 697-2454) Do not confuse with Alpine Press in Liberty Lake, WA.

†**Alpine Pubns,** *(Alpine Pubns., Inc.; 0-931866; 1-57779),* 225 S. Madison Ave., Loveland, CO 80537 Tel 970-667-9317; Fax: 970-667-9157; Toll Free: 800-777-7257 (orders only)
E-mail: alpinepubl@aol.com
Web site: http://www.alpinepub.com
Dist(s): **Baker & Taylor** *(Baker & Taylor Bks.)*
Wstrn Intl *(Western International, Inc.); CIP.*

AltaMira Pr, *(AltaMira Pr.; 0-7619; 0-910050; 0-942063; 0-7425; 0-7591),* Div. of Rowman & Littlefield Publishing Group, Orders Addr.: 15200 NBN Way, Blue Ridge Summit, PA 17214 Tel 717-794-3800 (phone/fax); Toll Free Fax: 800-338-4550; Toll Free: 800-462-6420; Edit Addr.: 1630 N. Main St., No. 367, Walnut Creek, CA 94596 (SAN 299-4054) Tel 925-938-7243; Fax: 925-933-9720
E-mail: explore@altamirapress.com
Web site: http://www.altamirapress.com
Dist(s): **Natl Bk Netwk** *(National Bk. Network)* **Rowman** *(Rowman & Littlefield Pubs., Inc.).*

Altan Pub, *(Altan Publishing; 0-9625402),* 1614 SE 38th Ave., Portland, OR 97214-5204 Tel 503-663-6024.

Altarfire Pub, *(Altarfire Publishing; 0-9655558; 1-930975),* 1835 Oak Terr., Newcastle, CA 95658 Tel 916-663-1510; Fax: 916-663-2030
E-mail: margie@altarfire.com
Web site: http://www.altarfire.com.

Alternat Hlth, *(Alternative Health Pr.; 0-9640393),* Div. of Pinkus Productions, 3350 Hardscrabble Rd., N., Minnetrista, MN 55364 Tel 612-472-8044; Fax: 612-472-8352; Toll Free: 800-497-7441
E-mail: winkus@ibm.net.

Alternat Treatment, *(Alternative Treatment Information Network; 0-9639818),* 1244 Ozeta Terr., Los Angeles, CA 90069 Tel 310-278-5642.

AlternMed Bks, *(AlternativeMedicine.com Bks.; 0-9636334; 1-887299),* 21-1/2 Main St., Tiburon, CA 94920 Tel 415-789-8700; Fax: 415-789-9138; Toll Free: 800-515-4325
E-mail: info@alternativemedicine.com
Web site: http://www.alternativemedicine.com.

Alverstone Med, *(Alverstone Medical Products; 0-9651278),* 6330 W. 80th Pl., Los Angeles, CA 90045 Tel 310-337-7658; Fax: 310-645-7476.

Alyson Bks Imprint of Alyson Pubns

Alyson Pubns, *(Alyson Pubns.; 0-932870; 1-55583),* Div. of Liberation Pubns., Inc., 6922 Hollywood Blvd., Suite 1000, Los Angeles, CA 90028 (SAN 213-6546) Tel 323-860-6065; Fax: 323-467-0152; Toll Free: 800-464-4574 (orders only) ; *Imprints:* Alyson Bks (Alyson Books)
E-mail: mail@alyson.com
Web site: http://www.alyson.com
Dist(s): **Consort Bk Sales** *(Consortium Bk. Sales & Distribution).*

Am Acad Facial, *(American Academy of Facial Plastic & Resonstructive Surgery; 0-9651231),* 310 S. Henry St., Alexandria, VA 22314 Tel 703-299-9291; Fax: 703-299-8898; Toll Free: 800-332-3223.

Am Acad Hospice, *(American Academy of Hospice & Palliative Medicine; 1-889296),* a/o Dept. Communications, 4700 W. Lake Ave., Glenview, IL 60025-1468 Tel 847-375-4712; Fax: 703-435-4390.

Am Acad Nursing Imprint of Am Nurses Pub

Am Acad Ophthal, *(American Academy of Ophthalmology; 1-56055),* 655 Beach St., Suite 300, San Francisco, CA 94109-1336 (SAN 688-7473) Tel 415-561-8540; Fax: 415-561-8533.

Am Acad Osteopathy, *(American Academy of Osteopathy; 0-940668),* 3500 DePauw Blvd., Suite 1080, Indianapolis, IN 46268-1136 (SAN 218-5296) Tel 317-879-1881; Fax: 317-879-0563
E-mail: AAOSJN@aol.com
Web site: http://www.academyofosteopathy.org.

Am Acad Pediat, *(American Academy of Pediatrics; 0-910761; 0-915473; 1-58110),* 141 Northwest Point Blvd., Elk Grove Village, IL 60007-1098 (SAN 265-3540) Tel 847-434-4000; Fax: 847-434-8000; Toll Free: 800-433-9016
E-mail: KIDSDOCS@aap.org
Web site: http://www.aap.org
Dist(s): **Medical Information Systems Inc** *(Medical Information Systems, Inc.).*

Am Animal Hosp Assoc, *(American Animal Hospital Assn.; 0-941451; 0-9616498; 1-58326),* 12575 W. Bayaud Ave., Lakewood, CO 80228 (SAN 224-4799) Tel 303-986-2800; Fax: 303-986-1700; Toll Free: 800-883-6301 ; *Imprints:* AAHA Pr (A A H A Press)
E-mail: marykay.kozyra@aahanet.org
Dist(s): **Matthews Medical Bk Co** *(Matthews Medical Bk. Co.).*

Am Anthro Assn, *(American Anthropological Assn.; 0-913167; 1-931303),* 4350 N. Fairfax Dr., Suite 640, Arlington, VA 22203-1620 (SAN 202-4284) Tel 703-528-1902; Fax: 703-528-3546
E-mail: tclifford@aaanet.org; egraves@aaanet.org
Web site: http://www.aaanet.org; http://www.ameranthassn.org.

Am Antiquarian, *(American Antiquarian Society; 0-912296; 0-944026; 1-929545),* 185 Salisbury St., Worcester, MA 01609 (SAN 206-474X) Tel 508-752-5221; Fax: 508-754-9069
E-mail: library@mwa.org
Web site: http://www.americanantiquarian.org
Dist(s): **Oak Knoll** *(Oak Knoll Pr.).*

Am Art Therapy, *(American Art Therapy Assn.; 1-882147),* 1202 Allanson Rd., Mundelein, IL 60060-3825 (SAN 688-7686) Tel 708-949-6064; Fax: 708-566-4580.

Am Articulat, *(American Articulation Assocs.; 0-924799),* Orders Addr.: P.O. Box 500, El Cajon, CA 92022-0500 Tel 619-442-6202; Fax: 619-440-1289; Edit Addr.: 11768 Shadow Glen Rd., El Cajon, CA 92020
E-mail: accent@home.com
Web site: http://www.accentenglish.com
Dist(s): **Baker & Taylor** *(Baker & Taylor Bks.).*

Am Assembly, *(American Assembly; 0-936904),* Affil. of Columbia Univ., 475 Riverside Dr., Suite 456, New York, NY 10115 (SAN 209-6471) Tel 212-870-3500; Fax: 212-870-3555
E-mail: amassembly@columbia.edu
Web site: http://www.americanassembly.org.

†**Am Assn Blood,** *(American Assn. of Blood Banks; 0-914404; 0-915355; 1-56395),* 8101 Glenbrook Rd., Bethesda, MD 20814-2749 (SAN 201-1573) Tel 301-907-6977; 301-215-6598; Fax: 301-907-6895 ; *Imprints:* AABB Pr (A A B B Press)
E-mail: aabb@aabb.org; sales@aabb.org
Web site: http://www.aabb.org; *CIP.*

Am Assn Cereal Chem, *(American Assn. of Cereal Chemists; 0-913250; 1-891127),* 3340 Pilot Knob Rd., Saint Paul, MN 55121-2097 (SAN 204-7934) Tel 651-454-7250; Fax: 651-454-0766; Toll Free: 800-328-7560
E-mail: aacc@scisoc.org
Web site: http://www.scisoc.org/aacc.

Am Assn Clinical Chem, *(American Assn. for Clinical Chemistry, Inc.; 0-915274; 1-890883),* Orders Addr.: 2101 L St., NW, Suite 202, Washington, DC 20037-1526 (SAN 214-2813) Tel 202-857-0717; Fax: 202-887-5093; Toll Free: 800-892-1400 ; *Imprints:* AACC Pr (AACC Press)
E-mail: info@aacc.org
Web site: http://www.aacc.org.

Am Assn Coun Dev, *See* **Am Coun Assn**

Am Assn Diabetes Ed, *(American Assn. of Diabetes Educators; 1-881876),* 100 W. Monroe St., 4th Flr., Chicago, IL 60603 (SAN 224-3091) Tel 312-424-2426; Fax: 312-424-2427; Toll Free: 800-338-3633
Web site: http://www.aadenet.org.

Am Assn Higher Ed, *(American Assn. for Higher Education; 1-56377),* Orders Addr.: P.O. Box 1932, Merrifield, VA 22116-1932; Edit Addr.: 1 Dupont Cir., Suite 360, Washington, DC 20036-1110 (SAN 236-3089) Tel 202-293-6440; Fax: 202-293-0073
Web site: http://www.aahe.org.

Am Assn Homes, *(American Assn. of Homes & Services for The Aging; 0-943774; 1-930599),* Div. of Vendor Relations, 901 E St. NW, Suite 500, Washington, DC 20004-2037 (SAN 260-3918) Tel 202-783-2422; Fax: 202-783-2255
E-mail: krainman@aahsa.org
Web site: http://www.aahsa.org.

†**Am Assn Mental,** *(American Assn. on Mental Retardation; 0-940898),* 444 N. Capitol St. NW, Suite 846, Washington, DC 20001 (SAN 206-961X) Tel 202-387-1968; Fax: 202-387-2193; Toll Free: 800-424-3688
E-mail: aamn@pmds.com
Web site: http://www.aamr.org; *CIP.*

Am Assn Neuro, *(American Assn. of Neurological Surgeons; 0-9624246; 1-879284),* 5550 MeadowBrook Dr., Rolling Meadows, IL 60008 (SAN 266-4828) Fax: 847-378-0681; Toll Free: 888-566-2667
E-mail: info@aans.org; jal@aans.org
Web site: http://www.neurosurgery.org; http://www.aans.org
Dist(s): **Blackwell Sci** *(Blackwell Science, Inc.)* **J Majors Co** *(Majors, J. A. Co.).*

Am Assn Physics, *(American Assn. of Physics Teachers; 0-917853; 1-931024),* One Physics Ellipse, College Park, MD 20740-3845 Tel 301-209-3322; Fax: 301-209-0845
E-mail: aapt-exec@aapt.org
Web site: http://www.aapt.org.

Am Assn Strat, *(American Assn. of Stratigraphic Palynologists Foundation; 0-931871),* Mobil Research DRL, P.O. Box 819047, Dallas, TX 75381-9047 (SAN 686-0524) Tel 972-851-8481.

Am Assoc Med, *(American Assn. for Medical Transcription; 0-935229),* 3460 Oakdale Rd., Suite M, Modesto, CA 95355-9690 (SAN 696-0715) Tel 209-551-0883; Fax: 209-551-9317; 3460 Oakdale Rd., Suite M, Modesto, CA 95355 (SAN 696-5202)
E-mail: aamt@sna.com
Web site: http://www.aamt.org.

Am Astronaut Soc Imprint of Univelt Inc

Am Bd Med Spec, *(American Board of Medical Specialties; 0-934277),* 1007 Church St., Suite 404, Evanston, IL 60201-5913 (SAN 228-0477) Tel 847-491-9091; Fax: 847-328-3596.

Am Bd Ophthal, *(American Board of Ophthalmology; 0-9632791),* 111 Presidential Blvd., Suite 241, Bala Cynwyd, PA 19004 Tel 415-461-4145.

Am Bd Pediatrics, *(American Board of Pediatrics; 1-885046),* 111 Silver Cedar Ct., Chapel Hill, NC 27514 Tel 919-929-0461; Fax: 919-929-9255.

Am Biog Ctr, *(American Biographical Ctr.; 0-9601168),* P.O. Box 473, Williamsburg, VA 23187 (SAN 210-0266) Tel 804-725-2234 (phone/fax)
Web site: http://www.inna.net/biocenter
Dist(s): **Creative Dev Ctr** *(Creative Development Ctr.).*

Am Brain Tumor, *(American Brain Tumor Assn.; 0-944093; 0-9616451),* 2720 River Rd., Suite 146, Des Plaines, IL 60018-4110 (SAN 224-280X) Tel 847-827-9910; Fax: 847-827-9918; Toll Free: 800-886-2282
E-mail: info@abta.org
Web site: http://www.abta.org.

Am Busn Direct, *(American Business Directories; 0-7687; 0-944316; 0-945041; 1-56105),* Div. of infoUSA Inc./American Business Directories, 5711 S. 86th Cir., Omaha, NE 68127 (SAN 246-0165) Tel 402-596-4600; Fax: 402-331-5481; Toll Free: 800-555-6124; P.O. Box 27347, Omaha, NE 68127
E-mail: sales@directoriesUSA.com; directory@infoUSA.com
Web site: http://www.directories USA.com.

Am Cancer NY, *(American Cancer Society, Inc.; 0-944235),* 1599 Clifton Rd., NE, Atlanta, GA 30329-4251 (SAN 227-6941) Tel 404-320-3333; Fax: 404-325-9341
Web site: http://www.cancer.org
Dist(s): **Blackwell Sci** *(Blackwell Science, Inc.).*

†**Am Ceramic,** *(American Ceramic Society, The; 0-916094; 0-934706; 0-944904; 1-57498),* Orders Addr.: P.O. Box 6136, Westerville, OH 43086-6136; Edit Addr.: 735 Ceramic Pl., Westerville, OH 43081-8720 (SAN 201-6958) Tel 614-890-4700; Fax: 614-899-6109
E-mail: customersrvc@acers.org
Web site: http://www.ceramics.org
Dist(s): **World Scientific Pub** *(World Scientific Publishing Co., Inc.); CIP.*

†**Am Chemical,** *(American Chemical Society; 0-8412),* 1155 16th St., NW, Washington, DC 20036 (SAN 201-2626) Tel 202-872-4600; Toll Free: 800-227-5558
E-mail: help@acs.org; service@acs.org
Web site: http://www.acs.org; http://www.ChemCenter.org
Dist(s): **OUP** *(Oxford Univ. Pr., Inc.); CIP.*

Am Chest Phys, *(American College of Chest Physicians; 0-916609),* 3300 Dundee Rd., Northbrook, IL 60062-2348 (SAN 227-7123) Tel 847-498-1400; Fax: 847-498-5460
E-mail: registration@chestnet.org; accp@chestnet.org
Web site: http://www.chestnet.org.

Am Chiro Assn, *(American Chiropractic Assn.; 0-9606618),* 1701 Clarendon Blvd., Arlington, VA 22209 (SAN 215-6180) Tel 703-276-8800; Toll Free: 800-368-3083.

Am Coll Apothecaries, *(American College of Apothecaries; 0-910769),* P.O. Box 341266, Memphis, TN 38184-1266 (SAN 217-0868) Tel 901-383-8119; Fax: 901-383-8882
E-mail: aca@acainfo.org
Web site: http://www.aca@acainfo.org.

Am Coll Cardiology, *(American College of Cardiology; 1-882764; 1-892895; 1-58397),* 9111 Old Georgetown Rd., Bethesda, MD 20814 (SAN 266-6928) Tel 301-897-5400; Fax: 301-897-9745; Toll Free: 800-253-4636
E-mail: resource@acc.org; publications@acc.org
Web site: http://www.acc.org.

Am Coll Hlth, *(American College Health Assn.; 1-877918),* P.O. Box 28937, Baltimore, MD 21240-8937 (SAN 204-8019) Tel 410-859-1500; Fax: 410-859-1510
E-mail: acha@access.digex.net
Dist(s): **Heldref Pubns** *(Heldref Pubns.).*

Am Coll Obstetric, *(American College of Obstetricians & Gynecologists; 0-915473),* Orders Addr.: P.O. Box 4500, Kearneysville, WV 25430-4500 Toll Free: 800-762-2264; Edit Addr.: 409 12th St., SW, Washington, DC 20024 (SAN 284-9623) Tel 202-638-5577; Fax: 202-484-1595
Web site: http://www.acog.org.

Am Coll Phys Execs, *(American College of Physician Executives; 0-924674; 0-9605218),* 4890 W. Kennedy Blvd., Suite 200, Tampa, FL 33609 (SAN 688-7449) Tel 813-287-2000; Fax: 813-287-8993; Toll Free: 800-562-8088
E-mail: acpe@acpe.org
Web site: http://www.acpe.org.

Am Coll Radiology, *(American College of Radiology; 1-55903),* 1891 Preston White Dr., Reston, VA 20191 (SAN 224-4462) Tel 703-648-9820; Fax: 703-620-4730; Toll Free: 800-227-5463
Web site: http://www.acr.org.

Am Coll Sports Med, *(American College of Sports Medicine; 1-885377),* Orders Addr.: P.O. Box 1440, Indianapolis, IN 46206-1440 (SAN 266-7231) Tel 317-637-9200; Fax: 317-634-7817; Edit Addr.: 401 W. Michigan St., Indianapolis, IN 46202-3233 (SAN 694-9479)
E-mail: publications@acsm.org
Web site: http://www.acsm.org.

Am Coll Surgeons, *(American College of Surgeons; 0-9620370; 1-880696),* 633 N. Saint Clair St., Chicago, IL 60611-3211 (SAN 224-4659) Tel 312-202-5000; Fax: 312-202-5001
E-mail: postmaster@facs.org
Web site: http://www.facs.org.

Am College Rheum, *(American College of Rheumatology; 0-9654316),* 1800 Century Pl., Suite 250, Atlanta, GA 30345 Tel 404-633-3777; Fax: 404-633-1870
E-mail: acr@rheumatology.org
Web site: http://www.rheumatology.org.

Am Conf Govt Indus Hygienist, *(American Conference of Governmental Industrial Hygienists; 0-936712; 1-882417),* Kemper Woods Ctr., 1330 Kemper Meadow Dr., Cincinnati, OH 45240 (SAN 204-8035) Tel 513-742-2020; Fax: 513-742-3355
E-mail: http://www.acgih.org
Web site: publishing@acgih.org.

Am Correctional, *(American Correctional Assn.; 0-929310; 0-942974; 1-56991),* 4380 Forbes Blvd., Lanham, MD 20706-4322 (SAN 204-8051) Tel 301-918-1800; Fax: 301-918-1886; Toll Free: 800-222-5646 (ext. 1860)
E-mail: chantew@aca.org
Web site: http://www.corrections.com/aca.

Am Coun Assn, *(American Counseling Assn.; 0-911547; 1-55620),* 5999 Stevenson Ave., Alexandria, VA 22304-3300 (SAN 291-9141) Tel 703-823-9800; Fax: 703-823-0252; Toll Free: 800-347-6647; 800-422-2648 (Book orders)
Web site: http://www.counseling.org.

Am Council Drug Ed, *(American Council for Drug Education, Inc.; 0-942348),* 164 W. 74th St., New York, NY 10023-2301 (SAN 239-7099) Tel 212-758-8060; Fax: 212-758-6475; Toll Free: 800-488-3784.

Am Dental, *(American Dental Assn.; 0-910074),* 211 E. Chicago Ave., Chicago, IL 60611 (SAN 202-4519) Tel 312-440-2500
Web site: http://www.ada.org.

Am Diabetes, *(American Diabetes Assn.; 0-945448; 1-58040),* Orders Addr.: 1701 N. Beauregard St., Alexandria, VA 22311 Toll Free Fax: 800-998-3103 (orders); Toll Free: 800-323-4900 (orders)
E-mail: lboswell@diabetes.org
Web site: http://www.diabetes.org
Dist(s): **McGraw-Hill Trade** *(McGraw-Hill Trade).*

Am Dietetic Assn, *(American Dietetic Assn.; 0-88091),* Orders Addr.: P.O. Box 97215, Chicago, IL 60678-7215 (SAN 665-6439); Edit Addr.: 216 W. Jackson Blvd., Suite 800, Chicago, IL 60606-6995 (SAN 228-1341) Tel 312-899-0040; Fax: 312-899-1757; Toll Free: 800-877-1600 (ext. 5000)
Web site: http://www.eatright.org.

Am Educ Systs, *(American Educational Systems),* Div. of Book Clearing House, 46 Purdy St., Harrison, NY 10528 (SAN 631-0109) Tel 914-835-0015; Fax: 914-835-0398; Toll Free: 800-431-1579
E-mail: bookch@aol.com.

†Am Enterprise, *(American Enterprise Institute for Public Policy Research; 0-8447),* 1150 17th St., NW, Washington, DC 20036-6670 (SAN 202-4527) Tel 202-862-5800; Fax: 202-862-7178; Toll Free: 800-862-5801 ; *Imprints:* AEI Pr (A E I Press)
E-mail: info@aei.org
Web site: http://www.aei.org
Dist(s): **Pub Resources Inc** *(Publisher Resources, Inc.); CIP.*

Am Equine Pract, *(American Assn. of Equine Practitioners; 0-9659590),* 4075 Iron Works Pike, Lexington, KY 40511 (SAN 224-4802) Tel 606-233-0147; Fax: 606-233-1968; Toll Free: 800-443-0177
E-mail: aaepoffice@aol.com
Web site: http://www.aaep.org.

Am Faculty Pr, *(American Faculty Pr., Inc.; 0-912834),* 44 Lake Shore Dr., Rockaway, NJ 07866 (SAN 201-2650) Tel 973-627-2727.

Am Fisheries Soc, *(American Fisheries Society; 0-913235; 1-888569),* Orders Addr.: P.O. Box 1020, Sewickley, PA 15143 Tel 412-741-5700 (book ordering); Fax: 412-741-0609 (book ordering); Edit Addr.: 5410 Grosvenor Ln., Suite 110, Bethesda, MD 20814-2199 (SAN 284-964X) Tel 301-897-8616; Fax: 301-897-5080
E-mail: afspubs@pbd.com; main@fisheries.org
Web site: http://www.fisheries.org.

Am for the Arts, *(Americans for the Arts; 0-915400; 1-879903),* Orders Addr.: One East 53rd St., New York, NY 10022 Tel 212-223-2787; Fax: 212-980-4857; Edit Addr.: 1000 Vermont Ave., NW, 12th Flr., Washington, DC 20005 (SAN 207-3706) Tel 202-311-2830; Fax: 732-225-1562; Toll Free: 800-321-4510 (ext. 241)
E-mail: info@artsusa.org
Web site: http://www.artsusa.org.

Am Foun Blind, *(American Foundation for the Blind Pr.; 0-89128),* 11 Penn Plaza, Suite 300, New York, NY 10001-2006 (SAN 201-2677) Tel 212-502-7600 (Head office); Fax: 412-741-0609; Toll Free: 800-232-3044 (ordering)
E-mail: afborder@abdintl.com; afbinfo@afb.org
Web site: http://www.afb.org.

†Am Geophysical, *(American Geophysical Union; 0-87590),* 2000 Florida Ave., NW., Washington, DC 20009 Tel 202-462-6900; Fax: 202-328-0566; Toll Free: 800-966-2481
E-mail: orders@agu.org
Web site: http://www.agu.org*; CIP.*

Am Guidance, *(American Guidance Service, Inc.; 0-7854; 0-88671; 0-913476; 0-942277; 1-56269),* 4201 Woodland Rd., Circle Pines, MN 55014-1796 (SAN 201-694X) Tel 763-786-4343; Fax: 763-786-9077; Toll Free: 800-328-2560
E-mail: ags@mr.net
Web site: http://www.agsnet.com.

Am Health Consults, *(American Health Consultants; 0-9603332; 1-931107),* Subs. of Medical Economics, 3525 Piedmont Rd., NE, Bldg. 6, Suite 400, Atlanta, GA 30305 (SAN 222-2655) Tel 404-262-7447; Fax: 404-262-5475; Toll Free: 800-559-1032
Web site: http://www.ahcpub.com.

Am Heart, *(American Heart Assn., Inc.; 0-87493),* 7272 Greenville Ave., Dallas, TX 75231-4596 (SAN 202-4551) Tel 214-373-6300; Toll Free: 800-242-8721
E-mail: dallasdivision@heart.com
Web site: http://www.americanheart.org
Dist(s): **Beet** *(Beet, Channing L. Co., Inc.)*
Laerdal Med Corp *(Laerdal Medical Corp.)*
WorldPoint *(WorldPoint/EEC).*

Am Heartworm Soc, *(American Heartworm Society; 0-940275),* P.O. Box 667, Batavia, IL 60510-0667 (SAN 664-2276) Tel 708-844-9676.

Am HistoLabs, *(American HistoLabs, Inc.; 0-9649737),* 7605-F Airpark Rd., Gaithersburg, MD 20879 Tel 301-330-1200; Fax: 301-330-6059
E-mail: ahl@erols.com.

Am Hlth Info, *(American Health Information Management Assn.; 1-58426),* 233 N. Michigan Ave., Suite 2150, Chicago, IL 60601-5519 (SAN 224-4489) Tel 312-233-1100; Fax: 312-233-1090
Web site: http://www.ahima.org.

Am Hlth Lawyers, *(American Health Lawyers Assn.; 0-918945),* 1025 Connecticut Ave., NW, Suite 600, Washington, DC 20036-5428 (SAN 225-0969).

Am Hospital, *(American Hospital Assn.; 0-87258),* Orders Addr.: c/o AHA Services, Inc., P.O. Box 92683, Chicago, IL 60675-2683 (SAN 295-2955) Tel 312-422-3000; Fax: 312-422-4505; Toll Free: 800-242-2626
Web site: http://www.aha.org/.

Am Indus Hygiene, *(American Industrial Hygiene Assn.; 0-932627; 1-931504),* 2700 Prosperity Ave., Suite 250, Fairfax, VA 22031 (SAN 224-3970) Tel 703-849-8888; Fax: 703-207-3561
E-mail: infonet@aiha.org
Web site: http://www.aiha.org.

Am Inst Bio Sci, *(American Institute of Biological Sciences; 0-936829),* 1444 I St., NW, Washington, DC 20001 (SAN 225-1469) Tel 202-628-1500.

Am Inst Chinese Herbs, *(American Institute of Chinese Herbs; 0-9655166),* Div. of TSUNG Corp., Orders Addr.: P.O. Box 50663, Irvine, CA 92619-0663 Tel 714-786-0828; Edit Addr.: 15642 Sand Canyon Rd., Irvine, CA 92612-9998.

†Am Inst CPA, *(American Institute of Certified Public Accountants; 0-87051),* Harborside Financial Ctr., 201 Plaza Three, Jersey City, NJ 07311-3881 (SAN 202-4578) Tel 201-938-3772; Fax: 201-938-3780; Toll Free: 888-777-7077 (order dept.)
E-mail: lmorales@AICPA.org
Web site: http://www.aicpa.org*; CIP.*

Am Inst Hist Pharm, *(American Institute of the History of Pharmacy; 0-931292),* 425 N. Charter St., Madison, WI 53706-1508 (SAN 204-5257) Tel 608-262-5378; Fax: 608-262-3397
E-mail: aihp@macc.wisc.edu; books@aihp.org.

Am Inst Nutrition, *See* **Am Soc Nutr Sci**

†Am Inst Physics, *(American Institute of Physics; 0-7354; 0-88318; 1-56396),* Orders Addr.: 2 Huntington Quadrangle, Suite 1NO1, Melville, NY 11747-4502 (SAN 201-162X) Tel 516-576-2477; Fax: 516-576-2450; Edit Addr.: 1 Physics Ellipse, College Park, MD 20740-3843 Tel 301-209-3100; Fax: 301-209-0843
E-mail: aipinfo@aip.org
Web site: http://www.aip.org/
Dist(s): **Spr-Verlag** *(Springer-Verlag New York, Inc.); CIP.*

Am Inst Prevent, *(American Institute for Preventive Medicine; 0-9635612),* 30445 Northwestern Hwy., Suite 350, Farmington Hills, MI 48334 Tel 248-539-1800; Fax: 248-539-1808; Toll Free: 800-345-2476.

Am Inst Res, *(American Institutes for Research; 0-89785),* Orders Addr.: P.O. Box 1113, Palo Alto, CA 94302 (SAN 202-442X) Tel 650-493-3550; Fax: 650-858-0958; Edit Addr.: 1791 Arstradero Rd., Palo Alto, CA 94304 (SAN 215-9368)
E-mail: info-jcfrc@air.org
Web site: http://www.air-dc.org.

Am Inst Ultrasound, *(American Institute of Ultrasound in Medicine; 1-930047),* 14750 Sweitzer Ln., Suite 100, Laurel, MD 20707-5906 (SAN 224-4756) Tel 301-498-4100 (ext. 235); Fax: 301-498-4450; Toll Free: 800-638-5352
E-mail: publications@aium.org
Web site: http://www.aium.org.

Am Journal Nurse, *(American Journal of Nursing Co., Educational Services Div.; 0-937126),* 345 Hudson St., 16th Flr., New York, NY 10014 (SAN 202-4616) Tel 212-886-1200; Toll Free: 800-225-5256
Web site: http://www.l.com.

Am Law Inst, *(American Law Institute; 0-8318),* 4025 Chestnut St., Philadelphia, PA 19104-3099 (SAN 204-756X) Tel 215-245-1654 (Library); 215-243-7000 (Customer Service); 215-243-1600; Fax: 215-243-0319; Toll Free: 800-253-6397
E-mail: publications@ali-aba.org
Web site: http://www.ali-aba.org; http://www.ali.org.

Am Lib Pub Co, *(American Library Publishing Co.; 0-934598; 0-935495),* Orders Addr.: P.O. Box 4272, Sedona, AZ 86340-4272 (SAN 201-9868) Tel 520-282-4922.

Am Lite Co, *(American Lite Co.; 0-9624515),* 2637 NW 65th St., Oklahoma City, OK 73116 Tel 405-848-6024.

Am Literary Pr, *(American Literary Pr., Inc.; 1-56167),* 8019 Belair Rd., Suite 10, Baltimore, MD 21236-3711 Tel 410-882-7700; Fax: 410-882-7703; Toll Free: 800-873-2003
E-mail: amerlit@erols.com
Web site: http://www.erols.com/amerlit
Dist(s): **Baker & Taylor** *(Baker & Taylor Bks.)*
Childrens Lib Poetry *(Children's Library of Poetry)*
Temme Haus *(Temme Haus Pr.).*

Am Lung Assn, *(American Lung Assn.; 0-915116),* 1740 Broadway, New York, NY 10019 (SAN 211-3503).

Am Map, *(American Map Corp.; 0-8416),* Subs. of Langenscheidt Pubs., Inc., 46-35 54th Rd., Maspeth, NY 11378 (SAN 202-4624) Tel 718-784-0055; Fax: 718-784-0640; Toll Free: 800-432-6277.

†**Am Math,** *(American Mathematical Society; 0-8218),* Orders Addr.: P.O. Box 6248, Providence, RI 02940-6248 (SAN 201-1654) Tel 401-455-4000; Fax: 401-331-3842; Toll Free: 800-321-4267; Edit Addr.: 201 Charles St., Providence, RI 02904 (SAN 250-3263)
E-mail: cust-serv@ams.org
Web site: http://www.ams.org; *CIP.*

Am Med Assts, *(American Assn. of Medical Assistants; 0-942732),* 20 N. Wacker Dr., Suite 1575, Chicago, IL 60606 (SAN 224-3520) Tel 312-899-1500.

Am Med Info Assn, *(American Medical Informatics Assn.; 0-9647743),* 4915 St. Elmo Ave., Suite 401, Bethesda, MD 20814 Tel 301-657-1291; Fax: 301-657-1296
E-mail: mail@mail.amia.org
Web site: http://www.amia.org.

Am Med Record Assn, *See* **Am Hlth Info**

Am Med Sales, *(American Medical Sales Schl., Inc.; 1-882328),* Orders Addr.: P.O. Box 800605, Dallas, TX 75380-0605 Fax: 972-241-6778; Toll Free: 800-658-4620; Edit Addr.: 4240 Allencrest Ln., Dallas, TX 75244 Tel 972-233-8059.

Am Media, *(American Media; 0-912986),* 910 La Cresta Dr., Thousand Oaks, CA 91362 (SAN 202-4632) Tel 805-496-1649; Fax: 805-381-0191; Toll Free: 800-595-6596 Do not confuse with American Media, Inc., West Des Moines, IA
E-mail: info@realityzone.com
Web site: http://www.realityzone.com
Dist(s): **JIST Pubng** *(JIST Publishing).*

Am Meteorological, *(American Meteorological Society; 0-933876; 1-878220),* 45 Beacon St, Boston, MA 02108-3693 (SAN 225-2139) Tel 617-227-2425; Fax: 617-742-8718
Web site: http://www.ametsoc.org/ams.

Am Nephrology, *(American Nephrology Nurses' Assn.; 0-9653379),* E. Holly Ave., Box 56, Pitman, NJ 08071-0056 Tel 609-256-2320; Fax: 609-589-7463; Toll Free: 888-600-2662
E-mail: anna@mail.ajj.com
Web site: http://www.nurse.com/~anna
Dist(s): **Jannetti Pubns** *(Jannetti Pubns., Inc.).*

Am Nurses Fnd Imprint of Am Nurses Pub

†**Am Nurses Pub,** *(American Nurses Publishing; 1-55810),* Orders Addr.: 1650 Blugrass Lakes Pkwy., Alpharetta, GA 30004 Fax: 770-442-9742; Toll Free: 800-637-0323; Edit Addr.: 600 Maryland Ave. SW, Suite 100 W., Washington, DC 20024-2571 (SAN 204-5176) Tel 202-651-7212; Fax: 202-651-7003; Toll Free: 800-274-4262 ; *Imprints:* Am Acad Nursing (American Academy of Nursing) Am Nurses Fnd (American Nurses Foundation)
E-mail: ancc@ana.org
Web site: http://www.nursingworld.org; http://www.nursesbooks.org
Dist(s): **PBD Inc** *(PBD, Inc.); CIP.*

Am Occup Therapy, *(American Occupational Therapy Assn., Inc.; 0-910317; 1-56900),* 4720 Montgomery Ln., Bethesda, MD 20824-1220 (SAN 224-4705) Tel 301-652-2682; Fax: 301-652-7711; Toll Free: 800-729-2682 (member line)
Web site: http://www.aota.org.

Am Occupat Ther, *(American Occupational Therapy Certification Board; 0-9639373),* 800 S. Frederick Ave., No. 200, Gaithersburg, MD 20877-4150 Tel 301-990-7979; Fax: 301-869-8492.

Am Oil Chemists, *(American Oil Chemists' Society; 0-935315; 1-893997),* Orders Addr.: P.O. Box 3489, Champaign, IL 61826 (SAN 225-1558) Tel 217-359-2344; Fax: 217-351-8091; Toll Free: 800-336-2627; Edit Addr.: 2211 W. Bradley Ave., Champaign, IL 61821
E-mail: general @aocs.org; publications@aocs.org; orders@aocs.org
Web site: http://www.aocs.org
Dist(s): **AOAC Intl** *(AOAC International).*

Am Opthlmc Admin, *(American Society of Ophthalmic Administrators; 1-929196),* 4000 Legato Rd., Suite 850, Fairfax, VA 22033 Tel 703-591-2220; Fax: 703-591-0614; Toll Free: 800-451-1339
E-mail: lsantiago@ascrs.org
Web site: http://www.ascrs.org.

Am Ornithologists, *(American Ornithologists Union; 0-943610),* National Museum of Natural History, Washington, DC 20560-0116 (SAN 225-2252) Tel 202-357-2051; Fax: 202-633-8084
E-mail: aou@nmnh.si.edu
Web site: http://www.aou.org.

Am Overseas Bk Co, *(American Overseas Bk. Co., Inc.),* 550 Walnut St., Norwood, NJ 07648 (SAN 169-4863) Tel 201-767-7600; Fax: 201-784-0263
E-mail: books@aobc.com
Web site: http://www.aobc.com.

Am Petroleum, *(American Petroleum Institute Pubns. & Distribution Section; 0-89364),* 1220 L St., NW, Washington, DC 20005 (SAN 204-5141) Tel 202-682-8375
Web site: http://www.api.org.

Am Phar & Ex, *(American Society for Pharmacology & Experimental Therapeutics; 0-9609094),* 9650 Rockville Pike, Bethesda, MD 20014 (SAN 267-3223) Tel 301-530-7060; Fax: 301-530-7061
E-mail: aspetinfo@faseb.org
Web site: http://www.faseb.org/aspet.

Am Pharm Assn, *(American Pharmaceutical Assn.; 0-914768; 0-917330; 1-58212),* 2215 Constitution Ave., NW, Washington, DC 20037 (SAN 202-4446) Tel 202-628-4410; Fax: 202-783-2351; Toll Free: 800-878-0729
E-mail: webmaster@mail.aphanet.org
Web site: http://www.aphanet.org
Dist(s): **J Majors Co** *(Majors, J. A. Co.).*

Am Philos, *(American Philosophical Society; 0-87169),* Orders Addr.: P.O. Box 40098, Philadelphia, PA 19106 (SAN 206-9016) Tel 215-440-3427 (Call Eileen Massi for all ordering); Fax: 215-440-3450; Edit Addr.: 104 S. Fifth St., Philadelphia, PA 19106 (SAN 661-9398)
E-mail: emassi@amphilsoc.org
Web site: http://www.amphilsoc.org/.

Am Phys Therapy Assn, *(American Physical Therapy Assn.; 0-912452; 1-887759; 1-931369),* 1111 N. Fairfax St., Alexandria, VA 22314-1488 (SAN 202-4683) Tel 703-684-2782; Fax: 703-684-7343; Toll Free: 800-999-2782
Web site: http://www.apta.org.

Am Phytopathol Soc, *(American Phytopathological Society; 0-89054),* 3340 Pilot Knob Rd., Saint Paul, MN 55121-2097 (SAN 212-0704) Tel 651-454-7250; Fax: 651-454-0766; Toll Free: 800-328-7560
E-mail: aps@scisoc.org
Web site: http://www.apsnet.org.

†**Am Psychiatric,** *(American Psychiatric Pr., Inc.; 0-88048; 0-89042; 1-882103; 1-58562),* Div of The American Psychiatric Publishing Group, Inc., 1400 K St., NW, 11th Flr., Washington, DC 20005 (SAN 293-2288) Tel 202-682-6262; Fax: 202-789-2648 (orders only); 202-682-6341; Toll Free: 800-368-5777 (orders only)
Web site: http://www.appi.org; *CIP.*

†**Am Psychol,** *(American Psychological Assn.; 0-912704; 0-945354; 1-55798; 1-59147),* Orders Addr.: P.O. Box 92984, Washington, DC 20090-2984 (SAN 685-3137) Tel 202-336-5510 (orders) ; 202-336-6123 (TDD/TTY); 202-336-5500; Fax: 202-336-5502 (orders); Toll Free: 800-374-2721; Edit Addr.: 750 First St., NE, Washington, DC 20002-4242
E-mail: apabooks@apa.org
Web site: http://www.apa.org; *CIP.*

Am Pub Health, *(American Public Health Assn. Pubns.; 0-87553),* Div. of American Public Health Assn., 800 I St., NW, Washington, DC 20001 (SAN 202-4713) Tel 202-777-2742; Fax: 202-777-2534
E-mail: comments@apha.org
Web site: http://www.apha.org/contact/
Dist(s): **AOAC Intl** *(AOAC International).*

Am Registry Path, *(American Registry of Pathology; 1-881041),* 14th St. & Alaska Ave. NW, Bldg. 54, Rm. 1077, Washington, DC 20306-6000 Tel 202-576-2043; Fax: 202-576-0941
E-mail: bookstore@afip.osd.mil; AASINFO@afip.osd.mil
Web site: http://www.afip.org/ARP/arp.html.

Am Roentgen, *(American Roentgen Ray Society; 1-890705),* 44211 Slatestone Ct., Leesburg, VA 20176-5109 (SAN 267-243X).

Am Safety, *See* **Mangan Comns**

Am Sch Athens, *(American Schl. of Classical Studies at Athens; 0-87661),* 6-8 Charlton St., Princeton, NJ 08540-5232 (SAN 201-1697) Tel 609-683-0800; Fax: 609-924-0578
E-mail: pat@ascsa.org; ascsa@ascsa.org; publications@vax.museum.upenn.edu
Web site: http://www.ascsa.org; http://www.upenn.edu/museum_pubs/frames.html
Dist(s): **David Brown** *(Brown, David Bk. Co.).*

Am Sch Health, *(American Schl. Health Assn.; 0-917160),* Orders Addr.: P.O. Box 708, Kent, OH 44240 (SAN 208-5240) Tel 330-678-1601; Fax: 330-678-4526; Edit Addr.: 7263 State Rte. 43, Kent, OH 44240 (SAN 662-7161)
E-mail: asha@ashaweb.org
Web site: http://www.ashaweb.org.

Am Sleep Disorders, *(American Sleep Disorders Assn.; 0-9657220),* 6301 Bandel Rd., NW, Suite 101, Rochester, MN 55901-8798
E-mail: asda@asda.org.

Am Soc Addict Med, *(American Society of Addiction Medicine; 1-880425),* 4601 N. Park Ave., No. U101, Chevy Chase, MD 20815-4519 Tel 301-656-3920; Fax: 301-656-3815.

Am Soc Ag Eng, *(American Society of Agricultural Engineers; 0-916150; 0-929355; 1-892769),* 2950 Niles Rd., Saint Joseph, MI 49085-9659 (SAN 223-6087) Tel 616-429-0300; Fax: 616-429-3852; Toll Free: 800-371-2723
E-mail: landeckasae.org; hq@asae.org
Web site: http://www.asae.org
Dist(s): **Motorbooks Intl** *(Motorbooks International Wholesalers & Distributors).*

Am Soc Aging, *(American Society on Aging; 0-9640387),* 833 Market St., Suite 511, San Francisco, CA 94103 Tel 415-974-9600; Fax: 415-974-0300; Toll Free: 800-537-9728
E-mail: info@asa.asaging.org
Web site: http://www.housecall.com/oac/asa; http://www.asaging.org.

†**Am Soc Civil Eng,** *(American Society of Civil Engineers; 0-7844; 0-87262),* 1801 Alexander Bell Dr., Reston, VA 20191-4400 (SAN 204-7594) Tel 703-295-6300; Fax: 703-295-6211; Toll Free: 800-548-2723
E-mail: marketing@asce.org
Web site: http://www.pubs.asce.org; *CIP.*

Am Soc Clin Hyp Pr, *(American Society of Clinical Hypnosis Pr.; 1-886610),* Div. of The American Society of Clinical Hypnosis, 1320 University St., Seattle, WA 98101 Tel 206-325-5700; Fax: 206-328-5005.

†**Am Soc Clinical,** *(ASCP Pr.; 0-89189),* Div. of American Society of Clinical Pathologists, 2100 W. Harrison St., Chicago, IL 60612 (SAN 207-9429) Tel 312-738-1336; Fax: 312-738-1619; Toll Free: 800-621-4142
Web site: http://www.ascp.org/press; *CIP.*

Am Soc Consult Phar, *(American Society of Consultant Pharmacists; 0-934322),* 1321 Duke St., Alexandria, VA 22314-3563 (SAN 223-7350) Tel 703-739-1300; Fax: 703-739-1500.

Am Soc Electroencephalograph, *See* **ASET**

Am Soc Hlth-Syst, *(American Society of Health-System Pharmacists; 0-930530; 1-879907; 1-58528),* 7272 Wisconsin Ave., Bethesda, MD 20814 (SAN 204-5052) Tel 301-657-3000 (main); 301-657-4383 (customer serv.); Fax: 301-657-1641; Toll Free Fax: 800-665-2747
E-mail: custserv@ashp.org
Web site: http://www.ashp.org.

Am Soc Hosp Pharm, *See* **Am Soc Hlth-Syst**

Am Soc Mammalogists, *(American Society of Mammalogists; 0-943612),* Brigham Young Univ., Dept. of Zoology, Provo, UT 84602 (SAN 225-204X) Tel 801-378-2492.

Am Soc Microbio, *See* **ASM Pr**

Am Soc Nutr Sci, *(American Society for Nutritional Sciences; 0-943029),* Div. of Constituent Society of the Federation of American Societies for Experimental Biology, 9650 Rockville Pike, Bethesda, MD 20814 (SAN 228-135X) Tel 301-530-7050; Fax: 301-571-1892
E-mail: jnutrition@asns.fuseb.org
Web site: http://www.nutrition.org.

Am Soc of Plan, *(American Society of Plant Physiologists; 0-943088),* 15501 Monona Dr., Rockville, MD 20855-2768 (SAN 240-3366) Tel 301-251-0560; Fax: 301-279-2996
E-mail: aspp@aspp.org
Web site: http://aspp.org.

Am Social Health, *(American Social Health Assn.; 1-885833),* Div. of Communications Design, Orders Addr.: P.O. Box 13827, Research Triangle Park, NC 27709 (SAN 224-4772) Tel 919-361-8422; Toll Free: 800-783-9877; Edit Addr.: 100 Capitola Dr., Suite 200, Durham, NC 27713 Tel 919-361-8400; Fax: 919-361-8425
Web site: http://www.ashestd.org.

Am Somerset, *(American Somerset, Inc.; 0-932823),* 3820 166th Ave., SE, Bellevue, WA 98008-5849 (SAN 688-6191).

Am Speech Lang Hearing, *(American Speech-Language Hearing Assn.; 0-910329; 1-58041),* 10801 Rockville Pike, Rockville, MD 20852 (SAN 224-4608) Tel 301-897-5700; Fax: 301-897-7355; Toll Free: 888-498-6699
E-mail: productsales@asha.org
Web site: http://www.asha.org.

Am Therapeutic, *(American Therapeutic Recreation Assn.; 1-889435),* Orders Addr.: P.O. Box 15215, Hattiesburg, MS 39404-5215 Tel 601-264-3413; Fax: 601-264-3337; Toll Free: 800-553-0304; Edit Addr.: 48 Liberty Pl., Suite 2, Hattiesburg, MS 39402.

Am Trend Pub, *(American Trend Publishing Co.; 0-941388),* 645 Emporia Rd., Boulder, CO 80303 (SAN 238-9401) Tel 303-499-4582; Fax: 303-494-1631
E-mail: 72037.1331@compuserv.com.

Am Trust Pubns, *(American Trust Pubns.; 0-89259),* 745 McClintock Dr., Suite 114, Burr Ridge, IN 60521-0857 (SAN 664-6158)
Dist(s): **Islamic Bk Service** *(Islamic Bk. Service).*

Am U Beirut, *(American Univ. of Beirut Pubns.),*850 Third Ave., 18th Flr., New York, NY 10022 Tel 212-583-7678
E-mail: supress@syr.edu
Web site: http://www.sumweb.syr.edu/su_press/
Dist(s): **Syracuse U Pr** *(Syracuse Univ. Pr.).*

Am Urological, *(American Urological Assn., Inc.; 0-9649702; 0-9709327),* 1120 N. Charles St., Baltimore, MD 21201-5559 Tel 410-727-1100; Fax: 410-223-4375 ; *Imprints:* CHAUAC (Centennial History of the AUA Committe)
E-mail: khahn@auanet.org; aua@auanet.org
Web site: http://www.auanet.org.

Am Vet Pubns, *(American Veterinary Pubns., Inc.; 0-939674),* 11830 Westline Industrial Dr., Saint Louis, MO 63146-3313 (SAN 277-6545).

Am Veterinary Med Assn, *(American Veterinary Medical Assn.; 1-882691),* 1931 N. Meacham Rd., Suite 100, Schaumburg, IL 60173-4360 (SAN 224-4837) Tel 847-925-8070; Fax: 847-925-1329; Toll Free: 800-248-2862
Web site: http://www.avma.org.

Am Water Wks Assn, *(American Water Works Assn.; 0-89867; 1-58321),* 6666 W. Quincy Ave., Denver, CO 80235-3098 (SAN 212-8241) Tel 303-794-7711; Fax: 303-794-7310; Toll Free: 800-926-7337 (customer service/orders)
Web site: http://www.awwa.org.

Am Welding, *(American Welding Society; 0-87171),* 550 NW LeJeune Rd., Miami, FL 33126 (SAN 201-1700) Tel 305-443-9353; Fax: 305-443-7559
Web site: http://www.aws.org/.

Am Wellness, *(American Wellness Co.; 0-9647559),* 636 Honey Locust Way, Lexington, KY 40503 Tel 606-257-6050; Fax: 606-323-4728.

AMA, *(American Medical Assn.; 0-89970; 1-57947),* Orders Addr.: 1650 Bluegrass Lakes Pkwy., Alpharetta, GA 30004; Edit Addr.: 515 N. State St., Chicago, IL 60610 (SAN 206-8516) Tel 312-464-5000; Fax: 312-464-5600; Toll Free: 800-621-8335 (customer service, orders)
Web site: http://www.ama-assn.org
Dist(s): **Majors Scientific Bks Inc** *(Majors Scientific Bks., Inc.)*
Matthews Bk Co *(Matthews Bk. Co.)*
Rittenhouse *(Rittenhouse Bk. Distributors).*

†AMACOM, *(AMACOM; 0-7612; 0-8144),* Orders Addr.: P.O. Box 169, Saranac Lake, NY 12983 (SAN 227-3578) Tel 518-891-5510; Fax: 518-891-2372; Toll Free: 800-250-5308 (orders & customer service); Edit Addr.: 1601 Broadway, New York, NY 10019-7420 (SAN 201-1670) Tel 518-891-1500; Fax: 518-903-8168
E-mail: cust_serv@amanet.org
Web site: http://www.amacombooks.org
Dist(s): **Product Pr** *(Productivity Pr.)*
netLibrary CO *(netLibrary, Inc.); CIP.*

Amadeus CA, *(Amadeus Pr.; 0-9631493),* Orders Addr.: P.O. Box 13011, Long Beach, CA 90803 (SAN 297-6153) Tel 562-438-5054 (phone/fax); Edit Addr.: 215 Prospect Ave., Long Beach, CA 90803
E-mail: amadeuspr@compuserve.com
Web site: http://www.ourworld.compuserve.com /homepages/amadeuspress
Dist(s): **Baker & Taylor** *(Baker & Taylor Bks.).*

Amadeus Multi Tech, *(Amadeus Multimedia Technologies, Ltd.; 1-928852),* One Bridge St., Suite 93, Irvington, NY 10533 Tel 914-591-0028; Fax: 914-591-0083; Toll Free: 800-651-3988
E-mail: amadeus@webaxis.com
Web site: http://www.amadeusmultimedia.com.

Amalie Pub, *See* **Swan Park**

Amber-Allen Pub, *(Amber-Allen Publishing; 1-878424),* P.O. Box 6657, San Rafael, CA 94903-0657 Tel 415-499-4657; Fax: 415-499-3174; Toll Free: 800-624-8855
E-mail: info@amberallen.com
Web site: http://www.amberallen.com
Dist(s): **New Leaf Dist** *(New Leaf Distributing Co., Inc.)*
Publishers Group *(Publishers Group West).*

Amer Acad Ortho Surg, *(American Academy of Orthopaedic Surgeons; 0-89203),* 6300 N. River Rd., Rosemont, IL 60018 (SAN 228-2097) Fax: 847-823-8033; Toll Free: 800-626-6726 (customer service)
E-mail: meeting@aaos.org; custserv@aaos.org; member@aaos.org; placement@aaos.org; webhelp@aaos.org
Web site: http://www.aaos.org/.

Amer Acad Periodontology, *(American Academy of Periodontology; 0-9624699),* 737 N. Michigan Ave., Suite 800, Chicago, IL 60611 Tel 312-787-5518; Fax: 312-787-3670.

Amer Alpine Club, *(American Alpine Club; 0-930410),* 710 Tenth St., Suite 100, Golden, CO 80401-1022 (SAN 223-6001) Tel 303-384-0110; Fax: 303-384-0111
E-mail: aacpress@americanalpineclub.org
Web site: http://www.americanalpineclub.org
Dist(s): **Mountaineers** *(Mountaineers Bks., The).*

Amer Artificial, *See* **AAAI Pr**

Amer Bar Assn, *(American Bar Assn.; 0-89707; 1-57073; 1-59031),* 750 N. Lake Shore Dr., Chicago, IL 60611 (SAN 211-4798) Tel 312-988-5561; Fax: 312-988-6030 ; *Imprints:* ABA Antitrust (Section of Antitrust Law)
E-mail: service@abanet.org
Web site: http://www.abanet.org
Dist(s): **Jossey-Bass** *(Jossey-Bass, Inc. Pubs.).*

Amer Bd Hypnotherapy, *(American Board of Hypnotherapy Pr.; 0-9624829),* 16842 Von Karman Ave., No. 475, Irvine, CA 92606 Tel 714-251-4632; Toll Free: 800-634-9766
E-mail: aih@lxnetcom.com
Web site: http://www.hypnosis.com.

Amer Bone, *(American Bone Research Group; 0-9704323),* Orders Addr.: P.O. Box 660, Merrick, NY 11566 Tel 516-867-0500; Fax: 516-623-1296; Edit Addr.: 209 Merrick Ave., Merrick, NY 11566
E-mail: osteo@sportspt.com
Web site: http://www.sportspt.com.

Amer Bookworks, *(American Bookworks Corp.; 0-9622813; 1-884965),* 309 Florida Hill Rd., Ridgefield, CT 06877 Tel 203-438-0345; Fax: 203-438-0379.

Amer Botanical, *(American Botanical Council; 0-9655555),* Orders Addr.: P.O. Box 144345, Austin, TX 78714-4345; Edit Addr.: 11540 Spicewood Pkwy., Austin, TX 78750
E-mail: abc@herbalgram.org
Web site: http://www.herbalgram.org
Dist(s): **Lppncott W & W** *(Lippincott Williams & Wilkins).*

Amer Busn Pub Imprint of Hlth Res Pub

Amer Cancer Soc OR, *(American Cancer Society, Oregon Div.; 0-9617128),* 0330 SW Curry St., Portland, OR 97201 (SAN 662-6750) Tel 503-295-6422.

Amer Chronic, *(American Chronic Pain Assn., Inc.; 0-9673878),* Orders Addr.: P.O. Box 850, Rocklin, CA 95677 Tel 916-632-0922; Fax: 916-632-3208; Edit Addr.: 4150 Roble Way, Rocklin, CA 95677
E-mail: acpa@pacbell.net
Web site: http://www.theacpa.org.

Amer Col Occ, *(American College of Occupational & Environmental Medicine; 1-885190),* 1114 N. Arlington Heights Rd., Arlington Heights, IL 60004-4770
E-mail: rwp@cstone.net.

Amer Coll Legal, *(American College of Legal Medicine Foundation; 0-9629575),* 2 E. Chase St., Baltimore, MD 21202 Tel 410-576-4548; Fax: 410-223-4402.

Amer Coll of Clin, *(American College of Clinical Pharmacy; 1-880401),* 3101 Broadway, Suite 380, Kansas City, MO 64111 (SAN 688-8879) Tel 816-531-2177; Fax: 816-531-4990
E-mail: Kpovilonis@accp.com
Web site: http://www.accp.com.

Amer Coll Phys, *(American College of Physicians; 0-943126; 1-930513),* Orders Addr.: c/o R1140, ACP-ASIM, P.O. Box 7777, Philadelphia, PA 19174; Edit Addr.: 190 N. Independence Mall West, Philadelphia, PA 19106-1572 (SAN 240-8120) Tel 215-351-2600; Fax: 215-351-2425; Toll Free: 800-523-1546
Web site: http://www.acponline.org
Dist(s): **Blackwell Sci** *(Blackwell Science, Inc.)*
Johns Hopkins *(Johns Hopkins Univ. Pr.)*
Majors Scientific Bks Inc *(Majors Scientific Bks., Inc.)*
Matthews Medical Bk Co *(Matthews Medical Bk. Co.)*
Rittenhouse *(Rittenhouse Bk. Distributors).*

Amer College, *(American College, The; 0-943590; 1-57996; 1-58293),* 270 S. Bryn Mawr Ave., Bryn Mawr, PA 19010 Tel 610-526-1321; Fax: 610-526-1310
Web site: http://www.amercoll.edu
Dist(s): **Maple-Vail Bk** *(Maple-Vail Bk. Manufacturing Group, The)*
PBDI *(Professional Bk. Dist., Inc.).*

Amer ComVision Inc, *(American ComVision, Inc.; 0-923680),* 9974 Scripps Ranch Blvd., Suite 21, San Diego, CA 92131-1899 (SAN 251-7981) Tel 619-566-8537.

Amer Frnds, *(American Friends of Beth Hatefutsoth; 0-9653735),* 633 Third Ave., Flr. 21, New York, NY 10017-6706.

Amer Health Pr, *(American Health Pr.; 0-942767),* 7935 216th SW, Suite E, Edmonds, WA 98020 (SAN 667-7363) Tel 206-776-9355.

Amer Herbal, *(American Herbal Pharmacopoeia; 1-929425),* P.O. Box 5159, Santa Cruz, CA 95063 Fax: 831-475-6219 (phone & fax)
E-mail: herbal@got.net
Web site: http://www.herbal-aph.org.

Amer Hlth Heritage, *(American Health Heritage; 0-9619896),* Orders Addr.: P.O. Box 2215, Lancaster, OH 43130 (SAN 246-845X) Tel 614-653-2973; Edit Addr.: 616 N. Columbus St., Lancaster, OH 43130 (SAN 246-8468).

Amer Hlthcare Radiol, *(American Healthcare Radiology Administrators; 0-9634176),* 111 Boston Post Rd., Suite 105, Sudbury, MA 01776 Tel 978-443-7591; Fax: 978-443-8046.

Amer Inst Res Ctr, *See* **Amer Institute Res**

Amer Institute Res, *(American Institute for Research; 1-887995),* 60 E. 100 S., Suite 201, Provo, UT 84606 Tel 801-377-0570; Fax: 801-377-0655; Toll Free: 800-748-4922
E-mail: alcarter@airnews.com
Web site: http://www.airnews.com.

Amer Lawyer Media, *(American Lawyer Media; 0-9677396; 1-58852; 0-9705970),* 105 Madison Ave., New York, NY 10016 Tel 212-313-9343; Fax: 212-410-8110 ; *Imprints:* Law Journal Pr (Law Journal Press) Do not confuse with American Lawyer Media, Philadelphia, PA
E-mail: ebrooks@amlaw.com
Web site: http://www.lawcatalog.com
Dist(s): **IPG Chicago** *(Independent Pubs. Group).*

Amer Life League, *(American Life League, Inc.; 1-890712),* Orders Addr.: P.O. Box 1350, Stafford, VA 22555 Tel 540-659-4171; Fax: 540-659-2586; Edit Addr.: 1179 Courthouse Rd., Stafford, VA 22555
E-mail: jbrown@all.org
Web site: http://www.all.org.

Amer Med Pub, *(American Medical Publishing Co., Inc.; 1-887272),* Orders Addr.: P.O. Box 604885, Bayside, NY 11360-4885 Tel 718-263-3784; Toll Free: 800-263-3782; Edit Addr.: 113-14 72nd Rd., Flushing, NY 11375.

Amer Med Res, *(American Medical Response; 0-9615819),* 517 S. Division, Grand Rapids, MI 49503 (SAN 696-6152) Tel 616-459-8197.

Amer Media, *(American Media, Inc.; 1-884926),* 4900 University Ave., West Des Moines, IA 50266-6769 Tel 515-224-0919; Toll Free Fax: 800-305-8997; Toll Free: 800-963-3426 Do not confuse with American Media, Westlake Village, CA
E-mail: ami@ammedia.com
Web site: http://www.amimedia.com.

Amer Music Therapy, *(American Music Therapy Asssoc.; 1-884914),* 8455 Colesville Rd., Suite 1000, Silver Spring, MD 20910-3392 Tel 301-589-3300; Fax: 301-589-5175
E-mail: info@namt.com
Web site: http://www.namt.com/namt/; http://www.musictherapy.org.

Amer Natural Hygiene, *(American Natural Hygiene Society, Inc.; 0-914532),* Div. of American Natural Hygiene Society, Orders Addr.: P.O. Box 30630, Tampa, FL 33630 Fax: 813-855-8052; Edit Addr.: 11816 Race Track Rd., Tampa, FL 33626 (SAN 202-4314) Tel 813-855-6607
E-mail: anhs@anhs.org
Web site: http://www.anhs.org.

Amer Nutri-Tech, *(American Nutri-Tech, Inc.; 0-9624150),* Orders Addr.: P.O. Box 1317, Amelia Island, FL 32034; Edit Addr.: 844 Laura St., Amelia Island, FL 32034 Tel 904-261-3719.

Amer Psych Assn, *(American Psychiatric Assn.; 0-89042),* Div. of American Psychiatric Pr., Inc., Orders Addr.: 1400 K St., NW, Washington, DC 20005 (SAN 228-3492) Tel 202-682-6000; Toll Free: 888-357-7924
E-mail: apa@psych.org
Web site: http://psych.org
Dist(s): **Am Psychiatric** *(American Psychiatric Pr., Inc.).*

Amer Psych Soc Inc, *(American Psychiatric Society, Inc.; 0-9710235),* 454 Cajon St., Redlands, CA 92373 Tel 909-792-7538; Fax: 909-307-7948
E-mail: sdave5150@aol.com.

Amer Pubng, *(American Publishing Corp.; 0-9638596),* 13751 Benson Ave., Chino, CA 91710 Tel 909-464-0500; Fax: 909-464-0502
E-mail: americanpub@earthlink.net
Web site: http://www.emarketupdate.com.

Amer Spectator, *(American Spectator; 0-9629072),* Orders Addr.: P.O. Box 549, Arlington, VA 22216-0549 Tel 703-243-3733; Fax: 703-243-6814; Edit Addr.: 2020 N. 14th St., Suite 750, Arlington, VA 22216.

Amer Statist, *(American Statistical Assn.; 1-883276; 1-931586),* 1429 Duke St., Alexandria, VA 22314-3402 Tel 703-684-1221; Fax: 703-684-2037; Toll Free: 888-231-3473
E-mail: asainfo@amstat.org
Web site: http://www.amstat.org.

Amer West Pubs, *(America West Pubs. & Distributors; 0-922356),* P.O. Box 2208, Carson City, NV 89702 (SAN 251-2300) Tel 702-885-0700; Fax: 877-726-2632; Toll Free: 800-729-4131
Dist(s): **New Leaf Dist** *(New Leaf Distributing Co., Inc.).*

Amera-Chem, *(Amera-Chem, Inc.; 0-9635626),* P.O. Box 518, Grand Junction, CO 81502 Tel 970-285-9152; Toll Free: 800-772-2539.

Amereon Ltd, *(Amereon, Ltd.; 0-8488; 0-88411; 0-89190),* Orders Addr.: P.O. Box 1200, Mattituck, NY 11952 (SAN 201-2413) Tel 631-298-5100; Fax: 631-298-5631; Edit Addr.: 800 Wickham Ave., Mattituck, NY 11952 ; *Imprints:* J M C & Co (Carroll, J. M. Company)
E-mail: amereon@nvbb.net.

Ameri Botan, *(American Botanicals; 0-9663398),* Orders Addr.: P.O. Box 158, Eolia, MO 63344 Tel 573-485-2300; Fax: 573-485-3801
E-mail: AMBOTNELS@AOL.COM.

American Academic Assn for Peace in the Middle East, *(American Academic Assn. for Peace in the Middle East),*
Dist(s): **U Pr of Amer** *(University Pr. of America).*

†**American College of Emergency Physicians,** *(American College of Emergency Physicians),* P.O. Box 619911, Dallas, TX 75261 (SAN 266-6960) Tel 202-638-5577; Fax: 202-580-2816
E-mail: pubsorders@acep.org
Web site: http://www.acep.org; *CIP.*

American Host, *(American Host; 0-9658300),* 3788 Elliott St., Suite 21, San Diego, CA 92106 Tel 619-226-4671.

American Pr, *(American Pr.; 0-89641),* 28 State St., Suite 1100, Boston, MA 02109 (SAN 210-7007) Do not confuse with companies with the same or similar name in Washington, DC, Tacoma, WA
E-mail: ampress@flash.net.

Ameripress, *(Ameripress; 0-9640421; 0-9709873),* 8777 E. Via de Ventura, Suite 175, Scottsdale, AZ 85258 Tel 480-596-3442; Fax: 480-596-4054; Toll Free: 800-225-3864
E-mail: barryasmus@aol.com
Web site: http://www.barryasmus.com.

Amherst Educ, *(Amherst Educational Publishing; 1-883998),* P.O. Box 6000, Amherst, MA 01004 Tel 413-253-7837; Fax: 413-253-7024; Toll Free: 800-865-5549.

Amherst Sci Pubs, *(Amherst Scientific Pubs.; 1-884940),* Div. of Association for the Environmental Health of Soils (AEHS), 150 Fearing St., Suite 21, Amherst, MA 01002 Tel 413-549-5170; Fax: 413-549-0579; Toll Free: 888-540-2347
E-mail: info@aehs.com
Web site: http://www.aehs.com.

Amicas Pubns, *(Amicas Pubns.; 0-942539),* 18 Ninth St., NE, No. 206, Washington, DC 20002-6042 (SAN 667-3554) Tel 202-547-8715
E-mail: fins2000@mindspring.com.

Amira Alchemy, *(Amira Alchemy; 0-9666688),* 22310 NW 62 Ave., Alachua, FL 32615-7076 Tel 904-418-1054
E-mail: amira@herbalchemy.com
Web site: http://herbalchemy.com.

Amistad Imprint of HarperTrade

Amok Bks, *(Amok Bks.; 1-878923),* 739 Onarga Ave., Los Angeles, CA 90042-1217 Tel 213-663-8618; Fax: 213-666-8105
E-mail: amok@primenet.com
Dist(s): **SCB Distributors** *(SCB Distributors)*
Subterranean Co *(Subterranean Co.).*

AMRITA Pr, *(AMRITA Pr.; 1-893553),* 53 Washington St. Ext., Middlebury, VT 05753 (SAN 299-7886) Tel 802-382-8845 (phone/fax).

†**AMS Pr,** *(AMS Pr., Inc.; 0-404),* 56 E. 13th St., New York, NY 10003-4686 (SAN 106-6706) Tel 212-777-4700; Fax: 212-995-5413 Do not confuse with companies with the same or similar name in Los Angeles, CA, Pittsburgh, PA
E-mail: amserve@earthlink.net; *CIP.*

AMSA Pubns, *(AMSA Pubns.; 1-878642),* Div. of American Medical Student Assn., 1902 Association Dr., Reston, VA 22091 (SAN 224-313X) Tel 703-620-6600; Fax: 703-620-5873.

Amsterdam U Pr (NLD) *(90-5356) Dist. by* **U of Mich Pr.**

An All American, *(An All American Medical Hall of Fame, L.L.C.; 0-9650659),* 605 Thunderbird Ct., No. D, Chesterfield, MO 63017 Tel 314-469-6539
Dist(s): **Matthews Medical Bk Co** *(Matthews Medical Bk. Co.).*

An LaBarre, *(LaBarre, An),* 105 Auburn Folsom Rd., Auburn, CA 95603 Tel 530-885-3233.

ANA, *See* **Am Nurses Pub**

Anabolics, *See* **W Llewellyn**

ANADEM, *See* **Anadem Pubng**

Anadem Pubng, *(Anadem Publishing, Inc.; 0-9646891; 1-890018),* 3620 N. High St., Suite 201, Columbus, OH 43214 Tel 614-262-2539; Fax: 614-262-6630; Toll Free: 800-633-0055
E-mail: anadem@erinet.com
Web site: http://www.anadem.com.

†**Analytic Pr,** *(Analytic Pr.; 0-88163),* Orders Addr.: 10 Industrial Ave., Mahwah, NJ 07430-2262 (SAN 267-5455) Tel 201-358-9477; Fax: 201-760-3735 (orders only); 201-358-4700; Toll Free: 800-926-6579 (orders only); Edit Addr.: 101 West St., Hillsdale, NJ 07642 Tel 201-358-9477; Fax: 201-358-4700
E-mail: TAPBooks@analyticpress.com; tap@analyticpress.com
Web site: http://www.analyticpress.com; *CIP.*

Ananse Pr, *(Ananse Pr.; 0-9605670),* Orders Addr.: P.O. Box 22565, Seattle, WA 98122 (SAN 216-3292) Tel 206-325-8205; Fax: 206-328-4371; 1504 32nd Ave. S., Seattle, WA 98144 (SAN 241-6123)
E-mail: gumbomedia@earthlink.net; gumbomedia@yahoo.com
Web site: http://home.usaa.net/~gumbomedia/ananse/index.htm.

Ananta Prnting, *(Ananta Printing & Publishing; 1-884295),* 2827 S. Rodeo Gulch, No. 10, Soquel, CA 95073 Tel 408-464-9045; Fax: 408-464-9047.

Anaphase II, *(Anaphase II; 0-945962),* 2739 Wightman St., San Diego, CA 92104-3526 (SAN 248-1707) Tel 619-688-1959; Fax: 619-423-3311
Dist(s): **Baker & Taylor** *(Baker & Taylor Bks.)*
Bookpeople *(Bookpeople).*

Anarek Pubns, *(Anarek Pubns.; 0-9633902),* Orders Addr.: P.O. Box 1822, Cordova, TN 38018 Tel 901-757-5723; Edit Addr.: 909 Rocky Hills Cove, N., Cordova, TN 38018.

Anatech MI, *(Anatech, Ltd.; 0-9645197),* 1020 Harts Lake Rd., Battle Creek, MI 49015 Tel 616-964-6450; Fax: 616-964-8084; Toll Free: 800-262-8324
E-mail: anatech@net.link.net
Web site: http://www.net-link.net/anatech.

Anatomical Chart, *(Anatomical Chart Co.; 0-9603730; 1-889241; 1-58779),* Div. of Springhouse Corp., 8221 Kimball Ave., Skokie, IL 60076-2956 (SAN 223-5315) Tel 847-679-4700; Fax: 847-676-0211; Toll Free: 800-621-7500 (ext. 217)
E-mail: accinfo@anatomical.com
Web site: http://www.anatomical.com.

Anchor Bks, *(Anchor Bks.; 0-9634774),* P.O. Box 54, Two Harbors, MN 55616 Do not confuse with Anchor Bks. an imprint of Doubleday.

Anchor NY Imprint of Vintage Anchor

†**Ancient City Pr,** *(Ancient City Pr., Inc.; 0-941270; 1-58096),* Orders Addr.: P.O. Box 5401, Santa Fe, NM 87502 (SAN 164-5552) Tel 505-982-8195; Toll Free Fax: 800-622-8667; Toll Free: 800-249-7737
Dist(s): **U of NM Pr** *(Univ. of New Mexico Pr.); CIP.*

Ancora Pubns, *(Ancora Pubns.; 0-9663990; 1-930875),* Orders Addr.: P.O. Box 36941, Tucson, AZ 85740-6941 Tel 520-887-8004; Edit Addr.: 2305 W. Ruthrauff Rd., No. G12, Tucson, AZ 85705
E-mail: Ancorapub@aol.com.

And Bks, *(And Bks.; 0-89708),* 702 S. Michigan, Suite 836, South Bend, IN 46601 (SAN 213-9502) Tel 219-232-3134; Fax: 219-288-4141
E-mail: andbooks@ripco.com
Dist(s): **Distributors** *(Distributors, The).*

Andent Inc, *(Andent, Inc.; 0-914555),* 1000 North Ave., Waukegan, IL 60085 (SAN 291-8560) Tel 847-223-5077.

Anderson Laguna, *(Anderson Pr.; 0-9647571),* Orders Addr.: P.O. Box 6873, Laguna Niguel, CA 92607-6873 Tel 714-499-0244; Fax: 714-499-2768; Edit Addr.: 15 Marseille, Laguna Niguel, CA 92677 Do not confuse with Anderson Pr., Ann Arbor, MI.

†**Anderson Pub Co,** *(Anderson Publishing Co.; 0-87084; 1-58360),* 2035 Reading Rd., Cincinnati, OH 45202-1576 (SAN 661-9436) Tel 513-421-4142; Fax: 513-562-8116; Toll Free: 800-582-7295 Do not confuse with companies with the same name in Burley, ID, Anacortes, WA
E-mail: mail@andersonpublishing.com
Web site: http://www.andersonpublishing.com; *CIP.*

Andersons Pubns, *(Anderson's Pubns.; 0-931353),* 196 Wikiup Dr., Suite F, Santa Rosa, CA 95403-7757 (SAN 693-7829) Tel 707-575-1280; Fax: 707-579-9070
E-mail: anderpub@sonic.net
Web site: http://www.manandwomanbalance.com.

And-Or Bks, *(And/Or Bks.; 0-915904; 1-57951),* Affil. of Ronin Publishing, P.O. Box 2246, Berkeley, CA 94702 (SAN 206-9458)
Dist(s): **Publishers Group** *(Publishers Group West).*

Andover Townsman, *(Andover Townsman; 0-9655817),* P.O. Box 1986, Andover, MA 01810 Tel 978-475-1943; Fax: 978-470-2819
E-mail: jprice@andovertownsman.com
Web site: http://www.andovertownsman.com.

Andrew Hall Cutler Imprint of Minerva Labs

†**Andrew Mtn Pr,** *(Andrew Mountain Pr.; 0-916897; 0-9603840),* P.O. Box 340353, Hartford, CT 06134 (SAN 658-0130); *CIP.*

†**Andrews McMeel,** *(Andrews McMeel Publishing; 0-8362; 0-7407),* Div. of Andrews McMeel Universal Co., Orders Addr.: P.O. Box 419150, Kansas City, MO 64141; Edit Addr.: 4520 Main St., Kansas City, MO 64111 (SAN 202-540X) Tel 816-932-6600; Fax: 816-932-6749; Toll Free Fax: 800-437-8683; Toll Free: 800-826-4216 ; *Imprints:* Cader Bks (Cader Books)
E-mail: marketplace@uexpress.com
Web site: http://www.uexpress.com/corporate/amp/; http://www.AndrewsMcMeel.com; *CIP.*

Andrews Pubns, *(Andrews Pubns.; 0-9636246; 1-890155),* 175 Strafford Ave., Bldg. 4, Suite 140, Wayne, PA 19087 (SAN 227-3764) Tel 610-225-0510; Fax: 610-225-0501; Toll Free Fax: 800-220-1640; Toll Free: 800-345-1101
E-mail: customer@andrewspub.com
Web site: http://www.andrewspub.com.

Andrsn Cont Educ, *(Anderson Continuing Education; 0-942028),* Orders Addr.: P.O. Box 276297, Sacramento, CA 95827-6297 (SAN 238-4434) Tel 916-856-5050; Fax: 916-856-5066; Toll Free: 800-532-2332; Edit Addr.: 3268 Ramos Cir., Sacramento, CA 95827 (SAN 661-9428).

Anesthesia Pr, *(Anesthesia Pr.; 0-9623307),* 1161 21st Ave., S., T-4216 MCN, Nashville, TN 37232-2125 Tel 615-322-4000; Fax: 615-936-2801.

Anew View, *(Anew View; 0-9701223),* 2554 Lincoln Blvd., No. 711, Marina Del Rey, CA 90291 Tel 310-827-8170; Fax: 310-821-5251; Toll Free: 800-974-7717
E-mail: snowcat711@mediane.net
Web site: http://anew-view.com.

Angel Pr MA, *See* **Angel River Pr**

Angel River Pr, *(Angel River Pr.; 0-9645757),* P.O. Box 1038, North Cambridge, MA 02140-0009 Tel 617-497-9431; Fax: 617-547-6970; Toll Free: 800-726-4173
Web site: http://www.tiac.nst/users/healfast; http://www.healfaster.com
Dist(s): **Baker & Taylor** *(Baker & Taylor Bks.)*
New Leaf Dist *(New Leaf Distributing Co., Inc.).*

Angels Work, *(Angels' Work; 0-9632553),* 9350 SE Dundee Ct., Portland, OR 97266 Tel 503-771-9412; Fax: 503-229-8016.

Angelwood Pr, *(Angelwood Pr.; 0-9638390),* c/o Publishers Distribution Service, 6893 Sullivan Rd., Grawn, MI 49637 (SAN 630-5717) Tel 616-276-5196; Fax: 616-276-5197; Toll Free: 800-345-0096 (orders only).

Angle Publishing Co Inc, *See* **Welcome Rain**

Animal Hlth, *(Animal Health Pubns., LC; 0-9701159),* P.O. Box 28, Preston, ID 83263 Toll Free: 877-424-7838
E-mail: admin@infouets.com
Web site: http://www.infovets.com.

Anmol (IND) *(81-7488; 81-261; 81-7041) Dist. by* **S Asia.**

Ann Arbor Bks Imprint of U of Mich Pr

Ann Arbor Div Imprint of Acad Therapy

Ann3ess (GBR) *(1-901688; 0-7548) Dist. by* **Natl Bk Netwk.**

Ann3ess (GBR) *(1-901688; 0-7548) Dist. by* **AOL Time Warner.**

Anne-Maries Peaceful Connect, *(Anne-Marie's Peaceful Connections; 0-9655557),* P.O. Box 561212, Rockledge, FL 32956-1212 Tel 407-632-3197
E-mail: am.chloe@juno.com.

Anness Pub, *(Anness Publishing, Inc.; 1-886890),* 27 W. 20th St., Suite 504, New York, NY 10011-3707 (SAN 299-0563) Tel 212-807-6739; Fax: 212-807-6813; Toll Free: 800-354-9657 ; *Imprints:* Lorenz Bks (Lorenz Books)
Dist(s): **AOL Time Warner** *(AOL Time Warner Bk. Group).*

†Annual Reviews, *(Annual Reviews, Inc.; 0-8243),* 4139 El Camino Way, P.O. Box 10139, Palo Alto, CA 94303-0139 (SAN 201-1816) Tel 650-493-4400; Fax: 650-424-0910; Toll Free: 800-523-8635 (including California, Alaska, Hawaii & Canada)
E-mail: service@annurev.org
Web site: http://www.AnnualReviews.org; *CIP.*

Anodyne Imprint of Lowell Hse

ANR Pubns CA, *(ANR Pubns.; 0-931876; 1-879906),* 6701 San Pablo Ave., Oakland, CA 94608-1239 (SAN 211-4771) Tel 510-642-2431; Fax: 510-643-5470; Toll Free: 800-994-8849
E-mail: danrcs@ucdavis.edu
Web site: http://www.danrcs.ucdavis.edu.

Antarctic Pr, *(Antarctic Pr.; 0-930655),* P.O. Box 7134, Bellevue, WA 98008 (SAN 684-2631) Tel 425-885-6853; Fax: 425-867-3905 Do not confuse with Antarctic Pr., San Antonio, TX.

Antares, *(Antares; 1-886112),* 10657 Countess Dr., Dallas, TX 75229 Tel 646-514-8260 (phone/fax)
E-mail: WDMasters@aol.com.

†Anthroposophic, *(Anthroposophic Pr., Inc.; 0-8334; 0-88010; 0-89345; 0-910142; 1-58420; 1-85584; 0-9701097),* Orders Addr.: P.O. Box 960, Herndon, VA 20172-0960 Tel 703-661-1594 (orders); Fax: 702-661-1501; Toll Free Fax: 800-277-7947 (orders); Toll Free: 800-856-8664 (orders); Edit Addr.: P.O. Box 799, Great Barrington, MA 01230 Tel 413-528-8233; Fax: 413-528-8826; Fulfillment Addr.: 22883 Quicksilver Dr., Dulles, VA 20166 (SAN 253-9519) Tel 703-661-1529; Fax: 703-996-1010 ; *Imprints:* Lindisfarne (Lindisfarne Books)
E-mail: service@anthropress.org
Web site: http://www.lindisfarne.org; http://www.bellpondbooks.com; http://www.anthropress.org
Dist(s): **Bookpeople** *(Bookpeople)*
New Leaf Dist *(New Leaf Distributing Co., Inc.)*
Red Wheel ME *(Red Wheel); CIP.*

Anti Aging Pr, ***(Anti-Aging Pr.; 0-9632907; 1-886369),*** **Orders Addr.: P.O. Box 141489, Coral Gables, FL 33114 (SAN 297-6986) Tel 305-662-3928; Fax: 305-661-4123; Toll Free: 800-769-6864; Edit Addr.: 4185 Pamona Ave., Miami, FL 33114**
E-mail: julia2@gate.net
Dist(s): **Baker & Taylor** ***(Baker & Taylor Bks.)***
Brodart ***(Brodart Co.)***
New Leaf Dist ***(New Leaf Distributing Co., Inc.)***
Quality Bks IL ***(Quality Bks., Inc.)***
Unique Bks Inc ***(Unique Bks., Inc.).***

Antietam, *(Antietam Pubns.; 0-936772),* P.O. Box 37, Chewsville, MD 21721-0037 (SAN 223-5080).

Antimicrob Ther, *(Antimicrobial Therapy, Inc.; 0-933775; 1-930808),* P.O. Box 70, Hyde Park, VT 05655 (SAN 692-6991) Tel 802-888-2855; Fax: 802-888-2874; 229 Main St., Hyde Park, VT 05655
E-mail: info@sanfordguide.com
Web site: http://www.sanfordguide.com.

Antioch New Eng, *(Antioch New England Graduate Schl.; 1-881245),* 40 Avon St., Keene, NH 03431-3516 Tel 603-357-3122 (ext. 222); Fax: 603-357-0718
E-mail: antiochne.bookstore@antiochne.edu
Web site: http://www.antiochne.edu.

Antiquarium, *(Antiquarium; 0-9603990),* 166 Humiston Dr., Bethany, CT 06525 (SAN 201-6850) Tel 203-393-2723.

Antique Collect, *(Antique Collectors' Club; 0-902028; 0-907462; 1-85149),* 91 Market Street Industrial Park, Wappingers Falls, NY 12590; Orders Addr.: 91 Market St. Industrial Park, Wappingers Falls, NY 12590 (SAN 630-7787) Tel 845-297-0003; Fax: 845-297-0068; Toll Free: 800-252-5231 (orders)
E-mail: info@antiquecc.com
Web site: http://www.antiquecc.com; http://www.antiquecc.com.

Antler Pub, *(Antler Publishing; 0-929658),* Orders Addr.: P.O. Box 43394, Tucson, AZ 85733 (SAN 249-8901) Tel 520-881-0492; Edit Addr.: 3033 E. Third St., Tucson, AZ 85716 (SAN 249-891X)
Dist(s): **Baker & Taylor** *(Baker & Taylor Bks.).*

Anxiety Disorders, *(Anxiety Disorders Assn. of America; 0-935943),* 11900 Parklawn Dr., Suite 100, Rockville, MD 20852-2624 (SAN 696-8015) Tel 301-231-9350; Fax: 301-231-7392
E-mail: anxdis@adaa.com
Web site: http://www.adaa.org.

AOAC Intl, *(AOAC International; 0-935584),* 481 N. Frederick Ave. Suite 500, Gaithersburg, MD 20877-2417 (SAN 260-3411) Tel 301-924-7077; Fax: 301-924-7089; Toll Free: 800-379-2622
E-mail: aoac@aoac.org
Web site: http://www.aoac.org.

AOCS Pr, *See* **Am Oil Chemists**

AOL Time Warner, *(AOL Time Warner Bk. Group; 0-446),* 1271 Avenue of the Americas, New York, NY 10020 Tel 212-522-7381; Fax: 800-222-6902; Toll Free: 800-222-6747.

A-One Chinese, *See* **Dr Chens**

AORN, *(AORN, Inc.; 0-939583; 1-888460),* 2170 S. Parker Rd., Suite 300, Denver, CO 80231-5711 (SAN 224-3814) Tel 303-755-6300; Fax: 303-750-3441; Toll Free: 800-755-2676
Web site: http://www.aorn.org
Dist(s): **J Majors Co** *(Majors, J. A. Co.).*

APA, *(Adlerian Psychology Assocs., Ltd.; 0-918287),* P.O. Box 1450, Port Townsend, WA 98368 (SAN 657-2502) Tel 312-337-5066; Fax: 312-337-9319
E-mail: adlerpsy@ix.netcom.com.

APCO Inst, *(APCO Institute; 1-57927),* 351 N. Williamson Blvd., Daytona Beach, FL 32114-1112 Tel 904-322-2500; Fax: 904-322-9766; Toll Free: 888-272-6911
E-mail: institute@apco911.org
Web site: http://www.apco911.org.

APEA, *(Advanced Practice Education Assocs.; 1-892418),* 103 Darwin Cir., Lafayette, LA 70508 Tel 318-981-0502; Fax: 318-981-0509; Toll Free: 800-899-4502
E-mail: jmdoucet@apea.com
Web site: http://www.apea.com.

†Aperture, *(Aperture Foundation, Inc.; 0-89381; 0-912334; 0-900406; 1-931788),* Orders Addr.: 20 E. 23rd St., New York, NY 10010 (SAN 201-1832) Tel 212-505-5555; Fax: 212-979-7759; Edit Addr.: 16365 James Madison Hwy., Gordonsville, VA 22942 (SAN 631-5011) Tel 540-672-7600; Fax: 540-672-7540
E-mail: editorial@aperture.org; customerservice@aperture.org
Web site: http://www.aperture.org
Dist(s): **FS&G** *(Farrar, Straus & Giroux, LLC); CIP.*

APG Trade, *(APG Trade West),* 1501 County Hospital Rd., Nashville, TN 37218-2501.

APH Pubng (IND) *(81-7024) Dist. by* **Nataraj Bks.**

APLIC Intl, *(APLIC International; 0-933438),* c/o Family Health International Library, P.O. Box 13950, Research Triangle Park, NC 27709 (SAN 205-1486) Tel 215-898-5375
Web site: http://www.med.jhu.edu/ccp/aplic/aplic.html.

Apollo Managed, *(Apollo Managed Care Consultants; 1-893826),* 860 Ladera Ln., Santa Barbara, CA 93108 Tel 805-969-2606; Fax: 805-969-3749
E-mail: mail@apollomanagedcare.com
Web site: http://www.apollomanagedcare.com; http://www.e-medicaldirectory.com.

Apollo Pub OR, *(Apollo Publishing; 0-9640599),* Orders Addr.: P.O. Box 30729, Seattle, WA 98103-0729; Edit Addr.: 223 15th Ave., Seaside, OR 97138 Tel 503-738-8256 Do not confuse with companies with similar name in Port Orchard, WA, Marietta, GA.

Apollyon Pr, *(Apollyon Pr.; 0-9632626),* P.O. Box 16052, Seattle, WA 98116-0052 Tel 206-932-7928; Fax: 206-937-5276.

APPA VA, *(APPA: The Assn. of Higher Education Facilities Officers; 0-913359; 1-890956),* 1643 Prince St., Alexandria, VA 22314-2818 (SAN 223-7776) Tel 703-684-1446; Fax: 703-549-2772
E-mail: steve@appa.org
Web site: http://www.appa.org.

Apple a Day, *(Apple A Day, Inc.; 0-9642510),* 213 Tenth Ave., W., West Fargo, ND 58078 Tel 701-282-6826; Fax: 701-281-0823
Dist(s): **Bookmen Inc** *(Bookmen, Inc.).*

Apple Lange Med Imprint of McGraw

Apple Pr, *(Apple Pr.; 0-941905; 0-9602238),* 5536 SE Harlow, Milwaukie, OR 97222 (SAN 212-8489) Tel 503-659-2475 Do not confuse with companies with the same or similar name in Greencastle, PA, Manchester Center, VT
Dist(s): **Nutri-Books Corp** *(Nutri-Bks. Corp.)*
Royal Pubns Inc *(Royal Pubns., Inc.).*

Apple Pubg Co, *(Apple Publishing Co., Ltd.; 0-9695272; 1-896817),* 4936 Lake Terrell Rd., Ferndale, WA 98248 Toll Free: 800-668-2775.

Apple-a-Day, *(Apple-a-Day Pr.; 0-929167),* 3654 Bee Caves Suite D, Austin, TX 78746 (SAN 248-8221) Tel 512-328-3996; Fax: 512-328-0812
E-mail: apple-a-day@jacktips.com
Web site: http://www.jacktips.com
Dist(s): **New Leaf Dist** *(New Leaf Distributing Co., Inc.)*
Partners-West *(Partners/West).*

†Appleton & Lange, *(Appleton & Lange; 0-8385; 0-87041; 0-87488; 0-87619; 0-89303),* P.O. Box 120041, Stamford, CT 06912-0041 (SAN 209-1488) Toll Free: 800-947-7700 (Pearson) ; *Imprints:* Medical Exam (Medical Examination Publishing Company)
E-mail: customer.service@mcgraw-hill.com
Web site: http://www.books.mcgraw-hill.com/medical/appleton; *CIP.*

Appleton Comms, *(Appleton Communications, Inc.; 1-56757),* P.O. Box 36443, Grosse Pointe, MI 48236 (SAN 298-6019) Tel 313-882-1293; Fax: 313-882-9238
Web site: http://www.appletonpub.com.

Appleton Davies, *See* **Davies Pubng**

Appleton-Century-Crofts Imprint of P-H

†Applewood, *(Applewood Bks.; 0-918222; 1-55709),* 128 The Great Rd., Bedford, MA 01730 (SAN 210-3419) Tel 781-271-0055; Fax: 781-271-0056; Toll Free: 800-277-5312
E-mail: applewood@awb.com
Web site: http://www.awb.com
Dist(s): **Consort Bk Sales** *(Consortium Bk. Sales & Distribution); CIP.*

Applied Arts, *(Applied Arts Pubs.; 0-911410),* Div. of Sowers Printing Co., Box 479, Lebanon, PA 17042 (SAN 204-4838) Tel 717-272-9442; Fax: 717-274-2928.

Applied Measurement, *(Applied Measurement Professionals, Inc.; 0-9624754),* 8310 Nieman Rd., Lenexa, KS 66214 Tel 913-541-0400; Fax: 913-541-0156.

Applied Therapeutics, *(Applied Therapeutics, Inc.; 0-915486),* c/o Maureen Connors, Lippincott Williams & Wilkins, P.O. Box 1600, Hagerstown, MD 21740-5176 Tel 800-638-3030
Dist(s): **Lppncott W & W** *(Lippincott Williams & Wilkins).*

†Appraisal Inst, *(Appraisal Institute, The; 0-922154),* Orders Addr.: c/o CBI Corporation, 859 Fiene Dr., Addison, IL 60101 Fax: 630-628-1669; Toll Free: 888-570-4545; Edit Addr.: 875 N. Michigan Ave., Suite 2400, Chicago, IL 60611-1980 Tel 312-335-4100; 312-335-4453; Fax: 312-335-4222
E-mail: info@appraisalinstitute.org
Web site: http://www.appraisalinstitute.com; *CIP.*

APU Pub Grp, *(APU Publishing Group; 1-878647),* Orders Addr.: P.O. Box 1137, Edgewood, MD 21040 Tel 410-538-7400; Fax: 410-538-7468.

AQC Resource, *(AQC Resource; 1-887212),* 175 N. Buena Vista Ave., San Jose, CA 95126 Tel 408-295-4102; Fax: 408-293-8889; Toll Free: 800-995-8702
E-mail: resourcebook@earthlink.net
Web site: http://www.resource-books.com.

Aqrn Pr (GBR) *(0-85030; 1-85538) Dist. by* **HarperCollins Pubs.**

Aqrn Pr (GBR) *(0-85030; 1-85538) Dist. by* **Harper SF.**

Aqua Quest, *(Aqua Quest Pubns., Inc.; 0-9623389; 1-881652),* Orders Addr.: P.O. Box 700, Locust Valley, NY 11560-0700 Tel 516-759-0476; Fax: 516-759-4519; Toll Free: 800-933-8989
E-mail: info@aquaquest.com; sales@aquaquest.com
Web site: http://www.aquaquest.com
Dist(s): **Natl Bk Netwk** *(National Bk. Network).*

Aquarius Hse, *(Aquarius Hse. Pr., The; 1-882888),* Div. of Relationship Training Ctr. International, Inc., P.O. Box 1241, Vista, CA 92085 Tel 760-758-7628
E-mail: AquariusHouse@aol.com
Web site: http://www.aquariushousepress.com.

ARA Pubns, *See* **Raintree Pubns**

Arapahoe Mental Hlth Ctr, *(Arapahoe Mental Health Ctr., Inc.; 0-9624700),* 5500 S. Sycamore St., Litteton, CO 80120 Tel 303-761-0620.

Arc Imprint of Hungry Minds

ARC Pub, *(ARC Publishing, Inc.; 0-9633540),* 7009 Woodthrush Dr., Concord, OH 44077-2310.

Arc Res, *(Arc Research Co.; 0-9636183),* 11595 State Rd. 70, Grantsburg, WI 54840-7135 Tel 715-689-2153; Fax: 715-689-2277 Do not confuse with A R C Research Foundation, Rockville, MD.

†Arcade Pub Inc, *(Arcade Publishing, Inc.; 1-55970; 1-58996),* Orders Addr.: c/o Time Warner Trade Publishing, 3 Center Plaza, Boston, MA 02108 (SAN 630-7248) Toll Free Fax: 800-890-0875; Toll Free: 800-759-0190; Edit Addr.: 141 Fifth Ave., New York, NY 10010 (SAN 252-2012) Tel 212-475-2633; Fax: 212-353-8148
E-mail: arcadeinfo@arcadepub.com
Web site: http://www.arcadepub.com
Dist(s): **AOL Time Warner** *(AOL Time Warner Bk. Group)*
TWI *(Time Warner Interactive); CIP.*

Arcadia AZ, *(Arcadia Pr.; 1-881185),* Orders Addr.: P.O. Box 8697, Scottsdale, AZ 85252-8697; Edit Addr.: 6270 N. 78th St., No. 340, Scottsdale, AZ 85250 Do not confuse with companies with the same name in New York, NY, Greenville, NH
E-mail: crcjct@ix.netcom.com
Web site: http://www.vegsource.org/parenting.

Arcadia Pr NH, *(Arcadia Pr.; 0-9649236),* Orders Addr.: P.O. Box 205, Greenville, NH 03048 Tel 603-878-1561; Fax: 603-878-0811; Toll Free: 800-398-8851; Edit Addr.: 161 Merriam Hill Rd., Greenville, NH 03048 Do not confuse with companies with the same name in New York, NY, Scottsdale, AZ
E-mail: larcadia@compuserve.com
Dist(s): **Baker & Taylor** *(Baker & Taylor Bks.)*
Bookpeople *(Bookpeople)*
Koen Bk Distributors *(Koen Bk. Distributors)*
Quality Bks IL *(Quality Bks., Inc.)*
Unique Bks Inc *(Unique Bks., Inc.).*

Arcadia Publng, *(Arcadia Publishing; 0-7524; 0-7385; 1-58973),* Div. of Tempus Publishing, Inc., 2 Cumberland St., Charleston, SC 29401 Tel 843-853-2070; Fax: 843-853-0044; Toll Free: 888-313-2665
E-mail: publishing@arcadiapublishing.com; sales@arcadiapublishing.com
Web site: http://www.arcadiapublishing.com.

Arcane Publns, *(Arcane Pubns., Inc.; 0-9641510),* Orders Addr.: P.O. Box 5592, Scottsdale, AZ 85261-5592; Edit Addr.: 7955 N. Via Azul, Scottsdale, AZ 85258 Tel 602-998-7370.

Archangel Pr, *(Archangel Pr.; 1-877718),* Orders Addr.: P.O. Box 23348, Ventura, CA 93002; Edit Addr.: 1363 Spinnaker Dr., No. 57, Ventura, CA 93001 Tel 805-642-1872 Do not confuse with companies with the same name in San Diego, CA, Kaysville, UT.

Archedigm Pubns, *(Archedigm Pubns.; 0-944135),* Subs. of Archedigm, Inc., Orders Addr.: P.O. Box 1109, Olney, MD 20830-1109 Tel 301-774-5536 (phone/fax)
E-mail: archedigm@aol.com.

Archeolog Soc, *(Archeological Society of Virginia Pr. of The Archeological Society of Virginia; 1-884626),* P.O. Box 70395, Richmond, VA 23255-0395 Tel 804-273-9291; Fax: 804-273-0885
E-mail: asv@archeology.org
Web site: http://www2.dgsys.com/~asv.

Archipelago Pubg, *(Archipelago Publishing; 0-9674988),* 716 Princeton Blvd, Suite 11, Lowell, MA 01851 Tel 978-458-3999; Toll Free: 888-350-1978 Do not confuse with Archipelago Publishing in Friday Harbor, WA
E-mail: turtle@kittynet.com
Web site: http://www.kittynet.com/turtle/.

ARCsoft, *(ARCsoft Pubs.; 0-86668),* 1698 Fairside Ct., Florence, KY 41042-7024 (SAN 216-2210).

Ardent Media, *(Ardent Media, Inc.; 0-8290; 0-89197; 0-9664902),* Affil. of Irvington Pubs., Orders Addr.: P.O. Box 286, New York, NY 10276-0286 Fax: 212-861-0998; Toll Free: 800-218-1535.

Ardor Scrib, *(Ardor Scribendi; 1-893357),* 145 E. 32nd St., 10th Flr., New York, NY 10016 (SAN 253-6633) Tel 212-889-6225; Fax: 212-889-8268
E-mail: ardorscribendi@aol.com
Web site: http://www.arborscribendi.com.

†ARE Pr, *(A.R.E. Pr.; 0-87604),* Orders Addr.: 215 67th St., Virginia Beach, VA 23451-2061 Tel 757-428-3588; Fax: 757-422-6921; Toll Free: 888-273-3400
E-mail: arepress@edgarcayce.org; tradesales@edgarcayce.org
Web site: http://www.edgarcayce.org
Dist(s): **Baker & Taylor** *(Baker & Taylor Bks.)*
Brodart *(Brodart Co.)*
DeVorss *(DeVorss & Co.)*
Midwest Lib Serv *(Midwest Library Service)*
New Concepts Bks & Tapes *(New Concepts Bks. & Tapes Distributors)*
New Leaf Dist *(New Leaf Distributing Co., Inc.)*
Red Wheel ME *(Red Wheel); CIP.*

Arena (GBR) *(1-85742) Dist. by* **Ashgate Pub Co.**

Ares, *(Ares Pubs., Inc.; 0-89005),* 14273 W. First Dr., Golden, CO 80401-5274 (SAN 205-6011) Tel 303-279-8435; Fax: 303-279-8572
E-mail: order.arespublishers@att.net
Web site: http://www.arespublishers.com.

Argee Pub, *(Argee Publishing Co.; 0-931084),* 29382 Buckhaven, Lagune Niguel, CA 92677 (SAN 211-8815) Tel 949-249-3755.

Argonaut Pr, *(Argonaut Pr.; 1-882206),* 369 11th St., San Francisco, CA 94103-4313 Tel 415-896-6383
Dist(s): **Publishers Group** *(Publishers Group West).*

Argosy, *(Argosy; 0-87266),* 116 E. 59th St., New York, NY 10022 (SAN 203-4875).

Argus Pub, *(Argus Publishing; 0-9659196),* 325 Sylvan Ave., Englewood Cliffs, NJ 07632 Tel 201-871-5871; Fax: 201-871-9304; Toll Free: 888-668-6455
E-mail: notmilk@earthlink.net
Web site: http://www.notmilk.com.

Argyll Pubng (GBR) *(1-874640; 1-902831) Dist. by* **St Mut.**

ARI CO, *(Allergy Respiratory Institute of Colorado; 0-9622943),* 5800 E. Evans Ave., Denver, CO 80222 Tel 303-756-3614; Fax: 303-757-1518.

Ariadne CA, *(Ariadne Pr.; 0-929497; 1-57241),* 270 Goins Ct., Riverside, CA 92507 (SAN 249-5791) Tel 909-684-9202; Fax: 909-779-0449 Do not confuse with Ariadne Pr., Rockville, MD
E-mail: bookinfo@ariadnepress.com
Web site: http://www.ariadnepress.com.

Aribet Bks, *(Aribet Bks.; 0-9644064),* P.O. Box 15640, West Palm Beach, FL 33416-5640 Fax: 561-791-3204
E-mail: aribetbks@aol.com.

Ariel GA, *(Ariel Pr.; 0-89804),* Subs. of Light, 4255 Trotters Way, No. 13A, Alpharetta, GA 30004 (SAN 219-8460) Tel 770-664-4886; Fax: 770-664-4974; Toll Free: 800-336-7769 ; *Imprints:* Enthea Pr (Enthea Press) Do not confuse with companies with the same or similar name in Berkeley, CA, Muscaline, IA
Dist(s): **Alliance Bk Co** *(Alliance Bk. Co.).*

Ariel Starr, *(Ariel Starr Productions, Ltd.; 1-889122),* P.O. Box 17, Demarest, NJ 07627 Tel 201-784-9148; Fax: 201-541-8796
E-mail: darkbird@aol.com
Dist(s): **Baker & Taylor** *(Baker & Taylor Bks.)*
Bookazine Co Inc *(Bookazine Co., Inc.)*
New Leaf Dist *(New Leaf Distributing Co., Inc.).*

Aries Rising, *(Aries Rising Pr.; 0-917211),* Orders Addr.: P.O. Box 29532, Los Angeles, CA 90029 (SAN 662-2313); Edit Addr.: 2132 Alcyona Dr., Los Angeles, CA 90068 (SAN 655-9573) Tel 323-462-6458 (phone/fax)
E-mail: alanrcan@aol.com
Dist(s): **Baker & Taylor** *(Baker & Taylor Bks.).*

Aristos Pub Hse, *(Aristos Publishing Hse./Geier Learning Systems; 0-927634),* Div. of John Geier & Assocs., Inc., 10650 County Rd. 81, Maple Grove, MN 55369 Tel 612-493-3374; Fax: 612-493-3794.

Armellini, *(Armellini, Inc.; 0-9675953),* 11151 S. Sandusky, Tulsa, OK 74137 Tel 918-298-1810; Fax: 918-299-7491
E-mail: toby.Armellini@prodigy.net.

Arno Press, *(Arno Press; 0-405),* 3 Park Ave., New York, NY 10016
Dist(s): **Ayer** *(Ayer Co. Pubs., Inc.).*

Arnold Arboretum, *(Arnold Arboretum of Harvard Univ.; 1-878297),* 125 Arborway, Jamaica Plain, MA 02130 Tel 617-524-1718; Fax: 617-524-1418.

Aroc Pub, *(Aroc Publishing; 0-945654),* 4068 S. 43rd St., Milwaukee, WI 53220-2773 (SAN 247-5391).

Aronson, *(Aronson, Jason Pubs.; 0-7657; 0-87668; 1-56821),* Orders Addr.: P.O. Box 1539, Fort Lee, NJ 07024-2539 (SAN 665-6536) Fax: 201-840-7242; Toll Free: 800-782-0015; Edit Addr.: 230 Livingston St., Northvale, NJ 07647 (SAN 201-0127) Tel 201-767-4093; Fax: 201-767-4330 Do not confuse with companies with similar name in Highmount, NY, Arcade, NY, Santa Monica, CA
E-mail: editor@aronson.com
Web site: http://www.aronson.com
Dist(s): **IPG Chicago** *(Independent Pubs. Group).*

Arpen Pr, *(Arpen Pr.; 0-9664985),* P.O. Box 400-135, Cambridge, MA 02140 Tel 617-661-8589; Fax: 617-661-8597
E-mail: najarian@mediaone.net.

Arrow Pr, *See* **Bright Bks CA**

Arroway, *(Arroway Pubs.; 0-9600284),* 40 San Jacinto Way, San Francisco, CA 94127-2033 (SAN 203-4913)
Dist(s): **R Co Hinkel Inc** *(Hinkel, A. R. Co., Inc.).*

Arrowhead AZ, *(Arrowhead Pr., Inc. (AZ); 0-910973),* 3131 W. Clarendon Ave., Phoenix, AZ 85017 (SAN 267-6672) Tel 602-263-8808; Fax: 602-265-6164 Do not confuse with Arrowhead Pr., Sitka, AK.

Arrowood Pr, *(Arrowood Pr.; 0-88486),* Div. of BBs Publishing Corp., 386 Park Ave., S., Suite 1200, New York, NY 10016-8804 (SAN 661-8758) Tel 212-679-4200; Fax: 212-679-4234
Dist(s): **Publishers Group** *(Publishers Group West).*

Arrowstar Pub, *(Arrowstar Publishing; 0-935151),* Orders Addr.: P.O. Box 100134, Denver, CO 80210-0134 (SAN 695-3379) Tel 303-715-9292; Fax: 303-733-8625
E-mail: wholeearthmoto@hotmail.com
Dist(s): **Baker & Taylor** *(Baker & Taylor Bks.).*

ARS Pub, *(Ars Publishing Co.; 0-941616),* P.O. Box 6276, Stockton, CA 95206-0276 (SAN 239-1422) Tel 209-465-8243.

Art Bks Intl (GBR) *(0-901033) Dist. by* **Partners Pubs Grp.**

Art Endeavors, *(Artistic Endeavors Publishing/Schore; 1-884390),* 609 Heights at Cape Ann, Gloucester, MA 01930-5348 (SAN 298-0673) Do not confuse with Artistic Endeavors in Stamford, CT.

Art Therapy, *(Art Therapy Pubns.; 0-9611462),* Orders Addr.: Mill Village, Craftsbury Common, VT 05827 (SAN 665-6544) Tel 802-586-2215.

Arthritis Trust, *(Arthritis Trust of America; 0-9615437),* 7111 Sweetgum Rd., Suite A, Fairview, TN 37062 (SAN 696-0677) Tel 615-799-1002 (phone/fax)
E-mail: taf@telalink.net
Web site: http://www.telalink.net/~taf.

Arthur James (GBR) *(0-85305) Dist. by* **Morehouse Pub.**

Arthur James (GBR) *(0-85305) Dist. by* **St Mut.**

Artspace Bks, *(Artspace Bks.; 0-9631095; 1-891273),* 33 Filbert Ave., Sausalito, CA 94965 Tel 415-331-3031; Fax: 415-332-7119
Dist(s): **Dist Art Pubs** *(Distributed Art Pubs./D.A.P.).*

ASCD, *(Association for Supervision & Curriculum Development; 0-87120),* 1703 N. Beauregaurd St., Alexandria, VA 22311 (SAN 201-1352) Tel 703-578-9600; Fax: 703-575-5400; Toll Free: 800-933-2723
E-mail: member@ascd.org
Web site: http://www.ascd.org
Dist(s): **netLibrary CO** *(netLibrary, Inc.).*

Ascelapias Pub, *(Ascelapias Publishing; 0-9662564),* 15228 SW Teal Blvd., Beaverton, OR 97007 Tel 503-816-2616; Fax: 503-579-8822
E-mail: csa@teleport.com.

ASCLA, *(Association of Specialized Cooperative Library Agencies),* 50 E. Huron St., Chicago, IL 60611 (SAN 233-4658) Tel 312-280-4399; Fax: 312-944-8085; Toll Free: 800-545-2433 (ext. 4399).

Asclepiad, *(Asclepiad Pubns.; 0-935718),* 3396 Breckland Ct., Ann Arbor, MI 48103-9733 (SAN 213-7240).

ASET, *(American Society of Electroneurodiagnostic Technologists; 1-57797),* Orders Addr.: 204 W. Seventh St., Carroll, IA 51401-2317 (SAN 224-2796) Tel 712-792-2978; Fax: 712-792-6962
E-mail: aset@netins.net
Web site: http://www.aset.org.

ASFE, *(ASFE; 1-58074),* 8811 Coleville Rd., Suite G106, Silver Spring, MD 20910 (SAN 224-0769) Tel 301-565-2733; Fax: 301-589-2017
E-mail: info@asfe.org
Web site: http://www.asfe.org.

Ash Tree, *(Ash Tree Publishing; 0-9614620; 1-888123),* Orders Addr.: P.O. Box 64, Woodstock, NY 12498 (SAN 691-8964) Tel 845-246-8081 (phone/fax); Edit Addr.: 416 Fishcreek Rd., Saugerties, NY 12477
E-mail: susunweed@hotmail.com
Web site: http://www.susunweed.com
Dist(s): **Baker & Taylor** *(Baker & Taylor Bks.)*
Bookpeople *(Bookpeople)*
New Leaf Dist *(New Leaf Distributing Co., Inc.)*
Nutri-Books Corp *(Nutri-Bks. Corp.)*
Partners Pubs Grp *(Partners Pubs. Group, Inc.).*

ASHAM, *(Asociacion de Hispanistas de las Americas; 0-943503),* 3600 SW Ninth Terr., No. 4, Miami, FL 33135 (SAN 668-5080) Tel 305-448-6590.

Ashbrook Pr, *See* **Ashbrook Pub**

Ashbrook Pub, *(Ashbrook Publishing; 0-9629950),* 10089 Bartholomew Rd., Chagrin Falls, OH 44023 Tel 216-543-8369; Fax: 440-543-8369
E-mail: elcrary@alltel.net.

Ashbury Pr, *(Ashbury Pr.; 0-9673445),* 736 Ashbury St., San Francisco, CA 94117-4014 Tel 415-665-5920
E-mail: info@ashburypress.com
Web site: http://www.ashburypress.com.

Ashgate Pub (GBR) *(0-566; 0-86078; 1-84014; 1-85521; 1-85928; 1-85972; 0-7546) Dist. by* **Ashgate Pub Co.**

†Ashgate Pub Co, *(Ashgate Publishing Co.; 0-566),* Subs. of Ashgate Publishing, Ltd., Orders Addr.: 2252 Ridge Rd., Brookfield, VT 05036-9704 Tel 802-276-3162; Fax: 802-276-3837; Toll Free: 800-535-9544 (Orders - US & Canada); Edit Addr.: 131 Main St., Burlington, VT 05401-5600 (SAN 213-4446) Tel 802-865-7641; Fax: 802-865-7847; Toll Free: 800-535-9544 (US & Canada)
E-mail: editor@ashgate.com; orders@ashgate.com
Web site: http://www.ashgatechem.com; http://www.gowerpub.com; http://www.gowertraining.co.uk/; http://www.ashgate.com*; CIP.*

Ashgrove Pr (GBR) *(0-906798; 1-85398) Dist. by* **Words Distrib.**

Ashish Pub Hse (IND) *(81-7024; 81-7648) Dist. by* **S Asia.**

Ashish Pub Hse (IND) *(81-7024; 81-7648) Dist. by* **Nataraj Bks.**

Ashley Bks, *(Ashley Bks., Inc.; 0-87949),* Orders Addr.: 4600 W. Commercial Blvd., Fort Lauderdale, FL 33319 (SAN 201-1409); Edit Addr.: P.O. Box 223580, Hollywood, FL 33022-3580.

Ashwin Pubns, *(Ashwins Pubns.; 0-9620939),* Orders Addr.: P.O. Box 1686, Ojai, CA 93023 (SAN 250-1384) Tel 805-646-6622; Edit Addr.: 1114 McNell Rd., Ojai, CA 93023 (SAN 250-1392)
E-mail: ashwins@aol.com
Dist(s): **New Leaf Dist** *(New Leaf Distributing Co., Inc.).*

Asia Bk Corp, *(Asia Bk. Corp. of America; 0-940500),* 45-77 157th St., Flushing, NY 11355 (SAN 214-493X) Tel 718-762-7204; Fax: 718-460-5030.

Asian Educ Servs (IND) *(81-206) Dist. by* **S Asia.**

Asian Humanities, *(Asian Humanities Pr.; 0-89581),* Div. of Jain Publishing Co., Inc., P.O. Box 3523, Fremont, CA 94539 Tel 510-659-8272; Fax: 510-659-0501
E-mail: mail@jainpub.com
Web site: http://www.jainpub.com.

Asian Prod Organ (JPN) *(92-833) Dist. by* **Bernan Associates.**

Asia-Pacific Res, *(Asia/Pacific Research Ctr.; 0-9653935; 1-931368),* Div. of The Institute for International Studies, c/o Stanford University, Rm. E301, Encina Hall, Stanford, CA 94305-6055 Tel 650-723-7453; Fax: 650-723-6530
E-mail: asia-pacific-research-center@stanford.edu
Web site: http://aparc.stanford.edu.

Asklepios Imprint of Pagan Pr

Askon Pub, *(Askon Publishing Co.; 0-931609),* Subs. of Askon Corp., 3000 Bluff Crest Ln., Abilene, TX 79601-4801 (SAN 683-678X) Tel 915-695-1505.

Aslan Pub, *(Aslan Publishing; 0-944031),* Owned by Renaissance Book Services Corp., 2490 Black Rock Tpke., No. 342, Fairfield, CT 06432 (SAN 242-6129) Tel 203-372-0300; Fax: 203-374-4766; Toll Free: 800-786-5427 Do not confuse with Aslan Publishing, Alpharetta, GA
E-mail: info@AslanPublishing.com
Web site: http://www.AslanPublishing.com
Dist(s): **Assoc Pubs Grp** *(Associated Pubs. Group).*

ASM, *(ASM International; 0-87170),* 9639 Kinsman Rd., Materials Park, OH 44073-0002 (SAN 204-7586) Tel 440-338-5151; Fax: 440-338-4634; Toll Free: 800-336-5152 (ext. 5900) Do not confuse with ASM International, Inc., Fort Lauderdale, FL
E-mail: Cust-Srv@asminternational.org
Web site: http://www.asminternational.org/.

ASM Pr, *(ASM Pr.; 0-914826; 1-55581),* Orders Addr.: P.O. Box 605, Herndon, VA 20172 Tel 703-661-1593; Fax: 703-661-1501; Toll Free: 800-546-2416; Edit Addr.: 1752 N St., NW, Washington, DC 20036 (SAN 202-1153) Tel 202-737-3600; Fax: 202-942-9342
E-mail: books@asmusa.org
Web site: http://www.asmpress.org.

ASME, *(American Society of Mechanical Engineers; 0-7918),* 22 Law Dr., P.O. Box 2300, Fairfield, NJ 07007-2300 (SAN 201-1379) Tel 973-882-1176; Fax: 973-882-1717; Toll Free: 800-843-2763
E-mail: infocentral@asme.org
Web site: http://www.asme.org.

ASME Pr, *(ASME Pr.; 0-7918),* Div. of American Society of Mechanical Engineers, Orders Addr.: 22 Law Dr., P.O. Box 2350, Fairfield, NJ 07007-2350 (SAN 665-6498); Edit Addr.: 3 Park Ave., New York, NY 10016 (SAN 201-1379) Tel 212-591-7000; Fax: 212-591-7292; Toll Free: 800-843-2763 (customer service)
Web site: http://www.asme.org/pubs/asmepress.

†Aspen Law, *(Aspen Law & Business; 0-13; 0-316),* Orders Addr.: 7201 McKinney Cir., Frederick, MD 21704 Fax: 301-695-7931; Toll Free: 800-638-8437; Edit Addr.: 1185 Avenue of the Americas, New York, NY 10036 Tel 212-597-0200; Fax: 212-597-0338; Toll Free Fax: 800-901-9075; Toll Free: 800-234-1660 (customer service); 800-447-1717 (sales dept.)
E-mail: customer.service@aspenpubl.com
Web site: http://www.aspenpublishers.com*; CIP.*

Aspen Leaf Pr, *(Aspen Leaf Pr.; 0-9632963),* 383 Ponderosa Ln., Woodland Park, CO 80863 Tel 719-687-5795 (phone/fax).

†Aspen Pub, *(Aspen Pubs., Inc.; 0-444; 0-7896; 0-8342; 0-87189; 0-87622; 0-89443; 0-912862),* Subs. of Wolters Kluwer U.S. Corp., 200 Orchard Ridge Dr., Suite 200, Gaithersburg, MD 20878 (SAN 203-4999) Tel 301-417-7500; Fax: 301-695-7931; Toll Free: 800-638-8437 (orders); 800-234-1660 (customer service)
E-mail: customer.service@aspenpubl.com
Web site: http://www.aspenpub.com*; CIP.*

ASQ Qual Pr, *(ASQ Quality Pr.; 0-87389),* Div. of American Society for Quality, 611 E. Wisconsin Ave., P.O. Box 3005, Milwaukee, WI 53201-3005 (SAN 683-5244) Tel 414-272-8575; Fax: 414-272-1734; Toll Free: 800-248-1946
E-mail: cs@asq.org
Web site: http://www.asq.org/.

ASQC Qual Pr, *See* **ASQ Qual Pr**

ASSE, *(American Society of Safety Engineers; 0-939874; 1-885581),* 1800 E. Oakton St., Des Plaines, IL 60018-2187 (SAN 201-7032) Tel 847-699-2929; Fax: 847-768-3434
Web site: http://www.asse.org.

Assn Adv Med Instrn, *(Assn. for the Advancement of Medical Instrumentation; 0-910275; 1-57020),* 1110 N. Glebe Rd., Suite 220, Arlington, VA 22201-5762 (SAN 224-3407) Tel 703-525-4890; Fax: 703-525-1067; Toll Free: 800-332-2264
Web site: http://www.aami.org.

Assn Am Med Coll, *(Association of American Medical Colleges; 1-57754),* 2450 N St., NW, Washington, DC 20037 Tel 202-828-0400; Fax: 202-828-1125
Web site: http://www.aamc.org.

Assn Asian Studies, *(Association for Asian Studies, Inc.; 0-924304),* 1021 E. Huron, Ann Arbor, MI 48104 Tel 734-665-4847; Fax: 734-665-3801.

Assn Birth Psych, *(Association for Birth Psychology; 0-9612182),* 444 E. 82nd St., New York, NY 10028 (SAN 289-114X) Tel 212-988-6617.

Assn Brain Tumor, *See* **Am Brain Tumor**

Assn Brit Dispen Opticians (GBR) *(0-900099) Dist. by* **St Mut.**

Assn Exper Ed, *(Association for Experiential Education; 0-929361),* 2305 Canyon Blvd., Suite 100, Boulder, CO 80302-5651 (SAN 225-7742) Tel 303-440-8844; Fax: 303-440-9581
E-mail: publications@aee.org
Web site: http://www.aee.org
Dist(s): **Am Camping** *(American Camping Assn.)*
Kendall-Hunt *(Kendall/Hunt Publishing Co.)*
Project Advent *(Project Adventure, Inc.).*

Assn Farmwrker, *(Association of Farmworker Opportunity Programs; 1-886567),* 1611 N. Kent St., Suite 910, Arlington, VA 22209 Tel 703-528-4141; Fax: 703-528-4145
E-mail: afopmull@aol.com; afopstaff@aol.com.

Assn Hist Chiro, *(Association for the History of Chiropractic, Inc.; 0-9659131),* 1000 Brady St., Davenport, IA 52803 Tel 319-884-5894; Fax: 319-884-5897; Toll Free: 800-722-3648
E-mail: Wiesr_g@palmer.edu.

Assn I M&R, *(Association for Investment Management & Research; 0-938367; 1-879087),* Orders Addr.: c/o PBD Worldwide Fulfillment Services, P.O. Box 931788, Atlanta, GA 31193-1788 Tel 770-442-8633; Fax: 770-442-9742
E-mail: info@aimr.org; aimrpubs@pbd.com
Web site: http://www.aimr.org
Dist(s): **PBD Inc** *(PBD, Inc.).*

Assn Med Illus, *(Association of Medical Illustrators; 1-883486),* 2965 Flowers Rd. S., Suite 105, Atlanta, GA 30341-5520 Tel 770-454-7933; Fax: 770-458-3314
E-mail: billjust@mindspring.com
Dist(s): **Serbin Commns** *(Serbin Communications, Inc.).*

Assn Modern Psy, *(Association for Modern Psychoanalysis; 0-9624534),* c/o Sara Sheftel, 225 W. 86th St., Apt. 1104, New York, NY 10024-4333 Tel 212-724-0159.

Assn Oper Rm Nurses, *See* **AORN**

Assn Pediatric, *(Association of Pediatric Oncology Nurses; 0-9666193),* 4700 W. Lake Ave., Glenview, IL 60025-1485 Tel 847-375-4727; Fax: 847-375-4777
E-mail: info@apon.org
Web site: http://www.apon.org/.

Assn Phys Plant Admin, *See* **APPA VA**

Assn Soil & Found Engrs, *See* **ASFE**

Assn Surgical, *(Association of Surgical Technologists; 0-926805),* 7108-C S. Alton Way, Suite 100, Englewood, CO 80112-2106 Tel 303-694-9130; Fax: 303-694-9169
E-mail: ast@ast.org
Web site: http://www.ast.org.

Assoc Official, *See* **AOAC Intl**

Assoc Publ, *(Association Publishing; 0-9668380),* 100 Oxmoor Rd., Suite 110, Birmingham, AL 35209 Tel 205-941-4623; Fax: 205-942-8390.

Assoc Pubs FL, *(Associated Pubs.; 1-56665; 1-877711),* Orders Addr.: P.O. Box 140103, Gainesville, FL 32614-0103 (SAN 202-4535) Tel 352-371-4071; Fax: 352-378-6045 (orders) Do not confuse with Associated Pubs., West Palm Beach, FL.

Assoc Pubs Grp, *(Associated Pubs. Group; 1-881511),* Div. of Hambleton-Hill, 1501 County Hospital Rd., Nashville, TN 37218 (SAN 630-818X) Tel 615-254-2450; Fax: 615-254-2405; Toll Free: 800-327-5113
E-mail: sswift@agpbooks.com
Web site: http://www.apgbooks.com.

Assoc Univ Prs, *(Associated Univ. Presses; 0-8453),* 440 Forsgate Dr., Cranbury, NJ 08512 (SAN 281-2959) Tel 609-655-4770; Fax: 609-655-8366 ; *Imprints:* Cornwall Bks (Cornwall Books)
E-mail: aup440@aol.com
Web site: http://arts.fdu.edu/aup/.

Assocs in Med, *(Associates in Medical Marketing Co., Inc.; 1-884065),* 3 Terry Dr., Suite 201, Newtown, PA 18940 Tel 215-860-9600; Fax: 215-860-9558 ; *Imprints:* Hndbks Hlth Care (Handbooks in Health Care Company)
E-mail: custserv@HHCbooks.com; custserv@handbooksinhealthcare.com
Web site: http://www.HHCbooks.com.

Astara, *(Astara, Inc.; 0-918936),* P.O. Box 5003, Upland, CA 91786-5003 (SAN 207-6446) Tel 909-981-4941; Fax: 909-920-9541; Toll Free: 800-964-4941
E-mail: info@astara.org; mail@astara.org
Web site: http://www.astara.org
Dist(s): **Bookpeople** *(Bookpeople)*
New Leaf Dist *(New Leaf Distributing Co., Inc.).*

Astarte Shell Pr, *(Astarte Shell Pr.; 0-9624626; 1-885349),* HC 63, Box 89, Bath, ME 04530-9503 Tel 207-828-1992; Fax: 207-442-7260; Toll Free: 800-349-0941
E-mail: INTP@Biddeford.com
Web site: http://www.HighwayTech.comAstarteShell
Dist(s): **Snow Pocket Distrib** *(Snow Pocket Distributors).*

ASTM, *(American Society for Testing & Materials; 0-8031),* 100 Barr Harbor Dr., West Conshohocken, PA 19428-2959 (SAN 201-1344) Tel 610-832-9500; Fax: 610-832-9635; P.O. Box C700, West Conshohocken, PA 19428-2959
E-mail: service@astm.org
Web site: http://www.astm.org.

Astor-Honor, *(Astor-Honor, Inc.; 0-8392),* 16 E. 40th St., Third Flr., New York, NY 10016 (SAN 203-5022) Tel 212-840-8800; Fax: 212-840-7246.

ASTP, *(American Society of Transplant Physicians; 0-9660150),* 236 Rte. 38, Suite 100, Moorestown, NJ 08057-3276
E-mail: astp@slackinc.com
Web site: http://www.astp.org/.

Astragal Pr, *(Astragal Pr.; 0-9618088; 1-879335; 1-931626),* Orders Addr.: P.O. Box 239, Mendham, NJ 07945-0239 (SAN 666-590X) Tel 973-543-3045; Fax: 973-543-3044; Edit Addr.: 5 Cold Hill Rd., Suite 12, Mendham, NJ 07945
E-mail: astragalpress@attglobal.net
Web site: http://www.astragalpress.com.

Astrolog Pub (ISR) *(965-494) Dist. by* **IPG Chicago.**

Astrolog Pub (ISR) *(965-494) Dist. by* **Assoc Pubs Grp.**

ATCC, *(American Type Culture Collection; 0-930009),* 10801 University Blvd., Manassas, VA 20110-2204 (SAN 224-2923) Tel 703-365-2700; Fax: 703-365-2701; Toll Free: 800-638-6597
E-mail: sales@atcc.org
Web site: http://www.atcc.org.

Athelia-Henrietta, *(Athelia-Henrietta Pr.; 0-9638787; 1-890157),* Div. of R. Francis Entertainment, Inc., 1194 Nostrand Ave., Brooklyn, NY 11225 Tel 718-493-4500; Fax: 718-467-0099
E-mail: atheliaheriettapress@yahoo.com
Dist(s): **Baker & Taylor** *(Baker & Taylor Bks.)*
BookWorld *(BookWorld Services, Inc.)*
Bookpeople *(Bookpeople)*
Koen Bk Distributors *(Koen Bk. Distributors)*
New Leaf Dist *(New Leaf Distributing Co., Inc.)*
Quality Bks IL *(Quality Bks., Inc.).*

Athena Bks, *(Athena Bks.; 0-9645750),* Orders Addr.: P.O. Box 2282, Gilroy, CA 95021-2282 Tel 408-842-4719; Fax: 408-842-1019; Edit Addr.: 7155 Revere Pl., Gilroy, CA 95020.

Atheneum Yung Read, *(Atheneum Books for Young Readers; 0-02; 0-684; 0-689),* 1230 Avenue of the Americas, New York, NY 10020
Web site: http://www.simonsays.com/
Dist(s): **BookWorld** *(BookWorld Services, Inc.).*

ATL Pr Sci, *(ATL Pr., Scientific Pubs., Inc.; 1-882360),* P.O. Box 4563, Shrewsbury, MA 01545-7563 (SAN 297-8334) Tel 508-898-2290; Fax: 508-898-2063; Toll Free: 800-835-7543
E-mail: atlpinc@aol.com
Web site: http://www.bookzone.com/ATLPress/
Dist(s): **Baker & Taylor** *(Baker & Taylor Bks.)*
Coutts Library Service Inc *(Coutts Library Service, Inc.)*
Follett Library *(Follett Library Resources)*
J Majors Co *(Majors, J. A. Co.)*
Quality Bks IL *(Quality Bks., Inc.).*

Atlantic Info Services Inc, *(Atlantic Information Services, Inc.; 0-929156; 1-931467),* 1100 17th St., NW, Suite 300, Washington, DC 20036-4601 (SAN 248-7705) Tel 202-775-9008; Fax: 202-331-9542; Toll Free: 800-521-4323
E-mail: customerserv@aispub.com; garnold@aispub.com
Web site: http://www.aishealth.com.

Atlantic Pub Co, *(Atlantic Publishing Co.; 0-937866),* P.O. Box 67, Tabor City, NC 28463 (SAN 215-6237) Tel 910-653-3153; Fax: 910-653-9440; Toll Free: 800-334-8301 Do not confuse with companies with the same or similar name in Aurora, IL , Neosho, MO , Lakeland FL , Ocala, FL , Combs, KY.

Atlntc Mnthly Imprint of Grove-Atltic

ATMA, *(ATMA; 0-9620108),* 10235 Cornelius Pass, Portland, OR 97231 (SAN 247-7033) Tel 503-690-9513 (phone/fax)
E-mail: atma@teleport.com
Web site: http://www.teleport.com/~atma.

Atsmorts Pub, *(Atsmorts Publishing; 0-9620355),* 2323 Rambling Rd., Kalamazoo, MI 49008-1636 (SAN 245-6443) Tel 616-381-4890.

Attent Span Advan, *(Attention Span Advancement Registry Service; 0-9606990),* 1940 Fifth Ave., Sacramento, CA 95818 (SAN 238-910X).

Attention Span Bks, *(Attention Span Bks.; 0-9646653),* P.O. Box 788, Niwot, CO 80544-0788 Tel 303-530-4777; Toll Free: 800-927-2469
E-mail: gdenton@ix.netcom.com
Web site: http://www.brainlash.com
Dist(s): **Baker & Taylor** *(Baker & Taylor Bks.)*
Tattered Cover *(Tattered Cover Bookstore).*

Auburn Hse Imprint of Greenwood

Auckland Univ (NZL) *(1-86940) Dist. by* **Paul & Co Pubs.**

Audio-Forum, *See* **J Norton Audio-Forum**

AudioText, *(AudioText; 1-884612),* Orders Addr.: P.O. Box 418, Barker, TX 77413 Tel 281-398-9381; Fax: 281-398-9481.

Augsburg Imprint of Augsburg Fortress

†Augsburg Fortress, *(Augsburg Fortress Pubs., Publishing Hse. of The Evangelical Lutheran Church in America; 0-8006; 0-8066),* Orders Addr.: P.O. Box 1209, Minneapolis, MN 55440-1209 (SAN 169-4081) Tel 612-330-3300; Fax: 612-330-3455; Toll Free: 800-328-4648 (orders only); Edit Addr.: 100 S. Fifth St., Suite 700, Minneapolis, MN 55440-1209 (SAN 169-4081) ; *Imprints:* Fortress Pr (Fortress Press) Augsburg (Augsburg)
E-mail: info@augsburgfortress.org; productinfo@augsburgfortress.org; subscriptions@augsburgfortress.org; customerservice@augsburgfortress.com
Web site: http://www.augsburgfortress.org; *CIP.*

Augustana Coll, *(Augustana College Library; 0-910182),* 3435 9 1/2 Ave., Rock Island, IL 61201 (SAN 203-5073) Tel 309-794-7266; Fax: 309-794-7640
E-mail: alijm@augustana.edu; alirg@augustana.edu
Web site: http://www.augustana.edu/library.

†Aunt Lute Bks, *(Aunt Lute Bks.; 0-918040; 0-933216; 1-879960),* Div. of Aunt Lute Foundation, Orders Addr.: P.O. Box 410687, San Francisco, CA 94141 Tel 415-826-1300; Fax: 415-826-8300; Edit Addr.: 2180 Bryant St., San Francisco, CA 94110-2128
E-mail: books@auntlute.com
Web site: http://www.auntlute.com
Dist(s): **Bookpeople** *(Bookpeople)*
Consort Bk Sales *(Consortium Bk. Sales & Distribution)*
SPD-Small Pr Dist *(SPD-Small Pr. Distribution); CIP.*

Aura Pub Co, *(Aura Publishing Co.; 0-9615513),* 22 Surrey Ln., San Rafael, CA 94903 (SAN 696-1878) Tel 415-492-8034; Fax: 415-492-0893 Do not confuse with Aura Publishing Co., Boston, MA.

Auromere, *(Auromere, Inc.; 0-89744),* 2621 W. US Hwy. 12, Lodi, CA 95242-9200 (SAN 169-0043) Fax: 209-339-3715; Toll Free: 800-735-4691
E-mail: sasp@lodinet.com
Web site: http://www.auromere.com
Dist(s): **DeVorss** *(DeVorss & Co.)*
New Leaf Dist *(New Leaf Distributing Co., Inc.)*
Red Wheel ME *(Red Wheel).*

Aurora Assocs, *(Aurora Assocs., Inc.; 0-931211),* 1015 18th St., NW, Suite 400, Washington, DC 20036 (SAN 681-9672) Tel 202-463-0950.

Aurora KS, *(Aurora Publishing Co.; 0-9622118),* Orders Addr.: P.O. Box 1729, Garden City, KS 67846-1729 Fax: 316-275-5026; Edit Addr.: 523 N. Main St., Garden City, KS 67846 Do not confuse with companies with the same or similar names in Ft. Lauderdale, FL, Arlington, VA, Los Altos Hills, CA, West Palm Beach, FL.

Aurora Press, *(Aurora Pr., Inc.; 0-943358),* P.O. Box 573, Santa Fe, NM 87504 (SAN 240-5881) Tel 505-989-9804; Fax: 505-982-8321; Toll Free: 800-423-7087 Do not confuse with companies with the same or similar name in Sarasota, FL, Columbia, MD
E-mail: aurorep@aol.com
Dist(s): **Bookpeople** *(Bookpeople)*
DeVorss *(DeVorss & Co.)*
Gem Guides Bk *(Gem Guides Bk. Co.)*
New Leaf Dist *(New Leaf Distributing Co., Inc.)*
Nutri-Books Corp *(Nutri-Bks. Corp.)*
Red Wheel ME *(Red Wheel).*

Aurora VA, *(Aurora Publishing; 0-9622150),* 5653 Seventh St., N., Arlington, VA 22205 Tel 703-841-1142; Fax: 703-841-1141 Do not confuse with companies with the same or similar names in Ft. Lauderdale, FL, Arlington, VA, Los Altos Hills, CA, West Palm Beach, FL, Garden City, KS.

Aurum Press Ltd (GBR) *(1-85410; 0-948149; 0-906053; 1-902538) Dist. by* **London Brdge.**

Aust Council Educ Res (AUS) *(0-85563; 0-86431) Dist. by* **St Mut.**

Aust Council Educ Res (AUS) *(0-85563; 0-86431) Dist. by* **Stylus Pub VA.**

Austin & Winfield, *(Austin & Winfield, Pubs., Inc.; 1-57292; 1-880921),* 7831 Woodmont Ave., No. 345, Bethesda, MD 20814 Toll Free: 800-992-8784
E-mail: austinisp1@aol.com
Web site: http://www.interscholars.com
Dist(s): **Rowman** *(Rowman & Littlefield Pubs., Inc.)*
U Pr of Amer *(University Pr. of America).*

Austin Univ Forestry, *(Austin, Stephen F. State Univ., Schl. of Forestry; 0-938361),* Orders Addr.: P.O. Box 6109, Nacogdoches, TX 75962 (SAN 659-7459); Edit Addr.: North St. & E. College Ave., Nacogdoches, TX 75962 (SAN 659-7467) Tel 409-468-3304.

Auth Village Pubns, *(Auth Village Pubns.; 0-9659365),* 5018 Braymer Ave., Camp Springs, MD 20746-3818 Tel 301-423-4530.

Authors Coop, *(Authors Cooperative, Inc.; 0-9623311; 1-888830),* Orders Addr.: c/o Cambridge Ctr. for Behavioral Studies, 336 Baker Ave., Boston, MA 02199-0053 Tel 978-369-2227; Fax: 978-369-8584; Edit Addr.: 1700 Ben Franklin Dr., Suite 9E, Sarasota, FL 34236-2374
E-mail: authcoop@home.com; store@behavior.org; authorscooperative@behavior.org
Web site: http://www.authorscooperatve.com
Dist(s): **Sunshine MA** *(Sunshine Bks., Inc.).*

Authors Pub NA Imprint of Elton-Wolf Pub

Auto Review Pub, *(Auto Review Publishing; 0-9624958),* 5 Rowan Oak Ln., Columbia, IL 62236-4148 Tel 618-281-3311
E-mail: autrev@aol.com.

Autodidactics, *(Autodidactics, Inc.; 0-9660784),* Orders Addr.: P.O. Box 14659, Akron, OH 44321 Tel 330-670-0679; Fax: 330-665-3163; Toll Free: 877-236-2665; Edit Addr.: 1245 S. Cleve-mass Rd., No. 3, Akron, OH 44321 Do not confuse with Autodidactics, Pr., Wasilla, AK.

Automat Diag, *(Automated Diagnostic Documentation, Inc.; 0-9639689),* 515 Beacon Blvd., Grand Haven, MI 49417 Tel 616-846-2910; Fax: 616-846-1390; Toll Free: 800-257-6298.

Autonomy Pub, *(Autonomy Publishing Corp.; 0-9636451),* P.O. Box 901, Larchmont, NY 10538 (SAN 298-122X) Tel 914-834-5412
E-mail: books@buildingyourself.com
Web site: http://www.buildingyourself.com.

AV Text Corp, *See* **Mstque Pubns**

Avalanche Pub, *(Avalanche Publishing, Ltd.; 0-9641719),* 2940 Thedford Rd., Bloomfield Hills, MI 48304-2060 Tel 248-375-2937.

Avalon NY, *(Avalon New York),* 841 Broadway, 4th Flr., New York, NY 10003 Tel 212-614-7880; Fax: 212-614-7887 ; *Imprints:* Thunders Mouth (Thunder's Mouth Press)
Web site: http://www.marlowe.com
Dist(s): **Publishers Group** *(Publishers Group West)*
netLibrary CO *(netLibrary, Inc.).*

Avalon Travel, *(Avalon Travel Publishing; 0-918373; 0-935701; 0-9603322; 1-56691; 1-57354),* 5855 Beaudry St., Emeryville, CA 94608 (SAN 221-7406) Tel 510-595-3664; Fax: 510-595-4228; Toll Free: 800-285-4078
E-mail: info@travelmatters.com
Web site: http://www.travelmatters.com
Dist(s): **Publishers Group** *(Publishers Group West).*

Avantage, *(Avantage Pubns.; 0-9630339),* 4230 Clover Knoll Ct., Carmichael, CA 95608-6734 Tel 916-944-7454.

Avanti, *(Avanti Publishing; 0-9629063),* Orders Addr.: P.O. Box 237, Clifton Heights, PA 19018 Tel 610-626-9124; Edit Addr.: 420 N. Springfield Rd., Clifton Heights, PA 19018 Do not confuse with companies with same or similar name in Munising, MI, Fort Lauderdale, FL.

Ave Maria, *(Ave Maria Pr.; 0-87793),* P.O. Box 428, Notre Dame, IN 46556-0428 (SAN 201-1255) Tel 219-287-2831; Fax: 219-239-2904; Toll Free Fax: 800-282-5681; Toll Free: 800-282-1865
E-mail: avemariapress.1@nd.edu
Web site: http://www.avemariapress.com.

Avebry (GBR) *(0-86127; 1-85628; 1-85972) Dist. by* **Ashgate Pub Co.**

Avebury Technical (GBR) *(0-291) Dist. by* **Ashgate Pub Co.**

Avena Pubg, *(Avena Publishing; 0-9670978),* Orders Addr.: 4821 Sunnyview Dr., Saint Louis, MO 63128 Tel 314-487-1974
E-mail: ravena@prodigy.net
Web site: http://pages.prodigy.net/ravena.

Avery Imprint of Putnam Pub Group

Avery Color, *(Avery Color Studios, Inc.; 0-932212; 1-892384),* 511 D Ave., Gwinn, MI 49841 (SAN 211-1470) Tel 906-346-3908; Fax: 906-346-3015; Toll Free: 800-722-9925
E-mail: avery@portup.com
Dist(s): **Partners Pubs Grp** *(Partners Pubs. Group, Inc.)*
R Hale & Co *(Hale, Robert & Co., Inc.).*

Avian Cetacean, *(Avian-Cetacean Pr.; 0-9628186),* Orders Addr.: P.O. Box 15643, Wilmington, NC 28408 Tel 910-392-5537 (phone/fax); Edit Addr.: 1616 Jetty's Reach, Wilmington, NC 28409
E-mail: avian@aol.com
Dist(s): **Sandlapper Pub Co** *(Sandlapper Publishing Co., Inc.).*

Aviation Info, *(Aviation Information Resources, Inc.; 1-891726),* 3800 Camp Creek Pkwy., Suite 18-100, Atlanta, GA 30331 Tel 404-592-6500; Fax: 404-592-6515; Toll Free Fax: 800-247-3297; Toll Free: 800-247-2777; 800-538-5627
E-mail: sales@airapps.com
Web site: http://www.airapps.com; http://www.jet-jobs.com
Dist(s): **Aviation** *(Aviation Bk. Co.)*
Sportsman s Market Inc *(Sportsman's Market, Inc.).*

Avicon, *(Avicon, Inc.; 0-9644732),* 3871 Sandlewood Dr., Okemos, MI 48864-3627 Tel 517-349-2840
E-mail: schwarl7@pilot.msu.edu.

Avid Reader, *(Avid Reader Pr.; 0-9700150),* Div. of VWI Corp., 2765 Wrondel Way, Suite 1, Reno, NV 89502-4377 Fax: 512-288-0317; Toll Free: 800-643-3389
Web site: http://www.visiontherapy.com.

Avocet Pub, *(Avocet Publishing; 0-9625645),* 1132 Princeton Dr., Wilmington, NC 28403 Tel 910-762-4945.

Avon Bks Imprint of Morrow Avon

Avondale Lab, *(Avondale Laboratories, Inc.; 0-9634721),* 304 N. Barrington Ave., Los Angeles, CA 90049-2925 (SAN 297-8040).

AVSC Int, *See* **EngenderHlth**

Aware Tribe, *(Aware Tribe, Inc.; 0-9626135),* R.D. 1, Box 223, Colton, NY 13625.

Awareness Prods, *(Awareness Productions; 0-9637649),* 9885 W. Haskett Ln., Dayton, OH 45424-1603 (SAN 298-0037) Tel 937-845-3617 (phone/fax)
E-mail: fyocum@ix.netcom.com
Web site: http://www.awarenessproductions.com.

Awareness Pubns, *(Awareness Pubns.; 0-9617549),* Orders Addr.: P.O. Box 300792, Houston, TX 77230-0792 (SAN 664-4376); Edit Addr.: 14126 Norway, Houston, TX 77047 (SAN 664-4384) Tel 713-434-2845.

Ayd Medical Comm, *(Ayd Medical Communications; 0-931858),* 1130 E. Cold Spring Ln., Baltimore, MD 21239 (SAN 222-4712).

Aye-Aye Arts, *(Aye-Aye Arts; 0-9627257; 1-890985),* Orders Addr.: P.O. Box 1122, Christiansted, VI 00821-1122
E-mail: rvvaughn@worldnet.att.net
Web site: http://www.vaughn-art.com; http://www.caribbean-art.net
Dist(s): **Wilbert Williams** *(Wilbert/Williams).*

Ayer, *(Ayer Co. Pubs., Inc.; 0-88143),* Orders Addr.: 6 Lower Mill Rd., North Stratford, NH 03590 Fax: 603-922-3348 (Ordering) ; Toll Free: 888-267-7323 (Ordering); Edit Addr.: c/o IDS, 195 McGregor St., Manchester, NH 03102 (SAN 211-6936) Fax: 603-922-3348; Toll Free: 888-267-7323
Web site: http://www.scry.com/ayer.

AYNI Pr, *(AYNI Pr.; 0-9658466),* Orders Addr.: P.O. Box 335, Saint Helena, CA 94574 (SAN 299-3597) Tel 707-963-1822; Fax: 707-963-7892; Edit Addr.: 1451 Library Ln., Saint Helena, CA 94574
E-mail: BuyHSchool@aol.com.

AYSL, *(AYSL Corp.; 0-9634979),* Orders Addr.: P.O. Box 181, Glen Rock, NJ 07452 Tel 201-445-7068; Fax: 201-493-1126; Edit Addr.: 35 Cumberland Rd., Glen Rock, NJ 07452.

Ayurveda Holistic, *(Ayurveda Holistic Ctr. Pr.; 0-9658042),* 82A Bayville Ave., Bayville, NY 11709 (SAN 299-5042) Tel 516-628-8200; Toll Free: 888-568-2515
E-mail: mail@ayurvedahc.com
Web site: http://ayurvedahc.com/press.html
Dist(s): **IPG Chicago** *(Independent Pubs. Group)*
New Leaf Dist *(New Leaf Distributing Co., Inc.).*

Ayurvedic Pr, *(Ayurvedic Pr.; 1-883725),* Div. of Ayurvedic Institute, Orders Addr.: P.O. Box 23445, Albuquerque, NM 87192-1445 Tel 505-291-9698; Fax: 505-294-7572; Edit Addr.: 11311 Menaul NE, Suite A, Albuquerque, NM 87112
Web site: http://www.ayurveda.com
Dist(s): **Bookpeople** *(Bookpeople)*
New Leaf Dist *(New Leaf Distributing Co., Inc.).*

AZ Bariatric Phy, *(Arizona Bariatric Physicians, P.C.; 0-9618415),* 207 W. Clarendon Ave., Apt. 14F, Phoenix, AZ 85013-3438 (SAN 667-6839) Tel 602-248-7852.

AZ Heart Inst, *(Arizona Heart Institute Foundation; 0-9635767),* 2632 N. 20th St., Phoenix, AZ 85006 Tel 602-266-2200; Fax: 602-240-5819; Toll Free: 800-835-2920.

Azure Zephyr, *(Azure Zephyr Pubns.; 0-9614833),* 9395 Harritt Rd., No. 105, Lakeside, CA 92040 (SAN 696-7000).

B Acad & Prof (GBR) *(0-7514) Dist. by* **Aspen Pub.**

B Berkel, *(Berkel, Boyce N.; 0-9603184),* 2245 N. McMullen Booth Rd., Clearwater, FL 34619-1420 (SAN 213-4667).

B C Garrison, *(Garrison, Burgus C.; 0-9633245),* 26181 Allentown Dr., Sun City, CA 92586-2164 Tel 909-679-9103 (phone/fax)
E-mail: burgus@personalmedrecords.com
Web site: http://www.personalmedrecords.com
Dist(s): **Baker & Taylor** *(Baker & Taylor Bks.).*

B Davis, *See* **Murdock Pubng**

B Dolphin Pub, *(Blue Dolphin Publishing, Inc.; 0-931892; 1-57733),* Orders Addr.: P.O. Box 8, Nevada City, CA 95959 (SAN 223-2480) Tel 530-265-6925; Fax: 530-265-0787; Toll Free: 800-643-0765; Edit Addr.: 12428 Nevada City Hwy., Grass Valley, CA 95945 (SAN 696-009X)
E-mail: bdolphin@netshel.net
Web site: http://www.bluedolphinpublishing.com
Dist(s): **Baker & Taylor** *(Baker & Taylor Bks.)*
Booklines Hawaii *(Booklines Hawaii, Ltd.)*
Bookpeople *(Bookpeople)*
Koen Bk Distributors *(Koen Bk. Distributors)*
Koen Pacific *(Koen Pacific)*
New Concepts Bks & Tapes *(New Concepts Bks. & Tapes Distributors)*
New Leaf Dist *(New Leaf Distributing Co., Inc.)*
Quality Bks IL *(Quality Bks., Inc.)*
Red Wheel ME *(Red Wheel)*
Vision Dists *(Vision Distributors).*

B Hallum, *(Hallum, Boen; 0-9608854),* 4977 Lockbourne Rd., Columbus, OH 43207 (SAN 241-0265) Tel 614-491-4639.

B J Pubns MD, *(BJ Pubns.; 0-924385),* 79-32 211th St., Bayside, NY 11364 Tel 718-464-9391 Do not confuse with BJ Publications, Riverside, CA.

B J Scott, *(Scott, Billie J.; 0-9638862),* 4400 El Parque, Las Vegas, NV 89102-3502 Tel 702-871-0261.

B Jensen, *(Jensen, Bernard Pub.; 0-932615; 0-9608360),* 24360 Old Wagon Rd., Escondido, CA 92027 (SAN 240-690X) Tel 760-749-2727; Fax: 760-749-1248; Toll Free: 877-536-7363 (877-JENSEN3)
E-mail: info@bernardjensenintl.com
Web site: http://www.bernardjensenintl.com.

B L Enter, *(B L Enterprises, LLC; 0-9701963),* 1315 Madison St., No. 225, Seattle, WA 98104 Tel 206-329-6565; Fax: 206-328-4441
E-mail: lungdz@home.com
Web site: http://www.lungdz.com/.

B L Publishing, *(BL Publishing; 0-9671655),* 3614 N. Raven Wash Dr., Tucson, AZ 85745 Tel 520-743-1711 (orders)
E-mail: Levinejm@aol.com.

B L Pubns, *(BL Pubns.; 0-9642703; 1-890766),* 14325 Barnes Dr., Detroit Lakes, MN 56501 Tel 218-846-2519; Fax: 218-846-2520; Toll Free: 877-266-5711 (877-BOOKS11)
E-mail: blpub@tekstar.com
Dist(s): **Alliance Bk Co** *(Alliance Bk. Co.)*
Baker & Taylor *(Baker & Taylor Bks.)*
New Leaf Dist *(New Leaf Distributing Co., Inc.)*
Nutri-Books Corp *(Nutri-Bks. Corp.)*
Quality Bks IL *(Quality Bks., Inc.).*

B Melger, *(Melger, Boyd; 0-9622463),* 2819 Cunningham Ave., San Jose, CA 95148-1106 Tel 408-270-3816.

B Mooney, *See* **Med-Travel Bks**

B Ranney, *(Ranney, Brooks; 0-9618939),* P.O. Box 590, Yankton, SD 57078 (SAN 242-4649) Tel 605-665-3596.

B Starnes, *(Starnes, Ben; 0-9661288),* Orders Addr.: P.O. Box 72, Paint Lick, KY 40461 Tel 606-925-2076; Edit Addr.: Hwy. 52, Paint Lick, KY 40461.

B T B (GBR) *(0-7134) Dist. by* **Intl Spec Bk.**

B Wilkerson Ctr Pr, *See* **Vanderbilt Wilkerson**

Baby Adjusters, *(Baby Adjusters; 0-9638642),* 1935 Shelburne Rd., Shelburne, VT 05482-7171.

Baby Hearts, *(Baby Hearts Pr.; 0-9652508),* Orders Addr.: 3910 Sierra Blanca, Temple, TX 76502 Toll Free: 888-222-4649
E-mail: ajaworski@aol.com
Web site: http://www.babyhearts.com.

Baby Steps Pr, *(Baby Steps Pr.; 0-9631666),* P.O. Box 1917, Beaverton, OR 97075-1917 Tel 503-641-1361; Fax: 503-526-0709; Toll Free: 888-994-0569
E-mail: lucky1951@aol.com
Web site: http://members.aol.com/atkeystone/baby/steps.html
Dist(s): **Baker & Taylor** *(Baker & Taylor Bks.)*
Koen Bk Distributors *(Koen Bk. Distributors)*
Partners-West *(Partners/West).*

Back Bay Imprint of Little

Back Talk Systs, *(Back Talk Systems, Inc.; 0-9631711),* 14998 W. Sixth Ave., Suite 500, Golden, CO 80401-5025.

Backhuys Pubs (NLD) *(3-8263; 90-73348; 90-5782) Dist. by* **Balogh.**

Backwoods Bks, *(Backwoods Bks.; 0-938833),* Orders Addr.: P.O. Box 25, Ohiopyle, PA 15470 (SAN 661-700X) Tel 724-329-5336; Fax: 724-329-0521
E-mail: marci@dcl.net
Web site: http://www.ohiopyle.com/author.

Bader Assoc Inc, *(Bader & Assoc., Inc.; 0-915963),* 1101 King St., Suite 444, Alexandria, VA 22314-2944 (SAN 293-9649) Tel 301-468-1610; Fax: 301-770-4919.

Baffin Bks, *(Baffin Bks., Inc.; 0-9665105),* 46-01 Broadway, Astoria, NY 11103 Tel 718-278-7676; Fax: 718-278-0354; Toll Free: 800-637-4644
E-mail: gdsmdpc@juno.com.

Baggetts, *(Baggetts Investigative Enterprises, Ltd.; 0-9666111),* Orders Addr.: P.O. Box 448, Ringgold, LA 71068 Tel 318-894-9370; Edit Addr.: 233 Haynes Rd., Ringgold, LA 71068
E-mail: oleirv@juno.com.

BainBridgeBooks, *(BainBridgeBooks; 1-891696),* 311 Bainbridge St., Philadelphia, PA 19147 Tel 215-925-5083; Fax: 215-925-7412; 215-925-1912 Do not confuse with Bainbridge Books, Jacksboro, TX
E-mail: order@transpub.comatlabtic
Web site: http://www.transatlanticpub.com
Dist(s): **Trans-Atl Phila** *(Trans-Atlantic Pubns., Inc.).*

Baja Bks, *(Baja Bks.; 0-9602838; 0-9615829; 1-882196),* Orders Addr.: P.O. Box 4151, Santa Barbara, CA 93140; Edit Addr.: 3774 Pescadero Dr., Santa Barbara, CA 93105 (SAN 213-0122) Tel 805-962-4029; Fax: 805-563-9709; Toll Free: 800-962-4028
E-mail: info@speedylanguage.com
Web site: http://www.speedylanguage.com
Dist(s): **BridgeWay** *(BridgeWay Bks.)*
Publishers Group *(Publishers Group West).*

Baker Bks, *(Baker Bks.; 0-8010; 0-913686),* Div. of Baker Bk. Hse., Orders Addr.: P.O. Box 6287, Grand Rapids, MI 49516-6287 (SAN 299-1500) Toll Free Fax: 800-398-3111; Toll Free: 800-877-2665 (orders only); Edit Addr.: 6030 E. Fulton, Ada, MI 49301 (SAN 201-4041) Tel 616-676-9185; Fax: 616-676-9573
E-mail: orders@bakerbooks.com
Web site: http://www.bakerbooks.com.

Baker Pub, *(Baker Publishing; 0-913193),* Orders Addr.: 16245 Armstead St., Granada Hills, CA 91344-3009 Tel 818-366-9847.

Baker Pubns (GBR) *(0-906006; 0-9505502) Dist. by* **New Leaf Dist.**

Baker-Hill, *(Baker-Hill Publishing; 0-9630158),* 303 16th St., Suite 16, Denver, CO 80202-5657 (SAN 297-4622) Tel 303-798-7574; Fax: 303-798-8081.

Balaban Intl Sci Serv, *(Balaban International Science Services; 0-86689),* 1175 Lake Blvd., Apt. 143, Davis, CA 95616-5651.

Balance Enter, *(Balance Enterprises, Inc.; 1-888614),* 120 Bethpage Rd., Suite 310, Hicksville, NY 11801-1515 Tel 516-822-3183; Fax: 516-822-3184; Toll Free: 800-789-4225
E-mail: BalanceEnt@aol.com.

Balanced Way, *(Balanced Way; 0-9653664),* Orders Addr.: P.O. Box 785, Fernandina Beach, FL 32035-0785 Tel 904-261-0323; Edit Addr.: 307B S. Seventh St., Fernandina Beach, FL 32034.

Balboa Pub, *(Balboa Publishing Corp.; 0-935902),* 1323 San Anselmo Ave., San Anselmo, CA 94960-2244 (SAN 220-035X) Tel 415-453-8886; Fax: 415-453-8888
E-mail: shapedown@aol.com
Web site: http://www.just-for-kids.org.

Ball Dynam, *(Ball Dynamics International, Inc.; 0-9645341; 0-9704291),* 14215 Mead St., Longmont, CO 80504 Tel 970-535-9090; Fax: 970-535-9548; Toll Free Fax: 877-223-2962; Toll Free: 800-752-2255
E-mail: dayna@balldynamics.com
Web site: http://www.balldynamics.com.

Ball Well, *(Ballantine Wellspring; 0-345; 1-4000),* Div. of Ballantine Publishing Group, Orders Addr.: 1540 Broadway, New York, NY 10036 Toll Free: 800-223-6834; 400 Hahn Rd., Westminster, MD 21157 Tel 410-848-1900; Toll Free: 800-726-0600.

Ballantine, *See* **Ballantine Pub Grp**

Ballantine Imprint of Ballantine Pub Grp

Ballantine Epiphany Imprint of Ballantine Pub Grp

†**Ballantine Pub Grp,** *(Ballantine Publishing Group; 0-345; 0-449; 0-8041; 0-87637; 1-4000),* Div. of Random Hse., Inc., Orders Addr.: 400 Hahn Rd., Westminster, MD 21157 (SAN 202-5515) Tel 410-848-1900; Toll Free Fax: 800-767-4465; Toll Free: 800-726-0600 (customer service); 800-733-3000 (orders); Edit Addr.: 1540 Broadway, 11th Flr., New York, NY 10036 (SAN 214-1175) Tel 212-782-9000; Fax: 212-940-7539; Toll Free: 800-733-3000 ; *Imprints:* Ballantine Epiphany (Ballantine Epiphany) Ballantine (Ballantine Books)
E-mail: bfi@randomnhouse.com
Web site: http://www.randomhouse.com
Dist(s): **Continental Bk** *(Continental Bk. Co., Inc.)*
Fawcett *(Fawcett); CIP.*

Ballena Pr, *(Ballena Pr.; 0-87919),* Orders Addr.: P.O. Box 2510, Novato, CA 94948 (SAN 669-0181) Tel 415-883-3530; Fax: 415-883-4280; Edit Addr.: 823 Valparaiso Ave., Menlo Park, CA 94025 (SAN 201-4076) Tel 650-323-9261; Fax: 650-324-1290.

Ballistic Pubns, *(Ballistic Pubns.; 0-9643577),* P.O. Box 772, El Segundo, CA 90245 Tel 310-322-9229; Fax: 310-322-0780
Web site: http://www.pw2.netcom.com/~dmacp/index.html.

Balogh, *(Balogh International, Inc.; 1-878762; 1-891770),* 1911 N. Duncan Rd., Champaign, IL 61822 (SAN 297-2344) Tel 217-355-9331; Fax: 217-355-9413
E-mail: balogh@balogh.com
Web site: http://www.balogh.com.

Banana Bk, *(Banana Bk. Co.; 0-9625049),* 11314 Davison Ln., Tavares, FL 32778-4840 Tel 352-343-6468
E-mail: bananabyte@aol.com.

Bananknotcom, *(Bananaknot.com; 0-9675257),* P.O. Box 9315, Chico, CA 95928
E-mail: petjournal@bananaknot
Web site: http://www.bananaknot.com.

Bandido Bks, *(Bandido Bks.; 1-929693),* 9806 Heaton Ct., Orlando, FL 32817 Tel 407-657-9707; Fax: 407-677-9796
E-mail: publish@bandidobooks.com
Web site: http://www.bandidobooks.com.

Banis & Assocs, *See* **Sci & Human Pr**

Banks-Baldwin, *(Banks-Baldwin Law Publishing Co. (A West Publishing Affiliated Co.); 0-8322),* 6111 Oak Tree Blvd., P.O. Box 318063, Cleveland, OH 44131-8063 (SAN 204-5370) Tel 216-520-5600; Fax: 216-520-5655; Toll Free: 800-362-4500 (in USA & Canada)
Web site: http://www.westpub.com/Practice/oh/bbhome.htm.

Banner Pr Intl, *(Banner Pr. International; 0-916650),* P.O. Box 21195, New York, NY 10129 (SAN 212-0119) Tel 212-459-4525 Do not confuse with companies with the same name in Austin, TX, Minneapolis, MN
Dist(s): **Liberation Distributors** *(Liberation Distributors).*

†**Bantam,** *(Bantam Bks.; 0-553; 0-593; 0-7704; 1-4000),* Div. of Bantam Dell Publishing Group, Orders Addr.: 400 Hahn Rd., Westminster, MD 21157 (SAN 201-3983) Tel 410-848-1900; Toll Free: 800-726-0600; Edit Addr.: 1540 Broadway, New York, NY 10036-4094 (SAN 201-3975) Tel 212-354-6500; Fax: 212-492-8941; Toll Free Fax: 800-233-3294; Toll Free: 800-223-6834 (Bulk orders); 800-726-0600 (Orders/Customer service) ; *Imprints:* Spectra (Spectra)
E-mail: bantampublicity@randomhouse.com
Web site: http://www.bantam.com
Dist(s): **Continental Bk** *(Continental Bk. Co., Inc.); CIP.*

†**Bantam Dell,** *(Bantam Dell Publishing Group; 0-440; 0-553; 0-593; 0-7704; 1-4000),* Div. of Random House, Inc., Orders Addr.: 400 Hahn Rd., Westminster, MD 21157 Tel 410-848-1900; Toll Free: 800-726-0600; Edit Addr.: 1540 Broadway, New York, NY 10036-4094 Tel 212-354-6500; Fax: 212-492-8941; *CIP.*

Banyan Pr HI, *(Banyan Pr.; 0-9623265),* 1188 Bishop St., No. 807, Honolulu, HI 96813 Tel 808-521-1744; Fax: 808-521-4846.

Barcelona Pubs, *(Barcelona Pubs.; 0-9624080; 1-891278),* 4 White Brook Rd., Lower Village, Gilsum, NH 03448 (SAN 298-6299) Tel 603-357-0236; Fax: 603-357-2073; Toll Free: 800-345-6665
E-mail: orders@pathwaybook.com; pbs@pathwaybook.com
Web site: http://www.barcelonapublishers.com
Dist(s): **MMB Music** *(MMB Music, Inc.)*
Pathway Bk Serv *(Pathway Bk. Service).*

Barcena & Co, *(Barcena & Co.; 0-9643995),* Div. of D & V Products, Orders Addr.: c/o D & V Products, Inc./West Coast Marketing, P.O. Box 522-1711, Claremont, CA 91711 (SAN 298-9689) Tel 626-299-3054; Fax: 818-960-0027; Toll Free: 888-223-7482; Edit Addr.: 800 N. Monterey St., Unit 303, Alhambra, CA 91801-1525
Dist(s): **J Majors Co** *(Majors, J. A. Co.)*
Matthews Medical Bk Co *(Matthews Medical Bk. Co.)*
Rittenhouse *(Rittenhouse Bk. Distributors).*

Barcharts, *(Barcharts, Inc.; 1-57222),* 1141 S. Rogers Cir., No. 11, Boca Raton, FL 33487 (SAN 299-5026) Tel 561-989-3666; Fax: 561-989-3722; Toll Free: 800-226-7799
E-mail: studyaid@barcharts.com
Web site: http://www.quickstudycharts.com.

Barclay Pr, *(Barclay Pr.; 0-913342),* Div. of Northwest Yearly Meeting of Friends Church, 110 S. Elliott Rd., Newberg, OR 97132-2120 (SAN 201-7520) Tel 503-538-7345; Fax: 503-538-7033; Toll Free: 800-962-4014
E-mail: info@barclaypress.com
Web site: http://www.barclaypress.com.

Bard Coll Pubns, *(Bard College Pubns. Office; 0-941276; 1-931493),* Annandale Rd., Annandale-on-Hudson, NY 12504-5000 Tel 845-758-7872 (7418); Fax: 845-758-7554 ; *Imprints:* Levy Econ Inst Bard (Levy Economics Institute of Bard College, The)
E-mail: rosasco@bard.edu; info@levy.org
Web site: http://www.bard.edu; http://www.levy.org
Dist(s): **Dist Art Pubs** *(Distributed Art Pubs./D.A.P.).*

Barez Pub, *(Barez Publishing; 0-9624701),* 8690 Aero Dr., Suite M332, San Diego, CA 92123 Tel 760-344-1101.

Barge Chiropract, *(Barge Chiropractic Publishing, Inc.; 1-885048),* Orders Addr.: 322 Cameron Ave., LaCrosse, WI 54601 Tel 608-784-4639; Fax: 608-784-3279; Toll Free: 800-882-5470
Dist(s): **CCC** *(Cleveland Chiropractic College)*
Clevelnd Chiropractic *(Cleveland Chiropractic College)*
Intl Chiropractors Assn *(International Chiropractors Assn.)*
Palmer College *(Palmer College of Chiropractice).*

Barksdale Foun, *(Barksdale Foundation; 0-918588),* Orders Addr.: P.O. Box 187, Idyllwild, CA 92549 (SAN 210-1718) Tel 909-659-4676; Fax: 909-659-4678
E-mail: info@barksdale.org; selfesteem@barksdale.org
Web site: http://www.barksdale.org.

Barmarrae Bks, *(Barmarrae Bks.; 0-9646151),* 4432 NW 23rd Ave., Suite 8, Gainesville, FL 32606 Tel 352-332-0057; Fax: 352-378-1441; Toll Free: 888-276-7780.

Barnes Publns, *(Barnes Pubns.; 0-9654168),* 5932A Hwy. 51, Colonial Pl., Suite 2, Horn Lake, MS 38637 Tel 662-342-4400; Fax: 520-563-2087
E-mail: barneschiro@aol.com.

†**Barricade Bks,** *(Barricade Bks., Inc.; 0-934878; 0-942637; 0-9623032; 1-56980),* 185 Bridge Plaza N., Suite 308A, Fort Lee, NJ 07024 (SAN 299-1780) Tel 201-944-7600; Fax: 201-944-6363; Toll Free: 800-592-6657
E-mail: customerservice@barricadebooks.com
Web site: http://www.barricadebooks.com; *CIP.*

Barrington MA, *(Barrington Pr.; 0-9616920),* 28 Lakewood Rd., Newton Highlands, MA 02161 (SAN 661-3942) Tel 617-969-9346.

†**Barron,** *(Barron's Educational Series, Inc.; 0-7641; 0-8120),* 250 Wireless Blvd., Hauppauge, NY 11788-3917 (SAN 201-453X) Tel 631-434-3311; Fax: 631-434-3723; 631-434-3217 (orders); Toll Free: 800-645-3476 Do not confuse with BARRONS, Monroe, WA
E-mail: info@barronseduc.com; barrons@barronseduc.com
Web site: http://www.barronseduc.com
Dist(s): **Continental Bk** *(Continental Bk. Co., Inc.)*
Lectorum Pubns *(Lectorum Pubns., Inc.)*
Prodn Assocs *(Production Assocs.)*
netLibrary CO *(netLibrary, Inc.); CIP.*

Barrytown Ltd, *(Barrytown, Ltd.; 1-58177; 1-886449),* Station Hill Rd., Barrytown, NY 12507 Tel 914-758-5840; Fax: 914-758-8163
E-mail: publishers@stationhill.org
Web site: http://www.stationhill.org
Dist(s): **Consort Bk Sales** *(Consortium Bk. Sales & Distribution)*
SPD-Small Pr Dist *(SPD-Small Pr. Distribution).*

Bartleby Pr, *(Bartleby Pr.; 0-910155),* 11141 Georgia Ave., Suite A-3, Silver Spring, MD 20902 (SAN 241-2098) Tel 301-949-2443; Fax: 301-949-2205; Toll Free: 800-953-9929.

Basal Books, *(Basal Bks.; 0-916961),* Div. of Basal-Tech, Inc., 726 Lafayette Ave, Cincinnati, OH 45220-1053 (SAN 292-3289) Tel 513-751-2723; Fax: 513-751-0280 Do not confuse with Basal Bks., Mansfield, OH
E-mail: orders@basaltech.com
Web site: http://www.basaltech.com.

†**Basic,** *(Basic Bks.; 0-465),* A Member of Perseus Books Group, Orders Addr.: 5500 Central Ave., Boulder, CO 80301-2877 Fax: 303-449-3356 (customer service); Toll Free: 800-386-5656 (customer service); Edit Addr.: 10 E. 53rd St., New York, NY 10022-5299 (SAN 201-4521) Tel 212-207-7600; Fax: 212-207-7703
E-mail: westview.orders@perseusbooks.com
Web site: http://www.perseusbooksgroup.com
Dist(s): **Cobblestone Pub Co** *(Cobblestone Publishing Co.)*
HarperCollins Pubs *(HarperCollins Pubs.); CIP.*

Basic Trauma, *(Basic Trauma Life Support International, Inc.; 0-9647418),* 1 S. 280 Summit Ave., Ct. B-2, Oakbrook Terrace, IL 60181 Tel 708-495-6404; Toll Free: 800-495-2857.

Basil Blackwell, *See* **Blackwell Pubs**

Baskin Pub OR, *(Baskin Publishing Co.; 0-9635500),* P.O. Box 21058, Eugene, OR 97402-0348 (SAN 297-8342).

Bath Univ Pr (GBR) *(0-86197; 0-900843) Dist. by* **Intl Spec Bk.**

Bathroom Reader, *(Bathroom Reader Pr.; 1-879682),* P.O. Box 1117, Ashland, OR 97520 Tel 541-488-4642; Fax: 541-482-6159
E-mail: brmail@mind.net; bathread@mind.net
Web site: http://www.bathroomreader.com
Dist(s): **Publishers Group** *(Publishers Group West).*

Baton Rouge Tourette Grp, *(Baton Rouge Tourette Support Group; 0-9625194),* 895 Dubois Dr., Baton Rouge, LA 70808 Tel 225-766-4002; Fax: 225-766-9755.

†**Battelle,** *(Battelle Pr.; 0-935470; 1-57477),* Div. of Battelle Memorial Institute, 505 King Ave., Columbus, OH 43201-2693 (SAN 213-4640) Tel 614-424-6393; Fax: 614-424-3819; Toll Free: 800-451-3543
E-mail: press@battelle.org
Web site: http://www.battelle.org/bookstore
Dist(s): **Univelt Inc** *(Univelt, Inc.); CIP.*

Batterers Anon, *(Batterers Anonymous Pr.; 0-9612754),* 1850 N. Riverside Ave., Suite 220, Rialto, CA 92376-8082 (SAN 289-730X) Tel 909-355-1100; Fax: 909-421-3092.

Bauhan, *(Bauhan, William L. Inc.; 0-87233),* P.O. Box 443, Dublin, NH 03444-0443 (SAN 204-384X) Tel 877-832-3738; Fax: 603-563-8026
E-mail: info@bauhauhanpublishing.com
Web site: http://www.bauhanpublishing.com.

Bay Dr Pubns, *(Bay Drive Pubns.; 0-9667388),* 1258 W. Bay Dr., Suite E, Largo, FL 33770.

Bay Pr, *(Bay Pr., Inc.; 0-941920),* 115 W. Denny Way, Seattle, WA 98119 (SAN 237-9902) Tel 206-284-5913; Fax: 206-284-1218 Do not confuse with Bay Pr., Albany, CA
E-mail: BayPress@aol.com
Web site: http://www.baypressinc.com/baypress/.

Bayrock, *(Bayrock Pr.; 0-9630439; 1-886622),* 10400 W. Overland Rd., No. 330, Boise, ID 83709 Tel 208-376-2266; Fax: 208-377-4202.

Baytree Pubn, *(Baytree Pubn. Co.; 0-944393),* P.O. Box 713, Nicasio, CA 94946-0713 (SAN 243-7163) Tel 415-662-2534; Fax: 415-662-2539
E-mail: gompertz@nbn.com.

†Baywood Pub, *(Baywood Publishing Co., Inc.; 0-89503),* 26 Austin Ave., P.O. Box 337, Amityville, NY 11701 (SAN 206-9326) Tel 631-691-1270; Fax: 631-691-1770; Toll Free: 800-638-7819 (orders only)
E-mail: info@baywood.com; baywood@baywood.com
Web site: http://baywood.com; *CIP.*

BBC (GBR) *(0-563) Dist. by* **Parkwest Pubns.**

BBCS, *(BBCS (Bits & Bytes Computer Services); 0-9636781),* Div. of BBCS Publishing, P.O. Box 23133, Eugene, OR 97402-0425 Tel 541-683-0671; Fax: 541-683-0675
E-mail: bbcs@pond.net
Dist(s): **Baker & Taylor** *(Baker & Taylor Bks.).*

BCC, *(Business Communications Co., Inc.; 0-89336; 1-56965),* 25 Van Zant St., Norwalk, CT 06855 (SAN 207-706X) Tel 203-853-4266; Fax: 203-853-0348
E-mail: info@bccresearch.com
Web site: http://www.buscom.com.

BDD LT Grp, *(Bantam Doubleday Dell Large Print Group, Inc.; 0-385),* Orders Addr.: 2451 S. Wolf Rd., Des Plaines, IL 60018 Toll Free: 800-323-9872 (orders); 800-258-4233 (EDI ordering); Edit Addr.: 1540 Broadway, New York, NY 10036-4094 Tel 212-354-6500; Toll Free: 800-223-5780
Dist(s): **Large Print Library** *(Large Print Library Discounter)*
T T Beeler *(Beeler, Thomas T. Publisher).*

Bea Pubg, *(Bea Publishing; 0-9671388),* 3205 VanAllen Cir., Greensboro, NC 27410-001 Tel 336-605-9779; Fax: 336-605-0021
E-mail: camaro46@aol.com.

Beacon Hill, *(Beacon Hill Pr. of Kansas City; 0-8341),* Div. of Nazarene Publishing Hse., 2923 Troost, Kansas City, MO 64109 (SAN 241-6328) Tel 816-931-1900; Fax: 816-753-4071; Toll Free: 800-877-0700 (orders only)
E-mail: inquiry@bhillkc.com; nphdirect@nph.com; orders@nph.com
Web site: http://www.nph.com; http://www.bhillkc.com.

Beacon Hlth, *(Beacon Health Products; 0-9641190),* 24722 Mendocino Ct., Laguna Hills, CA 92653 Tel 714-643-8462.

Beacon Pr, *(Beacon Pr.; 0-8070),* 25 Beacon St., Boston, MA 02108-2892 (SAN 201-4483) Tel 617-742-2110; Fax: 617-723-3097
Web site: http://www.beacon.org
Dist(s): **Continental Bk** *(Continental Bk. Co., Inc.)*
HM *(Houghton Mifflin Co.)*
Shens Bks *(Shen's Bks.)*
netLibrary CO *(netLibrary, Inc.).*

†Bear & Co, *(Bear & Co.; 0-939680; 1-879181; 1-59143),* Orders Addr.: One Park St., Rochester, VT 05767 (SAN 216-7174) Tel 802-767-3174; Fax: 802-767-3726; Toll Free: 800-246-8648 Do not confuse with Bear & Co. in Bedford, NH
E-mail: info@innertraditions.com; jeanie@innertraditions.com
Web site: http://www.innertraditions.com; *CIP.*

Beat the Fat, *(Beat the Fat; 0-9638671),* 2458 Calle Aquamarina, San Clemente, CA 92673-3904 Fax: 714-498-9284; Toll Free: 800-366-2151.

BeautyArt Pr, *(BeautyArt Pr.; 0-9666345),* 851 Meadows Rd., Suite 222, Boca Raton, FL 33486 Tel 561-395-5508; Fax: 561-395-1839; Toll Free: 800-232-5508
E-mail: info@www.drman.com
Web site: http://www.drman.com
Dist(s): **BookWorld** *(BookWorld Services, Inc.).*

Beavers Pond, *(Beaver's Pond Pr., Inc.; 1-890676; 1-931646),* 5125 Danen's Dr., Edina, MN 55439-1465 Tel 952-829-8818; Fax: 952-944-4065
E-mail: adamspo@aol.com
Web site: http://www.beaverspondpress.com
Dist(s): **Bookman Bks** *(Bookman Bks.).*

Beck Pr, *(Beck Pr., Inc.; 0-9660972),* 1628 E. Southern Ave., Suite 9-112, Tempe, AZ 85282 Tel 602-829-7678; Fax: 602-829-9199
E-mail: cstorad@asu.edu.

Beckley Cardy, *(Beckley Cardy Group; 1-58100),* 100 Paragon Pkwy., Mansfield, OH 44903 Tel 419-589-2100; Fax: 419-589-1416; Toll Free: 888-222-1332
Web site: http://www.BeckleyCardy.com.

Beebe Bks, *(Beebe Bks.; 1-878924),* 5430 34th Ave., S., Apt. 207, Minneapolis, MN 55417-2151 Tel 612-729-2714.

Beech Leaf, *(Beech Leaf Pr.; 0-939294),* Orders Addr.: P.O. Box 127, Kalamazoo, MI 49004-0127 (SAN 665-6633) Tel 616-381-1574; Fax: 616-381-2557
Dist(s): **Kalamazoo Nature Ctr Inc** *(Kalamazoo Nature Ctr., Inc.).*

Beechwood Hlthbks, *(Beechwood Healthbooks, Inc.; 0-916363),* 2026 Beechwood, Wilmette, IL 60091 (SAN 295-7604) Toll Free: 800-767-5215
Web site: http://www.beechwoodhealthbooks.com.

Beekman Pubs, *(Beekman Pubs., Inc.; 0-8464),* P.O. Box 888, Woodstock, NY 12498 (SAN 170-1622) Tel 914-679-2300; Fax: 914-679-2301; Toll Free: 888-233-5626
E-mail: manager@beekmanpublishers.com; beekman@beekmanpublishers.com
Web site: http://www.beekman.net.

Beeler LP Bks Imprint of T T Beeler

Begell Hse, *(Begell Hse. Pubs., Inc.; 1-56700),* 145 Madison Ave.,, New York, NY 10016 Tel 212-725-1999; Fax: 212-213-8368
E-mail: begelhouse@worldnet.att.net; orders@begellhouse.com
Web site: http://www.begellhouse.com.

Begos & Rosenberg, *(Begos & Rosenberg Pubs.; 0-941062),* Cedar Hill, Annandale-on-Hudson, NY 12504 (SAN 281-7594) Tel 518-398-5897.

Behav Med Assocs, *(Behavioral Medicine Assocs., Inc.; 0-9639747),* P.O. Box 90507, San Diego, CA 92169 Tel 858-488-9848; Fax: 858-488-9849.

Behav Sci Ctr Pubs, *(Behavioral Science Ctr., Pubs., Inc.; 0-938837),* 2316 Kemper Ln., Cincinnati, OH 45206-2611 (SAN 661-6895) Tel 513-221-8545; Fax: 513-861-2724; Toll Free: 800-966-1231.

Behavior Sci Systs, *(Behavior Science Systems, Inc.; 0-936787),* Orders Addr.: P.O. Box 580274, Minneapolis, MN 55458 (SAN 699-8976); Edit Addr.: 4553 Vincent Ave., S., Minneapolis, MN 55410 (SAN 699-8984) Tel 612-929-6220.

Behavioral Hlth Indus News, *See* **Open Minds PA**

Behavioral Sci, *(Behavioral Science Research Pr., Inc.; 0-935907),* 12803 Demetra Dr., Suite 100, Dallas, TX 75234 (SAN 696-6896) Tel 972-243-8543; Fax: 972-243-6349
Dist(s): **Publishers Group** *(Publishers Group West).*

Behavioral Studies, *(Behavioral Studies Pr.; 0-911958),* P.O. Box 5323, Beverly Hills, CA 90210 (SAN 202-3903) Tel 310-472-2662.

Behaviordyne, *(Behaviordyne, Inc.; 1-879858),* 2166 The Alameda, San Jose, CA 95126-1144 Toll Free: 800-627-2673.

Beijing Foreign Lang (CHN) *(7-119) Dist. by* **China Bks.**

Beil, *(Beil, Frederic C. Pub., Inc.; 0-913720; 1-929490),* 609 Whitaker St., Savannah, GA 31401 (SAN 240-9909) Tel 912-233-2446 (phone/fax)
E-mail: beilbook@beil.com
Web site: http://www.beil.com.

Being Bks, *(Being Bks.; 0-938292),* 19834 Gresham St., Northridge, CA 91324 (SAN 215-7292) Tel 818-341-0283; 818-891-9661
Dist(s): **Baker & Taylor** *(Baker & Taylor Bks.)*
Bookpeople *(Bookpeople).*

Believers Bkshelf, *(Believers Bookshelf, Inc.; 0-88172; 0-941202),* Box 261, Sunbury, PA 17801 (SAN 211-7746).

Belknap Imprint of HUP

Bella Pubns, *See* **Chem Toxicol Inst**

Belle Curve, *(Belle Curve Records, Inc.; 1-893601),* Orders Addr.: P.O. Box 18387, Boulder, CO 80301-8387 Tel 303-546-6211; Fax: 303-546-6360; Toll Free: 888-357-5867
E-mail: info@bellcurve.com
Web site: http://www.bellecurve.com.

Belleraphon, *(Belleraphon Pr.; 0-9613906),* 18829 Farmington Rd, Livonia, MI 48152 (SAN 683-2318) Tel 248-478-7860.

Belletrist, *(Belletrist Publishing Co.; 0-9648656),* Orders Addr.: P.O. Box 11506, South Bend, IN 46634 Tel 219-287-6580; Fax: 219-234-6860; Toll Free: 800-477-7869 (orders only); Edit Addr.: 2709 S. Twyckenham Dr., South Bend, IN 46634
E-mail: bellpub@earthlink.net
Web site: http://www.worldprofit.com/health/mbaigot.htm
Dist(s): **Baker & Taylor** *(Baker & Taylor Bks.)*
Koen Bk Distributors *(Koen Bk. Distributors).*

Bellowing Ark Pr, *(Bellowing Ark Pr.; 0-944920),* Orders Addr.: P.O. Box 55564, Shoreline, WA 98155 (SAN 245-7849) Tel 206-440-0791.

Bellwether-Cross, *(Bellwether-Cross Publishing; 0-9628440; 1-881795),* Orders Addr.: P.O. Box 139, East Dubuque, IL 61025-0139; Edit Addr.: 18319 Hwy. 20 W, East Dubuque, IL 61025 Tel 815-747-6255; Fax: 815-747-3770; Toll Free: 888-516-5096
E-mail: kharris@shepherd.clrs.com.

Bench Mark Bks, *(Bench Mark Bks.; 0-9627194),* Orders Addr.: P.O. Box 106, Tuckahoe, NY 10707; Edit Addr.: 33 Deerfield Ave., Tuckahoe, NY 10707 Tel 914-969-0400.

Benchmark Bks, *(Benchmark Bks.; 0-942246),* 2600 Mission St., Suite 200, San Marino, CA 91108-1676 (SAN 240-0839) Tel 626-799-1111; Fax: 626-799-3921 Do not confuse with companies with the same name Benchmark Books in Estes Park, CO, Fairfax, VA
Dist(s): **Pathway Bk Serv** *(Pathway Bk. Service).*

Benchmark CT, *(Benchmark Pubns., Inc.; 0-9647121),* 65 Locust Ave., New Canaan, CT 06840-4725 Tel 203-966-6653; Fax: 203-972-7129; Toll Free: 800-559-6653 Do not confuse with Benchmark Pubns., Inc., Chapel Hill, NC.

Benchmark Homeopathic, *(Benchmark Homeopathic Pubns.; 0-9653187),* 14947 Forward Pass, San Antonio, TX 78248-0918 Tel 210-492-8013 (phone/fax)
E-mail: benchmarkpub@stic.net
Web site: http://www.stic.net/users/benchmarkpub.

Bender, *(Bender, Matthew & Co., Inc.; 0-327; 0-8205),* Subs. of Reed Elsevier plc, Orders Addr.: 2 Park Ave., New York, NY 10016 (SAN 202-330X) Tel 212-448-2000; Toll Free: 800-223-1940; 800-422-2022
E-mail: nyo.library@bender.com
Web site: http://www.bender.com.

Benedet Pbng, *(Benedet Publishing Co.; 0-9637917),* 935 B 14th St., San Francisco, CA 94114 Tel 415-281-3380
E-mail: rosalindbenedet@msn.com
Web site: http://www.nccc.org/ComEd/reading.html.

Benef Explan-Shelton Mktg, *See* **Shelton Mktg**

Beneficial Bks Imprint of Lust

Bengal Tiger, *(Bengal Tiger Pr.; 1-884600),* 20176 Village 20, Camarillo, CA 93012 Tel 805-388-1068.

†Benjamin-Cummings, *(Benjamin-Cummings Publishing Co.; 0-201; 0-321; 0-582; 0-8053; 0-8465),* Subs. of Addison Wesley Longman, Inc., Orders Addr.: 1 Jacob Way, Reading, MA 01867 (SAN 206-7862) Tel 781-944-3700; Fax: 781-944-9351; Toll Free: 800-922-0579; Edit Addr.: 1301 Sansome St., San Francisco, CA 94111-1122 (SAN 200-2353) Tel 415-402-2500
E-mail: question@aol.com
Web site: http://www.awl.com/bc/; *CIP.*

Benjamins North Am, *See* **J Benjamins Pubng Co**

Benline Pr, *(Benline Pr.; 0-9642443),* 118 N. 60th Ave. E., Duluth, MN 55804 Tel 218-525-1834; Fax: 218-525-9200; Toll Free: 800-296-7163
E-mail: trudycar@aol.com
Web site: http://www.benline.com.

Berco Pubng, *(Berco Publishing, Inc.; 0-9666956),* P.O. Box 22233, Fort Lauderdale, FL 33335 Toll Free: 888-560-6683 (ext.8314)
E-mail: bercopublishing@hotmail.com
Web site: http://bercopublishing.com
Dist(s): **Baker & Taylor** *(Baker & Taylor Bks.)*
Spring Arbor Dist *(Spring Arbor Distributors Inc.).*

Berg Pubs (GBR) *(0-85496; 0-907582; 1-85973) Dist. by* **NYU Pr.**

†Berg Pubs, *(Berg Pubs., Inc.; 0-85496; 0-907582; 1-85973),* 838 Broadway, 3rd Flr., New York, NY 10003 (SAN 658-1293); *CIP.*

Bergin & Garvey Imprint of Greenwood

Bergner Comm, *See* **Timing CA**

Berkeley Planning Assocs, *(Berkeley Planning Assocs.; 0-9620825),* 440 Grand Ave., Oakland, CA 94610 (SAN 249-8731) Tel 510-465-7884.

Berkeley Sci, *(Berkeley Scientific Pubns.; 0-910224),* 415 Minden Way, Wynnewood, PA 19096 (SAN 211-7231) Tel 303-355-2675.

Publisher Symbol Index

†**Berkley Pub,** *(Berkley Publishing Group; 0-425; 0-515),* Div. of Penguin Putnam, Inc., Orders Addr.: 405 Murray Hill Pkwy., East Rutherford, NJ 07073 Toll Free: 800-788-6262 (individual consumer sales); 800-847-5515 (orders); 800-631-8571 (customer service); Edit Addr.: 375 Hudson St., New York, NY 10014 (SAN 201-3991) Tel 212-366-2000; Fax: 212-366-2385 ; *Imprints:* Perigee Bks (Perigee Books) Body Pr-Perigree (Body Press/Perigree) HP Books (H P Books)
E-mail: online@penguinputnam.com
Web site: http://www.penguinputnam.com
Dist(s): **Penguin Putnam** *(Penguin Putnam, Inc.)*
Warner Publishing Services *(Warner Publishing Services); CIP.*

Berkshire Hse, *(Berkshire Hse. Pubs., Inc.; 0-912944; 0-930145; 0-936399; 1-58157),* 480 Pleasant St., Suite 5, Lee, MA 01238 (SAN 698-1666) Tel 413-243-0303; Fax: 413-243-4737; Toll Free: 800-321-8526
E-mail: info@berkshirehouse.com
Web site: http://www.berkshirehouse.com
Dist(s): **Baker & Taylor** *(Baker & Taylor Bks.)*
Koen Bk Distributors *(Koen Bk. Distributors)*
Natl Bk Netwk *(National Bk. Network).*

Bernan Associates, *(Bernan Assocs.; 0-400; 0-527; 0-89059),* Div. of Kraus Organization, The, Orders Addr.: 4611-F Assembly Dr., Lanham, MD 20706-4391 (SAN 169-3182) Tel 301-459-7666; Fax: 301-459-0056; Toll Free Fax: 800-865-3450; Toll Free: 800-274-4888
E-mail: order@bernan.com; query@bernan.com
Web site: http://www.bernan.com.

Bernel Bks, *(Bernel Bks.; 0-9641887),* Div. of Bernel Co., LLC, 1 Militia Dr., Lexington, MA 02173-4703 Tel 781-674-2056; Fax: 781-674-2059
Dist(s): **R Hale & Co** *(Hale, Robert & Co., Inc.)*
Taylor & Francis *(Taylor & Francis, Inc.).*

Berrett-Koehler, *(Berrett-Koehler Pubs., Inc.; 1-57675; 1-58376; 1-881052),* 235 Montgomery St., Suite 650, San Francisco, CA 94104 Tel 415-288-0260; Fax: 415-362-2512; Toll Free: 800-929-2929
E-mail: bkpub@bkpubl.com
Web site: http://www.bkconnection.com
Dist(s): **Publishers Group** *(Publishers Group West)*
netLibrary CO *(netLibrary, Inc.).*

Bertelsmann (MEX) *(968-11) Dist. by* **Libros Fronteras.**

Bess Pr, *(Bess Pr., Inc.; 0-935848; 1-57306; 1-880188),* 3565 Harding Ave., Honolulu, HI 96816 (SAN 239-4111) Tel 808-734-7159; Fax: 808-732-3627; Toll Free: 800-910-2377
E-mail: info@besspress.com
Web site: http://www.besspress.com
Dist(s): **Aha Punana Leo** *(Aha Punana Leo)*
Shens Bks *(Shen's Bks.).*

Best Pub Co, *(Best Publishing Co.; 0-941332; 1-930536),* Orders Addr.: P.O. Box 30100, Flagstaff, AZ 86003-0100 (SAN 238-9509) Tel 520-527-1055; Fax: 520-526-0370; Toll Free: 800-468-1055; Edit Addr.: 2355 N. Steves Blvd., Flagstaff, AZ 86004
E-mail: divebooks@bestpub.com
Web site: http://www.bestpub.com.

BEST Research, *(B.E.S.T. Research, Inc.; 0-944994),* 1000 W. Poplar, Rogers, AR 72756 (SAN 246-0092) Tel 501-631-2749; Fax: 501-631-8201; Toll Free: 800-874-1478
E-mail: moreinfo@morter.com.

BEST WAY, *(BEST WAY to Health, Inc.; 0-9678916),* P.O. Box 463, Conyers, GA 30012 Tel 770-761-6349 (phone/fax)
E-mail: bestwaytohealth@yahoo.com.

Best Years Inc, *(Best Years, Inc.; 1-892870),* Div. of the Sparta Ecumenical Council on Senior Citizen Housing, 44 Carriup Ln., Sparta, NJ 07871 Tel 973-729-4311 ext. 29; Fax: 973-729-2750
E-mail: knoll@warick.com
Web site: http://www.best-years.com.

†**Bethany Hse,** *(Bethany Hse. Pubs.; 0-7642; 0-87123; 1-55661; 1-56179),* Div. of Bethany Fellowship, Inc., 11400 Hampshire Ave., S., Minneapolis, MN 55438-2455 (SAN 201-4416) Tel 612-829-2500; Fax: 612-829-2768; Toll Free: 800-328-6109
E-mail: cs@bethanyhouse.com
Web site: http://www.bethanyhouse.com
Dist(s): **Anchor Distributors** *(Anchor Distributors)*
Appalachian Bible *(Appalachian Bible Co.)*
Baker & Taylor *(Baker & Taylor Bks.)*
Brodart *(Brodart Co.)*
Follett Library *(Follett Library Resources)*
Permabound *(Permabound Bks.)*
Rvrside Bk & Bible *(Riverside Bk. & Bible Resource)*
Spring Arbor Dist *(Spring Arbor Distributors Inc.)*
T T Beeler *(Beeler, Thomas T. Publisher); CIP.*

Bethany Prods, *(Bethany Productions; 1-879058),* Div. of Bethany Christian Services, 901 Eastern Ave., NE, Grand Rapids, MI 49503-1295 Tel 616-459-6273; Fax: 616-459-0343; Toll Free: 800-238-4269.

Betrwy Bks Imprint of F & W Pubns Inc

Better Baby, *See* **Inst Achieve Human Pot**

Better Government, *(Better Government Assn.; 0-9641280),* 28 E. Jackson Blvd., Chicago, IL 60604 Tel 312-641-1181; Fax: 312-641-2513.

Better H Prog, *(Better Health Programs; 0-933161),* 2107 Van Ness Ave., Suite 408, San Francisco, CA 94109 (SAN 692-2597) Tel 415-775-5921.

Better Hlth, *(Better Health Publishing; 0-9661346),* 6434 Dawnmist Ln., Charlotte, NC 28269 (SAN 299-6154) Tel 704-875-6966; Fax: 704-948-7119; Toll Free: 888-919-6636
E-mail: bhpublishing@hotmail.com
Web site: http://www.womensbooks.com.

Better Hlth Bks, *(Better Health Bks.; 1-884030),* 7405 Winding Way, Fair Oaks, CA 95628 Tel 916-966-7395; Fax: 916-966-7398.

Better Life Pr, *(Better Life Pr.; 0-9663788),* Div. of Better Life Publishing Co., LLC, 1011Boren Ave., Suite 323, Seattle, WA 98106 Tel 206-323-0116; Fax: 206-323-2300 Do not confuse with Better Life Pr. in North Reading, MA
Dist(s): **IPG Chicago** *(Independent Pubs. Group).*

Betwn Lines (CAN) *(0-919946; 0-921284; 1-896357) Dist. by* **U of Toronto Pr.**

Beulah Land, *See* **Mann Daniel**

Beynch Pr, *(Beynch Pr.; 0-941383),* 1928 SE Ladd Ave., Portland, OR 97214 (SAN 666-6280) Tel 503-232-0433; Fax: 503-239-4984
Web site: http://www.justalyce.com
Dist(s): **Baker & Taylor** *(Baker & Taylor Bks.)*
Metamorphous Pr *(Metamorphous Pr., Inc.)*
New Leaf Dist *(New Leaf Distributing Co., Inc.).*

Beyond Words Pub, *(Beyond Words Publishing, Inc.; 0-941831; 1-58270; 1-885223; 1-892485),* 20827 NW Cornell Rd., Suite 500, Hillsboro, OR 97124-9808 (SAN 666-4210) Tel 503-531-8700; Fax: 503-531-8773; Toll Free: 800-284-9673
E-mail: sales@beyondword.com; info@beyondword.com
Web site: http://www.beyondword.com
Dist(s): **Publishers Group** *(Publishers Group West).*

Bezkorovainy, *(Bezkorovainy, Anatoly; 0-9607600),* 4242 W. Touhy Ave., Lincolnwood, IL 60646 (SAN 218-4672) Tel 312-942-5429.

BGC Pub Co, *(BGC Publishing Co.; 0-9620061),* 194 Lexington Pkwy. N., No. 3, Saint Paul, MN 55104-6454 (SAN 247-5057) Tel 612-646-5277.

BHB Intl, *(BHB International, Inc.),* Orders Addr.: 108 E. N. First St., Suite G, Seneca, SC 29678 (SAN 631-0915) Tel 864-885-9444; Fax: 864-885-1090
E-mail: bhbbooks@aol.com
Web site: http://www.bhbinternational.com.

Bibli O Phile Pub Co, *(Bibli O'Phile Publishing Co.; 0-942104),* 200 W. 58th St., No. 2C, New York, NY 10019-1432 (SAN 238-6437) Tel 212-888-1008; Fax: 212-486-9530; Toll Free: 800-255-1660
Dist(s): **Penguin Putnam** *(Penguin Putnam, Inc.).*

Bibliographic Pr, *(Bibliographic Pr., The; 0-930429),* P.O. Box 5433, Flushing, NY 11354 (SAN 670-9788).

Bick Pub Hse, *(Bick Publishing Hse.; 1-884158),* 307 Neck Rd., Madison, CT 06443 Tel 203-245-0073; Fax: 203-245-5990
E-mail: bickpubhse@aol.com
Web site: http://www.bickpubhouse.com
Dist(s): **Baker & Taylor** *(Baker & Taylor Bks.)*
BookWorld *(BookWorld Services, Inc.).*

Biddle Pub, *(Biddle Publishing Co.; 1-879418),* Orders Addr.: P.O. Box 1305, Brunswick, ME 04011 Tel 207-833-5016; Toll Free: 888-315-0582 (orders)
Web site: http://www.biddle-audenreed.com
Dist(s): **Baker & Taylor** *(Baker & Taylor Bks.).*

Bienestar, *(Bienestar, Inc.; 1-892039),* Orders Addr.: P.O. Box 47, Mount Tremper, NY 12457 Tel 914-688-2878; Fax: 914-688-5546; Toll Free: 888-692-4363; Edit Addr.: 1556 Wittenberg Rd., Mount Tremper, NY 12457
E-mail: bienestar3@aol.com
Web site: http://www.bienestarinc.com.

Big Bend Bks, *See* **Muriel S Pascoe**

Big Blue Bks, *(Big Blue Bks.; 0-916969),* 13239 Vanguard Way, Lakeside, CA 92040 (SAN 655-5772) Tel 619-443-6397.

Big Tree Bks Imprint of Easy Money Pr

Bigelow Charter, *(Bigelow Charter Services; 1-882537),* 1831 N. Bel Aire Dr., Burbank, CA 91504 Tel 818-558-7099; Fax: 818-558-7299; Toll Free: 800-225-2308.

Bimark, *(Bimark, Inc.; 1-884033),* 95 Bedar Ln., Suite 12, Englewood, NJ 07631 Tel 201-894-5314; Fax: 201-498-7227.

Binford Mort, *(Binford & Mort Publishing; 0-8323),* Orders Addr.: P.O. Box 91580, Portland, OR 97291; Edit Addr.: 5245 NE Elam Young Pkwy., Suite C, Hillsboro, OR 97124 (SAN 201-4386) Tel 503-844-4960; Fax: 503-844-4959; Toll Free: 888-221-4514
Web site: http://www.binfordandmort.com/
Dist(s): **Baker & Taylor** *(Baker & Taylor Bks.)*
Maverick Dist *(Maverick Distributors)*
Partners-West *(Partners/West).*

Bink Productions, *(Bink Productions, Inc.; 0-9658297),* P.O. Box 270157, San Diego, CA 92198 Tel 619-613-1100
E-mail: tdservices@aol.com.

Bio Concepts (AUS) *Dist. by* **St Mut.**

Bio Psych, *(Biological Psychiatry Institute; 0-9668886),* 5133 N. Central Ave., Suite 107, Phoenix, AZ 85012 Tel 602-279-1026; Fax: 602-279-0848.

Bio Pubns, *(Biological Pubns.; 1-879361),* 6529 W. Fond Du Lac Ave., Milwaukee, WI 53218 Tel 414-464-7680.

Bio Sonic Ent, *(Bio Sonic Enterprises, Ltd.; 0-9640604),* 132 E. 85th St., No. 2-1, High Falls, NY 12440 Tel 212-334-8392; 914-687-4767; Fax: 212-274-9325; Toll Free: 800-925-0159
Dist(s): **Bookpeople** *(Bookpeople)*
New Leaf Dist *(New Leaf Distributing Co., Inc.).*

Bio-Comns Pr, *(Bio-Communications Pr.; 0-942333),* Div. of Ctr. for the Improvement of Human Functioning International, Inc., 3100 N. Hillside, Wichita, KS 67219 (SAN 667-1063) Tel 316-682-3100; Fax: 316-682-5054
Web site: http://www.brightspot.org.

Bio-Dynamic Farm, *(Bio-Dynamic Farming & Gardening Assn., Inc.; 0-938250),* Orders Addr.: P.O. Box 29135, San Francisco, CA 94129-0135 (SAN 224-9871) Tel 415-561-7797; Fax: 415-561-7796; Toll Free: 888-516-7797; Edit Addr.: Bldg. 1002B, Thoreau Ctr., San Francisco, CA 94129-0135
E-mail: biodynamic@aol.com
Web site: http://www.biodynamics.com
Dist(s): **Chelsea Green Pub** *(Chelsea Green Publishing)*
New Leaf Dist *(New Leaf Distributing Co., Inc.)*
Small Changes Inc *(Small Changes, Inc.).*

Bioenergetics Pr, *See* **MPC Pr**

Bioethics Cnslt, *(Bioethics Consultation Group, Inc.; 1-882674),* 2322 Sixth St., Suite 103, Berkeley, CA 94710 Tel 510-486-0626; Fax: 510-540-7643
E-mail: bcg@ix.netcom.com.

Biofeedback Ctr, *(Biofeedback Ctr. Pr., The; 1-890669),* 3310 Smith Dr., Reno, NV 89509 Tel 775-825-0334; Toll Free: 800-310-7584
E-mail: el-kid@msn.com
Web site: http://www.stresslesslife.com
Dist(s): **Stoelting Co** *(Stoelting Co.).*

Biomat Pub Co, *(Biomateria Publishing Co., Inc.; 0-9609098),* P.O. Box 523, Stony Brook, NY 11790 (SAN 241-2748) Tel 516-383-1140
E-mail: ferruzd@sunysuffolk.edu.

Biomed Genl, *(Biomed General; 1-893549),* Orders Addr.: P.O. Box 272007, Concord, CA 94518 Tel 925-602-6140; Fax: 925-363-7798; Edit Addr.: 5801 Christie Ave., Suite 280, Emeryville, CA 94608 Tel 510-450-1657; Fax: 510-450-1336; Toll Free: 888-724-6633
E-mail: info@biomedgeneral.com
Web site: http://www.biomedbooks.com.

Biomed Pr, *(Biomedical Pr., Inc.; 1-883865),* 1899 SW 17th St., Boca Raton, FL 33486 Tel 407-391-5331; Fax: 407-750-1542.

Biomedical Pubns, *(Biomedical Pubns.; 0-9626523),* Div. of Chemical Toxicology Institute, P.O. Box 8229, Foster City, CA 94404
E-mail: biopub@altavista.com
Web site: http://www.biomedicalpublications.com
Dist(s): **BookMasters** *(BookMasters, Inc.).*

Bion Pub, *(Bion Publishing; 0-945196),* Orders Addr.: P.O. Box 10, Ojai, CA 93024 (SAN 246-5930) Tel 805-646-2865; Fax: 805-646-1506; Edit Addr.: 323 E. Matilija, No. 110-151, Ojai, CA 93023 (SAN 246-5949) Tel 805-646-3096
Dist(s): **Price Pottenger** *(Price Pottenger Foundation).*

Biopress (GBR) *(0-948737) Dist. by* **Balogh.**

Bio-Probe, *(Bio-Probe, Inc.; 0-941011),* 5508 Edgewater Dr., Orlando, FL 32810 (SAN 665-2891) Tel 407-290-9670; Fax: 407-299-4149; Toll Free: 800-282-9670
E-mail: bpinfo@bioprobe.com
Web site: http://www.bioprobe.com.

BioPsych Pr, *(BioPsychology Pr.; 0-9631937),* 76 Devoe Rd., Chappaqua, NY 10514 Tel 212-263-5740.

Bio-Pub, *(Bio-Publishing Co.; 0-916833),* P.O. Box 24906, Winston-Salem, NC 27114-4906 (SAN 654-3758) Tel 910-760-0944.

Bios Sci (GBR) *(1-85996; 1-872748) Dist. by* **Spr-Verlag.**

Bios Sci (GBR) *(1-85996; 1-872748) Dist. by* **Bks Intl VA.**

Biota Pubns, *(Biota Pubns.; 0-9649044),* 4700 Ridgedale Dr., Plano, TX 75024-2434
E-mail: biota@onramp.net
Web site: http://www.biota.com.

Biotech, *(Biotech Publishing; 1-880319),* Div. of Plant Something Different, Inc., Orders Addr.: P.O. Box 1032, Angleton, TX 77516-1032 Tel 281-369-2044; Toll Free: 800-659-3078
E-mail: services@biotechpub.com
Web site: http://www.biotechpub.com.

BioTechniques Imprint of Eaton Pub Co

Biotest, *(Biotest, Inc.; 1-893720),* Orders Addr.: 2137 Martinique Ln., Oxnard, CA 93035 Tel 805-984-7415; Fax: 805-984-7245; Edit Addr.: 2073 N. Oxnard Blvd., No. 300, Oxnard, CA 93030.

Birdcage Bks, *(Birdcage Bks; 1-889613),* 2310 Bowdoin St., Palo Alto, CA 94306 Tel 650-424-1763; Fax: 650-424-1701; 7560 Old Bridge Rd., Leavenworth, WA 98826
E-mail: info@birdcagebooks.com
Web site: http://www.birdcagebooks.com
Dist(s): **Publishers Group** *(Publishers Group West).*

Birkhauser, *(Birkhauser Boston; 0-8176; 3-7643),* Div. of Springer-Verlag GmbH & Co. KG, Orders Addr.: P.O. Box 2485, Secaucus, NJ 07094 (SAN 241-6344) Tel 201-348-4033; Edit Addr.: 675 Massachusetts Ave., Cambridge, MA 02139 (SAN 213-2869) Tel 617-876-2333; Toll Free: 800-777-4643 (customer service)
Web site: http://www.birkhauser.com
Dist(s): **Spr-Verlag** *(Springer-Verlag New York, Inc.).*

Birkhauser (CHE) *(3-7643) Dist. by* **Princeton Arch.**

Birkhauser (CHE) *(3-7643) Dist. by* **Spr-Verlag.**

Birth & Parenting, *(Birth & Parenting Pubns.; 0-9615484),* 876 Chapel Hill Rd., Charlottesville, VA 22901 (SAN 696-1134).

Bison Books Imprint of U of Nebr Pr

Bistai Pr, *(Bista'i Pr.; 0-9711097),* Orders Addr.: P.O. Box 748, Cuba, NM 87013 Tel 505-289-0288; Edit Addr.: 227 Los Pinos Rd., Cuba, NM 87013.

Bittersweet Bay, *(Bittersweet Bay Bks., LLC; 0-9705937),* Orders Addr.: P.O. Box 8, Evanston, IL 60204-0008 Tel 847-328-8610; Fax: 847-866-7206; Toll Free: 888-408-7748; Edit Addr.: 1132 Grant St., Evanston, IL 60201
E-mail: bittersweet@etpost.net
Web site: http://www.bittersweetbay.com.

BJB Pub, *(BJB Publishing; 0-9645178),* 16212 Bothell Way SE, Suite F171, Mill Creek, WA 98012-1219 Tel 425-337-3414; Fax: 425-338-0456; Toll Free: 800-799-3414
E-mail: bjbservices@prodigy.net
Web site: http://www.pages.prodigy.com/bjbservices
Dist(s): **Baker & Taylor** *(Baker & Taylor Bks.)*
Brodart *(Brodart Co.)*
Koen Bk Distributors *(Koen Bk. Distributors)*
Quality Bks IL *(Quality Bks., Inc.)*
Unique Bks Inc *(Unique Bks., Inc.).*

Bk Pub Co WA, *(Book Publishing Co.; 0-939737),* 201 Westlake Ave., N., Seattle, WA 98109 (SAN 663-7175) Tel 206-343-5700; Fax: 206-343-3038; Toll Free: 800-537-7881 Do not confuse with Book Publishing Co., Summertown, TN.

Bk Sales Inc, *(Book Sales, Inc.; 0-7858; 0-89009; 1-55521),* Orders Addr.: 114 Northfield Ave., Edison, NJ 08837 (SAN 169-488X) Tel 732-225-0530; Fax: 212-779-6058; 732-225-2257; Toll Free: 800-526-7257; Edit Addr.: 276 Fifth Ave., Suite 206, New York, NY 10001 (SAN 299-4062) Tel 212-779-4972; Fax: 212-779-6058
E-mail: bsiny@hotmail.com
Web site: http://www.booksales.com
Dist(s): **Continental Bk** *(Continental Bk. Co., Inc.).*

Bks Intl VA, *(Books International, Incorporated; 1-891078),* Orders Addr.: P.O. Box 605, Herndon, VA 20172-0605 (SAN 131-761X) Tel 703-661-1500; Fax: 703-661-1501
E-mail: mgreenwald@sorosny.org
Dist(s): **Intl Pubs Mktg** *(International Publishers Marketing).*

Bks Nippan, *(Books Nippan; 0-945814; 1-56970),* Div. of Nippan Shuppan Hanbai, U.S.A., Inc., 1123 Dominguez St., Suite K, Carson, CA 90746 (SAN 111-817X) Tel 310-604-9701; Fax: 310-604-1134; Toll Free: 800-562-1410
E-mail: distribution@emanga.com
Web site: http://www.booksnippan.com/.

Bks of Discov, *(Books of Discovery; 0-9658534),* P.O. Box 6107, Boulder, CO 80306 Fax: 303-545-2664; Toll Free: 800-775-9227
E-mail: bodytrail@aol.com.

Bks of Sci, *(Books of Science; 0-916615),* 10850 Green Mountain Cir., Columbia, MD 22044 (SAN 296-4589) Tel 410-730-8391
E-mail: Bosci@mindspring.com.

Bks of Value, *(Books of Value; 0-9603174),* 2458 Chislehurst Dr., Los Angeles, CA 90027 (SAN 210-5896) Tel 213-664-8981.

Black Belt Communs, *See* **River City Pub**

Black Dog Pub, *(Black Dog Publishing Co.; 0-9656231),* 127 Longfields Way, Downingtown, PA 19335 Tel 610-269-0479 (phone/fax)
E-mail: NewWavePh@aol.com
Web site: http://www.members.aol.com/blackdogpharma.

Black Forest Pr, *(Black Forest Pr.; 1-58275; 1-881116),* Div. of Black Forest Enterprises, Orders Addr.: P.O. Box 6342, Chula Vista, CA 91909-6342 Fax: 619-498-8540; Toll Free: 888-808-5440; Edit Addr.: 914 Nolan Way, Chula Vista, CA 91911-2408 (SAN 298-8445) Tel 619-656-8048
E-mail: bfp@blackforestpress.com
Web site: http://www.blackforestpress.com
Dist(s): **Baker & Taylor** *(Baker & Taylor Bks.)*
Herveys Bklink *(Hervey's Booklink & Cookbook Warehouse)*
Partners-West *(Partners/West).*

Black Mksgaard (DNK) *(87-16) Dist. by* **Iowa U Pr.**

Black Rose (CAN) *(0-919618; 0-919619; 0-920057; 0-921689; 1-55164; 1-895431) Dist. by* **Consort Bk Sales.**

Black Swan Pr, *(Black Swan Pr./Surrealist Editions; 0-941194),* P.O. Box 6424, Evanston, IL 60204 (SAN 211-593X) Tel 773-465-7774
Dist(s): **C H Kerr** *(Kerr, Charles H. Publishing Co.)*
SPD-Small Pr Dist *(SPD-Small Pr. Distribution).*

Black T T, *(Black Think Tank; 0-9613086),* 1801 Bush St., Suite 118, San Francisco, CA 94109 (SAN 293-969X) Tel 415-474-1707; Fax: 415-771-3485.

Blackbirch Pr Imprint of Gale

Blackstaff Pr (IRL) *(0-85640) Dist. by* **Dufour.**

Blackstone Pr (GBR) *(1-85431; 1-84174) Dist. by* **Gaunt.**

Blackstone Pr (GBR) *(1-85431; 1-84174) Dist. by* **Intl Spec Bk.**

Blackwell Hlthcare Imprint of Blackwell Sci

†Blackwell Pubs, *(Blackwell Pubs.; 0-631; 0-7456; 0-85012; 1-55786; 1-57718; 1-878975),* Orders Addr.: P.O. Box 20, Williston, VT 05495-0020 Tel 802-862-0095; Fax: 802-864-7626; Toll Free Fax: 800-864-7626; Toll Free: 800-216-2522; Edit Addr.: 350 Main St., 6th Flr., Malden, MA 02148-5018 (SAN 680-5035) Tel 781-388-8200; Fax: 781-388-8210
E-mail: books@blackwellpub.com
Web site: http://www.blackwellpub.com
Dist(s): **Am Intl Dist** *(American International Distribution Corp.)*
netLibrary CO *(netLibrary, Inc.); CIP.*

†Blackwell Sci, *(Blackwell Science, Inc.; 0-632; 0-86542),* Subs. of Blackwell Scientific Ltd, Orders Addr.: Commerce Pl., 350 Main St., Malden, MA 02148-5018 (SAN 215-2029) Tel 617-388-8250; Fax: 781-388-8255; Toll Free: 800-759-6102; 800-215-1000 (orders) ; *Imprints:* Blackwell Hlthcare (Blackwell Healthcare)
E-mail: csbooks@blacksci.com
Web site: http://www.blacksci.co.uk/usa
Dist(s): **Iowa U Pr** *(Iowa Univ. Pr.)*
netLibrary CO *(netLibrary, Inc.); CIP.*

Blair, *(Blair, John F. Pub.; 0-89587; 0-910244),* 1406 Plaza Dr., Winston-Salem, NC 27103 (SAN 201-4319) Tel 336-768-1374; Fax: 336-768-9194; Toll Free: 800-222-9796
E-mail: blairpub@blairpub.com
Web site: http://www.blairpub.com.

Blanchard & Loeb, *(Blanchard & Loeb Pubs.; 1-930138),* 865 Belfry Dr., Blue Bell, PA 19422 Tel 215-643-2359; Fax: 215-643-4865; Toll Free: 800-625-2666
E-mail: service@blanchardloeb.com
Web site: http://www.blanchardloeb.com
Dist(s): **Spr-Verlag** *(Springer-Verlag New York, Inc.).*

Blanchards Bks, *(Blanchard's Bks.; 0-9700529),* 10907 SE Azar Dr., Portland, OR 97266 Tel 503-698-5582 (phone/fax)
E-mail: dblanc@teleport.com.

Blanchards Brook, *(Blanchard's Brook; 0-9624399),* P.O. Box 8531, Medford, OR 97504 Tel 541-858-8916.

Blanco, *(Blanco Consulting; 0-9702555),* 3107 Timberwolf Ave., High Point, NC 27265 Tel 336-841-0082 (phone/fax)
E-mail: blanco231@aol.com
Web site: http://www.blancoconsulting.homestead.com.

Blast Bks, *(Blast Bks.; 0-922233),* Orders Addr.: P.O. Box 51, New York, NY 10276 (SAN 251-1576) Tel 212-674-6367
Dist(s): **Publishers Group** *(Publishers Group West).*

Blckbrry Crtns, *(Blackberry Creations; 0-9627724),* P.O. Box 92141, Milwaukee, WI 53202-0141 Tel 414-272-0661.

Blckwell Science (GBR) *(0-632; 0-86542) Dist. by* **Iowa U Pr.**

Blckwell Wissenschafts (DEU) *(3-8263; 3-89412) Dist. by* **Balogh.**

Blewstone Pr, *(Blewstone Pr.; 0-930961),* Div. of Allergenco, Orders Addr.: P.O. Box 8571, San Antonio, TX 78208 (SAN 678-8777) Tel 210-822-4116.

BLHY Growth Pubns, *(BLHY Growth Pubns., Inc.; 0-9664761),* 2521 Far Hills Ave., Dayton, OH 45419 Tel 937-294-3680; Fax: 937-293-5287.

BLL Pubng, *(BLL Publishing; 0-9643737),* Orders Addr.: P.O. Box 84900, Phoenix, AZ 85071 Tel 602-252-4477; Fax: 602-943-2363; Toll Free: 800-528-0559
Web site: http://www.johnleemd.com.

Blmsbury Pub (GBR) *(0-7475) Dist. by* **Trafalgar.**

Bloch, *(Bloch Publishing Co.; 0-8197),* 118 E. 28th St., Suite 501-503, New York, NY 10016-8413 (SAN 214-204X) Tel 212-532-3977; Fax: 212-779-9169
E-mail: BlochPub@worldnet.att.net
Web site: http://www.blochpub.com/.

Blom Pubns (GBR) *(0-405) Dist. by* **Ayer.**

Blood & Marrow, *(Blood & Marrow Transplant Information Network; 0-9647352),* 2900 Skokie Valley Rd., Suite B, Highland Park, IL 60035 Tel 847-433-3313; Fax: 847-433-4599; Toll Free: 888-597-7674
E-mail: help@bmtnews.org
Web site: http://www.bmtnews.org.

Blood-Horse, *(Blood-Horse, Inc., The; 0-936032; 0-939049; 1-58150),* Subs. of Thoroughbred Owners & Breeders Assn., Orders Addr.: P.O. Box 4038, Lexington, KY 40544-4038 (SAN 203-5294) Tel 859-278-2361; Fax: 859-276-4450; Toll Free: 800-866-2361; Edit Addr.: 1736 Alexandria Dr, Lexington, KY 40504
E-mail: info@eclipsepress.com; admin@bloodhorse.com
Web site: http://www.eclipsepress.com; http://www.bloodhorse.com
Dist(s): **IPG Chicago** *(Independent Pubs. Group)*
Natl Bk Netwk *(National Bk. Network).*

Bloomberg NJ, *(Bloomberg Pr.; 1-57660),* Orders Addr.: P.O. Box 888, Princeton, NJ 08542-0888 (SAN 298-6132) Tel 609-279-4670; Fax: 609-279-7155; Toll Free Fax: 800-458-6515; Toll Free: 800-388-2749 (ext.4670); Edit Addr.: 100 Business Pk. Dr., Princeton, NJ 08542-0888
E-mail: press@bloomberg.net
Web site: http://www.bloomberg.com
Dist(s): **Norton** *(Norton, W.W. & Co., Inc.).*

†Blue Bird Pub, *(Blue Bird Publishing; 0-933025; 0-9615578),* 10820 Farragut Hills Blvd., Knoxville, TN 37922 (SAN 200-5603) Tel 865-777-5218; Fax: 865-777-5219
E-mail: bluebird@bluebird1.com
Web site: http://www.bluebird1.com
Dist(s): **IPG Chicago** *(Independent Pubs. Group); CIP.*

Blue Danube Pub, *(Blue Danube Publishing; 0-9634791),* 3430 Oak Creek Cir., Dallas, TX 75227-5637 Fax: 972-247-2604; 32 Lariat Dr., Frisco, TX 75034 Tel 972-241-7031.

Blue Lamm, *(Blue Lamm Publishing; 0-9672532),* P.O. Box 87242, San Diego, CA 92138-7242 Fax: 619-223-8376
E-mail: renee@esordi.com
Web site: http://www.esordi.com/bluelamm; http://www.youhaveavisitor.com.

Blue Path Pr, *(Blue Path Pr., Inc.; 1-887109),* 367 Skyline Orchard Dr., Suite E, Hockessin, DE 19707 Tel 302-239-9046; Fax: 302-234-2840.

Blue Poppy Pr, *(Blue Poppy Pr.; 0-936185; 1-891845),* 5441 Western Ave., No. 2, Boulder, CO 80301 (SAN 697-0168) Tel 303-245-8337; Fax: 303-245-8362; Toll Free: 800-487-9296 (orders only)
E-mail: info@bluepoppy.com; bluepp@compuserve.com; bpeinc1@compuserve.com
Web site: http://www.bluepoppy.com
Dist(s): **Bookpeople** *(Bookpeople)*
New Leaf Dist *(New Leaf Distributing Co., Inc.)*
Redwing Bk Co *(Redwing Bk. Co.).*

Blue Skies, *(Blue Skies Pr.; 0-9667222),* P.O. Box 783, Lynbrook, NY 11563 Tel 516-596-3239; Fax: 516-596-0646; Toll Free: 888-414-3239
E-mail: fscoblete@earthlink.net
Dist(s): **Baker & Taylor** *(Baker & Taylor Bks.).*

Blue Turtle, *(Blue Turtle Publishing Co.; 0-9634662; 1-929977),* 2905 Echo Canyon Rd., Cornville, AZ 86325 Tel 520-634-9298 (phone/fax)
E-mail: docbones@sedona.net
Web site: http://www.medicinegurden.com
Dist(s): **New Leaf Dist** *(New Leaf Distributing Co., Inc.).*

Bluebelle Med Co, *(Bluebelle Medical Co., The; 0-9621594),* P.O. Box 1305, Woodland Hills, CA 91365 (SAN 252-1741) Tel 804-355-7996.

Bluestar Communs, *(Bluestar Communications Corp.; 1-885394),* c/o Words Distributing Company, 7900 Edgewater Dr., Oakland, CA 94621; Edit Addr.: 162 Camino Don Miguel, Orinda, CA 94563 Tel 925-368-0440; Fax: 925-368-0368; Toll Free: 866-625-7827 (866-6-bluestar)
E-mail: orders@bluestar.com
Web site: http://www.bluestar.com
Dist(s): **Words Distrib** *(Words Distributing Co.).*

Bluewood Bks, *(Bluewood Bks.; 0-912517),* Div. of The Siyeh Group, Inc., P.O. Box 689, San Mateo, CA 94010 (SAN 265-3214) Tel 650-548-0754; Fax: 650-548-0654
E-mail: Bluewoodb@aol.com
Dist(s): **LPC Group** *(LPC Group)*
Login Pubs Consort *(Login Pubs. Consortium).*

Bluwaters Pr, *(Bluwaters Pr.; 0-9665584),* Orders Addr.: P.O. Box 878, Mesilla, NM 88046 Tel 505-647-1408 (phone/fax); Toll Free: 888-541-5381; Edit Addr.: 1905 Sheryl Way, Las Cruces, NM 88001
E-mail: bwaters@totacc.com
Web site: http://www.totacc.com/user/bwaters/.

BMB Pub Co, *(BMB Publishing Co.; 0-930924; 0-9600164),* P.O. Box 390931, Cambridge, MA 02139-0021 (SAN 201-4270) Tel 617-492-5762.

BMJ Pub (GBR) *(0-7279) Dist. by* **AIDC.**

BMT Newsletter, *See* **Blood & Marrow**

B&N Imports, *(Barnes & Noble Bks.-Imports; 0-389),* Div. of Rowman & Littlefield Pubs., Inc., 4720 Boston Way, Lanham, MD 20706 (SAN 206-7803) Tel 301-459-3366; Toll Free: 800-462-6420.

BNA, *(Bureau of National Affairs, Inc., (BNA), The; 1-55871),* Orders Addr.: 9435 Key West Ave., Rockville, MD 20850 Fax: 301-294-6651; Toll Free: 800-372-1033; 800-468-3234 (in Canada); Edit Addr.: 1231 25th St., NW, Washington, DC 20037 Tel 202-452-4200; Fax: 202-452-4226
E-mail: customercare@bna.com
Web site: http://www.bna.com.

BNA Books, *(BNA Bks.; 0-87179; 1-57018),* Div. of Bureau of National Affairs, Inc., Orders Addr.: P.O. Box 7814, Edison, NJ 08818-7814 (SAN 661-9649) Fax: 732-346-1624; Toll Free: 800-960-1220
E-mail: books@bna.com
Web site: http://www.bna.com/bnabooks.

BNA PLUS, *(BNA PLUS; 1-55871),* Div. of The Bureau of National Affairs, Inc., 1231 25th St., NW, Washington, DC 20037 Tel 202-452-4323; Fax: 202-452-4644; Toll Free: 800-452-7773
E-mail: bnaplus@bna.com
Web site: http://www.bna.com.

Boabab Pub, *(Boabab Publishing, Inc.; 0-9662831),* 304 Newbery St., PMB 169, Boston, MA 02115 Tel 617-249-2022; Fax: 617-249-2023
E-mail: sales@boabab.com
Web site: http://www.boabab.com.

Boardroom, *(Boardroom Bks.; 0-88723; 0-932648),* Div. of Boardroom Reports, Inc., Box 2614, 55 Railroad Ave., Greenwich, CT 06836 (SAN 211-5956) Tel 203-625-5900.

†Bob Jones Univ, *(Jones, Bob Univ. Pr.; 0-89084; 1-57924; 1-59166),* 1700 Wade Hampton Blvd., Greenville, SC 29614 (SAN 223-7512) Tel 864-242-5731; Fax: 864-298-8398; Toll Free Fax: 800-525-8398; Toll Free: 800-845-5731
E-mail: bjup@bjup.com
Web site: http://www.bjup.com; *CIP.*

Bobbs Imprint of Macmillan

Body Care, *(Body Care Publishing; 0-9638201),* P.O. Box 5981, Lake Charles, LA 70606 Toll Free: 800-269-8460.

Body Ecol Diet, *See* **Body Ecology**

Body Ecology, *(Body Ecology; 0-9638458),* 1266 West Paces Ferry Rd., Suite 505, Atlanta, GA 30327 Toll Free: 800-511-2660
E-mail: bodyeco@aol.com.

Body Positive, *(Body Positive; 0-9653952),* 19 Fulton St., Suite 308B, New York, NY 10038 Tel 212-566-7333; Fax: 212-566-4539
Web site: http://www.hunter_pubs.com.au.

Body Pr-Perigee Imprint of Berkley Pub

Body Pr-Perigee Imprint of Penguin Putnam

BodyGuide, *(BodyGuide; 0-9655679),* Div. of MountainHeart, Inc., Orders Addr.: P.O. Box 575, Crested Butte, CO 81224 Tel 970-349-0473 (phone/fax); Toll Free: 800-673-0539
E-mail: cragmc@crestedbutte.net
Web site: http://www.user.gunnison.com/~cragmc/MRG.html.

Bodysmart Pubns, *(Bodysmart Pubns.; 0-9649741),* 14309 Lennell Dr., Minnetonka, MN 55345 Tel 612-542-9480.

Bodyworks Pubs, *(Bodyworks Pubs.; 0-9635503),* Orders Addr.: P.O. Box 10635, Palm Desert, CA 92255-0635; Edit Addr.: 74801 Holsely Ln., Palm Desert, CA 92260 Tel 760-360-0978.

Boehme Wkshps, *(Boehme Workshops; 1-879801),* 8642 N. 66th St., Brown Deer, WI 53223 Tel 414-355-8744; Fax: 414-355-6837; Toll Free: 888-463-4668
E-mail: boehme8642@aol.com
Web site: http://www.hoehmeworkshops.com.

Bogners Limited, *(Bogner's, Ltd.; 0-943323),* P.O. Box 260, Crofton, NE 68730 (SAN 668-2537).

Bohemian Brigade, *(Bohemian Brigade Bookshop & Publishing Co.; 1-877791),* 7347 Middlebrook Pike, Knoxville, TN 37909 Tel 423-694-8227.

Boitumelo Pub Imprint of Creat Logic

Bokar Cnslts, *(Bokar Consultants (US), Inc.; 0-9633703),* 455 N. Tegner St., No. 27, Wickenburg, AZ 85390 Tel 520-684-2867.

Boland Hlthcare, *(Boland Healthcare, Inc.; 0-9652717),* 1551 Solano Ave., 2nd Flr., Berkeley, CA 94707 Tel 510-524-4521; Fax: 510-524-4607
Dist(s): **Aspen Pub** *(Aspen Pubs., Inc.).*

†Bolchazy-Carducci, *(Bolchazy-Carducci Pubs.; 0-86516),* 1000 Brown St., Unit 101, Wauconda, IL 60084 (SAN 219-7685) Tel 847-526-4344; Fax: 847-526-2867; Toll Free: 800-392-6453
E-mail: info@bolchazy.com
Web site: http://www.bolchazy.com; *CIP.*

BOLD Bks, *(BOLD Bks.; 0-932588),* 1565 Madison St., Suite 308, Oakland, CA 94612-4511 (SAN 212-1034) Tel 510-763-4324.

Bollingen Imprint of Princeton U Pr

Bond Pub MN, *(Bond Publishing Co.; 0-9635576),* Div. of Business Newsletter, Inc., 537 E. Vine St., Owatonna, MN 55060 Tel 507-455-3220; Toll Free: 800-374-6888.

Bone Hollow, *(Bone Hollow Arts; 0-942561),* 759 President St., No. 2H, Brooklyn, NY 11215 (SAN 667-2086) Tel 718-638-3264
E-mail: isca4art2b@aol.com.

Bonne Chance, *(Bonne Chance Pr.; 0-9638398),* 209 River Bluff Rd., Cleveland, SC 29635 Tel 803-878-8577
Dist(s): **Baker & Taylor** *(Baker & Taylor Bks.)*
Brodart *(Brodart Co.).*

Bonneville Bks Imprint of CFI Dist

Bonnie Prudden, *(Prudden, Bonnie Pr.; 0-902146),* 4725 E. Sunrise Dr., No. 346, Tucson, AZ 85718-4534 (SAN 212-825X) Tel 413-298-3066; Toll Free: 800-221-4634.

Bontrager Pub, *(Bontrager Publishing Co.; 0-9641723),* Div. of Media Production Specialists, Inc., 12342 Cougar Dr., Sun City West, AZ 85375-3345.

Bonus Books, *(Bonus Bks., Inc.; 0-929387; 0-931028; 0-933893; 1-56625),* 160 E. Illinois St., Chicago, IL 60611 (SAN 630-0804) Tel 312-467-0580; Fax: 312-467-9271
E-mail: bb@bonus-books.com; webmaster@bonus-books.com
Web site: http://www.bonus-books.com.

Book Bin, *(Book Bin - Pacifica, The; 0-9621818),* 228 SW Third St., Corvallis, OR 97333-4630 Tel 541-752-0045; Fax: 541-754-4115
E-mail: seasia@bookbin.com.

Book Guild Ltd (GBR) *(1-85776; 0-86332) Dist. by* **Trans-Atl Phila.**

†Book Pub Co, *(Book Publishing Co., The; 0-913990; 0-9630243; 1-57067; 0-9669317; 0-9673108),* P.O. Box 99, Summertown, TN 38483 (SAN 202-439X) Tel 931-964-3571; Fax: 931-964-3518; Toll Free: 888-260-8458 Do not confuse with Book Publishing Co., Seattle, WA
E-mail: bookpub@bookpubco.com
Web site: http://www.bookpubco.com
Dist(s): **Baker & Taylor** *(Baker & Taylor Bks.)*
Bookpeople *(Bookpeople)*
Borders Inc *(Borders, Inc.)*
New Leaf Dist *(New Leaf Distributing Co., Inc.)*
Nutri-Books Corp *(Nutri-Bks. Corp.)*
Treas Chest Bks *(Treasure Chest Bks.); CIP.*

Bookery, *(Bookery; 0-930822),* 6899 Riata Dr., Redding, CA 96002 (SAN 211-8904) Tel 530-365-8068; Fax: 530-365-8082 Do not confuse with The Bookery, Ithaca, NY
Dist(s): **Baker & Taylor** *(Baker & Taylor Bks.).*

Book-Lab, *(Book-Lab; 0-87594),* Orders Addr.: P.O. Box 230206, New York, NY 10023-0206 Tel 212-874-5534; Fax: 212-874-3105; Toll Free: 800-654-4081
E-mail: BookLabpub@aol.com.

Booklight Inc, *(Booklight, Inc.; 1-930051),* 1 Union Sq., W. Suite 201, New York, NY 10003 Tel 212-414-2275; Fax: 212-414-2412
E-mail: info@booklight.com
Web site: http://www.booklightinc.com.

Bookmark CA, *(Bookmark, The; 0-930227),* Orders Addr.: P.O. Box 801143, Santa Clarita, CA 91380-1143 (SAN 694-6410) Tel 661-298-7767; Fax: 661-250-9227; Toll Free: 800-220-7767; Edit Addr.: 26536 Golden Valley Rd., No. 610, Saugus, CA 91350 (SAN 699-6035) Toll Free: 800-220-7767 Do not confuse with other companies with the same name in Marietta, GA, Knightstown, IN
E-mail: order@thebookmark.com
Web site: http://www.thebookmark.com.

Bookmates Intl, *(Bookmates International, Inc.; 0-933082),* P.O. Box 9883, Fresno, CA 93795-0883 (SAN 212-8799) Tel 562-925-0149; Toll Free: 888-925-0149 (phone/fax)
E-mail: atfm@aol.com.

BookPartners, *(BookPartners, Inc.; 0-9622269; 1-58151; 1-885221),* Orders Addr.: P.O. Box 68, Newberg, OR 97132 (SAN 298-4393) Tel 503-554-1997; Fax: 503-554-1998; Toll Free: 800-895-7323; Edit Addr.: 120 S. Elliot St., Newberg, OR 97132
E-mail: info@bookpartners.com; bpbooks@teleport.com
Web site: http://www.bookpartners.com.

Bookpeople, *(Bookpeople; 0-914728),* 7900 Edgewater Dr., Oakland, CA 94621 (SAN 168-9517) Tel 510-632-4700; Fax: 510-632-1281; Toll Free Fax: 800-999-4650
E-mail: custserv@bponline.com; bpeople@bponline.com
Web site: http://www.bponline.com.

Books For Midwives Pr (GBR) *(1-898507) Dist. by* **Balogh.**

Books For Midwives Pr (GBR) *(1-898507) Dist. by* **Buttrwrth-Heinemann.**

Books West CA, *(Books West; 0-9619383),* P.O. Box 27364, San Diego, CA 92198 (SAN 244-6065) Do not confuse with Books West, Boulder, CO.

Booksmythe, *(Booksmythe; 0-945585),* 17216 Saticoy St., No. 360, Van Nuys, CA 91406-2103 (SAN 247-3585) Tel 818-343-1648; Fax: 818-343-0274; Toll Free: 800-788-0064
E-mail: russ@booksmythe.com
Web site: http://www.booksmythe.com
Dist(s): **J Majors Co** *(Majors, J. A. Co.)*
Matthews Bk Co *(Matthews Bk. Co.)*
Rittenhouse *(Rittenhouse Bk. Distributors).*

Bookstein Pub, *(Bookstein Publishing; 0-9660645),* 3243-38 Caminito Eastbluff, La Jolla, CA 92037
Dist(s): **J Majors Co** *(Majors, J. A. Co.)*
Matthews Bk Co *(Matthews Bk. Co.)*
Rittenhouse *(Rittenhouse Bk. Distributors).*

Bookstore Pr, *(Bookstore Pr.; 0-912846),* Patterson's Wheeltrack, Freeport, ME 04032 (SAN 201-4211) Tel 207-865-6495.

BookWorld, *(BookWorld Services, Inc.; 1-884962),* 1933 Whitfield Pk. Loop, Sarasota, FL 34243 (SAN 173-0568) Tel 941-758-8094; Fax: 941-753-9396; Toll Free Fax: 800-777-2525; Toll Free: 800-444-2524 (orders only)
E-mail: central@bookworld.com; sales@bookworld.com
Web site: http://www.bookworld.com.

BookWorld Dist, *See* **BookWorld**

Boolarong Pubns (AUS) *Dist. by* **St Mut.**

Borage Bks, *(Borage Bks.; 0-9650976),* 3762 W. 11th Ave., No. 188, Eugene, OR 97402 Tel 541-683-8720; Fax: 541-345-9249
E-mail: orders@boragebooks.com
Web site: http://www.boragebooks.com
Dist(s): **Baker & Taylor** *(Baker & Taylor Bks.)*
New Leaf Dist *(New Leaf Distributing Co., Inc.)*
Nutri-Books Corp *(Nutri-Bks. Corp.).*

Bordalice, *(Bordalice Publishing, Inc.; 0-9666323),* 218 Murray Ave., Delmar, NY 12054 Tel 518-439-7284 (phone/fax)
E-mail: svare@cnsunix.albany.edu.

Borden, *(Borden Publishing Co.; 0-87505),* 2623 San Fernando Rd., Los Angeles, CA 90065 (SAN 201-419X) Tel 323-223-4267
E-mail: bordenpublishing@aol.com.

Borderlnds NH, *(Borderlands Pr.; 1-880325),* Orders Addr.: P.O. Box 1529, Grantham, NH 03753-1529 Tel 603-863-9879; Fax: 603-863-9886; Toll Free: 800-528-3310; Edit Addr.: 6 Winter Hill, Grantham, NH 03753 Do not confuse with companies with the same name in Gulf Breeze, FL, San Antonio, TX
E-mail: scribe@srnet.com
Dist(s): **Allnce Hse** *(Alliance Hse., Inc.)*
Baker & Taylor *(Baker & Taylor Bks.)*
Bookpeople *(Bookpeople)*
Brodart *(Brodart Co.)*
Capital City *(Capital City)*
Diamond Comic Distributors Inc *(Diamond Comic Distributors, Inc.).*

Borneo Res, *(Borneo Research Council, Inc.; 0-9629568; 1-929900),* Orders Addr.: P.O. Box A, Phillips, ME 04966 Tel 207-639-3939; Fax: 207-639-3636; Edit Addr.: Dill Rd., Phillips, ME 04966
E-mail: firebird@somtel.com.

Boston Am, *(Boston America Corp.; 1-889647),* 125 Walnut St., Watertown, MA 02472 Tel 617-923-1111; Fax: 617-923-8839
E-mail: sales@bostonamerica.com
Web site: htttp://www.bostonamerica.com.

Boston Chinese Med, *(Boston Chinese Medicine; 0-9625651),* c/o Margaret A. Naeser, 8 Whittier Pl., Apt. 19-C, Boston, MA 02114 Tel 617-720-4448
E-mail: MNaeser@aol.com
Dist(s): **Bookpeople** *(Bookpeople)*
New Leaf Dist *(New Leaf Distributing Co., Inc.)*
Spanda Med Co *(Spanda Medical Co.).*

Boston Medical, *(Boston Medical Publishing, Inc.; 1-890369; 1-58409),* Orders Addr.: 4780 Linden St., Lincoln, NE 68516; Edit Addr.: 237 S. 70th St., Suite 206, Lincoln, NE 68510 Tel 402-484-6118; Fax: 402-484-6552; Toll Free: 888-626-2737
Web site: http://www.bmppearls.com
Dist(s): **J Majors Co** *(Majors, J. A. Co.)*
Matthews Bk Co *(Matthews Bk. Co.)*
Rittenhouse *(Rittenhouse Bk. Distributors).*

Boston Univ Ctr Psy Rehab, *(Boston Univ., Ctr. for Psychiatric Rehabilitation; 1-878512),* 940 Commonwealth Ave., W., Boston, MA 02215 Tel 617-353-3550; Fax: 617-353-7700
Web site: http://www.web.bu.edu/sarpsych.

Botanica CA, *(Botanica Pr.; 0-9618470; 1-884360),* 4731 E. Fork Rd., Williams, OR 97544-9714 (SAN 668-5315) Tel 408-457-9095; Toll Free: 800-209-6885
Dist(s): **IPG Chicago** *(Independent Pubs. Group).*

Boulder Psychother, *(Boulder Psychotherapists' Pr., Inc.; 0-9645263),* Div. of Boulder Psychotherapist's Guild, Inc., 350 Broadway, Suite 210, Boulder, CO 80303 Tel 303-444-1036; Fax: 303-494-3837.

Bowker, *See* **Bowker LLC**

---

†Bowker LLC, ***(Bowker, R. R. LLC; 0-8352; 0-911255),*** **Subs. of Cambridge Information Group, Inc, Orders Addr.: P.O. Box 1001, Summit, NJ 07902-1001 Toll Free: 888-269-5372; Edit Addr.: 630 Central Ave., New Providence, NJ 07974 (SAN 214-1191) Tel 908-464-6800; Fax: 908-464-3553; Toll Free: 800-521-8110; 800-278-2991 subscriptions to: Publishers Weekly, School Library Journal, Library Journal (in Ohio: 614-383-3141)**
E-mail: info@bowker.com
Web site: http://www.bowker.com; *CIP.*

Bowling Gr Pr, *(Bowling Green Pr.; 0-9614621; 1-880064),* Orders Addr.: P.O. Box 582, Bowling Green, OH 43402 (SAN 691-9138) Tel 419-352-0493; Fax: 419-352-3698; Edit Addr.: 1435 Rosewood Dr., Bowling Green, OH 43402 (SAN 242-0295).

Bowling Green Univ Popular Press, *See* **Bowling Grn St Univ**

Bowling Grn St Univ, *(Bowling Green State Univ. Popular Pr.; 0-87972),* Orders Addr.: Popular Pr. Jerome Library, Rm. 100 Bowling Green State Univ., Bowling Green, OH 43403 (SAN 201-4165) Tel 419-372-7865; Fax: 419-372-8095; Toll Free: 800-515-5118 (orders only)
E-mail: crichar@bgnet.bgsu.edu; popularpress@bgnet.bgsu.edu
Web site: http://www.bgsu.edu/offices/press/.

Bowman Gray Schl, *See* **Wake Forest Univ**

Bowtie Press, *(BowTie Pr.; 0-9629525; 1-889540),* Div. of Fancy Pubns., Inc., Orders Addr.: P.O. Box 6050, Mission Viejo, CA 92690-0050 (SAN 298-5888) Tel 949-855-8822; Fax: 949-855-3045; Edit Addr.: 3 Burroughs, Irvine, CA 92718-2804 (SAN 298-5896)
Web site: http://www.bowtiepress.com
Dist(s): **Natl Bk Netwk** *(National Bk. Network).*

Boxergenics, *(Boxergenics Pr.; 1-888926),* Div. of Dr. E's Sports Science, Inc., Sports Science Ctr., 335 Billingsley Rd., Charlotte, NC 28211 Tel 704-334-4663; Fax: 704-343-0811; Toll Free: 800-774-6284.

Boxtree (GBR) *(0-7522; 1-85283) Dist. by* **Trans-Atl Phila.**

Boxweed Pubng, *(Boxweed Publishing; 0-9647407),* P.O. Box 20345, Saint Simon's Island, GA 31522 Tel 912-634-0150.

†Boxwood, *(Boxwood Pr.; 0-910286; 0-940168),* 183 Ocean View Blvd., Pacific Grove, CA 93950 (SAN 201-4149) Tel 813-375-9110; Fax: 813-375-0430
E-mail: boxwood@boxwoodpress.com
Web site: http://www.boxwoodpress.com; *CIP.*

Boydell & Brewer, *(Boydell & Brewer, Inc.; 0-85115; 0-85991; 0-86193; 0-907239; 1-870252),* Div. of Boydell & Brewer, Ltd. (UK), Orders Addr.: P.O. Box 41026, Rochester, NY 14604-4126 Tel 716-275-0419; Fax: 716-271-8778; Edit Addr.: 668 Mount Hope Ave., Rochester, NY 14620 ; *Imprints:* Boydell Pr (Boydell Press) Royal Historical Soc (Royal Historical Society)
E-mail: boydell@boydell.co.uk; camdenhouse@compuserve.com; 104572.1422@compuserve.com; urpress@mail.rochester.edu
Web site: http://www.boydell.co.uk.

Boydell Pr Imprint of Boydell & Brewer

Boykin, *(Boykin, James H.; 0-9603342; 1-880833),* 1260 NW 122nd St., Miami, FL 33167-2827 (SAN 215-0603) Tel 305-681-7663.

†Boynton Cook Pubs, *(Boynton/Cook Pubs.; 0-86709),* Div. of Reed Elsevier, Inc., Orders Addr.: 88 Post Rd. W., Box 5007, Westport, CT 06881-5007; Edit Addr.: 361 Hanover St., Portsmouth, NH 03801 (SAN 216-6186) Tel 603-431-7894; Fax: 603-431-7840; Toll Free: 800-793-2154
E-mail: custserv@BoyntonCook.com; info@heineman.com
Web site: http://www.boyntoncook.com
Dist(s): **Greenwood** *(Greenwood Publishing Group, Inc.); CIP.*

BPS Bks Imprint of Stylus Pub VA

BR Pub (IND) *(81-7018; 81-7646; 81-7343) Dist. by* **S Asia.**

BRADCOMM, *(BRADCOMM, Inc.; 0-913019),* P.O. Box 2178, Bowie, MD 20718-2178 (SAN 282-9835) Tel 301-262-5331; Fax: 301-262-8018; Toll Free: 877-893-1720
E-mail: Bradcominc@aol.com.

Bradford Bks Imprint of MIT Pr

Bradford Commun, *See* **BRADCOMM**

Bradford Pubns, *(Bradford Pubns.; 0-9630738),* 4350 E. Venture Pl., Meridian, ID 83642 Tel 208-658-6266; Fax: 208-659-6265.

Bradt Pubns (GBR) *(1-898323; 1-84162) Dist. by* **Globe Pequot.**

Brady Compu Bks, *See* **Brady Pub**

Brady Pub, *(Brady Publishing; 0-8359; 0-87618; 0-87619; 0-89303; 0-913486; 1-56686; 0-7440),* Div. of Macmillan USA, 201 W. 103rd St., Indianapolis, IN 46290 (SAN 219-6298) Tel 317-581-3500; Fax: 317-705-6290; Toll Free Fax: 800-835-3202; Toll Free: 800-428-5331 (orders); 800-571-5840
Web site: http://www.mcp.com/brady
Dist(s): **Mac USA** *(Macmillan USA).*

Brain Injury Assoc, *(Brain Injury Assn., Inc.; 0-927093),* 105 N. Alfred St., Alexandria, VA 22214 Tel 703-236-6000; Fax: 703-236-6001
E-mail: FamilyHelpline@biausa.org
Web site: http://www.biausa.org/i.

Brain Trauma, *(Brain Trauma Foundation; 0-9703144),* 523 E., 72nd St., 8th Flr., New York, NY 10021 Tel 212-772-0608; Fax: 212-772-0352
E-mail: quinn@braintrauma.org; info@braintrauma.org
Web site: http://www.braintrauma.org.

Branden Bks, *(Branden Bks.; 0-8283),* P.O. Box 812094, Wellesley, MA 02482 (SAN 201-4106) Tel 781-235-3634; Fax: 781-790-1056
E-mail: branden@branden.com
Web site: http://www.branden.com.

Branden Pub Co, *See* **Branden Bks**

Brandes-Miesner, *See* **Sun Bear**

Brandon Hse, *(Brandon Hse., Inc.; 0-913412),* P.O. Box 240, Bronx, NY 10471 (SAN 201-4092).

Brandt Pub, *(Brandt Publishing; 0-9616716),* 10209 N. 56th St., Scottsdale, AZ 85253 (SAN 659-4964) Tel 602-991-4860 (phone/fax)
E-mail: info@brandtpublishing.com
Web site: http://www.BrandtPublishing.com.

BRAT Pub, *(BRAT Publishing; 1-880257),* 369 Montezuma, Suite 203, Santa Fe, NM 87501 Tel 505-662-9200; Fax: 505-662-4044; Toll Free: 800-359-2728
E-mail: marvel@trail.com
Dist(s): **B&N Imports** *(Barnes & Noble Bks.-Imports)*
Baker & Taylor *(Baker & Taylor Bks.)*
Health Comm *(Health Communications, Inc.).*

Braziller, *(Braziller, George Inc.; 0-8076),* 171 Madison Ave., Suite 1103, New York, NY 10016 (SAN 201-9310) Tel 212-889-0909; Fax: 212-689-5405
Dist(s): **Norton** *(Norton, W.W. & Co., Inc.).*

Break on Through, *(Break on Through Pr.; 1-891173),* 1309 N. 73rd St., No. 201, Scottsdale, AZ 85260 Tel 404-978-3107; Fax: 413-425-6489
Web site: http://www.breakonthroughpress.com.

Breakthrgh NY, *(Breakthrough Pubns., Inc.; 0-914327),* 500 Executive Blvd., Suite 302, Ossining, NY 10562 (SAN 287-4946) Tel 914-762-5111; Fax: 914-762-4818; Toll Free: 800-824-5000 Do not confuse with Breakthrough Pubns., Inc., Spokane, WA
E-mail: webmaster@booksonhorses.com.

Breakthru Pub, ***(Breakthru Publishing; 0-942540),*** **421 Emerson, No. 1, Houston, TX 77006 (SAN 293-2407) Tel 713-789-8600; Fax: 713-789-4966; Toll Free: 800-227-1152**
Dist(s): **Publishers Group** ***(Publishers Group West).***

Brennyman Bks, *(Brennyman Bks.; 0-9654036),* P.O. Box 2629, Akron, OH 44309 Tel 330-882-4690.

Publisher Symbol Index

Publisher Symbol Index

Brentwood Fndt, *(Brentwood Foundation, The; 0-9678781),* 800 Superior Ave., NE, Cleveland, OH 44114 Tel 216-622-8200
E-mail: terrik@apk.net.

Briarwood VA, *(Briarwood Pubns.; 1-892614),* 150 W. College St., Rocky Mount, VA 24151 (SAN 299-8068) Tel 540-483-3606; Fax: 540-489-4692 ext. 51 Do not confuse with Briarwood Pubns., Terre Haute, IN
E-mail: bturner@swva.net
Web site: http://www.briarwoodva.com.

Brick Tower, *(Brick Tower Pr.; 1-883283),* 1230 Park Ave., No. 10A, New York, NY 10128 Tel 212-427-7139 (phone/fax); Toll Free: 800-682-7425
E-mail: bricktower@aol.com
Web site: http://www.bricktowerpress.com
Dist(s): **Baker & Taylor** *(Baker & Taylor Bks.)*
Bookmen Inc *(Bookmen, Inc.)*
Brodart *(Brodart Co.).*

Bridge Commns Inc, *(Bridge Communications, Inc.; 0-9621645),* 1450 Pilgrim Rd., Birmingham, MI 48009-1006 (SAN 251-7256) Tel 248-646-1020; Fax: 248-644-8546
E-mail: bridgecomm@aol.com
Web site: http://bridge-comm.com
Dist(s): **Baker & Taylor** *(Baker & Taylor Bks.)*
Follett Library *(Follett Library Resources).*

Bridge Pub, *See* **Bridge-Logos**

Bridge Pubns Inc, *(Bridge Pubns., Inc.; 0-88404; 1-57318; 1-58460; 1-4031),* 4751 Fountain Ave., Los Angeles, CA 90029 (SAN 208-3884) Tel 323-953-3320; Fax: 323-953-3328; Toll Free: 800-722-1733
E-mail: info@bridgepub.com
Web site: http://www.bridgepub.com
Dist(s): **Baker & Taylor** *(Baker & Taylor Bks.)*
Bookazine Co Inc *(Bookazine Co., Inc.)*
Brodart *(Brodart Co.)*
Lndmrk Audiobks *(Landmark Audiobooks).*

Bridge Resources, *(Bridge Resources; 1-57895),* Div. of Presbyterian Church, 100 Witherspoon St., Louisville, KY 40202-1396 Tel 502-569-5496; Fax: 502-569-8329
Web site: http://www.bridgeresources.org.

BridgeCity Bks, *(BridgeCity Bks.; 0-9623683),* 1717 SW Park Ave., Apt. 616, Portland, OR 97201-3238 Tel 503-220-4171; Fax: 503-220-4081; Toll Free: 800-884-4171
E-mail: jackdyost@aol.com.

Bridgeline Bks, *See* **Bridgeline Pr**

Bridgeline Pr, *(Bridgeline Pr.; 1-888843),* 455 Frietas Pkwy., Suite 144, San Rafael, CA 94903 Tel 415-507-9848 (phone/fax); Toll Free: 800-585-1488.

Bridge-Logos, *(Bridge-Logos Pubs.; 0-88270; 0-912106),* Orders Addr.: 17310 NW 32nd Ave., Newberry, FL 32669 Toll Free Fax: 800-935-6467 (orders only); Toll Free: 800-631-5802 (orders only); Edit Addr.: P.O. Box 141630, Gainesville, FL 32614 (SAN 253-5254) Tel 352-472-7900; Fax: 352-472-7908
E-mail: editor@bridgelogos.com; info@bridgelogos.com; mail@bridgelogos.com
Web site: http://www.bridgelogos.com
Dist(s): **Anchor Distributors** *(Anchor Distributors)*
Appalachian Bible *(Appalachian Bible Co.)*
Baker & Taylor *(Baker & Taylor Bks.)*
Riverside-World *(Riverside World)*
Spring Arbor Dist *(Spring Arbor Distributors Inc.).*

Bridgeport Bks, *(Bridgeport Bks.; 1-888824),* Div. of Griffin Publishing Co., 544 W. Colorado St., Glendale, CA 91204 (SAN 631-5046) Tel 818-244-1470; Fax: 818-244-7408; Toll Free: 800-472-9741
E-mail: griffinbooks@earthlink.net
Web site: http://www.griffinpublishing.com
Dist(s): **Assoc Pubs Grp** *(Associated Pubs. Group).*

Bridger Hse, *(Bridger Hse. Pubns., Inc.; 0-9640104; 1-893157),* Orders Addr.: P.O. Box 2208, Carson City, NV 89702 Tel 775-885-0700; Fax: 775-891-0704; Toll Free Fax: 877-726-2632; Toll Free: 800-729-4131; Edit Addr.: 675 Fairview Dr., No. 246, Carson City, NV 89701
E-mail: bridger@nohoax.com
Web site: http://www.nohoax.com
Dist(s): **New Leaf Dist** *(New Leaf Distributing Co., Inc.).*

Bridgestone Bks Imprint of Capstone Pr

Bridgeview, *(Bridgeview Bks.; 0-9613365),* 1065 Central Blvd., Hayward, CA 94542 (SAN 657-0755) Tel 510-889-6355.

Bridging The Gap, *(Bridging The Gap Communications; 0-9638875),* 1014 Sycamore Dr., Decatur, GA 30030 Fax: 404-373-0480; Toll Free: 800-721-6990.

Bridgtte Rose, *(Bridgette Rose; 0-9664485),* 1374 Alpine Dr., Olean, NY 14760.

BrierNet, *(BrierNet; 0-9657526),* 5208 Alta Vista St., San Diego, CA 92109-1303; 17770 Valle Verde Rd., Poway, CA 92064.

Brigham, *(Brigham Young Univ.; 0-8425),* 205 UPB, Provo, UT 84602 (SAN 201-9337) Tel 801-378-2809; Fax: 801-378-3374 ; *Imprints:* Friends of the Library (Friends of the Library)
E-mail: diane_foerster@byu.edu
Web site: http://www.upb.byu.edu
Dist(s): **BYU Print Srvs** *(Brigham Young Univ. Print Services)*
U Ch Pr *(Univ. of Chicago Pr.).*

Bright Bks CA, *(Bright Bks.; 0-9617317),* 113 S. Fork Way, Folsom, CA 95630-2082 (SAN 663-8201) Do not confuse with companies with the same name in Akron, IN, Austin, TX.

Bright Ideas Pr, *(Bright Ideas Pr.; 0-9651025),* Div. of E. Excel International, 1198 N. Spring Creek Pl., Springville, UT 84663 Tel 801-489-4588; Fax: 801-489-4489; Toll Free: 800-733-3744.

Bright Mtn Bks, *(Bright Mountain Bks., Inc.; 0-914875),* 138 Springside Rd., Asheville, NC 28803 (SAN 289-0674) Tel 828-684-8840; Fax: 828-681-1790; Toll Free: 800-437-3959
E-mail: booksbmb@aol.com.

Bright Sky, *(Bright Sky Pr.; 0-9704729; 0-9709987; 1-931721),* Orders Addr.: P.O. Box 416, Albany, TX 76430 Tel 915-762-3909; Fax: 915-762-3690; Edit Addr.: 340 S. Second St., Albany, TX 76430 Do not confuse with Breakaway Bks., Halcottsville, NY
E-mail: carolcates@brightskypress.com
Web site: http://www.brightskypress.com
Dist(s): **Sterling** *(Sterling Publishing Co., Inc.).*

†Brill Academic Pubs, *(Brill Academic Pubs., Inc.; 0-391; 0-916846; 90-04),* Subs. of Brill Academic Publishing Co., The Netherlands, 112 Water St., Suite 400, Boston, MA 02109 (SAN 121-6201) Tel 617-263-2323; Fax: 617-263-2324; Toll Free: 800-962-4406
E-mail: cs@brillusa.com
Web site: http://www.brill.nl
Dist(s): **Bks Intl VA** *(Books International, Incorporated); CIP.*

Bristol Hse, *(Bristol Hse., Ltd.; 0-917851; 1-885224),* P.O. Box 4020, Anderson, IN 46013 (SAN 225-4638) Tel 765-644-0856; Fax: 765-622-1045; Toll Free: 800-451-7323.

Bristol Hunter, *(Bristol Hunter Publishing Co.; 0-943843),* 90 Keswick Rd., Amherst, NY 14226 (SAN 242-4134) Tel 716-834-5128.

Bristol Pub Ent CA, *(Bristol Publishing Enterprises, Inc.; 0-911954; 1-55867),* Orders Addr.: P.O. Box 1737, San Leandro, CA 94577 (SAN 202-9197) Tel 510-895-4461; Fax: 510-895-4459; Toll Free: 800-346-4889; Edit Addr.: 14692 Wicks Blvd., San Leandro, CA 94577 (SAN 248-3874) ; *Imprints:* Nitty Gritty Ckbks (Nitty Gritty Cookbooks)
E-mail: aidan@bristolcookbooks.com; hannah@bristolcookbooks.com; sally@bristolcookbooks.com
Web site: http://www.bristolcookbooks.com.

Brit Ag for Adopt & Fost (GBR) *Dist. by* **St Mut.**

Brit Inst Lrning (GBR) *(1-873791; 0-906054; 1-902519) Dist. by* **Taylor & Francis.**

Brit Psychol Soc (GBR) *(0-901715; 1-85433) Dist. by* **P H Brookes.**

Brit Psychol Soc (GBR) *(0-901715; 1-85433) Dist. by* **Routledge.**

British Am Bks, *(British American Bks.; 0-89979),* P.O. Box 302, Willits, CA 95490 (SAN 201-9353) Tel 707-459-5424.

British Amer Pub, *(British American Publishing, Ltd.; 0-945167),* 4 British American Blvd., Latham, NY 12110 (SAN 246-3008) Tel 518-786-6000; Fax: 518-786-6001
Dist(s): **Midpt Trade** *(Midpoint Trade Bks., Inc.).*

British Textile Tech (GBR) *(0-900820; 0-903669; 0-9500275) Dist. by* **St Mut.**

Britton Inc, *(Britton, Inc.; 0-9611782),* 507 Main St., Hingham, MA 02043 (SAN 285-225X) Tel 617-749-9175.

Bro Life Inc, *(Brotherhood of Life, Inc.; 0-914732),* P.O. Box 46306, Las Vegas, NV 89114-6306 (SAN 111-3674) Fax: 702-319-5577
E-mail: brotherhoodoflife@hotmail.com
Web site: http://www.brotherhoodoflife.com
Dist(s): **Bookpeople** *(Bookpeople)*
New Leaf Dist *(New Leaf Distributing Co., Inc.).*

Broadfoot, *(Broadfoot Publishing Co.; 0-916107; 1-56837),* 1907 Buena Vista Cir., Wilmington, NC 28411 (SAN 294-9075) Tel 910-686-4816; Fax: 919-686-4379; Toll Free: 800-537-5243 (orders only)
E-mail: bropubco@wilmington.net
Web site: http://broadfoot.wilmington.net.

Broadway BDD, *(Broadway Bks.; 0-385; 0-553; 0-7679; 1-4000),* Div. of Doubleday Broadway Publishing Group, Orders Addr.: 400 Hahn Rd., Westminster, MD 21157 Tel 410-848-1900; Toll Free: 800-726-0600; Edit Addr.: 1540 Broadway, New York, NY 10036 Tel 212-354-6500; Fax: 212-782-8338; Toll Free: 800-223-6834
Web site: http://www.bdd.com.

Brookcliff Pubs, *(Brookcliff Pubs., Inc.; 0-9626185),* 24262 Stantonsburg Rd., PMB 325, Greenville, NC 27834-7210 Tel 252-413-6356.

†Brookings, *(Brookings Institution Pr.; 0-8157),* 1775 Massachusetts Ave., NW, Washington, DC 20036-2188 (SAN 201-9396) Tel 202-797-6258; Fax: 202-797-6004; Toll Free: 800-275-1447
E-mail: brookinfo@brook.edu; bibooks@brook.edu
Web site: http://www.brookings.edu; *CIP.*

†Brookline Bks, *(Brookline Bks., Inc.; 0-914797; 1-57129),* Orders Addr.: P.O. Box 1047, Cambridge, MA 02238 (SAN 289-0690) Tel 617-868-0360; Fax: 617-868-1772; Toll Free: 800-666-2665; Edit Addr.: 29 Ware St., Cambridge, MA 02138 ; *Imprints:* Lumen Eds (Lumen Editions)
E-mail: brooklinebks@delphi.com
Web site: http://www.brooklinebooks.com/
Dist(s): **LPC Group** *(LPC Group); CIP.*

†Brooks-Cole, *(Brooks/Cole Publishing Co.; 0-534; 0-8185),* Div. of Thomson Learning, Orders Addr.: 7625 Empire Dr., Florence, KY 41042-2978 (SAN 200-2663) Tel 606-525-2230; Toll Free: 800-354-9706 (orders); Edit Addr.: 511 Forest Lodge Rd., Pacific Grove, CA 93950 (SAN 202-3369) Tel 831-373-0728; Fax: 831-375-6414
E-mail: info@brookscole.com
Web site: http://www.brookscole.com
Dist(s): **Thomson Learn** *(Thomson Learning); CIP.*

Bros Grinn, *(Brothers Grinn Publishing; 0-9627601),* 1815 Ravine St., Janesville, WI 53545 Tel 608-755-5180; Fax: 608-755-5190.

Brother Bills, *(Brother Bill's Publishing Co.; 0-9640154),* 918 13th St., SE, Rochester, MN 55904 Tel 507-289-1185; Fax: 507-288-4313.

Brown & Benchmark, *(Brown & Benchmark; 0-697; 0-936157),* Div. of Times Mirror Higher Education Group, Inc., 25 Kessel Ct., Madison, WI 53711 Tel 608-273-0040; Toll Free: 800-338-5578
E-mail: customer.service@mcgraw-hill.com
Web site: http://www.mhhe.com.

Brown Spath, *(Brown-Spath & Assocs.; 1-929955),* P.O. Box 721, Forest Grove, OR 97116-0721 Tel 503-357-9185; Fax: 503-357-9267
E-mail: sales@brownspath.com
Web site: http://www.brownspath.com.

Brunner-Mazel, *See* **Brunner-Routledge**

†Brunner-Routledge, *(Brunner-Routledge; 0-87630; 1-58391),* Div. of Taylor & Francis, Orders Addr.: 7625 Empire Dr., Florence, KY 41042 Toll Free Fax: 800-248-4724; Toll Free: 800-634-7064; Edit Addr.: 325 Chestnut St., 8th Flr., Philadelphia, PA 19106 (SAN 164-9167) Tel 215-625-8900; Fax: 215-625-2940
E-mail: info@taylorandfrancis.com; bkorders@taylorandfrancis.com
Web site: http://www.brunner-routledge.com; http://www.taylorandfrancis.com
Dist(s): **Taylor & Francis** *(Taylor & Francis, Inc.); CIP.*

Bruno Pr, *(Bruno Pr.; 0-945032),* Div. of Behavior Therapy Ctr., Inc., 2627 General Pershing St., New Orleans, LA 70115 (SAN 245-8616) Tel 504-899-2367; Fax: 504-899-5263; Toll Free: 800-775-4138
E-mail: scrignar@communique.net
Web site: http://www.communique.net/~scrignar.

Brynmill Pr Ltd (GBR) *(0-907839; 0-9502723) Dist. by* **St Mut.**

Brynwood Publishing Co, *(Brynwood Publishing Co.; 0-937615),* 13567 Brynwood Ln., Fort Myers, FL 33912 (SAN 659-0527) Tel 941-369-2117.

BSA Pub, *(B.S.A. Publishing; 0-9625114),* Div. of Behavioral Science Assocs., 359 E. Hildebrand, San Antonio, TX 78212 Tel 210-824-3391; 9201 W. 44th Ave., Wheat Ridge, CO 80033 Tel 303-423-1288.

BSAVA (GBR) *(0-905214) Dist. by* **Iowa U Pr.**

Btler Pub, *(Butler Publishing; 0-916992),* Div. of Doug Butler Enterprises, Inc., P.O. Box 1390, LaPorte, CO 80535 (SAN 206-3999) Tel 970-482-7518; Fax: 970-482-8621; Toll Free: 800-728-3826.

Bubba Pr, *(Bubba Pr.; 0-9607240),* P.O. Box 5037, Vacaville, CA 95696-5037 (SAN 239-4138) Tel 510-943-5340.

Buccaneer Bks, *(Buccaneer Bks., Inc.; 0-89966; 0-89967; 0-89968; 1-56849),* P.O. Box 168, Cutchogue, NY 11935 (SAN 209-1542) Tel 631-734-5724; Fax: 631-734-7920
E-mail: BuccBooks@aol.com
Web site: http://www.BuccaneerBooks.com
Dist(s): **Natl Bk Netwk** *(National Bk. Network).*

Bucknell U Pr, *(Bucknell Univ. Pr.; 0-8387),* 440 Forsgate Dr., Cranbury, NJ 08512 Tel 609-655-4770
Web site:
http://www.department.bucknell.edu/univ_press/
Dist(s): **Assoc Univ Prs** *(Associated Univ. Presses)*
B & T International *(Baker & Taylor International).*

Budlong, *(Budlong Pr. Co.; 0-910304),* 4311 N. Normandy, Chicago, IL 60634 (SAN 202-4837).

Buffalo SNS, *(Buffalo Society of Natural Sciences; 0-944032),* 1020 Humboldt Pkwy., Buffalo, NY 14211 (SAN 242-4460) Tel 716-896-5200; Fax: 716-897-6723
E-mail: rebrew@sciencebuff.org
Web site: http://www.buffalomuseumofscience.org.

Build Servs Info Assn (GBR) *(0-86022) Dist. by* **St Mut.**

†Bull Pub, *(Bull Publishing Co.; 0-915950; 0-923521; 0-945946),* Orders Addr.: P.O. Box 1377, Boulder, CO 80306-1377 Tel 303-545-6350; Fax: 303-545-6354; Toll Free: 800-676-2855
E-mail: bullpublishing@msn.com
Web site: http://www.bullpub.com
Dist(s): **Publishers Group** *(Publishers Group West); CIP.*

Bullfrog Films, *(Bullfrog Films, Inc.; 1-56029),* Orders Addr.: P.O. Box 149, Oley, PA 19547-0149 (SAN 653-2136) Tel 610-779-8226; Fax: 610-370-1978; Toll Free: 800-543-3764 (800-543-FROG); Edit Addr.: 372 Dautrich Rd., Reading, PA 19606
E-mail: video@bullfrogfilms.com
Web site: http://www.bullfrogfilms.com
Dist(s): **Follett Audio** *(Follett Audiovisual Resources)*
Natl Video Res *(National Video Resources, Inc.).*

Bum Prodns, *(Bum Productions; 0-9656454),* 9690 Rockhaven Pl., Dallas, TX 75243 Tel 214-813-2637.

Bur For At-Risk, *(Bureau For At-Risk Youth; 1-56688),* Orders Addr.: P.O. Box 760, Plainview, NY 11803-0760; Edit Addr.: 135 Dupont St., Plainview, NY 11803-0760 (SAN 631-063X) Tel 516-349-5520; Fax: 516-349-5521; Toll Free Fax: 800-262-1886; Toll Free: 800-999-6884
E-mail: info@at-risk.com
Web site: http://www.at-risk.com.

Buraff Pubns, *See* **LRP Publications**

Burd St Pr Imprint of White Mane Pub

Burn Hart, *(Burn, Hart & Co., Pubs.; 0-918060),* Box 1772, Thousand Oaks, CA 91358 (SAN 210-1823)
Dist(s): **Shens Bks** *(Shen's Bks.).*

Burnell Co, *(Burnell Co./Pubs., Inc., The; 0-916973),* P.O. Box 304, Mankato, MN 56002 (SAN 655-587X) Tel 507-625-4302; Fax: 507-345-3816.

---

†Burnham Inc, *(Burnham, Inc.; 0-8304; 0-88229; 0-911012),* 111 N. Canal St., Suite 955, Chicago, IL 60606 (SAN 202-9065) Tel 312-930-9446; Fax: 312-930-5903
E-mail: publishers@burnhaminc.com
Web site: http://www.burnhaminc.com; *CIP.*

Buros Inst Mental, *(Buros Institute of Mental Measurements; 0-910674),* Div. of Univ. of Nebraska-Lincoln, Orders Addr.: 312 N. 14th St., Lincoln, NE 68588-0484 (SAN 662-4022) Toll Free: 800-755-1105; Edit Addr.: Univ. of Nebraska-Lincoln, 135 Bancroft, Lincoln, NE 68588-0348 (SAN 698-1895) Tel 402-472-6203; Fax: 402-472-6214; Toll Free: 800-526-2617
Dist(s): **U of Nebr Pr** *(Univ. of Nebraska Pr.).*

Burtis Ent, *(Burtis Enterprises, Pubs.; 0-939530),* 1085 SW 330th Ct., Federal Way, WA 98023-5327 (SAN 216-6593).

BusinessWatch, *(BusinessWatch.com Inc.; 0-912665),* 1908 Colton Blvd., Billings, MT 59102-2316 (SAN 282-7573) Tel 406-323-0131
E-mail: edbks@businesswatch.com.

Busn Imprint of P-H

Busn & Med (GBR) *Dist. by* **St Mut.**

Busn Concepts, *(Business Concepts, Inc.; 1-57327),* 734 Monte Dr., Santa Barbara, CA 93110 Tel 805-569-1363; Fax: 805-569-0861 ; *Imprints:* M Pr CA (M Press).

Busn Ctr Acad (JPN) *Dist. by* **Intl Spec Bk.**

Busn Info Srvs, *See* **Capitol Publns**

Busn Intl Corp, *See* **Economist Intell**

Busn Legal Reports, *(Business & Legal Reports; 1-55645),* P.O. Box 6001, Old Saybrook, CT 06475-6001 (SAN 661-504X).

Busn Living Pubns, *(Business of Living Pubns.; 1-879518),* Orders Addr.: P.O. Box 8388, Corpus Christi, TX 78468-8388 Tel 361-852-8515; Edit Addr.: 4630 Coventry Ln., Corpus Christi, TX 78411-4930
E-mail: dstiefel@mail.interconnect.net
Dist(s): **Baker & Taylor** *(Baker & Taylor Bks.).*

†Busn News, *(Business News Publishing Co.; 0-912524; 1-885863),* Orders Addr.: P.O. Box 2039, Mansfield, OH 44905; Edit Addr.: 755 W. Big Beaver Rd., No. 1000, Troy, MI 48084; *CIP.*

Butte Pubns, *(Butte Pubns., Inc.; 1-884362),* P.O. Box 1328, Hillsboro, OR 97123-1328 (SAN 299-8866) Tel 503-648-9791; Fax: 503-693-9526; Toll Free: 866-312-8883
E-mail: service@buttepublications.com
Web site: http://www.buttepublications.com.

Butternut & Blue, *(Butternut & Blue; 0-935523),* 3411 Northwind Rd., Baltimore, MD 21234 (SAN 696-1576) Tel 410-256-9220; Fax: 410-256-8423
E-mail: bbcwbks.mdo.net
Web site: http://www.dealersweb.com/Butternut.htm.

Butterwrth CAN Ltd (CAN) *(0-408; 0-409; 0-433) Dist. by* **Gaunt.**

†Buttrwrth-Heinemann, *(Butterworth-Heinemann; 0-240; 0-250; 0-407; 0-408; 0-409; 0-433; 0-434; 0-480; 0-7506; 0-86729; 0-87591; 0-914236; 0-932376; 0-9626521; 1-55558; 1-56372),* Subs. of Reed Elsevier plc, 225 Wildwood Ave., Unit B, Woburn, MA 01801 (SAN 206-3964) Tel 781-904-2500; Fax: 781-904-2640; Toll Free Fax: 800-446-6520 (orders); Toll Free: 800-366-2665 (orders) ; *Imprints:* Focal (Focal Press) Prgamon Press (Pergamon Press Textbooks) Newnes (Newnes)
E-mail: custserv@bhusa.com; sales@bhusa.com; orders@bhusa.com
Web site: http://www.bh.com
Dist(s): **Sams Tech Pub** *(Sams Technical Publishing); CIP.*

C & R Pubns, *(C & R Pubns., Inc.; 0-9679474),* Orders Addr.: P.O. Box 478, Revere, MA 02151-9963 Tel 781-485-0880; Fax: 781-485-0800; Edit Addr.: 750 Washington Ave., Suite 7, Brookdale Plaza, Revere, MA 02151.

C A B I Pub, *(CABI Publishing; 0-85198; 0-85199),* 10 E. 40th St., Suite 3203, New York, NY 10016 Tel 212-481-7018; Fax: 212-686-7993; Toll Free Fax: 800-528-4841
E-mail: orders@cabi.org; cabi-nao@cabi.org
Web site: http://www.cabi.org
Dist(s): **OUP** *(Oxford Univ. Pr., Inc.).*

C A Inc, *(C.A., Inc.; 0-9654622),* 11 W. 42nd St., 15th Flr., New York, NY 10036 Tel 212-789-2407; Fax: 212-575-4986.

C Bohling Pub, *(Bohling, Corey Publishing; 0-9625478),* 14741 Vista Verdi Rd., Davis, FL 33325 Tel 954-236-2577
E-mail: Bohling@ibm.net
Web site: http://www.Evolution1.com.

C C Cone, *(Cone, Clyde C.; 0-9621961),* 6249 Willow Springs Dr., Morrison, CO 80465-2133 Tel 303-424-1003.

†C C Thomas, *(Thomas, Charles C. Pub., Ltd.; 0-398),* 2600 S. First St., Springfield, IL 62794-9265 (SAN 201-9485) Tel 217-789-8980; Fax: 217-789-9130; Toll Free: 800-258-8980
E-mail: books@ccthomas.com
Web site: http://www.ccthomas.com; *CIP.*

C Coats Bestsellers, *(Coats', Carolyn Bestsellers; 1-878722),* Orders Addr.: P.O. Box 560532, Orlando, FL 32856; Edit Addr.: 1336 Windsong Rd., Orlando, FL 32809 Tel 407-855-0780.

C Cole, *See* **C Communs**

C Communs, *(Cole Communications; 1-890961),* 20042 Beach Blvd., Suite 130, Huntington Beach, CA 92648-3072 Tel 714-536-0305; Fax: 714-960-3997
E-mail: carolcole@worldnet.att.net.

C D Stampley Ent, *(Stampley, C.D. Enterprises, Inc.; 0-915741; 1-58087),* Orders Addr.: P.O. Box 33172, Charlotte, NC 28233 (SAN 294-1325) Tel 704-333-6631; Fax: 704-336-6932; Edit Addr.: 1135 N. Tryon St., Charlotte, NC 28206
E-mail: cdstampley@hotmail.com
Dist(s): **Lectorum Pubns** *(Lectorum Pubns., Inc.)*
Midpt Trade *(Midpoint Trade Bks., Inc.).*

C Drago, *(Drago, Carl; 0-9655930),* 1836 South Ave., La Crosse, WI 54601 Tel 608-782-7300; Fax: 608-791-4460.

C E Hugenberger, *(Hugenberger, Charles E.; 1-885057),* 721 20th St., SE, Cleveland, TN 37311-7704 Tel 530-288-3503.

C E Logan, *(Logan, Cordell E.; 0-9636519),* 1994 W. Carriage Ave., Riverton, UT 84065 Tel 801-562-2211.

C F Sexauer, *(Sexauer, Charles F.; 0-9607148),* 13904 Fiji Way, Suite 132, Venice, CA 90292 (SAN 239-0337) Tel 310-822-9148; Fax: 310-822-7567.

C G Jung Foun, *(Jung, C.G. Foundation Pubns.; 0-913430),* 28 E. 39th St., New York, NY 10016 (SAN 207-0391) Tel 212-697-6433.

C H Bessey, *(Bessey, Carol Hossner; 0-9670579),* 4258 E. 1400 N., Ashton, ID 83420 Tel 208-652-3373.

C H Organ, *(Organ, Claude H. Jr.; 0-9617380),* Dept. of Surgery, 1411 E. 31st St., Oakland, CA 94602 (SAN 663-8899) Tel 510-437-4965; Fax: 510-534-5639.

C I Pubns CA Imprint of Colgan Inst

C I T A Intl, *(CITA International (Chemical Industrial Technology & Application); 0-937425),* Div. of Erde International (U.S.A.), 3464 W. Earll Dr., Suites E & F, Phoenix, AZ 85017-5260 (SAN 658-9952) Tel 602-447-0480; Fax: 602-447-0305.

C J Adams, *See* **Exeter Hse**

C J Howie, *(Howie, C.J. Co.; 1-885275),* 1695 Quigley Rd., Columbus, OH 43227-3433 Tel 614-237-5474.

C Kent Agency, *(Kent, Christine Agency; 1-877691),* P.O. Box 8498, Van Nuys, CA 91409 (SAN 630-4206) Tel 818-776-8040; Fax: 818-776-0082
Web site: http://www.homepathy-md.com.

C Kroll, *(Kroll, Cecelia; 0-9614913),* 685 Lucas Ave., Apt. 820, Los Angeles, CA 90017-1911 (SAN 693-4544) Tel 213-622-2184.

C L Meinert, *(Meinert, Curtis L.; 0-9646424),* c/o Johns Hopkins Univ., 615 N. Wolfe St., Rm. 5010, Baltimore, MD 21205 Tel 410-955-8197; Fax: 410-955-0932
E-mail: cctmail@phir.sph.jhu.edu.

C L Vidano Pub, *(Vidano, Carl L. Publishing Co.; 0-9616606),* 1676 St. Malo Way, Henderson, NV 89014-7502 (SAN 659-8102).

C Lincoln, *(Lincoln, Carol; 0-9677836),* 10730 Rampart Dr. E., Puyallup, WA 98374-2066 Tel 253-845-9297
E-mail: Busbuster@aol.com.

C Manuals Trust, *(Clark Manuals Trust; 1-881914),* 1327 E. Vinedo Ln., Tempe, AZ 85284 Tel 480-838-1750
E-mail: lcphm@asuvm.inre.asu.edu.

C N Aronson, *(Aronson, Charles N. Writer-Pub.; 0-915736),* 11520 Bixby Hill Rd., Arcade, NY 14009-1701 (SAN 207-6144) Tel 716-496-6002 Do not confuse with companies with similar name in Highmount, NY, Northvale, NJ, Santa Monica, CA.

C Riggs-Bergesen, *See* **Other Worldly**

C S Houston, *(Houston, Charles S.; 0-9612246),* 77 Ledge Rd., Burlington, VT 05401 (SAN 220-2727) Tel 802-863-6441
E-mail: chouston@zoo.uvm.edu.

C Schiappacasse, *(Schiappacasse, Chuck; 0-9635913),* 3905 Gregory Dr., Northbrook, IL 60062 Tel 847-635-6849 (phone/fax)
Dist(s): **Anchor Distributors** *(Anchor Distributors)*
Spring Arbor Dist *(Spring Arbor Distributors Inc.).*

C Scribners Sons Imprint of Gale

C V Perrill, *(Perrill, Charles V. MD; 0-9701415),* 3520 Gwinn St., Pemney Farms, FL 32079 Tel 904-284-5507; Fax: 352-373-7241.

C W Daniel (GBR) *(0-85032; 0-85207; 0-85435; 0-85978) Dist. by* **Natl Bk Netwk.**

C W Henderson, *(Henderson, Charles W.; 0-9631698),* Orders Addr.: P.O. Box 5528, Atlanta, GA 30307 Tel 404-377-8895; Edit Addr.: 206 Rogers St., NE, Suite 126, Atlanta, GA 30317
Dist(s): **EBSCO** *(EBSCO Industries, Inc.).*

C W Kischer, *(Kischer, C. Ward; 0-9660344),* 6249 Camino Miraval, Tucson, AZ 85718 Tel 520-299-0521; Fax: 520-626-2097.

C Wilks, *(Wilk, Chester; 0-9701625),* 5130 W. Belmont Ave., Chicago, IL 60641 Tel 773-725-4878
Web site: http://chetwilk.com.

C Zimet, *(Zimet, Carol; 0-9639659),* 942 Stratford Ct., Westbury, NY 11590 Tel 516-334-1330.

CA College Health Sci, *(California College for Health Sciences; 0-933195; 1-57781),* 2423 Hoover Ave., National City, CA 91950 Tel 619-477-4800; Fax: 619-477-4360; Toll Free: 800-221-7374
E-mail: ahp@cchs.edu
Web site: http://www.cchs.edu/AHP.

Publisher Symbol Index

CA Health Pubns, *(California Health Pubns.; 0-9623581; 1-930469),* 6201 Florio St., Oakland, CA 94618 Tel 510-428-0937; Fax: 510-428-9235; Toll Free: 800-452-1008
E-mail: jeanh@breema.com
Web site: http://www.breema.com
Dist(s): **Baker & Taylor** *(Baker & Taylor Bks.)*
Bookpeople *(Bookpeople)*
New Leaf Dist *(New Leaf Distributing Co., Inc.).*

CA HlthCare Fnd, *(California HealthCare Foundation; 1-929008),* 476 Ninth St., Oakland, CA 94607 Tel 510-238-1040; Fax: 510-238-1388
E-mail: sharp@chcf.org
Web site: http://www.chcf.org.

CA Inc, *See* **C A Inc**

CA Med Pubns, *(California Medical Pubns.; 0-9615638),* P.O. Box 890160, Temcula, CA 92589 (SAN 695-8788) Tel 909-699-3915.

CA Public Emp Retire, *(California Public Employees' Retirement System; 0-9633681),* Orders Addr.: P.O. Box 942719, Sacramento, CA 94229-2719 Tel 916-326-3900; Fax: 916-326-3905; Edit Addr.: 400 P St., Sacramento, CA 95814.

CA Res Bureau, *(California Research Bureau; 1-58703),* Orders Addr.: P.O. Box 942837, Sacramento, CA 94237-0001 Tel 916-653-7843; Fax: 916-653-1764; Edit Addr.: 900 N. St., Suite 300, Sacramento, CA 95814
E-mail: tdangberg@library.ca.gov; crb@library.ca.gov
Web site: http://www.library.ca.gov.com.

CA St Libry, *See* **CA Res Bureau**

CA State Library Fndtn, *(California State Library Foundation; 0-929722; 1-893834),* 1225 Eighth St., Suite 345, Sacramento, CA 95814 (SAN 250-300X) Tel 916-447-6331; Fax: 916-447-0125.

Caballero Pr, *(Caballero Pr.; 0-9601346),* 1936 Caballero Way, Las Vegas, NV 89109 (SAN 210-6825) Tel 702-735-3406.

Cabell Cty Med Soc, *(Cabell County Medical Society; 0-9616839),* 1340 Hal Green Blvd., Huntington, WV 25701 (SAN 661-2792) Tel 304-522-3450.

Cache River Pr, *(Cache River Pr.; 0-9627422; 1-889899),* 2850 Oak Grove Rd., Vienna, IL 62995 Tel 618-658-3033; Fax: 618-658-4028; Toll Free: 888-862-2243
E-mail: sertoli@cacheriverpress.com
Web site: http://www.cacheriverpress.com
Dist(s): **Partners Pubs Grp** *(Partners Pubs. Group, Inc.).*

Cader Bks Imprint of Andrews McMeel

Caduceus Pr, *(Caduceus Pr.; 0-9658029),* 1614 Lynwood Ln., Albany, GA 31707 Tel 912-432-1536 Do not confuse with Caduceus Pr., Inc., Trenton, NJ
E-mail: vmiller@dmail.dartnet.peachnet.edu.

†CAI, *(Community Associations Institute; 0-941301; 0-944715),* 225 Reinekers Ln., Suite 300, Alexandria, VA 22314-2875 (SAN 666-2137) Tel 703-548-8600; Fax: 703-836-6907
Web site: http://www.caionline.org; *CIP.*

Caliana Pub, *(Caliana Publishing Co.; 0-9661143),* 8111 Moonlight Bay Dr., Baileys Harbor, WI 54202 Tel 920-739-5269; 328 Norhtridge Rd., Santa Barbara, CA 93105 Tel 805-687-2295.

Calif Acad, *(California Academic Pr., The; 1-891557),* 217 La Cruz Ave., Millbrae, CA 94030 Tel 650-697-5628; Fax: 650-692-0141
E-mail: info@calpress.com
Web site: http://www.calpress.com.

Calif Education, *(California Dept. of Education; 0-8011),* P.O. Box 271, Sacramento, CA 95812-0271 (SAN 268-5868) Tel 916-445-7608; Fax: 916-323-0823; Toll Free: 800-995-4099
Web site: http://www.cde.ca.gov/cdepress.

Calif Fin Pubns, *(California Financial Pubns.; 0-930926),* P.O. Box 306, Cardiff, CA 92007 (SAN 211-6588) Tel 760-942-2919.

Calif Health, *See* **Calif Fin Pubns**

Calli Callul, *See* **Hughes Henshaw**

Calliope Bks, *(Calliope Bks.; 0-9620187),* 2115 Chadbourne Ave., Madison, WI 53705 (SAN 247-9370) Tel 608-238-9258
E-mail: wcoleman@facstaff.wisc.edu
Web site: http://www.execpc.com/~calliope.

Calvary Pr, *(Calvary Pr.; 0-9604138),* 400 S. Bennett St., Southern Pines, NC 28387 (SAN 223-4505) Do not confuse with companies with the same name in Amityville, NY, Lumberton, NC.

Calyx Bks, *(Calyx Bks.; 0-934971),* Div. of Calyx, Inc., Orders Addr.: P.O. Box B, Corvallis, OR 97339 (SAN 695-1171) Tel 541-753-9384; Fax: 541-753-0515; Toll Free: 888-336-2665; Edit Addr.: 216 SW Madison, No. 7, Corvallis, OR 97333 (SAN 242-0643)
E-mail: calyx@proaxis.com
Web site: http://www.calyxpress.com
Dist(s): **Bookpeople** *(Bookpeople)*
Consort Bk Sales *(Consortium Bk. Sales & Distribution)*
Koen Bk Distributors *(Koen Bk. Distributors)*
SPD-Small Pr Dist *(SPD-Small Pr. Distribution).*

CAM Pub, *(CAM Pub.; 0-9631426),* Orders Addr.: P.O. Box 1277, West Palm Beach, FL 33402 Tel 407-642-7777; Edit Addr.: 1561 Florida Mango Rd., West Palm Beach, FL 33406.

Camaro Pub, *(Camaro Publishing Co.; 0-913290; 0-929733),* 90430 World Way Ctr., Los Angeles, CA 90009 (SAN 201-7865) Tel 310-837-7500.

Cambdge Ctr Behav, *(Cambridge Ctr. for Behavioral Studies; 1-881317),* 336 Baker Ave., Concord, MA 01742-2107 Tel 978-369-2227; Fax: 978-369-8584
E-mail: store@behavior.org
Web site: http://www.behavior.org.

Cambridge Cottage, *(Cambridge Cottage Pr.; 1-892869),* 1315-I Tustin, Suite 255, Orange, CA 92869 Tel 714-685-9450 (phone/fax)
E-mail: cameottpress@earthlink.net
Web site: http://www.camcottpress@earthlink.net.

†Cambridge U Pr, *(Cambridge Univ. Pr.; 0-521; 0-511),* Orders Addr.: 110 Midland Ave., Port Chester, NY 10573-4930 (SAN 281-3769) Tel 914-937-9600; Fax: 914-937-4712; Toll Free: 800-872-7423 (orders, returns, credit & accounting); Edit Addr.: 40 W. 20th St., New York, NY 10011-4211 (SAN 200-206X) Tel 212-924-3900; Fax: 212-691-3239
E-mail: orders@cup.org; information@cup.org; customer_service@cup.org
Web site: http://www.cup.org
Dist(s): **netLibrary CO** *(netLibrary, Inc.); CIP.*

Camden Hse, *(Camden Hse.; 0-938100; 1-57113; 1-879751),* Orders Addr.: 668 Mt. Hope Ave., Rochester, NY 14620 Tel 716-275-0419; Fax: 716-271-8778; Edit Addr.: P.O. Box 41026, Rochester, NY 14604-4126
E-mail: CamdenHouse2@Compuserve.com
Web site: http://www.boydell.co.uk/CAMDEN.HTM
Dist(s): **Boydell & Brewer** *(Boydell & Brewer, Inc.).*

Cameltrotters, *(Cameltrotters Publishing; 0-9666110),* Orders Addr.: P.O. Box 3022, La Jolla, CA 92038-3022 Tel 619-235-9393 (phone/fax); Toll Free: 800-494-5341 (pager); Edit Addr.: 1455 Second Ave., No. 310, San Diego, CA 92101-3026
E-mail: atborgeas@aol.com.

Camex, *(Camex, Inc.; 0-932565),* 535 Fifth Ave., New York, NY 10017 (SAN 687-4746) Tel 212-682-8400.

Camino Bks, *(Camino Bks., Inc.; 0-940159),* Orders Addr.: P.O. Box 59026, Philadelphia, PA 19102-9026 (SAN 664-225X) Tel 215-413-1917; Fax: 215-413-3255
E-mail: camino@caminobooks.com
Web site: http://www.caminobooks.com.

Can7 Govern Pub (CAN) *(0-315; 0-660; 0-662) Dist. by* **Intl Spec Bk.**

Cancer Care, *(Cancer Care, Inc.; 0-9606494),* 1180 Sixth Ave., New York, NY 10036 (SAN 225-9087) Tel 212-221-3300.

Cancer Treatment, *(Cancer Treatment Research Foundation; 0-9638263),* 3455 Salt Creek Ln., Suite 200, Arlington Heights, IL 60005-1090 Tel 847-342-7450; Fax: 847-342-7320
Web site: http://www.ctrf.org.

Candida, *(Candida Corp.; 1-891545),* 220 South State St., Suite 1310, Chicago, IL 60604 Tel 312-431-1601; Fax: 312-431-1605
E-mail: rmateles@candida.com.

Candle Bks, *(Candle Bks., Inc.; 0-9609644),* 1010 Grey Oak, San Antonio, TX 78213 (SAN 262-0065) Tel 210-342-5880.

†Candlewick Pr, *(Candlewick Pr.; 0-7636; 1-56402),* Div. of Walker Bks., London, England, 2067 Massachusetts Ave., Cambridge, MA 02140 Tel 617-661-3330; Fax: 617-661-0565 Do not confuse with Candlewick Pr., Crystal Lake, IL
E-mail: bigbear@candlewick.com; salesinfo@candlewick.com
Web site: http://www.candlewick.com/
Dist(s): **Lectorum Pubns** *(Lectorum Pubns., Inc.)*
Penguin Putnam *(Penguin Putnam, Inc.); CIP.*

Canfield Pubng, *(Canfield Publishing; 0-9647749),* 253 Passaic Ave., Fairfield, NJ 07004-2524.

Canine Eye Reg, *(Canine Eye Registration Foundation; 0-9635163),* Div. of Veterinary Medical Data Base, Purdue Univ., SCC-A, West Lafayette, IN 47907 Tel 765-494-8179; Fax: 765-494-9981.

Canoe Press, *(Canoe Pr.; 0-9613768),* Orders Addr.: P.O. Box 174, Oak Park, IL 60303 (SAN 685-4117) Tel 708-386-1968; Edit Addr.: 333 N. Euclid Ave., Oak Park, IL 60302-2109 (SAN 678-9633) Fax: 708-386-2080 Do not confuse with Canoe Pr., Traverse City, MI.

Canon Comns, *(Canon Communications, LLC; 0-9618649; 1-884551),* 11444 W. Olympic Blvd., Suite 900, Los Angeles, CA 90064 (SAN 668-5420) Tel 310-445-4251; Fax: 310-445-4259
Web site: http://www.cancom.com.

Canongate Books (GBR) *(0-86241; 0-903937; 1-84195) Dist. by* **Grove-Atltic.**

Canyonlands, *(Canyonlands Natural History Assn.; 0-937407),* 3031 S. Hwy. 191, Moab, UT 84532-3629 (SAN 659-0764) Tel 435-259-6003; Fax: 435-259-8263.

Canyonlnds Pubng, *(Canyonlands Publishing, Inc.; 0-9639381),* 75 W. Calle De Las Tiendas, Suite 133B, Green Valley, AZ 85614-4270 Do not confuse with Canyonlands Publishing Group, Provo, UT
Dist(s): **Commun Skill** *(Communication Skill Builders/Therapy Skill Builders).*

Capall Bann Pubng (GBR) *(1-898307; 1-86163) Dist. by* **Holmes Pub.**

CAPE Center, *(C.A.P.E. Ctr.; 0-944454),* 4621 Ross Ave., YWCA Bldg., Dallas, TX 75204-4994 (SAN 243-7333) Tel 214-821-4784; Fax: 972-699-8147
E-mail: EBKRAUSE@prodigy.net.

Capital Com Inc, *(Capital Communications, Inc.; 0-9647700),* P.O. Box 10338, Sarasota, FL 34278-0338 Tel 941-342-9088; Fax: 941-377-3120; Toll Free: 800-546-8378
E-mail: capital@investors.org
Web site: http://www.investors.org.

CapitalHlth Pub, *(CapitalHealth Publishing, Inc.; 1-890074),* 175 Lancaster St., Albany, NY 12210-1940 Tel 518-465-1686; Fax: 518-465-2953
E-mail: mwaldman@caphealth.com
Web site: http://caphealth.com/chphome.html.

Capitol Enquiry, *(Capitol Enquiry, Inc.; 0-917982),* 1228 N St., No. 10, Sacramento, CA 95814-5610 (SAN 211-5077) Tel 916-442-1434; Fax: 916-442-1260 ; *Imprints:* Cougar Books (Cougar Books)
E-mail: info@capenq.com
Web site: http://www.capenq.com.

Capitol Publns, *(Capitol Pubns., Inc.; 1-884561),* 1101 King St., Suite 444, Alexandria, VA 22314 Fax: 703-739-6517; Toll Free: 800-655-5597
Web site: http://www.grantscape.com.

Capitol VA, *(Capitol Publishing Group; 0-937925; 1-56925),* Div. of Capitol Pubns., Inc., 1101 King St., Suite 444, Alexandria, VA 22314-2968 (SAN 659-4980) Fax: 703-739-6517; Toll Free: 800-327-7203
Dist(s): **Aspen Pub** *(Aspen Pubs., Inc.).*

Capp Pubng, *(Capp Publishing, Inc.; 0-9638937),* Orders Addr.: P.O. Box 1988, Salt Lake City, UT 84110 Tel 801-328-8917; Edit Addr.: 1237 E 100 South, Salt Lake City, UT 84102
E-mail: cappub@inquo.net.

Capstone Pr, *(Capstone Pr., Inc.; 0-7368; 1-56065),* Orders Addr.: P.O. Box 669, Mankato, MN 56002-0669 (SAN 254-1815) Tel 507-388-6650; Fax: 507-625-4662; Toll Free Fax: 888-262-0705; Toll Free: 800-747-4992; Edit Addr.: 6117 Blue Circle Dr., Suite 150, Minnetonka, MN 55343 ; *Imprints:* Pebble Bks (Pebble Books) Bridgestone Bks (Bridgestone Books) LifeMatters Bks (LifeMatters Books) Do not confuse with Capstone Pr., Inc. in Decatur, IL
Web site: http://www.capstone-press.com
Dist(s): **American Econo** *(American Econo Clad)*
Continental Bk *(Continental Bk. Co., Inc.).*

CARC, *(Creative Arts Rehabilitation Ctr.; 0-9606876),* 17 E. 97th St., Apt. 6C, New York, NY 10029-6969 (SAN 217-3484).

Carden Jennings, *(Carden Jennings Publishing Co., Ltd.; 1-891524),* 1224 W. Main St., Suite 200, Charlottesville, VA 22903 Tel 804-817-2000; Fax: 804-817-2020
Web site: http://www.cjp.com.

Cardiac Self Assessmnt, *(Cardiac Self Assessment; 0-9653568; 0-9711137),* 1605 S. Clinton Rd., Spokane, WA 99216 Tel 509-926-0344 (phone/fax)
E-mail: westodd@iea.com
Web site: http://www.iea/~westodd.

Cardiothoracic Rsch, *(Cardiothoracic Research & Education Foundation; 0-9623617),* 100 E. Wood St., No. 300, Spartanburg, SC 29303-3059 Tel 864-583-4420; Fax: 864-542-1045.

Care Comm Inc, *See* **Care Educ Grp**

Care Educ Grp, *(Care Education Group, Inc.; 0-916499),* 2 Salt Creek Ln., Suite 100, Hinsdale, IL 60521 (SAN 295-5180) Tel 630-323-1900; Fax: 630-323-2123.

Care Solutions, *(Care Solutions, Inc.; 0-9631939; 1-887203),* 500 Sugar Mill Rd., Suite 100B, Atlanta, GA 30350-2843.

Career Pr Inc, *(Career Pr., Inc.; 1-56414),* Orders Addr.: 3 Tice Rd., Franklin Lakes, NJ 07417-1322 (SAN 694-3640) Tel 201-848-0310; Fax: 201-848-1727; Toll Free: 800-227-3371 (outside New Jersey); Edit Addr.: P.O. Box 687, Franklin Lakes, NJ 07417 ; *Imprints:* New Page Bks (New Page Books)
E-mail: Bbrienza@nisusa.net
Web site: http://www.careerpress.com; http://www.newpagebooks.com.

Career Pub, *(Career Publishing, Inc.; 0-89262),* Orders Addr.: P.O. Box 5486, Orange, CA 92863-5486 (SAN 208-581X) Tel 714-771-5155; Fax: 714-532-0180; Toll Free: 800-854-4014; Edit Addr.: 910 N. Main St., Orange, CA 92867-5403 (SAN 658-0246) Do not confuse with Career Publishing, Inc., Mundelein, IL
E-mail: careerpub@worldnet.att.net
Web site: http://www.careerpublishing.com
Dist(s): **Thomson Learn** *(Thomson Learning).*

Career Pub IL, *(Career Publishing, Inc.; 0-911744),* 905 Allanson Rd., Mundelein, IL 60060 (SAN 202-5132) Tel 847-949-0011; Fax: 847-566-8552 Do not confuse with Career Publishing, Inc., Orange, CA
E-mail: gree 933@attglobal.net.

Carelife Pubng, *(Carelife Publishing; 0-9648529),* P.O. Box 4196, West Hills, CA 91308-4196 Tel 818-360-0864
E-mail: carelife@webTV.net.

Caremore Pubns, *(Caremore Pubns.; 1-887454),* Div. of Caremore Corporation, 1213 16th St., N., Saint Petersburg, FL 33705 Tel 813-894-5333; Fax: 813-821-1684; Toll Free: 800-435-2999 (orders only)
Dist(s): **Quality Bks IL** *(Quality Bks., Inc.).*

CareWise, *(CareWise, Inc.; 1-886444),* a/o Mktg., 1501 Fourth Ave., Suite 800, Seattle, WA 98101-1629 Tel 206-749-1100; Fax: 206-749-1125; Toll Free: 800-755-2136
E-mail: www.carewiseline.com
Web site: http://www.carewise@carewiseinc.com.

Caribe Betania, *(Caribe/Betania Editores; 0-8499; 0-88113; 0-89922),* Div. of Thomas Nelson, Inc., 402 BNA Dr., Bldg. 100, Suite 600, Nashville, TN 37217 (SAN 240-6349) Fax: 615-883-9376; Toll Free: 800-322-7423
E-mail: info@editorialcaribe.com; sales@editorialcaribe.com
Web site: http://www.editorialcaribe.com
Dist(s): **Luciano Bks** *(Luciano Bks.)*
Pan De Vida Dists *(Pan De Vida Distributors)*
Penial Prod *(Peniel Productions).*

CaribMed, *(CaribMed, Inc.; 0-9663087),* 4n 212 Eighth Ave., Addison, IL 60101 Tel 312-682-8852; Fax: 630-834-8627
E-mail: info@caribmed.com
Web site: http://www.caribmed.com.

Caring, *(Caring, Inc.; 0-911163),* P.O. Box 400, Milton, WA 98354 (SAN 268-6597) Tel 206-922-8607.

Caring Pub, *(Caring Publishing; 0-9628363; 1-886450),* Div. of The National Assn. for Home Care, 228 Seventh St., SE, Washington, DC 20003 (SAN 272-8389) Tel 202-547-7424; Fax: 202-547-7518
Dist(s): **Assoc Pubs Grp** *(Associated Pubs. Group).*

Carlisle Pr, *(Carlisle Pr.; 0-9627369),* P.O. Box 747, Mechanicsburg, PA 17055 Tel 717-697-1642 Do not conufse with companies with the same name in Benbrook, TX, Sedona, AZ, Sugarcreek, OH
E-mail: carlislepress@pa.net
Dist(s): **Baker & Taylor** *(Baker & Taylor Bks.)*
Brodart *(Brodart Co.)*
Quality Bks IL *(Quality Bks., Inc.).*

Carlisle Pub, *(Carlisle Publishing, Inc.; 0-910177),* P.O. Box 3055, Amherst, MA 01004-3055 (SAN 240-9739) Do not confuse with Carlisle Publishing Company in Fremont, CA.

Carlton Bks Ltd (GBR) *(1-85868; 1-84222) Dist. by* **Natl Bk Netwk.**

Carmania Bks, *(Carmania Bks.; 1-884702),* P.O. Box 1272, Santa Monica, CA 90406-1272 (SAN 298-1300) Tel 310-453-7504
E-mail: carmaniabk@aol.com
Dist(s): **Baker & Taylor** *(Baker & Taylor Bks.)*
Bookpeople *(Bookpeople)*
Quality Bks IL *(Quality Bks., Inc.)*
Unique Bks Inc *(Unique Bks., Inc.).*

Carnegie Coun Policy, *See* **Carnegie Fnd Advan Teach**

†Carnegie Fnd Advan Teach, *(Carnegie Foundation for the Advancement of Teaching; 0-931050),* 555 Middlefield Rd., Menlo Park, CA 94025-3443 (SAN 211-5506) Tel 650-566-5100; Fax: 650-326-0278
E-mail: publications@carnegiefoundation.org
Web site: http://www.carnegiefoundation.org
Dist(s): **Jossey-Bass** *(Jossey-Bass, Inc. Pubs.); CIP.*

Carnegie Inst, *(Carnegie Institution of Washington; 0-87279),* Pubn. Office, 1530 P St., NW, Washington, DC 20005 (SAN 201-9663) Tel 202-939-1121; Fax: 202-387-8092
E-mail: jstrom@pst.ciw.edu
Web site: http://www.carnegieinstitution.org.

Carnelian Bay, *(Carnelian Bay Castle Pr., LLC; 1-889356),* P.O. Box 7100, Santa Monica, CA 90406-7100 Tel 310-822-1004; Fax: 310-822-3551; Toll Free: 800-777-7930
E-mail: welive@earthlink.net
Web site: http://www.home.earthlink.net/~welive
Dist(s): **BookMasters** *(BookMasters, Inc.)*
STCS Publisher Distrib *(STCS Pub. Distribution Services).*

Carolando, *(Carolando Pr., Inc.; 0-940542),* 6545 W. North Ave., Oak Park, IL 60302 (SAN 219-3426) Tel 708-383-6480; Fax: 708-383-6827
E-mail: info@carolando.com
Web site: http://www.carolando.com.

Carolina Acad Pr, *(Carolina Academic Pr.; 0-89089),* 700 Kent St., Durham, NC 27701 (SAN 210-7848) Tel 919-489-7486; Fax: 919-493-5668; Toll Free: 800-489-7486
E-mail: cap@cap-press.com
Web site: http://www.cap-press.com.

Carolina Pacific, *(Carolina Pacific Publishing; 0-945490),* Div. of John Ross & Assocs., 16350 SE Bel Air Dr., Clackamas, OR 97015 (SAN 247-1825) Tel 503-658-8754.

†Carolina Pop Ctr, *(Univ. of North Carolina at Chapel Hill, Carolina Population Ctr.; 0-89055),* Population Pubns., University Sq., Campus Box 8120, Chapel Hill, NC 27516-3997 (SAN 201-7687) Tel 919-966-2152; Fax: 919-966-6638; *CIP.*

Carolina Pr, *See* **Healthnet Pr**

Carroll & Graf, *(Carroll & Graf Pubs., Inc.; 0-7867; 0-88184),* 19 W. 21st St., Suite 601, New York, NY 10010-6806 (SAN 264-6560) Tel 212-627-8590; Fax: 212-627-8490; Toll Free: 800-788-3123 (Bookstore orders only)
Web site: http://www.carrollandgraf.com
Dist(s): **Continental Bk** *(Continental Bk. Co., Inc.)*
Publishers Group *(Publishers Group West).*

Carrot Top Nutrition, *(Carrot Top Nutrition Resources; 0-9622157),* Orders Addr.: P.O. Box 460172, Aurora, CO 80046-0172 Tel 303-690-3650 (phone/fax); Edit Addr.: 7266 S. Ireland Cir., Aurora, CO 80016
E-mail: CTNR@aol.com
Web site: http://members.aol.com/ctnr/.

Carswell, *(Carswell),* Div. of The Thomson Corp., 28 Glen Ave., Millburn, NJ 07041 Toll Free Fax: 973-313-1245; Toll Free: 888-307-1355
E-mail: steve.roses@carswell.com.

Carswell (CAN) *(0-459; 0-88820) Dist. by* **Carswell.**

CAS, *(Competence Assurance Systems; 0-89147),* Div. of Whole Brain Corp., P.O. Box 81, Cambridge, MA 02238 (SAN 208-0001).

Cas Con Grad Med, *(Castle Connolly Graduate Medical Publishing, LLC; 0-9707305),* 133 E 58th St., Suite 1101, New York, NY 10022 Tel 212-644-9696; Fax: 212-202-4972; Toll Free: 866-240-0573 Do not confuse with Castle Connolly Graduate Medical in New York, NY
E-mail: mwolf@ccgmp.com
Web site: http://www.ccgmp.com.

Casa Bautista, *(Casa Bautista de Publicaciones; 0-311),* Div. of Southern Baptist Convention, Orders Addr.: P.O. Box 4255, El Paso, TX 79914 (SAN 220-0139) Tel 915-566-9656; Fax: 915-562-6502; Toll Free: 800-755-5958
E-mail: epena@casabautista.org
Web site: http://www.casabautista.org.

CasAnanda, *(CasAnanda Publishing; 1-889131),* P.O. Box 7207, Bayonet Point, FL 34674 Tel 727-819-1082; Fax: 727-863-0564
Web site: http://www.casananda.com.

Case Sftware, *(Case Software; 1-880989),* 5601 Forest Manor Dr., Greensboro, NC 27410 Tel 336-286-9099; Fax: 336-288-4924.

Casenotes Pub, *(Casenotes Publishing Co., Inc.; 0-87457),* 1640 Fifth St., Suite 208, Santa Monica, CA 90401 (SAN 688-931X) Tel 310-395-6500; Fax: 310-458-2020; Toll Free: 800-726-6662
E-mail: casenotes@westworld.com
Web site: http://www.casenotes.com/.

Cash-Callahan, *See* **Race Pt Pr**

Cassandra Pr, *(Cassandra Pr.; 0-945946; 0-9615875),* P.O. Box 150868, San Rafael, CA 94915-0868 (SAN 697-0389) Tel 415-382-8507 Do not confuse with Cassandra Pr. in Sanatoga, PA
Dist(s): **Bookpeople** *(Bookpeople)*
Integral Yoga Pubns *(Integral Yoga Pubns.)*
New Leaf Dist *(New Leaf Distributing Co., Inc.)*
Nutri-Books Corp *(Nutri-Bks. Corp.)*
Red Wheel ME *(Red Wheel).*

Cassell (GBR) *(0-304; 1-86047; 1-84188) Dist. by* **Sterling.**

Castelli Studios, *(Castelli Studios; 0-9702806),* Orders Addr.: 211 Buckskill Rd., East Hampton, NY 11937-3273 Tel 631-329-3813; Fax: 631-329-2842
E-mail: orders@multiple-personality.com; jcastelli@hamptons.com
Web site: http://www.multiple-personality.com.

Castillo Intl, *See* **All Stars Project**

Castle Connolly Med, *(Castle Connolly Medical, Ltd.; 1-883769),* 42 W. 24th St., New York, NY 10010 (SAN 298-0347) Tel 212-367-8400; Fax: 212-367-0964; Toll Free: 800-399-3627 Do not confuse with Castle Connolly Graduate Medical Publishing in New York , NY
E-mail: info@castleconnolly.com
Web site: http://www.americastopdoctors.com
Dist(s): **IPG Chicago** *(Independent Pubs. Group).*

Castle Consult, *(Castle Consulting; 0-9644520),* 7725 Moe Rd., Lolo, MT 59847 Tel 406-273-6080; Fax: 406-273-0111.

Castle Hills, *(Castle Hills First Baptist Church Pr.; 0-945641),* 2220 NW Military Hwy., San Antonio, TX 78213 (SAN 247-3895) Tel 210-342-8833
E-mail: info.desk@chfbc.org.

Castle Peak, *(Castle Peak Media Group; 0-9642259),* 626 S. Shilling Ave., Blackfoot, ID 83221 Tel 208-785-4414; Fax: 208-782-3625; Toll Free: 800-715-0111.

CAT Pub, *(CAT Publishing Co.; 0-929655; 0-943437; 1-56226),* P.O. Box 492337, Redding, CA 96049-2337 (SAN 668-4920) Tel 530-222-6050; Fax: 530-222-6115; Toll Free: 800-767-0511
E-mail: publish@c-zone.net
Web site: http://www.ctpublishing.com/.

Catacombs Pr, *(Catacombs Pr., The; 0-9656313),* P.O. Box 261642, Encino, CA 91426 Tel 818-996-2585; Fax: 818-966-7226
E-mail: readmore1@juno.com
Web site: http://www.nutriscreen.com.

Catalyst FL, *(Catalyst; 0-9620549),* P.O. Box 20572, Sarasota, FL 34276-3572 (SAN 249-0226) Tel 941-366-0222 Do not confuse with companies with the same name in Newport News, VA, McKinney TX, Kentfield, CA
Dist(s): **Baker & Taylor** *(Baker & Taylor Bks.).*

Cath Free Choice, *(Catholics for a Free Choice; 0-915365),* 1436 U St., NW, Suite 301, Washington, DC 20009-3997 (SAN 291-1116) Tel 202-986-6093; Fax: 202-332-7995
E-mail: cffc@catholicsforchoice.org
Web site: http://www.catholicsforchoice.org.

Cath Health, *(Catholic Health Assn. of the U.S.; 0-87125),* 4455 Woodson Rd., Saint Louis, MO 63134-3797 (SAN 201-968X) Tel 314-427-2500; Fax: 314-427-0029
E-mail: rstephe@chausa.com
Web site: http://www.chausa.org.

Cathedral Holy Spirit, *(Cathedral of the Holy Spirit; 0-917595),* Div. of Chapel Hill Harvester Church, 4650 Flat Shoals Rd., Decatur, GA 30034 (SAN 657-1484) Tel 404-243-5020; Fax: 404-243-5927; Toll Free: 800-241-4702.

Cathie Kyle (GBR) *(1-85626) Dist. by* **Trafalgar.**

Publisher Symbol Index

Catholic Bk Pub, *(Catholic Bk. Publishing Co.; 0-89942),* 77 West End Rd., Totowa, NJ 07512-1405 (SAN 204-3432) Tel 973-890-2400; Fax: 973-890-2410; Toll Free: 800-892-6657 ; *Imprints:* Resurrection Pr (Resurrection Press)
E-mail: resurpress@aol.com
Web site: http://www.catholicbkpub.com
Dist(s): **Moshy Brothers Inc** *(Moshy Brothers, Inc.)*
Riverside-World *(Riverside World)*
Spring Arbor Dist *(Spring Arbor Distributors Inc.).*

Catholic Ctr at Tufts Univ, *(Catholic Ctr. at Tufts Univ., The; 0-9677471),* 58 Winthrop St., Medford, MA 02155 Tel 781-391-7272; Fax: 781-396-8779
E-mail: dolear01@tufts.edu.

†Cato Inst, *(Cato Institute; 0-932790; 1-882577; 1-930865),* **1000 Massachusetts Ave., NW, Washington, DC 20001-5403 (SAN 212-6095) Tel 202-842-0200; Fax: 202-842-3490; Toll Free: 800-767-1241**
E-mail: cato@cato.org
Web site: http://www.cato.org
Dist(s): **Natl Bk Netwk *(National Bk. Network); CIP.***

CattleDog Pubng, *(CattleDog Publishing; 0-9641518),* Orders Addr.: P.O. Box 4516, Davis, CA 95617-4516 Tel 916-757-2383; Edit Addr.: 3215 Trawler Pl., Davis, CA 95616.

Cavco Pubns, *(Cavco Pubns.; 0-932137),* Div. of Quintiles, Inc., 3936 W. Greenleaf Ave., Lincolnwood, IL 60645-2526.

Cave Bks MO, *(Cave Bks.; 0-939748),* Affil. of Cave Research Foundation, Orders Addr.: 4700 Amberwood Dr., Dayton, OH 45424 (SAN 699-5195) Tel 937-233-3561; Edit Addr.: 756 Harvard Ave., Saint Louis, MO 63130 (SAN 216-7220) Tel 314-862-7646
E-mail: info@cavemanbooks.com; editor@cavemanbooks.com
Web site: http://www.cavebooks.com.

Cavendish Pubng (GBR) *(1-85941; 1-874241; 1-84941) Dist. by* **Gaunt.**

Caverne Pub, *(Caverne Publishing; 0-937844),* 7 W. Garden Green, Port Heneme, CA 93041-1815 Tel 805-984-7827; Fax: 805-984-8400
E-mail: cavpub@earthlink.net
Web site: http://www.cavpub.com.

CBCCU Amer, *(Central Bureau, Catholic Central Union of America; 0-9626257; 1-887567),* 3835 Westminster Pl., Saint Louis, MO 63108-3472 Tel 314-371-1653
E-mail: centbur@juno.com
Web site: http://www.socialjusticereview.org.

C&C Communs, *(C&C Communications; 0-9636487),* 4627 Ocean Blvd., No. 112, San Diego, CA 92109 Tel 619-483-8569; Fax: 619-581-6640 Do not confuse with CC Communications in Endicott, NY
E-mail: ccichf@san.rr.com.

CC Services, *(Creative Computer Services; 0-944252),* 202 Rustic Hill Ln., Amherst, OH 44001-1948 (SAN 242-990X) Tel 216-985-1735.

CCH Access, *See* **CCH INC**

CCH INC, *(CCH, INC; 0-8080),* Div. of Wolters Kluwer U.S., 2700 Lake Cook Rd., Riverwoods, IL 60015 Tel 847-267-7000; Toll Free: 800-248-3248
Web site: http://www.cch.com
Dist(s): **LPC Group** *(LPC Group).*

CECOM Pub, *(CECOM Publishing; 0-9624764),* 617 Spitfire Ln., Oak Harbor, WA 98277-9105 Tel 360-679-0864.

Cedarwinds, *(Cedarwinds Publishing Co.; 0-915297),* 1305 Park Dr., Medway, OH 45341 (SAN 212-1700) Tel 904-224-9261; Fax: 513-849-1624; Toll Free: 800-548-2388
E-mail: balbert@aol.com
Dist(s): **Midpt Trade** *(Midpoint Trade Bks., Inc.).*

Cedrus Corp, *(Cedrus Corp.; 0-9661842),* Orders Addr.: P.O. Box 27553, Phoenix, AZ 85061 Tel 602-631-9044; Fax: 602-631-9047; Toll Free: 800-233-7871; Edit Addr.: 532 E. Maryland Ave., Suite B3, Phoenix, AZ 85012
E-mail: info@cedrus.com
Web site: http://www.cedrus.com.

CEEM Inc, *(CEEM Inc.; 1-883337),* 12110 Sunset Hills Rd., Suite 100, Reston, VA 20190 Fax: 703-250-5313; Toll Free: 800-745-5565
E-mail: order@ceem.com
Web site: http://www.ceem.com/.

†Celestial Arts, *(Celestial Arts Publishing Co.; 0-89087; 0-912310; 1-58761),* Div. of Ten Speed Pr., Orders Addr.: P.O. Box 7123, Berkeley, CA 94707 (SAN 159-8333) Tel 510-559-1600; Fax: 510-559-1637; Toll Free: 800-841-2665; Edit Addr.: 999 Harrison St., Berkeley, CA 94710 Fax: 510-524-1052
E-mail: order@tenspeed.com
Web site: http://www.tenspeed.com; *CIP.*

Celestial Gifts, *(Celestial Gifts; 0-935882),* Orders Addr.: 8505 Charter Club Cir., Chester, MD 21619 (SAN 219-1431) Tel 941-433-9200; Fax: 941-433-9220
Web site: http://www.nsdi.net/dr_rondalrymple/inner.html
Dist(s): **Baker & Taylor** *(Baker & Taylor Bks.)*
Distributors *(Distributors, The)*
New Leaf Dist *(New Leaf Distributing Co., Inc.).*

Celilo Pubns, *(Celilo Pubns.; 0-9614529),* 3021 SW Florida St., Portland, OR 97219 (SAN 689-738X) Tel 503-244-4548.

Celo Valley Bks, *(Celo Valley Bks.; 0-923687),* 346 Seven Mile Ridge Rd., Burnsville, NC 28714 (SAN 251-7973) Tel 828-675-5918.

CEN3 (GBR) *(0-7126) Dist. by* **Trafalgar.**

Centaur Bks, *(Centaur Bks.; 1-891530),* 731 Makaleka Ave., Apt. C, Honolulu, HI 96816-6002 Tel 808-739-1415; Fax: 808-733-7808 Do not confuse with Centaur Books, Royal Oak, MI
E-mail: sybrnes@chaminade.edu
Web site: http://www.naturalhawaii.com/centaur.htm.

Center Creative Life, *(Ctr. for Creative Life Pubns.; 0-9614588),* 200 Tower Ave., Bismarck, ND 58501-3510 (SAN 691-7747) Tel 701-222-2572.

Center Pr, *(Center Pr.; 0-934320),* 2045 Francisco St., Berkeley, CA 94709 (SAN 213-0351) Tel 510-845-8373; Fax: 510-841-3884 Do not confuse with companies with the same name in Encino, CA, Santa Fe, NM.

Center Reprod, *(Ctr. for Reproductive Law & Policy, The; 1-890671),* 120 Wall St., 18th Flr., New York, NY 10005 Tel 917-637-3600; Fax: 917-673-3666
E-mail: publications@crlp.org; info@crlp.org
Web site: http://www.crlp.org.

Centering Corp, *(Centering Corp.; 1-56123),* P.O. Box 4600, Omaha, NE 68104-0600 (SAN 298-1815) Tel 402-553-1200; Fax: 402-553-0507
E-mail: centering@centering.org; j1200@aol.com
Web site: http://www.centering.org
Dist(s): **Baker & Taylor** *(Baker & Taylor Bks.).*

CenterWatch, *(CenterWatch, Inc.; 0-9673029; 1-930624),* Subs. of Medical Economics Company, 22 Thomson Pl., 36T1, Boston, MA 02110 Tel 617-856-5900; Fax: 617-856-5901
E-mail: cw.marketing@centerwatch.com
Web site: http://www.centerwatch.com.

Central Pt, *(Central Point Publishing; 0-9630479),* P.O. Box 264, Grapeview, WA 98546-0264 Tel 360-275-9302; Fax: 360-275-9324
Dist(s): **Nutri-Books Corp** *(Nutri-Bks. Corp.).*

CentraLink, *(CentraLink; 1-887452),* 1110 MarWest St., Suite E, Tiburon, CA 94920-1870 Tel 415-435-9848; Fax: 415-435-9092.

†Century Foundation, *(Century Foundation, The; 0-87078),* Div. of Twentieth Century Fund, Inc., 41 E. 70th St., New York, NY 10021 (SAN 205-4647) Tel 212-535-4441; Fax: 212-535-7534
E-mail: info@tcf.org
Web site: http://www.tcf.org; http://www.socsec.org
Dist(s): **Brookings** *(Brookings Institution Pr.); CIP.*

CEPA Gall, *(CEPA Gallery; 0-939784),* 617 Main St., Suite 201, Buffalo, NY 14203 (SAN 216-8839) Tel 716-856-2717; Fax: 716-270-0184
E-mail: cepa@aol.com
Web site: http://cepa.buffnet.net.

Cequal, *(Cequal, Inc.; 1-881206),* 1328 16th St., Santa Monica, CA 90404 Tel 310-458-1102; Fax: 310-458-0444; Toll Free: 800-860-3949
E-mail: info@cequal.com
Web site: http://ww.ecqual.com
Dist(s): **SCB Distributors** *(SCB Distributors).*

Ceres Pr, *(Ceres Pr.; 0-9606138; 1-886101),* P.O. Box 87, Woodstock, NY 12498 (SAN 217-0949) Tel 914-679-5573; Toll Free: 888-804-8848 Do not confuse with Ceres Pr., Stamford, CT
E-mail: cem620@aol.com
Web site: http://www.heathiestdiet.com
Dist(s): **Baker & Taylor** *(Baker & Taylor Bks.)*
Bookpeople *(Bookpeople)*
Integral Yoga Pubns *(Integral Yoga Pubns.)*
Koen Bk Distributors *(Koen Bk. Distributors)*
New Leaf Dist *(New Leaf Distributing Co., Inc.)*
Nutri-Books Corp *(Nutri-Bks. Corp.).*

Certi Board, *(Certification Board Perioperative Nursing; 0-9670222; 0-9717619),* 2170 S. Parker Rd., Suite 295, Denver, CO 80231 Tel 303-369-9566; Fax: 303-695-8464; Toll Free: 888-257-2667
E-mail: moneale@certboard.org
Web site: http://www.certboard.org.

CES Assocs, *(CES Assocs.; 0-916780),* 112 S. Grant St., Hinsdale, IL 60521 (SAN 208-6107) Tel 630-654-2596; Fax: 630-654-2713
E-mail: cessassoc@aol.com
Web site: http://www.cesassoc.com.

CeShore Pubg, *(Ce Shore Publishing Co.; 1-58501),* Div. of Lee Shore Agency, Ltd., The Sterling Bldg., 440 Friday Rd., Pittsburgh, PA 15209 Tel 412-821-6211; Fax: 412-821-6997; Toll Free: 888-542-2665 (888-542-BOOK)
E-mail: ceshor@aol.com
Dist(s): **Partners Pubs Grp** *(Partners Pubs. Group, Inc.).*

CFH Animals IS, *(Concern for Helping Animals in Israel (CHAI); 0-9631596),* Orders Addr.: P.O. Box 3341, Alexandria, VA 22302 Tel 703-658-9650; Fax: 703-941-6132; Edit Addr.: 3914 Brenda Ln., Annandale, VA 22003.

CFI Dist, *(Cedar Fort, Inc./CFI Distribution; 0-934126; 1-55517),* 925 N. Main St., Springville, UT 84663-1051 (SAN 170-2858) Tel 801-489-4084; Fax: 801-489-9432; Toll Free Fax: 800-388-3727; Toll Free: 800-759-2665 ; *Imprints:* Bonneville Bks (Bonneville Books)
E-mail: sales@cedarfort.com; marketing@cedarfort.com; cedarfort@cedarfort.com; editorial@cedarfort.com
Web site: http://www.cedarfort.com.

Chalifoux Pub, *(Chalifoux Publishing; 0-9625549),* 6 Wellesley Ave., Wellesley, MA 02181 Tel 617-235-1747.

Challenge Bks, *(Challenge Bks.; 0-9671338),* 13320 SE 43rd Pl., Bellevue, WA 98006 Tel 425-641-4540; Fax: 425-641-7637
E-mail: pwom@aol.com.

Challenger CA, *(Challenger Pr.; 0-9625341),* Div. of Wallace & Assoc., Orders Addr.: P.O. Box 919, Solvang, CA 93464 Tel 805-688-2434; Fax: 805-686-1340; Toll Free: 800-726-0061; Edit Addr.: 540 Alisal Rd., Suite 3, Solvang, CA 93463
Dist(s): **Distributors** *(Distributors, The).*

Champagne Pr, *(Champagne Pr.; 0-9612146),* 2870 N. Towne Ave., Apt. 35, Pomona, CA 91767-2061 (SAN 290-6996) Do not confuse with Champagne Pr., San Leandro, CA.

†Chandler & Sharp, *(Chandler & Sharp Pubs., Inc.; 0-88316),* 11A Commercial Blvd., Novato, CA 94949 (SAN 205-6127) Tel 415-883-2353; Fax: 415-883-4280; *CIP.*

Chandler Hse, *(Chandler Hse. Pr.; 0-9636277; 1-886284),* 335 Chandler St., Worcester, MA 01602 Tel 508-756-7644; Fax: 508-756-9425; Toll Free: 800-642-6657 ; *Imprints:* Tatnuck (Tatnuck Bookseller Press)
E-mail: clairecs@tatnuck.com
Web site: http://www.chandlerhousepress.com
Dist(s): **Baker & Taylor** *(Baker & Taylor Bks.)*
Brodart *(Brodart Co.).*

Channel One, *(Channel One Communications, Inc.; 1-881343),* 30 Pleasant St., Needham, MA 02192 Tel 781-444-8540; Fax: 781-444-8189
Dist(s): **Baker & Taylor** *(Baker & Taylor Bks.)*
Distributors *(Distributors, The)*
Light Pubng *(Light Publishing)*
New Leaf Dist *(New Leaf Distributing Co., Inc.).*

Chans Corp, *(Chan's Corp.; 0-914322),* 5266 E. Pomoma Blvd., Los Angeles, CA 90023 (SAN 201-8764) Tel 213-721-0746.

Chap & Hall CRC Imprint of CRC Pr

Chap & Hall NY Imprint of Chapman & Hall

Chapel & Croft, *(Chapel & Croft Publishing; 0-9645171; 1-891128),* 5930 E. Pima, Suite 144, Tucson, AZ 85712 Tel 520-751-0390; Fax: 520-886-0008; Toll Free: 800-982-8196.

†Chapman & Hall, *(Chapman & Hall; 0-412; 1-86036),* 115 Fifth Ave., 4th Flr., New York, NY 10003-1004 Tel 212-260-1354; Toll Free: 800-842-3636 ; *Imprints:* Chap & Hall NY (Chapman & Hall)
E-mail: kluwer@wkap.com; services@wkap.com
Web site: http://www.chaphall.com; http://www.chaphall.com/chaphall/; *CIP.*

Chapman Univ Imprint of Seven Locks Pr

Charing Cross, *(Charing Cross Publishing Co.; 0-89074),* 3699 Wilshire Blvd., Suite 700, Los Angeles, CA 90010-2726 (SAN 206-4944) Tel 213-382-3335; Fax: 213-480-7712.

Charles, *(Charles Pr. Pubs.; 0-914783),* Subs. of Oxbridge Corp., Orders Addr.: P.O. Box 15715, Philadelphia, PA 19103 (SAN 203-638X) Tel 215-496-9925; Edit Addr.: 117 S. 17th St., Suite 310, Philadelphia, PA 19103 (SAN 241-6530) Tel 215-496-9616; Fax: 215-496-9637
E-mail: mailbox@charlespresspub.com
Web site: http://www.charlespresspub.com
Dist(s): **Baker & Taylor** *(Baker & Taylor Bks.)*
Brodart *(Brodart Co.)*
Koen Bk Distributors *(Koen Bk. Distributors).*

Charles Pub, *(Charles Publishing Co.; 0-912880),* 1308 Stewart St., Oceanside, CA 92054 (SAN 201-9779) Tel 760-433-5757; Fax: 760-433-3636
E-mail: NTMcharlespub@aol.com; charlespublishing@hotmail.com
Dist(s): **Baker & Taylor** *(Baker & Taylor Bks.)*
U of NM Pr *(Univ. of New Mexico Pr.).*

CHASER, *(Congenital Heart Anomalies; Support, Education & Resources; 0-9658918),* 2112 N. Wilkins Rd., Swanton, OH 43558 Tel 419-825-5575; Fax: 419-825-2880
E-mail: CHASER@compuserve.com; myer106w@wonder.em.cdc.gov
Web site: http://www.csun.edu/hfmth006/chaser/.

Chatham River Pr Imprint of Random Hse Value

Chattanga Grp, *(Chattanooga Group, Inc.; 1-879971),* Orders Addr.: P.O. Box 489, Hixson, TN 37343 Tel 423-870-2281; Fax: 423-875-5497; Toll Free: 800-592-7329.

CHAUAC Imprint of Am Urological

CHC Pub, *See* **Healing Within Prods**

Checkmark Imprint of Facts on File

Cheever Pub, *(Cheever Publishing, Inc.; 0-915708),* P.O. Box 700, Bloomington, IL 61702 (SAN 207-9410) Tel 309-378-2961; Fax: 309-378-4420; Toll Free: 800-787-8444
E-mail: acntlvng@aol.com
Web site: http://www.accentonliving.com.

†**Chelsea Hse,** *(Chelsea Hse. Pubs.; 0-7910; 0-87754; 1-55546),* Div. of Main Line Bk. Co., 1974 Sproul Rd., Suite 400, Broomall, PA 19008-0914 (SAN 206-7609) Tel 610-353-5166; Fax: 610-359-1439; Toll Free: 800-848-2665 ; *Imprints:* Chelsea Juniors (Chelsea Juniors)
E-mail: info@chelseahouse.com
Web site: http://www.chelseahouse.com
Dist(s): **Baker & Taylor** *(Baker & Taylor Bks.)*
Brodart *(Brodart Co.)*
Follett Library *(Follett Library Resources)*
Wolverine Distrib *(Wolverine Distributing, Inc.); CIP.*

Chelsea Juniors Imprint of Chelsea Hse

Chem Educ Res, *(Chemical Education Resources, Inc.; 0-87540),* Orders Addr.: P.O. Box 357, Palmrya, PA 17078 (SAN 297-1909) Tel 717-838-3165; Fax: 717-838-6275; Edit Addr.: 220 S. Railroad St., Palmrya, PA 17078
E-mail: cer@microserve.net
Web site: http://www.CERlabs.com.

Chem Heritage Fnd, *(Chemical Heritage Foundation; 0-941901),* 315 Chestnut St., Philadelphia, PA 19106-2702 (SAN 666-0193) Tel 215-925-2222; Fax: 215-925-1954; Toll Free: 888-224-6006
E-mail: booksales@chemheritage.org; skatz@chemheritage.org; aliciab@chemheritage.org
Web site: http://www.chemheritage.org.

†**Chem Pub,** *(Chemical Publishing Co., Inc.; 0-8206),* 527 Third Ave., No. 427, New York, NY 10016-4168 (SAN 203-6444) Tel 212-779-0090; Fax: 212-889-1537; Toll Free: 800-786-3659
E-mail: chempub@aol.com
Web site: http://www.ChemicalPublishing.com; *CIP.*

Chem Toxicol Inst, *(Chemical Toxicology Institute; 0-9626523),* Orders Addr.: P.O. Box 8299, Foster City, CA 94404 Tel 419-281-1802; Fax: 650-573-6698
E-mail: biopub@altavista.com
Web site: http://www.biomedicalpublications.com
Dist(s): **BookMasters** *(BookMasters, Inc.).*

Chem-Orbital, *(Chem-Orbital; 0-930376),* P.O. Box 134, Park Forest, IL 60466 (SAN 213-3466) Tel 708-747-3717; Fax: 708-747-3657
E-mail: jir@interaccess.com
Web site: http://www.jir.com.

Cheng & Tsui, *(Cheng & Tsui Co.; 0-646; 0-88727; 0-917056),* 25 West St., Boston, MA 02111-1213 (SAN 169-3387) Tel 617-988-2401; Fax: 617-426-3669
E-mail: service@cheng-tsui.com; ct@world.std.com
Web site: http://www.cheng-tsui.com.

Cherbo Pub Grp, *(Cherbo Publishing Group, Inc.; 1-882933),* 5535 Balboa Blvd., No. 108, Encino, CA 91316 Tel 818-783-0040; Fax: 818-783-0044; Toll Free: 800-854-9880
E-mail: cherbopub@aol.com
Web site: http://www.cherbopub.com.

†**Cherokee,** *(Cherokee Publishing Co.; 0-87797),* Orders Addr.: P.O. Box 1730, Marietta, GA 30061-1730 (SAN 650-0404) Tel 404-467-4189; Fax: 404-237-1062; Toll Free: 800-653-3952; Edit Addr.: 800 Miami Cir., NE, Suite 100, Atlanta, GA 30324-3055 Do not confuse with Cherokee Publishing Co., Antioch, CA
E-mail: books@mgci.com; *CIP.*

Cheryn Intl, *See* **Rophe Pr**

Chess Pub, *(Chess Pubns., Inc.; 0-935273),* 232 E. University Pkwy., Baltimore, MD 21218 (SAN 695-7404) Tel 410-243-5943; Fax: 410-467-5973; Toll Free: 800-467-5943.

Cheval Intl, *(Cheval International; 0-9640610; 1-885351),* 7600 Anderson Rd., Black Hawk, SD 57718 Tel 605-787-6486; Fax: 605-787-6203
E-mail: cheval@rapidnet.com
Web site: http://www.chevalinternational.com
Dist(s): **B&N Imports** *(Barnes & Noble Bks.-Imports)*
Baker & Taylor *(Baker & Taylor Bks.).*

Chevron Pub, *(Chevron Publishing Corp.; 1-883581),* 5018 Dorsey Hall Dr., Suite 104, Ellicott City, MD 21042 Tel 410-740-0065; Fax: 410-740-9213.

Chi Horticult, *(Chicago Horticultural Society/Chicago Botanic Garden; 0-939914),* 1000 Lake Cook Rd., Glencoe, IL 60022 (SAN 216-7980) Tel 847-835-5440; Fax: 847-835-1421
Web site: http://www.chicago-botanic.org.

Chi Rho Pr, *(Chi Rho Pr.; 1-888493),* Div. of Mid-Atlantic District, Universal Fellowship of Metropolitan Community Churches, Orders Addr.: P.O. Box 7864, Gaithersburg, MD 20898 Tel 301-926-1208 (phone/fax)
E-mail: mail@chirhopress.com; orders@chirhopress.com
Web site: http://www.chirhopress.com.

Chicago Ling, *(Chicago Linguistic Society; 0-914203),* Affil. of Univ. of Chicago, 1010 E. 59th St., Chicago, IL 60637 (SAN 241-9297) Tel 773-702-8529; 773-702-8522; Fax: 773-834-0924
E-mail: linguistic@uchicago.edu
Web site: http://www.humanities.uchicago.edu/linguistics
Dist(s): **Slavica** *(Slavica Pubs., Inc.).*

†**Chicago Review,** *(Chicago Review Pr., Inc.; 0-914090; 0-914091; 1-55652),* 814 N. Franklin St., Chicago, IL 60610 (SAN 213-5744) Tel 312-337-0747; Fax: 312-337-5985; Toll Free: 800-888-4741 (orders only)
E-mail: orders@ipgbook.com; frontdesk@ipgbook.com
Web site: http://www.ipgbook.com
Dist(s): **Cobblestone Pub Co** *(Cobblestone Publishing Co.)*
Gryphon Hse *(Gryphon Hse., Inc.)*
IPG Chicago *(Independent Pubs. Group); CIP.*

Chicago Spectrum, *(Chicago Spectrum Pr.; 1-58374; 1-879260; 1-886094),* Div. of Evanston Publishing Inc., 4824 Brownsboro Ctr., Louisville, KY 40207 Tel 502-899-1919; Fax: 502-896-0246; Toll Free: 888-266-5780 (888-BOOKS-80); 800-594-5190
E-mail: info@evanstonpublishing.com; EvanstonPB@aol.com
Web site: http://www.EvanstonPublishing.com
Dist(s): **Baker & Taylor** *(Baker & Taylor Bks.)*
Partners-West *(Partners/West).*

Chick Pubns, *(Chick Pubns., Inc.; 0-937958; 0-7589),* P.O. Box 3500, Ontario, CA 91761-1019 (SAN 211-7770) Tel 909-987-0771; Fax: 909-941-8128; Toll Free: 800-932-3050
E-mail: orderdesk@chick.com
Web site: http://www.chick.com.

Child Hosp LA, *(Children's Hospital of Los Angeles; 0-9623727),* 4650 Sunset Blvd., Mailstop 29, Los Angeles, CA 90027 Tel 323-669-4681; Fax: 323-664-0868
E-mail: jwelborne@chla,usc.edu
Web site: http://www.childrenshospital.org.

Child Hospice VA, *(Children's Hospice International; 0-932321),* 2202 Mount Vernon Ave., No. 3C, Alexandria, VA 22301-1314 (SAN 687-0570) Tel 703-684-0330; Fax: 703-684-0226; Toll Free: 800-242-4453; P.O. Box 756, Davidson, NC 28036 Tel 704-491-2833
E-mail: chi@chionline.com
Web site: http://www.chionline.com.

†**Child Welfare,** *(Child Welfare League of America, Inc.; 0-87868; 1-58760),* 440 First St., NW, 3rd Flr., Washington, DC 20001-2085 (SAN 201-9876) Tel 202-638-2952; Fax: 301-206-9789 (orders only); 202-638-4004; Toll Free: 800-407-6273 (orders only) ; *Imprints:* CWLA Pr (C W L A Press)
E-mail: cwla@pmds.com
Web site: http://www.cwla.org
Dist(s): **Baker & Taylor** *(Baker & Taylor Bks.)*
Koen Bk Distributors *(Koen Bk. Distributors); CIP.*

Childbirth Graphics, *(Childbirth Graphics, Ltd.; 0-943114),* P.O. Box 21207, Waco, TX 76702-1207 (SAN 240-3587).

†**Childrens,** *(Children's Pr.; 0-516),* Div. of Grolier Publishing, Orders Addr.: P.O. Box 1796, Danbury, CT 06816 Toll Free Fax: 800-374-4329; Toll Free: 800-621-1115; Edit Addr.: 90 Sherman Tpke., Danbury, CT 06816 (SAN 201-9264) Tel 203-797-3500; Fax: 203-797-3657
Web site: http://www.publishing.grolier.com/
Dist(s): **Shens Bks** *(Shen's Bks.); CIP.*

Childrens Defense, *(Children's Defense Fund; 0-938008; 1-881985),* 25 E St., NW, Washington, DC 20001 (SAN 216-1133) Tel 202-628-8787; Fax: 202-662-3510; Toll Free: 800-275-2222.

Childrens Hospital of Philadelphia, *(Children's Hospital of Philadelphia, The; 0-9617370),* 34th St. & Civic Ctr. Blvd., Philadelphia, PA 19104 (SAN 663-7949) Tel 215-590-1099; Fax: 215-590-3299.

Childs Hosp, *(Project CHAMP, Children's National Medical Ctr.; 0-9634295),* Div. of Children's Hospital, 111 Michigan Ave., NW, Washington, DC 20010-2970 Tel 202-884-5450; Fax: 202-939-5989.

Childs Med Ventures, *(Children's Medical Ventures, Inc.; 0-9666425),* 541 Main St., Suite 220, South Weymouth, MA 02190 Tel 781-337-3449; Fax: 781-337-5938; Toll Free: 800-377-3449
E-mail: info@childmed.com
Web site: http://www.childmed.com.

Childswork, *(Childswork/Childsplay; 1-882732; 1-58815),* Div. of The Guidance Channel, Orders Addr.: P.O. Box 760, Plainview, NY 11803-0760 Tel 516-349-5520; Fax: 516-349-5521; Toll Free Fax: 800-262-1886; Toll Free: 800-962-1141; 135 Dupont St., Plainview, NY 11803-0760
E-mail: karens@at-risk.com; info@childswork.com
Web site: http://www.childswork.com.

Chilmark Hse, *(Chilmark Hse.; 0-937532),* 5600 Wisconsin Ave., Suite 209, Chevy Chase, MD 20815 (SAN 215-9457).

†**China Bks,** *(China Bks. & Periodicals, Inc.; 0-8351),* 2929 24th St., San Francisco, CA 94110-4126 (SAN 145-0557) Tel 415-282-2994; Fax: 415-282-0994
E-mail: info@chinabooks.com
Web site: http://www.chinabooks.com
Dist(s): **Shens Bks** *(Shen's Bks.); CIP.*

China Hlthways, *(China Healthways Institute; 1-889983),* 115 N. El Camino Real, San Clemente, CA 92672 Tel 714-361-3976; Fax: 714-498-0947; Toll Free: 800-743-5608
E-mail: chi@exo.com
Web site: http://exo.com/~chi/.

China Intl Bk (CHN) *Dist. by* **Distribks Inc.**

Chinese Univ (HKG) *(962-201) Dist. by* **Coronet Bks.**

Chinese Univ (HKG) *(962-201) Dist. by* **U of Mich Pr.**

Chinmaya Pubns, *(Chinmaya Pubns.; 1-880687),* 1218 Saint Matthew, Los Altos, CA 94024 Fax: 650-961-7878
E-mail: publications@chinmaya.org
Web site: http://www.chinmaya.org/publications
Dist(s): **Bookpeople** *(Bookpeople)*
New Leaf Dist *(New Leaf Distributing Co., Inc.).*

Chiron Pubns, *(Chiron Pubns.; 0-933029; 1-888602),* 400 Linden Ave., Wilmette, IL 60091 (SAN 689-1659) Tel 847-256-7551; Fax: 847-256-2202; Toll Free: 800-397-8109
Dist(s): **Continuum** *(Continuum International Publishing Group, Inc.)*
In Between *(In Between Bks.).*

Chiropract Paradigm, *(Chiropractic Paradigm; 0-9637924),* 1103 Russell Pkwy., Warner Robins, GA 31088 Tel 912-922-4091; Fax: 912-929-8822; Toll Free: 800-336-2013
Web site: http://www.medianet.ca/nsca/health.htm.

Chiropractic Jrnl, *(Chiropractic Journal, The; 0-9647168),* 2950 N. Dobson Rd., Suite 1, Chandler, AZ 85224 Fax: 602-732-9313; Toll Free: 800-347-1011
Dist(s): **Baker & Taylor** *(Baker & Taylor Bks.)*
SCB Distributors *(SCB Distributors).*

Chis Enterprise, *(Chi's Enterprise, Inc.; 0-9657847),* 1435 N. Brasher St., Anaheim, CA 92807 Tel 714-777-1542; Fax: 714-777-7186; Toll Free: 800-457-5708
E-mail: veinlite@mindspring.com
Web site: http://www.chi-health.com/chi.htm.

Chldrns Fnd, *(Children's Foundation; 1-884093),* 725 Fifteenth St. NW, Suite 505, Washington, DC 20005-2109 Tel 202-347-3300; Fax: 202-347-3382
Web site: http://www.childrensfoundation.net.

Chllnger, *(Challenger Corp.; 1-58016; 1-889244),* 5530 Summer Ave., Memphis, TN 38134 Tel 901-385-1840; Fax: 901-385-8380; Toll Free: 888-242-5536
E-mail: steveh@chall.com
Web site: http://www.chall.com.

†CHOICE, *(CHOICE; 0-930659),* 1233 Locust St., 3rd Flr., Philadelphia, PA 19107 (SAN 260-3969) Tel 215-985-3355; *CIP.*

Chr Legal, *(Christian Legal Society; 0-944561),* 4208 Evergeen Ln., Suite 222, Annandale, VA 22003 (SAN 224-0947) Tel 703-642-1070; Fax: 703-642-1075.

Chr Marriage, *(Christian Marriage Enrichment; 0-938786),* P.O. Box 2468, Orange, CA 92859-0468 (SAN 216-1141).

Chrch Grwth VA, *(Church Growth Institute; 0-941005; 1-57052),* Div. of Ephesians Four Ministries, Orders Addr.: P.O. Box 9176, Oxnard, CA 93031; Edit Addr.: P.O. Box 7000, Forest, VA 24551 Tel 804-525-0022; Fax: 804-525-0608; Toll Free Fax: 800-860-3109 (orders only); Toll Free: 800-553-4769
E-mail: cgimail@churchgrowth.org
Web site: http://www.churchgrowth.org
Dist(s): **Spring Arbor Dist** *(Spring Arbor Distributors Inc.).*

**Chris Mass, *(Christopher Publishing Hse.; 0-8158),* 24 Rockland St., Hanover, MA 02339 (SAN 202-1625) Tel 781-826-7474; Fax: 781-826-5556
E-mail: cph@atigroupinc.com
Web site: http://atigroupinc.com.**

Chrisolith Bks, *(Chrisolith Bks.; 0-916085),* 2907 Belmont Blvd, Nashville, TN 37212 (SAN 294-7099) Tel 615-329-4182.

Christ for the Nations, *(Christ for the Nations, Inc.; 0-89985),* P.O. Box 769000, Dallas, TX 75376-9000 (SAN 211-7800) Tel 214-376-1711; Fax: 214-302-6228; Toll Free: 800-933-2364
E-mail: info@cfni.org
Web site: http://www.cfni.org
Dist(s): **Anchor Distributors** *(Anchor Distributors).*

Christ Found, *See* **Pts of Light Distributing**

Christ Growth Pubs, *(Christian Growth Pubs., Inc.; 0-940445),* P.O. Box 88, Santa Margarita, CA 93453-0088 (SAN 664-3655).

Christ Med & Dental Assns, *(Christian Medical & Dental Assns.; 0-9666809; 0-9706631),* Orders Addr.: P.O. Box 7500, Bristol, TN 37621 Tel 423-844-1000; Fax: 423-844-1005; Toll Free: 888-230-2637; Edit Addr.: 501 Fifth St., Bristol, TN 37620 (SAN 253-6102)
E-mail: main@cmdahome.org; alicia@cmdahome.org
Web site: http://www.cmdahome.org.

Christ Med & Dental Soc, *See* **Christ Med & Dental Assns**

Christian Pub, *(Christian Publishing Services, Inc.; 0-88144),* Subs. of Harrison Hse. Pubs., P.O. Box 55388, Tulsa, OK 74155-1388 (SAN 260-0285) Tel 918-494-5966
Dist(s): **Harrison Hse** *(Harrison Hse., Inc.).*

Christian Servs Pub, *(Christian Services Publishing; 1-879854),* Div. of Christian Services Network, 1959 Longs Hill Rd., El Cajon, CA 92021 Tel 619-444-0695; Fax: 619-579-0685; Toll Free: 800-636-7276 Do not confuse with Christian Services, Damascus, MD.

Christian Vet, *(Christian Veterinary Mission; 1-886532),* Div. of World Concern, P.O. Box 526, Ocilla, GA 31774 Tel 912-468-7711 (phone/fax)
E-mail: missionvet@aol.com.

Christopher Pubns, *(Christopher Pubns.; 1-879436),* Orders Addr.: P.O. Box 412, Springville, UT 84663 Tel 801-489-4254; Fax: 801-489-8341; Toll Free: 800-372-8255; Edit Addr.: 25W200 South, Suite 16, Springville, UT 84663 Do not confuse with Christopher Pubns., Atlanta, GA
E-mail: publications@snh.cc
Web site: http://www.snh.cc
Dist(s): **New Leaf Dist** *(New Leaf Distributing Co., Inc.)*
Royal Pubns Inc *(Royal Pubns., Inc.).*

Chrlston Ultrasnd, *(Charleston Ultrasound Institute; 0-9651644),* 954 Nabors Dr., Charleston, SC 29412 Tel 803-762-6539.

Chron Guide, *(Chronicle Guidance Pubns., Inc.; 0-912578; 1-55631),* Orders Addr.: P.O. Box 1190, Moravia, NY 13118-1190 (SAN 202-1641) Tel 315-497-0330; Fax: 315-497-3359; Toll Free: 800-622-7284; Edit Addr.: 66 Aurora St., Moravia, NY 13118
E-mail: CustomerService@ChronicleGuidance.com
Web site: http://www.chronicleguidance.com.

Chronic Fatigue, *See* **T Schlosser**

†Chronicle Bks, *(Chronicle Bks. LLC; 0-8118; 0-87701; 0-938491),* Div. of Chronicle Publishing Co., 85 Second St., San Francisco, CA 94105 (SAN 202-165X) Tel 415-537-4200; Fax: 415-537-4460; Toll Free Fax: 800-858-7787; Toll Free: 800-722-6657 (orders only)
E-mail: frontdesk@chroniclebooks.com
Web site: http://www.chroniclebooks.com
Dist(s): **Continental Bk** *(Continental Bk. Co., Inc.)*
Lectorum Pubns *(Lectorum Pubns., Inc.)*
Shens Bks *(Shen's Bks.); CIP.*

Chubb Commun, *(Chubb Communications, Inc.; 1-888026),* 3433 Sea Ledge Ln., Santa Barbara, CA 93109 Tel 805-687-5188; Fax: 805-687-5165.

Chugh Pubns (IND) *Dist. by* **S Asia.**

Church (GBR) *(0-443; 0-7000) Dist. by* **Saunders.**

Churchill Ctr, *(Churchill Ctr., Inc.; 0-943879),* Orders Addr.: P.O. Box 96, Contoocook, NH 03229 Tel 603-746-3452; Fax: 603-746-6963; Edit Addr.: P.O. Box 385, Contoocook, NH 03229 (SAN 242-2344) Tel 603-746-4433; Fax: 603-746-4260
E-mail: wsc1874@msn.com
Web site: http://www.winstonchurchill.org.

Churchill PC, *(Churchill PC Systems; 0-932223),* 2948 Dothan Ln., Dallas, TX 75229 (SAN 686-6069) Tel 972-247-5390.

CICRCL Pr, *(CICRCL Pr.; 1-882056),* P.O. Box 63720, Colorado Springs, CO 80962-3720 (SAN 248-3017) Tel 719-282-1753; Fax: 719-282-1853
E-mail: cicrcl@weinholds.org.

CIP Comms, *(CIP Communications; 0-9631938),* 967 North Point St., San Francisco, CA 94109 Tel 415-434-2175; Fax: 415-393-8083.

Circle Pr CA, *(Circle Pr.; 0-9621646),* 16444 Bolsa Chica St., Space 40, Huntington Beach, CA 92649 (SAN 251-7280) Do not confuse with companies with same name in New York, NY, Hamden, CT.

Circuit Writer, *(Circuit Writer; 0-9617971),* 2522 Waterford Rd., Auburn, AL 36830-4114 (SAN 666-2447).

CIS Comm, *(CIS Communications, Inc.; 0-935063; 1-56062),* 180 Park Avenue, Lakewood, NJ 08701 (SAN 694-5953) Tel 732-905-3000; Fax: 732-367-6666.

Citadel Pr Imprint of Kensgtn Pub Corp

Citilites Pr, *(Citilites Pr.; 0-9714865),* P.O. Box 425, Fulton, MD 20759-9652.

City Hope, *(City of Hope, Dept. Library Services; 0-940876),* 1500 E. Duarte Rd., Duarte, CA 91010 (SAN 209-1267) Tel 626-301-8497; Fax: 626-357-1929
E-mail: library@coh.org
Web site: http://www.cityofhope.org.

**†City Lights, *(City Lights Bks.; 0-87286),* 261 Columbus Ave., San Francisco, CA 94133 (SAN 202-1684) Tel 415-362-1901; Fax: 415-362-4921
E-mail: staff@citylights.com
Web site: http://www.citylights.com
Dist(s): Consort Bk Sales *(Consortium Bk. Sales & Distribution)*
SPD-Small Pr Dist *(SPD-Small Pr. Distribution)*
Subterranean Co *(Subterranean Co.); CIP.***

Civic Res Inst, *(Civic Research Institute, Inc.; 1-887554),* Orders Addr.: P.O. Box 585, Kingston, NJ 08528-0585 Tel 609-683-4450; Fax: 609-683-7291; Edit Addr.: 2067 Broadway, Suite 50, New York, NJ 10023 Tel 212-875-0414; Fax: 212-875-0167
E-mail: civres2@aol.com
Web site: http://www.crihealthcarepubs.com; http://www.civicresearchinstitute.com.

CIVICUS, *(CIVICUS: World Alliance for Citizen Participation; 0-9644001; 1-929842),* 919 18th St., NW, 3rd Flr., Washington, DC 20006 Tel 202-331-8518; Fax: 202-331-8774
E-mail: info@civicus.org
Web site: http://www.civicus.org.

Civil Society, *(Civil Society Publishing; 0-9671803),* P.O. Box 1663, Ames, IA 50010-1663
E-mail: noadnz@iastate.edu
Web site: http://www.mobbing-usa.com
Dist(s): **BookMasters** *(BookMasters, Inc.).*

Civis (CHE) *Dist. by* **U of Mich Pr.**

CIVIS-Civitas, *(CIVIS/Civitas; 0-9610016),* Div. of Buchrerlag CIVIS Pubns., Orders Addr.: P.O. Box 26, Swain, NY 14884 (SAN 268-5647) Tel 607-545-6213; Toll Free: 800-604-4884; Edit Addr.: 1 Main St., Swain, NY 14884.

Ckbk Morris Pr, *See* **Morris Pubng**

CKRB Pub, *(CKRB Publishing Co.; 0-9618671),* 1970 E. 16th St., Apt. N306, Newport Beach, CA 92663-5930 (SAN 668-5536).

CL Prodns, *(CL Productions; 1-887398),* 136 Verano Loop, Santa Fe, NM 87505-8350 Tel 505-466-2996; Toll Free: 800-203-3597.

Claitors, *(Claitor's Publishing Div.; 0-87511; 1-57980),* 3165 S. Acadian, P.O. Box 261333, Baton Rouge, LA 70826-1333 (SAN 206-8346) Tel 504-344-0476; Fax: 504-344-0480; Toll Free: 800-274-1403
E-mail: claitors@claitors.com
Web site: http://www.claitors.com
Dist(s): **Bernan Associates** *(Bernan Assocs.)*
Brodart *(Brodart Co.)*
Midpt Trade *(Midpoint Trade Bks., Inc.).*

CLAO Inc, *(CLAO, Inc.; 1-929652),* Orders Addr.: P.O. Box 24850, New Orleans, LA 70184-4850 Tel 504-835-3937; Fax: 504-833-5884; Edit Addr.: 721 Papworth Ave., Suite 206, Metairie, LA 70005
E-mail: tprterson@clao.org
Web site: http:///www.clao.org
Dist(s): **Kendall-Hunt** *(Kendall/Hunt Publishing Co.).*

Claremont Grad, *(Claremont Graduate Univ., Ctr. for Developmental Studies in Education; 0-941742),* 150 E. Tenth St., Claremont, CA 91711-6160 (SAN 239-1813) Tel 909-621-8075; Fax: 909-621-8734
E-mail: antonia.darde@cgu.edu.

Claremont Inst, *(Claremont Institute; 0-930783),* 250 W. First St. Suite 330, Claremont, CA 91711-4744 (SAN 677-6191) Tel 909-621-6825; Fax: 909-626-8724 ;
Imprints: Dr for Respons Gun (Doctors for Responsible Gun Ownersip)
Web site: http://www.claremont.org.

**Clarence Bass, *(Bass, Clarence Ripped Enterprises; 0-9609714),* 528 Chama NE, Albuquerque, NM 87108 (SAN 268-229X) Tel 505-266-5858; Fax: 505-266-9123
E-mail: cncbass@aol.com
Web site: http://www.cbass.com.**

Clarendon Pr Imprint of OUP

Clarian Hlth, *(Clarian Health; 0-9603164; 1-884742),* P.O. Box 1367, Indianapolis, IN 46206-1367 (SAN 221-7392) Tel 317-929-8021; Fax: 317-929-8397
Dist(s): **Ambulatory Innovat** *(Ambulatory Innovations, Inc.).*

Clark & Westman-Magnolia, *(Clark & Westman/Magnolia Hse.; 0-913145),* 1820 Dartmouth Ave., W., Seattle, WA 98199 (SAN 265-3915) Tel 206-283-1160; Fax: 206-283-5282
E-mail: eleg@aol.com.

Clark Pubs, *(Clark Pubs.; 0-9641197),* 133 Chestnut St., Amherst, MA 01002 Tel 941-255-0431
E-mail: ellusmith@aol.com
Dist(s): **Baker & Taylor** *(Baker & Taylor Bks.)*
Brodart *(Brodart Co.)*
North Country *(North Country Bks., Inc.)*
Quality Bks IL *(Quality Bks., Inc.).*

†Clark U Pr, *(Clark Univ. Pr.; 0-914206),* 950 Main St., Worcester, MA 01610 (SAN 205-6135) Tel 508-793-7278; Fax: 508-793-8839
E-mail: swapner@clarku.edu
Web site: http://www.clarku.edu; *CIP.*

Clarke Pub, *(Clarke Publishing; 0-9627883),* 191 University Bldg., Suite 249, Denver, CO 80206 Tel 303-377-4372
E-mail: DrIMichael@aol.com.

Clarkson Potter Imprint of Crown Pub Group

Classic Bks, *(Classic Bks.; 1-58201; 0-7426),* Orders Addr.: P.O. Box 130, Murrieta, CA 92564-0130 Tel 888-265-3547; Fax: 888-265-3550.

Classical Pubng (IND) *(81-7054) Dist. by* **S Asia.**

Classics India Pubns (IND) *(81-85132) Dist. by* **S Asia.**

Clean Data, *(Clean Data, Inc.; 1-881011),* a/o Chris Herndl, 2327 Englert Dr., No. 301, Durham, NC 27713 Tel 919-544-8752; Fax: 919-544-8558
E-mail: Ibondos@cleandata.com.

Clearwtr Pools Pub Co, *(Clearwater Pools Publishing Co.; 0-9619258),* P.O. Box 242, Carbondale, CO 81623 (SAN 243-573X) Tel 970-925-4149.

Cleis Pr, *(Cleis Pr.; 0-939416; 1-57344),* P.O. Box 14684, San Francisco, CA 94114-0684 (SAN 284-9976) Tel 415-575-4700; Fax: 415-575-4705; Toll Free: 800-780-2279
E-mail: cleis@cleispress.com
Web site: http://www.cleispress.com
Dist(s): **Baker & Taylor** *(Baker & Taylor Bks.)*
Bookpeople *(Bookpeople)*
Publishers Group *(Publishers Group West).*

Clerc Bks Imprint of Gallaudet Univ Pr

Cleveland Clinic, *(Cleveland Clinic Foundation; 0-9615424),* 9500 Euclid Ave., Cleveland, OH 44195-5058 (SAN 696-3196) Tel 216-444-3751; Fax: 216-444-9111
E-mail: Matarel@cesmtp.uf.org.

Cliff Imprint of Hungry Minds

Cliff Street Imprint of HarperTrade

CliffTop, *(CliffTop Publishing Co.; 0-9654882),* Orders Addr.: P.O. Box 44847, Eden Prairie, MN 55344 Tel 612-942-7658; Edit Addr.: 8621 Basswood Rd., Eden Prairie, MN 55344.

Clifton Pub, *(Clifton Publishing; 0-9652878),* 6109 Fox Run, Fairfax, VA 22030-5949 Tel 703-502-3994; Fax: 703-502-1878
E-mail: sales@cliftonpublishing.com
Web site: http://www.cliftonpublishing.com.

Cline-Fay Inst, *See* **Love & Logic**

Clinical Design, *(Clinical Design Group; 1-889160),* 2128 W. Evergreen Ave., Chicago, IL 60622 Tel 773-489-5721; Fax: 773-489-4281.

Clinical Hearing Consults, *(Clinical Hearing Consultants; 0-9614656),* 8732 E. Fairmount Ave., Scottsdale, AZ 85251-5055 (SAN 692-2031).

Clinical Lab Mgmnt Assn, *(Clinical Laboratory Management Assn.; 0-9625414; 1-892942),* 989 Old Eagle School Rd., Suite 815, Wayne, PA 19087-1704 Tel 610-995-9580; Fax: 610-995-9568
Web site: http://www.clma.org.

Clinical Psych, *(Clinical Psychology Publishing Co., Inc.; 0-88422),* Div. of John Wiley & Sons, Inc., 605 Third Ave., New York, NY 10158-0001 (SAN 201-7679).

Cloud Chief, *(Cloud Chief Publishing; 0-9636602),* P.O. Box 2344, Norman, OK 73070-2344 Tel 405-447-4008
E-mail: ww@telepath.com
Dist(s): **New Leaf Dist** *(New Leaf Distributing Co., Inc.)*
Nutri-Books Corp *(Nutri-Bks. Corp.).*

Cloverdale, *See* **Wyndham Hall**

Clown Ambassador, *See* **Clown Natural Hlth**

Clown Natural Hlth, *(Clown of Natural Health; 0-9648663),* 3131 Palo Verde Ave., Long Beach, CA 90808-4056 Tel 562-377-1141
E-mail: holitte5353@aol.com.

Clunie Pr (GBR) *(0-902965) Dist. by* **Other Pr LLC.**

CMAS Bks, *(CMAS Bks.; 0-9665356),* Div. of MIB, Inc., 160 University Ave., Westwood, MA 02090-2307 Tel 781-329-4500; Fax: 781-329-3379
Web site: http://www.mib.com.

CMDC Systs, *(CMDC Systems, Inc.; 0-9656032),* 1119 Ridglea Way, Boulder, CO 80303 Tel 303-499-5324; Fax: 303-499-5303; Toll Free: 888-367-9004
E-mail: danb@cmdcsystems.com
Web site: http://www.cmdcsystems.com.

CMI, *(CMI; 0-9670444),* 6400 N. Keating, Lincolnwood, IL 60646 Tel 847-679-8336; Fax: 773-465-0154
E-mail: karen6258@aol.com
Web site: http://www.homefirst.com.

Cmmn Man Inst, *(Common Man Institute; 0-944402),* 12665 Hwy. 59, N., Gillette, WY 82716-9801 (SAN 243-5535) Tel 307-682-2626.

CNC Med Physics, *(CNC Medical Physics Services; 0-9638266),* 2 Woodledge Ln., North Easton, MA 02356 Tel 508-238-2250 (phone/fax); 4513 Vernon Blvd., Madison, WI 53705-4964
E-mail: cncmed@juno.com.

CNC of Naprapathy, *(Chicago National College of Naprapathy Pr.; 0-9637136),* 3330 N. Milwaukee Ave., Chicago, IL 60641 (SAN 297-9802) Tel 773-282-2686; Fax: 773-282-2688; Toll Free: 800-262-6620.

CnE Varieties, *(CnE Varieties, Inc.; 0-9602118),* 3560 Hetzel Dr., Parma, OH 44134 (SAN 212-3754) Tel 440-843-1537; Fax: 440-843-3618
E-mail: varieties@msn.com.

CNS, *(CNS Pubns., Inc.; 0-926544),* Orders Addr.: 130 Third St., Box 96, Ashland, OR 97520 Tel 541-488-2805; Fax: 541-482-9252; Toll Free: 800-888-0617
E-mail: cns@mind.net
Web site: http://www.cnsproductions.com.

Cnslts in Care, *(Consultants in Care; 0-9640767),* 86 Shady Glen Rd., Memphis, TN 38120-2020.

Cnslts Psych Nursing, *(Consultants in Psychiatric Nursing, Inc.; 0-9627287),* 20 Ladd St., Portsmouth, NH 03801-4080 Fax: 603-433-6341.

Cntct Assocs Intl, *(Contact Assocs. International, Ltd.; 0-911059),* 600 Middle Rd., Bayport, NY 11705 (SAN 269-3526) Tel 516-472-2020.

CO Hist Soc, *(Colorado History Society; 0-942576),* Colorado Heritage Ctr., 1300 Broadway, Denver, CO 80203 (SAN 239-6297) Tel 303-866-4993.

Coast Pub OR, *(Coast Publishing; 0-9627341),* Orders Addr.: P.O. Box 3399, Coos Bay, OR 97420 (SAN 297-2905); Edit Addr.: 873 Vista Ct., Reedsport, OR 97467 Tel 541-271-3418; Fax: 541-271-3220 Do not confuse with Coast Publishing, Carmel, CA
Dist(s): **Baker & Taylor** *(Baker & Taylor Bks.).*

Cobb & Henry Pubs, *(Cobb & Henry Pubs.; 0-943539),* 1 Sutton Pl., Hampton, VA 23666 (SAN 668-5390) Tel 757-827-7213; Fax: 757-827-1060; Toll Free: 800-972-3273.

Coburn Pr, *(Coburn Pr.; 0-9631814),* P.O. Box 635, Dixfield, ME 04224-0635 Tel 207-562-7092
E-mail: jsrogers@aqate.net
Web site: http://www.real-food.com.

†Codex Pr, *(Codex Pr.; 0-935548),* P.O. Box 1686, Taos, NM 87571 (SAN 213-7925) Tel 505-751-3229
E-mail: codexbooks@earthlink.net
Web site: http://www.codexpress.org*; CIP.*

Coffee Break, *(Coffee Break Pr.; 0-933992),* P.O. Box 103, Burley, WA 98322 (SAN 212-341X) Tel 206-851-4074.

Cogito Bks Imprint of Med Physics Pub

Cogito Lrning, *(Cogito Learning Media, Inc.; 1-58032; 1-888902),* 235 Montgomery St., Flr. 27, San Francisco, CA 94104-3114 Tel 415-765-1900; Fax: 415-785-1902; Toll Free: 800-938-4465
E-mail: support@cogitomedia.com; think@cogitomedia.com
Web site: http://www.cogitomedia.com
Dist(s): **Natl Bk Netwk** *(National Bk. Network).*

Cognizant Comm, *(Cognizant Communication Corp.; 1-882345),* 3 Hartsdale Rd., Elmsford, NY 10523 Tel 914-592-7720; Fax: 914-592-8981
E-mail: cogcomm@aol.com
Web site: http://www.cognizantcommunication.com.

Coker Pub, *(Coker Publishing Hse.; 0-933012),* P.O. Box 81017, Chicago, IL 60681-0017 (SAN 284-9984).

Coker Publishing, *(Coker Publishing, LLC; 0-9655304),* 11660 Alpharetta Hwy., No. 710, Roswell, GA 30076 Tel 678-832-2000; Fax: 678-832-2016; Toll Free: 800-345-5829
E-mail: kaystanley@cokergroup.com
Web site: http://www.cokergroup.com.

†Col U Pr, *(Columbia Univ. Pr.; 0-231),* 61 W. 62nd St., New York, NY 10023 (SAN 212-2472) Tel 212-459-0600; Fax: 212-459-3678 ; *Imprints:* King's Crown Paperbacks (King's Crown Paperbacks)
Web site: http://www.columbia.edu/cu/cup
Dist(s): **Continental Bk** *(Continental Bk. Co., Inc.); CIP.*

Col U Sch Nursing, *(Columbia Univ. Schl. of Nursing; 0-9631670),* Div. of Columbia Univ., 630 W. 168th St., New York, NY 10032 Tel 212-305-3254; Fax: 212-305-6937.

Colco Pub, *(Colco Publishing; 0-9618345),* 5110 Yarwell, Houston, TX 77096 (SAN 667-3139) Tel 281-723-6111.

†Cold Spring Harbor, *(Cold Spring Harbor Laboratory Pr.; 0-87969),* Orders Addr.: 500 Sunnyside Blvd., Woodbury, NY 11797 (SAN 203-6185) Tel 516-422-4100; Fax: 516-422-4097; Toll Free: 800-843-4388
E-mail: cshpress@cshl.org
Web site: http://www.cshlpress.com*; CIP.*

Cole Valley Pr, *(Cole Valley Pr.; 0-9644089),* 915 Cole St. Suite 345, San Francisco, CA 94117 Tel 415-665-3027.

Coleman Pub, *(Coleman Publishing, Inc.; 0-87418; 0-942494),* 16363 Camini Ln., Fort Lauderdale, FL 33326 (SAN 238-1508) Tel 954-389-8076.

Colgan Inst, *(Colgan Institute; 0-9624840; 1-886736),* 523 Encinitas Blvd., Suite 204, Encinitas, CA 92024 Tel 760-632-7722; Fax: 760-632-7375 ; *Imprints:* C I Pubns CA (C I Publications).

Coll & U Personnel, *See* **CUPA-HR**

Coll Admin Pubns, *(College Administration Pubns., Inc.; 0-912557),* Orders Addr.: 830-D Fairview Rd., Asheville, NC 28803-1081 (SAN 240-8155) Tel 828-277-8777; Toll Free: 800-367-9577
E-mail: cap@collegepubs.com
Web site: http://www.collegepubs.com.

Coll Am Pathol, *(College of American Pathologists; 0-930304),* 325 Waukegan Rd., Northfield, IL 60093 (SAN 224-4160) Tel 847-832-7000; Fax: 847-832-8166; Toll Free: 800-323-4040.

Collective Creations, *(Collective Creations By Fisher; 0-9629201),* 262 Morada Ln., Santa Barbara, CA 93105 Tel 805-687-7611.

College Bd, *(College Board, The; 0-87447),* Orders Addr.: Two College Way, Forrester Center, WV 25438 (SAN 203-5685) Toll Free Fax: 800-525-5562; Toll Free: 800-323-7155 (for Visa, Mastercard, American Express, & Discover); Edit Addr.: 45 Columbus Ave., New York, NY 10023-6992 (SAN 203-5677) Tel 212-713-8000; Fax: 212-713-8309
Web site: http://www.collegboard.com
Dist(s): **H Holt & Co** *(Holt, Henry & Co., LLC)*
VHPS *(VHPS Holtzbrinck Pubs.).*

College Book, *(College Bk. Pubs., LLC; 0-9669823),* Orders Addr.: P.O. Box 483, East Hanover, NJ 07936 Tel 973-428-9454; Edit Addr.: 9 Heather Dr., East Hanover, NJ 07936.

College Pr Pub, *(College Pr. Publishing Co., Inc.; 0-89900),* Box 1132, 223 W. Third St., Joplin, MO 64802-1132 (SAN 211-9951) Tel 417-623-6280; Fax: 417-623-8250; Toll Free: 800-289-3300
E-mail: info@collegepress.com
Web site: http://www.collegepress.com
Dist(s): **Riverside-World** *(Riverside World)*
Spring Arbor Dist *(Spring Arbor Distributors Inc.).*

Collets (GBR) *Dist. by* **St Mut.**

Collins Pubns, *(Collins Pubns.; 0-9632857),* Orders Addr.: 3233 Grand Ave., Suite N-294, Chino Hills, CA 91709 (SAN 297-648X) Tel 909-590-2471; Fax: 909-628-9330
E-mail: collins@collinspub.com
Web site: http://www.collinspub.com
Dist(s): **Baker & Taylor** *(Baker & Taylor Bks.)*
Brodart *(Brodart Co.).*

Collins SF, *(Collins Pubs. San Francisco; 0-00),* Div. of HarperCollins Pubs., Inc., 10 E. 53rd St., New York, NY 10022 (SAN 247-5529) Tel 212-207-7000; Fax: 415-616-4777; Toll Free: 800-242-7737 (Bookstores)
Web site: http://www.harpercollins.com.

Colns (AUS) *(0-207; 0-7322) Dist. by* **Consort Bk Sales.**

Colo Cowboy, *(Colorado Cowboy Productions; 0-9641773),* 77 Clarkson St., Denver, CO 80218 Tel 303-781-7587.

Colon & Rectal Care, *(Colon & Rectal Care, Inc.; 0-9625295),* 7430 N. Shadeland Ave., Indianapolis, IN 46250 Tel 317-841-8090; Fax: 317-577-7538.

†Colonial Williamsburg, *(Colonial Williamsburg Foundation; 0-87935; 0-910412),* P.O. Box 3532, Williamsburg, VA 23187-3532 (SAN 128-4630) Fax: 757-565-8999 (orders only); Toll Free: 800-446-9240 (orders only)
Web site: http://www.colonialwilliamsburg.com
Dist(s): **Antique Collect** *(Antique Collectors' Club)*
Baker & Taylor *(Baker & Taylor Bks.)*
Koen Bk Distributors *(Koen Bk. Distributors); CIP.*

Color Coded Charting, *(Color Coded Charting & Filing Systems; 0-9605902),* 7759 California Ave., Riverside, CA 92504 (SAN 211-1888) Tel 909-688-0800.

Colorado Hlth, *(Colorado HealthNet; 0-9678647),* 1900 Baseline Rd., Boulder, CO 80302 Fax: 303 442-1194
E-mail: smccray@coloradohealthnet.org
Web site: http://www.coloradohealthnet.org.

Columbia College Chi, *(Columbia College Chicago; 0-932026),* 600 S. Michigan Ave., Chicago, IL 60640 (SAN 244-7932) Tel 312-344-8101 (phone/fax)
E-mail: tnawrocki@popmail.colum.edu
Web site: http://www.columbiacollegechicago.edu
Dist(s):* Login Pubs Consort *(Login Pubs. Consortium).

Columbia HCA Hlthcare, *(Columbia/HCA Healthcare Corp.; 0-9656835),* 1 Park Plaza, Bldg. 1-4E, Nashville, TN 37203 Tel 615-344-5703; Fax: 615-344-1128.

Columbia Pacific U Pr, *(Columbia Pacific Univ. Pr.; 0-945864),* 105 Digital Dr., Novato, CA 94949-5734 (SAN 248-0859) Tel 415-459-1650
E-mail: enquiries@cpuniv.edu.

†Columbia Pub, *(Columbia Publishing Co., Inc.; 0-914366),* 2 Hopkins Plaza, No. 900, Baltimore, MD 21201-2930 (SAN 201-8977) Tel 410-366-7070; Fax: 410-366-8687
Dist(s): **Bookpeople** *(Bookpeople); CIP.*

Columbine Imprint of Fawcett

Columbus Hlth, *(Columbus Health Dept.; 1-888492),* 181 Washington Blvd., Columbus, OH 43215 Tel 614-645-6252; Fax: 614-645-5888
E-mail: JSHUANG@Freenet.Columbus.oh.us.

Publisher Symbol Index

Columella Pr, *(Columella Pr.; 0-9605972),* P.O. Box 40098, Phoenix, AZ 85067 (SAN 216-7247) Tel 602-943-3770
E-mail: smilstein@webtv.net.

Colwell Syst, *(Colwell Systems; 0-940012),* Subs. of Deluxe Check Printer, Inc., 201 Kenyon Rd., Champaign, IL 61820 (SAN 208-1431) Tel 217-351-5400; Toll Free: 800-637-1140; 800-252-6960 (in Illinois).

Combined Bks, *See* **Combined Pub**

Combined Pub, *(Combined Publishing; 0-938289; 1-58097),* 476 W. Elm, P.O. Box 307, Conshohocken, PA 19428 Tel 610-828-2595; Fax: 610-828-2603; Toll Free: 800-418-6065
E-mail: combined@combinedpublishing.com
Web site: http://www.combinedpublishing.com
Dist(s): **Casemate Pubs** *(Casemate Pubs. & Bk. Distributors)*
Whitehurst & Clark *(Whitehurst & Clark).*

CoMed Comm, *(CoMed Communications; 0-943035),* Div. of Ted Thomas Assocs., Inc., 210 W. Washington Sq., Philadelphia, PA 19106-3512 (SAN 667-9307) Tel 215-592-7500.

Comfort Hse Pubs, *(Comfort Hse. Pubs.; 0-9622252),* Orders Addr.: P.O. Box 20973, Oklahoma City, OK 73156; Edit Addr.: 2521 NW 114th Terr., Oklahoma City, OK 73120 Tel 405-843-0595.

Comm Assn Inst, *See* **CAI**

†**Comm Econ Dev,** *(Committee for Economic Development; 0-87186),* 477 Madison Ave., New York, NY 10022 (SAN 202-1765) Tel 212-688-2063; Fax: 212-758-9068
E-mail: info@ced.org
Web site: http://www.ced.org; *CIP.*

Comm Europ Commun (BEL) *(92-825; 92-826; 92-827; 92-828) Dist. by* **Bernan Associates.**

Comm Intervention, *(Community Intervention, Inc.; 0-945485; 0-9613416),* 529 S. Seventh St., Suite 570, Minneapolis, MN 55415 (SAN 656-9706) Tel 612-332-6537; Toll Free: 800-328-0417.

Comm Nuclear Respon, *(Committee for Nuclear Responsibility, Inc.; 0-932682),* Orders Addr.: P.O. Box 421993, San Francisco, CA 94142-1933 (SAN 212-1530) Tel 415-776-8299 (phone/fax)
E-mail: policy@x-raysandhealth.org; cnr123@webtv.net
Web site: http://www.x-raysandhealth.org.

Comm Sec (GBR) *(0-85092) Dist. by* **Stylus Pub VA.**

Comm Serv Soc NY, *(Community Service Society of New York; 0-88156),* 105 E. 22nd St., New York, NY 10010 (SAN 204-3149) Tel 212-614-5314; Fax: 212-260-6218
Web site: http://www.cssny.org.

Comm Unltd, *(Communications Unlimited),* 1333 W. 120th Ave., No. 101, Denver, CO 80234-2709 (SAN 209-5459) Tel 303-450-2787.

Comm Unltd CA, *(Communication Unlimited; 0-910167; 0-9708621),* P.O. Box 6405, Santa Maria, CA 93456 (SAN 682-2568) Tel 805-937-8711; Toll Free Fax: 800-937-3035; Toll Free: 800-563-1454 ; *Imprints:* Dental Commun (Dental Communication Unlimited) Medical Comm (Medical Communication Unlimited)
E-mail: sops@fix.net
Web site: http://www.sops.com
Dist(s): **Baker & Taylor** *(Baker & Taylor Bks.).*

Command Spanish, *(Command Spanish; 1-888467),* P.O. Box 1091, Petal, MS 39465 Tel 601-582-8378; Fax: 601-582-5177
E-mail: info@commandspanish.com
Web site: http://www.commandspanish.com.

Common Courage, *(Common Courage Pr.; 0-9628838; 1-56751),* Orders Addr.: Box 702, Monroe, ME 04951 (SAN 299-223X) Tel 207-525-0900; Fax: 207-525-3068; Toll Free: 800-497-3207; Edit Addr.: 1 Red Barn Rd., Monroe, ME 04951
E-mail: orders-info@commoncouragepress.com
Web site: http://www.commoncouragepress.com
Dist(s): **LPC Group** *(LPC Group)*
SPD-Small Pr Dist *(SPD-Small Pr. Distribution).*

Commonwealth Imprint of S Asia

Commonwealth (IND) *(81-7169; 81-900026; 81-900046; 81-900066; 81-900069; 81-900077) Dist. by* **S Asia.**

†**Commun Skill,** *(Communication Skill Builders/Therapy Skill Builders; 0-7616; 0-88450),* Div. of The Psychological Corp., A Harcourt Co., 555 Academic Ct., San Antonio, TX 78204-2498 (SAN 201-7768) Toll Free Fax: 800-232-1223; Toll Free: 800-228-0752 ; *Imprints:* Thrpy Skill Bldrs (Therapy Skill Builders)
Web site: http://www.harcourt.com/; *CIP.*

Communs Skills, *(Communication Skills, Inc.; 1-884225),* 49 Richmondville Ave., Westport, CT 06880 Tel 203-227-1244; Fax: 203-226-8820; Toll Free: 800-824-2398.

Comn Studies, *(Communication Studies; 0-931814),* 6145 Anita St., Dallas, TX 75214-2612 (SAN 211-5530) Tel 214-823-1981
E-mail: crtimmins@yahoo.com
Web site: http://www.citybiz.com/drtimmins.

Comp Occup, *(Comprehensive Occupational; 1-883023),* P.O. Box 12770, Tucson, AZ 85732-2770 Tel 520-882-5852; Fax: 520-760-1566
E-mail: Peate@u.arizona.edu.

Comp Options, *See* **Present Dynam**

Comp Pr, *(Competency Pr.; 0-910307; 0-9602800; 1-56078),* Orders Addr.: P.O. Box 95, White Plains, NY 10605 (SAN 223-5579) Tel 914-948-6783; Fax: 914-961-7622; Edit Addr.: 9 Pine Brook Dr., White Plains, NY 10605.

Comp Res Assocs, *(Computer Resource Assocs. ,Inc.; 0-9658803),* 1110 Torrey Pines Rd., La Jolla, CA 92037 Tel 619-551-9308; Fax: 619-551-9956
E-mail: rjuarez@cra-usa.com
Web site: http://www.cra-usa.com.

†**Compact Books,** *(Compact Bks.; 0-936320),* 2131 Hollywood Blvd., Suite 204, Hollywood, FL 33020 (SAN 215-0670) Tel 954-925-5242
E-mail: lifetime@shadow.net
Web site: http://www.lifetimebooks.com; *CIP.*

Compact Clinicals, *(Compact Clinicals; 1-887537),* 7205 NW Waukomis Dr., Kansas City, MO 64151 Tel 816-587-0044; Fax: 816-587-7198; Toll Free: 800-408-8830
E-mail: ccdeanma@aol.com
Dist(s): **J Majors Co** *(Majors, J. A. Co.)*
Midpt Trade *(Midpoint Trade Bks., Inc.).*

Compass Imprint of Wheeler Pub

Compass Point, *(Compass Point Bks.; 0-7565),* 3722 W. 50th St., No.115, Minneapolis, MN 55410 (SAN 254-2013) Toll Free Fax: 877-371-1539; Toll Free: 877-371-1536
E-mail: custserv@compasspointbooks.com
Web site: http://www.compasspointbooks.com
Dist(s): **netLibrary CO** *(netLibrary, Inc.).*

Comp-based Patient Rec, *(Computer-based Patient Record Institute, Inc.; 0-9649285),* 1000 E. Woodfield Rd., Suite 102, Schaumburg, IL 60173 Tel 301-657-5918; Fax: 301-657-1296; 4915 Saint Elmo, Suite 401, Bethesda, MD 20814.

CompCare Pubns, *See* **Comp Occup**

Complement Med, *(Complementary Medicine Publishing Co.; 0-9638267),* Orders Addr.: P.O. Box 80085, Portland, OR 97280-1085 Fax: 503-452-1239; Toll Free: 800-952-2219; Edit Addr.: 5112 SW Garden Home Rd., Portland, OR 97280-0067.

Complmtry Medcne, *(Complementary Medicine Pr.; 0-9673034),* 44 Linden St., Brookline, MA 02445 Tel 617-738-4664; Fax: 617-738-4620; Toll Free: 800-873-3946
E-mail: cmp@redwingbooks.com
Dist(s): **Redwing Bk Co** *(Redwing Bk. Co.).*

Comprehen Cancer, *(Comprehensive Cancer Ctr. Communications; 0-9652910),* 205 Wallace Tumor Institute, 1824 Sixth Ave., S., Birmingham, AL 35294-3300 Tel 205-934-0282; Fax: 205-975-2432
E-mail: LeslieC@ccc.uab.edu
Web site: http://www.cancer.ccc.uab.edu.

Comprehen Health Educ, *(Comprehensive Health Education Foundation; 0-935529; 1-57021),* 22419 Pacific Hwy. S., Seattle, WA 98198-5106 (SAN 696-3668) Tel 206-824-2907; Fax: 206-824-3072; Toll Free: 800-323-2433
E-mail: chefstaff@chef.org
Web site: http://www.chef.org/.

Comprehensive Hlth, *(Comprehensive Health; 0-9636491),* 27701 Murrietta Rd., No. 30, Sun City, CA 92586 Fax: 909-679-8148; Toll Free: 888-244-4420
E-mail: rmotter@aol.com
Web site: http://www.crtadvised.com
Dist(s): **Bookpeople** *(Bookpeople).*

COMPress, *(COMPress; 0-88720; 0-933694),* Div. of Queue, Inc., 338 Commerce Dr., Fairfield, CT 06430 (SAN 284-9887) Tel 203-335-0908; Fax: 203-336-2481; Toll Free: 800-232-2224.

Comput in Occupat, *See* **Amer Col Occ**

Computational Mech MA, *(Computational Mechanics, Inc.),* 25 Bridge St., Billerica, MA 01821 (SAN 653-6425) Tel 978-667-5841; Fax: 978-667-7582
E-mail: marketing@compmech.com; info@compmech.com
Web site: http://www.compmech.com; http://www.witpress.com.

Comstock Bon, *(Comstock Bonanza Pr.; 0-933994),* 18919 William Quirk Dr., Grass Valley, CA 95945-8611 (SAN 223-694X) Tel 530-273-6220
Dist(s): **Wells** *(Wells, Philip V.).*

Comstock Edns, *(Comstock Editions, Inc.; 0-89174),* Orders Addr.: P.O. Box 2510, Novato, CA 94948 (SAN 207-6462); Edit Addr.: P.O. Box 191493, San Francisco, CA 94119 (SAN 207-6454) Tel 415-332-3216
Dist(s): **Todd Commns** *(Todd Communications).*

Conari Press, *(Conari Pr.; 0-943233; 1-57324),* 2550 Ninth St., Suite 101, Berkeley, CA 94710 (SAN 668-1085) Tel 510-649-7185; Fax: 510-649-7190; Toll Free: 800-685-9595 (orders)
E-mail: conari@conari.com
Web site: http://www.conari.com
Dist(s): **Publishers Group** *(Publishers Group West)*
netLibrary CO *(netLibrary, Inc.).*

Concept (IND) *(81-7022; 81-88686) Dist. by* **S Asia.**

Concept Arts, *See* **Two Blond Gdes**

Concordia, *(Concordia Publishing Hse.; 0-570; 0-7586),* Subs. of Lutheran Church Missouri Synod, 3558 S. Jefferson Ave., Saint Louis, MO 63118-3968 (SAN 202-1781) Tel 314-268-1000; Fax: 314-268-1360; Toll Free Fax: 800-490-9889 (orders only); Toll Free: 800-325-0191; 800-325-3040 (orders only)
E-mail: cphorder@cph.org
Web site: http://www.cph.org
Dist(s): **Natl Bk Netwk** *(National Bk. Network).*

Concpt Prodns, *(Concept Productions; 0-9664486),* 13858 Thomasville Ct., Jacksonville, FL 32223 Tel 904-262-1116
Dist(s): **Baker & Taylor** *(Baker & Taylor Bks.).*

Condor UT, *(Condor Bks.; 0-913238),* Orders Addr.: P.O. Box 2510, Novato, CA 94948 (SAN 201-3037) Tel 415-883-3530; Fax: 415-883-4280; Edit Addr.: 785 Lee Mountain Rd., Sedona, AZ 86351-8918 (SAN 206-7021) Tel 520-684-3890 (phone/fax) Do not confuse with Condor Bks., Lake Oswego, OR.

Confront Pubns, *(Confront Pubns., Inc.; 0-9658941),* 5106 Old Harding Rd., Franklin, TN 37064 Tel 615-646-1030.

†**Congr Quarterly,** *(Congressional Quarterly, Inc.; 0-87187; 1-56802),* 1255 22nd St., NW, Suite 400, Washington, DC 20037 (SAN 202-1803) Tel 202-887-8500; Fax: 202-887-6706; Toll Free Fax: 800-380-3810 (orders); Toll Free: 800-638-1710 (orders only)
E-mail: customerservice@cqpress.com
Web site: http://www.cqpress.com; *CIP.*

Conservatory, *(Conservatory Pr., The; 0-941401),* P.O. Box 7149, Baltimore, MD 21218 (SAN 667-7878) Fax: 410-889-3978
Dist(s): **Baker & Taylor** *(Baker & Taylor Bks.)*
RIE *(RIE).*

Consort Bk Sales, *(Consortium Bk. Sales & Distribution),* Orders Addr.: 1045 Westgate Dr., Suite 90, Saint Paul, MN 55114-1065 (SAN 200-6049) Tel 651-221-9035; Fax: 651-221-0124; Toll Free: 800-283-3572 (orders)
E-mail: consortium@cbsd.com
Web site: http://www.cbsd.com.

Consortium RI, *(Consortium Publishing; 0-940139),* 640 Weaver Hill Rd., West Greenwich, RI 02817-2261 (SAN 664-2667) Tel 401-397-9838; Fax: 401-392-1926.

Constable & Co (GBR) *(0-09) Dist. by* **Trafalgar.**

Consult Serv NW, *(Consultant Services Northwest, Inc.; 0-9617216),* 6521 36th Ave. NE, Seattle, WA 98115-7427 (SAN 663-4249) Tel 206-524-1950.

Consultant Pr, *(Consultant Pr., Ltd., The; 0-913069),* P.O. Box 54, Rhinebeck, NY 12572 (SAN 217-3603) Tel 845-876-7712; Fax: 212-873-7065
E-mail: consulinfo@aol.com
Web site: http://consultantpress.com.

†**Consulting Psychol,** *(Consulting Psychologists Pr., Inc.; 0-89106),* 3803 E. Bayshore Rd., Palo Alto, CA 94303 (SAN 201-7849) Tel 650-969-8901; Fax: 650-969-8608; Toll Free: 800-624-1765 ; *Imprints:* Davies-Black Pub (Davies-Black Publishing)
Web site: http://www.daviesblack.com; http://www.cpp-db.com
Dist(s): **Natl Bk Netwk** *(National Bk. Network); CIP.*

Consumer Info Pubns, *(Consumer Information Pubns.; 0-940062),* 35426 Jomar Ave., Zephyrhills, FL 33541-4639 (SAN 220-2395).

Consumer Press, *(Consumer Pr.; 0-9628336; 1-891264),* 13326 SW 28th St., Suite 102, Fort Lauderdale, FL 33330-1102 (SAN 297-7788) Tel 954-370-9153; Fax: 954-370-5722 ; *Imprints:* Womens Pubns (Women's Publications, Incorporated)
E-mail: bookguest@aol.com
Web site: http://members.aol.com/bookguest.

†**Consumer Reports,** *(Consumer Reports Bks.; 0-89043),* Div. of Consumers Union of U. S., Inc., 101 Truman Ave., Yonkers, NY 10703 (SAN 224-1048) Tel 914-378-2000; Fax: 914-378-2925; Toll Free: 800-500-9760 (book dept.)
Web site: http://www.consumerreports.org/
Dist(s): **Natl Bk Netwk** *(National Bk. Network); CIP.*

Consumer Research, *(Consumer Research Council of America; 0-9676546),* 2020 Pennsylvania Ave., NW, No.300-A, Washington, DC 20006 Tel 202-835-9698; Fax: 202-835-9739
E-mail: consumerreachcouncil@yahoo.com.

Consumers Union, *(Consumers Union of U. S., Inc.; 0-89043),* Orders Addr.: 540 Barnum Ave., Bridgeport, CT 06608 (SAN 661-9800); Edit Addr.: 101 Truman Ave., Yonkers, NY 10703 (SAN 269-3518) Tel 914-378-2000.

Consumertronics, *(Consumertronics; 0-934274),* P.O. Box 23097, Albuquerque, NM 87192-1097 (SAN 212-7369) Tel 505-321-1073; Fax: 505-275-5637
E-mail: wizguru@tsc-global.com
Web site: http://users.aol.com/wizguru/hi-tech.html; http://www.TSC-Global.com.

Cont Dental Educ, *(Univ. of Washington, Continuing Dental Education; 1-880291),* Box 357137, Seattle, WA 98195 Tel 206-543-5448; Fax: 206-543-6465.

Contemp Psycho, *(Contemporary Psychoanalytic Bks.; 0-9629993),* Div. of William Alanson White Institute, 20 W. 74th St., New York, NY 10023 Tel 212-873-0725; Fax: 212-362-6967
E-mail: Fantonoff@Psychoananlysis.net
Web site: http://www.wawhite.org.

Contemporary Imprint of McGraw-Hill Trade

Contented Hrts, *(Contented Hearts, Inc.; 0-9637562),* 11490 E. G Ave., Galesburg, MI 49053 Tel 616-665-4420
Dist(s): **Baker & Taylor** *(Baker & Taylor Bks.).*

Context Bks, *(Context Bks.; 1-893956),* 368 Broadway, Suite 314, New York, NY 10013 Tel 212-233-4880; Fax: 212-964-1810; Toll Free: 888-240-6032
E-mail: info@contextbooks.com; simnyc@interport.net
Web site: http://www.contextbooks.com
Dist(s): **Publishers Group** *(Publishers Group West).*

Context Pr, *(Context Pr.; 1-878978),* 933 Gear St., Reno, NV 89503-2729 Toll Free: 888-427-2665 Do not confuse with Context Pr., Berkeley, CA
E-mail: manager@contextpress.com; centextpress2000@hotmail.com
Web site: http://www.contextpress.com.

Context Pubns, *(Context Pubns.; 0-932654),* Orders Addr.: P.O. Box 2909, Rohnert Park, CA 94927-6506 (SAN 212-8977) Tel 707-576-1700; Fax: 707-575-6830
E-mail: inquiries@contextpub.com; nexus@sonic.net
Web site: http://www.contextpub.com.

Continental Bk, *(Continental Bk. Co., Inc.; 0-9626800),* Eastern Div., 80-00 Cooper Ave., Bldg. No. 29, Glendale, NY 11385 (SAN 169-5436) Tel 718-326-0560; Fax: 718-326-4276; Toll Free: 800-364-0350; Western Div., 625 E. 70th Ave., No. 5, Denver, CO 80229 (SAN 630-2882) Tel 303-289-1761; Fax: 303-289-1764 Do not confuse with Continental Book Company, Denver, CO
E-mail: esl@continentalbook.com; bonjour@continentalbook.com; tag@continentalbook.com; hola@continentalbook.com
Web site: http://www.continentalbook.com.

†**Continuum,** *(Continuum International Publishing Group, Inc.; 0-304; 0-7201; 0-8044; 0-8264),* Orders Addr.: 22883 Quicksilver Dr., Dulles, VA 20166 (SAN 253-3391) Fax: 703-661-1501; Toll Free: 800-561-7704; Edit Addr.: 370 Lexington Ave., New York, NY 10017-6503 (SAN 213-8220) Tel 212-953-5858; Fax: 212-953-5944
E-mail: info@continuum-books.com
Web site: http://www.continuum-books.com; *CIP.*

Continuum Pr, *(Continuum Pr.; 0-9633554),* P.O. Box 3125, Idyllwild, CA 92549-3125 Tel 909-659-4827.

Convalescnt Cnslts, *(Convalescent Consultants; 1-890118),* 5723 Ensign Ave., North Hollywood, CA 91601 Tel 818-760-4655; Fax: 818-760-4577; Toll Free: 800-341-0404 ; *Imprints:* QualityCare Pub (QualityCare Publishing, Limited).

Conversation Pr, *(Conversation Pr., Inc.; 0-9634395),* 1011 Oak St., Winnetka, IL 60093 Tel 847-446-7561; Fax: 847-441-5617; Toll Free: 800-848-5224
E-mail: convpress@aol.com.

Cook Communs Minist, *(Cook Communications Ministries; 0-7459; 0-7814; 0-88207; 0-89191; 0-89693; 0-912692; 1-55513; 1-56476; 983-45027; 983-45018; 983-45031),* 4050 Lee Vance View, Colorado Springs, CO 80918 Tel 719-536-0100; Fax: 719-536-3269; Toll Free: 800-708-5550; 55 Woodslee Ave., Paris, ON N3L 3E5 Toll Free Fax: 800-461-8575; Toll Free: 800-263-2664 Do not confuse with Cook Communications Ministries International, same address
E-mail: bergerj@cookministries.org
Web site: http://www.cookministries.com.

Cook Vision, *(Cook Vision Therapy Ctrs.; 0-9632657),* 1395 S. Marietta Pkwy., Suite 102, Bldg. 400, Marietta, GA 30067 Tel 770-419-0400.

Cooper & Harrison, *(Cooper & Harrison Pubns.; 1-885506),* Div. of Nova Therapy Systems, Inc., 717 E. Loyola Dr., Tempe, AZ 85282-3836 Tel 602-967-8194; Toll Free: 800-573-7067.

Cooper Ent, *(Cooper Enterprises; 0-9638533),* Orders Addr.: P.O. Box 601, Maysville, OK 73057; Edit Addr.: 207 Oak St., Maysville, OK 73057 Tel 405-867-5723.

Cooper Pub, *(Cooper Publishing; 0-9636312),* Div. of Happiness Holdings, Ltd., 250 H St., P.O. Box 2187, Blaine, WA 98231 Tel 604-597-4757; Fax: 604-597-8304; Toll Free: 800-663-8272.

Cooper Pubng, *(Cooper Publishing Group; 1-884125),* Orders Addr.: P.O. Box 1129, Traverse Ciry, MI 49686; Edit Addr.: 2694 Garfield Rd., N., Suite 26, Traverse City, MI 49686 Tel 231-933-9958; Fax: 231-933-9964
E-mail: icooper100@aol.com.

†**Cooper Sq,** *(Cooper Square Pubs., Inc.; 0-8154; 0-87833),* Member of Rowman & Littlefield Publishing Group, 150 5th Ave., Suite 817, New York, NY 10011 (SAN 281-5621) Tel 212-366-0410; Fax: 212-229-2619; Toll Free: 800-462-6420 (orders)
E-mail: custservrl@rowman.com
Web site: http://www.rowmanlittlefield.com/
Dist(s): **Natl Bk Netwk** *(National Bk. Network); CIP.*

Copernicus Imprint of Spr-Verlag

Copley Pub, *(Copley Publishing Group, Inc.; 0-87411; 1-58152; 1-58390),* 138 Great Rd, Acton, MA 01720 (SAN 687-4959) Tel 978-263-9090; Fax: 978-263-9190; Toll Free: 800-562-2147
E-mail: textbook@copleypublishing.com; publish@copleycustom.com
Web site: http://www.copleyeditions.com; http://www.copleycustom.com.

Copper Beech Bks Imprint of Millbrook Pr

Copyright Mgmt, *See* **Courier Custom**

Cor Bks, *(Cor Bks.; 0-9706790),* 5161 E. Arapahoe Rd., Suite 330, Littleton, CO 80122 Tel 303-694-2789; Fax: 303-721-9878; Toll Free: 800-976-1193
E-mail: rlaw@lawbrothersgroup.com.

Cor Hlthcare, *(Cor Healthcare Resources; 0-9645360),* Orders Addr.: P.O. Box 40959, Santa Barbara, CA 93140-0949 Tel 805-564-2177; Fax: 805-564-2146; Edit Addr.: 2040 Alameda Padre Sierra, Suite 220, Santa Barbara, CA 93103
E-mail: christman@corhealth.com
Web site: http://www.corhealth.com.

Coraco, *(Coraco; 0-917628),* 1017 S. Arlington Ave., Los Angeles, CA 90019 (SAN 203-5898) Tel 213-737-1066; Fax: 213-737-0212.

Corbin Hse, *(Corbin Hse.; 0-9621446),* 2457 Collins Ave., Suite 1403, Miami Beach, FL 33140-4769 (SAN 251-3234) Tel 305-532-8578
Dist(s): **Baker & Taylor** *(Baker & Taylor Bks.)*
Brodart *(Brodart Co.).*

Corectec, *(Corectec; 1-880890),* Orders Addr.: P.O. Box 7275, Athens, GA 30604-7275 Tel 706-613-8537; Fax: 706-613-1526; Edit Addr.: 109 Lenox Pl., Athens, GA 30606 Tel 770-613-8537.

Cor-Ed Pub, *(Cor-Ed Publishing Co.; 0-9630510),* 810 E. University Ave., Gainesville, FL 32601 Tel 904-376-0060; Fax: 904-371-4828; Toll Free: 800-749-4278.

Cornell CIS RDC, *(Cornell Univ., Ctr. for International Studies, Rural Development Committee; 0-86731),* 170 Uris Hall, Ithaca, NY 14853 (SAN 217-510X) Tel 607-255-6370; Fax: 607-254-5000.

Cornell East Asia Pgm, *(Cornell Univ. East Asia Program; 0-939657; 1-885445),* 140 Uris Hall, Cornell Univ., Ithaca, NY 14853-7601 (SAN 219-3604) Tel 607-255-5071; Fax: 607-255-1388
E-mail: ceas@cornell.edu
Web site: http://www.einaudi.cornell.edu/eastasia/EastAsia Series.html.

Cornell Food, *(Cornell Food & Nutrition Policy Programs; 1-56401),* Div. of Nutritional Sciences, College of Human Ecology, Cornell Univ., MVR Hall, Cornell Univ., Ithaca, NY 14853 Tel 607-255-8093; Fax: 607-255-0178
E-mail: pkm6@cornell.edu
Web site: http://www.human.cornell.edu/dns/cfnpp.html.

†**Cornell Maritime,** *(Cornell Maritime Pr., Inc.; 0-87033),* P.O. Box 456, Centreville, MD 21617 (SAN 203-5901) Tel 410-758-1075; Fax: 410-758-6849; Toll Free: 800-638-7641
E-mail: cornell@crosslink.net
Web site: http://www.cornellmaritimepress.com/
Dist(s): **R Hale & Co** *(Hale, Robert & Co., Inc.); CIP.*

Cornell U Div Nutrit Scis, *(Cornell Univ., Div. of Nutritional Sciences; 0-9655240),* 3MBA MVR Hall, Ithaca, NY 14853 Tel 607-255-1703; Fax: 607-255-0178
E-mail: vik1@cornell.edu.

†**Cornell U Pr,** *(Cornell Univ. Pr.; 0-8014; 0-87546),* Orders Addr.: P.O. Box 6525, Ithaca, NY 14851 (SAN 281-5680) Tel 607-277-2211; Toll Free Fax: 800-688-2877; Edit Addr.: Sage House, 512 E. State St., Ithaca, NY 14851 (SAN 202-1862) Tel 607-277-2338 ; *Imprints:* ILR Press (ILR Press)
E-mail: orders@plymbridge.com; cservs@plymbridge.com; cupress-sales@cornell.edu; cupressinfo@cornell.edu
Web site: http://www.cornellpress.cornell.edu
Dist(s): **CUP Services** *(CUP Services); CIP.*

Corner Hse, *(Corner Hse. Historical Pubns.; 0-87928),* Orders Addr.: P.O. Box 207, Gansevoort, NY 12831; Edit Addr.: 14 Catherine St., Gansevoort, NY 12831 Tel 518-798-3039; Fax: 518-798-0217
E-mail: sales@cornerhousebooks.com; cornerhouse@cityusa.net
Web site: http://www.cornerhousebooks.com.

Cornerstn FL, *(Cornerstone Publishing; 0-9629875),* 4524 Curry Ford Rd., Suite 211, Orlando, FL 32812 Tel 407-872-1418 Do not confuse with companies with the same or similar names in South Chicago Heights, IL, San Diego, CA, Minneapolis, MN, Wichita, KS.

Cornwall Bks Imprint of Assoc Univ Prs

Coronado Pr, *(Coronado Pr., Inc.; 0-87291),* P.O. Box 3232, Lawrence, KS 66044 (SAN 201-7776) Tel 913-843-5988; Fax: 913-842-3611.

Coronet Bks, *(Coronet Bks.; 0-89563; 91-7916),* 311 Bainbridge St., Philadelphia, PA 19147 (SAN 210-6043) Tel 215-925-2762; Fax: 215-925-1912 Do not confuse with Coronet Bks. & Pubns., Eagle Point, OR
E-mail: rsmolin@ix.netcom.com; order@coronetbooks.com
Web site: http://www.coronetbooks.com.

Corp Jobs Outlk, *See* **Plunkett Res**

Corp Res Grp, *(Corporate Research Group, Inc.; 0-9662321),* 524 North Ave., No. 302, New Rochelle, NY 10801 Tel 914-235-6000; Fax: 914-235-6002; Toll Free: 800-500-6467
E-mail: corprsrch@aol.com
Web site: http://www.managedcaretoday.com.

Cortlandt Grp, *(Cortlandt Group; 0-9634124),* 7 Skyline Dr., Hawthorne, NY 10532-2179 Tel 914-347-3800; Fax: 914-347-3801
E-mail: KGerosa@Cortgroup.com.

Corwin Pr, *(Corwin Pr., Inc.; 0-7619; 0-8039; 1-879179),* Subs. of Sage Pubns., Inc., 2455 Teller Rd., Thousand Oaks, CA 91320-2218 Tel 805-499-9734; 805-499-9774 (customer service); Fax: 805-499-0871; 805-499-5323
E-mail: orders@corwinpress.com
Web site: http://www.corwinpress.com.

Cosmo Therapy, *(Cosmo - Therapy Dr. Gumbel Pr.; 0-9714327),* 1210 Cherry Ln., Blue Bell, PA 19422-1802 (SAN 254-2986) Tel 610-275-3371; Fax: 610-292-0957
E-mail: cosmo-therapy@erols.com.

Cottage CA, *See* **Elder Bks**

Cottage Sq Pr, *(Cottage Square Pr.; 0-9633234),* 706 Rome Dr., Los Angeles, CA 90065 Tel 213-223-8688; Fax: 626-289-1321.

Cougar Books Imprint of Capitol Enquiry

Coulee Press Imprint of Adastra Pub

Coun Commun Serv, *(Council of Community Services; 1-888334),* 2012 21st Ave. S., Nashville, TN 37212 Tel 615-385-2221; Fax: 615-385-2157.

†**Coun Exc Child,** *(Council for Exceptional Children; 0-86586),* 1920 Association Dr., Reston, VA 20191-1589 (SAN 203-5952) Tel 703-264-9455; Fax: 703-620-2521; Toll Free: 888-232-7733
E-mail: Internet: cecpubs@cec.sped.org; suzannek@cec.sped.org; *CIP.*

Coun Oak Bks, *(Council Oak Bks.; 0-933031; 1-57178),* Div. of Council Oak Publishing Co., Inc., Orders Addr.: 1350 E. 15th St., Tulsa, OK 74120-5801 (SAN 689-5522) Tel 918-587-6454; Fax: 918-583-4995; Toll Free: 800-247-8850 (orders only); Edit Addr.: 1290 Chestnut St., Suite 2, San Francisco, CA 94109 Tel 415-931-6868; Fax: 415-931-5353
E-mail: kevincob@pacbell.net
Web site: http://www.counciloakbooks.com
Dist(s): **Baker & Taylor** *(Baker & Taylor Bks.)*
Gryphon Hse *(Gryphon Hse., Inc.)*
Koen Bk Distributors *(Koen Bk. Distributors)*
Penguin Putnam *(Penguin Putnam, Inc.)*
SPD-Small Pr Dist *(SPD-Small Pr. Distribution).*

Coun of Ethical, *(Council of Ethical Organizations; 0-9656061),* 214 S. Payne St., Alexandria, VA 22314-3530 Tel 703-683-7916; Fax: 703-299-8836
E-mail: Councile@aol.com
Web site: http://www.corporateethics.com.

Coun on Competitiveness, *(Council on Competitiveness; 1-889866),* 1401 H St., NW, Suite 650, Washington, DC 20005 Tel 202-682-4292; Fax: 202-682-5150
Web site: http://www.compete.org.

Coun Renal Nutrit, *(Council on Renal Nutrition Northern California/Northern Nevada; 1-883146),* Orders Addr.: 1542 Queenstown Ct., Sunnyvale, CA 94087 Tel 408-236-4137; Edit Addr.: 6397 Thornhill Dr., Oakland, CA 94611.

†**Coun Res Values,** *(Council for Research in Values & Philosophy; 1-56518),* Orders Addr.: P.O. Box 261, Washington, DC 20064 Toll Free: 800-659-9962
E-mail: cua-rvp@cua.edu
Web site: http://www.crvp.org; *CIP.*

Coun State Govts, *(Council of State Governments, The; 0-87292),* 2760 Research Park Dr., Lexington, KY 40578-1910 (SAN 225-1264) Tel 859-244-8000; Fax: 859-244-8001; Toll Free: 800-800-1910 (orders only)
E-mail: statenews@csg.org; info@csg.org
Web site: http://www.statenews.org.

Council of Europe (FRA) *(92-871) Dist. by* **Manhattan Pub Co.**

Counsel & Consult, *(Counseling & Consulting Services (CCS) Pubns.; 0-910819),* 4020 Moorpark Ave., Suite 204, San Jose, CA 95117 (SAN 262-0146) Tel 408-246-1128; Fax: 408-246-1011.

Counsel & Stress, *(Counseling & Stress Research Ctr.; 0-912561),* 94 Broad St., New London, CT 06320 (SAN 283-9466) Tel 860-447-9935.

Counsel Voice, *(Counselor's Voice Pubs.; 0-9618024),* 11811 E. Terra Dr., Scottsdale, AZ 85259 (SAN 666-4970).

Countrpnt Commns, *(CounterPoint Communications; 0-9666067),* P.O. Box 230927, Encinitas, CA 92023-0927 Tel 760-436-0183 (phone/fax)
E-mail: rdf@cpc-com.com.

Country Bazaar, *(Country Bazaar Publishing & Distributing; 0-936744),* Honey, Inc. Bldg., 1241 Highway 62 W., Berryville, AR 72616 (SAN 215-1669) Tel 870-423-3131.

†**Countryman,** *(Countryman Pr.; 0-88150; 0-914378; 0-942440),* Div. of W. W. Norton & Co., Inc., P.O. Box 748, Woodstock, VT 05091-0748 (SAN 206-4901) Tel 802-457-4826 Toll Free: 800-245-4151 (Orders only)
E-mail: countrymanpress@wwnorton.com
Web site: http://www.countrymanpress.com
Dist(s): **Norton** *(Norton, W.W. & Co., Inc.); CIP.*

Countway Lib Med Imprint of Watson Pub Intl

Couple to Couple, *(Couple to Couple League, The; 0-926412; 0-9601036),* Orders Addr.: P.O. Box 111184, Cincinnati, OH 45211 (SAN 208-1490) Tel 513-471-2000; Fax: 513-557-2449; Toll Free: 800-745-8252 (orders only); Edit Addr.: 4290 Delhi Pike, Cincinnati, OH 45238 (SAN 669-0564)
E-mail: ccli@ccli.org
Web site: http://www.ccli.org.

Courier Custom, *(Courier Custom Publishing, Inc.; 1-58692),* Div. of Courier Corp., 15 Wellman Ave., North Chelmsford, MA 01863-1334 Tel 978-251-6066; Fax: 978-251-6240; Toll Free Fax: 877-516-2874; Toll Free: 800-228-8637
E-mail: info@courier.com
Web site: http://www.custombook.com.

Course Tech, *(Course Technology, Inc.; 0-534; 0-619; 0-7600; 0-7895; 0-87709; 0-87835; 0-89426; 0-928763; 1-56527; 1-878748),* Div. of Thomson Learning, Orders Addr.: 7625 Empire Dr., Florence, KY 41042 (SAN 631-2144) Tel 606-525-6620; Fax: 606-647-5023; Toll Free Fax: 800-340-7450 (corp. customer sevice); Edit Addr.: One Main St., Cambridge, MA 02142 (SAN 298-8933) Tel 617-225-2595; Fax: 617-494-8008; Toll Free: 800-648-7450 (customer services)
E-mail: tucker_malenfant@course.com
Web site: http://www.course.com
Dist(s): **Thomson Learn** *(Thomson Learning).*

Covenant Hse Bks, *(Covenant Hse. Bks.; 0-925591),* 1301 Witt Hollow Rd., Sevierville, TN 37862 Tel 865-428-5176; Fax: 865-908-6116
E-mail: DDennis479@aol.com.

Cover Pub, *(Cover Publishing Co.; 0-912912),* P.O. Box 1092, Tampa, FL 33601 (SAN 203-6037) Tel 813-237-0266; Fax: 813-238-1819; Toll Free: 800-441-8398
E-mail: coverpub@gte.net
Web site: http://www.theMDsite.com.

Cowles Creative, *See* **Creat Pub Intl**

Cowles Mag, *See* **Intertec Pub Bks**

Cox Pubns, *See* **BusinessWatch**

Coyote Press, *(Coyote Pr.; 1-55567),* P.O. Box 3377, Salinas, CA 93912 (SAN 699-6752) Tel 831-422-4912; Fax: 831-422-4913 Do not confuse with companies with the same name in Eugene, OR, Altamonte Springs, FL
E-mail: coyote@coyotepress.com; coyote@dedot.com
Web site: http://www.coyotepress.com.

CPA Washington, *(Ctr. for Policy Alternatives; 0-89788),* 1875 Connecticut Ave. NW, Suite 710, Washington, DC 20009 (SAN 235-8255) Tel 202-387-6030; Fax: 202-986-2539.

CPG Pub, *(CPG Publishing Co.; 1-882149),* Div. of Montanari & Assocs., Inc., Orders Addr.: P.O. Box 50062, Phoenix, AZ 85076 Fax: 858-755-6681; Toll Free: 800-578-5549; Edit Addr.: 6260 S. Kings Ranch Rd., Gold Canyon, AZ 85219 Tel 858-755-6001 Do not confuse with C P G Publishing, Inc. in Carle Place, NY.

CPM Whole Hlth, *(CPM Whole Health; 0-9647445),* 51 Homer St., Newton, MA 02459-1511 Tel 617-734-0399; Fax: 617-332-0123.

CPS Inc, *(C.P.S.,Inc.; 0-918863),* P.O. Box 83, Larchmont, NY 10538 (SAN 670-0004) Tel 914-833-1633.

†**CQ Pr,** *(CQ Pr.; 0-87187; 1-56802),* Div. of Congressional Quarterly, Inc., 1414 22nd St., NW, Washington, DC 20037 Tel 202-887-8500; Fax: 202-822-6583; Toll Free: 800-638-1710 (orders) ; *Imprints:* CQ Pr Coll (C Q Press College) CQ Pr Lib Ref (C Q Press Library Reference)
Web site: http://www.cqpress.com; *CIP.*

CQ Pr Coll Imprint of CQ Pr

CQ Pr Lib Ref Imprint of CQ Pr

Crakel Pubns, *(Crakel Pubns.; 0-9642711),* Orders Addr.: P.O. Box 51701, Irvine, CA 92619 Tel 714-249-8651; Fax: 714-495-6753; Toll Free: 800-708-7623; Edit Addr.: 17 Cala Moreya, Laguna Niguel, CA 92677 Tel 714-249-8661
E-mail: crakel@ix.netcom.com
Web site: http://www.andreas.com/crakel.

Cram Pubs (CAN) *(2-9801489) Dist. by* **Seven Hills Bk.**

Cramer Prods, *(Cramer Products, Inc.; 1-889366),* Orders Addr.: P.O. Box 1001, Gardner, KS 66030 Tel 913-856-7511; Fax: 913-884-5626; Toll Free: 800-255-6621; Edit Addr.: 153 W. Warren, Gardner, KS 66030
E-mail: info@cramersportsmed.com
Web site: http://www.cramersportsmed.com.

Crane Russak Imprint of Taylor & Francis

†**CRC Pr,** *(CRC Pr. LLC; 0-8493; 0-87819; 1-58488),* Subs. of Information Ventures, LLC, 2000 Corporate Blvd., NW, Boca Raton, FL 33431 (SAN 202-1994) Tel 561-994-0555; Fax: 561-989-8732 (outside USA); Toll Free Fax: 800-374-3401 (inside USA); Toll Free: 800-272-7737 ; *Imprints:* Chap & Hall CRC (Chapman & Hall/CRC) Parthenon Pbng (Parthenon Publishing)
E-mail: orders@crcpress.com
Web site: http://www.crcpress.com; *CIP.*

CRC Reprint Imprint of Franklin

CRCS Pubns CA, *(CRCS Pubns.; 0-916360),* P.O. Box 1460, Sebastopol, CA 95473 (SAN 200-626X) Tel 707-829-0735; Fax: 707-793-9434
Dist(s): **Bookpeople** *(Bookpeople)*
SCB Distributors *(SCB Distributors).*

†**Creat Arts Bk,** *(Creative Arts Bk. Co.; 0-88739; 0-916870),* 833 Bancroft Way, Berkeley, CA 94710 (SAN 208-4880) Tel 510-848-4777; Fax: 510-848-4844; Toll Free: 800-848-7789
E-mail: staff@creativeartsbooks.com
Web site: http://www.creativeartsbooks.com
Dist(s): **Baker & Taylor** *(Baker & Taylor Bks.)*
Bookazine Co Inc *(Bookazine Co., Inc.)*
Bookpeople *(Bookpeople)*
Koen Bk Distributors *(Koen Bk. Distributors)*
New Leaf Dist *(New Leaf Distributing Co., Inc.)*
SPD-Small Pr Dist *(SPD-Small Pr. Distribution); CIP.*

Creat Concpt Child, *See* **Arcadia AZ**

Creat Core, *(Creative Core, Inc.; 1-57654),* Orders Addr.: P.O. Box 424, Algonquin, IL 60102 Fax: 847-854-2464; Edit Addr.: 1421 Lowe Dr., Algonquin, IL 60102 Tel 847-854-1111; Toll Free: 800-223-9473 ; *Imprints:* Creative Core (Creative Core)
E-mail: opplan@opplan.com
Web site: http://www.c-coreinc.com.

Creat Des Srvs, *(Creative Design Services; 1-880715),* P.O. Box 61263, King of Prussia, PA 19406-1263 Tel 610-640-9449; Fax: 610-648-0257
E-mail: fdbk@cdspub.com; info@cdspub.com
Web site: http://www.cdspub.com.

Creat Educ Imprint of Creative Co

Creat Educ Found, *(Creative Education Foundation, Inc.; 0-930222),* 1050 Union Rd., No. 4, Buffalo, NY 14224 (SAN 685-3218) Tel 716-675-3181; Fax: 716-675-3209; Toll Free: 800-447-2774
E-mail: cefhg@cef-cpsi.org
Web site: http://www.cef-cpsi.org.

Creat Hlth & Spirit, *(Creative Health & Spirit; 0-9656432),* Orders Addr.: P.O. Box 385, Manhattan Beach, CA 90267 (SAN 299-2124) Tel 310-546-8523; Fax: 310-545-4364; Toll Free: 800-555-5453; Edit Addr.: 728 Rosecrans Ave., Manhattan Beach, CA 90266 (SAN 299-2124)
E-mail: chsp@mindspring.com
Web site: http://www.healthylife.net.

Creat Ideas, *(Creative Ideas, Inc.; 0-9631030),* 5201 Five Points Rd., Indianapolis, IN 46239 Tel 317-887-7762; Fax: 317-887-7739 Do not confuse with Creative Ideas, Inc., Jacksonville, IL.

Creat Logic, *(Creative Logic Co.; 0-9661161),* 296 Toyon Rd., Ukiah, CA 95482 Tel 707-463-3663; Fax: 707-463-0835 ; *Imprints:* Boitumelo Pub (Boitumelo Publishing, Incorporated)
E-mail: info@boitumelo.com
Web site: http://www.boitumelo.com
Dist(s): **J Majors Co** *(Majors, J. A. Co.).*

Creat Opportunities, *(Creative Opportunities Publishing Co.; 0-9660704),* P.O. Box 2461, Orangevale, CA 95662 Tel 916-987-2161; Fax: 916-987-1378; Toll Free: 800-617-7667 Do not confuse with Creative Opportunities, Inc., Laguna Niguel, CA
Dist(s): **Quality Bks IL** *(Quality Bks., Inc.).*

Creat Pub Intl, *(Creative Publishing International, Inc.; 0-86573; 0-942802; 1-55971; 1-58923),* 5900 Green Oak Dr., Minnetonka, MN 55343 (SAN 289-7148) Tel 952-936-4700; Fax: 952-933-1456; Toll Free: 800-328-0590
E-mail: hnahvi@creativepub.com
Web site: http://www.howtobookstore.com
Dist(s): **Andrews McMeel** *(Andrews McMeel Publishing).*

Creation House, *(Creation Hse.; 0-88419),* Div. of Strang Communications Co., 600 Rinehart Rd., Lake Mary, FL 32746-4872 (SAN 677-5640) Tel 407-333-0600; Fax: 407-333-7118; Toll Free: 800-283-8494
E-mail: Webmaster@Strang.com
Web site: http://www.strang.com
Dist(s): **Anchor Distributors** *(Anchor Distributors)*
Appalachian Bible *(Appalachian Bible Co.)*
Baker & Taylor *(Baker & Taylor Bks.)*
Dake Publishing *(Dake Publishing)*
Harrison Hse *(Harrison Hse., Inc.)*
Riverside-World *(Riverside World)*
Spring Arbor Dist *(Spring Arbor Distributors Inc.).*

Creative Arts, *(Creative Arts & Multi-Media, Inc.; 0-9676182),* 3674 Touriga Dr., Pleasanton, CA 94566 Tel 925-846-6264; Fax: 925-417-8754
E-mail: eckn@aol.com
Web site: http://www.kesed.com.

Creative Attic, *(Creative Attic, Inc., The; 0-9653955),* P.O. Box 187, Canterbury, NH 03224 Tel 603-783-9103; Fax: 603-783-0118; Toll Free: 888-566-6539
E-mail: the5kids@aol.com
Dist(s): **Baker & Taylor** *(Baker & Taylor Bks.).*

Creative Co, *(Creative Co., The; 0-87191; 0-88682; 1-56660; 1-56846),* 123 S. Broad St., P.O. Box 227, Mankato, MN 56001 Tel 507-388-6273; Fax: 507-388-2746; Toll Free: 800-445-6209 ; *Imprints:* Creat Educ (Creative Education) Do not confuse with The Creative Co., Lawrenceburg, IN
E-mail: CreativeCo@aol.com.

Creative Core Imprint of Creat Core

Creative Educ, *(Creative Educators; 0-9641523),* 26072 Perdido Beach Blvd., Apt. 602-E, Orange Beach, AL 36561-3137.

Creative Hlth, *(Creative Health Concepts; 0-941549),* 855 Independence, Springfield, IL 62702 (SAN 666-2838) Tel 217-546-5189.

Creative Learning, *(Creative Learning Pr., Inc.; 0-936386; 1-931280),* Orders Addr.: P.O. Box 320, Mansfield Center, CT 06250 (SAN 298-4601) Tel 860-429-8118; Fax: 860-429-7783
E-mail: custoerservice@creativelearningpress.com; clp@creativelearningpress.com
Web site: http://www.creativelearningpress.com.

Creative Market, *(Creative Market Development; 1-892972),* 3450 SW 108th Ave., Beaverton, OR 97005-1831 Tel 503-641-1916; Fax: 503-644-9231
E-mail: delong@teleport.com.

Creative Nursing, *(Creative Nursing Management, Inc.; 0-9621520; 1-886624),* 1701 E. 79th St., Suite 1, Minneapolis, MN 55425-1151 (SAN 251-5466) Tel 612-854-9015; Fax: 612-854-1866; Toll Free: 800-728-7766; 800-264-3246
E-mail: chcm@chcm.com
Web site: http://www.chcm.com
Dist(s): **J Majors Co** *(Majors, J. A. Co.)*
Matthews Medical Bk Co *(Matthews Medical Bk. Co.).*

Creative Street, *(Creative Street, Inc.; 1-882079),* 3719 Washington Blvd., Indianapolis, IN 46205 (SAN 248-2304) Tel 317-926-9671.

†**Creative Therapeutics,** *(Creative Therapeutics, Inc.; 0-933812),* 155 County Rd., P.O. Box 522, Cresskill, NJ 07626-0522 (SAN 212-6508) Tel 201-567-7295; Fax: 201-567-3036; Toll Free: 800-544-6162
E-mail: ct39@erols.com
Web site: http://www.rgardner.com; *CIP.*

Creative Walking, *(Creative Walking, Inc.; 0-939041),* P.O. Box 50296, Clayton, MO 63105 (SAN 662-6521) Tel 314-721-3600; Fax: 314-721-0303.

†**Creighton U Pr,** *(Creighton Univ. Pr.; 1-881871),* California at 24th St., Omaha, NE 68178 Tel 402-280-2192; Fax: 402-280-2143
E-mail: spencr@creighton.edu
Web site: http://www.mockingbird.creighton.edu/ncw/cup.htm
Dist(s): **BookMasters** *(BookMasters, Inc.)*
Fordham *(Fordham Univ. Pr.)*
U of Nebr Pr *(Univ. of Nebraska Pr.); CIP.*

Crescent Pub Grp, *See* **TechDoc**

Crest Imprint of Fawcett

Cricket Commun, *(Cricket Communications; 0-9643606),* 1441 SW Clay St., Suite 209, Portland, OR 97201-6090 Tel 503-228-8421
E-mail: grillo@hevanet.com.

Cricket Sci, *(Cricket Science; 0-9634298),* 1611 Shane Dr., Pocatello, ID 83204 Tel 208-232-5548 (phone/fax); Toll Free: 800-232-5548 (phone/fax)
E-mail: robert@cricketscience.com
Web site: http://www.cricketscience.com.

Crisis Prevent, *(Crisis Prevention Institute, Inc.; 0-9651733),* 3315-K N. 124th St., Brookfield, WI 53005 Tel 414-783-5787; Fax: 414-783-5906; Toll Free: 800-558-8976
E-mail: info@crisisprevention.com
Web site: http://www.execpc.com/~cpi; http://www.crisisprevention.com.

†**Crisp Pubns,** *(Crisp Pubns., Inc.; 0-931961; 1-56052),* Orders Addr.: 1200 Hamilton Ct., Menlo Park, CA 94025 (SAN 686-0400) Tel 650-323-6100; Fax: 650-323-5800; Toll Free: 800-442-7477; Edit Addr.: c/o JV Midwest, 451 Blackhawk Trail, Eldridge, IA 52738
E-mail: postmaster@crisp-pub.com
Web site: http://www.crisplearning.com; *CIP.*

Criterion Pr, *(Criterion Pr.; 0-9609428),* P.O. Box 1014, Torrance, CA 90505 (SAN 260-0382) Tel 310-326-3503 Do not confuse with Criterion Pr., Cranbury, NJ.

Critical Care Pr, *(Critical Care Pr., Inc.; 0-910271),* Orders Addr.: P.O. Box 3465, New Orleans, LA 70177 (SAN 241-4899); Edit Addr.: 899 Martin Behrman Ave., Metairie, LA 70005 (SAN 241-6727) Tel 504-836-1594.

Critical Pr, *(Critical Pr., Inc.; 1-883831),* P.O. Box 333, Gardiner, NY 12525 Tel 914-255-8252
E-mail: gunk@mhv.net
Web site: http://www1.mhv.net/~gunk
Dist(s): **Bernhard DeBoer Inc** *(DeBoer, Bernhard Inc.)*
Dist Art Pubs *(Distributed Art Pubs./D.A.P.).*

Crnerstone GA, *(Cornerstone Productions, Inc.; 1-883427; 1-58470),* Div. of RAS Cardo Reggae Legends, P.O. Box 831955, Stone Mountain, GA 30083.

Crockett Pub Co, *(Crockett Publishing Co.; 0-915131),* 140 W. 1485 N., Orem, UT 84057 (SAN 289-9094) Tel 801-225-8873
Dist(s): **Sounds of Zion** *(Sounds of Zion).*

Cromlech Bks, *(Cromlech Bks., Inc.; 0-9618059),* Nobska Rd., Box 145, Woods Hole, MA 02543 (SAN 666-1025) Tel 508-540-1185.

Croner, *(Croner Pubns.; 0-87514),* 10951 Sorrento Valley Rd., Suite 1D, San Diego, CA 92121-1613 (SAN 203-8706) Tel 619-546-1894; Toll Free: 800-441-4033.

†**Cross River Pubns,** *(Cross River Pubns.; 0-945288),* Div. of T. C. Thomsen & Assocs., P.O. Box 1713, Shelter Island, NY 11964-1713 (SAN 246-3067) Tel 516-749-3074; Fax: 516-749-1029
Dist(s): **Baker & Taylor** *(Baker & Taylor Bks.); CIP.*

Cross Trng, *(Cross Training Publishing; 1-887002; 1-929478),* Orders Addr.: P.O. Box 1541, Grand Island, NE 68802 (SAN 298-7406) Tel 308-384-5762; Fax: 308-384-9974; Toll Free: 800-430-8588; Edit Addr.: 317 W. Second St., Grand Island, NE 68801
E-mail: crosstrainingpub@computer-concepts.com
Web site: http://www.crosstrainingpub.com.

†**Cross-Cultrl NY,** *(Cross-Cultural Communications; 0-89304),* 239 Wynsum Ave., Merrick, NY 11566-4725 (SAN 208-6212) Tel 516-868-5635; *CIP.*

†**Crossing Pr,** *(Crossing Pr., Inc., The; 0-89594; 0-912278; 1-58091),* Orders Addr.: 1201 Shaffer Rd., Suite B, Santa Cruz, CA 95060 (SAN 202-2060) Tel 831-420-1110; Fax: 831-420-1114; Toll Free: 800-777-1048 (orders only)
E-mail: katie@crossingpress.com
Web site: http://www.crossingpress.com
Dist(s): **Baker & Taylor** *(Baker & Taylor Bks.)*
Bookpeople *(Bookpeople)*
Koen Bk Distributors *(Koen Bk. Distributors)*
New Leaf Dist *(New Leaf Distributing Co., Inc.)*
Publishers Group *(Publishers Group West); CIP.*

Crossings Pr, *(Crossings Pr.; 0-9614119; 0-9712452),* 202 Park Ave., Marshall, MN 56258 Tel 507-532-3647; Fax: 507-537-6147
Dist(s): **Plains Press** *(Plains Pr.).*

†**Crossroad NY,** *(Crossroad Publishing Co.; 0-8245),* 481 Eighth Ave., Suite 1550, New York, NY 10001 (SAN 287-0118) Tel 212-868-1801; Fax: 212-868-2171; Toll Free: 800-395-0690
E-mail: ask@crossroadpublishing.com
Web site: http://www.crossroadpublishing.com
Dist(s): **ACTA Pubns** *(ACTA Pubns.)*
Abingdon *(Abingdon Pr.)*
Natl Bk Netwk *(National Bk. Network); CIP.*

Crossroads Imprint of African Studies Assn

†**Crossway Bks,** *(Crossway Bks.; 0-89107; 1-58134),* Div. of Good News Pubs., 1300 Crescent St., Wheaton, IL 60187 (SAN 211-7991) Tel 630-682-4300; Fax: 630-682-4785; Toll Free: 800-323-3890 (sales only)
Web site: http://www.crosswaybooks.org
Dist(s): **L I M Prodns** *(LIM Productions, LLC); CIP.*

Crown Imprint of Crown Pub Group

Crown Hse (GBR) *(1-899836) Dist. by* **LPC Group.**

Crown MA, *(Crown Pubns., Inc.; 0-925703),* Orders Addr.: P.O. Box 87, Southbridge, MA 01550-0087 Tel 508-248-3994 Do not confuse with companies with same or similar names in Westlake Village, CA, Powell, TN
Dist(s): **Spring Arbor Dist** *(Spring Arbor Distributors Inc.).*

†**Crown Pub Group,** *(Crown Publishing Group, Inc.; 0-517; 0-609; 0-676; 1-4000),* Div. of Random Hse., Inc., Orders Addr.: 400 Hahn Rd., Westminster, MD 21157 Tel 410-848-1900; Toll Free Fax: 800-659-2436; Toll Free: 800-733-3000; 800-726-0600; Edit Addr.: 299 Park Ave., New York, NY 10171 (SAN 200-2639) Tel 212-751-2600; Fax: 212-572-2165 ; *Imprints:* Crown (Crown) Three Riv Pr (Three Rivers Press) Clarkson Potter (Clarkson Potter)
E-mail: customerservice@randomnhouse.com
Web site: http://www.randomhouse.com/
Dist(s): **Shens Bks** *(Shen's Bks.); CIP.*

Crowood Pr (GBR) *(0-946284; 1-85223; 1-86126) Dist. by* **Trafalgar.**

Crozer-Keystone, *(Crozer-Keystone Health System; 0-9662274),* 100 W. Sproul Rd., No. HP-II, Springfield, PA 19064-2027.

CRRB, *(Court Reporter Reference Bks.; 1-881149),* 25512 Banff Ln., Suite 1114, Punta Gorda, FL 33983 Tel 210-805-7094; Toll Free: 888-958-2772
E-mail: monettebenwah@sprynet.com
Web site: http://www.CRRBooks.com.

Crystal Spgs Imprint of Staff Dev Educ

Crystal VA, *(Crystal Publishing; 0-9641059),* Div. of The Crystal Cos., 6107 Leopold Cir., Richmond, VA 23234-5829 Tel 804-320-7210; Fax: 809-272-6609; Toll Free: 800-627-9782 Do not confuse with Crystal Publishing in Grawn, MI.

CSA Pr, *(CSA Pr.; 0-87707),* Orders Addr.: P.O. Box 7, Lakemont, GA 30552-0007 (SAN 658-0408); Edit Addr.: Lake Rabun Rd., Lakemont, GA 30552-0001 (SAN 207-7329) Tel 706-782-4723; Fax: 706-782-4560.

†**CSIS,** *(Ctr. for Strategic & International Studies; 0-89206),* 1800 K St., NW, Washington, DC 20006 (SAN 281-4021) Tel 202-775-3119; Fax: 202-775-3199
E-mail: books@csis.org
Web site: http://www.csis.org; *CIP.*

CSLI, *(CSLI Pubns.; 0-937073; 1-57586; 1-881526),* Stanford Univ., Ventura Hall, Stanford, CA 94305-4115 (SAN 658-5582) Tel 650-723-1839; Fax: 650-725-2166
E-mail: pubs@csli.standford.edu
Web site: http://www.cslipublications.stanford.edu
Dist(s): **U Ch Pr** *(Univ. of Chicago Pr.).*

†**CSS OH,** *(CSS Publishing Co.; 0-7880; 0-89536; 1-55673),* Orders Addr.: P.O. Box 4503, Lima, OH 45802-4503 (SAN 207-0707) Tel 419-227-1818; Fax: 419-228-9184; Toll Free: 800-241-4056; Edit Addr.: 517 S. Main St., Lima, OH 45804-4503 ; *Imprints:* Fairway Pr (Fairway Press)
E-mail: editor@csspub.com; csspub@csspub.com; info@csspub.com
Web site: http://www.csspub.com
Dist(s): **BookWorld** *(BookWorld Services, Inc.)*
Spring Arbor Dist *(Spring Arbor Distributors Inc.); CIP.*

CT Pub, *See* **CAT Pub**

CTA Resrch Corp, *(CTA Research Corp.; 0-9635231),* 1734 Jasmine Ave., No. 18, Fairfield, IA 52556-9005 Tel 515-472-7522.

CTB Intl, *(CTB International Publishing, Inc.; 0-9623391; 1-887566),* Orders Addr.: P.O. Box 218, Maplewood, NJ 07040-0218 Tel 973-379-7749; Fax: 973-379-1158; Edit Addr.: 33 Bleeker St., Millburn, NJ 07041
Web site: http://www.ctbintl.com.

Ctr Adv Psychic Res, *(Ctr. for Advanced Psychic Research & Development, The; 0-9611788),* P.O. Box 1268, Riverhead, NY 11901 (SAN 285-2284) Tel 516-727-4270; Fax: 516-727-2868.

†**Ctr Amer Arche,** *(Ctr. for American Archeology Pr.; 0-942118),* Orders Addr.: P.O. Box 366, Kampsville, IL 62053 (SAN 694-9517) Tel 618-653-4688; Fax: 618-653-4232; *CIP.*

Ctr Analysis Public Issues, *(Ctr. for Analysis of Public Issues; 0-943136),* 164 Nassau St., Flr. 2, Princeton, NJ 08542-7005 (SAN 209-3227) Tel 609-924-9750; Fax: 609-924-0363.

†**Ctr Appl Res,** *(Ctr. for Applied Research in Education, The; 0-87628),* Subs. of Prentice Hall Ptr, Orders Addr.: P.O. Box 11071, Des Moines, IA 50381-1071 (SAN 241-6492) Fax: 515-284-2607; Toll Free: 800-288-4745; Edit Addr.: 240 Frisch Ct., Paramus, NJ 07652-5240 (SAN 206-6424) Tel 201-909-6200
Web site: http://vig.prenhall.com/
Dist(s): **Continental Bk** *(Continental Bk. Co., Inc.); CIP.*

Ctr Applications Psych, *(Ctr. for Applications of Psychological Type, Inc.; 0-935652),* 2815 NW 13th St., Suite 401, Gainesville, FL 32609 (SAN 213-9162) Tel 352-375-0160; Fax: 352-378-0503; Toll Free: 800-777-2278
E-mail: development@capt.org
Web site: http://www.capt.org.

Ctr Applied Psy, *See* **Childswork**

Ctr Bio-Gerontology, *(Ctr. for Bio-Gerontology, The; 0-937777),* P.O. Box 11097, Pensacola, FL 32524 (SAN 659-3208) Tel 904-484-0595; Fax: 904-474-5255.

Ctr Bkstore, *(Center Bookstore, The; 1-888196),* 16161 Ventura Blvd., No. 802, Encino, CA 91436 Tel 818-881-5959; Fax: 818-881-1613; Toll Free: 800-367-3454
Dist(s): **Baker & Taylor** *(Baker & Taylor Bks.)*
Bookpeople *(Bookpeople)*
New Leaf Dist *(New Leaf Distributing Co., Inc.).*

Ctr Cancer T & R, *See* **Palmetto Richland**

†**Ctr Chinese Studies,** *(Ctr. for Chinese Studies Pubns.; 0-89264),* Univ. Michigan, 202 S. Thayer St., Ann Arbor, MI 48104-1608 (SAN 208-2772) Tel 734-998-7181; Fax: 734-998-7263
E-mail: ccs.publications@umich.edu
Web site:
http://www.umich.edu/~iinet/ccs/ccspubs.htm
Dist(s): **U of Mich Pr** *(Univ. of Michigan Pr.); CIP.*

Ctr Counsel Hlth Resc, *(Ctr. for Counseling & Health Resources, Inc.; 0-9628408),* 611 Main, P.O. Box 700, Edmonds, WA 98020 Tel 425-771-5166; Fax: 425-670-2807.

Ctr Emp Med, *(Ctr. for Empirical Medicine; 0-916386),* 4221 45th St., NW, Washington, DC 20016 (SAN 207-5512) Tel 310-378-4597; Fax: 310-378-7026
E-mail: emptherapies@earthlink.net
Web site: http://www.empiricaltherapies.com.

Ctr Energy Envir, *See* **CEEM Inc**

Ctr Env Des Res, *(Ball State Univ., Ctr. for Environmental Design, Research & Service; 0-912431),* Ball State Univ., College of Archit. Planning AB104 Ctr. for Env. Design, Res. & Svc., Muncie, IN 47306 (SAN 265-1890) Tel 765-285-5859; Fax: 765-285-3726.

Ctr for Clin Res, *(Ctr. for Clinical Research Practice; 0-9663593),* 40 Washington St., Suite 130, Wellesley, MA 02481 Tel 781-431-7577; Fax: 781-237-0330
E-mail: ldoran@ccrp.com
Web site: http://www.ccrp.com
Dist(s): **Am Health Consults** *(American Health Consultants).*

Ctr for Hlth, *(Ctr. for Health Design; 0-9638938),* 4550 Alhambra Way, Martinez, CA 94553 Tel 510-370-0345; Fax: 510-228-4018.

Ctr for World Studies, *(Center For World Indigenous Studies; 1-893710),* 1001 Cooper Pt., Rd., SW, Suite 140-214, Olympia, WA 98502 Tel 360-754-1990; Fax: 360-786-5034
E-mail: cwisfwi@halcyon.com; lekorn@wco.com
Web site: http://www.halcyon.com/fwdp/.

Ctr Hlth Affairs, *(Ctr. for Health Affairs, Greater Cleveland Hospital Assn.; 0-942393),* 1226 Huron Rd., Cleveland, OH 44115 (SAN 667-1012) Tel 216-696-6900.

Ctr Hlthcare, *See* **Dorland Hlthcare**

Ctr Hlthcare IPS, *(Ctr. for Healthcare Industry Performance Studies; 1-882733),* 1550 Old Henderson Rd., Suite S277, Columbus, OH 43220-3626 Fax: 614-457-1113; Toll Free: 800-859-2447.

Ctr Hospice Care, *(Ctr. for Hospice Care; 0-9622089),* Affil. of St. Barnabas Health Care System, Three High St., Glen Ridge, NJ 07028 Tel 973-429-0300; Fax: 973-429-9274.

Ctr Human Natural Ntrtn, *(Ctr. for Human Natural Nutrition; 0-9628298),* 1614 Victory Blvd., Suite 114, Glendale, CA 91201-2946.

Ctr Intl Ed U of MA, *(Univ. of Massachusetts, Ctr. for International Education; 0-932288; 1-889536),* 285 Hills S., Amherst, MA 01003 (SAN 212-9329) Tel 413-545-0465; Fax: 413-545-1263.

Ctr Lake Superior, *See* **Lke Superior Res**

Ctr Learning, *(Ctr. for Learning, The; 1-56077),* Orders Addr.: P.O. Box 910, Villa Maria, PA 16155 Tel 724-964-8083; Toll Free Fax: 888-767-8080; Toll Free: 800-767-9090 (ordering); Edit Addr.: 21590 Center Ridge Rd., Rocky River, OH 44116 (SAN 248-2029) Tel 440-331-1404; Fax: 440-331-5414
E-mail: cfl@stratos.net
Web site: http://www.centerforlearning.org.

Ctr Marital Sexual, *(Ctr. for Marital & Sexual Studies; 0-9600626),* 5311 E. El Prado Ave., Long Beach, CA 90815-3905 (SAN 203-8587) Tel 310-597-4425.

Ctr Nursing Excell, *(Ctr. for Nursing Excellence; 0-9636792),* Pennswood Village, Suite 6, Newtown, PA 18940 Tel 215-579-0777.

Ctr Office Tech, *(Ctr. for Office Technology; 1-879887),* 301 N. Fairfax St., Suite 102, Alexandria, VA 22314-2633 Tel 703-276-1174; Fax: 703-276-1177.

Ctr on Budget, *(Ctr. on Budget & Policy Priorities; 1-57291),* 777 N. Capitol St., NE, Suite 705, Washington, DC 20002 Tel 202-408-1080; Fax: 202-408-1056.

Ctr Orang Asli (MYS) *(983-40042) Dist. by* **OR St Zoology.**

Ctr Partially, *(Ctr. for the Partially Sighted; 0-9622368),* 12301 Wilshire Blvd., Suite 600, Los Angeles, CA 90025-1021.

Ctr Phlebotomy Ed, *See* **HealthStar Pr**

Ctr Pr CA, *(Center Pr., The; 0-9626888; 1-889198),* Orders Addr.: P.O. Box 6936, Thousand Oaks, CA 91360; Edit Addr.: 200 Kirsten Lee Dr., Westlake Village, CA 91361 Tel 818-889-7071; Fax: 818-889-7072 Do not confuse with The Center Pr., Grapevine, TX
E-mail: center@centerbooks.com
Web site: http://www.centerbooks.com
Dist(s): **Baker & Taylor** *(Baker & Taylor Bks.)*
Login Pubs Consort *(Login Pubs. Consortium)*
Quality Bks IL *(Quality Bks., Inc.).*

Ctr Pr NM, *(Center Pr.; 0-916185),* 2070 Calle Contento, Santa Fe, NM 87505-5406 (SAN 294-913X) Tel 505-438-3979 Do not confuse with companies with the same name in Berkeley, CA, Encino, CA.

Ctr Prof Develop, *(Ctr. for Professional Development, Inc.; 0-9633550),* 524 S. Cascade, Suite 1, Colorado Springs, CO 80903 Tel 719-471-4110; Fax: 719-471-9519 Do not confuse with Center for Professional Development in Rochester, NY.

Ctr Public Rep, *(Ctr. for Public Representation, Inc.; 0-932622),* P.O. Box 260049, Madison, WI 53726-0049 (SAN 223-2855) Tel 608-251-4008; Fax: 608-251-1263.

Ctr Res Ambulatory, *See* **MGMA Ctr**

Ctr Respon Psych, *(Ctr. for Responsive Psychology; 1-55524),* Brooklyn College, CUNY, Brooklyn, NY 11210 (SAN 225-7165) Tel 718-780-5960.

Ctr Responsive Law, *(Ctr. for Study of Responsive Law; 0-936758),* P.O. Box 19367, Washington, DC 20036 (SAN 281-403X) Tel 202-387-8030.

Ctr Sacred Healing, *(Ctr. for Sacred Healing Arts Publishing Co.; 0-936901),* 207 E. 95th St., Brooklyn, NY 11212-2151 (SAN 658-5558).

Ctr Sci Info, *(Ctr. for Science Information; 0-912005),* 45 Mission Trail Rd., Woodside, CA 94062-3544 (SAN 264-6056) Tel 415-553-8772; Fax: 415-566-1048.

Ctr Sci Study, *(Ctr. for the Scientific Study of Religion; 0-913348),* 5757 University Ave., Chicago, IL 60637-9990 (SAN 203-8749) Tel 773-752-5757 (ext 214); Fax: 773-752-5925.

Ctr Self Suff, *(Ctr. for Self-Sufficiency Publishing; 0-910811),* P.O. Box 416, Denver, CO 80201-0416 (SAN 698-1828) Tel 303-575-5676; Fax: 970-292-2136
E-mail: mail@breadpudding.net
Web site: http://www.centerforselfsufficiency.com
Dist(s): **Prosperity & Profits** *(Prosperity & Profits Unlimited, Distribution Services).*

Ctr S&SE Asian, *(Univ. of Michigan, Ctr. for South & Southeast Asian Studies; 0-89148),* 130 Lane Hall, Ann Arbor, MI 48109 (SAN 206-491X) Tel 313-763-5790; Fax: 313-936-2948
Dist(s): **U of Mich Pr** *(Univ. of Michigan Pr.).*

Ctr Study Aging, *(Ctr. for the Study of Aging, Inc.; 0-937829),* 706 Madison Ave., Albany, NY 12208-3604 (SAN 659-4344) Tel 518-465-6927; Fax: 518-462-1339.

Ctr Study Language, *See* **CSLI**

Ctr Study Serv, *(Ctr. for the Study of Services; 0-9611432; 1-888124),* 733 15th St. NW, Suite 820, Washington, DC 20005 (SAN 287-2862) Tel 202-347-7283; Fax: 202-347-4000; Toll Free: 800-213-7283
E-mail: checkbook@checkbook.org
Web site: http://www.checkbook.org.

Ctr Thanatology, *(Ctr. for Thanatology Research & Education, Inc.; 0-930194),* 391 Atlantic Ave., Brooklyn, NY 11217-1701 (SAN 210-7414) Tel 718-858-3026; Fax: 718-852-1846
E-mail: rhalporn@pipeline.com
Web site: http://www.thanatology.org.

Ctr Trad Orthodox, *(Ctr. for Traditionalist Orthodox Studies; 0-911165),* Orders Addr.: c/o St. Gregory Palamas Monastery, 1307 Sawyers Bar Rd., PMB 398, Etna, CA 96027 (SAN 287-0029) Tel 530-467-3228; Fax: 530-467-5828
Web site: http://www.sisqtel.net/~sgpm/ctos.

Ctr Traditional Acupuncture, *(Ctr. for Traditional Acupuncture, Inc.; 0-912379),* American City Bldg., Suite 100, Columbia, MD 21044 (SAN 265-2137) Tel 410-997-3770; Fax: 410-964-3544
Dist(s): **Bookpeople** *(Bookpeople)*
New Leaf Dist *(New Leaf Distributing Co., Inc.)*
Redwing Bk Co *(Redwing Bk. Co.).*

Ctr Women Policy, *(Ctr. for Women Policy Studies; 1-877966),* 1211 Connecticut Ave., NW, Suite 312, Washington, DC 20036-2701 Tel 202-872-1770; Fax: 202-296-8962
E-mail: lwolfe@centerwomenpolicy.org
Web site: http://www.centerwomenpolicy.org.

Ctrl Bur voor Schimmel (NLD) *(90-70351) Dist. by* **Lubrecht & Cramer.**

CTS, *(CTS; 0-917429),* 131 Rolling Ave., Rockville, MD 20852 (SAN 656-1454) Tel 301-468-4800; Fax: 301-468-2309; Toll Free: 800-433-8015
E-mail: support@ctsguides.com
Web site: http://www.ctsguides.com.

CUCFP&FH, *(Columbia Univ., Ctr. for Population & Family Health; 0-9620952),* 60 Haven Ave., New York, NY 10032 (SAN 250-2860) Tel 212-305-6960; Fax: 212-305-7024.

Cum Index Nursing, *(CINAHL; 0-910478),* 1509 Wilson Terr., Glendale, CA 91206 (SAN 217-2356) Tel 818-409-8005; Fax: 818-546-5679; Toll Free: 800-959-7167
E-mail: jlevy@cinahl.com
Web site: http://www.cinahl.com.

Cummngs & Hath, *(Cummings & Hathaway; 0-943025; 1-57981),* 395 Atlantic Ave., East Rockaway, NY 11518 (SAN 667-9668) Fax: 516-593-1401; Toll Free: 800-344-7579
E-mail: info@sterlingpierce.com.

CUP Services, *(CUP Services),* 750 Cascadilla St., Ithaca, NY 14851 (SAN 630-6519) Tel 607-277-2211; Fax: 607-277-6292; Toll Free: 800-666-2211.

CUPA-HR, *(CUPA-HR; 0-910402; 1-878240),* 1233 20th St. NW, Suite 301, Washington, DC 20036 (SAN 236-5170) Tel 202-429-0311; Fax: 202-429-0149
Web site: http://www.cupahr.org.

Current Clin Strat, *(Current Clinical Strategies Publishing; 0-9626030; 1-881528; 1-929622),* 27071 Cabot Rd., Suite 126, Laguna Hills, CA 92653-7011 (SAN 298-4490) Tel 949-348-8404; Fax: 949-348-8405; Toll Free Fax: 800-965-9420; Toll Free: 800-331-8227
E-mail: info@ccspublishing.com
Web site: http://www.ccspublishing.com/ccs
Dist(s): **J Majors Co** *(Majors, J. A. Co.)*
Matthews Medical Bk Co *(Matthews Medical Bk. Co.)*
Rittenhouse *(Rittenhouse Bk. Distributors).*

Current Concept, *(Current Conceptions, Inc.; 0-9657648),* 1615 NE Eastgate Blvd., Pullman, WA 99163 Tel 509-334-5193; Fax: 509-335-7237.

Current Dist (IND) *Dist. by* **St Mut.**

Current Lit Pubns, *(Current Literature Pubns., Inc.; 0-914899),* 1513 E St., Bellingham, WA 98225 (SAN 289-0976) Tel 360-676-2298; Fax: 360-676-8814; Toll Free: 800-735-8970.

†**Current Med,** *(Current Medicine Current Medicine; 1-57340; 1-878132),* 400 Market St., 7th Flr., Philadelphia, PA 19106 Tel 215-574-2266; Fax: 215-574-2270; Toll Free: 800-427-1796
E-mail: info@phl.cursci.com
Dist(s): **Saunders** *(Saunders, W. B. Co.); CIP.*

Current Science, *See* **Rapid Science**

Curzon Pr Ltd (GBR) *(0-7007) Dist. by* **UH Pr.**

Cutters Rig Bks, *(Cutter's Rig Bks.; 0-9655207),* 10752 NE Bill Point Dr., Bainbridge Island, WA 98110 Tel 206-842-7813; Fax: 206-382-1965; Toll Free: 800-266-5564.

CWLA Pr Imprint of Child Welfare

CWRU Dept Surgery, *(Case Western Reserve Univ., Dept. of Surgery; 0-9616613),* 4845 Bunita Beach Rd., Bonita Springs, OH 33723 (SAN 660-9910) Tel 216-658-2620.

CyberAge Bks Imprint of Info Today Inc

CyPr NY, *(CyPress; 0-930269),* 235 Lexington Ave., North Babylon, NY 11704-5308.

Cypress Creek Pubns, *(Cypress Creek Pubns.; 0-937755),* 146 Cypress Bend Pl., Florence, AL 35630-0700 (SAN 659-3356).

Cyrus Pr Imprint of Waterside Prodns

D & C Pub (GBR) *(0-7153) Dist. by* **F & W Pubns Inc.**

D A Dahlin, *(Dahlin, Donald A.; 1-883243),* 824 W. Gurley St., Apt. 130, Prescott, AZ 86305-3652.

D Armstrong, *(Armstrong, D. Co., Inc.),* 7638 Antoine St., Houston, TX 77088 (SAN 210-0320) Tel 713-820-2715.

D B Taraporevala (IND) *Dist. by* **Asia Bk Corp.**

D Baird Pubs (GBR) *(1-900131; 1-903296) Dist. by* **Trafalgar.**

D Brannan, *(Brannan, Dan Pubns.; 0-9650228),* 4320 Ann Dr., Alton, IL 62002-5706 Tel 803-985-1300.

D C S Pubg, *(D C S Publishing; 0-9672352),* 33 W. Huron, Suite. 809, Chicago, IL 60610 Tel 312-944-4433; Fax: 312-944-4436
Dist(s): **Global Dist Co** *(Global Distributing Co.).*

D DiPasquale, *(DiPasquale, David; 0-9640918),* 710 N. Ocean Blvd., Pompano Beach, FL 33062 Tel 954-785-9595.

D E Donel, *(Donel, D.E. Co.; 0-913657),* P.O. Box 376, Loma Linda, CA 92354 (SAN 286-0929) Tel 909-796-5598.

D I Weiss, *(Weiss, David I.; 0-9618049),* Orders Addr.: P.O. Box 1705, Brookline, MA 02146 (SAN 666-2552) Tel 617-277-7547; Edit Addr.: 17 Parkman St., Brookline, MA 02146 (SAN 666-2560).

D K Ink Imprint of DK Pub Inc

D L OBrien, *See* **Hlth & Life**

D L Stewart, *(Stewart, Deborah L.; 0-9678177),* P.O. Box 594, Skiatook, OK 74070
E-mail: dls@nursingnownotes.com
Web site: http://www.nursingnownotes.com.

D L Thompson, *(Thompson, Diana L.; 0-9638347),* 6720 14th Ave., SW, Seattle, WA 98106 Tel 206-768-1556; Fax: 206-768-6276
E-mail: soapsage@home.com
Dist(s): **All You Knead** *(All You Knead).*

D Leonard Pubns, *(Leonard, Dennis Pubns.; 1-880809),* Heritage Christian Center, 9495 E. Florida Ave., Denver, CO 80231 Tel 303-369-5870; Fax: 303-752-3665
E-mail: dlpublishing@aol.com.

D Lynns Wrld, *(Diane-Lynn's World; 0-9705699),* 732 Thompson Ave., Roselle, NJ 07203-2211 Tel 908-245-4273; Fax: 908-245-4277
E-mail: A-S-D-F@worldnet.att.net.

D M Grant, *(Grant, Donald M. Pub., Inc.; 0-937986; 1-880418),* Orders Addr.: P.O. Box 187, Hampton Falls, NH 03844 (SAN 281-7535) Tel 603-778-7191 (phone/fax); Toll Free: 800-476-0510 (orders only); Edit Addr.: 19 Surrey Ln., Hampton Falls, NH 03844
E-mail: mail@grantbooks.com
Web site: http://www.grantbooks.com
Dist(s): **Baker & Taylor** *(Baker & Taylor Bks.)*
Bookazine Co Inc *(Bookazine Co., Inc.)*
Dreamhaven *(Dreamhaven Bks.).*

D M Whiteside, *(Whiteside, Dora M. Pub.; 0-938353),* 501 Juniper Dr., Prescott, AZ 86303 (SAN 659-9133) Tel 520-445-7245.

D Ostrander, *(Ostrander, Dan; 0-9653302),* 8927 W. 18th St., N., Wichita, KS 67212-5390 Tel 316-729-6900; Fax: 316-722-0090.

D R Senechek, *See* **Senyczak Pubns**

D S L Ltd, *(DSL, Ltd.; 1-889959),* 1218 Noridge, Port Washington, WI 53074-1367 Tel 414-284-2542; Fax: 414-284-7039
E-mail: ruthsova@execpc.com.

D S M, *(DSM PathWorks, Inc.; 0-9670354),* P.O. Box 33, Saint Mary's, IA 50241 Tel 641-297-2314
E-mail: pathwork@netins.net.

D Siebert Co, *(Siebert, Doug Co., Inc., The; 0-9631005),* 2457A S. Hiawassee Rd., No. 196, Orlando, FL 32835-6349 Toll Free: 800-367-3684.

D Singer Ent, *(Singer, David Enterprises, Inc.; 0-9636712),* 1130 Cleveland St., Suite 210, Clearwater, FL 34615 Tel 813-443-7008; Fax: 813-449-1353; Toll Free: 800-326-1797.

D Steinkopff (DEU) *(3-7985) Dist. by* **Spr-Verlag.**

D Thom, *See* **JELD Pub**

D Vine, *(Vine, David; 0-9703471),* 400 Arthur Godfrey Rd., Suite 403, Miami Beach, FL 33140 Tel 305-538-1115; Fax: 305-538-1129.

D W V, *(DWV Enterprises; 0-9642715),* 3050 Hillsdale Dr., Augusta, GA 30909 Tel 706-721-2971; Fax: 706-721-7248
E-mail: amvan@mail.mcg.edu.

†**Da Capo,** *(Da Capo Pr., Inc.; 0-306),* A Member of Perseus Books Group, Orders Addr.: 5500 Central Ave., Boulder, CO 80301 Fax: 303-449-3356 (customer service); Toll Free: 800-386-5656 (customer service); Edit Addr.: 11 Cambridge Ctr., Cambridge, MA 02142 Tel 617-252-5200; Fax: 617-252-5285
E-mail: westview.orders@perseusbooks.com
Web site: http://www.perseusbooksgroup.com
Dist(s): **HarperCollins Pubs** *(HarperCollins Pubs.); CIP.*

Dafina Imprint of Kensgtn Pub Corp

Damico, *(D'amico, Paul M.; 0-9607270),* P.O. Box 967, Livingston Manor, NY 12758 (SAN 239-4200) Tel 914-439-4990; Toll Free: 800-872-3048.

Damien-Dutton Soc, *(Damien-Dutton Society for Leprosy Aid, Inc.; 0-9606330),* 616 Bedford Ave., Bellmore, NY 11710 (SAN 217-1694) Tel 516-221-5829; 516-221-9588; Fax: 516-221-5909.

Dancng Jester, *(Dancing Jester Pr.; 1-887003),* 3411 Garth Rd., Suite 208, Baytown, TX 77521 Tel 713-427-9560; Fax: 713-427-8685
E-mail: djpress@aol.com.

Dar Al-Fikr, *(Dar Al-Fikr Al-Mouaser; 1-57547),* 3520 Forbes Ave., No. A259, Pittsburgh, PA 15213 Tel 412-441-7768; Fax: 412-441-8189
E-mail: fikr@fikr.com
Web site: http://www.fikr.com.

DARE, *(Dare, Inc.; 0-943690),* 3628 Grant Ave., Rockford, IL 61103 (SAN 238-2695) Tel 815-877-8511.

Darnell & Piper, *(Darnell, Jeanie & Buddy Piper; 0-9633475),* 5349 Newcastle Ave., Suite 32, Encino, CA 91316 Tel 818-996-4818; Fax: 818-344-9813; Toll Free: 800-743-0707.

Dart Pub Services, *See* **Nissi Pubns**

Dartmth Pub (GBR) *(1-85521) Dist. by* **Ashgate Pub Co.**

Data Pharm, *See* **Work-Loss Data**

Databks, *See* **Chandler Hse**

Datar Pub, *(Datar Publishing Co.; 0-931572; 1-57732),* P.O. Box 510222, Saint Louis, MO 63151-0222 (SAN 211-4135) Tel 314-416-4613; Fax: 314-416-4600; Toll Free: 800-633-8378
Web site: http://www.webexam.com.

Daughters Utah, *(Daughters of Utah Pioneers; 0-9658406),* 300 N. Main St., Salt Lake City, UT 84103-1699 (SAN 240-8465) Tel 801-538-1050; Fax: 801-538-1119.

David Brown, *(Brown, David Bk. Co.; 0-946897),* Orders Addr.: P.O. Box 511, Oakville, CT 06779 (SAN 630-9461) Tel 860-945-9329; Fax: 860-945-9468; Toll Free: 800-791-9354
E-mail: david.brown.bk.co@snet.net
Web site: http://www.oxbowbooks.com.

David Diagnostics, *See* **Baffin Bks**

David Fulton (GBR) *(1-85346; 1-84312) Dist. by* **Taylor & Francis.**

Davies Pubng, *(Davies Publishing, Inc.; 0-941022),* 32 S. Raymond Ave., Suite 4, Pasadena, CA 91105-1935 (SAN 217-3255) Tel 626-792-3046; Fax: 626-792-5308; Toll Free: 877-792-0005
E-mail: daviescorp@aol.com.

Davies-Black Pub Imprint of Consulting Psychol

Davila Assocs, *(Davila Assocs., Inc.; 0-941787),* Orders Addr.: P.O. Box 920142, Norcross, GA 30010 (SAN 666-4555) Tel 770-491-6306; Edit Addr.: 1350 Dogwood Ln., Tucker, GA 30084 (SAN 666-4563) Tel 404-491-6306
E-mail: ldavila@peachnet.campuscwix.net
Web site: http://www.ReadingMedicalRecords.net.

Davis & Geck, *(Davis & Geck; 0-9620916),* Div. of American Cyanamid Co., c/o American Cyanamid Co., 1 Cyanamid Plaza, Wayne, NJ 07470 (SAN 250-0957) Tel 973-831-4494.

Davis Ascs PA, *See* **N M Davis**

†**Davis Co,** *(Davis, F. A. Co.; 0-8036),* 1915 Arch St., Philadelphia, PA 19103 (SAN 295-3250) Tel 215-440-3001; Fax: 215-440-3016; Toll Free: 800-323-3555
E-mail: orders@fadavis.com
Web site: http://www.fadavis.com
Dist(s): **J Majors Co** *(Majors, J. A. Co.)*
Majors Scientific Bks Inc *(Majors Scientific Bks., Inc.)*
Matthews Medical Bk Co *(Matthews Medical Bk. Co.)*
Rittenhouse *(Rittenhouse Bk. Distributors); CIP.*

Davis Horwood Intl, *(Davis Horwood International Pubs., Ltd. (DHI); 1-930114),* 1464 Garner Station Blvd., Suite 413, Raleigh, NC 27603-3634 Tel 919-773-1645
E-mail: barrie@shadoweb.net
Web site: http://www.davishorwoodintlpub.com.

Dawn Eve Prod, *(Dawn Eve Productions; 0-9654257),* 3340 Sixth Ave., San Diego, CA 92103 Tel 619-295-4529; Fax: 619-295-8339.

Dawn Pubns TX, *(Dawn Pubns.; 0-942341),* 2103 N. Memorial Ct., Pasadena, TX 77502 (SAN 667-0865) Tel 713-944-2339; Toll Free: 888-657-8633 Do not confuse with Dawn Pubns., Nevada City, CA.

Dawn Sign, *(Dawn Sign Pr.; 0-915035; 1-58121),* 6130 Nancy Ridge Dr., San Diego, CA 92121-3223 (SAN 289-9183) Tel 858-625-0600; Fax: 858-625-2336; Toll Free: 800-549-5350
E-mail: comments@dawnsign.com
Web site: http://www.dawnsignpress.com
Dist(s): **Gryphon Hse** *(Gryphon Hse., Inc.)*
IPG Chicago *(Independent Pubs. Group).*

Dawud Ujamma, *(Ujamma, Dawud; 1-884938),* Sub. of Ujamaa Enterprises, 103 Eastwyck Rd., Decatur, GA 30032 Tel 404-244-7094
E-mail: aol@D1vjamaa.

Daye Pr, *(Daye Pr., Inc.; 0-918772),* P.O. Box 8021, Athens, GA 30603 (SAN 210-4180) Tel 706-549-3081; Fax: 706-548-3225
E-mail: baxter@negia.net.

Dayton Labs, *(Dayton Laboratories; 0-916750),* 3235 Dayton Ave., Lorain, OH 44055 (SAN 208-1946) Tel 440-246-1397
E-mail: dayton@erienet.net.

DBS Prodns, *(DBS Productions; 1-879471),* Orders Addr.: P.O. Box 1894, Charlottesville, VA 22903 (SAN 297-4452) Tel 804-293-5502 (phone/fax); Toll Free: 800-745-1581; Edit Addr.: 2508A Fontaine Ave., Charlottesville, VA 22903 (SAN 297-4460)
E-mail: info@dbs-sar.com
Web site: http://www.dbs-sar.com
Dist(s): **Emerg Response Inst** *(Emergency Response Institute, Inc.)*
Natl Assn Search & Rescue *(National Assn. for Search & Rescue)*
OSU Fire Protect *(OSU Fire Protection Pubns.).*

DCarlin Pub, *(D'Carlin Publishing; 0-939342),* Orders Addr.: P.O. Box 12521, Reno, NV 89510 (SAN 216-2369) Tel 702-828-3429; Edit Addr.: 1800 Manzanita Ln., Reno, NV 89509.

D&D Publns, *(D&D Pubns.; 0-9648370),* 3009 West Sahurro Dr., Phoenix, AZ 85008 Tel 602-504-0307 Do not confuse with D & D Pubns., Lawrence, KS
E-mail: .

DDDD Pubns, *(DDDD Pubns.; 0-9635341; 1-885519),* 9715 Foster, Saint Louis, MO 63114 (SAN 631-2675) Tel 314-427-3329
Dist(s): **Baker & Taylor** *(Baker & Taylor Bks.).*

†**De Gruyter,** *(De Gruyter, Walter Inc.; 0-89925; 1-56445; 3-11),* Subs. of Walter de Gruyter & Co. (GW), 200 Saw Mill River Rd., Hawthorne, NY 10532 (SAN 201-3088) Tel 914-747-0110; Fax: 914-747-1326
E-mail: customerservice@degruyterny.com
Web site: http://www.degruyter.com; *CIP.*

De Novo Pr, *(De Novo Pr.; 0-912357),* 2819 Piedmont Ave., Berkeley, CA 94705 (SAN 265-1173) Tel 510-849-9382 (phone/fax)
E-mail: lonny@sirius.com
Web site: http://www.photowords.com.

De Novo TX, *(De Novo, Inc.; 0-9631020; 0-9678268),* Div. of C-Six Diagnostics, Inc., 2922 University Blvd., Houston, TX 77005-3452 Tel 713-793-7102; Fax: 713-793-1213
E-mail: grodey@bena.tmc.edu.

De Young Pr, *(De Young Pr.; 0-936128),* 516 S. Washington St., Stark, KS 66775 (SAN 212-7652) Tel 316-754-3462
E-mail: deyoung@ekt.net.

Deaconess Fnd, *(Deaconess Foundation, The; 0-9642849),* 6150 Oakland Ave., Saint Louis, MO 63139 Tel 314-768-3013; Fax: 314-768-3118.

Deaconess Pr, *See* **Fairview Press**

DeafBlind Srvcs, *(DeafBlind Services, Inc.; 0-9626896),* 726 2nd St., NE, Minneapolis, MN 55413 Tel 612-362-8454; Fax: 612-362-8437.

Deakin Univ (AUS) *(0-7300) Dist. by* **St Mut.**

Dean Bks, *(Dean Bks.; 0-9619243),* 6 Hagen Ct., Coram, NY 11727 (SAN 243-8097) Tel 516-698-5442.

Dean Fnd for HRE, *See* **Madison Inst of Med**

†**Dearborn,** *(Dearborn Trade, A Kaplan Professional Co.; 0-7931; 0-88462; 0-913864; 0-936894; 0-942103; 1-57410),* 155 N. Wacker Dr., Chicago, IL 60606-1719 (SAN 211-2280) Tel 312-836-4400; Fax: 312-836-1021; Toll Free: 800-621-9621
Web site: http://www.dearborn.com
Dist(s): **Continental Bk** *(Continental Bk. Co., Inc.)*
Urban Land *(Urban Land Institute); CIP.*

Dearborn Finan, *See* **Dearborn**

Dechema (DEU) *(3-921567; 3-926959) Dist. by* **Scholium Intl.**

Decker Art, *(Decker Art Services; 0-9670709),* Orders Addr.: P.O. Box 101403, Anchorage, AK 99510 Tel 907-272-1589; Fax: 907-272-5395; Edit Addr.: 621 W. Sixth Ave., Anchorage, AK 99501
E-mail: julied@alskalife.net
Dist(s): **Todd Commns** *(Todd Communications)*
U of Wash Pr *(Univ. of Washington Pr.).*

Dee Maria Pub, *(Dee Maria Publishing; 0-9660414),* P.O. Box 293, Cranbury, NJ 08512 Tel 609-655-3683.

Deep & Deep Pubns (IND) *(81-7100; 81-7629; 81-86505) Dist. by* **S Asia.**

Degge Grp, *(Degge Group, Ltd., The; 0-9632020),* 1616 N. Fort Myer Dr., Suite 1430, Arlington, VA 22209 Tel 703-276-0067; Fax: 703-276-0069
E-mail: deggegroup@aol.com
Web site: http://www.deggegroup.com.

Degnon Assocs, *(Degnon Assocs., Inc.; 0-9656837),* 6728 Old McLean Village Dr., McLean, VA 22101-3906 Tel 703-556-9222; Fax: 703-556-8729
E-mail: info@degnon.org
Web site: http://www.degnon.org.

†Dekker, *(Dekker, Marcel Inc.; 0-8247),* 270 Madison Ave., New York, NY 10016 (SAN 201-3118) Tel 212-696-9000; Fax: 212-685-4540; Toll Free: 800-228-1160
E-mail: bookorders@dekker.com; sjones@dekker.com
Web site: http://www.dekker.com; *CIP.*

DEKR (CAN) *(0-941158; 1-55009; 1-55664) Dist. by* **Blackwell Sci.**

†Delacorte, *(Delacorte Pr.; 0-385; 0-87459; 1-4000),* Div. of Bantam Dell Publishing Group, A unit of Random Hse., Inc., Orders Addr.: 400 Hahn Rd., Westminster, MD 21157 Tel 410-848-1900; Toll Free: 800-726-0600; Edit Addr.: 1540 Broadway, New York, NY 10036-4094 (SAN 201-0097) Tel 212-782-9000; Fax: 212-765-3869; Toll Free: 800-323-9872
Web site: http://www.randomhouse.com; *CIP.*

Delft U Pr (NLD) *(90-407; 90-6275; 90-298) Dist. by* **Coronet Bks.**

Delgado, *(Delgado; 1-879084),* 25422 Trabuco Rd., Suite 105, No.141, Lake Forest, CA 92630 Tel 949-289-5232; Fax: 949-552-8751; Toll Free: 888-517-7421 ; *Imprints:* Health Wellness Studios (Health Wellness Studios)
E-mail: growyoungandslim@yahoo.com.

†Dell, *(Dell Publishing; 0-440; 1-4000),* Div. of Bantam Dell Publishing Group, Orders Addr.: 400 Hahn Rd., Westminster, MD 21157 Tel 410-848-1900; Toll Free: 800-726-0600; Edit Addr.: 1540 Broadway, New York, NY 10036-4094 (SAN 201-0097) Tel 212-782-9000; Fax: 212-492-9698; Toll Free: 800-223-6834 Bulk orders; 800-223-5780 Orders only; 800-323-9872 Customer service ; *Imprints:* Dell Trade Pbks (Dell Trade Paperbacks) LE (Laurel Editions) Delta Trade (Delta Trade Paperbacks) Dial Pr (Dial Press)
Web site: http://www.randomhouse.com
Dist(s): **Shens Bks** *(Shen's Bks.); CIP.*

Dell Trade Pbks Imprint of Dell

†Delmar, *(Delmar Thomson Learning; 0-7668; 0-8273; 0-916032; 0-944132; 1-56930; 1-4018),* Div. of Thomson Learning, Orders Addr.: P.O. Box 15015, Albany, NY 12212-5015 (SAN 206-7544) Tel 518-348-2300; Fax: 518-464-0393; Toll Free: 800-998-7498; Edit Addr.: 3 Columbia Cir., Albany, NY 12203-5015 (SAN 658-0440)
E-mail: cbutler@delmar.com
Web site: http://www.delmar.com
Dist(s): **Gryphon Hse** *(Gryphon Hse., Inc.)*
Thomson Learn *(Thomson Learning); CIP.*

Delphi Assocs, *(Delphi Assocs. 2000; 0-9643894),* 220 N.E. Landings Ct., Lee's Summit, MO 64064 Tel 816-373-9199.

Delphi Pub, *(Delphi Publishing; 1-929475),* 1282 Rte. 376, Wappingers Falls, NY 12590 Tel 914-226-2262; Fax: 914-226-2264
E-mail: fmdahl@frontiernet.net.

Delphic Associates, *(Delphic Assocs., Inc.; 1-55831),* 7700 Leesburg Pike, No. 218, Falls Church, VA 22043 (SAN 244-5522) Tel 703-761-4357; Fax: 703-556-0494
Web site: http://www.nvtemp.com.

Delta Pubng, *(Delta Publishing Co.; 0-9658242; 0-9704344),* 6714 Beach Blvd., Buena Park, CA 90621 Tel 714-523-8900; Fax: 714-523-3068
E-mail: naet@earthlink.net
Web site: http://www.naet.com.

Delta Pubs, *See* **Delta Pubng**

Delta Soc, *(Delta Society; 0-9627802; 1-889785),* 289 Perimeter Rd., E., Renton, WA 98055-1329 Tel 425-226-7357; Fax: 425-235-1076; Toll Free: 800-869-6898
E-mail: deltasociety@cis.copmuserve.com.

Delta Trade Imprint of Dell

Demeter Pr, *(Demeter Pr.; 1-885365),* Div. of Lapp & Assocs., P.O. Box 2583, Del Mar, CA 92014-5583.

Demos Medical, ***(Demos Medical Publishing, Inc.; 0-939957; 1-888799),*** **386 Park Ave. S., Suite 201, New York, NY 10016 (SAN 663-8635) Tel 212-683-0072; Fax: 212-683-0118; Toll Free: 800-532-8663**
E-mail: orderdept@demospub.com; info@demospub.com
Web site: http://www.demosmedpub.com
Dist(s): **SCB Distributors** ***(SCB Distributors).***

Demos Vermande, *See* **Demos Medical**

Denali Desgns, *(Denali Designs; 0-9648669),* Orders Addr.: P.O. Box 80503, Fairbanks, AK 99708-0503 Tel 907-456-1011; Fax: 907-456-3579; Edit Addr.: 2070 Nottingham Dr., Fairbanks, AK 99708
Dist(s): **Todd Commns** *(Todd Communications).*

Denise D, *(Davis, Denise; 0-9668415),* Orders Addr.: P.O. Box 43264, Cincinnati, OH 45243-0264 Tel 513-271-9258; Edit Addr.: 4940 Taft Rd., Cincinnati, OH 45243.

Dennis-Landman, *(Dennis-Landman Pubs.; 0-930422),* 1150 18th St., Santa Monica, CA 90403 (SAN 210-9352) Tel 310-828-0680.

Denta Pr, *(Denta Pr.; 0-9622139),* 18540 Long Lake Dr., Boca Raton, FL 33496-1937.

Dental Commun Imprint of Comm Unltd CA

Dental Store, *(Dental Store, Ltd.; 0-9640863),* 1061 S. Roselle Rd., Schaumburg, IL 60193-3900 Tel 847-301-0400; Fax: 847-301-7576
E-mail: shulkin@dentalstore.com
Web site: http://www.dentalstore.com.

Dental-Info, *(Dental-Info; 0-9607518),* Affil. of American Dental Institute, 2509 N. Campbell, No. 9, Tucson, AZ 85719 (SAN 239-4340)
Dist(s): **New Leaf Dist** *(New Leaf Distributing Co., Inc.).*

Denver Metro Chamber, *(Denver Metro Chamber of Commerce; 1-57975),* 1445 Market St., Denver, CO 80202 Tel 303-534-8500; Fax: 303-534-3200
E-mail: TiffanyMartinez@den-chamber.org
Web site: http://www.den-chamber.org.

DePauw Univ, *(DePauw Univ.; 0-936631),* 300 E. Seminary St., Greencastle, IN 46135 (SAN 699-6973) Tel 765-658-4629; Fax: 765-658-4625.

Dept Intl Health, *(Johns Hopkins Univ., Dept. of International Health; 0-912888),* 615 N. Wolfe St., Baltimore, MD 21205 (SAN 202-3520).

DER Prods, *(DER Productions; 0-9635454),* 5732 Nottingham Dr., Oakland, CA 94611-2163 Tel 510-531-4897; Fax: 510-531-4895.

Derma Found Pr, *(Dermatopathology Foundation Pr., Inc.; 0-9618536),* Orders Addr.: P.O. Box 377, Canton, MA 02021 (SAN 668-0798) Tel 617-821-0648; Edit Addr.: 291 Turnpike St., Canton, MA 02021 (SAN 668-0801).

Derricott Dental, *(Derricott Dental Management; 0-9640156),* 710 Glen Creek Rd., Salem, OR 97304 Tel 503-362-8727.

Descriptive Psych Pr, *(Descriptive Psychology Pr.; 0-9625661; 1-891700),* Div. of Society for Descriptive Psychology, 1019 Baldwin Ave., Ann Arbor, MI 48104 Tel 734-663-5435; Fax: 734-663-2806
E-mail: dpp@mediaone.net.

†Deseret Bk, *(Deseret Bk. Co.; 0-87579; 0-87747; 1-57345; 1-59038),* Div. of Deseret Management Corp., Orders Addr.: P.O. Box 30178, Salt Lake City, UT 84130 (SAN 150-763X) Tel 801-534-1515; 801-517-3165 (Wholesale Dept.); Fax: 801-517-3338; Toll Free: 800-453-3876; Edit Addr.: 40 E. South Temple, Salt Lake City, UT 84111
E-mail: dbwhsale@deseretbook.com; wholesale@deseretbook.com
Web site: http://www.deseretbook.com; *CIP.*

Desert City Pr, *(Desert City Pr.; 0-9642504),* P.O. Box 9994, Phoenix, AZ 85068-9994 Tel 602-943-0040; Toll Free: 800-266-5564
E-mail: gsmdcp@aol.com.

Desert Min, *(Desert Ministries, Inc.; 0-914733),* 2430 Mirow Pl., Charlotte, NC 28270 (SAN 657-6036) Tel 561-832-0207; Fax: 704-814-9247
E-mail: dmicathie@aol.com
Web site: http://www.desmin.org
Dist(s): **Spring Arbor Dist** *(Spring Arbor Distributors Inc.).*

Desert State, *(Desert State Publishing; 0-9655969),* 9702 E. Michigan, Sun Lakes, AZ 85248.

Design to Prnt, *(Design to Printing; 0-9653431),* 124 New Milford Tpke., New Preston, CT 06777 Tel 860-868-9423
E-mail: design.to.printing@snet.net.

Destiny Bks Imprint of Inner Tradit

Destiny Image Pubs, *(Destiny Image Pubs.; 0-7684; 0-914903; 1-56043; 0-9716036),* Orders Addr.: P.O. Box 310, Shippensburg, PA 17257-0310 (SAN 289-1050); Edit Addr.: 167 Walnut Bottom Rd., Shippensburg, PA 17257 (SAN 253-4339) Tel 717-532-3040; Fax: 717-532-9291; Toll Free: 800-722-6774
Web site: http://www.destinyimage.com
Dist(s): **Anchor Distributors** *(Anchor Distributors)*
Appalachian Bible *(Appalachian Bible Co.)*
Riverside-World *(Riverside World)*
Spring Arbor Dist *(Spring Arbor Distributors Inc.).*

Detrick Lawrence, *(Detrick Lawrence; 0-945790),* Orders Addr.: P.O. Box 1928, Edgartown, MA 02539; Edit Addr.: 140 Cooke St., Edgartown, MA 02539 (SAN 247-6126) Tel 508-627-8844; Fax: 508-627-8863; Toll Free: 800-842-0999
E-mail: info@efilmgroup.com
Web site: http://www.efilmgroup.com
Dist(s): **Emergency Film Group** *(Emergency Film Group).*

Detselig Ents (CAN) *(0-920490; 1-55059) Dist. by* **Temeron Bks.**

DevCom, *(DevCom; 1-887174),* Div. of MDDM, Inc., 114 Main St., Kingston, NJ 08528 Toll Free: 800-733-8266
Dist(s): **J Majors Co** *(Majors, J. A. Co.).*

Devel Play Trng Assocs, *See* **V A Brody**

†Devil Mountain Bks, *(Devil Mountain Bks.; 0-915685),* P.O. Box 4115, Walnut Creek, CA 94596 (SAN 292-4803) Tel 925-939-3415; Fax: 925-937-4883
E-mail: cbsturges@aol.com
Dist(s): **SPD-Small Pr Dist** *(SPD-Small Pr. Distribution); CIP.*

†Devin, *(Devin-Adair Pubs., Inc.; 0-8159),* Orders Addr.: P.O. Box A, Old Greenwich, CT 06870 (SAN 112-062X) Tel 203-531-7755; Fax: 718-359-8568 *CIP.*

Devon Pub, *(Devon Publishing Co., Inc., The; 0-941402),* 2700 Virginia Ave., NW, Washington, DC 20037 (SAN 238-9703) Tel 202-337-5197
Dist(s): **Baker & Taylor** *(Baker & Taylor Bks.).*

DeVorss, *(DeVorss & Co.; 0-87516),* Orders Addr.: P.O. Box 550, Marina del Rey, CA 90294-0550 (SAN 168-9886) Tel 310-822-8940; Fax: 310-821-6290; Toll Free: 800-843-5743; Edit Addr.: 1046 Princeton Dr., Marina del Rey, CA 90292
E-mail: devors@earthlink.net; service@devorss.com
Web site: http://www.devorss.com
Dist(s): **New Leaf Dist** *(New Leaf Distributing Co., Inc.).*

DeWitt & Sheppard, *(DeWitt & Sheppard Pubs.; 0-932365),* P.O. Box 5603, Tacoma, WA 98405 (SAN 687-3758) Tel 206-272-7588.

Dexter KS, *(Dexter Publishing; 0-9628012),* Div. of Dexter Industries, 2326 Sayles Blvd., Abilene, TX 79605-6141 Tel 915-692-0378
Dist(s): **F I T** *(F.A.I.T.H. Ministries).*

DFC Seminars, *(DFC Seminars, Inc.; 0-9637470),* 837 Mackall Ave., McLean, VA 22101-1615 Tel 703-734-8267; Fax: 703-734-0410; 931 Mackall Ave., McLean, VA 22103-3042.

†Dharma Pub, *(Dharma Publishing; 0-89800; 0-913546),* 2910 San Pablo Ave., Berkeley, CA 94702 (SAN 201-2723) Tel 510-548-5407; Fax: 510-548-2230; Toll Free: 800-873-4276
E-mail: info@dharma-publishing.com; Dharma-Publishing@Nyingma.org
Web site: http://www.dharmapress.com
Dist(s): **Bookpeople** *(Bookpeople)*
New Leaf Dist *(New Leaf Distributing Co., Inc.); CIP.*

DiaBetes Care Ctr, *(DiaBetes Care Ctr.; 1-890203),* 1222 14th Ave. S., Suite 306, Birmingham, AL 32505-5340.

Diabetes Educ, *(Diabetes Education & Support Ctr.; 0-9632453),* 2812 E. Bijou, Colorado Springs, CO 80909 Tel 719-473-6472; Fax: 719-473-6488
Dist(s): **Baker & Taylor** *(Baker & Taylor Bks.)*
Blackwell Corp *(Blackwell Corp.).*

Diadem Pub, *(Diadem Publishing; 0-939977),* 524 Gatlinburg Dr., Chatham, IL 62629 (SAN 663-8775) Tel 217-483-3326.

Diagnon Bioqual, *(Diagnon/Bioqual; 0-9632658),* 9600 Medical Ctr. Dr., Rockville, MD 20850-3300 Tel 301-251-2801; Fax: 301-251-1260.

Diagnostic & Cell, *(Diagnostic & Cell Research Institute; 0-9627824),* 2713 N. 43rd St., Waco, TX 76710 Tel 254-772-6388.

Diagnostic Solns, *(Diagnostic Solutions Management; 0-945628),* 402 Florence Ave., Southgate, KY 41071-3208 (SAN 247-445X) Tel 513-745-3022.

For full information on wholesalers and distributors, refer to the Wholesaler and Distributor Symbol Index

Diagnostic X-Ray, *(Diagnostic X-Ray Lab; 0-9670506),* 1711 Balsam Lane, Villanova, PA 19085 Tel 215-563-2024; Fax: 215-563-8450.

Dial Pr Imprint of Dell

Dialectic Pubng, *(Dialectic Publishing, Incorporated; 1-877589),* 3805 NE 167th St., North Miami Beach, FL 33160 Tel 305-945-5359; Fax: 305-945-5329
E-mail: dpublish@cris.com
Web site: http://www.acupunk.com
Dist(s): **New Leaf Dist** *(New Leaf Distributing Co., Inc.).*

Dialyrn, *(Dialyrn; 1-56488),* Div. of Total Renal Care, Inc., 825 S. Eighth St., Suite 400, Minneapolis, MN 55404 Tel 612-347-5949; Fax: 612-347-6192.

Diamond Bks CA, *(Diamond Bks.; 0-936713),* Orders Addr.: P.O. Box 10114, Berkeley, CA 94709 (SAN 630-5717); Edit Addr.: P.O. Box 10114, Berkeley, CA 94709 (SAN 699-878X) Tel 510-841-1283; Fax: 510-704-0158 Do not confuse with Diamond Bks., Salt Lake City, UT
E-mail: almaaspub@earthlink.net
Web site: http://www.ridhwan.org
Dist(s): **Bookpeople** *(Bookpeople)*
New Leaf Dist *(New Leaf Distributing Co., Inc.)*
Shambhala Pubns *(Shambhala Pubns., Inc.).*

Diamond Communications, *(Diamond Communications, Inc.; 0-912083; 1-888698),* Orders Addr.: P.O. Box 88, South Bend, IN 46624 (SAN 264-7346) Tel 219-299-9278; Fax: 219-299-9296; Toll Free Fax: 800-338-4550; Toll Free: 800-462-6420; Edit Addr.: 15200 NBN Way, Blue Ridge Summit, PA 17214
E-mail: custserve@nbnbooks.com; jalangford@rowman.com; shill@diamondbooks.com
Web site: http://www.nbnbooks.com; http://www.diamondbooks.com
Dist(s): **Natl Bk Netwk** *(National Bk. Network).*

Diamond Farm Bk, *(Diamond Farm Bk. Pubs.; 0-9506932),* Div. of Yesteryear Toys & Books, Inc., Orders Addr.: P.O. Box 537, Alexandria Bay, NY 13607 (SAN 674-9054) Tel 613-475-1771; Fax: 613-475-3748; Toll Free: 800-481-1353.

Diamond L Pub, *(Diamond L Publishing Co.; 0-9644682),* RR 1, Box 8169, Chandler, OK 74834 Tel 405-258-4073; Fax: 405-258-4086
E-mail: diamondl@swbell.net; miracle@diamondlequestrian.com
Web site: http://www.diamondlequestrian.com.

DIANE Pub, *(DIANE Publishing Co.; 0-7881; 0-941375; 1-56806; 0-7567),* Orders Addr.: P.O. Box 1428, Collingdale, PA 19023-8428 (SAN 667-1217) Tel 610-461-6200; Fax: 610-461-6130; Toll Free: 800-782-3833; Edit Addr.: 330 Pusey Ave., Suite 3, Collingdale, PA 19023
E-mail: dianepub@erols.com.

DIASPORA PR AM, *(DIASPORA PR. OF AMERICA; 0-9652860; 1-889601),* Div. of Development News, P.O. Box 200981, Boston, MA 02120-0018 Tel 617-298-1254 (phone/fax)
E-mail: diploman@mailexcite.com; princeyemi36@hotmail.com
Web site: http//members.tripod.com/yemiweb.

Didactic Syst, *(Didactic Systems, Inc.; 0-89401),* P.O. Box 457, Cranford, NJ 07016 (SAN 209-1739) Tel 908-789-2194; Fax: 908-789-0038
E-mail: didacticra@aol.com.

Diemer-Smith, *(Diemer, Smith Publishing Co., Inc.; 0-941138),* 1038 E Bastanchurym, No. 165, Fullerton, CA 92835 Fax: 714-256-5987; Toll Free: 800-821-4561
E-mail: JuneS2006@aol.com; DSPUB1999@aol.com
Web site: http://www.junestephenson.com.

Digits Intl, *(Digits International-Reflexology Institute; 0-9623429; 1-884727),* 27636 Ynez Rd. L7, No. 232, Temecula, CA 92591 Tel 909-694-0225; Fax: 909-694-5910.

Dilligaf Pubng, *See* **ebooksonthe**

Dillman Pub, *(Dillman Publishing; 0-9619221),* 2009 Bechtel Rd., Indianapolis, IN 46260 (SAN 243-6906) Tel 317-872-8987.

Dimensions, *(Dimensions Publishing; 0-9635791),* Orders Addr.: P.O. Box 7488, Redlands, CA 92375 Tel 909-864-4631; Fax: 909-797-3393; Toll Free: 800-578-5041; Edit Addr.: 7450 Bear Creek Ct., Higland, CA 92346 Tel 909-335-6406.

†Dine College Pr, *(Dine College Pr.; 0-912586),* Dine College Press, Tsaile, AZ 86556 (SAN 201-9582) Tel 520-724-6635; Fax: 520-724-6637
Web site: http://wwwcrystal.ncc.cc.nm.us
Dist(s): **Bookpeople** *(Bookpeople)*
Five Star AZ *(Five Star Pubns., Inc.); CIP.*

Dinshah Hlth Soc, *(Dinshah Health Society; 0-933917),* P.O. Box 707, Malaga, NJ 08328 (SAN 693-0220) Tel 856-692-4686
E-mail: dinshahhealth@aol.com
Web site: http://www.wj.net/dinshah
Dist(s): **New Leaf Dist** *(New Leaf Distributing Co., Inc.).*

Dioscorides Imprint of Timber

Dirigo Bks, *(Dirigo Bks., Inc.; 0-9623199),* 127 Elm St., Kingston, MA 02364-1925; Cushman Hill Rd., North Woodstock, ME 04219 Tel 207-665-2133.

Disc Enter Ltd, *(Discovery Enterprises, Ltd.; 1-57960; 1-878668),* 31 Laurelwood Dr., Carlisle, MA 01741 (SAN 297-2611) Tel 978-287-5401; Fax: 978-287-5402; Toll Free: 800-729-1720
E-mail: ushistorydocs@aol.com; del1jbw@aol.com
Dist(s): **Baker & Taylor** *(Baker & Taylor Bks.)*
Brodart *(Brodart Co.)*
Follett Library *(Follett Library Resources).*

Discov Bks, *(Discovery Bks.; 1-884981),* 1092 SW Second Ave., Ontario, OR 97914 Tel 541-889-5109 Do not confuse with Discovery Bks., Owls Heads, NY.

Discov CO, *(Discovery Pr.; 1-881292),* 2365 Pinhigh Ct., Colorado Springs, CO 80907 (SAN 297-892X) Tel 719-278-3708; Fax: 719-278-3709 Do not confuse with companies with the same name in Flushing, NY, Minneapolis, MN, Old San Juan, PR, Capistrano Beach, CA, Burbank, CA, Pacific Grove, CA, Point Pleasant, WV
E-mail: heart2heart@xc.org
Web site: http://www.sexaddict.com.

Discovery Hse Pubs, *(Discovery Hse. Pubs.; 0-929239; 1-57293),* Div. of R B C Ministries, Orders Addr.: P.O. Box 3566, Grand Rapids, MI 49501 (SAN 248-8949) Tel 616-942-9218; Fax: 616-957-5741; Toll Free: 800-653-8333; Edit Addr.: 3000 Kraft Ave., SE, Grand Rapids, MI 49512 (SAN 248-8957)
E-mail: dhp@rbc.org
Web site: http://www.dhp.org
Dist(s): **Barbour Pub** *(Barbour Publishing, Inc.).*

Distance Learning, *(Distance Learning Systems Indiana, Inc.; 0-9700638; 0-9710886),* Orders Addr.: 4271 N. High School Rd., Indianapolis, IN 46254 Tel 317-280-0000; Fax: 317-280-8888; Toll Free: 888-955-3276; Fulfillment Addr.: a/o J & A Fulfillment, 4271 N. High School Rd., Indianapolis, IN 46254
E-mail: ann@dlsii.com
Web site: http://www.dlsii.com.

Distinctive Pub, *(Distinctive Publishing Corp.; 0-942963),* 1888 NW 21st St., 2nd Flr., Pompano Beach, FL 33069 Do not confuse with Distinctive Publishing, Sandy, UT.

Distribks Inc, *(Distribooks, Inc.),* Div. of Midwest European Pubns., Inc., 8120 N. Ridgeway, Skokie, IL 60076 (SAN 630-9763) Tel 847-676-1596; Fax: 847-676-1195
E-mail: info@distribooks.com.

Dive Rescue, *(Dive Rescue International, Inc.; 0-929905),* 201 N. Link Ln., Fort Collins, CO 80524-2712 (SAN 250-7188) Tel 970-482-0887; Fax: 970-482-0893; Toll Free: 800-248-3483
E-mail: diveaccting@webaccess.net
Web site: http://www.diverescueintl.com.

Diveena Pubns, *(Diveena Pubns.; 0-9675624),* Orders Addr.: P.O. Box 413, Chelmsford, MA 01824 Tel 978-256-4262; Fax: 978-250-1938; Edit Addr.: 10 Armand Dr., Chelmsford, MA 01824
E-mail: davids@tiac.net.

Diversity Okla, *(Diversity Pr.; 0-936715),* P.O. Box 25, Idabel, OK 74745 (SAN 699-9131) Tel 580-286-3148 Do not confuse with Diversity Pr., Cambridge, MA
E-mail: diversitypress@netscape.net
Web site: http://www.diversitypress.com.

DJBA Inc, *See* **IVE Inc**

DJT Pub, *(D J T Publishing; 0-9637770),* Orders Addr.: P.O. Box 231352, Encinitas, CA 92023-1352 Tel 760-632-9047; Fax: 760-634-2095; Edit Addr.: 709 Snapdragon St., Encinitas, CA 92024
Dist(s): **Unique Bks Inc** *(Unique Bks., Inc.).*

†DK Pub Inc, *(Dorling Kindersley Publishing, Inc.; 0-673; 0-7513; 0-7894; 1-56458; 1-879431; 0-7566),* Div. of Pearson Learning, 375 Hudson St., New York, NY 10014 (SAN 253-0791) Tel 212-213-4800; Fax: 212-213-5240; Toll Free: 877-342-5357 (orders only) ;
Imprints: D K Ink (D K Ink)
E-mail: Annemarie.Cancienne@dk.com
Web site: http://www.dk.com
Dist(s): **Continental Bk** *(Continental Bk. Co., Inc.)*
Pub Resources Inc *(Publisher Resources, Inc.)*
R Hale & Co *(Hale, Robert & Co., Inc.)*
Shens Bks *(Shen's Bks.)*
Sunburst Comm *(Sunburst Communications, Inc.); CIP.*

D&MD Reports Imprint of International Business

DMS Pubs, *(DMS Pubs; 0-9623549),* P.O. Box 1817, Santa Monica, CA 90406 Tel 310-454-1238; Fax: 310-459-7667
E-mail: ah431@lafn.org.

Dncng Bear AR, *(Dancing Bear Publishing, Ltd.; 0-9653996),* 1 Longmeadow, Pine Bluff, AR 71603 Tel 501-534-1738.

Do It Now, *(Do It Now Foundation; 0-89230),* Orders Addr.: P.O. Box 27568, Tempe, AZ 85285 (SAN 225-9265) Tel 480-736-0599; Fax: 480-736-0771; Edit Addr.: 2750 S. Hardy Dr., Suite 2, Tempe, AZ 85282 (SAN 669-0661)
E-mail: doitnow123@earthlink.net; info@doitnow.org
Web site: http://www.doitnow.org.

Dock Pub Co, *(Dock Publishing Co.; 0-944478),* Div. of Brittony Rose Trading Co., 11631 Regio Ct., Dublin, CA 94568-1370 (SAN 243-6000).

Doctors Advice, *(Doctors Advice Pr.; 0-9669272),* 217 The Esplanade, S., Venice, FL 34285 Tel 941-412-0087; Fax: 941-483-4240; Toll Free: 877-988-2020.

Docubase, *See* **CMDC Systs**

DOE, *(U.S. Dept. of Energy; 0-87079),* DOE Office of Scientific & Technical Information P.O. Box 62, Oak Ridge, TN 37831 (SAN 210-7996) Tel 865-576-1188; Fax: 865-576-2865
Web site: http://www.osti.gov
Dist(s): **Natl Tech Info** *(National Technical Information Service, U.S. Dept. of Commerce).*

Dolphin Books, *See* **Seargeant Pub**

DOMA Pr, *(DOMA Pr.; 0-917816),* Orders Addr.: P.O. Box 564, Lisle, IL 60532 (SAN 210-0681) Tel 630-969-0734; Fax: 630-969-0282
E-mail: sladekmj@aol.com
Web site: http://hometown.aol.com.

Domel, *(Domel, Inc.; 0-9636345),* Orders Addr.: P.O. Box 3829, Albuquerque, NM 87190 Tel 505-898-0099; Fax: 505-897-2900; Edit Addr.: 801 Ranchitos, NW, Albuquerque, NM 87114
Web site: http://www.domelsica.com/.

Dominion Pr, *(Dominion Pr.; 0-912132),* Div. of Invisible Ministry, P.O. Box 4608, Salem, OR 97302-8608 (SAN 203-8935) Tel 503-362-9634 Do not confuse with Dominion Press in The Woodlands, TX.

Don Quixote Ed, *(Don Quixote Editions; 0-9709558),* 1400 S. Sixth St., Suite 301, McAllen, TX 78501 Tel 956-631-0344; Fax: 956-630-6736; Toll Free: 800-240-4661
E-mail: firigoyen@juno.com
Web site: http://www.firigoyen.yournd.com.

Donning Co, *(Donning Co. Pubs.; 0-89865; 0-915442; 1-57864),* Subs. of Walsworth Publishing Co., Inc., 184 Business Park Dr., No. 106, Virginia Beach, VA 23462-6533 (SAN 211-6316) Tel 757-497-1789; Fax: 757-497-2542; Toll Free: 800-296-8572
E-mail: dcpr3@pilot.infi.net
Web site: http://www.donning.com
Dist(s): **Schiffer** *(Schiffer Publishing, Ltd.).*

Do-Not Pr (GBR) *(1-899344) Dist. by* **Dufour.**

Doody Pubng, *(Doody Publishing; 1-885234),* 1101 Lake St., Suite 306, Oak Park, IL 60301 Tel 708-386-9500; Fax: 708-386-0860; Toll Free: 800-219-9500
E-mail: steve@doody.com
Web site: http://www.doody.com.

DOQ Srvs, *See* **Patient Adv Educ Res**

Dorland Hlthcare, *(Dorland Healthcare Information; 0-9624105; 1-880874),* 1500 Walnut St., Suite 1000, Philadelphia, PA 19102 Tel 215-875-1212; Fax: 215-735-3966; Toll Free: 800-784-2332
E-mail: info@dorlandhealth.com
Web site: http://www.dorlandhealth.com.

Dorling Kindersley, *See* **DK Pub Inc**

Dorrance, *(Dorrance Publishing Co., Inc.; 0-8059),* **643 Smithfield St., Pittsburgh, PA 15222 (SAN 201-3363) Tel 412-288-4543; Fax: 412-288-1786; Toll Free: 800-788-7654**
E-mail: dorrorder@dorrancepublishing.com
Web site: http://www.dorrancepublishing.com.

---

†Dorset Hse Pub, *(Dorset Hse. Publishing; 0-932633),* 353 W. 12th St., New York, NY 10014 (SAN 687-794X) Tel 212-620-4053; Fax: 212-727-1044; Toll Free: 800-342-6657
E-mail: info@dorsethouse.com
Web site: http://www.dorsethouse.com; *CIP.*

Dorset Pr MA, *(Dorset Pr.; 0-9656102),* P.O. Box 620026, Newton Lower Falls, MA 02462 Tel 617-969-5286; Fax: 617-243-6453.

Dotolo Inst, *(Dotolo Institute, Inc.; 0-9660627),* 2875 MCI Dr., Pinellas Park, FL 33782-6105 Toll Free: 800-237-8458
E-mail: Rdotolo@Dotoloresearch.com
Web site: http://www.Dotoloresearch.com.

Double Helix, *(Double Helix Pr.; 0-930578),* 1300 Tigertail Rd., Los Angeles, CA 90049 (SAN 211-0083) Tel 213-472-6452.

†Doubleday, *(Doubleday; 0-385; 1-4000),* Div. of Doubleday Broadway Publishing Group, Orders Addr.: 400 Hahn Rd., Westminster, MD 21157 (SAN 281-6083) Tel 410-848-1900; Toll Free: 800-726-0600; Edit Addr.: 1540 Broadway, New York, NY 10036-4094 (SAN 201-0089) Tel 212-354-6500; Fax: 212-492-9700; Toll Free: 800-223-6834 Bulk orders; 800-223-5780 Orders only; 800-323-9872 Customer service ; *Imprints:* Main St Bks (Main Street Books)
Web site: http://www.doubledaybookclub.com
Dist(s): **Continental Bk** *(Continental Bk. Co., Inc.); CIP.*

Doublem Bks, *(Doublem Bks.; 1-889080),* 228 Gleneagles Dr., Atlantis, FL 33462-6610 Tel 561-965-1111.

Doublenight Pr, *(Doublenight Pr.; 0-9644416),* 9617 Brecksville Rd., Brecksville, OH 44141-2903 (SAN 298-4989) Tel 440-526-6573.

Doug Butler, *See* **Btler Pub**

Douglas Pubns, *(Douglas Pubns.; 0-87228),* 2807 N. Parham Rd., Suite 200, Richmond, VA 23294 Tel 804-762-9600; Fax: 804-217-8999; Toll Free: 800-223-1797
E-mail: info@douglaspublications.com
Web site: http://www.douglaspublications.com.

Douglass Pubs, *(Douglass Pubs.; 0-935392),* P.O. Box 3270, Alexandria, VA 22302 (SAN 211-7037) Tel 703-379-1255
E-mail: dougpubh@ix.netcom.com
Web site: http://www.dougpubh@ix.netcom.com.

Dove & Orca, *(Dove & Orca; 0-9668528),* 611 W. Walnut St., Long Beach, NY 11561 Tel 516-432-9498 (phone/fax); Toll Free: 800-247-6553
Dist(s): **BookMasters** *(BookMasters, Inc.).*

Dove Audio, *See* **NewStar Media**

Dove Audio Imprint of NewStar Media

Dove Pr TX, *(Dove Pr.; 1-879667),* 388 Leisure Valley Rd., West, TX 76691-9709 Tel 254-829-0521; Fax: 254-829-0521
E-mail: Shilohacre@aol.com.

†Dover, *(Dover Pubns., Inc.; 0-486),* Orders Addr.: 31 E. Second St., Mineola, NY 11501 (SAN 201-338X) Tel 516-294-7000; Fax: 516-742-5049 (orders only); Toll Free: 800-223-3130 (Orders only)
Web site: http://www.doverpublications.co,
Dist(s): **Continental Bk** *(Continental Bk. Co., Inc.)*
Shens Bks *(Shen's Bks.)*
T T Beeler *(Beeler, Thomas T. Publisher); CIP.*

Dowd Hlthgrp, *(Dowd Healthgroup; 0-9630260),* 3732 Fairway Dr., Cameron Park, CA 95682 (SAN 297-472X) Tel 530-677-5954; Fax: 530-677-6733.

Dowden Pub, *(Dowden Publishing Co., Inc.; 0-9628716; 1-888892),* 110 Summit Ave., Montvale, NJ 07645 Tel 201-391-9100; Fax: 201-391-2778; Toll Free: 800-707-7040.

Dowling College Imprint of Global Pubns

DPA Assocs, *(DPA Associates, Inc.; 1-929162),* P.O. Box 22569, Kansas City, MO 64113-0569 Tel 816-942-8088; Fax: 816-943-1481; Toll Free: 800-245-0372
E-mail: gericne@compuserve.com
Dist(s): **KAHSA** *(KAHSA).*

Dr Chens, *(Dr. Chen's Acupuncture Clinic; 0-9645339),* 6215 50th St., Kenosha, WI 53144-1725 Tel 414-652-8886.

Dr Chris Pubns, *See* **Christopher Pubns**

Dr for Respons Gun Imprint of Claremont Inst

Dr Goodhlth, *(Doctor Goodhealth Pubns.; 0-9640710),* 18741 La Casita Ave., Yorba Linda, CA 92886-2645.

†Dr Hills Technol, *(Dr. Hills Technologies; 0-916438),* P.O. Box 644, Boulder Creek, CA 95006 (SAN 212-9965) Tel 831-338-2544; Fax: 831-338-3223; Toll Free: 877-947-4231
E-mail: chills@scruznet.com
Web site: http://www.scruz.net/~chills/
Dist(s): **Baker & Taylor** *(Baker & Taylor Bks.)*
New Leaf Dist *(New Leaf Distributing Co., Inc.); CIP.*

Dr L Cozen Pub, *(Cozen, Dr. Lewis Pub.; 0-9637929),* 1133 S. Alfred Dr., Los Angeles, CA 90035 Tel 213-653-5735.

Dr Pai Pubns, *(Dr. Pai Pubns.; 0-9667295),* c/o Public Health-Preventive Cardiology, 38 Somar Dr., Lewistown, PA 17044 Tel 717-248-5411; Fax: 717-248-0717 ; *Imprints:* Left Front (Left Front Shirt Pocket Publications)
E-mail: drpai@netscape.net,drusa.com,drpai.com.

Dr Schulzes Schl, *See* **Natural Healing Pubns**

Dr Shipps Lab, *(Dr. Shipp's Laboratories; 0-9635578),* 351 N. Foothill Rd., Beverly Hills, CA 90210 Tel 310-550-0107; Fax: 310-550-1664; Toll Free: 800-442-0107.

Dragon Pr VA, *(Dragon Pr.; 0-9679881),* 607 River Rd., Newport News, VA 23601-3910 Fax: 757-595-4118 Do not confuse with companies with same name in Marina Del Ray CA, Stockton, NJ
E-mail: stgeorgelee@aol.com
Web site: http://www.producer.com
Dist(s): **General Distrib Services** *(General Distribution Services, Inc.).*

Dragonfire, *(Dragonfire Productions, LLC; 0-9658807),* 145 Bledsoe Park Rd., Gallatin, TN 37066 Tel 615-452-1028 (phone/fax)
Dist(s): **Barnes & Noble Inc** *(Barnes & Noble, Inc.)*
Partners Pubs Grp *(Partners Pubs. Group, Inc.).*

Drama Thrpy Inst, *(Drama Therapy Institute of Los Angeles; 1-888657),* 1315 Westwood Blvd., Los Angeles, CA 90024-4901 Tel 310-478-7188.

DRC Graphics Serv, *(DRC Graphics Service; 0-9614887),* P.O. Box 4594, Portland, OR 97208 (SAN 693-2347) Tel 503-452-9338.

Dreenan Pr, *(Dreenan Pr. Ltd.; 0-88376),* Subs. of Young Discovery Library, c/o Young Discovery Library, 217 Main St., Ossining, NY 10562 Tel 914-945-0600; Fax: 914-945-0875; Toll Free: 800-343-7854.

Drelwood Comns, *(Drelwood Communications; 0-937766),* 1754 NE Mesford Rd., No. 63, Poulsbo, WA 98370 (SAN 215-756X) Tel 360-697-9381
E-mail: deana.m.healy@worldnet.att.net.

Drelwood Pubns, *See* **Drelwood Comns**

DrPEN, *(DrPEN, Inc.; 0-615; 0-9708511; 0-9717626),* P.O. Box 29040, Richmond, VA 23242-0040 Tel 804-740-1878 (phone/fax); Toll Free: 888-301-3615
E-mail: kfergusson@drpen.com
Web site: http://www.drpen.com
Dist(s): **Rittenhouse** *(Rittenhouse Bk. Distributors).*

Drug & Market Dev, *(Drug & Market Development Pubns.; 1-57936),* Div. of International Business Communications, P.O. Box 5194, Westborough, MA 01581-5194 Tel 508-616-5566; Fax: 508-616-5544
E-mail: cust.serv@drugandmarket.com
Web site: http://www.drugandmarket.com.

Drug Identif, *See* **Amera-Chem**

Drug Info Serv Co, *(Drug Information Service Co. (D.I.S.C.O.); 0-9626339),* 4841 Catclaw Dr., Abilene, TX 79606-4165 Tel 915-698-2302.

Drugs Dont Wrk, *(Drugs Don't Work; 0-9650675),* Div. of Phoenix Hse., 33 W. 60th St., 5th Flr., New York, NY 10023 Tel 212-757-2100; Fax: 212-757-2208; Toll Free: 800-883-3784.

Drumbeat Imprint of Longman

DRx, *(DRx; 0-9651040; 1-57577),* 240 Alta Vista Ave., Los Altos, CA 94022 Tel 650-948-6293
E-mail: DRxMail@metrika.com
Dist(s): **ISHK** *(ISHK).*

Dry Bones Pr, *(Dry Bones Pr.; 1-883938; 1-931333),* P.O. Box 1437, Roseville, CA 95678 Tel 415-707-2129 (phone/fax)
E-mail: drybones@drybones.com; DryBonesPress@egroups.com
Web site: http://www.drybones.com
Dist(s): **Spring Arbor Dist** *(Spring Arbor Distributors Inc.).*

†Dryden Pr, *(Dryden Pr.; 0-03; 0-15; 0-8498),* Div. of Thomson Corp., The, Orders Addr.: 6277 Sea Harbor Dr., Orlando, FL 32887 (SAN 250-0086) Toll Free: 800-782-4479 (orders, inquires); 800-544-6678 (customer service); Edit Addr.: 301 Commerce St., Suite 3700, Fort Worth, TX 76012 (SAN 281-613X) Tel 817-334-7500; Fax: 817-334-7844; Toll Free: 800-447-9479 Do not confuse with Dryden Pr., Jackson Center, OH
Web site: http://www.thomson.com; *CIP.*

Dshkn McG-Hill Imprint of McGrw-H Hghr Educ

dttm, *(dttm; 1-929410),* Orders Addr.: P.O. Box 195, Bronson, MI 49028 Tel 517-369-9639; Edit Addr.: 220 E. Chicago, Bronson, MI 49028
E-mail: dttm@CBPU.com.

Duffey Pubng, *(Duffey Publishing, Inc.; 0-9642103),* 1827 N. Rock Springs Rd., Atlanta, GA 30324 Tel 404-266-2600; Fax: 404-262-3198.

†Dufour, *(Dufour Editions, Inc.; 0-8023),* P.O. Box 7, Chester Springs, PA 19425-0007 (SAN 201-341X) Tel 610-458-5005; Fax: 610-458-7103; Toll Free: 800-869-5677
E-mail: dufour8023@aol.com
Web site: http://go.to/Dufour; http://members.aol.com/Dufour8023/index.html; *CIP.*

†Duke, *(Duke Univ. Pr.; 0-8223),* P.O. Box 90660, Durham, NC 27708-0660 (SAN 201-3436) Tel 919-687-3600; Fax: 919-688-4574
E-mail: orders@dukepress.edu; subscriptions@dukepress.edu
Web site: http://www.dukeupress.edu; *CIP.*

†Dumbarton Oaks, *(Dumbarton Oaks; 0-88402),* Orders Addr.: P.O. Box 4866, Baltimore, MD 21211 (SAN 665-6870) Tel 410-516-6954; Fax: 410-516-6998; Edit Addr.: 1703 32nd St., NW, Washington, DC 20007 (SAN 293-2547) Tel 202-339-6431; Fax: 202-625-6805
E-mail: publications@doaks.org
Web site: http://www.doaks.org/publications.html; *CIP.*

Dummies Tech Imprint of Hungry Minds

DuMont Buchverlag GmbH & Co (DEU) *(3-7701) Dist. by* **Advanced Global.**

Dunbar Bks, *(Dunbar Bks.; 0-9625297),* 8856 Sutter Cir., No. 526B, Huntington Beach, CA 92646 Tel 714-891-0033; Toll Free: 800-484-2759
E-mail: RN4etoh@aol.com.

Duncan & Duncan, *See* **APU Pub Grp**

Duncliffs Intl, *(Duncliff's International; 0-911663),* 5122 Katella Ave, Suite 305, Los Alamitos, CA 90720-2831 (SAN 264-018X).

Dundas-Devonhills Assoc, *(Dundas-Devonhills Assoc. Pubs.; 1-880011),* P.O. Box 90531, Tucson, AZ 85752-0531.

†Duquesne, *(Duquesne Univ. Pr.; 0-8207),* Orders Addr.: 750 Cascadilla St., Box 6525, Ithaca, NY 14851-6525 (SAN 249-2857) Tel 607-277-2211; Edit Addr.: 600 Forbes Ave., Pittsburgh, PA 15282 (SAN 658-0491) Tel 412-396-6610; Fax: 412-396-5984
Web site: http://www.dug.edu/dupress.html
Dist(s): **CUP Services** *(CUP Services); CIP.*

Dutt Imprint of Dutton Plume

Dutton Plume, *(Dutton/Plume; 0-525),* Div. of Penguin Putnam, Inc, Orders Addr.: 405 Murray Hill Pkwy., East Rutherford, NJ 07073-2136 Toll Free: 800-631-8571 (reseller customer service); 800-788-6262 (individual consumer sales); 800-526-0275 (reseller sales); Edit Addr.: 375 Hudson St., New York, NY 10014 Tel 212-366-2000; Fax: 212-366-2666 ; *Imprints:* Dutt (Dutton) Plume (Plume)
E-mail: online@penguinputnam.com
Web site: http://www.penguinputnam.com
Dist(s): **Penguin Putnam** *(Penguin Putnam, Inc.).*

Duxbury, *(Duxbury; 0-534),* Div. of Thomson Learning, Orders Addr.: a/o 1BCST059, 7625 Empire Dr., Florence, KY 41042-2919 Fax: 606-647-5020; Toll Free: 800-423-0563; Edit Addr.: 511 Forest Lodge Rd., Pacific Grove, CA 93950
E-mail: info@duxbury.com
Web site: http://www.duxbury.com
Dist(s): **Thomson Learn** *(Thomson Learning).*

Dyco Inc, *(Dyco, Inc.; 0-937224),* 6225 E. Saguaro Vista Ct., Cave Creek, AZ 85331 (SAN 216-1257) Tel 602-585-4386.

Dymphna Pr, *(Dymphna Pr.; 0-9634975),* Orders Addr.: P.O. Box 44, Belmont, MA 02178; Edit Addr.: 31 Willow St., Belmont, MA 02178 Tel 617-489-2126.

Dynamic Trn & Pub, *See* **Nucci-Saunders Pubns**

Dyslimbia Pr, *(Dyslimbia Pr., Inc.; 1-928947),* 109 NE 19th Dr., Okeechobee, FL 34972-1933 Tel 941-467-8771; Fax: 941-467-1883
Web site: http://www.biologicalunhappiness.com.

Dystonia Med Res, *See* **Natl Spasmodic Dysphonia**

E A (GBR) *(0-340; 0-7122; 0-7131; 0-85264) Dist. by* **OUP.**

E A (GBR) *(0-340; 0-7122; 0-7131; 0-85264) Dist. by* **St Martin.**

E A Sforza, *(Sforza, Eula Awbrey; 0-9636567),* 1229 Reading Ct., Wheaton, IL 60187 Tel 630-682-0592.

E B Lindemann, *(Lindemann, Elizabeth B.; 0-9618299),* 80 Lyme Rd., Apt. 346, Hanover, NH 03755-1218 (SAN 667-3996) Tel 603-643-1797.

E B Stanbury, *(Stanbury, Elise B.; 0-9668386),* 4 Fellows Rd., Ipswich, MA 01938-2702
E-mail: anneelise@jano.com.

E Bowers Pub, *(Bowers, Eddie Publishing Company, Inc.; 0-912855; 0-945483; 1-57879),* Orders Addr.: P.O. Box 130, Peosta, IA 52068; Edit Addr.: 18551 Pilot Grove Rd., Peosta, IA 52068-0130 Tel 319-876-3119; Fax: 319-876-3206 E-mail: eddiebowerspub@aol.com.

E Elgar, *(Elgar, Edward Publishing, Inc.; 1-84064; 1-85278; 1-85898; 1-84376),* Orders Addr.: c/o Custom Services, P.O. Box 574, Williston, VT 05495 Tel 802-862-0095; Fax: 802-864-7626; Toll Free: 800-390-3149; Edit Addr.: 136 West St. Suite 202, Northampton, MA 01060 (SAN 299-4615) Tel 413-584-5551; Fax: 413-584-9933 E-mail: tgorvine@e-elgar.com; eep.orders@aidcvt.com; rhenning@e-elgar.com Web site: http://www.e-elgar.co.uk *Dist(s):* **Am Intl Dist** *(American International Distribution Corp.)* **netLibrary CO** *(netLibrary, Inc.).*

E J Brill, *See* **Brill Academic Pubs**

E J Dwyer (AUS) *(0-85574; 1-86429) Dist. by* **Morehouse Pub.**

E K Kiwuwa, *(Kiwuwa, Edward Khiwa; 0-9643899),* Orders Addr.: P.O. Box 818, Guthrie, OK 73044 Tel 405-282-1890; Edit Addr.: 100 E. College Ave., Guthrie, OK 73044.

E Lewis Found, *(Lewis, Elvirita Forum; 0-924840),* P.O. Box 4110, Sparks, NV 89432 Tel 702-358-2768; Fax: 702-358-2783.

E M D Ent, *(E.M.D. Enterprises; 0-9638677),* 2082 Michelson Dr., Irvine, CA 92612 Tel 949-252-9277.

†E Mellen, *(Mellen, Edwin Pr., The; 0-7734; 0-88946; 0-935106),* P.O. Box 450, Lewiston, NY 14092-0450 (SAN 207-110X) Tel 716-754-2788 (order); 716-754-2266; Fax: 716-754-1860 (main/order) E-mail: cs@wzrd.com; mellen@wzrd.com Web site: http://www.mellenpress.com *Dist(s):* **Continuum** *(Continuum International Publishing Group, Inc.); CIP.*

E S Cleckley, *(Cleckley, Emily S.; 0-9621519),* 3024 Fox Spring Rd., Augusta, GA 30909 (SAN 251-5296) Tel 706-733-3443.

E T Pub Co, *(E.T. Publishing Co.; 0-9625203),* Orders Addr.: P.O. Box 16727, Milwaukee, WI 53216; Edit Addr.: 4351 N. 47th St., Milwaukee, WI 53216 Tel 414-444-8004.

E Temas de Hoy (ESP) *(84-7880; 84-86675) Dist. by* **Planeta.**

E V White, *(White, Eugene V.; 0-9602034),* P.O. Box 286, Berryville, VA 22611-0286 (SAN 212-5838) Tel 540-955-2280.

E Werner Pubns, *(Werner, Eliot Pubns.; 0-9712427),* P.O. Box 268, Clinton Corners, NY 12514 Tel 845-266-4241 E-mail: ewerner@vh.net Web site: http://www.eliotwerner.com.

EA Enas, *(Enas, Enas A.; 0-9616232),* 1935 Green Trails Dr., Lisle, IL 60532 (SAN 658-5752) Tel 312-961-0279.

Eagan Pr, *(Eagan Pr.; 0-9624407; 1-887568; 1-891127),* Affil. of American Assn. of Cereal Chemists, 3340 Pilot Knob Rd., Saint Paul, MN 55121-2097 Tel 651-454-7250; Fax: 651-454-0766; Toll Free: 800-328-7560 E-mail: aacc@scisoc.org Web site: http://www.scisoc.org/aacc.

Eagle Pub & Comms, *(Eagle Publishing & Communications; 1-881566),* 3350 Scott Blvd., Bldg. 30, Santa Clara, CA 95054-3104 Tel 408-246-2600; Fax: 408-246-2700; Toll Free: 800-944-9491 E-mail: info@managementtools.com.

Eagle Wing Bks, *(Eagle Wing Bks., Inc.; 0-940829),* Orders Addr.: P.O. Box 9972, Memphis, TN 38190 (SAN 665-1046) Tel 901-785-8278; Fax: 901-785-7592; Edit Addr.: 5077 E. Shore Dr., Memphis, TN 38109 (SAN 665-1054) E-mail: ewibooks@aol.com Web site: http://www.eaglewingbooks.com *Dist(s):* **Bookpeople** *(Bookpeople)* **New Leaf Dist** *(New Leaf Distributing Co., Inc.)* **Quality Bks IL** *(Quality Bks., Inc.).*

EagleBooks WI, *(Eagle Bks.; 1-882987),* P.O. Box 253, Hales Corners, WI 53130 Tel 414-425-2189; Fax: 414-425-4807; Toll Free: 800-252-0133 Do not confuse with Eagle Books, Carthage, MO.

Eaglecliff, *(Eaglecliff; 1-885879),* Div. of Eaglecliff Publications Group, 556 N. Crestway, Wichita, KS 67208 Tel 316-687-6330 E-mail: eaglecliff@southwind.net.

†Eakin Press, *(Eakin Pr.; 0-89015; 1-57168),* P.O. Drawer 90159, Austin, TX 78709-0159 (SAN 207-3633) Tel 512-288-1771; Fax: 512-288-1813; Toll Free: 800-880-8642 E-mail: sales@eakinpress.com; tom@eakinpress.com Web site: http://www.eakinpress.com *Dist(s):* **Baker & Taylor** *(Baker & Taylor Bks.)* **Follett Library** *(Follett Library Resources)* **Herveys Bklink** *(Hervey's Booklink & Cookbook Warehouse)* **Wolverine Distrib** *(Wolverine Distributing, Inc.); CIP.*

Earth Healing, *(Earth Healing Products; 0-9630373),* P.O. Box 11, Dennis, MA 02638 Tel 508-385-2055; Toll Free: 800-356-9315 E-mail: jpmurphy@neaccess.net *Dist(s):* **Baker & Taylor** *(Baker & Taylor Bks.)* **New Leaf Dist** *(New Leaf Distributing Co., Inc.)* **Nutri-Books Corp** *(Nutri-Bks. Corp.).*

Earth Nation, *(Earth Nation Publishing; 0-945111),* Div. of Church of the Earth Nation, Inc., 4271 N. Indian Hill Rd., Nashville, IN 47448 (SAN 246-2761) Tel 812-988-0873 E-mail: dwightsands@hotmail.com *Dist(s):* **Bookpeople** *(Bookpeople)* **New Leaf Dist** *(New Leaf Distributing Co., Inc.).*

Earth Works, *See* **Bathroom Reader**

Earthen Vessel Prodns, *(Earthen Vessel Production, Inc.; 1-887400),* 3620 Greenwood Dr., Kelseyville, CA 95451 Tel 707-277-7087; Fax: 707-277-7088; Toll Free: 800-233-6367 E-mail: request@earthsn.com; books@earthern.com Web site: http://www.earthen.com.

Earthpulse Pr, *(Earthpulse Pr.; 0-9648812; 1-890693),* Orders Addr.: P.O. Box 201393, Anchorage, AK 99520-1393 Tel 907-694-1277; Fax: 907-696-1277; Toll Free: 888-690-1277; Edit Addr.: 16419 Marcus St., Eagle River, AK 99577 E-mail: drnick@alaska.net Web site: http://www.earthpulse.com *Dist(s):* **AK Pr Dist** *(AK Pr. Distribution)* **Adventures Unltd** *(Adventures Unlimited Pr.)* **Baker & Taylor** *(Baker & Taylor Bks.)* **Bookmen Inc** *(Bookmen, Inc.)* **Bookpeople** *(Bookpeople)* **New Leaf Dist** *(New Leaf Distributing Co., Inc.).*

Earthtones Pr, *(Earthtones Pr.; 0-945668),* P.O. Box 411, Vashon, WA 98070 (SAN 247-381X) Tel 206-463-2796; Fax: 206-463-5353; Toll Free: 800-788-1770 *Dist(s):* Baker & Taylor *(Baker & Taylor Bks.)* Bookpeople *(Bookpeople)* New Leaf Dist *(New Leaf Distributing Co., Inc.)* Nutri-Books Corp *(Nutri-Bks. Corp.).*

Earth-Wise, *(Earth-Wise Pubns.; 0-9655793),* P.O. Box 723, Silver Spring, MD 20918 Tel 301-681-4829; Fax: 301-681-9892 E-mail: mrecords@aya.yale.edu; earthwise_greenglobe@compuserve.com Web site: http://www.erols.com/grglobe/.

EASE, *(EASE; 0-9636607),* P.O. Box 8032, Minneapolis, MN 55408 Tel 612-825-7681; Fax: 612-226-5641; Toll Free: 800-470-4769 E-mail: brdrmc@bitstream.com *Dist(s):* **Bookmen Inc** *(Bookmen, Inc.).*

East & West Pubns, *(East & West Pubns.; 0-935886),* 234 Avery Heights, Hartford, CT 06106-4200 (SAN 206-099X) Tel 860-953-5851.

East Eur Monographs, *(Eastern European Monographs; 0-88033; 0-914710),* Orders Addr.: 136 S. Broadway, Irvington-on-Hudson, NY 10533 (SAN 212-2480) Tel 914-591-9111; Fax: 914-591-9201; Toll Free: 800-944-8648; Edit Addr.: P.O. Box 10039, Bradenton, FL 34282 Tel 941-753-4782 (phone/fax) *Dist(s):* **Col U Pr** *(Columbia Univ. Pr.).*

East Eur Quarterly, *See* **East Eur Monographs**

East Gate Bk Imprint of M E Sharpe

East Hall Pr, *(East Hall Pr.; 1-878326),* Affil. of Augustana College, Augustana College, English Dept., Rock Island, IL 61201 Tel 309-794-7280.

East Hlth Dev, *(East Health Development Group; 0-9641605),* P.O. Box 947, Tustin, CA 92781 Tel 714-973-7962; Toll Free: 800-400-8644.

East Ridge Pr, *(East Ridge Pr.; 0-914896),* 161 Ridge Rd., Hankins, NY 12741 (SAN 201-2871) E-mail: eastridge@fcc.net *Dist(s):* **East Ridge Bookstore** *(East Ridge Bookstore).*

East Wash Univ, *(Eastern Washington Univ. Pr.; 0-910055),* Orders Addr.: MS 1, 705 W. First Ave., Spokane, WA 99201 (SAN 244-7967) Toll Free: 800-508-9095; Edit Addr.: Eastern Washington Univ. EWU, MS-1, 705 W. First Ave., Spokane, WA 99201 (SAN 241-2977) Tel 509-623-4286; Fax: 509-623-4283 E-mail: webadmin@mail.ewu.edu Web site: http://www.ewu.edu/ *Dist(s):* **U of Wash Pr** *(Univ. of Washington Pr.).*

Eastern Book (IND) *(81-7012) Dist. by* **St Mut.**

Eastern Corp, *(Eastern Corp.; 1-58311),* Div. of Eastern Co. for Pubns., 3915 Annandale Rd., Annandale, VA 22003 Tel 703-941-5488; Fax: 703-941-0120.

†Eastern National, *(Eastern National; 0-915992; 1-888213; 1-59091),* 470 Maryland Dr., Suite 1, Fort Washington, PA 19446 (SAN 630-4044) Web site: http://www.easternnational.org; *CIP.*

Eastern National Park & Monument, *See* **Eastern National**

Eastern Pr, *(Eastern Pr.; 0-939758),* P.O. Box 881, Bloomington, IN 47402-0881 (SAN 216-3713) Tel 812-339-3985.

EastGate Pubs, *(EastGate Pubs.; 0-941717),* 4137 Primavera Rd., Santa Barbara, CA 93110 (SAN 666-3036) Tel 805-683-5375 (phone/fax) E-mail: egbobgan@aol.com.

Eastland, *(Eastland Pr.; 0-939616),* Orders Addr.: 1240 Activity Dr., No. D, Vista, CA 92083 (SAN 665-6900) Tel 760-598-9695; Fax: 760-598-6083; Toll Free Fax: 800-241-3329; Toll Free: 800-453-3278; Edit Addr.: P.O. Box 99749, Seattle, WA 98199 (SAN 216-6216) Tel 206-217-0204; Fax: 206-217-0205; Toll Free: 800-453-3278 (sales office) E-mail: orders@eastlandpress.com; info@eastlandpress.com Web site: http://www.eastlandpress.com *Dist(s):* **Matthews Medical Bk Co** *(Matthews Medical Bk. Co.)* **Redwing Bk Co** *(Redwing Bk. Co.).*

Easton CA, *(Easton Publishing; 0-9629285),* 1195 Shenandoah Rd., San Marino, CA 91108-1041 Tel 626-568-3045.

Eastwind Pub, *See* **Bellwether-Cross**

Easy Money Pr, *(Easy Money Pr.; 0-9654563; 1-929714),* Orders Addr.: P.O. Box 50755, Irvine, CA 92604 Tel 949-551-2991; Fax: 949-733-2530; Edit Addr.: 24 W. Yale Loop, Irvine, CA 92604 ; *Imprints:* Big Tree Bks (Big Tree Books) E-mail: EasymoneyPress@yahoo.com *Dist(s):* **Baker & Taylor** *(Baker & Taylor Bks.).*

Eaton Pub Co, *(Eaton Publishing Co./Bio Techniques Bks. Div.; 1-881299),* 154 E. Central St., Natick, MA 01760 Tel 508-655-8282; Fax: 508-653-2706; Toll Free: 800-655-8285 ; *Imprints:* BioTechniques (BioTechniques Books) E-mail: rdavis@biotechniques.com; christine@biotechniques.com.

Ebewos Afr-Am, *(Ebewo's African-American Publishing & Distribution Co.; 0-9634998),* 2219 W. Minister, Parlin, NJ 08859 Fax: 732-316-0327.

Ebner & Sons, *(Ebner & Sons; 0-9626895),* 3714 48th Ave., NE, Seattle, WA 98105.

ebooksonthe, *(ebooksonthe.net; 0-9639070; 0-9701020; 1-931207),* Orders Addr.: P.O. Box 35, Ellsworth, ME 04605 Tel 207-667-6515 (phone/fax) E-mail: publisher@ebooksonthe.net Web site: http://www.ebooksonthe.net *Dist(s):* **BookWorld** *(BookWorld Services, Inc.).*

EBTS, *(EBTS, Inc.; 0-9634461),* 133 Court St., Ellsworth, ME 04605.

Ebury Pr (GBR) *(0-09; 0-7126; 0-85223) Dist. by* **Trafalgar.**

ECA Assoc, *(ECA Assocs.; 0-938818),* Orders Addr.: P.O. Box 15004, Chesapeake, VA 23328-0004 (SAN 215-9503) Tel 757-547-5542; P.O. Box 20186, New York, NY 10025 (SAN 215-9511) E-mail: eca@melanet.com.

ECHO Inc, *(ECHO, Inc. (Educational Concerns for Hunger Organization); 0-9610184; 0-9653360),* 17430 Durrance Rd., North Fort Myers, FL 33917-2239 Tel 941-543-3246; Fax: 941-543-5317 E-mail: echo@echonet.org Web site: http://www.~c.org/echo; http://www.echonet.org.

Echocardio, *(Echocardiography.org; 1-893508),* 17 E. Wharf Rd., Madison, CT 06443 E-mail: terencerafferty@hotmail.com.

Echolalia Pr, *(Echolalia Pr.; 0-9650733),* 707 Wheeler St., Santa Rosa, CA 95404-5054 Tel 707-575-3330 E-mail: AWSELIGMAN@aol.com *Dist(s):* **Books Now** *(Books Now).*

ECLAT Bks, *(ECLAT Bks.; 0-9625706),* Div. of R. K. Interstellar Industries, Inc., 3172 N. Rainbow Blvd., Suite 315, Las Vegas, NV 89108 Tel 702-255-7919.

Eclectic Inst, *(Eclectic Institute, The; 0-9659135),* 36350 Industrial Way, Sandy, OR 97055-7377.

Eclectic Med, *(Eclectic Medical Pubns.; 0-9623518; 1-888483),* 36350 SE Industrial Way, Sandy, OR 97055 Tel 503-668-4120; Toll Free Fax: 888-655-4372; Toll Free: 877-867-4372
E-mail: emp@eclecticherb.com
Web site: http://www.eclecticherb.com/emp.

Eclectic Pr NC, *See* **Holographic Hlth**

Economics Pr, *(Economics Pr., Inc., The; 0-910187),* 12 Daniel Rd., Fairfield, NJ 07004-2565 (SAN 204-1774) Tel 973-227-1224; Fax: 973-227-9742; Toll Free: 800-526-2554
E-mail: edit@epinc.com.

Economist Intell, *(Economist Intelligence Unit; 0-85058; 0-87180),* 111 W. 57th St., New York, NY 10019 (SAN 237-7896) Tel 212-554-0600; Fax: 212-586-1181; Toll Free: 800-938-4685.

ECRI, *(ECRI; 0-941417),* 5200 Butler Pike, Plymouth Meeting, PA 19462 (SAN 224-1234) Tel 610-825-6000; Fax: 610-834-7366
E-mail: info@ecri.org; ekuserk@ecri.org
Web site: http://www.ecri.org.

ECW (CAN) *(0-920763; 0-920802; 1-55022) Dist. by* **General Distrib Services.**

Ed & Psych, *(Ed & Psych Assocs.; 0-9638072),* 2071 S. Atherton St., Suite 900, State College, PA 16801
E-mail: mww10@psu.edu.

Ed Activities, *(Educational Activities, Inc.; 0-7925; 0-89525; 0-914296; 1-55737),* Orders Addr.: P.O. Box 392, Freeport, NY 11520; Edit Addr.: 1937 Grand Ave., Baldwin, NY 11510 (SAN 207-4400) Tel 516-223-4666; Fax: 516-623-9282; Toll Free: 800-645-3739
E-mail: learn@edact.com
Web site: http://www.edact.com.

Ed Commns NY, *(Educational Communications; 0-9672263),* P.O. Box 802, Mount Kisco, NY 10549-0802 Tel 914-242-3782; Fax: 914-242-3784
Dist(s): **J Majors Co** *(Majors, J. A. Co.)*
Matthews Bk Co *(Matthews Bk. Co.)*
Rittenhouse *(Rittenhouse Bk. Distributors).*

ED Inc, *(Education Design, Inc.; 0-9613138; 0-9622255),* Orders Addr.: P.O. Box 22275, Denver, CO 80222-0275 (SAN 294-7722) Tel 303-745-5996; Fax: 303-745-5856; Edit Addr.: 5925 E. Evans, Denver, CO 80222 Tel 303-692-9758.

Ed Law Assn, *(Education Law Assn. (ELA); 1-56534),* 300 College Pk. - 0528, Dayton, OH 45469 (SAN 226-6105) Tel 937-229-3589; Fax: 937-229-3845
E-mail: ela@udayton.edu
Web site: http://www.educationlaw.org.

Ed Media Corp, *(Educational Media Corp.; 0-932796; 1-930572),* Orders Addr.: P.O. Box 21311, Minneapolis, MN 55421 (SAN 665-6919); Edit Addr.: 4256 Central Ave. NE, Minneapolis, MN 55421-2920 (SAN 212-4203) Tel 763-781-0088; Fax: 763-781-7753; Toll Free: 800-966-3382
E-mail: emedia@educationalmedia.com
Web site: http://www.educationalmedia.com
Dist(s): **Baker & Taylor** *(Baker & Taylor Bks.)*
Bookmen Inc *(Bookmen, Inc.).*

Ed Pub Serv, *(Educators Publishing Service, Inc.; 0-8388),* 31 Smith Pl., Cambridge, MA 02138-1089 (SAN 201-8225) Tel 617-547-6706; Fax: 617-547-0412; Toll Free: 800-225-5750
E-mail: robinm@epsbooks.com; epsbooks@epsbooks.com
Web site: http://www.epsbooks.com.

Ed Sherman, *(Sherman, Edmund; 0-9701446),* 15 Lake Shore Dr., Watervliet, NY 12189 Tel 518-783-0675
E-mail: ared42039@aol.com
Dist(s): **BookMasters** *(BookMasters, Inc.).*

Ed Solutions, *(Educational Solutions, Inc.; 0-87825),* 99 University Pl., 6th Flr., New York, NY 10003-4555 (SAN 205-6186) Tel 212-674-2988 Do not confuse with Educational Solutions, Stafford, TX.

Ed Studies Pr, *(Educational Studies Pr.; 1-879528),* Nthrn Ill. Univ., College of Education, DeKalb, IL 60115 Tel 815-753-9362; Fax: 815-753-0369; Toll Free: 800-348-7543
E-mail: dsmith@niu.edu.

EDA Pubg, *(EDA Publishing; 0-944796),* P.O. Box 2184, Rancho Santa Fe, CA 92067 (SAN 245-4580) Tel 619-586-7626.

EDC Pubng, *(EDC Publishing; 0-7460; 0-88110; 1-58086; 0-7945),* Div. of Educational Development Corp., Orders Addr.: P.O. Box 470663, Tulsa, OK 74147-0663 (SAN 658-0505); Edit Addr.: 10302 E. 55th Pl., Tulsa, OK 74146-6515 (SAN 107-5322) Tel 918-622-4522; Fax: 918-665-7919; Toll Free: 800-475-4522 ; *Imprints:* Usborne (Usborne)
E-mail: edc@edcpub.com
Web site: http://www.edcpub.com
Dist(s): **Continental Bk** *(Continental Bk. Co., Inc.)*
Lectorum Pubns *(Lectorum Pubns., Inc.).*

Edconco Pr, *(Edconco Pr.; 0-9673892),* P.O. Box 357, Grass Valley, CA 95945 (SAN 299-9676) Tel 530-268-2580; Fax: 530-268-9570
E-mail: edconco@oro.net
Web site: http://www.prostatecanconoptious.com.

Edens Work, *See* **Laugh Cat**

Edgell Commns Inc, *See* **Advanstar Commns**

Edgewood KY, *(Edgewood Pr., Inc.; 0-938820),* 37000 Fox Glen, Farmington Hills, MI 48331-4305 (SAN 240-0170) Do not confuse with companies with the same name in Cambridge, MA, Clare, MI.

Ediciones, *(Ediciones Universal; 0-89729),* Orders Addr.: P.O. Box 450353, Miami, FL 33245-0353 (SAN 658-0548); Edit Addr.: 3090 SW Eighth St., Miami, FL 33135 (SAN 207-2203) Tel 305-642-3355; Fax: 305-642-7978
E-mail: ediciones@ediciones.com
Web site: http://www.ediciones.com.

Ediciones Cientificas (ESP) *(84-458) Dist. by* **P H Brookes.**

Ediciones Cientificas (MEX) *(968-435) Dist. by* **Continental Bk.**

Ediciones Diaz (ESP) *(84-7978) Dist. by* **IBD Ltd.**

Edinburgh U Pr (GBR) *(0-7486; 0-85224) Dist. by* **Col U Pr.**

Edit Betania, *See* **Caribe Betania**

Edit Concepts, *(Editorial Concepts, Inc.; 0-939193),* 3081 SW 129th Ave., Miami, FL 33175 (SAN 662-8958) Tel 305-446-7900; Fax: 305-446-6322
E-mail: edicon@gate.net
Web site: http://www.booksinspanish.com
Dist(s): **Lectorum Pubns** *(Lectorum Pubns., Inc.)*
Spanish Periodical & Bk Sales *(Spanish Periodical & Bk. Sales, Inc.).*

Editio Cantor Verlag (DEU) *(3-87193) Dist. by* **Balogh.**

Editorial Amer, *(Editorial America, S. A.; 0-944499; 1-56259),* 6355 NW 36th St., Miami, FL 33166 (SAN 243-7384) Tel 305-871-6400; Fax: 305-871-8769
Dist(s): **Spanish Periodical & Bk Sales** *(Spanish Periodical & Bk. Sales, Inc.).*

Editorial Unilit, *(Editorial Unilit; 0-7899; 0-945792; 1-56063),* Div. of Spanish Hse., Inc., 1360 NW 88th Ave., Miami, FL 33172-3093 (SAN 247-5979) Tel 305-592-6136; Fax: 305-592-0087; Toll Free: 800-767-7726
E-mail: sales1@unidial.com
Web site: http://www.editorialunilit.com/
Dist(s): **Harrison Hse** *(Harrison Hse., Inc.).*

EDITS Pubs, ***(EDITS Pubs.),*** **P.O. Box 7234, San Diego, CA 92167 (SAN 208-4600) Tel 619-222-1666; Fax: 619-226-1666; Toll Free: 800-416-1666**
E-mail: edits@k-online.com
Web site: http://www.edits.net.

Edmark GA, *See* **St Bart Pr Ltd**

Edmonston Publ, *(Edmonston Publishing, Inc.; 0-9622393; 1-892059),* Orders Addr.: P.O. Box 38, Hamilton, NY 13346 Tel 315-824-1965 (phone/fax); Edit Addr.: 1841 Preston Hill Rd., Hamilton, NY 13346
E-mail: shop@edmonstonpublishing.com
Web site: http://www.edmonstonpublishing.com
Dist(s): **Baker & Taylor** *(Baker & Taylor Bks.)*
North Country *(North Country Bks., Inc.).*

Edna FourCZNS, *(Edna 4CZNS, Inc.; 0-9631972),* Orders Addr.: P.O. Box 2224, Sparks, NV 89432 Fax: 702-358-3940; Edit Addr.: 323 11th St., Sparks, NV 89431 Tel 702-358-0905.

EDRA, ***(Environmental Design Research Assn.; 0-939922),*** **1800 Canyon Pk. Cir., Bldg. 4 Suite 403, Edmond, OK 73013 (SAN 216-8103) Tel 405-330-4863**
Web site: http://www.telepath.com/edra/.

Educ Dev Ctr, *(Education Development Ctr., Inc.; 0-89292),* Orders Addr.: P.O. Box 1020, Sewickley, PA 15143-1020 Tel 412-741-1968; Fax: 412-741-0609; Toll Free: 800-793-5076; Edit Addr.: 55 Chapel St., Newton, MA 02458-1060 (SAN 207-821X) Tel 617-618-2215; Fax: 617-630-8402; Toll Free: 800-225-4276
E-mail: jwcordone@edu.org
Web site: http://www.edc.org
Dist(s): **Juvenile Justice** *(Juvenile Justice Clearinghouse/NCJRS).*

†Educ Equity Con, *(Educational Equity Concepts, Inc.; 0-931629),* 114 E. 32nd St., Suite 701, New York, NY 10016 (SAN 683-7328) Tel 212-243-1110; Fax: 212-725-0947
E-mail: 75507.1306@compuserve.com
Web site: http://www.onisland.com/eec
Dist(s): **Gryphon Hse** *(Gryphon Hse., Inc.); CIP.*

†Educ Found, *(Educational Foundation of the National Restaurant Assn.; 0-915452; 1-58280; 1-883904),* 250 S. Wacker Dr., Suite 1400, Chicago, IL 60606-5834 (SAN 224-747X) Tel 312-715-1010; Fax: 312-715-0220; Toll Free: 800-765-2122
Web site: http://www.foodtrain.org; *CIP.*

Educ Hands, *(Educating Hands, Inc., Publishing; 0-9649356),* Div. of Educating Hands, Inc., 120 SW Eighth St., Miami, FL 33130 Tel 305-285-6991; Fax: 305-857-0298; Toll Free: 800-999-6991.

Educ Intl Pr, *(Educator's International Pr., Inc.; 0-9658339; 1-891928),* Orders Addr.: 18 Colleen Rd., Troy, NY 12180 Tel 518-271-9886; Fax: 518-266-9422
E-mail: sarah@edint.com
Web site: http://www.edint.com.

Educ Opportunities, *See* **Saunders Grp**

Educ Res Consortium, *(Education Resource Consortium, Inc.; 0-931263),* 2366 Park Blvd., Upland, CA 91784-1060 (SAN 681-9796).

Educ Res Hlth, *(Educational Resources in HealthCare, Inc.; 0-9638759),* P.O. Box 574, Jamestown, RI 02835 Tel 401-884-6185.

Educ Systems, *(Educational Systems, Inc.; 0-9629655),* 2252 Overton Rd., Augusta, GA 30904 Tel 404-738-6775.

Educ Systs Assocs Inc, *(Educational Systems Assocs., Inc.; 1-878276),* Orders Addr.: P.O. Box 96, Kearney, NE 68848-0096 Tel 308-234-6261; Edit Addr.: 1410 W. 36th St., Kearney, NE 68847
E-mail: edsys@kearney.net
Web site: http://www.kearney.net/~edsys.

†Educ Tech Pubns, *(Educational Technology Pubns, Inc.; 0-87778),* Orders Addr.: P.O. Box 1564, Englewood Cliffs, NJ 07632-0564 Toll Free: 800-952-2665 (orders only); Edit Addr.: 700 Palisade Ave., Englewood Cliffs, NJ 07632 (SAN 201-3738) Tel 201-871-4007; Fax: 201-871-4009
E-mail: EdTecPubs@aol.com
Web site: http://www.bookstoread.com/etp; *CIP.*

Educ Testing Serv, *(Educational Testing Service; 0-88685),* P.O. Box 6108, Princeton, NJ 08541-6108 (SAN 238-034X) Tel 609-771-7243; Fax: 609-771-7385 Do not confuse with Educational Testing Service in Washington, DC
Web site: http://www.ets.org
Dist(s): **IPG Chicago** *(Independent Pubs. Group).*

Educ Tsting Cnslts, *(Educational Testing Consultants, Inc.; 1-57774),* P.O. Box 510222, Saint Louis, MO 63151-0222 Tel 314-416-4600 (phone/fax); Toll Free: 800-633-8378
E-mail: info@webexam.com
Web site: http://www.webexam.com.

EduCare Pub, *(EduCare Publishing; 1-886665),* P.O. Box 280305, Columbia, SC 29228 Tel 803-796-6100; Fax: 803-796-4150; Toll Free: 800-849-9271
E-mail: educare@ix.netcom.com
Web site: http://www.cancerhelp.com/ed/
Dist(s): **Baker & Taylor** *(Baker & Taylor Bks.)*
Prof Bks Inc *(Professional Bks., Inc.)*
Quality Bks IL *(Quality Bks., Inc.)*
Unique Bks Inc *(Unique Bks., Inc.).*

Edutainment, *(Edutainment Productions, Inc.; 1-882799),* Orders Addr.: P.O. Box 840011, New Orleans, LA 70184-0011 Tel 504-486-9863; Fax: 504-727-3545; Edit Addr.: 6405 Colbert St., New Orleans, LA 70124.

†Eerdmans, *(Eerdmans, William B. Publishing Co.; 0-8028),* 255 Jefferson Ave., SE, Grand Rapids, MI 49503-4554 (SAN 220-0058) Tel 616-459-4591; Fax: 616-459-6540; Toll Free: 800-253-7521 (orders)
E-mail: info@eerdmans.com; customerservice@eerdmans.com; sales@eerdmans.com
Web site: http://www.eerdmans.com; *CIP.*

Ehde Pub Co, *(Ehde Publishing Co.; 0-936188),* 112 W. Chipwood Dr., Gulfport, MS 39503 (SAN 214-0071).

EHE Network, *(Exceptional Human Experience Network (EHE Network); 0-944446),* 414 Rockledge Rd., New Bern, NC 28562-9553 (SAN 692-9656) Tel 252-636-8734; Fax: 252-636-8371
Web site: http://www.ehe.org.

Ehret Lit, *(Ehret Literature Publishing Co.; 1-884772),* P.O. Box 24, Dobbs Ferry, NY 10522-0024 Tel 914-961-6540 (phone/fax)
E-mail: books@arnoldehrret.com
Web site: http://www.arnoldehret.org.

Eidetics, *(Eidetics; 0-9624044),* 1200 Soldiers Field Rd., Boston, MA 02134-1004 Tel 617-254-4100; Toll Free: 800-635-3495.

EIH Pubng, *(EIH Publishing; 1-929661),* Div. of Eastern Institute of Hypnotheraphy, Orders Addr.: P.O. Box 249, Goshen, VA 24439-0249 Tel 540-997-0325; Fax: 540-997-0324; Toll Free: 800-296-6463; Edit Addr.: 956 Knob Rd., Goshen, VA 24439
E-mail: hyptrainer@aol.com
Web site: http://members.aol.com.

Eileen Bks, *(Eileen Bks.; 0-9635627),* 2151 45th St., Suite 302, West Palm Beach, FL 33407 Tel 407-844-0801.

Eiron, *(Eiron, Inc),* P.O. Box 40072, Washington, DC 20016-0072 Tel 202-966-3240; Fax: 202-244-0913
E-mail: eironinc@aol.com
Web site: http://www.wdn.com/yellowdog.

El Rey Pub, *(El Rey Publishing Co.; 1-878575),* P.O. Box 14128, San Antonio, TX 78214-0128 Tel 210-922-6665; Fax: 210-922-5712.

Elder Bks, *(Elder Bks.; 0-943873),* Orders Addr.: P.O. Box 490, Forest Knolls, CA 94933 (SAN 242-3731) Tel 415-488-9002; Fax: 415-488-4720; Toll Free: 800-909-2673
E-mail: info@elderbooks.com
Web site: http://elderbooks.com
Dist(s): **Baker & Taylor** *(Baker & Taylor Bks.)*
Midpt Trade *(Midpoint Trade Bks., Inc.)*
Quality Bks IL *(Quality Bks., Inc.)*
Unique Bks Inc *(Unique Bks., Inc.).*

Eldersong, *(Eldersong Pubns., Inc.; 1-879633),* Orders Addr.: P.O. Box 74, Mount Airy, MD 21771 Tel 301-829-0533; Fax: 301-829-5249; Toll Free: 800-397-0533; Edit Addr.: 108 E. Ridgeville Blvd., Suite D, Mount Airy, MD 21771
E-mail: eldrsong@erols.com; info@eldersong.com
Web site: http://www.eldersong.com.

Electrochem Soc, *(Electrochemical Society, Inc.; 1-56677),* 65 S. Main St., Pennington, NJ 08534-2896 (SAN 210-7236) Tel 609-737-1902; Fax: 609-737-2743
E-mail: books@electrochem.org
Web site: http://www.electrochem.org.

†Element MA, *(Element Bks., Inc.; 0-906540; 1-85230; 1-86204; 1-901881),* 160 N. Washington St., Boston, MA 02114 Fax: 617-248-0909
E-mail: publishers@elementboston.com
Dist(s): **Natl Bk Netwk** *(National Bk. Network)*
Penguin Putnam *(Penguin Putnam, Inc.); CIP.*

Elephants Eye Imprint of Overlook Pr

Eli Mail, *(Eli Mail-Order, Inc.; 0-9602230),* P.O. Box 81, Brooklyn, NY 11208 (SAN 212-3509).

Elijim Pubns, *(Elijim Pubns.),* 2536 Clay St., San Francisco, CA 94115 Tel 415-563-2211.

Eliot Pr, *(Eliot Pr.; 0-9628976),* 262 Eliot St., Natick, MA 01760 Tel 508-655-8123.

Elite Pub IN, *(Elite Publishing Co., Inc.; 0-935589),* 2940 S. Harding St., Indianapolis, IN 46225 (SAN 696-3773) Tel 317-783-0489.

Elliots Bks, *(Elliot's Bks.; 0-911830),* P.O. Box 6, Northford, CT 06472 (SAN 204-1529) Tel 203-484-2184; Fax: 203-484-7644
E-mail: outofprintbooks@mindspring.com.

Elliott Clark Imprint of River City Pub

Ellipse Pub, *See* **SOFITS**

†Elsevier, *(Elsevier Science; 0-08; 0-444; 0-7204; 0-916086; 1-85617),* Orders Addr.: P.O. Box 945, New York, NY 10159-0945 (SAN 251-2564) Toll Free: 888-437-4636; Edit Addr.: 655 Ave. of the Americas, New York, NY 10010-5107 (SAN 200-2051) Tel 212-633-3730; Fax: 212-633-3680 ; *Imprints:* Excerpta Medica (Excerpta-Medica) North Holland (North-Holland) Pergamon Pr (Pergamon Press)
E-mail: usinfo-f@elsevier.com
Web site: http://www.elsevier.com; http://www.elsevier.nl; *CIP.*

Elsevier (GBR) *(0-08; 0-85334; 1-85166; 1-85861) Dist. by* **Elsevier.**

Elsevier (NLD) *Dist. by* **Elsevier.**

Elsvr Adv Tech (GBR) *(0-904705; 0-946395; 0-948577; 1-85617) Dist. by* **Elsevier.**

Elton-Wolf Pub, *(Elton-Wolf Publishing; 1-58619),* 2505 Second Ave., Suite 515, Seattle, WA 98121 Tel 206-748-0345; Fax: 206-748-0343 ; *Imprints:* Authors Pub NA (Author's Publishing of North America)
E-mail: hcox@elton-wolf.com
Web site: http://www.elton-wolf.com.

Elysian Arts, *(Elysian Arts; 0-927425),* P.O. Box 4043, Malibu, CA 90264 Tel 310-457-3164; Fax: 310-457-3396.

Elysium Pubng, *(Elysium Publishing, Inc.; 0-9648228),* 116 Knollwood Terr., Albany, NY 12203 Tel 518-452-3060.

Emalyn Pr, *(Emalyn Pr.; 0-9662216),* 5355 Henry Hudson Pkwy., Riverdale, NY 10741 Tel 718-543-1755.

†EMC-Paradigm, *(EMC/Paradigm Publishing; 0-7638; 0-8219; 0-88436; 0-912022; 1-56118),* Div. of EMC Corp., 875 Montreal Way, Saint Paul, MN 55102-4245 (SAN 201-3800) Tel 651-290-2800; Fax: 651-290-2828
E-mail: publish@emcp.com; educate@emcp.com
Web site: http://www.emcp.com
Dist(s): **Continental Bk** *(Continental Bk. Co., Inc.); CIP.*

eMedguides, *(eMedguides.com, Inc.; 0-9676811; 0-9700525; 0-9716450),* 15 Roszel Rd., Princeton, NJ 08540
Dist(s): **Matthews Medical Bk Co** *(Matthews Medical Bk. Co.).*

Emerald House Group Inc, *(Emerald Hse. Group, Inc.; 1-889893),* 427 Wade Hampton Blvd., Greenville, SC 29609 Tel 864-235-2434; Fax: 864-235-2491; Toll Free: 800-209-8570
E-mail: info@emeraldhouse.com
Web site: http://www.emeraldhouse.com.

Emerald Ink, *(Emerald Ink Publishing; 1-885373),* 9700 Almeda-Genoa Rd., No. 502, Houston, TX 77075-2400 Tel 713-946-8900; Fax: 713-946-6066; Toll Free: 800-324-5663
E-mail: emerald@emeraldink.com
Web site: http://www.emeraldink.com.

Emerald NV, *(Emerald Publishing; 0-9615757),* P.O. Box 11830, Reno, NV 89510 (SAN 696-3846) Tel 702-324-2624 Do not confuse with companies with the same name in Sterling Heights, IL, Harlingen, TX
Dist(s): **Nutri-Books Corp** *(Nutri-Bks. Corp.).*

Emerg Nurses IL, *(Emergency Nurses Assn.; 0-935890),* 915 Lee St., Des Plains, IL 60016-6569 (SAN 269-9036) Tel 847-460-4000; Fax: 847-460-4001; Toll Free: 800-900-9659
Web site: http://www.ena.org.

Emerg Response Inst, *(Emergency Response Institute, Inc.; 0-913724),* 4537 Foxhall Dr., NE, Olympia, WA 98516 (SAN 204-6490) Tel 360-491-7785.

Emerg Trng Assocs, *(Emergency Training Associates; 1-887321),* 105 Glenn Hill Ct., Union Bridge, MD 21791 Tel 410-775-7663; Fax: 410-775-0691; Toll Free: 800-367-0382
E-mail: lou@emsbooks.com.

Emerson, *(Emerson Bks., Inc.; 0-87523),* 121 N. Hampton Dr., White Plains, NY 10603 (SAN 201-3819) Tel 914-761-2643.

EMI Medical, *(EMI Medical Services, Inc.; 0-9655671),* 3130 NW 111th Ave., Coral Springs, FL 33065 Tel 954-341-9381; Fax: 954-341-0641; Toll Free: 800-604-9224 (South Florida only).

EMIS (GBR) *(1-85811) Dist. by* **Gaunt.**

EMIS, *(EMIS, Inc.; 0-917634; 0-929240),* P.O. Box 820062, Dallas, TX 75382-0062 (SAN 248-7586) Tel 214-349-0077; Fax: 214-349-2266; Toll Free: 800-225-0694
E-mail: emis@redriverok.com
Web site: http://www.emispub.com.

EMMPS, *(EMMPS, Inc.; 0-9659200),* 1203 S. Maple St., Northfield, MN 55057 Tel 507-645-0223; Fax: 507-645-7066; Toll Free: 888-645-0223
E-mail: info@emmps.com
Web site: http://www.emmps.com
Dist(s): **Bookmen Inc** *(Bookmen, Inc.).*

Emotions Anony Intl, *(Emotions Anonymous International; 0-9607356),* Orders Addr.: P.O. Box 4245, Saint Paul, MN 55104-0245 (SAN 239-5495) Tel 612-647-9712; Fax: 612-647-1593; Edit Addr.: 2233 University Ave., Suite 402, Saint Paul, MN 55114 (SAN 669-0734)
E-mail: eaisc@mtn.org
Web site: http://www.mtn.org/EA.

EMP Intl, *(EMP International; 0-940430),* 500 S. Danebo Ave., Eugene, OR 97402 Tel 541-344-7099; Fax: 541-344-7429; Toll Free: 800-800-7099
E-mail: emp@medicfirstaid.com
Web site: http://www.medicfirstaid.com.

Empathy Pubng, *(Empathy Publishing, L.L.C.; 0-9710104),* 1331 Canterbury Ln., Fullerton, CA 92831-1042 (SAN 253-7729) Tel 714-402-0738; Fax: 714-526-0575; Toll Free: 877-633-0738
E-mail: empii@home.com
Dist(s): **Biblio Dist** *(Biblio Distribution Ctr.).*

Empire CA, *(Empire Publishing; 0-9627734),* 1322 Fifth Ave., Suite 203, San Diego, CA 92101 Do not confuse with companies with the same name in Lancaster, CA, Denver, CO, Madison, NC.

Empire Pub Srvs, *(Empire Publishing Service; 1-58690),* P.O. Box 1344, Studio City, CA 91614-0344 (SAN 630-5687) Tel 818-784-8918.

†Empl Benefit Res Inst, *(Employee Benefit Research Institute; 0-86643),* Orders Addr.: P.O. Box 4866, Baltimore, MD 21211 (SAN 662-0035) Tel 410-516-6946; Fax: 410-516-6998; Edit Addr.: 2121 K St., NW, Suite 600, Washington, DC 20037-1896 (SAN 216-2423) Tel 202-659-0670; Fax: 202-775-6312
E-mail: info@ebri.org
Web site: http://www.ebri.org; *CIP.*

Employee Benefits, *See* **Empl Benefit Res Inst**

Empower Press, *(Empowerment Pr.; 0-9660451),* Div. of E.Y. Enterprise, Orders Addr.: P.O. Box 1895, Cedar Hill, TX 75106 Fax: 972-293-9879; Edit Addr.: 5009 Trail Lake Dr., Plamo, TX 75093 Tel 972-403-9083; Fax: 972-608-0743 Do not confuse with companies with the same name in South Jordan, UT, Jacksonville Beach, FL ,Los Angeles, CA, Gardnerville, NV
E-mail: info@empowermentpress.com; sales@empowermentpress.com
Web site: http://www.empowermentpress.com.

Empowering People, *(Empowering People, Inc.; 0-9606896; 0-9701190),* P.O. Box 1926, Provo, UT 84603 (SAN 237-9953) Tel 801-763-9096; Fax: 801-763-9452; Toll Free: 800-456-7770
E-mail: brad@empoweringpeople.com
Web site: http://www.empoweringpeople.com.

EMPR, *(EMPR, Inc.; 0-9660472),* P.O. Box 14684, Chicago, IL 60614-0684 Tel 773-348-8248
E-mail: orbeth@ibm.net.

Emrani Publns, *(Emrani Pubns.; 0-9654687),* 253 26th St., Suite 242, Santa Monica, CA 90402 Tel 304-453-3486.

Emron, *(Emron, Inc.; 0-9651745),* Div. of IMS Health, 100 Campus Rd., Totowa, NJ 07512 Tel 973-720-6011; Fax: 908-647-8558; Toll Free: 800-367-6613
E-mail: dhaweeny@us.imshealth.com.

EMS Advan, *(E.M.S. Advantage; 0-9658618),* Orders Addr.: P.O. Box 188, Placerville, CA 95667-0188 Tel 530-622-2752; Fax: 530-622-7329; Toll Free Fax: 800-250-9308; Toll Free: 800-250-9307; Edit Addr.: 685 Placerville Dr., Placerville, CA 95667
E-mail: info@emsadvantage.com
Web site: http://www.emsadvantage.com.

EMT Inc, *See* **Beechwood Hlthbks**

Encino Pr, *(Encino Pr.; 0-88426),* 510 Baylor St., Austin, TX 78703 (SAN 201-3843) Tel 512-476-6821; Fax: 512-476-9393.

Encouraging Words, *(Encouraging Words Publishing; 0-9628806),* Orders Addr.: P.O. Box 4600, Incline Village, NV 89450-4600; Edit Addr.: RFR 1178 E. Clark Lake Rd., Lake Hubert, MN 56459 Tel 218-963-4941
Dist(s): **Indpndnt Pubs** *(Independent Pubs. Marketing).*

Endocrine Res, *(Endocrine Research & Education, Inc.; 0-9637943),* Cedars-Sinai Medical Ctr., 8700 Beverly Blvd., N. Tower Rm. 2015, Los Angeles, CA 90048 Tel 310-855-4691; Fax: 310-967-0119
Web site: http://www.pituitary.com/Referrals/Endocrinologists/CA/ShlomoMelmed.htm.

Endocrine Soc, *(Endocrine Society; 1-879225),* 4350 East West Hwy., Suite 500, Bethesda, MD 20814-4410 (SAN 224-3172) Tel 301-941-0200; Fax: 301-941-0259; Toll Free: 888-363-6329
E-mail: cang@endo-society.org; endostaff@endo-society.org
Web site: http://www.endo-society.org.

Energeia Pub, *(Energeia Publishing, Inc.; 0-9626591; 1-57967; 1-884241),* Orders Addr.: 1307 Fairmount Ave., S., Salem, OR 97302-4313 Tel 503-362-1480; Fax: 503-362-2123; Toll Free: 800-639-6048; Edit Addr.: 1040 Commercial St., SE, Suite 265, Salem, OR 97302
E-mail: Energ123@aol.com.

Energy Essentials, *(Energy Essentials Publishing; 0-9678931),* Div. of KD Did, Inc., 22917 Pacific Coast Hwy, Suite 375, Malibu, CA 90265 Tel 310-456-1597; Fax: 310-456-1322; Toll Free: 888-456-1597
E-mail: norris@pixelgate.net
Web site: http://www.energyessentials.com.

Energy Pubns, *(Energy Pubns.; 0-9620527),* c/o Family Health News, 9845 NE Second Ave., Miami Shores, FL 33138 (SAN 249-1990) Tel 305-759-8710; Toll Free: 800-284-6263 Do not confuse with Energy Pubns., in Newport Beach, CA
Dist(s): **Baker & Taylor** *(Baker & Taylor Bks.)*
Distributors *(Distributors, The)*
New Leaf Dist *(New Leaf Distributing Co., Inc.)*
Nutri-Books Corp *(Nutri-Bks. Corp.).*

Enfield Pubs NH, *(Enfield Publishing & Distribution Co., Inc.; 0-9656184; 1-893598),* Orders Addr.: P.O. Box 699, Enfield, NH 03748 Tel 603-632-7377; Fax: 603-632-5611; Edit Addr.: May St., Enfield, NH 03748
E-mail: enfield@connriver.net
Web site: http://www.enfielddistribution.com.

†**Eng Mgmt Pr,** *(Engineering & Management Pr.; 0-89806),* Div. of Institute of Industrial Engineers, 25 Technology Pk., Norcross, GA 30092-2988 (SAN 213-2338) Tel 770-449-0460; Fax: 770-441-3295; Toll Free: 800-494-0460
E-mail: cmagee@www.iienet.org
Web site: http://www.iienet.org
Dist(s): **Baker & Taylor** *(Baker & Taylor Bks.); CIP.*

EngenderHlth, *(EngenderHealth; 0-9604536; 1-885063),* 440 Ninth Ave., New York, NY 10001 Tel 212-561-8000; Fax: 212-561-8068 (secondary fax); 212-561-8067 (main fax number)
E-mail: info@engenderhealth
Web site: http://www.engenderhealth.org.

Engin Systms Sol, *(Engineering Systems Solutions, Inc.; 0-9674834),* 5726 Industry Ln., Frederick, MD 21704 Tel 301-698-1177; Fax: 301-698-8750 ; *Imprints:* Medawellcom (Medawell.com Publishing)
E-mail: abacchus@essworld.net
Web site: http://www.essworld.net.

English Press, *(English Pr. Pubns.; 0-9663819),* P.O. Box 742945, Dallas, TX 75374 Tel 214-349-4441; Fax: 214-349-4241.

Ennsthaler (AUT) *(3-85068) Dist. by* **Am Educ Systs.**

†**Enslow Pubs,** *(Enslow Pubs., Inc.; 0-7660; 0-89490),* Orders Addr.: P.O. Box 398, Berkeley Heights, NJ 07922-0398 (SAN 213-7518) Tel 908-771-9400; Fax: 908-771-0925; Toll Free: 800-398-2504; Edit Addr.: 40 Industrial Rd., Berkeley Heights, NJ 07922-0398
E-mail: mail@enslow.com
Web site: http://www.enslow.com
Dist(s): **Bollett** *(Bollett Library Resources); CIP.*

Ensminger, *(Ensminger Publishing Co.; 0-941218),* 648 W. Sierra Ave., P.O. Box 429, Clovis, CA 93612 (SAN 239-4375) Tel 209-299-2263; Fax: 209-299-2098.

Ensoulment Educ, *(Ensoulment Education Institute Pr.; 0-9661982),* P.O. Box 3758, Long Beach, CA 90803 Tel 562-433-7499; Toll Free: 800-219-7552.

Entelek, *(Entelek, Inc.; 0-87567),* P.O. Box 242, Gloucester, MA 01931-0242 (SAN 201-3924) Tel 978-282-7439; Fax: 978-281-7071
E-mail: voyage@cove.com; voyage@entelek.com
Web site: http://www.entelek.com.

Enterprise Calif, *(Enterprise Pubns.; 0-918558),* 9339 Orizaba Ave., Downey, CA 90240-2742 (SAN 207-222X).

Enterprise Pr, *(Enterprise Pr.; 0-9604726),* 8600 Fenner Rd., Laingsburg, MI 48848 (SAN 214-2406) Tel 517-651-2953; Fax: 517-651-5573.

Enthea Pr Imprint of Ariel GA

Environ Comms, *(Environmental Communications; 0-9633720),* 200 E. End Ave., Apt. 3N, New York, NY 10128.

Environ Design, *(Environmental Design & Research Ctr.; 0-915250),* 26799 Elena Rd., Los Altos Hills, CA 94022 (SAN 285-0125) Tel 650-948-8383; Fax: 650-917-8168
E-mail: Kaiman_Lee@yahoo.com
Web site: http://www.technology-revolution.com.

Environ Health, *(Environmental Health Consultants; 0-9640831),* 117 Agate Way, Williamston, MI 48895 Tel 517-655-1697; Fax: 517-655-4027
E-mail: waited@msu.edu.

Environ Hlth Watch & H C R Ctr, *(Environmental Health Watch & Housing Resoure Ctr.; 0-9624845),* 4115 Bridge Ave., Cleveland, OH 44113 Tel 216-961-4646.

EO Acupuncture, *(EO Acupuncture Clinic; 0-9640207),* 31 S. First Ave., Arcadia, CA 91006-3651.

EPF, *(Employment Policy Foundation; 0-916559),* 1015 15th St., NW, Suite 1200, Washington, DC 20005 Tel 202-789-8685; Fax: 202-789-8684
E-mail: info@epf.org
Web site: http://www.epf.org.

Epidemiology, *(Epidemiology Resources, Inc.; 0-917227),* 1 Newton Executive Pk., Newton Lower Falls, MA 02162-1450 (SAN 656-0342) Tel 617-244-1200; Fax: 617-244-9669.

Epilepsy Foundation of America, *(Epilepsy Foundation of America; 0-916570),* 4351 Garden City Dr., Landover, MD 20785 (SAN 269-9443) Tel 301-459-3700; Fax: 301-577-2684; Toll Free: 800-332-1000
Web site: http://ww.eta.org/.

EPower & Assocs, *(EPower & Assocs.; 1-883307),* P.O. Box 2346, Brentwood, TN 37024-2346 Tel 615-371-1320; Fax: 206-374-5475; Toll Free: 800-453-4205
E-mail: powere@mindspring.com
Web site: http://www.epower-assoc.com.

EPS Excel Pub, *(EPS Excel Publishing Services; 0-9632735),* Orders Addr.: P.O. Box 86, Wilmette, IL 60091 Tel 847-251-1582 (phone/fax); Edit Addr.: 1729 Forest Ave., Wilmette, IL 60091
E-mail: epsexcps@aol.com
Web site: http://www.meditationsandreligion.com
Dist(s): **Baker & Taylor** *(Baker & Taylor Bks.).*

Equine Res, *(Equine Research, Inc.; 0-935842),* Orders Addr.: P.O. Box 8618, Tyler, TX 75711-8618 (SAN 221-1785) Tel 903-894-9203; Fax: 903-894-4137; Toll Free: 800-848-0225; Edit Addr.: 15931 FM2493 Unit A, Tyler, TX 75703
E-mail: sales@equine-research-inc.com
Web site: http://www.equine-research-inc.com.

Equinox Pr, *(Equinox Pr.; 1-881025),* 144 St. John's Pl., Brooklyn, NY 11217 Tel 718-636-4433; Fax: 718-636-0186; Toll Free: 800-980-1234
E-mail: info@cancerdecisions.com
Web site: http://www.cancerdecisions.com
Dist(s): **Natl Bk Netwk** *(National Bk. Network).*

Equisrvs Pubng, *(Equiservices Publishing; 0-9640072),* 4343 Garfoot Rd., Cross Plains, WI 53528 Tel 608-798-4910
E-mail: equipub@aol.com
Web site: http://www.globaldialog.com/~equiservices.

Erg Aerobics, *(Erg Aerobics, Inc.; 0-9664090),* 24 Fifth Ave., Suite 1222, New York, NY 10011 Tel 212-388-1917; Toll Free: 800-689-9199
E-mail: perryergaerobics@yahoo.com
Web site: http://www.ergaerobics.com.

Ergonome, *(Ergonome, Inc.; 1-884388),* 145 W. 96th St., Suite 800, New York, NY 10025 Tel 212-222-9600; Fax: 212-222-6699.

Ergotec Assn, *(Ergotec Assn., Inc.; 0-9622907),* P.O. Box 9571, Arlington, VA 22219 Fax: 703-516-4576.

†**Eriksson,** *(Eriksson, Paul S. Pub.; 0-8397),* Box 125, Forest Dale, VT 05745 (SAN 201-6702) Tel 802-247-4210; Fax: 802-247-4256
Dist(s): **IPG Chicago** *(Independent Pubs. Group); CIP.*

ESCOM Sci Pubs (NLD) *(90-72199) Dist. by* **Kluwer Academic.**

Eskay, *(Eskay, Inc.; 0-9639757),* 524 NW 142nd St., Edmond, OK 73013-1921.

ESP, *(ESP, Inc.; 0-8209),* Orders Addr.: P.O. Box 839, Tampa, FL 33601-0839; Edit Addr.: 1212 N. 39th St., Suite 444, Tampa, FL 33605-5890 (SAN 241-497X) Do not confuse with E S P Inc., Woodlands, TX
E-mail: epublish@tampalay.rr.com
Web site: http://www.espbooks.com.

ESP TX, *(ESP, Inc.; 0-9626444),* P.O. Box 7439, Woodlands, TX 77387-7439 Tel 713-292-9400 Do not confuse with ESP, Inc., Largo, FL.

Esperance Pub, *See* **William Penzer**

Esperanza Pubns, *(Esperanza Pubns.; 0-9626194),* 530 E. 76th St., Apt. 16D, New York, NY 10021-3148.

ESS Pubns, *(ESS Pubns.; 0-9628229),* E. Stroudsburg Univ., DeNike Bldg., East Stroudsburg, PA 18301 Tel 717-424-3330.

Essential Med Info Syst Inc, *See* **EMIS**

Essential Science, *(Essential Science Publishing; 0-943685),* 1216 S. 1580 W., Suite A, Orem, UT 84058 Tel 801-224-6228; Fax: 801-224-6229; Toll Free: 800-336-6308
E-mail: info@essentialscience.net
Web site: http://www.essentialscience.net.

Estrn Prlyzed Vet, *(Eastern Paralyzed Veterans Assn.; 0-9708873),* 75-20 Astoria Blvd., Jackson Heights, NY 11370 Tel 718-803-3782; Fax: 718-803-0414
E-mail: info@epva.org
Web site: http://www.epva.org
Dist(s): **Demos Medical** *(Demos Medical Publishing, Inc.).*

†**ETC Pubns,** *(ETC Pubns.; 0-88280),* 700 E. Vereda del Sur, Palm Springs, CA 92262 (SAN 124-8766) Tel 760-325-5352; Fax: 760-325-8841; Toll Free: 800-382-7869; *CIP.*

Eternal Gold, *(Eternal Gold Pubs.; 0-9665465),* Orders Addr.: P.O. Box 4633, Rocky Mount, NC 27803 Tel 252-442-4244; Edit Addr.: 1026 Sycamore St., Rocky Mount, NC 27803.

Etheridge Minist, *(Etheridge, G. & M. Ministries, Inc.; 0-937417),* P.O. Box 564, Sikeston, MO 63801-0564 (SAN 658-8581) Tel 573-471-9344.

Ethis Commns, *(Ethis Communications, Inc.; 0-9666621),* 258 W. 99th St., Suite 2, New York, NY 10025 Fax: 212-749-4471
E-mail: eyecareMD@aol.com.

ETNA Communs, *(ETNA Communications, LLC; 0-9659973),* 1300 W. Belmont, Suite 205, Chicago, IL 60657-3240 Tel 773-880-1354; Fax: 773-880-1376
E-mail: ETNAcomm@aol.com.

ETR Assocs, *(ETR Assocs.; 0-941816; 1-56071),* Orders Addr.: P.O. Box 1830, Santa Cruz, CA 95061-1830 (SAN 216-2881) Tel 408-438-4060; Fax: 408-438-4284; Toll Free: 800-321-4407; Edit Addr.: 4 Carbonero Way, Scotts Valley, CA 95066.

Eucalyptus Pr, *(Eucalyptus Pr.; 0-9611980),* P.O. Box 7073, Kansas City, MO 64113 (SAN 287-7430).

Euphonia Pub, *(Euphonia Publishing; 0-9651182),* Orders Addr.: P.O. Box 404, Laconia, NH 03247 Toll Free: 800-879-4214 (book orders only); Edit Addr.: 104 S. Tamilynn Cir., Cary, NC 27513.

†**Eureka Pubns,** *(Eureka Pubns.; 0-942848),* Box 372, Mantua, NJ 08051 (SAN 240-2165) Tel 609-468-4145; *CIP.*

Eurekah, *(Eurekah.Com, Inc.; 1-58706),* 810 S. Church St., Georgetown, TX 78626 Tel 512-863-7762; Fax: 512-863-0081; Toll Free: 800-736-9948
Web site: http://www.eurekah.com
Dist(s): **Landes Bioscience** *(Landes Bioscience).*

Euromed Communs (GBR) *Dist. by* **St Mut.**

Euromonitor PLC (GBR) *(0-86338; 0-903706) Dist. by* **Gale.**

European Amer, *(European American Publishing; 1-885610),* 1882 White Memorial Church Rd., Willow Springs, NC 27592 (SAN 298-3214) Tel 919-639-2890; Toll Free: 800-836-1175
E-mail: somapsych@msn.com.

Evangel Missions, *See* **Evangelism & Missions**

Evangelism & Missions, *(Evangelism & Missions Information Service (EMIS); 0-9617751; 1-879089),* Orders Addr.: P.O. Box 794, Wheaton, IL 60189 (SAN 225-4670) Tel 630-752-7158; Fax: 630-752-7155; Edit Addr.: 500 N. College Ave., No. 300, Wheaton, IL 60187 (SAN 669-0793)
E-mail: emis@wheaton.edu
Web site: http://www.wheaton.edu/bgc/emis.

Evans Bk, *See* **Evans Bk Dist**

Evans Bk Dist, *(Evans Bk. Distribution & Pubs., Inc.; 0-9654884; 1-56684),* 805 W. 1700 S., Salt Lake City, UT 84104 Tel 801-975-1315.

Evergreen MA, *(Evergreen Publishing Co.; 0-9601070),* 277 Farnum St., North Andover, MA 01845-5699 (SAN 221-5594) Tel 978-683-1128 Do not confuse with companies with the same or similar names in Monterey Park, CA, Aurora, CO, Seffner, FL, Evergreen, CO, Seattle, WA.

Everyday Learn, *(Everyday Learning Corp.; 0-9630009; 1-57039; 1-877817),* 2 Prudential Plaza, Suite 1200, Chicago, IL 60601 Tel 312-540-0210; Fax: 312-540-5848; Toll Free: 800-382-7670
Web site: http://www.everydaylearning.com.

Everyday Mathtools, *See* **Everyday Learn**

†**EW Ctr HI,** *(East-West Ctr.; 0-86638),* 1601 East-West Rd., Honolulu, HI 96848-1601 (SAN 210-802X) Tel 808-944-7111; Fax: 808-944-7376
E-mail: ewcinfo@EastWestCenter.org
Web site: http://www.ewc.hawaii.edu/pubs; *CIP.*

Excelsior Music Pub Co, *See* **Zinn Pub Grp**

Except Bks NM, *(Exceptional Bks., Ltd.; 0-944482),* 798 47th St., Los Alamos, NM 87544 (SAN 243-5772) Tel 505-662-6601
Dist(s): **Falcon Pub Inc** *(Falcon Publishing, Inc.).*

Excerpta Medica Imprint of Elsevier

†**Excerpta Princeton,** *(Excerpta Medica-Princeton),* 105 Raider Blvd., Belle Mead, NJ 08502 (SAN 209-5041); *CIP.*

Excptnl Parent, *(Exceptional Parent Pr.; 0-930958),* 555 Kinderkamack Rd., Oradell, NJ 07649-1517 (SAN 211-5611) Tel 201-634-6550; Fax: 201-947-9376; Toll Free: 800-535-1910
E-mail: eplibrary@aol.com
Web site: http://www.eparent.com.

†Exec Ent Pubns, *(Executive Enterprises Pubns. Co., Inc.; 0-7816; 0-88057; 0-917386; 1-55840),* 1 Ramada Plaza, New Rochelle, NY 10801-5766 (SAN 208-953X); *CIP.*

Exec Knowledge, *(Executive Knowledgeworks; 0-943353),* 4083 Ames Rd., Crystal Lake, IL 60012-1424 (SAN 668-5455).

†Exec Reports, *(Executive Reports Corp.; 0-13),* Subs. of Prentice Hall, Inc., Orders Addr.: Dept. 200-B, Englewood Cliffs, NJ 07632 (SAN 204-1308) Tel 201-767-5059; Edit Addr.: 240 Frisch Ct., Paramus, NJ 07652-5240 (SAN 204-1294); *CIP.*

Exelrod Pr, *(Exelrod Pr.; 0-917388),* P.O. Box 2303, Pleasant Hill, CA 94523-0003 (SAN 208-1555) Tel 925-228-0344; Fax: 510-228-7443.

Exeter Grp, *(Exeter Group, The; 0-9665523),* 425 Madison Ave., Suite 1801, New York, NY 10017 Tel 212-644-1017; Fax: 212-644-6762.

Exeter Hse, *(Exeter Hse. Bks.; 0-9610008; 1-880683),* P.O. Box 8134, Reading, PA 19603 (SAN 266-0865) Tel 610-779-8149; 610-775-0464; Fax: 610-376-7756
E-mail: info@exeterhousebools.com; exhouseboo@aol.com
Web site: http://www.exeterhousebooks.com
Dist(s): **Koen Bk Distributors** *(Koen Bk. Distributors).*

Expectancy Data, *(Expectancy Data; 0-9667944),* Subs. of John O. Ward & Associates, Inc., 8340 Mission Rd., Suite 235, Prairie Village, KS 66206 Tel 913-381-9420; Fax: 913-648-5740
E-mail: krueger@johnwardeconomics.com
Web site: http://www.expectancydata.com.

Expedit Advisory Ctr (GBR) *(0-907649) Dist. by* **St Mut.**

Exploration Pr, *(Exploration Pr.; 0-913552),* Div. of Chicago Theological Seminary, 5757 S. University Ave., Chicago, IL 60637-1507 (SAN 203-851X) Tel 773-752-5757; Fax: 773-752-1905
E-mail: info@chgosem.edu
Web site: http://www.chgosem.edu.

Exten Inc, *(Exten, Inc.; 0-9661764),* Orders Addr.: P.O. Box 1508, Buffalo, NY 14240-1508 Tel 716-895-2214; Fax: 716-895-2216; Toll Free: 800-551-5004; Edit Addr.: 50 Stradtman St., Buffalo, NY 14240
E-mail: exteninc@mindspring.com.

Extend Learn, *See* **Extend Studies**

Extend Studies, *(Extended Studies; 0-9665049),* Div. of Texas Tech Univ., Orders Addr.: P.O. Box 42191, Lubbock, TX 79409-2191 Tel 806-742-2352; Fax: 806-742-0405; Toll Free: 800-692-6877; Edit Addr.: 15th St. & Akron Ave., Lubbock, TX 79409-2191
E-mail: d.nash@coed.ttu.edu; distlearn@ttu.edu
Web site: http://www.dce.ttu.edu/dl/.

Extension Pr Imprint of Lowell Hse

Extracorporeal Life Support, *(Extracorporeal Life Support Organization; 0-9656756),* 1327 Jones Dr., Suite 101, Ann Arbor, MI 48105 Tel 734-998-6600; Fax: 734-998-6602
Web site: http://www.elso.med.umich.edu.

Eye Ctr N CA, *(Eye Ctr. of Northern Califonia; 0-9633665),* 6500 Fairmount Ave., El Cerrito, CA 94530 Tel 510-525-2800; Fax: 510-524-1887; Toll Free: 800-553-2266.

F & W Pubns Inc, *(F&W Pubns., Inc.; 0-89134; 0-89879; 0-932620; 1-55870; 1-58180; 1-58297; 1-884910),* Orders Addr.: 3637 Woodburn Ave., Cincinnati, OH 45207; Edit Addr.: 1507 Dana Ave., Cincinnati, OH 45207 (SAN 287-0274) Tel 513-531-2690; Fax: 513-531-4082; Toll Free Fax: 888-590-4082; Toll Free: 800-289-0963 ; *Imprints:* Wrtrs Digest Bks (Writer's Digest Books) Betrwy Bks (Betterway Books)
E-mail: marciaj@fwpubs.com
Web site: http://www.fwpublications.com.

F A Countway, *(Countway, Francis A. Library of Medicine),* 10 Shattuck St., Boston, MA 02115 (SAN 206-4057) Tel 617-432-2134; Fax: 617-4320693
E-mail: countref@warren.med.harvard.edu
Web site: http://www.countway.harvard,edu/countway/home.html.

F A Thorpe (GBR) *(0-7089; 0-85456) Dist. by* **Ulverscroft US.**

F C B, *(FCB Pubns.; 0-9713098),* Orders Addr.: P.O. Box 725, Brandon, SD 57005 Tel 605-339-9738; Edit Addr.: 48176 Kim Cir., Brandon, SD 57005
E-mail: fboulden@u.s.west.net.

F C Grosso, *(Grosso, Federiw C. DDS, PhD, MFT; 0-9654534),* 2020 Alameda Padre Serra, Suite 217, Santa Barbara, CA 93103-1756 Tel 805-962-3628; Fax: 805-692-2143
E-mail: fcgt@fgrosso.com
Web site: http://www.fgrosso.com.

F Cass Pubs (GBR) *(0-7146; 0-85303) Dist. by* **Intl Spec Bk.**

F E Peacock Pubs, *(Peacock, F.E. Pubs., Inc.; 0-87581),* 115 W. Orchard St., Itasca, IL 60143-1780 (SAN 202-876X) Tel 630-775-9000; Fax: 630-775-9003
E-mail: fepeacock@aol.com
Web site: http://www.fepeacock.com.

F Fell Pubs Inc, *(Fell, Frederick Pubs., Inc.; 0-8119; 0-88391; 0-9672469),* 2131 Hollywood Blvd., Suite 305, Hollywood, FL 33020 Tel 954-925-0555; Fax: 954-925-5244.

F Fergeson, *(Fergeson, F. Productions; 0-935510),* 7090 E. Roberts, Mount Zion, IL 62549 (SAN 214-3704) Tel 217-864-5620.

F I Comm, *(F.I. Communications; 0-89533),* 45 Alhambra Ct., Portola Valley, CA 94028-7722 (SAN 201-8489) Tel 650-851-0254.

F I Intl, *(F.I. International; 1-930241),* 42 San Roque Rd., Santa Barbara, CA 93105-2835 Tel 805-687-1832
E-mail: fiinter@silcom.com
Web site: http://www.silcom.com/~fiinter.

F Lincoln (GBR) *(0-7112; 0-906459) Dist. by* **St Mut.**

F M Roberts, *(Roberts, F.M. Enterprises; 0-912746),* P.O. Box 608, Dana Point, CA 92629-0608 (SAN 201-4688) Tel 714-493-1977; Fax: 714-493-7124.

F Morrow, *(Morrow, Felix Pub.; 0-9615659),* 13 Welwyn Rd., Great Neck, NY 11021 (SAN 696-1029) Tel 516-482-1044.

F Pyrczak, *See* **Pyrczak Pub**

F R Parker, *(Parker, F.R. Publishing Co.; 0-9654700; 1-893091),* P.O. Box A, New Foundland, PA 18445 Tel 570-424-8563; Fax: 570-476-7372
E-mail: parker.f@worldnet.att.net..

F S C Pubng, *(FSC Publishing; 1-930069),* 6013 Moss Rose Ct., Brentwood, TN 37027 Tel 615-371-2900; Fax: 615-377-0291; Toll Free: 800-371-3114 (phone/fax)
E-mail: info@fosterseminars.com
Web site: http://www.fosterseminars.com.

F S H, *(F.S.H., Inc.; 1-880864),* 4524 S. Cameron Ave., Tampa, FL 33611 Tel 813-839-6006.

F Thibodeau, *(Thibodeau, Faith; 0-9671168),* 7 Simpson Rd., Saco, ME 04072 Tel 207-284-4537 (phone/fax)
E-mail: NurtRx@gwi.net.

F W Barnes, *(Barnes, Frederick W.; 0-9653311),* 355 Blackstone Blvd., Apt. 343, Providence, RI 02906 Tel 401-421-7931.

F W Ernst, *(Ernst, Frederick W.; 0-9651454),* 7 Woodmere Dr., Dothan, AL 36301 Tel 334-792-7237; Fax: 334-792-2208
Dist(s): **Partners Pubs Grp** *(Partners Pubs. Group, Inc.).*

F Watts, *(Watts, Franklin; 0-531),* Div. of Grolier Publishing, 90 Sherman Tpke., Danbury, CT 06816 (SAN 285-1156) Tel 203-797-3500; Fax: 203-797-3657; Toll Free: 800-621-1115
Web site: http://www.publishing.grolier.com/.

FA Services, *(Fertility Awareness Services; 0-9628284),* P.O. Box 986, Corvallis, OR 97339 Tel 541-753-8530.

FAAO, *(Foundation of the American Academy of Ophthalmology; 0-926866),* 655 Beach St., San Francisco, CA 94109-1336 Tel 415-561-8500; Fax: 415-561-8533
Web site: http://www.eyenet.org.

†Faber & Faber, *(Faber & Faber, Inc.; 0-571),* Affil. of Farrar, Straus & Giroux, LLC, Orders Addr.: c/o Van Holtzbrinck Publishing Services, 16365 James Madison Hwy., Gordonsville, VA 22942 Fax: 540-572-7540; Toll Free: 888-330-8477; Edit Addr.: 19 Union Sq., W, New York, NY 10003-3304 (SAN 218-7256) Tel 212-741-6900; Fax: 212-633-9385
Dist(s): **Continental Bk** *(Continental Bk. Co., Inc.)* **VHPS** *(VHPS Holtzbrinck Pubs.); CIP.*

Fabiano (ITA) *(88-87333) Dist. by* **SLACK Inc.**

Face Value, *(Face Value; 0-9646774),* P.O. Box 45854, Los Angeles, CA 90045 Fax: 310-338-1537.

Facticity Tr, *(Facticity Trainings, Inc.; 0-9628686; 1-887367),* P.O. Box 22814, Seattle, WA 98122 Tel 425-462-4369
E-mail: ragini@facticity.com
Web site: http://www.facticity.com.

Factor Pr, *(Factor Pr.; 0-9626531; 1-887650),* Orders Addr.: P.O. Box 8888, Mobile, AL 36689 (SAN 631-466X) Tel 334-380-0606; Fax: 334-380-0606; Toll Free: 800-304-0077; Edit Addr.: 5354 Gaillard Dr., Mobile, AL 36608 Toll Free: 800-304-0077
E-mail: factorpress@zebra.net
Dist(s): **BookWorld** *(BookWorld Services, Inc.).*

Facts & Comparisons, *(Facts & Comparisons; 0-932686; 1-57439),* Subs. of Wolters Kluwer U.S. Corp., 111 West Port Plaza, Suite 300, Saint Louis, MO 63146 Tel 314-216-2100; Fax: 314-878-5563; Toll Free: 800-223-0554
E-mail: editor@fandc.com; sales@drugfacts.com
Web site: http://www.factsandcomparisons.com
Dist(s): **Lppncott W & W** *(Lippincott Williams & Wilkins).*

Facts on Demand, *(Facts on Demand Pr.; 1-889150),* Affil. of BRB Pubns., P.O. Box 27869, Tempe, AZ 85285-7869 Tel 602-829-7475; Fax: 620-829-8505; Toll Free Fax: 800-929-4981; Toll Free: 800-929-3811
E-mail: brb@brbpub.com
Web site: http://www.brbpub.com
Dist(s): **Natl Bk Netwk** *(National Bk. Network).*

†Facts on File, *(Facts on File; 0-8160; 0-87196),* 132 W. 31st St., 17th Flr., New York, NY 10001-2006 (SAN 201-4696) Tel 212-967-8800; Fax: 212-967-9196; 212-967-8107; Toll Free: 800-322-8755 ; *Imprints:* Checkmark (Checkmark)
E-mail: lharris@factsonfile.com
Web site: http://www.factsonfile.com; *CIP.*

FAFCTPC, *(First Aid for Children & Teens Publishing Co.; 0-9622812),* 211 Trysail Ct., Foster City, CA 94404 Tel 650-574-7179; Fax: 650-574-0455.

Fair Winds Pr, *(Fair Winds Pr.; 1-931412),* Div. of Rockport Publishers, 33 Commerical St., Gloucester, MA 01930 Tel 978-282-9590; Fax: 978-283-2742; Sheridan Hse., 112-116A Western Rd., Hove, BN3 1DD
E-mail: questions@rockpub.com
Web site: http://www.rockpub.com
Dist(s): **Tuttle Pubng** *(Tuttle Publishing).*

†Fairleigh Dickinson, *(Fairleigh Dickinson Univ. Pr.; 0-8386),* 285 Madison Ave., Madison, NJ 07940 Tel 973-443-8564; Fax: 973-443-8364
E-mail: fdupress@fdu.edu
Web site: http://www.fdu.edu/newspubs/fdupress.html
Dist(s): **Assoc Univ Prs** *(Associated Univ. Presses)* **B & T International** *(Baker & Taylor International); CIP.*

FairMail Serv, *(FairMail Service, Inc.; 0-9601262),* 417 Cleveland Ave., Plainfield, NJ 07060 (SAN 210-4210) Tel 973-754-7770.

†Fairmont Pr, *(Fairmont Pr., Inc.; 0-88173; 0-915586),* 700 Indian Trail, Lilburn, GA 30047 (SAN 207-5946) Tel 770-925-9388; Fax: 770-381-9865
E-mail: fpinfo@fairmontprinting.com
Web site: http://www.fairmonprinting.com
Dist(s): **Assn Energy Eng** *(Association of Energy Engineers); CIP.*

Fairview Press, *(Fairview Pr.; 0-925190; 1-57749),* 2450 Riverside Ave., Minneapolis, MN 55545 (SAN 298-170X) Tel 612-672-4180; Fax: 612-672-4980; Toll Free: 800-544-8207 Do not confuse with Fairview Pr., in Silver Spring, MD
E-mail: press@webx.fairview.org
Web site: http://www.fairviewpress.org
Dist(s): **Natl Bk Netwk** *(National Bk. Network).*

Fairway Pr Imprint of CSS OH

Faith Lib Pubns, *(Faith Library Pubns., Inc.; 0-89276),* P.O. Box 50126, Tulsa, OK 74150-0126 (SAN 208-2578) Tel 918-258-1588; Fax: 918-251-8016
E-mail: admin@rhema.org
Web site: http://www.rhema.org/
Dist(s): **Harrison Hse** *(Harrison Hse., Inc.).*

Faith One, *(Faith One Publishing; 1-883798),* Div. of Crenshaw Christian Ctr., Orders Addr.: P.O. Box 90000, Los Angeles, CA 90009 Tel 323-758-3777; Fax: 323-565-4160; Edit Addr.: 7901 S. Vermont Ave., Los Angeles, CA 90044 Tel 213-565-4135.

Faith Pub & Media, *(Faith Publishing & Media Co.; 0-9631880),* 2920 N First St., Abilene, TX 79603-7110 Tel 915-672-8537; Fax: 915-672-8532; Toll Free: 800-547-2272.

Faith Ridge, *(Faith Ridge; 0-9633796),* Div. of Afirms Software, Inc., 2211 Pane Rd., Koloa, HI 96756.

Falcon Pr Intl, *(Falcon Pr. International; 1-884459),* P.O. Box 4113, Mountain View, CA 94040 Tel 415-941-6691; Fax: 650-941-4436; Toll Free: 800-884-4436
E-mail: health@vitabooks.com
Web site: http://www.vitabooks.com.

Falcon Pub Inc, *(Falcon Publishing, Inc.; 0-934318; 0-934641; 0-937959; 0-9609452; 1-56044; 1-57540; 1-58592),* Div. of Globe Pequot Press, Orders Addr.: P.O. Box 1718, Helena, MT 59624 (SAN 221-1726) Fax: 406-442-0384; Toll Free Fax: 800-968-3550; Toll Free: 800-582-2665; Edit Addr.: 48 Last Chance Gulch, Helena, MT 59601 Do not confuse with companies with similar names in Ben Lomond,CA, Venice, CA, Long Island City, NY, Wauwatosa, WI, Palo Alto, CA, Grand Prairie, TX
E-mail: falconbk@ix.netcom.com
Web site: http://www.falcon.com
Dist(s): **Baker & Taylor** *(Baker & Taylor Bks.)*
Koen Bk Distributors *(Koen Bk. Distributors)*
Peregrine Outftrs *(Peregrine Outfitters)*
Sunbelt Pubns *(Sunbelt Pubns., Inc.).*

Falmer Pr Imprint of Taylor & Francis

Fam By Design, *(Families By Design; 0-9703525),* P.O. Box 2812, Glenwood Springs, CO 81602 Tel 970-984-2222; Fax: 970-984-0422
E-mail: ncthomas@rof.net.

Fam Health Media, *(Family Health Media; 0-931470),* 1811 N. Jay, Aberdeen, SD 57401 (SAN 211-965X) Tel 605-229-5990.

Fam Hlth Pubns, *(Family Health Pubns.; 1-878726),* 3963 North M-63, Benton Harbor, MI 49022 Tel 616-849-0359; Fax: 616-849-0862; Toll Free: 800-488-3878
E-mail: joann@familyhealthpub.com
Web site: http://www.familyhealthpub.com
Dist(s): **Angelas Bkshelf** *(Angela's Bookshelf)*
New Leaf Dist *(New Leaf Distributing Co., Inc.)*
Royal Pubns Inc *(Royal Pubns., Inc.)*
TEACH Servs *(TEACH Services, Inc.).*

Fam USA Found, *(Families U.S.A. Foundation; 0-9617893),* 1334 G St., NW, Washington, DC 20005 (SAN 665-5254) Tel 202-628-3030; Fax: 202-347-2417.

Family Amer Fnd, *(Family of the Americas Foundation, Inc.; 0-9633125),* P.O. Box 1170, Dunkirk, MD 20754-1170 Tel 301-627-3346; Fax: 301-627-0847; Toll Free: 800-443-3395
E-mail: family@upbeat.com
Web site: http://www.familyplanning.net.

Family Friends, *See* **Wisdom of Pain**

Family Mtrs, *(Family Matters; 0-910529),* Div. of Parent Scene, 990 Red Hill Valley Rd., Cleveland, TN 37323 (SAN 260-244X) Tel 423-339-0500
E-mail: 74532.333@compuserve.com.

Family Process, *(Family Process Pr.; 0-9615519),* Div. of Family Process, Inc., P.O. Box 23980, Rochester, NY 14692 (SAN 696-4249) Tel 716-244-2770; Fax: 716-244-3942
Dist(s): **Norton** *(Norton, W.W. & Co., Inc.).*

Family Pubns, *(Family Pubns.; 0-931128),* P.O. Box 940398, Maitland, FL 32794-0398 (SAN 211-3147) Tel 407-539-1411; Fax: 407-539-2862 Do not confuse with Family Publications, Glens Falls, NY
Dist(s): **Baker & Taylor** *(Baker & Taylor Bks.)*
New Leaf Dist *(New Leaf Distributing Co., Inc.).*

†**Family Relat,** *(Family Relations Foundation; 0-9614218),* P.O. Box 462, Sebastopol, CA 95473 (SAN 687-1097) Tel 707-823-0876; *CIP.*

Family Respte, *(Family Respite Ctr.; 0-9678646),* 2036 Westmoreland St., Falls Church, VA 22046 Tel 703-532-8899; Fax: 703-532-9134
E-mail: respite@erols.com.

FAO (ITA) *(92-5) Dist. by* **Bernan Associates.**

Far Estrn Univ, *See* **P S Chua**

Far West Edns, *(Far West Editions; 0-914480),* P.O. Box 27901-113, San Francisco, CA 94127 (SAN 207-0456) Tel 415-255-5911; Fax: 415-255-1372.

Farah Consult, *(Farah Consulting; 0-9678437),* 8755 Bame Rd., Colfax, NC 27235 Tel 336-664-9218; Fax: 336-299-7630
E-mail: drandyfarah@yahoo.com.

Farming Pr (GBR) *(0-85236) Dist. by* **Diamond Farm Bk.**

Farmworker Hlth, *(Farmworker Health Services, Inc.; 0-9702892),* 1234 Massachusetts Ave., NW, Suite C-1017, Washington, DC 20005 Tel 202-347-7377; Fax: 202-347-6385
E-mail: oscargom@aol.com
Web site: http://www.farmworkerhealth.org.

Fast Horse, *(Fast Horse Pr.; 0-9707109),* Div. of Medical Device Assistance, Inc., P.O. Box 246, Front Royal, VA 22630 (SAN 253-6617) Tel 540-636-6740; Fax: 540-636-6878; Toll Free: 888-571-1148
E-mail: info@fasthorsepress.com; info@fdainsideandout.org
Web site: http://www.fdainsideandout.org.

FastMark, *(FastMark, Inc.; 1-887562),* 125 University Ave., Suite 250, Palo Alto, CA 94301 Tel 415-327-7700; Fax: 415-327-7734; Toll Free: 800-406-2035 ; *Imprints:* Accordia Pr (Accordia Press)
E-mail: info@fastmark.com; FastGuide@Fastmark.com
Web site: http://www.fastmark.com.

Fat Control, *(Fat Control Inc.; 0-918275),* P.O. Box 10117, Towson, MD 21204 (SAN 682-2711).

Fat Free Ent, *See* **Fat Free Living**

Fat Free Living, *(Fat Free Living, Inc.; 0-9636876; 1-893694),* 15202 N. 50th Pl., Scottsdale, AZ 85254 Tel 602-996-6300; Fax: 602-996-9897; Toll Free: 888-328-3731
E-mail: fatfree@dancis.com
Web site: http://www.fatfreeliving.com
Dist(s): **Herveys Bklink** *(Hervey's Booklink & Cookbook Warehouse).*

Faulkner & Gray, *(Faulkner & Gray, Inc.; 0-9624775; 1-57987; 1-881393),* Div. of Thomson Professional Publishing, 11 Penn Plaza, 17th Flr., New York, NY 10001 Tel 212-967-7000; Fax: 212-239-4993; Toll Free: 800-535-9422; 300 S. Wacker Dr. Suite 1800, Chicago, IL 60606 Tel 312-913-1334; Fax: 312-913-6135
Web site: http://wwwfaulknergray.com.

†**Fawcett,** *(Fawcett; 0-345; 0-449; 0-8041; 1-4000),* Div. of Ballantine Publishing Group, Orders Addr.: 400 Hahn Rd., Westminster, MD 21157 Tel 410-848-1900; Toll Free: 800-762-0600; Edit Addr.: 201 E. 50th St., New York, NY 10022 (SAN 201-4572) Tel 212-572-2713; Fax: 212-572-6046; Toll Free: 800-733-3000 (orders); 800-726-0600 (customer service) ; *Imprints:* Columbine (Columbine) Crest (Crest Books)
E-mail: customerservice@randomnhouse.com
Web site: http://www.randomhouse.com
Dist(s): **Shens Bks** *(Shen's Bks.); CIP.*

FBI Lab, *(Federal Bureau of Investigation, Laboratory Div.; 0-932115),* 935 Pennsylvania Ave., NW, Rm. 3865, Washington, DC 20535 (SAN 686-4740) Tel 202-324-4384.

FC&A Pub, *(FC&A Publishing; 0-915099; 1-890957),* 103 Clover Green, Peachtree City, GA 30269-1695 (SAN 289-7946) Tel 770-487-6307; Fax: 770-631-4357; Toll Free: 800-226-8024
E-mail: customerservice@fca.com; charlotte_carpenter@fca.com
Web site: http://www.fca.com
Dist(s): **Baker & Taylor** *(Baker & Taylor Bks.)*
Quality Bks IL *(Quality Bks., Inc.).*

FDM Distributor, *(F.D.M. Distributor; 0-9615720),* 7807 Hohman Ave., Munster, IN 46321 (SAN 696-4168) Tel 219-836-8107.

FE Chronic Pain, *(Freedom Enterprises in Chronic Pain; 0-9637353),* 1061 Lovell Ave., Saint Paul, MN 55113-4419 Tel 612-487-3611
Dist(s): **Adventure Pubns** *(Adventure Pubns.).*

Fear Free, *(Fear Free Foundation; 0-939637),* P.O. Box 251030, Glendale, CA 91225 (SAN 663-575X) Tel 818-242-7227.

Fed Focus, *(Federal Focus, Inc.; 0-9654148),* 11 Dupont Cir., NW, Suite 700, Washington, DC 20036 Tel 202-797-6368; Fax: 202-939-6969
Web site: http://www.fedfocus.org/.

Federal Bar, *(Federal Bar Assn.; 1-56986),* 2215 M St., NW, Washington, DC 20037 (SAN 223-7784) Tel 202-785-1614; Fax: 202-785-1568
E-mail: pubs@fedbar.org
Web site: http://www.fedbar.org.

Federal St Pr, *(Federal Street Pr.; 1-892859),* Div. of Merriam Webster, Inc., 47 Federal St. Box 281, Springfield, MA 01102 Fax: 610-965-2983; Toll Free: 877-886-2830
E-mail: info@federalstreetpress.com.

Federation Pr (AUS) *(1-86287) Dist. by* **Gaunt.**

Federlin, *(Federlin, Tom; 0-9603136),* 47 Cardinal Ct., Saratoga Springs, NY 12866 (SAN 213-4934) Tel 518-587-3704.

Feedback Rsch, *(Feedback Research; 1-889713),* P.O. Box 1329, Jacksonville, OR 97530 Tel 541-899-8088; Fax: 541-899-7344; Toll Free: 800-927-8071
E-mail: info@feed-back.com
Web site: http://www.feed-back.com.

†**Feldheim,** *(Feldheim, Philipp Inc.; 0-87306; 1-58330),* 200 Airport Executive Pk., Nanuet, NY 10954 (SAN 106-6307) Tel 845-356-2282; Fax: 845-425-1908; Toll Free: 800-237-7149
E-mail: mike613@netvision.net.il
Web site: http://www.feldheim.com; *CIP.*

Feline Pr, *(Feline Pr.; 0-9625150),* Orders Addr.: P.O. Box 357219, Gainesville, FL 32605 Tel 352-371-6439 (phone/fax); Edit Addr.: 1930 NW 40th Terr., Gainesville, FL 32605; P.O. Box 1173, Sarasota, FL 34230 Do not confuse with Feline Pr. Inc., Sarasota, FL
E-mail: jlcastner@aol.com.

†**Feminist Pr,** *(Feminist Pr. at The City Univ. of New York; 0-912670; 0-935312; 1-55861),* 365 Fifth Ave., New York, NY 10016 (SAN 213-6813) Tel 212-817-7915; Fax: 212-817-2988
E-mail: lglazer@gc.cuny.edu
Web site: http://www.feministpress.org
Dist(s): **Consort Bk Sales** *(Consortium Bk. Sales & Distribution)*
Continental Bk *(Continental Bk. Co., Inc.); CIP.*

Fence Crk Pubng, *(Fence Creek Publishing, LLC; 0-9651916; 1-889325),* Orders Addr.: P.O. Box 136, Madison, CT 06443 Tel 203-245-5174; Fax: 203-245-1193; Edit Addr.: 9 Linden Lane, Madison, CT 06443
E-mail: fencecreek@aol.com
Dist(s): **Blackwell Sci** *(Blackwell Science, Inc.).*

Fenix Pr, *(Fenix Pr.; 0-9664016),* 2927 SE Main St., Portland, OR 97214 Tel 503-234-4949
E-mail: mgrange@hevanet.com.

Fer1nwd Publ Co (CAN) *(1-55266; 1-895686) Dist. by* **Eiron.**

Feral Hse, *(Feral Hse.; 0-922915),* P.O. Box 13067, Los Angeles, CA 90013 (SAN 251-5423) Tel 213-689-4502; Fax: 213-689-4728; Toll Free: 800-967-7885
E-mail: info@feralhouse.com
Web site: http://www.feralhouse.com
Dist(s): **Publishers Group** *(Publishers Group West).*

Ferguson-Florissant, *(Ferguson-Florissant Schl. District/Early Education; 0-939418),* 1005 Waterford Dr., Florissant, MO 63033 (SAN 216-5740) Tel 314-831-8809; Fax: 314-831-1525.

Fern Ridge Pr, *(Fern Ridge Pr.; 0-9615332),* 1927 McLean Blvd., Eugene, OR 97405 (SAN 695-0868) Tel 541-485-8243; Fax: 541-687-7701; Toll Free: 800-816-5679
E-mail: lgold@efn.org
Dist(s): **Baker & Taylor** *(Baker & Taylor Bks.).*

Fernhurst Bks (GBR) *(0-906754; 1-898660) Dist. by* **Motorbooks Intl.**

Fernhurst Bks (GBR) *(0-906754; 1-898660) Dist. by* **St Mut.**

Fertil Solns, *(Fertility Solutions, Inc.; 0-9660540),* 13000 Shaker Blvd., Cleveland, OH 44120 Tel 216-491-0030; Fax: 216-491-0032; Toll Free: 800-959-7656
E-mail: sarfsi@aol.com
Web site: http://fertilitysolutions.com.

FES Info Ctr, *(FES Information Ctr.; 1-888470),* Div. of Cleveland FES Ctr., 11000 Cedar Ave., Suite 230, Cleveland, OH 44106-3052 Tel 216-231-3257; Fax: 216-231-3258; Toll Free: 800-666-2353
E-mail: fes_info@po.cwru.edu
Web site: http://www.fes.cwru.edu
Dist(s): **Univ Bkstore** *(University Bookstore).*

Fetters InfoMgmt, *See* **FimCo Bks**

Fibromyalgia Educ, *(Fibromyalgia Educational Systems, Inc.; 0-9665774),* 500 Bushaway Rd., Wayzata, MN 55391 Tel 419-843-3153; Fax: 419-843-3155
E-mail: jawk80@aol.com
Web site: http://www.fmsedsys.com.

Fibromyalgia Solns, *(Fibromyalgia Solutions; 0-9660190),* 305 E. Ninth St., Kearney, MO 64060 Tel 816-903-5427; Fax: 816-903-9029
E-mail: karl@fibrosolutions.com
Web site: http://www.fibrosolutions.com.

Field & Wood Inc Medical, *(Field & Wood, Inc., Medical Pubs.; 0-938607),* P.O. Box 975, Blue Bell, PA 19422-0239 (SAN 661-3519) Tel 610-828-4010
Dist(s): **Norton** *(Norton, W.W. & Co., Inc.).*

Fieldside Pub, *(Fieldside Publishing; 0-9619628),* 15 Windsor Ct., No. A, Keene, NH 03431-1737 (SAN 245-9450) Tel 603-525-6652.

Fifty Gates, *(50 Gates Publishing Co.; 0-9647831),* P.O. Box 6090, Malibu, CA 90264 (SAN 693-4285) Tel 310-457-1218; Fax: 310-457-3790
Dist(s): **Baker & Taylor** *(Baker & Taylor Bks.)*
Bookpeople *(Bookpeople)*
Koen Bk Distributors *(Koen Bk. Distributors)*
New Leaf Dist *(New Leaf Distributing Co., Inc.)*
Quality Bks IL *(Quality Bks., Inc.).*

FimCo Bks, *(FimCo Bks.; 0-929599),* 4531 Ayers St., No. 220, Corpus Christi, TX 78415 (SAN 249-7786) Tel 361-857-8049; Fax: 361-814-2243
E-mail: lfetters@caller.infi.net.

Finacial Inst, *See* **Guardian Pub**

Finan Exec, *(Financial Executives Research Foundation; 0-910586; 1-885065),* Orders Addr.: P.O. Box 6996, Alpharetta, GA 30239-6996 Tel 770-751-1986; Fax: 770-442-9742; Toll Free: 800-680-3373; Edit Addr.: 10 Madison Ave., Box 1938, Morristown, NJ 07962-1938 (SAN 206-4111) Tel 973-898-4600; Fax: 973-898-4649
E-mail: RFerling@fei.org
Web site: http://www.fei.org
Dist(s): **E Elgar** *(Elgar, Edward Publishing, Inc.)*
PBD Inc *(PBD, Inc.).*

Finan Srcebk Pub, *(Financial Sourcebook Publishing; 0-9661060),* 417 Saint Joseph St., P.O. Box 40, Suttons Bay, MI 49682 Tel 616-271-2811; Fax: 616-271-4087; Toll Free: 800-632-5528
E-mail: pubfimg@traverse.com.

Finan Strats Pr, *(Financial Strategies Pr., Inc.; 0-9642896),* c/o Gordon & Friedler, 15 Broad St., Suite 1700, Boston, MA 02109 Tel 617-720-1212
Dist(s): **Publishers Group** *(Publishers Group West).*

FIND MN, *See* **DeafBlind Srvcs**

Findhorn Pr (GBR) *(0-905249; 1-899171; 0-906191; 0-9504268) Dist. by* **Words Distrib.**

Findhorn Pr (GBR) *(0-905249; 1-899171; 0-906191; 0-9504268) Dist. by* **Lantern Books.**

FIND-SVP, *(FIND SVP; 0-931634; 0-941285; 1-56241),* 625 Ave. of the Americas, New York, NY 10011-2002 (SAN 212-6680) Tel 212-645-4500; Fax: 212-645-7681; Toll Free: 800-298-5699.

Fine Comms, *(Fine Communications; 1-56731),* Div. of Fine Creative Media, Inc., 2 Lincoln Sq., 60 W. 66th St., 2nd Flr., New York, NY 10023 Tel 212-595-3500; Fax: 212-595-3779 ; *Imprints:* MJF Bks (M J F Books)
E-mail: scott@mjfbooks.com.

Finnigan Clinic, *(Finnigan Clinic; 0-9662786),* 1307 Violet, SE, Olympia, WA 98503 Tel 360-459-7800; Fax: 360-459-1216
E-mail: heffey@aol.com.

Finnish Acad (FIN) *(951-653; 951-717; 951-41; 951-710; 951-746) Dist. by* **Intl Spec Bk.**

Fire Eng, *(Fire Engineering Bks. & Videos; 0-912212),* Div. of PennWell Corp., Orders Addr.: P.O. Box 21288, Tulsa, OK 74101 (SAN 281-7136) Fax: 918-831-9555; Toll Free: 800-752-9768; Edit Addr.: 1421 S. Sheridan Rd., Tulsa, OK 74112 (SAN 281-7128)
E-mail: sales@pennwell.com
Web site: http://www.pennwell-store.com.

Fire Protect Pubns, *See* **IFSTA**

Firebird NY, *(Firebird Pubns., Inc.; 0-8285),* 4956 Boiling Brook Pkwy., Rockville, MD 20852 Tel 301-881-5973; Fax: 301-852-6546; Toll Free: 800-854-9595
E-mail: kamkin@kamkin.com
Web site: http://www.kamkin.com.

†Firebrand Bks, *(Firebrand Bks.; 0-932379; 1-56341),* 141 The Commons, Ithaca, NY 14850 (SAN 687-3855) Tel 607-272-0000; Toll Free: 800-663-1766
E-mail: firebrand@firebrandbooks.com
Web site: http://www.firebrandbooks.com
Dist(s): **LPC Group** *(LPC Group); CIP.*

Firefly Bks Limited, *(Firefly Bks., Ltd.; 0-920668; 1-55209; 1-895565; 1-896284; 1-55297),* Orders Addr.: P.O. Box 1338, Buffalo, NY 14205 (SAN 630-611X) Toll Free Fax: 800-565-6034; Toll Free: 800-387-5085
E-mail: fireflybooks@globalserv.net
Web site: http://www.fireflybooks.com/
Dist(s): **Lectorum Pubns** *(Lectorum Pubns., Inc.).*

Fireside Imprint of S&S Trade Pap

First Class Bks, *(First Class Bks., Inc.; 1-880246),* 113 E. Magnesium Rd., Suite C, Spokane, WA 99208 Tel 509-466-6847; Fax: 509-466-6896; Toll Free: 800-524-6911
E-mail: fcb@icehouse.net
Dist(s): **Baker & Taylor** *(Baker & Taylor Bks.).*

First Data, *(First Data Bank; 0-9626616),* 530 Maryville Centre Dr., Saint Louis, MO 63141-5814 Tel 314-275-8848; Fax: 314-432-0573; Toll Free: 800-366-4737.

First Med Pub, *See* **Inst Knowledge**

First Prsn Pr, *(First Person Pr.; 0-9635307),* 25 Allen Rd., Swampscott, MA 01907 Tel 617-593-4362; Fax: 617-599-0081.

First Pubs Grp, *(First Pubs Group, Ltd.; 0-9704254),* Orders Addr.: P.O. Box 481, State College, PA 16804-0481 Tel 814-238-9400; Fax: 814-238-8600; Edit Addr.: 220 Reese Rd., State College, PA 16801
Web site: http:// firstpublishers.com.

First Teacher, *(First Teacher Pr.; 0-9615005; 1-878727),* 28 Tamarack Rd., Weston, MA 02193 Tel 617-893-7274.

First-Care, *(First-Care Co.; 1-882822),* Div. of Alan W. MacCarthy, Jr., Corp., P.O. Box 427, Pala, CA 92059 Tel 760-742-1536; 37457 Magee Rd., Pala, CA 92059.

Fischer Pub, *(Fischer Publishing; 0-915421),* Orders Addr.: P.O. Box 116, Canfield, OH 44406 (SAN 291-1574) Tel 330-533-1232; Edit Addr.: 7851 Herbert Rd., Canfield, OH 44406.

†Fisher Bks, *(Fisher Bks.; 1-55561),* Div. of Perseus Books Group, Orders Addr.: 5500 Central Ave., Boulder, CO 80301 Toll Free: 800-386-5656; Edit Addr.: 11 Cambridge Ctr., Cambridge, MA 02142 (SAN 698-1410) Tel 617-252-5200; Fax: 617-252-5275
E-mail: orders@fisherbooks.com
Web site: http://www.fisherbooks.com
Dist(s): **HarperCollins Pubs** *(HarperCollins Pubs.)*
Motorbooks Intl *(Motorbooks International Wholesalers & Distributors); CIP.*

Fisons Corp, *(Fisons Corp.; 0-914132),* 2 Preston Ct., Bedford, MA 01730 (SAN 220-5459) Tel 617-275-1000.

Fit Info Tech, *(Fitness Information Technology, Inc.; 0-9627926; 1-885693),* P.O. Box 4425, Morgantown, WV 26504-4425 Tel 304-599-3483; Fax: 304-599-3482; Toll Free: 800-477-4348
E-mail: fit@fitinfotech.com
Web site: http://www.fitinfotech.com
Dist(s): **BookWorld** *(BookWorld Services, Inc.).*

FIT Pub, *See* **G Landry**

Fithian Pr, *(Fithian Pr.; 0-931832; 1-56474),* Div. of Daniel & Daniel Pubs., Inc., P.O. Box 1525, Santa Barbara, CA 93102 (SAN 211-6103) Tel 805-962-1780; Fax: 805-962-8835; Toll Free: 800-662-8351 (orders only)
E-mail: dandd@danielpublishing.com
Web site: http://www.danielpublishing.com
Dist(s): **SCB Distributors** *(SCB Distributors).*

FITNE, *(FITNE, Inc.; 1-888418),* Div. of Electronic Vision, Inc., 5 Depot St., Athens, OH 45701 Tel 614-592-2511; Fax: 614-592-2650.

Fitness Ojai, *(Fitness Pubns.; 0-9618805),* Orders Addr.: P.O. Box 863, Ojai, CA 93024 (SAN 253-6048) Tel 805-646-0350; Fax: 805-646-2815; Edit Addr.: 1991 Country Pl., Ojai, CA 93203 (SAN 242-651X)
E-mail: fitpub@cs.com
Dist(s): **Baker & Taylor** *(Baker & Taylor Bks.).*

Fitzgerald Sci, *(Fitzgerald Science Pr., Inc.; 1-891786),* 4814 Auburn Ave., Suite 2, Bethesda, MD 20814 Tel 301-654-6884; Fax: 703-661-1501 (orders); 301-654-6886; Toll Free: 800-869-4409 (orders)
E-mail: info@fitzscipress.com
Web site: http://www.fitzscipress.com.

Fitzroy Dearborn, *(Fitzroy Dearborn Pubs., Inc.; 1-57958; 1-884964),* 919 N. Michigan Ave., Suite 760, Chicago, IL 60611 Tel 312-587-0131; Fax: 312-587-1049; Toll Free: 800-850-8102
E-mail: fitzroy@aol.com
Web site: http://www.fitzroydearborn.com.

Five Star Pub Imprint of Hatherleigh

Five Wisdoms Pubns, *(Five Wisdoms Pubns.; 0-9655210),* 9322 21st Ave., NW, Seattle, WA 98117 Tel 206-783-1838
E-mail: jelias@sprynet.com
Web site: http://www.home.sprynet.com/~jelias
Dist(s): **Bookpeople** *(Bookpeople)*
Metamorphous Pr *(Metamorphous Pr., Inc.)*
New Leaf Dist *(New Leaf Distributing Co., Inc.)*
Partners Pubs Grp *(Partners Pubs. Group, Inc.).*

FL Cryonics Assn, *See* **Life Ext Media**

Flagship Pubns, *(Flagship Pubns.; 1-885397),* Div. of Flagship Consulting, 720 Chelsea Ln., Tipp City, OH 45371-8651 Tel 513-335-0797.

Flaming Hooker Pr, *(Flaming Hooker Pr.; 0-9615223),* Div. of Markin Medical Research, Orders Addr.: P.O. Box 9106, Virginia Beach, VA 23450 (SAN 662-3441); Edit Addr.: 1236 Ginger Crescent, Virginia Beach, VA 23456 (SAN 695-152X) Tel 757-427-0220.

Flaming Sparrow, *See* **Foreworks**

Flash Anatomy Inc, *(Flash Anatomy, Inc.; 1-878576),* Div. of Bryan Edwards, a Publishing Company, Inc., 2040 S. Santa Cruz, Suite 115, Anaheim, CA 92805 Tel 714-634-0264; Toll Free: 800-222-1775
E-mail: contact@bryanedwards.com
Web site: http://www.bryanedwards.com.

Fleur-Di-Lee, *(Fleur-Di-Lee; 0-911579),* 5969 Donna, Tarzana, CA 91356 (SAN 264-0422).

Flinn Scientific, *(Flinn Scientific, Inc.; 1-877991),* Orders Addr.: P.O. Box 219, Batavia, IL 60510 (SAN 630-1800) Tel 630-879-6900; Fax: 630-879-6962; Toll Free: 800-452-1261; Edit Addr.: 770 N. Raddant Rd., Batavia, IL 60510
E-mail: flinn@flinnsci.com
Web site: http://www.flinnsci.com.

Floris Bks (GBR) *(0-86315; 0-903540) Dist. by* **Anthroposophic.**

Flower Essence, *(Flower Essence Society; 0-9631306),* Div. of Earth-Spirit, Inc., P.O. Box 459, Nevada City, CA 95959 Tel 916-265-9163; Fax: 916-265-6467; Toll Free: 800-548-0075
E-mail: mail@flowersociety.org
Dist(s): **Bookpeople** *(Bookpeople)*
New Leaf Dist *(New Leaf Distributing Co., Inc.)*
Nutri-Books Corp *(Nutri-Bks. Corp.).*

Flower Valley Pr, *(Flower Valley Pr., Inc.; 0-9620543; 1-886388),* P.O. Box 952, Glen Echo, MD 20812 (SAN 249-0277) Tel 301-654-1996; Fax: 301-654-1905; Toll Free: 800-735-5197
E-mail: dbress@flowervalleypress.com
Web site: http://www.dbress@flowervalleypress.com.

FLPB Pr, *(Fat Little Pudding Boys Pr.; 0-9647895),* 1221 SE 11th St., Lee's Summit, MO 64081 Tel 816-525-4826.

Fly Eagle, *(Flying Eagle Publishing Co.; 0-9663702),* Div. of Flying Eagle Enterprises, Inc., 3125 S. Mendenhall, No. 422, Memphis, TN 38115-2827 Tel 901-366-4945; Fax: 901-365-9430; Toll Free: 888-366-5247.

Flyana, *(Flyana Rhyme, Inc.; 0-9630198; 1-892997),* P.O. Box 248, Anahola, HI 96703 Tel 808-828-1919
E-mail: diana@flyana.com
Web site: http://www.flyana.com
Dist(s): **Baker & Taylor** *(Baker & Taylor Bks.)*
Booklines Hawaii *(Booklines Hawaii, Ltd.)*
New Leaf Dist *(New Leaf Distributing Co., Inc.)*
Nutri-Books Corp *(Nutri-Bks. Corp.).*

Flying Fox Pr, *(Flying Fox Pr., The; 0-9617225),* 4700 Jamestown Rd., Bethesda, MD 20816 (SAN 663-3692) Tel 301-229-8160.

Flying Pig, *(Flying Pig Pubns.; 1-888342),* Div. of Homeworks Midwifery Service, 491 Lincoln Ave., Elgin, IL 60120 Tel 847-931-5222; Fax: 847-931-0438.

FMJ Intl (GBR) *Dist. by* **St Mut.**

FMSG, *(FMSG Publishing Co.; 1-886468),* Orders Addr.: c/o A.J. Majors, P.O. Box 819074, Dallas, TX 75381-9074 Tel 904-774-5277; Fax: 904-774-5563
E-mail: fmsgco@n-jcenter.com
Dist(s): **J Majors Co** *(Majors, J. A. Co.)*
Matthews Bk Co *(Matthews Bk. Co.)*
Rittenhouse *(Rittenhouse Bk. Distributors).*

Fnd Behav Hlth, *(Foundation for Behavioral Health; 0-9637577),* 561 Keystone Ave., No. 212, Reno, NV 89503-4304 Tel 602-423-7717; Fax: 602-451-0369
E-mail: cummfound@aol.com.

Fnd Blood Res, *(Foundation for Blood Research; 0-9653655),* Orders Addr.: P.O. Box 190, Scarborough, ME 04070-0190 Tel 207-883-4131; Fax: 207-883-1527; Toll Free: 800-639-8605; Edit Addr.: 69 US Rte. 1, Scarborough, ME 04074
E-mail: jbeaudoi@fbr.org.

Fnd Chiro Educ Res, *(Foundation for Chiropractic Education & Research; 0-9631715),* 704 E. Fourth St., Des Moines, IA 50309 Tel 515-282-7118; Fax: 515-282-3347; Toll Free: 800-622-6309
E-mail: fcernow@aol.com
Web site: http://www.fcer.org.

Fnd Chiropractic Educ, *(Foundation for the Advancement of Chiropractic Education; 1-890419),* Orders Addr.: P.O. Box 1052, Levittown, PA 19058 Tel 215-946-6815; Toll Free: 800-397-9722; Edit Addr.: 1405 Frosty Hollow Rd., Levittown, PA 19056
E-mail: face@f-a-c-e.com
Web site: http://www.f-a-c-e.com.

Fnd NY St Nurses, *(Foundation of the New York State Nurses Assn., Inc.; 1-886511),* 2113 Western Ave., Guilderland, NY 12084 Tel 518-456-7858; Fax: 518-452-3760.

Focal Imprint of Buttrwrth-Heinemann

Publisher Symbol Index

Focus Pub-R Pullins, *(Focus Publishing/R. Pullins Co., Inc.; 0-941051; 1-58510),* Orders Addr.: P.O. Box 390, Jaffrey, NH 03452 Tel 603-532-7454; Toll Free: 800-848-7236; Edit Addr.: P.O. Box 369, Newburyport, MA 01950 (SAN 665-2646) Tel 978-462-7288; Fax: 978-462-9035; Toll Free: 800-848-7236; 311 Merrimac St., Newburyport, MA 01950 (SAN 665-2654)
E-mail: pullins@pullins.com
Web site: http://www.pullins.com.

Focused Treat, *(Focused Treatment Systems; 0-9661673),* Orders Addr.: P.O. Box 530, Glen Echo, MD 20812-0530 Tel 301-320-0529 (phone/fax); Toll Free: 800-728-6799; Edit Addr.: 5204 Sangamore Rd., Bethesda, MD 20816-2322
E-mail: info@sagetalk.com
Web site: http://www.sagetalk.com.

FOI Services, *(FOI Services, Inc.; 0-9622958; 1-880626),* 11 Firstfield Rd., Gaithersburg, MD 20878-1703 Tel 301-975-9400; Fax: 301-975-0702
E-mail: infofoi@foiservices.com
Web site: http://www.foiservices.com.

Folk-Life, *(Folk-Life Bks.; 0-914917),* Orders Addr.: P.O. Box 128, Princeton, LA 71067 (SAN 289-1336) Tel 318-949-3915; Edit Addr.: 3330 Hwy 80E, Haughton, LA 71037 (SAN 289-1344).

Fondo CA, *(Fondo de Cultura Economica USA; 968-16; 950-557; 956-7083; 9972-663),* 2293 Verus St., San Diego, CA 92154 Tel 619-429-0827; Fax: 619-429-0455; Toll Free: 800-532-3872
E-mail: sales@fceusa.com; fceusa@fceusa.com
Web site: http://www.fceusa.com
Dist(s): **Latin Am Bk Source** *(Latin American Bk. Source, Inc.).*

Font & Ctr Pr, *(Font & Ctr. Pr.; 1-883280),* Orders Addr.: P.O. Box 95, Weston, MA 02493-0005 Tel 781-647-9756; Fax: 781-788-9643; Toll Free: 800-647-8658; Edit Addr.: 69 Pinecroft Rd., Weston, MA 02493
E-mail: info@fontandcenter.com
Web site: http://www.fontandcenter.com.

†**Food & Nut Pr,** *(Food & Nutrition Pr., Inc.; 0-917678),* 6527 Main St., Trumbull, CT 06611-1338 (SAN 221-1475) Tel 203-261-8587; Fax: 203-261-9724
E-mail: 72400.3517@compuserve.com; *CIP.*

Food Addicts, *(Food Addicts Anonymous; 0-9638074),* 4623 Forest Hill Blvd., Suite 109-4, West Palm Beach, FL 33415 Tel 407-967-3871
Web site: http://foodaddictsanonymous.org/.

Food Allergy, *(Food Allergy & Anaphylaxis Network; 1-882541),* 10400 Eaton Pl. Suite 107, Fairfax, VA 22030-2208 Tel 703-691-3179; Fax: 703-691-2713; Toll Free: 800-929-4040
E-mail: faan@foodallergy.org
Web site: http://www.foodallergy.org.

Food Products, *See* **Haworth Jrnl Co-Edits**

Ford Headache, *See* **Intl Headache**

Fordham, *(Fordham Univ. Pr.; 0-8232),* University Box L, Bronx, NY 10458 (SAN 201-6516) Tel 718-817-4780; Fax: 718-817-4785
E-mail: mnoonan@fordham.edu
Web site: http://www.bookmasters.com/fordhampress/
Dist(s): **BookMasters** *(BookMasters, Inc.).*

Forefront Pub, *(Forefront Publishing; 0-9674933),* 5 River Rd., PMB 113, Wilton, CT 06897-0940 Tel 203-834-0631; Fax: 203-834-0940
E-mail: ZAPDO1B@prodigy.com.

Foreign Policy, *(Foreign Policy Assn.; 0-87124),* 470 Park Ave. S., 2nd Flr., New York, NY 10016-6819 (SAN 212-9426) Tel 212-481-8100; Fax: 212-481-9275; Toll Free: 800-628-5754; 800-477-5836 (orders)
Web site: http://www.fpa.org.

Forensic Imaging Inst, *(Forensic Imaging Institute; 0-9677866),* 2284 S. Victoria Ave., Suite 1-G, Ventura, CA 93003 Tel 805-642-0381; Fax: 805-656-3205
E-mail: cmbowers@aol.com
Web site: http://www.firms.findlaw.com/cmbowers.

Forest Hist Soc, *(Forest History Society, Inc.; 0-89030),* 701 William Vickers Ave., Durham, NC 27701 (SAN 201-6524) Tel 919-682-9319; Fax: 919-682-2349.

Forever Truth, *See* **Windsor Hse Pub Grp**

Foreworks, *(Foreworks; 0-943292),* P.O. Box 82289, Portland, OR 97282 (SAN 240-6519) Tel 503-653-2614; Fax: 503-786-2492 (4:00 - 8:00 A.M. PST)
E-mail: index@foreworks.com
Web site: http://www.foreworks.com.

Forge Bks Imprint of T Doherty Assocs

Formur Intl, *(Formur International; 0-89378),* 4200 Laclede Ave., Saint Louis, MO 63108 (SAN 207-5768) Tel 314-533-9600.

Fortkamp, *(Fortkamp Publishing Co.; 1-879175),* P.O. Box 3087, Washington, DC 20010-3087 Fax: 202-842-7401; Toll Free: 1-800-437-3223 (Messages and Orders)
E-mail: bookstore@catholicworker.com
Web site: http://www.catholicworker.com/bookstore.

Fortress Pr Imprint of Augsburg Fortress

Forum Pubns, *See* **Cortlandt Grp**

Foster Parents, *(Foster Parents Plan International, Inc.; 0-918397),* 155 Plan Way, Warwick, RI 02886-1011 (SAN 657-341X).

Foulsham UK (GBR) *(0-572) Dist. by* **Assoc Pubs Grp.**

Foun Am Comm, *(Foundation for American Communications; 0-910755),* 75 S. Grand Ave., No. 85, Pasadena, CA 91105-1602 (SAN 270-2746).

Foun Bks, *(Foundation Bks., Inc.; 0-934988),* P.O. Box 22828, Lincoln, NE 68542-2828 (SAN 201-6567) Tel 402-438-7080; Fax: 402-438-7099
Dist(s): **Baker & Taylor** *(Baker & Taylor Bks.)*
Bookmen Inc *(Bookmen, Inc.).*

Foun Econ Ed, *(Foundation for Economic Education, Inc.; 0-910614; 1-57246),* 30 S. Broadway, Irvington-on-Hudson, NY 10533-1861 (SAN 311-3515) Tel 914-591-7230; Fax: 914-591-8910; Toll Free: 800-452-3518
E-mail: fee@fee.org
Web site: http://www.fee.org.

Foun Human Under, *(Foundation of Human Understanding, The; 0-933900),* Orders Addr.: P.O. Box 1000, Grants Pass, OR 97528 (SAN 213-9545) Tel 541-597-4360; Fax: 541-597-2191; Toll Free: 800-877-3227; Edit Addr.: 1607 Williams Hwy., Grants Pass, OR 97527
E-mail: fhu1963@cdsnet.net
Web site: http://www.fhu.com.

Found Care Mgmt, *(Foundation for Care Management; 1-891814),* 10323 NE 126th Pl., Kirkland, WA 98034 Tel 425-820-9625; Fax: 425-820-1060
E-mail: fcm@medcare.org
Web site: http://www.medcare.org.

Foundation Ctr, *(Foundation Ctr., The; 0-87954; 1-931923),* 79 Fifth Ave., New York, NY 10003-3076 (SAN 207-5687) Tel 212-807-3670; Fax: 212-807-3677
Web site: http://www.fdncenter.org.

Foundation Hse, *(Foundation Hse. Pubns., Inc.; 0-935427),* Div. of The Emissaries, 5569 N. County Rd. 29, Loveland, CO 80538 (SAN 630-0634) Tel 970-679-4302; 970-679-4229; Fax: 970-679-4233
E-mail: emissaries@emnet.org
Web site: http://www.emissaries.org.

†**Foundation Pr,** *(Foundation Pr.; 0-88277; 1-56662; 1-58778),* Div. of West Group, Orders Addr.: 11 Penn Plaza, New York, NY 10001 (SAN 281-7225) Tel 212-760-8700; Fax: 212-760-8740; Toll Free: 877-888-1330; Edit Addr.: 610 Opperman Dr., Eagan, MN 55123-1396 (SAN 202-9618) Do not confuse with companies with similar names in Dunn, NC, Chattanooga, TN
E-mail: gerry.gelke@Westgroup.com
Web site: http://www.FDPress.com; *CIP.*

Fountain AL, *(Fountain Pr.; 0-9622607),* 2055 E. South Blvd., Suite 410, Montgomery, AL 36116-2004 Tel 334-284-9595 Do not confuse with companies with the same name in Indianola, IA, Delaware, OH.

Four Cts Pr (IRL) *(1-85182; 0-906127) Dist. by* **Intl Spec Bk.**

Four Geez, *(Four Geez Pr.; 0-9637068),* 1911 Douglas Blvd., Suite 85-131, Roseville, CA 95661-3707 Tel 916-781-3440; Fax: 916-781-3814
E-mail: GGolomb@ns.net
Web site: http://www.readersndex.com/fourgeez.

Four Leaf Pr, *(Four Leaf Pr.; 0-9637578),* P.O. Box 23502, Eugene, OR 97402 Tel 541-485-4938 (phone/fax); Toll Free: 800-322-1883
E-mail: fourleafpr@aol.com
Web site: http://www.autism.com/fourleafpress
Dist(s): **Baker & Taylor** *(Baker & Taylor Bks.).*

Four Seasons, *(Four Seasons Pubs.; 0-9656811; 1-891929),* Orders Addr.: P.O. Box 6467, Titusville, FL 32782 Tel 407-267-9800; Fax: 407-267-8076; P.O. Box 51, Titusville, FL 32781; Edit Addr.: 350 N. Washington Ave., Suite 3M, Titusville, FL 32782
E-mail: fourseasons@gnc.net
Web site: http://www.fourseasonspub.net
Dist(s): **Baker & Taylor** *(Baker & Taylor Bks.).*

Four Winds OR, *(Four Winds Publishing; 0-9628608),* 6267 SW Miles Ct., Portland, OR 97219 Tel 503-246-9424; Fax: 503-246-9497; Toll Free: 800-484-9653 (ext. 1944) Do not confuse with Four Winds Publishing, Fair Oaks, CA
Dist(s): **Baker & Taylor** *(Baker & Taylor Bks.)*
New Leaf Dist *(New Leaf Distributing Co., Inc.)*
New Life Dist *(New Life Distributors).*

Fowler & Wells, *See* **Good Commun Inc**

FPT VA, *(Foundation for Physical Therapy, Inc.; 0-9628807),* 1055 N. Fairfax St., Suite 350, Alexandria, VA 22314-1488 Tel 703-684-5984; Fax: 703-706-8519; Toll Free: 800-875-1378
Web site: http://www.foundation@apta.org.

Fr & Eur, *(French & European Pubns., Inc.; 0-320; 0-7859; 0-8288),* Rockefeller Ctr. Promenade, 610 Fifth Ave., New York, NY 10020-2497 (SAN 206-8109) Tel 212-581-8810; Fax: 212-265-1094
E-mail: frenchbookstore@aol.com; livresny@aol.com
Web site: http://www.frencheuropean.com.

Fr Lib LA Cty Med, *(Friends of the Library of Los Angeles County Medical Assn.; 0-9607646; 0-9631270),* 341 S. Westmoreland, Los Angeles, CA 90020 Tel 213-388-0121.

Franciscan Pr, *(Franciscan Pr.; 0-8199),* Orders Addr.: Dept. NL Quincy Univ., 1800 College Ave., Quincy, IL 62301-2699 Tel 217-228-5670; Fax: 217-228-5672; Edit Addr.: Quincy Univ., 1800 College Ave., Quincy, IL 62301-2699 ; *Imprints:* Frncscn Herld (Franciscan Herald Press)
E-mail: coopebe@quincy.edu
Web site: http://quincy.edu/fpress/index-html.

Frank B Brady, *(Brady, Frank B.; 0-9614639),* P.O. Box 4653, Annnapolis, MD 21403-6653 (SAN 691-9219) Tel 410-263-8388.

Franklin, *(Franklin Bk. Co., Inc.),* 7804 Montgomery Ave., Elkins Park, PA 19027 (SAN 121-4160) Tel 215-635-5252; Fax: 215-635-6155 ; *Imprints:* CRC Reprint (C R C Press Reprints)
E-mail: service@franklinbook.com
Web site: http://www.franklinbook.com.

Franklin Bks, *(Franklin Bks.; 0-9620490),* 11815 W. Somerset Dr., Franklin, WI 53132 (SAN 249-0323) Tel 414-529-2285.

Franklin Comp, *See* **Franklin Elect**

Franklin Elect, *(Franklin Electronics Pubs., Inc.; 0-945731; 1-56712; 1-59074),* 1 Franklin Plaza, Burlington, NJ 08016-4907 (SAN 277-1292) Tel 609-386-2500; Fax: 609-387-2666; Toll Free: 800-762-5382.

Franklin Pubs, *(Franklin Pubs.; 0-916503),* P.O. Box 1338, Bryn Mawr, PA 19010 (SAN 295-4141) Tel 610-525-1225
E-mail: bodychem@dynanet.com
Dist(s): **Nutri-Books Corp** *(Nutri-Bks. Corp.)*
Publishers Group *(Publishers Group West).*

†**Fraser Pub Co,** *(Fraser Publishing Co.; 0-87034; 0-918632),* Div. of Fraser Management Assocs., Inc., Orders Addr.: Box 494, Burlington, VT 05402 (SAN 213-9537) Toll Free: 800-253-0900; Edit Addr.: 309 S. Willard St., Burlington, VT 05401 (SAN 110-8646) Tel 802-658-0324; Fax: 802-658-0260
E-mail: info@fraserbooks.com
Web site: http://www.fraserbooks.com; *CIP.*

Free Assoc Bks (GBR) *(0-946960; 1-85343) Dist. by* **Intl Spec Bk.**

Free Begin Pr, *(Free Beginning Pr.; 0-930707),* 10 Hillshire Ln., Norwood, MA 02062-3009 (SAN 677-2145) Tel 617-769-5931.

†**Free Pr,** *(Free Pr., The; 0-02; 0-669; 0-671; 0-684; 0-7432),* Div. of Simon & Schuster Trade, Orders Addr.: 100 Front St., Riverside, NJ 08075 Toll Free Fax: 800-943-9831; Toll Free: 800-223-2336; Edit Addr.: 1230 Avenue of the Americas, New York, NY 10020 (SAN 200-2450) Tel 212-698-7000; Toll Free: 800-223-2348 (customer service)
E-mail: Consumer.CustomerService@simonandschuster.com
Web site: http://www.simonsays.com
Dist(s): **S&S Trade** *(Simon & Schuster Trade)*
T T Beeler *(Beeler, Thomas T. Publisher)*
Wheeler Pub *(Wheeler Publishing, Inc.); CIP.*

†**Free Spirit Pub,** *(Free Spirit Publishing, Inc.; 0-915793; 1-57542),* 217 Fifth Ave., N., Suite 200, Minneapolis, MN 55401-1299 (SAN 293-9584) Tel 612-338-2068; Fax: 612-337-5050; Toll Free: 800-735-7323
E-mail: help4kids@freespirit.com
Web site: http://www.freespirit.com
Dist(s): **Baker & Taylor** *(Baker & Taylor Bks.)*
Bookmen Inc *(Bookmen, Inc.)*
Quality Bks IL *(Quality Bks., Inc.); CIP.*

Freedom FL, *(Freedom Pubns.; 1-879805),* P.O. Box 944, Ringgold, GA 30736.

Freedom Pr Inc, *(Freedom Pr., Inc.; 1-893910),* 1801 Chart Trail, Topanga, CA 90290 Tel 310-455-2995; Fax: 310-455-8962; 310-455-3203; Toll Free: 800-959-9797
E-mail: info@freedompressonline.com
Web site: http://freedompressonline.com
Dist(s): **BookWorld** *(BookWorld Services, Inc.)*
Nutri-Books Corp *(Nutri-Bks. Corp.).*

Freefall Fact, *(Freefall Factory, The; 0-9665418),* 4017 San Mateo, North Las Vegas, NV 89030 Tel 702-645-4204; Fax: 702-645-0814
E-mail: freefall@lvdi.net.

Freeman Family, *(Freeman Family Trust Pubns.; 0-9665706),* P.O. Box 402, Tustin, CA 92781.

Freemor, *(Freemor Publishing; 0-9659478),* Orders Addr.: P.O. Box 157, Whitehall, MI 49461 Tel 616-894-2243; Fax: 616-894-5141; Edit Addr.: 608 E. Colby St., Whitehall, MI 49461.

Freeperson, *(Freeperson Pr.; 0-918236),* Div. of TH-EC, Inc., 1516 Grant Ave., Suite 212, Novato, CA 94945 (SAN 209-438X) Tel 415-897-0336; Fax: 415-892-4388.

Freestone Pub Co, *(Freestone Publishing Co.; 0-913512),* P.O. Box 398, Monroe, UT 84754 (SAN 206-4154) Tel 435-527-3738
E-mail: freestone@hubwest
Dist(s): **Bookpeople** *(Bookpeople)*
New Leaf Dist *(New Leaf Distributing Co., Inc.).*

Fremont Rideout Found, *(Fremont Rideout Foundation; 0-9667500),* Div. of Fremont Rideout Health Group, 989 Plumas St., Yuba City, CA 95991 Tel 530-751-4280; Fax: 530-751-4226.

†Freundlich, *(Freundlich Bks.; 0-88191),* Div. of Lawrence Freundlich Pubns., Inc., 333 E. 30th St., Apt. 5-K, New York, NY 10016 (SAN 264-7419) Tel 212-686-4122; *CIP.*

Frieda Carrol, *(Frieda Carrol Communications; 1-890928),* P.O. Box 416, Denver, CO 80201-0416 Tel 303-575-5676; Fax: 970-292-2136
E-mail: mail@besomebodybeyourself.com
Web site: http://www.contentprovidermedia.com
Dist(s): **Prosperity & Profits** *(Prosperity & Profits Unlimited, Distribution Services).*

Friends Karen, *(Friends of Karen, Inc.; 0-9619785),* Orders Addr.: P.O. Box 217, Croton Falls, NY 10519 (SAN 246-6074) Tel 914-277-4547; Edit Addr.: Sun Valley Dr., Croton Falls, NY 10519 (SAN 246-6082).

Friends of the Library Imprint of Brigham

Friends Ohio St U Lib, *(Friends of the Ohio State Univ. Libraries; 0-88215),* Div. of Ohio State Libraries, Rm. 112, Main Lib., 1858 Neil Ave. Mall, Columbus, OH 43210 (SAN 202-814X) Tel 614-292-3387.

Frncscn Herld Imprint of Franciscan Pr

Frnds & Relatives, *(Friends & Relatives of Institutionalized Aged, Inc.; 0-9652790),* 11 John St., Suite 601, New York, NY 10038 Tel 212-732-5667; Fax: 212-732-6945
E-mail: friany@aol.com
Web site: http://www.fria.org
Dist(s): **Bookazine Co Inc** *(Bookazine Co., Inc.).*

Frnds Hosp, *(Friends Hospital; 0-9642252),* 4641 Roosevelt Blvd., Philadelphia, PA 19124-2399 Tel 215-831-4763; Fax: 215-289-9260
E-mail: soultoukis@hslc.org.

Frog Ltd CA, *(Frog, Ltd.; 1-883319; 1-58394),* Div. of North Atlantic Bks., Orders Addr.: P.O. Box 12327, Berkeley, CA 94712 Tel 510-559-8277; Fax: 510-559-8279; Toll Free: 800-337-2665 (orders only)
E-mail: orders@northatlanticbooks.com
Web site: http://www.northatlanticbooks.com
Dist(s): **Publishers Group** *(Publishers Group West).*

Front Row, *(Front Row Experience; 0-915256),* 540 Discovery Bay Blvd., Discovery Bay, CA 94514 (SAN 207-1274) Tel 925-634-5710; Toll Free: 800-524-9091 (credit card/established credit orders & information)
E-mail: service@frontrowexperience.com
Web site: http://www.frontrowexperience.com.

Frontal Lobe, *(Frontal Lobe; 0-931400),* 836 Starlite Ln., Los Altos, CA 94024 (SAN 211-9013) Tel 650-941-8561
E-mail: masonc@ix.netcom.com
Web site: http://www.netcom.com/~masonc.

Frontline Pub, *(Frontline Publishing Corp.; 0-9653629; 0-9716483),* Orders Addr.: P.O. Box 441002, Somerville, MA 02144 Tel 617-625-7188; Fax: 617-625-7446; Toll Free: 800-348-0605; Edit Addr.: 17 Herbert St., Somerville, MA 02144
E-mail: cgreland@frontlinepub.com
Web site: http://www.frontlinepub.com.

Frontrunners, *(Frontrunners Board Review/Frontrunners Publishing; 0-9677025),* Orders Addr.: 360-A W. Merrick Rd., P.O. Box 221, Valley Stream, NY 11580 Tel 516-285-0758; Edit Addr.: 39 Lyon St., Valley Stream, NY 11580
E-mail: abimexam@aol.com
Dist(s): **Baker & Taylor** *(Baker & Taylor Bks.)*
Rittenhouse *(Rittenhouse Bk. Distributors).*

Frost & Sullivan, *(Frost & Sullivan Market Intelligence; 0-7889; 0-86621; 0-916483; 1-56753),* 2525 Charleston Rd., Mountain View, CA 94043 (SAN 215-8698) Tel 650-961-9000; Fax: 650-961-5042
E-mail: webmaster@frost.com
Web site: http://www.frost.com.

FSCOD, *(Federation of Special Care Organizations in Dentistry; 0-9657191),* 211 E. Chicago Ave., Suite 948, Chicago, IL 60611 Tel 312-440-2660; Fax: 312-440-2824.

†FS&G, *(Farrar, Straus & Giroux, LLC; 0-374),* Orders Addr.: c/o Von Holtzbrinck Publishing Services, 16365 James Madison Hwy., Gordonsville, VA 22942 (SAN 631-5011) Tel 540-672-7600; Toll Free Fax: 800-672-2054; Toll Free: 888-330-8477; Edit Addr.: 19 Union Sq., W., New York, NY 10003 (SAN 206-782X) Tel 212-741-6900; Fax: 212-633-9385 ; *Imprints:* Noonday (Noonday Books)
E-mail: sales@fsgee.com
Web site: http://www.fsbassociates.com/fsg/index.htm
Dist(s): **Continental Bk** *(Continental Bk. Co., Inc.)*
Shens Bks *(Shen's Bks.)*
iPublishcom *(iPublish.com); CIP.*

Fujisawa Health, *(Fujisawa Healthcare, Inc.; 0-9702446),* 3 Parkway, N., Deerfield, IL 60015 Tel 847-317-1077; Fax: 847-317-8229; Toll Free: 800-727-7003
E-mail: goldman-garrity@fujisawa.com
Web site: http://fujisawa.com.

Fulcrum Inc, *See* **Fulcrum Pub**

†Fulcrum Pub, *(Fulcrum Publishing; 0-912347; 1-55591; 1-56373),* 16100 Table Mountain Pkwy., Suite 300, Golden, CO 80403 (SAN 200-2825) Tel 303-277-1623; Fax: 303-279-7111; Toll Free Fax: 800-726-7112; Toll Free: 800-992-2908
E-mail: dianneh@fulcrum-books.com
Web site: http://www.fulcrum-books.com
Dist(s): **Continental Bk** *(Continental Bk. Co., Inc.)*
Wolverine Distrib *(Wolverine Distributing, Inc.); CIP.*

Full of Life, *(Full of Life Pubns.; 0-942501),* P.O. Box 31025, Sante Fe, NM 87594 (SAN 667-237X) Fax: 505-982-4011
E-mail: drluc@nets.com
Web site: http://www.LMhomespathy.com.

Fund Adv Sci, *(Fund for the Advancement of Science & Mathematics Education in North Carolina; 0-9631387),* 1219 Broad St., Durham, NC 27705 Tel 919-286-3366; Fax: 919-286-5960
E-mail: liles@academic.ncssm.edu
Web site: http://www.infoserver.ncssm.edu.

Funmakers, *(Funmakers, Ltd.; 0-9634399),* P.O. Box 1560, Dearborn, MI 48121 Tel 313-438-3337.

Fut Educ, *See* **Fut Horizons**

Fut Horizons, *(Future Horizons, Inc.; 1-885477),* 721 W. Abram St., Arlington, TX 76013-6995 Tel 817-277-0727; Fax: 817-277-2270; Toll Free: 800-489-0727
E-mail: info@futurehorizons-autism.com; edfuture@onramp.net
Web site: http://www.FutureHorizons-autism.com.

Futa Bk Pubs, *(Futa Bk. Pubs.; 0-9654416),* 233 S. Wacker Dr., Box 91, Chicago, IL 60606 Tel 312-993-0430; Fax: 312-993-9140
E-mail: ojmoses@earthlink.net
Dist(s): **MyoData** *(MyoData).*

Futura Media Imprint of Futura Pub

†Futura Pub, *(Futura Publishing Co., Inc.; 0-87993),* 135 Bedford Rd., Armonk, NY 10504-0418 (SAN 201-582X) Tel 914-273-1014; Fax: 914-273-1015; Toll Free: 800-877-8761; P.O. Box 418, Armonk, NY 10504-0418 ; *Imprints:* Futura Media (Futura Media Services, Incorporated)
E-mail: kecheverria@futuraco.com
Web site: http://www.futuraco.com
Dist(s): **J Majors Co** *(Majors, J. A. Co.)*
Matthews Bk Co *(Matthews Bk. Co.)*
NA Blackwell *(Blackwell North America)*
Rittenhouse *(Rittenhouse Bk. Distributors); CIP.*

Future Amer Pubng, *See* **Who You Are**

Future Md Pub, *See* **AlternMed Bks**

Future of Freedom, *(Future of Freedom Foundation, The; 0-9640447; 1-890687),* 11350 Random Hills Rd., Suite 800, Fairfax, VA 22030 Tel 703-934-6101; Fax: 703-352-8678
E-mail: info@fff.org; fffva@compuserve.com
Web site: http://www.fff.org.

Futuro Ohio, *(Futuro Co., The; 0-9617392),* Subs. of The Kendall Co., 5801 Mariemont Ave., Cincinnati, OH 45227 (SAN 663-6101) Tel 513-271-3400; Toll Free: 800-543-4452.

†FWEW, *(Four Walls Eight Windows; 0-941423; 1-56858),* 39 W. 14th St., No. 503, New York, NY 10011 (SAN 667-6103) Tel 212-206-8965; Fax: 212-206-8799; Toll Free: 800-788-3123 (orders)
E-mail: edit@4w8w.com
Web site: http://www.4w8w.com
Dist(s): **Publishers Group** *(Publishers Group West); CIP.*

G & B Science Imprint of Gordon & Breach

G & R Pub, *(G&R Publishing; 1-56383),* Orders Addr.: 507 Industrial St., Waverly, IA 50677 Tel 319-352-5391; Fax: 319-352-5338; Toll Free Fax: 800-886-7496; Toll Free: 800-383-1679
E-mail: gandr@gandrpublishing.com; gifts@cqproducts.com
Web site: http://www.gandrpublishing.com; http://www.cqproducts.com
Dist(s): **CQ Products** *(CQ Products).*

G Agell, *(Agell, Gun; 0-9640299),* Orders Addr.: P.O. Box 1090, Eatonville, WA 98328 Fax: 360-832-6606; Edit Addr.: 38209 62nd Ave. E., Eatonville, WA 98328 Tel 360-832-4404
Dist(s): **Baker & Taylor** *(Baker & Taylor Bks.)*
Bookpeople *(Bookpeople)*
New Concepts Bks & Tapes *(New Concepts Bks. & Tapes Distributors)*
New Leaf Dist *(New Leaf Distributing Co., Inc.)*
Nutri-Books Corp *(Nutri-Bks. Corp.)*
Unique Bks Inc *(Unique Bks., Inc.).*

G B Magruder, *(Magruder, G. Brock; 0-9622095),* 1911 N. Mills Ave., Orlando, FL 32803-1432 Tel 407-843-5191.

G Brummel Pub, *(Brummel Publishing Co.; 0-9613041),* Orders Addr.: P.O. Box 198, Jamaica, NY 11419 (SAN 295-3765) Tel 718-836-3639; Edit Addr.: 116-10 103rd Ave., Richmond Hill, NY 11419 (SAN 295-3773) Tel 718-835-1155.

G Burton, *(Burton, Gail; 0-9703256),* P.O. Box 25283, Woodbury, MN 55125 Tel 651-501-3807
E-mail: gburton@candidafix.com
Web site: http://www.candidafix.com.

G E M, *(GEM/McCuen Pubns., Inc.; 0-86596),* 411 Mallalieu Dr., Hudson, WI 54016-1395 (SAN 691-909X) Tel 715-386-7113 (phone/fax); Toll Free: 800-290-6128
E-mail: gem@spacestar.net
Web site: http://www.spacestar.com/users/gem.

G E Sella, *(Sella, Gabriel E.; 1-884325),* 92 N. Fourth St., Suite 12, Martins Ferry, OH 43935 Tel 740-633-4485; Fax: 740-633-4141
E-mail: paris10@aol.com
Web site: http://www.gesellamd.com.

G Eby Research, *(Eby, George Research, Inc.; 0-9638967),* P.O. Box 91508, Austin, TX 78709-1506.

G Handwerk, *(Handwerk, Gordon Pubs.; 0-940524),* P.O. Box 685, Madison, NJ 07940 (SAN 217-1791) Tel 973-377-8232.

G J Shugar, *(Shugar, Gershon J.; 1-891671),* 140 Hepburn Rd., No. 15M, Clifton, NJ 07012 (SAN 299-6065) Tel 973-778-0089; Fax: 973-779-4098.

G Johnson, *(Johnson Jr., George; 0-9649826),* 217 Mill Race Dr., Chapel Hill, NC 27514-3130 Tel 919-966-3391; Fax: 919-966-2898.

G Kurasz, *(Kurasz, Grace; 0-9628432),* 2011 St. George Ave., Rahway, NJ 07065 Tel 732-574-0385.

G L B, *See* **GLB Worldwide**

G Landry, *(Landry, Greg M.S.; 0-929363),* 2805 Newkirk Ave., Wilmington, NC 28412-6527
E-mail: Greg@Landry.com.

G M Worthington, *(Worthington, George Marshall; 0-9623474),* 1343 Bullock Ln., Houston, TX 77055-4103.

G Miller, *(Miller, Gordon; 0-9659594),* 2001 Commercial St., SE, Salem, OR 97302 Tel 503-363-1500.

G O Wuzor, *(Wuzor, Geoffrey O.; 0-9647631),* Orders Addr.: P.O. Box 56693, Washington, DC 20040 Tel 202-462-5063; Fax: 202-462-2646; Edit Addr.: 2833 Georgia Ave. NW, No. 205, Washington, DC 20001.

Publisher Symbol Index

G Ohsawa, *(Ohsawa, George Macrobiotic Foundation; 0-918860),* P.O. Box 3998, Chico, CA 95927-3998 (SAN 207-7663) Tel 530-533-7702; Fax: 530-533-7908
E-mail: foundation@gomf.macrobiotic.net
Web site: http://www.gomf.macrobiotic.net
Dist(s): **New Leaf Dist** *(New Leaf Distributing Co., Inc.)*
Nutri-Books Corp *(Nutri-Bks. Corp.).*

G Olms Pubs, *(Olms, Georg Pubs.; 3-487),* Orders Addr.: 18 E. Main St., Port Jervis, NY 12771 Tel 845-856-5990 (phone/fax); Edit Addr.: Empire State Bldg., Suite 3304, 350 Fifth Ave., New York, NY 10118-0069 Toll Free: 800-920-9334
E-mail: olms@georg-olms.hi.eunet.de
Dist(s): **Lubrecht & Cramer** *(Lubrecht & Cramer, Ltd.)*
Trafalgar *(Trafalgar Square).*

G Stone Servs, *(Stone, Gary Services; 0-930427),* R.R. 1, Box 61-A, Savoy, TX 75479-9707 (SAN 670-9931) Tel 903-965-7724
E-mail: gstone@airmail.net.

G Thieme (DEU) *(3-13; 3-89373) Dist. by* **Thieme Med Pubs.**

Gabriel Rose, *(Gabriel Rose Pr., Inc.; 0-9649301),* 7221 Aloma Ave., Suite 500, Winter Park, FL 32792-7137 Tel 407-539-2849; 9045 Lake Hope Dr., Maitland, FL 32751.

Galahad Bks, *(Galahad Bks.; 0-88365; 1-57866),* Div. of BBS Publishing Corp., 386 Park Ave. S., Suite 1200, New York, NY 10016 Tel 212-679-4200; Fax: 212-679-4234.

Galaxy IN, *(Galaxy Pr.; 0-9654901),* P.O. Box 58, Hammond, IN 46325 Tel 312-646-5001 Do not confuse with Galaxy Pr. in Hollywood, CA or Saint Albans, WV
Dist(s): **Distributors** *(Distributors, The).*

Galde Pr, *(Galde Pr., Inc.; 1-880090; 1-931942),* Orders Addr.: P.O. Box 460, Lakeville, MN 55044-460 Tel 952-891-5991; Fax: 952-891-6091; Toll Free: 800-777-3454 (orders only)
E-mail: pgalde@galdepress.com
Web site: http://www.galdepress.com.

†**Gale,** *(Gale Group; 0-13; 0-7876; 0-8103; 0-936474; 1-57302; 1-878623),* Subs. of The Thomson Corp., Orders Addr.: P.O. Box 9187, Farmington Hills, MI 48333-9187 Toll Free Fax: 800-414-5043; Toll Free: 800-877-4253; Edit Addr.: 27500 Drake Rd., Farmington Hills, MI 48331-3535 (SAN 213-4373) Tel 248-699-4253 ; *Imprints:* UXL (UXL) Macmillan Ref (Macmillan Reference USA) C Scribners Sons (Charles Scribner's Sons) Saint James (Saint James Press) Thorndike (Thorndike Press) Blackbirch Pr (Blackbirch Press, Incorporated) Lucent Books (Lucent Books) Greenhaven Pr (Greenhaven Press, Incorporated) PSM (Primary Source Microfilm)
E-mail: galeord@galegroup.com
Web site: http://www.galegroup.com; *CIP.*

Gale Pubng, *(Gale Publishing; 0-9675896),* Div. of Neely Enterprises, 8939 Jewella Ave., No. 108-138, Shreveport, LA 71118 Tel 318-868-4298; Fax: 318-868-4631
E-mail: webmaster@galepublishing.com
Web site: http://galepublishing.com.

Galen AZ, *(Galen Pr., Ltd.; 1-883620),* Orders Addr.: P.O. Box 64400, Tucson, AZ 85728-4400 (SAN 254-1823) Tel 520-577-8363; Fax: 520-529-6459; Toll Free: 800-442-5369 (orders only) Do not confuse with Galen Pr. in Madison, NJ
E-mail: sales@galenpress.com; info@galenpress.com
Web site: http://www.galenpress.com
Dist(s): **Baker & Taylor** *(Baker & Taylor Bks.)*
J Majors Co *(Majors, J. A. Co.)*
Matthews Medical Bk Co *(Matthews Medical Bk. Co.)*
Rittenhouse *(Rittenhouse Bk. Distributors).*

Galen Pr DC Imprint of Lkng Glass Pubns

†**Gallaudet Univ Pr,** *(Gallaudet Univ. Pr.; 0-913580; 0-930323; 1-56368),* 800 Florida Ave., NE, Washington, DC 20002-3695 (SAN 205-261X) Tel 202-651-5488; Fax: 202-651-5489; Toll Free Fax: 800-621-8476; Toll Free: 888-630-9347 (TTY) ; *Imprints:* Clerc Bks (Clerc Books)
E-mail: david.gunton@gallaudet.edu
Web site: http://www.gupress.gallaudet.edu
Dist(s): **Chicago Distribution Ctr** *(Chicago Distribution Ctr.)*
U Ch Pr *(Univ. of Chicago Pr.); CIP.*

Gallopade Intl, *(Gallopade International; 0-635; 0-7933; 0-935326; 1-55609),* 665 Highway 74 South Suite 600, Peachtree City, GA 30269 (SAN 213-8441) Tel 770-631-4222; Toll Free Fax: 800-871-2979; Toll Free: 800-536-2438
E-mail: info@gallopade.com
Web site: http://www.gallopade.com.

Gallopade Pub Group, *See* **Gallopade Intl**

Gamala Pub Co, *(Gamala Publishing Co.; 0-9626952),* Orders Addr.: P.O. Box 740971, Houston, TX 77274 Fax: 713-496-4022; Edit Addr.: 1001 S. Dairy-Ashford, Suite 206, Houston, TX 77077 Tel 713-496-0188.

Gannel Pubns, *(Gannel Pubns.; 0-9626382),* 4740 Bradley Blvd., Chevy Chase, MD 20815 Tel 301-654-1064.

Garant Uitgevers (BEL) *(90-5350) Dist. by* **Gaunt.**

†**Gardner Pr,** *(Gardner Pr., Inc.; 0-89876),* Box 32266, Palm Beach Gardens, FL 33420-2266 (SAN 214-1906) Fax: 561-627-6191 Do not confuse with Gardner Pr., Klamath Falls, OR*; CIP.*

Gargoyle Pub, *(Gargoyle Pubs.; 0-9644983),* P.O. Box 472530, San Francisco, CA 94147 Tel 415-921-6888
E-mail: lapinpsy@sirius.com
Web site: http://wwwsirius.com/~lapinpsy.

Garkakee, *(Garkakee Pr.; 0-9636536),* 1315 Brookside Dr., No. D2, Hurst, TX 76053-3942.

†**Garland,** *(Garland Publishing, Inc.; 0-8153; 0-8240),* Member of Taylor & Francis, Inc., 29 W. 35th St., Flr. 10, New York, NY 10001-2299 Tel 212-216-7800; Fax: 212-564-7854; Toll Free: 800-627-6273 (orders)
E-mail: info@garland.com
Web site: http://www.garlandscience.com; http://www.garlandpub.com
Dist(s): **Taylor & Francis** *(Taylor & Francis, Inc.)*
netLibrary CO *(netLibrary, Inc.); CIP.*

Garland Pub, *See* **Garland**

Garrett FL, *(Garrett Publishing, Inc.; 1-880539),* 384 S. Military Trail, Deerfield Beach, FL 33442-3007 Tel 954-480-8543; Fax: 954-698-0057; Toll Free: 800-333-2069 Do not confuse with companies with the same name in Fair Oaks, CA, Lockhart, TX, Granada Hills, CA
E-mail: Barbara@garrettpub.com
Web site: http://www.garrettpub.com
Dist(s): **Baker & Taylor** *(Baker & Taylor Bks.)*
Made E-Z *(Made E-Z Products, Inc.).*

Garson Associates, *(Garson Assocs.; 0-9614591),* 172 Babylon Tpke., Merrick, NY 11566 (SAN 691-7763) Tel 516-868-9833.

Gateways Bks & Tapes, *(Gateways Bks. & Tapes; 0-89556),* Div. of Institute for the Development of the Harmonious Human Being, Inc., P.O. Box 370, Nevada City, CA 95959 (SAN 211-3635) Tel 530-272-0180; Fax: 530-272-0184; Toll Free: 800-869-0658
E-mail: orders@gatewaysbooksandtapes.com; info@gatewaysbooksandtapes.com
Web site: http://www.gatewaysbooksandtapes.com.

Gatewood Pr, *(Gatewood Pr.; 0-9639027),* 17140 Kinnear Rd., NE, Bainbridge Island, WA 98110-3021 Tel 914-246-1361; Fax: 914-246-1378
Dist(s): **Taylor & Taylor** *(Baker & Taylor Bks.).*

†**Gaunt,** *(Gaunt, Inc.; 0-912004; 1-56169),* 3011 Gulf Dr., Holmes Beach, FL 34217-2199 (SAN 202-9413) Tel 941-778-5211; Fax: 941-778-5252; Toll Free: 800-942-8683 (US & Canada)
E-mail: info@gaunt.com; sales@gaunt.com
Web site: http://www.gaunt.com*; CIP.*

Gavilan Hills, *(Gavilan Hills Publishing; 0-9631117),* 17305 Santa Rosa Mine Rd., Perris, CA 92370 Tel 909-943-1658; Fax: 909-657-3998.

†**Gay Sunshine,** *(Gay Sunshine Pr., Inc.; 0-917342; 0-940567),* P.O. Box 410690, San Francisco, CA 94141 (SAN 208-0915) Tel 415-626-1935; Fax: 415-626-1802
Web site: http://www.gaysunshine.com
Dist(s): **Bookazine Co Inc** *(Bookazine Co., Inc.)*
Bookpeople *(Bookpeople)*
Koen Bk Distributors *(Koen Bk. Distributors); CIP.*

Gazette Intl, *(Gazette International Networking Institute; 0-931301),* 4207 Lindell Blvd., No. 110, Saint Louis, MO 63108-2915 (SAN 683-2539) Tel 314-534-0475; Fax: 314-534-5070
E-mail: gini_intl@msw.com.

GBSP (NLD) *(90-5699) Dist. by* **Gordon & Breach.**

GDS Communs, *(GDS Communications; 0-9638425),* 2380 Riverdale Dr., N., Miramar, FL 33625 Tel 954-431-2566; Fax: 954-431-5445.

Gearhart-Edwards, *(Gearhart-Edwards Pr.; 0-936400),* 2917 N. Summit Ave., Milwaukee, WI 53211 (SAN 214-0217) Tel 414-962-9580.

Gebruder Borntraeger (DEU) *(3-443) Dist. by* **Balogh.**

Gefen Bks, *(Gefen Bks.; 0-86343; 965-229),* 12 New St., Hewlett, NY 11557-2012 Tel 516-295-2805; Fax: 516-295-2739; Toll Free: 800-477-5257
E-mail: gefenbooks@compuserve.com
Web site: http://www.israelbooks.com.

Gefen Pub Hse (ISR) *(965-229) Dist. by* **Gefen Bks.**

Geist & Russell, *(Geist & Russell Cos., Ltd.; 1-884228),* 833 N. Johnson St., Iowa City, IA 52245 Tel 319-337-4874; Toll Free: 800-581-2724 (phone/fax)
E-mail: cholly@inav.net
Web site: http://www.geistbooks.com.

Gemin-Ideas Pr, *(Gemin-Ideas Pr.; 0-9625347),* 5400 Friedrich Ln., No. 77, Austin, TX 78744-2751 Tel 512-447-0459.

Gems Pubng, *(Gems Publishing USA; 0-9651544),* 12 Walnut St., Framingham, MA 01701 Tel 508-872-0066; Fax: 508-872-0020; Toll Free: 888-880-4367
E-mail: orent@1000gems.com
Web site: http://www.1000gems.com.

Gen Hall, *(General Hall, Inc.; 0-930390; 1-882289),* 5 Talon Way, Dix Hills, NY 11746 (SAN 211-1306) Tel 631-243-0155; Fax: 631-254-3894.

Gen Welfare Pubns, *(General Welfare Pubns.; 0-87312),* 3571 Sudberry Rd., Camberon Park, CA 95682 (SAN 240-4753) Tel 916-677-1610.

Genassist, *(Genassist, Inc.; 0-9644243),* Div. of H. S. Wexler & Assocs., 8101 E. Belleview Ave., Suite J, Bldg. 3, Denver, CO 80237 Tel 303-694-4665; Fax: 303-694-3473; Toll Free: 800-359-9412.

Gene Therapy, *(Gene Therapy Pr.; 1-892245),* 249 Matadero Ave., Palo Alto, CA 94306 Tel 650-813-9264; Fax: 650-424-9594
E-mail: boulikas@worldnet.att.net
Dist(s): **Majors Scientific Bks Inc** *(Majors Scientific Bks., Inc.).*

General Distrib Services, *(General Distribution Services, Inc.),* 4500 Witmer Industrial, E., Niagara Falls, NY 14305-1386 (SAN 630-7949) Toll Free Fax: 800-481-6207; Toll Free: 800-805-1083
E-mail: cservice@genpub.com
Web site: http://genpub.com.

Generic Human Studies, *(Generic Human Studies Publishing; 0-942055),* P.O. Box 6535, Malibu, CA 90265 (SAN 666-3753).

Genesis Comns, *(Genesis Communications, L L C; 0-945704),* 1200 Riverside Dr., Tuscaloosa, AL 35401-1139 (SAN 247-7580)
E-mail: 74561.3705@compuserve.com.

Genesis Pub PA, *(Genesis Publishing Co.; 0-940967),* 663 Exton Commons, Exton, PA 19341-2446 (SAN 664-7812) Tel 610-648-0876 Do not confuse with companies with the same name in La Mesa, CA, Bedford, MA, North Andover, MA.

Genetics Heritage, *(Genetics Heritage Pr.; 0-9653362),* 02 Sunrise Dr., Placitas, NM 87043 Tel 505-867-1712
E-mail: mgbooks@flash.net.

Genium Pub, *(Genium Publishing Corp.; 0-931690; 1-890911),* 1171 Riverfront Ctr., Amsterdam, NY 12010-4600 (SAN 213-5027) Tel 518-842-1843; Fax: 518-842-4111; Toll Free: 800-243-6486
E-mail: sales@genium.com; genium@genium.com
Web site: http://www.genium.com
Dist(s): **AOAC Intl** *(AOAC International).*

Genl Dist Srvs, *See* **General Distrib Services**

†**Genl Med Pub,** *(General Medical Pubs.; 0-935236),* P.O. Box 210, Venice, CA 90294-0210 (SAN 215-689X) Tel 310-392-4911*; CIP.*

Genmark DC, *(Genmark; 0-9664774),* P.O. Box 23931, Washington, DC 20026-3931 Tel 301-680-0876 (phone/fax) Do not confuse with Genmark, Martinez, CA.

†**Genotype,** *(Genotype; 0-936618),* 15042 Montebello Rd., Cupertino, CA 95014 (SAN 214-3089)*; CIP.*

Geo U Kennedy Inst, *(Georgetown Univ., Kennedy Institute of Ethics; 0-9614448; 1-883913),* P.O. Box 571212, Washington, DC 20057-1212 (SAN 689-3775) Tel 202-687-8099; 202-687-8089; 202-687-3885; Fax: 202-687-6770; Toll Free: 800-633-3849
E-mail: kicoures@georgetown.edu; medethx@gunet.georgetown.edu
Web site: http://bioethics.georgetown.edu.

Geocom Ltd, *(Geocom, Ltd.; 0-945669),* 160 Washington, SE, No. 233, Albuquerque, NM 87108 (SAN 247-4824) Tel 505-268-2042.

Georgetown U Med, *(Georgetown Univ. Medical Ctr.; 0-9652807),* Dept. of Medicine, 5 PHC, 3800 Reservoir Rd., NW, Washington, DC 20007-2197 Tel 202-687-8646; Fax: 202-687-7797.

†**Georgetown U Pr,** *(Georgetown Univ. Pr.; 0-87840; 1-58901),* Orders Addr.: P.O. Box 50370, Baltimore, MD 21211-4370 Tel 410-516-6995; Fax: 410-516-6998; Toll Free: 800-246-9606 (orders); Edit Addr.: 3700 O St., NW, Washington, DC 20007 (SAN 203-4247) Tel 202-687-5889; Fax: 202-687-6340
E-mail: gupress@gusun.georgetown.edu
Web site: http://www.georgetown.edu/publications/gup/; *CIP.*

Georgian Intl, *(Georgian International, Ltd., Inc.; 0-9611392),* 3300 Oakland Park Blvd., E., Fort Lauderdale, FL 33308-7217 (SAN 662-2054).

Geri-Active, *(Geri-Active Consultants; 0-9621846),* 8920 Crest Oak Ln., Saint Louis, MO 63126-1915; 9426 Crockett Dr., Saint Louis, MO 63132 Tel 314-768-5615
Dist(s): **Act Prod Intl** *(Activity Products International).*

Geri-Rehab, *(Geri-Rehab, Inc.; 0-941930),* 170 Hibbler Rd., Lebanon, NJ 08833 (SAN 239-4383) Tel 973-735-8918.

Geronima, *(Geronima Pr.; 0-943164),* P.O. Box 224, Audubon, IA 50025-0224 (SAN 240-7191) Tel 712-563-3799 (phone/fax)
E-mail: electtype@aol.com.

Gestalt Journal, *(Gestalt Journal Pr.; 0-939266),* P.O. Box 990, Highland, NY 12528-0990 (SAN 216-5317) Tel 845-691-7192; Fax: 775-599-3950 (Prefered order method)
E-mail: tgjournal@gestalt.org
Web site: http://www.gestalt.org.

Get Well Fnd, *(Get Well Foundation; 0-9638285),* 8001 Capwell Dr., Oakland, CA 94621 Tel 510-635-9778; Fax: 510-639-9140
Web site: http://www.pma-online.org/list/6159.cfm.

G&G Pub, *(G&G Publishing; 0-9660563),* 3 Westridge Dr., Hampton, NH 03842 Tel 603-929-0219; Fax: 603-433-6992
Dist(s): **Bryant Altman** *(Bryant Altman Map, Inc.).*

Gibbs Assocs, *(Gibbs Assocs.; 0-943909),* P.O. Box 706, Boulder, CO 80306-0706 (SAN 242-6668) Tel 303-444-6032 (phone/fax)
E-mail: bgibb@csn.org
Web site: http://www.csn.net/~bgibbs.

†Gibbs Smith Pub, *(Smith, Gibbs Pub.; 0-87905; 1-58685; 0-9676662),* Orders Addr.: P.O. Box 667, Layton, UT 84041 (SAN 201-9906) Tel 801-544-9800; Fax: 801-544-5582; Toll Free Fax: 800-213-3023 (orders); Toll Free: 800-748-5439 (orders); Edit Addr.: 1877 E. Gentile St., Layton, UT 84040
E-mail: info@gibbs-smith.com; text@gibbs-smith.com
Web site: http://www.gibbs-smith.com
Dist(s): **Wolverine Distrib** *(Wolverine Distributing, Inc.)*
Wrldwide Media Srv *(Worldwide Media Service, Inc.); CIP.*

Gibson, *(Gibson, C. R. Co.; 0-7667; 0-8378; 0-937970; 0-7053),* Div. of Thomas Nelson, Inc., Orders Addr.: P.O. Box 14100, Nashville, TN 37214; Edit Addr.: 501 Nelson Place, Nashville, TN 37214 Tel 615-889-9000; Fax: 615-885-3863; Toll Free: 800-251-4000
E-mail: customerservice@crgibson.com
Web site: http://www.crgibson.com/.

Giddings Studio Pub, *(Giddings Studio Publishing; 0-9615226; 1-889326),* 5913 Greenridge Cir., Fort Collins, CO 80525 (SAN 695-1406) Tel 970-226-8587; Fax: 970-204-0543
E-mail: fdgid@colostate.edu.

Gieben (NLD) *(90-5063; 90-70265) Dist. by* **J Benjamins Pubng Co.**

Gifted Educ Pr, *(Gifted Education Pr.; 0-910609),* Orders Addr.: P.O. Box 1586, Manassas, VA 20108; Edit Addr.: 10201 Yuma Ct., Manassas, VA 20109 (SAN 694-132X) Tel 703-369-5017; Toll Free: 800-484-1406 (code 6857)
E-mail: mfisher345@home.com; mdfish@cais.com
Web site: http://GIFTEDEDPRESS.COM.

Gifted Psych Pr, *See* **Great Potential Pr**

GIFTGO, *(GIFTGO; 0-9660543),* Orders Addr.: P.O. Box 5429, Santa Barbara, CA 93109 Tel 805-569-2729; Edit Addr.: 3101 Las Gaviotas Dr., Santa Barbara, CA 93109.

Gila River, *(Gila River Designs; 0-89741),* Div. of Desert Laboratories, Inc., P.O. Box 124, Oracle, AZ 85623 (SAN 204-2169) Tel 520-896-2395.

Gilgal Pubns, *(Gilgal Pubns.; 0-916895),* P.O. Box 3399, Sunriver, OR 97707 (SAN 655-8801) Tel 541-593-8418; Fax: 541-593-5604.

Gillman-Marcuse, *(Gillman-Marcuse, Inc.; 0-9620349),* 1518 Walnut St., Suite 1401, Philadelphia, PA 19102 (SAN 248-2908) Tel 215-732-2020.

Ginn Pr, *See* **Pearson Custom**

Girl Scouts USA, *(Girl Scouts of the USA; 0-88441),* 420 Fifth Ave., New York, NY 10018 (SAN 203-4611) Tel 212-852-8000; Fax: 212-852-6511
Web site: http://www.gsusa.org/.

Glacier Publng, *(Glacier Publishing; 0-9650315),* 40 Oak St., Southington, CT 06489 Tel 860-621-7644; Fax: 860-585-9283
Dist(s): **Bookazine Co Inc** *(Bookazine Co., Inc.).*

Glad Pubn, *(Glad Pubn.; 0-9629091),* 966 Palmwood Dr., Sparks, NV 89434 Tel 702-356-7856.

Glass Pub Co, *(Glass Publishing Co.; 0-9614759),* 106 Wickford Way St., San Antonio, TX 78213-2640 (SAN 676-5947).

GLB Worldwide, *(GLB Worldwide; 1-889823),* P.O. Box 6495, Kaneohe, HI 96744 Tel 808-239-1579; Toll Free Fax: 888-326-3701; Toll Free: 800-224-3701
E-mail: glb@glbworld.com
Web site: http://www.glbworld.com.

Gldn Gate Pub, *(Golden Gate Publishing; 0-9636736),* P.O. Box 2043, Saratoga, CA 95070 (SAN 298-1548) Tel 408-741-0622; Fax: 408-741-0492.

Gldn Quill NV, *(Golden Quill Publishing; 0-9646913),* P.O. Box 275, Gardnerville, NV 89410 Tel 702-265-2904; Fax: 702-265-7587 Do not confuse with Golden Quill Publishing,San Diego, CA.

Gldn Temple, *See* **KRI**

Gleisners Bk, *See* **WFP**

Glenbridge Pub, *(Glenbridge Publishing, Ltd.; 0-944435),* 19923 E. Long Ave., Aurora, CO 80016 (SAN 243-5403) Tel 720-870-8381; Fax: 720-870-5598; Toll Free: 800-986-4135 (orders only)
E-mail: glenbr@eazy.net
Web site: http://www.glenbridgepublishing.com
Dist(s): **Baker & Taylor** *(Baker & Taylor Bks.).*

†Glencoe, *(Glencoe/McGraw-Hill; 0-02; 0-07),* Div. of The McGraw-Hill Cos., 8787 Orion Pl., Columbus, OH 43240-4027
Web site: http://www.glencoe.com; *CIP.*

Glendon Assn, *(Glendon Assn; 0-9676684),* 5383 Hollister Ave., Suite 230, Santa Barbara, CA 93111 Tel 805-681-0415; Fax: 805-681-0425; Toll Free: 800-663-5281
E-mail: glendon@glendon.org
Web site: http://www.glendon.org.

Glendor Bks, *(Glendor Bks.; 0-9626143),* 115 Clover Dr., Monaca, PA 15061-2611 Tel 650-266-6413; 291 Sixth St., Ambridge, PA 15003 Tel 415-266-6413.

Global Bks (GBR) *(1-86034) Dist. by* **Midpt Trade.**

Global Comm Netwk, *(Global Communication Network, Inc.; 0-9632313),* 12100 187th Ave., Bristol, WI 53104-9229.

Global Environ, *(Global Environment Facility; 1-884122),* 1818 H St. NW, Rm. G6146, Washington, DC 20433 Tel 202-473-0508; Fax: 202-522-3240
Web site: http://www.gefweb.org
Dist(s): **World Bank** *(World Bank, The, Office of the Publisher).*

Global Eyes, *(Global Eyes International Pr.; 0-9662973),* 343 Soquel Ave., No. 92, Santa Cruz, CA 95062 Fax: 408-459-7732.

Global Hlth, *(Global Health Solutions, Inc.; 0-9629942),* 8472A Tyco Rd., Vienna, VA 22182 Tel 703-848-2333; Fax: 703-848-0028; Toll Free: 800-759-3999
E-mail: info@watercure.com; shipping@watercure,com
Web site: http://www.watercure.org; http://www.watercure.com
Dist(s): **Baker & Taylor** *(Baker & Taylor Bks.)*
Bookpeople *(Bookpeople)*
New Leaf Dist *(New Leaf Distributing Co., Inc.)*
Nutri-Books Corp *(Nutri-Bks. Corp.).*

Global MI, *(Global Publishing; 0-9649707),* P.O. Box 1210, Birmingham, MI 48012-1210 Tel 248-443-2222 Do not confuse with Global Publishing, Decatur, GA.

Global Pub NJ, *(Global Publishing Co., Inc.; 0-9625118; 1-879771),* Div. of World Scientific Publishing Co., 1060 Main St., River Edge, NJ 07661 Tel 201-837-8858; Fax: 201-837-8859; Toll Free: 800-227-7562 Do not confuse with companies of the same name in Los Angeles, CA, Scottsdale, AZ, Eugene, OR, Costa Mesa, CA, Sauk Rapids, MN.

Global Pubns, *(Global Pubns. (SSIPS); 0-9633277; 1-883058; 1-58684),* Institute of Global Cultural Studies, Binghamton Univ., Binghamton, NY 13902-6000 Tel 607-777-6104; 607-777-4495; Fax: 607-777-2642; 607-777-6132 ; *Imprints:* Dowling College (Dowling College Press)
E-mail: skafrawi@binghamton.edu
Web site: http://www.globalpublicationspress.com
Dist(s): **Hesteria Recs** *(Hesteria Records & Publishing Co.).*

Global Twnty-One Fnd, *See* **Sharif Ent**

Global Vil CA, *(Global Village Pr.; 0-9632977),* 2118 Wilshire Blvd., No. 262, Santa Monica, CA 90403-5784 (SAN 297-6692) Tel 310-204-4018 Do not confuse with Global Village Pr., Huntington, NY.

Global Village, *(Global Village Publishing; 0-9623434),* 10601-A Tierrasanta Blvd., Suite 336, San Diego, CA 92124 (SAN 200-3376) Tel 619-279-1515.

Globe Fearon, *(Globe Fearon Educational Publishing; 0-13; 0-8224; 0-8359; 0-87065; 0-88102; 0-912925; 0-915510; 1-55555; 1-55675),* Div. of Pearson Education Corporate Communications, Orders Addr.: 4350 Equity Dr., P.O. Box 2649, Columbus, OH 43216-2649 Toll Free Fax: 800-393-3156; Toll Free: 800-321-3106 (customer service); 800-848-9500; Edit Addr.: One Lake St., Upper Saddle River, NJ 07458
Web site: http://www.globefearon.com/
Dist(s): **Cambridge Bk** *(Cambridge Bk. Co.)*
IFSTA *(IFSTA).*

†Globe Pequot, *(Globe Pequot Pr., The; 0-7627; 0-87106; 0-88742; 0-914788; 0-933469; 0-934802; 1-56440; 1-57034),* Div. of Morris Communications Corp., Orders Addr.: P.O. Box 480, Guilford, CT 06437-0480 (SAN 201-9892) Toll Free Fax: 800-820-2329 (in Connecticut); Toll Free: 800-243-0495 (24 hours); Edit Addr.: 246 Goose Ln., Guilford, CT 06437 Tel 203-458-4500; Fax: 203-458-4604 ; *Imprints:* Lyons (Lyons Press)
E-mail: info@globe-pequot.com; adessaint@globe-pequot.com
Web site: http://www.globe-pequot.com
Dist(s): **AMC Books** *(Appalachian Mountain Club Bks.); CIP.*

GlobeTekne Res, *See* **Eaglecliff**

Glovebox Guidebks, *(Glovebox Guidebooks of America, L.L.P.; 1-881139),* 1112 Washburn Pl., E., Saginaw, MI 48602-2997 Tel 989-792-8363 (phone/fax); Toll Free: 800-289-4843
E-mail: baileybill@aol.com
Dist(s): **Baker & Taylor** *(Baker & Taylor Bks.)*
Booksource *(Booksource, The)*
Borders Inc *(Borders, Inc.)*
Distributors *(Distributors, The)*
Koen Bk Distributors *(Koen Bk. Distributors)*
Partners Pubs Grp *(Partners Pubs. Group, Inc.).*

Gloyd Grp Inc, *(Gloyd Group, Inc.; 0-9678005),* 3 Penny Lane Ct., Willmington, DE 19803 Tel 302-761-9650; Fax: 302-761-9680
E-mail: drKGloyd@aol.com.

GN Comns, *See* **Real Est News**

†Godine, *(Godine, David R. Pub., Inc.; 0-87923; 1-56792),* Orders Addr.: P.O. Box 450, Jaffrey, NH 03452 Tel 603-532-4100; Fax: 603-532-5940; Toll Free Fax: 800-226-0934; Toll Free: 800-344-4771; Edit Addr.: 9 Hamilton Pl., Boston, MA 02108 (SAN 213-4381) Tel 617-451-9600; Fax: 617-350-0250
E-mail: info@godine.com
Web site: http://www.godine.com
Dist(s): **B & T International** *(Baker & Taylor International); CIP.*

Golden Adult Imprint of St Martin

Golden Harp, *(Golden Harp; 0-9623165),* P.O. Box 1073, Mendocino, CA 95460-1073 Tel 707-964-6740 (phone/fax)
E-mail: goldharp@jps.net
Web site: http://www.net/goldharp/jharp/html
Dist(s): **Music Design Inc** *(Music Design, Inc.)*
New Leaf Dist *(New Leaf Distributing Co., Inc.).*

Golden Lght, *(Golden Light Pr.; 0-9640635),* Orders Addr.: P.O. Box 415, Englewood, OH 45322-0415; Edit Addr.: 2219 E. Rahn Rd., Kettering, OH 45440 Tel 937-434-7017 Do not confuse with Golden Light Pr., West Palm Beach, FL
E-mail: goldenlightpress3@juno.com; rxrwg6@juno.com.

Golden Meridian, *(Golden Meridian Pr.; 0-9657336),* 738 Monroe, River Forest, IL 60305 Tel 708-848-4651; Fax: 708-343-1335.

Golden Point Prod, *(Golden Point Productions; 0-9624716),* P.O. Box 685, Crestone, CO 81131-0685 Tel 719-256-4551 (phone/fax)
E-mail: rokryder@fone.net
Web site: http://www.creative-harmonics.org
Dist(s): **Bookpeople** *(Bookpeople)*
New Leaf Dist *(New Leaf Distributing Co., Inc.).*

Golden Psych, *(Golden Psych Pr.; 0-9645528),* c/o Weiss Psychologists, Ltd., 4202 N. 32nd St., Suite H, Phoenix, AZ 85018 Tel 602-954-6998.

Golden Sufi Ctr, *(Golden Sufi Ctr., The; 0-9634574; 1-890350),* Orders Addr.: P.O. Box 428, Inverness, CA 94937 Tel 415-663-8773; Fax: 415-663-9128
E-mail: goldensufi@aol.com
Web site: http://www.goldensufi.org
Dist(s): **Words Distrib** *(Words Distributing Co.).*

Golden Tri Org, *(Golden Triangle Organization, Inc., The; 0-9657889),* 4660 La Jolla Village Dr., No. 500, San Diego, CA 92122 Tel 619-535-4814; Fax: 619-535-4890; Toll Free: 888-225-4814
E-mail: dmiller@goldentriangle.com
Web site: http://www.goldentriangle.com/dmiller.

†Golden West Pub, *(Golden West Pubs.; 0-914846; 1-885590; 1-58581),* 4113 N. Longview Ave., Phoenix, AZ 85014-4949 (SAN 207-5652) Tel 602-265-4392; Fax: 602-279-6901; Toll Free: 800-658-5830 Do not confuse with Golden West Pubs. Unlimited, Fresno, CA
E-mail: goldwest1@mindspring.com
Web site: http://www.goldenwestpublishers.com; *CIP.*

Gomer Pr (GBR) *(0-85088; 0-86383; 1-85902) Dist. by* **St Mut.**

Gondolier, *(Gondolier Pr.; 0-935824),* P.O. Box 7586, Carmel, CA 93921 (SAN 214-0233) Tel 408-626-9080; Fax: 408-624-5126.

Good Commun Inc, *(Good Communications, Inc.; 0-937776),* P.O. Box 10069, Austin, TX 78766 (SAN 277-6804) Tel 512-454-6090; Fax: 512-454-3420; Toll Free: 800-968-1738
E-mail: help@gooddogmagazine.com
Web site: http://www.gooddogmagazine.com.

Good Ideas MI, *See* **Univ Scripts**

Good Sign NY, *(Good Sign; 0-9640929),* 3554 Carlisle Pl., Bronx, NY 10467-6017 Tel 718-519-7896.

Good Things, *See* **P A B Bks**

Good Year Imprint of Pearson Learn

Goodheart, ***(Goodheart-Willcox Pub., The; 0-87006; 1-56637; 1-59070),*** **18604 W. Creek Dr., Tinley Park, IL 60477 (SAN 203-4387) Tel 708-687-5000; Fax: 708-687-5068; Toll Free: 800-323-0440**
E-mail: custserv@goodheartwillcox.com
Web site: http://goodheartwillcox.com.

Goodlife CA, *See* **Select Bks CA**

†Gordian, *(Gordian Pr., Inc.; 0-87752),* P.O. Box 40304, Staten Island, NY 10304 (SAN 201-6389) Tel 718-273-4700 (phone & fax)
E-mail: roger4700@aol.com; *CIP.*

†Gordon & Breach, *(Gordon & Breach Publishing Group; 0-19; 0-677; 0-905203; 1-872501; 2-88124; 2-88449; 2-903928; 2-919875; 3-364; 3-7186; 90-5699; 90-5700; 90-5701; 90-5702; 90-5703; 90-5704; 90-5708; 976-641; 976-8097; 90-5755; 90-5706; 90-5707; 90-5709),* Div. of Taylor & Francis, Inc., Orders Addr.: 7625 Empire Dr., Florence, KY 41042 Toll Free Fax: 800-248-4724; Toll Free: 800-634-7064; Edit Addr.: 2 Gateway Ctr., Newark, NJ 07102-0301 (SAN 201-6370) Tel 973-643-7500; Fax: 973-643-7676; Toll Free: 800-545-8398 ; *Imprints:* Harwood Acad Pubs (Harwood Academic Publishers) Abacus (Abacus Press) G & B Science (Gordon & Breach Science Publishers)
E-mail: ncarter@taylorandfrances.com
Web site: http://www.gbhap.com; *CIP.*

Gordon Bks, *(Gordon Bks.; 0-9671605),* 567 Amber Ct., Livermore, CA 94550 Tel 925-443-6213
E-mail: dbgordon@ix.netcom.com.

†Gordon Pr, *(Gordon Pr. Pubs.; 0-8490; 0-87968),* P.O. Box 459, New York, NY 10004 (SAN 201-6362) Tel 212-969-8419; Fax: 718-624-8419; *CIP.*

Gordon Soules Bk, *(Soules, Gordon Bk. Pubs., Ltd.; 0-919574),* 1916 Pike Pl., Suite 620, Seattle, WA 98101 (SAN 208-2845) Tel 604-922-6588; Fax: 604-688-5442
E-mail: books@gordonsoules.com
Web site: http://www.gordonsoules.com.

Gospel Lght, *(Gospel Light Pubns.; 0-8307),* 2300 Knoll Dr., Ventura, CA 93003 (SAN 299-0873) Tel 805-644-9721; Fax: 805-289-0200; Toll Free: 800-446-7735 (orders only) Do not confuse with companies with similar names in Brooklyn, NY, Delight, AR
E-mail: info@gospellight.com; pamweston@gospellight.com
Web site: http://www.gospellight.com
Dist(s): **Christian Bk Distributors** *(Christian Bk. Distributors).*

Gosport Pubng, *(Gosport Publishing, Inc.; 0-9641170),* 7737 SW Freeway, Suite 780, Houston, TX 77074 Tel 713-988-5514; Fax: 713-988-9515.

Gov Insts, *(Government Institutes; 0-86587),* Div. of ABS Group, Inc., 4 Research Pl., Suite 200, Rockville, MD 20850-3226 (SAN 214-3801) Tel 301-921-2300 (General); 301-921-2323 (Customer Service); Fax: 301-921-0373 (General); 301-921-0264 (Customer Service)
E-mail: giinfo@govinst.com
Web site: http://www.govinst.com; http://www.governmentinstitutes.com.

Gower (GBR) *(0-566) Dist. by* **Ashgate Pub Co.**

GP Courseware, *(GP Courseware; 0-87683; 0-9663133),* 1347 W. Washington Blvd., No. 3C, Chicago, IL 60607 (SAN 294-0264) Tel 312-543-0974
E-mail: info@genphysics.com
Web site: http://generalphysics.com/courses/about.asp.

GP Pub, *See* **GP Courseware**

Gr Arts Ctr Pub, *(Graphic Arts Ctr. Publishing Co.; 0-88240; 0-912856; 0-932575; 1-55868),* Orders Addr.: P.O. Box 10306, Portland, OR 97296-0306 (SAN 201-6338) Tel 503-226-2402; Fax: 503-223-1410 (executive & editorial); Toll Free Fax: 800-355-9685 (sales office); Toll Free: 800-452-3032 ; *Imprints:* Alaska NW Bks (Alaska Northwest Books)
E-mail: sales@gacpc.com
Web site: http://www.gacpc.com.

Grace Ch-St Louis, *(Grace Church/Saint Louis; 0-933643),* 2695 Creve Coeur Mill Rd., Maryland Heights, MO 63043 (SAN 692-6495) Tel 314-291-6647; Fax: 314-291-0918.

Graceway, *(Graceway Publishing Co., Inc.; 0-932126),* P.O. Box 670159, Flushing, NY 11367-0159 Fax: 516-498-2029; Toll Free: 800-440-0499
E-mail: ibf@ibf.org
Web site: http://www.ibf.org.

Gracie Ent, *(Gracie Enterprises, Inc.; 0-9606398),* P.O. Box 506, Chula Vista, CA 92012 (SAN 226-7934) Tel 619-421-8055.

Grads of For Nursing, *(Commission on Graduates of Foreign Nursing Schls.; 0-9630592; 0-9715483),* 3600 Market St., Suite 400, Philadelphia, PA 19104-2651
Web site: http://www.cgfns.org.

Gran Farnum, *(Farnum, Gran Printing & Publishing, Inc.; 0-9649593),* 3401 Grand Ave., Glenwood Springs, CO 81601 Tel 970-945-9605; Fax: 970-945-7492.

Granite Pub, *(Granite Publishing, LLC; 0-926524; 0-9632310; 1-893183),* P.O. Box 1429, Columbus, NC 28722 Tel 828-894-3088; Fax: 828-894-8454; Toll Free: 800-366-0264 Do not confuse with companies with same or similar names in Madison, WI, Orem, UT
E-mail: brian@5thworld.com
Web site: http://www.5thworld.com
Dist(s): **Bookpeople** *(Bookpeople).*

Grant Hse Pr, *(Grant Hse. Pr.; 0-9625624),* Orders Addr.: P.O. Box 229, Geneva, IL 60134; Edit Addr.: 127 Hamilton St., Geneva, IL 60134 Tel 708-232-4994; Fax: 708-232-6001.

Grant-DeHoog, *(Grant/DeHoog Pub.; 0-9627678),* P.O. Box 75057, Seattle, WA 98125 Tel 425-548-4533; Fax: 425-885-2849.

Graphic Pub Williamsbrg, *(Graphic Publishing of Williamsburg; 0-9631949),* Div. of PrintShack & Datamat, 1315 Jamestown Rd., Suite 201, Williamsburg, VA 23185 Tel 757-229-6230; Fax: 757-229-7044.

Gratefuldeb, *(Gratefuldeb Publishing; 0-9663353),* Orders Addr.: P.O. Box 811, Waianae, HI 96792; Edit Addr.: 95-1064 Puneki St., Mililani, HI 96789
E-mail: gratefuldeb@worldnet.att.net.

Grayson Pub, *(Grayson Publishing; 1-890056),* Div. of STOUT Ventures, 22, 918 N. Woodcrest Ln., Kildeer, IL 60047-7844 Tel 847-550-0092; Fax: 847-550-0098; Toll Free: 800-656-3296
E-mail: Chris@StoutVentures.com
Web site: http://www.StoutVentures.com.

Graywind Pubns, *(Graywind Pubns., Inc.; 1-880659),* 555 Academic Ct., San Antonio, TX 78204-2455.

†Graywolf, *(Graywolf Pr.; 0-915308; 1-55597),* 2402 University Ave., Suite 203, Saint Paul, MN 55114 (SAN 207-1665) Tel 651-641-0077; Fax: 651-641-0036
E-mail: wolves@graywolfpress.org
Web site: http://www.graywolfpress.org
Dist(s): **Consort Bk Sales** *(Consortium Bk. Sales & Distribution)*
SPD-Small Pr Dist *(SPD-Small Pr. Distribution); CIP.*

Greasewood, *(Greasewood Pr.; 0-9649759; 0-9710267),* c/o Dept. of Pathology/350, Univ. of Nevada Schl. of Medicine, Reno, NV 89557 Tel 775-784-4068; Fax: 775-784-1636
E-mail: lmulvey@med.unr.edu
Web site: http://www.unr.edu/med/dept/pathology
Dist(s): **U of Nev Pr** *(Univ. of Nevada Pr.).*

Great Begin CA, *(Great Beginnings Bks.; 0-9708893),* 2515 Clement St., No. 1, San Francisco, CA 94121-1844 Tel 415-387-2764 (phone/fax)
E-mail: gregjirak@earthlink.net.

Great Comm Pubns, *(Great Commission Pubns.; 0-934688),* Subs. of Orthodox Presbyterian Church, Orders Addr.: P.O. Box P, Willow Grove, PA 19090-0920 (SAN 215-1502) Tel 215-956-0123; Toll Free: 800-695-3387.

†Great Ocean, *(Great Ocean Pubs.; 0-915556),* 294 Lone Pine Rd., Marshall, NC 28701-9714 (SAN 207-527X) Tel 828-658-9877
E-mail: greatocean@mindspring.com
Dist(s): **Midpt Trade** *(Midpoint Trade Bks., Inc.); CIP.*

†Great Potential Pr, *(Great Potential Pr., Inc.; 0-910707),* P.O. Box 5057, Scottsdale, AZ 85261 (SAN 260-2385) Tel 602-954-4200; Fax: 602-954-0185
E-mail: info@greatpotentialpress.com; GiftedBook@earthlink.net
Web site: http://www.greatpotentialpress.com
Dist(s): **Baker & Taylor** *(Baker & Taylor Bks.)*
Bookmen Inc *(Bookmen, Inc.); CIP.*

Great Pyramid, *(Great Pyramid Pr.; 0-9605822),* 205 Simmons Pl., Augusta, GA 30904 (SAN 220-1704) Tel 770-860-9633.

†Green, *(Green, Warren H. Inc.; 0-87527),* 8356 Olive Blvd., Saint Louis, MO 63132 (SAN 201-4939) Tel 314-991-1335; Fax: 314-997-1788; Toll Free: 800-537-0655
E-mail: whgreen@inlink.com
Web site: http://www.whgreen.com; *CIP.*

Greenaire Pr, *(Greenaire Pr.; 0-9660267),* 3600 S. Harbor Blvd., No. 138, Oxnard, CA 93035 Tel 805-985-8832; Fax: 203-222-0171
E-mail: writebooks@aol.com.

Greene Pubns, *(Greene Pubns.; 0-9608892),* 2820 Midwick Dr., Alhambra, CA 91803 (SAN 241-1180) Tel 213-413-2150 Do not confuse with Greene Pubns., Inc. in Alahambra, CA.

Greenhaven Pr Imprint of Gale

Greenlawn Pr, *(Greenlawn Pr.; 0-937779),* Div. of LaSalle Co., Orders Addr.: 237 N. Michigan St., South Bend, IN 46601 Tel 219-234-6021; Fax: 219-289-3316; Toll Free: 800-348-2227; Edit Addr.: 107 S. Greenlawn Ave., South Bend, IN 46617 (SAN 659-2309) Tel 219-234-5088; Fax: 219-236-6633
Dist(s): **Riverside-World** *(Riverside World).*

Greenlf Bks, *(Greenleaf Bks.; 0-934676),* Greenleaf Books, Canton, ME 04221 (SAN 203-4514) Tel 207-388-2860.

Greensward Pr, *(Greensward Pr.; 0-930165),* P.O. Box 640472, San Francisco, CA 94164-0472 (SAN 670-7149) Tel 415-928-4142
Dist(s): **Bookpeople** *(Bookpeople)*
Cancer Control Soc *(Cancer Control Society)*
New Leaf Dist *(New Leaf Distributing Co., Inc.).*

Greenwich Med (GBR) *(1-900151; 1-84110) Dist. by* **OUP.**

Greenwich Med (GBR) *(1-900151; 1-84110) Dist. by* **JAMCO Dist.**

Greenwich Pub Group, *(Greenwich Publishing Group, Inc.; 0-944641),* 243 Hamburg Rd., Lyme, CT 06371 (SAN 244-4933) Tel 860-434-8880; Fax: 860-434-8887
E-mail: info@greenwichpublishing.com
Web site: http://www.greenwichpublishing.com.

Greenwich Univ Pr (GBR) *(1-874529; 1-86166) Dist. by* **NYU Pr.**

---

†Greenwood, ***(Greenwood Publishing Group, Inc.; 0-275; 0-313; 0-8371; 0-86569; 0-89789; 0-89930; 1-56720),*** **Orders Addr.: P.O. Box 5007, Westport, CT 06881-5007 (SAN 213-2028) Fax: 203-222-1502 (customer service and sales) ; Toll Free: 800-225-5800 (orders only); Edit Addr.: 88 Post Rd., W., Westport, CT 06881-5007 Tel 203-226-3571; Fax: 203-222-1502; 203-226-2540 ;** ***Imprints:*** **Quorum Bks (Quorum Books) Bergin & Garvey (Bergin & Garvey) Greenwood Pr (Greenwood Press) Auburn Hse (Auburn House) Praeger Pubs (Praeger Publishers) Praeger Trade (Praeger Trade) Aburn Hse Paperback (Auburn House Paperback) Ablex (Ablex Publishing Corporation) Oryx (Oryx Press) Do not confuse with Greenwood Publishing in Glenview, IL**
E-mail: customer-service@greenwood.com; sales@greenwood.com
Web site: http://www.greenwood.com
Dist(s): **Natl Bk Netwk** ***(National Bk. Network); CIP.***

Greenwood Pr Imprint of Greenwood

Greenwood-Gene, *(Greenwood Genetic Ctr.; 1-879554),* 1 Gregor Mendel Cir., Greenwood, SC 29646 Tel 803-223-9411; Fax: 803-227-1614; Toll Free: 800-473-9411.

Gregg Revivals (GBR) *(0-7512) Dist. by* **Ashgate Pub Co.**

Gregorc Assocs, *(Gregorc Assocs., Inc.; 0-934481),* 15 Doubleday Rd., Columbia, CT 06237 (SAN 693-885X) Tel 860-228-0093 (phone/fax).

†Grey Hse Pub, *(Grey Hse. Publishing, Inc.; 0-939300; 1-891482; 1-930956),* 185 Millerton Rd., Millerton, NY 12546 Tel 518-789-8700; Fax: 518-789-0556; Toll Free: 800-562-2139 ; *Imprints:* Sedgwick Pr (Sedgwick Press)
E-mail: books@greyhouse.com
Web site: http://www.greyhouse.com*; CIP.*

Grey Spider, *(Grey Spider Pr.; 0-9652272; 1-58249),* 37607 Cape Horn Rd., Sedro-Woolley, WA 98284 Tel 360-826-5306 (phone/fax).

Greycliff Pub, *(Greycliff Publishing Co.; 0-9626663; 1-890373),* Orders Addr.: P.O. Box 1273, Helena, MT 59624 (SAN 663-0804) Tel 406-443-1888 (orders); Fax: 406-443-0788 (orders); Toll Free: 800-874-4171 (orders)
E-mail: orders@greycliff.com
Web site: http://greycliff.com
Dist(s): **Alpenbooks** *(Alpenbooks)*
Baker & Taylor *(Baker & Taylor Bks.)*
Benjamin News *(Benjamin News Group)*
Books West CO *(Books West)*
Brodart *(Brodart Co.)*
Partners Pubs Grp *(Partners Pubs. Group, Inc.)*
Partners-West *(Partners/West)*
Peregrine Outftrs *(Peregrine Outfitters).*

Greyden Pr, *(Greyden Pr.; 0-9632238; 1-57074),* 2020 Builders Pl., Columbus, OH 43204-4885 (SAN 298-0282) Tel 614-488-2525; Fax: 614-488-2817
E-mail: sales@greydenpress.com
Web site: http://www.greydenpress.com.

Greyrock, *(Greyrock Publishing; 0-9673715),* P.O. Box 272964, Fort. Collins, CO 80525 Tel 970-226-1725 (phone & fax)
E-mail: GreyrockP@aol.com.

Greystone Pubng, *(Greystone Publishing, Inc.; 0-9652203),* P.O. Box 27127, Greenville, SC 29616-1127 Tel 864-476-2126; Fax: 864-476-6012; Toll Free: 800-881-0804.

Grief & Grief, *See* **G&G Pub**

Griefwork Ctr, *(Griefwork Ctr., Inc.; 1-892906),* P.O. Box 5104, Kendall Park, NJ 08824 Tel 732-422-0400; Fax: 732-422-4609
E-mail: Griefwork2@aol.com
Web site: http://www.griefworkcenter.com.

Grinnen-Barrett Pub Co, *(Grinnen-Barrett Publishing Co.; 0-9613063),* Orders Addr.: P.O. Box 779, Brookline, MA 02446 (SAN 294-8184) Tel 617-232-1993; Edit Addr.: 36 Winchester St., No. 8, Brookline, MA 02446 (SAN 665-8393)
E-mail: miriam3608@cs.com; miriamae@ix.netcom.com; maerick@bics.bwh.harvard.edu
Web site: http://www.morningsickness.org.

Grnlf Ent, *(Greenleaf Enterprises, Inc.; 0-9665319; 1-929774),* Div. of Greenleaf Book Group LLC, Orders Addr.: 660 Elmwood Point, Aurora, OH 44202 Tel 330-995-9700; Fax: 330-995-9704; Toll Free: 800-932-5420; Edit Addr.: 7600 Thistle Ln., Novelty, OH 44072
E-mail: email@greenleafbookgroup
Web site: http://www.greenleafbookgroup.com.

Grnwd Resch, *(Greenwood Research Bks. & Software; 1-890121),* 1036 Murray Ct., Wichita, KS 67212-4031 Tel 316-722-4954; Fax: 530-325-3469
E-mail: grnwdrsch@hotmail.com.
Web site: http://grnwd.tripod.com.

Grolier Educ, *(Grolier Educational; 0-7172),* Div. of Grolier Publishing, 6 Park Lawn Dr., Bethel, CT 06801 (SAN 205-3195) Tel 203-797-3500; Fax: 203-797-3428; Toll Free: 800-243-7256
E-mail: specref0@grolier.com
Web site: http://publishing.grolier.com.

†Group Pub, *(Group Publishing, Inc.; 0-7644; 0-931529; 0-936664; 1-55945),* Orders Addr.: P.O. Box 485, Loveland, CO 80539 (SAN 214-4689) Tel 970-669-3836; Fax: 970-679-4373; Toll Free: 800-635-0404; 800-447-1070 (consumer orders only); 800-541-5200 (trade orders only); Edit Addr.: 1515 Cascade Ave., Loveland, CO 80538 (SAN 662-1376)
E-mail: innovatr@grouppublishing.com
Web site: http://www.grouppublishing.com
Dist(s): **Appalachian Bible** *(Appalachian Bible Co.)*
Riverside-World *(Riverside World)*
Spring Arbor Dist *(Spring Arbor Distributors Inc.); CIP.*

Grove Imprint of Grove-Atltic

Grove Educ Tech, *(Grove Educational Technologies; 0-936735),* 6435 Yamhill St., SE, Portland, OR 97215-2027 (SAN 699-9840); 27 Hy Pl., Lake Grove, NY 11755 (SAN 699-9859)
E-mail: geta@juno.com.

†Grove-Atltic, *(Grove/Atlantic, Inc.; 0-8021; 0-87113; 1-55584),* 841 Broadway, 4th Flr., New York, NY 10003-4793 (SAN 201-4890) Tel 212-614-7850; Fax: 212-614-7886; Toll Free: 800-521-0178 ; *Imprints:* Grove (Grove Press) Atlntc Mnthly (Atlantic Monthly Press)
Dist(s): **Continental Bk** *(Continental Bk. Co., Inc.)*
Publishers Group *(Publishers Group West); CIP.*

Groves dict Music, *See* **Groves Dictionaries**

†Groves Dictionaries, *(Groves Dictionaries, Inc.; 0-935859; 0-943818; 1-56159; 1-884446),* Div. of Macmillan Pubs., Ltd. UK, Orders Addr.: P.O. Box 2224, Williston, VT 05495 Toll Free: 800-972-9892; Edit Addr.: 345 Park Ave., S., 10th Flr., New York, NY 10010-1707 (SAN 211-9579) Tel 212-689-9200 (phone/fax); Toll Free: 800-221-2123
E-mail: grove@grovereference.com
Web site: http://www.grovereference.com*; CIP.*

Grow Families, *(Growing Families International; 1-883035),* 1846 Angus Ave., Simi Valley, CA 93063 (SAN 298-7767) Tel 805-582-9800.

Growing Images, *(Growing Images; 0-9601200),* P.O. Box 2510, Novato, CA 94948 (SAN 661-9770) Tel 907-456-4400.

Growth Publ, *(Growth Publishing; 1-893505),* Div. of Growth Central LLC, 750 Columbus Ave., Suite 9S, New York, NY 10025 Tel 212-749-3684; Fax: 212-749-7872
E-mail: growth@growthgroups.com
Web site: http://www.growthcentral.com/publishing.htm.

Growth Unltd, *(Growth Unlimited, Inc.; 0-916927; 0-9601334),* 31 East Ave., S., Battle Creek, MI 49017-5501 (SAN 210-8976) Tel 616-964-4821; Fax: 616-964-4071; Toll Free: 800-441-7676
E-mail: artfettig@aol.com
Web site: http://www.imasource.com.

Grp Adv Psych, *(Group for the Advancement of Psychiatry; 0-87318),* Div. of American Psychiatric Pr., Inc., Orders Addr.: 1400 K St. NW, 11th Flr., Washington, DC 20005 (SAN 228-3492) Tel 202-682-6261; Fax: 202-789-2648 orders; Toll Free: 800-368-5777
Web site: http://www.appi.org
Dist(s): **Am Psychiatric** *(American Psychiatric Pr., Inc.).*

Grune & Strat Imprint of Saunders

Grunt, *(Grunt; 0-9644558),* 13227 N. Mimosa Dr., No. 121, Fountain Hills, AZ 85268 Tel 602-816-9673.

Gryphon Hse, *(Gryphon Hse., Inc.; 0-87659; 1-58904),* Orders Addr.: P.O. Box 207, Beltsville, MD 20704-0207 (SAN 169-3190) Tel 301-595-9500; Fax: 301-595-0051; Toll Free: 800-638-0928; Edit Addr.: 10726 Tucker St., Beltsville, MD 20705
E-mail: info@ghbooks.com
Web site: http://www.gryphonhouse.com
Dist(s): **Consort Bk Sales** *(Consortium Bk. Sales & Distribution)*
IPG Chicago *(Independent Pubs. Group).*

GSI Pubns, *(GSI Pubns.; 0-9627701; 1-887306),* Div. of Gordon Systems, Inc., Orders Addr.: P.O. Box 746, DeWitt, NY 13214 Tel 315-446-4849; Fax: 315-446-2012; Toll Free: 800-550-2343; Edit Addr.: 301 Ambergate Rd., DeWitt, NY 13214
E-mail: addgsi@aol.com
Web site: http://www.gsi-add.com
Dist(s): **Baker & Taylor** *(Baker & Taylor Bks.).*

Guardian Pub, *(Guardian Publishing; 1-890415),* 269 S. Beverly Dr., No. 810, Beverly Hills, CA 90212 Tel 310-208-1088; Fax: 310-208-7506; Toll Free: 800-554-7233
E-mail: fipub@aol.com.

Guide Inc, *(Guide, Inc., The; 0-9661654),* Orders Addr.: P.O. Box 969, Hightstown, NJ 08520 Tel 609-448-8021; Fax: 609-448-8075; Edit Addr.: 38 Meadow Dr., Hightstown, NJ 08520.

Guided Imagery, *See* **US Pub FL**

Guidelines Pr, *(Guidelines Pr.; 0-932570),* 1307 S. Killian Dr., Lake Park, FL 33403 (SAN 212-0984) Tel 407-842-9411.

Guiding Light, *(Guiding Light Pubns., Inc.; 0-9704431),* Orders Addr.: P.O. Box 6478, Louisville, KY 40206; Edit Addr.: 111 Blankenlaker Ln., Louisville, KY 40207.

Guild Pr Emmis Pubng, *(Guild Press Emmis Publishing; 0-9617367; 1-57860; 1-878208),* 10665 Andrade Dr., Zionsville, IN 46077-9230 (SAN 663-7965) Tel 317-733-4175; Fax: 317-733-4176; Toll Free: 800-913-9563
E-mail: info@guildpress.com; sales@quildpress.com
Web site: http://www.guildpress.com
Dist(s): **Distributors** *(Distributors, The)*
Herveys Bklink *(Hervey's Booklink & Cookbook Warehouse)*
Maus Tales *(Maus Tales)*
Partners Pubs Grp *(Partners Pubs. Group, Inc.).*

Guild Pr IN, *See* **Guild Pr Emmis Pubng**

†Guild Psy, *(Guild for Psychological Studies Publishing Hse.; 0-917479),* P.O. Box 29385, San Francisco, CA 94129-0385 (SAN 656-0687) Tel 415-561-2385; Fax: 415-561-2386
E-mail: guildsf@aol.com
Web site: http://www.guildsf.org*; CIP.*

Guilford Pubns, *(Guilford Pubns., Inc.; 0-89862; 1-57230),* 72 Spring St., New York, NY 10012 (SAN 212-9442) Tel 212-431-9800; Fax: 212-966-6708; Toll Free: 800-365-7006
E-mail: info@guilford.com
Web site: http://www.guilford.com
Dist(s): **Red Toad Rd** *(Red Toad Road Co.).*

Gurze Bks, *(Gurze Bks.; 0-936077),* Orders Addr.: P.O. Box 2238, Carlsbad, CA 92018 (SAN 697-0818) Tel 760-434-7533; Fax: 760-434-5476; Toll Free: 800-756-7533; Edit Addr.: 3420 Woodland Way, Carlsbad, CA 92018 (SAN 697-0826)
E-mail: qzcati@aol.com; gurze@aol.com
Web site: http://www.gurze.com
Dist(s): **Publishers Group** *(Publishers Group West)*
Quality Bks IL *(Quality Bks., Inc.).*

Gustav Fischer (DEU) *(3-437; 3-334) Dist. by* **Lubrecht & Cramer.**

Guttmacher Inst, *(Guttmacher, Alan Institute; 0-939253),* 120 Wall St., 21st Flr., New York, NY 10005 (SAN 225-9648) Tel 212-248-1111; Fax: 212-248-1951
E-mail: info@agi-usa.org; buyit@AGI-USA.org
Web site: http://www.agi-usa.org.

GW Medical, *(G.W. Medical Publishing, Inc.; 1-878060),* 2601 Metro Blvd., Saint Louis, MO 63043-2411 Tel 314-298-0330; Fax: 314-298-2820; Toll Free: 800-600-0330
E-mail: info@gwmedical.com
Web site: http://www.gwmedical.com.

GWC Inc, *(GWC, Inc.; 1-56168; 1-886865),* Orders Addr.: P.O. Box 5023, Cahokia, IL 62206 Tel 618-337-9300; Fax: 618-337-7880; Toll Free: 800-851-5406; Edit Addr.: 530 Falling Spring Rd., Cahokia, IL 62206
E-mail: info@gwcinc.com
Web site: http://www.gwcinc.com.

GWU Ctr Int Hlth, *See* **PAHO**

GWU Ctr WAS, *(George Washington Univ., Ctr. for Washington Area Studies; 1-888028),* 2201 G St. NW, Funger Hall 507, Washington, DC 20052 (SAN 247-4816) Tel 202-994-5758; Fax: 202-994-5844
E-mail: cwas@www.gwu.edu
Web site: http://www.gwu.edu/~cwas.

Gyan Publishing Hse (IND) *(81-212; 81-85199; 81-86423) Dist. by* **Nataraj Bks.**

Gylantic Pub, *(Gylantic Publishing Co.; 1-880197),* Orders Addr.: P.O. Box 2792, Littleton, CO 80161-2792; Edit Addr.: 6024 S. Pearl St., Littleton, CO 80121 Tel 303-797-6093
Dist(s): **Baker & Taylor** *(Baker & Taylor Bks.).*

H & H Ltd, *(H&H, Ltd.; 0-9670685),* P.O. Box 816, Lone Star, TX 75668-0816 Fax: 903-639-2461
E-mail: chazman@texramp.net.

H & H Pub, *(H&H Publishing Co., Inc.; 0-943202),* 1231 Kapp Dr., Clearwater, FL 33765 (SAN 240-5350) Tel 727-442-7760; Fax: 727-442-2195; Toll Free: 800-366-4079 Do not confuse with H&H Publishing Co. in Amarillo, TX
E-mail: hhservice@hhpublishing.com
Web site: http://www.hhpublishing.com.

H & H Pub WA, *(H&H Pubns.; 0-9674718),* 16921 76th Ave., W., Edmonds, WA 98026 Tel 206-543-1413; Fax: 425-743-1908
E-mail: jhorn@cmc.net
Web site: http://hanstenandhorn.com.

H A W M, *(H.A.W.M.; 0-9663791),* P.O. Box 462, Orfield, PA 18069-0462 Tel 610-826-2352.

H Allen & Assocs, *(Allen, Hubert & Assocs.; 0-9641694),* 720-25 Tramway Ln., NE, Albuquerque, NM 87122 Tel 505-797-3520; Fax: 505-797-3521
E-mail: hubertaallen@compuserve.com.

H Blackburn, *(Blackburn, Henry; 1-887268),* c/o Univ. of Minnesota, Div. of Epidemiology, 1300 S. Second St., Suite 300, Minneapolis, MN 55454 Tel 612-626-8816; Fax: 612-624-0315.

H E W, *(H E W Enterprises; 0-9665600),* 305 Birch Ave., Grandview, WA 98930 Tel 509-882-1790 Do not confuse with H E W Enterprizes, Mesa, AZ
Dist(s): **H&O Pioneer** *(H&O Pioneer Barns).*

H F Boggiano, *(Boggiano, H. F.; 0-9654469),* Boggiano Dr., El Paso, TX 79912 Tel 915-581-0908; Fax: 915-747-6553
E-mail: mhagan@vlep.edu.

H F Hlth Syst, *(Henry Ford Health System; 0-9659494),* 1 Ford Pl., Detroit, MI 48202 Tel 313-874-4282; Fax: 313-874-5442
E-mail: ppaintel@nfhs.org
Web site: http://www.sladen.hfhs.org.

H Hamilton (GBR) *(0-241) Dist. by* **Trafalgar.**

†**H Holt & Co,** *(Holt, Henry & Co., LLC; 0-03; 0-8050),* 115 W. 18th St., 5th Flr., New York, NY 10011 (SAN 200-6472) Tel 212-886-9200; Fax: 212-633-0748 ;
Imprints: Owl (Owl Paperback Books) Times Bks (Times Books)
E-mail: info@hholt.com
Web site: http://www.henryholt.com
Dist(s): **Penguin Putnam** *(Penguin Putnam, Inc.)*
VHPS *(VHPS Holtzbrinck Pubs.)*
Weston Woods *(Weston Woods Studios, Inc.); CIP.*

H Holt Bks Young Read, *(Holt, Henry Bks. for Young Readers; 0-8050),* 115 W. 18th St., New York, NY 10011 Tel 212-886-9200; Fax: 212-633-0748 ;
Imprints: Owlet Pbks (Owlet Paperbacks for Young Readers)
Web site: http://www.henryholt.com
Dist(s): **VHPS** *(VHPS Holtzbrinck Pubs.).*

H Hultgren, *See* **Hultgren Pubns**

H J Kaiser, *(Kaiser, Henry J. Family Foundation; 0-944525),* 2400 Sand Hill Rd., Menlo Park, CA 94025 (SAN 242-9616) Tel 650-854-9400; Fax: 415-854-4800.

H J Kramer Inc, *(Kramer, H.J. Inc.; 0-915811),* P.O. Box 1082, Tiburon, CA 94920 (SAN 294-0833) Tel 415-435-5367; Fax: 415-435-5364
E-mail: hjkramer@jps.net
Dist(s): **Bookpeople** *(Bookpeople)*
New Leaf Dist *(New Leaf Distributing Co., Inc.)*
New Wrld Lib *(New World Library)*
Publishers Group *(Publishers Group West)*
Shens Bks *(Shen's Bks.).*

H L Levin, *(Levin, Hugh Lauter Assocs.; 0-88363),* 2507 Post Rd., Southport, CT 06490 (SAN 201-6109) Tel 203-254-7733; Fax: 203-254-7586
E-mail: inquiries@hlla.com
Web site: http://www.hlla.com
Dist(s): **Publishers Group** *(Publishers Group West).*

H Lamb, *(Lamb, Howard; 0-9609150),* P.O. Box 1001, Belvedere Tiburon, CA 94920-0949 (SAN 241-3906).

H M Curran, *(Curran, Helen M.; 0-9642185),* 56B Calle Cadiz, Laguna Hills, CA 92653 Tel 714-458-8510
Dist(s): **New Leaf Dist** *(New Leaf Distributing Co., Inc.).*

H M Erickson, *(Erickson, Harold M.; 0-9640626),* 347 Twin Lakes Dr., Santa Rosa, CA 95409 Tel 707-538-3836.

H P Sgambato, *(Sgambato, Hubert Pacifico Publishing Enterprises; 0-9621636),* 440 E. Baltimore Ave., Clifton Heights, PA 19018 (SAN 251-7043) Tel 610-259-3590.

H P Three, *(HP3 Healthcare Concepts, Inc.; 0-9713305),* 60 W. Broad St., Suite 304, Bethlehem, PA 18018 Tel 610-332-2990; Fax: 610-332-2993; Toll Free: 877-774-7853
E-mail: info@hp3.net
Web site: http://www.hp3.net.

H Shaw Pubs Imprint of Waterbrook Pr

H Smith, *(Smith, Hilary; 0-9621110),* Box 72, Alumni Hse., Peacham, VT 05862 (SAN 250-5509) Tel 802-592-3500.

H Sq Co, *(H Squared Co.; 0-927054),* 315 Whitney Ave., New Haven, CT 06511 Tel 203-562-3159; Fax: 203-865-8163
E-mail: askh2@juno.com
Dist(s): **Forms Worms Inc** *(Forms & Worms, Inc.).*

H Stern, *(Stern, Henry; 0-9646379),* 841 Chapman Ln., Petaluma, CA 94952-1669 Tel 707-766-9848.

H W Bks, *(Whitney, Harvey Bks. Co.; 0-929375; 0-9606488),* P.O. Box 42696, Cincinnati, OH 45242 (SAN 217-2143) Tel 513-793-3555; Fax: 513-793-3600; Toll Free: 877-742-7631
E-mail: hwb@hwbooks.com; customerserv@HWBooks.com
Web site: http://www.hwbooks.com.

H W Parker, *(Parker, Homer W.; 0-922958),* 1601 Woodrock Dr., Round Rock, TX 78681 (SAN 251-5350) Tel 512-255-0702.

Haase Hse, *See* **Easy Money Pr**

Hacienda Pub, *(Hacienda Publishing, Inc.; 0-9641077),* 5791 Kentucky Downs Dr., Macon, GA 31210 Tel 912-757-9873; Fax: 912-757-9725; Toll Free: 800-757-9873
E-mail: hfaria@mindspring.com
Web site: http://www.haciendapub.com
Dist(s): **Baker & Taylor** *(Baker & Taylor Bks.)*
J Majors Co *(Majors, J. A. Co.)*
Quality Bks IL *(Quality Bks., Inc.).*

†**Hackett Pub,** *(Hackett Publishing Co., Inc.; 0-87220; 0-915144; 0-915145),* Orders Addr.: P.O. Box 44937, Indianapolis, IN 46244-0937 (SAN 201-6044) Tel 317-635-9250; Fax: 317-635-9292; Toll Free Fax: 800-783-9213
E-mail: customer@hackettpublishing.com
Web site: http://www.hackettpublishing.com; *CIP.*

Haer Inst, *(Haer Institute for Electro Physiological Research; 0-940090),* Orders Addr.: P.O. Box 337, Brunswick, ME 04011 (SAN 220-2255) Tel 207-729-1601.

Hagin Ministries, *See* **Faith Lib Pubns**

Hahnemann Clinic, *(Hahnemann Clinic Publishing; 0-9635368),* 13974 Glenn Pines Rd., Grass Valley, CA 95945 Tel 530-477-7397 (phone/fax).

Halcyon Imprint of Natl Book

Halcyon TX, *(Halcyon Pr.; 0-9621114),* 3219 McKinney Ave., Dallas, TX 75204 (SAN 250-4227) Tel 214-720-0607 Do not confuse with companies with same or similar name in Hendersonville, NC, Flushing, NY, Houston, TX.

Hale-Van Ruth, *(Hale-Van Ruth; 0-9623691),* 2424 Huntington Dr., Pittsburgh, PA 15241 Tel 412-833-3614.

Half Halt Pr, *(Half Halt Pr.; 0-939481),* Orders Addr.: P.O. Box 67, Boonsboro, MD 21713-0067 (SAN 663-270X) Tel 301-733-7119; Fax: 301-733-7408; Toll Free: 800-822-9635
E-mail: hhpress@aol.com
Web site: http://www.halfhaltpress.com.

Hall Reference Imprint of Macmillan

Hallum Pub, *(Hallum Publishing Co.; 0-9653658),* Pop Warner Suite, 1533 Madrono Ave., Palo Alto, CA 94306 Tel 415-328-4005; Toll Free: 800-484-4871
E-mail: tbyrd@best.com
Web site: http://www.best.com/tbyrd.

†**Halo Bks,** *(Halo Bks.; 0-9622874; 1-879904),* Orders Addr.: P.O. Box 150, Glen Ellen, CA 95442 Tel 707-933-9093; Fax: 415-434-3441; Edit Addr.: 534 Pacific Ave., San Francisco, CA 94133 (SAN 200-3147) Tel 415-981-5144; Fax: 415-434-3441
E-mail: halobks@prodigy.net
Dist(s): **BookWorld** *(BookWorld Services, Inc.); CIP.*

†**Halsted Pr,** *(Halsted Pr.; 0-470),* Div. of John Wiley & Sons, Inc., 605 Third Ave., New York, NY 10158-0012 (SAN 202-2680) Tel 212-850-6000; Fax: 212-850-6816; Toll Free: 800-225-5945 (customer service)
E-mail: info@qm.wiley.com
Web site: http://www.wiley.com
Dist(s): **netLibrary CO** *(netLibrary, Inc.); CIP.*

Halyburton, *(Halyburton Pr.; 0-916717),* Orders Addr.: P.O. Box 2973, Ann Arbor, MI 48106 (SAN 653-7480); Edit Addr.: 1446 Karlin Ct., East Lansing, MI 48823 (SAN 653-7499) Tel 517-332-7129.

†**Hambledon Press,** *(Hambledon Pr.; 0-907628; 1-85285),* P.O. Box 162, Rio Grande, OH 45674-0162 (SAN 677-4946) Tel 740-245-9624; *CIP.*

Hamilton Pubns, *(Hamilton Pubns.; 0-940059),* Orders Addr.: P.O. Box 3222, Boulder, CO 80307-3222 (SAN 663-9461) Tel 303-499-3183; Edit Addr.: 2825 Colby Dr., Boulder, CO 80303.

Hamlyn Pub (GBR) *(0-600; 0-601) Dist. by* **Sterling.**

Hamp Court Pr, *(Hampton Court Pr.; 0-9617667),* 112 Pitchkettle Point Cir., Suffolk, VA 23434-7558 (SAN 664-9424).

Hampton Pr NJ, *(Hampton Pr., Inc.; 1-57273; 1-58283; 1-881303),* 23 Broadway, Cresskill, NJ 07626 Tel 201-894-1686; Fax: 201-894-8732; Toll Free: 800-894-8955
E-mail: HamptonPr1@aol.com
Web site: http://www.hamptonpress.com
Dist(s): **Baker & Taylor** *(Baker & Taylor Bks.)*
NA Blackwell *(Blackwell North America).*

Hampton Roads Pub Co, *(Hampton Roads Publishing Co., Inc.; 0-9624375; 1-57174; 1-878901),* 1125 Stoney Ridge Rd., Charlottesville, VA 22902 (SAN 299-8874) Tel 804-296-2772; Fax: 804-296-1441; Toll Free: 800-766-8009
E-mail: hrpc@hrpub.com; vcolburn@hrpub.com
Web site: http://www.hrpub.com
Dist(s): **Aramark WA** *(Aramark)*
Baker & Taylor *(Baker & Taylor Bks.)*
Book Warehse *(Book Warehouse)*
Bookazine Co Inc *(Bookazine Co., Inc.)*
Bookmen Inc *(Bookmen, Inc.)*
Bookpeople *(Bookpeople)*
Booksource *(Booksource, The)*
Brodart *(Brodart Co.)*
Integral Yoga Pubns *(Integral Yoga Pubns.)*
Koen Bk Distributors *(Koen Bk. Distributors)*
Koen Pacific *(Koen Pacific)*
Levy Home Entertainment *(Levy Home Entertainment)*
New Concepts Bks & Tapes *(New Concepts Bks. & Tapes Distributors)*
New Leaf Dist *(New Leaf Distributing Co., Inc.)*
Nutri-Books Corp *(Nutri-Bks. Corp.)*
Partners Pubs Grp *(Partners Pubs. Group, Inc.)*
Partners-West *(Partners/West)*
Quality Bks IL *(Quality Bks., Inc.)*
Red Wheel ME *(Red Wheel)*
Treas Chest Bks *(Treasure Chest Bks.)*
Unique Bks Inc *(Unique Bks., Inc.)*
Vision Dists *(Vision Distributors).*

†**Hancock House,** *(Hancock Hse. Pubs.; 0-88839; 0-919654),* 1431 Harrison Ave., Blaine, WA 98230-5005 (SAN 665-7079) Tel 604-538-1114; Fax: 604-538-2262; Toll Free Fax: 800-983-2262; Toll Free: 800-938-1114
E-mail: sales@hancockhouse.com
Web site: http://www.hancockhouse.com
Dist(s): **Todd Commns** *(Todd Communications); CIP.*

Hands Across Sea, *(Hands Across The Sea; 0-9679053),* P.O. Box 346, Old Bethpage, NY 11804 Tel 516-433-5430 (phone/fax)
E-mail: handsacrossthesea@worldnet.att.net
Web site: http://www.home.att.net/~handsacrossthesea.

Hands Jesus, *(Hands for Jesus; 1-891125),* P.O. Box 18655, Milwaukee, WI 53218 Tel 414-536-0863; Fax: 414-536-0823.

Hanford Mead, *(Hanford Mead Pubs., Inc.; 0-9643158),* P.O. Box 8051, Santa Cruz, CA 95061-8051 (SAN 253-9195) Tel 831-459-6855; Fax: 831-426-4474
E-mail: kyleat@hanfordmead.com
Web site: http://www.hanfordmead.com
Dist(s): **Bookpeople** *(Bookpeople)*
New Leaf Dist *(New Leaf Distributing Co., Inc.).*

Hanley & Belfus, *(Hanley & Belfus, Inc.; 0-932883; 1-56053),* 210 S. 13th St., Philadelphia, PA 19107 (SAN 689-0032) Tel 215-546-7293; Fax: 215-790-9330; Toll Free: 800-962-1892
E-mail: info@hanleyandbelfus.com
Web site: http://www.hanleyandbelfus.com
Dist(s): **Lppncott W & W** *(Lippincott Williams & Wilkins).*

Hanlit Pubns, *(Hanlit Pubns., Inc.; 1-880165),* 270 W. 19th St., New York, NY 10011 Tel 212-989-7200; Fax: 212-633-8022.

Hanna Kroeger, *(Hanna Kroeger Pubns.; 1-883713),* 805 Walnut St., Boulder, CO 80302 Tel 303-443-0261; Fax: 303-443-0108; Toll Free: 800-225-8787
E-mail: khp@kroegerherb.com; rick@kroegerherb.com
Web site: http://www.kroegerherb.com
Dist(s): **Integral Yoga Pubns** *(Integral Yoga Pubns.)*
New Leaf Dist *(New Leaf Distributing Co., Inc.)*
Nutri-Books Corp *(Nutri-Bks. Corp.).*

Hannibal Bks, *(Hannibal Bks.; 0-929292),* Div. of KLMK Communications, Inc., P.O. Box 461592, Garland, TX 75046-1592 Tel 972-487-5710; Fax: 972-487-7960; Toll Free: 800-742-0723; 800-747-0738
E-mail: hannibalbooks@earthlink.net; orders@hannibalbooks.com
Web site: http://www.hannibalbooks.com
Dist(s): **Spring Arbor Dist** *(Spring Arbor Distributors Inc.).*

Hanrow, *(Hanrow Pr.; 0-9703549),* Div. of Hanrow House Corp., Orders Addr.: P.O. Box 675551, Rancho Santa Fe, CA 92067 Tel 858-759-1020; Fax: 858-756-2922
E-mail: heg101@msn.com
Web site: http://www.hanrowpress.com; http://www.purposeandmeaningoflife.com.

Hanser-Gardner, *(Hanser-Gardner Pubns.; 1-56990),* 6915 Valley Ave., Cincinnati, OH 45244-3029 (SAN 297-9683) Tel 513-527-8977; Fax: 513-527-8950; Toll Free Fax: 800-953-8805; Toll Free: 800-950-8977
E-mail: mskavlem@gardnerweb.com
Web site: http://www.hansergardner.com.

Happiness Pr, *(Happiness Pr.; 0-916508),* Div. of Celtic Ocean International, Inc., 273 Fairway Dr., Asheville, NC 28805 (SAN 208-6719) Tel 828-299-9005; Fax: 828-299-1640; Toll Free: 800-867-7258
E-mail: topsalt@aol.com
Web site: http://www.celtic-seasalt.com.

Happiness Unltd, *(Happiness Unlimited Pubns.; 0-939372),* 228 N. Donnawood Dr., Suite 204, Virginia Beach, VA 23452 (SAN 220-1550) Tel 757-431-1317; Fax: 757-431-1503; Toll Free: 800-777-3529
E-mail: teplitz@compuserve.com
Web site: http://www.teplitz.com.

Hara Pub, *(Hara Publishing Group; 1-883697),* Orders Addr.: P.O. Box 507, Lynnwood, WA 98046 (SAN 631-4953) Tel 425-398-3679; Fax: 425-672-8597; Edit Addr.: 18728 Bothell Way, NE, Bothell, WA 98011 Tel 425-775-7868; P.O. Box 19732, Seattle, WA 98109 Tel 425-775-7868; Fax: 425-398-1380
E-mail: harapub@foxinternet.net
Web site: http://www.harapublishing.com.

Har-Anand Pubns (IND) *(81-241) Dist. by* **S Asia.**

Harbin Springs, *(Harbin Springs Publishing; 0-944202),* 18424 Harbin Springs Rd., Box 82, Middletown, CA 95461 (SAN 243-184X) Tel 707-987-0477; Fax: 707-987-0616.

Harbinger Med Pr NC, *(Harbinger Medical Pr.; 0-9612242),* 1100 S. Stratford Rd., Suite 530A, Winston-Salem, NC 27103 (SAN 291-834X) Tel 910-659-6250; Fax: 910-659-6239.

Harbor Pr, *(Harbor Pr., Inc.; 0-936197),* Orders Addr.: P.O. Box 1656, Gig Harbor, WA 98335 (SAN 696-8953) Tel 253-851-5190; Fax: 253-851-5191; Edit Addr.: 5713 Wollochet Dr. NW, Gig Harbor, WA 98335 (SAN 696-8961) Do not confuse with companies with the same name in Friday Harbor, WA, Austin, TX, Ardmore, PA
E-mail: young2327@mindspring.com
Web site: http://www.harborpress.com
Dist(s): **Natl Bk Netwk** *(National Bk. Network).*

†Harbor Pub, *(Harbor Publishing Co.; 0-937638),* 610 Cooke St., Apt. 218, Honolulu, HI 96813-6010 (SAN 656-8882) Do not confuse with Harbor Publishing, Redding, CT; *CIP.*

HarBrace, *See* **Harcourt**

†Harcourt, *(Harcourt Trade Pubs.; 0-15; 0-534),* Div. of Reed Elsevier plc, Orders Addr.: 6277 Sea Harbor Dr., Orlando, FL 32887 (SAN 200-285X) Tel 619-699-6707; Toll Free Fax: 800-235-0256; Toll Free: 800-543-1918 (trade orders, inquiries, claims); Edit Addr.: 525 B St., Suite 1900, San Diego, CA 92101-4495 (SAN 200-2736) Tel 619-231-6616 ; *Imprints:* Harvest Bks (Harvest Books)
E-mail: apbcs@harcourtbrace.com
Web site: http://www.harcourtbooks.com; *CIP.*

Harcourt (AUS) *(0-7295) Dist. by* **Saunders.**

Harcourt Childs Bks, *(Harcourt Children's Bks.; 0-15),* Div. of Reed Elsevier plc, Orders Addr.: 6277 Sea Harbor Dr., Orlando, FL 32887 Toll Free Fax: 800-235-0256; Toll Free: 800-543-1918; Edit Addr.: 15 E. 26th St., 15th Flr., New York, NY 10010 Tel 212-592-1000 ; *Imprints:* Harcourt Pbk (Harcourt Paperbacks)
Dist(s): **Harcourt** *(Harcourt Trade Pubs.)*
Shens Bks *(Shen's Bks.).*

Harcourt Coll Pubs, *(Harcourt College Pubs.; 0-03; 0-15),* Div. of Thomson Corp., The, Orders Addr.: 6277 Sea Harbor Dr., Orlando, FL 32887 (SAN 250-0086) Toll Free: 800-782-4479 (orders, inquiries); 800-245-8744 (customer service); Edit Addr.: 301 Commerce St., Suite 3700 City Center Tower Two, Fort Worth, TX 76102 (SAN 297-4789) Tel 817-334-7500; Fax: 817-334-7844
E-mail: wlittle@harbrace.com
Web site: http://www.harcourtcollege.com/.

Harcourt Pbk Imprint of Harcourt Childs Bks

Harcourt Prof, *(Harcourt Professional Publishing; 0-15),* 525 B St., Suite 1900, San Diego, CA 92101 Tel 619-699-6716.

†Harcrt Hlth Sci Grp, *(Harcourt Health Sciences Group; 0-03; 0-15; 0-443; 0-7216),* 11830 Westline Industrial Dr., Saint Louis, MO 63146 Tel 314-872-8370; Toll Free Fax: 800-535-9935 ; *Imprints:* Grune & Strat (Grune & Stratton, Incorporated)
Web site: http://www.harcourt-international.com; *CIP.*

HARKEN!, *(HARKEN!; 0-615),* Orders Addr.: P.O. Box 1428, Centreville, VA 20122-8428 Tel 703-803-8819; Edit Addr.: 13908 Gunners Pl., Centreville, VA 20121
Web site: http://www.holisticparadigm.com.

†Harlan Davidson, *(Davidson, Harlan Inc.; 0-88295),* 773 Glenn Ave., Wheeling, IL 60090-6000 (SAN 201-2375) Tel 847-541-9720; Fax: 847-541-9830
E-mail: abeeparker@aol.com
Web site: http://www.harlandavidson.com; *CIP.*

Harlo Press, *(Harlo Pr.; 0-8187),* 50 Victor Ave., Detroit, MI 48203 (SAN 202-2745) Tel 313-883-3600
Dist(s): **Mustrd Seed Pubns** *(Mustard Seed Pubns.).*

Harmony Bks, *(Harmony Bks.; 0-517; 0-609; 0-8129; 1-4000),* Div. of Crown Publishing Group, Orders Addr.: 400 Hahn Rd., Westminster, MD 21157 Tel 410-848-1900; Toll Free: 800-726-0600; Edit Addr.: 299 Park Ave., New York, NY 10171 Tel 212-751-2600; Toll Free: 800-726-0600 ; *Imprints:* Three Riv Pr (Three Rivers Press)
Web site: http://www.randomhouse.com
Dist(s): **Lectorum Pubns** *(Lectorum Pubns., Inc.).*

Harmony Publng, *(Harmony Publishing; 0-9653612),* Orders Addr.: P.O. Box 110331, Cleveland, OH 44111 Tel 216-883-3159 (phone/fax); Edit Addr.: 6514 Hosmor Ave., Cleveland, OH 44105
E-mail: harmonypbl@aol.com
Web site: http://www.ryu.com/harmony.

Harp PBks Imprint of HarperCollins Pubs

HarpBusn Imprint of HarpInfo

HarpC (GBR) *(0-00; 0-261) Dist. by* **Trafalgar.**

Harper Ref Imprint of HarperCollins Pubs

†Harper SF, *(HarperSanFrancisco; 0-06; 0-85924; 0-86683),* Div. of HarperCollins General Bks. Group, 353 Sacramento St., Suite 500, San Francisco, CA 94111 (SAN 215-3734) Tel 415-477-4400; Fax: 415-477-4444; Toll Free: 800 242-7737 (customer service)
Web site: http://www.harpercollins.com
Dist(s): **HarperCollins Pubs** *(HarperCollins Pubs.); CIP.*

HarperCollins Gen Bks, *(HarperCollins General Bks. Group; 0-06),* 10 E. 53rd St., New York, NY 10022-5299 Fax: 212-207-7826 ; *Imprints:* Rayo (Rayo)
Dist(s): **HarperCollins Pubs** *(HarperCollins Pubs.).*

†HarperCollins Pubs, *(HarperCollins Pubs.; 0-00; 0-06; 0-688; 0-690; 0-694; 0-7322),* Div. of News Corp., Orders Addr.: 1000 Keystone Industrial Pk., Scranton, PA 18512-4621 (SAN 215-3742) Tel 570-941-1500; Toll Free Fax: 800-822-4090; Toll Free: 800-242-7737 (orders only); Edit Addr.: 10 E. 53rd St., New York, NY 10022-5299 (SAN 200-2086) Tel 212-207-7000 ; *Imprints:* Harp PBks (HarperPaperback Books) Torch (HarperTorchbooks) Harper Ref (Harper Reference) HarperFlamingo (HarperFlamingo) ReganBooks (ReganBooks)
Web site: http://www.harpercollins.com
Dist(s): **CMG** *(Comag Marketing Group)*
Consort Bk Sales *(Consortium Bk. Sales & Distribution)*
Continental Bk *(Continental Bk. Co., Inc.)*
Shens Bks *(Shen's Bks.)*
T T Beeler *(Beeler, Thomas T. Publisher)*
Wheeler Pub *(Wheeler Publishing, Inc.); CIP.*

HarperFlamingo Imprint of HarperCollins Pubs

HarperTrade, *(HarperTrade; 0-06; 0-688),* Div. of HarperCollins General Bks. Group, 10 E. 53rd St., New York, NY 10022 Tel 212-207-7000; Fax: 217-207-7633; Toll Free: 800-242-7737 (orders) ; *Imprints:* Cliff Street (Cliff Street Books) Perennial (Perennial) Quil (Quill) Amistad (Amistad Press)
Web site: http://www.harpercollins.com/
Dist(s): **Continental Bk** *(Continental Bk. Co., Inc.)*
HarperCollins Pubs *(HarperCollins Pubs.).*

HarpInfo, *(HarperInformation; 0-06),* Div. of HarperCollins General Bks. Group, 10 E. 53rd St., New York, NY 10022-5299 Tel 212-207-7000 ; *Imprints:* HarpBusn (HarperBusiness) HarpRes (HarperResource)
Web site: http://www.harpercollins.com/
Dist(s): **HarperCollins Pubs** *(HarperCollins Pubs.).*

HarpR, *See* **Harper SF**

HarpRes Imprint of HarpInfo

HarpTorch Imprint of Morrow Avon

Harrington Park Imprint of Haworth Pr

†Harrison Hse, *(Harrison Hse., Inc.; 0-89274; 1-57794),* Orders Addr.: P.O. Box 35035, Tulsa, OK 74153 (SAN 208-676X) Tel 918-494-5944; Fax: 918-494-3665; Toll Free: 800-888-4126; Edit Addr.: 2448 E. 81st St., Suite 4400, Tulsa, OK 74137
Web site: http://www.harrisonhouse.com
Dist(s): **Anchor Distributors** *(Anchor Distributors)*
Appalachian Bible *(Appalachian Bible Co.)*
Riverside-World *(Riverside World)*
Spring Arbor Dist *(Spring Arbor Distributors Inc.); CIP.*

Harsand Pr, *(Harsand Pr.; 0-9612310),* 996 E. Church Rd., Cambridge, WI 53523-9470 (SAN 287-7309) Toll Free: 800-451-0643 (outside Wisconsin)
Dist(s): **Baker & Taylor** *(Baker & Taylor Bks.)*
Harsand Distributing *(Harsand Distributing).*

Hart Mktg, *(Hart Marketing; 0-9631828),* Orders Addr.: P.O. Box 274, Great Neck, NY 11022; Edit Addr.: 1 Welwyn Rd., Great Neck, NY 11022 Tel 516-466-5479.

Hart Pub (GBR) *(1-901362; 1-84113) Dist. by* **Intl Spec Bk.**

†Hartley & Marks, *(Hartley & Marks, Inc.; 0-88179),* P.O. Box 147, Point Roberts, WA 98281 (SAN 264-0880) Tel 604-739-1771; Fax: 604-738-1913; Toll Free: 800-277-5887
E-mail: info@hartleyandmarks.com
Dist(s): **Publishers Group** *(Publishers Group West); CIP.*

Hartman Pub, *(Hartman Publishing, Inc.; 1-888343),* 8529 Indian School Rd., NE, Suite A, Albuquerque, NM 87112 Tel 505-291-1274; Fax: 505-291-1284; Toll Free Fax: 800-474-6106; Toll Free: 800-999-9534
E-mail: orders@hartmanonline.com; help@hartmanonline.com
Web site: http://www.hartmanonline.com.

Hart-Whitlow Pubs, *(Hart-Whitlow Pubs.; 0-9637951),* 1845 Brandywine Dr., Lenoir City, TN 37772 Tel 865-986-8553
E-mail: dickins@utk.edu.

†Harvard Common Pr, *(Harvard Common Pr.; 0-87645; 0-916782; 1-55832),* 535 Albany St., Boston, MA 02118 (SAN 208-6778) Tel 617-423-5803; Fax: 617-695-9794; Toll Free: 888-657-3755
E-mail: orders@harvardcommonpress.com
Web site: http://www.harvardcommonpress.com
Dist(s): **Natl Bk Netwk** *(National Bk. Network); CIP.*

Harvard Educ Rev, *(Harvard Educational Review; 0-916690),* Gutman Library Suite 349, 6 Appian Way, Cambridge, MA 02138 (SAN 208-3426) Tel 617-495-3432; Fax: 617-496-3584; Toll Free: 800-513-0763 Do not confuse with Harvard Education Letter, Cambridge, MA
E-mail: hepg@harvard.edu
Web site: http://gseweb.harvard.edu/~hepg.

Harvard Terrace HC, *(Harvard Terrace Health Care; 0-9631469),* 321 Indian Hill Dr., Buffalo Grove, IL 60089-1902.

Harvard Ukrainian, *(Harvard Ukrainian Research Institute; 0-916458),* 1583 Massachusetts Ave., Cambridge, MA 02138 (SAN 208-967X) Tel 617-495-4053; 617-496-8768; Fax: 617-495-8097
E-mail: huri@fas.harvard.edu
Web site: http://www.huri.harvard.edu
Dist(s): **HUP** *(Harvard Univ. Pr.).*

Harvest, *(Harvest Publishing; 0-9638366),* P.O. Box 33270, Northglenn, CO 80233-3270 Tel 303-404-9612; Fax: 303-404-9542 Do not confuse with Harvest Publishing, Traverse City, MI
Web site: http://bookzone.com/freethruhealth/order.html.

Harvest Bks Imprint of Harcourt

Harvest Hse, *(Harvest Hse. Pubs.; 0-7369; 0-89081; 1-56507),* 990 Owens Loop, N., Eugene, OR 97402-9173 (SAN 207-4745) Tel 541-343-0123; Fax: 541-342-6410; Toll Free: 888-501-6991
Web site: http://www.harvesthousepubl.com.

Harwood Acad Pubs Imprint of Gordon & Breach

Haskell, *See* **M S G Haskell Hse**

Hastings, *See* **Hastings Hse**

†Hastings Ctr, *(Hastings Ctr.; 0-916558),* Route 9D, Garrison, NY 10524 (SAN 208-6980) Tel 914-424-4040; Fax: 914-424-4545
E-mail: mail@thehastingscenter.org
Web site: http://www.thehastingscenter.org; *CIP.*

Hastings Hse, *(Hastings Hse. Daytrips Pubs.; 0-8038),* 2601 Wells Ave., Suite 161, Fern Park, FL 32730 Tel 203-838-4083; Fax: 203-838-4084; Toll Free: 800-206-7822
E-mail: hhousebks@aol.com
Web site: http://www.daytripsbooks.com; http://www.hastingshousebooks.com
Dist(s): **Midpt Trade** *(Midpoint Trade Bks., Inc.)* **Natl Bk Netwk** *(National Bk. Network).*

Hatch Creek, *(Hatch Creek Publishing; 0-9663946),* Orders Addr.: 4911 Baker Street Extension, No. 29, Ashville, NY 14710 Tel 716-763-1009
E-mail: bonnie@hatchcreek; bcrand@cecomet.net
Web site: http://www.hatchcreek.com.

Hatherleigh, *(Hatherleigh Co., Ltd., The; 1-57826; 1-886330),* 5-22 46th Ave., Suite 200, Long Island City, NY 11101-5215 (SAN 298-878X) Tel 212-832-1584; Fax: 212-832-1502; Toll Free: 800-367-2550 ; *Imprints:* Red Brick (Red Brick Press) Five Star Pub (Five Star Publishing)
E-mail: info@hatherleigh.com
Web site: http://www.hatherleigh.com; http://www.getfitnow.com
Dist(s): **Norton** *(Norton, W.W. & Co., Inc.).*

Hatier Pub, *(Hatier Publishing),* Subs. of Groupe Hatier International, c/o Schoenhof's Foreign Bks., 486 Green St., Cambridge, MA 02139 (SAN 122-7963) Tel 617-547-8855; Fax: 617-547-8551
E-mail: hatier@schoenhofs.com
Web site: http://www.schoenhofs.com.

Haven Pubns, *(Haven Pubns.; 0-930586),* G.P.O. Box 8101, New York, NY 10116-8101 (SAN 220-6293) Tel 212-663-1787.

Hawaii Hlth Pubs, *(Hawaii Health Pubs.; 0-9646538),* 1415 Victoria St., Suite 1106, Honolulu, HI 96822-3663 Tel 808-536-4006; Toll Free: 800-408-7884
E-mail: ruthheidrich@juno.com
Web site: http://www.ironlady.com.

Hawkes Pub Inc, *See* **Liahona Pub Trust**

Haworth Clinical Imprint of Haworth Pr

Haworth Herbal Pr Imprint of Haworth Pr

Haworth Info Pr Imprint of Haworth Pr

†**Haworth Jrnl Co-Edits,** *(Haworth Pr. Journal Co-Editions; 1-56022),* Affil. of Haworth Pr., 10 Alice St., Binghamton, NY 13904-1580 (SAN 211-0156) Tel 607-722-5857; Fax: 607-722-6362; 607-722-1424; Toll Free Fax: 800-895-0582; Toll Free: 800-429-6784 (800-HAWORTH)
E-mail: getinfo@haworthpressinc.com
Web site: http://www.haworthpressinc.com; *CIP.*

Haworth Pastrl Imprint of Haworth Pr

†**Haworth Pr,** *(Haworth Pr., Inc., The; 0-7890; 0-86656; 0-917724; 1-56022; 1-56023; 1-56024),* 10 Alice St., Binghamton, NY 13904-1580 (SAN 211-0156) Tel 607-722-5857; Fax: 607-722-6362; 607-722-1424; Toll Free Fax: 800-895-0582; Toll Free: 800-429-6784 ; *Imprints:* Pharmctl Prods (Pharmaceutical Products Press) Hawrth Medical (Haworth Medical Press) Haworth Pastrl (Haworth Pastoral Press) Maltreatment & Trauma Pr (Haworth Maltreatment & Trauma Press, The) Haworth Info Pr (Haworth Information Press, The) Harrington Park (Harrington Park Press) Haworth Clinical (Haworth Clinical Practice Press) Haworth Herbal Pr (Haworth Herbal Press, The) PPP (P P P) HSWPP (Haworth Social Work Practice Press, The) Integrative Healing Pr (Haworth Integrative Healing Press, The)
E-mail: getinfo@haworthpressinc.com
Web site: http://www.haworthpressinc.com
Dist(s): **Barnes & Noble Inc** *(Barnes & Noble, Inc.)* **Bookazine Co Inc** *(Bookazine Co., Inc.)* **Bookpeople** *(Bookpeople)* **Borders Inc** *(Borders, Inc.)* **Distributors** *(Distributors, The)* **Koen Bk Distributors** *(Koen Bk. Distributors)* **Matthews Medical Bk Co** *(Matthews Medical Bk. Co.)* **New Leaf Dist** *(New Leaf Distributing Co., Inc.)* **Quality Bks IL** *(Quality Bks., Inc.)* **Rittenhouse** *(Rittenhouse Bk. Distributors)* **SPD-Small Pr Dist** *(SPD-Small Pr. Distribution)* **Unique Bks Inc** *(Unique Bks., Inc.)* **Waldenbooks Co Inc** *(Waldenbooks Co., Inc.); CIP.*

Hawrth Medical Imprint of Haworth Pr

Hawthorn Press (GBR) *(0-9507062; 1-869890; 1-903458) Dist. by* **Anthroposophic.**

Hawthorne Educ Servs, *(Hawthorne Educational Services; 1-878372),* 800 Gray Oak, Columbia, MO 65201 Tel 573-874-1710; Fax: 573-442-9509; Toll Free: 800-542-1673 (orders only)
E-mail: adina_laird@hes-inc.com
Web site: http://www.hes-inc.com.

†**Hay House,** *(Hay Hse., Inc.; 0-937611; 0-945923; 1-56170; 1-891751; 1-58825; 1-4019),* Orders Addr.: P.O. Box 5100, Carlsbad, CA 92018-5100 (SAN 630-477X) Tel 760-431-7695 (ext.112); Fax: 760-431-6948; Toll Free Fax: 800-650-5115 (orders only); Toll Free: 800-654-5126 (orders only); Edit Addr.: 2776 Loker Ave., W., Carlsbad, CA 92008 ; *Imprints:* Hay Hse Lifestyles (Hay House Lifestyles)
E-mail: jkramer@hayhouse.com
Web site: http://www.hayhouse.com; *CIP.*

Hay Hse Lifestyles Imprint of Hay House

Hayden-McNeil, *(Hayden-McNeil Publishing, Inc.; 0-7380; 1-57182; 1-881592),* 47461 Clipper St., Plymouth, MI 48170-2470 Tel 734-455-7900; Fax: 734-455-3901
E-mail: orders@hupublishing.com
Web site: http://www.hmpub.com.

Hayes, *(Hayes Publishing Co., Inc.; 0-910728),* 6304 Hamilton Ave., Cincinnati, OH 45224 (SAN 277-6154) Tel 513-681-7559; Fax: 513-681-9298
E-mail: hayespub@aol.com
Web site: http://www.hayespub.tripod.com/catalog/orders.

Haymkt-Doyma, *(Haymarket-Doyma, Inc.; 0-937716),* Affil. of Medical Pubns., 170 Broadway, Rm. 1612, New York, NY 10038-4154 (SAN 658-4020) Tel 212-766-4300.

Haypenny Pr, *(Haypenny Pr.; 0-929885),* 32 Forest St., New Britain, CT 06052-1425 (SAN 250-9571) Fax: 860-832-9566
E-mail: ipsiverba@aol.com.

†**Hazelden,** *(Hazelden Information & Educational Services; 0-89486; 0-89638; 0-935908; 0-942421; 1-56246; 1-56838),* 15251 Pleasant Valley Rd., P.O. Box 176, Center City, MN 55012-0176 (SAN 209-4010) Tel 651-257-4010; Fax: 651-213-4577; Toll Free: 800-328-0094 ; *Imprints:* HazeldenJohnson Inst (Hazelden/Johnson Institute) Hazelden-Pittman (Hazelden-Pittman Archives Press)
E-mail: bgreydanus@hazelden.org
Web site: http://www.hazelden.org; *CIP.*

HazeldenJohnson Inst Imprint of Hazelden

Hazelden-Pittman Imprint of Hazelden

Hazelwood Pr, *(Hazelwood Pr., The; 0-9643012),* 2633 Hazelwood Rd., Lancaster, PA 17601 Tel 717-569-8864
E-mail: jascoll@supernet.com.

HBJ College Pubs, *See* **Harcourt Coll Pubs**

HC Info Res, *(HC Information Resources; 0-9649926; 1-930488),* Orders Addr.: P.O. Box 2109, Fallbrook, CA 92088-2109 Tel 760-451-1020; Fax: 619-839-3166; Toll Free Fax: 800-290-1967; Toll Free: 800-801-8050; Edit Addr.: 125 S. Main, Suite E, Box 2109, Fallbrook, CA 92028
E-mail: hcinfo@hcinfo.com
Web site: http://www.hcinfo.com.

HCF NRF, *(HCF Nutrition Research Foundation, Inc.; 0-922859),* Orders Addr.: P.O. Box 22124, Lexington, KY 40522 (SAN 251-4575) Tel 606-276-3119; Edit Addr.: 258 Plaza Dr., Suite 208, Lexington, KY 40503 (SAN 251-4583).

HCI Pr, *(HCI Pr.; 0-938863),* P.O. Box 780316, Orlando, FL 32878-1225
E-mail: hcihilsher@aol.com.

HCIA, *See* **Solucient**

HCS Pubns, *(HCS Pubns.; 0-9639835),* Orders Addr.: P.O. Box 781982, Dallas, TX 75378 Tel 214-357-7864; Fax: 214-357-7883; Edit Addr.: 11218 Wonderland, Suite A, Dallas, TX 75229
Dist(s): **Baker & Taylor** *(Baker & Taylor Bks.)* **J Majors Co** *(Majors, J. A. Co.)* **Rittenhouse** *(Rittenhouse Bk. Distributors).*

HDI Pubs, *(HDI Pubs.; 1-882855),* P.O. Box 131401, Houston, TX 77219 Tel 713-682-8700; Fax: 713-956-2288; Toll Free: 800-321-7037
E-mail: cwhaynes@hdipub.com
Dist(s): **Baker & Taylor** *(Baker & Taylor Bks.).*

HDSO Wkshps, *See* **Fibromyalgia Solns**

Head & Neck, *(American Head & Neck Society; 0-9675702),* 203 Lothrop St., Suite 519, Pittsburgh, PA 15213 Tel 412-674-2227; Fax: 412-647-8944
E-mail: rlwa@med.pitt.edu.

Headline Bk Pub (GBR) *(0-7472) Dist. by* **Trafalgar.**

Heal Arts VT Imprint of Inner Tradit

Healing Arts Comns, *(Healing Arts Communications; 0-9653873; 0-9705556),* Orders Addr.: P.O. Box 1440, Jacksonville, OR 97530 Tel 541-858-9664; Fax: 541-858-6696; Toll Free: 888-846-7008; Edit Addr.: 33 N. Central, No. 211, Medford, OR 97501
E-mail: info@Homecarecompanion.com; Marion@Homecarecompanion.com
Web site: http://www.homecarecompanion.com.

Healing Arts Therapies, *(Healing Arts Therapies; 0-9656189),* 6680 Alhambra Ave., No. 265, Martinez, CA 94553-6105 Tel 510-937-9566; Fax: 510-932-5776.

Healing Bks, *(Healing Bks., Inc.; 0-9659267),* 180 W. Germantown Pike, Suite B1, Norristown, PA 19401 Tel 610-277-1990; Fax: 610-277-2007; Toll Free: 800-637-8977
E-mail: uei@bellatlantic.net
Web site: http://www.nervepain.com.

Healing Connect, *(Healing Connection, The; 1-888674),* 62 Windsor Mews, Cherry Hill, NJ 08002-2435 Tel 609-667-7705; Fax: 609-482-5929.

Healing Place CA, *(Healing Place Productions; 0-9707950),* 1835A S. Centre City Pkwy., No. 417, Escondido, CA 92025-6504 Tel 760-739-9530; Fax: 760-739-9186 Do not confuse with Healing Place Productions, Inc. in Baton Rouge, LA
E-mail: kate@about-books.com.

Healing Wisdom, *(Healing Wisdom Pubns.; 0-9647080),* Div. of Klabin Computer & Marketing Consultants, Ltd., Inc., 2067 Broadway, Suite 700, New York, NY 10023 Tel 212-877-3632; Fax: 212-580-4329; Toll Free: 800-933-9440.

Healing Within Prods, *(Healing Within Products; 0-9616184),* Orders Addr.: P.O. Box 1013, Larkspur, CA 94977-1013 (SAN 658-327X); Edit Addr.: 84 Berkeley Ave., San Anselmo, CA 94960-1449 (SAN 658-3261) Tel 415-454-6677 Do not confuse with Healing Within in Hartwell, GA
Dist(s): **Assoc Pubs Grp** *(Associated Pubs. Group).*

Health & Allied, *(Health & Allied Science Pubs.; 0-943589),* Orders Addr.: P.O. Box 6036, Rutland, VT 05702-6036 (SAN 668-646X).

Health Act Pr, *(Health Action Pr.; 0-913571),* Subs. of Center for Health Action, 6439 Taggart Rd., Delaware, OH 43015 (SAN 285-2691) Tel 614-548-5340; Fax: 614-548-0388.

†**Health Admin Pr,** *(Health Administration Pr.; 0-910701; 0-914904; 1-56793),* Div. of Foundation of the American College of Healthcare Executives, Orders Addr.: 1 North Franklin, Chicago, IL 60606-3491 (SAN 241-7154) Tel 312-845-9869; Fax: 312-424-0703; Edit Addr.: 1 North Franklin, Suite 1700, Chicago, IL 60606-3491 (SAN 207-0464) Tel 312-424-2800; Fax: 312-424-0014
Web site: http://www.ache.org/hap.html; *CIP.*

Health Care NJ, *(Health Care Communications, Inc.; 0-945986),* 1 Bridge Plaza, Suite 350, Fort Lee, NJ 07024 (SAN 248-1014) Tel 201-947-5545; Fax: 201-947-8406.

Health Choice, *(Health Choice Productions; 0-9655715),* 2554 Lincoln Blvd., Suite 484, Marina Del Rey, CA 90291 Tel 310-841-5163; Fax: 310-821-9478.

†**Health Comm,** *(Health Communications, Inc.; 0-922352; 0-932194; 0-941405; 1-55874; 1-880257; 0-7573),* 3201 SW 15th St., Deerfield Beach, FL 33442-8157 (SAN 212-100X) Tel 954-360-0909; Fax: 954-360-0034; Toll Free: 800-851-9100 Do not confuse with Health Communications, Inc., Edison, NJ
E-mail: hci@hcibooks.com
Web site: http://www.hcibooks.com
Dist(s): **Continental Bk** *(Continental Bk. Co., Inc.)* **Lndmrk Audiobks** *(Landmark Audiobooks); CIP.*

Health Digest, *(Health Digest Bks.; 1-882657),* Orders Addr.: P.O. Box 1100, Cannon Beach, OR 97110-1100 Tel 760-731-1292; Fax: 760-731-1225; Edit Addr.: 620 N. Elm St., Cannon Beach, OR 97110.

Health Dimensions, *(Health Dimensions of New Jersey; 1-878294),* 1086 Teaneck Rd., Teaneck, NJ 07666-4838 Tel 201-224-3700; Fax: 201-224-9468.

Health Ed & Life Exp Res, *(Health Education & Life Expansion Research; 0-9607142),* Box 70309, Los Angeles, CA 90070 (SAN 238-9878) Tel 213-738-9940.

Health Ed Consults, *(Health Education Consultants; 1-891330),* Orders Addr.: P.O. Box 22593, Kansas City, MO 64113 Tel 913-831-1393; Fax: 913-831-7605; Edit Addr.: 4600 Madison, Suite 600, Kansas City, MO 64112 Do not confuse with Health Education Consultants, Lakewood, OH
E-mail: hec@sky.net
Web site: http://health-ed-consultants.org.

Health Ed Pubns, *(Health Educator Pubns., Inc.; 0-932887),* 63 Gould Rd., Orono, ME 04473 (SAN 689-0059) Tel 207-262-0123
E-mail: DOakesDO@aol.com
Web site: http://www.healthedpub.com.

Health Ed Res Intl, *(Health Education Resources-International; 1-882136),* 10407 Barwood Dr., Houston, TX 77043 (SAN 248-5648) Tel 281-468-7828.

Health Ed Train, *(Health Education Training & Administration Consortium, Inc., The; 0-911067),* 86 Versailles, Cincinnati, OH 45240-3856 (SAN 270-711X) Tel 513-851-5210.

Health Facts Pub, *(Health Facts Publishing; 0-9626145),* Subs. of Consumer Health Information Research Institute, 300 E. Pink Hill Rd., Independence, MO 64057-3220 Tel 816-753-8850.

Health Hope, *See* **Health Digest**

Health Info Pr Imprint of Practice Mgmt Info

Health InfoNet Inc, *(Health InfoNet, Inc.; 1-57810; 1-885274),* 231 Market Pl., No. 331, San Ramon, CA 94583 Tel 925-358-4370; Fax: 925-358-4377; Toll Free: 800-446-1947
E-mail: HINBooks@aol.com; logo47@aol.com
Web site: http://www.hinbooks.com.

Health Ins Assn Am, *(Health Insurance Assn. of America; 1-879143),* 555 13th St. NW, Suite 600 E., Washington, DC 20004-1109 (SAN 224-8131) Tel 202-824-1840; Fax: 202-824-1800; Fulfillment Addr.: 9050 Junction Dr., Annapolis Junction, MD 20701 Tel 301-317-4422; Fax: 301-206-9789; Toll Free: 800-828-0111
Web site: http://www.hiaa.org.

Health Life, *(Health for Life; 0-944831),* Div. of JPR Enterprises, 13352 Beach Ave., Marina del Rey, CA 90292 (SAN 245-7296) Tel 310-306-0777; Fax: 310-305-7672; Toll Free: 800-874-5339.

Health Now, *(Health Now; 0-9638768),* P.O. Box 60126, Sunnyvale, CA 94088-0126 Fax: 800-242-5665; Toll Free: 888-752-9457.

Health Plus, *(Health Plus, Pubs.; 0-932090),* Div. of Airola, Inc., P.O. Box 1027, Sherwood, OR 97140 (SAN 211-4984) Tel 503-625-0589; Fax: 503-625-1525
E-mail: airola@cyberhighway.net
Web site: http://www.cyberhighway.net/~airola
Dist(s): **Baker & Taylor** *(Baker & Taylor Bks.)*
Nutri-Books Corp *(Nutri-Bks. Corp.).*

Health Pr (GBR) *(1-899541; 1-903734) Dist. by* **JAMCO Dist.**

Health Press, *(Health Pr.; 0-929173),* P.O. Box 1388, Santa Fe, NM 87504 (SAN 248-5036) Tel 505-474-0303; Fax: 505-424-0444
E-mail: goodbooks@healthpress.com
Web site: http://www.healthpress.com.

Health Pubng, *See* **Time Inc Health**

Health Res Las Vegas, *(Health Research; 0-9601978),* Box 19420, Las Vegas, NV 89132 (SAN 212-2553) Tel 702-733-8476.

Health Sci Imprint of Addison-Wesley

Health Sci Comm, *(Health Sciences Communications Assn.),* 6728 Old McLean Village Dr., McLean, VA 22101-3906 (SAN 224-2915) Tel 314-725-4722.

Health Studies, *(Health Studies Institute, Inc.; 1-879772),* P.O. Box 6808, Deerfield Beach, FL 33442-6808 Tel 954-917-1950; Fax: 954-917-1988; Toll Free: 800-700-3454
E-mail: hsimail@healthstudies.com; rauzin@healthstudies.com
Web site: http://www.healthstudies.com
Dist(s): **J Majors Co** *(Majors, J. A. Co.).*

Health Trend, *(Health Trend Publishing; 0-9619329),* P.O. Box 7390, Menlo Park, CA 94026 (SAN 243-8941) Tel 415-462-1881 Do not confuse with companies with similar names in Marion, MA, Bethesda, MD.

Health Water Res, *(Healthy Water Research; 0-9617432),* P.O. Box 173, Portsmouth, NH 03802-0173 (SAN 200-8378) Tel 207-439-7647; Fax: 207-439-0936
E-mail: mfox@nh.ultranet.com; mfox@healthywater.com
Web site: http://www.healthywater.com.

Health Wealth Found, *(Health Is Wealth Foundation, Inc.; 0-9701658),* 19106 Clover Meadow Pl., Gaithersburg, MD 20879 Tel 301-916-8982 (phone/fax); Toll Free: 800-204-0511
E-mail: hiwfound@aol.com.

Health Wellness Studios Imprint of Delgado

Healthcare Info, *(Healthcare Information & Management Systems Society; 0-9704287; 0-9715301),* 230 E. Ohio St., Suite 500, Chicago, IL 60611 Tel 312-664-4467; Fax: 312-664-6143
E-mail: himss@himss.org
Web site: http://www.himss.org.

Healthcare Pr, *(Healthcare Pr.; 0-9613775),* Orders Addr.: P.O. Box 4488, Rollingbay, WA 98061 (SAN 678-9749) Tel 206-842-5243; Edit Addr.: 11504 Logg Rd., NE, Bainbridge Island, WA 98110 (SAN 241-9904)
E-mail: eringland@aol.com.

Healthcare Sys, *(Healthcare Technology Systems, LLC; 0-9702974),* 7617 Mineral Point Rd., Suite 300, Madison, WI 53713 Tel 608-827-2481; Fax: 608-827-2444; Toll Free: 800-316-2414
E-mail: brank@healthtechsys.com
Web site: http://www.healthtechsys.com.

HealthComm, *See* **HealthComm Intl**

HealthComm Intl, *(HealthComm International, Inc.; 0-9624859),* Orders Addr.: P.O. Box 1729, Gig Harbor, WA 98335 Tel 253-851-3943; Fax: 253-851-9749; Edit Addr.: 5800 Soundview Dr., Gig Harbor, WA 98335 (SAN 299-3996).

HealthFirst Pr, *(HealthFirst Pr.; 0-9666373),* 311 Miller Ave., Mill Valley, CA 94941 Tel 415-487-6131; Fax: 415-487-6195.

HealthMasters, *(HealthMasters; 0-9632923),* 2800 Fourth St., N., No. 124, Saint Petersburg, FL 33704-2102.

HealthNet Pages, *(HealthNet Pages, Inc.; 1-879657),* Div. of South Florida Rehab & Healthcare Directory, 53106 Commerce Pkwy., Miramar, FL 33025-3943 Tel 305-948-3001; Fax: 305-948-3943; Toll Free: 800-486-7352 ; *Imprints:* Nedmar Graphics (Nedmar Graphics, Incorporated).

Healthnet Pr, *(Healthnet Pr.; 0-9616475),* Orders Addr.: P.O. Box 24906, Winston-Salem, NC 27114 (SAN 666-7058); Edit Addr.: P.O. Box 24906, Winston-Salem, NC 27114-4906 (SAN 659-3194) Tel 336-764-3378.

HealthScan, *(HealthScan, Inc.; 0-941932),* 908 Pompton Ave., Unit A2, Cedar Grove, NJ 07009-1252 (SAN 238-4612) Tel 973-239-3139.

HealthSouth, *(HealthSouth Corp.; 1-891525),* 9119 Cinnamon Hill, San Antonio, TX 78240 ; *Imprints:* HealthSouth Pr (HealthSouth Press)
E-mail: rsenelick@aol.com
Web site: http://www.healthsouth.com
Dist(s): **Partners Pubs Grp** *(Partners Pubs. Group, Inc.).*

HealthSouth Pr Imprint of HealthSouth

Healthspirit Pr, *(Healthspirit Pr.; 0-9671247),* Orders Addr.: P.O. Box 806, Clayton, GA 30525 (SAN 299-9250) Tel 706-782-9682; Fax: 706-782-1532; Edit Addr.: 156 N. Main St., Clayton, GA 30525
E-mail: woodard.md@healthspirit.com.

HealthStar Pr, *(HealthStar Pr.; 0-9700588),* P.O. Box 151, Ramsey, IN 47166 Tel 812-633-2297; Fax: 812-633-2346; Toll Free: 866-213-3937
E-mail: phlebotomy@phlebotomy.com
Web site: http://www.phlebotomy.com.

HealthTrac, *(HealthTrac, Inc.; 1-879919),* Orders Addr.: P.O. Box 13599, Tallahassee, FL 32317 Tel 850-561-8722; Fax: 850-561-3422; Toll Free: 800-533-5259; Edit Addr.: 1812 Riggins Rd., Suite B, Tallahassee, FL 32308 Tel 904-877-5110.

Healthwealth, *(Healthwealth International; 0-9614029),* 517 NW 103rd Ave., Fort Lauderdale, FL 33324-1625 (SAN 683-5538) Tel 954-472-0505
E-mail: hlthwlth@aol.com
Web site: http://www.hlthwlth.com.

Healthwise, *(Healthwise, Inc.; 0-9612690; 1-877930),* Orders Addr.: P.O. Box 1989, Boise, ID 83701 (SAN 289-2367) Tel 208-345-1161; Fax: 208-345-1897; Toll Free: 800-706-9646; Edit Addr.: 2601 N. Bogus Basin Rd., Boise, ID 83702 (SAN 289-2375)
E-mail: moreinfo@healthwise.org
Web site: http://www.healthwise.com.

Healthworks, *(Healthworks, Inc.; 0-938480),* 5596 Colstin Rd., Hornbrook, CA 96044-9712 (SAN 215-7721).

HealthWorld, *(HealthWorld, Inc.; 0-9624780),* 1675 Rollins Rd., Suite B3, Burlingame, CA 94010-2320.

HealthWrights, *(HealthWrights; 0-9655585),* 964 Hamilton Ave., Palo Alto, CA 94301 Tel 415-325-7500; Fax: 415-325-1080
E-mail: jweston@healthwrights.org
Web site: http://www.healthwrights.org.

Healthy Wealthy & Wise, *(Healthy, Wealthy & Wise; 0-9657027),* 371 Tamworth Dr., Clemmons, NC 27012 Tel 336-764-5950.

Healthyculture, *(Healthyculture.com; 0-941703),* 115 Dunder Rd., Burlington, VT 05401 (SAN 681-8234) Tel 802-862-8855; Fax: 802-862-6389; Toll Free: 800-800-3004 (phone/fax, orders only)
E-mail: Info@healthyculture.com
Web site: http://www.healthyculture.com.

Hear Again, *(Hear Again; 0-9664780),* 1200 Madison Ave., Austin, TX 78767 Tel 512-479-9300; Fax: 512-472-1558
E-mail: hearagain@beacon.moontower.com
Web site: http://www.hearagainpublishing.com.

Hear You Are, *See* **The Davis Ctr**

Hearcare, *(Hearcare, Inc.; 0-9632001),* a/o John G. Clark, 5963 Glenway Ave., Cincinnati, OH 45238-2040 Tel 513-661-4327.

Hearing & Speech, *(Hearing & Speech Institute; 0-9618297; 1-883204),* 3515 SW Veterans Hospital Rd., Portland, OR 97201 (SAN 667-402X) Tel 503-228-6479; Fax: 503-228-4248; Toll Free: 877-702-2828
Web site: http://www.hearingandspeech.org
Dist(s): **Butte Pubns** *(Butte Pubns., Inc.)*
Imaginart Intl *(Imaginart International, Inc.).*

†Hearst Bks, *(Hearst Bks.; 0-688; 0-87851; 0-910990; 0-910992),* Div. of Hearst Communications, Inc., Orders Addr.: P.O. Box 1219, Fairfield, NJ 07007 (SAN 202-5779) Tel 973-227-7200; Toll Free: 800-237-0657; Edit Addr.: 1350 Avenue of Americas, New York, NY 10019 (SAN 202-2842) Tel 212-261-6500; Fax: 212-261-6599; *CIP.*

Heart Gallery, *(Heart Gallery Pr.; 1-928888),* 603 Seventh St., S., Suite 400, Saint Petersburg, FL 33701 Tel 727-824-8346; Fax: 727-824-8312; 900 Central Ave., Saint Petersburg, FL 33705
E-mail: mcurran@sagonet.net.

Heart in Hand Inc, *(Heart in Hand, Inc.; 0-9619445),* Orders Addr.: P.O. Box 170, Clifton, VA 22024 (SAN 244-6308); Edit Addr.: 7145 Main St., Clifton, VA 22024 (SAN 244-6316) Tel 703-830-4111.

Heart-Bound Bks, *(Heart-Bound Bks.; 0-9629092),* 4020 Meadowridge Dr., Charlotte, NC 28226.

Heartland Inst, *(Heartland Institute; 0-9632027),* 19 S. La Salle St., Suite 903, Chicago, IL 60603-1405 Tel 312-377-4000
E-mail: think@heartland.org
Web site: http://www.heartland.org
Dist(s): **Natl Bk Netwk** *(National Bk. Network).*

Hearts Desire, *(Heart's Desire; 0-9642424),* P.O. Box 187, Madison, NH 03849-0187 Tel 603-367-4374; Fax: 603-447-3655.

HeartWatchers Pr, *(HeartWatchers Pr.; 0-9619796),* Div. of HeartWatchers International, Inc., 32505 Woodsdale Ln., Solon, OH 44139-1340 (SAN 246-2451) Tel 216-349-1197.

Heaton Pubns, *(Heaton Pubns.; 1-881057),* 600 College St., Albertville, AL 35950 Tel 205-878-0986; Fax: 205-891-3508; Toll Free Fax: 800-553-5635; Toll Free: 800-221-2469
E-mail: sales@heaton.org
Web site: http://www.heaton.org.

Heaven Earth, *See* **HEAVEN-ON-EARTH**

HEAVEN-ON-EARTH, *(HEAVEN-ON-EARTH-NOW.COM; 1-892177),* Orders Addr.: P.O. Box 398, Hanalei, HI 96714; Edit Addr.: 258 S. Hummingbird Ln., Rocky Point, NC 28457 ; *Imprints:* Lightning Source (Lightning Source) Do not confuse with companies with same or similar names in Westminster, CA, Washington, DC, Indianapolis, IN, Baraboo, WI, Hanalei, HI, Anahola, HI
E-mail: i-am@heaven-on-earth-now.com
Web site: http://www.IAMLOVE.TV; http://www.heaven-on-earth-now.com.

HEBS, *(Human Ecology Balancing Sciences; 0-945262),* P.O. Box 21091, Sedona, AZ 86341 (SAN 246-1854) Tel 520-203-0689; Fax: 520-203-0987
E-mail: hebs@sedona.net
Web site: http://www.wellatlast.com
Dist(s): **Baker & Taylor** *(Baker & Taylor Bks.)*
New Leaf Dist *(New Leaf Distributing Co., Inc.).*

Hefty Pr, *(Hefty Pr., The; 0-9653999),* 10480 SW 70th Ave., Miami, FL 33156 Tel 305-661-8849; Fax: 305-661-1613
E-mail: Rdowd01@msn.com
Dist(s): **BookWorld** *(BookWorld Services, Inc.).*

Heian Intl, *(Heian International Publishing, Inc.; 0-89346),* 1815 W. 205th St., Suite 301, Torrance, CA 90501-1518 (SAN 213-2036) Tel 310-782-6268; Fax: 310-782-6269
E-mail: heianemail@heian.com
Web site: http://www.heian.com
Dist(s): **Cheng & Tsui** *(Cheng & Tsui Co.)*
Shens Bks *(Shen's Bks.)*
Weatherhill *(Weatherhill, Inc.).*

Heidenreich, *(Heidenreich Hse.; 0-9600428),* 5012 Oak Point Way, Fair Oaks, CA 95628 (SAN 204-0395) Tel 916-961-3297.

†**Heinemann,** *(Heinemann; 0-325; 0-435),* Div. of Greenwood Publishing Group, Inc., Orders Addr.: P.O. Box 5007, Westport, CT 06881-5007 Toll Free: 800-793-2154; Edit Addr.: 88 Post Rd., W., Westport, CT 06881-5007 (SAN 210-5829) Tel 603-431-7894; Fax: 603-431-7840
E-mail: info@heinemann.com
Web site: http://www.heinemann.com
Dist(s): **Natl Bk Netwk** *(National Bk. Network); CIP.*

Heinemann Ed, *See* **Heinemann**

Heinemann Lib, *(Heinemann Library; 0-431; 1-57572; 1-58810; 1-4034),* Div. of Reed Elsevier, Orders Addr.: P.O. Box 1650, Crystal Lake, IL 60039-1650 Toll Free Fax: 888-844-5329; Toll Free: 888-454-2279; Edit Addr.: 100 N. LaSalle St., Suite 300, Chicago, IL 60602 Tel 312-827-1000; Fax: 312-845-1030; Toll Free: 888-475-7038
E-mail: sheryl.gafka@rigby.com; sgafka@rigby-edue.com
Web site: http://www.heinemannlibrary.com/
Dist(s): **Lectorum Pubns** *(Lectorum Pubns., Inc.).*

Heirloom Memories, *(Heirloom Memories, Inc.; 0-9663273),* 351 Carrera Dr., Mill Valley, CA 94941 Tel 415-381-2900; Fax: 415-381-3160; Toll Free: 800-762-2986
E-mail: rubyshoe@sirius.com
Web site: http://www.heirloommemories.com.

Helen Keller Intl, *(Keller, Helen International; 0-915173),* 90 West St. No. 2, New York, NY 10006 (SAN 224-2699) Tel 212-943-0890; Fax: 212-943-1220
Web site: http://www.hki.org/world.html.

Helix Pr, *(Helix Pr.; 0-914587),* 4410 Hickey, Corpus Christi, TX 78413 (SAN 289-2669) Tel 512-852-8834.

Helm Seminars, *(Helm Seminars; 0-9631033),* Orders Addr.: P.O. Box 2105, Lake Dallas, TX 75065 Tel 940-497-3558; Edit Addr.: 5 Hickory Hills Blvd., Lake Dallas, TX 75065.

Help Yourself, *(Help Yourself Pubns.; 0-9652193),* 1280 S. Alhambra Cir., Apt. 2301, Coral Gables, FL 33146-3132.

Hem Of His Garment, *(Hem Of His Garment; 0-9641901),* P.O. Box 14883, Surfside Beach, SC 29587-4883 Tel 843-650-8249.

Hemed Bks, *See* **Lambda Pubs**

†**Hemisp Pub,** *(Hemisphere Publishing Corp.; 0-89116; 1-56032),* Member of Taylor & Francis Group, Orders Addr.: 325 Chestnut St., 8th Flr., Philadelphia, PA 19106 Fax: 215-269-0363; Toll Free: 800-821-8312
Dist(s): **McGraw** *(McGraw-Hill Cos., The)*
Taylor & Francis *(Taylor & Francis, Inc.); CIP.*

Henderson Pr, *(Henderson Pr.; 0-9620330),* 5 Bee, S. Main, Henderson, KY 42420 (SAN 248-2762) Tel 502-826-2586.

†**Hendrickson MA,** *(Hendrickson Pubs., Inc.; 0-913573; 0-917006; 0-943575; 1-56563),* Orders Addr.: P.O. Box 3473, Peabody, MA 01961-3473 (SAN 285-2772) Tel 978-532-6546; Fax: 978-531-8146; Toll Free: 800-358-3111; Edit Addr.: 140 Summit St., Peabody, MA 01960-3203 (SAN 663-6594) Fax: 978-573-8414 Do not confuse with Hendrickson Group, Sandy Hook, CT
E-mail: pmurdoch@hendrickson.com
Web site: http://www.hendrickson.com; *CIP.*

Henninger Prod, *(Henninger Productions; 0-9703265),* 2601-A Wilson Blvd., Arlington, VA 22201 Tel 703-243-3444; Fax: 703-243-4023 ; *Imprints:* Time Life (Time Life Video)
Web site: http://www.henninger.com.

†**Herald Press,** *(Herald Pr.; 0-8361),* Div. of Mennonite Publishing Hse., Inc., 616 Walnut Ave., Scottdale, PA 15683-1999 (SAN 202-2915) Tel 724-887-8500; Fax: 724-887-3111; Toll Free: 800-245-7894 (orders only) Do not confuse with Herald Pr., Charlotte, NC
E-mail: hp@mph.org
Web site: http://www.mph.org
Dist(s): **Baker & Taylor** *(Baker & Taylor Bks.)*
Spring Arbor Dist *(Spring Arbor Distributors Inc.); CIP.*

†**Herald Pub Hse,** *(Herald Publishing Hse.; 0-8309),* P.O. Box 390, Independence, MO 64051-0390 Tel 816-252-5010; Fax: 816-252-3976; Toll Free: 800-767-8181; 1001W. Walnut St., Independence, MO 64051-0390 (SAN 111-7556) ; *Imprints:* Indep Pr (Independence Press)
E-mail: hhmark@heraldhouse.org
Web site: http://www.heraldhouse.org; *CIP.*

Herb Studies, *See* **Herb Studies Library**

Herb Studies Library, *(Herbal Studies Library; 0-9620838; 1-879687),* Orders Addr.: P.O. Box 225336, San Francisco, CA 94122-5336 Tel 415-564-6785; Fax: 415-564-6799; Edit Addr.: 219 Carl St., San Francisco, CA 94117-3804 (SAN 249-8480) ; *Imprints:* J R Herb Pubns (Rose, Jeanne Herbal Publications)
E-mail: hydrosol@yahoo.com
Web site: http://aromaticplantproject.com/jeannerose/.

Herbal Free, *(Herbal Free Pr., Ltd.; 0-9639297),* P.O. Box 1883, Brattleboro, VT 05302-1883 (SAN 298-5292) Tel 802-254-1337; Fax: 802-254-0396; Toll Free: 800-903-9104.

†**HERC Pubng,** *(H E R C, Publishing; 0-916999),* Orders Addr.: P.O. Box 30090, Lincoln, NE 68503 (SAN 655-6418) Tel 402-486-0622; Fax: 402-486-0626; *CIP.*

Herit Global, *(Heritage Global Publishing; 0-9669096),* 908 Innergary Pl., Valrico, FL 33594 (SAN 299-8092).

Herit Pubns, *(Heritage Pubns.; 1-882545),* Orders Addr.: P.O. Box 71, Virginia Beach, VA 23458 Tel 757-428-0100; Fax: 757-428-3632; Toll Free: 800-329-2292 Do not confuse with companies with the same name in Gunterville AL, Arkville NY, Kirkwood, MO, Hendrum, MN
Dist(s): **New Leaf Dist** *(New Leaf Distributing Co., Inc.).*

Herit Pubs AZ, *(Heritage Pubs., Inc.; 0-929690),* 5312 N. 12th St., Suite 302, Phoenix, AZ 85014 (SAN 249-9460) Tel 602-277-4780; Fax: 602-277-1659; Toll Free: 800-972-8507
E-mail: info@heritagepublishers.com; heritage@amug.org
Web site: http://www.heritagepublishers.com.

Heritage Assocs, *(Heritage Assocs., Inc.; 0-910467),* Orders Addr.: P.O. Box 6291, Albuquerque, NM 87197 (SAN 260-0706); Edit Addr.: 447 Gavilan, NW, Albuquerque, NM 87106 (SAN 662-0353) Tel 505-268-0155 Do not confuse with companies with the similar or same name in Polson, MT, Fort Valley, VA, Salt Lake City, UT.

Heritage Bk, *(Heritage Bks., Inc.; 0-7884; 0-917890; 1-55613),* 1540 E Pointer Ridge Pl., Bowie, MD 20716-1800 (SAN 209-3367) Tel 301-390-7708; Toll Free Fax: 800-276-1760; Toll Free: 800-398-7709
E-mail: heritagebooks@pipeline.com
Web site: http://www.heritagebooks.com.

Heritage Cinn, *(Heritage Communications; 0-9618291),* 12055 Cooperwood Ln., Cincinnati, OH 45242 (SAN 667-0679) Tel 513-771-2230; Fax: 513-771-5241
E-mail: heritcom@aol.com
Web site: http://www.niblickgolf.com; http://www.cincinnatismiles.com.

Heritage MO, *(Heritage Pubns., Inc.; 0-9625674),* 111 W. Jewel Ave., Kirkwood, MO 63122 Tel 314-822-3796 Do not confuse with companies with the same name in Gunterville, Al, Virginia Beach, VA, Arkville, NY, Hendrum, MN, Hendrum, MN.

Heritage West, *(Heritage West Bks.; 0-9623048),* P.O. Box 357, Keene, CA 93531 Tel 661-823-1888 (phone/fax)
E-mail: orders@heritagewestbooks.com; customerservice@heritagewestbooks.com
Web site: http://www.heritagewestbooks.com
Dist(s): **Amer West Books** *(American West Bks.)*
Baker & Taylor *(Baker & Taylor Bks.)*
Sunbelt Pubns *(Sunbelt Pubns., Inc.).*

Herm Barr Pub, *(Herm-Barr Publishing Co.; 0-944785),* 118 Elmora Ave., Elizabeth, NJ 07202 (SAN 245-4165) Tel 201-354-1000.

HES & DE GRAAF (NLD) *(90-6004; 90-6194) Dist. by* **Coronet Bks.**

†**Hesperian Found,** *(Hesperian Foundation, The; 0-942364),* 1919 Addison St., Suite 304, Berkeley, CA 94704-1144 (SAN 239-8567) Tel 510-845-1447; Fax: 510-845-9141; 510-845-0539; Toll Free: 888-729-1796 Do not confuse with Hesperian Pr., Davenport, IA
E-mail: hesperian@hesperian.org
Web site: http://www.hesperian.org; *CIP.*

Heuston Consult, *(Heuston Consulting, Inc.; 0-9675465),* 9280 E. Thompson Peak Pkwy., Suite 27, Scottsdale, AZ 85255 Tel 480-563-1022; Fax: 480-502-2029
E-mail: mcheu@aol.com.

Hewitt Homeschl Res Imprint of Hewitt Res Fnd

Hewitt Res Fnd, *(Hewitt Research Foundation, Inc.; 0-913717; 1-57896),* Orders Addr.: P.O. Box 9, Washougal, WA 98671 (SAN 286-1852) Tel 360-835-8708; Fax: 360-835-8697; Toll Free: 800-348-1750; Edit Addr.: 2103 B St., Washougal, WA 98671 ; *Imprints:* Hewitt Homeschl Res (Hewitt Homeschooling Resources)
E-mail: hewitths@aol.com
Web site: http://www.homeeducation.org.

Hezel Assocs, *(Hezel Assocs.; 1-889794),* 1201 E. Fayette St., Syracuse, NY 13210 Tel 315-422-3512; Fax: 315-422-3513; Toll Free: 800-466-3512
E-mail: info@hezel.com
Web site: http://www.hezel.com.

HFSI Inc, *(Human Factors in Space Institute, Inc.; 0-9622456),* P.O. Box 25260, Washington, DC 20007-8260.

HI St Primary, *(Hawaii State Primary Care Assn.),* 345 Queen St., Suite 702, Honolulu, HI 96813 Tel 808-536-8442
Dist(s): **UH Pr** *(Univ. of Hawaii Pr.).*

Hibiscus FL, *(Hibiscus Pr.; 0-9647763),* P.O. Box 77066, Coral Springs, FL 33077 (SAN 298-9506) Tel 813-528-8851; Fax: 813-528-8466; Toll Free: 800-356-9315
E-mail: bjd@aol.com
Dist(s): **Quality Bks IL** *(Quality Bks., Inc.)*
Unique Bks Inc *(Unique Bks., Inc.).*

hic pubng, *(h.i.c. publishing; 0-9700443),* P.O. Box 3026, Peterborough, NH 03458 Tel 603-924-6524 (phone/fax).

Hickory Corners, *(Hickory Corners Pr.; 0-925634),* 8324 N. 37th St., Richland, MI 49083 Tel 616-629-9922.

Hickory Grove Pr, *(Hickory Grove Pr.; 0-9628509),* 2030 Whipple Ave. NW, No. 166, Canton, OH 44708-2360 Do not confuse with Hickory Grove Pr., Bellevue, IA.

†**Hid Valley MD,** *(Hidden Valley Pr.; 0-935710),* 7051 Poole Jones Rd., Frederick, MD 21702 (SAN 213-5094) Tel 301-662-6726; Fax: 301-696-1847
E-mail: HVPress@aol.com; *CIP.*

Hidden Springs, *(Hidden Springs Pr.; 1-885113),* P.O. Box 29613, Los Angeles, CA 90029 Tel 213-664-0007; Fax: 213-664-6782; Toll Free: 800-848-5505.

Higginson Bk Co, *(Higginson Bk. Co.; 0-7404; 0-8328),* 148 Washington St., Salem, MA 01970 (SAN 247-9400) Tel 978-745-7170; Fax: 978-745-8025
E-mail: higginsn@cove.com
Web site: http://higginsonbooks.com.

High Desert Mus, *(High Desert Museum, The; 0-9663487),* 59800 S. Hwy. 97, Bend, OR 97702 Tel 541-382-4754; Fax: 541-382-5256
E-mail: tcooper@highdesert.org
Web site: http://www.highdesert.org.

High Light Pub, *(High Light Publishing; 0-9636297),* Orders Addr.: P.O. Box 13778, Albuquerque, NM 87192-3778 Tel 505-821-6883; Edit Addr.: 8420 San Diego Ave., NE, Albuquerque, NM 87122
Dist(s): **Baker & Taylor** *(Baker & Taylor Bks.).*

High Noon Bks, *(High Noon Bks.; 0-87879; 1-57128),* Div. of Academic Therapy Pubns., Inc., 20 Commercial Blvd., Novato, CA 94949-6191 Tel 415-883-3314; Fax: 415-883-3720; Toll Free: 800-422-7249
E-mail: atpub@aol.com
Web site: http://www.atpub.com.

High Oaks Pub, *(High Oaks Publishing Co.; 0-9645773),* Div. of Ctr. Urology of Toledo, Inc., 2000 Regency Ct., Suite 200, Toledo, OH 43623-3075 Tel 419-531-1722; Fax: 419-531-1728.

High Tide Pr, *(High Tide Pr.; 0-9653744; 1-892696),* 3650 W. 183rd St., Homewood, IL 60430-2603 Tel 708-206-2054; Fax: 708-206-2044; Toll Free: 888-487-7377; 800-869-3979 Do not confuse with The Trinity Foundation, Hobbs, NM
E-mail: managing.editor@hightidepress.com; editor1@hightidepress.com
Web site: http://www.hightidepress.com.

Highfield Pubns (GBR) *Dist. by* **St Mut.**

Highlights Opthal (PAN) *(958-95544) Dist. by* **SLACK Inc.**

†**High-Scope,** *(High/Scope Pr.; 0-929816; 0-931114; 1-57379),* Div. of High/Scope Educational Research Foundation, 600 N. River St., Ypsilanti, MI 48198-2898 (SAN 211-9617) Tel 734-485-2000; Fax: 734-485-0704; Toll Free Fax: 800-442-4329 (orders); Toll Free: 800-407-7377 (orders only)
E-mail: info@highscope.org
Web site: http://www.highscope.org; *CIP.*

†**Hill & Wang,** *(Hill & Wang; 0-374; 0-8090),* Div. of Farrar, Straus & Giroux, LLC, 19 Union Sq., W., New York, NY 10003 (SAN 201-9299) Tel 212-741-6900; Fax: 212-633-9385
Dist(s): **VHPS** *(VHPS Holtzbrinck Pubs.); CIP.*

Hill Content Pubng (AUS) *(0-85572) Dist. by* **Seven Hills Bk.**

Hillbilly Bks, *(Hillbilly Bks.; 0-9647202),* Orders Addr.: P.O. Box 430, Old Hickory, TN 37138-2212 Tel 615-391-9988; Edit Addr.: 518 Knapp Farm Dr., Hermitage, TN 37076-1377.

Hillgarth Pr, *(Hillgarth Pr.; 0-940106),* P.O. Box 1440, Lake Placid, NY 12946 (SAN 220-2832) Tel 212-758-6389 (phone/fax); 518-523-1360
E-mail: russellk@sprynet.com
Web site: http://www.lifetalk.org.

Hills Med, *(Hills Medical/Sports),* 4201 Bee Cave Rd., Suite B112, Austin, TX 78746 (SAN 264-097X).

Hillsboro Pr Imprint of Providence Hse

Hilson Res, *(Hilson Research, Inc.; 1-885738),* 82-28 Abingdon Rd., P.O. Box 150239, Kew Gardens, NY 11415-0239 Tel 718-805-0063; Fax: 718-849-6238; Toll Free: 800-926-2258
E-mail: hilsonres@aol.com
Dist(s): **Baker & Taylor** *(Baker & Taylor Bks.).*

Hilton Pubg, *(Hilton Publishing Inc.; 0-9675258; 0-9716067),* Orders Addr.: P.O. Box 737, Roscoe, IL 61073 Tel 815-885-1070; Edit Addr.: 7192 Cauletti Dr., Loves Park, IL 61111
E-mail: info@hiltonpub.com
Web site: http://www.hiltonpub.com
Dist(s): **IPG Chicago** *(Independent Pubs. Group).*

Himalayan Bks (IND) *Dist. by* **St Mut.**

Himalayan Inst, *(Himalayan Institute Pr.; 0-89389; 1-887645),* Div. of Himalayan International Institute of Yoga Science & Philosophy, R.R. 1, Box 405, Honesdale, PA 18431 (SAN 207-5067) Tel 570-253-5551; Fax: 570-253-6360; Toll Free: 800-822-4547
E-mail: alena@himalayaninstitute.org; hibooks@himalayaninstitute.org
Web site: http://www.himalayaninstitute.org
Dist(s): **Baker & Taylor** *(Baker & Taylor Bks.)*
Bookpeople *(Bookpeople)*
New Leaf Dist *(New Leaf Distributing Co., Inc.).*

Himalayan Pubs, *See* **Himalayan Inst**

HIN, *See* **Health InfoNet Inc**

Hindustan (IND) *(81-7075) Dist. by* **S Asia.**

Hippocrates Pubns, *(Hippocrates Pubns.; 0-9622373),* Div. of Hippocrates Health Institute, 1443 Palmdale Ct., West Palm Beach, FL 33411 Tel 407-471-8876
Web site: http://www.hippocrates.org.

Hisarlik Pr (GBR) *(1-874312) Dist. by* **Intl Spec Bk.**

Hispanic Seminary, *(Hispanic Seminary of Medieval Studies; 0-940639; 0-942260; 1-56954),* 613 W. 155th St., New York, NY 10032-7501 (SAN 207-9836).

Hist Saranac, *(Historic Saranac Lake; 0-9615159),* P.O. Box 1030, Saranac Lake, NY 12983 (SAN 694-387X) Tel 518-891-0971
Web site: http://www.historicsaranaclake.org.

Hist Soc Carroll, *(Historical Society of Carroll County; 0-9614125; 1-886742),* 210 E. Main St., Westminster, MD 21157-5225 (SAN 686-4724) Tel 410-848-6494
E-mail: hscc@carr.org
Web site: http://www.carr.org/hscc.

HISTECH, *(HISTECH, Inc.; 1-56993),* 1477 Harwell Ave., Crofton, MD 21114-2138 Tel 410-721-0853.

Hi-Time Pflaum, *See* **Pflaum Pubng Grp**

HIV Coalition, *(HIV Coalition, The; 0-9639390),* 990 Criss Cir., Elk Grove Village, IL 60007 Tel 847-228-5200; Fax: 847-228-5451
E-mail: hivco@theramp.net.

HK Univ Pr (HKG) *(962-209; 0-85656) Dist. by* **Coronet Bks.**

HK Univ Pr (HKG) *(962-209; 0-85656) Dist. by* **Intl Spec Bk.**

Hlistic Hlth Assn, *(Holistic Health Assn. of the Princeton Area, The; 0-9651767),* 360 Nassau St., Princeton, NJ 08540 Tel 609-924-8711; Fax: 609-924-3836
Web site: http://www.holisticliving.org
Dist(s): **Baker & Taylor** *(Baker & Taylor Bks.)*
Koen Bk Distributors *(Koen Bk. Distributors).*

Hlth & Hap, *(Health & Happiness Bks.; 1-893637),* 1414 Barcelona Dr., Knoxville, TN 37923 Tel 865-539-1601 (phone/fax)
E-mail: mkuman@hotmail.com
Web site: http://www.angelfire.com/ok2/hahahbooks.

Hlth & Human Imprint of USGPO

Hlth & Life, *(Health & Life Dynamics; 0-9633361),* 2720 Pleasant Grove Rd., Lansing, MI 48910 Tel 517-882-6605; Fax: 517-882-1668.

Hlth Care Creat, *(Health Care Creative Services; 0-923109),* Subs. of Health Care Equipment Services, 8248 Lackland Rd., Saint Louis, MO 63114-4509 (SAN 251-5989) Tel 314-968-1616.

Hlth Care Excell, *(Health Care Excellence; 0-9664061),* 331 W. Dixie Ave., Suite 200, Elizabethtown, KY 42701 Tel 270-769-0418; Fax: 502-737-6293; Toll Free: 888-684-3645
E-mail: mikjones@ne.infi.net.

Hlth Care Systs, *(Health Care Systems, Inc.; 0-9643160),* 18 Country Rd., Westport, CT 06880-2525 Tel 203-834-1416.

Hlth Data Concepts, *(Health Data Concepts, Inc.; 1-884103),* 6 Mount Vernon St., Suite 226, Winchester, MA 01890 Tel 617-648-8449.

Hlth Edu Lit, *(Health Education Literary Pub.; 1-883257),* P.O. Box 948, Westbury, NY 11590 Tel 516-997-1777; Fax: 516-997-9555
Dist(s): **Assoc Pubs Grp** *(Associated Pubs. Group).*

Hlth Educ Consults, *(Health Education Consultants; 0-9622034),* 1284 Manor Pk., Lakewood, OH 44107 Tel 216-521-1766 Do not confuse with Health Education Consultants, Kansas City, MO.

Hlth Educ Netwk, *(Health Education Network, Inc.; 1-882515),* 11104 Glen Arm Rd., Glen Arm, MD 21057 Tel 410-668-7718; Toll Free: 800-690-1150
Web site: http://www.healthed.net.

Hlth Educ Res, *(Health Education Resources, LLC; 0-9653928),* Orders Addr.: P.O. Box 621030, Littleton, CO 80162-1030; Edit Addr.: 7273 W. Otero Ave., Littleton, CO 80123 Tel 303-933-2339.

Hlth Facility, *(Health Facility Pubs., Inc.; 1-881556),* 11721 Village Ln., Suite 100, Jacksonville, FL 32223 Tel 904-268-6092
E-mail: medspace@mediaone.net
Web site: http://www.jacksonville.net/~medspace/hsp.html.

Hlth Freedom, *See* **Smart Pubns CA**

Hlth Frontiers, *(Health Frontiers; 0-9602790),* 44500 66th Ave. Way, Kenyon, MN 55946 (SAN 212-9752) Tel 507-789-6725; 216-368-6321.

Hlth Interact, *(Health Interaction Assocs., Inc.; 0-9640405),* 9 Conifer Dr., Branford, CT 06405 Tel 203-483-4729
Dist(s): **BookMasters** *(BookMasters, Inc.).*

Hlth Kinesiol Pubns, *(Health Kinesiology Pubns.; 0-945509),* 649 Irving St., San Francisco, CA 94122 (SAN 247-0454) Tel 415-664-1464.

Hlth Lead Assoc, *(Health Leadership Assocs., Inc.; 1-878028),* P.O. Box 59153, Potomac, MD 20859 Tel 301-983-2405; Fax: 301-983-2693; Toll Free: 800-435-4775
E-mail: hlacert@erols.com
Web site: http://www.healthleadership.com
Dist(s): **J Majors Co** *(Majors, J. A. Co.)*
Matthews Medical Bk Co *(Matthews Medical Bk. Co.)*
Rittenhouse *(Rittenhouse Bk. Distributors).*

Hlth Mngmnt Pubns, *(Health Management Pubns., Inc.; 0-9628084; 1-893446),* 950 W. Valley Rd., Suite 2800, Wayne, PA 19087-1824 Tel 610-688-8220; Fax: 610-688-8050; Toll Free: 800-237-7285.

Hlth Monitor, *(Health Monitor Pr.; 0-9635998),* P.O. Box 2700, Southampton, NY 11969 Tel 516-287-3140; Fax: 516-287-3136.

Hlth Mrkts Res, *(Health Markets Research; 0-9627640),* 851 Moana Ct., Palo Alto, CA 94306 Tel 650-948-1960; Fax: 650-948-7827
E-mail: HMRPUB@aol.com
Web site: http://www.hmtpub@aol.com.

Hlth Prof Inst, *(Health Professions Institute; 0-934385),* Orders Addr.: P.O. Box 801, Modesto, CA 95353 Tel 209-551-2112; Fax: 209-551-0404; Edit Addr.: 2105 Lancey Dr., Suite 1, Modesto, CA 95355 (SAN 693-806X)
E-mail: hpi@hpisum.com
Web site: http://www.hpisum.com.

†**Hlth Prof Pr,** *(Health Professions Pr.; 1-878812),* Div. of Paul H. Brookes Publishing Co., Inc., Orders Addr.: P.O. Box 10624, Baltimore, MD 21285-0624 (SAN 297-7338) Tel 410-337-9585; Fax: 410-337-8539; Toll Free: 888-337-8808; Edit Addr.: 409 Washington Ave., Baltimore, MD 21204 Tel 410-337-9505; Toll Free: 888-337-8539
E-mail: custserv@healthpropress.com
Dist(s): **Baker & Taylor** *(Baker & Taylor Bks.)*
J Majors Co *(Majors, J. A. Co.); CIP.*

Hlth Pub SF, *See* **Psychol Educ Pubns**

Hlth Quest, *(Health Quest Pubns.; 1-883201),* 520 Washington, No. 420, Marina Del Rey, CA 90292 Tel 310-822-2722; Fax: 310-306-1058 Do not confuse with Health Quest Publications, Modesto, CA.

Hlth Res Pub, *(Health Resources Publishing; 1-882364),* Orders Addr.: P.O. Box 559, Allenwood, NJ 08720 (SAN 253-7001) Tel 732-292-1100; Fax: 732-292-1111; Edit Addr.: 1913 Atlantic Ave., Suite F4, Manasquan, NJ 08736 Toll Free Fax: 888-329-6242; Toll Free: 800-516-4343 ; *Imprints:* Amer Busn Pub (American Business Publishing)
E-mail: info@healthrespubs.com
Web site: http://www.healthresourcesonline.com.

Hlth Research, *(Health Research; 0-7873),* P.O. Box 850, Pomeroy, WA 99347 Tel 509-843-2385; Fax: 509-843-2387; Toll Free: 888-844-2386
E-mail: publish@pomeroy-wa.com
Web site: http://www.healthresearchbooks.com.

Hlth Sci, *(Health Science; 0-87790),* Div. of Live Food Products, Inc., Bragg Live Food, Inc., Box 7, Santa Barbara, CA 93102 (SAN 208-1016) Tel 805-968-1020; Fax: 805-968-1001; Toll Free: 800-446-1990
E-mail: info@bragg.com; books@bragg.com
Web site: http://www.bragg.com
Dist(s): **Natl Bk Netwk** *(National Bk. Network)*
Royal Pubns Inc *(Royal Pubns., Inc.).*

Hlth TREND, *(Health T.R.E.N.D. (Todays Relaxation Exercise & Nutrition Developments); 0-9633536),* 14 Register Rd., Marion, MA 02738 Tel 508-697-1200; Fax: 508-748-3039 Do not confuse with companies with similar names in Marion, MA, Bethesda, MD.

Hlth Trends, *(Health Trends; 1-887324),* 4405 East-West Highway, Suite 406, Bethesda, MD 20814 Tel 301-652-8937; Fax: 301-907-6790; Toll Free: 800-945-8816 Do not confuse with companies with similar names in Menlo Park, CA, Marion, MA
E-mail: admin@htrinc.com
Web site: http://www.htrinc.com.

Hlth Unltd, *(Health Unlimited; 0-9654904),* 18242 Burbank Blvd., Unit 4, Tarzana, CA 91356-2512.

Hlth Valley Foods, *(Health Valley Foods Co.; 0-9633608),* 16100 Foothill Blvd., Irwindale, CA 91706 Tel 626-334-3241; Fax: 626-969-9176; Toll Free: 800-334-3204.

Hlthcare Alternatives, *See* **Power of One**

Hlthcare Comput, *(Healthcare Computing Pubns., Inc.; 0-9637397; 0-9672843),* 462 Second St., Brooklyn, NY 11215-2503 Tel 718-499-5910; Fax: 718-768-3260
E-mail: hcpstaff@healthcarecomputing.com
Web site: http://www.healthcarecomputing.com.

HlthCare Consult, *(HealthCare Consultants, Inc.; 1-879249),* 1054 Claussen Rd., Suite 307, Augusta, GA 30907 Tel 706-724-2078.

†**Hlthcare Fin Mgmt,** *(Healthcare Financial Management Educational Foundation; 0-930228; 1-882198),* Two Westbrook Corp. Ctr., Suite 700, Westchester, IL 60154 (SAN 207-5911) Tel 708-531-9600; Toll Free: 800-252-4362; *CIP.*

Hlthcare Mktg & Comns, *(Healthcare Marketing & Communications, Inc.; 0-9622718),* Orders Addr.: P.O. Box 811, Cadillac, MI 49601 Fax: 616-775-2511; Edit Addr.: 107 N. Mitchell St., Cadillac, MI 49601 Tel 616-775-4708.

HlthQuest Pubs, *(HealthQuest Pubs.; 0-9639238),* 1101 Standiford Ave., Suite C-3, Modesto, CA 95350 Tel 209-577-4888; Fax: 209-577-3557
Web site: http://www.mcol.com.

HlthRd Prods, *(HealthRoad Productions; 0-9653493),* P.O. Box 2176, Stateline, NV 89449 Tel 415-461-9600; Fax: 415-454-1087
E-mail: healthrd@nbn.com
Web site: http://www.healthroad.com.

HlthSavers Pr, *(HealthSavers Pr.; 0-927839),* Orders Addr.: P.O. Box 683, Herndon, VA 22070; Edit Addr.: 1850 Golf View Ct., Reston, VA 22090 Tel 703-471-4734.

Hlthspan, *(Healthspan Comns.; 0-9643673),* 2726 Land Park Dr., Sacramento, CA 95818 Tel 916-443-2120; Fax: 916-443-2424
E-mail: haring@hspan.com.

HlthWise Pubns Imprint of Piccadilly Bks

Publisher Symbol Index

Hlthy Healing, *(Healthy Healing Pubns.; 1-884334),* Orders Addr.: P.O. Box 436, Carmel Valley, CA 93924 Tel 831-659-8324; Fax: 831-659-8326; Toll Free: 888-447-2939; Edit Addr.: 300 Country Club Hts., Carmel Valley, CA 93924
Web site: http://www.HealthyHealing.com
Dist(s): **Crystal Star Herbal** *(Crystal Star Herbal Nutrition)*
Nutri-Books Corp *(Nutri-Bks. Corp.)*
Royal Pubns Inc *(Royal Pubns., Inc.)*
Words Distrib *(Words Distributing Co.).*

Hlthy Heart, *(Healthy Heart Pubs.; 0-9654590),* 3135 Imperial Blvd., Springfield, OH 45503 Tel 937-325-1155; Fax: 937-325-6611.

Hlthy Hse, *(Healthy Hse. Institute, The; 0-9637156; 1-929903),* 430 N. Sewell Rd., Bloomington, IN 47408 Tel 812-332-5073 (phone/fax)
E-mail: healthy@bloomington.in.us
Web site: http://www.hhinst.com
Dist(s): **Bookpeople** *(Bookpeople)*
Distributors *(Distributors, The).*

Hlthy Weight Jrnl Imprint of Hlthy Wght Network

Hlthy Wght Network, *(Healthy Weight Network; 0-918532),* 402 S. 14th St., Hettinger, ND 58639 Tel 701-567-2646; Fax: 701-567-2602 ; *Imprints:* Hlthy Weight Jrnl (Healthy Weight Journal)
E-mail: hwj@healthyweight.net
Web site: http://www.healthyweight.net
Dist(s): **IPG Chicago** *(Independent Pubs. Group).*

Hlthy Wght Pub, *See* **Hlthy Wght Network**

†HM, *(Houghton Mifflin Co.; 0-395; 0-87466; 0-87477; 0-89919; 0-9631591; 1-57630; 1-881527; 0-618),* Orders Addr.: 181 Ballardvale St., Wilmington, MA 01887 (SAN 215-3793) Tel 978-661-1300; Toll Free: 800-225-3362; P.O. Box 7050, Wilmington, MA 01887-7050; Edit Addr.: 215 Park Ave., S., New York, NY 10003 (SAN 282-4043) Tel 212-420-5800; Fax: 212-420-5855 ; *Imprints:* AHD & Ref (American Heritage Dictionaries & Reference Books) Mariner Bks (Mariner Books)
Web site: http://www.hmco.com
Dist(s): **Chelsea Green Pub** *(Chelsea Green Publishing)*
Cheng & Tsui *(Cheng & Tsui Co.)*
Continental Bk *(Continental Bk. Co., Inc.)*
Shens Bks *(Shen's Bks.)*
netLibrary CO *(netLibrary, Inc.); CIP.*

HM College Div, *See* **HM Trade Div**

HM Soft Schl Col Div, *(Houghton Mifflin Software, Schl. & College Div.; 0-395),* 222 Berkeley St., Boston, MA 02116-3764 (SAN 215-3793) Tel 617-725-5000
E-mail: hrassist@hmco.com
Web site: http://www.hmco.com.

HM Trade Div, *(Houghton Mifflin Co. (Trade Div.); 0-669),* 222 Berkeley St., Boston, MA 02116 (SAN 200-2388) Tel 617-351-5000; Fax: 617-227-5409; 215 Park Ave., S., New York, NY 10003 (SAN 282-4043) Tel 212-420-5800; Fax: 212-420-5855
Web site: http://www.hmco.com/
Dist(s): **netLibrary CO** *(netLibrary, Inc.).*

HMR Pubns Grp, *(HMR Pubns. Group, Inc.; 0-9627545),* 3180 Presidential Dr., Suite K, Atlanta, GA 30340-3900 Tel 770-457-6105; Fax: 770-457-4606.

Hndbks Hlth Care Imprint of Assocs in Med

Hoard & Sons Co, *(Hoard, W.D. & Sons Co.; 0-932147),* P.O. Box 801, Fort Atkinson, WI 53538-0801 (SAN 686-4341) Tel 920-563-5551; Fax: 920-563-7298 ; *Imprints:* Hoards Dairyman (Hoard's Dairyman)
Web site: http://www.hoards.com.

Hoards Dairyman Imprint of Hoard & Sons Co

Hodder & Stought Ltd (GBR) *(0-340; 0-450; 0-7122; 0-7131) Dist. by* **Trafalgar.**

Hodder & Stought Ltd (GBR) *(0-340; 0-450; 0-7122; 0-7131) Dist. by* **Lubrecht & Cramer.**

Hogg Found, *(Hogg Foundation for Mental Health; 0-943463),* P.O. Box 7998, Austin, TX 78713-7998 (SAN 204-8337) Tel 512-471-5041; Fax: 512-471-9608.

†Hogrefe & Huber Pubs, *(Hogrefe & Huber Pubs.; 0-88937),* Orders Addr.: P.O. Box H388, Kirkland, WA 98083-2487 Tel 425-820-1500; Fax: 425-823-8324; Toll Free: 800-228-3749; Edit Addr.: 218 Main St., Suite 485, Kirkland, WA 98073 (SAN 293-2792)
E-mail: hh@hhpub.com
Web site: http://www.hhpub.com
Dist(s): **Baker & Taylor** *(Baker & Taylor Bks.)*
BookMasters *(BookMasters, Inc.)*
Coutts Library Service Inc *(Coutts Library Service, Inc.)*
Majors Scientific Bks Inc *(Majors Scientific Bks., Inc.)*
Matthews Medical Bk Co *(Matthews Medical Bk. Co.)*
Rittenhouse *(Rittenhouse Bk. Distributors); CIP.*

Hohm Pr, *(Hohm Pr.; 0-934252; 1-890772),* Div. of Hohm, Inc., P.O. Box 2501, Prescott, AZ 86302 (SAN 221-0924) Tel 520-778-9189; Fax: 520-717-1779; Toll Free: 800-381-2700 (orders only)
E-mail: staff@hohmpress.com; pinedr@goodnet.com
Web site: http://www.hohmpress.com
Dist(s): **SCB Distributors** *(SCB Distributors).*

Holcomb Hath, *(Holcomb Hathaway, Inc.; 1-890871),* 6207 N. Cattle Track Rd., Suite 5, Scottsdale, AZ 85250 Tel 480-991-7881; Fax: 480-991-4770
E-mail: sales@hh-pub.com
Web site: http://www.hh-pub.com.

Holden-Day, *(Holden-Day, Inc.; 0-8162),* 1259 SW 14th St., Boca Raton, FL 33486-5311 (SAN 202-2990) Tel 407-750-9229.

Holistic Educ Pr, *See* **Psychology Pr**

Holloway, *(Holloway Hse. Publishing Co.; 0-87067; 1-58520),* 8060 Melrose Ave., Los Angeles, CA 90046 (SAN 206-8451) Tel 323-653-8060; Fax: 323-655-9452
E-mail: psi@loop.com
Web site: http://www.hollowayhousebooks.com
Dist(s): **All Am Dist Corp** *(All America Distributors Corp.).*

†Hollowbrook, *(Hollowbrook Publishing; 0-88072; 0-89341),* Div. of Hollowbrook Communications, Inc., 236 S. Third St., Unit 242, Montrose, CO 81401 Fax: 970-249-2041; *CIP.*

†Holmes & Meier, *(Holmes & Meier Pubs., Inc.; 0-8419),* Orders Addr.: 41 Monroe Tpke., Trumbull, CT 06611 Tel 800-698-7781; Fax: 800-557-5601; Edit Addr.: 160 Broadway E. Bldg, 9th Flr.,, New York, NY 10038 (SAN 201-9280) Tel 212-374-0100; Fax: 212-374-1313
E-mail: info@holmesandmeier.com
Web site: http://www.holmesandmeier.com
Dist(s): **H&M Dist** *(H & M Distribution); CIP.*

Holmes Pub, *(Holmes Publishing Group, LLC; 0-916411; 1-55818),* Orders Addr.: P.O. Box 623, Edmonds, WA 98020-0623 (SAN 655-8321) Tel 425-771-2701; Fax: 425-771-5651; Edit Addr.: 406 Main, Suite 116, Edmonds, WA 98020 (SAN 243-282X) ; *Imprints:* Sure Fire (Sure Fire Press) Do not confuse with Holmes Publishing Co., Philadelphia, PA
E-mail: jdh@jdholmes.com.

Holographic Hlth, *(Holographic Health Pr.; 0-9619595),* 119 Pigeon St., Waynesville, NC 28786 (SAN 245-484X) Tel 828-456-6231; Fax: 828-452-0879; Toll Free: 800-566-1522 Do not confuse with companies with same or similar names in New York, NY, Portland, OR, Carson City, NV.

Holt R&W, *(Holt, Rinehart & Winston; 0-03),* Div. of Harcourt, Inc., Orders Addr.: 6277 Sea Harbor Dr., Orlando, FL 32887-0001 Tel 407-345-3800; Fax: 407-352-3395; Toll Free Fax: 800-235-0256; Toll Free: 800-544-6678; Edit Addr.: 1120 S. Capital of Texas Hwy. No. II-100, Austin, TX 78746-6487 (SAN 297-4711) Tel 512-314-6500; Toll Free: 800-479-9799; 800-992-1627
E-mail: holtinfo@hrw.com
Web site: http://www.hrw.com
Dist(s): **Continental Bk** *(Continental Bk. Co., Inc.).*

†Holy Cross Orthodox, *(Holy Cross Orthodox Pr.; 0-916586; 0-917651; 1-885652),* Div. of Hellenic College, Inc., 50 Goddard Ave., Brookline, MA 02445 (SAN 208-6840) Tel 617-731-3500 (ext. 1230); Fax: 617-850-1460; Toll Free: 800-245-0599
Dist(s): **Baker & Taylor** *(Baker & Taylor Bks.); CIP.*

Home Care Univ, *(Home Care Univ.; 1-930304),* Div. of National Assn. for Home Care, 228 Seventh St., SE, Washington, DC 20003 Tel 202-547-3576; Fax: 202-547-4322
E-mail: caring@NAHC.org
Web site: http://www.homecareuniversity.org.

Home Merciful SFCC, *(Home of the Merciful Saviour for Crippled Children; 0-9613558),* 4400 Baltimore Ave, Philadelphia, PA 19104 (SAN 669-8581) Tel 215-222-2566; Fax: 215-222-1889
E-mail: admin@hmsschool.org
Web site: http://www.hmsschool.org.

Home Mgmt, *(Home Management, Employment Skills & Entrepreneurship Institute, Inc.; 0-9638634),* Orders Addr.: P.O. Box 86, Cheyney, PA 19319 Fax: 610-399-6660; Edit Addr.: 129 Locksley Rd., Cheyney, PA 19319 Tel 610-459-1299.

Homefront Graphics, *(Homefront Graphics; 0-939374),* 2275 Featherhill Rd., Santa Barbara, CA 93108-1518 (SAN 216-4892).

Homestead Bk, *(Homestead Bk., Inc.; 0-930180),* Orders Addr.: P.O. Box 31608, Seattle, WA 98103 (SAN 662-037X); Edit Addr.: 6101 22nd Ave., NW, Seattle, WA 98107 (SAN 169-8796) Tel 206-782-4532; Fax: 206-784-9328; Toll Free: 800-426-6777 (orders only) ; *Imprints:* Sun Magic (Sun Magic)
Web site: http://www.homesteadbook.com.

†Hoover Inst Pr, *(Hoover Institution Pr.; 0-8179),* Stanford Univ., Stanford, CA 94305-6010 (SAN 202-3024) Tel 650-723-3373; Fax: 650-723-8626; Toll Free: 800-935-2882
E-mail: digest@hoover.stanford.edu
Web site: http://www.hoover.org; *CIP.*

Hope Homes Pubs, *(Hope Homes Pubs.; 1-878228),* 5519 S. Justice St., Chicago, IL 60636 Tel 312-925-8680.

Hope Pr CA, *(Hope Pr.; 1-878267),* Orders Addr.: P.O. Box 188, Duarte, CA 91009-0188 (SAN 200-3244) Tel 626-303-0644; Fax: 626-358-3520; Toll Free: 800-321-4039; Edit Addr.: 1110 Mill Run, Monvaia, CA 91016 Do not confuse with Hope Pr., Pittsville, WI
E-mail: dcomings@mail.earthlink.com
Web site: http://www.hopepress.com.

Hope Pub Hse, *(Hope Publishing Hse.; 0-932727),* Affil. of Southern California Ecumenical Council, Orders Addr.: P.O. Box 60008, Pasadena, CA 91116 (SAN 688-4849) Tel 626-792-6123; Fax: 626-792-2121; Toll Free: 800-326-2671 (orders only); Edit Addr.: 696 S. Madison Ave., Pasadena, CA 91106
E-mail: hopepub@loop.com
Web site: http://www.hope-pub.com.

Hope Springs, *(Hope Springs Pr.; 0-9639531),* 500 Hope Springs Ln., Manakin-Sabot, VA 23103 Tel 804-784-5025; Fax: 804-784-5484
E-mail: webpartners@webpointers.com
Web site: http://www.firstaidyourself.org; http://www.awty.webpointers.com.

HopeLines, *(HopeLines; 0-9657755),* P.O. Box 306, Penfield, NY 14526 Tel 716-377-0079
E-mail: Cynjoy@frontiernet.com.

Horatius Pr, *(Horatius Pr.; 1-888456),* Orders Addr.: P.O. Box 241527, Omaha, NE 68124-5527 Tel 402-399-1767; Fax: 402-391-8079; Edit Addr.: 1315 S. 79th St., Omaha, NE 68124
E-mail: horatiuspress@att.net.

Horizon Consltng, *(Horizon Consulting Group, Inc.; 0-9678758),* Orders Addr.: P.O. Box 7238, Jacksonville, FL 32238 Tel 904-573-2232; Fax: 425-988-1163; Edit Addr.: 5722 Ft. Sumter Rd., Jacksonville, FL 32210
E-mail: harvey@mediaone.net.

Horizon Herbs, *(Horizon Herbs; 0-9700312),* P.O. Box 69, Williams, OR 97544 Tel 541-846-6704; Fax: 541-846-6233
E-mail: Herbseed@chatlink.com
Web site: http://www.chatlink.com/~herbseed.

Horizon Sci (GBR) *(1-898486) Dist. by* **Intl Spec Bk.**

Horticult Pubns, *See* **N F Childers**

Horwood Pub (GBR) *(1-898563) Dist. by* **Paul & Co Pubs.**

Hosp & Hlthcare, *(Hospital & Healthcare Compensation Service; 0-939326; 1-893772),* Subs. of John R. Zabka Assocs., Inc., P.O. Box 376, Oakland, NJ 07436 (SAN 217-1090) Tel 201-405-0075; Fax: 201-405-2110
E-mail: info@hhcsinc.com; hhcsinc@aol.com
Web site: http://www.hhcsinc.com.

Hosp Compensation, *See* **Hosp & Hlthcare**

Hosp For Joint Diseases, *(Hospital for Joint Diseases; 0-9642813),* Div. of NYU Medical Ctr., 301 E. 17th St., New York, NY 10003 Tel 212-598-6530; Fax: 212-260-1203.

Hosp Pubns, *(Hospitality Pubns., Inc.; 0-932235),* P.O. Box 448, Okemos, MI 48805 (SAN 686-5801) Tel 517-676-4030.

†**Hosp Res & Educ,** *(Hospital Research & Educational Trust; 0-87914),* Affil. of American Hospital Assn., Orders Addr.: 4444 W. Ferdinand, Chicago, IL 60626 (SAN 662-040X); Edit Addr.: One N. Franklin, Chicago, IL 60606 (SAN 206-9121) Tel 312-280-6620; Toll Free: 800-242-2626; *CIP.*

Hospice Education, *(Hospice Education Institute; 0-9623438),* 190 Westbrook Rd., Essex, CT 06426-1510 Tel 860-767-1620; Fax: 860-767-2746.

Hospice Fndt Amer, *(Hospice Foundation of America; 1-893349),* 2001 S. St., NW Suite 300, Miami Beach, FL 33139 Tel 202-638-5419; Fax: 202-638-5312; Toll Free: 800-854-3402
E-mail: hfa@hospicefoundation.org
Web site: http://www.hospicefoundation.org
Dist(s): **Brunner-Routledge** *(Brunner-Routledge).*

Hospice Montclair, *See* **Ctr Hospice Care**

Hospice of Bldr Cty, *(Hospice of Boulder County; 0-9655182),* 2825 Marine St., Boulder, CO 80303-1079 Tel 303-449-7740; Fax: 303-449-6961.

Houston Law Review, *(Houston Law Review; 0-913797),* Univ. of Houston Law Ctr., Houston, TX 77004 (SAN 226-5427) Tel 713-749-3195.

Hover, *(Hover Co., The; 0-934414),* 14713 La Mesa Dr., La Mirada, CA 90638 (SAN 213-747X) Tel 714-521-3046
E-mail: hoverthc@earthlink.net.

Hovnanian, *(Hovnanian, Ralph R.; 0-9607774),* 2128 Prospect Ave., Evanston, IL 60201 (SAN 241-5399) Tel 847-869-4346.

How To Bks (GBR) *(1-85703) Dist. by* **Midpt Trade.**

Howard & Assocs, *(Howard & Assocs.; 0-935801),* Orders Addr.: P.O. Box 263, Fortuna, CA 95540 (SAN 696-8384); Edit Addr.: 639 11th St., Suite C, Fortuna, CA 95540 (SAN 696-8392) Tel 707-725-2987.

Howard U Inst UAR, *(Howard Univ., Institute for Urban Affairs & Research; 1-56669),* 2900 Van Ness St., NW, Washington, DC 20008 Tel 202-806-8770; Fax: 202-806-8782.

†**Howard U Pr,** *(Howard Univ. Pr.; 0-88258),* 2225 Georgia Ave., Suite 218, Washington, DC 20001 (SAN 202-3067) Tel 202-238-2570; Fax: 202-588-9849
E-mail: eborden@howard.edu
Web site: http://www.founders.howard.edu/HUPRESS
Dist(s): **Baker & Taylor** *(Baker & Taylor Bks.); CIP.*

Howarth Pr, *(Howarth Pr., Inc., The; 0-939533),* 3426 Aston St., Annandale, VA 22003-1445 (SAN 663-4362); 7306 Brad St., Falls Church, VA 22042 (SAN 663-4370) Tel 703-573-8521.

Howell Imprint of Hungry Minds

Howln Moon, *(Howln Moon Pr.; 1-888994),* P.O. Box 238, Eliot, ME 03903 Toll Free: 888-349-9438 (orders only)
E-mail: bmueller@howlnmoonpress.com.

HP Books Imprint of Berkley Pub

HRAFP, *(Human Relations Area Files Pr., Inc.; 0-87536),* Affil. of Yale Univ., 755 Prospect St., New Haven, CT 06511-1225 (SAN 200-4348) Tel 203-764-9401; Fax: 203-764-9404.

HRS, *(HRS, Inc.; 0-9639267),* P.O. Box 891, Dana Point, CA 92629-0891 Tel 714-661-5840.

Hrt to Hrt Med, *(Heart to Heart Medical Ctr.; 0-9660950),* 175 Airport Blvd., Santa Rosa, CA 95403 Tel 707-524-9640; Fax: 707-524-9649; Toll Free: 888-707-9640
E-mail: hth@hthmc.com.

HR&W Schl Div, *See* **Holt R&W**

Hse BonGiovanni, *(House of BonGiovanni; 0-912981),* 5712 Herbert Rd., Canfield, OH 44406 (SAN 283-0442) Tel 330-702-1978 (phone/fax)
E-mail: guyBon@aol.com.

Hse of Steno, *(House of Steno, Inc.; 1-883952),* 1701 California St., Redding, CA 96001-1906 Tel 530-241-6051; Fax: 530-241-3257; Toll Free: 800-479-6062
E-mail: sking@steno.com
Web site: http://www.steno.com.

Hse White Birches, *(House of White Birches, Inc.; 1-882138),* Orders Addr.: P.O. Box 9025, Big Sandy, TX 75755 Toll Free Fax: 888-848-4414; Toll Free: 800-829-5865; Edit Addr.: 306 E. Parr Rd., Berne, IN 46711 (SAN 248-8310) Tel 219-589-4000; Fax: 219-589-8093
E-mail: customer_servive@whitebirches.com
Web site: http://www.whitebirches.com.

HSMP Pr, *(HSMP Pr.; 0-9629868),* 176 Heatherstone Rd., Amherst, MA 01003 Tel 413-545-2347; Fax: 413-545-3958
E-mail: craker.pssci.umas.edu.

HSWPP Imprint of Haworth Pr

Huber-Copeland Pub, *(Huber/Copeland Publishing; 0-934293),* P.O. Box 665, Mattoon, IL 61938 (SAN 693-2657) Tel 317-872-4472.

Huebner Foun Insur, *(Huebner, S.S. Foundation for Insurance Education; 0-918930),* 430 Vance Hall, 3733 Spruce St., Philadelphia, PA 19104-6301 (SAN 211-6405) Tel 215-898-9631; Fax: 215-573-2218
E-mail: harowitl@wharton.upenn.edu
Web site: http://www.rider.wharton.upenn.edu/~sshuebne.

Hughes Henshaw, *(Hughes Henshaw Pubns.; 0-9617223; 1-892693),* Orders Addr.: 7196 W. Fourth Ave., Lakewood, CO 80226-1642 (SAN 663-3927) Tel 303-237-5905; Fax: 303-233-6545
E-mail: hugheshenshaw@aol.com; hugheshenshaw@home.com
Web site: http://www.hugheshenshaw.com.

Hughes Pr, *(Hughes Pr.; 0-912560),* 2400 Virginia Ave. NW, Suite C501, Washington, DC 20037-2612 (SAN 210-9360) Tel 202-293-2686 Do not confuse with Hughes Pr., Warren, OH.

Hultgren Pubns, *(Hultgren Pubns.; 0-9655183),* 827 San Francisco Ct., Stanford, CA 94305-1021 Tel 650-857-9574; Fax: 650-493-4225
E-mail: hultgren@highaltitudemedicine.com
Web site: http://www.highaltitudemedicine.com.

Human Energy Pr, *(Human Energy Pr.; 0-941523),* 422 First St., Suite D, Eureka, CA 95501 (SAN 666-542X) Tel 707-269-0806.

Human Esteem Pub, *(Human Esteem Publishing; 0-9613559),* 424 N. Larchmont Blvd., Los Angeles, CA 90004 (SAN 669-8646) Tel 213-463-6424; Fax: 213-663-7568.

Human Factors, *(Human Factors & Ergonomics Society; 0-945289),* Orders Addr.: P.O. Box 1369, Santa Monica, CA 90406-1369 (SAN 270-8590) Tel 310-394-1811; Fax: 310-394-2410; Edit Addr.: 1124 Montana Ave., No. B, Santa Monica, CA 90403 (SAN 680-0424)
E-mail: hfes@compuserve.com
Web site: http://www.hfes.org.

†**Human Kinetics,** *(Human Kinetics Pubs.; 0-7360; 0-87322; 0-88011; 0-918438; 0-931250),* Orders Addr.: P.O. Box 5076, Champaign, IL 61825-5076 (SAN 211-7088) Tel 217-351-5076 (ext. 2423); Fax: 217-351-2674; Toll Free: 800-747-4457; Edit Addr.: 1607 N. Market St., Champaign, IL 61820 (SAN 658-0866) Fax: 217-351-2674 ; *Imprints:* YMCA USA (Y M C A of the U. S. A.)
E-mail: humank@hkusa.com
Web site: http://www.humankinetics.com; http://www.hkusa.com
Dist(s): **Follett Audio** *(Follett Audiovisual Resources)*
Lppncott W & W *(Lippincott Williams & Wilkins); CIP.*

Human Netwrks, *(Human Networks, Inc.; 0-933933),* 210 Crest St., Ann Arbor, MI 48103-4315 (SAN 693-0506) Tel 313-665-1220 Do not confuse with Human Networks in Solon, OH.

Human Policy Pr, *(Human Policy Pr.; 0-937540),* P.O. Box 127, Syracuse, NY 13210 (SAN 213-8476) Tel 315-443-3851; Fax: 315-443-4338; Toll Free: 800-894-0826
E-mail: thechp@sued.syr.edu
Web site: http://soeweb.syr.edu/thechp/.

Human Res Inst, *See* **Healthyculture**

Human Rsch, *(Human Research Pubs.; 0-9618277),* 1987 S. McClelland St., Salt Lake City, UT 84105 (SAN 667-058X) Tel 208-322-3546
E-mail: gdaniel6587@qwest.net.

†**Humana,** *(Humana Pr.; 0-89603; 1-58829),* 999 Riverview Dr., Suite 208, Totowa, NJ 07512 (SAN 212-3606) Tel 973-256-1699; Fax: 973-256-8341
E-mail: humana@humanapr.com
Web site: http://www.humanapress.com; *CIP.*

Humanics Ltd, *See* **Humanics Pub Grp**

†**Humanics Pub Grp,** *(Humanics Publishing Group; 0-89334),* Orders Addr.: P.O. Box 7400, Atlanta, GA 30357-0400 (SAN 208-3833) Tel 404-874-1930; Fax: 404-874-1976; Toll Free: 800-874-8844; Edit Addr.: 1197 Peachtree St., Suite 533B, Atlanta, GA 30361 (SAN 658-0882) Do not confuse with Humanics ErgoSystems, Inc., Reseda, CA
E-mail: humanics@mindspring.com
Web site: http://www.humanicslearning.com; http://www.humanicsdealer.com; http://www.humanicspub.com
Dist(s): **Baker & Taylor** *(Baker & Taylor Bks.)*
Bookpeople *(Bookpeople)*
Borders Inc *(Borders, Inc.)*
New Leaf Dist *(New Leaf Distributing Co., Inc.); CIP.*

Humanitarian, *(Humanitarian Publishing Co.; 0-916285),* P.O. Box 220, Quakertown, PA 18951-0220 (SAN 295-8422) Tel 215-538-5300; Fax: 215-536-9099; Toll Free: 877-652-3535 (orders only)
Web site: http://www.philpub.com.

Humanity Bks Imprint of Prometheus Bks

Hummingbrd Assocs, *(Hummingbird Assocs.; 0-9647903),* Orders Addr.: P.O. Box 10279, Bainbridge Island, WA 98110 Tel 206-842-2661; Fax: 206-842-6952; Toll Free: 800-552-7558; Edit Addr.: 10009 Edgecombe Pl., NE, Bainbridge Island, WA 98110.

Hummingbrd WA, *(Hummingbird Pubns.; 0-9631446),* Orders Addr.: P.O. Box 10279, Bainbridge Island, WA 98110 Fax: 206-842-6952; Toll Free: 800-552-7558; Edit Addr.: 10009 Edgecombe Pl., NE, Bainbridge Island, WA 98110 Tel 206-842-2661 Do not confuse with companies with the same name in Edmond, OK, Santa Fe, NM.

Humor Bks, *(Humor Bks.; 0-9633921; 1-885694),* 620 SW 23rd Rd., Miami, FL 33129 Tel 305-854-6616; Fax: 305-860-9559
Dist(s): **Baker & Taylor** *(Baker & Taylor Bks.).*

Hundley & Assocs, *(Hundley & Assocs.; 0-9635430),* 12221 Merit Dr., Suite 465, Dallas, TX 75251 Tel 972-233-6343; Fax: 972-233-3187.

Hungry Minds, *(Hungry Minds, Inc.; 0-02; 0-7645; 1-55828; 1-56884; 1-878058),* Div. of John Wiley & Sons, Inc., Orders Addr.: 10475 Crosspoint Blvd., Indianapolis, IN 46256 (SAN 299-089X) Tel 416-293-8464; 317-572-3000; Fax: 317-572-4000; Toll Free: 800-667-1115 (Canadian customers); 800-434-3422 (Volume purchases); 800-762-2974 ; *Imprints:* Dummies Tech (Dummies Technology Press) Cliff (Cliffs Notes, Incorporated) Unoffic Guide (Unofficial Guide) Arc (Arco) Webs New Wrld (Webster's New World) Spectrm (Spectrum) Howell (Howell Books)
E-mail: siteemail@idgbooks.com
Web site: http://www.idgbooks.com
Dist(s): **Bryant Altman** *(Bryant Altman Map, Inc.)*
Continental Bk *(Continental Bk. Co., Inc.)*
Sams Tech Pub *(Sams Technical Publishing)*
Wiley *(Wiley, John & Sons, Inc.).*

Hunter Bks, *(Hunter Bks.; 0-917726; 1-878209),* 201 McClellan Rd., Kingwood, TX 77339-2710 (SAN 209-2611) Tel 281-358-7575; Fax: 281-358-4130; Toll Free: 800-683-3024.

Hunter Coll CEP, *(Hunter College, Centro de Estudios Puertorriquenos; 1-878483),* 695 Park Ave., New York, NY 10021 Tel 212-772-5686; Toll Free: 800-772-5688
Web site: http://www.hunter.any.edu.

Hunter House, *(Hunter Hse. Pubns.; 0-9662769),* Div. of Hunter & Assocs., 1132 21st St., SE, Cedar Rapids, IA 52403 Tel 319-362-4777; Fax: 319-369-9853
E-mail: hunter.c@mcleodusa.net.

Hunter Hse, *(Hunter Hse., Inc.; 0-89793),* P.O. Box 2914, Alameda, CA 94501-0914 (SAN 281-7969) Tel 510-865-5282; Fax: 510-865-4295; Toll Free: 800-266-5592
E-mail: hhi@hunterhouse.com; info@hunterhouse.com
Web site: http://www.hunterhouse.com
Dist(s): **Gryphon Hse** *(Gryphon Hse., Inc.)*
P G Weiss *(Weiss, Paul G.)*
Publishers Group *(Publishers Group West)*
Quality Bks IL *(Quality Bks., Inc.)*
Unique Bks Inc *(Unique Bks., Inc.).*

Huntington Hse, *(Huntington Hse. Pubs.; 0-910311; 1-56384),* Orders Addr.: P.O. Box 53788, Lafayette, LA 70505 (SAN 241-5208) Tel 337-237-7049; Fax: 337-237-7060; Toll Free: 800-749-4009; Edit Addr.: 104 Row 2, Suite A1 & A2, Lafayette, LA 70508 ; *Imprints:* Vital Issue Pr (Vital Issue Press)
E-mail: joycedwyer@cs.com
Web site: http://www.huntingtonhousebooks
Dist(s): **Anchor Distributors** *(Anchor Distributors)*
Appalach Bk Dist *(Appalachian Bk. Distributors)*
BookWorld *(BookWorld Services, Inc.)*
Riverside-World *(Riverside World)*
Spring Arbor Dist *(Spring Arbor Distributors Inc.).*

†**HUP,** *(Harvard Univ. Pr.; 0-674; 0-916724; 0-935617; 0-945454),* Orders Addr.: 79 Garden St., Cambridge, MA 02138 (SAN 200-2043) Tel 617-495-2600; Fax: 617-495-5898; Toll Free Fax: 800-962-4983; Toll Free: 800-448-2242 (customer service) ; *Imprints:* Belknap (Belknap Press)
E-mail: contact_hup@harvard.edu
Web site: http://www.hup.harvard.edu
Dist(s): **Univelt Inc** *(Univelt, Inc.); CIP.*

Hutchinson Cancer Res Ctr, *(Hutchinson, Fred Cancer Research Ctr.; 0-945278),* 1124 Columbia St., Seattle, WA 98104 (SAN 246-0726) Tel 206-467-4586.

HUWEI Cnslts (CHN) *Dist. by* **Am Overseas Bk Co.**

HWD Pub, *(HWD Publishing; 0-9637360),* P.O. Box 220, Veneta, OR 97487 Toll Free: 800-935-7323
Dist(s): **Baker & Taylor** *(Baker & Taylor Bks.)*
Bookpeople *(Bookpeople)*
New Leaf Dist *(New Leaf Distributing Co., Inc.)*
Quality Bks IL *(Quality Bks., Inc.).*

Hyde Assocs, *(Hyde Assocs., Inc.; 0-9637057),* Orders Addr.: P.O. Box 490034, Key Biscayne, FL 33149-0034 Tel 305-361-5900; Fax: 305-361-9955; Edit Addr.: 641 Hampton Ln., Key Biscayne, FL 33149
Dist(s): **BookMasters** *(BookMasters, Inc.)*
Soc Auto Engineers *(Society of Automotive Engineers, Inc.).*

Hygeia Pubng, *(Hygeia Publishing; 0-9647537),* Orders Addr.: P.O. Box 1119, Cardiff, CA 92007 Tel 760-753-4174; Fax: 760-943-1894; Edit Addr.: 65-1231 Opelo Rd., Kamuein, HI 96743
Dist(s): **Nutri-Books Corp** *(Nutri-Bks. Corp.).*

†Hyperion, *(Hyperion; 0-7868; 1-56282; 1-4013),* Div. of Disney Bk. Publishing, Inc., A Walt Disney Co., 77 W. 66th St., 11th Flr., New York, NY 10023-6298 Tel 212-456-0100; Fax: 212-456-0108
Web site: http://www.hyperionbooks.com
Dist(s): **AOL Time Warner** *(AOL Time Warner Bk. Group)*
Little *(Little, Brown & Co.)*
Warner Bks *(Warner Bks., Inc.)*
iPublishcom *(iPublish.com); CIP.*

I B T (GBR) *(1-85043; 1-86064) Dist. by* **St Martin.**

I Henry Pubns (GBR) *(0-86025) Dist. by* **Empire Pub Srvs.**

I L Livingston, *(Livingston, Ivor L.; 0-9631535),* 3701 Martins Dairy Cir., Olney, MD 20832-6620 Tel 301-570-5093.

I Levin, *(Levin, Irving Assocs.,Inc.; 1-930625),* 72 Park St., Suite 104, New Canaan, CT 06840 Tel 203-966-4343; Fax: 203-966-8510; Toll Free: 800-248-1668
E-mail: general@levinassociates.com
Web site: http://www.levinassociates.com.

I Lvl Imprint of Acrpls Bks GA

I Negroni, *(Negroni, Iraida; 0-9620054),* Georgetown St., No. 272, University Gardens, Rio Piedras, PR 00927 (SAN 247-4166) Tel 809-751-3173.

I Omoike Bks, *(Omoike, Isaac Bks.; 0-9632236),* P.O. Box 44801, Fort Washington, MD 20749-0801 Tel 225-387-2393.

---

†I R Dee, *(Dee, Ivan R. Pub.; 0-929587; 1-56663),* Orders Addr.: 15200 NBN Way, Blue Ridge Summit, PA 17214 Tel 717-794-3800; Fax: 717-794-3803; Toll Free Fax: 800-338-4550; Toll Free: 800-462-6420; Edit Addr.: 1332 N. Halsted St., Chicago, IL 60622-2694 (SAN 249-535X) Tel 312-787-6262; Fax: 312-787-6269
E-mail: elephant@ivanrdee.com
Web site: http://www.ivanrdee.com
Dist(s): **Natl Bk Netwk** *(National Bk. Network); CIP.*

IAAS Pubs, *(IAAS Pubs., Inc.; 1-879893),* 7676 New Hampshire Ave., Suite 330, Langley Park, MD 20783 Tel 301-499-6308.

IAD Pr (AUS) *(0-949659; 1-86465; 0-9596206) Dist. by* **Intl Spec Bk.**

IAEA (AUT) *(92-0) Dist. by* **Bernan Associates.**

IAP (GBR) *Dist. by* **Elsevier.**

IAQ Pubns, *(IAQ Pubns., Inc.; 0-9633003; 1-890773),* 7920 Norfolk Ave., Suite 1900, Bethesda, MD 20814 Tel 301-913-0115; Fax: 301-913-0119
Web site: http://www.iaqpubs.com.

IatroSoft Corp, *(IatroSoft Corp.; 0-9665627),* 121 Washington Ave., S., Suite 1607, Minneapolis, MN 55401-2132 Tel 612-414-6697; Fax: 612-359-0223
E-mail: kolan@iatrosoft.com
Web site: http://www.iatrosoft.com.

IBC Tech Srvs (GBR) *Dist. by* **St Mut.**

IBC USA, *See* **Drug & Market Dev**

IBD Ltd, *(i.b.d., Ltd.; 0-88431),* 24 Hudson St., Kinderhook, NY 12106 (SAN 630-7779) Tel 518-758-1755; Fax: 518-758-6702
E-mail: lankhof@ibdltd.com
Web site: http://www.ibdltd.com.

IBS Intl, *(I.B.S. International; 0-89564),* 3144 Dove St., San Diego, CA 92103 (SAN 210-3001).

IC Hope, *(IC Hope, Ltd.; 0-9667750),* P.O. Box 360965, Cleveland, OH 44136 Tel 440-582-9502; Fax: 440-582-9503; Toll Free: 877-597-5766
E-mail: ICHopeLtd@aol.com
Web site: http://www.angelfire.com/biz2/ichope/index.html.

ICA Pub Co, *(ICA Publishing Co.; 1-879774),* Div. of ICA, Inc., 1020 N. Commerce, Stockton, CA 95202 Tel 209-460-0622; Fax: 209-938-0416
E-mail: goss09@aol.com
Dist(s): **Academic Bk Ctr Inc** *(Academic Bk. Ctr., Inc.)*
Baker & Taylor *(Baker & Taylor Bks.)*
Yankee Ped Bkshop *(Yankee Peddler Bookshop).*

ICAN LA, *(ICAN; 0-9643622),* Orders Addr.: P.O. Box 4409, Gulfshores, AL 36547 Tel 334-967-4850; Fax: 334-967-4870; Toll Free: 800-234-0575
E-mail: contact@icanpublishing.com; rayfield@gulftel.com
Web site: http://www.icanpublishing.com.

ICAN Pr, *See* **Black Forest Pr**

ICDC Pubng, *(ICDC Publishing, Inc.; 1-881159),* 4123 Lankershim Blvd., North Hollywood, CA 91602-2020 Tel 818-487-1199; Fax: 818-769-3100.

Ichthys Bks, *(Ichthys Bks.; 0-930711),* 8464 Carter St., Overland Park, KS 66212-4417 (SAN 677-2390) Do not confuse with Ichthys Bks., Vienna, VA.

ICNR Newtown, *(International Ctr. for Nutritional Research, Inc.; 0-9617838),* 303 Corporate Dr., E., Langhorne, PA 19047-8009 (SAN 665-3812) Tel 215-968-4781; Fax: 215-968-8904.

Icon Lrning Systs, *(Icon Learning Systems, LLC; 0-914168; 1-929007),* 295 North St., Teterboro, NJ 07608 Fax: 201-727-0099; Toll Free: 800-631-1181
E-mail: mjahn.icon@medimedia.com
Web site: http://www.netterart.com.

ICPC, *(Intercultural Communication Publishing Corp.; 0-9628364),* Orders Addr.: P.O. Box 1444, Voorhees, NJ 08043-7444 Tel 609-767-4408.

ICPSR, *(Inter-University Consortium for Political & Social Research; 0-89138),* Affil. of Univ. of Michigan Institute for Social Research, P.O. Box 1248, Ann Arbor, MI 48106-1248 (SAN 207-7450) Tel 734-998-9900; Fax: 734-998-9889
E-mail: netmail@icpsr.umich.edu
Web site: http://www.icpsr.wmich.edu.

Idarius Pr, *(Idarius Pr.; 0-9649304),* 2-B Lorraine St., Ukiah, CA 95482 Tel 707-463-3739; Fax: 707-468-0205
E-mail: bidarius@saber.net.

IDC Pubng, *(IDC Publishing; 1-885115),* Div. of Institute for Research & Education Health System Minnesota, 3800 Park Nicollet Blvd., Minneapolis, MN 55416-2699 Toll Free: 888-637-2675
Web site: http://www.idcpublishing.com.

Ide Hse, *(Ide Hse., Inc.; 0-86663),* 22497 Swordfish Dr., Boca Raton, FL 33428-4609 (SAN 216-146X) Tel 561-477-3364; Fax: 561-477-2534
Web site: http://www.idehouse.com.

Idea Group Pub, *(Idea Group Publishing; 1-878289; 1-930708; 1-59140),* 1331 E. Chocolate Ave., Hershey, PA 17033 Tel 717-533-8845; Fax: 717-533-8661; Toll Free: 800-345-4332
E-mail: jtravers@idea-group.com
Web site: http://www.idea-group.com
Dist(s): **IPG Chicago** *(Independent Pubs. Group).*

IDEALS PA, *(Institute for the Development of Emotional Life Skills (IDEALS); 0-932990),* Box 391, State College, PA 16804 (SAN 224-358X) Tel 301-231-6162; Fax: 301-231-6151.

Idelson Gnocchi Pub, *(Idealson-Gnocchi Pub.; 1-928649),* Div. of Idelson-Gnocchi Editore, 12255 NW Hwy. 255-A, Reddick, FL 32686 Tel 352-591-1136; Fax: 352-591-1189
E-mail: candotti@worldnet.att.net
Web site: http://idelson-gnocchi.com
Dist(s): **J Majors Co** *(Majors, J. A. Co.).*

IDG Bks, *See* **Hungry Minds**

IDI Pub, *(IDI Publishing; 1-880906),* Div. of Infectious Diseases, Inc., 17121 Lakewood Dr., Omaha, NE 68123-3954 Tel 402-292-6070 (phone/fax).

IDRC-CRDI (CAN) *(0-88936; 1-55250) Dist. by* **Stylus Pub VA.**

IDS Pubng, *(IDS Publishing Corp.; 0-9642598),* Orders Addr.: P.O. Box 389, Worthington, OH 43085 Tel 614-885-2323; Edit Addr.: 868 Cherryfield Ave., Columbus, OH 43235.

Idyll Arbor, *(Idyll Arbor, Inc.; 0-937663; 1-882883; 1-930461),* Orders Addr.: P.O. Box 720, Ravensdale, WA 98051 Tel 425-432-3231; Fax: 425-432-3726; Edit Addr.: 25119 SE 262nd St., Ravensdale, WA 98051
E-mail: sales@idyllarbor.com
Web site: http://www.Idyllarbor.com.

Idylwild Bks, *(Idylwild Bks.; 0-9613054),* Orders Addr.: P.O. Box 246, Ojai, CA 93024 (SAN 295-3870)
E-mail: light@idylwildbooks.com
Dist(s): **New Leaf Dist** *(New Leaf Distributing Co., Inc.).*

†IEEE Comp Soc, *(IEEE Computer Society Pr.; 0-7695; 0-8186),* Div. of IEEE, Orders Addr.: a/o Customer Service Dept., P.O. Box 1331, Piscataway, NJ 08855-1331 Tel 800-701-4333 (800-701-IEEE); 732-981-0060 (Outside the USA); Fax: 732-981-9667; 445 Hoes Lane, Piscataway, NJ 08855; Edit Addr.: 10662 Los Vaqueros Cir., Los Alamitos, CA 90720 (SAN 631-0877) Tel 714-821-8380; Fax: 714-821-4010; Toll Free: 800-272-6657
E-mail: cs.book@computer.org
Web site: http://www.computer.org
Dist(s): **Inst Electrical** *(Institute of Electrical & Electronics Engineers, Inc.); CIP.*

†IEEE Standards, *(IEEE Standards Office; 0-7803; 1-55937; 0-7381),* Div. of Institute of Electrical & Electronics Engineers, Inc., Orders Addr.: P.O. Box 1331, Piscataway, NJ 08855-1331 (SAN 250-6130) Tel 732-562-3822; Fax: 732-562-1571; Toll Free: 800-678-4333; Edit Addr.: 445 Hoes Ln., Piscataway, NJ 08855 Tel 732-562-3966; 908-562-3966
E-mail: customer.service@ieee.org
Web site: http://www.ieee.org; *CIP.*

IEST, *(Institute of Environmental Sciences & Technology; 0-915414; 1-877862),* 940 E. Northwest Hwy., Mount Prospect, IL 60056 (SAN 209-2077) Tel 847-255-1561; Fax: 847-255-1699
E-mail: iest@iest.org; publicationsales@iest.org
Web site: http://www.iest.org.

IFSTA, *(IFSTA; 0-87939),* Orders Addr.: c/o Oklahoma State Univ., Fire Protection Pubns., 930 N. Willis, Stillwater, OK 74078-8045 Tel 405-744-5723; Fax: 405-744-8204; Toll Free: 800-654-4055 (orders only)
Web site: http://www.ifsta.org/.

†Igaku-Shoin, *(Igaku-Shoin Medical Pubs.; 0-89640; 4-260),* Subs. of Igaku-Shoin, Ltd. (Japan), 60 Madison Ave., Suite 1107, New York, NY 10010-1600 (SAN 211-5689) Tel 212-779-0123; Fax: 212-779-0322; Toll Free: 800-765-0800
Dist(s): **Lppncott W & W** *(Lippincott Williams & Wilkins); CIP.*

Ignatius Pr, *(Ignatius Pr.; 0-89870; 1-58617),* Div. of Guadalupe Assocs., Inc., Orders Addr.: P.O. Box 1339, Fort Collins, CO 80522-1339 Tel 970-221-3920; Fax: 970-221-3964; Toll Free Fax: 800-278-3566; Toll Free: 800-651-1531 (credit card orders, no minimum, individual orders); 877-320-9276 (bookstore orders); Edit Addr.: 2515 McAllister St., San Francisco, CA 94118 (SAN 214-3887) Tel 415-387-2324; Fax: 415-387-0896
E-mail: info@ignatius.com
Web site: http://www.ignatius.com
Dist(s): **Baker & Taylor** *(Baker & Taylor Bks.)*
Midpt Trade *(Midpoint Trade Bks., Inc.)*
Riverside-World *(Riverside World)*
Spring Arbor Dist *(Spring Arbor Distributors Inc.).*

Iguana Med Bks, *(Iguana Medical Bks.; 0-9643482),* P.O. Box 23772, Milwaukee, WI 53223-0772 Tel 414-254-4097; Fax: 414-354-8930
E-mail: hgollup@ah.com.

IHA, *(Institute for Healthcare Advancement; 0-9701245),* 15111 E. Whittier Blvd., Suite 460, Whittier, CA 90603-2181 Tel 562-693-9721; Fax: 562-907-1963; Toll Free: 800-434-4633
E-mail: nprushton@aol.com
Web site: http://www.iha4health.org.

IHC Home Health, *(IHC Home Health Agency; 0-9622967),* Div. of Intermountain Health Care, 2250 S. 1300 W., No. A, Salt Lake City, UT 84119-1475 Tel 801-484-8700.

IHEMI, *(International Health Economics & Management Institute; 0-914943),* Southern Illinois Univ. at Edwardsville, Box 1101, Edwardsville, IL 62026-1101 (SAN 289-2626) Tel 618-692-2291.

IHS Health Grp, *(IHS Health Group; 0-935184; 1-57491),* Orders Addr.: 15 Inverness Way, E., Englewood, CO 80112-5776 (SAN 295-3374) Tel 303-662-9101; Toll Free: 877-295-9240
E-mail: interpharm@interpharm.com
Web site: http://www.interpharm.com.

IL Coll Optometry, *(Illinois College of Optometry; 0-9652759),* 3241 S. Michigan Ave., Chicago, IL 60616 Tel 312-225-1700; Fax: 312-949-7670
E-mail: brenard@eyecare.ico.edu.

†Ill St Museum, *(Illinois State Museum Society; 0-89792),* Spring & Edwards, Springfield, IL 62706 (SAN 201-5137) Tel 217-782-7388; Fax: 217-782-1254
E-mail: editor@museum.state.il.us
Web site: http://www.museum.state.il.us; *CIP.*

Illumination CA, *(Illumination Pr.; 0-9708299),* P.O. Box 269, Santa Monica, CA 90406 Tel 310-451-1143; Fax: 310-451-4044 Do not confuse with companies with same name in Mansfield, MA, Montclair, VA
E-mail: illuminationprs@aol.com
Web site: http://illuminationpress.com
Dist(s): **IPG Chicago** *(Independent Pubs. Group).*

ILOC, *(ILOC, Inc.; 1-882531),* Orders Addr.: P.O. Box 232, Granville, OH 43023 Tel 740-587-2658; Fax: 740-587-2679; Edit Addr.: 905 River Rd., Granville, OH 43023
Dist(s): **J Majors Co** *(Majors, J. A. Co.)*
Rittenhouse *(Rittenhouse Bk. Distributors).*

ILR Press Imprint of Cornell U Pr

ILSI, *(International Life Sciences Institute/ILSI Pr.; 0-935368; 0-944398; 1-57881),* 1126 16th St., NW, Suite 300, Washington, DC 20036-4810 (SAN 224-3911) Tel 202-659-0074; Fax: 202-659-8654; Toll Free: 800-538-9601
E-mail: ilsi@ilsi.org
Web site: http://www.ilsi.org.

ILSI-NF, *See* **ILSI**

Image Ad Vantage, *(Image Ad Vantage; 0-9649106),* 1420 Yellowstone Ave., Billings, MT 59102-5340 Tel 307-674-5343.

Image Pr TX, *(Image Pr.; 0-9640099),* 2602 Plum Hollow, San Antonio, TX 78258-4420 Tel 210-497-5361 Do not confuse with Image Pr., Topeka, KS.

Imaginart Intl, *(Imaginart International, Inc.; 0-9609464; 1-883315),* 307 Arizona St., Bisbee, AZ 85603 (SAN 260-2067) Tel 520-432-5741; Fax: 520-432-5134; Toll Free Fax: 800-737-1376 (U.S. & Canada only); Toll Free: 800-828-1376 (U.S. & Canada only)
E-mail: imaginart@compuserve.com
Web site: http://www.imaginartonline.com.

Imaginart Pr, *See* **Imaginart Intl**

IMMEL Pubng (GBR) *(0-907151; 1-898162) Dist. by* **Trans-Atl Phila.**

IMPACC ME, *See* **IMPACC USA**

IMPACC USA, *(IMPACC USA; 1-879864),* P.O. Box 1247, Greenville, ME 04441-1247 Tel 207-695-3354; Fax: 207-695-2330; Toll Free: 800-762-7720 Do not confuse with IMPACC Assocs., Inc. in Gwynedd Valley, PA
E-mail: info@impaccusa.com
Web site: http://www.impaccusa.com.

Impact Bks MO, *See* **Impact Christian**

Impact Christian, *(Impact Christian Bks., Inc.; 0-89228),* 2124 Broadway, PMB 389, New York, NY 10023 (SAN 214-0330) Tel 212-581-5543; Toll Free: 800-451-2708 (wats-orders only)
E-mail: impactchristianbooks@juno.com
Web site: http://www.impactchristianbooks//
Dist(s): **Spring Arbor Dist** *(Spring Arbor Distributors Inc.).*

Impact Commun, *(Impact Communications, Inc.; 0-9645991),* 330 Madison Ave., 21st Flr., New York, NY 10017 Tel 212-490-2300; Fax: 212-557-4729; Toll Free: 800-922-0949.

Impact FL, *See* **Spec Pr FL**

†Impact Pubs CA, ***(Impact Pubs., Inc.; 0-915166; 1-886230),* P.O. Box 6016, Atascadero, CA 93422 (SAN 202-6864) Tel 805-466-5917; Fax: 805-466-5919; Toll Free: 800-246-7228**
E-mail: info@impactpublishers.com
Web site: http://www.impactpublishers.com; *CIP.*

IMPAKT Communs, *(IMPAKT Communications, Inc.; 0-9647489; 1-890694),* Orders Addr.: P.O. Box 12496, Green Bay, WI 54307-2496 Tel 920-434-3838; Fax: 920-434-8884; Toll Free: 800-477-2995; Edit Addr.: 2251 Hutson Rd., Green Bay, WI 54307-2496
E-mail: info@impakt.com
Web site: http://www.impakt.com
Dist(s): **Prima Pub** *(Prima Publishing).*

Imperial College (GBR) *(1-86094) Dist. by* **World Scientific Pub.**

Imprint Pubns, *(Imprint Pubns., Inc.; 1-879176),* 230 E. Ohio St., Suite 300, Chicago, IL 60611 Tel 312-337-9268; Fax: 312-337-9622
E-mail: orders@imprint-chicago.com; imppub@imprint-chicago.com
Web site: http://www.imprint-chicago.com/contactus.htm.

In Ctr Global, *(Indiana Ctr. on Global Change & World Peace; 1-881157),* Div. of Indiana Univ., 201 N. Indiana Ave., Bloomington, IN 47405-3603 Tel 812-855-0756; Fax: 812-855-6271
E-mail: orugs@indiana.edu
Web site: http://www.indiana.edu/~rugs/ctrdir/icgcwp.html.

In The Pink, *(In The Pink Institute, Inc.; 0-9659154),* 8160 Grapevine Rd., Marshall, NC 28753 Tel 828-689-0009
E-mail: inthepinkherbs@juno.com.

IN U Dept Health, *(Indiana Univ. Dept. of Health & Safety Education, Office of Pubns. & Editorial Services; 0-941636),* HPER Bldg., Rm. 116, Bloomington, IN 47405 (SAN 239-233X) Tel 812-335-7975.

IN U Schl Soc Wrk, *(Indiana Univ. Schl. of Social Work; 0-9643817),* 902 W. New York St., Indianapolis, IN 46202-5156 Tel 317-274-6713; Fax: 317-274-8630.

IN Univ Schl Dentstry, *(Indiana Univ. Schl. of Denistry; 0-9655149),* 1121 W. Michigan St., Rm. 104, Indianapolis, IN 46202-5186 Tel 317-274-8135; Fax: 317-274-7188.

Incinerat Consults, *(Incinerator Consultants, Inc.; 0-9621774),* 11204 Longwood Grove Dr., Reston, VA 20194 (SAN 252-2128) Tel 703-437-1790; Fax: 703-437-9048
E-mail: cbrunner@clark.net
Web site: http://www.clark.net/pub/cbrunner.

Incremental Motion, *(Incremental Motion Control Systems Society; 0-931538),* Orders Addr.: P.O. Box 2772, Champaign, IL 61825 (SAN 211-4259) Tel 217-356-1523; Fax: 217-356-2356.

Ind Eng Mgmt Pr, *See* **Eng Mgmt Pr**

†Ind Hist Soc, *(Indiana Historical Society; 0-87195),* 450 W. Ohio St., Indianapolis, IN 46202-3269 (SAN 201-5234) Tel 317-232-1882; 317-233-3156; Fax: 317-233-0857; Toll Free: 800-447-1830
E-mail: ghanlin@indianahistory.org
Web site: http://www.indianahistory.org
Dist(s): **Ind U Pr** *(Indiana Univ. Pr.); CIP.*

†Ind U Pr, *(Indiana Univ. Pr.; 0-253),* 601 N. Morton St., Bloomington, IN 47404-3797 (SAN 202-5647) Tel 812-855-4203; Fax: 812-855-7931
E-mail: iuporder@indiana.edu
Web site: http://www.Indiana.edu/~iupress
Dist(s): **B & T International** *(Baker & Taylor International); CIP.*

Indelble Ink, *(Indelible Ink; 0-9638436),* P.O. Box 563, Rockton, IL 61072-3102 Tel 815-624-2253.

Indep Pr Imprint of Herald Pub Hse

Independ Prod, *(Independent Production Fund; 1-930783),* 45 W. 45th St., Suite 808, New York, NY 10036 Tel 212-221-6310; Fax: 212-302-1854; Toll Free: 800-727-2470
E-mail: tlevine@tobylevine.com; lzbar@aol.com.

Independent Inst, *(Independent Institute; 0-945999),* 100 Swan Way, Suite 200, Oakland, CA 94621-1428 (SAN 135-2938) Tel 510-632-1366; Fax: 510-568-6040; Toll Free: 800-927-8733
E-mail: info@indenpendent.org; orders@independent.org
Web site: http://www.independent.org
Dist(s): **Seven Hills Bk** *(7 Hills Bk. Distributors).*

†Independent Scholars Asia Inc, *(Independent Scholars of Asia, Inc.; 0-945875),* 2321 Russell, No. 3C, Berkeley, CA 94705-1959 (SAN 248-000X) Tel 510-849-3791
E-mail: riheinze@juno.com
Web site: http://www.hypersphere.com/isa; *CIP.*

Indiana Africa, *(Indian Univ., African Studies Program; 0-941934),* Indiana Univ., 221 Woodburn Hall, Bloomington, IN 47405 (SAN 238-6135) Tel 812-855-8625; Fax: 812-855-6734
E-mail: afrist@indiana.edu; jecole@indiana.edu
Web site: http://www.indiana.edu/~ afrist/.

Indigo Pr AR, *(Indigo Pr.; 0-9641214),* Orders Addr.: P.O. Box 968, West Fork, AR 72774-0968 Tel 501-839-3944; Fax: 501-839-8384; Toll Free: 888-294-8127; Edit Addr.: 14081 S. Hwy. 170, West Fork, AR 72774 Do not confuse with Indigo Pr.LC, Sanibel, FL
E-mail: t_roloff@hotmail.com
Dist(s): **Baker & Taylor** *(Baker & Taylor Bks.)*
Bookazine Co Inc *(Bookazine Co., Inc.)*
Quality Bks IL *(Quality Bks., Inc.).*

Indus Pub, *(Indus Publishing Corp.; 1-890838),* 7052 Pokey Moonshine, Wayland, NY 14572 Tel 716-728-5752; Fax: 716-728-9756
E-mail: scura@aol.com
Dist(s): **Assoc Pubs Grp** *(Associated Pubs. Group).*

Infant Hearing Resc, *See* **Hearing & Speech**

Infection Control, *(Infection Control Pubns.; 0-936751),* 1150 E. Nicholls Rd., Fruit Heights, UT 84037 (SAN 699-8836) Tel 801-544-2146; Toll Free: 800-426-6588.

Infinite Des, *(Infinite Design, Inc.; 0-9670573),* Orders Addr.: P.O. Box 610717, Dallas, TX 75261-0717 Tel 817-318-5552 (phone/fax); Toll Free: 877-434-4620; Edit Addr.: 2400 State Hwy. 121, No. 1201, Dallas, TX 75261-0717.

Infinity Impress, *(Infinity Impressions, Ltd.; 1-879339),* 51 Dean Rd., Mendham, NJ 07945 Tel 973-543-9231; Fax: 973-543-9211.

Infinity NY, *(Infinity Pr.; 0-9621975),* 360 Montauk Hwy., West Islip, NY 11795 Tel 516-422-1110 Do not confuse with companies with the same name in Takoma Park, MD, Rochester, NY, Seattle, WA, Watkinsville, GA, Taos, NM.

Infnty Pub, *(Infinity Publishing; 0-9651590),* 7721 17th Ave., NE, Seattle, WA 98115 Tel 206-525-8434; Fax: 206-525-5388 Do not confuse with companies with same name in Lansing IL, Darien, IL, West Palm Beach, FL
E-mail: Jusihnds@aol.com.

Info Better Liv, *See* **PIBL**

Info Guides, *(Information Guides; 0-938329),* Orders Addr.: P.O. Box 0531, Hermosa Beach, CA 90254 (SAN 661-4337); Edit Addr.: 32 18th St., Hermosa Beach, CA 90254 (SAN 661-4345) Tel 310-379-1094; Fax: 310-379-1925; Toll Free: 800-347-3257.

Info Inst, *(Information Institute; 0-939823),* P.O. Box 638, Vienna, VA 22183-0638 (SAN 663-8392).

Info Prods, *(Information Products; 0-937978),* P.O. Box 389, Awhahnee, CA 93601-0389 (SAN 214-0349) Tel 209-642-2330 Do not confuse with Information Products, Lompoc, CA.

Info Res Cons, *(Information Resource Consultants; 0-931821; 1-55804),* 1556 Walpole Dr., Chesterfield, MO 63017 (SAN 685-2874) Tel 636-530-7966 (phone/fax); Toll Free: 800-858-7966
E-mail: sgill1@mindspring.com
Web site: http://www.slgill.com.

Info Resources, *(Information Resources Pr.; 0-87815),* Div. of Herner & Co., 5640 Nicholson Ln., Suite 300, Rocksville, MD 20852 (SAN 202-6961) Fax: 301-984-8527; Toll Free: 800-451-7363.

Info Today Inc, *(Information Today, Inc.; 0-910965; 0-938734; 1-57387),* 143 Old Marlton Pike, Medford, NJ 08055-8750 (SAN 215-8841) Tel 609-654-6266; Fax: 609-654-4309; Toll Free: 800-300-9868 ;
Imprints: CyberAge Bks (CyberAge Books)
E-mail: custserv@infotoday.com
Web site: http://www.infotoday.com
Dist(s): **IPG Chicago** *(Independent Pubs. Group).*

Info Tomorrow, *(Information for Tomorrow; 0-9657674),* 4121 Warner St., Kensington, MD 20895 Tel 301-581-9488; Fax: 301-581-0090; Toll Free: 800-506-6587
E-mail: kinsella@cua.edu
Web site: http://www.informationfortomorrow.com.

Info USA, *(Information U.S.A., Inc.; 1-878346),* Orders Addr.: P.O. Box E, Kensington, MD 20895-0418 Tel 301-924-0556; Fax: 301-929-8907; Toll Free: 800-955-7693
Dist(s): **Baker & Taylor** *(Baker & Taylor Bks.)*
Distributors *(Distributors, The).*

Info Ventures Inc, *(Information Ventures, Inc.; 0-9617314),* 42 S. 15th St., Suite 700, Philadelphia, PA 19102-2299 (SAN 663-7485) Tel 215-569-2300; Fax: 215-569-2575
E-mail: emf-link@infoventures.com; IVI@infoventures.com
Web site: http://www.infoventures.com.

Infobriefings, *(Infobriefings, Inc.; 0-9662096),* P.O. Box 1299, Highland Park, NJ 08904 Tel 732-249-2002; Fax: 732-249-3786
E-mail: infobrief@earthlink.net.

Infoconnect, *(Infoconnect, Ltd.; 0-9630843),* Orders Addr.: P.O. Box 427, Burbank, CA 91503-0427; Edit Addr.: 1180 Matmor Rd., No. 165, Woodland, CA 95695 Tel 916-666-5671.

Infolink New York, *(Infolink; 0-9659104),* 31 Albany Post Rd., Montrose, NY 10548-0306 Tel 914-736-1565; Fax: 914-736-3806; Toll Free: 800-743-5465 Do not confuse with companies with the same name in Croton-on-Hudson, NY, Yucca Valley, CA.

InfoPlus, *(InfoPlus; 0-9648684),* 1000 Fair Oaks Ave., No. 224, South Pasadena, CA 91030 Tel 626-403-0416.

InforMed OR, *(InforMed; 1-890495),* Div. of Creative Ventures, Inc., Orders Addr.: P.O. Box 1001, Lake Oswego, OR 97034 Tel 503-624-8014; Fax: 503-639-1369; Edit Addr.: 7110 SW Fir Loop, Suite 110, Tigard, OR 97223.

Ingenix Inc, *(Ingenix, Inc.; 1-56329; 1-56337),* 2525 Lake Park Blvd., West Valley City, UT 84120 (SAN 630-5482) Tel 801-982-3453; Toll Free: 800-765-6095
E-mail: jeni.smith@ingenix.com; chris.smith@ingenix.com
Web site: http://www.ingenix.com
Dist(s): **J Majors Co** *(Majors, J. A. Co.)*
Matthews Medical Bk Co *(Matthews Medical Bk. Co.)*
Rittenhouse *(Rittenhouse Bk. Distributors).*

Ingenix Pub Grp, *See* **Ingenix Inc**

Ingham Pub, *(Ingham Publishing, Inc.; 0-9611804; 1-891130),* Orders Addr.: P.O. Box 12642, Saint Petersburg, FL 33733-2642 Tel 813-343-4811; Fax: 813-381-2807; Edit Addr.: 5650 First Ave., N., Saint Petersburg, FL 33710 (SAN 112-8930)
E-mail: ftreflex@concentric.net.

Inkslingers Res, *(InkSlingers Research & Writing Services, Inc.; 1-893360),* 5800 Lumberdale Rd., Suite 94, Houston, TX 77092 Tel 713-956-0110; Fax: 713-956-1014
Web site: http://www.slingink.com.

Inkwell Prods, *(Inkwell Productions; 0-9658158),* 3370 N. Hayden Rd., No. 123-276, Scottsdale, AZ 85251 Tel 480-315-9636; Fax: 480-315-9641
E-mail: speciality@home.com.

Inner City Bks (CAN) *(0-919123; 1-894574) Dist. by* **BookWorld.**

†Inner Growth Bks, *(Inner Growth Bks.; 0-914073),* P.O. Box 520, Chiloquin, OR 97624 (SAN 287-5829) Tel 541-783-3126
E-mail: arraj@innerexplorations.com
Web site: http://innerexplorations.com*; CIP.*

Inner Passages, *(Inner Passages Publishing; 0-9663271),* Orders Addr.: P.O. Box 8827, Colorado Springs, CO 80908-8227 Fax: 719-495-3865; Edit Addr.: 7575 Pinery Cir., Colorado Springs, CO 80908-2838
Web site: http://www.readersndex.com/innerpassages.

Inner Path, *(Inner Path Publishing Co., The; 0-9651506),* 15 Paradise Plaza, Box 299, Sarasota, FL 34239 Tel 941-955-5410; Fax: 941-366-7182; Toll Free: 800-444-2524; 2105 11th Pl., Sarasota, FL 34239
Web site: http://www.bookworld.com/innevpath/index.html
Dist(s): **Quality Bks IL** *(Quality Bks., Inc.).*

Inner Search Found, *(Inner Search Foundation; 0-9621790),* 1314 Alps Dr., McLean, VA 22102-1502 (SAN 252-2276) Tel 703-448-3362; Fax: 703-448-0814
E-mail: innersearch@mindspring.com
Dist(s): **Bookpeople** *(Bookpeople)*
Distributors International *(Distributors International)*
New Leaf Dist *(New Leaf Distributing Co., Inc.).*

Inner Trad Imprint of Inner Tradit

†Inner Tradit, *(Inner Traditions International, Ltd.; 0-89281; 1-879181),* Orders Addr.: P.O. Box 388, Rochester, VT 05767; Edit Addr.: One Park St., Rochester, VT 05767 (SAN 208-6948) Tel 802-767-3174; Fax: 802-767-3726; Toll Free: 800-246-8648 ; *Imprints:* Destiny Bks (Destiny Books) Heal Arts VT (Healing Arts Press) Park St Pr (Park Street Press) Inner Trad (Inner Traditions)
E-mail: jeanie@InnerTraditions.com; orders@innertraditions.com
Web site: http://www.InnerTraditions.com
Dist(s): **Bookazine Co Inc** *(Bookazine Co., Inc.)*
Bookpeople *(Bookpeople)*
Integral Yoga Pubns *(Integral Yoga Pubns.)*
Koen Bk Distributors *(Koen Bk. Distributors)*
Lotus Pr *(Lotus Pr.)*
New Leaf Dist *(New Leaf Distributing Co., Inc.)*
Nutri-Books Corp *(Nutri-Bks. Corp.)*
Red Wheel ME *(Red Wheel)*
Unique Bks Inc *(Unique Bks., Inc.)*
Wrldwide Media Srv *(Worldwide Media Service, Inc.); CIP.*

InnerVision, *(Inner Vision Publishing Co.; 0-917483),* Orders Addr.: P.O. Box 1117, Virginia Beach, VA 23451-0117 (SAN 656-0709) Tel 757-460-5422; Fax: 757-460-5452; Edit Addr.: 4407 Ocean View Ave., Virginia Beach, VA 23455
Dist(s): **New Leaf Dist** *(New Leaf Distributing Co., Inc.).*

Innisfree Pr, *(Innisfree Pr.; 0-931055; 1-880913),* 136 Roumfort Rd., Philadelphia, PA 19119 Tel 215-247-4085; Fax: 215-247-2343; Toll Free: 800-367-5872 (religious trade); 800-283-3572 (general)
E-mail: InnisfreeP@aol.com
Web site: http://www.innifreepress.com
Dist(s): **Consort Bk Sales** *(Consortium Bk. Sales & Distribution).*

Innovat Med, *(Innovative Medical Education Consortium, Inc.; 0-9641386),* 1601 Lincoln Ave., Vancouver, WA 98660-2758 Tel 360-699-1179; Fax: 360-699-1944; Toll Free: 800-205-4632
Dist(s): **Baker & Taylor** *(Baker & Taylor Bks.)*
Bookpeople *(Bookpeople)*
Brodart *(Brodart Co.).*

Innovat Pub & Graph, *(Innovative Publishing & Graphics; 0-9632231),* 417 S. Dearborn St., Suite 800, Chicago, IL 60605 Tel 312-431-0900; Fax: 312-431-0990 Do not confuse with Innovative Publishing in Brooklyn, NY.

Innovat Systems, *(Innovative Systems for Rehabilitation; 0-929538),* P.O. Box 3192, Boulder, CO 80307-3192 (SAN 249-6216) Tel 303-443-7363; Fax: 303-443-9844
E-mail: bjheadley@aol.com
Dist(s): **Orthopedic Phys** *(Orthopedic Physical Therapy Products (OPTP)).*

Innvtve Med, *(Innovative Medical Communications; 0-9653045),* 1013 Ridgewood Ct., West Des Moines, IA 50265 Fax: 515-223-9389; Toll Free: 800-409-9706
E-mail: orders@telemedprimer.com
Web site: http://www.telemedprimer.com.

Inpsyte, *(Inpsyte; 0-9637450),* Div. of Bi-Polar, Inc., Orders Addr.: P.O. Box 160220, Austin, TX 78716-0220 Tel 512-327-2656; Fax: 512-327-7516; Toll Free: 800-899-5115; Edit Addr.: 423 Brady Ln., Austin, TX 78746
E-mail: info@inpsyte.com
Web site: http://www.inpsyte.com.

Inquiry Pr, *(Inquiry Pr.; 0-918112),* 1880 N. Eastman, Midland, MI 48640 (SAN 208-1164) Tel 517-631-0009; Fax: 517-631-8801.

Ins Career Dev, *See* **ICDC Pubng**

Insight TX, *See* **Apple-a-Day**

Insignia Publng, *(Insignia Publishing Co.; 0-9652400),* 1429 G St., NW, Suite 535, Washington, DC 20005 (SAN 298-993X) Tel 301-540-4413; Fax: 301-540-3795; Toll Free: 800-606-2665
E-mail: InsigniaPC@aol.com
Web site: http://www.InsigniaUSA.com
Dist(s): **Baker & Taylor** *(Baker & Taylor Bks.).*

Inspir Univ, *(Inspiration Univ.; 0-945793),* P.O. Box 118, Walton, NY 13856-0118 (SAN 247-5634) Fax: 540-885-1230
Dist(s): **New Leaf Dist** *(New Leaf Distributing Co., Inc.).*

Inst Achieve Human Pot, *(Institute for the Achievement of Human Potential; 0-936676; 0-944349),* Div. of Institutes for the Achievement of Human Potential, 8801 Stenton Ave., Wyndmoor, PA 19038 (SAN 215-7314) Tel 215-233-2050 (ext. 288); Fax: 215-233-9312; 215-233-1530
E-mail: institutes@iahp.org; iahp@earthlink.net
Web site: http://www.iahp.org.

Inst Afro-Am Schol, *See* **IAAS Pubs**

Inst Chinese Med, *(Institute of Chinese Medicine; 0-9639715),* 602 San Gabriel Blvd., Rosemead, CA 91770 Tel 818-280-8811
Dist(s): **Redwing Bk Co** *(Redwing Bk. Co.).*

Inst Drug-Free Wrkpl, *(Institute for a Drug-Free Workplace; 1-889437),* 1225 I St., NW, Suite 1000, Washington, DC 20005-3914 Tel 202-842-7400; Fax: 202-842-0022
Web site: http://www.drugfreeworkplace.org.

Inst Economic Affairs (GBR) *(0-255) Dist. by* **Coronet Bks.**

Inst Educ Lead, *(Institute for Educational Leadership; 0-937846),* 1001 Connecticut Ave., NW, Suite 310, Washington, DC 20036 (SAN 225-7823) Tel 202-822-8405; Fax: 202-872-4050.

Inst Electrical, *(Institute of Electrical & Electronics Engineers, Inc.; 0-7803; 0-87942; 0-7381),* Orders Addr.: c/o IEEE Service Ctr., P.O. Box 1331, Piscataway, NJ 08855-1331 (SAN 203-8072) Toll Free Fax: 800-716-6447; Toll Free: 800-716-3447 (ext. 025); Edit Addr.: 445 Hoes Ln., Piscataway, NJ 08855 (SAN 203-8064) Tel 732-562-3967; Fax: 732-981-9334; Toll Free: 800-678-4333
E-mail: ieeepress@ieee.org
Web site: http://www.ieee.org/organizations/pubs/press.

Inst Evolutionary, *(Institute for Evolutionary Research; 0-938710),* Orders Addr.: 1621 Freeway Dr., Suite 220, Mount Vernon, WA 98273 (SAN 662-0477) Tel 360-428-5737; Fax: 360-428-5710
Dist(s): **Bookpeople** *(Bookpeople).*

Inst Fmly Ctr, *(Institute for Family-Centered Care; 0-9642014; 0-9677733),* 7900 Wisconsin Ave., Suite 405, Bethesda, MD 20814 Tel 301-652-0281; Fax: 301-652-0186
E-mail: ifcc@aol.com
Web site: http://www.familycenteredcare.org.

Inst Fnd Trning, *See* **Inpsyte**

Inst Food & Develop, *(Institute for Food & Development Policy/Food First Bks.; 0-935028),* 398 60th St., Oakland, CA 94618-1212 (SAN 213-327X) Tel 510-654-4400; Fax: 510-654-4551
E-mail: foodfirst@foodfirst.org
Web site: http://www.foodfirst.org
Dist(s): **LPC Group** *(LPC Group).*

Inst for Health Real, *(Institute for Health Realities, Inc.; 0-9620479),* Orders Addr.: P.O. Box 49308, Colorado Springs, CO 80949-9308 (SAN 248-6784) Tel 719-598-4968; Fax: 719-548-1785; Toll Free: 800-414-3438; Edit Addr.: 5245 Centennial Blvd., Suite 100, Colorado Springs, CO 80919
E-mail: baqueen@qwest.net
Web site: http://www.healthrealities.org.

Inst for Hlthcare, *(Institute for Healthcare Improvement; 1-890070),* 135 Francis St., Boston, MA 02215 Tel 617-754-4800; Fax: 617-754-4848
Web site: http://www.ihi.org.

Inst for Psycho-Imag, *(Institute for Psycho-Imagination Therapy; 0-9638685),* 111 N. La Cienega Blvd., Beverly Hills, CA 90211 Tel 310-652-2922.

Inst Global Cultl, *See* **Global Pubns**

Inst Hist Rev, *See* **Legion Survival**

Inst Knowledge, *(Institute of Knowledge, The; 1-886974),* 4 Duck Hawk Ct., Suite 2001, Hackettstown, NJ 07840-3307 Tel 908-979-1779 (phone/fax).

Inst Logo, *See* **V Frankl Inst**

Inst Mgmt & Labor, *(Rutgers Univ., Institute of Management & Labor Relations; 0-941312),* Cook Campus, Industrial Relations & Human Resources Dept., P.O Box 231, Ryders Ln., New Brunswick, NJ 08903 (SAN 215-8779).

Inst Mgmt Account, *(Institute of Management Accountants; 0-86641),* 10 Paragon Dr., P.O. Box 433, Montvale, NJ 07645-1760 (SAN 207-2637) Tel 201-573-9000; Fax: 201-573-0559; Toll Free: 800-638-4427
E-mail: ima@imanet.org; imacma@imanet.org
Web site: http://www.imanet.org
Dist(s): **St Lucie Pr** *(St. Lucie Pr.).*

Inst Mind Behavior, *(Institute of Mind & Behavior; 0-930195),* Orders Addr.: P.O. Box 522, New York, NY 10014 (SAN 691-9618) Tel 212-595-4853
Web site: http://kramer.ume.maine.edu./~jmb/.

Inst of Physics Pubng, *(Institute of Physics Publishing; 0-7503; 0-85274; 0-85498),* The Public Ledte Bldg., Suite 1035 150 S. Independence Mall, W., Philadelphia, PA 19106 (SAN 298-2315) Tel 215-627-0880; Fax: 215-627-0879; Toll Free: 800-632-0880
E-mail: book.enquiries@iop.org
Web site: http://bookmark.iop.org
Dist(s): **Am Intl Dist** *(American International Distribution Corp.).*

Inst of Prev Med, *(Institute of Preventive Medicine; 1-879131),* 95 E. Main St., Suite 101, Denville, NJ 07834 Tel 973-586-4111; Fax: 973-586-8466.

Inst of Pro Edu, *(Institute of Professional Education-Louisiana State Univ. Health Science Ctr.; 0-9704788),* Div. of LSUHSC Foundation, 1600 Canal St., Suite 1034, New Orleans, LA 70112 Tel 504-568-5272; Fax: 504-568-3920; Toll Free: 800-648-5272
E-mail: cme@isuhsc.edu.

Inst of Science, *(Institute of Science; 1-892506),* 1158 26th St., No. 323, Santa Monica, CA 90403-0382 Tel 310-281-6760; Fax: 310-453-7707
E-mail: mail@instituteofscience.com
Web site: http://www.instituteofs_ience.com.

Inst Personality & Ability, *(Institute for Personality & Ability Testing, Inc.; 0-918296),* 1801 Woodfield Dr., Savoy, IL 61874 (SAN 209-3197) Tel 217-352-4739; Fax: 217-352-9674; Toll Free: 800-225-4728
E-mail: custservice@ipat.com
Web site: http://www.ipat.com.

Inst Phobic Awareness, *(Institute for Phobic Awareness, The; 0-9627373),* Orders Addr.: P.O. Box 1180, Palm Springs, CA 92263; Edit Addr.: 1472 San Jacinto Way, Palm Springs, CA 92262 Tel 760-322-2673; Fax: 760-416-0175.

Inst Polynesian, *(Institute for Polynesian Studies, The; 0-939154),* Div. of Brigham Young Univ.- Hawaii, Box 1979, Brigham Young Univ., Hawaii Campus, Laie, HI 96762-1274 (SAN 219-1911) Tel 808-293-3667; Fax: 808-293-3664
E-mail: robertsd@byuh.edu
Dist(s): **UH Pr** *(Univ. of Hawaii Pr.).*

Inst Psych Inc, *(Institute of Psychorientology; 0-913343),* Orders Addr.: P.O. Box 2249, Laredo, TX 78044-2249 (SAN 283-118X) Tel 210-722-6391.

Inst Pub ILCI, *See* **Intl Loss Cntrl**

Inst Rational-Emotive, *(Institute for Rational-Emotive Therapy),* 45 E. 65th St., New York, NY 10021-6593 Tel 212-535-0822; Fax: 212-249-3582; Toll Free: 800-323-4738.

Inst Res Metapsychol, *(Institute for Research in Metapsychology; 1-887927),* 431 Burgess Dr., Menlo Park, CA 94025 Tel 415-327-0920; Fax: 415-325-0389.

†**Inst Soc Res,** *(Univ. of Michigan, Institute for Social Research; 0-87944),* 426 Thompson, Ann Arbor, MI 48106-1248 (SAN 210-6035) Tel 734-764-8354; *CIP.*

Inst Southern Studies, *(Institute for Southern Studies; 0-943810),* Orders Addr.: P.O. Box 531, Durham, NC 27702 (SAN 669-1080); Edit Addr.: 2009 Chapel Hill Rd., Durham, NC 27707 (SAN 219-192X) Tel 919-419-8311; Fax: 919-419-8315.

Inst Spine, *(Institute for Spine & Biomedical Research; 1-879952),* Div. of TBI, Inc., Orders Addr.: P.O. Box 447, Brookline Village, MA 02147 Toll Free: 800-848-7236; Edit Addr.: 6300 W. Parker Rd., Suite 100, Plano, TX 75093 Tel 972-608-5150; Fax: 972-608-5183.

Inst Study Man, *(Institute for the Study of Man, Inc.; 0-941694),* 1133 13th St., NW, No. C2, Washington, DC 20005 (SAN 213-523X) Tel 202-371-2700; Fax: 202-371-1523
E-mail: iejournal@aol.com.

Inst Subs Abuse Res, *(Institute for Substance Abuse Research; 0-935847),* Subs. of Security Consultant Services, Inc., 21124 Edinborough Pl., Leesburg, FL 34748-7523 (SAN 699-7759) Tel 352-315-0538
Dist(s): **Schaefer Ed Found** *(Schaefer Education Foundation).*

Inst Womens Policy Rsch, *(Institute for Women's Policy Research; 1-878428),* 1707 L St., NW, Suite 750, Washington, DC 20036-4226.

†**Instant Improve,** *(Instant Improvement, Inc.; 0-941683),* 135 W 26th St., 3rd Flr., New York, NY 10001-6833 (SAN 666-0045) Tel 212-439-6904; Fax: 212-439-6902; *CIP.*

Insti Study Aware, *(Institute for the Study of Human Awareness; 0-937067),* P.O. Box 1478, Lake Villa, IL 60046-1478 (SAN 658-6112) Tel 612-424-8392.

Institute Classical, *See* **Totality Pr**

Institute Government, *(Institute of Government; 1-56011),* CB 3330 UNC at Chapel Hill, Chapel Hill, NC 27599-3330 (SAN 204-8752) Tel 919-966-4119; Fax: 919-962-2707
E-mail: khunt@iogmail.iog.unc.edu
Web site: http://ncinfo.iog.unc.edu.

Instruct Tech, *(Instructional Technologies, Inc.; 0-935115),* P.O. Box 6146, Plymouth, MI 48170-0146 (SAN 695-2666) Tel 313-565-7053.

Insur Info, *(Insurance Information Institute; 0-932387),* 110 William St., New York, NY 10038 (SAN 271-1192) Tel 212-669-9200; Fax: 212-732-1916
Dist(s): **Whitehurst & Clark** *(Whitehurst & Clark).*

InSync Commn, *(InSync Communications, LLC; 0-9673439; 1-929902),* Orders Addr.: 2445 River Tree Cir., Sanford, FL 32771 (SAN 254-1270) Tel 407-688-1156; Fax: 407-688-1135; Toll Free: 866-602-1476
E-mail: info@insyncpress.com
Web site: http://www.insyncpress.com
Dist(s): **Midpt Trade** *(Midpoint Trade Bks., Inc.).*

Int Med Res, *(International Medical Research, Inc.; 0-9636432),* 2900 Saturn St., No. B, Brea, CA 92621-6203.

Int Soc Comp App, *(International Society for Computers & Their Applications; 1-880843),* 975 Walnut St., Suite 132, Cary, NC 27511-4216 Tel 919-467-5559; Fax: 919-467-3430
E-mail: isca@ipass.net
Web site: http://www.isca-hq.org.

Int Soc Mini Micro, *See* **Int Soc Comp App**

Int Soc Pros & Orth, *(International Society for Prosthetics & Orthotics; 0-9633698),* 1650 King St., Suite 500, Alexandria, VA 22314 Tel 703-836-7118.

Integ Pr, *(Integration Pr.; 0-925525; 0-9609928),* 180 N. Oakland, Pasadena, CA 91101 (SAN 665-715X) Tel 626-584-5528.

Integral Pr, *(Integral Pr.; 0-9636001),* 2554 Lincoln Blvd., No. 373, Marina del Rey, CA 90291 Tel 310-305-9911; Fax: 425-732-0236
E-mail: info@brodietech.com
Web site: http://www.brodietech.com/meme.htm.

†**Integral Yoga Pubns,** *(Integral Yoga Pubns.; 0-932040),* Satchidananda Ashram-Yogaville, Rte. 1, Box 1720, Buckingham, VA 23921 (SAN 285-0338) Tel 804-969-1706; Fax: 804-969-1463; Toll Free: 800-262-1008 (orders)
Web site: http://www.yogaville.org/pubs.html
Dist(s): **Bookpeople** *(Bookpeople)*
New Leaf Dist *(New Leaf Distributing Co., Inc.); CIP.*

Integrated Pr, *(Integrated Pr.; 0-9610310),* 200 W. 79th St., Apt. 8B, New York, NY 10024-6214 (SAN 263-2403); 526 Comstock Dr., Tiburon, CA 94920 Tel 415-435-3223.

Integrated Res Servs, *(Integrated Research Services, Inc.; 0-943277),* 66 Club Rd., Suite 370, Eugene, OR 97401 (SAN 668-1913) Tel 541-683-9278.

Integrative Healing Pr Imprint of Haworth Pr

Integrative Med, *(Integrative Medicine, Inc.; 1-892014),* Orders Addr.: P.O. Box 4344, Tallahassee, FL 32315 Tel 508-892-1562; Fax: 508-892-3164; Edit Addr.: 3583 Doris Dr., Tallahassee, FL 32303
E-mail: IntMedInc@aol.com.

Integratv Med Commn, *(Integrative Medicine Communications; 0-9670772; 1-930256),* 1029 Chestnut St., Newton, MA 02464 Tel 617-641-2300; Fax: 617-641-2301; Toll Free: 877-462-7088
Web site: http://onemedicine.com
Dist(s): **Lppncott W & W** *(Lippincott Williams & Wilkins).*

Intell Hearing, *(Intelligent Hearing Systems; 1-886887),* 7356 SW. 48th St., Miami, FL 33155 Tel 305-668-6102; Fax: 305-668-6103; Toll Free: 800-447-9783
E-mail: sales@ihsys.com
Web site: http://www.ihsys.com/home
Dist(s): **Alexander Graham** *(Bell, Alexander Graham Assn. for the Deaf)*
Singular Publishing *(Singular Publishing Group, Inc.).*

Intellect (GBR) *(1-871516; 1-84150) Dist. by* **Intl Spec Bk.**

Intellicard, *(Intellicard; 1-888411),* Orders Addr.: P.O. Box 8255, Yakima, WA 98908 Tel 509-965-9266; Fax: 509-965-5447; Edit Addr.: 8902 Tieton Dr., Yakima, WA 98908
Web site: http://www.intelli-card.com.

Inter Print Pubs, *See* **Interstate**

Inter Thomson, *See* **Thomson Learn**

Interact Cnslting, *(Interactive Consulting, Inc.; 0-9641617),* Orders Addr.: P.O. Box 66, East Norwich, NY 11732 Tel 516-922-2167; Fax: 516-922-3830; Edit Addr.: 7 Deusenberg Dr., East Norwich, NY 11732.

Interact Media, *(Interactive Media),* 1218 Roosevelt Ave., Glenview, IL 60025 Tel 847-724-7609; Fax: 847-724-7614 Do not confuse with Interactive Media Corp. in North Stonington, CT.

Interaction Bk Co, *(Interaction Bk. Co.; 0-939603),* 7208 Cornelia Dr., Edina, MN 55435 (SAN 663-5970) Tel 952-831-9500; Fax: 952-831-9332.

Intercept UK (GBR) *(0-946707; 1-898298) Dist. by* **Spr-Verlag.**

†**Intercult Pr,** *(Intercultural Pr., Inc.; 0-933662; 1-877864; 1-931930),* Div. of Nicholas Brealey Publishing, Ltd., P.O. Box 700, Yarmouth, ME 04096 (SAN 212-6699) Tel 207-846-5168; Fax: 207-846-5181; Toll Free: 800-370-2665
E-mail: books@interculturalpress.com
Web site: http://www.interculturalpress.com; *CIP.*

Interdata, *(Interdata; 1-58239),* 1741 Kekamek, NW, Poulsbo, WA 98370 Tel 360-779-1511; Fax: 360-697-4696; Toll Free: 800-818-0140
E-mail: interdata@export-leads.com
Web site: http://www.export-leads.com.

Interdimens Sci, *(Interdimensional Sciences, Inc.; 0-943975),* Orders Addr.: P.O. Box 128, Lakemont, GA 30552 (SAN 242-6838) Tel 706-782-2524; Fax: 706-782-6127; Edit Addr.: Lake Rabun Rd., Lakemont, GA 30552 (SAN 243-301X)
E-mail: petkell@alltel.net
Web site: http://www.betar.com.

Interlink Pub, *(Interlink Publishing Group, Inc.; 0-940793; 1-56656),* 46 Crosby St., Northampton, MA 01060-1804 (SAN 664-8908) Tel 413-582-7054; Fax: 413-582-6731; Toll Free: 800-238-5465
E-mail: info@interlinkbooks.com; editor@interlinkbooks.com
Web site: http://www.interlinkbooks.com.

Intermed Tech (GBR) *(0-946688; 1-85339; 0-903031) Dist. by* **Stylus Pub VA.**

Intermtn Hlth Care, *(Intermountain Health Care; 0-9646476),* 36 S. State St., 22nd Flr., Salt Lake City, UT 84111 Tel 801-442-5703; Fax: 801-442-5702.

Internal Med, *(Internal Medicine PREPP; 0-9678841),* P.O. Box 7145, Orange, CA 92863-7145 Fax: 714-516-1270
E-mail: Intmedprepp@hotmail.com
Web site: http://www.imprepp.com.

International Business, *(International Business Communications; 1-57936),* One Research Dr., Westborough, MA 01581 Tel 508-616-5566; Fax: 508-616-5544 ; *Imprints:* D&MD Reports (D&MD Reports)
Web site: http://www.drugandmarket.com.

Internatl Pub Hse, *(International Publishing Hse.; 1-879144),* 1657 Kanawha Dr., Stone Mountain, GA 30087 Tel 770-496-0809; Fax: 770-496-0417 Do not confuse with International Publishing Hse., New York, NY.

Interpacific Pr, *(Interpacific Pr.; 1-57946),* Div. of Health-Pro Mex., Inc., P.O. Box 7597, Chula Vista, CA 91912 Tel 760-414-1341; Fax: 760-414-1953; Toll Free: 800-950-6505
E-mail: interpac@ix.netcom.com
Web site: http://Contrerashospital.com
Dist(s): **Nutri-Books Corp** *(Nutri-Bks. Corp.).*

Interpharm, *See* **IHS Health Grp**

Interplast, *(Interplast, Inc.; 0-9703998),* 300-B Pioneer Way, Mountain View, CA 94041-1506 Tel 650-962-0123; Fax: 650-962-1619; Toll Free: 888-467-5278
E-mail: ipnews@interplast.org
Web site: http://www.interplast.org.

Interpret Lab Data, *(Interpretive Laboratory Data, Inc.; 0-945577),* Orders Addr.: P.O. Box 2250, Myrtle Beach, SC 29578 (SAN 247-3615); Edit Addr.: 618B 36th Ave. N., Myrtle Beach, SC 29577 (SAN 247-3623) Tel 803-448-3055.

Interprint (IND) *(81-85017) Dist. by* **St Mut.**

Interscience (GBR) *Dist. by* **Wiley.**

Interstate, *(Interstate Pubs., Inc.; 0-8134),* P.O. Box 50, Danville, IL 61834-0050 (SAN 206-6548) Tel 217-446-0500; Fax: 217-446-9706; Toll Free: 800-843-4774
E-mail: info-ipp@ippinc.com
Web site: http://www.ippinc.com.

Intersystems Pubns, *(Intersystems Pubns.; 0-914105),* 22945 Guidotti Dr., Salinas, CA 93908 (SAN 237-9619) Tel 408-484-9092.

Intertec Pub, *See* **Primedia Bus Mag Med**

Intertec Pub Bks, *(Intertec Publishing Bks.; 0-918110; 0-936889; 0-9639479),* Orders Addr.: 11 Riverbend Dr., S., Stamford, CT 06907 Tel 203-358-4236; Fax: 203-358-5812; Toll Free: 800-828-1133
E-mail: book_orders@intertec.com
Web site: http://www.intertecmediabooks.com.

†**InterVarsity,** *(InterVarsity Pr.; 0-8308; 0-87784),* Div. of InterVarsity Christian Fellowship of the USA, Orders Addr.: P.O. Box 1400, Downers Grove, IL 60515 (SAN 202-7089) Tel 630-734-4000; Fax: 630-734-4200; Toll Free: 800-843-9487 (orders); 800-843-1019 (customer service); 800-873-0143 (electronic ordering); 800-843-7225 (other depts.)
E-mail: mail@ivpress.com
Web site: http://www.ivpress.com
Dist(s): **Baker & Taylor** *(Baker & Taylor Bks.)*
Rvrside Bk & Bible *(Riverside Bk. & Bible Resource); CIP.*

Intervention Instruct Inc, *(Intervention Instruction, Inc.; 0-9654994),* 432 N. Clark St., No. 202, Chicago, IL 60610-4517 Tel 312-467-7100; Fax: 312-467-7105.

Publisher Symbol Index

Interweave, *(Interweave Pr., Inc.; 0-934026; 1-883010; 1-931499),* 201 E. Fourth St., Loveland, CO 80537-5655 (SAN 214-3151) Tel 970-669-7672; Fax: 970-669-6117; Toll Free: 800-272-2193
E-mail: betsya@interweave.com; lindas@interweave.com
Web site: http://www.interweave.com
Dist(s): **IPG Chicago** *(Independent Pubs. Group).*

Intl Assn Paratuber, *(International Assn. for Paratuberculosis, Inc.; 0-9633043),* 44 Francis St., Rehoboth, MA 02769 Tel 508-252-6895.

Intl Assn Psych, *(International Assn. of Psychosocial Rehabilitation Services; 0-9655843),* 10025 Governor Warfield Pkwy., No. 301, Columbia, MD 21044-3357 Tel 410-730-7190; Fax: 410-730-5965.

Intl Assn Study Pain, *(International Assn. for the Study of Pain/IASP Pr.; 0-931092),* 909 NE 43rd St., Suite 306, Seattle, WA 98105 Tel 206-547-6409; Fax: 206-547-1703
E-mail: iasp@locke.hs.washington.edu; iasppress@juno.com
Web site: http://www.painbooks.org.

Intl Assn Trichologists, *(International Assn. of Trichologists; 0-9614548),* 37320 22nd St., Kalamazoo, MI 49009 (SAN 224-4586) Tel 616-375-4430.

†Intl Bk Ctr, *(International Bk. Ctr., Inc.; 0-86685; 0-917062),* 2007 Laurel Dr., P.O. Box 295, Troy, MI 48099 (SAN 169-4014) Tel 248-879-8436; Fax: 810-254-7230
E-mail: ibc@ibcbooks.com
Web site: http://www.ibcbooks.com*; CIP.*

Intl Bk Distr (IND) *(81-7089) Dist. by* **St Mut.**

Intl Bks & Periodicals (IND) *Dist. by* **St Mut.**

Intl Business Pubns, *(International Business Pubns., USA; 0-7397; 0-9646241; 1-57751),* Orders Addr.: P.O. Box 15343, Washington, DC 20003 Tel 202-546-2103; Fax: 202-546-3275; Edit Addr.: 705 Eighth St., SE, Suite 400, Washington, DC 20003 Do not confuse with International Business Pubn., Inc. in Cincinnati, OH
E-mail: rusric@erols.com
Web site: http://world.mirhouse.com.

Intl Cannabinoid, *(International Cannabinoid Research Society; 0-9658053),* Dept. of Psychology, Univ. of Vermont, Burlington, VT 05405 Tel 802-865-0970
E-mail: icrs@together.net
Web site: http://www.129.49.19.42/icrs/icrs.main.htm/.

†Intl Childbirth, *(International Childbirth Education Assn.; 0-934024; 0-937604),* P.O. Box 20048, Minneapolis, MN 55420 (SAN 224-3962) Tel 612-854-8660 ; *Imprints:* Pennypr (Pennypress)*; CIP.*

Intl Chiropractors Assn, *(International Chiropractors Assn.; 1-886190),* 1110 N. Glebe Rd., Suite 1000, Arlington, VA 22201 (SAN 224-1617) Tel 703-528-5000; Fax: 703-528-5023; Toll Free: 800-423-4690.

Intl Chlamydia, *(International Chlamydia Symposium; 0-9664383),* 1001 Potrero Ave., Bldg. 30, Rm. 416, San Francisco, CA 94110 Tel 415-824-5115; Fax: 415-821-8940
E-mail: eeks@itsa.ucsf.edu.

Intl Churchill Soc, *See* **Churchill Ctr**

†Intl Comm Rad Meas, *(International Commission on Radiation Units & Measurements; 0-913394),* 7910 Woodmont Ave., Suite 800, Bethesda, MD 20814 (SAN 202-7127) Tel 301-657-2652; Fax: 301-907-8768; Toll Free: 800-657-2652
E-mail: icru@icru.org
Web site: http://www.icru.org*; CIP.*

Intl Coun Nurses, *(International Council of Nurses; 0-9658360),* 600 Maryland Ave., SW, Suite 100W, Washington, DC 20024 Tel 202-651-7000; Toll Free: 800-274-4262
E-mail: icn@uni2a.unige.ch
Web site: http://www.nursingworld.org
Dist(s): **Am Nurses Pub** *(American Nurses Publishing).*

Intl Ediemme (ITA) *Dist. by* **Scholium Intl.**

Intl Educ Improve, *(International Educational Improvement Ctr. Pr.; 1-884169),* Orders Addr.: 5081 Townpoint Rd., Suffolk, VA 23435 Tel 757-488-5104.

Intl Fnd Gynecol, *(International Foundation for Gynecologic Cancer Detection & Prevention; 0-9642179),* 5301 Westbard Cir., No. 5, Bethesda, MD 20816 Tel 301-654-0445; Fax: 301-907-9764.

Intl Found Biosocial Dev, *(International Foundation for Biosocial Development & Human Health; 0-934314),* Orders Addr.: 6 Lomond Ave., Spring Valley, NY 10977 (SAN 214-0381) Tel 914-624-8516 (phone/fax)
E-mail: ivana8@aol.com; biosocmed@aol.com.

Intl Found Employ, *(International Foundation of Employee Benefit Plans; 0-89154),* Orders Addr.: P.O. Box 69, Brookfield, WI 53008-0069 (SAN 317-9214) Tel 262-786-6710; Fax: 262-786-8780; Toll Free: 888-334-3327
E-mail: books@ifebp.org
Web site: http://www.ifebp.org.

Intl Gen Semantics, *(International Society for General Semantics; 0-918970),* P.O. Box 728, Concord, CA 94522 (SAN 203-8161) Tel 925-798-0311; Fax: 925-798-0312
E-mail: isgs@generalsemantics.org
Web site: http://www.generalsemantics.org.

Intl Headache, *(International Headache Management, Inc.; 0-9636292),* 3918 Montclair Rd., Suite 102, Birmingham, AL 35213 Tel 205-871-2243; Fax: 205-879-4399
Web site: http://www.fordheadacheclinic.com/.

Intl Health, *(International Health & Healing Publishing; 0-9700530),* 28607 N. 152nd St., Scottsdale, AZ 85262 Tel 480-471-2244 (phone/fax)
E-mail: bchik@aol.com.

Intl Hlth MD, *(International Health; 1-878290),* Div. of Clearfield Co., 200 E. Eager St., Baltimore, MD 21202 Tel 410-837-8271; Fax: 410-752-8492; Toll Free: 800-296-6687 Do not confuse with International Health Pubns., San Diego, CA.

Intl Inst Rural, *(International Institute of Rural Reconstruction; 0-942717; 1-930261),* 475 Riverside Dr., Rm. 725, New York, NY 10115 (SAN 225-9710) Tel 212-870-2992
E-mail: iirr@cav.pworld.net.ph
Web site: http://www.cav.pworld.net..ph/llrr.

Intl Labour Office, *(International Labour Office; 92-2; 92-9014),* 1828 L St., NW, Suite 600, Washington, DC 20036-5121 (SAN 203-817X) Tel 202-653-7652; Fax: 202-653-7687; Fulfillment Addr.: P.O. Box 753, Waldorf, MD 20604-0753 Tel 301-638-3152; Fax: 301-843-0159
E-mail: ilopubs@tascol.com; crow@ilo.org
Web site: http://www.us.ilo.org; http://www.ilo.org/publns
Dist(s): **Bernan Associates** *(Bernan Assocs.)*
Brookings *(Brookings Institution Pr.)*
Gale *(Gale Group).*

Intl Loss Cntrl, *(International Loss Control Institute, Inc.; 0-88061),* 3805 Crestwood Pkwy., NW, No. 200, Duluth, GA 30136-5049 (SAN 240-9887) Toll Free: 800-486-4524.

Intl Maritime Org (GBR) *(0-900496; 92-801) Dist. by* **St Mut.**

Intl Marriage, *(International Marriage Encounter, Inc.; 0-936098),* 955 Lake Dr., Saint Paul, MN 55120 (SAN 215-6830) Tel 651-454-6434; Fax: 651-452-0466; Toll Free: 800-627-7424
E-mail: info@marriagemagazine.org
Web site: http://www.marriagemagazine.org.

Intl Masters Pub, *(International Masters Pubs., Inc.; 1-886614; 1-892207; 1-930560),* Div. of International Masters Publishers, AB, 225 Park Ave., S., New York, NY 10003 Tel 212-353-6400; Fax: 212-353-7105
E-mail: thomas.nolan@imp-usa.com
Web site: http://www.imponline.com.

Intl Med Pub, *(International Medical Publishing, Inc.; 0-9634063; 1-883205; 1-58808),* Orders Addr.: P.O. Box 479, McLean, VA 22101 Tel 703-356-2037; Fax: 703-734-8987; Edit Addr.: 1516 Mintwood Dr., McLean, VA 22101
E-mail: medicalpublishing@ediabetes.com
Web site: http://www.medicalpublishing.com
Dist(s): **Majors Scientific Bks Inc** *(Majors Scientific Bks., Inc.)*
Matthews Medical Bk Co *(Matthews Medical Bk. Co.)*
Rittenhouse *(Rittenhouse Bk. Distributors).*

Intl Med Srvs, *(International Medical Services Directory Publishing Co.; 0-9635675),* 3590 NW 54th St., Suite 6, Fort Lauderdale, FL 33309 Tel 954-486-0699; Fax: 954-733-8108.

Intl Med Volntrs, *(International Medical Volunteers Assn.; 0-9649425),* P.O. Box 205, Woodville, MA 01784-0205 Tel 508-435-7377; Fax: 508-497-9568
E-mail: info@imva.org
Web site: http://www.imva.org.

Intl Mgmt Pubns, *(International Management Pubns.; 1-880136),* 13380 Oak Hill Ln., Brookfield, WI 53005-4955 Toll Free: 800-827-6770
E-mail: office@burrus.com
Web site: http://www.burrus.com.

Intl Myeloma, *(International Myeloma Foundation; 0-9633186),* 12650 Riverside Dr., Suite 206, North Hollywood, CA 91607-3421 Tel 818-487-7455; Fax: 818-487-7454; Toll Free: 800-452-2873
E-mail: theIMF@myeloma.org
Web site: http://www.myeloma.org.

Intl Myopia, *(International Myopia Prevention Assn.; 0-9608476),* 1054 Gravel Hill Rd., Ligonier, PA 15658 (SAN 228-1848) Tel 724-238-2101.

Intl Phys PONW, *(International Physicians for the Prevention of Nuclear War; 0-7167; 0-945257; 0-9634455; 3-88454; 1-893368; 5-85941),* 727 Massachusetts Ave., Cambridge, MA 02139 Tel 617-868-5050; Fax: 617-868-2560
E-mail: ippnwbos@ippnw.org
Web site: http://www.ippnw.org.

Intl Plan Parent, *(International Planned Parenthood Federation; 0-916683),* 120 Wall St., 9th Flr., New York, NY 10005 (SAN 271-5171) Tel 212-248-6400.

Intl Promotions, *(International Promotions/Promotion Publishing; 1-57901),* 3368 F Governor Dr., Suite 144, San Diego, CA 92122 Fax: 619-490-1455; Toll Free: 800-231-1776 (orders)
E-mail: promopub@worldnet.att.net
Web site: http://www.promotionpub.com.

Intl Psych Pr, *(International Psychological Pr., Inc.; 0-915662),* 1514 Mendota Way, Carmichael, CA 95608 (SAN 207-3722) Tel 916-973-8788.

†Intl Pubns Serv, *(International Pubns. Service; 0-8002),* Div. of Taylor & Francis, Inc., Orders Addr.: 325 Chestnut St., 8th Flr., Levittown, PA 19057-4700 Tel 215-785-5800; Fax: 215-785-5515; Toll Free: 800-821-8312
E-mail: bkorders@tandfpa.com*; CIP.*

Intl Pubs Co, *(International Publishers Co., Inc.; 0-7178),* 239 W. 23rd St., 5th Flr., New York, NY 10011 (SAN 202-5655) Tel 212-366-9816; Fax: 212-366-9820
E-mail: service@intpubnyc.com
Web site: http://www.intpubnyc.com.

Intl Pubs Mktg, *(International Publishers Marketing),* Orders Addr.: 22883 Quicksilver Dr., Dulles, VA 20166 (SAN 253-3375) Toll Free: 800-758-3756; Edit Addr.: P.O. Box 605, Herndon, VA 20172-0605 Fax: 703-661-1501.

Intl Qual, *(International Quality Pr.; 1-57172),* Div. of Compliance Quality International, 110 Mill St., No. 9, Middletown, PA 17057-1729.

Intl Rescue Comm, *(International Rescue Committee; 0-9637711),* 122 E. 42nd St., 12th Flr., New York, NY 10168-1289 (SAN 271-5406) Tel 212-551-3000
Web site: http://www.intrescom.org.

Intl Risk Mgt, *(International Risk Management Institute, Inc.; 0-938358; 1-886813),* 12222 Merit Dr., Suite 1450, Dallas, TX 75251-2276 Tel 972-960-7693; Fax: 972-371-5120 Do not confuse with International Risk Management, Inc., Loganville, GA
E-mail: info@IRMI.com
Web site: http://www.IRMI.com.

Intl Scholars, *(International Scholars Pubns.; 1-57309; 1-85607; 1-883255),* 4720 Boston, Lanham, MD 20706 Tel 301-459-3366; Fax: 301-459-5357; Toll Free Fax: 800-338-4550; Toll Free: 800-462-6420
E-mail: info@interscholars.com
Web site: http://www.interscholars.com
Dist(s): **Natl Bk Netwk** *(National Bk. Network)*
Rowman *(Rowman & Littlefield Pubs., Inc.)*
U Pr of Amer *(University Pr. of America).*

Intl Spec Bk, *(International Specialized Bk. Services; 0-7130),* 5824 NE Hassalo St., Portland, OR 97213-3644 (SAN 169-7129) Tel 503-287-3093; Fax: 503-280-8832; Toll Free: 800-944-6190
E-mail: info@isbs.com
Web site: http://www.isbs.com.

Intl Toxicol, *(International Toxicology, Inc.; 0-9644990),* P.O. Box 2144, Eugene, OR 97402-0041.

Intl Transactional, *(International Transactional Analysis Assn.; 0-89489),* 436 14th St., Suite 1301, Oakland, CA 94612-2710 (SAN 224-4365) Tel 510-625-7720; Fax: 510-625-7725
E-mail: itaa@itaa-net.org
Web site: http://www.itaa-net.org.

Intl Univ Line, *(International Univ. Line; 0-9636817),* P.O. Box 2525, La Jolla, CA 92038 Tel 858-581-3506; Fax: 858-581-9073
E-mail: info@iul-press.com.

†Intl Univ Pr, *(International Univ. Pr.; 0-89697),* 1301 S. Noland Rd., Independence, MO 64055 (SAN 271-6291) Tel 816-461-3633*; CIP.*

†Intl Univs Pr, *(International Universities Pr., Inc.; 0-8236; 1-887841),* 59 Boston Post Rd., P.O. Box 1524, Madison, CT 06443-1524 (SAN 202-7186) Tel 203-245-4000; Fax: 203-245-0775; Toll Free: 800-835-3487 (orders only) ; *Imprints:* Psychosocial (Psychosocial Press)
E-mail: office@iup.com
Web site: http://www.iup.com*; CIP.*

Intl Vet Acup, *(International Veterinary Acupuncture Society; 0-9616627),* P.O. Box 1478, Longmont, CO 80502-1478 (SAN 689-6979)
E-mail: ivasoffice@aol.com.

Inverted-A, *(Inverted-A, Inc.; 0-938245),* 900 Monarch Way, Northport, AL 35473-2663 (SAN 661-4213) Tel 417-457-6652
E-mail: amnfn@well.com.

Invictus LA, *(Invictus Publishing Co.; 0-940019),* 4417 Lorino St., Metairie, LA 70006 (SAN 664-1474) Tel 504-455-5895; Fax: 504-455-5740 Do not confuse with Invictus Publishing Corp. in Scarsdale, NY.

Invisible-Red Hill, *(Invisible City/Red Hill Pr.; 0-88031),* P.O. Box 2853, San Francisco, CA 94126 (SAN 205-6429) Tel 510-527-1018
Dist(s): **SPD-Small Pr Dist** *(SPD-Small Pr. Distribution).*

IOMA, *(Institute of Management & Administration, IOMA; 1-58673),* 29 W. 35th St., New York, NY 10001 Tel 212-244-0360 (ext. 232); Fax: 212-564-0465
E-mail: subserve@ioma.com
Web site: http://www.ioma.com.

IOS Pr (NLD) *(90-5199) Dist. by* **IOS Press.**

IOS Press, *(IOS Pr., Inc.; 90-5199; 0-9673355; 1-58603),* 5795-G Burke Centre Pkwy., Burke, VA 22015 Tel 703-323-5554; Fax: 703-323-3668
E-mail: iosbooks@iospress.com
Web site: http://www.iospress.nl.

Iowa St U Pr, *See* **Iowa U Pr**

†**Iowa U Pr,** *(Iowa Univ. Pr.; 0-8138),* 2121 S. State Ave., Ames, IA 50014-8300 (SAN 202-7194) Tel 515-292-0140; Fax: 515-292-3348
E-mail: orders@isupress.com
Web site: http://www.iowastatepress.com; *CIP.*

IPAS, *(IPAS; 1-882220),* Div. of Information & Pubns., 303 E. Main St., P.O. Box 999, Carrboro, NC 27510 Tel 919-967-7052; Fax: 919-929-0258; Toll Free: 800-334-8446
E-mail: ipas@ipas.org
Web site: http://www.ipas.org.

IPG Chicago, *(Independent Pubs. Group),* Subs. of Chicago Review Pr., 814 N. Franklin, Chicago, IL 60610 (SAN 202-0769) Tel 312-337-0747; Fax: 312-337-5985; Toll Free: 800-888-4741
E-mail: lreardon@ipgbook.com
Web site: http://www.ipgbook.com.

IPM Hse, *(IPM Hse.; 0-9668385),* P.O. Box 277668, Sacramento, CA 95827 Tel 916-962-1065; Fax: 916-441-4730
E-mail: ipmgt@msn.com; sns123@aol.com
Dist(s): **St Mut** *(State Mutual Bk. & Periodical Service, Ltd.).*

IPSB Pubns, *(IPSB Pubns.; 0-9618179),* 1366 Hornblend St., San Diego, CA 92109 (SAN 666-8348) Tel 619-272-4142.

Ipswich Pr, *(Ipswich Pr., The; 0-938864),* P.O. Box 291, Ipswich, MA 01938 (SAN 218-4826) Tel 978-356-0541; Fax: 978-412-0079.

IQ Design, *(IQ Design, Inc.; 0-615),* 1055 E 5825 S., Ogden, UT 84405 Tel 801-698-2750; Fax: 801-650-3664
E-mail: printcop@home.com
Web site: http://www.iois.net.

IRFD, *(IRFD Pubns. (Institute for Reasearch of Food-related Disease); 0-9628681),* Orders Addr.: P.O. Box 150-007, San Rafael, CA 94915-0007 Tel 415-453-1709; Fax: 415-453-7158; Edit Addr.: 129 Reservoir Rd., San Rafael, CA 94901
Web site: http://www.foodforhumans.com
Dist(s): **Bookpeople** *(Bookpeople)*
New Leaf Dist *(New Leaf Distributing Co., Inc.).*

Irish Acad Pr (IRL) *(0-7165) Dist. by* **Intl Spec Bk.**

Irish Bks Media, *(Irish Bks. & Media, Inc.; 0-937702),* Orders Addr.: 1433 E. Franklin Ave., Minneapolis, MN 55404-2135 (SAN 111-8870) Tel 612-871-3505; Fax: 612-871-3358; Toll Free: 800-229-3505 Do not confuse with Irish Bks. in New York, NY
E-mail: Irishbook@aol.com
Web site: http://www.irishbook.com.

IRRC Inc DC, *(Investor Responsibility Research Ctr., Inc.; 0-931035; 1-879775),* 1350 Connecticut Ave. NW, Suite 700, Washington, DC 20036 (SAN 271-6631) Tel 202-833-0700; Fax: 202-833-3555
Web site: http://www.store.irrc.org.

†**Irvington,** *(Irvington Pubs.; 0-512; 0-8290; 0-8422; 0-89197),* Orders Addr.: P.O. Box 286, New York, NY 10276-0286 Fax: 212-861-0998; Toll Free Fax: 800-455-5520; Toll Free: 800-472-6037; *CIP.*

Irwin Law (CAN) *(1-55221) Dist. by* **Gaunt.**

Irwn McGrw-H Imprint of McGrw-H Hghr Educ

Irwn Prfssnl Imprint of McGraw-Hill Educ Grp

Isa Mira, *(Isa Mira Co.; 0-9679932),* 5114 Pt. Fosdick Dr., NW., PMB 275, Gig Harbor, WA 98335 Tel 206-624-4544; Fax: 206-374-2230; Toll Free: 888-465-2619
E-mail: EcovePress@aol.com
Web site: http://elfincovepress.com
Dist(s): **Elfin Cove Pr** *(Elfin Cove Pr.).*

ISB Edns, *(ISB Editions; 0-9619497),* 515 SW 18th Terr., Miami, FL 33145 (SAN 245-4459).

ISC Div Wellness, *(ISC Div. of Wellness; 0-929736),* Orders Addr.: P.O. Box 8798, Lakeland, FL 33806 (SAN 250-3042); Edit Addr.: 1035 S. Florida Ave., No. 208, Lakeland, FL 33806 (SAN 250-3050) Tel 941-686-8934.

ISCD, *(ISCD Pr.; 1-930858),* Div. of Good Shepherd Foundation, Orders Addr.: P.O. Box 1880, Pahoa, HI 96778 Tel 808-935-5563; Fax: 808-965-1842; Edit Addr.: Government Rd., Pahoa, HI 96778
E-mail: iscd@gte.net
Web site: http://www.iscdpress.com.

ISHK, *(ISHK; 0-86304; 0-900860; 1-883536),* Div. of Institute for the Study of Human Knowledge, Orders Addr.: P.O. Box 381069, Cambridge, MA 02238-1069 (SAN 226-4536) Tel 617-497-4124; Fax: 617-876-2976; Toll Free Fax: 800-223-4200; Toll Free: 800-222-4745; Edit Addr.: P.O. Box 176, Los Altos, CA 94023 Tel 650-948-9428 ; *Imprints:* Malor Bks (Malor Books)
E-mail: ishkbooks@aol.com; ishkorders@aol.com
Web site: http://www.ishkbooks.com
Dist(s): **Baker & Taylor** *(Baker & Taylor Bks.)*
Bookpeople *(Bookpeople)*
Borders Inc *(Borders, Inc.)*
New Leaf Dist *(New Leaf Distributing Co., Inc.).*

ISIS Lrg Prnt (GBR) *(0-7531; 1-85089; 1-85695) Dist. by* **Transaction Pubs.**

Isis Med (GBR) *(1-899066; 1-901865) Dist. by* **Bks Intl VA.**

Islamic Texts (GBR) *(0-946621) Dist. by* **Intl Spec Bk.**

Island Heritage, *(Island Heritage Publishing; 0-89610; 0-931548),* Div. of The Madden Corp., 99880 Iwaena St., Aiea, HI 96701 (SAN 211-1403) Tel 808-487-7299; Fax: 808-488-2279; Toll Free: 800-468-2800
E-mail: hawaii4u@islandheritage.com
Web site: http://www.islandheritage.com/.

Island Pr, *(Island Pr.; 0-933280; 1-55963),* Div. of Ctr. for Resource Economics, Orders Addr.: P.O. Box 7, Covelo, CA 95428 (SAN 665-7206) Tel 707-983-6432; Fax: 707-983-6414; Toll Free: 800-828-1302; Edit Addr.: 1718 Connecticut Ave., NW, Suite 300, Washington, DC 20009-1148 (SAN 241-7332) Tel 202-232-7933; Fax: 202-234-1328; Toll Free: 800-828-1302 Do not confuse with Island Pr., Olathe, KS
E-mail: service@islandpress.com; orders@islandpress.org
Web site: http://www.islandpress.org
Dist(s): **Penguin Putnam** *(Penguin Putnam, Inc.).*

Island Pr KS, *(Island Pr.; 0-9661831),* Div. of Iles Pubns., 1065 Wyckford Rd., Olathe, KS 66061 Tel 913-782-7472; Fax: 913-782-7138 Do not confuse with Island Pr., Washington, DC
E-mail: bobiles@home.com
Web site: http://www.medwriting.com.

Isle Botanica, *(Isle Botanica; 0-9645426),* 2814 Kalawao St., Honolulu, HI 96822-1576 Tel 808-945-9334 (phone/fax)
E-mail: whistler@hawaii.edu.

Isomed, *(Isomed, Inc.; 0-9621736),* P.O. Box 22248, Portland, OR 97269-2248 (SAN 252-127X) Tel 503-653-2008; Fax: 503-659-0350.

ISU-CIKARD, *(Iowa State Univ., Ctr. for Indigenous Knowledge for Agriculture & Rural Development; 0-945271; 1-882116),* 319 Printing & Publications Bldg., Iowa State Univ., Ames, IA 50011 (SAN 246-6392) Tel 515-294-5247; Fax: 515-294-2945.

ISU-TSCP, *See* **ISU-CIKARD**

ITBP (GBR) *(1-86152) Dist. by* **Thomson Learn.**

ITCP, *(International Thomson Computer Pr.; 1-85032),* Orders Addr.: 7625 Empire Dr., Florence, KY 41042-2978 Tel 606-525-6600; Fax: 606-525-7778; Toll Free: 800-842-3636; Edit Addr.: 20 Park Plaza, 13th Flr., Boston, MA 02116 Fax: 617-695-1615
E-mail: itcp@itp.thomson.com
Web site: http://www.itcpmedia.com
Dist(s): **Thomson Learn** *(Thomson Learning).*

ITEST Faith, *(ITEST Faith/Science Pr.; 0-9625431; 1-885583),* Div. of Institute for Theological Encounter With Science & Technology, 3601 Lindell Blvd., Saint Louis, MO 63108 Tel 314-977-2703; Fax: 314-977-7264
E-mail: postigm@slu.edu
Web site: http://itest.slu.edu.

Ithaca House, *(Ithaca Hse.; 0-87886),* P.O. Box 4556, Ithaca, NY 14852 Tel 607-275-9658
E-mail: ithacahouse@juno.com.

ITServices, *(ITServices; 0-9628840; 1-890302),* 3301 Alta Arden, No. 2, Sacramento, CA 95825 Tel 916-483-1085; Fax: 916-483-1431
E-mail: kirk@clinicalpearls.com.

IVE Inc, *(IVE, Inc.; 0-9623160; 1-883992),* 2974 S. 900 E., Bountiful, UT 84010-4437 Tel 801-298-8996; Fax: 801-298-8784.

Ivory Tower CA, *(Ivory Tower Pubns.; 0-9655573),* 675 Forest Ave., Palo Alto, CA 94301 Tel 415-325-6445 Do not confuse with Ivory Tower Pubns., East Patchogue, NY.

Ivy Books, *(Ivy Bks.; 0-345; 0-449; 0-8041; 1-4000),* Div. of Ballantine Publishing Group, Orders Addr.: 400 Hahn, Westminster, MD 21157 Tel 410-848-1900; Toll Free: 800-726-0600; Edit Addr.: 201 E. 50th St., New York, NY 10022 (SAN 661-7832) Tel 212-572-2572; Fax: 212-572-4912; Toll Free: 800-733-3000 (orders); 800-726-0600 (customer service/credit)
E-mail: customerservice@randomhouse.com
Web site: http://www.randomhouse.com/.

IWRC, *(International Wildlife Rehabilitation Council; 1-884196),* 4437 Central Pl., Suite B4, Suisun City, CA 94585 Tel 707-864-1761; Fax: 707-864-3106
E-mail: iwrc@inreach.com
Web site: http://www.iwrc-online.org.

J & J Baby Prod, *See* **J & J Consumer Prods**

J & J Consumer Prods, *(Johnson & Johnson Consumer Products, Inc.; 0-931562),* Orders Addr.: P.O. Box 71687, Chicago, IL 60694 (SAN 241-7340); Edit Addr.: 199 Grandview Rd., Skillman, NJ 08558 (SAN 211-5131) Tel 908-874-2679; Toll Free: 800-526-3967.

J & L Prods, *(J&L Products; 0-9642926),* 2034 Via Solona, San Clemente, CA 92673-3738.

J & R Pub, *(J&R Publishing Co.; 0-9616771),* 3908 Dunn Ave., Sebring, FL 33872 (SAN 661-3381) Tel 941-471-0887 Do not confuse with J&R Publishing, Atascadero, CA.

J & S Pub VA, *(J&S Publishing Co., Inc.; 0-9632873; 1-888308),* 1300 Bishop Ln., Alexandria, VA 22302 Tel 703-823-9833; Fax: 703-823-9834 Do not confuse with J&S Publishing in Prescott, AZ
E-mail: jandspub@ix.netcom.com
Web site: http://www.jandspub.com
Dist(s): **J Majors Co** *(Majors, J. A. Co.)*
Matthews Medical Bk Co *(Matthews Medical Bk. Co.)*
Rittenhouse *(Rittenhouse Bk. Distributors).*

J A Allen (GBR) *(0-85131) Dist. by* **Trafalgar.**

J A Allen (GBR) *(0-85131) Dist. by* **St Mut.**

J A Easley, *See* **Stratford NC**

J B Pr, *See* **Quit Smart**

J B Universal, *(JB Universal Pr., Inc.; 0-9715079),* 130-14 133rd Ave., South Ozone Park, NY 11420 (SAN 254-3338) Fax: 718-738-7763.

J Bellis, *See* **SIMAX**

J Benjamins Pubng (NLD) *(90-272) Dist. by* **J Benjamins Pubng Co.**

J Benjamins Pubng Co, *(Benjamins, John Publishing Co.; 0-915027; 1-55619; 1-58811),* Subs. of John Benjamins BV, Orders Addr.: P.O. Box 27519, Philadelphia, PA 19118-0519 (SAN 219-7677) Tel 215-836-1200; Fax: 215-836-1204; Toll Free: 800-562-5666 (orders); Edit Addr.: 821 Bethlehem Pike, Erdenheim, PA 19038
E-mail: paul@benjamins.com; service@benjamins.com
Web site: http://www.benjamins.com.

J Block, *(Block, Jed; 0-9672728),* 4300 Knollwood Ln., Appleton, WI 54915 Tel 920-735-6061; Fax: 920-735-6067
E-mail: jed@athenet.net
Web site: http://www.jedblock.com.

J Burnett, *(Burnett, Joanne; 0-9647389),* 4616 N. Avenida del Cazador, Tucson, AZ 85718-6806.

J C & A L Fawcett, *(Fawcett, J.C. & A.L., Inc.; 0-941567),* 38-01 23rd Ave., Long Island City, NY 11105 (SAN 666-6019) Tel 718-204-0900.

J C Crighton Pub, *(Crighton, John C. Pub.; 0-9639699),* 3710 Lenoir St., Columbus, MO 65201 Tel 314-876-5885.

J C Press, *(JC Pr.; 0-9654654),* 3508 Market St., Suite 420, Philadelphia, PA 19104 Tel 215-222-1818; Fax: 215-222-5325.

J Clarke Co Ltd (GBR) *(0-227) Dist. by* **Parkwest Pubns.**

J Curtis KS, *(Curtis, John; 0-9627130),* P.O. Box 1222, Manhattan, KS 66502 Tel 913-776-3863 Do not confuse with J Curtis Pubns., Scottsdale, AZ.

J Donald (GBR) *(0-85976) Dist. by* **St Mut.**

J E A Enter, *See* **Jjea enter**

J E Jensen, *(Jensen, Jack E.; 0-9633870),* 9180 Old Katy Rd., No. 200, Houston, TX 77055 Tel 713-984-1400; Fax: 713-984-0544.

J E Smallwood, *(Smallwood, James E.; 0-9702165),* 3612 Willow Bluff Dr., Raleigh, NC 27604-6059 Tel 919-790-0298; Fax: 919-513-6465
E-mail: ed_smallwood@ncsu.edu.

J F Whitley, *(Whitley, Joe F. Pub.; 0-937577),* 3729 Canyon Dr., Coeur D'Alene, ID 83815-8043 (SAN 659-1345) Tel 208-664-2329; 208-765-1127.

J Fankhauser, *(Fankhauser, Jerry; 0-9617006),* 7676 Woodway Dr., Suite 235, Houston, TX 77063 (SAN 662-5517) Tel 713-787-9057
Dist(s): **New Leaf Dist** *(New Leaf Distributing Co., Inc.).*

J Goodman & Assocs, *(Goodman, John & Assocs.; 0-9625207),* 8668 Spring Mountain Rd., Las Vegas, NV 89117 Tel 702-871-9200; Fax: 702-838-5613; Toll Free: 800-542-5435
E-mail: ljudd@jga-net.com
Web site: http://www.jga-net.com.

J Grekin, *(Grekin, Jacqueline; 0-9659685),* 36708 Tanglewood Ln., Farmington Hills, MI 48331-1946.

J Grubb Taylor, *(Taylor, Janet Grubb; 0-9628434),* 2310 W. 11th St., Wilmington, DE 19805.

J H D Communs, *(Day, J.H. Communications, Inc.; 0-9648369),* 625 E. Pointe Ct., SW, Vero Beach, FL 32962-5598.

J H Hoffmann, *(Hoffman, J. Henry; 0-9614287),* 6889 Beverly Glen Ave., Las Vegas, NV 89110-4101 (SAN 687-4509).

J H Hunt, *(Hunt, John H.; 0-9665422),* 11 Gross Point Rd., Orland, ME 04472 Tel 207-469-3614.

J J Keller, *(Keller, J.J. & Assocs., Inc.; 0-934674; 1-57943; 1-877798; 1-59042),* Orders Addr.: P.O. Box 368, Neenah, WI 54957-0368 (SAN 201-5056) Tel 920-722-2848; Toll Free: 800-558-5011 (orders, customer service); Edit Addr.: 3003 W. Breezewood Ln., Neenah, WI 54957
E-mail: sales@jjkeller.com
Web site: http://www.jjkeller.com.

J Kakkis, *(Kakkis, Joyce; 0-9709399),* 6398 Rochelle Ln., Long Beach, CA 90815
E-mail: pafot@aol.com
Web site: http://www.estrogenevangelist.com.

J L Denser, *(Denser, J.L.; 0-9629513),* 831 Hillcrest Blvd., Millbrae, CA 94030 Tel 650-552-9330
E-mail: denser@slip.net
Dist(s): **Bookpeople** *(Bookpeople).*

J L Lu, *(Lu, J. L.; 0-9601768),* 2736 W. Illinois, Dallas, TX 75233 (SAN 211-9137).

J L Prods, *(JL Productions; 0-9610564),* 93 Medford St., Arlington, MA 02174 (SAN 264-1321) Tel 617-641-2852.

J Libbey Med (GBR) *(0-86196) Dist. by* **Buttrwrth-Heinemann.**

J M C & Co Imprint of Amereon Ltd

J M McCartney, *(McCartney, Joan M. Pub.; 0-9609788),* 18 Carroll Dr., Somerville, NJ 08876 (SAN 269-5634).

J M Ryan, *(Ryan, J. Michael Publishing; 1-887064),* 24 Crescent Dr. N., Andover, NJ 07821 Tel 973-786-7777; Fax: 973-786-7776.

J M Sattler, *(Sattler, Jerome M. Pubs., Inc.; 0-9618209; 0-9702671),* Orders Addr.: P.O. Box 3557, La Mesa, CA 91944-3557 (SAN 666-8259) Tel 619-460-3667; Fax: 619-460-2489; Edit Addr.: 8080 La Mesa Blvd., No. 206, La Mesa, LA 91941
E-mail: jsattler@psychology.sdsu.edu
Web site: http://www.zweb.com.sattler.

J Macy Foun, *(Macy, Josiah Jr. Foundation; 0-914362; 0-9614362),* 44 E. 64th St., New York, NY 10021 (SAN 287-2544) Tel 212-486-2424; Fax: 212-644-0765
E-mail: nickrjmacy@aol.com
Web site: http://www.josiahmacyfoundation.org/.

J Majors Co, *(Majors, J. A. Co.),* Orders Addr.: 1401 Lakeway Dr., Lewisville, TX 75057 (SAN 169-8117) Tel 972-353-1100; Fax: 972-353-1300; Toll Free: 800-633-1851
E-mail: dallas@majors.com
Web site: http://www.majors.com.

J Martin, *(Martin's, Julie Miracle System; 0-9702723),* P.O. Box 3852, Costa Mesa, CA 92628 Tel 714-376-6081
E-mail: writejuliem@yahoo.com
Web site: http://www.jmmiraclesystempress.com.

J Melek, *(Melek, Jacques; 0-942330),* P.O. Box 1273, Alta Loma, CA 91701 (SAN 241-5607) Tel 909-987-5929 ; *Imprints:* Sunbright Bks (Sunbright Books).

J Miller, *(Miller, Joan; 0-9613786),* 2520 Windy Hill Rd., Suite 106, Marietta, GA 30067 (SAN 678-9986) Tel 770-952-3308; Fax: 770-952-3309
E-mail: joanmiller@mindspring.com
Web site: http://mindspring.com/~joanmiller.

J Miller Assocs, *See* **JMA Pubns**

J Muir Chirop, *(Muir, John Chiropractic Ctr.; 0-9645301),* 1776 Ygnacio Valley Rd., Suite 201, Walnut Creek, CA 94598 Tel 510-939-2225; Fax: 510-939-8017.

J Norton Audio-Forum, *(Norton Pubs., Inc., Jeffrey /Audio-Forum; 0-88432; 1-57970),* 96 Broad St., Guilford, CT 06437-2612 (SAN 213-957X) Tel 203-453-9794; Fax: 203-453-9774; Toll Free Fax: 888-453-4329; Toll Free: 800-243-1234
E-mail: info@audioforum.com
Web site: http://www.audioForum.com.

J O Pubns, *(Osteen, John Pubns.; 0-912631),* Orders Addr.: P.O. Box 23297, Houston, TX 77228
Web site: http://www.lakewood-church.org
Dist(s): **Anchor Distributors** *(Anchor Distributors)*
Harrison Hse *(Harrison Hse., Inc.).*

J P Gustafson, *(Gustafson, James P.; 0-9662185),* 6001 Research Pk. Blvd., Madison, WI 53719-1176 Tel 608-263-6059; Fax: 608-263-0265.

J Pangloss, *See* **Rachelle Simon**

J Patelson Mus, *(Patelson, Joseph Music Hse., Ltd.; 0-915282),* 160 W. 56th St., New York, NY 10019 (SAN 203-9028) Tel 212-757-5587.

J Patterson, *(Patterson, Jeanne Vision & Health Ctr.; 0-9666126),* 2103 Pleasant Dr., Cambridge, WI 53523-9614 Tel 608-423-4358.

J Pohl Assocs, *(Pohl, J. Assocs.; 0-939332),* 1706 Berkwood Dr., Pittsburgh, PA 15243 (SAN 220-181X) Tel 412-279-5000; Fax: 412-279-9404.

J R Herb Pubns Imprint of Herb Studies Library

J R Pierce, *(Pierce, Jon Robert; 0-9630559),* 2010 Bushy Creek Rd., Apt. 501, Greer, SC 29650-2669.

J S Eye Inst, *(Univ. of California, Los Angeles, Jules Stein Eye Institute; 0-9630545),* 100 Stein Plaza, UCLA, Box 957008, Los Angeles, CA 90095-7008 Tel 310-825-4148.

J Stanfield, *(Stanfield, James Co.; 1-56304),* P.O. Box 41058, Santa Barbara, CA 93140 Tel 805-897-1185; Fax: 805-565-3918; Toll Free: 800-421-6534
E-mail: maindesk@stanfield.com
Web site: http://www.stanfield.com.

J Striano Bks, *(Striano, Judi Bks.; 0-943659),* 225 Central Park W., No. 820, New York, NY 10024 (SAN 668-7350) Tel 212-873-9053.

J T Willis, *(Willis, Jay Thomas; 0-9618486),* 4902 Bay View Rd., Richton Park, IL 60471-3110 (SAN 668-1638).

J Thoma Bks Imprint of Nelson

J V Cook, *(Cook, Jaunita Vaughan; 0-9649121),* 2217 Wayside Ct., Deer Park, TX 77536 Tel 713-479-2500; Fax: 713-479-7979
Dist(s): **Herveys Bklink** *(Hervey's Booklink & Cookbook Warehouse).*

J Van Impe, *(Van Impe, Jack Ministries; 0-934803; 1-884137; 1-928954),* 1718 Northfield Dr., Rochester Hills, MI 48309 (SAN 697-3620) Tel 248-852-2244; Fax: 248-852-2692
E-mail: jvim@jvim.com
Web site: http://www.jvim.com
Dist(s): **W Pubng Grp** *(W Publishing Group).*

J Vaughan Assocs, *(Vaughan, Joe Assocs./Pubs.; 0-9636863),* Orders Addr.: P.O. Box 8524, Prairie Village, KS 66208-0524; Edit Addr.: 6727 Granada Rd., Prairie Village, KS 66208-1636 Tel 913-384-6966; Fax: 913-384-6967
Dist(s): **Baker & Taylor** *(Baker & Taylor Bks.)*
Booksource *(Booksource, The).*

J W Cooper Cnslt, *(Cooper, J.W. Consultant Pr.; 0-9635702),* 1200 Colliers Creek Rd., Watkinsville, GA 30677 Tel 706-769-7586.

J W Edwards, *(Edwards, J.W. Inc.; 0-910546; 1-886569),* 2500 S. State St., Ann Arbor, MI 48104 (SAN 223-0348) Tel 313-769-1000.

J Wong, *(Wong, John; 0-9635700),* 196 Harvard Ave., Suite 2, Allston, MA 02134 Tel 617-254-5805.

Jacobs Pub, *(Jacobs Publishing, Inc.; 0-9615234),* 11405 N. Pensylvania St., No. 102, Carmel, IN 46032 (SAN 692-4905) Tel 317-815-9400; Fax: 317-573-2299
E-mail: lori@rjco.com.

Jade Pr, *(Jade Pr.; 0-9644862),* Orders Addr.: P.O. Box 822, Bedford, MA 01730 Tel 781-862-8658; Edit Addr.: 5 Manning St., Lexington, MA 02173.

Jaguar Ed (ESP) *(84-89960; 84-922423) Dist. by* **Libros Fronteras.**

†Jai Pr, *(Jai Pr., Inc.; 0-7623; 0-89232; 1-55938),* Subs. of Elsevier Science, Orders Addr.: P.O. Box 811, Stamford, CT 06904-0811; Edit Addr.: 100 Prospect St., Stamford, CT 06904-0811 (SAN 208-4082) Tel 203-323-9606; Fax: 203-357-8446
E-mail: order@jaipress.com
Web site: http://www.JAIPRESS.com; *CIP.*

Jalice Pubs, *(Jalice Pubs.; 0-9627375),* P.O. Box 455, Notre Dame, IN 46556 Tel 219-232-9534; Fax: 219-232-8968.

Jalmar Pr, *(Jalmar Pr.; 0-915190; 0-935266; 1-880396; 1-931061),* Subs. of B. L. Winch & Assocs., 24426 S. Main St., Suite 702, Carson, CA 90745 (SAN 113-3640) Tel 310-816-3085; Fax: 310-816-3092; Toll Free: 800-662-9662 (orders)
E-mail: jalmarpress@att.net
Web site: http://jalmarpress.com
Dist(s): **B L Winch** *(Winch, B. L. & Assocs.)*
Baker & Taylor *(Baker & Taylor Bks.)*
Brodart *(Brodart Co.).*

Jalor Med, *(JaLor Medical References; 0-9670164),* 12204 Bridgehead Pl., Glen Allen, VA 23059 Tel 804-364-5747; Fax: 804-364-5748; 570-472-3774 (PA office); Toll Free: 800-831-9624
E-mail: spiascik@erols.com
Web site: http://jalormedical.com
Dist(s): **Millenium Mktg** *(Millenium Marketing).*

Jalsa Pubs, *(Jalsa Pubs.; 0-9662282),* 870 Coral Ridge Dr., Suite 104, Coral Springs, FL 33071 Tel 954-255-0483; Fax: 954-255-5254; Toll Free: 800-647-1735.

Jalsco Inc, *(Jalsco, Inc.; 0-9617818),* 893 Markley Woods Way, Cincinnati, OH 45230 (SAN 665-3170).

Jamarda NC, *(Jamarda Resources; 0-9663552),* 1315 Excelsior St., Winston-Salem, NC 27101 Tel 336-722-7139; Fax: 336-722-8467
E-mail: info@jamardaresources.com
Web site: http://www.jamardaresources.com.

JAMCO Dist, *(JAMCO Distribution),* 1401 Lakeway Dr., Lewisville, TX 75057 Fax: 972-353-1300; Toll Free: 800-538-1287
E-mail: jamco@majors.com.

James C Smith, *(Smith, James C.; 0-9646206),* 1103 Russell Pkwy., Warner Robins, GA 31088 Tel 912-922-4091; Fax: 912-929-8822.

James Pubns NY, *(James Pubns.; 0-9615267),* Box 545, Guilderland, NY 12084 (SAN 695-1783) Tel 518-479-0929; Fax: 518-479-1044 Do not confuse with James Pubns. in West Palm Beach, Fl.

Jane Pubns, *(Jane Pubns.; 0-9649093),* P.O. Box 948, Virginia Beach, VA 23451
E-mail: janepub@aol.com.

Janelle Pubns, *(Janelle Pubns., Inc.; 0-9626739; 1-890265),* Orders Addr.: P.O. Box 811, De Kalb, IL 60115-0811 Tel 815-756-2300; Fax: 815-756-4799; Toll Free: 800-888-8834; Edit Addr.: 1189 Twombley Rd., De Kalb, IL 60115
E-mail: info@janellepublications.com
Web site: http://www.janellepublications.com.

Janice Prodn, *(Janice Production, Inc.; 0-9660549),* 7530 S. Constance, Chicago, IL 60649 Tel 773-288-5660
E-mail: jgillespie6@juno.com.

Jannetti Pubns, *(Jannetti Pubns., Inc.; 0-9655310),* Div. of Anthony J. Jannetti, Inc., East Holly Ave., Box 56, Pitman, NJ 08071-0056 Tel 856-256-2300; Fax: 856-256-2345
E-mail: Thomask@mail.ajj.com
Web site: http://www.inurse.com.

Janson Pubns, *(Janson Pubns.; 0-939765; 1-889597),* 2 Prudential Plaza, No. 1200, Chicago, IL 60601-5524 (SAN 663-7663) Toll Free: 800-322-6284.

Janus Pubng (GBR) *(1-85756) Dist. by* **Paul & Co Pubs.**

Japan Pubns USA, *(Japan Pubns. (U.S.A.), Inc.; 0-87040; 1-57883),* Subs. of Japan Pubns., Inc. (Tokyo, Japan), 160 Spruce Knob Rd., Middletown Springs, VT 05757-4432 (SAN 680-0513) Tel 802-235-2814; c/o Kodansha America, Inc., 114 Fifth Ave., 18th Flr., New York, NY 10011 (SAN 201-0526) Tel 212-727-6460; Toll Free: 800-788-6262 (booksellers 1-800-631-8571)
Dist(s): **OUP** *(Oxford Univ. Pr., Inc.).*

JARR UK (GBR) *(0-7117; 0-85306) Dist. by* **Seven Hills Bk.**

Jason Pr, *(Jason Pr.; 0-9633198),* 111 Lake Shore Dr., Rancho Mirage, CA 92270-4055 Do not confuse with Jason Pr. in Shrewsbury, MA.

JayJo Bks, *(JayJo Bks., LLC; 0-9639449; 1-891383),* Orders Addr.: P.O. Box 760, Plainview, NY 11803-0760 (SAN 178-5435) Tel 516-349-5520; Fax: 800-262-1886; Toll Free: 800-999-6884; Edit Addr.: 135 Dupont St., Plainview, NY 11803-0760
E-mail: jayjobook@guidancechannel.com
Web site: http://www.jayjo.com
Dist(s): **Quality Bks IL** *(Quality Bks., Inc.)*
Unique Bks Inc *(Unique Bks., Inc.).*

Jaypee Brothers (IND) *(81-7179) Dist. by* **SLACK Inc.**

JB Enterp, *(J B Enterprises; 0-9674306),* 122 N. Buckingham, Aurora, IL 60506 Fax: 630-859-7275 Do not confuse with J B Enterprises, Talent, OR
E-mail: JohnNelson@email.msn.com.

JBK Pub, *(JBK Publishing, Inc.; 0-945892),* 1863 SW Montgomery Dr., Portland, OR 97201-2438 (SAN 247-9494) Tel 503-248-0717.

JBS Pub, *(JBS Publishing; 0-9644344),* 5431 Lucy Dr., Waldorf, MD 20601-3217 Tel 301-843-8350; Fax: 301-645-0944 Do not confuse with JBS Publishing, Inc, Marathon, FL
E-mail: beelady@olg.com.

JDV Pub, *See* **Booksmythe**

JELD Pub, *(JELD Publishing; 0-9631918),* 11320 SE Lincoln St., Portland, OR 97216 Tel 503-520-8859; Fax: 503-627-0919
E-mail: Drdwthom@aol.com.

Je-Lynn Pubns, *(Je-Lynn Pubns.; 0-9650555),* 1621 W. Edgerton Ave., Suite H, Milwaukee, WI 53221 Tel 414-281-4245; Fax: 414-382-6332
E-mail: jelynn3@aol.com
Web site: http://members.aol.com/jelynn3/gift.html.

Jems Comm, *(Jems Communications; 0-936174),* Div. of Reed Elsevier Plc, Orders Addr.: P.O. Box 2789, Carlsbad, CA 92018 (SAN 241-550X); Edit Addr.: 1947 Camino Vida Roble, Ste. 200, Carlsbad, CA 92008 (SAN 663-6454)
Web site: Http://www.jems.com.

†Jen Hse Pub Co, *(Jen Hse. Publishing Co.; 0-910841),* 119 Cherry Valley Rd., Reisterstown, MD 21136 (SAN 262-7604) Tel 410-526-3805
E-mail: jenhouse@erols.com; *CIP.*

Jeremiah Pr, *(Jeremiah Pr.; 0-9631517; 1-883520),* 5840 Windrift Ln., Boca Raton, FL 33433-5426 Tel 561-368-2322.

Jessica Kingsley (GBR) *(1-85302; 1-84310) Dist. by* **Taylor & Francis.**

Jesus Bks, *See* **BOLD Bks**

Jewel Pubns, *(Jewel Pubns.; 0-917728),* 2417 Hazelwood Ave., Fort Wayne, IN 46805 (SAN 209-3049) Tel 219-483-6625 Do not confuse with Jewel Pubns., Dallas, TX.

JHPIEGO, *(JHPIEGO Corp.; 0-929817),* Affil. of Johns Hopkins Univ., 1615 Thames St., Suite 310, Baltimore, MD 21231-3492 (SAN 250-5673) Fax: 410-614-0586
E-mail: info@jhpiego.org
Web site: http://www.jhpiego.org.

JHPIERH, *See* **JHPIEGO**

†JIST Pubng, *(JIST Publishing; 0-942784; 1-56370; 1-57112),* 8902 Otis Ave., Indianapolis, IN 46216-1033 (SAN 240-2351) Tel 317-613-4200; Fax: 317-613-4307; Toll Free Fax: 800-547-8329; Toll Free: 800-648-5478
E-mail: info@jist.com; generaldelivery@jist.com
Web site: http://www.jist.com; *CIP.*

JIST Works, *See* **JIST Pubng**

JJ Pub FL, *(JJ Publishing; 0-9604610),* 1312 Arthur St., Hollywood, FL 33019 (SAN 220-0090) Tel 954-929-3559 (phone/fax).

Jjea enter, *(J+j.e.a. enterprises; 0-9639102),* 2487 Pleasant Valley Rd., Jackson, WI 53037 Tel 414-677-2140; Fax: 414-677-4274.

JLW Pub, *(JLW Pubns.; 0-9644624),* Orders Addr.: P.O. Box 141, Wyckoff, NJ 07481 Tel 973-838-2267; Fax: 973-838-2994; Toll Free: 800-484-1398 (ext. 5146); Edit Addr.: 571 Greenhill Rd., Kinnelon, NJ 07405
Dist(s): **Majors Scientific Bks Inc** *(Majors Scientific Bks., Inc.)*
Matthews Medical Bk Co *(Matthews Medical Bk. Co.)*
Rittenhouse *(Rittenhouse Bk. Distributors).*

JMA Pubns, *(JMA Pubns.; 0-9658190),* Div. of Miller & Assocs., 1427 N. Seventh St., Lebanon, PA 17046-4307 Tel 717-228-2302
E-mail: janemiller@msn.com
Web site: http://www.횡janeswords.com
Dist(s): **Baker & Taylor** *(Baker & Taylor Bks.)*
Koen Bk Distributors *(Koen Bk. Distributors).*

JMJ Publng, *(JMJ Publishing; 0-9652174),* 1042 Longfellow Dr., Canton, MI 48187 Tel 313-981-6775; Fax: 313-534-5923.

Jo Ann Heltzel, *(Heltzel, Jo Ann; 0-9633041),* 3714 York Cir., Woodbury, MN 55125 Tel 612-738-6506.

Jobs for Future, *(Jobs for the Future; 1-887410),* 88 Broad St., 8th Flr., Boston, MA 02110-3407 Tel 617-728-4446; Fax: 617-728-4857
E-mail: info@jff.org
Web site: http://www.jff.org.

JODA, *(JODA Communications, Ltd.; 1-56583),* P.O. Box 793, Germantown, WI 53022-0793 Tel 414-250-0719; Fax: 414-255-8180.

Joelle Pub, *(Joelle Publishing; 0-942723),* Orders Addr.: P.O. Box 91229, Santa Barbara, CA 93190-1229 (SAN 667-2574); Edit Addr.: 1276 Mountain View Rd., Santa Barbara, CA 93109 (SAN 667-2582) Tel 805-962-9887; Fax: 805-965-0332
Dist(s): **Quality Bks IL** *(Quality Bks., Inc.)*
Seven Hills Bk *(7 Hills Bk. Distributors).*

Johmax Bks Inc, *(Johmax Bks., Inc.; 0-912095),* 108 Spring Ave., Chestertown, MD 21620 (SAN 264-7559) Tel 410-778-9041; Fax: 410-778-7318
E-mail: parkerbb@dmv.com
Web site: http://www.chestertown.com/parker/parker.html.

John Bastyr, *(Bastyr, John College Pubns.; 0-9618764),* 14500 Juanita Dr., NE, Bothell, WA 98011-4966 (SAN 242-3081).

†John Jay Pr, *(John Jay Pr.; 0-89444),* 899 Tenth Ave., New York, NY 10019 (SAN 210-2196) Tel 212-237-8442; Fax: 212-237-8486; *CIP.*

John Libby (GBR) *(0-86196) Dist. by* **Buttrwrth-Heinemann.**

John Murray (GBR) *(0-7195) Dist. by* **Trafalgar.**

John Wright (GBR) *(0-7236; 0-85608) Dist. by* **Macmillan.**

John Wright (GBR) *(0-7236; 0-85608) Dist. by* **Buttrwrth-Heinemann.**

†Johns Hopkins, *(Johns Hopkins Univ. Pr.; 0-8018),* Div. of Johns Hopkins Univ., 2715 N. Charles St., Baltimore, MD 21218-4319 (SAN 202-7348) Tel 410-516-6900; Fax: 410-516-6998; Toll Free: 800-537-5487
E-mail: bkinfo@chaos.press.jhu.edu
Web site: http://muse.jhu.edu/; http://www.press.jhu.edu; *CIP.*

Johnson Bks, *(Johnson Bks.; 0-917895; 0-933472; 1-55566),* Div. of Johnson Publishing Co., 1880 S. 57th Ct., Boulder, CO 80301 (SAN 201-0313) Tel 303-443-9766; Fax: 303-443-1106; Toll Free: 800-258-5830
E-mail: JohnsonBks@aol.com; books@jpcolorado.com
Web site: http://www.jpcolorado.com/
Dist(s): **Books West CO** *(Books West).*

Johrei Fellow, *(Johrei Fellowship; 0-9629183),* Div. of Church of World Messianity, 1971 W. 190th St., Suite 280, Torrance, CA 90504.

†Joint Comm Hlthcare, *(Joint Commission on Accreditation of Healthcare Organizations; 0-86688),* Dept. of Pubns., 1 Renaissance Blvd., OakBrook Terrace, IL 60181 (SAN 210-8194) Tel 630-792-5430; Fax: 630-792-4430; *CIP.*

Joint Pub (HKG) *(962-04) Dist. by* **Cheng & Tsui.**

Jola Pubns, *(Jola Pubns.; 1-878373),* 2933 Second St. N., Minneapolis, MN 55411-1605 Tel 612-529-5001; Fax: 612-521-2289.

Jolance Pr, *(Jolance Pr.; 0-9645952),* 259 Riverside Pkwy., Fort Thomas, KY 41075 Tel 606-781-4881; Fax: 513-977-4894
Dist(s): **Distributors** *(Distributors, The).*

Jon Carpenter (GBR) *(1-897766) Dist. by* **Paul & Co Pubs.**

†Jones & Bartlett, *(Jones & Bartlett Pubs., Inc.; 0-7637; 0-86720),* 40 Tall Pine Dr., Sudbury, MA 01776-2256 (SAN 285-0893) Tel 978-443-5000; Fax: 978-443-8000; Toll Free: 800-832-0034 ; *Imprints:* N L N Bart (N L N Press)
E-mail: info@jbpub.com
Web site: http://www.jbpub.com
Dist(s): **Natl Bk Netwk** *(National Bk. Network); CIP.*

Jones Med, *(Jones Medical Pubns.; 0-930010),* Orders Addr.: 35 E. Wacker Dr., Chicago, IL 60601 (SAN 665-7222) Toll Free: 800-621-9262; Edit Addr.: 355 Los Cerros Dr., Greenbrae, CA 94904 (SAN 210-4466) Tel 415-461-3749.

Jones Riv Pr, *(Jones River Pr.; 0-9628738; 1-888964),* Div. of News Ink, P.O. Box 6039, Plymouth, MA 02362 Tel 508-747-3899; Fax: 508-747-9784; Toll Free: 800-498-3899
Web site: http://www.jones-river-press.com.

Jones Strain, *(Jones Strain Counterstrain Inc.; 0-9645135),* 1501 Tyrell Ln., Boise, ID 83706 Tel 208-343-4080; Fax: 208-344-7430.

Jonorm Pub, *See* **Jonorm Pubs**

Jonorm Pubs, *(Jonorm Pubs.; 0-9630413),* 3020 Leesbourg Trail, Woodstock, GA 30189-3422 Tel 770-924-2577.

Jordan Res, *(Jordan Research & Development International; 0-9639610),* 201 N. State Rd. 7, Margate, FL 33063 Tel 305-973-3001.

Jormax Pubng, *(Jormax Publishing, Inc.; 0-9641332; 1-888309),* 6605 Tracy Ave., Edina, MN 55439-1359.

Jos A Jackson, *(Jackson, Joseph A.; 0-9702208),* 66 Old Stockbridge Rd., Lenox, MA 01240 Tel 413-637-1436; Fax: 413-637-0338 ; *Imprints:* Socarean Pr (Socarean Press)
E-mail: eldercare@earthlink.net
Web site: http://www.eldercareadvisors.com.

Josara Pub, *(Josara Publishing; 0-9660419),* 69 Indian Hill Rd., Mount Kisco, NY 10549 Tel 914-241-7408; Fax: 914-242-4924
E-mail: nintrator@aol.com
Web site: http://www.pregnancyrx.com
Dist(s): **Pathway Bk Serv** *(Pathway Bk. Service).*

Joseph Henry Pr Imprint of Natl Acad Pr

†Jossey-Bass, *(Jossey-Bass, Inc. Pubs.; 0-471; 0-7879; 0-87589; 0-88390; 0-89384; 1-55542),* Div. of John Wiley & Sons, Orders Addr.: 432 Elizabeth Ave., Somerset, NJ 08875 Tel 732-469-4400; Fax: 732-302-2300; Edit Addr.: 350 Sansome St., San Francisco, CA 94104-1342 Tel 415-433-1740; Fax: 415-433-0499; Toll Free: 800-956-7739; 888-378-2537 (customer service) ; *Imprints:* Pffr & Co (Pfeiffer & Company)
E-mail: webperson@jbp.com
Web site: http://www.josseybass.com
Dist(s): **netLibrary CO** *(netLibrary, Inc.); CIP.*

Jostens Pub, *See* **Cherbo Pub Grp**

Journey Pubns, *(Journey Pubns.; 0-918038),* P.O. Box 423, Woodstock, NY 12498 (SAN 209-570X) Tel 914-657-8434 Do not confuse with companies with the same name in Savannah, GA, Metairie, LA.

Journeyman, *See* **Journeyworks Pub**

Journeys Together, *(Journeys Together; 0-9619040),* 609 Shields St., San Francisco, CA 94132-2701.

Journeyworks Pub, *(Journeyworks Publishing; 1-56885),* P.O. Box 8466, Santa Cruz, CA 95061-8466 Tel 408-423-1400; Fax: 408-423-8102; Toll Free Fax: 800-775-5853; Toll Free: 800-775-1998.

Joy Pub SJC, *(Joy Publishing; 0-939513),* Div. of California Clock Co., P.O. Box 9901, Fountain Valley, CA 92708 (SAN 663-3544) Tel 714-545-4321; Fax: 714-708-2099; Toll Free: 800-454-8228 Do not confuse with Joy Publishing in College Station, TX,
E-mail: mail@joypublishing.com
Web site: http://www.joypublishing.com
Dist(s): **BookWorld** *(BookWorld Services, Inc.)*
Spring Arbor Dist *(Spring Arbor Distributors Inc.).*

Joy Pubns MD, *(Joy Pubns.; 0-923081),* 133A Lee Dr., Annapolis, MD 21403 (SAN 251-6039) Tel 410-268-3752; Toll Free: 800-542-1400 Do not confuse with companies with the same name in Santa Maria, CA, Gardena, CA, Stoneham, MA
E-mail: joypub@aol.com
Web site: http://www.members.aol.com/joypub
Dist(s): **Baker & Taylor** *(Baker & Taylor Bks.)*
New Leaf Dist *(New Leaf Distributing Co., Inc.).*

Joyce Homecare, *(Joyce Homecare, Inc.; 0-9642138),* 13 S. Point Rd., Fairview Heights, IL 62208.

Joyce Media, *(Joyce Media, Inc.; 0-917002),* P.O. Box 57, Acton, CA 93510 (SAN 208-7197) Tel 805-269-1169; Fax: 805-269-2139
E-mail: joycemed@pacbell.net
Web site: http://joycemedia.com.

Joy-Full Pubng, *(Joy-Full Publishing Co.; 0-9668742),* Orders Addr.: P.O. Box 591661, Houston, TX 77259-1661 Tel 281-218-8773
E-mail: joy_full@earthlink.net
Web site: http://www.joy-full.com.

JPC Pubng, *(JPC Publishing; 0-9659476),* 3300 P G A Blvd., Suite 600, Palm Beach Gardens, FL 33410 Tel 561-627-3810; Fax: 561-624-3871.

†JPS Phila, *(Jewish Pubn. Society; 0-8276; 965-7157),* Orders Addr.: 22883 Quicksilver Dr., Sterling, VA 20166 (SAN 253-9446) Tel 703-661-1165; Fax: 703-661-1501; Toll Free: 800-355-1165; Edit Addr.: 2100 Arch St., 2nd Flr., Philadelphia, PA 19103 Tel 215-832-0601; Fax: 215-568-2017; Toll Free: 800-234-3151
E-mail: marketing@jewishpub.org
Web site: http://www.jewishpub.org
Dist(s): **Gefen Bks** *(Gefen Bks.); CIP.*

Publisher Symbol Index

Jrnl Applied Behavior Analysis, *(Journal of Applied Behavior Analysis; 1-882018),* Univ. of Kansas, Dept. Human Development, Lawrence, KS 66045 (SAN 248-3351) Tel 913-843-0008.

Jrny Editions, *(Journey Editions; 1-58290; 1-885203),* Div. of Charles E. Tuttle Co., Inc., Orders Addr.: R.R. 1, Box 231-5, North Clarendon, VT 05759-9700 Tel 802-773-8930; Fax: 802-773-6993; Toll Free: 800-526-2778; Edit Addr.: 153 Milk St., 5th Flr., Boston, MA 02109 Tel 617-951-4080; Fax: 617-951-4045; Toll Free: 800-247-1060 Do not confuse with Journey Editions in Saint Paul, MN
Web site: http://www.tuttle-periplus.com
Dist(s): **Tuttle Pubng** *(Tuttle Publishing).*

Jrny Pub TX, *(Journey Publishing; 0-9654728),* 6610 Stewart Rd., Suite 16, Galveston, TX 77551 Tel 409-763-5373; Fax: 409-762-3772 Do not confuse with companies with the same name in North Pole, AR, Los Angeles, CA, Winston Salem, NC, Nashville, TN
E-mail: journeypub@aol.com.

†**Judson,** *(Judson Pr.; 0-8170),* Div. of American Baptist Churches, U.S.A., P.O. Box 851, Valley Forge, PA 19482-0851 (SAN 201-0348) Tel 610-768-2118; Fax: 610-768-2107; Toll Free: 800-331-1053
Web site: http://www.judsonpress.com
Dist(s): **Appalachian Bible** *(Appalachian Bible Co.)*
Riverside-World *(Riverside World)*
Spring Arbor Dist *(Spring Arbor Distributors Inc.); CIP.*

Julstro Pubns, *(Julstro Pubns.; 1-929632),* 112 Grotke Rd., Chestnut Ridge, NY 10977 Tel 914-620-0672; Fax: 914-620-9520.

Junius-Vaughn, *See* **St Aedans Pr & Bk**

Jupiter Pub, *(Jupiter Publishing; 0-9622374),* One Tweitter Ct., Oakland, CA 94619 Tel 510-530-6351; Fax: 510-530-0103.

Just Peachy, *(Just Peachy Pr.; 0-9700026),* Orders Addr.: P.O. Box 4100, Scottsdale, AZ 85261-4100 Tel 480-315-1655; Fax: 480-661-0149
E-mail: justpeachypress@att.net.

Just Pub Hse, *(Just Publishing Hse.; 0-9618532),* 2265 Starlight Ct., Apt. 282, Melbourne, FL 32904-8130 (SAN 668-0976) Tel 407-259-8213.

Juta & Co (ZAF) *(0-7021) Dist. by* **Gaunt.**

Juta & Co (ZAF) *(0-7021) Dist. by* **Intl Spec Bk.**

Juvenescent, *(Juvenescent Research Corp.; 0-9600148; 1-884996),* 807 Riverside Dr., Apt. 1F, New York, NY 10032 (SAN 206-7250) Tel 212-795-3749
Web site: http://www.juvenescent.qpg.com
Dist(s): **Barnes & Noble Inc** *(Barnes & Noble, Inc.).*

K Brandt, *(Brandt, Kevin; 1-928813),* 332 Park St., Sterling, CO 80751-3937
E-mail: savbra@henge.com
Web site: http://www.stopsmokingbook.com.

K Bursell, *(Bursell, Kaare; 0-9700262),* 1041 Kains Ave., Albany, CA 94706-2260 Tel 510-559-8057; Fax: 510-528-3027
E-mail: kaareb@creative.net
Web site: http://www.alchemycalpages.com.

K F Haug Pubs (DEU) *(3-7760) Dist. by* **Medicina Bio.**

K Kelroy, *(Kelroy, Karen; 0-9661509),* 6500 Libra Ln., Racine, WI 53406
Dist(s): **Commitments Bkstore** *(Commitments Bookstore).*

K Kvaale, *(Kvaale, Kathy),* 1748 Sixth St., S., Fargo, ND 58103-4907.

K LaTour, *(LaTour, Kathy; 0-9612870),* P.O. Box 141182, Dallas, TX 75214 (SAN 291-2511) Tel 214-827-2753.

K Milner, *(Milner, Kathleen; 1-886903),* 13812 N. 42nd Pl., Phoenix, AZ 85032 Tel 602-404-1689; Fax: 602-404-1685
Web site: http://www.kathleenmilner.com
Dist(s): **Bookpeople** *(Bookpeople)*
New Leaf Dist *(New Leaf Distributing Co., Inc.)*
Red Wheel ME *(Red Wheel).*

K Poole, *(Poole, Karuna; 0-9643629),* 3212 25th St., Seattle, WA 98144 Tel 206-722-0878; Fax: 206-722-2911
E-mail: karunap@aol.com.

K S H Pubns, *(KSH Pubns.; 0-9672076),* 11445 E. Via Linda, Suite 2 -122, Scottsdale, AZ 85259 Tel 602-391-3322 (phone/fax)
E-mail: kshpublications@hotmail.com
Web site: http://www.medicalrecordbook.com.

K&A Pubns, *(K&A Pubns.; 0-9616230),* P.O. Box 22075, San Diego, CA 92192 (SAN 658-5981) Tel 619-455-6578 Do not confuse with K & A Pubns. in Pleasanton, CA.

Kabel Pubs, *(Kabel Pubs.; 0-930329; 1-57529),* 11225 Huntover Dr., Rockville, MD 20852-3613 (SAN 670-8323) Tel 301-468-6463 (phone/fax); Toll Free: 800-543-3167
E-mail: kabelcomp@erols.com
Web site: http://www.erols.com/kabelcomp/index2.html.

Kairos Bks, *(Kairos Bks., Inc.; 0-9608410),* P.O. Box 3247, Davenport, IA 52808-3247 (SAN 240-6942) Tel 563-326-5970; Fax: 563-326-2225 Do not confuse with companies with the same name in Portland, OR, Columbus, OH.

Kali Pr, *(Kali Pr.; 0-9628882; 1-890941),* Orders Addr.: P.O. Box 1031, Port Townsend, WA 98368-1031 Tel 360-385-1933; Fax: 360-385-1180; Toll Free: 888-999-5254; Edit Addr.: 211 Taylor, Suite 35A, Port Townsend, WA 98368-1031
E-mail: sales@kalipress.com
Web site: http://www.kalipress.com
Dist(s): **Bookpeople** *(Bookpeople)*
New Leaf Dist *(New Leaf Distributing Co., Inc.).*

Kalyx.com, *(Kalyx.com; 0-9650253),* P.O. Box 417, Camden, NY 13316 Tel 315-245-3000; Fax: 315-245-5700
E-mail: info@kalyx.com.

Kapala Corp, *(Kapala Corp.; 0-914833),* 1515 State St., Suite 1, Santa Barbara, CA 93101 (SAN 289-3339) Tel 805-963-5454; Fax: 805-965-3318.

Kapala Pr, *See* **Kapala Corp**

Kaplan, *(Kaplan Bks.; 0-684; 0-7432),* Affl. of Simon & Schuster Trade, Orders Addr.: 100 Front St., Riverside, NJ 08075 Fax: 856-824-2289; Toll Free Fax: 800-943-9831; Toll Free: 800-223-2348; Edit Addr.: 1230 Avenue of the Americas, 1st Flr., New York, NY 10020 Tel 212-698-7000; Fax: 212-698-7007
E-mail: kaplan@simonandschuster.com
Web site: http://www.SimonSays.com.

Kappeler Inst Pub, *(Kappeler Institute Publishing; 0-942958),* Div. of Kappeler Institute for the Science of Being, Orders Addr.: c/o Joel Jessen, P.O. Box 99735, Seattle, WA 98199-0735 (SAN 240-1185) Tel 206-286-1617; Fax: 206-286-1675
E-mail: mail@kappelerinstitute.org
Web site: http://www.kappelerinstitute.org
Dist(s): **Rare Bk Co** *(Rare Bk. Co.).*

Kardinal Pubng, *(Kardinal Publishing; 0-9650689),* 915 Murle Ln., Loveland, OH 45140 Tel 513-683-9233.

Karma Pubng, *(Karma Publishing; 0-9647794),* 58 Brookhaven Dr., East Providence, RI 02914-4006 Tel 401-435-7044 Do not confuse with Karma Publishing Co., Monessen, PA.

Karnac Bks (GBR) *(0-946439; 0-9501647; 0-9507146; 1-85575) Dist. by* **Other Pr LLC.**

Kashan Pub, *(Kashan Publishing; 0-9622669),* 9050 County Rd., No. 11, Maple Plain, MN 55359 Tel 612-972-3762
E-mail: kafhan@worldnet.att,net
Web site: http://www.members.aol.com/symptoms5.

Katan Pubns, *(Katan Pubns.; 0-9622460),* 1019 W. Lafayette Ave., Jacksonville, IL 62650-1860 Tel 217-243-3029.

Katydid, *(Katydid Publishing; 1-888349),* Div. of The Mug Joint, Inc., 3418 SE. Bright St., Muncie, IN 47302 Tel 765-284-3929; Fax: 765-284-0074
E-mail: chirsch@mugjoint.com
Web site: http://www.mugjoint.com/katydid.

Katydid Press, *See* **Katydid**

Kazi Pubns, *(Kazi Pubns., Inc.; 0-933511; 0-935782; 1-56744),* 3023 W. Belmont Ave., Chicago, IL 60618 (SAN 162-3397) Tel 773-267-7001; Fax: 773-267-7002 ; *Imprints:* Library of Islam (Library of Islam, Limited)
E-mail: info@kazi.org
Web site: http://www.kazi.org.

KBA Pub, *(KBA Publishing; 1-880931),* Div. of KBA, Box 116, Rockwall, TX 75087.

KC Press, *(KC Pr.; 0-9667080),* Subs. of Med-Legal.net, 1828 45th Ave., Suite 104, Osceola, WI 54020-5403 Tel 715-755-3555 (phone/fax)
E-mail: kcpress@med-legal.net
Web site: http://www.med-legal.net.

Keats Pubng Imprint of McGraw-Hill Trade

Keep Hope Alive, *(Keep Hope Alive; 1-887831),* P.O. Box 27041, West Allis, WI 53227 Tel 262-548-4344; Fax: 414-329-0653
E-mail: keephope@execpc.com
Web site: http://www.keephope.net
Dist(s): **Alamo Sq Dist** *(Alamo Square Distributors)*
Nutri-Books Corp *(Nutri-Bks. Corp.).*

Keep it Simple, *(Keep it Simple Bks.; 0-9636255; 0-9710309),* P.O. Box 431, Murphys, CA 95247 (SAN 298-0061) Tel 209-728-0420; Fax: 209-728-0568
E-mail: kisjune@mlode.com
Web site: http://www.keepitsimplebooks.com
Dist(s): **Words Distrib** *(Words Distributing Co.).*

Kegan Paul Intl (GBR) *(0-7103) Dist. by* **Col U Pr.**

Kehayoff Verlag (DEU) *(3-929078; 3-934296) Dist. by* **Prestel Pub NY.**

Keithley Asyst, *See* **Keithley Instruments**

Keithley Instruments, *(Keithley Instruments; 0-924729),* Div. of Keithley Instruments, Inc., 28775 Aurora Rd., Solon, OH 44139-1891 (SAN 246-4055) Toll Free: 800-348-0033.

†**Kelley,** *(Kelley, Augustus M. Pubs.; 0-678),* Orders Addr.: P.O. Box 1048, Fairfield, NJ 07004-1048 (SAN 206-9768) Tel 212-685-7202 (phone/fax); *CIP.*

Kelly Fnd, *(Kelly Foundation; 1-883094),* 2801 W. Roosevelt Rd., Little Rock, AR 72204 Tel 501-663-6553; Toll Free: 800-245-6428
E-mail: kellyadm@kellyfdn.com.

Kelsey Enterprises, *See* **Cheval Intl**

Kempler Inst, *(Kempler Institute; 0-9600808),* P.O. Box 2185, Laguna Hills, CA 92654 Tel 949-472-4155
E-mail: kemplerinstusa@net-star.net.

Kendall-Hunt, *(Kendall/Hunt Publishing Co.; 0-7872; 0-8403; 0-7575),* Orders Addr.: P.O. Box 1840, Dubuque, IA 52004-1840; Edit Addr.: 4050 Westmark Dr., Dubuque, IA 52002 (SAN 203-9184) Tel 319-589-1000; Fax: 319-589-1046; Toll Free Fax: 800-772-9165; Toll Free: 800-228-0810
E-mail: orders@kendallhunt.com
Web site: http://www.kendallhunt.com.

Kenilworth Pr (GBR) *(0-600; 0-901366; 1-872082; 1-872119) Dist. by* **Half Halt Pr.**

Kennedy Carlisle, *(Kennedy Carlisle Publishing Co.; 0-9643348),* P.O. Box 2247, San Francisco, CA 94126 (SAN 298-7848) Tel 415-675-5630; Fax: 415-674-8339
E-mail: act4health@aol.com.

Kensgtn Pub Corp, *(Kensington Publishing Corp.; 0-7860; 0-8217; 1-55817; 1-57566; 0-7582),* 850 Third Ave., New York, NY 10022-6222 Tel 212-407-1500; Fax: 212-935-0699; Toll Free: 800-221-2647 ; *Imprints:* Citadel Pr (Citadel Press) Zebra Kensgtn (Zebra Books) Pinncle Kensgtn (Pinnacle Books) Knsington (Kensington Books) Dafina (Dafina) Twin Streams (Twin Streams)
E-mail: jmclean@kensingtonbooks.com
Web site: http://www.kensingtonbooks.com
Dist(s): **Penguin Putnam** *(Penguin Putnam, Inc.)*
Wrldwide Media Srv *(Worldwide Media Service, Inc.).*

Kensington Hse Publishing Ltd, *(Kensington Hse. Publishing, Ltd.; 1-878518),* 19 Lowell St., Bethpage, NY 11714 Tel 516-731-2260; Fax: 516-731-2438.

Kent Fine Art, *See* **Kent Gallery**

Kent Gallery, *(Kent Gallery; 1-878607),* 67 Prince St., New York, NY 10012 Tel 212-966-4500; Fax: 212-966-7820
E-mail: kent@kentgallery.com
Web site: http:///www.kentgallery.com
Dist(s): **Dist Art Pubs** *(Distributed Art Pubs./D.A.P.).*

†**Kent St U Pr,** *(Kent State Univ. Pr.; 0-87338),* Orders Addr.: c/o BookMasters, Inc., 30 Amberwood Pkwy., Ashland, OH 44805 Tel 419-281-1802; Fax: 419-281-6883; Toll Free: 800-247-6553; Edit Addr.: 307 Lowry Hall, Kent, OH 44242-0001 (SAN 201-0437) Tel 330-672-7913; Fax: 330-672-3104
Web site: http://bookmasters.com ksu-press
Dist(s): **BookMasters** *(BookMasters, Inc.); CIP.*

Kerr Lib, *(Kerr Library Special Collections; 0-9629082),* Oregon State Univ., KLib 422, Corvallis, OR 97331 Tel 541-737-2075; Fax: 541-737-3453.

Kerr Pubns, *(Kerr Pubns., Inc.; 0-9628237),* Orders Addr.: P.O. Box 976, Forsyth, MT 59327-0976; Edit Addr.: 307 Rapel, Hysham, MT 59038 Tel 406-342-5626.

†**Kesend Pub Ltd,** *(Kesend, Michael Publishing, Ltd.; 0-935576),* Orders Addr.: Raritan Industrial Pk., 100 Newfield Ave., Edison, NJ 08837 Tel 732-225-2727; Fax: 732-225-1562; Toll Free: 800-488-8040; Edit Addr.: 1025 Fifth Ave., New York, NY 10028 (SAN 213-6902) Tel 212-249-5150; Fax: 212-249-2129
E-mail: mkpublishing@yahoo.com; *CIP.*

Kessinger Pub, *(Kessinger Publishing Co.; 0-7661; 0-922802; 1-56459),* Orders Addr.: P.O. Box 160, Kila, MT 59920 (SAN 251-4621) Tel 406-756-0167; Fax: 406-257-5051; Edit Addr.: 1550 Roger's Ln., Kila, MT 59920
E-mail: books@kessinger-publishing.com
Web site: http://www.kessinger-publishing.com.

Keswick Hse, *(Keswick Hse.; 0-9653024),* Orders Addr.: P.O. Box 992535, Redding, CA 96099-2535 (SAN 299-1314) Tel 916-244-2472; Fax: 916-244-1649; Edit Addr.: 15812 Rock Creek Rd., Redding, CA 96001 (SAN 299-1322)
E-mail: KeswickH@aol.com
Web site: http://www.snowcrest.net/keswick.

Ketman Pubng, *See* **Wooster Bk**

Kevco Pubg, *(Kevco Publishing; 0-9643635),* 2002 Burnt Rd., Tustin, CA 92781 (SAN 298-4253) Tel 714-838-9771; Fax: 714-838-9924
E-mail: TYCO33@aol.com.

Key Porter (CAN) *(0-88619; 0-919493; 0-919630; 1-55013; 1-55263; 1-85375; 1-55356) Dist. by* **Firefly Bks Limited.**

Key-Logic, *(Key-Logic Publishing; 1-879671),* 124 Quail Hollow Dr., San Jose, CA 95128-4540 Tel 408-377-5525.

Keystone Pr, *(Keystone Pr.; 0-940701),* Orders Addr.: P.O. Box 6163, Bradenton, FL 34281 (SAN 665-2433) Tel 941-753-5179; Edit Addr.: 6515 Massachusetts St., Bradenton, FL 34207.

KG-EKG, *(KG/EKG Pr.; 0-9663389; 1-930553),* 2330 SW Williston Rd., No. 2515, Gainesville, FL 32608 Tel 352-336-3240; Fax: 352-332-9154
E-mail: ekgpress@gnv.fdt.net
Web site: http://www.kg-ekgpress.com.

Khalifahs Booksellers, *(Khalifah's Booksellers & Assocs.; 1-56411),* 26070 Barhams Hill Rd., Drewyville, VA 23844 (SAN 630-6748) Tel 757-328-7200 (cell phone); 434-658-4934 (phone/fax)
E-mail: khalifah@meckcom.net
Web site: http//www.ubusbooks.com; http//www.kbabooks.com.

Khera Pubns, *(Khera Pubns., Ltd.; 0-9640719),* Orders Addr.: P.O. Box 1722, Snohomish, WA 98291 Fax: 425-334-5928; Edit Addr.: 3026 139th Ave., NE, Snohomish, WA 98290.

Kidsrights, *(Kidsrights; 1-55864),* 3700 Progress Blvd., Mount Dora, FL 32757 (SAN 248-0891) Tel 904-483-1100 Do not confuse with Kidsrights, Charlotte, NC.

Kiefer Enterprises, *(Kiefer Enterprises International Pr.; 0-9645934),* 22320 Albatross Cir., Farmington, MN 55024 Tel 651-460-8205; Fax: 651-463-3862
Dist(s): **Bookmen Inc** *(Bookmen, Inc.).*

Kilpatrick Pubng, *(Kilpatrick Publishing Co.; 0-9701671),* 205 Laurel Rd., Athens, TX 75751 Fax: 903-675-6823
E-mail: JRKilpatrickMYO@asol.com.

Kindred Pr, *See* **Kindred Prods**

Kindred Prods, *(Kindred Productions; 0-919797; 0-921788),* Orders Addr.: 315 S. Lincoln St., Hillsboro, KS 67063 (SAN 202-2915) Tel 316-947-3151; Fax: 316-947-3266; Toll Free: 800-545-7322
E-mail: kindred@mbconf.ca
Web site: http://www.mbconf.org/kindred.htm
Dist(s): **Spring Arbor Dist** *(Spring Arbor Distributors Inc.).*

Kingdom Pubs, *See* **Cathedral Holy Spirit**

King's Crown Paperbacks Imprint of Col U Pr

Kirban, *See* **Second Comng Inc**

KISS, *(Keep It Simple Solutions; 0-9660319),* Orders Addr.: P.O. Box 136, Lafayette Hill, PA 19444-0136 Tel 215-233-5055; Fax: 215-233-5711; Toll Free: 888-385-5477; Edit Addr.: 779 Germantown Pike, Lafayette Hill, PA 19444
Dist(s): **Baker & Taylor** *(Baker & Taylor Bks.)*
Koen Bk Distributors *(Koen Bk. Distributors).*

Kisses from Heaven, *(Kisses from Heaven, Inc.; 0-9659509),* P.O. Box 6742, Lee's Summit, MO 64064 Tel 913-791-1959; Fax: 816-537-8739.

KITLV Pr (NLD) *(90-6718) Dist. by* **Book Bin.**

Kjos, *(Kjos, Neil A. Music Co.; 0-8497; 0-910842),* Orders Addr.: P.O. Box 178270, San Diego, CA 92177-8270 Tel 858-270-9800; Fax: 858-270-3507; Toll Free: 800-854-1592; Edit Addr.: 4380 Jutland Dr., San Diego, CA 92117-3698 (SAN 201-0488)
E-mail: email@kjos.com
Web site: http://www.kjos.com.

Kluwer Acad Imprint of Kluwer Academic

Kluwer Acad Hman Sci Imprint of Kluwer Academic

†Kluwer Academic, *(Kluwer Academic Pubs.; 0-412; 0-7923; 0-85200; 0-89838; 1-55608; 90-5576; 90-440; 1-4020),* Subs. of Wolters Kluwer N.V., Orders Addr.: P.O. Box 358, Hingham, MA 02018-0358 (SAN 662-0647) Tel 781-871-6600; Fax: 781-871 6528; Edit Addr.: 101 Philip Dr. Assinippi Park, Norwell, MA 02061 (SAN 211-481X); a/o Kluwer Academic/Plenum Pubs., 233 Spring St., 7th Flr., New York, NY 10013-1522 Tel 212-620-8000 ; *Imprints:* Kluwer Plenum (Kluwer Academic/Plenum Publishers) Kluwer Acad (Kluwer Academic Publishers) Kluwer Acad Hman Sci (Kluwer Academic/Human Science Press)
E-mail: kluwer@wkap.com
Web site: http://www.wkap.nl
Dist(s): **Aspen Pub** *(Aspen Pubs., Inc.)*
Lppncott W & W *(Lippincott Williams & Wilkins); CIP.*

Kluwer Academic (NLD) *(0-85200; 90-247; 90-277; 0-7462; 90-6193; 90-286) Dist. by* **Kluwer Academic.**

†Kluwer Law Intl, *(Kluwer Law International; 90-411; 90-6544),* 675 Massachusetts Ave., Cambridge, MA 02139 Tel 617-354-0140; Fax: 617-354-8595
E-mail: sales@kluwerlaw.com
Web site: http://www.kluwerlaw.com/; *CIP.*

Kluwer Law Tax Pubs, *See* **Kluwer Law Intl**

Kluwer Plenum Imprint of Kluwer Academic

KM Enterprises, *(KM Enterprises; 0-945947),* 6829 Canoga Ave., Suite 5, Canoga Park, CA 91303 (SAN 248-1790) Tel 818-710-6868; Fax: 818-710-6855.

KMK Assocs, *(KMK Assocs.; 0-9630002),* P.O. Box 60246, Palo Alto, CA 94306 Tel 650-326-7947; Fax: 415-941-8573
E-mail: haceneb@ix.netcom.com
Web site: http://www.Kirstens.com/KMK-Associates/publishing.html
Dist(s): **Bookazine Co Inc** *(Bookazine Co., Inc.).*

†Knopf, *(Knopf, Alfred A. Inc.; 0-375; 0-394; 0-676; 0-679),* Div. of The Knopf Publishing Group, Orders Addr.: 400 Hahn Rd., Westminster, MD 21157 (SAN 202-5515) Tel 410-848-1900; Toll Free Fax: 800-659-2436; Toll Free: 800-733-3000 (orders); Edit Addr.: 299 Park Ave., New York, NY 10171 (SAN 202-5825) Tel 212-751-2600; Fax: 212-572-2593; Toll Free: 800-726-0600 ; *Imprints:* KnopfC (Knopf College Department)
E-mail: customerservice@randomhouse.com
Web site: http://www.randomhouse.com/knopf
Dist(s): **Continental Bk** *(Continental Bk. Co., Inc.)*
Penguin Putnam *(Penguin Putnam, Inc.); CIP.*

KnopfC Imprint of Knopf

Know Unltd, *(Knowledge Unlimited, Inc.; 1-55933),* P.O. Box 52, Madison, WI 53701 (SAN 290-0017) Tel 608-836-6660; Fax: 608-831-1570; Toll Free: 800-356-2303 Do not confuse with companies of the same name in Palatine, IL, Ephraim, UT, Bedford Hills, NY
Web site: http://www.ku.com.

Knowldge Unltd, *(Knowledge Unlimited Publishing; 0-9639451),* P.O. Box 707, Bedford Hills, NY 10507-0707 Tel 914-793-6330; Toll Free: 800-667-5157 (orders) Do not confuse with companies with the same name in Ephraim, UT, Madison, WI, Palatine, IL
E-mail: KUP@Manic-Depression.com
Web site: http://www.manic-depression.com.

Knowledge Bank, *(Knowledge Bank Pubs., Inc.; 0-939036),* 601 Oak Haven Dr., Falls Church, VA 22046-2627 (SAN 224-1765) Tel 703-938-2814.

Knowledge Hse, *(Knowledge Hse. Pubs.; 1-931078),* 1455 Lakeside Dr., Waukegon, IL 60085 Tel 847-473-4798; Fax: 847-473-4780.

Knsington Imprint of Kensgtn Pub Corp

†Knwldg Ideas & Trnds, *(Knowledge, Ideas & Trends, Inc.; 1-879198),* 1131-0 Tolland Tpke., PMB 175, Manchester, CT 06040 Tel 860-646-0745; Fax: 860-646-3931; Toll Free: 800-826-0529 (orders only)
E-mail: slbkit@aol.com
Web site: http://www.booktrends.com
Dist(s): **Baker & Taylor** *(Baker & Taylor Bks.)*
Bookpeople *(Bookpeople)*
LPC Group *(LPC Group); CIP.*

†Kodansha, *(Kodansha America, Inc.; 0-87011; 1-56836),* 575 Lexington Ave., 23rd Flr., New York, NY 10022-6102 (SAN 201-0526) Tel 917-322-6200; Fax: 212-935-6929; Toll Free: 800-451-7556 ; *Imprints:* Kodansha Globe (Kodansha Globe)
E-mail: Kabooks@aol.com
Dist(s): **OUP** *(Oxford Univ. Pr., Inc.); CIP.*

Kodansha Globe Imprint of Kodansha

Kodansha Intl (JPN) *(4-7700) Dist. by* **Kodansha.**

Kodansha Ltd (JPN) *(4-06) Dist. by* **Bks Nippan.**

Kodiak Media, *(Kodiak Media Group; 0-9637813),* Orders Addr.: P.O. Box 1029A, Wilsonville, OR 97070 (SAN 297-9993) Fax: 503-625-4087.

Koeltz Sci Bks (DEU) *(3-87429; 3-87921) Dist. by* **Lubrecht & Cramer.**

Koeltz Sci Bks, *See* **Balogh**

Kogan Pg (GBR) *(0-7494; 0-85038; 1-85091) Dist. by* **Nichols Pub.**

Konark Pubs (IND) *(81-7398) Dist. by* **S Asia.**

Konemann, *(Konemann; 3-89508; 3-8290),* 137 W. 19th St., New York, NY 10011 Tel 212-367-8855; Fax: 212-367-8866; Toll Free: 888-317-8855
E-mail: mchin@konemann.com
Dist(s): **Baysde Ent Dist** *(Bayside Entertainment Distribution)*
Daedalus Bks *(Daedalus Bks.)*
Koen Bk Distributors *(Koen Bk. Distributors)*
Lectorum Pubns *(Lectorum Pubns., Inc.)*
Mel Bay *(Mel Bay Pubns., Inc.).*

Kopy Xpress, *(Kopy Xpress; 0-9651073),* 106 S. Heber St., Beckley, WV 25801 Tel 304-252-2751; Fax: 304-252-2752.

Kosei Pub Co (JPN) *(4-333) Dist. by* **Tuttle Pubng.**

Kraus, *See* **Periodicals Srv**

†Kregel, *(Kregel Pubns.; 0-8254),* Div. of Kregel, Inc., Orders Addr.: P.O. Box 2607, Grand Rapids, MI 49501-2607 (SAN 206-9792) Tel 616-451-4775; Fax: 616-451-9330; Toll Free: 800-733-2607; Edit Addr.: 733 Wealthy St., SE., Grand Rapids, MI 49503-5553 (SAN 298-9115)
E-mail: kregelbooks@kregel.com
Web site: http://kregel.com
Dist(s): **Appalach Bk Dist** *(Appalachian Bk. Distributors)*
Riverside-World *(Riverside World)*
Spring Arbor Dist *(Spring Arbor Distributors Inc.); CIP.*

KRI, *(KRI; 0-9639847; 0-9639991),* Rte. 2, Box 4, Shady Ln., Espanola, NM 87532 Tel 505-753-0562; Fax: 505-753-5982
E-mail: satkerpal@roadrunner.com
Dist(s): **Ancient Healing** *(Ancient Healing Ways).*

†Krieger, *(Krieger Publishing Co.; 0-88275; 0-89464; 0-89874; 1-57524),* P.O. Box 9542, Melbourne, FL 32902-9542 (SAN 202-6562) Tel 321-724-9542; Fax: 321-951-3671; Toll Free: 800-724-0025
E-mail: info@krieger-publishing.com
Web site: http://www.krieger-publishing.com
Dist(s): **Univelt Inc** *(Univelt, Inc.); CIP.*

Krishna Pr, *(Krishna Pr.),* Div. of Gordon Pr., Orders Addr.: P.O. Box 459, New York, NY 10004 (SAN 202-6570).

Kroeger Herb, *See* **Hanna Kroeger**

KS Bar, *(Kansas Bar Assn.; 0-942357; 1-890452),* Orders Addr.: P.O. Box 1037, Topeka, KS 66601-1037 (SAN 237-7314) Tel 785-234-5696; Fax: 785-234-3813; Edit Addr.: 1200 SW Harrison St., Topeka, KS 66601.

KS Bar CLE, *See* **KS Bar**

†Ktav, *(Ktav Publishing Hse., Inc.; 0-87068; 0-88125),* Orders Addr.: P.O. Box 6249, Hoboken, NJ 07030 (SAN 201-0038) Tel 201-963-9524; Fax: 201-963-0102; Toll Free Fax: 800-626-7517 (orders); Edit Addr.: 900 Jefferson St., Hoboken, NJ 07030 (SAN 200-8866)
E-mail: orders@ktav.com; editor@ktav.com; staff@ktav.com
Web site: http://www.ktav.com
Dist(s): **Baker & Taylor** *(Baker & Taylor Bks.); CIP.*

Kugler (NLD) *(90-6299) Dist. by* **Lib Res.**

Kujichagulia Pr, *(Kujichagulia Pr.; 0-9644932),* 9506 Ridgeview Dr., Columbia, MD 21046 Tel 410-880-4354.

†Kumarian Pr, *(Kumarian Pr., Inc.; 0-931816; 1-56549; 1-887208),* 1294 Blue Hills Ave., Bloomfield, CT 06002 (SAN 212-5978) Tel 860-243-2098; Fax: 860-243-2867; Toll Free: 800-289-2664
E-mail: Kpbooks@aol.com
Web site: http://www.kpbooks.com
Dist(s): **Berrett-Koehler** *(Berrett-Koehler Pubs., Inc.); CIP.*

K-W Pubns, *(K-W Pubns.; 0-929894),* P.O. Box 26455, San Diego, CA 92196 (SAN 250-7064) Tel 858-566-6489; Fax: 858-271-1425; Toll Free: 800-450-2665
Web site: http://www.kwpub.com; http://www.intubations.com; http://www.bookzone.com/kwpub.

L A Blazek, *(Blazek, L. A. Consulting & Publishing; 0-9649995),* 4903 N. Hoyne, Chicago, IL 60625 Tel 312-275-6879.

L A Wells, *(Wells, L.A. Co.; 0-9616256),* 2025 Chatsworth Blvd., San Diego, CA 92107 (SAN 658-7275) Tel 619-224-8286.

L C Cantrell, *(Cantrell, Lana Corrine; 0-9620749),* 8215 Belden Blvd., Cottage Grove, MN 55016 (SAN 249-6720) Tel 612-459-1142.

L C Ellsworth, *(Ellsworth, Lorna Cecelia; 0-9618870),* 13701 Kismet Ave., Sylmar, CA 91342-1765 (SAN 242-5513).

L C Gitzen, *(Gitzen, Louise C.; 0-9632708),* 161 Forest Ln., Menlo Park, CA 94025 Tel 415-328-3379.

L Canyon Bks, *(Laurel Canyon Bks.; 0-9648850),* 53 Ninth Ave., Sea Cliff, NY 11579-1117.

L Daro Prodns, *(Daro, Lorren Productions; 0-9706608),* P.O. Box 9, Cobb, CA 95426-0009 Fax: 707-928-5529
E-mail: lorrendaro@earthlink.net
Web site: http://bigdictionary.com
Dist(s): **BookWorld** *(BookWorld Services, Inc.).*

L Davis Pr, *(Davis, L. Pr., Inc.; 0-933485; 0-9607902),* 1125 Oxford Pl., Schenectady, NY 12308 (SAN 238-1540) Tel 518-374-5636; Fax: 518-346-5781.

L E Stevens, *See* **White Bush Pub**

†L Erlbaum Assocs, *(Erlbaum, Lawrence Assocs., Inc.; 0-8058; 0-86377; 0-89859),* 10 Industrial Ave., Mahwah, NJ 07430-2262 (SAN 213-960X) Tel 201-236-9500; Fax: 201-236-0072; Toll Free: 800-926-6579 (orders only)
E-mail: orders@erlbaum.com
Web site: http://www.erlbaum.com; *CIP.*

L Greenfield, *(Greenfield, Louise; 0-9617947),* 19970 Lathers Ave., Livonia, MI 48152 (SAN 666-6353) Tel 248-474-1955.

L M Becker, *See* **Caliana Pub**

†L P Pubns, *(LP Pubns.; 0-916192; 1-931619),* Div. of Teleos Institute, 7119 E. Shea Blvd., Suite 109, PMB 418, Scottsdale, AZ 85254-6107 (SAN 207-2513) Tel 480-948-1800; Fax: 480-948-1870
E-mail: teleosinst@aol.com
Web site: http://www.consciousnesswork.com; *CIP.*

L Pietro, *(Pietro, Laura; 0-9704186),* Orders Addr.: P.O. Box 471, Breckenridge, CO 80424 Tel 719-836-2676; Fax: 970-453-3219; Toll Free: 800-789-7669 (ext. 7235); Edit Addr.: 232 Ute Trail, Alma, CO 80420
E-mail: lp-petey@hotmail.com.

L R Frank, *(Frank, Leonard Roy; 0-9601376),* 2300 Webster St., No. 603, San Francisco, CA 94115 (SAN 212-0917) Tel 415-922-3029
E-mail: lfrank@igc.org.

†L Rienner, *(Rienner, Lynne Pubs., Inc.; 0-89410; 0-931477; 1-55587; 1-58826),* 1800 30th St., Suite 314, Boulder, CO 80301-1026 (SAN 683-1869) Tel 303-444-6684; Fax: 303-444-0824
E-mail: sglover@rienner.com; cservice@rienner.com
Web site: http://www.rienner.com; *CIP.*

L Smith Ent, *(Smith, Lynn Enterprises; 0-9633706),* 6717 Donerail Trail, Tallahassee, FL 32308-1601 Tel 904-668-4342.

L Y A N Pub, *(LYAN Publishing; 0-9655414),* Orders Addr.: 2232 S. Nellis Blvd., Box 194, Las Vegas, NV 89104 Tel 702-641-6692; Edit Addr.: 1282 N. Ringe, Las Vegas, NV 89110.

La Jolla Cancer Res, *(La Jolla Cancer Research Foundation; 0-9647206),* 10901 N. Torrey Pines Rd., La Jolla, CA 92037 Tel 619-455-6480; Fax: 619-646-3199.

†La Leche, *(La Leche League International; 0-912500),* P.O. Box 4079, Schaumburg, IL 60168-4079 (SAN 201-0585) Tel 847-519-7730; Fax: 847-519-0035; Toll Free: 800-525-3243
E-mail: llli@llli.org
Web site: http://www.lalecheleague.org; *CIP.*

La Maison Du Dict (FRA) *(2-85608) Dist. by* **IBD Ltd.**

†La State U Pr, *(Louisiana State Univ. Pr.; 0-8071),* P.O. Box 25053, Baton Rouge, LA 70894-5053 (SAN 202-6597) Tel 225-388-6295; Fax: 225-388-6461; Toll Free Fax: 800-305-4416 (orders); Toll Free: 800-861-3477 (orders)
E-mail: lsuprss@lsu.edu
Web site: http://lsupress.lsu.edu; *CIP.*

La Vida Bks, *(La Vida Bks. & Software; 0-9664575),* 7046 Broadway, No. 315, Lemon Grove, CA 91945 Tel 619-266-1283
E-mail: jclogan@pacbell.net.

Labelmaster, *(Labelmaster; 0-940394),* Div. of American Labelmark Co., Inc., 5724 N. Pulaski Rd., Chicago, IL 60646 (SAN 665-7192) Tel 773-478-0900; Fax: 773-478-6054; Toll Free: 800-621-5805
E-mail: sales@labelmaster.com
Web site: http://www.labelmaster.com.

Labor Dept Imprint of USGPO

LabPro Pr, *(LabPro Pr.; 0-9629216),* Orders Addr.: P.O. Box 156, Thousand Palms, CA 92276 Tel 760-343-0170; Edit Addr.: 30-300 Via Las Palmas, Thousand Palms, CA 92276.

Labrys Pr, *(Labrys Pr.; 1-891145),* Div. of Matrix Midwifery Enterprises, Ltd., 7528 NE Oregon St., Portland, OR 97213 Tel 503-255-3378; Fax: 503-255-1474
E-mail: info@midwiferybooks.com
Web site: http://wwwmidwiferybooks.com.

LABS, *(Laboratory for Applied Behavioral Science; 0-943300),* 41 Gifford Rd., Somerset, NJ 08873 (SAN 239-4499) Tel 201-545-8269.

Lactation Assocs Pub, *(Lactation Assocs. Publishing Co.; 0-9623529),* P.O. Box 773, Franklin, VA 23851 Fax: 757-569-1447; Toll Free: 800-397-5833
E-mail: lapco@gc.net.

Ladd Foundation, *See* **Davila Assocs**

Lady Bug, *(Lady Bug Pr.; 0-9630730),* 6622 SE 108th, Portland, OR 97266 Tel 503-760-5750.

Laennec Pub, *(Laennec Publishing, Inc.; 1-886128),* 253 Passaic Ave., Fairfield, NJ 07004 Tel 973-239-4300; Toll Free: 800-528-0797
Dist(s): **Canfield Pubng** *(Canfield Publishing).*

Laerdal Med Corp, *(Laerdal Medical Corp.; 0-9665371),* 167 Myers Corners Rd., Wappingers Falls, NY 12590 Tel 914-297-7770; Fax: 914-298-4545; Toll Free Fax: 800-227-1143; Toll Free: 888-562-4242
E-mail: cdespo@compuserve.com.

LAF Pub, *(L.A.F. Publishing; 0-9645587),* 31839 N. 66th St., Cave Creek, AZ 85331-5791 Tel 602-488-0612; Fax: 602-488-6197
E-mail: lafpub@aol.com.

Lafayette NH, *(Lafayette Publishing; 0-9648173),* Div. of Fowler Chiropractic Office, Inc., 549 Lafayette Rd., Seabrook, NH 03874 Tel 603-474-2525; Fax: 508-388-7172; c/o H. N. Fowler, Sr., 30 Merrill St., Amesbury, MA 01913 Do not confuse with Lafayette Publishing Co., Galveston, TX.

Lagumo Corp, *(Lagumo Corp.; 1-878117),* c/o Glenda Eoyang, 50 E. Golden Lake Rd., Circle Pines, MN 55014.

Laing Res Servs, *(Laing Research Services; 0-938106),* Div. of Laing Communications, Inc., 16250 NE 80th St., Redmond, WA 98052-3821 (SAN 240-0901) Tel 206-869-6313.

Lake Hill Pr, *(Lake Hill Pr.; 0-9634819),* 920 Summit Ave., Saint Louis, MO 63119 Tel 314-962-8529; Fax: 314-962-8281
E-mail: rickstoff@compuserve.com.

Lakeshore Counsel, *(Lakeshore Counseling Services; 0-922639),* 15281 Lake Michigan Dr., West Olive, MI 49460 (SAN 251-3641) Tel 616-846-3502.

Lakeside Pr, *(Lakeside Pr.; 1-879653),* 5124 Mayfield Rd., No. 191, Lyndhurst, OH 44124 Tel 216-464-2005; Fax: 216-442-3565 Do not confuse with companies with the same name in Anacortes, WA, Tamarac, FL.

Lambda Pubs, *(Lambda Pubs., Inc.; 0-915361; 1-55774),* 3709 13th Ave., Brooklyn, NY 11218-3622 (SAN 291-0640) Tel 718-972-5449; Fax: 718-972-6307
E-mail: judaica@email.msn.com.

LaMont Pubng, *(LaMont Publishing; 0-9712175),* P.O. Box 125 A, Redding, KS 66868 Tel 620-699-3378
E-mail: suemarie@osprey.net.

Lamp Light Pr Imprint of Prosperity & Profits

Lampus Pr, *(Lampus Pr.; 0-9609002),* 19611 Antioch Rd., White City, OR 97503 (SAN 240-8643) Tel 541-826-7418
E-mail: lampus@wizzards.net
Dist(s): **New Leaf Dist** *(New Leaf Distributing Co., Inc.).*

Lanahan Pubs, *(Lanahan Pubs., Inc.; 0-9652687; 1-930398),* 324 Hawthorne Rd., Baltimore, MD 21210-2303 Tel 410-366-2434; Fax: 410-366-8798; Toll Free Fax: 888-345-7257; Toll Free: 866-345-1949
E-mail: lanahan@aol.com.

Land Pub FL, *(Land Publishing Corp.; 0-9618098),* Orders Addr.: P.O. Box 26983, Fort Lauderdale, FL 33320 (SAN 666-3532); Edit Addr.: 7875 NW 57th St., Tamarac, FL 33320 (SAN 666-3540) Do not confuse with Land Publishing, Los Alamos, NM.

Landauer, *(Landauer, Inc.; 0-9639768),* 2 Science Rd., Glenwood, IL 60425 Tel 708-755-7000; Fax: 708-755-7016.

Landes Bioscience, *(Landes Bioscience; 0-941432; 1-57059; 1-879702),* 810 S. Church St., Georgetown, TX 78626 Tel 512-863-7762; Fax: 512-863-0081; Toll Free: 800-736-9948
E-mail: orders@landesbioscience.com
Web site: http://www.landesbioscience.com
Dist(s): **J Majors Co** *(Majors, J. A. Co.)*
Matthews Medical Bk Co *(Matthews Medical Bk. Co.)*
Rittenhouse *(Rittenhouse Bk. Distributors).*

Landing Pr, *(Landing Pr., The; 0-943912),* 17 Sherwood Way, Landing, NJ 07850 (SAN 241-1296) Tel 973-398-7027.

Landover Pub, *(Landover Publishing; 0-9626604),* P.O. Box 53295, Lubbock, TX 79453 Tel 806-793-2406.

Lang E N T Pub, *(Lang E.N.T. Publishing; 0-943023),* Orders Addr.: P.O. Box 6846, Jefferson City, MO 65109 (SAN 667-9900) Tel 573-893-5545; Edit Addr.: 2110 Julie Ln., Jefferson City, MO 65109 (SAN 667-9919).

Lange Prodns, *(Lange Productions; 0-9663610),* 7661 Curson Terr., Los Angeles, CA 90046 Tel 213-874-4730; Fax: 213-874-3318; Toll Free: 888-526-4388
E-mail: langevideo@aol.com
Web site: http://www.langeproductions.com
Dist(s): **Jones & Bartlett** *(Jones & Bartlett Pubs., Inc.).*

Langer Found BSMR, *(Langer Foundation for Biomechanics & Sports Medicine Research; 0-9620848),* 450 Commack Rd., Deer Park, NY 11729 (SAN 250-278X) Tel 516-667-1200; Toll Free: 800-233-2687.

Lantern Books, *(Lantern Bks.; 1-930051; 1-59056),* Div. of Booklight, Inc., One Union Sq., W., Suite 201, New York, NY 10003-3303 Tel 212-414-2275; Fax: 212-414-2412
E-mail: info@booklightinc.com
Web site: http://www.booklightinc.com.

Lao Tse Pr, *(Lao Tse Pr., Ltd.; 1-887078),* 1020 SW Broadway Dr., Portland, OR 97201 Tel 503-222-3395; Fax: 503-222-3782
E-mail: kjobe@igc.org; laotse@e-z.net
Web site: http://www.laotse.com
Dist(s): **Words Distrib** *(Words Distributing Co.).*

Lar Pubg, *(Lar Publishing; 0-9669115),* 5501 N. 19th Ave., Suite 420, Phoenix, AZ 85022 Tel 602-249-1033 (ext. 106); Fax: 602-336-4650
E-mail: ortho@dancris.com
Dist(s): **J Majors Co** *(Majors, J. A. Co.).*

Larata Pr, *(Larata Pr., LLC; 0-9654985),* 238 Zipfeldburg Rd., Box 729, Rhinebeck, NY 12572 Tel 914-876-6330; Fax: 914-876-6650
E-mail: laratapress@aol.com
Web site: http://www.larata.com.

†Laredo, *(Laredo Publishing Co., Inc.; 1-56492),* 8907 Wilshire Blvd., No. 102, Beverly Hills, CA 90211 Tel 310-358-5288; Fax: 310-358-5282; Toll Free: 800-547-5113
E-mail: info@laredopublishing.com
Web site: http://www.laredopublishing.com; *CIP.*

†Larksdale, *(Larksdale; 0-89896),* P.O. Box 801222, Houston, TX 77280 (SAN 220-0643) Tel 713-461-7200; Fax: 713-467-4770 (purchase orders); Toll Free: 877-461-7200; *CIP.*

Larson Pubns, *(Larson Pubns.; 0-943914),* 4936 Rte. 414, Burdett, NY 14818 (SAN 241-130X) Tel 607-546-9342; Fax: 607-546-9344; Toll Free: 800-828-2197 Do not confuse with Larson Pubns., Joliet, IL
E-mail: larson@lightlink.com
Web site: http://www.larsonpublications.org
Dist(s): **Baker & Taylor** *(Baker & Taylor Bks.)*
Bookpeople *(Bookpeople)*
Natl Bk Netwk *(National Bk. Network)*
New Leaf Dist *(New Leaf Distributing Co., Inc.)*
Red Wheel ME *(Red Wheel).*

Lasenda, *(Lasenda Pubs.; 0-918916),* 1590 Via Chaparral, Fallbrook, CA 92028 (SAN 210-4504) Tel 760-723-1407.

Laser Inst, *(Laser Institute of America; 0-912035),* P.O. Box 781029, Orlando, FL 32878-1029 (SAN 225-2007) Tel 407-380-1553; Fax: 407-380-5588; Toll Free: 800-345-2737
E-mail: lia@laserinstitute.org
Web site: http://www.laserinstitute.org.

Last Gasp, *(Last Gasp Eco-Funnies, Inc.; 0-86719),* Orders Addr.: P.O. Box 410067, San Francisco, CA 94141-0067 (SAN 216-8308); Edit Addr.: 777 Florida St., San Francisco, CA 94110-2025 (SAN 170-3242) Tel 415-824-6636; Fax: 415-824-1836; Toll Free: 800-366-5121
E-mail: lastgasp@hooked.net
Dist(s): **Bookpeople** *(Bookpeople)*
Publishers Group *(Publishers Group West)*
SPD-Small Pr Dist *(SPD-Small Pr. Distribution).*

Latin Assoc, *See* **Hillgarth Pr**

Latitude Twenty Imprint of UH Pr

Laugh Cat, *(Laughing Cat, The; 0-937226),* RFD 1, Box 540A, Franklin, ME 04634 (SAN 219-998X)
E-mail: editor@zoofence.com
Web site: http://www.zoofence.com.

Launch Pr, *(Launch Pr.; 0-9613205; 1-877872),* P.O. Box 3050, Fairfax, VA 20855 (SAN 295-0154) Toll Free: 800-251-8336
Dist(s): **Self esteem shop** *(Self esteem shop II).*

Laurel Glen Pub Imprint of Advantage Pubs

Laurel Hse NJ, *(Laurel Hse. Publishing Co., Inc.; 0-9621697),* 135 Gaither Dr., Suite E, Mount Laurel, NJ 08054 (SAN 251-8155) Tel 609-273-8478.

LaVonne Pr, *(LaVonne Pr.; 1-878743),* 5481 S. Cornell, Suite B, Chicago, IL 60615 Tel 312-288-3708.

Law & Econ U Miami, *(Univ. of Miami, Law & Economics Ctr.; 0-916770),* P.O. Box 248000, Coral Gables, FL 33124 (SAN 208-9017) Tel 305-284-6174.

Law & Psych, *(Law & Psychology Pr.; 0-9603630; 1-879689),* Orders Addr.: P.O. Box 24219, Los Angeles, CA 90024 (SAN 281-871X) Tel 310-475-2108; Fax: 310-474-5938; Edit Addr.: 1830 Westholme Ave., Suite 301, Los Angeles, CA 90025
Web site: http://www.lawpsychpress.com.

Law Journal Pr Imprint of Amer Lawyer Media

Lawbk Exchange, *(Lawbook Exchange, Ltd., The; 0-9630106; 1-886363; 1-58477),* 965 Jefferson Ave., Union, NJ 07083-8605 Tel 908-686-1998; Fax: 908-686-3098; Toll Free: 800-422-6686
E-mail: law@lawbookexchange.com
Web site: http://www.lawbookexchange.com
Dist(s): **Baker & Taylor** *(Baker & Taylor Bks.).*

LawPak, *(LawPak, Inc.; 1-879421),* P.O. Box 221, Terrace Park, OH 45174-1045 (SAN 174-0784) Tel 513-831-3900; Fax: 513-831-1620; Toll Free: 800-552-9725
Web site: http://www.elawpak.com
Dist(s): **Baker & Taylor** *(Baker & Taylor Bks.).*

Lawrence & Wishart (GBR) *(0-85315) Dist. by* **NYU Pr.**

Lawton-Teague, *(Lawton-Teague Pubns.; 0-932516),* P.O. Box 12353, Oakland, CA 94604 (SAN 211-2485)
Dist(s): **Bookpeople** *(Bookpeople).*

†**Lawyers & Judges,** *(Lawyers & Judges Publishing Co., Inc.; 0-913875; 1-930056),* Orders Addr.: P.O. Box 30040, Tucson, AZ 85751-0040 (SAN 202-2354) Tel 520-323-1500; Fax: 520-323-0055; Toll Free Fax: 800-330-8795; Toll Free: 800-209-7109; Edit Addr.: 917 N. Swan Rd., Suite 300, Tucson, AZ 85711
E-mail: sales@lawyersandjudges.com
Web site: http://www.lawyersandjudges.com*; CIP.*

LBJ Sch Pub Aff, *(Johnson, Lyndon B. Schl. of Public Affairs; 0-89940),* c/o University of Texas at Austin, P.O. Box Y, Austin, TX 78713-8925 (SAN 223-0410) Tel 512-471-4218; Fax: 512-475-8867
E-mail: pubsinfo@uts-cc.utexas.edu
Web site: http://www.utexas.edu/lbj/pubs/.

LDF Pubns, *(LDF Pubns.; 0-9633923),* 11114 Lawson Ln., Culpeper, VA 22701 Tel 540-825-0339; Fax: 540-829-6527; Toll Free: 800-258-6992.

Ldrship Intl, *(Leadership International Library; 0-9665347),* 306 N. Mulberry St., Suite 3, Richmond, VA 23220-4026 Tel 804-355-6932; Fax: 804-358-4737
E-mail: Mrrollings@worldnet.alt.nej.

LE Imprint of Dell

Le Jacq Commns, *(Le Jacq Communications, Inc.; 0-9626020; 1-929660),* 777 W. Putnam Ave., Greenwich, CT 06830 Tel 203-531-0450; Fax: 203-531-0533
E-mail: atownsend@lejacq.com.

Le Lettere (ITA) *(88-7166) Dist. by* **IBD Ltd.**

Leader OH, *(Leader Co., Inc., The; 1-886898),* 931 N. Main St., Suite 101, North Canton, OH 44720 Tel 330-494-6988; Fax: 330-494-6989; Toll Free: 800-899-6117
Dist(s): **BookWorld** *(BookWorld Services, Inc.).*

League Women Voters TX, *(League of Woman Voters of Texas, & League of Women Voters of Texas Education Fund; 0-915757),* 1212 Guadalupe, No. 107, Austin, TX 78701 (SAN 294-121X) Tel 512-472-1100.

Learn Made, *(Learning Made Easy; 0-9659975),* Orders Addr.: P.O. Box 249, Ashland, AL 36251 Tel 205-354-4477; Fax: 205-354-3360; Toll Free: 800-243-2474; Edit Addr.: 7031 County Rd. 18, Talladega, AL 35160.

Learn Pubns, *(Learn Pubns., Inc.; 0-9643582),* P.O. Box 6703, McLean, VA 22106 Fax: 703-538-6689; Toll Free: 800-762-0991.

Learned Info, *See* **Info Today Inc**

Learning Inc, *(Learning, Inc.; 0-913692),* Learning Pl., 353 Seawall Rd., Manset, ME 04679 (SAN 201-5714) Tel 207-244-5015
Dist(s): **Door Hse** *(Door Hse.).*

Learning Proc Ctr, *(Learning Process Ctr.; 0-931657),* 222 W. 24th St., National City, CA 92050 (SAN 683-5589) Tel 619-477-1200; Toll Free: 800-221-7374.

Learning Pubns, *(Learning Pubns., Inc.; 0-918452; 1-55691),* Orders Addr.: P.O. Box 1338, Holmes Beach, FL 34218-1338 (SAN 688-3990) Toll Free: 800-222-1525; Edit Addr.: 5351 Gulf Dr., Holmes Beach, FL 34217 (SAN 208-1695) Tel 941-778-6651; Fax: 941-778-6818
E-mail: info@learningpublications.com
Web site: http://www.learningpublications.com.

Leathers Pub, *(Leathers Publishing; 0-9646898; 1-890622; 1-58597),* Div. of Ad Ctr., 4500 College Blvd., Overland Park, KS 66211-1760 Tel 913-498-2625; Fax: 913-498-1561; Toll Free: 888-888-7696
E-mail: leatherpub@aol.com
Web site: http://www.leatherspublishing.com.

Leaves of Healing, *(Leaves of Healing; 0-9602850),* P.O. Box 126, Joshua Tree, CA 92252 (SAN 222-2078)
E-mail: chops@leavesofhealing.com
Web site: http://www.leavesofhealing.com
Dist(s): **Baker & Taylor** *(Baker & Taylor Bks.)*
Bookpeople *(Bookpeople)*
New Leaf Dist *(New Leaf Distributing Co., Inc.)*
Unique Bks Inc *(Unique Bks., Inc.).*

Ledero Pr, *(Ledero Pr.; 0-9627775),* U.T. Box 35099, Galveston, TX 77555-5099 Tel 409-772-2091; Fax: 409-772-5144.

Lee Pub AZ, *(Lee Publishing; 0-9627703),* Orders Addr.: P.O. Box 5444, Scottsdale, AZ 85261 Tel 480-483-6953; Edit Addr.: 7246 E. Loma Ln., Scottsdale, AZ 85258 Do not confuse with companies with the same or similar names in Ridgecrest, CA, Burbank, CA, Nashua, NH, Richmond, VA, Sunnyvale, CA.

Leela Pr, *(Leela Pr., Inc.; 0-9629835; 1-887906),* 4026 River Rd., Faber, VA 22938 Tel 804-361-1130; Fax: 804-361-9199
E-mail: jscher@leelapress.com
Dist(s): **Baker & Taylor** *(Baker & Taylor Bks.)*
Bookpeople *(Bookpeople)*
New Leaf Dist *(New Leaf Distributing Co., Inc.)*
Red Wheel ME *(Red Wheel)*
Sathya Sai Bk Ctr *(Sathya Sai Bk. Ctr. of America).*

Lees-Haley Psych, *(Lees-Haley Psychological Corp.; 0-9668410),* 21331 Costanso St., Woodland Hills, CA 91364 Tel 818-887-2874; Fax: 818-887-9034
E-mail: plh@ix.netcom.com.

Leetes Isl, *(Leete's Island Bks.; 0-918172),* P.O. Box 3131, Branford, CT 06405-1731 (SAN 210-2285)
E-mail: Pneill@compuserve.com
Web site: http://www.leetesisland.com
Dist(s): **IPG Chicago** *(Independent Pubs. Group).*

Left Front Imprint of Dr Pai Pubns

Left Front Shirt, *See* **Dr Pai Pubns**

Lega Bks, *(Lega Bks.),* Div. of Charing Cross Publishing Co., 3699 Wilshire Blvd., Suite 700, Los Angeles, CA 90010-2726 (SAN 212-5218) Tel 213-382-3335.

Legacy OH Imprint of Temple Pubg

Legal Coun Elderly, *(Legal Counsel for the Elderly; 0-933945),* Div. of American Assn. of Retired People, Orders Addr.: P.O. Box 96474, Washington, DC 20090-6474 (SAN 669-408X) Tel 202-434-2197; Fax: 202-434-6466; Edit Addr.: 601 E St., NW, Washington, DC 20049 (SAN 657-4963)
E-mail: aalbright@aarp.org
Web site: http://www.aarp.org/ntltrpro/trproject.html.

Legendary Pub, *(Legendary Publishing Co.; 0-9625040; 1-887747),* Orders Addr.: P.O. Box 7706, Boise, ID 83707-1706 (SAN 297-231X) Tel 208-376-9814 (phone/fax); Toll Free: 877-909-1016 (orders only)
E-mail: dproctor@rmci.net
Web site: http://www.legendarypublishing.com
Dist(s): **New Leaf Dist** *(New Leaf Distributing Co., Inc.)*
Partners Pubs Grp *(Partners Pubs. Group, Inc.)*
Partners-West *(Partners/West)*
Sunbelt Pubns *(Sunbelt Pubns., Inc.)*
Unique Bks Inc *(Unique Bks., Inc.).*

Legion Survival, *(Legion for the Survival of Freedom, Inc.; 0-939484),* P.O. Box 2719, Newport Beach, CA 92659 (SAN 220-1275) Tel 949-631-1490; Fax: 949-631-0981 ; *Imprints:* Noontide Pr (Noontide Press)
E-mail: orders@noontidepress.com; ihr@ihr.org
Web site: http://www.ihr.org; http://www.noontidepress.com.

Legis, *(Legis Pr.; 0-9670004),* 3646 E. Ray Rd., Suite B16-52, Phoenix, AZ 85044 Fax: 480-496-9983; Toll Free: 877-485-0345
E-mail: PG980C@aol.com.

Legovac, *(Legovac, Inc.; 1-878135),* Orders Addr.: P.O. Box 150784, Altamonte Springs, FL 32715-0784 Tel 407-830-1380; Fax: 407-332-1210; Edit Addr.: 625 Mariner Way, Altamonte Springs, FL 32701.

Lehigh Univ Pr, *(Lehigh Univ. Pr.; 0-934223),* c/o Associated University Presses, 440 Forsgate Dr., Cranbury, NJ 08512 (SAN 281-2959) Tel 609-655-4770; Fax: 609-655-8366
E-mail: inlup@lehigh.edu.

Lemar Pubs, *(Lemar Pubs.; 0-9639269),* 110 E. Savannah Ave., Suite B-103, McAllen, TX 78503-1240 Tel 210-687-4878; Toll Free: 800-483-3223
Web site: http://www.lemarpublishers.com.

Lenox Pub Co, *(Lenox Publishing Co.; 0-9657783),* Orders Addr.: P.O. Box 134, Lenox, MA 01240-0134 Tel 413-637-4826; Fax: 413-637-3397; Toll Free: 888-261-9641; Edit Addr.: 73 Main St., Lenox, MA 01240 Toll Free: 888-261-9648 Do not confuse with Lenox Publishing Co., Atlanta, GA
Web site: http://www.lenoxpublishing.com.

Leo Cooper (GBR) *(0-85052) Dist. by* **Trans-Atl Phila.**

†**LEpervier Pr,** *(L'Epervier Pr.; 0-934332),* 1326 62nd NE, Seattle, WA 98115 (SAN 281-8779)
Dist(s): **SPD-Small Pr Dist** *(SPD-Small Pr. Distribution); CIP.*

LEPS Pr, *See* **Ed Studies Pr**

Lester St Pub, *(Lester Street Publishing; 0-9634440),* Orders Addr.: P.O. Box 41484, Tucson, AZ 85717-1484 Tel 520-326-0104; Toll Free: 800-370-0104; Edit Addr.: 2920 N. Forgeus Ave., Tucson, AZ 85716
E-mail: 74462.2350@compuserve.com.

Leuven Univ (BEL) *(90-6186; 90-5867) Dist. by* **Coronet Bks.**

Levin Family, *(Levin Family Publishing; 0-9642777),* R.D. 4, Box 808, Green River Rd., Brattleboro, VT 05301 Tel 802-257-1482; Fax: 802-254-4670.

Levy Econ Inst Bard Imprint of Bard Coll Pubns

Lewis Pub CA, *(Lewis Publishing; 0-9664069),* 352 1/2 N. Gardner St., Los Angeles, CA 90036 Tel 213-936-6699 ; *Imprints:* Symbols Power (Symbols of Power) Do not confuse with Lewis Publishing, El Cajon, CA.

†**Lewis Pubs,** *(Lewis Pubs.; 0-87371; 1-56670),* Subs. of CRC Pr., Inc., Orders Addr.: 2000 Corporate Blvd., NW, Boca Raton, FL 33431 (SAN 202-1994) Fax: 561-998-9114; Toll Free Fax: 800-374-3401; Toll Free: 800-272-7737
E-mail: orders@crcpress.com; enquiries@crcpress.com
Web site: http://www.crcpress.com
Dist(s): **Battelle** *(Battelle Pr.)*
CRC Pr *(CRC Pr. LLC)*
NSF Intl *(N S F International); CIP.*

†**Lewis-Sloan,** *(Lewis-Sloan Publishing Co.; 0-915114),* 207 E. Richardson Ave., Summerville, SC 29483-6334 (SAN 201-0852)*; CIP.*

Lexi-Comp, *(Lexi-Comp, Inc.; 0-916589; 1-930598),* 1100 Terex Rd., Hudson, OH 44236 (SAN 296-4473) Tel 330-650-6506; Fax: 330-656-4307; Toll Free: 800-837-5394
E-mail: brad@lexi.com
Web site: http://www.lexi.com
Dist(s): **J Majors Co** *(Majors, J. A. Co.)*
Matthews Medical Bk Co *(Matthews Medical Bk. Co.)*
Rittenhouse *(Rittenhouse Bk. Distributors).*

LEXIS Law Pub, *See* **LEXIS Pub**

Publisher Symbol Index

LEXIS Pub, *(LEXIS Publishing; 0-327; 0-406; 0-409; 0-672; 0-87215; 0-87473; 0-88063; 0-930273; 1-55834; 1-56257),* Div. of Reed Elsevier, Orders Addr.: P.O. Box 7587, Charlottesville, VA 22906-7587 Tel 804-972-7600; Fax: 804-972-7686; Toll Free Fax: 800-643-1280; Toll Free: 800-446-3410; Edit Addr.: 701 E. Water St., Charlottesville, VA 22902 ; *Imprints:* MICHIE (MICHIE) Do not confuse with Lexis Publishing, Malabar, FL
E-mail: Custserv@Michie.com
Web site: http://www.lexislawpublishing.com.

Leyland Pubns, *(Leyland Pubns.; 0-943595),* P.O. Box 410690, San Francisco, CA 94141 (SAN 668-663X) Tel 415-626-1935; Fax: 415-626-1802
Web site: http://www.leylandpublications.com
Dist(s): **Bookazine Co Inc** *(Bookazine Co., Inc.)*
Bookpeople *(Bookpeople)*
Koen Bk Distributors *(Koen Bk. Distributors).*

LF Pub VA, *(LF Publishing; 1-877631),* P.O. Box 6812, San Jose, CA 95150 Tel 408-429-5987; 831-688-3920; Fax: 408-429-5993
Dist(s): **Baker & Taylor** *(Baker & Taylor Bks.).*

LFDV Inc, *(Lupus Foundation of Delaware Valley, Inc.; 0-9659530),* P.O. Box 740, Gladwyne, PA 19035-0740.

LGR Prod, *See* **LGR Pubg Inc**

LGR Pubg Inc, *(LGR Publishing, Inc.; 0-9657610),* 3219 NW C St., Richmond, IN 47374 Tel 765-939-8924 (phone/fax)
E-mail: mcphd@infocom.com; jwilde@indiana.edu
Dist(s): **Baker & Taylor** *(Baker & Taylor Bks.).*

LHC Pubs, *(LHC Pubs.; 0-9636998),* Orders Addr.: P.O. Box 4343, Logan, UT 84323-4343 Tel 435-752-3160; Edit Addr.: 45 S. 1300 E., Logan, UT 84321.

LIAAC, *(Long Island Assn. for AIDS Care, Inc. (LIAAC); 1-881305),* Orders Addr.: P.O. Box 2859, Huntington Station, NY 11746 Tel 516-385-2451; Fax: 516-423-2788; Edit Addr.: 755 Park Ave., Huntington, NY 11743.

Liahona Pub Trust, *(Liahona Publishing Trust; 0-89036),* 869 E. 4500 S., Salt Lake City, UT 84107-3049 (SAN 205-6232) Tel 801-262-5555; Fax: 801-263-3233.

Liaison Coun, *(Liaison Council on Certification for the Surgical Technologist; 0-9622332),* Div. of Association of Surgical Technologists, 7790 E. Arapahoe Rd., Suite 240, Englewood, CO 80112-1274 Tel 303-694-9130; Fax: 303-694-9169; Toll Free: 800-637-7433.

Lib Art Soc Sci, *See* **Lib Soc Sci**

Lib Co Phila, *(Library Co. of Philadelphia; 0-914076),* 1314 Locust St., Philadelphia, PA 19107 (SAN 201-4955) Tel 215-546-3181; Fax: 215-546-5167
E-mail: nscalessa@librarycompany.org; refdept@librarycompany.org
Web site: http://www.librarycompany.org.

†Lib Congress, *(Library of Congress; 0-8444),* Div. of U.S. Government, Orders Addr.: P.O. Box 371954, Pittsburgh, PA 15250-7954 Tel 202-512-1800; Fax: 202-512-2250; Edit Addr.: c/o Cataloging Distribution Serv., Customer Serv. Section 101 Independence Ave., SE, Washington, DC 20541-4912 (SAN 205-6593) Tel 202-707-5093; 202-707-0204 Sales Shop, Library of Congress
E-mail: wwwadmin@gpo.gov
Web site: http://www.access.gpo.gov; http://www.loc.gov/loc/pub/celebrate
Dist(s): **Bernan Associates** *(Bernan Assocs.)*
Johns Hopkins *(Johns Hopkins Univ. Pr.)*
Oak Knoll *(Oak Knoll Pr.)*
U Pr of New Eng *(University Pr. of New England)*
USGPO *(U.S. Government Printing Office); CIP.*

†Lib Res, *(Library Research Assocs., Inc.; 0-89824; 0-912526),* 474 Dunderberg Rd., Monroe, NY 10950-3703 (SAN 201-0887) Tel 845-783-1144; Fax: 845-782-3953; Toll Free: 800-914-3379; *CIP.*

Lib Soc Sci, *(Library of Social Science; 0-915042),* 92-30 56th Ave., No. 3E, Elmurst, NY 11373-4604 (SAN 207-589X) Tel 718-393-1075; Fax: 718-393-1068.

Liberty Pub, *(Liberty Publishing Co., Inc.; 0-89709),* P.O. Box 4248, Deerfield Beach, FL 33442-4248 (SAN 211-030X) Tel 954-360-9000 Do not confuse with companies with the same name in Port Townsend, WA, San Francisco, CA
E-mail: jblittle@bellsouth.net
Web site: http://www.bullsorbears.com/; http://www.horseracingusa.com.

LibertyTree Pr, *See* **Independent Inst**

Libra, *(Libra Pubs., Inc.; 0-87212),* 3089C Clairemont Dr., PMB 383, San Diego, CA 92117 (SAN 201-0909) Tel 858-571-1414 (phone & fax).

Libra & Gemini, *(Libra & Gemini Pubns., Inc.; 0-9630670),* 10703 Paulwood, Houston, TX 77071 Tel 281-981-6321; Fax: 281-790-5053.

Libra Press Chi, *See* **HCI Pr**

Library of America, *(Library of America, The; 0-940450; 1-883011; 1-931082),* Div. of Literary Classics of the U. S., Inc., 14 E. 60th St., New York, NY 10022 (SAN 286-9918) Tel 212-308-3360; Fax: 212-750-8352
E-mail: info@loa.org
Web site: http://www.loa.org
Dist(s): **Penguin Putnam** *(Penguin Putnam, Inc.).*

Library of Islam Imprint of Kazi Pubns

Library Research Assocs, *(Library Research Assocs.; 0-9670497),* 440 E. Calaveras Blvd., Milpitas, CA 95035-5412 Tel 408-258-5832; Fax: 408-946-0779.

Library Solns, *(Library Solutions Pr.; 1-882208),* 2137 Oregon St., Berkeley, CA 94705 Tel 916-939-2018; Fax: 916-939-9626
E-mail: sales@library-solutions.com
Web site: http://www.library-solutions.com.

Libreria Univ, *(Libreria Universal, Inc.; 1-881375),* 55 N. Post St., P.O. Box 1480, Mayaguez, PR 00680 Tel 787-832-6041; Fax: 787-832-8477
E-mail: colom@coqui.net.

Libros Imprint of S&S Trade Pap

Libros Fronteras, *(Libros Sin Fronteras),* P.O. Box 2085, Olympia, WA 98507 Tel 360-357-4332; Fax: 360-357-4964
E-mail: info@librossinfronteras.com
Web site: http://www.librossinfronteras.com.

†Libs Unl, *(Libraries Unlimited, Inc.; 0-87287; 1-56308; 1-59158),* 6931 S. Yosemite St., Englewood, CO 80112 (SAN 202-6767) Tel 303-770-1220; Fax: 303-220-8843; Toll Free: 800-237-6124
E-mail: lubooks@lu.com
Web site: http://www.lu.com
Dist(s): **Shens Bks** *(Shen's Bks.); CIP.*

Life Care, *(Life Care Concepts, Inc.; 1-893865),* 457 W. 22nd St., Suite B, New York, NY 10011 Tel 212-366-1016; Fax: 212-243-1063; Toll Free: 800-401-2233
E-mail: rshaker@cancerresources.com
Web site: http://www.cancerresources.com.

Life Cycle Bks, *(Life Cycle Bks.; 0-919225),* P.O. Box 792, Lewiston, NY 14092-0792 (SAN 692-7173).

Life Ext Media, *(Life Extension Media; 0-9658777),* 1881 NE 26th St., Suite 237, Fort Lauderdale, FL 33305 Tel 954-561-7909; Fax: 954-561-8335; Toll Free: 800-544-4440
E-mail: customerservice@lef.org; generalquestions@lef.org
Web site: http://www.lef.org.com
Dist(s): **BookWorld** *(BookWorld Services, Inc.).*

Life Ext Terres, *(LETS (Life Extension Terrestrial Shielding); 0-9665962),* 2130 W. Monte Vista Rd., Phoenix, AZ 85009 Tel 602-254-4404; Fax: 602-254-4369.

Life Goes On, *(Life Goes On Productions; 1-891409),* 720 Farmington Ave., West Hartford, CT 06119-1734 Tel 860-236-5555; Fax: 860-236-2299
E-mail: lifegoeson@kathleencairns.com
Web site: http://www.kathleencairns.com.

Life Office, *(Life Office Management Assn.; 0-915322; 0-939921; 1-57974),* 2300 Windy Ridge Pkwy., Suite 600, Atlanta, GA 30339-8443 (SAN 207-2548) Tel 770-951-1770; Fax: 770-984-0441
E-mail: education@loma.org
Web site: http://www.loma.org
Dist(s): **PBD Inc** *(PBD, Inc.).*

Life Res Found, *(Life Research Foundation, Inc.; 0-9618919),* P.O. Box 653, McMinnville, OR 97128 (SAN 242-7362) Tel 503-472-4748.

Life Shadows, *(Life Shadows Pubns.; 0-9654678),* 1623 Parkview Dr., Lockhart, TX 78644 Tel 512-376-9958.

Life Skills WI, *See* **JODA**

Life Style Prods, *(Life Style Productions; 0-9654001),* 97 Antigua Ct., Coronado, CA 92118 Tel 619-429-7422.

LifeCare Inc, *(LifeCare, Inc.; 1-58559),* Orders Addr.: P.O. Box 2783, Westport, CT 06880 Tel 203-291-3521; Fax: 203-291-3571; Toll Free: 800-873-4636; Edit Addr.: 400 Nyala Farm Rd., Westport, CT 06880
E-mail: akarl@lifecare.com
Web site: http://www.lifecare.com.

LifeCare.com, *See* **LifeCare Inc**

Lifecircle, *(Lifecircle Publishing; 0-935815),* Affil. of The Better Life Assn., PMB 113, 566 White Pond Dr., C, Akron, OH 44320-1116 (SAN 699-6388) Tel 330-865-9225 (phone/fax); Toll Free: 800-542-1923 (phone/fax)
E-mail: betrlife@juno.com.

Lifeknox Pub, *(Lifeknox Publishing; 0-9625908),* 7904 NE Sixth, Suite B293, Vancouver, WA 98665 Tel 360-693-9303
E-mail: lifeknox@aol.com
Web site: http://www.lifeknox.com.

Lifeline Inst, *(Lifelines Institute; 0-9666839),* 2222 Hyde St., Suite 1, San Francisco, CA 94109 Tel 415-929-8150; Fax: 415-563-1062; Toll Free: 888-664-3543
E-mail: compasskit@aol.com
Web site: http://www.lifelinesinst.com
Dist(s): **Bookpeople** *(Bookpeople).*

LifeLine Press Imprint of Regnery Pub

LifeMatters Bks Imprint of Capstone Pr

LifeRhythm, *(LifeRhythm; 0-940795),* Orders Addr.: P.O. Box 806, Mendocino, CA 95460 (SAN 664-886X) Tel 707-937-1825; Fax: 707-937-3052; Edit Addr.: 42271 Little Lake Rd., Mendocino, CA 95460 (SAN 664-8878)
E-mail: books@liferhythm.com
Web site: http://www.liferythm.com
Dist(s): **Baker & Taylor** *(Baker & Taylor Bks.)*
Bookpeople *(Bookpeople)*
New Leaf Dist *(New Leaf Distributing Co., Inc.)*
Red Wheel ME *(Red Wheel).*

Lifeservs Pr, *(Lifeservices Pr.; 0-9660988),* Orders Addr.: P.O. Box 4314, Boca Raton, FL 33429 Tel 561-392-1538; Toll Free: 888-445-8856; Edit Addr.: 8 Royal Palm Way, Boca Raton, FL 33432
E-mail: Tiffywiff2@aol.com
Dist(s): **New Leaf Dist** *(New Leaf Distributing Co., Inc.).*

Lifesounds, *(Lifesounds, Inc.; 0-9627583),* 7921 S. Valentia St., Englewood, CO 80112 Tel 303-530-2678.

LifeStar, *(LifeStar; 1-884180),* 2244 S. Olive St., Denver, CO 80224 Tel 303-753-9355; Fax: 303-753-9675; Toll Free Fax: 888-468-1536; Toll Free: 888-468-1535
E-mail: lifestar@rmi.net
Web site: http://quantum-I.com
Dist(s): **Metamorphous Pr** *(Metamorphous Pr., Inc.).*

Lifestyle Inst, *(Lifestyle Institute; 0-9622182),* Orders Addr.: P.O. Box 4735, Ruidoso, NM 88355; Edit Addr.: 1204 Mechem, No. 10, Ruidoso, NM 88345 Tel 505-258-3046; Fax: 505-258-1068
E-mail: drbartnett@drbartnett.com
Web site: http://www.drbartnett.com.

Lifestyles Four, *(Lifestyles 4-Heart Pr.; 1-878319),* Orders Addr.: P.O. Box 974, Lake Oswego, OR 97034 (SAN 253-5378) Tel 503-697-7572 (phone/fax); Toll Free: 800-863-6000; Edit Addr.: 616 Fourth St., Lake Oswego, OR 97034
Web site: http://www.rondagates.com.

LifeTime OR, *(LifeTime Publishing; 0-9627954),* 6914 SE 18th Ave., Portland, OR 97202-5723 Tel 503-232-5699 Do not confuse with Life Time Pub., Austin, TX.

LifeWays Pr, *(LifeWays Pr.; 0-9659224),* 443 Richmond Park, W., Apt. 532D, Cleveland, OH 44143-1821 Tel 216-646-9129; Toll Free: 800-646-5731 (ext. 4619).

Light & Life Comm, *(Light & Life Communications; 0-89367),* P.O. Box 535002, Indianapolis, IN 46253-5002 (SAN 206-8419) Tel 317-244-3660; Fax: 317-248-9055; Toll Free: 800-348-2513.

Light Tech Comns Servs, *See* **Light Tech Pubng**

Light Tech Pubng, *(Light Technology Publishing; 0-929385; 1-891824),* Orders Addr.: P.O. Box 3870, Flagstaff, AZ 86003 (SAN 249-1389) Tel 520-526-1345; Fax: 520-714-1132; Toll Free: 800-450-0985; Edit Addr.: 4030 E. Huntington Dr., Flagstaff, AZ 86004
E-mail: sedonajo@sedonajo.com
Web site: http://www.sedonajournal.com
Dist(s): **New Leaf Dist** *(New Leaf Distributing Co., Inc.).*

Lightening Bolt, *See* **Adi Gaia Esalen**

Lightening Up Pr, *(Lightening Up Pr.; 0-9620960),* P.O. Box 325, Woodstock, VT 05091-0325 (SAN 250-2054)
E-mail: ebragdon@aol.com
Dist(s): **Spiritual Emerg Netwk** *(Spiritual Emergence Network).*

Lighthouse, *(Lighthouse Publishing; 0-945272),* Orders Addr.: P.O. Box 40, Gladstone, OR 97027 (SAN 246-697X) Tel 503-557-2277; Fax: 503-557-2278; Edit Addr.: 1420 Windsor Dr., Gladstone, OR 97027 (SAN 246-6988) Do not confuse with companies with the same or similar name in Ashby, MN, Birmingham, MI, Cary, NC, Deer Lodge, TN,Malibu, CA, North Haven, CT, Sacramento, CA, Middletown, OH, Corona, CA, St. Mary's, OH
E-mail: lightpub@spiritone.com
Web site: http://www.aolighthouse.com
Dist(s): **Baker & Taylor** *(Baker & Taylor Bks.)*
Partners-West *(Partners/West).*

Lighthouse Inst, *(Lighthouse Institute; 0-938475),* 720 W. Chestnut St., Bloomington, IL 61701-2814 (SAN 661-3160) Tel 309-827-6026; Fax: 309-829-4661; Toll Free: 888-547-8271
E-mail: jthomas@chestnut.org
Web site: http://www.chestnut.org.

Lighthouse NYC, *(Lighthouse, Inc., The; 0-9603444; 1-888504),* 111 E. 59th St., New York, NY 10022 (SAN 221-7414) Tel 212-821-9200.

Lighthse MA, *(Lighthouse Pr.; 0-9621799),* P.O. Box 602, Marblehead, MA 01945 Fax: 978-745-1855; Toll Free: 800-225-9886 Do not confuse with companies with the same or similar names in York, ME, La Junta, CO, Rochester, NY, Deerfield Beach, FL, San Mateo, CA, Sanford, MI, Minneapolis, MN, Millersburg, OH, Nashville TN
E-mail: nsarles@mediaone.net.

Light&Life Pub Co MN, *(Light & Life Publishing Co.; 0-937032; 1-880971),* 4808 Park Glen Rd., Minneapolis, MN 55416 (SAN 213-8565) Tel 612-925-3888; Fax: 612-925-3918
E-mail: info@light-n-life.com
Web site: http://www.light-n-life.com.

LightLines, *(LightLines Publishing; 1-890405),* Orders Addr.: P.O. Box 5067, Portsmouth, NH 03802-5067 Toll Free: 800-828-3730; Edit Addr.: 72 Mirona Rd., Suite 10, Portsmouth, NH 03801-5366 Tel 603-433-5784; Fax: 603-766-5786 Do not confuse with Lightlines Publishing Co., Palm Desert, CA
E-mail: weboflight@aol.com
Web site: http://www.weboflight.com/publish.htm
Dist(s): **New Leaf Dist** *(New Leaf Distributing Co., Inc.).*

Lightning Powder, *(Lightning Powder Co., Inc.; 0-9622305),* 1230 Hoyt St., SE, Salem, OR 97302 Tel 503-585-9900; Fax: 503-588-0398; Toll Free: 800-852-0300
Web site: http://www.redwop.com.

Lightning Source Imprint of HEAVEN-ON-EARTH

Liguori Pubns, *(Liguori Pubns.; 0-7648; 0-89243),* 1 Liguori Dr., Liguori, MO 63057-9999 (SAN 202-6783) Tel 636-464-2500; Fax: 636-464-8449; Toll Free Fax: 800-325-9526; Toll Free: 800-325-9521 (orders) ; *Imprints:* Liguori Triumph (Liguori/Triumph)
E-mail: liguori@liguori.org
Web site: http://www.liguori.org
Dist(s): **ACTA Pubns** *(ACTA Pubns.)*
Baker & Taylor *(Baker & Taylor Bks.).*

Liguori Triumph Imprint of Liguori Pubns

Lilac Pub, *(Lilac Publishing; 0-9635782),* P.O. Box 665, Saint Charles, MO 63302-0665 Tel 314-947-6469
E-mail: Barfield@aol.com.

Lillenas, *(Lillenas Publishing Co.; 0-8341),* Div. of Nazarene Publishing Hse., P.O. Box 419527, Kansas City, MO 64141 (SAN 298-7619) Tel 816-931-1900; Fax: 816-753-4071; Toll Free: 800-877-0700 (Orders Only)
E-mail: music@lillenas.com
Web site: http://www.lillenas.com
Dist(s): **Riverside-World** *(Riverside World)*
Spring Arbor Dist *(Spring Arbor Distributors Inc.).*

Linacre Centre (GBR) *(0-906561) Dist. by* **St Augustines Pr.**

Lincoln Pubng, *(Lincoln Publishing, Inc.; 1-884929),* Orders Addr.: P.O. Box 1499, Lake Oswego, OR 97035-0499 Tel 503-699-1000; Fax: 503-699-2000; Toll Free: 800-266-5748
Dist(s): **IPG Chicago** *(Independent Pubs. Group).*

Lincoln-Bradley, *(Lincoln-Bradley Publishing Group; 1-879111),* Div. of Creative Living, Inc., Orders Addr.: P.O. Box 808, Gatlinburg, TN 37738 (SAN 297-3162) Tel 423-436-4150; Fax: 423-436-4762; Toll Free: 800-422-6946; Edit Addr.: 420 Mountain Dr., Gatlinburg, TN 37738.

Lincoln-Herndon Pr, *(Lincoln-Herndon Pr.; 0-942936),* 818 S. Dirksen Pkwy., Springfield, IL 62703 (SAN 240-3188) Tel 217-522-2732; Fax: 217-544-8738; Toll Free: 800-243-8884
E-mail: lhp@cityscape.net
Web site: http://www.lincolnherndon.com
Dist(s): **Baker & Taylor** *(Baker & Taylor Bks.)*
Distributors *(Distributors, The).*

Lindisfarne Imprint of Anthroposophic

LinguiSystems, *(LinguiSystems, Inc.; 0-7606; 1-55999),* 3100 Fourth Ave., East Moline, IL 61244-9700 Tel 309-755-2300; Fax: 309-755-2377; Toll Free: 800-577-4555; 800-776-4332
E-mail: kmicka@linguisystems.com
Web site: http://www.linguisystems.com.

Linholm, *(Linholm Corp.; 0-9618935),* 913 W. Alder St., Louisville, CO 80027 (SAN 242-5335) Tel 888-339-2229
E-mail: linholm@aol.com
Dist(s): **R Berrie** *(Berrie, Russ & Co., Inc.).*

Link Pub, *(Link Publishing; 0-9637670),* P.O. Box 15562, San Antonio, TX 78212-8762 Tel 210-601-2038 Do not confuse with Link Publishing, Virginia Beach, VA
E-mail: sales@linkpublishing.com
Web site: http://www.linkpublishing.com.

Link Pub VA, *(Link Publishing; 0-9658409),* 4356 Bonney Rd., Suite 2-103, Virginia Beach, VA 23452 Tel 757-498-0014; Fax: 757-498-0290; Toll Free: 800-922-0866 Do not confuse with Link Publishing, San Antonio, TX
E-mail: LLMiles@ix.netcom.com.

Linscotts Direct, *(Linscott's Directory; 0-9604920; 1-892153),* 4877 Grange Rd., Santa Rosa, CA 95404 (SAN 214-4018) Tel 707-544-9555; Fax: 415-389-6025
E-mail: linscottsdirectory@compuserve.com.

LInstitut Francais (FRA) *(2-7099) Dist. by* **Balogh.**

Linstok Pr, *(Linstok Pr., Inc.; 0-932130),* 4020 Blackburn Ln., Burtonsville, MD 20866 (SAN 207-6195) Tel 301-421-0268; Fax: 301-421-0270; Toll Free: 800-475-4756
E-mail: signmedia@aol.com
Web site: http://www.signmedia.com.

Lion Pr & Vid, *(Lion Pr. & Video; 0-936635),* Orders Addr.: P.O. Box 92541, Rochester, NY 14692 (SAN 699-685X) Tel 716-381-6410; Fax: 716-381-7439; Toll Free: 800-597-3068 (orders only); Edit Addr.: 19 Greentree, Pittsford, NY 14534 (SAN 699-6841) Do not confuse with companies with similar names in Allison Park, PA, Forest Hills, NY
E-mail: aleone@frontiernet.net
Web site: http://ourworld.compuserve.com/homepages/lionpress.

†**Lion USA,** *(Lion Publishing; 0-7459; 0-85648),* Div. of Chariot Victor Publishing, 4050 Lee Vance View, Colorado Springs, CO 80918-7102 (SAN 663-611X) Tel 719-536-0100; Toll Free: 800-437-4337
Web site: http://www.cookministries.com/
Dist(s): **Cook Communs Minist** *(Cook Communications Ministries); CIP.*

Liposuction Inst Am, *(Liposuction Institute of America; 0-9621284),* 1700 W. Central Rd., Arlington Heights, IL 60005 (SAN 250-9377) Tel 312-259-6161.

Lippnctt Imprint of Lppncott W & W

Lisa Drew Imprint of Scribner

Listening Inst, *(Listening Institute; 0-9635378),* Div. of National Market Makers, Inc., Orders Addr.: P.O. Box 2188, Venice, CA 90294-2188 Tel 310-815-8181; Fax: 310-815-9953; Toll Free: 800-758-7327; Edit Addr.: 1808 Pier Ave., Santa Monica, CA 90405.

Lita Lee, *(Lee, Lita; 1-880358),* 2852 Willamette St., No. 397, Eugene, OR 97405-3240.

Litarvan Lit, *(Litarvan Literature; 0-937557),* 4410 Leesburg Cir., Idaho Falls, ID 83404 (SAN 658-8603).

Literary Frontiers Pubs, *(Literary Frontiers Pubs.; 0-939636),* P.O. Box 54101, New York, NY 11354 (SAN 216-6321) Tel 718-445-2836.

Lith Res & Studies, *(Lithuanian Research & Studies Ctr.; 0-929700),* 5600 S. Claremont Ave., Chicago, IL 60636-1039 (SAN 249-9541) Tel 773-434-4545; Fax: 773-434-9363
E-mail: lithuanianresearch@ameritech.net.

Little (GBR) *(0-316) Dist. by* **Trafalgar.**

†**Little,** *(Little, Brown & Co.; 0-316; 0-8212),* Div. of Time Warner Trade Publishing, Orders Addr.: 3 Center Plaza, Boston, MA 02108-2084 (SAN 630-7248) Tel 617-227-0730; Toll Free Fax: 800-286-9471; Toll Free: 800-759-0190; Edit Addr.: Time & Life Bldg., 1271 Avenue of the Americas, New York, NY 10020 (SAN 200-2205) Tel 212-522-8700; Fax: 212-522-2067; Toll Free: 800-343-9204 ; *Imprints:* Back Bay (Back Bay)
E-mail: cust.service@littlebrown.com
Web site: http://www.littlebrown.com
Dist(s): **AOL Time Warner** *(AOL Time Warner Bk. Group)*
Continental Bk *(Continental Bk. Co., Inc.)*
Hastings Bks *(Hastings Bks.)*
Rounder Kids Mus Dist *(Rounder Kids Music Distribution)*
Shens Bks *(Shen's Bks.)*
T T Beeler *(Beeler, Thomas T. Publisher)*
Warner Bks *(Warner Bks., Inc.)*
iPublishcom *(iPublish.com); CIP.*

Little Bkrm, *(Little Bookroom; 0-9641262; 1-892145),* 5 Saint Luke's Pl., New York, NY 10014 Tel 212-691-3321; Fax: 212-691-2011
Dist(s): **NY Rev Bks** *(New York Review of Bks., Inc., The)*
Publishers Group *(Publishers Group West).*

Little Brown (GBR) *(0-349; 0-356; 0-7515) Dist. by* **Trafalgar.**

Little Brwn Med Div Imprint of Lppncott W & W

Little Red Hen, *(Little Red Hen, Inc.; 0-933046),* P.O. Box 4260, Pocatello, ID 83201 (SAN 212-7571) Tel 208-232-1847 Do not confuse with Little Red Hen Pubn., Inc., Las Vegas, NV.

Little Treasure, *(Little Treasure Pubns., Inc.; 0-9639838),* 47 Westtown Rd., Thornton, PA 19373 Tel 610-399-9057; Fax: 610-399-9437.

Little Tree Pr, *(Little Tree Pr.; 1-888474),* Orders Addr.: P.O. Box 1692, Copperas Cove, TX 76522 Tel 254-547-6158; Edit Addr.: 807 Kubitz Rd., Copperas Cove, TX 76522
E-mail: littletree@softwarepub.com.

Little Whte Buffalo, *(Little White Buffalo Publishing Cottage; 0-9658545),* 12345 Lake City Way, NE, PMB 204, Seattle, WA 98125 (SAN 299-3511) Tel 425-771-2744; Fax: 425-673-9325
E-mail: sanano@zipcon.net
Web site: http://www.whidbey.com/onedegreebeyond; http://www.onedegreebeyond.com
Dist(s): **New Leaf Dist** *(New Leaf Distributing Co., Inc.).*

†**Littlefield,** *(Littlefield Adams Quality Paperbacks; 0-8226),* Div. of Rowman & Littlefield Pubs., Inc., 4720 Boston Way, Lanham, MD 20706 (SAN 202-6791) Tel 301-459-3366; Fax: 301-459-2118
E-mail: jlyons@rowman.com
Dist(s): **Natl Bk Netwk** *(National Bk. Network)*
Rowman *(Rowman & Littlefield Pubs., Inc.); CIP.*

†**Liturgical Pr,** *(Liturgical Pr., The; 0-8146),* Div. of Order of St. Benedict, Inc., Orders Addr.: St. Johns Abbey, Collegeville, MN 56321-7500 (SAN 202-2494) Tel 320-363-2213; Fax: 320-363-3299; Toll Free Fax: 800-445-5899; Toll Free: 800-858-5450
E-mail: sales@litpress.org
Web site: http://www.litpress.org; *CIP.*

Liv from Vis, *(Living from Vision; 1-884246),* Orders Addr.: P.O. Box 1530, Stanwood, WA 98292 Tel 360-387-5713; Fax: 360-387-9846; Toll Free: 800-758-7836; Edit Addr.: 1837 S. Cascade View Dr., Camano Island, Stanwood, WA 98292
E-mail: dolphinlove@sos.net
Web site: http://www.livingfromvision.com
Dist(s): **APG Trade** *(APG Trade West)*
Bookpeople *(Bookpeople)*
New Leaf Dist *(New Leaf Distributing Co., Inc.).*

Liv Lang, *(Living Language; 0-517; 0-609; 1-4000),* Member of The Random Hse. Information Group, Orders Addr.: 400 Hahn Rd., Westminster, MD 21157 Tel 410-848-1900; Toll Free: 800-726-0600; Edit Addr.: 280 Park Ave., New York, NY 10017 Tel 212-751-2600; Fax: 212-940-7400; Toll Free: 800-726-0600
Web site: http://www.fodors.com/language/
Dist(s): **Random** *(Random Hse., Inc.).*

Liv Resources, *(Living Resources Pr.; 0-9674218),* P.O. Box 221, Columbia, MD 21045-0221 Tel 301-596-5018; Fax: 410-997-2805; Toll Free: 800-358-3507
E-mail: drhurd@drhurd.com
Web site: http://www.lrpress.com; http://www.drhurd.com.

Liv Wellness, *(Living Wellness, Inc.; 0-9631405),* Orders Addr.: P.O. Box 279, Koloa, Kauai, HI 96756 Tel 808-332-5941; Toll Free: 800-338-6977; Edit Addr.: 4671 Kua Rd., Kalaheo, HI 96741
E-mail: drdeal@aloha.net
Web site: http://planet-hawaii.com/drdeal/.

Live Oak, *(Live Oak Pr., The; 0-931095; 0-931378),* Orders Addr.: P.O. Box 60036, Palo Alto, CA 94306 (SAN 299-1748) Tel 650-853-0197; Edit Addr.: 2620 Emerson St., Palo Alto, CA 94306 Do not confuse with companies with same or similar names in Orlando, FL, Austin, TX.
E-mail: info@liveoakpress.com
Web site: http://www.liveoakpress.com.

Live Oak CA, *(Live Oak Publishing; 0-9629517),* Orders Addr.: P.O. Box 8329, Woodland, CA 95776; Edit Addr.: 18595 County Rd. 97, Woodland, CA 95695 Tel 916-668-6415.

†Liveright, *(Liveright Publishing Corp.; 0-87140),* Subs. of W. W. Norton Co., Inc., 500 Fifth Ave., New York, NY 10110 (SAN 201-0976) Tel 212-354-5500; Fax: 212-869-0856; Toll Free Fax: 800-458-6515; Toll Free: 800-233-4830
Web site: http://www.wwnorton.com
Dist(s): **Norton** *(Norton, W.W. & Co., Inc.); CIP.*

Liverpool Univ Pr (GBR) *(0-85323) Dist. by* **Intl Spec Bk.**

Livia Pr CT, *(Livia Pr.; 0-9637045),* P.O. Box 983, Ridgefield, CT 06877 Tel 718-358-9432 Do not confuse with Livia Pr., Albany, CA.

Living Planet Pr, *(Living Planet Pr.; 0-9626072; 1-879326),* 3408 34th Pl., NW, Washington, DC 20016-3136.

Lke Superior Res, *(Lake Superior Research Institute; 0-9614968),* Div. of Univ. of Wisconsin-Superior, Univ. of Wisconsin-Superior, Superior, WI 54880 (SAN 693-7306) Tel 715-394-8315; Fax: 715-394-8107
E-mail: jbarnes@staff.uwsuper.edu
Web site: http://staff.uwsuper.edu/biology/lsri/lsri.htm.

Lkng Glass Pubns, *(Looking Glass Pubns.; 0-936485),* P.O. Box 19161, Sarasota, FL 34276 (SAN 698-0988) Tel 941-925-7048 ; *Imprints:* Galen Pr DC (Galen Press) Do not confuse with companies with the same or similar name in Annapolis, MD , Riverside, CT , Quincy, IL , Roswell, GA , Tucson, AZ
E-mail: lgp@webcom.com
Dist(s): **Bookpeople** *(Bookpeople).*

†Llewellyn Pubns, *(Llewellyn Pubns.; 0-7387; 0-87542; 1-56718; 1-892485),* Div. of Llewellyn Worldwide, Ltd., Orders Addr.: P.O. Box 64383, Saint Paul, MN 55164-0383 (SAN 201-100X) Tel 651-291-1970; Fax: 651-291-1908; Toll Free: 800-843-6666; Edit Addr.: 84 S. Wabasha, Saint Paul, MN 55107
E-mail: nweditor@llewellyn.com
Web site: http://www.llewellyn.com
Dist(s): **Bookpeople** *(Bookpeople)*
Koen Bk Distributors *(Koen Bk. Distributors)*
Lectorum Pubns *(Lectorum Pubns., Inc.)*
Natl Bk Netwk *(National Bk. Network)*
New Leaf Dist *(New Leaf Distributing Co., Inc.); CIP.*

LM Pubns, *(LM Pubns.; 0-935596),* Orders Addr.: P.O. Box 482, Provo, UT 84604 Tel 801-374-1858; Fax: 801-374-1858; Toll Free: 888-554-3727; Edit Addr.: 509 E. 2100 N., Box 482, Provo, UT 84604 (SAN 213-0653) Tel 801-374-1858; Fax: 801-374-1858; Toll Free: 888-554-3727
E-mail: lmp@vitalvillage.net; LeArta@VitalVillage.net; info@vitalvillage.net
Web site: http://www.vitalvillage.net
Dist(s): **Q W Inc** *(QW, Inc.).*

LMA Publishing, *(LMA Publishing; 1-892426),* Div. of Lifestyle Management Assocs., 111 Grove St., Apt. 1, West Roxbury, MA 02132 Tel 617-325-6752 (phone/fax)
E-mail: pentzj@ix.netcom.com
Web site: http://www.lifestylemanagement.com.

Load N Go Pr, *(Load N Go Pr.; 0-9626357),* P.O. Box 175, Kiamesha Lake, NY 12751 Tel 914-794-3772; Toll Free: 800-522-8528.

Lockwood Pr, *(Lockwood Pr.; 0-9627939),* 9361 F Montgomery Rd., Cincinnati, OH 45242-7738 Tel 513-793-9949; Toll Free: 800-793-6553.

Loft Pr, *(Loft Pr., Inc.; 0-9630797; 1-893846),* Orders Addr.: P.O. Box 126, Fort Valley, VA 22652 Tel 540-933-6210; Fax: 540-933-6523
E-mail: books@loftpress.com
Web site: http://www.loftpress.com.

Logical Hlth, *(Logical Health Care Solutions; 0-9702957),* Orders Addr.: 1991 Hacienda Dr., El Cajon, CA 92020; Edit Addr.: P.O. Box 712823, Santee, CA 92072 Tel 619-562-3447; Fax: 619-562-1414
E-mail: l.obrien@logicalhealth.com
Web site: http://www.logicalhealth.com.

Login Fulfillment Services, *See* **LPC Group**

Login Pubs Consort, *(Login Pubs. Consortium; 0-9648574),* 1436 W. Randolph St., 2nd Flr., Chicago, IL 60607 (SAN 630-5733) Tel 312-432-7650; Fax: 312-733-3107; Toll Free: 800-626-4330
E-mail: lpc-info@lb.com
Web site: http://www.coolbooks.com.

LOMA, *See* **Life Office**

Loma Lnda U Neur, *(Loma Linda Univ. Neurology Assocs. Medical Group, Inc.; 0-9655186),* 11370 Anderson St., Suite 2400, Loma Linda, CA 92553 Tel 909-824-4907; Fax: 909-478-4207.

Lompico Cr Pr, *(Lompico Creek Pr.; 0-9619311),* Orders Addr.: P.O. Box 1403, Felton, CA 95018-1403 (SAN 243-7767) Tel 831-335-7696; Edit Addr.: 12480 Lompico Rd., Felton, CA 95018
E-mail: editor@sasquatch.com
Web site: www.loveisageless.com.

London Brdge, *(London Bridge),* Div. of General Distribution Services, Orders Addr.: 4500 Witmer Industrial EST, Niagara Falls, NY 14305-1386 (SAN 630-7949) Toll Free: 800-805-1083.

London Hse, *(London Hse.; 0-930171),* Div. of The McGraw-Hill Cos., 9701 W. Higgins Rd., Rosemont, IL 60018-4703 (SAN 670-7262) Tel 708-292-1900.

Lone Star Bks, *(Lone Star Bks.; 1-58907),* 4720 Boston Way, Lanham, MD 20706 Tel 301-731-9545.

Long Life Pr, *(Long Life Pr.; 0-9634020),* 8824 Easthaven Ct., New Port Richey, FL 34655-5246 Do not confuse with Long Life Press, Company, Rome, ME.

Longevity Herb Pr, *(Longevity Herb Pr.; 0-9624868),* Div. of Washington State is Longevity Herb Co., 1549 W. Jewett Blvd., White Salmon, WA 98672 Tel 509-493-2626
E-mail: avery@gorge.net.

Longleaf Pr NC, *(Longleaf Pr.; 0-9657319),* Orders Addr.: P.O. Box 4224, Chapel Hill, NC 27515 Tel 919-942-5232; Edit Addr.: 700 Emory Dr., Chapel Hill, NC 27514 Do not confuse with Longleaf Pr., Hattiesburg, MS.

†Longman, *(Longman Publishing Group; 0-13; 0-321; 0-582; 0-8013),* Div. of Addison Wesley Longman, Inc., The Longman Bldg., 10 Bank St., White Plains, NY 10606-1951 (SAN 202-6856) Tel 914-993-5000; Fax: 914-997-8115 800-922-0579 (college, bkstores, customer service only) ; *Imprints:* Drumbeat (Drumbeat)
E-mail: orders@mcp.com
Web site: http://store.awl.com
Dist(s): **Coronet Bks** *(Coronet Bks.)*
Trans-Atl Phila *(Trans-Atlantic Pubns., Inc.); CIP.*

Longmuir Jones Pub, *(Longmuir/Jones Publishing, Inc.; 0-9625440; 1-884542),* Orders Addr.: P.O. Box 1346, Murray, KY 42071-1346; Edit Addr.: Rte. 1, Box 231-B, Carlton Rd., Almo, KY 42020 Tel 502-753-5740.

Longstreet, *(Longstreet Pr., Inc.; 0-929264; 1-56352),* Subs. of Cox Newspapers, Inc., 2140 Newmarket Pkwy., Suite 122, Marietta, GA 30067 (SAN 248-7640) Tel 770-980-1488; Fax: 770-859-9894; Toll Free: 800-927-1488
E-mail: rrichardson@longstreetpress.net
Dist(s): **Natl Bk Netwk** *(National Bk. Network).*

Longwood Ctr, *(Longwood Ctr. for the Visual Arts; 1-890327),* Div. of Longwood College, 129 N. Main St., Farmville, VA 23901 (SAN 279-4136) Tel 804-395-2206; Fax: 804-392-6441
Web site: http://www.lwc.edu.

Longwood Div Imprint of Allyn

Longwood Fine, *See* **Longwood Ctr**

Loompanics, *(Loompanics Unlimited; 0-915179; 1-55950),* Orders Addr.: P.O. Box 1197, Port Townsend, WA 98368 (SAN 206-4421) Tel 360-385-5087; Fax: 360-385-7785; Toll Free: 800-380-2230 (credit card orders only)
E-mail: service@loompanics.com
Web site: http://www.loompanics.com
Dist(s): **Baker & Taylor** *(Baker & Taylor Bks.)*
Bookpeople *(Bookpeople)*
Homestead Bk *(Homestead Bk., Inc.)*
Last Gasp *(Last Gasp Eco-Funnies, Inc.)*
Left Bank *(Left Bank Distribution).*

Lorenz Bks Imprint of Anness Pub

Lorenzo Prema, *(Lorenzo Prema; 0-941122),* 310 West End Ave., New York, NY 10023 (SAN 217-4170) Tel 212-874-7692.

Lost Coast, *(Lost Coast Pr.; 1-882897),* 155 Cypress St., Fort Bragg, CA 95437 Tel 707-964-9520; Fax: 707-964-7531; Toll Free: 800-773-7782
E-mail: forms@cypresshouse.com
Web site: http://www.cypresshouse.com
Dist(s): **Baker & Taylor** *(Baker & Taylor Bks.)*
Continental Bk *(Continental Bk. Co., Inc.)*
New Leaf Dist *(New Leaf Distributing Co., Inc.)*
Partners-West *(Partners/West).*

Lotus Light, *See* **Lotus Pr**

Lotus Pr, *(Lotus Pr.; 0-910261; 0-914778; 0-914955; 0-940676; 0-940985; 0-941524),* Div. of Lotus Brands, Inc., P.O. Box 325, Twin Lakes, WI 53181 (SAN 239-1120) Tel 262-889-8561; Fax: 262-889-8591; Toll Free: 800-824-6396 ; *Imprints:* Shangri-La (Shangri-La) Do not confuse with companies with the same or similar name in Lotus, CA, Westerville, OH, Bokeelia, FL, Brattleboro, VT, Detroit, MI, Tobyhanna, PA
E-mail: lotuspress@lotuspress.com
Web site: http://www.lotuspress.com
Dist(s): **Natl Bk Netwk** *(National Bk. Network).*

Love & Logic, *(Love & Logic Institute, Inc.; 0-944634; 1-930429),* 2207 Jackson St., Golden, CO 80401-2300 (SAN 244-5867) Tel 303-278-7552; Fax: 303-278-3894; Toll Free Fax: 800-455-7557; Toll Free: 800-338-4065 (orders)
E-mail: carolt@loveandlogic.com
Web site: http://www.loveandlogic.com
Dist(s): **Midpt Trade** *(Midpoint Trade Bks., Inc.)*
Penton Overseas *(Penton Overseas, Inc.).*

†Love Line Bks, *(Love Line Bks.; 0-915972; 0-9600688),* P.O. Box 989, Coos Bay, OR 97420-0220 (SAN 281-9082) Tel 541-269-2812; Fax: 541-267-5312
Dist(s): **Bookpeople** *(Bookpeople)*
New Leaf Dist *(New Leaf Distributing Co., Inc.)*
Publishers Group *(Publishers Group West); CIP.*

Love Lives Imprint of Triple U Enterprises

Love Pub Co, *(Love Publishing Co.; 0-89108),* 9101 E. Kenyon Ave., Suite 2200, Denver, CO 80237 (SAN 205-2482) Tel 303-221-7333; Fax: 303-221-7444 Do not confuse with companies with the same name in Belmont, NC, Indiantown, FL, Bossier, LA
E-mail: lovepublishing@compuserve.com
Web site: http://www.lovepublishing.com.

Lovejoy Hospice, *(Lovejoy Hospice; 0-9654910),* 400 NE E St., Grants Pass, OR 97526-2324 Tel 541-474-1193; Fax: 541-474-3035.

Low Fat Pr, *(Low Fat Pr.; 0-9629675),* 625 Pecan Dr., Mesquite, TX 75149-4029 Fax: 617-523-8486; 7 Queen Anne Rd., Hopkinton, MA 01748 Tel 508-435-9492.

Low Price (IND) *(81-7536; 81-85395; 81-85418; 81-85557; 81-86142) Dist. by* **S Asia.**

†Lowell Hse, *(Lowell Hse.; 0-7373; 0-8092; 0-929923; 1-56565),* 2020 Avenue of the Stars, Suite 300, Los Angeles, CA 90067-4704 (SAN 250-863X) Tel 310-552-7555; Fax: 310-552-7573 ; *Imprints:* Anodyne (Anodyne) Extension Pr (Extension Press); *CIP.*

Lowell Hse Juvenile, *(Lowell Hse. Juvenile; 0-7373; 0-929923; 1-56565),* 2020 Avenue of the Stars, No. 300, Los Angeles, CA 90067 (SAN 250-863X) Tel 310-552-7555; Fax: 310-552-7573 ; *Imprints:* Roxbury Pk Juvenile (Roxbury Park Juvenile)
Web site: http://www.lowellh.com.

†Lowell Pr, *(Lowell Pr., The, Gallion Communications; 0-913504; 0-932845),* P.O. Box 411877, Kansas City, MO 64141-1877 (SAN 207-0774) Tel 816-753-4545; Fax: 816-753-4057; Toll Free: 800-736-7660 Do not confuse with Lowell Pr. in Eugene, OR
E-mail: plowell@gri.net; *CIP.*

Loyal Pubng, *(Loyal Publishing; 1-929125),* Orders Addr.: P.O. Box 1892, Sisters, OR 97759 Tel 541-549-8890; Fax: 541-549-8879; Edit Addr.: 251 W. Barclay Dr., Sisters, OR 97759
E-mail: jmilliken@loyalpublishing.com
Web site: http://loyalpublishing.com.

†Loyola Pr, *(Loyola Pr.; 0-8294),* 3441 N. Ashland Ave., Chicago, IL 60657 (SAN 211-6537) Tel 773-281-1818; Fax: 773-281-0555; Toll Free: 800-621-1008
E-mail: customerservice@loyolapress.com
Web site: http://www.loyolapress.com
Dist(s): **Baker & Taylor** *(Baker & Taylor Bks.)*
Bookazine Co Inc *(Bookazine Co., Inc.)*
Partners Pubs Grp *(Partners Pubs. Group, Inc.)*
Riverside-World *(Riverside World)*
Spring Arbor Dist *(Spring Arbor Distributors Inc.); CIP.*

Loyola U Crim, *(Loyola Univ., Criminal Justice Dept.; 0-942854),* 820 N. Michigan Ave., Chicago, IL 60611 (SAN 693-6962) Tel 312-915-7568; Fax: 312-915-7650
Web site: http://www.luc.edu/depts/crim_jus/.

LPC Group, *(LPC Group),* c/o CDS, 193 Edwards Dr., Jackson, TN 38305 (SAN 630-5644) Fax: 312-432-7603; Toll Free Fax: 800-334-3892; Toll Free: 800-243-0138
E-mail: fm@lb.com
Web site: http://www.coolbooks.com.

†Lppncott W & W, *(Lippincott Williams & Wilkins; 0-316; 0-397; 0-683; 0-7817; 0-8121; 0-88167; 0-89004; 0-89313; 0-911216; 1-881063),* Subs. of Wolters Kluwer U.S. Corp., Orders Addr.: P.O. Box 1600, Hagerstown, MD 21741 Tel 301-714-2300; Fax: 301-824-7390; Toll Free: 800-638-3030; Edit Addr.: 530 Walnut St., Philadelphia, PA 19106-3780 (SAN 201-0933) Tel 215-521-8300; Fax: 215-521-8902; Toll Free: 800-638-3030 ; *Imprints:* Lippncott (Lippincott) Little Brwn Med Div (Little, Brown Medical Division)
E-mail: custserv@lww.com
Web site: http://www.lww.com
Dist(s): **Continental Bk** *(Continental Bk. Co., Inc.)*
Univelt Inc *(Univelt, Inc.); CIP.*

Lppncott-Raven, *See* **Lppncott W & W**

Lrng Tools, *(Learning Tools; 0-940221),* 3060 Racetrack View Dr., Del Mar, CA 92014-2462 (SAN 664-1733).

Lrng Tools-Bilicki Pubns, *See* **Lrng Tools**

Lrning Cnnect, *(Learning Connection, The; 0-9624688),* 12510 Kaibab Ct., Colorado Springs, CO 80908 Tel 719-495-3400; Toll Free: 800-299-7323.

Lrning Res Intl, *(Learning Resources International, Inc.; 0-942835),* Orders Addr.: 7416 La Jara Ct., NE, Albuquerque, NM 87109-3850 (SAN 667-7657) Tel 505-822-8951
E-mail: mishalea@aol.com
Web site: http://www.fetalmonitoring.com.

Lrning Thrgh Ent, *(Learning Through Entertainment; 1-883681),* P.O. Box 8300-611, Dallas, TX 75205
Dist(s): **Video Distributors Inc** *(Video Distributors, Inc.).*

LrningExprss, *(LearningExpress, LLC; 1-57685),* 900 Broadway, Suite 604, New York, NY 10003 Tel 212-995-2566; Fax: 212-995-5512; Toll Free: 800-295-9556
E-mail: info@learnatest.com; customerservice@learnatest.com
Web site: http://www.learnatest.com
Dist(s): **Thomson Learn** *(Thomson Learning).*

LRP Publications, *(LRP Pubns.; 1-882594),* Orders Addr.: P.O. Box 980, Horsham, PA 19044-0980 Toll Free: 800-341-7874; Edit Addr.: 747 Dresher Rd., Horsham, PA 19044
E-mail: custserve@lrp.com
Web site: http://www.lrp.com.

†LRP Pubns, *(LRP Pubns.; 0-934753; 1-57834),* Orders Addr.: P.O. Box 980, Horsham, PA 19044-0980 (SAN 237-8329) Tel 215-784-0941; Fax: 215-784-9014; Toll Free: 800-341-7874; Edit Addr.: 747 Dresher Rd., Suite 500, Horsham, PA 19044*; CIP.*

Lublin Graph, *(Lublin Graphics, Inc.; 0-941393),* 323 Railroad Ave., Greenwich, CT 06830-6306 (SAN 665-5661) Tel 203-622-8777; Toll Free: 800-243-4004.

Lubrecht & Cramer, *(Lubrecht & Cramer, Ltd.; 0-934454; 0-945345),* 18 E. Main St., Port Jervis, NY 12771; Edit Addr.: P.O. Box 3110, Port Jervis, NY 12771 (SAN 214-1256) Tel 914-856-5990; Toll Free: 800-920-9334; 350 Fifth Ave., Suite 3304, New York, NY 10118-0069
E-mail: lubrecht@ny.frontiernet.net; books@lubrechtcramer.com
Web site: http://www.lubrechtcramer.com.

Lucent Books Imprint of Gale

Lucis, *(Lucis Publishing Co.; 0-85330),* Div. of Lucis Trust, 120 Wall St., 24th Flr., New York, NY 10005 (SAN 201-1085) Tel 212-292-0707; Fax: 212-292-0808
E-mail: newyork@lucistrust.org
Web site: http://www.lusictrust.org/lusicpub/; http://www.alicebailey.org/lusicpub/.

Luckenbooth, *(Luckenbooth Pr.; 0-9643837),* P.O. Box 3082, Newport Beach, CA 92659-0646 Tel 949-722-8977
E-mail: LamazeBaby@aol.com.

Ludann Co, *(Ludann Co.; 0-929689),* P.O. Box 127, Lowell, MI 49331-0127 (SAN 249-9967) Toll Free: 800-367-1553
Web site: http://www.ladann.com.

Lugano Bks, *See* **Hanrow**

Lumen Eds Imprint of Brookline Bks

Lupus Found Am, *(Lupus Foundation of America, Inc.; 0-9608660; 1-879990),* 1300 Piccard Dr., Suite 200, Rockville, MD 20850-4303 (SAN 240-7094) Tel 301-670-9292; Fax: 301-670-9486; Toll Free: 800-558-0121.

LuraMedia, *See* **Innisfree Pr**

Lust, *(Lust, Benedict Pubns.; 0-87904),* Orders Addr.: P.O. Box 128, Paso Robles, CA 93447 (SAN 201-1107) Tel 805-226-8771; Fax: 805-226-8772; Toll Free: 800-522-5878; Edit Addr.: 2917 Union Rd., Paso Robles, CA 93446 ; *Imprints:* Beneficial Bks (Beneficial Books)
E-mail: blp1896@tcsn.net
Web site: http://www.lustforlife.net
Dist(s): **New Leaf Dist** *(New Leaf Distributing Co., Inc.)*
Royal Pubns Inc *(Royal Pubns., Inc.).*

†Lustrum Pr, *(Lustrum Pr.; 0-912810),* 714 Broadway, New York, NY 10003 (SAN 281-9562)*; CIP.*

Luthers, *(Luthers; 1-877633),* 1009 N. Dixie Freeway, New Smyrna Beach, FL 32168-6221 (SAN 200-3961) Tel 386-423-1600 (phone/fax)
E-mail: luthers@n-jcenter.com.

Lutterwrth (GBR) *(0-7188) Dist. by* **Parkwest Pubns.**

LWVUS, *(League of Women Voters of the United States; 0-89959),* 1730 M St., NW, Washington, DC 20036 (SAN 207-5288) Tel 202-429-1965; Fax: 202-429-0854
E-mail: lwv@lwv.org
Web site: http://www.lwv.org.

Lxngtn Bks, *(Lexington Bks.; 0-7391),* Orders Addr.: c/o Rowman & Littlefield Publishing Group, 15200 NBN Way, Blue Ridge Summit, PA 17214 Tel 717-794-3800; Toll Free Fax: 800-338-4550; Toll Free: 800-462-6420; Edit Addr.: 4720 Boston Way, Lanham, MD 20706 Tel 301-459-3366; Fax: 301-429-5748
E-mail: sleigh@rowman.com
Web site: http://www.lexingtonbooks.com
Dist(s): **Natl Bk Netwk** *(National Bk. Network)*
Rowman *(Rowman & Littlefield Pubs., Inc.).*

Lyceum IL, *(Lyceum Bks., Inc.; 0-925065),* 5758 S. Blackstone Ave., Chicago, IL 60637 Tel 773-643-1902; Fax: 773-643-1903
E-mail: lyceum@lyceumbooks.com
Web site: http://www.lyceumbooks.com.

LYCO Pub, *(LYCO Publishing),* 3636 Drummond, Houston, TX 77025 (SAN 240-9631) Tel 713-668-0194.

Lymphoedema (AUS) *(0-646) Dist. by* **Medicina Bio.**

Lynnwrd Pr, *(Lynnword Pr.; 0-9653659),* P.O. Box 1732, Evanston, IL 60201 Tel 847-866-9630; Fax: 847-733-0665
E-mail: lynnword@aol.com.

Lyons Imprint of Globe Pequot

M & H Enter, *(M&H Enterprises; 0-936997),* 679 Pestana Dr., Galt, CA 95632-2179 (SAN 658-3180) Tel 209-745-6653.

M & S Pr, *(M&S Pr.; 0-87730),* Orders Addr.: P.O. Box 2594, Providence, RI 02906 (SAN 203-9591) Tel 401-421-1050; Fax: 401-272-0831
E-mail: dsiegel@msrarebooks.com.

M & W Prods, *(M&W Productions; 0-9640082),* Orders Addr.: R.R. 1, Box 618, Sperry, OK 74073-9689; Edit Addr.: 9623 N. Yale, Sperry, OK 74073 Tel 918-288-6899.

M A Haske, *(Haske, Mary Ann; 0-9619475),* 24204 Drayton Landing Dr., Worton, MD 21678-9792 (SAN 244-9838) Tel 410-778-2779.

M A Taylor, *(Taylor, Mark A.; 0-9664171),* 18071 N. 91st Dr., Peoria, AZ 85382 Tel 602-933-1264.

M B Glass Assocs, *(Glass, Michael B. & Assocs., Inc.; 0-940429),* 735 Calebs Path/Glaro Bldg., Hauppauge, NY 11788 (SAN 664-3574).

M Borofka, *(Borofka, Michael; 0-9640856),* Orders Addr.: P.O. Box 221021, Carmel, CA 93922 (SAN 298-2552); Edit Addr.: 25005 Outlook Dr., Carmel, CA 93922 Tel 408-624-2825.

M Boyars Pubs, *(Boyars, Marion Pubs., Inc.; 0-7145; 0-905223),* 237 E. 39th St., No. 1A, New York, NY 10016-2110 (SAN 284-981X) Tel 212-697-1599; Fax: 212-808-0664; Toll Free: 800-283-3572 (orders only)
Dist(s): **Consort Bk Sales** *(Consortium Bk. Sales & Distribution).*

M C Greene, *(Greene, Mary Cooper; 0-9619979),* R.D. 2, P.O. Box 76, Springboro, PA 16435 (SAN 247-3631) Tel 814-587-6089.

M C S ME, *(MCS Information Exchange; 0-9675619),* 2 Oakland St., Brunswick, ME 04011 Tel 207-725-8570
Web site: http://members.xoom.com/Ibutterfly/mcsvideo.

M Chace Mem Fund, *(Chace, Marian Memorial Fund of the American Dance Therapy Assn.; 1-881766),* 2000 Century Plaza, Columbia, MD 21044 Tel 410-997-4040; Fax: 410-997-1608.

M D Mortiere, *See* **Clifton Pub**

M Dunitz Imprint of Scovill Paterson

M E D S Inc, *(MEDS, Inc. Publishing (Medical Education Development Services, Inc.); 1-56533),* 4000 Blackburn Ln., Suite 260, Burtonsville, MD 20866 Tel 301-476-9666; Fax: 301-476-9677; Toll Free: 800-200-9191
E-mail: info@medspub.com
Web site: http://www.medspub.com
Dist(s): **Baker & Taylor** *(Baker & Taylor Bks.)*
J Majors Co *(Majors, J. A. Co.)*
Matthews Bk Co *(Matthews Bk. Co.)*
Rittenhouse *(Rittenhouse Bk. Distributors)*
Yankee Ped Bkshop *(Yankee Peddler Bookshop).*

M E Pinkham, *(Pinkham, Mary Ellen; 0-941298),* P.O. Box 39221, Edina, MN 55439-0221 (SAN 212-0429).

†M E Sharpe, *(Sharpe, M.E. Inc.; 0-7656; 0-87332; 1-56324),* 80 Business Park Dr., Armonk, NY 10504 (SAN 202-7100) Tel 914-273-1800; Fax: 914-273-2106; Toll Free: 800-541-6563 ; *Imprints:* East Gate Bk (East Gate Book)
E-mail: mesinfo@usa.net
Web site: http://www.mesharpe.com*; CIP.*

†M Evans, *(Evans, M. & Co., Inc.; 0-87131; 1-59077),* 216 E. 49th St., New York, NY 10017 (SAN 203-4050) Tel 212-688-2810; Fax: 212-486-4544
E-mail: mevans@sprynet.com
Web site: http://www.mevans.com/
Dist(s): **Natl Bk Netwk** *(National Bk. Network); CIP.*

M F Connors, *(Connors, Mary Frances; 0-9702600),* P.O. Box 40235, San Francisco, CA 94140-0235
E-mail: msings@mindspring.com.

M F R Treatment Ctrs, *(M F R Treatment Centers & M F R Seminars; 1-929894),* 222 W. Lancaster Ave., Paoli, PA 19301 (SAN 253-5696) Tel 610-644-0136; Toll Free: 800-327-2425
E-mail: fascia@erols.com
Web site: http://myofascialrelease.com.

M F Sohn Pubns, *(Sohn, Mark F. Pubns.; 0-9616911; 1-883207),* 103 Honeysuckle Dr., Pikeville, KY 41501 (SAN 661-5228) Tel 606-437-6467; Fax: 606-437-7837
E-mail: sohn@kymtnnet.org.

M G M A, *(Medical Group Management Assn. (MGMA); 0-933948; 1-56829),* 104 Inverness Terr., E., Englewood, CO 80112-5306 (SAN 221-3982) Tel 303-799-1111; Fax: 303-397-1823; Toll Free Fax: 800-329-4633; Toll Free: 888-608-5601
E-mail: infocenter@mgma.com
Web site: http://www.mgma.com
Dist(s): **Jossey-Bass** *(Jossey-Bass, Inc. Pubs.).*

M George, *(George, Marian; 0-9623843),* 1221 S. Laura Cir., Maryville, MO 64468 Tel 816-582-4462.

M Goens Pub, *(Goens, Mary Pub.; 0-9623993),* 3921 Steck Ave., No. 110-A, Austin, TX 78759-8647 Tel 512-343-6013
Dist(s): **DeVorss** *(DeVorss & Co.).*

M Hickey Min, *(Hickey, Marilyn Ministries; 1-56441),* 8081 E. Orchard Rd., Greenwood, CO 80111 (SAN 298-7090) Tel 303-770-0400; Fax: 303-796-1322; Toll Free: 800-743-1324
E-mail: marionn@mhmin.org
Web site: http://mhmin.org
Dist(s): **Harrison Hse** *(Harrison Hse., Inc.).*

M J Utley, *(Utley, Marguerite Jones; 0-9643328),* P.O. Box 1923, DeSoto, TX 75123-1923 Tel 972-223-2783; Fax: 972-223-6696
E-mail: mjutle@aol.com
Web site: http://www.obdiv.com/narco.

M Joseph (GBR) *(0-7181) Dist. by* **Trafalgar.**

M K Jadav, *(Jadav, Manhar K.; 0-9709184),* 38945 Grays Airport Rd., Lady Lake, FL 32159 Tel 352-259-5490; Fax: 352-259-5491
E-mail: mkjadav@aol.com
Web site: http://indiaabsolutezeropopulation.com.

M Kennedy Enter, *(Kennedy, Mitchell Enterprises; 0-9661893),* 2308 Thomas Pl., Fort Worth, TX 76107 Tel 817-731-2347; Fax: 817-731-3306
E-mail: MKenn29941@aol.com.

M Kincheloe, *(Kincheloe, Marsha; 0-9622832),* 25 Scampini Sq., Barre, VT 05641 Tel 802-479-2420.

M L Wave, *(M.L. Wavecrest Publishing; 0-9675782),* Div. of Victory Consulting, 9801 Fall Creek Rd., Suite 130, Indianapolis, IN 46256 Tel 317-826-9550; Fax: 317-826-8395
E-mail: wavecrest_pub@vcstrategies.com
Web site: http://vcstrategies.com/wavecrestpub..

M Lee Smith, *(Smith, M. Lee Pubs. LLC; 0-925773; 0-9605796),* Orders Addr.: P.O. Box 5094, Brentwood, TN 37024-5094 (SAN 226-403X) Tel 615-373-7517; Fax: 615-373-5183; Toll Free: 800-274-6774; Edit Addr.: 5201 Virginia Way, Brentwood, TN 37024-5094
E-mail: custserv@mleesmith.com
Web site: http://www.mleesmith.com.

M Liebert, *(Liebert, Mary Ann Inc.; 0-913113),* 2 Madison Ave., Larchmont, NY 10538 (SAN 283-2259) Tel 914-834-3100; Fax: 914-834-3688.

M Lowenfeld (GBR) *(0-9521788) Dist. by* **Intl Spec Bk.**

M M Bruce, *(Bruce, Martin M.; 0-935198),* 22516 Caravelle Cir., Boca Raton, FL 33433-5909 (SAN 203-6819) Tel 561-393-2428; Fax: 561-362-6185
E-mail: brucepubl@aol.com.

M M Fain, *(Fain, Max M.; 0-9618960),* P.O. Box 426, Lineville, AL 36266-0426 (SAN 242-8091).

M Manoharial (IND) *(81-215; 81-87586) Dist. by* **Coronet Bks.**

M Mincolla, *See* **Pennyroyal Pr**

M Morris Assocs, *(Morris, Mark Assocs.; 0-945837),* P.O. Box 2097, Topeka, KS 66601 (SAN 247-8528) Tel 785-286-8101; Fax: 785-286-8173
Dist(s): **Hills Pet Products Inc** *(Hill's Pet Products, Inc.).*

M Nijhoff (NLD) *(90-247) Dist. by* **Kluwer Academic.**

M Orndorff, *See* **Garkakee**

M Pr CA Imprint of Busn Concepts

M Quitno Pr Imprint of Morgan Quitno Corp

M Rosenfeld, *(Rosenfeld, Michael Gallery; 1-930416),* 24 W. 57th St., New York, NY 10019 Tel 212-247-0082; Fax: 212-247-0402
E-mail: info@rosenfeldart.com
Web site: http://www.rosenfeldart.com.

M S G Haskell Hse, *(M.S.G. Haskell Hse.; 0-8383),* Orders Addr.: P.O. Box 190420, Brooklyn, NY 11219-0009 (SAN 202-2818) Tel 718-435-7878; Fax: 718-633-7050.

M S W Pubng, *(M.S.W. Publishing Co.; 0-9640903),* P.O. Box 5332, Ocala, FL 34478 Tel 352-694-1055; Fax: 352-694-5200
Dist(s): **Baker & Taylor** *(Baker & Taylor Bks.).*

M Tecton Pub, *(Tecton, Mike Publishing; 0-922070; 1-58203),* 1469 Spring Vale Ave., McLean, VA 22101 (SAN 251-0960) Tel 703-893-7945; 703-356-5800; Fax: 703-893-7945
E-mail: mtecton@erols.com
Web site: http://www.miketectonpublishing.com.

M Ward, *(Ward, Marcia; 0-9613444),* 406 Main St., Johnson City, NY 13790 (SAN 657-1050) Tel 607-797-0875.

MA-AH Pub, *(MA/AH Publishing; 0-89126),* Div. of Sunflower Univ. Pr., 1531 Yuma, Box 1009, Manhattan, KS 66505-1009 (SAN 208-0230) Tel 785-539-1888; Fax: 785-559-2233; Toll Free: 800-258-1232
Web site: http://www.sunflower-univ-press.org
Dist(s): **Sunflower U Pr** *(Sunflower Univ. Pr.).*

Mac Bks, *(Macmillan Bks.; 0-02),* Div. of Hungry Minds, Inc., 201 W. 103rd St., Indianapolis, IN 46290 (SAN 219-6298) Toll Free: 800-428-5331 (orders); 800-858-7674 (customer service)
Dist(s): **Continental Bk** *(Continental Bk. Co., Inc.).*

Mac Comp Pub, *See* **Mac USA**

MAC Pub, *(MAC Publishing; 0-910223),* Div. of Claudja, Inc., PMB 346, 321 High School Rd. NE, Bainbridge Island, WA 98110 Tel 206-842-6303; Fax: 206-842-6235; Toll Free: 800-698-0148 (orders/inquiries)
E-mail: cblack@nwlink.com
Web site: http://www.claudiablack.com.

Mac USA, *(Macmillan USA; 0-02; 0-672; 0-7357; 0-7897; 1-57595; 0-7431),* Div. of Pearson Education Corporate Communications, 201 W. 103rd St., Indianapolis, IN 46290-1097 (SAN 219-6298) Tel 317-581-3575; Fax: 317-581-3611; Toll Free: 800-428-5331 (orders); 800-858-7674 (customer service)
E-mail: international@macmillanusa.com
Web site: http://www.mcp.com/pu
Dist(s): **Sams Tech Pub** *(Sams Technical Publishing).*

Mack Pub, *(Mack Publishing Co.; 0-912734),* 1991 Northampton St., Easton, PA 18042 (SAN 203-9508) Tel 610-250-7241; Fax: 610-250-7202.

Macmill Educ (AUS) *(0-7329) Dist. by* **Paul & Co Pubs.**

†**Macmillan,** *(Macmillan Publishing Co., Inc.; 0-02; 0-87605; 0-89256),* Orders Addr.: 200 Old Tappan Rd., Old Tappan, NJ 07675 (SAN 202-5574) Toll Free: 800-428-5331 (Order dept.) ; *Imprints:* Bobbs (Bobbs-Merrill Company) Rawson Assocs (Rawson Associates) Hall Reference (Hall Reference Books)
E-mail: ssonline_feeback@simonsays.com
Web site: http://www.simonsays.com
Dist(s): **Mountain Pr** *(Mountain Pr. Publishing Co., Inc.); CIP.*

Macmillan (GBR) *(0-333) Dist. by* **Trans-Atl Phila.**

Macmillan Coll Imprint of P-H

Macmillan Ed (GBR) *(0-333) Dist. by* **Scholium Intl.**

Macmillan Info, *(Macmillan Information; 0-02),* Div. of Macmillan Publishing Co., Inc., 135 Mt. Zion Rd., Lebanon, IN 46052 (SAN 202-599X)
Web site: http://www.mcp.com/.

Macmillan Ref Imprint of Gale

MacMurray & Beck, *(MacMurray & Beck, Inc.; 1-878448),* 4101 E. Louisiana Ave., Suite 100, Denver, CO 80246 (SAN 200-3562) Tel 303-753-7565; Fax: 303-753-7566; Toll Free: 800-774-3777
E-mail: koffler@macmurraybeck.com
Web site: http://www.macmurraybeck.com.

Macro Bks, *(Macro Bks.; 0-913080),* P.O. Box 26880, Tempe, AZ 85285-6880 (SAN 207-0480) Tel 423-274-0945; Fax: 423-274-9843
E-mail: macrosociety@attglobal.net
Web site: http://www.macrosociety.com.

MacroPrintBks Imprint of Sci & Human Pr

Mad River, *(Mad River Pr.; 0-916422),* 141 Carter Ln., Eureka, CA 95503 (SAN 207-530X) Tel 707-443-2947 (phone/fax) Do not confuse with Mad River Pr., Richmond, MA
E-mail: mrpbooks@humboldt1.com.

Madison Ave Pub, *(Madison Avenue Publishing Co.; 0-9613697),* Div. of Humanetics Educational Service, Inc., 809 N. Madison, Dallas, TX 75208 (SAN 681-8269) Tel 214-946-8450; Toll Free: 800-527-1522.

Madison Bks UPA, *(Madison Bks., Inc.; 0-8128; 0-8191; 0-911572; 1-56833; 1-879511),* Div. of Rowman & Littlefield Publishers, Inc., 4720 Boston Way, Lanham, MD 20706 (SAN 246-7356) Tel 800-462-6420; 301-459-3366; Fax: 301-429-5748; Toll Free Fax: 800-338-4550 ; *Imprints:* Scrbrough Hse (Scarborough House)
Web site: http://www.univpress.com/
Dist(s): **Natl Bk Netwk** *(National Bk. Network)*
Rowman *(Rowman & Littlefield Pubs., Inc.).*

Madison Inst of Med, *(Madison Institute of Medicine; 1-890802),* 7617 Mineral Point Rd., Suite 300, Madison, WI 53717 Tel 608-827-2470; Fax: 608-827-2479
E-mail: mim@healthtechsys.com
Web site: http://www.deancare.com/info/info11.htm.

Madjec Jet, *(Madjec Jet Publishing Co.; 1-892589),* P.O. Box 120, North Freedom, WI 53951 Tel 608-522-4385; Fax: 608-522-4141
E-mail: madjecjet@jvlnet.com
Web site: http://www.madjecjet.com.

Magalhaes Sci Pr, *(Magalhaes Scientific Pr.; 0-9663292),* Orders Addr.: P.O. Box 461, Cheektowaga, NY 14225 Tel 716-656-8511; Fax: 716-668-5178; Edit Addr.: 93 Lynnette Ct., Cheektowaga, NY 14227.

Magellan Pub, *(Magellan Publishing Co.; 0-9628241),* 7035 Hwy. 6 S., No. 176, Houston, TX 77083 Tel 713-341-9703; Fax: 713-879-7666.

Magills Choice Imprint of Salem Pr

Magnes Mus, *(Magnes, Judah L. Museum; 0-943376),* 2911 Russell St., Berkeley, CA 94705 (SAN 214-2511) Tel 510-549-6950; Fax: 510-849-3673
E-mail: pfpr@magnesmuseum.org
Web site: http://www.magnesmuseum.org/.

Magnoart Pubns, *(Magnoart Pubns.; 0-918935),* Subs. of Magnoart Studio, 3280 Percival Ave., Coconut Grove, FL 33133 (SAN 670-0993) Tel 305-447-8660
E-mail: Gmagno5@cs.com
Web site: http://www.gmagno.htmlplanet.com; http://www.gmagno.scriptmania.com.

Magnolia St Pub, *(Magnolia Street Pubs.; 0-9613309; 1-890374),* 1250 W. Victoria, Chicago, IL 60660 (SAN 653-8843) Tel 773-561-2121; Fax: 773-477-6096.

Magoos Umbrella, *(Magoo's Umbrella; 0-932904),* 3766 Fontvelle Ct., San Jose, CA 95127-2147 (SAN 212-2197).

Maier Pubns, *(Maier Pubns.; 0-9626513),* 12013 Royal Portrush Dr., Charlotte, NC 28277-9639 Fax: 704-844-0868.

Main St Bks Imprint of Doubleday

Mainely Phys, *(Mainely Physical Therapy; 1-890989),* Orders Addr.: P.O. Box 7242, Scarborough, ME 04070-7242 Tel 207-885-0304; Fax: 207-883-8377; Toll Free: 866-783-9267; Edit Addr.: 6 Woodgate Rd., Scarborough, ME 04074
E-mail: ptexams@cybertours.com
Web site: http://www.ptexams.com
Dist(s): **J Majors Co** *(Majors, J. A. Co.)*
Matthews Bk Co *(Matthews Bk. Co.).*

Mainstream Pubng (GBR) *(0-906391; 1-85158; 1-84018) Dist. by* **Trafalgar.**

Majesty Pr, *(Majesty Pr.; 0-9654601),* 4040 Del Rey Ave., No. 7, Marina Del Rey, CA 90292-5600 Tel 310-301-8481.

Making Med Wk, *(Making Medicine Work, Inc.; 0-9631700),* 850 Biesterfield Rd., Suite 3002, Elk Grove Village, IL 60007 Tel 708-364-4717; Fax: 708-364-0191; Toll Free: 800-848-4977.

Maklu Uitgev (BEL) *(90-6215) Dist. by* **Gaunt.**

Malki Mus Pr, *(Malki Museum Pr.; 0-939046),* Div. of Malki Museum, Inc., P.O. Box 578, Banning, CA 92220-0004 (SAN 281-9724) Tel 909-849-5415 (orders)
Web site: http://www.the-pass.com/malki/.

Maloine (FRA) *Dist. by* **IBD Ltd.**

Maloof Enter, *(Maloof Enterprises; 1-891361),* 23166 Los Alisos, Suite 114, Mission Viejo, CA 92691 Tel 949-581-6543; Fax: 949-581-3029
Web site: http://www.drmaloof.com.

Malor Bks Imprint of ISHK

Malprac Reporting, *See* **Med Litigation**

Maltreatment & Trauma Pr Imprint of Haworth Pr

Manak Pubns Pvt Ltd (IND) *(81-85445; 81-86562) Dist. by* **Nataraj Bks.**

Manas-Sys, *(Manas-Systems; 0-9610076),* Box 5153, Fullerton, CA 92635 (SAN 272-2062) Tel 714-870-1064; Fax: 714-870-6970.

Manchester Group, *(Manchester Group, Ltd., The; 0-9605792),* 3400 25th Ave. W., No. 102, Seattle, WA 98199-2250 (SAN 220-1747) Tel 206-282-2057.

Manchester Univ Pr (GBR) *(0-7190) Dist. by* **St Martin.**

Mancorp Pub, *(Mancorp Publishing, Inc.; 0-931541),* P.O. Box 21492, Tampa, FL 33622 (SAN 682-286X) Tel 813-288-0406; Fax: 813-281-2361
E-mail: mancorp@gte.net
Web site: http://home1.gte.net/mancorp
Dist(s): **BookWorld** *(BookWorld Services, Inc.).*

Mandala Holistic, *(Mandala Holistic Health; 0-939410),* P.O. Box 1233, Del Mar, CA 92014 (SAN 216-5783) Tel 619-481-7751.

Mandeville LA, *(Mandeville Pr.; 0-914829; 1-893020),* Div. of M S I A (The Movement of Spiritual Inner Awareness), Orders Addr.: P.O. Box 513935, Los Angeles, CA 90051 (SAN 289-1395) Tel 323-737-4055; Fax: 323-737-5680; Edit Addr.: 3500 W. Adams Blvd., Los Angeles, CA 90018
Web site: http://www.mandevillepress.org
Dist(s): **Assoc Pubs Grp** *(Associated Pubs. Group)*
IPG Chicago *(Independent Pubs. Group).*

Mandil Pub Co, *(Mandil Publishing Co.; 0-9666861),* P.O. Box 642, Stockton, CA 92604 Tel 209-333-2336 (phone/fax).

Mandrake Pr (GBR) *(1-872736; 1-872189) Dist. by* **Holmes Pub.**

Manfld U Rural, *(Mansfield Univ., Rural Services Institute; 0-940299),* Doane Ctr., Mansfield, PA 16933 (SAN 664-2462) Tel 717-662-4808; Fax: 717-662-4120.

Mangan Comns, *(Mangan Communications, Inc.; 0-9669664),* 317 W. Fourth St., Davenport, IA 52801-1204 Tel 563-326-5837; Fax: 563-323-0804
E-mail: safetyinfo@mancomm.com
Web site: http://www.mancomm.com.

Manhattan Pub Co, *(Manhattan Publishing Co.),* Div. of U.S. & Europe Bks., Inc., P.O. Box 850, Croton-on-Hudson, NY 10520 (SAN 113-7476) Tel 914-271-5194; Fax: 914-271-5856
Web site: http://www.manhattanpublishing.com.

Manifest Pubns, *(Manifest Pubns.; 0-9627896; 1-929354),* Orders Addr.: P.O. Box 429, Carpinteria, CA 93014 Tel 805-684-4905; Fax: 805-684-3100; Edit Addr.: 6816 Shepard Mesa Rd., Carpinteria, CA 93013
E-mail: publisher@manifestpub.com; editor@manifestpub.com
Web site: http://www.manifestpub.com
Dist(s): **Sunbelt Pubns** *(Sunbelt Pubns., Inc.).*

Manisha Pr, *(Manisha Pr.; 0-9650621),* 14797 Dix Toledo, Southgate, MI 48195 Tel 313-281-4851; Fax: 313-281-4998; Toll Free: 800-382-1190.

Manisses Communs, *(Manisses Communications Group, Inc.; 1-884937),* Orders Addr.: P.O. Box 9758, Providence, RI 02940-9758 Tel 401-831-6020; Fax: 401-861-6370; Toll Free: 800-333-7771; Edit Addr.: 208 Governor St., Providence, RI 02906.

Mann Daniel, *(Mann, Daniel MD; 0-9661010),* 715 Lake St., Suite 600, Oak Park, IL 60301 Tel 708-848-7789; Fax: 708-848-7763; Toll Free: 800-797-7656
E-mail: drhauser@caringmedical.com
Web site: http://www.caringmedical.com
Dist(s): **BookWorld** *(BookWorld Services, Inc.).*

Manohar (IND) *(81-7304; 81-85952) Dist. by* **S Asia.**

Manor Health, *(Manor Health Care Corp.; 0-917025),* 10770 Columbia Pike, Silver Spring, MD 20901 (SAN 655-4059) Tel 301-593-9600; Toll Free: 800-637-1400.

Manor Hse Pub, *(Manor Hse. Publishing; 0-942383),* Coddingtown Ctr., Box 6768, Santa Rosa, CA 95406 (SAN 666-9840) Tel 707-542-7995; Toll Free: 888-860-8399 Do not confuse with companies with the same name in Cape May, NJ, Alexandria, VA.

Manson Pubng (GBR) *(1-874545; 1-84076) Dist. by* **Iowa U Pr.**

Manticore Europe Imprint of Manticore Pubs

†**Manticore Pubs,** *(Manticore Pubs.; 0-87304; 1-896918; 1-900887),* Orders Addr.: P.O. Box 711, Lewiston, NY 14092 Tel 905-945-7221; Fax: 905-945-8486; Toll Free: 888-263-1877 ; *Imprints:* Manticore Europe (Manticore Europe)
E-mail: results@manticore.ca
Web site: http://www.Manticore.ca; *CIP.*

Mantra Pr, *(Mantra Pr. International; 1-891676),* 6278 N. Federal Hwy., Suite 412, Fort Lauderdale, FL 33308 Tel 954-796-5008; Fax: 954-796-5009.

Manu Pub, *(Manu Publishing; 0-9652319),* Orders Addr.: P.O. Box 561, Pacific Palisades, CA 90272-0561 Tel 310-281-9770; Fax: 310-454-7841; Edit Addr.: 1027 Embury St., Pacific Palisades, CA 90272
Dist(s): **PSI Ful** *(P S I Fulfillment).*

Many Voices Pr, *(Many Voices Pr.; 0-9637277),* P.O. Box 2639, Cincinnati, OH 45201-2639 Tel 513-751-8020; Fax: 513-751-8060
E-mail: LynnW@manyvoicespress.com; lynnwatmv@aol.com
Web site: http://www.manyvoicespress.com.

Manzana, *(Manzana Pubns. & Program Services; 0-9660225),* Orders Addr.: P.O. Box 8122, Roanoke, VA 24012; Edit Addr.: 2620 Avenham Ave., SW, Roanoke, VA 24012 Tel 540-581-0852
E-mail: manzana@rev.net.

MAP Intl, *(MAP International; 1-879148),* Orders Addr.: P.O. Box 50, Brunswick, GA 31521-0050 Fax: 912-265-6170; Toll Free: 800-225-8550; Edit Addr.: 2200 Glynco Pkwy., Brunswick, GA 31521 Tel 912-265-6010
Dist(s): **Amrcns Snd AIDS** *(Americans for a Sound A I D S/H I V Policy).*

Maps Pub, *(Maps Publishing, Inc.; 1-886722),* 6203 Woodlake Ctr., San Antonio, TX 78244-3006 Tel 210-523-2424; Fax: 210-647-4554; Toll Free: 800-845-7638.

Mar Co Prods, *(MAR*CO Products, Inc.; 1-57543; 1-884063),* Orders Addr.: 1443 Old York Rd., Warminster, PA 18974 Tel 215-956-0313; Fax: 215-956-9041; Toll Free: 800-448-2197
E-mail: csfunk@marcoproducts.com
Web site: http://www.store.yahoo.com/marcoproducts; http://www.marcoproducts.com.

Marathon Intl Bk, *(Marathon International Bk. Co.; 0-915216; 1-928877),* P.O. Box 40, Madison, IN 47250-0040 (SAN 206-443X) Tel 812-273-4672; Fax: 812-273-4672
E-mail: jwortham@seidata.com.

MARC Pubns Imprint of World Vision Intl

†**March of Dimes,** *(March of Dimes Birth Defects Foundation; 0-86525),* 1275 Mamaroneck Ave., White Plains, NY 10605 (SAN 205-7441) Tel 914-428-7100; *CIP.*

Marciel Pub & Print, *(Marciel Publishing & Printing; 1-879331),* W. 4914 Richland Ave., Spokane, WA 99204 Tel 509-838-0061; Toll Free: 800-729-2315.

MarCin Enter, *(MarCin Enterprises; 0-9641671),* 1412 S. Douglas, Springfield, IL 62704 Tel 217-546-6833.

Mare Pub Dist, *(Mare Publishing & Distribution; 0-9632212),* Orders Addr.: P.O. Box 230311, Brooklyn, NY 11223; Edit Addr.: 1974 82nd St., Brooklyn, NY 11214 Tel 718-256-7928.

Mariah Manage, *(Mariah Management; 0-9662099),* 1153 Bergen Park Way, No. M438, Evergreen, CO 80439 Tel 303-526-5009; Fax: 303-526-7559; 29659 US Hwy. 40 W., Golden, CO 80401.

Mariel Pubns, *(Mariel Pubns.; 0-910919),* 196 Eddy Glover Blvd., New Britain, CT 06053 (SAN 272-2291) Tel 860-229-7382.

Mariner Bks Imprint of HM

Mark Sugar, *(Sugar, Mark; 0-9632757),* 4329 Avocado St., Los Angeles, CA 90027-2102.

Markbks, *(Markbooks; 0-911107),* P.O. Box 3230, Boulder, CO 80307 (SAN 272-2526).

Marketscope Bks, *(Marketscope Bks.; 0-934061),* 119 Richard Ct., Aptos, CA 95003 (SAN 692-9095) Tel 831-688-7535 (phone/fax)
E-mail: marketscope@webtv.net
Dist(s): **Sunbelt Pubns** *(Sunbelt Pubns., Inc.).*

Marlowe & Co, *(Marlowe & Co.; 1-56924),* 841 Broadway, 4th Flr., New York, NY 10003 Tel 212-614-7880; Fax: 212-614-7887
E-mail: avalonpub@aol.com
Web site: http://www.marlowepub.com
Dist(s): **Publishers Group** *(Publishers Group West)*
netLibrary CO *(netLibrary, Inc.).*

Marquette, *(Marquette Univ. Pr.; 0-87462),* P.O. Box 1881, Milwaukee, WI 53201-1881 Tel 414-288-1564; Fax: 414-288-3300
Web site: http://www.mu.edu/MUPRESS/
Dist(s): **BookMasters** *(BookMasters, Inc.).*

Marquis, *(Marquis Who's Who; 0-8379; 0-87876),* Div. of Reed Elsevier, Inc., 121 Chanlon Rd., New Providence, NJ 07974 (SAN 202-6120) Tel 908-464-6800; Fax: 908-464-3553; Toll Free: 800-521-8110
E-mail: serge.sarkis@renp.com
Web site: http://www.marquiswhoswho.com/.

Marrelli, *(Marrelli & Assocs., Inc.; 0-9647801),* Orders Addr.: P.O. Box 629, Boca Grande, FL 33921-0629 Tel 941-697-2900; Fax: 941-697-2901; Toll Free: 800-993-6397; Edit Addr.: 2800 Placida Rd., Suite 104, Englewood, FL 34224.

Marrelli Pubng, *See* **Marrelli**

Martin Dayton, *(Dayton, Martin; 0-9664838),* 18600 Collins Ave., Sunny Isles Beach, FL 33160 Tel 305-931-8484; Fax: 305-936-1849
E-mail: mddomddo@pol.net.

Martin Dunitz (GBR) *(0-948269; 1-85317; 0-906348; 1-84184) Dist. by* **Blackwell Sci.**

Martin Dunitz (GBR) *(0-948269; 1-85317; 0-906348; 1-84184) Dist. by* **Mosby Inc.**

Martin Dunitz (GBR) *(0-948269; 1-85317; 0-906348; 1-84184) Dist. by* **Thieme Med Pubs.**

Martino Pubng, *(Martino Publishing; 1-57898; 1-888262),* P.O. Box 373, Mansfield Center, CT 06250 Tel 860-429-4569; Fax: 860-429-4619; Toll Free: 800-771-2665
E-mail: martino@martinopublishing.com
Web site: http://www.martinopublishing.com
Dist(s): **Oak Knoll** *(Oak Knoll Pr.).*

Mary Bks, *(Mary Bks./Prelude Pr.; 0-931580; 1-929767),* 5806 Elizabeth Ct., Allen Park, MI 48101-2622 Fax: 313-928-3247
E-mail: marymac2000@aol.com
Web site: http://www.mcwilliams.com.

Maryland Pub, *See* **Olde Maryland**

MAS, *(MAS, Inc.; 0-9620723; 1-892537),* 111 S. Whittier St., Wichita, KS 67207 (SAN 249-8502) Tel 316-689-4225; Fax: 316-733-6091.

MAS Mktg, *(MAS Marketing; 0-9673193),* Orders Addr.: P.O. Box 4459, Helena, MT 59604 Tel 406-442-4016; Fax: 406-449-4814; Toll Free: 800-992-9111; Edit Addr.: 2513 Hertiage, Helena, MT 59601.

Mass CLE, *(Massachusetts Continuing Legal Education, Inc.; 0-944490; 1-57589),* 10 Winter Pl., Boston, MA 02108-4751 (SAN 226-3033) Tel 617-350-7006; Fax: 617-482-9498; Toll Free: 800-966-6253
Web site: http://www.mcle.org.

Mass Med Pub Div, *(Massachusetts Medical Society, Publishing Div., The; 0-910133; 0-9608238),* 10 Shattuck St., Boston, MA 02115 (SAN 666-6671) Toll Free: 800-445-8080
E-mail: support@massmed.org
Web site: http:www/mms.org.

Massage-Muscle, *(Massage/Muscle Therapy Productions; 0-9662677),* 608 Main St., Bolton, MA 01740 Tel 978-779-2994; Fax: 978-779-0448
E-mail: mmt@ma.ultranet.com
Web site: http://members.aol.com/bsmttank/equine.htm.

Masson (FRA) *(2-225) Dist. by* **IBD Ltd.**

Mast Hlth Grp, *(Mast Health Group; 0-9633017),* 2001 Thoroughbred Dr., Virginia Beach, VA 23456-6624.

Master Bks, *(Master Bks.; 0-89051),* P.O. Box 727, Green Forest, AR 72638-0727 (SAN 205-6119) Tel 870-438-5288; Fax: 870-438-5120; Toll Free: 800-999-3777
E-mail: nlp@newleafpress
Web site: http://www.masterbooks.net.

Masterco Pr, *(Masterco Pr., Inc.; 0-912164),* P.O. Box 7382, Ann Arbor, MI 48107 (SAN 205-8774) Tel 313-428-8300; Toll Free: 800-666-4626.

Mateel Pr, *(Mateel Pr.; 0-9637599),* Orders Addr.: P.O. Box 1014, Redway, CA 95560; Edit Addr.: New Harn's Store, Bell Springs Rd., Garberville, CA 95440 Tel 707-923-2766.

Material Dev, *See* **TRR**

†**Materials Res,** *(Materials Research Society; 0-931837; 1-55899),* 506 Keystone Dr., Warrendale, PA 15086 (SAN 686-0125) Tel 724-779-3003; Fax: 724-779-8313
E-mail: info@mrs.org
Web site: http://www.mrs.org; *CIP.*

Maternity Ctr, *(Maternity Ctr. Assn.; 0-912758),* 281 Park Ave. S., 5th Flr., New York, NY 10010 (SAN 203-9729) Tel 212-777-5000; Fax: 212-777-9320
E-mail: mcabirth@aol.com
Web site: http://www.maternity.org/i.

Matreya, *(Matreya, Inc.),* 500 Tressler St., Pleasant Gap, PA 16823.

Maval Med Educ, *See* **Maval Pub**

Maval Pub, *(Maval Publishing, Inc.; 1-884083; 1-59134),* Div. of Maval Printing Co., 567 Harrison St., Denver, CO 80206-4534 Tel 303-320-1835; Fax: 303-320-1546
E-mail: maval@maval.com
Web site: http://www.maval.com
Dist(s): **Majors Scientific Bks Inc** *(Majors Scientific Bks., Inc.)*
Matthews Medical Bk Co *(Matthews Medical Bk. Co.).*

Max Pubns, *(Max Pubns.; 0-9633577),* 825 Malvern Hill, Alpharetta, GA 30202 Tel 770-664-0825; Fax: 770-740-0188.

Maximedia NM, *(Maximedia; 0-9639456),* Orders Addr.: P.O. Box 668, Questa, NM 87556; Edit Addr.: 255 Echo Forest Rd., Questa, NM 87556 Tel 505-586-1554.

Maxishare, *(Maxishare; 1-930605),* Div. of Children's Health System, Orders Addr.: P.O. Box 2041, Milwaukee, WI 53201 Fax: 414-266-3428; Toll Free: 800-444-7747; Edit Addr.: 10310A W. Watertown Polk Rd., Wauwatosa, WI 53226
E-mail: maxishare@shw.org
Web site: http://www.maxishare.com.

Mayer-Johnson, *(Mayer-Johnson Co.; 0-9609160; 1-884135),* Orders Addr.: P.O. Box 1579, Solana Beach, CA 92075-1579 (SAN 241-4007) Tel 858-550-0084; Fax: 858-550-0449; Edit Addr.: 6650 Flanders Dr., Suite F, San Diego, CA 92121 Tel 858-550-0084; 800-588-4548
E-mail: mayerj@mayer-johnson.com
Web site: http://www.mayer-johnson.com.

†**Mayfield Pub,** *(Mayfield Publishing Co.; 0-7674; 0-87484; 1-55934),* Div. of McGraw-Hill Companies, 1280 Villa St., Mountain View, CA 94041-1176 (SAN 202-8972) Tel 650-960-3222; Fax: 650-960-0328; Toll Free: 800-433-1279
E-mail: mjensen@mayfieldpub.com
Web site: http://www.mayfieldpub.com
Dist(s): **McGraw** *(McGraw-Hill Cos., The); CIP.*

Mayo Fndtn Med Ed & Res, *(Mayo Foundation for Medical Education & Research; 0-9627865; 1-893005),* 200 First St., SW, Rochester, MN 55905 Tel 507-284-8878; Fax: 507-266-0230; Toll Free: 800-297-1185
E-mail: development@mayo.edu
Web site: http://www.mayo.edu.

MB Pubs, *(MB Pubs.; 0-9650827),* 716 Mount Curve Blvd., Saint Paul, MN 55116-1159 Tel 612-699-4468; Fax: 612-699-4959
Dist(s): **Baker & Taylor** *(Baker & Taylor Bks.)*
Bookpeople *(Bookpeople)*
Distributors *(Distributors, The)*
Koen Bk Distributors *(Koen Bk. Distributors)*
New Leaf Dist *(New Leaf Distributing Co., Inc.)*
Nutri-Books Corp *(Nutri-Bks. Corp.)*
Quality Bks IL *(Quality Bks., Inc.).*

MBA Pub, *(MBA Publishing; 0-945795),* Div. of Macduff/Bunt Assocs., Orders Addr.: 925 East St., Walla Walla, WA 99362 (SAN 247-5677) Tel 509-529-0244; Fax: 509-529-8865
E-mail: mba@bmi.net.

MBG Indust Inc, *(MBG Industries, Inc.; 1-890215),* 9800 NW 47th Dr., Coral Springs, FL 33076-2602 Tel 954-344-0018; Fax: 954-796-0889.

MBI Pubg, *(MBI Publishing Co.; 0-7603; 0-87938; 0-912612),* Orders Addr.: c/o Motorbooks International Wholesalers & Distributors, P.O. Box 1, Osceola, WI 54020 (SAN 699-5462) Tel 800-826-6600; Edit Addr.: 729 Prospect Ave., Osceola, WI 54020 (SAN 169-9164) Tel 715-294-3345; Fax: 715-294-4448; Toll Free: 800-458-0454
E-mail: mbibks@motorbooks.com
Web site: http://www.motorbooks.com
Dist(s): **Motorbooks Intl** *(Motorbooks International Wholesalers & Distributors).*

Mc Gowan Pubns, *(Mc Gowan Pubns.; 1-928752),* P.O. Box 1375, Amherst, MA 01004-1375 Fax: 413-259-1744; Toll Free: 800-897-0999
E-mail: mcgconsl@pipeline.com
Web site: http://mcgowanpubs.com.

Mc Keith Pr (GBR) *(0-901260; 1-873566; 1-898683) Dist. by* **Cambridge U Pr.**

†**McBooks Pr,** *(McBooks Pr.; 0-935526; 1-59013),* 120 W. State St., Ithaca, NY 14850-9423 (SAN 213-8573) Tel 607-272-2114; Fax: 607-273-6068; Toll Free: 888-266-5711
E-mail: mcbooks@mcbooks.com
Web site: http://www.mcbooks.com
Dist(s): **LPC Group** *(LPC Group); CIP.*

McCall-Faure, *(McCall-Faure Pr.; 0-9605084),* 4203 W. 179th St., Torrance, CA 90504 Tel 310-833-7863.

McClanahan Pub, *(McClanahan Publishing Hse., Inc.; 0-913383),* P.O. Box 100, Kuttawa, KY 42055 (SAN 285-8371) Tel 270-388-9388; Fax: 270-388-6186; Toll Free: 800-544-6959
E-mail: books@kybooks.com
Web site: http://www.kybooks.com
Dist(s): **Barron White** *(White, Barron)*
Partners Pubs Grp *(Partners Pubs. Group, Inc.).*

McCland & Stewart, *(McClelland & Stewart/Tundra Bks.; 0-7710),* P.O. Box 1030, Plattsburgh, NY 12901 Tel 416-598-1114; Fax: 416-598-4002
Web site: http://www.mcclelland.com
Dist(s): **Random** *(Random Hse., Inc.).*

McConnell, *(McConnell, R.A.; 0-9610232),* 430 Kennedy Ave., Pittsburgh, PA 15214 (SAN 272-1600) Tel 412-321-1213
Web site: http://www.ramcconnell.com/
Dist(s): **Distributors** *(Distributors, The).*

†**McCutchan,** *(McCutchan Publishing Corp.; 0-8211),* Orders Addr.: 3220Blume Dr., No. 197, Richmond, CA 94806 (SAN 658-1188); Edit Addr.: 3220 Blume Dr., No. 197, Richmond, CA 94806 (SAN 203-9486) Tel 510-758-5510; Fax: 510-758-6078; Toll Free: 800-227-1540
E-mail: mccutchanpublish@aol.com
Web site: http://www.mccutchanpublishing.com; *CIP.*

†**McFarland & Co,** *(McFarland & Co., Inc. Pubs.; 0-7864; 0-89950),* P.O. Box 611, Jefferson, NC 28640 (SAN 215-093X) Tel 336-246-4460; Fax: 336-246-5018; Toll Free: 800-253-2187 (orders only)
E-mail: editorial@mcfarlandpub.com
Web site: http://www.mcfarlandpub.com; *CIP.*

McG-Queens Univ Pr (CAN) *(0-7709; 0-7735; 0-88629; 0-88911; 1-55240) Dist. by* **CUP Services.**

McGrath NH, *(McGrath; 0-8434),* c/o IDS, Lower Mill Rd., North Stratford, NH 03590
Dist(s): **Ayer** *(Ayer Co. Pubs., Inc.).*

†**McGraw,** *(McGraw-Hill Cos., The; 0-02; 0-07),* Orders Addr.: 860 Taylor Station Rd., Blacklick, OH 43004-0545 (SAN 200-254X) Fax: 614-755-5645; Toll Free: 800-338-3987 (college); 800-525-5003 (subscriptions); 800-352-3566 (books - US/Canada orders); 800-722-4726 (orders & customer service); P.O. Box 545, Blacklick, OH 43004-0545 ; *Imprints:* Apple Lange Med (Appleton & Lange Medical)
E-mail: customer.service@mcgraw-hill.com
Web site: http://www.ebooks.mcgraw-hill.com/; http://www.mcgraw-hill.com
Dist(s): **Sams Tech Pub** *(Sams Technical Publishing); CIP.*

McGraw-Hill Educ Grp, *(McGraw-Hill Education Group; 0-07; 0-7602; 0-8306; 0-911314; 0-917253; 1-55738),* Orders Addr.: P.O. Box 545, Blacklick, OH 43004-0545 (SAN 200-254X) Fax: 614-755-5645; Toll Free: 800-722-4726; Edit Addr.: Two Penn Plaza, New York, NY 10121 Tel 212-904-5423; Fax: 212-904-6096; c/o Grand Rapids Distribution Center, 3195 Wilson NW, Grand Rapids, MI 49544 (SAN 253-6420) Fax: 614-755-5611 ; *Imprints:* Irwn Prfssnl (Irwin Professional Publishing)
Web site: http://www.pbg.mcgraw-hill.com/
Dist(s): **IPG Chicago** *(Independent Pubs. Group)*
Jossey-Bass *(Jossey-Bass, Inc. Pubs.)*
Urban Land *(Urban Land Institute)*
netLibrary CO *(netLibrary, Inc.).*

McGraw-Hill HPD, *See* **McGraw-Hill Med Pub**

McGraw-Hill Interamer (ESP) *(84-486) Dist. by* **McGraw.**

McGraw-Hill Med Pub, *(McGraw-Hill Medical Publishing Div.; 0-07),* Div. of The McGraw-Hill Cos., Orders Addr.: P.O. Box 545, Blacklick, OH 43004-0545 (SAN 200-254X) Fax: 614-755-5645 (customer service); Toll Free: 800-722-4726 (bookstores & libraries); 800-262-4729 (customer service)
E-mail: customerservice@mcgraw-hill.com
Web site: http://www.mghmedical.com.

McGraw-Hill Prof, *See* **McGraw-Hill Educ Grp**

McGraw-Hill Prof, *(McGraw-Hill Professional; 0-07),* Orders Addr.: P.O. Box 545, Blacklick, OH 43004-0545 Fax: 614-755-5645; Toll Free: 800-722-4726; Edit Addr.: 2 Penn Plaza, New York, NY 10121 Tel 212-904-2000 ; *Imprints:* Contemporary (Contemporary Books) Tch Yourself (Teach Yourself)
Dist(s): **McGraw-Hill Trade** *(McGraw-Hill Trade).*

McGraw-Hill Trade, *(McGraw-Hill Trade; 0-07; 0-658),* Div. of McGraw-Hill Professional, Orders Addr.: P.O. Box 545, Blacklick, OH 43004-0545 Tel 800-722-4726; Fax: 614-755-5645; Edit Addr.: 2 Penn Plaza, New York, NY 10121 Tel 212-904-2000 ; *Imprints:* Schaums Outline (Schaum's Outline Series) Ragged Mtn (Ragged Mountain Press) Contemporary (Contemporary Books) Tch Yourself (Teach Yourself) Keats Pubng (Keats Publishing) VGM Career Bks (VGM Career Books) Mstrs Press (Masters Press) Passport Bks (Passport Books)
Web site: http://www.books.mcgraw-hill.com.

McGrw-H College Imprint of McGrw-H Hghr Educ

McGrw-H Hghr Educ, *(McGraw-Hill Higher Education; 0-07),* Div. of the McGraw-Hill Professional Publishing Group, Orders Addr.: P.O. Box 545, Blacklick, OH 43004-0545 (SAN 200-254X); Edit Addr.: 1333 Burr Ridge Pkwy., Burr Ridge, IL 60521 ; *Imprints:* WCB McGr Hill (WCB/McGraw-Hill) Irwn McGrw-H (Irwin/McGraw-Hill) Dshkn McG-Hill (Dushkin/McGraw-Hill) McGrw-H College (McGraw-Hill College)
Web site: http://www.mhhe.com.

McGrw-H Primis Cstm, *(McGraw-Hill Primis Custom Publishing; 0-390),* A Unit of McGraw-Hill Higher Education, Div. of the McGraw-Hill Cos. Educational & Professional Publishing Group, 148 Princeton-Hightstown Rd., Hightstown, NJ 08520-1450 Tel 609-426-5721; Toll Free: 800-962-9342.

McGuire & Beckley, *(McGuire & Beckley Bks.; 0-9635890),* Orders Addr.: P.O. Box 770445, Cleveland, OH 44107; Edit Addr.: 1298 Thoreau Rd., Cleveland, OH 44107 Tel 216-521-2316.

MCK, *(MCK; 0-9660594),* 5201 Five Points Rd., Indianapolis, IN 46239 Tel 317-862-2138; Fax: 317-865-2952.

†**McKay,** *(McKay, David Co., Inc.; 0-679; 0-88326; 0-89440),* Subs. of Random Hse., Inc., Orders Addr.: 400 Hahn Rd., Westminster, MD 21157 (SAN 202-5515) Tel 410-848-1900; Toll Free: 800-733-3000 (orders only); Edit Addr.: 201 E. 50th St., MD 4-6, New York, NY 10022 (SAN 200-240X) Tel 212-751-2600; Fax: 212-872-8026; *CIP.*

MCL Assocs, *(MCL Assocs.; 0-930696),* **P.O. Box 26, McLean, VA 22101-0026 (SAN 281-9589) Tel 703-356-5979.**

McLean County, *(McLean County Historical Society; 0-943788),* 200 N. Main St., Bloomington, IL 61701 (SAN 241-0362) Tel 309-827-0428; Fax: 309-827-0100
E-mail: gregkoos@mchistory.org
Web site: http://www.mchistory.org.

McLean Research Assocs, *See* **Spectrum Biosci**

McMahon Grp, *(McMahon Group; 0-9641623),* 545 W. 45th St. 8th flr., New York, NY 11238 Tel 212-957-5300; Fax: 212-620-5928.

MCP Hahn Schl, *(MCP Hahnemann School of Medicine; 0-9658774; 0-9658980),* Div. of Allegheny Univ. of the Health Sciences, 2900 Queen Ln., Philadelphia, PA 19129 Tel 215-991-8450; Fax: 215-843-0253
E-mail: mcphuHelp@drexel.edu
Web site: http://www.mcphu.edu.

†**McPherson & Co,** *(McPherson & Co.; 0-914232; 0-929701),* Orders Addr.: P.O. Box 1126, Kingston, NY 12402 (SAN 203-0624) Tel 845-331-5807; Toll Free: 800-613-8219
E-mail: bmcpher@ulster.net
Web site: http://www.mcphersonco.com
Dist(s): **SPD-Small Pr Dist** *(SPD-Small Pr. Distribution); CIP.*

McRay, *(McRay Co.; 0-9636311),* 780 N. Arm Dr., Mound, MN 55364 Tel 612-475-4003; Fax: 612-472-5969.

MCS Pubns KY, *(MCS Pubns.; 0-933811),* P.O. Box 486, Murray, KY 42071 (SAN 692-7742) Tel 502-753-7750.

MD Vet Med Assn, *(Maryland Veterinary Medical Assn.; 0-9615658),* Box 439, Fallston, MD 21047 (SAN 695-9563) Tel 410-879-9108.

MDTA Pr, *(MDTA Pr.; 0-929517),* Div. of Management Development & Training Assocs., 11 Cedarford Ct., Palm Coast, FL 32137-8949 (SAN 249-5902) Tel 813-787-5530.

Meadow Mtn Pr, *(Meadow Mountain Pr.; 0-9647692),* Div. of Meadow Mountain Productions., 1375 Coney Island Ave., Suite 136, Brooklyn, NY 11230 (SAN 287-7023) Tel 718-338-1559; Fax: 718-258-4566; Toll Free: 800-444-2524 (orders).

†**Meadowbrook,** *(Meadowbrook Pr.; 0-88166; 0-915658),* 5451 Smetana Dr., Minnetonka, MN 55343 (SAN 207-3404) Tel 612-930-1100; Fax: 612-930-1940; Toll Free: 800-338-2232
E-mail: mballard@meadowbrookpress.com
Web site: http://www.meadowbrookpress.com
Dist(s): **S&S Childrens** *(Simon & Schuster Children's Publishing)*
S&S Trade *(Simon & Schuster Trade); CIP.*

Meadowlark Springs, *(Meadowlark Springs Productions; 0-9703371),* Orders Addr.: P.O. Box 4460, Marbleton, WY 83113 Tel 307-276-5454; Fax: 307-276-5276; Edit Addr.: 353 Mickelson Ln., Big Piney, WY 83113
E-mail: wtclose@trib.com.

Meckler Corp, *See* **Mecklermedia**

†**Mecklermedia,** *(Mecklermedia Corp.; 0-88736; 0-913672; 0-930466; 1-57207),* 16 Thorndal Cir., Westport, CT 06820-5421 (SAN 211-0334)
E-mail: info@mecklermedia.com; *CIP.*

MecPublishing, *(MecPublishing; 0-9672285),* Orders Addr.: P.O. Box 22, Morgantown, PA 19543 Tel 610-286-9926; Edit Addr.: 125 W. Main St., Morgantown, PA 19543.

Med Acupuncture, *(Medical Acupuncture Pubs.; 1-57250),* Orders Addr.: P.O. Box 815, Berkeley, CA 94701 Fax: 510-841-3250; Edit Addr.: 2520 Milvia St., Berkeley, CA 94704.

Med Ad Hall Fame, *(Medical Advertising Hall of Fame; 0-9667793),* 200 Madison Ave., 9th Flr., New York, NY 10016 Tel 212-251-7900; Fax: 212-689-1062
E-mail: patconno@aol.com; ron.pantello@hview.com.

Med Alternat, *(Medical Alternative Pr.; 0-9660882),* 4173 Fieldbrook Rd., West Bloomfield, MI 48323 Tel 248-851-3372; Fax: 248-851-0421; Toll Free: 888-647-5616 Do not confuse with Medical Alternative Pr., Colleyville, TX
Web site: http://www.drbrownstein.com.

Med Assn Atlanta, *(Medical Assn. of Atlanta; 0-9647461),* 875 W. Peachtree St., NW, Atlanta, GA 30309 Tel 408-881-1020; Fax: 404-872-0601.

Med Cnslt Grp, *(Medical Consulting Group; 0-9631819),* P.O. Box 1558, Arlington, MA 02474 Tel 781-646-6466; Fax: 781-646-4666; Toll Free: 800-851-8518 (orders only)
E-mail: mcg@mcgbooks.com
Web site: http://www.mcgbooks.com
Dist(s): **Majors Scientific Bks Inc** *(Majors Scientific Bks., Inc.)*
Matthews Bk Co *(Matthews Bk. Co.)*
Rittenhouse *(Rittenhouse Bk. Distributors).*

Med Coll of OH Pr, *(Medical College of Ohio Pr.; 0-944742),* Div. of Medical College of Ohio, Toledo, 3000 Arlington Ave., Toledo, OH 43614 (SAN 244-9919) Tel 419-383-4267; Fax: 419-385-6351.

Med Coll PA ASCWM, *(Medical College of Pennsylvania, Archives & Special Collections on Women in Medicine; 0-944542),* 3200 Henry Ave., Conference Ctr., Philadelphia, PA 19129 (SAN 243-9255) Tel 215-842-4700; Fax: 215-843-0349
E-mail: archivesmcphu@drexel.edu.

Med Communications, *(Medical Communications & Services Assn.; 0-917054),* 10223 NE 58th St., Kirkland, WA 98033 (SAN 203-9796) Tel 425-828-4263; Toll Free: 888-272-7022
E-mail: jayswakefield@yahoo.com.

†Med Econ, *(Medical Economics Co.; 0-87489; 0-942036; 1-56363; 1-880080),* 5 Paragon Dr., Montvale, NJ 07645-1742 (SAN 253-0562) Tel 201-358-7522; 201-358-7500; Fax: 201-358-7450; Toll Free Fax: 877-737-3535; Toll Free: 800-442-6657 ; *Imprints:* PDR (Physician's Desk Reference (PDR))
E-mail: medec@aol.com; linda.levine@medec.com
Web site: http://www.pdr.net; *CIP.*

Med Econ Data, *See* **Med Econ**

Med Ed Az, *(Med Ed, Inc.; 0-9628311),* P.O. Box 40696, Mesa, AZ 85282 Tel 602-345-1943; Fax: 602-831-1165.

Med Educ, *See* **Med Nurs Educ**

Med Group Mgmt, *See* **M G M A**

Med Info Internatl, *(Medical Information International; 0-9620473),* Orders Addr.: P.O. Box 241, Creswell, OR 97426-0241 (SAN 248-6636) Tel 541-895-2314 (phone/fax); Edit Addr.: 82099 Lost Creek Rd., Dexter, OR 97431 (SAN 248-6644) Tel 541-937-2226
E-mail: medinfoint@aol.com.

Med Info Srvs, *See* **CTA Resrch Corp**

Med Ins Servs, *(Medical Insurance Services; 0-9643510),* P.O. Box 238, Lynn, NC 28750-0238 Tel 828-859-5692 (phone/fax)
E-mail: clarkcon@aol.com.

Med Lang Dev, *(Medical Language Development; 0-9663470),* 33H Foxboro Ct., Princeton, NJ 08540-1729 Tel 609-924-4748
E-mail: georgecmt@aol.com
Web site: http://www.workingfrom.homestead.com.

Med Learn, *(Medical Learning, Inc.; 1-889115; 1-931136),* 245 E. Sixth St., Suite 502, Saint Paul, MN 55101 Fax: 651-229-0835; Toll Free: 800-252-1578
E-mail: slappen@medlearn.com; lmaxwell@medlearn.com
Web site: http://www.medlearn.com.

Med Letter, *(Medical Letter, Inc., The; 0-9660510),* 1000 Main St., 2nd Flr., New Rochelle, NY 10801-7537 (SAN 223-7938) Tel 914-235-0500; Fax: 914-576-1733; Toll Free: 800-211-2769
E-mail: custserv@themedicalletter.org
Web site: http://www.medletter.com.

Med Lib Assn, *(Medical Library Assn., Inc.; 0-912176),* 65 E. Wacker Pl., Suite 1900, Chicago, IL 60601-7298 Tel 312-419-9094; Fax: 312-419-8950
Web site: http://www.mlanet.org.

Med Litigation, *(Medical Litigation; 0-9626905),* One Gateway Ctr., Newark, NJ 07102-5315.

Med Manor Bks, *(Medical Manor Bks.; 0-934232),* Subs. of Manor Hse. Pubns., Inc., 3501 Newberry Rd., Philadelphia, PA 19154 (SAN 217-2526) Tel 215-637-9255; Fax: 215-632-2176; Toll Free: 800-343-8464
E-mail: medmanor@bellatlantic.net
Web site: http://www.diet-step.com
Dist(s): **Baker & Taylor** *(Baker & Taylor Bks.)*
BookWorld *(BookWorld Services, Inc.)*
Bookpeople *(Bookpeople)*
Distributors *(Distributors, The)*
Koen Bk Distributors *(Koen Bk. Distributors)*
Quality Bks IL *(Quality Bks., Inc.)*
Unique Bks Inc *(Unique Bks., Inc.).*

Med Nurs Educ, *(Medical & Nursing Education Consultants; 0-937142),* Box 67159, Century City, Los Angeles, CA 90067 (SAN 209-2891) Tel 310-475-5141 (phone/fax).

Med Physics Pub, *(Medical Physics Publishing; 0-944838; 1-930524),* 4513 Vernon Blvd., Madison, WI 53705-4964 (SAN 245-7407) Tel 608-262-4021; Fax: 608-265-2121; Toll Free: 800-442-5778 ; *Imprints:* Cogito Bks (Cogito Books)
E-mail: junej@medicalphysics.org
Web site: http://www.medicalphysics.org.

Med Plastics Lab Inc, *(Medical Plastics Laboratory, Inc.; 0-9713433),* Div. of Laerdal Medical Corp., Orders Addr.: P.O. Box 38, Gatesville, TX 76528 Tel 254-865-7221; Fax: 254-865-1150; Toll Free: 800-433-5539; Edit Addr.: 226 FM 116, Gatesville, TX 76528
E-mail: marketing@mpltx.com
Web site: http://www.medicalplastics.com.

Med Prod, *(Medical Productions, Inc.; 0-933745),* Orders Addr.: P.O. Box 270776, Houston, TX 77277-0776 (SAN 692-8544) Fax: 713-666-3299; Edit Addr.: 5308C Elm, Houston, TX 77081 (SAN 692-5979) Tel 713-666-4269.

Med Res Assocs, *(Medical Research Assocs. Pubns.; 0-930835),* Subs. of AV-Nurse International, P.O. Box 1247, Ballwin, MO 63022 (SAN 677-685X) Tel 314-569-7763.

Med Res Modern, *(Medical Research Modernization Committee; 0-9623858),* Orders Addr.: P.O. Box 2751, New York, NY 10163-2751 Tel 212-579-3477; Fax: 216-283-6702
E-mail: staufman@aol.net
Web site: http://www.mrmcmed.org.

Med Risk Mgmt, *(Medical Risk Management, Inc.; 1-884269),* 8 Greenway Plaza, Suite 1120, Houston, TX 77046 Tel 713-629-4700; Fax: 713-629-8080; Toll Free: 800-728-2375.

Med Sci Pub, *(Medical Science Publishing International, Inc.; 0-9638210),* 403 Main St., Port Washington, NY 11050 Tel 516-944-7340; Fax: 516-944-8663.

Med Software, *(Medical Software Co.; 0-88672),* Div. of Computer Medica Corp., 860 Fifth Ave., New York, NY 10021 (SAN 265-1661) Tel 212-794-2000; 860 Fifth Ave., Apt. 10E, New York, NY 10021 (SAN 667-4593) Tel 212-794-9588.

Med Staff Pr, *(Medical Staff Pr., LLC; 0-9653101),* 3319 Park Ridge Dr., NE, Grand Rapids, MI 49525-7037 (SAN 299-0474) Tel 616-363-8655; Toll Free: 800-826-4944
E-mail: civilmed@aol.com
Web site: http://www.iserv.net/~civilmed
Dist(s): **Baker & Taylor** *(Baker & Taylor Bks.)*
Brodart *(Brodart Co.)*
Partners Pubs Grp *(Partners Pubs. Group, Inc.)*
Quality Bks IL *(Quality Bks., Inc.)*
Unique Bks Inc *(Unique Bks., Inc.).*

Med Surveill, *(Medical Surveillance, Inc.; 0-942447),* Orders Addr.: P.O. Box 480, Willow Grove, PA 19090 (SAN 667-2922) Tel 215-784-0976; Fax: 215-657-1475; Toll Free: 800-417-3189
E-mail: medsurvellance@aol.com
Web site: http://medicalsurvellance.com.
Dist(s): **Majors Scientific Bks Inc** *(Majors Scientific Bks., Inc.)*
Rittenhouse *(Rittenhouse Bk. Distributors).*

Med Tribune, *(Medical Tribune, Inc.; 0-931861),* 444 Park Ave. S., Rm. 503, New York, NY 10016-7321 (SAN 686-0559) Tel 212-674-8500.

Medawellcom Imprint of Engin Systms Sol

MedBooks, *(MedBooks; 0-923369),* 101 W. Buckingham Rd., Richardson, TX 75081-4802 (SAN 252-0788) Tel 972-643-1809; Fax: 972-994-0215; Toll Free: 800-443-7397.

Medex Pr, *See* **HlthSavers Pr**

Med-Facts, *(Med-Facts, Inc.; 1-884006),* 16240 San Fernando Mission Blvd., Granada Hills, CA 91344 Tel 818-363-5156; Toll Free: 800-633-3227.

Medfo, *(Medfo Publishing; 1-930822),* Div. of Medfo Inc., 6110 Ninth St., N., Saint Petersburg, FL 33703 Fax: 727-527-6961
E-mail: jplshaw@aol.com
Web site: http://antiagingrevolution.com.

Medford Press Imprint of Plexus Pub

Medhumor, *(Medhumor Pubns.; 0-9700287),* 1127 High Ridge Rd., Suite 332, Stamford, CT 06905 Tel 203-406-4298; Fax: 203-323-9036
E-mail: info@mdhumor.com
Web site: http://www.passtheboards.com; http://www.mdhumor.com.

Media Ctr, *(Media Ctr., Schl. of Veterinary Medicine, Tuskegee Univ.; 0-9645067),* A102 Patterson Hall, Tuskegee, AL 36088 Tel 205-727-8308; Fax: 205-727-8177.

Media Institute, *(Media Institute, The; 0-937790),* 1000 Potomac St., NW, Suite 301, Washington, DC 20007 (SAN 215-966X) Tel 202-298-7512; Fax: 202-337-7092
E-mail: tmi@clark.net
Web site: http://www.mediainst.org.

Media Mktg Group, *(Media Marketing Group; 0-933474),* P.O. Box 611, DeKalb, IL 60115 (SAN 241-7790) Tel 815-895-6842
Dist(s): **Baker & Taylor** *(Baker & Taylor Bks.).*

Media Pub, *(Media Publishing; 0-939644),* Div. of Trozzolo Resources, Inc., 802 Broadway St., Suite 300, Kansas City, MO 64105-1528 (SAN 216-6372) Tel 816-842-8111; Fax: 816-842-8188; Toll Free: 800-347-2665 ; *Imprints:* Midgrd Press (Midgard Press) Do not confuse with Media Publishing, Miami, FL
Dist(s): **Baker & Taylor** *(Baker & Taylor Bks.).*

Media Syncresis, *See* **Ajna Media**

Medic Pub, *(Medic Publishing Co.; 0-934230),* P.O. Box 89, Redmond, WA 98073 (SAN 210-8313) Tel 425-881-2883; Fax: 425-867-8939 Do not confuse with Medic Publishing, Gaston, SC.

Medic Pub SC, *(Medic Publishing; 0-9656879),* Orders Addr.: P.O. Box 760, Gaston, SC 29053 Tel 803-796-9131; Fax: 803-874-1242; Edit Addr.: 201 Mill St., Saint Matthews, SC 29135 Do not confuse with Medic Publishing Co., Redmond, WA
E-mail: ccems@ix.netcom.com.

Medical Alumni Association of Univ, *(Medical Alumni Assn. of the Univ. of Maryland, Inc.; 0-9619119),* 522 W. Lombard St., Baltimore, MD 21201-1636 (SAN 243-5195) Tel 410-706-7454; Fax: 410-706-3658
E-mail: maa@medalumni.umartland.edu
Web site: http://www.medicalalumni.org.

Medical Arts, *(Medical Arts Publishing Co.; 0-913092),* P.O. Box 36600, Grosse Pointe, MI 48236 (SAN 202-2184) Tel 313-886-5160; Fax: 313-886-4288.

Medical Comm Imprint of Comm Unltd CA

Medical Exam Imprint of Appleton & Lange

Medical Info, *(Medical Information Systems, Inc.; 1-891953),* 25 Horseshoe Ln., Stamford, CT 06903 Tel 203-322-1164; Fax: 203-595-9069; Toll Free: 800-595-8649 Do not confuse with Medical Information Systems, Port Washington, NY
Web site: http://medicalinfosystems.com.

Medical Info Assocs, *(Medical Information Assocs.; 0-9656764),* 401 Hickorywood Blvd., Morrisville, NC 27560 Tel 919-468-9960.

Medical Mgmt, *See* **Robert D Keene**

Medical Priority, *(Medical Priority Consultants, Inc.; 0-9658890),* 139 E. South Temple, Suite 500, Salt Lake City, UT 84111 Tel 801-363-9127; Fax: 801-363-9144; Toll Free: 800-363-9127
E-mail: info@MedicalPriority.com.

Medical Recs, *(Medical Records Institute; 0-9640667; 1-893378),* Orders Addr.: 567 Walnut St., Newton, MA 02460 Tel 617-964-3923; Fax: 617-964-3926; Edit Addr.: 567 Walnut St., Newton, MA 02460
E-mail: cust_serv@medrecinst.com
Web site: http://www.medrecinst.com.

Medical Srvs, *(Medical Services Research Group; 0-9643336),* 1407 Union Ave., Suite 200, Memphis, TN 38104 Tel 901-726-6808; Fax: 901-726-9028.

Medical Trading Ctr, *(Medical Trading Ctr.; 0-9667937),* 2 French St., East Brunswick, NJ 08816 Tel 732-238-7583
E-mail: morrisbl@bellatlantic.net.

Medicina Bio, *(Medicina Biologica),* 2937 NE Flanders St., Portland, OR 97232 (SAN 113-0226) Tel 503-287-6775; Fax: 503-235-3520
E-mail: med_bio@imagina.com.

Medicine Grp USA, *(Medicine Group USA, Inc., The; 0-944036; 1-57130),* 5 Neshaminy Interplex, Suite 103, Trevose, PA 19053 (SAN 242-7486) Tel 215-244-8840; Fax: 215-244-8850; Toll Free: 800-220-8358
E-mail: reception@cincint-inc.com.

Medi-Ed Pr, *(Medi-Ed Pr.; 0-936741),* 5 White Pl., Bloomington, IL 61701 (SAN 699-9530) Tel 309-827-4620; Fax: 309-829-3378; Toll Free: 800-500-8205.

Medieval & Renaissance NY, *See* **MRTS**

†Medieval Inst, *(Medieval Institute Pubns.; 0-918720; 1-58044; 1-879288),* Medieval Institute Publications Walwood Hall, Western Michigan Univ., 1903 W. Michigan Ave., Kalamazoo, MI 49008-5432 (SAN 212-2928) Tel 616-387-8755; Fax: 616-387-8750
E-mail: cynthia.seedorff@wmich.edu; seiler@wmich.edu
Web site: http://www.wmich.edu/medieval/mip; *CIP.*

Medilex Co, *(Medilex Co., The; 0-916763),* Subs. of Robert Stephan Jr. PC, 371 E. Monte Vista, Phoenix, AZ 85004 (SAN 654-3340) Tel 602-241-1400.

Med-Info Bks, *(Medical-Info Bks.; 0-916093),* 2929 SE Ocean Blvd., Apt. 127-7, Stuart, FL 34996 (SAN 294-6114).

MediPress, *(MediPress; 0-9636979),* P.O. Box 5154, Coeur D'Alene, ID 83814-1952 (SAN 298-5462) Fax: 208-765-6924; Toll Free: 800-775-5300
E-mail: healinglights@icehouse.net.

MediPro Mgmt, *(MediPro Management/Pubns.; 0-9631623),* 100 Highland Ave., Millinocket, ME 04462-1517 Tel 207-723-4820.

Medi-Record, *(Medi-Record International, Inc.; 0-9632430),* 9031 S. Fawcett Ave., Tacoma, WA 98444-6248 Tel 206-473-5636; 10507 Gravelly Lake Dr. SW, Suite 15A-307, Tacoma, WA 98498 Tel 206-537-7714.

MediSci Pubs, *(MediScience Pubs.; 0-938869),* P.O. Box 256, Deerfield, IL 60015 (SAN 662-5304) Tel 708-564-1040.

MedLaw Bks Inc, *(MedLaw Bks., Inc.; 0-9660525),* Orders Addr.: P.O. Box 4007, Eire, PA 16512-4007; Edit Addr.: 4204 French St., Erie, PA 16504 Tel 814-868-0900; Fax: 814-868-1485.

MedLaw Inc, *See* **MedLaw Bks Inc**

Med-Legal.net, *See* **KC Press**

MedMaster, *(MedMaster, Inc.; 0-940780),* Orders Addr.: P.O. Box 640028, Miami, FL 33164 (SAN 219-7960) Tel 954-962-8414; Fax: 954-962-4508; Toll Free: 800-335-3480; Edit Addr.: 3337 Hollywood Oaks Dr., Fort Lauderdale, FL 33312
E-mail: stgoldberg@aol.com.

Med-Natl Consult, *(Med-National Consulting Group; 1-892923),* 1010 Central Pkwy., S., San Antonio, TX 78232 Tel 210-490-4515; Fax: 210-490-5742; Toll Free: 800-725-6364
E-mail: drjimspring@sprintmail.com
Web site: http://www.mnconsultinggroup.com.

Medpharm Sci Pubs (DEU) *(3-88763) Dist. by* **Medicina Bio.**

MedPoint Pr, *(MedPoint Pr.; 0-9677909),* Orders Addr.: P.O. Box 701, Springvale, ME 04083 Tel 207-324-9088; Edit Addr.: 11 Marginal Way, Springvale, ME 04083
E-mail: dfs@medpointpress.com
Web site: http://www.medpointpress.com.

MedPress, *(MedPress; 0-9671107),* Orders Addr.: P.O. Box 691546, San Antonio, TX 78269 Tel 210-699-9007; Fax: 210-641-6334; Edit Addr.: 11238 Jade Green, San Antonio, TX 78249 Toll Free: 888-633-9898
E-mail: info@medpress.com
Web site: http://www.medpress.com.

MEDSTAT Systs, *(MEDSTAT Systems, Inc.; 0-9641308),* 777 E. Eisenhower Pkwy., Ann Arbor, MI 48108 Tel 313-913-3469; Fax: 313-913-3500.

MedStudy, *(MedStudy Corp.; 0-9640788; 0-9708767),* Orders Addr.: P.O. Box 6008, Woodland Park, CO 80866 Tel 719-687-8382; Fax: 719-687-8386; Toll Free: 800-841-0547; Edit Addr.: 400 W. Midland, Suite 250, Woodland Park, CO 80863
E-mail: dgantos@medstudy.com
Web site: http//:www.medstudy.com.

Medsurg, *(Medsurg Assocs.; 0-9710958),* Orders Addr.: P.O. Box 1454, Coatesville, PA 19320 Tel 610-383-5610; Fax: 610-383-9038; Edit Addr.: 203 E. Lincoln Hwy., Coatesville, PA 19320
E-mail: jstephe@earthlink.net
Web site: http://www.healthyhajj.com.

Medtext, *(Medtext; 0-9629279),* 15W560 89th St., Hinsdale, IL 60521 Tel 708-325-3277; Fax: 708-887-1446
Dist(s): **Baker & Taylor** *(Baker & Taylor Bks.)*
Brodart *(Brodart Co.).*

MEDTEXT Med, *(MEDTEXT Medical Publishing Co.; 0-9635538; 1-889344),* 409 N. Pacific Coast Hwy., Suite 384, Redondo Beach, CA 90277 Tel 310-379-1263; Fax: 310-379-5183; Toll Free: 800-232-8398.

Med-Travel Bks, *(Med-Travel Bks.; 0-9638226),* 301 Ripple Rd., River Ridge, LA 70123 Tel 504-866-3582; Fax: 504-738-3085
Dist(s): **Baker & Taylor** *(Baker & Taylor Bks.)*
Quality Bks IL *(Quality Bks., Inc.).*

Meeta Goswami, *(Meeta/Goswami; 0-9667122),* Montefiore Med. Ctr., 111 E. 210th St., Bronx, NY 10467 Tel 718-920-6799; Fax: 718-654-9580
E-mail: wgoswami@aol.com.

Melbourne Univ Pr (AUS) *(0-522) Dist. by* **Paul & Co Pubs.**

†**Melius Pub,** *(Melius Publishing, Inc.; 0-937603; 0-9610130),* Div. of Video Resources, Inc., 118 River Rd., Pierre, SD 57501 (SAN 262-7477) Tel 605-224-1929; Toll Free: 800-882-5171; *CIP.*

Melrose (GBR) *(0-900332; 0-948875; 0-9501016) Dist. by* **Taylor & Francis.**

Memoirs Unltd, *(Memoirs Unlimited; 1-889833),* 21 Lothrop St., Beverly, MA 01915 Tel 978-921-0747; Fax: 978-927-8195
E-mail: memoirs@mediaone.net.

Memory Skills, *(Memory Skills; 0-9627777),* 1439 E. Park Pl., Ann Arbor, MI 48104 Tel 313-764-2556.

MemoryMinder, *(MemoryMinder Journals, Inc.; 0-9637968),* Orders Addr.: P.O. Box 23108, Eugene, OR 97402 Tel 541-342-2300; Fax: 541-342-6000; Toll Free: 800-888-3392
Web site: http://www.memoryminder.com
Dist(s): **New Leaf Dist** *(New Leaf Distributing Co., Inc.).*

MemoryMinder Journals, *See* **MemoryMinder**

†**Menasha Ridge,** *(Menasha Ridge Pr., Inc.; 0-89732),* 2000 First Ave., N., Suite 1400, Birmingham, AL 35203 (SAN 219-7294) Tel 205-322-0439; Fax: 205-326-1012; Toll Free: 800-247-9437
E-mail: info@menasharidge.com
Web site: http://www.menasharidge.com
Dist(s): **Globe Pequot** *(Globe Pequot Pr., The); CIP.*

Mendocino Found Health, *(Mendocino Foundation for Health Education, The; 0-9615167),* P.O. Box 1377, Mendocino, CA 95460 (SAN 694-308X) Tel 707-964-0425.

Menieres Aust (AUS) *Dist. by* **St Mut.**

Ment Imprint of NAL

Menta Pubns, *(Menta Pubns.; 0-935688; 0-9657303),* P.O. Box 632, Alexandria, LA 71309
E-mail: rhh43@aztec.asu.edu.

Mental Hlth KY, *(Mental Health Assn. of Northern Kentucky; 1-889022),* 605 Madison Ave., Covington, KY 41011 Tel 606-431-1077; Fax: 606-292-2485
E-mail: mhnky@aol.com.

Mer Imprint of NAL

Mercat Pr Bks (GBR) *Dist. by* **St Mut.**

†**Mercer Univ Pr,** *(Mercer Univ. Pr.; 0-86554),* 6316 Peake Rd., Macon, GA 31210-3960 (SAN 220-0716) Tel 478-301-2880; Fax: 478-301-2264; Toll Free: 800-637-2378 (Ext. 2880 orders only); 800-342-0841 (Ext. 2880 in Georgia)
E-mail: mupressorders@mercer.edu
Web site: http://www.mupress.org; *CIP.*

Mercie Pub, *(Mercie Publishing; 0-9644355),* 9030 Napfield Dr., Spring, TX 77379 Tel 281-370-3724.

†**Merck,** *(Merck & Co., Inc.; 0-911910),* P.O. Box 2000, Rahway, NJ 07065 (SAN 202-6236) Tel 732-594-4600; Fax: 732-388-9778
Web site: http://www.merck.com; *CIP.*

Merck-Sharp-Dohme, *(Merck Sharp & Dohme International; 0-911910),* Professional Communications Dept., West Point, PA 19486 (SAN 212-1921).

†**Mercury Hse,** *(Mercury Hse.; 0-916515; 1-56279),*
E-mail: mercury@hooked.net
Web site: http://www.wenet.net/~mercury
Dist(s): **Consort Bk Sales** *(Consortium Bk. Sales & Distribution)*
Continental Bk *(Continental Bk. Co., Inc.); CIP.*

Mercury Pub, *(Mercury Publishing; 0-935717),* 1032 Canada Rd., Woodside, CA 94062 (SAN 695-9288) Tel 415-851-3515 Do not confuse with Mercury Publishing, Coral Springs, FL.

Mercy & Truth, *(Mercy & Truth Pubs.; 0-9615494),* Rte. 1, P.O. Box 503, Osceola, WI 54020 (SAN 696-379X) Tel 715-294-2052.

Mercy Ambulance, *See* **Amer Med Res**

Meriah-Morgan, *(Meriah-Morgan Pr.; 1-882678),* 8452 Fredricksburg Rd., Suite 144, San Antonio, TX 78229 Tel 512-492-1969; Fax: 512-492-5638.

Meridian Hill, *(Meridian Hill Pubns.; 0-940206),* 2435 Vance St., Lakewood, CO 80215 (SAN 220-3413) Tel 303-237-0755.

Meridian VA, *(Meridian Pubns.; 0-9657903),* Orders Addr.: P.O. Box 7987, Hampton, VA 23666 Tel 757-850-2963 Do not confuse with companies with the same name in Santa Monica, CA, Fort Lauderdale, FL
E-mail: dudley_delany@yahoo.com
Web site:
http://www.geocities.com/dudley_delany/meridian.html
Dist(s): **Baker & Taylor** *(Baker & Taylor Bks.)*
Matthews Medical Bk Co *(Matthews Medical Bk. Co.)*
New Leaf Dist *(New Leaf Distributing Co., Inc.).*

Merit Pub Intl, *(Merit Publishing International, Inc.; 1-873413),* 8260 NW 49th Manor, Coral Springs, FL 33067 Tel 954-755-4280; Fax: 954-755-4287
E-mail: meritpi@aol.com
Web site: http://www.meritpublishing.com
Dist(s): **Alliance Bk Co** *(Alliance Bk. Co.).*

Merkur Pubng, *(Merkur Publishing, Inc.; 0-9693820; 1-885928),* P.O. Box 171306, Salt Lake City, UT 84117 Tel 801-272-9008 (phone/fax); Toll Free: 800-204-2473 (USA only)
E-mail: merkurbook@aol.com
Web site: http://www.merkurpublishing.com
Dist(s): **Bro Life Inc** *(Brotherhood of Life, Inc.)*
New Leaf Dist *(New Leaf Distributing Co., Inc.)*
Partners-West *(Partners/West)*
Red Wheel ME *(Red Wheel).*

Merriam-Eddy, *(Merriam-Eddy Co., Inc.; 0-914562),* P.O. Box 25, South Waterford, ME 04081 (SAN 202-6252).

†**Merriam-Webster Inc,** *(Merriam-Webster, Inc.; 0-87779),* Subs. of Encyclopaedia Britannica, Inc., 47 Federal St., P.O. Box 281, Springfield, MA 01102 (SAN 202-6244) Tel 413-734-3134 (ext. 152); Fax: 413-731-5979; Toll Free: 800-828-1880
E-mail: mgeoghegan@Merriam-Webster.com; sales@Merriam-Webster.com
Web site: http://www.WordCentral.com; http://www.Merriam-Webster.com; *CIP.*

Merrill Coll Imprint of P-H

MES FX Pub, *(MES/FX Publishing; 0-9632877),* Orders Addr.: P.O. Box 21179, Cleveland, OH 44121; Edit Addr.: 2318 S. Overlook Rd., Cleveland Heights, OH 44106-3107 Tel 216-231-2581.

Mesa Pr, *(Mesa Pr.; 0-941938),* 5835 S. Kimbark Ave., Chicago, IL 60637 (SAN 215-3270) Tel 773-702-1596; Fax: 773-834-0326
E-mail: mesa@uchicago.edu
Web site: http://www.winsteps.com.

MESD Pr, *(MESD Pr.; 1-880118),* 11611 NE Ainsworth Cir., Portland, OR 97220 Tel 503-257-1582; Fax: 503-257-1519.

MET Pr, *(MET Pr.; 0-9647250),* Orders Addr.: P.O. Box 4577, East Lansing, MI 48826-4577 Tel 517-351-5248; Fax: 517-332-4196; Edit Addr.: 906 Lantern Hill Dr., East Lansing, MI 48823.

META Pubns, *(META Pubns.; 0-916990),* P.O. Box 1910, Capitola, CA 95010-1910 (SAN 208-7448) Tel 831-464-0254; Fax: 831-464-0517
E-mail: metapub@prodigy.net.

Metabolic Medicine, *(College of Metabolic Medicine; 0-9669422),* Orders Addr.: P.O. Box 103, Winfield, KS 67156 Tel 316-221-2035; 817-535-5681; Fax: 316-229-8840; Toll Free: 888-477-3618; Edit Addr.: 414 W. 12th St., Winfield, KS 67156.

Metamind Ent, *(Metamind Enterprises, Inc.; 0-9660843),* P.O. Box 5548, Savannah, GA 31416 Tel 912-598-8320; Fax: 912-598-4900
E-mail: enigma@syscom.com
Web site: http://www.metamind.net.

Metamorphic, *(Metamorphic Enterprises; 0-9634612),* 11135 Pima Rd., Dewey, AZ 86327-3623.

†**Metamorphous Pr,** *(Metamorphous Pr., Inc.; 0-943920; 1-55552),* Orders Addr.: P.O. Box 10616, Portland, OR 97296-0616 (SAN 110-8786) Tel 503-228-4972; Fax: 503-223-9117; Toll Free: 800-937-7771 (orders only); Edit Addr.: 2950 NW 29th Ave., Portland, OR 97210
E-mail: metabooks@metamodels.com
Web site: htp://www.metamodels.com; *CIP.*

Meth Hosp IN, *See* **Clarian Hlth**

Methuselah Bks, *(Methuselah Bks.; 0-937092),* 5325 Smith Ave., Richmond, VA 23228-6115 (SAN 214-4174).

MetriTech, *(MetriTech, Inc.; 0-9635895),* P.O. Box 6479, Champaign, IL 61826-6479 Tel 217-398-4868; Fax: 217-398-5798; Toll Free: 800-747-4868
E-mail: mtinfo@metritech.com
Web site: http://www.metritech.com.

Metro Deaf Senior, *(Metro Hearing Impaired Seniors, Inc.; 0-9613623),* 413 Wacouta St., Suite 300, Saint Paul, MN 55101-1648 (SAN 670-8757) Tel 612-647-9565.

Metron Pubns, *(Metron Pubns.; 0-940268),* P.O. Box 1213, Princeton, NJ 08542 (SAN 217-5401) Tel 609-430-0915 (phone/fax); Toll Free: 800-463-6474
E-mail: shape@mars.superlink.net
Web site: http://www.Grazian-archivel.com.

Meyer Rehab Inst, *See* **Munroe-Meyer Inst**

Meyerbooks, *(Meyerbooks; 0-916638),* Orders Addr.: P.O. Box 427, Glenwood, IL 60425 (SAN 208-998X) Tel 708-757-4950; Edit Addr.: 235 W. Main St., Glenwood, IL 60425 (SAN 658-1234).

Meyers Pub, *(Meyers Publishing; 0-937119),* 6025 NW 45th Way, Coconut Creek, FL 33073-1993 (SAN 658-5965) Tel 407-479-3566.

MGMA Ctr, *(MGMA Ctr. for Research; 0-933948),* Affil. of Medical Group Management Assn., 104 Inverness Terr., E., Englewood, CO 80112-5306 (SAN 230-9459) Tel 303-799-1111; Fax: 303-643-4429 Web site: http://www.mgma.com.

Mgmt Advantage, *(Management Advantage, Inc., The; 1-879876),* Orders Addr.: P.O. Box 3708, Walnut Creek, CA 94598-0708 Tel 925-671-0404; Fax: 925-825-3930; Toll Free: 888-671-0404 E-mail: info@management-advantage.com; tmainc@management-advantage.com Web site: http://www.management-advantage.com.

Mgmt Sci Health, *(Management Sciences for Health; 0-913723),* Orders Addr.: 165 Allandale Rd., Boston, MA 02130; Edit Addr.: 891 Centre St., Boston, MA 02130 Tel 617-524-7766; Fax: 617-524-1363 E-mail: bookstore@msh.org; development@msh.org Web site: http://www.msh.org.

†Mho & Mho, *(Mho & Mho Works; 0-917320),* Box 33135, San Diego, CA 92163 (SAN 238-7999) Tel 619-280-3488 E-mail: poo@cts.com Web site: http://www.ralphmag.org/mho.html; *CIP.*

Miami Univ Art, *(Miami Univ. Art Museum; 0-940784),* 801S.Patterson Ave., Oxford, OH 45056 (SAN 219-6042) Tel 513-529-2232; Fax: 513-529-6555.

†Micah Pubns, *(Micah Pubns.; 0-916288),* 255 Humphrey St., Marblehead, MA 01945 (SAN 209-1577) Tel 781-631-7601; Fax: 781-639-0772; Toll Free: 877-268-9963 E-mail: micah@micahbooks.com Web site: http://www.micahbooks.com *Dist(s):* **Jonathan David** *(Jonathan David Pubs., Inc.); CIP.*

Micamar Pub, *(Micamar Publishing; 0-937373),* Orders Addr.: P.O. Box 56, Barneveld, WI 53507 (SAN 658-9200) Tel 608-924-2101; Edit Addr.: 7910 Lakeview Rd., Barneveld, WI 53507 (SAN 658-9219).

†Mich St U Pr, *(Michigan State Univ. Pr.; 0-87013; 0-937191),* 1405 S. Harrison Rd. Suite 25, East Lansing, MI 48823-5202 (SAN 202-6295) Tel 517-355-9543; Fax: 517-432-2611 E-mail: msupress@msu.edu Web site: http://web.msu.edu/press *Dist(s):* **Academic Bk Ctr Inc** *(Academic Bk. Ctr., Inc.)* **Baker & Taylor** *(Baker & Taylor Bks.)* **Barnes & Noble Inc** *(Barnes & Noble, Inc.)* **Brodart** *(Brodart Co.)* **Coutts Library Service Inc** *(Coutts Library Service, Inc.)* **Emery-Pratt Co** *(Emery-Pratt Co.)* **Falcon Pub Inc** *(Falcon Publishing, Inc.)* **Gazelle Books** *(Gazelle Bks.)* **Midwest Lib Serv** *(Midwest Library Service)* **NA Blackwell** *(Blackwell North America)* **Yankee Bk Peddler Inc** *(Yankee Bk. Peddler, Inc.); CIP.*

Michaelis Med, *(Michaelis Medical Publishing Corp.; 1-884084),* 2274 S. 1300 E., Suite 68-288, Salt Lake City, UT 84106 *Dist(s):* **Majors Scientific Bks Inc** *(Majors Scientific Bks., Inc.)* **Matthews Medical Bk Co** *(Matthews Medical Bk. Co.)* **Quality Bks IL** *(Quality Bks., Inc.)* **Rittenhouse** *(Rittenhouse Bk. Distributors).*

Michelle Pub, *(Michelle Publishing Co.; 0-9626001),* 2317 Silas Deane Hwy., Rocky Hill, CT 06067 Tel 860-721-8800.

MICHIE Imprint of LEXIS Pub

Microscope Pubns, *(Microscope Pubns.; 0-904962),* Div. of McCrone Research Institute, 2820 S. Michigan Ave., Chicago, IL 60616-3292 (SAN 209-9594) Tel 312-842-7100; Fax: 312-842-1078 E-mail: lkrummick@mcri.org Web site: http://www.mcri.org.

Microtek Pubs, *See* **Ron L Dawson**

Microwave, *(Microwave News; 0-9610580),* Orders Addr.: P.O. Box 1799, New York, NY 10163 (SAN 264-2107); Edit Addr.: 155 E. 77th St., New York, NY 10021 (SAN 665-7389) Tel 212-517-2800.

Mid Am Pr, *(Mid-America Pr.; 0-9604672),* 3986 Central Ave., NE, Columbia Heights, MN 55421 (SAN 220-0724) Tel 612-781-5166.

Midewiwin, ***(Midewiwin Pr.; 0-9620884),*** **797 Goodrich Ave., Saint Paul, MN 55105-3344 (SAN 250-0728) Tel 651-224-7039 E-mail: wilso004@maroon.tc.umn.edu.**

Midgrd Press Imprint of Media Pub

Midpt Trade, *(Midpoint Trade Bks., Inc.),* Orders Addr.: 1263 Southwest Blvd., Kansas City, KS 66103 (SAN 631-3736) Tel 913-831-2233; Fax: 913-362-7401; Toll Free: 800-742-6139 (consumer orders); Edit Addr.: 27 W. 20th St., No. 1102, New York, NY 10011 (SAN 631-1075) Tel 212-727-0190; Fax: 212-727-0195; P.O. Box 411037, Kansas City, MO 64141-1037 (SAN 253-8539) Tel 913-362-7400; Fax: 913-362-7401 E-mail: midpointny@aol.com Web site: http://midpt.com.

Midtown Pub, *(Midtown Publishing Co.; 0-9656880),* 5821 Gall Blvd., Zephyrhills, FL 33541 Tel 813-782-6280; Fax: 813-780-6972.

Midway Reprint Imprint of U Ch Pr

Midwifery Today, *(Midwifery Today, Inc.; 1-890446),* Orders Addr.: P.O. Box 2672, Eugene, OR 97402 Tel 541-344-7438; Fax: 541-344-1422; Toll Free: 800-743-0974; Edit Addr.: 1372 S. Bertelsen St., Eugene, OR 97402 E-mail: Midwifery@aol.com Web site: http://www.midwiferytoday.com.

†Milady Pub, *(Milady Publishing Co.; 0-8273; 0-87350; 1-56253),* Div. of Delmar Pubs., Orders Addr.: P.O. Box 15015, Albany, NY 12212-5015 Tel 518-464-3500; Fax: 518-464-0357; Toll Free: 800-347-7707; Edit Addr.: 3 Columbia Cir., Albany, NY 12212-5015 (SAN 202-635X) Web site: http://www.thomsonlearning.com *Dist(s):* **B I G** *(B.I.G. (Business, Industry & Government))* **Thomson Learn** *(Thomson Learning); CIP.*

Milbank Memorial, *(Milbank Memorial Fund; 0-9629870; 1-887748),* 645 Madison Ave., New York, NY 10022 Tel 212-355-8400; Fax: 212-355-8599 E-mail: mmf@milbank.org Web site: http://www.milbank.org.

Miles River, *(Miles River Pr.; 0-917917),* 400 Madison St., Suite 1309, Alexandria, VA 22314 (SAN 657-0550) Tel 703-683-1500 (orders); Fax: 703-683-0827 (orders); Toll Free: 800-767-1501 (orders) E-mail: milesriverpress@aol.com Web site: http://www. milesriverpress.com.

Milkweed Ed, *(Milkweed Editions; 0-915943; 1-57131),* 1011 Washington Ave. S., Suite 300, Minneapolis, MN 55415-1246 (SAN 294-0671) Tel 612-332-3192; Fax: 612-215-2550; Toll Free: 800-520-6455 E-mail: market@milkweed.org Web site: http://www.worldashome.org; http://www.milkweed.org *Dist(s):* **Publishers Group** *(Publishers Group West)* **Todd Commns** *(Todd Communications).*

Mill Valley Med, *(Mill Valley Medical Pubs.; 0-9643644),* 1336 El Camino Real, No. 245, Millbrae, CA 94030-1411 Toll Free: 800-996-6324 (phone/fax).

†Millbrook Pr, *(Millbrook Pr., Inc.; 0-7613; 1-56294; 1-878841),* 2 Old New Milford Rd., Dept. LS, Brookfield, CT 06804 (SAN 299-9390) Tel 203-740-2220; Fax: 203-740-2223; Toll Free: 800-462-4703 ; *Imprints:* Copper Beech Bks (Copper Beech Books) Do not confuse with Mill Brook Pr., Highland Park, NJ Web site: http://www.millbrookpress.com; *CIP.*

Millenn Pub, *See* **Prog Wellness Res**

Millennium Bks (AUS) *(1-86429) Dist. by* **Morehouse Pub.**

Millers Pr, *(Miller's Pr., The; 0-9628401),* 2010 Kirkwood Rd., Cuba City, WI 53807 Tel 608-873-9891.

Million Dollar, *(Million Dollar Round Table Ctr. for Productivity; 1-891042),* 325 W. Touhy Ave., Park Ridge, IL 60068-4265 (SAN 224-8328) Tel 847-692-6378; Fax: 847-518-0696; Toll Free: 800-879-6378 E-mail: ordercfp@mdrtcfp.org Web site: http://www.mdrtcfp.org; http:// www.agents-online.com.

Millpond Pr, *(Millpond Pr.; 0-9701270),* P.O. Box 2524, Mill Valley, CA 94942-2524 Fax: 415-459-8656; Toll Free: 800-852-4890 E-mail: millpondpress@aol.com *Dist(s):* **Grnlf Ent** *(Greenleaf Enterprises, Inc.).*

Milusik Pr, *(Milusik Pr.; 0-9628475),* P.O. Box 18, Ogunquit, ME 03907-0018 Tel 207-646-5431 (phone/fax) E-mail: pala@maine.rr.com.

Milw Acad Med, *(Milwaukee Academy of Medicine Pr.; 0-9617070),* Orders Addr.: P.O. Box 26509, Milwaukee, WI 53226 (SAN 662-8923); Edit Addr.: 8701 Watertown Plank Rd., Milwaukee, WI 53226 (SAN 662-8931) Tel 414-464-4460.

Mind Prods Assocs, *(Mind Productions & Assocs.; 0-935257),* P.O. Box 11221, Tallahassee, FL 32302-3221 (SAN 695-5304) Tel 850-222-1764; Fax: 850-224-5331; Toll Free: 800-662-6463 E-mail: mindpro@mindpro.com Web site: http://www.mindpro.com.

Mind Rivers, *(Mind Rivers; 0-9640822),* 924 N. Daysville, Oregon, IL 61061 Tel 815-732-7150 *Dist(s):* **Bookpeople** *(Bookpeople)* **New Leaf Dist** *(New Leaf Distributing Co., Inc.).*

Mind-Matter-Motion, *(Mind Matter Motion; 0-9608910),* P.O. Box 2759, Rancho Mirage, CA 92270 (SAN 262-0790) Fax: 760-836-9347.

MindWrks, *(MindWorks Pr.; 1-886554),* 350 Chadbourne Rd., Suisun City, CA 94585-9636 Tel 707-429-7181; Fax: 707-429-8210; Toll Free: 800-626-2720 *Dist(s):* **BookWorld** *(BookWorld Services, Inc.).*

Minerva Labs, *(Minerva Laboratories; 0-9676168),* 3006 230th Ln., SE, No. X103, Sammamish, CA 98075 ; *Imprints:* Andrew Hall Cutler (Andrew Hall Cutler) E-mail: AndyCutler@aol.com Web site: http://hometown.aol.com/noamalgam.

MinervaPress, *(MinervaPress; 0-9637795),* Div. of Heartmates, Inc., Orders Addr.: P.O. Box 16202, Minneapolis, MN 55416 Tel 612-929-3331; Fax: 612-929-6395; Toll Free: 800-946-3331; Edit Addr.: 2828 Xenwood Ave., S., Minneapolis, MN 55416 E-mail: heartmates@outtech.com Web site: http://www.heartmates.com.

MiniMed Tech, *(MiniMed Technologies; 0-9647837),* 12744 San Fernando Rd., Sylmar, CA 91342 Tel 818-362-5958; Fax: 818-364-0968; Toll Free: 800-933-3322.

†Minn Hist, *(Minnesota Historical Society Pr.; 0-87351),* 345 Kellogg Blvd., W., Saint Paul, MN 55102-1906 (SAN 202-6384) Tel 651-296-2264; Fax: 651-297-1345 E-mail: kevin.morrissey@mnhs.org Web site: http://www.mnhs.org/mhspress *Dist(s):* **Wolverine Distrib** *(Wolverine Distributing, Inc.); CIP.*

Minn Soc Prev Blind, *See* **Sight & Hearing**

Minot Pubg, *(Minot Publishing Co.; 0-9670221),* 280 Higman Pk., Benton Harbor, MI 49022 Tel 616-925-0257 (phone/fax) E-mail: odden@qtm.net.

Mir Collection, *(Mir Collection Publishing Hse.; 0-9658114; 1-893552),* Div. of The International Emigre Assn., 8700 25th Ave., Suite 6G, Brooklyn, NY 11214 Tel 718-449-6245 E-mail: leonora@ultinet.net.

Mirkov Pubns, *(Mirkov Pubns., Inc.; 0-9648508),* Orders Addr.: P.O. Box 81971, Pittsburgh, PA 15217 Tel 412-521-1959; Fax: 412-521-2903; Toll Free: 800-851-8303; Edit Addr.: 1531 S. Negley Ave., Pittsburgh, PA 15217 E-mail: mgoldman@torah.com Web site: http://www.Mirkov.com *Dist(s):* **Koen Bk Distributors** *(Koen Bk. Distributors).*

Missing Diag, *(Missing Diagnosis, Inc.; 0-9615758),* Orders Addr.: P.O. Box 26508, Birmingham, AL 35226 (SAN 662-359X) Tel 205-328-6483 (phone/fax); Edit Addr.: 2614 Highland Ave., Birmingham, AL 35205 (SAN 695-8966) Tel 205-326-0642.

†MIT Pr, *(MIT Pr.; 0-262),* 5 Cambridge Ctr., Suite 4, Cambridge, MA 02142-1493 (SAN 202-6414) Tel 617-253-5646; 617-625-8569 (orders); Fax: 617-253-6779; 617-625-6660 (orders); Toll Free: 800-356-0343 (orders) ; *Imprints:* Bradford Bks (Bradford Books) E-mail: mitpress-orders@mit.edu Web site: http://mitpress.mit.edu; *CIP.*

Mitchell Beazley (GBR) *(0-85533; 1-84000; 1-85732; 0-86134) Dist. by* **Antique Collect.**

Mitchell Beazley (GBR) *(0-85533; 1-84000; 1-85732; 0-86134) Dist. by* **Sterling.**

Mitchell WA, *(Mitchell Publishing; 1-879909),* c/o Mitchell Law Office, West 28 Augusta, Spokane, WA 99205 Tel 509-327-5181 Do not confuse with companies with the same or similar names in Medicine Lodge, KS, Medina, NY, San Francisco, CA.

Mittal Pubs Dist (IND) *Dist. by* **S Asia.**

MJF Bks Imprint of Fine Comms

MKS Inc, *(MKS, Inc.; 0-913087),* 1259 El Camino Real, Suite 1500, Menlo Park, CA 94025 (SAN 134-5605) Tel 650-854-3922; Fax: 650-854-5779; Toll Free: 800-445-4325
E-mail: HopeMKS@aol.com
Web site: http://www.mksalaman.com
Dist(s): **Bay To Bay Dist** *(Bay To Bay Distribution).*

Mktdata Ent, *(Marketdata Enterprises, Inc.; 0-9632529; 1-891084),* 2807 W. Busch Blvd. Suite 110, Tampa, FL 33618-4518 Tel 813-931-3900; Fax: 813-931-3802
E-mail: mktdata5@aol.com
Web site: http://www.marketdataenterprises.com.

Mktg Methods Pr, *(Marketing Methods Pr.; 0-9624798),* Div. of Marketing Methods, L. C., 2811 N. Seventh Ave., Phoenix, AZ 85007 Tel 602-266-9344; Fax: 602-266-9478; Toll Free: 800-745-5047
Dist(s): **Baker & Taylor** *(Baker & Taylor Bks.)*
Quality Bks IL *(Quality Bks., Inc.).*

MLP Ent, *(MLP Enterprises; 0-939020),* Orders Addr.: P.O. Box 18918, Philadelphia, PA 19119-0418 (SAN 650-0420); Edit Addr.: 236 E. Durham St., Philadelphia, PA 19119 (SAN 214-4077) Tel 215-248-3218.

MLR Pub, *(MLR Publishing Co.; 0-926700),* Div. of MLR Enterprises, 229 S. 18th St., Philadelphia, PA 19103 Tel 215-790-7000; Fax: 215-790-7005; Toll Free: 800-637-4464.

Mlti-Media Prodns, *(Multi-Media Productions, Inc.; 1-878938),* 4913 Lake Arrowhead Dr., Waco, TX 76710 Tel 254-776-7142 Do not confuse with Multi-Media Productions in Maple Glen, PA.

ML-Verlag (DEU) *(3-88136) Dist. by* **Medicina Bio.**

MMB Music, *(MMB Music, Inc.; 0-918812; 1-58106),* Orders Addr.: 3526 Washington Ave. Contemporary Arts Bldg., Saint Louis, MO 63103-1019 (SAN 298-3281) Tel 314-531-9635; Fax: 314-531-8384; Toll Free: 800-543-3771
E-mail: mmbmusic@mmbmusic.com
Web site: http://www.mozarteffect.com.

MN-Commonwlth, *(Minnesota-Commonwealth Fund, Inc.; 0-9650378),* c/o Natalie Westreich, 1779 Emerson Ave. S., Minneapolis, MN 55403 Tel 612-377-9798; Fax: 612-377-3885.

Mnstry Pubns, *(Ministry Pubns.; 0-914271; 1-892843),* Div. of Ministry of the Word, Inc., Orders Addr.: P.O. Box 12222, Scottsdale, AZ 85267 (SAN 287-5926) Tel 480-948-4050; Fax: 480-922-1338; Toll Free: 800-573-4105; Edit Addr.: 10909 E. Kalil Dr., Scottsdale, AZ 85259 Toll Free: 800-573-4405
E-mail: Minword12@aol.com
Web site: http://www.thechristian.org
Dist(s): **Chr Lit** *(Christian Literature Crusade, Inc.).*

Mnstry Wrd, *See* **Mnstry Pubns**

Mntn Pr MA, *(Mountain Pr.; 0-9625313),* P.O. Box 592, Dalton, MA 01227 Do not confuse with companies with the same name in Dover, DE, Redding, CA, La Canada, CA, Princeton, NJ, Signal Mountain, TN.

MO Arch Soc, *(Missouri Archaeological Society; 0-943414),* P.O. Box 958, Columbia, MO 65205-0958 (SAN 238-8316) Tel 573-882-3544; Fax: 573-882-9410
E-mail: GalenM@missouri.edu
Web site: http://www.missouri.edu/~moarch/.

Mobium Pr, *(Mobium Pr.; 0-916371),* Div. of Mobium Corp. for Design & Communication, 222 Merchandise Mart Plz., No. 2000, Chicago, IL 60654-1016 (SAN 295-7256) Tel 312-527-0500.

---

†Modern Lang, ***(Modern Language Assn. of America; 0-87352),*** **26 Broadway, 3rd Fl., New York, NY 10004-1789 (SAN 202-6422) Tel 646-576-5000; Fax: 646-458-0030**
E-mail: info@mla.org
Web site: http://www.mla.org
Dist(s): **Baker & Taylor** ***(Baker & Taylor Bks.)***
NACSCORP Inc ***(NACSCORP, Inc.); CIP.***

Modern Learn Pr, *(Modern Learning Pr.; 0-935493; 1-56762),* P.O. Box 167, Rosemont, NJ 08556 Tel 609-397-2214; Fax: 609-397-3467; Toll Free Fax: 888-558-7350; Toll Free: 800-627-5867.

Modern Signs, *(Modern Signs Pr., Inc.; 0-916708),* Orders Addr.: P.O. Box 1181, Los Alamitos, CA 90720 (SAN 282-0056) Tel 562-493-4168; Toll Free: 800-572-7332; Edit Addr.: 10443 Los Alamitos Blvd., Los Alamitos, CA 90720 (SAN 282-0048) Tel 562-596-8548; Fax: 562-795-6614
E-mail: modsigns@aol.com
Web site: http://www.modsigns.com.

Mokelumne, *See* **Hlth Research**

Molysdatur Pubns, *(Molysdatur Pubns.; 1-882042),* P.O. Box 2510, Novato, CA 94948-2510 (SAN 248-3068) Tel 415-883-3530; Fax: 415-883-4280.

Mombaccus Pubng, *(Mombaccus Publishing; 0-9650380),* Box 321, Cooper Sta., New York, NY 10276-0321 Tel 212-627-7252; Fax: 212-242-5052
Web site: http://www.theinstitute.org
Dist(s): **Bookpeople** *(Bookpeople).*

Monaco & Assocs, *(Monaco & Assocs., Inc.; 1-882322),* 4125 Gage Center Dr., Suite 204, Topeka, KS 66604 Tel 785-272-5501; Fax: 785-272-5152; Toll Free: 800-798-1309
E-mail: busmgr@monacoassociates.com
Web site: http://www.monacoassociates.com.

Monarch Butterfly, *(Monarch Butterfly Productions; 1-880790),* 910 Kahili St., Kailua, HI 96734-4045 Tel 808-262-7740.

Monkestee Pr, *(Monkestee Pr.; 0-9634417),* 708 Bedfordshire Rd., Louisville, KY 40222-5513 Tel 502-423-7665; Fax: 502-588-8904.

Mont Pac Inst, *See* **Monterey Pacific**

Mont Sci Pubns, *(Montgomery Scientific Pubns.; 0-935643),* P.O. Box 2704, Durham, NC 27715 (SAN 696-1614) Fax: 919-489-1235.

Mont Urgent CC, *See* **Van Slyke Bray**

Montage Media Corp, *(Montage Media Corp.; 0-9673009),* 1000 Wyckoff Ave., Mahwah, NJ 07430 Tel 201-891-3200 (ext. 127); Fax: 201-891-2626
Web site: http://Montagemedia.com.

Monte Sano, *(Monte Sano Publishing; 0-9659392),* P.O. Box 824, Madison, AL 35758 (SAN 299-6782) Tel 205-922-9963; Fax: 205-922-0499; Toll Free: 800-508-9461
E-mail: marcia@msano.com; info@msano.com
Web site: http://www.msano.com
Dist(s): **Baker & Taylor** *(Baker & Taylor Bks.).*

Monterey Pacific, *(Monterey Pacific Pubs.; 1-880710),* P.O. Box 1619, Bandon, OR 97411 Tel 650-994-6570; Fax: 650-994-6579
E-mail: ingram@uci.net
Dist(s): **Baker & Taylor** *(Baker & Taylor Bks.).*

Montgomery Media, *(Montgomery Media, Inc.; 0-929807),* 740 N. Plankinton Ave., Suite 210, Milwaukee, WI 53203-2403 (SAN 250-5711) Tel 414-223-4266.

†Monthly Rev, *(Monthly Review Pr.; 0-85345; 1-58367),* Div. of Monthly Review Foundation, Inc., 122 W. 27th St., New York, NY 10001 (SAN 202-6481) Tel 212-691-2555; Fax: 212-727-3676; Toll Free: 800-670-9499
Web site: http://www.monthlyreview.org
Dist(s): **Bookpeople** *(Bookpeople)*
NYU Pr *(New York Univ. Pr.); CIP.*

Monument Pr, *(Monument Pr.; 0-930383),* 22497 Swordfish Dr., Boca Raton, FL 33428-4609 (SAN 670-7742) Tel 561-477-3364; Fax: 561-477-2534
E-mail: publishers_associates@yahoo.com
Dist(s): **Pubs Assoc** *(Publishers Assocs.).*

†Moody, *(Moody Pr.; 0-8024),* Div. of Moody Bible Institute, 820 N. LaSalle Blvd., Chicago, IL 60610 (SAN 202-5604) Tel 312-329-2102; Fax: 312-329-2019; Toll Free: 800-678-8812
Web site: http://www.moodypress.org
Dist(s): **Bob Jones Univ** *(Jones, Bob Univ. Pr.); CIP.*

Moon River, *(Moon River Publishing; 1-878143),* Div. of The Tape Hse., 2646 Palma Dr., No.357, Ventura, CA 93003 Tel 805-644-3137; Fax: 805-644-4927; Toll Free: 800-522-7735 Do not confuse with Moon River Publishing, Savannah, GA.

Moon Trvl Hdbks, *See* **Avalon Travel**

Moonfall Pr VA, *(Moonfall Pr.; 0-9619930; 0-9623183; 1-930387),* 7845 Glenister Dr., Springfield, VA 22152 Tel 703-912-9774; Fax: 703-866-9207
E-mail: info@moonfallpress.com
Web site: http://www.moonfallpress.com
Dist(s): **Baker & Taylor** *(Baker & Taylor Bks.)*
Barnes & Noble Inc *(Barnes & Noble, Inc.).*

Moontree Pub, *(Moontree Publishing; 1-881350),* 1141 Masterpiece Dr., Oceanside, CA 92057-6806 Tel 760-630-4848; Fax: 760-630-1818.

Moore & Assocs, *See* **Pub Partners**

Moore Fnd, *(Moore Foundation, The; 0-9713590),* Orders Addr.: P.O. Box 1, Camas, WA 98607 (SAN 631-5208) Tel 360-835-5500; Fax: 360-835-5392; Toll Free: 800-891-5255; Edit Addr.: 101 Moore Falls Rd., Washougal, WA 98671
E-mail: moorefnd@pacifier.com
Web site: http://www.moorefoundation.com.

Moose Moun, *(Moose Mountain Digital Pr.; 0-9707836),* 29 Moose Mountain Lodge Rd., Etna, NH 03750 Tel 603-643-2877; Fax: 603-643-6293
E-mail: lish.huggins@dartmouth.edu
Dist(s): **Lutz Services** *(Lutz Services).*

Moran Assocs, *See* **SafetyCertified**

Moray Pr, *(Moray Pr.; 0-9636528),* 1356 S. Devon, Springfield, MO 65809 Tel 417-889-4951; Fax: 417-865-6111.

†Morehouse Pub, *(Morehouse Publishing; 0-8192),* Orders Addr.: P.O. Box 1321, Harrisburg, PA 17105-1321 (SAN 202-6511) Tel 717-541-8130; Fax: 717-541-8128; Toll Free: 800-877-0012
E-mail: morehouse@morehousegroup.com
Web site: http://www.morehousegroup.com
Dist(s): **Intl Pubs Mktg** *(International Publishers Marketing); CIP.*

Morgan Fnd Pubs, *(Morgan Foundation Pubs.: International Published Innovations; 1-885679),* c/o Dr. Morgan, 310 Ladera Ln., No. 404, Mangilao, GU 96913 Tel 671-734-8064; Fax: 815-550-4456
E-mail: rmorgan@ite.net.

†Morgan Kaufmann, *(Morgan Kaufmann Pubs.; 0-12; 0-934613; 1-55860),* Div. of Academic Pr., A Harcourt Science & Technology Co., Orders Addr.: 6277 Sea Harbor Dr., Orlando, FL 32887 (SAN 630-253X) Tel 407-345-3800; Fax: 407-345-4060; Toll Free Fax: 800-874-6418; Toll Free: 800-321-5068; 800-745-7323; Edit Addr.: 340 Pine St., 6th Flr., San Francisco, CA 94104 Tel 415-392-2665; Fax: 415-982-2665
E-mail: mkp@mkp.com; orders@mkp.com
Web site: http://www.mkp.com; *CIP.*

Morgan Quitno Corp, *(Morgan Quitno Corp.; 0-7401; 0-9625531; 1-56692),* Orders Addr.: P.O. Box 1656, Lawrence, KS 66044-8656 Tel 785-841-3534; Fax: 785-841-3568; Toll Free: 800-457-0742; Edit Addr.: 512 E. Ninth St., Lawrence, KS 66044 ; *Imprints:* M Quitno Pr (Morgan Quitno Press)
E-mail: sales@morganquitno.com; info@morganquitno.com
Web site: http://www.statestats.com; http://www.morganquitno.com.

Morgana Pubns, *(Morgana Pubns.; 0-9630177),* P.O. Box 5403, Evanston, IL 60204-5403 Tel 708-634-6085.

Morgan-Rand, *See* **Volt Directory**

Morgantown Print & Bind, *(Morgantown Printing & Binding Co.; 0-930284),* P.O. Box 850, Morgantown, WV 26505 (SAN 213-1188) Tel 304-292-3368.

Morpheus Intl, *(Morpheus International; 0-9623447; 1-883398),* 9250 Wilshire Blvd., LL15, Beverly Hills, CA 90212-3352 Tel 310-859-2557; Fax: 310-859-7455
Web site: http://morpheusart.com; http://morpheusint.com
Dist(s): **Publishers Group** *(Publishers Group West).*

Morris Pubng, *(Morris Publishing; 0-7392; 0-9631249; 1-57502; 1-885591),* Subs. of Morris Pr. & Office Supplies, 3212 E. Hwy. 30, P.O. Box 2110, Kearney, NE 68847 Tel 308-236-7888; Fax: 308-237-0263; Toll Free: 800-650-7888 Do not confuse with companies with the same or similar name in Sarveta, PA, Plymouth Meeting, PA, Beecher City, IL, Urbana, IL, San Francisco, CA
E-mail: publish@morrispublishing.com
Web site: http://morrispublishing.com.

Morrow Avon, *(Morrow/Avon; 0-06; 0-380; 0-688),* Div. of HarperCollins General Bks. Grp., 1350 Ave. of the Americas, New York, NY 10019 Tel 212-261-6788; Fax: 570-941-1599 (customer service); Toll Free: 800-242-7737 (orders) ; *Imprints:* Wm Morrow (Morrow, William & Company) Avon Bks (Avon Books) HarpTorch (HarperTorch)
Web site: http://www.harpercollins.com/hc/
Dist(s): **HarperCollins Pubs** *(HarperCollins Pubs.)*
IPG Chicago *(Independent Pubs. Group)*
Shens Bks *(Shen's Bks.).*

Morson Pub, *(Morson Publishing; 1-878423),* Div. of Morson Corp., 8184 Highland Dr., Suite C-4, Sandy, UT 84093-6481.

Morton Pub, *(Morton Publishing Co.; 0-89582),* 925 W. Kenyon Ave., Unit 12, Englewood, CO 80110 (SAN 210-9174) Tel 303-761-4805; Fax: 303-762-9923
E-mail: morton@morton-pub.com
Web site: http://www.morton-pub.com.

Mosaic, *(Mosaic Pr.; 0-88962),* Orders Addr.: PMB 145, 4500 Witmer Industrial Estates, Niagara Falls, NY 14305 Tel 905-825-2130 (phone/fax); Toll Free: 800-387-8992
E-mail: mosaicpress@on.aibn.com
Web site: http://w3.one.net~kirwin/mp.htm
Dist(s): **Midpt Trade** *(Midpoint Trade Bks., Inc.).*

Mosaic Pr OH, *(Mosaic Pr.; 0-88014),* 358 Oliver Rd., Cincinnati, OH 45215 (SAN 219-6077) Tel 513-761-5977; Fax: 513-821-1270; Toll Free: 800-932-4044 Do not confuse with Mosaic Pr., Philadelphia, PA
E-mail: mirwin@cinci.rr.com
Web site: http://w3.one.net/~kirwin/mp.htm.

Mosby Consmer Hlth, *(Mosby Consumer-Health & Safety; 1-57857),* Div. of Times-Mirror, 6810 Deerpath Rd., Suite 200, Elkridge, MD 21075-6276.

†Mosby Inc, *(Mosby, Inc.; 0-323; 0-7234; 0-8016; 0-8151; 0-88416; 0-941158; 1-55664; 1-56815),* Div. of Harcourt, Inc., A Harcourt Health Sciences Co., Orders Addr.: 6227 Sea Harbor Dr., Orlando, FL 32887 Toll Free Fax: 800-235-0256; Toll Free: 800-543-1918; Edit Addr.: 11830 Westline Industrial Dr., Saint Louis, MO 63146 (SAN 200-2280) Toll Free: 800-325-4177
Web site: http://www.mosby.com/
Dist(s): **PennWell Corp** *(PennWell Corp.); CIP.*

†Mosby Multi-Media, *(Mosby/Multi-Media; 0-8016; 0-940122),* Div. of Times Mirror Co., 11830 Westline Industrial Dr., Saint Louis, MO 63141 (SAN 220-2913) Tel 314-872-8370; Toll Free: 800-325-4177; *CIP.*

Mosby Yr, *See* **Mosby Inc**

Mosby-Doyma Libros (ESP) *(84-7592; 84-8086; 84-8174; 84-85285) Dist. by* **Mosby Inc.**

Mosby-Doyma Libros (ESP) *(84-7592; 84-8086; 84-8174; 84-85285) Dist. by* **Saunders.**

Motamed Med Pub, *(Motamed Medical Publishing Co.; 0-910161),* 7141 N. Kedzie Ave., Suite 1504, Chicago, IL 60645 (SAN 241-2276) Tel 773-761-6667.

Mothering Magazine, *(Mothering Magazine; 0-914257),* Orders Addr.: P.O. Box 1690, Santa Fe, NM 87504 (SAN 287-5616) Tel 505-984-8116; Fax: 505-986-8335; Toll Free: 800-984-8116; Edit Addr.: 649 Harkle Rd., Suite F, Santa Fe, NM 87505
E-mail: info@mothering.com
Web site: http;//www.mothering.com.

Motherly Way, *(Motherly Way Enterprises; 0-9671428),* P.O. Box 11, Marylhurst, OR 97036-0011 Tel 503-329-1987; Fax: 503-636-0515
E-mail: motherly@teleport.com
Web site: http://www.motherlyway.com.

Motilal Bnarsidass (IND) *(81-208) Dist. by* **S Asia.**

Motilal Bnarsidass (IND) *(81-208) Dist. by* **St Mut.**

Motion Palpat Inst, *(Motion Palpation Institute; 0-924889),* 3197 Linwood Ave., Cincinnati, OH 45208-2962 Tel 513-321-8484.

Motion Pubns, *(Motion Pubns.; 0-9679446),* 3485 Heron Lake Ln., Box 2551, Elk Grove, CA 95758 Toll Free: 800-351-8000
E-mail: mpublishing@email.com
Web site: http://www.terryoneal.com.

Motivat Inst Phila, *(Motivation Institute of Philadelphia; 1-891251),* P.O. Box 12315, Philadelphia, PA 19119-0315 Tel 215-224-1783 (phone/fax)
E-mail: hugnothit@aol.com.

†Motorbooks Intl, *(Motorbooks International Wholesalers & Distributors; 0-7603; 0-87938; 0-912612; 1-85010),* Div. of Chronicle Publishing, 729 Prospect Ave., Osceola, WI 54020 (SAN 169-9164) Tel 715-294-3345; Fax: 715-294-4448; Toll Free: 800-458-0454
E-mail: mbibks@win.bright.net
Web site: http://www.motorbooks.com; *CIP.*

Mount Hope Pub, *(Mount Hope Publishing Co., Inc.; 0-9640886),* c/o Elizabeth Wende Breast Clinic, 1351 Mt. Hope Ave., Rm. 110, Rochester, NY 14620-3992 Tel 716-442-8432.

†Mountaineers, *(Mountaineers Bks., The; 0-89886; 0-916890; 0-938567),* Div. of Mountaineers, Orders Addr.: 1001 SW Klickitat Way, Suite 201, Seattle, WA 98134-1162 (SAN 212-8756) Tel 206-223-6303; Fax: 206-223-6306; Toll Free: 800-568-7604
E-mail: mbooks@mountaineersbooks.org
Web site: http://www.mountaineersbooks.org
Dist(s): **Heinecken Assoc** *(Heinecken & Assoc., Ltd.)*
Karel Dutton *(Karel/Dutton Group)*
Nor East Bk Sls *(Nor' East Book Sales)*
Ryen R E Assoc *(Ryen/RE Assocs.); CIP.*

Mouton (DEU) *(0-89925; 0-938198; 3-11; 90-279) Dist. by* **De Gruyter.**

Mouvement Pubns, *(Mouvement Pubns.; 0-932392),* 109 Forest Glen, Longmeadow, MA 01106 (SAN 211-7460) Tel 413-567-5898; Fax: 413-565-2678.

Movable Type, *See* **Equinox Pr**

†Moyer Bell, *(Moyer Bell; 0-918825; 1-55921),* 54 Phillips St., Wickford, RI 02852 (SAN 630-1762) Tel 401294-0106; Fax: 401-294-1076; Toll Free: 888-789-1945
E-mail: info@moyerbell.com
Web site: http://www.moyerbell.com
Dist(s): **Publishers Group** *(Publishers Group West)*
Wittenborn Art *(Wittenborn Art Bks.); CIP.*

MPC Pr, *(MPC Pr.; 0-9613177),* Div. of Bioenergetics, Inc., P.O. Box 55094, Madison, WI 53705 (SAN 295-6624) Tel 608-238-6681; Fax: 608-251-0658; Toll Free: 800-203-4028
E-mail: mpcpress@pobox.com
Dist(s): **Baker & Taylor** *(Baker & Taylor Bks.)*
Bookazine Co Inc *(Bookazine Co., Inc.).*

MRLN (GBR) *(0-85036) Dist. by* **Paul & Co Pubs.**

Mrngstar Pubns, *(Morningstar Pubns.; 0-9623812),* 44 Rim Rd., Boulder, CO 80302-9766 Tel 303-444-6072; Fax: 303-473-9997; Toll Free: 800-435-1670 Do not confuse with Morningstar Pubns., Inc. in Charlotte, NC
E-mail: dstclaire@mindspring.com.

Mrningstar Pubng, *(Morningstar Publishing Co.; 0-9642387),* P.O. Box 671427, Chugiak, AK 99567-1427 Tel 541-389-0078
E-mail: akstork@aol.com.

†MRTS, *(MRTS; 0-86698),* Orders Addr.: P.O. Box 6525, Ithaca, NY 14851 Tel 607-277-2211; Fax: 607-277-6292; Toll Free: 800-666-2211; Edit Addr.: P.O. Box 872508, Tempe, AZ 85287-2508 (SAN 216-6119) Tel 480-727-6503; Fax: 480-727-6505
E-mail: mrts@asu.edu
Web site: http://www.asu.edu/clas/acmrs/mrts
Dist(s): **Cornell U Pr** *(Cornell Univ. Pr.); CIP.*

MSP Communs, *(MSP Communications; 0-9641908; 1-892845),* 220 S. Sixth St., Suite 500, Minneapolis, MN 55402 Tel 612-339-7571; Fax: 612-339-5806
E-mail: edit@mspcommunications.com
Web site: http://www.mspcommunications.com
Dist(s): **Bookmen Inc** *(Bookmen, Inc.).*

Mstque Pubns, *(Mystique Pubns., L.A.; 0-914865),* P.O. Box 02, Los Angeles, CA 90036 (SAN 289-0577) Tel 213-656-7745.

Mstrs Press Imprint of McGraw-Hill Trade

Mt SA Coll Philos, *(Mount San Antonio College/Philosophy Group; 1-56543),* 1100 N. Grand Ave., Walnut, CA 91789 Tel 909-594-5611 Ext. 4593; Toll Free: 800-672-2463 Ext. 4593
E-mail: dlane@ibm.mtsac.edu
Web site: http://www.mtsac.edu/~dlane.

MTA Pub, *(MTA Publishing; 0-9622533),* Div. of Michael Thomas Agency, 830 Potomac Cir., Unit 150, Aurora, CO 80011-6751 Tel 303-699-9161.

MTL Pubns, *(MTL Pubns.; 0-9702211),* P.O. Box 645, Lake Havasu City, AZ 86405 Fax: 520-855-7152
E-mail: marypat@ctaz.com.

Mtn Gem Pubng, *(Mountain Gem Publishing; 0-9638245),* 344 N. 15th Ave., No. 2C, Pocatello, ID 83201 Tel 208-233-1592.

Mtn Greenery, *(Mountain Greenery Pr.; 0-9635457),* RFD 1, Box 4856, Camden, ME 04843 Tel 207-236-3726.

Mtn Home Pub, *(Mountain Home Publishing; 0-944649),* P.O. Box 829, Ingram, TX 78025 (SAN 244-4658) Tel 210-367-4492; Toll Free: 800-527-3044.

Mtn Weed Pub, *(Mountain Weed Publishing; 0-9638638),* Div. of Mountain Weed Co., P.O. Box 212, Conner, MT 59827 Tel 406-821-4090
E-mail: animals@bitterroot.net
Dist(s): **New Leaf Dist** *(New Leaf Distributing Co., Inc.).*

Mulberry Hill, *(Mulberry Hill Pr.; 0-9637139),* Orders Addr.: 2710 S. Washington St., Englewood, CO 80110 (SAN 297-9659) Tel 303-781-8974; Fax: 303-806-9313
E-mail: hjelmstd@csd.net
Web site: http://www.bookzone.com/mulberry
Dist(s): **Baker & Taylor** *(Baker & Taylor Bks.).*

Mulberry Tree, *(Mulberry Tree Pr., The; 0-9610684),* 22 Auburn Ct., No. D, Alexandria, VA 22305-2935 (SAN 264-7672).

Multigrowth, *(Multigrowth Resources; 0-9630847),* 12345 Jones Rd., No. 101, Houston, TX 77070 Tel 281-890-5334; Fax: 281-894-8611.

Multilingual Matters (GBR) *(0-905028; 1-85359) Dist. by* **U of Toronto Pr.**

Multimed Virt, *See* **Echocardio**

Multinatl Busn Serv, *(Multinational Businesses Services, Inc.; 0-9655476),* 11 Dupont Cir., NW, Suite 700, Washington, DC 20036 Tel 202-293-5886; Fax: 202-939-6969.

Multnomah Bks Imprint of Multnomah Pubs

Multnomah Pubs, *(Multnomah Pubs., Inc.; 0-88070; 0-930014; 0-945564; 1-57673; 1-885305; 1-58860; 1-59052),* Orders Addr.: P.O. Box 1720, Sisters, OR 97759 (SAN 247-123X) Tel 541-549-1144; Fax: 541-549-8048; Toll Free: 800-929-0910; Edit Addr.: 204 W. Adams, Sisters, OR 97759 ; *Imprints:* Multnomah Bks (Multnomah Books)
E-mail: djacobson@multnomahbooks.com
Web site: http://multnomahbooks.com
Dist(s): **Christian Bk Distributors** *(Christian Bk. Distributors)*
GL Services *(GL Services)*
Zondervan *(Zondervan Publishing Hse.).*

Munroe-Meyer Inst, *(Munroe-Meyer Institute for Genetics & Rehabilitation; 1-889843),* Div. of Univ. of Nebraska, Orders Addr.: c/o Media Ctr., 985450 Nebraska Medical Ctr., Omaha, NE 68198-5450 Tel 402-559-7467; Fax: 402-559-5737; Toll Free: 800-656-3937
E-mail: mmimedia@unmc.edu
Web site: http://www.unmc.edu/mmi.

Mura Pub Co, *(Mura Publishing Co., Inc.; 0-929602),* P.O. Box 3170, Honolulu, HI 96802-3170 (SAN 249-7557).

Murdock Pubng, *(Murdock Publishing Co./Black & White Enterprises; 0-9668865),* R. R. 1, Box 191 A, Tannersville, PA 18372 Tel 717-688-9039.

Muriel S Pascoe, *(Pascoe, Muriel S.; 0-9628963),* 7 Clydehurst Dr., Webster Groves, MO 63119-2011 Tel 314-962-4878 (phone/fax).

Murrayhollow, *(Murrayhollow Pubs.; 0-9610242),* Murrayhollow Rd., Shushan, NY 12873 (SAN 264-2263) Tel 518-854-3305.

Mus Texas, *(Museum of Texas Tech Univ. Assn.; 0-911618),* Box 43191, Lubbock, TX 79409-3191 (SAN 206-667X) Tel 806-742-2443; Fax: 806-742-0399.

Muscle Joint, *(Muscle Joint Nerve, LLC; 0-9706580),* 136-89 41st Ave., Flushing, NY 11355 Tel 212-545-7075; Fax: 212-545-7116
E-mail: lowhaijin@aol.com
Web site: http://musclejointnerve.com
Dist(s): **Bk Clearing Hse** *(Book Clearing Hse.)*
CyberRead Pubng *(CyberRead Publishing).*

MuscleMag Intl (CAN) *(1-55210) Dist. by* **BookWorld.**

Museum NM Pr, *(Museum of New Mexico Pr.; 0-89013),* Orders Addr.: 1720 Lomas Blvd., NE, Albuquerque, NM 87131 (SAN 202-2575) Tel 505-277-2346; Toll Free Fax: 800-622-8667
E-mail: llury@lvr.state.nm.us
Dist(s): **U of NM Pr** *(Univ. of New Mexico Pr.).*

Mustang Pub, *(Mustang Publishing; 0-914457),* Orders Addr.: P.O. Box 770426, Memphis, TN 38177 (SAN 289-6702) Tel 901-684-1200; Fax: 901-684-1256; Toll Free: 800-250-8713
E-mail: MustangPub@aol.com
Web site: http://www.mustangpublishing.com
Dist(s): **Natl Bk Netwk** *(National Bk. Network).*

Mustard Seed, *(Mustard Seed Pubns.; 0-9632392),* 9904 Gunforge Rd., Perry Hall, MD 21128-9518 Tel 410-256-6835.

Mxwll Pub, *(Maxwell Publishing Co.; 0-9645191),* P.O. Box 21503, Oklahoma City, OK 73156-1503 Tel 405-751-7785; Fax: 405-751-7987
E-mail: mxwell@flash.net
Dist(s): **J Majors Co** *(Majors, J. A. Co.)*
Matthews Bk Co *(Matthews Bk. Co.)*
Rittenhouse *(Rittenhouse Bk. Distributors).*

My Life, *(My Life Changes; 0-9701970),* 14080 Nacogdoches Rd., No. 281, San Antonio, TX 78247-1944 Tel 210-653-8963; Fax: 210-653-0692
E-mail: ptravers@stic.net
Web site: http://www.mylifechanges.com.

Mycological, *(Mycological Society of San Francisco, Inc.; 0-918942),* P.O. Box 882163, San Francisco, CA 94188 (SAN 210-3621) Tel 415-759-0495.

Mycotaxon Ltd, *(Mycotaxon, Ltd.; 0-930845),* P.O. Box 264, Ithaca, NY 14851 (SAN 677-6051) Tel 607-273-0508; Fax: 607-273-4357
E-mail: info@mycotaxon
Web site: http://www.mycotaxon.com.

Myers Inc, *(Myers, S. D. Inc.; 0-939320),* 180 South Ave., Talmadge, OH 44278 (SAN 216-2725) Toll Free: 800-444-9580
E-mail: mike_horning@sdmyers.com.

Myers Resear Inst, *(Myers Research Institute; 0-9676343),* 27100 Cedar Rd., Beachwood, OH 44122 Tel 216-831-6500; Fax: 216-595-7331
E-mail: ckalman@myersri.com.

Publisher Symbol Index

MyoData, *(MyoData; 0-924728),* Orders Addr.: P.O. Box 89698, Tucson, AZ 85752-9698 (SAN 631-4139) Tel 520-744-8000; Fax: 520-744-3558; Toll Free: 800-533-5121 ; *Imprints:* TMJ Stress Ctr (TMJ & Stress Center)
E-mail: tmjinfo@myodata.com
Web site: http://www.myodata.com.

Myopia Internatl Res Fndtn, *(Myopia International Research Foundation, Inc.; 1-879037),* 1265 Broadway, Rm. 608, New York, NY 10001 Tel 212-684-2777.

Myrin Institute, *See* **Orion Society**

Mystic Planet, *(Mystic Planet; 0-9622539),* P.O. Box 357274, Gainesville, FL 32635 Tel 352-378-8764
E-mail: mystic@mysticplanet.com
Web site: http://www.mysticplanet.com/
Dist(s): **The Dream Zone** *(Dream Zone, The).*

N AM Nursing, *See* **Nursecom Inc**

N Am Soc Adlerian, *(North American Society of Adlerian Psychology; 0-926164),* 65 E. Wacker Pl., No. 400, Chicago, IL 60601-3703 (SAN 274-1571) Tel 312-629-8801; Fax: 312-629-8859
E-mail: nasap@msn.com
Web site: http://www.ncf.carleton.ca/~ak996/; http://www.alfredadler.org.

N Amer Men, *(North American Menopause Society, The; 0-9701251),* Orders Addr.: P.O. Box 94527, Cleveland, OH 44101 Tel 440-442-7550; Fax: 440-442-2660; Toll Free: 800-774-5342; Edit Addr.: 5900 Landerbrook Dr., Suite 195, Mayfield Heights, OH 44124
E-mail: info@menopause.org
Web site: http://www.menopause.org.

N Amricn Inst Audtry, *(North American Institute for Auditory Prosthetics; 0-9715385),* 1525 B Farmers Ln., Santa Rosa, CA 95405.

N Breslau, *(Breslau, Nathan Publishing Co.; 0-9610716),* 918 A. Savannas Point Dr., Fort Pierce, FL 33450 (SAN 264-6544) Tel 407-466-3439.

N C A Inst, *See* **Satyam Pub**

N C Coop Ext, *(N C Cooperative Extension Service/N C State Univ.; 0-9659498),* Div. of North Carolina State Univ., Orders Addr.: Box 7605, NCSU, Raleigh, NC 27695-7605 Tel 919-515-9157; Fax: 919-513-0159; Edit Addr.: Lampe Dr., Raleigh, NC 27695
E-mail: susan_baker@ncsu.edu
Web site: http://www.ces.ncsu.edu.

N C D Pubg, *(NCD Publishing; 0-9679718),* Orders Addr.: P.O. Box 741594, Dallas, TX 75374-1594 (SAN 253-5084) Tel 972-494-9497; Fax: 972-205-9979; Toll Free: 800-484-9410; Edit Addr.: 2302 St. Albens Pl., Garland, TX 75040
E-mail: drpbj@ncdpublishing.com
Web site: http://www.ncdpublishing.com.

N C State Univ, *(North Carolina State Univ., College of Veterinary Medicine; 0-9651794),* 4700 Hillsborough St., Raleigh, NC 27606 Tel 919-829-4267; Fax: 919-829-4465.

N Century Pubng, *(New Century Publishing; 1-884348),* 5225 Blakeslee Ave., Apt. 439, North Hollywood, CA 91601-3248 Do not confuse with companies with the same name in San Francisco, CA, Maryville, TN, New York, NY.

N Cihylik, *See* **H A W M**

N Crowley, *(Crowley, Nancy; 0-9640358),* 394 E. 4750 N., Provo, UT 84604 Tel 801-785-3738; Fax: 801-226-3624.

N F Childers, *(Childers, Dr. Norman F. Pubns.; 0-938378),* 3906 NW 31st Pl., Gainesville, FL 32606 (SAN 216-1389) Tel 352-372-5077; Fax: 352-392-5653
E-mail: NORMA@circa.ufl.edu.

†N Ill U Pr, *(Northern Illinois Univ. Pr.; 0-87580),* 310 N. Fifth St., DeKalb, IL 60115-2854 (SAN 202-8875) Tel 815-753-1826; Fax: 815-753-1845
E-mail: bberg@niu.edu
Web site: http://www.niu.edu/univ_press/; *CIP.*

N L Clark, *See* **Clark Pubs**

N L N Bart Imprint of Jones & Bartlett

N Late Pub, *(Late, N. Pub.; 0-9641448),* 910 Portland Pl., No. 7, Boulder, CO 80304 Tel 303-440-0193.

N M Davis, *(Davis, Neil M. Assocs.; 0-931431),* 1143 Wright Dr., Huntingdon Valley, PA 19006 (SAN 683-1729) Tel 215-947-1752; Fax: 215-938-1937
E-mail: med@neilmdavis.com
Web site: http://www.neilmdavis.com.

N Montessori, *(Nienhuis Montessori U.S.A., Inc.; 1-879341),* Div. of Nienhuis Group Zelhem, Holland, 320 Pioneer Way, Mountain View, CA 94041-1576 (SAN 200-2817) Tel 415-964-2735; Fax: 415-964-8162; Toll Free: 800-942-8697.

N Nedley, *See* **Nedley Publishing**

†N Point Pr, *(North Point Pr.; 0-374; 0-86547),* Div. of Farrar, Straus & Giroux, LLC, 19 Union Sq., W., New York, NY 10003 (SAN 220-133X) Tel 212-741-6900; Fax: 212-633-9385; *CIP.*

N S Kline Inst, *(Kline, Nathan S. Institute; 0-936934),* Information Sciences Div., Bldg. 37, Orangeburg, NY 10962 (SAN 239-6041) Tel 914-359-0002.

N Shore Asthma, *(North Shore Asthma Clinic; 0-9678835),* 1950 Sheridan Rd., Suite 202, Highland Park, IL 60035 Tel 847-266-3580; Fax: 847-266-3582
E-mail: drsorensen@whydoiwheeze.com
Web site: http://www.whydoIwheeze.com.

N Star Pubns, *(North Star Pubns., Inc.; 0-9655067; 1-880823),* P.O. Box 227, East Sandwich, MA 02537-0227 (SAN 298-0002) Tel 508-420-6188; Fax: 508-420-6570; Toll Free: 800-742-6139 Do not confuse North Star Pubns., Provo, UT
E-mail: norbook@aol.com
Web site: http://readersndex.com/northstar
Dist(s): **Midpt Trade** *(Midpoint Trade Bks., Inc.).*

N Van Duong, *(Van Duong, Nguyen; 0-9637303),* 938 26th St., Santa Monica, CA 90403 Tel 310-828-6649.

N Verrier, *See* **Verrier Pub**

N Watson Imprint of Watson Pub Intl

N X Phuong, *(Phuong, Ngo Xuan; 0-9635459),* 7891 Westminster Blvd., Westminster, CA 92683 Tel 714-891-7775; Fax: 714-891-2596.

NAAHP Inc, *(National Assn. of Advisors for the Health Professions, Inc.; 0-911899),* P.O. Box 1518, Champaign, IL 61824-1518 (SAN 264-679X) Tel 217-355-0063; Fax: 217-355-1287.

Nadex Pub (CAN) *(0-9685665) Dist. by* **New Centry Pr.**

NAGNA, *(National Assn. of Geriatric Nursing Assistants (NAGNA); 0-9662101),* 1706 E. Fourth St., Joplin, MO 64801-1807 Tel 417-623-6049; Fax: 417-623-2230; Toll Free: 800-784-6049.

Nakaii Pubg, *(Nakaii Publishing; 1-892930),* Orders Addr.: P.O. Box 706, Eureka, MT 59917 Tel 406-882-4177; Edit Addr.: 150 Grave Creek Rd., Eureka, MT 59917
E-mail: sita@interbel.net.

NAL, *(NAL; 0-451; 0-452; 0-453; 0-525; 0-8015),* Div. of Penguin Putnam, Inc., Orders Addr.: 405 Murray Hill Pkwy., East Rutherford, NJ 07073 Toll Free: 800-788-6262 (individual consumer sales); 800-526-0275 (reseller sales); 800-631-8571 (reseller customer service); Edit Addr.: 375 Hudson St., New York, NY 10014-3657 Tel 212-366-2000; Fax: 212-366-2666; Toll Free: 800-331-4624 (Customer service) ; *Imprints:* Sig (Signet Books) Ment (Mentor) Mer (Meridian Books) Plume (Plume)
E-mail: online@penguinputnam.com
Web site: http://www.penguinputnam.com
Dist(s): **Penguin Putnam** *(Penguin Putnam, Inc.).*

NAL-Dutton, *See* **NAL**

Nancy Eos, *(Eos, Nancy; 0-9644923),* 1233 Cornell Rd., Muskegon, MI 49441-3832 Tel 517-522-4880.

Nandel Pub Co, *See* **Covenant Hse Bks**

NAPSAC, *(National Assn. of Parents & Professionals for Safe Alternatives in Childbirth, International; 0-917314),* Rte. 4, Box 646, Marble Hill, MO 63764 (SAN 208-7766) Tel 573-238-2010; Toll Free: 800-758-8629.

NAPSAC Reprods, *(NAPSAC Reproductions; 0-934426),* Rte. 4, Box 646, Marble Hill, MO 63764 (SAN 222-4607) Tel 573-238-4273; Fax: 573-238-2010; Toll Free: 800-578-8629
E-mail: napsac@clas.net.

Nat Acad Practice, *(National Academies of Practice; 1-883848),* P.O. Box 1037, Edgewood, MD 21040-0337.

Nat Assn Bds Exam, *(National Assn. of Boards of Examiners of Long Term Care Administrators; 0-9635064),* 1444 I St., NW, Suite 700, Washington, DC 20005-2210 Tel 202-712-9040; Fax: 202-216-9646
E-mail: nab@bostromdc.com
Web site: http://www.nabweb.org.

Nat Assn Insurance, *(National Assn. of Insurance Commissioners; 0-89382),* 120 W. 12th St., Suite 1100, Kansas City, MO 64105-1925 (SAN 225-0780) Tel 816-842-3600; Fax: 816-471-7004
Web site: http://www.naic.org.

Nat Council on Womens Health, *(National Council on Women's Health, Inc., The; 0-9678633),* 1300 York Ave., New York, NY 10021 Tel 212-746-6967; Fax: 212-746-8691
E-mail: sdb2002@mail.med.cornell.edu
Web site: http://www.ncwh.org.

Nat Ctr Educ, *(National Ctr. for Education in Maternal & Child Health; 1-57285),* Div. of Georgetown Univ., 2000 15th St. N, Suite 701, Arlington, VA 22201-2617 Tel 703-524-7802; Fax: 703-524-9335.

Nat Hlth Res, *(Natural Health Resource Ctr., Inc.; 0-9649166),* 14 Hawk Dr., Bedford, NH 03110-4803 Tel 603-471-0094
E-mail: BarbaraSharp@compuserve.com.

Nat Learn, *(National Learning Corp.; 0-8293; 0-8373),* 212 Michael Dr., Syosset, NY 11791 (SAN 206-8869) Tel 516-921-8888; Fax: 516-921-8743; Toll Free: 800-645-6337.

Nat Med Assn, *(National Medical Assn., Section on Radiology; 0-9651714),* c/o Kathleen Herd, Radiology, Washington Adventist Hosp., 7600 Carroll Ave., Takoma Park, MD 20912 Tel 301-891-5109; Fax: 301-891-5253.

Nat Med Chest, *See* **LM Pubns**

Nat Sleep Alert, *(National Sleep Alert, Inc.; 0-9635137),* 1240 Iroquois Ave., Apt. 406, Naperville, IL 60563-8540 Tel 630-420-7673; Fax: 630-420-7835.

Nataraj Bks, *(Nataraj Bks.; 1-881338),* Orders Addr.: P.O. Box 5076, Springfield, VA 22150 (SAN 696-6527) Tel 703-455-4996; Fax: 703-912-9052; Edit Addr.: 7073 Brookfield Plaza, Springfield, VA 22150
E-mail: nataraj@erols.com
Web site: http://www.natarajbooks.com; http://www.erols.com/nataraj.

National Alliance, *(National Alliance of Breast Cancer Organizations, Inc.; 0-9703468),* 9 E. 37th St., 10th Flr., New York, NY 10016 Fax: 212-689-1213; Toll Free: 888-806-2226
E-mail: nabcoinfo@aol.com
Web site: http://www.nabco.org.

National Direct, *(National Directory CYF; 1-885461),* 14 Inverness Dr. E., D144, Englewood, CO 80112 Tel 303-662-8716; Toll Free Fax: 800-845-6452; Toll Free: 800-343-6681 Do not confuse with National Directories in Jacksonville, FL
E-mail: natldircyf@aol.com
Web site: http://www.childrenyouthfamilydir.com.

Native Sun Pubs, *(Native Sun Pubs., Inc.; 0-9625169; 1-879289),* Orders Addr.: P.O. Box 13394, Richmond, VA 23225 Tel 804-233-7768; Edit Addr.: 1021 Hioaks Rd., Richmond, VA 23225.

Natl Abort Fed, *(National Abortion Federation; 0-9601326),* 1755 Massachusetts Ave., NW, Suite 600, Washington, DC 20036 (SAN 222-089X) Tel 202-667-5881; Fax: 202-667-5890.

†Natl Acad Pr, *(National Academy Pr.; 0-309),* 2101 Constitution Ave., NW HA 384, Washington, DC 20418 (SAN 202-8891) Tel 202-334-3180; Fax: 202-334-2793; Toll Free: 800-624-6242 (orders only) ; *Imprints:* Joseph Henry Pr (Joseph Henry Press)
E-mail: zjones@nas.edu
Web site: http://www.nap.edu
Dist(s): **World Scientific Pub** *(World Scientific Publishing Co., Inc.); CIP.*

Natl Acup Fndt, *(National Acupuncture Foundation; 0-9670262),* Orders Addr.: P.O. Box 2271, Gig Harbor, WA 98335-4271 Tel 253-851-6538; Fax: 253-851-6883; Edit Addr.: 14637 Starr Rd., SE, Olalla, WA 98359-9537
Dist(s): **NA&OMA** *(Natl. Acupuncture & Oriental Medicine Alliance).*

Natl Assn Accts, *See* **Inst Mgmt Account**

Natl Assn Child Ed, *(National Assn. for the Education of Young Children; 0-912674; 0-935989; 1-928896),* 1509 16th St., NW, Washington, DC 20036-1426 (SAN 202-8905) Tel 202-232-8777; Fax: 202-234-6415; Toll Free: 800-424-2460
E-mail: lthompson@naeyc.org
Web site: http://www.naeyc.org.

Natl Assn Deaf, *(National Assn. of the Deaf; 0-913072),* 814 Thayer Ave., Silver Spring, MD 20910 (SAN 159-4974) Tel 301-587-6282; Fax: 301-587-4873
E-mail: sales@nad.org
Web site: http://www.nad.org.

Natl Assn Ortho Nurse, *(National Assn. of Orthopaedic Nurses, The; 1-892665),* East Holly Ave., Box 56, Pitman, NJ 08071-0056 Tel 609-256-2310; Fax: 609-589-7463; Toll Free: 800-289-6266
Web site: http://www.iNurse.com/~naon
Dist(s): **A J Jannetti** *(Jannetti, Inc., Anthony J.).*

Natl Assn Schl Psych, *(National Assn. of Schl. Psychologists; 0-932955),* 4340 East-West Hwy., Suite 402, Bethesda, MD 20814 (SAN 688-9077) Tel 301-657-0270; Fax: 301-657-0275
E-mail: nasp@naspweb.org; publications@naspweb.org
Web site: http://www.uncg.edu/~ericcas2/nasp; http://www.naspweb.org.

†**Natl Assn Soc Wkrs,** *(National Assn. of Social Workers/NASW Pr.; 0-87101),* Orders Addr.: P.O. Box 431, Annapolis Junction, MD 20701 Fax: 301-206-7989; Toll Free: 800-227-3590; Edit Addr.: 750 First St. NE, Suite 700, Washington, DC 20002-4241 (SAN 202-893X) Tel 202-408-8600; Fax: 202-336-8312; Toll Free: 800-638-8799
E-mail: press@naswdc.org
Web site: http://www.naswpress.org; *CIP.*

Natl Assn Sport, *(National Assn. for Sport & Physical Education (NASPE); 0-88314),* Subs. of American Alliance for Health, Physical Education, Recreation & Dance, 1900 Association Dr., Reston, VA 22091 (SAN 272-6866) Tel 703-476-3460; Fax: 703-476-8316; Toll Free: 800-213-7193
E-mail: naspe@aahperd.org
Dist(s): **AAHPERD** *(American Alliance for Health, Physical Education, Recreation & Dance).*

Natl Ataxia Found, *(National Ataxia Foundation; 0-943218),* 2600 Fernbrook Ln., Suite 119, Minneapolis, MN 55447 (SAN 228-0957) Tel 612-553-0020; Fax: 612-553-0167
E-mail: naf@mr.net
Web site: http://www.ataxia.org.

Natl Biomedical, *(National Biomedical Research Foundation; 0-912466),* Georgetown Univ., Medical Ctr., 3900 Reservoir Rd., NW, Washington, DC 20007 (SAN 203-7106) Tel 202-687-2121; Fax: 202-687-1662
E-mail: pirmail@nbrf.georgetown.edu
Web site: http://www.nbrf.georgetown.edu.

Natl Bk Netwk, *(National Bk. Network),* 15200 NBN Way, Blue Ridge Summit, PA 17214 (SAN 630-0065) Tel 717-794-3800; Toll Free Fax: 800-338-4550; Toll Free: 800-462-6420; Edit Addr.: 4720 Boston Way, Lanham, MD 20706 Tel 301-459-3366; Fax: 301-459-1705
Web site: http://www.nbnbooks.com.

Natl Board Cert Occp Ther, *(National Board for Certification in Occupational Therapy, Inc.; 0-9677436),* 800 S. Frederick Ave., Suite 200, Gaithersburg, MD 20877-4150 Tel 301-990-7979; Fax: 301-869-8492
Web site: http://www.nbcot.org.

Natl Book, *(National Bk. Co.; 0-89420),* Div. of Educational Research Assocs., P.O. Box 8795, Portland, OR 97207-8795 (SAN 212-4661) Tel 503-228-6345; Fax: 503-228-3961 ; *Imprints:* Halcyon (Halcyon House) Do not confuse with National Book Company, Scranton, PA
E-mail: info@halcyon.org.

†**Natl Bur Econ Res,** *(National Bureau of Economic Research, Inc.; 0-87014),* 1050 Massachusetts Ave., Cambridge, MA 02138 (SAN 203-7114) Tel 617-868-3900; Fax: 617-868-2742
E-mail: orders@nber.org
Web site: http://www.nber.org
Dist(s): **Cambridge U Pr** *(Cambridge Univ. Pr.)*
MIT Pr *(MIT Pr.)*
OUP *(Oxford Univ. Pr., Inc.)*
U Ch Pr *(Univ. of Chicago Pr.)*
Univ Microfilms *(University Microfilms, Inc.)*
Wiley *(Wiley, John & Sons, Inc.); CIP.*

Natl Cath Educ, *(National Catholic Educational Assn.; 1-55833),* 1077 30th St., NW, Suite 100, Washington, DC 20007-3852 (SAN 676-8636) Tel 202-337-6232; Fax: 202-333-6706
E-mail: pubs@ncea.org
Web site: http://www.ncea.org.

Natl Childrens Bur (GBR) *(1-874579; 1-900990) Dist. by* **Paul & Co Pubs.**

Natl Coal Advocates, *(National Coalition of Advocates for Students; 1-880002),* 100 Boylston St., Suite 737, Boston, MA 02116 Tel 617-357-8507; Fax: 617-375-9549.

Natl Coll Chiro, *(National College of Chiropractic; 0-9615849),* 200 E. Roosevelt Rd., Lombard, IL 60148 (SAN 696-6470) Tel 630-889-6524; Fax: 630-889-6482; Toll Free: 800-826-6285
E-mail: dana5140@aol.com
Web site: http://www.national.chiropractic.edu.

Natl Comm Assn, *(National Communication Assn. (NCA); 0-944811),* 1765 N St., NW, Washington, DC 20036-2801 (SAN 202-0726) Tel 703-750-0533; Fax: 703-914-9471
Web site: http://www.natcom.org.

Natl Comm Clin Lab Stds, *See* **NCCLS**

Natl Comm Mental, *(National Council of Community Mental Health Ctrs.; 1-883066),* 12300 Twinbrook Pkwy., Suite 320, Rockville, MD 20852 (SAN 224-3628) Tel 301-984-6200; Fax: 301-881-7159.

Natl Comm Philan, *(National Committee for Responsive Philanthropy; 1-891465),* 2001 S St., NW, Suite 620, Washington, DC 20009 (SAN 273-2114) Tel 202-387-9177; Fax: 202-332-5084
E-mail: info@ncrp.org
Web site: http://www.ncrp.org.

Natl Conf State Legis, *(National Conference of State Legislatures; 0-941336; 1-55516; 1-58024),* 1560 Broadway, Suite 700, Denver, CO 80202-5140 (SAN 225-1000) Tel 303-830-2200; Fax: 303-863-8003
E-mail: rita.morris@ncsl.org
Web site: http://www.ncsl.org.

†**Natl Coun Aging,** *(National Council on the Aging, The; 0-910883),* 409 Third St. SW, Suite 200, Washington, DC 20024 (SAN 675-3361) Tel 202-479-1200; Fax: 202-479-0735; *CIP.*

Natl Coun Family, *(National Council on Family Relations; 0-916174),* 3989 Central Ave. NE, Suite 550, Minneapolis, MN 55421 (SAN 689-1764) Tel 763-781-9331; Fax: 763-781-9348; Toll Free: 888-781-9331
E-mail: ncfr3989@ncfr.org
Web site: http://www.ncfr.org.

Natl Ct Report, *(National Court Reporters Assn.; 1-881859),* 8224 Old Courthouse Rd., Vienna, VA 22182-3808 Tel 703-556-6272; Fax: 703-556-6291
E-mail: msic@ncrahq.org
Web site: http://www.ncraonline.org
Dist(s): **Baker & Taylor** *(Baker & Taylor Bks.).*

Natl Ctr CIP, *See* **ZERO TO THREE**

†**Natl Ctr Health Stats,** *(National Ctr. for Health Statistics; 0-8406),* 6525 Belcrest Rd., Rm. 1064, Hyattsville, MD 20782 (SAN 206-6033) Tel 301-436-8500
Web site: http://www.cdc.gov/nchs/
Dist(s): **Natl Tech Info** *(National Technical Information Service, U.S. Dept. of Commerce)*
USGPO *(U.S. Government Printing Office); CIP.*

Natl Ctr Pol, *(National Ctr. for Policy Analysis; 0-943802; 1-56808),* 12655 N. Central Expwy, Suite 720, Dallas, TX 75243 (SAN 241-0869) Tel 972-386-6272; Fax: 972-386-0924
Web site: http://www.ncpa.org.

†**Natl Ctr St Courts,** *(National Ctr. for State Courts; 0-89656),* Orders Addr.: P.O. Box 580, Williston, VT 05495-0580 (SAN 210-928X) Tel 757-253-2000; Fax: 757-220-0449; Edit Addr.: 300 Newport Ave., Williamsburg, VA 23187-8798
E-mail: webmaster@ncsc.dni.us; ncscorders@aidevt.com
Web site: http://www.ncsc.dni.us/
Dist(s): **Am Intl Dist** *(American International Distribution Corp.); CIP.*

Natl Easter Seal, *(National Easter Seal Society; 0-933851),* 230 W. Monroe St., Suite 1800, Chicago, IL 60606 (SAN 225-9419) Tel 312-726-6200
Web site: http://www.easter-seals.org.

Natl Educ Serv, *(National Educational Service; 1-879639),* 304 W. Kirkwood Ave., Suite 2, Bloomington, IN 47404-5132 Tel 812-336-7700; Fax: 812-336-7790; Toll Free: 800-733-6786
E-mail: nes@nesonline.com
Web site: http://www.nesonline.com.

Natl Environ Health, *(National Environmental Health Assn.; 0-944111),* 720 S. Colorado Blvd., Suite 970, South Tower, Denver, CO 80246 (SAN 224-3180) Tel 303-756-9090; Fax: 303-691-9490
E-mail: staffeneh@neha.org
Web site: http://www.neha.org.

Natl Fire Prot, *(National Fire Protection Assn.; 0-87765),* Batterymarch Pk., Quincy, MA 02269 (SAN 202-8948) Tel 617-770-3000; Fax: 617-770-0700; Toll Free: 800-344-3555
Web site: http://www.nfpa.org
Dist(s): **IFSTA** *(IFSTA).*

Natl Forensic, *(National Forensic Ctr.; 0-9602962; 1-880694),* Div. of Forensic Services Directory, Inc., Orders Addr.: P.O. Box 3161, Princeton, NJ 08543 (SAN 241-7928) Tel 609-883-0550; Fax: 609-883-7622; Toll Free: 800-526-5177; Edit Addr.: 17 Temple Terr., Lawrenceville, NJ 08648 (SAN 212-7792).

†**Natl Geog,** *(National Geographic Society; 0-7922; 0-87044),* Orders Addr.: P.O. Box 1640, Washington, DC 20013-1640 Tel 301-921-1200; Edit Addr.: 1145 17th St., NW, Washington, DC 20036 (SAN 202-8956) Tel 202-857-7000; Fax: 301-921-1575; Toll Free: 800-647-5463; 800-548-9797 (TTD users only)
Web site: http://nationalgeographic.com
Dist(s): **Follett Audio** *(Follett Audiovisual Resources)*
Lectorum Pubns *(Lectorum Pubns., Inc.)*
Publishers Group *(Publishers Group West)*
S&S Trade *(Simon & Schuster Trade)*
Shens Bks *(Shen's Bks.); CIP.*

Natl Governor, *(National Governors' Assn.; 1-55877),* Orders Addr.: P.O. Box 421, Annapolis Junction, MD 20701 Tel 301-498-3738; Fax: 301-206-9789; Edit Addr.: 444 N. Capitol St., NW, Suite 267, Washington, DC 20001 (SAN 226-5222) Tel 202-624-5332; Fax: 202-624-5313
E-mail: badams@pmds.com
Web site: http://www.nga.org.

Natl Hall Humor, *(National Hall of Humor; 1-882082),* P.O. Box 453, Brahan, MN 55006 (SAN 248-3378) Tel 612-444-7341
Dist(s): **Bookmen Inc** *(Bookmen, Inc.).*

Natl Head Injury, *See* **Brain Injury Assoc**

Natl Health Coun, *(National Health Council; 0-929852),* 1730 M St., NW, Suite 500, Washington, DC 20036 (SAN 224-3261) Tel 202-785-3910; Fax: 202-785-5923
E-mail: holmes@nhcouncil.org
Web site: http://www.nhcouncil.org.

Natl Health Lawyers, *See* **Am Hlth Lawyers**

Natl Hospice, *(National Hospice Organization; 0-931207),* 1700 Diagonal Rd., Suite 300, Alexandria, VA 22314-2848 (SAN 689-2205) Tel 703-837-1500; Fax: 703-525-5762; Toll Free: 800-658-8898 (Hospice Helpline)
E-mail: info@nhpco.org
Web site: http://www.nhpco.org.

Natl Inst Nurse, *(National Institute of Nurse Education; 0-9701171),* 4960 Almaden Expressway, No. 227, San Jose, CA 95118 Fax: 508-462-0214
E-mail: cehrs4rns@hotmail.com
Web site: http://cehours4rns.com.

Natl Inst Soc Work (GBR) *(0-902789; 1-899942) Dist. by* **St Mut.**

Natl Kidney, *(National Kidney Foundation, Inc.; 0-9629721; 1-931472),* 30 E. 33rd St., New York, NY 10016 (SAN 224-3431) Tel 212-889-2210; Fax: 212-689-9261; Toll Free: 800-622-9010
E-mail: info@kidney.org
Web site: http://www.kidney.org.

†**Natl Lawyers Guild,** *(National Lawyers Guild; 0-9602188),* 126 University Pl., 5th Flr., New York, NY 10003-4538 (SAN 212-5307) Do not confuse with companies with the same name in Philadelphia, PA & San Jose, CA; *CIP.*

Natl League Nurse, *(National League for Nursing Pr. (NLN Pr.); 0-7637; 0-88737),* 61 Broadway, 33rd Flr., New York, NY 10006-2701 (SAN 203-7130) Tel 978-443-5000 ; *Imprints:* NLN Pr (N L N Press)
Web site: http://www.nlnpress.jbpub.com
Dist(s): **J Majors Co** *(Majors, J. A. Co.)*
Jones & Bartlett *(Jones & Bartlett Pubs., Inc.)*
Matthews Bk Co *(Matthews Bk. Co.)*
Yankee Ped Bkshop *(Yankee Peddler Bookshop).*

Natl Marfan Foun, *(National Marfan Foundation, The; 0-918335),* 382 Main St., Port Washington, NY 11050 (SAN 657-2855) Tel 516-883-8712; Fax: 516-883-8040; Toll Free: 800-862-7326
E-mail: staff@marfan.org
Web site: http://www.marfan.org.

Natl Middle Schl, *(National Middle Schl. Assn.; 1-56090),* 4151 Executive Pkwy., Suite 300, Westerville, OH 43081-3867 (SAN 225-8455) Tel 614-895-4730; Fax: 614-895-4750; Toll Free: 800-528-6672.

Natl Mus Am, *(National Museum of American History, Smithsonian Institution; 0-929847),* Constitution Ave. & 12th St., NW, Rm. MBB66, Washington, DC 20560 (SAN 279-7941) Tel 202-357-1965
Dist(s): **Univ Pub Assocs** *(University Publishing Assocs., Inc.).*

Natl Opinion Res, *(National Opinion Research Ctr. (NORC); 0-932132),* Affil. of Univ. of Chicago, 1155 E. 60th St., Rm. 281, Chicago, IL 60637 (SAN 205-7735) Tel 773-256-6204; Fax: 773-753-7886
E-mail: cloud@norcmail.uchicago.edu
Web site: http://www.norc.uchicago.edu.

Natl Org Orthopaedic Nurse, *See* **Natl Assn Ortho Nurse**

Natl Paperback, *(National Paperback Bks., Inc.; 0-89826),* Orders Addr.: 3102 Schaad Rd., Knoxville, TN 37921 (SAN 211-5344) Tel 423-947-5243; Fax: 423-947-4320.

Natl Planning, *(National Planning Assn.; 0-89068),* 1424 16th St., NW, Washington, DC 20036 (SAN 207-0030) Tel 202-265-7685.

Natl Prac Inst, *(National Practice Institute; 1-55917),* 701 Fourth Ave. S., No. 1710, Minneapolis, MN 55415-1634 (SAN 217-2577) Tel 612-338-1977; Fax: 612-349-6561; Toll Free: 800-328-4444.

Publisher Symbol Index

Natl Res Ctr, *(National Resource Ctr. for Youth Services; 1-878848),* 4502 E. 41st St., Bldg 4W, Tulsa, OK 74135 (SAN 630-401X) Tel 918-660-3700; Fax: 918-660-3737
E-mail: pcorreia@ou.edu
Web site: http://www.nrcys.ou.edu.

Natl Resource Ctr, *(National Resource Ctr.; 0-9677724),* 8100 26th Ave. S., Suite 120, Bloomington, MN 55425 Tel 612-858-8999; Fax: 612-858-8982 Do not confuse with National Resource Center, Coral Springs, FLA
Web site: http://www.ncccconline.org.

Natl Ret Fed Emps, *(National Assn. of Retired Federal Employees; 0-9631168),* 606 N. Washington St., Alexandria, VA 22314 (SAN 225-0764) Tel 703-838-7760.

Natl Safety Coun, *(National Safety Council; 0-87912),* 1121 Spring Lake Dr., Itasca, IL 60143-3201 (SAN 203-7157) Tel 630-285-1121; Fax: 630-285-1315; Toll Free: 800-621-7619
Web site: http://www.nsc.org.

Natl Ski Patrol, *(National Ski Patrol System, Inc.; 0-929752),* 133 S. Van Gordon St., Lakewood, CO 80228 (SAN 689-5166) Tel 303-988-1111; Fax: 303-988-3005
Web site: http://www.nsp@nsp.org.

Natl Spasmodic Dysphonia, *(National Spasmodic Dysphonia; 0-9659941),* Div. of Dystoria Medical Research Foundation, 1 E. Wacker Dr., Suite 2430, Chicago, IL 60601-1905 Tel 312-755-0198; Fax: 312-803-0138; Toll Free: 800-795-6732
E-mail: info@dystonia-foundation.org
Web site: http://www.dystonia-foundation.org/.

Natl Stroke Assn, *(National Stroke Assn.; 0-9624876),* 96 Inverness Dr., E., Suite I, Englewood, CO 80112-5112 Tel 303-649-9299; Toll Free: 800-787-6537.

Natl Tech Info, *(National Technical Information Service, U.S. Dept. of Commerce; 0-934213),* Orders Addr.: 5285 Port Royal Rd., Springfield, VA 22161 (SAN 205-7255) Tel 703-605-6000; Fax: 703-605-6900; Toll Free: 800-553-6847
E-mail: orders@ntis.gov; info@ntis.gov
Web site: http://www.ntis.gov
Dist(s): **Bernan Associates** *(Bernan Assocs.).*

Natl Textbk Co Imprint of NTC Contemp Pub Co

Natl Tinn Fund, *(National Tinnitus Fund; 0-9612648),* P.O. Box 5081, Springfield, MO 65801 (SAN 289-3428) Tel 417-831-0436.

Natl Trop Bot, *(National Tropical Botanical Garden; 0-915809),* P.O. Box 340, Lawai Kauai, HI 96765 (SAN 293-8979) Tel 808-332-7324; Fax: 808-332-9765
E-mail: acctg@ntbg.org
Dist(s): **UH Pr** *(Univ. of Hawaii Pr.).*

Natl Wellness Inst, *(National Wellness Institute; 0-940981),* Orders Addr.: 1045 Clark St., Suite 210, Stevens Point, WI 54481 (SAN 665-4312) Tel 715-342-2969; Fax: 715-342-2979.

Natl Writ Pr, *(National Writers Pr., The; 0-88100),* Div. of National Writers Assn., 3140 S. Peoria St., No. 294, Aurora, CO 80014 (SAN 240-320X) Tel 720-851-1944; Fax: 303-841-2607
E-mail: AnitaEdits@aol.com
Web site: http://www.nationalwriters.com.

Natural CA, *(Natural Pr.; 0-9625499),* Box 611, Dana Point, CA 92629 Tel 714-497-9459; Toll Free: 800-549-3907 Do not confuse with Natural Pr., Manitowoc, WI
Dist(s): **Baker & Taylor** *(Baker & Taylor Bks.)*
New Leaf Dist *(New Leaf Distributing Co., Inc.).*

Natural Energy, *(Natural Energy Works; 0-9621855),* P.O. Box 1148, Ashland, OR 97520-0039 Tel 541-552-0118 phone/fax
E-mail: demeo@mind.net
Web site: http://www.orgonelab.org/.

Natural Healing Pubns, *(Natural Healing Pubns.; 0-9671567),* P.O. Box 3628, Santa Monica, CA 90408 Tel 310-576-0710; Fax: 310-576-6575; Toll Free: 877-832-2463
E-mail: johnr@dssnh.com.

Natural Hygiene, *See* **Amer Natural Hygiene**

Natural Med, *(Natural Medicine; 0-9661285),* Orders Addr.: P.O. Box 3441, Grass Valley, CA 95945 Tel 916-273-3674; Fax: 916-273-5193; Edit Addr.: 1097 E. Main, Suite C, Grass Valley, CA 95945
E-mail: DRL@NaturalMedicine
Web site: http://www.NaturalMedicine.com.

Natural Pr, *(Natural Pr.; 0-939956),* P.O. Box 730, Manitowoc, WI 54221-0730 (SAN 287-0215) Tel 920-758-2500 Do not confuse with Natural Pr., San Clemente, CA
Dist(s): **Nutri-Books Corp** *(Nutri-Bks. Corp.).*

Natural Prod, *(Natural Products Co.; 0-9614234; 1-888755),* Orders Addr.: P.O. Box 1251, Occidental, CA 95465 Fax: 707-874-1910
Dist(s): **Bookpeople** *(Bookpeople).*

Nature Pubg Grp, *(Nature Publishing Group; 1-56159),* Div. of Groves Dictionaries, Inc., 345 Park Ave., S., New York, NY 10010 Tel 212-726-0200; Fax: 212-689-9711
E-mail: grove@grovereference.com
Dist(s): **Holtzbrinck** *(Holtzbrinck Online Publishing).*

Naturegraph, *(Naturegraph Pubs., Inc.; 0-87961; 0-911010),* P.O. Box 1047, Happy Camp, CA 96039 (SAN 202-8999) Tel 530-493-5353; Fax: 530-493-5240; Toll Free: 800-390-5353
E-mail: nature@sisqtel.net
Web site: http://www.naturegraph.com
Dist(s): **New Leaf Dist** *(New Leaf Distributing Co., Inc.)*
Rutgers U Pr *(Rutgers Univ. Pr.)*
Sunbelt Pubns *(Sunbelt Pubns., Inc.).*

Natures Pubng, *(Nature's Publishing, Ltd.; 0-9640539; 1-928820),* Orders Addr.: P.O. Box 380361, Murdock, FL 33938-0361 Tel 941-426-1929; Fax: 941-426-6871; Edit Addr.: 5621 Reisterstown Rd., Northport, FL 34287 Tel 941-426-1929; Toll Free: 800-950-1929
E-mail: NPath1@aol.com.

Navajo Coll Pr, *See* **Dine College Pr**

†Naval Inst Pr, *(Naval Institute Pr.; 0-87021; 1-55750; 1-59114),* Orders Addr.: 2062 Generals Hwy., Annapolis, MD 21401 (SAN 662-0930) Tel 410-268-6110; Fax: 410-295-1042; Toll Free: 800-233-8764; Edit Addr.: 291 Wood Rd., Beach Hall, Annapolis, MD 21402-5034 (SAN 202-9006)
E-mail: psappington@usni.org
Web site: http://www.navalinstitute.org; *CIP.*

Navarang (IND) *(81-7013) Dist. by* **S Asia.**

NavPress, *(NavPress Publishing Group; 0-89109; 1-57683),* Orders Addr.: P.O. Box 35001, Colorado Springs, CO 80935 Tel 719-598-1212; Fax: 719-260-7223
Web site: http://www.navpress.com.

Naya Prokash (IND) *(81-85109; 81-85421) Dist. by* **S Asia.**

NC Ctr Healing, *(North Carolina Ctr. for Healing Touch; 1-889293),* 413 Waterside Dr., Carrboro, NC 27510 Tel 919-942-5214; Fax: 919-968-0994
E-mail: maryjo@mindspring.com.

†NCBC, *(National Catholic Bioethics Ctr., The; 0-935372),* 159 Washington St., Boston, MA 02135 (SAN 282-1729) Tel 732-787-1900; Fax: 617-787-4900; *CIP.*

NCCL (GBR) *Dist. by* **St Mut.**

NCCLS, *(NCCLC; 1-56238),* 940 W. Valley Rd., Suite 1400, Wayne, PA 19087 (SAN 224-344X) Tel 610-688-0100; Fax: 610-527-8399.

†NCCP, *(National Ctr. for Children in Poverty; 0-926582),* 154 Haven Ave., New York, NY 10032 Tel 212-304-7100; Fax: 212-544-4200
E-mail: nccp@columbia.edu
Web site: http://www.NCCP.org; *CIP.*

NCLS Inc, *(National Clearinghouse for Legal Services, Inc.; 0-941077),* 205 W. Monroe St., 2nd Flr., Chicago, IL 60606-5013 (SAN 226-2169) Toll Free: 800-621-3256.

NCM Pubs, *(NCM Pubs, Inc.; 0-9643884),* 200 Varick St., New York, NY 10014 Tel 212-691-9100; Fax: 212-645-2571.

†NCRP Pubns, *(National Council on Radiation Protection & Measurements; 0-913392; 0-929600),* 7910 Woodmont Ave., Suite 800, Bethesda, MD 20814-3095 (SAN 677-1254) Tel 301-657-2652; Fax: 301-907-8768; Toll Free: 800-229-2652
E-mail: ncrp@ncrp.com
Web site: http://www.ncrp.com; *CIP.*

†NCUP, *(NCUP, Inc.; 0-8084),* 69 Velina Dr., Albany, NY 12203 (SAN 203-6223) Tel 518-869-3734; Fax: 518-218-1717; *CIP.*

NDE Pub (CAN) *(1-55321; 0-9684749) Dist. by* **IPG Chicago.**

NDI Mktg Grp, *See* **Falcon Pr Intl**

NDTA, *(Neuro-Developmental Treatment Assn.; 0-9621991),* 401 N. Michigan Ave., Chicago, IL 60611-4267 Tel 312-321-5151; Fax: 312-321-6869; Toll Free: 800-869-9295.

†NE U Pr, *(Northeastern Univ. Pr.; 0-930350; 1-55553),* Orders Addr.: 750 Cascadilla St., Ithaca, NY 14851 (SAN 630-6519) Tel 607-277-2211; Fax: 607-277-6292; Toll Free: 800-666-2211; Edit Addr.: 360 Huntington Ave., 416 Columbus Pl., Boston, MA 02115 (SAN 205-3764) Tel 617-373-5480; Fax: 617-373-5483
E-mail: univpress@nunet.neu.edu
Web site: http://www.neu.edu/nupress; *CIP.*

†NEA, *(National Education Assn.; 0-8106),* Orders Addr.: 9050 Junction Dr., Annapolis Junction, MD 20701 Tel 301-617-7830; Fax: 301-206-9789; Edit Addr.: P.O. Box 2035, Annapolis Junction, MD 20701 (SAN 203-7262) Tel 202-822-7202; Fax: 202-822-7206; Toll Free: 800-229-4200
E-mail: neapl@pmds.com
Web site: http://www.nea.org/books; *CIP.*

†Neal-Schuman, *(Neal-Schuman Pubs., Inc.; 0-918212; 1-55570),* 100 Varick St., New York, NY 10013 (SAN 210-2455) Tel 212-925-8650; Fax: 212-219-8916; Toll Free Fax: 800-584-2414
E-mail: info@neal-schuman.com
Web site: http://www.neal-schuman.com; *CIP.*

Necro Publns, *(Necro Pubns.; 1-889186),* Orders Addr.: P.O. Box 540298, Orlando, FL 32854-0298 Tel 407-839-0463; Fax: 407-551-0220
E-mail: necrodave@cfl.rr.com
Web site: http://www.necropublications.com.

Nedley Publishing, *(Nedley Publishing; 0-9661979),* 1010 14th St., NW, Ardmore, OK 73401 Tel 580-226-8007; Fax: 580-223-1108; Toll Free: 888-778-4445
E-mail: Neil@BrightOK.net
Web site: http://www.proofpositive.net.

Nedmar Graphics Imprint of HealthNet Pages

Nehemiah Pubng, *(Nehemiah Publishing House; 0-9644135),* 12730 Carmel Country Rd., No. 120, San Diego, CA 92130 Tel 619-259-9230 Do not confuse with Nehemiah Publishing in Omaha, NE.

Neighborhood Bible, *(Neighborhood Bible Studies, Inc.; 1-880266),* 56 Main St., P.O. Box 222, Dobbs Ferry, NY 10522-0222 Tel 914-693-3273; Fax: 914-693-4345; Toll Free: 800-369-0307
E-mail: nbstudies@aol.com
Web site: http://www.neighborhoodbiblestudy.org.

†Nelson, *(Nelson, Thomas Inc.; 0-7852; 0-8407; 0-8499; 0-86605; 0-89840; 0-918956; 1-4003),* Orders Addr.: P.O. Box 141000, Nashville, TN 37214-1000 (SAN 209-3820) Tel 615-889-9000; Fax: 615-391-5225; Toll Free: 800-251-4000; Edit Addr.: 501 Nelson Pl., Nashville, TN 37214 ; *Imprints:* J Thoma Bks (Thoma, Janet Books)
E-mail: thomasnelson.com
Web site: http://www.thomasnelson.com
Dist(s): **Christian Bk Distributors** *(Christian Bk. Distributors); CIP.*

Nelson Ref & Elec Pub, *(Nelson Reference & Electronic Publishing; 0-7852; 0-8407; 0-8499),* P.O. Box 141000, Nashville, TN 37214-1000.

Nelson Thornes (GBR) *(0-17; 0-7487; 0-85950; 1-873732) Dist. by* **Aspen Pub.**

Nelson Thornes (GBR) *(0-17; 0-7487; 0-85950; 1-873732) Dist. by* **Intl Spec Bk.**

Nelson Thornes (GBR) *(0-17; 0-7487; 0-85950; 1-873732) Dist. by* **Trans-Atl Phila.**

Nelson-Hall, *See* **Burnham Inc**

Nelsons Bks, *(Nelson's Bks.; 0-9612188),* P.O. Box 2302, Santa Cruz, CA 95063 (SAN 289-4858) Tel 831-465-9148.

Neofax, *(Neofax-PC, Inc.; 1-888703),* P.O. Box 20554, Raleigh, NC 27619 Tel 919-250-7645; Fax: 919-250-8135; Toll Free: 800-386-9159
Dist(s): **Blackwell Sci** *(Blackwell Science, Inc.).*

Neo-Tech Pub, *(Neo-Tech Publishing Co.; 0-911752),* P.O. Box 60906, Boulder City, NV 89006-0906 (SAN 202-3156) Tel 702-891-0303; Fax: 702-795-8393
E-mail: cservice@neo-tech.com
Web site: http://www.neo-tech.com; http://www.neo-tech.com/front/cservice.html.

Nest Egg Pr, *(Nest Egg Pr.; 0-9631221),* 2721 NE Clackamas St., Portland, OR 97232-1730 Tel 503-460-3374
E-mail: user912724@aol.com.

Net Worth, *(Net Worth, Inc.; 0-9645633),* Orders Addr.: P.O. Box 471462, Forestville, MD 20753-1462 Tel 301-445-8546; Edit Addr.: 7203 Willow Hill Dr., Seat Pleasant, MD 20743.

NetGuide Pubg, *See* **SurfLess**

Network Pubns, *See* **ETR Assocs**

Network Three Thous, *(Network 3000 Publishing; 0-9635085; 0-9709321),* Orders Addr.: 3432 Denmark, No. 108, Eagan, MN 55123 Tel 952-707-1898 (phone/fax); Toll Free: 800-398-4642
E-mail: khogan1652@aol.com
Web site: http://www.kevinhogan.com
Dist(s): **Baker & Taylor** *(Baker & Taylor Bks.).*

Neuro Diabetic, *(Neuro Diabetic Concepts; 0-9657143),* Orders Addr.: P.O. Box 608, Blue Bell, PA 19422 Tel 215-646-4556; Fax: 215-646-5455; Toll Free: 800-968-0665; Edit Addr.: 795 Boehm Church Rd., Blue Bell, PA 19422
E-mail: martinm747@aol.com
Web site: http://www.beatbiabe.com.

Neuroinfo, *(Neuroinformatics, Inc.; 0-9664949),* 1763 E. Marlton Pike, Suite 201, Cherry Hill, NJ 08003 Tel 609-489-5532; Fax: 215-489-7525; Toll Free: 800-569-0320
E-mail: neuroinformatics@yahoo.com
Web site: http://www.neuroinformatics.net.

Neuropsych Pr, *(Neuropsychology Pr.; 0-934515),* 2920 S. Fourth St., Tucson, AZ 85713-4819 (SAN 693-8256) Tel 520-882-2022.

NeuroSci Soc NY, *(Neuroscience Society of New York; 0-944809),* 750 Lexington Ave., 23rd Flr., New York, NY 10022-1200 (SAN 244-9579) Tel 212-695-2740.

Neurotechtonics, *(Neurotechtonics, Inc.; 0-9650204),* Orders Addr.: P.O. Box 176, Park Forest, IL 60466 Tel 708-534-3869; Fax: 708-534-2640; Edit Addr.: 1213 Blackhawk Dr., University Park, IL 60466-3321
E-mail: nurotekinc@aol.com
Dist(s): **New Leaf Dist** *(New Leaf Distributing Co., Inc.).*

Neva Pr, *(Neva Pr., Inc.; 0-9637603),* Orders Addr.: P.O. Box 347, Branford, CT 06405; Edit Addr.: 305 Crown St., New Haven, CT 06511 Tel 203-272-5338
E-mail: nevapress@snet.net
Web site: http://www.nevapress.com.

Nevada Policy, *(Nevada Policy Research Institute; 1-886306),* P.O. Box 20312, Reno, NV 89515-0312 Tel 702-786-9600; Fax: 702-786-9604; Toll Free: 800-786-9602
E-mail: info@npri.org
Web site: http://www.npri.org.

Never-Give-Up Weight, *(Never-Give-Up Weight Loss/Control Program; 1-878502),* Orders Addr.: P.O. Box 16, Snohomish, WA 98290; Edit Addr.: 6430 157th Dr., SE, Snohomish, WA 98290 Tel 360-568-1636.

New Age FL Pub, *(New Age Publishing Co.; 0-934619),* P.O. Box 01-1549, Miami, FL 33101 (SAN 694-0226) Tel 305-534-8437; Fax: 305-446-9206
Dist(s): **New Leaf Dist** *(New Leaf Distributing Co., Inc.).*

New Age Gainesville, *See* **Mystic Planet**

New Atlantean, *(New Atlantean Pr.; 1-881217),* Orders Addr.: P.O. Box 9638, Santa Fe, NM 87504 (SAN 297-617X) Tel 505-983-1856 (phone/fax); Edit Addr.: 1 Camino Delilah, Santa Fe, NM 87501
E-mail: global@new-atlantean.com
Dist(s): **Baker & Taylor** *(Baker & Taylor Bks.)*
Midpt Trade *(Midpoint Trade Bks., Inc.)*
New Leaf Dist *(New Leaf Distributing Co., Inc.)*
Nutri-Books Corp *(Nutri-Bks. Corp.).*

New Atlantis, *(New Atlantis Pr.; 0-9615480),* 32 Sunset Hill Rd., Bethel, CT 06801-2919 (SAN 695-9083).

New Cent Pub CT, *(New Century Pubs. 2000; 0-9701110; 0-9702964),* P.O. Box 36, East Canaan, CT 06024 Tel 860-824-5301; Fax: 860-824-0309
E-mail: safe@snet.net
Dist(s): **SAFE GOODS** *(SAFE GOODS/New Century Publishing 2000).*

New Centry Pr, *(New Century Pr.; 1-890035),* 1055 Bay Blvd., Suite C, Chula Vista, CA 91911-1628 Tel 619-476-7400; Fax: 619-476-7474; Toll Free: 800-519-2465 (orders)
E-mail: sales@newcenturypress.com
Web site: http://www.newcenturypress.com.

New Decade Inc, *See* **Next Decade**

New Destiny Ed, *(New Destiny Educational Products, Inc.; 0-9674969),* 188 Rte. 101, Suite 314 The American Office, Bedford, NH 03110 Fax: 603-471-6362.

New Energy, *(New Energy Dynamics; 1-892241),* Orders Addr.: P.O. Box 963, Greensburg, PA 15601; Edit Addr.: 860 Harrison City Rd., Suite 5A, Greensburg, PA 15601 Tel 724-832-7459; Fax: 724-838-7638
E-mail: jacpal@westol.com.

New Energy Pr, *(New Energy Pr.; 0-9642979),* 1225 LaSalle, No. 1604, Minneapolis, MN 55403 Tel 612-342-0104
Dist(s): **Adventure Pubns** *(Adventure Pubns.)*
Baker & Taylor *(Baker & Taylor Bks.)*
Bookmen Inc *(Bookmen, Inc.).*

New Eng & Reg All, *See* **OceanSide Pubns**

New Engld Schl Homeopthy, *(New England Schl. of Homeopathy Pr.; 0-9654004),* 356 Middle St., Amherst, MA 01002 Tel 413-256-5949; Fax: 413-256-6223
E-mail: nesh@nesh,com
Web site: http://www.nesh.com.

New Falcon Pubns, *(New Falcon Pubns.; 0-941404; 0-9622452; 1-56184),* 1739 E. Broadway Rd., No. 1-277, Tempe, AZ 85282 (SAN 262-0243) Tel 602-708-1409; Fax: 602-708-1410; Fulfillment Addr.: c/o JV Company, 1585 Linda Way, Sparks, NV 89431
E-mail: info@newfalcon.com
Web site: http://www.newfalcon.com
Dist(s): **Baker & Taylor** *(Baker & Taylor Bks.)*
Bookpeople *(Bookpeople)*
New Leaf Dist *(New Leaf Distributing Co., Inc.)*
Red Wheel ME *(Red Wheel).*

New Forums, *(New Forums Pr.; 0-913507; 1-58107),* Orders Addr.: P.O. Box 876, Stillwater, OK 74076 (SAN 285-8673) Tel 405-372-6158; Fax: 405-377-2237; Toll Free: 800-606-3766; Edit Addr.: 1018 S. Lewis, Stillwater, OK 74074
E-mail: newforums@aol.com.; dougdollar@newforums.com
Web site: http://www.newforums.com
Dist(s): **Booksource** *(Booksource, The).*

New Frntr Pub, *(New Frontier Publishing; 0-9625448),* Orders Addr.: P.O. Box 246654, Sacramento, CA 95824; Edit Addr.: 4311 Stockton Blvd., Sacramento, CA 95820 Tel 916-455-5381.

New Futures, *(New Futures, Inc.; 0-945886),* 5400 Cutler Ave. NE, Albuquerque, NM 87110 (SAN 247-9524) Tel 505-883-5680; Fax: 505-880-3977.

New Harbinger, *(New Harbinger Pubns.; 0-934986; 1-57224; 1-879237),* 5674 Shattuck Ave., Oakland, CA 94609 (SAN 205-0587) Tel 510-652-2002; 510-652-0215; Fax: 510-652-5472; Toll Free: 800-748-6273
E-mail: nhhelp@newharbinger.com
Web site: http://www.newharbinger.com
Dist(s): **Publishers Group** *(Publishers Group West)*
Red Toad Rd *(Red Toad Road Co.).*

New Holland Pubs (GBR) *(1-85368; 1-85974) Dist. by* **Sterling.**

New Horizon NJ, *(New Horizon Pr. Pubs., Inc.; 0-88282),* Orders Addr.: P.O. Box 669, Far Hills, NJ 07931 (SAN 677-119X) Tel 908-604-6311; Fax: 908-604-6330; Toll Free: 800-533-7978 (orders only)
E-mail: nhp@newhorizonpressbooks.com
Web site: http://www.newhorizonpressbooks.com
Dist(s): **Natl Bk Netwk** *(National Bk. Network).*

New Idea Pr, *(New Idea Pr., Inc.; 0-9617099),* 532 W. Lois Way, Louisville, CO 80027 (SAN 662-5002) Tel 303-666-5687; 1736 36th St., Boulder, CO 80308-3683 (SAN 662-5010) Tel 303-494-4488
Dist(s): **Baker & Taylor** *(Baker & Taylor Bks.).*

New Leaf Dist, *(New Leaf Distributing Co., Inc.; 0-9627209),* Div. of Al-Wali Corp., 401 Thornton Rd., Lithia Springs, GA 30122-1557 (SAN 169-1449) Tel 770-948-7845; Fax: 770-944-2313; Toll Free Fax: 800-326-1066; Toll Free: 800-326-2665
E-mail: NewLeaf@NewLeaf-dist.com
Web site: http://www.NewLeaf-dist.com.

New Liberty Pubns, *(New Liberty Pubns.; 1-879204),* 405 W. 48th St., Rm. 2R, New York, NY 10036 Tel 212-459-2614
Dist(s): **Baker & Taylor** *(Baker & Taylor Bks.).*

New Life GA, *(New Life Publishing; 0-9643554),* P.O. Box 344, Roswell, GA 30077-0344 Tel 770-921-6038 Do not confuse with companies with the same name in Detroit, MI, Summerlin, NV, Burnet, TX
E-mail: newlfpubl@aol.com
Web site: melodymccloud.com.

New Manticore, *See* **Manticore Pubs**

New Med, *(New Medical Pr.; 0-9701022),* 2403 Lyndhurst Dr., Champaign, IL 61820 Tel 217-351-9009 (phone/fax)
E-mail: msmeone@uiuc.edu
Web site: http://www.fivestarsupport.com
Dist(s): **General Distrib Services** *(General Distribution Services, Inc.).*

New Mill Pr, *(New Mill Pr.; 0-9715707),* 35 Evergreen Ave., Rye, NY 10580.

New Nurse, *(New Nurse, Pub., The; 0-914698),* P.O. Box 803, Plattsburgh, NY 12901 (SAN 206-6041)
Dist(s): **Baker & Taylor** *(Baker & Taylor Bks.).*

New Orient Media, *See* **Creat Core**

New Page Bks Imprint of Career Pr Inc

New Press NY, *(New Pr., The; 1-56584),* 450 W. 41st St., 6th Flr., New York, NY 10036 Tel 212-629-8802; Fax: 212-629-8617; Toll Free Fax: 800-458-6515; Toll Free: 800-233-4830
E-mail: thenewpress.com
Web site: http://www.thenewpress.com
Dist(s): **Norton** *(Norton, W.W. & Co., Inc.).*

New Readers, *(New Readers Pr.; 0-88336; 1-56420),* Div. of Laubach Literacy International, Orders Addr.: P.O. Box 888, Syracuse, NY 13210 (SAN 202-1064) Fax: 315-422-6369; Toll Free: 800-448-8878; Edit Addr.: 1320 Jamesville Ave., Syracuse, NY 13210 Tel 315-422-9121
E-mail: nrp@laubach.org
Web site: http://www.newreaderspress.com.

New Resour, *(New Resources Pr.; 0-9701555),* 865 College Ave., Columbus, OH 43209-2309 (SAN 253-2832) Tel 614-237-4556; Fax: 614-237-5333
E-mail: editor@newresourcespress.com
Web site: http://newresourcespress.com
Dist(s): **BookWorld** *(BookWorld Services, Inc.).*

New Right Watch, *See* **Violence Policy Ctr**

New Soc Pubs, *(New Society Pubs., Ltd.; 0-86571),* P.O. Box 976, North Kingston, RI 02852 Tel 401-885-3482; Fax: 401-885-7996; Toll Free Fax: 800-567-7311; Toll Free: 800-567-6772
E-mail: info@newsociety.com
Web site: http://www.newsociety.com
Dist(s): **Consort Bk Sales** *(Consortium Bk. Sales & Distribution).*

New South Wales Univ Pr (AUS) *(0-86840; 0-909465; 0-7334; 0-908237) Dist. by* **Intl Spec Bk.**

New South Wales Univ Pr (AUS) *(0-86840; 0-909465; 0-7334; 0-908237) Dist. by* **U of Wash Pr.**

New Technology, *(New Technology Publishing, Inc.; 1-882431),* 6 West Blvd., P.O. Box 1737, Onset, MA 02558 Tel 508-291-1111; Fax: 508-291-1704; Toll Free Fax: 800-452-7632; Toll Free: 800-672-7632
E-mail: sales@newtechpub.com
Web site: http://www.HealthyResources.com
Dist(s): **Baker & Taylor** *(Baker & Taylor Bks.)*
Quality Bks IL *(Quality Bks., Inc.)*
Unique Bks Inc *(Unique Bks., Inc.).*

New View Pubns, *(New View Pubns.; 0-944337),* P.O. Box 3021, Chapel Hill, NC 27516 (SAN 243-4644) Tel 919-942-8491; Fax: 919-942-3760; Toll Free: 800-441-3604
E-mail: nview@aol.com
Web site: http://www.nvpi.com
Dist(s): **AMP Distrib** *(AMP Distributors)*
Baker & Taylor *(Baker & Taylor Bks.)*
Quality Bks IL *(Quality Bks., Inc.)*
Unique Bks Inc *(Unique Bks., Inc.).*

New Voice, *(New Voice Pubns.; 0-9661735),* P.O. Box 14113, Irvine, CA 92623 Tel 949-551-3397; Fax: 949-552-9041
E-mail: marcus@newvoice.net
Web site: http://www.newvoice.net
Dist(s): **BookMasters** *(BookMasters, Inc.)*
IPG Chicago *(Independent Pubs. Group).*

†**New Win Pub,** *(New Win Publishing, Inc.; 0-8329; 0-87691),* P.O. Box 5159, Clinton, NJ 08809 (SAN 217-1201) Tel 908-735-9701; Fax: 908-735-9703
Dist(s): **Continental Bk** *(Continental Bk. Co., Inc.); CIP.*

New Wind, *(New Wind Publishing; 0-9651412; 1-929777),* Orders Addr.: 5315 Spilman Ave., Sacramento, CA 95819-1733
E-mail: info@NewWindPub.com
Web site: http://NewWindPub.com
Dist(s): **Majors Scientific Bks Inc** *(Majors Scientific Bks., Inc.)*
Matthews Medical Bk Co *(Matthews Medical Bk. Co.)*
Rittenhouse *(Rittenhouse Bk. Distributors).*

New World Pr (CHN) *(7-80005) Dist. by* **China Bks.**

†**New Wrld Lib,** *(New World Library; 0-931432; 0-945934; 1-57731; 1-878424; 1-880032),* 14 Pamaron Way, Novato, CA 94949 (SAN 211-8777) Tel 415-884-2100; Fax: 415-884-2199; Toll Free: 800-972-6657 (retail orders only) Do not confuse with New World Library Publishing Co., Los Altos, CA
E-mail: escort@nwlib.com
Web site: http://www.newworldlibrary.com
Dist(s): **Bookpeople** *(Bookpeople)*
Lndmrk Audiobks *(Landmark Audiobooks)*
New Leaf Dist *(New Leaf Distributing Co., Inc.)*
Publishers Group *(Publishers Group West)*
netLibrary CO *(netLibrary, Inc.); CIP.*

Newark Beth, *(Newark Beth Israel Medical Ctr.; 0-937714),* 201 Lyons Ave., Newark, NJ 07112 (SAN 215-3297) Tel 973-926-7000.

Newbreed Imprint of Adebara & Honeycomb

Newbridge Comms, *See* **Newbridge Educ**

Newbridge Educ, *(Newbridge Educational Publishing; 1-56784; 1-58273; 1-4007),* Div. of Haights Cross Communications, Orders Addr.: P.O. Box 5267, Clifton, NJ 07015 Tel 973-614-8763; Toll Free: 800-729-1463; Edit Addr.: 333 E. 38th St., 8th Flr., New York, NY 10016
E-mail: kristinl@newbridgeeducational.com
Web site: http://www.newbridgeeducational.com.

Newconcept Pr, *(Newconcept Pr., Inc.; 0-931231),* 10 Industrial Ave., Mahwah, NJ 07430-2262 (SAN 689-1705) Tel 212-265-6284; Fax: 212-265-6659; Toll Free: 800-926-6579
E-mail: orders@erlbaum.com
Web site: http://www.erlbaum.com
Dist(s): **Baker & Taylor** *(Baker & Taylor Bks.).*

Newhouse Pr, *(Newhouse Pr.; 0-918050),* Orders Addr.: P.O. Box 76145, Los Angeles, CA 90076 (SAN 209-2697) Tel 213-382-1463; Edit Addr.: 146 N. Rampart Blvd., Los Angeles, CA 90026 (SAN 209-2689) Tel 213-383-1089.

Newmark Pub, *(Newmark Publishing Co.; 0-938539),* P.O. Box 603, South Windsor, CT 06074 (SAN 661-4760) Tel 860-282-7265; Toll Free: 800-280-7265.

---

†Newmarket, *(Newmarket Pr.; 0-937858; 1-55704),* Div. of Newmarket Publishing & Communications Corp., 18 E. 48th St., New York, NY 10017 (SAN 217-2585) Tel 212-832-3575; Fax: 212-832-3629; Toll Free Fax: 800-458-6515 (trade orders); Toll Free: 800-233-4830 (trade orders)
E-mail: mailbox@newmarketpress.com
Web site: http://www.newmarketpress.com
Dist(s):* Norton *(Norton, W.W. & Co., Inc.)
Wrldwide Media Srv *(Worldwide Media Service, Inc.); CIP.*

Newnes Imprint of Buttrwrth-Heinemann

Newport Pub Hse, *(Newport Publishing Hse.; 1-882013),* 12200 E. State Rte. 69, Lot 1, Dewey, AZ 86327-4502 (SAN 248-1235); 410 Acacia, Corona del Mar, CA 92625 (SAN 248-1243) Tel 714-675-8995.

Newpt Media, *(Newport Media Concepts, Inc.; 1-889972),* Orders Addr.: 1 Ave. at Port Imperial, No. 1123, West New York, NJ 07093-8303 (SAN 299-1519) Tel 201-865-8929; Fax: 212-208-4409; Toll Free: 800-732-3344
E-mail: adm@NewportBooks.com; books@NewportBooks.com
Web site: http://www.NewportMedia Concepts.com; http://www.NewportBooks.com.

NewSage Press, *(NewSage Pr.; 0-939165),* P.O. Box 607, Troutdale, OR 97060-0607 (SAN 662-8370) Tel 503-695-2211; Fax: 503-695-5406; Toll Free: 877-695-2211
E-mail: newsage@teleport.com
Web site: http://www.newsagepress.com
Dist(s): **Publishers Group** *(Publishers Group West).*

Newspaper Agcy, *(Newspaper Agency, Inc., The; 0-9607254),* P.O. Box 674, Commack, NY 11725 (SAN 239-2690).

NewStar Media, *(NewStar Media, Inc.; 0-7871; 1-55800),* 8955 Beverly Blvd., Los Angeles, CA 90048 (SAN 297-2913) Tel 310-786-1600; Fax: 310-247-2924; Toll Free: 800-368-3007 ; *Imprints:* Dove Audio (Dove Audio)
E-mail: customerservice@audiouniverse.com
Web site: http://www.newstarmedia.com; http://www.audiouniverse.com
Dist(s): **Lectorum Pubns** *(Lectorum Pubns., Inc.)*
Lndmrk Audiobks *(Landmark Audiobooks)*
Penguin Putnam *(Penguin Putnam, Inc.).*

Next Decade, *(Next Decade, Inc.; 0-9626003; 0-9700908),* 39 Old Farmstead Rd., Chester, NJ 07930 Tel 908-879-6625; Fax: 908-879-2920; Toll Free: 800-595-5440
E-mail: nexdec@aol.com; barbara@nextdecade.com
Web site: http://www.nextdecade.com
Dist(s): **IPG Chicago** *(Independent Pubs. Group).*

Next Step Pr, *(Next Step Pr.; 1-892876),* Sub. of New Wisdom, Inc., 1201 Delta Glen Ct., Vienna, VA 22182-1320 Tel 703-757-7945; Fax: 703-757-7946
E-mail: Wyattwooodsmall@compuserve.com
Web site: http://www.peoplepatterns.com.

Next Step Pubns, *(Next Step Pubns.; 0-942783),* 420 S. Beach St., Ormond Beach, FL 32174-7069 (SAN 667-7312).

NFID, *(National Foundation for Infectious Diseases, The; 0-9614520),* 4733 Bethesda Ave., Suite 750, Bethesda, MD 20814-5228 (SAN 689-7762) Tel 301-656-0003; Fax: 301-907-0878
E-mail: nfid@aol.com
Web site: http://www.nfid.org/nfid.

NFSEP, *See* **EPF**

NH Breast Cancer, *(New Hampshire Breast Cancer Coalition; 0-9644254),* 18 Belle Ln., Lee, NH 03824 Tel 603-659-3482; Fax: 603-862-4685.

Nia Consult, *See* **N C D Pubg**

†Nichols Pub, *(Nichols Publishing Co.; 0-89397),* P.O. Box 6036, East Brunswick, NJ 08816-6036 (SAN 212-0291) Tel 732-297-2862; Fax: 732-940-0549; *CIP.*

---

†Nicolas-Hays, *(Nicolas-Hays, Inc.; 0-89254),* Orders Addr.: P.O. Box 612, York Beach, ME 03910 (SAN 202-9588) Tel 207-363-4393; Fax: 207-363-5799; Toll Free: 800-423-7087 (orders only); Edit Addr.: P.O. Box 2039, York Beach, ME 03910
E-mail: nhi@weiserbooks.com
Web site: http://www.weiserbooks.com
Dist(s):* Baker & Taylor *(Baker & Taylor Bks.)
Bookpeople *(Bookpeople)*
New Leaf Dist *(New Leaf Distributing Co., Inc.)*
Red Wheel ME *(Red Wheel); CIP.*

Nicolin Flds, *(Nicolin Fields Publishing, Inc.; 0-9637077; 1-892066),* 3 Red Fox Rd., North Hampton, NH 03862 Tel 603-964-1727; Fax: 603-964-4221; Toll Free: 800-431-1579 (orders only)
E-mail: nfp@nh.ultranet.com; nfp@nh.ultranet.com
Web site: http://wwwnicolinfields.com
Dist(s): **Alpenbooks** *(Alpenbooks)*
Peregrine Outftrs *(Peregrine Outfitters)*
Quality Bks IL *(Quality Bks., Inc.)*
U Pr of New Eng *(University Pr. of New England).*

NICU Ink, *(NICU Ink Bk. Pubs.; 0-9622975; 1-887571),* Subs. of Neonatal Network, 1410 Neotomas Ave., Suite 107, Santa Rosa, CA 95405-7533 Tel 707-569-1415; Fax: 707-569-0786; Toll Free: 888-642-8465 (For book orders only)
E-mail: mbj@neonatalnetwork.com
Web site: http://www.neonatalnetwork.com.

Nieves Pr, *(Nieves Pr.; 0-9612008),* P.O. Box 4564, Albuquerque, NM 87196-4564 (SAN 286-8385) Tel 505-255-3547.

Night Owl Prod, *See* **R Bridges Enter**

Nightngale Rose, *(Nightingale Rose Pubns.; 1-889755),* Div. of Nightingale Counseling Ctr., 16960 E. Bastanchury Rd., Suite J, Yorba Linda, CA 92886 Tel 714-993-5343; Fax: 714-993-3467; Toll Free: 800-943-5728
Web site: http://www.nightingalerose.com.

Nine-Heart-Nine, *(9-Heart-9 Publishing; 0-9639877),* 1058 Devonshire Dr., San Diego, CA 92107-4038.

Ninth St Ctr, *(Ninth Street Ctr., Inc.; 0-932961),* 151 First Ave., Suite 25, New York, NY 10003 (SAN 695-6777) Tel 212-228-5153.

Nissi Pubns, *(Nissi Pubns.; 0-944372),* 1409 Rider Cir., Grapevine, TX 76051-4965 (SAN 243-4148) Tel 817-488-4481
E-mail: nissi@nissipub.com
Web site: http://www.nissipub.com.

Nitty Gritty Ckbks Imprint of Bristol Pub Ent CA

NLB, *(New Lifestyle Bks.; 0-942658),* 30 Uchee Pines Rd., Seale, AL 36875 (SAN 239-5053) Tel 334-855-4708; Fax: 334-855-3952; Toll Free: 800-542-5695
Dist(s): **Angelas Bkshelf** *(Angela's Bookshelf)*
Nelsons Bks *(Nelson's Bks.).*

NLN Pr Imprint of Natl League Nurse

NMCI Pubns, *(NMCI Pubns.; 1-885077),* Div. of National MultiCultural Institute, 3000 Connecticut Ave. NW, Suite 438, Washington, DC 20008-2556 Tel 202-483-0700; Fax: 202-483-5233
E-mail: nmci@nmci.org
Web site: http://www.nmci.org.

NNCC, *(NNCC, Inc.; 0-615; 0-9700484),* 100 Precision Ct., Lancaster, KY 40444 Tel 606-792-4456; Fax: 606-792-6405; Toll Free: 800-755-6901
E-mail: nncc@kih.net
Web site: http://www.nnccusa.com.

No Ariz Univ, *(Northern Arizona Univ., Institute for Human Development; 1-888557; 1-930563),* Orders Addr.: P.O. Box 5630, Flagstaff, AZ 86011 Tel 520-523-4791; Fax: 520-523-9127; Toll Free: 800-553-0714; Edit Addr.: c/o Northern Arizona Univ. Campus, Bldg. 27A, Riordan Rd., Flagstaff, AZ 86011
E-mail: ihd.uap@nau.edu
Web site: http://www.nau.edu./~ihd.

No Barriers, *(No Barriers Publishing; 0-9654568),* 2340 S. Oceanshore Dr., Flagler Beach, FL 32136 Tel 616-344-6038; Fax: 616-344-5473; Toll Free: 800-828-3057
E-mail: trbian@aol.com
Web site: http://NutriGlobe.com
Dist(s): **Quality Bks IL** *(Quality Bks., Inc.).*

Noah Pub, *(Noah Publishing Co.; 1-879933),* 1315 W. Mallon Ave., Spokane, WA 99201-2038.

Noble House, *(Noble Hse.; 0-9653085),* Orders Addr.: P.O. Box 852, Jensen Beach, FL 34958 Tel 407-334-0466; Edit Addr.: 2640 NE Indian River Dr., Jensen Beach, FL 34957 Do not confuse with Noble Hse., Baltimore, MD.

Noble Pr, *(Noble Pr., Inc., The; 0-9622683; 1-879360),* 636 N. Orleans St., No. 2SO, Chicago, IL 60610-3609 (SAN 200-3236) Tel 312-642-1168; Fax: 312-642-7682; Toll Free: 800-486-7737 Do not confuse with Noble Press, Inc., Coral Springs, FL.

Noetic Pr CA, *(Noetic Pr., The; 0-9678687),* 610 16th St., Suite 506, Oakland, CA 94612-1229 Tel 510-832-6059 (phone/fax); 120 Village Sq., MS 49, Orinda, CA 94563-2502
E-mail: noeticj@mindspring.com
Web site: http://www.mindspring.com/'noeticj.

Noise Control, *(Noise Control Foundation; 0-931784),* P.O. Box 2469, Poughkeepsie, NY 12603 (SAN 215-2193) Tel 914-462-4006; Fax: 914-463-0201
E-mail: inceusa@aol.com.

Nolo com, *(Nolo.com; 0-87337; 0-917316),* 950 Parker St., Berkeley, CA 94710 (SAN 206-7935) Tel 510-549-1976; Fax: 510-548-5902; Toll Free: 800-992-6656; 800-955-4775 (trade orders only)
E-mail: cs@nolo.com
Web site: http://www.nolo.com.

Nolo Pr, *See* **Nolo com**

NOLPE, *See* **Ed Law Assn**

Non-Fictitious, *(Non-Fictitious Pr.; 0-9622762),* 7201 Northeast Dr., Austin, TX 78723-1424.

Nook Pubs, *(Nook Pubs., The; 0-938339),* 6700 Jefferson Paige Rd., No. 349, Shreveport, LA 71119 (SAN 661-2849) Tel 318-525-0541 (phone/fax).

Noonday Imprint of FS&G

Noontide Pr Imprint of Legion Survival

NORC, *See* **Natl Opinion Res**

Nordic Africa (SWE) *(91-7106) Dist. by* **Transaction Pubs.**

Norfolk & Wstrn HS, *(Norfolk & Western Historical Society, Inc.; 0-9633254; 0-9704794),* Orders Addr.: P.O. Box 13908, Roanoke, VA 24038-3908 Tel 540-342-0575; Fax: 540-342-0972; Edit Addr.: 2101 Salem Ave., Roanoke, VA 24016
Web site: http://www.nwhs.org.

†Norman SF, *(Norman Publishing; 0-930405),* Div. of Jeremy Norman & Co., Inc., P.O. Box 2566, San Anselmo, CA 94979-2566 (SAN 122-3380) Tel 415-456-6507; Fax: 415-456-6511; Toll Free: 800-544-9359
E-mail: orders@jnorman.com
Web site: http://www.normanpublishing.com; http://www.historyofscience.com; http://www.historyofmedicine.com; *CIP.*

Normed Verlag, *(Normed Verlag, Inc.; 0-926592),* 291 Audubon Rd., Englewood, NJ 07631 Tel 201-569-5386 (phone/fax)
E-mail: renatek@attglobal.net; hoshang.khambatta@normed.net.

Norris Ln Pr, *(Norris Lane Pr.; 0-9637280),* 24829 Norris Ln., Junction City, OR 97448-9559 Tel 541-998-3285; Fax: 541-998-1873
Web site: http://www.FinalExit.org.

†North Atlantic, *(North Atlantic Bks.; 0-913028; 0-938190; 0-942941; 1-55643; 1-883319),* Div. of The Society of the Study of Native Art & Science, Orders Addr.: P.O. Box 12327, Berkeley, CA 94712 (SAN 203-1655) Tel 510-559-8277; Fax: 510-559-8279; Toll Free: 800-337-2665 (orders only); Edit Addr.: 1456 Fourth St., Berkeley, CA 94710
E-mail: orders@northatlanticbooks.com
Web site: http://www.northatlanticbooks.com
Dist(s): **Nutri-Books Corp** *(Nutri-Bks. Corp.)*
Publishers Group *(Publishers Group West)*
SPD-Small Pr Dist *(SPD-Small Pr. Distribution); CIP.*

North Holland Imprint of Elsevier

North Ridge Pr, *(North Ridge Pr.; 0-9629614),* 5700 Boone Ave., N., Minneapolis, MN 55428 Tel 763-473-5999; Fax: 763-536-9311; Toll Free: 888-473-5999
E-mail: lisa_pattee@northridgepress.com
Web site: http://www.northridgepress.com
Dist(s): **Bookmen Inc** *(Bookmen, Inc.).*

North Scale Co, *(North Scale Institute Publishing Co.; 0-916299),* Orders Addr.: P.O. Box 11467, Atlanta, GA 30310 (SAN 295-7418); Edit Addr.: 2205 Taraval St., San Francisco, CA 94116 (SAN 295-7426) Tel 415-759-9491.

North Shore Pr, *(North Shore Pr.; 0-9637802; 1-891576),* 7902 W. Waters, Suite G, Tampa, FL 33615 Tel 813-880-7546; Fax: 813-249-5210; Toll Free: 800-488-7336.

†North Star, *(North Star Pr. of St. Cloud; 0-87839),* P.O. Box 451, Saint Cloud, MN 56302-0451 (SAN 203-7491) Tel 320-253-1636; Fax: 320-240-9075; Toll Free: 888-820-1636
E-mail: nspress@cloudnet.com
Dist(s): **Adventure Pubns** *(Adventure Pubns.)*
Bookmen Inc *(Bookmen, Inc.)*
Skandisk *(Skandisk, Inc.); CIP.*

Northbrook Pub, *(Northbrook Publishing Co., Inc.; 0-9614018),* 1352 Estate Ln., Lake Forest, IL 60045-3624 (SAN 683-6348) Tel 708-735-0055.

Northern Bk Centre (IND) *(81-7211; 81-85119) Dist. by* **S Asia.**

Northern Maple, *See* **Nrthrn Expressions**

Northpeak Pubng, *(Northpeak Publishing; 0-9664862),* Div. of Northwind Business Consultants, Inc., Orders Addr.: P.O. Box 6832, Traverse City, MI 49696-6832 Tel 231-929-7370; Fax: 231-935-3104; Edit Addr.: 2329 River Rd., W., Traverse City, MI 49696-6832
Web site: http://www.llh-net.com/startabiz/.

Northwestern U Pr, *(Northwestern Univ. Pr.; 0-8101),* Orders Addr.: 11030 S. Langley Ave., Chicago, IL 60628 (SAN 202-5299) Tel 773-568-1550; Fax: 773-660-2235; Toll Free Fax: 800-621-8476; Toll Free: 800-621-2736; Edit Addr.: 625 Colfax St., Evanston, IL 60208-4210 (SAN 202-5787) Tel 847-491-5313; Fax: 847-491-8150
E-mail: nupress@northwestern.edu
Web site: http://www.nupress.northwestern.edu
Dist(s): **U Ch Pr** *(Univ. of Chicago Pr.).*

†Norton, *(Norton, W.W. & Co., Inc.; 0-393; 0-920256),* Orders Addr.: 800 Keystone Industrial Pk., Scranton, PA 18512 (SAN 157-1869) Tel 570-346-2020; Toll Free Fax: 800-548-6515; Toll Free: 800-233-4830 (book orders only); Edit Addr.: 500 Fifth Ave., New York, NY 10110-0017 (SAN 202-5795) Tel 212-354-5500; Fax: 212-869-0856; Toll Free: 800-223-2584 ; *Imprints:* Norton Medical Bks (Norton Medical Books) Norton Paperbks (Norton Paperbacks)
E-mail: webmaster@wwnorton.com
Web site: http://www.wwnorton.com/trade; http://www.wwnorton.com
Dist(s): **Continental Bk** *(Continental Bk. Co., Inc.)*
Peoples Pub Grp *(Peoples Publishing Group, Inc., The)*
U Pr of New Eng *(University Pr. of New England)*
netLibrary CO *(netLibrary, Inc.); CIP.*

Norton Medical Bks Imprint of Norton

Norton Paperbks Imprint of Norton

†Norwalk Pr, *(Norwalk Pr.; 0-89019),* P.O. Box 12260, Prescott, AZ 86304-2260 (SAN 207-4052) Tel 928-445-5567 (phone/fax)*; CIP.*

Nostalgia CA, *(Nostalgia Pr.; 0-9628676),* 2150 Eucalyptus Ave., Escondido, CA 92029 Tel 619-489-5372.

NotaBell Imprint of Purdue U Pr

Nottingham Univ Pr (GBR) *(1-897676) Dist. by* **St Mut.**

Nova Kroshka Bks Imprint of Nova Sci Pubs

Nova Media, *(Nova Media, Inc.; 0-9618567; 1-884239),* 1724 N. State St., Big Rapids, MI 49307-9073 (SAN 668-0372) Tel 231-796-4637 (phone/fax)
E-mail: Trund@nov.com
Web site: http://www.nov.com.

Nova Pubng, *(Nova Publishing Corp.; 0-9639560),* 11607 Nebel St., Rockville, MD 20852 Tel 301-231-8228; Fax: 301-816-0816; Toll Free: 800-637-0067.

†Nova Sci Pubs, *(Nova Science Pubs., Inc.; 0-941743; 1-56072; 1-59033),* 227 Main St., Suite 100, Huntington, NY 11743-6682 (SAN 666-0266) Tel 631-424-6682; Fax: 631-425-5933 ; *Imprints:* Nova Kroshka Bks (Nova Kroshka Books) Nova Troitsa Bks (Nova Troitsa Books)
E-mail: novasci1@aol.com
Web site: http://nexusworld.com/nova
Dist(s): **Baker & Taylor** *(Baker & Taylor Bks.); CIP.*

Nova Troitsa Bks Imprint of Nova Sci Pubs

Nova U Fam Ctr, *(Nova Univ. Family Ctr.; 1-879744),* 3301 College Ave., Fort Lauderdale, FL 33314 Tel 954-475-7450; Fax: 954-452-1451; Toll Free: 800-836-8326
Dist(s): **Gryphon Hse** *(Gryphon Hse., Inc.).*

Novateur Med, *(Novateur MedMedia, LLC; 0-9663441),* 39 Terry Hill Rd., R.R. 11, Carmel, NY 10512 Tel 914-228-4565
E-mail: novateur@aol.com.

Novel Pen, *(Novel Pen, The; 0-9648511),* 210 Windy Hills, Hamilton, IL 62341 Tel 217-847-2816; Fax: 319-524-9785.

November Bks, *(November Bks.; 0-941098),* 203 Hitchcock Way, Santa Barbara, CA 93110 (SAN 217-409X) Tel 805-569-5779.

†Noyes, *(Noyes Data Corp.; 0-8155),* 169 Kinderkamack Rd., Suite 5, Park Ridge, NJ 07656-1338 (SAN 209-2840)*; CIP.*

NP-Chilton, *(NP/Chilton; 0-8019),* 1025 Andrew Dr., West Chester, PA 19380-4273 Tel 610-738-9280; Fax: 610-738-9370; Toll Free: 800-695-1214
Dist(s): **Natl Bk Netwk** *(National Bk. Network)*
Thomson Learn *(Thomson Learning).*

NPeducationcom, *(NPeducation.com; 0-9679170),* P.O. Box 396, Wallingford, PA 19086 Tel 215-289-0569; Fax: 978-336-0794
E-mail: inquiries@npeducation.com
Web site: http://www.npeducation.com.

NPP Bks, *(NPP Bks.; 0-916182),* P.O. Box 1491, Ann Arbor, MI 48106-1491 (SAN 208-1067) Tel 734-971-7363.

Nrth Amer Compendiums, *(North American Compendiums, Inc.; 1-889750),* 942 Miltary St., Port Huron, MI 48060 Tel 810-985-5028; Fax: 810-985-5190; Toll Free: 800-350-0627
E-mail: pam@netbase.net
Dist(s): **Iowa U Pr** *(Iowa Univ. Pr.).*

Nrth Country Pr, *(North Country Pr.; 0-945980),* Div. of Maine Fulfillment Corp., R.R. 1, Box 1395, Unity, ME 04988 (SAN 247-9680) Tel 207-948-2208; Fax: 207-948-2717; Toll Free: 800-722-2169 Do not confuse with North Country Pr., White Cloud, MI
E-mail: ncp@uninet.net
Web site: http://www.midcoast.com/~ncp/.

Nrthrn Expressions, *(Northern Expressions; 0-9626683),* 2399 W. School Lake Rd., Maple City, MI 49664 Tel 616-334-3360.

Nrthrn NV Amputee, *(Northern Nevada Amputee Support; 0-9654069),* 710 Marian Way, Sparks, NV 89431 Tel 702-358-8449; Fax: 702-358-5789
E-mail: NNASG@aol.com
Web site: http://www.powernet.net/~nnasg/.

NRW Assocs, *(NRW Assocs.; 0-9631990),* 3063 Hawks Landing Dr., Tallahassee, FL 32308-7224.

NSU Pr LA, *(Northwestern State Univ. of Louisiana Pr.; 0-917898),* P.O. Box 5305, Natchitoches, LA 71497 (SAN 209-973X) Tel 318-357-4586.

NTC Business Bks Imprint of NTC Contemp Pub Co

NTC Contemp Pub Co, *(NTC/Contemporary Publishing Co.; 0-658; 0-8092; 0-8325; 0-8442; 0-88499; 0-89061; 0-913327; 0-940279; 0-941263; 0-9630646; 1-56626; 1-56943; 1-57028),* Subs. of Tribune Education (Tribune Co.), 4255 W. Touhy Ave., Lincolnwood, IL 60712 (SAN 169-2208) Tel 847-679-5500; Fax: 847-679-2494; Toll Free Fax: 800-998-3103; Toll Free: 800-323-4900 ; *Imprints:* Natl Textbk Co (National Textbook Company) NTC Business Bks (N T C Business Books)
E-mail: ntcpub@tribune.com
Web site: http://www.ntc-cb.com
Dist(s): **Continental Bk** *(Continental Bk. Co., Inc.)*
Shens Bks *(Shen's Bks.).*

Nthwest Shline Pub, *(Northwest Shoreline Publishing; 0-9666728),* P.O. Box 7104, Shoreline, WA 98133.

NTL Inst, *(NTL Institute; 0-9610392),* 300 N. Lee St., No. 300, Alexandria, VA 22314-2607 (SAN 223-9485) Tel 703-548-8840; Fax: 703-684-1256; Toll Free: 800-277-4685
Web site: http://www.ntl.org.

Ntl Nurses Bus, *(National Nurses in Business Assn.; 0-9629419),* 8 Cedar Ct., Petaluma, CA 94952-2020 Fax: 707-763-1706.

Ntl Pubs Blck Imprint of P-H

Nucci-Saunders Pubns, *(Nucci - Saunders' Pubns.; 1-877738),* Orders Addr.: P.O. Box 16747, Seattle, WA 98116 Tel 206-932-0632; Fax: 206-932-0511; Edit Addr.: 3052 60th Ave., SW, Seattle, WA 98116 Tel 206-932-0632; Fax: 206-932-0511
E-mail: JCSaunders@aol.com.

NuLife Pubg, *(NuLife Publishing; 0-9642982),* 30 Vista De Oro, Placitas, NM 87043 Tel 505-857-0000; Fax: 505-867-7664.

Nurse Saver, *(Nurse Saver, Inc.; 0-9663913),* P.O. Box 83706, Vancouver, WA 98687 Tel 360-891-8808.

Nursecom Inc, *(Nursecom, Inc.; 0-9637042; 0-9706400),* 1211 Locust St., Philadelphia, PA 19107 Tel 215-545-3334; Fax: 215-545-8107; Toll Free: 888-580-8373
E-mail: nursecomwebsite
Web site: http://www.nursecominc.com.

Nursing Ed Consultants, *(Nursing Education Consultants; 0-9628210; 1-892155),* Orders Addr.: P.O. Box 763593, Dallas, TX 75376-3593 Tel 972-223-1356; Fax: 972-223-2663; Toll Free: 800-933-7277; Edit Addr.: 436 Ten Mile Dr., Desoto, TX 75115
E-mail: jozerwekh@aol.com
Dist(s): **Majors Scientific Bks Inc** *(Majors Scientific Bks., Inc.)*
Rittenhouse *(Rittenhouse Bk. Distributors).*

Nursing Knowledge, *(Nursing Knowledge, Inc.; 0-9622174),* 2540 Severn Ave., No. 206, Metairie, LA 70002-5941 Tel 504-887-0401; Fax: 504-887-0051; Toll Free: 800-359-5114
E-mail: nursknow@aol.com.

Nursing Spect, *(Nursing Spectrum; 1-930745),* Div. of Gannett Satellite Information Network, Inc., 2002 Renaissance Blvd., Suite 120, King of Prussia, PA 19406 Tel 610-275-4100; Fax: 610-275-4303; Toll Free Fax: 800-285-8880; Toll Free: 800-866-0919
E-mail: ce@nursingspectrum.com
Web site: http://www.nursingspectrum.com.

NutrAnalysis Inc, *(NutrAnalysis, Inc.; 0-9667211),* 677 Spartanburg Hwy., Suite 153, Lake Lure, NC 28746 Tel 828-692-0779; Fax: 828-625-8081; Toll Free: 800-377-7879
E-mail: ssalik@nutranalysis.com
Web site: http://www.nutranalysis.com.

Nutrek Pr, *(Nutrek Pr.; 0-9642534),* Div. of Nutrek, Inc., P.O. Box 5, Brookline, MA 02146-0001 Tel 617-739-4887; Fax: 617-277-0306
Web site: http://www.efafood.com.

Nutri Tapes, *(Nutri Tapes & Pubns., Inc.; 1-891036),* 10175 Joerschke Dr., Suite 335, Grass Valley, CA 95945 Tel 530-272-4247; Fax: 530-272-9085; Toll Free: 800-565-7192.

Nutrifit Cnslt, *See* **Nutrifit Pub**

Nutrifit Pub, *(Nutrifit Publishing; 1-880347),* Orders Addr.: P.O. Box 690452, Houston, TX 77269-0452 Tel 281-955-5326; Fax: 281-955-2574; Toll Free: 888-421-5326
E-mail: dininglean@aol.com
Web site: http://www.dininglean.com
Dist(s): **Baker & Taylor** *(Baker & Taylor Bks.)*
Bk Marketing Plus *(Book Marketing Plus)*
Quality Bks IL *(Quality Bks., Inc.).*

Nutrisci Pubs, *(Nutriscience Pubs., Inc.; 0-9647856),* 121 Ethel Rd. W., Unit 6, Piscataway, NJ 08854 Tel 732-777-1111; Fax: 732-777-1443.

Nutrit Educ, *(Nutrition Education Assn. Inc.; 0-916243),* Orders Addr.: P.O. Box 20301, Houston, TX 77225 (SAN 294-9830) Tel 713-665-2946; Edit Addr.: 3647 Glen Haven, Houston, TX 77025 (SAN 294-9849).

Nutrit Intl, *(Nutrition International Co.; 0-9640678),* Orders Addr.: P.O. Box 50632, Irvine, CA 92619-0632 Fax: 714-854-6170; Edit Addr.: 6 Siverfern Dr., Irvine, CA 92715 Tel 714-854-4855.

Nutrit Res, *(Nutritional Research, LLC; 0-9672346),* 2533 N. Carson St., Suite 2985, Carson City, NV 89706 Tel 412-341-2703; Fax: 412-341-6761; Toll Free: 877-341-2703
E-mail: info@nutritionalresearch.net
Web site: http://www.nutritionalresearch.net.

Nutrit Times, *(Nutrition Times Pr., Inc.; 0-9638372),* Orders Addr.: P.O. Box 700512, Tulsa, OK 74170-0512; Edit Addr.: 8777 S. Toledo, Tulsa, OK 74137 Tel 918-495-1137; Fax: 918-477-7790
E-mail: 7patrick@concentric.net
Dist(s): **BookMasters** *(BookMasters, Inc.)*
BookWorld *(BookWorld Services, Inc.).*

Nutrit Unltd Pubns, *(Nutrition Unlimited Pubns.; 0-929622),* Orders Addr.: P.O. Box 660701, Arcadia, CA 91006-0701 (SAN 250-1422) Tel 626-355-6513; Fax: 213-728-7401; Edit Addr.: 1444 Oaklawn Rd., Arcadia, CA 91006 (SAN 250-1430).

Nutrition Ed, *(Nutrition Education Ctr.; 0-915187),* Subs. of C. L. Gerwick & Assocs., Inc., 9500 Nall Ave., Suite 404, Overland Park, KS 66207 (SAN 289-7776) Tel 913-383-3464; Fax: 913-383-3729; Toll Free: 888-383-3464.

Nutrition Encounter, *(Nutrition Encounter; 0-944501),* Orders Addr.: P.O. Box 5847, Novato, CA 94948 (SAN 243-685X) Tel 415-883-5154; Fax: 415-883-9051; Edit Addr.: 61 Bahama Reef, Novato, CA 94948
E-mail: sikam@earthlink.net; betty@well.com
Web site: http://www.bettykamen.com
Dist(s): **Baker & Taylor** *(Baker & Taylor Bks.)*
Bookpeople *(Bookpeople)*
New Leaf Dist *(New Leaf Distributing Co., Inc.)*
Nutri-Books Corp *(Nutri-Bks. Corp.)*
Quality Bks IL *(Quality Bks., Inc.).*

Nutrition Wks, *(Nutrition Works; 0-9633990),* 1630 Shady Brook, Fullerton, CA 92631 Tel 714-447-4947.

Nutrtnl Data Resces, *(Nutritional Data Resources; 0-9665665),* 4462 S. 84th, Omaha, NE 68127 Tel 402-397-8408; Fax: 402-397-5340; Toll Free: 888-288-7920
E-mail: douglasringer@hotmail.com.

NW Ctr Homeopathic, *See* **Picnic Pt Pr**

NW Family Srvs, *(Northwest Family Services; 1-880220),* 4805 NE Glisan St., Portland, OR 97213 Tel 503-230-6377; Fax: 503-232-5967.

NW Wilderness, *(Northwest Wilderness Bks.; 1-883183),* 11507 24th Ave., NE, Seattle, WA 98125-5211 Tel 206-363-1756.

NY Acad Med, *(New York Academy of Medicine; 0-924143),* 2 E. 103rd St., New York, NY 10029 (SAN 252-2306) Tel 212-822-7250; Fax: 212-722-7650.

†NY Acad Sci, *(New York Academy of Sciences; 0-89072; 0-89766; 1-57331),* 2 E. 63rd St., New York, NY 10021 (SAN 203-753X) Tel 212-838-0230; Fax: 212-838-5226; Toll Free: 800-843-6927
E-mail: publications@nyas.org
Web site: http://www.nyas.org
Dist(s): **Johns Hopkins** *(Johns Hopkins Univ. Pr.); CIP.*

†NY Botanical, *(New York Botanical Garden Pr.; 0-89327),* New York Botanical Garden Press, Bronx, NY 10458-5126 (SAN 205-7085) Tel 718-817-8721; Fax: 718-817-8842
Web site: http://www.nybg.org; *CIP.*

NY Chiro Coll, *(New York Chiropractic College; 0-938470),* 2360 State Rte. 89, Seneca Falls, NY 13148-0800 (SAN 216-1680) Tel 315-568-3000.

NY Genealogical & Biographical, *(New York Genealogical & Biographical Society, The; 1-877692),* 122 E. 58th St., New York, NY 10022-1939 (SAN 223-9361) Tel 212-755-8532; Fax: 212-754-4218
E-mail: publications@nygbs.org
Web site: http://www.nygbs.org.

NY Neurosci Pr, *(New York Neuroscience Pr., Inc.; 0-9655600),* Penthouse, 19 W. 34th St., New York, NY 10001 Tel 212-947-7111; Fax: 212-239-0948.

†NY Pub Lib, *(New York Public Library; 0-87104),* Pubns. Office, 6th Flr., 8 W. 40th St., New York, NY 10018 (SAN 202-926X) Tel 212-512-0202; Fax: 212-704-8620
Web site: http://www.nypl.org; *CIP.*

NY Rev Bks, *(New York Review of Bks., Inc., The; 0-940322; 1-59017),* 1755 Broadway, 5th Flr., New York, NY 10019-3780 (SAN 220-3448) Tel 212-757-8070; Fax: 212-333-5374
E-mail: mail@nybooks.com
Web site: http://www.nybooks.com
Dist(s): **Publishers Group** *(Publishers Group West).*

NY Univ Med Ctr, *(New York Univ. Medical Ctr., NYU School of Medicine; 0-9651593),* 550 First Ave., New York, NY 10016 Tel 212-263-7300; Fax: 212-263-6534.

NYCCWMH, *(New York City Coalition for Women's Mental Health; 0-9616028),* 320 W. 86th St., No 2B, New York, NY 10024 (SAN 697-9203) Tel 212-787-1766.

Nychthemeron Pr, *(Nychthemeron Pr.; 0-9649338),* P.O. Box 912, Menlo Park, CA 94026-0912 Tel 415-725-6416; Fax: 415-725-7341.

†NY-NJ Trail Confer, *(New York-New Jersey Trail Conference, Inc.; 0-9603966; 1-880775),* Orders Addr.: P.O. Box 2250, New York, NY 10116 (SAN 213-9421); Edit Addr.: 232 Madison Ave., Suite 401, New York, NY 10016; *CIP.*

NYS Bar, *(New York State Bar Assn.; 0-942954; 1-57969),* 1 Elk St., Albany, NY 12207 (SAN 226-1952) Tel 518-463-3200; Fax: 518-463-8844; Toll Free: 800-582-2452
Web site: http://www.nysba.org
Dist(s): **Direct Cinema** *(Direct Cinema, Ltd.).*

NYS Task Force, *(New York State Task Force on Life & the Law; 1-881268),* Div. of New York State Dept. of Health, 5 Penn Plaza, Rm. 301, New York, NY 10001-1803 Tel 212-613-4303; Fax: 212-613-4351.

†NYU Pr, *(New York Univ. Pr.; 0-8147),* Div. of New York Univ., 838 Broadway, 3rd Flr., New York, NY 10003-4812 (SAN 658-1293) Tel 212-998-2575; Fax: 212-995-3833; Toll Free: 800-996-6987
E-mail: orders@nyupress.nyu.edu
Web site: http://www.nyupress.nyu.edu
Dist(s): **Slavica** *(Slavica Pubs., Inc.); CIP.*

O M Pinkston, *See* **Pinkston**

O R Manager, *(OR Manager, Inc.; 0-945970),* P.O. Box 5303, Santa Fe, NM 87502-5303 (SAN 248-3416) Tel 505-982-0510; Fax: 505-983-0790; Toll Free: 800-442-9918.

†Oak Knoll, *(Oak Knoll Pr.; 0-938768; 1-884718; 1-58456),* 310 Delaware St., New Castle, DE 19720 (SAN 216-2776) Tel 302-328-7232; Fax: 302-328-7274; Toll Free: 800-996-2556
E-mail: oakknoll@oakknoll.com
Web site: http://www.oakknoll.com; *CIP.*

†Oaklawn Pr, *(Oaklawn Pr., Inc.; 0-916198),* 1318 Fair Oaks Ave., South Pasadena, CA 91030 (SAN 208-0621) Tel 626-799-0880; *CIP.*

Oakvale Pr, *(Oakvale Pr.; 0-9638888),* The Quadrangle, 3300 Darby Rd., No. 3101, Haverford, PA 19041-1069 Tel 610-642-1158; Toll Free: 800-356-9315.

OAS, *(Organization of American States; 0-8171; 0-8270),* OAS Bookshop, 1889 F St., NW, Washington, DC 20006 (SAN 206-8877) Tel 202-458-3535
E-mail: pspranger@oas.org
Web site: http://www.oas.org/.

OCA, *(Obsessive Compulsive Anonymous World Servs., Inc.; 0-9628066),* P.O. Box 215, New Hyde Park, NY 11040 Tel 516-739-0662; Fax: 212-768-4679
Dist(s): **Hazelden** *(Hazelden Information & Educational Services).*

OCC, *(OCC (Oxford Clinical Communications); 0-9660389),* 41 University Dr., Newton, PA 18940 Tel 215-493-5883; Fax: 215-493-5963.

†Oceana, *(Oceana Pubns., Inc.; 0-379),* 75 Main St., Dobbs Ferry, NY 10522-1601 (SAN 202-5744) Tel 914-693-8100; Fax: 914-693-0402; Toll Free: 800-831-0758
E-mail: orders@oceanalaw.com
Web site: http://www.oceanalaw.com; *CIP.*

Oceanco Ltd, *(Oceanco, Ltd.; 0-9622584),* Orders Addr.: P.O. Box 970562, Boca Raton, FL 33497-0562; Edit Addr.: 188H Salisbury, West Palm Beach, FL 33417 Tel 407-640-0047
Web site: http://divesales.com/.

Oceanides Pr, *(Oceanides Pr.; 0-9624424),* 1111 Kearny St., San Francisco, CA 94133 Tel 415-981-4880.

OceanSide Pubns, *(OceanSide Pubns.; 0-936587),* 95 Pitman St., Providence, RI 02906 (SAN 698-0856) Tel 401-331-2510; Fax: 401-331-5138
E-mail: oceanside@oceansidepubl.com
Web site: http://www.oceansidepubl.com.

Octagon Pr (GBR) *(0-86304; 0-900860) Dist. by* **ISHK.**

Octagon Press I S H K Book Service, *See* **ISHK**

Octavia Ohio, *(Octavia Pr.; 0-940601),* 12127 Sperry Rd., Chesterland, OH 44026-2230 (SAN 665-0236) Tel 440-729-3252; Fax: 440-729-2003 ; *Imprints:* Wilson St Press (Wilson Street Press) Do not confuse with Octavia Pr., Miami Beach, FL.

October, *(October Hse.; 0-8079),* 29 Bunny Rd., Preston, CT 06365-8705 (SAN 203-7610) Tel 860-535-3725.

Odense Univ (DNK) *(87-7492; 87-7838) Dist. by* **Intl Spec Bk.**

OECD, *(Organization for Economic Cooperation & Development),* 2001 L St., NW, Suite 650, Washington, DC 20036-4922 (SAN 202-1277) Tel 202-785-6323; Fax: 202-785-0350; Toll Free: 800-456-6323
E-mail: washington.contact@oecd.org
Web site: http://www.oecdwash.org.

OEM Health, *(OEM Health Information, Inc.; 0-9623864; 1-883595),* 8 West St., Beverly Farms, MA 01915-2226 Tel 978-921-7300; Fax: 978-921-0304; Toll Free: 800-533-8046 ; *Imprints:* OEM Pr (O E M Press)
Web site: http://www.oempress.com.

OEM Pr Imprint of OEM Health

OEPF, *(Optometric Extension Program Foundation; 0-943599),* 1921 Carnegie Ave., Suite 3L, Santa Ana, CA 92705-5510 (SAN 274-3094) Tel 949-250-8070; Fax: 949-250-8157
E-mail: smc.oep@worldnet.att.net
Web site: http://www.oep.org.

Of Course Pubns, *(Of Course Pubns., Inc.; 0-935255),* P.O. Box 4944, Clearwater, FL 33758 (SAN 695-507X) Tel 727-531-6666; Fax: 727-539-1344.

Off Air Force, *See* **AFH & MP**

Offbeat Imprint of Snta Monica

OH Distinct Pub, *(Ohio Distinctive Publishing, Inc.; 0-9647934),* 6500 Fiesta Dr., Columbus, OH 43235 Tel 614-459-0453; Fax: 614-457-2488
E-mail: tim@ohio-distinctive.com
Web site: http://www.hoio-distinctive.com.

Ohana Grp, *(Ohana Group; 0-9632599),* 19800 Seventh St., E., Sonoma, CA 95476 Tel 707-996-9163.

Ohio Bio Survey, *(Ohio Biological Survey; 0-86727),* Div. of Ohio State Univ College of Biological Sciences, c/o Ohio State Univ., Museum of Biological Diversity, 1315 Kinnear Rd., Columbus, OH 43212-1192 (SAN 217-0787) Tel 614-292-9645; Fax: 614-688-4322
Web site: http://www.obs.biosci.ohio-state.edu.

†Ohio St U Pr, *(Ohio State Univ. Pr.; 0-8142),* 1070 Carmack Rd., Columbus, OH 43210 (SAN 202-8158) Tel 614-292-6930; 773-568-1550 (orders); Fax: 614-292-2065; Toll Free Fax: 800-621-8476 (orders); Toll Free: 800-621-2736 (orders)
E-mail: ohiostatepress@osu.edu
Web site: http://www.ohiostatepress.org
Dist(s): **U Ch Pr** *(Univ. of Chicago Pr.); CIP.*

†Ohio U Pr, *(Ohio Univ. Pr.; 0-8214),* Orders Addr.: 11030 S. Langley Ave., Chicago, IL 60628 (SAN 202-5280) Tel 773-568-1559; Fax: 773-660-2235; Toll Free Fax: 800-621-8476; Toll Free: 800-621-2736; Edit Addr.: Scott Quadrangle, Athens, OH 45701 (SAN 282-0773) Tel 740-593-1154; Fax: 740-593-4536
E-mail: arnold@ohiou.edu
Web site: http://www.ohiou.edu/oupress/
Dist(s): **U Ch Pr** *(Univ. of Chicago Pr.); CIP.*

Ohio Vet, *(Ohio Veterinary Medical Assn.; 0-9613273),* 3168 Riverside Dr., Columbus, OH 43221-2540 (SAN 297-0449) Tel 614-486-7253.

Oily Pr (GBR) *(0-9514171) Dist. by* **Matreya.**

OK St Dept Hlth Injury, *(Oklahoma State Dept. of Health, Injury Prevention Service; 1-889728),* 1000 NE Tenth St., Oklahoma City, OK 73117-1299 Tel 405-271-3430; Fax: 405-271-5149.

Okpaku Communications, *(Okpaku Communications Corp.; 0-89388),* Div. of Third Pr. Review of Bks. Co., 222 Forest Ave., New Rochelle, NY 10804 (SAN 202-5701) Tel 914-632-2355; Fax: 914-632-2320
E-mail: okpaku@aol.com.

Old Barn Entrprs, *(Old Barn Enterprises, Inc.; 0-9624737; 1-879009),* 600 Kelly Rd., Carthage, NC 28327 (SAN 631-3450) Tel 910-947-2587; Fax: 910-947-5112.

Old Cookbooks HT Hicks, *(Old Cookbooks; 0-932965),* 151 W. Crystal Lake Ave., Westmont, NJ 08108-3416 (SAN 689-9935) Tel 609-854-2844.

Old Ct Pr, *(Old Court Pr.; 0-9649391),* P.O. Box 4031, Brookings, OR 97415 Do not confuse with Old Court Pr., Winter Park, FL.

Old Mountain, *(Old Mountain Pr.; 1-884778; 1-931575),* 2542 S. Edgewater Dr., Fayetteville, NC 28303 Tel 910-484-5887; Fax: 910-484-7639
Web site: http://www.oldmp.com.

Old Theology Bk Hse, *(Old Theology Bk. Hse.; 0-9612964),* P.O. Box 120342, New Brighton, MN 55112-0016 (SAN 293-4965)
E-mail: viskichi@aol.com.

Olde & Oppenheim, *(Olde & Oppenheim Pubs.; 0-944861),* 3219 N. Margate Pl., Chandler, AZ 85224 (SAN 245-4769) Tel 602-839-2280; Fax: 602-897-0685.

Olde Maryland, *(Olde Maryland Publishing Co.; 0-911071),* 10 Jack Frost Ln., Baltimore, MD 21204 (SAN 272-2690) Tel 410-823-3460.

Olde Soldier Bks, *(Olde Soldier Bks., Inc.; 0-942211; 1-56013),* 18779B N. Frederick Rd., Gaithersburg, MD 20879 (SAN 668-3738) Tel 301-963-2929.

†Olive Pr Pubns, *(Olive Pr. Pubns.; 0-933380),* P.O. Box 99, Los Olivos, CA 93441 (SAN 212-5331) Tel 805-688-2445 (phone/fax); *CIP.*

Oliver Pr MN, *(Oliver Pr., Inc.; 1-881508),* 5707 W. 36th St., Minneapolis, MN 55416-2510 Tel 952-926-8981; Fax: 952-926-8965; Toll Free: 800-865-4837
E-mail: info@oliverpress.com
Web site: http://www.oliverpress.com.

Olken Pubns, *(Olken Pubns.; 0-934818),* 2830 Kennedy St., Livermore, CA 94550 (SAN 203-7939) Tel 510-447-5177.

Olmstead Pr, *(Olmstead Pr.; 1-58754),* Div. of LPC Group, 22 Broad St., Suite 34, Milford, CT 06460 Tel 203-878-6417; Fax: 203-874-2308; Toll Free: 800-243-0138
E-mail: mo@lpcgroup.com
Dist(s): **LPC Group** *(LPC Group).*

For full information on wholesalers and distributors, refer to the Wholesaler and Distributor Symbol Index

Ololon Pubns, *(Ololon Pubns.; 0-9607332),* P.O. Box 569, Lumberton, NC 28359 (SAN 239-2712) Tel 910-738-9396; Fax: 910-738-9395.

OM Literature, *(OM Literature),* P.O. Box 1047, Waynesboro, GA 30830-2047 Tel 706-554-5827; Fax: 706-554-7444; Toll Free: 800-733-5907 Web site: http://www.doneomlit.om.org.

Omb, *(Ombudsman Pr., Inc.; 0-930175),* 8825 Auburn Valley Rd., Auburn, CA 95602-9256 (SAN 210-3184) Tel 530-269-3230.

Omedic, *See* **Isomed**

Omega Pubns OR, *(Omega Pubns.; 0-86694; 0-931608),* P.O. Box 4130, Medford, OR 97501 (SAN 220-1534) Tel 541-826-4512; Fax: 541-826-1023; Toll Free: 800-345-0175 Do not confuse with companies with the same name in Indianapolis, IN, New Lebanon, NY.

Omenana, *(Omenana; 0-943324),* 1345 N. Kingsley Dr., Apt. 308, Los Angeles, CA 90027-5769 (SAN 240-5571).

OMERI, *(Orthopedic Massage Education & Research Institute (OMERI); 0-9661196),* Orders Addr.: P.O. Box 1468, Bend, OR 97709 Tel 541-317-9855; Fax: 541-317-9856; Toll Free: 888-340-1614; Edit Addr.: 237 NW Saint Helens Pl., Bend, OR 97701 E-mail: wlowe@omeri.com Web site: http://www.omeri.com.

Omni Pr Imprint of Quiet Lion Pr

Omni Recovery, *(Omni Recovery, Inc.; 0-9628703),* P.O. Box 50033, Minneapolis, MN 55403 Tel 612-698-2721.

†Omnigraphics Inc, *(Omnigraphics, Inc.; 0-7808; 1-55888),* Orders Addr.: P.O. Box 625, Holmes, PA 19043 Toll Free Fax: 800-875-1340 (orders & customer service); Toll Free: 800-234-1340 (orders & customer service); Edit Addr.: 615 Griswold St., Detroit, MI 48226 (SAN 249-2520) Tel 313-961-1340; Fax: 313-961-1383 E-mail: info@omnigraphics.com Web site: http://www.omnigraphics.com; *CIP.*

On A Shoestring, *(On A Shoestring),* P.O. Box 831537, Richardson, TX 75083-1537 Tel 972-235-5069 (phone/fax); Toll Free: 800-687-5541 E-mail: eileeny@sprintmail.com Web site: http://www.insicknessandinhealth.com.

Oncology Educ, *(Oncology Educational Services; 0-9663138),* 2601 Southfield Trail Dr., Apt. E, Saint Louis, MO 63129-6154.

Oncology Nursing, *(Oncology Nursing Pr., Inc.; 1-890504),* Subs. of Oncology Nursing Society, 501 Holiday Dr., Pittsburgh, PA 15220-2749 (SAN 689-8041) Tel 412-921-7373 (ext. 218); Fax: 412-921-2131 E-mail: onpress@ons.org Web site: http://www.ons.org.

One Eight Inc, *(One 8, Inc.; 0-935081),* P.O. Box 2075, Forks, WA 98331 (SAN 695-0132) Tel 360-374-7500; Fax: 360-374-9014 *Dist(s):* **New Leaf Dist** *(New Leaf Distributing Co., Inc.).*

One Hundred One, *See* **Break on Through**

One Lambda, *(One Lambda, Inc.; 0-945756),* 21001 Kittridge St., Canoga Park, CA 91303-2801 (SAN 247-4875) Tel 310-478-1001; Fax: 310-478-1004; Toll Free: 800-822-8824.

One More Pr, *(One More Pr.; 0-941361),* Affil. of Ki2 Enterprises, Orders Addr.: P.O. Box 1885, Lake Oswego, OR 97035 Tel 503-697-7964; Fax: 503-636-5293; Edit Addr.: 15800 SW Lower Boones Ferry Rd., No. A14, Lake Oswego, OR 97035.

One Peaceful World, *(One Peaceful World Pr.; 0-9628528; 1-882984),* Orders Addr.: P.O. Box 10, Becket, MA 01223 (SAN 631-2519) Tel 413-623-2322; Fax: 413-623-6042; Toll Free: 888-322-4095; Edit Addr.: 308 Leland Rd., Becket, MA 01223 E-mail: opw@macrobiotics.org Web site: http://www.macrobiotics.org *Dist(s):* **BookWorld** *(BookWorld Services, Inc.).*

One Plus One, *(One Plus One; 1-885899),* P.O. Box 1557, North Baldwin, NY 11510 (SAN 298-3583).

OnGuard, *(OnGuard; 1-56916),* Div. of Emergency Resource, Inc., 4015 S. Lincoln Ave., Suite 500, Loveland, CO 80537-7537 Tel 970-203-1300; Fax: 970-203-1311; Toll Free: 800-544-3473 E-mail: info@onguard.com Web site: http://www.onguard.com.

Ontarolina, *(Ontarolina Publishing Co.; 0-9666162),* Orders Addr.: P.O. Box 3293, Burlington, NC 27215 Tel 336-227-0000; Fax: 336-227-0426; Toll Free: 800-551-9721; Edit Addr.: 2263 Crescent Dr., No. 12, Graham, NC 27253 E-mail: socrnuz@netpath.net.

Oolichan Bks (CAN) *(0-88982) Dist. by* **General Distrib Services.**

†Open Court, *(Open Court; 0-02; 0-8126; 0-87548; 0-89688; 0-912050),* Div. of S R A/McGraw-Hill, 332 S. Michigan Ave., Suite 1100, Chicago, IL 60604 Tel 312-939-1500; Fax: 510-528-3444 (orders); 312-939-8150; Toll Free: 800-788-3123 (orders) E-mail: opencourt@caruspub.com Web site: http://www.opencourtbooks.com *Dist(s):* **Publishers Group** *(Publishers Group West)* **SRA McGraw** *(SRA/McGraw-Hill); CIP.*

Open Minds PA, *(Open Minds; 1-878586),* 10 York St. Suite 200, Gettysburg, PA 17325 Tel 717-334-1329; Fax: 717-334-0538 Do not confuse with companies with same or similar names in Columbus, OH, Honolulu, HI E-mail: openminds@openminds.com Web site: http://www.openminds.com.

Open Soc Fund, *See* **Open Soc Inst**

Open Soc Inst, *(Open Society Institute; 0-9641568; 1-891385),* 400 W. 59th St., No. 4, New York, NY 10019 Tel 212-887-0668; Fax: 212-245-3429 E-mail: mgreenwald@sorosny.org Web site: http://www.soros.org.

Open Spaces, *(Open Spaces; 0-9654977),* Orders Addr.: P.O. Box 4313, Arcata, CA 95518 Tel 707-441-9940; Fax: 707-839-4664; Toll Free: 800-345-5859; Edit Addr.: 1210 G St., Arcata, CA 95521 E-mail: hb@humboldt1.com *Dist(s):* **J Majors Co** *(Majors, J. A. Co.)* **Rittenhouse** *(Rittenhouse Bk. Distributors).*

OPEN TX, *(OPEN, Inc. (Offender Preparation & Education Network, Inc.); 1-878436),* Orders Addr.: P.O. Box 566025, Dallas, TX 75356-6025 Tel 972-271-1971; Fax: 972-278-5884; Toll Free: 800-966-1966; Edit Addr.: 1308 Kynn Dr., Garland, TX 75041 *Dist(s):* **Greystone Educ Mat** *(Greystone Educational Materials)* **Kindred Pub** *(Kindred Publishing).*

Open Univ TX, *(Open Univ. Pr.; 1-878556),* Orders Addr.: P.O. Box 541541, Houston, TX 77254 Tel 713-528-1999.

Optical Resolution, *(Optical Resolution Information Ctr.; 0-9601918),* 28 Morley Ln., Bloomfield, NJ 07003-4309 (SAN 212-3770) Tel 718-920-0100.

Optical Soc, *(Optical Society of America; 0-936659; 0-9600380; 1-55752),* 2010 Massachusetts Ave., NW, Washington, DC 20036 (SAN 203-7750) Tel 202-223-8130; Fax: 202-223-1096 Web site: http://www.osa.org.

Optima (GBR) *(0-356) Dist. by* **Trafalgar.**

Optimal HealthSpan, *(Optimal HealthSpan Publishing; 1-891410),* 1580 Shadowridge Dr., No. 122, Vista, CA 92083 Tel 760-727-7411; Fax: 760-727-7118 E-mail: mlb@optimalhealthspan.com Web site: http://www.optimalhealthspan.com.

Optimal Hlth Pr, *(Optimal Health Pr.; 0-9671597),* 55 Crow Hill Rd., Mount Kisco, NY 10549 Tel 914-666-2943 (phone/fax).

Optimization Soft, *(Optimization Software, Inc.; 0-911575),* 10800 Savona Rd., Los Angeles, CA 90077-2307 (SAN 664-5453) Tel 310-472-2910 E-mail: Aries@optipub.bizland.com Web site: http://www.optipub.bizland.com.

OpUniv Pr (GBR) *(0-335) Dist. by* **Taylor & Francis.**

Opus Communs, *(Opus Communications; 1-57839; 1-885829),* Div. of HCPro, Inc., Orders Addr.: P.O. Box 1168, Marblehead, MA 01945; Edit Addr.: 200 Hoods Ln., Marblehead, MA 01945 Tel 781-639-1872; Fax: 781-639-2982; Toll Free Fax: 800-639-8511; Toll Free: 800-650-6787 E-mail: customer_service@opuscomm.com Web site: http://www.hemarketplace.com *Dist(s):* **J Majors Co** *(Majors, J. A. Co.)* **Matthews Bk Co** *(Matthews Bk. Co.).*

OR Med Pr, *(Oregon Medical Pr.; 0-9648280),* 315 Tenth Ave., N., Princeton, MN 55371 Tel 763-389-0768; Fax: 612-395-5239; Toll Free: 800-610-0768 E-mail: sales@ompress.com Web site: http://www.ompress.com.

OR St Zoology, *(Oregon State Univ., Dept. of Zoology),* Oregon State Univ., Corvallis, OR 97331-2914 Tel 541-737-5355; Fax: 541-737-0501 E-mail: baera@bcc.orst.edu.

Oramedics Intl, *(Oramedics International Pr.; 0-933420),* Rte 1, Box 102, Lake Linden, MI 49945 (SAN 221-9670).

Orange Caregiver, *(Orange Caregiver Resource Ctr.; 0-9644874),* Div. of St. Jude Medical Ctr., 251 E. Imperial Hwy., Suite 460, Fullerton, CA 92635 Tel 714-680-0122; Fax: 714-870-9708.

†Orbis Bks, *(Orbis Bks.; 0-88344; 1-57075),* Div. of The Catholic Foreign Mission Society of America, Inc., P.O. Box 308, Maryknoll, NY 10545-0308 (SAN 202-828X) Tel 914-941-7590 (ext. 2487); Fax: 914-945-0670; Toll Free: 800-258-5838 E-mail: orbisbooks@maryknoll.org Web site: http://www.orbisbooks.com; *CIP.*

Ordinary Man, *(Ordinary Man Publishing Co.; 0-936407),* 3717 S. Taft Hill, Suite 271, Fort Collins, CO 80526 (SAN 697-9297) Tel 970-223-5780 E-mail: omp@jymis.com.

Oreg Mus Sci & Indus, *(Oregon Museum of Science & Industry; 0-9617645),* 1945 SE Water Ave., Portland, OR 97214-3354 (SAN 665-3499) Tel 503-797-4000; Fax: 503-797-4500.

†Oreg St U Pr, *(Oregon State Univ. Pr.; 0-87071),* Oregon State Univ., 101 Waldo Hall, Corvallis, OR 97331 (SAN 202-8328) Tel 541-737-3166; Fax: 541-737-3170 E-mail: osu.press@orst.edu Web site: http://osu.orst.edu/dept/press *Dist(s):* **U of Ariz Pr** *(Univ. of Arizona Pr.); CIP.*

OReilly & Assocs, *(O'Reilly & Assocs., Inc.; 0-937175; 1-56592; 0-596),* Orders Addr.: 1005 Gravenstein Hwy., N., Sebastopol, CA 95472 (SAN 658-5973) Tel 707-829-0515; Fax: 707-829-0104; Toll Free: 800-998-9938 (US & Canada inquiries); 800-889-8969 (US & Canada credit card orders); Edit Addr.: 90 Sherman St., Cambridge, MA 02140 Tel 617-499-7406; Fax: 617-661-1116; Toll Free: 800-775-7731 ; *Imprints:* Patient-Centered (Patient-Centered Guides) E-mail: order@oreilly.com; nuts@ora.com Web site: http://www.oreilly.com; http://www.editions-oreilly.fr; http://oreilly.co.uk; http://oreilly.com.tw; http://www.ora.com *Dist(s):* **netLibrary CO** *(netLibrary, Inc.).*

Org for Econ (FRA) *(92-64; 92-821; 0-9501741) Dist. by* **OECD.**

†Orient Heal Arts, *(Oriental Healing Arts Institute; 0-941942),* 1945 Palo Verde Ave., Suite 208, Long Beach, CA 90815 (SAN 238-6038) Tel 310-431-3544; *CIP.*

Origin Bks, *(Origin Bks.; 0-945817),* 3900 Ford Rd., No. 19D, Philadelphia, PA 19131 (SAN 247-8420).

Original Bks, *(Original Bks., Inc.; 0-944558),* P.O. Box 5161, Torrance, CA 90510 (SAN 243-8739) Tel 310-539-7015; Fax: 310-377-0511 Do not confuse with Original Books in Silver Spring, MD E-mail: originalbooks@morelight.net Web site: http://www.westworld.com/~poorjob/origbks *Dist(s):* **New Leaf Dist** *(New Leaf Distributing Co., Inc.).*

Original Pubns, *(Original Pubns.; 0-942272),* Subs. of Maximo Inc., 22 E. Mall, Plainview, NY 11803 (SAN 133-0225) Tel 516-454-6809; Fax: 516-454-6829; Toll Free: 888-622-8581.

Orion (GBR) *(0-575; 0-7528; 1-85797; 1-85881) Dist. by* **Trafalgar.**

Orion Assocs, *See* **Back Talk Systs**

Orion Society, *(Orion Society, The; 0-913098),* 187 Main St., Great Barrington, MA 01230-1601 (SAN 204-0182) Tel 413-528-4422; Fax: 413-528-0676; Toll Free: 888-909-6568 E-mail: orion@orionsociety.org Web site: http://www.oriononline.org.

Ortho Diag, *(Ortho Diagnostic Systems, Inc.; 0-910771),* Rte. 202, N., Raritan, NJ 08869 (SAN 260-2393) Tel 201-218-1300.

Orthopedic Phys, *(Orthopedic Physical Therapy Products (OPTP)),* Orders Addr.: P.O. Box 47009, Minneapolis, MN 55447-0009 Tel 612-553-0452; Fax: 612-553-9355; Toll Free: 800-367-7393; Edit Addr.: 3700 Annaplis Ln., No. 175, Minneapolis, MN 55447-5435 E-mail: optp@worldnet.att.net Web site: http://www.optp.com.

Oryx Imprint of Greenwood

Osteogenesis Imper, *(Osteogenesis Imperfecta Foundation; 0-9642189),* 804 W. Diamond Ave., Suite 210, Gaithersburg, MD 20878 Tel 301-947-0083; Fax: 301-947-0456; Toll Free: 800-981-2663 E-mail: bonelink@oif.org Web site: http://www.oif.org.

OSU Nisonger, *(Ohio State Univ. Nisonger Ctr., The; 0-9658966),* 1581 Dodd Dr., Columbus, OH 43210-1296 Tel 614-688-8214; Fax: 614-688-4908 E-mail: proj.med@osu.edu *Dist(s):* **Am Assn Mental** *(American Assn. on Mental Retardation).*

Other Pr LLC, *(Other Pr., LLC, The; 1-892746; 1-59051),* 377 W. 11th St., New York, NY 10014 Tel 212-924-3344; Fax: 212-414-9654 Do not confuse with Other Press in Jersey City, NJ
E-mail: info@otherpress.com
Web site: http://www.otherpress.com.

Other Stuff, *(Other Stuff; 0-9647865),* 123 Hooks Ln., Canonsburg, PA 15317-1835 Tel 412-746-2529.

Other Worldly, *(Other Worldly Publishing; 0-9640440),* 131 E. 7th St., New York, NY 10009 Tel 212-260-9188; Fax: 212-614-9108.

Oughten Hse, *(Oughten Hse. Foundation, Inc.; 1-880666),* P.O. Box 1059, Coarsegold, CA 93614 (SAN 169-1449) Tel 559-641-7950; Fax: 559-641-7952
E-mail: info@oughtenhouse.com
Web site: http://www.oughtenhouse.com
Dist(s): **Bookpeople** *(Bookpeople)*
Koen Pacific *(Koen Pacific)*
New Leaf Dist *(New Leaf Distributing Co., Inc.)*
Partners Bk Dist *(Partners Bk. Distributing, Inc.).*

OUP, *(Oxford Univ. Pr., Inc.; 0-19; 0-904147; 0-947946; 1-85221),* Orders Addr.: 2001 Evans Rd., Cary, NC 27513 (SAN 202-5892) Tel 919-677-0977 (general voice); Fax: 919-677-1303 (customer service); Toll Free: 800-445-9714 (customer service - inquiry); 800-451-7556 (customer service - orders); Edit Addr.: 198 Madison Ave., New York, NY 10016-4314 (SAN 202-5884) Tel 212-726-6000 (general voice); Fax: 212-726-6440 (general fax) ; *Imprints:* Clarendon Pr (Clarendon Press)
E-mail: orders@oup-usa.org; custserv@oup-usa.org
Web site: http://www.oup-usa.org
Dist(s): **ACTA Pubns** *(ACTA Pubns.)*
Cobblestone Pub Co *(Cobblestone Publishing Co.)*
Continental Bk *(Continental Bk. Co., Inc.)*
IPG Chicago *(Independent Pubs. Group)*
Shens Bks *(Shen's Bks.)*
netLibrary CO *(netLibrary, Inc.).*

Our Earths, *(Our Earth's Natural Secrets, Inc.; 0-9663568),* P.O. Box 10035, Green Bay, WI 54307-0035 Tel 920-497-3670; Fax: 920-497-3675; Toll Free: 800-546-1797
E-mail: oens@netnet.net.

OurStory, *(OurStory; 0-9663758),* 187 Stone Wall Ln., Charlotte, VT 05445 Tel 802-425-2389
E-mail: kidsbks@aol.com.

Outcomes Unltd, *(Outcomes Unlimited Pr., Inc.; 0-925640),* 75 Cambridge Rd., Asheville, NC 28804 Tel 704-258-1001
E-mail: drdossey@compscape.com
Web site: http://www.comscape.com/drdossey/
Dist(s): **BookWorld** *(BookWorld Services, Inc.)*
Bright Horizons Specialty Distributors Inc *(Bright Horizons Specialty Distributors, Inc.).*

Outlet Bk Co, *See* **Random Hse Value**

Over Cliff, *(Over the Cliff Pubns., Inc.; 0-9661147),* 768 Walker Rd., No. 720, Great Falls, VA 22066 Tel 703-757-7960; Fax: 703-759-1521; Toll Free: 888-447-0024
E-mail: ovrclifva@aol.com
Web site: http://www.overcliff.com.

Overeaters Anym, *(Overeaters Anonymous, Inc.; 0-9609898; 1-889681),* Orders Addr.: P.O. Box 44020, Rio Rancho, NM 87174-4020 (SAN 237-2134) Tel 505-891-2664; Fax: 505-891-4320; Edit Addr.: 6075 Zenith Ct., NE, Rio Rancho, NM 87124-6424
E-mail: overeatr@technet.nm.org
Web site: http://www.overeatersanonymous.org.

†Overlook Pr, *(Overlook Pr., The; 0-87951; 1-58567; 1-59020),* 141 Wooster St., New York, NY 10012 (SAN 202-8360) Tel 212-673-2210; Fax: 212-673-2296 ; *Imprints:* Elephants Eye (Elephant's Eye)
Web site: http://www.overlookpress.com
Dist(s): **Natl Bk Netwk** *(National Bk. Network)*
Penguin Putnam *(Penguin Putnam, Inc.); CIP.*

Overseas, *(Overseas Academic Opportunities; 1-930459),* 72 Franklin Ave., Ocean Grove, NJ 07756 Tel 732-774-1040 (phone/fax)
E-mail: mrwaffle@usa.net.

Overseas Pub, *(Overseas Publishing Co.; 0-9626615),* 14350 Phinney Ave., N., Seattle, WA 98133-6849.

Owl Imprint of H Holt & Co

Owlet Pbks Imprint of H Holt Bks Young Read

Owlet Pubns, *(Owlet Pubns.; 0-916209),* 7611 Tenth Ave., Brooklyn, NY 11228 (SAN 294-9946) Tel 718-965-6400
E-mail: avdefina@aol.com.

Ox Bow, *(Ox Bow Pr.; 0-918024; 1-881987),* P.O. Box 4045, Woodbridge, CT 06525 (SAN 210-2501) Tel 203-387-5900; Fax: 203-387-0035
E-mail: oxbow@gte.net
Web site: http://www.oxbowpress-books.com.

Oxfam Pub (GBR) *(0-85598; 971-91752) Dist. by* **Stylus Pub VA.**

Oxfam Pubns (GBR) *(0-85598) Dist. by* **St Mut.**

Oxford IBH (IND) *Dist. by* **S Asia.**

Oxford Inst, *(Oxford Institute; 0-944335),* 455 Barclay Cir., Rochester, MI 48307-4512 (SAN 243-3982) Tel 248-853-8260.

Oxford Pr Inc, *(Oxford Pr., Inc.; 0-9614854),* 6917 Collins Ave., Miami Beach, FL 33141 (SAN 693-0514) Tel 305-866-7771.

Oxmoor Hse, *(Oxmoor Hse., Inc.; 0-8487),* Div. of Southern Progress Corp., 2100 Lakeshore Dr., Birmingham, AL 35209 Tel 205-877-6000; Fax: 205-877-6790; Toll Free: 800-633-4910
E-mail: oxmoorhouse@spc.com
Web site: http://www.oxmoorhouse.com/
Dist(s): **Leisure AR** *(Leisure Arts, Inc.)*
Little *(Little, Brown & Co.).*

P & R Pubng, *(P&R Publishing; 0-87552),* Orders Addr.: P.O. Box 817, Phillipsburg, NJ 08865-0817 (SAN 205-3918) Tel 908-454-0505; Fax: 908-859-2390; Toll Free: 800-631-0094 Do not confuse with P & R Publishing Co. in Sioux Center, IA
E-mail: tara@prpbooks.com
Web site: http://www.prpbooks.com.

P A B Bks, *(P.A.B. Bks., Inc.; 0-942023),* 610 W. Main St., Greenfield, IN 46140-2059 (SAN 666-3885) Tel 317-326-4608.

P A Castheley, *(Casthely, Pierre A.; 0-9623083),* 293 Coventry Ct., Ramsey, NJ 07446-1271.

P Avery, *(Avery, Phyllis; 1-880598),* 2422 Hutchinson St., Vista, CA 92084 Tel 760-630-8288.

P B Pubng, *(Peanut Butter Publishing; 0-89716),* 2505 Second Ave., Suite 515, Seattle, WA 98121 (SAN 212-7881) Tel 206-748-0345; Fax: 206-748-0343; Toll Free: 888-281-5965
E-mail: pnutpub@aol.com
Web site: http://www.pbpublishing.com.

P Chapman (GBR) *(1-85396) Dist. by* **Sage.**

P D Hays, *(Hays, Peter D.; 1-885554),* 342 1/2 W. Eighth, Eugene, OR 97401 Tel 541-485-6254.

P Diamond, *(P Diamond Enterprises; 1-888875),* Orders Addr.: P.O. Box 3473, Joplin, MO 64803-3473 Tel 417-782-6885; Edit Addr.: 1520 Kentucky, Joplin, MO 64804.

†P E Randall Pub, *(Randall, Peter E. Pub.; 0-914339; 1-931807),* Orders Addr.: P.O. Box 4726, Portsmouth, NH 03802; Edit Addr.: 5 Greenlead Woods Dr., No. 102, Portsmouth, NH 03802 (SAN 223-0496) Tel 603-431-5667; Fax: 603-431-3566
E-mail: deidre@perpublisher.com
Web site: http://www.perpublisher.com
Dist(s): **U Pr of New Eng** *(University Pr. of New England); CIP.*

P Gaines Co, *(Gaines, P. Co.; 0-936284),* P.O. Box 2253, Oak Park, IL 60303 (SAN 214-0209) Tel 708-524-9033; Fax: 708-524-9038; Toll Free: 800-578-3853.

P H Brookes, *(Brookes, Paul H. Publishing Co.; 0-933716; 1-55766),* Orders Addr.: P.O. Box 10624, Baltimore, MD 21285-0624 (SAN 212-730X) Tel 410-337-9580; Fax: 410-337-8539; Toll Free: 800-638-3775; Edit Addr.: 409 Washington Ave., Suite 500, Towson, MD 21204 (SAN 666-6485)
E-mail: custserv@brookespublishing.com
Web site: http://www.brookespublishing.com.

P I Industries, *(P.I. Industries Publishing Co.; 0-916976),* Orders Addr.: P.O. Box 2285, Fort Collins, CO 80521 (SAN 208-7995) Tel 970-224-9381; Edit Addr.: 330 S. Loomis Ave., Fort Collins, CO 80521 (SAN 663-6543).

†P Juul Pr, *(Juul, Peter Pr., Inc.; 0-915456),* P.O. Box 40605, Tucson, AZ 85717 (SAN 207-513X) Tel 520-622-0048; *CIP.*

P Lang (CHE) *(3-906750; 3-906751; 3-906752; 3-906753; 3-906754; 3-906755; 3-906756; 3-906757; 3-906758; 3-906759; 3-906760; 3-906761; 3-906762; 3-906763; 3-906764; 3-906765; 3-906766; 3-906767; 3-906768; 3-906769) Dist. by* **P Lang Pubng.**

†P Lang Pubng, *(Lang, Peter Publishing, Inc.; 0-8204; 3-631),* Subs. of Verlag Peter Lang AG (SZ), 275 Seventh Ave., 28th Flr., New York, NY 10001-6708 (SAN 241-5534) Tel 212-647-7700; Fax: 212-647-7707; Toll Free: 800-770-5264
E-mail: patty@plang.com
Web site: http://www.peterlang.com; *CIP.*

P M C & B, *(Piazza, Melmed, Canner & Berkowitz; 0-9635237),* 112 Prospect St., Stamford, CT 06901-1267 Tel 203-348-2465; Fax: 203-964-9509.

P Migaly, *(Migaly, Peter; 0-9647363),* 417C Glen Malcolm Dr., Glenshaw, PA 15116-2728 Tel 412-486-4621; Toll Free: 800-997-8678 (credit card orders only)
E-mail: migaly@e-help.com
Web site: http://www.e-help.com
Dist(s): **Baker & Taylor** *(Baker & Taylor Bks.).*

P Owen Ltd (GBR) *(0-7206) Dist. by* **Dufour.**

P P Pubs (GBR) *(0-86187; 0-903804; 1-85567) Dist. by* **Continuum.**

P Ray-Mart, *(Raymond-Martimbeau, Pauline; 1-880693),* 5439 Glen Lakes Dr., Dallas, TX 75231-4307 Tel 214-691-2331; Fax: 214-369-5019.

P Roberts, *(Roberts, Phyllis A. Publishing Co.; 0-9657819),* 3526 38th St., Des Moines, IA 50310 Tel 515-279-7239.

P S Chua, *(Chua, Philip S.; 0-9641472),* 1830 Mirmar Rd., Munster, IN 46321 Tel 219-769-2340; Fax: 219-972-1734
E-mail: philschua@pol.net.

P T Pugliese, *(Pugliese, Peter T.; 0-9630211),* Orders Addr.: P.O. Box 307, Bernville, PA 19506 Tel 610-921-5955; Fax: 610-921-8257; Edit Addr.: Rte. 183, Bernville, PA 19506.

P Topp, *(Topp, Patricia; 0-9667369),* 22429 Milner Rd., Saint Clair Shores, MI 48081 Tel 810-774-1224
E-mail: topphat1@aol.com
Dist(s): **Anchor Point** *(Anchor Point Assocs.)*
New Leaf Dist *(New Leaf Distributing Co., Inc.).*

P Walsh Pr, *(Walsh, Patrick Pr.; 0-86700),* 2017 S. Ventura, Tempe, AZ 85282 (SAN 216-6135) Tel 602-968-1549 ; *Imprints:* Synergy Bks (Synergy Books).

PA Bar Inst, *(Pennsylvania Bar Institute; 1-57804),* 5080 Ritter Rd., Mechanicsburg, PA 17055-6903 (SAN 226-8329) Tel 717-796-0804; Fax: 717-796-2348; Toll Free: 800-932-4637
E-mail: sswope@pbi.org
Web site: http://www.pbi.org.

Pa Hist & Mus, *(Pennsylvania Historical & Museum Commission; 0-89271; 0-911124),* Commonwealth Keystone Bldg., Plaza Level, 400 North St., Harrisburg, PA 17120-0053 (SAN 282-1532) Tel 717-783-2618; Fax: 717-787-8312; Toll Free: 800-747-7790
Web site: http://www.phmc.state.pa.us.

PA Podiatric, *(Pennsylvania Podiatric Medical Assn.; 0-9639030),* 757 Poplar Church Rd., Camp Hill, PA 17011 Tel 717-763-7665; Fax: 717-761-4091; Toll Free: 800-841-3668
E-mail: papodassoc@aol.com
Web site: http://www.ppma.org.

†Pa St U Pr, *(Pennsylvania State Univ. Pr.; 0-271),* 820 N. University Dr., USB-1 Suite C, University Park, PA 16802 (SAN 213-5760) Tel 814-865-1327; Fax: 814-863-1408; Toll Free: 800-326-9180 (orders only)
E-mail: ajs23@psu.edu
Web site: http://www.psupress.org; *CIP.*

Pac Ctr Thermal, *(Pacific Ctr. of Thermal-Fluids Engineering; 0-9652469; 1-930746),* Orders Addr.: 2385 S. Kihei Rd., KBR, No. 308, Maui, HI 96753 Tel 734-746-9910; Fax: 734-995-4735; Edit Addr.: c/o Wen-Jei Yang, 3925 Waldenwood Dr., Ann Arbor, MI 48105
E-mail: wjyang@engin.umich.edu.

Pac Inst Conflict, *(Pacific Institute for the Study of Conflict & Aggression; 0-9649535),* Orders Addr.: P.O. Box 819, Kamuela, HI 96743 Tel 808-885-9800; Fax: 808-885-6776; Edit Addr.: 65-1230 Mamalahoa Hwy., Suite C-21, Kamuela, HI 96743.

Pace Pr MA, *(Pace Pr.; 1-881814),* 89 Massachusetts Ave., Boston, MA 02115 Tel 617-247-9141.

†Pacific Bks, *(Pacific Bks., Pubs.; 0-87015),* P.O. Box 558, Palo Alto, CA 94302-0558 (SAN 202-8468) Tel 650-965-1980; Fax: 650-965-0776; *CIP.*

Pacific Meridian, *(Pacific Meridian Ctr.; 1-928702),* Orders Addr.: P.O. Box 2808, San Buenaventura, CA 93002-2808 (SAN 254-0576); Edit Addr.: 301 Los Cabos Ln., San Buenaventura, CA 93001-2812
E-mail: pacificmeridian@aol.com
Web site: http://www.pacificmeridiancenter.com.

Pacific Odyssey, *(Pacific Odyssey; 0-9623293),* 140 N. Louise St., Glendale, CA 91206-4226 Tel 626-301-1604; Fax: 818-551-7845.

†**Pacific Pr Pub Assn,** *(Pacific Pr. Publishing Assn.; 0-8163),* P.O. Box 5353, Nampa, ID 83653-5353 (SAN 202-8409) Tel 208-465-2500; Fax: 208-465-2531; Toll Free: 800-447-7377
E-mail: anisey@pacificpress.com
Web site: http://www.adventistbookcenter.com
Dist(s): **Riverside-World** *(Riverside World)*
Spring Arbor Dist *(Spring Arbor Distributors Inc.); CIP.*

Pacific Santa Barbara, *(Pacific Pr. Santa Barbara; 0-911094),* P.O. Box 219, Pierce City, MO 65723 (SAN 202-1161) Tel 417-476-5514; Fax: 417-476-2089; Toll Free: 800-381-7712
E-mail: andelins@softnet.com.

Pacific View Pr, *(Pacific View Pr.; 1-881896),* 2864 Harrison St., San Francisco, CA 94110 Tel 510-849-4216; 415-285-8538; Fax: 510-843-5835; 415-285-2620
E-mail: pvp@sirius.com
Web site: http://www.pacificviewpress.com
Dist(s): **Cheng & Tsui** *(Cheng & Tsui Co.)*
China Bks *(China Bks. & Periodicals, Inc.)*
Shens Bks *(Shen's Bks.).*

Pacific Word, *(Pacific Word Publishing; 0-9636421),* 117 E. High St., Kendallville, IN 46755-1109 Tel 415-856-2885.

PACT Pubns, *(PACT Pubns., Inc.; 0-9637044; 1-888753),* Div. of Private Agencies Collaborating Together, Inc., 1200 18th St. NW, Suite 350, Washington, DC 20036 Tel 202-466-5666; Fax: 202-466-5669
E-mail: books@pactpub.org
Web site: http://www.pactpub.com.

†**Pagan Pr,** *(Pagan Pr.; 0-943742),* Box 1902, Provincetown, MA 02657-0245 (SAN 241-0540) Tel 508-487-8369 ; *Imprints:* Asklepios (Asklepios)
E-mail: john_lauritsen@post.harvard.edu
Dist(s): **Alamo Sq Dist** *(Alamo Square Distributors); CIP.*

Pagano Organization, *(Pagano Organization; 0-9628847),* Orders Addr.: P.O. Box 1215, Englewood Cliffs, NJ 07632; Edit Addr.: 35 Hudson Terr., Englewood Cliffs, NJ 07632 Tel 201-947-0606.

PageMill Pr, *(PageMill Pr.; 1-879290),* Div. of Circulus Publishing Group, Inc., 2716 Ninth St., Berkeley, CA 94710 Tel 510-848-3600; Fax: 510-848-1326
E-mail: rok27@aol.com
Dist(s): **Publishers Group** *(Publishers Group West).*

PAHO, *(Pan American Health Organization (PAHO); 0-9636369; 92-75),* Orders Addr.: P.O. Box P O Box 27, Annapolis Junction, MD 20701-0027 Tel 301-617-7806; Fax: 301-206-9789; Edit Addr.: 525 23rd St., NW, Washington, DC 20037 Tel 202-974-3000; Fax: 202-994-3663
E-mail: paho@pmds.com; sales@paho.org
Web site: http://www.paho.org.

†**Paideia Pubs,** *(Paideia Pubs.; 0-913993),* P.O. Box 343, Ashfield, MA 01330 (SAN 287-7511) Tel 413-628-3838
E-mail: products@edpsych.com; paideia@javanet.com
Web site: http://www.edpsych.com/; *CIP.*

Pain & Stress, *(Pain & Stress Pubns.; 0-9625914; 1-889391),* Orders Addr.: 5282 Medical Dr., No. 160, San Antonio, TX 78229-6023 Tel 210-614-7246; Fax: 210-614-4336; Toll Free: 800-669-2256; Edit Addr.: P.O. Box 291101, San Antonio, TX 78229-1701
E-mail: psctr@stic.net; mrc@texas.net
Web site: http://www.painstresscenter.com
Dist(s): **Nutri-Books Corp** *(Nutri-Bks. Corp.).*

Pain & Stress Mgt, *See* **Pain Stress & Sleep**

Pain Mgmt, *(Pain Management Innovations; 0-9678176),* P.O. Box 931, Evergreen, CO 80437 Tel 303-674-2381
E-mail: mail@painmgtinnovations.com
Web site: http://www.painmgtinnovations.com.

Pain Resc Ltd, *See* **Innovat Systems**

Pain Review, *(Pain Review, Inc.; 1-884401),* 261 E. 1700 N., Centerville, UT 84014-1043.

Pain Stress & Sleep, *(Pain Stress & Sleep Management; 0-9622041),* 421 N. Otter Branch Dr., Glendora, NJ 08029 Tel 856-939-4484; Fax: 856-939-6158; P.O. Box 856, Marlton, NJ 08029.

Paladin Hse, *(Paladin Hse. Pubs.; 0-88252),* P.O. Box 123, Zenda, WI 53195-0123 (SAN 203-7041) Tel 414-275-2050; Fax: 414-275-9688
E-mail: farleyct@genevaonline.com.

†**Paladin Pr,** *(Paladin Pr.; 0-87364; 1-58160; 1-891268),* Orders Addr.: c/o Gunbarrel Tech Center, 7077 Winchester Cir., Boulder, CO 80301 (SAN 662-1066) Tel 303-443-7250; Fax: 303-442-8741
E-mail: sales@paladin-press.com; editorial@paladin-press.com
Web site: http://www.flying-machines.com; http://www.sycamoreisland.com; http://www.paladin-press.com; *CIP.*

Palladian Law (GBR) *(1-902558) Dist. by* **Gaunt.**

Palmetto Richland, *(Palmetto Richland Memorial Hospital; 1-889863),* 7 Richland Medical Pk. Dr., Columbia, SC 29203 Tel 803-434-4760; Fax: 803-434-7291 (orders); 803-434-3095; Toll Free: 800-775-2287
E-mail: arts.healing@rmh.edu
Web site: http://www.sccancercenter.org.

Palomino Pr, *(Palomino Pr.; 0-9610036),* 86-07 144th St., Briarwood, NY 11435-3119 (SAN 241-5739) Tel 718-297-5053
Dist(s): **Baker & Taylor** *(Baker & Taylor Bks.)*
Brodart *(Brodart Co.)*
Quality Bks IL *(Quality Bks., Inc.).*

Pamphleteers, *(Pamphleteer's Pr.; 0-9630587; 1-890102),* Orders Addr.: P.O. Box 3374, Stony Creek, CT 06405 Tel 800-473-9781; Fax: 203-483-1429; Edit Addr.: 28 School St., Stony Creek, CT 06405 Tel 203-483-8820; Fax: 203-483-9457.

Pan (GBR) *(0-330) Dist. by* **Trans-Atl Phila.**

Pan Am Intl Ozone, *(Pan American Group/International Ozone; 0-918650),* 31 Strawberry Hill Ave., Stamford, CT 06902 (SAN 271-5082) Tel 203-348-3542; Fax: 203-967-4845.

Pan Ishtar, *(Pan/Ishtar Unlimited; 0-941698),* P.O. Box 216, Edgewood, TX 75117 (SAN 239-2747) Tel 903-896-1700; Fax: 903-896-7770
E-mail: astralal@vzinet.com
Web site: http://www.vzinet.com/esplab.

Panda Ink, *(Panda Ink; 0-9658291),* 2211 NW. Military Hwy., Suite 116, San Antonio, TX 78213-1849
Web site: http://www.intx.net/strilce.

Panda Press VA, *(Panda Pr.; 0-9616700),* 4111 Watkins Trail, Annandale, VA 22003 (SAN 659-6711) Tel 703-256-2461; Fax: 703-750-2782 Do not confuse with Panda Pr., Wilmington, DE
E-mail: joytobias@aol.com.

Pandora (GBR) *(0-04; 0-86358; 0-9698762) Dist. by* **NYU Pr.**

Pandora (GBR) *(0-04; 0-86358; 0-9698762) Dist. by* **Harper SF.**

†**Panel Pubs,** *(Panel Pubs.; 0-7355; 0-916592; 1-56706; 1-878375),* Div. of Aspen Pubs., Inc., Subs. of Wolters Kluwer U.S. Corp., Orders Addr.: 7201 McKinney Cir., Frederick, MD 21704 Fax: 301-695-7931; Toll Free: 800-638-8437; Edit Addr.: 1185 Avenue of the Americas, 37th Flr., New York, NY 10036 (SAN 204-921X) Tel 212-597-0200; Fax: 212-597-0334
Web site: http://www.aspenpublishers.com; *CIP.*

†**Panjandrum,** *(Panjandrum Bks.; 0-915572),* 6156 Wilkinson Ave., North Hollywood, CA 91606-4518 (SAN 282-1257) Tel 818-985-7259
Dist(s): **Baker & Taylor** *(Baker & Taylor Bks.)*
Bookpeople *(Bookpeople)*
Coutts Library Service Inc *(Coutts Library Service, Inc.)*
New Leaf Dist *(New Leaf Distributing Co., Inc.); CIP.*

Panorama Van Nuys, *(Panorama Publishing Co.; 0-937671),* 18607 Ventura Blvd., No. 310, Tarzana, CA 91356 (SAN 659-2627) Tel 818-758-2751; Toll Free: 800-634-5620
Web site: http://www.hypnosismotivation.com.

Panos Pubns (GBR) *(1-870670) Dist. by* **Paul & Co Pubs.**

†**Pantheon,** *(Pantheon Bks.; 0-375; 0-394; 0-676; 0-679),* Div. of Random Hse., Inc., Orders Addr.: 400 Hahn Rd., Westminster, MD 21157 (SAN 202-5515) Tel 410-848-1900; Toll Free: 800-733-3000 (orders); Edit Addr.: 299 Park Ave, New York, NY 10171 (SAN 202-862X) Fax: 212-572-6030; Toll Free: 800-638-6460 (customer service)
Web site: http://www.pantheonbooks.com
Dist(s): **Continental Bk** *(Continental Bk. Co., Inc.); CIP.*

Papyrus Pr, *(Papyrus Pr.; 0-9633087),* 826 Hartzell St., Pacific Palisades, CA 90272 Tel 310-454-0920.

Par Rad, *(Par Rad Publishing Co.; 1-880359),* 22132 Wren Way, Lake Forest, CA 92630-1862 Tel 949-770-4233 (phone/fax)
E-mail: profsrxray@aol.com; bparelli@aol.com.

Parabola Bks, *(Parabola Bks.; 0-930407),* 656 Broadway, New York, NY 10012-2317 (SAN 219-5763) Tel 212-505-6200; Fax: 212-979-7325; Toll Free: 800-560-6984
E-mail: parabola@panix.com
Web site: http://www.parabola.org/
Dist(s): **Baker & Taylor** *(Baker & Taylor Bks.)*
Bookpeople *(Bookpeople)*
IPG Chicago *(Independent Pubs. Group)*
New Leaf Dist *(New Leaf Distributing Co., Inc.)*
Weiser Bks *(Weiser Bks.).*

Parabola Mag, *See* **Parabola Bks**

Paracelsus Pr, *(Paracelsus Pr.; 0-9651435),* 9396 N. Scarlet Canyon Dr., Tucson, AZ 85743-5138 Tel 520-744-0430; Fax: 520-744-0428 Do not confuse with Paracelsus Pr. in Silver City, NM.
E-mail: ggoldberg@sprintmail.com.

Paraclete MA, *(Paraclete Pr.; 0-941478; 1-55725),* Subs. of Creative Joys, Inc., Orders Addr.: P.O. Box 1568, Orleans, MA 02653 (SAN 282-1508) Tel 508-255-4685; Fax: 508-255-5705; Toll Free: 800-451-5006; Edit Addr.: 36 Southern Eagle Cartway, Brewster, MA 02631 (SAN 664-6239)
E-mail: srmercy@paracletepress.com; miao@paracletepress.com
Web site: http://www.paraclete-press.com.

Paradgm Pubns Imprint of Redwing Bk Co

†**Paradigm MN,** *(Paradigm Publishing, Inc.; 0-7638; 1-56118),* 300 York Ave., Saint Paul, MN 55101 Do not confuse with companies with the same or similar names in Oklahoma City, OK, Laguna Park, TX, Chicago, IL, Midvale, UT, Saint Cloud, FL, MacFarland, WI; *CIP.*

†**Paradigm Publns,** *(Paradigm Pubns.; 0-912111),* 44 Linden St., Brookline, MA 02445 (SAN 264-7745) Tel 617-738-4664; Fax: 617-738-4620; Toll Free: 800-873-3946 Do not confuse with Paradigm Pubns., Pocatello, ID
E-mail: info@paradigm-pubs.com
Web site: http://www.paradigm-pubs.com
Dist(s): **Redwing Bk Co** *(Redwing Bk. Co.)*
Words Distrib *(Words Distributing Co.); CIP.*

Paradise Cay Pubns, *(Paradise Cay Pubns.; 0-939837),* P.O. Box 29, Arcata, CA 95518-0029 (SAN 663-690X) Tel 707-822-9063; Fax: 707-822-9163; Toll Free: 800-736-4509 (orders only)
E-mail: paracay@humboldt1.com
Web site: http://www.paracay.com
Dist(s): **Baker & Taylor** *(Baker & Taylor Bks.)*
IPG Chicago *(Independent Pubs. Group)*
R Hale & Co *(Hale, Robert & Co., Inc.).*

Paradise Pr FL, *(Paradise Pr., Inc.; 1-57657; 1-884907),* 1575 N. Park Dr., Suite 100, Weston, FL 33326-3230 Tel 954-476-5900; Fax: 954-476-0062 Do not confuse with companies with the same or similar names in Crested Butte, CO, Santa Monica, CA.

Paradise Sacramento, *(Paradise Pubns.; 0-9633816),* 1717 I St., Sacramento, CA 95814-3001 Tel 916-922-8797 Do not confuse with companies with the same name in Paradise, PA, Sayville NY .

Paradox Bks, *(Paradox Bks.; 0-9640827),* 2027 Rose St., Sarasota, FL 34239 Tel 941-365-1988 (phone/fax) Do not confuse with Paradox Books, South Orange, NJ.

Paradox CO, *(Paradox Publishing; 0-9633305),* Orders Addr.: P.O. Box 3289, Winter Park, CO 80482 Tel 970-726-4707; Fax: 970-726-5645 Do not confuse with companies with the same name in Ludlow, MA, Lancaster, CA, Florissant, MO, Wexford, PA.

†**Paragon Hse,** *(Paragon Hse. Pubs.; 0-88702; 0-89226; 0-913729; 0-943852; 1-55778),* 2700 University Ave., W., Suite 200, Saint Paul, MN 55114-1016 (SAN 286-1704) Tel 651-644-3087; Fax: 651-644-0997; Toll Free Fax: 800-494-0997; Toll Free: 800-447-3709
E-mail: paragon@paragonhouse.com
Web site: http://www.paragonhouse.com
Dist(s): **Continuum** *(Continuum International Publishing Group, Inc.); CIP.*

Parallax Pr, *(Parallax Pr.; 0-938077; 1-888375),* Affil. of the Community of Mindful Living, Orders Addr.: P.O. Box 7355, Berkeley, CA 94707 (SAN 663-4494) Tel 510-525-0101; Fax: 510-525-7129; Toll Free: 800-863-5290; Edit Addr.: 850 Talbot Ave., Albany, CA 94706
E-mail: parapress@aol.com
Web site: http://www.parallax.org
Dist(s): **SCB Distributors** *(SCB Distributors)*
SPD-Small Pr Dist *(SPD-Small Pr. Distribution).*

Paralyzed Vets, *(Paralyzed Veterans of America; 0-929819),* 801 18th St., NW, Washington, DC 20006-3517 (SAN 250-4626) Tel 202-872-1300; Fax: 202-785-4452; Toll Free: 800-424-8200 (TDD 800-795-4327).

Paramont Pub, *(Paramont Publishing Co.; 0-9623178),* 5044 Royal Palm Dr., Fremont, CA 94538 Tel 510-659-8162.

Paramount Bks, *(Paramount Bks.; 0-929753; 0-9616024),* P.O. Box 1371, Provo, UT 84603-1371 (SAN 249-3217) Tel 801-375-1053
Dist(s): **Granite UT** *(Granite Publishing & Distribution, LLC).*

Paraninfo (ESP) *(84-283) Dist. by* **Distribks Inc.**

Parapsych Foun, *(Parapsychology Foundation; 0-912328; 1-931747),* 228 E. 71st St., New York, NY 10021 (SAN 203-6851) Tel 212-628-1550; Fax: 212-628-1559
E-mail: info@parapsychology.org
Web site: http://www.parapsychology.org.

Parapsych Sources, *See* **EHE Network**

Parasitology, *(Parasitology; 0-9665807),* Orders Addr.: P.O. Box T2, San Antonio, TX 78209 Tel 210-829-3154; Fax: 210-829-3153; Edit Addr.: c/o Univ. of Incarnate Word, 4301 Broadway, San Antonio, TX 78209
E-mail: sullivan@universe.uiwtx.edu
Web site: http://www.geocities.com/sunsetstrip/venue/2851/parasitology.html.

Parent AIDS, *(Parent AIDS Education Project; 0-9629938),* Div. of Cornell Univ., Cornell Univ. Human Service Studies, 184 MVR Hall, Ithaca, NY 14853 Fax: 607-255-1533; Cornell Univ., Martha Van Rensselaer Hall Rm. 184, Ithaca, NY 14853 Tel 607-255-1942.

Parent Scene, *See* **Family Mtrs**

Parent Tching Pubns, *(Parenting & Teaching Pubns., Inc.; 1-879276),* 16686 Meadowbrook Ln., Wayzata, MN 55391 Tel 612-473-1793; Fax: 612-475-1448; Toll Free: 800-837-8336
E-mail: ander007@tc.umn.edu
Dist(s): **Bookmen Inc** *(Bookmen, Inc.).*

Parents Pipeline, *(Parents' Pipeline, Inc.; 0-9631049),* 4 Sound Shore Dr., Greenwich, CT 06830 Tel 203-661-0338; Fax: 203-661-0438
E-mail: parentppln@aol.com.

Parexel Intl, *(Parexel International Corp.; 0-9625962; 1-882615),* 195 West Street, Waltham, MA 02154 Tel 617-487-9900; Fax: 617-466-8497; Toll Free: 800-937-7795
Web site: http://www.parexel.com.

Parissound, *(Parissound Publishing; 0-9648974),* Div. of K-Enterprises, Inc., 30 Tamalpais Ave., Larkspur, CA 94939 (SAN 299-2663) Tel 415-925-6060; Fax: 415-924-5379; Toll Free: 888-544-5433
E-mail: Parissound@aol.com
Web site: http://www.parissound.com
Dist(s): **Baker & Taylor** *(Baker & Taylor Bks.)*
Bookpeople *(Bookpeople)*
New Leaf Dist *(New Leaf Distributing Co., Inc.).*

Park City Pr, *(Park City Pr.),* Div. of Sunflower Publishing, Inc., P.O. Box 25, Glenwood Landing, NY 11547 (SAN 287-2838).

Park Hurst Pubs, *(Park Hurst Pubs.; 1-885132),* Orders Addr.: P.O. Box 6636, Louisville, KY 40207; Edit Addr.: 206 Cambridge Sta. Rd., Louisville, KY 40223 Tel 502-245-2816.

Park Nicollet, *(Park Nicollet Pr.; 0-9655104),* Div. of Institute for Research & Education Health System Minnesota, 3800 Park Nicollet Blvd., Minneapolis, MN 55416-2699 Tel 612-993-1982; Fax: 612-993-1302.

Park Ridge Ctr, *(Park Ridge Ctr., The; 0-945482),* 211 E. Ontario St., Suite 800, Chicago, IL 60611 (SAN 247-1698) Tel 312-266-2222; Fax: 312-266-6086
Dist(s): **ACTA Pubns** *(ACTA Pubns.).*

Park St Pr Imprint of Inner Tradit

Parker Publishing Co Imprint of P-H

Parkinsonian, *(Parkinsonian Pubns.; 0-9642109),* 4801 Richmond Rd., Tyler, TX 75703 Tel 903-509-0054; Fax: 903-509-3211.

Parkview Pub OH, *(Parkview Publishing; 0-9657038),* Orders Addr.: P.O. Box 09784, Columbus, OH 43209-0784 Tel 614-258-4848; Fax: 614-258-7272; Toll Free: 888-599-6463; Edit Addr.: 281 S. Parkview Ave., Columbus, OH 43209 Do not confuse with Parkview Publishing Co., Fort Collins, CO
E-mail: ss@parkviewpub.com
Web site: http://www.parkviewpub.com
Dist(s): **IPG Chicago** *(Independent Pubs. Group).*

Parkwest Pubns, *(Parkwest Pubns., Inc.; 0-88186),* 451 Communipaw Ave., Jersey City, NJ 07304 (SAN 264-6846) Tel 201-432-3257; Fax: 201-432-3708
E-mail: parkwest@parkwestpubs.com
Web site: http://www.parkwestpubs.com.

Partera Pr, *(Partera Pr.; 0-9659873),* 123 Wellesley, SE, Albuquerque, NM 87106 Tel 505-254-4884; Fax: 505-255-7890; Toll Free: 800-717-6813
Dist(s): **IPG Chicago** *(Independent Pubs. Group).*

Parthenon Pbng Imprint of CRC Pr

Partners Bk Dist, *See* **Partners Pubs Grp**

Partners Pubs Grp, *(Partners Pubs. Group, Inc.),* Orders Addr.: P.O. Box 580, Holt, MI 48842 Tel 517-694-3205; Fax: 517-694-0617; Toll Free: 800-336-3137; Edit Addr.: 2325 Jarco Dr., Holt, MI 48842 (SAN 631-3418).

Passages, *(Passages, Inc.; 0-9614334),* 200 W. Dickson, Fayetteville, AR 72701 (SAN 687-6625).

Passport Bks Imprint of McGraw-Hill Trade

Pate Pub, *(Pate Publishing Co., Inc.; 0-9625083),* 6408 Wilburn Dr., Capitol Heights, MD 20743-3348 Tel 301-350-6020 Do not confuse with Pate Publishing in Detroit, MI
Dist(s): **BkMstrs TX** *(BookMasters).*

Paternoster Pr (GBR) *(0-85364; 1-84227) Dist. by* **OM Literature.**

Pathfinder CA, *(Pathfinder Publishing of California; 0-934793),* 3600 Harbor Blvd., Suite 82, Oxnard, CA 93035 (SAN 694-2571) Tel 805-984-7756; Fax: 805-985-3267; Toll Free: 800-977-2282 Do not confuse with companies with the same or similar names in Minneapolis, MN, Greenwich, CT, Glendale, AZ, Buellton, CA
E-mail: bmosbrook@earthlink.net
Web site: http://www.pathfinderpublishing.com
Dist(s): **IPG Chicago** *(Independent Pubs. Group)*
Quality Bks IL *(Quality Bks., Inc.)*
Unique Bks Inc *(Unique Bks., Inc.).*

†Pathfinder Fund, *(Pathfinder Fund; 0-933853),* 9 Galen St., Suite 217, Watertown, MA 02172-4501 (SAN 225-9664) Tel 617-924-7200; *CIP.*

Pathfinder WA, *(Pathfinder Pr.; 0-9647936),* 25224 NE Jolma Rd., Battle Ground, WA 98604 Tel 360-687-4319 Do not confuse with companies with the same or similar names in New York, NY, Alameda, CA, Elicott City, MD
E-mail: kebja@earthlink.net
Dist(s): **Baker & Taylor** *(Baker & Taylor Bks.)*
Partners-West *(Partners/West).*

Paths of Life, *(Paths of Life Pr.; 0-9637493),* Orders Addr.: P.O. Box 24, Honeoye Falls, NY 14472 Tel 716-624-3210; Toll Free: 800-673-2859; Edit Addr.: 321 Cheese Factory Rd., Honeoye Falls, NY 14472.

Pathway Bks, *(Pathway Bks.; 0-935538),* P.O. Box 27790, Golden Valley, MN 55427-0790 (SAN 213-4241) Tel 612-694-9434; Toll Free: 800-958-3375 (Pin 32) Do not confuse with Pathway Books, Gilsum, NH
E-mail: shermjim@aol.com
Web site: http://www.caregiver911.com.

Pathways Pr NM, *(Pathways Pr.; 0-9657169),* Div. of Ctr. for Self Healing, 912 Baca St., Santa Fe, NM 87501-3522 Tel 505-983-1120 Do not confuse with companies with the same name in Palo Alto, CA, El Cajon, CA.

Patient Adv Educ Res, *(P. A. E. R.; 1-889014),* P.O. Box 9397, Erie, PA 16506 Tel 814-836-9243 (phone/fax)
Web site: http://www.paer.org/.

Patient Med Progs, *(Patient Medical Programs, Inc.; 0-9637123),* Orders Addr.: P.O. Box 40354, Bellevue, WA 98015 Fax: 206-641-3202; Toll Free: 800-608-7585; Edit Addr.: 712 S. 11th Ave., Yakima, WA 98902.

Patient Pr, *(Patient Pr.; 0-9701545),* 6475 Perimeter Dr., Box 110, Dublin, OH 43016 (SAN 253-3685) Tel 614-799-1444; Fax: 614-799-1448 Do not confuse with Patient Press, Kendall Park, NJ
E-mail: dlangenf@columbus.rr.com.

Patient-Centered Imprint of OReilly & Assocs

Patter Pubns, *(Patter Pubns.; 0-9643366),* Orders Addr.: P.O. Box 204, Burlington, IA 52601-0204 (SAN 298-5020) Tel 319-752-0039; Fax: 208-361-8889; Edit Addr.: 301 Maple St., No. 21, Burlington, IA 52601 (SAN 298-5039)
E-mail: patter@willinet.net; patterpub@yahoo.com.

†Patterson Smith, *(Smith, Patterson Publishing Corp.; 0-87585),* 23 Prospect Terr., Montclair, NJ 07042 (SAN 202-8735) Tel 973-744-3291; Fax: 973-744-4501
E-mail: patsmith@voicenet.com; *CIP.*

Patton Pub, *(Patton Publishing Co.; 0-9628886),* 15601 Woodland Dr., No. 201, Dearborn, MI 48120 Tel 313-271-7833; Fax: 313-336-9033 Do not confuse with Patton Publishing in Morrison, CO.

Paul & Co Pubs, *(Paul & Co. Pubs. Consortium, Inc.),* Div. of Independent Publishers Group, Orders Addr.: 814 N. Franklin St., Chicago, IL 60610 Tel 312-337-0747; Fax: 312-337-5985; Toll Free: 800-888-4741; Edit Addr.: P.O. Box 442, Concord, MA 01742 (SAN 630-5318) Tel 978-369-3049; Fax: 978-369-2385
E-mail: frontdesk@ipgbook.com
Web site: http://www.ipgbook.com
Dist(s): **IPG Chicago** *(Independent Pubs. Group).*

†Pauline Bks, *(Pauline Bks. & Media; 0-8198),* 50 St. Paul's Ave., Boston, MA 02130-3491 (SAN 203-8900) Tel 617-522-8911; Fax: 617-524-8035; Toll Free: 800-876-4463 (orders only)
E-mail: mjudge@pauline.org
Web site: http://www.PAULINE.org
Dist(s): **Alba** *(Alba Hse.); CIP.*

†Paulist Pr, *(Paulist Pr.; 0-8091; 1-58768),* 997 MacArthur Blvd., Mahwah, NJ 07430-2096 (SAN 202-5159) Tel 201-825-7300 (ext. 232); Fax: 201-825-8345; Toll Free Fax: 800-836-3161; Toll Free: 800-218-1903
E-mail: info@paulispress.com; mwhiton@paulistpress.com
Web site: http://www.paulistpress.com
Dist(s): **Baker & Taylor** *(Baker & Taylor Bks.)*
Bookazine Co Inc *(Bookazine Co., Inc.)*
Riverside-World *(Riverside World)*
Spring Arbor Dist *(Spring Arbor Distributors Inc.); CIP.*

Pause Pub Co, *(Pause Publishing Co.; 0-9669829),* 912 W. Fourth St., Mosinee, WI 54455 Tel 715-693-1699; Fax: 715-693-9535.

Paw Print Pub, *(Paw Print Publishing Co.; 1-883785),* Div. of Mielchevaerk, Inc., 4429 Morse Ave., Studio City, CA 91604-1427 (SAN 297-9543) Do not confuse with companies with the same or similar name in Mooresville, NC, Columbia, SC, Castro Valley, CA, Boca Raton, FL
Dist(s): **SCB Distributors** *(SCB Distributors).*

Pawprint Pr, *(Pawprint Pr.; 0-9622100; 1-879238),* 8001 Crescent Rd., Norfolk, VA 23505 Tel 757-480-2826.

PAX Pr, *(PAX Pr.; 1-882632),* Div. of Beneficial Designs, Inc., Orders Addr.: P.O. Box 8317, Santa Cruz, CA 95061 Fax: 408-423-8450; Edit Addr.: 5858 Empire Grade, Santa Cruz, CA 95061 Tel 408-429-8476.

†PB, *(Pocket Bks.; 0-671; 0-7434),* Div. of Simon & Schuster, Inc., Orders Addr.: 100 Front St., Riverside, NJ 08075 (SAN 200-2442) Toll Free Fax: 800-943-9831; Toll Free: 800-223-2336; Edit Addr.: 1230 Ave. of the Americas, New York, NY 10020 (SAN 202-5922) Tel 212-698-7000 ; *Imprints:* WSP (Washington Square Press) Pocket Star Bks (Pocket Star Books) PB Hardcover (Pocket Books Hardcover) PB Trade Paper (Pocket Books Trade Paperback) Star Trek (Star Trek) Pocket Books (Pocket Books)
E-mail: ssonline_feedback@simonsays.com
Web site: http://www.simonsays.com
Dist(s): **Replica Bks** *(Replica Bks.)*
T T Beeler *(Beeler, Thomas T. Publisher); CIP.*

PB Hardcover Imprint of PB

PB Trade Paper Imprint of PB

PC Pubns, *(PC Pubns.; 0-9631222),* Orders Addr.: P.O. Box 1593, Piscataway, NJ 08855-1593 (SAN 297-5327) Tel 732-699-0733; Fax: 732-699-0882; Edit Addr.: 437 Rivercrest Dr., Piscataway, NJ 08854 (SAN 297-5319) Do not confuse with PC Pubns., Ann Arbor, MI.

PDA, *(Parenteral Drug Assn.; 0-939459),* 7500 Old Georgetown Rd., No. 620, Bethesda, MD 20814-6133 (SAN 260-3233) Tel 301-986-0293; Fax: 301-986-0296.

PDC Pr, *(PDC Pr., Inc.; 0-9662475),* Div. of PDC Pr., Orders Addr.: P.O. Box 548, Buffalo, NY 14231 Tel 716-633-1991; Fax: 716-633-2435; Toll Free: 888-292-1991; Edit Addr.: 13 Hopkins Rd., Williamsville, NY 14221
E-mail: PDCPress@Lookmom.com
Web site: http://www.Lookmom.com.

PDR Imprint of Med Econ

PDS Pub Mo, *See* **First Data**

†Peabody Harvard, *(Peabody Museum of Archaeology & Ethnology, Harvard Univ., Pubns. Dept.; 0-87365),* 11 Divinity Ave., Cambridge, MA 02138 (SAN 203-1426) Tel 617-496-9922; Fax: 617-495-7535
E-mail: tjcullen@fas.harvard.edu
Web site: http://www.harvard.edu/publications
Dist(s): **U of NM Pr** *(Univ. of New Mexico Pr.); CIP.*

Peacehaven, *(Peacehaven Pubns.; 0-917610),* Div. of Peacehaven, Inc., HCR 72, Box 235, Jasper, AR 72641 (SAN 241-8371) Tel 870-446-5793
E-mail: jself@eritter.net.

Peachpit Pr, *(Peachpit Pr.; 0-201; 0-938151; 1-56609),* Div. of Pearson Education, 1249 Eighth St., Berkeley, CA 94710 (SAN 630-110X) Tel 510-524-2178; Fax: 510-524-2221; Toll Free: 800-283-9444
E-mail: mimiv@peachpit.com
Web site: http://www.peachpit.com
Dist(s): **Addison-Wesley** *(Addison-Wesley Longman, Inc.)*
Baker & Taylor *(Baker & Taylor Bks.)*
Bookazine Co Inc *(Bookazine Co., Inc.)*
Koen Bk Distributors *(Koen Bk. Distributors)*
Koen Pacific *(Koen Pacific)*
Partners-West *(Partners/West).*

Peachtree Prof, *(Peachtree Professional Education, Inc.; 0-9655979),* Orders Addr.: P.O. Box 471199, Tulsa, OK 74147 Tel 918-663-6541; Fax: 918-622-8032; Toll Free: 800-390-9536; Edit Addr.: 7217 E. 55th Pl., Tulsa, OK 74147
E-mail: rnongard@aol.com
Web site: http://home.earthline.net/nptree.

†**Peachtree Pubs,** *(Peachtree Pubs., Ltd.; 0-931948; 0-934601; 1-56145),* 1700 Chattahoochee Ave., Atlanta, GA 30318-2112 (SAN 212-1999) Tel 404-876-8761; Fax: 404-875-2578; Toll Free Fax: 800-875-8909; Toll Free: 800-241-0113
E-mail: peachtree@mindspring.com
Web site: http://www.peachtree-online.com
Dist(s): **Lectorum Pubns** *(Lectorum Pubns., Inc.)*
Shens Bks *(Shen's Bks.); CIP.*

Peak Pr, *(Peak Pr.; 0-9605376; 0-9679688),* 2402 Westgate, Suite 200, Houston, TX 77019-6608 (SAN 239-8834) Tel 713-528-6680; Fax: 713-528-6577; Toll Free: 800-270-1303 Do not confuse with Peak Pr., Colorado Springs, CO
Dist(s): **BookWorld** *(BookWorld Services, Inc.).*

Peak Pubns CA, *(Peak Pubns.; 0-9650590),* Div. of Creative Solutions, P.O. Box 451067, Los Angeles, CA 90048 (SAN 299-0253) Tel 323-655-8777; Fax: 323-655-7509; Toll Free: 800-600-8207.

Pearce Pub, *(Pearce Pubs., Inc.; 1-883122),* Orders Addr.: P.O. Box 4923, Timonium, MD 21094-4923 Tel 410-453-9462; Fax: 410-453-9461; Toll Free: 800-662-2354
E-mail: cpearce@home.com
Web site: http://www.pearcepub.com.

Pearl Ctr Nat Med, *See* **Yehs Ctr Nat Med**

Pearl Pub Hse, *(Pearl Publishing Hse.; 1-879405),* 1142 N. 64th St., Philadelphia, PA 19151 Tel 215-877-4458; Fax: 215-877-7439 Do not confuse with companies with the same or similar names in Northfield, IL, Cottonwood, AZ, Surprise, AZ, Costa Mesa, CA, Lawrenceville, GA
E-mail: order@pearlpublishing; akili@pearlpublishing.com
Web site: http://www.pearlpublishing.com/.

Pearl Pub IL, *(Pearl Publishing; 0-9655023),* 540 Frontage Rd., Suite 2045, Northfield, IL 60093 Tel 847-441-5470; Fax: 847-441-5754; Toll Free: 888-845-8585 Do not confuse with companies with the same or similar names in Cottonwood, AZ, Surprise, AZ, Costa Mesa, CA, Philadelphia, PA, Lawrenceville, GA, San Diego, CA, Elgin, IL
E-mail: stopdiets@aol.com
Web site: http://www.stopdiets.com.

Pearlman Pr, *(Pearlman Pr.; 0-9664927),* 15724 Cherry Blossom Ln., North Potomac, MD 20878 Tel 301-869-8091
E-mail: rpearl@erols.com.

Pearson Custom, *(Pearson Custom Publishing; 0-536; 0-8087),* Div. of Simon & Schuster Higher Education Publishing Group, 75 Arlington St., Suite 300, Boston, MA 02116 (SAN 214-0225) Tel 617-848-6300; Fax: 617-848-6333; Toll Free: 800-428-4466 (orders only)
E-mail: pcp@pearsoncustom.com
Web site: http://www.pearsoncustom.com.

Pearson Educ, *(Pearson Education Corporate Communications; 0-582),* Orders Addr.: 135 S. Mount Zion Rd., Lebanon, IN 46052 Toll Free Fax: 800-882-8583; Toll Free: 800-428-5331; Edit Addr.: One Lake St., Upper Saddle, NJ 07458 Tel 201-236-3342; Fax: 201-236-6549
Web site: http://www.pearsoned.com
Dist(s): **Gaunt** *(Gaunt, Inc.).*

Pearson Learn, *(Pearson Learning),* Div of Pearson Education, Orders Addr.: 4350 Equity Dr., P. O. Box 2649, Columbus, OH 43216-2649 Toll Free Fax: 800-393-3156; Toll Free: 800-321-3016; Edit Addr.: 299 Jefferson Rd., Parsippany, NJ 07054 Toll Free: 800-526-9907 (Customer Service) ; *Imprints:* Good Year (Good Year Books)
Web site: http://www.pearsonlearning.com.

Pebble Bch Pr, *See* **Four Geez**

Pebble Bks Imprint of Capstone Pr

†**Pediatric Projects,** *(Pediatric Projects, Inc.; 0-912599),* P.O. Box 571555, Tarzana, CA 91357 (SAN 282-8146) Tel 818-705-3660; Toll Free: 800-947-0947
E-mail: medpubl@earthlink.net
Web site: http://www.pediatricmentalhealth.org*; CIP.*

†**Pedipress,** *(Pedipress, Inc.; 0-914625),* Orders Addr.: 125 Red Gate Ln., Amherst, MA 01002 (SAN 287-7570) Tel 413-549-7798; Fax: 413-549-4095; Toll Free: 800-611-6081
E-mail: info@pedipress.com
Web site: http://www.pedipress.com
Dist(s): **Baker & Taylor** *(Baker & Taylor Bks.); CIP.*

Pegasus Pr, *(Pegasus Pr.; 1-889818),* Univ. of North Carolina, Asheville, NC 28804 Tel 828-232-5143; Fax: 828-232-5146
E-mail: pegpress@mindspring.com
Web site: http://www.pegasuspress.org.

Pegus Pr, *(Pegus Pr.; 0-941218),* 648 W. Sierra Ave., Box 429, Clovis, CA 93612 (SAN 241-5763) Tel 209-299-2263.

†**Pelican,** *(Pelican Publishing Co., Inc.; 0-88289; 0-911116; 1-56554; 1-58980),* Orders Addr.: P.O. Box 3110, Gretna, LA 70054 (SAN 212-0623) Tel 504-368-1175; Fax: 504-368-1195; Toll Free: 800-843-1724; 1000 Burmaster St., Gretna, LA 70053 Do not confuse with companies with the same or similar names in Lowell, MA, Dallas, TX
E-mail: promo@pelicanpub.com; office@pelicanpub.com
Web site: http://www.e-pelican.com; http://www.bedandbreakfastguide.com; http://www.pelicanpub.com
Dist(s): **Continental Bk** *(Continental Bk. Co., Inc.)*
Shens Bks *(Shen's Bks.); CIP.*

Pelican Pr CA, *(Pelican Pr.; 0-9652561),* Orders Addr.: P.O. Box 1766, Aptos, CA 95001-1766 Tel 831-688-5561; Edit Addr.: 544 Beach Dr., Aptos, CA 95003 Do not confuse with companies with the same name in Santa Barbara, CA, Belvedere, CA, Albion, CA, Prather, CA
E-mail: pelicanpress@altavista.com.

Pelizza & Assocs, *(Pelizza & Assocs.; 0-9614872),* P.O. Box 225, North Chatham, NY 12132-0225 (SAN 693-2266) Tel 518-766-4849; Toll Free: 800-375-6467
E-mail: john@pelizza.com
Web site: http://www.pelizza.com.

Peltec Pubng, *(Peltec Publishing Co., Inc.; 0-9642316),* 4400 N. Federal Hwy., Suite 210, Boca Raton, FL 33431 Tel 407-998-5665; Fax: 407-394-2336.

PEMA Pubns, *(PEMA Pubns., Inc.; 0-9640430),* P.O. Box 186, Spring Green, WI 53588-0186 Tel 608-643-3649 (voice mail); Fax: 608-831-9632
Dist(s): **Bookmen Inc** *(Bookmen, Inc.).*

Pendergrass Pub, *(Pendergrass Publishing Co., Inc.; 0-88323),* P.O. Box 52, Phoenix, NY 13135 (SAN 203-0861) Tel 315-695-7261; Toll Free: 800-853-9379.

Pendle Hill, *(Pendle Hill Pubns.; 0-87574),* Pendle Hill, 338 Plush Mill Rd., Wallingford, PA 19086 (SAN 202-8794) Tel 610-566-4507; Fax: 610-566-3679; Toll Free: 800-742-3150
E-mail: bookstore@pendlehill.org
Web site: http://www.bookstore@pendlehill.org
Dist(s): **Morehouse Pub** *(Morehouse Publishing).*

†**Pendragon NY,** *(Pendragon Pr.; 0-918728; 0-945193; 1-57647),* Div. of Camelot Publishing Co., Inc., P.O. Box 190, Hillsdale, NY 12529-0190 (SAN 213-1463); 52 White Hill Ln., Hillsdale, NY 12529-5839 Tel 518-325-6100; Fax: 518-325-6102
E-mail: penpress@Taconic.net
Web site: http://www.bmtsinc.com/pdragon; http://www.pendragonpress.com*; CIP.*

Penguin, *See* **Penguin Putnam**

Penguin Bks Imprint of Viking Penguin

Penguin Compass Imprint of Penguin Putnam

Penguin Putnam, *(Penguin Putnam, Inc.; 0-14),* Div. of The Penguin Group owned by Pearson plc, Orders Addr.: 405 Murray Hill Pkwy., East Rutherford, NJ 07073-2136 (SAN 282-5074) Fax: 201-933-2903 (customer service); Toll Free Fax: 800-227-9604; Toll Free: 800-788-6262 (individual consumer sales); 800-526-0275 (reseller sales); 800-631-8571 (reseller customer service); Edit Addr.: 375 Hudson St., New York, NY 10014 Tel 212-366-2000; Fax: 212-366-2666 ; *Imprints:* Body Pr-Perigree (Body Press/Perigree) HP Books (H P Books) Grosset-Putnam (Grosset/Putnam) Penguin Bks (Penguin Books) Price Stern (Price Stern Sloan) G P Putnam (G. P. Putnam's Sons) Avery (Avery) Penguin Compass (Penguin Compass)
Web site: http://www.penguinputnam.com.

Peninsula Pubns, *(Peninsula Pubns.; 0-914372),* 26030 New Bridge Dr., Los Altos Hills, CA 94022 (SAN 202-8816) Tel 415-948-1405.

Penn Science, *(Pennsylvania Academy of Science; 0-945809; 0-9606670),* Dept. of Biology, Lafayette College, Easton, PA 18042 (SAN 219-6220) Tel 610-330-5464; Fax: 610-330-5705
E-mail: leibelw@lafayette.edu.

PennWell Bks, *See* **PennWell Corp**

PennWell Corp, *(PennWell Corp.; 0-87814),* Div. of Information Products Group, Orders Addr.: P.O. Box 21288, Tulsa, OK 74121 (SAN 282-1567) Tel 918-831-9421; Edit Addr.: 1421 S. Sheridan, Tulsa, OK 74112 (SAN 282-1559) Tel 918-835-3161; Fax: 918-831-9555; Toll Free Fax: 877-218-1348; Toll Free: 800-752-9764 (orders only)
E-mail: renaew@pennwell.com
Web site: http://www.pennwell-store.com.

Pennypr Imprint of Intl Childbirth

Pennyroyal Pr, *(Pennyroyal Pr., Inc.; 0-9632811),* P.O. Box 153, Cohasset, MA 02025 Tel 617-383-6554; Fax: 617-383-1047.

PenRose Pub, *(PenRose Publishing Co.; 0-9632687),* Orders Addr.: P.O. Box 620, Mystic Island, NJ 08087 Tel 609-296-1401; Fax: 609-294-1987; Edit Addr.: 55 Beach Dr., Mystic Island, NJ 08087.

People for Reason, *(People for Reason in Science & Medicine; 1-886605),* 2446 Clearbrook Ln., Anaheim, CA 92804 Tel 714-995-4889.

Peoples Med Soc, *(People's Medical Society; 0-9627334; 1-882606),* 462 Walnut St., Allentown, PA 18102 Tel 610-770-1670; Fax: 610-770-0607
Dist(s): **IPG Chicago** *(Independent Pubs. Group).*

PEPI, *(Pyramid Educational Products, Inc.; 1-928598),* Div of Pyramid Educational Consultants, Incorporated, 5 C Garfield Way, Newark, DE 19713 Tel 302-894-9155; Fax: 302-894-9156
Web site: http://www.pyramidproducts.com.

Per Aspera, *(Per Aspera Bks.; 0-9652322),* 45 W. 73rd St., New York, NY 10023 Tel 212-362-7904; Fax: 212-721-4936.

Pere Marquette, *(Pere Marquette Pr.; 0-934640),* P.O. Box 495, Alton, IL 62002 (SAN 206-3042) Tel 618-462-5415; Fax: 618-462-8909
E-mail: education@accessus.net
Web site: http://www.firstreader.com.

Perelandra Ltd, *(Perelandra, Ltd.; 0-927978; 0-9617713),* Orders Addr.: P.O. Box 3603, Warrenton, VA 20188 (SAN 665-0198) Tel 540-937-2153; Fax: 540-937-3360; Toll Free: 800-960-8806
E-mail: email@perelandra-ltd.com
Web site: http://www.perelandra-ltd.com
Dist(s): **Bookpeople** *(Bookpeople)*
New Leaf Dist *(New Leaf Distributing Co., Inc.).*

Perennial Imprint of HarperTrade

Perf Resource Pr, *(Performance Resource Pr., Inc.; 0-944246; 0-9610026),* Subs. of Performance Resource Corp., 1270 Rankin, Suite F, Troy, MI 48083-2843 (SAN 274-5127) Tel 248-588-7733; Fax: 248-588-6633; Toll Free: 800-453-7733.

Perf Strategies, *(Performance Strategies, Inc.; 0-9632885),* 1801 Lavaca St., Apt. 13-G, Austin, TX 78701-1332 Tel 512-474-1774; Fax: 512-477-7205
Web site: http://www.perfstrat.com/.

Perfusion Res, *(Perfusion Research & Education Foundation; 0-9643233),* 2123 FM 1960 W., No. 168, Houston, TX 77090 Tel 281-791-4793; Fax: 281-791-4993.

Pergamon Pr Imprint of Elsevier

Perigee Bks Imprint of Berkley Pub

Perinatal Loss, *(Perinatal Loss - Grief Watch; 0-9615197),* Div. of Metanoia Peace Community United Methodist Church, 2116 NE 18th Ave., Portland, OR 97212 (SAN 694-2911) Tel 503-284-7426; Fax: 503-282-8985
E-mail: order@tearsoup.com; webmaster@tearsoup.com; info@tearsoup.come
Web site: http://www.griefwatch.com; http://www.tearsoup.com.

Peringian & Assocs, *(Peringian & Assocs., Inc.; 0-9622773),* P.O. Box 1175, Birmingham, MI 48012 Tel 248-647-2880
E-mail: peringia@juno.com.

†**Periodicals Srv,** *(Periodicals Service Co.; 0-527; 0-8115; 3-262; 3-601),* 11 Main St., Germantown, NY 12526 (SAN 164-8608) Tel 518-537-4700; Fax: 518-537-5899
E-mail: psc@backsets.com
Web site: http://www.backsets.com*; CIP.*

Peripat Club, *(Peripatetic Club; 0-9641132),* Orders Addr.: P.O. Box 367, Stoddard, NH 03464 Tel 603-446-7908; Fax: 603-446-7750; Edit Addr.: Upton Pond, Stoddard, NH 03464.

Publisher Symbol Index

Peripatetic Pub, *(Peripatetic Pub., The; 0-9658750),* 491 Bow Line Dr., Naples, FL 34103 Tel 941-649-8765; Fax: 941-649-6184; Toll Free: 800-554-5695 E-mail: findlater@worldnet.att.net.

Periplus (HKG) *(0-945971; 962-593; 0-7946) Dist. by* **Tuttle Pubng.**

Permanent Pr, *(Permanent Pr., The; 0-932966; 1-57962; 1-877946),* Affil. of Second Chance Pr., 4170 Noyac Rd., Sag Harbor, NY 11963 (SAN 212-2995) Tel 516-725-1101; Fax: 516-725-8215 Do not confuse with companies with the same name in Santurce, PR, San Francisco, CA, Brooklyn, NY, Santa Fe, NM E-mail: info@thepermanentpress.com Web site: http://www.thepermanentpress.com.

Pers & Prof Growth, *(Personal & Professional Growth Organization; 1-880793),* 7454 Kendall St., Arvada, CO 80003-2860 Tel 303-420-8192.

†Persea Bks, *(Persea Bks., Inc.; 0-89255),* 853 Broadway, Suite 604, New York, NY 10003 (SAN 212-8233) Tel 212-779-7668; Fax: 212-689-5405 E-mail: info@perseabooks.com Web site: http://www.perseabooks.com *Dist(s):* **Norton** *(Norton, W.W. & Co., Inc.); CIP.*

Perseus Bks, *See* **Perseus Pubng**

Perseus Bks Grp, *(Perseus Bks. Group),* Orders Addr.: 5500 Central Ave., Boulder, CO 80301 Fax: 303-449-3356 (customer service); Toll Free: 800-386-5656 (customer service); Edit Addr.: 10 E. 53rd St., New York, NY 10022 Tel 212-207-7817 Web site: http://www.perseusbooksgroup.com *Dist(s):* **HarperCollins Pubs** *(HarperCollins Pubs.).*

Perseus Pubng, *(Perseus Publishing; 0-7382),* A Member of Perseus Bks. Grp., Orders Addr.: 5500 Central Ave., Boulder, CO 80301 Fax: 303-449-3356; Toll Free: 800-386-5656; Edit Addr.: c/o Perseus Books Publishing, 11 Cambridge Ctr., Cambridge, MA 02142 Tel 617-252-5200; Fax: 617-252-5285 ; *Imprints:* Plen Insight (Plenum Insight) Plenum Trade (Plenum Trade) E-mail: westview.orders@perseusbooks.com Web site: http://www.perseusbooks.com *Dist(s):* **HarperCollins Pubs** *(HarperCollins Pubs.).*

Personality Res, *(Personality Resources, LLC; 1-929112),* 14232 Marsh Ln., Suite 303, Addison, TX 75001 Tel 972-247-8988; Fax: 972-484-7116; Toll Free: 888-247-4656.

Perspect Indiana, *(Perspectives Pr., Inc.; 0-944934; 0-9609504),* P.O. Box 90318, Indianapolis, IN 46290-0318 (SAN 262-5059) Tel 317-872-3055 E-mail: ppress@iquest.net Web site: http://www.perspectivespress.com *Dist(s):* **Quality Bks IL** *(Quality Bks., Inc.).*

Perspective Chicago, *(Perspective Pr.; 0-9603382),* 629 Deming Pl., Rm. 702, Chicago, IL 60614 (SAN 208-3191) Tel 312-871-4820.

Pet Care Bks, *(Pet Care Bks.; 0-9644637),* Orders Addr.: P.O. Box 3536, Pinedale, CA 93650-3536 Tel 209-278-4288; Fax: 209-297-7622; Edit Addr.: 771 W. Sierra, Clovis, CA 93612.

Peter Smith, *(Smith, Peter Pub., Inc.; 0-8446),* 5 Lexington Ave., Magnolia, MA 01930 (SAN 206-8885) Tel 978-525-3562; Fax: 978-525-3674 *Dist(s):* **Continental Bk** *(Continental Bk. Co., Inc.).*

†Petersons, *(Peterson's; 0-7689; 0-87866; 1-56079),* Div. of Thomson Learning, Orders Addr.: P.O. Box 67005, Lawrenceville, NJ 08648-6105 (SAN 200-2167) Toll Free: 800-338-3282; Edit Addr.: 202 Carnegie Ctr., Princeton, NJ 08540 (SAN 297-5661) E-mail: info@petersons.com Web site: http://www.petersons.com; *CIP.*

†Petrocelli, *(Petrocelli Bks.; 0-89433),* 174 Brookstone Dr., Princeton, NJ 08540-2404 (SAN 211-3848) Tel 609-921-2548 *Dist(s):* **TAB Bks** *(TAB Bks.); CIP.*

Petroglyph, *(Petroglyph Pr., Ltd.; 0-912180),* 160 Kamehameha Ave., Hilo, HI 96720-2834 (SAN 204-9457) Tel 808-935-6006; Fax: 808-935-1553; Toll Free: 888-666-8644 E-mail: reedbook@interpac.net Web site: http://www.basicallybooks.com *Dist(s):* **Booklines Hawaii** *(Booklines Hawaii, Ltd.).*

Pfeifer-Hamilton, *(Pfeifer-Hamilton Pubs.; 0-938586; 1-57025),* 210 W. Michigan St., Duluth, MN 55802-1908 Tel 218-727-0500; Fax: 218-727-0620; Toll Free: 800-247-6789 E-mail: books@phpublisher.com Web site: http://www.phpublisher.com.

Pffr & Co Imprint of Jossey-Bass

Pflaum Pubng Grp, *(Pflaum Publishing Group; 0-89837; 0-937997),* Orders Addr.: 2621 Dryden Rd., Dayton, OH 45439 (SAN 661-2539) Toll Free Fax: 800-370-4450; Toll Free: 800-543-4383 (customer service); Edit Addr.: N90 W16890 Roosevelt Dr., Menomonee Falls, WI 53051 Tel 262-502-4222; Fax: 262-502-4224; Toll Free: 888-558-2292 E-mail: kac@hi-time.com Web site: http://www.pflaum.com *Dist(s):* **ACTA Pubns** *(ACTA Pubns.).*

†P-H, *(Prentice Hall PTR; 0-02; 0-13),* Div. of Pearson Education Corp. Commun., Orders Addr.: 200 Old Tappan Rd., Old Tappan, NJ 07675 (SAN 200-2442) Fax: 416-447-2819 (orders - Canada); Toll Free Fax: 800-445-6991 (government orders); 800-835-5327 (individual single copy orders - US); Toll Free: 800-567-3800 (orders - Canada); 800-223-1360 (individual single copy orders - US); 800-922-0579 (government orders); Edit Addr.: 240 Frisch Ct., Paramus, NJ 07652-5240 ; *Imprints:* Appleton-Century-Crofts (Appleton-Century-Crofts) Busn (Business & Professional Division) Parker Publishing Co (Parker Publishing Company) Reward (Reward Books) Ntl Pubs Blck (National Publishers of the Black Hills, Incorporated) Macmillan Coll (Macmillan College) Prentice Hall (Prentice Hall) Merrill Coll (Merrill College) Web site: http://www.prenhall.com *Dist(s):* **Cambridge Bk** *(Cambridge Bk. Co.)* **Continental Bk** *(Continental Bk. Co., Inc.)* **IFSTA** *(IFSTA); CIP.*

PH Pr, *(Prentice Hall Pr.; 0-13; 0-7352),* Div. of Pearson Education, Orders Addr.: 200 Old Tappan Rd., Old Tappan, NJ 07675; Edit Addr.: 240 Frisch Ct., Paramus, NJ 07652 Tel 201-909-6200; Fax: 201-909-6360; Toll Free: 800-288-4745; 800-223-2336 (customer service) E-mail: pearsoned@eds.com Web site: http://www.phdirect.com *Dist(s):* **Penguin Putnam** *(Penguin Putnam, Inc.).*

PH School, *(Prentice Hall (Schl. Div.); 0-13),* Div. of Pearson Education, Orders Addr.: 4350 Equity Dr., Columbus, OH 43216-2649 Fax: 614-771-7361; Toll Free: 800-848-9500; P.O. Box 2649, Columbus, OH 43216-2649; Edit Addr.: 160 Gould St. (Northeast Region), Needham Heights, MA 02194-2310 Tel 617-455-1300; 500 S. Polk St., Suite 6 (Great Lakes Region), Greenwood, IN 46143 Tel 317-882-9816 Web site: http://www.phschool.com/.

Pharm Info, *(Pharmaceutical Information Assocs., Ltd.; 0-9631310),* 2761 Trenton Rd., Levittown, PA 19056 Tel 215-949-0490; Fax: 215-949-2594 E-mail: pialtd@ix.netcom.com Web site: http://www.pialtd.com.

Pharmaceutical Pr (GBR) *(0-85369) Dist. by* **Rittenhouse.**

Pharmasft Med, *See* **Pharmasft Pub**

Pharmasft Pub, *(Pharmasoft Publishing; 0-9636219),* 21 Tascocita Cir., Amarillo, TX 79124 Tel 806-358-8138; Fax: 806-356-9480; Toll Free: 800-378-1317 E-mail: kami@iBreastfeeding.com Web site: http://www.iBreastfeeding.com.

Pharmavet Pub, *(Pharmavet Publishing; 0-9626619),* Orders Addr.: P.O. Box 10881, White Bear Lake, MN 55110 Tel 612-625-5231; Edit Addr.: 5314 Carolyn Ln., White Bear Lake, MN 55110.

Pharmctl Prods Imprint of Haworth Pr

Pharmedica Pr, *(Pharmedica Pr.; 1-890076),* 257 Rte. 80, Killingworth, CT 06419 Tel 860-663-4060; Fax: 860-663-4069; Toll Free: 800-835-7633 E-mail: mace@pharmedica.com Web site: http://www.pharmedica.com.

Pharmsource, *(Pharmsource Information Services, Inc.; 0-9701533),* 4903 Tarheel Way, Annadale, VA 22003 Tel 703-323-4971; Fax: 703-503-4506 E-mail: info@pharmsource.com Web site: http://www.pharmsource.com; http://www.clinicaltrialsadvisor.com.

Phidippides, *(Phidippides Publishing; 0-9647187),* Div. of Galloway Productions, 4651 Roswell Rd., No. I-802, Atlanta, GA 30342 Tel 404-257-1033 (ext. 10); Fax: 404-252-3971; Toll Free: 800-200-2771 E-mail: gallowayprod@mindspring.com.

Phila Mag, *(Philadelphia Magazine; 0-9635666),* Div. of Metrocorp, 1818 Market St., Philadelphia, PA 19103 Tel 215-564-7700; Fax: 215-656-3500.

Phila Scis Group, *(Philadelphia Sciences Group; 0-924236),* 11232 Midlothian Tpke., Suite 325, Richmond, VA 23235-9620 (SAN 252-2365) Tel 804-744-5233.

Phillips Pub MA, *(Phillips Publishing Co.; 0-941219),* 289 Rogers Ave., West Springfield, MA 01089-1921 (SAN 665-2425) Tel 413-781-7731 Do not confuse with companies with similar names in Potomac, MD, Broomfield, CO.

Philos Pub, *(Philosophical Publishing Co.; 0-932785; 1-891485),* Div. of Beverly Hall Corp., Orders Addr.: P.O. Box 220, Quakertown, PA 18951; Edit Addr.: 5916 Clymer Rd., Quakertown, PA 18951 (SAN 295-8430) Tel 215-538-5300; Fax: 215-536-9099; Toll Free: 877-652-3535 Web site: http://www.philpub.com.

†Philos Res, *(Philosophical Research Society, Inc.; 0-89314),* 3910 Los Feliz Blvd., Los Angeles, CA 90027 (SAN 205-3829) Tel 323-663-2167; Fax: 323-663-9443; Toll Free: 800-548-4062 E-mail: info@prs.org Web site: http://www.prs.org *Dist(s):* **New Leaf Dist** *(New Leaf Distributing Co., Inc.); CIP.*

Philosophia Pr, *(Philosophia; 3-88405),* Orders Addr.: P.O. Box 605, Herndon, VA 22070-0605 (SAN 131-761X) Tel 703-435-7064; Fax: 703-689-0660; Toll Free: 800-359-7340.

Phobia Soc Am, *See* **Anxiety Disorders**

Phoenix Chicago, *See* **Healthwealth**

Phoenix Medical, *(Phoenix Medical Communication; 0-938633),* 6113 E. Quail Track Dr., Cave Creek, AZ 85331-6809 (SAN 661-5821) Tel 602-867-2241.

†Phoenix Pub, *(Phoenix Publishing; 0-914016; 0-914659),* P.O. Box 652, Sugar Hill, NH 03585 (SAN 691-4209) Tel 603-823-8531; Fax: 207-985-3298 Do not confuse with companies with the same or similar name in Newark, NJ, Fairfield, FL, Alpharetta, GA, Custer, WA, Rocklin, CA, Tolono, IL, Redmond, WA, Missoula, MT, Bloomington, IN, Miami, FL, East Lansing, MI, Marina del Ray, CA, Marina del Ray, CA E-mail: info@phoenixpublishing.com; orders@phoenixpublishing.com Web site: http://www.phoenixpublishing.com; *CIP.*

Phoenix Pubg, *(Phoenix Publishing; 1-928812),* Orders Addr.: P.O. Box 8231, Missoula, MT 59807 Fax: 406-721-1978; Toll Free: 800-549-8371; Edit Addr.: 309 SW Higgins, Missoula, MT 59803 Do not confuse with companies with the same or similar names in Redmond, WA, W. Kennebunk, ME, Rocklin, CA, Bloomington, IN, Miami, FL, Fairfield, FL, Tolono, IL, Newark, NJ, Lansing, MI, Alpharetta, GA, Custer, WA, Marina del Ray, CA E-mail: phoenixi@phoenixpub.com.

Phoenix Pubng Co, *(Phoenix Publishing Co.),* P.O. Box 8231, Missoula, MT 59807 Tel 406-549-8371 Do not confuse with companies with the same name in Miami, FL, Bloomington, IN, Marina Del Ray, CA.

Phoenix Seattle, *(Phoenix Project, The; 0-9636594),* Orders Addr.: P.O. Box 84151, Seattle, WA 98124 (SAN 247-784X) Tel 206-329-1371; Fax: 206-624-4961; Edit Addr.: 212 Pioneer Bldg., 600 First Ave., Seattle, WA 98104 E-mail: brain@headinjury.com Web site: http://www.headinjury.com.

Phoenix Soc, *(Phoenix Society, The),* 2153 Wealthy St., SE, No. 215, East Grand Rapids, MI 49506 (SAN 225-9796) Tel 616-458-2773; Fax: 616-458-2831; Toll Free: 800-888-2876 E-mail: info@phoenix-society.org Web site: http://www.phoenix-society.org.

Phoenix WA, *(Phoenix Publishing, Inc.; 0-919345),* P.O. Box 3829, Blaine, WA 98231 (SAN 695-5517) Tel 360-366-2204; Fax: 360-380-1859 Do not confuse with companies with the same name in Sugar Hill, NH, Newark, NJ, Fairfield, FL, Roswell, GA, Rocklin, CA, Tolono, IL or Phoenix Publishing Services, Lewisville, TX., Marina del Ray, CA E-mail: info@phoenixpublishing.com Web site: http://www.phoenixplublishing.com *Dist(s):* **Words Distrib** *(Words Distributing Co.).*

Photo Gallery, *(Photographic Gallery of Fine Art Bks.; 1-889169),* Orders Addr.: P.O. Box 370175, San Diego, CA 92137 Tel 619-221-0340; Fax: 619-223-5744; Edit Addr.: 3665 Hyacinth Dr., San Diego, CA 92106 *Dist(s):* **Baker & Taylor** *(Baker & Taylor Bks.).*

Phunn Pubs, *(Phunn Pubs.; 0-931762),* P.O. Box 6, Viroqua, WI 54665-0006 (SAN 212-128X) Tel 608-637-8742.

Phy Human Rights, *(Physicians for Human Rights; 1-879707),* 100 Boylston St., No. 702, Boston, MA 02116-4610 Tel 617-695-0041; Fax: 617-695-0307 E-mail: phrusa@phrusa.org Web site: http://www.phrusa.org.

Phys Dis Servs, *(Physicians' Disability Services, Inc.; 1-878140),* P.O. Box 827, Arnold, MD 21012 Tel 410-431-5279; Fax: 410-431-5485 E-mail: dfacts@earthlink.net Web site: http://www.disabilityfacts.com.

Phys Law Rev, *(Physicians Law Review; 0-9631342),* 210 Saint Michael Ct., Oak Brook, IL 60521-2556.

Phys Postgrad, *(Physicians Postgraduate Pr., Inc.; 0-933171),* P.O. Box 752870, Memphis, TN 38175-2870 (SAN 692-3208) Tel 901-751-3800; Fax: 907-751-3444.

Phys Sci Pub, *(Physicians & Scientists Publishing Co.; 0-924428),* Orders Addr.: P.O. Box 435, Glenview, IL 60025 Tel 847-559-0605; Fax: 847-559-0699; Edit Addr.: 2540 Osage Dr., Glenview, IL 60025
E-mail: info@medpub.com
Web site: http://www.medpub.com
Dist(s): **Koen Bk Distributors** *(Koen Bk. Distributors).*

Phys Weight, *(Physicians Weight Management Group; 0-9637877),* 10120 Fair Oaks Blvd., Suite D, Fair Oaks, CA 95628-7137.

Physica-Verlag (DEU) *(3-7908) Dist. by* **Spr-Verlag.**

Physicians Pr, *(Physician's Pr.; 0-9633886; 1-890114),* 555 S. Woodward, Suite 1409, Birmingham, MI 48009 Tel 248-645-6443; Fax: 248-642-4949
Dist(s): **Natl Bk Netwk** *(National Bk. Network).*

Physicians Rec, *(Physicians' Record Co.; 0-917036),* 3000 S. Ridgeland Ave., Berwyn, IL 60402 (SAN 205-3853) Tel 708-749-3111; Fax: 708-749-0171; Toll Free: 800-323-9268
E-mail: prco@physiciansrecord.com
Web site: http://www.physiciansrecord.com.

Phytotech Database, *(Phytotech Database Publishing; 0-9657310),* 1620 Olive Ave., Richmond, CA 94805 Tel 510-215-9525 (phone/fax)
E-mail: belanger@jps.net
Web site: http://www.jps.net/belanger
Dist(s): **Redwing Bk Co** *(Redwing Bk. Co.).*

Piatkus Bks (GBR) *(0-7499; 0-86188) Dist. by* **London Brdge.**

PIBL, *(PIBL (Products & Information For Better Living); 1-883558),* 1321 N. Vermont Ave., Suite A, Los Angeles, CA 90027.

Piccadilly Bks, *(Piccadilly Bks., Ltd.; 0-941599),* P.O. Box 25203, Colorado Springs, CO 80936 (SAN 665-9969) Tel 818-789-4980 ; *Imprints:* HlthWise Pubns (HealthWise Publications)
Web site: http://www.piccadillybooks.com
Dist(s): **Empire Pub Srvs** *(Empire Publishing Service)*
Players Pr *(Players Pr., Inc.).*

Piccin Nuova (ITA) *(1-57235; 88-299) Dist. by* **Gordon & Breach.**

Piccin Nuova (ITA) *(1-57235; 88-299) Dist. by* **Scholium Intl.**

Picnic Pt Pr, *(Picnic Point Pr.; 0-9640654),* 131 Third Ave., N., Suite B, Edmonds, WA 98020 (SAN 298-5306) Tel 206-233-1155; Fax: 425-670-0319.

Pictorial Hist, *(Pictorial Histories Publishing Co., Inc.; 0-929521; 0-933126; 1-57510),* 713 S. Third St., Missoula, MT 59801 (SAN 212-4351) Tel 406-549-8488; Fax: 406-728-9280; Toll Free Fax: 888-763-8360; Toll Free: 888-763-8350
E-mail: phpc@montana.com
Web site: http://www.pictorialhistoriespublishing.com
Dist(s): **Motorbooks Intl** *(Motorbooks International Wholesalers & Distributors).*

Pierian, *(Pierian Pr.; 0-87650),* P.O. Box 1808, Ann Arbor, MI 48106 (SAN 204-8949) Tel 734-434-5530; Fax: 734-434-6409; Toll Free: 800-678-2435
E-mail: pubinfo@pierianpress.com
Web site: http://www.pierianpress.com.

Pierson Pubs, *(Romaine Pierson Pubs., Inc.; 0-935466),* 1065 Old Country Rd., Suite 213, Westbury, NY 11590-5628 (SAN 213-3660) Tel 516-883-6350.

Pilgrim OH, *(Pilgrim Pr., The/United Church Pr.; 0-8298),* Div. of United Church Board for Homeland Ministries, Orders Addr.: 230 Sheldon Rd., Berea, OH 44017 Fax: 216-732-3713; Toll Free: 800-537-3394; Edit Addr.: 700 Prospect Ave. E., Cleveland, OH 44115-1100 Tel 216-736-3764; Fax: 216-736-2207
E-mail: ucpress@ucc.org; pilgrim@ucc.org
Web site: http://www.ucpress.com; http://www.pilgrimpress.com.

Pilgrim Pubns, *(Pilgrim Pubns.; 1-56186),* Orders Addr.: P.O. Box 66, Pasadena, TX 77501 (SAN 206-3069) Tel 713-477-4261; Fax: 713-477-7561; Edit Addr.: 1609 Preston, Pasadena, TX 77503
E-mail: pilgrimpub@juno.com
Web site: http://www.members.gnm.com/pilgrimpub.

†Pilot Bks, *(Pilot Bks.; 0-87576),* 127 Sterling Ave., Greenport, NY 11944-0893 (SAN 202-0017) Tel 516-477-1094; Fax: 516-477-0978; Toll Free: 800-797-4568 Do not confuse with Pilot Books, Vienna, VA
E-mail: feedback@pilotbooks.com
Web site: http://www.pilotbooks.com
Dist(s):* Midpt Trade *(Midpoint Trade Bks., Inc.); CIP.

Pimpernel Pr, *(Pimpernel Pr.; 0-9651383),* Orders Addr.: P.O. Box 33110, San Diego, CA 92163-3110 Tel 619-266-4080 (phone/fax); Edit Addr.: 1818 Tulip St., San Diego, CA 92105-5150
Web site: http://www.peaceafterabortion.com.

Pine Hill Pr, *(Pine Hill Pr., Inc.; 1-57579),* 4000 W. 57th St., Sioux Falls, SD 57106 Tel 605-362-9200; Fax: 605-362-9222; Toll Free: 800-676-4228 Do not confuse with Pine Hill Pr., Lafayette, CA
E-mail: print@pinehillpress.com
Web site: http://www.pinehillpress.com
Dist(s): **BookWorld** *(BookWorld Services, Inc.).*

Pine NY, *(Pine Pubns.; 0-9657910),* 2947 Jerusalem Ave., Wantagh, NY 11793-2020 Tel 516-781-0707 (phone/fax) Do not confuse with Pine Pubns., Sanibel, FL.

Pine Orchard, *(Pine Orchard, Inc.; 0-9645727; 1-930580),* Orders Addr.: 2607 Southeast Blvd., No. B150, Spokane, WA 99223-4942 (SAN 253-4258) Tel 509-534-9401; Fax: 509-534-9430; Toll Free: 877-354-7433 ; *Imprints:* Ulyssian Pubns (Ulyssian Publications)
E-mail: orders@pineorchard.com; pineorch@pineorchard.com
Web site: http://www.pineorchard.com
Dist(s): **Amazon Com** *(Amazon.Com).*

Pine Orchard Pr, *See* **Pine Orchard**

Pine Ridge Publns, *(Pine Ridge Pubns., Inc.; 0-9652954),* 1051 W. Burma Rd., Bloomington, IN 47404 Tel 812-876-7211; Fax: 812-876-9117
E-mail: skip@pine-ridge-publication.com
Web site: http://www.pine-ridge-publication.com.

Pine Rm Pr, *See* **Mark Sugar**

Pinegrove Publishing, *(Pinegrove Publishing; 0-9635865),* Orders Addr.: P.O. Box 557, Winona Lake, IN 46590-0557 Tel 219-267-6033; Fax: 219-267-8875; Edit Addr.: 59 EMS Ln., No. C28C, Warsaw, IN 46580
E-mail: 71334.331@compuserve.com.

Pinegrove Pubns, *See* **Pinegrove Publishing**

Pink Hse, *(Pink Hse. Productions; 0-9648176),* P.O. Box 80312, Charleston, SC 29416-0312 Tel 843-763-0860; Fax: 803-763-0466
E-mail: pinkhse@aol.com.

Pinkston, *(Pinkston's Pr.; 0-9627055),* 7124 S. Richmond St., Chicago, IL 60629 Tel 773-737-7333.

Pinnacle FL, *See* **Capital Com Inc**

Pinncle Kensgtn Imprint of Kensgtn Pub Corp

Pinon Press, *(Pinon Pr.; 0-89109; 1-57683),* Div. of NavPress Publishing Group, Orders Addr.: P.O. Box 35007, Colorado Springs, CO 80935 Tel 719-548-9222; Fax: 719-260-7223; Toll Free: 800-366-7788 (orders only); Edit Addr.: 7899 Lexington Dr., Colorado Springs, CO 80920 Do not confuse with Pinon Press Los Alamos, NM
Web site: http://www.navpress.org
Dist(s): **Spring Arbor Dist** *(Spring Arbor Distributors Inc.).*

Pioneer Inst, *(Pioneer Institute for Public Policy Research; 0-929930),* 85 Devonshire St., 8th Flr., Boston, MA 02109 (SAN 250-8982) Tel 617-723-2277; Fax: 617-723-1880
E-mail: pioneer@pioneerinstitute.org
Web site: http://www.pioneerinstitute.org.

Pioneer Pubns, *(Pioneer Pubns., Inc.; 1-881547),* Div. of Pioneer Pubns., Inc., 12345 Jones Rd., Suite 103, Houston, TX 77070-4843 Tel 281-469-9627; Fax: 281-469-2648 Do not confuse with companies with the same or similar names in Broomfield, CO, Las Vegas, NV, Victoria, BC, Tecumseh, OK, Englewood, CO, Kearney, NE, Fresno, CA, Oregon City, OR, Carrollton, MS, Big Timber, MT.

PIP, *(Partners in Publishing; 0-937660),* P.O. Box 50347, Tulsa, OK 74150 (SAN 209-6323) Tel 918-835-8258 (phone/fax) Do not confuse with Partners In Publishing, LLC, Broomfield, CO
E-mail: plmfieldin@aol.com.

Pit Tumor Netwk, *(Pituitary Tumor Network Assn.; 0-9660141),* 16350 Ventura Blvd., Suite 231, Encino, CA 91436 (SAN 299-4356) Tel 805-499-9973; Fax: 805-499-1523
E-mail: mnl@pituitary.com
Web site: http://www.pituitary.com.

Pithy Parodies, *(Pithy Parodies, LLC; 0-9655003),* Orders Addr.: P.O. Box 787, Meridian, ID 83680-0787 Tel 208-727-6343; Toll Free: 888-727-6343; Edit Addr.: 242 N. Eighth St., Suite 200, Boise, ID 83702.

Pitman Pub (GBR) *(0-273) Dist. by* **Trans-Atl Phila.**

Pitspopany, *(Pitspopany Pr.; 0-943706; 1-930143),* Orders Addr.: 40 E. 78th St., Suite 16D, New York, NY 10021-1830 (SAN 238-373X) Tel 212-472-4959; Fax: 212-472-6253; Toll Free: 800-232-2931
E-mail: pop@netvision.net.il
Web site: http://www.pitspopany.com
Dist(s): **Baker & Taylor** *(Baker & Taylor Bks.)*
Bookazine Co Inc *(Bookazine Co., Inc.).*

Pixel Pr, *(Pixel Pr.; 0-9620354),* Orders Addr.: P.O. Box 3151, Tequesta, FL 33469-0151 (SAN 248-4927) Tel 561-744-8775; Fax: 561-747-4407; Edit Addr.: 319 Ridge Rd., Jupiter, FL 33477 (SAN 248-4935) Tel 407-744-8775.

Pizzazz Pr, *(Pizzazz Pr.; 0-939390),* 5114 Chicago, Omaha, NE 68132 (SAN 220-1801) Tel 402-556-1371.

PJD Pubns, *(PJD Pubns., Ltd.; 0-915340; 0-9600290),* P.O. Box 966, Westbury, NY 11590 (SAN 202-0068) Tel 516-626-0650; Fax: 516-626-5546.

PKR Foundation, *(PKR Foundation; 0-9614567),* 4901 Main St., Suite 200, Kansas City, MO 64112-2674 (SAN 691-8433) Tel 816-931-2600; Fax: 816-931-8655; Toll Free: 800-753-2873
E-mail: 75713.2275@compuserve.com
Web site: http://www.kumc.edu/pkrf/.

Pkway Pubs, *(Parkway Pubs., Inc.; 0-9635752; 1-887905),* P.O. Box 3678, Boone, NC 28607 Tel 828-265-3993; Fax: 828-265-3993; Toll Free: 800-821-9155
E-mail: sales@parkwaypublishers.com; parkwaypub@hotmail.com
Web site: http://www.parkwaypublishers.com
Dist(s): **Baker & Taylor** *(Baker & Taylor Bks.).*

†Plan Parent, *(Planned Parenthood Federation of America, Inc.; 0-934586; 1-930996),* 810 Seventh Ave., New York, NY 10019 (SAN 205-1281) Tel 212-245-1845 (phone/fax); Toll Free: 800-829-7732
E-mail: communications@ppfa.org
Web site: http://www.plannedparenthood.org; *CIP.*

Planeta, *(Planeta Publishing Corp.; 0-9715256),* 939 Crandon Blvd., Key Biscayne, FL 33149 Tel 305-361-0053; Fax: 305-361-0054; Toll Free: 800-407-4770
E-mail: mnormanppc@aol.com.

Planning Innovat, *(Planning Innovations; 0-9662512),* P.O. Box 99, Lake City, MN 55041 Tel 612-345-5964; Fax: 651-345-6427.

Platinum Pen Pubs, *(Platinum Pen Pubs., Inc.; 0-912815),* Orders Addr.: P.O. Box 11127, Kansas City, MO 64119 (SAN 265-394X) Tel 816-741-2894.

Platinum Pr, *(Platinum Pr., Inc.; 1-879582),* Div. of Bobley-Harmann Publishing & Marketing Co., 311 Crossways Park Dr., Woodbury, NY 11797 Tel 516-364-1800; Fax: 516-364-1899.

Platte River Pr, *(Platte River Pr.; 0-926719),* 1120 W. Colorado Ave., Colorado Springs, CO 80904-4330 Tel 719-528-8147.

Players Pr, *(Players Pr., Inc.; 0-88734),* P.O. Box 1132, Studio City, CA 91614-0132 (SAN 239-0213) Tel 818-789-4980.

Pleasant Vally GA, *(Pleasant Valley Pubns.; 0-9678059),* Div. of Pleasant Valley Church, Inc., 4178 Hwy 74, W., Thomaston, GA 30286 Tel 706-646-2074; Fax: 706-646-2864; Toll Free: 800-453-5775
E-mail: pvcm@alltel.net.

Plen Insight Imprint of Perseus Pubng

Plenary Systs, *(Plenary Systems, Inc.; 0-926218),* P.O. Box 724, Terrell, TX 75160-0724 (SAN 655-4954) Tel 972-564-6565; Fax: 972-564-0202; Toll Free: 800-841-1070
E-mail: psi-rick@swbell.net.

†Plenum, *(Plenum Publishing Corp.; 0-306; 0-87705; 0-89885),* Div. of Kluwer Academic Pubs., 233 Spring St., New York, NY 10013-1578 (SAN 201-9248) Tel 212-620-8000; Fax: 212-463-0742; Toll Free: 800-221-9369
E-mail: info@plenum.com
Web site: http://www.plenum.com; *CIP.*

Plenum Trade Imprint of Perseus Pubng

Plexus Pub, *(Plexus Publishing, Inc.; 0-937548; 0-9666748),* 143 Old Marlton Pike, Medford, NJ 08055 (SAN 212-436X) Tel 609-654-6500; Fax: 609-654-4309 ; *Imprints:* Medford Press (Medford Press)
E-mail: patp@plexuspub.com
Web site: http://www.plexuspublishing.com
Dist(s): **IPG Chicago** *(Independent Pubs. Group)*
Koen Bk Distributors *(Koen Bk. Distributors).*

PLI, *(Practising Law Institute; 0-87224; 1-4024),* 810 Seventh Ave., 26th Flr., New York, NY 10019 (SAN 203-0136) Toll Free: 800-260-4754
Web site: http://www.pli.edu.

Plume Imprint of Dutton Plume

Publisher Symbol Index

Plumosa Pr, *(Plumosa Pr.; 0-9638492),* 700 W. Waters Ave., Tampa, FL 33604 Tel 813-932-5391; Fax: 813-932-5392; Toll Free: 800-932-5391
E-mail: drmichael@mindspring.com
Web site: http://www.oxytank.com/book.htm
Dist(s): **New Leaf Dist** *(New Leaf Distributing Co., Inc.).*

Plunkett Res, *(Plunkett Research, Ltd.; 0-9638268; 1-891775),* P.O. Drawer 541737, Houston, TX 77254-1737 Tel 713-932-0000; Fax: 713-932-7080
E-mail: info@plunkettresearch.com
Web site: http://www.plunkettresearch.com.

Pluto GBR (GBR) *(0-7453; 0-86104; 0-902818; 0-904383; 1-85305) Dist. by* **Stylus Pub VA.**

Plymouth Pr, *(Plymouth Pr.; 0-935540; 0-9605760),* 101 Panton Rd., Vergennes, VT 05491 Tel 802-877-2150; Fax: 802-877-2116; Toll Free Fax: 800-350-3272; Toll Free: 800-350-1007 Do not confuse with Plymouth Pr., Ltd. in Plymouth, MI
E-mail: plymouth@together.net
Web site: http://www.plymouthpress.com.

Plymouth VT, *(Plymouth Pr., Ltd.; 1-882663),* 101 Panton Rd., Vergennes, VT 05491 Tel 802-877-2150; Fax: 802-877-2116; Toll Free: 800-350-1007 Do not confuse with Plymouth Pr. in Miami Beach, FL
E-mail: plymouth@together.net
Web site: http://www.plymouthpress.com.

PNB Pub, *(PNB Pub.; 0-9629115),* P.O. Box 11391, Chicago, IL 60611 Tel 312-943-1719; Fax: 312-943-0123
Dist(s): **Baker & Taylor** *(Baker & Taylor Bks.)*
Brodart *(Brodart Co.)*
Partners Pubs Grp *(Partners Pubs. Group, Inc.)*
Quality Bks IL *(Quality Bks., Inc.).*

Pneumatikos Counsel Inst, *(Pneumatikos Counseling Institute, Publishing Div.; 0-929564),* 1040 W. 18th Ave., Eugene, OR 97402-4035 (SAN 249-7271) Tel 541-484-4804.

Pnguin Bks Ltd (GBR) *(0-14) Dist. by* **Trafalgar.**

Pocahontas Pr, *(Pocahontas Pr., Inc.; 0-936015),* 832 Hutcheson Dr., P.O. Drawer F, Blacksburg, VA 24063-1020 (SAN 630-124X) Tel 540-951-0467; Fax: 540-961-2847; Toll Free: 800-446-0467
E-mail: mchollim@vt.edu
Dist(s): **Baker & Taylor** *(Baker & Taylor Bks.)*
Coutts Library Service Inc *(Coutts Library Service, Inc.)*
Koen Bk Distributors *(Koen Bk. Distributors)*
Quality Bks IL *(Quality Bks., Inc.).*

Pocket Books Imprint of PB

Pocket Brain, *(Pocket Brain Publishing; 0-9668187),* Orders Addr.: 3758 Cambridge Ct., Loveland, OH 45140-5505 Tel 513-697-8824; Edit Addr.: P.O. Box 498947, Cincinnati, OH 45249
E-mail: Pearls@pol.net
Web site: http://home.fuse.net/pearls/homepage.

Pocket Essentials (GBR) *(1-903047) Dist. by* **Trafalgar.**

Pocket Power, *(Pocket Power; 0-945893),* 11922 Paseo Lucido, San Diego, CA 92128-6263.

Pocket Star Bks Imprint of PB

Pogment Pr, *(Pogment Pr., The; 0-938823),* 11939 Escalante Ct, Reston, VA 22091 (SAN 661-7468) Tel 703-758-0258.

Points of Light, *(Points of Light Foundation; 1-58534),* 1400 I St., NW, Suite 800, Washington, DC 20005 Fax: 202-729-8105
E-mail: lgarcia@pointsoflight.org
Web site: http://www.pointsoflight.org.

Pol Studies, *(Policy Studies Organization; 0-918592; 0-944285),* 711 Ashton Ln., S., Champaign, IL 61820 (SAN 210-1343) Tel 217-352-5094; Fax: 217-352-3037
E-mail: s-nagel@uiuc.edu
Web site: http://www.staff.uiuc.edu/~s-nagel.

Polaris Pub, *(Polaris Publishing; 0-9669791),* P.O. Box 11252, Glendale, CA 91226 Tel 818-956-3736; Fax: 626-576-7727.

Police Beat Pr, *(Police Beat Pr.; 0-942724),* 45 Albert St., S., No. 1, Saint Paul, MN 55105-2250 (SAN 240-1231) Tel 612-699-4750.

Polinym Pr, *(Polinym Pr.; 0-942287),* 33 Berry Oaks Ln., Saint Louis, MO 63122-1908 (SAN 666-8151) Tel 314-968-0986.

Polity Pr (GBR) *(0-7456) Dist. by* **Blackwell Pubs.**

Pollywog Pr, *(Pollywog Pr., The; 0-9663067),* 3803 Villa Terr., San Diego, CA 92104 Tel 619-688-0973; Fax: 619-688-1322
E-mail: jstinson@adnc.com
Web site: http://www.rxforliving.com.

Poltergeist, *(Poltergeist Pr.; 0-9603918),* 706 S. Morain St., Kennewick, WA 99336 (SAN 213-5477) Tel 509-735-4078.

Ponderosa Press, *(Ponderosa Pr.; 0-9659513),* 1525 Eighth Ave., W., Spokane, WA 99204 Tel 509-838-8473; Fax: 509-838-2372 Do not confuse with companies with the same name in Colorado Springs, CO, Yosemite, CA, Fredericksburg, TX, Hackensack, MN, Riesel, TX.

Ponte Vedra Pub, *(Ponte Vedra Publishing; 0-9654996),* Orders Addr.: P.O. Box 773, Ponte Vedra Beach, FL 32004-0773 Tel 904-398-8950; Fax: 904-396-4911; Edit Addr.: 7045 Cypress Brook Dr., S., Ponte Vedra, FL 32082
E-mail: wagemaker@aol.com
Web site: http://www.mentaldisorders.com.

Poolbeg Pr (IRL) *(0-905169; 0-907085; 1-85371; 1-84223) Dist. by* **Dufour.**

Pope John Ctr, *See* **NCBC**

Pope Paul Sixth, *(Pope Paul VI Institute Pr.; 0-9626485),* Div. of Pope Paul VI Institute for the Study of Human Reproduction, 6901 Mercy Rd., Omaha, NE 68106 Tel 402-390-9167; Fax: 402-390-9851.

Popular E Commerce, *(Popular E Commerce, Inc.; 0-87380),* P.O. Box 1901, Boerne, TX 78006 Tel 830-537-3411.

Popular Prakashan (IND) *(81-7154) Dist. by* **Asia Bk Corp.**

Popular Prakashan (IND) *(81-7154) Dist. by* **S Asia.**

†Population Coun, *(Population Council; 0-87834),* 1 Dag Hammarskjold Plaza, New York, NY 10017 (SAN 225-1582) Tel 212-339-0514; Fax: 212-755-6052
E-mail: pubinfo@popcouncil.org
Web site: http://www.popcouncil.org; *CIP.*

†Porcupine Pr, *(Porcupine Pr., Inc.; 0-87991),* 1500 Walnut St., Suite 1300, Philadelphia, PA 19102-3507 Tel 215-735-0101; Fax: 215-546-0664 Do not confuse with Porcupine Pr., Inc., Cedarburg, WI
Web site: http://www.angelfire.com/mi2/Daporky; *CIP.*

Portage Pub, *(Portage Publishing Co.; 0-9637330),* 2041 Ganyard Rd., Akron, OH 44313-6021 Tel 216-864-7676; Fax: 216-864-1055.

Porter & Assocs, *(Porter & Assocs.; 1-882740),* Orders Addr.: P.O. Box 1740, Bend, OR 97709 Fax: 541-383-0129; Toll Free: 800-758-8861; Edit Addr.: 2117 NE Kim Ln., Bend, OR 97701
E-mail: porter@bendcable.com
Dist(s): **J Majors Co** *(Majors, J. A. Co.)*
Matthews Medical Bk Co *(Matthews Medical Bk. Co.)*
Rittenhouse *(Rittenhouse Bk. Distributors).*

Portfolio Pr, *See* **Portfolio Pr Corp**

Portfolio Pr Corp, *(Portfolio Press Corp.; 0-942620),* Orders Addr.: 130 Wineow St., Suite 3, Cumberland, MD 21502 (SAN 238-5554) Tel 301-724-2795; Fax: 301-724-2796; Toll Free: 877-737-1200; Edit Addr.: 1107 Broadway, 12th Flr., New York, NY 10010 (SAN 238-5554) Tel 212-989-8700; Fax: 212-691-3073
E-mail: portfolio@hereintown.net
Web site: http://www.portfoliopress.com.

Portfolio Pub, *(Portfolio Publishing Co., Inc.; 0-943255),* Orders Addr.: P.O. Box 986, Saratoga, WY 82331-0986 (SAN 668-3576) Tel 713-363-3577; Fax: 713-292-9722.

Portunus Pubng, *(Portunus Publishing Co.; 0-9641330; 1-886440),* 27875 Berwick Dr., Carmel, CA 93923 Tel 831-622-0604; Fax: 310-399-5644
E-mail: service@portunus.net
Dist(s): **Lectorum Pubns** *(Lectorum Pubns., Inc.).*

Positive Pr AZ, *(Positive Pr., The; 0-9655381),* Orders Addr.: P.O. Box 32668, Tucson, AZ 85751-2668 (SAN 299-2744); Edit Addr.: 905 LaGrange St., West Lafayette, IN 47906 Do not confuse with companies with the same name in Chico, CA, La Grange, IL, Sharon, IL
E-mail: TNKPOS@aol.com.

Positive Support, *(Positive Support Seminars; 1-885335),* 28641 Elbamar Dr., Grosse Ile, MI 48138 Tel 734-675-6200; Fax: 734-675-6247; Toll Free: 800-676-3806
E-mail: bertie@wdl.net
Web site: http://www.bookzone.com/bookzone/10000641.html.

Post Apollo Pr, *(Post-Apollo Pr., The; 0-942996),* 35 Marie St., Sausalito, CA 94965 (SAN 240-429X) Tel 415-332-1458; Fax: 415-332-8540
E-mail: tpapress@dnai.com
Web site: http://www.dnai.com/~tpapress/
Dist(s): **SPD-Small Pr Dist** *(SPD-Small Pr. Distribution).*

Postcard Activist, *(Postcard Activist; 1-879096),* 42 Hollywood Dr., Hastings-On-Hudson, NY 10706-1206 Tel 914-699-0200.

Postgraduate Med Rev Ed, *(Postgraduate Medical Review Education; 0-9626486; 1-884588),* 407 Lincoln Rd., Suite 12I, Miami Beach, FL 33139 Tel 305-538-4444; Fax: 305-538-9544; Toll Free: 800-433-3539.

Potential Unltd, *(Potential Unlimited Publishing Foundation; 0-9650700),* Orders Addr.: P.O. Box 218, Stratham, NH 03885-0218 Fax: 603-772-9695; Edit Addr.: 12 Evergreen Way, Stratham, NH 03885; 151 Portsmouth Ave., Stratham, NH 03885 ; *Imprints:* PUP Bks (P U P Books)
E-mail: abby.messner@eudoramail.com.

Potes Poets, *(Potes & Poets Pr., Inc.; 0-937013; 1-893541),* 181 Edgemont Ave., Elmwood, CT 06110-1005 (SAN 658-6759) Tel 860-233-2023
Dist(s): **SPD-Small Pr Dist** *(SPD-Small Pr. Distribution).*

Poultry Sci, *(Poultry Science Assn.; 0-9649811),* 1111 N. Dunlap Ave., Savoy, IL 61874 Tel 217-356-3182; Fax: 217-398-4119
E-mail: psa@assochq.org
Web site: http://www.psa.uiuc.edu.

Power NY, *(Power Pubns.; 0-9627246; 1-888315),* 56 McArthur Ave., Staten Island, NY 10312 Tel 718-948-4938; Fax: 718-317-0858; Toll Free: 800-331-6534 Do not confuse with companies with the same name in Tyler, TX, Mountain City, GA
E-mail: afeduprn@aol.com
Web site: http://www.greatnurses.com.

Power of One, *(Power of One Publishing; 0-9628770),* c/o Renew Life, 2076 Sunnydale Dr., Clearwater, FL 33765-1204 Toll Free: 800-830-4778
E-mail: susan@healthcarealternatives.net
Web site: http://www.healthcarealternatives.net; http://www.powerofonepublishing.com.

PowerKids Pr Imprint of Rosen Group

PPI (GBR) *Dist. by* **Elsevier.**

PPI (GBR) *Dist. by* **McGraw.**

PPI Pubng, *(PPI Publishing; 1-57515),* P.O. Box 292-239, Kettering, OH 45429 Tel 937-294-5057; Fax: 937-294-9442; Toll Free: 800-773-6825
Dist(s): **Baker & Taylor** *(Baker & Taylor Bks.).*

PPL (GBR) *Dist. by* **Elsevier.**

PPP Imprint of Haworth Pr

†Pr Assocs, *(Press Assocs., Inc.; 0-918763),* 815 15th St., NW, Suite 1102, Washington, DC 20005 (SAN 657-3738) Tel 202-638-0444; Fax: 202-638-0955; *CIP.*

Pract Field, *(Practice Field Publishing; 0-9648264; 1-930869),* 2048 Lake Michigan Dr., NW, Grand Rapids, MI 49504 Tel 616-791-6399; Fax: 616-791-6380
E-mail: lindadeleeuw@cpmrc.com
Web site: http://www.cpmrc.com.

Practical Allergy, *(Practical Allergy Research Foundation; 0-9616318; 1-880509),* Orders Addr.: P.O. Box 60, Buffalo, NY 14223-0060 (SAN 658-6813) Tel 716-875-5578; Fax: 716-875-5399; Toll Free: 800-787-8780; Edit Addr.: 1421 Colvin Blvd., Buffalo, NY 14223.

Practical Footcare, *(Practical Footcare Pubs.; 1-885421),* Orders Addr.: P.O. Box 114, Churchton, MD 20733 Tel 703-329-0186; Toll Free: 800-284-6307
E-mail: oasdi@compuserve.com.

†Practice Mgmt Info, *(Practice Management Information Corp.; 1-57066; 1-878487; 1-885987),* 4727 Wilshire Blvd., Suite 300, Los Angeles, CA 90010 Tel 323-954-0224 (corporate office, editorial); Fax: 323-954-0253 (corporate offfice, editorial); Toll Free: 800-633-4215 (customer service); 800-633-7467 (sales) ; *Imprints:* Health Info Pr (Health Information Press)
E-mail: pmiceditor@lainet.com
Web site: http://www.medicalbookstore.com
Dist(s): **J Majors Co** *(Majors, J. A. Co.)*
Matthews Medical Bk Co *(Matthews Medical Bk. Co.); CIP.*

Praeger Pubs Imprint of Greenwood

Praeger Trade Imprint of Greenwood

Pratt Inst, *(Pratt Institute Creative Arts Therapy Review; 1-884870),* E. 3, Willoughby Ave., Brooklyn, NY 11205 Tel 718-636-3428; Fax: 718-636-3785.

PRC Pub, *(PRC Publishing; 0-944183),* Div. of Professional Reports Corp., 3976 Fulton Dr., NW, Canton, OH 44718 (SAN 243-0959) Tel 330-492-6063; Fax: 330-492-6176; Toll Free: 800-336-0083.

Prctnrs Pub Co, *(Practitioners Publishing Co.; 0-7646; 1-56433),* Div. of Thomson Professional & Regulatory, Inc., Orders Addr.: P.O. Box 966, Fort Worth, TX 76101-0966 Tel 817-332-3709; Fax: 817-336-2433; Toll Free: 800-323-8724; Edit Addr.: 3221 Collinsworth, Fort Worth, TX 76107
E-mail: Linda_Lusk@ppctx.com
Web site: http://www.ppc.com.

Prdox Pubng (CAN) *(0-9695822) Dist. by* **New Centry Pr.**

Precept Pr, *(Precept Pr.; 0-931028; 0-944496),* Div. of Bonus Bks., Inc., 160 E. Illinois St., Chicago, IL 60611 (SAN 238-8413) Tel 312-467-0424; Fax: 312-467-9271; Toll Free: 800-225-3775
E-mail: bb@bonus-books.com
Web site: http://www.bonus-books.com
Dist(s): **J Majors Co** *(Majors, J. A. Co.)*
Tanager Pub Co *(Tanager Publishing Co.).*

Prefer Pub Co, *(Preferred Publishing Co.; 0-9665067),* 3013 Fountainview Dr. Suite 100, Houston, TX 77057 (SAN 299-6502) Tel 713-266-8178; Fax: 713-334-9454.

Prema Bks, *See* **Lorenzo Prema**

Premier Pub CO, *(Premier Publishing; 0-942933),* 8 Red Birch, Littleton, CO 80127 (SAN 667-8246) Tel 303-978-0122 Do not confuse with companies with same or similar names in Wamego, KS, Baton Rouge, LA, DuBois, PA, Stratford, CT, Smyrna, GA, Bethesda, MD, Fresno, CA, Palatine, IL, Las Vegas, NV, San Diego, CA, Branson, MO, Worthington, OH.

Prentice ESL, *(Prentice Hall, ESL Dept.; 0-13; 0-88345),* 240 Frisch Ct., Paramus, NJ 07652-5240 (SAN 200-2175) Tel 201-236-7000; Fax: 201-592-0904; Toll Free: 800-922-0579
Web site: http://vig.prenhall.com/
Dist(s): **Continental Bk** *(Continental Bk. Co., Inc.).*

Prentice Hall Imprint of P-H

PREP Pubng, *(PREP Publishing; 1-885288),* Div. of PREP, Inc., 1110 1/2 Hay St., PMB 66, Fayetteville, NC 28305 Tel 910-483-6611; Fax: 910-483-2439; Toll Free: 800-533-2814
E-mail: preppub@aol.com
Web site: http://www.prep-pub.com
Dist(s): **Baker & Taylor** *(Baker & Taylor Bks.).*

Presby & Reformed, *See* **P & R Pubng**

Present Dynam, *(Presentation Dynamics, Inc.; 0-9614937; 1-928564),* Orders Addr.: 774 Mays Blvd., Suite 10-143, Incline Village, NV 89451-9607 (SAN 693-5311) Tel 775-832-8210; Fax: 702-920-8313
E-mail: pdi@knock-knock.com
Web site: http://www.bodymind.net; http://www.testinfo.net
Dist(s): **Majors Scientific Bks Inc** *(Majors Scientific Bks., Inc.)*
Matthews Bk Co *(Matthews Bk. Co.)*
Rittenhouse *(Rittenhouse Bk. Distributors).*

Press Gang Pubs (CAN) *(0-88974) Dist. by* **LPC Group.**

Prestel Pub NY, *(Prestel Publishing; 3-7913),* 175 Fifth Ave., Suite 402, New York, NY 10010 Tel 212-995-2720; Fax: 212-995-2733
E-mail: sales@prestel-usa.com
Web site: http://www.prestel.com
Dist(s): **BPI Commns** *(B. P. I. Communications).*

Preston Publng, *(Preston Publishing Co., Inc.; 0-9652442),* 18 Wilson Rd., Brewster, NY 10509 Tel 914-278-6773; Toll Free: 800-275-3800.

Preston Pubns, *(Preston Pubns., Inc.; 0-912474),* P.O. Box 48312, Niles, IL 60714 (SAN 205-3926) Tel 847-647-2900; Fax: 847-647-1155; 6600 W. Touhy Ave., Niles, IL 60714-0312 Do not confuse with Preston Pubns., Marion, MA
Web site: http://www.prestonpub.com.

Pretext Pr, *(Pretext Pr.; 0-9654873),* P.O. Box 988, North Branford, CT 06471 Tel 203-481-0145.

Prevention Ctr, *(West Virginia Univ., Prevention Research Ctr.; 0-9665085),* P.O. Box 6300, Morgantown, WV 26506-6300 Tel 304-293-1823; Fax: 304-293-8624
E-mail: ebarnett@wvu.edu.

Prevention Educ, *(Prevention Education Counseling System Research; 0-9660855),* 1617 Ridge Rd., Leavenworth, KS 66048 Tel 913-772-1926; Toll Free: 800-772-1926.

Prgamon Press Imprint of Buttrwrth-Heinemann

Price-Pottenger, *(Price-Pottenger Nutrition Foundation; 0-916764),* 2667 Camino Del Rio S., Suite 109, San Diego, CA 92108-3763 (SAN 208-1849) Tel 619-582-4168.

Prima Health Imprint of Prima Pub

Prima Health Prof, *See* **Hlth Prof Inst**

Prima Lifesty Imprint of Prima Pub

†Prima Pub, *(Prima Publishing; 0-7615; 0-914629; 1-55958; 1-4000),* Orders Addr.: P.O. Box 1260, Rocklin, CA 95677 Toll Free: 800-632-8676; Edit Addr.: 3000 Lava Ridge Ct., Roseville, CA 95661 (SAN 289-5609) Tel 916-787-7000; Fax: 916-787-7001 ; *Imprints:* Prima Health (Prima Health) Prima Lifesty (Prima Lifestyles) TNP (TNP.com)
E-mail: sales@primapub.com
Web site: http://www.primapublishing.com
Dist(s): **IPG Chicago** *(Independent Pubs. Group)*
Random *(Random Hse., Inc.); CIP.*

Primary Research, *(Primary Research; 0-9626749; 1-57440),* 850 Seventh Ave., Suite 1200, New York, NY 10019 Tel 212-764-1579; Fax: 212-397-5056; 30 Lincoln Plaza, Suite 14-N, New York, NY 10023
E-mail: primarydat@aol.com.

Prime Natl Pub, *(Prime National Publishing Corp.; 0-932834),* 470 Boston Post Rd., Weston, MA 02193 (SAN 212-3053) Tel 617-899-2702; Fax: 617-899-4900.

Primedia Bus Mag Med, *(Primedia Business Magazines & Media; 0-87288; 0-89287; 0-918371),* Orders Addr.: P.O. Box 12901, Overland Park, KS 66282-2901 (SAN 670-8463) Tel 913-341-1300; Fax: 913-967-1901; Toll Free: 800-262-1954; Edit Addr.: 9800 Metcalf, Overland Park, KS 66212
Web site: http://www.intertec.com
Dist(s): **SCB Distributors** *(SCB Distributors).*

Princess Pub, *(Princess Publishing; 0-943367),* P.O. Box 25406, Portland, OR 97298 (SAN 668-4718) Tel 503-297-1565; Fax: 503-292-2752 Do not confuse with Princess Publishing in Marlton, NJ
E-mail: matschek@teleport.com.

Princeton Arch, *(Princeton Architectural Pr.; 0-907259; 0-910413; 0-9636372; 1-56898; 1-878271; 1-885232),* 37 E. Seventh St., New York, NY 10003 (SAN 260-1176) Tel 212-995-9620; Fax: 212-995-9454; Toll Free: 800-722-6657
E-mail: sales@papress.com
Web site: http://www.papress.com
Dist(s): **Chronicle Bks** *(Chronicle Bks. LLC).*

Princeton Bk Co, *(Princeton Bk. Co. Pubs.; 0-87127; 0-916622),* Orders Addr.: P.O. Box 831, Hightstown, NJ 08520-0831 (SAN 630-1568) Tel 609-426-0602; Fax: 609-426-1344; Toll Frcc: 800-220-7149; Edit Addr.: 614 Rte. 130, Hightstown, NJ 08520 (SAN 244-8076)
E-mail: pbc@dancehorizons.com; elysian@aosi.com
Web site: http://www.dancehorizons.com
Dist(s): **IPG Chicago** *(Independent Pubs. Group).*

Princeton Hlth, *(Princeton Health Pr.; 0-933665),* 115 Wall St., Princeton, NJ 08540 (SAN 692-5391) Tel 609-921-6360; Fax: 609-921-3593; Toll Free: 800-636-3415
E-mail: sales@phplifeskills.com
Web site: http://www..lifeskillstraining.com.

†Princeton U Pr, *(Princeton Univ. Pr.; 0-691),* Orders Addr.: California-Princeton Fulfillment Services, 1445 Lower Ferry Rd., Ewing, NJ 08618 Tel 800-777-4726; Fax: 800-999-1958; Edit Addr.: 41 William St., Princeton, NJ 08540 (SAN 202-0254) Tel 609-258-4900; Fax: 609-258-6305 ; *Imprints:* Bollingen (Bollingen)
E-mail: webmaster@pupress.princeton.edu
Web site: http://www.pup.princeton.edu
Dist(s): **Cal Prin Full Svc** *(California Princeton Fulfillment Services)*
Continental Bk *(Continental Bk. Co., Inc.); CIP.*

Prinit Pr, *(Prinit Pr.; 0-932970),* 211 NW Seventh St., Richmond, IN 47374-4051 (SAN 212-680X) Tel 765-966-7130; Fax: 765-966-7131; Toll Free: 800-478-4885
Web site: http://www.printpress.com.

Print Hse (IND) *(81-85453; 81-7533; 81-85880; 81-85009) Dist. by* **St Mut.**

Printed Horse, *(Printed Horse, The; 0-912830),* P.O. Box 1908, Fort Collins, CO 80522 (SAN 210-4377) Tel 970-482-2286.

Printed Page, *See* **Genesis Comns**

Printers Devil, *(Printers' Devil, The; 0-915497),* SCI Dept. of State Embassy, No. DELHI, Washington, DC 20521-9000 (SAN 274-8029).

Prion (GBR) *(1-85375) Dist. by* **Trafalgar.**

Prion Bks, *See* **Service Press**

Priority Consult, *(Priority Consulting, Inc.; 0-9667727),* Div. of Priority Publishing, 125 Creekway Bend, Southlake, TX 76092 Tel 817-975-5244; Fax: 817-656-5510.

Priority Press, *(Priority Pr., Ltd.; 0-9621007),* Orders Addr.: P.O. Box 306, Yardley, PA 19067 (SAN 250-5029) Tel 215-321-9488; Edit Addr.: 2111 Yardley-Morrisville Rd., Yardley, PA 19067 (SAN 250-5037).

Prism Coll, *(Prism Collective; 1-890662),* Orders Addr.: P.O. Box 1042, Webster, NY 14580-7742 Tel 716-872-6657; Fax: 716-787-0314; Toll Free: 800-875-6740; Edit Addr.: 13 Summit Knolls Dr., Webster, NY 14580-2847.

Prism MD, *(Prism Pr.; 0-9665068),* 7839 Ellenham Rd., Baltimore, MD 21204-3545 Tel 410-828-5649; Fax: 410-339-3456 Do not confuse with companies with the same or similar name in Gladwin, MI, New York, NY, Edison, NJ, Houston, TX, Dayton, NJ, Minneapolis, MN, Detroit, MI, Boulder, CO.

Prisma Bks, *(Prisma Bks., Inc.; 0-910235),* 2016 Kenwood Pkwy., Minneapolis, MN 55405 (SAN 241-4384) Tel 612-377-0555.

†Pritchett & Hull, *(Pritchett & Hull Assocs., Inc.; 0-939838),* 3440 Oakcliff Rd., NE, Suite 110, Atlanta, GA 30340 (SAN 216-9258) Tel 770-451-0602; Fax: 770-454-7130; Toll Free: 800-241-4925
Web site: http://www.p-h.com/; *CIP.*

Prk Nicollet, *(Park Nicollet Medical Foundation; 1-884153),* 5000 W. 39th St., Minneapolis, MN 55416 Tel 612-927-3454; Fax: 612-927-3033
Dist(s): **Bookmen Inc** *(Bookmen, Inc.).*

Prncton Gamma-Tech, *(Princeton Gamma-Tech, Inc.; 0-9641455),* Div. of Outokumpu Mintec Group, CN 863, Princeton, NJ 08542-0863 Tel 609-924-7310; Fax: 609-924-1729.

Pro Exam Review, *(Professional Examination Review System; 1-878199),* 1020 Kidder Rd., Carencro, LA 70520 Tel 318-896-4780.

Pro Resource, *(Professional Resource Exchange, Inc.; 0-943158; 1-56887),* P.O. Box 15560, Sarasota, FL 34277-1560 (SAN 241-8290) Tel 941-343-9601; Fax: 941-343-9201; Toll Free: 800-443-3364 (orders only) ; *Imprints:* Prof Resc Pr (Professional Resource Press)
E-mail: editorial@prpress.com; orders@prpress.com; mail@prpress.com
Web site: http://www.prpress.com.

PRO-ACT Pub, *(PRO-ACT Publishing; 1-880610),* Div. of PRO-ACT Continuing Education, 20601 Michale St., Winnetka, CA 91306-1253 (SAN 297-5483) Tel 818-718-1129; Fax: 818-718-1344.

Process Pr (GBR) *(1-899209) Dist. by* **Intl Spec Bk.**

Proctor Pubns, *(Proctor Pubns.; 1-882792; 1-928623),* Div. of Proctor Publications, LLC, Orders Addr.: P.O. Box 2498, Ann Arbor, MI 48106-2498 Tel 734-480-9900; Fax: 734-480-9811; Toll Free: 800-343-3034; Edit Addr.: 1832 Midvale, Ypsilanti, MI 48197
E-mail: DPro153922@aol.com
Web site: http://www.proctorpublications.com
Dist(s): **Baker & Taylor** *(Baker & Taylor Bks.)*
Follett Library *(Follett Library Resources)*
Partners Pubs Grp *(Partners Pubs. Group, Inc.)*
Quality Bks IL *(Quality Bks., Inc.).*

Prodist Imprint of Watson Pub Intl

†Product Pr, *(Productivity Pr.; 0-527; 0-915299; 1-56327),* Orders Addr.: P.O. Box 13390, Portland, OR 97213-0390 (SAN 290-036X) Tel 503-235-0600; Fax: 503-235-0909; Toll Free Fax: 800-394-6286; Toll Free: 800-394-6868 (orders); Edit Addr.: 541 NE 20th Ave., Portland, OR 97232
E-mail: service@productivityinc.com
Web site: http://www.productivityinc.com; *CIP.*

Productivity Inc, *See* **Product Pr**

†PRO-ED, *(PRO-ED, Inc.; 0-88744; 0-89079; 0-933014; 0-936104; 0-944480),* 8700 Shoal Creek Blvd., Austin, TX 78757-6897 (SAN 222-1349) Tel 512-451-3246; Fax: 512-451-8542; Toll Free Fax: 800-397-7633; Toll Free: 800-897-3202
E-mail: info@proedinc.com
Web site: http://www.proedinc.com; *CIP.*

Prof & Tech Pub, *(Professional & Technical Publishing, Inc.; 1-878212),* 370 Seventh Ave., No 316, New York, NY 10001-3900 Tel 212-633-8975.

Prof Audience, *(Professional Audience Communications, Inc.; 0-9662849),* Orders Addr.: P.O. Box 243, Yardley, PA 19067 Tel 215-493-7400; Fax: 215-493-9804; Edit Addr.: 1578 Silo Rd., Yardley, PA 19067
E-mail: dntlpblshr@aol.com.

Prof Bks Future Health, *(Professional Bks./Future Health, Inc.; 0-933478),* Orders Addr.: P.O. Box 3246, Jackson, TN 38301 (SAN 205-3977) Tel 901-660-5027; Fax: 901-660-5029; Edit Addr.: 45 Conrad Dr., No. 100, Jackson, TN 38305 (SAN 662-7374)
Dist(s): **Publishers Group** *(Publishers Group West).*

Prof Comms, *(Professional Communications, Inc.; 0-9632400; 1-884735),* Orders Addr.: P.O. Box 10, Caddo, OK 74729-0010 Tel 580-367-9838; Fax: 580-367-9989; Toll Free: 800-337-9838; Edit Addr.: Rte. 1, Box 251, Caddo, OK 74729 Do not confuse with companies with the same or similar names in Ann Arbor, MI, Madison, WI
E-mail: profcomm@netcommander.com
Web site: http://www.pcibooks.com.

Prof Human Being, *(Professional Human Being Group; 0-9637814),* R.D. 21, Box 117, Dover, PA 17315 Tel 717-843-2215.

Prof Phys Pub, *(Professional Physicians Publishing & Health Services, Inc.; 1-887742),* c/o Myca, Inc., 9639 Hillcroft, No. 117, Houston, TX 77096 Tel 713-772-3277; Fax: 713-774-0482.

Prof Pr NC, *(Professional Pr.; 1-57087; 1-880365),* Orders Addr.: P.O. Box 4371, Chapel Hill, NC 27515-4371 Fax: 919-942-8020; Toll Free: 800-277-8960; Edit Addr.: 314 Warren Way, Chapel Hill, NC 27516 Do not confuse with Professional Pr., New York, NY
E-mail: tag@geldermann.com
Dist(s): **Sunbelt Pubns** *(Sunbelt Pubns., Inc.).*

Prof Preference, *See* **Comprehensive Hlth**

Prof Pride, *(Professional Pride; 1-882960),* 1812 Pease Ave., Sumner, WA 98390 Tel 206-891-9084; Fax: 253-863-3568; Toll Free: 800-830-8228
E-mail: terri@911trainer.com; train911@accessone.com
Web site: http://www.professionalpride.com.

Prof Prnting & Pub, *(Professional Printing & Publishing; 0-929442; 1-877735),* Orders Addr.: P.O. Box 5758, Bossier City, LA 71171-5758 (SAN 248-2177) Tel 318-746-6880; Fax: 318-746-6995; Toll Free: 800-551-8783; Edit Addr.: 601 Barksdale Blvd., Bossier City, LA 71111 (SAN 249-3403)
E-mail: order@ppandp.com
Web site: http://www.pandp.com.

Prof Reports Corp, *See* **PRC Pub**

Prof Resc Pr Imprint of Pro Resource

Prof Resource, *(Professional Resource Pubns.; 0-9639023),* Div. of New Perspectives of Indiana, Inc., Orders Addr.: P.O. Box 501485, Indianapolis, IN 46256 Tel 317-465-9688; Fax: 317-465-9689; Edit Addr.: 6308-B Rucker Rd., Indianapolis, IN 46220.

Professionl NY, *See* **J Striano Bks**

Profile Press, *(Profile Pr.; 0-942267),* 111 Cloister Ct., Chapel Hill, NC 27515-4054 (SAN 667-0172) Tel 919-967-9400; Fax: 919-408-0643; Toll Free: 800-390-2638 Do not confuse with Profile Pr., Arlington, VA
E-mail: profiler@intrex.net
Web site: http://www.drivers.com/pol.

Prog Human Environ, *(Program for the Human Environment; 0-9646419),* Div. of Rockefeller Univ., 1230 York Ave., New York, NY 10021-6399 Tel 212-327-7917; Fax: 212-327-7519.

†**Prog Studies,** *(Programmed Studies, Inc.; 0-917194),* 6 Top Gallant Cir., Savannah, GA 31411 (SAN 207-7434) Tel 912-598-9220
E-mail: affiliatesignnalpha@aol.com; *CIP.*

Prog Wellness Res, *(Program for Wellness Restoration; 0-9662231),* 1112 Jackson Blvd., Houston, TX 77006 Tel 713-520-6630; Fax: 713-526-5883; Toll Free: 800-350-2392 Do not confuse with Millennium Publishing Co., MacLean, VA
E-mail: powertx@aol.com
Web site: http://www.medibolics.com.

Proj Renaissance, *(Project Renaissance; 0-931865),* P.O. Box 332, Gaithersburg, MD 20884-0332 (SAN 686-0567) Tel 301-948-1122; Fax: 301-977-4712
E-mail: win@thebestweb.com
Web site: http://www.winwenger.com.

Project Advent, *(Project Adventure, Inc.; 0-934387),* 701 Cabot St., Beverly, MA 01915 (SAN 693-8078) Tel 978-524-4500; Fax: 978-524-4501
E-mail: sdresser@pa.org
Web site: http://www.pa.org.

Project Impact, *(Project Impact Government Training Service; 0-9622478),* Div. of State of Minnesota, 480 Cedar St., No. 401, Saint Paul, MN 55101-2240 Tel 612-222-7409; Fax: 612-223-5307.

Promethean Pr, *(Promethean Pr.; 0-916859),* P.O. Box 6827, Ithaca, NY 14851 (SAN 654-2468) Tel 607-257-3278.

†**Prometheus Bks,** *(Prometheus Bks., Pubs.; 0-87975; 1-57392; 1-59102),* 59 John Glenn Dr., Amherst, NY 14228-2197 (SAN 202-0289) Tel 716-691-0133; Fax: 716-691-0137; Toll Free: 800-421-0351 ; *Imprints:* Humanity Bks (Humanity Books)
E-mail: mhall@prometheusmail.com
Web site: http://www.prometheusbooks.com; *CIP.*

Prometheus Pubg, *(Prometheus Publishing, Inc.; 0-9660427),* 950 E. Broad St., Columbus, OH 43205 Tel 614-258-8000; Fax: 614-258-8900; Toll Free: 800-607-9006
E-mail: prome@infinet.com.

Prominnt Pr, *(Prominent Pr.; 0-9668997),* Div. of KVP Communications, Inc., 6828 E. Thunderbird Rd., Scottsdale, AZ 85254 Tel 602-951-4331; Fax: 602-607-7912
E-mail: kamshel@aol.com.

Pronet Pr, *(Pronet Pr.; 0-9638856),* Orders Addr.: P.O. Box 486, Naperville, IL 60560; Edit Addr.: 2100 Manchester Rd., No. 900, Wheaton, IL 60187 Tel 708-653-5588.

Prosperity & Profits, *(Prosperity & Profits Unlimited, Distribution Services),* P.O. Box 416, Denver, CO 80201-0416 (SAN 200-4682) Tel 303-575-5676; Fax: 970-292-2136 ; *Imprints:* Lamp Light Pr (Lamp Light Press)
E-mail: mail@breadpudding.net; mail@contentprovidermedia.com.

Prostate Cancer, *See* **Seneca Hse**

Proste Cancer, *(Prostate Cancer Resource Network, Inc.; 0-9651827),* Orders Addr.: 2803 Fruitville Rd., Sarasota, FL 34237 Tel 941-365-5599; Fax: 941-955-5828; Toll Free: 800-915-1001
Web site: http://www.pcrn.org.

Prosveta USA, *(Prosveta, U.S.A.; 0-911857),* P.O. Box 1176, New Smyrna Beach, FL 32170-1176 (SAN 264-3235) Tel 904-428-1465 (phone/fax)
E-mail: Info@prosveta.com
Web site: http://www.prosveta-usa.com.

Protex Pr, *(Protex Pr.; 0-9714503),* 11645 Wilshire Blvd., No. 120, Los Angeles, CA 90025 Tel 310-231-7000; Fax: 310-231-7227 Do not confuse with Darrow Publishing in Lancaster, PA
E-mail: lawdoc@marcdarrow.com
Web site: http://www.jointrehab.com.

Providence Hse, *(Providence Hse. Pubs.; 1-57736; 1-881576),* 238 Seaboard Ln., Franklin, TN 37067 Tel 615-771-2020; Fax: 615-771-2002; Toll Free: 800-321-5692 ; *Imprints:* Hillsboro Pr (Hillsboro Press)
E-mail: books@providencehouse.com
Web site: http://www.providencehouse.com.

Provideo Ent, *(Provideo Entertainment Corp.; 0-945744),* P.O. Box 7846, Eugene, OR 97401-0032 (SAN 247-6630).

PRP NY, *(Princeton Review Publishing Corp.; 0-375; 0-679; 1-884536),* Div. of Random House Information Group, Orders Addr.: 400 Hahn Rd., Westminster, MD 21157 Tel 410-848-1900; Toll Free: 800-726-0600; Edit Addr.: 2315 Broadway, New York, NY 10024 Tel 212-874-8282; Fax: 212-874-0775; Toll Free: 800-273-8439
Web site: http://www.review.com
Dist(s): **Random** *(Random Hse., Inc.).*

PRR, *(PRR, Inc.; 0-9641823; 1-891483),* 48 S. Service Rd., Suite 310, Melville, NY 11747 Tel 631-777-3800; Fax: 631-777-3952; Toll Free: 800-777-0965
E-mail: linda@cancernetwork.com
Web site: http://www.cancernetwork.com.

Prsnl Footprint, *(Personal Footprint Pubns.; 0-9627591),* 3704 Hampton Brook Dr., Hamburg, NY 14075 Tel 716-649-3004.

Prsnl Pathways, *(Personal Pathways Pr.; 0-929841),* 4015 Falls Ridge Dr., Alpharetta, GA 30022 (SAN 250-4391) Tel 770-410-1140; Fax: 770-410-0698
Dist(s): **Baker & Taylor** *(Baker & Taylor Bks.)*
New Leaf Dist *(New Leaf Distributing Co., Inc.).*

Prtlnd Habilitat, *(Portland Habilitation Ctr., Inc.; 0-9635238),* 5312 NE 148th Ave., Portland, OR 97230-3438 Tel 503-261-1266; Fax: 503-256-8665; Toll Free: 800-874-7917.

†**PS Assocs Croton,** *(Policy Studies Assocs.; 0-936826),* P.O. Box 337, Croton-on-Hudson, NY 10520 (SAN 214-4417) Tel 914-271-6500; Toll Free: 800-316-2739
E-mail: cipany@igc.apc.org
Web site: http://www.cipa-apex.org; *CIP.*

PSGA, *(Parkinson Support Groups of America; 0-945520),* 11376 Cherry Hill Rd., No 204, Beltsville, MD 20705 (SAN 247-1965) Tel 301-937-1545.

PSI & Assocs, *(PSI & Assocs.; 0-938261; 1-55993),* 9745 SW 125th Terr., Miami, FL 33176-4941 (SAN 659-834X) Tel 305-255-7959.

PSI Pr PA, *(PSI Pr.; 0-9625500),* 1025 Miller Ln., Harrisburg, PA 17110-2899 Tel 717-236-0080
E-mail: psinet@voicenet.com
Dist(s): **Baker & Taylor** *(Baker & Taylor Bks.)*
Bookpeople *(Bookpeople)*
New Leaf Dist *(New Leaf Distributing Co., Inc.).*

PSM Imprint of Gale

PSRF Pub, *(PSRF Publishing; 0-9618734),* P.O. Box 23220, San Diego, CA 92193 (SAN 668-7644) Tel 760-751-8841.

Psych & Consul Assocs, *(Psychology & Consulting Assocs. Pr.; 0-930626),* c/o Jesse Thomas, 2740 First Ave., San Diego, CA 92103 (SAN 211-3856) Tel 619-233-4562; Fax: 760-568-4060.

†**Psych Assess,** *(Psychological Assessment Resources, Inc.; 0-911907),* Orders Addr.: P.O. Box 998, Odessa, FL 33556 (SAN 665-8199); Edit Addr.: 16204 N. Florida Ave., Lutz, FL 33549 (SAN 264-6897) Tel 813-968-3003; Fax: 813-968-2598; Toll Free: 800-331-8378
E-mail: custserv@parinc.com; nfazioli@parinc.com
Web site: http://www.parinc.com
Dist(s): **JIST Pubng** *(JIST Publishing)*
Psychol Corp *(Psychological Corp., The); CIP.*

Psych Bks, *(Psychiatric Bks.; 0-9615865),* Orders Addr.: P.O. Box 10578, Rockville, MD 20850; Edit Addr.: 13305 Cleveland Dr., Rockville, MD 20850 (SAN 696-6233) Tel 301-762-0334.

†**Psych Dimensions,** *(Psychological Dimensions, Inc.; 0-88437),* 301 E. 87th St., Suite 21A, New York, NY 10128 (SAN 204-3866) Tel 212-289-5158; *CIP.*

Psych Qtly, *(Psychoanalytic Quarterly, Inc.; 0-911194),* 175 Fifth Ave., New York, NY 10010 (SAN 205-4043) Tel 212-982-9358.

Psyche Pr NY, *(Psyche Pr.; 0-9622885; 1-885809),* 517 Amsterdam Ave., New York, NY 10024 Tel 212-721-4466.

Psychegenics, *See* **Proj Renaissance**

Psychgy Srce, *(Psychology Source Consultants; 0-9703594),* P.O. Box 1083, Collins, MS 39428
E-mail: phdpsych@aol.com
Web site: http://psychologysourceconsultants.safeshopper.com.

Psychic Bks, *(Psychic Bks.; 0-930984),* 9711 Shamrock Ln., Lakeside, CA 92040-3010 (SAN 219-2586) Tel 619-561-9361.

Psychogenic Disease, *(Psychogenic Disease Publishing Co.; 0-87312),* 3571 Sudbury Rd., Cameron Park, CA 95682-8205 (SAN 203-4239).

Psychol Conslt Pub, *See* **Diagnostic Solns**

Psychol Educ Pubns, *(Psychological & Educational Pubns., Inc.; 0-931421),* P.O. Box 520, Hydesville, CA 95547-0520 (SAN 683-5422) Tel 415-340-9669; Fax: 800-447-0907; Toll Free: 800-523-5775.

Psychol Pr (GBR) *(0-86377; 1-84169) Dist. by* **Taylor & Francis.**

Psychology Pr, *(Psychology Pr.; 0-9627232; 1-885580),* P.O. Box 328, Brandon, VT 05733-0328 Tel 802-247-8312; Toll Free: 800-639-4122 (orders only)
E-mail: csj@great-ideas.org; info@great-ideas.org
Web site: http://www.great-ideas.org.

Psychometric, *(Psychometric Affiliates; 0-9606044),* P.O. Box 807, Murfreesboro, TN 37133-0807 (SAN 203-1205) Tel 615-890-6296 (phone/fax).

Psychosocial Imprint of Intl Univs Pr

Psychosynth Pr, *(Psychosynthesis Pr.; 0-9611444),* Orders Addr.: P.O. Box 1602, Bayfield, CO 81122 (SAN 283-1589) Tel 970-884-7590
E-mail: psychosynthesis@ecoliteracyproject.org
Web site: http://www.ecoliteracyproject.org.

PsychStat, *(PsychStat; 0-9631763),* 2605 Goldfinch Dr., Cedar Park, TX 78613-5113 Tel 512-257-8600.

Pts of Light Distributing, *(Points of Light Distributing; 0-910315),* P.O. Box 10, Port Angeles, WA 98362 (SAN 241-4872) Tel 360-928-2139.

PTS Pubng, *(PTS Publishing Co.; 0-9639841),* Div. of Parkview Therapy Services, Inc., 1 Bethany Rd., Bldg. 6, Suite 81, Hazlet, NJ 07730 Tel 732-888-4880; Fax: 732-739-0071.

Pub Citizen, *(Public Citizen; 0-937188; 1-58231),* 1600 20th St., NW, Washington, DC 20009 (SAN 239-4774) Tel 202-588-1000; Fax: 202-588-7798
E-mail: slittle@citizen.org
Web site: http://www.citizen.org.

Pub Media Ctr, *(Public Media Ctr.; 0-915287),* 466 Green St., San Francisco, CA 94133 (SAN 290-0378) Tel 415-434-1403; Fax: 415-986-6779.

Pub Mgmt Assoc, *See* **R E Fellows**

Pub Partners, *(Publication Partners, Inc.; 0-923944),* P.O. Box 21216, Saint Paul, MN 55121-0216 (SAN 252-1512).

Pub Strategy, *(Public Strategy Co.; 0-9635808),* 2000 Huntington Bldg., Cleveland, OH 44115 Tel 216-696-4700; Fax: 216-696-6569.

Public Agenda, *(Public Agenda; 1-889483),* 6 E. 39th St., 9th Flr., New York, NY 10016-0112 Tel 212-686-6610; Fax: 212-889-3461
E-mail: info@publicagenda.org; paresearch@aol.com
Web site: http://www.publicagenda.org.

Public Statistics, *(Public Statistics Institute; 0-9651259),* 4521 Campus Dr., Suite 130, Irvine, CA 92612 Tel 714-640-2171; Fax: 714-640-0332.

PublicAffairs NY, *(PublicAffairs, LLC; 1-891620; 1-58648),* A Member of Perseus Books Group, 250 W. 57th St., Suite 1321, New York, NY 10107 Tel 212-397-6666; Fax: 212-397-4277; Toll Free: 877-782-1234
E-mail: westview.orders@perseusbooks.com; pubaff@interport.net
Web site: http://www.publicaffairsbooks.com
Dist(s): **HarperCollins Pubs** *(HarperCollins Pubs.).*

Publicare Pr, *See* **Prof Prnting & Pub**

Publishers Consult, *(Publishers Consultants; 0-88310),* Box 1908, Fort Collins, CO 80522 (SAN 203-2449) Tel 970-482-2286.

†**Publitec,** *(Publitec Editions; 0-913581),* 1762 Glenneyre St., Laguna Beach, CA 92651-3222 (SAN 285-3663) Tel 949-497-6100 (phone/fax)
E-mail: mmrowe@worldnet.att.net
Dist(s): **Distributors** *(Distributors, The)*
New Leaf Dist *(New Leaf Distributing Co., Inc.)*
Quality Bks IL *(Quality Bks., Inc.)*
Unique Bks Inc *(Unique Bks., Inc.); CIP.*

Pubns Chldrn, *(Pubns. for Children's Healing; 0-9678523),* Orders Addr.: P.O. Box 240, Devon, PA 19333 Tel 610-964-1697; Fax: 610-964-8013; Edit Addr.: 193 Church Rd., Devon, PA 19333
Web site: http://www.healingyourchild.com.

Pubns for Achieving, *(Publications for Achieving Total Health; 0-9638869),* Div. of Total Health Nutrients, Inc., 664 Rte. 518, Skillman, NJ 08558-2508 Tel 609-921-1842; Fax: 609-921-6092.

Pubns Intl Ltd, *(Publications International, Ltd.; 0-7853; 0-88176; 1-56173),* 7373 N. Cicero Ave., Lincolnwood, IL 60646 (SAN 263-9823) Tel 847-676-3470; Fax: 847-676-3671; Toll Free: 800-745-9299
Web site: http://www.consumerguide.com
Dist(s): **Pan Amer Pub** *(Pan American Publishing, Inc.)*
Penguin Putnam *(Penguin Putnam, Inc.)*
Pubs Clearing Hse *(Publishers Clearing Hse.).*

Pubns Puertorriquenas, *(Publicaciones Puertorriquenas, Inc.; 0-929441; 1-881713; 1-881720),* Calle Mayaguez, No. 104, Hato Rey, 00919 (SAN 249-4272) Tel 787-759-9673; Fax: 787-250-6498
E-mail: pubpr@tld.net
Web site: http://www.tld.net/users/pubpr/2/.

Pubs Pr UT, *(Publishers Pr.; 0-916095),* 1900 W. 2300, S., Salt Lake City, UT 84119 (SAN 219-3884) Tel 801-972-6600 Do not confuse with Publishers Pr., Portland, OR.

PuffinBks Imprint of Viking Penguin

Puget Snd, *(Puget Sound Pub.; 0-9653591),* 10408 SW 268th St., Vashon, WA 98070 Tel 206-463-5965.

Puget Sound, *(Puget Sound Pr.; 0-9660092; 1-930809),* 6523 California Ave., SW, PMB 292, Seattle, WA 98136-1833 Tel 206-768-9432 (phone/fax)
E-mail: psp@pugetsoundpress.com
Web site: http://www.pugetsoundpress.com
Dist(s): **Baker & Taylor** *(Baker & Taylor Bks.)*
Partners-West *(Partners/West)*
Quality Bks IL *(Quality Bks., Inc.).*

PUP Bks Imprint of Potential Unltd

†**Purdue U Pr,** *(Purdue Univ. Pr.; 0-911198; 1-55753; 90-74134),* Orders Addr.: P.O. Box 388, Ashland, OH 44805; Edit Addr.: 1207 SCC-E, West Lafayette, IN 47907-1207 (SAN 203-4026) Tel 765-494-2038; Fax: 765-496-2442 ; *Imprints:* NotaBell (NotaBell) Do not confuse with Purdue Univ. Pubns., same address
E-mail: libpup@omni.cc.purdue.edu
Web site: http://www.thepress.purdue.edu/; *CIP.*

Purdue U Pubns, *(Purdue Univ., Office of Pubns.; 0-931682),* South Campus Cts., Bldg. D, West Lafayette, IN 47907 (SAN 215-2649) Tel 765-494-2040; Fax: 765-494-0793 Do not confuse with Purdue Univ. Pr., same address.
E-mail: mchunt@purdue.edu
Web site: http://www.directory.purdue.edu/.

Push the Envelope, *(Pushing the Envelope Pubns.; 0-9649938),* 1278 Glenneyre St., No. 313, Laguna Beach, CA 92651-3103 (SAN 298-895X) Fax: 714-497-1498
E-mail: pushenpub@aol.com
Web site: http://www.Korpi.com/Dying101/.

Pussywillow Pub, *(Pussywillow Publishing Hse.; 0-934739),* 621 Leisure World, Mesa, AZ 85206-3153 (SAN 694-1702) Tel 480-641-9049; Fax: 480-854-1222
Dist(s): **Baker & Taylor** *(Baker & Taylor Bks.).*

†**Putnam Pub Group,** *(Putnam Publishing Group, The; 0-399; 0-698; 0-89828),* Div. of Penguin Putnam, Inc., Orders Addr.: 405 Murray Hill Pkwy., East Rutherford, NJ 07073-2136 Toll Free Fax: 800-227-9604; Toll Free: 800-788-6262 (individual consumer sales); 800-631-8571 (reseller customer service); 800-526-0275 (reseller sales); Edit Addr.: 375 Hudson St., New York, NY 10014 (SAN 202-5531) Tel 212-366-2000; Fax: 212-366-2643 ; *Imprints:* Riverhead Books (Riverhead Books (Hardcovers)) Tarcher Putnam (Tarcher/Putnam) Avery (Avery)
E-mail: online@penguinputnam.com
Web site: http://www.penguinputnam.com
Dist(s): **Continental Bk** *(Continental Bk. Co., Inc.)*
Hastings Bks *(Hastings Bks.)*
Lectorum Pubns *(Lectorum Pubns., Inc.)*
Lndmrk Audiobks *(Landmark Audiobooks)*
Penguin Putnam *(Penguin Putnam, Inc.)*
Rounder Kids Mus Dist *(Rounder Kids Music Distribution)*
Shens Bks *(Shen's Bks.)*
T T Beeler *(Beeler, Thomas T. Publisher); CIP.*

P-W Perspect, *(Prader-Willi Perspectives; 0-9646533),* Div. of Visible Ink Public Relations, 40 Holly Ln., Roslyn Heights, NY 11577 Tel 516-621-2445; Fax: 516-484-7154; Toll Free: 800-358-0682.

PWJ Pubg, *(PWJ Publishing; 0-939221),* Orders Addr.: P.O. Box 238, Tehama, CA 96090 (SAN 662-670X) Tel 530-384-1341; Edit Addr.: 8619 Sherwood Blvd., Los Molinos, CA 96055 (SAN 662-6718)
E-mail: pwj@tco.net.

†**PWS Pubs,** *(PWS Pubs.; 0-534; 0-87150; 0-87872),* Div. of International Thomson Publishing Education Group, Orders Addr.: 7625 Empire Dr., Florence, KY 41042-2978 (SAN 200-2663) Tel 859-525-2230; Toll Free: 800-354-9706
Dist(s): **Thomson Learn** *(Thomson Learning); CIP.*

PWS-KENT Pub, *See* **PWS Pubs**

Pyramid Educ Inc, *(Pyramid Education, Inc.; 1-881242),* 186 S. Belvedere Blvd., Memphis, TN 38104 Tel 901-725-4940.

Pyramid Pub TN, *See* **Pyramid Educ Inc**

Pyrczak Pub, *(Pyrczak Publishing; 0-9623744; 1-884585),* P.O. Box 39731, Los Angeles, CA 90039 Tel 323-660-7600; Fax: 818-246-1277
E-mail: pyrpublish@hotmail.com.

Q Pr (CAN) *(1-895564) Dist. by* **Stackpole.**

Q Pubng VA, *(Q Publishing LLC; 0-9665228; 1-931169),* 2226 Maple St., Virginia Beach, VA 23451 Tel 757-481-5210; Fax: 757-481-3448; Toll Free: 888-311-5210.

Q S O V, *(QSOV; 0-9669830),* 5431 S. Shawnee Dr., Sierra Vista, AZ 85650 Tel 520-803-0586; Fax: 520-803-0729
E-mail: ancient@compuserve.com.

QED Ft Bragg, *(QED Pr.; 0-936609),* 155 Cypress St., Fort Bragg, CA 95437 (SAN 248-966X) Tel 707-964-9520; Fax: 707-964-7531; Toll Free: 800-773-7782
E-mail: qedpress@mcn.org
Web site: http://www.cypresshouse.com/catalog.html
Dist(s): **Baker & Taylor** *(Baker & Taylor Bks.)*
Bookpeople *(Bookpeople)*
Quality Bks IL *(Quality Bks., Inc.)*
Unique Bks Inc *(Unique Bks., Inc.).*

QMP Imprint of Quality Med Pub

QPC (JPN) *(4-87417) Dist. by* **Quint Pub Co.**

QRP Bks Imprint of Quail Ridge

Quadrangle Res, *(Quadrangle Research, Inc.; 0-9637094),* Orders Addr.: P.O. Box 12873, Research Triangle Park, NC 27709 Tel 919-489-9588; Edit Addr.: 17 Running Brook Ct., Durham, NC 27713-9497.

Quail Prods, *(Quail Productions; 0-9610764),* Orders Addr.: P.O. Box 322, Livingston, NJ 07039 (SAN 264-6323) Tel 973-992-5865; Edit Addr.: 37 Belmont Dr., Livingston, NJ 07039 (SAN 264-6331).

Quail Ridge, *(Quail Ridge Pr., Inc.; 0-937552; 1-893062),* Orders Addr.: P.O. Box 123, Brandon, MS 39043 (SAN 214-2201) Tel 601-825-2063; Fax: 601-825-3091; Toll Free: 800-343-1583 ; *Imprints:* QRP Bks (Q R P Books)
E-mail: agoode@quailridge.com
Web site: http://www.quailridge.com
Dist(s): **Bright Horizons Specialty Distributors Inc** *(Bright Horizons Specialty Distributors, Inc.)*
D Gibson *(Gibson, Dot Pubns.)*
Forest Sales & Dist *(Forest Sales & Distributing Co.)*
Herveys Bklink *(Hervey's Booklink & Cookbook Warehouse)*
Partners Pubs Grp *(Partners Pubs. Group, Inc.)*
Southwest Cookbk *(Southwest Cookbook Distributors).*

Quail Valley, *(Quail Valley Pubns.; 0-934249),* 19234 Vanowen St., Reseda, CA 91335 (SAN 693-1944) Tel 818-705-1157.

Qual Cont Systs Srvs, *(Quality Control Systems & Services; 1-881006),* P.O. Box 3411, San Clemente, CA 92674 Tel 949-388-7686; Fax: 949-388-7696
E-mail: qcss@qcss.com
Web site: http://www.qcss.com/
Dist(s): **Baker & Taylor** *(Baker & Taylor Bks.)*
Coutts Library Service Inc *(Coutts Library Service, Inc.).*

Quality Med Pub, *(Quality Medical Publishing, Inc.; 0-942219; 1-57626),* 11970 Borman Dr., Suite 222, Saint Louis, MO 63146-4137 (SAN 666-8755) Tel 314-878-7808; Fax: 314-878-9937; Toll Free: 800-423-6865; 800-348-7808 (customer service) ; *Imprints:* QMP (QMP)
E-mail: qmp@qmp.com
Web site: http://www.qmp.com
Dist(s): **Lppncott W & W** *(Lippincott Williams & Wilkins)*
Majors Scientific Bks Inc *(Majors Scientific Bks., Inc.)*
Matthews Medical Bk Co *(Matthews Medical Bk. Co.)*
Rittenhouse *(Rittenhouse Bk. Distributors).*

Quality Metric, *(Quality Metric, Inc.; 1-891810),* 640 George Washington Hwy., Suite 201, Lincoln, RI 02865 Tel 401-334-8800; Fax: 401-334-8801
Web site: http://www.qmetric.com.

QualityCare Pub Imprint of Convalescnt Cnslts

Quantum Bks, *(Quantum Bks.; 0-912845),* 6 Knoll Ln., Suite D, Mill Valley, CA 94941 (SAN 283-1449) Tel 415-388-1006; Fax: 415-388-2257
Dist(s): **Assoc Pubs Grp** *(Associated Pubs. Group).*

Quantum Hlth Pr, *(Quantum Health Pr., LLC; 0-9678443),* Orders Addr.: P.O. Box 1637, Fairfield, CT 06432 Tel 203-396-0342; Fax: 203-372-5773; Toll Free: 888-277-1328; Edit Addr.: 85 Meadowcrest Dr., Fairfield, CT 06432-1312
E-mail: QHPress@yahoo.com.

Quantum Inst Inc, *(Quantum Institute, Inc.; 0-9670362),* 101 Grand Ave., Suite 11, Capiola, CA 95010 Tel 831-464-0564; Fax: 831-479-8233
Dist(s): **Words Distrib** *(Words Distributing Co.).*

Quarry Pr (CAN) *(0-919627; 1-55082) Dist. by* **SCB Distributors.**

†**Quarterdeck,** *(Quarterdeck Pr.; 0-918546),* Affil. of Yoga Transformations, 2336 Ross Ln., Medford, OR 97501 (SAN 209-990X) Tel 541-770-6035; Fax: 541-734-2389; *CIP.*

Quarterman, *(Quarterman Pubns., Inc.; 0-88000),* P.O. Box 156, Lincoln, MA 01773 (SAN 203-3992) Tel 617-259-8047.

Que, *(Que; 0-7897; 0-88022; 1-56529),* Div. of Macmillan USA, 201 W. 103rd St., Indianapolis, IN 46290-1094 (SAN 219-6298) Tel 317-581-3500; Toll Free: 800-428-5331 (orders); 800-858-7674 (customer service) ; *Imprints:* Ziff-Davis Pr (Ziff-Davis Press) Do not confuse with Que Software, also a division of Macmillan Computer Publishing, same address
E-mail: customerservice@macmillanUSA.com
Web site: http://www.mcp.com/que
Dist(s): **Mac USA** *(Macmillan USA)*
Sams Tech Pub *(Sams Technical Publishing).*

Queen Co Hlth Comns, *See* **Inst for Health Real**

Queenship Pub, *(Queenship Publishing Co.; 1-57918; 1-882972),* Orders Addr.: P.O. Box 220, Goleta, CA 93116 Tel 805-692-0043; Fax: 805-967-5843; Toll Free: 800-647-9882
E-mail: qship@impulse.net
Web site: http://www.queenship.org
Dist(s): **Spring Arbor Dist** *(Spring Arbor Distributors Inc.).*

Quest Imprint of Theos Pub Hse

Questar Pubs, *See* **Multnomah Pubs**

Questover Bks, *(Questover Bks.; 0-9663653),* Orders Addr.: P.O. Box 933, Epping, NH 03042 Tel 603-679-2432 (phone/fax); Edit Addr.: 225 Old Nottingham Rd., Epping, NH 03042
E-mail: QuestDCL@aol.com
Web site: http://www.questover.com.

Quick Am Pub, *(Quick American Publishing Co.; 0-932551),* Div. of Quick Trading Co., Orders Addr.: 1635 E. 22nd St., Oakland, CA 94606-4047 (SAN 687-4843) Tel 510-533-0605; Fax: 510-535-0437
E-mail: qtc@quicktrading.com
Web site: http://www.quicktrading.com
Dist(s): **Bookpeople** *(Bookpeople)*
Last Gasp *(Last Gasp Eco-Funnies, Inc.)*
Publishers Group *(Publishers Group West).*

Quicksilv Pr, *(Quicksilver Pr.; 0-9643870),* Div. of Morning Glory Pr., 211 W. 92nd St., Suite 71, New York, NY 10025 Tel 212-874-6526; Fax: 212-579-3224; Toll Free: 800-423-6722 Do not confuse with companies with the same name in San Francisco, CA, Foothill Ranch, CA.

QuickSource Pr, *(QuickSource Pr.; 1-886515),* Div. of Benjamin Projects Network, Inc., 10 Pelham Ave., Nanuet, NY 10954-3428 (SAN 298-5314) Tel 914-627-6511; Fax: 914-627-6512; Toll Free: 800-576-4342.

Quiet Lion Pr, *(Quiet Lion Pr.; 1-882550),* 7215 SW LaView Dr., Portland, OR 97219 Tel 503-771-1907 ; *Imprints:* Omni Pr (Omni Press)
E-mail: quietlion@mindspring.com
Dist(s): **SPD-Small Pr Dist** *(SPD-Small Pr. Distribution).*

Quil Imprint of HarperTrade

Quill Pubns GA, *(Quill Pubns. GA; 0-932281),* Orders Addr.: P.O. Box 8193, Columbus, GA 31908 (SAN 686-6123) Tel 706-323-9313; Edit Addr.: 3908 Hamilton Rd., Columbus, GA 31904.

†Quint Pub Co, *(Quintessence Publishing Co., Inc.; 0-86715; 0-931386; 1-85097; 1-883695),* 551 Kimberly Dr., Carol Stream, IL 60188 (SAN 215-9783) Tel 630-682-3223; Fax: 630-682-3288; Toll Free: 800-621-0387
E-mail: service@quintbook.com
Web site: http://www.quintpub.com
Dist(s): **IPG Chicago** *(Independent Pubs. Group); CIP.*

Quintessenz Verlags (DEU) *(3-87652; 3-8148) Dist. by* **Quint Pub Co.**

Quintin Pub RI, *(Quintin Pubns.; 1-58211; 1-886560),* 22 Delta Dr., Pawtucket, RI 02860-4555 Tel 401-723-6797; Fax: 401-726-0327; Toll Free: 800-747-6687
E-mail: sales@quintinpublications.com; bobquint@aol.com
Web site: http://www.quintinpublications.com.

Quit Smart, *(Quit Smart Stop Smoking Resources, Inc.; 0-9614881; 1-880781),* Orders Addr.: P.O. Box 99016, Durham, NC 27708 (SAN 693-1227) Tel 919-644-0736; Toll Free: 888-737-6278; Edit Addr.: 4614 Arrowhead Trail, Hillsborough, NC 27278
E-mail: shipley@mindspring.com
Web site: http://www.QuitSmart.com
Dist(s): **New Leaf Dist** *(New Leaf Distributing Co., Inc.).*

Quixote Pr IA, *(Quixote Pr.; 1-57166; 1-878488),* 1854 345th Ave., Wever, IA 52658-9597 Tel 319-372-7480; Fax: 319-372-7485; Toll Free: 800-571-2665 Do not confuse with Quixote Pr., Houston, TX
E-mail: heartsntummies@hotmail.com
Dist(s): **Badger Periodicals Distributors** *(Badger Periodicals Distributors)*
Bookmen Inc *(Bookmen, Inc.).*

Quorum Bks Imprint of Greenwood

Quotidian, *(Quotidian, Inc.; 0-934391),* HC 68 Box 16, Cushing, ME 04563-9502 (SAN 693-8094).

R & D, *(R&D Laboratories, Inc.; 0-9670439),* 4640 Admiralty Way Suite 710, Marina del Rey, CA 90292 Tel 310-305-8053; Fax: 310-305-8103.

R A Hasan, *(Hasan, Rashed A. & Michael D. Pappas; 0-9704158),* P.O. Box 99148, Troy, MI 48099-9914 Tel 248-417-3890; Fax: 419-251-5330
E-mail: rashedh48@hotmail.com
Web site: http://www.mdmeetingguide.com.

R A McCaffrey, *(McCaffrey, Roger A. Publishing; 0-9661325; 0-9717721),* Orders Addr.: P.O. Box 1209, Ridgefield, CT 06877 Tel 970-490-2735
Dist(s): **Roman Cath Bks** *(Roman Catholic Bks.).*

R A Moss, *(Moss, Robert A.; 0-9638848),* P.O. Box 591, Travelers Rest, SC 29690 Tel 864-292-2242; Fax: 864-834-9402
E-mail: duffy4562@aol.com
Web site: http://www.emotionalrestructuring.com.

R A Rapaport, *(Rapaport, R.A. Publishing, Inc.; 0-9631701),* 150 W. 22nd St., New York, NY 10011 Tel 212-989-0200; Fax: 212-989-4786; Toll Free: 800-366-3303 (book orders)
E-mail: staff@diabetes-self-mgmt.com
Web site: http://www.diabetes-self-mgmt.com.

R Altschuler, *(Altschuler, Richard & Assocs., Inc.; 1-884092),* 100 W. 57th St., No. 2M, New York, NY 10019 (SAN 299-2949) Tel 212-397-7233; Fax: 212-397-6090
E-mail: icra@aol.com
Web site: http://www.richardaltschuler.com
Dist(s): **U of Nebr Pr** *(Univ. of Nebraska Pr.).*

R B Collier Pleneurethics, *(Collier, Richard Bangs Pleneurethics Society; 1-882152),* 5900 S. 12th, Tacoma, WA 98465 Tel 206-566-5100.

†R B Luce, *(Luce, Robert B. Pubs.; 0-88331),* Div. of Renaisance Book Services Corp., 2490 Black Rock Tpke., Fairfield, CT 06432 Tel 203-372-0300; Fax: 203-374-4766; Toll Free: 800-786-5427
E-mail: info@aslanpublishing.com
Web site: http://www.aslanpublishing.com; *CIP.*

R Barfield, *See* **Lilac Pub**

R Benedet, *See* **Benedet Pbng**

R Bridges Enter, *(Bridges, Roy G. Enterprises; 0-9666974),* P.O. Box 17102, Indianapolis, IN 46217-0102 Tel 317-784-7266; Fax: 317-788-9986
E-mail: royb@iquest.net.

R Colbert, *(Colbert, Roman; 0-9630253),* 2808 Castle Bar Dr., Las Vegas, NV 89134-8915 Tel 702-255-8005.

R Conklin, *See* **CliffTop**

R D Anderson, *See* **Andrsn Cont Educ**

R D Reed Pubs, *(Reed, Robert D. Pubs.; 1-885003; 1-931741),* 750 La Playa St., Suite 647, San Francisco, CA 94121-3262 Tel 650-994-6570; Fax: 650-994-6579; Toll Free: 800-774-7336
E-mail: 4bobreed@msn.com
Web site: http://www.rdrpublishers.com
Dist(s): **Midpt Trade** *(Midpoint Trade Bks., Inc.).*

R Dean Pr, *(Robbie Dean Pr.; 0-9630608; 1-889743),* 2910 E. Eisenhower Pkwy., Ann Arbor, MI 48108 Tel 313-973-9511; Fax: 313-973-9475
E-mail: fairyha@aol.com.

R E Fellows, *(Fellows, RE Publishing; 0-939968),* 2014 Siegle Dr., Lemon Grove, CA 91945 (SAN 216-8537) Tel 619-465-3841.

R F Gottier, *(Gottier, Richard F.; 0-9625671),* Orders Addr.: P.O. Box 737, Kitty Hawk, NC 27949; Edit Addr.: 16 Mallard Dr., Kitty Hawk, NC 27949 Tel 919-261-3517.

R F Quinn, *(Quinn, R.F. Publishing Co.; 0-9632839; 0-9653346),* Orders Addr.: P.O. Box 2786, Carlsbad, CA 92018-2786 Tel 760-720-4764; Fax: 760-720-9111; Toll Free: 800-283-3998; Edit Addr.: 2725 Jefferson St, Suite 2B, Carlsbad, CA 92008
E-mail: rfqmpls@aol.com
Web site: http://www.ldirect.com/quinn
Dist(s): **Baker & Taylor** *(Baker & Taylor Bks.)*
Bookazine Co Inc *(Bookazine Co., Inc.)*
Bookmen Inc *(Bookmen, Inc.)*
New Leaf Dist *(New Leaf Distributing Co., Inc.)*
Nutri-Books Corp *(Nutri-Bks. Corp.)*
Royal Pubns Inc *(Royal Pubns., Inc.)*
Tree Life NE *(Tree of Life Northeast Distributors)*
Tree of Life Midwest *(Tree of Life Midwest).*

R G Landes, *See* **Landes Bioscience**

R G Rockman, *(Rockman, R.G. Pubns.; 0-9630916),* 240 N. Fenway Dr., Fenton, MI 48430-2635 Tel 810-750-6128; Fax: 810-750-9832
Dist(s): **Baker & Taylor** *(Baker & Taylor Bks.)*
Borders Inc *(Borders, Inc.)*
Little Professor Bk Ctrs *(Little Professor Bk. Ctrs., Inc.).*

R Gumbiner, *(Gumbiner, Robert; 0-9645847),* 5456 The Toledo, Long Beach, CA 90803 Tel 310-433-5459; Fax: 310-439-2473.

R H Kapilian, *(Kapilian, Ralph H. Pub.; 0-916311),* 30 Lake St., Brighton, MA 02135 (SAN 295-9232) Tel 617-254-3054.

R Hale Ltd (GBR) *(0-7090; 0-7198) Dist. by* **Trafalgar.**

R Heffner Vocat, *(Heffner, R. Vocational Counseling Service; 0-9653317),* P.O. Box 1391, Tualatin, OR 97062 Tel 503-620-3882.

R I Williams, *(Williams, Russell I.; 0-9613013),* 414 E. 23rd St., Cheyenne, WY 82001 (SAN 294-2941) Tel 307-634-7905.

R J Kitson Pubng, *(Kitson, R.J. Publishing; 0-9639767),* 4400 NE 29th Ave., Lighthouse Point, FL 33064 Tel 954-946-7905
Dist(s): **Baker & Taylor** *(Baker & Taylor Bks.).*

R J Quintin, *See* **Quintin Pub RI**

R K Pubns (GBR) *Dist. by* **St Mut.**

R K Woltz, *(Woltz, Raymond K.; 0-9613447),* 1355 Hermes Ave., Leucadia, CA 92024 (SAN 657-1115) Tel 760-753-0055.

R L Harvin, *See* **Rebecca Entpses**

R L Whiteside, *(Whiteside, Robert L.; 0-9623385),* 191 Alohilani St., Pukalani, HI 96768 Tel 808-572-9613; Fax: 808-871-8109.

R M Khalilullah, *(Khalilullah, Dr. Riza M.; 1-930329),* 3330 W, 147th St., Suite 105, Hawthorne, CA 90250 Tel 323-349-1922 (phone/fax).

R Mass Ltd (ISR) *(965-09) Dist. by* **Lambda Pubs.**

R Meerdink Co Ltd, *(Meerdink, Russell Co., Ltd., The; 0-929346),* 1555 S. Park Ave., Neenah, WI 54956 (SAN 249-1680) Tel 920-725-0955; Fax: 920-725-0709; Toll Free: 800-635-6499
E-mail: editor@horseinfo.com
Web site: http://www.horseinfo.com.

R Peat, *(Peat, Raymond PH.D.; 0-9702913),* Orders Addr.: P.O. Box 5764, Eugene, OR 97405 Tel 503-345-9855; Fax: 541-683-4279; Toll Free: 800-783-6120; Edit Addr.: 3300 Wilamette St., Eugene, OR 97405
E-mail: raypeat@efn.org.

R Ross, *(Ross, Rosemary; 0-9647382),* P.O. Box 273003, Houston, TX 77277-3003 Tel 713-662-0561; Fax: 713-662-7430.

R S Lourie Ctr, *(Lourie, Reginald S. Ctr. for Infants & Young Children; 1-880341),* 11710 Hunters Ln., Rockville, MD 20852 Tel 301-984-4444; Fax: 301-881-8043.

R S Rauch, *(Rauch, Robert S.; 0-9624076),* 91 Cherry St., Milford, CT 06460 Tel 203-874-5577.

R Sevier, *See* **Wesley Pub Co**

R Spiegel, *See* **SRG Pubng**

R Steiner Col, *(Steiner, Rudolf College Pr./St. George Pubns.; 0-916786; 0-945803),* 9200 Fair Oaks Blvd., Fair Oaks, CA 95628 (SAN 208-8371) Tel 916-961-3722; Fax: 916-961-3032 ; *Imprints:* Saint George Pubns (Saint George Publications)
E-mail: rsc@steinercollege.org.

R Steiner Pr (GBR) *(0-85440; 1-85584) Dist. by* **Anthroposophic.**

R Stevenson Conslt, *(Stevenson, Robert Consultant; 0-9606252),* 525 Princeton Cir., W., Fullerton, CA 92631 (SAN 217-5878).

R Tanner Assocs Inc, *(Tanner, Ralph Assocs., Inc.; 0-942078),* 122 N. Cortez St., Suite 102, Prescott, AZ 86301 (SAN 239-9857) Tel 520-778-4162.

R W Johnson Found, *(Johnson, Robert Wood Foundation, The; 0-942054),* P.O. Box 2316, Princeton, NJ 08540-2316 (SAN 238-4639) Tel 609-452-8701
Web site: http://www.rwjf.org.

R Weaver, *See* **Specialty Pub**

R Westerman, *(Westerman, Robert Dean; 0-9629983),* 7931 Jefferson Hwy., Baton Rouge, LA 70809 Tel 504-927-3442; Fax: 504-927-3457.

Rabkin-Silverman, *(Rabkin/Silverman),* 3644 Creekside Dr., Ann Arbor, MI 48105 Tel 313-995-3513
Dist(s): **Baker & Taylor** *(Baker & Taylor Bks.)*
NACSCORP Inc *(NACSCORP, Inc.).*

Race Pt Pr, *(Race Point Pr.; 0-9633145),* Orders Addr.: P.O. Box 770, Provincetown, MA 02657-0770 Tel 508-487-9597; Fax: 508-487-7902; Edit Addr.: 15 Standish Way, Provincetown, MA 02657 (SAN 299-1136)
E-mail: jennison@racepointpress.com
Web site: http://www.racepointpress.com.

†Rachelle Simon, *(Simon, Rachelle; 0-934710),* 331 Vista Pacifica, Santa Barbara, CA 93109-2133 (SAN 213-9669) Tel 805-965-4259; Fax: 805-965-1959; *CIP.*

Radcliffe Med Pr (GBR) *(1-870905; 1-85775) Dist. by* **Balogh.**

Radcliffe Med Pr Imprint of Scovill Paterson

Radiol Res & Educ Found, *(Radiology Research & Education Foundation; 0-9646199),* Harry K. Genant, M.D., Department of Radiology, Box 0682, University of California, San Francisco, CA 94143-0628 Tel 415-476-4864; Fax: 415-476-8901.

Radiology Pub, *(Radiology Publishing; 0-9644594),* Div. of Wisconsin Radiology Services, 700 Regent St., Suite 303, Madison, WI 53715 Tel 608-233-2668; Fax: 608-255-1760; Toll Free: 800-628-7927
Web site: http://www.oasmennon@inxpress.net.

Rae John, *(Rae John Pubs.; 0-939438; 0-9605226),* 1442A Walnut, No. 222, Berkeley, CA 94709-1405 (SAN 220-1739) Tel 916-783-1942; Fax: 570-540-1057
E-mail: lori@bookandhammer.com.

For full information on wholesalers and distributors, refer to the Wholesaler and Distributor Symbol Index

Ragged Mtn Imprint of McGraw-Hill Trade

Ragweed (CAN) *(0-920304; 0-921556; 0-921881) Dist. by* **U of Toronto Pr.**

RAINBO, *(Research, Action & Information Network For Bodily Integrity Of Women (RAINBO); 1-893136),* 915 Broadway, Suite 1109, New York, NY 10010-7108 Tel 212-477-3318; Fax: 212-477-4154
E-mail: rainbo@aol.com
Web site: http://www.rainbo.org
Dist(s): **Women Ink** *(Women Ink).*

Rainbow Books, *(Rainbow Bks., Inc.; 0-935834; 1-56825),* P.O. Box 430, Highland City, FL 33846-0430 (SAN 213-5515) Do not confuse with Rainbow Bks., Inc. in Amsterdam, NY
E-mail: rbibooks@aol.com
Dist(s):* Baker & Taylor *(Baker & Taylor Bks.)
Bk Clearing Hse *(Book Clearing Hse.)*
Quality Bks IL *(Quality Bks., Inc.)*
Unique Bks Inc *(Unique Bks., Inc.).*

Rainlight Bk, *(Rainlight Bks.; 1-887020),* Orders Addr.: P.O. Box 411, Neskowin, OR 97149-0411 Fax: 503-392-3009; Edit Addr.: 7995 Slab Creek Rd., Neskowin, OR 97149-0411 ; *Imprints:* Sanicula Pr (Sanicula Press)
Dist(s): **Distributors** *(Distributors, The)*
Quality Bks IL *(Quality Bks., Inc.).*

Rainmaker Pr, *(Rainmaker Pr.; 1-889346),* Div. of Olcott & Assocs., Orders Addr.: P.O. Box 2343, Appleton, WI 54913 Tel 920-730-5566; Fax: 920-730-5601; Edit Addr.: 1412 N. Superior St., Appleton, WI 54913.

Raintree Pubns, *(Raintree Pubns.; 0-9635964),* P.O. Box 1338, Fort Bragg, CA 95437 Tel 707-964-4380; Fax: 707-964-1868; Toll Free: 800-422-5963.

†Raintree Steck-V, *(Raintree Steck-Vaughn Pubs.; 0-8114; 0-8172; 0-8393; 0-7398),* Div. of Reed Elsevier plc, Orders Addr.: P.O. Box 690789, Orlando, FL 32819-0789 Tel 512-343-8227; Fax: 512-795-3699; Toll Free Fax: 800-699-9459; Toll Free: 800-531-5015; Edit Addr.: 15 E. 26th St., New York, NY 10010 (SAN 658-1757) Tel 646-935-3702; Fax: 646-935-3713
E-mail: tlefebre@steckvaughn.com
Web site: http://www.raintreesteckvaughn.com
Dist(s): **Shens Bks** *(Shen's Bks.); CIP.*

Rama Pub Co, *(Rama Publishing Co.; 0-913071),* P.O. Box 793, Carthage, MO 64836 (SAN 283-3875) Tel 417-358-1093 Do not confuse with Rama Publishing, Buffalo, NY.

Ramsey Found, *(Ramsey Foundation; 0-9629302),* 640 Jackson St., Saint Paul, MN 55101-2595 Tel 612-221-2928; Fax: 612-225-5191.

†Rand Corp, *(Rand Corp., The; 0-8330),* Orders Addr.: P.O. Box 2138, Santa Monica, CA 90407-2138 (SAN 218-9291) Tel 310-393-0411; Fax: 310-451-6996; Edit Addr.: 1700 Main St., Santa Monica, CA 90407-2138 (SAN 665-763X)
E-mail: jwarren@rand.org
Web site: http://www.rand.org
Dist(s): **Natl Bk Netwk** *(National Bk. Network); CIP.*

Random (GBR) *(0-09; 0-224; 0-7126) Dist. by* **Trafalgar.**

†Random, *(Random Hse., Inc.; 0-345; 0-375; 0-394; 0-553; 0-676; 0-679; 0-87665; 0-929661; 1-58836; 1-4000),* Div. of Bertelsmann AG, Orders Addr.: 400 Hahn Rd., Westminster, MD 21157 (SAN 202-5515) Tel 410-848-1900; Toll Free Fax: 800-659-2436; Toll Free: 800-726-0600 (customer service/orders); Edit Addr.: 1540 Broadway, New York, NY 10036 (SAN 202-5507) Tel 212-782-9000; Fax: 212-302-7985
E-mail: customerservice@randomhouse.com
Web site: http://www.randomhouse.com
Dist(s): **Continental Bk** *(Continental Bk. Co., Inc.)*
Cookbook Collection Inc *(Cookbook Collection, Inc.)*
Shens Bks *(Shen's Bks.)*
T T Beeler *(Beeler, Thomas T. Publisher)*
Urban Land *(Urban Land Institute); CIP.*

Random Hse Chldrns, *(Random Hse. Children's Publishing; 0-375; 0-676; 0-679; 1-58836; 1-4000),* Div. of Random Hse., Inc., Orders Addr.: 400 Hahn Rd., Westminster, MD 21157 Tel 410-848-1900; Toll Free: 800-726-0600; Edit Addr.: 1540 Broadway, New York, NY 10036 (SAN 202-5507) Tel 212-782-8491; Fax: 212-782-9577; Toll Free: 800-200-3552
E-mail: kids@random.com;
pmuller@randomhouse.com
Dist(s): **IPG Chicago** *(Independent Pubs. Group).*

Random Hse Lrg Prnt, *(Random Hse. Large Print; 0-375; 0-679; 1-4000),* Div. of Random House, Orders Addr.: 400 Hahn Rd., Westminster, MD 21157 Tel 410-848-1900; Toll Free Fax: 800-659-2436; Toll Free: 800-733-3000 (customer service/orders); Edit Addr.: 201 E. 50th St., New York, NY 10022 (SAN 202-5825) Fax: 212-572-8797
E-mail: editor@randomhouse.com;
customerservice@randomhouse.com
Web site: http://www.randomhouse.com
Dist(s): **Large Print Library** *(Large Print Library Discounter)*
T T Beeler *(Beeler, Thomas T. Publisher).*

†Random Hse Value, *(Random Hse. Value Publishing, Inc.; 0-517; 0-609; 0-87000; 1-4000),* Div. of Random Hse., Inc., Orders Addr.: 400 Hahn Rd., Westminster, MD 21157 Toll Free: 800-733-3000 (orders); 800-726-0600 (customer service, credit, electronic ordering dept.); Edit Addr.: 201 E. 50th St., New York, NY 10022 Tel 212-572-2400 ; *Imprints:* Chatham River Pr (Chatham River Press)
Web site: http://www.randomhouse.com*; CIP.*

Random Ref & Info, *(Random Hse. Reference & Information Publishing; 0-375; 0-679; 1-4000),* Div. of Random Hse. Information Group, Orders Addr.: 400 Hahn Rd., Westminster, MD 21157 Tel 410-848-1900; Toll Free: 800-726-0600; Edit Addr.: 280 Park Ave., New York, NY 10022 Tel 212-751-2600; Toll Free: 800-726-0600
E-mail: customerservice@randomhouse.com
Web site: http://www.randomhouse.com/
Dist(s): **Random** *(Random Hse., Inc.).*

Random Trade, *(Random House Adult Trade Group; 0-375; 0-679; 0-8129; 1-4000),* Orders Addr.: 400 Hahn Rd., Westminster, MD 21157 Tel 410-848-1900; Toll Free: 800-726-0600; Edit Addr.: 299 Park Ave., New York, NY 10171 Tel 212-751-2600; Fax: 212-572-4949; Toll Free: 800-726-0600
Dist(s): **Random** *(Random Hse., Inc.).*

Range Light, *(Range of Light Publishing; 0-9658001),* P.O. Box 2000-153, South Lake Tahoe, CA 96151 Tel 530-541-1999; Fax: 530-544-5306
E-mail: kimball@sierra.net
Web site: http://www.ggweb.com/books/rangeoflight
Dist(s): **Bookpeople** *(Bookpeople)*
Sunbelt Pubns *(Sunbelt Pubns., Inc.).*

Ranrai Pub, *(Ranrai Publishing; 0-9622066),* 13511 117th Ave., NE, Kirkland, WA 98034 Tel 425-821-4287
E-mail: jlrbanners@juno.com
Web site: http://www.rainwaterbooks.com.

Rapha Pub, *(Rapha Publishing; 0-945276),* Div. of Rapha, Inc., 2323 Clear Lake City Blvd., Suite 180-300, Houston, TX 77062 (SAN 248-3726) Tel 713-488-3836; Fax: 713-488-8879; Toll Free: 800-460-4673 Do not confuse with Rapha Publishing in Upper Marlboro, MD.

Rapid Science, *(Rapid Science Pubs.; 1-85922; 1-870485),* 227 E. Washington Sq., 1st Flr., Philadelphia, PA 19106-3713 Tel 215-574-2300; Fax: 215-574-2292; Toll Free: 800-552-5866 (orders only).

Rappahannock Bks, *(Rappahannock Bks.; 1-892105),* 7004 Tapps Ford Rd., Amissville, VA 20106 Tel 540-364-9518
E-mail: rwaldrip@earthlink.net;
lwaldrip@mnsinc.com.

Rational Isl, *(Rational Island Pubs.; 0-911214; 0-913937; 1-885357; 1-893165; 1-58429),* Orders Addr.: P.O. Box 2081, Seattle, WA 98111 (SAN 204-6725) Tel 206-284-0311; Fax: 206-284-8429; Edit Addr.: 719 Second Ave., N., Seattle, WA 98109 (SAN 662-1201)
E-mail: litsales@rc.org
Web site: http://www.rc.org/.

Ratna Pustak Bhandar (NPL) *Dist. by* **St Mut.**

Ratnl Self-Help Aids, *See* **Tangrm Bks**

Rattle OK Pubns, *(Rattle OK Pubns.; 0-9626210; 1-883965),* Orders Addr.: P.O. Box 5614, Napa, CA 94581 (SAN 297-5475) Tel 707-253-9641; Edit Addr.: 533 Soscol Ave., No. 81, Napa, CA 94559
Dist(s): **Gryphon Hse** *(Gryphon Hse., Inc.).*

Raven Ent, *(Raven Entertainment, Inc.; 0-9655450),* Orders Addr.: P.O. Box 242, Damascus, MD 20872 Tel 301-482-1548; Fax: 301-482-1549; Edit Addr.: 8808 Garfield Dr., Gaithersburg, MD 20882
E-mail: ravenent@erols.com
Web site: http://www.ravenentertainment.com.

Raven Pr ID, *(Raven Pr.; 0-9708696),* 612 S. 11th St., Coeur d' Alene, ID 83814 Tel 208-676-9490; Fax: 208-765-2724 Do not confuse with companies with same or similar name in Fairbank, AK, Lancaster, CA, Fort Collins, CO, Melbourne, FL
E-mail: trishuwa@aol.com
Dist(s): **Chelsea Green Pub** *(Chelsea Green Publishing).*

Raven Pubs, *(Raven Pubs.; 0-9621726),* Orders Addr.: P.O. Box 242275, Charlotte, NC 28224-9798 (SAN 252-0532) Tel 704-552-2477; Edit Addr.: 7302 Quail Meadow Ln., Charlotte, NC 28210
E-mail: oxygenbook@aol.com
Web site: http://www.OxygenBook.com.

Ravenwood Pub, *(Ravenwood Publishing; 1-892038),* 4421 Ravenwood Ave., Sacramento, CA 95821 Tel 916-974-0764
E-mail: dlinton@ravenwoodpub.com
Web site: http://www.ravenwoodpub.com.

Rawat Pubns (IND) *(81-7033) Dist. by* **S Asia.**

Rawson Assocs Imprint of Macmillan

Rayo Imprint of HarperCollins Gen Bks

Rayve Prodns, *(Rayve Productions, Inc.; 1-877810),* Orders Addr.: P.O. Box 726, Windsor, CA 95492 (SAN 248-4250) Tel 707-838-6200; 707-544-7424 (phone/fax); Fax: 707-838-2220; Toll Free: 800-852-4890
E-mail: rayvepro@aol.com
Web site: http://www.rayveproductions.com
Dist(s): **Baker & Taylor** *(Baker & Taylor Bks.)*
Book Wholesalers *(Book Wholesalers, Inc.)*
Brodart *(Brodart Co.)*
Follett Library *(Follett Library Resources)*
J Majors Co *(Majors, J. A. Co.)*
Quality Bks IL *(Quality Bks., Inc.)*
Sunbelt Pubns *(Sunbelt Pubns., Inc.)*
Unique Bks Inc *(Unique Bks., Inc.).*

Raztec Entrprises, *(Raztec Enterprises; 0-9656921),* 520 Franklin Ave., Suite L21, Garden City, NY 11530 Tel 516-877-5074; Fax: 516-562-4794.

R-C Pubns, *(R-C Pubns., Inc.; 0-933311),* P.O. Box 35425, Phoenix, AZ 85069 (SAN 692-6061) Tel 602-242-9276.

†RD Assn, *(Reader's Digest Assn., Inc., The; 0-7621; 0-89577; 0-86438),* Orders Addr.: Reader's Digest Rd., Pleasantville, NY 10570 (SAN 282-2091) Toll Free: 800-234-9000
Web site: http://www.readersdigest.com
Dist(s): **IPG Chicago** *(Independent Pubs. Group)*
Penguin Putnam *(Penguin Putnam, Inc.); CIP.*

RDLE INST Bkstre, *(RODALE INSTITUTE Bookstore; 0-9652477),* 611 Siegfriedale Rd., Kutztown, PA 19530 Tel 610-683-6009; Fax: 610-683-8548; Toll Free: 800-832-6285
E-mail: ribooks@fast.net
Web site: http://www.rodaleinstitute.org.

†Ready Ref Pr, *(Ready Reference Pr.; 0-916270; 1-57333),* Orders Addr.: P.O. Box 5249, Santa Monica, CA 90405 (SAN 218-9305) Tel 310-475-4895; Toll Free: 800-424-5627; Edit Addr.: 1652 N. Pepper Dr., Pasadena, CA 90409*; CIP.*

Real Est News, *(Real Estate News Corp.; 0-9637713),* 3525 W. Peterson Ave., Chicago, IL 60659 Tel 312-866-9900.

†Real People, *(Real People Pr.; 0-911226),* Orders Addr.: P.O. Box F, Moab, UT 84532 (SAN 203-3879) Tel 435-259-7578; Fax: 435-259-4042 Do not confuse with Real People Publishing in Newark, CA
Web site: http://www.realpeoplepress.com
Dist(s): **Baker & Taylor** *(Baker & Taylor Bks.)*
Bookpeople *(Bookpeople)*
Distributors *(Distributors, The); CIP.*

Realizing Potential, *(Realizing Potentials Pr.; 0-9670829),* Orders Addr.: P.O. Box 1014, New Lenox, IL 60541-1014; Edit Addr.: 321 W. Maple, Suite 203, New Lenox, IL 60451 Tel 815-463-1823; Fax: 815-463-0804
E-mail: drwellness@prodigy.net
Web site: http://drwellness.net
Dist(s): **BookWorld** *(BookWorld Services, Inc.).*

Real-Life Pubns, *(Real-Life Pubns.; 0-9631846),* 8124 33rd Place N., Minneapolis, MN 55427-1921 (SAN 297-5971) Tel 612-544-5471 (phone/fax).

Rebecca Entpses, *(Rebecca Enterprises; 0-9641477),* 1001 Hargrove St., Henderson, NC 27536 Tel 252-438-8849; Fax: 252-438-3762
E-mail: lharvin@mindspring.com.

Rebel Records, *(Rebel Records, Inc.; 0-9664166),* 1413 Mill St., Camden, SC 29020-2934 Tel 803-432-7682; Fax: 803-425-8555
E-mail: coding@rebrecords.com
Web site: http://www.rebrecords.com.

Rebus, *(Rebus, Inc.; 0-929661; 0-9617311),* 632 Broadway, New York, NY 10012 (SAN 663-7019) Tel 212-505-2255; Fax: 212-505-5462
Dist(s): **Natl Bk Netwk** *(National Bk. Network).*

Rebus Pr Ltd (GBR) *(1-900877) Dist. by* **Intl Spec Bk.**

Recov Couples, *(Recovering Couples Anonymous; 0-9637495),* Orders Addr.: P.O. Box 11872, Saint Louis, MO 63105 Tel 314-830-2600; Fax: 314-830-2670
E-mail: info@recovering-couple.org
Web site: http://www.recovering-couples.org.

Recovery Pubns, *(Recovery Pubns.; 0-9613185),* P.O. Box 57233, Lincoln, NE 68505-7233 (SAN 295-9372) Tel 402-475-3172
E-mail: dgensign@aol.com.

Red Apple Pub, *(Red Apple Publishing; 1-880222),* 15010 113th St., KPN, Gig Harbor, WA 98329-5014 Tel 253-884-1450; Fax: 253-884-1451
E-mail: peggy@redapplepublishing.com
Web site: http://www.redapplepublishing.com.

Red Brick Imprint of Hatherleigh

†Red Crane Bks, *(Red Crane Bks., Inc.; 1-878610),* 2008 Rosina St., Suite B, Santa Fe, NM 87505 Tel 505-988-7070; Fax: 505-989-7476; Toll Free: 800-922-3392
E-mail: publish@redcrane.com
Web site: http://www.redcrane.com
Dist(s): **Consort Bk Sales** *(Consortium Bk. Sales & Distribution)*
Continental Bk *(Continental Bk. Co., Inc.); CIP.*

Red Cross St Paul, *(American Red Cross, Saint Paul Area Chapter; 0-9605584),* 100 S. Robert St., Saint Paul, MN 55107 (SAN 240-8392) Tel 612-291-6789.

Red Dragon VA, *(Red Dragon Pr.; 0-9637704; 1-891387),* 433 Old Town Ct., Alexandria, VA 22314-3545 Tel 703-683-5877 (phone/fax) Do not confuse with Red Dragon Press, Wilmot, WI
Web site: http://www.reddragonpress.com
Dist(s): **Qa Ent** *(Qa Enterprises).*

Red Lantern Pr, *(Red Lantern Pr.; 0-9618099),* 27920 Arlington Dr., Southfield, MI 48076 (SAN 666-1149) Tel 248-353-1221.

Red Lion, *(Red Lion Bks.; 0-940162),* 12 Ryder Ct., Dixville, NY 11746 (SAN 217-4898) Tel 516-586-1072.

Red Maple Pubg, *(Red Maple Publishing; 1-893309),* Orders Addr.: P.O. Box 291, Jefferson, OH 44047 Tel 440-576-9483; Edit Addr.: 2 E. Jefferson St., Jefferson, OH 44047.

Red Rose Pr, *(Red Rose Pr.; 0-9609888; 1-889891),* 12755 Byron Ave., Granada Hills, CA 91344 (SAN 282-2121) Tel 818-368-8586; Fax: 818-368-8506; Toll Free: 800-789-7673 Do not confuse with Red Rose Press in Scottsdale, AZ
E-mail: debkro@excite.com
Web site: http://home.earthlink.net/~rowsbud
Dist(s): **Baker & Taylor** *(Baker & Taylor Bks.)*
Bookpeople *(Bookpeople)*
New Leaf Dist *(New Leaf Distributing Co., Inc.).*

Red Rvr Nutritn, *See* **Apple a Day**

Red Sea NY, *(Red Sea; 1-887478),* 114 Oak St., Patchogue, NY 11772 Tel 516-475-1142; Fax: 516-475-9673 ; *Imprints:* WiseAcre (WiseAcre Books)
E-mail: wiseacre@redsea.com
Web site: http://users.aol.com/wiseacrebk/.

Red Sea Pr, *(Red Sea Pr.; 0-932415; 1-56902),* 11 Princess Rd., Suites D, E & F, Lawrenceville, NJ 08648 (SAN 630-1983) Tel 609-844-9583; Fax: 609-844-0198
E-mail: africawpress@nyo.com
Web site: http://www.africanworld.com/.

Red Toad Rd, *(Red Toad Road Co.; 1-889287),* Orders Addr.: P.O. Box 642, Havre de Grace, MD 21078 Tel 410-939-4092; Fax: 410-939-5614; Edit Addr.: 223 Heather Way, Havre de Grace, MD 21078
E-mail: redtoadroad@aol.com
Web site: http://www.amazon.com/shops/redtoadroad.

---

†Red Wheel ME, *(Red Wheel; 0-87728; 1-57863; 1-59003),* Div. of Weiser Bks., P.O. Box 612, York Beach, ME 03910-0612 (SAN 202-9588) Tel 207-363-4393; Fax: 207-363-5799; Toll Free: 800-423-7087 (orders only)
E-mail: customerservice@redwheelweiser.com
Web site: http://www.redwheelweiser.com; http://www.weiserbooks.com
Dist(s):* Abyss Dist *(Abyss Distribution)
Baker & Taylor *(Baker & Taylor Bks.)*
Bookpeople *(Bookpeople)*
Koen Bk Distributors *(Koen Bk. Distributors)*
New Leaf Dist *(New Leaf Distributing Co., Inc.); CIP.*

Red Wing Pubng, *(Red Wing Publishing Hse.; 0-9640193),* 9861 Palmer Ln., Denver, CO 80221 Tel 303-280-5665
E-mail: sommers2@uswest.net.

Redding Pr, *(Redding Pr.; 0-9658879),* Orders Addr.: c/o Mary Mahony, P.O. Box 366, Belmont, MA 02178 Fax: 617-489-9476; Toll Free: 800-267-6012; Edit Addr.: 405 Concord Ave., Belmont, MA 02178
E-mail: msmahony@channel.com
Web site: http://www.channel.com/users/msmahony
Dist(s): **Baker & Taylor** *(Baker & Taylor Bks.)*
Koen Bk Distributors *(Koen Bk. Distributors)*
Quality Bks IL *(Quality Bks., Inc.).*

Redwing Bk Co, *(Redwing Bk. Co.),* 44 Linden St., Brookline, MA 02445 (SAN 163-3597) Tel 617-738-4664; Fax: 617-738-4620; Toll Free: 800-873-3946 ; *Imprints:* Paradgm Pubns (Paradigm Publications)
E-mail: bob@redwingbooks.com
Web site: http://www.redwingbooks.com.

Reed Grp Ltd, *(Reed Group, Ltd.; 1-889010),* 4041 Hanover Ave., 2nd Flr., Boulder, CO 80305 Tel 303-247-1860; Fax: 303-247-1863; Toll Free: 800-347-7443
E-mail: reedmda@rgl.net
Web site: http://www.presleyreed.com.

Reed Publns, *See* **Reed Grp Ltd**

Reedswain, *(Reedswain, Inc.; 0-9651020; 1-890946; 1-59164),* Orders Addr.: 612 Pughtown Rd., Spring City, PA 19475 Tel 610-469-6911; Fax: 610-469-9588; Toll Free: 800-331-5191
E-mail: bryan@reedswain.com
Web site: http://www.reedswain.com.

†Ref Pubns, *(Reference Pubns., Inc.; 0-917256),* 218 St. Clair River Dr., P.O. Box 344, Algonac, MI 48001-0344 (SAN 208-4392) Tel 810-794-5722; Fax: 810-794-7463
E-mail: referencepub@juno.com*; CIP.*

Ref Rsch Serv, *(Reference & Research Services; 0-937855; 1-892068),* 511 Lincoln St., Santa Cruz, CA 95060 (SAN 659-5774) Tel 831-426-4479; Fax: 831-426-4429
E-mail: refres_2000@yahoo.com.

Reflex Res Proj, *(Reflexology Research Project; 0-9606070),* P.O. Box 35820, Albuquerque, NM 87176-5820 (SAN 216-9312) Tel 505-344-9392; Fax: 505-344-0246; Toll Free: 888-777-9911
E-mail: footc@aol.com
Web site: http://www.reflexology-research.com
Dist(s): **Baker & Taylor** *(Baker & Taylor Bks.)*
New Leaf Dist *(New Leaf Distributing Co., Inc.)*
Nutri-Books Corp *(Nutri-Bks. Corp.)*
Redwing Bk Co *(Redwing Bk. Co.).*

†Reg Baptist, *(Regular Baptist Pr.; 0-87227),* Div. of General Assn. of Regular Baptist Churches, 1300 N. Meacham Rd., Schaumburg, IL 60173-4806 (SAN 205-2229) Tel 847-843-1600 (foreign orders); Fax: 847-843-3757; Toll Free: 800-727-4440 (orders only)
E-mail: rbp@garbc.org
Web site: http://www.garbc.org/*; CIP.*

Regal Pubns, *See* **Univ Publng Hse**

ReganBooks Imprint of HarperCollins Pubs

Regency Imprint of Scholarly

Regency Pr (GBR) *(0-7212) Dist. by* **St Mut.**

Regenics Pr, *(Regenics Pr.; 0-9644918),* Orders Addr.: P.O. Box 1944, Sonoma, CA 95476-1944 Tel 707-939-0379; Edit Addr.: 18020 Comstock Way, Sonoma, CA 95476-1944
Dist(s): **Bookpeople** *(Bookpeople)*
Quality Bks IL *(Quality Bks., Inc.).*

Regent Pr, *(Regent Pr.; 0-916147; 1-889059; 1-58790),* 6020-A Adeline St., Oakland, CA 94608 (SAN 294-9717) Tel 510-547-7602; Fax: 510-547-6357 Do not confuse with Regent Pr., Oxnard, CA
E-mail: regent1@mindspring.com
Web site: http://www.sirius.com/~regent
Dist(s): **AK Pr Dist** *(AK Pr. Distribution)*
Bookpeople *(Bookpeople)*
Koen Bk Distributors *(Koen Bk. Distributors)*
Southern Bk Service *(Southern Bk. Service).*

Regents U CA, *(Regents of the Univ. of California, UCLA Div. of Geriatrics, The; 0-9661178),* 10945 Le Conte Ave., Suite 2339, Los Angeles, CA 90095-1687 Tel 310-825-8253; Fax: 310-794-2199 Do not confuse with The Regents of the University of California in Davis CA.

Regional Sci Res Inst, *(Regional Science Research Institute; 1-55869),* 34 Exeter Rd., East Windsor, NJ 08520-1128 (SAN 239-3794).

Regnery Gateway, *See* **Regnery Pub**

†Regnery Pub, *(Regnery Publishing, Inc., An Eagle Publishing Co.; 0-89526),* Subs. of Phillips Publishing International, One Massachusetts Ave., NW, Suite 600, Washington, DC 20001 (SAN 210-5578) Tel 202-216-0600; Fax: 202-216-0612 ; *Imprints:* LifeLine Press (LifeLine Press)
E-mail: info@regnery.com
Web site: http://www.regnery.com/
Dist(s): **Continental Bk** *(Continental Bk. Co., Inc.)*
Natl Bk Netwk *(National Bk. Network); CIP.*

Regnts College, *(Regents College; 1-889403),* 7 Columbia Cir., Albany, NY 12203-5159 Tel 518-464-8500; Fax: 518-464-8777.

Regulatory Info Ctr, *(Regulatory Information Ctr.; 0-9648291),* 12713 Franklin Farm Rd., Herndon, VA 22071-1914 Tel 703-476-7177; Fax: 703-476-6545.

Rehab Nursing, *(Rehabilitation Nursing Foundation of the Assn. of Rehabilitation Nurses, The; 1-884278),* Div. of Association of Rehabilitation Nurses, 4700 W. Lake Ave., Glenview, IL 60025 Tel 847-375-4710; Fax: 847-375-6310; Toll Free: 800-229-7530.

Rehab P & T, *(Rehabilitation Pubns. & Therapies, Inc.; 0-9630294),* P.O. Box 767171, Roswell, GA 30076-7171 Tel 706-234-6447; Fax: 706-234-8922.

RehabTech, *(RehabTech Assocs., Inc.; 0-9635859),* 3640 Dry Creek Ct., Ellicott City, MD 21043 Tel 410-750-0353; Fax: 410-465-4072.

Reiki Plus, *(Reiki Plus Pubns.; 0-9634690),* 707 Barcelona Rd., Key Largo, FL 33037 (SAN 253-7230) Tel 305-451-9881; Fax: 305-451-9841
E-mail: reikiplus@mindspring.com
Web site: http://www.reikiplus.com
Dist(s): **Assoc Pubs Grp** *(Associated Pubs. Group).*

Reiman Assocs, *See* **Reiman Pubns**

Reiman Pubns, *(Reiman Pubns., L.P.; 0-89821),* 5400 S. 60th St., Greendale, WI 53129 (SAN 208-4368) Tel 414-423-0100; Fax: 414-423-8463; Toll Free: 800-682-9019
Web site: http://www.reimanpub.com/.

Relative Val, *(Relative Value Studies, Inc.; 1-879298; 1-929061),* 1675 Larimer St., Suite 410, Denver, CO 80202-1520 Tel 303-534-0506; Fax: 303-534-0577; Toll Free: 800-824-2133
E-mail: stacyl@rvsdata.com; info@rvsdata.com
Web site: http://www.rvsdata.com.

Relaxed Bks, *(Relaxed Bks.; 0-9615140),* 165 Church St., Winfield, IL 60190-1245 (SAN 694-2091) Tel 630-462-1768; Fax: 630-462-7064; Toll Free: 800-421-2717
E-mail: seelight@juno.com.

†Religious Educ, *(Religious Education Pr., Inc.; 0-89135),* 5316 Meadow Brook Rd., Birmingham, AL 35242 (SAN 207-3951) Tel 205-991-1000; Fax: 205-991-9669
E-mail: releduc@ix.netcom.com
Web site: http://www.bham.net/releduc/
Dist(s): **Baker & Taylor** *(Baker & Taylor Bks.)*
Spring Arbor Dist *(Spring Arbor Distributors Inc.)*
iUniverse Inc *(iUniverse, Inc.); CIP.*

Remco Inc, *(Remco, Inc.; 0-9623535),* 1711 Tyvale Ct., Vienna, VA 22182-2374 Tel 703-790-9061
E-mail: smoky@erols.com.

Remedica (GBR) *(1-901346) Dist. by* **Gordon & Breach.**

Remembrance, *(Remembrance Pr., The; 0-9617210),* Div. of Rosemary Hse., Inc., 120 S. Market St., Mechanicsburg, PA 17055 (SAN 663-2777) Tel 717-697-5111.

Remington NJ, *(Remington Pr.; 0-9626830),* 454 Foothill Rd., Bridgewater, NJ 08807 Tel 201-722-7108 Do not confuse with companies with the same name in Denver, CO, Radnor, PA.

Remnant Pubns, *(Remnant Pubns.; 1-883012),* 649 E. Chicago Rd., Coldwater, MI 49036-9497 Tel 517-279-1304; Fax: 517-279-1804; Toll Free: 800-423-1319
E-mail: remnant@charter.net
Web site: http://www.remnantpublications.com
Dist(s): **Spring Arbor Dist** *(Spring Arbor Distributors Inc.).*

Renaiss AZ, *(Renaissance Publishing; 0-9637144),* Div. of Renaissance Knowledge Systems, Inc., 8634 S. Willow Dr., Tempe, AZ 85284 Tel 602-820-0514 Do not confuse with companies with the same or similar names in Sonoma, CA, Omaha, NE, Redmond, WA, Indianapolis, IN, Taylor, MI, Longview, TX.

Renaissance, *(Renaissance Bks.; 1-58063),* Div. of Renaissance Media, 5858 Wilshire Blvd., Suite 200, Los Angeles, CA 90036 Tel 323-939-1840; Fax: 323-939-6436; Toll Free: 800-266-2834 Do not confuse with Renaissance Books, Kernersville, NC
E-mail: pubbooks@aol.com
Web site: http://www.renaissancebks.com/
Dist(s): **St Martin** *(St. Martin's Pr., LLC)*
VHPS *(VHPS Holtzbrinck Pubs.).*

Reniew Pubng, *(Reniew Publishing Co.; 0-9641828),* 8 Howe Cir., Randolph, MA 02368 Tel 617-963-8697; Fax: 508-376-1919.

Replica Bks, *(Replica Bks.; 0-7351),* Div. of Baker & Taylor, Orders Addr.: 1200 US Hwy., 22 E., Bridgewater, NJ 07060 Tel 908-541-7393; Fax: 908-541-7875; Toll Free: 800-775-1800; Edit Addr.: P.O. Box 6885, Bridgewater, NJ 08807-0885
E-mail: btinfo@baker-taylor.com; frosts@btol.com
Web site: http://www.replicabooks.com.

†Reprint, *(Reprint Co.; 0-87152),* 611 Perrin Dr., P.O. Box 5401, Spartanburg, SC 29304 (SAN 203-3828) Tel 864-579-4433; *CIP.*

Reprint Servs, *See* **Rprt Serv**

Res & Educ, *(Research & Education Assn.; 0-7386; 0-87891),* 61 Ethel Rd., W., Piscataway, NJ 08854 (SAN 204-6814) Tel 732-819-8880; Fax: 732-819-8808; Toll Free: 800-822-0830
Web site: http://www.rea.com.

Res Appl Inc, *(Resource Applications, Inc.; 0-932491; 1-55702),* 7794 Grow Dr., Pensacola, FL 32514-7072 (SAN 687-4061) Toll Free: 800-826-1877.

Res Ctr Child, *(Research Ctr. for Children, Youth, & Families/Achenbach System of Empirically Based Assesment (ASEBA); 0-938565; 0-9611898),* 1 S. Prospect St., Rm. 6-436, Burlington, VT 05401-3456 (SAN 286-2123) Tel 802-656-8313; Fax: 802-656-2602
E-mail: aseba@uvm.edu
Web site: http://aseba.uvm.edu.

Res for Aging, *(Resources for Aging, Inc.; 0-9645965; 1-929035),* 1265 Erie Ave., North Tonawanda, NY 14120 Tel 716-693-3554; Toll Free: 888-243-4636
E-mail: rfasherry@aol.com
Web site: http://www.ageinfo.com.

Res Press, *(Research Pr.; 0-87822),* Orders Addr.: P.O. Box 9177, Champaign, IL 61826-9177 (SAN 282-2490) Toll Free: 800-519-2707; Edit Addr.: 2612 N. Mattis Ave., Champaign, IL 61822 (SAN 282-2482) Tel 217-352-3273; Fax: 217-352-1221 Do not confuse with Research Pr., Prairie Village, KS
E-mail: rp@researchpress.com
Web site: http://www.researchpress.com.

Res Pubns CA, *(Re:Source Pubns.; 0-9642329),* 4767 York Blvd., Los Angeles, CA 90042 Tel 213-255-3382; Toll Free: 800-231-1776 Do not confuse with Resource Pubns. in San Jose, CA
E-mail: susanbc@aol.com
Web site: http://www.quickpage.com/k/keepyour
Dist(s): **Baker & Taylor** *(Baker & Taylor Bks.)*
Bookpeople *(Bookpeople)*
Nutri-Books Corp *(Nutri-Bks. Corp.).*

Resc Rehab, *(Resources for Rehabilitation; 0-929718),* 33 Bedford St., No. 19A, Lexington, MA 02420 (SAN 250-0566) Tel 781-862-6455; Fax: 781-861-7517
E-mail: orders@rfr.org
Web site: http://www.rfr.org.

Research Better, *(Research for Better Schls.; 1-56602),* 444 N. Third St., Philadelphia, PA 19123 (SAN 275-0473) Tel 215-574-9300; Fax: 215-574-0133
E-mail: info@rbs.org
Web site: http://www.rbs.org.

Research Ent, *(Research Enterprises, Inc.; 1-883021),* 1185 Faulkingham Rd., Merritt Island, FL 32952 Tel 407-453-6033; Fax: 407-453-9664.

Research Triangle, *(Research Triangle Publishing; 1-884570),* Orders Addr.: P.O. Box 1130, Fuquay Varina, NC 27526 Fax: 919-557-2161; Toll Free: 800-941-0020; Edit Addr.: 503 N. Ennis St., Fuquay Varina, NC 27526
E-mail: info@tripub.com
Web site: http://www.RTPWeb.com/BooksExpress.

Resource Dynamics, *(Resource Dynamics, Inc.; 0-9623925),* 9728 163rd Pl., NE, Redmond, WA 98052-3135 Do not confuse with Resource Dynamics, Inc., Henderson, NV.

†Resource Pubns, *(Resource Pubns., Inc.; 0-89390),* 160 E. Virginia St., No. 290, San Jose, CA 95112-5876 (SAN 209-3081) Tel 408-286-8505; Fax: 408-287-8748; Toll Free: 888-273-7782 Do not confuse with Resource Pubns. in Los Angeles, CA
E-mail: info@rpinet.com
Web site: http://www.rpinet.com
Dist(s): **Empire Pub Srvs** *(Empire Publishing Service)*
Feldheim *(Feldheim, Philipp Inc.); CIP.*

†Resources Future, *(Resources for the Future; 0-915707; 1-891853),* Orders Addr.: P.O. Box 4852, Baltimore, MD 21211-2190 (SAN 200-5166) Tel 410-516-6955; Fax: 410-516-6998; Edit Addr.: 1616 P St., NW, Rm. 414, Washington, DC 20036-1400 (SAN 213-1544) Tel 202-328-5000; Fax: 202-328-5024
E-mail: rffpress@rff.org
Web site: http://www.rff.org
Dist(s): **Johns Hopkins** *(Johns Hopkins Univ. Pr.)*
netLibrary CO *(netLibrary, Inc.); CIP.*

Respirator Support, *(Respirator Support Services; 0-9626831),* 2028 Virts Ln., Jefferson, MD 21755-8801 Tel 301-834-6008.

Resurge Pr, *(Resurge Pr.; 0-9616747),* 1717 Kirby Pkwy., Suite 100, Memphis, TN 38120-4331 (SAN 661-4612) Tel 901-751-0350; Fax: 901-751-9977
E-mail: Dnmartin46@aol.com.

Resurrection Pr Imprint of Catholic Bk Pub

Rev Exist Psych, *(Review of Existential Psychology & Psychiatry; 0-914857),* P.O. Box 23220, Seattle, WA 98102 (SAN 289-3940) Tel 206-524-3880.

Revelation Hse, *(Revelation Hse. Pubs., Inc.; 0-9604852),* P.O. Box 73175, Metairie, LA 70033 (SAN 217-1295) Tel 504-454-3141; Fax: 504-454-3141
E-mail: revhouse@aol.com.

†Revell, *(Revell, Fleming H. Co.; 0-8007; 0-922066; 1-58743),* Div. of Baker Bk. Hse., Orders Addr.: P.O. Box 6287, Grand Rapids, MI 49516-6287 (SAN 299-1500) Toll Free Fax: 800-398-3111; Toll Free: 800-877-2665; Edit Addr.: 6030 E. Fulton, Ada, MI 49301 (SAN 201-4041) Tel 616-676-9185; Fax: 616-676-9573 ; *Imprints:* Spire (Spire)
E-mail: sharlow@bakerbooks.com
Web site: http://www.bakerbooks.com; *CIP.*

†Review & Herald, *(Review & Herald Publishing Assn.; 0-8280),* 55 W. Oak Ridge Dr., Hagerstown, MD 21740 (SAN 203-3798) Tel 301-393-3000
Web site: http://www.reviewandherald.com/
Dist(s): **Shens Bks** *(Shen's Bks.)*
Spring Arbor Dist *(Spring Arbor Distributors Inc.); CIP.*

†Revisionist Pr, *(Revisionist Pr.; 0-87700),* G.P.O. Box 022009, Brooklyn, NY 11202-0043 (SAN 203-378X) Tel 212-332-0009; *CIP.*

Reward Imprint of P-H

Rhema Pubng, *(Rhema Publishing Co., Inc.; 0-9642497),* 977 Mill Creek Run, Suwanee, GA 30024 Tel 770-932-6991 Do not confuse with companies with similar name in Miami, FL, Flint, MI
Web site: http://members.aol.com/keninga/index.htm.

Rhodes & Easton, *(Rhodes & Easton; 0-9649401; 1-890394),* 400 W. Front St., 4th Flr., Traverse City, MI 49684 Tel 231-933-0445; Fax: 231-933-0448; Toll Free: 800-706-4636
E-mail: mclweley@bookpublishing.com
Web site: http://www.bookpublishing.com
Dist(s): **Baker & Taylor** *(Baker & Taylor Bks.)*
Partners Pubs Grp *(Partners Pubs. Group, Inc.)*
TSBI *(TSBI, Inc.).*

Rhythmic Med, *(Rhythmic Medicine; 1-886051),* 11445 Craig, Overland Park, KS 66210 Tel 913-696-1990; Fax: 913-696-1994.

RID Pubns, *(Registry of Interpreters for the Deaf, Inc.; 0-916883; 0-9602220),* 8630 Fenton St., Suite 324, Silver Spring, MD 20910-3803 (SAN 216-1796) Tel 301-608-0050; Fax: 301-608-0508
E-mail: views@rid.org
Web site: http://www.rid.org.

Rideout Pub, *(Rideout Publishing Co.; 0-9651484),* 4118 Montrose Ct., Orlando, FL 32812 Tel 407-859-8638; Fax: 407-826-9524.

Ridgeback Pr, *(Ridgeback Pr., Inc.; 0-9643754),* 305 Vineyard Town Ctr., No. 171, Morgan Hill, CA 95037 Tel 408-683-2008.

Ridgeview, *(Ridgeview Publishing Co.; 0-917930; 0-924922),* Box 686, Atascadero, CA 93423 (SAN 209-9993) Tel 805-466-7252.

Riegel Pub, *(Riegel Publishing; 0-944871),* P.O. Box 3241, San Clemente, CA 92674 (SAN 245-3916) Tel 714-582-7562.

Rigby Interact Lib, *See* **Heinemann Lib**

Riggs Inst Pr, *(Riggs Institute Pr.; 0-942311),* 4185 SW 102nd St., Beaverton, OR 97005 (SAN 298-1726) Tel 503-646-9459
E-mail: riggs@riggsinst.org.

Rinella Edit, *(Rinella Editorial Services; 0-940267),* 817 W. Cuyler, No. 3W, Chicago, IL 60613 (SAN 200-4135) Tel 773-281-0975; Fax: 773-281-1310; Toll Free: 800-982-0839
E-mail: joseph@laiacona.org.

Rising Star Publns, *(Rising Star Pubns., Inc.; 1-888770),* 353 High St., Closter, NJ 07624 Tel 201-784-9711; Toll Free: 800-716-7827 Do not confuse with Rising Star Pubns., Seattle, WA.

RiskCare, *(RiskCare; 1-893929),* Orders Addr.: P.O. Box 8742, Harrisburg, PA 17105-8742; Edit Addr.: 777 E. Park Dr., Harrisburg, PA 17111 Tel 717-558-7520; Fax: 717-558-9804; Toll Free: 800-492-7898
E-mail: info@rskcare.com
Web site: http://www.rskcare.com.

Ritchie Unltd, *(Ritchie Unlimited Pubns.; 0-939656),* 1427 Anderson Rd., Springfield, OR 97477 (SAN 216-6461) Tel 541-741-0794 (phone/fax)
E-mail: ralph-ritchie@worldnet.att.net.

Rittenhouse, *(Rittenhouse Bk. Distributors; 0-87381),* Orders Addr.: 511 Feheley Dr., King of Prussia, PA 19406 (SAN 213-4454) Tel 610-277-1414; Fax: 610-227-0390; Toll Free Fax: 800-223-7488; Toll Free: 800-345-6425
Web site: http://www.rittenhouse.com.

River City Pub, *(River City Publishing; 0-913515; 0-9622815; 1-57966; 1-880216; 1-881320),* 1719 Mulberry St, PMB 551, Montgomery, AL 36106 (SAN 631-4910) Tel 334-265-6753; Fax: 334-265-8880; Toll Free: 877-408-7078 ; *Imprints:* Elliott Clark (Elliott & Clark) Starrhill Press (Starrhill Press)
E-mail: sales@rivercitypublishing.com
Web site: http://www.rivercitypublishing.com.

†Rivercross Pub, *(Rivercross Publishing, Inc.; 0-944957; 1-58141),* 6214 Wynfield Ct., Orlando, FL 32819 (SAN 245-6826) Tel 407-876-7720; Fax: 407-876-7758; Toll Free: 800-451-4522
Web site: http://www.rivercross.com; *CIP.*

Riverhead Books Imprint of Putnam Pub Group

Riverhse Lit Creat, *(Riverhouse Literary Creations, Inc.; 0-9638111),* 11524 Mississippi Dr., N., Champlin, MN 55316-2507 Tel 612-422-9681.

Rivers Oram (GBR) *(0-04; 0-86358; 1-85489) Dist. by* **NYU Pr.**

Riverstone, *(Riverstone Pr.; 0-9601130),* 434 W. Roscoe, Suite 14-D, Chicago, IL 60657 (SAN 210-2641) Tel 773-472-2501 Do not confuse with companies with similar names in Meridian, ID, Golden, CO
E-mail: ashafton@aol.com.

Rivijon Pr, *(Rivijon Pr.; 0-942937),* 1093 Aia Beach Blvd., No. 390, Saint Augustine, FL 32084 (SAN 667-8300).

†Rizzoli Intl, *(Rizzoli International Pubns., Inc.; 0-8478),* Subs. of RCS Rizzoli Editore Corp., 300 Park Ave., S., 3rd Flr., New York, NY 10010 (SAN 111-9192) Tel 212-387-3400; Fax: 212-387-3535
Dist(s): **St Martin** *(St. Martin's Pr., LLC)*
VHPS *(VHPS Holtzbrinck Pubs.); CIP.*

RJ Assocs, *(R/J Assocs.; 0-9602090),* 564 Tyler Ave., Livermore, CA 94550 (SAN 212-1352) Tel 510-443-7140.

R&M Pub Co, *(R&M Publishing Co.; 0-936026),* P.O. Box 1276, Holly Hill, SC 29059 (SAN 213-6392) Tel 706-738-0360 Do not confuse with the same or similar name in Foresthill, CA, Las Vegas, NV, Minnetonka, MN.

RMI, *(RMI Corp.; 0-910117),* 30 Boston Post Rd., Wayland, MA 01778-2400 (SAN 240-835X).

Rnd Table Pr, *(Round Table Pr.; 1-882275),* Orders Addr.: P.O. Box 475, Southeastern, PA 19399; Edit Addr.: 261 Dayleview Rd., Berwyn, PA 19312 Tel 610-647-4235 Do not confuse with Round Table Pr., Boulder, CO.

Rndrs Wllns, *(Renders Wellness; 0-9711551),* 1540 Mays Landing Rd., Egg Harbor Township, NJ 08234 Tel 609-927-2292; Fax: 609-927-4414
E-mail: erendersnd@aol.com
Web site: http://www.naturalhealingdr.com
Dist(s): **Biblio Dist** *(Biblio Distribution Ctr.)*
Natl Bk Netwk *(National Bk. Network).*

RNIX, *(RNIX Co.; 0-9641407),* 6631 Lakehurst Ave., Dallas, TX 75230 Tel 214-368-1224.

Roadrunner Tech, *See* **Gila River**

Rob Briggs, *(Briggs, Robert Assocs.; 0-931191; 0-9609850),* P.O. Box 407, West Linn, OR 97068 (SAN 268-4632) Tel 503-655-7579; Fax: 503-657-4349
E-mail: rbawest@europa.com
Web site: http://www.skysociety.com
Dist(s): **Pubs Services** *(Publishers Services).*

Robbe Health Intl, *(Robbe Health International, Inc.; 0-9712221),* 5265 Cedar Lake Rd., No. 6-25, Boynton Beach, FL 33437 Tel 561-364-1719; Fax: 561-733-2130
Web site: http://www.robbehealth.com.

Robert D Keene, *(Keene, Robert D.; 1-58383),* 11405 Old Roswell Rd., Alpharetta, GA 30004-1863 (SAN 299-8696) Tel 770-475-1220; Fax: 770-442-9761; Toll Free: 800-334-5724
E-mail: thor96@aol.com; greg@ipractice.md
Web site: http://www.institute.md.

Roberts Pub Co, *(Roberts Publishing Co.; 0-931764),* 738 32nd St., S. E., Grand Rapids, MI 49548 Tel 616-245-1560; Fax: 616-245-1561 Do not confuse with companies with same or similar name in Green Lake, WI, Sacramento, CA, Harveys Lake, PA
E-mail: robertspublishingco@juno.com
Web site: http://www.scoliosishelp.com; http://www.scoliosishelp.org.

Roberts Rinehart, *(Rinehart, Roberts Pubs.; 0-911797; 0-943173; 1-57098; 1-57140; 1-879373),* Orders Addr.: 4720 Boston Way, Lanhan, MD 20706 Tel 301-459-3366; Toll Free Fax: 800-238-4650; Toll Free: 800-462-6420; Edit Addr.: c/o Rowman & Littlefield Publishing Group, 5360 Manhattan Cir., No. 101, Boulder, CO 80303 (SAN 264-3510) Tel 303-543-7835
E-mail: books@robertsrinehart.com
Web site: http://www.robertsrinehart.com
Dist(s): **Natl Bk Netwk** *(National Bk. Network)*
netLibrary CO *(netLibrary, Inc.).*

Robin & Russ, *(Robin & Russ Handweavers, Inc.; 1-56659),* 533 N. Adams St., McMinnville, OR 97128 (SAN 207-284X) Tel 503-472-5760; Fax: 503-472-8220; Toll Free: 800-932-8391.

Robson Bks (GBR) *(0-86051; 0-903895; 1-86105) Dist. by* **Parkwest Pubns.**

Rocin, *(Rocin Pr.; 0-9608304),* Div. of Rocin Laboratories, Inc., 120 Central Pk. S., Apt. 1F, New York, NY 10019-1508 (SAN 240-9550) Tel 212-355-0109.

Rock Found, *(Rock Foundations Pr.; 0-9673755),* Orders Addr.: P.O. Box 2307, Huntington, NY 11743 Tel 516-421-3372; Fax: 516-421-6340; Edit Addr.: 63 Glenna Little Trail, Huntington, NY 11743
E-mail: abandonment@erols.com
Web site: http://www.abandonmentrecovery.com
Dist(s): **Partners Pubs Grp** *(Partners Pubs. Group, Inc.).*

†**Rockefeller,** *(Rockefeller Univ. Pr.; 0-87470),* 1114 First Ave., New York, NY 10021 (SAN 203-3747) Tel 212-327-8572; Fax: 212-327-7944
Dist(s): **Paul & Co Pubs** *(Paul & Co. Pubs. Consortium, Inc.); CIP.*

Rockford Pr, *(Rockford Pr.; 0-9630940),* P.O. Box 8, Thousand Palms, CA 92276 Fax: 909-302-0949; Toll Free: 800-574-2437
Web site: http://www.drday.com.

Rockin Enter, *(Rockin Enterprises, Inc.; 0-9616081),* 211 E. Ontario, Suite 1110, Chicago, IL 60611 (SAN 698-0759) Tel 312-266-8505.

Rockport Pubs, *(Rockport Pubs.; 0-935603; 1-56496),* 33 Commercial St., Gloucester, MA 01930-5089 (SAN 696-236X) Tel 978-282-9590; Fax: 978-283-2742
E-mail: questions@rockpub.com
Web site: http://www.rockpub.com
Dist(s): **Advanced Global** *(Advanced Global Distribution Services)*
F & W Pubns Inc *(F&W Pubns., Inc.).*

Rocky Mtn Homeopathics, *(Rocky Mountain Homeopathics; 0-9619203),* Orders Addr.: P.O. Box 10265, Sedona, AZ 86336 (SAN 243-6337) Tel 520-282-9362; Fax: 520-282-1933; Edit Addr.: 100 El Camino, Sedona, AZ 86336
E-mail: life@sedona.net
Web site: http://www.alternative-health-4u.com
Dist(s): **New Leaf Dist** *(New Leaf Distributing Co., Inc.)*
Nutri-Books Corp *(Nutri-Bks. Corp.).*

Rocky Run, *(Rocky Run Publishing; 0-9636565),* Orders Addr.: P.O. Box 456, McLean, VA 22101; Edit Addr.: 1110 Cedrus Ln., McLean, VA 22102 Tel 703-759-0241
E-mail: rockyrunllc@aol.com.

†**Rodale Pr Inc,** *(Rodale Pr., Inc.; 0-87596; 0-87857; 1-57954),* 33 E. Minor St., Emmaus, PA 18098 (SAN 200-2477) Tel 610-967-5171; Fax: 215-967-8963; Toll Free: 800-527-8200 ; *Imprints:* Rodale Reach (Rodale Reach)
Web site: http://www.rodalepress.com
Dist(s): **Penguin Putnam** *(Penguin Putnam, Inc.)*
St Martin *(St. Martin's Pr., LLC)*
VHPS *(VHPS Holtzbrinck Pubs.); CIP.*

Rodale Reach Imprint of Rodale Pr Inc

Rodef Shalom Pr, *(Rodef Shalom Pr.; 0-929699),* 4905 Fifth Ave., Pittsburgh, PA 15213 (SAN 249-955X) Tel 412-621-6566; Fax: 412-621-5475
E-mail: wjacob@Pgh.net.

Rodmell Pr, *(Rodmell Pr.; 0-9627138; 1-930485),* 2147 Blake St., Berkeley, CA 94704-2715 Tel 510-841-3123; Fax: 510-841-3191; Toll Free: 800-841-3123
E-mail: rodmellprs@aol.com
Dist(s): **SCB Distributors** *(SCB Distributors).*

Rodopi, *(Rodopi; 90-5183; 90-420; 90-6203),* Orders Addr.: One Rockefeller Plaza, Suite 1420, New York, NY 10020 Tel 212-265-6360; Fax: 212-265-6402; Toll Free: 800-225-3998 (within the U.S.)
E-mail: orders-queries@rodopi.nl
Web site: http://www.rodopi.nl.

Roman Cath Bks, *(Roman Catholic Bks.; 0-912141; 1-929291),* Div. of Catholic Media Apostolate, Orders Addr.: P.O. Box 2286, Fort Collins, CO 80522 Tel 970-490-2735; Fax: 970-493-8781; Edit Addr.: P.O. Box 993, Ridgefield, CT 06877 (SAN 264-7877)
E-mail: bookpub@compuserve.com
Web site: http://www.booksforcatholics.com.

Romping Feet, *(Romping Feet Greetings; 1-886730),* Orders Addr.: P.O. Box 55332, Sherman Oaks, CA 91413 Tel 818-761-5494; Fax: 818-752-4212; Edit Addr.: 5055 Coldwater Canyon Ave., No. 207, Sherman Oaks, CA 91423.

Ron L Dawson, *(Dawson, Ron L.; 0-9647141),* 6720 Emerald St., Boise, ID 83704 Tel 208-375-9458; Fax: 208-378-0563.

Ronin Pub, *(Ronin Publishing; 0-914171; 1-57951),* P.O. Box 522, Berkeley, CA 94701 (SAN 287-5365) Tel 510-420-3669; Fax: 510-420-3672 Do not confuse with Ronin Publishing in Cambridge, MA
E-mail: orders@roninpub.com
Web site: http://www.roninpub.com
Dist(s): **Publishers Group** *(Publishers Group West).*

RonJon Pub, *(RonJon Publishing, Inc.; 1-56870),* 1001 S. Mayhill Rd., Denton, TX 76208 Tel 940-383-3060; Fax: 940-387-0505; Toll Free: 800-262-3060
E-mail: sales@ronjonpublishing.com
Web site: http://www.ronjonpublishing.com.

Rophe Pr, *(Rophe Pr.; 0-9650670),* 15227 Medella Cir., Rancho Murieta, CA 95683 Tel 775-852-0621
E-mail: cheryn@cheryn.com
Web site: http://www.cheryn.com.

Roscoe Pound Inst, *(Roscoe Pound Institute; 0-933067),* Affil. of Assn. of Trial Lawyers of America, 1050 31st St., NW, Washington, DC 20007 (SAN 689-7894) Tel 202-965-0355; Fax: 202-944-2843; Toll Free: 800-424-2725
E-mail: pound@atlahq.org
Web site: http://www.atla.org/rpf.ht.

Rose & Nefr Pr, *(Rose & Nefr Pr.; 1-877934),* 7307 W. Franklin Ave., Saint Louis Park, MN 55426 Tel 612-541-9827.

Rosebud Pubns, *(Rosebud Pubns.; 0-9663040),* Div. of Rosegud Management Group, Inc., 2371D Via Mariposa, W., Laguna Hills, CA 92653 Tel 714-829-0809; Fax: 714-829-0805 Do not confuse with Rosebud Publications, Baltimore, MD
Dist(s): **Ecology Res Intl** *(Ecology Resources International).*

†**Rosen Group,** *(Rosen Publishing Group, Inc., The; 0-8239),* a/o Dept. C234561, 29 E. 21st St., New York, NY 10010 (SAN 203-3720) Tel 212-777-3017; Fax: 212-777-0277; Toll Free: 800-237-9932 ; *Imprints:* PowerKids Pr (PowerKids Press)
E-mail: ginas@rosenpub.com
Web site: http://www.rosenpublishing.com
Dist(s): **Shens Bks** *(Shen's Bks.); CIP.*

†**Ross Bks,** *(Ross Bks.; 0-89496; 0-931272),* P.O. Box 4340, Berkeley, CA 94704 (SAN 209-5912) Tel 510-841-2474; Fax: 510-841-2695; Toll Free: 800-367-0930
E-mail: staff@rossbooks.com; sales@rossbooks.com
Web site: http://www.rossbooks.com; http://www.baldar.com; http://www.hdoinfo.com; *CIP.*

Ross Pub Co, *(Ross Publishing Co.; 0-9615202),* 1245 Sleepy Hollow Ln., Rockledge, FL 32955 (SAN 694-2903) Tel 407-633-0042.

Rothman Imprint of W S Hein

Rothrock & DAmore, *(Rothrock, R. & G. D'Amore; 0-9632602),* P.O. Box 1355, Morrisville, PA 19067 Tel 215-736-1266; Fax: 215-736-1986
Dist(s): **Baker & Taylor** *(Baker & Taylor Bks.).*

Roundtable Pr, *(Roundtable Pr.; 0-934512),* 4 Linden Sq., Wellesley, MA 02482-4709 (SAN 282-2628) Tel 781-235-5320; Fax: 781-237-2842; Toll Free: 800-726-5320 (orders) Do not confuse with Roundtable Pub., Malibu, CA.

Roundtable Pub, *(Roundtable Publishing; 0-915677),* P.O. Box 6488, Malibu, CA 90264-6488 (SAN 237-9260) Tel 310-457-8433 Do not confuse with Roundtable Publishing, Mesa, AZ.

Rourke Pr, *(Rourke Pr., Inc.; 1-57103),* Div. of Rourke Publishing Group, P.O. Box 3328, Vero Beach, FL 32964 Tel 561-234-6001; Fax: 561-234-6622.

Route Sixty-Six, *(Route 66 Publishing, Ltd.; 0-9644293),* Orders Addr.: P.O. Box 25222, Albuquerque, NM 87125-5222 Tel 505-266-6128; Fax: 505-341-2608; Toll Free: 800-687-2665
E-mail: bren&ric@aol.com.

†**Routledge,** *(Routledge; 0-04; 0-413; 0-415; 0-7100; 0-86861; 0-87830),* Mem. of Taylor & Frances Group, Orders Addr.: 7625 Empire Dr., Florence, KY 41042 (SAN 631-2144) Toll Free Fax: 800-248-4724 (orders, customer serv.); Toll Free: 800-634-7064 (orders, customer serv.); Edit Addr.: 29 W. 35th St., New York, NY 10001-2299 Tel 212-216-7800; Fax: 212-564-7854 ; *Imprints:* Routledge Thoemms (Routledge/Thoemms Press) Spon (Spon Press)
E-mail: info@routledge-ny.com; cserve@routledge-ny.com
Web site: http://www.routledge-ny.com
Dist(s): **Taylor & Francis** *(Taylor & Francis, Inc.)*
netLibrary CO *(netLibrary, Inc.); CIP.*

Routledge Thoemms Imprint of Routledge

Rovern Pr, *(Rovern Pr.; 0-943150),* 180 Birch St., Willimantic, CT 06226-2108 (SAN 240-7620) Tel 860-456-1500; Toll Free: 800-391-2929.

Rowe Rehab, *(Rowe Rehabilitation & Consultation; 0-9666080),* P.O. Box 703, Brookings, SD 57006 Tel 605-692-3903
E-mail: rrehab@brookings.net.

†**Rowman,** *(Rowman & Littlefield Pubs., Inc.; 0-8476; 0-87471; 0-7425),* Div. of University Press of America, P.O. Box 191, Blue Ridge Summit, PA 17214-0191 Tel 717-794-3800; Fax: 717-794-3801; Orders Addr.: 15200 NBN Way, Blue Ridge Summit, PA 17214 Toll Free Fax: 800-338-4550; Toll Free: 800-462-6420; 67 Mowat Ave., Suite 241, Toronto, ON M6K 3E3 Tel 416-534-1660; Fax: 416-534-3699; Edit Addr.: 4720 Boston Way, Lanham, MD 20706 (SAN 203-3704) Tel 301-459-3366; Fax: 301-459-2118
E-mail: Rogers@univpress.com
Web site: http://www.rowmanlittlefield.com
Dist(s): **Natl Bk Netwk** *(National Bk. Network)*
Univ Pub Assocs *(University Publishing Assocs., Inc.); CIP.*

Roxbury Pk Juvenile Imprint of Lowell Hse Juvenile

Roxbury Pub Co, *(Roxbury Publishing Co.; 0-935732; 1-891487; 1-931719),* Orders Addr.: P.O. Box 491044, Los Angeles, CA 90049-9044 (SAN 213-6422) Tel 310-473-3312; Fax: 310-473-4490; Edit Addr.: 2034 Cotner Ave., 3rd Flr., Los Angeles, CA 90025
E-mail: roxbury@roxbury.net
Web site: http://www.roxbury.net.

Royal Botnic Grdns (GBR) *(0-947643; 1-900347; 0-85521; 1-84246) Dist. by* **Balogh.**

Royal Coll Psych (GBR) *(0-902241; 1-901242) Dist. by* **Balogh.**

Royal Historical Soc Imprint of Boydell & Brewer

Royal Netherlands Acad (NLD) *(0-444) Dist. by* **Elsevier.**

Royal Soc Chem (GBR) *(0-85186; 0-85404; 0-85990; 0-901886; 1-870343) Dist. by* **Spr-Verlag.**

Royal Soc of Medicine Pr Ltd (GBR) *(0-905958; 0-9501555; 1-85315) Dist. by* **Balogh.**

Royal Tropical (NLD) *(90-6832) Dist. by* **Stylus Pub VA.**

†**Rprt Serv,** *(Reprint Services Corp.; 0-7812; 0-932051),* P.O. Box 890820, Temecula, CA 92589-0820 (SAN 686-2640) Tel 909-296-3388; Fax: 909-767-0133; Toll Free: 800-273-6635
Web site: http://www.reprintservices.com; *CIP.*

RSA Pubns, *(RSA Pubns.; 0-9630191),* Div. of Radiation Safety Assocs., Inc., Orders Addr.: P.O. Box 19, Hebron, CT 06248 Tel 860-228-0824; Fax: 860-228-4402; Edit Addr.: 19 Pendleton Dr., Hebron, CT 06248.

Rsch Assocs, *See* **Meyers Pub**

RTR Publng, *See* **Red Toad Rd**

Rubbers Bros Comics, *(Rubbers Bros. Comics, The AIDS Prevent Pubns. & Seminars; 1-880058),* Orders Addr.: c/o Peter Mozeleski, 601 Starkey Rd., No. 77, Largo, FL 33771-2862 Tel 727-531-8410; Edit Addr.: c/o Paul Mozeleski, 72 Grand Ave., Vernon, CT 06066 Tel 860-870-3804.

Rube Pubns, *(Rube Pubns., Inc.; 0-911603),* Orders Addr.: P.O. Box 665, Port Jefferson, NY 11777 (SAN 696-5083) Tel 516-331-4990; Edit Addr.: 1 Buena Vista Rd., Port Jefferson, NY 11777 (SAN 263-9939).

Rudd Fuller, *See* **Parents Pipeline**

Rudi Pub, *(Rudi Publishing; 0-945213),* 12 Geary St., Suite 508, San Francisco, CA 94108 (SAN 246-5973) Tel 415-392-6940; Fax: 415-392-6942; Toll Free: 800-999-6901
E-mail: rudi3@ix.netcom.com
Web site: http://www.rudipublishing.com.

Rudra Pr, *(Rudra Pr.; 0-915801),* P.O. Box 13310, Portland, OR 97213-0390 (SAN 294-1260) Tel 503-231-0346; Fax: 503-236-9878; Toll Free: 800-876-7798
E-mail: sharon@europa.com
Web site: http://www.rudrapress.com.

Ruka Pubns, *(Ruka Pubns.; 0-915178),* 4300 N. Rodeo Qulch Rd., Soquel, CA 95073 (SAN 207-768X) Tel 408-475-0865.

†Running Pr, *(Running Pr. Bk. Pubs.; 0-7624; 0-89471; 0-914294; 1-56138),* 125 S. 22nd St., Philadelphia, PA 19103-4399 (SAN 204-5702) Tel 215-567-5080; Fax: 215-568-2919; Toll Free Fax: 800-453-2884; Toll Free: 800-345-5359 customer service
E-mail: support@runningpress.com
Web site: http://www.runningpress.com
Dist(s): **Hungry Minds** *(Hungry Minds, Inc.); CIP.*

Russ Info & Busn Ctr, *See* **Intl Business Pubns**

Russell Sage, *(Russell Sage Foundation; 0-87154),* 112 E. 64th St., New York, NY 10021 (SAN 202-1862) Tel 212-750-6038; Fax: 212-371-4761; Toll Free: 800-666-2211
E-mail: pubs@rsage.org
Web site: http://www.russellsage.org
Dist(s): **CUP Services** *(CUP Services).*

Russo (RUS) *(5-88037; 5-88721) Dist. by* **Coronet Bks.**

Rutgers Ctr Alcohol, *(Rutgers Ctr. of Alcohol Studies Pubns.; 0-911290),* Div. of Alcohol Research Documentation, Inc., Rutgers State Univ. of New Jersey, 607 Allison Rd., Piscataway, NJ 08854-8001 (SAN 203-3658) Tel 732-445-2190; Fax: 732-445-3500
E-mail: chrouse@rci.rutgers.edu
Web site: http://www.rci.rutgers.edu/~cas2.

†Rutgers U Pr, *(Rutgers Univ. Pr.; 0-8135),* 100 Joyce Kilmer Ave., Piscataway, NJ 08854-8099 (SAN 253-2115) Tel 732-445-7762; Fax: 732-445-7039; Toll Free Fax: 888-471-9014; Toll Free: 800-446-9323 (orders)
Web site: http://rutgerspress.rutgers.edu; *CIP.*

Rutledge Bks, *(Rutledge Bks., Inc.; 0-9643937; 1-58244; 1-887750),* 107 Mill Plain Rd., Suite 302, Danbury, CT 06811 Tel 203-778-5925; Fax: 203-798-7272; Toll Free: 800-278-8533
E-mail: rutbooks@aol.com
Web site: http://www.rutledgebooks.com
Dist(s): **Baker & Taylor** *(Baker & Taylor Bks.).*

Rutledge Hill Pr, *(Rutledge Hill Pr.; 0-934395; 1-55853; 1-4016),* 501 Nelson Pl., Nashville, TN 37214 Tel 615-889-9000; Toll Free: 800-251-4000
E-mail: NelsonDirect@ThomasNelson.com
Web site: http://www.rutledgehillpress,com.

Ryan Research, *(Ryan Research International; 0-942158),* 51 Skymountain Cir., Chico, CA 95928-6309 (SAN 239-9776) Tel 916-343-2373.

Ryandic Pub, *(Ryandic Publishing, Inc.; 0-9625272),* 656 Riverpark Cir., Longwood, FL 32779 Tel 407-897-1801.

S & D, *(Smith & Daniel; 0-9630463; 1-889668),* 7324 Atlantic Blvd., Jacksonville, FL 32211 Tel 904-724-9113; Fax: 904-724-9119; Toll Free: 800-330-1325.

S & J Books, *(S&J Bks.; 0-9609608),* Orders Addr.: P.O. Box 276092, Boca Raton, FL 33427-6092 (SAN 260-2598) Tel 561-395-4231.

S & J Unltd, *(S&J Unlimited; 1-881201),* Orders Addr.: P.O. Box 1249, Orville, WA 98844-1249.

S&S Trade, *(Simon & Schuster Trade; 0-671; 0-684; 0-689; 0-914676; 0-7432),* Div. of Simon & Schuster, Inc., Orders Addr.: 100 Front St., Riverside, NJ 08075 (SAN 200-2442) Toll Free Fax: 800-943-9831; Toll Free: 800-223-2348 (customer service); 800-223-2336 (ordering); Edit Addr.: 1230 Avenue of the Americas, New York, NY 10020 (SAN 200-2450) Tel 212-698-7000; Fax: 212-698-7007; Toll Free: 800-897-7650 (customer financial services)
E-mail: ssonline_feedback@simonsays.com; consumer.customerservice@simonandschuster.com
Web site: http://www.simonandschuster.com/ebooks; http://www.oasis.simonandschuster.com; http://www.simonsays.com
Dist(s): **IPG Chicago** *(Independent Pubs. Group)*
Large Print Library *(Large Print Library Discounter)*
Penguin Putnam *(Penguin Putnam, Inc.)*
Rdrs Digest *(Reader's Digest Children's Publishing, Inc.)*
T T Beeler *(Beeler, Thomas T. Publisher).*

S&S Trade Pap, *(Simon & Schuster Trade Paperbacks; 0-684),* Div. of Simon & Schuster Trade, Orders Addr.: 100 Front St., Riverside, NJ 08075 Toll Free Fax: 800-943-9831; Toll Free: 800-223-2336; Edit Addr.: 1230 Avenue of the Americas, New York, NY 10020 Tel 212-698-7000; Fax: 212-698-7007 ; *Imprints:* Fireside (Fireside) Libros en Espanol (Libros en Espanol) Scribner Pap Fic (Scribner Paperback Fiction) Touchstone (Touchstone Books)
Web site: http://www.simonandschuster.com.

S Asia, *(South Asia Bks.; 0-8364; 0-88386),* P.O. Box 502, Columbia, MO 65205 (SAN 207-4044) Tel 573-474-0116; Fax: 573-474-8124 ; *Imprints:* Commonwealth (Commonwealth)
E-mail: sabooks@juno.com
Web site: http://www.southasiabooks.com.

S Bayle, *(Bayle, Susan; 0-9667440),* 424 W. Johnson Rd., Scottville, MI 49454 Tel 616-757-9308
E-mail: sbayle@t-one.net
Web site: http://www.t-one./~sbayle.

S Breer, *(Breer, Sally; 0-9665981),* Orders Addr.: P.O. Box 344, Sparkill, NY 10976 (SAN 253-8253) Tel 914-359-6254; Fax: 914-365-3117; Edit Addr.: 80 Sparkill Ave., Tappan, NY 10983-2211
E-mail: breerflax@aol.com.

S C Becker, *(Becker, Susan Cope; 0-9660058),* 2555 Newtown Rd., Cincinnati, OH 45244 Tel 513-231-9446; Fax: 513-231-9448; Toll Free: 800-775-9446
E-mail: scope2000@aol.com
Dist(s): **Baker & Taylor** *(Baker & Taylor Bks.)*
Dogwise Pubng *(Dogwise Publishing)*
Four-M Enterp *(Four-M Enterprises, Inc.).*

S C K Pubns, *(SCK Pubns.; 0-9653000),* P.O. Box 2125, Church Hill, TN 37642 Tel 423-357-8166.

S D A Pub, *(S.D.A. Publishing Co.; 0-9634084),* 20243 Vaughan, Detroit, MI 48219 (SAN 297-7516) Tel 313-533-2206.

S Dawson Pubs, *(Dawson, Sheffield Pub., Ltd.; 0-9668202),* 23 Murray Rd., Greenwood Lake, NY 10925 Tel 914-477-3303; Fax: 914-477-8541
E-mail: rapproth@aol.com.

S Deal Assoc, *(Deal, S. Assocs.; 0-930006),* 5128 Neeper Valley Rd., Manitou Springs, CO 80829-3862 (SAN 210-4105) Tel 719-685-9166 (phone/fax)
Dist(s): **R Hale & Co** *(Hale, Robert & Co., Inc.).*

S F I M M S Pr, *(SFIMMS Pr.; 0-615; 0-9701841),* 4104 24th St., Box 504, San Francisco, CA 94114 Fax: 415-750-5919; 415-456-5664; Toll Free: 800-746-8817
E-mail: sfimms@wenet.net
Web site: http://www.wenet.net/~sfimms.

S F Vanni, *(Vanni, S.F.; 0-913298),* 30 W. 12th St., New York, NY 10011-8691 (SAN 220-0031) Tel 212-675-6336.

S Freud RT&PF, *(Freud, S. Romanian Translation & Pubn. Fund, Inc.; 1-883881),* One Marine Midland Plaza, E. Tower, 4th Flr., Binghamton, NY 13901-3216.

S Fried, *See* **TALKAIDS**

S Hunter, *(Hunter, Skip; 0-9649873),* P.O. Box 61, Clemson, SC 29633 Tel 803-654-3800; Fax: 803-654-4006.

†S Ill U Pr, *(Southern Illinois Univ. Pr.; 0-8093),* Div. of Southern Illinois Univ., Orders Addr.: P.O. Box 3697, Carbondale, IL 62902-3697 (SAN 203-3623) Tel 618-453-6624; Fax: 618-453-1221; Toll Free: 800-346-2680; Edit Addr.: 200 McLafferty Rd., Carbondale, IL 62902-3623 Toll Free Fax: 800-346-2681
Web site: http://www.siu.edu/~siupress; *CIP.*

S K Kakar, *(Kakar, Sharwan Kumar; 0-9638976),* 37 June Ave., Bayville, NY 11709 Tel 516-628-1845.

S Karger, *(Karger, S. AG; 3-8055),* 26 W. Avon Rd., Farmington, CT 06085 (SAN 281-8531) Tel 860-675-7834; Fax: 860-675-7302; Toll Free: 800-828-5479; Allschwilerstr 10, Basel, 4009 Tel 0761 452070; Fax: 0761 4520714
E-mail: karger@snet.net.
Web site: http://www.karger.com.

S L C Pubns, *(S.L.C. Pubns.; 0-9653267),* 1612 Blaine Ave., Salt Lake City, UT 84105 Tel 801-483-2911; Fax: 801-483-2059.

S M Derrick, *(Derrick, Sara M.),* 1323 Johnson St., Sandusky, OH 44870 (SAN 283-9881) Tel 419-625-1893.

S M P F Inc, *(Scientific & Medical Pubns. of France, Inc.),* 100 E. 42nd St., Suite 1002, New York, NY 10017 (SAN 169-5940) Tel 212-983-6278.

S Masley, *See* **Vitality Bks**

S N A P, *(S.N.A.P., Inc.; 1-881671),* Orders Addr.: P.O. Box 574, San Anselmo, CA 94979; Edit Addr.: 72 Yolanda Dr., San Anselmo, CA 94960 Tel 415-453-6029 (phone/fax).

S Paul (GBR) *(0-09) Dist. by* **Trafalgar.**

S R Sprague, *(Sprague, Stephen R.; 0-9713426),* P.O. Box 140676, Staten Island, NY 10314-0676
E-mail: spraguecml@aol.com.

S Rubenfeld, *(Rubenfeld, Sheldon; 0-9660398),* 3122 Robinhood, Houston, TX 77005 Tel 713-661-6999; Fax: 713-661-7007
E-mail: zlotty@aol.com.

S Schupp, *(Schupp, S.; 0-9617405),* 27539 Londick, Burr Oak, MI 49030 (SAN 663-9801) Tel 616-384-7657.

S Stafford, *(Stafford, Shirley; 0-9607580),* 12424 Oliva Rd., San Diego, CA 92128-3124 (SAN 239-9806).

S Wilson, *(Wilson, Stuart; 0-9626846),* 616 Allview Pl., Laguna Beach, CA 92651 Tel 949-497-1825.

SA Literature, *(SA Literature; 0-9622887),* Orders Addr.: P.O. Box 111910, Nashville, TN 37222-1910 Tel 615-331-6230; Fax: 615-331-6901; Edit Addr.: 4813 Nolensville Rd., Suite 114, Nashville, TN 37222
Web site: http://www.sa.org.

SAA Pubn Dept (IND) *(81-7058; 81-7060) Dist. by* **Lotus Pr.**

SABA Bks, *(SABA Bks.; 0-9705464),* P.O. Box 5265, Bluewater Bay, FL 32578-5265 Tel 850-897-8261; Fax: 850-897-8271
E-mail: sallieburdine@aol.com
Dist(s): **BookWorld** *(BookWorld Services, Inc.).*

Sabolich Pros & Res, *(Sabolich Prosthetic & Research Ctr.; 0-9637331),* 4301 N. Classen, Oklahoma City, OK 73118 Tel 405-525-4000; Fax: 405-530-3672; Toll Free: 800-522-4428.

Sacrum Pr, *(Sacrum Pr.; 0-937543),* 145 Woodhaven Ridge, Athens, GA 30606 (SAN 659-1329) Tel 706-546-0378.

Sadhana Pubns, *(Sadhana Pubns.; 0-9656208),* Orders Addr.: P.O. Box 365, Floresville, TX 78114; Edit Addr.: 1903 Third St., Floresville, TX 78114 Tel 830-393-4182
Dist(s): **Lotus Pr** *(Lotus Pr.).*

Saetes & Saetes, *(Saetes & Saetes; 0-9646038),* 914 29th St., Sacramento, CA 95816 Tel 916-441-4826; Fax: 916-441-6427.

SAFE GOODS, *(SAFE GOODS/New Century Publishing 2000; 1-884820),* Orders Addr.: 60 Bullock Dr., Unit 6, Markham, ON L3P 3P2 Tel 860-824-5301; Fax: 860-824-0309; Toll Free: 888-628-8731; 561 Shunpike Rd., Sheffield, MA 01257
E-mail: info@SafeGoodsPub.com; safe@snet.net
Web site: http://www.safegoodspub.com
Dist(s): **Distributors** *(Distributors, The)*
Koen Bk Distributors *(Koen Bk. Distributors)*
New Leaf Dist *(New Leaf Distributing Co., Inc.)*
Nutri-Books Corp *(Nutri-Bks. Corp.).*

Safe Place Pub, *(Safe Place Publishing; 0-9626323),* Orders Addr.: P.O. Box 4411, Scottsdale, AZ 85261; Edit Addr.: 8260 E. Arabian Trail, Suite 257, Scottsdale, AZ 85261 Tel 602-991-8499.

Safer Soc, *(Safer Society Pr.; 1-884444),* Orders Addr.: P.O. Box 340, Brandon, VT 05733-0340 Tel 802-247-3132; Fax: 802-247-4233; Edit Addr.: 8-10 Conant Sq., Brandon, VT 05733-1121
Web site: http://www.safersociety.org.

Safety Now, *(Safety Now Co., Inc.; 0-917066),* P.O. Box 567, Jenkintown, PA 19046 (SAN 208-8355) Tel 215-884-0210.

SafetyCertified, *(SafetyCertified; 0-9632296; 1-890966),* 1202 Kongsley Ave., Orange Park, FL 32073 Tel 904-278-5155; Fax: 904-278-5494; Toll Free: 800-597-2040
E-mail: mmoran@safetycertified.com
Web site: http://www.safetycertified.com.

Sagacity Pr, *(Sagacity Pr.; 0-9648589),* 2800 NW 25th, Oklahoma City, OK 73107 Tel 405-947-3667 (phone/fax).

Sagamore Pub, *(Sagamore Publishing, Inc.; 0-915611; 1-57167; 1-58382),* 804 N. Neil St., Champaign, IL 61820-3015 (SAN 292-5788) Tel 217-359-5940; Fax: 217-359-5975; Toll Free: 800-327-5557 (orders only)
E-mail: books@sagamorepub.com
Web site: http://www.coacheschoice-pub.com; http://www.sagamorepub.com.

†Sage, *(Sage Pubns., Inc.; 0-7619; 0-8039),* 2455 Teller Rd., Thousand Oaks, CA 91320-2218 (SAN 204-7217) Tel 805-499-0721; Fax: 805-499-0871 ; *Imprints:* Sage Prdcls Pr (Sage Periodicals Press)
E-mail: info@sagepub.com
Web site: http://www.sagepub.com
Dist(s): **Baker & Taylor** *(Baker & Taylor Bks.)*
Red Toad Rd *(Red Toad Road Co.)*
Yankee Bk Peddler Inc *(Yankee Bk. Peddler, Inc.); CIP.*

Sage Femme Pr, *(Sage Femme Pr.; 0-9673688),* 4100 W St., NW, No. 313, Washington, DC 20007 Tel 202-338-9623; P.O. Box 32124, Washington, DC 20007
E-mail: masson@erols.com.

Sage Prdcls Pr Imprint of Sage

Sage Pubng, *(Sage Publishing Productions; 0-9643340),* Orders Addr.: P.O. Box 2561, Mill Valley, CA 94942-2561 Tel 415-383-0659 (phone/fax)
E-mail: lhorn@ricochet.net.

Sagebrush UT, *(Sagebrush Pr.; 0-9703130),* 225 Tenth Ave., Salt Lake City, UT 84103-2529 Tel 801-363-6124 Do not confuse with companies with same name in Cedarville,CA, Morongo Valley, CA
E-mail: paulg@aros.net
Web site: http://www.sagebrushpress.com
Dist(s): **IPG Chicago** *(Independent Pubs. Group).*

Saguaro Pub AZ, *(Saguaro Publishing; 0-9659847),* P.O. Box 457, Litchfield Park, AZ 85340 Tel 623-935-1515 (phone/fax); Toll Free: 888-561-3095 Do not confuse with companies with the same name in Denver, CO, Phoenix, AZ
E-mail: saguaropub@aol.com
Web site: http://members.aol.com/saguaropub/website/htmls/home.html
Dist(s): **Brodart** *(Brodart Co.)*
Partners Pubs Grp *(Partners Pubs. Group, Inc.)*
Quality Bks IL *(Quality Bks., Inc.)*
Unique Bks Inc *(Unique Bks., Inc.).*

Sahuaro Pr, *(Sahuaro Pr.; 0-9660066),* 11675 N. 83rd Pl., Scottsdale, AZ 85260-5657 Tel 602-998-2183
E-mail: ngn@amug.org.

Saifer, *(Saifer, Albert Pub.; 0-87556),* P.O. Box 7125, Watchung, NJ 07060 (SAN 204-7225).

Saint George Pubns Imprint of R Steiner Col

Saint James Imprint of Gale

†Salem Pr, *(Salem Pr., Inc.; 0-89356; 1-58765),* Two University Plaza, Suite 121, Hackensack, NJ 07601 (SAN 241-841X) Tel 201-968-9899; Fax: 201-968-1411; Toll Free: 800-221-1592 ; *Imprints:* Magills Choice (Magill's Choice)
E-mail: csr@salempress.com
Web site: http://www.salempress.com
Dist(s): **netLibrary CO** *(netLibrary, Inc.); CIP.*

Sally Milner (AUS) *(0-646; 1-86351) Dist. by* **Seven Hills Bk.**

Sally Milner (AUS) *(0-646; 1-86351) Dist. by* **Sterling.**

Samhita Enterprises, *(Samhita Enterprises, Inc.; 1-57582),* 183 Saint Paul St., Suite 301, Rochester, NY 14604 Fax: 716-546-4746; Toll Free: 800-784-2773
E-mail: ayurveda@samhita.com
Web site: http://samhita.com.

Samhita Prodns, *(Samhita Productions; 1-929297),* 1537 Union St., Schenectady, NY 12309 Tel 518-377-1149; Fax: 518-393-6301; Toll Free: 888-603-9171
E-mail: mavhc@aol.com
Web site: http://www.allhealthyfamily.com.

Sams, *(Sams; 0-672; 0-8104),* Div. of Macmillan USA, 201 W. 103rd St., Indianapolis, IN 46290-1097 (SAN 219-6298) Tel 317-581-3500; Toll Free: 800-428-5331 (orders)
Web site: http://www.macmillan.com
Dist(s): **Mac USA** *(Macmillan USA)*
Sams Tech Pub *(Sams Technical Publishing).*

San Francisco Pr, *(San Francisco Pr., Inc.; 0-911302),* 660 Spruce St., Berkeley, CA 94707 (SAN 207-4990)
E-mail: SFPress_Inc@Yahoo.com.

Sanctuary Comns, *See* **Sanctuary Unltd**

Sanctuary Unltd, *(Sanctuary Unlimited; 0-9620318),* P.O. Box 25, Dennisport, MA 02639 (SAN 248-6962) Tel 508-790-8485
Dist(s): **New Leaf Dist** *(New Leaf Distributing Co., Inc.).*

Sandbird Pub, *(Sandbird Publishing Group of Chapel Hill, The; 0-9615111),* P.O. Box 56, Carrboro, NC 27510-0056 (SAN 694-1540) Tel 919-968-3249.

SandKey, *(SandKey Co., Inc.; 0-9618821; 1-887202),* Orders Addr.: P.O. Box 3068, Syracuse, NY 13220 (SAN 242-4037) Tel 315-455-7862; Fax: 315-454-8119; Toll Free: 800-846-6687 Do not confuse with Prestige Pubs., Portland, OR
E-mail: orders@prestigepublishing.com
Web site: http://www.prestigepublishing.com.

Sandness, *(Sandness, Robert C.; 0-9614076),* 321 Beaumont, Las Vegas, NV 89106 (SAN 685-9712) Tel 702-382-3796.

Sandra Pubns, *(Sandra Pubns.; 0-9635824),* Div. of Business Builders Consulting Group, Inc., 39 Brenton Ave., Providence, RI 02906 Tel 401-751-0120; Fax: 401-751-7955; Toll Free: 800-346-3287.

Sandridge Pub, *(Sandridge Publishing Co.; 0-945080),* P.O. Box 5006, Bloomington, IN 47407 (SAN 245-825X) Tel 812-339-2825; Fax: 812-339-0540
Dist(s): **Quality Bks IL** *(Quality Bks., Inc.).*

Sanicula Pr Imprint of Rainlight Bk

Sankofa Pr, *(Sankofa Pr.; 0-9654009),* Orders Addr.: P.O. Box 3144, Jacksonville, FL 32206 Tel 904-355-0126 (phone/fax); Edit Addr.: 239 W. 40th St., Jacksonville, FL 32206
E-mail: sankofa@leading.net
Web site: http://www.users.southeast.net/~sankofa.

Sankofa Prods, *See* **Sankofa Pr**

Santa Fe Health, *(Santa Fe Health Education Project; 0-9622933),* P.O. Box 577, Santa Fe, NM 87504-0577 Tel 505-982-3236.

Santee Pub, *(Santee Publishing Co.; 0-9661796),* Orders Addr.: 615 E. Lexington Ave., El Cajon, CA 92020 Tel 619-687-4209; Edit Addr.: 202 S. Ivory Ave., El Cajon, CA 92019-1983 Tel 619-441-2821 (phone/fax)
E-mail: miyarespip@aol.com.

Sanuk, *(SANUK, Inc.; 1-878394),* P.O. Box 140777, Lakewood, CO 80214 Tel 303-616-0197.

Saphrograph, *(Saphrograph Corp.; 0-87557),* 4910-12 Fort Hamilton Pkwy., Brooklyn, NY 11219 (SAN 110-4128) Tel 718-331-1233; Fax: 718-372-8890.

Sarasota Press, *(Sarasota Pr.; 1-55356),* Div. of Key Porter Bks., 4808 S. Tamiami Trail, PMB 205, Sarasota, FL 34231-4352 Tel 941-758-8094; Fax: 941-753-9396; Toll Free Fax: 800-777-2525; Toll Free: 800-444-2524
Dist(s): **BookWorld** *(BookWorld Services, Inc.).*

Sarasota Sci, *(Sarasota Scientific Pr.; 0-9614464),* 2519 Sesame St., Sarasota, FL 34231 (SAN 689-433X) Tel 941-922-0604.

Sarat (IND) *Dist. by* **S Asia.**

Sargasso Ent, *(Sargasso Enterprises; 0-9635554),* 14 Wildwood St., Winchester, MA 01890 Tel 781-729-9037; Fax: 781-729-2726
E-mail: cak@sargasso.ne.mediaone.net
Web site: http://www.krumme.com
Dist(s): **Baker & Taylor** *(Baker & Taylor Bks.)*
Unique Bks Inc *(Unique Bks., Inc.).*

SAS Inc, *(SAS, Inc.; 0-9659846),* 2883 Farmington Cir., SW, Canton, OH 44706 Tel 330-478-1632 Do not confuse with companies with the same or similar name in Cary, NC, Knoxville, TN
Web site: http://www.Bookwire.com.

SAS Inst, *See* **SAS Publ**

SAS Publ, *(SAS Publishing; 0-917382; 1-55544; 1-58025; 1-59047),* SAS Campus Dr., Cary, NC 27513-2414 (SAN 208-8347) Tel 919-677-8000; Fax: 919-677-4444; Toll Free: 800-727-3228 (book orders only) Do not confuse with companies with the same or similar name in Canton, OH, Knoxville, TN
E-mail: pubs@sas.com
Web site: http://www.sas.com/pubs.

Sasquatch Bks, *(Sasquatch Bks.; 0-912365; 1-57061),* 615 Second Ave., Suite 260, Seattle, WA 98104 (SAN 289-0208) Tel 206-467-4300 (ext 300); Fax: 206-467-4301; Toll Free: 800-775-0817
E-mail: books@sasquatchbooks.com
Web site: http://www.sasquatchbooks.com
Dist(s): **Publishers Group** *(Publishers Group West).*

Saturn Press, *(Saturn Pr., Inc.; 1-885843),* 17639 Foxborough Ln., Boca Raton, FL 33496 Tel 561-477-6602; Fax: 561-477-7909 Do not confuse with Saturn Press in Ann Arbor, MI
E-mail: drlevison@saturnpress.com
Web site: http://www.saturnpress.com.

Satyam Pub, *(Satyam Publishing; 0-9641323),* 396 Ventura Ave., Palu Alto, CA 94306-3453 Tel 707-224-2909.

†Saunders, *(Saunders, W. B. Co.; 0-03; 0-15; 0-7216),* Div. of Harcourt, Inc., A Harcourt Health Sciences Co., Orders Addr.: 6277 Sea Harbor Dr., Orlando, FL 32887 (SAN 244-8106) Toll Free: 800-654-2452; Edit Addr.: 150 S. Independence Mall W. The Public Ledger Bldg., Suite 1250, Philadelphia, PA 19106-3412 (SAN 203-266X) Tel 215-238-5500 ; *Imprints:* Grune & Strat (Grune & Stratton, Incorporated)
Web site: http://www.wbsaunders.com; *CIP.*

Saunders Ents, *(Saunders Enterprises; 0-9666146),* 1700 N. Racine St., Appleton, WI 54911 Tel 920-733-9178.

Saunders Grp, *(Saunders Group, Inc., The; 0-9616461; 1-879190),* 4250 Norex Dr., Chaska, MN 55318-3047 (SAN 630-2750) Tel 612-368-9214; Fax: 612-368-9249; Toll Free: 800-456-1289
E-mail: sales@thesaundersgroup.com
Web site: http://www.thesaundersgroup.com.

SBC SBC, *(SBC/SBC, Inc.; 0-9621398),* 826 Glendover, Lexington, KY 40502 (SAN 251-1711) Tel 859-266-6317; Fax: 859-266-3949.

Scandia Pubs, *(Scandia Pubs.; 0-937242),* Orders Addr.: 11594 Willamette Meridian NW, Silverdale, WA 98383 (SAN 282-2806) Tel 360-337-7688; Fax: 360-337-7602
E-mail: dorieerick@cs.com.

Scanning Microscopy, *(Scanning Microscopy International; 0-931288),* P.O. Box 66507, AMF O'Hare, Chicago, IL 60666 (SAN 213-5868) Fax: 847-985-6698
E-mail: 73211.647@compuserve.com.

†Scarecrow, *(Scarecrow Pr., Inc.; 0-8108; 1-57886),* Div. of Rowman & Littlefield Publishing Group, Orders Addr.: 15200 NBN Way, Blue Ridge Summit, PA 17214 Tel 717-794-3800; Fax: 717-794-3803; Toll Free Fax: 800-338-4550; Toll Free: 800-462-6420; Edit Addr.: 4720 Boston Way, Lanham, MD 20706-4310 (SAN 203-2651) Tel 301-459-3366; Fax: 301-459-1705; Toll Free Fax: 800-338-4550; Toll Free: 800-462-6420
E-mail: orders@scarecrowpress.com
Web site: http://www.scarecrowpress.com
Dist(s): **Rowman** *(Rowman & Littlefield Pubs., Inc.); CIP.*

SCB, *(SCB/J. Elliott; 0-9658646),* Orders Addr.: P.O. Box 2574, Kingston, NY 12402 Tel 914-338-6368; Fax: 914-339-5881; Edit Addr.: 10 Guyton St., Kingston, NY 12401-1704
E-mail: jelliotsoy@aol.com
Dist(s): **New Leaf Dist** *(New Leaf Distributing Co., Inc.).*

SCB Distributors, *(SCB Distributors),* 15608 S. New Century Dr., Gardena, CA 90248-2129 (SAN 630-4818) Tel 310-532-9400; Fax: 310-532-7001; Toll Free: 800-729-6423 (orders only)
E-mail: aaron@scbdistributors.com; info@scbdistributors.com
Web site: http://www.scbdistributors.com.

SCCM Fullerton, *(Society of Critical Care Medicine; 0-936145),* 701 Lee St., Suite 200, Des Plains, IL 60016 (SAN 275-5505) Tel 847-827-6869
Web site: http://www.sccm.org.

†Schaumburg Pubns, *(Schaumburg Pubns., Inc.; 0-935690),* 1432 S. Mohawk, Schaumburg, IL 60193 (SAN 214-221X) Tel 847-352-2441; *CIP.*

Schaums Outline Imprint of McGraw-Hill Trade

†Schenkman Bks Inc, *(Schenkman Bks., Inc.; 0-87047; 0-87073),* 118 Main St., P.O. Box 119, Rochester, VT 05767 (SAN 203-2643) Tel 802-767-3702; Fax: 802-767-9528
E-mail: schenkma@sover.net
Web site: http://www.sover.net/~schenkma/
Dist(s): **Academic Bk Ctr Inc** *(Academic Bk. Ctr., Inc.)*
Baker & Taylor *(Baker & Taylor Bks.)*
New Leaf Dist *(New Leaf Distributing Co., Inc.); CIP.*

Schiffer, *(Schiffer Publishing, Ltd.; 0-7643; 0-88740; 0-916838),* 4880 Lower Valley Rd., Atglen, PA 19310 (SAN 208-8428) Tel 610-593-1777; Fax: 610-593-2002 ; *Imprints:* Whitford (Whitford Press)
E-mail: schifferii@aol.com
Web site: http://www.schifferbooks.com.

Schl Hse Pubns, *See* **Maier Pubns**

Schl Nat Med, *(School of Natural Medicine-Wisdome Pr.; 1-57093),* Orders Addr.: 3106 Umatilla St., Denver, CO 80211 Tel 303-455-8048; Fax: 303-964-8624; Edit Addr.: PMB 403, 2888 Bluff St., Boulder, CO 80301-1227 (SAN 298-0223) Tel 303-443-4882; Fax: 303-443-8276; Toll Free: 888-593-6173
E-mail: farida@purehealth.com
Web site: http://www.purehealth.com
Dist(s): **Baker & Taylor** *(Baker & Taylor Bks.)*
Bookpeople *(Bookpeople)*
New Leaf Dist *(New Leaf Distributing Co., Inc.)*
Nutri-Books Corp *(Nutri-Bks. Corp.).*

Schlutersche Verlags (DEU) *(3-87706) Dist. by* **Iowa U Pr.**

†Schocken, *(Schocken Bks., Inc.; 0-8052),* Div. of The Knopf Publishing Group, Orders Addr.: 400 Hahn Rd., Westminster, MD 21157 (SAN 202-5515) Tel 410-848-1900; Toll Free: 800-733-3000 (orders); Edit Addr.: 299 Park Ave., New York, NY 10171 (SAN 213-7585) Tel 212-572-2559; Fax: 212-572-6030
Web site: http://www.randomhouse.com/knopf/schocken/
Dist(s): **Pantheon** *(Pantheon Bks.); CIP.*

†Schol Am Res, *(School of American Research Pr.; 0-933452; 1-930618),* Orders Addr.: P.O. Box 2188, Santa Fe, NM 87504-2188 (SAN 212-6222) Tel 505-954-7261; Fax: 505-954-7241; Toll Free: 888-390-6070; Edit Addr.: 660 Garcia St., Santa Fe, NM 87504
E-mail: bkorders@sarsf.org
Web site: http://www.sarweb.org*; CIP.*

†Schol Facsimiles, *(Scholars' Facsimiles & Reprints; 0-8201),* Subs. of Academic Resources Corp., 410 Lenawee Dr., Ann Arbor, MI 48104 (SAN 203-2627) Tel 734-741-0344
E-mail: nm320@columbia.edu*; CIP.*

Scholar Educ Systs, *(Scholar Educational Systems, Inc.; 0-9655384),* 1550 Crofton Pkwy., Crofton, MD 21114 Tel 410-721-5466; Fax: 410-721-5466
Dist(s): **Majors Scientific Bks Inc** *(Majors Scientific Bks., Inc.)*
Rittenhouse *(Rittenhouse Bk. Distributors).*

†Scholarly, *(Scholarly Pr., Inc.; 0-403),* P.O. Box 160, Saint Clair Shores, MI 48080 (SAN 209-0473) Tel 810-231-3728 (phone/fax) ; *Imprints:* Regency (Regency Press)
Dist(s): **North Amer Bk** *(North American Bk. Distributors); CIP.*

†Scholarly Res Inc, *(Scholarly Resources, Inc.; 0-8420),* 104 Greenhill Ave., Wilmington, DE 19805-1897 (SAN 203-2619) Tel 302-654-7713; Fax: 302-654-3871; Toll Free: 800-772-8937 ; *Imprints:* SR Bks (S R Books)
E-mail: sr@scholarly.com; sales@scholarly.com; market@scholarly.com
Web site: http://www.scholarly.com
Dist(s): **Baker & Taylor** *(Baker & Taylor Bks.); CIP.*

Scholars Libr, *(Scholars Library; 0-9701997),* 328 Temperance Ave., Clovis, CA 93611 Tel 559-291-1458.

†Scholastic Inc, *(Scholastic, Inc.; 0-439; 0-590),* Subs. of SI Holdings, Inc., Orders Addr.: 2931 E. McCarty St., Jefferson City, MO 65101 Tel 573-636-5271; Toll Free Fax: 800-724-4716 (orders); Edit Addr.: 555 Broadway, New York, NY 10012-3999 (SAN 202-5442) Tel 212-343-6100; Fax: 212-343-6802; Toll Free: 800-325-6149 (customer service)
Web site: http://www.scholastic.com
Dist(s): **HarperCollins Pubs** *(HarperCollins Pubs.)*
Shens Bks *(Shen's Bks.); CIP.*

Scholium Intl, *(Scholium International, Inc.; 0-333; 0-87936),* P.O. Box 1519, Port Washington, NY 11050-0306 (SAN 169-5282) Tel 516-767-7171; Fax: 516-944-9824
E-mail: info@scholium.com
Web site: http://www.scholium.com.

Schoolsearch Pr, *(Schoolsearch Pr.; 0-9620326),* 127 Marsh St., Belmont, MA 02178 (SAN 248-2606) Tel 617-489-5785.

Schreiber Pub, *(Schreiber Publishing, Inc.; 1-887563),* 51 Monroe St., Suite 101, Rockville, MD 20850 (SAN 298-6876) Tel 301-424-7737; Fax: 301-424-2336; Toll Free: 800-822-3213
E-mail: spbooks@aol.com
Web site: http://www.schreibernet.com
Dist(s): **Baker & Taylor** *(Baker & Taylor Bks.)*
Natl Bk Netwk *(National Bk. Network)*
Quality Bks IL *(Quality Bks., Inc.).*

Schwarz Pub, *(Schwarz Publishing; 1-887417),* c/o Aletheia Institute, P.O. Box 2400, Mendocino, CA 95460-2400 Tel 707-937-0602; Fax: 707-937-0624
E-mail: aletheia@mcn.org
Web site: http://www.holisticu.org
Dist(s): **New Leaf Dist** *(New Leaf Distributing Co., Inc.).*

Sci & Behavior, *(Science & Behavior Bks., Inc.; 0-8314),* Orders Addr.: P.O. Box 60519, Palo Alto, CA 94306 (SAN 204-7349) Tel 650-965-0954; Fax: 650-965-8998; Toll Free: 800-547-9982; Edit Addr.: 2225 Grant Rd., No. 3, Los Altos, CA 94024
E-mail: sbbks@netgate.net
Web site: http://www.sbbks.com
Dist(s): **Baker & Taylor** *(Baker & Taylor Bks.)*
Bookpeople *(Bookpeople).*

Sci & Human Pr, *(Science & Humanities Pr.; 1-888725),* Subs. of Banis & Assocs., Orders Addr.: P.O. Box 7151, Chesterfield, MO 63006-7151 (SAN 299-8459) Tel 636-394-4950; Fax: 636-394-1381; Edit Addr.: 1023 Stuyvesant Ln., Manchester, MO 63011-3601 Tel 636-394-4950; Fax: 636-394-1381 ; *Imprints:* MacroPrintBks (MacroPrintBooks)
E-mail: sales@sciencehumanitiespress.com; pub@macroprintbooks.com; banis@banis-associates.com
Web site: http://www.stressmyth.com; http://www.normajeanebook.com; http://www.route66book.com; http://www.accessible-travel.com; http://www.banis-associates.com; http://www.sciencehumanitiespress.com; http://www.macroprintbooks.com
Dist(s): **T T Beeler** *(Beeler, Thomas T. Publisher).*

Sci Am Medicine, *(Scientific American Medicine; 0-89454),* Div. of Scientific American, Inc., 415 Madison Ave., New York, NY 10017 (SAN 678-0636) Tel 212-451-8824; Fax: 212-980-3062.

Sci Hist Imprint of Watson Pub Intl

Sci of Mind, *(Science of Mind Publishing; 0-911336; 0-917849),* Div. of United Church of Religious Science, Orders Addr.: P.O. Box 75127, Los Angeles, CA 90075-0127 (SAN 203-2570) Tel 213-388-2181; Fax: 213-388-1926; Edit Addr.: 3251 W. Sixth St., Los Angeles, CA 90075-0127
Web site: http://www.scienceofmind.com
Dist(s): **DeVorss** *(DeVorss & Co.).*

Sci People, *(Science for the People; 0-9607314),* P.O. Box 364, Somerville, MA 02143-0005 (SAN 218-3544).

Sci Pr (CHN) *(7-03) Dist. by* **Lubrecht & Cramer.**

Sci Pr NY, *(Science Pr. New York, Ltd.; 1-880132),* 84-04 58th Ave., Elmhurst, NY 11373 Tel 718-476-0238; Fax: 718-476-0273
E-mail: spnyltd@aol.com.

†Sci Ware, *(Scientific Software International, Inc.; 0-89498),* 7383 N. Lincoln Ave., Suite 100, Lincolnwood, IL 60712-1704 (SAN 209-9691) Tel 847-675-0720; Fax: 847-675-2140; Toll Free: 800-247-6113 (USA and Canada only)
E-mail: info@ssicentral.com
Web site: http://www.ssicentral.com*; CIP.*

Science Pubs, *(Science Pubs., Inc.; 1-57808; 1-881570; 1-886106),* Orders Addr.: c/o Enfield Distribution Co., P.O. Box 699, Enfield, NH 03748 Tel 603-632-7377; Fax: 603-632-5611; Edit Addr.: May St., Enfield, NH 03748
E-mail: info@scipub.net; enfield@connriver.net
Web site: http://www.scipub.net.

Scientific (GBR) *Dist. by* **St Mut.**

Scientific Pubs (IND) *Dist. by* **St Mut.**

Scinta, *(Scinta, Inc.; 0-917251),* 2421 Homestead Dr., Silver Spring, MD 20902 (SAN 656-1934) Tel 301-593-9478.

SciTech Pubs, *(SciTech Pubs., Inc.; 0-925760),* 56 Espanono Rd., Lake Hopatcong, NJ 07849 Do not confuse with Scitech Publishing, Inc., Mendham, NJ.

Sci-Thru-Media, *(Science-Thru-Media, Inc.; 0-918473),* Orders Addr.: P.O. Box 663, Millwood, NY 10546 (SAN 657-7156) Toll Free: 800-462-3883; Edit Addr.: 10 Taconic Rd., Millwood, NY 10546
E-mail: staff@sciencethrumedia.com.

SCJP Imprint of Truman St Univ

Scolar Pr (GBR) *(0-85417; 0-85967; 1-84014; 1-85928) Dist. by* **Ashgate Pub Co.**

Scopcraeft, *(Scopcraeft Pr.; 1-881604),* Orders Addr.: P.O. Box 1091, Portales, NM 88130 Tel 505-359-0901; Edit Addr.: 1400 S. Main Ave., Portales, NM 88130-6666 Tel 505-562-2532.

Scott-Townsend Pubs, *(Scott-Townsend Pubs.; 1-878465),* Subs. of Council for Social & Economic Studies, P.O. Box 34070, Washington, DC 20043 Tel 202-371-2700; Fax: 202-371-1523
E-mail: socecon@aol.com.

Scovill Paterson, *(Scovill, Paterson, Inc.; 1-879040),* P.O. Box 1725, Jacksonville, OR 97530-1725 ; *Imprints:* Radcliffe Med Pr (Radcliffe Medical Press) M Dunitz (Dunitz, Martin).

†SCP, *(Saunders College Publishing; 0-03),* Orders Addr.: 6277 Sea Harbor Dr., Orlando, FL 32887 (SAN 250-0086) Tel 407-345-2525; Toll Free: 800-782-4479 (orders); 800-544-6678 (customer service); Edit Addr.: The Public Ledger Bldg., 150 S. Independence Mall W., Suite 1250, Philadelphia, PA 19106-3412 (SAN 282-2768) Tel 215-238-5500
Web site: http://www.hbcollege.com*; CIP.*

SCP Rochester, *(Specialty Cookbooks Pubs.; 0-9623225),* 65 Gladmar Dr., Rochester, NY 14622 Tel 716-467-9867.

Scrbrough Hse Imprint of Madison Bks UPA

SCRDP, *(Stanford Ctr. for Research in Disease Prevention (SCRDP); 1-879552),* Div. of Health Promotion Resource Ctr., 730 Welch Rd., Suite B, Palo Alto, CA 94304 Tel 650-723-0003; Fax: 650-498-7775
E-mail: askscrdp@med.stanford.edu
Web site: http://www.med.stanford.edu/school/smysp/main.html.

Scribe Write, *(Scribe Write Bks.; 0-939909),* Subs. of Scribe Write, 102 Rolling Green Pl., Missoula, MT 59803 (SAN 661-454X) Tel 406-721-1424.

Scribner, *(Scribner; 0-684; 0-7432),* Div. of Simon & Schuster Trade, Orders Addr.: 100 Front St., Riverside, NJ 08075 Toll Free Fax: 800-943-9831; Toll Free: 800-223-2336; Edit Addr.: 1230 Avenue of the Americas, New York, NY 10020 ; *Imprints:* Lisa Drew (Drew, Lisa Books)
E-mail: ssonline_feedback@simonsays.com
Web site: http://www.simonsays.com/ebooks; http://www.simonsays.com
Dist(s): **S&S Trade** *(Simon & Schuster Trade).*

Scribner Pap Fic Imprint of S&S Trade Pap

Scripts Pub, *(Scripts Publishing; 1-889826),* Orders Addr.: 10603 N. W. 49th Pl., Coral Springs, FL 33076 Tel 954-341-8565; 954-346-8906; Fax: 954-753-6761
E-mail: pathamilto@aol.com
Web site: http://www.hometown.aol.com/pathamilto/myhomepage/howto.html.

Scrub Hill, *(Scrub Hill Pr., Inc.; 0-9645467),* 46 S. Glebe Rd., Suite 301, Arlington, VA 22204 Tel 301-469-8854 (phone/fax)
E-mail: johndavidgordon@erols.com
Web site: http://www.scrubhillpress.com
Dist(s): **J Majors Co** *(Majors, J. A. Co.)*
Matthews Medical Bk Co *(Matthews Medical Bk. Co.)*
Rittenhouse *(Rittenhouse Bk. Distributors).*

Scty Gastro, *(Society of Gastroenterology Nurses & Assocs./SGNA; 0-9702133),* 401 N. Michigan Ave., Suite 2400, Chicago, IL 60611-4267 Tel 312-321-5165; Fax: 312-527-6658; Toll Free: 800-245-7462
E-mail: SGNA@sba.com
Web site: http://www.sgna.org.

SDSU Coll Hlth Hum Servs, *(San Diego State Univ., College of Health & Human Services; 1-879167),* 5500 Campanile Dr., San Diego, CA 92182-4124 Tel 619-594-7102; Fax: 619-594-7103
E-mail: tshuman@mail.sdsu.edu.

†SDSU Press, *(San Diego State Univ. Pr.; 0-916304; 1-879691),* 5500 Campanile Dr., San Diego, CA 92182-8141 (SAN 202-0637) Tel 619-594-6220
E-mail: sheila.d@sdsu.edu*; CIP.*

SDSU Univ Ctr on Aging, *See* **SDSU Coll Hlth Hum Servs**

Sea Island, *(Sea Island Information Group; 1-877610),* 11022 Belton St., Upper Marlboro, MD 20772-1402 Tel 301-350-1360.

Sea to Sea, *(Sea to Sea Cookery; 0-9610600),* c/o Goodkind, S. Daisy Ln., Irvington, NY 10533 (SAN 264-6919) Tel 914-591-7558.

Seahorse Press, *(Seahorse Pr.; 0-9656501),* P.O. Box 38, Bath, ME 04530-1617 Fax: 207-442-7445; Toll Free: 888-442-7445
E-mail: SeahorsePress@gwi.net
Web site: http://www.gwi.net/SeahorsePress.

SEAK, *(SEAK, Inc.; 0-9652197; 1-892904),* Orders Addr.: P.O. Box 729, Falmouth, MA 02540 Tel 508-457-5486; 508-548-7023; Fax: 508-540-8304; Edit Addr.: 316 Gifford St., Falmouth, MA 02540
E-mail: cjtodd@seak.com; mbison126@aol.com
Web site: http://www.seak.com.

Seal Pr Feminist, *See* **Seal Pr WA**

†**Seal Pr WA,** *(Seal Pr.; 0-931188; 1-58005; 1-878067),* 3131 Western Ave., Suite 410, Seattle, WA 98121-1028 (SAN 215-3416) Tel 206-283-7844; Fax: 206-285-9410; Toll Free: 800-788-3123 Do not confuse with Seal Pr. in Cypress, CA
E-mail: leslie.miller@avalonpub.com; sealpress@sealpress.com
Web site: http://www.sealpress.com
Dist(s): **Publishers Group** *(Publishers Group West); CIP.*

Seargeant Pub, *(Seargeant Publishing; 0-9657867),* Orders Addr.: P.O. Box 1849, Visalia, CA 93279 Tel 209-738-8085; Fax: 209-738-9183; Toll Free: 888-236-1999; Edit Addr.: 36273A RD 112, Visalia, CA 93291
E-mail: sseargeant@aol.com
Web site: http://www.dolphinbooks.com
Dist(s): **Baker & Taylor** *(Baker & Taylor Bks.).*

SeaStar Pub, *(SeaStar Publishing Co.; 1-886583),* P.O. Box 741413, Dallas, TX 75240-8311
Dist(s): **Baker & Taylor** *(Baker & Taylor Bks.)*
Quality Bks IL *(Quality Bks., Inc.).*

Seattle-King Cty Dept, *(Seattle-King County Dept. of Public Health; 1-893234),* 400 Yesler Way 13th Flr., Seattle, WA 98104 Tel 206-296-4902; Fax: 206-205-5281
E-mail: barbara.warner@metrokc.gov.

SEBT, *See* **SevenStar Comm**

Second Comng Inc, *(Second Coming, Inc.; 0-912582),* 650 Willow Valley Sq., Suite K107, Lancaster, PA 17602-4872 (SAN 201-047X) Tel 717-464-6282; Fax: 717-464-6117
E-mail: salemk@aol.com
Web site: http://www.kirban.org
Dist(s): **AMG Pubs** *(AMG Pubs.).*

Sedgwick Pr Imprint of Grey Hse Pub

See Do Pr, *(See-Do Pr.; 0-9607836),* 3620 Greenwood Dr., Kelseyville, CA 95451 (SAN 238-1974) Tel 707-277-7087; Fax: 707-277-7088; Toll Free: 800-233-6367.

See Sharp Pr, *(See Sharp Pr.; 0-9613289; 1-884365),* P.O. Box 1731, Tucson, AZ 85702-1731 (SAN 653-8134) Tel 520-628-8720 (phone/fax)
E-mail: cb@seesharpress.com
Web site: http://www.seesharppress.com
Dist(s): **LPC Group** *(LPC Group).*

Select Bks CA, *(Select Bks.; 0-9632556),* 1451 Grant Rd., Suite 102, Mountain View, CA 94040 Tel 650-966-1144; Fax: 650-966-1609 Do not confuse with companies with the same name in Starke, FL, Evanston, IL, San Francisco, CA, New York, NY
E-mail: glccorp@aol.com.

Selena Pr, *(Selena Pr.; 0-938451),* 1010 Southwood Dr., Fargo, ND 58103 (SAN 660-9880) Tel 701-235-2890.

Self Hlth Care, *(Self Health Care Systems; 1-883989),* 1800 S. Robertson Blvd., No. 239, Los Angeles, CA 90035 Fax: 310-202-1170; Toll Free: 800-900-4325; 8927 W. 25th St., Los Angeles, CA 90034 Tel 310-202-1170
Dist(s): **Distributors** *(Distributors, The)*
New Leaf Dist *(New Leaf Distributing Co., Inc.).*

Self Realization, *(Self-Realization Fellowship; 0-87612),* 3880 San Rafael Ave., Los Angeles, CA 90065 (SAN 204-5788) Tel 323-342-0336; Fax: 323-342-0237; Toll Free: 888-773-8680 (orders only)
Web site: http://www.srfpublishers.org/; http://www.srf-yogananda.org.

Self-Prog Control, *(Self-Programmed Control Pr.; 0-9601926),* 11949 Jefferson Blvd., Suite 104, Culver City, CA 90230 (SAN 665-7796) Tel 310-306-3917; Toll Free: 800-728-2256
E-mail: stresscard@aol.com
Web site: http://www.lifelines.com/spc.

†**Semaphore Bks,** *(Semaphore Bks.; 1-879601),* 30 Old Harbor Rd., Chatham, MA 02633-2315 Fax: 508-945-1290; *CIP.*

Semiotexte, *(Semiotexte/Smart Art; 1-58435),* 2571 W. Fifth St., Los Angeles, CA 90057 Tel 216-487-5203; Fax: 216-487-5204
Dist(s): **Autonomedia** *(Autonomedia)*
MIT Pr *(MIT Pr.)*
SPD-Small Pr Dist *(SPD-Small Pr. Distribution).*

Seneca Hse, *(Seneca Hse. Pr.; 0-9640088),* P.O. Box 966, New Port Richey, FL 34656 Tel 727-847-1619; Fax: 727-848-2494; 727-842-9841; Toll Free: 800-915-1001
E-mail: kaltenba@gte.net
Web site: http://www.pcrn.org; http://www.pcaguide.com.

Sensory Integration, *(Sensory Integration International; 1-882068),* 1602 Cabrillo Ave., Torrance, CA 90501-2819 (SAN 248-3106) Tel 310-320-9986; Fax: 310-320-9934.

Sentinel Pubg, *See* **Berco Pubng**

Senyczak Pubns, *(Senyczak Pubns.; 0-9657466),* 450 Sutter St., Suite 1400, San Fransico, CA 94108 Tel 415-788-4535; Fax: 415-392-7608; Toll Free: 800-572-2027
Web site: http://www.senechek.com.

Serala Pr, *See* **Lompico Cr Pr**

Serenity NY, *(Serenity Pubns.; 1-885909),* 41 Hemlock Ave., Newton, NJ 07860 Tel 973-786-5761 Do not confuse with Serenity Pubns. in Lakeside AZ.

Serentec Pr, *See* **Davis Horwood Intl**

Serono Symposia USA, *(Serono Symposia USA, Inc.; 1-878601),* 100 Longwater Cir., Norwell, MA 02061 Tel 781-982-9000; Fax: 781-982-9481; Toll Free: 800-283-8088.

Serpents Tail, *(Serpent's Tail; 1-85242),* 904 W. Univ. Pkwy., Baltimore, MD 21210-2716
E-mail: stail@echonyc.com
Web site: http://www.serpentstail.com
Dist(s): **Consort Bk Sales** *(Consortium Bk. Sales & Distribution).*

†**Servant,** *(Servant Pubns.; 0-89283; 1-56955),* Div. of Servant Ministries, Inc., Orders Addr.: P.O. Box 8617, Ann Arbor, MI 48107-8617 (SAN 208-9246) Tel 734-677-6490; Toll Free Fax: 800-315-8505; Edit Addr.: 1143 Highland Dr., Suite E, Ann Arbor, MI 48108 (SAN 208-9238) Fax: 734-677-6685; Toll Free: 800-458-8505 ; *Imprints:* Vine Bks (Vine Books)
E-mail: dgriffin@servantpub.com
Web site: http://www.servantpub.com/
Dist(s): **Anchor Distributors** *(Anchor Distributors)*
Appalachian Bible *(Appalachian Bible Co.)*
Baker & Taylor *(Baker & Taylor Bks.)*
Brodart *(Brodart Co.)*
Riverside-World *(Riverside World)*
Spring Arbor Dist *(Spring Arbor Distributors Inc.); CIP.*

Service Press, *(Service Pr.; 0-9629372),* 3747 E. Joy Rd., Ann Arbor, MI 48105-9608 Tel 734-769-6971
Dist(s): **Distributors** *(Distributors, The).*

SethNet Pub, *(SethNet Publishing; 1-889828),* Div. of Seth Network International, Orders Addr.: P.O. Box 1620, Eugene, OR 97440 Tel 541-683-6731; Fax: 541-683-1084; Edit Addr.: 1840 Willamette, Suite 100, Eugene, OR 97401.

†**Seton Med Ctr,** *(Seton Medical Ctr.; 0-9616516),* Div. of Catholic Healthcare West, 1900 Sullivan Ave., Suite 1105, Daly City, CA 94015-2229 (SAN 659-5847) Tel 650-991-6464; Fax: 650-991-6098
E-mail: dburnham@chw.edu; *CIP.*

Setter Pubns, *(Setter Pubns.; 0-9655196),* Orders Addr.: P.O. Box 144, Bowie, TX 76230 Tel 940-872-5097; Edit Addr.: Rte. 1, Box 20X, Bowie, TX 76230.

Seven Galaxy, *(Seven Galaxy Pubns.; 1-890016),* Orders Addr.: P.O. Box 330, Belmont, MA 02178 (SAN 299-5832) Tel 617-661-1961; Fax: 617-868-3870; Edit Addr.: 2302 Massachusetts Ave., Cambridge, MA 02140 (SAN 299-5824)
Web site: http://www.m7749k@aol.com.

Seven Hills Bk, *(7 Hills Bk. Distributors; 0-911403),* 1531 Tremont St., Cincinnati, OH 45214-1458 (SAN 169-6629) Tel 513-471-4300; Fax: 513-471-4311; Toll Free Fax: 888-777-7799; Toll Free: 800-545-2005
E-mail: customerservice@sevenhillsbooks.com
Web site: http://www.sevenhillsbooks.com.

†**Seven Locks Pr,** *(Seven Locks Pr.; 0-929765; 0-932020; 0-9615964; 1-931643),* 3100 W. Warner Ave., Suite 8, Santa Ana, CA 92704 (SAN 211-9781) Tel 714-545-2526; Fax: 714-545-1572; Toll Free: 800-354-5348 ; *Imprints:* Chapman Univ (Chapman University Press)
E-mail: sevenlocks@aol.com
Web site: http://sevenlockspress.com
Dist(s): **Baker & Taylor** *(Baker & Taylor Bks.)*
Koen Bk Distributors *(Koen Bk. Distributors); CIP.*

Seven Stories, *(Seven Stories Pr.; 1-58322; 1-888363),* 140 Watts St., New York, NY 10013 Tel 212-226-8760; Fax: 212-226-1411; Toll Free: 800-596-7437
E-mail: info@sevenstories.com
Web site: http://www.sevenstories.com
Dist(s): **Continental Bk** *(Continental Bk. Co., Inc.)*
Publishers Group *(Publishers Group West).*

SevenStar Comm, *(SevenStar Communications Group; 0-937064; 1-887575),* 13315 Washington Blvd., Suite 200, Los Angeles, CA 90066 (SAN 217-2704) Tel 310-302-1207; Fax: 310-302-1208; Toll Free: 800-578-9526 (orders only) ; *Imprints:* Yo San Bks (Yo San Books)
E-mail: taostar@taostar.com
Web site: http://www.sevenstarcom.com
Dist(s): **BookWorld** *(BookWorld Services, Inc.)*
Bookpeople *(Bookpeople)*
Christian Dist *(Christian Distribtuion Services, Inc.)*
Distributors *(Distributors, The)*
New Leaf Dist *(New Leaf Distributing Co., Inc.).*

Seventh Ray, *(Seventh Ray Pr.; 1-882834),* P.O. Box 442, Poulsbo, WA 98370 Tel 360-697-2777; Fax: 360-779-9677; Toll Free: 888-329-4325 (phone/fax)
E-mail: orders@seventhraypress.com; seventhray@email.msn.com
Web site: http://www.seventhraypress.com; http://www.kitchendoctor.com.

Sexual Health Mag, *(Sexual Health Magazine, Inc.; 0-9666416),* 2515 E. Hwy. No. 54, Durham, NC 27713 Tel 919-544-7997; Fax: 919-361-1907; 2200 Century Plaza, Durham, NC 27713
E-mail: charlesebel@mindspring
Web site: http://www./sexhealth.com.

Sexual Hlth, *(Sexual Health Network, LLC, The; 0-9659185),* 3 Mayflower Ln., Huntington, CT 06484 Tel 203-924-4623
E-mail: mitch@sexualhealth.com
Web site: http://www.sexualhealth.com.

SF Comns, *(S.F. Communications, Inc.),* 3959 Electric Rd., Suite 155, Roanoke, VA 24018 (SAN 630-4737) Tel 540-772-4500; Fax: 540-772-4505; Toll Free: 800-322-3834
E-mail: Adschaal@travelknowledge.com
Web site: http://www.TravelKnowledge.com.

SF Study Ctr, *(San Francisco Study Ctr.; 0-936434; 1-888956),* 1095 Market St., Rm. 602, San Francisco, CA 94103 (SAN 214-4654) Tel 415-626-1650; Fax: 415-626-7276; Toll Free: 888-281-3757 ; *Imprints:* Study Ctr Pr (Study Center Press)
E-mail: sfsc@sirius.com
Web site: http://www.studycenter.org.

SGC Biomedical, *(SGC Biomedical Engineering; 0-925395),* 10641 Allen Dr., Garden Grove, CA 92840-3143 Tel 714-284-9424.

Shad Board, *(Shad Board; 1-886465),* 4403 E. Clearwater Pkwy., Paradise Valley, AZ 85253 Tel 602-596-1605
E-mail: haddadmnd@primenet.com.

Shades of Gray, *(Shades of Gray Bks.; 0-9636710),* 283 Yank Ct., Lakewood, CO 80228-1305 Tel 303-694-7400; Toll Free: 800-368-1307.

Shadow & Light, *(Shadow & Light; 0-9625231),* 1749 Vine St., Berkeley, CA 94703 Tel 510-527-7932 (phone/fax)
E-mail: gp@askdrgayle.com
Web site: http://www.askdrgayle.com
Dist(s): **Bookpeople** *(Bookpeople).*

Shadow Pubns, *(Shadow Pubns.; 0-9639152),* P.O. Box 5683, Athens, GA 30604-5683 Tel 706-613-1899 Do not confuse with companies with the same name in Bid Bend, WI, Winchester, MA, San Antonio, TX, Bend, OR.

Shallowater, *(Shallowater Pr.; 0-9648404),* Orders Addr.: P.O. Box 1151, Shallowater, TX 79363-1151 Tel 806-873-3617; Edit Addr.: 3815 50th St., No. 36, Lubbock, TX 79413
E-mail: sales@shallowater.com
Web site: http://www.shallowater.com.

†**Shambhala Pubns,** *(Shambhala Pubns., Inc.; 0-87773; 1-56957; 1-57062; 1-59030),* Horticultural Hall, 300 Massachusetts Ave., Boston, MA 02115 (SAN 203-2481) Tel 617-424-0030; Fax: 617-236-1563
E-mail: editors@shambhala.com
Web site: http://www.shambhala.com
Dist(s): **Random** *(Random Hse., Inc.)*
Sounds True *(Sounds True, Inc.); CIP.*

Shane CA, *(Shane Pubns.; 0-9628235),* P.O. Box 3873, San Rafael, CA 94912-3873 Tel 415-472-4458.

Shangri-La Imprint of Lotus Pr

Shapiro Kuba, *(Shapiro, Kuba, Harmon & Burks; 0-9624335),* 1106 Pipestem Pl., Rockville, MD 20854 Tel 703-255-3595; Fax: 301-424-6558.

Shared Experiences, *(Shared Experiences Publishing; 0-9624133),* P.O. Box 433, Miranda, CA 95553-0433.

Sharif Ent, *(Sharif Enterprises, Inc.; 0-9637036),* 14808 S. 46th Pl., Phoenix, AZ 85044-6871 Tel 602-225-2248; Fax: 602-225-0985
E-mail: asus@ix.netcom.com.

Sharing, *(Sharing; 1-891117),* 212 E. Seventh St., Mount Carmel, PA 17851-2211 Tel 570-339-2567.

Sharp Legis, *(Sharp Legislative Resources; 0-9659713),* 8819 Ridge Rd., Bethesda, MD 20817 Tel 301-469-4997; Fax: 301-469-8411 E-mail: Nursharp@aol.com.

Sharp Pub, *(Sharp Publishing; 0-9629350),* 2767 Highland Dr., Carlsbad, CA 92008 Tel 760-729-3838 Do not confuse with Sharp Publishing, Park City, UT.

Shaw Spelling, *(Shaw/Spelling Assocs., Inc.; 0-9626972),* 1180 S. Beverly Dr., Suite 401, Los Angeles, CA 90035-1156 Tel 310-458-2011; Fax: 310-394-8852 *Dist(s):* **Publishers Group** *(Publishers Group West).*

SHE, *(S.H.E.; 0-9704354),* P.O. Box 571078, Miami, FL 33257-1078 Tel 876-960-1521; Fax: 876-754-2713 E-mail: chooselife-irisdx-ja@hotmail.com.

Sheba Pr, *(Sheba Pr., Ltd.; 1-880613),* P.O. Box 59637, Potomac, MD 20859-9637 Tel 703-734-1956; Fax: 301-469-9227.

She-Bear Pubs, *(She-Bear Pubs.; 0-9655435),* Orders Addr.: P.O. Box 503, Ellicottville, NY 14731 Tel 716-257-9332; Edit Addr.: 8275 Crumb Hill Rd., East Otto, NY 14729.

Sheed & Ward WI, *(Sheed & Ward; 0-934134; 1-55612; 1-58051),* Orders Addr.: 1444 US Rte. 42, Mansfield, OH 44903 Tel 800-266-5564; Fax: 419-281-6883; Edit Addr.: 7373 S. Lovers Ln. Rd., Franklin, WI 53132 (SAN 207-7396) Tel 414-529-6400; Fax: 414-529-6419; 30 Amberwood Pkwy., Ashland, OH 44805 E-mail: jereditor@aol.com; sheed@execpc.com Web site: http://www.sheedandward.com.

Sheffield Acad (GBR) *(0-905774; 1-85075; 1-84127) Dist. by* **CUP Services.**

Sheldon Pr (GBR) *(0-85969) Dist. by* **Intl Pubs Mktg.**

Sheltering Arms, *(Sheltering Arms Hospital; 0-9623370),* 1311 Palmyra Ave., Richmond, VA 23227 Tel 804-254-6515.

Shelton Mktg, *(Shelton Marketing Services, Inc.; 0-9633516),* Orders Addr.: P.O. Box 17526, Nashville, TN 37217-0526 Tel 615-361-1152; Fax: 615-361-1845; Toll Free: 800-844-4893; Edit Addr.: 1420 Donelson Pike, Suite A-11, Nashville, TN 37217-2927.

Shelton Pubns, *(Shelton Pubns.; 0-9617594),* 6507 Lakebend Way, Greensboro, NC 27410-8415 (SAN 665-0082) Do not confuse with Shelton Pubns., Sausalito, CA.

†Shepards, *(Shepard's; 0-07; 0-7698; 1-57911), Dist(s):* **Brodart** *(Brodart Co.); CIP.*

Shepards-McGraw, *See* **Shepards**

†Sheridan, *(Sheridan Hse., Inc.; 0-911378; 0-924486; 1-57409),* 145 Palisade St., Dobbs Ferry, NY 10522 (SAN 204-5915) Tel 914-693-2410; Fax: 914-693-0776; Toll Free: 888-743-7425 (orders only) E-mail: Sheribks@aol.com Web site: http://www.sheridanhouse.com; *CIP.*

Shiloh Med, *(Shiloh Medical Pubns.; 0-9643914),* P.O. Box 377, Oakfield, ME 04763 Tel 207-757-7294 (phone/fax) E-mail: rahansen@sms-witness.org Web site: http://www.sms-witness.org.

Shiloh Press, *(Shiloh Pr.; 1-889868),* P.O. Box 18723, West Palm Beach, FL 33416 Tel 561-753-7737 Do not confuse with Shiloh Pr., Long Island, ME.

Shire Pr, *(Shire Pr.; 0-918828),* 26873 Hester Creek Rd., Los Gatos, CA 95033-9242 (SAN 293-3942) Tel 408-353-4253 E-mail: shirepress@aol.com *Dist(s):* **SCB Distributors** *(SCB Distributors).*

Shoeless Pub, *(Shoeless Publishing Co.; 0-87208; 0-9644574),* P.O. Box 2545, Fort Myers Beach, FL 33932 Tel 941-463-1337; Fax: 941-463-4929.

Shoreys Bkstore, *(Shorey's Bookstore; 0-8466),* P.O. Box 77316, Seattle, WA 98177-0316 (SAN 204-5958) Tel 206-633-2990 E-mail: shorey@serv.net Web site: http://www.serv.net/shorey.

Sidney Scott Ross, *(Ross, Sidney Scott; 0-9602028),* 94 Joyce Rd., Eastchester, NY 10709-1432 (SAN 212-1379).

Sidran Pr, *(Sidran Pr.; 0-9629164; 1-886968),* Div. of Sidran Traumatic Foundation, 200 E. Joppa Rd., Suite 207, Baltimore, MD 21286 Tel 410-825-8888; Fax: 410-337-0747; Toll Free: 888-825-8249 (orders only) E-mail: sidran@sidran.org Web site: http://www.sidran.org *Dist(s):* **Baker & Taylor** *(Baker & Taylor Bks.)* **Bookpeople** *(Bookpeople)* **Quality Bks IL** *(Quality Bks., Inc.).*

SIDS Educ Srvs, *(SIDS Educational Services, Inc.; 0-9641218),* 2905 64th Ave., Cheverly, MD 20785 Tel 301-773-9671; Fax: 301-322-9822 E-mail: sidses@aol.com *Dist(s):* **Baker & Taylor** *(Baker & Taylor Bks.).*

SIECUS, *(Sex Information & Education Council of the U. S.; 0-9609212),* 130 W. 42nd St., Suite 350, New York, NY 10036 (SAN 224-2435) Tel 212-819-9770; Fax: 212-819-9776 E-mail: siecus@siecus.org Web site: http://www.siecus.org.

Siemens Pacesetter, *(Siemens Pacesetter, Inc.; 0-9626364),* 12884 Bradley Ave., Sylmar, CA 91342 Tel 818-362-6822; Fax: 818-362-8093; Toll Free: 800-777-2237.

†Sierra, *(Sierra Club Bks.; 0-375; 0-87156; 1-57805),* Member of Crown Publishing Group, 85 Second St., 2nd Flr., San Francisco, CA 94105 (SAN 203-2406) Tel 415-977-5500; Fax: 415-977-5792 E-mail: books@sierraclub.org Web site: http://www.sierraclub.org/books *Dist(s):* **AOL Time Warner** *(AOL Time Warner Bk. Group)* **Gibbs Smith Pub** *(Smith, Gibbs Pub.)* **Random** *(Random Hse., Inc.); CIP.*

Sierra Pub Co, *(Sierra Publishing Co.; 0-918493),* 2930 Weston Way, Rancho Cordova, CA 95670-5525 (SAN 676-9578) Tel 916-366-7724 Do not confuse with Sierra Publishing Co., Clovis, CA.

Sierra Sunrise Pub, *(Sierra Sunrise Pub., Inc.; 1-887263),* 14622 Ventura Blvd., Suite 800, Sherman Oaks, CA 91403 Tel 818-386-9102 E-mail: Sierra@LifeOnNet.org *Dist(s):* **Baker & Taylor** *(Baker & Taylor Bks.)* **Seven Hills Bk** *(7 Hills Bk. Distributors).*

Sig Imprint of NAL

Sight & Hearing, *(Sight & Hearing Assn.; 0-9612370),* 674 Transfer Rd., Saint Paul, MN 55114-1402 (SAN 289-5358) Tel 612-645-2546; Fax: 612-645-2742; Toll Free: 800-992-0424 Web site: http://www.sightandhearing.org.

Sigler & Flanders, *(Sigler & Flanders, Inc.; 1-880579),* Orders Addr.: P.O. Box 3578, Lawrence, KS 66046 Tel 913-749-5259; Fax: 785-841-6297; Toll Free: 800-446-6293; Edit Addr.: 1420C Kasold Dr., Lawrence, KS 66049.

Sigma Theta Tau, *(Sigma Theta Tau International, Ctr. for Nursing Pr.; 0-9656391; 1-930538),* 550 W. North St., Indianapolis, IN 46202 (SAN 224-5345) Tel 317-634-8171; Fax: 317-634-8188; Toll Free: 888-634-7575 E-mail: jeff@stti.iupui.edu Web site: http://www.nursingsociety.org.

Signal Bks, *(Signal Bks.; 0-930095),* Subs. of Computer Textual Services, Inc., 403 Oak Ave., Carrboro, NC 27510-1749 (SAN 670-1795).

Signum-Verlag (DEU) *(3-927731) Dist. by* **Gallaudet Univ Pr.**

Sigo Pr, *(Sigo Pr.; 0-938434; 1-879041),* P.O. Box 1435, Fort Collins, CO 80522 (SAN 216-3020) Tel 970-221-2055; Fax: 970-221-1785; Toll Free: 800-338-0446 E-mail: sigopress@hotmail.com Web site: http://www.sigopress.com.

SIIS, *(Spring Institute for International Studies; 0-940723),* 1610 Emerson St., Denver, CO 80218-1412 (SAN 664-9742) Tel 303-571-5008; Fax: 303-571-5102 E-mail: springinst@earthlink.net Web site: http://www.springinstitute.com.

Silent Partners, *(Silent Partners, Inc.; 1-878353),* 8727 Shoal Creek Blvd., Austin, TX 78757-6815 Tel 512-458-1191; Fax: 512-458-1234 Do not confuse with Silent Partners in College Station, TX E-mail: info@silentpartners.com Web site: http://www.silentpartners.com.

Silent Walker Pub, *(Silent Walker Publishing; 0-9620364),* P.O. Box 80098, Los Angeles, CA 90080-0098 (SAN 248-7004) Tel 310-271-9931.

Silk Pages Pub, *(Silk Pages Publishing; 0-9645815),* 7030 Gullwood Rd., Lakeshore, MN 56468 Tel 218-963-3591.

†Silver, *(Silver, Burdett & Ginn, Inc.; 0-382; 0-663),* Div. of Simon & Schuster, Inc., Orders Addr.: 4350 Equity Dr., P.O. Box 2649, Columbus, OH 43216 Fax: 614-771-5841; Toll Free: 800-848-9500; Edit Addr.: P.O. Box 480, Parsippany, NJ 07054 (SAN 204-5982); 108 Wilmot Rd., Suite 380, Midwest Div., Deerfield, IL 60015 (SAN 111-6517) Tel 708-945-1240 E-mail: customerservice@scottforesman.com Web site: http://www.scottforesman.com/; *CIP.*

Silver Cherner, *(Silver & Cherner, Ltd.; 0-9645024),* 10221 N. 32nd St., Suite D, Phoenix, AZ 85028-3849 Tel 602-996-2220; Fax: 602-996-2330 E-mail: uhaeditor@aol.com.

Silver Lake Col Pr, *(Silver Lake College Pr.; 0-9625034),* 2406 S. Alverno Rd., Manitowoc, WI 54220 Tel 920-684-6691.

Silver Press, *(Silver Pr. Co.; 0-9640442),* 69 E. Wilson Bridge Rd., No. A, Worthington, OH 43085-2357 Tel 614-459-1999; Fax: 614-457-8741.

Silvercat Pubns, *(Silvercat Pubns.; 0-9624945; 1-893067),* 4070 Goldfinch St., Suite C, San Diego, CA 92103 Tel 619-299-6774; Fax: 619-299-9119; Toll Free: 888-299-9119 E-mail: info@silvercat.com.

Silverton Bks, *(Silverton Bks.; 0-9629528),* 3359 Garden Ave., Los Angeles, CA 90039-2130 Tel 213-666-2846; Fax: 213-660-3247 E-mail: silvertonb@aol.com.

SIMAX, *(SIMAX; 0-9655109),* 8904 Carlisle Rd., Wyndmoor, PA 19038 Tel 610-989-7144; Fax: 215-836-9148; Toll Free: 800-356-9315 E-mail: jbellis@RSIProgram.com Web site: http://www.RSIProgram.com; http://www.UsabilityInstitute.com.

Simmons & Hall Pub, *(Simmons & Hall Publishing; 0-943723),* 4419 Prairie Willow Ct., Concord, CA 94521-4440 (SAN 242-343X) Tel 510-686-9041.

Simon & Schuster, *(Simon & Schuster; 0-684; 0-689),* Div. of Simon & Schuster Trade, 1230 Avenue of the Americas, New York, NY 10020 Tel 212-698-7000; Fax: 212-698-7007 Web site: http://www.oasis.simonandschuster.com.

Simple Life Bks, *(Simple Life Bks.; 0-9642335),* Orders Addr.: P.O. Box 84, Ojo Caliente, NM 87549; Edit Addr.: 19 Hwy. 414, Ojo Caliente, NM 87549 Tel 505-583-2470.

†Sinauer Assocs, *(Sinauer Assocs., Inc.; 0-87893),* 23 Plumtree Rd., P.O. Box 407, Sunderland, MA 01375-0407 (SAN 203-2392) Tel 413-549-4300; Fax: 413-549-1118 E-mail: publish@sinauer.com Web site: http://www.sinauer.com; *CIP.*

Single-Knight, *(Single-Knight; 0-9622483),* 1818 Lower Mountain Rd., Furlong, PA 18925-1215 (SAN 200-3104).

Singlish Pub, *(Singlish Pubn. Society, The; 1-888822),* 14140 Sherwood, Oak Park, MI 48237 Tel 248-546-4255; Fax: 248-874-1047 E-mail: singlishps@aol.com Web site: http://www.singlishps.com.

†Singular Publishing, *(Singular Publishing Group, Inc.; 0-7693; 1-56593; 1-879105),* Div. of Delmar Publishers, 401 W. A St., Suite 325, San Diego, CA 92101-7904 (SAN 297-455X) Tel 619-238-6777; Fax: 619-238-6789; Toll Free: 800-521-8545 E-mail: singpub@mail.cerfnet.com Web site: http://www.singpub.com *Dist(s):* **BookWorld** *(BookWorld Services, Inc.)* **Thomson Learn** *(Thomson Learning); CIP.*

SIRS Mandarin, *See* **SIRS Pubng**

†SIRS Pubng, *(SIRS Publishing, Inc.; 0-89777; 0-9678914),* P.O. Box 272348, Boca Raton, FL 33427-2348 (SAN 222-8920) Tel 561-994-0079; Fax: 561-994-4704; Toll Free: 800-232-7477 ; *Imprints:* Upton Bks (Upton Books) E-mail: custserve@sirs.com; monicag@sirs.com Web site: http://www.sirs.com *Dist(s):* **Baker & Taylor** *(Baker & Taylor Bks.)* **Brodart** *(Brodart Co.)* **Distributors** *(Distributors, The); CIP.*

Six Ponies Pr, *(6 Ponies Pr; 0-9656350),* P.O. Box 783, Kaysville, UT 84037-0783 Tel 801-593-9269; Fax: 801-593-9367.

Sjogrens Syndrome, *(Sjogren's Syndrome Foundation, Inc.; 0-9621157),* 333 N. Broadway, Jericho, NY 11753-2007 (SAN 250-9091) Tel 516-933-6365; Fax: 516-933-6368 Web site: http://www.sjogrens.com.

SKF Bks, *(SKF Bks.; 0-9657565),* 413B 19th St., No. 322, Lynden, WA 98264 Tel 604-534-6956; Fax: 604-534-9527 E-mail: skfreeman@aol.com Web site: http://www.skfbooks.com/aml; http://www.skfbooks.com/tml.

Skin Cancer Fndtn, *(Skin Cancer Foundation; 0-9627688),* 245 Fifth Ave., Suite 2402, New York, NY 10016 Tel 212-725-5176; Fax: 212-725-5751.

Sky Blue Pr, *(Sky Blue Pr.; 0-9652364),* 3438 Kilmer, Troy, MI 48083 Tel 248-619-9918 E-mail: paul@skybluepress.com; sara@skybluepress.com; skybluepress@skybluepress.com Web site: http://www.skybluepress.com.

SkyLght, *See* **SkyLght Prof Dev**

SkyLght Prof Dev, *(SkyLight Professional Development; 0-932935; 1-57517; 1-4029),* Div. of Pearson Education, 2626 S. Clearbrook Dr., Arlington Heights, IL 60005-5310 (SAN 690-0135) Tel 847-290-6600; Fax: 847-290-6609; Toll Free: 800-348-4474
E-mail: info@skylightedu.com
Web site: http://www.skylightedu.com.

SLACK Inc, *(SLACK, Inc.; 0-913590; 0-943432; 1-55642),* 6900 Grove Rd., Thorofare, NJ 08086-9447 (SAN 201-8632) Tel 856-848-1000; Fax: 856-853-5991; Toll Free: 800-257-8290
E-mail: jstewart@slackinc.com; orders@slackinc.com
Web site: http://www.slackbooks.com
Dist(s): **B&N Imports** *(Barnes & Noble Bks.-Imports)*
Baker & Taylor *(Baker & Taylor Bks.)*
Coutts Library Service Inc *(Coutts Library Service, Inc.)*
Emery-Pratt Co *(Emery-Pratt Co.)*
H Holt & Co *(Holt, Henry & Co., LLC)*
J Majors Co *(Majors, J. A. Co.)*
Matthews Medical Bk Co *(Matthews Medical Bk. Co.)*
Rittenhouse *(Rittenhouse Bk. Distributors).*

Slapering Hol, *(Slapering Hol Pr.; 0-9624178; 0-9700277),* Div. of The Hudson Valley Writers' Center, 300 Riverside Dr., Sleepy Hollow, NY 10591 Tel 914-332-4469; Fax: 914-332-5953
Web site: http://www.writerscenter.org.

Sleep Disorders, *See* **Nychthemeron Pr**

Sleepng Bear, *(Sleeping Bear Pr.; 1-57504; 1-886947; 1-58536),* Orders Addr.: P.O. Box 20, Chelsea, MI 48118 (SAN 253-8466) Tel 734-475-4411; Fax: 734-475-0787; Toll Free: 800-487-2323; Edit Addr.: 310 N. Main, Suite 300, Chelsea, MI 48118
E-mail: customerservice@sleepingbearpress.com
Web site: http://www.sleepingbearpress.com
Dist(s): **Baker & Taylor** *(Baker & Taylor Bks.)*
Keith Distributors *(Keith Distributors)*
Partners Pubs Grp *(Partners Pubs. Group, Inc.)*
Shens Bks *(Shen's Bks.)*
Southern Bk Service *(Southern Bk. Service)*
Urban Land *(Urban Land Institute).*

Smart Apple, *(Smart Apple Media; 1-58340; 1-887068),* Orders Addr.: P.O. Box 206, North Mankato, MN 56003 Tel 507-388-6273 (ext. 260); 507-388-2601; Fax: 507-388-2746; 507-386-0061; Toll Free: 800-445-6209; Edit Addr.: 1980 Lookout Dr., North Mankato, MN 56003
E-mail: CreativeCo@aol.com
Dist(s): **Creative Co** *(Creative Co., The).*

Smart Choices, *(Smart Choices; 0-9634276),* Orders Addr.: P.O. Box 799003, LB241, Dallas, TX 75379 Fax: 972-733-4767; Edit Addr.: 17194 Preston Rd., No. 123-241, Dallas, TX 75248 Tel 972-867-4699.

Smart Pubns CA, *(Smart Pubns.; 0-9627418; 1-890572),* P.O. Box 4667, Petaluma, CA 94954-4667 Tel 707-769-8308; Fax: 707-763-3944
E-mail: info@smart-publications.com
Web site: http://www.smart-publications.com
Dist(s): **Alive Bks** *(Alive Bks.)*
Bookpeople *(Bookpeople)*
Nutri-Books Corp *(Nutri-Bks. Corp.)*
Publishers Group *(Publishers Group West)*
Royal Pubns Inc *(Royal Pubns., Inc.).*

SmartMedicine, *(SmartMedicine Pr.; 0-9648991),* 2817 E. Park Dr., Seattle, WA 98112 (SAN 253-4037) Tel 206-768-5356; Fax: 206-768-5331
Dist(s): **Pathway Bk Serv** *(Pathway Bk. Service).*

SMC Publng, *(SMC Publishing; 1-889423),* 6532 Killarrey Ave., Garden Grove, CA 92845 Tel 714-565-9741; Fax: 714-892-1990; Toll Free: 800-915-7911 Do not confuse with SMC Publishing, Houston, TX
E-mail: mail04740@pop.net.

SMH Med Ctr, *See* **Uncharted Ctry Pub**

Smith Hse Pr, *(Smith Hse. Pr.; 0-9615221),* 2700 Rice St., Saint Paul, MN 55113 Tel 612-490-9408
E-mail: smithhse@aol.com
Dist(s): **Baker & Taylor** *(Baker & Taylor Bks.)*
Bookmen Inc *(Bookmen, Inc.)*
King Distributors *(King Distributors)*
Natl Bk Netwk *(National Bk. Network).*

Smith Pubs, *See* **Smithmark**

Smith Vet Srvs, *(Smith Veterinary Services; 1-885780),* P.O. Box 254, Leavenworth, WA 98826 Tel 509-763-2052; Fax: 509-763-2112
Web site: http://www.smithvet.com
Dist(s): **Baker & Taylor** *(Baker & Taylor Bks.).*

Smithfield Pr, *See* **Princeton Hlth**

Smithmark, *(Smithmark Pubs., Inc.; 0-7651; 0-8317),* Div. of US Media Holdings, 115 W. 18th St.. 5th Flr., New York, NY 10011-4113 (SAN 176-0912) Tel 212-519-1300; Fax: 212-519-1310; Toll Free: 800-932-0070 (customer service); Raritan Plaza 111, Fieldcrest Ave., Edison, NJ 08837 (SAN 658-1625) Tel 732-225-6499 (phone/fax); Toll Free Fax: 800-732-8688
Dist(s): **AOL Time Warner** *(AOL Time Warner Bk. Group)*
Continental Bk *(Continental Bk. Co., Inc.).*

†Smithsonian, *(Smithsonian Institution Pr.; 0-87474; 1-56098; 1-58834),* Div. of Smithsonian Institution, Orders Addr.: P.O. Box 960, Herndon, VA 20172-0960 Tel 202-287-3738 (ext. 375); Fax: 202-287-3637; Toll Free: 800-782-4612 (customer service & orders); 22883 Quicksilver Dr., Dulles, VA 20166 (SAN 253-3383); Edit Addr.: 470 L'Enfant Plaza, Suite 7100, Washington, DC 20560-0950 (SAN 206-8044)
E-mail: inquiries@sipress.si.edu
Web site: http://www.si.edu/organiza/offices/sipress
Dist(s): **Continental Bk** *(Continental Bk. Co., Inc.)*
Univelt Inc *(Univelt, Inc.)*
Wittenborn Art *(Wittenborn Art Bks.)*
netLibrary CO *(netLibrary, Inc.); CIP.*

Smooth Stone Pr, *(Smooth Stone Pr.; 0-9619401),* P.O. Box 19875, Saint Louis, MO 63144 (SAN 244-4259) Tel 314-968-2596
Dist(s): **Baker & Taylor** *(Baker & Taylor Bks.)*
Bookpeople *(Bookpeople)*
Koen Bk Distributors *(Koen Bk. Distributors)*
New Leaf Dist *(New Leaf Distributing Co., Inc.)*
Nutri-Books Corp *(Nutri-Bks. Corp.).*

†SMU Press, *(Southern Methodist Univ. Pr.; 0-87074),* Orders Addr.: c/o Texas A&M Univ. Pr., 4354 TAMU, College Sta., TX 77843-4354 Toll Free Fax: 888-617-2421; Toll Free: 800-826-8911; Edit Addr.: P.O. Box 750415, Dallas, TX 75275-0415 (SAN 203-3615) Tel 214-768-1432; Fax: 214-768-1428
Web site: http://www.tamu.edu/upress
Dist(s): **Tex A&M Univ Pr** *(Texas A&M Univ. Pr.); CIP.*

†Smyth & Helwys, *(Smyth & Helwys Publishing, Inc.; 0-9628455; 1-57312; 1-880837),* 6316 Peake Rd., Macon, GA 31210-3960 (SAN 298-7732) Tel 478-301-2117; Fax: 478-301-2264; Toll Free: 800-747-3016
E-mail: market@helwys.com
Web site: http://www.helwys.com*; CIP.*

Snakebite, *(Snakebite Publishing; 0-9639911),* P.O. Box 413, Midway, FL 32343-0413 Tel 850-539-4292 (phone/fax).

Snd Wave Energy, *(Sound Wave Energy Pr.; 0-9650387),* Div. of Sound Wave Energy, P.O. Box 3969, Pagosa Springs, CO 81147 Tel 970-264-6469; Fax: 970-264-2696; Toll Free: 888-267-2309.

Sngapore Univ Pr (SGP) *(9971-69; 981-04) Dist. by* **Coronet Bks.**

†Snow Lion Pubns, *(Snow Lion Pubns., Inc.; 0-937938; 1-55939),* Orders Addr.: P.O. Box 6483, Ithaca, NY 14851-6483 (SAN 250-328X) Tel 607-273-8519; Fax: 607-273-8508; Toll Free: 800-950-0313; Edit Addr.: 605 W. State St., Ithaca, NY 14851
E-mail: editors@snowlionpub.com; tibet@snowlionpub.com
Web site: http://www.snowlionpub.com
Dist(s): **Bookpeople** *(Bookpeople)*
Natl Bk Netwk *(National Bk. Network)*
New Leaf Dist *(New Leaf Distributing Co., Inc.); CIP.*

Snow Lotus, *(Snow Lotus Pr., Inc.; 0-9623477; 1-890029),* P.O. Box 1824, Boulder, CO 80306 Tel 303-443-9289; Fax: 303-433-6361
Dist(s): **Bookpeople** *(Bookpeople)*
New Leaf Dist *(New Leaf Distributing Co., Inc.)*
Nutri-Books Corp *(Nutri-Bks. Corp.)*
Red Wheel ME *(Red Wheel)*
Redwing Bk Co *(Redwing Bk. Co.).*

Snta Monica, *(Santa Monica Pr.; 0-9639946; 1-891661),* P.O. Box 1076, Santa Monica, CA 90406-1076 (SAN 298-1459) Tel 310-230-7759; Fax: 310-230-7761; Toll Free: 800-784-9553 ; *Imprints:* Offbeat (Offbeat Press)
E-mail: books@santamonicapress.com
Web site: http://www.santamonicapress.com
Dist(s): **Baker & Taylor** *(Baker & Taylor Bks.)*
IPG Chicago *(Independent Pubs. Group)*
Quality Bks IL *(Quality Bks., Inc.).*

Soc Actuaries, *(Society of Actuaries; 0-938959),* 475 N. Martingale Rd., Suite 800, Schaumburg, IL 60173-2226 (SAN 224-8387) Tel 847-706-3526; Fax: 847-706-3599
E-mail: bhaynes@soa.org
Web site: http://soa.org.

†Soc Auto Engineers, *(Society of Automotive Engineers, Inc.; 0-7680; 0-89883; 1-56091),* 400 Commonwealth Dr., Warrendale, PA 15096 (SAN 232-5721) Tel 724-776-4970; Fax: 724-776-0790
E-mail: sae@sae.org
Web site: http://www.sae.org*; CIP.*

Soc Computer Sim, *(Society for Computer Simulation International; 0-911801; 1-56555),* 4838 Ronson Ct., Suite L, San Diego, CA 92111 (SAN 225-1973) Tel 858-277-3888; Fax: 858-277-3930
E-mail: info@scs.org
Web site: http://www.scs.org.

Soc Dev Educ, *See* **Staff Dev Educ**

Soc Healthcare Strategy, *(Society for Healthcare Strategy & Market Development; 0-9676441),* Div. of American Hospital Assn., 1 N. Franklin, Chicago, IL 60606 Tel 312-422-3888; Fax: 312-422-4579
E-mail: stratsoc@aha.org
Web site: http://www.stratsociety.org.

Soc Human Resc Mgmt, *(Society for Human Resource Management; 0-939900; 1-58644),* Orders Addr.: 1650 Bluegrass Lake Pkwy., Alpharetta, GA 30004-7714 Tel 770-442-8633; Fax: 770-442-9742; Toll Free: 800-444-5006; Edit Addr.: 1800 Duke St., Alexandria, VA 22314 (SAN 224-8964) Tel 703-535-6154; Fax: 703-836-0367; Toll Free: 800-283-7476
E-mail: shrmstore@shrm.org
Web site: http://www.shrm.org
Dist(s): **IPG Chicago** *(Independent Pubs. Group).*

Soc Indus-Appl Math, *(Society for Industrial & Applied Mathematics; 0-89871),* 3600 University City Science Ctr., Philadelphia, PA 19104-2688 (SAN 206-5207) Tel 215-382-9800; Fax: 215-386-7999; Toll Free: 800-447-7426
E-mail: siam@siam.org
Web site: http://www.siam.org.

Soc Laparo Surg, *(Society of Laparoendoscopic Surgeons, Inc.; 0-9663768),* 7330 SW 62nd Pl., Suite 410, Miami, FL 33143-4825 Tel 305-665-9959; Fax: 305-667-4123; Toll Free: 800-446-2659; Dept of Surgical Education St Elizabeth Health Center 1044 Belmont Ave, Youngs Town, OH 44501-1750
E-mail: publications@sos.org; info@sls.org
Web site: http://www.sls.org.

Soc Mem Sloan-Kettering, *(Society of Memorial Sloan-Kettering Cancer Ctr., The; 0-9653303),* 1233 York Ave., New York, NY 10021 Tel 212-639-7972; Fax: 212-472-2514.

†Soc Nuclear Med, *(Society of Nuclear Medicine, Inc.; 0-932004),* 1850 Samuel Morse Dr., Reston, VA 20190-5316 (SAN 212-5625) Tel 703-708-9000; Fax: 703-708-9018
E-mail: mmckenna@snm.org
Web site: http://www.snm.org
Dist(s): **Matthews Medical Bk Co** *(Matthews Medical Bk. Co.); CIP.*

Soc Nutrition Ed, *(Society for Nutrition Education; 0-910869),* 1001 Connecticut Ave., NW, Suite 528, Washington, DC 20036-5546 (SAN 225-8552) Tel 202-452-8534.

Soc Sci Study Sex, *(Society for the Scientific Study of Sexuality, The; 0-9628266; 1-888986),* Orders Addr.: P.O. Box 418, Allentown, PA 18105 Fax: 610-530-2485.

Soc Tchrs Fam Med, *(Society of Teachers of Family Medicine; 0-942295),* 11400 Tomahawk Creek Pkwy., Leawood, KS 66211 (SAN 224-3199) Tel 913-906-6000; Fax: 913-906-6096; Toll Free: 800-274-2237
E-mail: admstaff@stfm.org
Web site: http://www.stfm.org.

Soc Thor Surgeons, *(Society of Thoracic Surgeons; 0-9626174),* 401 N. Michigan Ave., Chicago, IL 60611-4267.

SoCal Med Pr, *(SoCal Medical Pr.; 0-9633747),* 999 N. Pacific St., Apt. B101, Oceanside, CA 92054-2079 Tel 760-433-9240; Fax: 760-434-0234
E-mail: hmoriarty@hotmail.com.

Socarean Pr Imprint of Jos A Jackson

Social Change Pr, *(Social Change Pr.; 0-9644437),* 46 Bell Hollow Rd., Putnam Valley, NY 10579 Tel 914-526-2873; Fax: 914-526-2905 Do not confuse with Social Change Pr., Sun City, AZ
E-mail: socngpress@aol.com
Web site: http://members.aol.com/socngpress
Dist(s): **Aletheia** *(Aletheia Pubns., Inc.).*

Society for Neuroscience, *(Society for Neuroscience; 0-916110),* 11 Dupont Cir., NW, Suite 500, Bethesda, MD 20036 (SAN 208-8606) Tel 202-462-6688; Fax: 202-462-5175 Do not confuse with Society for Neuroscience in Washington, DC
Web site: http://www.sfn.org.

Society Prom Christ Know (GBR) *(0-281; 0-9501987) Dist. by* **Intl Pubs Mktg.**

Society Pubng, *See* **Sync Society Pubng**

†Society Vascular Surgery, *(Society for Vascular Surgery, The; 0-9612978),* 13 Elm St., Manchester, MA 01944 (SAN 292-6741) Tel 508-526-8330; Fax: 508-526-4018
E-mail: sus@prrl.com
Web site: http://www.vascsurg.org; *CIP.*

SOCO Pubns, *(S.O.C.O. Pubns.; 0-910119),* 276 Ward Rd., Mohawk, NY 13407 (SAN 241-5720) Tel 315-866-7445
E-mail: copress@borg.com.

SOFITS, *(SOFITS Publishing; 1-879752),* P.O. Box 1131, Harrison, AR 72602 Tel 870-743-2552; Fax: 870-743-4211; Toll Free: 800-929-7889 (orders only)
E-mail: coredk@alltel.net
Web site: http://www.seniorhumor.com.

Soft Words, *(Soft Words Publishing; 0-9637149),* 1503 Kingsroyal Blvd., Pueblo, CO 81005-1889.

Solar Crown, *(Solar Crown Publishing; 1-885569),* Orders Addr.: P.O. Box 922621, Sylmar, CA 91392; Edit Addr.: 12089 Lopez Canyon, No. 201, Sylmar, CA 91342 Tel 818-896-1769.

Solomon Bks, *(Solomon Bks., Inc.; 0-9625508),* 3095 Elmwood Ave., Buffalo, NY 14217 Tel 716-874-5155; Fax: 716-874-0746.

Solucient, *(Solucient LLC; 1-57372; 1-880678),* 300 E. Lombard St., Baltimore, MD 21202 Tel 410-576-9600; Fax: 410-783-0575; Toll Free: 800-568-3282; 1800 Sherman Ave., Evanston, IL 60201 Tel 847-570-3969; Fax: 847-570-3950
Web site: http://www.solucient.com.

Solum Verlag (NOR) *(82-560) Dist. by* **Intl Spec Bk.**

SOM Pub, *(SOM Publishing Co.; 0-944386),* 163 Moon Valley Rd., Windyville, MO 65783 (SAN 159-5423) Tel 417-345-8411; Fax: 417-345-6668
E-mail: som@som.org
Web site: http://www.som.org
Dist(s): **Baker & Taylor** *(Baker & Taylor Bks.)*
Bookpeople *(Bookpeople)*
New Leaf Dist *(New Leaf Distributing Co., Inc.).*

Somerleyton Pr, *(Somerleyton Pr.; 0-9674623),* 545 N. Woodlawn, Wichita, KS 67208-3600 Tel 316-683-7800
E-mail: somerleyton@jnutra.com.

Somerset Bks, *(Somerset Bks. Publishing; 0-9658528),* Orders Addr.: P.O. Box 213, Bellevue, WA 98009 Fax: 425-277-3903; Toll Free: 888-449-1979; Edit Addr.: 17519 149th Ave. SE, No. D1, Renton, WA 98058
E-mail: bodycare@somerset-co.com
Web site: http://www.somerset-co.com
Dist(s): **New Leaf Dist** *(New Leaf Distributing Co., Inc.)*
Quality Bks IL *(Quality Bks., Inc.).*

Somnos Programs, *(Somnos Programs; 0-9651214),* Div. of D. G. Catron, M.D., P.A., P.O. Box 11691, Knoxville, TN 37939-1691.

Sonoma County Med, *(Sonoma County Medical Assn.; 0-9677244),* 3033 Cleveland Ave, Santa Rosa, CA 95403-2183 Tel 707-525-4325; Fax: 707-525-4289
E-mail: sosborn@scma.org; scma@scma.org
Web site: http://www.scma.org.

Son-Rise Pubns, *(Son-Rise Pubns. & Distribution Co.; 0-936369),* 52 Greenfield Rd., New Wilmington, PA 16142 (SAN 698-0031) Tel 724-946-9057; Fax: 724-946-8700; Toll Free: 800-358-0777
Web site: http://www.softspace.com/steelvalley; http://www.sonrisepublications.com
Dist(s): **Baker & Taylor** *(Baker & Taylor Bks.).*

Sonters Pubng, *(Sonters Publishing, Ink; 0-9639154),* Orders Addr.: P.O. Box 109, Washington, MO 63090; Edit Addr.: 24 Forest Hills Dr., Washington, MO 63090 Tel 636-239-5450; Fax: 636-239-9937
E-mail: sonpub@fidnet.com.

Sopris, *(Sopris West; 0-944584; 1-57035),* 4093 Specialty Pl., Longmont, CO 80504 (SAN 243-945X) Tel 303-651-2829; Fax: 303-776-5934; Toll Free Fax: 888-819-7767 (orders only); Toll Free: 800-547-6747 (orders only)
E-mail: webmaster@sopriswest.com
Web site: http://www.sopriswest.com.

SOS Clinton, *(SOS of Clinton, N.Y.; 0-9627964),* Orders Addr.: P.O. Box 10, Clinton, NY 13323-0010 Tel 315-863-8691; Fax: 315-853-3966; Edit Addr.: 12 1/2 W. Park Row, Clinton, NY 13323
E-mail: bozmoran@borg.com.

SOS Pubns NJ, *(SOS Pubns.; 0-9625505; 1-887052),* 43 DeNormandie Ave., Fair Haven, NJ 07704 Tel 732-530-3199; Fax: 732-530-5896 Do not confuse with SOS Pubns., Springfield, OR
E-mail: sosjs@netlabs.net
Web site: http://www.netlabs.net/hp/sosjs.

Soulprint Pubng, *(Soulprint Publishing Co.; 0-9641576),* 1300 Adams Ave., No.29G, Costa Mesa, CA 92626 Tel 714-241-8999 (phone/fax)
E-mail: bevjinn@aol.com.

Soulstar Creations, *(Soulstar Creations; 0-9625000),* 1001 Garnet Ave., No. 200, San Diego, CA 92109 Tel 619-270-0845.

Sound Nutri, *(Sound Nutrition; 0-9609226),* P.O. Box 55, Hurricane, UT 84737-0055 (SAN 241-4597) Tel 435-635-4206; Fax: 435-635-2110
E-mail: mreug@redrock.net
Dist(s): **New Leaf Dist** *(New Leaf Distributing Co., Inc.)*
Nutri-Books Corp *(Nutri-Bks. Corp.).*

Soundview Pubns, *(Soundview Pubns., Inc.; 0-9626646; 1-885385),* 7100 Peachtree Dunwoody Rd. NE, No. 100, Atlanta, GA 30328-1689 Toll Free: 800-728-2288.

Source Pubng, *(Source Publishing of Western North Carolina, Inc.; 0-9651216),* 153 Skyview Cir., Asheville, NC 28804 Tel 704-252-7482; Fax: 704-285-0979.

†Sourcebks, *(Sourcebooks, Inc.; 0-942061; 0-9629162; 0-9629803; 1-57071; 1-57248; 1-883518; 1-887166; 1-4022),* 1935 Brookdale Rd., Suite 139, Naperville, IL 60563 (SAN 666-7864) Tel 630-961-3900; Fax: 630-961-2168; Toll Free: 800-432-7444
E-mail: info@sourcebooks.com
Web site: http://www.sourcebooks.com/
Dist(s): **Continental Bk** *(Continental Bk. Co., Inc.); CIP.*

Sourcebook, *(Sourcebook Project, The; 0-915554; 0-9600712),* P.O. Box 107, Glen Arm, MD 21057 (SAN 201-7652) Tel 410-668-6047
Web site: http://www.science-frontiers.com.

†South End Pr, *(South End Pr.; 0-89608),* Orders Addr.: c/o Consortium Book Sales & Distribution, 1045 Westgate Dr., Saint Paul, MN 55114-3572 Fax: 651-221-0124; Edit Addr.: 7 Brookline St., No. 1, Cambridge, MA 02139-4146 (SAN 211-979X) Tel 617-547-4002; Fax: 617-547-1333; Toll Free Fax: 800-334-3892; Toll Free: 800-283-3572
E-mail: southend@igc.org
Web site: http://www.southendpress.org
Dist(s): **Consort Bk Sales** *(Consortium Bk. Sales & Distribution); CIP.*

Southall Res, *(Southall Research; 0-9639682),* 7095 Hollywood Blvd., Suite 713, Hollywood, CA 90028 Tel 213-465-3221; Fax: 213-467-6642; Toll Free: 800-228-4425
E-mail: contact@hyssopherd.com
Web site: http://www.hyssopherb.com.

Southern IL Univ Sch, *(Southern Illinois Univ., Schl. of Medicine; 0-931369),* P.O. Box 19622, Springfield, IL 62794-9622 (SAN 663-6667) Tel 217-782-5665; Fax: 217-524-0192
Web site: http://www.pbli.org.

Southern Inst Pr, *(Southern Institute Pr.; 0-9615502),* Orders Addr.: P.O. Box 529, Indian Rocks Beach, FL 34635 (SAN 695-9237) Tel 813-596-4891; Edit Addr.: 13663 Kimberly Oaks Cir., Largo, FL 34644 (SAN 244-8386)
E-mail: sunnlp@intl-nlp.com
Web site: http://www.intl-nlp.com.

Southern U Pr, *(Southern Univ. Pr.; 0-87651),* P.O. Box 131298, Birmingham, AL 35213-6298 (SAN 204-6148) Tel 205-251-5113; Fax: 205-251-2222.

Southlnd Tutor, *(Southland Tutorials; 1-888628),* 289 Revere St., Upland, CA 91784-1364 Toll Free: 800-233-5150
Dist(s): **Majors Scientific Bks Inc** *(Majors Scientific Bks., Inc.)*
Technical Bk Co *(Technical Bk. Co.).*

Southpaw Pr, *(Southpaw Pr.; 0-9658600),* 1653 S. 2500 E., New Harmony, UT 84657 Tel 435-865-1785; Fax: 435-865-1786 Do not confuse with Southpaw Press in Longmont, CO
E-mail: mp@southpawpress.com
Web site: http://
www.herpesnomove.southpawpress.com.

Souvenir Pr Ltd (GBR) *(0-285) Dist. by* **IPG Chicago.**

Soyfoods Center, *(Soyfoods Ctr.; 0-933332; 1-928914),* Orders Addr.: P.O. Box 234, Lafayette, CA 94549 (SAN 212-8411) Tel 925-283-2991; Fax: 925-283-9091.

SP Press Intl, *(SP Pr. International, Inc.; 0-9617129),* 7806 Honeybee Ct., Bethesda, MD 20817 (SAN 662-6939) Tel 301-365-2739.

Sp1 France Editions (FRA) *(2-287; 3-540) Dist. by* **Spr-Verlag.**

SpaceLabs, *(SpaceLabs Medical, Inc.; 0-9627449; 1-882588),* Div. of Westmark International, Orders Addr.: P.O. Box 97013, Redmond, WA 98073 Tel 425-882-3700; Fax: 425-885-4877; Toll Free: 800-251-9910; Edit Addr.: 15220 NE 40th St., Redmond, WA 98052.

SPAN Intl Train, *(SPAN International Training; 1-886786; 1-891017),* 4226 Greenbriar Dr., Nixa, MO 65714 Tel 417-724-2881; Fax: 417-724-2883; Toll Free: 888-589-6757.

SPAN Pub, *(SPAN Publishing, Inc.; 1-880245),* Div. of Span Publishing, Inc., Orders Addr.: P.O. Box 365, Stevens Point, WI 54481-0365 (SAN 226-3572) Tel 715-345-2772; Fax: 715-345-7288; Toll Free: 800-647-7579.

Span-Text Bks, *(Span-Text Bks.; 0-9638926),* P.O. Box 35412, Fayetteville, NC 28303-0412 Tel 910-867-6735 (phone/fax).

Sparhawk Health, *(Sparhawk Health Pubns.; 0-9705025),* P.O. Box 35725, Brighton, MA 02135
E-mail: akay777@aol.com.

Sparrow Hawk Pr, *(Sparrow Hawk Pr.; 0-945027),* 11 Summit Ridge Dr., Tahlequah, OK 74464 (SAN 245-663X) Tel 918-456-3421; Fax: 918-458-5501; Sparrow Hawk Village, Tahlequah, OK 74464 (SAN 245-6648) Toll Free: 800-386-7161
E-mail: lccc@sanctasophia.org
Web site: http://www.sanctasophia.org
Dist(s): **Baker & Taylor** *(Baker & Taylor Bks.)*
Bookpeople *(Bookpeople)*
Distributors *(Distributors, The)*
New Concepts Bks & Tapes *(New Concepts Bks. & Tapes Distributors)*
New Leaf Dist *(New Leaf Distributing Co., Inc.)*
Quality Bks IL *(Quality Bks., Inc.).*

SPB Acad Pub (NLD) *(90-5103) Dist. by* **Balogh.**

Spec Clin Srvs, *(Specialized Clinical Services, Inc.; 1-883202),* 15102 Redhill Ave., Tustin, CA 92780 Tel 714-259-0106; Fax: 714-259-1838; Toll Free: 800-488-6424.

Spec Pr FL, *(Specialty Pr., Inc.; 0-9621629; 1-886941),* 300 NW 70th Ave., Suite 102, Plantation, FL 33317 (SAN 251-6977) Tel 954-792-8100; Fax: 954-792-8545; Toll Free: 800-233-9273 Do not confuse with Specialty Pr., Inc., in Ocean, NJ
E-mail: sales@addwarehouse.com
Web site: http://www.addwarehouse.com
Dist(s): **Baker & Taylor** *(Baker & Taylor Bks.)*
IPG Chicago *(Independent Pubs. Group).*

Specialist Journals, *(Specialist Journals; 0-911131),* Div. of Nature Publishing Group, 345 Park Ave., S., New York, NY 10010-1707 (SAN 274-7995) Tel 212-726-9333; Fax: 212-696-0052
E-mail: sjsupport@nature.com
Web site: http://www.nature.com.

Specialized Solns, *(Specialized Solutions, Inc.; 0-9663920; 1-893596),* 3910 Riga Blvd., Tampa, FL 33619 Fax: 813-621-8823; Toll Free Fax: 877-200-5959; Toll Free: 800-942-1660
E-mail: susan@specializedsolutions.com
Web site: http://www.specializedsolutions.com.

Specialty Cards, *(Specialty Cards; 0-9642193; 1-930393),* 5116 E. 88th St., Tulsa, OK 74137 Tel 918-493-6232; Fax: 918-493-2101 (phone/fax); Toll Free: 888-360-3206
E-mail: orders@specialtycards.com
Web site: http://www.specialtycards.com.

Specialty Pub, *(Specialty Publishing; 0-9636688),* P.O. Box 739, Bentonville, AR 72712 Toll Free: 800-701-6101 Do not confuse with Specialty Publishing Co., La Crosse, WI.

Specific Pr, *(Specific Pr.; 0-930846),* 1523 Franklin St., San Francisco, CA 94109 (SAN 222-8556) Tel 415-928-1133.

Speck Pub, *(Speck Publishing Co.; 0-9654202),* Orders Addr.: P.O. Box 965, Granite Falls, NC 28630 Tel 704-396-3168; Fax: 704-396-8783; Edit Addr.: 9 Forest Ave., Granite Falls, NC 28630.

Spect Ln Pr, *(Spectacle Lane Pr., Inc.; 0-930753),* P.O. Box 1237, Mount Pleasant, SC 29465-1237 Tel 843-971-9165; Fax: 843-971-9165; Toll Free: 888-669-8114
E-mail: jaskar44@aol.com
Dist(s): **Dot Gibson Dist** *(Dot Gibson Distribution).*

Spectra Imprint of Bantam

Spectra Pub Co, *(Spectra Publishing Co., Inc.; 0-915667),* P.O. Box 966, Silverthorne, CO 80498 (SAN 292-6814) Tel 970-468-6439; Fax: 970-468-6446
E-mail: spec_pubco@aol.com.

Spectrm Imprint of Hungry Minds

Spectrum Biosci, *(Spectrum Bioscience, Inc.; 0-9642976),* 2020 F St., NW, No. 505, Washington, DC 20006-4216 (SAN 298-3826) Tel 202-467-0572
E-mail: kjdillon@nmaa
Web site: http://www.biophoton.com.

Speech Bin, *(Speech Bin, Inc., The; 0-937857),* 1965 25th Ave., Vero Beach, FL 32960 (SAN 630-1657) Tel 561-770-0007; Fax: 561-770-0006
E-mail: info@speechbin.com
Web site: http://www.speechbin.com.

Speech Commun Assn, *See* **Natl Comm Assn**

Speech Found Am, *See* **Stuttering Fnd Am**

†Speller, *(Speller, Robert & Sons, Pubs., Inc.; 0-8315),* Orders Addr.: P.O. Box 411, New York, NY 10159 (SAN 203-2295) Tel 212-473-0333; P.O. Box 461, New York, NY 10108 (SAN 203-2309)*; CIP.*

Spencer Bks, *(Spencer Bks.; 1-889793),* Div. of Positive Medicine, Inc., 235 E. 42nd St., 15th Flr., New York, NY 10017 Fax: 212-973-7279; Toll Free: 800-774-3313
Web site: http://www.positiveprofiles.com
Dist(s): **Rittenhouse** *(Rittenhouse Bk. Distributors).*

SPI, *See* **DOMA Pr**

SPI, *(SPI Bks.; 0-944007; 1-56171),* 99 Spring St., 3rd Flr., New York, NY 10012 Tel 212-431-5011; Fax: 212-431-8646
E-mail: ian@spibooks.com
Web site: http://www.spibooks.com
Dist(s): **Assoc Pubs Grp** *(Associated Pubs. Group).*

SPIE, *(SPIE-International Society for Optical Engineering; 0-8194; 0-89252),* Orders Addr.: P.O. Box 10, Bellingham, WA 98227-0010 (SAN 224-1706) Tel 360-676-3290; Fax: 360-647-1445; Edit Addr.: 1000 20th St., Bellingham, WA 98225 (SAN 669-1323)
E-mail: spie@spie.org
Web site: http://www.spie.org/bookstore.

Spinal Pubns Ltd (NZL) *(0-9597746) Dist. by* **Orthopedic Phys.**

Spire Imprint of Revell

Spirit Dance, *(Spirit Dance Publishing; 1-880782),* P.O. Box 82, Howey In The Hills, FL 3437-0082 Fax: 904-735-0033; Toll Free: 800-223-5333.

Spirit Pr, *(Spirit Pr.; 0-944296),* 1005 Granite Ridge Dr., Santa Cruz, CA 95065 (SAN 243-2544) Tel 408-426-7971 Do not confuse with companies with the same name in Porrtland, OR, Raleigh, NC.

SpiritPassage, *(SpiritPassage; 1-929341),* 4 Agua Viviendo, Santa Fe, NM 87508 Tel 505-466-6520 (phone/fax)
E-mail: SpiritPass@aol.com; mail@spiritpassage.org
Web site: http://www.SpiritPassage.org.

Spiritpoint Pr, *(Spiritpoint Pr.; 1-887270),* 851 Mt. Vernon Ct., Naperville, IL 60563 Tel 630-420-1887; Fax: 630-963-0341; Toll Free: 800-750-6649; 2736 Maple Ave., Downers Grove, IL 60515
E-mail: maryannako@aol.com
Web site: http://www.namepower101.com.

Spon Imprint of Routledge

Spondylitis Assn, *(Spondylitis Assn. of America; 1-881941),* P.O. Box 5872, Sherman Oaks, CA 91413 Toll Free: 800-777-8189.

Spoon River, *(Spoon River Pr., The; 0-930358),* 2319-C W. Rohmann Ave., Peoria, IL 61604 (SAN 211-5190) Tel 309-672-2665; Fax: 309-672-7853 Do not confuse with Spoon River Poetry Pr..

SPORT Found, *(SPORT Foundation; 0-9629739),* P.O. Box 1026, Vista, CA 92085-1026 Tel 760-931-5947; Fax: 760-931-9013.

Sports Hlth, *(Sports Health Education; 0-9630564),* 202 W. Hills Way, Woodstock, GA 30189-6756.

Sports Med Bks Inc, *(Sports Medicine Bks., Inc.; 0-914363),* 876 Guy Lombardo Ave., Freeport, NY 11520 (SAN 289-6818) Tel 516-546-1425.

Sports Touch, *(Sports Touch Publishing; 1-878069),* P.O. Box 8154, Belleville, IL 62222 Tel 618-233-9886.

Spring Jrnl, *(Spring Journal; 1-882670),* Box 583, Putnam, CT 06260 Tel 860-974-3428; Fax: 860-974-3195
E-mail: spring@springpub.com
Web site: http://www.springpub.com
Dist(s): **Continuum** *(Continuum International Publishing Group, Inc.).*

Spring Pubns, *(Spring Pubns., Inc.; 0-88214),* 299 E. Quassett Rd., Woodstock, CT 06281 (SAN 203-2244) Tel 860-974-3428; Fax: 860-974-3195
E-mail: spring@springpub.com
Web site: http://www.springpub.com
Dist(s): **Continuum** *(Continuum International Publishing Group, Inc.).*

†Springer Pub, *(Springer Publishing Co., Inc.; 0-8261),* 536 Broadway, 11th Flr., New York, NY 10012-3955 (SAN 203-2236) Tel 212-431-4370; Fax: 212-941-7842
E-mail: springer@springerpub.com
Web site: http://www.springerpub.com*; CIP.*

†Springhouse Corp, *(Springhouse Corp.; 0-87434; 0-916730; 1-58255),* Member of Wolters Kluwer, Orders Addr.: P.O. Box 908, Springhouse, PA 19477-0908 Tel 215-646-8700; Fax: 215-646-4508; Toll Free: 800-346-7844
E-mail: sph.publishing@springnet.com
Web site: http://www.springnet.com
Dist(s): **J Majors Co** *(Majors, J. A. Co.)*
Lppncott W & W *(Lippincott Williams & Wilkins)*
Matthews Bk Co *(Matthews Bk. Co.)*
Rittenhouse *(Rittenhouse Bk. Distributors); CIP.*

†Spr-Verlag, *(Springer-Verlag New York, Inc.; 0-387; 0-8176; 3-211; 3-540; 3-7908; 4-431; 1-85233),* Subs. of Springer-Verlag GmbH & Co. KG, Orders Addr.: P.O. Box 2485, Secaucus, NJ 07096-2485 (SAN 665-7842) Tel 201-348-4033; Fax: 201-348-4505; Toll Free: 800-777-4643; Edit Addr.: 175 Fifth Ave., New York, NY 10010 (SAN 203-2228) Tel 212-460-1500; Fax: 212-473-6272 ; *Imprints:* Copernicus (Copernicus) AIP Pr (A I P Press)
E-mail: service@springer-ny.com; orders@springer.de
Web site: http://www.springer.de/; http://www.springer-ny.com*; CIP.*

Spr-Verlag (SGP) *(981-3083; 981-4021) Dist. by* **Spr-Verlag.**

Spr-Verlag (GBR) *(1-85233) Dist. by* **Spr-Verlag.**

Spr-Verlag (ITA) *(88-470) Dist. by* **Spr-Verlag.**

Spurge ink, *(Spurge ink!; 1-888232),* Affil. of Knowledge Exchange, LLC, 16350 Ventura Blvd., Suite 362, Encino, CA 92436 Tel 818-705-1269; Fax: 818-708-8764
E-mail: info@spurgeink.com
Web site: http://www.spurgeink.com
Dist(s): **Natl Bk Netwk** *(National Bk. Network).*

Spyglass Pubns, *(Spyglass Pubns.; 0-9627559),* 8242 Spyglass Cir., Orland Park, IL 60462 Tel 708-349-8369.

Square One, *(Square One Pubs.; 0-7570),* 16 Frist St., Garden City Park, NY 11040 Tel 516-535-2010; Fax: 516-535-2014
E-mail: sq1info@aol.com
Web site: http://squareonepublishers.com.

Sr Assist Essent, *(Senior Assistance For Essentials (S.A.F.E.); 0-9652930),* 3079 Hathaway Ct., Atlanta, GA 30341-4641 Tel 770-496-1523.

SR Bks Imprint of Scholarly Res Inc

SRG Pubng, *(SRG Publishing; 0-9637824),* 1360 Swordfish St., Foster City, CA 94404-1956 Tel 650-573-7177; Fax: 650-573-6166; Toll Free: 800-938-0942
E-mail: rolfnyoga@aol.com
Web site: http://www.rolfnyoga.com.

Sri Satguru Pubns (IND) *(81-7030) Dist. by* **S Asia.**

SRIS (GBR) *(0-7123; 0-7141; 0-946655) Dist. by* **L Erlbaum Assocs.**

St Aedans Pr & Bk, *(St. Aedan's Pr. & Bk. Distributors, Inc.; 0-940198),* P.O. Box 335, Hillsdale, NJ 07642-0385 (SAN 217-1139) Tel 201-664-0127
E-mail: junius1920@yahoo.com
Web site: http://www.juniusbooks.com.

St Andrew Press (GBR) *(0-7152; 0-86153) Dist. by* **St Mut.**

St Augustines Pr, *(St. Augustine's Pr., Inc.; 1-890318; 1-58731),* P.O. Box 2285, South Bend, IN 46680 Tel 219-291-3500; Fax: 219-291-3700; Toll Free: 888-997-4994
E-mail: bruce@staugustine.net
Web site: http://www.staugustine.net
Dist(s): **Chicago Distribution Ctr** *(Chicago Distribution Ctr.)*
U Ch Pr *(Univ. of Chicago Pr.).*

St Bart Pr Ltd, *(St. Barthelemey Pr., Ltd.; 1-887617),* 2971 Flowers Rd., S., Suite 100, Atlanta, GA 30341 Tel 770-451-1922; Fax: 770-457-9808; Toll Free: 800-451-1923
E-mail: fullerws@aol.com
Web site: http://www.stbarthelemypress.com.

St George Bk Serv, *See* **R Steiner Col**

St Georges Pr, *(St. Georges Pr.; 1-883855),* 991 Colonial Village N., New Castle, DE 19720 Tel 302-328-4150.

St Lucie Pr, *(St. Lucie Pr.; 0-9634030; 1-57444; 1-878205; 1-884015),* Div. of CRC Pr., 2000 Corporate Blvd., NW, Boca Raton, FL 33431-7372 (SAN 297-9489) Tel 561-274-9906; Fax: 561-274-9927; Toll Free: 800-272-7737
E-mail: information@slpress.com
Web site: http://www.slpress.com.

St Lukes Hosp, *(St. Luke's Hospital of Kansas City; 0-9657425),* 4401 Wornall Rd., Kansas City, MO 64111 Tel 816-932-2000; Fax: 816-932-5990.

†St Martin, *(St. Martin's Pr., LLC; 0-312; 0-8050; 0-940687; 0-9603648; 1-55927; 1-58063; 1-58238),* Div. of V H P S, Inc., Orders Addr.: c/o VHPS, 16365 James Madison Hwy., Gordonville, VA 22942 Tel 540-672-7600; Toll Free Fax: 800-672-2054; Toll Free: 888-330-8477; Edit Addr.: 175 Fifth Ave., New York, NY 10010 (SAN 200-2132) Tel 212-726-0200 (College Div.); 212-674-5151 (Trade Div.); Fax: 212-686-9491 (College Div.); 212-674-3179 (Trade Div.); Toll Free: 800-470-4767 (College Div.); 800-221-7945 (Trade Div.) ; *Imprints:* St Martin Griffin (Saint Martin's Griffin) St Martins Paperbacks (Saint Martin's Paperbacks) Thomas Dunne (Dunne, Thomas Books) Golden Adult (Golden Books Adult Publishing Group) Whitman Coin (Whitman Coin Products)
E-mail: webmaster@stmartins.com; enquiries@stmartins.com
Web site: http://www.smpcollege.com; http://www.stmartins.com
Dist(s): **CMG** *(Comag Marketing Group)*
Shens Bks *(Shen's Bks.)*
VHPS *(VHPS Holtzbrinck Pubs.); CIP.*

St Martin Griffin Imprint of St Martin

St Martins Paperbacks Imprint of St Martin

St Mut, *(State Mutual Bk. & Periodical Service, Ltd.; 0-7855; 0-89771),* Orders Addr.: P.O. Box 1199, Bridgehampton, NY 11932-1199.

St Paul Bks, *See* **Pauline Bks**

St Paul Pubns (GBR) *(0-85439) Dist. by* **St Mut.**

†Stackpole, *(Stackpole Bks.; 0-8117; 1-881982),* 5067 Ritter Rd., Mechanicsburg, PA 17055 (SAN 202-5396) Tel 717-796-0411; Fax: 717-796-0412
E-mail: sales@stackpolebooks.com
Web site: http://www.stackpolebooks.com
Dist(s): **Penn Capitol Presrv** *(Pennsylvania Capitol Preservation Committee); CIP.*

Staff Dev Educ, *(Staff Development for Educators; 0-9627389; 1-884548),* Div. of Highlights for Children, 75 Jaffrey Rd., Box 500, Peterborough, NH 03458 Tel 603-924-9621; Fax: 603-924-6688; Toll Free Fax: 800-337-9929; Toll Free: 800-321-0401 ; *Imprints:* Crystal Spgs (Crystal Springs Books)
E-mail: jay@sde.com
Web site: http://www.sde.com.

Standard Arts, *(Standard Arts Pr.; 0-911426),* 2324 Butler Rd., P.O. Box 121, Butler, MD 21023 (SAN 204-6318) Tel 410-771-4698.

Stanford Bkstore, *(Stanford Bookstore Palo Alto; 0-9638338),* 135 University Ave., Palo Alto, CA 94301 (SAN 103-3913) Tel 415-327-3680; Fax: 415-322-2021
Web site: http://www.stanfordbookstores.com.

†Stanford U Pr, *(Stanford Univ. Pr.; 0-8047),* Stanford Univ. Pr., Stanford, CA 94305-2235 (SAN 203-3526) Tel 650-723-9434; Fax: 650-725-3457
Web site: http://www.sup.org
Dist(s): **Cambridge U Pr** *(Cambridge Univ. Pr.); CIP.*

Star Industries, *(Star Industries, Inc.; 0-9628220),* Orders Addr.: P.O. Box 1027, Melrose, MA 02176; Edit Addr.: 99R Washington St., Melrose, MA 02176 Tel 617-662-2220.

Star Mtn Pr, *(Star Mountain Pr.; 0-9653755),* P.O. Box 1845, Ann Arbor, MI 48106 Tel 313-665-3171.

Star Orange Park, *(Star Pubns.; 0-9622992),* 596 Aberdeen Ct., Orange Park, FL 32073 Tel 904-272-9598 Do not confuse with companies with the same name in Rancho Palos Verdes, CA, Kansas City, MO, Chico, CA, San Jose, CA, Colorado Springs, CO.

Star Pr, *(Star Pr.; 0-937038),* P.O. Box 835, Friday Harbor, WA 98250 (SAN 226-8035) Tel 360-378-5871.

Star Pub CA, *(Star Publishing Co.; 0-89863),* 940 Emmett Ave., Belmont, CA 94002 (SAN 212-6958) Tel 650-591-3505; Fax: 650-591-3898 Do not confuse with companies with similiar names in Galion, OH, Saint Louis, MO, Boynton Beach, FL, Vancouver, WA, Raleigh, NC, Carmichael, CA, San Rafael, CA, Orange, CA
E-mail: mail@starpublishing.com
Web site: http://www.starpublishing.com.

Star Trek Imprint of PB

Star Valley, *(Star Valley Pubns.; 0-911223),* P.O. Box 421, Noti, OR 97461 (SAN 287-7562) Tel 541-935-0832.

Starburst, *(Starburst Pubs.; 0-914984; 1-892016),* Orders Addr.: P.O. Box 4123, Lancaster, PA 17604 Tel 717-293-0939; Fax: 717-293-1945; Toll Free: 800-441-1456 (orders only)
E-mail: starburst@starburstpublishers.com
Web site: http://www.starburstpublishers.com
Dist(s): **Anchor Distributors** *(Anchor Distributors)*
Appalachian Bible *(Appalachian Bible Co.)*
Baker & Taylor *(Baker & Taylor Bks.)*
Brodart *(Brodart Co.)*
Natl Bk Netwk *(National Bk. Network)*
Nutri-Books Corp *(Nutri-Bks. Corp.)*
Quality Bks IL *(Quality Bks., Inc.)*
Riverside-World *(Riverside World)*
Spring Arbor Dist *(Spring Arbor Distributors Inc.)*
Unique Bks Inc *(Unique Bks., Inc.).*

Stargazer, *(Stargazer Publishing Co.; 0-9643853; 0-9713756),* Orders Addr.: P.O. Box 77002, Corona, CA 92877-0100 Tel 909-898-4619; Fax: 909-898-4633; Toll Free: 800-606-7895; Edit Addr.: 958 Stanislaus Dr., Corona, CA 92881 (SAN 298-6566)
E-mail: stargazer@stargazerpub.com
Web site: http://www.stargazerpub.com.

Starkey Labs, *(Starkey Laboratories, Inc.; 0-9601970),* Orders Addr.: P.O. Box 9457, Minneapolis, MN 55440 Tel 612-941-6401; Fax: 612-828-9262; Toll Free: 800-328-8602; Edit Addr.: 6700 Washington Ave., S., Eden Prairie, MN 55344 (SAN 215-1111).

Starpoint Ent, *(Starpoint Enterprises, Ltd.; 0-9641810),* P.O. Box 15, Jericho, NY 11753 (SAN 298-3354) Tel 516-626-2801; 800-922-7337 (ext. 120)
E-mail: honeybs4u@aol.com
Web site: http://www.amberrose.com.

Starr Publ, *(Starr Publishing; 0-9659188),* 2486 Nobility Ave., Melbourne, FL 32934 Tel 407-259-9301 Do not confuse with companies with the same name in Aurora, CO, Newcastle, ME, Las Vegas, NV, Wynnewood, PA.

Starrhill Press Imprint of River City Pub

Stat Nursing, *(Stat Nursing Consultants; 0-9640556),* 6003 Deer Run Dr., Trafford, PA 15085 Tel 412-856-1590.

State Art, *(State of the Art, Inc.; 1-881782),* 4455 Connecticut Ave. NW, Suite B200, Washington, DC 20008-2328 Tel 202-797-0818; Fax: 202-232-2261 Do not confuse with State of the Art, Ltd., Denver, CO.

†State U NY Pr, *(State Univ. of New York Pr.; 0-7914; 0-87395; 0-88706),* Orders Addr.: c/o CUP Services, P.O. Box 6525, Ithaca, NY 14851 (SAN 203-3496) Tel 607-277-2211; Fax: 607-277-6292; Edit Addr.: 90 State St., Suite 700, Albany, NY 12207 (SAN 658-1730) Tel 518-472-5000; Fax: 518-472-5038
E-mail: info@sunypress.edu; orderbook@cupscrve.org
Web site: http://www.sunypress.edu
Dist(s): **Baker & Taylor** *(Baker & Taylor Bks.)*
Pegasus Pr *(Pegasus Pr.); CIP.*

Statesman-Exam, *(Statesman-Examiner, Inc.; 0-940151),* P.O. Box 271, Colville, WA 99114-0271 (SAN 664-2691) Tel 509-684-4567; Fax: 509-684-3849.

Statford CA, *See* **MKS Inc**

†Station Hill Pr, *(Station Hill Pr.; 0-88268; 0-930794),* Station Hill Rd., Barrytown, NY 12507 (SAN 214-1485) Tel 845-758-5840; Fax: 845-758-8163
E-mail: buun@stationhill.org
Web site: http://www.stationhill.org/
Dist(s): **BookWorld** *(BookWorld Services, Inc.)*
Bookpeople *(Bookpeople)*
Consort Bk Sales *(Consortium Bk. Sales & Distribution)*
SPD-Small Pr Dist *(SPD-Small Pr. Distribution)*
Writers & Bks *(Writers & Bks.); CIP.*

Statnry Office (GBR) *(0-10; 0-11; 0-337) Dist. by* **Bernan Associates.**

Statnry Office (GBR) *(0-10; 0-11; 0-337) Dist. by* **Balogh.**

Steck-V, *See* **Raintree Steck-V**

Steerforth Pr, *(Steerforth Pr.; 1-883642; 1-58642),* 105-106 Chelsea St., P.O. Box 70, South Royalton, VT 05068 Tel 802-763-2808; Fax: 802-763-2818
E-mail: helga@steerforth.com; info@steerforth.com
Web site: http://www.steerforth.com
Dist(s): **Publishers Group** *(Publishers Group West).*

Steiner Book Centre (CAN) *(0-919924) Dist. by* **Anthroposophic.**

Stenotype Educ, *(Stenotype Educational Products, Inc.; 0-938643),* P.O. Box 959, Melrose, FL 32666 (SAN 661-6356); P.O. Box 1235, Melrose, FL 32666 (SAN 661-6364)
Web site: http://www.stened.com.

Step Out On Faith, *(Step Out On Faith Publishing Co.; 0-9672052),* P.O. Box 921, Slidell, LA 70459 Tel 504-645-8803; Toll Free: 877-246-4126 Do not confuse with Montgomery Publishing Co., Atlanta, GA
E-mail: gmwalker@bellsouth.net
Dist(s): **Walkers Ent** *(Walker's Enterprises).*

Steppstone Pr, *(Steppingstone Pr., Inc.; 0-9642338),* Orders Addr.: P.O. Box 1025, Boise, ID 83701 (SAN 298-3214); Edit Addr.: 3113 Fallingbrook Ln., Boise, ID 83706 Tel 208-345-2864.

Sterling (IND) *Dist. by* **Asia Bk Corp.**

†Sterling, *(Sterling Publishing Co., Inc.; 0-8069; 1-4027),* 387 Park Ave., S., New York, NY 10016-8810 (SAN 211-6324) Tel 212-532-7160; Fax: 212-213-2495; Toll Free Fax: 800-775-8736 (warehouse) Do not confuse with companies with similar names in Falls Church, VA, Fallbrook, CA, Lewisville, TX
E-mail: custservice@sterlingpub.com
Web site: http://www.sterlingpub.com; *CIP.*

Sterling Hse, *See* **SterlingHse**

SterlingHse, *(SterlingHouse Pubs.; 1-56315),* Div. of Lee Shore Agency, The Sterling Bldg., 440 Friday Rd., Pittsburgh, PA 15209-2114 Tel 412-821-6211; Fax: 412-821-6997; Toll Free: 888-542-2665
E-mail: sterlingho@aol.com
Web site: http://www.sterlinghousepublisher.com
Dist(s): **Partners Pubs Grp** *(Partners Pubs. Group, Inc.).*

Stern-Greco, *(Stern/Greco; 0-9674422),* Elm Ct., Sands Point, NY 11050 Tel 516-767-1661 (phone/fax)
E-mail: sternshome@aol.com.

Stethophonics, *(Stethophonics; 0-9626835),* Div. of Pulmonology Services, Inc., 21 Wayside Rd., Westborough, MA 01581 Tel 617-522-5800; Fax: 617-522-4156
E-mail: info@stethographics.com
Web site: http://www.stethographics.com.

Stevenson Intl, *See* **R Stevenson Conslt**

Stillpoint Pr, *(Stillpoint Pr.; 0-9639791),* 133 E. De la Guerra St., Suite 362, Santa Barbara, CA 93101 Tel 805-681-0040; Fax: 805-681-0070 Do not confuse with companies with the same or similar names in New York, NY, Mount Laurel, NJ.

Stipes, *(Stipes Publishing L.L.C.; 0-87563; 1-58874),* Orders Addr.: P.O. Box 526, Champaign, IL 61824 (SAN 206-8664) Tel 217-356-8391; Fax: 217-356-5753; Edit Addr.: 202-204 W. University Ave., Champaign, IL 61824
E-mail: stipes@soltec.com
Web site: http://www.stipes.com.

Stockton Pr, *See* **Specialist Journals**

Stoddart Publ (CAN) *(0-7736; 0-7737; 0-919292) Dist. by* **General Distrib Services.**

St-of-the-Art Tech, *(State-of-the-Art Technologies, Inc.; 0-9650767),* 4019 W. Rosecrans Ave., Hawthorne, CA 90250 Tel 310-675-9121 Toll Free: 800-963-3429
E-mail: medicinechief@aol.com
Web site: http://www.medicinehouse.com.

Stokesville Pub, *(Stokesville Publishing Co.; 0-936030),* P.O. Box 14401, Atlanta, GA 30324 (SAN 211-3333) Tel 404-365-8975.

Stoma Pr, *(Stoma Pr., Inc.; 0-89939),* 13231 42nd Ave., NE., Seattle, WA 98125 (SAN 222-8432) Tel 206-365-2665.

Stone Age Pr, *(Stone Age Pr. of Alaska; 0-9615808),* 1649 Bannister Dr., Anchorage, AK 99508-4058 (SAN 696-5938) Tel 907-279-3740.

Stone House Pr Inc, *(Stone House Pr., Inc; 0-9675060),* RR 1, Box 247, Richville, MN 56576 Tel 218-495-2855; Fax: 218-495-3035
E-mail: joliejim@djam.com.

Stonebrdge Pubng, *(Stonebridge Publishing, Ltd.; 0-9639303),* 15 Lake Rd., Great Neck, NY 11020 Tel 516-482-2485; Fax: 516-482-2480; Toll Free: 800-334-7323.

Stonefly Pub, *(Stonefly Publishing; 0-9624083),* Div. of Stonefly Industries, Inc., Orders Addr.: P.O. Box 4264, Bryan, TX 77805; Edit Addr.: 2704 Broadmoor, Bryan, TX 77805 Tel 409-776-1868; Fax: 409-731-1331.

Stonehaven Pubs, *(Stonehaven Pubs.; 0-937775),* Orders Addr.: P.O. Box 367, Lena, IL 61048 (SAN 659-347X); Edit Addr.: 602 Oak St., Lena, IL 61048 (SAN 659-3488) Tel 815-369-2823 Do not confuse with Stonehaven Pubs., Fort Worth, TX
E-mail: millievic.com.

Stonehorse, *(Stonehorse Pr.; 0-9639632),* 3908 E. 80th St., Tulsa, OK 74136 Tel 918-488-9530
E-mail: jeacarlton@aol.com.

Stony Pt Christian, *(Stony Point Christian Pubns.; 0-9661484),* 316 Terrace Lawn, Taylorsville, NC 28681 Tel 828-632-8215 (phone/fax)
E-mail: tjcraig@bellsouth.net; spchristianpub@i-america.net; tcraig@twave.net
Web site: http://www.spchristianpub.org.

†Storey Bks, *(Storey Bks.; 0-88266; 1-58017),* Orders Addr.: P.O. Box 445, Pownal, VT 05261; Edit Addr.: R.R. 1, Box 105, Pownal, VT 05261-9718 (SAN 203-4158) Fax: 802-823-5819; Toll Free Fax: 800-865-3429; Toll Free: 800-793-9396
E-mail: info@storey.com
Web site: http://www.storeybooks.com
Dist(s): **Workman Pub** *(Workman Publishing Co., Inc.); CIP.*

Storey Comm Inc, *See* **Storey Bks**

Storm Peak, *(Storm Peak Pr.; 0-9641357; 1-928990),* 2629 Nob Hill Ave., N., Seattle, WA 98109 Tel 206-286-1332; Fax: 206-286-1314
Dist(s): **Baker & Taylor** *(Baker & Taylor Bks.).*

Stough Inst, *(Stough Institute, Inc., The; 0-940830),* 200 E. 66th St., Suite A1105, New York, NY 10021 (SAN 219-8193) Tel 212-308-7138.

Strafford Pubns, *(Strafford Pubns., Inc.; 0-9616858; 1-887986),* Orders Addr.: P.O. Box 13729, Atlanta, GA 30324-0729 (SAN 661-5953) Tel 404-881-1141; Fax: 404-881-0074; Toll Free: 800-926-7926 (Customer service); Edit Addr.: 590 Dutch Valley Rd., NE, Atlanta, GA 30324-0729
E-mail: custserv@straffordpub.com.

Stratford NC, *(Stratford Bks.; 0-9621194; 1-891137),* 3064 Old Sides Mill Rd., Winston-Salem, NC 27103 (SAN 250-765X) Tel 336-768-9236 Do not confuse with Stratford Bks. in Princeton, NJ.

Strauss Pub, *(Strauss Publishing Co.; 0-9625324),* Orders Addr.: P.O. Box 654, Ardsley, NY 10502 Tel 914-693-1705; Edit Addr.: 39 Prospect Ave., Ardsley, NY 10502.

Strawberry Fields Pr, *(Strawberry Fields Pr.; 0-942033),* 920 Shorey Rd., Chehalis, WA 98532 (SAN 666-3184) Tel 360-748-9657.

Strawberry GA, *(Strawberry Patch; 0-9618306; 1-887987),* Orders Addr.: P.O. Box 52404, Atlanta, GA 30355-0404 (SAN 667-3031) Tel 404-261-2197; Fax: 404-841-9586; Toll Free: 800-875-7242; Edit Addr.: 273 Eureka Dr., Atlanta, GA 30305-4214 Do not confuse with Strawberry Pr., New York, NY
E-mail: dipfeifer@aol.com
Web site: http://www.strawberrypatch.net.

†Strawberry Hill, *(Strawberry Hill Pr.; 0-89407),* 3848 SE Division St., Portland, OR 97202-1641 (SAN 238-8103); *CIP.*

Stray Dog, *(Stray Dog Pr.; 0-9664082),* P.O. Box 1099, Calistoga, CA 94515 Tel 707-963-8364
E-mail: mickiv@napanet.net
Web site: http://www.dogchefs.com.

Stress Less, *(Stress Less Publishing, Inc.; 1-885044),* 5115 N. Scottsdale, Scottsdale, AZ 85250 Fax: 602-945-1579; Toll Free: 800-794-7066.

†Strong Mus, *(Strong Museum, The; 0-940365),* 1 Manhattan Sq., Rochester, NY 14607 (SAN 281-1847); *CIP.*

STT, *(S T T/ Scientific & Technical Translations; 0-9702353),* 351 Pleasant St., No. 210, Northampton, MA 01060 Tel 817-390-7400
E-mail: stt-pub@usa.net.

Stuart Titles Ltd (GBR) *(0-948474) Dist. by* **St Mut.**

Stuart Victor, *(Stuart Victor Publishing; 0-9653155),* Orders Addr.: P.O. Box 60322, Phoenix, AZ 85082-0322 Tel 602-244-0422; Edit Addr.: 2015 N. 47th Pl., Phoenix, AZ 85008
E-mail: stuartvictor@inficad.com
Web site: http://www.inficad.com/~stuartvictor/
Dist(s): **Bookpeople** *(Bookpeople)*
New Leaf Dist *(New Leaf Distributing Co., Inc.).*

Student Coll, *(Student College Aid; 0-932495),* 7950 N. Stadium Dr., Apt. 229, Houston, TX 77030-4421 (SAN 687-4320) Tel 713-796-2209; Fax: 713-796-9963
E-mail: edwherros@aol.com.

Studios West, *See* **Ritchie Unltd**

Study Ctr Pr Imprint of SF Study Ctr

Sturge Weber, *(Sturge-Weber Foundation; 0-9670484),* Orders Addr.: P.O. Box 418, Mount Freedom, NJ 07970-0418 Tel 973-895-4445; Fax: 973-895-4846; Edit Addr.: 2 W. Hanover Ave., Suite 208, Mount Freedom, NJ 07970-0418
E-mail: sws@sturge-weber.com
Web site: http://www.sturge-weber.com.

Stuttering Fnd Am, *(Stuttering Foundation of America; 0-933388; 1-930244),* Orders Addr.: P.O. Box 11749, Memphis, TN 38111-0749 (SAN 282-3330) Tel 901-452-7343; Fax: 901-452-3931; Toll Free: 800-992-9392; Edit Addr.: 3100 Walnut Grove Rd., Suite 603, Memphis, TN 38111-3530 (SAN 282-3349)
E-mail: stutter@vantek.net
Web site: http://www.stutteringhelp.org.

Stuttman, *See* **Websters Unified**

Stylus Pub VA, *(Stylus Publishing, LLC; 1-57922),* Orders Addr.: P.O. Box 605, Herndon, VA 20172-0605; Edit Addr.: 22883 Quicksilver Dr., Sterling, VA 20166-2012 (SAN 299-1853) Tel 703-661-1581; Fax: 703-661-1501 ; *Imprints:* BPS Bks (B P S Books) Trentham Bks (Trentham Books) Do not confuse with companies with the same name in Sunnyvale, CA, Quakertown, PA
E-mail: stylusmail@presswarehouse.com
Web site: http://styluspub.com
Dist(s): **LPC Group** *(LPC Group).*

Successful Living, *(Successful Living Pr.; 0-937743),* 804 Northey Dr., Sacramento, CA 95833 (SAN 659-3526) Tel 916-927-7942; 727 56th St., Sacramento, CA 95818 (SAN 659-3534).

Sudz Pub, *(Sudz Publishing; 0-9623114),* Orders Addr.: P.O. Box 1199, Pilot Point, TX 76258 Tel 940-686-9208; Edit Addr.: 1222 S. Hwy. 377, Pilot Point, TX 76258.

Sugar Mtn, *(Sugar Mountain Productions; 1-893667; 1-930591),* P.O. Box 351, East Burke, VT 05832 Fax: 781-863-1076 Do not confuse with companies with same or similar names in Warner, NH, Seattle, WA
E-mail: ezra53a@aol.com.

Sugarday Bks, *(Sugarday Bks.; 0-9659646),* 2901 Barracks Rd., Charlottesville, VA 22901 Tel 804-296-1558; Fax: 804-296-0615
E-mail: sugarday@aol.com
Web site: http://www.sugarday.com.

Sugden, *(Sugden, Sherwood & Co.; 0-89385),* 315 Fifth St., Peru, IL 61354 (SAN 210-5659) Tel 815-223-2520; Fax: 815-223-4486
E-mail: philomon1@netscape.net
Dist(s): **Open Court** *(Open Court).*

Sullivan & Foster, *(Sullivan & Foster Publishing; 1-890410),* Div. of Entagon Communications, Inc., Orders Addr.: P.O. Box 246, New York, NY 10024 Tel 212-501-8181; Fax: 212-501-8926; Toll Free: 800-717-2669; Edit Addr.: 173 W. 81st St., Lower Level, New York, NY 10024.

Sulzburger & Graham Pub, *(Sulzburger & Graham Publishing, Ltd.; 0-910328; 0-943519; 0-945819; 1-57613),* 793 Arbuckle Ave., Woodmere, NY 11598-2723 (SAN 247-9664) Tel 212-947-0100; Fax: 212-947-0360; Toll Free: 800-366-7086 (orders).

Summers Pr, *(Summers Pr.; 0-9625969; 1-56759),* Div. of Aspen Pubs., Inc., Orders Addr.: P.O. Box 822068, Fort Worth, TX 76182 Toll Free: 800-743-6491; Edit Addr.: 950 Westbank Dr., Suite 204, Austin, TX 78746-6684 Tel 512-329-9140; Fax: 512-367-2029
E-mail: getlegal@summerspress.com
Web site: http://www.summerspress.com.

Summers Pub, *(Summers Publishing; 0-916109),* 200 Chester St., Jefferson City, MO 65101-4023 (SAN 294-9083)
Dist(s): **Cowley Distributing Inc** *(Cowley Distributing, Inc.).*

†**Summit Bks,** *(Summit Bks.; 0-671),* Div. of Simon & Schuster, Inc., 1230 Ave. of the Americas, New York, NY 10020 (SAN 206-1244) Tel 212-698-7000; Fax: 212-698-7501; Toll Free: 800-223-2336 Do not confuse with companies with the same name in Toledo, OH, Tempe, AZ
Web site: http://www.simonsays.com/; *CIP.*

Summit CA, *(Summit Publishing; 0-945806),* P.O. Box 6583, Malibu, CA 90264-6583 (SAN 247-6770) Tel 805-374-2272 Do not confuse with Summit Publishing, Fort Worth, TX
E-mail: web@summitpub.com
Web site: http://www.summitpub.com
Dist(s): **Publishers Group** *(Publishers Group West).*

†**Summit TX,** *(Summit Publishing Group - Legacy Bks.; 0-9626219; 1-56530),* 3649 Conflans Rd., No. 103, Irving, TX 75061 (SAN 631-1253) Tel 972-399-8856; Fax: 972-313-9060 Do not confuse with Summit Publishing, Los Angeles, CA
E-mail: info@summitbooks.com
Web site: http://www.summitbooks.com
Dist(s): **BookWorld** *(BookWorld Services, Inc.); CIP.*

†**Sun & Moon CA,** *(Sun & Moon Pr.; 0-940650; 1-55713),* 6026 Wilshire Blvd., Los Angeles, CA 90036 (SAN 630-3234) Tel 323-857-1115; Fax: 323-857-0143
E-mail: djmess@sunmoon.com
Web site: http://www.sunmoon.com
Dist(s): **Consort Bk Sales** *(Consortium Bk. Sales & Distribution)*
SPD-Small Pr Dist *(SPD-Small Pr. Distribution); CIP.*

Sun Bear, *(Sun Bear Pr.; 0-9666367),* 4822 Santa Monica Ave., No. 158, San Diego, CA 92107 Tel 619-523-6698
E-mail: sunbear@att.net
Web site: http://www.home@att.net/~sunbear.

Sun Coast Hosp, *(Sun Coast Hospital Foundation, Inc.; 0-9649148),* P.O. Box 2084, Largo, FL 34644 Tel 813-587-0023; Fax: 813-587-0219.

Sun Eagle Pub, *(Sun Eagle Publishing; 0-944346),* 855 E. Commercial Blvd., Fort Lauderdale, FL 33335 (SAN 243-4369) Tel 954-771-3685.

Sun Life, *(Sun Life; 0-937930),* 2399 Cool Springs Rd., Thaxton, VA 24174 (SAN 240-8333) Tel 540-586-4898.

Sun Magic Imprint of Homestead Bk

Sun Pub, *(Sun Publishing Co.; 0-89540; 0-914172),* P.O. Box 5588, Santa Fe, NM 87502-5588 (SAN 206-1325) Tel 505-471-5177; Fax: 505-473-4458 Do not confuse with companies with the same or similar name in Bend, OR, South Easton, MA, Denver, CO, Atlanta, GA, Cleveland, TN
E-mail: sunbooks@aol.com
Web site: http://www.sunbooks.com
Dist(s): **Baker & Taylor** *(Baker & Taylor Bks.)*
Bookhouse *(Bookhouse, The)*
Bookpeople *(Bookpeople)*
Brodart *(Brodart Co.)*
Coos Bay Distributors *(Coos Bay Distributors)*
Coutts Library Service Inc *(Coutts Library Service, Inc.)*
Distributors *(Distributors, The)*
E B S Inc Bk *(EBS, Inc. Bk. Service)*
Emery-Pratt Co *(Emery-Pratt Co.)*
New Leaf Dist *(New Leaf Distributing Co., Inc.).*

Sunbelt Med Pubs, *(Sunbelt Medical Pubs.; 0-924381),* Orders Addr.: P.O. Box 13512, Tallahassee, FL 32317-3512 Tel 850-386-8918; Fax: 850-893-7738; Edit Addr.: 6515 Aqueduct Ct., Tallahassee, FL 32308 Tel 904-386-8918; Fax: 904-893-7738.

Sunbelt Media, *See* **Eakin Press**

Sunbright Bks Imprint of J Melek

Sun-Coyote Pr, *(Sun-Coyote Pr.; 0-925048),* 1302 East St., No. 48, Emporia, KS 66801 Tel 316-342-8643.

Sundeep Prak (IND) *(81-85067; 81-85055; 81-7574) Dist. by* **S Asia.**

Sunflower Ink, *See* **SunInk Pubn**

Sunflower U Pr, *(Sunflower Univ. Pr.; 0-89745),* Subs. of Journal of the West, Inc., 1531 Yuma, Box 1009, Manhattan, KS 66505-1009 (SAN 218-5075) Tel 785-539-1888; Fax: 785-539-2233; Toll Free: 800-258-1232 (orders)
Web site: http://www.sunflower-univ-press.org.

SunInk Pubn, *(SunInk Pubn.; 0-931104),* 37931 Palo Colorado Rd., Carmel, CA 93923 (SAN 212-9728) Tel 408-625-0588; Fax: 408-625-3770
E-mail: sunink@ricmasten.com
Web site: http://www.ricmasten.com.

Sunnyside, *(Sunnyside Publishing Co.; 0-934650),* Box 29, 51 Willow St., Lynn, MA 01903 (SAN 213-1757) Tel 781-593-2718.

Sunrise Hlth, *(Sunrise Health Coach; 0-9653171),* Orders Addr.: P.O. Box 12091, Panama City, FL 32401-9091 Tel 904-747-8669; Fax: 904-769-1436; Toll Free: 800-464-7034; Edit Addr.: 415 S. Bonita Ave., Panama City, FL 32401-9091.

Sunrise Internat, *(Sunrise International; 0-9637222),* 6345 Clinton Hwy., Knoxville, TN 37912 Tel 423-947-7774
Dist(s): **Baker & Taylor** *(Baker & Taylor Bks.)*
Unique Bks Inc *(Unique Bks., Inc.).*

SunRise Pbl, *(SunRise Publishing; 0-9644552; 1-57636),* Orders Addr.: P.O. Box 1001, Orem, UT 84059 Tel 801-224-7270; Fax: 801-225-2106; Toll Free: 888-732-2470; Edit Addr.: 961 S. Orem Blvd., Orem, UT 84058
E-mail: brian@sunrisebooks.com
Web site: http://www.selfpublish-lds.com
Dist(s): **Granite UT** *(Granite Publishing & Distribution, LLC)*
Origin Bk Sales *(Origin Bk. Sales, Inc.)*
Village Mktg *(Village Marketing).*

Sunrise Pr, *See* **Empowering People**

Sunrise Pubs, *(Sunrise Pubs.; 0-9621168),* 123 Second Ave., No. P6, Salt Lake City, UT 84103 (SAN 250-6432) Tel 801-595-8155 Do not confuse with Sunrise Publishers, Parowan, UT
Dist(s): **Covenant Comms** *(Covenant Communications, Inc.).*

Sunrise River Pr, *(Sunrise River Pr.; 0-9624814),* 11481 Kost Dam Rd., North Branch, MN 55056 Tel 651-583-3239; Fax: 651-583-2023; Toll Free: 800-895-4585.

Sunset Intl, *(Sunset International; 0-9648088),* P.O. Box 825, Uniontown, OH 44685-0825.

SunShine CO, *(SunShine Pr. Pubns., Inc.; 0-9615743; 1-888604),* P.O. Box 333, Hygiene, CO 80533-0333 (SAN 696-0510) Fax: 303-772-3556 (phone/fax) Do not confuse with Sunshine Pr., Malibu, CA
E-mail: sunshinepress@sunshinepress.com
Web site: http://www.sunshinepress.com
Dist(s): **Baker & Taylor** *(Baker & Taylor Bks.)*
Books West CO *(Books West)*
New Leaf Dist *(New Leaf Distributing Co., Inc.).*

Sunshine Sentinel, *(Sunshine Sentinel Pr., Inc.; 0-9633260; 1-884243),* Orders Addr.: P.O. Box 17799, West Palm Beach, FL 33416-7799 Tel 561-588-7628; Fax: 561-547-8008; Toll Free: 800-814-9800; Edit Addr.: 6708 Pamela Ln., West Palm Beach, FL 33405
E-mail: sunsentpress@aol.com
Web site: http://www.sunsentpress.com
Dist(s): **B&N Imports** *(Barnes & Noble Bks.-Imports)*
Baker & Taylor *(Baker & Taylor Bks.)*
Health Press *(Health Pr.)*
Quality Bks IL *(Quality Bks., Inc.).*

†**Sunstone Pr,** *(Sunstone Pr.; 0-86534; 0-913270),* Orders Addr.: 239 Johnson St., Santa Fe, NM 87504-2321; Edit Addr.: P.O. Box 2321, Santa Fe, NM 87504-2321 (SAN 214-2090) Tel 505-988-4418; Fax: 505-988-1025; Toll Free: 800-243-5644 (orders only)
E-mail: jsmith@sunstonepress.com
Web site: http://www.sunstonepress.com
Dist(s): **Baker & Taylor** *(Baker & Taylor Bks.)*
Bookpeople *(Bookpeople)*
Brodart *(Brodart Co.)*
New Leaf Dist *(New Leaf Distributing Co., Inc.)*
Quality Bks IL *(Quality Bks., Inc.)*
Treas Chest Bks *(Treasure Chest Bks.); CIP.*

SUNY Buff Music, *(State Univ. of New York at Buffalo Music Dept.; 0-931111),* 222 Baird Hall, Buffalo, NY 14260 (SAN 678-9498) Tel 716-636-2765
Web site: http://wings.buffalo.edu/AandL/music/.

Supcon Intl, *(Supcon International; 0-9634567; 1-884736),* P.O. Box 5275, Woodridge, IL 60517-0275 Tel 630-910-1551; Fax: 630-910-1561
E-mail: syshen@megsinet.net
Web site: http://www.globalwarming.net.

Supreme Pub, *(Supreme Publishing; 0-9626875),* Orders Addr.: P.O. Box 90242, Lafayette, LA 70509-0242 (SAN 297-3049) Tel 318-232-5530; Edit Addr.: 111 Wilkins, Lafayette, LA 70501
Dist(s): **Quality Bks IL** *(Quality Bks., Inc.).*

Sure Fire Imprint of Holmes Pub

SurfLess, *(SurfLess, LLC; 1-893957),* PMB 155, 5284 Randolph Rd., Rockville, MD 2852-2116 Fax: 603-925-8755
E-mail: info@surfless.com
Web site: http://www.surfless.com.

Surgical Laser, *(Surgical Laser Technologies, Inc.; 1-883765),* 147 Keystone Dr., Montgomeryville, PA 18936-9638 Tel 215-619-3600; Fax: 215-619-3208; Toll Free: 800-366-4758.

Surrey Beatty & Sons (AUS) *Dist. by* **St Mut.**

**Surrey Bks, *(Surrey Bks.; 0-940625; 0-9609516; 1-57284),* 230 E. Ohio, Suite 120, Chicago, IL 60611 (SAN 275-8857) Tel 312-751-7330; Fax: 312-751-7334; Toll Free: 800-326-4430
E-mail: SurreyBk@aol.com
Web site: http://www.surreybooks.com
Dist(s): Publishers Group *(Publishers Group West).***

Surrey Park Pr, *(Surrey Park Pr.; 0-9625540),* Orders Addr.: P.O. Box 2887, La Jolla, CA 92038-2887 (SAN 297-2158) Tel 619-454-9333; Fax: 619-454-9397; Edit Addr.: 7946 Ivanhoe, No. 107, La Jolla, CA 92037
E-mail: johntaddey@aol.com
Dist(s): **Baker & Taylor** *(Baker & Taylor Bks.)*
New Leaf Dist *(New Leaf Distributing Co., Inc.).*

Susquehanna U Pr, *(Susquehanna Univ. Pr.; 0-941664; 0-945636; 1-57591),* Affil. of Associated Univ. Presses, Orders Addr.: 440 Forsgate Dr., Cranbury, NJ 08512 (SAN 281-2959) Tel 609-655-4770; Fax: 609-655-8366
Web site: http://www.susqu.edu/su_press
Dist(s): **B & T International** *(Baker & Taylor International).*

Sutton Libs & Arts (GBR) *Dist. by* **St Mut.**

Sutton Publng, *(Sutton Publishing; 0-7509; 0-86299; 0-904387),* Subs. of Sutton Publishing, Ltd., 260 Fifth Ave., 6th Flr., New York, NY 10001 Toll Free: 800-758-3756 (orders) Do not confuse with companies with same names in Old Greenwich, CT, Eugene, OR
E-mail: Suttonus@mindspring.com
Web site: http://www.suttonpublishing.co.uk/
Dist(s): **Natl Bk Netwk** *(National Bk. Network).*

S-W Pub, *See* **S-W Thomson**

†**S-W Thomson,** *(South-Western Thomson Learning; 0-324; 0-538),* Subs. of Thomson Learning, 5191 Natorp Blvd., Mason, OH 45040 (SAN 202-7518) Tel 513-229-1000; Toll Free: 800-354-9706 (orders only)
E-mail: billhendee@itped.com
Web site: http://www.swcollege.com
Dist(s): **ITCP** *(International Thomson Computer Pr.)*
Thomson Learn *(Thomson Learning); CIP.*

†**Swallow,** *(Swallow Pr.; 0-8040),* Ohio Univ. Pr., Scott Quadrangle, Athens, OH 45701 (SAN 202-5663) Tel 740-593-1158; Fax: 740-593-4536; Toll Free: 800-621-2736
E-mail: arnold@ohio.edu
Web site: http://www.ohio~.edu/oupress/
Dist(s): **Ohio U Pr** *(Ohio Univ. Pr.)*
U Ch Pr *(Univ. of Chicago Pr.); CIP.*

Swan Park, *(Swan Park Publishing Co.; 0-9631071),* 5436 N. Dean Rd., Orlando, FL 32817-3241 (SAN 297-6773).

Swan Pub, *(Swan Publishing Co.; 0-943629),* 1059 County Rd. 100, Burnet, TX 78611 (SAN 668-6974) Tel 512-756-6800; Fax: 512-756-0102
E-mail: swanbooks@ghg.net
Web site: http://www.swan-pub.com
Dist(s): **Baker & Taylor** *(Baker & Taylor Bks.)*
Herveys Bklink *(Hervey's Booklink & Cookbook Warehouse)*
Quality Bks IL *(Quality Bks., Inc.).*

Swanstone Pr, *(Swanstone Pr.; 0-9643530),* 15127 NE 24th St., Suite 136, Redmond, WA 98052 Tel 206-644-1401
E-mail: LIZCH@TheChildbirthKit.com
Web site: http://www.TheChildbirthKit.com.

Swedenborg, *(Swedenborg Foundation, Inc.; 0-87785),* 320 N. Church St., West Chester, PA 19380 (SAN 111-7920) Tel 610-430-3222; Fax: 610-430-7982; Toll Free: 800-355-3222 (customer service)
E-mail: info@swedenborg.com
Web site: http://www.Swedenborg.com
Dist(s): **Words Distrib** *(Words Distributing Co.).*

†**Swedenborg Sci Assn,** *(Swedenborg Scientific Assn.; 0-915221),* Orders Addr.: P.O. Box 757, Bryn Athyn, PA 19009 (SAN 289-8454) Tel 215-914-2977; Fax: 215-914-2986
E-mail: ssa@newchurch.edu; *CIP.*

Sweetlight, *(Sweetlight Bks.; 0-9604462; 1-877714),* 16625 Heitman Rd., Cottonwood, CA 96022 (SAN 215-1154) Tel 916-529-5392
E-mail: swtlight@snowcrest.net
Web site: http://www.snowcrest.net/swtlight
Dist(s): **Baker & Taylor** *(Baker & Taylor Bks.)*
Bookpeople *(Bookpeople)*
New Leaf Dist *(New Leaf Distributing Co., Inc.).*

Sweinbinder, *(Sweinbinder Pubns., LLC; 0-9664873),* Orders Addr.: P.O. Box 11988, Atlanta, GA 30355 Tel 404-299-9724; Fax: 404-233-5662; Edit Addr.: 4453 Mount Paran Pkwy., Atlanta, GA 30327
E-mail: msdavismd@aol.com.

Swets (NLD) *(90-265) Dist. by* **Ashgate Pub Co.**

Swets & Zeitlinger, *(Swets & Zeitlinger Pubs.; 90-70430),* Orders Addr.: P.O. Box 582, Downingtown, PA 19335-9998.

SWI, *(S W I; 0-9606246; 1-880776),* P.O. Box 5028, University Park, NM 88003 (SAN 220-3553) Tel 505-525-1370; Fax: 505-525-1394; 5803 Leasburg Dr., Las Cruces, NM 88005
E-mail: nutconsult@zianet.com.

Sycamore Pub, *(Sycamore Publishing Co.; 0-9625233),* 511 Forest Lodge Rd., Pacific Grove, CA 93950-5040 Do not confuse with Sycamore Publishing Co., Lafayette, IN.

Sylvan Creek Pr, *(Sylvan Creek Pr.; 0-9621761),* 420 Elk St., Grangeville, ID 83530 (SAN 252-0710) Tel 208-983-0427; Fax: 208-983-2595; Toll Free: 800-727-9174.

Sylvan Inst, *(Sylvan Institute; 0-918428),* 330 Lei Dr., Palm Springs, CA 92264 (SAN 209-6838) Tel 760-327-6875.

Sylvan Pr WA, *(Sylvan Pr.; 0-9625638),* 1122 E. Pike St., Suite 746, Seattle, WA 98122 Tel 206-292-1069; Fax: 206-633-2902
Dist(s): **Bookpeople** *(Bookpeople)*
Homestead Bk *(Homestead Bk., Inc.)*
New Leaf Dist *(New Leaf Distributing Co., Inc.)*
Royal Pubns Inc *(Royal Pubns., Inc.).*

Symbolic Prods, *(Symbolic Productions; 0-9640559),* Orders Addr.: P.O. Box 6705, Moraga, CA 94556 (SAN 298-265X) Tel 510-631-0360; Edit Addr.: 1980 Ascot Dr., Moraga, CA 94556 (SAN 298-2668)
E-mail: angelus@valve.net
Web site: http://www.angelhealth.com
Dist(s): **Baker & Taylor** *(Baker & Taylor Bks.)*
New Leaf Dist *(New Leaf Distributing Co., Inc.).*

Symbols Power Imprint of Lewis Pub CA

Symphonic Lion, *(Symphonic Lion Publishing; 0-9703224),* P.O. Box 69085, Tucson, AZ 85737-0010 Tel 520-877-2842; Fax: 520-324-3744
E-mail: arslanphd@aol.com.

Sync Society Pubng, *(Syncreny Society Publishing; 0-940683),* Subs. of Syncreny Society International Church, P.O. Box 3965, Lihue, HI 96766 Fax: 615-834-5411
E-mail: syncsoc@syncreny.org
Web site: http://www.syncreny.org.

Synchrony Pub, *(Synchrony Publishing; 0-9653648),* 3934 Nelson Dr., Palo Alto, CA 94306-4523 Tel 570-792-2207; Fax: 650-852-0493.

Synerg CA, *(Synergetic Pr.),* Div. of Global Ecotechnics Corp., Orders Addr.: P.O. Box 2510, Novato, CA 94948 (SAN 201-3037) Tel 415-883-3530; Fax: 415-883-4280; Edit Addr.: 7 Silver Hills Rd., Santa Fe, NM 87505-4488 Tel 505-424-0237; Fax: 505-424-3336
E-mail: biospheres@compuserve.com
Web site: http://www.synergeticpress.com
Dist(s): **Pubs Services** *(Publishers Services).*

Synergy Bks Imprint of P Walsh Pr

Synergy Pr, *(Synergy Pr.; 0-9616548),* 3420 Holly Rd., Annandale, VA 22003 (SAN 659-5405) Tel 703-573-0909; Fax: 703-698-0372 Do not confuse with Synergy Pr., Saint Petersburg, FL .

Synesis Pr, *(Synesis Pr.; 0-925572),* Orders Addr.: P.O. Box 1843, Bend, OR 97709 (SAN 200-3481) Tel 541-382-6517; Fax: 541-382-0750; Edit Addr.: 21651 Dale Rd., Bend, OR 97701 (SAN 200-3503); 569 NE Clay, Bend, OR 97701 (SAN 200-349X).

Synthesis Pr, *(Synthesis Pr.; 0-9617972),* P.O. Box 231624-1624, Escinitas, CA 92023-1624 (SAN 666-2005) Tel 760-634-7755
Dist(s): **New Leaf Dist** *(New Leaf Distributing Co., Inc.).*

Syracuse U Cont Ed, *(Syracuse Univ. Pubns. in Continuing Education; 0-87060),* 820 Comstock, Syracuse, NY 13244 (SAN 202-7577) Tel 315-423-4172.

Syracuse U Foreign Comp, *(Syracuse Univ., Foreign & Comparative Studies Program; 0-915984),* 209 Maxwell Hall, Dept. of Anthropology, Syracuse, NY 13244-1090 (SAN 220-0082) Tel 315-443-2200; Fax: 315-443-4860.

†**Syracuse U Pr,** *(Syracuse Univ. Pr.; 0-8156),* 621 Skytop Rd., Suite 110, Syracuse, NY 13244-5290 (SAN 206-9776) Tel 315-443-2597; Fax: 315-443-5545
E-mail: supress@syr.edu
Web site: http://www.sumweb.syr.edu/su_press/
Dist(s): **Gryphon Hse** *(Gryphon Hse., Inc.)*
Penguin Putnam *(Penguin Putnam, Inc.); CIP.*

Systemic Therapy, *(Systemic Therapy Pr.; 0-9626461),* 1741 James Ave., Saint Paul, MN 55105-2114 Tel 612-641-0119.

Systems Co, *(Systems Co., Inc.; 0-937041; 1-56216),* Orders Addr.: P.O. Box 339, Carlsborg, WA 98324 (SAN 699-7880); Edit Addr.: 185 Ferngully Ln., Sequim, WA 98382 Tel 360-683-6860.

Systems DC, *(Systems DC; 0-929721),* 275 W. Abriendo Ave., Pueblo, CO 81004 (SAN 250-0310) Tel 719-543-3617; Fax: 719-543-2357; Toll Free: 800-221-6262.

SYTAC Health Publishing, *See* **SYTAC Pub**

SYTAC Pub, *(SYTAC Publishing; 0-9656065),* Orders Addr.: P.O. Box 7853, Cave Creek, AZ 85327-7853 Tel 602-563-1362; Edit Addr.: 4504 E. Creosote Dr., Cave Creek, AZ 85331
E-mail: sytac.pubuswest.net.

T & T Clark (GBR) *(0-567) Dist. by* **Bks Intl VA.**

T Bradford, *See* **Bradford Pubns**

T Doherty Assocs, *(Doherty, Tom Assocs., LLC; 0-312; 0-7653; 0-8125),* 175 Fifth Ave., New York, NY 10010 ; *Imprints:* Forge Bks (Forge Books) Tor Books (Tor Books)
Dist(s): **St Martin** *(St. Martin's Pr., LLC)*
VHPS *(VHPS Holtzbrinck Pubs.).*

T E D Assocs, *(T.E.D. Assocs.; 0-916598),* 2000 Commonwealth Ave., No. 315, Auburndale, MA 02166-2004 (SAN 208-8835) Tel 617-277-8446.

T H Coleman, *(Coleman, Thomas H.; 0-9653110),* 180 Humboldt St., Denver, CO 80218 Tel 303-733-5253.

T H I N K Pr, *(T.H.I.N.K. Productions; 0-9641656),* Orders Addr.: P.O. Box 99, Big Bend, CA 96011-0099 Fax: 707-838-9630; Toll Free: 800-808-4465; Edit Addr.: 8890 Lakewood Dr., Windsor, CA 95492.

T Holtzclaw, *(Holtzclaw, Teri Kai; 0-9712601),* 1594 Harts Mill Rd., Atlanta, GA 30319
E-mail: drtkholt@aol.com
Web site: http://www.humaninvestment.net.

T J Designs, *(T.J. Designs; 0-939287),* 1237 Laguna Ln., San Luis Obispo, CA 93405 (SAN 659-4565) Tel 805-545-8430
Dist(s): **Rittenhouse** *(Rittenhouse Bk. Distributors).*

T J Pubs, *(TJ Pubs., Inc.; 0-932666),* 817 Silver Spring Ave., No. 206, Silver Spring, MD 20910 (SAN 299-5263) Tel 301-585-4440; Fax: 301-585-5930; Toll Free: 800-999-1168
E-mail: tjpubinc@aol.com
Dist(s): **Baker & Taylor** *(Baker & Taylor Bks.)*
Brodart *(Brodart Co.).*

T J Terry, *(Terry, T.J.; 1-887258),* P.O. Box 49225, Jacksonville Beach, FL 32240-9225 Tel 904-738-4488
E-mail: tjterry@sprynet.com
Web site: http://home.sprynet.com/sprynet/tjterry.

T L C Med Pub, *(TLC Medical Publishing; 1-890045),* Div. of Total Learning Concepts, Inc., 441 Stuart St., Sixth Flr, Boston, MA 02116-5019 Tel 617-262-3336; Fax: 617-267-8231; Toll Free: 800-282-4852
E-mail: info@tlconline.com
Web site: http://www.tlconline.com.

T L Emmons, *(Emmons, T. Louis; 0-9643151),* 1031 Nuuanu Ave., Apt. 1005, Honolulu, HI 96817-5603.

T Peters & Co, *(Peters, Tim & Co., Inc.; 1-879874),* Orders Addr.: P.O. Box 370, Peapack, NJ 07977 Tel 908-234-2050; Fax: 908-234-1961; Toll Free: 800-543-2230; Edit Addr.: 87 Main St., Peapack, NJ 07977
E-mail: tpc@biocomics.com
Web site: http://www.wellbook.com; http://www.biocomics.com; http://www.captainbio.com.

T Schlosser, *(Thea Schlosser; 0-9653215),* 17131 Village 17, Camarillo, CA 93012 Tel 805-383-1043; Fax: 805-384-1077; Toll Free: 800-266-5564
E-mail: cfidsmedia@aol.com
Web site: http://www.misc.wanted.com.

T T Beeler, *(Beeler, Thomas T. Publisher; 1-57490),* 22 King St., Hampton Falls, NH 03844-2414 Tel 603-772-1175; Fax: 603-778-9025; Toll Free: 800-818-7574 ; *Imprints:* Beeler LP Bks (Beeler Large Print Books)
E-mail: tbeeler@beelerpub.com
Web site: http://www.beelerpub.com.

T T Nguyen, *See* **N X Phuong**

T W Rutledge, *(Rutledge, Thomas W.; 0-9627963),* 331 22nd Ave. N., Suite 1, Nashville, TN 37203 Tel 615-327-3423; Fax: 615-792-5781.

TA Assocs, *(TA Assocs.; 0-9617020),* 815 Indian Rd., Glenview, IL 60025 (SAN 662-8648) Tel 708-729-5133.

Table Top, *(Table Top Publishing; 0-9655549),* Orders Addr.: P.O. Box 1944, Twin Falls, ID 83303 Tel 208-734-2504; Fax: 208-734-3213; Edit Addr.: 401 Second St., N., No. 101, Twin Falls, ID 83303.

Tactilitics, *(Tactilitics, Inc.; 0-9637866),* 4760 Walnut St., Suite 105, Boulder, CO 80301 Tel 303-442-7746; Fax: 303-442-5337; Toll Free: 800-866-4544.

Tafnews, *(Tafnews Pr.; 0-911520; 0-911521),* Div. of Track & Field News, 2570 El Camino Real, Suite 606, Mountain View, CA 94040 (SAN 202-7593) Tel 650-948-8188; Fax: 650-948-9445
E-mail: biz@trackandfieldnews.com
Web site: http://www.trackandfieldnews.com.

Tagari Pubns (AUS) *(0-908228) Dist. by* **RDLE INST Bkstre.**

Tahrike Tarsile Quran, *(Tahrike Tarsile Quran, Inc.; 0-940368; 1-879402),* 80-08 51st Ave., Elmhurst, NY 11373 (SAN 658-1870) Tel 718-446-6472; Fax: 718-446-4370
E-mail: ttq@n-site.com
Web site: http://www.koranusa.org
Dist(s): **Publishers Group** *(Publishers Group West).*

Tale Weaver, *(Tale Weaver; 0-942139),* 8033 W. Sunset Blvd., No. 2612, Los Angeles, CA 90046-2401 (SAN 666-7570).

Talk Leaves, *(Talking Leaves Pr.; 0-9632574),* 210 White Rd., Watsonville, CA 95076 Tel 408-685-2804
Web site: http://wwwdirrid.com.

Talk Miramax Bks, *(Talk Miramax Bks.; 0-7868),* Div. of Disney Bk. Publishing, Inc., A Walt Disney Co., 118 W. 20th St., New York, NY 10011-3602 Tel 212-830-5858
Dist(s): **AOL Time Warner** *(AOL Time Warner Bk. Group).*

TALKAIDS, *(TALKAIDS, Inc.; 0-9659046),* P.O. Box 112, New York, NY 10113 Tel 212-465-2646; Fax: 212-675-7291
E-mail: TALKAIDS@aol.com.

Tall Oaks Pub, *(Tall Oaks Publishing, Inc.; 0-927188),* P.O. Box 621669, Littleton, CO 80162 (SAN 294-8583) Tel 303-973-6700; Fax: 303-973-5327.

Tallgrass Pubs, *(Tallgrass Pubs., LLC; 0-9645982),* 4559 W. Red Rock Dr., Larkspur, CO 80118 Tel 303-681-3033; Fax: 303-681-2999
E-mail: acupressure4all@earthlink.net
Web site: http://www.tallgrasspublishers.com.

Tamarack Bks, *(Tamarack Bks., Inc.; 0-9634839; 1-886609),* Orders Addr.: P.O. Box 190313, Boise, ID 83719-0313 (SAN 297-8792) Tel 208-387-2656; Fax: 208-387-2650; Toll Free: 800-962-6657; Edit Addr.: 3200A Overland Rd., Boise, ID 83705
E-mail: sales@tamarackbooks.com
Web site: http://www.tamarackbooks.com.

Tamarack Hse, *(Tamarack Hse.; 0-9621546),* 1574 Tamarack Trail, Decatur, GA 30033 (SAN 251-5385) Tel 404-982-9758.

Tangelwuld, *(Tangelwuld Pr.; 0-934667),* Orders Addr.: 22497 Swordfish Dr., Boca Raton, FL 33428-4609 (SAN 695-8982) Fax: 561-477-2534
E-mail: tangelwuld@yahoo.com
Web site: http://www.publishers-associates.com
Dist(s): **Pubs Assoc** *(Publishers Assocs.).*

Tangrm Bks, *(Tangram Bks. & Coffee Shop; 0-932838),* 7811 Roundabout Way, Springfield, VA 22153-1830 Fax: 512-392-0063; 314 N. LBJ, San Marcos, TX 78666 Tel 512-392-0002
Web site: http://www.the-igview.com.

Taoist Pubs, *(Taoist Pubs.; 0-9608030),* 2222 Hempstead Dr., Troy, MI 48083 Tel 248-680-8688.

Taote Pub, *(Taote Publishing; 0-9626124),* P.O. Box 22660, Honolulu, HI 96823 Tel 808-671-5708; Fax: 808-671-5750
E-mail: pekelo@lava.net
Dist(s): **Baker & Taylor** *(Baker & Taylor Bks.)*
Booklines Hawaii *(Booklines Hawaii, Ltd.).*

Tapestry Bks, *(Tapestry Bks.; 0-9653409),* P.O. Box 359, Ringoes, NJ 08551 Tel 908-806-6695; Fax: 908-788-2999; Toll Free: 800-765-2367
E-mail: info@tapestrybooks.com
Web site: http://www.tapestrybooks.com/.

Tapestry Pr, *(Tapestry Pr.; 0-929283),* 925 N. Main St., Springville, UT 84663-1051 (SAN 248-8809) Do not confuse with companies with the same or similar name in Acton, MA, Springville, UT, Biloxi, MS.

†**Taplinger,** *(Taplinger Publishing Co., Inc.; 0-8008),* P.O. Box 175, Marlboro, NJ 07746 Tel 201-432-3257; Fax: 201-432-3708
E-mail: info@parkwestpubs.com
Web site: http://www.parkwestpubs.com/
Dist(s): **Parkwest Pubns** *(Parkwest Pubns., Inc.); CIP.*

Taproot Bks, *See* **Kalyx.com**

Tarascon Pub, *(Tarascon Publishing; 1-882742),* Div. of Tarascon, Inc., Orders Addr.: Box 1159, Loma Linda, CA 92354 Tel 909-794-0220; Fax: 909-748-0469; Toll Free Fax: 877-929-9926; Toll Free: 800-929-9926; Edit Addr.: 721 Nevada St., Suite 305, Redlands, CA 92373
E-mail: info@tarascon.com; beth@tarascon.com
Web site: http://www.tarascon.com
Dist(s): **J Majors Co** *(Majors, J. A. Co.)*
Matthews Medical Bk Co *(Matthews Medical Bk. Co.)*
Rittenhouse *(Rittenhouse Bk. Distributors).*

Tarcher Putnam Imprint of Putnam Pub Group

Targum Pr, *(Targum Pr., Inc.; 0-944070; 1-56871),* 22700 W. Eleven Mile Rd., Southfield, MI 48034 (SAN 242-8997) Tel 248-355-2266; Toll Free Fax: 888-298-9992
E-mail: targum@elronet.co.il
Web site: http://www.targum.com
Dist(s): **Feldheim** *(Feldheim, Philipp Inc.).*

Taschen Amer, *(Taschen America, LLC; 1-886155; 3-8228),* Div. of Benedikt Taschen Verlag GmbH., 230 Fifth Ave., Suite 1411, New York, NY 10001 (SAN 253-0937) Tel 212-683-3377; Fax: 212-683-5858; Toll Free: 888-827-2436
E-mail: p.sommers@taschen-america.com
Web site:
http://www.taschen-america.com/main/main2.htm
Dist(s): **Client Dist Srvs** *(Client Distribution Services)*
Continental Bk *(Continental Bk. Co., Inc.).*

Taterhill, *(Taterhill Pr.; 0-9616792),* P.O. Box 100, Santa Cruz, CA 95063 (SAN 661-0692) Tel 408-458-9004
Dist(s): **Baker & Taylor** *(Baker & Taylor Bks.)*
Bookpeople *(Bookpeople)*
New Leaf Dist *(New Leaf Distributing Co., Inc.).*

Tatnuck Imprint of Chandler Hse

Tattersall Pr, *(Tattersall Pr.; 0-9639890),* Orders Addr.: P.O. Box 712, Elkhart, IN 46515-0712; Edit Addr.: 1920 Grant St., Elkhart, IN 46514 Tel 219-264-6692
Dist(s): **Winters IN** *(Winters Publishing).*

Tay Francis Ltd (GBR) *(0-7484; 0-85066; 0-905273; 1-85000) Dist. by* **Taylor & Francis.**

†**Taylor & Francis,** *(Taylor & Francis, Inc.; 0-335; 0-8448; 0-85066; 0-89116; 0-903796; 0-905273; 1-56032; 1-85000),* Orders Addr.: 7625 Empire Dr., Florence, KY 41042 Toll Free Fax: 800-248-4724; Toll Free: 800-634-7064; Edit Addr.: 325 Chestnut St., Philadelphia, PA 19106 (SAN 241-9246) Tel 215-625-8900; Fax: 215-625-2940; 29 W. 35th St., New York, NY 10001 Tel 212-216-7800; Fax: 212-564-7854 ; *Imprints:* Falmer Pr (Falmer Press) Crane Russak (Crane Russak & Company, Incorporated)
E-mail: info@taylorandfrancis.com
Web site: http://www.taylorandfrancis.com
Dist(s): **netLibrary CO** *(netLibrary, Inc.); CIP.*

Taylor Hill, *(Taylor Hill Publishing, Ltd.; 0-9702904),* 34 Brompton Rd., Garden City, NY 11530-4226 (SAN 253-3294) Tel 516-248-9092 (phone/fax) Do not confuse with Taylor Hill Publishing in Bay City,TX
E-mail: sales@taylorhill.org
Web site: http://www.cancerbook.com.

†**Taylor Pub,** *(Taylor Publishing Co.; 0-87833),* Subs. of Insilco, 4720 Boston Way, Lanham, MD 20706 Toll Free: 800-462-6420 Do not confuse with companies with the same or similar names in Rochester, MI, Bellingham, WA, St. Petersburg, FL, Owatonna, MN, Eureka, CA
Web site: http://www.taylorpub.com
Dist(s): **Natl Bk Netwk** *(National Bk. Network); CIP.*

TBI Press, *See* **Inst Spine**

TBL, *(Technical Bks. for the Layperson, Inc. (TBL); 1-881818),* P.O. Box 391, Lake Grove, NY 11755-0391 (SAN 297-7184) Tel 540-877-1477 (phone/fax)
E-mail: tbl@shental.net.

TC Enter, *(TC Enterprise; 0-9700076),* 39 Hawk Feather Cir., Madison, WI 53717-2744 Fax: 608-833-7204
E-mail: tcook@agingmedicine.com
Web site: http://www.agingmedicine.com.

T-C Pr CA, *(T/C Pr.; 0-938648),* P.O. Box 36006, Los Angeles, CA 90036 (SAN 297-7435) Tel 323-938-6923 (phone/fax)
E-mail: geps222@aol.com.

T-C Pubns CA, *See* **T-C Pr CA**

TCFP-PPP, *See* **Century Foundation**

Tch Yourself Imprint of McGraw-Hill Trade

Tchr Create Mat, *(Teacher Created Materials, Inc.; 0-87673; 1-55734; 1-57690; 0-7439),* 6421 Industry Way, Westminster, CA 92683-3608 (SAN 665-5270) Tel 714-891-7895; Fax: 714-892-0283; Toll Free: 800-662-4321
E-mail: ppulido@teachercreated.com
Web site: http://www.teachercreated.com.

†**Tchrs Coll,** *(Teachers College Pr., Teachers College, Columbia Univ.; 0-8077),* Orders Addr.: P.O. Box 20, Williston, VT 05495-0020 (SAN 248-3904) Fax: 802-864-7626; Toll Free: 800-575-6566; Edit Addr.: 1234 Amsterdam Ave., New York, NY 10027 (SAN 282-3985) Tel 212-678-3929; Fax: 212-678-4149
E-mail: tcpress@www.tc.columbia.edu
Web site: http://www.teacherscollegepress.com
Dist(s): **B & T International** *(Baker & Taylor International)*
Continental Bk *(Continental Bk. Co., Inc.); CIP.*

TCNFPC, *(Twin Cities Natural Family Planning Ctr., Inc.; 0-9616827),* 69 Exchange St., W., Saint Paul, MN 55102 (SAN 661-1273) Tel 612-340-9830.

TDC Pubng, *(TDC Publishing; 0-9640594),* Div. of TDC Group, 211 S. Main St., Suite 220, Dayton, OH 45402-2411 Tel 937-461-2000; Fax: 937-461-2150 Do not confuse with TDC Publishing in Miami, FL.

Teach Servs, *See* **TEACH Servs**

TEACH Servs, *(TEACH Services, Inc.; 0-945383; 1-57258),* 254 Donovan Rd., Brushton, NY 12916 (SAN 246-9863) Tel 518-358-3494; Fax: 518-358-3028; Toll Free: 800-367-1844
E-mail: info@teachservicesinc.com
Web site: http://www.teachservicesinc.com.

Teach-em, *(Teach'em; 0-931028; 0-944496; 1-56625),* Div. of Bonus Bks., Inc., 160 E. Illinois St., Chicago, IL 60611 (SAN 211-2787) Tel 312-467-0580; Fax: 312-467-9271; Toll Free: 800-225-3775
E-mail: bb@bonus-books.com
Web site: http://www.bonus-books.com.

†**Teacher Ideas Pr,** *(Teacher Ideas Pr.; 0-87287; 0-931510; 1-56308),* Div. of Libraries Unlimited, Inc., P.O. Box 6633, Englewood, CO 80155-6633 (SAN 202-6767) Tel 303-770-1220; Fax: 303-220-8843; Toll Free: 800-237-6124
E-mail: lu-books@lu.com
Web site: http://www.lu.com; *CIP.*

Teaching Res, *(Teaching Research Pubns.; 0-944232),* 345 N. Monmouth Ave., Monmouth, OR 97361 (SAN 211-1861) Tel 503-838-8792; Fax: 503-838-8150
E-mail: dbp@wou.edu
Web site: http://www.tr.wou.edu/tr/dbp.

Teague Hse Pr, *(Teague Hse. Pr.; 0-9653697),* Orders Addr.: P.O. Box 24258, Ventura, CA 93002 Tel 805-653-0924; Fax: 805-648-6706; Edit Addr.: 1776 Marisol Dr., Ventura, CA 93001
E-mail: stophiv@aol.com
Dist(s): **Sunbelt Pubns** *(Sunbelt Pubns., Inc.).*

Team Surgery, *(Team Surgery; 0-9666043),* 3900 Padeo Del Sol, No. 332, Santa Fe, NM 87505 Tel 505-438-2844; Fax: 505-424-1144
E-mail: briley@teamsurgery.com
Web site: http://www.teamsurgery.com.

Tecg Document Srvs, *See* **Bink Productions**

Tech Bks Layperson, *See* **TBL**

Tech Comm (GBR) *(0-946655; 1-85953) Dist. by* **St Mut.**

Tech Data, *(Tech Data Pubns.; 0-937816),* Div. of Lith-O-Lux Corp., 9814 W. Menadota Dr., Peoria, AZ 85382-4147 (SAN 216-0129) Tel 623-825-3551; Fax: 625-825-9884.

Tech Group, *(Technology Group, The; 0-939856; 1-877884),* P.O. Box 21172, El Sobrante, CA 94820-1172 (SAN 220-195X) Tel 510-262-6991; Fax: 510-262-6990
E-mail: whtmagick@aol.com
Web site: http://www.techgroupbooks.com.

Tech Insights, *(Technical Insights/John Wiley & Sons, Inc.; 0-914993; 1-56217),* 605 Third Ave., New York, NY 10158 (SAN 665-8326) Tel 212-850-8600; Fax: 212-850-8643
E-mail: tiinfo@insights.com
Web site: http://www.wiley.com/technical_insights.

Tech Marketing, *(Technology Marketing Corp.; 0-936840),* 1 Technology Plaza, Norwalk, CT 06854-1924 (SAN 212-4629) Tel 203-852-6800; Fax: 203-853-2845; Toll Free: 800-243-6002.

TechDoc, *(TechDoc, Inc.; 0-9658864),* 7 Waltham St., Newark, DE 19713 Tel 302-368-2239; Fax: 302-368-2234
E-mail: KMHEALTH@ix.netcom.com.

Techkits, *(Techkits, Inc.; 0-918662),* P.O. Box 105, Demarest, NJ 07627 (SAN 210-3753) Tel 201-768-7334 (phone/fax); Toll Free: 800-201-0547.

Tecolote Pubns, *(Tecolote Pubns.; 0-938711),* Orders Addr.: 4918 Del Monte Ave., San Diego, CA 92107-3209 (SAN 661-5058) Tel 619-222-6066; Fax: 619-223-5832
E-mail: tecopubs@earthlink.com.

Tektran, *(Tektran, Inc.; 0-9661128),* Orders Addr.: P.O. Box 665, Edmonds, WA 98020 Tel 425-776-4556; Fax: 425-771-1178; Edit Addr.: 1030 Carol Way, Edmonds, WA 98020
E-mail: sales@tektran.com
Web site: http://www.tektran.com.

Tel-A-Train, *(Tel-A-Train, Inc.; 1-56355),* P.O. Box 4752, Chattanooga, TN 37421 Tel 423-266-0113; Fax: 423-267-2555; Toll Free: 800-251-6018
Web site: http://www.telatrain.com.

Telesis CA, *(Telesis II of California, Inc.; 1-56117),* 409 Camino Del Rio S., Suite 205, San Diego, CA 92108-3506 Tel 619-497-0193; Fax: 619-497-0582; Toll Free: 800-542-2966.

Telford Pr, *(Telford Pr., The; 0-936923),* P.O. Box 287, Caldwell, NJ 07006 (SAN 658-3652).

Teller Press, *(Teller Pr.; 0-9650712),* P.O. Box 2275, Boulder, CO 80306-2275 Tel 303-273-5567.

Telos Pubns, *(Telos Pubns.; 0-9664624; 0-9712144),* P.O. Box 4457, Huntington Beach, CA 92605-4457 Tel 714-668-1818; Fax: 714-668-1100; Toll Free: 866-416-8973
E-mail: kris@16types.com
Web site: http://www.telospublications.com.

†TelShare Pub Co, *(Telshare Publishing Co., Inc.; 0-910287),* 823 N. Olive Ave., West Palm Beach, FL 33401 (SAN 241-4651) Tel 561-655-1231; Fax: 561-655-4820; Toll Free: 800-343-9707
Dist(s): **Gryphon Hse** *(Gryphon Hse., Inc.); CIP.*

Temenos Found, *(Temenos Foundation; 0-9629561),* 37 Kawananakoa Pl., Honolulu, HI 96817 Tel 808-528-2433; Fax: 808-528-2434
E-mail: temenos@lava.net.

Temeron Bks, *(Temeron Bks., Inc.; 1-895510),* P.O. Box 896, Bellingham, WA 98227 Tel 360-738-4016.

Temple Lodge (GBR) *(0-904693; 1-902636) Dist. by* **Anthroposophic.**

Temple Pubg, *(Temple Publishing Group, LLC; 1-58446),* 18515 Underwood Ave., Cleveland, OH 44119 (SAN 253-679X) Tel 216-738-1759; Fax: 216-738-1762 ; *Imprints:* Legacy OH (Legacy Books)
E-mail: PubTemple@aol.com
Web site: http://www.templepublishing.com
Dist(s): **Baker & Taylor** *(Baker & Taylor Bks.).*

Temple Treasures Pubns, *(Temple Treasures Pubns.; 0-9625716),* Orders Addr.: P.O. Box 35625, Tulsa, OK 74153 Tel 918-663-4929; Fax: 918-838-0496; Edit Addr.: 3033 S. 72nd East Ave., Tulsa, OK 74129.

†Temple U Pr, *(Temple Univ. Pr.; 0-87722; 1-56639),* 1601 N. Broad St., University Services Bldg., Rm. 305, Philadelphia, PA 19122-6099 (SAN 202-7666) Tel 215-204-8787; Fax: 215-204-4719; Toll Free: 800-447-1656
E-mail: tempress@astro.ocis.temple.edu
Web site: http://www.temple.edu/tempress
Dist(s): **Baker & Taylor** *(Baker & Taylor Bks.)*
Koen Bk Distributors *(Koen Bk. Distributors); CIP.*

Temple Univ Schl Med, *(Temple Univ., Schl. of Medicine, Office of Development and Alumni Affairs; 0-9711095),* 3340 N. Broad St., 2nd Flr., Philadelphia, PA 19140 Tel 215-707-4850; Fax: 215-707-1650; Toll Free: 800-331-2839
E-mail: jwalke00@thunder.ocis.temple.edu.

Templeton Fnd, *(Templeton Foundation Pr.; 1-890151),* Div. of John Templeton Foundation, 5 Radnor Corporate Ctr., Suite 120 100 Matsonford Rd., Radnor, PA 19087 Tel 610-971-2670; Fax: 610-971-2672; Toll Free: 800-561-3367
E-mail: tfp@templeton.org; mphelan@templeton.org
Web site: http://www.templetonpress.org/press
Dist(s): **U Ch Pr** *(Univ. of Chicago Pr.).*

Tempus Pubng (GBR) *(0-7524; 0-7385) Dist. by* **Arcadia Publng.**

†Ten Speed Pr, *(Ten Speed Pr.; 0-89815; 0-913668; 1-58008),* Orders Addr.: P.O. Box 7123, Berkeley, CA 94707 (SAN 202-7674) Fax: 510-559-1629 (orders); Toll Free: 800-841-2665
E-mail: order@tenspeed.com
Web site: http://www.tenspeed.com
Dist(s): **IPG Chicago** *(Independent Pubs. Group); CIP.*

Ten Talents, *(Ten Talents; 0-9603532),* P.O. Box 313, Murphy, OR 97533 (SAN 207-9364) Tel 541-472-1113 (phone/fax); Toll Free Fax: 877-442-4425
E-mail: tentalents@cyberhouse.org
Web site: http://www.cyerhouse.org/public/tentalents
Dist(s): **Ctry Life Natrl Fds** *(Country Life Natural Foods)*
Nelsons Bks *(Nelson's Bks.)*
Nutri-Books Corp *(Nutri-Bks. Corp.).*

Tennenhouse Prof Pubns, *(Tennenhouse Professional Pubns.; 1-930548),* 427 County View Dr., Mill Valley, CA 94941-4089
E-mail: info@tennenhouse.com
Web site: http://www.tennenhouse.com.

Tenpo Syst Study (JPN) *(4-87246) Dist. by* **Bks Nippan.**

Terra Firma NM, *(Terra Firma Publishing Co.; 1-930263),* Div. of Intellitek, Inc., Orders Addr.: P.O. Box 1100, Tesuque, NM 87574 Tel 505-984-2598; Fax: 505-984-2802; Toll Free: 800-416-1192; Edit Addr.: 23B County Rd., No. 78, Santa Fe, NM 87501
E-mail: Intellitek@aol.com.

Terra Publng, *(Terra Publishing; 0-9661066),* Orders Addr.: 4103 Plaza Ln., Fairfax, VA 22033-3019 (SAN 299-335X) Tel 703-263-2468 Do not confuse with companies with the same name in Jefferson, KY, Ann Arbor, MI
E-mail: greeze@juno.com
Web site: http://www.unassistedhomebirth.com.

Tesla Bk Co, *(Tesla Bk. Co.; 0-914119; 0-9603536),* P.O. Box 121873, Chula Vista, CA 91912-6573 (SAN 241-8703) Tel 619-585-8487; Toll Free: 800-398-2056
E-mail: bfeuling@teslabook.com.

Tesseract SD, *(Tesseract Pubns.; 1-877649),* P.O. Box 164, Canton, SD 57013-0164 Tel 775-417-7146 (phone/fax)
E-mail: ta_shi@dtgnet.com
Web site: http://www.tesseractpublications.com.

Teton New, *(Teton New Media; 1-893441; 1-59161),* Orders Addr.: P.O. Box 4833, Jackson, WY 83001 Tel 307-732-0028; Fax: 307-734-0841; Toll Free: 877-306-9793; Edit Addr.: 4125 S. Hwy. 89, No. 1, Jackson, WY 83001
E-mail: croantree@tetonnm.com
Web site: http://www.tetonnm.com.

Tetra Pr, *(Tetra Pr.; 1-56465; 3-89356; 3-923880),* Div. of Warner-Lambert Co., 3001 Commerce St., Blacksburg, VA 24060 Tel 540-951-5400; Fax: 540-951-5415; Toll Free: 800-526-0650
Dist(s): **Voyageur Pr** *(Voyageur Pr., Inc.).*

Tetrahedron, *See* **Tetrahedron Pub**

Tetrahedron Pub, *(Tetrahedron Publishing Group; 0-923550; 0-9609386),* Orders Addr.: 206 N. Fourth Ave., Suite 147, Sandpoint, ID 83864; Edit Addr.: P.O. Box 2033, Sandpoint, ID 83864-0906 (SAN 260-2717) Tel 208-265-2575; Fax: 208-265-2775; Toll Free: 888-508-4787 (orders)
E-mail: tetra@tetrahedron.org
Web site: http://www.tetrahedron.org
Dist(s): **Baker & Taylor** *(Baker & Taylor Bks.)*
New Leaf Dist *(New Leaf Distributing Co., Inc.).*

†Tex A&M Univ Pr, *(Texas A&M Univ. Pr.; 0-89096; 1-58544),* 4354 TAMU John H. Lindsey Bldg., Lewis St., College Station, TX 77843-4354 (SAN 658-1919) Tel 979-845-1436; Fax: 979-847-8752; Toll Free Fax: 888-617-2421 (orders); Toll Free: 800-826-8911 (orders)
E-mail: wjl@tampress.tamu.edu
Web site: http://www.tamu.edu/upress/; *CIP.*

†Tex Christian, *(Texas Christian Univ. Pr.; 0-87565; 0-912646),* P.O. Box 298300, Fort Worth, TX 76129 (SAN 202-7690) Tel 817-257-7822; Fax: 817-257-5075
E-mail: j.alter@tcu.edu
Web site: http://www.prs.tcu.edu/prs
Dist(s): **Tex A&M Univ Pr** *(Texas A&M Univ. Pr.); CIP.*

Tex Med Pr, *(Texas Medical Pr., Inc.; 0-9615085),* Orders Addr.: P.O. Box 1409, Texarkana, TX 75504 (SAN 694-0641) Tel 214-792-7151; Edit Addr.: 21 Northridge Cir., Texarkana, TX 75504 (SAN 699-5993) Tel 214-792-1315.

†Tex St Hist Assn, *(Texas State Historical Assn.; 0-87611),* 2-306 Richardson Hall, University Sta., Austin, TX 78712 (SAN 202-7704) Tel 512-471-1525; Fax: 512-471-1551; Toll Free: 800-687-8132
Web site: http://www.dla.utexas.edu/texhist/index.html; http://www.tsha.utexas.edu/
Dist(s): **Tex A&M Univ Pr** *(Texas A&M Univ. Pr.); CIP.*

†Tex Tech Univ Pr, *(Texas Tech Univ. Pr.; 0-89672),* Affil. of Texas Tech Univ., Orders Addr.: P.O. Box 41037, Lubbock, TX 79409-1037 (SAN 218-5989) Tel 806-742-2982; Fax: 806-742-2979; Toll Free: 800-832-4042; Edit Addr.: 2903 Fourth St., Lubbock, TX 79409-1037
E-mail: ttup@ttu.edu
Web site: http://www.ttup.ttu.edu; *CIP.*

Texas Histopages, *(Texas Histopages, Inc.; 0-9701785),* P.O. Box 4737, Austin, TX 78765 Fax: 512-479-8549
E-mail: histopages@austin.rr.com
Web site: http://www.histopages.com.

†TFC Bks NY, *(Twenty-First Century Bks., Inc.; 0-7613; 0-8050; 0-941477),* Div. of The Millbrook Pr., Inc., Orders Addr.: 2 Old New Milford Rd., Brookfield, CT 06804 (SAN 666-0827) Tel 203-740-2220; Fax: 203-740-2223 (fax orders); Toll Free: 800-462-4703 (orders) Do not confuse with Twenty-First Century Bks., Inc., Lafayette, LA
Web site: http://www.millbrookpress.com; *CIP.*

†TFH Pubns, *(TFH Pubns., Inc.; 0-7938; 0-86622; 0-87666; 1-85279),* Orders Addr.: One TFH Plaza, Third & Union Aves., Neptune City, NJ 07753 (SAN 202-7720) Tel 732-988-8400; Fax: 732-988-5466; Toll Free: 800-631-2188 (outside New Jersey); Edit Addr.: P.O. Box 427, Neptune, NJ 07753 (SAN 658-1862)
E-mail: info@tfh.com
Web site: http://www.tfh.com
Dist(s): **K K & B** *(Kampmann, Kump & Bell, LLC)*
Midpt Trade *(Midpoint Trade Bks., Inc.); CIP.*

Thameside Pr, *(Thameside Pr.; 1-929298; 1-930643),* Orders Addr.: P.O. Box 206, North Mankato, MN 56003; Edit Addr.: 1980 Lookout Dr., North Mankato, MN 56003 Tel 507-388-6273; 507-388-2601; Fax: 507-388-1364; 507-388-2746; Toll Free: 800-445-6209
E-mail: creativeco@aol.com
Dist(s): **Creative Co** *(Creative Co., The)*
Smart Apple *(Smart Apple Media).*

Thaneros Pr, *(Thaneros Pr.),* P.O. Box 773, Lone Pine, CA 93545 (SAN 631-0117) Tel 760-876-5762 (phone/fax).

Thatch Tree, *(Thatch Tree Pubns.; 0-9709909),* 2250 N. Rock Rd., Suite 118-169, Wichita, KS 67226 Tel 316-687-6629
E-mail: thatchtreepub@aol.com; evajess@kscable.com
Web site: Http://www.breastbook.com
Dist(s): **Baker & Taylor** *(Baker & Taylor Bks.).*

The Davis Ctr, *(The Davis Ctr. for Hearing, Speech & Learning, Inc.; 0-9622326),* 4 Musconetcong Ave., Stanhope, NJ 07874-2936
E-mail: hearyouare@aol.com
Web site: http://www.thedaviscenter.com/.

The Garden, *See* **Hlth Frontiers**

The Terraces, *(The Terraces; 0-9632545),* 1170 S. State St., Ephrata, PA 17522 Tel 717-859-4100; Fax: 717-859-2131; Toll Free: 800-441-7345.

†Theophrastus, *(Theophrastus; 0-913728),* 1340 Main Rd., Tiverton, RI 02878-4456 (SAN 202-7771) Tel 401-635-4348; *CIP.*

†Theos Pub Hse, *(Theosophical Publishing Hse.; 0-8356; 81-7059; 0-7229),* Div. of Theosophical Society in America, 306 W. Geneva Rd., P.O. Box 270, Wheaton, IL 60189-0270 (SAN 202-5698) Tel 630-665-0130; Fax: 630-665-8791; Toll Free: 800-669-9425 ; *Imprints:* Quest (Quest Books)
E-mail: questbooks@aol.com
Web site: http://www.theosophical.org
Dist(s): **Natl Bk Netwk** *(National Bk. Network); CIP.*

Theraptc Res, *(Therapeutic Research Faculty; 0-9676136),* Orders Addr.: P.O. Box 8190, Stockton, CA 95208 Tel 209-472-2240; Fax: 209-472-2249; Toll Free: 800-995-8712; Edit Addr.: 3120 W. March Ln., Stockton, CA 95219
E-mail: mail@pletter.com
Web site: http://www.naturaldatabase.com.

Theraputic Assoc, *(Theraputic Assocs., Inc.; 1-888629),* 15060 Ventura Blvd., No. 240, Sherman Oaks, CA 91403 Tel 818-377-2588; Fax: 818-377-2595.

Therapy Careers, *See* **Peringian & Assocs**

Therapy Wrks, *(TherapyWorks, Inc.; 0-9643041),* 4901 Butte Pl., NW, Albuquerque, NM 87120 Tel 505-897-3478; Fax: 505-899-4071
Web site: http://www.alertprogram.com.

Theresevision, *(Theresevision Pubns.; 0-9653861),* Orders Addr.: P.O. Box 39, Bensalem, PA 19020 Tel 215-333-2408; Fax: 215-332-5370; Toll Free: 800-518-3758; Edit Addr.: 3336 Aldine St., Philadelphia, PA 19136
Dist(s): **Brodart** *(Brodart Co.).*

†Thieme Med Pubs, *(Thieme Medical Pubs., Inc.; 0-86577; 0-913258; 1-58890),* Subs. of Georg Thieme Verlag Stuttgart, 333 Seventh Ave., 5th Flr., New York, NY 10001 (SAN 169-5983) Tel 212-760-0888; Fax: 212-947-1112; Toll Free: 800-782-3488 (orders only)
E-mail: Info@Thieme.com; custserv@thieme.de
Web site: http://www.thieme.com
Dist(s): **J Majors Co** *(Majors, J. A. Co.)*
Matthews Medical Bk Co *(Matthews Medical Bk. Co.)*
Rittenhouse *(Rittenhouse Bk. Distributors); CIP.*

Thinking Pubns, *(Thinking Pubns.; 0-930599; 0-9610370; 1-888222),* Div. of McKinley Cos., Inc., Orders Addr.: P.O. Box 163, Eau Claire, WI 54702-0163 (SAN 264-4320) Tel 715-832-2488; Fax: 715-832-9082; Toll Free: 800-225-4769; 800-225-4709 (in U.S. & Canada); Edit Addr.: 424 Galloway St., Eau Claire, WI 54703
E-mail: custserv@ThinkingPublications.com
Web site: http://www.thnkingpublications.com.

Third Line Pr, *(Third Line Pr.; 0-9618550; 1-891710),* 4751 Viviana Dr., Tarzana, CA 91356 (SAN 668-1220) Tel 818-996-0076; Fax: 818-774-1575; Toll Free: 800-916-0076
E-mail: tlpinfo@werbach.com
Web site: http://www.third-Line.com.

Third Party Pub, *(3rd Party Publishing Co.; 0-89914),* Div. of Third Party Assocs., Inc., P.O. Box 13306, Oakland, CA 94661-0306 (SAN 127-7294) Tel 510-339-2323; Fax: 510-339-6729; Toll Free: 888-339-2323
E-mail: paulmico@tpaserver.com
Web site: http://www.tpaserver.com.

Third Rail Pr NY, *(Third Rail Pr., Inc.; 0-9702744),* P.O. Box 356, New York, NY 10276 Tel 212-505-0980; Fax: 212-674-5113 Do not confuse with companies with the same or similar name in Santa Monica, CA, Brooklyn, NY
E-mail: mlevin@igc.org.

Third Side Pr, *(3rd Side Pr., Inc.; 1-879427),* 2250 W. Farragut, Chicago, IL 60625-1863 Tel 773-271-3029; Fax: 773-271-0459
E-mail: ThirdSide@aol.com
Dist(s): **Consort Bk Sales** *(Consortium Bk. Sales & Distribution).*

Third World, *(Third World Press; 0-88378),* P.O. Box 19730, Chicago, IL 60619 (SAN 202-778X) Tel 773-651-0700; Fax: 773-651-7286
Web site: http://www.thirdworldpress.com.

Thoemmes Pr, *(Thoemmes Pr.; 1-85506),* Orders Addr.: P.O. Box 605, Herndon, VA 20172-0605 Tel 703-661-1500; Toll Free: 800-561-7704; Edit Addr.: 22883 Quicksilver Dr., Dulles, VA 20166.

Thomas Dunne Imprint of St Martin

Thomas Nelson Pubs, *(Nelson, Thomas Pubs.; 0-7852; 0-8407),* Orders Addr.: P.O. Box 141000, Nashville, TN 37214-1000
Web site: http://ThomasNelsonPublishers.com.

Thomas Publications, *(Thomas Pubns.; 0-939631; 1-57747),* 3245 Fairfield Rd., Gettysburg, PA 17325 (SAN 663-7213) Tel 717-642-6600; Fax: 717-642-5555; Toll Free: 800-840-6782 Do not confuse with companies with the same name in Austin, TX, La Crescenta, CA
E-mail: thomaspub@blazenet.net
Web site: http://www.thomaspublications.com.

†Thompson Co Inc, *(Thompson & Co., Inc.; 0-918351),* 4600 Longfellow Ave., Minneapolis, MN 55414-1524 (SAN 657-3843) Tel 612-722-4235; Fax: 612-722-4488; Toll Free: 800-257-6933 Do not confuse with Thompson Co. in Huntington, TX
E-mail: blt@skypoint.com; *CIP.*

Thomson Learn, *(Thomson Learning),* 7625 Empire Dr., Florence, KY 41042 (SAN 631-2144) Tel 859-525-6620; Fax: 859-525-0978; Toll Free: 800-347-7707 (customer service); 800-842-3636 (orders)
Web site: http://www.thomsonlearning.com.

Thorndike Imprint of Gale

Thornsbury Bailey Brown, *(Thornsbury Bailey & Brown; 0-945253),* P.O. Box 5169, Arlington, VA 22205 (SAN 246-2192) Tel 703-532-2210.

Thorsons (GBR) *(0-00; 0-7225; 0-85030; 1-85538; 0-85269) Dist. by* **Natl Bk Netwk.**

Thoth NV, *(Thoth, Inc.; 0-918993),* 2533 N. Carson St., No. 751, Carson City, NV 89706.

Three Copper, *(3 Copper Pennies Publishing; 0-9656066),* Orders Addr.: P.O. Box 41647, Los Angeles, CA 90041 (SAN 299-3090) Tel 323-255-2433; Fax: 626-792-7435; Edit Addr.: 1580 Yosemite, Suite 9, Los Angeles, CA 90041 (SAN 299-3082)
E-mail: threecupen@aol.com.

Three D Comp, *(ThreeD-Computing, Inc.; 0-9702897),* 900 Hideaway Pl., DeSoto, TX 75115-5213 Tel 972-223-2904; Fax: 972-223-7278
E-mail: info@3d-computing.com
Web site: http://www.3d-computing.com.

Three Riv Pr Imprint of Harmony Bks

Three Star Pr, *(3 Star Pr.; 0-9645127),* CSU - AMPS Project Occupational Therapy Dept., Fort Collins, CO 80523 Tel 970-491-6299; Fax: 970-491-3782 Do not confuse with Three Star Pr., Dickson, TN
E-mail: ampsi@cahs.colostate.edu
Web site: http://www.colostate.edu/Programs/AMPS.

Three Wishes, *(3 Wishes Pr.; 0-9622281),* P.O. Box 81033, Pittsburgh, PA 15217 Tel 412-521-1057.

Thriving Pubns, *(Thriving Pubns.; 0-9625872),* 9600 Potomac Dr., Fort Washington, MD 20744 Tel 301-567-8333.

Thrpy Skill Bldrs Imprint of Commun Skill

Thunderbird, *See* **Relaxed Bks**

Thunders Mouth Imprint of Avalon NY

Tichenor Pub, *(Tichenor Publishing; 0-89917; 1-56581; 0-7421),* Div. of T.I.S., Inc., 5005 N. State Rd. 37 Business, Bloomington, IN 47404-1626 (SAN 283-8818) Tel 812-332-3307; Fax: 812-331-7690; Toll Free: 800-367-4002
E-mail: tich@tisbook.com
Web site: http://www.tisbook.com/~tichpubs.

Tiffin Pr ME, *(Tiffin Pr. of Maine; 0-9646018),* Div. of Tiffin Pr., P.O. Box 549, Orono, ME 04473 Tel 207-866-3080
E-mail: joanmacc@aol.com.

†Timber, *(Timber Pr., Inc.; 0-88192; 0-917304; 0-931146; 0-931340; 1-57467),* 133 SW Second Ave., Suite 450, Portland, OR 97204-3527 (SAN 216-082X) Tel 503-227-2878; Fax: 503-227-3070; Toll Free: 800-327-5680 ; *Imprints:* Dioscorides (Dioscorides Press)
E-mail: orders@timberpress.com; publicity@timberpress.com
Web site: http://www.timberpress.com; *CIP.*

Timberline Pr, *(Timberline Pr., Inc.; 0-9608284),* P.O. Box 1056, Gig Harbor, WA 98335 (SAN 240-4559) Tel 206-858-6227 Do not confuse with companies with the same or similar name in Fulton, MO, Media, PA, Boise, ID, Denvor, CO, Bozeman, MT.

Timbritom, *(Timbritom; 0-9665934),* 32380 Mayfair Ln., Beverly Hills, MI 48025 Tel 248-646-7672; Fax: 248-593-4895.

Time Inc Health, *(Time Inc. Health; 0-9644119),* Div. of Time Publishing Ventures, Inc., Two Embarcadero Ctr., Suite 600, San Francisco, CA 94111 Tel 415-248-2700; Fax: 415-248-2779
E-mail: health_editors@time-inc.com.

Time Life Imprint of Henninger Prod

Time Warner, *See* **AOL Time Warner**

---

†Timeless Bks, *(Timeless Bks.; 0-931454),* Div. of Association for the Development of Human Potential, P.O. Box 3543, Spokane, WA 99220-3543 (SAN 211-6502) Tel 509-838-6652 (phone/fax); Toll Free: 800-251-9273
E-mail: info@timeless.org
Web site: http://www.timeless.org
Dist(s):* Baker & Taylor *(Baker & Taylor Bks.)
Bookpeople *(Bookpeople)*
New Leaf Dist *(New Leaf Distributing Co., Inc.); CIP.*

---

†Time-Life, *(Time-Life, Inc.; 0-7835; 0-8094),* Div. of Time Warner Co., Orders Addr.: Three Center Plaza, Boston, MA 02108-2084 Toll Free Fax: 800-308-1083; 800-286-9471; Toll Free: 800-277-8844; 800-759-0190; Edit Addr.: 2000 Duke St., Alexandria, VA 22314 (SAN 202-7836) Tel 703-838-7000; Fax: 703-838-7090; Toll Free: 800-621-7026
Web site: http://timelifeedu.com
Dist(s): **AOL Time Warner** *(AOL Time Warner Bk. Group)*
Time-Life Publng *(Time-Life Publishing Warehouse)*
Wrldwide Media Srv *(Worldwide Media Service, Inc.); CIP.*

Time-Life Bks (GBR) *(0-7054; 0-7370; 0-7835; 0-8094; 0-900658) Dist. by* **AOL Time Warner.**

Time-Life Educ, *(Time-Life Education, Inc.; 0-7054; 0-7370; 0-7835; 0-8094),* Orders Addr.: P.O. Box 85026, Richmond, VA 23285-5026 Toll Free Fax: 800-449-2011; Edit Addr.: 2000 Duke St., Alexandria, VA 22314 Tel 703-838-7000; Fax: 703-518-4124; Toll Free: 800-449-2010
E-mail: education@timelifecs.com
Web site: http://www.timelifeedu.com/
Dist(s): **AOL Time Warner** *(AOL Time Warner Bk. Group).*

Times Academic (SGP) *(981-210; 981-232) Dist. by* **Intl Spec Bk.**

Times Bks Imprint of H Holt & Co

Timing CA, *(Timing Pubns.; 1-886893),* 659 E. Kiowa, Flagstaff, AZ 86001 Tel 520-525-9461; Fax: 520-525-9474; Toll Free: 800-584-6464
E-mail: timing@igc.apc.org
Web site: http://www.northlink.com/timing.

Tiny Thought, *(Tiny Thought Pr.; 0-925928),* 1427 S. Jackson St., Louisville, KY 40217 Tel 502-637-6870; Fax: 502-634-1693; Toll Free: 800-456-3208
E-mail: aprint6870@aol.com.

Tiresias Pr, *(Tiresias Pr., Inc.; 0-913292),* 116 Pinehurst Ave., New York, NY 10033 (SAN 202-7879) Tel 212-568-9570 (phone/fax)
E-mail: dorothyalewis@aol.com.

TJU Pr, *See* **Truman St Univ**

T-L Custom Pub, *(Time-Life Custom Publishing; 0-7054; 0-7370),* Div. of Time Life, Inc., Orders Addr.: 3 Center Plaza, Boston, MA 02108-2084 (SAN 200-7746) Toll Free Fax: 800-308-1083; Toll Free: 800-277-8844; 34 Armstrong Ave., Georgetown, ON L76 4R9 Tel 888-595-3009; Toll Free Fax: 888-595-3008; Edit Addr.: 2000 Duke St., Alexandria, VA 22314 Tel 703-838-7218; Fax: 703-838-7045
E-mail: jennifer_ward@time-inc.com
Dist(s): **AOL Time Warner** *(AOL Time Warner Bk. Group).*

TLM Cnslting, *(TLM Consulting; 0-9654891),* Orders Addr.: P.O. Box 293, Monticello, IL 61856 Tel 217-762-9372; Edit Addr.: 200 W. Washington St., Monticello, IL 61856.

TMJ Stress Ctr Imprint of MyoData

TN Valley Pub, *(Tennessee Valley Publishing; 1-882194),* P.O. Box 52527, Knoxville, TN 37950-2527 Tel 423-584-5235; Fax: 423-584-0113; Toll Free: 800-762-7079
E-mail: info@typ1.com
Web site: http://www.tvp1.com.

TNP Imprint of Prima Pub

Today Tomorrow (IND) *(81-7019) Dist. by* **Lubrecht & Cramer.**

Together Lifeworks, *(Together Lifeworks Co.; 1-887796),* P.O. Box 38114, Blawnox, PA 15238 Tel 412-781-1092; Fax: 412-781-1096
E-mail: sheilakirk@aol.com.

Tolley Pubng (GBR) *(0-85459; 1-86012) Dist. by* **St Mut.**

Tolvan Co, *(Tolvan Co.; 0-916774),* 108 Idlewild St., Kaukauna, WI 54130-1312 (SAN 208-8924).

†Top Mtn Pub, *(Top of the Mountain Publishing; 0-914295; 1-56087),* P.O. Box 2244, Pinellas Park, FL 33780-2244 (SAN 287-590X) Tel 727-391-3958; Fax: 727-391-4598
E-mail: orders@abcinfo.com
Web site: http://www.abcinfo.com; http://www.10-10-net.com
Dist(s): **Baker & Taylor** *(Baker & Taylor Bks.)*
Brodart *(Brodart Co.)*
Emery-Pratt Co *(Emery-Pratt Co.)*
New Leaf Dist *(New Leaf Distributing Co., Inc.); CIP.*

Topiary Pubg, *(Topiary Publishing; 0-9667162),* R.R. 2, Box 91, Mount Vernon, IL 62864 (SAN 299-7282) Tel 618-246-1222; Fax: 618-242-1813; Toll Free: 800-584-7670.

Topping Inst, *(Topping International Institute, Inc.; 0-935299),* 2622 Birchwood Ave., No. 7, Bellingham, WA 98225-1462 (SAN 696-1932) Tel 360-647-2703 (phone/fax); Toll Free: 888-859-5863.

Tor Books Imprint of T Doherty Assocs

Torch Imprint of HarperCollins Pubs

Torchlght Pub, *(Torchlight Publishing; 0-9635309; 1-887089),* Orders Addr.: 49334 Stagecoach Dr., Box 52, Badger, CA 93603 Tel 559-337-2200; Fax: 559-337-2354; Toll Free: 888-867-2458 Do not confuse with Torchlight Publishing in Colorado Springs, CO
E-mail: torchlight@spiralcomm.net
Web site: http://www.torchlight.com.

Torrey PP, *(Torrey Pines Pr.; 1-884804),* 1030 W. Upas St., San Diego, CA 92103 Tel 619-497-0900 Do not confuse with Torrey Pines Assoc. in La Jolla, CA
Web site: http://www.diabetesnet.com.

Torstar, *(Torstar Pubns.; 1-929942),* Div. of Harlequin Enterprises, 99 Hawley Ln., Suite 1440 Merritt 8 Corp Pk., Stratford, CT 06614 Tel 203-378-1250; Fax: 203-375-9867
E-mail: jkilmurray@erols.com.

Tortoise NV, *(Tortoise Bks., Inc.; 0-9627160),* 127 Victory Rd., Henderson, NV 89015 (SAN 297-2980)
Dist(s): **J Majors Co** *(Majors, J. A. Co.)*
Matthews Medical Bk Co *(Matthews Medical Bk. Co.).*

Tortoise Press, *(Tortoise Pr.; 0-9642682),* 1310 San Miguel Ave., Santa Barbara, CA 93109 Tel 805-962-5431; Fax: 805-965-9761
E-mail: mbono@earthlink.net.

Totality Pr, *(Totality Pr.; 0-9663388),* 1336D Oak Ave., Saint Helena, CA 94574 Tel 707-963-7796; Fax: 707-963-6131
E-mail: ichinfo@classicalhomoeopathy.org
Web site: http://www.classicalhomoeopathy.org.

Totem Bks, *(Totem Bks.; 1-84046),* Subs. of Icon Bks., Ltd., 457 Broome St., New York, NY 10013 Tel 212-431-9368
E-mail: peterelek@theliteraryagency.com
Dist(s): **Natl Bk Netwk** *(National Bk. Network).*

Touchstone Imprint of S&S Trade Pap

Tous Bks, *See* **J Burnett**

†**TQS Pubns,** *(TQS Pubns., Eclectic Chicano Literature; 0-88412; 0-89229),* Div. of Tonatiuh/Quinto Sol International, Inc., P.O. Box 9275, Berkeley, CA 94709 (SAN 203-3984) Tel 510-655-8036; Fax: 510-601-6938
Web site: http://www.tqsbooks.com
Dist(s): **Baker & Taylor** *(Baker & Taylor Bks.)*
Continental Bk *(Continental Bk. Co., Inc.); CIP.*

Traces Inst, *(Traces Institute Pubns.; 0-934185),* 535 Fenchurch St., Suite 102, Norfolk, VA 23510-2812 (SAN 693-3874) Toll Free: 800-280-0122.

Trad Acupuncture, *(Traditional Acupuncture Institute, Inc., The; 0-912381),* 10227 Wincopin Cir., Columbia, MD 21044-3422 (SAN 265-2366) Tel 410-997-4888; Fax: 410-964-3544; Toll Free: 800-735-2968 (credit card orders).

Trafalgar, *(Trafalgar Square; 0-943955; 1-57076),* Orders Addr.: P.O. Box 257, North Pomfret, VT 05053 (SAN 213-8859) Tel 802-457-1911; Fax: 802-457-1913; Toll Free: 800-423-4525; Edit Addr.: Howe Hill Rd., North Pomfret, VT 05053 ; *Imprints:* Trafalgar Sq Pub (Trafalgar Square Publishing)
E-mail: tsquare@sover.net
Web site: http://www.trafalgarsquarebooks.com.

Trafalgar Sq Pub Imprint of Trafalgar

TranceTime, *(TranceTime Publishing; 1-929957),* 910 Florin Rd., Suite 107, Sacramento, CA 95831
E-mail: info@trancetime.com
Web site: http://www.trancetime.com.

Tranquil Pr, *(Tranquility Pr.; 0-9614923),* 600 Parkview Dr., Apt. 708, Hallandale, FL 33009-2973 (SAN 693-465X) Tel 954-454-8082 Do not confuse with Tranquility Pr., Austin, TX
Dist(s): **New Leaf Dist** *(New Leaf Distributing Co., Inc.).*

Trans T Pub (CHE) *(0-87849) Dist. by* **Enfield Pubs NH.**

†**Transaction Pubs,** *(Transaction Pubs.; 0-7658; 0-87855; 0-88738; 1-56000),* Orders Addr.: 390 Campus Dr., Somerset, NJ 08873 Fax: 732-748-9801; Toll Free: 888-999-6778; Edit Addr.: Rutgers-The State Univ. of NJ 35 Berrue Cir., Piscataway, NJ 08854-8042 (SAN 202-7941) Tel 732-445-2280; Fax: 732-445-3138; Toll Free: 888-999-6778
E-mail: trans@transactionpub.com
Web site: http://www.Transactionpub.com; *CIP.*

Transatl Arts, *(Transatlantic Arts, Inc.; 0-693),* P.O. Box 6086, Albuquerque, NM 87197 (SAN 202-7968) Tel 505-898-2289 Do not confuse with Trans-Atlantic Pubns., Inc., Philadelphia, PA.
E-mail: books@transatlantic.com
Web site: http://www.transatlantic.com/direct.

Trans-Atl Phila, *(Trans-Atlantic Pubns., Inc.),* 311 Bainbridge St., Philadelphia, PA 19147 (SAN 694-0234) Tel 215-925-5083; Fax: 215-925-1912 Do not confuse with Transatlantic Arts, Inc., Albuquerque, NM
E-mail: order@transatlanticpub.com
Web site: http://www.transatlanticpub.com
Dist(s): **Baker & Taylor** *(Baker & Taylor Bks.).*

Transcope, *(Transcope, Inc.; 0-9655606),* 6680 Traverse Rd., Thompsonville, MI 49683 Tel 231-269-4473
E-mail: doc@ERbook.net
Web site: http://www.ERbook.net.

Transform Inc, *(Transformations, Inc.; 0-9604856),* Orders Addr.: 4200 W. Good Hope Rd., Milwaukee, WI 53209 (SAN 662-085X) Tel 414-351-5770; Fax: 414-351-5760; Edit Addr.: 2728 N. Prospect Ave., Milwaukee, WI 53211 (SAN 215-8906) Tel 414-962-0213
E-mail: mornings7@aol.com
Web site: http://www.transformationsusa.com.

Transform WA, *(Transformational Tools Made Simple; 0-9649990),* Orders Addr.: P.O. Box 3633, Federal Way, WA 98063; Edit Addr.: 10819 Matthews, Anderson Island, WA 98303 Tel 253-884-3422
E-mail: arlenea3@aol.com
Dist(s): **New Leaf Dist** *(New Leaf Distributing Co., Inc.).*

Transforming Pr, *(Transforming Pr.; 0-9656218),* Orders Addr.: P.O. Box 9369, Santa Rosa, CA 95405 (SAN 299-1837) Tel 209-962-6403 (phone/fax); Edit Addr.: 4730 Alta Vista Ave., Santa Rosa, CA 95404 (SAN 299-1845)
E-mail: transformp@aol.com
Web site: http://www.sonic.net/hypno.

Transit Press, *(Transitions Pr.; 1-884537),* Orders Addr.: P.O. Box 618, Wadsworth, OH 44282 Tel 330-336-0403; Toll Free: 800-886-5735; Edit Addr.: 1153 Clark Rd., Wadsworth, OH 44281 Do not confuse with Transitions Press, Appleton, WI
E-mail: WLWeston@aol
Dist(s): **B&N Imports** *(Barnes & Noble Bks.-Imports)*
New Leaf Dist *(New Leaf Distributing Co., Inc.).*

TransMedia Group, *(TransMedia Group; 1-890819),* 240 W. Palmetto Park Blvd., Suite 300, Boca Raton, FL 33432 Tel 561-750-9800 Do not confuse with Transmedia, Honolulu, HI
E-mail: tmadden@transmediagroup.com
Dist(s): **Partners Pubs Grp** *(Partners Pubs. Group, Inc.).*

†**Transnatl Pubs,** *(Transnational Pubs., Inc.; 0-941320; 1-57105),* 410 Saw Mill River Rd., Ardsley, NY 10502 (SAN 226-2967) Tel 914-693-5100; Fax: 914-693-4430; Toll Free: 800-914-8186
E-mail: info@transnationalpubs.com
Web site: http://www.transnationalpubs.com; *CIP.*

Transplant Creat, *(Transplant Creations, L.C.; 0-9707183),* 5597 Seminary Rd., Suite 2210, Falls Church, VA 22041 Tel 703-820-4582; Fax: 703-820-4583
E-mail: mvanhoef@mindspring.com
Web site: http://www.transplantcreations.com.

†**Transport Res Bd,** *(Transportation Research Board; 0-309),* Div. of National Academy of Sciences, Orders Addr.: Box 289, Washington, DC 20055; Edit Addr.: 2101 Constitution Ave., NW, Washington, DC 20418 (SAN 225-2554) Tel 202-334-3214
E-mail: bpost@nas.edu; spetrite@library.berkeley.edu
Web site: http://www.nas.edu/trb/about/pubindex.html; http://www.nationalacademiesorg/trb; *CIP.*

Travel Med, *(Travel Medicine, Inc.; 0-923947),* 351 Pleasant St., No. 312, Northampton, MA 01060 (SAN 251-8236) Tel 413-584-0381; Fax: 413-584-6656; Toll Free: 800-872-8633
E-mail: travmed@travmed.com
Web site: http://www.travmed.com/.

TreCavalli Pr, *(TreCavalli Pr.; 0-9620635),* P.O. Box 49-1271, Los Angeles, CA 90049-1271 (SAN 249-5090) Tel 310-207-6147
E-mail: trecavpr@hotmail.com
Dist(s): **Academic Bk Ctr Inc** *(Academic Bk. Ctr., Inc.)*
Baker & Taylor *(Baker & Taylor Bks.).*

Tree Life Pubns, *(Tree of Life Pubns.; 0-930852),* P.O. Box 126, Joshua Tree, CA 92252 (SAN 222-5395) Tel 760-366-3695; Fax: 760-366-3596 Do not confuse with Tree of Life Pubns., Houston, TX
Dist(s): **Baker & Taylor** *(Baker & Taylor Bks.)*
Bookpeople *(Bookpeople).*

Tree of Light, *(Tree of Light Institute; 1-890855),* Orders Addr.: 1201 W. Center, Suite A, Provo, UT 84601; Edit Addr.: P.O. Box 1028, Roosevelt, UT 84066-1028 Tel 801-429-0041; Fax: 801-429-0043; Toll Free: 888-416-2887
E-mail: treelite@itsnet.com.

Treehouse, *(Treehouse Enterprises; 0-935571),* 810 Saturn St., No. 16, Jupiter, FL 33477-4456 (SAN 696-2025) Tel 407-575-0547 Do not confuse with Tree House Pr., Shelter Island, NY or Treehouse Pr., Chagrin Falls, OH
Dist(s): **New Leaf Dist** *(New Leaf Distributing Co., Inc.).*

Trends Res Inst, *(Trends Research Institute; 0-9648167),* 121 Main St., Cold Spring, NY 10516 Tel 914-876-6700; Fax: 914-758-5252.

Trentham Bks Imprint of Stylus Pub VA

†**Triad Pub FL,** *(Triad Publishing Co.; 0-937404),* Imprint of Triad Communications, Inc., P.O. Drawer 13355, Gainesville, FL 32604 (SAN 205-4574) Tel 352-373-5800; Fax: 352-373-1488; Toll Free Fax: 800-854-4947; Toll Free: 800-525-6902 (orders) Do not confuse with Triad Publishing Co., La Crescenta CA
E-mail: lorna@triadpublishing.com
Web site: http://www.triadpublishing.com; *CIP.*

TRIAD Svcs, *See* **Pink Hse**

Trillium Pr, *(Trillium Pr.; 0-89824),* Div. of Royal Fireworks Publishing Co., Orders Addr.: P.O. Box 399, Unionville, NY 10988 (SAN 212-4637) Tel 914-726-4444 (ordering info.); Fax: 914-726-3824; Edit Addr.: First Ave., Unionville, NY 10988 Do not confuse with companies with the same name in Saint Albans, WV, Tucson, AZ
E-mail: rfpress@frontiernet.net.

Trineurogenics, *(Trineurogenics, Inc.; 1-890243),* 455 N. Indian Rocks Rd., Belleair Bluffs, FL 33770 Tel 813-585-6333; Fax: 813-581-6107; Toll Free: 800-522-8114
E-mail: cadler@sixsteps.com
Web site: http://www.sixsteps.com.

Tringa Pr, *(Tringa Pr.; 0-9615255; 1-889458),* 2074 Highland Pkwy., Saint Paul, MN 55116 (SAN 694-4027) Tel 651-699-7184
E-mail: help@tringa.com
Web site: http://www.tringa.com.

Tri-Oak, *(Tri-Oak Education; 0-9609732),* 3698 Armstrong Valley Rd., Murfreesboro, TN 37130 (SAN 262-1002) Tel 615-890-8940; Fax: 615-896-1624.

Triple U Enterprises, *(Triple U Enterprises; 1-57876),* P.O. Box 2141, Ponca City, OK 74602-2141 Tel 580-762-3244 (phone/fax) ; *Imprints:* Love Lives (Love Lives)
E-mail: tripleu@poncacity.net.

Triple U Prods, *See* **Triple U Enterprises**

Trisib Pubng, *(Trisib Publishing; 0-9647823),* 19 Grotto Ct., Germantown, MD 20874 Tel 301-972-2197; Fax: 703-421-1418; Toll Free: 800-423-7804.

Triumph Pr, *(Triumph Pr., Inc.; 0-931515),* P.O. Box 93, Hillsboro, KS 67063 (SAN 682-3157) Tel 913-965-2245.

Trning Res, *(Training Resource Network, Inc. (TRN); 1-883302),* P.O. Box 439, Saint Augustine, FL 32085-0439 (SAN 299-2647) Tel 904-823-9800 (order); Fax: 904-823-3554; Toll Free: 866-823-9800
E-mail: info@trninc.com
Web site: http://www.trninc.com
Dist(s): **Baker & Taylor** *(Baker & Taylor Bks.).*

TRR, *(The Rehabilitation Resource; 0-916671),* Div. of Stout Vocational Rehabilitation Institute, Stout Vocational Rehabilitation Institute, Univ. of Wisconsin-Stout, Menomonie, WI 54751 (SAN 297-1917) Tel 715-232-1342; Fax: 715-232-2356.

Truman St Univ, *(Truman State Univ. Pr.; 0-943549; 1-931112),* 100 E. Normal St., Kirksville, MO 63501-4221 (SAN 253-4231) Tel 660-785-7299; Fax: 660-785-4480; Toll Free: 800-916-6802 ; *Imprints:* SCJP (Sixteenth Century Journal Publishers, Incorporated)
E-mail: tsup@truman.edu
Web site: http://www.tsup.truman.edu
Dist(s): **Rowman** *(Rowman & Littlefield Pubs., Inc.).*

Trunkey Pub, *(Trunkey Publishing Co.; 1-887620),* 2841 NE 21st Ct., Fort Lauderdale, FL 33305-3617 Tel 954-565-8608; Fax: 954-565-8609
E-mail: Money127@aol.com
Dist(s): **Baker & Taylor** *(Baker & Taylor Bks.)*
Unique Bks Inc *(Unique Bks., Inc.).*

Truth Forum, *(Truth Forum; 0-916387),* 496 Halbert Ln., Waco, TX 76705-5440 (SAN 295-8058) Tel 254-776-9972.

TSG Ent Pubns, *See* **TSG Pub Found**

TSG Pub Found, *(T.S.G. Publishing Foundation, Inc.; 0-929874),* Orders Addr.: 28641 N. 63rd Pl., Cave Creek, AZ 85331 (SAN 250-6718) Tel 480-502-1909; Fax: 480-502-0713
E-mail: info@tsg-publishing.com
Web site: http://www.tsg-publishing.com
Dist(s): **Baker & Taylor** *(Baker & Taylor Bks.)*
New Leaf Dist *(New Leaf Distributing Co., Inc.).*

TTM Pub, *(TTM Publishing; 0-9635819),* 1740 Spruce Ln., Colorado Springs, CO 80906 Tel 719-448-9800; Fax: 719-448-0417; Toll Free: 800-987-9277
E-mail: ttmpublishing@compuserve.com.

Tucker IL, *(Tucker Pubns., Inc.; 0-923950),* 5823 Queens Cove, Lisle, IL 60532 (SAN 252-0362) Tel 630-969-3809; Fax: 630-969-3895 Do not confuse with Tucker Pubns., Fayetteville, TN.

Tuckwell Pr (GBR) *(1-86232; 1-898410) Dist. by* **General Distrib Services.**

Turning Pt WA, *(Turning Point Pr.; 0-9625720),* P.O. Box 1542, North Bend, WA 98045-1542 Do not confuse with companies with the same name in Rancho Cucamonga, CA, Kansas City, MO, Port Townsend, WA, Santa Barbara, CA.

Turpin & Assocs, *(Turpin, John C. & Assocs.; 0-939506),* 1825 E. Faunsdale Dr., Sandy, UT 84092-3817 (SAN 216-700X) Tel 801-572-0999.

Turtleback, *(Turtleback Bks.; 0-606),* Orders Addr.: P.O. Box 14260, Madison, WI 53714-0260 Toll Free Fax: 800-828-0401; Toll Free: 800-448-8939; Edit Addr.: 2810 Crossroads Dr., Suite 2700, Madison, WI 5378-7942 Fax: 608-241-0666 Do not confuse with Turtleback Bks., Friday Harbor, WA. Turtleback Books are available only to schools and libraries. Not available to the retail market.
E-mail: turtleback@demco.com
Web site: http://www.turtlebackbooks.com/
Dist(s): **Demco** *(Demco Media, Ltd.).*

Tuskegee U CAENS, *(Tuskegee Univ., College of Agricultural, Environmental & Natural Sciences (CAENS); 0-9625021; 1-891196),* 107 Campbell Hall, Tuskegee, AL 36088 Tel 334-727-8035; Fax: 334-724-4451
E-mail: mloretan@acd.tuck.edu.

Tuttle Pubng, *(Tuttle Publishing; 0-8048; 4-900737),* Orders Addr.: 364 Innovation Dr., North Clarendon, VT 05759-9700 Tel 802-773-8930; Toll Free: 800-526-2778; Edit Addr.: 153 Milk St., 5th Flr., Boston, MA 02109 (SAN 213-2621) Tel 617-951-4080; Fax: 617-951-4045
E-mail: info@tuttlepublishing.com
Web site: http://www.tuttlemartialarts.com; http://www.tuttlepublishing.com
Dist(s): **Cheng & Tsui** *(Cheng & Tsui Co.)*
Continental Bk *(Continental Bk. Co., Inc.)*
Shens Bks *(Shen's Bks.).*

TV Bks, *(TV Bks., L.L.C.; 1-57500),* 1619 Broadway, 9th Flr., New York, NY 10019 Tel 212-603-1824; Fax: 212-245-7281
E-mail: mail@tvbooks.com
Web site: http://www.tvbooks.com
Dist(s): **HarperCollins Pubs** *(HarperCollins Pubs.)*
S&S Trade *(Simon & Schuster Trade).*

Twen Fir Cent, *(21st Century Pubns.; 0-933278),* Orders Addr.: P.O. Box 702, Fairfield, IA 52556-0702 (SAN 170-3226) Tel 515-472-5105; Fax: 515-472-8443; Toll Free: 800-593-2665; Edit Addr.: 401 N. Fourth St., Fairfield, IA 52556 Do not confuse with Twenty First Century Pubns., Tolland, CT
E-mail: books21st@lisco.com
Web site: http://www.21stbooks.com.

Twenty Fst CT, *(21st Century Pubns.; 0-9610708),* 190 Old Stafford Rd., Tolland, CT 06084 (SAN 264-8032) Tel 860-872-4083 Do not confuse with Twenty First Century Pubns., Fairfield, IA.

Twenty-Third, *(23rd Pubns./Bayard; 0-89622; 1-58595),* Orders Addr.: P.O. Box 180, Mystic, CT 06355 (SAN 210-9204) Tel 860-536-2611; Fax: 860-572-0788; Toll Free Fax: 800-572-0788; Toll Free: 800-321-0411
E-mail: ttpubs@aol.com
Web site: http://www.twentythirdpublications.com.

Twin Enterp, *(Twin Enterprises, Inc.; 0-9704385),* P.O. Box 150, Grafton, MA 01519 Fax: 508-887-8812
E-mail: info@twinenterprises.com
Web site: http://www.twinenterprises.com.

Twin Peaks Pr, *(Twin Peaks Pr.; 0-933261),* P.O. Box 129, Vancouver, WA 98666-0129 (SAN 692-4034) Tel 360-694-2462; Fax: 360-696-3210
E-mail: twinpeak@pacifier.com
Web site: http://www.pacifier.com/~twinpeak/.

Twin Streams Imprint of Kensgtn Pub Corp

Twenty-Fifth Cent Pr, *(25th Century Pr.; 1-56721),* Div. of Rio Grande Technology, 100 E. Washington St., Suite 102, Charleston, WV 25301; 7102 Ilfield Rd., SW, Albuquerque, NM 87105 Tel 505-873-2220; Fax: 505-877-4443
E-mail: editor@25c.com.

Two As, *See* **Two As Pub**

Two As Pub, *(Two A's Publishing, Inc.; 0-915001),* 809-B Cuesta Dr., No. 200, Mountain View, CA 94040 (SAN 289-4564) Tel 650-964-2981.

Two Blond Gdes, *(The Two Blondes Guides; 0-9660181),* Orders Addr.: P.O. Box 525, Peterborough, NH 03458 Tel 603-525-4434; Fax: 603-525-4329; Toll Free: 800-862-5042 (access code 23); Edit Addr.: 1 Fairfield Rd., Hancock, NH 03449.

Two Pillars, *(Two Pillars Pr.; 0-9648754),* 22588 Westview Ave., Golden, CO 80401 Tel 303-526-9095.

TWT Pubng, *(TWT Publishing; 1-57691),* P.O. Box 685, Pelham, NH 03076 Tel 603-635-8066; Fax: 603-635-9381; Toll Free: 800-497-1807
E-mail: twtpub@ma.ultranet.com
Web site: http://www.ultranet.com/~twtpub/twtpub.htm
Dist(s): **New Leaf Dist** *(New Leaf Distributing Co., Inc.).*

TX AES, *(Texas Agricultural Experiment Station; 0-926195),* Div. of Texas A&M Univ. System, 6500 Amarillo Blvd., W., Amarillo, TX 79106 Tel 806-359-5401; Fax: 806-358-9718
Web site: http://www.taeswww.tamu.edu.

TX A&M Thermodyn, *(Texas A&M Univ., Thermodynamics Research Ctr.; 1-883400),* Div. of Texas Engineering Experiment Station, Texas A&M Univ., 916 Richardson Petroleum Engineering Bldg., College Station, TX 77843-3111 Tel 409-845-4940; Fax: 409-847-8590.

TX Med Assn, *(Texas Medical Assn.; 0-9640262; 1-893621),* 401 W. 15th St., Austin, TX 78701-1680 Tel 512-370-1300; Fax: 512-370-1630; Toll Free: 800-880-1300
E-mail: anne_g@texmed.org
Web site: http://www.texmed.org.

TX Psych Found, *(Texas Psychological Foundation; 0-9630867),* Div. of Texas Psychological Assn., 6633 E. Hwy. 290, Suite 305, Austin, TX 78723 Tel 512-454-2449; Fax: 512-454-2469.

Tycooly Pub Imprint of Weidner & Sons

†Tyndale Hse, *(Tyndale Hse. Pubs.; 0-8423),* Orders Addr.: P.O. Box 80, Wheaton, IL 60189-0080 (SAN 206-7749) Tel 630-668-8310; Fax: 630-668-3245; Toll Free: 800-323-9400; Edit Addr.: 351 Executive Dr., Wheaton, IL 60189
E-mail: Timothy_Olson@tyndale.com
Web site: http://www.tyndale.com
Dist(s): **Appalach Bk Dist** *(Appalachian Bk. Distributors)*
Christian Bk Distributors *(Christian Bk. Distributors)*
Riverside-World *(Riverside World)*
Spring Arbor Dist *(Spring Arbor Distributors Inc.)*
T T Beeler *(Beeler, Thomas T. Publisher); CIP.*

Type & Temperament, *(Type & Temperament, Inc.; 1-878287),* Orders Addr.: P.O. Box 200, Gladwyne, PA 19035-0200 Tel 610-527-2330; Fax: 610-527-1722; Toll Free: 800-447-8973; Edit Addr.: 270 N. Ithan Ave., Villanova, PA 19085
E-mail: wdgmurray@aol.com
Web site: http://www.typemperament.com.

Tyrell & Jerem, *(Tyrell & Jerem Pr.; 1-882522),* Orders Addr.: P.O. Box 20089, Cincinnati, OH 45220 Tel 513-751-4352; Fax: 513-961-0835; Edit Addr.: 407 Resor Ave., Cincinnati, OH 45220.

U Auckland (NZL) *(0-86869; 981-4021; 0-908689) Dist. by* **Spr-Verlag.**

U Buffalo Sch Dental, *(University at Buffalo Schl. of Dental Medicine; 0-9639893),* Div. of State Univ. of New York, 355 Squire Hall, 3435 Main St., Buffalo, NY 14214 Tel 716-829-2056; Fax: 716-833-3517.

U C Books, *(U.C. Bks.; 0-9656505),* Div. of Uncommon Communications, Inc., P.O. Box 51662, Pacific Grove, CA 93950-9998 (SAN 299-2671) Tel 831-372-3770; Fax: 831-372-3771; Toll Free: 888-411-2075
E-mail: mike@ucbooks.com
Web site: http://www.beyondglasses.com
Dist(s): **IPG Chicago** *(Independent Pubs. Group).*

†U CA Pr, *(Univ. of California Pr.; 0-520),* Orders Addr.: 1445 Lower Ferry Rd., Ewing, NJ 08618 Tel 609-883-1759; Edit Addr.: 2120 Berkeley Way, Berkeley, CA 94720 Tel 520-642-4247; Fax: 520-643-7127
E-mail: orders@cpfs.pupress.princeton.edu; ucpress.comments@ucop.edu
Web site: http://www.ucpress.edu
Dist(s): **Brookings** *(Brookings Institution Pr.)*
Cal Prin Full Svc *(California Princeton Fulfillment Services); CIP.*

U CA Riverside, *(Univ. of California, Riverside; 1-891168),* Div. of Vice Chancellor Administration, UCR, 900 University Ave., E., Riverside, CA 92521 Tel 909-787-4444; Fax: 909-787-3686
E-mail: allas.johnson@ucr.edu
Web site: http://www.ucrservice.ucr.edu/Phome.htm.

U Cal Hist Sci Tech, *(Univ. of California, Office for History of Science & Technology; 0-918102; 0-9672617),* 543 Stephens Hall, No. 2350, Berkeley, CA 94720-2350 (SAN 210-1394) Tel 510-642-4581; Fax: 510-643-5321
E-mail: Office@ohst7.berkeley.edu
Web site: http://ohst7.berkley.edu.

U Cal LA Indus Rel, *(Univ. of California, Institute of Industrial Relations; 0-89215),* c/o Schl. of Public Policy & Social Research, 6350B Public Policy Bldg., Box 951478, Los Angeles, CA 90095-1478 (SAN 205-4698) Tel 310-794-5955; Fax: 310-794-6410.

†U Ch Pr, *(Univ. of Chicago Pr.; 0-226; 0-89065; 0-943056; 1-892850),* Div. of Univ. of Chicago, Orders Addr.: 11030 S. Langley Ave., Chicago, IL 60628 (SAN 202-5280) Tel 773-568-1550; Fax: 773-660-2235; Edit Addr.: 1427 E. 60th St., Chicago, IL 60637 (SAN 202-5299) Tel 773-702-7700; Fax: 773-702-9756 ; *Imprints:* Midway Reprint (Midway Reprint)
E-mail: general@press.uchicago.edu; kh@press.uchicago.edu
Web site: http://www.press.uchicago.edu
Dist(s): **netLibrary CO** *(netLibrary, Inc.); CIP.*

U Chi Pritzker Schl, *(Univ. of Chicago Pritzker Schl. of Medicine, The; 1-891539),* Div. of Hartford Geriatrics Initiative, 5841 S. Maryland Ave., MC-6098, Chicago, IL 60637 Tel 773-702-9327; Fax: 773-702-3538.

†U Delaware Pr, *(Univ. of Delaware Pr.; 0-87413),* 326 Hullihen Hall, Newark, DE 19716 (SAN 203-4476) Tel 302-831-1149
E-mail: udpress@udel.edu
Web site: http://www.udpress.udel.edu/udpress/index.html
Dist(s): **Assoc Univ Prs** *(Associated Univ. Presses)*
B & T International *(Baker & Taylor International); CIP.*

†U IA Pubns Dept, *(Univ. of Iowa, Pubns. Dept.; 0-87414),* a/o Pubns. Order Dept., 2222 Old Hwy. 218 S., Iowa City, IA 52242-1602 (SAN 282-4876) Tel 319-335-1727; Toll Free: 800-235-2665 Do not confuse with Univ. of Iowa Pr., same address; *CIP.*

U KS Nat Hist Mus, *(Univ. of Kansas, Natural History Museum; 0-89338),* 1345 Jayhawk Blvd., Lawrence, KS 66045-7561 (SAN 206-0957) Tel 913-864-4540; Fax: 913-864-5335
Web site: http://ron.nhm.ukans.edu/.

U MA W M Trotter Inst, *(Univ. of Massachusetts, William Monroe Trotter Institute; 1-878358),* Harbor Campus, Dorchester, MA 02125 Tel 617-929-8630.

U Maine Pr, *(Univ. of Maine Pr.; 0-89101),* 5717 Corbett Hall, Rm. 326, Orono, ME 04469 (SAN 207-2971) Tel 207-581-1408; Fax: 207-581-1490
E-mail: umpress@umit.maine.edu
Web site: http://www.umaine.edu/umpress.

U MI Mus Zool, *(Univ. of Michigan Museum of Zoology; 0-9628499),* 1109 Geddes, Ann Arbor, MI 48109-1079 Tel 313-764-0476.

U Miami N-S Ctr, *(Univ. of Miami, North/South Ctr. Pr.; 0-935501; 1-57454),* Orders Addr.: P.O. Box 248205, Coral Gables, FL 33146-3027 (SAN 695-8834) Tel 305-284-8914; 305-284-8908; Fax: 305-284-5089; Edit Addr.: 1500 Monza Ave., Coral Gables, FL 33124-3027
E-mail: nscenter@miami.edu
Web site: http://www.miami.edu/nsc/
Dist(s): **L Rienner** *(Rienner, Lynne Pubs., Inc.).*

U Mich Mus Anthro, *(Univ. of Michigan, Museum of Anthropology, Pubns. Dept.; 0-915703; 0-932206),* 4009 Museums Bldg., 1109 Geddes, Ann Arbor, MI 48109 (SAN 203-0489) Tel 734-764-0482; Fax: 734-763-7783
E-mail: shorv@umich.edu
Web site: http://www.umma.lsa.umich.edu/pub.

†U Museum Pubns, *(Univ. Museum Pubns.; 0-924171; 0-934718; 1-931707),* Univ. of Pennsylvania, 33rd & Spruce Sts., Philadelphia, PA 19104 (SAN 207-9283) Tel 215-898-4124; Fax: 215-573-2497; Toll Free: 800-306-1941
E-mail: publications@museum.upenn.edu
Web site: http://www.upenn.edu/museum_pubs; *CIP.*

U N I C E F, *(UNICEF (United Nations Children's Fund); 0-940065; 92-806),* 3 UN Plaza, New York, NY 10017 (SAN 664-0338) Tel 212-503-0320
E-mail: netmaster@unicef.org
Web site: http://www.unicef.org/
Dist(s): **Balogh** *(Balogh International, Inc.)*
Bernan Associates *(Bernan Assocs.)*
UN *(United Nations Pubns.).*

U NC School Med, *(Univ. of North Carolina, Schl. of Medicine, Dept. of Surgery; 0-9653036),* Box 7050, 136 Burnett-Womack Bldg., Chapel Hill, NC 27599-7050 Tel 919-942-4320; Fax: 919-966-6009.

U NE CPAR, *(Univ. of Nebraska at Omaha, Ctr. for Public Affairs Research; 1-55719),* 6001 Dodge St., Omaha, NE 68182 (SAN 665-4339) Tel 402-595-1231; Fax: 402-595-2366
E-mail: melanie_hayes@mail.unomaha.edu
Web site: http://www.unomaha.edu.

U NE Ctr Public Affairs, *See* **U NE CPAR**

U NV Oral Hist, *(Univ. of Nevada Oral History Program; 1-56475),* Univ. of Nevada, MS324, Reno, NV 89557-0099 Tel 775-784-6932 (orders); Fax: 775-784-1365 (orders)
E-mail: ohp@unr.nevada.edu
Web site: http://www.unr.edu/artsci/oralhist/ohweb/oralhist.htm
Dist(s): **CMIL** *(Ctr. for Media & Independent Learning).*

†**U of Ala Pr,** *(Univ. of Alabama Pr.; 0-8173),* Orders Addr.: 11030 S. Langley, Chicago, IL 60628 (SAN 630-6047); Edit Addr.: P.O. Box 870380, Tuscaloosa, AL 35487-0380 (SAN 202-5272) Tel 205-348-5180; Fax: 205-348-9201
E-mail: jkramer@uapress.ua.edu
Web site: http://www.uapress.ua.edu
Dist(s): **U Ch Pr** *(Univ. of Chicago Pr.); CIP.*

U of Alaska Pr, *(Univ. of Alaska Pr.; 0-912006; 1-889963),* P.O. Box 756240, Fairbanks, AK 99775-6240 (SAN 203-3011) Tel 907-474-5831; Fax: 907-474-5502; Toll Free: 888-252-6657
E-mail: fypress@uaf.edu
Web site: http://www.uaf.edu/uapress
Dist(s): **Todd Commns** *(Todd Communications).*

†**U of Ariz Pr,** *(Univ. of Arizona Pr.; 0-8165),* 355 S. Euclid Ave., Suite 103, Tucson, AZ 85719 (SAN 205-468X) Tel 520-621-1441; Fax: 520-621-8899
E-mail: orders@uapress.arizona.edu
Web site: http://www.uapress.arizona.edu
Dist(s): **Continental Bk** *(Continental Bk. Co., Inc.)*
Many Feathers Bks & Maps *(Many Feathers Bks. & Maps)*
U of A Crit Lang *(Univ of Arizona Critical Languages Program); CIP.*

†**U of Ark Pr,** *(Univ. of Arkansas Pr.; 0-938626; 1-55728),* 201 Ozark Ave., Fayetteville, AR 72701 (SAN 239-3972) Tel 501-575-3246; Fax: 501-575-6044; Toll Free: 800-626-0090
E-mail: uaprinfo@cavern.uark.edu
Web site: http://www.uark.edu/~uaprinfo; http://www.uapress.com
Dist(s): **Baker & Taylor** *(Baker & Taylor Bks.)*
Yankee Ped Bkshop *(Yankee Peddler Bookshop); CIP.*

†**U of Ga Pr,** *(Univ. of Georgia Pr.; 0-8203),* 330 Research Dr., Suite B100, Athens, GA 30602-4901 (SAN 203-3054) Tel 706-369-6130; Fax: 706-369-6131
E-mail: books@ugapress.uga.edu
Web site: http://www.uga.edu; *CIP.*

U of Healing, *See* **UNIPress**

†**U of Ill Pr,** *(Univ. of Illinois Pr.; 0-252),* Orders Addr.: P.O. Box 4856, Baltimore, MD 21211; Edit Addr.: 1325 S. Oak St., Champaign, IL 61820 (SAN 202-5310) Tel 217-333-0950; Fax: 217-244-8082
E-mail: uipress@uiuc.edu
Web site: http://www.uiuc.edu/providers/uipress; http://www.press.uillinois.edu; *CIP.*

†**U of Iowa Pr,** *(Univ. of Iowa Pr.; 0-87745; 1-58729),* Div. of The University of Iowa, Orders Addr.: c/o Chicago Distribution Ctr. 11030 S. Langley Ave., Chicago, IL 60628 (SAN 282-4876) Toll Free Fax: 800-621-8476; Toll Free: 800-621-2736; Edit Addr.: 100 Kuhl Hse. 119 W. Parker Rd., Iowa City, IA 52242-1000 (SAN 202-5280) Tel 319-335-2000; Fax: 319-335-2055 Do not confuse with Univ. of Iowa, Pubns. Dept. at same address
E-mail: holly-carver@uiowa.edu
Web site: http://www.uiowa.edu/~uipress
Dist(s): **U Ch Pr** *(Univ. of Chicago Pr.)*
netLibrary CO *(netLibrary, Inc.); CIP.*

U of KY Libs, *(Univ. of Kentucky Libraries; 0-917519),* 127 King Library N. Univ. of Kentucky, Lexington, KY 40506-0059 (SAN 656-1098) Tel 606-257-1466.

†**U of Mass Pr,** *(Univ. of Massachusetts Pr.; 0-87023; 1-55849),* Orders Addr.: P.O. Box 429, Amherst, MA 01004 (SAN 203-3089) Tel 413-545-2219 (orders); 413-545-2217 (editorial); Fax: 413-545-1226; Toll Free Fax: 800-488-1144
E-mail: orders@umpress.umass.edu
Web site: http://www.umass.edu/umpress; *CIP.*

U of MD Physical Therapy, *(Univ. of Maryland Schl. of Medicine, Dept. of Physical Therapy; 0-9627560),* 32 S. Greene St., Baltimore, MD 21201 Tel 410-706-7720; Fax: 410-706-6387.

†**U of Miami Pr,** *(Univ. of Miami Pr.; 0-87024),* Raritan Industrial Park, 100 Newfield Ave., Edison, NJ 08837 Tel 732-225-2727
E-mail: rfuerst@miami.edu; *CIP.*

U of Mich Inst Labor, *(Univ. of Michigan, Institute of Labor & Industrial Relations; 0-87736),* Univ. of Michigan, Victor Vaughan Bldg., 1111 E. Catherine, Ann Arbor, MI 48109 (SAN 662-1716) Tel 734-647-0699; Fax: 734-763-0913
E-mail: swines@umich.edu
Web site: http://www.umich.edu/~ilir.

†**U of Mich Pr,** *(Univ. of Michigan Pr.; 0-472),* Orders Addr.: P.O. Box 1104, Ann Arbor, MI 48106-1104 (SAN 282-4884) Tel 734-764-4388; Fax: 734-936-0456; Edit Addr.: 839 Greene St., Ann Arbor, MI 48106 ; *Imprints:* Ann Arbor Bks (Ann Arbor Books)
E-mail: um.press@umich.edu
Web site: http://www.press.umich.edu/; *CIP.*

†**U of Minn Pr,** *(Univ. of Minnesota Pr.; 0-8166),* Affil. of Univ. of Minnesota, 111 Third Ave. S., Suite 290, Minneapolis, MN 55401-2520 (SAN 213-2648) Tel 612-627-1970; Fax: 612-627-1980; Toll Free: 800-621-2736 (customer service only)
E-mail: ump@staff.tc.umn.edu
Web site: http://www.upress.umn.edu
Dist(s): **Chicago Distribution Ctr** *(Chicago Distribution Ctr.)*
Continental Bk *(Continental Bk. Co., Inc.)*
U Ch Pr *(Univ. of Chicago Pr.); CIP.*

†**U of Mo Pr,** *(Univ. of Missouri Pr.; 0-8262),* 2910 LeMone Blvd., Columbia, MO 65201 (SAN 203-3143) Tel 573-882-0180; Fax: 573-884-4498; Toll Free: 800-828-1894 (orders only)
E-mail: order@ext.missouri.edu
Web site: http://www.system.missouri.edu/upress
Dist(s): **East-West Export Bks** *(East-West Export Bks.)*
netLibrary CO *(netLibrary, Inc.); CIP.*

†**U of NC Pr,** *(University of North Carolina Pr.; 0-8078),* P.O. Box 2288, Chapel Hill, NC 27515-2288 (SAN 203-3151) Tel 919-966-3561; Fax: 919-966-3829; Toll Free: 800-848-6224 (orders)
E-mail: uncpress@unc.edu
Web site: http://www.uncpress.unc.edu
Dist(s): **Replica Bks** *(Replica Bks.)*
netLibrary CO *(netLibrary, Inc.); CIP.*

†**U of Nebr Pr,** *(Univ. of Nebraska Pr.; 0-8032),* P.O. Box 880484, Lincoln, NE 68588-0484 (SAN 202-5337); 233 N. Eighth St., Lincoln, NE 68588-0255 Tel 402-472-3581 ; *Imprints:* Bison Books (Bison Books)
E-mail: pressmail@unl.edu
Web site: http://www.nebraskapress.unl.edu
Dist(s): **Continental Bk** *(Continental Bk. Co., Inc.); CIP.*

†**U of Nev Pr,** *(Univ. of Nevada Pr.; 0-87417),* Mail Stop 166, Reno, NV 89557 (SAN 203-316X) Tel 775-784-6573; Fax: 775-784-6200; Toll Free: 877-682-6657 (orders only)
E-mail: ceh@unr.edu
Web site: www.nvbooks.nevada.edu
Dist(s): **netLibrary CO** *(netLibrary, Inc.); CIP.*

†**U of NM Pr,** *(Univ. of New Mexico Pr.; 0-8263),* 3721 Spirit Dr., SE, Albuquerque, NM 87106-5631 Tel 505-277-4810 (orders); Fax: 505-277-3350; Toll Free Fax: 800-622-8667; Toll Free: 800-249-7737 (orders only); Edit Addr.: 1720 Lomas Blvd., NE, Albuquerque, NM 87131-1591 (SAN 213-9588) Tel 505-277-2346; Fax: 505-277-9270
E-mail: unmpress@unm.edu
Web site: http://www.unmpress.com
Dist(s): **Baker & Taylor** *(Baker & Taylor Bks.)*
Continental Bk *(Continental Bk. Co., Inc.)*
Treas Chest Bks *(Treasure Chest Bks.); CIP.*

†**U of Notre Dame Pr,** *(Univ. of Notre Dame Pr.; 0-268),* Orders Addr.: 11030 S. Langley Ave., Chicago, IL 60628 (SAN 202-5280) Tel 773-568-1550; Toll Free Fax: 800-621-8476; Toll Free: 800-621-2736; Edit Addr.: 310 Flanner Hall, Notre Dame, IN 46556 (SAN 203-3178) Tel 219-631-6346; Fax: 219-631-8148
E-mail: undpress.1@nd.edu
Web site: http://www.undpress.nd.edu
Dist(s): **Chicago Distribution Ctr** *(Chicago Distribution Ctr.)*
U Ch Pr *(Univ. of Chicago Pr.)*
netLibrary CO *(netLibrary, Inc.); CIP.*

†**U of Okla Pr,** *(Univ. of Oklahoma Pr.; 0-8061),* Orders Addr.: 4100 28th Ave., NW, Norman, OK 73069-8218 (SAN 203-3194) Tel 405-325-2000; Fax: 405-364-5798; Toll Free: 800-627-7377; Edit Addr.: 1005 Asp Ave., Norman, OK 73019-6051 Fax: 405-325-4000
Web site: http://www.ou.edu/oupress
Dist(s): **Continental Bk** *(Continental Bk. Co., Inc.)*
netLibrary CO *(netLibrary, Inc.); CIP.*

†**U of Pa Pr,** *(Univ. of Pennsylvania Pr.; 0-8122; 0-940663),* Orders Addr.: P.O. Box 4836, Baltimore, MD 21211 Tel 410-516-6948; Fax: 410-516-6998; Edit Addr.: 4200 Pine St., Philadelphia, PA 19104-4011 (SAN 202-5345) Tel 215-898-6261; Fax: 215-898-0404; Toll Free: 800-445-9880
E-mail: custserv@pobox.upenn.edu
Web site: http://www.upenn.edu/pennpress; *CIP.*

†**U of Pittsburgh Pr,** *(Univ. of Pittsburgh Pr.; 0-8229),* 3400 Forbes Ave., Eureka Bldg., Fifth Flr., Pittsburgh, PA 15260 (SAN 203-3216) Tel 412-383-2456; Fax: 412-383-2466
E-mail: press+@pitt.edu
Web site: http://pitt.edu/~press
Dist(s): **Cornell U Pr** *(Cornell Univ. Pr.); CIP.*

†**U of PR Pr,** *(Univ. of Puerto Rico Pr.; 0-8477),* Subs. of Univ. of Puerto Rico, Orders Addr.: P.O. Box 23322, Rio Piedras, PR 00931-3322 (SAN 208-1245) Tel 787-758-6932; Fax: 787-753-9116
Web site: http://www.press.uchicago.edu/journals/presses/puerto_ri
Dist(s): **Lectorum Pubns** *(Lectorum Pubns., Inc.)*
Libros Fronteras *(Libros Sin Fronteras); CIP.*

U of Rochester, *(Univ. of Rochester-Strong Memorial Hospital; 0-9641841),* 601 Elmwood Ave., Box 660, Rochester, NY 14642 Tel 716-275-2420; Fax: 716-273-1118.

†**U of SC Pr,** *(Univ. of South Carolina Pr.; 0-87249; 1-57003),* Orders Addr.: 718 Devine St., Columbia, SC 29208 Tel 803-777-1774; Fax: 803-777-0026; Toll Free Fax: 800-868-0740; Toll Free: 800-768-2500; Edit Addr.: 937 Assembly St., Carolina Plaza, 8th Flr., Columbia, SC 29208 (SAN 203-3224) Tel 803-777-5243; Fax: 803-777-0160; Toll Free Fax: 800-868-0740; Toll Free: 800-768-2500
E-mail: cdibble@sc.edu
Web site: http://www.sc.edu/uscpress/; *CIP.*

U of SW LA Ctr LA Studies, *See* **Univ LA Lafayette**

†**U of Tenn Pr,** *(Univ. of Tennessee Pr.; 0-87049; 1-57233),* Div. of Univ. of Tennessee & Member of Assn. of American Univ. Presses, Orders Addr.: 11030 S. Langley, Chicago, IL 60628 (SAN 202-5280) Tel 773-568-1550; Toll Free Fax: 800-621-8471; Toll Free: 800-621-2736 (orders only); Edit Addr.: 110 Conference Ctr. Bldg., Knoxville, TN 37996-0325 (SAN 212-9930) Tel 865-974-3321; Fax: 865-974-3724
E-mail: sstephens@utk.edu; gadair@utk.edu
Web site: http://www.sunsite.utk.edu/utpress
Dist(s): **U Ch Pr** *(Univ. of Chicago Pr.); CIP.*

†**U of Tex Pr,** *(Univ. of Texas Pr.; 0-292),* Orders Addr.: P.O. Box 7819, Austin, TX 78713-7819 (SAN 212-9876) Tel 512-471-7233; Fax: 512-320-0668; Toll Free: 800-252-3206; Edit Addr.: University of Texas at Austin, Austin, TX 78713-7819
E-mail: utpress@utpress.ppb.utexas.edu
Web site: http://www.utexas.edu/utpress
Dist(s): **Continental Bk** *(Continental Bk. Co., Inc.)*
Urban Land *(Urban Land Institute); CIP.*

U of Tokyo (JPN) *(0-86008) Dist. by* **Col U Pr.**

†**U of Toronto Pr,** *(Univ. of Toronto Pr.; 0-7727; 0-8020),* 2250 Military Rd., Tonawanda, NY 14150 Toll Free Fax: 800-221-9985
E-mail: utpbooks@utpress.utoronto.ca
Web site: http://www.upress.utoronto.ca; *CIP.*

†**U of Utah Pr,** *(Univ. of Utah Pr.; 0-87480),* 1795 E. South Campus Dr., Rm. 101, Salt Lake City, UT 84112-9402 (SAN 220-0023) Tel 801-581-6771; Fax: 801-581-3365; Toll Free: 800-773-6672
E-mail: info@upress.utah.edu
Web site: http://www.upress.utah.edu
Dist(s): **Baker & Taylor** *(Baker & Taylor Bks.)*
Treas Chest Bks *(Treasure Chest Bks.); CIP.*

U of VT Psych, *See* **Res Ctr Child**

†**U of Wash Pr,** *(Univ. of Washington Pr.; 0-295; 1-902716),* Orders Addr.: P.O. Box 50096, Seattle, WA 98145-5096 (SAN 212-2502); Edit Addr.: 1326 Fifth Ave., Suite 555, Seattle, WA 98101 Tel 206-543-8870; Fax: 206-685-3460; Toll Free Fax: 800-669-7993; Toll Free: 800-441-4115; 1126 N. 98th St., Seattle, WA 98103
E-mail: uwpord@u.washington.edu
Web site: http://www.washington.edu/uwpress
Dist(s): **Shens Bks** *(Shen's Bks.)*
Urban Land *(Urban Land Institute)*
netLibrary CO *(netLibrary, Inc.); CIP.*

U of Wis CEFM, *(Univ. of Wisconsin - Madison, Ctr. for Excellence in Family Studies; 0-9639334),* 1300 Linden Dr., Madison, WI 53706-1575 Tel 608-262-4847; Fax: 608-262-5335.

Publisher Symbol Index

U of Wis Ctr Arch-Urban, *(Univ. of Wisconsin-Milwaukee, Ctr. for Architecture & Urban Planning Research; 0-938744; 1-886437),* P.O. Box 413, Milwaukee, WI 53201 Tel 414-229-2878; Fax: 414-229-6976
E-mail: caupr@uwm.edu.

†**U of Wis Pr,** *(Univ. of Wisconsin Pr.; 0-299),* Orders Addr.: c/o Chicago Dist Ctr., 11030 S Langley Ave, Chicago, IL 60628 (SAN 501-0039) Tel 773-568-1550; Fax: 773-660-2235; Toll Free Fax: 800-621-8476 (orders only); Toll Free: 800-621-2736 (orders only); Edit Addr.: 1930 Monroe St., Madison, WI 53711 Tel 608-263-1110; Fax: 608-263-1132
E-mail: uwiscpress@macc.wisc.edu
Web site: http://www.wisc.edu/wisconsinpress/
Dist(s): **Chicago Distribution Ctr** *(Chicago Distribution Ctr.)*
I Brecht Soc *(International Brecht Society)*
Max Kade *(Kade, Max Institute for German American Studies)*
Sheridan *(Sheridan Hse., Inc.)*
U Ch Pr *(Univ. of Chicago Pr.); CIP.*

†**U Pr of Amer,** *(University Pr. of America; 0-7618; 0-8191; 1-879691),* Orders Addr.: 15200 NBN Way, P.O. Box 190, Blue Ridge Summit, PA 17214-0190 (SAN 253-2387) Toll Free Fax: 800-338-4550; Toll Free: 800-462-6420; Edit Addr.: 4720 Boston Way, Lanham, MD 20706 (SAN 200-2256) Tel 301-459-3366; Fax: 301-459-2118; Toll Free: 800-462-6420
Web site: http://www.univpress.com
Dist(s): **Natl Bk Netwk** *(National Bk. Network)*
Rowman *(Rowman & Littlefield Pubs., Inc.); CIP.*

†**U Pr of KS,** *(University Pr. of Kansas; 0-7006),* 2501 W. 15th St., Lawrence, KS 66049 (SAN 203-3267) Tel 785-864-4154; 785-864-4155 (orders); Fax: 785-864-4586
E-mail: jpigza@ukans.edu
Web site: http://www.kansaspress.ku.edu; *CIP.*

†**U Pr of KY,** *(University Pr. of Kentucky; 0-8131; 0-912839; 0-916968),* Orders Addr.: P.O. Box 11578, Lexington, KY 40576-1578 Tel 859-257-8400; Fax: 859-257-8481; Toll Free: 800-839-6855; Edit Addr.: 663 S. Limestone St., Lexington, KY 40508-4008 (SAN 203-3275) Tel 859-257-5200; Fax: 859-323-4981; Toll Free Fax: 800-870-4981
E-mail: leilas@pop.uky.edu
Web site: http://www.kentuckypress.com
Dist(s): **CUP Services** *(CUP Services)*
netLibrary CO *(netLibrary, Inc.); CIP.*

†**U Pr of Miss,** *(University Pr. of Mississippi; 0-87805; 1-57806),* 3825 Ridgewood Rd., Jackson, MS 39211-6492 (SAN 203-1914) Tel 601-432-6205; Fax: 601-432-6217; Toll Free: 800-737-7788 (orders only)
E-mail: press@ihl.state.ms.us
Web site: http://www.upress.state.ms.us; *CIP.*

†**U Pr of New Eng,** *(University Pr. of New England; 0-87451; 0-915032; 1-891507; 1-58465),* Orders Addr.: 23 S. Main St., Hanover, NH 03755-2048 (SAN 203-3283) Tel 603-643-7100; Fax: 603-643-1540; Toll Free: 800-421-1561 (orders only) ; *Imprints:* Wesleyan Univ Pr (Wesleyan University Press)
E-mail: University.Press@Dartmouth.edu
Web site: http://www.upne.com; *CIP.*

†**U Pr of Va,** *(University Pr. of Virginia; 0-8139; 0-912759; 1-57814),* Orders Addr.: P.O. Box 400318, Charlottesville, VA 22904-4318 (SAN 202-5361) Tel 804-924-3468; Fax: 804-982-2655
E-mail: upress@virginia.edu
Web site: http://www.upress.virginia.edu
Dist(s): **BookWorld** *(BookWorld Services, Inc.)*
U Pr of New Eng *(University Pr. of New England); CIP.*

†**U Press Fla,** *(Univ. Pr. of Florida; 0-8130),* 15 NW 15th St., Gainesville, FL 32611-0279 (SAN 207-9275) Tel 352-392-1351; Fax: 352-392-7302; Toll Free: 800-226-3822
E-mail: info@upf.com
Web site: http://www.upf.com
Dist(s): **netLibrary CO** *(netLibrary, Inc.); CIP.*

U Rchstr Med & Dntstry, *(Univ. of Rochester, Schl. of Medicine & Dentistry; 1-892273),* 1000 S. Ave., Rochester, NY 14620 Tel 716-275-4310; Fax: 716-244-9562.

U Scranton Pr, *(Univ. of Scranton Pr.; 0-940866; 1-58966),* Orders Addr.: c/o Univ. of Scranton Pr., St. Thomas Hall, Linden & Monroe Sts., Scranton, PA 18510 (SAN 281-2959) Toll Free Fax: 800-941-8804; Toll Free: 800-941-3081; Edit Addr.: Linden & Monroe Sts., Scranton, PA 18510 (SAN 688-4067) Tel 570-941-7955; Fax: 570-941-4309
E-mail: sinclairj2@uofs.edu
Web site: http://www.scrantonpress.com
Dist(s): **Assoc Univ Prs** *(Associated Univ. Presses)*
U of Toronto Pr *(Univ. of Toronto Pr.).*

U TX MB Microb, *(Univ. of Texas Medical Branch, Dept. of Microbiology; 0-9631172),* Rte. J19, Galveston, TX 77550 Tel 409-772-4923; Fax: 409-772-5065; 11th St. & Mechanic Ave., Galveston, TX 77555-1019
E-mail: sabaron@utmb.edu
Web site: http://gsbs.utmb.edu/microbook.

U WI Clearinghse, *(Univ. of Wisconsin-Madison, Wisconsin Clearinghouse; 1-882145),* 1552 University Ave., Madison, WI 53705 Tel 608-263-2797; Fax: 608-262-6346; Toll Free: 800-322-1468
E-mail: klglunz@facstaff.wisc.edu
Web site: http://www.uhs.wisc.edu/wch.

U Wis Sch Lib, *(Univ. of Wisconsin-Madison, Schl. of Library & Information Studies; 0-936442),* 600 N. Park St., Madison, WI 53706 (SAN 219-9874) Tel 608-263-2900; Fax: 608-263-4849
E-mail: uw-slis@slis.wisc.edu
Web site: http://www.slis.wisc.edu.

†**UAHC,** *(UAHC Pr.; 0-8074),* 633 Third Ave., New York, NY 10017 (SAN 203-3291) Tel 212-650-4121; Fax: 212-650-4119; Toll Free: 888-489-8242
E-mail: rabrams@uahc.org; press@uahc.org
Web site: http://www.uahcpress.com; *CIP.*

UASM, *(Univ. of Alabama, Schl. of Medicine; 0-9621672),* 301 MEB, Birmingham, AL 35294 (SAN 251-8783) Tel 205-934-4807
Web site: http://main.uab.edu/uasom/new/.

UBC Pr, *(Univ. of British Columbia Pr.; 0-7748; 0-88865),* Orders Addr.: Univ. of WA Pr., Box 50096, Seattle, WA 98145-5096 Toll Free: 800-441-4115 (trade orders & returns only)
E-mail: custserv@raincoast.com; info@ubcpress.ubc.ca
Web site: http://www.ubcpress.ubc.ca/
Dist(s): **U of Wash Pr** *(Univ. of Washington Pr.).*

UBS Pubs (IND) *(81-7476; 81-85273; 81-85674; 81-85944; 81-86112; 81-87374) Dist. by* **S Asia.**

UC Ctr UR&PS, *(Univ. of Chicago, Ctr. for Urban Research & Policy Studies; 0-9626755),* 1155 E. 60th St., Chicago, IL 60637 Tel 773-702-0081
Dist(s): **U of Ill Pr** *(Univ. of Illinois Pr.).*

UCL Pr Ltd (GBR) *(1-85728; 1-84142; 0-203) Dist. by* **Taylor & Francis.**

UCLA Lat Am Ctr, *(Univ. of California, Latin American Ctr.; 0-87903),* 10353 Bunche Hall, Box 951447, Los Angeles, CA 90095-1447 (SAN 201-0704) Tel 310-825-6634; Fax: 310-206-6859
E-mail: latinamctr@isop.ucla.edu
Web site: http://www.isop.ucla.edu/lac.

UCLA Tissue, *(UCLA Tissue Typing Laboratory; 0-9604606; 1-880318),* 1000 Veteran Ave., Los Angeles, CA 90095-1652 (SAN 282-4752) Tel 310-825-7651; Fax: 310-206-3216.

UCSF Schl Nursing, *(Univ. of California, San Francisco, Schl. of Nursing; 0-943671),* Orders Addr.: P.O. Box 0608, San Francisco, CA 94143-0608 (SAN 242-3596) Tel 415-476-4992; Fax: 415-476-6042; Edit Addr.: 521 Parnassus Ave., Rm. N535C, San Francisco, CA 94143-0608 (SAN 242-360X)
Web site: http://www.nurseweb.ucsf.edu/www/books.htm.

†**UH Pr,** *(Univ. of Hawaii Pr.; 0-8248; 0-87022),* Orders Addr.: 2840 Kolowalu St., Honolulu, HI 96822-1888 (SAN 202-5353) Tel 808-956-8255; Fax: 808-988-6052 ; *Imprints:* Latitude Twenty (Latitude Twenty Book)
E-mail: uhpmkt@hawaii.edu; uhpbooks@hawaii.edu
Web site: http://www.uhpress.hawaii.edu; *CIP.*

UI Pub, *(UI Publishing; 0-9627157),* Div. of Upledger Institute, 11211 Prosperity Farms Rd., Palm Beach Gardens, FL 33410 Tel 561-622-4334; Fax: 561-622-4771; Toll Free: 800-233-5880
E-mail: upledger@upledger.com.

Ulverscroft US, *(Ulverscroft Large Print Bks., Ltd.; 0-7089),* Orders Addr.: P.O. Box 1230, West Seneca, NY 14224-1230; Edit Addr.: 1881 Ridge Rd., West Seneca, NY 14224-1230 (SAN 208-3035) Tel 716-674-4270; Fax: 716-674-4195; Toll Free: 800-955-9659
E-mail: g.haddon@ulverscroft.co.uk
Web site: http://www.ulverscroft.co.uk.

Ulysses Pr, *(Ulysses Pr.; 0-915233; 1-56975),* Orders Addr.: P.O. Box 3440, Berkeley, CA 94703-3440 (SAN 289-8764) Tel 510-601-8301; Fax: 510-601-8307; Toll Free: 800-377-2542; Edit Addr.: 3286 Adeline St., Suite 1, Berkeley, CA 94703 (SAN 289-8772)
E-mail: ulysses@ulyssespress.com
Web site: http://www.ulyssespress.com
Dist(s): **Publishers Group** *(Publishers Group West).*

Ulyssian Pubns Imprint of Pine Orchard

UM CHGD, *(Univ. of Michigan, Ctr. for Human Growth & Development; 0-929921),* 300 N. Ingalls, Ann Arbor, MI 48109-0406 (SAN 250-104X) Tel 734-647-1111; Fax: 734-936-9288
E-mail: needhamp@izzy.net; cgs_editorial@umich.edu
Web site: http://www.needhampress.com
Dist(s): **Needham Pr** *(Needham Pr., Inc.).*

Umea U Bibl (SWE) *(91-7174) Dist. by* **Coronet Bks.**

UMI Schl Dentsy, *(Univ. of Michigan, Schl. of Dentistry, Office of Continuing Dental Education; 0-9645852),* 1011 N. University, Rm. 1205, Ann Arbor, MI 48109-1078 Tel 313-763-5070; Fax: 313-936-3065.

UN, *(United Nations Pubns.; 0-680; 0-89714; 92-1; 92-808; 952-9520),* 2 United Nations Plaza, Sales Section, Publishing Div., Rm. DC2-853, New York, NY 10017 (SAN 206-6718) Tel 212-963-7680 UN Bookshop; 212-963-8302; Fax: 212-963-4910 UN Bookshop; 212-963-3489; Toll Free: 800-553-3210 UN Bookshop; 800-253-9646 (bookshop orders)
E-mail: publications@un.org
Web site: http://www.un.org/pubs
Dist(s): **Balogh** *(Balogh International, Inc.)*
Bernan Associates *(Bernan Assocs.).*

Unarius Acad Sci, *(Unarius Academy of Science Pubns.; 0-932642; 0-935097),* 145 S. Magnolia Ave., El Cajon, CA 92020-4522 (SAN 168-9614) Tel 619-444-7062; Fax: 619-444-9637; Toll Free: 800-475-7062
E-mail: uriel@unarius.org
Web site: http://www.unarius.org.

Uncharted Ctry Pub, *(Uncharted Country Publishing; 1-877950),* 408 South Baldwin St., Madison, WI 53703-4805 Tel 608-280-9730; Fax: 608-280-9736; Toll Free: 800-488-4940
E-mail: ucp@taichihealth.com
Web site: http://www.taichihealth.com
Dist(s): **Rom Dance Ntwrk** *(Rom Dance Network).*

Undena Pubns, *(Undena Pubns.; 0-89003),* Orders Addr.: 3064 Holline Ct., Lancaster, CA 93535-4910 Tel 661-946-2726 (phone/fax).

Undersea & Hyperbaric, *(Undersea & Hyperbaric Medical Society; 0-930406),* 10531 Metropolitan Ave., Kensington, MD 20895 (SAN 224-4764) Tel 301-942-2980; Fax: 301-942-7804
E-mail: ann@uhms.org
Web site: http://www.uhms.org.

Undersea Med, *See* **Undersea & Hyperbaric**

Underwood Bks, *(Underwood Bks., Inc.; 0-88733; 0-934438; 1-887424),* P.O. Box 1609, Grass Valley, CA 95945 Tel 530-274-7997; Fax: 530-274-7179
Dist(s): **Publishers Group** *(Publishers Group West).*

Underwrtrs Labs, *(Underwriters Laboratories, Inc.; 0-7629; 1-55989),* 333 Pfingsten Rd., Northbrook, IL 60062-2096 Tel 847-272-8800 ext. 43950; Toll Free: 800-854-7179
Web site: http://www.ul.com.

Unicor Medical, *(Unicor Medical, Inc.; 1-56781),* 4160 Carmichael Rd., Suite 102, Montgomery, AL 36106 Tel 334-260-8150; Fax: 334-272-1046; Toll Free Fax: 800-305-8030; Toll Free: 800-825-7421
E-mail: sales@unicormed.com
Web site: http://www.unicormed.com.

UNIPress, *(UNIPress; 0-940480),* Div. of God Unlimited/University of Healing, 1101 Far Valley Rd., Campo, CA 91906-3213 (SAN 211-7983) Tel 619-478-5111; Fax: 619-478-5013; Toll Free Fax: 888-499-8545; Toll Free: 888-463-8654 Do not confuse with Unipress, Bellevue, WA
E-mail: godellen@mei.ws; unihealing@fda.net
Web site: http://www.university-of-healing.edu.

UniPsych Pr, *(UniPsych Pr.; 1-883945),* Div. of Bradman Consulting Services, Inc., 7777 Davie Rd., Ext. 302, Hollywood, FL 33024-2515 Toll Free: 800-272-3626.

UNIPUB, *See* **Bernan Associates**

Unique Pubns, *(Unique Pubns.; 0-86568; 1-892515),* Subs. of CFW Enterprises, Inc., 4201 Vanowen Pl., Burbank, CA 91505 (SAN 214-3313) Tel 818-845-2656; Fax: 818-845-7761; Toll Free Fax: 800-249-7761; Toll Free: 800-332-3330.

UniStar Pubng, *(UniStar Publishing, Inc.; 1-885854),* Orders Addr.: P.O. Box 27740, Las Vegas, NV 89126; Edit Addr.: 3132 W. Post Rd., Las Vegas, NV 89118 Fax: 805-823-7535
Dist(s): **Desert News Co** *(Desert News Co.).*

†**Unitarian Univ,** *(Unitarian Universalist Assn.; 0-933840; 1-55896),* 25 Beacon St., Boston, MA 02108-2800 (SAN 225-4840) Tel 617-742-2100; Fax: 617-742-7025; Toll Free: 800-215-9076
Web site: http://www.uua.org; *CIP.*

United Cereb Palsy, *(United Cerebral Palsy Assn. of California, Inc.; 0-9632338),* Div. of United Cerebral Palsy Assn., Inc., 3 Buena Vista, Carmel Valley, CA 93924 Tel 408-659-0382 Do not confuse with companies with similar names in New York, NY, Petaluma, CA.

†**United Hosp Fund,** *(United Hospital Fund; 0-934459; 1-881277),* 350 Fifth Ave., 23rd Flr., New York, NY 10118-2399 (SAN 206-1473) Tel 212-494-0700; Fax: 212-494-0823
Web site: http://www.uhfnyc.org; *CIP.*

United Network, *(United Network for Organ Sharing; 1-886651),* Orders Addr.: P.O. Box 13770, Richmond, VA 23225-8770 Tel 804-330-8500; Fax: 804-330-8593; Edit Addr.: 1100 Boulders Pkwy., Suite 500, Richmond, VA 23225-8770
Web site: http://www.unos.org.

United Path Pr, *(United Pathologists Pr.; 1-893941),* 1142 Audaz Ln., SW, Rochester, MN 55902 Fax: 507-292-0231; Toll Free: 800-214-6628
E-mail: bostwick@millcomm.com.

United Prof Pubns, *(United Professional Pubns.; 0-944375),* Orders Addr.: P.O. Box 1126, Redlands, CA 92373 (SAN 243-4385); Edit Addr.: 201 Brookside Ave., Redlands, CA 92373 (SAN 243-4393) Tel 714-793-0822.

United Res CA, *(United Research Publishers; 0-9614924; 1-887053),* Div. of Solor Products, Inc., 2816 Atadero Ct., Carlsbad, CA 92009-9201 (SAN 693-5834) Tel 760-930-8937; Fax: 760-930-4291 Do not confuse with United Research, Black Mountain, NC
Web site: http://www.unitedresearchpubs.com.

United Sr Hlth Co-op, *(United Seniors Health Cooperative; 0-944847),* 409 Third St., SW, No. 200, Washington, DC 20024-3212 (SAN 245-4106) Tel 202-479-6973; Fax: 202-479-6660; Toll Free: 800-637-2604
Web site: http://www.ushc-online.org.

United Way SD, *(United Way of San Diego County; 0-9629793),* Orders Addr.: P.O. Box 881307, San Diego, CA 92168 Tel 619-531-4799; Fax: 619-531-4801; Edit Addr.: 7947 Mission Ctr. Ct.,, San Diego, CA 92108.

Univ AZ Surg, *(University of Arizona, Surgery, Lymphology; 0-9711731),* Orders Addr.: P.O. Box 245063, Tucson, AZ 85724 Tel 520-626-6118; Fax: 520-626-0822; Edit Addr.: 1501 N. Campbell Ave., Rm. 4406, Tucson, AZ 85724
E-mail: lymph@u.arizona.edu.

Univ CT Hlth, *(Univ. of Connecticut Health Ctr.; 1-891509),* 263 Farmington Ave., MC 5215, Farmington, CT 06030 Tel 860-679-3956; Fax: 860-679-1307.

Univ Edtns Imprint of Aegina Pr

Univ Exeter Pr (GBR) *(0-85989; 0-900771; 0-902414; 0-9501308) Dist. by* **David Brown.**

†**Univ Fla Food,** *(Univ. of Florida, Institute of Food & Agricultural Sciences; 0-916287),* P.O. Box 110810, Gainesville, FL 32611-0810 (SAN 295-6055) Tel 352-392-2411; Fax: 352-392-7902; *CIP.*

Univ Florida Lib, *(Univ. of Florida, Libraries; 0-929595),* U of Fla., Libraries West, Gainesville, FL 32611 (SAN 287-7104) Tel 904-392-0345.

Univ Health Ctr, *(Univ. of Oklahoma Health/Science Ctr., Dept. of Family Medicine; 0-9617230; 1-931528),* Orders Addr.: P.O. Box 26901, Oklahoma City, OK 73104 (SAN 663-6322) Tel 405-271-8000 (ext. 32211); Fax: 405-271-2784; Edit Addr.: 900 NE Tenth St., Oklahoma City, OK 73104
E-mail: howard-stein@ouhsc.edu
Dist(s): **Soc Tchrs Fam Med** *(Society of Teachers of Family Medicine).*

Univ KY Vet Sci, *(Univ. of Kentucky, Dept. of Veterinary Science; 0-9626367),* 108 Gluck Equine Research Ctr., Lexington, KY 40546 Tel 606-257-3765; Fax: 606-323-1059.

Univ LA Lafayette, *(Univ. of Louisiana at Lafayette, Ctr. for Louisiana Studies; 0-940984; 1-887366),* P.O. Box 40831, Lafayette, LA 70504 (SAN 630-9755) Tel 337-482-6027; Fax: 337-482-6028
E-mail: labiche@louisiana.edu
Web site: http://www.louisiana.edu.

Univ Med Pr, *(Universal Medical Pr., Inc.; 0-9643425; 1-890131),* 18127 E. Hwy. 26, Linden, CA 95236-9710
E-mail: info@ump.com
Web site: http://www.ump.com.

†**Univ Microfilms,** *(University Microfilms, Inc.; 0-608; 0-7837; 0-8357),* Div. of Bell & Howell, Orders Addr.: P.O. Box 1307, Ann Arbor, MI 48106 (SAN 241-8797); Edit Addr.: 300 N. Zeeb Rd., Ann Arbor, MI 48106 (SAN 212-2464) Tel 313-761-4700; Fax: 313-665-5022; Toll Free: 800-521-0600; 800-343-5299 (in Canada)
Web site: http://www.umi.com; *CIP.*

Univ Mus of U PA, *See* **U Museum Pubns**

Univ Natal Pr (ZAF) *(0-86980; 0-620) Dist. by* **Intl Spec Bk.**

Univ Nottingham (GBR) *(0-85358; 0-900572) Dist. by* **St Mut.**

Univ of New Mexico Schl, *(Univ. of New Mexico, Schl. of Medicine, Biomedical Communications),* Orders Addr.: c/o Health Science Ctr., P.O. Box 719, Albuquerque, NM 87131 Tel 505-277-3633.

Univ of West Aust Pr (AUS) *(0-85564; 0-86422; 0-909751; 1-875560; 1-876268) Dist. by* **Intl Spec Bk.**

Univ OK Archeol, *(Univ. of Oklahoma, Oklahoma Archeological Survey; 1-881346),* Orders Addr.: 111 E. Chesapeake St., Norman, OK 73019-5111 Tel 405-325-7211; Fax: 405-325-7604; Toll Free: 800-523-7363 (ext. 7211)
E-mail: lealbert@ou.edu.

Univ Otago Pr (NZL) *(0-908569; 1-877133; 1-877276) Dist. by* **Intl Spec Bk.**

Univ Pr, *(Universal Pr.; 0-9631966),* P.O. Box 92, Big Flat, AR 72617-0092.

Univ Pr CA, *(Univ. Pr., California; 0-9700733; 0-9716445),* 677 Elm St., San Jose, CA 95126 Do not confuse with companies with the same name in Hudson, WI, Flushing, NY, San Francisco, CA, Missoula, MT, Wolf City, TX
E-mail: Brain-Mind@Brain-Mind.com
Web site: http://www.brain-mind.com.

Univ Pr Colo, *(University Pr. of Colorado; 0-87081),* Orders Addr.: c/o Univ. Press of Colorado, 4100 28th Ave., NW, Norman, OK 73069-8218 Toll Free Fax: 800-735-0476; Toll Free: 800-627-7377; Edit Addr.: 5589 Arapahoe Ave., No. 206C, Boulder, CO 80303 (SAN 658-0343) Tel 720-406-8849
Web site:
http://bcn.boulder.co.us/capuspress/presshome.html
Dist(s): **U of Okla Pr** *(Univ. of Oklahoma Pr.).*

Univ Pub Group, *(University Publishing Group, Inc.; 1-55572),* Orders Addr.: 17100 Cole Rd., Suite 312, Hagerstown, MD 21740 (SAN 699-7171) Tel 301-582-2200; Fax: 301-582-2406; Toll Free: 800-654-8188
E-mail: orders@upgbooks.com; editorial@upgbooks.com
Web site: http://www.upgbooks.com.

Univ Publng Hse, *(University Publishing Hse., Inc.; 1-57002; 1-877767),* P.O. Box 1664, Mannford, OK 74044-1664 Tel 918-865-4726 (phone/fax)
E-mail: upub@juno.com.

Univ Queensland Pr (AUS) *(0-7022) Dist. by* **Intl Spec Bk.**

Univ Rochester Pr, *(Univ. of Rochester Pr.; 1-58046; 1-878822),* Div. of Boydell & Brewer, Inc., P.O. Box 41026, Rochester, NY 14604-4126 Tel 716-275-0419; Fax: 716-271-8778
E-mail: urpress@mail.rochester.edu; 104572.1422@compuserve.com
Web site: http://www.boydell.co.uk
Dist(s): **Boydell & Brewer** *(Boydell & Brewer, Inc.).*

Univ SC Inst Pub Affairs, *(Univ. of South Carolina, Institute of Public Affairs; 0-917069),* Carolina Plaza, Univ. of SC, Columbia, SC 29208 (SAN 655-4849) Tel 803-777-8156; Fax: 803-777-4575
E-mail: dobson@iopa.sc.edu.

Univ Sci Bks, *(University Science Bks.; 0-935702; 1-891389),* Orders Addr.: c/o Books International, 22841 Quicksilver Dr., Dulles, VA 20166 Tel 703-661-1572; Fax: 703-661-1501; Edit Addr.: 55D Gate Five Rd., Sausalito, CA 94965 (SAN 213-8085) Tel 415-332-5390; Fax: 415-332-5393; 648 Broadway, Suite 902, New York, NY 10012 Tel 212-253-1367; Fax: 212-253-1419
E-mail: univscibks@igc.org; bjellis@igc.org
Web site: http://www.uscibooks.com.

Univ Sci Publns, *(Universal Scientific Pubns. Co., Inc., The; 0-88078),* P.O. Box 4307, Orange, CA 92613 (SAN 220-309X) Tel 213-723-1776.

Univ Scripts, *(University Scripts; 0-9642134),* 1953 Boulder Dr., Ann Arbor, MI 48104-4165 Tel 734-973-6682.

Univ South ME, *(Univ. of Southern Maine; 0-939561),* P.O. Box 9300, Portland, ME 04103 (SAN 663-4281) Tel 207-780-4094; Fax: 207-780-4860; Toll Free: 800-800-4876.

Univ Tampa, *(Univ. of Tampa; 1-879852),* 401 W. Kennedy Blvd., Tampa, FL 33606 Tel 813-253-6266; Fax: 813-258-7593
E-mail: utpress@alpha.utampa.edu
Web site: http://www.utpress.utampa.edu.

Univ TX Med Humanities, *(Univ. of Texas Medical Branch, Institute for the Medical Humanities; 0-9621294),* 301 University Blvd., Galveston, TX 77555-1311 (SAN 250-9482) Tel 409-772-2376.

Univ UT Sch Med, *(Univ. of Utah, Schl. of Medicine; 0-940193),* Dept. of Family & Preventive Medicine, 50 N. Medical Dr., Salt Lake City, UT 84132 (SAN 664-3213) Tel 801-581-7234.

**Univelt Inc, *(Univelt, Inc.; 0-87703; 0-912183),* Orders Addr.: P.O. Box 28130, San Diego, CA 92198-0130 (SAN 170-3099) Tel 760-746-4005; Fax: 760-746-3139; Edit Addr.: 740 Metcalf St., Suite 13, Escondido, CA 92025-1671 (SAN 658-2095) ; *Imprints:* Am Astronaut Soc (American Astronautical Society)
E-mail: 76121.1532@compuserve.com
Web site: http://univelt.staigerland.com.**

Universal Res MA, *(Universal Research; 0-942951),* 539 E. Bixby Rd., Suite 144, Long Beach, CA 90807 (SAN 668-6524) Tel 213-694-2233; Fax: 310-632-4406.

Universe, *(Universe Publishing; 0-7893; 0-87663; 1-55550),* Div. of Rizzoli International Pubns., Inc., 300 Park Ave. S., 3rd Flr., New York, NY 10010 (SAN 202-537X) Tel 212-387-3400; Fax: 212-387-3535 Do not confuse with similar names in North Hollywood, CA, Englewood, NJ, Mendocino, CA
Dist(s): **Andrews McMeel** *(Andrews McMeel Publishing)*
St Martin *(St. Martin's Pr., LLC)*
VHPS *(VHPS Holtzbrinck Pubs.).*

Universe Pub Co, *(Universe Publishing Co.; 0-935484),* 185 Demarest Ave., Englewood, NJ 07631 (SAN 214-3321) Tel 201-567-4296; Fax: 201-567-6488 Do not confuse with similar names in North Hollywood, CA, New York, NY, Mendocino, CA
Web site: http://www.erdelyonline.com.

Univrsl Pubng, *(Universal Publishing Co.; 1-885917),* P.O. Box 15424, Newport Beach, CA 92659 Tel 714-723-5748.

Univs Fed Animal Welfare (GBR) *(0-900767; 1-900630) Dist. by* **St Mut.**

Unoffic Guide Imprint of Hungry Minds

Untd Bros & Sis, *See* **Khalifahs Booksellers**

UNTX Pr, *(Univ. of North Texas Pr.; 0-929398; 1-57441),* Orders Addr.: 4354 Tamus, College Station, TX 77843-4354 (SAN 249-4299) Fax: 888-617-2421; Toll Free: 800-826-8911 (orders only); Edit Addr.: P.O. Box 311336, Denton, TX 76203 (SAN 249-4280) Tel 940-565-2142; Fax: 940-565-4590
E-mail: kdevinney@unt.edu; poates@unt.edu; rchrisman@unt.edu
Web site: http://www.unt.edu/untpress
Dist(s): **Tex A&M Univ Pr** *(Texas A&M Univ. Pr.).*

Upper Room Bks, *(Upper Room Bks.; 0-8358),* Div. of The Upper Room, 1908 Grand Ave., Nashville, TN 37212 (SAN 203-3364) Tel 615-340-7256; Fax: 615-340-7266; Toll Free: 800-972-0433 (customer service, orders); 1650 Bluegrass Lakes Pkwy., Alphretta, GA 30201 Do not confuse with Upper Room Education for Parenting, Inc. in Derry, NH
E-mail: kwatts@upperroom.org
Web site: http://www.upperroom.org.

Uppsala Universitet (SWE) *(91-506; 91-554) Dist. by* **Coronet Bks.**

Upshur Pr, *(Upshur Pr.; 0-912975),* 216 E. Battle Ave., Tarboro, NC 27886-3010 (SAN 297-4762) Tel 919-823-3340
E-mail: istallone@ncwc.edu
Dist(s): **Baker & Taylor** *(Baker & Taylor Bks.)*
Koen Bk Distributors *(Koen Bk. Distributors).*

Upstream Pr TX, *(Upstream Pr.; 0-9701058),* P.O. Box 1128, Glen Rose, TX 76043 Fax: 254-897-7047; Toll Free: 877-401-9100 Do not confuse with Upstream Press, Hope, RI
E-mail: info@upstreampress.com
Web site: http://www.upstreampress.com.

Uptime Sprts Nutrit, *(Uptime Sports Nutrition/Medical Industries; 0-9656924),* Orders Addr.: P.O. Box 90659, Santa Barbara, CA 93190-0659 Tel 805-564-3494; Fax: 805-564-4879; Toll Free: 800-441-5656; Edit Addr.: 310 E. Haley St., Santa Barbara, CA 93101
E-mail: Uptime@up-time.com
Web site: http://www.up-time.com.

Upton Bks Imprint of SIRS Pubng

Urban & Schwarz (AUT) *(3-541; 3-85327) Dist. by* **IBD Ltd.**

†**Urban Inst,** *(Urban Institute Pr.; 0-87766),* 2100 M St., NW, Washington, DC 20037 (SAN 203-3380) Tel 202-261-5687; Fax: 202-467-5775; Toll Free: 877-847-7377
E-mail: pubs@ui.urban.org
Web site: http://www.uipress.org; *CIP.*

URSA Cos, *See* **Ursa Pub Co Inc**

Ursa Pub Co Inc, *(Ursa Publishing Co., Inc.; 1-893808),* 8707 Short Hill Rd., Suite A, Rome, NY 13440 Tel 315-338-9858; Fax: 315-338-0834
E-mail: Ursa2000@aol.com.

US Catholic, *See* **US States Conference**

†**US HHS,** *(U.S. Dept. of Health & Human Services; 1-55672),* Office of Minority Health 5515 Security Ln., Rockwall 2 Bldg. Suite 1000, 10th Flr., Rockville, MD 20857 (SAN 663-4346) Tel 301-443-5084; *CIP.*

US Pharmacopeia, *(United States Pharmacopeia; 0-913595; 1-889788),* Div. of Information Technology, 12601 Twinbrook Pkwy., Rockville, MD 20852 (SAN 220-2794) Tel 301-881-0666; Fax: 301-816-8301; Toll Free: 800-877-6733
Web site: http://www.usp.org.

US Pub FL, *(United States Publishing; 1-880698),* Box 504, Captain Cook, HI 96704 Tel 808-328-8283; Fax: 808-328-8289
Dist(s): **Bookpeople** *(Bookpeople)*
New Leaf Dist *(New Leaf Distributing Co., Inc.).*

US States Conference, *(United States Conference of Catholic Bishops; 1-55586; 1-57455),* 3211 Fourth St., NE, Washington, DC 20017-1194 (SAN 207-5350) Tel 202-541-3090; Fax: 202-541-3089; Toll Free: 800-235-8722
Web site: http://www.usccb.org.

Usborne Imprint of EDC Pubng

USC Biomedical, *(Univ. of Southern California, Biomedical Simulations Resource; 0-941639),* c/o Biomedical Simulations Resource, Schl. of Engineering, OHE 500, Los Angeles, CA 90089-1451 (SAN 666-1726) Tel 213-740-0342; Fax: 213-740-0343
E-mail: marcos@bmsrs.usc.edu
Web site: http://www.usc.edu/dept/biomed/BMSR.

USF SGC, *(Univ. of South Florida, Suncoast Gerontology Ctr.; 0-9622070),* MDC 50, 12901 Bruce B. Downs Blvd., Tampa, FL 33612 Tel 813-974-4355; Fax: 813-974-4251
E-mail: jpaul@comf.med.usf.edu
Web site: http://www.med.usf.edu/suncoast/alzheimer/.

USFI, *(USFI; 0-9643211),* 1801 Royal Ln., Suite 810, Dallas, TX 75229-3169 Tel 972-444-8381; Fax: 972-402-8139; Toll Free: 800-422-2898
E-mail: tarrington@usfi-dallas.com.

†**USGPO,** *(U.S. Government Printing Office; 0-16; 0-18),* Orders Addr.: P.O. Box 371954, Pittsburgh, PA 15250-7954 (SAN 658-0785) Tel 202-512-1800; Fax: 202-512-2250; Toll Free: 866-512-1800; Edit Addr.: USGPO Stop SSMB, Washington, DC 20401 (SAN 206-152X) Tel 202-512-1705 (bibliographic information only); 202-512-2268 (book dealers only); Fax: 202-512-1655 ; *Imprints:* Hlth & Human (Health and Human Services Department) Labor Dept (Labor Department)
E-mail: rdavis@gpo.gov; orders@gpo.gov
Web site: http://bookstore.gpo.gov; http://www.access.gpo.gov/su_docs
Dist(s): **Bernan Associates** *(Bernan Assocs.); CIP.*

USPC, *See* **US Pharmacopeia**

UWI IRE, *(Univ. of Wisconsin System, Institute on Race & Ethnicity; 0-942672),* c/o University of Wisconsin, P.O. Box 413, Milwaukee, WI 53201 Tel 414-229-6701; Fax: 414-229-4581
Web site: http://www.uwm.edu/Dept/IRE.

UXL Imprint of Gale

V A Brody, *(Brody, Viola A.; 0-9646232),* 519 Plaza Seville Ct., No. 38, Treasure Island, FL 33706 Tel 813-360-2062; Fax: 813-360-7174.

V Frankl Inst, *(Frankl, Viktor Institute of Logotherapy; 0-917867),* Div. of Institute of Logotherapy, P.O. Box 15211, Albilene, TX 79698-5211 (SAN 657-095X) Tel 915-692-9597; Fax: 915-677-8351.

V Gollancz (GBR) *(0-575) Dist. by* **Trafalgar.**

V Gollancz (GBR) *(0-575) Dist. by* **Sterling.**

V H A, *(VHA, Inc.; 0-9629192),* 200 Berwyn Pk., Suite 202, Berwyn, PA 19312 Tel 610-296-2558; Fax: 610-296-8850 Do not confuse with VHA, Inc., Irving, TX
Web site: http://www.vha.com.

†**V Mason Clinic,** *(Mason, Virginia Clinic; 0-9601944),* 1015 Seneca St., Seattle, WA 98111 (SAN 213-8972)
Web site: http://www.vmmc.org; *CIP.*

V W I Corp, *See* **Avid Reader**

V Young, *(Young, Victor A.; 0-9603694),* 548 S. Main St., Red Lion, PA 17356 (SAN 213-5736) Tel 717-244-6816.

Vac Wrk Pubns (GBR) *(0-907638; 1-85458; 0-901205) Dist. by* **Petersons.**

Vadare, *(Vadare Publishing Co.; 0-933725; 0-9610782),* 4 Burnham Ln., Dix Hills, NY 11746 (SAN 265-1491) Tel 516-581-4422; Toll Free: 800-645-1112.

Valaske Pub, *(Valaske Publishing; 0-9616601),* 24065 Squires Rd., Columbia Station, OH 44028-9637 (SAN 659-5448).

Valdenmar, *(Valdenmar Publishing; 0-9632105),* 9812 W. 121st Terr., Overland Park, KS 66213 Tel 913-897-2768.

Valentine & Assocs, *(Valentine & Assocs.; 0-9638351),* 22647 Ventura Blvd., Suite 197, Woodland Hills, CA 91367 Tel 818-704-6735.

Valentine Commun, *(Valentine Communications Corp.; 0-9648325),* Orders Addr.: P.O. Box 11089, Naples, FL 33941 Tel 941-353-9688; Fax: 941-353-2365; Edit Addr.: 2900 14th St. N., Suite 12, Naples, FL 33940.

Valhalla Rehab, *(Valhalla Rehabilitation Pubns., Ltd.; 0-911681),* 21 Roosevelt Dr., Valhalla, NY 10595 (SAN 262-1053) Tel 914-948-1004.

Validated Biosysts, *(Validated Biosystems, Inc.; 0-9653515),* 5751 N. Kolb Rd., Suite 25203, Tucson, AZ 85750 Tel 520-299-7786; Fax: 520-299-8218
E-mail: info@validated.com
Web site: http://www.validated.com
Dist(s): **BookMasters** *(BookMasters, Inc.).*

Valkyrie Pub Hse, *(Valkyrie Publishing Hse.; 0-912589; 0-912760; 0-934616),* 8245 26th Ave., N., Saint Petersburg, FL 33710 (SAN 203-1671) Tel 727-345-8864
Dist(s): **Baker & Taylor** *(Baker & Taylor Bks.)*
Brodart *(Brodart Co.).*

Valley Hill Pub, *(Valley Hill Publishing Co.; 0-9619238),* Orders Addr.: P.O. Box 5021, Lakeland, FL 33807 (SAN 243-525X); Edit Addr.: 1210 Valley Hill, W., Lakeland, FL 33807 (SAN 243-5268) Tel 941-646-0165; Fax: 941-648-3573
E-mail: hartman.r@popmail.firn.edu.

Valley Pr IN, *(Valley Pr.; 0-927935),* P.O. Box 14134, Bradenton, FL 34280-4134 Do not confuse with companies with the same name in Porterville, CA, Lyndhurst, NJ, Green Bay, WI, Mill Valley, CA
Dist(s): **Act Prod Intl** *(Activity Products International)*
Baker & Taylor *(Baker & Taylor Bks.)*
Goldn Horiz *(Golden Horizons, Inc.)*
Incent Lrning *(Incentives For Learning)*
Nasco Math *(Nasco Math Eighty-Six)*
Potentials Development *(Potentials Development, Inc.)*
Prof Prnting & Pub *(Professional Printing & Publishing)*
S & S Worldwide *(S & S Worldwide).*

Valley Presbyterian, *(Valley Presbyterian Hospital; 0-9605718),* Orders Addr.: P.O. Box 9102, Van Nuys, CA 91409-9102 (SAN 216-4701); Edit Addr.: 15107 Vanowen St., Van Nuys, CA 91405 (SAN 251-2629) Tel 818-902-2973.

†**Valley Publishing,** *(Valley Publishing; 0-9612990),* 333 Michigan Dr., Lower Burrell, PA 15068 (SAN 292-7209) Tel 412-337-0635 Do not confuse with companies with same or similar names in Richmond, VA, Paradise Valley, AZ, Sheffield, PA; *CIP.*

Value Quest Grp, *(Value Quest Group, Inc.; 0-9632949),* Div. of Edward Walter Assocs., 10841 Bill Point Bluff, NE, Bainbridge Island, WA 98110-2105 Tel 206-842-4821.

Valverde Pubns, *(Valverde Pubns.; 0-9641088),* HC 70, Box 19Z, Pecos, NM 87552-9602.

Van der Kar Pr, *(Van der Kar Pr., The; 0-9645352),* Orders Addr.: P.O. Box 189, Malibu, CA 90265 Tel 310-457-6966; Fax: 310-457-2996; Edit Addr.: 27313 Old Chimney Rd., Malibu, CA 90265
E-mail: vanderkar@interline.net
Web site: http://www.vanderkar.com
Dist(s): **Baker & Taylor** *(Baker & Taylor Bks.)*
Bookpeople *(Bookpeople)*
Distributors *(Distributors, The)*
New Leaf Dist *(New Leaf Distributing Co., Inc.)*
Nutri-Books Corp *(Nutri-Bks. Corp.).*

Van Hoy Pubs, *(Van Hoy Pubs.; 1-886149),* P.O. Box 636, Greenville, PA 16125-0636 Tel 724-347-1580
E-mail: yasgur@juno.com
Web site: http://www.pathway.net/aardvark
Dist(s): **Baker & Taylor** *(Baker & Taylor Bks.)*
New Leaf Dist *(New Leaf Distributing Co., Inc.).*

Van Ness Pub, *(Van Ness Publishing; 0-9645713),* 1422 N. Allen, Mesa, AZ 85203 Tel 602-890-2170; Fax: 602-890-2182; Toll Free: 800-529-8836
E-mail: freedom1@extremezone.com
Web site:
http://www.bookzone.com/bookzone/10000378.html
Dist(s): **New Leaf Dist** *(New Leaf Distributing Co., Inc.)*
Partners Pubs Grp *(Partners Pubs. Group, Inc.).*

Van Slyke Bray, *(Van Slyke & Bray Pubs.; 0-9635435),* 4152-C Carmichael Rd., Montgomery, AL 36106 Tel 334-272-4445; Fax: 334-272-2464.

†**Van Vactor & Goodheart,** *(Van Vactor & Goodheart; 0-941324),* 24 Lee St., Cambridge, MA 02139 (SAN 282-5007) Tel 617-497-5277; Fax: 617-876-7232; *CIP.*

Van Valkenburgh, *(Van Valkenburgh, Paul; 0-9617425),* Orders Addr.: P.O. Box 3611, Seal Beach, CA 90740 (SAN 665-9527); Edit Addr.: 6903 Anaheim Rd., Long Beach, CA 90815 (SAN 663-9186) Tel 310-598-5378
E-mail: pvanvalken@aol.com
Web site: http://www.wryt.com.

Vandalay Pubs, *(Vandalay Pubs.; 0-9657467),* P.O. Box 847, Scottsdale, AZ 85252 Tel 310-379-0609; Fax: 310-374-8260; Toll Free: 800-247-6553; 800-345-0096 (orders)
E-mail: stephc@peoplepc.com
Dist(s): **BookMasters** *(BookMasters, Inc.)*
Quality Bks IL *(Quality Bks., Inc.).*

Vandamere, *(Vandamere Pr.; 0-918339),* Subs. of AB Assocs., P.O. Box 5243, Arlington, VA 22205 (SAN 657-3088) Tel 703-538-5750; Fax: 703-536-9644; Toll Free: 800-551-7776.

Vanderbilt Press, *(Vanderbilt Pr.; 0-9656686),* P.O. Box 2866, Huntington Station, NY 11746 (SAN 299-2639) Tel 516-499-1569; Fax: 516-499-0955; Toll Free: 800-714-1328
E-mail: Rabbit@mail.htp.com.

†**Vanderbilt U Pr,** *(Vanderbilt Univ. Pr.; 0-8265),* Div. of Vanderbilt Univ., VU Station B 351813 112 21st Ave., S., No. 201, Nashville, TN 37235 (SAN 202-9308) Tel 615-322-3585; Fax: 615-343-8823; Toll Free: 800-627-7377 (orders)
E-mail: vupress@vanderbilt.edu
Web site: http://www.vanderbilt.edu/VUPress
Dist(s): **U of Okla Pr** *(Univ. of Oklahoma Pr.); CIP.*

Vanderbilt Wilkerson, *(Vanderbilt Bill Wilkerson Ctr. Pr.; 0-9631439),* 1114 19th Ave., S., Nashville, TN 37212-2197 Tel 615-936-5000; Fax: 615-936-5013; Toll Free: 877-844-3840
E-mail: georgia.m.walker@vanderbilt.edu
Web site: http://www.vandervbilt.edu/billwilkersoncenter.

Vanessapress, *(Vanessapress; 0-940055),* P.O. Box 82761, Fairbanks, AK 99708-2761 (SAN 696-5040) Tel 907-452-5070
Web site:
http://www.mospuitonet.com/~inkworks/vanessa.html
Dist(s): **Alaska News Agency Inc** *(Alaska News Agency, Inc.)*
Todd Commns *(Todd Communications)*
Wizard Works *(Wizard Works).*

VanPress, *(VanPress; 0-942223),* Orders Addr.: P.O. Box 508, Ogden, UT 84401 (SAN 666-8801) Tel 801-393-1015; Edit Addr.: 1430 Boughton St., Ogden, UT 84403 (SAN 666-881X).

Vantage, ***(Vantage Pr., Inc.; 0-533),*** **516 W. 34th St., New York, NY 10001 (SAN 206-8893) Tel 212-736-1767; Fax: 212-736-2273; Toll Free: 800-882-3273**
Web site: http://www.vantagepress.com
Dist(s): **Dr Leisure *(Dr. Leisure).***

Vantage Info, *(Vantage Information; 0-914791),* 3516 Castlegate Wynd, Lexington, KY 40502-7701 (SAN 655-1459) Tel 859-266-9412.

Variorum (GBR) *(0-86078; 0-902089) Dist. by* **Ashgate Pub Co.**

Varsity Pubs, *See* **Pelizza & Assocs**

Vector Counsel, *(Vector Counseling Institute; 0-913596),* 1129 E. State St., Sedro-Woolley, WA 98284 (SAN 205-4752) Tel 360-856-2414.

Vedanta Ctr, *(Vedanta Ctr. Pubs.; 0-911564),* Div. of Vedanta Centre, Inc., 130 Beechwood St., Cohasset, MA 02025-2108 (SAN 206-7781) Tel 781-383-0940; Fax: 781-383-8237
E-mail: vcpublish@aol.com
Web site: http://anandaashrama.org/.

Vegetarian Resc, *(Vegetarian Resource Group, The; 0-931411),* P.O. Box 1463, Baltimore, MD 21203 (SAN 630-172X) Tel 410-366-8343; Fax: 410-366-8804
E-mail: vrg@vrg.org
Web site: http://www.vrg.org
Dist(s): **Bookpeople** *(Bookpeople)*
New Leaf Dist *(New Leaf Distributing Co., Inc.).*

Ventajas, *(Ventajas; 1-892380),* 6547 Sperryville Pike, Boston, VA 22713 Tel 540-825-5337; Fax: 540-825-9615
E-mail: services@socialworkinfo.com
Web site: http://www.socialworkinfo.com.

Venture NJ, *(Venture Publishing Co.; 0-9646611),* 28 Stone Fence Rd., Allendale, NJ 07401-1849 Tel 201-934-9676 Do not confuse with companies with similar names in Washington, DC, Andover, MA, State College, PA.

Venture Pub PA, *(Venture Publishing, Inc.; 0-910251; 1-892132),* 1999 Cato Ave., State College, PA 16801 (SAN 240-897X) Tel 814-234-4561; Fax: 814-234-1651 Do not confuse with companies with the same name in Andover, MA, Ho-Ho-Kus, NJ
E-mail: vpublish@venturepublish.com
Web site: http://www.venturepublish.com.

Veracruz Pubs, *(Veracruz Pubs.; 1-879219),* Orders Addr.: P.O. Box 5262, Tucson, AZ 85703 Tel 520-628-1135; Edit Addr.: 1531 N. Hualpai, Tucson, AZ 85745.

Verav Med, *(Verav Medical Pubs.; 0-9630864),* Div. of Univ. of Rochester, Dept. Obstetrics/Gynecology, 601 Elmwood Ave., Rochester, NY 14642-8668 Tel 716-275-1907.

Veritas Ed Pub, *(Veritas-Editor-Pub.; 0-9619117),* 557A Trigo St., San Juan, PR 00907 (SAN 243-167X) Tel 809-723-3183.

Veritas Pubns (IRL) *(1-85390) Dist. by* **Irish Bks Media.**

Veritas Pubns (IRL) *(1-85390) Dist. by* **St Mut.**

Vermilion (GBR) *(0-09; 0-7126; 0-85223) Dist. by* **Trafalgar.**

Vernal Equinox, *(Vernal Equinox Pr.; 0-942380),* P.O. Box 1175, Fairfax, CA 94978 (SAN 240-1762) Tel 415-258-9308
E-mail: perceval@gtcinternet.com.

Verrier Pub, *(Verrier Publishing; 0-9636480),* P.O. Box 208, Lafayette, CA 94549 Tel 925-284-5813; Fax: 925-284-4248
Web site: http://www.primalwound.com.

Verso, *(Verso; 0-86091; 0-902308; 1-85984),* 180 Varick St., New York, NY 10014-4606 Tel 212-807-9680; Fax: 212-807-9152; Toll Free: 800-233-4830
E-mail: versoinc@aol.com
Web site: http://www.versobooks.com
Dist(s): **Norton** *(Norton, W.W. & Co., Inc.).*

Very Healthy Ent, *(Very Healthy Enterprises, Inc.; 0-9615452),* Orders Addr.: P.O. Box 4728, Inglewood, CA 90309 (SAN 696-2254) Toll Free: 800-222-9932; Edit Addr.: 322 1/2 E. Beach, Inglewood, CA 90302 (SAN 242-0716) Tel 310-672-3269.

Vestibular, *(Vestibular Disorders Assn.; 0-9632611),* Orders Addr.: P.O. Box 4467, Portland, OR 97208-4467 Tel 503-229-7705; Fax: 503-229-8064; Toll Free: 800-837-8428
E-mail: veda@vestibular.org
Web site: http://www.vestibular.org.

Vet Lrn Syst, *(Veterinary Learning Systems; 1-884254),* 275 Phillips Blvd., Trenton, NJ 08618-1496 Tel 609-882-5600; Fax: 609-882-6357; Toll Free: 800-426-9119
E-mail: books.vls@medimedia.com
Web site: http://www.vetlearn.com
Dist(s): **J Majors Co** *(Majors, J. A. Co.).*

Vet Ophthal Notes, *(Veterinary Ophthalmology Notes; 0-9646143),* 1701 S. Whitcomb St., Fort Collins, CO 80526 Tel 303-482-7061.

Vet Practice, *(Veterinary Practice Publishing Co.; 0-9603534; 1-890417),* Div. of Fancy Pubns., Orders Addr.: P.O. Box 4457, Santa Barbara, CA 93117 (SAN 221-6906) Tel 714-855-8802; Fax: 714-855-3045; Edit Addr.: 7 Ashley Ave., S., Santa Barbara, CA 93103
E-mail: vppc@worldnet.att.net.

Veterinary Hlthcare, *(Veterinary Healthcare Communications; 0-935078),* Subs. of Medical Economics Co., Inc., 8033 Flint St., Lenexa, KS 66214 (SAN 209-0074) Tel 913-492-4300; Fax: 913-492-4157; Toll Free: 800-255-6864
Web site: http://www.vetmedpub.com.

Veterinary Med, *See* **Veterinary Hlthcare**

Veterinary Textbks, *(Veterinary Textbooks; 0-9601152),* 36 Woodcrest Ave., Ithaca, NY 14850 (SAN 207-2998) Tel 607-272-1860.

VGM Career Bks Imprint of McGraw-Hill Trade

VHA Inc, *(VHA, Inc.; 0-9667828),* Orders Addr.: P.O. Box 140909, Irving, TX 75014-0909 Tel 972-830-0000; Fax: 972-830-0562; Edit Addr.: 220 E. Las Colinas Blvd., Irving, TX 75039-5500 Do not confuse with VHA, Inc., Berwyn, PA
E-mail: feedback@vha.com
Web site: http://www.vha.com.

VICER Pub, *(VICER Publishing; 3-902104),* c/o Dr. Kaye, Dept. of Anesthesiology, Texas Tech Univ., Lubbock, TX 79340.

VICER Pubg (AUT) *(3-902104) Dist. by* **VICER Pub.**

Vicktor, *(Vicktor, Inc.; 0-9625327),* 8201 Greensboro Dr., Suite 500, McLean, VA 22102-3810 Tel 703-218-8400.

Victory Hse, *(Victory Hse., Inc.; 0-932081),* P.O. Box 700238, Tulsa, OK 74170 (SAN 686-2667) Tel 918-747-5009; Fax: 918-747-1970; Toll Free: 800-262-2631
Dist(s): **Anchor Distributors** *(Anchor Distributors)*
Appalach Bk Dist *(Appalachian Bk. Distributors)*
Rvrside Bk & Bible *(Riverside Bk. & Bible Resource)*
Spring Arbor Dist *(Spring Arbor Distributors Inc.).*

Victory Pubns, *(Victory Pubns.; 0-936261),* P.O. Box 372, Lehi, UT 84043 (SAN 697-3442) Tel 801-572-7611; Fax: 801-571-6545 Do not confuse with companies with the same or similar names in Palm Coast, FL, Racine, WI .

Vida Life Pubs, *See* **Vida Pubs**

Vida Pub, *(Vida Publishing, Inc.; 0-9632547),* Orders Addr.: P.O. Box 300946, Fern Park, FL 32730-0946 Tel 407-894-3504; Edit Addr.: 233 Northway Rd., Reisterstown, MD 21136 Do not confuse with Vida Publishing in Willow Street, PA
Dist(s): **Baker & Taylor** *(Baker & Taylor Bks.).*

Vida Pubs, *(Vida Pubs.; 0-8297; 0-943258),* 8325 NW 53rd St., Suite 100, Miami, FL 33166 Fax: 305-463-9295; Toll Free: 800-843-2548
E-mail: vidapubsales@harpercollins.com
Web site: http://www.editorialvida.com
Dist(s): **Zondervan** *(Zondervan Publishing Hse.).*

Viewpt Pr, *(Viewpoint Pr.; 0-9659473),* 19 Longwood Dr., Portland, ME 04102 Tel 207-772-5944
E-mail: ttomchnk@mcbvi.org.

Vikas (IND) *(81-259; 0-7069) Dist. by* **S Asia.**

Viking Imprint of Viking Penguin

†**Viking Penguin,** *(Viking Penguin; 0-14; 0-670),* Div. of Penguin Putnam, Inc., Orders Addr.: 405 Murray Hill Pkwy, East Rutherford, NJ 07073 (SAN 282-5074) Toll Free: 800-788-6262 (individual consumer sales); 800-631-8571 (reseller customer service); 800-526-0275 (reseller sales) ; Edit Addr.: 375 Hudson St., New York, NY 10014-3657 (SAN 298-0258) Tel 212-366-2000; Fax: 212-366-2952; Toll Free: 800-331-4624 ; *Imprints:* Viking (Viking) Penguin Bks (Penguin Books) PuffinBks (Puffin Books)
E-mail: publicity@warnerbooks.com
Web site: http://www.penguinputnam.com/
Dist(s): **Cheng & Tsui** *(Cheng & Tsui Co.)*
Continental Bk *(Continental Bk. Co., Inc.)*
Penguin Putnam *(Penguin Putnam, Inc.)*
Shens Bks *(Shen's Bks.)*
Trafalgar *(Trafalgar Square); CIP.*

Village Healer, *(Village Healer Pr., The; 0-9678988),* 23996 Dory Dr., Laguna Niguel, CA 92677 Tel 310-714-4040
E-mail: bpolydor@mba2000.hbs.edu
Web site: http://www.vhp.com
Dist(s): **Natl Bk Netwk** *(National Bk. Network).*

Villard Books, *(Villard Bks.; 0-375; 0-679; 1-4000),* Div. of Random Hse. Trade Publishing Group, Orders Addr.: 400 Hahn Rd., Westminster, MD 21157 Tel 410-848-1900; Toll Free: 800-726-0600; Edit Addr.: 299 Park Ave., New York, NY 10171 Tel 212-751-2600; Fax: 212-572-4949; Toll Free: 800-726-0600
Web site: http://www.villard.com
Dist(s): **Random** *(Random Hse., Inc.).*

Vin Bks, *(Vintage Bks.; 0-375; 0-394; 0-679),* Div. of Knopf Publishing Group, Orders Addr.: 400 Hahn Rd., Westminster, MD 21157 Tel 410-848-1900; Toll Free Fax: 800-659-2436; Toll Free: 800-733-3000; Edit Addr.: 299 Park Ave., 7th Flr., New York, NY 10171 Tel 212-751-2600; Toll Free: 800-726-0600
Web site: http://www.randomhouse.com/vintage/.

Vine Bks Imprint of Servant

Vineyard Minist, *(Vineyard Ministries International; 0-9651509),* Orders Addr.: P.O. Box 68025, Anaheim, CA 92817 Fax: 714-777-1257; Edit Addr.: 5300 E. La Palma Ave., Anaheim, CA 92807.

Vintage (IND) *(81-85326) Dist. by* **S Asia.**

Vintage Anchor, *(Vintage Anchor Publishing; 0-385),* Orders Addr.: 400 Hahn Rd., Westminster, MD 21157 Tel 410-848-1900; Toll Free: 800-726-0600; Edit Addr.: 201 E. 50th St., New York, NY 10022 Tel 212-571-2600 ; *Imprints:* Anchor NY (Anchor Books).

Vinton, *(Vinton Publishing; 0-9621388),* 13033 Ridgedale Dr., No. 134, Minnetonka, MN 55305-18074 (SAN 277-710X) Tel 612-472-7400; Fax: 612-472-5252; Toll Free: 800-221-4331 Do not confuse with Vinton Publishing Co. in Las Vegas, NV.

Vinton Pubng, *(Vinton Publishing Co.; 1-885026),* P.O. Box 94075, Las Vegas, NV 89193 Tel 702-262-9747; Fax: 702-739-0461; Toll Free: 800-897-9747 Do not confuse with Vinton Publishing in Mound, MN
E-mail: winters04@aol.com
Web site: http://www.sirjasonwinters.com.

Violence Policy Ctr, *(Violence Policy Ctr.; 0-927291),* 1140 19th St., NW, Suite 600, Washington, DC 20036-6608 Tel 202-822-8200; Fax: 202-822-8205
Web site: http://www.vpc.org.

Virgin Bks (GBR) *(0-426; 0-7535; 0-86369; 1-85227; 0-907080) Dist. by* **London Brdge.**

Vis Nurse Amer, *(Visiting Nurse Assns. of America; 0-9658572),* 11 Beacon St., Suite 910, Boston, MA 02108 Tel 617-523-4042; Fax: 617-227-4843; Toll Free: 888-866-8773 Do not confuse with Visiting Nurse Assn., Denver, CO
E-mail: vnaa.org.

Vishwa, *(Vishwa Dharma Pubns.; 0-942508),* 14 Driftwood, No. 2, Marina del Rey, CA 90292 (SAN 238-2075).

Visible Ink Pr, *(Visible Ink Pr.; 0-7876; 0-8103; 1-57859),* 42015 Ford Rd., No. 208, Canton, MI 48187-3669 Tel 734-667-3211; Fax: 253-276-7704
E-mail: inquiries@visibleink.com
Web site: http://www.visibleink.com.

Vision Care Intl, *(Vision Care International Ministries, Inc.; 0-9626292),* 8600 Foundry St., Box 2005, Savage, MD 20763 Tel 301-498-2325; Savage Mill, Box 2005, Savage, MD 20763.

Vision Dev Ctr, *See* **Lrning Cnnect**

Vision Pub, *(Vision Publishing; 0-9631567),* 29209 Northwestern Hwy., No. 592, Southfield, MI 48034 Tel 248-948-8112 Do not confuse with companies with the same name in Sandy, UT, Huntsville, AL, Carson, CA,Ramona, CA, Griffen, GA, Phoenix, MD, Detroit, MI.

Vision Publng, *(Vision Publishing; 0-9651783),* Orders Addr.: P.O. Box 11166, Carson, CA 90746-1166 Tel 310-537-0791; Edit Addr.: 20123 Harlan Ave., Carson, CA 90746 Do not confuse with companies with the same name in Sandy, UT, Huntsville, AL, Ramona, CA, Southfield, MI, Griffen, GA, Phoenix, MD, Detroit, MI.

†**VisionExtension,** *(VisionExtension; 0-929780),* 1921 Carnegie Ave., Suite 3L, Santa Ana, CA 92705-5510 (SAN 250-3875) Tel 949-250-8070; Fax: 949-250-8157
E-mail: smc.oep@worldnet.att.net; *CIP.*

Visions-Srvs, *(Visions/Services for the Blind & Visually Impaired; 1-890786),* 500 Greenwich St., 3rd Flr., New York, NY 10013 Toll Free: 888-245-8333
E-mail: al@visionsvcb.org
Web site: http://www.cilpubs.com.

Visit Nurse, *(Visiting Nurse Service, Inc.; 1-880504),* Div. of Community Health Ventures, Inc., 1200 McArthur Dr., Akron, OH 44320 Tel 330-745-1601; Fax: 330-848-6211; Toll Free: 800-362-0031
Dist(s): **Alimed** *(Alimed, Inc.)*
Imaginart Intl *(Imaginart International, Inc.)*
Psychol Corp *(Psychological Corp., The).*

Vista, *(Vista Publishing, Inc.; 1-880254),* 422 Morris Ave., Suite 1, Long Branch, NJ 07740 Tel 732-229-6500; Fax: 732-229-9647; Toll Free: 800-634-2498
E-mail: info@vistapubl.com
Web site: http://www.vistapubl.com.

Vista Pr of Am, *See* **DIASPORA PR AM**

Publisher Symbol Index

Visual Educ, *(Visual Education; 1-55637),* Div. of Graphic Paper Products Corp., Orders Addr.: P.O. Box 1666, Springfield, OH 45501 (SAN 660-9775) Tel 937-328-2854; Fax: 937-324-5697; Toll Free: 800-243-7070; Edit Addr.: 581 W. Leffel Ln., Springfield, OH 45501 (SAN 660-9783)
E-mail: sales@vis-ed.com
Web site: http://www.vis-ed.com.

Visual Mentor, *(Visual Mentor, The; 1-886728),* 40 Trace Ln., Half Moon Bay, CA 94019 Tel 415-726-9152; Fax: 415-726-2756
E-mail: info@visual-mentor.com
Dist(s): **Sunburst Comm** *(Sunburst Communications, Inc.).*

Vita Pr, *(Vita Pr. International (VPI); 0-9659474),* Orders Addr.: P.O. Box 399, Grambling, LA 71245 Tel 318-251-1107 (phone/fax); Toll Free: 888-596-8482; Edit Addr.: 2300 Rusty Ln., No. 38, Ruston, LA 71270
E-mail: atakyen@hotmail.com.

Vital Health, *(Vital Health Publishing; 1-890612; 1-890995),* Orders Addr.: P.O. Box 544, Bloomingdale, IL 60108 Tel 630-876-0426 (phone/fax)
E-mail: vitalhealth@compuserve.com
Web site: http://www.vitalhealth.net.

Vital Issue Pr Imprint of Huntington Hse

Vital Signs, *(Vital Signs Unlimited, Inc.; 0-9638043),* P.O. Box 2502, Tunica, MS 38676 Tel 501-224-6363; Fax: 501-224-6371; Toll Free: 800-844-2257
Web site: http://www.vsu.com.

Vitaliity Corp, *(Vitaliity Corp. of America; 0-9639683),* 4425 Oakley Greene, Sarasota, FL 34235-2330 Tel 941-953-2969.

Vitality Bks, *(Vitality Bks.; 0-9659977),* 2681 Crystal Cir., Dunedin, FL 34698 Fax: 727-789-1746
E-mail: chefmail@drmasley.com
Web site: http://www.drmasley.com
Dist(s): **Partners Pubs Grp** *(Partners Pubs. Group, Inc.).*

Vitality Dr, *(Vitality Doctor; 0-9704348),* 1700 S. College Ave., Suite C, Fort Collins, CO 80525 (SAN 253-9489) Tel 970-224-0774; Fax: 970-224-0783
E-mail: conquerfatique@aol.com
Web site: http://www.conquerfatique.com.

Vitality Hse Int Inc, *(Vitality Hse. International, Inc.; 0-912547),* 3707 N. Canyon Rd., Suite 2A, Provo, UT 84604-4585 (SAN 265-2935) Tel 801-373-5100; Fax: 801-373-5370.

Vitality Pr, *(Vitality Pr.; 0-9652544),* Div. of E. J. Conley Investments, Inc., G-3494 Beecher Rd., Flint, MI 48532 Tel 810-733-1565; Fax: 810-230-7855 Do not confuse with Vitality Press in Carol Stream, IL
E-mail: vitality@cfids.com
Web site: http://www.cfids.com
Dist(s): **BookWorld** *(BookWorld Services, Inc.).*

VNR Imprint of Wiley

Vocat Consult, *(Vocational Consultants Pr.; 0-9664026),* P.O. Box 682, Lake Zurich, IL 60047 Tel 847-438-1309 (phone/fax)
E-mail: vcpbooks@aol.com.

†**Volcano Pr,** *(Volcano Pr., Inc.; 0-912078; 1-884244),* Orders Addr.: P.O. Box 270, Volcano, CA 95689 (SAN 220-0015) Tel 209-296-4991; Fax: 209-296-4995; Toll Free: 800-879-9636; Edit Addr.: 21496 National St., Volcano, CA 95689
E-mail: info@volcanopress.com
Web site: http://www.volcanopress.com
Dist(s): **Baker & Taylor** *(Baker & Taylor Bks.)*
Bookpeople *(Bookpeople)*
New Leaf Dist *(New Leaf Distributing Co., Inc.)*
Quality Bks IL *(Quality Bks., Inc.); CIP.*

Volt Directory, *(Volt Directory Marketing, Ltd.; 0-913061; 0-925133),* One Sentry Pkwy., Suite 1000, Blue Bell, PA 19006 (SAN 283-2135) Tel 610-825-7720; Fax: 610-941-6874; Toll Free: 800-458-8658
E-mail: thanusey@volt.com
Web site: http://internettollfree.com; http://www.voltdirectory.com/.

Volunteer Mgmt, *(Volunteer Management Assocs.; 0-9603362),* 320 S. Cedar Brook Rd., Boulder, CO 80304 (SAN 221-6914) Tel 303-447-0558; Fax: 303-447-1749; Toll Free: 800-944-1470
E-mail: Rosemaryw@compuserve.com
Web site: http://www.volunteermanagement.com.

VPI1 (CAN) *(0-9686022) Dist. by* **Allnce Hse.**

VSP (NLD) *(90-6764) Dist. by* **Coronet Bks.**

VU Univ Pr (NLD) *(90-5383; 90-6256) Dist. by* **Paul & Co Pubs.**

VUB Univ Pr (BEL) *(90-5487; 90-70289) Dist. by* **Paul & Co Pubs.**

VWB (DEU) *(3-86135) Dist. by* **Thaneros Pr.**

W & C Cole Found, *(Cole, Warren & Clara Foundation; 0-9628799),* 55 E. Erie St., Chicago, IL 60611 Tel 312-202-5000; Fax: 312-202-5001.

W Austin Pr, *(Austin, William Pr.; 0-9663686),* 5594 SR441, Suite 128, Orlando, FL 32810 Tel 407-884-5749; Toll Free Fax: 800-638-0028; Toll Free: 800-638-0026.

W B Patterson, *(Patterson, W.B.; 0-9606968),* 3080 Alaneo Pl., Wailuku, Maui, HI 96793 (SAN 205-4914) Tel 808-244-5437.

W B Saunders (GBR) *(0-7020) Dist. by* **Saunders.**

W C H Architects, *(Watkins Carter Hamilton Architects, Inc.; 0-9636950),* 6575 W. Loop S., Suite 300, Bellaire, TX 77401 Tel 713-665-5665; Fax: 713-665-6213.

W C Uy, *(Uy, William C.; 0-9704843),* P.O. Box 1090, Hockessin, DE 19707 Fax: 302-239-9518
E-mail: DrWCUy@yahoo.com.

†**W E Upjohn,** *(Upjohn, W.E. Institute for Employment Research; 0-88099; 0-911558),* 300 S. Westnedge Ave., Kalamazoo, MI 49007-4686 (SAN 236-9486) Tel 616-343-4330 (orders); 616-343-5541; Fax: 616-343-7310 (orders); 616-343-3308
E-mail: publications@we.upjohninst.org
Web site: http://www.upjohninst.org; *CIP.*

†**W H Freeman,** *(Freeman, W. H. & Co.; 0-7167),* Div. of Bedford Freeman & Worth Publishing Group, LLC, Orders Addr.: 16365 James Madison Hwy., Gordonsville, VA 22942 (SAN 631-5011) Tel 540-672-7600; Toll Free Fax: 800-672-2054; Toll Free: 888-330-8477 (orders & customer service); Edit Addr.: 41 Madison Ave., 37th Flr., New York, NY 10010 (SAN 290-6864) Tel 212-576-9400; Fax: 212-689-2383
E-mail: webmaster@whfreeman.com
Web site: http://www.whfreeman.com
Dist(s): **VHPS** *(VHPS Holtzbrinck Pubs.); CIP.*

W Hamilton, *(Hamilton, William; 0-9676296),* 40 Shakespeare St., Daly City, CA 94014-1052 (SAN 253-7524) Tel 650-757-0842; Fax: 650-757-7000
E-mail: whamilton1@earthlink.net
Web site: http://www.fightingforyourlife.com.

W Harris, *See* **Hawaii Hlth Pubs**

W J Staab, *(Staab, Wayne J.; 1-881148),* 512 E. Canterbury Ln., Phoenix, AZ 85022 Tel 602-942-4939; Fax: 602-942-1486
E-mail: wstaab@aol.com.

W K Allen, *(Allen, William K.; 0-9624897),* 3220 E. Livingstone Ave., Columbus, OH 43227 Tel 614-231-1072.

W Kernodle, *(Kernodle, William; 0-9631533),* c/o Tucker Clinic, 7149 Jahnke Rd., Richmond, VA 23225 Tel 804-320-7881; Fax: 804-320-2050; Toll Free: 800-444-2524 (orders only).

W Laurier U Pr (CAN) *(0-88920; 0-921821) Dist. by* **Wilfrid Laurier.**

W Llewellyn, *(Llewellyn, William; 0-9679304),* P.O. Box 1162, Sound Beach, NY 11789 Tel 617-770-0616; Fax: 617-249-0127
E-mail: anabolix_web@hotmail.com.

W M Mercer, *(Mercer, William M. Inc.; 1-880754),* Div. of Marsh & McLennan Cos., Inc., 1500 Meidinger Tower, 9th Flr., Louisville, KY 40202 Tel 502-561-4542; Fax: 502-561-4747; Toll Free: 800-477-4541
Dist(s): **IPG Chicago** *(Independent Pubs. Group).*

W Mast, *(Mast, William; 0-9648937),* 18850 E. 114th St. S., Broken Arrow, OK 74011 Tel 918-587-3277.

W P Smedley, *(Smedley, W.P. Co.; 0-938279),* 9 Hamilton Rd., Dallas, PA 18612-9134 (SAN 659-820X).

W Pawluk, *(Pawluk, William; 0-9664227),* Orders Addr.: P.O. Box 366, Rancocas, NJ 08073 Tel 609-267-9085; Fax: 609-267-8615; Edit Addr.: 325 Centerton Rd., Rancocas, NJ 08073
E-mail: wpaw@home.com.

W Pubng Grp, *(W Publishing Group; 0-8499; 0-87680),* Div. of Thomas Nelson, Inc., P.O. Box 141000, Nashville, TN 37214-1000 (SAN 203-283X) Tel 615-902-3400; Fax: 615-902-3200 Do not confuse with Word Publishing Co. in Greenville, MS
Web site: http://www.wordpublishing.com; http://www.thomasnelson.com
Dist(s): **Christian Bk Distributors** *(Christian Bk. Distributors).*

W R Scaife, *(Scaife, William R. Pub.; 0-9619508),* Orders Addr.: P.O. Box 98094, Atlanta, GA 30359 (SAN 245-4807) Tel 770-987-2863; Edit Addr.: 101 Maypop Ln., Decatur, GA 30035 (SAN 245-4815).

W S Dawson, *(Dawson, W. S. Co.; 0-910581; 1-57000; 1-878515),* 801 Cathedral Dr., Virginia Beach, VA 23455 (SAN 297-6641) Tel 757-490-2504; Fax: 757-490-3494
E-mail: N2504@exis.net.

W S Hein, *(Hein, William S. & Co., Inc.; 0-8377; 0-87452; 0-89941; 0-930342; 1-57588),* 1285 Main St., Buffalo, NY 14209-1987 (SAN 210-9212) Tel 716-882-2600; Fax: 716-883-8100; Toll Free: 800-828-7571 ; *Imprints:* Rothman (Rothman, Fred B. & Company)
E-mail: mail@wshein.com
Web site: http://www.wshein.com.

W S Sullwold, *(Sullwold, William S. Publishing; 0-88492),* 18 Pearl St., Taunton, MA 02780 (SAN 203-1744) Tel 508-823-0924.

W Shepperd, *(Shepperd, Walter; 0-9660256),* 3429 Jacks Valley Rd., Carson City, NV 89705 Tel 702-267-3531; Fax: 800-487-2551
E-mail: wrshepperd@juno.com.

W Stephens, *(Stephens III, Westeron; 0-9644215),* 230 N. McLean Blvd., Elgin, IL 60123.

W W Gaunt, *See* **Gaunt**

W W Keen James, *(James, W.W. Keen; 0-9628197),* 378 Cottage St., New Bedford, MA 02740-5249 Tel 401-453-5714.

W W Whitman, *(Whitman, Wendell W. Co.; 1-885653),* 302 E. Winona Ave., Warsaw, IN 46580 Tel 219-267-3941; Fax: 219-267-2614; Toll Free: 800-421-2401
Web site: http://www.wwhitman.com.

W Zuckschwerdt (DEU) *(3-88603) Dist. by* **Scholium Intl.**

WA Advocates, *(Washington Advocates for the Mentally Ill; 0-926980),* 802 NW 70th St., Seattle, WA 98117-5135 Tel 206-783-9264; Fax: 206-784-0957; Toll Free: 800-782-9264
Web site: http://www.nami-wami.com.

WA Public Health, *(Washington State Public Health Assn.; 0-9662376),* Div. of American Public Health Assn. (APHA), Orders Addr.: P.O. Box 27007, Seattle, WA 98125-1407 Tel 206-362-4728; Fax: 206-362-4587; Edit Addr.: 107 Hemlock Dr., Chehalis, WA 98532
E-mail: kathy@wspha.org
Web site: http://www.wspha.org/.

Waclion, *(Waclion International, Inc.; 0-9679935),* P.O. Box 163205, Miami, FL 33116-3205 Tel 305-279-8180; Fax: 305-274-8168.

†**Wadsworth Pub,** *(Wadsworth Publishing Co.; 0-534),* Div. of Thomson Learning, Orders Addr.: 7625 Empire Dr., Florence, KY 41042-2978 (SAN 200-2663) Tel 859-525-2230; Toll Free: 800-354-9706; Edit Addr.: 10 Davis Dr., Belmont, CA 94002 (SAN 200-2213) Tel 650-595-2350; Fax: 606-525-0978
Web site: http://www.wadsworth.com
Dist(s): **Thomson Learn** *(Thomson Learning); CIP.*

Wagner Design, *(Wagner Design; 0-9653526),* 18629 Topham St., Tarzana, CA 91335-6804.

Wagner Pub, *(Wagner Publishing; 0-9621652),* 29636 Middlebelt Rd., Unit 2601, Farmington Hills, MI 48334-2357 (SAN 251-7396) Do not confuse with companies with the same name in Omaha, NE, Clifton Park, NY.

Waianae Coast CHC, *(Waianae Coast Comprehensive Health Ctr.; 0-9646023),* 86-260 Farrington Hwy., Waianae, HI 96792 Tel 808-696-7081; Fax: 808-696-7093.

Wakan Tanka, *(Wakan Tanka, Inc.; 0-9660484),* 11 S. 706 Lillian Ct., Naperville, IL 60564 Tel 630-904-0895; Fax: 630-904-0854
Dist(s): **Dogwise Pubng** *(Dogwise Publishing).*

Wake Forest Univ, *(Wake Forest Univ., Schl. of Medicine; 0-9644070),* Department of Biomedical Communications, Medical Center Blvd., Winston-Salem, NC 27157 Tel 336-716-4298; Fax: 336-716-2808.

Wakefield Pr (AUS) *(0-949268; 1-86254) Dist. by* **BHB Intl.**

Walgrn Drug, *(Walgreen Drug Stores Historical Foundation; 0-9648458),* 200 Wilmot Rd., MS No. HF, Deerfield, IL 60015 Tel 708-940-3033; Fax: 708-940-2824.

†**Walker & Co,** *(Walker & Co.; 0-8027),* 435 Hudson St., New York, NY 10014-3941 (SAN 202-5213) Tel 212-727-8300; Fax: 212-727-0984; Toll Free Fax: 800-218-9367; Toll Free: 800-289-2553 (orders)
E-mail: orders@walkerbooks.com
Web site: http://www.walkerbooks.com
Dist(s): **Empire Pub Srvs** *(Empire Publishing Service)*
Shens Bks *(Shen's Bks.)*
T T Beeler *(Beeler, Thomas T. Publisher); CIP.*

Walkers Pubg, *See* **Step Out On Faith**

Walk-In Counseling, *(Walk-In Counseling Ctr.; 0-9624337),* 2421 Chicago Ave., S., Minneapolis, MN 55404 Tel 612-870-0565.

Wallcur Inc, *See* **WI Pubns Inc**

Walter J Johnson, *(Johnson, Walter J. Inc.; 0-8472),* 1 New York Plaza 28th Flr., New York, NY 10004-1901 (SAN 209-1828).

Walther Cnslt, *(Walther Consultancy; 1-885327),* Orders Addr.: P.O. Box 29011, Greensboro, NC 27429-9011; Edit Addr.: 1013 N. Elm St., Suite A2, Greensboro, NC 27401-1423 Tel 336-379-0240
E-mail: waltcon@nr.infi.net.

Wal-Zac Ent, *(Wal-Zac Enterprises; 0-9634973),* 1574 Temple Ave., Mayfield Heights, OH 44124 Tel 216-464-7200; Fax: 216-464-0020.

Warde Pubs, *(Warde Pubs., Inc.; 1-886346),* 3000 Alpine Rd., Portola Valley, CA 94028 Tel 415-854-3389; Toll Free: 800-699-2733
E-mail: jwarde@wardepub.com.

†**Warner Bks,** *(Warner Bks., Inc.; 0-445; 0-446),* Div. of Time Warner Trade Publishing, Orders Addr.: c/o Little Brown & Co., 3 Center Plaza, Boston, MA 02108-2084 Fax: 800-286-9471; Toll Free: 800-759-0190; Edit Addr.: 1271 Avenue of the Americas, New York, NY 10020 (SAN 281-8892) Tel 212-522-7200
Web site: http://www.warnerbooks.com
Dist(s): **Little** *(Little, Brown & Co.)*
T T Beeler *(Beeler, Thomas T. Publisher)*
Todd Commns *(Todd Communications)*
iPublishcom *(iPublish.com); CIP.*

Warren Comns, *(Warren Communications; 0-945949),* Orders Addr.: PMB 508, Suite B, San Diego, CA 92154-4731 (SAN 248-0239) Tel 011 5266 801052 (Tijuana); Edit Addr.: 1636 32nd St., San Diego, CA 92102 (SAN 248-0247).

†**Warren Gorham & Lamont,** *(Warren, Gorham & Lamont, Inc.; 0-7913; 0-88262; 0-88712),* 90 Fifth Ave., New York, NY 10011 Tel 212-645-4800; Fax: 201-816-3581
E-mail: customer_services@riag.com
Web site: http://www.riahome.com/; *CIP.*

Warthog Pr, *(Warthog Pr.; 0-942292),* 29 South Valley Rd., West Orange, NJ 07052 (SAN 219-5399) Tel 201-731-9269.

Wash Bk Trad, *(Washington Bk. Trading Co.; 0-915168),* P.O. Box 1676, Arlington, VA 22210 (SAN 216-7115) Tel 703-525-6873
E-mail: washbook@aol.com.

Wash Busn Info, *(Washington Business Information, Inc.; 0-914176),* 300 N. Washington St., Suite 200, Falls Church, VA 22046-3431 (SAN 201-890X) Tel 703-538-7600; Fax: 703-538-7676
E-mail: customerservice@fdanews.com
Web site: http://www.fdanews.com.

Wash Emerg Squad, *(Washington Emergency Squad; 0-9604020),* 19 W. Washington Ave., Washington, NJ 07882 (SAN 221-6477) Tel 201-689-2111.

†**Wash Sea Grant,** *(Washington Sea Grant Program; 0-934539),* c/o Univ. of Washington, 3716 Brooklyn Ave., NE, Seattle, WA 98105-6716 (SAN 693-7861) Tel 206-543-6600; Fax: 206-685-0380; Toll Free: 800-583-6235
E-mail: seagrant@u.washington.edu
Web site: http://www.wsg.washington.edu; *CIP.*

†**Wash St U Pr,** *(Washington State Univ. Pr.; 0-87422),* P.O. Box 645910, Pullman, WA 99164-5910 (SAN 206-6688) Tel 509-335-3518; Fax: 509-335-8568; Toll Free: 800-354-7360
E-mail: wsupress@wsu.edu; emory@wsu.edu
Web site: http://www.wsu.edu/wsupress
Dist(s): **Baker & Taylor** *(Baker & Taylor Bks.)*
Benjamin News *(Benjamin News Group)*
Partners-West *(Partners/West); CIP.*

Wash U Ctr Psychobiol, *(Washington Univ., Ctr. for Psychobiology of Personality; 0-9642917),* 4940 Children's Pl., Saint Louis, MO 63110 Tel 314-362-7005; Fax: 314-362-5594.

Waterbrook Pr, *(WaterBrook Pr.; 0-87788; 1-57856; 1-4000),* Div. of Random Hse., Inc., Orders Addr.: 400 Hahn Rd., Westminster, MD 21157 Tel 410-848-1900; Toll Free: 800-726-0600; Edit Addr.: 2375 Telstar Dr., Suite 160, Colorado Springs, CO 80920 (SAN 299-4682) Tel 719-590-4999; Fax: 719-590-8977; Toll Free Fax: 800-294-5686; Toll Free: 800-603-7051 ; *Imprints:* H Shaw Pubs (Shaw, Harold Publishers) Do not confuse with WaterBrook Pr., Great Falls, VA
Dist(s): **Appalach Bk Dist** *(Appalachian Bk. Distributors)*
B&T Entertainment *(Baker & Taylor Entertainment)*
Follett Audio *(Follett Audiovisual Resources)*
Riverside-World *(Riverside World)*
Spring Arbor Dist *(Spring Arbor Distributors Inc.).*

Waters Pub, *(Waters Publishing; 0-930107),* P.O. Box 442, Brevard, NC 28712 (SAN 670-2309) Tel 704-884-4495.

Waterside Prodns, *(Waterside Productions, Inc.; 0-9627145),* 2191 San Elijo Ave., Cardiff, CA 92007 Tel 760-632-9190; Fax: 760-632-9295 ; *Imprints:* Cyrus Pr (Cyrus Press).

†**Watson Pub Intl,** *(Watson Publishing International; 0-88135),* P.O. Box 493, Canton, MA 02021 (SAN 689-8386) Tel 781-828-8450; Fax: 781-828-8915 ; *Imprints:* Prodist (Prodist) Sci Hist (Science History Publications) N Watson (Watson, Neale Academic Publications (NWAP)) Countway Lib Med (Countway Library of Medicine)
E-mail: acadsvc@aol.com
Web site: http://www.watsonpublishing.com; *CIP.*

Waveland Pr, *(Waveland Pr., Inc.; 0-88133; 0-917974; 1-57766),* P.O. Box 400, Prospect Heights, IL 60070 (SAN 209-0961) Tel 847-634-0081; Fax: 847-634-9501
E-mail: info@waveland.com
Web site: http://www.waveland.com.

**†Wayne St U Pr, *(Wayne State Univ. Pr.; 0-8143),* Leonard N. Simons Bldg., 4809 Woodward Ave., Detroit, MI 48201-1309 (SAN 202-5221) Tel 313-577-6120; Fax: 313-577-6131; Toll Free: 800-978-7323 (customer orders)
Web site: http://www.wsupress.wayne.edu**; *CIP.*

WBB (CAN) *(0-9696200) Dist. by* **Interact Media.**

WCB McGr Hill Imprint of McGrw-H Hghr Educ

†**Weatherhill,** *(Weatherhill, Inc.; 0-8348),* 41 Monroe Tpke., Trumbull, CT 06611-1315 (SAN 202-9529) Tel 203-459-5090; Fax: 203-459-5095; Toll Free: 800-437-7840
E-mail: weatherhill@weatherhill.com
Web site: http://www.weatherhill.com; *CIP.*

WebMD, *(WebMD Reference; 0-9703902),* 825 Third Ave. 15th Flr., New York, NY 10022 Tel 646-521-9200
Web site: http://www.webmd.com.

Webs New Wrld Imprint of Hungry Minds

Websters Unified, *(Webster's Unified, Inc.; 0-87475),* Orders Addr.: P.O. Box 2001, Tarrytown, NY 10591-9001 (SAN 202-7453) Tel 914-366-8880; Fax: 914-366-8881.

Wehawken Bk, *See* **Ctr Emp Med**

Weidenfeld & Nicolson (GBR) *(0-297; 0-575; 0-303) Dist. by* **Trafalgar.**

Weidner & Sons, *(Weidner & Sons Publishing; 0-86346; 0-907567; 1-85148),* Div. of Weidner Publishing Group, P.O. Box 2178, Riverton, NJ 08077 (SAN 659-4557) Tel 856-486-1755; Fax: 856-486-7583 ; *Imprints:* Tycooly Pub (Tycooly Publishing U. S. A.)
E-mail: weidner@waterw.com
Web site: http://www.weidnerpublishing.com.

Weigh of Life, *(Weigh of Life; 0-9639799),* 16450 Fairway Woods Dr., No. 601, Fort Myers, FL 33908 Tel 941-482-0556.

Weight Loss, *(Weight Loss & Fitness Facts; 0-9638588),* 513 Biscayne Cove, Clinton, MS 39056
Dist(s): **Baker & Taylor** *(Baker & Taylor Bks.).*

Wein & Wein, *(Wein & Wein Pubs.; 0-9629358),* 2122 Brookfield Dr., Thousand Oaks, CA 91362 Tel 805-493-1379.

Weiser, *See* **Red Wheel ME**

WEKA Pub, *(WEKA Publishing, Inc.; 0-929321),* 25 County Center Rd., No. B15, White Plains, NY 10607-1503 (SAN 248-9902) Toll Free: 800-222-9352.

WELCOA, *(Wellness Councils of America (WELCOA); 0-9628334; 0-9713563),* 9802 Nicholas St., Suite 315, Omaha, NE 68114-2106 Tel 402-827-3590; Fax: 402-827-3594
E-mail: wellworkplace@welcoa.org
Web site: http://www.welcoa.org.

Welcome Home, *(Welcome Home Star Babies; 0-9624690),* Orders Addr.: P.O. Box 6513, Santa Fe, NM 87502-6513; Edit Addr.: 1570 Pacheco, Suite A1, Santa Fe, NM 87501 Tel 505-757-6377.

Welcome Rain, *(Welcome Rain Pubs.; 1-56649),* 532 LaGuardia Pl., No. 473, New York, NY 10012 (SAN 299-9528)
Dist(s): **IPG Chicago** *(Independent Pubs. Group)*
Natl Bk Netwk *(National Bk. Network).*

Weldon Pub, *(Weldon Publishing; 0-9635407),* P.O. Box 4146, Prescott, AZ 86302 Tel 520-771-2369
Dist(s): **Baker & Taylor** *(Baker & Taylor Bks.)*
New Leaf Dist *(New Leaf Distributing Co., Inc.).*

Well Aware, *(Well Aware About Health; 0-943562),* 834 E. Camino De Fray Marcos, Tucson, AZ 85718-1914 (SAN 238-4140) Tel 520-297-2960.

Well Being, *(Well Being 2000 Pr.; 0-9671059),* Orders Addr.: P.O. Box 159002, Nashville, TN 37215 Tel 615-320-1100; Fax: 615-383-4571; Edit Addr.: c/o Richard P. Pinson, 2023 Castleman Dr., Nashville, TN 37215-6123
E-mail: rpinson@wb2k.com.

Wellingham-Jones, *See* **PWJ Pubg**

Wellington Pr, *(Wellington Pr.; 0-910959; 1-57501),* Div. of Felder Bks. & Games, 9601-30 Miccosukee Rd., Tallahassee, FL 32308-9662 (SAN 264-4878) Tel 904-878-6500; Fax: 850-893-3442 (orders); Toll Free: 877-390-4425 (orders only) Do not confuse with companies with the same name in Minneapolis, MN, Cheyenne, WY, Eau Claire, WI, South Nyack, NY
E-mail: peacegames@aol.com
Web site: http://www.peacegames.com
Dist(s): **Baker & Taylor** *(Baker & Taylor Bks.).*

Wellington Pubns, *(Wellington Pubns.; 0-915915),* P.O. Box 223159, Carmel, CA 93922 (SAN 294-1104) Tel 831-624-7871; Fax: 831-624-7994
E-mail: staff@wellingtonpublications.com
Web site: http://www.wellingtonpublications.com.

Wellness, *(Wellness Publishing, Inc.; 0-9641843),* 1323 SE 17th St., No. 694, Fort Lauderdale, FL 33316 Tel 954-462-4239; Fax: 954-728-8855; Toll Free: 888-616-4321 Do not confuse with companies with the same or similar name in Rock Port, TX, Omaha, NE, Santa Barbara, CA, Chula Vista, CA, Holland, MI.

Wellness Assocs, *(Wellness Assocs.; 0-9625882),* 123 Wildwood Trail, Afton, VA 22920 Tel 804-361-2361; Fax: 804-361-2353
E-mail: info@thewellspring.com
Web site: http://www.TheWellspring.com.

Wellness Ctr, *(Wellness Ctr. for Research & Education, Inc., The; 0-9652947),* 1216 State St., No. 407, Santa Barbara, CA 93101 Tel 805-962-6484; Fax: 805-962-6648
E-mail: t4joy@earthlink.net
Web site: http://www.wellnesscenter.net
Dist(s): **Baker & Taylor** *(Baker & Taylor Bks.)*
Nutri-Books Corp *(Nutri-Bks. Corp.).*

Wellness Inst, *(Wellness Institute, Inc.; 0-9617202; 1-58741),* 1007 Whitney Ave., Gretna, LA 70056 (SAN 663-382X) Tel 504-361-1845; Fax: 504-365-0114 Do not confuse with Wellness Institute in Tallahassee, FL
E-mail: publisher@selfhelpbooksnow.com
Web site: http://www.selfhelpbooksnow.com.

Wellness Pubns, *(Wellness Pubns.; 0-934957),* Orders Addr.: P.O. Box 2397, Holland, MI 49422; Edit Addr.: 930 S. Shore Dr., Holland, MI 49422-2397 (SAN 694-468X) Tel 616-335-2721; Toll Free: 800-543-0815 Do not confuse with companies with the same or similar name in Rockport, TX, Omaha, NE, Ft. Lauderdale, FL, Santa Barbara, CA, Chula Vista, CA,
Web site: http://www.lifeskillstraining.org
Dist(s): **Baker & Taylor** *(Baker & Taylor Bks.).*

Wellpower, *(Wellpower Pubns.; 0-917073),* 107 W. Chicago St., Brooklyn, MI 49230 (SAN 655-5659) Tel 517-592-3275.

Welstar Pubns, *(Welstar Pubns.; 0-938503),* Div. of Occupational Hygiene Ctr. of New York, Inc., 20 Colonel Robert Magaw Pl., New York, NY 10033 (SAN 660-9791) Tel 212-928-7528.

WeR Pr, *See* **CRRB**

Werbel Pub, *(Werbel Publishing Co., Inc.; 1-884803),* 686 Deer Park Ave., Dix Hills, NY 11746-6219 (SAN 219-0486) Tel 631-243-0032; Fax: 631-243-0069; Toll Free: 800-293-7235
E-mail: werbel@erols.com
Web site: http://www.werbel.com.

Wesley Pub Co, *(Wesley Publishing Co.; 0-9652703),* 2704 Blue Quail Pass, Edmond, OK 73013 Tel 405-340-3436
E-mail: rwsevier@home.com.

Wesleyan Univ Pr Imprint of U Pr of New Eng

West Group, *(West Group; 0-7620; 0-8321; 0-8366; 0-87632),* Orders Addr.: 610 Opperman Dr., Saint Paul, MN 55123-1396 Tel 651-687-7000; Fax: 651-687-5664; Toll Free: 800-328-9352
E-mail: beckie.burmeister@westgroup.com; gavin.phillips@westgroup.com
Web site: http://www.westgroup.com; http://www.westgroup.com.

West Pharm Soc, *(Western Pharmacology Society, Inc.; 1-930061),* c/o University of Arizona, College of Medicine, Dept. of Pharmacology, 1501 N. Campbell Ave., Tucson, AZ 85724-5050 Tel 520-626-7843; Fax: 520-626-6883
E-mail: huxtable@u.arizona.edu.

West Pine Pub, *(West Pine Publishing Co.; 0-929593),* 912 W. Pine St., Hattiesburg, MS 39401 (SAN 249-7069) Tel 601-582-1977; Fax: 601-582-9639 Do not confuse with West Pine Publishing in Saint Louis, MO.

†**West Pub,** *(West Publishing Co., College & Schl. Div.; 0-314; 0-8299),* Div. of Thomson, 610 Opperman Dr., Eagan, MN 55123 (SAN 202-9618) Tel 651-687-7000; Fax: 651-687-6857 (orders, pricing & availability); 651-687-5827; Toll Free: 800-328-4880; 800-328-9424 (Law & College Dept.); 800-328-2209 (bookstore customer service)
E-mail: customer.service@westgroup.com
Web site: http://www.lawschool.westlaw.com; http://www.westgroup.com
Dist(s): **Gale** *(Gale Group)*
Thomson Learn *(Thomson Learning); CIP.*

West Tex Mus, *See* **Mus Texas**

West Va U Pr, *(West Virginia Univ. Pr.; 0-937058),* P.O. Box 6295, Morgantown, WV 26506-6295 (SAN 205-5163) Tel 304-293-3107; Fax: 304-293-6638
E-mail: press24@wvu.edu
Web site: http://www.as.wvu.edu/press; http://www.vandaliapress.com; http://www.wvupress.com.

Westcliff Pubns, *(Westcliff Pubns.; 0-932896),* 1441 Avocado, No. 408, Newport Beach, CA 92660 (SAN 212-2448) Tel 714-720-1135.

Western Bk Journ, *(Western Bk. Journal Pr.; 0-936029),* 6560 SW McCarran Blvd. Suite A, Reno, NV 89509 (SAN 206-2305) Tel 775-787-1110; Fax: 775-786-1354.

Western Practnr Res, *See* **Open Spaces**

Western Psych, *(Western Psychological Services; 0-87424),* Div. of Manson Western Corp., 12031 Wilshire Blvd., Los Angeles, CA 90025 (SAN 160-8002) Tel 310-478-2061; Fax: 310-478-7838; Toll Free: 800-648-8857
E-mail: weinberg@wpspublish.com
Web site: http://www.wpspublish.com.

Western Reflections, *(Western Reflections Publishing Co.; 1-890437),* P.O. Box 1647, Montrose, CO 81402 Tel 970-249-7180; Fax: 970-249-7181; Toll Free: 800-993-4490
E-mail: westref@ouraycolorado.net
Web site: http://www.westernreflectionspub.com
Dist(s): **Baker & Taylor** *(Baker & Taylor Bks.)*
Books West CO *(Books West)*
Partners-West *(Partners/West)*
Quality Bks IL *(Quality Bks., Inc.)*
Treas Chest Bks *(Treasure Chest Bks.).*

Western Res Pr, *(Western Reserve Pr., Inc.; 0-912400),* 1436 Hidden Hemlock Dr., Austinburg, OH 44010-9756 (SAN 205-5201) Tel 216-964-2728.

Western Schls, *(Western Schls.; 1-57801),* Div. of SC Corp., 21 Bristol Dr., South Easton, MA 02375 Tel 508-238-0199 (ext. 2300); Fax: 508-238-5473.

Westgard Qual, *(Westgard Quality Corp.; 1-886958),* 7614 Gray Fox Trail, Madison, WI 53717-1857 Tel 207-646-1553; 112 Shore Rd., Ogunquit, ME 03907
E-mail: westgard@westgard.com
Web site: http://www.westgard.com.

†**Westminster John Knox,** *(Westminster John Knox Pr.; 0-664; 0-8042),* Div. of Presbyterian Publishing Corp., Orders Addr.: 100 Witherspoon St., Louisville, KY 40202-1396 (SAN 202-9669) Tel 502-569-5058; 502-569-5052 (outside U.S. for ordering); Fax: 502-569-5113 (outside U.S. for faxed orders); Toll Free Fax: 800-541-5113 (toll-free U.S. faxed orders); Toll Free: 800-523-1631
E-mail: ppc@ctr.pcusa.org; BFalvey@ctr.pcus.org; SHardin@ctr.pcusa.org
Web site: http://www.wjk.org
Dist(s): **Presbyterian Pub** *(Presbyterian Publishing Corp.); CIP.*

†**Westview,** *(Westview Pr.; 0-8133; 0-86531; 0-89158),* A Member of Perseus Books Group, 5500 Central Ave., Boulder, CO 80301-2877 (SAN 219-970X) Tel 303-444-3541; Fax: 303-449-3356; Toll Free: 800-386-5656
E-mail: westview.orders@perseusbooks.com
Web site: http://www.perseusbooksgroup.com
Dist(s): **HarperCollins Pubs** *(HarperCollins Pubs.); CIP.*

Westwood Pub Co, *(Westwood Publishing Co.; 0-930298),* 700 S. Central Ave., Glendale, CA 91204 (SAN 211-8769) Tel 818-242-1159; Fax: 818-247-9379
Web site: http://www.gilboyne.com.

Weve Got Your Number, *See* **Spiritpoint Pr**

WEWMG, *(West End Women's Medical Group; 0-9662827),* Orders Addr.: P.O. Box 9257, Incline Village, NV 89452 Tel 702-827-0616; Fax: 702-831-8937; Edit Addr.: 5915 Tyrone Rd., Reno, NV 89502
E-mail: eurugl@aol.com.

WFP, *(White Feather Pr.; 1-880357),* P.O. Box 1209, Laytonville, CA 95454 Tel 707-984-6048; Fax: 707-984-8045 Do not confuse with White Feather Press in Aurora, CO
E-mail: reiki@mcn.org
Web site: http://www.mendonet.com/reiki
Dist(s): **Baker & Taylor** *(Baker & Taylor Bks.)*
New Leaf Dist *(New Leaf Distributing Co., Inc.).*

Whalehall Inc, *(Whalehall, Inc.; 0-9617918),* 277 West End Ave., Apt. 15A, New York, NY 10023 (SAN 665-9691) Tel 212-787-5897
Dist(s): **Baker & Taylor** *(Baker & Taylor Bks.)*
Redwing Bk Co *(Redwing Bk. Co.).*

Whales Tale Pr, *(Whales' Tale Pr.; 1-882195),* 106 Welwyn Ct., Lake Bluff, IL 60044-1152
Web site: http://homepage.interaccess.com/~tfal/whales-tale.

Whatever Pubns, *See* **Four Winds OR**

Wheeler Pub, *(Wheeler Publishing, Inc.; 1-56895; 1-58724),* Orders Addr.: P.O. Box 531, Accord, MA 02018-0531 (SAN 253-228X); Edit Addr.: 405 VFW Dr., Rockland, MA 02370-1160 Tel 781-871-9170; Fax: 781-871-9173; Toll Free: 800-588-8881 (orders) ; *Imprints:* Compass (Compass Press)
E-mail: custsvc@wheelerpub.com.

Whi Stone, *(White Stone Publishing; 0-9630069),* 3489 Ashwood Ave., Los Angeles, CA 90066 Tel 310-397-7214
E-mail: lmallord@aol.com
Web site: http://www.whitestone.homepage.com.

Whitaker Hse, *(Whitaker Hse.; 0-88368),* 30 Hunt Valley Cir., New Kensington, PA 15068 (SAN 203-2104) Tel 724-334-7000; Fax: 724-334-1200; Toll Free Fax: 800-765-1960; Toll Free: 800-444-4484
E-mail: marketing@anchordistributors.com
Dist(s): **Anchor Distributors** *(Anchor Distributors).*

Whitaker Pub, *(Whitaker Publishing; 0-9620899),* 19 Jersey St., Denver, CO 80220 (SAN 250-1244) Tel 303-333-5233.

Whitcomb Pub, *(Whitcomb Publishing, Inc.; 0-9626978),* 5049 Paces Lakes Dr., Dallas, GA 30132-4819 Tel 770-443-2399 Do not confuse with Whitcomb Publishing in Springfield, MA.

White Bush Pub, *(White Bush Publishing Co.; 0-9661514),* 2932 Saint Mary's Way, Salt Lake City, UT 84108 Tel 801-583-0719; Fax: 801-582-0706.

White Dove Ent, *(White Dove Enterprises; 0-9636771),* Orders Addr.: P.O. Box 326, New Philadelphia, OH 44663 Tel 216-339-3021; Edit Addr.: Box 2685, State Rte. 416, SE, New Philadelphia, OH 44663-6866.

White Mane Pub, *(White Mane Publishing Co., Inc.; 0-942597; 1-57249),* Orders Addr.: P.O. Box 152, Shippensburg, PA 17257 (SAN 667-1926) Tel 717-532-2237; Fax: 717-532-6110; Toll Free: 888-948-6263 ; *Imprints:* Burd St Pr (Burd Street Press)
E-mail: marketing@whitemane.com
Web site: http://www.whitemane.com/.

White Rose Bks, *(White Rose Bks.; 0-9660486),* 30 Clark Ridge, Hockessin, DE 19707-1516 Tel 302-234-7940
E-mail: wrkbks@aol.com.

Whiteaker Pr, *(Whiteaker Pr., Inc.; 0-9653800),* 2006 1/2 S. Spokane St., Seattle, WA 98144 Tel 206-725-7889; Toll Free: 800-489-9095
E-mail: cmaurol@aol.com
Dist(s): **Baker & Taylor** *(Baker & Taylor Bks.)*
Bookpeople *(Bookpeople)*
SPD-Small Pr Dist *(SPD-Small Pr. Distribution)*
Words Distrib *(Words Distributing Co.).*

White-Boucke, *(White-Boucke Publishing; 0-9625006; 1-888580),* Orders Addr.: P.O. Box 400, Lafayette, CO 80026 Tel 303-604-0661; Fax: 303-604-0662
E-mail: ordering@white-boucke.com
Web site: http://www.white-boucke.com
Dist(s): **Baker & Taylor** *(Baker & Taylor Bks.)*
Bookazine Co Inc *(Bookazine Co., Inc.)*
Brodart *(Brodart Co.)*
Quality Bks IL *(Quality Bks., Inc.).*

Whitehall Pr, *(Whitehall Pr.-Budget Pubns.; 0-916565),* Whitehall, 1325 Jordan Mill Pond Rd., Sandersville, GA 31082 (SAN 295-5512) Tel 912-552-7455.

Whitewing Pr, *(Whitewing Pr.; 0-9639519; 1-888965),* Orders Addr.: P.O. Box 65539, Tucson, AZ 85728-5539 Tel 520-293-6580
E-mail: whitewingpress@mindspring.com.

Whitford Imprint of Schiffer

Whiting & Birch (GBR) *(1-86177; 1-871177) Dist. by* **Paul & Co Pubs.**

Whitman Coin Imprint of St Martin

Whitman Walker, *(Whiman-Walker Clinic, Inc., The; 0-9619604),* 1407 S St., NW, Washington, DC 20011 (SAN 237-9775) Tel 202-797-3500.

†**Whitmore,** *(Whitmore Publishing Co.; 0-87426),* 1144 Riverview Ln., West Conshohocken, PA 19428-2964 (SAN 203-2112)*; CIP.*

Whitston Pub, *(Whitston Publishing Co., Inc.; 0-87875),* 1717 Central Ave., Suite 201, Albany, NY 12205-4759 (SAN 203-2120) Tel 518-452-1900; Fax: 518-452-1777
E-mail: whitston@capital.net; jwolcott@nycap.rr.com
Web site: http://www.whitston.com.

Whittier Pubns, *(Whittier Pubns., Inc.; 1-57604; 1-878045),* 64 Alabama Ave., Island Park, NY 11558-1116 Tel 516-432-8120; Fax: 516-889-0341; Toll Free: 800-897-8398 (800-897-TEXT)
E-mail: info@whitbooks.com.

Who You Are, *(Who You Are International, Inc.; 0-9651842; 1-929737),* 8510 Elmore Ave., Webster, MN 55088 Tel 507-744-5875; Fax: 507-744-5876
Dist(s): **Bookmen Inc** *(Bookmen, Inc.)*
JayMar Servs *(JayMar Services, LLC).*

Whole Hlth Bks, *(Whole Health Bks.; 0-9644616),* 41 Crossroads Plaza, Suite 300, West Hartford, CT 06117 Tel 860-233-3000.

Whole Person, *(Whole Person Assocs., Inc.; 0-938586; 1-57025),* 210 W. Michigan St., Duluth, MN 55802-1908 (SAN 282-5430) Tel 218-727-0500; Fax: 218-727-0505; Toll Free: 800-247-6789
E-mail: books@wholeperson.com
Web site: http://www.wholeperson.com.

Whole World, *(Whole World Publishing, Inc.; 0-938184),* 400 Lake Cook Rd., No. 207, Deerfield, IL 60015 (SAN 217-1422) Tel 312-945-8050; Toll Free: 800-323-4305.

Wholeness Pr, *(Wholeness Pr.; 0-9665195),* 20 Sunnyside Ave., No. 334, Mill Valley, CA 94941 Tel 415-381-5000; Fax: 415-381-0543
E-mail: holos@laskow.net
Web site: http://www.laskow.net.

Whurr Pub (GBR) *(1-897635; 1-86156; 1-870332) Dist. by* **Taylor & Francis.**

WI Dept Pub Instruct, *(Wisconsin Dept. of Public Instruction; 1-57337),* Orders Addr.: Drawer 179, Milwaukee, WI 53293-0179 Tel 608-266-2188; Fax: 608-267-9110; Toll Free: 800-243-8782; Edit Addr.: 125 S. Webster St., Box 7841, Madison, WI 53702 Web site: http://www.dpi.state.wi.us.

WI Pubns Inc, *(W.I. Pubns., Inc.; 0-918082),* 7720 Clairemont Mesa Blvd., San Diego, CA 92111-1533 (SAN 209-3642) Tel 858-565-4366; Fax: 858-571-2067; Toll Free: 800-565-4331
Web site: http://www.wipublications.com
Dist(s): **J Majors Co** *(Majors, J. A. Co.)*
Matthews Bk Co *(Matthews Bk. Co.)*
Rittenhouse *(Rittenhouse Bk. Distributors).*

Wide Range, *(Wide Range Pr.; 0-9630709),* 4006-3B Calle Sonora Oeste, Laguna Hills, CA 92653 Tel 714-855-9723.

Wide World-Tetra, *(Wide World Publishing/Tetra; 0-933174; 1-884550),* P.O. Box 476, San Carlos, CA 94070 (SAN 211-1462) Tel 650-593-2839; Fax: 650-595-0802
E-mail: wwpbl@aol.com
Web site: http://www.wideworldpublishing.com
Dist(s): **Baker & Taylor** *(Baker & Taylor Bks.)*
Booklines Hawaii *(Booklines Hawaii, Ltd.)*
Bookpeople *(Bookpeople)*
Publishers Group *(Publishers Group West).*

Wieser & Wieser, *(Wieser & Wieser, Inc.; 0-914373),* 25 E. 21st St., Flr. 6, New York, NY 10010-6207 (SAN 289-6958) Tel 212-260-0860.

For full information on wholesalers and distributors, refer to the Wholesaler and Distributor Symbol Index

Wild Foods Co, *(Wild Foods Co.; 0-936699),* Orders Addr.: P.O. Box 206, Youngstown, AZ 85363 (SAN 248-4048) Fax: 602-933-5022; Edit Addr.: 11141 Arizona Ave., Youngtown, AZ 85363.

Wildcat Pubs, *(Wildcat Publishing Co., Inc.; 0-941968),* P.O. Box 366, Greens Farms, CT 06436 (SAN 238-2776) Tel 203-255-0680
Dist(s): **Natl Bk Netwk** *(National Bk. Network).*

Wilderness Med, *(Wilderness Medical Assocs.; 0-9704646),* 189 Dudley Rd., Bryant Pond, ME 04219 Tel 207-665-2707; Fax: 207-665-2747; Toll Free: 888-945-6633
E-mail: office@wildmed.com
Web site: http://www.wildmed.com.

---

†Wilderness Pr, *(Wilderness Pr.; 0-89997; 0-911824),* 1200 Fifth St., Berkeley, CA 94710-1306 (SAN 203-2139) Tel 510-843-1666; Fax: 510-548-1696; Toll Free: 800-443-7227
E-mail: mail@wildernesspress.com
Web site: http://www.wildernesspress.com
Dist(s):* Alpenbooks *(Alpenbooks)
Baker & Taylor *(Baker & Taylor Bks.)*
Bookpeople *(Bookpeople)*
Peregrine Outftrs *(Peregrine Outfitters)*
Quality Bks IL *(Quality Bks., Inc.)*
Rivers & Mnts *(Rivers & Mountains)*
Sunbelt Pubns *(Sunbelt Pubns., Inc.); CIP.*

Wildlife, *See* **A Natural Path**

†Wiley, *(Wiley, John & Sons, Inc.; 0-471; 0-8260; 0-937721; 0-939246; 1-56561; 1-57313; 3-527),* Orders Addr.: 1 Wiley Dr., Somerset, NJ 08875-1272 Tel 732-469-4400; Fax: 732-302-2300; Toll Free: 800-225-5945 (orders); Edit Addr.: 605 Third Ave., 4th Flr., New York, NY 10158-0012 (SAN 200-2272) Tel 212-850-6276 (Retail and Wholesale); 212-850-6000; Fax: 212-850-8641 (Retail and Wholesale) ; 212-850-6088 ; *Imprints:* Wiley-Interscience (Wiley-Interscience) Wiley-Liss (Wiley-Liss) Wiley-VCH (Wiley-VCH) Wiley Heyden (Wiley Heyden) VNR (Van Nostrand Reinhold) Wiley-IEEE (Wiley-IEEE Press)
E-mail: bookinfo@wiley.com; compbks@wiley.com
Web site: http://www.wiley.com; http://www.wiley.com/compbooks/; http://www.interscience.wiley.com
Dist(s): **AOAC Intl** *(AOAC International)*
ASM *(ASM International)*
Am Soc Civil Eng *(American Society of Civil Engineers)*
Aspen Pub *(Aspen Pubs., Inc.)*
IPG Chicago *(Independent Pubs. Group)*
Peoples Pub Grp *(Peoples Publishing Group, Inc., The)*
Shens Bks *(Shen's Bks.)*
Urban Land *(Urban Land Institute)*
netLibrary CO *(netLibrary, Inc.); CIP.*

Wiley Heyden Imprint of Wiley

Wiley-IEEE Imprint of Wiley

Wiley-Interscience Imprint of Wiley

Wiley-Liss Imprint of Wiley

Wiley-VCH Imprint of Wiley

Wilfrid Laurier, *(Wilfrid Laurier Univ. Pr.; 0-88920),* Box 277, 4408 Milestrip Rd., Blasdell, NY 14219-2599 Tel 519-884-0710; Fax: 519-725-1399
E-mail: press@wlu.ca
Web site: http://www.wlu.ca/~wwwpress/home.html.

Wilhelmina, *(Wilhelmina Bks.; 0-9631125),* Orders Addr.: SVL Box 8354, Victorville, CA 92392 Tel 760-961-7666; Fax: 760-961-8666; Toll Free: 800-390-0916; Edit Addr.: 21620 Bear Valley Rd., Apple Valley, CA 92308 Tel 619-240-9231.

†Wilkerson Pub Co, *(Wilkerson, J. L. Publishing Co.; 0-915253),* P.O. Box 948, Westbury, NY 11590 (SAN 289-8950) Tel 516-334-6297; *CIP.*

Willapa Bay, *(Willapa Bay Co., Inc., The; 1-884255),* 5223 NE 187th St., Lake Forest Park, WA 98155-4345 Tel 206-364-5696; Fax: 206-364-5992; Toll Free: 800-403-1424.

Willett Pub Co, *(Willett Publishing Co.; 0-915005),* 710 Bluff St., Glencoe, IL 60022 (SAN 289-4688) Tel 847-835-0900.

William Andrew, *(William Andrew Publishing; 0-8155; 1-884207; 1-891121),* 13 Eaton Ave., Norwich, NY 13815 Tel 607-337-5000; Fax: 607-337-5090; 1 Kattelville Rd., Suite 8, Bighamton, NY 13901 Tel 607-648-4770; Fax: 530-688-6497; Toll Free: 800-932-7045
E-mail: publishing@williamandrew.com
Web site: http://www.williamandrew.com.

William Carey Lib, *(Carey, William Library Pubs.; 0-87808),* Orders Addr.: 129 Mobilization Dr., Waynesboro, GA 30830 (SAN 208-2101) Tel 706-554-1594; Fax: 706-554-7444; Toll Free: 866-732-6657; Edit Addr.: 1705 N. Sierra Bonita, Pasadena, CA 91104
E-mail: inquiry@wclbooks.com.

William Penzer, *(Penzer, William N.; 0-9622658),* 150 S. University Dr., Plantation, FL 33324 Tel 954-475-1371; Fax: 954-475-1466
Web site: http://www.williampenzerphd.com.

Willow Pub, *(Willow Publishing Co.; 0-9606948),* Orders Addr.: P.O. Box 6636, San Antonio, TX 78209 (SAN 205-9401) Tel 210-822-5263 (phone/fax)
Dist(s): **Nutri-Books Corp** *(Nutri-Bks. Corp.).*

Willowgreen Pubng, *(Willowgreen Publishing; 1-885933),* 10351 Dawsons Creek Blvd., Fort Wayne, IN 46825 Tel 219-490-2222; Fax: 219-497-9622
Web site: http://www.willowgreen.com.

Willyshe Pub, *(Willyshe Publishing Co., Inc.; 0-936112),* 112 Mountain Rd., Linthicum Heights, MD 21090 (SAN 213-9499) Tel 410-789-0241.

Wilshire, *(Wilshire Bk. Co.; 0-87980),* 12015 Sherman Rd., North Hollywood, CA 91605-3781 (SAN 168-9932) Tel 818-765-8579; Fax: 818-765-2922
E-mail: mpowers@mpowers.com
Web site: http://www.mpowers.com.

†Wilson, *(Wilson, H. W.; 0-8242),* 950 University Ave., Bronx, NY 10452-4224 (SAN 203-2961) Tel 718-588-8400 (Ext. 2244); Fax: 718-681-1511 (Outside of the U.S. & Canada); Toll Free: 800-367-6770
E-mail: intlsales@hwwilson.com
Web site: http://www.hwwilson.com; *CIP.*

Wilson & Assocs, *(Wilson & Assocs.; 0-9633599),* 12804 47th Ave., NW, Gig Harbor, WA 98332 Tel 206-858-7492; Fax: 253-858-7491 Do not confuse with Wilson & Associates, Alvin, TX.

Wilson Pubng, *(Wilson Publishing; 0-9638590),* 20031 York Rd., Bothell, WA 98012 Tel 206-486-4316 Do not confuse with companies with the same name in Los Angeles, CA, Carson, CA.

Wilson St Press Imprint of Octavia Ohio

Windrose Pubs CA, *(Windrose Pubs.; 0-941819),* 890 S. Park Pl., El Cajon, CA 92021 (SAN 665-9934) Do not confuse with Windrose Productions, Port Townsend, WA.

Windsor Hse Pub Grp, *(Windsor Hse. Publishing Group, The; 1-881636),* 802 N. Milam, Fredericksburg, TX 78642 Tel 830-990-2620 (phone/fax)
E-mail: windhou@fbg.net.

Windsor Profess, *(Windsor Professional Information; 1-893190),* 11835 Carmel Mountain Rd., Suite 1304, San Diego, CA 92128 Tel 619-487-2945; Fax: 619-487-3279.

WinePress Pub, *(WinePress Publishing; 0-9622413; 1-57921; 1-883893),* Orders Addr.: P.O. Box 428, Enumclaw, WA 98022 Tel 360-802-9758; Fax: 360-802-9992; Toll Free: 800-326-4674
E-mail: info@winepresspub.com; Books4Him@aol.com; jhughes@winepresspub.com
Web site: http://www.winepresspub.com
Dist(s): **Appalach Bk Dist** *(Appalachian Bk. Distributors)*
Baker & Taylor *(Baker & Taylor Bks.)*
Spring Arbor Dist *(Spring Arbor Distributors Inc.).*

Wingborne-Diaconal, *(Wingborne-Diaconal Productions; 0-9629755),* 445 Hill 'n Dale Dr. N., York, PA 17403 Tel 717-845-3374
E-mail: laurahess1@juno.com.

†Wingbow Pr, *(Wingbow Pr.; 0-914728),* Div. of Bookpeople, 7900 Edgewater Dr., Oakland, CA 94621 Tel 510-632-4700; Fax: 510-632-1281
Dist(s): **Words Distrib** *(Words Distributing Co.); CIP.*

Winged Eagle Pr, *(Winged Eagle Pr.; 0-9626009),* Orders Addr.: P.O. Box 901, Auburn, WA 98071-0901; Edit Addr.: 21002 Edwards Rd., E., Sumner, WA 98390.

Wingers Pub, *See* **Zoological Educ**

Wings ME, *(Wings Pr.; 0-939736),* P.O. Box 809, Union, ME 04862 (SAN 216-7689) Tel 207-785-4355 Do not confuse with companies with the same or similar name in Northhampton, MA, San Antonio, TX, Lusk, WY.

Wings Pub, *(Wings Publishing; 1-882332),* 1 Clifford Ct., South Paris, ME 04281 Tel 207-743-8173
E-mail: bev@megalink.net.

Winkler Pub, *(Winkler Publishing Co.; 0-9610522),* 2520 W. First St., Grand Island, NE 68803-5308 (SAN 264-5009) Tel 308-382-1361.

Winner Enter, *(Winner Enterprises; 0-932855),* 670 Nighthawk Cir., Winter Springs, FL 32708 (SAN 691-2923) Tel 407-696-2103 (phone/fax)
E-mail: info@winnerenterprises.com
Web site: http://www.techware.com/winner.

WINNEWS, *(Women's International Network News Quarterly; 0-942096),* 187 Grant St., Lexington, MA 02420 (SAN 237-9740) Tel 781-862-9431; Fax: 781-862-1734
E-mail: winnews@igc.org
Web site: http://feminist.com/win.htm.

Winning Artist, *(Winning Artist Sounds Productions & Publishing (W.A.S.P.P.); 0-9638949),* 3131 Hyde Park Blvd., Los Angeles, CA 90043 Tel 213-971-3378.

Winning St Paul, *(Winning Pubns.; 0-9617124; 1-884367),* 2372 Leibel St., Saint Paul, MN 55110-2308 (SAN 662-6831) Tel 651-407-8547; Fax: 651-407-8179; Toll Free: 800-553-6458 Do not confuse with companies with the same or similar names in Oakland, CA, Nashville, TN
E-mail: paule@usinternet.com
Web site: http://www.taxhelponline.com.

†Winrock Intl, *(Winrock International Institute for Agricultural Development; 0-933595; 1-57360),* 38 Winrock Dr., Morrilton, AR 72110-9370 Tel 501-727-5435; Fax: 501-727-5242
Web site: http://www.winrock.org; *CIP.*

Winsted Pubns, *(Winsted Pubns.; 0-9630213),* 2055 Winsted Ct., Ann Arbor, MI 48103 Tel 313-665-3789
Dist(s): **New Leaf Dist** *(New Leaf Distributing Co., Inc.).*

Winter Pub Co, *(Winter Publishing Co.; 0-938372),* Orders Addr.: P.O. Box 36536, Tucson, AZ 85740 (SAN 220-1100); Edit Addr.: 6632 N. Willowbrook Dr., Tucson, AZ 85704 (SAN 220-1119) Tel 520-742-4104; Fax: 520-742-2833.

Winters KS, *(Winters Publishing; 0-9661900),* Orders Addr.: P.O. Box 782041, Witchita, KS 67278; Edit Addr.: 9350 E. Corporate Hills Dr., Wichita, KS 67278 Tel 316-371-0635 Do not confuse with Winter Publishing, Greensburg, IN
E-mail: samw@kscable.com
Web site: http://www.wavetherapy.com
Dist(s): **Pleiades Proj** *(Pleiades Project).*

Wipf & Stock, *(Wipf & Stock Pubs.; 0-9653517; 1-57910),* 150 W. Broadway, Eugene, OR 97401-3004 Tel 541-344-1528; Fax: 541-344-1506
E-mail: wspub@academicbooks.com
Web site: http://www.academicbooks.com.

Wis Inst Drug Abuse, *(Wisconsin Institute on Drug Abuse; 0-9615363),* Div. of Tellurian Community, Inc., 300 Femrite Dr., Madison, WI 53716 (SAN 695-2690) Tel 608-222-7311.

†Wisdom MA, *(Wisdom Pubns.; 0-86171),* 199 Elm St., Somerville, MA 02144 (SAN 246-022X) Tel 617-776-7416 (ext. 24); Fax: 617-776-7841; Toll Free Fax: 800-338-4550 (orders only); Toll Free: 800-462-6420 (orders only)
E-mail: marketing@wisdompubs.org
Web site: http://www.wisdompubs.org
Dist(s): **Natl Bk Netwk** *(National Bk. Network); CIP.*

Wisdom of Pain, *(Wisdom of Pain; 0-9609324),* P.O. Box 99952, Louisville, KY 40269-0952 (SAN 240-849X).

Wisdom Pubng, *(Wisdom Publishing Co.; 1-57569),* 3330 Earhart Dr., Suite 213, Carrollton, TX 75006-5041 Tel 972-404-8125; Fax: 972-404-8821
Web site: http://www.wisdompublishing.com.

Wise Acres, *(Wise Acres; 1-881517),* P.O. Box 1168, Creswell, OR 97426-0279 Tel 541-895-5152
E-mail: lfiore@rio.com.

Wise Pub, *(Wise Publishing Co.; 0-915766),* Orders Addr.: 5625 Wilhelmina Ave., Woodland Hills, CA 91367 (SAN 203-1876) Tel 818-883-7527; Fax: 818-883-9212 Do not confuse with companies with the same or similar name in Indianapolis, IN, Mansfield, TX.

Wise Woman Herbals, *See* **Wise Acres**

WiseAcre Imprint of Red Sea NY

WiseGuide Pub, *(WiseGuide Publishing; 0-9659599),* 44 Holly Dr., Short Hills, NJ 07078-1318 Tel 973-376-5385; Fax: 973-376-0199
E-mail: Multiactor@aol.com
Web site: http://www.homel.gte.net/rgwinter
Dist(s): **BookMasters** *(BookMasters, Inc.)*
Koen Bk Distributors *(Koen Bk. Distributors).*

Publisher Symbol Index

WiseWord Pub, *(WiseWord Publishing; 0-9627762),* Orders Addr.: 351 Wayne Ave., Oakland, CA 94610 (SAN 253-326X) Tel 510-839-4800; Fax: 510-836-0477; Toll Free: 800-398-0034
E-mail: mgordon@hypnotherapycenter.com
Web site: http://www.extraordinaryhealing.com; http://www.hypnotherapycenter.com
Dist(s): **Quest MA** *(Quest, The)*
SPD-Small Pr Dist *(SPD-Small Pr. Distribution).*

Wishland Inc, *(Wishland, Inc.; 0-9632091; 1-893623),* Orders Addr.: P.O. Box 41504, Mesa, AZ 85274 Tel 480-346-3104; Fax: 480-998-1530; Edit Addr.: 8260 E. Gelding Dr., Suite 101, Scottsdale, AZ 85267
Dist(s): **Barnes & Noble Inc** *(Barnes & Noble, Inc.)*
IPG Chicago *(Independent Pubs. Group)*
New Leaf Dist *(New Leaf Distributing Co., Inc.)*
Nutri-Books Corp *(Nutri-Bks. Corp.).*

Wishland Pub Inc, *See* **Wishland Inc**

WIT Pr (GBR) *(0-905451; 0-931215; 0-945824; 1-56252; 1-85312) Dist. by* **Computational Mech MA.**

Witherby & Co (GBR) *(0-900886; 1-85609; 0-948691; 0-907591; 0-906270) Dist. by* **St Mut.**

Witness CA, *(Witness, Inc.; 1-883858),* Orders Addr.: P.O. Box 597, Clayton, CA 94517 Tel 925-672-5979; Fax: 925-672-8230; Edit Addr.: 5733 Verna Way, Clayton, CA 94517
E-mail: jwbooks@juno.com
Web site: http://www.witnessinc.com
Dist(s): **Jeremiah Films** *(Jeremiah Films).*

WIU CBER, *(Western Illinois Univ., Ctr. for Business & Economic Research; 0-931497),* c/o Dept. of Economics, 442 Stipes Hall, Macomb, IL 61455 (SAN 683-2180) Tel 309-298-1153
E-mail: info@wiu.edu
Web site: wiu.edu.

Wizards, *(Wizards Bookshelf; 0-913510),* P.O. Box 6600, San Diego, CA 92166 (SAN 203-2872) Tel 619-258-0049; Fax: 619-258-0139
Web site: http://www.wizbooks-blavatsky.com
Dist(s): **DeVorss** *(DeVorss & Co.)*
New Leaf Dist *(New Leaf Distributing Co., Inc.).*

Wld Assn Vet, *(World Assn. of Veterinary Anatomists),* c/o Purdue Univ., 1249 Lynn Hall, West Lafayette, IN 47907 Tel 765-494-2386.

WLP Botsford, *See* **Lifestyle Inst**

Wm Caxton, *(Caxton, Wm Ltd.; 0-940473),* P.O. Box 220, Ellison Bay, WI 54210-0220 (SAN 135-1303) Tel 920-854-2955.

Wm Morrow Imprint of Morrow Avon

Wntergrn, *(Wintergreen Pr.; 0-9609456; 1-883525),* 3630 Eileen St., Maple Plain, MN 55359 (SAN 694-101X) Tel 612-476-1303
E-mail: wpress@aol.com.

Wolfe Publishing (GBR) *(0-7234) Dist. by* **Mosby Inc.**

Wolff New Media, *(Wolff New Media, LLC; 1-889670),* 666 Fifth Ave., No. 289, New York, NY 10103-0001 Tel 212-308-8100; Fax: 212-308-8837
Dist(s): **Fodors Travel** *(Fodor's Travel Pubns., Inc.)*
Natl Bk Netwk *(National Bk. Network).*

Wom & Child Hlth, *(Women's & Children's Health Policy Ctr.; 1-893692),* Div. of Johns Hopkins Schl. of Public Health, 624 N. Broadway, Baltimore, MD 21205 Tel 410-502-5443; Fax: 410-955-2303
E-mail: hgrason@jhsph.edu
Web site: http://www.med.jhu.edu/wchpc
Dist(s): **Ntl Maternal** *(National Maternal & Child Health Clearinghouse).*

Wom Hlth Educ, *(Women's Health Education Project; 0-9643861),* 333 E. 68th St., No. 1E, New York, NY 10021-5693 Tel 212-987-0066; Fax: 212-987-3278.

Women & Addiction, *(Women & Addiction Counseling & Educational Services; 0-9663144),* 43522 Modena Dr., Temecula, CA 92592-9235 Tel 909-303-0236 (phone/fax); Toll Free: 877-926-6636
E-mail: info@women-addiction.com
Web site: http://www.women-addiction.com.

Women in Process, *(Women in Process, Seminars & Pubs.; 1-886563),* 82 Chapel Hill Dr., Napa, CA 94559 Tel 707-253-7325; Fax: 707-224-2529.

Womens Auxiliary Cancer, *(Women's Auxiliary of the American Cancer Society; 0-9607282),* Affil. of American Cancer Society, 241 Fourth Ave., Pittsburgh, PA 15222 (SAN 239-3506) Tel 412-261-4352; Fax: 412-261-2501.

Womens Hlth, *See* **MCP Hahn Schl**

Womens Hlthcare Pr, *(Women's Healthcare Pr.; 0-9626223),* 500 Davis, Suite 700, Evanston, IL 60201 Tel 847-869-1200; Fax: 847-328-9056; Toll Free: 800-543-3854.

Womens Pr (CAN) *(0-88961) Dist. by* **U of Toronto Pr.**

Womens Press (GBR) *(0-7043) Dist. by* **Trafalgar.**

Womens Pubns Imprint of Consumer Press

Wood Lib-Mus, *(Wood Library-Museum of Anesthesiology; 0-9614932; 1-889595),* Subs. of American Society of Anesthesiologists, 520 N. Northwest Hwy., Park Ridge, IL 60068-2573 (SAN 693-4048) Tel 847-825-5586; Fax: 847-825-1692.

Wood N Barnes, *(Wood 'N Barnes; 1-885473),* Div. of Jean Barnes Bks., 2717 NW 50th, Oklahoma City, OK 73112 (SAN 298-9433) Tel 405-942-6812; Fax: 405-946-4074; Toll Free: 800-678-0621
E-mail: wnb@barnesbooks.com
Web site: http://www.woodnbarnes.com.

†**Woodbine House,** *(Woodbine Hse.; 0-933149; 1-890627),* 6510 Bells Mill Rd., Bethesda, MD 20817 (SAN 630-4052) Tel 301-897-3570; Fax: 301-897-5838
E-mail: info@woodbinehouse.com
Web site: http://www.woodbinehouse.com
Dist(s): **Penguin Putnam** *(Penguin Putnam, Inc.); CIP.*

Woodbridge Pr, *(Woodbridge Pr. Publishing Co.; 0-88007; 0-912800),* Orders Addr.: P.O. Box 209, Santa Barbara, CA 93102 (SAN 212-9892) Tel 805-965-7039; Fax: 805-963-0540; Toll Free: 800-237-6053; Edit Addr.: 815 De La Vina St., Santa Barbara, CA 93101
E-mail: woodpress@aol.com
Web site: http://www.woodbridgepress.com.

Woodburn Pr, *(Woodburn Pr.; 0-9612798),* 402 Workman Ln., Bellefonte, PA 16823-6431 (SAN 289-906X) Tel 814-234-1833.

Woodhead Pubng (GBR) *(1-85573) Dist. by* **Am Educ Systs.**

Woodholme Hse, *(Woodholme Hse. Pubs.; 0-9656342; 1-891521),* 131 Village Square I Village of Cross Keys, Baltimore, MD 21210 Tel 410-532-5018; Fax: 410-532-9741; Toll Free: 800-488-0051
E-mail: info@woodholmehouse.com
Dist(s): **Koen Bk Distributors** *(Koen Bk. Distributors)*
Wash Bk Distrib *(Washington Bk. Distributors).*

†**Woodland,** *(Woodland Publishing Co., Inc.; 0-934104),* Box 85, Wayzata, MN 55391 (SAN 213-1900) Tel 612-473-2725
E-mail: roofus2005@aol.com; *CIP.*

Woodland Hlth Bks, *See* **Woodland UT**

Woodland UT, *(Woodland Publishing, Inc.; 0-913923; 1-58054; 1-885670),* Orders Addr.: P.O. Box 160, Pleasant Grove, UT 84062 (SAN 286-9063) Tel 801-785-8100; Fax: 801-785-8511; Toll Free: 800-777-2665; Edit Addr.: 1030 W. 500 N., Lindon, UT 84042.

Woodstock Books, *(Woodstock Bks.; 0-9640096),* 120 W. Main St., Box 70, Plainville, CT 06062-0070 Tel 860-793-0728; Fax: 860-747-6144
E-mail: woodstkbks@aol.com
Dist(s): **Bookazine Co Inc** *(Bookazine Co., Inc.).*

Woodstone Bks, *(Woodstone Bks.; 0-939866),* 2888 Bluff St., No. 34, Boulder, CO 80301 (SAN 216-9436) Tel 303-449-8100.

Wooster Bk, *(Wooster Bk. Co., The; 1-888683; 1-59098),* 205 W. Liberty St., Wooster, OH 44691-4831 Tel 330-262-1688; Fax: 330-264-9753; Toll Free: 800-882-6651 (800-WUBook-1)
E-mail: mail@woosterbook.com
Web site: http://www.woosterbook.com.

Word Among Us, *(Word Among Us Pr.; 0-932085),* 9639 Dr. Perry Rd., No. 126, Ijamsville, MD 21754 (SAN 686-4651) Tel 301-831-1262; Fax: 301-831-1188; Toll Free: 800-775-9673
E-mail: jeffsmith@wau.org; theresa@wau.org
Web site: http://www.wau.org
Dist(s): **Spring Arbor Dist** *(Spring Arbor Distributors Inc.).*

Word Assn, *(Word Association Pubs.; 1-891231),* 205 Fifth Ave., Tarentum, PA 15084 Tel 724-226-1255; Fax: 724-226-3974; Toll Free: 800-827-7903
E-mail: publish@wordassociation.com
Web site: http://www.WordAssociation.com.

Word Pub, *See* **W Pubng Grp**

Words & Pict, *(Words & Pictures By; 0-9647480),* Orders Addr.: P.O. Box 482, East Brunswick, NJ 08816 Tel 732-254-9262; Fax: 732-257-1992; Edit Addr.: 18 Churchill Rd., East Brunswick, NJ 08816 Do not confuse with Words & Pictures, Oakland, CA.

Words Distrib, *(Words Distributing Co.; 0-914728),* Div. of Bookpeople, 7900 Edgewater Dr., Oakland, CA 94621 (SAN 154-7763) Tel 510-632-4700; Fax: 510-632-1281; Toll Free: 800-999-4650; 800-593-9673 (orders)
Dist(s): **Bookpeople** *(Bookpeople).*

Wordscope Inc, *(Wordscope, Inc.; 0-930121),* 2562 Wellington Ct., Evanston, IL 60201-4975 (SAN 670-3194) Tel 847-328-4512.

Wordsworth KS, *(Wordsworth; 0-945530),* 702 NE 24th St., Newton, KS 67114-9275 (SAN 247-0640) Tel 316-283-6708 Do not confuse with companies with the same name in Ridgewood, NJ, Cody, WY
E-mail: publisher@books-wordsworth.com
Web site: http://www.books-wordsworth.com.

†**Work in Amer,** *(Work in America Institute, Inc.; 0-89361),* 700 White Plains Rd., Scarsdale, NY 10583-5058 (SAN 208-9262) Tel 914-472-9600; Fax: 914-472-9606; Toll Free: 800-787-0707; *CIP.*

†**Workers Comp Res Inst,** *(Workers Compensation Research Institute; 0-935149; 1-931906),* 955 Massachusetts Ave., Cambridge, MA 02139 (SAN 695-2291)
Web site: http://wcrinet.org; *CIP.*

Workfit Consult, *(Workfit Consultants, L.L.C.; 0-9668792),* 50 Cherry Hill Rd., Parsippany, NJ 07054 Tel 973-683-0162; Fax: 973-335-8429
E-mail: margie@workfitonline.com
Web site: http://www.workfitonline.com.

Work-Loss Data, *(Work-Loss Data Institute; 1-880891),* 500 N. Shoreline Blvd., Suite 1101N, Corpus Christi, TX 78471 Tel 361-883-5000; Fax: 361-883-7025; Toll Free: 800-488-5548.

†**Workman Pub,** *(Workman Publishing Co., Inc.; 0-7611; 0-89480; 0-911104; 1-56305),* 708 Broadway, New York, NY 10003 (SAN 203-2821) Tel 212-254-5900; Fax: 212-254-8098; Toll Free: 800-722-7202
E-mail: mged@workman.com
Web site: http://www.workmanweb.com; http://www.workman.com
Dist(s): **ACTA Pubns** *(ACTA Pubns.)*
Cookbook Collection Inc *(Cookbook Collection, Inc.)*
Wrldwide Media Srv *(Worldwide Media Service, Inc.); CIP.*

†**World Bank,** *(World Bank, The, Office of the Publisher; 0-8213),* Orders Addr.: P.O. Box 960, Herndon, VA 20172-0960; Edit Addr.: 1818 H St., NW, Rm. U11-063, Washington, DC 20433 (SAN 219-0648) Tel 703-661-1580; 202-473-1153 (Review or Desk Copies); Fax: 703-661-1501; Toll Free: 800-645-7247
E-mail: books@worldbank.org
Web site: http://www.worldbank.org/publications
Dist(s): **Balogh** *(Balogh International, Inc.)*
Johns Hopkins *(Johns Hopkins Univ. Pr.)*
OUP *(Oxford Univ. Pr., Inc.); CIP.*

World Bk, *(World Bk., Inc.; 0-7166),* Div. of Scott Fetzer Co., 233 N. Michigan, Suite 2000, Chicago, IL 60601 (SAN 201-4815) Tel 312-729-5800; Fax: 312-729-5614; 312-729-5600; Toll Free Fax: 800-433-9330 (school & library orders); Toll Free: 800-967-5325; 800-975-3250 (school & library orders)
E-mail: Janet.Peterson@worldbook.com
Web site: http://www.worldbook.com.

World Class Enterprises, *(World Class Enterprises, Inc.; 0-933079),* 3209 Jackqueln Dr., Albany, GA 31705 (SAN 689-8149) Tel 912-436-7434.

World Development, *(World Development Group, Inc.; 0-9666866),* 5272 River Rd., Bethesda, MD 20816 Tel 301-652-1818; Fax: 301-632-1250.

World Health, *(World Health Organization; 92-4),* Orders Addr.: 49 Sheridan Ave., Albany, NY 12210 (SAN 221-6310) Tel 518-436-9686; Fax: 518-436-7433
E-mail: publications@who.ch
Web site: http://www.who.ch
Dist(s): **Balogh** *(Balogh International, Inc.)*
Bernan Associates *(Bernan Assocs.).*

World Hlth Found, *(World Health Foundation; 0-944213),* 3900 Birch St., Suite 203, Newport Beach, CA 92660-2227 (SAN 243-0479) Toll Free: 800-968-8418.

World Neigh, *(World Neighbors; 0-942716),* 4127 NW 122nd St., Oklahoma City, OK 73120-8869 (SAN 276-8283) Tel 405-752-9700; Fax: 405-752-9393; Toll Free: 800-242-6387
E-mail: info@wn.org
Web site: http://www.wn.org.

World Resources Inst, *(World Resources Institute; 0-915825; 1-56973),* Orders Addr.: P.O. Box 4852, Baltimore, MD 21211 (SAN 693-9899); Edit Addr.: 10 G St., NE 8th Flr., Washington, DC 20002 (SAN 294-2968) Tel 410-516-6963; Fax: 410-516-6998; Toll Free: 800-822-0504
E-mail: publications@wri.org
Web site: http://www.wristore.com; http://www.wri.org
Dist(s): **Brookings** *(Brookings Institution Pr.).*

World Scientific Pub, *(World Scientific Publishing Co., Inc.; 981-02),* 1060 Main St., River Edge, NJ 07661 (SAN 241-9920) Tel 201-487-9655; Fax: 201-487-9656; Toll Free: 800-227-7562
Web site: http://www.worldscientific.com/index.cgi.

World Vision Intl, *(World Vision International; 0-918261; 1-887983),* 800 W. Chestnut Ave., Monrovia, CA 91016-3198 (SAN 225-4719) ; *Imprints:* MARC Pubns (MARC Publications)
E-mail: marcpubs@wvi.org; wvpp@wvi.org
Web site: http://www.wvi.org; http://www.marcpublications.com; http://www.wvpublications.com.

WorldComm, *(WorldComm; 1-56664),* Div. of Creativity, Inc., 65 Macedonia Rd., Alexander, NC 28701 Tel 828-252-9515; Fax: 828-255-8719; Toll Free: 800-472-0438 (phone/fax)
E-mail: sales@abooks.com
Web site: http://www.abooks.com.

Worldwatch Inst, *(Worldwatch Institute; 0-916468; 1-878071),* 1776 Massachusetts Ave., NW, Washington, DC 20036 (SAN 209-2727) Tel 202-452-1999; Fax: 202-296-7365; Toll Free: 800-555-2028
E-mail: worldwatch@worldwatch.org
Web site: http://www.worldwatch.org.

Worldwide Educ, *(Worldwide Educational Resources, Inc.; 0-9675498),* 1604 E. Sheena Dr., Phoenix, AZ 85022 Tel 602-504-0154; Fax: 602-504-3643
E-mail: SHULMAN@INFINET-IS.com.

World-Wide Tampa, *See* **Wrld Tampa**

Worth, *(Worth Pubs., Inc.; 0-312; 0-87901; 1-57259),* Div. of Bedford, Freeman & Worth Publishing Group, LLC, Orders Addr.: 16365 James Madison Hwy., Gordonsville, VA 22942 (SAN 631-5011) Tel 540-672-7600; Fax: 540-672-7052; Toll Free Fax: 800-672-2054; Toll Free: 888-330-8477; Edit Addr.: 41 Madison Ave., 36th Flr., New York, NY 10010-2202 (SAN 205-5546) Tel 212-576-9400; Fax: 212-561-8281; Toll Free: 800-903-3019
Web site: http://www.worthpublishers.com
Dist(s): **St Martin** *(St. Martin's Pr., LLC)*
VHPS *(VHPS Holtzbrinck Pubs.).*

Wrds Lght Intl, *(Words of Light International Publishing; 1-887480),* Orders Addr.: P.O. Box 238, Templeton, MA 01468 (SAN 298-6264) Tel 978-249-4336
E-mail: wordsoflight@netzero.net
Web site: http://www.angelfire.com/art/wordsoflight.

Wrdsworth Edits (GBR) *(1-85326; 1-84022) Dist. by* **Combined Pub.**

Wrdswrth Communs, *(Wordsworth Comn. Serv.; 0-9643981),* P.O. Box 20202, Albuquerque, NM 87154-0202 Tel 505-296-4056.

Wright CA, *See* **IRFD**

Wright Pubg, *(Wright Publishing; 0-9675536),* P.O. Box 10095, Torrance, CA 90505 Tel 949-824-3760; Fax: 949-824-4015 Do not confuse with companies with the same name in New York, NY, West Seneca, NY, Virginia Beach, VA, Fayetteville, GA, Los Angeles, CA
E-mail: kwwright@uci.edu.

Wrightson Biomed (GBR) *(1-871816) Dist. by* **Taylor & Francis.**

Write Imprint of Write Stuff Syndicate

Write Prodns, *(Write Productions; 0-9657924),* P.O. Box 3533, South Attleboro, MA 02703-0058 Tel 401-724-7241; Fax: 401-724-5221.

Write Stuff Syndicate, *(Write Stuff Syndicate, Inc.; 0-945903),* 1001S. Andrew Ave., 2nd Flr., Fort Lauderdale, FL 33316 (SAN 248-0360) Tel 954-462-6657; Fax: 954-463-2220; Toll Free: 800-900-2665 ; *Imprints:* Write (Write Stuff)
E-mail: legends@writestuffbooks.com
Web site: http://www.writestuffbooks.com.

Writers & Readers, *(Writers & Readers Publishing, Inc.; 0-86316; 0-904613; 0-906386; 0-906495),* 457 Washington St., New York, NY 10013-1344 (SAN 665-813X) Tel 212-982-3158; Fax: 212-777-4924
Dist(s): **Publishers Group** *(Publishers Group West).*

Writers & Res, *(Writers & Research, Inc.; 0-9647035),* 4810 St. Paul Blvd., Rochester, NY 14617 Tel 716-266-4630; Fax: 716-544-1838.

Writers Inc, *(Writers' Inc.; 0-9627854),* 11240 Cherry Hill Rd., No. 302, Beltsville, MD 20705 Tel 301-937-3959; Fax: 301-937-1168 Do not confuse with Writer, Inc., Boston, MA
E-mail: writers_inc@mindspring.com
Web site: http://www.writersincusa.com.

Writers Wrld, *(Writer's World Pr.; 0-9631441),*
E-mail: writersworld@juno.com
Web site: http://www.writersworldpress.com
Dist(s): **Baker & Taylor** *(Baker & Taylor Bks.)*
Koen Bk Distributors *(Koen Bk. Distributors)*
Partners Pubs Grp *(Partners Pubs. Group, Inc.)*
Quality Bks IL *(Quality Bks., Inc.).*

Writeway Servs, *(Writeway Services; 0-9623117),* 25123 SE 146th St., Issaquah, WA 98027-3651 Tel 425-391-9605; Fax: 425-391-9606.

Wrld Bank, *(World Bank),* 1818 H St., NW, Washington, DC 20433 Tel 703-661-1580; Fax: 703-661-1501
E-mail: books@worldbank.org
Web site: http://www.worldbank.org.

Wrld Changing, *(World Changing Bks.; 0-9636589),* 489 Ocean View Dr., Hilo, HI 96720 Tel 808-934-7942 (phone/fax); Toll Free: 800-736-3922.

Wrld Chiropractic, *See* **Chiropractic Jrnl**

Wrld Hlth Pubns, *(World Health Pubns.; 0-9604268),* P.O. Box 408, Penryn, CA 95663 Tel 916-663-1661; Fax: 916-663-3657.

Wrld Tampa, *(World Pubns.; 0-911977),* P.O. Box 24339, Tampa, FL 33623 (SAN 276-9492) Tel 813-620-4517; Fax: 813-620-9096 Do not confuse with companies with similar names in Kingwood, TX, Winter Park, FL, North Dighton, MA.

Wrld-Wide Bks, *(World-Wide Bks.; 0-9614296),* 2027 Grand Canal Blvd., 20, Stockton, CA 95207 (SAN 687-4606) Tel 209-957-9601.

WrLock (GBR) *(0-7063) Dist. by* **Sterling.**

WRS Group, *(WRS Group, Inc.; 0-941539; 1-56796),* Orders Addr.: P.O. Box 21207, Waco, TX 76702-1207 (SAN 666-086X) Tel 254-776-6461; Fax: 254-776-0530; Toll Free: 800-299-3366; Edit Addr.: 5045 Franklin Ave., Waco, TX 76710 (SAN 666-0878)
E-mail: sales@wrsgroup.com
Web site: http://www.wrsgroup.com.

Wrtrs Digest Bks Imprint of F & W Pubns Inc

WSP Imprint of PB

WV Busn Pub, *(West Virginia Business Publishing Corp.; 0-937683),* Orders Addr.: P.O. Box 2521, Charleston, WV 25329-2521 (SAN 659-3666) Tel 304-345-8283; Fax: 304-342-5925; Edit Addr.: 1550 Kanawha Blvd., E., Charleston, WV 25311 (SAN 659-3674).

WV Soc Osteo Med, *(West Virginia Society of Osteopathic Medicine, Inc.; 0-9617546),* P.O. Box 5266, Charleston, WV 25361-0266 (SAN 664-4864) Tel 304-345-9836.

Wyatt Co, *(Wyatt Co.; 0-9630189),* 6707 Democracy Blvd., Suite 800, Bethesda, MD 20817-1129 Tel 301-581-4600; Fax: 301-581-4688.

Wyndham Hall, *(Wyndham Hall Pr.; 0-932269; 1-55605),* 5050 Kerr Rd., Lima, OH 45806 (SAN 686-6743) Tel 419-648-9124
E-mail: mark@wyndhamhallpress.com; whpbooks@wcoil.com
Web site: http://www.wyndhamhallpress.com.

WynnHart Pr, *(WynnHart Pr.; 0-9645035),* 6770 W Highway 89A, Unit 184, Sedona, AZ 86336-9505.

Wysteria Ltd, *(Wysteria, Ltd.; 0-9651162; 0-9677839),* Orders Addr.: P.O. Box 1250, Bellmore, NY 11710 Tel 516-377-9877; Fax: 516-867-3488; Toll Free: 888-997-8300; Edit Addr.: 55 N. Ocean Ave., Freeport, NY 11520
E-mail: Wysteria@Wysteria.com
Web site: http://www.Wysteria.com.

Xandex Pr, *(Xandex Pr., The; 1-888716),* Orders Addr.: P.O. Box 41103, Eagle Rock, CA 90041 Tel 323-441-9331 (phone/fax).

Xlibris Corp, *(Xlibris Corp.; 0-7388; 0-9663501; 1-4010),* 436 Walnut St., 11th Flr., Philadelphia, PA 19106 (SAN 299-5522) Tel 215-923-4686; Fax: 215-923-4685; Toll Free: 888-795-4274
E-mail: info@xlibris.com; orders@xlibris.com
Web site: http://www.xlibris.com
Dist(s): **Baker & Taylor** *(Baker & Taylor Bks.)*
BookWorld *(BookWorld Services, Inc.).*

Y M Fox, *(Fox, Yvonne Mart; 0-9643703),* 9454 Wilshire Blvd., Suite 650, Beverly Hills, CA 90212 Tel 323-934-9949; Fax: 323-935-7954.

Y Morris Carib, *(Morris, Yvon Carib Indian Publishing; 1-888139),* P.O. Box 236, Lemon Grove, CA 91946 Fax: 619-475-0058.

Y W DMD Med, *(Yale Wasserman DMD Medical Pubs., Ltd.; 1-881072),* 3036 S. 92nd St., West Allis, WI 53227 Tel 414-327-5545; Fax: 414-327-7777; Toll Free: 800-669-3337
Web site: http://www.NDAS.com.

†Yale U Pr, *(Yale Univ. Pr.; 0-300),* Orders Addr.: P.O. Box 209040, New Haven, CT 06520-9040 (SAN 203-2759) Tel 203-432-0940; Toll Free: 800-987-7323; Edit Addr.: 302 Temple St., New Haven, CT 06511 (SAN 203-2740) Tel 203-432-0960; Fax: 203-432-0948
E-mail: yupmkt@yale.edu
Web site: http://www.yale.edu/yup/index.html; http://www.yale.edu/yup/
Dist(s): **Cheng & Tsui** *(Cheng & Tsui Co.); CIP.*

Yehs Ctr Nat Med, *(Yeh's Ctr. of Natural Medicine, Inc.; 0-9652967),* 195 N. Second Ave., Upland, CA 91786 Tel 909-946-6444; Fax: 909-946-1099; Toll Free: 800-728-0187
E-mail: janet@yehcenter.com.

Yeoman Bks, *See* **Lagumo Corp**

Yes Intl, *See* **Yes Intl Pubs**

Yes Intl Pubs, *(Yes International Pubs.; 0-936663),* 1317 Summit Ave., Saint Paul, MN 55105-2602 (SAN 699-6787) Tel 651-645-6808; Fax: 651-645-0335
E-mail: yes@yespublishers.com
Web site: http://www.yespublishers.com
Dist(s): **Bookmen Inc** *(Bookmen, Inc.)*
Bookpeople *(Bookpeople)*
New Leaf Dist *(New Leaf Distributing Co., Inc.)*
Quality Bks IL *(Quality Bks., Inc.).*

Yes You Can Pr, *(Yes You Can Pr.; 1-878639),* P.O. Box 337, Desert Hot Springs, CA 92240 (SAN 297-3294) Tel 760-251-1103; Fax: 760-251-5064
E-mail: mandy@mandyevans.com
Web site: http://www.mandyevans.com
Dist(s): **Baker & Taylor** *(Baker & Taylor Bks.)*
Distributors *(Distributors, The).*

Yip Fun Li, *(Li, Yip Fun; 0-9649931),* Orders Addr.: P.O. Box 111, Monterey Park, CA 91754 Tel 626-573-8892; Edit Addr.: 3423 Twin Ave., Rosemead, CA 91770.

Yllw Brick Rd, *See* **Pitspopany**

YMAA Pubn, *(YMAA Pubn. Ctr.; 0-940871; 1-886969),* 4354 Washington St., Roslindale, MA 02131 (SAN 665-2077) Tel 617-323-7215; Fax: 617-323-7417; Toll Free: 800-669-8892
E-mail: ymaa@aol.com
Web site: http://www.ymaa.com
Dist(s): **Natl Bk Netwk** *(National Bk. Network).*

YMCA USA Imprint of Human Kinetics

Yng Ideas, *(Young Ideas; 0-9643420),* 7002 Bradford Dr., Amarillo, TX 79109-6496 Tel 806-353-8436; Fax: 806-354-2810; Toll Free: 800-213-2229.

Yo San Bks Imprint of SevenStar Comm

Yoga, *(Yoga Pubn. Society; 0-911662),* P.O. Box 600190, Jacksonville, FL 32260 (SAN 203-2724) Tel 904-287-0088
Dist(s): **DeVorss** *(DeVorss & Co.)*
New Leaf Dist *(New Leaf Distributing Co., Inc.).*

Yokibics, *(Yokibics, Inc.; 0-9635563),* P.O. Box 606, Oyster Bay, NY 11771-0606 (SAN 297-8393).

†York Pr, *(York Pr., Inc.; 0-912752),* P.O. Box 504, Timonium, MD 21094 (SAN 203-2708) Tel 410-560-1557; Fax: 410-560-6758; Toll Free: 800-962-2763
E-mail: info@yorkpress.com
Web site: http://www.yorkpress.com; *CIP.*

Young, *(Young, Thomas; 0-9614151),* P.O. Box 539, Bellaire, TX 77402 (SAN 686-418X) Tel 713-667-3356.

Youth Advocate, *(Youth Advocate Program International; 0-9663709),* Div. of National Youth Advocate Program, 4545 42nd St., NW Suite 209, Washington, DC 20016 Tel 202-244-1986; Fax: 202-244-6396
E-mail: yapi@igc.org
Web site: http://www.yapi.org.

Yuchi Pines, *See* **NLB**

Yuin Univ Pr, *(Yuin Univ. Pr.; 0-915649),* 2007 E. Compton Blvd., Compton, CA 90221 (SAN 292-742X) Tel 310-609-2704; Fax: 310-609-1415.

YWCA, *(Young Women's Christian Assn. of the U.S.A.; 1-878263),* 350 Fifth Ave., Suite 301, New York, NY 10118-0399 (SAN 207-9674) Tel 212-273-7800; Fax: 212-677-9716.

Z Hashemi, *(Hashemi, Zia; 0-9645956),* 1109 Yardley Ln., Wilmington, NC 28412-8428 Toll Free: 800-507-9376.

Zackback, *(Zackback International, Inc.; 0-9660169),* Orders Addr.: P.O. Box 9100, Rochester, MN 55903 Tel 507-252-9293; Fax: 507-252-5150; Toll Free: 800-748-8464; Edit Addr.: 1532 Tenth St., SE, Suite 10C, Rochester, MN 55904
E-mail: zmail@zackback.com
Web site: http://www.zackback.com.

Zahourek Systs, *(Zahourek Systems, Inc.; 1-887087),* 2198 W. 15th St., Loveland, CO 80538 Tel 303-667-9047; Fax: 303-667-5025.

Zanichelli (ITA) *(88-08) Dist. by* **IBD Ltd.**

Zanni Pubs, *(Zanni Pubs.; 0-9623475),* 5175 Montiel, Jamul, CA 92035 Tel 619-445-2415.

Zebra Kensgtn Imprint of Kensgtn Pub Corp

Zed Books (GBR) *(0-86232; 0-905762; 1-85649; 1-84277) Dist. by* **St Martin.**

Zeig Tucker, *See* **Zeig Tucker Theisen**

Zeig Tucker Theisen, *(Zeig, Tucker & Theisen, Inc.; 1-891944),* 3614 N. 24th St., Phoenix, AZ 85016 (SAN 254-0096) Tel 602-957-1270; Toll Free: 877-850-0442
E-mail: ZeigTucker@aol.com; jkzphd@aol.com
Web site: http://www.zeigtucker.com
Dist(s): **Tapeworm** *(Tapeworm Video Distributor, Inc.).*

Zephyr Med Enter, *(Zephyr Medical Enterprise; 0-9621879),* 5311 Aldea Ave., Encino, CA 91316 Tel 818-981-1300; Fax: 818-501-6639.

Zephyr Pub Corp, *(Zephyr Publishing Corp.; 0-9627099),* P.O. Box 3077, Minneapolis, MN 55337
Do not confuse with Zephyr Publishing in Glen Rock, NJ
Dist(s): **Baker & Taylor** *(Baker & Taylor Bks.)*
Bookmen Inc *(Bookmen, Inc.).*

Zephyr Pubns, *See* **Zephyr Pub Corp**

Zero Prods (GBR) *(1-898863) Dist. by* **Kazi Pubns.**

ZERO TO THREE, *(ZERO TO THREE:National Ctr. for Infants, Toddlers & Families; 0-943657),* 734 15th St. NW, Suite 1000, Washington, DC 20005-1013 (SAN 242-5084) Tel 202-638-1144; Fax: 202-638-0851; Toll Free: 800-899-4301
E-mail: n.guadagno@zerotothree.org
Web site: http://www.zerotothree.org.

Ziff-Davis Pr Imprint of Que

Zimmerman & Assocs, *See* **EagleBooks WI**

Zinn Pub Grp, *(Zinn Publishing Group; 0-87165; 0-935016),* Div. of Zinn Communications, Inc., 35-19 215th Pl., Bayside, NY 11361 (SAN 241-693X) Tel 718-428-6121; Fax: 718-428-2857
Dist(s): **Assoc Pubs Grp** *(Associated Pubs. Group)*
BookWorld *(BookWorld Services, Inc.)*
Empire Pub Srvs *(Empire Publishing Service).*

Zom Log, *(Zombie Logic Pr.; 0-9670191),* Orders Addr.: P.O. Box 319, Byron, IL 61010 Tel 815-234-5347; Edit Addr.: 420 E. Third St., Byron, IL 61010
E-mail: dobe1968@aol.com
Web site: http://members.aol.com/dobe1968/page/index.htm.

†Zondervan, *(Zondervan Publishing Hse.; 0-310; 0-937336),* Div. of HarperCollins Pubs., c/o Zondervan, Order Processing-B36, 5300 Patterson Ave., SE, Grand Rapids, MI 49530 (SAN 203-2694) Tel 616-698-6900; Fax: 616-698-3439; Toll Free Fax: 800-934-6381 (fax orders); Toll Free: 800-727-1309 (orders & customer service)
E-mail: zprod@zph.com
Web site: http://www.zondervan.com
Dist(s): **Baker & Taylor** *(Baker & Taylor Bks.)*
Christian Bk Distributors *(Christian Bk. Distributors)*
HarperCollins Pubs *(HarperCollins Pubs.)*
Spring Arbor Dist *(Spring Arbor Distributors Inc.); CIP.*

Zone Bks, *(Zone Bks.; 0-942299; 1-890951),* Div. of Urzone, Inc., 611 Broadway, Suite 608, New York, NY 10012 (SAN 666-864X) Tel 212-529-5674; Fax: 212-260-4572
E-mail: mitpress-orders@mit.edu; mitpress-order-inq@mit.edu; info@hup-mitpress.co.uk; cs-books@wiley.co.uk; urzone@aol.com
Dist(s): **MIT Pr** *(MIT Pr.).*

Zoological Educ, *(Zoological Education Network, Inc.; 0-9636996; 0-9706395),* Orders Addr.: P.O. Box 541749, Lake Worth, FL 33454-1749 Tel 561-641-6745; Fax: 561-641-0234; Toll Free: 800-981-4782; Edit Addr.: 5700 Lake Worth Rd., Suite 107, Lake Worth, FL 33463
E-mail: info@zen-inc.com
Web site: http://www.exoticdvm.com; http://www.zen-inc.com.

Zoological Soc, *(Zoological Society of San Diego; 0-911461),* Orders Addr.: P.O. Box 551, San Diego, CA 92112 (SAN 276-931X) Tel 619-231-1515; Fax: 619-231-0249; Edit Addr.: 2920 Zoo Dr., San Diego, CA 92101 Tel 619-557-3999; Fax: 619-557-3971.

Zorba Pr, *(Zorba Pr.; 0-927379),* 209 E. Jay St., Ithaca, NY 14850 (SAN 200-3740) Tel 607-277-9783
E-mail: info@ZorbaPress.com
Web site: http://www.zorbapress.com.

WHOLESALER & DISTRIBUTOR SYMBOL INDEX

A & M Church, *(A & M Church Supplies),* 220 E. Genesee Ave., Saginaw, MI 48607-1228 (SAN 157-0145) Tel 517-753-4672; Fax: 517-753-4799; Toll Free: 800-345-4694.

A B S Corp, *See* **Budgetext**

A C Hood, *(Hood, Alan C. & Co., Inc.; 0-911469),* P.O. Box 775, Chambersburg, PA 17201 (SAN 270-8221) Tel 717-267-0867; Fax: 717-267-0572.

A C Vroman, *(Vroman's, A. C.; 0-9639197),* 695 E. Colorado Blvd., Pasadena, CA 91101 (SAN 169-0027) Tel 626-449-5320; Fax: 626-792-7308.

A H A Inc, *(AHA, Inc.; 0-918545),* P.O. Box 8405, Santa Cruz, CA 95061-8405 (SAN 295-5059) Tel 408-458-9119.

A J Jannetti, *(Jannetti, Inc., Anthony J.),* E. Holly Ave., Box 56, Pitman, NJ 08071-0058 Tel 856-256-2300; Fax: 856-589-7463
E-mail: thomask@ajj.com
Web site: http://www.ajj.com.

A K J Bk Fare, *See* **AKJ Educ Servs**

AAHPERD, *(American Alliance for Health, Physical Education, Recreation & Dance; 0-88314),* Orders Addr.: P.O. Box 385, Oxon Hill, MD 20750-0385 (SAN 202-3237) Tel 301-839-9808; Fax: 301-567-9553; Toll Free: 800-321-0789; Edit Addr.: 1900 Association Dr., Reston, VA 22091 Toll Free: 800-213-7193
Web site: http://www.aahperd.org.

Abel Love Inc, *(Abel Love, Inc.),* Orders Addr.: P.O. Box 2250, Newport News, VA 23609 (SAN 158-4081) Tel 757-877-2939; Toll Free: 800-520-2939; Edit Addr.: 935 Lucas Creek Rd., Newport News, VA 23608 Fax: 804-877-2939.

Abingdon, *(Abingdon Pr.; 0-687),* Div. of United Methodist Publishing Hse., Orders Addr.: P.O. Box 801, Nashville, TN 37202-3919 (SAN 201-0054) Tel 615-749-6409; Fax: 615-749-6056; Toll Free Fax: 800-836-7802; Toll Free: 800-251-3320; Edit Addr.: 201 Eighth Ave., S., Nashville, TN 37202 (SAN 699-9956)
E-mail: info@abingdon.org
Web site: http://www.abingdon.org.

Abyss Dist, *(Abyss Distribution),* 48 Chester Rd., Middlefield, MA 012343-0078 (SAN 630-9925) Tel 413-623-2155; Fax: 413-623-2156
E-mail: AbyssDist@aol.com.

Acad Book, *(Academic Bk. Services, Inc.),* 5490 Fulton Industrial Blvd., Atlanta, GA 30336 (SAN 631-0591) Tel 404-344-8317; Fax: 404-349-2127.

Academic Bk Ctr Inc, *(Academic Bk. Ctr., Inc.),* 5600 NE Hassalo St., Portland, OR 97213-3640 (SAN 169-7145) Tel 503-287-6657; Fax: 503-284-8859; Toll Free: 800-547-7704
E-mail: orders@acbc.com
Web site: http://www.abc.com.

Academi-Text Medical Wholesalers, *(Academi-Text Medical Wholesalers),* 333 N. Superior, Toledo, OH 43604 (SAN 135-2415) Tel 419-255-9755; Fax: 419-255-9606; Toll Free: 800-552-8398 (out of state).

Act Prod Intl, *(Activity Products International),* P.O. Box 12476, Omaha, NE 68112-0476 (SAN 630-2025) Tel 402-457-3500; Fax: 402-457-3535; Toll Free: 800-541-9152
Web site: http://www.sapa.com/apl.com.

ACTA Pubns, *(ACTA Pubns.; 0-87946; 0-914070; 0-915388),* 4848 N. Clark St., Chicago, IL 60640-4711 (SAN 204-7489) Tel 773-271-1030; Fax: 773-271-7399; Toll Free Fax: 800-397-0079; Toll Free: 800-397-2282
E-mail: acta@one.org.

Action Products International Inc, *(Action Products International, Inc.),* 344 Cypress Rd., Ocala, FL 34472-3108 (SAN 630-8805) Tel 352-687-4961; Toll Free: 800-772-2846
E-mail: sales@apii.com.

Adams Bk Co Inc, *(Adams Bk. Co., Inc.),* 537 Sackett St., Brooklyn, NY 11217 (SAN 107-7171) Tel 718-875-5464; Fax: 718-852-3212; Toll Free: 800-221-0909
E-mail: sales@adamsbook.com
Web site: http://www.adamsbook.com.

Adams News, *(Adams News),* 1555 W. Galer St., Seattle, WA 98119 (SAN 169-8842) Tel 206-284-7617; Fax: 206-284-7599; Toll Free: 800-533-7617.

Addison-Wesley, *(Addison-Wesley Longman, Inc.; 0-201; 0-321; 0-582; 0-8053; 0-9654123),* Div. of Pearson Education Corp. Commun., Orders Addr.: 200 Old Tappan Rd., Old Tappan, NJ 07675 (SAN 299-4739) Toll Free: 800-922-0579; Edit Addr.: 75 Arlington St., Boston, MA 02116 (SAN 200-2000) Tel 617-848-6000; Toll Free: 800-447-2226
E-mail: pearsoned@eds.com; orderdeptnj@pearsoned.com
Web site: http://www.awl.com.

Adlers Foreign Bks, *(Adler's Foreign Bks., Inc.; 0-8417),* 915 Foster St., Evanston, IL 60201 (SAN 111-3089) Tel 847-864-0664; Fax: 847-864-0804; Toll Free: 800-235-3771
E-mail: info@afb-adlers.com
Web site: http://www.afb-adlers.com.

Advanced Global, *(Advanced Global Distribution Services),* 5880 Oberlin Dr., San Diego, CA 32121 Toll Free Fax: 800-499-3822; Toll Free: 800-284-3580.

Adventure Pubns, *(Adventure Pubns.; 0-934860; 1-885061),* Orders Addr.: P.O. Box 269, Cambridge, MN 55008 (SAN 212-7199) Tel 763-689-9800; Fax: 763-689-9039; Toll Free Fax: 877-725-0088; Toll Free: 800-678-7006.

Adventures Unltd, *(Adventures Unlimited Pr.; 0-932813; 0-908477; 1-931882),* Orders Addr.: P.O. Box 74, Kempton, IL 60946 (SAN 630-1126) Tel 815-253-6390; Fax: 815-253-6300; Edit Addr.: 303 Main St., Kempton, IL 60946 (SAN 250-3484)
E-mail: auphq@frontiernet.net
Web site: http://www.adventuresunlimitedpress.com; http://www.adventuresunlimited.co.nz.

Advertising Specialties Inc, *(Advertising Specialties, Inc.),* 4920 River Rd., Pascagoula, MS 39567 (SAN 108-6316) Tel 601-769-7904.

Affiliated Bk Distributor, *(Affiliated Bk. Distributor),* Div. of North Shore Distributors, Inc., 1200 N. Branch St., Chicago, IL 60622 (SAN 169-2267).

Afro-American Bk Distributor, *(Afro-American Bk. Distributor),* 2537 Prospect, Houston, TX 77004 (SAN 169-8257).

AgeAdvantAge, *See* **Rom Dance Ntwrk**

Agritech Pub, *(Agritech Publishing Group, Inc.),* Div. of Agritech Corp., 95 Court St., Units A&B, Exeter, NH 03833-2621 (SAN 174-612X) Tel 603-773-9823.

Aha Punana Leo, *(Aha Punana Leo; 0-9645646; 1-58191; 1-890270),* 928 Nuuanu Ave., No. 403, Honolulu, HI 96817 Tel 808-523-3992; Fax: 808-523-8158
E-mail: haawina@leoki.uhh.hawaii.edu
Web site: http://www.ahapunanaleo.org.

AIDC, *(AIDC),* 50 Winter Sport Ln., Williston, VT 05495 Tel 802-862-0095; Fax: 802-864-4672-; Toll Free: 800-488-2665.

AIMS Intl, *(AIMS International Bks., Inc.; 0-922852),* 7709 Hamilton Ave., Cincinnati, OH 45231-3103 (SAN 630-270X) Tel 513-521-5590; Fax: 513-521-5592; Toll Free: 800-733-2067
E-mail: aimsbooks@juno.com.

A-K News Co, *See* **Aramark Magazine**

AK Pr Dist, *(AK Pr. Distribution; 1-873176; 1-902593),* 674 A 23rd St., Oakland, CA 94612-1163 (SAN 298-2234) Tel 510-208-1700; Fax: 510-208-1701
E-mail: orders@akpress.org; akpress@akpress.org
Web site: http://www.akpress.org.

AKJ Educ Servs, *(AKJ Educational Services, Inc.),* 5609-2A Fishers Ln., Rockville, MD 20852 (SAN 170-5431) Tel 301-770-4030; Fax: 301-770-2338; Toll Free: 800-770-2338
E-mail: info@akjedsvcs.com
Web site: http://www.akjedsvcs.com.

Alabama Bk Store, *(Alabama Bk. Store),* Orders Addr.: P.O. Box 1279, Tuscaloosa, AL 35401-1626 Tel 205-758-4532; Fax: 205-758-5525; Toll Free: 800-382-2665 (orders only); Edit Addr.: 1015 University Blvd., Tuscaloosa, AL 35403-1279 (SAN 100-0063)
E-mail: ABS@AlabamaBook.com
Web site: http://www.AlabamaBook.com.

Alamo Sq Dist, *(Alamo Square Distributors),* P.O. Box 14543, San Francisco, CA 94114 (SAN 298-1289) Tel 415-863-7410; Fax: 415-863-7456
E-mail: alamosqdist@earthlink.net.

Alba, *(Alba Hse.; 0-8189),* Div. of Society of St. Paul, 2187 Victory Blvd., Staten Island, NY 10314-6603 (SAN 201-2405) Tel 718-761-0047; Fax: 718-761-0057; 718-698-8390; Toll Free: 800-343-2522
E-mail: albabooks@aol.com
Web site: http://www.albahouse.org.

Aletheia, *(Aletheia Pubns., Inc.; 0-9639260; 1-929129),* 46 Bell Hollow Rd., Putnam Valley, NY 10579 Tel 914-526-2873; Fax: 914-526-2905
E-mail: alethpub@aol.com
Web site: http://members.aol.com/alethpub.

Alexander Graham, *(Bell, Alexander Graham Assn. for the Deaf; 0-88200),* 3417 Volta Pl., NW, Washington, DC 20007 (SAN 203-6924) Tel 202-337-5220; Fax: 202-337-8270
Web site: http://wwww.agbell.org.

Alfonsi Enterprises, *(Alfonsi Enterprises),* 8621 Gavinton Ct., Dublin, OH 43017-9615 (SAN 169-4227).

Alimed, *(Alimed, Inc.),* 297 High St., Dedham, MA 02026 (SAN 631-5054) Tel 617-329-2900; Fax: 617-329-8392.

Alive Bks, *(Alive Bks.; 0-920470),* Div. of Canadian Health Reform Products, Ltd., 8110-357 250 H St., Blaine, WA 98230 Tel 604-435-1919; Fax: 604-435-4888; Toll Free: 800-663-6513
E-mail: orders@lalivebooks.com.

All Am Dist Corp, *(All America Distributors Corp.),* 8431 Melrose Pl., Los Angeles, CA 90069-5382 (SAN 168-972X) Tel 213-651-2650; Fax: 213-655-9452
E-mail: psi@loop.com.

All You Knead, *(All You Knead),* 1518 Broadway, Seattle, WA 98122 Tel 206-328-3412; Fax: 206-328-3453; Toll Free Fax: 800-952-5375
Web site: http://www.allyouknead.com.

Allentown News Agency Inc, *(Allentown News Agency, Inc.),* Orders Addr.: P.O. Box 446, Allentown, PA 18105; Edit Addr.: 719-723 Liberty St., Allentown, PA 18105 (SAN 169-7226) Tel 610-432-4441; Fax: 610-432-2708.

Alliance Bk Co, *(Alliance Bk. Co.),* 5045 Southland Dr., Woodstock, GA 30188 Tel 770-592-0770; Fax: 770-592-6083; Toll Free: 877-767-0057
E-mail: alliancebk@mindspring.com.

Allnce Hse, *(Alliance Hse., Inc.; 0-9665234),* 220 Ferris Ave., Suite 201, White Plains, NY 10603 Tel 914-328-5456; Fax: 914-946-1929
E-mail: alliancehs@aol.com.

Alonso Bk & Periodical Services, *(Alonso Bk. & Periodical Services, Inc.),* 7670 Richmond Hwy., Alexandria, VA 22306 (SAN 170-7035) Tel 703-765-1211.

Alpenbooks, *(Alpenbooks; 0-9669795),* 3616 South Rd., C-1, Mukilteo, WA 98275 (SAN 113-5309) Tel 425-290-8587; Fax: 425-290-9461; Toll Free: 800-290-9898
E-mail: cserve@alpenbooks.com
Web site: http://www.alpenbooks.com.

Alph & Omga Dist, *(Alpha & Omega Distributor),* P.O. Box 36640, Colorado Springs, CO 80936-3664 (SAN 169-0515).

Alpine News Distributors, *(Alpine News Distributors),* Div. of Mountain States Distributors, 0105 Marand Rd., Glenwood Springs, CO 81601 (SAN 159-6462) Tel 970-945-2269; Fax: 970-945-2260.

Am Assn Mental, *(American Assn. on Mental Retardation; 0-940898),* 444 N. Capitol St. NW, Suite 846, Washington, DC 20001 (SAN 206-961X) Tel 202-387-1968; Fax: 202-387-2193; Toll Free: 800-424-3688
E-mail: aamn@pmds.com
Web site: http://www.aamr.org.

Am Buddhist Shim Do, *(American Buddhist Shim Gum Do Assn., Inc.; 0-9614427),* 203 Chestnut Hill Ave., Brighton, MA 02135 (SAN 113-2873) Tel 617-787-1506; Fax: 617-787-2708
E-mail: marystackhouse@shimgumdo.org
Web site: http://www.shimgumdo.org.

Am Busn Syst, *(American Business Systems, Inc.),* 315 Littleton Rd., Chelmsford, MA 01824 (SAN 264-8229) Tel 508-250-9600; Fax: 508-250-8027; Toll Free: 800-356-4034.

Am Camping, *(American Camping Assn.; 0-87603),* 5000 State Rd. 67, N., Martinsville, IN 46151-7902 (SAN 201-2596) Tel 765-342-8456 (General Info.); Fax: 765-349-6357 (orders); Toll Free: 800-428-2267 (orders)
E-mail: bookstore@aca-camps.org
Web site: http://www.acacamps.org.

Am Educ Comp, *See* **Am Education**

Am Educ Systs, *(American Educational Systems),* Div. of Book Clearing House, 46 Purdy St., Harrison, NY 10528 (SAN 631-0109) Tel 914-835-0015; Fax: 914-835-0398; Toll Free: 800-431-1579
E-mail: bookch@aol.com.

Am Education, *(American Education Corp., The; 0-87570; 1-58636),* 7506 N. Broadway, Suite 505, Oklahoma City, OK 73116-9016 (SAN 654-6250) Tel 405-840-6031; Fax: 405-848-3960; Toll Free: 800-222-2811
Web site: http://www.amered.com.

Am Health Consults, *(American Health Consultants; 0-9603332; 1-931107),* Subs. of Medical Economics, 3525 Piedmont Rd., NE, Bldg. 6, Suite 400, Atlanta, GA 30305 (SAN 222-2655) Tel 404-262-7447; Fax: 404-262-5475; Toll Free: 800-559-1032
Web site: http://www.ahcpub.com.

Am Intl Dist, *(American International Distribution Corp.),* Orders Addr.: P.O. Box 80, Williston, VT 05495-0020 Tel 802-862-0095 (Ext. 115); Fax: 802-864-7749; Toll Free: 800-426-4742; Edit Addr.: 50 Winter Sport Ln., Williston, VT 05495 (SAN 630-2238) Toll Free: 800-488-2665.

Am Nurses Pub, *(American Nurses Publishing; 1-55810),* Orders Addr.: 1650 Blugrass Lakes Pkwy., Alpharetta, GA 30004 Fax: 770-442-9742; Toll Free: 800-637-0323; Edit Addr.: 600 Maryland Ave. SW, Suite 100 W., Washington, DC 20024-2571 (SAN 204-5176) Tel 202-651-7212; Fax: 202-651-7003; Toll Free: 800-274-4262
E-mail: ancc@ana.org
Web site: http://www.nursingworld.org; http://www.nursesbooks.org.

Am Overseas Bk Co, *(American Overseas Bk. Co., Inc.),* 550 Walnut St., Norwood, NJ 07648 (SAN 169-4863) Tel 201-767-7600; Fax: 201-784-0263
E-mail: books@aobc.com
Web site: http://www.aobc.com.

Am Pharm Assn, *(American Pharmaceutical Assn.; 0-914768; 0-917330; 1-58212),* 2215 Constitution Ave., NW, Washington, DC 20037 (SAN 202-4446) Tel 202-628-4410; Fax: 202-783-2351; Toll Free: 800-878-0729
E-mail: webmaster@mail.aphanet.org
Web site: http://www.aphanet.org.

Am Psychiatric, *(American Psychiatric Pr., Inc.; 0-88048; 0-89042; 1-882103; 1-58562),* Div of The American Psychiatric Publishing Group, Inc., 1400 K St., NW, 11th Flr., Washington, DC 20005 (SAN 293-2288) Tel 202-682-6262; Fax: 202-789-2648 (orders only); 202-682-6341; Toll Free: 800-368-5777 (orders only)
Web site: http://www.appi.org.

Am Soc Agron, *(American Society of Agronomy; 0-89118),* 677 S. Segoe Rd., Madison, WI 53711-1086 (SAN 107-5683) Tel 608-273-8080; Fax: 608-273-2021
Web site: http://www.agronomy.org.

Am Soc Civil Eng, *(American Society of Civil Engineers; 0-7844; 0-87262),* 1801 Alexander Bell Dr., Reston, VA 20191-4400 (SAN 204-7594) Tel 703-295-6300; Fax: 703-295-6211; Toll Free: 800-548-2723
E-mail: marketing@asce.org
Web site: http://www.pubs.asce.org.

Amarillo Periodical Distributors, *(Amarillo Periodical Distributors),* P.O. Box 3823, Lubbock, TX 70404 (SAN 156-4986) Tel 806-745-6000.

Amazon Com, *(Amazon.Com; 1-58060),* Orders Addr.: P.O. Box 80387, Seattle, WA 98108-0387 (SAN 156-143X) Tel 206-622-2335; Fax: 206-622-2405; 1 Centerpoint Blvd., non-carton, New Castle, DE 19720 (SAN 155-3992); 1 Centerpoint Blvd., carton, New Castle, DE 19720 (SAN 156-1405); 520 S. Brandon, non-carton, Seattle, WA 98108 (SAN 152-6642); 520 S. Brandon, carton, Seattle, WA 98108 (SAN 156-1383); 1600 E. Newlands Dr., carton, Fernley, NV 89408 (SAN 156-5982); 1600 E. Newlands Dr., non-carton, Fernley, NV 89408 (SAN 156-6008); Edit Addr.: 520 Pike St., Seattle, WA 98101 (SAN 155-3984); P.O. Box 81226, Seattle, WA 98108-1226
E-mail: catalog-dept@amazon.com
Web site: http://www.amazon.com.

Ambassador Bk Service, *See* **Ambassador Bks & Media**

Ambassador Bks & Media, *(Ambassador Bks. & Media),* 42 Chasner St., Hempstead, NY 11550 (SAN 120-064X) Tel 516-489-4011; Fax: 516-489-5661; Toll Free: 800-431-8913
E-mail: ambassador@absbook.com
Web site: http://www.absbook.com.

Ambulatory Innovat, *(Ambulatory Innovations, Inc.),* 6455 Dover Rd., Indianapolis, IN 46220 Fax: 317-255-4399; Toll Free: 800-367-9180.

AMC Books, *(Appalachian Mountain Club Bks.; 0-910146; 1-878239; 1-929173),* 5 Joy St., Boston, MA 02108 (SAN 203-4808) Tel 617-523-0636; 617-523-0655; Fax: 617-523-0722; Toll Free: 800-262-4455
E-mail: bdesher@amcinfo.org
Web site: http://www.outdoors.org.

Amer Mktg Pub, *See* **Chrstian Pub Netwrk**

Amer West Books, *(American West Bks.),* 8386 N. Madsen Ave., Clovis, CA 93611 (SAN 630-8570) Tel 209-322-5917; Fax: 209-322-5967; Toll Free: 800-497-4909 Do not confuse with American West Bks., Albuquerque, NM
E-mail: JBM12@CSUFresno.edu.

American Econo, *(American Econo Clad),* Orders Addr.: P.O. Box 1777, Topeka, KS 66601; Edit Addr.: 2101 N. Topeka Blvd., Topeka, KS 66601.

American Kennel, *(American Kennel Club Museum of the Dog; 0-9615072),* 1721 S. Mason Rd., Saint Louis, MO 63131 (SAN 110-8751) Tel 314-821-3647; Fax: 314-821-7381.

American Micro Media, *(American Micro Media),* 19 N. Broadway, Box 306, Red Hook, NY 12571 (SAN 653-9920) Tel 914-758-5567.

Americana Souvenirs & Gifts, *(Americana Souvenirs & Gifts; 1-890541),* 302 York St., Gettysburg, PA 17325-1996 (SAN 169-7366) Tel 717-334-6251; Fax: 717-334-9174; Toll Free: 800-692-7436.

Americas Hobby Ctr, *(America's Hobby Ctr.),* 146 W. 22nd St., New York, NY 10011 (SAN 111-0403) Tel 212-675-8922.

Ames News Agency Inc, *(Ames News Agency, Inc.),* 2110 E. 13th St., Ames, IA 50010 (SAN 169-2550).

AMG Pubs, *(AMG Pubs.; 0-89957),* Subs. of CLW Communications Group, Inc., Orders Addr.: P.O. Box 22000, Chattanooga, TN 37422 Tel 423-894-6060; Fax: 423-894-9511; Toll Free Fax: 800-265-6690; Toll Free: 800-266-4977; Edit Addr.: 6815 Shallowford Rd., Chattanooga, TN 37421 (SAN 211-3074) Toll Free Fax: 800-395-2682
E-mail: sales@AMGpublishers.com; info@amgpublishers.com
Web site: http://www.amgpublishers.com; http://www.followinggod.com.

Amoskeag News, *(Amoskeag News Agency),* 92 Allard Dr., Manchester, NH 03102 (SAN 169-4537) Tel 603-623-5343.

AMP Distrib, *(AMP Distributors),* Deerfield Rd., P.O. Box 205, Whippany, NJ 07981 Fax: 973-597-1637.

Amrcns Snd AIDS, *(Americans for a Sound A I D S/H I V Policy; 0-9629009),* Orders Addr.: P.O. Box 17433, Washington, DC 20041 (SAN 630-5075) Fax: 703-471-8409; Edit Addr.: 905 Monroe St., Herndon, VA 22070 Tel 703-471-7350.

AMS Pr, *(AMS Pr., Inc.; 0-404),* 56 E. 13th St., New York, NY 10003-4686 (SAN 106-6706) Tel 212-777-4700; Fax: 212-995-5413 Do not confuse with companies with the same or similar name in Los Angeles, CA, Pittsburgh, PA
E-mail: amserve@earthlink.net.

ANA, *See* **Am Nurses Pub**

Anchor Distributors, *(Anchor Distributors),* 30 Hunt Valley Cir., New Kensington, PA 15068 (SAN 631-077X) Tel 724-334-7000; Fax: 724-334-1200; Toll Free: 800-444-4484
E-mail: marketing@whitakerhouse.com.

Anchor Point, *(Anchor Point Assocs.),* 259 S. 500 E., Salt Lake City, UT 84102-2017 Tel 801-534-1022.

Ancient Healing, *(Ancient Healing Ways),* P.O. Box 130, Espanola, NM 87532 Fax: 505-747-9718; Toll Free: 877-753-5351.

Ander-Austin News, *(Anderson/Austin News Co., LLC),* P.O. Box E, Johnson City, IL 62951-0184 (SAN 169-8036).

Andersn News, *See* **H Kopplemann**

Anderson News Co, *(Anderson News Co.),* 4415 Industrial Dr., P.O. Box 7337, Roanoke, VA 24019 (SAN 168-9223) Tel 540-992-5356; Fax: 540-992-5093; 6355 N. Palafox St., Pensacola, FL 32503 (SAN 168-9363) Tel 904-477-0920; 2541 Westcott Blvd., Knoxville, TN 37931 (SAN 169-7927) Tel 423-966-7575; 3945 Volunteer Dr., Chattanooga, TN 37416 (SAN 169-7862) Tel 423-894-3945; 6301 Forbing Rd., Little Rock, AR 72219 (SAN 106-956X) Tel 501-562-7360; 3777 Hartsfield Rd., Tallahassee, FL 32303 (SAN 169-1309) Tel 904-575-8070; 1857 W. Grant, P.O. Box 5465, Tucson, AZ 85705 (SAN 168-9401) Tel 520-622-2831; 125 Regional Park Dr., Kingsport, TN 37660 (SAN 241-6131) Tel 423-349-7145; 390 Exchange St., Box 1624, New Haven, CT 06506 (SAN 241-6158) Tel 203-777-5545; 5000 Moline St., Denver, CO 80239-2622 (SAN 169-0523) Tel 303-321-1111; 1709 N. East St., Flagstaff, AZ 86002 (SAN 168-9290) Tel 520-774-6171; Fax: 520-779-1958; 4935 Covington Way, Memphis, TN 38128 (SAN 169-7943); P.O. Box 22968, Chattanooga, TN 37422; P.O. Box 36003, Knoxville, TN 37930-6003; P.O. Box 280077, Memphis, TN 38168-0077; P.O. Box 6660, Pensacola, FL 32503.

Anderson Stephen, *(Anderson Stephen News Co., LLC),* 1919 Garfield Ave., Parkersburg, WV 26101 (SAN 169-9008) Tel 304-428-1441; Fax: 304-428-2190.

Anderson-Austin, *(Anderson-Austin News Co., LLC),* 808 Newtown Cir., No. B, Lexington, KY 40511-1230 (SAN 169-2836) Tel 606-254-2765; Fax: 606-254-3328.

Anderson-Stephan, *(Anderson/Stephan News Co.),* P.O. Box 487, Scott Depot, WV 25560 (SAN 169-8923) Tel 304-757-8831; Fax: 304-757-8833; Toll Free: 800-344-5680.

Andrews McMeel, *(Andrews McMeel Publishing; 0-8362; 0-7407),* Div. of Andrews McMeel Universal Co., Orders Addr.: P.O. Box 419150, Kansas City, MO 64141; Edit Addr.: 4520 Main St., Kansas City, MO 64111 (SAN 202-540X) Tel 816-932-6600; Fax: 816-932-6749; Toll Free Fax: 800-437-8683; Toll Free: 800-826-4216
E-mail: marketplace@uexpress.com
Web site: http://www.uexpress.com/corporate/amp/; http://www.AndrewsMcMeel.com.

Andrsn News Tacoma, *(Anderson News - Tacoma),* 9914 32nd Ave., S., Lakewood, WA 98499 (SAN 108-1322) Tel 253-581-1940; Fax: 253-584-5941; Toll Free: 800-552-2000 (in Washington).

Andrson News, *(Anderson News - Orlando Bk. Annex),* 3840 Vineland Rd., Orlando, FL 32811-6427 (SAN 169-1201) Tel 407-841-8738; Fax: 407-839-4043; Toll Free: 800-338-3988.

Andrzejewskis MCS, *See* **A & M Church**

Angelas Bkshelf, *(Angela's Bookshelf; 1-881545),* 3039 S. Bagley, Ithaca, MI 48847 Tel 517-875-4985; Fax: 517-875-4988; Toll Free: 800-882-6443.

Angeles Mart, *(Los Angeles Mart, The),* 1933 S. Broadway, Suite 665, Los Angeles, CA 90007 (SAN 168-9797) Tel 213-748-6449; Fax: 714-523-0796.

answers period, *(answers period, inc.; 0-917875),* Orders Addr.: P.O. Box 427, Goliad, TX 77963 (SAN 112-6431) Tel 361-645-2268; Toll Free: 800-852-4752
Web site: http://www.answersbook.com.

Antex Data, *(Antex Data Systems; 0-925340),* Div. of International Antex, Inc., 1380 Borregas Ave., Sunnyvale, CA 94089-1004 (SAN 652-866X).

Anthroposophic, *(Anthroposophic Pr., Inc.; 0-8334; 0-88010; 0-89345; 0-910142; 1-58420; 1-85584; 0-9701097),* Orders Addr.: P.O. Box 960, Herndon, VA 20172-0960 Tel 703-661-1594 (orders); Fax: 702-661-1501; Toll Free Fax: 800-277-7947 (orders); Toll Free: 800-856-8664 (orders); Edit Addr.: P.O. Box 799, Great Barrington, MA 01230 Tel 413-528-8233; Fax: 413-528-8826; Fulfillment Addr.: 22883 Quicksilver Dr., Dulles, VA 20166 (SAN 253-9519) Tel 703-661-1529; Fax: 703-996-1010
E-mail: service@anthropress.org
Web site: http://www.lindisfarne.org; http://www.bellpondbooks.com; http://www.anthropress.org.

Antipodes Bks, *(Antipodes Bks. & Beyond),* 9707 Fairway Ave., Silver Spring, MD 20901-3001 Tel 301-602-9519; Fax: 301-565-0160
E-mail: Antipode@antipodesbooks.com
Web site: http://www.antipodesbooks.com.

Antiquarian Bookstore, *(Antiquarian Bookstore, The),* 1070 Lafayette Rd., Portsmouth, NH 03801 (SAN 158-9938) Tel 603-436-7250.

Antique Collect, *(Antique Collectors' Club; 0-902028; 0-907462; 1-85149),* 91 Market Street Industrial Park, Wappingers Falls, NY 12590; Market Street Industrial Park, Wappinger's Falls, NY 12590; Orders Addr.: 91 Market St. Industrial Park, Wappingers Falls, NY 12590 (SAN 630-7787) Tel 845-297-0003; Fax: 845-297-0068; Toll Free: 800-252-5231 (orders)
E-mail: info@antiquecc.com
Web site: http://www.antiquecc.com; http://www.antiquecc.com.

AOAC Intl, *(AOAC International; 0-935584),* 481 N. Frederick Ave. Suite 500, Gaithersburg, MD 20877-2417 (SAN 260-3411) Tel 301-924-7077; Fax: 301-924-7089; Toll Free: 800-379-2622
E-mail: aoac@aoac.org
Web site: http://www.aoac.org.

AOL Time Warner, *(AOL Time Warner Bk. Group; 0-446),* 1271 Avenue of the Americas, New York, NY 10020 Tel 212-522-7381; Fax: 800-222-6902; Toll Free: 800-222-6747.

A-One Bk Distributors Inc, *(A-One Bk. Distributors, Inc.),* 2100-4 Arctic Ave., Bohemia, NY 11716-2430 (SAN 630-7981) Tel 516-589-3377; Fax: 516-589-9161.

APG Trade, *(APG Trade West),* 1501 County Hospital Rd., Nashville, TN 37218-2501.

Apollo, *(Apollo Bks.; 0-938290),* 91 Market St., Wappingers Falls, NY 12590-2333 (SAN 170-0928).

Apollo Library Bk Supplier, *(Apollo Library Bk. Supplier),* 865 Kent Ln., Philadelphia, PA 19115 (SAN 159-8031).

Appalach Bk Dist, *(Appalachian Bk. Distributors),* Orders Addr.: 522 Princeton Rd., Johnson City, TN 37601 (SAN 630-7388) Tel 423-282-9475; Fax: 423-282-9110; Toll Free: 800-759-2779; Edit Addr.: 506 Princeton Rd., Johnson City, TN 37601.

Appalachian Bible, *(Appalachian Bible Co.; 1-889049),* Orders Addr.: 522 Princeton Rd., Johnson City, TN 37605 (SAN 169-7889) Tel 423-282-9475; Fax: 423-282-9110; Toll Free: 800-289-2772; Edit Addr.: P.O. Box 1573, Johnson City, TN 37601
E-mail: appainc@aol.com.

Appalachian Inc, *See* **Appalachian Bible**

Apple Bk Co, *(Apple Bk. Co.),* Div. of Scholastic Bk. Fairs, Inc., P.O. Box 217156, Charlotte, NC 28221-0156 Tel 704-596-6641; Fax: 704-599-1738; Toll Free: 800-331-1993; 5901 N. Northwoods Busn. Pkwy., Charlotte, NC 28269 (SAN 108-4569).

ARA Services Inc, *(ARA Services, Magazine & Bk. Div.; 0-9620756),* 1333 30th St., Suite D, San Diego, CA 92154-3404 (SAN 200-7401) Tel 619-275-3090; 16150 W. Lincoln, New Berlin, WI 53151 (SAN 200-8327) Tel 414-786-5650; P.O. Box 2399, Yakima, WA 98907 (SAN 169-8893) Tel 509-248-7810; P.O. Box 4067, Spokane, WA 99202 (SAN 169-8850); 7000 N. Robinson, Oklahoma City, OK 73125 (SAN 281-2827) Tel 405-843-9383; 909 W. 23rd St., Tulsa, OK 74107 (SAN 169-7013); P.O. Box 25489, Oklahoma City, OK 73125 (SAN 249-2709); P.O. Box 448, Brainerd, MN 56401 (SAN 169-4049).

Arabic & Islamic Univ Pr, *(Arabic & Islamic Univ. Pr.),* 4283 Fountain Ave., Los Angeles, CA 90029 (SAN 107-6299) Tel 213-665-1000; Fax: 213-665-3107.

Aramark Mag & Bk Servs, *(Aramark Magazine & Bk. Services, Inc.),* Box 2240, Norfolk, VA 23501 (SAN 169-8680) Do not confuse with Aramark Magazine & Book Co., Oklahoma City, OK.

Aramark Magazine, *(Aramark Magazine & Bk. Co.),* P.O. Box 25489, Oklahoma City, OK 73125 (SAN 169-6971) Tel 405-843-9383; Fax: 405-843-0379 Do not confuse with Aramark Magazine & Bk. Services, Inc., Norfolk, VA.

Aramark WA, *(Aramark),* 18825 67th Ave., NE, Arlington, WA 98223-9656 (SAN 631-3507) Tel 360-435-2524; Fax: 360-435-6805 Do not confuse with Aramark, Albuquerque, NM.

Arbit, *(Arbit Bks., Inc.; 0-930038),* 8050 N. Port Washington Rd., Milwaukee, WI 53217 (SAN 169-913X) Tel 414-352-4404.

Ardic Bk Distributors Inc, *(Ardic Bk. Distributors, Inc.),* 331 High St., 2nd Flr., Burlington, NJ 08016-4411 (SAN 170-5415).

Argus International Corp, *(Argus International Corp.),* Subs. of ICS International Group, Skypark Business Pk., P.O. Box 4082, Irvine, CA 92716-4082 (SAN 681-9761) Tel 714-552-8494 (phone/fax).

Aries Pr, *(Aries Pr.; 0-933646),* P.O. Box 30081, Chicago, IL 60630 (SAN 111-9168) Tel 312-725-8300.

Aries Prod, *(Aries Productions, Inc.; 0-910035),* Orders Addr.: P.O. Box 29396, Sappington, MO 63126 (SAN 669-0009); Edit Addr.: 9633 Cinnabar Dr., Sappington, MO 63126 (SAN 241-2004) Tel 314-849-3722
E-mail: uspsisquad@aol.com
Web site: http://ww.ussisquad.com.

Arizona Periodicals Inc, *(Arizona Periodicals, Inc.),* P.O. Box 5780, Yuma, AZ 85366-5780 (SAN 168-941X) Tel 520-782-1822.

Arkansas Bk Co, *(Arkansas Bk. Co.),* 1207 E. Second St., Little Rock, AR 72202-2732 (SAN 168-9460) Tel 501-375-1184.

Arlington Card Co Bk Dept, *(Arlington Card Co., Bk. Dept.),* 140 Gansett Ave., Cranston, RI 02910 (SAN 108-5794) Tel 401-942-3188.

Arrowhead Magazine Co Inc, *(Arrowhead Magazine Co., Inc.),* P.O. Box 5947, San Bernardino, CA 92412 (SAN 169-0094) Tel 909-799-8294; Fax: 909-799-3774; 1055 Cooley Ave., San Bernardino, CA 92408 (SAN 249-2717) Tel 909-370-4420.

Ars Obscura, *(Ars Obscura; 0-9623780),* P.O. Box 4424, Seattle, WA 98104-0424 (SAN 113-5368) Tel 206-324-9792.

Art Inst Chi, *(Art Institute of Chicago; 0-86559),* Orders Addr.: a/o Museum Shop Mail Order Dept., 1224 W. Van Buren, 3rd Flr., Chicago, IL 60607 Tel 312-563-5150; Fax: 312-563-1973 (attn: Museum Shop); Edit Addr.: 111 S. Michigan Ave., Chicago, IL 60603-6110 (SAN 204-479X) Tel 312-443-3540; Fax: 312-443-1334
Web site: http://www.artic.edu.

Artisoft, *(Artisoft, Inc.; 0-927538),* 1 S. Church Ave., Suite 2200, Tucson, AZ 85745 (SAN 287-458X) Tel 520-670-7100; Fax: 520-670-7101; Toll Free: 800-233-5564.

ARVEST, *(ARVEST),* P.O. Box 200248, Denver, CO 80220 (SAN 159-8694) Tel 303-388-8486; Fax: 303-355-4213; Toll Free: 800-739-0761
E-mail: copy@concentric.net.

Ashgate Pub Co, *(Ashgate Publishing Co.; 0-566),* Subs. of Ashgate Publishing, Ltd., Orders Addr.: 2252 Ridge Rd., Brookfield, VT 05036-9704 Tel 802-276-3162; Fax: 802-276-3837; Toll Free: 800-535-9544 (Orders - US & Canada); Edit Addr.: 131 Main St., Burlington, VT 05401-5600 (SAN 213-4446) Tel 802-865-7641; Fax: 802-865-7847; Toll Free: 800-535-9544 (US & Canada)
E-mail: editor@ashgate.com; orders@ashgate.com
Web site: http://www.ashgatechem.com; http://www.gowerpub.com; http://www.gowertraining.co.uk/; http://www.ashgate.com.

Asia Bk Corp, *(Asia Bk. Corp. of America; 0-940500),* 45-77 157th St., Flushing, NY 11355 (SAN 214-493X) Tel 718-762-7204; Fax: 718-460-5030.

ASM, *(ASM International; 0-87170),* 9639 Kinsman Rd., Materials Park, OH 44073-0002 (SAN 204-7586) Tel 440-338-5151; Fax: 440-338-4634; Toll Free: 800-336-5152 (ext. 5900) Do not confuse with ASM International, Inc., Fort Lauderdale, FL
E-mail: Cust-Srv@asminternational.org
Web site: http://www.asminternational.org/.

Aspen Pub, *(Aspen Pubs., Inc.; 0-444; 0-7896; 0-8342; 0-87189; 0-87622; 0-89443; 0-912862),* Subs. of Wolters Kluwer U.S. Corp., 200 Orchard Ridge Dr., Suite 200, Gaithersburg, MD 20878 (SAN 203-4999) Tel 301-417-7500; Fax: 301-695-7931; Toll Free: 800-638-8437 (orders); 800-234-1660 (customer service)
E-mail: customer.service@aspenpubl.com
Web site: http://www.aspenpub.com.

Aspen West Pub, *(Aspen West Publishing; 0-9615390; 1-885348),* 8535 S. 700 W., Unit C, Sandy, UT 84070 (SAN 112-7993) Tel 801-565-1370; Fax: 801-565-1373; Toll Free: 800-222-9133 (orders only)
E-mail: kent@aspenwest.com
Web site: http://www.aspenwest.com.

Assn Energy Eng, *(Association of Energy Engineers),* Orders Addr.: P.O. Box 1026, Liburn, GA 30048 Tel 770-925-9558; Fax: 770-381-9865; Edit Addr.: 4025 Pleasantdale Rd., Suite 420, Atlanta, GA 30340 (SAN 207-5946) Tel 770-447-5083.

Assoc Official, *See* **AOAC Intl**

Assoc Pubs Grp, *(Associated Pubs. Group; 1-881511),* Div. of Hambleton-Hill, 1501 County Hospital Rd., Nashville, TN 37218 (SAN 630-818X) Tel 615-254-2450; Fax: 615-254-2405; Toll Free: 800-327-5113
E-mail: sswift@agpbooks.com
Web site: http://www.apgbooks.com.

Assoc Univ Prs, *(Associated Univ. Presses; 0-8453),* 440 Forsgate Dr., Cranbury, NJ 08512 (SAN 281-2959) Tel 609-655-4770; Fax: 609-655-8366
E-mail: aup440@aol.com
Web site: http://arts.fdu.edu/aup/.

Associated Libraries Inc, *(Associated Libraries, Inc.),* 50 Cardinal Lane, Suite 138, Warminster, PA 18974-5107 (SAN 169-7528) Tel 215-672-7750.

Astran, *(Astran, Inc.),* 591 SW Eighth St., Miami, FL 33130-3413 (SAN 169-1082) Tel 305-858-4300; Fax: 305-858-0405; Toll Free: 800-431-4957
Web site: http://www.astranbooks.com.

ATEXINC, *(ATEXINC, Corp.; 0-9702332),* 13104 Canterbury Rd., Leawood, KS 66209 (SAN 631-774X) Tel 913-663-3703; Fax: 913-663-1881 Do not confuse with Atex, Inc., Bedford, MA
E-mail: atexinc@aol.com
Web site: http://www.atexinc.com.

Atlas News Co, *(Atlas News Co.),* Div. of Hudson News Co., P.O. Box 779, Boylston, MA 01505-0779 (SAN 169-3360).

Atlas Pub Co, *(Atlas Publishing Co.; 0-930575),* 1464 36th St., Ogden, UT 84403 (SAN 110-3873) Tel 801-627-1043.

Aubrey Bks, *(Aubrey Bks. International, Ltd.),* 721 Ellsworth Dr., No. 203, Silver Spring, MD 20910-4436 (SAN 113-3411) Tel 301-588-5496; Fax: 301-588-5249
E-mail: accents@iamdigex.net.

Audio Bk, *(Audio Bk. Co.; 0-89926),* 125 N. Aspen Ave., Suite 2, Azusa, CA 91702 (SAN 158-1414) Fax: 626-969-6099; Toll Free: 800-423-8273
E-mail: sales@audiobookco.com
Web site: http://www.audiobookco.com.

Audubon Prints & Bks, *(Audubon Prints & Bks.),* 9720 Spring Ridge Ln., Vienna, VA 22182 (SAN 111-820X).

Augsburg Fortress, *(Augsburg Fortress Pubs., Publishing Hse. of The Evangelical Lutheran Church in America; 0-8006; 0-8066),* Orders Addr.: P.O. Box 1209, Minneapolis, MN 55440-1209 (SAN 169-4081) Tel 612-330-3300; Fax: 612-330-3455; Toll Free: 800-328-4648 (orders only); Edit Addr.: 100 S. Fifth St., Suite 700, Minneapolis, MN 55440-1209 (SAN 169-4081)
E-mail: info@augsburgfortress.org; productinfo@augsburgfortress.org; subscriptions@augsburgfortress.org; customerservice@augsburgfortress.com
Web site: http://www.augsburgfortress.org.

Augusta News Co, *(Augusta News Co.),* 25 Second St., Apt. 124, Hallowell, ME 04347-1481 (SAN 169-3026).

Auromere, *(Auromere, Inc.; 0-89744),* 2621 W. US Hwy. 12, Lodi, CA 95242-9200 (SAN 169-0043) Fax: 209-339-3715; Toll Free: 800-735-4691
E-mail: sasp@lodinet.com
Web site: http://www.auromere.com.

Austin Management Group, *(Austin Management Group),* Orders Addr.: P.O. Box 3206, Paducah, KY 42002-3206 (SAN 135-3349); Edit Addr.: 1051 Husbands Rd., Paducah, KY 42003 (SAN 249-6844) Tel 502-442-1052.

Auto-Bound Inc, *(Auto-Bound, Inc.),* 909 Marina Village Pkwy., No. 67B, Alameda, CA 94501-1048 (SAN 170-0782) Tel 510-521-8630; Fax: 510-521-8755; Toll Free: 800-523-5833.

Autonomedia, *(Autonomedia; 0-936756; 1-57027),* Orders Addr.: P.O. Box 568, Brooklyn, NY 11211-0568; Edit Addr.: 55 S. 11th St., Brooklyn, NY 11211-0568 (SAN 221-3869) Tel 718-963-2603
E-mail: info@autonomedia.org
Web site: http://www.autonomedia.org.

Avanti Enterprises Inc, *(Avanti Enterprises, Inc.),* 18901 Springfield, Flossmoor, IL 60422 (SAN 158-3727) Tel 708-799-6464; Fax: 708-799-8713; Toll Free: 800-799-6464.

Avenue Bks, *(Avenue Bks.),* 2270 Porter Way, Stockton, CA 95207-3339 (SAN 122-4158).

Avery BookStores Inc, *(Avery BookStores, Inc.),* 308 Livingston St., Brooklyn, NY 11217 (SAN 169-510X).

Aviation, *(Aviation Bk. Co.; 0-911720; 0-911721; 0-916413),* 7201 Perimeter Rd., S., No. C, Seattle, WA 98108-3812 (SAN 120-1530) Tel 206-767-5232; Fax: 206-763-3428; Toll Free: 800-423-2708
E-mail: sales@aviationbook.com.

Avonlea Bks Inc, *(Avonlea Bks., Inc.),* Orders Addr.: P.O. Box 74, White Plains, NY 10602-0074 (SAN 680-4446) Tel 914-946-5923; Fax: 914-761-3119; Toll Free: 800-423-0622
E-mail: avonlea@bushkin.com
Web site: http://www.bushkin.com.

Ayer, *(Ayer Co. Pubs., Inc.; 0-88143),* Orders Addr.: 6 Lower Mill Rd., North Stratford, NH 03590 Fax: 603-922-3348 (Ordering) ; Toll Free: 888-267-7323 (Ordering); Edit Addr.: c/o IDS, 195 McGregor St., Manchester, NH 03102 (SAN 211-6936) Fax: 603-922-3348; Toll Free: 888-267-7323
Web site: http://www.scry.com/ayer.

B&N Imports, *(Barnes & Noble Bks.-Imports; 0-389),* Div. of Rowman & Littlefield Pubs., Inc., 4720 Boston Way, Lanham, MD 20706 (SAN 206-7803) Tel 301-459-3366; Toll Free: 800-462-6420.

B&T Entertainment, *(Baker & Taylor Entertainment),* Corporate Headquarters: 8140 N. Lehigh Ave., Morton Grove, IL 60053 (SAN 631-1156) Tel 847-965-8060; Fax: 847-965-8093; Toll Free: 800-775-2600; 7000 N. Austin Ave., Niles, IL 60714 (SAN 630-4311) Tel 847-647-0800; Fax: 847-647-7396; Toll Free: 800-775-2800; 1825 Monetary Ln., Suite 112, Carrollton, TX 75006 Tel 972-242-3098; Fax: 972-242-8375; Toll Free: 800-775-3300; 2501 SW 31st Ave., Pembroke Park, FL 33009 Tel 954-983-9055; Fax: 954-983-9350; Toll Free: 800-775-3400; 800-775-4300; 2150 Boggs Rd., Suite 640, Duluth, GA 30096 Tel 770-813-3253; Fax: 770-813-9460; Toll Free: 800-775-2600 (Orders only); 960 Turnpike St., Canton, MA 02021 Tel 781-821-2730; Fax: 781-821-1983; Toll Free: 800-775-2600; 3150 N. 24th St., Suite A210, Phoenix, AZ 85016 Tel 602-954-8558; Fax: 602-954-8870; Toll Free: 800-775-3300; 2709 Water Ridge Pkwy., Suite 500, Charlotte, NC 28217 Tel 704-329-9063; Fax: 704-329-9065; Toll Free: 800-775-2600; 8936 Comanche Ave., Chatsworth, CA 91311 Tel 818-886-0200; Fax: 818-886-0646; Toll Free: 800-775-4200; 3005 S. Parker Rd., Suite 318, Aurora, CO 80014 Tel 303-369-9229; Fax: 303-369-9669; Toll Free: 800-775-3300; Campbells Run Busn. Ctr., 100 Business Center Dr., Pittsburgh, PA 15205 Tel 412-787-8890; Fax: 412-787-0368; Toll Free: 800-775-2600; 5769 NE Columbia Blvd., Portland, OR 97218 Tel 503-249-8397; Fax: 503-282-5904; Toll Free: 800-775-3300; 1120 US Hwy. 22 E., Bridgewater, NJ 08807 Tel 908-541-7401; Fax: 908-541-7857; Toll Free: 800-775-2600
E-mail: info@btent.com
Web site: http://www.btent.com.

B & T International, *(Baker & Taylor International),* 1120 US Hwy. 22 E., Box 6885, Bridgewater, NJ 08807 (SAN 200-6804) Tel 908-541-7000; Fax: 908-729-4037.

B&T Video, *See* **B&T Entertainment**

B I G, *(B.I.G. (Business, Industry & Government)),* P.O. Box 15015, Albany, NY 12212-5015 (SAN 631-5194).

B L Winch, *(Winch, B. L. & Assocs.; 0-935266),* P.O. Box 1185, Torrance, CA 90505 (SAN 247-2716) Tel 310-816-3085; Fax: 310-816-3092; Toll Free: 800-662-9662 (orders only)
E-mail: czippi@att.net
Web site: http://www.ierc.com.

B McCaslin, *(McCaslin, Boyce),* 9 Colonial Village Ct., No. A, Webster Groves, MO 63119-2730 (SAN 110-8298) Tel 314-968-3296.

Badger Periodicals Distributors, *(Badger Periodicals Distributors),* 2420 W. Fourth, Appleton, WI 54914 (SAN 169-9024) Tel 920-731-9521.

Baggins Bks, *(Baggins Bks.),* 3560 Meridian St., Bellingham, WA 98225-1731 (SAN 156-501X).

Baker & Taylor, *(Baker & Taylor Bks.; 0-8480),* Orders Addr.: Commerce Service Ctr., 251 Mt. Olive Church Rd., Commerce, GA 30599-9988 (SAN 169-1503) Tel 404-335-5000; Toll Free: 800-775-1800 (orders); 800-775-1200 (customer service); Reno Service Ctr., 1160 Trademark Dr., Reno, NV 89511 (SAN 169-4464) Tel 775-850-3800; Fax: 775-850-3826 (customer service); Toll Free Fax: 800-775-7480 (orders); Edit Addr.: National Sales Hdqtrs., 5 Lakepointe Plaza, Suite 500, 2709 Water Ridge Pkwy., Charlotte, NC 28217 (SAN 169-5606) Fax: 704-329-8989; Toll Free: 800-775-1800 (information); 1120 US Hwy. 22, E., Bridgewater, NJ 08807 (SAN 169-4901) Toll Free: 800-775-1500 (customer service); Momence Service Ctr., 5012 S. Gladiolus St., Momence, IL 60954-1799 (SAN 169-2100) Tel 815-472-2444 (international customers); Fax: 815-472-9886 (international customers); Toll Free: 800-775-2300 (customer service, academic libraries)
E-mail: btinfo@btol.com
Web site: http://www.btol.com.

Bal Mus Lith Col, *(Balzekas Museum of Lithuanian Culture),* 6500 S. Pulaski Rd., Chicago, IL 60629 (SAN 110-8522) Tel 773-582-6500; Fax: 773-582-5133.

Ballantine, *See* **Ballantine Pub Grp**

Ballantine Pub Grp, *(Ballantine Publishing Group; 0-345; 0-449; 0-8041; 0-87637; 1-4000),* Div. of Random Hse., Inc., Orders Addr.: 400 Hahn Rd., Westminster, MD 21157 (SAN 202-5515) Tel 410-848-1900; Toll Free Fax: 800-767-4465; Toll Free: 800-726-0600 (customer service); 800-733-3000 (orders); Edit Addr.: 1540 Broadway, 11th Flr., New York, NY 10036 (SAN 214-1175) Tel 212-782-9000; Fax: 212-940-7539; Toll Free: 800-733-3000
E-mail: bfi@randomhouse.com
Web site: http://www.randomhouse.com.

Balogh, *(Balogh International, Inc.; 1-878762; 1-891770),* 1911 N. Duncan Rd., Champaign, IL 61822 (SAN 297-2344) Tel 217-355-9331; Fax: 217-355-9413
E-mail: balogh@balogh.com
Web site: http://www.balogh.com.

Banner of Truth, *(Banner of Truth, The; 0-85151),* Orders Addr.: P.O. Box 621, Carlisle, PA 17013 Tel 717-249-5747; Fax: 717-249-0604; Toll Free: 800-263-8085; Edit Addr.: 63 E. Louther St., Carlisle, PA 17013 (SAN 112-1553)
E-mail: info@banneroftruth.org
Web site: http://www.banneroftruth.co.uk.

Barbour & Co, *See* **Barbour Pub**

Barbour Pub, *(Barbour Publishing, Inc.; 0-916441; 1-55748; 1-57748; 1-58660),* P.O. Box 719, Uhrichsville, OH 44683 (SAN 295-7094) Tel 740-922-6045; Fax: 740-922-5948; Toll Free Fax: 800-220-5948; Toll Free: 800-852-8010
E-mail: info@barbourbooks.com
Web site: http://www.barbourbooks.com.

Barnes & Noble Inc, *(Barnes & Noble, Inc.; 0-7607; 0-88029; 1-4028),* 122 Fifth Ave., New York, NY 10011 (SAN 141-3651) Tel 212-633-3300
E-mail: staylor@bn.com.

Barron White, *(White, Barron),* 4704 Buckner Ln., Paducah, KY 42001 Tel 270-443-1205.

Basic Crafts Co, *(Basic Crafts Co.),* 6001 66th Ave., No. 10, Riverdale, MD 20737-1717 (SAN 169-5622) Toll Free: 800-847-4127 (outside New York).

Basin Distributing Co, *(Basin Distributing Co.),* 7208 E. Main St., Farmington, NM 87402-5132 (SAN 169-0558).

Basin News Co, *(Basin News Co.),* 1051 Husband Rd., Paducah, KY 42001 (SAN 169-2860).

Batavia Periodicals, *(Batavia Periodicals),* Orders Addr.: P.O. Box 1211, Rochester, NY 14603-1211 (SAN 169-5045).

Battelle, *(Battelle Pr.; 0-935470; 1-57477),* Div. of Battelle Memorial Institute, 505 King Ave., Columbus, OH 43201-2693 (SAN 213-4640) Tel 614-424-6393; Fax: 614-424-3819; Toll Free: 800-451-3543
E-mail: press@battelle.org
Web site: http://www.battelle.org/bookstore.

Bay News, *(Bay News, Inc.),* 3333 NW 35th Ave., Portland, OR 97210 (SAN 169-7153) Tel 503-219-3001; Fax: 503-241-1877.

Bay To Bay Dist, *(Bay To Bay Distribution),* 453 Ravendale Dr., Suite A, Mountain View, CA 94043 (SAN 631-0931) Tel 650-691-0108; Fax: 650-691-0663; Toll Free: 800-647-5749
E-mail: Bay2Bay@aol.com
Web site: http://www.BaytoBay@aol.com.

Bayou Bks, *(Bayou Bks.),* 1005 Monroe St., Gretna, LA 70053 (SAN 120-1913) Tel 504-368-1171; Toll Free: 800-843-1724.

Baysde Dist, *See* **Baysde Ent Dist**

Baysde Ent Dist, *(Bayside Entertainment Distribution; 0-7691),* 885 Riverside Pkwy., West Sacramento, CA 95605 (SAN 631-1261) Tel 916-371-2800; Fax: 916-371-1995; Toll Free: 800-525-5709
E-mail: stecon@baysidedist.com.

BCM Pubn, *(BCM Pubns., Inc.; 0-86508),* 237 Fairfield Ave., Upper Darby, PA 19082-2206 (SAN 211-7762) Tel 610-352-7177; Fax: 610-352-5561; Toll Free: 800-226-4685
E-mail: info@bcmintl.org; 103046.613@compuserve.com
Web site: http://www.bcmintl.org.

Beaver News Co Inc, *(Beaver News Co., Inc.),* 230 W. Washington St., Rensselaer, IN 47978 (SAN 630-8864).

Becks Bk Store, *(Beck's Bk. Store),* 4520 N. Broadway, Chicago, IL 60640 (SAN 159-8139) Tel 773-784-7963; Fax: 773-784-0066
E-mail: rsvltrd@aol.com
Web site: http://www.aol.members/becks.html.

Beechwood Pubns Inc, *(Beechwood Pubns., Inc.),* P.O. Box 1158, Kennett Square, PA 19348 (SAN 107-5853) Tel 610-444-5991; Fax: 215-566-4178.

Beekman Pubs, *(Beekman Pubs., Inc.; 0-8464),* P.O. Box 888, Woodstock, NY 12498 (SAN 170-1622) Tel 914-679-2300; Fax: 914-679-2301; Toll Free: 888-233-5626
E-mail: manager@beekmanpublishers.com; beekman@beekmanpublishers.com
Web site: http://www.beekman.net.

Beet, *(Beet, Channing L. Co., Inc.),* 200 State Rd., South Deerfield, MA 01373-0200 Fax: 800-499-6464; Toll Free: 800-611-6083.

Before Columbus Foundation, *(Before Columbus Foundation),* 655 13th St., Suite 300, The Raymond Hse., Oakland, CA 94612 (SAN 159-2955) Tel 510-268-9775.

Beijing Bk Co Inc, *(Beijing Bk. Co., Inc.),* 701 E. Linden Ave., Linden, NJ 07036-2495 (SAN 169-5673) Tel 908-862-0909; Fax: 908-862-4201.

Bell Magazine, *(Bell Magazine),* Orders Addr.: P.O. Box 1957, Monterey, CA 93940 (SAN 159-7221); Edit Addr.: 3 Justin Ct., Monterey, CA 93940 (SAN 169-0353) Tel 408-642-4668.

Belle News Agency, *(La Belle News Agency),* 814 University Blvd., Steubenville, OH 43952 (SAN 169-6858).

Benjamin News, *(Benjamin News Group),* P.O. Box 16147, Missoula, MT 59806 (SAN 631-6476) Tel 406-721-7801; Fax: 406-721-7802.

Benjamins North Am, *See* **J Benjamins Pubng Co**

Bennett & Curran, *(Bennett & Curran, Inc.; 1-879607),* 1545 W. Tufts Ave., Suite M, Englewood, CO 80110-5575 Tel 303-783-2255; Fax: 303-783-2256
E-mail: Jeff@bennettandcurran.com.

Berkeley Educational Paperbacks, *(Berkeley Educational Paperbacks),* 2480 Bancroft Way, Berkeley, CA 94704 (SAN 168-9509) Tel 510-848-7907.

Berkley Pub, *(Berkley Publishing Group; 0-425; 0-515),* Div. of Penguin Putnam, Inc., Orders Addr.: 405 Murray Hill Pkwy., East Rutherford, NJ 07073 Toll Free: 800-788-6262 (individual consumer sales); 800-847-5515 (orders); 800-631-8571 (customer service); Edit Addr.: 375 Hudson St., New York, NY 10014 (SAN 201-3991) Tel 212-366-2000; Fax: 212-366-2385
E-mail: online@penguinputnam.com
Web site: http://www.penguinputnam.com.

Bernan Associates, *(Bernan Assocs.; 0-400; 0-527; 0-89059),* Div. of Kraus Organization, The, Orders Addr.: 4611-F Assembly Dr., Lanham, MD 20706-4391 (SAN 169-3182) Tel 301-459-7666; Fax: 301-459-0056; Toll Free Fax: 800-865-3450; Toll Free: 800-274-4888
E-mail: order@bernan.com; query@bernan.com
Web site: http://www.bernan.com.

Bernard H Hamel Spanish Bk, *(Hamel, Bernard H. Spanish Bk. Corp.),* 10977 Santa Monica Blvd., Los Angeles, CA 90025 (SAN 111-8862) Tel 310-475-0453; Fax: 310-473-6132
E-mail: spanish@primenet.com
Web site: http://www.BernardHamel.com; http://www.SpanishBooksUSA.com.

Bernhard DeBoer Inc, *(DeBoer, Bernhard Inc.),* 113 E. Centre St., Nutley, NJ 07110 (SAN 282-1990) Tel 973-667-9300; Fax: 973-667-0086
E-mail: stout@javanet.com
Web site: http://www.javanet.com/-stout/pannus.

Berrett-Koehler, *(Berrett-Koehler Pubs., Inc.; 1-57675; 1-58376; 1-881052),* 235 Montgomery St., Suite 650, San Francisco, CA 94104 Tel 415-288-0260; Fax: 415-362-2512; Toll Free: 800-929-2929
E-mail: bkpub@bkpubl.com
Web site: http://www.bkconnection.com.

Best Continental Bk Co Inc, *(Best Continental Bk. Co., Inc.),* P.O. Box 615, Merrifield, VA 22116 (SAN 107-3737) Tel 703-280-1400.

Beyda & Assoc Inc, *(Beyda & Assocs., Inc.),* 6943 Valjean Ave., Van Nuys, CA 91406 (SAN 169-0426) Tel 818-988-3102; Fax: 818-994-8724; Toll Free: 800-422-3932 (orders only)
E-mail: sales@beydabooks.com.

Biblio Dist, *(Biblio Distribution Ctr.),* Div. of Littlefield, Adams & Co., 4720 Boston Way, Lanham, MD 20706 (SAN 211-724X) Tel 301-306-0400; Fax: 301-459-2118.

Biddy Bks, *(Biddy Bks.),* 1235 168 Model Rd., Manchester, TN 37355 (SAN 157-8561) Tel 931-728-6967.

Bilingual Ed Serv, *(Bilingual Educational Services, Inc.; 0-86624; 0-89075),* 2514 S. Grand Ave., Los Angeles, CA 90007 (SAN 218-4680) Tel 213-749-6213; Fax: 213-749-1820; Toll Free: 800-448-6032
E-mail: bes@besbooks.com; Sales@besbooks.com
Web site: http://www.besbooks.com.

Bilingual Pubns, *(Bilingual Pubns. Co., The),* 270 Lafayette St., New York, NY 10012 (SAN 164-8993) Tel 212-431-3500; Fax: 212-431-3567 Do not confuse with Bilingual Pubns., in Denver, CO
E-mail: lindagoodman@juno.com.

Bill Cole Enterprises Inc, *(Cole, Bill Enterprises, Inc.),* P.O. Box 60, Randolph, MA 02368-0060 (SAN 685-6373) Tel 617-986-2653.

Birdlegs, *(Birdlegs Christian Apparel),* P.O. Box 189, Duluth, GA 30136-0189 (SAN 631-3280) Toll Free: 800-545-0790.

Bk Box Inc, *(Book Box, Inc.),* 3126 Purdue Ave., Los Angeles, CA 90066 (SAN 243-2285) Tel 310-391-2313.

Bk Buy Back, *(Book Buy Back),* 5150 Candlewood St., No. 6, Lakewood, CA 90712 (SAN 631-7251) Tel 562-461-9355; Fax: 562-461-9445.

Bk Clearing Hse, *(Book Clearing Hse.),* 46 Purdy St., Harrison, NY 10528 (SAN 125-5169) Tel 914-835-0015; Fax: 914-835-0398; Toll Free: 800-431-1579
E-mail: bookch@aol.com.

Bk Dist Ctr, *(Book Distribution Ctr., Inc.),* Orders Addr.: P.O. Box 64631, Virginia Beach, VA 23467 (SAN 134-8019) Tel 757-456-0005; Fax: 757-552-0837; Edit Addr.: 4617 N. Witchduck Rd., Virginia Beach, VA 23455 (SAN 169-8672)
E-mail: sales@bookdist.com
Web site: http://www.bookdist.

Bk Dynamics Inc, *(Book Dynamics, Inc.; 0-9612440),* 18 Kennedy Blvd., East Brunswick, NJ 08816 (SAN 169-5649) Tel 732-545-5151; Fax: 732-545-5959; Toll Free: 800-441-4510.

Bk Fairs of Covina, *(Book Fairs of Covina),* 1030 Bonita Ave., La Verne, CA 91750 (SAN 630-6225) Tel 909-593-0697; 2988 First St., Suite F, La Verne, CA 91750 (SAN 299-2434).

Bk Home, *(Book Home, The),* 119 E. Dale St., Colorado Springs, CO 80903-4701 (SAN 249-3055) Tel 719-634-5885.

Bk Margins Inc, *(Book Margins, Inc.),* 7100 Valley Green Rd., Fort Washington, PA 19034-2206 (SAN 106-7788) Tel 215-223-5300
E-mail: paul.gross@bookmargins.com
Web site: http://www.bookmargins.com.

Bk Marketing Plus, *(Book Marketing Plus),* 406 Post Oak Rd., Fredericksburg, TX 78624 (SAN 630-6543) Tel 830-997-4776; Fax: 830-997-9752; Toll Free: 800-356-2445.

Bk Mart, *(Book Mart, The),* 1153 E. Hyde Pk., Inglewood, CA 90302 (SAN 168-969X).

Bk Sales Inc, *(Book Sales, Inc.; 0-7858; 0-89009; 1-55521),* Orders Addr.: 114 Northfield Ave., Edison, NJ 08837 (SAN 169-488X) Tel 732-225-0530; Fax: 212-779-6058; 732-225-2257; Toll Free: 800-526-7257; Edit Addr.: 276 Fifth Ave., Suite 206, New York, NY 10001 (SAN 299-4062) Tel 212-779-4972; Fax: 212-779-6058
E-mail: bsiny@hotmail.com
Web site: http://www.booksales.com.

Bk Service Unlimited, *(Book Service Unlimited),* P.O. Box 31108, Seattle, WA 98103-1108 (SAN 169-877X) Toll Free: 800-347-0042.

Bk Services International, *(Book Services International),* Orders Addr.: P.O. Box 1434-SMS, Fairfield, CT 06430 (SAN 157-9541) Tel 203-374-4939; Fax: 203-384-6099; Toll Free: 800-243-2790.

Bk Shelf, *(Book Shelf, The),* 919 Central Ave., Fort Dodge, IA 50501 (SAN 169-2658) Tel 515-573-3535.

Bk World, *(Book World),* 311 Sagamore Pkwy., N., Lafayette, IN 47904 (SAN 135-4051) Tel 765-448-1131 Do not confuse with companies with the same or similar name in Sun Lakes, AZ, Roanoke, VA.

Bklegger CA, *(Booklegger, The; 0-936421),* Orders Addr.: P.O. Box 2626, Grass Valley, CA 95945 (SAN 697-9548); Edit Addr.: 13100 Grass Valley Ave., Suite D, Grass Valley, CA 95945 (SAN 120-6125) Tel 530-272-1556; Fax: 530-272-2133; Toll Free Fax: 800-250-2199; Toll Free: 800-262-1556
E-mail: order@booklegger.com
Web site: http://www.booklegger.com/.

BkMstrs TX, *(BookMasters),* 6745 FM 2738, Burleson, TX 76028-1167 (SAN 630-8406) Do not confuse with BookMasters Inc., Ashland, OH
E-mail: bookmast@gte.net
Web site: http://www.home1.gte.net/bookmast.

Bks & Research Inc, *(Books & Research, Inc.),* 32 Main St., Hastings On Hudson, NY 10706-1602 (SAN 130-1101) Fax: 914-478-1315
E-mail: brinc@ix.netcom.com
Web site: http://www.books-and-research.com.

Bks Intl VA, *(Books International, Incorporated; 1-891078),* Orders Addr.: P.O. Box 605, Herndon, VA 20172-0605 (SAN 131-761X) Tel 703-661-1500; Fax: 703-661-1501
E-mail: mgreenwald@sorosny.org.

Bks Nippan, *(Books Nippan; 0-945814; 1-56970),* Div. of Nippan Shuppan Hanbai, U.S.A., Inc., 1123 Dominguez St., Suite K, Carson, CA 90746 (SAN 111-817X) Tel 310-604-9701; Fax: 310-604-1134; Toll Free: 800-562-1410
E-mail: distribution@emanga.com
Web site: http://www.booksnippan.com/.

Bks to Grow On, *(Books to Grow On),* 826 S. Aiken Ave., Pittsburgh, PA 15232 (SAN 128-438X); 210 S. Highland Ave., Pittsburgh, PA 15206 Fax: 412-621-5324.

Black Box, *(Black Box Corp.),* 1000 Park Dr., Lawrence, PA 15055 (SAN 277-1985) Tel 412-746-5500; Fax: 412-746-0746.

Black Magazine Agency, *(Black Magazine Agency),* Box 1018, Logansport, IN 46947 (SAN 107-0819) Tel 219-753-2429; Fax: 219-753-5480; Toll Free: 800-782-9787.

Blackburn News Agency, *(Blackburn News Agency),* P.O. Box 1039, Kingsport, TN 37662 (SAN 169-7900).

Blackwell Corp, *(Blackwell Corp.),* P.O. Box 2169, Vienna, VA 22183-2169 (SAN 630-5601).

Blackwell Sci, *(Blackwell Science, Inc.; 0-632; 0-86542),* Subs. of Blackwell Scientific Ltd, Orders Addr.: Commerce Pl., 350 Main St., Malden, MA 02148-5018 (SAN 215-2029) Tel 617-388-8250; Fax: 781-388-8255; Toll Free: 800-759-6102; 800-215-1000 (orders)
E-mail: csbooks@blacksci.com
Web site: http://www.blacksci.co.uk/usa.

Bloomington News Agency, *(Bloomington News Agency),* P.O. Box 3757, Bloomington, IL 61702-3757 (SAN 169-1732).

Blue Cat, *(Blue Cat; 0-932679; 0-936200),* 469 Barbados, Walnut, CA 91789 (SAN 214-0322) Tel 909-594-3317.

Blue Mount SPS Studios, *(Blue Mountain Arts (R) by SPS Studios, Inc.; 0-88396; 1-58786),* Orders Addr.: P.O. Box 4549, Boulder, CO 80306 (SAN 299-9609) Tel 303-449-0536; Fax: 303-417-6496; Toll Free Fax: 800-256-1213; Toll Free: 800-473-2082
E-mail: ordersbma@mindspring.com.

Blue Rdge News, *(Blue Ridge News, Inc.),* 101 E. Patrick St., Frederick, MD 21701-5629 (SAN 169-3158) Tel 301-694-8440.

Blue Ridge News Co, *(Blue Ridge News Co.),* 21 Westside Dr., No. B, Asheville, NC 28806-2846 (SAN 169-6335).

Bluefield News Agency Inc, *(Bluefield News Agency, Inc.),* P.O. Box 947, Bluefield, WV 24701 (SAN 169-8915).

Bob Jones Univ, *(Jones, Bob Univ. Pr.; 0-89084; 1-57924; 1-59166),* 1700 Wade Hampton Blvd., Greenville, SC 29614 (SAN 223-7512) Tel 864-242-5731; Fax: 864-298-8398; Toll Free Fax: 800-525-8398; Toll Free: 800-845-5731
E-mail: bjup@bjup.com
Web site: http://www.bjup.com.

Boley International Subscription Agency Inc, *(Boley International Subscription Agency, Inc.),* 1001 Fries Mill Rd., Blackwood, NJ 08012 (SAN 159-6225) Tel 609-629-2500.

Bollett, *(Bollett Library Resources),* 1340 Ridgeview Dr., McHenry, IL 60050 Tel 815-759-1700; Fax: 815-759-9552.

Bonneville News Co, *(Bonneville News Co.),* 965 Beardsley Pl., Salt Lake City, UT 84119 (SAN 169-8516) Tel 801-972-5454; Fax: 801-972-1075; Toll Free: 800-748-5453.

Book Company, *(Book Co., The),* 145 S. Glencoe St., Denver, CO 80222-1152 (SAN 200-2809).

Book Dist Ctr, *(Book Distribution Ctr.; 0-941722),* Div. of Free Islamic Literatures, Inc., Orders Addr.: P.O. Box 35844, Houston, TX 77235 (SAN 241-6395); Edit Addr.: P.O. Box 31669, Houston, TX 77231 (SAN 226-2770).

Book Gallery, *(Book Gallery; 1-878382),* P.O. Box 50700, Tulsa, OK 74150-0700 (SAN 630-9321) Tel 918-587-6847; Toll Free: 800-444-6847.

Book Hse, *(Book Hse., Inc., The),* 208 W. Chicago St., Jonesville, MI 49250-0125 (SAN 169-3859) Tel 517-849-2117; Fax: 517-849-9716; Toll Free Fax: 800-858-9716; Toll Free: 800-248-1146
E-mail: bhinfo@thebookhouse.com.

Book Warehse, *(Book Warehouse),* 5154 NW 165th St., Hialeah, FL 33014-6335.

Book Wholesalers, *(Book Wholesalers, Inc.; 0-7587),* Div. of Follett Corp., 1847 Mercer Rd., Lexington, KY 40511-1001 (SAN 135-5449) Tel 606-231-9789; Fax: 606-233-4740; Toll Free Fax: 800-888-6319; Toll Free: 800-888-4478
E-mail: jcarrico@bwibooks.com
Web site: http://bwibooks.com.

Bookazine Co Inc, *(Bookazine Co., Inc.),* 75 Hook Rd., Bayonne, NJ 07002 (SAN 169-5665) Tel 201-339-7777; Fax: 201-339-7778; Toll Free: 800-221-8112.

Bookhouse, *(Bookhouse, The),* 10505 N. May Ave., Oklahoma City, OK 73120-2611 (SAN 200-8467) Tel 405-755-0020.

Bookline, *(Bookline),* Div. of Michiana News Service, Inc., 2232 S. 11th St., Niles, MI 49120 (SAN 169-3948) Tel 616-684-3013; Fax: 616-684-8740.

Booklines Hawaii, *(Booklines Hawaii, Ltd.; 1-929844; 1-58849),* 94-527 Puahi St., Waipahu, HI 96797 (SAN 630-6624) Tel 808-676-0116; Fax: 808-676-0634; Toll Free: 877-828-4852
E-mail: cynthiar@booklines.com
Web site: http://www.booklineshawaii.com.

Bookman Bks, *(Bookman Bks.),* 138 Elena St., Santa Fe, NM 87501 (SAN 630-933X) Tel 505-982-5964.

Bookmark Inc, *(Bookmark, Inc., The),* 14643 W. 95th St., Lenexa, KS 66215 (SAN 131-4017) Tel 913-894-1288; Fax: 913-894-1842; Toll Free: 800-642-1288.

BookMasters, *(BookMasters, Inc.; 0-917889),* Orders Addr.: P.O. Box 388, Mansfield, OH 44903 (SAN 631-3566) Tel 419-281-1802; Fax: 419-281-6883; Toll Free: 800-247-6553; 30 Amberwood Pkwy., Ashland, OH 44805 Fax: 419-281-6886 Do not confuse with BookMasters, Burleson, TX
E-mail: order@bookmaster.com; info@bookmasters.com
Web site: http://www.bookmasters.com.

Bookmen Inc, *(Bookmen, Inc.),* Orders Addr.: 525 N. Third St., Minneapolis, MN 55401 (SAN 169-409X) Tel 612-359-5757; Fax: 612-341-2903; Toll Free Fax: 800-266-5636; Toll Free: 800-328-8411 (customer service)
Web site: http://www.bookmen.com.

Bookpeople, *(Bookpeople; 0-914728),* 7900 Edgewater Dr., Oakland, CA 94621 (SAN 168-9517) Tel 510-632-4700; Fax: 510-632-1281; Toll Free Fax: 800-999-4650
E-mail: custserv@bponline.com; bpeople@bponline.com
Web site: http://www.bponline.com.

Books Now, *(Books Now),* 6600 W. Charleston Blvd., Las Vegas, NV 89102 (SAN 631-1458) Tel 702-258-3338; Fax: 702-258-3411
Web site: http://www.booksnow.com.

Books West CO, *(Books West),* 5757 Arapahoc Ave., Unit D2, Boulder, CO 80303 (SAN 631-4724) Tel 303-449-5995; Fax: 303-449-5951; Toll Free: 800-378-4188 Do not confuse with Books West, San Diego, CA
E-mail: wnack@rmi.net.

Booksellers Order Service, *(Booksellers Order Service),* 828 S. Broadway, Tarrytown, NY 10591-5112 (SAN 106-5181) Tel 914-591-2665; Fax: 914-591-2720; Toll Free: 800-637-0037.

Booksmith Promotional Co, *(Booksmith Promotional Co.),* 100 Paterson Plank Rd., Jersey City, NJ 07307 (SAN 664-5364) Tel 201-659-2768; Fax: 201-659-3631.

Booksource, *(Booksource, The; 0-7383; 0-911891; 0-9641084; 1-890760),* 1230 Macklind Ave., Saint Louis, MO 63110-1432 (SAN 169-4324) Tel 314-647-0600; Fax: 314-647-2622; Toll Free: 800-444-0435
E-mail: vstadts@freewwweb.com
Web site: http://www.booksource.com.

BookWorld, *(BookWorld Services, Inc.; 1-884962),* 1933 Whitfield Pk. Loop, Sarasota, FL 34243 (SAN 173-0568) Tel 941-758-8094; Fax: 941-753-9396; Toll Free Fax: 800-777-2525; Toll Free: 800-444-2524 (orders only)
E-mail: central@bookworld.com; sales@bookworld.com
Web site: http://www.bookworld.com.

BookWorld Dist, *See* **BookWorld**

Bookworm, *(Bookworm, The),* 417 Monmouth Dr., Cherry Hill, NJ 08002 (SAN 120-9531) Tel 609-667-5884.

Bookworm Bookfairs, *(Bookworm Bookfairs),* 968 Farmington Ave., W., West Hartford, CT 06107 (SAN 156-5621).

Bookworm ME, *(Bookworm),* 14 Griffin St., Northport, ME 04849-4446 (SAN 170-8074).

Borders Inc, *(Borders, Inc.),* 100 Phoenix Ave., Ann Arbor, MI 48104 (SAN 169-3662) Tel 313-913-1100.

Bound to Stay Bound Bk, *(Bound to Stay Bound Bk.),* 1880 W. Morton Rd., Jacksonville, IL 62650 (SAN 169-1996) Tel 217-245-5191; Fax: 217-245-0424; Toll Free Fax: 800-747-2872; Toll Free: 800-637-6586
E-mail: btsb@btsb.com
Web site: http://www.btsbbooks.com.

Bowers & Merena, *(Bowers & Merena Galleries, Inc.; 0-943161),* Orders Addr.: P.O. Box 1224, Wolfeboro, NH 03894 (SAN 168-9746) Tel 603-569-5095; Fax: 603-569-5319; Toll Free: 800-222-5993; Edit Addr.: 61 S. Main St., Wolfeboro, NH 03894 (SAN 668-2561).

Bowker, *See* **Bowker LLC**

Bowker LLC, *(Bowker, R. R. LLC; 0-8352; 0-911255),* Subs. of Cambridge Information Group, Inc, Orders Addr.: P.O. Box 1001, Summit, NJ 07902-1001 Toll Free: 888-269-5372; Edit Addr.: 630 Central Ave., New Providence, NJ 07974 (SAN 214-1191) Tel 908-464-6800; Fax: 908-464-3553; Toll Free: 800-521-8110; 800-278-2991 subscriptions to: Publishers Weekly, School Library Journal, Library Journal (in Ohio: 614-383-3141)
E-mail: info@bowker.com
Web site: http://www.bowker.com.

Boydell & Brewer, *(Boydell & Brewer, Inc.; 0-85115; 0-85991; 0-86193; 0-907239; 1-870252),* Div. of Boydell & Brewer, Ltd. (UK), Orders Addr.: P.O. Box 41026, Rochester, NY 14604-4126 Tel 716-275-0419; Fax: 716-271-8778; Edit Addr.: 668 Mount Hope Ave., Rochester, NY 14620
E-mail: boydell@boydell.co.uk; camdenhouse@compuserve.com; 104572.1422@compuserve.com; urpress@mail.rochester.edu
Web site: http://www.boydell.co.uk.

BPI Commns, *(B. P. I. Communications),* Div. of Prestel Publishing, 575 Prospect Ave., Lakewood, NJ 08701 (SAN 631-7758) Tel 732-363-5679; Fax: 732-363-0338; Toll Free: 888-463-6110.

Brauninger News Co, *(Brauninger News Co.),* Orders Addr.: Box 290, Trenton, NJ 08602-0290 (SAN 169-4936) Tel 609-396-1500; Fax: 609-394-2594
E-mail: philfriend@worldnet.att.net.

Brazos Periodical Distributors, *(Brazos Periodical Distributors),* Box 4131, Bryan, TX 77805 (SAN 169-8060).

Bridge Pubns Inc, *(Bridge Pubns., Inc.; 0-88404; 1-57318; 1-58460; 1-4031),* 4751 Fountain Ave., Los Angeles, CA 90029 (SAN 208-3884) Tel 323-953-3320; Fax: 323-953-3328; Toll Free: 800-722-1733
E-mail: info@bridgepub.com
Web site: http://www.bridgepub.com.

BridgeWay, *(BridgeWay Bks.; 0-9675977),* Div. of BridgeWay Enterprises, P.O. Box 343, Louisville, CO 80027 Tel 720-890-4009; Fax: 954-212-8338
E-mail: webmaster@bridgewayonline.com
Web site: http://www.bridgewayonline.com.

Bright Horizons Specialty Distributors Inc, *(Bright Horizons Specialty Distributors, Inc.),* 138 Springside Rd., Asheville, NC 28803 (SAN 110-4101) Tel 704-684-8840; Fax: 704-681-1790; Toll Free: 800-437-3959 (orders only).

Brisco Pubns, *(Brisco Pubns.; 0-9603576),* P.O. Box 2161, Palos Verdes Peninsula, CA 90274 (SAN 133-0268) Tel 310-534-4943; Fax: 310-534-8437.

Bristol-Myers Squibb, *(Bristol-Myers Squibb),* Rte. 206 & Provinceline Rd., Princeton, NJ 08540.

Bro Life Inc, *(Brotherhood of Life, Inc.; 0-914732),* P.O. Box 46306, Las Vegas, NV 89114-6306 (SAN 111-3674) Fax: 702-319-5577
E-mail: brotherhoodoflife@hotmail.com
Web site: http://www.brotherhoodoflife.com.

Brodart, *(Brodart Co.; 0-87272),* Orders Addr.: 500 Arch St., Williamsport, PA 17705 (SAN 169-7684) Tel 570-326-2461; Fax: 570-326-1479; Toll Free Fax: 800-999-6799; Toll Free: 800-233-8467
Web site: http://www.brodart.com.

Brookings, *(Brookings Institution Pr.; 0-8157),* 1775 Massachusetts Ave., NW, Washington, DC 20036-2188 (SAN 201-9396) Tel 202-797-6258; Fax: 202-797-6004; Toll Free: 800-275-1447
E-mail: brookinfo@brook.edu; bibooks@brook.edu
Web site: http://www.brookings.edu.

Brunner News Agency, *(Brunner News Agency),* 217 Flanders Ave., P.O. Box 598, Lima, OH 45801 (SAN 169-6777) Tel 419-225-5826; Fax: 419-225-5537; Toll Free: 800-998-1727
E-mail: brunnews@aol.com
Web site: http://www.readmoreshallmark.com.

Brunner-Mazel, *See* **Brunner-Routledge**

Brunner-Routledge, *(Brunner-Routledge; 0-87630; 1-58391),* Div. of Taylor & Francis, Orders Addr.: 7625 Empire Dr., Florence, KY 41042 Toll Free Fax: 800-248-4724; Toll Free: 800-634-7064; Edit Addr.: 325 Chestnut St., 8th Flr., Philadelphia, PA 19106 (SAN 164-9167) Tel 215-625-8900; Fax: 215-625-2940
E-mail: info@taylorandfrancis.com; bkorders@taylorandfrancis.com
Web site: http://www.brunner-routledge.com; http://www.taylorandfrancis.com.

Bryant Altman, *(Bryant Altman Map, Inc.),* Endicott St., Bldg. 26, Norwood, MA 02062 (SAN 630-2475) Tel 781-762-3339; Fax: 781-769-9080
E-mail: JPG63@aol.com.

BTP Dist, *(B T P Distribution),* 4135 Northgate Blvd., Suite 5, Sacramento, CA 95834-1226 (SAN 631-2489) Tel 916-567-2496; Fax: 916-441-6749.

Buckeye News Co, *(Buckeye News Co.),* 6800 W. Central Ave., Suite F, Toledo, OH 43617-1157 (SAN 169-6874).

Budget Bk Service Inc, *(Budget Bk. Service, Inc.),* Div. of LDAP, Inc., 386 Park Ave. S., Suite 1913, New York, NY 10016-8804 (SAN 169-5762) Tel 212-679-4200; Fax: 212-679-2247.

Budget Marketing Inc, *(Budget Marketing, Inc.),* P.O. Box 1805, Des Moines, IA 50306 (SAN 285-8754).

Budgetext, *(Budgetext),* Orders Addr.: P.O. Box 1487, Fayetteville, AR 72702 (SAN 111-3321) Tel 501-443-9205; Fax: 501-442-3064; Toll Free: 800-643-3432; Edit Addr.: 1936 N. Shiloh Dr., Fayetteville, AR 72704 (SAN 249-3330)
E-mail: wmorgan@absc.com
Web site: http://www.budgetext.com.

Burlington News Agency, *(Burlington News Agency),* Hercules Dr., P.O. Box 510, Colchester, VT 05446-0510 (SAN 169-8583) Tel 802-655-7000.

Burns News Agency, *(Burns News Agency),* P.O. Box 1211, Rochester, NY 14603-1211 (SAN 169-5320).

Butte Pubns, *(Butte Pubns., Inc.; 1-884362),* P.O. Box 1328, Hillsboro, OR 97123-1328 (SAN 299-8866) Tel 503-648-9791; Fax: 503-693-9526; Toll Free: 866-312-8883
E-mail: service@buttepublications.com
Web site: http://www.buttepublications.com.

Buttrwrth-Heinemann, *(Butterworth-Heinemann; 0-240; 0-250; 0-407; 0-408; 0-409; 0-433; 0-434; 0-480; 0-7506; 0-86729; 0-87591; 0-914236; 0-932376; 0-9626521; 1-55558; 1-56372),* Subs. of Reed Elsevier plc, 225 Wildwood Ave., Unit B, Woburn, MA 01801 (SAN 206-3964) Tel 781-904-2500; Fax: 781-904-2640; Toll Free Fax: 800-446-6520 (orders); Toll Free: 800-366-2665 (orders)
E-mail: custserv@bhusa.com; sales@bhusa.com; orders@bhusa.com
Web site: http://www.bh.com.

Byrrd Ent Inc, *(Byrrd Enterprises, Inc.; 1-886715),* 1302 Lafayette Dr., Alexandria, VA 22308 (SAN 169-8605) Tel 703-765-5626; Fax: 703-768-4086; Toll Free: 800-628-0901.

BYU Print Srvs, *(Brigham Young Univ. Print Services),* 205 UPB, Provo, UT 84602 (SAN 201-9337) Tel 801-378-2809; Fax: 801-378-3374
E-mail: denise@upb.byu.edu
Web site: http://www.upb.byu.edu.

C & B Bk Hse, *(C & B Bk. Hse.),* 21 Oak Ridge Rd., Monroe, CT 06468 (SAN 159-8279).

C & H News Co, *(C & H News Co.),* P.O. Box 2768, Corpus Christi, TX 78403-2768 (SAN 169-8249).

C & W Zabel Co, *(Zabel, C. & W. Co.),* Orders Addr.: P.O. Box 953, East Brunswick, NJ 08816-0953 (SAN 169-4731) Tel 732-254-1000; Fax: 732-254-0121; Edit Addr.: 24 Rebel Run Dr., East Brunswick, NJ 08816 (SAN 241-6441) Tel 201-947-3300.

C D Distributing Inc, *(CD Distributing, Inc.),* P.O. Box 4965, Missoula, MT 59806-4965 (SAN 169-4367) Fax: 406-454-0415.

C H Kerr, *(Kerr, Charles H. Publishing Co.; 0-88286),* 1740 W. Greenleaf Ave., Chicago, IL 60626 (SAN 207-7043) Tel 773-465-7774
Web site: http://www.spdbooks.org.

C Levy Co, *(Levy, Charles Co.),* 1200 N. North Branch St., Chicago, IL 60622 (SAN 159-835X) Tel 312-440-4400.

Cal Prin Full Svc, *(California Princeton Fulfillment Services),* 1445 Lower Ferry Rd., Ewing, NJ 08618 (SAN 630-639X) Tel 609-883-1759 (ext. 536); Toll Free: 800-777-4726
E-mail: donnaw@cpfs.pupress.princeton.edu.

Calico Subscription Co, *(Calico Subscription Co.),* P.O. Box 640337, San Jose, CA 95164-0337 (SAN 285-9173) Tel 408-432-8700; Fax: 408-432-8813; Toll Free: 800-952-2542.

Cambridge Bk, *(Cambridge Bk. Co.; 0-8428),* Div. of Simon & Schuster, Inc., 4350 Equity Dr., Box 249, Columbus, OH 43216 (SAN 169-5703) Toll Free: 800-238-5833
Web site: http://www.simonsays.com/.

Cambridge U Pr, *(Cambridge Univ. Pr.; 0-521; 0-511),* Orders Addr.: 110 Midland Ave., Port Chester, NY 10573-4930 (SAN 281-3769) Tel 914-937-9600; Fax: 914-937-4712; Toll Free: 800-872-7423 (orders, returns, credit & accounting); Edit Addr.: 40 W. 20th St., New York, NY 10011-4211 (SAN 200-206X) Tel 212-924-3900; Fax: 212-691-3239
E-mail: orders@cup.org; information@cup.org; customer_service@cup.org
Web site: http://www.cup.org.

Cancer Control Soc, *(Cancer Control Society; 0-943080),* 2043 N. Berendo St., Los Angeles, CA 90027 (SAN 216-2296) Tel 213-663-7801.

Canfield Pubng, *(Canfield Publishing; 0-9647749),* 253 Passaic Ave., Fairfield, NJ 07004-2524.

Canyonlands Pubns, *(Canyonlands Pubns.; 0-9702595),* Orders Addr.: P.O. Box 16175, Bellemont, AZ 86015-6175 (SAN 114-3824) Tel 520-779-3888; Fax: 520-779-3778; Toll Free: 800-283-1983; Edit Addr.: 4860 N. Ken Morey, Bellemont, AZ 86015
E-mail: books@infomagic.com.

Cape News Co, *(Cape News Co.),* P.O. Box 568680, Rockledge, FL 32955 (SAN 169-0949) Tel 407-636-5909.

Capital Business Systems, *(Capital Business Systems),* Div. of Capital Business Service, Orders Addr.: P.O. Box 2088, Napa, CA 94558 (SAN 698-3146) Tel 707-252-8844; Fax: 707-252-6368; Edit Addr.: 2033 First St., Napa, CA 94558.

Capital City, *(Capital City),* 2537 Daniels St., Madison, WI 53704-6772 (SAN 200-5328) Tel 608-223-2000; Fax: 608-223-2010.

Capital News Co, *(Capital News Co.),* 961 Palmyra, Jackson, MS 39203 (SAN 169-4219) Tel 601-355-8341; Fax: 601-352-1343.

Capitol News Agency, *(Capitol News Agency),* P.O. Box 7771, Richmond, VA 23231 (SAN 169-8699); 5203 Hatcher St., Richmond, VA 23231-0271 (SAN 249-2768) Tel 804-222-7252.

Capitol Preserv, *See* **Penn Capitol Presrv**

Capper Pr, *(Capper Pr.),* 1503 SW 42nd, Topeka, KS 66609 (SAN 285-8886) Tel 913-274-4324; Fax: 913-274-4305; Toll Free: 800-678-5779 (ext. 4324).

Cards Bks N Things, *(Cards Bks. N Things),* 1446 St., Rd. 2 West, La Porte, IN 46350 (SAN 159-8295).

Carl B Noelke, *(Noelke, Carl B.),* 529 Main, Box 563, La Crosse, WI 54602 (SAN 111-8315) Tel 608-782-8544.

Carolina Biological, *(Carolina Biological Supply Co., Pubns. Dept.; 0-89278),* 2700 York Rd., Burlington, NC 27215-3398 (SAN 249-2784) Tel 336-584-0381; Fax: 910-584-3399; Toll Free Fax: 800-222-7112; Toll Free: 800-334-5551
E-mail: carolina@carolina.com
Web site: http://www.carolina.com.

Carolina Cassette, *(Carolina Cassette Distributors),* Orders Addr.: P.O. Box 429, New Bern, NC 28560 (SAN 110-8395) Fax: 919-638-1291; Edit Addr.: 2600 Oaks Rd., New Bern, NC 28560 (SAN 659-2155) Tel 919-638-5583.

Carolina News Co, *(Carolina News Co.),* Orders Addr.: P.O. Box 10, Fayetteville, NC 28302 (SAN 169-6394); Edit Addr.: 245 Tillinghast St., Fayetteville, NC 28302 (SAN 249-2792) Tel 910-483-4135.

Carswell, *(Carswell),* Div. of The Thomson Corp., 28 Glen Ave., Millburn, NJ 07041 Toll Free Fax: 973-313-1245; Toll Free: 888-307-1355
E-mail: steve.roses@carswell.com.

Cascade News Inc, *(Cascade News, Inc.),* 1055 Commerce Ave., Longview, WA 98632 (SAN 169-8761) Tel 360-425-2450; Fax: 360-425-2451.

Casemate Pubs, *(Casemate Pubs. & Bk. Distributors; 0-9711709),* 2114 Darby Rd., 2nd Flr., Havertown, PA 19083 Tel 610-853-9131; Fax: 610-853-9146
E-mail: casemate@casematepublishing.com
Web site: http://www.casematepublishing.com.

Casino Distributors, *(Casino Distributors),* Orders Addr.: P.O. Box 849, Pleasantville, NJ 08232 (SAN 169-457X) Tel 609-646-4165; Edit Addr.: 10 Canale Dr., Pleasantville, NJ 08234 (SAN 249-3276).

Casper Magazine Agency, *(Casper Magazine Agency),* P.O. Box 2340, Casper, WY 82602 (SAN 159-8325).

Cassette Bk, *See* **Audio Bk**

Catholic Bookrack Service, *(Catholic Bookrack Service),* 700 E. Elm St., La Grange, IL 60525 (SAN 169-2178) Tel 708-482-0044; Fax: 708-482-9644.

Catholic Literary Guild Inc, *(Catholic Literary Guild, Inc.),* 200 Hamilton Ave., White Plains, NY 10601 (SAN 285-8908) Tel 914-949-4444.

Cave of the Winds, *(Cave of the Winds),* P.O. Box 826, Manitou Springs, CO 80829 Tel 719-685-5444
Web site: http://www.caveofthewinds.com.

CBLS, *(CBLS Pubs.),* 119 Brentwood St., Marietta, OH 45750 (SAN 169-5517) Tel 703-758-2539; Fax: 703-758-1518; 2600 Seskey Glen Ct., Herndon, VA 20171 Tel 614-374-9458; Fax: 614-374-8029.

CCC, *(Cleveland Chiropractic College),* 590 N. Vermont Ave., Los Angeles, CA 90004 Tel 323-660-6166.

Celestial Arts, *(Celestial Arts Publishing Co.; 0-89087; 0-912310; 1-58761),* Div. of Ten Speed Pr., Orders Addr.: P.O. Box 7123, Berkeley, CA 94707 (SAN 159-8333) Tel 510-559-1600; Fax: 510-559-1637; Toll Free: 800-841-2665; Edit Addr.: 999 Harrison St., Berkeley, CA 94710 Fax: 510-524-1052
E-mail: order@tenspeed.com
Web site: http://www.tenspeed.com.

Cent AZ Dist, *(Central Arizona Distributing),* 4932 W. Pasadena Ave., Glendale, AZ 85301 (SAN 170-6128) Tel 602-939-6511.

Centennl Pbns, *(Centennial Pubns.),* 1400 Ash Dr., Fort Collins, CO 80521 (SAN 630-494X) Tel 970-493-2041 Do not confuse with Centennial Pubns., Grand Junction, CO.

Central Illinois Periodicals, *(Central Illinois Periodicals),* P.O. Box 3757, Bloomington, IL 61701 (SAN 630-8945) Tel 309-829-9405.

Central News of Sandusky, *(Central News of Sandusky),* 5716 McCartney Rd., Sandusky, OH 44870-1538 (SAN 169-684X).

Centralia News Co, *(Centralia News Co.),* 232 E. Broadway, Centralia, IL 62801 (SAN 159-8341) Tel 618-532-5601.

Ceramic Bk & Literature Service, *See* **CBLS**

CFI Dist, *(Cedar Fort, Inc./CFI Distribution; 0-934126; 1-55517),* 925 N. Main St., Springville, UT 84663-1051 (SAN 170-2858) Tel 801-489-4084; Fax: 801-489-9432; Toll Free Fax: 800-388-3727; Toll Free: 800-759-2665
E-mail: sales@cedarfort.com; marketing@cedarfort.com; cedarfort@cedarfort.com; editorial@cedarfort.com
Web site: http://www.cedarfort.com.

Champaign-Urbana News Agency, *(Champaign-Urbana News Agency),* Orders Addr.: P.O. Box 793, Champaign, IL 61824 (SAN 630-8953); Edit Addr.: 503 Kenyon, Champaign, IL 61820.

Charleston News Co, *(Charleston News Co.),* 3296 Ashley Phosphate Rd., No. B, Charleston, SC 29418-8484 (SAN 169-7757).

Chelsea Green Pub, *(Chelsea Green Publishing; 0-930031; 1-890132; 1-931498; 88-86283),* Orders Addr.: P.O. Box 428, White River Junction, VT 05001 (SAN 669-7631) Tel 802-295-6300; Fax: 802-295-6444; Toll Free: 800-639-4099; Edit Addr.: 205 Gates-Briggs Bldg., Main St., White River Junction, VT 05001
Web site: http://www.chelseagreen.com.

Cheng & Tsui, *(Cheng & Tsui Co.; 0-646; 0-88727; 0-917056),* 25 West St., Boston, MA 02111-1213 (SAN 169-3387) Tel 617-988-2401; Fax: 617-426-3669
E-mail: service@cheng-tsui.com; ct@world.std.com
Web site: http://www.cheng-tsui.com.

Chicago Distribution Ctr, *(Chicago Distribution Ctr.),* 11030 S. Langley Ave., Chicago, IL 60628 (SAN 630-6047) Tel 773-568-1550; Fax: 773-660-2235; Toll Free: 800-621-2736; 800-621-8471 (credit & collections).

Chico News Agency, *(Chico News Agency),* P.O. Box 690, Chico, CA 95927 (SAN 168-9533) Tel 916-895-3865.

Childrens Lib Poetry, *(Children's Library of Poetry),* P.O. Box 831, Dearborn Heights, MI 48127 Tel 313-563-3030; Fax: 313-563-6888
E-mail: poetrylibrary@aol.com.

Childrns Bkfair, *(Children's Bookfair Co., The),* 700 E. Grand Ave., Chicago, IL 60611-3472 (SAN 630-6705) Tel 312-477-7323; 837 W. Altgeld St., Chicago, IL 60614 (SAN 630-6713).

China Bks, *(China Bks. & Periodicals, Inc.; 0-8351),* 2929 24th St., San Francisco, CA 94110-4126 (SAN 145-0557) Tel 415-282-2994; Fax: 415-282-0994
E-mail: info@chinabooks.com
Web site: http://www.chinabooks.com.

China Cultural Ctr, *(China Cultural Ctr.),* 970 N. Broadway, Suite 103, Los Angeles, CA 90012 (SAN 111-8161) Tel 213-489-3827; Fax: 213-489-3080.

China Institute Gallery, *(China Institute Gallery, China Institute in America; 0-9654270),* 125 E. 65th St., New York, NY 10021 (SAN 110-8743) Tel 212-744-8181; Fax: 212-628-4159
E-mail: gallery@chinainstitute.org
Web site: http://www.chinainstitute.org.

Chinese American Co, *(Chinese American Co.),* 44 Kneeland St., Boston, MA 02111 (SAN 159-7248) Fax: 617-451-2318.

Chivers N Amer, *(Chivers North America; 0-7540; 0-7927; 0-89340; 1-55504),* Orders Addr.: P.O. Box 1450, Hampton, NH 03843-1450 (SAN 208-4864) Tel 603-926-8744; Fax: 603-929-3890; Toll Free: 800-621-0182; Edit Addr.: 1 Lafayette Rd., Hampton, NH 03843.

Chr Lit, *(Christian Literature Crusade, Inc.; 0-87508),* Div. of CLC Publications, Orders Addr.: P.O. Box 1449, Fort Washington, PA 19034-8449 Tel 215-542-1242; Fax: 215-542-7580; Toll Free: 800-659-1240; Edit Addr.: 701 Pennsylvania Ave., Fort Washington, PA 19034 (SAN 169-7358)
E-mail: joinclc@juno.com
Web site: http://www.clcusa.org.

Christian Bk Distributors, *(Christian Bk. Distributors),* Orders Addr.: P.O. Box 7000, Peabody, MA 01961-7000 (SAN 630-5458) Tel 978-977-5000; Fax: 978-977-5010
Web site: http://www.christianbook.com.

Christian Dist, *(Christian Distribtuion Services, Inc.),* 1230 Heil Quaker Blvd., Lavergne, TN 37086 Tel 615-793-5955; Fax: 615-793-5973.

Christian Printing Service, *(Christian Printing Service),* 4861 Chino Ave., Chino, CA 91710-5132 (SAN 108-2647) Tel 714-871-5200.

Christine Pegram, *(Pegram, Christine),* 1901 Upper Cove Terr., Sarasota, FL 33581 (SAN 110-0254) Tel 941-921-2467.

Chronicle Bks, *(Chronicle Bks. LLC; 0-8118; 0-87701; 0-938491),* Div. of Chronicle Publishing Co., 85 Second St., San Francisco, CA 94105 (SAN 202-165X) Tel 415-537-4200; Fax: 415-537-4460; Toll Free Fax: 800-858-7787; Toll Free: 800-722-6657 (orders only)
E-mail: frontdesk@chroniclebooks.com
Web site: http://www.chroniclebooks.com.

Chrstian Pub Netwrk, *(Christian Publishing Network; 0-9628406),* P.O. Box 405, Tulsa, OK 74101 (SAN 631-2756) Tel 918-296-4673 (918-296-HOPE); Toll Free: 888-688-8125
E-mail: vpsales@olp.net.

Church of Scient Info, *(Church of Scientology Information Service-Pubns.; 0-915598),* c/o Bridge Pubns., Inc., 1414 N. Catalina, Los Angeles, CA 90029 (SAN 268-9774).

Church Richards Co, *(Church Richards Co.),* 10001 Roosevelt Rd., Westchester, IL 60154 (SAN 285-8975) Toll Free: 800-323-0227.

Circa Pubns Inc, *(Circa Pubns., Inc.),* 415 Fifth Ave., Pelham, NY 10803-0408 (SAN 169-6122) Tel 914-738-5570; Toll Free: 800-582-5952 (orders only).

Circle Bk Service, *(Circle Bk. Service; 0-87397),* P.O. Box 626, Tomball, TX 77377 (SAN 158-2526) Tel 281-255-6824; Fax: 281-255-8158; Toll Free: 800-227-1591
E-mail: orders@circlebook.com
Web site: http://www.circlebook.com.

City News Agency, *(City News Agency),* Orders Addr.: P.O. Box 561129, Charlotte, NC 28256-1129 (SAN 169-782X); Edit Addr.: P.O. Box 2069, Newark, OH 43055 (SAN 169-6947); 220 Cherry Ave., NE, Canton, OH 44702-1198 (SAN 169-6602); 303 E. Lasalle St., South Bend, IN 46617 (SAN 159-9992); 417 S. McKinnley, Harrisburg, IL 62946 (SAN 169-1961).

Clarks Out of Town News, *(Clarks Out of Town News),* 303 S. Andrews Ave., Fort Lauderdale, FL 33301 (SAN 159-8384) Tel 954-467-1543.

Classroom Read, *(Classroom Reading Service),* 9830 Norwalk Blvd., Suite 174, Santa Fe Springs, CA 90670 (SAN 131-3959) Tel 562-906-1366; Fax: 562-906-1370; Toll Free: 800-422-6657
E-mail: crsbooks@aol.com.

Clevelnd Chiropractic, *(Cleveland Chiropractic College),* 6401 N. Rockhill Rd., Kansas City, MO 64131 Tel 816-501-0100.

Client Dist Srvs, *(Client Distribution Services),* 425 Madison Ave., New York, NY 10017 (SAN 631-760X) Tel 212-223-2969; Fax: 212-223-1504 Do not confuse with Client Distribution Services, Jackson, TN.
E-mail: skail@cds.aeneas.com.

Clover Bk Service, *(Clover Bk. Service),* 1220 S. Monroe St., Covingtons, LA 70433-3639 (SAN 106-472X) Tel 504-875-0038.

CMG, *(Comag Marketing Group),* 1790 Broadway, Suite 401, New York, NY 10019 (SAN 169-5800) Tel 212-841-8365; Fax: 212-977-9401.

CMIL, *(Ctr. for Media & Independent Learning),* 2000 Center St., 4th Flr., Berkeley, CA 94704 Tel 510-642-0460; Fax: 510-643-9271.

CNS Judaica, *(CNS Judaica),* 13 Van Ness Pl., Caldwell, NJ 07006-7329 (SAN 158-6254).

Cobblestone Pub Co, *(Cobblestone Publishing Co.; 0-382; 0-942389; 0-9607638),* Div. of Cricket Magazine Group, 30 Grove St., Suite C, Peterborough, NH 03458 (SAN 237-9937) Tel 603-924-7209; Fax: 603-924-7380; Toll Free: 800-821-0115.

Cochran News Agency Inc, *(Cochran News Agency, Inc.),* P.O. Box 1110, Wichita Falls, TX 76307 (SAN 169-8486).

Cogan Bks, *(Cogan Bks.; 0-940688),* 15020 Desman Rd., La Mirada, CA 90638 (SAN 168-9649) Tel 714-523-0309; Fax: 714-523-0796; Toll Free: 800-733-3630.

Col U Pr, *(Columbia Univ. Pr.; 0-231),* 61 W. 62nd St., New York, NY 10023 (SAN 212-2472) Tel 212-459-0600; Fax: 212-459-3678
Web site: http://www.columbia.edu/cu/cup.

Collector Bks, *(Collector Bks.; 0-89145; 1-57432),* Div. of Schroeder Publishing Co., Inc., Orders Addr.: P.O. Box 3009, Paducah, KY 42003 (SAN 157-5368) Tel 270-898-6211; 270-898-7903; Fax: 270-898-8890; 270-898-1173; Toll Free: 800-626-5420 (orders only); Edit Addr.: 5801 Kentucky Dam Rd., Paducah, KY 42003 (SAN 200-7479)
E-mail: Info@collectorbooks.com; info@AQSquilt.com
Web site: http://www.AQSquilt.com; http://www.collectorbooks.com.

College Bk Co of California, *(College Bk. Co. of California, Inc.),* 6590 Darrin Way, Cypress, CA 90630 (SAN 269-0802) Tel 714-894-4791.

Colmbia News Agcy, *(Columbia County News Agency, Inc.),* 135 Warren St., Hudson, NY 12534 (SAN 169-5339) Tel 518-828-1017.

Colonial Williamsburg, *(Colonial Williamsburg Foundation; 0-87935; 0-910412),* P.O. Box 3532, Williamsburg, VA 23187-3532 (SAN 128-4630) Fax: 757-565-8999 (orders only); Toll Free: 800-446-9240 (orders only)
Web site: http://www.colonialwilliamsburg.com.

Colorado Periodical Distributor Inc, *(Colorado Periodical Distributor, Inc.),* 1227 Pitkin St., Grand Junction, CO 81502 (SAN 169-0582) Tel 970-242-3865; Fax: 970-242-3760.

Comm Tech, *(Communications Technology, Inc.; 0-918232),* P.O. Box 209, Rindge, NH 03461 (SAN 159-8198) Tel 603-899-6957.

Commitments Bkstore, *(Commitments Bookstore),* 3701 Durand Ave., Racine, WI 53405 Toll Free: 800-765-5815.

Commn Ground Dist, *(Common Ground Distributors, Inc.),* Orders Addr.: P.O. Box 25249, Asheville, NC 28813-1249 Toll Free: 800-654-0626; Edit Addr.: 115 Fairview Rd., Asheville, NC 28803-2307 (SAN 113-8006) Tel 828-274-5575; Fax: 828-274-1955
E-mail: orders@comground.com.

Commun Skill, *(Communication Skill Builders/Therapy Skill Builders; 0-7616; 0-88450),* Div. of The Psychological Corp., A Harcourt Co., 555 Academic Ct., San Antonio, TX 78204-2498 (SAN 201-7768) Toll Free Fax: 800-232-1223; Toll Free: 800-228-0752
Web site: http://www.harcourt.com/.

Comp & Tech Bks, *(Computer & Technical Bks.),* 7508 Colfax Ave., N., Brooklyn Park, MN 55444 (SAN 630-8120) Tel 612-566-4464.

Conde Nast Pubns, *(Conde Nast Pubns., Inc.; 1-878494),* 4 Times Square, 20th Flr., New York, NY 10036 (SAN 285-905X) Tel 212-880-8800; Fax: 212-880-8289.

Consort Bk Sales, *(Consortium Bk. Sales & Distribution),* Orders Addr.: 1045 Westgate Dr., Suite 90, Saint Paul, MN 55114-1065 (SAN 200-6049) Tel 651-221-9035; Fax: 651-221-0124; Toll Free: 800-283-3572 (orders)
E-mail: consortium@cbsd.com
Web site: http://www.cbsd.com.

Consulting Psychol, *(Consulting Psychologists Pr., Inc.; 0-89106),* 3803 E. Bayshore Rd., Palo Alto, CA 94303 (SAN 201-7849) Tel 650-969-8901; Fax: 650-969-8608; Toll Free: 800-624-1765
Web site: http://www.daviesblack.com; http://www.cpp-db.com.

Contemporary Arts, *(Contemporary Arts Pr.; 0-931818),* Div. of La Mamelle, Inc., P.O. Box 3123, San Francisco, CA 94119-3123 (SAN 170-5423) Tel 415-282-0286.

Continental Bk, *(Continental Bk. Co., Inc.; 0-9626800),* Eastern Div., 80-00 Cooper Ave., Bldg. No. 29, Glendale, NY 11385 (SAN 169-5436) Tel 718-326-0560; Fax: 718-326-4276; Toll Free: 800-364-0350; Western Div., 625 E. 70th Ave., No. 5, Denver, CO 80229 (SAN 630-2882) Tel 303-289-1761; Fax: 303-289-1764 Do not confuse with Continental Book Company, Denver, CO
E-mail: esl@continentalbook.com; bonjour@continentalbook.com; tag@continentalbook.com; hola@continentalbook.com
Web site: http://www.continentalbook.com.

Continuum, *(Continuum International Publishing Group, Inc.; 0-304; 0-7201; 0-8044; 0-8264),* Orders Addr.: 22883 Quicksilver Dr., Dulles, VA 20166 (SAN 253-3391) Fax: 703-661-1501; Toll Free: 800-561-7704; Edit Addr.: 370 Lexington Ave., New York, NY 10017-6503 (SAN 213-8220) Tel 212-953-5858; Fax: 212-953-5944
E-mail: info@continuum-books.com
Web site: http://www.continuum-books.com.

Cook Communs Minist, *(Cook Communications Ministries; 0-7459; 0-7814; 0-88207; 0-89191; 0-89693; 0-912692; 1-55513; 1-56476; 983-45027; 983-45018; 983-45031),* 4050 Lee Vance View, Colorado Springs, CO 80918 Tel 719-536-0100; Fax: 719-536-3269; Toll Free: 800-708-5550; 55 Woodslee Ave., Paris, ON N3L 3E5 Toll Free Fax: 800-461-8575; Toll Free: 800-263-2664 Do not confuse with Cook Communications Ministries International, same address
E-mail: bergerj@cookministries.org
Web site: http://www.cookministries.com.

Cookbook Collection Inc, *(Cookbook Collection, Inc.; 0-929410),* 2500 E. 195th St., Belton, MO 64012 (SAN 200-6359) Tel 816-322-2122; Fax: 816-322-8086
Web site: http://www.cookbookstore.com.

Coos Bay Distributors, *(Coos Bay Distributors),* 131 N. Schoneman St., Coos Bay, OR 97420 (SAN 169-7064).

Copper Island News, *(Copper Island News),* 1010 Wright St., Marquette, MI 49855-1834 (SAN 169-3824).

Cornell U Pr, *(Cornell Univ. Pr.; 0-8014; 0-87546),* Orders Addr.: P.O. Box 6525, Ithaca, NY 14851 (SAN 281-5680) Tel 607-277-2211; Toll Free Fax: 800-688-2877; Edit Addr.: Sage House, 512 E. State St., Ithaca, NY 14851 (SAN 202-1862) Tel 607-277-2338
E-mail: orders@plymbridge.com; cservs@plymbridge.com; cupress-sales@cornell.edu; cupressinfo@cornell.edu
Web site: http://www.cornellpress.cornell.edu.

Coronet Bks, *(Coronet Bks.; 0-89563; 91-7916),* 311 Bainbridge St., Philadelphia, PA 19147 (SAN 210-6043) Tel 215-925-2762; Fax: 215-925-1912 Do not confuse with Coronet Bks. & Pubns., Eagle Point, OR
E-mail: rsmolin@ix.netcom.com; order@coronetbooks.com
Web site: http://www.coronetbooks.com.

Coun Oak Bks, *(Council Oak Bks.; 0-933031; 1-57178),* Div. of Council Oak Publishing Co., Inc., Orders Addr.: 1350 E. 15th St., Tulsa, OK 74120-5801 (SAN 689-5522) Tel 918-587-6454; Fax: 918-583-4995; Toll Free: 800-247-8850 (orders only); Edit Addr.: 1290 Chestnut St., Suite 2, San Francisco, CA 94109 Tel 415-931-6868; Fax: 415-931-5353
E-mail: kevincob@pacbell.net
Web site: http://www.counciloakbooks.com.

Country News Distributor, *(Country News Distributors),* Div. of Bakers, Inc., Putney Rd., Box 8127, Brattleboro, VT 05304 (SAN 169-8575) Tel 802-254-2373; Fax: 802-257-0228.

Countryside Bks, *(Countryside Bks.; 0-88453),* 2410 Northside Dr., Clearwater, FL 33761-2216 (SAN 107-4415) Tel 813-796-7337.

Coutts Library Service Inc, *(Coutts Library Service, Inc.),* 1823 Maryland Ave., Box 1000, Niagara Falls, NY 14302-1000 (SAN 169-5401) Tel 716-282-8627; Fax: 905-356-5064; Toll Free: 800-772-4304
E-mail: coutts@wizbang.coutts.on.ca.

Cove Distributors, *(Cove Distributors),* 6325 Erdman Ave., Baltimore, MD 21205 (SAN 158-9814) Toll Free: 800-622-5656 (Orders).

Covenant Comms, *(Covenant Communications, Inc.; 1-55503; 1-57734; 1-59156),* Orders Addr.: P.O. Box 416, American Fork, UT 84003-0416 (SAN 169-8540) Tel 801-756-9966; Fax: 801-756-1049; Toll Free: 800-662-9545; Edit Addr.: 920 E. State Rd., Suite F, American Fork, UT 84003 Do not confuse with Covenant Communications in American Fork, UT
E-mail: lindao@covenant-lds.com
Web site: http://www.covenant-lds.com.

Cowley Distributing Inc, *(Cowley Distributing, Inc.),* 732 Heisinger Rd., Jefferson City, MO 65109 (SAN 169-426X) Tel 573-636-6511; Fax: 573-636-6262; Toll Free: 800-346-5950 (orders).

Cox Subscriptions Inc, *(Cox Subscriptions, Inc.),* 411 Marcia Dr., Goldsboro, NC 27530 (SAN 107-0061) Tel 919-735-1001; Fax: 919-734-3332; Toll Free: 800-553-8088.

CQ Products, *(CQ Products),* 507 Industrial St., Waverly, IA 50677 (SAN 631-5216) Tel 319-352-2086; Fax: 319-352-5338
E-mail: gifts@cqproducts.com
Web site: http://www.cqproducts.com.

CRC Pr, *(CRC Pr. LLC; 0-8493; 0-87819; 1-58488),* Subs. of Information Ventures, LLC, 2000 Corporate Blvd., NW, Boca Raton, FL 33431 (SAN 202-1994) Tel 561-994-0555; Fax: 561-989-8732 (outside USA); Toll Free Fax: 800-374-3401 (inside USA); Toll Free: 800-272-7737
E-mail: orders@crcpress.com
Web site: http://www.crcpress.com.

Creative Co, *(Creative Co., The; 0-87191; 0-88682; 1-56660; 1-56846),* 123 S. Broad St., P.O. Box 227, Mankato, MN 56001 Tel 507-388-6273; Fax: 507-388-2746; Toll Free: 800-445-6209 Do not confuse with The Creative Co., Lawrenceburg, IN
E-mail: CreativeCo@aol.com.

Creative Dev Ctr, *(Creative Development Ctr.),* P.O. Box 395, North, VA 23128 Tel 804-725-2234 (phone/fax).

Creative Homeowner, *(Creative Homeowner Pr.; 0-932944; 1-58011; 1-880029),* Div. of Federal Marketing Corp., 24 Park Way, Upper Saddle River, NJ 07458-9960 (SAN 213-6627) Tel 201-934-7100; Fax: 201-934-7541; Toll Free: 800-631-7795
E-mail: info@chp-publiser.com
Web site: http://www.chp-publisher.com.

Crescent Imports Pubns, *(Crescent Imports & Pubns.; 0-933127),* P.O. Box 7827, Ann Arbor, MI 48107-7827 (SAN 111-3976) Tel 734-665-3492; Fax: 734-677-1717; Toll Free: 800-521-9744
E-mail: crescentus@aol.com
Web site: http://www.crescentimports.com.

Crescent International Inc, *(Crescent International, Inc.),* 2238 Otranto Rd., Charleston, SC 29418 (SAN 110-0777) Tel 803-797-6363; Fax: 803-797-6367.

Cromland, *(Cromland, Inc.),* 1995 Highland Ave., Suite 200, Bethlehem, PA 18020 (SAN 108-2833) Tel 610-997-3000; Fax: 610-997-8880; Toll Free: 800-944-5554 (U.S. & Canada)
E-mail: info@cromland.com
Web site: http://www.cromland.com.

CrossLife Express, *(CrossLife Expressions; 0-9636049; 1-57838),* Div. of Exchanged Life Ministries, Inc., 10610 E. Bethany Dr., Suite A, Aurora, CO 80014 (SAN 169-0590) Tel 303-750-0440; Fax: 303-750-1228; Toll Free: 800-750-6818
E-mail: info@crosslifebooks.com
Web site: http://www.crosslifebooks.com.

Crowley Inc, *(Crowley, Inc.),* 16120 U.S. Hwy. 19 N., Suite 220, Clearwater, FL 34624-6862 (SAN 285-9130) Tel 813-531-5889.

Crown Agents Service Ltd, *(Crown Agents Service, Ltd.),* 3100 Massachusetts Ave., NW, Washington, DC 20008 (SAN 285-919X).

Crystal Star Herbal, *(Crystal Star Herbal Nutrition),* 4069 Wedgeway Ct., Earth City, MO 63045 (SAN 630-9801) Toll Free: 800-736-6015.

Ctrl KY News Dist, *See* **Anderson-Austin**

Ctry Life Natrl Fds, *(Country Life Natural Foods),* P.O. Box 489, Pullman, MI 498450 (SAN 631-2772) Tel 616-236-5011; Toll Free: 800-456-7694.

Cultural Hispana Ameriketako, *(Cultural Hispana/Ameriketako Liburuak),* Orders Addr.: P.O. Box 7729, Silver Spring, MD 20907 (SAN 159-2823); Edit Addr.: 1413 Crestridge Dr., Silver Spring, MD 20910 (SAN 249-3063) Tel 301-585-0134
E-mail: mokordo@erols.com
Web site: http://www.coloquio.com/libros.html.

Cummins News Co, *(Cummins News Co.),* Orders Addr.: Box 1695, Danville, IL 61834 (SAN 169-1910); Edit Addr.: P.O. Box 1937, Bloomington, IN 47402 (SAN 169-2305) Tel 812-332-4775.

CUP Services, *(CUP Services),* 750 Cascadilla St., Ithaca, NY 14851 (SAN 630-6519) Tel 607-277-2211; Fax: 607-277-6292; Toll Free: 800-666-2211.

Curley Pub, *See* **Chivers N Amer**

Cybernetics Tech Corp, *(Cybernetics Technology Corp.; 0-923458),* 1370 Port Washington Blvd., Port Washington, NY 11050-2628 (SAN 295-933X) Tel 516-883-7676.

CyberRead Pubng, *(CyberRead Publishing; 1-931921),* 11700 Mukilteo Speedway, Suite 201, Mukilteo, WA 98275 Tel 425-315-1434; Fax: 425-315-8835
E-mail: info@cyberread.com
Web site: http://www.cyberread.com.

Cypress Co, *(Cypress Bk. Co., Inc.; 0-934643),* Subs. of China International Bk. Trading Corp., 3450 Third St., Unit 4B, San Francisco, CA 94124 (SAN 112-1162).

D & H News Co, *(D & H News Co., Inc.),* 79 Albany Post Rd., Montrose, NY 10548 (SAN 169-5533) Tel 914-737-3152.

D Gibson, *(Gibson, Dot Pubns.; 0-941162),* Orders Addr.: P.O. Box 117, Waycross, GA 31502-0117 (SAN 200-4143) Tel 912-285-2848; Fax: 912-285-0349; Toll Free: 800-336-8095; Edit Addr.: 383 Bonneyman Rd., Blackshear, GA 31516 (SAN 200-9676)
E-mail: info@dotgibson.com
Web site: http://www.dotgibson.com.

Dade County Newsdealers Supply Co, *(Dade County Newsdealers Supply Co.),* P.O. Box 155, Miami, FL 33152 (SAN 159-8457).

Daedalus Bks, *(Daedalus Bks.),* 9645 Gerwig Ln., Columbia, MD 21046-1520 (SAN 158-9202) Tel 410-309-2700
E-mail: tstock@daedalus-books.com; custserv@daedalus-books.com
Web site: http://www.daedalus-books.com.

Dake Bible, *See* **Dake Publishing**

Dake Publishing, *(Dake Publishing; 0-9655968; 1-55829),* Orders Addr.: P.O. Box 1050, Lawrenceville, GA 30046 (SAN 212-0828) Tel 770-963-1611; Fax: 770-963-7700; Toll Free: 800-241-1239; Edit Addr.: 764 Martins Chapel Rd., Lawrenceville, GA 30246 (SAN 243-2684)
E-mail: derrick@dake.com
Web site: http://www.dake.com.

Dakota Bks, *(Dakota Bks.; 0-9632861),* P.O. Box 1551, Santa Cruz, CA 95061 (SAN 630-9445) Tel 831-477-7174 (phone/fax)
E-mail: office@dakota-books.com
Web site: http://www.dakota-books.com.

Dakota News Inc, *(Dakota News, Inc.),* 221 Petro Ave., Box 1310, Sioux Falls, SD 57101 (SAN 169-7854) Tel 605-336-3000; Fax: 605-336-7279; Toll Free: 800-658-5498.

Darcy Williamson, *See* **Southrn Cross Pubs**

Darr Subscription Agency, *(Darr Subscription Agency),* Rte. 1, Box 5, Centralia, KS 66415 (SAN 285-9149) Tel 785-857-3741; Fax: 785-857-3746; Toll Free: 800-850-3741
E-mail: lgriff@midusa.net.

David Brown, *(Brown, David Bk. Co.; 0-946897),* Orders Addr.: P.O. Box 511, Oakville, CT 06779 (SAN 630-9461) Tel 860-945-9329; Fax: 860-945-9468; Toll Free: 800-791-9354
E-mail: david.brown.bk.co@snet.net
Web site: http://www.oxbowbooks.com.

Dawson Subscription Service, *See* **Faxon Illinois**

Day Schl Magazine Service, *(Day School Magazine Service),* Orders Addr.: P.O. Box 262, Brooklyn, NY 11219 (SAN 285-9157) Tel 718-871-1486; Fax: 718-435-2342
E-mail: Elciv@juno.com.

De Gruyter, *(De Gruyter, Walter Inc.; 0-89925; 1-56445; 3-11),* Subs. of Walter de Gruyter & Co. (GW), 200 Saw Mill River Rd., Hawthorne, NY 10532 (SAN 201-3088) Tel 914-747-0110; Fax: 914-747-1326
E-mail: customerservice@degruyterny.com
Web site: http://www.degruyter.com.

De Vore Group Carla Bks, *(De Vore Group/Carla Bks. & More),* Orders Addr.: P.O. Box 10276, San Juan, PR 00922 (SAN 159-8309) Tel 809-721-7645; Fax: 809-722-9216; Edit Addr.: 1409 Ave. Ponce De Leon, San Juan, PR 00907-4023 (SAN 249-2776).

De Wolfe & Fiske Co, *(De Wolfe & Fiske Co.),* 300 Turnpike, Canton, MA 02021 (SAN 169-3409).

DeHoff Christian, *(DeHoff Christian Bookstore),* 749 NW Broad St., Murfreesboro, TN 37129 (SAN 184-4202) Tel 615-893-8322; Fax: 615-896-7447; Toll Free: 800-695-5385.

Dehoff Pubns, *See* **DeHoff Christian**

Delmar News Agency Inc, *(Delmar News Agency, Inc.),* P.O. Box 7169, Newark, DE 19714-7169 (SAN 169-0892) Tel 302-455-9922; Toll Free: 800-441-7025.

DeLong Subscription Agency, *(DeLong Subscription Agency),* P.O. Box 806, Lafayette, IN 47902 (SAN 285-9246) Toll Free: 800-992-2092.

Deltiologists Am, *(Deltiologists of America; 0-913782),* P.O. Box 8, Norwood, PA 19074 (SAN 170-3072) Tel 610-485-8572.

Demco, *(Demco Media, Ltd.; 0-606),* Affil. of Demco, Inc., Orders Addr.: P.O. Box 14260, Madison, WI 53714-0260; Edit Addr.: 2810 Crossroads Dr., Suite 2700, Madison, WI 53718-7942 (SAN 111-1167) Fax: 608-241-0666; Toll Free Fax: 800-828-0401 (orders); Toll Free: 800-448-8939 (Turtleback customer orders/service) Do not confuse with Demco, Inc., Madison, WI. Demco Media titles are available only to schools and libraries. Not available to the retail market.
E-mail: mediacustserv@demco.com
Web site: http://www.demcomedia.com.

Demos Medical, *(Demos Medical Publishing, Inc.; 0-939957; 1-888799),* 386 Park Ave. S., Suite 201, New York, NY 10016 (SAN 663-8635) Tel 212-683-0072; Fax: 212-683-0118; Toll Free: 800-532-8663
E-mail: orderdept@demospub.com; info@demospub.com
Web site: http://www.demosmedpub.com.

Demos Vermande, *See* **Demos Medical**

DeRus Fine Arts, *(DeRu's Fine Arts; 0-939370),* 9100 E. Artesia Blvd., Bellflower, CA 90706 (SAN 159-3862) Tel 562-920-1312; Fax: 562-920-3077
E-mail: derusgal@aol.com.

Deseret Bk, *(Deseret Bk. Co.; 0-87579; 0-87747; 1-57345; 1-59038),* Div. of Deseret Management Corp., Orders Addr.: P.O. Box 30178, Salt Lake City, UT 84130 (SAN 150-763X) Tel 801-534-1515; 801-517-3165 (Wholesale Dept.); Fax: 801-517-3338; Toll Free: 800-453-3876; Edit Addr.: 40 E. South Temple, Salt Lake City, UT 84111
E-mail: dbwhsale@deseretbook.com; wholesale@deseretbook.com
Web site: http://www.deseretbook.com.

Desert News, *(Desert News),* 3242 S. Richey St., Tucson, AZ 85713 (SAN 114-3875) Tel 520-747-0428.

Desert News Co, *(Desert News Co.),* 206 East Ave., K4, Lancaster, CA 93535 (SAN 249-2849) Tel 805-945-4571; Fax: 805-945-9799; Toll Free: 800-266-4571.

Devin, *(Devin-Adair Pubs., Inc.; 0-8159),* Orders Addr.: P.O. Box A, Old Greenwich, CT 06870 (SAN 112-062X) Tel 203-531-7755; Fax: 718-359-8568.

DeVorss, *(DeVorss & Co.; 0-87516),* Orders Addr.: P.O. Box 550, Marina del Rey, CA 90294-0550 (SAN 168-9886) Tel 310-822-8940; Fax: 310-821-6290; Toll Free: 800-843-5743; Edit Addr.: 1046 Princeton Dr., Marina del Rey, CA 90292
E-mail: devors@earthlink.net; service@devorss.com
Web site: http://www.devorss.com.

Diamond Comic Distributors Inc, *(Diamond Comic Distributors, Inc.),* 1966 Greenspring Dr., Suite 300, Timonium, MD 21093 (SAN 110-9502) Tel 410-560-7100; Fax: 410-560-7148; Toll Free: 800-452-6642
E-mail: service@diamondcomics.com
Web site: http://www.diamondcomics.com.

Dillon Bk, *(Dillon Bk.),* Subs. of Harold Dillon, Inc., 460 S. Marion Pkwy., Apt. 851B, Denver, CO 80209-2508 (SAN 169-0493) Tel 303-442-5323; Toll Free: 800-525-0842.

Direct Cinema, *(Direct Cinema, Ltd.; 1-55974),* Orders Addr.: P.O. Box 10003, Santa Monica, CA 90410-1003 (SAN 653-256X) Tel 310-636-8200; Fax: 310-636-8228; Toll Free: 800-525-0000; Edit Addr.: 3200 Airport Ave., No. 6, Santa Monica, CA 90405
E-mail: dcivideo@aol.com; sales@directcinemalimited.com; info@directcinemalimited.com
Web site: http://www.directcinema.com.

Discount Bk Distributors, *(Discount Bk. Distributors),* 1854 Wallace School Rd., No. E, Charleston, SC 29407-4822 (SAN 107-2250) Tel 843-556-6582.

Dist Art Pubs, *(Distributed Art Pubs./D.A.P.; 1-881616; 1-891024),* Orders Addr.: 575 Prospect St., Lakewood, NJ 08701 Fax: 732-363-0338; Toll Free: 800-338-2665; Edit Addr.: 155 Sixth Ave., 2nd Flr., New York, NY 10013-1507 (SAN 630-6446) Tel 212-627-1999; Fax: 212-627-9484
E-mail: dap@dapinc.com
Web site: http://www.artbook.com/.

Distribks Inc, *(Distribooks, Inc.),* Div. of Midwest European Pubns., Inc., 8120 N. Ridgeway, Skokie, IL 60076 (SAN 630-9763) Tel 847-676-1596; Fax: 847-676-1195
E-mail: info@distribooks.com.

Distribuidora Escolar Inc, *(Distribuidora Escolar, Inc.),* 2250 SW 99th Ave., Miami, FL 00165-7569 (SAN 169-1104).

Distributors, *(Distributors, The; 0-942520),* 702 S. Michigan, South Bend, IN 46601 (SAN 169-2488) Tel 219-232-8500; Fax: 312-803-0887; Toll Free: 800-348-5200.

Distributors International, *(Distributors International),* Div. of Dennis-Landman Pubs., 1150 18th St., Santa Monica, CA 90403 (SAN 129-8089) Tel 310-828-0680
E-mail: info@moviecraft.com
Web site: http://www.moviecraft.com.

Dixie News Co, *(Dixie News Co.),* P.O. Box 561129, Charlotte, NC 28256-1129 (SAN 169-636X) Tel 704-376-0140; Fax: 704-335-8604; Toll Free: 800-532-1045.

D&J Bk Dist, *(D&J Bk. Distributors; 1-883080),* 229-21B Merrick Blvd., Laurelton, NY 11413 (SAN 630-5091) Tel 718-949-5400; Fax: 718-949-6161; Toll Free: 800-446-4707.

Dog Museum, *See* **American Kennel**

Dogwise Dog, *See* **Dogwise Pubng**

Dogwise Pubng, *(Dogwise Publishing; 1-929242),* P.O. Box 2778, Wentachee, WA 98807 (SAN 631-1415) Tel 509-663-9115; Fax: 509-662-7233; Toll Free: 800-776-2665
E-mail: mail@dogwise.com
Web site: http://www.dogwise.com.

Donars, *(Donars Spanish Bks.),* P.O. Box 808, Lafayette, CO 80026 (SAN 108-1586) Tel 303-666-9175; Toll Free: 800-552-3316
E-mail: donars@prolynx.com.

Dot Gibson Dist, *(Dot Gibson Distribution),* Div. of Dot Gibson Pubns., P.O. Box 117, Waycross, GA 31502 Tel 912-285-2848.

Downtown Bk, *(Downtown Bk. Ctr., Inc.; 0-941010),* 247 SE First St., Suites 236-237, Miami, FL 33131 (SAN 169-1112) Tel 305-377-9941
E-mail: raxdown@aol.com.

Dr Leisure, *(Dr. Leisure; 0-9638802; 1-887471),* P.O. Box 1137, Kihei, HI 96753 Tel 808-879-4160
E-mail: drleisure@drleisure.com
Web site: http://www.drleisure.com.

Dreamhaven, *(Dreamhaven Bks.; 0-9630944; 1-892058),* 912 W. Lake St., Minneapolis, MN 55408 (SAN 630-0154) Tel 612-823-6161; Fax: 612-823-6062; Toll Free: 800-379-0657
E-mail: dreamhvn@visi.com
Web site: http://www.visi.com/~dreamhvn.

Drown News Agency, *(Drown News Agency),* 15172 Golden West Cir., Westminster, CA 92683 (SAN 169-0450).

Durkin Hayes Pub, *(Durkin Hayes Publishing Ltd.; 0-88625; 0-88646; 1-55204),* 2221 Niagara Falls Blvd., Niagara Falls, NY 14304-1696 (SAN 630-9518) Tel 716-731-9177; Fax: 716-731-9180; Toll Free: 800-962-5200
E-mail: info@dhaudio.com
Web site: http://www.dhaudio.com.

Duval News Co, *(Duval News Co.),* Orders Addr.: P.O. Box 61297, Jacksonville, FL 32203 (SAN 169-1015); Edit Addr.: 5638 Commonwealth Ave., Jacksonville, FL 32205 (SAN 249-2865) Tel 904-783-2350.

Duval-Bibb, *(Duval-Bibb Publishing Co.; 0-937713),* Orders Addr.: P.O. Box 24168, Tampa, FL 33623-4168 (SAN 111-8641) Tel 813-281-0091; Fax: 813-282-0220; Edit Addr.: 5300 W. Cypress St., Suite 250, Tampa, FL 33607-1712 (SAN 659-3127)
E-mail: ReeseCopp@aol.com.

E A & Prince Sons, *(Prince, E. A. & Sons),* Box 436, Anderson, SC 29622 (SAN 169-7749) Fax: 803-224-4380.

E A L Enterprises Inc, *(EAL Enterprises, Inc.),* Div. of Ambassador Bk. Service, 42 Chasner St., Hempstead, NY 11550 (SAN 169-6645) Toll Free: 800-431-8913.

E B S C O, *(EBSCO Subscription Services),* 5724 Hwy. 280 E., Birmingham, AL 35242-6818 (SAN 285-9394) Tel 205-991-6000; Fax: 205-991-1479
E-mail: jacomo@ebsco.com
Web site: http://www.ebsco.com.

E B S Inc Bk, *(EBS, Inc. Bk. Service),* 290 Broadway, Lynbrook, NY 11563 (SAN 169-5487) Tel 516-593-1195; Fax: 516-596-2911.

E Elgar, *(Elgar, Edward Publishing, Inc.; 1-84064; 1-85278; 1-85898; 1-84376),* Orders Addr.: c/o Custom Services, P.O. Box 574, Williston, VT 05495 Tel 802-862-0095; Fax: 802-864-7626; Toll Free: 800-390-3149; Edit Addr.: 136 West St. Suite 202, Northampton, MA 01060 (SAN 299-4615) Tel 413-584-5551; Fax: 413-584-9933
E-mail: tgorvine@e-elgar.com; eep.orders@aidcvt.com; rhenning@e-elgar.com
Web site: http://www.e-elgar.co.uk.

E Louis Hinrichs, *(Hinrichs, E. Louis),* P.O. Box 1090, Lompoc, CA 93438-1090 (SAN 133-1493) Tel 805-736-7512
E-mail: booklompoc@aol.com.

Eagle Business Systems, *(Eagle Business Systems; 0-928210),* P.O. Box 1240, El Toro, CA 92630-1240 (SAN 285-7510) Tel 714-859-9622.

Eagle Feather Trading Post Inc, *(Eagle Feather Trading Post, Inc.),* Orders Addr.: 168 W. 12th St., Ogden, UT 84404 (SAN 630-8996) Tel 801-393-3991; Fax: 801-745-0903; Toll Free: 800-547-3364 (orders only).

Eaglecrafts, *(Eaglecrafts),* Orders Addr.: 168 W. 12th St., Ogden, UT 84404 (SAN 630-6381) Tel 801-393-3991; Fax: 801-745-0903; Toll Free: 800-547-3364 (orders only)
E-mail: porsturbo@aol.com.

East Kentucky News Inc, *(East Kentucky News, Inc.),* 416 Teays Rd., Paintsville, KY 41240 (SAN 169-2879) Tel 606-789-8169.

East Ridge Bookstore, *(East Ridge Bookstore),* 161 Ridge Rd., Hankins, NY 12741 (SAN 282-6453).

Eastern Bk Co, *(Eastern Bk. Co.),* Orders Addr.: P.O. Box 4540, Portland, ME 04112-4540 Fax: 207-774-0331; Toll Free Fax: 800-214-3895; Toll Free: 800-937-0331; Edit Addr.: 131 Middle St., Portland, ME 04112 (SAN 169-3050)
E-mail: info@ebc.com
Web site: http://www.ebc.com.

Eastern News Distributors, *(Eastern News Distributors),* Subs. of Hearst Corp., 250 W. 55th St., New York, NY 10019 (SAN 169-5738) Tel 212-649-4484; Fax: 212-265-6239; Toll Free: 800-221-3148; 1 Media Way, 12406 Rte. 250, Milan, OH 44846-9705 (SAN 200-7711); 227 W. Trade St., Charlotte, NC 28202 (SAN 631-600X) Tel 704-348-8427
E-mail: enews@hearst.com.

Eastern Subscription Agency, *(Eastern Subscription Agency),* 5413 Wynnefield Ave., Philadelphia, PA 19131 (SAN 285-9467).

Easton News Co, *(Easton News Co.),* 2601 Dearborn St., Easton, PA 18042 (SAN 169-7315).

Eastview, *(Eastview Editions; 0-89860),* P.O. Box 247, Bernardsville, NJ 07924 (SAN 169-4952) Tel 908-204-0535.

East-West Export Bks, *(East-West Export Bks.),* c/o Univ. of Hawaii Pr., 2840 Kolowalu St., Honolulu, HI 96822 (SAN 202-5353) Tel 808-956-8830; Fax: 808-988-6052
E-mail: royden@hawaii.edu
Web site: http://www.2.hawaii.edu/uhpress/eweb.

Eastwind Bks & Arts, *(Eastwind Bks. & Arts, Inc.),* 1435-A Stockton St., San Francisco, CA 94133 (SAN 127-3159) Tel 415-772-5888; Fax: 415-772-5885
E-mail: info@eastwindsf.com
Web site: http://www.eastwindsf.com.

Eau Claire News Co Inc, *(Eau Claire News Co., Inc.),* 8100 Partridge Rd., Eau Claire, WI 54703-9646 (SAN 169-9059) Tel 715-835-5437.

EBSCO, *(EBSCO Industries, Inc.; 0-913956; 1-888751),* Orders Addr.: P.O. Box 1943, Birmingham, AL 35201-1943 (SAN 201-3584) Tel 205-991-6600; Fax: 205-995-1636; Toll Free: 800-826-3024; Edit Addr.: 5724 Hwy. 280 E., Birmingham, AL 35242
Web site: http://www.ebsco.com.

Ecology Res Intl, *(Ecology Resources International; 0-9671357),* 4847 Hopyard Rd., PMB 4380, Pleasanton, CA 94588 Tel 925-461-9096; Fax: 925-461-1705
E-mail: eri@home.com.

Econo-Clad Bks, *(Econo-Clad Bks.; 0-613; 0-7857; 0-8085; 0-8335; 0-88103),* Div. of American Cos., Inc., Orders Addr.: P.O. Box 1777, Topeka, KS 66601 (SAN 169-2763) Tel 913-233-4252; Toll Free: 800-255-3502; Edit Addr.: 2101 N. Topeka Blvd., Topeka, KS 66608-1830 (SAN 249-2687)
Web site: http://www.sagebrushcorp.com.

Economical Wholesale Co, *(Economical Wholesale Co.),* 6 King Philip Rd., Worcester, MA 01606 (SAN 169-3646).

Ed Media Corp, *(Educational Media Corp.; 0-932796; 1-930572),* Orders Addr.: P.O. Box 21311, Minneapolis, MN 55421 (SAN 665-6919); Edit Addr.: 4256 Central Ave. NE, Minneapolis, MN 55421-2920 (SAN 212-4203) Tel 763-781-0088; Fax: 763-781-7753; Toll Free: 800-966-3382
E-mail: emedia@educationalmedia.com
Web site: http://www.educationalmedia.com.

Ediciones Norte, *(Ediciones del Norte; 0-910061),* P.O. Box 5130, Hanover, NH 03755 (SAN 241-2993).

Editorial Cernuda Inc, *(Editorial Cernuda, Inc.),* 1040 27th Ave., SW, Miami, FL 33135 (SAN 158-8850) Tel 305-264-9400.

Edna Hibel Studio, *(Hibel, Edna Studio),* P.O. Box 9967, Riviera Beach, FL 33419 (SAN 111-1574) Tel 407-848-9633; Toll Free: 800-275-3426.

Educ Guide, *(Education Guide, Inc.; 0-914880),* P.O. Box 421, Randolph, MA 02368 (SAN 201-4580) Tel 617-376-0066; Fax: 617-376-0067.

Educational Bk Distributors, *(Educational Bk. Distributors),* P.O. Box 2510, Novato, CA 94948 (SAN 158-2259) Tel 415-883-3530; Fax: 415-883-4280; Toll Free: 800-761-5501
E-mail: PblshrSvcs@aol.com.

Edu-Tech Corp, *(Edu-Tech Corp., The),* 65 Bailey Rd., Fairfield, CT 06432 (SAN 157-5392) Tel 203-374-4212; Fax: 203-374-8050; Toll Free: 800-338-5463
E-mail: edutcorp@aoc.com.

Edward Wston Fine Arts, *(Weston, Edward Fine Arts),* P.O. Box 3098, Chatsworth, CA 91313-3098 (SAN 168-9967) Tel 818-885-1044; Fax: 818-885-1021.

Egypt News, *(Egypt News),* Orders Addr.: P.O. Box E, Johnston City, IL 62951 (SAN 169-2046) Tel 618-983-6976; Fax: 618-983-5611.

Eisenbrauns, *(Eisenbrauns, Inc.; 0-931464; 1-57506),* Orders Addr.: P.O. Box 275, Winona Lake, IN 46590-0275 (SAN 200-7835) Tel 219-269-2011; Fax: 219-269-6788; Edit Addr.: 600 N. Bay Dr., Warsaw, IN 46580
E-mail: orders@eisenbrauns.com
Web site: http://www.eisenbrauns.com.

Elders Bk Store, *(Elder's Bk. Store),* 2115 Elliston Pl., Nashville, TN 37203 (SAN 112-6091) Tel 615-327-1867.

Elfin Cove Pr, *(Elfin Cove Pr.; 0-944958),* 1481 130th Ave., NE, Belleuve, WA 98005 (SAN 245-8578) Tel 425-467-6565; Fax: 425-467-6564
E-mail: ecovepress@aol.com
Web site: http://www.elfincovepress.com.

Elizabeth City News Agency, *(Elizabeth City News Agency),* 504-508 E. Elizabeth St., Elizabeth City, NC 27909 (SAN 169-6386).

Ellis News Co, *(Ellis News Co.),* Affil. of L-S Distributors, 130 E. Grand Ave., South San Francisco, CA 94080 (SAN 169-0183) Tel 415-873-2094; Fax: 415-873-4222; Toll Free: 800-654-7040 (orders only).

ELS Educ Servs, *(ELS Educational Services; 0-87789; 0-89285; 0-89318),* Orders Addr.: 200 Old Tappan Rd., Old Tappan, NJ 07675; Edit Addr.: 1357 Second St., Santa Monica, CA 90401-1102 (SAN 281-6326).

Elsevier, *(Elsevier Science; 0-08; 0-444; 0-7204; 0-916086; 1-85617),* Orders Addr.: P.O. Box 945, New York, NY 10159-0945 (SAN 251-2564) Toll Free: 888-437-4636; Edit Addr.: 655 Ave. of the Americas, New York, NY 10010-5107 (SAN 200-2051) Tel 212-633-3730; Fax: 212-633-3680
E-mail: usinfo-f@elsevier.com
Web site: http://www.elsevier.com; http://www.elsevier.nl.

Emerg Response Inst, *(Emergency Response Institute, Inc.; 0-913724),* 4537 Foxhall Dr., NE, Olympia, WA 98516 (SAN 204-6490) Tel 360-491-7785.

Emergency Film Group, *(Emergency Film Group),* P.O. Box 1928, Edgartown, MA 02539-1928 (SAN 630-737X) Tel 508-627-8844; Fax: 508-627-8863; Toll Free: 800-842-0999
E-mail: sales@efilmgroup.com
Web site: http://www.efilmgroup.com.

Emery-Pratt Co, *(Emery-Pratt Co.),* Orders Addr.: 1966 W. Main St., Owosso, MI 48867-1397 (SAN 170-1401) Tel 989-723-5291; Fax: 989-723-4677; Toll Free Fax: 800-523-6379; Toll Free: 800-762-5683 (library orders only); 800-248-3887 (customer service only) Distributor to Libraries & Hospitals
E-mail: custserv@emery-pratt.com
Web site: http://www.emery-pratt.com.

Empire Comics, *(Empire Comics),* 375 Stone Rd., Rochester, NY 14616 (SAN 110-943X) Tel 716-442-0371; Fax: 716-442-7807
E-mail: empires@frontiernet.net.

Empire News of Jamestown, *(Empire News of Jamestown),* Foot Ave. & Extension St., Box 2029, Sta. A, Jamestown, NY 14701 (SAN 169-5371).

Empire Pub Srvs, *(Empire Publishing Service; 1-58690),* P.O. Box 1344, Studio City, CA 91614-0344 (SAN 630-5687) Tel 818-784-8918.

Empire State News, *(Empire State News Corp.),* Orders Addr.: P.O. Box 1167, Buffalo, NY 14240-1167 Tel 716-681-1100; Fax: 716-681-1120; Toll Free: 800-414-6247; Edit Addr.: 2800 Walden Ave., Cheektowaga, NY 14225-4772 (SAN 169-5177)
Web site: http://www.esnc.com.

Enrica Fish Medical Bks, *(Fish, Enrica Medical Bks.),* 814 Washington Ave., SE, Minneapolis, MN 55414 (SAN 157-8588) Tel 612-623-0707; Fax: 612-623-0539; Toll Free: 800-728-8398.

Enrichment Reading Corp of America, *(Enrichment Reading Corp. of America),* 518 S. Hubbard St., Horicon, WI 53032-1717 (SAN 159-8546).

Entrep Start Busn Store, *(Entrepreneur Start a Business Store),* 9114 River Look Ln., Fair Oaks, CA 95628-6565 (SAN 133-1485) Fax: 916-863-0361.

Epic Bk Promo, *(Epic Book Promotions),* 914 Nolan Way, Chula Vista, CA 91911-2408 Tel 619-498-8547; Fax: 619-498-8540
E-mail: gvjack@pacbell.net.

Epson Mid-Atlantic, *(Epson Mid-Atlantic),* Subs. of Epson America, Inc., 8 Neshaminy Interplex, Suite 319, Trerose, PA 19053 (SAN 285-7243) Tel 215-245-2180.

Eriksson Enterprises, *(Eriksson Enterprises),* 850 E. 1050 N., Bountiful, UT 84010 (SAN 110-5892) Tel 801-292-8320.

ETD Gulf Coast, *(ETD Gulf Coast Division),* 3600 75th Terr., Pinellas Park, FL 33781-2704 (SAN 108-6707).

ETD KroMar Temple, *(ETD KroMar Temple),* P.O. Box 535695, Grand Prairie, TX 75053-5625 (SAN 169-8435) Tel 254-778-5261; Fax: 254-778-5267.

ETX Dist, *(East Texas Distributing),* 7171 Grand Blvd., Houston, TX 77054 (SAN 169-8265) Tel 713-748-2520; Fax: 713-748-2504.

European Bk Co Inc, *(European Bk. Co., Inc.),* 925 Larkin St., San Francisco, CA 94109 (SAN 169-0191) Tel 415-474-0626; Fax: 415-474-0630; Toll Free: 877-746-3666
E-mail: info@europeanbook.com.

European Pr Service - PBD, *(European Press Service - PBD America Wholesalers),* 30 Edison Dr., Wayne, NJ 07470-4713 (SAN 630-7825).

Excaliber Pub, *(Excaliber Publishing Co.; 1-881353),* 7954 W. Bury Ave., San Diego, CA 92126 (SAN 297-6412) Tel 619-695-3091; Fax: 619-695-3095.

Excalibur Hobbies Ltd, *(Excalibur Hobbies, Ltd.),* 100 Federal St., Boston, MA 02110-1802 (SAN 158-2755).

Exciting Times, *(Exciting Times),* 4667 W. Rosecrans, Hawthorne, CA 90250 (SAN 114-4642).

Executive Bks, *(Executive Bks.; 0-937539),* Div. of Life Management Services, Inc., 206 W. Allen St., Mechanicsburg, PA 17055-6240 (SAN 156-5419) Tel 717-766-9499; Fax: 717-766-6565; Toll Free: 800-233-2665
E-mail: jason@executivebooks.com
Web site: http://www.executivebooks.com.

E-Z Legal, *See* **Made E-Z**

F & F Books, *(Flora & Fauna Bks.),* P.O. Box 15718, Gainesville, FL 32604 (SAN 133-1221) Tel 352-373-5630; Fax: 352-373-3249
E-mail: ffbks@aol.com
Web site: http://www.ffbooks.com.

F & W Pubns Inc, *(F&W Pubns., Inc.; 0-89134; 0-89879; 0-932620; 1-55870; 1-58180; 1-58297; 1-884910),* Orders Addr.: 3637 Woodburn Ave., Cincinnati, OH 45207; Edit Addr.: 1507 Dana Ave., Cincinnati, OH 45207 (SAN 287-0274) Tel 513-531-2690; Fax: 513-531-4082; Toll Free Fax: 888-590-4082; Toll Free: 800-289-0963
E-mail: marciaj@fwpubs.com
Web site: http://www.fwpublications.com.

F E C News Distributing, *(FEC News Distributing),* 2201 Fourth Ave., N., Lake Worth, FL 33461-3835 (SAN 169-1341) Tel 407-547-3000; Fax: 407-547-3080.

F M Roberts, *(Roberts, F.M. Enterprises; 0-912746),* P.O. Box 608, Dana Point, CA 92629-0608 (SAN 201-4688) Tel 714-493-1977; Fax: 714-493-7124.

F O Schwarz, *(Schwarz, F. A. O.),* 500 Pierce St., Somerset, NJ 08873-1270 (SAN 170-8554).

Fairfield Bk Service Co, *(Fairfield Bk. Service Co.),* 150 Margherita Lawn, Stratford, CT 06615 (SAN 131-0976) Tel 203-375-7607.

Fairfield County News Co Inc, *(Fairfield County News Co., Inc., Paperback Div.),* 387 Warren St., Bridgeport, CT 06604-5096 (SAN 169-0663).

FaithWorks NBN, *(FaithWorks/NBN),* 9247 Hunterboro Dr., Brentwood, TN 37027 Tel 615-221-6442 (phone/fax); Toll Free: 877-323-4550 Do not confuse with Faithworks in Bronx NY
Web site: http://www.faithworksonline.com.

Falcon Pub Inc, *(Falcon Publishing, Inc.; 0-934318; 0-934641; 0-937959; 0-9609452; 1-56044; 1-57540; 1-58592),* Div. of Globe Pequot Press, Orders Addr.: P.O. Box 1718, Helena, MT 59624 (SAN 221-1726) Fax: 406-442-0384; Toll Free Fax: 800-968-3550; Toll Free: 800-582-2665; Edit Addr.: 48 Last Chance Gulch, Helena, MT 59601 Do not confuse with companies with similar names in Ben Lomond,CA, Venice, CA, Long Island City, NY, Wauwatosa, WI, Palo Alto, CA, Grand Prairie, TX
E-mail: falconbk@ix.netcom.com
Web site: http://www.falcon.com.

Falkyn Inc, *(G-Jo Institute/Deer Haven Hills, Inc.; 0-916878),* Orders Addr.: P.O. Box 548, Columbus, NC 28722-0548; Edit Addr.: P.O. Box 1460, Columbus, NC 28722-1460 (SAN 111-0004).

Falkynor Bks, *See* **Falkyn Inc**

Fall River News Co Inc, *(Fall River News Co., Inc.),* 144 Robeson St., Fall River, MA 02720-4925 (SAN 169-3425) Tel 508-679-5266.

Fam Hist World, *(Family History World),* P.O. Box 129, Tremonton, UT 84337 (SAN 159-673X) Fax: 801-250-6727; Toll Free: 800-377-6058
E-mail: genealogy@utahlinx.com
Web site: http://www.genealogical-institute.com.

Fam Reading Svc, *(Family Reading Service),* 1601 N. Slappey Blvd., Albany, GA 31701-1431 (SAN 169-1376).

Far West Bk Serv, *(Far West Bk. Service),* 3515 NE Hassalo, Portland, OR 97232 (SAN 107-6760) Tel 503-234-7664; Fax: 503-231-0573; Toll Free: 800-964-9378.

Fawcett, *(Fawcett; 0-345; 0-449; 0-8041; 1-4000),* Div. of Ballantine Publishing Group, Orders Addr.: 400 Hahn Rd., Westminster, MD 21157 Tel 410-848-1900; Toll Free: 800-762-0600; Edit Addr.: 201 E. 50th St., New York, NY 10022 (SAN 201-4572) Tel 212-572-2713; Fax: 212-572-6046; Toll Free: 800-733-3000 (orders); 800-726-0600 (customer service)
E-mail: customerservice@randomnhouse.com
Web site: http://www.randomhouse.com.

Faxon, *(Faxon Co., The; 0-87305),* 15 Southwest Park, Westwood, MA 02090-1725 (SAN 159-8619) Tel 781-329-3350; Fax: 781-329-9875; Toll Free: 800-766-0039
E-mail: helpdesk@faxon.com; pubservices@faxon.com
Web site: http://www.faxon.com.

Faxon Illinois, *(Faxon Illinois Service Ctr.),* Affil. of Dawson Holdings PLC, 1001 W. Pines Rd., Oregon, IL 61061-9570 (SAN 286-0147) Tel 815-732-9001; Toll Free: 800-852-7404
E-mail: postmaster@dawson.com
Web site: http://www.faxon.com.

Fayette Cty News Agcy, *(Fayette County News Agency),* Orders Addr.: P.O. Box 993, Uniontown, PA 15401; Edit Addr.: Cherry Tree Square 42 Matthew Dr., Uniontown, PA 15401 (SAN 169-765X).

Feldheim, *(Feldheim, Philipp Inc.; 0-87306; 1-58330),* 200 Airport Executive Pk., Nanuet, NY 10954 (SAN 106-6307) Tel 845-356-2282; Fax: 845-425-1908; Toll Free: 800-237-7149
E-mail: mike613@netvision.net.il
Web site: http://www.feldheim.com.

FEP, *(FEP, A Booksource Co.),* 1230 Macklind Ave., Saint Louis, MO 63110 (SAN 169-1317) Tel 314-647-0600; Fax: 314-647-6850; Toll Free: 800-444-0435
Web site: http://www.booksource.com.

Fiddlecase Bks, *(Fiddlecase Bks.),* HC 63 Box 104, East Alstead, NH 03602 (SAN 200-7495) Tel 603-835-7889.

Fiesta Bk, *(Fiesta Bk. Co.; 0-88473),* P.O. Box 490641, Key Biscayne, FL 33149 (SAN 201-8470) Tel 305-858-4843.

Fiesta Pub, *See* **Fiesta Bk**

Fine Assoc, *(Fine Assocs.),* 1 Farragut Sq., S., Washington, DC 20006 (SAN 169-0914).

Finn News Agency Inc, *(Finn News Agency, Inc.),* 4415 State Rd. 327, Auburn, IN 46706-9542 (SAN 169-2356).

Fire Protect Pubns, *See* **IFSTA**

Firebird Dist, *(Firebird Distributing, LLC),* 2030 First St., Unit 5, Eureka, CA 95501 (SAN 631-1229) Tel 707-444-1434; Fax: 707-444-8537; Toll Free: 800-353-3575
E-mail: griffins@northcoast.com.; sales@firebirddistributing .com
Web site: http://www.firebirddistributing.com.

Fischer Inc NY, *(Fischer, Carl Inc.; 0-8258),* 65 Bleeker St., New York, NY 10012-2420 (SAN 107-4245) Tel 212-772-0900; Fax: 212-477-6996; Toll Free: 800-762-2328
E-mail: cf-info@carlfischer.com
Web site: http://www.carlfischer.com.

Five Star AZ, *(Five Star Pubns., Inc.; 0-9619853; 1-877749; 1-58985),* Orders Addr.: P.O. Box 6698, Chandler, AZ 85246-6698 (SAN 246-7429) Tel 480-940-8182; Fax: 480-940-8787; Toll Free: 800-545-7827; Edit Addr.: 4696 W. Tyson St., Chandler, AZ 85226-2903
E-mail: info@fivestarsupport.com
Web site: http://www.bookproducer.com.

Flannery Co, *(Flannery Co.),* 13123 Aerospace Dr., Victorville, CA 92394 (SAN 168-9754) Tel 760-246-8995; Fax: 760-246-8595; Toll Free: 800-456-3400.

Florida Classics, *(Florida Classics Library; 0-912451),* P.O. Drawer 1657, Port Salerno, FL 34992-1657 (SAN 265-2404) Tel 561-546-9380 (orders); Fax: 561-546-7545 (orders).

Florida Schl Bk Depository, *(Florida Schl. Bk. Depository),* 1125 N. Ellis Rd., P.O. Box 6578, Jacksonville, FL 32236 (SAN 161-8423).

Flury & Co, *(Flury & Co.),* 322 First Ave S., Seattle, WA 98104 (SAN 107-5748) Tel 206-587-0260.

Fodor, *See* **Fodors Travel**

Fodors Travel, *(Fodor's Travel Pubns., Inc.; 0-609; 0-676; 0-679; 1-878867; 1-4000),* Div. of Random Hse., Information Group, Orders Addr.: 400 Hahn Rd., Westminster, MD 21157 Tel 410-848-1900; Toll Free: 800-726-0600; Edit Addr.: 280 Park Ave., Tenth Flr., New York, NY 10017 Tel 212-572-8784; Fax: 212-572-2248
Web site: http://www.fodors.com.

Follett Audio, *(Follett Audiovisual Resources),* 220 Exchange Dr., Suite A, Crystal Lake, IL 60014 (SAN 631-7316) Tel 815-455-1555; Fax: 815-455-7090; Toll Free: 888-281-1216.

Follett Educ Srvs, *(Follett Educational Services),* Orders Addr.: 1433 Internationale Pkwy., Woodridge, IL 60517 (SAN 631-7901) Tel 800-621-4272; Fax: 630-972-4673; Edit Addr.: 5563 S. Archer Ave., Chicago, IL 60638 (SAN 169-1899).

Follett Library, *(Follett Library Resources; 0-329),* Div. of the Follett Corp., 1340 Ridgeview Dr., McHenry, IL 60050 (SAN 169-1902) Tel 815-759-1700; Toll Free: 800-435-6170.

Fondo Cultural Latinoamericano, *(Fondo Cultural Latinoamericano),* Box 1784, San Diego, CA 92112 (SAN 159-8627).

Fordham, *(Fordham Univ. Pr.; 0-8232),* University Box L, Bronx, NY 10458 (SAN 201-6516) Tel 718-817-4780; Fax: 718-817-4785
E-mail: mnoonan@fordham.edu
Web site: http://www.bookmasters.com/fordhampress/.

Forest Sales & Dist, *(Forest Sales & Distributing Co.; 0-9712183),* 4157 Saint Louis St., New Orleans, LA 70119 (SAN 157-5511) Tel 504-486-3331; Fax: 504-486-6223; Toll Free: 800-347-2106
E-mail: tbooks2@juno.com.

Forms Worms Inc, *(Forms & Worms, Inc.),* 3800 Williston Rd., No. 100, Minnetonka, MN 55345-2130 (SAN 631-5143).

Forsyth Travel, *(Forsyth Travel Library, Inc.; 0-9614539),* 1750 E. 131st St., P.O. Box 480800, Kansas City, MO 64148-0800 (SAN 169-2755) Tel 816-942-9050; Fax: 816-942-6969; Toll Free: 800-367-7984 (orders only)
E-mail: forsyth@gvi.net
Web site: http://www.forsyth.com.

Four-M Enterp, *(Four-M Enterprises, Inc.),* 1280 Pacific St., Union City, CA 94587 (SAN 631-5097) Tel 510-489-8722; Fax: 510-489-8331
E-mail: orders@4mdogbooks.com; books4m@aol.com.

Fr & Eur, *(French & European Pubns., Inc.; 0-320; 0-7859; 0-8288),* Rockefeller Ctr. Promenade, 610 Fifth Ave., New York, NY 10020-2497 (SAN 206-8109) Tel 212-581-8810; Fax: 212-265-1094
E-mail: frenchbookstore@aol.com; livresny@aol.com
Web site: http://www.frencheuropean.com.

Franklin, *(Franklin Bk. Co., Inc.),* 7804 Montgomery Ave., Elkins Park, PA 19027 (SAN 121-4160) Tel 215-635-5252; Fax: 215-635-6155
E-mail: service@franklinbook.com
Web site: http://www.franklinbook.com.

Franklin Readers Service, *(Franklin Readers Service),* P.O. Box 662, Dunn Loring, VA 22027-0662 (SAN 285-9599).

Franklin Square Overseas, *(Franklin Square Overseas),* 17-19 Washington St., Tenafly, NJ 07670-2084 (SAN 285-9637) Tel 201-569-2500; Fax: 201-569-5141
E-mail: esstn@ebsco.com.

Fraser Pub Co, *(Fraser Publishing Co.; 0-87034; 0-918632),* Div. of Fraser Management Assocs., Inc., Orders Addr.: Box 494, Burlington, VT 05402 (SAN 213-9537) Toll Free: 800-253-0900; Edit Addr.: 309 S. Willard St., Burlington, VT 05401 (SAN 110-8646) Tel 802-658-0324; Fax: 802-658-0260
E-mail: info@fraserbooks.com
Web site: http://www.fraserbooks.com.

Fred Biermann Bookseller, *(Biermann, Fred Bookseller),* Rte. 7, Box 414, Springfield, MO 65802 (SAN 108-0407) Tel 417-866-6983.

Fris News Co, *(Fris News Co.),* 194 River Ave., Holland, MI 49423 (SAN 159-8643).

FS&G, *(Farrar, Straus & Giroux, LLC; 0-374),* Orders Addr.: c/o Von Holtzbrinck Publishing Services, 16365 James Madison Hwy., Gordonsville, VA 22942 (SAN 631-5011) Tel 540-672-7600; Toll Free Fax: 800-672-2054; Toll Free: 888-330-8477; Edit Addr.: 19 Union Sq., W., New York, NY 10003 (SAN 206-782X) Tel 212-741-6900; Fax: 212-633-9385
E-mail: sales@fsgee.com
Web site: http://www.fsbassociates.com/fsg/index.htm.

Fulcrum Inc, *See* **Fulcrum Pub**

Fulcrum Pub, *(Fulcrum Publishing; 0-912347; 1-55591; 1-56373),* 16100 Table Mountain Pkwy., Suite 300, Golden, CO 80403 (SAN 200-2825) Tel 303-277-1623; Fax: 303-279-7111; Toll Free Fax: 800-726-7112; Toll Free: 800-992-2908
E-mail: dianneh@fulcrum-books.com
Web site: http://www.fulcrum-books.com.

Fulmont News Co, *(Fulmont News Co.),* Affil. of Rubin Periodical Group, P.O. Box 1211, Rochester, NY 14603-1211 (SAN 169-5029) Tel 518-843-2421.

Fultz News Agency, *(Fultz News Agency),* 2008 Woodbrook, Denton, TX 76205 (SAN 169-8168).

G Borchardt Inc, *(Borchardt, G. Inc.),* 136 E. 57th St., New York, NY 10022 (SAN 285-8614) Tel 212-753-5785; Fax: 212-838-6518.

G Freihofer, *(Freihofer, A. G.),* 175 Fifth Ave., New York, NY 10010 (SAN 285-9602) Tel 272-460-7500; Fax: 272-473-6272.

G H Arrow Co, *(Arrow, G. H. Co.),* P.O. Box 676, Bala Cynwyd, PA 19004 (SAN 111-3771) Tel 215-227-3211.

G Kurian, *(Kurian, George Reference Bks.; 0-914746),* Orders Addr.: P.O. Box 519, Baldwin Place, NY 10505 (SAN 203-1981); Edit Addr.: 3689 Campbell Ct., Yorktown Heights, NY 10598 (SAN 110-6236) Tel 914-962-3287.

G Paulsen Co, *(Paulsen, G. Co.),* 27 Sheep Davis Rd., Pembroke, NH 03275 (SAN 169-4499) Tel 603-225-9787.

Galahad Bks, *(Galahad Bks.; 0-88365; 1-57866),* Div. of BBS Publishing Corp., 386 Park Ave. S., Suite 1200, New York, NY 10016 Tel 212-679-4200; Fax: 212-679-4234.

Gale, *(Gale Group; 0-13; 0-7876; 0-8103; 0-936474; 1-57302; 1-878623),* Subs. of The Thomson Corp., Orders Addr.: P.O. Box 9187, Farmington Hills, MI 48333-9187 Toll Free Fax: 800-414-5043; Toll Free: 800-877-4253; Edit Addr.: 27500 Drake Rd., Farmington Hills, MI 48331-3535 (SAN 213-4373) Tel 248-699-4253
E-mail: galeord@galegroup.com
Web site: http://www.galegroup.com.

Galesburg News Agency Inc, *(Galesburg News Agency, Inc.),* 5 E. Simmons St., Galesburg, IL 61401 (SAN 169-1945).

Galveston News Agency, *(Galveston News Agency),* P.O. Box 7608, San Antonio, TX 78207-0608 (SAN 169-8230).

GAM Pubn, *(GAM Pubn.),* P.O. Box 25, Sterling, VA 20167 (SAN 158-7218) Tel 703-450-4121; Fax: 703-450-5311.

Gamboge Intl Inc, *(Gamboge International, Inc.),* 18 Brittany Ave., Trumbull, CT 06611 (SAN 631-046X) Tel 203-261-2130; Fax: 203-452-0180
E-mail: gamboge@pcaet.com.

Gannon, *(Gannon Distributing Co.; 0-88307),* 100 La Salle Cir., No. A, Santa Fe, NM 87505-6916 (SAN 201-5889).

Gardners Bk Service, *(Gardner's Bk. Service),* 16461 N. 25th Ave., Phoenix, AZ 85023-3111 (SAN 106-9322) Tel 602-863-6000; Fax: 602-863-2400 (orders only); Toll Free: 800-851-6001 (orders only)
E-mail: gbsbooks@bgsbooks.com
Web site: http://www.gbsbooks.com.

Garrett Ed Corp, *(Garrett Educational Corp.; 0-944483; 1-56074),* Orders Addr.: P.O. Box 1588, Ada, OK 74820 (SAN 169-6955) Tel 580-332-6884; Fax: 580-332-1560; Toll Free: 800-654-9366; Edit Addr.: 130 E. 13th St., Ada, OK 74820 (SAN 243-2722)
E-mail: mail@garrettbooks.com
Web site: http://www.garrettbooks.com.

Gasman News Agency, *(Gasman News Agency),* 2211 Third Ave., S., Escanaba, MI 49829 (SAN 169-3794).

Gaunt, *(Gaunt, Inc.; 0-912004; 1-56169),* 3011 Gulf Dr., Holmes Beach, FL 34217-2199 (SAN 202-9413) Tel 941-778-5211; Fax: 941-778-5252; Toll Free: 800-942-8683 (US & Canada)
E-mail: info@gaunt.com; sales@gaunt.com
Web site: http://www.gaunt.com.

Gazelle Books, *(Gazelle Bks.; 1-891211),* 17965 Hooker Creek Rd., Cottonwood, CA 96022-1545 Tel 530-347-1057
E-mail: gazelbook@nstate.net.

GCPI, *(Generic Computer Products, Inc.; 0-918611),* P.O. Box 790, Marquette, MI 49855 (SAN 284-8856) Tel 906-226-7600; Fax: 906-226-8309.

Gefen Bks, *(Gefen Bks.; 0-86343; 965-229),* 12 New St., Hewlett, NY 11557-2012 Tel 516-295-2805; Fax: 516-295-2739; Toll Free: 800-477-5257
E-mail: gefenbooks@compuserve.com
Web site: http://www.israelbooks.com.

Gem Guides Bk, *(Gem Guides Bk. Co.; 0-935182; 0-937799; 1-889786),* 315 Cloverleaf Dr., Suite F, Baldwin Park, CA 91706 (SAN 221-1637) Tel 626-855-1611; Fax: 626-855-1610
E-mail: gembooks@aol.com
Web site: http://www.gemguidesbooks.com.

Gemini Enterprises, *(Gemini Enterprises),* P.O. Box 8251, Stockton, CA 95208 (SAN 128-1402).

Genealog Sources, *(Genealogical Sources, Unlimited; 0-913857),* 407 Ascot Ct., Knoxville, TN 37923-5807 (SAN 170-8058) Tel 865-690-7831.

Genealogy Digest, *(Genealogy Digest),* 960 N. 400 E., North Salt Lake, UT 84054-1920 (SAN 110-389X); 420 S. 425 W., Bountiful, UT 84010 (SAN 243-2439).

General Distrib Services, *(General Distribution Services, Inc.),* 4500 Witmer Industrial, E., Niagara Falls, NY 14305-1386 (SAN 630-7949) Toll Free Fax: 800-481-6207; Toll Free: 800-805-1083
E-mail: cservice@genpub.com
Web site: http://genpub.com.

Genl Dist Srvs, *See* **General Distrib Services**

Genl Med Pub, *(General Medical Pubs.; 0-935236),* P.O. Box 210, Venice, CA 90294-0210 (SAN 215-689X) Tel 310-392-4911.

Geographia, *(Geographia Map Co., Inc.; 0-88433),* 231 Hackensack Plank Rd., Weehawken, NJ 07087 (SAN 132-5566) Tel 201-863-3866; Fax: 201-863-5977.

Gerard Hamon Inc, *See* **Lafayette Bks**

Gerold International Booksellers Inc, *(Gerold International Booksellers, Inc.),* 35-23 Utopia Pkwy., Flushing, NY 11358 (SAN 129-959X) Tel 718-358-4741; Fax: 718-358-3688.

Gibbs Smith Pub, *(Smith, Gibbs Pub.; 0-87905; 1-58685; 0-9676662),* Orders Addr.: P.O. Box 667, Layton, UT 84041 (SAN 201-9906) Tel 801-544-9800; Fax: 801-544-5582; Toll Free Fax: 800-213-3023 (orders); Toll Free: 800-748-5439 (orders); Edit Addr.: 1877 E. Gentile St., Layton, UT 84040
E-mail: info@gibbs-smith.com; text@gibbs-smith.com
Web site: http://www.gibbs-smith.com.

Gilmore-Howard, *(Gilmore-Howard),* P.O. Box 1268, Arlington, TX 76004-1268 (SAN 157-485X).

GL Services, *(GL Services),* 4588 Interstate Dr., Cincinnati, OH 45246 Tel 805-677-6815.

Global Dist Co, *(Global Distributing Co.),* P.O. Box 750234, Topeka, KS 66675 Toll Free: 800-769-8025.

Global Eng Latin, *(Global Engineering Documents-Latin America),* 3909 NE 163rd St., Suite 110, North Miami Beach, FL 33160 (SAN 630-7868) Tel 305-944-1099; Fax: 305-944-1028
E-mail: global.csa@ihs.com
Web site: http://www.ihs.com/global/.

Global Info Centres, *See* **Global Eng Latin**

Globe Pequot, *(Globe Pequot Pr., The; 0-7627; 0-87106; 0-88742; 0-914788; 0-933469; 0-934802; 1-56440; 1-57034),* Div. of Morris Communications Corp., Orders Addr.: P.O. Box 480, Guilford, CT 06437-0480 (SAN 201-9892) Toll Free Fax: 800-820-2329 (in Connecticut); Toll Free: 800-243-0495 (24 hours); Edit Addr.: 246 Goose Ln., Guilford, CT 06437 Tel 203-458-4500; Fax: 203-458-4604
E-mail: info@globe-pequot.com; adessaint@globe-pequot.com
Web site: http://www.globe-pequot.com.

Goldn Horiz, *(Golden Horizons, Inc.; 0-9667653),* Orders Addr.: P.O. Box 193, Sullivan, IL 61951 Tel 217-728-8182; Fax: 217-728-8690; Toll Free: 800-218-8182; Edit Addr.: R.R. 3, Box 364, Sullivan, IL 61951 (SAN 631-5542) Do not confuse with companies with similar names in San Gabriel, CA, Seattle, WA.

Good News Magazine Distributors, *(Good News Magazine Distributors),* 85 Crescent Ave., New Rochelle, NY 10801 (SAN 113-7271) Toll Free: 800-624-7257.

Gopher News Co, *(Gopher News Co.),* 420 First Ave., NW, Rochester, MN 55901 (SAN 169-4138) Tel 507-282-8641 (phone/fax).

Gordon & Breach, *(Gordon & Breach Publishing Group; 0-19; 0-677; 0-905203; 1-872501; 2-88124; 2-88449; 2-903928; 2-919875; 3-364; 3-7186; 90-5699; 90-5700; 90-5701; 90-5702; 90-5703; 90-5704; 90-5708; 976-641; 976-8097; 90-5755; 90-5706; 90-5707; 90-5709),* Div. of Taylor & Francis, Inc., Orders Addr.: 7625 Empire Dr., Florence, KY 41042 Toll Free Fax: 800-248-4724; Toll Free: 800-634-7064; Edit Addr.: 2 Gateway Ctr., Newark, NJ 07102-0301 (SAN 201-6370) Tel 973-643-7500; Fax: 973-643-7676; Toll Free: 800-545-8398
E-mail: ncarter@taylorandfrances.com
Web site: http://www.gbhap.com.

Gosp Mission, *(Gospel Mission, Inc.),* Orders Addr.: P.O. Box 318, Choteau, MT 59422 (SAN 170-3196) Tel 406-466-2311; Edit Addr.: 316 First St., NW, Choteau, MT 59422 (SAN 243-2455).

Gould Athletic Supply, *(Gould Athletic Supply),* 3156 N. 96th St., Milwaukee, WI 53222-3499 (SAN 169-9148).

Goyescas Corp of Florida, *(Goyescas Corp. of Florida),* 2155 NW 26th Ave., Miami, FL 33142 (SAN 169-1120).

Graham Maughan Publishing Co, *(Maughan, Graham Publishing Co.),* 50 E. 500, S., Provo, UT 84601-3203 (SAN 110-3903) Tel 801-377-3335; Toll Free: 800-234-3335.

Graham Services Inc, *(Graham Services, Inc.),* 180 James Dr., E., Saint Rose, LA 70087-9481 (SAN 169-2895) Tel 504-467-5863; Fax: 504-464-6196; Toll Free: 800-457-7323 (in Los Angeles only)
E-mail: gsi@aol.com.

Granite UT, *(Granite Publishing & Distribution, LLC; 1-890558; 1-930980),* 868 N. 1430 W., Orem, UT 84057 (SAN 631-0605) Tel 801-229-9023; Fax: 801-229-1924; Toll Free: 800-574-5779 Do not confuse with companies with same or similar names in Madison, WI, Columbus, NC
E-mail: granitepd@aol.com.

Great Lakes Readers Service, *(Great Lakes Reader's Service, Inc.),* Orders Addr.: P.O. Box 1078, Detroit, MI 48231 (SAN 285-9912) Tel 313-965-4577; Fax: 313-965-2445.

Green Gate Bks, *(Green Gate Bks.),* 1162 Latham Ave., Lima, OH 45805 (SAN 169-6785) Tel 419-222-3816; Fax: 419-227-3816; Toll Free: 800-228-3816
E-mail: ggb@wcoil.com
Web site: http://www.greengatebooks.com.

Greenville News Co Inc, *(Greenville News Co., Inc.),* P.O. Box 1313, Greenville, MS 38702 (SAN 169-4197).

Greenwood, *(Greenwood Publishing Group, Inc.; 0-275; 0-313; 0-8371; 0-86569; 0-89789; 0-89930; 1-56720),* Orders Addr.: P.O. Box 5007, Westport, CT 06881-5007 (SAN 213-2028) Fax: 203-222-1502 (customer service and sales) ; Toll Free: 800-225-5800 (orders only); Edit Addr.: 88 Post Rd., W., Westport, CT 06881-5007 Tel 203-226-3571; Fax: 203-222-1502; 203-226-2540 Do not confuse with Greenwood Publishing in Glenview, IL
E-mail: customer-service@greenwood.com; sales@greenwood.com
Web site: http://www.greenwood.com.

Grey Owl Indian Craft Co, *(Grey Owl Indian Craft Co., Inc.),* 132-05 Merrick Blvd., P.O. Box 468, Jamaica, NY 11434 (SAN 132-9979) Tel 718-341-4000.

Greystone Educ Mat, *(Greystone Educational Materials; 1-881639),* Orders Addr.: P.O. Box 86, Scandia, MN 55073 Tel 651-433-4502; Fax: 651-433-4269; Toll Free: 800-733-0671.

Grnlf Ent, *(Greenleaf Enterprises, Inc.; 0-9665319; 1-929774),* Div. of Greenleaf Book Group LLC, Orders Addr.: 660 Elmwood Point, Aurora, OH 44202 Tel 330-995-9700; Fax: 330-995-9704; Toll Free: 800-932-5420; Edit Addr.: 7600 Thistle Ln., Novelty, OH 44072
E-mail: email@greenleafbookgroup
Web site: http://www.greenleafbookgroup.com.

Grolier Americana, *(Grolier Americana),* 1111 Crandon Blvd., Apt. C501, Key Biscayne, FL 33149-2734 (SAN 108-1764) Tel 305-551-6711.

Grt Nrthrn Dists, *(Great Northern Distributors, Inc.),* 634 South Ave., Rochester, NY 14620-1316 (SAN 169-7676) Tel 717-342-8159.

Gryphon Hse, *(Gryphon Hse., Inc.; 0-87659; 1-58904),* Orders Addr.: P.O. Box 207, Beltsville, MD 20704-0207 (SAN 169-3190) Tel 301-595-9500; Fax: 301-595-0051; Toll Free: 800-638-0928; Edit Addr.: 10726 Tucker St., Beltsville, MD 20705
E-mail: info@ghbooks.com
Web site: http://www.gryphonhouse.com.

Guardian Bk Co, *(Guardian Bk. Co.),* 8464 Brown St., Ottawa Lake, MI 49267 (SAN 163-7355) Tel 313-856-1765; Fax: 313-854-7638.

Gulf Coast Periodicals, *See* **ETD Gulf Coast**

Gulf States Bk Fairs, *See* **Gulf States Educ Bks**

Gulf States Educ Bks, *(Gulf States Educational Bks.),* Orders Addr.: 368 Laurel Dr., Satsuma, AL 36572 (SAN 158-7870) Toll Free: 800-533-1189.

H Holt & Co, *(Holt, Henry & Co., LLC; 0-03; 0-8050),* 115 W. 18th St., 5th Flr., New York, NY 10011 (SAN 200-6472) Tel 212-886-9200; Fax: 212-633-0748
E-mail: info@hholt.com
Web site: http://www.henryholt.com.

H Kopplemann, *(Kopplemann, H. P. Inc.),* P.O. Box 145, Hartford, CT 06141-0145 (SAN 169-0744).

H P K Educational Resource, *(HPK Educational Resource Ctr.; 0-89895),* Div. of H. P. Koppelmann, Inc., 140 Van Block Ave., Hartford, CT 06141 (SAN 169-071X) Tel 860-549-6210; Toll Free: 800-243-7724.

Hackensack News Co Inc, *(Hackensack News Company, Incorporated),* 760 First St., Harrison, NJ 07029-2303 (SAN 169-4626).

Ham Radio s Bookstore, *See* **Radio Bkstore**

Hamakor Judaica Inc, *(Hamakor Judaica, Inc.),* 6153 Mulford, Unit D, Niles, IL 60714 (SAN 169-1791) Tel 847-966-4040; Fax: 847-966-4033; Toll Free: 800-552-4088.

Hamilton News Co Ltd, *(Hamilton News Co., Ltd.),* Hannay Ln., Glenmont, NY 12077 (SAN 169-5312).

Hammond Pub, *(Hammond Publishing Co., Inc.; 1-883882),* P.O. Box 279, G7166 N. Saginaw St., Mount Morris, MI 48458 (SAN 185-142X) Tel 810-686-8881; Fax: 810-686-0561; Toll Free: 800-521-3440 (orders only)
E-mail: hammondpub@juno.com.

Handleman, *(Handleman),* 2050 S. Santa Cruz St., No. 1100, Anaheim, CA 92805-6816 (SAN 106-4886) Tel 626-912-8182.

Handler News Agency, *(Handler News Agency),* P.O. Box 27007, Omaha, NE 68127-0007 (SAN 169-4405).

Hans E Rohr, *(Rohr, Hans E.),* 76 State St., Newburyport, MA 01950-6616 (SAN 113-8804).

HarBrace, *See* **Harcourt**

Harcourt, *(Harcourt Trade Pubs.; 0-15; 0-534),* Div. of Reed Elsevier plc, Orders Addr.: 6277 Sea Harbor Dr., Orlando, FL 32887 (SAN 200-285X) Tel 619-699-6707; Toll Free Fax: 800-235-0256; Toll Free: 800-543-1918 (trade orders, inquiries, claims); Edit Addr.: 525 B St., Suite 1900, San Diego, CA 92101-4495 (SAN 200-2736) Tel 619-231-6616
E-mail: apbcs@harcourtbrace.com
Web site: http://www.harcourtbooks.com.

HarperCollins Pubs, *(HarperCollins Pubs.; 0-00; 0-06; 0-688; 0-690; 0-694; 0-7322),* Div. of News Corp., Orders Addr.: 1000 Keystone Industrial Pk., Scranton, PA 18512-4621 (SAN 215-3742) Tel 570-941-1500; Toll Free Fax: 800-822-4090; Toll Free: 800-242-7737 (orders only); Edit Addr.: 10 E. 53rd St., New York, NY 10022-5299 (SAN 200-2086) Tel 212-207-7000
Web site: http://www.harpercollins.com.

Harrisburg News Co, *(Harrisburg News Co.),* Orders Addr.: P.O. Box 60307, Harrisburg, PA 17106 Fax: 717-232-1573; Edit Addr.: 980 Briars Dale Rd., Harrisburg, PA 17109 (SAN 169-7420) Tel 717-561-8377.

Harrison Hse, *(Harrison Hse., Inc.; 0-89274; 1-57794),* Orders Addr.: P.O. Box 35035, Tulsa, OK 74153 (SAN 208-676X) Tel 918-494-5944; Fax: 918-494-3665; Toll Free: 800-888-4126; Edit Addr.: 2448 E. 81st St., Suite 4400, Tulsa, OK 74137
Web site: http://www.harrisonhouse.com.

Harry L Epply Bk Co, *(Epply, Harry L. Bk. Co.),* 155 N. Gardner St., Scottsburg, IN 47170 (SAN 159-8554).

Harry-Young Pubn Services Agency Inc, *(Harry-Young Pubn. Services Agency, Inc.),* 6261 Manchester Blvd., Buena Park, CA 90621-2259 (SAN 110-8832).

Harsand Distributing, *(Harsand Distributing),* P.O. Box 515, Holmen, WI 54636 (SAN 242-1232) Toll Free: 800-321-0643.

Harvard Assocs, *(Harvard Assocs., Inc.; 0-924346),* 10 Holworthy St., Cambridge, MA 02138 (SAN 170-2939) Tel 617-492-0660; Fax: 617-492-4610; Toll Free: 800-774-5646
E-mail: info@harvassoc.com
Web site: http://www.harvassoc.com.

Harvard Univ Art Museums Shop, *(Harvard Univ. Art Museums Shop),* 32 Quincy St., Cambridge, MA 02138 (SAN 111-3372) Tel 617-495-8286; Fax: 617-496-2359
E-mail: appleyar@fas.harvard.edu
Web site: http://www.artmuseums.harvard.edu.

Harvest Distributors, *See* **ARVEST**

Hastings Bks, *(Hastings Bks.; 0-940846),* 116 N. Wayne Ave., Wayne, PA 19087 (SAN 205-048X).

Hawaiian Magazine Distributor, *(Hawaiian Magazine Distributor),* 3375 Koapaka St., No. D180, Honolulu, HI 98619-1865 (SAN 169-1619).

Hazelden, *(Hazelden Information & Educational Services; 0-89486; 0-89638; 0-935908; 0-942421; 1-56246; 1-56838),* 15251 Pleasant Valley Rd., P.O. Box 176, Center City, MN 55012-0176 (SAN 209-4010) Tel 651-257-4010; Fax: 651-213-4577; Toll Free: 800-328-0094
E-mail: bgreydanus@hazelden.org
Web site: http://www.hazelden.org.

Health Comm, *(Health Communications, Inc.; 0-922352; 0-932194; 0-941405; 1-55874; 1-880257; 0-7573),* 3201 SW 15th St., Deerfield Beach, FL 33442-8157 (SAN 212-100X) Tel 954-360-0909; Fax: 954-360-0034; Toll Free: 800-851-9100 Do not confuse with Health Communications, Inc., Edison, NJ
E-mail: hci@hcibooks.com
Web site: http://www.hcibooks.com.

Health Press, *(Health Pr.; 0-929173),* P.O. Box 1388, Santa Fe, NM 87504 (SAN 248-5036) Tel 505-474-0303; Fax: 505-424-0444
E-mail: goodbooks@healthpress.com
Web site: http://www.healthpress.com.

Hearst Corp, *See* **CMG**

Heartlnd Bk KS, *(Heartland Bk. Co.),* 10195 N. Lake Ave., Olathe, KS 66061 (SAN 631-2497) Tel 913-829-1784.

Heffernan Schl Supply, *(Heffernan School Supply),* 2111 West Ave., San Antonio, TX 78201-2822 (SAN 166-8722).

Heimburger Hse Pub, *(Heimburger Hse. Publishing Co.; 0-911581),* 7236 W. Madison St., Forest Park, IL 60130 (SAN 264-0929) Tel 708-366-1973 (phone/fax)
E-mail: heimburgerhouse@heimburgerhouse.com
Web site: http://www.heimburgerhouse.com.

Heinecken Assoc, *(Heinecken & Assoc., Ltd.),* 1733 N. Mohawk, Chicago, IL 60614 Toll Free Fax: 800-947-5694; Toll Free: 800-449-0138.

Heinemann, *(Heinemann; 0-325; 0-435),* Div. of Greenwood Publishing Group, Inc., Orders Addr.: P.O. Box 5007, Westport, CT 06881-5007 Toll Free: 800-793-2154; Edit Addr.: 88 Post Rd., W., Westport, CT 06881-5007 (SAN 210-5829) Tel 603-431-7894; Fax: 603-431-7840
E-mail: info@heinemann.com
Web site: http://www.heinemann.com.

Heinemann Ed, *See* **Heinemann**

Heirloom Bible Pubs, *(Heirloom Bible Pubs.),* Orders Addr.: P.O. Box 118, Wichita, KS 67201-0118 (SAN 630-2793) Fax: 316-267-1850; Toll Free: 800-676-2448; Edit Addr.: 1199 E. Central, Wichita, KS 67214 Tel 316-267-3211.

Heldref Pubns, *(Heldref Pubns.; 0-916882),* Div. of The Helen Dwight Reid Educational Foundation, 1319 18th St. NW, Washington, DC 20036-1802 (SAN 208-0788) Tel 202-296-6267; Fax: 202-296-5149; Toll Free: 800-365-9753.

Helena News Agency, *(Helena News Agency),* 26 N. Last Chance Gulch St., Helena, MT 59601-4122 (SAN 169-4375).

Helix, *(Helix),* 310 S. Racine St., Chicago, IL 60607 (SAN 111-915X) Tel 312-421-6000; Fax: 312-421-1586.

Herald Pub Hse, *(Herald Publishing Hse.; 0-8309),* P.O. Box 390, Independence, MO 64051-0390 Tel 816-252-5010; Fax: 816-252-3976; Toll Free: 800-767-8181; 1001W. Walnut St., Independence, MO 64051-0390 (SAN 111-7556)
E-mail: hhmark@heraldhouse.org
Web site: http://www.heraldhouse.org.

Herbert Furse-Bookman, *(Herbert Furse-Bookman),* 1461 Baffin Rd., Glenview, IL 60025 (SAN 159-8724).

Herit Bkstore, *(Heritage Bookstore),* Orders Addr.: 2101 W. Chesterfield Blvd., Suite A101, Springfield, MO 65807-8672 (SAN 111-7696).

Herveys Bklink, *(Hervey's Booklink & Cookbook Warehouse),* P.O. Box 831870, Richardson, TX 75083 (SAN 630-9747) Tel 214-221-2711; Fax: 214-221-2715; Toll Free: 800-413-3300.

Hesteria Recs, *(Hesteria Records & Publishing Co.),* 124 Hagar Ct., Santa Cruz, CA 95064 Tel 831-459-2575; Fax: 831-457-2917
E-mail: alissa@aainnovators.com
Web site: http://www.aainnovators.com.

Hi Jolly Library Service, *(Hi Jolly Library Service),* 150 N. Gay St., Susanville, CA 96130-3902 (SAN 133-5944).

Hill City News Agency Inc, *(Hill City News Agency, Inc.),* 3228 Odd Fellow Rd., Lynchburg, VA 24501 (SAN 169-8656) Tel 804-845-4231; Fax: 804-845-0864.

Hills Pet Products Inc, *(Hill's Pet Products, Inc.),* P.O. Box 148, Topeka, KS 66601 (SAN 630-1932) Tel 913-354-8523.

Hillsboro News, *(Hillsboro News),* Orders Addr.: P.O. Box 25738, Tampa, FL 33622-5738 (SAN 169-1325) Tel 813-622-8087; Edit Addr.: 7002 Park E. Blvd., Tampa, FL 33610 (SAN 249-3071).

Himber Bks, *(Himber Bks.),* Div. of F. C. Himber & Son's, Inc., 1380 W. Second Ave., Eugene, OR 97402 (SAN 169-7099) Tel 541-686-8003; Toll Free: 800-888-5904.

Hinshaw Music, *(Hinshaw Music Textbook Div.),* Orders Addr.: P.O. Box 571816, Houston, TX 77257-1816.

Hist Cherry Hill, *(Historic Cherry Hill; 0-943366),* 523 1/2 S. Pearl St., Albany, NY 12202 (SAN 110-8859) Tel 518-434-4791; Fax: 518-434-4806.

Historic Aviation Bks, *(Historic Aviation Bks.),* 121 Fifth Ave., Suite 300, New Brighton, MN 55112 (SAN 129-5284) Tel 651-635-0100; Fax: 651-635-0700.

HM, *(Houghton Mifflin Co.; 0-395; 0-87466; 0-87477; 0-89919; 0-9631591; 1-57630; 1-881527; 0-618),* Orders Addr.: 181 Ballardvale St., Wilmington, MA 01887 (SAN 215-3793) Tel 978-661-1300; Toll Free: 800-225-3362; P.O. Box 7050, Wilmington, MA 01887-7050; Edit Addr.: 215 Park Ave., S., New York, NY 10003 (SAN 282-4043) Tel 212-420-5800; Fax: 212-420-5855
Web site: http://www.hmco.com.

H&M Dist, *(H & M Distribution),* 41 Monroe Tpke., Trumbull, CT 06611 Tel 800-698-7781; Fax: 203-459-5095.

H&O Pioneer, *(H&O Pioneer Barns; 0-9637155),* 305 Birch St., Grandview, WA 98930 Tel 509-882-1799.

Holiday Enterprises Inc, *(Holiday Enterprises, Inc.),* 3328 US Hwy. 123, Greenville, SC 29602 (SAN 169-779X) Tel 803-269-4311.

Holtzbrinck, *(Holtzbrinck Online Publishing),* Orders Addr.: P.O. Box 2244, Williston, VT 05495 Fax: 802-864-7626; Toll Free: 800-972-9892
E-mail: gdi.orders@aidcvt.com.

Holyoke News Co Inc, *(Holyoke News Co., Inc.),* 720 Main St., P.O. Box 990, Holyoke, MA 01041 (SAN 169-3468) Tel 413-534-4537; Fax: 413-538-7161; Toll Free: 800-628-8372
E-mail: sales@holyoke-news.com.

Homestead Bk, *(Homestead Bk., Inc.; 0-930180),* Orders Addr.: P.O. Box 31608, Seattle, WA 98103 (SAN 662-037X); Edit Addr.: 6101 22nd Ave., NW, Seattle, WA 98107 (SAN 169-8796) Tel 206-782-4532; Fax: 206-784-9328; Toll Free: 800-426-6777 (orders only)
Web site: http://www.homesteadbook.com.

Hotho & Co, *(Hotho & Co.),* 916 Norwood St., Fort Worth, TX 76107-2994 (SAN 169-8192) Tel 817-335-1833.

Houston Paperback Distributor, *(Houston Paperback Distributor),* 4114 Gairloch Ln., Houston, TX 77025-2912 (SAN 169-8273).

Howard Smith Brokerage Inc, *(Smith, Howard Brokerage, Inc.),* 1100 Penn Ctr. Blvd., Apt. 216, Pittsburgh, PA 15235-5328 (SAN 286-0023).

Howell Pr VA, *(Howell Pr.; 0-943231; 0-9616878; 1-57427),* 1713-2D Allied Ln., Charlottesville, VA 22903-5336 (SAN 661-6607) Tel 804-977-4006; Fax: 804-971-7204; Toll Free Fax: 888-971-7204; Toll Free: 800-868-4512
E-mail: custserv@howellpress.com
Web site: http://www.howellpress.com.

Hubbard, *(Hubbard),* P.O. Box 100, Defiance, OH 43512 (SAN 169-6726).

Hudsn Valley News Dists, *(Hudson Valley News Distributors),* P.O. Box 1236, Newburgh, NY 12550 (SAN 169-6084) Tel 914-562-3399; Fax: 914-562-6010.

Hudson County News Co, *(Hudson County News Co.),* 1305 Paterson Plank Rd., North Bergen, NJ 07047 (SAN 169-4782) Tel 201-867-3600.

Hungry Minds, *(Hungry Minds, Inc.; 0-02; 0-7645; 1-55828; 1-56884; 1-878058),* Div. of John Wiley & Sons, Inc., Orders Addr.: 10475 Crosspoint Blvd., Indianapolis, IN 46256 (SAN 299-089X) Tel 416-293-8464; 317-572-3000; Fax: 317-572-4000; Toll Free: 800-667-1115 (Canadian customers); 800-434-3422 (Volume purchases); 800-762-2974
E-mail: siteemail@idgbooks.com
Web site: http://www.idgbooks.com.

HUP, *(Harvard Univ. Pr.; 0-674; 0-916724; 0-935617; 0-945454),* Orders Addr.: 79 Garden St., Cambridge, MA 02138 (SAN 200-2043) Tel 617-495-2600; Fax: 617-495-5898; Toll Free Fax: 800-962-4983; Toll Free: 800-448-2242 (customer service)
E-mail: contact_hup@harvard.edu
Web site: http://www.hup.harvard.edu.

I Brecht Soc, *(International Brecht Society; 0-9623206),* c/o Marc Silberman, Univ. of Wisconsin, German Dept., 818 Van Hisc Hall, Madison, WI 53706 Tel 608-262-2192; Fax: 608-262-4747.

IBD Ltd, *(i.b.d., Ltd.; 0-88431),* 24 Hudson St., Kinderhook, NY 12106 (SAN 630-7779) Tel 518-758-1755; Fax: 518-758-6702
E-mail: lankhof@ibdltd.com
Web site: http://www.ibdltd.com.

ICG Muse, *(ICG Muse, Inc.),* 73 Spring St., Suite 206, New York, NY 10012 (SAN 631-7200) Tel 212-343-1119; Fax: 212-343-1116.

ID International Bk Service, *(ID International Bk. Service),* 126 Old Ridgefield Rd., Wilton, CT 06897-3017 (SAN 630-8074) Tel 203-834-2272; Fax: 203-762-9725
E-mail: orders@idintl.com.

Idaho News Agency, *(Idaho News Agency),* 2710 Julia St., Coeur D'Alene, ID 83814 (SAN 169-1651) Tel 208-664-3444.

Ideal Foreign Bks Inc, *(Ideal Foreign Bks., Inc.),* 132-10 Hillside Ave., Richmond Hill, NY 11418 (SAN 169-6173) Tel 718-297-7477; Fax: 718-297-7645; Toll Free: 800-284-2490 (orders only).

IDG Bks, *See* **Hungry Minds**

IFSTA, *(IFSTA; 0-87939),* Orders Addr.: c/o Oklahoma State Univ., Fire Protection Pubns., 930 N. Willis, Stillwater, OK 74078-8045 Tel 405-744-5723; Fax: 405-744-8204; Toll Free: 800-654-4055 (orders only)
Web site: http://www.ifsta.org/.

IHS Health Grp, *(IHS Health Group; 0-935184; 1-57491),* Orders Addr.: 15 Inverness Way, E., Englewood, CO 80112-5776 (SAN 295-3374) Tel 303-662-9101; Toll Free: 877-295-9240
E-mail: interpharm@interpharm.com
Web site: http://www.interpharm.com.

Illinois News Service, *See* **News Grp IL**

Image Process, *(Image Processing Software, Inc.; 0-924507),* 6409 Appalachian Way, Madison, WI 53705 (SAN 265-5977) Tel 608-233-5033; 4414 Regent St., Madison, WI 53705 (SAN 249-3020).

Imaginart Intl, *(Imaginart International, Inc.; 0-9609464; 1-883315),* 307 Arizona St., Bisbee, AZ 85603 (SAN 260-2067) Tel 520-432-5741; Fax: 520-432-5134; Toll Free Fax: 800-737-1376 (U.S. & Canada only); Toll Free: 800-828-1376 (U.S. & Canada only)
E-mail: imaginart@compuserve.com
Web site: http://www.imaginartonline.com.

Imaginart Pr, *See* **Imaginart Intl**

Imperial News Co Inc, *(Imperial News Co., Inc.),* 5131 Post Rd., Dublin, OH 43017-1160 (SAN 169-5509) Fax: 516-752-8515.

Imported Bks, *(Imported Bks.),* Orders Addr.: St., Dallas, TX 75208 (SAN 169-8095) Tel 214-941-6497.

In Between, *(In Between Bks.; 0-935430),* P.O. Box 790, Sausalito, CA 94966 (SAN 213-6236) Tel 415-383-8447; Fax: 415-381-3513; 415-381-1938
E-mail: inbetweenbooks@atthebutterflytree.com
Web site: http://www.atthebutterflytree.com.

Incent Lrning, *(Incentives For Learning; 1-56872),* 111 Center Ave., Suite I, Pacheco, CA 94553 Tel 925-682-2428; Fax: 925-682-2645; Toll Free: 888-238-2379.

Incor Periodicals, *(Incor Periodicals),* 32150 Hwy. 34, Tangent, OR 97389-9704 (SAN 169-7072) Tel 541-926-8889; Fax: 541-926-9553.

Ind U Pr, *(Indiana Univ. Pr.; 0-253),* 601 N. Morton St., Bloomington, IN 47404-3797 (SAN 202-5647) Tel 812-855-4203; Fax: 812-855-7931
E-mail: iuporder@indiana.edu
Web site: http://www.Indiana.edu/~iupress.

Independent Inst, *(Independent Institute; 0-945999),* 100 Swan Way, Suite 200, Oakland, CA 94621-1428 (SAN 135-2938) Tel 510-632-1366; Fax: 510-568-6040; Toll Free: 800-927-8733
E-mail: info@indenpendent.org; orders@independent.org
Web site: http://www.independent.org.

Indiana Periodicals Inc, *(Indiana Periodicals, Inc.),* 2120 S. Meridian St., Indianapolis, IN 46225 (SAN 169-2380) Tel 317-786-1488; Fax: 317-782-4999.

Indpndnt Magzne, *(Independent Magazine Co.),* 2970 N. Ontario St., Burbank, CA 91504-2016 (SAN 159-8783).

Indpndnt Pubs, *(Independent Pubs. Marketing),* 6824 Oaklawn Ave., Edina, MN 55435 (SAN 630-5725) Tel 612-920-9044; Fax: 612-920-7662; Toll Free: 800-669-9044
Web site: http://www.Stjohns.ipm.worldnet.att.net.

Ingham Pub, *(Ingham Publishing, Inc.; 0-9611804; 1-891130),* Orders Addr.: P.O. Box 12642, Saint Petersburg, FL 33733-2642 Tel 813-343-4811; Fax: 813-381-2807; Edit Addr.: 5650 First Ave., N., Saint Petersburg, FL 33710 (SAN 112-8930)
E-mail: ftreflex@concentric.net.

Ingram Bk Co, *(Ingram Bk. Co.),* Subs. of Ingram Industries, Inc., Orders Addr.: 1 Ingram Blvd., P.O. Box 3006, La Vergne, TN 37086-1986 (SAN 169-7978) Tel 615-793-5000 (ext. 3-2622, customer service, ext. 81-367 Electronic Orders); Fax: 615-793-3976 (Electronic Orders); Toll Free Fax: 800-876-0186 (orders); 877-663-5367 (Canadian); Toll Free: 800-937-8000 (orders only); 800-937-8200 (customer service); 800-234-6737 (Canadian Electronic Orders); 800-677-5116 (Canadian Electronic Orders); 800-281-0687 (Canadian Orders) Do not confuse with Ingram Pr., Sacramento, CA
E-mail: ics-sales@ingrambook.com; flashback@ingrambook.com
Web site: http://www.ingrambook.com.

Ingram Software, *(Ingram Software),* Subs. of Ingram Distribution Group, Inc., 1759 Wehrle, Williamsville, NY 14221 (SAN 285-760X) Toll Free: 800-828-7250; 900 W. Walnut Ave., Compton, CA 90220 (SAN 285-7073).

Inst Electrical, *(Institute of Electrical & Electronics Engineers, Inc.; 0-7803; 0-87942; 0-7381),* Orders Addr.: c/o IEEE Service Ctr., P.O. Box 1331, Piscataway, NJ 08855-1331 (SAN 203-8072) Toll Free Fax: 800-716-6447; Toll Free: 800-716-3447 (ext. 025); Edit Addr.: 445 Hoes Ln., Piscataway, NJ 08855 (SAN 203-8064) Tel 732-562-3967; Fax: 732-981-9334; Toll Free: 800-678-4333
E-mail: ieeepress@ieee.org
Web site: http://www.ieee.org/organizations/pubs/press.

Int Mag Srv, *(International Magazine Service),* Div. of Periodical Pubs. Service Bureau, 1 N. Superior St., Sandusky, OH 44870 (SAN 285-9955) Tel 419-626-0623.

Int Period Dist, *(International Periodical Distributors),* 674 Via de la Valle, Suite 204, Solana Beach, CA 92075 (SAN 250-5290) Tel 619-481-5928; Toll Free: 800-999-1170; 800-228-5144 (in Canada).

Int Rdrs Leag, *(International Readers League),* Div. of Periodical Pubs. Service Bureau, 1 N. Superior St., Sandusky, OH 44870 (SAN 285-9971) Tel 419-626-0633.

Integral Yoga Pubns, *(Integral Yoga Pubns.; 0-932040),* Satchidananda Ashram-Yogaville, Rte. 1, Box 1720, Buckingham, VA 23921 (SAN 285-0338) Tel 804-969-1706; Fax: 804-969-1463; Toll Free: 800-262-1008 (orders)
Web site: http://www.yogaville.org/pubs.html.

Inter Thomson, *See* **Thomson Learn**

Interactv Knowlg, *See* **netLibrary CO**

Intermntn Periodcl Dists, *See* **Majic Enterprises**

Interpharm, *See* **IHS Health Grp**

Interstate Distributors, *(Interstate Distributors),* 199 Commander Shea Blvd., Quincy, MA 02171 (SAN 170-4885) Tel 617-328-9500; Toll Free: 800-365-6430.

Interstate Periodical Distributors, *(Interstate Periodical Distributors),* P.O. Box 2237, Madison, WI 53701 (SAN 169-9105) Tel 608-271-3600; Fax: 608-277-2410; Toll Free: 800-752-3131.

Intertech Bk Services Inc, *(Intertech Bk. Services, Inc.),* 25971 Sarazen Dr., South Riding, VA 20152-1741 (SAN 630-5253).

Intl Chiropractors Assn, *(International Chiropractors Assn.; 1-886190),* 1110 N. Glebe Rd., Suite 1000, Arlington, VA 22201 (SAN 224-1617) Tel 703-528-5000; Fax: 703-528-5023; Toll Free: 800-423-4690.

Intl Ntwrkng Assn, *(International Networking Assn.),* 4130 Citrus Ave., Suite 5, Rocklin, CA 95677 (SAN 631-1857).

Intl Pubns Serv, *(International Pubns. Service; 0-8002),* Div. of Taylor & Francis, Inc., Orders Addr.: 325 Chestnut St., 8th Flr., Levittown, PA 19057-4700 Tel 215-785-5800; Fax: 215-785-5515; Toll Free: 800-821-8312
E-mail: bkorders@tandfpa.com.

Intl Pubs Mktg, *(International Publishers Marketing),* Orders Addr.: 22883 Quicksilver Dr., Dulles, VA 20166 (SAN 253-3375) Toll Free: 800-758-3756; Edit Addr.: P.O. Box 605, Herndon, VA 20172-0605 Fax: 703-661-1501.

Intl Spec Bk, *(International Specialized Bk. Services; 0-7130),* 5824 NE Hassalo St., Portland, OR 97213-3644 (SAN 169-7129) Tel 503-287-3093; Fax: 503-280-8832; Toll Free: 800-944-6190
E-mail: info@isbs.com
Web site: http://www.isbs.com.

Intl Svce Co, *(International Service Co.),* International Service Bldg., 333 Fourth Ave., Indialantic, FL 32903-4295 (SAN 169-5134) Tel 407-724-1443 (phone/fax).

Intrepid Gp, *(Intrepid Group, Inc., The),* 1331 Red Cedar Cir., Fort Collins, CO 80524 (SAN 631-5429) Tel 970-493-3793; Fax: 970-493-8781
E-mail: intrepid@fril.com.

IntSystems, *(Internet Systems, Inc.),* Subs. of Internet Systems, Inc., 20250 Century Blvd., Germantown, MD 20874 (SAN 129-9611) Tel 301-540-5100; Fax: 301-540-5522; Toll Free: 800-638-8725
Web site: http://www.pwl.com/Internet.

Iowa & Illinois News, *(Iowa & Illinois News),* 8645 Northwest Blvd., Davenport, IA 52806-6418 (SAN 169-2607).

Iowa St U Pr, *See* **Iowa U Pr**

Iowa U Pr, *(Iowa Univ. Pr.; 0-8138),* 2121 S. State Ave., Ames, IA 50014-8300 (SAN 202-7194) Tel 515-292-0140; Fax: 515-292-3348
E-mail: orders@isupress.com
Web site: http://www.iowastatepress.com.

IPG Chicago, *(Independent Pubs. Group),* Subs. of Chicago Review Pr., 814 N. Franklin, Chicago, IL 60610 (SAN 202-0769) Tel 312-337-0747; Fax: 312-337-5985; Toll Free: 800-888-4741
E-mail: lreardon@ipgbook.com
Web site: http://www.ipgbook.com.

Irish Bks Media, *(Irish Bks. & Media, Inc.; 0-937702),* Orders Addr.: 1433 E. Franklin Ave., Minneapolis, MN 55404-2135 (SAN 111-8870) Tel 612-871-3505; Fax: 612-871-3358; Toll Free: 800-229-3505 Do not confuse with Irish Bks. in New York, NY
E-mail: Irishbook@aol.com
Web site: http://www.irishbook.com.

ISHK, *(ISHK; 0-86304; 0-900860; 1-883536),* Div. of Institute for the Study of Human Knowledge, Orders Addr.: P.O. Box 381069, Cambridge, MA 02238-1069 (SAN 226-4536) Tel 617-497-4124; Fax: 617-876-2976; Toll Free Fax: 800-223-4200; Toll Free: 800-222-4745; Edit Addr.: P.O. Box 176, Los Altos, CA 94023 Tel 650-948-9428
E-mail: ishkbooks@aol.com; ishkorders@aol.com
Web site: http://www.ishkbooks.com.

Islamic Bk Service, *(Islamic Bk. Service),* 2622 E. Main St., Plainfield, IN 46168 (SAN 169-2453) Tel 317-839-8150; Fax: 317-839-2511.

Island Heritage, *(Island Heritage Publishing; 0-89610; 0-931548),* Div. of The Madden Corp., 99880 Iwaena St., Aiea, HI 96701 (SAN 211-1403) Tel 808-487-7299; Fax: 808-488-2279; Toll Free: 800-468-2800
E-mail: hawaii4u@islandheritage.com
Web site: http://www.islandheritage.com/.

ITCP, *(International Thomson Computer Pr.; 1-85032),* Orders Addr.: 7625 Empire Dr., Florence, KY 41042-2978 Tel 606-525-6600; Fax: 606-525-7778; Toll Free: 800-842-3636; Edit Addr.: 20 Park Plaza, 13th Flr., Boston, MA 02116 Fax: 617-695-1615
E-mail: itcp@itp.thomson.com
Web site: http://www.itcpmedia.com.

iUniverse Inc, *(iUniverse, Inc.; 0-9665514; 1-58348; 0-9668591; 1-893652; 0-595),* 5220 S. 16th St., Suite 200, Lincoln, NE 68512 Tel 402-323-7800; Fax: 402-323-7824; Toll Free: 877-823-9235
E-mail: pubservices@iuniverse.com; custservice@iuniverse.com
Web site: http://www.iuniverse.com.

iUniversecom, *See* **iUniverse Inc**

J & L Bk Co, *(J&L Bk. Co.),* Orders Addr.: P.O. Box 3548, Spokane, WA 99220 (SAN 129-6817) Fax: 509-535-3360; Toll Free: 800-288-9756; Edit Addr.: 1710 Trent, Spokane, WA 99220 (SAN 243-2145).

J B Armstrong News Agency, *See* **News Group NC**

J Benjamins Pubng Co, *(Benjamins, John Publishing Co.; 0-915027; 1-55619; 1-58811),* Subs. of John Benjamins BV, Orders Addr.: P.O. Box 27519, Philadelphia, PA 19118-0519 (SAN 219-7677) Tel 215-836-1200; Fax: 215-836-1204; Toll Free: 800-562-5666 (orders); Edit Addr.: 821 Bethlehem Pike, Erdenheim, PA 19038
E-mail: paul@benjamins.com; service@benjamins.com
Web site: http://www.benjamins.com.

J League Greensboro, *(Junior League of Greensboro Pubns.; 0-9605788),* 220 State St., Greensboro, NC 27408 (SAN 112-9597).

J Levine Religious Supplies, *(Levine, J. Religious Supplies),* 5 W. 30th St., New York, NY 10001 (SAN 169-5878) Tel 212-695-6888; Fax: 212-643-1044
E-mail: sales@levine.judica.com.

J Majors Co, *(Majors, J. A. Co.),* Orders Addr.: 1401 Lakeway Dr., Lewisville, TX 75057 (SAN 169-8117) Tel 972-353-1100; Fax: 972-353-1300; Toll Free: 800-633-1851
E-mail: dallas@majors.com
Web site: http://www.majors.com.

JAMCO Dist, *(JAMCO Distribution),* 1401 Lakeway Dr., Lewisville, TX 75057 Fax: 972-353-1300; Toll Free: 800-538-1287
E-mail: jamco@majors.com.

James & Law Co, *(James & Law Co.),* Orders Addr.: P.O. Box 2468, Clarksburg, WV 26302-2468 (SAN 169-894X); Edit Addr.: Middletown Mall I-79 & U. S. 250, Fairmont, WV 26554 (SAN 169-8966) Tel 304-624-7401.

James C Strelow, *(Strelow, James C.),* 9440 El Blanco Ave., Fountain Valley, CA 92708 (SAN 132-4144) Tel 714-962-3697.

Jannetti Pubns, *(Jannetti Pubns., Inc.; 0-9655310),* Div. of Anthony J. Jannetti, Inc., East Holly Ave., Box 56, Pitman, NJ 08071-0056 Tel 856-256-2300; Fax: 856-256-2345
E-mail: Thomask@mail.ajj.com
Web site: http://www.inurse.com.

Janway, *(Janway),* 11 Academy Rd., Cogan Station, PA 17728 (SAN 108-3708) Tel 717-494-1239; Fax: 717-494-1350; Toll Free: 800-877-5242.

JayMar Servs, *(JayMar Services, LLC),* P.O. Box 210752, Nashville, TN 37221 Tel 615-673-6938; Fax: 615-673-0540; 1331 Red Cedar Cir., Fort Collins, CO 80524 Tel 970-493-3793; Fax: 970-493-8781
E-mail: JayMarLLC@aol.com
Web site: http://www.JayMarSvcs.com.

Jean Karr & Co, *(Karr, Jean & Co.),* 10116 Crestbury Pl., Bethesda, MD 20817 (SAN 169-0922) Tel 202-529-6789.

Jeanies Classics, *(Jeanies Classics; 0-9609672),* Orders Addr.: 2123 Oxford St., Rockford, IL 61103 (SAN 271-7409); Edit Addr.: 2123 Oxford St., Rockford, IL 61103 (SAN 271-7395) Tel 815-968-4544.

Jeans Dulcimer Shop, *(Jean's Dulcimer Shop & Crying Creek Pubs.),* P.O. Box 8, Hwy. 32, Cosby, TN 37722 (SAN 249-9282) Tel 423-487-5543.

Jech Distributors, *(Jech Distributors),* 674 Via De La Valle, No. 204, Solana Beach, CA 92075-2462 (SAN 107-0258) Tel 619-452-7251.

Jellyroll Prodns, *See* **Osborne Enterps**

Jeremiah Films, *(Jeremiah Films; 1-57618; 1-878993),* Orders Addr.: P.O. Box 1710, Hemet, CA 92546 Tel 909-652-1006; Fax: 909-652-5848; Toll Free: 800-828-2290; Edit Addr.: 43400 Cactus Valley Rd., Hemet, CA 92544
E-mail: orders@jeremiahfilms.com
Web site: http://www.jeremiahfilms.com.

Jeremiah Pubs, *See* **Jeremiah Films**

Jim Swenson, *(Swenson, Jim),* 2610 Riverside Ln., NE, Rochester, MN 55901 (SAN 285-9505).

JIST Pubng, *(JIST Publishing; 0-942784; 1-56370; 1-57112),* 8902 Otis Ave., Indianapolis, IN 46216-1033 (SAN 240-2351) Tel 317-613-4200; Fax: 317-613-4307; Toll Free Fax: 800-547-8329; Toll Free: 800-648-5478
E-mail: info@jist.com; generaldelivery@jist.com
Web site: http://www.jist.com.

JIST Works, *See* **JIST Pubng**

Johns Hopkins, *(Johns Hopkins Univ. Pr.; 0-8018),* Div. of Johns Hopkins Univ., 2715 N. Charles St., Baltimore, MD 21218-4319 (SAN 202-7348) Tel 410-516-6900; Fax: 410-516-6998; Toll Free: 800-537-5487
E-mail: bkinfo@chaos.press.jhu.edu
Web site: http://muse.jhu.edu/; http://www.press.jhu.edu.

Johnson News Agency, *(Johnson News Agency),* P.O. Box 9009, Moscow, ID 83843 (SAN 169-1678).

Jonathan David, *(Jonathan David Pubs., Inc.; 0-8246),* 68-22 Eliot Ave., Middle Village, NY 11379 (SAN 169-5274) Tel 718-456-8611; Fax: 718-894-2818
E-mail: jondavpub@aol.com
Web site: http://www.jdbooks.com.

Jones & Bartlett, *(Jones & Bartlett Pubs., Inc.; 0-7637; 0-86720),* 40 Tall Pine Dr., Sudbury, MA 01776-2256 (SAN 285-0893) Tel 978-443-5000; Fax: 978-443-8000; Toll Free: 800-832-0034
E-mail: info@jbpub.com
Web site: http://www.jbpub.com.

Joseph Adelman, *(Adelman, Joseph),* 217-17 82nd Ave., Jamaica, NY 11427 (SAN 285-8002) Tel 212-465-1711.

Joseph T Reilly Church Goods, *(Reilly, Joseph T. Church Goods),* 184 Rockaway Ave., Valley Stream, NY 11580-5824 (SAN 114-3492).

Joshua Morris, *See* **Rdrs Digest**

Jossey-Bass, *(Jossey-Bass, Inc. Pubs.; 0-471; 0-7879; 0-87589; 0-88390; 0-89384; 1-55542),* Div. of John Wiley & Sons, Orders Addr.: 432 Elizabeth Ave., Somerset, NJ 08875 Tel 732-469-4400; Fax: 732-302-2300; Edit Addr.: 350 Sansome St., San Francisco, CA 94104-1342 Tel 415-433-1740; Fax: 415-433-0499; Toll Free: 800-956-7739; 888-378-2537 (customer service)
E-mail: webperson@jbp.com
Web site: http://www.josseybass.com.

Joyce Media, *(Joyce Media, Inc.; 0-917002),* P.O. Box 57, Acton, CA 93510 (SAN 208-7197) Tel 805-269-1169; Fax: 805-269-2139
E-mail: joycemed@pacbell.net
Web site: http://joycemedia.com.

Juvenile Justice, *(Juvenile Justice Clearinghouse/ NCJRS),* c/o U.S. Dept. of Justice, P.O. Box 6000, Rockville, MD 20849 Tel 301-519-5500; Fax: 301-519-5212; Toll Free: 800-638-8736
E-mail: askncjrs@ncjrs.org
Web site: http://www.ncjrs.org.

K K & B, *(Kampmann, Kump & Bell, LLC),* Orders Addr.: 27 W. 20th St., Suite 1102, New York, NY 10011 Tel 212-727-0190; Fax: 212-727-0195
E-mail: midpointny@aol.com.

Kable News Co Inc, *(Kable News Co., Inc.),* Subs. of AMREP Corp., 641 Lexington Ave., 6th Flr., New York, NY 10022 (SAN 169-5835) Tel 212-705-4600; Toll Free: 800-223-6640
E-mail: info@kable.com.

KAHSA, *(KAHSA),* 217 SE Eighth St., Topeka, KS 66603
E-mail: kahsainto@kahsa,org
Web site: http://www.kahsa.org.

Kalamazoo Nature Ctr Inc, *(Kalamazoo Nature Ctr., Inc.),* 7000 N. Westnedge Ave., P.O. Box 127, Kalamazoo, MI 49004-0127 (SAN 268-2478) Tel 616-381-1574; Fax: 616-381-2557.

Kalispell News Agency, *(Kalispell News Agency),* P.O. Box 4965, Missoula, MT 59806-4965 (SAN 169-4383) Toll Free: 800-955-1266.

Kane-Miller Bk, *(Kane/Miller Bk. Pubs.; 0-916291; 1-929132),* Orders Addr.: P.O. Box 8515, La Jolla, CA 92038 (SAN 295-8945) Tel 858-456-0540; Fax: 858-456-9641; Toll Free: 800-968-1930
E-mail: jason@kanemiller.com
Web site: http://www.kanemiller.com; http://www.everyonepoops.com.

Kansas City Periodical Distributing, *(Kansas City Periodical Distributing),* Orders Addr.: P.O. Box 14948, Lenexa, KS 66285-4948 (SAN 107-9433); Edit Addr.: 9605 Dice Ln., Lenexa, KS 66215 Tel 913-541-8600.

Kansas State Reading Circle, *(Kansas State Reading Circle),* 715 W. Tenth St., C-170, Topeka, KS 66601 (SAN 169-2771).

Karel Dutton, *(Karel/Dutton Group),* P.O. Box 210490, San Francisco, CA 94121 Tel 415-668-0829; Fax: 415-668-2463.

Kaybee Montessori Inc, *(Kaybee Montessori, Inc.),* 4717 Chesapeake St., NW, Washington, DC 20016 (SAN 133-1256) Tel 202-362-1172.

Kazi Pubns, *(Kazi Pubns., Inc.; 0-933511; 0-935782; 1-56744),* 3023 W. Belmont Ave., Chicago, IL 60618 (SAN 162-3397) Tel 773-267-7001; Fax: 773-267-7002
E-mail: info@kazi.org
Web site: http://www.kazi.org.

Keith Distributors, *(Keith Distributors),* 1055 S. Ballenger Hwy., Flint, MI 48532 (SAN 112-6377) Tel 801-238-9104; Fax: 810-238-9028; Toll Free: 800-373-2366.

Kendall-Hunt, *(Kendall/Hunt Publishing Co.; 0-7872; 0-8403; 0-7575),* Orders Addr.: P.O. Box 1840, Dubuque, IA 52004-1840; Edit Addr.: 4050 Westmark Dr., Dubuque, IA 52002 (SAN 203-9184) Tel 319-589-1000; Fax: 319-589-1046; Toll Free Fax: 800-772-9165; Toll Free: 800-228-0810
E-mail: orders@kendallhunt.com
Web site: http://www.kendallhunt.com.

Kent News Agency Inc, *(Kent News Agency, Inc.),* P.O. Box 661, Scottsbluff, NE 69361 (SAN 169-4448).

Keramos, *(Keramos),* P.O. Box 7500, Ann Arbor, MI 48107 (SAN 169-3670) Tel 313-439-1261.

Kerhulas News Co, *(Kerhulas News Co.),* P.O. Box 751, Union, SC 29379 (SAN 169-7838).

Ketab Corp, *(Ketab Corp.; 1-883819),* Orders Addr.: 1419 Westwood Blvd., Los Angeles, CA 90024 (SAN 107-7791) Tel 818-908-0808; Fax: 818-908-1457
E-mail: ketab@ketab.com
Web site: http://www.ketab.com.

Kewanee News Agency, *(Kewanee News Agency),* Main St., Kewanee, IL 61443 (SAN 159-8856).

Key Bk Serv, *(Key Bk. Service, Inc.; 0-934636),* P.O. Box 1434, Fairfield, CT 06430 (SAN 169-0671) Tel 203-374-4939; Fax: 203-384-6099.

KF Ent, *See* **Prodn Assocs**

Kidsbooks Inc, *(Kidsbooks, Inc.),* 220 Monroe Tpke., No. 560, Monroe, CT 06468-2247 (SAN 169-0795).

Kindred Pub, *(Kindred Publishing; 1-887411),* 732 Cieneguitas Rd., No. B, Santa Barbara, CA 93110-1134.

King Distributors, *(King Distributors),* 7600 W. 27th St., Suite A2, Saint Louis Park, MN 55426-3146 (SAN 630-2084).

King Electronics Distributing, *(King Electronics Distributing),* 1711 Southeastern Ave., Indianapolis, IN 46201-3990 (SAN 107-6795) Tel 317-639-1484; Fax: 317-639-4711.

Kings News Inc, *(Kings News, Inc.),* 1823 Fifth Ave., N., Grand Forks, ND 58203-3054 (SAN 169-6564) Tel 701-775-3925.

Kinokuniya Bookstores, *(Kinokuniya Bookstores of America Co., Ltd.),* 1581 Webster St., San Francisco, CA 94115 (SAN 121-8441) Tel 415-567-7625; Fax: 415-567-4109.

Kinokuniya Pubns Service of New, *(Kinokuniya Pubns. Service of New York),* 10 W. 49th St., New York, NY 10020 (SAN 157-5414) Tel 212-765-1465; Fax: 212-307-5593
E-mail: kinokuniya@kinokuniya.com
Web site: http://www.kinokuniya.com.

Kirkbride Bible, *(Kirkbride, B.B. Bible Co., Inc.; 0-88707; 0-934854),* P.O. Box 606, Indianapolis, IN 46206 (SAN 169-2372) Tel 317-633-1900; Fax: 317-633-1444; Toll Free: 800-428-4385
E-mail: hyperbible@aol.com
Web site: http://www.kirkbride.com.

Kitrick Management, *(Kitrick Management Co., Ltd.),* P.O. Box 15523, Cincinnati, OH 45215 (SAN 132-6236) Tel 513-782-2930; Fax: 513-782-2936
E-mail: bachb@aol.com.

Kleins Bklein, *(Klein's Booklein),* Orders Addr.: P.O. Box 968, Fowlerville, MI 48836 (SAN 631-3329) Tel 517-223-3964; Fax: 517-223-1314; Toll Free: 800-266-5534; Edit Addr.: One Klein Dr., Fowlerville, MI 48836 (SAN 631-3337).

KMR Ent, *(K. M. R. Enterprises; 0-9656379),* 5731 Pony Express Trail, Pollock Pines, CA 95726 (SAN 299-237X) Tel 530-644-1410.

Knopf, *(Knopf, Alfred A. Inc.; 0-375; 0-394; 0-676; 0-679),* Div. of The Knopf Publishing Group, Orders Addr.: 400 Hahn Rd., Westminster, MD 21157 (SAN 202-5515) Tel 410-848-1900; Toll Free Fax: 800-659-2436; Toll Free: 800-733-3000 (orders); Edit Addr.: 299 Park Ave., New York, NY 10171 (SAN 202-5825) Tel 212-751-2600; Fax: 212-572-2593; Toll Free: 800-726-0600
E-mail: customerservice@randomhouse.com
Web site: http://www.randomhouse.com/knopf.

Koeltz Sci Bks, *See* **Balogh**

Koen Bk Distributors, *(Koen Bk. Distributors),* Orders Addr.: 10 Twosome Dr., P.O. Box 600, Moorestown, NJ 08057 (SAN 169-4642) Tel 609-235-4444; Fax: 609-727-6914; Toll Free Fax: 800-225-3840; Toll Free: 800-257-8481
E-mail: kbdinfo@koen.com
Web site: http://www.koen.com.

Koen Pacific, *(Koen Pacific),* Orders Addr.: 18249 Olympic Ave., S., Tukwila, WA 98188-4722 (SAN 631-5593) Tel 206-575-7544; Fax: 206-575-7444; Toll Free: 800-995-4840
E-mail: info@koenpacific.com.

Kraus, *See* **Periodicals Srv**

Kurtzman Bk Sales Co, *(Kurtzman Bk. Sales Co.),* 17348 W. 12 Mile Rd., Southfield, MI 48076 (SAN 114-0787) Tel 248-557-7230; Fax: 248-557-8705; Toll Free: 800-869-0505.

Kuykendalls Pr Bookstore Div, *(Kuykendalls Pr., Bookstore Div.),* P.O. Box 627, Athens, AL 35612-0627 (SAN 168-9185).

L & M News Co, *(L & M News Co.),* P.O. Box 3788, Wilmington, NC 28406-0788 (SAN 169-6459).

L I M Prodns, *(LIM Productions, LLC; 1-929617),* 4466 Whyem Dr., Akron, OH 44319 Tel 330-645-4387; Fax: 330-644-1642; Toll Free: 877-628-4532
E-mail: customerservice@limproductions.com
Web site: http://www.limproductions.com.

L Rienner, *(Rienner, Lynne Pubs., Inc.; 0-89410; 0-931477; 1-55587; 1-58826),* 1800 30th St., Suite 314, Boulder, CO 80301-1026 (SAN 683-1869) Tel 303-444-6684; Fax: 303-444-0824
E-mail: sglover@rienner.com; cservice@rienner.com
Web site: http://www.rienner.com.

L Valladares & Son, *(Valladares, L. & Son),* 1200 Duval St., Key West, FL 33040 (SAN 159-981X).

La Cite, *(La Cite French Bks.),* Div. of The La Cite Group, Inc., 2306 Westwood Blvd., Los Angeles, CA 90064 (SAN 168-9789) Tel 310-475-0095; Fax: 310-470-0610
E-mail: lacite@aol.com.

Laerdal Med Corp, *(Laerdal Medical Corp.; 0-9665371),* 167 Myers Corners Rd., Wappingers Falls, NY 12590 Tel 914-297-7770; Fax: 914-298-4545; Toll Free Fax: 800-227-1143; Toll Free: 888-562-4242
E-mail: cdespo@compuserve.com.

Lafayette Bks, *(Lafayette Bks.),* P.O. Box 758, Mamaroneck, NY 10543-0758 (SAN 135-292X) Tel 914-833-0248.

Lakeport Distributors Inc, *(Lakeport Distributors, Inc.),* 139 W. 18th St., P.O. Box 6195, Erie, PA 16501 (SAN 169-734X).

Lambert Bk, *(Lambert Bk. Hse., Inc.; 0-89315),* 4139 Parkway Dr., Florence, AL 35630-6347 (SAN 180-5169) Tel 205-764-4098; 256-974-1529 (orders ask Stan Johnson); Fax: 205-766-9200; Toll Free: 800-551-8511.

Lancaster County News Co, *(Lancaster County News Co.),* 221 N. Queen St., Lancaster, PA 17603 (SAN 169-7412).

Landes Bioscience, *(Landes Bioscience; 0-941432; 1-57059; 1-879702),* 810 S. Church St., Georgetown, TX 78626 Tel 512-863-7762; Fax: 512-863-0081; Toll Free: 800-736-9948
E-mail: orders@landesbioscience.com
Web site: http://www.landesbioscience.com.

Landmark NY, *(Landmark Bk. Co.; 0-929194),* 131 Hicks St., Brooklyn, NY 11201-2318 (SAN 169-5843).

Large Print Library, *(Large Print Library Discounter; 1-56895),* Div. of Wheeler Publishing, Inc., 405 VFW Dr., Rockland, MA 02370 Fax: 781-871-9173; Toll Free: 800-429-9743.

Larry D Laster, *(Laster, Larry D.),* 2416 Maplewood Ave., Winston-Salem, NC 27103 (SAN 112-9600) Tel 919-724-7544.

Lash Distributors, *(Lash Distributors),* 7106 Geoffrey Way, Frederick, MD 21704 (SAN 169-3131).

Last Gasp, *(Last Gasp Eco-Funnies, Inc.; 0-86719),* Orders Addr.: P.O. Box 410067, San Francisco, CA 94141-0067 (SAN 216-8308); Edit Addr.: 777 Florida St., San Francisco, CA 94110-2025 (SAN 170-3242) Tel 415-824-6636; Fax: 415-824-1836; Toll Free: 800-366-5121
E-mail: lastgasp@hooked.net.

Latcorp Ltd, *(Latcorp, Ltd.),* 10 Norden Ln., Huntington Station, NY 11746 (SAN 159-8910) Tel 516-271-0548; Fax: 516-549-8849.

Latin Am Bk Source, *(Latin American Bk. Source, Inc.),* 289 Third Ave., Chula Vista, CA 91910 Tel 619-426-1226; Fax: 619-426-0212
Web site: http://www.latinbooks.com.

Lattas, *(Latta's),* 1502 Fourth Ave., P.O. Box 2668, Huntington, WV 25726 (SAN 169-8982) Fax: 304-525-5038; Toll Free: 800-624-3501.

Learning Collection, *(Learning Collection, The),* 5180 Smith Rd., Suite B, Denver, CO 80216-4431 (SAN 630-8287) Tel 303-722-9843.

Lebanon Valley News Co, *(Lebanon Valley News Co.),* 37 S. Eighth St., Lebanon, PA 17042 (SAN 169-7420).

Lectorum Pubns, *(Lectorum Pubns., Inc.; 0-9625162; 1-880507; 1-930332),* Subs. of Scholastic, Inc., 205 Chubb Ave., Lyndhurst, NJ 07071-3520 (SAN 169-586X) Tel 212-929-2833; Fax: 212-727-3035; Toll Free Fax: 877-532-8676; 877-532-8678; Toll Free: 800-345-5946
E-mail: info@lectorum.com
Web site: http://www.lectorum.com.

Lee Bks, *(Lee Bks.; 0-939818),* Div. of Lee S. Cole & Assocs., Inc., 524 San Anselmo Ave., No 215, San Anselmo, CA 94960-2614 (SAN 110-649X) Tel 415-456-4388; Fax: 415-456-7532; Toll Free: 800-828-3550 Do not confuse with other companies with the same or similar names in Jacksonville, FL, Columbia, SC
E-mail: lcs@lsc-associates.com
Web site: http://www.lsc-associates.com.

Left Bank, *(Left Bank Distribution; 0-939306)*, Orders Addr.: 92 Pike St., Box B, Seattle, WA 98101; Edit Addr.: 1004 Turner Way E., Seattle, WA 98112-3642 (SAN 216-5368) Tel 206-322-2868; Fax: 206-322-2868
E-mail: leftbank@leftbankbooks.com
Web site: http://www.leftbankbooks.com.

Leisure AR, *(Leisure Arts, Inc.; 0-942237; 1-57486)*, Div. of AOL/Time Warner, Inc., Orders Addr.: P.O. Box 55595, Little Rock, AR 72215 (SAN 666-9565) Tel 501-868-8800; Fax: 501-868-8937; Toll Free: 800-643-8030 (customer service); Edit Addr.: 5701 Ranch Dr., Little Rock, AR 72223 (SAN 666-9573) Tel 650-324-5586; Fax: 650-324-1532; Toll Free: 800-227-7346
E-mail: barker1@sunset.com
Web site: http://www.leisurearts.com.

Leman Pubns, *(Leman Pubns., Inc.; 0-943721; 0-9602970)*, Div. of Rodale Pr. Co., Box 4100, 741 Corporate Cir., Suite A, Golden, CO 80401-5622 (SAN 213-3415) Fax: 303-277-0370; Toll Free: 800-877-3775.

Leo Adler, *(Adler, Leo)*, P.O. Box 10308, Eugene, OR 97440-2308 (SAN 169-7021).

Leonard Rock Magazine Service, *(Rock, Leonard Magazine Service)*, 97 Irene Dr., Vernon, CT 06066-4005 (SAN 285-9688).

Lesnick News, *(Lesnick News)*, 3117 Maringo Rd., SE, Olympia, WA 98501-3427 (SAN 169-8877).

Levy Home Entertainment, *(Levy Home Entertainment)*, Div. of Charles Levy Co., 4201 Raymond Dr., Hillside, IL 60162 (SAN 169-197X) Tel 708-547-4400; Fax: 708-547-4503; Toll Free: 800-947-1967.

Lib Res, *(Library Research Assocs., Inc.; 0-89824; 0-912526)*, 474 Dunderberg Rd., Monroe, NY 10950-3703 (SAN 201-0887) Tel 845-783-1144; Fax: 845-782-3953; Toll Free: 800-914-3379.

Liberation Distributors, *(Liberation Distributors; 0-89928)*, P.O. Box 5341, Chicago, IL 60680 (SAN 169-880X) Tel 773-248-3442.

LibertyTree Pr, *See* **Independent Inst**

Library & Educ, *(Library & Educational Services)*, P.O. Box 146, Berrien Springs, MI 49103 Tel 616-695-1800; Fax: 616-695-8500
E-mail: libraryanded@juno.com.

Library Bk Selection Service, *(Library Bk. Selection Service)*, P.O. Box 277, 2714 McGraw Dr., Bloomington, IL 61704 (SAN 169-1740) Tel 309-663-1411; Fax: 309-664-0059.

Libros de Espana, *(Libros de Espana y America; 1-883110)*, 170-23 83rd Ave., Jamaica Hills, NY 11432 (SAN 170-5407) Tel 718-291-9891; Fax: 718-291-9830
E-mail: leabook@idt.net
Web site: http://www.leabooks.com.

Libros Fronteras, *(Libros Sin Fronteras)*, P.O. Box 2085, Olympia, WA 98507 Tel 360-357-4332; Fax: 360-357-4964
E-mail: info@librossinfronteras.com
Web site: http://www.librossinfronteras.com.

Light Impressions, *(Light Impressions Corp.; 0-87992)*, Orders Addr.: P.O. Box 940, Rochester, NY 14603-0940 (SAN 169-619X) Toll Free Fax: 800-826-5539; Toll Free: 800-828-6216; Edit Addr.: P.O. Box 22708, Rochester, NY 14692-2708
Web site: http://www.lightimpresionsdirect.com.

Light Pubng, *(Light Publishing; 1-884410)*, Div. of Association of Universal Light Volunteers, 1187 W. 132nd Ln., Crown Point, IN 46307-9282 (SAN 298-6914) Tel 219-662-7248; Fax: 219-663-9974; Toll Free: 800-603-7986.

Light&Life Pub Co MN, *(Light & Life Publishing Co.; 0-937032; 1-880971)*, 4808 Park Glen Rd., Minneapolis, MN 55416 (SAN 213-8565) Tel 612-925-3888; Fax: 612-925-3918
E-mail: info@light-n-life.com
Web site: http://www.light-n-life.com.

Lightn Source, *(Lightning Source, Inc.)*, 1246 Heil Quaker Blvd., LaVergne, TN 37086 (SAN 179-6976) Tel 615-213-4595; Fax: 615-213-4426.

Likely Story Bkfrs, *(Likely Story Bookfairs, A)*, 7210 SW 57th Ave., Suite 207-A, South Miami, FL 33143 (SAN 631-1210) Tel 305-668-9183; Fax: 305-667-3323.

Lilly News Agency, *(Lilly News Agency)*, P.O. Box 280077, Memphis, TN 38168-0077 (SAN 168-9452).

Limerock Bks Inc, *(Limerock Bks., Inc.)*, P.O. Box 57, New Canaan, CT 06840 (SAN 630-8708) Tel 203-322-5352; Fax: 203-322-2182
E-mail: limerockbk@aol.com
Web site: http://www.netpocus.com/limerock.

Linda Thomson, *(Thomson, Linda)*, P.O. Box 1225, Orem, UT 84059-1225 (SAN 110-3881) Tel 801-226-0155; Fax: 801-226-0166; Toll Free: 800-226-0155.

Lindsay News & Photo Service, *(Lindsay News & Photo Service, Inc.)*, 3025 Niagara St., MPO 948, Niagara Falls, NY 14303 (SAN 169-6092).

Lings International Bks, *(Ling's International Bks.)*, Orders Addr.: P.O. Box 82684, San Diego, CA 92138 (SAN 169-0116) Tel 619-292-8104; Fax: 619-292-8207; Edit Addr.: 7531 Convoy Ct., San Diego, CA 92111.

Literal Bk Distributors Bks, *(Literal Bk. Distributors: Bks. in Spanish)*, Orders Addr.: P.O. Box 7113, Langley Park, MD 20787; Edit Addr.: 7705 Georgia Ave. NW, Suite 102, Washington, DC 20012 (SAN 113-2784) Tel 202-723-8688; Fax: 202-882-6592; Toll Free: 800-366-8680.

Little, *(Little, Brown & Co.; 0-316; 0-8212)*, Div. of Time Warner Trade Publishing, Orders Addr.: 3 Center Plaza, Boston, MA 02108-2084 (SAN 630-7248) Tel 617-227-0730; Toll Free Fax: 800-286-9471; Toll Free: 800-759-0190; Edit Addr.: Time & Life Bldg., 1271 Avenue of the Americas, New York, NY 10020 (SAN 200-2205) Tel 212-522-8700; Fax: 212-522-2067; Toll Free: 800-343-9204
E-mail: cust.service@littlebrown.com
Web site: http://www.littlebrown.com.

Little Danias, *(Little Dania's Juvenile Promotions)*, Div. of Booksmith Promotional Co., 100 Paterson Plank Rd., Jersey City, NJ 07307 (SAN 169-5681) Tel 201-659-2317; Fax: 201-659-3631
E-mail: hochberga@aol.com.

Little Professor Bk Ctrs, *(Little Professor Bk. Ctrs., Inc.)*, 130 S. First St., Suite 300, Ann Arbor, MI 48104 (SAN 144-2503) Tel 313-994-1212; Fax: 313-994-9009.

LL Co, *(LL Co.; 0-937892)*, 1647 Manning Ave., Los Angeles, CA 90024 (SAN 110-0009) Tel 310-615-0116; Fax: 310-640-6863; Toll Free: 800-473-3699
E-mail: wallacelab@aol.com.

Lndmrk Audiobks, *(Landmark Audiobooks)*, 4865 Sterling Dr., Boulder, CO 80301 Fax: 303-443-3775
Web site: http://www.landmarkaudio.com.

Login Fulfillment Services, *See* **LPC Group**

Login Pubs Consort, *(Login Pubs. Consortium; 0-9648574)*, 1436 W. Randolph St., 2nd Flr., Chicago, IL 60607 (SAN 630-5733) Tel 312-432-7650; Fax: 312-733-3107; Toll Free: 800-626-4330
E-mail: lpc-info@lb.com
Web site: http://www.coolbooks.com.

Logos Prods, *(Logos Productions, Inc.; 0-9618891; 1-885361)*, 6160 Carmen Ave., E., Inver Grove Heights, MN 55076-4422 Tel 612-451-9945; Fax: 612-457-4617; Toll Free: 800-328-0200 Do not confuse with Logos Productions, Carmel, CA
E-mail: lpstaff@mn.uswest.net
Web site: http://www.1logos.com.

Long Beach Bks Inc, *(Long Beach Bks., Inc.)*, P.O. Box 179, Long Beach, NY 11561-0179 (SAN 164-632X) Tel 718-471-5934.

Looseleaf Law, *(Looseleaf Law Pubns., Inc.; 0-930137; 1-889031)*, Orders Addr.: P.O. Box 650042, Fresh Meadows, NY 11365 (SAN 135-0099) Tel 718-359-5559; Fax: 718-539-0941; Toll Free: 800-647-5547; Edit Addr.: 43-08 162nd St., Flushing, NY 11358
E-mail: llawpub@erols.com
Web site: http://www.looseleaflaw.com.

Lords Line, *(Lord's Line; 0-915952)*, 1065 Lomita Blvd., No. 434, Harbor City, CA 90710-1944 (SAN 169-0051).

Lotus Light, *See* **Lotus Pr**

Lotus Pr, *(Lotus Pr.; 0-910261; 0-914778; 0-914955; 0-940676; 0-940985; 0-941524)*, Div. of Lotus Brands, Inc., P.O. Box 325, Twin Lakes, WI 53181 (SAN 239-1120) Tel 262-889-8561; Fax: 262-889-8591; Toll Free: 800-824-6396 Do not confuse with companies with the same or similar name in Lotus, CA, Westerville, OH, Bokeelia, FL, Brattleboro, VT, Detroit, MI, Tobyhanna, PA
E-mail: lotuspress@lotuspress.com
Web site: http://www.lotuspress.com.

Louis Goldberg Library Bk Supplier, *(Goldberg, Louis Library Bk. Supplier)*, 45 Belvidere St., Nazareth, PA 18064 (SAN 169-7536) Tel 610-759-9458; Fax: 610-759-8134.

Louisville Dist, *See* **United Mag**

Louisvlle News Co, *(Louisville News Co.)*, P.O. Box 36, Columbia, KY 42728 (SAN 169-281X) Tel 502-384-3444; Fax: 502-384-9324.

LPC Group, *(LPC Group)*, c/o CDS, 193 Edwards Dr., Jackson, TN 38305 (SAN 630-5644) Fax: 312-432-7603; Toll Free Fax: 800-334-3892; Toll Free: 800-243-0138
E-mail: fm@lb.com
Web site: http://www.coolbooks.com.

Lppncott W & W, *(Lippincott Williams & Wilkins; 0-316; 0-397; 0-683; 0-7817; 0-8121; 0-88167; 0-89004; 0-89313; 0-911216; 1-881063)*, Subs. of Wolters Kluwer U.S. Corp., Orders Addr.: P.O. Box 1600, Hagerstown, MD 21741 Tel 301-714-2300; Fax: 301-824-7390; Toll Free: 800-638-3030; Edit Addr.: 530 Walnut St., Philadelphia, PA 19106-3780 (SAN 201-0933) Tel 215-521-8300; Fax: 215-521-8902; Toll Free: 800-638-3030
E-mail: custserv@lww.com
Web site: http://www.lww.com.

Lppncott-Raven, *See* **Lppncott W & W**

Lubrecht & Cramer, *(Lubrecht & Cramer, Ltd.; 0-934454; 0-945345)*, 18 E. Main St., Port Jervis, NY 12771; Edit Addr.: P.O. Box 3110, Port Jervis, NY 12771 (SAN 214-1256) Tel 914-856-5990; Toll Free: 800-920-9334; 350 Fifth Ave., Suite 3304, New York, NY 10118-0069
E-mail: lubrecht@ny.frontiernet.net; books@lubrechtcramer.com
Web site: http://www.lubrechtcramer.com.

Luciano Bks, *(Luciano Bks.)*, 13111 NW Le Jeune, Opa Locka, FL 33054 (SAN 631-2829) Tel 305-769-3103.

Ludington News Co, *(Ludington News Co.)*, 1600 E. Grand Blvd., Detroit, MI 48211-3195 (SAN 169-3751) Tel 313-929-7600.

Lutz Services, *(Lutz Services)*, 1523 Maple St., Hartford, VT 05047-0501 Tel 802-296-2715
E-mail: john@vtstamp.com.

L-W Inc, *(L-W, Inc.; 0-89538)*, P.O. Box 69, Gas City, IN 46933 (SAN 159-6292) Tel 765-674-6450; Fax: 765-674-3503; Toll Free: 800-777-6450
E-mail: catalogs@lwbooks.com; lwbooks@comteek.com
Web site: http://www.lwbooks.com.

M & J Bk Fair, *(M & J Bk. Fair Service)*, 2307 Sherwood Cir., Minneapolis, MN 55431 (SAN 169-4030).

M & M News Agency, *(M & M News Agency)*, Orders Addr.: P.O. Box 1129, La Salle, IL 61301 (SAN 169-2062) Fax: 815-223-2828; Toll Free: 800-245-6247.

M Stevens Indus, *(Stevens, Mark Industries)*, Div. of Christian World, Inc., 1215 N. Portland, Oklahoma City, OK 73107 (SAN 631-127X) Tel 405-948-1077; Fax: 405-948-1110; Toll Free: 800-654-6760.

Ma ayan, *See* **WellSpring MA**

Mac Comp Pub, *See* **Mac USA**

Mac USA, *(Macmillan USA; 0-02; 0-672; 0-7357; 0-7897; 1-57595; 0-7431)*, Div. of Pearson Education Corporate Communications, 201 W. 103rd St., Indianapolis, IN 46290-1097 (SAN 219-6298) Tel 317-581-3575; Fax: 317-581-3611; Toll Free: 800-428-5331 (orders); 800-858-7674 (customer service)
E-mail: international@macmillanusa.com
Web site: http://www.mcp.com/pu.

MacGregor News Agency, *(MacGregor News Agency)*, 1733 Industrial Park Dr., Mount Pleasant, MI 48858 (SAN 169-3921) Toll Free: 800-626-1982.

Macmillan, *(Macmillan Publishing Co., Inc.; 0-02; 0-87605; 0-89256)*, Orders Addr.: 200 Old Tappan Rd., Old Tappan, NJ 07675 (SAN 202-5574) Toll Free: 800-428-5331 (Order dept.)
E-mail: ssonline_feeback@simonsays.com
Web site: http://www.simonsays.com.

MacRaes Indian Bk Dist, *(MacRae's Indian Bk. Distributor)*, 1605 Cole St., P.O. Box 652, Enumclaw, WA 98022 (SAN 157-5473) Tel 360-825-3737.

Made E-Z, *(Made E-Z Products, Inc.; 1-56382)*, 384 S. Military Trail, Deerfield Beach, FL 33442 (SAN 253-8148) Tel 954-480-8933; Fax: 954-480-8906; Toll Free: 800-822-4566
E-mail: lschrift@madee-z.com
Web site: http://www.madee-z.com.

Madison Art, *(Madison Art Ctr., Inc.; 0-913883)*, 211 State St., Madison, WI 53703 (SAN 110-8875) Tel 608-257-0158; Fax: 608-257-5722
E-mail: mac@itis.com
Web site: http://www.madisonartcenter.org.

Magazine Distributors Inc, *(Magazine Distributors, Inc.)*, 15 Sparks St., Plainville, CT 06062 (SAN 169-0817).

Magazines Inc, *(Magazines, Inc.)*, 1135 Hammond St., Bangor, ME 04401 (SAN 169-3034) Tel 207-942-8237; Fax: 207-942-9226; Toll Free: 800-649-9224 (in Maine)
E-mail: pam@mint.net.

Mahoning Valley Distributing Agency Inc, *(Mahoning Valley Distributing Agency, Inc.),* 2556 Rush Blvd., Youngstown, OH 44507 (SAN 169-6920) Tel 330-788-6162; Fax: 330-788-9046.

Majic Enterprises, *(Majic Enterprises),* 313 E. Main St., Niles, MI 49120-2305 (SAN 169-8508).

Majors Scientific Bks Inc, *(Majors Scientific Bks., Inc.),* 1401 Lakeway Dr., Lewisville, TX 75057 Tel 972-353-1100; Fax: 972-353-1300; Toll Free: 800-633-1851
E-mail: dallas@majors.com
Web site: http://www.majors.com.

Manchester News Co Inc, *(Manchester News Co., Inc.),* P.O. Box 4838, Manchester, NH 03108-4838 (SAN 169-4480).

Manhattan Pub Co, *(Manhattan Publishing Co.),* Div. of U.S. & Europe Bks., Inc., P.O. Box 850, Croton-on-Hudson, NY 10520 (SAN 113-7476) Tel 914-271-5194; Fax: 914-271-5856
Web site: http://www.manhattanpublishing.com.

Manitowoc News Agency, *(Manitowoc News Agency),* 907 S. Eighth St., Manitowoc, WI 54220 (SAN 159-9046).

Mannings Bks & Prints, *(Manning's Bks. & Prints),* 580M Crespi Dr., Pacifica, CA 94044 (SAN 157-5384) Fax: 650-355-1851
E-mail: manningsbks@aol.com
Web site: http://www.printsoldandrare.com.

Many Feathers Bks & Maps, *(Many Feathers Bks. & Maps),* 2626 W. Indian School Rd., Phoenix, AZ 85017 (SAN 158-8877) Tel 602-266-1043; Toll Free: 800-279-7652.

Maple-Vail Bk, *(Maple-Vail Bk. Manufacturing Group, The; 0-9659704),* Orders Addr.: 60 Grumbacher Rd., York, PA 17405; Edit Addr.: P.O. Box 2695, York, PA 17405 Tel 717-764-5911; Fax: 717-764-4702
Web site: http://www.Maple-Vail.com.

Marco Bk Distributors, *(Marco Bk. Distributors; 0-88298),* P.O. Box 30108, Brooklyn, NY 11203-0108 (SAN 169-5142) Tel 718-774-0750; Fax: 718-774-0380; Toll Free: 800-842-4234.

Marcus Wholesale, *(Marcus Wholesale),* P.O. Box 1618, R49 E. Hwy. 4, Murphys, CA 95247 (SAN 185-0296).

Mardelva News Co Inc, *(Mardelva News Co., Inc.),* 8999 Ocean Hwy., Delmar, MD 21875 (SAN 169-3247) Tel 410-742-8613; Fax: 410-742-2616.

Mariuccia Iaconi Bk Imports, *(Iaconi, Mariuccia Bk. Imports; 0-9628720),* 970 Tennessee St., San Francisco, CA 94107 (SAN 161-1364) Tel 415-821-1216; Fax: 415-821-1596; Toll Free: 800-955-9577
E-mail: mibibook@ixnetcom.com
Web site: http://www.mibibook.com.

Marshall-Mangold Distribution Co Inc, *(Marshall-Mangold Distribution Co., Inc.),* 4805 Nelson Ave., Baltimore, MD 21215-2507 (SAN 169-3115) Toll Free: 800-972-2665.

Marshalltown News Agency, *(Marshalltown News Agency),* 1714 S. Center St., Marshalltown, IA 50158-4258 (SAN 169-2674).

Maruzen International Co Ltd, *(Maruzen International Co., Ltd.),* 1200 Harbor Blvd., 10th Flr., Weehawken, NJ 07087 (SAN 630-6012) Tel 201-865-4400.

Marvin Law Bk, *(Marvin Law Bk.),* 11020 27th Ave., S., Burnsville, MN 55337 (SAN 163-898X) Tel 612-644-2236.

Matthews Bk Co, *(Matthews Bk. Co.),* 11559 Rock Island Ct., Maryland Heights, MO 63043 (SAN 169-4316) Tel 314-432-1400; Fax: 314-432-7044; Toll Free: 800-633-2665
E-mail: blc@mattmccoy.com
Web site: http://www.mattmccoy.com.

Matthews Medical Bk Co, *(Matthews Medical Bk. Co.),* 11559 Rock Island Ct., Maryland Heights, MO 63043 (SAN 169-4316) Tel 314-432-1400; Fax: 314-432-7044; Toll Free: 800-633-2665.

Maus Tales, *(Maus Tales),* 77-490 Loma Vista, La Quinta, CA 92253 Fax: 760-564-6669
E-mail: maustales@aol.com.

Maverick Dist, *(Maverick Distributors; 1-884646),* Orders Addr.: Drawer 7289, Bend, OR 97708 (SAN 298-3222) Tel 541-382-2728; Fax: 541-382-8444; Toll Free: 800-333-8046; Edit Addr.: 525 NE Revere Ave., Bend, OR 97701.

Max Kade, *(Kade, Max Institute for German American Studies; 0-924119),* 901 University Bay Dr., Madison, WI 53703.

Maxwell Sci Intl, *(Maxwell Scientific International, Inc.; 0-8277),* Div. of Pergamon Pr., Inc., 1345 Ave. of the Americas, No. 1036C, New York, NY 10105-0302 (SAN 169-524X) Tel 914-592-9141.

MBS Textbook Exchange Inc, *(MBS Textbook Exchange, Inc.),* Orders Addr.: 2711 W. Ash, Columbia, MO 65203-4613 (SAN 140-7015) Tel 573-445-2243; Fax: 573-446-5254; Toll Free: 800-325-0929 (orders); 800-325-0530 (customer service)
Web site: http://www.mbsbooks.com.

McCoy Church Goods, *(McCoy Church Goods),* 1010 Howard Ave., San Mateo, CA 94401 (SAN 107-2315) Tel 415-342-0924.

McCrorys Bks, *See* **McCrorys Whlesale Bks**

McCrorys Whlesale Bks, *(McCrory's Wholesale Bks.),* Orders Addr.: P.O. Box 2032, Alexandria, LA 71301 (SAN 108-5999) Tel 318-448-8954; Toll Free: 800-734-3264; Edit Addr.: 1808 Rapides Ave., Alexandria, LA 71301.

McGraw, *(McGraw-Hill Cos., The; 0-02; 0-07),* Orders Addr.: 860 Taylor Station Rd., Blacklick, OH 43004-0545 (SAN 200-254X) Fax: 614-755-5645; Toll Free: 800-338-3987 (college); 800-525-5003 (subscriptions); 800-352-3566 (books - US/Canada orders); 800-722-4726 (orders & customer service); P.O. Box 545, Blacklick, OH 43004-0545
E-mail: customer.service@mcgraw-hill.com
Web site: http://www.ebooks.mcgraw-hill.com/; http://www.mcgraw-hill.com.

McGraw-Hill Trade, *(McGraw-Hill Trade; 0-07; 0-658),* Div. of McGraw-Hill Professional, Orders Addr.: P.O. Box 545, Blacklick, OH 43004-0545 Tel 800-722-4726; Fax: 614-755-5645; Edit Addr.: 2 Penn Plaza, New York, NY 10121 Tel 212-904-2000
Web site: http://www.books.mcgraw-hill.com.

McKnight Sales Co, *(McKnight Sales Co.),* P.O. Box 4138, Pittsburgh, PA 15202 (SAN 169-7587).

Meadville News Co Inc, *(Meadville News Co., Inc.),* 105 Mead Ave., Meadville, PA 16335-3597 (SAN 169-7455).

Med Physics Pub, *(Medical Physics Publishing; 0-944838; 1-930524),* 4513 Vernon Blvd., Madison, WI 53705-4964 (SAN 245-7407) Tel 608-262-4021; Fax: 608-265-2121; Toll Free: 800-442-5778
E-mail: junej@medicalphysics.org
Web site: http://www.medicalphysics.org.

Medical & Activities Sales, *See* **Act Prod Intl**

Medical Information Systems Inc, *(Medical Information Systems, Inc.),* 2 Seaview Blvd., Port Washington, NY 11050 (SAN 242-1720) Tel 516-621-7200 Do not confuse with Medical Information Systems, Inc., Stamford, CT.

Medicina Bio, *(Medicina Biologica),* 2937 NE Flanders St., Portland, OR 97232 (SAN 113-0226) Tel 503-287-6775; Fax: 503-235-3520
E-mail: med_bio@imagina.com.

Mel Bay, *(Mel Bay Pubns., Inc.; 0-7866; 0-87166; 1-56222),* Orders Addr.: Four Industrial Dr., Pacific, MO 63069; Edit Addr.: P.O. Box 66, Pacific, MO 63069-0066 (SAN 657-3630) Tel 636-257-3970; Fax: 636-257-5062; Toll Free: 800-863-5229
E-mail: catalog@melbay.com; email@melbay.com
Web site: http://www.melbay.com.

Melton Bk, *(Melton Bk. Co., Inc.),* P.O. Box 141000, Nashville, TN 37214-1000 (SAN 169-8133).

Merced News Co, *(Merced News Co.),* 1324 Coldwell Ave., Modesto, CA 95350-5702 (SAN 168-9894) Tel 209-722-5791.

Mercedes Bk Distributors Corp, *(Mercedes Bk. Distributors Corp.),* 62 Imlay St., Brooklyn, NY 11231 (SAN 169-5150) Tel 718-522-7110; Fax: 718-852-5341
E-mail: contact@.mdist.com.

Merkos, *(Merkos Pubns.),* 291 Kingston Ave., Brooklyn, NY 11213 (SAN 631-1040) Tel 718-778-0226; Fax: 718-778-4148.

Merle Distributing, *(Merle Distributing Co.),* 18161 E. Eight Mile Rd., Eastpointe, MI 48021-3219 (SAN 169-3778).

Merry Thoughts, *(Merry Thoughts; 0-88230),* 364 Adams St., Bedford Hills, NY 10507 (SAN 169-5061) Tel 914-241-0447; Fax: 914-241-0247.

Metamorphous Pr, *(Metamorphous Pr., Inc.; 0-943920; 1-55552),* Orders Addr.: P.O. Box 10616, Portland, OR 97296-0616 (SAN 110-8786) Tel 503-228-4972; Fax: 503-223-9117; Toll Free: 800-937-7771 (orders only); Edit Addr.: 2950 NW 29th Ave., Portland, OR 97210
E-mail: metabooks@metamodels.com
Web site: http://www.metamodels.com.

Metro Sys, *(Metro Systems),* 3381 Stevens Creek Blvd., Suite 209, San Jose, CA 95117 (SAN 631-1016) Tel 408-247-4050; Fax: 408-247-4236.

Metropolitan News Co, *(Metropolitan News Co.),* 47-25 34th, Long Island City, NY 11101 (SAN 159-9089) Do not confuse with Metropolitan News Co. in Los Angeles, CA.

Miami Bks Inc, *(Miami Bks., Inc.),* 17842 State Rd. 9, Miami, FL 33162 (SAN 106-8997) Tel 305-652-3231.

Miami Valley News Agency, *(Miami Valley News Agency),* 2127 Old Troy Pike, Dayton, OH 45404 (SAN 169-6718) Fax: 513-233-8544; Toll Free: 800-791-5137.

Mich News Srv, *(Michiana News Service),* 2232 S. 11th St., Niles, MI 49120 (SAN 110-5051) Tel 616-684-3013; Fax: 616-684-8740.

Michigan Church Supply, *(Michigan Church Supply),* P.O. Box 279, Mount Morris, MI 48458-0279 (SAN 184-413X) Toll Free: 800-521-3440.

Micklers Floridiana Inc, *(Micklers Floridiana, Inc.),* Orders Addr.: P.O. Box 621450, Oviedo, FL 32762-1450 (SAN 200-4356) Tel 407-365-6425; Edit Addr.: 181 W. Broadway, Oviedo, FL 32765.

Microdistributors International Inc, *(Microdistributors International, Inc.; 0-918025),* Subs. of Medcomp Technologies, Inc., 34 Maple Ave., P.O. Box 8, Armonk, NY 10504 (SAN 296-158X) Tel 914-273-6480.

Mid Penn Magazine Agency, *(Mid Penn Magazine Agency),* 100 Eck Cir., Williamsport, PA 17701 (SAN 169-7692).

Mid-Cal Periodical Distributors, *(Mid-Cal Periodical Distributors),* P.O. Box 245230, Sacramento, CA 95824-5230 (SAN 169-0078).

Midpt Trade, *(Midpoint Trade Bks., Inc.),* Orders Addr.: 1263 Southwest Blvd., Kansas City, KS 66103 (SAN 631-3736) Tel 913-831-2233; Fax: 913-362-7401; Toll Free: 800-742-6139 (consumer orders); Edit Addr.: 27 W. 20th St., No. 1102, New York, NY 10011 (SAN 631-1075) Tel 212-727-0190; Fax: 212-727-0195; P.O. Box 411037, Kansas City, MO 64141-1037 (SAN 253-8539) Tel 913-362-7400; Fax: 913-362-7401
E-mail: midpointny@aol.com
Web site: http://midpt.com.

Mid-South Magazine Agency Inc, *(Mid-South Magazine Agency, Inc.),* P.O. Box 4585, Jackson, MS 39296-4585 (SAN 286-0163) Toll Free: 800-748-9444.

Mid-State Periodicals Inc, *(Mid-State Periodicals, Inc.),* P.O. Box 3455, Quincy, IL 62305-3455 (SAN 169-2038) Tel 217-222-0833; Fax: 217-222-1256.

Mid-States Distributors, *(Mid-States Distributors),* 1201 Sheffler Dr., Chambersburg, PA 17201 (SAN 169-3166) Tel 717-263-2413; Fax: 717-263-7289.

Midtown Auto Bks, *(Midtown Auto Bks.),* 212 Burnet Ave., Syracuse, NY 13203 (SAN 169-6289).

Midwest European Pubns, *(Midwest European Pubns.),* 915 Foster St., Evanston, IL 60201 (SAN 169-1937) Tel 847-866-6289; Fax: 847-866-6290; Toll Free: 800-380-8919
E-mail: info@mep-eli.com
Web site: http://www.mep-eli.com.

Midwest Lib Serv, *(Midwest Library Service),* 11443 St. Charles Rock Rd., Bridgeton, MO 63044-2789 (SAN 169-4243) Tel 314-739-3100; Fax: 314-739-1326; Toll Free Fax: 800-962-1009; Toll Free: 800-325-8833.

Military History Assoc, *(Military History Assocs.),* 407B E. Sixth St., No. 200, Austin, TX 78701-3739 (SAN 111-7866).

Millenium Mktg, *(Millenium Marketing),* 800 E. Leigh St., Suite 110, Richmond, VA 23213 Fax: 804-827-0065; 804-827-0060
E-mail: gmi@vabiotech.com.

Miller Harness, *(Harness, Miller),* 235 Murray Hill Pkwy., East Rutherford, NJ 07073 (SAN 169-5789) Fax: 201-460-0334; Toll Free: 800-526-6310.

Milligan News Co Inc, *(Milligan News Co., Inc.),* 150 N. Autumn St., San Jose, CA 95110 (SAN 169-0272) Tel 408-286-7604; Fax: 408-298-0235; Toll Free: 800-873-2387.

Minerva Science Bookseller Inc, *(Minerva Science Bookseller, Inc.),* 175 Fifth Ave., New York, NY 10010 (SAN 286-0171).

Mississippi Library Media & Supply, *(Mississippi Library Media & Supply Co.),* P.O. Box 108, Brandon, MS 39043-0108 (SAN 169-4189) Tel 601-824-1900; Fax: 601-824-1999; Toll Free: 800-257-7566 (in Mississippi).

MIT Pr, *(MIT Pr.; 0-262),* 5 Cambridge Ctr., Suite 4, Cambridge, MA 02142-1493 (SAN 202-6414) Tel 617-253-5646; 617-625-8569 (orders); Fax: 617-253-6779; 617-625-6660 (orders); Toll Free: 800-356-0343 (orders)
E-mail: mitpress-orders@mit.edu
Web site: http://mitpress.mit.edu.

MMB Music, *(MMB Music, Inc.; 0-918812; 1-58106),* Orders Addr.: 3526 Washington Ave. Contemporary Arts Bldg., Saint Louis, MO 63103-1019 (SAN 298-3281) Tel 314-531-9635; Fax: 314-531-8384; Toll Free: 800-543-3771
E-mail: mmbmusic@mmbmusic.com
Web site: http://www.mozarteffect.com.

Mobile News Co, *(Mobile News Co.),* 1118 14th St., Tuscaloosa, AL 35401-3318 (SAN 168-924X) Tel 334-479-1435.

Moderna Poesia Inc, *(La Moderna Poesia, Inc.),* 5246 SW Eighth St., Miami, FL 33134 (SAN 169-1139) Tel 305-446-9884; Fax: 305-445-1635.

Modesto News Co, *(Modesto News Co.),* 1324 Coldwell Ave., Modesto, CA 95350-5702 (SAN 168-9908) Tel 209-577-5551.

Montfort Pubns, *(Montfort Pubns.; 0-910984),* Div. of Montfort Missionaries, 26 S. Saxon Ave., Bay Shore, NY 11706-8993 (SAN 169-5053) Tel 631-665-0726; Fax: 631-665-4349
Web site: http://www.montfortmissionaries.com.

Montgomery News Co, *(Montgomery News Co.),* 874 Martha St., Montgomery, AL 36104-3299 (SAN 168-9258).

Mook & Blanchard, *(Mook & Blanchard),* 546 S. Hofgaarden, La Puente, CA 91744 (SAN 168-9703) Tel 626-968-6424; Fax: 626-968-6877; Toll Free: 800-875-9911
E-mail: mookbook@ix.netcom.com
Web site: http://www.mookandblanchard.com.

Moon Over Mntn, *See* **Leman Pubns**

Morehouse Pub, *(Morehouse Publishing; 0-8192),* Orders Addr.: P.O. Box 1321, Harrisburg, PA 17105-1321 (SAN 202-6511) Tel 717-541-8130; Fax: 717-541-8128; Toll Free: 800-877-0012
E-mail: morehouse@morehousegroup.com
Web site: http://www.morehousegroup.com.

Morlock News Co Inc, *(Morlock News Co., Inc.),* 496 Duanesburg Rd., Schenectady, NY 12306 (SAN 169-6246).

Mosby Inc, *(Mosby, Inc.; 0-323; 0-7234; 0-8016; 0-8151; 0-88416; 0-941158; 1-55664; 1-56815),* Div. of Harcourt, Inc., A Harcourt Health Sciences Co., Orders Addr.: 6227 Sea Harbor Dr., Orlando, FL 32887 Toll Free Fax: 800-235-0256; Toll Free: 800-543-1918; Edit Addr.: 11830 Westline Industrial Dr., Saint Louis, MO 63146 (SAN 200-2280) Toll Free: 800-325-4177
Web site: http://www.mosby.com/.

Mosby Yr, *See* **Mosby Inc**

Moshy Brothers Inc, *(Moshy Brothers, Inc.),* 127 W. 25th St., New York, NY 10001 (SAN 169-5886) Tel 212-255-0613.

Mother Lode Distributing, *(Mother Lode Distributing),* 119 E. Theall St., Sonora, CA 95370-5798 (SAN 169-0361).

Motorbooks Intl, *(Motorbooks International Wholesalers & Distributors; 0-7603; 0-87938; 0-912612; 1-85010),* Div. of Chronicle Publishing, 729 Prospect Ave., Osceola, WI 54020 (SAN 169-9164) Tel 715-294-3345; Fax: 715-294-4448; Toll Free: 800-458-0454
E-mail: mbibks@win.bright.net
Web site: http://www.motorbooks.com.

Mountain Pr, *(Mountain Pr. Publishing Co., Inc.; 0-87842),* Orders Addr.: P.O. Box 2399, Missoula, MT 59806-2399 (SAN 202-8832) Tel 406-728-1900; Fax: 406-728-1635; Toll Free: 800-234-5308; Edit Addr.: 1301 S. Third West, Missoula, MT 59801 (SAN 662-0868)
E-mail: johnargyle@aol.com; mtnpress@montana.com
Web site: http://www.mountainpresspublish.com.

Mountain States News Distributor, *(Mountain States News Distributor),* P.O. Drawer P, Fort Collins, CO 80522 (SAN 169-0566) Tel 970-221-2330; Fax: 970-221-1251.

Mountaineers, *(Mountaineers Bks., The; 0-89886; 0-916890; 0-938567),* Div. of Mountaineers, Orders Addr.: 1001 SW Klickitat Way, Suite 201, Seattle, WA 98134-1162 (SAN 212-8756) Tel 206-223-6303; Fax: 206-223-6306; Toll Free: 800-568-7604
E-mail: mbooks@mountaineersbooks.org
Web site: http://www.mountaineersbooks.org.

MPHC, *(MPHC),* 870 Market St., Suite 720, San Francisco, CA 94102 Tel 415-362-2331; Fax: 415-362-2333
E-mail: mphill@pacbell.net.

Mr Paperback Pubs News Co, *(Mr. Paperback/ Publishers News Co.),* 6030 Fostoria Ave., Findlay, OH 45840 (SAN 169-393X) Tel 419-424-6774; Fax: 419-420-1805; Toll Free: 800-872-0031.

M-S News Co Inc, *(M-S News Co., Inc.),* P.O. Box 13278, Wichita, KS 67213-0278 (SAN 169-2798) Fax: 316-267-5405.

Mullare News Agency Inc, *(Mullare News Agency, Inc.),* P.O. Box 578, Brockton, MA 02401 (SAN 169-3379).

Multilingual Bks, *(Multilingual Bks.),* Orders Addr.: P.O. Box 440632, Miami, FL 33144 (SAN 169-1155) Tel 305-471-9847 Do not confuse with Multilingual Bks., Seattle, WA.

Mumford Lib Bks Inc, *(Mumford Library Bks., Inc.),* 7847 Bayberry Rd., Jacksonville, FL 32256 (SAN 156-7721) Fax: 904-730-8913; Toll Free: 800-367-3927.

Mumford Library Bk Sales, *See* **Mumford Lib Bks Inc**

Murrs Library Service, *(Murr's Library Service),* 4045 E. Palm Ln., No. 5, Phoenix, AZ 85008-3116 (SAN 107-3222) Fax: 602-273-1217; Toll Free: 888-273-0279.

Music Design Inc, *(Music Design, Inc.),* 4650 N. Port Washington Rd., Milwaukee, WI 53212 (SAN 200-7649) Tel 414-961-8380; Fax: 414-961-8381; Toll Free: 800-862-7232
E-mail: order@musicdesign.com
Web site: http://www.musicdesign.com.

Music Sales, *(Music Sales Corp.; 0-7119; 0-8256),* Orders Addr.: 445 Bellvale Rd., P.O. Box 572, Chester, NY 10918 (SAN 662-0876) Tel 845-469-2271; Fax: 845-469-7544; Toll Free Fax: 800-345-6842; Toll Free: 800-431-7187; Edit Addr.: 257 Park Ave., S., 20th Flr., New York, NY 10010 (SAN 282-0277) Tel 212-254-2100; Fax: 212-254-2103
Web site: http://www.musicsales.com.

Musicart West, *(Musicart West),* P.O. Box 1900, Orem, UT 84059-1900 (SAN 110-1250) Tel 801-225-0859; Toll Free: 800-950-1900 (orders only).

Mustrd Seed Pubns, *(Mustard Seed Pubns.),* P.O. Box 1360, San Antonio, TX 78295 Tel 830-216-7244
E-mail: goodmarine@aol.com.

MVP Wholesales, *(MVP Wholesales),* 9301 W. Hwy. 290, No. D, Austin, TX 78736-7817 (SAN 630-9550) Tel 512-416-1452; Toll Free: 800-328-7931 (phone/fax).

MyoData, *(MyoData; 0-924728),* Orders Addr.: P.O. Box 89698, Tucson, AZ 85752-9698 (SAN 631-4139) Tel 520-744-8000; Fax: 520-744-3558; Toll Free: 800-533-5121
E-mail: tmjinfo@myodata.com
Web site: http://www.myodata.com.

N Central Bk, *(North Central Bk. Distributors),* N57 W13636 Carmen Ave., Menomonee Falls, WI 53051 (SAN 173-5195) Tel 414-781-3299; Fax: 414-781-4432; Toll Free: 800-966-3299.

NA Blackwell, *(Blackwell North America; 0-913262; 0-916472; 0-946344),* Orders Addr.: 6024 SW Jean Rd., Bldg. G, Lake Oswego, OR 97034 (SAN 169-7048) Tel 503-684-1140; Fax: 503-639-2481; Toll Free: 800-547-6426 (in Oregon); Edit Addr.: 100 University Ct., Blackwood, NJ 08012 (SAN 169-4596) Tel 856-228-8900; Toll Free: 800-257-7341.

NACSCORP Inc, *(NACSCORP, Inc.),* Subs. of National Assn. of College Stores, Orders Addr.: 528 E. Lorain St., Oberlin, OH 44074-1298 (SAN 169-6823) Tel 440-775-7777; Toll Free Fax: 800-344-5059; Toll Free: 800-321-3883 (orders only); 800-458-9303 (backorder status only); 800-334-9882 (support programs/technical support)
E-mail: service@nacscorp.com; orders@nacscorp.com
Web site: http://www.nacscorp.com.

Najarian Music Co Inc, *(Najarian Music Co., Inc.),* 269 Lexington St., Waltham, MA 02452 (SAN 169-3344) Tel 781-899-2200; Fax: 781-899-0838.

NA&OMA, *(Natl. Acupuncture & Oriental Medicine Alliance),* 14637 Starr Rd., SE, Olalla, WA 98359 Tel 253-851-6896.

Napa Childrens Bk Co, *(Napa Children's Bk. Co.),* 1239 First St., Napa, CA 94559 (SAN 122-2732) Tel 707-224-3893; Fax: 707-224-1212.

Nasco Math, *(Nasco Math Eighty-Six),* 901 Janesville Ave., Fort Atkinson, WI 53538 (SAN 679-7512).

Nat Catholic Reading, *(National Catholic Reading Distributor),* 997 Macarthur Blvd., Mahwah, NJ 07430 (SAN 169-4855) Tel 201-825-7300; Fax: 201-825-8345; Toll Free: 800-218-1903
E-mail: paulistp@pipeline.com.

Nat Learn, *(National Learning Corp.; 0-8293; 0-8373),* 212 Michael Dr., Syosset, NY 11791 (SAN 206-8869) Tel 516-921-8888; Fax: 516-921-8743; Toll Free: 800-645-6337.

Nataraj Bks, *(Nataraj Bks.; 1-881338),* Orders Addr.: P.O. Box 5076, Springfield, VA 22150 (SAN 696-6527) Tel 703-455-4996; Fax: 703-912-9052; Edit Addr.: 7073 Brookfield Plaza, Springfield, VA 22150
E-mail: nataraj@erols.com
Web site: http://www.natarajbooks.com; http://www.erols.com/nataraj.

Nathaniel Dame & Co Inc, *(Dame, Nathaniel & Co., Inc.),* 318 Lincoln St., Lexington, MA 02173-7422 (SAN 169-3395).

National Bk Co, *(National Bk. Co.),* Keystone Industrial Pk., Scranton, PA 18512 (SAN 157-1869) Tel 717-346-2020; Toll Free: 800-233-4830 Do not confuse with National Book Company, Portland, OR.

National Health Federation, *(National Health Federation),* Box 688, Monrovia, CA 91016 (SAN 227-9266) Tel 626-357-2181; Fax: 818-303-0642
E-mail: nhf@earthlink.net
Web site: http://www.healthfreedom.net.

National Magazine Service, *(National Magazine Service),* Orders Addr.: P.O. Box 834, Mars, PA 16046 (SAN 169-7595); Edit Addr.: 535 Linden Way, Pittsburgh, PA 15202 Tel 412-898-0001.

National Sales Inc, *(National Sales Inc.),* 1818 W. 2300 South, Salt Lake City, UT 84119 (SAN 159-9127) Tel 801-972-2300; Fax: 801-972-2883.

Natl Assn Deaf, *(National Assn. of the Deaf; 0-913072),* 814 Thayer Ave., Silver Spring, MD 20910 (SAN 159-4974) Tel 301-587-6282; Fax: 301-587-4873
E-mail: sales@nad.org
Web site: http://www.nad.org.

Natl Assn Search & Rescue, *(National Assn. for Search & Rescue; 0-929788),* 4500 Southgate Pl., Suite 100, Chantilly, VA 22021-1714 (SAN 250-3352).

Natl Bk Netwk, *(National Bk. Network),* 15200 NBN Way, Blue Ridge Summit, PA 17214 (SAN 630-0065) Tel 717-794-3800; Toll Free Fax: 800-338-4550; Toll Free: 800-462-6420; Edit Addr.: 4720 Boston Way, Lanham, MD 20706 Tel 301-459-3366; Fax: 301-459-1705
Web site: http://www.nbnbooks.com.

Natl Org Srv, *(National Organization Service, Inc.),* 4515 Fleur Dr., Suite 301, Des Moines, IA 50321-2369 (SAN 107-1548) Fax: 515-256-8028; Toll Free: 800-747-3032.

Natl Rifle Assn, *(National Rifle Assn.; 0-935998),* a/o Office of the General Counsel, 11250 Waples Mill Rd., Fairfax, VA 22030 (SAN 213-859X) Tel 703-267-1269; Fax: 703-267-3985; Toll Free: 800-672-3888.

Natl Tech Info, *(National Technical Information Service, U.S. Dept. of Commerce; 0-934213),* Orders Addr.: 5285 Port Royal Rd., Springfield, VA 22161 (SAN 205-7255) Tel 703-605-6000; Fax: 703-605-6900; Toll Free: 800-553-6847
E-mail: orders@ntis.gov; info@ntis.gov
Web site: http://www.ntis.gov.

Natl Video Res, *(National Video Resources, Inc.; 1-884188),* 73 Spring St., Suite 606, New York, NY 10012 Tel 212-274-8080; Fax: 212-274-8081
Web site: http://www.nvr.org.

NC News, *(North Carolina News Co.),* P.O. Box 1051, Durham, NC 27702-1051 (SAN 169-6378) Tel 919-682-5779.

NC Sch Bk Depositry, *(North Carolina Schl. Bk. Depository, Inc.),* P.O. Box 950, Raleigh, NC 27602-0950 (SAN 169-6467) Tel 919-833-6615.

Needham Pr, *(Needham Pr., Inc.; 0-9635022),* P.O. Box 130530, Ann Arbor, MI 48113-0530 Tel 734-668-6666; Fax: 734-668-8339
E-mail: needham@izzy.net
Web site: http://www.needhampress.com.

Neighborhood Periodical Club Inc, *(Neighborhood Periodical Club, Inc.),* 653 Northland Blvd., Cincinnati, OH 45240-3215 (SAN 285-9262) Tel 513-851-8600; Fax: 513-851-8695.

Nelson News Agency, *(Nelson News Agency),* 726 First Ave., N., Fort Dodge, IA 50501 (SAN 169-264X).

Nelson News Inc, *(Nelson News, Inc.),* P.O. Box 27007, Omaha, NE 68127-0007 (SAN 169-443X) Tel 402-734-3333; Fax: 402-731-0516.

Nelsons Bks, *(Nelson's Bks.; 0-9612188),* P.O. Box 2302, Santa Cruz, CA 95063 (SAN 289-4858) Tel 831-465-9148.

Ner Tamid Bk Distributors, *(Ner Tamid Bk. Distributors),* P.O. Box 10401, Riviera Beach, FL 33419-0401 (SAN 169-135X) Tel 561-686-9095.

Net Productions, *(Net Productions),* 210 Elm Cir., Colorado Springs, CO 80906-3348 (SAN 159-9143).

netLibrary CO, *(netLibrary, Inc.; 0-585),* 3080 Center Green Dr., Boulder, CO 80301-2252 (SAN 253-9497) Tel 303-415-2548; Fax: 303-381-7000; 303-381-8999; Toll Free: 800-413-4557
E-mail: mgilbert@netlibrary.com
Web site: http://www.netlibrary.com.

New Alexandrian Bookstore, *(New Alexandrian Bookstore),* 110 N Cayuga St., Ithaca, NY 14850-4331 (SAN 159-4958) Tel 607-272-1163.

New Concepts Bks & Tapes, *(New Concepts Bks. & Tapes Distributors),* Orders Addr.: P.O. Box 55068, Houston, TX 77255 (SAN 114-2682) Tel 713-465-7736; Fax: 713-465-7106; Toll Free: 800-842-4807; Edit Addr.: 9722 Pine Lake, Houston, TX 77055 (SAN 630-7531).

New England Bk Service, *(New England Bk. Service, Inc.),* 1037 Prindle Rd., Charlotte, VT 05445 (SAN 170-0952) Tel 802-425-3841; Fax: 802-425-3158; Toll Free: 800-356-5772
E-mail: nebs@together.net.

New England Mobile Bk Fair, *(New England Mobile Bk. Fair),* 82 Needham St., P.O. Box 610159, Newton Highlands, MA 02461 (SAN 169-3530) Tel 617-527-5817; Fax: 617-527-0113.

New Era Publns MI, *(New Era Pubns., Inc.; 0-939830),* P.O. Box 130109, Ann Arbor, MI 48113-0109 (SAN 111-8757) Tel 734-663-1929 Do not confuse with New Era Pubns. in Happy Camp, CA.

New Jersey Bk Agency, *(New Jersey Bk. Agency),* Orders Addr.: P.O. Box 144, Morris Plains, NJ 07950 (SAN 106-861X) Tel 973-267-7093; Fax: 973-292-3177; Edit Addr.: 59 Leamoor Dr., Morris Plains, NJ 07950 (SAN 243-2307).

New Jersey Bks Inc, *(New Jersey Bks., Inc.),* 59 Market St., Newark, NJ 07102 (SAN 156-5443) Tel 973-624-8070; Toll Free: 800-772-3678.

New Leaf Dist, *(New Leaf Distributing Co., Inc.; 0-9627209),* Div. of Al-Wali Corp., 401 Thornton Rd., Lithia Springs, GA 30122-1557 (SAN 169-1449) Tel 770-948-7845; Fax: 770-944-2313; Toll Free Fax: 800-326-1066; Toll Free: 800-326-2665
E-mail: NewLeaf@NewLeaf-dist.com
Web site: http://www.NewLeaf-dist.com.

New Life, *(New Life Foundation; 0-911203),* P.O. Box 2230, Pine, AZ 85544-2230 (SAN 170-3986) Tel 520-476-3224; Fax: 520-476-4743; Toll Free: 800-293-3377 (wholesale only)
E-mail: info@anewlife.org
Web site: http://www.anewlife.org.

New London News Co, *(New London News Co.),* 25 Westwood Ave., New London, CT 06320-2726 (SAN 169-0752).

New World Resource Ctr, *(New World Resource Ctr.),* 2600 W. Fullerton Ave., Chicago, IL 60647-3008 (SAN 169-1848).

New Wrld Lib, *(New World Library; 0-931432; 0-945934; 1-57731; 1-878424; 1-880032),* 14 Pamaron Way, Novato, CA 94949 (SAN 211-8777) Tel 415-884-2100; Fax: 415-884-2199; Toll Free: 800-972-6657 (retail orders only) Do not confuse with New World Library Publishing Co., Los Altos, CA
E-mail: escort@nwlib.com
Web site: http://www.newworldlibrary.com.

New York Periodical Distributors, *(New York Periodical Distributors),* P.O. Box 29, Massena, NY 13662-0029 (SAN 169-6149).

Newborn Enterprises Inc, *(Newborn Enterprises, Inc.),* P.O. Box 1713, Altoona, PA 16603 (SAN 169-7242) Tel 814-944-3593; Fax: 814-944-1881; Toll Free: 800-227-0285 (in Pennsylvania).

News Group NC, *(News Group, The),* P.O. Box 25367, Winston-Salem, NC 27114 (SAN 169-6513) Fax: 910-765-8842 Do not confuse with companies with the same name in Columbus, SC, Anchorage, AK, Elizabeth, NC.

News Grp AK, *(News Group, The),* 325 W. Potter Dr., Anchorage, AK 99518 (SAN 168-9274) Tel 907-563-3251; Fax: 907-261-8523 Do not confuse with companies with the same name in Columbus, SC, Winston-Salem, NC, Elizabeth, NC.

News Grp IL, *(News Group - Illinois, The),* 1301 SW Washington St., Peoria, IL 61602 (SAN 169-216X) Tel 309-673-4549; Fax: 309-673-8883.

News Supply Co, *(News Supply Co.),* 216 S. La Huerta Cir., Carlsbad, NM 88220-9620 (SAN 159-9151).

Newsdealers Supply Co Inc, *(Newsdealers Supply Co., Inc.),* P.O. Box 3516, Tallahassee, FL 32315-3516 (SAN 168-9215).

NEWSouth Distributors, *(NEWSouth Distributors),* P.O. Box 2198, Ocala, FL 34470 (SAN 159-8732).

Newsstand Distributors, *(Newsstand Distributors),* 155 W. 14th St., Ogden, UT 84404 (SAN 169-8494) Fax: 810-621-7336; Toll Free: 800-283-6247; 800-231-4834 (in Utah).

Niagara County News, *(Niagara County News),* 70 Nicholls St., Lockport, NY 14094 (SAN 169-541X) Tel 716-433-6466.

Nonagon, *(Nonagon),* 1556 Douglas Dr., El Cerrito, CA 94530 (SAN 654-0503) Tel 510-237-5290.

Nor East Bk Sls, *(Nor' East Book Sales),* 440 Mendon Rd., N., Attleboro, MA 02760 Tel 508-761-5414; Fax: 508-761-6372.

Nor-Cal News Co, *(Nor-Cal News Co.),* 2040 Petaluma Blvd., P.O. Box 2508, Petaluma, CA 94953 (SAN 169-0035) Tel 707-763-2606; Fax: 707-763-3905.

North Amer Bk, *(North American Bk. Distributors),* P.O. Box 510, Hamburg, MI 48139 (SAN 630-4680) Tel 810-231-3728.

North Country, *(North Country Bks., Inc.; 0-925168; 0-932052; 0-9601158),* 311 Turner St., Utica, NY 13501 (SAN 110-828X) Tel 315-735-4877; Fax: 315-738-4342
E-mail: NCBOOKS@NTCNET.COM.

North Shore Distributors, *(North Shore Distributors),* 1200 N. Branch, Chicago, IL 60622 (SAN 169-2275).

North Shore News Co Inc, *(North Shore News Co., Inc.),* 150 Blossom St., Lynn, MA 01902 (SAN 169-3492).

North Texas Periodicals, *(North Texas Periodicals, Inc.),* Orders Addr.: P.O. Box 3823, Lubbock, TX 79452 Tel 806-745-6000; Fax: 806-745-7028; Edit Addr.: 118 E. 70th St., Lubbock, TX 79404 (SAN 169-8338)
E-mail: ntp@hts-online_net.

Northern News Co, *(Northern News Co.),* Harbor-Petoskey Rd., P.O. Box 543, Petoskey, MI 49770 (SAN 169-3964) Tel 616-347-3936; Fax: 616-347-6475; Toll Free: 800-632-7138 (Michigan only).

Northern Schl Supply Co, *(Northern Schl. Supply Co.),* P.O. Box 2627, Fargo, ND 58108 (SAN 169-6548) Fax: 800-891-5836.

Northern Sun, *(Northern Sun),* 2916 E. Lake St., Minneapolis, MN 55406 (SAN 249-9290) Tel 612-729-2001; Fax: 612-729-0149; Toll Free: 800-258-8579.

Northern Sun Merchandising, *See* **Northern Sun**

Northwest News Co Inc, *(Northwest News Co., Inc.),* Orders Addr.: P.O. Box 4965, Missoula, MT 59806 (SAN 660-9406); Edit Addr.: 1701 Ranklin St., Missoula, MT 59802-1629 (SAN 169-4391) Tel 406-721-7801.

Norton, *(Norton, W.W. & Co., Inc.; 0-393; 0-920256),* Orders Addr.: 800 Keystone Industrial Pk., Scranton, PA 18512 (SAN 157-1869) Tel 570-346-2020; Toll Free Fax: 800-548-6515; Toll Free: 800-233-4830 (book orders only); Edit Addr.: 500 Fifth Ave., New York, NY 10110-0017 (SAN 202-5795) Tel 212-354-5500; Fax: 212-869-0856; Toll Free: 800-223-2584
E-mail: webmaster@wwnorton.com
Web site: http://www.wwnorton.com/trade; http://www.wwnorton.com.

Norton News Agency, *(Norton News Agency),* 801 Cedar Cross Rd., Dubuque, IA 52003-7735 (SAN 169-2631); 1467 Service Dr., Winona, MN 55987 (SAN 156-4889).

NSF Intl, *(N S F International; 0-9675817),* 789 N. Dixboro Rd., Ann Arbor, MI 48105 Tel 734-913-5703; Fax: 734-827-7795
E-mail: conferences@nsf.org
Web site: http://www.nsf.org.

NTC Contemp Pub Co, *(NTC/Contemporary Publishing Co.; 0-658; 0-8092; 0-8325; 0-8442; 0-88499; 0-89061; 0-913327; 0-940279; 0-941263; 0-9630646; 1-56626; 1-56943; 1-57028),* Subs. of Tribune Education (Tribune Co.), 4255 W. Touhy Ave., Lincolnwood, IL 60712 (SAN 169-2208) Tel 847-679-5500; Fax: 847-679-2494; Toll Free Fax: 800-998-3103; Toll Free: 800-323-4900
E-mail: ntcpub@tribune.com
Web site: http://www.ntc-cb.com.

Ntl Maternal, *(National Maternal & Child Health Clearinghouse),* 2070 Chain Bridge Rd., Suite 450, Vienna, VA 22182-2536 Tel 703-356-1964.

Nueces News Agency, *(Nueces News Agency),* P.O. Box 2768, 209 N. Padre Island Dr., Corpus Christi, TX 78403 (SAN 169-8079).

Nueva Vida Distributors, *(Nueva Vida Distributors),* 3725 Montana Ave., El Paso, TX 79903-4503 (SAN 107-8615) Tel 915-755-2058.

Nutri-Books Corp, *(Nutri-Bks. Corp.),* Div. of Royal Pubns., Inc., 790 W. Tennessee Ave., P.O. Box 5793, Denver, CO 80223 (SAN 169-054X) Tel 303-778-8383; Fax: 303-744-9383; Toll Free: 800-279-2048 (orders only).

NW News, *(Northwest News),* 1560 NE First St., No. 13, Bend, OR 97701 (SAN 111-8587) Tel 541-382-6065; 3100 Merriman Rd., Medford, OR 97501 (SAN 169-7137) Tel 541-779-5225.

NY Rev Bks, *(New York Review of Bks., Inc., The; 0-940322; 1-59017),* 1755 Broadway, 5th Flr., New York, NY 10019-3780 (SAN 220-3448) Tel 212-757-8070; Fax: 212-333-5374
E-mail: mail@nybooks.com
Web site: http://www.nybooks.com.

NYU Pr, *(New York Univ. Pr.; 0-8147),* Div. of New York Univ., 838 Broadway, 3rd Flr., New York, NY 10003-4812 (SAN 658-1293) Tel 212-998-2575; Fax: 212-995-3833; Toll Free: 800-996-6987
E-mail: orders@nyupress.nyu.edu
Web site: http://www.nyupress.nyu.edu.

O G Waffle Bk Co, *(Waffle, O. G. Bk. Co. (The Bookhouse)),* P.O. Box 586, Marion, IA 52302 (SAN 112-8817) Tel 319-373-1832.

Oak Knoll, *(Oak Knoll Pr.; 0-938768; 1-884718; 1-58456),* 310 Delaware St., New Castle, DE 19720 (SAN 216-2776) Tel 302-328-7232; Fax: 302-328-7274; Toll Free: 800-996-2556
E-mail: oakknoll@oakknoll.com
Web site: http://www.oakknoll.com.

Octagon Press I S H K Book Service, *See* **ISHK**

Odyssey Distributing Co, *(Odyssey Distributing Co.),* 2010 Washington Ave., Santa Monica, CA 90403-3308 (SAN 157-0188).

Ohio Periodical Distributors, *(Ohio Periodical Distributors),* P.O. Box 145449, Cincinnati, OH 45250-5449 (SAN 169-6904) Fax: 513-853-6245; Toll Free: 800-777-2216.

Ohio U Pr, *(Ohio Univ. Pr.; 0-8214),* Orders Addr.: 11030 S. Langley Ave., Chicago, IL 60628 (SAN 202-5280) Tel 773-568-1559; Fax: 773-660-2235; Toll Free Fax: 800-621-8476; Toll Free: 800-621-2736; Edit Addr.: Scott Quadrangle, Athens, OH 45701 (SAN 282-0773) Tel 740-593-1154; Fax: 740-593-4536
E-mail: arnold@ohiou.edu
Web site: http://www.ohiou.edu/oupress/.

Oil City News Co, *(Oil City News Co.),* 112 Innis St., Oil City, PA 16301-2930 (SAN 169-7501).

Oklahoma Schl & Office Supply, *(Oklahoma School & Office Supply),* 605 W. Poplar St., Fort Gibson, OK 74434-8730 (SAN 169-6963).

Ollis Bk Corp, *(Ollis Bk. Corp.),* Orders Addr.: P.O. Box 258, Steger, IL 60475 (SAN 658-1323); Edit Addr.: 28 E. 35th St., Steger, IL 60475 (SAN 169-2224) Tel 312-755-5151; Fax: 708-755-5153; Toll Free: 800-323-0343.

Olson News Agency, *(Olson News Agency),* P.O. Box 129, Ishpeming, MI 49849 (SAN 169-3832).

OM Literature, *(OM Literature),* P.O. Box 1047, Waynesboro, GA 30830-2047 Tel 706-554-5827; Fax: 706-554-7444; Toll Free: 800-733-5907
Web site: http://www.doneomlit.om.org.

Omnibooks, *(Omnibooks),* 456 Vista Del Mar Dr., Aptos, CA 95003-4832 (SAN 168-9487) Tel 408-688-4098; Toll Free: 800-626-6671.

Ong Hing Kee, *(Ong Hing Kee),* 724 Jackson, San Francisco, CA 94133 (SAN 107-1084) Tel 415-956-0432.

Onondaga News Agency, *(Onondaga News Agency),* 474 E. Brighton Ave., Syracuse, NY 13210 (SAN 169-6297) Tel 315-475-3121.

Open Court, *(Open Court; 0-02; 0-8126; 0-87548; 0-89688; 0-912050),* Div. of S R A/McGraw-Hill, 332 S. Michigan Ave., Suite 1100, Chicago, IL 60604 Tel 312-939-1500; Fax: 510-528-3444 (orders); 312-939-8150; Toll Free: 800-788-3123 (orders)
E-mail: opencourt@caruspub.com
Web site: http://www.opencourtbooks.com.

Options GA, *(Options Unlimited),* 550 Swan Creek Ct., Suwanee, GA 30174 (SAN 631-3949) Tel 770-237-3282 Do not confuse with Options Unlimited, Inc., Green Bay, WI.

Orbit Bks Corp, *(Orbit Bks. Corp.),* 43 Timberline Dr., Poughkeepsie, NY 12603 (SAN 169-6157) Tel 914-462-5653; Fax: 914-462-8409.

Orca Bk Pubs, *(Orca Bk. Pubs.; 1-55143),* P.O. Box 468, Custer, WA 98240-0468 (SAN 630-9674) Tel 250-380-1229; Fax: 250-380-1892; Toll Free: 800-210-5277
E-mail: mcolgan@orcabook.com
Web site: http://www.orcabook.com.

Origin Bk Sales, *(Origin Bk. Sales, Inc.),* 415 N., Neil Armstrong Rd., International Ctr., Salt Lake City, UT 84116 (SAN 631-1407) Tel 801-972-8060; Fax: 801-972-6570; Toll Free Fax: 888-467-4442; Toll Free: 888-467-4446
E-mail: rsandack@originbooks.com; jasay@qwest.com.

Orthopedic Phys, *(Orthopedic Physical Therapy Products (OPTP)),* Orders Addr.: P.O. Box 47009, Minneapolis, MN 55447-0009 Tel 612-553-0452; Fax: 612-553-9355; Toll Free: 800-367-7393; Edit Addr.: 3700 Annaplis Ln., No. 175, Minneapolis, MN 55447-5435
E-mail: optp@worldnet.att.net
Web site: http://www.optp.com.

Osborne Enterps, *(Osborne Enterprises Publishing; 0-932117),* P.O. Box 255, Port Townsend, WA 98368 (SAN 242-7567) Tel 360-385-1200; Fax: 360-385-6572; Toll Free: 800-246-3255 (orders only) Web site: http://www.jerryosborne.com.

Osiander Bk Trade, *(Osiander Bk. Trade),* 7483H Candlewood Rd., Hanover, MD 21076-3102 (SAN 130-0970).

OSU Fire Protect, *(OSU Fire Protection Pubns.),* 9030 N. Willis, Stillwater, OK 74078 Toll Free: 800-654-4055.

Other Pr LLC, *(Other Pr., LLC, The; 1-892746; 1-59051),* 377 W. 11th St., New York, NY 10014 Tel 212-924-3344; Fax: 212-414-9654 Do not confuse with Other Press in Jersey City, NJ
E-mail: info@otherpress.com
Web site: http://www.otherpress.com.

OUP, *(Oxford Univ. Pr., Inc.; 0-19; 0-904147; 0-947946; 1-85221),* Orders Addr.: 2001 Evans Rd., Cary, NC 27513 (SAN 202-5892) Tel 919-677-0977 (general voice); Fax: 919-677-1303 (customer service); Toll Free: 800-445-9714 (customer service - inquiry); 800-451-7556 (customer service - orders); Edit Addr.: 198 Madison Ave., New York, NY 10016-4314 (SAN 202-5884) Tel 212-726-6000 (general voice); Fax: 212-726-6440 (general fax)
E-mail: orders@oup-usa.org; custserv@oup-usa.org
Web site: http://www.oup-usa.org.

Outbooks, *See* **Vistabooks**

Outdoorsman, *(Outdoorsman, The),* Orders Addr.: P.O. Box 268, Boston, MA 02134 (SAN 169-3352).

Ozark Magazine Distributing Inc, *(Ozark Magazine Distributing, Inc.),* 1630 N. Eldon, Springfield, MO 65801 (SAN 169-4332).

Ozark News Agency Inc, *(Ozark News Agency, Inc.),* P.O. Box 1150, Fayetteville, AR 72702 (SAN 168-9436).

P & G Wholesale, *(P & G Wholesale),* P.O. Box 1548, Fargo, ND 58102 (SAN 156-4536).

P D Meany, *(Meany, P.D. Pubs.; 0-88835),* 825 E. Roosevelt Rd., Unit 447, Lombard, IL 60148 Tel 905-804-0512; Fax: 905-804-0513
E-mail: mbooks@interlog.com
Web site: http://www.interlog.com/~mbooks/.

P D Music Headquarters Inc, *(P. D. Music Headquarters, Inc.),* Orders Addr.: P.O. Box 252, New York, NY 10014 (SAN 282-5880) Tel 212-242-5322.

P G Weiss, *(Weiss, Paul G.),* Myron Taylor Hall, Ithaca, NY 14853 (SAN 237-9236).

P H Brookes, *(Brookes, Paul H. Publishing Co.; 0-933716; 1-55766),* Orders Addr.: P.O. Box 10624, Baltimore, MD 21285-0624 (SAN 212-730X) Tel 410-337-9580; Fax: 410-337-8539; Toll Free: 800-638-3775; Edit Addr.: 409 Washington Ave., Suite 500, Towson, MD 21204 (SAN 666-6485)
E-mail: custserv@brookespublishing.com
Web site: http://www.brookespublishing.com.

Pacific Magazine-Book Wholesaler, *(Pacific Magazine-Bk. Wholesaler),* 1515 NW 51st St., Seattle, WA 98107 (SAN 274-3884) Tel 206-789-5333.

Pacific Period, *See* **Andrsn News Tacoma**

Pacific Trade Group, *(Pacific Trade Group),* 68-309 Crozier Dr., Waialua, HI 96791 (SAN 169-1635) Tel 808-636-2300; Fax: 808-636-2301.

Palgr, *See* **Palgr Mac**

Palgr Mac, *(Palgrave Macmillan; 0-312; 0-333; 1-4039),* Div. of Saint Martin's Press, LLC, 175 Fifth Ave., New York, NY 10010 Tel 212-982-9300; Fax: 212-777-6359; Toll Free: 800-221-7945
Web site: http://www.palgrave.com.

Palmer College, *(Palmer College of Chiropractice),* 90 E. Tasman Dr., San Jose, CA 95134 Tel 408-944-6000.

Palmer News Co Inc, *(Palmer News Co., Inc.),* 1050 Republican, P.O. Box 1400, Topeka, KS 66601 Tel 913-234-6679; Fax: 913-234-6338.

Palmer News Inc, *(Palmer News, Inc.),* 9605 Dice Ln., Lenexa, KS 66215 Tel 913-541-8600; Fax: 913-541-9413
E-mail: palmerco@oni.com.

Palmetto News Co, *(Palmetto News Co.),* 200 Sunbelt Ct., Greer, SC 29650-9349 (SAN 169-7803).

Palmyra Pubg Co, *(Palmyra Publishing Co.; 0-9666627),* P.O. Box 1164, Sioux Falls, SD 57101-1164 Tel 605-330-2707; Fax: 605-330-6009
E-mail: alyajim@sd.cybernex.net.

Pan Amer Pub, *(Pan American Publishing, Inc.; 1-889867),* 420 E. Ohio St., Suite 4-F, Chicago, IL 60611-3355 (SAN 299-1977) Tel 773-404-7282.

Pan De Vida Dists, *(Pan De Vida Distributors),* 312 N. Azusa Ave., Azusa, CA 91702 (SAN 631-0753) Tel 626-962-0203; Fax: 626-334-5842; Toll Free: 800-321-6633.

Pantheon, *(Pantheon Bks.; 0-375; 0-394; 0-676; 0-679),* Div. of Random Hse., Inc., Orders Addr.: 400 Hahn Rd., Westminster, MD 21157 (SAN 202-5515) Tel 410-848-1900; Toll Free: 800-733-3000 (orders); Edit Addr.: 299 Park Ave, New York, NY 10171 (SAN 202-862X) Fax: 212-572-6030; Toll Free: 800-638-6460 (customer service)
Web site: http://www.pantheonbooks.com.

Paperback Bks Inc, *See* **Bk Dist Ctr**

Paperbacks for Educators, *(Paperbacks for Educators; 0-9702376),* 426 W. Front St., Washington, MO 63090 (SAN 103-3379) Tel 636-239-1999; Fax: 636-239-4515; Toll Free Fax: 800-514-7323; Toll Free: 800-227-2591
E-mail: paperbacks@mail.usmo.com
Web site: http://www.any-book-in-print.com.

Parkwest Pubns, *(Parkwest Pubns., Inc.; 0-88186),* 451 Communipaw Ave., Jersey City, NJ 07304 (SAN 264-6846) Tel 201-432-3257; Fax: 201-432-3708
E-mail: parkwest@parkwestpubs.com
Web site: http://www.parkwestpubs.com.

Parliament News Co Inc, *(Parliament News Co., Inc.),* P.O. Box 910, Santa Clarita, CA 91380-9010 (SAN 168-9924).

Partners Bk Dist, *See* **Partners Pubs Grp**

Partners Pubs Grp, *(Partners Pubs. Group, Inc.),* Orders Addr.: P.O. Box 580, Holt, MI 48842 Tel 517-694-3205; Fax: 517-694-0617; Toll Free: 800-336-3137; Edit Addr.: 2325 Jarco Dr., Holt, MI 48842 (SAN 631-3418).

Partners-West, *(Partners/West),* 1901 Raymond Ave., SW, Suite C, Renton, WA 98055 (SAN 631-421X) Tel 425-227-8486; Fax: 425-204-1448; Toll Free: 800-563-2385.

Pathway Bk Serv, *(Pathway Bk. Service),* Div. of MLES, Inc., Orders Addr.: P.O. Box 89, Gilsum, NH 03448 Toll Free: 800-345-6665; Edit Addr.: 4 White Brook Rd., Gilsum, NH 03448 (SAN 170-0545) Tel 603-357-0236; Fax: 603-357-2073
E-mail: pbs@pathwaybook.com
Web site: http://www.pathwaybook.com.

Paul & Co Pubs, *(Paul & Co. Pubs. Consortium, Inc.),* Div. of Independent Publishers Group, Orders Addr.: 814 N. Franklin St., Chicago, IL 60610 Tel 312-337-0747; Fax: 312-337-5985; Toll Free: 800-888-4741; Edit Addr.: P.O. Box 442, Concord, MA 01742 (SAN 630-5318) Tel 978-369-3049; Fax: 978-369-2385
E-mail: frontdesk@ipgbook.com
Web site: http://www.ipgbook.com.

PB, *(Pocket Bks.; 0-671; 0-7434),* Div. of Simon & Schuster, Inc., Orders Addr.: 100 Front St., Riverside, NJ 08075 (SAN 200-2442) Toll Free Fax: 800-943-9831; Toll Free: 800-223-2336; Edit Addr.: 1230 Ave. of the Americas, New York, NY 10020 (SAN 202-5922) Tel 212-698-7000
E-mail: ssonline_feedback@simonsays.com
Web site: http://www.simonsays.com.

PBD Inc, *(PBD, Inc.),* 1650 Bluegrass Lakes Pkwy., Alpharetta, GA 30004 (SAN 126-6039) Tel 770-442-8633; Fax: 770-442-9742
Web site: http://www.pbd.com.

PBDI, *(Professional Bk. Dist., Inc.),* 1650 Bluegrass Lakes Pkwy., Alpharetta, GA 30004.

PCI Educ Pubg, *(PCI Educational Publishing; 1-884074; 1-58804),* 12029 Warfield, San Antonio, TX 78216-3231 Tel 210-377-1999; Fax: 210-377-1121; Toll Free Fax: 888-259-8284; Toll Free: 800-594-4263
E-mail: lboulet@pcicatalog.com
Web site: http://www.pcicatalog.com.

Pee Dee News Co, *(Pee Dee News Co.),* 2321 Lawrens Cir., Florence, SC 29501-9408 (SAN 169-7781).

Pegasus Pr, *(Pegasus Pr.; 1-889818),* Univ. of North Carolina, Asheville, NC 28804 Tel 828-232-5143; Fax: 828-232-5146
E-mail: pegpress@mindspring.com
Web site: http://www.pegasuspress.org.

Pekin News Agency, *(Pekin News Agency),* 1637 Monroe St., Madison, WI 53711-2021 (SAN 169-2151).

Pen Notes, *(Pen Notes, Inc.; 0-939564),* 61 Bennington Ave., Freeport, NY 11520 (SAN 107-3621) Tel 516-868-5753; Fax: 516-868-8441
E-mail: pennotes@worldnet.att.net.

Penguin, *See* **Penguin Putnam**

Penguin Putnam, *(Penguin Putnam, Inc.; 0-14),* Div. of The Penguin Group owned by Pearson plc, Orders Addr.: 405 Murray Hill Pkwy., East Rutherford, NJ 07073-2136 (SAN 282-5074) Fax: 201-933-2903 (customer service); Toll Free Fax: 800-227-9604; Toll Free: 800-788-6262 (individual consumer sales); 800-526-0275 (reseller sales); 800-631-8571 (reseller customer service); Edit Addr.: 375 Hudson St., New York, NY 10014 Tel 212-366-2000; Fax: 212-366-2666
Web site: http://www.penguinputnam.com.

Penial Prod, *(Peniel Productions),* 73 Smith Hill Rd., Monsey, NY 10952-4131 (SAN 631-2837).

Penmarch Pub, *(Penmarch Publishing),* 3932 S. Willow Ave., Sioux Falls, SD 57105 Toll Free: 800-282-2399.

Penn Capitol Presrv, *(Pennsylvania Capitol Preservation Committee; 0-9643048),* P.O. Box 202231, Harrisburg, PA 17120 Tel 717-783-6484; Fax: 717-772-0742.

Penn News Co, *(Penn News Co.),* 944 Franklin St., Johnstown, PA 15905 (SAN 169-7390).

PennWell Bks, *See* **PennWell Corp**

PennWell Corp, *(PennWell Corp.; 0-87814),* Div. of Information Products Group, Orders Addr.: P.O. Box 21288, Tulsa, OK 74121 (SAN 282-1567) Tel 918-831-9421; Edit Addr.: 1421 S. Sheridan, Tulsa, OK 74112 (SAN 282-1559) Tel 918-835-3161; Fax: 918-831-9555; Toll Free Fax: 877-218-1348; Toll Free: 800-752-9764 (orders only)
E-mail: renaew@pennwell.com
Web site: http://www.pennwell-store.com.

Penton Overseas, *(Penton Overseas, Inc.; 0-939001; 1-56015; 1-59125),* 2470 Impala Dr., Carlsbad, CA 92008 (SAN 631-0826) Tel 760-431-0060; Fax: 760-431-8110; Toll Free: 800-748-5804
E-mail: info@pentonoverseas.com
Web site: http://www.pentonoverseas.com.

Peoples Pub Grp, *(Peoples Publishing Group, Inc., The; 1-56256; 1-58984),* Orders Addr.: P.O. Box 513, Saddle Brook, NJ 07633 Tel 201-712-0090; Fax: 201-712-1016; Toll Free: 800-822-1080; Edit Addr.: 299 Market St., Saddle Brook, NJ 07663
E-mail: sales@peoplespublishing.com; customersupport@peoplespublishing.com; editorial@peoplespublishing.com; solvier@peoplespublishing.com
Web site: http://www.peoplespublishing.com/index.html.

Peregrine Outftrs, *(Peregrine Outfitters),* Orders Addr.: P.O. Box 1500, Williston, VT 05495 (SAN 631-1059) Tel 802-860-2977; Fax: 802-860-2978; Toll Free: 800-222-3088; Edit Addr.: 25 Omega Dr., Suite A, Williston, VT 05482.

Periodical Distributors Inc, *See* **North Texas Periodicals**

Periodical Marketing Services, *(Periodical Marketing Services),* 1065 Bloomfield Ave., Clifton, NJ 07012 (SAN 250-5304) Tel 201-342-6334.

Periodical Pubs Service Bureau, *(Periodical Pubs. Service Bureau),* 1 N. Superior St., Sandusky, OH 44870 (SAN 285-9351) Tel 419-626-0623.

Periodicals Srv, *(Periodicals Service Co.; 0-527; 0-8115; 3-262; 3-601),* 11 Main St., Germantown, NY 12526 (SAN 164-8608) Tel 518-537-4700; Fax: 518-537-5899
E-mail: psc@backsets.com
Web site: http://www.backsets.com.

Permabound, *(Permabound Bks.),* 617 E. Vandalia Rd., Jacksonville, IL 62650.

Perry Enterprises, *(Perry Enterprises; 0-941518),* 3907 N. Foothill Dr., Provo, UT 84604 (SAN 171-0281) Tel 801-226-1002.

Petterson Antiques, *(Petterson Antiques),* 201 King St., Charleston, SC 29401 (SAN 114-2399) Tel 803-723-5714.

Phillips News Co, *(Phillips News Co.),* P.O. Box 13278, Wichita, KS 67213-0278 (SAN 169-2704).

Philos Document, *(Philosophy Documentation Ctr.; 0-912632; 1-889680),* Orders Addr.: P.O. Box 7147, Charlottesville, VA 22906-7147 (SAN 218-6586) Tel 434-220-3300; Fax: 434-220-3301; Toll Free: 800-444-2419; Edit Addr.: 706 Forest St., Suite C, Charlottesville, VA 22903-5220
E-mail: order@pdcnet.org
Web site: http://www.pdcnet.org.

Piedmont News, *(Piedmont News),* P.O. Box 25367, Winston-Salem, NC 27114 (SAN 135-227X).

Pittsfield News Co Inc, *(Pittsfield News Co., Inc.),* 6 Westview Rd., Pittsfield, MA 01201 (SAN 124-2768) Tel 413-445-5682; Fax: 413-445-5683.

Pks & Hist, *(Parks & History Assn.; 1-887878),* 126 Raleigh St., SE, Washington, DC 20032 (SAN 170-8821) Tel 202-472-3083; Fax: 202-755-0469.

Plains Distribution Service, *(Plains Distribution Service),* P.O. Box 931, Moorhead, MN 56561 (SAN 169-6556).

Plains Press, *(Plains Pr.; 0-918461),* P.O. Box 6, Granite Falls, MN 56241 (SAN 677-0185) Tel 507-537-6463.

Planeta, *(Planeta Publishing Corp.; 0-9715256),* 939 Crandon Blvd., Key Biscayne, FL 33149 Tel 305-361-0053; Fax: 305-361-0054; Toll Free: 800-407-4770
E-mail: mnormanppc@aol.com.

Players Pr, *(Players Pr., Inc.; 0-88734),* P.O. Box 1132, Studio City, CA 91614-0132 (SAN 239-0213) Tel 818-789-4980.

Pleiades Proj, *(Pleiades Project; 1-885757),* Orders Addr.: P.O. Box 1270, Rancho Mirage, CA 92270-1941 Tel 760-770-9720; Toll Free: 800-934-6423; Edit Addr.: 511 E. Second St., Wichita, KS 67202
E-mail: pleja@earthlink.net
Web site: http://www.timelink.net/pleiades.

Plough, *(Plough Publishing Hse., The; 0-87486),* Rte. 381 N., Farmington, PA 15437 (SAN 202-0092) Tel 724-329-1100; Fax: 724-329-0914; Toll Free: 800-521-8011; Rte. 381 N., Farmington, PA 15437 (SAN 202-0092) Tel 724-329-1100; Fax: 724-329-0914; Toll Free: 800-521-8011
E-mail: plough@plough.com
Web site: http://www.plough.com.

PMG Bks, *(PMG Bks. Ltd.),* 321 Nolan St., San Antonio, TX 78202 (SAN 631-3183) Tel 210-226-0772; Fax: 210-224-5194.

Polybook Distributors, *(Polybook Distributors),* 22 S. Sixth Ave., P.O. Box 109, Mount Vernon, NY 10550 (SAN 169-5568) Tel 914-664-1633; Fax: 914-428-3953.

Pomona Valley News Agency, *(Pomona Valley News Agency),* 10736 Fremont Ave., Ontario, CA 91762 (SAN 169-0019) Tel 909-591-3885.

Popular Subscription Service, *(Popular Subscription Service),* P.O. Box 1566, Terre Haute, IN 47808 (SAN 285-9386) Tel 812-466-1258; Fax: 812-466-9443; Toll Free: 800-466-5038
E-mail: info@popularsubscriptionsvc.com
Web site: http://www.popularsubscriptionsvc.com.

Portland News Co, *(Portland News Co.),* Orders Addr.: P.O. Box 6970, Scarborough, ME 04070-6970 (SAN 169-3093) Toll Free: 800-639-1708 (in Maine); Edit Addr.: 10 Southgate Rd., Scarborough, ME 04074 Tel 207-883-1300.

Portsmouth News Agency, *(Portsmouth News Agency),* 3051 Walnut St., Portsmouth, OH 45662 (SAN 169-6831).

Pottstown News Co, *(Pottstown News Co.),* 557 W. High St., Pottstown, PA 19464 (SAN 169-7609) Tel 610-326-2450; Fax: 610-326-3599.

Pratz News Agency, *(Pratz News Agency),* Box 892, Deming, NM 88030 (SAN 159-9275).

Prebound Periodicals, *(Prebound Periodicals),* 2101 N. Topeka Blvd., Topeka, KS 66608 (SAN 285-8037) Tel 785-233-4252.

Premier Publishers, *(Premier Pubs., Inc.; 0-915665),* P.O. Box 330309, Fort Worth, TX 76163 (SAN 292-5966) Tel 817-293-7030; Fax: 817-293-3410.

Presbyterian Pub, *(Presbyterian Publishing Corp.; 0-664),* 100 Witherspoon St., Louisville, KY 40202-1396 Toll Free: 800-227-2872
E-mail: rpinotti@presbypub.com.

Price Pottenger, *(Price Pottenger Foundation),* 2667 Camino del Rio, S., No. 109, San Diego, CA 92108-3767 (SAN 631-7030) Tel 619-574-7763; Toll Free: 800-366-3748.

Prima Pub, *(Prima Publishing; 0-7615; 0-914629; 1-55958; 1-4000),* Orders Addr.: P.O. Box 1260, Rocklin, CA 95677 Toll Free: 800-632-8676; Edit Addr.: 3000 Lava Ridge Ct., Roseville, CA 95661 (SAN 289-5609) Tel 916-787-7000; Fax: 916-787-7001
E-mail: sales@primapub.com
Web site: http://www.primapublishing.com.

Princeton U Pr, *(Princeton Univ. Pr.; 0-691),* Orders Addr.: California-Princeton Fulfillment Services, 1445 Lower Ferry Rd., Ewing, NJ 08618 Tel 800-777-4726; Fax: 800-999-1958; Edit Addr.: 41 William St., Princeton, NJ 08540 (SAN 202-0254) Tel 609-258-4900; Fax: 609-258-6305
E-mail: webmaster@pupress.princeton.edu
Web site: http://www.pup.princeton.edu.

Printed Matter, *(Printed Matter, Inc.; 0-89439),* 77 Wooster St., New York, NY 10012 (SAN 169-5924) Tel 212-925-0464
E-mail: dplatzker@printedmatter.org.

Prodn Assocs, *(Production Assocs.; 1-887120),* 1206 W. Collins Ave., Orange, CA 92867 Tel 714-771-6519; Fax: 714-771-2456; Toll Free: 800-535-8368.

Product Pr, *(Productivity Pr.; 0-527; 0-915299; 1-56327),* Orders Addr.: P.O. Box 13390, Portland, OR 97213-0390 (SAN 290-036X) Tel 503-235-0600; Fax: 503-235-0909; Toll Free Fax: 800-394-6286; Toll Free: 800-394-6868 (orders); Edit Addr.: 541 NE 20th Ave., Portland, OR 97232
E-mail: service@productivityinc.com
Web site: http://www.productivityinc.com.

Productivity Inc, *See* **Product Pr**

PRO-ED, *(PRO-ED, Inc.; 0-88744; 0-89079; 0-933014; 0-936104; 0-944480),* 8700 Shoal Creek Blvd., Austin, TX 78757-6897 (SAN 222-1349) Tel 512-451-3246; Fax: 512-451-8542; Toll Free Fax: 800-397-7633; Toll Free: 800-897-3202
E-mail: info@proedinc.com
Web site: http://www.proedinc.com.

Prof Bk Dist Inc, *See* **PBD Inc**

Prof Bks Inc, *(Professional Bks., Inc.),* 215 California St., Newton, MA 02158 (SAN 631-4252) Fax: 617-630-9396; Toll Free: 800-210-7323.

Prof Prnting & Pub, *(Professional Printing & Publishing; 0-929442; 1-877735),* Orders Addr.: P.O. Box 5758, Bossier City, LA 71171-5758 (SAN 248-2177) Tel 318-746-6880; Fax: 318-746-6995; Toll Free: 800-551-8783; Edit Addr.: 601 Barksdale Blvd., Bossier City, LA 71111 (SAN 249-3403)
E-mail: order@ppandp.com
Web site: http://www.pandp.com.

Program Concepts, *See* **PCI Educ Pubg**

Project Advent, *(Project Adventure, Inc.; 0-934387),* 701 Cabot St., Beverly, MA 01915 (SAN 693-8078) Tel 978-524-4500; Fax: 978-524-4501
E-mail: sdresser@pa.org
Web site: http://www.pa.org.

Prosperity & Profits, *(Prosperity & Profits Unlimited, Distribution Services),* P.O. Box 416, Denver, CO 80201-0416 (SAN 200-4682) Tel 303-575-5676; Fax: 970-292-2136
E-mail: mail@breadpudding.net; mail@contentprovidermedia.com.

PSI Ful, *(P S I Fulfillment),* 8803 Tara Ln., Austin, TX 78737 (SAN 631-3914) Tel 512-288-5005
E-mail: orders@psifulfillment.com
Web site: http://www.psifulfillment.com.

Psychol Corp, *(Psychological Corp., The; 0-928317),* Div. of Reed Elsevier PLc, 555 Academic Ct., San Antonio, TX 78204-2498 (SAN 207-1509) Tel 210-299-1061; Fax: 210-270-0327.

Pub Resources Inc, *(Publisher Resources, Inc.),* 1224 Heil Quaker Blvd., P.O. Box 7001, La Vergne, TN 37086-7001 (SAN 630-5431) Tel 615-793-5090; Toll Free Fax: 800-774-6733; Toll Free: 800-937-5557
Web site: http://www.bk.com.

Pub Serv Inc, *See* **PSI Ful**

Pub Wholesale Assocs, *(Publishers Wholesale Assocs., Inc.),* Orders Addr.: P.O. Box 2078, Lancaster, PA 17608-2078 (SAN 630-7450) Fax: 717-397-9253; Edit Addr.: 231 N. Shippen St., Lancaster, PA 17608.

Public Lands, *(Public Lands Interpretive Assn.; 1-879343),* 6501 Fourth St., NW, No. 1, Albuquerque, NM 87107-5800 (SAN 133-3119) Tel 505-345-9498; Fax: 505-344-1543.

Publicare Pr, *See* **Prof Prnting & Pub**

Publishers Group, *(Publishers Group West),* Subs. of Publishers Group Inc., 1700 Fourth St., Berkeley, CA 94710 (SAN 202-8522) Tel 510-528-1444; Fax: 510-528-3444; Toll Free: 800-788-3123; 800-788-3122 (electronic orders)
Web site: http://www.pgw.com.

Publishers Media, *(Publishers Media; 0-934064),* 1447 Valley View Rd., Glendale, CA 91202-1716 (SAN 159-6683) Tel 818-548-1998.

Pubns Unlimited, *(Publications Unlimited),* 7512 Coconut Dr., Lake Worth, FL 33467-6511 (SAN 285-9432) Tel 407-434-4688.

Pubs Assoc, *(Publishers Assocs.),* P.O. Box 140361, Irving, TX 75014-0361 (SAN 200-6979) Tel 972-681-9190; Fax: 972-686-5332
Web site: http://www.idekocese.com.

Pubs Business Service Inc, *(Publishers Business Service, Inc.),* P.O. Box 25674, Chicago, IL 60625 (SAN 285-9459) Tel 312-561-5552.

Pubs Clearing Hse, *(Publishers Clearing Hse.),* 382 Channel Dr., Port Washington, NY 11050 (SAN 285-9440) Tel 516-883-5432.

Pubs Continental Sales Corp, *(Publishers Continental Sales Corp.),* 2601 E. Michigan St., Michigan City, IN 46360 (SAN 285-9475).

Pubs Services, *(Publishers Services),* Orders Addr.: P.O. Box 2510, Novato, CA 94948 (SAN 201-3037) Tel 415-883-3530; Fax: 415-883-4280.

Pulley Learning Assoc, *(Pulley Learning Assocs.),* 210 Alpine Meadow Rd., Winchester, VA 22602-6701 (SAN 133-1434).

Purple Unicorn, *(Purple Unicorn Bks.; 0-931998),* 1928 W. Kent Rd., Duluth, MN 55812-1154 (SAN 111-0071) Tel 218-525-4781 Do not confuse with Purple Unicorn in Augusta, ME.

Putnam Pub Group, *(Putnam Publishing Group, The; 0-399; 0-698; 0-89828),* Div. of Penguin Putnam, Inc., Orders Addr.: 405 Murray Hill Pkwy., East Rutherford, NJ 07073-2136 Toll Free Fax: 800-227-9604; Toll Free: 800-788-6262 (individual consumer sales); 800-631-8571 (reseller customer service); 800-526-0275 (reseller sales); Edit Addr.: 375 Hudson St., New York, NY 10014 (SAN 202-5531) Tel 212-366-2000; Fax: 212-366-2643
E-mail: online@penguinputnam.com
Web site: http://www.penguinputnam.com.

Q W Inc, *(QW, Inc.; 1-928547),* P.O. Box 463180, Mount Clemens, MI 48046-3180 Tel 810-954-2986; Fax: 810-954-1085; Toll Free: 800-838-8854
E-mail: janinerange@ameritech.net
Web site: http://qwincorporated.com.

Qa Ent, *(Qa Enterprises),* Orders Addr.: P.O. Box 19425, Alexandra, VA 22320-0425 (SAN 631-1636) Tel 703-683-5877 (phone/fax).

Quality Bk Fairs, *(Quality Book Fairs),* 110 W. Liberty St., Medina, OH 44256 (SAN 630-7752) Tel 330-725-6977; Fax: 330-723-5325.

Quality Bks IL, *(Quality Bks., Inc.; 0-89196),* 1003 W. Pines Rd., Oregon, IL 61061-9680 (SAN 169-2127) Tel 815-732-4450; Fax: 815-732-4499; Toll Free: 800-323-4241 (libraries only)
E-mail: quality.books@dawson.com.

Quality Schl Plan Inc, *(Quality Schl. Plan, Inc.),* P.O. Box 10203, Des Moines, IA 50381-0001 (SAN 285-953X).

Quest MA, *(Quest, The; 1-888861),* 3 Danforth Dr., Northboro, MA 01532 (SAN 299-2884) Tel 508-393-7131; Fax: 419-828-2070; Toll Free: 800-777-9149 (orders)
E-mail: thequest@att.net.

Qui-Jote Bk Inc, *(El Qui-Jote Bk., Inc.),* 12651 Monarch, Houston, TX 77047 (SAN 107-8666) Tel 713-433-3388.

R & W Distribution Inc, *(R & W Distribution, Inc.),* 87 Bright St., Jersey City, NJ 07302 (SAN 169-4723) Tel 201-333-1540; Fax: 201-333-1541
E-mail: rwmag@mail.idt.net.

R Berrie, *(Berrie, Russ & Co., Inc.),* 111 Bauer Dr., Oakland, NJ 07436
Web site: http://www.thepregnancycalendar.com.

R Co Hinkel Inc, *(Hinkel, A. R. Co., Inc.),* 18121 Parthenia St., No. C, Northridge, CA 91325-3301 (SAN 200-934X) Tel 818-775-2942; Fax: 818-775-2941; Toll Free: 800-982-1600
E-mail: bschuler@arhinkel.com.

R G Landes, *See* **Landes Bioscience**

R H Donnelley Co, *(Donnely, R. H. Co.),* 70 Seaview Ave., P.O Box 10250, Stamford, CT 06904 (SAN 285-9297) Tel 203-353-7000.

R H Flem Mus, *(Fleming, Robert Hull Museum; 0-934658),* Univ. of Vermont, Colchester Ave., Burlington, VT 05405 (SAN 110-8824).

R H Pub, *(Renaissance Hse. Pubs.; 0-935810; 0-939650; 1-55838),* Div. of Primer Pubs., 5738 N. Central Ave., Phoenix, AZ 85012 (SAN 220-0864) Tel 602-234-1574; Fax: 602-234-3062; Toll Free: 800-521-9221 (orders)
E-mail: bfessler@earthlink.net.

R Hale & Co, *(Hale, Robert & Co., Inc.),* 1803 132nd Ave., NE, Suite 4, Bellevue, WA 98005 (SAN 200-6995) Tel 425-881-5212; Fax: 425-881-0731; Toll Free: 800-733-5330.

Radio Bkstore, *(Radio Bookstore),* P.O. Box 209, Rindge, NH 03461-0209 (SAN 111-3496) Tel 603-899-6957 Do not confuse with Radio Bookstore Pr., Bellevue, WA.

Rainier News Inc, *(Rainier News, Inc.),* 3400-D Industry Dr., E., Fife, WA 98424-1853 (SAN 169-8745) Toll Free: 800-843-2995 (in Washington).

Random, *(Random Hse., Inc.; 0-345; 0-375; 0-394; 0-553; 0-676; 0-679; 0-87665; 0-929661; 1-58836; 1-4000),* Div. of Bertelsmann AG, Orders Addr.: 400 Hahn Rd., Westminster, MD 21157 (SAN 202-5515) Tel 410-848-1900; Toll Free Fax: 800-659-2436; Toll Free: 800-726-0600 (customer service/orders); Edit Addr.: 1540 Broadway, New York, NY 10036 (SAN 202-5507) Tel 212-782-9000; Fax: 212-302-7985
E-mail: customerservice@randomhouse.com
Web site: http://www.randomhouse.com.

Rare Bk Co, *(Rare Bk. Co.; 0-911212),* P.O. Box 6957, Freehold, NJ 07728 (SAN 205-0978) Tel 732-364-8043; Toll Free: 888-222-4899
E-mail: RareBookCS@aol.com.

Rdrs Digest, *(Reader's Digest Children's Publishing, Inc.; 0-88705; 0-89577; 1-57584; 1-57619; 0-7944),* Subs. of Reader's Digest Assn., Inc., Reader's Digest Rd., Pleasantville, NY 10570-7000 (SAN 283-2143) Tel 914-244-4800; Fax: 914-244-4841
Web site: http://www.readersdigestkids.com.

Read News Agency, *(Read News Agency),* 2501 Greensboro Ave., Tuscaloosa, AL 35401-6520 (SAN 168-9266) Tel 205-752-3515.

Readex Bk Exchange, *(Readex Bk. Exchange),* Box 1125, Carefree, AZ 85377 (SAN 159-9291).

Reading Circle, *(Reading Circle, The),* 1456 N. High St., Columbus, OH 43201-0458 (SAN 169-670X) Tel 614-299-9673; Fax: 614-299-1388.

Reading Peddler Bk Fairs, *(Reading Peddler Bk. Fairs),* 10580 3/4 W. Pico Blvd., Los Angeles, CA 90064 (SAN 157-9770) Tel 310-559-2665.

Readmor, *(Readmor),* Orders Addr.: P.O. Box 7264, Grand Rapids, MI 49508 (SAN 169-3875); Edit Addr.: 301 S. Rath Ave., Ludington, MI 49431 Tel 231-843-2537.

Readmore Academic Services, *(Readmore Academic Services),* Orders Addr.: P.O. Box 1459, Blackwood, NJ 08012 (SAN 630-5741) Tel 609-227-1100; Fax: 609-227-8322; Toll Free: 800-645-6595; Edit Addr.: 700 Black Horse Pike, Suite 207, Blackwood, NJ 08012.

Readmore Inc, *(Readmore, Inc.),* 22 Cortlandt St., New York, NY 10007 (SAN 159-9313) Tel 212-349-5540; Fax: 212-233-0746; Toll Free: 800-221-3306.

Red Sea Pr, *(Red Sea Pr.; 0-932415; 1-56902),* 11 Princess Rd., Suites D, E & F, Lawrenceville, NJ 08648 (SAN 630-1983) Tel 609-844-9583; Fax: 609-844-0198
E-mail: africawpress@nyo.com
Web site: http://www.africanworld.com/.

Red Toad Rd, *(Red Toad Road Co.; 1-889287),* Orders Addr.: P.O. Box 642, Havre de Grace, MD 21078 Tel 410-939-4092; Fax: 410-939-5614; Edit Addr.: 223 Heather Way, Havre de Grace, MD 21078
E-mail: redtoadroad@aol.com
Web site: http://www.amazon.com/shops/redtoadroad.

Red Wheel ME, *(Red Wheel; 0-87728; 1-57863; 1-59003),* Div. of Weiser Bks., P.O. Box 612, York Beach, ME 03910-0612 (SAN 202-9588) Tel 207-363-4393; Fax: 207-363-5799; Toll Free: 800-423-7087 (orders only)
E-mail: customerservice@redwheelweiser.com
Web site: http://www.redwheelweiser.com; http://www.weiserbooks.com.

Redwing Bk Co, *(Redwing Bk. Co.),* 44 Linden St., Brookline, MA 02445 (SAN 163-3597) Tel 617-738-4664; Fax: 617-738-4620; Toll Free: 800-873-3946
E-mail: bob@redwingbooks.com
Web site: http://www.redwingbooks.com.

Reference Bk Ctr, *(Reference Bk. Ctr.),* 175 Fifth Ave., New York, NY 10010 (SAN 159-9356) Tel 212-677-2160; Fax: 212-533-0826.

Regent Bk Co Inc, *(Regent Bk. Co., Inc.),* Orders Addr.: P.O. Box 750, Lodi, NJ 07644-0750 Tel 973-574-7600; Fax: 973-574-7605; Toll Free: 800-999-9554; Edit Addr.: 25 Saddle River Rd., South Hackensack, NJ 07606 (SAN 169-4715)
E-mail: info@regentbook.com
Web site: http://www.regentbook.com.

Reginald F Fennell Subscription Service, *(Fennell, Reginald F. Subscription Service),* 1002 W. Michigan Ave., Jackson, MI 49202 (SAN 159-6071) Tel 517-782-3132; Fax: 517-782-1109.

Replica Bks, *(Replica Bks.; 0-7351),* Div. of Baker & Taylor, Orders Addr.: 1200 US Hwy., 22 E., Bridgewater, NJ 07060 Tel 908-541-7393; Fax: 908-541-7875; Toll Free: 800-775-1800; Edit Addr.: P.O. Box 6885, Bridgewater, NJ 08807-0885
E-mail: btinfo@baker-taylor.com; frosts@btol.com
Web site: http://www.replicabooks.com.

Res Inst Am, *(Research Institute of America; 0-7811),* Div. of International Thomson Organization, Inc., Orders Addr.: 117 E. Stevens Ave., Valhalla, NY 10595-1264 (SAN 665-7672) Tel 914-749-5000; Fax: 914-666-4452; Toll Free: 800-431-9025; Edit Addr.: 395 Hudson St., New York, NY 10014 Tel 212-367-6300.

Res Soft Intl, *(Resource Software International, Inc.; 0-87539),* Affil. of Datamatics Management, 330 New Brunswick Ave., Fords, NJ 08863 (SAN 264-8628) Tel 732-738-8500; Fax: 732-738-9603; Toll Free: 800-673-0366
E-mail: info@datamaticsinc.com
Web site: http://www.tc-1.com.

Rex Heck News Co, *(Heck, Rex News Co.),* 327 W. Main, Clarksburg, WV 26301 (SAN 156-4676) Tel 304-624-7993.

Rhinelander News Agency, *(Rhinelander News Agency),* 314 Courtney, Crescent Lake, WI 54501 (SAN 159-9372) Tel 715-362-6397.

Richardson s Bks Inc, *(Richardson's Bks., Inc.),* 2014 Lou Ellen Ln., Houston, TX 77018 (SAN 169-829X) Tel 713-688-2244; Fax: 713-688-8420; Toll Free: 800-392-8562.

RIE, *(RIE; 0-9649888),* 24505 Old Ferry Rd., Spicewood, TX 78669 Tel 512-264-9018; Fax: 512-264-1901; Toll Free: 800-410-5571.

Rio Grande Bk Co, *(Rio Grande Bk. Co.),* P.O. Box 2795, McAllen, TX 78502-2795 (SAN 169-8354).

Rishor News Co Inc, *(Rishor News Co., Inc.),* 109 Mountain Laurel Dr., Butler, PA 16001-3921 (SAN 159-9402).

Rittenhouse, *(Rittenhouse Bk. Distributors; 0-87381),* Orders Addr.: 511 Feheley Dr., King of Prussia, PA 19406 (SAN 213-4454) Tel 610-277-1414; Fax: 610-227-0390; Toll Free Fax: 800-223-7488; Toll Free: 800-345-6425
Web site: http://www.rittenhouse.com.

Ritter Bk Co, *(Ritter Bk. Co.),* 7011 Foster Pl., Downers Grove, IL 60516-3446 (SAN 169-1856).

River Road Recipes Cookbook, *(River Road Recipes Cookbook),* 9523 Fenway Dr., Baton Rouge, LA 70809 (SAN 132-7852) Tel 504-924-0300; Fax: 504-927-2547; Toll Free: 800-204-1726.

Rivers & Mnts, *(Rivers & Mountains),* 862 San Antonio Rd., Palo Alto, CA 94303 (SAN 631-1938) Tel 415-424-1213; Fax: 415-424-1402; Toll Free: 800-243-5522.

Riverside-World, *(Riverside World; 0-934298; 1-55518),* Orders Addr.: P.O. Box 370, Iowa Falls, IA 50126 (SAN 169-2666) Tel 641-648-4271; Toll Free: 800-922-9777 (Telemarketing); 636 S. Oak St., Iowa Falls, IA 50126 (SAN 631-2063) Toll Free Fax: 800-822-4271; Toll Free: 800-247-5111
E-mail: orders@riversideworld.com
Web site: http://www.riversideworld.com.

Roadrunner Library Service, *(Roadrunner Library Service),* c/o Kerbs, 700 Highview Ave., Glen Ellyn, IL 60137-5504 (SAN 160-2373).

Robert Henry Adams, *(Adams, Robert Henry Fine Art; 0-9713010),* 715 N. Franklin St., Chicago, IL 60610 (SAN 159-6918) Tel 312-642-8700; Fax: 312-642-8785
E-mail: info@adamsfineart.com
Web site: http://www.adamsfineart.com.

Rockbottom Bks, *(Rockbottom Bks.),* Pentagon Towers, P.O. Box 398166, Minneapolis, MN 55439 (SAN 108-4402) Tel 612-831-2120.

Rockland Catskill Inc, *(Rockland Catskill, Inc.),* 26 Church St., Spring Valley, NY 10977 (SAN 169-6254) Tel 914-356-1222; Fax: 914-356-8415; Toll Free: 800-966-6247.

Rocky Mount News Agency, *(Rocky Mount News Agency),* 2 Great State Ln., Rocky Mount, NC 27801 (SAN 169-6483).

Rogue Valley News Agency Inc, *(Rogue Valley News Agnecy, Inc.),* 550 Airport Rd., Medford, OR 97504-4156 (SAN 169-7137).

Roig Spanish Bks, *(Roig Spanish Bks.),* 146 W. 29th St., No. 3W, New York, NY 10001-5303 (SAN 165-1021) Tel 212-695-6410; Fax: 212-695-6811
E-mail: roig@interport.net.

Rom Dance Ntwrk, *(Rom Dance Network),* P.O. Box 3332, Madison, WI 53703 (SAN 630-3773) Tel 608-280-9730; Fax: 608-280-9736; Toll Free: 800-488-4940 (orders)
E-mail: unchartedcountry@taichihealth.com
Web site: http://www.romdance.com.

Roman Cath Bks, *(Roman Catholic Bks.; 0-912141; 1-929291),* Div. of Catholic Media Apostolate, Orders Addr.: P.O. Box 2286, Fort Collins, CO 80522 Tel 970-490-2735; Fax: 970-493-8781; Edit Addr.: P.O. Box 993, Ridgefield, CT 06877 (SAN 264-7877)
E-mail: bookpub@compuserve.com
Web site: http://www.booksforcatholics.com.

Rome News Co Inc, *(Rome News Co., Inc.),* 12 Redmond Ct., Rome, GA 30161 (SAN 169-1546).

Rosenblums, *(Rosenblum's),* 2906 W. Devon Ave., Chicago, IL 60659 (SAN 169-1864) Tel 773-262-1700; Fax: 773-262-1930; Toll Free: 800-626-6536.

Rosenblum's Hebrew Bkstr, *See* **Rosenblums**

Rounder Kids Mus Dist, *(Rounder Kids Music Distribution),* Orders Addr.: P.O. Box 516, Montpelier, VT 05602 (SAN 630-6675) Tel 802-223-5825; Fax: 802-223-5303; Toll Free: 800-223-6357; Edit Addr.: 79 River Rd., Montpelier, VT 05602
E-mail: Pauls@rounder.com.

Rowman, *(Rowman & Littlefield Pubs., Inc.; 0-8476; 0-87471; 0-7425),* Div. of University Press of America, P.O. Box 191, Blue Ridge Summit, PA 17214-0191 Tel 717-794-3800; Fax: 717-794-3801; Orders Addr.: 15200 NBN Way, Blue Ridge Summit, PA 17214 Toll Free Fax: 800-338-4550; Toll Free: 800-462-6420; 67 Mowat Ave., Suite 241, Toronto, ON M6K 3E3 Tel 416-534-1660; Fax: 416-534-3699; Edit Addr.: 4720 Boston Way, Lanham, MD 20706 (SAN 203-3704) Tel 301-459-3366; Fax: 301-459-2118
E-mail: Rogers@univpress.com
Web site: http://www.rowmanlittlefield.com.

Roy Derstine Bk Co, *(Derstine, Roy Bk. Co.),* 14 Birch Rd., Kinnelon, NJ 07405 (SAN 130-822X) Tel 973-838-1109.

Royal Pubns Inc, *(Royal Pubns., Inc.; 0-918738),* Orders Addr.: P.O. Box 5793, Denver, CO 80217 (SAN 244-7193) Tel 303-778-8383; Toll Free: 800-279-2048 (orders only); Edit Addr.: 790 W. Tennessee Ave., Denver, CO 80223.

Rsrch Bks CT, *(Research Bks., Inc.),* 38 Academy St., P.O. Box 1507, Madison, CT 06443 Tel 203-245-3279; Fax: 203-245-1830
E-mail: info@researchbooks.com.

RTR Publng, *See* **Red Toad Rd**

Rubin Periodical Group, *(Rubin Periodical Group),* P.O. Box 1211, Rochester, NY 14603-1211 (SAN 106-6226) Tel 518-272-8400.

Rushmore News Inc, *(Rushmore News, Inc.),* 924 East St. Andrew, Rapid City, SD 57701 (SAN 169-7846) Tel 605-342-2617; Fax: 605-342-9091; Toll Free: 800-423-0501
E-mail: afreese911@aol.com.

Russell News Agency Inc, *(Russell News Agency, Inc.),* P.O. Box 158, Sarasota, FL 33578 (SAN 169-1287).

Russica Bk & Art Shop, *(Russica Bk. & Art Shop, Inc.),* 799 Broadway, New York, NY 10003 (SAN 165-1072) Tel 212-473-7480; Fax: 212-473-7486.

Rutgers U Pr, *(Rutgers Univ. Pr.; 0-8135),* 100 Joyce Kilmer Ave., Piscataway, NJ 08854-8099 (SAN 253-2115) Tel 732-445-7762; Fax: 732-445-7039; Toll Free Fax: 888-471-9014; Toll Free: 800-446-9323 (orders)
Web site: http://rutgerspress.rutgers.edu.

Rutland News Co, *(Rutland News Co.),* 634 South Ave., Rochester, NY 14620-1316 (SAN 169-8591).

Rvrside Bk & Bible, *(Riverside Bk. & Bible Resource),* 1500 Riverside Dr., Iowa Falls, IA 50126 Tel 515-648-4801; Toll Free Fax: 800-822-4271; Toll Free: 800-247-5111.

Ryen R E Assoc, *(Ryen/RE Assocs.),* 20 W. Ridgewood Ave., Ridgewood, NJ 07450 (SAN 282-731X) Tel 201-652-9770; Fax: 201-658-9780
E-mail: rhook@bellatlantic.net.

S & L Sales Co, *(S&L Sales Co., Inc.),* Orders Addr.: P.O. Box 2067, Waycross, GA 31502 (SAN 107-413X) Tel 912-283-0210; Fax: 912-283-0261; Toll Free: 800-243-3699 (orders only).

S&S Childrens, *(Simon & Schuster Children's Publishing; 0-02; 0-671; 0-684; 0-689),* Div. of Simon & Schuster, Inc., Orders Addr.: 100 Front St., Riverside, NJ 08075; Edit Addr.: 1230 Avenue of the Americas, New York, NY 10020 (SAN 200-2442) Tel 212-698-7000; Fax: 212-698-7007; Toll Free Fax: 800-943-9831 (orders/fax); Toll Free: 800-223-2336 (customer service)
E-mail: ss_feedback@simonsays.com
Web site: http://www.oasis.simonandschuster.com; http://www.SimonSaysKids.com.

S & S News &, *(S & S News & Greeting),* 5304 15th Ave., S., Minneapolis, MN 55417-1812 (SAN 159-9453) Tel 612-224-8227; Toll Free: 800-346-9892.

S&S Trade, *(Simon & Schuster Trade; 0-671; 0-684; 0-689; 0-914676; 0-7432),* Div. of Simon & Schuster, Inc., Orders Addr.: 100 Front St., Riverside, NJ 08075 (SAN 200-2442) Toll Free Fax: 800-943-9831; Toll Free: 800-223-2348 (customer service); 800-223-2336 (ordering); Edit Addr.: 1230 Avenue of the Americas, New York, NY 10020 (SAN 200-2450) Tel 212-698-7000; Fax: 212-698-7007; Toll Free: 800-897-7650 (customer financial services)
E-mail: ssonline_feedback@simonsays.com; consumer.customerservice@simonandschuster.com
Web site: http://www.simonandschuster.com/ebooks; http://www.oasis.simonandschuster.com; http://www.simonsays.com.

S & S Worldwide, *(S & S Worldwide),* P.O. Box 513, Colchester, CT 06415 Tel 860-537-3451; Fax: 860-537-2866.

S & W Distributors Inc, *(S & W Distributors, Inc.),* 1600-H E. Wendover Ave., Greensboro, NC 27405.

S Asia, *(South Asia Bks.; 0-8364; 0-88386),* P.O. Box 502, Columbia, MO 65205 (SAN 207-4044) Tel 573-474-0116; Fax: 573-474-8124
E-mail: sabooks@juno.com
Web site: http://www.southasiabooks.com.

S Goldman Otzar Hasefarim Inc, *(Goldman, S. Otzar Hasefarim, Inc.),* 125 Ditmas Ave., New York, NY 11218 (SAN 169-5770).

S M P F Inc, *(Scientific & Medical Pubns. of France, Inc.),* 100 E. 42nd St., Suite 1002, New York, NY 10017 (SAN 169-5940) Tel 212-983-6278.

S V E Suzie, *(S.A.V.E. Suzie & Vic Enterprises),* 303 N. Main, P.O. Box 30, Schulenburg, TX 78956 (SAN 630-6365) Tel 409-743-4145; Fax: 409-743-4147.

SAAN Corp, *(SAAN Corp.),* 189-01 Springfield Ave., Suite 201, Flossmoor, IL 60422 (SAN 631-0419) Tel 708-799-5225; Fax: 708-799-8713.

Saddleback Pubns, *(Saddleback Publishing, Inc.; 1-56254),* 3 Watson, Irvine, CA 92618-2716 Tel 949-860-2500; Fax: 949-860-2508; Toll Free: 800-637-8715
E-mail: info@sdlback.com
Web site: http://www.sdlback.com.

Safari Museum Pr, *(Safari Museum Pr.),* 111 N. Lincoln Ave., Chanute, KS 66720 (SAN 110-8840) Tel 314-431-2730.

SAFE GOODS, *(SAFE GOODS/New Century Publishing 2000; 1-884820),* Orders Addr.: 60 Bullock Dr., Unit 6, Markham, ON L3P 3P2 Tel 860-824-5301; Fax: 860-824-0309; Toll Free: 888-628-8731; 561 Shunpike Rd., Sheffield, MA 01257
E-mail: info@SafeGoodsPub.com; safe@snet.net
Web site: http://www.safegoodspub.com.

Sage, *(Sage Pubns., Inc.; 0-7619; 0-8039),* 2455 Teller Rd., Thousand Oaks, CA 91320-2218 (SAN 204-7217) Tel 805-499-0721; Fax: 805-499-0871
E-mail: info@sagepub.com
Web site: http://www.sagepub.com.

Sagebrush Pr, *(Sagebrush Pr.; 0-930704),* P.O. Box 87, Morongo Valley, CA 92256 (SAN 113-387X) Tel 760-363-7398 Do not confuse with companies with same name in Cedarville, CA, Salt Lake City, UT.

Saks News Inc, *(Saks News, Inc.),* P.O. Box 1857, Bismarck, ND 58502 (SAN 169-653X).

Sams Tech Pub, *(Sams Technical Publishing; 0-7906),* Orders Addr.: P.O. Box 681008, Indianapolis, IN 46268 Toll Free Fax: 800-552-3910; Toll Free: 800-428-7267; Edit Addr.: 5436 W. 78th St., Indianapolis, IN 46268 Tel 317-334-1256
Web site: http://www.samswebsite.com.

San Diego Museum of Art, *(San Diego Museum of Art; 0-937108),* Balboa Park, P.O. Box 2107, San Diego, CA 92112-2107 (SAN 121-3679) Tel 619-696-19703.

San Franciscana, *(San Francisciana; 0-934715),* P.O. Box 590955, San Francisco, CA 94159 (SAN 161-1607) Tel 415-751-7222.

San Val Inc, *(San Val, Inc.),* 1230 Macklind Ave., Saint Louis, MO 63110-1432 (SAN 159-947X) Tel 314-644-6100; Fax: 314-647-0979; Toll Free: 800-458-8438
E-mail: sanval@misn.com
Web site: http://www.sanval.com.

Sandlapper Pub Co, *(Sandlapper Publishing Co., Inc.; 0-87844),* Orders Addr.: P.O. Box 730, Orangeburg, SC 29115 (SAN 203-2678) Toll Free Fax: 800-337-9420 (orders); Toll Free: 800-849-7263 (orders); Edit Addr.: 1281 Amelia St., NE., Orangeburg, SC 29116 Tel 803-533-1658; Fax: 803-534-5223.

Santa Barb Botanic, *(Santa Barbara Botanic Garden; 0-916436),* 1212 Mission Canyon Rd., Santa Barbara, CA 93105 (SAN 208-8398) Tel 805-682-4726; Fax: 805-563-0352.

Santa Barb News, *(Santa Barbara News Agency),* 725 S. Kellogg Ave., Goleta, CA 93117-3806 (SAN 168-9665) Tel 805-564-5200.

Santa Monica Software Inc, *(Santa Monica Software, Inc.),* 30018 Zenith Point Rd., Malibu, CA 90265-4264 (SAN 630-6764) Tel 310-457-8381; Fax: 310-395-7635.

Saphrograph, *(Saphrograph Corp.; 0-87557),* 4910-12 Fort Hamilton Pkwy., Brooklyn, NY 11219 (SAN 110-4128) Tel 718-331-1233; Fax: 718-372-8890.

Saranac Lake News Co, *(Saranac Lake News Co.),* P.O. Box 1211, Rochester, NY 14603-1211 (SAN 169-6238).

Sathya Sai Bk Ctr, *(Sathya Sai Bk. Ctr. of America; 1-57836),* 305 W. First St., Tustin, CA 92780 (SAN 111-3542) Tel 714-669-0522; Fax: 714-669-9138.

Saunders, *(Saunders, W. B. Co.; 0-03; 0-15; 0-7216),* Div. of Harcourt, Inc., A Harcourt Health Sciences Co., Orders Addr.: 6277 Sea Harbor Dr., Orlando, FL 32887 (SAN 244-8106) Toll Free: 800-654-2452; Edit Addr.: 150 S. Independence Mall W. The Public Ledger Bldg., Suite 1250, Philadelphia, PA 19106-3412 (SAN 203-266X) Tel 215-238-5500
Web site: http://www.wbsaunders.com.

SC Bkstore, *(South Carolina Bookstore),* Orders Addr.: P.O. Box 4767, West Columbia, SC 29171 (SAN 131-2294) Tel 803-796-8200; Fax: 803-794-6927; Toll Free: 800-845-8200; Edit Addr.: 523 Jasper St., West Columbia, SC 29169 (SAN 243-2390).

SCB Distributors, *(SCB Distributors),* 15608 S. New Century Dr., Gardena, CA 90248-2129 (SAN 630-4818) Tel 310-532-9400; Fax: 310-532-7001; Toll Free: 800-729-6423 (orders only)
E-mail: aaron@scbdistributors.com; info@scbdistributors.com
Web site: http://www.scbdistributors.com.

Sch Aid, *(School Aid Co.; 0-87385),* 911 Colfax Dr., P.O. Box 123, Danville, IL 61832 (SAN 158-3719) Tel 217-442-6855; Toll Free: 800-447-2665.

Schaefer Ed Found, *(Schaefer Education Foundation),* Orders Addr.: 4400 PGA Blvd., Suite 700, Palm Beach Gardens, FL 33410-6555 (SAN 631-7138) Tel 561-622-0912; Fax: 561-622-5090; Edit Addr.: P.O. Box 14448, North Palm Beach, FL 33408-0448.

Schaeffer News Agency, *(Schaeffer News Agency),* P.O. Box 1211, Rochester, NY 14603-1211 (SAN 169-5037).

Schiffer, *(Schiffer Publishing, Ltd.; 0-7643; 0-88740; 0-916838),* 4880 Lower Valley Rd., Atglen, PA 19310 (SAN 208-8428) Tel 610-593-1777; Fax: 610-593-2002
E-mail: schifferii@aol.com
Web site: http://www.schifferbooks.com.

Schl Aids, *(School Aids),* 9335 Interline Ave., Baton Rouge, LA 70809-1910 (SAN 169-2909) Tel 504-926-4498.

Schl Bk Service, *(School Bk. Service),* 3650 Coral Ridge Dr., Suite 112, Coral Springs, FL 33065-2559 (SAN 158-6963) Tel 954-341-7207; Fax: 954-341-7303; Toll Free: 800-228-7361
E-mail: compedge@ix.netcom.com.

Schl of Metaphysics, *(School of Metaphysics),* HCR1, Box 15, Windyville, MO 65783 (SAN 159-5423) Tel 417-345-8411; Fax: 417-345-6668
E-mail: som@som.org
Web site: http://www.som.org.

Schmul Pub Co, *(Schmul Publishing Co., Inc.; 0-88019),* Orders Addr.: P.O. Box 716, Salem, OH 44460-0716 (SAN 180-2771) Tel 330-222-2249; Fax: 330-222-0001; Toll Free: 800-772-6657; Edit Addr.: 3583 Newgarden Rd., Salem, OH 44460
E-mail: spchale@valunet.com
Web site: http://www.wesleyanbooks.com.

Schoenhof, *(Schoenhof's Foreign Bks., Inc.; 0-87774),* Subs. of Editions Gallimard, 486 Green St., Cambridge, MA 02139 (SAN 212-0062) Tel 617-547-8855; Fax: 617-547-8551
E-mail: info@schoenhofs.com
Web site: http://www.schoenhofs.com.

Scholars Bookshelf, *(Scholar's Bookshelf; 0-945726),* 110 Melrick Rd., Cranbury, NJ 08512 (SAN 110-8360) Tel 609-395-6933
E-mail: books@scholarsbookshelf.com
Web site: http://www.scholarsbookshelf.

Scholastic Inc, *(Scholastic, Inc.; 0-439; 0-590),* Subs. of SI Holdings, Inc., Orders Addr.: 2931 E. McCarty St., Jefferson City, MO 65101 Tel 573-636-5271; Toll Free Fax: 800-724-4716 (orders); Edit Addr.: 555 Broadway, New York, NY 10012-3999 (SAN 202-5442) Tel 212-343-6100; Fax: 212-343-6802; Toll Free: 800-325-6149 (customer service)
Web site: http://www.scholastic.com.

Scholium Intl, *(Scholium International, Inc.; 0-333; 0-87936),* P.O. Box 1519, Port Washington, NY 11050-0306 (SAN 169-5282) Tel 516-767-7171; Fax: 516-944-9824
E-mail: info@scholium.com
Web site: http://www.scholium.com.

Schroeders Bk Haven, *(Schroeder's Bk. Haven),* 104 Michigan Ave., League City, TX 77573 (SAN 122-7998) Tel 281-332-5226; Fax: 281-332-1695; Toll Free: 800-894-5032
E-mail: schroedr@interloc.com.

Schulze News Co, *(Schulze News Co.),* 2451 Eastman Ave., Suite 13, Oxnard, CA 93030-5193 (SAN 169-0434) Tel 805-642-9759.

Schuylkill News Service, *(Schuylkill News Service),* 1764 W. Market St., Pottsville, PA 17901 (SAN 159-9518) Tel 717-622-7510.

Schwartz Bros, *(Schwartz Brothers, Inc.),* 822 Montgomery Ave., No. 204, Narberth, PA 19072-1937 (SAN 285-7529) Fax: 301-459-6418; Toll Free: 800-638-0243.

Seaboard Sub Agency, *(Seaboard Sub Agency),* 44 S. Fulton St., Allentown, PA 18102 (SAN 285-9718) Tel 610-435-8174; Fax: 610-435-0290.

Selective, *(Selective Bks., Inc.; 0-912584),* P.O. Box 1140, Clearwater, FL 34617 (SAN 204-577X) Tel 813-447-0100.

Self esteem shop, *(Self esteem shop II; 0-9670949),* Div. of Self Esteem Shop, 32851 Woodward Ave., Royal Oak, MI 48073 Tel 248-554-9432; Fax: 248-549-0442
E-mail: info@selfesteemship.com
Web site: http://www.selfesteemshop.com.

Semler News Agency, *(Semler News Agency),* Orders Addr.: P.O. Box 350, New Castle, PA 16101 (SAN 169-7471); Edit Addr.: P.O. Box 526, Morgantown, WV 26505 (SAN 169-8990).

Seneca News Agency, *(Seneca News Agency),* Box 631, Geneva, NY 14456 (SAN 169-5304) Tel 315-789-3551; Fax: 315-781-1015.

Sentai Distributors, *(Sentai Distributors),* 8839 Shirley Ave., Northridge, CA 91324 (SAN 168-9959) Tel 818-886-3113; Fax: 818-886-0423
Web site: http://www.plasticmodels.com.

Sepher-Hermon, *(Sepher-Hermon Press; 0-87203),* 1153 45th St., Brooklyn, NY 11219 (SAN 169-5959) Tel 718-972-9010; Fax: 718-972-6935.

Serbin Communs, *(Serbin Communications, Inc.; 0-9628858; 1-888318),* 511 Olive St., Santa Barbara, CA 93101 Tel 805-963-0439; Fax: 805-965-0496; Toll Free: 800-876-6425.

Serendpty Couriers, *(Serendipity Couriers, Inc.),* 470 Du Bois St., San Rafael, CA 94901-3911 (SAN 169-0329) Tel 415-459-4000; Fax: 415-459-0833; Toll Free: 800-459-4005 (Bay area only)
E-mail: dipity@14.netcom.com.

Service News Co, *(Service News Co.),* 1306 N. 23rd St.,, Wilmington, NC 28406 (SAN 169-6491); P.O. Box 5027, Macon, GA 31208 (SAN 169-152X); Pope's Island, Box D-629, New Bedford, MA 02742 (SAN 169-3514).

Seven Hills Bk, *(7 Hills Bk. Distributors; 0-911403),* 1531 Tremont St., Cincinnati, OH 45214-1458 (SAN 169-6629) Tel 513-471-4300; Fax: 513-471-4311; Toll Free Fax: 888-777-7799; Toll Free: 800-545-2005
E-mail: customerservice@sevenhillsbooks.com
Web site: http://www.sevenhillsbooks.com.

Shambhala Pubns, *(Shambhala Pubns., Inc.; 0-87773; 1-56957; 1-57062; 1-59030),* Horticultural Hall, 300 Massachusetts Ave., Boston, MA 02115 (SAN 203-2481) Tel 617-424-0030; Fax: 617-236-1563
E-mail: editors@shambhala.com
Web site: http://www.shambhala.com.

Sharon News Agency Co, *(Sharon News Agency Co.),* 527 Silver St., Sharon, PA 16146 (SAN 169-7633).

Shea Bks, *(Shea Bks.),* 1563 Solano Ave., Suite 206, Berkeley, CA 94707 (SAN 159-9720) Tel 510-528-5201; Fax: 510-528-4987.

Shelter Pubns, *(Shelter Pubns., Inc.; 0-936070),* Orders Addr.: P.O. Box 279, Bolinas, CA 94924 (SAN 122-8463) Tel 415-868-0280; Fax: 415-868-9053; Toll Free: 800-307-0131; Edit Addr.: 285 Dogwood Rd, Bolinas, CA 94924
E-mail: shelter@shelterpub.com
Web site: http://www.shelterpub.com.

Shens Bks, *(Shen's Bks.; 1-885008),* 40951 Fremont Blvd., Fremont, CA 94538 (SAN 138-2926) Tel 510-668-1898; Fax: 510-668-1057; Toll Free: 800-456-6660
E-mail: info@shens.com
Web site: http://www.shens.com.

Sher Distributing Co, *(Sher Distributing Co.),* 8 Vreeland Ave., Totowa, NJ 07512 (SAN 169-4820) Tel 973-256-4050; Toll Free: 800-289-4050.

Sheridan, *(Sheridan Hse., Inc.; 0-911378; 0-924486; 1-57409),* 145 Palisade St., Dobbs Ferry, NY 10522 (SAN 204-5915) Tel 914-693-2410; Fax: 914-693-0776; Toll Free: 888-743-7425 (orders only) E-mail: Sheribks@aol.com Web site: http://www.sheridanhouse.com.

Shinders Bk Co, *(Shinder's Bk. Co.),* 733 Hennepin Ave., Minneapolis, MN 55403 (SAN 125-6157) Tel 612-333-3628.

Shoppers Guide Pr, *(Shoppers Guide Pr.),* 706 N. Fifth, Alpine, TX 79830 (SAN 159-9550) Tel 915-837-7426.

Sierra News Co, *(Sierra News Co.),* 2136 Pony Express Ct., Stockton, CA 95215-7946 (SAN 169-4472).

Silky Way Inc, *(Silky Way, Inc.),* 1227 38th Ave., San Francisco, CA 94122-1334 (SAN 169-3328).

Silver, *(Silver, Burdett & Ginn, Inc.; 0-382; 0-663),* Div. of Simon & Schuster, Inc., Orders Addr.: 4350 Equity Dr., P.O. Box 2649, Columbus, OH 43216 Fax: 614-771-5841; Toll Free: 800-848-9500; Edit Addr.: P.O. Box 480, Parsippany, NJ 07054 (SAN 204-5982); 108 Wilmot Rd., Suite 380, Midwest Div., Deerfield, IL 60015 (SAN 111-6517) Tel 708-945-1240; 1925 Century Blvd. NE, Suite 14, Southeast Div., Atlanta, GA 30345 (SAN 111-6509); 8445 Freeport Pkwy., Suite 400, South Div., Irving, TX 75063 (SAN 108-0458) Tel 214-915-4200; 2001 The Alameda, West Div., San Jose, CA 95126 (SAN 111-6525) Tel 408-248-6854; 160 Gould St., East Div., Needham Heights, MA 02194-2310 E-mail: customerservice@scottforesman.com Web site: http://www.scottforesman.com/.

Silver Bow News Distributing Co, *(Silver Bow News Distributing Co., Inc.),* 219 E. Park St., Butte, MT 59701 (SAN 169-4359) Tel 406-782-6995.

Singular Publishing, *(Singular Publishing Group, Inc.; 0-7693; 1-56593; 1-879105),* Div. of Delmar Publishers, 401 W. A St., Suite 325, San Diego, CA 92101-7904 (SAN 297-455X) Tel 619-238-6777; Fax: 619-238-6789; Toll Free: 800-521-8545 E-mail: singpub@mail.cerfnet.com Web site: http://www.singpub.com.

Skandisk, *(Skandisk, Inc.; 0-9615394; 1-57534),* 6667 W. Old Shakopee Rd., Suite 109, Bloomington, MN 55438-2622 (SAN 695-4405) Tel 952-829-8998; Fax: 952-829-8992; Toll Free: 800-468-2424 (orders) E-mail: lhamnes@tomten-skandisk.com; skandisk@tomten-skandisk.com Web site: http://www.tomten-skandisk.com.

Slavica, *(Slavica Pubs., Inc.; 0-89357),* c/o Indiana University, 2611 E. Tenth St., Bloomington, IN 47408-2618 (SAN 208-8576) Tel 812-856-4186; Fax: 812-856-4187 E-mail: slavica@indiana.edu Web site: http://www.slavica.com.

Sleuth Pubns Ltd, *(Sleuth Pubns., Ltd.; 0-915341),* 3398 Washington, San Francisco, CA 94118 (SAN 130-9374) Tel 415-771-2689.

Small Pr Dist, *See* **SPD-Small Pr Dist**

Smart Apple, *(Smart Apple Media; 1-58340; 1-887068),* Orders Addr.: P.O. Box 206, North Mankato, MN 56003 Tel 507-388-6273 (ext. 260); 507-388-2601; Fax: 507-388-2746; 507-386-0061; Toll Free: 800-445-6209; Edit Addr.: 1980 Lookout Dr., North Mankato, MN 56003 E-mail: CreativeCo@aol.com.

Smith News Agency, *(Smith News Agency),* 118 S. Mitchell St., Cadillac, MI 49601 (SAN 169-3727).

Smith Pubs, *See* **Smithmark**

Smithmark, *(Smithmark Pubs., Inc.; 0-7651; 0-8317),* Div. of US Media Holdings, 115 W. 18th St.. 5th Flr., New York, NY 10011-4113 (SAN 176-0912) Tel 212-519-1300; Fax: 212-519-1310; Toll Free: 800-932-0070 (customer service); Raritan Plaza 111, Fieldcrest Ave., Edison, NJ 08837 (SAN 658-1625) Tel 732-225-6499 (phone/fax); Toll Free Fax: 800-732-8688.

Snow Pocket Distrib, *(Snow Pocket Distributors),* Orders Addr.: c/o Sowbel, P.O. Box 64, West Topsham, VT 05086 Tel 802-439-6875 E-mail: sotops@sover.net Web site: http://www.dragonflies.com.

Snyder Magazine Agency, *(Snyder Magazine Agency),* 4817 W. 62nd Terr., Shawnee Mission, KS 66205-3083 (SAN 285-9750) Tel 913-722-6766.

So Wis News, *(Southern Wisconsin News),* 4838 N. County Rd. Y, Milton, WI 53563 (SAN 169-9121) Tel 608-756-2376; Fax: 608-756-2357.

Soc Auto Engineers, *(Society of Automotive Engineers, Inc.; 0-7680; 0-89883; 1-56091),* 400 Commonwealth Dr., Warrendale, PA 15096 (SAN 232-5721) Tel 724-776-4970; Fax: 724-776-0790 E-mail: sae@sae.org Web site: http://www.sae.org.

Soc for Visual, *See* **SVE & Churchill**

Soc Studies Schl, *(Social Studies Schl. Service; 1-56004),* 10200 Jefferson Blvd., P.O. Box 802, Culver City, CA 90232-0802 (SAN 168-9592) Tel 310-839-2436; Fax: 310-839-2249; Toll Free: 800-421-4246 E-mail: sssservice@aol.com Web site: http://socialstudies.com.

Soc Tchrs Fam Med, *(Society of Teachers of Family Medicine; 0-942295),* 11400 Tomahawk Creek Pkwy., Leawood, KS 66211 (SAN 224-3199) Tel 913-906-6000; Fax: 913-906-6096; Toll Free: 800-274-2237 E-mail: admstaff@stfm.org Web site: http://www.stfm.org.

Sopris, *(Sopris West; 0-944584; 1-57035),* 4093 Specialty Pl., Longmont, CO 80504 (SAN 243-945X) Tel 303-651-2829; Fax: 303-776-5934; Toll Free Fax: 888-819-7767 (orders only); Toll Free: 800-547-6747 (orders only) E-mail: webmaster@sopriswest.com Web site: http://www.sopriswest.com.

Sort Card Co, *(Sort Card Co., The),* 400 S. Summit View Dr., Fort Collins, CO 80524-1424 (SAN 159-9607).

Sounds of Zion, *(Sounds of Zion; 1-886472),* 6973 S. 300 W., Midvale, UT 84047-1050 (SAN 200-7525) Tel 801-255-1991; Fax: 801-255-1998.

Sounds True, *(Sounds True, Inc.; 1-56455),* Orders Addr.: P.O. Box 8010, Boulder, CO 80306-8010 Tel 303-665-3151 (ext. 155 for audios & videos); Fax: 303-665-5292; Toll Free: 800-333-9185; Edit Addr.: 413 S. Arthur Ave., Louisville, CO 80027 E-mail: SoundsTrue@aol.com Web site: http://www.soundstrue.com.

Source Bks CA, *(Source Bks.; 0-940147),* P.O. Box 794, Trabuco Canyon, CA 92678 (SAN 248-2231) Tel 949-858-1420 (phone/fax); Toll Free: 800-695-4237 Do not confuse with Source Bks., Nashville, TN E-mail: studio185@earthlink.net.

South Central Bks Inc, *(South Central Bks., Inc.),* 1106 S. Strong Blvd., McAlester, OK 74501-6952 (SAN 108-1144) Tel 405-275-4522; Toll Free: 800-548-9858.

South Eastern Bk Co Inc, *(South Eastern Bk. Co., Inc.),* 3333 Hwy. 641 N., P.O. Box 309, Murray, KY 42071 (SAN 630-4869) Tel 270-753-0732; Fax: 270-759-4742; Toll Free Fax: 800-433-6966 (orders); Toll Free: 800-626-3952 (orders) E-mail: orders@sebook.com Web site: http://www.sebook.com.

Southeast Library Bindery Inc, *(Southeast Library Bindery, Inc.),* P.O. Box 35484, Greensboro, NC 27425-5484 (SAN 159-9445) Tel 336-931-0800 E-mail: 70304.3023@compuserve.com Web site: http://www.webmasters.net/bookbinding/.

Southeast Periodical & Bk Sales, *(Southeast Periodical & Bk. Sales, Inc.),* 10100 NW 25th St., Box 520155-Biscayne Annex, Miami, FL 33152 (SAN 169-1163).

Southeastern Educational Toy & Bk, *(Southeastern Educational Toy & Bk. Distributors),* Orders Addr.: P.O. Box 15129, Charlotte, NC 28211 (SAN 630-8104) Tel 704-364-6988; Edit Addr.: 4217 Park Rd., Charlotte, NC 28209 Tel 704-527-1921; Fax: 704-527-1653.

Southeastern Library Service, *(Southeastern Library Service),* Subs. of Haskins Hse., Box 44, Gainesville, FL 32602-0044 (SAN 159-9615) Tel 352-372-3823.

Southern Bk Service, *(Southern Bk. Service; 0-9663836),* 5154 NW 165th St., Palmetto Lakes Industrial Pk., Hialeah, FL 33014-6335 (SAN 169-0981) Tel 305-624-4545; Fax: 305-621-0425; Toll Free: 800-766-3254 Web site: http://southernbooks.com.

Southern Library Bindery Co, *(Southern Library Bindery Co.),* 2952 Sidco Dr., Nashville, TN 37204 (SAN 169-7986).

Southern Michigan News Co, *(Southern Michigan News Co.),* 2571 Saradan, P.O. Box 908, Jackson, MI 49204 (SAN 169-3697) Tel 517-784-7163; Toll Free: 800-248-2213 (in Michigan); 800-828-2140.

Southern Periodicals Inc, *(Southern Periodicals, Inc.),* P.O. Box 407, Rayne, LA 70578-0407 (SAN 113-2520); 102 Industrial Dr., Rayne, LA 70578.

Southern Tier News Co, *(Southern Tier News Co.),* P.O. Box 2128, Elmira Heights, NY 14903 (SAN 169-5223).

Southrn Cross Pubs, *(Southern Cross Pubns.),* 1734 W. Roseberry Rd., P.O. Box 717, Donnelly, ID 83615 (SAN 110-8549) Tel 208-325-8606; Fax: 208-325-3400 E-mail: scp@cyberhighway.net Web site: http://www.thoughtlines.com/southerncross/.

Southwest Cookbk, *(Southwest Cookbook Distributors),* Orders Addr.: P.O. Box 707, Bonham, TX 75418 (SAN 200-4925) Tel 903-583-8898; Fax: 903-583-2522; Toll Free: 800-725-8898 (orders); Edit Addr.: 1430 Texas Ave., Bonham, TX 75418 (SAN 630-8325).

Southwest News Co, *(Southwest News Co.),* Box 5465, Tucson, AZ 85704 (SAN 159-9631).

Southwestern Bk Distributors, *(Southwestern Bk. Distributors),* c/o Kerbs, 700 Highview Ave., Glen Ellyn, IL 60137-5504 (SAN 160-2373).

Sovereign News Co, *See* **Trans Wrld News**

Spama, *(Spama, Inc.),* 78 Lake St., Jersey City, NJ 07306-3407 (SAN 169-5967).

Spanda Med Co, *(Spanda Medical Co.),* 823 North St., Pittsfield, MA 01201-1503 (SAN 631-4090) Tel 413-442-0123; Fax: 413-448-2122; Toll Free: 800-772-6320 E-mail: info@spanda.com Web site: http://spanda.com/books.

Spanish & European Bookstore, *(Spanish & European Bookstore, Inc.),* 3102 Wilshire Blvd., Los Angeles, CA 90010 (SAN 135-7654) Tel 213-739-8899; Fax: 213-739-0087.

Spanish Bookstore-Wholesale, *(Spanish Bookstore-Wholesale, The),* 10977 Santa Monica Blvd., Los Angeles, CA 90025-4538 (SAN 168-9835) Tel 310-475-0453; Fax: 310-473-6132 E-mail: BernardHamel@SpanishbooksUSA.com Web site: http://www.BernardHamel.com.

Spanish Hse Distributors, *(Spanish Hse. Distributors),* 1360 NW 88th Ave., Miami, FL 33172-3093 (SAN 169-1171) Tel 305-592-6136; Fax: 305-592-0087; Toll Free: 800-767-7726.

Spanish Periodical & Bk Sales, *(Spanish Periodical & Bk. Sales, Inc.),* 10100 NW 25th St., Miami, FL 33172 (SAN 200-7576).

Spanishtech Inc, *(Spanishtech, Inc.),* Div. of Editor's Bureau, Ltd., Box 68, Westport, CT 06881 (SAN 289-9620) Tel 203-452-7655.

SPD-Small Pr Dist, *(SPD-Small Pr. Distribution; 0-914068),* 1341 Seventh St., Berkeley, CA 94710-1409 (SAN 204-5826) Tel 510-524-1668; Fax: 510-524-0852; Toll Free: 800-869-7553 (orders) E-mail: orders@spdbooks.org Web site: http://www.spdbooks.org.

Specialized Bk Service Inc, *(Specialized Bk. Service, Inc.),* 307 Autumn Ridge Rd., Fairfield, CT 06432-1003 (SAN 166-9788) Tel 203-377-6510; Fax: 203-377-4792.

Specialty Bk Services, *(Specialty Bk. Services),* 1150 N. San Francisco, Flagstaff, AZ 86001 (SAN 130-8114) Tel 520-779-7843.

Specialty Promotions, *(Specialty Promotions),* 6841 S. Cregier Ave., Chicago, IL 60649 (SAN 110-9987) Tel 773-493-6900.

Speedimpex, *(Speedimpex U.S.A., Inc.),* 35-02 48th Ave., Long Island City, NY 11101-2421 (SAN 169-5479) Tel 718-392-7477; Fax: 718-361-0815 E-mail: nsalvatore@speedimpex.com Web site: http://www.speedimpex.com.

Spencer Muse Art, *(Spencer Museum of Art; 0-913689),* Affil. of Univ. of Kansas, Univ. of Kansas 1301 Mississippi St., Lawrence, KS 66045-7500 (SAN 111-347X) Tel 785-864-4710; Fax: 785-864-3112 E-mail: spencerart@ku.edu Web site: http://www.ukans.edu/~sma.

Spiritual Emerg Netwk, *(Spiritual Emergence Network),* 930 Mission St., No. 7, Santa Cruz, CA 95060 Tel 408-426-0902 E-mail: sen@cruzio.com Web site: http://elfi.com/sen.

Sportsman s Market Inc, *(Sportsman's Market, Inc.; 0-912796),* Clermont County Airport, Batavia, OH 45103 (SAN 205-0803) Tel 513-732-2411.

Spring Arbor Dist, *(Spring Arbor Distributors Inc.),* Subs. of Ingram Industries Inc., 4271 Edison Ave., Chino, CA 91710; 7315 Innovation Blvd., Fort Wayne, IN 46818-1371; 201 Ingram Dr., Roseburg, OR 97470-7148; Newbury Rd., East Windsor, CT 06088; 25420 Weakley Rd., Petersburg, VA 23803; 11333 E. 53rd Ave., Denver, CO 80239-2108; Edit Addr.: 1 Ingram Blvd., La Vergne, TN 37086-1976 Fax: 615-213-5192; Toll Free: 800-395-4340; 800-395-7234 (customer service) E-mail: orders@springarbor.com.

Springwater Bks, *(Springwater Bks.),* Orders Addr.: P.O. Box 194, Springwater, NY 14560-0194 (SAN 111-8900); Edit Addr.: Main St. & East Ave., Springwater, NY 14560-0194 (SAN 243-2412) Tel 716-669-2450.

Spr-Verlag, *(Springer-Verlag New York, Inc.; 0-387; 0-8176; 3-211; 3-540; 3-7908; 4-431; 1-85233),* Subs. of Springer-Verlag GmbH & Co. KG, Orders Addr.: P.O. Box 2485, Secaucus, NJ 07096-2485 (SAN 665-7842) Tel 201-348-4033; Fax: 201-348-4505; Toll Free: 800-777-4643; Edit Addr.: 175 Fifth Ave., New York, NY 10010 (SAN 203-2228) Tel 212-460-1500; Fax: 212-473-6272
E-mail: service@springer-ny.com; orders@springer.de
Web site: http://www.springer.de/; http://www.springer-ny.com.

SPS Studios, *See* **Blue Mount SPS Studios**

Square Deal Records, *(Square Deal Records),* 303 Higuera St., San Luis Obispo, CA 93401-4209 (SAN 170-6799) Tel 805-543-3636; Fax: 805-543-3938; Toll Free: 800-253-4114
E-mail: sdrsslo@aol.com.

SRA McGraw, *(SRA/McGraw-Hill; 0-02; 0-383),* Div. of The McGraw-Hill Cos., Orders Addr.: 220 E. Danieldale Rd., DeSoto, TX 75115-2490 Fax: 214-228-1982; Toll Free: 800-843-8855; Edit Addr.: 8787 Orion Pl., Columbus, OH 43240-4027 Tel 614-430-6600; Fax: 614-430-6621; Toll Free: 800-468-5850
E-mail: sra@mcgraw-hill.com
Web site: http://www.mcgraw-hill.com/education/sra.html.

St Lucie Pr, *(St. Lucie Pr.; 0-9634030; 1-57444; 1-878205; 1-884015),* Div. of CRC Pr., 2000 Corporate Blvd., NW, Boca Raton, FL 33431-7372 (SAN 297-9489) Tel 561-274-9906; Fax: 561-274-9927; Toll Free: 800-272-7737
E-mail: information@slpress.com
Web site: http://www.slpress.com.

St Maries Gopher News, *(St. Marie's Gopher News Co.),* 9000 Tenth Ave., N., Minneapolis, MN 55427 (SAN 169-4103) Tel 612-546-5300; Fax: 612-546-1487.

St Martin, *(St. Martin's Pr., LLC; 0-312; 0-8050; 0-940687; 0-9603648; 1-55927; 1-58063; 1-58238),* Div. of V H P S, Inc., Orders Addr.: c/o VHPS, 16365 James Madison Hwy., Gordonville, VA 22942 Tel 540-672-7600; Toll Free Fax: 800-672-2054; Toll Free: 888-330-8477; Edit Addr.: 175 Fifth Ave., New York, NY 10010 (SAN 200-2132) Tel 212-726-0200 (College Div.); 212-674-5151 (Trade Div.); Fax: 212-686-9491 (College Div.); 212-674-3179 (Trade Div.); Toll Free: 800-470-4767 (College Div.); 800-221-7945 (Trade Div.)
E-mail: webmaster@stmartins.com; enquiries@stmartins.com
Web site: http://www.smpcollege.com; http://www.stmartins.com.

St Mary Seminary Bookstore, *(St. Mary Seminary Bookstore),* 28700 Euclid Ave., Wyckliffe, OH 44092 (SAN 169-667X) Tel 216-943-7600.

St Mut, *(State Mutual Bk. & Periodical Service, Ltd.; 0-7855; 0-89771),* Orders Addr.: P.O. Box 1199, Bridgehampton, NY 11932-1199.

Stackpole, *(Stackpole Bks.; 0-8117; 1-881982),* 5067 Ritter Rd., Mechanicsburg, PA 17055 (SAN 202-5396) Tel 717-796-0411; Fax: 717-796-0412
E-mail: sales@stackpolebooks.com
Web site: http://www.stackpolebooks.com.

Stanley Lewis & Assoc, *(Lewis, Stanley & Assocs.),* 35 W. 92nd St., No. 2C, New York, NY 10025-7639 (SAN 135-020X) Tel 212-229-9747.

Star Brght Bks, *(Star Bright Bks.; 1-887734),* 325 W. 38th St., Suite 511, New York, NY 10018-2915 Tel 212-564-3981; Fax: 212-564-3984; Toll Free: 800-788-4439
E-mail: starbrightbk@earthlink.net
Web site: http://www.starbrightbooks.com.

Starkmann Inc, *(Starkmann Inc.),* 38 River St., Winchester, MA 01890 (SAN 126-6128) Tel 781-721-1537; Fax: 781-721-2825
E-mail: biggs@starkmann.co.uk.

Starmaster Co, *(Starmaster Co.),* 6911 Haverhill Dr., Knoxville, TN 37909 (SAN 108-1217) Tel 423-588-6661.

State News Agency, *(State News Agency),* 2750 Griffith Rd., Winston Salem, NC 27103-6418 (SAN 169-6424).

STCS Publisher Distrib, *(STCS Pub. Distribution Services),* 452 N. Main St., Woodstown, NJ 08098 (SAN 631-3639) Tel 609-769-8008; Fax: 609-769-5390; Toll Free: 800-266-5564
E-mail: stcsbooks@aol.com
Web site: http://www.stcsbooks.com.

Sterling, *(Sterling Publishing Co., Inc.; 0-8069; 1-4027),* 387 Park Ave., S., New York, NY 10016-8810 (SAN 211-6324) Tel 212-532-7160; Fax: 212-213-2495; Toll Free Fax: 800-775-8736 (warehouse) Do not confuse with companies with similar names in Falls Church, VA, Fallbrook, CA, Lewisville, TX
E-mail: custservice@sterlingpub.com
Web site: http://www.sterlingpub.com.

Sterling Rock Falls News Agency, *(Sterling Rock Falls News Agency),* 30 W. Third St., Sterling, IL 61081 (SAN 169-2232).

Stoelting Co, *(Stoelting Co.),* 620 Wheat Ln., Wood Dale, IL 60191 (SAN 275-8172) Tel 630-860-9700; Fax: 630-860-9775; Toll Free: 800-860-9775
E-mail: psychtests@stoeltingco.com
Web site: http://www.stoeltingco.com.

Strauss Cnslts, *(Strauss Consultants),* 48 W. 25th St., 11th Flr., New York, NY 10010-2708 Toll Free Fax: 888-528-8273; Toll Free: 800-236-7918
E-mail: strausscon@aol.com.

Stylus Pub VA, *(Stylus Publishing, LLC; 1-57922),* Orders Addr.: P.O. Box 605, Herndon, VA 20172-0605; Edit Addr.: 22883 Quicksilver Dr., Sterling, VA 20166-2012 (SAN 299-1853) Tel 703-661-1581; Fax: 703-661-1501 Do not confuse with companies with the same name in Sunnyvale, CA, Quakertown, PA
E-mail: stylusmail@presswarehouse.com
Web site: http://styluspub.com.

Subscription Acct, *(Subscription Acct.),* 84 Needham, Newton Highlands, MA 02161 (SAN 285-9424).

Subscription Hse Inc, *(Subscription Hse., Inc.),* 209 Harvard St., Suite 407, Brookline, MA 02146-5005 (SAN 285-9343).

Subterranean Co, *(Subterranean Co.),* Orders Addr.: P.O. Box 160, Monroe, OR 97456 Tel 541-847-5274; Fax: 541-847-6018
E-mail: subco@clipper.net.

Success Education Association, *(Success Education Assn.),* Box 175, Roanoke, VA 24002 (SAN 159-9690).

Sun Life, *(Sun Life; 0-937930),* 2399 Cool Springs Rd., Thaxton, VA 24174 (SAN 240-8333) Tel 540-586-4898.

Sun News Co, *(Sun News Co.),* 3600 75th Terr., N., Pinellas Park, FL 34665 (SAN 169-1260).

Sunbelt Pubns, *(Sunbelt Pubns., Inc.; 0-916251; 0-932653; 0-9606704; 0-9620402),* 1250 Fayette St., El Cajon, CA 92020-1511 (SAN 630-0790) Tel 619-258-4911; Fax: 619-258-4916; Toll Free: 800-626-6579
E-mail: sunbeltpub@prodigy.net
Web site: http://www.sunbeltpub.com.

Sunburst Comm, *(Sunburst Communications, Inc.; 0-7805; 0-911831; 1-55636; 1-55826),* 101 Castleton St., Pleasantville, NY 10570 (SAN 213-5620) Tel 914-747-3310; Toll Free: 800-431-1934
E-mail: webmaster@nysunburst.com
Web site: http://www.sunburst.com.

Sundance Pub, *(Sundance Publishing; 0-7608; 0-88741; 0-940146; 1-56801),* Orders Addr.: P.O. Box 1326, Littleton, MA 01460 (SAN 169-3484) Tel 508-486-9201; Fax: 508-486-1053; Toll Free: 800-343-8204 Do not confuse with Sundance Publishing, Inc., Patchogue, NY
E-mail: info@sundancepub.com
Web site: http://www.sundancepub.com/.

Sunflower U Pr, *(Sunflower Univ. Pr.; 0-89745),* Subs. of Journal of the West, Inc., 1531 Yuma, Box 1009, Manhattan, KS 66505-1009 (SAN 218-5075) Tel 785-539-1888; Fax: 785-539-2233; Toll Free: 800-258-1232 (orders)
Web site: http://www.sunflower-univ-press.org.

Sunset Books, *(Sunset Bks./Sunset Publishing Corp.; 0-376),* Div. of Time Warner Co., 80 Willow Rd., Menlo Park, CA 94025-3691 Tel 650-321-3600; Fax: 650-324-1532; Toll Free: 800-227-7346 (except California); 800-321-0372 (in California)
Web site: http://sunsetbooks.com.

Sunshine Harbor, *(Sunshine Harbor),* 825 Glen Arden Way, Altamonte Springs, FL 32701 (SAN 159-6640) Tel 407-339-0401.

Sunshine MA, *(Sunshine Bks., Inc.; 0-9624017; 1-890948),* 49 River St., Suite 3, Waltham, MA 02453-8345 (SAN 299-8718) Tel 781-398-0754; Fax: 781-398-0761; Toll Free: 800-472-5425
E-mail: info@clickertraining.com
Web site: http://www.clickertraining.com.

Sunshine WA, *See* **Sunshine MA**

SVE & Churchill, *(S V E & Churchill Media; 0-7932; 0-89290; 1-56357),* 6677 N. Northwest Hwy., Chicago, IL 60631-1304 (SAN 208-3930) Tel 773-775-9550; Fax: 773-775-5091; Toll Free Fax: 800-624-1678; Toll Free: 800-829-1900
E-mail: custserv@svemedia.com
Web site: http://www.svemedia.com.

SW NCH Assn, *See* **Public Lands**

Swedenborg, *(Swedenborg Foundation, Inc.; 0-87785),* 320 N. Church St., West Chester, PA 19380 (SAN 111-7920) Tel 610-430-3222; Fax: 610-430-7982; Toll Free: 800-355-3222 (customer service)
E-mail: info@swedenborg.com
Web site: http://www.Swedenborg.com.

Swift News Agency, *(Swift News Agency),* Orders Addr.: P.O. Box 160, Poncha Springs, CO 81242 (SAN 282-3810); Edit Addr.: 338 E. Hwy. 50, Poncha Springs, CO 81242 (SAN 169-0639).

Symmes Syst, *(Symmes Systems; 0-916352),* 3977 Briarcliff Rd., NE, Atlanta, GA 30345-2647 (SAN 169-1465) Tel 404-876-7260.

Syracuse U Pr, *(Syracuse Univ. Pr.; 0-8156),* 621 Skytop Rd., Suite 110, Syracuse, NY 13244-5290 (SAN 206-9776) Tel 315-443-2597; Fax: 315-443-5545
E-mail: supress@syr.edu
Web site: http://www.sumweb.syr.edu/su_press/.

T T Beeler, *(Beeler, Thomas T. Publisher; 1-57490),* 22 King St., Hampton Falls, NH 03844-2414 Tel 603-772-1175; Fax: 603-778-9025; Toll Free: 800-818-7574
E-mail: tbeeler@beelerpub.com
Web site: http://www.beelerpub.com.

TAB Bks, *(TAB Bks.),* Div. of The McGraw-Hill Cos., 11 W. 19th St., New York, NY 10011 (SAN 202-568X)
E-mail: bookstore@mcgraw-hill.com; customer.service@mcgraw-hill.com
Web site: http://www.mcgraw-hill.com/.

Tallahassee News Co Inc, *(Tallahassee News Co., Inc.),* 3777 Hartsfield Rd., Tallahassee, FL 32303-1120 (SAN 169-1309).

Tanager Pub Co, *(Tanager Publishing Co.; 0-9661202),* Orders Addr.: P.O. Box 59647, San Jose, CA 95159-9647 Tel 408-249-8793; Edit Addr.: 1048 S. Winchester Blvd., No. 15, San Jose, CA 95128.

Tapeworm, *(Tapeworm Video Distributor, Inc.),* 27833 Avenue Hopkins, Unit 6, Valencia, CA 91355-3407 (SAN 630-8767) Tel 805-257-4904; Fax: 805-257-4820; Toll Free: 800-367-8437
E-mail: sales@tapeworm.com
Web site: http://www.tapeworm.com.

Tatnuck BookSeller, *(Tatnuck BookSeller, The),* 335 Chandler St., Worcester, MA 01602-3402 (SAN 169-3654) Tel 508-756-7644.

Tattered Cover, *(Tattered Cover Bookstore),* 2955 E. First Ave., Denver, CO 80206 (SAN 631-0214) Fax: 303-399-2279; Toll Free: 800-833-9327 (ext. 250).

Taylor & Francis, *(Taylor & Francis, Inc.; 0-335; 0-8448; 0-85066; 0-89116; 0-903796; 0-905273; 1-56032; 1-85000),* Orders Addr.: 7625 Empire Dr., Florence, KY 41042 Toll Free Fax: 800-248-4724; Toll Free: 800-634-7064; Edit Addr.: 325 Chestnut St., Philadelphia, PA 19106 (SAN 241-9246) Tel 215-625-8900; Fax: 215-625-2940; 29 W. 35th St., New York, NY 10001 Tel 212-216-7800; Fax: 212-564-7854
E-mail: info@taylorandfrancis.com
Web site: http://www.taylorandfrancis.com.

TBN Ent, *(TBN Enterprises; 0-935554),* Orders Addr.: P.O. Box 55, Alexandria, VA 22313 (SAN 206-2380) Tel 703-684-6111; Fax: 703-683-5486; Edit Addr.: 3000 S. Eads St., Arlington, VA 22202 (SAN 663-656X).

Teach Servs, *See* **TEACH Servs**

Technical Bk Co, *(Technical Bk. Co.),* 2056 Westwood Blvd., Los Angeles, CA 90025 (SAN 168-9851) Fax: 310-470-9810; Toll Free: 800-233-5150.

Techno Mecca CA, *(Techno Mecca, Inc.),* 4412 W. Pico Blvd., 2nd Flr., Los Angeles, CA 90019 (SAN 631-7812) Tel 213-353-3900; Fax: 213-353-3910
E-mail: tjtj@tmecca.com
Web site: http://www.tmecca.com.

Temme Haus, *(Temme Haus Pr.),* P.O. Box 1547, Stockton, CA 95201 (SAN 253-1925) Tel 209-463-2782
Web site: http://www.atlasbooks.com/marktplc/00483.htm.

Temple News Agency, *See* **ETD KroMar Temple**

Tesla Bk Co, *(Tesla Bk. Co.; 0-914119; 0-9603536),* P.O. Box 121873, Chula Vista, CA 91912-6573 (SAN 241-8703) Tel 619-585-8487; Toll Free: 800-398-2056
E-mail: bfeuling@teslabook.com.

Tex A&M Univ Pr, *(Texas A&M Univ. Pr.; 0-89096; 1-58544),* 4354 TAMU John H. Lindsey Bldg., Lewis St., College Station, TX 77843-4354 (SAN 658-1919) Tel 979-845-1436; Fax: 979-847-8752; Toll Free Fax: 888-617-2421 (orders); Toll Free: 800-826-8911 (orders)
E-mail: wjl@tampress.tamu.edu
Web site: http://www.tamu.edu/upress/.

Texas Art Supply, *(Texas Art Supply),* 2001 Montrose Blvd., Houston, TX 77006 (SAN 169-8303) Tel 713-526-5221; Fax: 713-524-7474; Toll Free: 800-888-9278
E-mail: info@texasart.com
Web site: http://www.texasart.com.

Texas Bk, *(Texas Bk.),* 2601 King, Greenville, TX 75401 (SAN 103-4308) Tel 903-455-6937.

Texas Bookman, *(Texas Bookman, The; 1-931040),* 8650 Denton Dr., Dallas, TX 75235 (SAN 106-875X) Tel 214-350-6648; Fax: 214-352-0726; Toll Free: 800-566-2665
E-mail: texas.bookman@halfpricebooks.com.

Texas Hill Country Cookbook, *(Texas Hill Country Cookbook),* P.O. Box 126, Round Mountain, TX 78663 (SAN 110-831X) Tel 210-825-3242; Fax: 210-825-3244; Toll Free: 800-231-3553.

Texas Library Bk Sales, *(Texas Library Bk. Sales),* 1408 West Koenig Lane, Austin, TX 78756 (SAN 169-8044) Tel 512-452-4140.

Texoma Periodical, *(Texoma Periodical),* P.O. Box 1812, Sherman, TX 75090 (SAN 113-1699).

Thames Bk Co, *(Thames Bk. Co.),* 1 Quarry Rd., Mystic, CT 06355-3200 (SAN 169-0760).

Thames Hudson, *(Thames & Hudson; 0-500),* 500 Fifth Ave., New York, NY 10110 Tel 212-354-3763; Fax: 212-398-1252; Toll Free: 800-233-4830 (orders)
E-mail: info@thames.wwnorton.com
Web site: http://www.thamesandhudsonusa.com.

The Dream Zone, *(Dream Zone, The),* 4000 Newberry Rd., Gainesville, FL 32607 Tel 352-372-5777.

Thieme Med Pubs, *(Thieme Medical Pubs., Inc.; 0-86577; 0-913258; 1-58890),* Subs. of Georg Thieme Verlag Stuttgart, 333 Seventh Ave., 5th Flr., New York, NY 10001 (SAN 169-5983) Tel 212-760-0888; Fax: 212-947-1112; Toll Free: 800-782-3488 (orders only)
E-mail: Info@Thieme.com; custserv@thieme.de
Web site: http://www.thieme.com.

Thinkers Pr, *(Thinkers' Pr., Inc.; 0-938650; 1-888710),* Orders Addr.: P.O. Box 8, Davenport, IA 52805-0008 Tel 319-323-1226; Fax: 319-323-0511; Toll Free: 800-397-7117 (orders only); Edit Addr.: 1101 W. Fourth St., Davenport, IA 52802 (SAN 162-7759)
E-mail: tpi@chessco.com
Web site: http://www.chessco.com.

Thomas Bros Maps, *(Thomas Brothers Maps; 0-88130; 1-58174),* Div. of Rand McNally & Co., 17731 Cowan, Irvine, CA 92614 (SAN 158-8192) Fax: 949-757-1564; Toll Free: 800-899-6277
Web site: http://www.thomas.com.

Thomas More Association, *(More, Thomas Assn.),* 205 W. Monroe St., Sixth Flr., Chicago, IL 60606-5097 (SAN 169-1880) Tel 312-609-8880; Toll Free: 800-835-8965.

Thomas Slatner & Co Inc, *(Slatner, Thomas & Co., Inc.),* 1127 Kennedy Blvd., North Bergen, NJ 07047-1839 (SAN 130-9862) Tel 201-865-6662; Fax: 201-865-6966.

Thompson Schl Bk Depository, *(Thompson Schl. Bk. Depository),* Orders Addr.: P.O. Box 60160, Oklahoma City, OK 73146 (SAN 159-9747); Edit Addr.: 39 NE 24th St., Oklahoma City, OK 73143.

Thomson Learn, *(Thomson Learning),* 7625 Empire Dr., Florence, KY 41042 (SAN 631-2144) Tel 859-525-6620; Fax: 859-525-0978; Toll Free: 800-347-7707 (customer service); 800-842-3636 (orders)
Web site: http://www.thomsonlearning.com.

ThreeM Sptsmans Vid, *(3M Sportsman's Video Collection),* 3M Ctr., Bldg. 223-4NE-05, Saint Paul, MN 55144-1000 (SAN 159-8929) Tel 612-733-7412; Fax: 612-736-7479; Toll Free: 800-940-8273 (orders only).

Tiffin News Agency, *(Tiffin News Agency),* 1024 S. Bon Aire Ave., Tiffin, OH 44883-2553 (SAN 169-6866).

Tiger Bk Dist, *(Tiger Bk. Distributors, Ltd.),* 328 S. Jefferson, Chicago, IL 60661 (SAN 631-0672) Tel 312-382-1160; Fax: 312-382-0323.

Time Warner, *See* **AOL Time Warner**

Time-Life Publng, *(Time-Life Publishing Warehouse),* 5240 W. 76th, Indianapolis, IN 43268-4137 (SAN 631-1504) Fax: 717-348-6409; Toll Free: 800-277-8844
Web site: http://www.timelifecs.com; http://www.timelifeedu.com.

TIS Inc, *(TIS, Inc.; 0-89917; 1-56581; 0-7421),* Orders Addr.: P.O. Box 669, Bloomington, IN 47402 Tel 812-332-3307; Fax: 812-331-7690; Toll Free: 800-367-4002; Edit Addr.: 5005 N. State Rd. 37 Business, Bloomington, IN 47404.

Titan Bookstore, *(Titan Bookstore),* P.O. Box 34080, Fullerton, CA 92634-9480 (SAN 106-4851).

Title Books, *(Title Bks., Inc.),* 3013 Second Ave. S, Birmingham, AL 35233 (SAN 168-9207) Tel 205-324-2596.

Tobias News Co, *(Tobias News Co.),* 130 18th St., Rock Island, IL 61201 (SAN 169-2186) Tel 309-788-7517.

Todd Commns, *(Todd Communications; 1-57833; 1-878100),* 203 W. 15th Ave., Suite 102, Anchorage, AK 99501 (SAN 298-6280) Tel 907-274-8633; Fax: 907-276-6858
E-mail: info@toddcom.com.

Total Information Inc, *(Total Information, Inc.),* 844 Dewey Ave., Rochester, NY 14613 (SAN 123-7373) Tel 716-254-0621.

TPI PA, *(Trinity Pr. International; 0-334; 1-56338),* Orders Addr.: P.O. Box 1321, Harrisburg, PA 17105-1321 Tel 717-541-8130; Fax: 717-541-8128; Toll Free: 800-877-0012; Edit Addr.: 4775 Linglestown Rd., Harrisburg, PA 17112 (SAN 253-8156)
E-mail: trinity@morehousegroup.com
Web site: http://www.trinitypressintl.com.

Tracor Technology Resources TTR Specialized, *(Tracor Technology Resources (TTR), Specialized Bk. Distributors),* 1601 Research Blvd., Rockville, MD 20850 (SAN 169-3220) Tel 301-251-4970.

Trafalgar, *(Trafalgar Square; 0-943955; 1-57076),* Orders Addr.: P.O. Box 257, North Pomfret, VT 05053 (SAN 213-8859) Tel 802-457-1911; Fax: 802-457-1913; Toll Free: 800-423-4525; Edit Addr.: Howe Hill Rd., North Pomfret, VT 05053
E-mail: tsquare@sover.net
Web site: http://www.trafalgarsquarebooks.com.

Trans Wrld News, *(Trans World News),* 3700 Kelley Ave., Cleveland, OH 44114-4533 (SAN 169-6688) Tel 216-391-4800; Fax: 216-391-9911; Toll Free: 800-321-9858.

Transaction Pubs, *(Transaction Pubs.; 0-7658; 0-87855; 0-88738; 1-56000),* Orders Addr.: 390 Campus Dr., Somerset, NJ 08873 Fax: 732-748-9801; Toll Free: 888-999-6778; Edit Addr.: Rutgers-The State Univ. of NJ 35 Berrue Cir., Piscataway, NJ 08854-8042 (SAN 202-7941) Tel 732-445-2280; Fax: 732-445-3138; Toll Free: 888-999-6778
E-mail: trans@transactionpub.com
Web site: http://www.Transactionpub.com.

Transamerican & Export News Co, *(Transamerican & Export News Co.),* 591 Camino de la Reina St., Suite 200, San Diego, CA 92108-3192 (SAN 169-0140) Tel 619-297-8065; Fax: 619-297-5353.

Trans-Atl Phila, *(Trans-Atlantic Pubns., Inc.),* 311 Bainbridge St., Philadelphia, PA 19147 (SAN 694-0234) Tel 215-925-5083; Fax: 215-925-1912 Do not confuse with Transatlantic Arts, Inc., Albuquerque, NM
E-mail: order@transatlanticpub.com
Web site: http://www.transatlanticpub.com.

Traveler Restaurant, *(Traveler Restaurant),* 741 Buckley Hwy., Union, CT 06076 (SAN 111-8218) Tel 860-684-4920.

Treas Chest Bks, *(Treasure Chest Bks.; 0-918080; 1-887896; 0-9700750),* Orders Addr.: P.O. Box 5250, Tucson, AZ 85703-0250 (SAN 209-3251) Tel 520-623-9558; Fax: 520-624-5888; Toll Free Fax: 800-715-5888; Toll Free: 800-969-9558; Edit Addr.: 1802 West Grand Rd., Suite 101, Tucson, AZ 85745 (SAN 209-3243)
E-mail: info@rionuevo.com
Web site: http://www.rionuevo.com/.

Treasure Chest, *See* **Treas Chest Bks**

Treasure Valley News, *(Treasure Valley News),* 11677 President Dr., Boise, ID 83713-8972 (SAN 108-187X) Tel 208-323-8480.

Tree Frog Trucking Co, *(Tree Frog Trucking Co.),* 318 SW Taylor St., Portland, OR 97204 (SAN 169-7188) Tel 503-227-4760; Fax: 503-227-0829.

Tree Life NE, *(Tree of Life Northeast Distributors),* 2501 71st St., North Bergen, NJ 07047 (SAN 631-0982) Tel 201-662-7200.

Tree of Life Midwest, *(Tree of Life Midwest),* P.O. Box 2629, Bloomington, IN 47402-2629 (SAN 169-7994) Toll Free: 800-999-4200.

Tri County News, *(Tri County News Co., Inc.),* 202 W. Point Ave., P.O. Box 1, Dunkirk, NY 14048 (SAN 108-8106).

Triang News, *(Triangle News Co., Inc.),* 3498 Grand Ave., Pittsburgh, PA 15225 (SAN 169-7447).

Tri-County News Co Inc, *(Tri-County News Co., Inc.),* 1376 W. Main St., Santa Maria, CA 93458 (SAN 169-0345) Tel 805-925-6541; Fax: 805-925-3565
E-mail: trico2000@aol.com
Web site: http://tri-countynews.com.

Trinidad News Service, *(Trinidad News Service),* 216 W. Main, Trinidad, CO 81082 (SAN 169-0647).

Tri-State News Agency, *(Tri-State News Agency),* P.O. Box 778, Johnson City, TN 37601 (SAN 169-7897) Tel 423-926-8159; 604 Rolling Hills Dr., Johnson City, TN 37601 (SAN 282-4744).

Tri-State Periodicals Inc, *(Tri-State Periodicals, Inc.),* Orders Addr.: P.O. Box 1110, Evansville, IN 47706-1110 (SAN 169-233X) Tel 812-867-7416; Edit Addr.: 9844 Heddon Rd., Evansville, IN 47711 (SAN 241-7537) Tel 812-867-7419.

Troy News Co Inc Educational, *(Troy News Co., Inc., Educational Div.),* P.O. Box 1211, Rochester, NY 14603-1211 (SAN 169-6300).

TSBI, *(TSBI, Inc.; 0-9643020),* P.O. Box 9249, Detroit, MI 48209 Tel 313-843-1910; Fax: 313-843-1912; Toll Free: 800-927-1901
E-mail: savingbond@aol.com
Web site: http://www.bondinformer.com.

Tulare County News, *(Tulare County News),* Box 831, Visalia, CA 93279 (SAN 169-0442) Fax: 209-734-5732.

Turner Subscription Agency, *(Turner Subscription Agency),* Subs. of Dawson Holdings PLC, 1005 W Pines Rd., Oregon, IL 61061-9681 (SAN 107-7112) Tel 815-732-4476; Fax: 815-732-4489; Toll Free: 800-847-4201
E-mail: postmaster@dawson.com.

Tuttle Pubng, *(Tuttle Publishing; 0-8048; 4-900737),* Orders Addr.: 364 Innovation Dr., North Clarendon, VT 05759-9700 Tel 802-773-8930; Toll Free: 800-526-2778; Edit Addr.: 153 Milk St., 5th Flr., Boston, MA 02109 (SAN 213-2621) Tel 617-951-4080; Fax: 617-951-4045
E-mail: info@tuttlepublishing.com
Web site: http://www.tuttlemartialarts.com; http://www.tuttlepublishing.com.

Twen Fir Cent, *(21st Century Pubns.; 0-933278),* Orders Addr.: P.O. Box 702, Fairfield, IA 52556-0702 (SAN 170-3226) Tel 515-472-5105; Fax: 515-472-8443; Toll Free: 800-593-2665; Edit Addr.: 401 N. Fourth St., Fairfield, IA 52556 Do not confuse with Twenty First Century Pubns., Tolland, CT
E-mail: books21st@lisco.com
Web site: http://www.21stbooks.com.

Twenty-First Century Antiques, *(21st Century Antiques),* Orders Addr.: P.O. Box 70, Hatfield, MA 01038 (SAN 110-8085); Edit Addr.: 11 1/2 Main St., Hatfield, MA 01038 (SAN 243-248X) Tel 413-247-9396.

TWI, *(Time Warner Interactive; 1-57251),* Div. of Time Warner Trade Publishing, 2210 W. Olive Ave., Burbank, CA 91506 (SAN 298-3230).

Twin City News Agency Inc, *(Twin City News Agency, Inc.),* P.O. Box 466, Lafayette, IN 47902-0466 (SAN 169-2402) Tel 765-742-1051.

U Ch Pr, *(Univ. of Chicago Pr.; 0-226; 0-89065; 0-943056; 1-892850),* Div. of Univ. of Chicago, Orders Addr.: 11030 S. Langley Ave., Chicago, IL 60628 (SAN 202-5280) Tel 773-568-1550; Fax: 773-660-2235; Edit Addr.: 1427 E. 60th St., Chicago, IL 60637 (SAN 202-5299) Tel 773-702-7700; Fax: 773-702-9756
E-mail: general@press.uchicago.edu; kh@press.uchicago.edu
Web site: http://www.press.uchicago.edu.

U of A Crit Lang, *(Univ of Arizona Critical Languages Program),* 1230 N. Park Ave., Suite 102, Tuscon, AZ 85719.

U of Ariz Pr, *(Univ. of Arizona Pr.; 0-8165),* 355 S. Euclid Ave., Suite 103, Tucson, AZ 85719 (SAN 205-468X) Tel 520-621-1441; Fax: 520-621-8899
E-mail: orders@uapress.arizona.edu
Web site: http://www.uapress.arizona.edu.

U of Ill Pr, *(Univ. of Illinois Pr.; 0-252),* Orders Addr.: P.O. Box 4856, Baltimore, MD 21211; Edit Addr.: 1325 S. Oak St., Champaign, IL 61820 (SAN 202-5310) Tel 217-333-0950; Fax: 217-244-8082
E-mail: uipress@uiuc.edu
Web site: http://www.uiuc.edu/providers/uipress; http://www.press.uillinois.edu.

U of Mich Pr, *(Univ. of Michigan Pr.; 0-472),* Orders Addr.: P.O. Box 1104, Ann Arbor, MI 48106-1104 (SAN 282-4884) Tel 734-764-4388; Fax: 734-936-0456; Edit Addr.: 839 Greene St., Ann Arbor, MI 48106
E-mail: um.press@umich.edu
Web site: http://www.press.umich.edu/.

U of Nebr Pr, *(Univ. of Nebraska Pr.; 0-8032),* P.O. Box 880484, Lincoln, NE 68588-0484 (SAN 202-5337); 233 N. Eighth St., Lincoln, NE 68588-0255 Tel 402-472-3581
E-mail: pressmail@unl.edu
Web site: http://www.nebraskapress.unl.edu.

U of Nev Pr, *(Univ. of Nevada Pr.; 0-87417),* Mail Stop 166, Reno, NV 89557 (SAN 203-316X) Tel 775-784-6573; Fax: 775-784-6200; Toll Free: 877-682-6657 (orders only)
E-mail: ceh@unr.edu
Web site: www.nvbooks.nevada.edu.

U of NM Pr, *(Univ. of New Mexico Pr.; 0-8263),* 3721 Spirit Dr., SE, Albuquerque, NM 87106-5631 Tel 505-277-4810 (orders); Fax: 505-277-3350; Toll Free Fax: 800-622-8667; Toll Free: 800-249-7737 (orders only); Edit Addr.: 1720 Lomas Blvd., NE, Albuquerque, NM 87131-1591 (SAN 213-9588) Tel 505-277-2346; Fax: 505-277-9270
E-mail: unmpress@unm.edu
Web site: http://www.unmpress.com.

U of Okla Pr, *(Univ. of Oklahoma Pr.; 0-8061),* Orders Addr.: 4100 28th Ave., NW, Norman, OK 73069-8218 (SAN 203-3194) Tel 405-325-2000; Fax: 405-364-5798; Toll Free: 800-627-7377; Edit Addr.: 1005 Asp Ave., Norman, OK 73019-6051 Fax: 405-325-4000
Web site: http://www.ou.edu/oupress.

U of Toronto Pr, *(Univ. of Toronto Pr.; 0-7727; 0-8020),* 2250 Military Rd., Tonawanda, NY 14150 Toll Free Fax: 800-221-9985
E-mail: utpbooks@utpress.utoronto.ca
Web site: http://www.upress.utoronto.ca.

U of Wash Pr, *(Univ. of Washington Pr.; 0-295; 1-902716),* Orders Addr.: P.O. Box 50096, Seattle, WA 98145-5096 (SAN 212-2502); Edit Addr.: 1326 Fifth Ave., Suite 555, Seattle, WA 98101 Tel 206-543-8870; Fax: 206-685-3460; Toll Free Fax: 800-669-7993; Toll Free: 800-441-4115; 1126 N. 98th St., Seattle, WA 98103
E-mail: uwpord@u.washington.edu
Web site: http://www.washington.edu/uwpress.

U Pr of Amer, *(University Pr. of America; 0-7618; 0-8191; 1-879691),* Orders Addr.: 15200 NBN Way, P.O. Box 190, Blue Ridge Summit, PA 17214-0190 (SAN 253-2387) Toll Free Fax: 800-338-4550; Toll Free: 800-462-6420; Edit Addr.: 4720 Boston Way, Lanham, MD 20706 (SAN 200-2256) Tel 301-459-3366; Fax: 301-459-2118; Toll Free: 800-462-6420
Web site: http://www.univpress.com.

U Pr of New Eng, *(University Pr. of New England; 0-87451; 0-915032; 1-891507; 1-58465),* Orders Addr.: 23 S. Main St., Hanover, NH 03755-2048 (SAN 203-3283) Tel 603-643-7100; Fax: 603-643-1540; Toll Free: 800-421-1561 (orders only)
E-mail: University.Press@Dartmouth.edu
Web site: http://www.upne.com.

Ubiquity Distributors Inc, *(Ubiquity Distributors, Inc.),* 607 Degraw St., Brooklyn, NY 11217 (SAN 200-7428) Tel 718-875-5491; Fax: 718-875-8047.

UH Pr, *(Univ. of Hawaii Pr.; 0-8248; 0-87022),* Orders Addr.: 2840 Kolowalu St., Honolulu, HI 96822-1888 (SAN 202-5353) Tel 808-956-8255; Fax: 808-988-6052
E-mail: uhpmkt@hawaii.edu; uhpbooks@hawaii.edu
Web site: http://www.uhpress.hawaii.edu.

Ultra Bks, *(Ultra Bks.),* P.O. Box 945, Oakland, NJ 07436 (SAN 112-9074) Tel 201-337-8787.

UN, *(United Nations Pubns.; 0-680; 0-89714; 92-1; 92-808; 952-9520),* 2 United Nations Plaza, Sales Section, Publishing Div., Rm. DC2-853, New York, NY 10017 (SAN 206-6718) Tel 212-963-7680 UN Bookshop; 212-963-8302; Fax: 212-963-4910 UN Bookshop; 212-963-3489; Toll Free: 800-553-3210 UN Bookshop; 800-253-9646 (bookshop orders)
E-mail: publications@un.org
Web site: http://www.un.org/pubs.

Unarius Acad Sci, *(Unarius Academy of Science Pubns.; 0-932642; 0-935097),* 145 S. Magnolia Ave., El Cajon, CA 92020-4522 (SAN 168-9614) Tel 619-444-7062; Fax: 619-444-9637; Toll Free: 800-475-7062
E-mail: uriel@unarius.org
Web site: http://www.unarius.org.

Underground Railroad, *(Underground Railroad, The),* 2769 Club House Rd., Mobile, AL 36605-4373 (SAN 630-7892) Tel 334-432-8811.

UNIPUB, *See* **Bernan Associates**

Unique Bks Inc, *(Unique Bks., Inc.),* 5010 Kemper Ave., Saint Louis, MO 63139 (SAN 630-0472) Tel 314-776-6695; Fax: 314-776-0841; Toll Free: 800-533-5446.

United Mag, *(United Magazine),* Orders Addr.: P.O. Box 36, Columbia, KY 42728-0036 (SAN 169-2852) Tel 502-384-3444; Fax: 502-384-9324; Edit Addr.: 361 Industrial Park Rd., Louisville, KY 42728-0036 (SAN 250-3336).

United News Co Inc, *(United News Co., Inc.),* 111 Lake St., P.O. Box 3426, Bakersfield, CA 93305 (SAN 169-7579) Tel 805-323-7864.

United Soc Shakers, *(United Society of Shakers; 0-915836),* 707 Shaker Rd., New Gloucester, ME 04260 (SAN 158-619X) Tel 207-926-4597; Fax: 207-926-3559
E-mail: sdlshakers@aol.com
Web site: http://www.shaker.lib.me.us.

United Subscription Service, *(United Subscription Service),* 527 Third Ave., No. 284, New York, NY 10016-4100 (SAN 286-0104).

Univ Bk Service, *(University Bk. Service),* Orders Addr.: P.O. Box 608, Grove City, OH 43123 (SAN 169-6912); Edit Addr.: 2297 Southwest Blvd., Suite A, Grove City, OH 43123 (SAN 282-4841) Toll Free: 800-634-4272.

Univ Bkstore, *(University Bookstore),* Case Western Reserve Univ., 11111 Euclid Ave., Cleveland, OH 44106-7102 (SAN 100-4743) Tel 216-368-1656; Fax: 216-368-5205.

Univ Microfilms, *(University Microfilms, Inc.; 0-608; 0-7837; 0-8357),* Div. of Bell & Howell, Orders Addr.: P.O. Box 1307, Ann Arbor, MI 48106 (SAN 241-8797); Edit Addr.: 300 N. Zeeb Rd., Ann Arbor, MI 48106 (SAN 212-2464) Tel 313-761-4700; Fax: 313-665-5022; Toll Free: 800-521-0600; 800-343-5299 (in Canada)
Web site: http://www.umi.com.

Univ Pub Assocs, *(University Publishing Assocs., Inc.; 0-8026),* 4720 Boston Way, Lanham, MD 20706 (SAN 630-1878) Tel 301-459-3366.

Univ Sci Bks, *(University Science Bks.; 0-935702; 1-891389),* Orders Addr.: c/o Books International, 22841 Quicksilver Dr., Dulles, VA 20166 Tel 703-661-1572; Fax: 703-661-1501; Edit Addr.: 55D Gate Five Rd., Sausalito, CA 94965 (SAN 213-8085) Tel 415-332-5390; Fax: 415-332-5393; 648 Broadway, Suite 902, New York, NY 10012 Tel 212-253-1367; Fax: 212-253-1419
E-mail: univscibks@igc.org; bjellis@igc.org
Web site: http://www.uscibooks.com.

Univelt Inc, *(Univelt, Inc.; 0-87703; 0-912183),* Orders Addr.: P.O. Box 28130, San Diego, CA 92198-0130 (SAN 170-3099) Tel 760-746-4005; Fax: 760-746-3139; Edit Addr.: 740 Metcalf St., Suite 13, Escondido, CA 92025-1671 (SAN 658-2095)
E-mail: 76121.1532@compuserve.com
Web site: http://univelt.staigerland.com.

Universal Subscription Service, *(Universal Subscription Service),* P.O. Box 35445, Houston, TX 77035 (SAN 287-4768).

Urban Land, *(Urban Land Institute; 0-87420),* 1025 Thomas Jefferson St. NW, Suite 500 W., Washington, DC 20007-5201 (SAN 203-3399) Tel 202-624-7000; Fax: 202-624-7140; Toll Free: 800-321-5011
E-mail: bookstore@uli.org
Web site: http://www.ULI.ORG.

US Games Syst, *(U.S. Games Systems, Inc.; 0-88079; 0-913866; 1-57281),* 179 Ludlow St., Stamford, CT 06902 (SAN 158-6483) Tel 203-353-8400; Fax: 203-353-8431; Toll Free: 800-544-2637
E-mail: usgames@aol.com
Web site: http://www.usgamesinc.com.

USGPO, *(U.S. Government Printing Office; 0-16; 0-18),* Orders Addr.: P.O. Box 371954, Pittsburgh, PA 15250-7954 (SAN 658-0785) Tel 202-512-1800; Fax: 202-512-2250; Toll Free: 866-512-1800; Edit Addr.: USGPO Stop SSMB, Washington, DC 20401 (SAN 206-152X) Tel 202-512-1705 (bibliographic information only); 202-512-2268 (book dealers only); Fax: 202-512-1655
E-mail: rdavis@gpo.gov; orders@gpo.gov
Web site: http://bookstore.gpo.gov; http://www.access.gpo.gov/su_docs.

Val Publishing, *(Val Publishing),* 16 S. Terrace Ave., Mount Vernon, NY 10551 (SAN 107-6876) Tel 914-664-7077.

Valiant, *(Valiant International Multi-Media Corp.),* 55 Ruta Ct., South Hackensack, NJ 07606 (SAN 652-8813) Tel 201-229-9800; Fax: 201-814-0418.

Valley Distributors Inc, *(Valley Distributors, Inc.),* 2947 Felton Rd., Norristown, PA 19401 (SAN 169-7498) Tel 610-279-7650; Fax: 610-279-9093; Toll Free: 800-355-2665 (orders only).

Valley News Service, *See* **Anderson Stephen**

Van Dyke News Agency, *(Van Dyke News Agency),* 2238 W. Pinedale Ave., Fresno, CA 93711-0453 (SAN 168-9630) Tel 209-291-7768; Fax: 209-291-7770.

Van Khoa Bks, *(Van Khoa Bks.),* 9200 Bolsa Ave., Suite 123, Westminster, CA 92683 (SAN 110-7534) Tel 714-892-0801
E-mail: vankhoa@vinet.com.

Vegas News Agency, *(Las Vegas News Agency),* 3933 Ali Baba Ln., Las Vegas, NV 89118 (SAN 110-4063) Tel 702-795-4600.

Verham News Corp, *(Verham News Corp.),* 75 Main St., West Lebanon, NH 03784 (SAN 169-4561) Fax: 603-298-8843.

VHPS, *(VHPS Holtzbrinck Pubs.; 0-374),* Orders Addr.: 16365 James Madison Hwy., Gordonsville, VA 22942 (SAN 631-5011) Tel 540-672-7600; Fax: 540-672-7540 (Customer Service); 800-672-2054 (Order Dept.); 540-672-7664; Toll Free: 888-330-8477; Edit Addr.: 175 Fifth Ave., New York, NY 10010 Tel 212-674-5151; Fax: 212-677-6487; Toll Free: 800-488-5233.

Victor Kamkin, *(Kamkin, Victor),* 4956 Boiling Brook Pkwy., Rockville, MD 20852 Tel 301-881-5973; Fax: 301-881-1637; Toll Free: 800-852-6546; 925 Broadway, New York, NY 10010 (SAN 113-7395) Tel 212-673-0776; Fax: 212-673-2473.

Video Distributors Inc, *(Video Distributors, Inc.),* Dixie Village Shopping Ctr., Gastonia, NC 28052 (SAN 630-7604) Tel 704-868-8670; Fax: 704-868-2519; Toll Free: 800-445-5142.

Village Mktg, *(Village Marketing),* 145 N. 400 W., Richfield, UT 84701 (SAN 631-6751). Tel 800-982-6683

Vinabind, *(Vinabind),* Box 340, Steelville, MO 65565 (SAN 159-9828).

Vincennes News Agency, *(Vincennes News Agency),* P.O. Box 1110, Evansville, IN 47706-1110 (SAN 169-2518).

Virginia Periodical Distributors, *See* **Aramark Mag & Bk Servs**

Vision Dists, *(Vision Distributors; 0-9626732),* Div. of Infinite Creations, Inc., Orders Addr.: P.O. Box 9839, Santa Fe, NM 87504 Tel 505-986-8221.

Vision Pr NM, *See* **Vision Dists**

Vistabooks, *(Vistabooks; 0-89646),* 0637 Blue Ridge Rd., Silverthorne, CO 80498-8931 (SAN 211-0849) Tel 970-468-7673 (phone/fax)
E-mail: vistabooks@compuserve.com
Web site: http://www.vistabooks.com.

Vitality Distributors, *(Vitality Distributors),* 940 NW 51st Pl., Fort Lauderdale, FL 33309 (SAN 169-0973) Toll Free: 800-226-8482.

Volcano Pr, *(Volcano Pr., Inc.; 0-912078; 1-884244),* Orders Addr.: P.O. Box 270, Volcano, CA 95689 (SAN 220-0015) Tel 209-296-4991; Fax: 209-296-4995; Toll Free: 800-879-9636; Edit Addr.: 21496 National St., Volcano, CA 95689
E-mail: info@volcanopress.com
Web site: http://www.volcanopress.com.

Voyageur Pr, *(Voyageur Pr., Inc.; 0-89658),* Orders Addr.: P.O. Box 338, Stillwater, MN 55082 Toll Free: 800-888-9653; Edit Addr.: 123 N. Second St., Stillwater, MN 55082 (SAN 287-2668) Tel 651-430-2210; Fax: 651-430-2211
E-mail: books@voyageurpress.com
Web site: http://www.voyageurpress.com.

W Bk Service, *(WA Bk. Service),* 26 Ranick Rd., Hauppauge, NY 11788 (SAN 107-2943) Tel 516-234-2255; Fax: 516-234-2268.

W E Falk, *(Falk, W. E.),* Orders Addr.: P.O. Box 693710, Miami, FL 33179 (SAN 169-118X) Tel 305-653-0088; Fax: 305-651-4097.

W Pubng Grp, *(W Publishing Group; 0-8499; 0-87680),* Div. of Thomas Nelson, Inc., P.O. Box 141000, Nashville, TN 37214-1000 (SAN 203-283X) Tel 615-902-3400; Fax: 615-902-3200 Do not confuse with Word Publishing Co. in Greenville, MS
Web site: http://www.wordpublishing.com; http://www.thomasnelson.com.

W R Watson & Staff, *(Watson, W. R. & Staff),* 150 Mariner Green Ct., Corte Madera, CA 94925 (SAN 286-0155) Tel 510-524-6156; Fax: 510-526-5023.

W W Gaunt, *See* **Gaunt**

W W Wickel Co Inc, *(Wickel, W. W. Co., Inc.),* 8970 Hanslik Ct., Naperville, IL 60564-5629 (SAN 135-1230) Tel 708-820-0044.

Wabash Valley News Agency, *(Wabash Valley News Agency),* 2200 N. Curry Pike, No. 2, Bloomington, IN 47404-1486 (SAN 169-250X).

Waldenbooks Co Inc, *(Waldenbooks Co., Inc.; 0-681),* Div. of Borders Group, Inc., 100 Phoenix Dr., Ann Arbor, MI 48108-2202 (SAN 200-8858).

Walker Art Ctr, *(Walker Art Ctr.; 0-935640),* Orders Addr.: Vineland Pl., Minneapolis, MN 55403 (SAN 206-1880) Tel 612-375-7638; Fax: 612-375-7565
E-mail: topher.elliott@walkerart.org.

Walkers Ent, *(Walker's Enterprises),* P.O. Box 871570, New Orleans, LA 70187.

Wallace s College Bk Co, *(Wallace's College Bk. Co.),* 928 Nandino Blvd., P.O. Box 11518, Lexington, KY 40576-1518 (SAN 169-2844) Tel 606-255-0886; Fax: 606-259-9892; Toll Free Fax: 800-433-9329 (orders only); Toll Free: 800-354-9590 (orders only); 800-354-9500
E-mail: orders@wallaces.com.

Walter J Johnson, *(Johnson, Walter J. Inc.; 0-8472),* 1 New York Plaza 28th Flr., New York, NY 10004-1901 (SAN 209-1828).

Warner Bks, *(Warner Bks., Inc.; 0-445; 0-446),* Div. of Time Warner Trade Publishing, Orders Addr.: c/o Little Brown & Co., 3 Center Plaza, Boston, MA 02108-2084 Fax: 800-286-9471; Toll Free: 800-759-0190; Edit Addr.: 1271 Avenue of the Americas, New York, NY 10020 (SAN 281-8892) Tel 212-522-7200
Web site: http://www.warnerbooks.com.

Warner Pr, *(Warner Pr. Pubs.; 0-87162),* Orders Addr.: P.O. Box 2499, Anderson, IN 46018-2499 (SAN 691-4241); Edit Addr.: 1200 E. Fifth St., Anderson, IN 46012 (SAN 111-8110) Tel 765-644-7721; Fax: 765-622-9511; Toll Free: 800-741-7721 (orders only)
E-mail: akelly@warnerpress.org
Web site: http://www.warnerpress.org.

Warner Publishing Services, *(Warner Publishing Services),* 1271 Avenue of the Americas, New York, NY 10020 (SAN 200-5522) Tel 212-522-8900.

Wash Bk Distrib, *(Washington Bk. Distributors),* 4930A Eisenhower Ave., Alexandria, VA 22304 (SAN 631-0095) Tel 703-212-9113; Fax: 703-212-9114; Toll Free: 800-699-9113
E-mail: washbook@juno.com
Web site: http://www.washbook.com.

Washington Toy Co, *(Washington Toy Co.),* 220 Ninth St., San Francisco, CA 94103 (SAN 107-1718) Tel 415-863-5965.

Waverly News Co, *(Waverly News Co.),* 17 State St., Newburyport, MA 01950 (SAN 169-3522).

Waymont Bk Co, *(Waymont Bk. Co.),* 136 Steuben St., Jersey City, NJ 07302 (SAN 630-768X) Tel 201-434-4268; Fax: 201-432-1293
E-mail: waymont@worldnet.att.net.

Weatherhill, *(Weatherhill, Inc.; 0-8348),* 41 Monroe Tpke., Trumbull, CT 06611-1315 (SAN 202-9529) Tel 203-459-5090; Fax: 203-459-5095; Toll Free: 800-437-7840
E-mail: weatherhill@weatherhill.com
Web site: http://www.weatherhill.com.

Weiner News Co, *(Weiner News Co.),* 1011 N. Frio, P.O. Box 7608, San Antonio, TX 78207 (SAN 169-8427) Tel 210-226-9333; Fax: 210-226-8679.

Weiser, *See* **Red Wheel ME**

Weiser Bks, *(Weiser Bks.; 0-87728; 1-57863),* P.O. Box 612, York Beach, ME 03910-0612 (SAN 202-9588) Tel 207-363-4393; Fax: 207-363-5799; Toll Free: 800-423-7087
E-mail: customerservice@redwheelweiser.com
Web site: http://www.weiserbooks.com.

Wells, *(Wells, Philip V.),* Haworth Hall, Univ. of Kansas, Lawrence, KS 66045 Tel 785-864-4619.

WellSpring MA, *(WellSpring Bks.),* P.O. Box 2765, Woburn, MA 01888-1465 (SAN 111-3399) Do not confuse with companies with the same or similar names in Albuquerque, NM, Ukiah, CA, Adelphia, NJ, Woburn, MA, Groton, VT.

Wenatchee News Agency, *(Wenatchee News Agency),* 434 Rock Island Rd., East Wenatchee, WA 98802-5360 (SAN 169-8885) Tel 509-662-3511.

West Texas News Co, *(West Texas News Co.),* Orders Addr.: 1214 Barranca, El Paso, TX 79935; Edit Addr.: P.O. Box 26488, El Paso, TX 79926 (SAN 169-8184) Tel 915-594-7586; Fax: 915-594-7589.

West Virginia Periodical Distributors, *See* **Anderson-Stephan**

Western Booksource Inc, *(Western Booksource, Inc.),* 4935 Metart Shwayn, Tillamook, OR 97141 (SAN 158-4332) Toll Free: 800-825-0100; 230 Fifth Ave., No. 1104, New York, NY 10001 Tel 212-889-9339; Fax: 212-889-9572.

Western Library Bks, *(Western Library Bks.),* 560 S. San Vicente Blvd., Los Angeles, CA 90048 (SAN 168-9878) Tel 213-653-8880.

Western Merchandisers, *(Western Merchandisers),* 2900 Airport Rd., Denton, TX 76207-2102 (SAN 156-4633).

Western Michigan, *See* **Readmor**

Western Res, *(Western Reserve Historical Society; 0-911704),* 10825 East Blvd., Cleveland, OH 44106 (SAN 110-8387) Tel 216-721-5722; Fax: 216-721-0645.

Weston Woods, *(Weston Woods Studios, Inc.; 0-7882; 0-89719; 1-55592; 1-56008),* Div. of Scholastic, Inc,, 12 Oakwood Ave., Norwalk, CT 06850 (SAN 630-3838) Tel 203-226-3355; Fax: 203-845-0498; Toll Free: 800-290-7531; 800-243-5020 (customer service)
E-mail: Leighcorra@aol.com
Web site: http://www.scholastic.com.

Westwater, *(Westwater Bks.; 0-916370),* Div. of Belknap Photographic Services, Inc., P.O. Box 2560, Evergreen, CO 80437 (SAN 208-3698) Tel 303-674-5410; Fax: 303-670-0586; Toll Free: 800-628-1326.

Wheeler Pub, *(Wheeler Publishing, Inc.; 1-56895; 1-58724),* Orders Addr.: P.O. Box 531, Accord, MA 02018-0531 (SAN 253-228X); Edit Addr.: 405 VFW Dr., Rockland, MA 02370-1160 Tel 781-871-9170; Fax: 781-871-9173; Toll Free: 800-588-8881 (orders)
E-mail: custsvc@wheelerpub.com.

Whitaker Dists, *See* **Anchor Distributors**

Whitehurst & Clark, *(Whitehurst & Clark),* 100 Newfield Ave., Edison, NJ 08837 (SAN 630-8716) Tel 732-225-2727; 732-417-9575; Fax: 732-225-1562; 732-417-1562; Toll Free: 800-488-8040.

Whiting News Co, *(Whiting News Co.),* 1417 119th St., Whiting, IN 46394 (SAN 169-2542).

Whitlock & Co, *(Whitlock & Co.),* 10001 Roosevelt Rd., Westchester, IL 60153 (SAN 285-9645).

Wholesale Distributors, *(Wholesale Distributors),* P.O. Box 126, Burlington, IA 52601 (SAN 145-8051) Tel 319-753-1683; Fax: 319-753-5988; Toll Free: 800-272-1556.

Wiener Pubs Inc, *(Wiener, Markus Pubs., Inc.; 0-910129; 1-55876),* Orders Addr.: P.O. Box 2240, Williston, VT 05495 Fax: 802-864-7626 (orders); Toll Free: 800-515-2475 (orders); Edit Addr.: 231 Nassau St., Princeton, NJ 08542 (SAN 282-5465) Tel 609-921-1141; Fax: 609-921-1140
E-mail: mwp.cs@aidcvt.com; wiener95@aol.com
Web site: http://www.markuswiener.com.

Wieser Educational, *(Wieser Educational, Inc.),* 30085 Comercio, Santa Margarita, CA 92688 (SAN 630-7361) Tel 714-858-4920; Fax: 714-858-0209; Toll Free: 800-880-4433
E-mail: info@wieser-ed.com
Web site: http://www.wieser-ed.com.

Wilbert Williams, *(Wilbert/Williams),* Orders Addr.: P.O. Box 2572, Kingshill, VI 008511 Tel 340-778-8081.

Wilcor International Bk Dept, *(Wilcor International Bk. Dept.),* 700 Broad St., Utica, NY 13501-1336 (SAN 107-7023) Tel 315-733-3542.

Wilcox & Follet Co, *See* **Follett Educ Srvs**

Wiley, *(Wiley, John & Sons, Inc.; 0-471; 0-8260; 0-937721; 0-939246; 1-56561; 1-57313; 3-527),* Orders Addr.: 1 Wiley Dr., Somerset, NJ 08875-1272 Tel 732-469-4400; Fax: 732-302-2300; Toll Free: 800-225-5945 (orders); Edit Addr.: 605 Third Ave., 4th Flr., New York, NY 10158-0012 (SAN 200-2272) Tel 212-850-6276 (Retail and Wholesale); 212-850-6000; Fax: 212-850-8641 (Retail and Wholesale) ; 212-850-6088
E-mail: bookinfo@wiley.com; compbks@wiley.com
Web site: http://www.wiley.com; http://www.wiley.com/compbooks/; http://www.interscience.wiley.com.

Wilfrid Laurier, *(Wilfrid Laurier Univ. Pr.; 0-88920),* Box 277, 4408 Milestrip Rd., Blasdell, NY 14219-2599 Tel 519-884-0710; Fax: 519-725-1399
E-mail: press@wlu.ca
Web site: http://www.wlu.ca/~wwwpress/home.html.

Wilshire, *(Wilshire Bk. Co.; 0-87980),* 12015 Sherman Rd., North Hollywood, CA 91605-3781 (SAN 168-9932) Tel 818-765-8579; Fax: 818-765-2922
E-mail: mpowers@mpowers.com
Web site: http://www.mpowers.com.

Wilson & Sons, *(Wilson & Sons),* P.O. Box 996, Bellevue, WA 98009 (SAN 129-0010) Tel 425-392-1965
E-mail: dchief@seanst.com.

Windham County News Co, *(Windham County News Co.),* P.O. Box 8127, Brattleboro, VT 05304 (SAN 159-9917) Tel 802-254-2373.

Wine Appreciation, *(Wine Appreciation Guild, Ltd.; 0-932664; 1-891267),* 360 Swift Ave., South San Francisco, CA 94080-6220 (SAN 169-0264) Tel 650-866-3020; Fax: 650-866-3513; Toll Free: 800-242-9462 (orders only)
E-mail: wineappreciation.com
Web site: http://www.wineappreciation.com.

Winebaum News Inc, *(Winebaum News, Inc.),* P.O. Box 1620, Raymond, NH 03077-3620 (SAN 169-4529).

Winters IN, *(Winters Publishing; 0-9625329; 1-883651),* Orders Addr.: P.O. Box 501, Greensburg, IN 47240 (SAN 298-1645) Tel 812-663-4948 (phone/fax); Toll Free: 800-457-3230; Edit Addr.: 705 E. Washington, Greensburg, IN 47240 Do not confuse with Winters Publishing, Wichita, KS.

Wittenborn Art, *(Wittenborn Art Bks.; 0-8150; 0-89648),* Orders Addr.: P.O. Box 2210, San Francisco, CA 94126 Toll Free: 800-660-6403; Edit Addr.: 1109 Geary Blvd., San Francisco, CA 94109 Tel 415-292-6500; Fax: 415-292-6594
E-mail: wittenborn@earthlink.net
Web site: http://www.art-books.com.

Wizard Works, *(Wizard Works; 0-9621543; 1-890692),* Orders Addr.: P.O. Box 1125, Homer, AK 99603-1125 Tel 907-235-8757 (phone/fax); Toll Free: 877-210-2665
E-mail: Wizard@xyz.net
Web site: http://www.xyz.net/~wizard.

Wolfe News Service Inc, *(Wolfe News Service, Inc.),* P.O. Box 5481, Syracuse, NY 13200-5481 (SAN 169-6319).

Wolper Sales Agency Inc, *(Wolper Sales Agency, Inc.),* 6 Centre Sq., Suite 302A, Easton, PA 18042-3606 (SAN 285-9785) Tel 610-559-9550; Fax: 610-559-9898.

Wolverine Distrib, *(Wolverine Distributing, Inc.; 0-941875),* P.O. Box 24, Basin, WY 82410-0024 (SAN 666-1211) Tel 307-568-2434; Fax: 307-568-3306; Toll Free: 800-967-1633
E-mail: wolverine@tctwest.net.

Wolverine Gallery, *See* **Wolverine Distrib**

Women Ink, *(Women Ink),* 777 United Nations Plaza, New York, NY 10017 (SAN 630-8309) Tel 212-687-8633; Fax: 212-661-2704
E-mail: wink@womenink.org
Web site: http://www.womenink.org.

Woodbine Pub, *(Woodbine Publishing Co., The),* 15621 Chemical Ln., No. B, Huntington Beach, CA 92649 (SAN 114-4243) Tel 714-894-9080; Fax: 714-894-4949; Toll Free: 800-451-4788
Web site: http://www.safaripress.com.

Woodcrafters Lumber Sales Inc, *(Woodcrafters Lumber Sales, Inc.),* 212 NE Sixth Ave., Portland, OR 97232 (SAN 112-6075) Tel 503-231-0226; Toll Free: 800-777-3709.

Word for Today, *(Word for Today, The; 0-936728; 1-931713),* Orders Addr.: P.O. Box 8000, Costa Mesa, CA 92628 (SAN 110-8379) Toll Free: 800-272-9673; Edit Addr.: 3232 W. MacArthur Blvd., Santa Ana, CA 92704 (SAN 214-2260) Tel 714-825-9673 Toll Free: 800-272-9637
E-mail: info@twft.com
Web site: http://www.twft.com.

Word of Life Distributors, *(Word of Life Distributors),* 2717 W. Olympic Blvd., Suite 103, Los Angeles, CA 90006 (SAN 108-433X) Tel 213-382-4538; Fax: 213-382-1154; Toll Free: 800-347-7057.

Word Pub, *See* **W Pubng Grp**

Words Distrib, *(Words Distributing Co.; 0-914728),* Div. of Bookpeople, 7900 Edgewater Dr., Oakland, CA 94621 (SAN 154-7763) Tel 510-632-4700; Fax: 510-632-1281; Toll Free: 800-999-4650; 800-593-9673 (orders).

Workman Pub, *(Workman Publishing Co., Inc.; 0-7611; 0-89480; 0-911104; 1-56305),* 708 Broadway, New York, NY 10003 (SAN 203-2821) Tel 212-254-5900; Fax: 212-254-8098; Toll Free: 800-722-7202
E-mail: mged@workman.com
Web site: http://www.workmanweb.com; http://www.workman.com.

World Bank, *(World Bank, The, Office of the Publisher; 0-8213),* Orders Addr.: P.O. Box 960, Herndon, VA 20172-0960; Edit Addr.: 1818 H St., NW, Rm. U11-063, Washington, DC 20433 (SAN 219-0648) Tel 703-661-1580; 202-473-1153 (Review or Desk Copies); Fax: 703-661-1501; Toll Free: 800-645-7247
E-mail: books@worldbank.org
Web site: http://www.worldbank.org/publications.

World Pubns, *(World Pubns., Inc.; 0-7669; 0-9640034; 1-57215; 0-7429),* Orders Addr.: P.O. Box 622, North Dighton, MA 02764; Edit Addr.: 455 Somerset Ave., Bldg. 2A, North Dighton, MA 02764 (SAN 631-7014) Tel 508-880-5555; Fax: 508-880-0469 Do not confuse with World Publications, Inc., Winter Park, FL
E-mail: sales@wrldpub.com
Web site: http://www.worldpub.com.

World Readers Service Inc, *(World Readers Service, Inc.),* 248 Sisson Ave., Hartford, CT 06153 (SAN 285-9653).

World Scientific Pub, *(World Scientific Publishing Co., Inc.; 981-02),* 1060 Main St., River Edge, NJ 07661 (SAN 241-9920) Tel 201-487-9655; Fax: 201-487-9656; Toll Free: 800-227-7562
Web site: http://www.worldscientific.com/index.cgi.

World Univ AZ, *(World Univ.; 0-941902),* P.O. Box 2470, Benson, AZ 85602 (SAN 239-7943) Tel 520-586-2985; Fax: 520-586-4764
E-mail: desertsanctuary@theriver.com
Web site: http://worlduniversity.org.

World Wide Pubs, *(World Wide Pubns.; 0-89066),* 1303 Hennepin Ave., Minneapolis, MN 55403-1780 (SAN 159-9941) Tel 612-338-0500; Fax: 612-338-3029; Toll Free: 800-788-0442.

WorldPoint, *(WorldPoint/EEC),* 151 S. Psingsten Rd., Suite E, Deerfield, IL 60015 Toll Free Fax: 888-281-2627; Toll Free: 888-322-8350.

Wright Bk Educational, *(Wright Bk./Educational),* 2195 Owendale Dr., Dayton, OH 45439 (SAN 159-9968).

Writers & Bks, *(Writers & Bks.; 0-9618487),* 740 University Ave., Rochester, NY 14607 (SAN 156-9678) Tel 716-473-2590.

Wrld Wisdom, *(World Wisdom, Inc.; 0-941532),* P.O. Box 2682, Bloomington, IN 47402-2682 (SAN 239-1406) Tel 812-332-1663; Fax: 812-332-1983
E-mail: mknason@worldwisdom.com
Web site: http://www.worldwisdom.com.

Wrld Wisdom Bks, *See* **Wrld Wisdom**

Wrldwide Media Srv, *(Worldwide Media Service, Inc.),* Affil. of Hudson County News Agency, 30 Montgomery St., Jersey City, NJ 07302-3821 (SAN 630-4826) Tel 201-332-7100; Fax: 201-332-0265; Toll Free: 800-345-6478
Web site: http://www.americanmagazine.com.

Wstrn Intl, *(Western International, Inc.; 0-9665194),* 1875 Oddie Blvd., Sparks, NV 89431-3559 (SAN 631-1695) Tel 775-359-4400; Fax: 775-359-4431; Toll Free: 800-634-6737.

Wyoming Periodical Distributor, *(Wyoming Periodical Distributor),* P.O. Box 2340, Casper, WY 82601 (SAN 169-9245).

X-S Bks Inc, *(X-S Bks., Inc.),* 81 Brookside Ave., Amsterdam, NY 12010-0740 (SAN 169-4634).

Yankee Bk Peddler Inc, *(Yankee Bk. Peddler, Inc.),* 999 Maple St., Contoocook, NH 03229 (SAN 169-4510) Tel 603-746-3102; Fax: 603-746-5628; Toll Free: 800-258-3774
E-mail: ybp@office.ybp.com
Web site: http://www.ybp.com.

Yankee News Co, *(Yankee News Co.),* P.O. Box 145, Hartford, CT 06141-0145 (SAN 169-0876).

Yankee Paperback & Textbook Co, *(Yankee Paperback & Textbook Co.),* P.O. Box 18880, Tucson, AZ 85731 (SAN 112-1073) Tel 520-325-7229 (phone/fax); Toll Free: 800-340-2665 (in Arizona, California, Nevada, Colorado, New Mexico and Utah only).

Yankee Ped Bkshop, *(Yankee Peddler Bookshop; 0-918426),* 2006 Ridge Rd., Ontario, NY 14519 (SAN 209-925X) Tel 315-524-4352; Fax: 315-524-3365.

Ye Olde Genealogie Shoppe, *(Ye Olde Genealogie Shoppe; 0-932924; 1-878311),* Orders Addr.: P.O. Box 39128, Indianapolis, IN 46239 (SAN 200-7010) Tel 317-862-3330; Toll Free: 800-419-0200 (orders); Edit Addr.: 9605 Vandergriff Rd., Indianapolis, IN 46239.

Young News Inc, *(Young News, Inc.),* 1600 E. Grand Blvd., Detroit, MI 48211-3144 (SAN 169-3999) Fax: 517-753-7774.

Zeitlin Periodicals Co Inc, *(Zeitlin Periodicals Co., Inc.),* 7917 Lark Meadow Ave., Las Vegas, NV 89131-4710 (SAN 160-8088).

Zondervan, *(Zondervan Publishing Hse.; 0-310; 0-937336),* Div. of HarperCollins Pubs., c/o Zondervan, Order Processing-B36, 5300 Patterson Ave., SE, Grand Rapids, MI 49530 (SAN 203-2694) Tel 616-698-6900; Fax: 616-698-3439; Toll Free Fax: 800-934-6381 (fax orders); Toll Free: 800-727-1309 (orders & customer service)
E-mail: zprod@zph.com
Web site: http://www.zondervan.com.

Zook News Agency, *(Zook News Agency),* 550 S. G St., No. 14, Arcata, CA 95521-6683 (SAN 168-9622).

Zubal Inc, *(Zubal, John T. Inc.; 0-939738),* 2969 W. 25th St., Cleveland, OH 44113 (SAN 165-5841) Tel 216-241-7640; Fax: 216-241-6966
Web site: http://www.zuba.com.

SERIALS

Subject Index

A

ABSTRACTING AND INDEXING SERVICES

see also BIBLIOGRAPHIES; and also Abstracting, Bibliographies, Statistics subheadings under specific subjects

A C C CURRENT JOURNAL REVIEW. see *MEDICAL SCIENCES—Abstracting, Bibliographies, Statistics*

A C O G CLINICAL REVIEW. see *MEDICAL SCIENCES—Abstracting, Bibliographies, Statistics*

A E T F A T INDEX; releve des travaux de phanerogamie systematique et des taxons nouveaux concernant l'Afrique au sud du Sahara et Madagascar. see *BIOLOGY—Abstracting, Bibliographies, Statistics*

A M E D. see *ALTERNATIVE MEDICINE—Abstracting, Bibliographies, Statistics*

A S F A MARINE BIOTECHNOLOGY ABSTRACTS. (Aquatic Sciences & Fisheries Abstracts) see *BIOLOGY—Abstracting, Bibliographies, Statistics*

A T PASES. (Adenosine Triphosphatases) see *BIOLOGY—Abstracting, Bibliographies, Statistics*

ABSEARCH A S H A. (American Speech - Language - Hearing Association) see *HANDICAPPED—Abstracting, Bibliographies, Statistics*

ABSTRACTS IN SOCIAL GERONTOLOGY; current literature on aging. see *GERONTOLOGY AND GERIATRICS—Abstracting, Bibliographies, Statistics*

ABSTRACTS OF BULGARIAN SCIENTIFIC LITERATURE. AGRICULTURE AND FORESTRY. VETERINARY MEDICINE. see *VETERINARY SCIENCE—Abstracting, Bibliographies, Statistics*

ABSTRACTS OF BULGARIAN SCIENTIFIC MEDICAL LITERATURE. see *MEDICAL SCIENCES—Abstracting, Bibliographies, Statistics*

ABSTRACTS OF CLINICAL CARE GUIDELINES. see *MEDICAL SCIENCES—Abstracting, Bibliographies, Statistics*

ABSTRACTS OF CURRENT LITERATURE IN TOXICOLOGY. see *ENVIRONMENTAL STUDIES—Abstracting, Bibliographies, Statistics*

ABSTRACTS OF ENTOMOLOGY. see *BIOLOGY—Abstracting, Bibliographies, Statistics*

ABSTRACTS OF MYCOLOGY. see *BIOLOGY—Abstracting, Bibliographies, Statistics*

ABSTRACTS ON HYGIENE AND COMMUNICABLE DISEASES. see *MEDICAL SCIENCES—Abstracting, Bibliographies, Statistics*

ACTA VETERINARIA JAPONICA. see *VETERINARY SCIENCE—Abstracting, Bibliographies, Statistics*

AFRICAN HEALTH ANTHOLOGY. see *MEDICAL SCIENCES—Abstracting, Bibliographies, Statistics*

AFRICAN INDEX MEDICUS. see *MEDICAL SCIENCES—Abstracting, Bibliographies, Statistics*

AGBIOTECH NEWS AND INFORMATION. see *BIOLOGY—Abstracting, Bibliographies, Statistics*

AGE.INFO CD-ROM. see *GERONTOLOGY AND GERIATRICS—Abstracting, Bibliographies, Statistics*

AGELINE. see *GERONTOLOGY AND GERIATRICS—Abstracting, Bibliographies, Statistics*

AGING. see *BIOLOGY—Abstracting, Bibliographies, Statistics*

AGROFORESTRY ABSTRACTS. see *AGRICULTURE—Abstracting, Bibliographies, Statistics*

AIDS ABSTRACTS; international literature on acquired immunodeficiency syndrome and related retroviruses. see *MEDICAL SCIENCES—Abstracting, Bibliographies, Statistics*

AIDS & CANCER RESEARCH. see *MEDICAL SCIENCES—Abstracting, Bibliographies, Statistics*

AIDS & T B WEEKLY ABSTRACTS FROM CONFERENCE PROCEEDINGS. (Tuberculosis) see *MEDICAL SCIENCES—Abstracting, Bibliographies, Statistics*

AIDS & T B WEEKLY ARTICLE SUMMARIES. (Tuberculosis) see *MEDICAL SCIENCES—Abstracting, Bibliographies, Statistics*

AIDSEARCH. see *MEDICAL SCIENCES—Abstracting, Bibliographies, Statistics*

ALT-HEALTH WATCH; alternative health & wellness. see *ALTERNATIVE MEDICINE—Abstracting, Bibliographies, Statistics*

AMERICAN DRUG INDEX. see *PHARMACY AND PHARMACOLOGY—Abstracting, Bibliographies, Statistics*

AMERICAN SOCIETY FOR MICROBIOLOGY. ABSTRACTS OF THE GENERAL MEETING. see *BIOLOGY—Abstracting, Bibliographies, Statistics*

ANIMAL BEHAVIOR ABSTRACTS. see *BIOLOGY—Abstracting, Bibliographies, Statistics*

ANIMAL BREEDING ABSTRACTS; a monthly abstract of world literature. see *AGRICULTURE—Abstracting, Bibliographies, Statistics*

ANNALES COLLEGII MEDICI UNIVERSITATIS IAGIELLONICAE CRACOVIENSIS. see *MEDICAL SCIENCES—Abstracting, Bibliographies, Statistics*

ANNALS OF BEHAVIORAL MEDICINE. see *MEDICAL SCIENCES—Abstracting, Bibliographies, Statistics*

APOPTOSIS. see *BIOLOGY—Abstracting, Bibliographies, Statistics*

APSTRACTS. see *BIOLOGY—Abstracting, Bibliographies, Statistics*

AQUATIC BIOLOGY, AQUACULTURE & FISHERIES RESOURCES. see *BIOLOGY—Abstracting, Bibliographies, Statistics*

ARTEMISA. see *MEDICAL SCIENCES—Abstracting, Bibliographies, Statistics*

ASTHMA UPDATE; a newsletter for people with asthma. see *MEDICAL SCIENCES—Abstracting, Bibliographies, Statistics*

AUSTRALIAN AND NEW ZEALAND DIRECTORY OF GENETICS SUPPORT GROUPS, SERVICES AND INFORMATION. see *BIOLOGY—Abstracting, Bibliographies, Statistics*

AUTOIMMUNE DISEASES. see *MEDICAL SCIENCES—Abstracting, Bibliographies, Statistics*

BIBLIOGRAPHIES AND INDEXES IN GERONTOLOGY. see *GERONTOLOGY AND GERIATRICS—Abstracting, Bibliographies, Statistics*

BIBLIOGRAPHIES AND INDEXES IN MEDICAL STUDIES. see *MEDICAL SCIENCES—Abstracting, Bibliographies, Statistics*

A

BIO-ELECTRONICS AND BIOSENSORS. see *BIOLOGY—Abstracting, Bibliographies, Statistics*

BIOCHEMISTRY AND BIOPHYSICS CITATION INDEX. see *BIOLOGY—Abstracting, Bibliographies, Statistics*

BIOCONTROL NEWS AND INFORMATION. see *AGRICULTURE—Abstracting, Bibliographies, Statistics*

BIOETHICS LITERATURE REVIEW. see *MEDICAL SCIENCES—Abstracting, Bibliographies, Statistics*

BIOLOGICAL ABSTRACTS; references, abstracts, and indexes to the world's life sciences research literature. see *BIOLOGY—Abstracting, Bibliographies, Statistics*

BIOLOGICAL ABSTRACTS CUMULATIVE INDEXES. see *BIOLOGY—Abstracting, Bibliographies, Statistics*

BIOLOGICAL ABSTRACTS - R R M; references and indexes to the world's life science reports, reviews, and meeting literature. (Reports, Reviews, Meetings) see *BIOLOGY—Abstracting, Bibliographies, Statistics*

BIOLOGICAL ABSTRACTS - R R M CUMULATIVE INDEX. (Reports, Reviews, and Meetings) see *BIOLOGY—Abstracting, Bibliographies, Statistics*

BIOLOGICAL & AGRICULTURAL INDEX. see *BIOLOGY—Abstracting, Bibliographies, Statistics*

BIOLOGICAL RHYTHMS. see *BIOLOGY—Abstracting, Bibliographies, Statistics*

BIOLOGY DIGEST. see *BIOLOGY—Abstracting, Bibliographies, Statistics*

BIOPHYSICAL SOCIETY. ANNUAL MEETING. ABSTRACTS. see *BIOLOGY—Abstracting, Bibliographies, Statistics*

BIOSIS EVOLUTIONS. see *BIOLOGY—Abstracting, Bibliographies, Statistics*

BIOSIS SEARCH GUIDE (YEAR). see *BIOLOGY—Abstracting, Bibliographies, Statistics*

BIOSIS SERIAL SOURCES. see *BIOLOGY—Abstracting, Bibliographies, Statistics*

BIOTECHNOLOGY ABSTRACTS. see *BIOLOGY—Abstracting, Bibliographies, Statistics*

BIOTECHNOLOGY INFORMATION. see *BIOLOGY—Abstracting, Bibliographies, Statistics*

BIOWORLD TODAY INDEX. see *BIOLOGY—Abstracting, Bibliographies, Statistics*

BLOOD COAGULATION FACTORS; current awareness service for researchers in life sciences. see *MEDICAL SCIENCES—Abstracting, Bibliographies, Statistics*

BOTANISK CENTRALBIBLIOTEK. FORTEGNELSE OVER LOEBENDE PERIODICA VED BOTANISK CENTRALBIBLITEK. see *BIOLOGY—Abstracting, Bibliographies, Statistics*

BOTTOM LINE (LANSING); on alcohol in society. see *DRUG ABUSE AND ALCOHOLISM—Abstracting, Bibliographies, Statistics*

BREASTFEEDING ABSTRACTS. see *MEDICAL SCIENCES—Abstracting, Bibliographies, Statistics*

BRITISH LIBRARY. DOCUMENT SUPPLY CENTRE. INDEX OF CONFERENCE PROCEEDINGS. see *MEETINGS AND CONGRESSES—Abstracting, Bibliographies, Statistics*

BRITISH NURSING INDEX; index of journal articles of interest to nurses, midwives and community staff. see *MEDICAL SCIENCES—Abstracting, Bibliographies, Statistics*

BYOIN KANRI KENKYUJO KENKYU SHUDANKAI ENDAI SHOROKU/NATIONAL INSTITUTE OF HOSPITAL ADMINISTRATION. ABSTRACTS OF THE MEETING. see *HEALTH FACILITIES AND ADMINISTRATION—Abstracting, Bibliographies, Statistics*

C A S BIOTECH UPDATES. ANTIBODY CONJUGATES. see *CHEMISTRY—Abstracting, Bibliographies, Statistics*

C A S BIOTECH UPDATES. BIOCHEMICAL IMMOBILIZATION & BIOCATALYTIC REACTORS. see *BIOLOGY—Abstracting, Bibliographies, Statistics*

C A S BIOTECH UPDATES. BIOSENSORS. see *BIOLOGY—Abstracting, Bibliographies, Statistics*

C A S BIOTECH UPDATES. CELL & TISSUE CULTURE. see *BIOLOGY—Abstracting, Bibliographies, Statistics*

C A S BIOTECH UPDATES. COMMERCIAL FERMENTATION. see *BIOLOGY—Abstracting, Bibliographies, Statistics*

C A S BIOTECH UPDATES. D N A & R N A PROBES. see *BIOLOGY—Abstracting, Bibliographies, Statistics*

C A S BIOTECH UPDATES. D N A FORMATION & REPAIR. see *BIOLOGY—Abstracting, Bibliographies, Statistics*

C A S BIOTECH UPDATES. ENVIRONMENTAL BIOTECHNOLOGY. see *ENVIRONMENTAL STUDIES—Abstracting, Bibliographies, Statistics*

C A S BIOTECH UPDATES. ENZYMES IN BIOTECHNOLOGY. see *BIOLOGY—Abstracting, Bibliographies, Statistics*

C A S BIOTECH UPDATES. GENETIC ENGINEERING. see *BIOLOGY—Abstracting, Bibliographies, Statistics*

C A S BIOTECH UPDATES. NUCLEIC ACID & PROTEIN SEQUENCES. see *BIOLOGY—Abstracting, Bibliographies, Statistics*

C A S BIOTECH UPDATES. PHARMACEUTICAL APPLICATIONS. see *BIOLOGY—Abstracting, Bibliographies, Statistics*

C A S BIOTECH UPDATES. PRODUCT PURIFICATION & SEPARATION. see *CHEMISTRY—Abstracting, Bibliographies, Statistics*

C A S BIOTECH UPDATES. SLOW-RELEASE PHARMACEUTICALS. see *PHARMACY AND PHARMACOLOGY—Abstracting, Bibliographies, Statistics*

C A SELECTS. see *CHEMISTRY—Abstracting, Bibliographies, Statistics*

C A SELECTS. AIDS AND RELATED IMMUNODEFICIENCIES. see *MEDICAL SCIENCES—Abstracting, Bibliographies, Statistics*

C A SELECTS. ALKOXYLATED OLEOCHEMICALS. see *PHARMACY AND PHARMACOLOGY—Abstracting, Bibliographies, Statistics*

C A SELECTS. ALLERGY AND ANTIALLERGIC AGENTS. see *MEDICAL SCIENCES—Abstracting, Bibliographies, Statistics*

C A SELECTS. ANIMAL LONGEVITY AND AGING. see *BIOLOGY—Abstracting, Bibliographies, Statistics*

C A SELECTS. ANTI-INFLAMMATORY AGENTS AND ARTHRITIS. see *MEDICAL SCIENCES—Abstracting, Bibliographies, Statistics*

C A SELECTS. ANTIARRHYTHMICS. see *MEDICAL SCIENCES—Abstracting, Bibliographies, Statistics*

C A SELECTS. ANTIBACTERIAL AGENTS. see *CHEMISTRY—Abstracting, Bibliographies, Statistics*

C A SELECTS. ANTIFUNGAL & ANTIMYCOTIC AGENTS. see *BIOLOGY—Abstracting, Bibliographies, Statistics*

C A SELECTS. ATHEROSCLEROSIS & HEART DISEASE. see *MEDICAL SCIENCES—Abstracting, Bibliographies, Statistics*

C A SELECTS. BETA-LACTAM ANTIBIOTICS. see *PHARMACY AND PHARMACOLOGY—Abstracting, Bibliographies, Statistics*

C A SELECTS. BIOGENIC AMINES & THE NERVOUS SYSTEM. see *MEDICAL SCIENCES—Abstracting, Bibliographies, Statistics*

C A SELECTS. BLOOD COAGULATION. see *MEDICAL SCIENCES—Abstracting, Bibliographies, Statistics*

C A SELECTS. CALCIUM CHANNEL BLOCKERS. see *PHARMACY AND PHARMACOLOGY—Abstracting, Bibliographies, Statistics*

C A SELECTS. COSMETIC CHEMICALS. see *BEAUTY CULTURE—Abstracting, Bibliographies, Statistics*

C A SELECTS. DRUG ANALYSIS BIOLOGICAL FLUIDS & TISSUES. see *PHARMACY AND PHARMACOLOGY—Abstracting, Bibliographies, Statistics*

C A SELECTS. DRUG & COSMETIC TOXICITY. see *PHARMACY AND PHARMACOLOGY—Abstracting, Bibliographies, Statistics*

C A SELECTS. DRUG INTERACTIONS. see *PHARMACY AND PHARMACOLOGY—Abstracting, Bibliographies, Statistics*

C A SELECTS. ELECTROCHEMICAL REACTIONS. see *CHEMISTRY—Abstracting, Bibliographies, Statistics*

C A SELECTS. ENZYME ASSAYS. see *CHEMISTRY—Abstracting, Bibliographies, Statistics*

C A SELECTS. FOOD, DRUGS, & COSMETICS - LEGISLATIVE & REGULATORY ASPECTS. see *FOOD AND FOOD INDUSTRIES—Abstracting, Bibliographies, Statistics*

C A SELECTS. FOOD TOXICITY. see *CHEMISTRY—Abstracting, Bibliographies, Statistics*

C A SELECTS. FREE RADICALS (BIOCHEMICAL ASPECTS). see *BIOLOGY—Abstracting, Bibliographies, Statistics*

C A SELECTS. HERBICIDES. see *AGRICULTURE—Abstracting, Bibliographies, Statistics*

C A SELECTS. INDOOR AIR POLLUTION. see *ENVIRONMENTAL STUDIES—Abstracting, Bibliographies, Statistics*

C A SELECTS. INORGANIC & ORGANOMETALLIC REACTION SYSTEMS. see *CHEMISTRY—Abstracting, Bibliographies, Statistics*

C A SELECTS. INSECTICIDES. see *AGRICULTURE—Abstracting, Bibliographies, Statistics*

C A SELECTS. LEUKOTRIENES. see *CHEMISTRY—Abstracting, Bibliographies, Statistics*

C A SELECTS. MEMBRANE SEPARATION. see *CHEMISTRY—Abstracting, Bibliographies, Statistics*

C A SELECTS. METALLO ENZYMES & METALLO COENZYMES. see *CHEMISTRY—Abstracting, Bibliographies, Statistics*

C A SELECTS. MONOCLONAL ANTIBODIES. see *BIOLOGY—Abstracting, Bibliographies, Statistics*

C A SELECTS. NEW ANTIBIOTICS. see *PHARMACY AND PHARMACOLOGY—Abstracting, Bibliographies, Statistics*

C A SELECTS. NOVEL PESTICIDES & HERBICIDES. see *ENGINEERING—Abstracting, Bibliographies, Statistics*

C A SELECTS. NUTRITIONAL ASPECTS OF CANCER. see *MEDICAL SCIENCES—Abstracting, Bibliographies, Statistics*

C A SELECTS. OCCUPATIONAL EXPOSURE & HAZARDS. see *OCCUPATIONAL HEALTH AND SAFETY—Abstracting, Bibliographies, Statistics*

C A SELECTS. OLEOCHEMICALS CONTAINING NITROGEN. see *CHEMISTRY—Abstracting, Bibliographies, Statistics*

C A SELECTS. OMEGA-3 FATTY ACIDS & FISH OIL. see *CHEMISTRY—Abstracting, Bibliographies, Statistics*

C A SELECTS. ORGANIC ANALYTICAL CHEMISTRY. see *CHEMISTRY—Abstracting, Bibliographies, Statistics*

C A SELECTS. ORGANIC OPTICAL MATERIALS. see *CHEMISTRY—Abstracting, Bibliographies, Statistics*

C A SELECTS. ORGANIC STEREOCHEMISTRY. see *CHEMISTRY—Abstracting, Bibliographies, Statistics*

617 CHN
CHINA MEDICAL ABSTRACTS (SURGERY). Text in English. q. USD 28.10 (effective 2000). abstr.
Document type: *Abstract/Index.* **Description:** Contains abstracts from over 70 major medical journals published in China and up-to-date news of technology and advances in general surgery, orthopedic surgery, neurosurgery, thoracic cardiovascular surgery, urogenital surgery, plastic surgery, treatment of burns, organ transplantation and anaesthesia.
Published by: Sun Yat-sen University of Medical Sciences, Zhongshan Ophthalmic Center, 54 Xianlie Rd, Guangzhou, Guangdong 510060, China. **Dist. by:** China Books & Periodicals, Inc, 2929 24th St, San Francisco, CA 94110. TEL 415-282-0994, 415-282-2994, info@chinabooks.com, http://www.chinabooks.com/.

A

CURRENT MEDICAL LITERATURE. HEALTH CARE OF OLDER PEOPLE. see *GERONTOLOGY AND GERIATRICS—Abstracting, Bibliographies, Statistics*

CURRENT MEDICAL LITERATURE. PSYCHIATRY REVIEWS; recent developments in psychiatric care for General Practitioners. see *MEDICAL SCIENCES—Abstracting, Bibliographies, Statistics*

CURRENT OPINION IN IMMUNOLOGY. see *MEDICAL SCIENCES—Abstracting, Bibliographies, Statistics*

CYSTIC FIBROSIS. see *MEDICAL SCIENCES—Abstracting, Bibliographies, Statistics*

CYTOSKELETON. see *BIOLOGY—Abstracting, Bibliographies, Statistics*

D N A PROBES. see *BIOLOGY—Abstracting, Bibliographies, Statistics*

DENTAL ABSTRACTS. see *MEDICAL SCIENCES—Abstracting, Bibliographies, Statistics*

DIABETES MELLITUS. see *MEDICAL SCIENCES—Abstracting, Bibliographies, Statistics*

DIGEST OF NEUROLOGY & PSYCHIATRY. see *MEDICAL SCIENCES—Abstracting, Bibliographies, Statistics*

016 JOR
DIRASAT. ANNUAL INDEX. Text in Arabic, English. 1974. a. back issues avail. **Document type:** *Abstract/Index, Academic/Scholarly.* **Description:** Indexes all the articles published in all the series of Dirasat journals.
Published by: University of Jordan, Deanship of Academic Research, Dean of Academic Research, Amman, Jordan. TEL 962-6-5355000 ext 3200, FAX 962-6-5355599, dirasata@ju.edu.jo, http://www.ju.edu.jo/research/dar. Ed. Nabil Shawagfeh.

DIRECTORY OF PUBLISHED PROCEEDINGS. SERIES M L S - MEDICAL, LIFE SCIENCES. see *MEDICAL SCIENCES—Abstracting, Bibliographies, Statistics*

DIRECTORY OF PUBLISHED PROCEEDINGS. SERIES S E M T - SCIENCE, ENGINEERING, MEDICINE AND TECHNOLOGY. see *SCIENCES: COMPREHENSIVE WORKS—Abstracting, Bibliographies, Statistics*

DRUG FILE UPDATE; a current awareness index to publications on drugs and doping in sport. see *SPORTS AND GAMES—Abstracting, Bibliographies, Statistics*

DRUG TARGETING. see *PHARMACY AND PHARMACOLOGY—Abstracting, Bibliographies, Statistics*

E & P HEALTH, SAFETY AND ENVIRONMENT. (Exploration and Production) see *PETROLEUM AND GAS—Abstracting, Bibliographies, Statistics*

E C M T STATISTICAL REPORT ON ROAD ACCIDENTS. see *TRANSPORTATION—Abstracting, Bibliographies, Statistics*

E-PSYCHE. see *PSYCHOLOGY—Abstracting, Bibliographies, Statistics*

EMBASE ALERT. see *MEDICAL SCIENCES—Abstracting, Bibliographies, Statistics*

EMBASE LIST OF JOURNALS INDEXED (YEAR). see *MEDICAL SCIENCES—Abstracting, Bibliographies, Statistics*

ENDOTHELIUM. see *BIOLOGY—Abstracting, Bibliographies, Statistics*

ENTOMOLOGY ABSTRACTS. see *BIOLOGY—Abstracting, Bibliographies, Statistics*

ENTREZ DOCUMENT RETRIEVAL SYSTEM. see *BIOLOGY—Abstracting, Bibliographies, Statistics*

ENVIROFICHE. see *BIOLOGY—Abstracting, Bibliographies, Statistics*

ENVIRONMENT ABSTRACTS. see *CONSERVATION—Abstracting, Bibliographies, Statistics*

ENVIRONMENTAL AND SAFETY TECHNOLOGY. see *ENVIRONMENTAL STUDIES—Abstracting, Bibliographies, Statistics*

ERGA. see *OCCUPATIONAL HEALTH AND SAFETY—Abstracting, Bibliographies, Statistics*

ERGONOMICS ABSTRACTS. see *ENGINEERING—Abstracting, Bibliographies, Statistics*

ERYTHROCYTES. see *MEDICAL SCIENCES—Abstracting, Bibliographies, Statistics*

EUROPEAN CONGRESS OF CARDIOLOGY. ABSTRACTS OF PAPERS. see *MEDICAL SCIENCES—Abstracting, Bibliographies, Statistics*

EXCEPTIONAL CHILD EDUCATION RESOURCES. see *EDUCATION—Abstracting, Bibliographies, Statistics*

EXCERPTA MEDICA. ABSTRACT JOURNALS. see *BIOLOGY—Abstracting, Bibliographies, Statistics*

EXCERPTA MEDICA. SECTION 1: ANATOMY, ANTHROPOLOGY, EMBRYOLOGY & HISTOLOGY. see *BIOLOGY—Abstracting, Bibliographies, Statistics*

EXCERPTA MEDICA. SECTION 10: OBSTETRICS AND GYNECOLOGY. see *MEDICAL SCIENCES—Abstracting, Bibliographies, Statistics*

EXCERPTA MEDICA. SECTION 11: OTORHINOLARYNGOLOGY. see *MEDICAL SCIENCES—Abstracting, Bibliographies, Statistics*

EXCERPTA MEDICA. SECTION 12: OPHTHALMOLOGY. see *MEDICAL SCIENCES—Abstracting, Bibliographies, Statistics*

EXCERPTA MEDICA. SECTION 13: DERMATOLOGY AND VENEREOLOGY. see *MEDICAL SCIENCES—Abstracting, Bibliographies, Statistics*

EXCERPTA MEDICA. SECTION 14: RADIOLOGY. see *MEDICAL SCIENCES—Abstracting, Bibliographies, Statistics*

EXCERPTA MEDICA. SECTION 15: CHEST DISEASES, THORACIC SURGERY AND TUBERCULOSIS. see *MEDICAL SCIENCES—Abstracting, Bibliographies, Statistics*

EXCERPTA MEDICA. SECTION 16: CANCER. see *MEDICAL SCIENCES—Abstracting, Bibliographies, Statistics*

EXCERPTA MEDICA. SECTION 17: PUBLIC HEALTH, SOCIAL MEDICINE AND EPIDEMIOLOGY. see *PUBLIC HEALTH AND SAFETY—Abstracting, Bibliographies, Statistics*

EXCERPTA MEDICA. SECTION 18: CARDIOVASCULAR DISEASES AND CARDIOVASCULAR SURGERY. see *MEDICAL SCIENCES—Abstracting, Bibliographies, Statistics*

EXCERPTA MEDICA. SECTION 19: REHABILITATION AND PHYSICAL MEDICINE. see *MEDICAL SCIENCES—Abstracting, Bibliographies, Statistics*

EXCERPTA MEDICA. SECTION 2: PHYSIOLOGY. see *MEDICAL SCIENCES—Abstracting, Bibliographies, Statistics*

EXCERPTA MEDICA. SECTION 20: GERONTOLOGY AND GERIATRICS. see *GERONTOLOGY AND GERIATRICS—Abstracting, Bibliographies, Statistics*

EXCERPTA MEDICA. SECTION 21: DEVELOPMENTAL BIOLOGY AND TERATOLOGY. see *BIOLOGY—Abstracting, Bibliographies, Statistics*

EXCERPTA MEDICA. SECTION 22: HUMAN GENETICS. see *BIOLOGY—Abstracting, Bibliographies, Statistics*

EXCERPTA MEDICA. SECTION 23: NUCLEAR MEDICINE. see *MEDICAL SCIENCES—Abstracting, Bibliographies, Statistics*

EXCERPTA MEDICA. SECTION 24: ANESTHESIOLOGY. see *MEDICAL SCIENCES—Abstracting, Bibliographies, Statistics*

EXCERPTA MEDICA. SECTION 25: HEMATOLOGY. see *MEDICAL SCIENCES—Abstracting, Bibliographies, Statistics*

EXCERPTA MEDICA. SECTION 26: IMMUNOLOGY, SEROLOGY AND TRANSPLANTATION. see *MEDICAL SCIENCES—Abstracting, Bibliographies, Statistics*

EXCERPTA MEDICA. SECTION 27: BIOPHYSICS, BIO-ENGINEERING AND MEDICAL INSTRUMENTATION. see *BIOLOGY—Abstracting, Bibliographies, Statistics*

EXCERPTA MEDICA. SECTION 28: UROLOGY AND NEPHROLOGY. see *MEDICAL SCIENCES—Abstracting, Bibliographies, Statistics*

EXCERPTA MEDICA. SECTION 29: CLINICAL AND EXPERIMENTAL BIOCHEMISTRY. see *BIOLOGY—Abstracting, Bibliographies, Statistics*

EXCERPTA MEDICA. SECTION 3: ENDOCRINOLOGY. see *MEDICAL SCIENCES—Abstracting, Bibliographies, Statistics*

EXCERPTA MEDICA. SECTION 30: CLINICAL AND EXPERIMENTAL PHARMACOLOGY. see *PHARMACY AND PHARMACOLOGY—Abstracting, Bibliographies, Statistics*

EXCERPTA MEDICA. SECTION 31: ARTHRITIS AND RHEUMATISM. see *MEDICAL SCIENCES—Abstracting, Bibliographies, Statistics*

EXCERPTA MEDICA. SECTION 32: PSYCHIATRY. see *MEDICAL SCIENCES—Abstracting, Bibliographies, Statistics*

EXCERPTA MEDICA. SECTION 33: ORTHOPEDIC SURGERY. see *MEDICAL SCIENCES—Abstracting, Bibliographies, Statistics*

EXCERPTA MEDICA. SECTION 35: OCCUPATIONAL HEALTH AND INDUSTRIAL MEDICINE. see *MEDICAL SCIENCES—Abstracting, Bibliographies, Statistics*

EXCERPTA MEDICA. SECTION 36: HEALTH POLICY, ECONOMICS AND MANAGEMENT. see *HEALTH FACILITIES AND ADMINISTRATION—Abstracting, Bibliographies, Statistics*

EXCERPTA MEDICA. SECTION 38: ADVERSE REACTIONS TITLES. see *PHARMACY AND PHARMACOLOGY—Abstracting, Bibliographies, Statistics*

EXCERPTA MEDICA. SECTION 4: MICROBIOLOGY: BACTERIOLOGY, MYCOLOGY, PARASITOLOGY AND VIROLOGY. see *BIOLOGY—Abstracting, Bibliographies, Statistics*

EXCERPTA MEDICA. SECTION 40: DRUG DEPENDENCE, ALCOHOL ABUSE AND ALCOHOLISM. see *DRUG ABUSE AND ALCOHOLISM—Abstracting, Bibliographies, Statistics*

EXCERPTA MEDICA. SECTION 46: ENVIRONMENTAL HEALTH AND POLLUTION CONTROL. see *ENVIRONMENTAL STUDIES—Abstracting, Bibliographies, Statistics*

EXCERPTA MEDICA. SECTION 48: GASTROENTEROLOGY. see *MEDICAL SCIENCES—Abstracting, Bibliographies, Statistics*

EXCERPTA MEDICA. SECTION 49: FORENSIC SCIENCE ABSTRACTS. see *MEDICAL SCIENCES—Abstracting, Bibliographies, Statistics*

EXCERPTA MEDICA. SECTION 5: GENERAL PATHOLOGY AND PATHOLOGICAL ANATOMY. see *BIOLOGY—Abstracting, Bibliographies, Statistics*

EXCERPTA MEDICA. SECTION 52: TOXICOLOGY. see *ENVIRONMENTAL STUDIES—Abstracting, Bibliographies, Statistics*

EXCERPTA MEDICA. SECTION 6: INTERNAL MEDICINE. see *MEDICAL SCIENCES—Abstracting, Bibliographies, Statistics*

EXCERPTA MEDICA. SECTION 7: PEDIATRICS AND PEDIATRIC SURGERY. see *MEDICAL SCIENCES—Abstracting, Bibliographies, Statistics*

EXCERPTA MEDICA. SECTION 8: NEUROLOGY AND NEUROSURGERY. see *MEDICAL SCIENCES—Abstracting, Bibliographies, Statistics*

EXCERPTA MEDICA. SECTION 9: SURGERY. see *MEDICAL SCIENCES—Abstracting, Bibliographies, Statistics*

A

L M S ALERT. PEPTIC ULCER DISEASE. (Literature Monitoring and Evaluation Service) see *MEDICAL SCIENCES—Abstracting, Bibliographies, Statistics*

L M S ALERT. PHARMACOECONOMICS. (Literature Monitoring and Evaluation Service) see *PHARMACY AND PHARMACOLOGY—Abstracting, Bibliographies, Statistics*

L M S ALERT. RHEUMATIC DISEASE. (Literature Monitoring and Evaluation Service) see *MEDICAL SCIENCES—Abstracting, Bibliographies, Statistics*

L M S ALERT. WOMEN'S HEALTH. (Literature Monitoring and Evaluation Service) see *WOMEN'S HEALTH—Abstracting, Bibliographies, Statistics*

LABORATORY HAZARDS BULLETIN. see *OCCUPATIONAL HEALTH AND SAFETY—Abstracting, Bibliographies, Statistics*

LEUCOCYTES. see *MEDICAL SCIENCES—Abstracting, Bibliographies, Statistics*

LIPOSOMES. see *BIOLOGY—Abstracting, Bibliographies, Statistics*

LITERATURE MONITORING AND EVALUATION SERVICE ALERT. ANTIBACTERIAL. see *MEDICAL SCIENCES—Abstracting, Bibliographies, Statistics*

LYSOSOMES AND ENDOCYTOSIS. see *BIOLOGY—Abstracting, Bibliographies, Statistics*

M E D I C. (Monthly Ethical Drug Index Complication) see *PHARMACY AND PHARMACOLOGY—Abstracting, Bibliographies, Statistics*

M I M S DISEASE INDEX. see *MEDICAL SCIENCES—Abstracting, Bibliographies, Statistics*

M I M S MEDICAL SPECIALITIES. (Monthly Index of Medical Specialties) see *MEDICAL SCIENCES—Abstracting, Bibliographies, Statistics*

MACROPHAGES. see *MEDICAL SCIENCES—Abstracting, Bibliographies, Statistics*

MAMMARY GLAND. see *BIOLOGY—Abstracting, Bibliographies, Statistics*

MEDICAL & PHARMACEUTICAL BIOTECHNOLOGY ABSTRACTS. see *MEDICAL SCIENCES—Abstracting, Bibliographies, Statistics*

MEDICAL CARE RESEARCH AND REVIEW. see *PUBLIC HEALTH AND SAFETY—Abstracting, Bibliographies, Statistics*

MEDICAL LITERATURE INDEXING SERVICES IN PAKISTAN. see *MEDICAL SCIENCES—Abstracting, Bibliographies, Statistics*

MEDICINAL AND AROMATIC PLANTS ABSTRACTS. see *MEDICAL SCIENCES—Abstracting, Bibliographies, Statistics*

MEDIFAX INDEX. see *MEDICAL SCIENCES—Abstracting, Bibliographies, Statistics*

MEDITSINSKI PREGLED. KLINIKA I PREDKLINIKA. see *MEDICAL SCIENCES—Abstracting, Bibliographies, Statistics*

MEDITSINSKI PREGLED. MEDITSINSKI MENIDZHMENT I ZDRAVNA POLITIKA. see *PUBLIC HEALTH AND SAFETY—Abstracting, Bibliographies, Statistics*

MICROBIOLOGY ABSTRACTS: SECTION A. INDUSTRIAL & APPLIED MICROBIOLOGY. see *BIOLOGY—Abstracting, Bibliographies, Statistics*

MICROBIOLOGY ABSTRACTS: SECTION B. BACTERIOLOGY. see *BIOLOGY—Abstracting, Bibliographies, Statistics*

MICROBIOLOGY ABSTRACTS: SECTION C. ALGOLOGY, MYCOLOGY AND PROTOZOOLOGY. see *BIOLOGY—Abstracting, Bibliographies, Statistics*

MITOCHONDRIA. see *BIOLOGY—Abstracting, Bibliographies, Statistics*

MOLECULAR BIOLOGY TECHNIQUES. see *BIOLOGY—Abstracting, Bibliographies, Statistics*

MONOCLONAL ANTIBODIES. see *BIOLOGY—Abstracting, Bibliographies, Statistics*

MULTICULTURAL EDUCATION ABSTRACTS. see *EDUCATION—Abstracting, Bibliographies, Statistics*

MYCOBACTERIA. see *BIOLOGY—Abstracting, Bibliographies, Statistics*

N T I S ALERTS: BIOMEDICAL TECHNOLOGY & HUMAN FACTORS ENGINEERING. see *MEDICAL SCIENCES—Abstracting, Bibliographies, Statistics*

N T I S ALERTS: HEALTH CARE. see *PHYSICAL FITNESS AND HYGIENE—Abstracting, Bibliographies, Statistics*

NEMATOLOGICAL ABSTRACTS. see *BIOLOGY—Abstracting, Bibliographies, Statistics*

NERVE CELL BIOLOGY. see *BIOLOGY—Abstracting, Bibliographies, Statistics*

NEUROPEPTIDES (SHEFFIELD). see *BIOLOGY—Abstracting, Bibliographies, Statistics*

NEUROPHYSIOLOGY. see *BIOLOGY—Abstracting, Bibliographies, Statistics*

NEUROPSYCHOLOGY ABSTRACTS. see *MEDICAL SCIENCES—Abstracting, Bibliographies, Statistics*

NIHON BOKIN BOBAI GAKKAI. NENJI TAIKAI YOSHISHU/SOCIETY FOR ANTIBACTERIAL AND ANTIFUNGAL AGENTS, JAPAN. ABSTRACTS OF THE MEETING. see *BIOLOGY—Abstracting, Bibliographies, Statistics*

NIHON IYAKU BUNKEN SHOROKUSHU/JAPAN PHARMACEUTICAL ABSTRACTS. see *PHARMACY AND PHARMACOLOGY—Abstracting, Bibliographies, Statistics*

NIHON JIKKEN DOBUTSU GAKKAI SOKAI KOEN YOSHISHU/JAPANESE ASSOCIATION FOR LABORATORY ANIMAL SCIENCE. ABSTRACTS OF GENERAL MEETING. see *BIOLOGY—Abstracting, Bibliographies, Statistics*

NIHON JINRUI IDEN GAKKAI TAIKAI SHOROKUSHU/ JAPAN SOCIETY OF HUMAN GENETICS. ABSTRACTS OF THE ANNUAL MEETING. see *BIOLOGY—Abstracting, Bibliographies, Statistics*

NIHON KAIBOGAKU BUNKENSHU/ABSTRACTS OF JAPANESE ANATOMY. see *MEDICAL SCIENCES—Abstracting, Bibliographies, Statistics*

NIHON SEIRI JINRUI GAKKAI TAIKAI SHOROKUSHU/JAPAN SOCIETY OF PHYSIOLOGICAL ANTHROPOLOGY. ABSTRACTS OF THE MEETING. see *BIOLOGY—Abstracting, Bibliographies, Statistics*

NIHON SENSHOKUTAI KENSA GAKKAI SHOROKUSHU/JAPANESE ASSOCIATION FOR CHROMOSOME ANALYSIS. ABSTRACT OF ANNUAL MEETING. see *BIOLOGY—Abstracting, Bibliographies, Statistics*

NITRIC OXIDE. see *BIOLOGY—Abstracting, Bibliographies, Statistics*

NO NO IGAKU SEIBUTSUGAKU KONWAKAI SHOROKU/ABSTRACTS OF CONFERENCE ON MEDICINE AND BIOLOGY OF THE BRAIN. see *BIOLOGY—Abstracting, Bibliographies, Statistics*

NOTIZIARIO BIBLIOGRAFICO DI AUDIOLOGIA O R L E FONIATRIA. see *MEDICAL SCIENCES—Abstracting, Bibliographies, Statistics*

NUCLEIC ACIDS ABSTRACTS. see *BIOLOGY—Abstracting, Bibliographies, Statistics*

NUTRITION ABSTRACTS AND REVIEWS. SERIES A: HUMAN AND EXPERIMENTAL. see *NUTRITION AND DIETETICS—Abstracting, Bibliographies, Statistics*

NUTRITION ABSTRACTS AND REVIEWS. SERIES B: LIVESTOCK FEEDS AND FEEDING. see *AGRICULTURE—Abstracting, Bibliographies, Statistics*

NYUSEN HINYU KENKYUKAI KOEN YOSHISHU/ SOCIETY FOR MAMMARY GLANDS AND LACTATION RESEARCH. ABSTRACTS OF THE MEETING. see *MEDICAL SCIENCES—Abstracting, Bibliographies, Statistics*

O R REPORTS. (Operating Room) see *HEALTH FACILITIES AND ADMINISTRATION—Abstracting, Bibliographies, Statistics*

OBSTETRIC ANESTHESIA DIGEST. see *MEDICAL SCIENCES—Anaesthesiology*

OCCUPATIONAL HEALTH & SAFETY CURRENT CONTENTS. see *OCCUPATIONAL HEALTH AND SAFETY—Abstracting, Bibliographies, Statistics*

ONCOGENES. see *MEDICAL SCIENCES—Abstracting, Bibliographies, Statistics*

ONCOGENES AND GROWTH FACTORS ABSTRACTS. see *MEDICAL SCIENCES—Abstracting, Bibliographies, Statistics*

OPHTHALMIC LITERATURE. see *MEDICAL SCIENCES—Abstracting, Bibliographies, Statistics*

OSTEOPOROSIS. see *MEDICAL SCIENCES—Abstracting, Bibliographies, Statistics*

OXYGEN RADICALS. see *BIOLOGY—Abstracting, Bibliographies, Statistics*

P H L S LIBRARY BULLETIN. see *BIOLOGY—Abstracting, Bibliographies, Statistics*

PAKISTAN VETERINARY INDEX. see *VETERINARY SCIENCE—Abstracting, Bibliographies, Statistics*

PANCREATIC AND SALIVARY SECRETION. see *BIOLOGY—Abstracting, Bibliographies, Statistics*

PARASITOLOGY (SHEFFIELD). see *BIOLOGY—Abstracting, Bibliographies, Statistics*

PEDIATRIC PRIMARY CARE; practical pediatrics for the pediatric practitioner. see *MEDICAL SCIENCES—Abstracting, Bibliographies, Statistics*

PESTICIDES ABSTRACTS. see *ENVIRONMENTAL STUDIES—Abstracting, Bibliographies, Statistics*

PHARMACOECONOMICS AND OUTCOMES NEWS; rapid alerts to world pharmacoeconomic news, views and practical application. see *PHARMACY AND PHARMACOLOGY—Abstracting, Bibliographies, Statistics*

PHILIPPINE INDEX MEDICUS. see *MEDICAL SCIENCES—Abstracting, Bibliographies, Statistics*

PHYSICAL EDUCATION INDEX. see *EDUCATION—Abstracting, Bibliographies, Statistics*

PHYSIOTHERAPY INDEX. see *MEDICAL SCIENCES—Abstracting, Bibliographies, Statistics*

PLANT BIOTECHNOLOGY. see *BIOLOGY—Abstracting, Bibliographies, Statistics*

PLANT BREEDING ABSTRACTS. see *AGRICULTURE—Abstracting, Bibliographies, Statistics*

PLATELETS (SHEFFIELD). see *BIOLOGY—Abstracting, Bibliographies, Statistics*

POHYBOVE USTROJI; pokroky ve vyzkumu diagnostice a terapii. see *MEDICAL SCIENCES—Orthopedics And Traumatology*

PROLACTIN. see *MEDICAL SCIENCES—Abstracting, Bibliographies, Statistics*

PROSTAGLANDINS - BIOLOGY. see *MEDICAL SCIENCES—Abstracting, Bibliographies, Statistics*

PROTEINS: POST-TRANSLATIONAL PROCESSING. see *BIOLOGY—Abstracting, Bibliographies, Statistics*

PROTOZOOLOGICAL ABSTRACTS. see *BIOLOGY—Abstracting, Bibliographies, Statistics*

PSICODOC. see *PSYCHOLOGY—Abstracting, Bibliographies, Statistics*

REFERATOVY VYBER Z PEDIATRIE/ABSTRACTS OF PEDIATRICS. see *MEDICAL SCIENCES—Abstracting, Bibliographies, Statistics*

REFERATOVY VYBER Z PORODNICTVI A GYNEKOLOGIE/ABSTRACTS OF OBSTETRICS AND GYNECOLOGY. see *MEDICAL SCIENCES—Abstracting, Bibliographies, Statistics*

REFERATOVY VYBER Z RADIODIAGNOSTIKY/ ABSTRACTS OF RADIOLOGY. see *MEDICAL SCIENCES—Abstracting, Bibliographies, Statistics*

REFERATOVY VYBER Z REVMATOLOGIE/ABSTRACTS OF RHEUMATOLOGY. see *MEDICAL SCIENCES—Abstracting, Bibliographies, Statistics*

REHABILITATION INDEX. see *MEDICAL SCIENCES—Abstracting, Bibliographies, Statistics*

RENAL PHYSIOLOGY. see *BIOLOGY—Abstracting, Bibliographies, Statistics*

RENIN, ANGIOTENSIN & KININS. see *BIOLOGY—Abstracting, Bibliographies, Statistics*

REPINDEX. see *ENVIRONMENTAL STUDIES—Abstracting, Bibliographies, Statistics*

REPRODUCTION. ABSTRACT SERIES. see *BIOLOGY—Abstracting, Bibliographies, Statistics*

016 USA
RESEARCH ALERT (PHILADELPHIA). Text in English. 1965. w. USD 280. **Document type:** *Academic/Scholarly, Bibliography.* **Description:** Reports on all newly published items that match personalized parameters within research specialties in the sciences, social sciences, arts and humanities.
Former titles (until 1989): Automatic Subject Citation Alert; A S C A Topics
Published by: Institute for Scientific Information, 3501 Market St., Philadelphia, PA 19104. TEL 215-386-0100, FAX 215-386-2911.

REVIEW OF AROMATIC AND MEDICINAL PLANTS. see *BIOLOGY—Abstracting, Bibliographies, Statistics*

REVIEW OF MEDICAL AND VETERINARY ENTOMOLOGY. see *MEDICAL SCIENCES—Abstracting, Bibliographies, Statistics*

REVIEW OF MEDICAL AND VETERINARY MYCOLOGY. see *BIOLOGY—Abstracting, Bibliographies, Statistics*

REVIEW OF PLANT PATHOLOGY; consisting of abstracts and reviews of current literature on plant pathology. see *BIOLOGY—Abstracting, Bibliographies, Statistics*

RIBOSOMES AND TRANSLATION. see *BIOLOGY—Abstracting, Bibliographies, Statistics*

RISK ABSTRACTS. see *ENVIRONMENTAL STUDIES—Abstracting, Bibliographies, Statistics*

SAFETY AND HEALTH AT WORK. see *OCCUPATIONAL HEALTH AND SAFETY—Abstracting, Bibliographies, Statistics*

SAGE FAMILY STUDIES ABSTRACTS. see *SOCIOLOGY—Abstracting, Bibliographies, Statistics*

SEA GRANT ABSTRACTS; publications from the nation's Sea Grant programs. see *BIOLOGY—Abstracting, Bibliographies, Statistics*

SECURITE ET SANTE AU TRAVAIL. see *OCCUPATIONAL HEALTH AND SAFETY—Abstracting, Bibliographies, Statistics*

SIGNAL TRANSDUCTION & CYCLIC NUCLEOTIDES. see *BIOLOGY—Abstracting, Bibliographies, Statistics*

SIGNAL'NAYA INFORMATSIYA. FIZIOLOGIYA I MORFOLOGIYA CHELOVEKA I ZHIVOTNYKH: KROV' I LIMFA. see *BIOLOGY—Abstracting, Bibliographies, Statistics*

SIGNAL'NAYA INFORMATSIYA. NEIROPEPTIDY. see *MEDICAL SCIENCES—Abstracting, Bibliographies, Statistics*

SIGNAL'NAYA INFORMATSIYA. TEKHNIKA BEZOPASNOSTI. SANITARNAYA TEKHNIKA. see *OCCUPATIONAL HEALTH AND SAFETY—Abstracting, Bibliographies, Statistics*

SIGNAL'NAYA INFORMATSIYA. TOKSIKOLOGIYA LEKARSTVENNAYA. see *PHARMACY AND PHARMACOLOGY—Abstracting, Bibliographies, Statistics*

SPECIAL EDUCATIONAL NEEDS ABSTRACTS. see *EDUCATION—Abstracting, Bibliographies, Statistics*

SPORTS DOCUMENTATION MONTHLY BULLETIN. see *EDUCATION—Abstracting, Bibliographies, Statistics*

SURVEY OF ANESTHESIOLOGY. see *MEDICAL SCIENCES—Abstracting, Bibliographies, Statistics*

SURVEY OF OPHTHALMOLOGY. see *MEDICAL SCIENCES—Abstracting, Bibliographies, Statistics*

TABACHNAYA ZAVISIMOST I KURENIE TABAKA. see *MEDICAL SCIENCES—Abstracting, Bibliographies, Statistics*

TECHNICAL LITERATURE ABSTRACTS: HEALTH & ENVIRONMENT. see *ENVIRONMENTAL STUDIES—Abstracting, Bibliographies, Statistics*

THANATOLOGY ABSTRACTS. see *PSYCHOLOGY—Abstracting, Bibliographies, Statistics*

THYROID HORMONES. see *MEDICAL SCIENCES—Abstracting, Bibliographies, Statistics*

TISSUE CULTURE. see *BIOLOGY—Abstracting, Bibliographies, Statistics*

TOBACCO ABSTRACTS; world literature on Nicotiana. see *TOBACCO—Abstracting, Bibliographies, Statistics*

TOXICOLOGY ABSTRACTS. see *ENVIRONMENTAL STUDIES—Abstracting, Bibliographies, Statistics*

TRANSMITTERS, RECEPTORS & SYNAPSES. see *PHARMACY AND PHARMACOLOGY—Abstracting, Bibliographies, Statistics*

TROPICAL DISEASES BULLETIN. see *MEDICAL SCIENCES—Abstracting, Bibliographies, Statistics*

TSETSE AND TRYPANOSOMIASIS INFORMATION QUARTERLY. see *MEDICAL SCIENCES—Abstracting, Bibliographies, Statistics*

U.S. CENTERS FOR DISEASE CONTROL. CONGENITAL MALFORMATIONS SURVEILLANCE. see *BIOLOGY—Abstracting, Bibliographies, Statistics*

U.S. NATIONAL CENTER FOR HEALTH STATISTICS. CATALOG OF PUBLICATIONS. see *PUBLIC HEALTH AND SAFETY—Abstracting, Bibliographies, Statistics*

UKRAINSKII REFERATIVNYI ZURNAL. SERIA 1. PRIRODNICHI NAUKI, MEDICINA/UKRAINIAN JOURNAL OF ABSTRACTS. SER. 1. PRIRODNICI NAUKI, MEDICINE. see *SCIENCES: COMPREHENSIVE WORKS—Abstracting, Bibliographies, Statistics*

UNIVERSITY OF TOKYO. INSTITUTE OF APPLIED MICROBIOLOGY. REPORTS. see *BIOLOGY—Abstracting, Bibliographies, Statistics*

VETERINARY BULLETIN; a monthly abstract journal on veterinary science. see *VETERINARY SCIENCE—Abstracting, Bibliographies, Statistics*

VIOLENCE & ABUSE ABSTRACTS; current literature in interpersonal violence. see *SOCIOLOGY—Abstracting, Bibliographies, Statistics*

VIROLOGY AND AIDS ABSTRACTS. see *BIOLOGY—Abstracting, Bibliographies, Statistics*

VISION (SHEFFIELD). see *MEDICAL SCIENCES—Abstracting, Bibliographies, Statistics*

WESTERN SOCIETY OF PERIODONTOLOGY. JOURNAL. PERIODONTAL ABSTRACTS. see *MEDICAL SCIENCES—Abstracting, Bibliographies, Statistics*

▼ **THE YEAR BOOK OF DERMATOLOGY AND DERMATOLOGIC SURGERY.** see *MEDICAL SCIENCES—Abstracting, Bibliographies, Statistics*

YIXUE WENZHAI/MEDICAL ABSTRACTS. see *MEDICAL SCIENCES—Abstracting, Bibliographies, Statistics*

ZHONGGUO YAOXUE WENZHAI/CHINESE PHARMACEUTICAL ABSTRACTS. see *ALTERNATIVE MEDICINE—Abstracting, Bibliographies, Statistics*

ZHONGGUO YIXUE WENZHAI (ERKEXUE)/CHINA MEDICAL ABSTRACTS (PEDIATRICS). see *MEDICAL SCIENCES—Abstracting, Bibliographies, Statistics*

ZHONGGUO YIXUE WENZHAI (JIHUA SHENGYU, FUCHAN KEXUE)/CHINA MEDICAL ABSTRACTS (BIRTH CONTROL AND GYNECOLOGY). see *MEDICAL SCIENCES—Abstracting, Bibliographies, Statistics*

ZHONGGUO YIXUE WENZHAI (KOUQIANG YIXUE)/CHINA MEDICAL ABSTRACTS (STOMATOLOGY). see *MEDICAL SCIENCES—Abstracting, Bibliographies, Statistics*

ZHONGGUO YIXUE WENZHAI (NEIKE XUE). see *MEDICAL SCIENCES—Abstracting, Bibliographies, Statistics*

ZHONGGUO YIXUE WENZHAI (WEISHENGXUE)/ CHINESE MEDICAL DIGEST (HYGIENICS). see *PHYSICAL FITNESS AND HYGIENE—Abstracting, Bibliographies, Statistics*

ZOOLOGICAL RECORD. see *BIOLOGY—Abstracting, Bibliographies, Statistics*

ACCOUNTING

see BUSINESS AND ECONOMICS—Accounting

ADULT EDUCATION

see EDUCATION—Adult Education

ADVERTISING AND PUBLIC RELATIONS

see also BUSINESS AND ECONOMICS—Marketing And Purchasing

659.1314 DEU ISSN 0173-1882
APOTHEKE HEUTE; Schaufenster - Werbung - Einrichtung - Marketing. Text in German. 1950. q. EUR 12.76 domestic; EUR 13.40 in Europe; EUR 15.28 elsewhere; EUR 3.50 newsstand/cover (effective 2002). **Document type:** *Journal, Trade.* **Description:** Explores store window-dressing and advertising in pharmacies.
Former titles: Schaufenster (Stuttgart) (0173-2110); Aktuelle Schaufenster (0568-7632)
Related titles: ◆ Supplement to: Deutsche Apotheker Zeitung. ISSN 0011-9857.
—BLDSC (1568.907000), GNLM.
Published by: Deutscher Apotheker Verlag, Postfach 101061, Stuttgart 70009, Germany. TEL 49-711-2582-0, FAX 49-711-2582290, daz@deutscher-apotheker-verlag.de, http://www.deutscher-apotheker-verlag.de. Ed. Peter Ditzel.

DIRECTORY OF ADVERTISING AGENCIES. see *BUSINESS AND ECONOMICS—Trade And Industrial Directories*

H M C NEWS. see *PHARMACY AND PHARMACOLOGY*

741.67 USA ISSN 8756-4513
HEALTHCARE ADVERTISING REVIEW; creative forum for the people who plan and create healthcare advertising programs. Text in English. 1985. bi-m. USD 259 (effective 1998). back issues avail. **Document type:** *Trade.* **Description:** Covers advertising and marketing programs successfully implemented in the health care industry, with emphasis on print advertising.
Related titles: Online - full text ed.: (from NewsNet, Gale Group, Factiva).
—CCC.
Published by: Business Word Inc., 5350 S. Roslyn St, Ste. 400, Greenwood Village, CO 80111-2145. TEL 303-290-8500, 800-328-3211, FAX 303-290-9025, plmoore@businessword.com, customer.service@businessword.com. Circ: 1,323 (paid).

741.67 150.19 USA ISSN 1057-7408
HF5415.32
JOURNAL OF CONSUMER PSYCHOLOGY. Text in English. 1992. bi-m. USD 55 in US & Canada to individuals; USD 85 elsewhere to individuals; USD 395 in US & Canada to institutions; USD 425 elsewhere to institutions (effective 2002). adv. *Refereed.* **Document type:** *Journal, Academic/Scholarly.* **Description:** Publishes original data and theoretical, methodological and review papers on the role of advertising in consumer psychology, the development and change of consumer attitudes, choice and decision processes.
Related titles: Online - full text ed.: ISSN 1532-7663. USD 49.50 to individuals; USD 355.50 to institutions (effective 2002) (from CatchWord Ltd., EBSCO Publishing, O C L C Online Computer Library Center, Inc., RoweCom Information Quest, Swets Blackwell, Institute for Scientific Information).
Indexed: Curr.Cont., PsycInfo, Psychol.Abstr. (1992-), SSCI, e-psyche.
—BLDSC (4965.214000), CatchWord, Infotrieve, ingenta. **CCC.**
Published by: (Society for Consumer Psychology), Lawrence Erlbaum Associates, Inc., 10 Industrial Ave, Mahwah, NJ 07430-2262. TEL 201-760-3735, 800-926-6579, FAX 201-236-0072, journals@erlbaum.com, http://www.erlbaum.com/Journals/journals/JCP/jcp.htm. Ed. Dawn Iacobucci. adv.: page USD 250; trim 7 x 10.

M P R EXCHANGE. see *HEALTH FACILITIES AND ADMINISTRATION*

MEDICAL NEWS REPORT. see *BUSINESS AND ECONOMICS—Marketing And Purchasing*

PHARMA-MARKETING JOURNAL. see *BUSINESS AND ECONOMICS—Marketing And Purchasing*

741.67 658 USA ISSN 1097-3389
PRACTICE BUILDERS. Key Title: Practice Builder Association's What's Working. Variant title: What's Working. Text in English. 1983. m. (except Nov.-Dec. combined). USD 194 (effective 2000). adv. back issues avail. **Document type:** *Newsletter.* **Description:** Covers innovative marketing and promotional strategies for healthcare professionals to help build their practices in an effective yet ethical way.
Formerly (until 199?): Practice Builder (0883-3036)
Address: 18351 Jamboree Rd, Irvine, CA 92715-1011. TEL 949-253-7900, FAX 949-252-1002, sam_jones@practicebuilders.com, http://www.practicebuilders.com. Ed. Michael Riley. Pub. S.L. Jones. R&P, Adv. contact S L Jones.

659.1 USA ISSN 0275-9632
PROFILES IN HEALTHCARE MARKETING; idea exchange for the people who plan and create healthcare marketing and PR campaigns. Text in English. 1984. bi-m. USD 294 (effective 2001). back issues avail.; reprints avail. **Document type:** *Trade.* **Description:** Provides up-close case studies of successful and not-so-successful hospital marketing and public relations campaigns. Includes reprints of actual ads, press releases, brochures, and story boards.
Related titles: Online - full text ed.: (from NewsNet).
—CCC.
Published by: Business Word Inc., 5350 S. Roslyn St, Ste. 400, Greenwood Village, CO 80111-2145. TEL 303-290-8500, 800-328-3211, FAX 303-290-9025, plmoore@businessword.com, customer.service@businessword.com, http://www.businessword.com. Ed. Pamela Moore. Circ: 700 (paid).

ADVERTISING AND PUBLIC RELATIONS—Abstracting, Bibliographies, Statistics

659.1021 ZAF
SOUTH AFRICA. STATISTICS SOUTH AFRICA. CENSUS OF PROFESSIONAL AND BUSINESS SERVICES - ADVERTISING PRACTITIONERS AND ALLIED SERVICES AND MARKETING RESEARCH SERVICES. Text in English. irreg., latest 1987. ZAR 10 (effective 2000). **Document type:** *Government.*
Former titles: South Africa. Statistics South Africa. Census of Business Services - Advertising Practitioners and Allied Services and Marketing Research Services; (until Aug. 1998): South Africa. Central Statistical Service. Census of Business Services - Advertising Practitioners and Allied Services and Marketing Research Services
Published by: Statistics South Africa/Statistieke Suid-Afrika, Private Bag X44, Pretoria 0001, South Africa. TEL 27-12-310-8911, FAX 27-12-310-8500, info@statssa.pwv.gov.za, http://www.statssa.gov.za.

AERONAUTICS AND SPACE FLIGHT

see also ENGINEERING—Mechanical Engineering; TRANSPORTATION—Air Transport

AIR MEDICAL JOURNAL. see *MEDICAL SCIENCES*

616.980711 USA ISSN 0067-2661
AVIATION MEDICAL EDUCATION SERIES. Text in English. 1965. irreg. **Document type:** *Monographic series, Government.*
Published by: U.S. Federal Aviation Administration, Aviation Medicine Office, 800 Independence Ave, Washington, DC 20591. TEL 202-655-4000.

FLIGHT PARAMEDIC NEWS. see *MEDICAL SCIENCES*

FLIGHT PHYSICIAN. see *MEDICAL SCIENCES*

629.132 GBR ISSN 0015-3737
FLIGHT SAFETY BULLETIN. Text in English. 1965. q. GBP 12; GBP 18 foreign (effective 2001). adv. bk.rev. illus, stat. back issues avail. *Refereed.* **Document type:** *Bulletin.* **Description:** Contains articles, statistics, and accident details of UK general aviation accidents and incidents. Aims to foster the development of general aviation and its safety by encouraging competence among pilots and operators.
Indexed: Environ.Sci.Poll.Mgmt., Pollut.Abstr., Saf.Sci.Abstr.
Published by: General Aviation Safety Council, Rochester Airport, Chatham, Kent ME5 9SD, United Kingdom. TEL 44-1634-200203, FAX 44-1634-200203, editor@gen-av-safety.demon.co.uk, johncampbell@gen-av-safety.demon.co.uk. Ed. Nigel Everett. Adv. contact Andrew Dent TEL 44-1993-891000. Circ: 14,500.

358.4 USA ISSN 0279-9308
UG633
FLYING SAFETY. Text in English. 1944. m. USD 45 (effective 2001). bk.rev. illus, charts. back issues avail.; reprint service avail. from PQC. **Document type:** *Government.* **Description:** Covers the many fields of flight, aircraft engineering, flight training, and safety both in the air and on the ground.
Formerly (until vol.37, 1981): Aerospace Safety (0001-9429)
Related titles: Microform ed.: (from MIM,PQC); Online - full text ed.: (from Northern Light Technology, Inc., ProQuest Information & Learning, Factiva).
Indexed: Air Un.Lib.Ind., Environ.Sci.Poll.Mgmt., Ind.U.S.Gov.Per., Pollut.Abstr., Ref.Zh., Risk Abstr., Saf.Sci.Abstr.
—BLDSC (3964.128000), ingenta, Linda Hall.
Published by: U.S. Air Force Safety Agency, 9700 Ave G, S E, Ste 282, Kirtland, NM 87117-5670. TEL 505-846-0936, FAX 505-846-2710, http://www-afsc.saia.af.mil/magazine/htdocs/afsc2.html. Ed. Maj James H Grigsby. Circ: 18,350. **Subscr. to:** U.S. Government Printing Office, Superintendent of Documents, PO Box 371954, Pittsburgh, PA 15250-7954. TEL 202-512-1800, FAX 202-512-2250, orders@gpo.gov, http://www.access.gpo.gov.

616.98021 CHN ISSN 1002-0837
HANGTIAN YIXUE YU YIXUE GONGCHENG/SPACE MEDICINE & MEDICAL ENGINEERING. Text in Chinese. 1988. bi-m. USD 17.40; CNY 5, USD 2.90 newsstand/cover (effective 2001). **Document type:** *Academic/Scholarly.*
Related titles: Online - full content ed.: (from WanFang Data Corp.).
Indexed: Eng.Ind., Int.Aerosp.Abstr.
—Linda Hall.
Published by: Hangtian Yixue Gongcheng Yanjiusuo, 5104 Xinxiang, Beijing 100094, China. Ed. Jinhe Wei. **Dist. by:** China International Book Trading Corp, 35, Chegongzhuang Xilu, Haidian District, Beijing 100044, China. TEL 86-1-68413849, FAX 86-1-68412048, cibtc@mail.cibtc.com.cn, http://www.cibtc.com.cn.

614.85 629.1 USA ISSN 1057-5545
HUMAN FACTORS & AVIATION MEDICINE. Text in English. 1957. bi-m. USD 240 worldwide to non-members; USD 120 worldwide to members (effective 2000). bk.rev. reprint service avail. from PQC. **Document type:** *Newsletter.* **Description:** Allows specialists, researchers, and physicians to present information critical to the training, performance and health of aviation professionals.
Former titles (until vol.34, no.6, 1987): Human Factors and Aviation Medicine Bulletin (0898-5723); (until vol.34, no.4, 1987): Human Factors Bulletin
Indexed: Ref.Zh.
Published by: Flight Safety Foundation, Inc., 601 Madison St, Ste 300, Alexandria, VA 22314-1756. TEL 703-739-6700, FAX 703-739-6708. Ed. Roger Rozelle. Circ: 2,200.

THE INTERNATIONAL JOURNAL OF AVIATION PSYCHOLOGY. see *TRANSPORTATION—Air Transport*

JOURNAL OF FLOW VISUALIZATION AND IMAGE PROCESSING. see *ENGINEERING—Mechanical Engineering*

629.45 GBR
▼ **JOURNAL OF HUMAN FACTORS AND AEROSPACE SAFETY.** Text in English. 2001. q. GBP 50 to individuals; GBP 120 to institutions (effective 2002). **Document type:** *Academic/Scholarly.*
Published by: Ashgate Publishing Ltd (Subsidiary of: Gower Publishing Co. Ltd.), Gower House, Croft Rd, Aldershot, Hants GU11 3HR, United Kingdom. TEL 44-1252-331551, FAX 44-1252-317446, info@ashgate.com, http://www.ashgate.com.

ZHONGHUA HANGKONG YIXUE ZAZHI/CHINESE JOURNAL OF AVIATION MEDICINE. see *MEDICAL SCIENCES*

AERONAUTICS AND SPACE FLIGHT—Abstracting, Bibliographies, Statistics

AEROSPACE MEDICINE AND BIOLOGY; a continuing bibliography. see *MEDICAL SCIENCES—Abstracting, Bibliographies, Statistics*

AGRICULTURE

see also AGRICULTURE—Crop Production And Soil; AGRICULTURE—Dairying And Dairy Products; AGRICULTURE—Feed, Flour And Grain; AGRICULTURE—Poultry And Livestock; FOOD AND FOOD INDUSTRIES; FORESTS AND FORESTRY; GARDENING AND HORTICULTURE

344.94043 AUS ISSN 1033-9280
A Q I S BULLETIN. Text in English. 1989. m. **Document type:** *Bulletin, Government.* **Description:** Summarizes information and news from A.Q.I.S. for individuals and organizations involved in quarantine and inspection matters.
Indexed: Ind.Vet., Rev.Appl.Entomol., Rev.Plant Path.
—CISTI.
Published by: Australian Quarantine and Inspection Service, GPO. Box 858, Canberra, ACT, Australia. TEL 61-2-6272-5156, FAX 61-2-6272-4494, carson.creagh@agis.gov.au, http://www.agis.gov.au. Ed., R&P Carson Creagh. Circ: 3,000.

ACCADEMIA DELLE SCIENZE DI SIENA DETTA DE FISIOCRITICI. ATTI. see *MEDICAL SCIENCES*

AGBIOTECH NEWS AND INFORMATION. see *BIOLOGY—Abstracting, Bibliographies, Statistics*

630 USA
CODEN: BRPOEF
AGBIOTECH REPORTER; agricultural research - business. Text in English. 1984. m., latest vol.18, no.6. USD 485 domestic; USD 545 foreign; USD 265 university and government individuals. adv. tr.lit. back issues avail.; reprints avail. **Document type:** *Newsletter, Trade.* **Description:** Current scientific and business news in the specific field of agricultural biotechnology.
Former titles (until 1993): Biotech Reporter (1069-4773); AgBiotechnology News (0899-3998); Agricultural Biotechnology News (0748-822X); Agricultural Biotechnology
Related titles: Online - full text ed.
Indexed: ASCA, Biotech.Cit.Ind. (coverage dropped), Curr.Biotech.Abstr., Telegen.
—CISTI.
Published by: Freiberg Publishing Company, Inc., 2302 W First St, Box 7, Cedar, IA 50613. TEL 319-277-3599, 800-959-3276, FAX 319-277-3783, bmcchane@cfu.net, kfreiberg@cfu.net, http://www.bioreporter.com. Ed. Andrew Apel. Pub. Bill Freiberg. Adv. contact Kathy Freiberg. Circ: 1,500.

A

630 570 IND ISSN 0970-1907
CODEN: ABRSEG
AGRICULTURAL AND BIOLOGICAL RESEARCH. Text in English. 1985. s-a. INR 750, USD 100 to individuals; INR 350, USD 50 to institutions (effective 2001). adv. *Refereed.* **Document type:** *Academic/Scholarly.*
Description: An international journal on agricultural and biological research including environmental and toxicological studies.
Indexed: Food Sci.& Tech.Abstr., Zoo.Rec.
—BLDSC (0742.710000).
Published by: Young Environmentalist Association, 64 Khurshed Bagh, Lucknow, Uttar Pradesh 226 004, India. TEL 91-522-226091, FAX 91-522-682610. Ed., R&P, Adv. contact Anil Mishra. page INR 2,000. Circ: 1,000.

AGRICULTURAL & VETERINARY CHEMICALS. see *AGRICULTURE—Crop Production And Soil*

AGROFORESTRY ABSTRACTS. see *AGRICULTURE—Abstracting, Bibliographies, Statistics*

631.091 BRA ISSN 0103-3816
CODEN: AGROE5
AGROTROPICA. Text in English, French, Portuguese, Spanish; Summaries in English. 1971. 3/yr. BRL 40, USD 60 (effective 2001). index, cum.index: 1971-1975. back issues avail.
Formerly (until 1989): Revista Theobroma (0370-7962)
Indexed: Abstr.Trop.Agri., Agri.Eng.Abstr., Agrindex, Agroforest.Abstr., Bibl.Agri., Biol.Abstr., Chem.Abstr., Excerp.Med., Food Sci.& Tech.Abstr., GeoRef, Hort.Abstr., Ind.Agri.Am.Lat.Caribe, Nutr.Abstr., Plant Breed.Abstr., Protozool.Abstr., Rev.Appl.Entomol., Rev.Plant Path., Seed Abstr., Soils & Fert., Trop.Oil Seeds Abstr., World Ag.Econ.& Rur.Soc.Abstr.
—BLDSC (0771.856000), CASDDS, CISTI, ingenta, Linda Hall.
Published by: Centro de Pesquisas do Cacau/Cacao Research Center, Caixa Postal 7, Itabuna, BA 45600-970, Brazil. TEL 55-73-214-3217, 55-73-2143220, FAX 55-73-2143218, TELEX 0732157 CLRC BR, agrotrop@cepec.gov.br, http://www.cepec.gov.br/agrotrop. Eds. Miguel Moreno Ruiz, Paulo Dos Santos Terra. Circ: 650. **Co-sponsor:** Comissao Executiva do Plano da Lavoura Cacaueira.

ANIMAL BREEDING ABSTRACTS; a monthly abstract of world literature. see *AGRICULTURE—Abstracting, Bibliographies, Statistics*

BANGLADESH JOURNAL OF BIOLOGICAL SCIENCES. see *BIOLOGY*

630.091 636.089 DEU ISSN 0301-567X
CODEN: BTLVBR
BEITRAEGE ZUR TROPISCHEN LANDWIRTSCHAFT UND VETERINAERMEDIZIN. Text in English, French, German, Spanish; Summaries in English, French, German, Spanish. 1963. q. adv. bk.rev. charts, illus. **Document type:** *Academic/Scholarly.* **Description:** Contains research and communications in the fields of agrarian economy and management, agriculture and plant cultivation, soil science, animal nutrition and husbandry, veterinary hygiene, forestry and forest economics.
Formerly (until 1973): Beitraege zur Tropischen und Subtropischen Landwirtschaft und Tropen Veterinaermedizin (0005-8203)
Indexed: Agroforest.Abstr., Anim.Breed.Abstr., Biodet.Abstr., Biol.Abstr., Chem.Abstr., Chem.Indus.Notes, Chem.Titles, Curr.Adv.Ecol.Sci., Curr.Cont. (coverage dropped), Dairy Sci.Abstr., Excerp.Med., Field Crop Abstr., Food Sci.& Tech.Abstr., GeoRef, Helminthol.Abstr., Herb.Abstr., Hort.Abstr., IDA, Ind.Med. (coverage dropped), Ind.Vet., Plant Breed.Abstr., Poult.Abstr., Rev.Med.& Vet.Mycol., Rev.Plant Path., Rice Abstr., Rural Recreat.Tour.Abstr., Seed Abstr., Soils & Fert., Vet.Bull., Weed Abstr., World Ag.Econ.& Rur.Soc.Abstr.
—CASDDS, CISTI, ingenta.
Published by: (Verband der Tropenlandwirte aus Witzenhausen e.V.), Verlag der Tropenlandwirt, Steinstr 19, Witzenhausen 37213, Germany. TEL 49-5542-981216, FAX 49-5542-981313, tropen@wiz.uni-kassel.de, http://www.wiz.uni-kassel.de/trop/. Circ: 650.

BIOCONTROL NEWS AND INFORMATION. see *AGRICULTURE—Abstracting, Bibliographies, Statistics*

BIOMETEOROLOGY BULLETIN. see *METEOROLOGY*

BIOTECHNOLOGY AND GENETIC ENGINEERING REVIEWS. see *BIOLOGY—Biotechnology*

BIOTECHNOLOGY IN AGRICULTURE AND FORESTRY. see *BIOLOGY—Biotechnology*

BIOTECHNOLOGY INDUSTRY GUIDE. see *BIOLOGY*

630 570 ESP
BOLETIN DE AGRICULTURA BIOLOGICO-DINAMICA. Text in Spanish. 1986. q. ESP 954. **Document type:** *Bulletin.*
Published by: Editorial Rudolf Steiner, Guipuzcoa, 11-1 izda, Madrid 28020, Spain. TEL 34-1-2531481. Ed. Antonio Malagon Golderos.

630 570 BRA ISSN 0006-8705
SB13 CODEN: BRGTAF
BRAGANTIA. Text in English, Portuguese; Abstracts in English. 1941. s-a. BRL 30 domestic; USD 70 foreign (effective 1999). bibl, charts, illus. index. back issues avail. **Document type:** *Government, Academic/Scholarly.*
Related titles: Online - full text ed.: (from SciELO).
Indexed: Abstr.Trop.Agri., AgBiotech, Agri.Eng.Abstr., Bibl.Agri., Biol.Abstr., Chem.Abstr., Chem.Indus.Notes, Chem.Titles, Cott.& Trop.Fibr.Abstr., Ecol.Abstr., Field Crop Abstr., Forest.Abstr., Geo.Abstr.P.G., Helminthol.Abstr., Herb.Abstr., Hort.Abstr., INIS Atomind., Maize Abstr., Nutr.Abstr., Plant Breed.Abstr., Plant Gen.Res.Abstr., Plant Grow.Reg.Abstr., Postharvest, Potato Abstr., Rev.Appl.Entomol., Rev.Plant Path., Rice Abstr., Seed Abstr., Soils & Fert., Soyabean Abstr., Sugar Ind.Abstr., Triticale Abstr., Trop.Oil Seeds Abstr., VITIS, Weed Abstr.
—CASDDS, CISTI, Linda Hall.
Published by: Instituto Agronomico, Servico de Divulgacao Tecnico-Cientifica, Centro, Caixa Postal 28, Sao Paulo, SP 13001-970, Brazil. TEL 55-19-2315422, ext. 118, FAX 55-19-2314943, editor@barao.iac.br, http://www.scielo.br/. Ed. Angela M C Furlani. Circ: 1,000.

636.082 JPN
CODEN: BRSCES
BREEDING SCIENCE. Text and summaries in English. 1951. q. JPY 6,500 (effective 1999). adv. back issues avail. *Refereed.* **Document type:** *Academic/Scholarly, Abstract/Index.*
Formerly: Japanese Journal of Breeding (0536-3683)
Related titles: Online - full text ed.: (from Institute for Scientific Information).
Indexed: ASCA, AgBiotech, Biol.Abstr., Chem.Abstr., Chem.Indus.Notes, Chem.Titles, Crop Physiol.Abstr., Curr.Adv.Plant Sci., Curr.Cont., Field Crop Abstr., Food Sci.& Tech.Abstr., Forest.Abstr., Helminthol.Abstr., Hort.Abstr., INIS Atomind., Int.Abstr.Biol.Sci., Maize Abstr., Ornam.Hort., Plant Breed.Abstr., Plant Gen.Res.Abstr., Plant Grow.Reg.Abstr., Plant Sci., Postharvest, Potato Abstr., Rev.Appl.Entomol., Rev.Plant Path., Rice Abstr., SSCI (coverage dropped), Seed Abstr., Sorghum & Millets Abstr., Soyabean Abstr., Triticale Abstr., Trop.Oil Seeds Abstr., Weed Abstr.
—BLDSC (2277.716000), CASDDS, CISTI, EMDOCS, IDS, ingenta.
Published by: Japanese Society of Breeding, c/o Faculty of Agriculture, University of Tokyo, Bunkyo-ku, Tokyo 113, Japan. TEL 81-3-5841-5065, FAX 81-3-5841-5063. Ed. Masahiro Nakagahra. Pub., R&P Atsushi Hirai TEL 81-3-5841-5084. Adv. contact Ryo Ohsawa. Circ: 2,000.

630 636.089 BGR ISSN 1310-0351
BULGARIAN JOURNAL OF AGRICULTURAL SCIENCE. Text in English. 1995. 6/yr. USD 190, DEM 340 (effective 2002). **Document type:** *Journal, Academic/Scholarly.* **Description:** Includes papers covering all areas of agriculture and veterinary science. Aimed at scientific researchers in Bulgaria and abroad.
Indexed: Abstr.Hyg., AgBiotech, Agri.Eng.Abstr., Anim.Breed.Abstr., Bio-Contr.News & Info., Crop Physiol.Abstr., Dairy Sci.Abstr., Field Crop Abstr., Food Sci.& Tech.Abstr., Forest.Abstr., Helminthol.Abstr., Herb.Abstr., Hort.Abstr., INIS Atomind., Ind.Vet., Irr.& Drain.Abstr., Maize Abstr., Nutr.Abstr., Ornam.Hort., Pig News & Info., Plant Breed.Abstr., Plant Gen.Res.Abstr., Plant Grow.Reg.Abstr., Postharvest, Potato Abstr., Poult.Abstr., Rev.Appl.Entomol., Rev.Med.& Vet.Mycol., Rev.Plant Path., Rice Abstr., Seed Abstr., Soils & Fert., Soyabean Abstr., Triticale Abstr., Vet.Bull., Weed Abstr., World Ag.Econ.& Rur.Soc.Abstr.
—BLDSC (2366.686500).
Published by: Akademiia na Selskostopanskite Nauki, Tsarigradsko shose 125, bldg 1, etazh 1, rm 215, Sofia 1113, Bulgaria. TEL 359-2-704042, FAX 359-2-709127, http://www.geocities.com/PicketFence/Garden/9151/Agrisci/ABOUT.htm. Ed. Dr. Ya. Profirov.

630 PHL ISSN 0116-7847
CODEN: CJANES
C M U JOURNAL OF SCIENCE. Text in English. 1979. q. PHP 60, USD 4. back issues avail.
Formerly (until vol.9, 1987): C M U Journal of Agriculture, Food and Nutrition (0115-4931)
Indexed: Bio-Contr.News & Info., Dairy Sci.Abstr., Field Crop Abstr., Herb.Abstr., Ind.Phil.Per., Ind.Vet., Maize Abstr., Pig News & Info., Potato Abstr., Rural Recreat.Tour.Abstr., Seed Abstr., Soils & Fert., Soyabean Abstr., World Ag.Econ.& Rur.Soc.Abstr.
—CCC.
Published by: Central Mindanao University, University Town, Musuan, Bukidnon 8710, Philippines. Ed. Herminio M Pava. Circ: 350.

630 636.08 BRA ISSN 0103-8478
S191 CODEN: CIRUEP
CIENCIA RURAL. Text and summaries in English, Portuguese. 1971. bi-m. USD 30 domestic; USD 45 foreign (effective 2001). adv. bk.rev. bibl, charts, illus. *Refereed.* **Document type:** *Journal, Government.*
Formerly (until 1990, vol.20): Centro de Ciencias Rurais. Revista (0085-5901)
Indexed: Abstr.Hyg., AgBiotech, Agri.Eng.Abstr., Anim.Breed.Abstr., Bio-Contr.News & Info., Chem.Abstr., Crop Physiol.Abstr., Dairy Sci.Abstr., Field Crop Abstr., Forest Prod.Abstr., Forest.Abstr., Helminthol.Abstr., Herb.Abstr., Hort.Abstr., Ind.Vet., Irr.& Drain.Abstr., Maize Abstr., Meteor.& Geoastrophys.Abstr., Nutr.Abstr., Ornam.Hort., Pig News & Info., Plant Breed.Abstr., Plant Gen.Res.Abstr., Plant Grow.Reg.Abstr., Postharvest, Potato Abstr., Poult.Abstr., Protozool.Abstr., Rev.Appl.Entomol., Rev.Arom.& Med.Plants, Rev.Med.& Vet.Mycol., Rev.Plant Path., Rice Abstr., Seed Abstr., Soils & Fert., Soyabean Abstr., Sugar Ind.Abstr., Triticale Abstr., Vet.Bull., Weed Abstr., Wild.Rev., World Ag.Econ.& Rur.Soc.Abstr., Zoo.Rec.
—CASDDS, CISTI.
Published by: Universidade Federal de Santa Maria, Centro de Ciencias Rurais, Campus Universitario, Santa Maria, RGS 97105-900, Brazil. TEL 55-55-220-8698, FAX 55-55-220-8695, TELEX 552230 UFSM BR, rudi@ccr.ufsm.br, http://www.ufsm.br/ccr/revista/. Ed., Adv. contact Rudi Weiblen. Circ: 1,200 (controlled).

570 630 USA ISSN 1067-585X
CODEN: CORFFN
CORNELL FOCUS. Text in English. 1968. 3/yr. free per issue. charts, illus. index. **Document type:** *Academic/Scholarly.*
Former titles (until vol.20, no.4, 1991): New York's Food and Life Sciences Quarterly (0361-5367); Farm Research (0028-7938)
Indexed: Aqua.Sci.& Fish.Abstr., Biol.Abstr., Biol.Dig., Dairy Sci.Abstr., Environ.Abstr., Environ.Ind., Environ.Sci.Poll.Mgmt., Field Crop Abstr., Food Sci.& Tech.Abstr., Herb.Abstr., Hort.Abstr., Irr.& Drain.Abstr., Nutr.Abstr., Plant Breed.Abstr., Pollut.Abstr., Potato Abstr., Rev.Plant Path., Rural Recreat.Tour.Abstr., Saf.Sci.Abstr., Sel.Water Res.Abstr., Soils & Fert., Sport Fish.Abstr., Weed Abstr., Wild.Rev., World Ag.Econ.& Rur.Soc.Abstr.
—BLDSC (3470.942400), CISTI, ingenta, Linda Hall.
Published by: Cornell University, Agricultural Experiment Station, 1150 Comstock Hall, College of Agriculture & Life Sciences, Ithaca, NY 14853. TEL 607-255-1876, FAX 607-255-9873. Ed. Elizabeth Bauman. Circ: 5,000 (controlled).

028.1 USA ISSN 1098-4399
E-STREAMS (CONTOOCOOK); electronic reviews of science and technology references covering engineering, agriculture, medicine and science. Text in English. 1998. m. free per issue. bk.rev. back issues avail. **Document type:** *Academic/Scholarly.*
Media: Online - full text. **Related titles:** Online - full text ed.
Published by: Yankee Book Peddler, Inc., 999 Maple St, Contoocook, NH 03229. TEL 603-746-3102, FAX 603-746-5628, estreams@ybp.com, http://www.e-streams.com. Ed. H Robert Malinowsky. Pub. Glen Secor. R&P Jennifer Goodrich.

630 570 COL ISSN 0304-2847
S15
FACULTAD NACIONAL DE AGRONOMIA MEDELLIN. REVISTA. Key Title: Revista Facultad Nacional de Agronomia. Text in English; Summaries in English, Spanish. 1939. s-a. COP 15,000 domestic; USD 20 foreign (effective 2000). cum.index: 1939-1981. back issues avail. **Document type:** *Academic/Scholarly.*

Indexed: Agri.Eng.Abstr., Anim.Breed.Abstr., Bio-Contr.News & Info., Biol.Abstr., Field Crop Abstr., Forest.Abstr., Helminthol.Abstr., Herb.Abstr., Hort.Abstr., Irr.& Drain.Abstr., Nutr.Abstr., Plant Breed.Abstr., Poult.Abstr., Rev.Appl.Entomol., Rev.Plant Path., Seed Abstr., Soils & Fert., Sugar Ind.Abstr., World Ag.Econ.& Rur.Soc.Abstr.
—Linda Hall.
Published by: Universidad Nacional de Colombia, Facultad de Ciencias Agropecuarias, Apartado 568, Medellin, Colombia. TEL 57-4-2607333 ext 106, FAX 57-4-2300420, rvergara@perseus.unalmed.edu.co. Ed. Miryam Ospina. Circ: 700 (controlled).

FOOD STRUCTURE. see *NUTRITION AND DIETETICS*

GAMMA FIELD SYMPOSIA. see *BIOLOGY—Biophysics*

630 636 VEN ISSN 0046-5399
GANAGRINCO; ganaderia - agricultura - industria - comercio. Text in Spanish; Summaries in English, Spanish. q. USD 6. adv. illus, charts.
Address: Ed. Rafael Salom, Apdo. de Correos 3318, Caracas 101, Venezuela. Circ: 2,000.

GARDEN TO KITCHEN NEWSLETTER. see *NUTRITION AND DIETETICS*

GINSENG REVIEW. see *PHARMACY AND PHARMACOLOGY*

630 300 636.089 IND ISSN 0379-4008
HARYANA AGRICULTURAL UNIVERSITY. JOURNAL OF RESEARCH. Text in English. 1971. q. INR 200, USD 60. adv. abstr, bibl, charts. **Document type:** *Academic/Scholarly.* **Description:** Contains original research articles and notes on agriculture, animal and veterinary sciences, basic sciences, social sciences and home science.
Indexed: Agroforest.Abstr., Biol.Abstr., Chem.Abstr., Chem.Indus.Notes, Chem.Titles, Cott.& Trop.Fibr.Abstr., Dairy Sci.Abstr., Field Crop Abstr., Food Sci.& Tech.Abstr., Helminthol.Abstr., Hort.Abstr., Ind.Vet., Maize Abstr., Nutr.Abstr., Ornam.Hort., Pig News & Info., Plant Breed.Abstr., Plant Grow.Reg.Abstr., Postharvest, Potato Abstr., Rev.Appl.Entomol., Rev.Plant Path., Rice Abstr., Rural Devel.Abstr., Seed Abstr., Soils & Fert., Sorghum & Millets Abstr., Triticale Abstr., Vet.Bull., Weed Abstr., World Ag.Econ.& Rur.Soc.Abstr., Zoo.Rec.
Published by: Haryana Agricultural University, Hisar, Haryana 125 004, India. Circ: 500.

HEALTHY HARVEST. see *PUBLIC HEALTH AND SAFETY*

HEBREW UNIVERSITY OF JERUSALEM. AUTHORITY FOR RESEARCH AND DEVELOPMENT. CURRENT RESEARCH. see *MEDICAL SCIENCES*

630 IND ISSN 0970-0595
CODEN: HJARAN
HIMACHAL JOURNAL OF AGRICULTURAL RESEARCH. Text and summaries in English. 1971. s-a. INR 75, INR 100 to institutional members (effective 2000). adv. bk.rev. *Refereed.* **Description:** Publishes research on agricultural, veterinary, animal and home sciences.
Indexed: Agri.Eng.Abstr., Anim.Breed.Abstr., Bio-Contr.News & Info., Biol.Abstr., Dairy Sci.Abstr., Field Crop Abstr., Herb.Abstr., Hort.Abstr., Indian Sci.Abstr., Maize Abstr., Nutr.Abstr., Postharvest, Rev.Appl.Entomol., Rev.Plant Path., Seed Abstr., Soils & Fert., Sugar Ind.Abstr., Triticale Abstr., Weed Abstr.
Published by: H.P. Agriculture University, Himachal Pradesh Krishi Vishvavidyalaya, c/o Hirday Paul Singh, Directorat of Research, Palanpur, Himachal Pradesh 176 062, India. TEL 91-189-30406, FAX 91-1894-30511, dr@hpkv.hp.nic.in. Ed. Hirday Paul Singh. Circ: 300 (paid).

HOKKAIDO KYOIKU DAIGAKU KIYO. DAI-2-BU, B. SEIBUTSUGAKU, CHIGAKU, NOGAKU-HEN/ HOKKAIDO UNIVERSITY OF EDUCATION. JOURNAL. SECTION 2 B. BIOLOGY, GEOLOGY, AND AGRICULTURE. see *BIOLOGY*

INDONESIAN BIOLOGICAL AND AGRICULTURAL INDEX/INDEKS BIOLOGI DAN PERTANIAN DE INDONESIA. see *AGRICULTURE—Abstracting, Bibliographies, Statistics*

INSTITUTE OF AGRICULTURE AND ANIMAL SCIENCE. JOURNAL. see *VETERINARY SCIENCE*

630 IND ISSN 0021-3713
J N K V V NEWS. Text in English. 1967. q. free per issue.
Published by: Jawaharlal Nehru Krishi Vishwa Vidyalaya, c/o Information and Public Relations Office, Jabalpur, Madhya Pradesh 482 004, India. Ed. S D N Tiwari. Circ: 1,100.

363.11963 USA ISSN 1074-7583
S565 CODEN: JASHFD
JOURNAL OF AGRICULTURAL SAFETY AND HEALTH. Text in English. 1995. q. USD 83 domestic to non-members; USD 90 foreign to non-members; USD 44 domestic to members; USD 49 foreign to members (effective 2001). bk.rev., video rev. abstr, illus. index. reprints avail. *Refereed.* **Document type:** *Trade.* **Description:** Focuses on the unique needs and concerns of safety and health as they relate to agriculture.
Indexed: Abstr.Hyg., Agri.Eng.Abstr., Agricola, Aqua.Sci.& Fish.Abstr., Dairy Sci.Abstr., Eng.Ind., Environ.Sci.Poll.Mgmt., Ergon.Abstr., Ind.Med., Pig News & Info., Pollut.Abstr., Postharvest, Potato Abstr., Rev.Appl.Entomol., Rev.Med.& Vet.Mycol., Rev.Plant Path., Risk Abstr., Saf.Sci.Abstr., Tox.Abstr., Weed Abstr., World Ag.Econ.& Rur.Soc.Abstr.
—BLDSC (4922.980000), CISTI, ingenta. **CCC.**
Published by: American Society of Agricultural Engineers, 2950, Niles, MI 49085-9659. TEL 616-429-0300, FAX 616-429-3852, hq@asae.org, http://asae.org. Ed. Pamela Devore Hansen. R&P Sandy Rutter. Circ: 400.

JOURNAL OF AGROMEDICINE; interface of human health & agriculture. see *OCCUPATIONAL HEALTH AND SAFETY*

JOURNAL OF ENVIRONMENTAL SCIENCE AND HEALTH. PART B: PESTICIDES, FOOD CONTAMINANTS, AND AGRICULTURAL WASTES. see *ENVIRONMENTAL STUDIES*

JOURNAL OF GINSENG RESEARCH. see *PHARMACY AND PHARMACOLOGY*

JOURNAL OF RANGE MANAGEMENT; covering the study, management, and use of rangeland ecosystems and range resources. see *BIOLOGY*

630 570 JPN ISSN 0452-2370
CODEN: KNGKAP
KOBE UNIVERSITY. FACULTY OF AGRICULTURE. SCIENCE REPORTS. Text in English, Japanese; Summaries in English. 1953. a. per issue exchange basis.
Indexed: Agri.Eng.Abstr., Anim.Breed.Abstr., Bio-Contr.News & Info., Biol.Abstr., Dairy Sci.Abstr., Field Crop Abstr., Food Sci.& Tech.Abstr., Forest Prod.Abstr., Forest.Abstr., Hort.Abstr., Nutr.Abstr., Plant Breed.Abstr., Plant Grow.Reg.Abstr., Ref.Zh., Rice Abstr., Wild.Rev., Zoo.Rec.
—BLDSC (8152.377000), CASDDS, CISTI.
Published by: Kobe Daigaku, Nogakubu/Kobe University, Faculty of Agriculture, 1 Rokko-Dai-cho, Nada-ku, Kobe-shi, Hyogo-ken 657-0013, Japan. FAX 078-871-8450. Circ: 800.

630 570 JPN ISSN 0389-0473
CODEN: KDGHBF
KOCHI DAIGAKU GAKUJUTSU KENKYU HOKOKU. NOGAKU/KOCHI UNIVERSITY. AGRICULTURAL SCIENCE. RESEARCH REPORTS. Text in English, Japanese; Summaries in English. 1952. a. free per issue. **Document type:** *Bulletin.*
Supersedes in part (in 1969): Kochi Daigaku Gakujutsu Kenkyu Hokoku. Shizen Kagaku 2 (0389-0236); Which superseded in part (in 1961): Kochi Daigaku Gakujutsu Kenkyu Hokoku (0452-246X)
Indexed: Biol.Abstr., GeoRef, Helminthol.Abstr., Hort.Abstr., Ornam.Hort., Rev.Plant Path.
—BLDSC (7762.399500), CASDDS.
Published by: Kochi Daigaku/Kochi University, 5-1 Akebono-cho 2-chome, Kochi-shi, Kochi-ken 780-8520, Japan. TEL 0888-44-0111, FAX 0888-64-5200.

630.711 636.089 DNK ISSN 0109-4998
KONGELIGE VETERINAER- OG LANDBOHOEJSKOLE. HAANDBOG. Text in Danish. 1982. a. DKK 30.
Formerly: Haandbog for Studerende ved Landbohoejskolen
Published by: Kongelige Veterinaer- og Landbohoejskole, Studerendes Raad, Copenhagen, Denmark. Ed. B Rasmussen. Circ: 1,500.

630 DEU ISSN 0023-9917
LEBENDIGE ERDE; Zeitschrift fuer Biologisch-Dynamische Wirtschaftsweise. Text in German. 1950. bi-m. DEM 45; DEM 50 foreign. adv. bk.rev. **Document type:** *Academic/Scholarly.*
Indexed: Ref.Zh.
Published by: Forschungsring fuer Biologisch-Dynamische Wirtschaftsweise e.V., Brandschneise 2, Darmstadt 64295, Germany. TEL 49-6155-84123, FAX 49-6155-846911. Adv. contact Birgit Johannssen. page DEM 620; trim 195 x 135. Circ: 8,500.

630 CAN ISSN 0848-8851
N B I A NEWSLETTER. Text in English, French. 1989. q. free per issue. bk.rev. back issues avail. **Document type:** *Newsletter.* **Description:** For professional agrologists in Atlantic Canada.
Published by: New Brunswick Institute of Agrologists, P O Box 20280, Fredericton, NB E3B 4Z7, Canada. TEL 506-452-3260, FAX 506-452-3316. Ed. Dr. Warren K Coleman. Circ: 200 (controlled).

630 570 JPN ISSN 1342-6648
NATIONAL INSTITUTE OF AGRO-ENVIRONMENTAL SCIENCES. ANNUAL REPORT. Text in English. 1995. a.
—Linda Hall.
Published by: National Institute for Agro-Environmental Sciences/Nogyo Kankyo Gijutsu Kenkyusho, 3-1-3 Kannondai, Tsukuba 305-8604, Japan. TEL 81-298-38-8148, FAX 81-298-38-8199.

630 FRA ISSN 0182-7146
NATURE ET PROGRES. Text in French. 1964. bi-m. FRF 190; FRF 27 newsstand/cover (effective 1998). adv. **Description:** Provides a forum to discuss the environment, agriculture and health issues.
Published by: Association Europeenne d'Agriculture et d'Hygiene Biologiques, 14, rue de Goncourt, Paris 75011, France. TEL 33-4-90310042, FAX 33-4-90324391, http://www.euronature.com. Ed. Didier Dillen. Pub., Adv. contact Marc Durand.

630 570 JPN ISSN 0911-9450
CODEN: NKGHEW
NOGYO KANKYO GIJUTSU KENKYUSHO HOKOKU/NATIONAL INSTITUTE OF AGRO-ENVIRONMENTAL SCIENCES. BULLETIN. Text in English, Japanese; Summaries in English. 1986. irreg. free per issue. back issues avail. **Document type:** *Bulletin, Academic/Scholarly.*
Indexed: Chem.Abstr., Chem.Indus.Notes, Chem.Titles, Ref.Zh., VITIS, Zoo.Rec.
—BLDSC (2640.020000), CASDDS, CISTI, Linda Hall.
Published by: National Institute for Agro-Environmental Sciences/Nogyo Kankyo Gijutsu Kenkyusho, 3-1-3 Kannondai, Tsukuba 305-8604, Japan. TEL 81-298-38-8148, FAX 81-298-38-8199. Circ: 1,700.

NUCLEUS. see *ENERGY—Nuclear Energy*

NUTRITION SOCIETY OF INDIA. PROCEEDINGS. see *NUTRITION AND DIETETICS*

630 PAK ISSN 1015-3055
SB610
PAKISTAN JOURNAL OF AGRICULTURE, AGRICULTURAL ENGINEERING AND VETERINARY SCIENCES. Text in English. 1985. s-a. USD 50 (effective 1998). adv. back issues avail. **Document type:** *Academic/Scholarly.* **Description:** Original research papers in agricultural and veterinary sciences, including agricultural engineering.
Indexed: Ecol.Abstr., IDA.
Published by: Sindh Agriculture University, Tandojam 70050, Pakistan. TEL 92-2233-5869, FAX 92-2233-5300. Ed., R&P Dr. Bherulal Devrajani TEL 92-2233-5460. Circ: 1,000.

630 BRA ISSN 0100-204X
CODEN: PEABBT
PESQUISA AGROPECUARIA BRASILEIRA/BRAZILIAN JOURNAL OF AGRICULTURAL RESEARCH. Text in Portuguese; Abstracts in English. 1966. m. BRL 48, USD 180 (effective 2000). adv. bk.rev. abstr, charts, illus. back issues avail. *Refereed.* **Document type:** *Academic/Scholarly.*
Formerly (until 1978): Pesquisa Agropecuaria. Serie Agronomia; Incorporates (in 1978): Pesquisa Agropecuaria Brasileira. Serie Veterinaria-Zootecnia; Which was formed by the 1977 merger of: Pesquisa Agropecuaria Brasileira. Serie Veterinaria; Pesquisa Agropecuaria Brasileira. Serie Zootenia
Related titles: Online - full text ed.: (from Institute for Scientific Information).

Indexed: ASCA, AgBiotech, Agri.Eng.Abstr., Agroforest.Abstr., Anim.Breed.Abstr., Bio-Contr.News & Info., Biol.Abstr., Cadscan, Chem.Abstr., Cott.& Trop.Fibr.Abstr., Crop Physiol.Abstr., Curr.Adv.Ecol.Sci., Curr.Cont., Dairy Sci.Abstr., Field Crop Abstr., Food Sci.& Tech.Abstr., Forest.Abstr., GeoRef, Helminthol.Abstr., Herb.Abstr., Hort.Abstr., INIS Atomind., Ind.Vet., Irr.& Drain.Abstr., Lead Abstr., Maize Abstr., Nutr.Abstr., Ornam.Hort., Pig News & Info., Plant Breed.Abstr., Plant Gen.Res.Abstr., Plant Grow.Reg.Abstr., Postharvest, Potato Abstr., Poult.Abstr., Rev.Appl.Entomol., Rev.Arom.& Med.Plants, Rev.Med.& Vet.Mycol., Rev.Plant Path., Rice Abstr., Risk Abstr., Rural Devel.Abstr., Seed Abstr., Soils & Fert., Sorghum & Millets Abstr., Soyabean Abstr., Sugar Ind.Abstr., Triticale Abstr., Trop.Oil Seeds Abstr., Vet.Bull., Weed Abstr., World Ag.Econ.& Rur.Soc.Abstr., Zincscan, Zoo.Rec.
—BLDSC (6428.230000), CASDDS, CINDOC, CISTI, IDS.
Published by: Empresa Brasileira de Pesquisa Agropecuaria, Servico de Producao e Informacao, Z Industrial (Guara), Caixa Postal 040315, Brasilia, DF 71204-970, Brazil. TEL 55-61-2739616, FAX 55-61-3405483, pab@spi.imbrapa.br. Ed. Allert Rosa Suhet. Adv. contact Lucio Brunale. Circ: 1,600 (controlled).

PHILIPPINE JOURNAL OF VETERINARY AND ANIMAL SCIENCES. see *VETERINARY SCIENCE*

PLANT BREEDING ABSTRACTS. see *AGRICULTURE—Abstracting, Bibliographies, Statistics*

PLANT CELL, TISSUE AND ORGAN CULTURE; an international journal on in vitro culture of higher plants. see *BIOLOGY—Cytology And Histology*

630 663 664 HRV ISSN 0352-1753
PODRAVKA; znanstveno-strucni casopis. Text in Croatian; Summaries in English. 1983. s-a. USD 10. back issues avail.
Indexed: Nutr.Abstr.
Published by: R.O. Istrazivanja i Razvoj, Marinkoivca 32, Koprivnica 43300, Croatia. TEL 043-827-144, FAX 043-827-169, TELEX 23348 YU POD KC. Ed. Ante Babic. Circ: 1,000.

POSTHARVEST BIOLOGY AND TECHNOLOGY. see *BIOLOGY—Biotechnology*

630 BRA ISSN 0034-737X
S15 CODEN: RCERA2
REVISTA CERES; orgao de divulgacao tecnico-cientifica em ciencias agrarias. Text in English, Portuguese, Spanish; Summaries in English. 1939. bi-m. USD 40 (effective 2002). abstr, bibl, charts, illus. index. back issues avail. *Refereed.* **Document type:** *Journal, Academic/Scholarly.* **Description:** Publishes research papers on agriculture and related fields.
Formerly (until 1944): Ceres (0366-5798)
Indexed: Agri.Eng.Abstr., Agroforest.Abstr., Anim.Breed.Abstr., Bio-Contr.News & Info., Biol.Abstr., Chem.Abstr., Chem.Indus.Notes, Chem.Titles, Crop Physiol.Abstr., Dairy Sci.Abstr., Field Crop Abstr., Food Sci.& Tech.Abstr., Forest.Abstr., Helminthol.Abstr., Herb.Abstr., Hort.Abstr., INIS Atomind., Irr.& Drain.Abstr., Maize Abstr., Nutr.Abstr., Plant Breed.Abstr., Plant Grow.Reg.Abstr., Postharvest, Poult.Abstr., Ref.Zh., Rev.Appl.Entomol., Rev.Arom.& Med.Plants, Rev.Plant Path., Rice Abstr., Seed Abstr., Soils & Fert., Soyabean Abstr., Sport Fish.Abstr., Sugar Ind.Abstr., Triticale Abstr., Weed Abstr., Wild.Rev., World Ag.Econ.& Rur.Soc.Abstr., Zoo.Rec.
—BLDSC (7848.000000), CASDDS, CINDOC, CISTI, Linda Hall.
Published by: Universidade Federal de Vicosa, Vicosa, MG 36570-000, Brazil. TEL 55-31-8992136, FAX 55-31-8992205, ceres@mail.ufv.br. Ed. Clibas Vieira. Circ: 1,100 (controlled).

636.082 POL ISSN 0137-1657
CODEN: RNZOD8
ROCZNIKI NAUKOWE ZOOTECHNIKI/ANNALS OF ANIMAL SCIENCE. Text in English, Polish; Summaries in English, German, Polish, Russian. 1974. q. USD 70 (effective 1998). back issues avail. **Document type:** *Academic/Scholarly.* **Description:** Covers breeding, feeding and feed science, technology, ethology and animal production economics.
Related titles: CD-ROM ed.; Online - full text ed.
Indexed: AgBiotech, Agri.Eng.Abstr., AgroLibrex, Anim.Breed.Abstr., Biol.Abstr., Dairy Sci.Abstr., Food Sci.& Tech.Abstr., Herb.Abstr., Ind.Vet., Maize Abstr., Nutr.Abstr., Pig News & Info., Plant Breed.Abstr., Postharvest, Poult.Abstr., Seed Abstr., Soils & Fert., Soyabean Abstr., Sport Fish.Abstr., Sugar Ind.Abstr., Triticale Abstr., Vet.Bull., Wild.Rev., World Ag.Econ.& Rur.Soc.Abstr.
—BLDSC (8015.703000), CASDDS, CISTI.
Published by: Instytut Zootechniki/Institute of Animal Production, Ul Sarego 2, Krakow 31047, Poland. TEL 48-12-2856777, FAX 48-12-2856733, TELEX PL 0322304 ZOOT, alaszczk@izoo.krakow.pl, http://saturn.ci.uw.edu.pl/psjc; http:/ciuw.warman.net.pl/alf/psjc. Ed. Andrzej Laszczka. R&P Danuta Rymut. Circ: 450.

SEOUL NATIONAL UNIVERSITY. FACULTY PAPERS. BIOLOGY AND AGRICULTURE SERIES. see *BIOLOGY*

630 639.2 636.089 SGP ISSN 0129-6485
S322.S55 CODEN: SJPIDP
SINGAPORE JOURNAL OF PRIMARY INDUSTRIES. Text in English. 1973. a. SGD 15 (effective 1999). adv. back issues avail.
Indexed: Anim.Breed.Abstr., Biol.Abstr., Chem.Abstr., Helminthol.Abstr., Hort.Abstr., Ind.Vet., Nutr.Abstr., Ornam.Hort., Pig News & Info., Plant Grow.Reg.Abstr., Poult.Abstr., Protozool.Abstr., Rev.Appl.Entomol., Rev.Plant Path., Soils & Fert., Sport Fish.Abstr., VITIS, Vet.Bull.
—BLDSC (8285.464000), CASDDS, CISTI.
Published by: Ministry of National Development, Primary Production Department, National Development Bldg, 5 Maxwell Rd 03-00, Singapore 069110, Singapore. FAX 65-2206068, TELEX RS-28851-PPD. Ed. Tan Hock Seng. Circ: 500.

630 SVN ISSN 0350-1655
SODOBNO KMETIJSTVO. Text in Slovenian. 1950. m. SIT 1,584, USD 107. adv.
Formerly: Socialisticno Kmetijstvo
Indexed: AgBiotech, Agri.Eng.Abstr., Anim.Breed.Abstr., Bio-Contr.News & Info., Crop Physiol.Abstr., Dairy Sci.Abstr., Field Crop Abstr., Forest.Abstr., Helminthol.Abstr., Herb.Abstr., Hort.Abstr., Ind.Vet., Irr.& Drain.Abstr., Maize Abstr., Nutr.Abstr., Ornam.Hort., Pig News & Info., Plant Breed.Abstr., Plant Gen.Res.Abstr., Plant Grow.Reg.Abstr., Postharvest, Potato Abstr., Poult.Abstr., Rev.Appl.Entomol., Rev.Plant Path., Russ.Acad.Sci.Bibl., Seed Abstr., Soils & Fert., Triticale Abstr., Vet.Bull., Weed Abstr., World Ag.Econ.& Rur.Soc.Abstr.
Published by: C Z P Kmecki Glas, Celovska 43, Box 47, Ljubljana 61001, Slovenia. TEL 061-328670, FAX 061-321-651. Ed. Rajko Ocepek. Circ: 1,000.

UNIVERSITATEA DIN CRAIOVA. ANALE. SERIA: BIOLOGIE, AGRONOMIE, HORTICULTURA. see *BIOLOGY*

630 636.089 TZA
UNIVERSITY OF DAR ES SALAAM. FACULTY OF AGRICULTURE, FORESTRY AND VETERINARY SCIENCE. ANNUAL RECORD OF RESEARCH. Text in English. 1979. a. USD 6. **Document type:** *Academic/Scholarly.*
Published by: Sokoine University of Agriculture, PO Box 3022, Mzumbe-morogoro, Tanzania. Ed. M Mgheni. Circ: 1,000.

630 570 JPN ISSN 1344-848X
S19 CODEN: BSKBAM
UNIVERSITY OF OSAKA PREFECTURE. COLLEGE OF AGRICULTURE. SCIENTIFIC REPORT. Text in Multiple languages. 1951. a. per issue exchange basis. **Document type:** *Academic/Scholarly.*
Former titles (until 1999): University of Osaka Prefecture. Bulletin. Series B: Agriculture and Life Sciences (1342-3266); (until 1997): University of Osaka Prefecture. Series B Agriculture and Life Sciences Bulletin (1342-4548); (until 1993): University of Osaka Prefecture. Bulletin. Series B: Agriculture and Biology (0366-3353); (until 1953): Naniwa University. Bulletin. Series B: Agricultural and Natural Science (0474-7852)
Indexed: Biol.Abstr., Chem.Abstr., Chem.Indus.Notes, Chem.Titles, Crop Physiol.Abstr., Field Crop Abstr., GeoRef, Hort.Abstr., INIS Atomind., Ind.Vet., Irr.& Drain.Abstr., Ornam.Hort., Plant Breed.Abstr., Plant Gen.Res.Abstr., Plant Grow.Reg.Abstr., Postharvest, Poult.Abstr., Rev.Appl.Entomol., Rev.Arom.& Med.Plants, Rev.Plant Path., Rice Abstr., Rural Recreat.Tour.Abstr., Sel.Water Res.Abstr., Soils & Fert., Vet.Bull., Weed Abstr., Zoo.Rec.
—BLDSC (8195.695000), CASDDS, CISTI.
Published by: University of Osaka Prefecture/Osaka-furitsu Daigaku, 1-1 Gakuen-cho, Sakai-shi, Osaka 593, Japan. TEL 0722-52-1161, FAX 0722-52-6798.

AGRICULTURE—Abstracting, Bibliographies, Statistics

AGBIOTECH NEWS AND INFORMATION. see *BIOLOGY—Abstracting, Bibliographies, Statistics*

016.63 GBR ISSN 0952-1453
AGROFORESTRY ABSTRACTS. Text in English. 1988. q. GBP 185, USD 365 (effective 2001). Index. **Document type:** *Abstract/Index.* **Description:** Covers all aspects of agroforestry. Includes agroforestry components and processes - trees, animals and crops; production, service, conservation, human ecology, and social and economic aspects; development issues; research and methodology.
Media: Online - full text. **Related titles:** CD-ROM ed.
Published by: (International Council for Research in Agroforestry (ICRAF)), CABI Publishing, Wallingford, Oxon OX10 8DE, United Kingdom. TEL 44-1491-832111, FAX 44-1491-829198, publishing@cabi.org. Ed. R E H Haynes. **U.S. subscr. to:** 10 E 40th St, Ste 3203, New York, NY 10016. TEL 212-481-7018, FAX 212-686-7993.

016.63 GBR ISSN 0003-3499
SF1
ANIMAL BREEDING ABSTRACTS; a monthly abstract of world literature. Text in English. 1933. m. GBP 695 to institutions; USD 1,240 in the Americas to institutions; GBP 710 to institutions includes single site internet access; USD 1,260 in the Americas to institutions includes single site internet access (effective 2002). adv. bk.rev. abstr. index. back issues avail.; reprint service avail. from SCH,PSC. **Document type:** *Abstract/Index.* **Description:** Covers animal breeding, genetics, reproduction, and production; includes research about immunogenetics, genetic engineering, and fertility improvement.
Related titles: Online - full text ed.: GBP 610 to institutions; USD 1,140 in the Americas to institutions (effective 2002) (from DIMDI, The Dialog Corporation, S T N International).
—BLDSC (0903.000000), Linda Hall.
Published by: CABI Publishing, Wallingford, Oxon OX10 8DE, United Kingdom. TEL 44-1491-832111, FAX 44-1491-829198, publishing@cabi.org, http://www.cabi.org/Publishing/Products/Journals/Abstract/ABA/Index.asp#a. Adv. contact S Harris. B&W page GBP 125; 170 x 267. Circ: 1,400. **U.S. subscr. to:** 10 E 40th St, Ste 3203, New York, NY 10016. TEL 212-481-7018, FAX 212-686-7993.

016.63 GBR ISSN 0143-1404
BIOCONTROL NEWS AND INFORMATION. Text in English. 1980. q. GBP 250 Includes single site Internet access; USD 435 in the Americas Includes single site Internet access; GBP 260 For Internet only; USD 455 in the Americas For Internet only (effective 2001). reprints avail. **Document type:** *Abstract/Index.*
Related titles: Online - full text ed.: (from DIMDI, The Dialog Corporation, S T N International, EBSCO Publishing).
Indexed: Helminthol.Abstr., Hort.Abstr., Rev.Appl.Entomol., Rev.Plant Path., Weed Abstr., Zoo.Rec.
—BLDSC (2071.100000), CISTI, Infotrieve, ingenta. **CCC.**
Published by: CABI Publishing, Wallingford, Oxon OX10 8DE, United Kingdom. TEL 44-1491-832111, FAX 44-1491-829198, publishing@cabi.org, http://www.cabi.org. **US subscr. to:** 10 E 40th St, Ste 3203, New York, NY 10016. TEL 212-481-7018, FAX 212-686-7993.

BIOLOGICAL & AGRICULTURAL INDEX. see *BIOLOGY—Abstracting, Bibliographies, Statistics*

016.632954 USA
CODEN: CSHEFW
C A SELECTS. HERBICIDES. Text in English. s-w. USD 250 to non-members; USD 75 to members (effective 1999). **Document type:** *Abstract/Index.* **Description:** Covers preparation, mechanism of action, and effects of herbicides; plant growth inhibitors and defoliants.
Former titles: C A Selects Plus. Herbicides (1084-0060); C A Selects. Herbicides (0160-9084)
Published by: Chemical Abstracts Service (Subsidiary of: American Chemical Society), 2540 Olentangy River Rd, Box 3012, Columbus, OH 43210-0012. TEL 614-447-3600, 800-753-4227, FAX 614-447-3751.

016.6329517 USA CODEN: CSPIFG
C A SELECTS. INSECTICIDES. Text in English. s-w. USD 250 to non-members; USD 75 to members (effective 1999). **Document type:** *Abstract/Index.* **Description:** Covers preparation, mechanism of action, and effects of insecticides; insect control and repellants.
Former titles: C A Selects Plus. Insecticides (1084-2373); C A Selects. Insecticides (0160-9092)
Published by: Chemical Abstracts Service (Subsidiary of: American Chemical Society), 2540 Olentangy River Rd, Box 3012, Columbus, OH 43210-0012. TEL 614-447-3600, 800-753-4227, FAX 614-447-3751.

016.57 IDN
INDONESIAN BIOLOGICAL AND AGRICULTURAL INDEX/INDEKS BIOLOGI DAN PERTANIAN DE INDONESIA. Text in English, Indonesian. 1969. bi-m. free per issue.
Former titles (until 1980): Index of Biology, Agriculture and Agro Economy (0216-0803); Indonesian Biological and Agricultural Index (0019-3593)
Indexed: Biol.& Agr.Ind. (coverage dropped).
Published by: National Library for Agricultural Science, Jalan Ir. Haji Juanda 20, Bogor, Indonesia. Ed. Sulastuti Sophia. Circ: 1,500.

016.6331 GBR ISSN 0309-135X
SF95
NUTRITION ABSTRACTS AND REVIEWS. SERIES B: LIVESTOCK FEEDS AND FEEDING. Text in English. 1931. m. GBP 540, USD 930 (effective 2000). back issues avail.; reprint service avail. from SCH,PSC. **Document type:** *Abstract/Index.* **Description:** Covers the analysis, technology, and biochemistry of feeds.
Supersedes in part: Nutrition Abstracts and Reviews (0029-6619)
Related titles: Online - full text ed.: (from DIMDI, The Dialog Corporation, S T N International).
Indexed: Dairy Sci.Abstr., Herb.Abstr., Maize Abstr., Nutr.Abstr., Pig News & Info.
—CISTI, Linda Hall. **CCC.**
Published by: CABI Publiching, Wallingford, Oxon OX10 8DE, United Kingdom. TEL 44-1491-832111, FAX 44-1491-829198, publishing@cabi.org, http://www.cabi.org. **U.S. subscr. to:** 10 E 40th St, Ste 3203, New York, NY 10016. TEL 212-481-7018, 800-528-4841, FAX 212-686-7993, cabi-nao@cabi.org.

016.63152 GBR ISSN 0032-0803
PLANT BREEDING ABSTRACTS. Text in English. 1930. m. GBP 1,095 Includes single site Internet access; USD 1,915 in the Americas Includes single site Internet access; GBP 1,120, USD 1,950 For Internet access only (effective 2001). adv. bk.rev. abstr. index. reprint service avail. from SCH,PSC. **Document type:** *Abstract/Index.* **Description:** Covers world literature on crop breeding and genetics. All species of economic importance are included.
Related titles: Online - full text ed.: (from DIMDI, The Dialog Corporation, S T N International).
Indexed: Russ.Acad.Sci.Bibl.
—BLDSC (6514.000000).
Published by: CABI Publishing, Wallingford, Oxon OX10 8DE, United Kingdom. TEL 44-1491-832111, FAX 44-1491-829198, publishing@cabi.org, http://www.cabi.org. Ed. S Harris. **US subscr. to:** 10 E 40th St, Ste 3203, New York, NY 10016. TEL 212-481-7018, 800-528-4841, FAX 212-686-7993, cabi-nao@cabi.org.

AGRICULTURE—Crop Production And Soil

see also AGRICULTURE—Feed, Flour And Grain; GARDENING AND HORTICULTURE; TOBACCO

631.8 GBR ISSN 0140-0657
AGRICULTURAL & VETERINARY CHEMICALS. Text in English. 1960. bi-m. GBP 25, USD 70 domestic; GBP 35 overseas. adv. bk.rev. charts, illus. **Document type:** *Newsletter.* **Description:** Covers news of interest to research chemists, managers of research stations, and converters and formulators of agricultural and veterinary chemicals.
Formerly (until no.26): Agricultural and Veterinary Chemicals and Agricultural Engineering (0002-1377)
Indexed: Chem.Abstr.
—CCC.
Published by: Chandler Publications Ltd., 187 Drury Ln, London WC2B 5QD, United Kingdom. Ed., Pub. Jack R.D. Heming. Circ: 2,000.

363.78 USA ISSN 8756-971X
RA640 CODEN: JAMAET
AMERICAN MOSQUITO CONTROL ASSOCIATION. JOURNAL. Text in English. 1940. q. USD 110 (effective 2002). adv. bk.rev. abstr, bibl, charts, illus. index. *Refereed.* **Description:** Provides information on the biology and control of mosquitoes and other vectors which affect the health of man and animals; the prevention of vector-borne disease and protection of human and animal health, with concern toward protection of the environment.
Incorporates (1969-1995): Mosquito Systematics (0091-3669); Supersedes (in 1985): Mosquito News (0027-142X)
Related titles: Microform ed.: 1940 (from PMC); Online - full text ed.: (from Institute for Scientific Information); Supplement: American Mosquito Control Association. Journal. Supplement. ISSN 1046-3607. 1988.
Indexed: AIDS & Cancer Res., ASCA, Abstr.Hyg., Agri.& Environ.Biotech.Abstr. (coverage dropped), Agri.Eng.Abstr., Agricola, Anim.Behav.Abstr. (coverage dropped), Aqua.Sci.& Fish.Abstr., Bio-Contr.News & Info., Biol.Abstr., Biotech.& Bioeng.Abstr. (coverage dropped), Chem.Abstr., Chem.Indus.Notes, Chem.Titles, Curr.Adv.Ecol.Sci., Curr.Cont., Derwent Biotech.Abstr., Entomol.Abstr., Environ.Sci.Poll.Mgmt., Forest Prod.Abstr., Forest.Abstr., Helminthol.Abstr., INIS Atomind., Ind.Med. (1985-), Ind.Sci.Rev., Ind.Vet., Microbiol.Abstr., Pollut.Abstr., Protozool.Abstr., Rev.Appl.Entomol., Rev.Arom.& Med.Plants, Rev.Med.& Vet.Mycol., Rice Abstr., Sci.Cit.Ind., Sel.Water Res.Abstr., So.Pac.Per.Ind., Sport Fish.Abstr., Trop.Dis.Bull., Vet.Bull., Virol.Abstr., Weed Abstr., Wild.Rev., Zoo.Rec.
—BLDSC (4689.125000), CASDDS, CISTI, GNLM, IDS, Infotrieve, ingenta, Linda Hall. **CCC.**
Published by: American Mosquito Control Association, PO Box 234, Eatontown, NJ 07724. TEL 732-932-0667, FAX 732-932-0930, amca@mosquito.org, http://www.mosquito.org. Ed. Dr. Ronald A Ward. Circ: 2,000.

632.8 USA
SB951.5
ARTHROPOD MANAGEMENT TESTS. Text in English. 1976. a. USD 40 domestic to individuals; USD 45 foreign to individuals; USD 45 domestic to institutions; USD 50 foreign to institutions (effective 2000). *Refereed.* **Document type:** *Journal, Academic/Scholarly.* **Description:** Presents the results of field and laboratory screenings performed with agricultural chemicals on a variety of crops.
Formerly (until 1995): Insecticide and Acaricide Tests (0276-3656)
Related titles: ♦ Online - full content ed.: Arthropod Management Tests Online.
Indexed: Derwent Biotech.Abstr., Rev.Appl.Entomol.
—BLDSC (1733.893500), CISTI, Infotrieve, Linda Hall. **CCC.**
Published by: Entomological Society of America, 9301 Annapolis Rd, Lanham, MD 20706. TEL 301-731-4535, FAX 301-731-4538, esa@entsoc.org, http://www.entsoc.org. Ed. K N Saxena.

630 AUS ISSN 0816-1089
CODEN: AJEAEL
AUSTRALIAN JOURNAL OF EXPERIMENTAL AGRICULTURE. Text in English. 1961. 8/yr. AUD 625; AUD 695 combined subscription for print & online eds. (effective 2002). adv. index. 144 p./no. back issues avail.; reprints avail. *Refereed.* **Document type:** *Journal, Academic/Scholarly.* **Description:** Publishes original research into applied agriculture, papers in animal production, animal-plant interactions, pasture and fodder crops, field crops, agroforestry, extension methodology and horticulture.
Formerly: Australian Journal of Experimental Agriculture and Animal Husbandry (0045-060X)
Related titles: Microform ed.: (from PQC); Online - full text ed.: AUD 475 (effective 2000) (from EBSCO Publishing, Swets Blackwell, Institute for Scientific Information).
Indexed: ASCA, AgBiotech, Agri.& Environ.Biotech.Abstr. (coverage dropped), Agri.Eng.Abstr., Agricola, Agroforest.Abstr., Anim.Breed.Abstr., Apic.Abstr., Bio-Contr.News & Info., Biol.& Agr.Ind. (coverage dropped), Biol.Abstr., Cadscan, Chem.Abstr., Chem.Indus.Notes, Chem.Titles, Crop Physiol.Abstr., Curr.Adv.Ecol.Sci., Curr.Cont., Dairy Sci.Abstr., Derwent Biotech.Abstr., Ecol.Abstr., Environ.Sci.Poll.Mgmt., Excerp.Med., Fababean Abstr., Field Crop Abstr., Food Sci.& Tech.Abstr., Forest Prod.Abstr., Forest.Abstr., Geo.Abstr.H.G., Geo.Abstr.P.G., Geol.Abstr., Helminthol.Abstr., Herb.Abstr., Hort.Abstr., IDA, INIS Atomind., Ind.Sci.Rev., Ind.Vet., Int.Abstr.Biol.Sci., Irr.& Drain.Abstr., Lead Abstr., Maize Abstr., Nutr.Abstr., Ornam.Hort., Pig News & Info., Plant Breed.Abstr., Plant Gen.Res.Abstr., Plant Grow.Reg.Abstr., Pollut.Abstr., Postharvest, Potato Abstr., Poult.Abstr., Rev.Appl.Entomol., Rev.Arom.& Med.Plants, Rev.Med.& Vet.Mycol., Rev.Plant Path., Rice Abstr., Rural Recreat.Tour.Abstr., Sci.Cit.Ind., Seed Abstr., Sel.Water Res.Abstr., Soils & Fert., Sorghum & Millets Abstr., Soyabean Abstr., Sugar Ind.Abstr., Triticale Abstr., Trop.Oil Seeds Abstr., Vet.Bull., Weed Abstr., World Ag.Econ.& Rur.Soc.Abstr., World Text.Abstr., Zincscan.
—BLDSC (1807.695000), CASDDS, CISTI, EMDOCS, IDS, Infotrieve, ingenta, Linda Hall. **CCC.**
Published by: (C S I R O Australia), C S I R O Publishing, 150 Oxford St, Collingwood, VIC 3066, Australia. TEL 61-3-96627614, FAX 61-3-9662-7611, chris.anderson@publish.csiro.au, http://www.publish.csiro.au/journals/ajea. Eds. C A Anderson, L L Muir. R&P C A Anderson. Circ: 850. **Co-sponsor:** Australian Agricultural Council.

631.4 DEU ISSN 0178-4765
BIO NACHRICHTEN. Text in German. 1979. 4/yr. membership. adv. bk.rev. **Document type:** *Newsletter.*
Published by: Biokreis Ostbayern e.V., Theresienstr 36, Passau 94032, Germany. TEL 0851-31696, FAX 0851-32332. Ed., Adv. contact Wolfgang Denk. Circ: 750.

632.9 GBR ISSN 0958-3157
SB975 CODEN: BSTCE6
BIOCONTROL SCIENCE AND TECHNOLOGY. Text in English. 1991. 6/yr. GBP 175, USD 307 to individuals; GBP 609, USD 1,067 to institutions (effective 2002). adv. bk.rev. index. back issues avail. *Refereed.* **Document type:** *Academic/Scholarly.* **Description:** Presents original research and reviews in the fields of biological pest, disease, and weed control, including basic research and applications of new techniques.
Related titles: Microfiche ed.; Online - full text ed.: ISSN 1360-0478 (from CatchWord Ltd., EBSCO Publishing, O C L C Online Computer Library Center, Inc., RoweCom Information Quest, ProQuest Information & Learning, Swets Blackwell, Institute for Scientific Information).
Indexed: ASCA, Agri.& Environ.Biotech.Abstr., Agricola, Bibl.Agri., Bio-Contr.News & Info., Biotech.Cit.Ind., Curr.Adv.Plant Sci., Curr.Cont., Derwent Biotech.Abstr., Ecol.Abstr., Entomol.Abstr., Environ.Sci.Poll.Mgmt., Field Crop Abstr., Food Sci.& Tech.Abstr., Forest Prod.Abstr., Forest.Abstr., Helminthol.Abstr., Hort.Abstr., Int.Abstr.Biol.Sci., Maize Abstr., Microbiol.Abstr., Ornam.Hort., Plant Sci., Postharvest, Potato Abstr., Ref.Zh., Rev.Appl.Entomol., Rev.Med.& Vet.Mycol., Rev.Plant Path., Rice Abstr., Sci.Cit.Ind., Seed Abstr., Soyabean Abstr., Triticale Abstr., Weed Abstr.
—BLDSC (2071.150000), CatchWord, CISTI, EMDOCS, IDS, Infotrieve. **CCC.**
Published by: Carfax Publishing Limited (Subsidiary of: Taylor & Francis Group), PO Box 25, Abingdon, Oxon OX14 3UE, United Kingdom. TEL 44-1235-401000, FAX 44-1235-401550, enquiries@carfax.co.uk, enquiry@tandf.co.uk, http://www.carfax.co.uk. Ed. C C Payne.

631.8 DEU ISSN 0178-2762
CODEN: BFSOEE
BIOLOGY AND FERTILITY OF SOILS. Text in English. 1985. 18/yr. EUR 2,448.80 domestic; EUR 2,420.20 in Germany; EUR 158.70 newsstand/cover foreign (effective 2002). back issues avail.; reprint service avail. from ISI. *Refereed.* **Document type:** *Journal, Academic/Scholarly.* **Description:** Covers fundamental and applied aspects of the biology and productivity of soils.
Related titles: Microform ed.: (from PQC); Online - full text ed.: ISSN 1432-0789 (from EBSCO Publishing, RoweCom Information Quest, Swets Blackwell, Springer LINK, Institute for Scientific Information).

A

Indexed: ASCA, AgBiotech, Agri.Eng.Abstr., Agricola, Agroforest.Abstr., Aqua.Sci.& Fish.Abstr., Bibl.Agri., Bio-Contr.News & Info., Biol.Abstr., Chem.Abstr., Chem.Indus.Notes, Chem.Titles, Crop Physiol.Abstr., Curr.Adv.Ecol.Sci., Curr.Adv.Plant Sci., Curr.Cont., Dairy Sci.Abstr., Ecol.Abstr., Environ.Sci.Poll.Mgmt., Excerp.Med., Fababean Abstr., Field Crop Abstr., Forest.Abstr., Geo.Abstr.P.G., Helminthol.Abstr., Herb.Abstr., Hort.Abstr., IDA, Ind.Sci.Rev., Int.Abstr.Biol.Sci., Irr.& Drain.Abstr., Maize Abstr., Microbiol.Abstr., Plant Breed.Abstr., Plant Grow.Reg.Abstr., Plant Sci., Pollut.Abstr., Protozool.Abstr., Rev.Appl.Entomol., Rev.Plant Path., Rice Abstr., Sci.Cit.Ind., Seed Abstr., Sel.Water Res.Abstr., Soils & Fert., Soyabean Abstr., Sugar Ind.Abstr., Triticale Abstr., Weed Abstr., Zoo.Rec.
—BLDSC (2086.998000), CASDDS, CISTI, EMDOCS, IDS, Infotrieve, ingenta, Linda Hall. **CCC.**
Published by: (International Society of Soil Science NLD), Springer-Verlag (Subsidiary of: BertelsmannSpringer), Tiergartenstr 17, Heidelberg 69121, Germany. TEL 49-6221-345-0, FAX 49-6221-345229, subscriptions@springer.de, http://link.springer.de/link/service/journals/00374/index.htm, http://www.springer.de. Ed. P Nannipieri. **Subscr. in N. America to:** Springer-Verlag New York Inc., PO Box 2485, Secaucus, NJ 07096-2485. TEL 212-460-1500, FAX 212-473-6272.

631 USA ISSN 1081-5228
BLUEBOOK UPDATE. Text in English. 1994. q. adv. **Document type:** *Newsletter.*
Related titles: ♦ Supplement to: (Year) Soya & Oilseed Bluebook. ISSN 1099-7970.
Published by: Soyatech, Inc., 7 Pleasant St, Box 84, Bar Harbor, ME 04609. TEL 207-288-4969, 800-424-SOYA, FAX 207-288-5264, data@soyatech.com, http://www.soyatech.com. Ed. Keri Hayes. R&P Peter Golbitz. Adv. contact Joy Froding. Circ: 6,000.

C A SELECTS. HERBICIDES. see *AGRICULTURE—Abstracting, Bibliographies, Statistics*

C A SELECTS. INSECTICIDES. see *AGRICULTURE—Abstracting, Bibliographies, Statistics*

632.9 USA ISSN 1047-8140
CODEN: CSAYEM
C A SELECTS. PESTICIDE ANALYSIS. Text in English. 1988. s-w. USD 275 (effective 2001). **Document type:** *Abstract/Index.* **Description:** Covers the analysis of pesticides (insecticides, herbicides, and fungicides) including chemical and physical analysis of preparations used for the control of plant and animal pests.
Formerly (until 1989): BIOSIS CAS Selects: Pesticide Analysis
Published by: Chemical Abstracts Service (Subsidiary of: American Chemical Society), 2540 Olentangy River Rd, Box 3012, Columbus, OH 43210-0012. TEL 614-447-3600, 800-753-4227, FAX 614-447-3751.

COMMON SENSE PEST CONTROL QUARTERLY. see *GARDENING AND HORTICULTURE*

631 DNK ISSN 0905-8478
DENMARK. KGL. VETERINAER- OG LANDBOHOEJSKOLE. FORSKNINGSRAPPORT/ RESEARCH REPORT. Text in Danish. irreg. free per issue.
Formerly: Denmark. Kgl. Veterinaer- og Landbohoejskole. Meddelelser (0105-2543)
—BLDSC.
Published by: Kgl. Veterinaer- og Landbohoejskole, Institut for Jordbrugsvidenskab, Sektion for Kulturteknik og Planteernaering, Thorvaldsens vej 40, Frederiksberg C 1871, Denmark. TEL 45-35-28-34-96, FAX 45-35-28-34-60.

FOOD & WATER JOURNAL. see *CONSUMER EDUCATION AND PROTECTION*

GLOBAL PESTICIDE CAMPAIGNER. see *ENVIRONMENTAL STUDIES—Toxicology And Environmental Safety*

632.9 USA ISSN 0738-968X
I P M PRACTITIONER; monitoring the field of pest management. (Integrated Pest Management) Text in English. 1979. m. USD 35 to individuals; USD 60 to institutions (effective 2000). adv. bk.rev. index. back issues avail. **Document type:** *Newsletter, Trade.* **Description:** Covers integrated pest management programs, methods, products and research.
Indexed: Agri.Eng.Abstr., Agricola, Bio-Contr.News & Info., Forest Prod.Abstr., Forest.Abstr., Gard.Lit. (1992-1994), Helminthol.Abstr., Hort.Abstr., Nutr.Abstr., Ornam.Hort., Postharvest, Poult.Abstr., Rev.Appl.Entomol., Rev.Med.& Vet.Mycol., Rev.Plant Path., Triticale Abstr., Weed Abstr.
—BLDSC (4567.390000).
Published by: Bio Integral Resource Center, PO Box 7414, Berkeley, CA 94707. TEL 510-524-2567, FAX 510-524-1758. Ed., R&P William Quarles. Circ: 5,000.

635.21 IND ISSN 0970-8235
INDIAN POTATO ASSOCIATION. JOURNAL. Text and summaries in English. 1974. q. INR 400, USD 40 (effective 2001). adv. bk.rev. 100 p./no. back issues avail. *Refereed.* **Document type:** *Journal, Academic/Scholarly, Abstract/Index.* **Description:** Disseminates the research work, development and technology on potato production to researchers, growers and potato industry.
Indexed: Agri.Eng.Abstr., Biol.Abstr., Crop Physiol.Abstr., Curr.Adv.Ecol.Sci., Field Crop Abstr., Helminthol.Abstr., Herb.Abstr., Hort.Abstr., Irr.& Drain.Abstr., Plant Breed.Abstr., Plant Grow.Reg.Abstr., Postharvest, Potato Abstr., Rev.Appl.Entomol., Rev.Plant Path., Seed Abstr., Soils & Fert., Soyabean Abstr., Triticale Abstr., Weed Abstr., World Ag.Econ.& Rur.Soc.Abstr.
—CISTI.
Published by: Indian Potato Association, Central Potato Research Institute, Simla, Himachal Pradesh 171 001, India. TEL 91-177-225073, FAX 91-177-224460, khurana@cpri.hp.nic.in. Ed., Adv. contact S M Paul Khurana. Circ: 750 (paid).

631 NLD ISSN 0926-6690
CODEN: ICRDEW
INDUSTRIAL CROPS AND PRODUCTS. Text in English. 1992. 6/yr. EUR 609 in Europe to institutions; JPY 80,800 in Japan to institutions; USD 681 elsewhere to institutions (effective 2002). bk.rev. abstr. back issues avail. *Refereed.* **Document type:** *Academic/Scholarly.* **Description:** Covers advances in the development, production, harvesting, storage and processing of nonfood crops for industrial uses, including applications of pharmaceuticals, lubricants, fuels, fibers, essential oils, biologically active materials, and uses for industrial crop by-products.
Related titles: Microform ed.: (from PQC); Online - full text ed.: (from ingenta, Swets Blackwell, ScienceDirect, Institute for Scientific Information).
Indexed: ASCA, AgBiotech, Agricola, Chem.Abstr., Chem.Indus.Notes, Chem.Titles, Crop Physiol.Abstr., Curr.Adv.Plant Sci., Curr.Cont., Ecol.Abstr., Environ.Abstr., Field Crop Abstr., Fluidex, Food Sci.& Tech.Abstr., Forest Prod.Abstr., Forest.Abstr., Geo.Abstr.P.G., Helminthol.Abstr., Herb.Abstr., Hort.Abstr., IDA, Int.Abstr.Biol.Sci., Irr.& Drain.Abstr., Nutr.Abstr., Ornam.Hort., Plant Breed.Abstr., Plant Gen.Res.Abstr., Plant Grow.Reg.Abstr., Plant Sci., Postharvest, Rev.Appl.Entomol., Rev.Arom.& Med.Plants, Rev.Plant Path., Seed Abstr., Soils & Fert., Sugar Ind.Abstr., Triticale Abstr., Weed Abstr., World Ag.Econ.& Rur.Soc.Abstr., World Text.Abstr.
—BLDSC (4448.357000), CASDDS, CISTI, EMDOCS, IDS, Infotrieve, ingenta. **CCC.**
Published by: (Association for the Advancement of Industrial Crops), Elsevier Science BV, PO Box 211, Amsterdam 1000 AE, Netherlands. TEL 31-20-485-2911, FAX 31-20-485-2457, http://www.elsevier.com/locate/indcrop. Eds. F S Nakayama, J T P Derksen. **Subscr. in Australasia and the Far East to:** Elsevier Science (Singapore) Pte Ltd, No.1 Temasek Ave, 17-01 Millenia Tower, Singapore 039192, Singapore. TEL 65-434-3727, FAX 65-337-2230; **Subscr. in Japan to:** Elsevier Science Inc - Japan Regional Office, 9-15 Higashi-Azabu 1-chome, Minato-ku, Tokyo 106-0044, Japan. TEL 81-3-5561-5033; **Subscr. in the Americas to:** Elsevier Science, PO Box 945, New York, NY 10159-0945. TEL 212-633-3730, FAX 212-633-3680, usinfo-f@elsevier.com.

630 571.4 POL ISSN 0236-8722
CODEN: INAGEX
INTERNATIONAL AGROPHYSICS; a quarterly journal on physics in agricultural and environmental sciences. Text in English. 1985-1989 (vol.5); resumed 1992. q. USD 140 (effective 2002). adv. bk.rev. 90 p./no. 2 cols./p. reprints avail. *Refereed.* **Document type:** *Trade.* **Description:** Focusses on physical properties and processes effecting plant production.
Indexed: Agri.Eng.Abstr., AgroAgen, AgroLibrex, Chem.Abstr., Crop Physiol.Abstr., Dairy Sci.Abstr., Ecol.Abstr., Field Crop Abstr., Geo.Abstr.P.G., GeoRef, Herb.Abstr., Hort.Abstr., INIS Atomind., Irr.& Drain.Abstr., Maize Abstr., Ornam.Hort., Plant Breed.Abstr., Plant Gen.Res.Abstr., Postharvest, Potato Abstr., Poult.Abstr., Rev.Arom.& Med.Plants, Seed Abstr., Soils & Fert., Soyabean Abstr., Triticale Abstr., Weed Abstr.
—BLDSC (4535.654000), CASDDS, CISTI, EMDOCS, Infotrieve, Linda Hall. **CCC.**
Published by: Polska Akademia Nauk, Instytut Agrofizyki/Polish Academy of Sciences, Institute of Agrophysics, Ul Doswiadczalna 4, PO Box 201, Lublin 20290, Poland. TEL 48-81-7445061, FAX 48-81-7445067, agrof@demeter.ipan.lublin.pl. Ed. Jan Glinski. Adv. contact Ewa Sikora. page USD 25.

632.9 GBR ISSN 0967-0874
SB950.A1 CODEN: TPMAD5
INTERNATIONAL JOURNAL OF PEST MANAGEMENT. Text in English. 1971 (vol.17). q. GBP 133, USD 220 to individuals; GBP 324, USD 534 to institutions (effective 2002). adv. bk.rev. charts, illus, stat. index. *Refereed.* **Document type:** *Trade.* **Description:** Covers all spheres of pre- and postharvest pest management, vector-borne diseases and public health, and the relationship of pest management to the wider aspects of farming systems and rural developments.
Former titles: Tropical Pest Management (0143-6147); P A N S (0030-7793)
Related titles: Online - full text ed.: ISSN 1366-5863 (from CatchWord Ltd., EBSCO Publishing, O C L C Online Computer Library Center, Inc., RoweCom Information Quest, Swets Blackwell, Institute for Scientific Information).
Indexed: ASCA, Agri.& Environ.Biotech.Abstr. (coverage dropped), Agricola, Agroforest.Abstr., Apic.Abstr., Aqua.Sci.& Fish.Abstr., Bibl.Agri., Bio-Contr.News & Info., Biodet.Abstr., Biol.Abstr., Biotech.& Bioeng.Abstr., Chem.Abstr., Chem.Indus.Notes, Chem.Titles, Cott.& Trop.Fibr.Abstr., Curr.Adv.Ecol.Sci., Curr.Cont., Derwent Biotech.Abstr., Ecol.Abstr., Entomol.Abstr., Environ.Per.Bibl. (1990-), Environ.Sci.Poll.Mgmt., Field Crop Abstr., Food Sci.& Tech.Abstr., Forest Prod.Abstr., Forest.Abstr., Geo.Abstr.H.G., Helminthol.Abstr., Hort.Abstr., IDA, Ind.Vet., Irr.& Drain.Abstr., Maize Abstr., Microbiol.Abstr., Ornam.Hort., Plant Breed.Abstr., Plant Gen.Res.Abstr., Plant Grow.Reg.Abstr., Postharvest, Rev.Appl.Entomol., Rev.Plant Path., Rice Abstr., Rural Devel.Abstr., Seed Abstr., So.Pac.Per.Ind., Soils & Fert., Sorghum & Millets Abstr., Soyabean Abstr., Triticale Abstr., Trop.Oil Seeds Abstr., Vet.Bull., Weed Abstr., World Ag.Econ.& Rur.Soc.Abstr., World Text.Abstr., Zoo.Rec.
—BLDSC (4542.452800), CASDDS, CatchWord, CISTI, IDS, Infotrieve, ingenta, Linda Hall. **CCC.**
Published by: Taylor & Francis Group, Taylor & Francis Ltd., 11 New Fetter Ln, London EC4P 4EE, United Kingdom. TEL 44-20-7583-9855, FAX 44-20-7842-2298, info@tandf.co.uk, http://www.tandf.co.uk. Ed. Mark A Jervis. Circ: 3,000. **Subscr. in N. America to:** Taylor & Francis Ltd., 325 Chestnut St, Suite 800, Philadelphia, PA 19016. TEL 800-354-1420, FAX 215-625-8914, info@tandf.co.uk, http://www.taylorandfrancis.com/.

630 570 IND ISSN 0379-5489
S589.5 CODEN: JNABDS
JOURNAL OF NUCLEAR AGRICULTURE AND BIOLOGY. Text in English. 1972. q. INR 200, USD 65 (effective 1991). adv. bk.rev. back issues avail. **Document type:** *Academic/Scholarly.*
Formerly: I S N A Newsletter
Indexed: Bio-Contr.News & Info., Biol.Abstr., Chem.Abstr., Chem.Titles, Crop Physiol.Abstr., Curr.Cont. (coverage dropped), Dairy Sci.Abstr., Excerp.Med., Field Crop Abstr., Herb.Abstr., Hort.Abstr., INIS Atomind., Ind.Vet., Irr.& Drain.Abstr., Nutr.Abstr., Ornam.Hort., Plant Breed.Abstr., Plant Grow.Reg.Abstr., Postharvest, Rev.Appl.Entomol., Rev.Plant Path., Rice Abstr., Seed Abstr., Soils & Fert., Soyabean Abstr., Sugar Ind.Abstr., Triticale Abstr., Vet.Bull., Weed Abstr.
—BLDSC (5022.848000), CASDDS, CISTI, ingenta, Linda Hall.
Published by: Indian Society for Nuclear Techniques in Agriculture and Biology, Nuclear Research Laboratory, Indian Agricultural Research Institute, New Delhi 110 012, India. Ed. M S Chatrath. R&P M.S. Chatrath. Adv. contact M S Sachdey. Circ: 400 (controlled).

632.9 USA
MIDWEST BIOLOGICAL CONTROL NEWS. Text in English. m. **Document type:** *Newsletter, Academic/Scholarly.* **Description:** Dedicated to providing information on the use of beneficial organisms for controlling insect and mite pests of the farm, garden, and home.
Related titles: Online - full text ed.

Published by: U S D A Extension Service smahr@entomology.wisc.edu, http://www.wisc.edu/entomology/mbcn/mbcn.html. Ed. Susan Rice Mahr.

MOSKOVSKII GOSUDARSTVENNYI UNIVERSITET. VESTNIK. SERIYA 16: BIOLOGIYA. see *BIOLOGY*

NIPPON NOGEIKAGAKU KAISHI/JAPAN SOCIETY FOR BIOSCIENCE, BIOTECHNOLOGY, AND AGROCHEMISTRY. JOURNAL. see *BIOLOGY—Biotechnology*

NIPPON NOYAKU GAKKAISHI. see *ENGINEERING—Chemical Engineering*

631.4 DEU ISSN 0031-4056
QL110 CODEN: PDBLAM
PEDOBIOLOGIA. Text in English. 1961. bi-m. EUR 153, GBP 114 to individuals; EUR 366, GBP 246 to institutions (effective 2002). adv. bk.rev. bibl, charts, illus. index. reprint service avail. from ISI. *Refereed.* **Document type:** *Journal, Academic/Scholarly.*
Description: Covers fundamental and applied aspects of soil biology.
Related titles: Online - full text ed.: (from Swets Blackwell, Institute for Scientific Information).
Indexed: ASCA, Agroforest.Abstr., Appl.Ecol.Abstr., Aqua.Sci.& Fish.Abstr., Biol.Abstr., Chem.Abstr., Chem.Titles, Curr.Adv.Biochem., Curr.Adv.Ecol.Sci., Curr.Cont., Ecol.Abstr., Entomol.Abstr., Environ.Abstr., Environ.Ind., Environ.Sci.Poll.Mgmt., Excerp.Med., Field Crop Abstr., Forest Prod.Abstr., Forest.Abstr., Geo.Abstr.H.G., Geo.Abstr.P.G., GeoRef, Helminthol.Abstr., Herb.Abstr., Hort.Abstr., IBR, INIS Atomind., Ind.Sci.Rev., Int.Abstr.Biol.Sci., Irr.& Drain.Abstr., Maize Abstr., Microbiol.Abstr., Potato Abstr., Protozool.Abstr., Rev.Appl.Entomol., Rev.Plant Path., Rice Abstr., Sci.Cit.Ind., Seed Abstr., Soils & Fert., Sugar Ind.Abstr., Triticale Abstr., Weed Abstr., Zoo.Rec.
—BLDSC (6417.750000), CASDDS, CISTI, EMDOCS, IDS, Infotrieve, ingenta, Linda Hall. **CCC.**
Published by: Urban & Fischer Verlag, Loebdergraben 14A, Jena 07743, Germany. TEL 49-3641-626444, FAX 49-3641-626500, info@urbanfischer.de, http://www.urbanfischer.de. Eds. John Lussenhop, Juergen Schauermann, Stefan Scheu. R&P Martin Huber TEL 49-3641-626430. Adv. contact Sabine Schroeter. page DEM 600; trim 240 x 170. Circ: 450.

631.8 USA ISSN 0048-3575
SB951 CODEN: PCBPBS
PESTICIDE BIOCHEMISTRY AND PHYSIOLOGY; an international journal. Text in English. 1971. 9/yr. USD 820 in US & Canada to institutions; USD 940 rest of world to institutions (effective 2001). adv. index. back issues avail. *Refereed.* **Document type:** *Academic/Scholarly.* **Description:** Discusses the modes of action of plant protection agents such as insecticides, fungicides, herbicides, and similar compounds including nonlethal pest control agents, biosynthesis of pheromones, hormones, and plant resistance agents.
Related titles: Online - full text ed.: (from EBSCO Publishing, O C L C Online Computer Library Center, Inc., RoweCom Information Quest, ingenta, Swets Blackwell, IDEAL Online Library, Institute for Scientific Information).
Indexed: ASCA, Abstr.Hyg., AgBiotech, Agri.& Environ.Biotech.Abstr. (coverage dropped), Agricola, Aqua.Sci.& Fish.Abstr., Aquacult.Abstr., BBCI, Bibl.Agri., Bio-Contr.News & Info., Biodet.Abstr., Biol.& Agr.Ind. (Feb.1983-), Biol.Abstr., Chem.Abstr., Chem.Titles, Cott.& Trop.Fibr.Abstr., Crop Physiol.Abstr., Curr.Adv.Ecol.Sci., Curr.Cont., Curr.Ref.Fish Res., Dairy Sci.Abstr., Derwent Biotech.Abstr., Energy Ind., Energy Info.Abstr., Entomol.Abstr., Environ.Per.Bibl., Environ.Sci.Poll.Mgmt., Excerp.Med., Field Crop Abstr., Helminthol.Abstr., Herb.Abstr., Hort.Abstr., INIS Atomind., Ind.Sci.Rev., Ind.Vet., Inpharma, Int.Abstr.Biol.Sci., Maize Abstr., Ornam.Hort., Pharm.&Out.News, Plant Breed.Abstr., Plant Grow.Reg.Abstr., Pollut.Abstr., Potato Abstr., Poult.Abstr., Reac., Rev.Appl.Entomol., Rev.Med.& Vet.Mycol., Rev.Plant Path., Rice Abstr., Sci.Cit.Ind., Sel.Water Res.Abstr., Soils & Fert., Soyabean Abstr., Sport Fish.Abstr., Tox.Abstr., Triticale Abstr., Trop.Dis.Bull., Vet.Bull., Weed Abstr., Wild.Rev., Zoo.Rec.
—BLDSC (6428.370000), ADONIS, CASDDS, CINDOC, CISTI, EMDOCS, IDS, ingenta, Linda Hall. **CCC.**
Published by: Academic Press, Inc., Journal Division (Subsidiary of: Harcourt Brace & Company), 525 B St, Ste 1900, San Diego, CA 92101-4495. TEL 619-230-1840, FAX 619-699-6800, apsubs@acad.com, http://www.academicpress.com/pest. Ed. Fumio Matsumura.

PESTICIDE LITIGATION MANUAL. see *ENVIRONMENTAL STUDIES—Toxicology And Environmental Safety*

PESTICIDES MONITOR; a monthly listing of UK approvals and other announcements on pesticides. see *ENVIRONMENTAL STUDIES—Toxicology And Environmental Safety*

571.959 USA ISSN 1520-9350
▼ **PESTICIDES, PEOPLE AND NATURE.** Text in English. 1999. s-a. USD 60 to individuals; USD 154 to institutions (effective 2001). **Document type:** *Academic/Scholarly.*
—BLDSC (6428.773400).
Published by: (Rachel Carson Council), Begell House Inc., 79 Madison Ave, Ste 1205, New York, NY 10016-7892. TEL 212-725-1999, FAX 212-213-8368, orders@begellhouse.com, http://www.begellhouse.com/ppn/ppn.html, http://www.begellhouse.com/index.html. Ed. David J McGarvey.

PLANT FOODS FOR HUMAN NUTRITION. see *NUTRITION AND DIETETICS*

PROGRESS IN PESTICIDE BIOCHEMISTRY AND TOXICOLOGY. see *ENGINEERING—Chemical Engineering*

RECOMMENDATIONS ON THE SAFE USE OF PESTICIDES IN SHIPS. see *ENVIRONMENTAL STUDIES—Toxicology And Environmental Safety*

SAFETY NEWS. see *WATER RESOURCES*

632.9 ESP ISSN 0213-6910
SPAIN. MINISTERIO DE AGRICULTURA, PESCA Y ALIMENTACION. BOLETIN DE SANIDAD VEGETAL: PLAGAS. Text in Spanish. 1975. q. ESP 3,500; ESP 4,500 foreign (effective 1998). **Document type:** *Academic/Scholarly.*
Formerly (until 1985): Spain. Ministerio de Agricultura, Pesca y Alimentacion. Servicio de Defensa Contra Plagas e Inspeccion Fitopatologica. Boletin (0210-8038)
Indexed: Bio-Contr.News & Info., Biodet.Abstr., Derwent Biotech.Abstr., Food Sci.& Tech.Abstr., Forest.Abstr., Helminthol.Abstr., Hort.Abstr., Maize Abstr., Nutr.Abstr., Ornam.Hort., Plant Breed.Abstr., Postharvest, Potato Abstr., Ref.Zh., Rev.Appl.Entomol., Rev.Arom.& Med.Plants, Rev.Plant Path., Seed Abstr., Soils & Fert., Triticale Abstr., Weed Abstr., Zoo.Rec.
—CINDOC, CISTI.
Published by: Ministerio de Agricultura Pesca y Alimentacion, Subdireccion General de Sanidad Vegetal, Centro de Publicaciones, Paseo Infanta Isabel, 1, Madrid 28014, Spain. TEL 34-1-3475551. Ed. Ramon Vazquez Hombrados. R&P Juan Carlos Palacios Lopez.

630.13 BEL ISSN 0771-3312
CODEN: TRPIEP
LE TROPICULTURA. Text in English, French, Spanish; Contents page in English. 1983. 4/yr. free. bk.rev. *Refereed.* **Document type:** *Journal, Academic/Scholarly.*
Indexed: Agri.Eng.Abstr., Anim.Breed.Abstr., Bio-Contr.News & Info., Curr.Ind.Stat., Dairy Sci.Abstr., Field Crop Abstr., Forest Prod.Abstr., Forest.Abstr., Helminthol.Abstr., Herb.Abstr., Hort.Abstr., Ind.Vet., Nutr.Abstr., Plant Breed.Abstr., Postharvest, Poult.Abstr., Protozool.Abstr., Rev.Appl.Entomol., Rev.Plant Path., Rice Abstr., Rural Devel.Abstr., Seed Abstr., Soils & Fert., Sport Fish.Abstr., Sugar Ind.Abstr., Triticale Abstr., Vet.Bull., Weed Abstr., Wild.Rev., World Ag.Econ.& Rur.Soc.Abstr.
—BLDSC (9057.040000), ingenta.
Published by: (Belgium Administration for Cooperation and Development), A G C D - A B O S, Rue du Trone 4, Bte 605, Brussels 1000, Belgium. TEL 32-2-519-0447. Ed. Guy Mergeai. R&P Marie-Josee Desmet TEL 32-2-519-0476. Circ: 2,500.

632.9 SWE ISSN 0042-2169
SB605.S9
VAEXTSKYDDSNOTISER. Text in Swedish; Summaries in English. 1937. q. SEK 300 (effective 1998). adv. bk.rev. bibl, charts, illus. index, cum.index. **Document type:** *Academic/Scholarly.* **Description:** Provides current information about plant protection, along with results from experiments and research.
Related titles: Supplement: Vaxtskyddsnotiser. Supplement. ISSN 0283-2437. 1986.
Indexed: Bio-Contr.News & Info., Biol.Abstr., Chem.Abstr., Field Crop Abstr., Food Sci.& Tech.Abstr., Forest.Abstr., Helminthol.Abstr., Herb.Abstr., Hort.Abstr., Maize Abstr., Ornam.Hort., Plant Breed.Abstr., Pollut.Abstr., Postharvest, Potato Abstr., Rev.Appl.Entomol., Rev.Plant Path., Seed Abstr., Soils & Fert., Triticale Abstr., Weed Abstr.
Published by: Sveriges Lantbruksuniversitet/Swedish University of Agricultural Sciences, Fack 7044, Uppsala 75007, Sweden. TEL 46-18-671000, FAX 46-18-672890. Ed. Jan Pettersson. R&P Mats W Pettersson. Adv. contact Inger Blomstedt.

WEED WORLD. see *DRUG ABUSE AND ALCOHOLISM*

AGRICULTURE—Dairying And Dairy Products

see also AGRICULTURE—Poultry And Livestock

ARCHIVOS DE ZOOTECNIA. see *AGRICULTURE—Poultry And Livestock*

DAIRY, FOOD AND ENVIRONMENTAL SANITATION; a publication for food safety professionals. see *FOOD AND FOOD INDUSTRIES*

JOURNAL OF FOOD PROTECTION. see *FOOD AND FOOD INDUSTRIES*

LACTIC ACID BACTERIA. see *BIOLOGY—Microbiology*

NATIONAL DAIRY COUNCIL. QUARTERLY REVIEW. see *NUTRITION AND DIETETICS*

REVISTA BRASILEIRA DE ZOOTECNIA/BRAZILIAN JOURNAL OF ANIMAL SCIENCE. see *VETERINARY SCIENCE*

AGRICULTURE—Feed, Flour And Grain

633.2 NLD ISSN 0377-8401
CODEN: AFSTDH
ANIMAL FEED SCIENCE AND TECHNOLOGY; an international scientific journal. Text in English. 1976. 28/yr. EUR 1,806 in Europe to institutions; JPY 240,100 in Japan to institutions; USD 2,019 elsewhere to institutions (effective 2002). adv. bk.rev. illus, bibl. index. *Refereed.* **Document type:** *Academic/Scholarly.*
Description: Publishes scientific papers dealing with the production, composition and nutritive value of feeds for animals.
Related titles: Microform ed.: (from PQC); Online - full text ed.: (from ingenta, Swets Blackwell, ScienceDirect, Institute for Scientific Information).
Indexed: ASCA, Agricola, Agroforest.Abstr., Anim.Breed.Abstr., Biodet.Abstr., Biol.Abstr., Chem.Abstr., Chem.Indus.Notes, Chem.Titles, Curr.Cont., Dairy Sci.Abstr., Field Crop Abstr., Food Sci.& Tech.Abstr., Forest Prod.Abstr., Forest.Abstr., Herb.Abstr., Ind.Sci.Rev., Ind.Vet., Maize Abstr., Nutr.Abstr., Pig News & Info., Plant Breed.Abstr., Plant Gen.Res.Abstr., Postharvest, Poult.Abstr., Ref.Zh., Rev.Med.& Vet.Mycol., Rev.Plant Path., Rice Abstr., Sci.Cit.Ind., Seed Abstr., Soils & Fert., Sorghum & Millets Abstr., Soyabean Abstr., Sport Fish.Abstr., Sugar Ind.Abstr., Triticale Abstr., Trop.Oil Seeds Abstr., Vet.Bull., Weed Abstr., Wild.Rev., World Ag.Econ.& Rur.Soc.Abstr.
—BLDSC (0903.550000), CASDDS, CISTI, IDS, Infotrieve, ingenta, Linda Hall. **CCC.**
Published by: Elsevier Science BV, PO Box 211, Amsterdam 1000 AE, Netherlands. TEL 31-20-485-2911, FAX 31-20-485-2457, nlinfo-f@elsevier.nl, http://www.elsevier.com/anifeedsci. Eds. P Uden, P H Robinson. **Subscr. in Australasia and the Far East to:** Elsevier Science (Singapore) Pte Ltd, No.1 Temasek Ave, 17-01 Millenia Tower, Singapore 039192, Singapore. TEL 65-434-3727, FAX 65-337-2230; **Subscr. in Japan to:** Elsevier Science Inc - Japan Regional Office, 9-15 Higashi-Azabu 1-chome, Minato-ku, Tokyo 106-0044, Japan. TEL 81-3-5561-5033; **Subscr. in the Americas to:** Elsevier Science, PO Box 945, New York, NY 10159-0945. TEL 212-633-3730.

ARCHIVOS DE ZOOTECNIA. see *AGRICULTURE—Poultry And Livestock*

338.1 DEU ISSN 0014-0228
ERNAEHRUNGSDIENST; unabhaengige Handels- und Boersenzeitung. Variant title: Agrarzeitung Ernaehrungsdienst. Text in German. 1946. 2/w. DEM 655.50; DEM 724.70 foreign (effective 1999). adv. bk.rev. charts, stat. **Document type:** *Trade.*
Related titles: Online - full text ed.: (from Factiva).
Indexed: CBNB (1997-), Rural Recreat.Tour.Abstr., World Ag.Econ.& Rur.Soc.Abstr.
Published by: Deutscher Fachverlag GmbH, Mainzer Landstr 251, Frankfurt Am Main 60326, Germany. TEL 49-69-75952052, FAX 49-69-75952050, info@dfv.de, http://www.dfv.de. Circ: 5,971.

A

636.085 GBR
HANDBOOK OF FEED ADDITIVES. Text in English. 1982. a. GBP 49 in United Kingdom; GBP 51 in Europe; GBP 54 elsewhere (effective 2000). adv. **Document type:** *Directory.* **Description:** Provides compendium of data sheets for additives available for use in livestock feeds and drinking waters. Products included are: medicines, zootechnicals, enzymes and micro-organisms, acidifiers, antioxidants, mould inhibitors and pigmenters.
Formerly (until 1998): Handbook of Medicinal Feed Additives (0957-2368)
—CISTI.
Published by: H G M Publications, HGM House, Nether End, Baslow, Bakewell, Derbys DE45 1SR, United Kingdom. TEL 44-1246-584000, 44-1246-584002, FAX 44-1246-584005, mail@hgmpubs.com, http://www.hgmpubs.com. Ed. Andrew D Mounsey. Pub. Howard Mounsey. Adv. contact Simon P Mounsey. Circ: 3,000.

AGRICULTURE—Poultry And Livestock

see also AGRICULTURE—Dairying And Dairy Products; VETERINARY SCIENCE

636 POL ISSN 0065-0935
SF1 CODEN: AASZBW
ACTA AGRARIA ET SILVESTRIA. SERIES ZOOTECHNICA. Text in Polish; Summaries in English, Russian. 1961. irreg. (1-2/yr.). price varies. bibl, charts. **Document type:** *Academic/Scholarly.* **Description:** Experimental studies on farm animal breeding, physiology, animal hygiene and environment as well as animal reproduction.
Formerly (until 1965): Acta Agraria et Silvestria. Seria Zootechniczna (0376-1568)
Indexed: Agri.Eng.Abstr., AgroLibrex, Anim.Breed.Abstr., Biol.Abstr., Chem.Abstr., Excerp.Med., Field Crop Abstr., Herb.Abstr., Ind.Vet., Irr.& Drain.Abstr., Maize Abstr., Nutr.Abstr., Pig News & Info., Poult.Abstr., Soils & Fert., Triticale Abstr., Vet.Bull., Zoo.Rec.
—CASDDS, KNAW.
Published by: (Polska Akademia Nauk/Polish Academy of Sciences, Oddzial w Krakowie, Komisja Nauk Rolniczych i Lesnych), Ossolineum Publishing House of the Polish Academy of Sciences, Pl Solny 14 a, Wroclaw 50062, Poland. TEL 48-71-343-6961, FAX 48-71-448-103. Ed. Thomas M Janowski.

ANIMAL BIOTECHNOLOGY. see *BIOLOGY—Biotechnology*

636 636.089 GRC
ANIMAL HUSBANDRY AND BREEDING. Text in Greek. 1986. q. back issues avail. **Document type:** *Academic/Scholarly.* **Description:** Covers livestock production and provides marketing information on new methods, technology and techniques, breeders, scientists and traders.
Published by: Agrotechnical Publications S.A., 24-26 Favierou St, Athens 104 38, Greece. TEL 30-1-5222-054, FAX 30-1-5246-628, TELEX 222264 STIM GR. Ed. Costas Colotouros. Circ: 8,000.

636.0852 CAN
ANIMAL NUTRITION ASSOCIATION OF CANADA. EASTERN NUTRITION CONFERENCE. PROCEEDINGS. Text in English; Abstracts in English, French. 1996. a. CND 40 to non-members; CND 30 to members. back issues avail. **Document type:** *Proceedings.* **Description:** Discusses animal nutrition research.
Formerly: Canadian Feed Industry Association. Eastern Nutrition Conference. Proceedings (1203-8881)
—BLDSC (3646.763000).
Published by: Animal Nutrition Association of Canada, 325 Dalhousie St, Ste 625, Ottawa, ON K1N 7G2, Canada. TEL 613-241-6421, FAX 613-241-7970, info@anac-anac.ca, cfia@cfia-aciaa.ca. Ed. Tracey McGrath.

636 NLD ISSN 0378-4320
CODEN: ANRSDV
ANIMAL REPRODUCTION SCIENCE. Text in Dutch. 1977. 20/yr. EUR 1,325 in Europe to institutions; JPY 176,000 in Japan to institutions; USD 1,483 elsewhere to institutions (effective 2002). back issues avail. *Refereed.* **Document type:** *Academic/Scholarly.* **Description:** Publishes scientific papers dealing with the study of reproduction of all animals which could be regarded as being useful to man.
Related titles: Microform ed.: (from PQC); Online - full text ed.: (from ingenta, Swets Blackwell, ScienceDirect, Institute for Scientific Information).
Indexed: ASCA, AgBiotech, Agri.Eng.Abstr., Agricola, Anim.Breed.Abstr., Bibl.Repro., Chem.Abstr., Chem.Indus.Notes, Chem.Titles, Curr.Adv.Ecol.Sci., Curr.Cont., Dairy Sci.Abstr., Derwent Biotech.Abstr., Excerp.Med., Focus on: Vet.Sci.& Med., Ind.Med. (1978-), Ind.Sci.Rev., Ind.Vet., Int.Abstr.Biol.Sci., Maize Abstr., Nutr.Abstr., Pig News & Info., Poult.Abstr., Protozool.Abstr., Sci.Cit.Ind., Soyabean Abstr., Sport Fish.Abstr., Vet.Bull., Weed Abstr., Wild.Rev., Zoo.Rec.
—BLDSC (0905.076000), CASDDS, CISTI, EMDOCS, IDS, Infotrieve, ingenta, Linda Hall. **CCC.**
Published by: Elsevier Science BV, PO Box 211, Amsterdam 1000 AE, Netherlands. TEL 31-20-485-2911, FAX 31-20-485-2457, nlinfo-f@elsevier.nl, http://www.elsevier.com/locate/anireprosci. Eds. J E Kinder, K L Macmillan. **Subscr. in Australasia and the Far East to:** Elsevier Science (Singapore) Pte Ltd, No.1 Temasek Ave, 17-01 Millenia Tower, Singapore 039192, Singapore. TEL 65-434-3727, FAX 65-337-2230; **Subscr. in Japan to:** Elsevier Science Inc - Japan Regional Office, 9-15 Higashi-Azabu 1-chome, Minato-ku, Tokyo 106-0044, Japan. TEL 81-3-5561-5033; **Subscr. in the Americas to:** Elsevier Science, PO Box 945, New York, NY 10159-0945. TEL 212-633-3730, FAX 212-633-3680.

APIS; the international journal bulletin for specialty livestock and pet-animal product development. see *VETERINARY SCIENCE*

ARCHIVES OF ANIMAL NUTRITION/ARCHIV FUER TIERERNAEHRUNG. see *VETERINARY SCIENCE*

637 ESP ISSN 0004-0592
SF1 CODEN: AZOTAW
ARCHIVOS DE ZOOTECNIA. Text and summaries in English, French, Spanish, Portuguese. 1952. q. ESP 6,000 domestic; USD 75 foreign (effective 2000 & 2001). bk.rev. abstr, bibl, charts, illus. index, cum.index: 1952-1999. back issues avail. *Refereed.* **Document type:** *Academic/Scholarly.* **Description:** Publishes experimental and research work on forage and pasture production, animal feeding, genetics, ethnology and reproduction and the optimization of systems in animal production. Its main emphasis is on the Mediterranean regions.
Indexed: AgBiotech, Agri.Eng.Abstr., Anim.Breed.Abstr., Aqua.Sci.& Fish.Abstr., Aquacult.Abstr., Bibl.Agri., Biol.Abstr., Chem.Abstr., Chem.Indus.Notes, Chem.Titles, Curr.Adv.Ecol.Sci., Dairy Sci.Abstr., Environ.Sci.Poll.Mgmt., Excerp.Med., Fababean Abstr., Field Crop Abstr., Food Sci.& Tech.Abstr., Helminthol.Abstr., Herb.Abstr., Ind.SST, Ind.Vet., Maize Abstr., Nutr.Abstr., Pig News & Info., Poult.Abstr., Rev.Appl.Entomol., Soyabean Abstr., Sport Fish.Abstr., Sugar Ind.Abstr., Triticale Abstr., Vet.Bull., Virol.Abstr. (coverage dropped), Wild.Rev., World Ag.Econ.& Rur.Soc.Abstr., Zoo.Rec.
—BLDSC (1658.000000), CASDDS, CINDOC, Linda Hall. **CCC.**
Published by: Instituto de Zootecnia, Facultad de Veterinaria, Avda Medina Azahara, 9, Cordoba 14005, Spain. TEL 34-57-218743, FAX 34-57-218667, pa1gocag@lucano.uco.es. Ed. Dr. A G Gomez Castro. Circ: 600.

636 660 KOR ISSN 1011-2367
CODEN: AJASEL
ASIAN - AUSTRALASIAN JOURNAL OF ANIMAL SCIENCES. Variant title: A J A S. Text in English. 1988. 10/yr., latest vol.14, 2001. USD 70 to individuals Non-AAAP member countries; USD 50 to individuals AAAP member countries; USD 120 to institutions Non-AAAP member countries; USD 70 to institutions AAAP member countries (effective 2001). adv. bk.rev. *Refereed.* **Document type:** *Academic/Scholarly.* **Description:** Disseminates research on the zoology of domestic farm animals, including diseases and environmental issues.
Related titles: Online - full text ed.: (from Institute for Scientific Information).
Indexed: ASCA, AgBiotech, Agri.Eng.Abstr., Agricola, Agroforest.Abstr., Anim.Breed.Abstr., Bibl.Agri., Biol.Abstr., Chem.Abstr., Chem.Indus.Notes, Chem.Titles, Curr.Cont., Dairy Sci.Abstr., Field Crop Abstr., Focus on: Vet.Sci.& Med., Food Sci.& Tech.Abstr., Forest.Abstr., Helminthol.Abstr., Herb.Abstr., Ind.Vet., Maize Abstr., Nutr.Abstr., Pig News & Info., Plant Breed.Abstr., Postharvest, Poult.Abstr., Protozool.Abstr., Rev.Appl.Entomol., Rev.Med.& Vet.Mycol., Rev.Plant Path., Rice Abstr., Rural Devel.Abstr., Rural Recreat.Tour.Abstr., SSCI (coverage dropped), Seed Abstr., Soils & Fert., Soyabean Abstr., Sugar Ind.Abstr., Triticale Abstr., Vet.Bull., Weed Abstr., World Ag.Econ.& Rur.Soc.Abstr.
—BLDSC (1742.389000), CASDDS, IDS, ingenta.
Published by: Asian - Australasian Association of Animal Production Societies, 806 Kwachon Officetel, 1-14 Pyullyang-dong, Kwachon-shi, Kyunggi-do 427-040, Korea, S.. TEL 82-2-502-0757, FAX 82-502-0758, inkhan@plaza.snu.ac.kr, inkhan@kornet.net, http://www.ajas.snu.ac.kr. Ed., R&P In K Han. Circ: 1,000. **Co-publisher:** Korean Society of Animal Science and Technology.

636 BGD ISSN 0379-430X
BANGLADESH JOURNAL OF ANIMAL SCIENCE. Text in English. 1968. s-a. BDT 100 to individuals; USD 10 foreign to individuals; BDT 200 to institutions; USD 15 foreign to institutions (effective 1999). adv. bk.rev. charts, stat. **Document type:** *Academic/Scholarly.* **Description:** Contains scholarly articles covering topics in animal husbandry.
Formerly: Animal Science Journal of Pakistan (0003-3588)
Indexed: Anim.Breed.Abstr., Biol.Abstr., Chem.Abstr.
—BLDSC (1861.640000), CISTI.
Published by: Bangladesh Husbandry Association, Bangladesh Agricultural University, Department of Animal Nutrition, Mymensingh 2202, Bangladesh. TEL 880-91-55695, FAX 880-91-55810. Ed., Pub., R&P, Adv. contact Abidur Reza. page BDT 7,500. Circ: 1,000.

636.293 THA ISSN 0857-1554
BUFFALO JOURNAL; an international journal of buffalo science. Text in English. 1985. 3/yr. USD 85 in S.E. Asia; USD 90 elsewhere. back issues avail. **Document type:** *Academic/Scholarly.* **Description:** Publishes research paper, reviews and comments on buffalo anatomy, breeding, diseases, genetics, management, nutrition, physiology, reproduction, and socio-economic problem.
Indexed: AgBiotech, Agroforest.Abstr., Anim.Breed.Abstr., Dairy Sci.Abstr., Food Sci.& Tech.Abstr., Helminthol.Abstr., Herb.Abstr., Ind.Vet., Maize Abstr., Nutr.Abstr., Poult.Abstr., Rev.Appl.Entomol., Rev.Med.& Vet.Mycol., Soyabean Abstr., Sugar Ind.Abstr., Triticale Abstr., Vet.Bull.
—BLDSC (2357.595000).
Published by: Chulalongkorn University, Research Centre for Bioscience in Animal Production, Faculty of Veterinary Science, Henri Dunant St, Bangkok 10330, Thailand. TEL 662-2518936, FAX 662-2189736, kmaneewa@netserv.chula.ac.th. Ed. M Kamonpatana.

636.089 KEN ISSN 0378-9721
CODEN: BAHADH
BULLETIN OF ANIMAL HEALTH AND PRODUCTION IN AFRICA/BULLETIN DES SANTE ET PRODUCTION ANIMALES EN AFRIQUE. Text and summaries in English, French. 1953. q. USD 15; USD 20 foreign. abstr, bibl, charts, illus. index. back issues avail. **Document type:** *Academic/Scholarly.* **Description:** Publishes articles on original research relevant to animal health and production activities that may lead to improvement of the livestock industry in Africa and better utilization of her animal resources.
Formerly: Bulletin of Epizootic Diseases of Africa (0525-1443)
Related titles: Supplement: Weekly Information Leaflets.
Indexed: Agri.Eng.Abstr., Anim.Breed.Abstr., Biol.Abstr., Curr.Cont. (coverage dropped), Helminthol.Abstr., INIS Atomind., Ind.Vet., Pig News & Info., Poult.Abstr., Rev.Appl.Entomol., Rev.Med.& Vet.Mycol., Sport Fish.Abstr., Vet.Bull., Wild.Rev., Zoo.Rec.
—CASDDS, GNLM.
Published by: Organization of African Unity, Inter-African Bureau of Animal Resources/Organisation de l'Unite Africaine, Bureau Interafricain des Resources Animales, PO Box 30786, Nairobi, Kenya. TEL 254-2-338544, FAX 254-2-332046, TELEX 22983. Ed. W N Masiga.

636 DNK ISSN 0105-6883
CODEN: BSHUDX
DENMARK. STATENS HUSDYRBRUGSFORSOEG. BERETNING/DENMARK. DANISH INSTITUTE OF ANIMAL SCIENCE. REPORT. Text in Danish; Summaries in English. 1883. irreg. price varies. **Document type:** *Government.*
Former titles (until 1975): Denmark. Forsoegslaboratoriet. Beretning (0005-8904); (until 1915): Denmark. Den Kongelige Veterinaer- og Landbohoejskoles Laboratorium for Landoekonomiske Forsoeg. Beretning (0105-2314)
Indexed: Agri.Eng.Abstr., Anim.Breed.Abstr., Dairy Sci.Abstr., Field Crop Abstr., Food Sci.& Tech.Abstr., Helminthol.Abstr., Herb.Abstr., Ind.Vet., Nutr.Abstr., Rural Recreat.Tour.Abstr., Soyabean Abstr., Sugar Ind.Abstr., Triticale Abstr., Vet.Bull., World Ag.Econ.& Rur.Soc.Abstr.
—CISTI.
Published by: Statens Husdyrbrugsforsoeg/Danish Institute of Animal Science, Research Center Foulum, PO Box 39, Tjele 8830, Denmark. TEL 45-8999-1900, FAX 45-8999-1919. Circ: 1,300.

636 DNK ISSN 0908-021X
DENMARK. STATENS HUSDYRBRUGSFORSOEG. FORSKNINGSRAPPORT/DENMARK. DANISH INSTITUTE OF ANIMAL SCIENCE. RESEARCH REPORT. Text in Danish. 1993. irreg. price varies. back issues avail. **Document type:** *Trade.*
Indexed: Agri.Eng.Abstr., Maize Abstr., Nutr.Abstr., Triticale Abstr.
—CISTI.
Published by: Statens Husdyrbrugsforsoeg/Danish Institute of Animal Science, Research Center Foulum, PO Box 39, Tjele 8830, Denmark. TEL 45-8999-1900, FAX 45-8999-1919.

636 JPN ISSN 0286-4754
EIYO SEIRI KENKYUKAIHO/JAPANESE SOCIETY FOR ANIMAL NUTRITION AND METABOLISM. PROCEEDINGS. Text in Japanese. 1956. s-a. JPY 3,000 (effective 2000). adv. **Document type:** *Academic/Scholarly.*
Published by: Kachiku Eiyo Seiri Kenkyukai/Japanese Society for Animal Nutrition and Metabolism, Miyazaki University, Faculty of Agriculture, Animal Science Division, Miyazaki 889-2192, Japan. TEL 81-985-58-7201, FAX 81-985-58-7201, a0c301u@cc.miyazaki-u.ac.jp. Ed. Ryoj Onodera.

EQUATOR; newsletter on veterinary aspects of international development cooperation. see *VETERINARY SCIENCE*

ETHOLOGY. see *BIOLOGY—Zoology*

ETHOLOGY ONLINE. see *BIOLOGY—Zoology*

FARM SCIENTIST. see *VETERINARY SCIENCE*

636 CHN ISSN 1002-6746
GUOWAI XUMU KEJI/FOREIGN ANIMAL HUSBANDRY SCIENCE AND TECHNOLOGY. Text in Chinese. 1974. bi-m. CNY 18 (effective 1997). **Document type:** *Academic/Scholarly.*
Published by: Zhongguo Nongye Kexueyuan, Xumu Yanjiusuo/Chinese Academy of Agricultural Sciences, Institute of Animal Husbandry, Yuanminyuan Lu, Haidian-qu, Beijing 100094, China. TEL 86-10-6258-1177, FAX 86-10-6258-2594. Ed. Nianfan Guo.

HANDBOOK OF FEED ADDITIVES. see *AGRICULTURE—Feed, Flour And Grain*

636.084 IND ISSN 0970-3209
CODEN: IJNUEA
INDIAN JOURNAL OF ANIMAL NUTRITION. Text in English. 1984. q. INR 700 domestic; USD 70 foreign (effective 2001). adv. bk.rev. 100 p./no. 1 cols./p. back issues avail. *Refereed.* **Document type:** *Journal, Academic/Scholarly.* **Description:** Contains animal nutrition research in ruminants, poultry and other monogastric animals.
Indexed: Agroforest.Abstr., Anim.Breed.Abstr., Dairy Sci.Abstr., Food Sci.& Tech.Abstr., Forest.Abstr., Herb.Abstr., Ind.Vet., Maize Abstr., Nutr.Abstr., Pig News & Info., Plant Breed.Abstr., Postharvest, Poult.Abstr., Rev.Appl.Entomol., Rev.Med.& Vet.Mycol., Rice Abstr., Sorghum & Millets Abstr., Soyabean Abstr., Sugar Ind.Abstr., Triticale Abstr., Trop.Oil Seeds Abstr., Vet.Bull., Weed Abstr.
—Linda Hall.
Published by: Animal Nutrition Society of India, National Dairy Research Institute, Karnal, Haryana 132 001, India. TEL 91-184-259057, FAX 91-184-250042, TELEX 0396-204 NDRI IN, pps@ndri.hry.nic.in. Ed. K K Singhal. Adv. contact Aruna Chhabra. B&W page INR 1,500. Circ: 700.

636 IND ISSN 0367-6722
SF1 CODEN: IALRBR
INDIAN JOURNAL OF ANIMAL RESEARCH; half-yearly research journal of animal, food, dairying and zoological sciences. Text in English. 1967. s-a. INR 300 domestic; USD 40 foreign (effective 2001). **Document type:** *Academic/Scholarly.* **Description:** Publishes results of original research work on various aspects of Animal sciences, viz., animal breeding, physiology, nutrition, diseases, production, fisheries and zoological sciences.
Formerly (until 1971): Indian Journal of Science and Industry. Section B. Animal Sciences (0367-830X); Supersedes in part (in 1970): Indian Journal of Science and Industry (0019-5618)
Indexed: Anim.Breed.Abstr., Biol.Abstr., Chem.Abstr., Dairy Sci.Abstr., Food Sci.& Tech.Abstr., Helminthol.Abstr., Herb.Abstr., Ind.Vet., Nutr.Abstr., Pig News & Info., Postharvest, Poult.Abstr., Protozool.Abstr., Rev.Appl.Entomol., Rev.Med.& Vet.Mycol., Rice Abstr., Small Anim.Abstr., Vet.Bull., Weed Abstr., World Ag.Econ.& Rur.Soc.Abstr.
—CASDDS, CISTI, ingenta, Linda Hall.
Published by: Agricultural Research Communication Centre, 1130 Sadar Bazar, Post Office Marg, Karnal, Haryana 132 001, India. TEL 91-184-255080. Ed. Dr. D D Sharma. Adv. contact R D Goel.

636.5 IND ISSN 0970-9738
INDIAN POULTRY INDUSTRY YEARBOOK. Text in English. 1974. a. USD 250. bk.rev. **Description:** Sourcebook on trade, technical and economic aspects of poultry. Lists 7,000 specialists and organizations by business and geographic locations.
Indexed: Anim.Breed.Abstr., Nutr.Abstr.
Published by: S.P. Gupta Pub., A-25 Priyadarshini Vihar, Patparganj Rd., New Delhi 110 092, India. TEL 91-11-224-3326, FAX 91-11-2243039. Ed. Sharad Gupta. adv.: B&W page USD 800; trim 15 x 20. Circ: 2,500 (paid).

636.5 IND ISSN 0019-6150
CODEN: IPRWD9
INDIAN POULTRY REVIEW. Text in English. 1969. m. USD 70 (effective 1995). adv. bk.rev. abstr, illus.
Indexed: Chem.Abstr., Indian Sci.Abstr.
—BLDSC (4427.850000), CASDDS.
Published by: Indian Poultry Lovers Association, 57-B Townshend Rd., Kolkata, West Bengal 700 025, India. TEL 4750838. Ed. G N Ghosh. Circ: 18,000.

636 179 660 IND ISSN 0970-2857
CODEN: IASCEK
INTERNATIONAL JOURNAL OF ANIMAL SCIENCES. Text in English. 1986. s-a. USD 100. adv. bk.rev. bibl, charts, illus. *Refereed.* **Document type:** *Academic/Scholarly.* **Description:** Publishes research and review articles in the field of animal health, animal biology, animal production, dairy science and biotechnology.
Formerly (until 1987): Farm Animals
Indexed: AgBiotech, Anim.Breed.Abstr., Biol.Abstr., Chem.Abstr., Dairy Sci.Abstr., Derwent Biotech.Abstr., Helminthol.Abstr., Ind.Vet., Maize Abstr., Nutr.Abstr., Pig News & Info., Poult.Abstr., Protozool.Abstr., Rev.Appl.Entomol., Rev.Arom.& Med.Plants, Rev.Med.& Vet.Mycol., Rice Abstr., Vet.Bull., World Ag.Econ.& Rur.Soc.Abstr., Zoo.Rec.
—BLDSC (4542.082000), Infotrieve. **CCC.**
Published by: Nitasha Publications, 921, Sector 14, Sonipat, Haryana 131 001, India. TEL 91-1662-32703. Ed., Pub., R&P, Adv. contact Sadhana Jindal.

JOURNAL OF APPLIED ANIMAL WELFARE SCIENCE. see *ANIMAL WELFARE*

LEBENSMITTEL- UND BIOTECHNOLOGIE; die oesterreichische Fachzeitschrift fuer Lebensmittelindustrie und -forschung. see *FOOD AND FOOD INDUSTRIES*

MAGAZYN - DROBIARSTWO. see *VETERINARY SCIENCE*

354.59 USA
MEAT AND POULTRY INSPECTION REGULATIONS; meat inspection, poultry inspection, rabbit inspection, voluntary inspection and certificate service of meat and poultry, humane slaughter of livestock. Text in English. 1990. base vol. plus m. updates. USD 297 (effective 2001); USD 290 foreign (effective 1995). **Document type:** *Government.* **Description:** Publishes the regulations for slaughter and processing of livestock and poultry, as well as certain voluntary services for more humane slaughter.
Published by: U.S. Department of Agriculture, Food Safety and Inspection Service, Rm 1140, South Bldg, 14th and Independence Ave, SW, Washington, DC 20250. TEL 202-720-2109, FAX 202-690-3023, http://www.fsis.usda.gov. **Subscr. to:** U.S. Government Printing Office, Superintendent of Documents, PO Box 371954, Pittsburgh, PA 15250-7954. TEL 202-512-1800, FAX 202-512-2250, orders@gpo.gov, http://www.access.gpo.gov.

636 NGA
NIGERIA. NATIONAL ANIMAL PRODUCTION RESEARCH INSTITUTE. JOURNAL; Journal of Animal Production Research. Abbreviated title: N A P R I Journal. Text in English. 1981. s-a., latest vol.16, 1996. USD 90 per issue (effective 2001). adv. bk.rev. cum.index. back issues avail. **Document type:** *Academic/Scholarly.*
Indexed: Poult.Abstr.
Published by: National Animal Production Research Institute, Ahmadu Bello University, PMB 1096, Zaria, Kaduna, Nigeria. napri@in@t-global.com. Ed. L O Eduvie. Circ: 1,000.

636.2 NLD ISSN 0030-2775
ONS VEE✱ ; maandblad voor de veehouderij. Text in Dutch. 1967 (vol.18). m. NLG 15.15. adv. illus.
Address: Past. van Akenstraat 8, Roosendaal, Netherlands.

636 PAK
PAKISTAN JOURNAL OF ANIMAL SCIENCES. Text in English. q. PKR 10, USD 1.25. adv. bibl, charts.
Published by: Society for the Advancement of Animal Sciences, c/o Veterinary Research Institute, Ghazi Rd., Lahore, 13, Pakistan.

THE PIG JOURNAL. see *VETERINARY SCIENCE*

636 ITA
PROFESSIONEALLEVATORE✱ . Text in Italian. 1984. 14/yr. ITL 50,000; ITL 100,000 foreign. adv.
Published by: Point Veterinaire Italie s.r.l, Via Francesco Melzi D'Eril, 26, Milan, MI 20154, Italy. TEL 39-2-336035, FAX 39-2-33606655. Ed. Dr. J P Dagneauz. Circ: 32,000.

636.089 ITA
RAZZA BRUNA. Text in Italian. 1961. bi-m. ITL 25,000; ITL 50,000 foreign (effective 1997). adv. **Document type:** *Bulletin, Academic/Scholarly.* **Description:** Presents general, technical, and economical information for breeders, especially for the Bruna breeders.
Published by: Associazione Nazionale Allevatori Razza Bruna (A.N.A.R.B.), Localita Ferlina, 204, Bussolengo, VR 37012, Italy. TEL 39-45-6701990, FAX 39-45-7156655, anarb.vr@pn.inet.it, http://www.ifinet.it/anarb. Ed. Giuseppe Perotti. Adv. contact Paola Fassini. B&W page ITL 70,000, color page ITL 1,000,000.

REVUE D'ELEVAGE ET DE MEDECINE VETERINAIRE DES PAYS TROPICAUX. see *VETERINARY SCIENCE*

636 ITA ISSN 0304-0607
CODEN: RZOVBM
RIVISTA DI ZOOTECNIA E VETERINARIA✱ ; rassegna di informazione e aggiornamento. Text in Italian; Summaries in English, French. 1924. bi-m. ITL 5,000. adv. bk.rev. abstr, bibl, charts, illus, stat. index, cum.index.
Formerly (until 1973): Rivista di Zootecnia (0035-6646)
Indexed: Agri.& Environ.Biotech.Abstr. (coverage dropped), Anim.Breed.Abstr., Biol.Abstr., Chem.Abstr., Dairy Sci.Abstr., Derwent Biotech.Abstr., Field Crop Abstr., Food Sci.& Tech.Abstr., Helminthol.Abstr., Herb.Abstr., Ind.Vet., Nutr.Abstr., Pig News & Info., Sport Fish.Abstr., Vet.Bull., Wild.Rev.
—BLDSC (7993.705000), CASDDS, CISTI, Linda Hall.
Published by: (Societa Farmaceutici Italia), Centralvet, Via Colleoni, 15, Agrate Brianza, MI 20041, Italy. Ed. Remo Faustini.

636.3 NLD ISSN 0921-4488
SF380 CODEN: SRUREW
SMALL RUMINANT RESEARCH. Text in English; Summaries in French, German, Spanish. 1980-1984; N.S. 1988. m. EUR 1,146 in Europe to institutions; JPY 152,000 in Japan to institutions; USD 1,281 elsewhere to institutions (effective 2002). bk.rev. reprints avail. *Refereed.* **Document type:** *Academic/Scholarly.* **Description:** Covers nutrition, physiology, anatomy, genetics, microbiology, ethology, product technology, socio-economics, management, veterinary medicine and husbandry engineering.
Formerly (until 1984): International Goat and Sheep Research (0197-7393)
Related titles: Microform ed.: N.S. (from PQC); Online - full text ed.: (from ingenta, Swets Blackwell, Institute for Scientific Information, ScienceDirect).
Indexed: ASCA, AgBiotech, Agri.Eng.Abstr., Agricola, Agroforest.Abstr., Anim.Breed.Abstr., Bibl.Agri., Biol.Abstr., Chem.Abstr., Curr.Cont., Dairy Sci.Abstr., Derwent Biotech.Abstr., Focus on: Vet.Sci.& Med., Food Sci.& Tech.Abstr., Forest Prod.Abstr., Helminthol.Abstr., Herb.Abstr., Ind.Vet., Maize Abstr., Nutr.Abstr., Protozool.Abstr., Rev.Appl.Entomol., Rev.Arom.& Med.Plants, Rev.Med.& Vet.Mycol., Rice Abstr., Rural Devel.Abstr., Rural Recreat.Tour.Abstr., Soyabean Abstr., Sugar Ind.Abstr., Triticale Abstr., Vet.Bull., Wild.Rev., World Ag.Econ.& Rur.Soc.Abstr.
—BLDSC (8310.140000), CASDDS, CISTI, IDS, Infotrieve, ingenta, Linda Hall. **CCC.**

A

A

Published by: (International Goat Association), Elsevier Science BV, PO Box 211, Amsterdam 1000 AE, Netherlands. TEL 31-20-485-2911, FAX 31-20-485-2457, nlinfo-f@elsevier.nl, http://www.elsevier.com/locate/smallrumres. Ed. D M Sherman. Circ: 500. **Subscr. in Australasia and the Far East to:** Elsevier Science (Singapore) Pte Ltd, No.1 Temasek Ave, 17-01 Millenia Tower, Singapore 039192, Singapore. TEL 65-434-3727, FAX 65-337-2230; **Subscr. in Japan to:** Elsevier Science Inc - Japan Regional Office, 9-15 Higashi-Azabu 1-chome, Minato-ku, Tokyo 106-0044, Japan. TEL 81-3-5561-5033; **Subscr. in the Americas to:** Elsevier Science, PO Box 945, New York, NY 10159-0945. TEL 212-633-3730, FAX 212-633-3680.

636 ZAF ISSN 0375-1589
CODEN: SAJAC9

SOUTH AFRICAN JOURNAL OF ANIMAL SCIENCE. Text in English. 1971. 3/yr. ZAR 228 to institutions; USD 82 foreign (effective 2000). adv. *Refereed.* **Document type:** *Academic/Scholarly.* **Description:** Publishes original contributions in animal science research.
Incorporates: South African Society of Animal Production. Proceedings. Handelinge (0081-2536); And (1958-1981): Agroanimalia (0302-7104); Which superseded in part (in 1969): South African Journal of Agricultural Science
Related titles: Online - full text ed.: (from Institute for Scientific Information).
Indexed: ASCA, Anim.Breed.Abstr., Aqua.Sci.& Fish.Abstr., Biol.Abstr., Chem.Abstr., Chem.Indus.Notes, Chem.Titles, Curr.Adv.Ecol.Sci., Curr.Cont., Dairy Sci.Abstr., Derwent Biotech.Abstr., Environ.Sci.Poll.Mgmt., Field Crop Abstr., Focus on: Vet.Sci.& Med., Food Sci.& Tech.Abstr., Helminthol.Abstr., Herb.Abstr., INIS Atomind., Ind.S.A.Per., Ind.Vet., Maize Abstr., Nutr.Abstr., Pig News & Info., Pollut.Abstr., Postharvest, Poult.Abstr., Ref.Zh., Rev.Med.& Vet.Mycol., Rural Devel.Abstr., Rural Recreat.Tour.Abstr., Soils & Fert., Sorghum & Millets Abstr., Soyabean Abstr., Sport Fish.Abstr., Sugar Ind.Abstr., Triticale Abstr., Vet.Bull., Wild.Rev., World Ag.Econ.& Rur.Soc.Abstr., Zoo.Rec.
—BLDSC (8338.650000), CASDDS, CISTI, IDS, Infotrieve, ingenta, Linda Hall. **CCC.**
Published by: (South African Society of Animal Science), South African Bureau for Scientific Publications, PO Box 11663, Pretoria, Hatfield 0028, South Africa. TEL 27-12-322-6404, FAX 27-12-320-7803, bspman@icon.co.za, http://www.safest.org.za/bsp. Ed., Adv. contact J G van der Walt. Circ: 700.

636.2 NLD
STIERENBOEK. Text in Dutch. s-a. NLG 195; BEF 3,700 in Belgium (effective 1999 & 2000). **Document type:** *Trade.* **Description:** Current genetic information on all available breeding bulls.
Former titles: Boerderij Stierenboek; Stierenboek
Published by: Elsevier Bedrijfsinformatie BV, Misset (Subsidiary of: Reed Elsevier plc), Postbus 4, Doetinchem 7000 BA, Netherlands. TEL 31-314-349371, FAX 31-314-363638, info@ebi.nl, http://www.ebi.nl. Circ: 2,000.

TROPICAL ANIMAL HEALTH AND PRODUCTION. see *VETERINARY SCIENCE*

TURK VETERINERLIK VE HAYVANCILIK DERGISI/TURKISH JOURNAL OF VETERINARY AND ANIMAL SCIENCES. see *VETERINARY SCIENCE*

636 ROM
CODEN: LSIVDF

UNIVERSITATEA AGRONOMICA ION IONESCU DE LA BRAD. LUCRARI STIINTIFICE. SERIA ZOOTECHNIE - MEDICINA VETERINARIA. Text in Romanian. 1957. a.
Formerly: Institutul Agronomic Ion Ionescu de la Brad. Lucrari Stiintifice. Seria Zootechnie - Medicina Veterinaria (0075-3513)
Indexed: Anim.Breed.Abstr., Biol.Abstr., Ind.Vet., Nutr.Abstr., Rev.Appl.Entomol., Rev.Med.& Vet.Mycol., VITIS, Vet.Bull.
—CASDDS, CISTI.
Published by: Universitatea Agronomica "Ion Ionescu de la Brad", Al. M. Sadoveanu 3, Jassy, Romania.

636 636.089 ROM ISSN 1221-3594
CODEN: BIAVDX

UNIVERSITATEA DE STIINTE AGRICOLE CLUJ-NAPOCA. BULETINUL. SERIA ZOOTEHNIE SI MEDICINA VETERINARA. Text in Romanian; Summaries in English, French. 1975. a. back issues avail.
Formerly (until 1992): Institutul Agronomic Cluj-Napoca. Buletinul. Seria Zootehnie si Medicina Veterinara (0557-4668); Supersedes in part (in 1977): Institutul Agronomic Cluj-Napoca. Buletinul (0378-0554)
Indexed: Biodet.Abstr., Biol.Abstr., Food Sci.& Tech.Abstr., Ind.Vet., Poult.Abstr., Protozool.Abstr., Rev.Appl.Entomol., Soyabean Abstr., Sport Fish.Abstr., Vet.Bull., Wild.Rev., Zoo.Rec.
—CASDDS, CISTI.
Published by: Universitatea de Stiinte Agricole Cluj-Napoca, Str. Manastur 3, Cluj-Napoca 3400, Romania. Ed. Alexandru Salontai. Circ: 500.

VETERINARIA E ZOOTECNIA. see *VETERINARY SCIENCE*

WORLD BUIATRICS CONGRESS. see *VETERINARY SCIENCE*

WORLD RABBIT SCIENCE. see *BIOLOGY—Zoology*

XUMU SHOUYI XUEBAO/ACTA VETERINARIA ET ZOOTECHNICA SINICA. see *VETERINARY SCIENCE*

ZHIVOTNOVOD DLYA VSEKH. see *VETERINARY SCIENCE*

636 CHN ISSN 0258-7033
CODEN: BM452

ZHONGGUO XUMU ZAZHI/CHINESE JOURNAL OF ANIMAL SCIENCE. Text in Chinese. 1963. bi-m. USD 0.70 per issue.
Indexed: AgBiotech, Anim.Breed.Abstr., Chem.Abstr., Dairy Sci.Abstr., Ind.Vet., Maize Abstr., Nutr.Abstr., Pig News & Info., Poult.Abstr., Rev.Med.& Vet.Mycol., Soyabean Abstr., Triticale Abstr., Trop.Oil Seeds Abstr., Vet.Bull.
—CASDDS, CISTI, Linda Hall.
Published by: Zhongguo Xumu Shouyi Xuehui/Chinese Society of Animal Husbandry and Veterinary Science, 33 Nong Feng Li, Dongdaqiao, Chaoyang-qu, Beijing 100020, China. TEL 86-1-65066533. Ed. Feng Yanglian.

AIR TRANSPORT

see *TRANSPORTATION—Air Transport*

ALLERGOLOGY AND IMMUNOLOGY

see *MEDICAL SCIENCES—Allergology And Immunology*

ALTERNATIVE MEDICINE

see also *MEDICAL SCIENCES*

A A M TERRA NUOVA; rivista ecoalternativa. (Agricoltura Alimentazione Medicina) see *ENVIRONMENTAL STUDIES*

615.822 USA
ACUPRESSURE NEWS. Text in English, French, German, Italian. 1987. a., latest vol.16. USD 2.50 (effective 2001). tr.mk. 8 p./no. 3 cols./p. back issues avail.; reprints avail. **Document type:** *Newsletter.* **Description:** Jin Shin Do Bodymind Acupressure combines gentle yet deep finger pressure on specific acu-points with body focusing techniques, to help physical and emotional tension and armoring.
Published by: Jin Shin Do Foundation, Acupressure Workshop, 1084 G San Miguel Canyon Rd, Watsonville, CA 95076. TEL 831-763-7702, FAX 831-763-1551, http://www.jinshindo.org. Ed. Iona Marsaa Teeguarden. Circ: 6,000 (paid and controlled).

615.892 615.845 USA ISSN 0360-1293
RM184 CODEN: AEREDS

ACUPUNCTURE AND ELECTRO-THERAPEUTICS RESEARCH; the international journal. Text in English. 1976. q. USD 220 domestic; USD 240 foreign (effective 2001). bk.rev. abstr, bibl, charts, illus, stat. index. back issues avail. *Refereed.* **Document type:** *Academic/Scholarly.* **Description:** Covers developments in basic and clinical research in acupuncture, electro-therapeutics and related fields. Fosters efforts to understand and improve these treatments and their use in diagnosis, prognosis, treatment and prevention of diseases in both Western and Oriental medicine.
Related titles: Microform ed.; Online - full text ed.: (from Institute for Scientific Information).
Indexed: AMED, ASCA, Bioeng.Abstr., Biol.Abstr., Biotech.& Bioeng.Abstr., CINAHL, Chem.Abstr., Comput.& Info.Sys., Curr.Adv.Ecol.Sci., Curr.Cont., Dent.Ind., Eng.Ind., Excerp.Med., Ind.Med. (1975-), Inpharma, Psychol.Abstr., Reac., Sci.Cit.Ind. (coverage dropped).
—BLDSC (0677.930000), CASDDS, CISTI, Ei, EMDOCS, GNLM, IDS, ingenta, KNAW. **CCC.**
Published by: (International College of Acupuncture and Electro-Therapeutics), Cognizant Communication Corporation, 3 Hartsdale Rd, Elmsford, NY 10523-3701. TEL 914-592-7720, FAX 914-592-8981, cogcomm@aol.com, http://www.cognizantcommunication.com. Ed. Dr. Yoshiaki Omura. Pub., R&P Robert N Miranda. Adv. contact Lori Miranda. Circ: 1,000.

615.89 GBR ISSN 0964-5284
CODEN: ACMEF

ACUPUNCTURE IN MEDICINE. Text in English. 1981. s-a. GBP 20 in Europe to non-members; GBP 25 elsewhere to non-members (effective 2001). adv. bk.rev. cum.index. 2 cols./p. back issues avail. *Refereed.* **Document type:** *Journal, Academic/Scholarly.* **Description:** Aimed at medical practitioners. Publishes the results of controlled trials, reviews, audits, case histories and speculative discussion concerning acupuncture and related techniques.
Related titles: Online - full text ed.
Indexed: AMED, CINAHL, Excerp.Med. (1996-), Ref.Zh.
—BLDSC (0677.935000), EMDOCS, GNLM.
Published by: British Medical Acupuncture Society, 12 Marbury House, Higher Whitley, Warrington, Ches WA4 4QW, United Kingdom. TEL 44-1925-730727, FAX 44-1925-730492, editor@medical-acupuncture.org.uk, admin@medical-acupuncture.org.uk, http://www.medical-acupuncture.co.uk/aimintro.htm. Eds. Dr. Jacqueline Filshie, Dr. Mike Cummings. R&P Dr. Mike Cummings. Adv. contact Julian Price. page GBP 225. Circ: 5,000.

610.95 615.892 NLD ISSN 1382-6883
ADVANCED TRADITIONAL CHINESE MEDICINE SERIES. Text mainly in English; Text occasionally in Chinese. 1996. irreg., latest vol.8, 1998. price varies. back issues avail. *Refereed.* **Document type:** *Monographic series, Academic/Scholarly.* **Description:** Publishes studies on the theory and practice of traditional Chinese medicine, including discussions of herbs, techniques, and clinical applications. Volumes include glossary of terminology in Pinyin and Chinese characters.
Indexed: Ind.Med. (coverage dropped).
Published by: I O S Press, Van Diemenstraat 94, Amsterdam 1013 CN, Netherlands. TEL 31-20-638-2189, FAX 31-20-620-3419, market@iospress.nl, http://www.iospress.nl/html/atcms.html. **Subscr. to:** I O S Press, Inc, 5795-G Burke Centre Pkwy, Burke, VA 22015. TEL 703-323-5554, FAX 703-323-3668, iosbooks@iospress.com. **Dist. by:** Ohmsha Ltd, 3-1 Kanda-Nishiki-cho, Chiyoda-ku, Tokyo 101-0054, Japan. TEL 81-3-3233-0641, FAX 81-3-3233-2426, http://www.ohmsha.co.jp.

ADVANCES IN MIND - BODY MEDICINE. see *MEDICAL SCIENCES*

ADVERSE EFFECTS OF HERBAL DRUGS. see *PHARMACY AND PHARMACOLOGY*

615.89 DEU ISSN 0720-6003
AERZTEZEITSCHRIFT FUER NATURHEILVERFAHREN. Text mainly in German; Summaries in English, French. 1959. m. DEM 98 domestic; DEM 12 newsstand/cover; DEM 143 foreign; DEM 73.50 domestic to students; DEM 118.50 foreign to students (effective 2001). adv. bk.rev. charts, illus. index, cum.index. back issues avail. **Document type:** *Magazine, Academic/Scholarly.*
Formerly: Physikalische Medizin und Rehabilitation (0031-9287)
Indexed: Excerp.Med., Ref.Zh.
—GNLM, Infotrieve. **CCC.**
Published by: (Zentralverband der Aerzte fuer Naturheilverfahren e.V.), Medizinisch Literarische Verlagsgesellschaft mbH, Postfach 1151-1152, Uelzen 29501, Germany. TEL 49-581-808151, FAX 49-581-808158, mlverlag@mlverlag.de, http://www.mlverlag.de. Circ: 12,500.

615.89 USA
AESCLEPIAN CHRONICLES. Text in English. 1995. m. back issues avail. **Document type:** *Newsletter.* **Description:** Promotes the role of holistic health practice and integral philosophy.
Related titles: Online - full text ed.
Published by: Synergistic Health Center, 1506 E Franklin St, Ste 104, Chapel Hill, NC 27514. TEL 919-932-7266, http://www.forthrt.com/~chronicl/homepage.html.

615.892 DEU ISSN 0340-3130
CODEN: AKUPE
AKUPUNKTUR: THEORIE UND PRAXIS. Text in German. 1973. q. DEM 49 domestic; DEM 65 foreign; DEM 36.75 domestic to students; DEM 52.75 foreign to students (effective 2001). adv. bk.rev. back issues avail. **Document type:** *Magazine, Academic/Scholarly.* **Description:** Publishes articles on scientific research in acupuncture and includes lists of courses and events.
Indexed: Excerp.Med.
—CCC.
Published by: Medizinisch Literarische Verlagsgesellschaft mbH, Postfach 1151-1152, Uelzen 29501, Germany. TEL 49-581-808151, FAX 49-581-808158, mlverlag@mlverlag.de, http://www.mlverlag.de. Ed., Pub. Dr. Thomas Weinschuetz. Circ: 10,500.

615.53 SWE ISSN 1100-7079
ALTERNATIV MEDICIN* . Text in Swedish. 1989. q.
Published by: Svenska Naturmedicinska Saellskapet, Storgatan 17, Vaexjoe 35231, Sweden.

615.89 USA ISSN 1076-2809
R733 CODEN: ACTHFZ
ALTERNATIVE & COMPLEMENTARY THERAPIES; a bimonthly publication for health care practitioners. Text in English. 1995. bi-m. USD 69 domestic to individuals; USD 184 foreign to individuals; USD 83 domestic to individuals print and online edition combined; USD 198 foreign to individuals print and online eds. combined; USD 229 domestic to institutions; USD 317 foreign to institutions; USD 275 domestic to institutions print and online edition combined; USD 363 foreign to institutions print and online edition combined (effective 2002). adv. back issues avail.; reprints avail. **Document type:** *Journal, Academic/Scholarly.* **Description:** Covers latest trends in the field of alternative medicine. Topics covered include a variety of nontraditional holistic health specialties.
Related titles: Online - full content ed.: USD 69 to individuals; USD 229 to institutions (effective 2002) (from EBSCO Publishing, Swets Blackwell); Online - full text ed.: (from CatchWord Ltd., RoweCom Information Quest).
Indexed: AMED, Excerp.Med., I.P.A.
—BLDSC (0803.581470), CISTI, GNLM, Infotrieve, ingenta. **CCC.**
Published by: Mary Ann Liebert, Inc. Publishers, 2 Madison Ave, Larchmont, NY 10538. TEL 914—834-3100, FAX 914-834-1388, info@liebertpub.com, www.liebertpub.com/act, http://www.alternativemed.com. Ed. Karen L Dean. Adv. contact Harriet Matysko.

615.89 USA
ALTERNATIVE MEDICINE ALERT. Text in English. 1997. m. USD 229 domestic; USD 259 foreign; USD 38 newsstand/cover (effective 2001). **Description:** Dedicated to providing clinically sound information on alternative medicine to medical professionals.
Published by: American Health Consultants (Subsidiary of: Medical Economics Co., Inc.), 3525 Piedmont Rd, N E, 6 Piedmont Center, Ste 400, Atlanta, GA 30305. TEL 404-262-5476, 800-688-2421, FAX 404-262-7837, 800-284-3291, custserv@ahcpub.com, http://www.ahcpub.com.

615.89 USA
ALTERNATIVE MEDICINE MAGAZINE. Text in English. 1994. bi-m. USD 20; USD 45 foreign (effective 1999). adv. bk.rev. illus. **Document type:** *Magazine, Consumer.* **Description:** Offers feature articles, departments, and digest summaries of information from doctor's journals, research, conferences and newsletters, covering the entire field of alternative medicine.
Formerly: Alternative Medicine Digest (1081-4000)
Indexed: CINAHL.
—ingenta.
Published by: Future Medicine Publishing, Inc., 1640 Tiburon Blvd., Ste. 2, Tiburon, CA 94920. TEL 415-435-1779, 800-333-4325, FAX 415-435-9448, http://www.alternativemedicine.com. Ed., R&P Tom Klaber TEL 415-789-1415. Pub. Burton Goldberg. Adv. contact Harold Abend. Circ: 170,000.

615.5 USA ISSN 1089-5159
CODEN: ALMRFP
ALTERNATIVE MEDICINE REVIEW; a journal of clinical therapeutics. Text in English. bi-m. USD 85; USD 100 foreign (effective 1999). bk.rev. abstr. *Refereed.* **Document type:** *Academic/Scholarly.* **Description:** Dedicated to providing accurate, timely and clinically relevant original articles, abstracts, and literature reviews to the practicing preventive health-care professional.
Indexed: AMED, CINAHL, Ind.Med. (coverage dropped), Rev.Arom.& Med.Plants.
—BLDSC (0803.588880), GNLM, Infotrieve. **CCC.**
Published by: Thorne Research Inc., PO Box 25, Dover, ID 83825. TEL 208-263-1337, FAX 208-265-2488, altmedrev@thorne.com, http://www.thorne.com/altmedrev. Ed. Kelly Czap. Pub. A F Czap.

615.89 USA
▼ **ALTERNATIVE MEDICINE SOURCEBOOK.** Text in English. 1999 (June). irreg., latest 1999. USD 78 per issue (effective 2001). charts. Index. **Description:** Contains basic Information for the layperson about non-traditional therapies, including acupuncture, homeopathy, herbal remedies, mega-vitamin regimes, and more, along with current research data.
Published by: Omnigraphics, Inc., 615 Griswold St, Detroit, MI 48226. TEL 313-961-1340, 800-234-1340, FAX 313-961-1383, 800-875-1340, info@omnigraphics.com, http://www.omnigraphics.com. Ed. Allan R Cook.

615.89 USA ISSN 1078-6791
R733 CODEN: ATHMF7
ALTERNATIVE THERAPIES IN HEALTH AND MEDICINE. Text in English. 1995. bi-m. USD 64 domestic to individuals; USD 88 foreign to individuals; USD 155 domestic to institutions; USD 215 foreign to institutions; USD 12 newsstand/cover domestic; USD 18 newsstand/cover foreign (effective 2002). adv. *Refereed.* **Document type:** *Journal, Academic/Scholarly.* **Description:** Explores the integration of alternative therapies with conventional medical practices.
Related titles: Online - full text ed.: (from ProQuest Information & Learning, Institute for Scientific Information).
Indexed: AMED, CINAHL, Curr.Cont., Environ.Sci.Poll.Mgmt., Ind.Med. (1995-), Inpharma, Int.Nurs.Ind., NRN, Pharm.&Out.News, Reac.
—BLDSC (0803.661500), GNLM, IDS, Infotrieve. **CCC.**
Published by: InnoVision Communications, 169 Saxony Rd, Ste 104, Encinitas, CA 92024. TEL 760-633-3910, FAX 760-633-3918, 866-828-2962, info@invcom.com. Ed. Dr. Larry Dossey. Pub. Bonnie Horrigan. R&P Beth Wos TEL 800-899-1712. Adv. contact Bob Vrooman. Circ: 15,000 (paid).

615.892 USA ISSN 0091-3960
CODEN: AJAPB9
AMERICAN JOURNAL OF ACUPUNCTURE. Text in English. 1972. q. USD 60 to individuals; USD 90 to institutions (effective 1999). adv. bk.rev. abstr, charts, illus. back issues avail.; reprint service avail. from ISI. *Refereed.* **Document type:** *Academic/Scholarly.* **Description:** Publishes papers spanning the full spectrum of acupuncture modalities from classical to modern variations plus correlations and combinations with Western medicine. Includes instruction on methods and treatment, research, case studies.
Indexed: AMED, ASCA, Biol.Abstr., Chic.Per.Ind., Curr.Cont. (coverage dropped), Dent.Abstr., Excerp.Med., Ind.Med. (1973-), Ind.Vet., Inpharma, Med.Care Rev., Oral Res.Abstr., Pharm.&Out.News, Pig News & Info., Reac., Sci.Cit.Ind. (coverage dropped), Vet.Bull.
—BLDSC (0820.945000), CISTI, EMDOCS, GNLM, IDS, ingenta, KNAW. **CCC.**
Address: 1840 41st Ave, Ste 102, Box 610, Capitola, CA 95010. TEL 831-475-1700, FAX 831-475-1439, readaja@attglobal.net, http://www.acupuncturejournal.com; http://www.readaja.com. Ed. W G Grace. Pub. Deborah Salisbury. Adv. contact P Scarborough. Circ: 4,800.

THE AMERICAN JOURNAL OF CHINESE MEDICINE. see *MEDICAL SCIENCES—Abstracting, Bibliographies, Statistics*

615.53 IND ISSN 0257-7941
R605
ANCIENT SCIENCE OF LIFE. Text in English. 1981. q. INR 140, USD 37 (effective 2001). adv. bk.rev. 85 p./no. 2 cols./p. back issues avail.; reprints avail. **Document type:** *Journal, Academic/Scholarly.* **Description:** Publishes research papers on Ayurveda, the Indian system of medicine, and allied disciplines. Also acts as an interdisciplinary medium on all aspects of medical health care.
Indexed: AMED, Forest Prod.Abstr., Forest.Abstr., Hort.Abstr., Rev.Med.& Vet.Mycol.
—BLDSC (0900.325500).
Published by: International Institute of Ayurveda, Ramanathapuram, P O Box 7102, Coimbatore, Tamil Nadu 641 045, India. TEL 313188, FAX 314953, ayurveda@vsnl.com, http://www.avpayurveda.org. Ed. S Vijayan. Pubs. Dr. G Gangadharan, Suresh Kunar. R&P P R Krishna Kumar. adv.: B&W page INR 2,500; 165 x 220. Circ: 2,000.

615.89 GBR ISSN 1470-4056
▼ **AROMATHERAPY.** Text in English. 1999. bi-m. GBP 13 domestic; GBP 27 in Europe; GBP 34 elsewhere (effective 2001). **Document type:** *Magazine, Consumer.* **Description:** Covers all aspects of aromatherapy; features include essential oils, home remedies, health, beauty and aromatherapy products.
Published by: W V Publications, 53-79 Highgate Rd, London NW5 1TW , United Kingdom. http://www.aromatherapymagazine.com/. Ed. Juliet Giles. Adv. contact Jason Grant.

615.89 AUS
AROMATHERAPY TODAY. Text in English. q. AUD 41.80 domestic; AUD 50 in New Zealand; GBP 18 in United Kingdom; GBP 20 in Europe; USD 40 in US & Canada; AUD 60 elsewhere (effective 2001). 52 p./no. **Document type:** *Magazine, Consumer.* **Description:** Covers all aspects of aromatherapy; each issue includes an extensive profile on a specific essential oil as well as regular features such as research reports, calendars of international and Australian aromatherapy conferences, and items of general interest about aromatherapy.
Address: PO BOX 211, Kellyville, NSW 2155, Australia. TEL 61-2-9894-9933, FAX 61-2-9894-0199, jkerr@aromatherapytoday.com, http://www.aromatherapytoday.com/.

615.89 USA
AROMATIC THYMES; explorations in aromatherapy. Text in English. q. USD 21.95; USD 35 in Canada & Mexico; USD 45 elsewhere (effective 1999). adv. bk.rev. back issues avail. **Document type:** *Consumer.* **Description:** Covers all aspects of aromatherapy to educate, inform and inspire the reader from a broad perspective.
Address: 18 4 East Dundee Rd, Barrington, IL 60010. TEL 847-304-0975, 877-480-6934, FAX 615-377-0525, aromatic@interaccess.com, http://www.aromaticthymes.com/. Ed. Pamela H Parsons. Adv. contact Kathy Morris. B&W page USD 1,000, color page USD 1,400; trim 10.88 x 8.38. Circ: 20,000.
Subscr. to: 307 Southgate Court, Brentwood, TN 37027.

▼ **ATKINS: A PASSION FOR HEALTHY LIVING.** see *NUTRITION AND DIETETICS*

615.3 AUS ISSN 1033-8330
AUSTRALIAN JOURNAL OF MEDICAL HERBALISM. Text in English. 1989. q. AUD 75. adv. bk.rev. abstr. index. *Refereed.* **Document type:** *Academic/Scholarly.* **Description:** Publishes material on all aspects of medical herbalism with emphasis on phytochemistry, pharmacology and clinical applications of medicinal plants.
Indexed: AMED, Plant Gen.Res.Abstr., Rev.Arom.& Med.Plants.
—BLDSC (1810.230000).
Published by: National Herbalists Association of Australia, Ste. 305, 3 Smail St, Broadway, NSW 2007, Australia. TEL 61-2-9211-6437, FAX 61-2-9211-6452, nhaa@nhaa.org.au. Ed., R&P, Adv. contact Anne Cowper. page AUD 250. Circ: 1,600.

615.88 AUS ISSN 1326-3390
AUSTRALIAN TRADITIONAL-MEDICINE SOCIETY. JOURNAL. Text in English. q. USD 143 to membership for accredited member; USD 66 to membership for associated member; USD 33 to membership for student member (effective 2001); plus a once only joining fee of $44.00 (all prices include GST).. adv. bk.rev. *Refereed.* **Document type:** *Academic/Scholarly.* **Description:** Presents articles on all aspects of the principles and practice of alternative medicine including Western herbal medicine.
Formerly (until 1995): A T O M S Journal (1324-647X)
Indexed: AMED, CINAHL, Nutr.Abstr.
—BLDSC (4707.607000).
Published by: Australian Traditional-Medicine Society Ltd., PO Box 1027, Meadowbank, NSW 2114, Australia. TEL 61-2-9809-1652, FAX 61-2-9807-8130, journal@atms.com.au, enquiries@atms.com.au, http://www.atms.com.au. Ed., R&P, Adv. contact Raymond Khoury. Circ: 6,000.

A

A

613 363.7 USA
AWARENESS MAGAZINE. Text in English. bi-m. USD 18 domestic; USD 36 foreign (effective 2000). **Document type:** *Magazine, Consumer.* **Description:** Devoted to improving your life and the life of our planet.
Related titles: Online - full text ed.
Published by: Awareness Publishing Group, Inc., 7441 Garden Grove Blvd Ste C, Garden Grove, CA 92841-4209. TEL 714-894-5133, 800-758-3223, FAX 714-890-1664, awarenessmag@earthlink.net, http://www.awarenessmag.com.

615.89 IND ISSN 0970-7158
AYURVEDA EDUCATION SERIES/AYURVEDA SHIKSHAN MALA. Text in English, Marathi. 1978. irreg., latest vol.65, 1997. price varies. charts. back issues avail. *Refereed.* **Document type:** *Monographic series, Academic/Scholarly.*
Related titles: CD-ROM ed.
Address: 36 Kothrud, Pune, Maharashtra 411 029, India. TEL 91-20-5463132, FAX 91-20-5383933, drph_k@yahoo.com. Ed. Dr. P H Kulkarni.

615.53 IND
AYURVEDA SAUKHYAM SERIES. Text in English, Sanskrit. 1980. irreg. price varies. index. **Document type:** *Monographic series.* **Description:** Includes fundamental principles of Ayurveda, anatomy, physiology, hygiene, various aspects of public health, and the treatment of diseases.
Published by: Concept Publishing Company, A 15-16 Commercial Block, Mohan Garden, New Delhi 110 059, India. TEL 91-11-564-8039, FAX 91-11-564-8053.

615.89 CHN ISSN 0476-0247
BEIJING ZHONGYI/BEIJING TRADITIONAL CHINESE MEDICINE. Text in Chinese. bi-m.
Indexed: Hort.Abstr.
Published by: (Beijing Zhongyi Xuehui), Beijing Zhongyi Zazhishe, A-7 Dongdan Santiao, Beijing 100005, China. TEL 6127766.

615.892 GBR ISSN 0260-5996
BRITISH ACUPUNCTURE ASSOCIATION. NEWSLETTER✱. Text in English. 1965. 2/yr. **Document type:** *Newsletter.*
Formerly (until 1976): Acupuncture Association. Newsletter (0307-4994)
Published by: British Acupuncture Association & Register, 34 Alderney St, London SW1V 4EW, United Kingdom.

615.89 GBR ISSN 0959-6879
BRITISH JOURNAL OF PHYTOTHERAPY. Text in English. 1990. s-a. GBP 27.50 to individuals; GBP 38 to institutions. adv. bk.rev. *Refereed.* **Document type:** *Academic/Scholarly.*
Indexed: AMED.
—BLDSC (2319.300000), GNLM.
Published by: College of Phytotherapy, Bucksteep Manor, Bodle St, Hailsham, E Sussex BN27 4RJ, United Kingdom. TEL 44-1323-834800, FAX 44-1323-834801, medherb@pavilion.co.uk, http://www.blazeweb.com/phytotherapy. Ed., Adv. contact Douglas Schar. R&P Pamela Bull. Circ: 600.

615.89 580 IND ISSN 0253-6889
CODEN: BMERDZ
BULLETIN OF MEDICO-ETHNO-BOTANICAL RESEARCH✱. Text in English; Summaries in Hindi. 1980. q. INR 60. adv. bk.rev. bibl, charts, illus. **Description:** Covers folk medicine, pharmacognosy, and phytochemistry. Examines the correlation between ancient insights and modern scientific thought.
Indexed: Hort.Abstr.
—CASDDS, CISTI.
Published by: Central Council for Research in Ayurveda and Siddha, c/o Sahitya Akademi - National Academy of Letters, Rabindra Bhavan, 35 Ferozshah Rd., New Delhi 110 001, India. TEL 11-669315. Ed. Dr. V N Pandey. Circ: 300.

615.321 CAN ISSN 0848-9629
CANADIAN JOURNAL OF HERBALISM. Text in English. 1979. q. CND 32.10 to individual members; CND 107 to institutional members (effective 2001). adv. bk.rev. reprints avail. **Document type:** *Consumer.* **Description:** Covers herbal medicine, complementary health care. Includes botanical and pharmacological profiles on specific plants, therapeutics and updates on legislation and quality control as well as environmental issues relating to health.
Formerly (until 1988): Ontario Herbalists Association. Journal
Published by: Ontario Herbalists Association, RR1, Port Burwell, ON N0J 1T0, Canada. Ed. Dr. Paul Saunders. Adv. contact Tara Hawley-Renault. Circ: 2,500.

CANNABIS CULTURE; marijuana & hemp around the world. see *LIFESTYLE*

CARE MAGAZINE; South Carolina's premeir waiting room publication. see *MEDICAL SCIENCES*

615.89 IND ISSN 0255-8726
CENTRAL COUNCIL FOR RESEARCH IN UNANI MEDICINE. ANNUAL REPORT✱. Text in English. 1978. a. **Document type:** *Government, Corporate.*
Published by: Ministry of Health & Family Welfare, Central Council for Research in Unani Medicine, Nirman Bhavan, Maulana Azad Rd., New Delhi 110 110, India.

615.89 DEU ISSN 0930-2786
CODEN: CHMEFE
CHINESISCHE MEDIZIN; theoretische Grundlagen, Diagnostik, Akupunktur, Arzneimittel, Taiji, Qigong. Text in German. 1986. q. EUR 102.33 domestic; EUR 108.33 foreign; EUR 60.27 domestic to students; EUR 66.27 foreign to students; EUR 28.04 newsstand/cover (effective 2002). adv. abstr. back issues avail. *Refereed.* **Document type:** *Journal, Academic/Scholarly.*
Related titles: Online - full text ed.: (from RoweCom Information Quest, Springer LINK).
—CISTI, GNLM.
Published by: (Societas Medicinae), Urban und Vogel Medien und Medizin Verlagsgesellschaft mbH (Subsidiary of: BertelsmannSpringer), Neumarkter Str 43, Munich 81673, Germany. TEL 49-89-43721411, FAX 49-89-43721410, verlag@urban-vogel.de, http://www.urban-vogel.de. Eds. C.H. Hempen, E Stueder-Wobmann. R&P Oliver Renn. Adv. contact Sibylle Schurr TEL 49-89-43721353. Circ: 1,600.
Subscr. to: Springer Auslieferungs Gesellschaft, Postfach 105160, Heidelberg 69041, Germany. TEL 49-6221-345244, FAX 49-6221-345244.

CHOJUGAKU KENKYU/RESEARCH OF LONGEVITY SCIENCE. see *GERONTOLOGY AND GERIATRICS*

615.89 JPN ISSN 0389-4843
CHUI RINSHO/CLINICAL JOURNAL OF TRADITIONAL CHINESE MEDICINE. Text in Japanese. 1980. q. JPY 1,600 per issue.
Published by: Toyo Gakujutsu Shuppansha, 1-5 Miyakubo 3-chome, Ichikawa-shi, Chiba-ken 272-0822, Japan.

615.892 GBR ISSN 1461-1449
CLINICAL ACUPUNCTURE AND ORIENTAL MEDICINE. Text in English. 1998. q. GBP 56 to individuals; GBP 116 to institutions (effective 2002). adv. *Refereed.* **Document type:** *Journal, Academic/Scholarly.* **Description:** Covers acupuncture and related therapies.
Related titles: Online - full text ed.
—BLDSC (3286.244300).
Published by: Churchill Livingstone (Subsidiary of: Harcourt Publishers Ltd.), Robert Stevenson House, 1-3 Baxter's Pl, Leith Walk, Edinburgh, Midlothian EH1 3AF, United Kingdom. TEL 44-131-556-2424, FAX 44-131-459-1177, cservice@harcourt.com, http://www.harcourt-international.com/journals/caom. Ed. Kevin Ergill. Adv. contact David Dunnachie. **Subscr. to:** Harcourt Publishers Ltd., Foots Cray High St, Sidcup, Kent DA14 5HP, United Kingdom. TEL 44-20-8308-5700, FAX 44-20-8309-0807.

615.899 USA
▼ **COLLEGE OF MAHARISHI VEDIC MEDICINE NEWS.** Text in English. 1999. bi-m. bk.rev. back issues avail. **Document type:** *Newsletter, Academic/Scholarly.* **Description:** Includes case histories of patients treated with Maharishi Vedic Medicine, as well as news of the faculty and students.
Formerly: Vedic Medicine News
Media: Online - full text.
Published by: Maharishi University of Management, College of Maharishi Vedic Medicine, Fairfield, IA 52557-1155. TEL 515-472-1194, 800-831-6523, FAX 515-472-1297, cshaw@mum.edu, http://www.mum.edu/CMVM/news.html. Ed. Craig Shaw.

700 535.84 GBR ISSN 1351-1696
COLOURAMA; world's premier colour magazine & directory. Text in English. 1970. a. GBP 4.50 domestic; GBP 5.50 foreign; GBP 3.75 newsstand/cover (effective 2000). adv. bk.rev. back issues avail. *Refereed.* **Document type:** *Directory.* **Description:** Concerns the power of color and vibrational healing, and related topics in complementary medicine.
Formerly (until 1993): Colour Circle
Published by: International Association of Colour, 46 Cottenham Rd, Histon, Cambs CB4 9ES, United Kingdom. TEL 44-1223-563403, FAX 44-1223-237113, michael@kgrevis.freeserve.co.uk. Ed., R&P, Adv. contact Michael Grevis. B&W page GBP 150, color page GBP 450; trim 210 x 297. Circ: 1,000.

COMMON GROUND HAWAII. see *PSYCHOLOGY*

615.89 USA
R733 CODEN: AHPRFC
COMPLEMENTARY HEALTH PRACTICE REVIEW. Text in English. 1995. 3/yr. USD 44 domestic to individuals; USD 52 foreign to individuals; USD 98 domestic to institutions; USD 106 foreign to institutions (effective 2001). adv. bk.rev., software rev., video rev., Website rev. abstr, bibl, illus. 80 p./no. back issues avail. *Refereed.* **Document type:** *Abstract/Index, Academic/Scholarly.* **Description:** Serves as a forum for alternative health care practitioners and traditional health care professionals who incorporate alternative methods into their practices (e.g. homeopathy, meditation, hypnotherapy, acupressure and acupuncture, chiropractic medicine, art therapy, and related disciplines and procedures). Includes news from NIH - OAM, and a calendar.
Formerly (until 2000): Alternative Health Practitioner (1076-1675)
Indexed: CINAHL, SOPODA, Sociol.Abstr.
—BLDSC (3364.203660), Infotrieve. **CCC.**
Published by: Springer Publishing Company, 536 Broadway, New York, NY 10012. TEL 212-431-4370, FAX 212-941-7842, springer@springerpub.com, http://www.springerpub.com. Ed. Rena Gordon. R&P Dorothy Kouwenberg. Adv. contact Bob Friel. B&W page USD 300.

COMPLEMENTARY MEDICINE FOR THE PHYSICIAN. see *MEDICAL SCIENCES*

COMPLEMENTARY THERAPIES IN MEDICINE. see *MEDICAL SCIENCES—Chiropractic, Homeopathy, Osteopathy*

COMPLEMENTARY THERAPIES IN NURSING & MIDWIFERY. see *MEDICAL SCIENCES—Nurses And Nursing*

615.89 158 USA ISSN 1099-9159
COUNTRY LIVING'S HEALTHY LIVING; the magazine that refreshes body, mind, and soul. Variant title: Healthy Living. Text in English. 1996. bi-m. USD 24 domestic; USD 42 foreign; USD 2.95 newsstand/cover; CND 3.95 newsstand/cover in Canada (effective 2000). adv. bk.rev. illus. **Document type:** *Magazine, Consumer.* **Description:** Brings clear, authoritative, new ways to create, boost, and maintain one's physical and emotional well-being.
Published by: Hearst Corporation, Hearst Special Publications, 1790 Broadway, New York, NY 10019. TEL 212-830-2900, FAX 212-586-3455, http://www.homearts.com/healthyliving, http://www.hearstcorp.com. Ed. Rachel Newman. Pub. Stacey Bettman. Adv. contact Kathleen Craven. page USD 12,500. Circ: 400,000 (paid).

COUNTRY ROAD CHRONICLES. see *NATIVE AMERICAN STUDIES*

DANCE MEDICINE & SCIENCE. see *MEDICAL SCIENCES—Physical Medicine And Rehabilitation*

615.89 IND ISSN 0970-3381
DEERGHAYU INTERNATIONAL. Text in English. 1984. q. INR 200; USD 10 foreign (effective 2001). adv. bk.rev. abstr. 32 p./no. 2 cols./p. back issues avail.; reprints avail. *Refereed.* **Document type:** *Journal, Academic/Scholarly.* **Description:** Contains case reports, research results and reviews on Indian medicine.
Published by: Ayurveda Education Series, 36 Kothrud, Pune, Maharashtra 411 029, India. TEL 91-20-5463132, FAX 91-20-5383933, roveda_gg@yahoo.com, roveda_99@yahoo.com. Ed. Dr. P H Kulkarni. Adv. contact Pavan Kulkarni. B&W page INR 2,000, color page INR 3,000; trim 267 x 203.

DELICIOUS!; guide to natural living. see *NUTRITION AND DIETETICS*

615.89 USA
DINSHAH HEALTH SOCIETY NEWSLETTER. Text in English. 1976. q. USD 3 (effective 2000). back issues avail. **Document type:** *Newsletter.* **Description:** Covers general health topics, including unorthodox methods of healing (primarily chromopathy).

Published by: Dinshah Health Society, PO Box 707, Malaga, NJ 08328. TEL 856-692-4686, http://www.wj.net/dinshah. Ed. Darius Dinshah. Circ: 4,075.

DIRECTION; a journal on the Alexander Technique. see *PHYSICAL FITNESS AND HYGIENE*

615.89 POL ISSN 1230-9370
DOMOWY DOKTOR; miesiecznik medycyny naturalnej. Text in Polish. 1993. m. PLZ 2.60 newsstand/cover. back issues avail. **Description:** Covers natural medicine.
Published by: Faktor Sp. z o.o., Ul Ksiecia Wladyslawa Opolskiego 3 a, Kety 32650, Poland. TEL 48-33-453888. Ed. Jozej Gaweda. Circ: 17,500.

615.53 USA ISSN 1069-6253
THE DOOR OPENER; Connecticut's holistic health and metaphysical networking magazine. Text in English. 1986. q. USD 12; USD 3 newsstand/cover (effective 2000). adv. back issues avail. **Document type:** *Consumer.* **Description:** Includes articles, calendar of events, and lists of resources covering holistic health and metaphysics in Connecticut.
Published by: An Open Door, 70 Valley Falls Rd., Vernon, CT 06066. TEL 860-875-4101, FAX 860-875-4101, anopendoor@aol.com, http://www.anopendoor.com. Ed., Pub., Adv. contact Jon Roe. R&P John Roe. page USD 290; trim 11 x 8.5. Circ: 2,300 (paid).

615.8 USA ISSN 1085-0880
DR. ANDREW WEIL'S SELF HEALING; creating natural health for your body and mind. Text in English. 1995. m. USD 29 domestic; USD 32 in Canada (effective 2000). bk.rev. index. back issues avail. **Document type:** *Newsletter.* **Description:** Covers natural health and well-being.
Related titles: Online - full text ed.
Published by: Thorne Communications, Inc., 42 Pleasant St, Watertown, MA 02472. TEL 617-926-0200, FAX 617-926-5562, http://www.drweilselfhealing.com. Ed. Dr. Andrew Weil. Pub. David Thorne. R&P Jessica Cerretani. Circ: 380,000 (paid). **Subscr. to:** PO Box 2057, Marion, OH 43305-2057.

615.89 GBR ISSN 1368-9797
DR. ATKINS' HEALTH REVELATIONS. Text in English. 1996. m. USD 39.95 in United States. back issues avail. **Document type:** *Newsletter, Consumer.* **Description:** Focuses on special diet to combat major diseases.
Published by: (Atkins Center for Complementary Medicine USA), Agora Ireland Publishing & Services, 11th Fl, Centre Point, 103 New Oxford St, London WC1A 1QQ, United Kingdom. TEL 44-20-7447-4018, FAX 44-20-7447-4041. Circ: 6,000.

615 610 GBR ISSN 1362-6035
EQUILIBRIUM. Text in English. 1995. q. **Description:** Aims to serve as an educational resource with information on various treatments, therapies, products and views on health. Includes articles on homeopathy, essential oils and extracts, physiotherapy, immunology, choosing a doctor etc.
Published by: Equilibrium Health Resources Ltd., c/o Julia Bard, Ed., Clarendon Centre, 16 Clarendon Rd, Hornsey, London N8 0DJ, United Kingdom. TEL 44-20-7241-2960, FAX 44-20-7241-2960, equilibr@dircon.co.uk.

ESALEN CATALOG. see *PSYCHOLOGY*

ETHNOBOTANY. see *BIOLOGY—Botany*

615.89 AUT ISSN 1609-4557
▼ **EUROPEAN JOURNAL OF ACUPUNCTURE.** Text in English. 2000. q. USD 75 domestic; USD 115 foreign; USD 35 newsstand/cover (effective 2001). adv. back issues avail. *Refereed.* **Document type:** *Journal, Academic/Scholarly.* **Description:** Improves communication and understanding in international acupuncture research and applications.
Related titles: Online - full text ed.: ISSN 1609-4565.
Published by: V I C E R Publishing, PO Box 14, Vienna A-1097, Austria. TEL 43-676-9568085, FAX 43-676-9568086, vicer@vicer.org, http://www.vicer.org. Ed., R&P Roland Hofbauer. adv.: B&W page USD 1,700, color page USD 2,200. Circ: 1,000 (paid and controlled).

EUROPEAN JOURNAL OF HERBAL MEDICINE. see *PHARMACY AND PHARMACOLOGY*

610.95 GBR ISSN 1351-6647
EUROPEAN JOURNAL OF ORIENTAL MEDICINE. Text in English. 1977; N.S. 1993. s-a. GBP 20 domestic; GBP 21 in Europe; GBP 26 elsewhere. adv. bk.rev. back issues avail. **Document type:** *Academic/Scholarly.* **Description:** Stimulates debate and scholarship in Chinese medicine and other traditions of Oriental medicine.
Former titles (until 1993): British Journal of Acupuncture (0143-4977); (until 1979): British Acupuncture Association. Journal (0142-2340)
Indexed: AMED.
—BLDSC (3829.733260), GNLM.
Address: 19 Trinity Rd, London N2 8JJ, United Kingdom. Circ: 700.

FITOTERAPIA; journal for the study of medicinal plants - rivista di studi ed applicazioni delle piante medicinali. see *BIOLOGY—Botany*

FOCUS ON ALTERNATIVE AND COMPLEMENTARY THERAPIES. see *PHARMACY AND PHARMACOLOGY*

615.8 CHE ISSN 1424-7364
FORSCHENDE KOMPLEMENTAERMEDIZIN UND KLASSISCHE NATURHEILKUNDE/RESEARCH IN COMPLEMENTARY AND NATURAL CLASSICAL MEDICINE. Text in English, German. 1994. bi-m. CHF 214, EUR 139 in Europe to institutions; CHF 231.40, USD 173 elsewhere to institutions (effective 2002). adv. back issues avail. *Refereed.* **Document type:** *Journal, Academic/Scholarly.* **Description:** Establishes a bridge of communication between complementary medicine and university research medicine on a scientific level.
Formerly: Forschende Komplementaermedizin (1021-7096)
Related titles: Online - full text ed.: ISSN 1421-9999. CHF 58, EUR 42, USD 45 to institutions (effective 2002) (from EBSCO Publishing, O C L C Online Computer Library Center, Inc., RoweCom Information Quest, Institute for Scientific Information).
Indexed: AMED, Curr.Cont., Ind.Med. (coverage dropped), Inpharma, Int.Nurs.Ind., Pharm.&Out.News, Reac., Rev.Arom.& Med.Plants.
—BLDSC (4008.991200), GNLM, IDS, KNAW.
Published by: S. Karger AG, Allschwilerstr 10, PO Box, Basel 4009, Switzerland. TEL 41-61-306-1111, FAX 41-61-306-1234, karger@karger.ch, http://www.online.karger.com/journals/fkm, http://www.karger.com. Adv. contact Christiane Opitz. Circ: 5,000.

FOUR CORNERS. see *NEW AGE PUBLICATIONS*

615.89 USA
FREE SPIRIT JOURNAL. Text in English. q. USD 20; USD 30 foreign. adv. **Document type:** *Bulletin.* **Description:** Features articles by and for alternative practitioners who use various aspects of clearing technology and operate independently.
Related titles: Online - full text ed.
Address: PO Box 4326, San Rafael, CA 94913-4326. TEL 415-492-0728, 800-799-3733, FAX 415-499-8441, http://www.freezone.org/f_spirit.htm. Ed. Hank Levin.

615.89 619 CHN ISSN 1000-338X
FUJIAN ZHONGYI YAO/FUJIAN JOURNAL OF TRADITIONAL CHINESE MEDICINE. Text in Chinese. 1956-1966; resumed 1981. bi-m. USD 1.20 per issue. adv. bk.rev.
Related titles: CD-ROM ed.
Indexed: ExtraMED, Plant Breed.Abstr.
—GNLM.
Published by: Fujian Zhongyi Xueyuan/Fujian Institute of Traditional Chinese Medicine, 282 Wusi Lu, Fuzhou, Fujian 350003, China. TEL 0591-7841296, FAX 0591-7842524. Ed. Yu Changrong. Circ: 16,000. **Dist. overseas by:** China International Book Trading Corp, 35 Chegongzhuang Xilu, Haidian District, Beijing 100044, China. **Co-sponsor:** Zhonghua Quanguo Zhongyi Xuehui Fujian Fenhui.

615.89 JPN
FUKUOKA ISHI KANPO KENKYUKAI KAIHO/FUKUOKA MEDICAL ASSOCIATION FOR KAMPO MEDICINE. Text in Japanese. 1980. m.
Published by: Fukuoka Ishi Kanpo Kenkyukai, 6-1 Wakahisa 2-chome, Minami-ku, Fukuoka-shi 815-0042, Japan.

FUNCTIONAL FOODS AND NUTRACEUTICALS; the magazine for the global supply market. see *NUTRITION AND DIETETICS*

615.89 JPN ISSN 0388-6719
CODEN: GTIGDO
GENDAI TOYO IGAKU/JOURNAL OF TRADITIONAL SINO-JAPANESE MEDICINE. Text in Japanese. 1980. q. JPY 1,800 per issue.
—CASDDS.
Published by: Igaku Shuppan Senta/Medical Publication Center Inc., 25-2 Asakusa-Bashi 1-chome, Taito-ku, Tokyo 111-0053, Japan.

GERSON HEALING NEWSLETTER. see *MEDICAL SCIENCES*

GINSENG REVIEW. see *PHARMACY AND PHARMACOLOGY*

GREATLIFE. see *NUTRITION AND DIETETICS*

615.89 USA
THE GREY FOX. Text in English. m. adv. **Document type:** *Newsletter.* **Description:** Covers alternative medicine in a simple and straightforward fashion with an emphasis on providing practical information that can be applied to making positive changes in everyone's lifestyle.
Media: Online - full text.
Published by: TGFox, Inc. marc@cide.com, http://www.tgfox.com. Ed. Ronald L Breazeale.

615.89 CHN
GUANGXI ZHONGYI YAO/GUANGXI TRADITIONAL CHINESE MEDICINE. Text in Chinese. bi-m.
Published by: Guangxi Zhongyi Xueyuan/Guangxi Institute of Traditional Chinese Medicine, 21 Mingxiu Donglu, Nanning, Guangxi 530001, China. TEL 32101. Ed. Ban Qiuwen. **Co-sponsor:** Zhonghua Quanguo Zhongyi Xuehui, Guangxi Fenhui.

GUOWAI YIXUE (ZHONGYI ZHONGYAO FENCE)/FOREIGN MEDICAL SCIENCES (TRADITIONAL CHINESE MEDICINE). see *MEDICAL SCIENCES*

615.89 USA
H L Q THREE RIVERS RESOURCE GUIDE FOR HOLISTIC LIVING. Text in English. 1980. a. USD 7; USD 9 foreign (effective 1997). adv. bk.rev. index. *Refereed.* **Document type:** *Directory.* **Description:** Focuses on personal health, social responsibility, global awareness, and self sufficiency.
Former titles: Three Rivers Wellness Directory (1060-006X); Former titles: H L Q Wellness Calendar; H L Q Magazine; Holistic Learning Quarterly
Published by: H L Q Associates, PO Box 86054, Pittsburgh, PA 15221-0054. TEL 412-242-9355, hlq@ttrfn.clpgh.org, http://trfn.clpgh.org/hlq. Ed. Allen Goodman. Pub. Priscilla Brown. Adv. contact Marlene Linden. Circ: 10,000 (paid).

H S R: HEALTH SUPPLEMENT RETAILER. see *NUTRITION AND DIETETICS*

HANF!; das Cannabis-Magazin. see *LIFESTYLE*

HANFBLATT; das Magazin fuer Hanfkultur. see *LIFESTYLE*

HEADS. see *LIFESTYLE*

615.537 USA
HEALING NEWS. Text in English. fortn. free per issue. **Document type:** *Newsletter.*
Media: Online - full text.
Published by: E G W Publishing Co., 1041 Shary Circle, Concord, CA 94518. TEL 925-671-9852, FAX 510-671-0692, hstevens@egw.com, http://www.naturalland.com/hlgv/hlgnc.htm.

HEALING RETREATS & SPAS. see *MEDICAL SCIENCES—Physical Medicine And Rehabilitation*

615.89 AUS
HEALTH & HEALING; journal of complementary medicine. Text in English. 1981. q. AUD 24.80 domestic; AUD 45.80 foreign (effective 2001). adv. bk.rev. abstr. 60 p./no. back issues avail. **Document type:** *Journal, Consumer.*
Formerly: Australasian Health and Healing (0812-3896)
—ingenta.
Published by: Trim-Keg Party Ltd, 29 Terrace St, PO Box 1424, Kingscliff, NSW 2487, Australia. TEL 61-2-6674-2407, FAX 61-2-6674-3633. Ed., R&P, Adv. contact Maurice Finkel. Circ: 12,000 (paid).

A

A

615.89 USA ISSN 0895-9986
HEALTH CONSCIOUSNESS; the international holistic magazine. Text in English. 1980. bi-m. USD 18; USD 32 foreign. adv. bk.rev. illus. back issues avail.
Description: Contains health news for both the lay and professional reader. Includes viewpoints from pioneers in alternative medicine.
Formerly: Kup's Komments
Indexed: AMED.
—BLDSC (4274.959800).
Published by: Dr. Roy B. Kupsinel, Ed. & Pub., Shangri La Ln, Box 550, Oviedo, FL 32765. TEL 407-365-6681, FAX 407-365-1834. Circ: 2,500.

615 USA ISSN 0888-7330
HEALTH WORLD. Variant title: New Editions, Health World. Text in English. 1982. q. USD 12; USD 30 foreign (effective 1997). adv. bk.rev. back issues avail.
Document type: *Consumer.* **Description:** Provides information on different health therapies, remedies, and practices around the world with emphasis on homeopathy, Chinese medicine, herbs, acupuncture and chiropractic.
Former titles (until 1986): Holistic Health (0882-8148); (until 1985): International Journal of Holistic Health and Medicine (0737-9560)
Related titles: Microform ed.: (from PQC); Online - full text ed.: (from ProQuest Information & Learning).
Published by: Health World, Inc., PO Box 4157, Burlingame, CA 94010. TEL 510-784-2318, FAX 510-781-0248, nehealth@dsp.com. Ed., Pub., R&P, Adv. contact Kumar Pati. Circ: 110,000.

615.89 USA ISSN 1082-6734
HEALTHINFORM✶ ; essential information on alternative health care. Text in English. 1995. m. USD 60 to individuals; USD 92 foreign to individuals; USD 54 to students. bk.rev. index. back issues avail. *Refereed.*
Document type: *Newsletter, Abstract/Index, Academic/Scholarly.* **Description:** Covers alternative and complementary medicine for health care professionals and consumers. Includes information on research conferences, proceedings, and grants.
Related titles: Fax ed.; Online - full text ed.: (from H. W. Wilson, Gale Group).
Indexed: AMED, Gen.Sci.Ind. (Jan.1999-).
Published by: Infolink, PO Box 640, Croton on Hudson, NY 10520-0640. TEL 914-736-1565, 800-743-LINK, FAX 914-736-3806, hininform@bestweb.com, http://www.healthinform.com. Ed. Katherine Mason-Page. Pub. Janet Gotkin. R&P Katherine Mason Page.

615.89 USA
HEALTHINFORM'S RESOURCE GUIDE TO ALTERNATIVE HEALTH✶ . Text in English. 1998. a. USD 49.95 to individuals; USD 79.95 to institutions.
Document type: *Directory.* **Description:** Lists more than 50 alternative and complementary therapies. Includes international listings of organizations, schools, journals, books, and Web sites.
Indexed: Gen.Sci.Ind. (Jan.1997-, dropped).
Published by: Infolink, PO Box 640, Croton on Hudson, NY 10520-0640. TEL 914-736-1565, 800-743-LINK, FAX 914-736-3806, hinform@bestweb.net, http://www.healthinform.com. Ed. Katherine Mason-Page. Pub. Janet Gotkin. R&P Katherine Mason Page.

▼ **HEALTHOLOGY.** see *PHYSICAL FITNESS AND HYGIENE*

615.8 613.7 USA ISSN 1079-4530
HEALTHY & NATURAL JOURNAL. Text in English. 1994. bi-m. USD 17.50 domestic; USD 35 in Canada; USD 45 elsewhere (effective 2001). adv. bk.rev. illus. back issues avail. **Document type:** *Consumer.* **Description:** Provides information on the latest developments in natural health, natural and organic foods, consumer activism, and the environment.
Published by: Measurements & Data Corp., 100 Wallace Ave, Ste 100, Sarasota, FL 34237-6041. TEL 941-366-1153, 800-883-8894, FAX 941-366-5743, hnnmag@healthyandnatural.com, editor@mac-mag.com. Ed. Debra Gorham. Pub. Robert Aronson. adv.: color page USD 4,370; trim 10.88 x 8. Circ: 215,000.

HEALTHY OPTIONS. see *PHYSICAL FITNESS AND HYGIENE*

615.89 CHN ISSN 1002-2619
HEBEI ZHONGYI/HEBEI TRADITIONAL MEDICINE. Text in Chinese. 1979. bi-m. CNY 3.20 per issue. adv. bk.rev. *Refereed.* **Document type:** *Academic/Scholarly.*
Published by: Hebei Yixue Kexueyuan, Qingbao Yanjiusuo/Hebei Academy of Medical Sciences, Information Institute, Department of Traditional Medicine, Zhongyi Fenhui, 241 Qingyuan St, Shijiazhuang, Hebei 050021, China. TEL 86-311-5812687, FAX 86-311-5809161, mazhi@public.sj.hj.cn. Ed. Jintang Xia. Pub. Dingwen Shi. R&P Zhi Ma. Adv. contact Weiguo Liu. Circ: 500.

615.89 DEU
HEILMITTEL AUS DER NATUR. Text in German. a.
Document type: *Bulletin, Consumer.*
Published by: Otto Hoffmanns Verlag GmbH, Arnulfstr 10, Munich 80335, Germany. TEL 49-89-545845-0, FAX 49-89-54584520. adv.: B&W page DEM 32,500, color page DEM 44,200; trim 175 x 112. Circ: 1,850,000 (controlled).

615.5 ISL
HEILSUHRINGURINN; timarit um hollefni og heilsuraekt. Text in Icelandic. 1978. s-a. ISK 1,000 (effective 2001). back issues avail. **Description:** Deals with issues in alternative medicine, orthomolecular medicine and natural hygiene.
Related titles: Magnetic Tape ed.
Address: Sidumula 27, Reykjavik 108, Iceland. TEL 354-568-9933. Circ: 2,000.

615.537 USA
HERBAL NEWS. Text in English. fortn. free per issue.
Document type: *Newsletter.*
Media: Online - full text.
Published by: E G W Publishing Co., 1041 Shary Circle, Concord, CA 94518. TEL 925-671-9852, FAX 510-671-0692, hstevens@egw.com, http://www.naturalland.com/hrbv/hrbnc.htm.

HERBALGRAM; the journal of the American botanical council & the herb research foundation. see *BIOLOGY—Botany*

615.89 AUT ISSN 1609-4573
▼ **HERBALS AND COMPLEMENTARY MEDICINE.** Text in English. 2000. q. USD 75 domestic; USD 115 foreign; USD 35 newsstand/cover (effective 2001). adv. back issues avail.; reprints avail. *Refereed.* **Document type:** *Journal, Academic/Scholarly.* **Description:** Publishes articles, case reports, reviews, and letters that improve communications in understanding herbal effects and all parts of complementary medicine.
Related titles: Online - full text ed.: ISSN 1609-4581.
Published by: V I C E R Publishing, PO Box 14, Vienna A-1097, Austria. TEL 43-676-9568085, FAX 43-676-9568086, vicer@vicer.org, http://www.vicer.org. Ed., R&P Roland Hofbauer. adv.: B&W page USD 1,700, color page USD 2,200. Circ: 1,000 (paid and controlled).

581.63 AUS ISSN 0729-560X
HERBOLOGY. Text in English. 1979. q. AUD 30 domestic; AUD 35 foreign (effective 2000). adv. bk.rev. charts. *Refereed.* **Document type:** *Academic/Scholarly.*
Description: Educates people in the use, taking and growing of herbs.
Published by: Australian Herb Society, PO Box 110, Mapleton, QLD 4560, Australia. TEL 61-7-54469243, FAX 61-7-54469277, aherbsoc@hotmail.com.au, http://www.maleny.net.au/sunweb/groups/aherbsoc.html. Ed., Adv. contact Denise Patterson. B&W page AUD 75; trim 6 x 8. Circ: 600.

615.89 USA ISSN 1086-1955
HERBS FOR HEALTH✶ . Text in English. 1996. bi-m. USD 24; USD 34 foreign. adv. illus. back issues avail.
Document type: *Consumer.* **Description:** Focuses on remedial and nutritional benefits of nature's herbs and spices.
—ingenta.
Published by: Herb Companion Press, LLC, 201 E 4th St, Loveland, CO 80537-5655. TEL 303-216-9220, FAX 303-216-9224, leah.karo@rodale.com. Ed. Erika Lenz. Pub. Logan Chamberlain. R&P Linda Ligon TEL 970-613-4614. Adv. contact Katie Wilson. **Subscr. to:** Agency Subscription Center, PO Box 14425, Des Moines, IA 50306-3425.

615.535 USA
HERBS TO YOUR HEALTH. Text in English. m. free per issue. **Document type:** *Newsletter.* **Description:** Presents information about herbs, vitamins, and other healthful botanicals.
Media: E-mail.
Address: shirbell@vcn.com. Ed. Shirley Bell.

HIGH TIMES; the magazine of the counter-culture. see *LIFESTYLE*

HOLISTIC HEALTH DIRECTORY. see *NEW AGE PUBLICATIONS*

HOLISTIC HEALTH SOURCEBOOK. see *NEW AGE PUBLICATIONS*

615.892 JPN ISSN 0287-6760
IDO NO NIPPON/JOURNAL OF JAPANESE ACUPUNCTURE & MOXIBUSTION. Text in Japanese. 1938. m. JPY 450 per issue.
Indexed: Ref.Zh.
Published by: Ido no Nipponsha, 1-45 Oppama-Hon-cho, Yokosuka-shi, Kanagawa-ken 237-0068, Japan.

INCANTESIMO. see *ASTROLOGY*

615.89 IND
INDIAN JOURNAL OF UNANI MEDICINE✶ ; devoted to interdisciplinary research in Unani medicine and allied sciences. Text in English. 1991. s-a. **Document type:** *Academic/Scholarly.*
Published by: Ministry of Health & Family Welfare, Central Council for Research in Unani Medicine, Nirman Bhavan, Maulana Azad Rd., New Delhi 110 110, India. Ed. Hakim Ummul Fazal.

615.89 IND ISSN 0971-314X
INDIAN MEDICINE/INDIYAN MEDISIN. Text in English, Telugu. 1971 (vol.20). m. INR 50. adv. bk.rev. charts.
Description: Covers alternative medicine with special emphasis on Ayurveda.
Published by: Indian Medicine Industries, Dubagunta Nivas, Vijayawada, Andhra Pradesh 520 002, India. Ed. Dr. D L Narayana. Circ: 2,000.

615.89 301 USA
INTERNATIONAL CONFERENCE ON THE STUDY OF SHAMANISM AND ALTERNATIVE MODES OF HEALING. PROCEEDINGS. Text in English. 1984. a. USD 20 (effective 2001). back issues avail. **Document type:** *Proceedings.* **Description:** Essays and discussion of interdisciplinary approaches to alternative healing and forms of shamanism.
Published by: Independent Scholars of Asia, Inc., 2321 Russell St, No 3C, Berkeley, CA 94705-1959. TEL 510-849-3791, FAX 510-849-3791, riheinze@juno.com, http://www.hypersphere.com/isa. Ed., Pub. Ruth-Inge Heinze. R&P Ruth Inge Heinze. Circ: 300 (paid).

615.89 616.97 GBR ISSN 1357-9452
INTERNATIONAL JOURNAL OF ALTERNATIVE & COMPLEMENTARY MEDICINE. Text in English. 1983. m. GBP 31.50 domestic to individuals; GBP 37 in Europe to individuals; GBP 45 elsewhere to individuals; GBP 24.50 domestic to students; GBP 29 in Europe to students; GBP 37.50 elsewhere to students (effective 2001). adv. video rev., bk.rev. illus, stat, tr.lit. back issues avail. *Refereed.* **Document type:** *Magazine, Trade.* **Description:** Contains news, articles, research, features, debate, treatment, masterclasses, case histories, comment, services, etc. Aimed at alternative and complementary practitioners, doctors, nurses.
Former titles (until 1991): Journal of Alternative & Complementary Medicine (0959-9886); (until 1987): Journal of Alternative Medicine (0950-5466)
Published by: Reasonhold Limited, 9 Rickett St, London SW6 1RU, United Kingdom. TEL 44-20-7385-0012, FAX 44-20-7385-4566. Ed., R&P Graeme Millar. Pub. Satpal Dulay. Adv. contact Julia March. B&W page GBP 575, color page GBP 850; trim 182 x 272. Circ: 5,000 (paid).

615.537 GBR ISSN 0962-4562
INTERNATIONAL JOURNAL OF AROMATHERAPY. Text in English. 1988. q. GBP 31 to individuals; GBP 96 to institutions (effective 2002). *Refereed.* **Document type:** *Journal, Academic/Scholarly.* **Description:** Covers the pursuit of health and well-being, whether mental, emotional or physical through aromatherapy treatment.
Related titles: Online - full text ed.
Indexed: AMED.
—BLDSC (4542.104400).
Published by: Churchill Livingstone (Subsidiary of: Harcourt Publishers Ltd.), Robert Stevenson House, 1-3 Baxter's Pl, Leith Walk, Edinburgh, Midlothian EH1 3AF, United Kingdom. TEL 44-131-556-2424, FAX 44-131-459-1177, cservice@harcourt.com, http://www.harcourt-international.com/journals/ijar. Ed. Bob Harris. **Subscr. to:** Harcourt Publishers Ltd., Foots Cray High St, Sidcup, Kent DA14 5HP, United Kingdom. TEL 44-20-8308-5700, FAX 44-20-8309-0807.

615.89 USA ISSN 1047-1979
RM184
INTERNATIONAL JOURNAL OF CLINICAL ACUPUNCTURE. Text in English. 1990. q. USD 135 domestic to individuals; USD 180 foreign to individuals; USD 355 domestic to institutions; USD 410 foreign to institutions (effective 2002). *Refereed.* **Document type:** *Journal, Academic/Scholarly.* **Description:** Emphasizes clinical results in acupuncture.
Indexed: AMED.
—BLDSC (4542.169500), GNLM, Infotrieve. **CCC.**
Published by: Allerton Press, Inc., 18 W 27th St, New York, NY 10001. TEL 212-924-3950, FAX 212-463-9684. Ed. Chen Shaozong.

615.85 USA ISSN 1522-6255
▼ **THE INTERNATIONAL JOURNAL OF INTEGRATIVE MEDICINE.** Text in English. 1999. bi-m. USD 73 in United States; USD 133 in Canada (effective 2000 & 2001); USD 64 domestic to individuals; USD 88 foreign to individuals; USD 135 domestic to institutions; USD 175 foreign to institutions; USD 12 newsstand/cover domestic; USD 18 newsstand/cover foreign (effective 2002). adv. bk.rev. charts, illus, abstr. 56 p./no. 2 cols./p. back issues avail. *Refereed.* **Document type:** *Magazine, Corporate, Academic/Scholarly.* **Description:** Covers clinical aspects of natural and integrative medicine for the healthcare professional.
Formerly (until 1998): American Journal of Natural Medicine (1521-4702)
Published by: InnoVision Communications, 169 Saxony Rd, Ste 104, Encinitas, CA 92024. TEL 760-633-3910, FAX 760-633-3918, 866-828-2962, info@invcom.com.

615.89 USA ISSN 1044-0003
INTERNATIONAL JOURNAL OF ORIENTAL MEDICINE/GUOJI HANFANG YIYAO ZAZHI. Text in Chinese, English. 1976. q. USD 60 domestic; USD 80 foreign (effective 2000). bibl. index. back issues avail. **Document type:** *Academic/Scholarly.*
Former titles (until 1989): Oriental Healing Arts International Bulletin (0888-9341); (until 1986): Oriental Healing Arts Institute of U S A. Bulletin (0278-5315)
—BLDSC (4542.435400), ingenta.
Published by: Oriental Healing Arts Institute, 1945 Palo Verde Ave, Ste 208, Long Beach, CA 90815. TEL 562-431-3544, FAX 949-380-2688, ohai@sunten.com. Ed. Dr. Qing Fu Hu. Circ: 500.

615.89 CHN ISSN 1001-9537
CODEN: CIYCD5
JIANGSU ZHONGYI/JIANGSU TRADITIONAL CHINESE MEDICINE. Text in Chinese. 1956. m. adv. bk.rev. **Document type:** *Academic/Scholarly.* **Description:** Covers Chinese herbal medicine, acupuncture, massage, qigong, and health care issues.
Published by: Jiangsu Sheng Weisheng Ting/Jiangsu Provincial Bureau of Public Health, 42 Zhongyang Lu, Nanjing, Jiangsu 210008, China. TEL 643684. Ed. Zhang Huaqiang. Adv. contact Yabo Huang. B&W page CNY 2,500, color page CNY 5,000. Circ: 100,000. **Dist. overseas by:** China International Book Trading Corp, 35 Chegongzhuang Xilu, Haidian District, Beijing 100044, China.

615.89 CHN
JILIN ZHONGYIYAO/JILIN TRADITIONAL CHINESE MEDICINE. Text in Chinese. bi-m.
Published by: Changchun Zhongyiyuan/Changchun Institute of Traditional Chinese Medicine, 15 Gongnong Dalu, Changchun, Jilin 130021, China. Ed. Gao Guangzhen.

615.8 615.5 USA ISSN 1075-5535
R733 CODEN: JACPFP
JOURNAL OF ALTERNATIVE & COMPLEMENTARY MEDICINE; research on paradigm, practice, and policy. Text in English. 1993. bi-m. USD 99 domestic to individuals; USD 119 foreign to individuals; USD 119 domestic to individuals print and online combined; USD 139 foreign to individuals print and online combined; USD 224 domestic to institutions; USD 283 foreign to institutions; USD 269 domestic to institutions print and online combined; USD 328 foreign to institutions print and online combined (effective 2002). Supplement avail.; back issues avail.; reprints avail. *Refereed.* **Document type:** *Journal, Academic/Scholarly.* **Description:** Acts as an interdisciplinary source for research in alternative medical therapies. The primary goal is the establishment of rigorous research methodologies.
Related titles: Online - full content ed.: USD 99 to individuals; USD 224 to institutions (effective 2002) (from Swets Blackwell); Online - full text ed.: (from CatchWord Ltd., Institute for Scientific Information, RoweCom Information Quest).
Indexed: AMED, Curr.Cont., I.P.A., Ind.Med. (1995-), Inpharma, Int.Nurs.Ind., NRN, Pharm.&Out.News, Reac., Rev.Arom.& Med.Plants, Sugar Ind.Abstr., Weed Abstr.
—BLDSC (4927.202300), CISTI, GNLM, IDS, ingenta. **CCC.**
Published by: Mary Ann Liebert, Inc. Publishers, 2 Madison Ave, Larchmont, NY 10538. TEL 914—834-3100, FAX 914-834-1388, info@liebertpub.com, http://www.liebertpub.com/acm. Eds. Jackie Wootton, Kim A Jobst.

615.535 CHE ISSN 1028-6020
▼ **JOURNAL OF ASIAN NATURAL PRODUCTS RESEARCH.** Text in English. 2000. q. GBP 74, USD 89, EUR 98 to individuals; GBP 254, USD 327, EUR 338 to institutions; GBP 411, USD 536, EUR 548 to corporations (effective 2002). **Document type:** *Journal, Academic/Scholarly.* **Description:** Presents scientific articles from the field of natural product research on Asian ethnic medicine.
Related titles: Online - full text ed.: (from Institute for Scientific Information).
Indexed: Aqua.Sci.& Fish.Abstr., BBCI, Biotech.& Bioeng.Abstr., Curr.Chem.React., Ind.Chem., RCI.
Published by: Gordon and Breach - Harwood Academic (Subsidiary of: Taylor & Francis Group), PO Box 531, Lausanne 1000, Switzerland. TEL 41-21-6411280, FAX 41-21-6411281, info@gbhap.com, http://www.gbhap.com. Ed. Xiao Tian Liang. **Subscr. addr. in US:** International Publishers Direct, PO Box 32160, Newark, NJ 07102. FAX 215-750-6343.

JOURNAL OF BODYWORK & MOVEMENT THERAPIES. see *MEDICAL SCIENCES—Physical Medicine And Rehabilitation*

615.53 USA
▼ **JOURNAL OF CANNABIS THERAPEUTICS**; studies in endogenous, herbal, and synthetic cannabinoids. Text in English. 2001. q. USD 60 to individuals; USD 81 in Canada to individuals; USD 87 elsewhere to individuals; USD 85 to institutions; USD 115 in Canada to institutions; USD 123 elsewhere to institutions; USD 125 to libraries; USD 169 in Canada to libraries; USD 181 elsewhere to libraries (effective Aug. 2001). adv. bk.rev. charts, illus. *Refereed.* **Document type:** *Journal, Academic/Scholarly.* **Description:** Discusses high-quality research in the experimental and clinical use of marijuana and other cannabinoids in physical and psychiatric medicine.
Related titles: Online - full text ed.: free with print ed. (effective 2001).
—BLDSC (4954.851500).
Published by: Haworth Press, Inc., 10 Alice St, Binghamton, NY 13904-1580. TEL 607-722-5857, 800-429-6784, FAX 607-722-6362, 800-895-0582, getinfo@haworthpressinc.com, http://www.haworthpress.com/journals/journallist.asp. Ed. Dr. Ethan Russo. Pub. William Cohen. R&P Ruthann Heath TEL 607-723-5857 ext 316. Adv. contact Jackie Blakeslee TEL 607-722-5857 ext 346. B&W page USD 315, color page USD 550; trim 6 x 8.5.

615.89 GBR ISSN 0143-8042
JOURNAL OF CHINESE MEDICINE. Text in English. 1979. 3/yr. GBP 27 in United Kingdom to individuals; GBP 29 in Europe to individuals; GBP 31 elsewhere to individuals (effective 2001). adv. bk.rev. back issues avail. **Document type:** *Academic/Scholarly.* **Description:** Covers the entire field of traditional Chinese medicine.
Related titles: CD-ROM ed.: 1998. GBP 123.38.
Indexed: AMED, Ref.Zh.
—BLDSC (4958.110000).
Address: 22 Cromwell Rd, Hove, E Sussex BN3 3EB, United Kingdom. TEL 44-1273-777760, FAX 44-1273-7485888, info@jcm.co.uk, http://www.jcm.co.uk. Ed., R&P Peter Deadman. Circ: 2,000. **Dist. in US by:** Eastland Press, 1240 Activity Dr, Ste D, Vista, CA 92083. TEL 800-453-3278, orders@eastlandpress.com.

▼ **JOURNAL OF HERBAL PHARMACOTHERAPY**; innovations in clinical & applied evidence-based herbal medicinals. see *MEDICAL SCIENCES—Internal Medicine*

JOURNAL OF INTERPROFESSIONAL CARE. see *MEDICAL SCIENCES*

615.89 200 USA ISSN 1079-8390
JOURNAL OF SPIRITUAL BODYWORK. Text in English. 1995. q. USD 25; USD 30 foreign (effective 1999). bk.rev. index. back issues avail. *Refereed.* **Document type:** *Academic/Scholarly.* **Description:** Provides information about different kinds of spiritual healing (including massage) to laymen, clergymen, and members of licensed professions concerned with the healing arts.
Media: Online - full text.
—CCC.
Published by: (Church for Spiritual Healing and Health), Spiritual Massage Healing Ministry, 6907 Sherman St, Philadelphia, PA 19119. TEL 215-842-0265, FAX 215-842-2388, aschatz@unix.temple.edu, http://www.healingandlaw.com. Ed., Pub., R&P Albert Schatz. Circ: 290 (paid).

615.89 JPN ISSN 0288-2485
KANPO IGAKU/CHINESE MEDICINE. Text in Japanese. 1977. m. JPY 450 per issue.
Published by: Kanpo Igakusha/Kanpo Medicine Publications, 12-7 Niban-cho, Chiyoda-ku, Tokyo 102-0084, Japan.

615.89 JPN ISSN 0385-6526
KANPO KENKYU/STUDY ON CHINESE MEDICINE. Text in Japanese. 1975. m. JPY 400 per issue.
Published by: Gekkan Kanpo Kenkyu, 5-23 Nakatsu 2-chome, Kita-ku, Osaka-shi 531-0071, Japan.

615.89 JPN ISSN 0451-307X
KANPO NO RINSHO/JOURNAL OF KAMPO MEDICINE. Text in Japanese. 1954. m. JPY 850 per issue (effective 1999). adv. **Description:** Looks to contribute to the development of East-Asian medicine.
—CCC.
Published by: Toa Igaku Kyokai/Association of East Asian Medicine, 1-5 Misaki-cho 2-chome, Chiyoda-ku, Tokyo 101-0061, Japan. TEL 03-3264-8410, FAX 03-3265-5995. Ed. Isao Tuchiya. R&P, Adv. contact Toa Igaku Kyokai. Circ: 1,600.

615.89 JPN ISSN 0914-6407
KANPO TO MEN'EKI ARERUGI* /KAMPO AND IMMUNO-ALLERGY. Text in Japanese; Summaries in English, Japanese. 1988. a. JPY 4,500.
Published by: Fama Intanashonaru/Pharma International, Inc., c/o Nibau-cho, TS Bldg, Chiyoda-ku, Tokyo 102, Japan.

615.89 JPN ISSN 0912-9545
KANSAI SHINKYU TANKI DAIGAKU NENPO/KANSAI COLLEGE OF ACUPUNCTURE MEDICINE. ANNUAL REPORT. Text in English, Japanese. 1985. a.
Published by: Kansai Shinkyu Tanki Daigaku, 990 Ogai-To, Sennan-gun, Kumatori-cho, Osaka-fu 590-0432, Japan.

615.89 JPN ISSN 0912-0718
KATSU/JAPAN INSTITUTE OF TRADITIONAL MEDICINE. NEWS. Text in Japanese. 1959. m. JPY 400 per issue.
Published by: Nihon Kanpo Igaku Kenkyujo, 2-20 Nihonbashi 2-chome, Chuo-ku, Tokyo 103-0027, Japan.

615.89 JPN
KEIRAKU CHIRYO/JAPANESE SOCIETY OF ACUPUNCTURE. JOURNAL. Text in Japanese. 1965. q. JPY 7,000. adv. bk.rev. *Refereed.* **Document type:** *Academic/Scholarly.*
Published by: Keiraku Chiryo Gakkai, 14-9 Jinnan 1-chome, Shibuya-ku, Tokyo 150-0041, Japan. TEL 81-3-3461-2426, FAX 81-3-3770-1675. Ed., Pub., R&P, Adv. contact Okabe Somei.

KRAUT UND RUEBEN; biologisches Gaertnern und naturgemaesses Leben. see *GARDENING AND HORTICULTURE*

▼ **L O H A S JOURNAL.** see *BUSINESS AND ECONOMICS*

615.88 POL ISSN 1233-9253
LEKARZ DOMOWY MEDYCYNY LUDOWEJ; miesiecznik lekarski. Text in Polish. 1995. bi-m. PLZ 2.50 newsstand/cover. back issues avail. **Description:** Covers folk herbal medicine.
Published by: Faktor Sp. z o.o., Ul Ksiecia Wladyslawa Opolskiego 3 a, Kety 32650, Poland. TEL 48-33-453888. Ed. Jozef Gaweda. Circ: 8,000.

615.89 615.328 CHN ISSN 1000-1719
R97.7.C5 CODEN: LZZAEJ
LIAONING ZHONGYI ZAZHI/LIAONING JOURNAL OF TRADITIONAL CHINESE MEDICINE. Text in Chinese. 1979. m. USD 0.70 per issue.

Indexed: Dent.Ind., Ind.Med. (coverage dropped).
Published by: Liaoning Zhongyi Xueyuan/Liaoning College of Traditional Chinese Medicine, 79 Congshan Donglu, Shenyang, Liaoning 110032a, China. **Dist. outside China by:** China International Book Trading Corp, 35 Chegongzhuang Xilu, Haidian District, Beijing 100044, China. **Co-sponsor:** Zhonghua Quanguo Zhongyi Xuehui Liaoning Fenhui.

615.89 USA
LIFE EXTENSION; the ultimate source for new health and medical findings from around the world. Text in English. m. USD 40 domestic; USD 47 in Canada; USD 60 elsewhere; USD 3.95, CND 4.95 newsstand/cover (effective 2000). adv. illus. **Document type:** *Magazine, Consumer.* **Description:** Provides information and articles on the latest in health and medical findings.
Published by: (Life Extension Foundation), Life Extension Media, 1100 W Commercial Blvd, Fort Lauderdale, FL 33309-3746. TEL 954-561-7909, FAX 954-561-8335, lemagazine@lef.org. Ed. Rocio Paola Yaffar. Adv. contact Mike Freeman. **Subscr. to:** Life Extension Foundation, PO Box 229120, Hollywood, FL 33022. TEL 800-841-5433.

615.535 CAN
LIFESTYLE AND WELLNESS. Text in English. q. CND 10.70 domestic; USD 15 in United States; CND 2.50 newsstand/cover (effective 2000). **Document type:** *Magazine, Consumer.*
Address: 2813 Victoria Park Ave, Scarborough, ON M1W 1A1, Canada. TEL 416-492-6598, sheilam@spirit.ca, http://www.starpages.com/lifestyle-wellness.

613 USA
LILIPOH; a quarterly guide to health, nutrition and the environment. Text in English. q. USD 24 domestic; USD 28 foreign (effective 2002). adv. **Document type:** *Consumer.* **Description:** Offers hope and courage in dealing with illnes as a phenomenon reflective of the soul and spirit as well as the body.
Indexed: Alt.Press Ind.
Published by: Lilipoh Inc, Box 649, Nyack, NY 10960. TEL 914-268-2627, FAX 914-268-2764, info@lilipoh.com, http://lilipoh.com. Pub. Christine Murphy.

LONGEVITY REPORT. see *GERONTOLOGY AND GERIATRICS*

MACROBIOTICS TODAY. see *NUTRITION AND DIETETICS*

651.89 CAN
A MAGAZINE OF PEOPLE AND POSSIBILITIES. Text in English. 1990. 5/yr. free. **Description:** Seeks to connect people and explore possibilities in a rich exchange of vital information about health, ecology, personal growth, professional development, creativity, and wellness.
Formerly (until 1995): In Touch (Calgary) (1188-3944)
Related titles: Online - full text ed.
Published by: Rebecca Ryan Resources, #611, 7620 Elbow Dr S W, Calgary, AB T2V 1K2, Canada. TEL 403-245-6815, hayv@intouchmag.com, http://www.intouchmag.com, www.rebeccaryan.com. Ed. Veronica M Hay.

615.89 GBR
MASSAGE AND HEALTH REVIEW. Text in English. 1991. 3/yr. AUD 21 (effective 2001). **Document type:** *Newsletter.*
Published by: Massage Therapy Institute of Great Britain, P.O. Box 2726, London NW2 3NR, United Kingdom. TEL 44-20-8208-1607, FAX 44-20-8208-1639. Ed. Safia Shah. Circ: 450.

615.822 USA ISSN 0895-0814
MASSAGE THERAPY JOURNAL. Text in English. 1946. q., latest vol.40. USD 25 in US & Canada; USD 70 elsewhere; USD 6.50 newsstand/cover (effective 2001). adv. bk.rev., music rev., video rev. tr.lit. back issues avail.; reprints avail. *Refereed.* **Document type:** *Trade.* **Description:** Feature articles and columns cover techniques, research, successful practices, business advice and industry news relating to massage therapy.
Formerly (until 1962): Massage Journal
Published by: American Massage Therapy Association, 820 Davis St, Ste 100, Evanston, IL 60201-4444. TEL 847-864-0123, FAX 847-864-1178, mschwarz@amtamassage.com, eberland@inet.automassage, http://www.amtamassage.org. Ed. Michael Schwanz. R&P Kelly Gospudarek. Adv. contact Christina Rompan TEL 847-869-5127 ext 113. color page USD 3,096; 7.125 x 9.875. Circ: 65,000 (paid).

615.89 FRA ISSN 0760-811X
MEDECINES NOUVELLES. Text in French. 1985. q. FRF 200; FRF 48 newsstand/cover (effective 2000). **Document type:** *Monographic series.* **Description:** Informs on the new medical therapies.
Formerly: Cahiers Pratiques de Medecine (1243-7042)
Published by: Societe J A G, BP 002, Blangy-le-Chateau 14130, France. TEL 33-2-31648505. Ed. Annie Cristinacce. Pub. Jean Jacques Rocca Cristinacce. Circ: 33,000.

MEDICINA NATURALE. see *MEDICAL SCIENCES—Chiropractic, Homeopathy, Osteopathy*

615.892 BGR
MEDITSINSKI PREGLED. AKUPUNKTURA/MEDICAL REVIEW. ACUPUNCTURE. Text in Bulgarian. 3/yr. USD 36 foreign (effective 2002). **Document type:** *Journal, Academic/Scholarly.* **Description:** Publishes original articles in the field of acupuncture and acupressure.
Published by: Meditsinski Universitet - Sofia, Tsentur za Informatsiia po Meditsina/Medical University - Sofia, Medical Information Center, 1 Sv Georgi Sofiiski ul, Sofia 1431, Bulgaria. TEL 359-2-9522342, FAX 359-2-9522393, http://www.medun.acad.bg. **Dist. by:** Sofia Books, Ul Silivria 16, Sofia 1404, Bulgaria. TEL 359-2-9586257, sofiabooks@hotmail.com, http://www.sofiabooks.hit.bg.

615.89 JPN ISSN 0912-2419
MEIJI SHINKYU IGAKU/MEIJI UNIVERSITY OF ORIENTAL MEDICINE. BULLETIN. Text in Japanese; Abstracts in English. 1986. s-a. dist. to libraries of medical schools & researchers of acupuncture only. 150 p./no. *Refereed.* **Document type:** *Journal, Academic/Scholarly.*
Published by: Meiji Shinkyu Daigaku/Meiji University of Oriental Medicine, Funai-gun, Hiyoshicho, Kyoto 629-0392, Japan. TEL 81-771-72-1181, FAX 81-771-72-0326, kiyou_edit@muom_meiji-u.ac.jp. Ed. Kenji Kawakita. Pub. Kinya Kuriyama. Circ: 350.

615.892 USA
MERIDIANS (COLUMBIA); redefining health. Text in English. q. USD 20 domestic; USD 30 foreign (effective 2000). bk.rev. illus. **Document type:** *Consumer.* **Description:** Contains detailed articles and information regarding acupuncture and related health care issues.
Formerly (until 1992): Journal of Traditional Acupuncture (0270-661X)
—BLDSC (5680.789880).
Published by: Traditional Acupuncture Institute, 10227 Wincopin Circle, Ste 100, Columbia, MD 21044. TEL 301-596-6006. Ed. Mary Ellen Zorbaugh. R&P John Wilson TEL 410-997-4888. Circ: 2,000.

615 USA ISSN 1092-8774
MISAHA NEWSLETTER. (Monterrey Institute for the Sutdy of Alternative Healing Arts) Text in English. 1993. q. USD 20 domestic; USD 25 foreign (effective 2001). bibl. 24 p./no. back issues avail. *Refereed.* **Document type:** *Newsletter, Journal, Academic/Scholarly.*
Related titles: Online - full text ed.
Published by: MISAHA, 3855 Via Nona Marie, Ste 102-C, Carmel, CA 93923. TEL 831-622-7975, FAX 831-625-9617, misaha@aol.com, http://www.whps.com/misaha. Ed. Savely Savva. Circ: 400.

615.89 IND ISSN 0971-684X
N A M A H; a journal of Sri Aurobindo International Institute for Integral Health and Research. (New Approaches to Medicine And Health) Text in English. 1993. q. INR 150 domestic; USD 25 foreign; INR 60 newsstand/cover domestic; USD 8 newsstand/cover foreign (effective 2001). bk.rev., Website rev. abstr, charts, illus. 50 p./no. back issues avail.; reprints avail. *Refereed.* **Document type:** *Journal, Academic/Scholarly.* **Description:** Reports on developments in new approaches in medicine and general health care.
Published by: Sri Aurobindo Society, Academy of the Future, Beach Office - EDP Section, 1 Rue Rangapillai St, Pondicherry, Tamil Nadu 605 001, India. TEL 91-413-334458, FAX 91-413-330682, mother@sriaurobindosociety.org.in, sasocty@md2.vsnl.net.in, saapress@eth.net, http://www.sriaurobindosociety.org.in. Eds. Dr. Alok Pandey, Dr. Soumitra Basu. Pub. Pradeep Narang. R&P A R Ganguly.

N C A H F NEWSLETTER; quality in the health marketplace. (National Council Against Health Fraud) see *PUBLIC HEALTH AND SAFETY*

362 USA ISSN 1081-5678
N H O NEWSLINE. Text in English. 1984. s-m. membership only. **Document type:** *Newsletter.* **Description:** Provides brief updates of regulatory and educational news and information of relevance to hospice administrators.
Former titles (until 1991): N H O Hospice News; N H O President's Letter
Published by: National Hospice Organization, 1700 Diagonal Rd, Ste 3000, Arlington, VA 222314. TEL 703-243-5900, FAX 703-525-5762, http://www.nho.org. Ed. Larry Beresford. Circ: 2,800 (controlled).

N O H A NEWS. see *NUTRITION AND DIETETICS*

615.89 JPN ISSN 0911-9760
NAGAKURA KANPO DAIJESUTO/NAGAKURA KANPO DIGEST. Text in Japanese. 1970. a.
Published by: Nagakura Seiyaku K.K./Nagakura Pharmaceutical Co., Ltd., 7-16 Shoten-Shita 1-chome, Nishinari-ku, Osaka-shi 557-0012, Japan.

615.89 DEU ISSN 1433-9935
NATUR UND GESUNDHEIT; aktuelle Informationen aus der Naturheilkunde. Text in German. 1997. m. (14/yr.). DEM 233.10 (effective 1999). adv. back issues avail. *Refereed.* **Document type:** *Newsletter, Consumer.* **Description:** Contains information on natural healing, alternative medicine, therapies and remedies.
Related titles: Online - full text ed.
Published by: F I D Verlag GmbH, Koblenzer Str 99, Bonn 53177, Germany. TEL 49-228-359585, FAX 49-228-361992, http://www.natur-und-gesundheit.de. Ed. Ingeborg Gernaj. Pub. Helmut Graf. R&P, Adv. contact Susanne Kolle. **Subscr. to:** Leser-Service, Postfach 1327, Neckarsulm 74150, Germany. TEL 49-7132-959205, FAX 49-7132-959209.

NATURAL BEAUTY & HEALTH. see *PHYSICAL FITNESS AND HYGIENE*

613 GBR
NATURAL HEALTH. Text in English. q. **Document type:** *Magazine, Consumer.* **Description:** Contains information and advice on how to lead a healthy and happy life.
Published by: Ultima Publishing Ltd., 46 Oxford St, London W1N 9FJ, United Kingdom. TEL 44-20-7436-6800, FAX 44-20-7636-6886, info@ultimapublishing.com, http://www.ultimapublishing.com.

613.7 USA ISSN 1067-9588
AP2
NATURAL HEALTH. Text in English. 1971. 9/yr. USD 23.90 domestic; USD 35.90 foreign; USD 4.95 newsstand/cover domestic; CND 5.95 newsstand/cover in Canada (effective 2000). adv. bk.rev. back issues avail.; reprint service avail. from PQC. **Document type:** *Magazine, Consumer.* **Description:** Guide to mind, body, and spirit self-care.
Former titles (until Nov. 1992): EastWest Natural Health (1061-4664); (until Jan. 1992): EastWest (0888-1375); (until 1986): East West Journal (0191-3700); (until 1978): EastWest (0149-0362); (until 1977): East West Journal (0149-7839)
Related titles: Microform ed.: (from PQC); Online - full text ed.: (from Gale Group, America Online, Inc., Factiva).
Indexed: AMED, Alt.Press Ind., CHNI, GeoRef, New Per.Ind., Per.Islam. (1991-).
—BLDSC (6037.930000), ingenta.
Published by: Weider Publications, 21100 Erwin St, Woodland Hills, CA 91367. TEL 818-884-6800, 800-340-8959, FAX 818-716-5626, cpellino@weiderpub.com, http://www.naturalhealthmag.com/. Ed. Rachel Streit. Pub. Will Marks. adv.: B&W page USD 12,540, color page USD 15,135. Circ: 300,000 (paid).

613.7 USA
▼ **NATURAL HEALTH HOLLYWOOD.** Text in English. 2001 (Oct.). a. USD 4.95 newsstand/cover; USD 5.95 newsstand/cover in Canada (effective 2001). **Document type:** *Magazine, Consumer.* **Description:** Contains celebrity choices and recommendations on natural health and beauty products and lifestyles.
Published by: Weider Publications, 21100 Erwin St, Woodland Hills, CA 91367. TEL 818-884-6800, 800-998-0731, FAX 818-716-5626.

NATURAL HEALTH REVIEW. see *PHYSICAL FITNESS AND HYGIENE*

NATURAL PARENT. see *CHILDREN AND YOUTH—About*

NATURAL PHARMACY. see *PHARMACY AND PHARMACOLOGY*

615.89 USA ISSN 1094-0189
R733
NATURAL REMEDIES. Text in English. 1997. bi-m. USD 3.99 newsstand/cover. **Document type:** *Consumer.* **Description:** Provides readers with natural, alternative and complementary solutions for better health and living.
Published by: Cowles Enthusiast Media, 4 Highridge Park, Stamford, CT 06905. TEL 203-322-2900, 800-829-3340, FAX 203-322-1966, norined@cowles.com, http://www.cowles.com. Ed. Norine Dworkin. Pub. Toni Apgar. adv.: B&W page USD 2,730, color page USD 3,500. Circ: 120,000.

615.89 USA ISSN 1082-0531
THE NATURAL WAY; For Better Health. Text in English. 1995. bi-m. USD 18; USD 3.50 newsstand/cover; USD 24 foreign (effective 1999). adv. bk.rev., software rev., video rev. back issues avail. **Document type:** *Consumer.* **Description:** Promotes natural methods of living, healing towards better health.
Related titles: E-mail ed.; Fax ed.; Online - full text ed.
Published by: The Publishing Group, 1 Bridge St Ste 125, Irvington, NY 10533. TEL 914-591-2011, FAX 914-591-2017, NatWay@aol.com. Ed., R&P Cathy Raymond. Pub. Warren Tabatch. Adv. contact Arthur Maxwell. B&W page USD 3,829, color page USD 5,208; trim 10.88 x 8.13. Circ: 150,000 (paid).

615.89 DEU ISSN 0028-081X
DER NATURARZT; Zeitschrift fuer naturgemaesse Lebens- und Heilweisen. Text in German. 1861. m. DEM 70. adv. bk.rev. charts, illus. index. **Document type:** *Consumer.*
Published by: Access Marketing GmbH, Alt Falkenstein 379, Koenigstein 61462, Germany. TEL 06174-9263-0, FAX 06174-926329. Circ: 70,000.

615.89 110 AUS ISSN 0815-7006
NATURE AND HEALTH. Text in English. 1977. bi-m. AUD 36 domestic; AUD 100 foreign (effective 2001). adv. bk.rev. **Document type:** *Consumer.* **Description:** Covers diverse health care topics: natural health, self-improvement body care, relationships, organic gardening, natural beauty and fitness, oriental herbs, whole foods, science, social change, and spirituality.
Former titles (until 1984): Nature and Health Australia (0815-6999); (until 1980): Nature and Health Quarterly (0158-9911)
—ingenta. **CCC.**
Published by: Yaffa Publishing Group, 17-21 Bellevue St, Surry Hills, NSW 2010, Australia. TEL 61-2-9281-2333, FAX 61-2-9281-2750, yaffa@yaffa.com.au, http://www.yaffa.com.au/. Ed. Pamela Allardice. Pub. Tracy Yaffa. Adv. contact Margaret Forbes. B&W page AUD 2,080, color page AUD 3,200; trim 210 x 273.

615.89 DEU ISSN 0177-6754
NATURHEILPRAXIS MIT NATURMEDIZIN; Fachzeitschrift fuer Naturheilkunde, Erfahrungsheilkunde und biologische Heilverfahren. Text in German. 1947. m. EUR 88.80 domestic; EUR 100.80 foreign; EUR 7.70 newsstand/cover (effective 2002). adv. bk.rev. illus. index. **Document type:** *Journal, Academic/Scholarly.*
Former titles (until 1984): N. Naturheilpraxis (0177-6746); (until 1983): Naturheilpraxis (0028-0941)
—GNLM. **CCC.**
Published by: Richard Pflaum Verlag GmbH und Co. KG, Lazarettstr 4, Munich 80636, West Germany. TEL 49-89-12607-0, FAX 49-89-12607202, unterstoeger@naturheilpraxis.de, richard.pflaum@pflaum.de, http://www.naturheilpraxis.de, http://www.pflaum.de. Ed. K F Liebau. Adv. contact Christine Keller. B&W page XEU 1,900, color page XEU 3,130; trim 185 x 256. Circ: 16,403.

615.89 USA ISSN 0028-100X
NATUROPATH* . Text in English. 1961. m. USD 7.50. adv. bk.rev. stat, tr.lit.
Published by: Naturopath Publishing Co., 141 N Steelhammer Dr, Silverton, OR 97381-1821. TEL 206-695-0213. Ed. Robert W Noble. Circ: 3,600.

NEW AGE JOURNAL SOURCEBOOK. see *NEW AGE PUBLICATIONS*

615.89 158 USA
NEXUS (BOULDER); Colorado's holistic journal. Text in English. 1980. bi-m. USD 21. adv. bk.rev. illus. **Document type:** *Newspaper.* **Description:** Publishes news and commentary pertaining to all aspects of holistic and alternative health care and related issues.
Address: 1680 Sixth St, Ste 6, Boulder, CO 80302. TEL 303-442-6662, FAX 303-442-7596, nexuspub@aol.com, http://www.nexuspub.com. Ed., Pub. Ravi Dykema. R&P, Adv. contact Margo Hayden. Circ: 54,000 (controlled).

NUTRITION FORUM. see *NUTRITION AND DIETETICS*

ONKRUID; voor aarde, lichaam en geest. see *NEW AGE PUBLICATIONS*

ORGANICA; a magazine of arts & activism. see *LITERATURE*

615.89 JPN
ORIENTAL MEDICINE. Text in Japanese. m. JPY 1,408 per issue. **Document type:** *Trade.* **Description:** Covers kampo medicine, acupuncture, moxibustion, manipulative therapeutics for physicians, herbal pharmacists, and manufacturers.
Published by: Midori - Shobo Co. Ltd. (Subsidiary of: Midori Group), Ikebukuro Nishiguchi Sky Bldg, 2-14-4 Ikebukuro, Toshima-ku, Tokyo 171-0014, Japan. TEL 03-35990-4441, FAX 03-3590-4446. Ed. Toshikazo Nakamura. Circ: 18,000.

DE ORTHOMOLECULAIRE KOERIER; Nederlands - Vlaams tijdschrift voor nutritionele geneeskunde. see *NUTRITION AND DIETETICS*

THE PANIC RELIEF NEWS. see *PSYCHOLOGY*

615.89 USA
▼ **PATHOS MAGAZINE.** Text in English. 1999. bi-m. USD 3.95 newsstand/cover. **Document type:** *Consumer.* **Description:** Covers alternative methods of health and healing.
Published by: Alexander Publishing, Inc., PO Box 550, Ronan, MT 59864. TEL 406-676-4825, FAX 406-676-4824, ibedell@pathosmag.com, http://www.pathosmag.com.

615.8 ZAF ISSN 1022-2170
PATHWAYS TO HEALTH. Text in English. 1993. m. ZAR 91 (effective 1999). adv. **Document type:** *Consumer.* **Description:** To discuss issues, concepts and trends related to the various "pathways to health" so that our readers can make informed and educated decisions as to the path they want to follow.
Published by: F A S Publications, PO Box 41632, Craighall, Gauteng 2024, South Africa. FAX 27-11-7876316, sophie@fas.co.za. Ed. Monica Fairall. Pub. Ian Hughes. R&P Sophie MacKensie TEL 27-11-7893740. Adv. contact Theresa de Jongh. page ZAR 8,380; trim 275 x 210. Circ: 20,000.

615.89 IND ISSN 0972-3293
PHYTOMEDICA. Text in English. 1978. s-a.
Formerly: Indian Journal of Indigenous Medicines (0971-5452)
Published by: Society for Phytomedica, Indian Herbs House, Sharda Nagar, Saharanpur 247 001, India. Ed. S. Misra.

POSITIVE HEALTH; integrated medicine for the 21st century. see *PHYSICAL FITNESS AND HYGIENE*

POTPOURRI FROM HERBAL ACRES. see *GARDENING AND HORTICULTURE*

615.89 POL ISSN 1231-6652
PRZEPISY MEDYCYNY LUDOWEJ; miesiecznik zdrowia. Text in Polish. 1994. bi-m. PLZ 2.50 newsstand/cover. back issues avail. **Description:** Covers folk medicine.
Published by: Gawenda Sp. z o.o., Ul Kiecia Wladyslawa Opolskiego 3 a, Kety 32650, Poland. TEL 48-33-453888. Ed. Jozef Gaweda. Circ: 22,500.

615.89 158 AUT ISSN 1605-4652
PULSAR; Zeitschrift fuer Gesundheit, Therapie und Innere Entwicklung. Text in German. 1989. m. ATS 350 (effective 2001). adv. bk.rev. illus. 68 p./no. 4 cols./p. **Document type:** *Newspaper, Consumer.*
Related titles: Online - full text ed.: ISSN 1605-1300.
Published by: Regenbogen Buchverlags GmbH, Wutschdorf 89, St. Ulrich A-8072, Austria. TEL 43-3135-809020, FAX 43-3135-809023, pulsar@aon.at, http://www.pulsar.at. Eds. Kurt Bach, Marlis Bach. Adv. contact Kurt Bach. B&W page ATS 16,512; 192 x 250. Circ: 18,000 (paid). **Subscr. to:** Pulsar, Florianigasse 5, Vienna, W 1080, Austria. TEL 43-1-406826310, FAX 43-1-4038422.

615.89 USA
RADIANCE TECHNIQUE JOURNAL. Text in English. 1980. s-a. membership. adv. bk.rev. back issues avail. **Document type:** *Newsletter.* **Description:** Features alumni sharing news of their use of The Radiance Technique; includes the latest articles on the subject. Also includes information on peace projects in the U.S. and abroad.
Former titles: T R T and R P A I Journal; Radiance Technique Newsletter; Radiance Technique Journal (1040-5836); Reiki Journal
Published by: The Radiance Technique International Association, Inc., PO Box 40570, St. Petersburg, FL 33743-0570. TEL 727-343-8212, TRTPeace@aol.com, http://www.trtia.org. R&P Shoshana Shay. Circ: 2,000 (paid).

615.89 NZL ISSN 1174-3530
RAINBOW NEWS; the spirit of aotearoa. Text in English. 1990. bi-m. NZD 21; NZD 4.20 newsstand/cover (effective 2001). music rev., bk.rev. back issues avail. **Document type:** *Magazine, Consumer.* **Description:** Covers holistic health, lifestyle, native, workshops, retreats, and events.
Formerly (until 1997): Rainbow Network (0114-328X)
Published by: Healthy Options Ltd., 100 Grage Rd, PO Box 13209, Tauranga, New Zealand. http://www.healthyoptions.co.nz. Ed., R&P, Adv. contact Toni Bourget. Pub. Janice-Ann Priest. Circ: 14,000.

615.89 DEU
REIKI MAGAZIN. Text in German. 1997. q. DEM 36; CHF 36 in Switzerland; ATS 280 in Austria. **Document type:** *Consumer.*
Published by: Juergen Kindler Verlag, Rossdorfer Str 46, Frankfurt Am Main 60385, Germany. TEL 49-69-446851, FAX 49-69-4990501, http://www.reiki-magazin.de. Ed. Juergen Kindler.

615.89 FRA ISSN 0337-6877
REVUE FRANCAISE D'ACUPUNCTURE. Text in French; Summaries in English. 1975. q. FRF 400 foreign. adv. bk.rev. cum.index: 1975-1977; 1978-1991; 1982-1984; 1985-1988; 1989-1993. back issues avail. *Refereed.* **Document type:** *Academic/Scholarly.* **Description:** Covers techniques in acupuncture medicine.
Related titles: Diskette ed.
—GNLM.
Published by: Association Francaise d'Acupuncture, Tour CIT, 3 rue de l'Arrivee, Paris Cedex 15 75749, France. TEL 33-1-43202626, FAX 33-1-43205446, afa-qibo@imginet.fr, http://members.aol.com:/lishishen/acupuncture. Ed. Gilles Andres. Adv. contact Isabelle Regne.

615.89 FRA ISSN 0758-2633
REVUE FRANCAISE DE MEDECINE TRADITIONELLE CHINOISE. Text in French. 1973. m. FRF 600 domestic; FRF 650 foreign (effective 2001). adv. bibl, illus.
Former title (until 1982): Mensuel du Medecin Acupuncteur (0301-6366)
Indexed: AMED.
—BLDSC (7904.201000).
Published by: Nguyen Van Nghi Ed. & Pub., 27 bd. d'Athenes, Marseille 13001, France. acudoc@wanadoo.fr.

615.535 613.7 ITA ISSN 1128-4366
▼ **SALUTE NATURALE**; la nuova via del vivere bene. Text in Italian. 1999. m. ITL 53,000 (effective 1999). adv. **Document type:** *Newspaper.* **Description:** Contains information about natural and holistic medicine.
Published by: Edizioni Riza, Via Luigi Anelli, 1, Milan, MI 20122, Italy. TEL 39-02-5830-1022, FAX 39-02-5831-8162, http://www.riza.net. Ed. Rosalba Pagano. Pub. Liliana Tieger. adv.: color page ITL 16,400,000. Circ: 150,000.

615.89 USA ISSN 1095-0656
R733
THE SCIENTIFIC REVIEW OF ALTERNATIVE MEDICINE. Text in English. 1997. s-a. USD 50 to individuals; USD 90 to institutions. bk.rev. back issues avail. *Refereed.* **Description:** Evaluates the claims of alternative medicine.
Indexed: CINAHL.
—BLDSC (8203.914000).
Published by: Prometheus Books Incorporated, 59 John Glenn Dr., Amherst, NY 14228. TEL 716-691-0133, 800-421-0351, FAX 716-691-0137, 76453.1565@compuserve.com; pbooks6205@aol.com. Ed. Dr. Wallace Sampson. Pub. Paul Kurtz.

A

291.22 HUN ISSN 1216-7827
BL2370.S5
SHAMAN; journal of the international society for shamanistic research. Text in English. 1993. s-a., latest vol.9, 2001. USD 40 to individuals; USD 50 to institutions (effective 2001). adv. bk.rev. abstr, bibl, charts, maps. 96 p./no. back issues avail. *Refereed.* **Document type:** *Journal, Academic/Scholarly.* **Description:** An international periodical for the shamanistic studies and as such publishes original articles on shamanism and neighboring fields. In addtion, the journal publishes brief accounts of work in progress, abstracts of dissertations and annoucements of coming events.
Related titles: Online - full content ed.
Indexed: A.I.C.P., Intl.Bibl.Soc.Sci.
Published by: Molnar & Kelemen Oriental Publishers, PO Box 1195, Szeged 6701, Hungary. TEL 36-1-3169947, FAX 36-1-3150461, customtr@elender.hu; molnar@folkscene.hu, http://www.arts.u-szeged/journal/shamen.html; http://www.folkscene.hu. Ed. Mihaly Hoppal. Pub., R&P, Adv. contact Adam Molnar.

615.89 615.328 CHN ISSN 0559-7269
SHANGHAI ZHONGYIYAO ZAZHI/REVISTA DE MEDICINA TRADICIONAL CHINA DE SHANGHAI/REVUE DE MEDECINE TRADITIONNELLE CHINOISE/SHANGHAI JOURNAL OF TRADITIONAL CHINESE MEDICINE. Text in Chinese. m. USD 0.80 per issue. **Document type:** *Academic/Scholarly.*
Published by: China International Book Trading Corp/Zhongguo Guoji Tushu Maoyi Zonggongsi, 35 Chegongzhuang Xilu, Haidian District, Beijing 100044, China. TEL 86-1-68413849, FAX 86-1-68412048, cibtc@mail.cibtc.com.cn, http://www.cibtc.com.cn.

615.89 CHN ISSN 1000-7156
SHANXI ZHONGYI/SHANXI JOURNAL OF TRADITIONAL CHINESE MEDICINE. Text in Chinese. 1985. bi-m. CNY 3.50 newsstand/cover (effective 2001). 64 p./no. **Document type:** *Academic/Scholarly.* **Description:** Covers the latest development, trends, theories and applications of traditional Chinese medicine.
Published by: (Shanxi Sheng Weisheng Ting), Shanxi Zhongyi Bianjibu, 23 Donghua Men, Taiyuan, Shanxi 030013, China. TEL 86-351-4173499. Ed. Bingyi Qi.

615.89 USA
SHARE GUIDE; the holistic health magazine. Text in English. 1989. bi-m., latest 2001, Jul./Aug. (on-line ed. w.). USD 14 domestic; USD 22 foreign (effective 2001). adv. bk.rev., music rev., software rev., video rev. tr.lit. 116 p./no. back issues avail. **Document type:** *Magazine, Consumer.* **Description:** A holistic health magazine focusing on alternative medicine, personal growth, and environmental awareness.
Related titles: CD-ROM ed.; Online - full text ed.: 1995.
Address: PO Box 420, Groton, CA 95444. TEL 707-829-0260, FAX 707-829-0261, share@shareguide.com, http://www.shareguide.com. Ed., R&P Janice Hughes. Pubs. Dennis Hughes, Janice Hughes. Adv. contact Dennis Hughes. B&W page USD 899, color page USD 1,500; trim 11 x 8.5. Circ: 30,000.

SHIZHEN GUOYAO YANJIU/SHIZHEN JOURNAL OF TRADITIONAL CHINESE MEDICINE RESEARCH. see *PHARMACY AND PHARMACOLOGY*

615.89 CHN ISSN 1000-3649
SICHUAN ZHONGYI/SICHUAN JOURNAL OF TRADITIONAL CHINESE MEDICINE. Text in Chinese. m.
Published by: Zhonghua Quanguo ZhongYi Xuehui, Sichuan Fenhui/Chinese National Society for Traditional Chinese Medicine, Sichuan Branch, 80, Wenmiao Xijie, Chengdu, Sichuan 610041, China. TEL 26595. Ed. Jin Jiajun.

615.852 291 USA ISSN 1080-3262
SPIRITUAL MASSAGE MINISTRY NEWSLETTER. Text in English. 1995. q. USD 25; USD 30 foreign (effective 1999). bk.rev. index. back issues avail. **Document type:** *Newsletter.* **Description:** Provides information about different types of spiritual healing to laymen, clergymen, and other professionals concerned with health and the healing arts.
Media: Online - full text.
Published by: Church for Spiritual Healing and Health, Spiritual Massage Healing Ministry, 6907 Sherman St, Philadelphia, PA 19119. TEL 215-842-0265, FAX 215-842-2388, aschatz@unix.temple.edu, http://ww.healingandlaw.com. Ed., Pub., R&P Rev. Albert Schatz. Circ: 300.

615.535 299 USA ISSN 1520-5444
SPIRITUALITY & HEALTH; the soul body connection. Text in English. 1998. q., latest vol.4. USD 20 domestic; USD 30 foreign; USD 4.95 newsstand/cover domestic; USD 6.75 newsstand/cover in Canada (effective 2001). adv. bk.rev., film rev., music rev., video rev. 72 p./no. **Document type:** *Magazine, Consumer.* **Description:** Chronicles the spiritual renaissance of the 21st century and the connection between spirituality and personal well-being in its broadest sense. Explores all aspects of personal growth including spiritual beliefs, music, media and the arts, and provides practical resources for individual exploration and practice.
Published by: Spirituality and Health Publishing, Inc., 74 Trinity Place, New York, NY 10006-2088. TEL 212-602-0705, FAX 212-602-0726, editor@spiritualityhealth.com, http://www.spiritualityhealth.com. Ed. Robert Owens Scott. Pub., Adv. contact Peter D Wild TEL 212-602-0772. R&P N Brockman TEL 212-602-0706. page USD 3,500; 8.5 x 11. Circ: 55,000 (paid); 10,000 (controlled). **Dist. by:** Ingram Periodicals, La Vergne, TN 37086.

615.89 SWE ISSN 1104-5477
SVENSK TIDSKRIFT FOER MEDICINSK AKUPUNKTUR. Text in Swedish. 1993. q. SEK 200; SEK 55 newsstand/cover (effective 2000 & 2001). **Document type:** *Trade.*
Published by: (Legitimerade Sjukskoeterskors Akupunkturfoerening), Via Media, Fack 640, Landskrona 26125, Sweden. TEL 46-418-10780, FAX 46-418-12394, viamedia@nornemark.com, http://www.nornemark.com/viamedia. Ed. Katarina Johansson. Circ: 2,100 (paid). **Co-sponsor:** Svensk Laekarefoerening foer Akupunktur.

TAI CHI & ALTERNATIVE HEALTH. see *ORIENTAL STUDIES*

615.537 ITA
TERAPIE NATURALI E ERBE. Text in Italian. 1984. m. ITL 70,000, USD 70. adv. **Document type:** *Academic/Scholarly.*
Former titles: Erbe e Terapie Naturali; Erbe Secondo Natura
Published by: Stampa Natura Solidarieta s.p.a., Via Antonio Bazzini, 40, Milan, MI 20131, Italy. TEL 39-2-26680654, FAX 39-2-26680664. Circ: 40,000.

TIJDSCHRIFT VOOR CREATIEVE THERAPIE. see *PSYCHOLOGY*

615.82 NLD ISSN 0928-0065
TIJDSCHRIFT VOOR INTEGRALE GENEESKUNDE. Text in Dutch; Summaries in Dutch, English. 1984. bi-m. NLG 95 (effective 1995). adv. bk.rev. back issues avail. *Refereed.* **Document type:** *Academic/Scholarly.* **Description:** Publishes studies of fundamental and applied research relating to complementary medicine, alternative medicine, homeopathy, health policy and developments in diagnosis and other branches of the medical sciences.
Published by: Stichting Tijdschrift voor Integrale Geneeskunde, Tooropstraat 181, Nijmegen 6521 NM, Netherlands. TEL 31-80-601688. Ed. Dr. C W Kramers.

615.89 USA ISSN 1525-4283
TOWNSEND LETTER FOR DOCTORS & PATIENTS. Text in English. 1983. m. (10/yr.). USD 49; USD 53 in Washington state; USD 79 in Canada & Mexico; USD 117 elsewhere (effective 2000). bk.rev. **Document type:** *Consumer.*
Formerly (until 1995): Townsend Letter for Doctors (1059-5864)
Indexed: AMED.
—BLDSC, ingenta.
Address: 911 Tyler St, Port Townsend, WA 98368-6541. TEL 360-385-6021, FAX 360-385-0699, tldp@olympus.net, http://www.tldp.com. Ed., Pub. Dr. Jonathan Collin. R&P, Adv. contact Barbara Smith. Circ: 6,000 (paid).

TRAGER NEWSLETTER. see *MEDICAL SCIENCES—Physical Medicine And Rehabilitation*

610 CAN
TURFSEER'S ALTERNATIVE HEALTH AND BUSINESS OPPORTUNITIES NEWSLETTER. Text in English. bi-m. **Document type:** *Newsletter.* **Description:** Focuses on drug-free natural healing and alternative medicine using natural remedies.
Media: Online - full text.
Address: Canada. Turfseer@aol.com, http://hartley.on.ca/turfseer. Pub. Lewis Papier.

613.7 613.2 CAN ISSN 1180-0291
VITALITY MAGAZINE; Toronto's monthly wellness journal. Text in English. 1989. m. (10/yr.). CND 30 domestic; CND 35 in United States; CND 40 elsewhere. adv. **Document type:** *Consumer.* **Description:** Covers holistic health, nutritional medicine, self development, news and reviews of events and services in Toronto.
Address: 356 Dupont St, Toronto, ON M5R 1V9, Canada. TEL 416-964-0528. Ed. Julia Woodford. Adv. contact Jody Hatt. Circ: 44,000 (controlled).

615.89 USA
VOICE OF NAPRAPATHY. Text in English. 1955. irreg., latest vol.82, 1988. back issues avail. **Description:** A forum for practitioners of naprapathy, a system of manipulation administered by the hands.
Published by: American Naprapathic Association, 5321 N Central Ave, Chicago, IL 60630. TEL 312-685-6020. Ed. Ray Webster. Circ: 5,000. **Subscr. to:** 5913 W Montrose Ave, Chicago, IL 60634. **Co-sponsor:** Illinois Naprapathic Association.

WEED WORLD. see *DRUG ABUSE AND ALCOHOLISM*

615.89 USA ISSN 1352-1241
WHAT DOCTORS DON'T TELL YOU* . Text in English. 1989. m. USD 39.95 to individuals; USD 79.95 to institutions. bk.rev. abstr. back issues avail. **Document type:** *Academic/Scholarly.* **Description:** Criticizes conventional medicine and shows its failings through scientific evidence.
Indexed: AMED.
—BLDSC (9309.679050).
Published by: Wallace Press, 3027 Lanier Dr NE, Atlanta, GA 30319-2710. Ed. Lynne McTaggart. Pub. Bryan Hubbard.

WHOLENESS. see *RELIGIONS AND THEOLOGY*

615.89 615.328 CHN ISSN 0256-7415
XINZHONGYI/NEW JOURNAL OF TRADITIONAL CHINESE MEDICINE. Text in Chinese. 1969. m. CNY 42 (effective 1999). **Document type:** *Academic/Scholarly.* **Description:** Covers theory and clinical practice of traditional Chinese medicine.
Published by: Guangzhou Zhongyiyao Daxue/Guangzhou University of Traditional Chinese Medicine, 12, Jichang Lu, Guangzhou, Guangdong 510405, China. TEL 86-20-86591233, FAX 86-20-8659-4735, xbgutcm@ihw.com.cn. Ed. Li Renxian. adv.: B&W page USD 5,000. Circ: 80,000. **Dist. overseas by:** China International Book Trading Corp, 35 Chegongzhuang Xilu, Haidian District, Beijing 100044, China.

615.53 CAN ISSN 1488-0253
YOUR LIFE - YOUR CHOICE. Text in English. 1997. s-m. free per issue. adv. back issues avail. **Document type:** *Newsletter.* **Description:** Discusses the choices available with alternative medicine.
Media: Online - full text. **Related titles:** E-mail ed.
Address: 188 Gammage St, London, ON N5Y 2B3, Canada. TEL 519-645-7797, yourlife@life-choices.com, http://www.life-choices.com. Ed., Pub., R&P Brigitte Synesael. Circ: 3,000.

615.89 615.328 CHN ISSN 0255-2914
R97.7.C5
YUNNAN ZHONGYI ZAZHI/YUNNAN JOURNAL OF TRADITIONAL CHINESE MEDICINE. Text in Chinese. 1980. bi-m. USD 0.80 per issue. adv. **Document type:** *Academic/Scholarly.* **Description:** Covers scientific researches, theories and clinical practices in traditional Chinese medicine, medical materials, acupuncture, and moxibustion.
Related titles: CD-ROM ed.
Indexed: ExtraMED.
Published by: Yunnan Sheng Zhongyi Zhongyao Yanjiusuo/Yunnan Research Institute of Traditional Chinese Medicine and Material Medica, Lianhua Chi, Kunming, Yunnan 650223, China. TEL 5154494. Ed. Zhang Zhen. Adv. contact Zhao Hua. **Dist. overseas by:** China International Book Trading Corp, 35 Chegongzhuang Xilu, Haidian District, Beijing 100044, China.

615.89 DEU ISSN 0044-3182
ZEITSCHRIFT FUER NATURHEILKUNDE. Text in German. 1949. m. DEM 54 (effective 1999). adv. bk.rev. **Document type:** *Consumer.*
Published by: Berufsverband der Heilpraktiker Nordrhein-Westfalen e.V., Koernerstr 59, Solingen 42659, Germany. Circ: 5,800.

615.89 615.328 CHN ISSN 0411-8421
ZHEJIANG ZHONGYI ZAZHI/ZHEJIANG JOURNAL OF TRADITIONAL CHINESE MEDICINE. Text in Chinese. 1956. m. CNY 3.50 per issue domestic (effective 2000). back issues avail. **Document type:** *Academic/Scholarly.*
Related titles: CD-ROM ed.
Indexed: ExtraMED.
Published by: Zhejiang-sheng Zhongyiyao Yanjiuyuan/Zhejiang Academy of Traditional Chinese Medicine, Tianmushan Lu 26 Hao, Hangzhou, Zhejiang 310007, China. TEL 86-571-8842882, FAX 86-571-8845196. Ed. Yi Cheng Chen. **Dist. overseas by:** China International Book Trading Corp, 35 Chegongzhuang Xilu, Haidian District, Beijing 100044, China.

ZHONGCAOYAO/CHINESE TRADITIONAL AND HERBAL DRUGS. see *MEDICAL SCIENCES*

615.89 CHN ISSN 1007-5798
ZHONGGUO MINJIAN LIAOFA/CHINA'S NATUROPATHY. Text in Chinese. 1993. m. USD 30; CNY 4.80, USD 2.50 newsstand/cover (effective 2001). **Document type:** *Academic/Scholarly.*
Related titles: Online - full content ed.: (from WanFang Data Corp.).
Published by: Zhongguo Zhongyiyao Chubanshe, Zhaoyang Qu, 7, Dongxing Lu, Beijing 100027, China. **Dist. by:** China International Book Trading Corp, 35, Chegongzhuang Xilu, Haidian District, Beijing 100044, China. TEL 86-1-68413849, FAX 86-1-68412048, cibtc@mail.cibtc.com.cn, http://www.cibtc.com.cn.

615.89 CHN ISSN 1005-2569
ZHONGGUO QIGONG KEXUE/CHINA QIGONG SCIENCE. Text in Chinese. 1994. m. USD 30; USD 2.50 newsstand/cover (effective 2001). **Document type:** *Academic/Scholarly.*
Published by: China International Book Trading Corp/Zhongguo Guoji Tushu Maoyi Zonggongsi cibtc@mail.cibtc.com.cn, http://www.cibtc.com.cn. **Dist. by:** 35, Chegongzhuang Xilu, Haidian District, Beijing 100044, China.

615.892 CHN
ZHONGGUO ZHENJIU/CHINESE ACUPUNCTURE AND MOXIBUSTION. Text in Chinese; Abstracts in English. 1981. m. USD 32.40 (effective 2001); USD 2.70 newsstand/cover.
Published by: (China Academy of Traditional Chinese Medicine), Zhongguo Zhenjiu Zazhishe, Dongzhimennei, Beijing 100700, China. TEL 86-1-84014607. **Dist. by:** China International Book Trading Corp, 35, Chegongzhuang Xilu, Haidian District, Beijing 100044, China. TEL 86-1-68413849, FAX 86-1-68412048, cibtc@mail.cibtc.com.cn, http://www.cibtc.com.cn. **Co-sponsor:** Chinese Society of Acupuncture and Moxibustion.

ZHONGGUO ZHONGYAO ZAZHI/CHINA JOURNAL OF CHINESE MATERIA MEDICA. see *PHARMACY AND PHARMACOLOGY*

ZHONGHUA QIGONG/CHINESE BREATH EXERCISE. see *PHYSICAL FITNESS AND HYGIENE*

615.8907 CHN ISSN 1003-305X
ZHONGYI JIAOYU/EDUCATION OF TRADITIONAL CHINESE MEDICINE. Text in Chinese. 1982. bi-m. **Document type:** *Academic/Scholarly.* **Description:** Covers all aspects of education of traditional Chinese medicine.
Published by: (Beijing Zhongyi Daxue/Beijing University of Traditional Chinese Medicine), Zhongyi Jiaoyu Bianjibu, 11 Beisanhuan Donglu, Beijing 100029, China. TEL 86-10-4225566, FAX 86-10-4220890. Ed. Liu Zhenmin. **Dist. overseas by:** China International Book Trading Corp, 35 Chegongzhuang Xilu, Haidian District, Beijing 100044, China.

615.89 615.328 CHN ISSN 1001-1668
ZHONGYI ZAZHI. Text in Chinese. 1955. m. USD 40.80 foreign; CNY 5.80 newsstand/cover domestic; USD 3.40 newsstand/cover foreign (effective 2001).
Formerly (until 1978): Xin Yiyaoxue Zazhi (0376-656X)
Related titles: English ed.: Journal of Traditional Chinese Medicine.
Indexed: Helminthol.Abstr., Ind.Med. (coverage dropped), Ref.Zh.
Published by: (Zhongguo Zhongyiyao Xuehui), China International Book Trading Corp/Zhongguo Guoji Tushu Maoyi Zonggongsi, 35 Chegongzhuang Xilu, Haidian District, Beijing 100044, China. TEL 86-1-68413849, FAX 86-1-68412048, cibtc@mail.cibtc.com.cn, http://www.cibtc.com.cn. **Co-publisher:** Zhongguo Zhongyi Yanjiuyuan.

ZHONGYI ZHENGGU/JOURNAL OF TRADITIONAL CHINESE ORTHOPEDICS AND TRAUMATOLOGY. see *MEDICAL SCIENCES—Orthopedics And Traumatology*

ALTERNATIVE MEDICINE—Abstracting, Bibliographies, Statistics

615.89 GBR
A M E D. Variant title: Allied and Complementary Medicine. (Related indexes are avail. in print format: Complementary Medicine Index (ISSN 0950-6667); Rehabilitation Index (ISSN 0955-0984); Podiatry Index (ISSN 1354-9979); Palliative Care Index (ISSN 0961-4591); Physiotherapy Index (ISSN 0950-6659); Occupational Therapy Index (0950-6675)) Text in English. q. GBP 595 for single user. index. **Document type:** *Abstract/Index.* **Description:** Covers the fields of allied and complementary medicine with references to articles from 400 journals. Coverage is strongly European with the majority of titles in English. Includes coverage of complementary medicine, physiotherapy, occupational therapy, rehabilitation and podiatry.
Media: Online - full content. **Related titles:** CD-ROM ed.
Published by: British Library, Health Care Information Service, British Library, Boston Spa, Wetherby, W Yorks LS23 7BQ, United Kingdom. TEL 44-1937-546039, FAX 44-1937-546458, phillipa.seaton@bl.uk.

016.613 USA
ALT-HEALTH WATCH; alternative health & wellness. Text in English. bi-m. **Document type:** *Abstract/Index.* **Description:** Focuses on the many perspectives of complementary, holistic and integrated approaches to healthcare and wellness. Offers a resource of nearly 50,000 articles.
Media: Online - full text.
Published by: EBSCO Publishing (Subsidiary of: EBSCO Industries, Inc.), 10 Estes St, Box 682, Ipswich, MA 01938. TEL 508-356-6500, 800-653-2726, http://www.epnet.com.

016.615 CHN ISSN 1003-3521
ZHONGGUO YAOXUE WENZHAI/CHINESE PHARMACEUTICAL ABSTRACTS. Text in Chinese. 1982. m. USD 250. adv. *Refereed.* **Document type:** *Abstract/Index, Academic/Scholarly.* **Description:** Published on the basis of the Traditional Chinese Medicines (TCMs) Contemporary Literature Database, as well as abstracts in modern drugs in China. Covers 420 current domestic medical journals.
Published by: Guojia Yiyao Guanli-ju, Keji Qingbao Yanjiusuo/State Pharmaceutical Administration of China, Science and Technology Information Research Institute, A-38 Beilishilu, Beijing 100810, China. TEL 86-10-6831-3344, FAX 86-10-6831-1978. Ed. Fengwen Guo.

ZHONGGUO YIXUE WENZHAI (ZHONGYI)/CHINA MEDICAL ABSTRACTS (TRADITIONAL MEDICINE SCIENCE). see *MEDICAL SCIENCES—Abstracting, Bibliographies, Statistics*

ANAESTHESIOLOGY

see MEDICAL SCIENCES—Anaesthesiology

ANALYTICAL CHEMISTRY

see CHEMISTRY—Analytical Chemistry

ANIMAL WELFARE

see also PETS

179 636.089 AUS ISSN 1039-9089
A N Z C C A R T NEWS. Variant title: Anzccart News. Text in English. 1988. q. free. bk.rev., Website rev. 20 p./no. back issues avail.; reprints avail. **Document type:** *Newsletter, Academic/Scholarly.*
Formerly (until 1993): A C C A R T News
Indexed: AgBiotech, Anim.Breed.Abstr., Ind.Vet., Pig News & Info.
Published by: Australian and New Zealand Council for the Care of Animals in Research and Teaching Limited, Dept. of Environmental Biology, University of Adelaide, Adelaide, SA 5005, Australia. TEL 61-8-8303-7586, FAX 61-8-8303-7587, anzccart@adelaide.edu.au, http://www.adelaide.edu.au/anzccart/. Ed. Dr. Robert Baker. Circ: 6,000.

179.3 179.4 USA ISSN 0274-7774
HV4701
THE A V MAGAZINE. Text in English. 1892. q. USD 20 to members (effective 1999). bk.rev. charts, illus. back issues avail.; reprints avail. **Document type:** *Academic/Scholarly, Consumer.* **Description:** Seeks to end experiments using animals and promote humane research by awarding grants for work not involving animals.
Formerly: A-V (0001-2831)
Indexed: W.R.C.Inf.
—ingenta.
Published by: American Anti-Vivisection Society, Noble Plaza, Ste 204, 801 Old York Rd, Jenkintown, PA 19046. TEL 215-887-0816, FAX 215-887-2088, aavsonline@aol.com, http://www.aavs.org/. Ed. Tina Nelson. Circ: 11,000.

179.3 179.4 GBR
ADVOCATES FOR ANIMALS. ANNUAL PICTORIAL REVIEW. Text in English. 1912. a., latest 2001. free per issue. adv. bk.rev. back issues avail. **Document type:** *Bulletin.*
Formerly (until 1990): Scottish Society for Prevention of Vivisection. Annual Pictorial Review (0080-8210)
Published by: Advocates for Animals, 10 Queensferry St, Edinburgh EH2 4PG, United Kingdom. TEL 44-131-225-6039, FAX 44-131-220-6377, advocates.animals@virgin.net, http://www.advocatesforanimals.org.uk. Ed., Pub., R&P, Adv. contact Les Ward. Circ: 10,000.

ALTEX. see *MEDICAL SCIENCES—Experimental Medicine, Laboratory Technique*

179.3 USA
ANIMAL WELFARE INFORMATION CENTER BULLETIN. Text in English. 1990. q. free per issue. **Document type:** *Bulletin, Government.* **Description:** Publishes articles on animal-welfare issues, along with other information of use to persons conducting biomedical research. Lists funding opportunities for related research.
Formerly: Animal Welfare Information Center Newsletter (1050-561X)
Related titles: Online - full text ed.
Indexed: Agricola, Ind.Vet.
—BLDSC (0905.135500).
Published by: (U.S. Department of Agriculture), U.S. Animal Welfare Information Center, National Agricultural Library, 10301 Baltimore Blvd, 5th Fl, Beltsville, MD 20705-2351. TEL 301-504-6212, FAX 301-504-7125, tallen@nal.usda.gov, http://netvet.wustl.edu/awic.htm. Ed., R&P Tim Allen TEL 301-504-5174. Circ: 6,200.

APIS; the international journal bulletin for specialty livestock and pet-animal product development. see *VETERINARY SCIENCE*

ASKO; dwumiesiecznik kynologiczny. see *PETS*

THE CIVIL ABOLITIONIST. see *MEDICAL SCIENCES*

ERSATZ- UND ERGAENZUNGSMETHODEN ZU TIERVERSUCHEN. see *MEDICAL SCIENCES—Experimental Medicine, Laboratory Technique*

179 636.8 GBR
F A B JOURNAL. Text in English. 1958. q. GBP 20 (effective 1999). adv. bk.rev. charts, illus, stat. back issues avail. **Document type:** *Academic/Scholarly, Consumer.* **Description:** Contains items of interest to veterinarians and breeders specializing in cats, as well as general-interest articles for cat lovers and owners.
Formerly: F A B Bulletin
Media: Duplicated (not offset).
Published by: Feline Advisory Bureau, Taeselbury, High St, Tisbury, Salisbury, Wilts SP3 6LD, United Kingdom. TEL 44-1747-871872, FAX 44-1747-871873, fab.fab@ukonline.co.uk, http://web.ukonline.co.uk/fab.fab.html. Ed., R&P, Adv. contact Claire Bessant. Circ: 3,500 (paid).

179.3 GBR ISSN 0268-4306
F R A M E NEWS. Text in English. 1979. irreg. (3-4/yr.). GBP 15, USD 25 (effective 1999). illus. **Document type:** *Newsletter.* **Description:** Discusses the organization's efforts to abolish the use of animals in laboratory testing. Reports general news in the area.
Formerly (until 1984): F R A M E Technical News (0143-8352)
Published by: Fund for the Replacement of Animals in Medical Experiments, Russell & Burch House, 96-98 N. Sherwood St, Nottingham NG1 4EE, United Kingdom. TEL 44-115-958-4740, FAX 44-115-950-3570, atla@frame.org.uk, http://www.frame.org.uk. Ed. Vivienne Hunter.

A

179.3 GBR
FRIENDS OF F R A M E. Text in English. m. illus. **Document type:** *Newsletter.* **Description:** Covers organization news and events for donors.
Published by: Fund for the Replacement of Animals in Medical Experiments, Russell & Burch House, 96-98 N. Sherwood St, Nottingham NG1 4EE, United Kingdom. TEL 44-115-958-4740, FAX 44-115-950-3570, atla@frame.org.uk, http://www.frame.org.uk. Ed. Vivienne P Hunter.

INTERNATIONAL JOURNAL OF ANIMAL SCIENCES. see *AGRICULTURE—Poultry And Livestock*

179.3 USA ISSN 1051-8827
INTERNATIONAL SOCIETY FOR ANIMAL RIGHTS REPORT. Text in English. 1959. q. USD 15. bk.rev. **Document type:** *Newsletter.*
Former titles (until Aug. 1983): Society for Animal Rights Report; N C S A W Report (0027-6340)
Published by: International Society for Animal Rights, Inc., 965 Griffin Pond Rd, Clarks Summit, PA 18411-9214. TEL 717-586-2200, FAX 717-586-9580, isar@aol.com, http://www.isar.com. Ed. Susan Altieri. Circ: 50,000.

179 USA ISSN 1088-8705
WMLC 93/1440
JOURNAL OF APPLIED ANIMAL WELFARE SCIENCE. Short title: J A A W S. Text in English. 1989. q. USD 45 in US & Canada to individuals; USD 75 elsewhere to individuals; USD 255 in US & Canada to institutions; USD 285 elsewhere to institutions (effective 2002). adv. bk.rev. illus. cum.index. back issues avail.; reprints avail. *Refereed.* **Document type:** *Journal, Academic/Scholarly.* **Description:** Publishes reports and articles on methods of experimentation, husbandry and care that demonstrably enhance the welfare of farm, laboratory, companion and wild animals.
Supersedes (in 1995): Humane Innovations and Alternatives (1062-4805); Which was formerly (until 1991): Humane Innovations and Alternatives in Animal Experimentation (0893-9535)
Related titles: Online - full text ed.: ISSN 1532-7604. USD 40.50 to individuals; USD 229.50 to institutions (effective 2002) (from CatchWord Ltd., EBSCO Publishing, O C L C Online Computer Library Center, Inc., RoweCom Information Quest, Swets Blackwell).
Indexed: Agri.Eng.Abstr., Agricola, Anim.Breed.Abstr., Ind.Vet., InterActions Bibl. (1992-), Pig News & Info., PsycInfo, Vet.Bull., Wild.Rev., Zoo.Rec., e-psyche.
—BLDSC (4616.316500), CatchWord. **CCC.**
Published by: (Psychologists for the Ethical Treatment of Animals, American Society for the Prevention of Cruelty to Animals), Lawrence Erlbaum Associates, Inc., 10 Industrial Ave, Mahwah, NJ 07430-2262. TEL 201-760-3735, 800-926-6579, FAX 201-236-0072, journals@erlbaum.com, http://www.erlbaum.com/Journals/journals/JAWS/jaws.htm. Eds. Kenneth Shapiro, Stephen Zawistowski. adv.: page USD 375; trim 5 x 8.

179.3 636.089 DEU ISSN 0948-4647
LEBENDIGE TIERWELT; tieraerztlicher Ratgeber fuer Tierfreunde. Text in German. 1994. q. DEM 15 (effective 2000). adv. bk.rev. back issues avail. **Document type:** *Magazine, Consumer.*
Published by: (Bundesverband Praktischer Tieraerzte e.V.), Schluetersche GmbH und Co. KG, Hans-Boeckler-Allee 7, Hannover 30173, Germany. TEL 49-511-8550-0, FAX 49-511-85502405, vertrieb@schluetersche.de, http://www.schluetersche.de. Circ: 80,100 (paid); 4,376 (controlled).

179.3 179.4 GBR
LORD DOWDING FUND FOR HUMANE RESEARCH. BULLETIN. Text in English. 1980 (no.14). s-a. per issue contribution. adv. illus. **Document type:** *Bulletin.* **Description:** Gives scientific reports on projects that will replace the use of live animals in medical research.
Published by: National Anti-Vivisection Society, 261 Goldhawk Rd, London W12 8EU, United Kingdom. TEL 44-20-8846-9777, FAX 44-20-8846-9712. Ed., R&P, Adv. contact Jan Creamer. Circ: 20,000.

PENDIK VETERINER MIKROBIYOLOJI DERGISI. see *VETERINARY SCIENCE*

PRIMATE EYE. see *ANTHROPOLOGY*

179.4 619 NLD ISSN 1380-4316
PROEFDIERVRIJ. Text in Dutch. 1977. q. NLG 30 to membership; NLG 12.50 to students (effective 2000). bk.rev. back issues avail. **Document type:** *Newsletter.* **Description:** Includes information about animal experimentation with the purpose to inform the public and to change their attitude in favor of animals and against vivisection.
Former titles (until 1994): Proefkonijn (0169-8915); (until 1985): Nederlands Bond tot Bestrijding van de Vivisectie. Berichten (0165-8778); Which was formed by the merger of (1971-1977): Androkles (0169-9989); (1971-1977): Androkles Bulletin (0169-9180); Incorporates (1992-1997): ProefkoneenNieuws (1382-9734); Incorporates (in 1999): Tegenbericht (1381-6438); Which was formerly (until 1995): Raegeermuis (0924-9400); (until 1990): Nieuwsbrief. Anti - Vivisectie - Stichting (0169-2704); (1930-1981): Mededelingen. Anti - Vivisectie - Stichting (0165-8816)
Address: Gevers Deynootweg 61, The Hague 2586 BJ, Netherlands. TEL 31-70-306-2468, info@proefdiervrij.nl, http://www.proefdiervrij.nl. Ed. Joop van Eijk. Circ: 5,500.

SANS LAISSE; magazine de l'education et des sports canins. see *PETS*

SATYA; magazine of vegetarianism, environmentalism, and animal advocacy. see *NUTRITION AND DIETETICS*

179.3 USA ISSN 0742-5260
SCIENTISTS CENTER FOR ANIMAL WELFARE. NEWSLETTER. Text in English. 1978. q. USD 40. bk.rev. index. back issues avail. **Document type:** *Newsletter.* **Description:** Directed to scientists, administrators, and regulatory agencies interested in current issues of animal welfare in research, testing, and education.
Published by: Scientists Center for Animal Welfare, 7833 Walker Dr, 340, Greenbelt, MD 20770-3229. TEL 301-345-3500, FAX 301-345-3503, scaw@erols.com. Ed., R&P Lee Krulisch. Circ: 5,000.

179.3 NLD ISSN 1063-1119
QL85 CODEN: SANIEL
SOCIETY & ANIMALS; social scientific studies of the human experience of other animals. Text in English. 1983; N.S. 1993. 3/yr. EUR 36, USD 42 to individuals; EUR 95, USD 110 to institutions (effective 2002). adv. bk.rev. illus. cum.index. back issues avail. *Refereed.* **Document type:** *Journal, Academic/Scholarly.* **Description:** Publishes original research studies describing and analyzing the ways in which animals figure in human life, in particular examining applied uses of animals in research, medicine, science and agriculture, animals in the popular culture, including animal symbolism and cultic rituals, wildlife and environmental issues, as well as sociopolitical and legal concerns.
Former titles (until 1993): P S Y E T A Bulletin; (until 1986): P S Y E T A Newsletter
Related titles: Online - full text ed.: N.S. (from EBSCO Publishing, RoweCom Information Quest, CatchWord Ltd., Swets Blackwell, Institute for Scientific Information).
Indexed: ASCA, Agricola, Crim.Just.Abstr., Curr.Cont., Focus on: Vet.Sci.& Med., InterActions Bibl., Intl.Bibl.Soc.Sci., Lang.& Lang.Behav.Abstr., PsycInfo, Ref.Zh., SOPODA, SSCI, Soc.Serv.Abstr., Sociol.Abstr., Wild.Rev., Zoo.Rec., e-psyche.
—BLDSC (8319.187500), IDS, Infotrieve, ingenta. **CCC.**
Published by: (Psychologists for the Ethical Treatment of Animals USA), Brill Academic Publishers, PO Box 9000, Leiden 2300 PA, Netherlands. TEL 31-71-53-53-500, FAX 31-71-53-17-532, cs@brill.nl, http://www.brill.nl/. Ed. Kenneth Shapiro. Circ: 400.

156 179 GBR ISSN 1363-464X
SOCIETY FOR COMPANION ANIMAL STUDIES. JOURNAL. Text in English. 1988. q. GBP 15 domestic; GBP 20 foreign (effective 2000). adv. **Document type:** *Newsletter.*
Indexed: InterActions Bibl. (1989-), e-psyche.
Published by: Society for Companion Animal Studies, 10b Leny Rd, Callander FK17 8BA, United Kingdom. TEL 44-1877-330996, FAX 44-1877-330996, http://www.vetweb.co.uk/sites/scas/scashome.htm. Ed., R&P, Adv. contact Anne Docherty. Circ: 600.

179 GBR
U F A W HANDBOOK ON THE CARE AND MANAGEMENT OF LABORATORY ANIMALS. Text in English. 1993 (6th ed.). base vol. plus irreg. updates. GBP 91, USD 185. **Document type:** *Journal, Trade, Academic/Scholarly.* **Description:** Provides guidance on practical animal husbandry, breeding, laboratory procedures and disease control for a wide variety of vertebrates.
Published by: Blackwell Science Ltd., Osney Mead, Oxford OX2 0EL, United Kingdom. TEL 44-1865-206206, FAX 44-1865-721205, journals.cs@blacksci.co.uk, http://www.blackwell-science.com.

THE VEGAN. see *NUTRITION AND DIETETICS*

THE VEGAN NEWS. see *NUTRITION AND DIETETICS*

ANTHROPOLOGY

see also ARCHAEOLOGY; FOLKLORE

ACTA ANATOMICA NIPPONICA/KAIBOGAKU ZASSHI. see *BIOLOGY*

AMERICAN JOURNAL OF PRIMATOLOGY. see *BIOLOGY—Zoology*

306.461 GBR ISSN 1364-8470
ANTHROPOLOGY & MEDICINE. Text in English. 1997 (vol.4). 3/yr. GBP 85, USD 141 to individuals; GBP 196, USD 324 to institutions (effective 2002). **Document type:** *Academic/Scholarly.* **Description:** Publishes original papers within the broad framework of medical anthropology and now addresses a world-wide audience.
Related titles: Online - full content ed.: ISSN 1469-2910 (from EBSCO Publishing, O C L C Online Computer Library Center, Inc., Swets Blackwell); Online - full text ed.: (from CatchWord Ltd., RoweCom Information Quest).
Indexed: A.I.C.P. (1993-), Anthropol.Lit., Indian Psychol.Abstr., Lang.& Lang.Behav.Abstr., PsycInfo, SOPODA, Soc.Serv.Abstr., Sociol.Abstr., e-psyche.
—BLDSC (1546.502740), CatchWord, Infotrieve. **CCC.**
Published by: Carfax Publishing Limited (Subsidiary of: Taylor & Francis Group), PO Box 25, Abingdon, Oxon OX14 3UE, United Kingdom. TEL 44-1235-401000, FAX 44-1235-401550, enquiries@carfax.co.uk, enquiry@tandf.co.uk, http://www.carfax.co.uk. Ed. Sushrut Jadhav.

301 USA ISSN 1053-4202
CODEN: ATCNEI
ANTHROPOLOGY OF CONSCIOUSNESS. Text in English. 1985. q. USD 42 to individuals; USD 56 to institutions (effective 1999). bk.rev. back issues avail. *Refereed.* **Document type:** *Academic/Scholarly.* **Description:** Provides an interdisciplinary forum addressing the cross-cultural dimension of human consciousness from empirical, experimental, and theoretical perspectives.
Former titles (until vol.5, 1989): A A S C Quarterly (1045-4330); A A S C Newsletter (0897-2672)
Indexed: Abstr.Anthropol., Anthropol.Lit., Lang.& Lang.Behav.Abstr., SOPODA, Soc.Serv.Abstr., Sociol.Abstr., e-psyche.
—BLDSC (1546.502770).
Published by: American Anthropological Association, Society for the Anthropology of Consciousness, 4350 N Fairfax Dr, Ste 640, Arlington, VA 22203-1620. TEL 703-528-1902, 71554.1033@compuserve.com, http://www.ameranthassn.org/sacpubs.htm. Ed. Lisa Ann Mertz. R&P Terry Clifford. Circ: 250 (paid).

ANTHROPOLOGY OF FOOD AND NUTRITION. see *FOOD AND FOOD INDUSTRIES*

APPLIED HUMAN SCIENCE; journal of physiological anthropology. see *BIOLOGY—Physiology*

ASCLEPIO; archivo iberoamericano de historia de la medicina. see *MEDICAL SCIENCES*

ASSOCIATION FOR THE STUDY OF PLAY NEWSLETTER. see *PSYCHOLOGY*

BIOETHICS FORUM. see *HUMANITIES: COMPREHENSIVE WORKS*

301 FRA ISSN 1279-7863
GN51
BIOMETRIE HUMAINE ET ANTHROPOLOGIE. Text in French; Summaries in English, French. 1932. s-a. FRF 270 domestic; FRF 300 foreign (effective 2000). adv. bk.rev. bibl, charts, illus. index. **Document type:** *Proceedings.*
Former titles (until 1997): Cahiers d'Anthropologie et Biometrie Humaine (0758-2714); (until 1983): Societe de Biometrie Humaine. Revue (0183-5688); Biometrie Humaine (0006-3428); Biotypologie
Indexed: A.I.C.P., Anthropol.Lit., Biol.Abstr., Chem.Abstr., Curr.Ind.Stat., Excerp.Med., GeoRef, Intl.Bibl.Soc.Sci., Nutr.Abstr., Psychol.Abstr., Ref.Zh.
—CISTI, GNLM, Linda Hall.
Published by: Societe de Biometrie Humaine, 28 rue de Charenton, Paris 75012, France. TEL 33-1-46330596, FAX 33-1-43408785. Ed. E A Cabanis. R&P Ms. Pineau. Adv. contact M Pineau. Circ: 600.

301 ITA ISSN 0392-2529
BIOPSYCHE; rivista di scienze antropologiche. Text in Italian. 1970. q. ITL 15,000. bk.rev. back issues avail.
Published by: Ispasa Societa Cooperativa, Corso Italia, 104, Catania, CT 95129, Italy. TEL 095-532181.

CARNEGIE MUSEUM OF NATURAL HISTORY. ANNALS. see *SCIENCES: COMPREHENSIVE WORKS*

CARNEGIE MUSEUM OF NATURAL HISTORY. BULLETIN. see *SCIENCES: COMPREHENSIVE WORKS*

CROSS-CULTURAL PSYCHOLOGY BULLETIN. see *PSYCHOLOGY*

CROSS-CULTURAL RESEARCH AND METHODOLOGY SERIES. see *PSYCHOLOGY*

CULTURE & PSYCHOLOGY. see *PSYCHOLOGY*

306.461 NLD ISSN 0167-4447
CODEN: CIHEET
CULTURE, ILLNESS AND HEALING; studies in comparative cross-cultural research. Text in English. 1980. irreg. price varies. *Refereed.* **Document type:** *Monographic series.*
Published by: Kluwer Academic Publishers Group (Subsidiary of: Wolters Kluwer N.V.), Spuiboulevard 50, PO Box 17, Dordrecht 3300 AA, Netherlands. FAX 31-78-639-2254, services@wkap.nl, http://www.wkap.nl. Eds. Allan Young, Margaret Lock. **Dist. by:** Journals Department, PO Box 322, Dordrecht 3300 AH, Netherlands. FAX 31-78-654-6474.

306.461 NLD ISSN 0165-005X
RC455.4.E8 CODEN: CMPSD2
CULTURE, MEDICINE AND PSYCHIATRY; an international journal of comparative cross-cultural research. Text in English. 1977. q. EUR 326, USD 327 to institutions for print or online ed.; EUR 391.20, USD 392.40 to institutions for print & online eds.combined (effective 2002). adv. bk.rev. illus. reprint service avail. from SWZ. *Refereed.* **Document type:** *Journal, Academic/Scholarly.* **Description:** Provides an international and interdisciplinary forum for the discussion of medical and psychiatric anthropology, cross-cultural psychiatry, and related cross-societal clinical and epidemiological studies.
Related titles: Microform ed.: (from PQC); Online - full text ed.: (from EBSCO Publishing, O C L C Online Computer Library Center, Inc., RoweCom Information Quest, Swets Blackwell, Kluwer Online, Institute for Scientific Information).
Indexed: ASCA, Abstr.Anthropol., AgeLine, Anthropol.Lit., Arts & Hum.Cit.Ind. (coverage dropped), Bibl.Asian Stud. (1977-1991), Biol.Abstr., Curr.Cont., E.I., Excerp.Med., IBZ, Ind.Med. (1977-), Indian Psychol.Abstr., Int.Nurs.Ind., Intl.Bibl.Soc.Sci., Lang.& Lang.Behav.Abstr., Mid.East: Abstr.& Ind., Phil.Ind., PsycInfo, Psychol.Abstr. (1977-), Ref.Zh., Risk Abstr., SOPODA, SSCI, Soc.Serv.Abstr., Sociol.Abstr., e-psyche.
—BLDSC (3491.669100), CISTI, GNLM, IDS, ingenta. **CCC.**
Published by: Kluwer Academic Publishers Group (Subsidiary of: Wolters Kluwer N.V.), Spuiboulevard 50, PO Box 17, Dordrecht 3300 AA, Netherlands. TEL 31-78-639-2392, FAX 31-78-654-2254, services@wkap.nl, http://www.wkap.nl/journalhome.htm/0165-005X. Eds. Anne E Becker, Byron J Good, Mary-Jo DelVecchio Good. **Subscr. in the Americas to:** Kluwer Academic - Plenum Publishers, 233 Spring St, New York, NY 10013-1578. TEL 212-620-8468, FAX 212-807-1047; **Subscr. to:** Journals Department, PO Box 322, Dordrecht 3300 AH, Netherlands. TEL 31-78-639-2392, FAX 31-78-654-6474.

306.461 DEU ISSN 0344-8622
RC455.4.E8
CURARE; Zeitschrift fuer Ethnomedizin - journal for ethnomedicine. Text in English, French, German. 1978. s-a. EUR 43 (effective 2002). back issues avail. **Document type:** *Journal, Academic/Scholarly.* **Description:** Forum of exchange and discussion concerning traditional medical systems, medical aid programs, health planning, and related issues.
Indexed: A.I.C.P. (1989-), Abstr.Hyg., Anthropol.Lit., E.I., IBZ, Intl.Bibl.Soc.Sci., Lang.& Lang.Behav.Abstr., SOPODA, Soc.Serv.Abstr., Sociol.Abstr., Trop.Dis.Bull.
—BLDSC (3493.435000), GNLM. **CCC.**
Published by: (Arbeitsgemeinschaft Ethnomedizin e.V.), V W B - Verlag fuer Wissenschaft und Bildung, Zossener Str 55, Berlin 10961, Germany. TEL 49-30-2510415, FAX 49-30-2511136, 100615.1565@compuserve.com, http://www.vwb-verlag.com. Circ: 1,000.

599.9 MEX
ESTUDIOS DE ANTROPOLOGIA BIOLOGICA. Text in Spanish. 1982. biennial. MXP 40 per issue (effective 2000). **Description:** Includes lectures and conferences given at the Physical Anthropology Congress "Juan Comas".
Published by: Universidad Nacional Autonoma de Mexico, Instituto de Investigaciones Antropologicas, Circuito Exterior, Ciudad Universitaria, Mexico, DF 04510, Mexico. TEL 52-5-622-9531, FAX 52-5-622-9651. Ed. Luis Alberto Vargas.

EVOLUTIONARY MONOGRAPHS. see *BIOLOGY*

FOOD AND FOODWAYS; explorations in the history and culture of human nutrition. see *NUTRITION AND DIETETICS*

FOOD AND NUTRITION IN HISTORY AND ANTHROPOLOGY. see *NUTRITION AND DIETETICS*

FRONTIERES; les vivants et les morts. see *PSYCHOLOGY*

301 PRT ISSN 0870-0168
GARCIA DE ORTA: SERIE DE ANTROPOBIOLOGIA. Text in English, French, Italian, Portuguese, Spanish. 1982. irreg., latest vol.9, 1996. price varies. back issues avail. **Document type:** *Academic/Scholarly.*
Indexed: A.I.C.P. (1987-1988), Anthropol.Lit., Documentatieblad, GeoRef, Intl.Bibl.Soc.Sci.
—GNLM.
Published by: Instituto de Investigacao Cientifica Tropical, Rua da Junqueira, 30, Lisbon 1349-007, Portugal. TEL 351-21-3622621, FAX 351-21-3631460, iict@iict.pt. Circ: 1,000. **Subscr. to:** Centro de Documentacao e Informacao, Rua de Jau, 47, Lisbon 1300, Portugal. TEL 351-21-3644846, FAX 351-21-3628218.

HISTORICAL BIOLOGY; an international journal of paleobiology. see *PALEONTOLOGY*

304.2 USA ISSN 0300-7839
GF1 CODEN: HMECAJ
HUMAN ECOLOGY (NEW YORK); an interdisciplinary journal. Text in English. 1972. q. USD 561, EUR 560 to institutions for print or online ed.; USD 673.20, EUR 672 to institutions for print & online eds. combined (effective 2002). adv. bk.rev. illus. Index. back issues avail.; reprints avail. *Refereed.* **Document type:** *Journal, Academic/Scholarly.* **Description:** Discusses the quality of the environment and the role of social and cultural factors and population density in the maintenance of ecosystems.
Related titles: Online - full text ed.: (from CatchWord Ltd., Gale Group, EBSCO Publishing, O C L C Online Computer Library Center, Inc., RoweCom Information Quest, ProQuest Information & Learning, Swets Blackwell, Factiva, Institute for Scientific Information).
Indexed: A.I.C.P. (1972-), Abstr.Anthropol., Agricola, Agroforest.Abstr., Anthropol.Lit., Appl.Ecol.Abstr., Bibl.Asian Stud. (1972-1998), Bio-Contr.News & Info., Biol.Abstr., Curr.Adv.Ecol.Sci., Curr.Cont., Deep Sea Res.& Oceanogr.Abstr., E.I., ERA, Ecol.Abstr., Energy Ind., Energy Info.Abstr., Energy Rev., Eng.Ind., Environ.Per.Bibl. (1972-), Environ.Sci.Poll.Mgmt., Excerp.Med., Forest Prod.Abstr., Forest.Abstr., Geo.Abstr.H.G., Geo.Abstr.P.G., IDA, IMFL, INIS Atomind., Ind.Vet., Irr.& Drain.Abstr., Lang.& Lang.Behav.Abstr., Maize Abstr., Mid.East: Abstr.& Ind., Mult.Ed.Abstr., NAA, Nutr.Abstr., P C I, Peace Res.Abstr., Pollut.Abstr., Protozool.Abstr., Psychol.Abstr., Ref.Zh., Rev.Arom.& Med.Plants, Rice Abstr., Rural Devel.Abstr., Rural Recreat.Tour.Abstr., Russ.Acad.Sci.Bibl., SOPODA, SSCI, Sage Urb.Stud.Abstr., Soc.Sci.Ind. (Nov.1982-), Soc.Serv.Abstr., Sociol.Abstr., Soils & Fert., Sport Fish.Abstr., Stud.Wom.Abstr., Vet.Bull., Weed Abstr., Wild.Rev., World Ag.Econ.& Rur.Soc.Abstr., Zoo.Rec.
—BLDSC (4336.055000), CatchWord, CISTI, Ei, GNLM, IDS, Infotrieve, ingenta, Linda Hall. **CCC.**
Published by: Kluwer Academic - Plenum Publishers (Subsidiary of: Wolters Kluwer N.V.), 233 Spring St, New York, NY 10013-1578. TEL 212-620-8000, 800-221-9369, FAX 212-463-0742, info@plenum.com, http://www.wkap.nl/journalhome.htm/0300-7839. Ed. Daniel G Bates. R&P Rose Luongo TEL 781-871-6311. **Subscr. outside the Americas to:** Kluwer Academic Publishers Group, Journals Department, PO Box 322, Dordrecht 3300 AH, Netherlands. TEL 31-78-639-2392, FAX 31-78-654-6474.

HUMAN ETHOLOGY BULLETIN. see *PSYCHOLOGY*

599.938 ITA ISSN 0393-9375
GN281
HUMAN EVOLUTION; international journal. Text in English; Summaries in English, French. 1986. q. ITL 150,000 to individuals; ITL 200,000 to institutions (effective 2000). adv. bk.rev. illus. Index. back issues avail.; reprints avail. **Description:** Multi-disciplinary forum on the study of human evolution. Reflects current interests in molecular evolution, genetics, palaeontology and biological variability considered in social, cultural and physical contexts.
Media: Magnetic Tape.
Indexed: A.I.C.P. (1986-), Anthropol.Lit., Bibl.Asian Stud. (1998), Curr.Cont. (coverage dropped), Excerp.Med., GeoRef, Russ.Acad.Sci.Bibl., Zoo.Rec.
—BLDSC (4336.071200), GNLM, ingenta, Linda Hall.
Published by: (International Institute for the Study of Man), Angelo Pontecorboli Editore, c/o Inst.d'Antropologia, Universita di Firenze, Via Del Proconsolo, 12, Florence, FI 50122, Italy. TEL 39-55-2398065, FAX 39-55-283358, antropos@cesit1.unifi.it, http://www.unifi.it/unifi/antrop/. Ed. A B Chiarelli. Circ: 700.

301 IND ISSN 0019-4387
GN1 CODEN: JIASDA
INDIAN ANTHROPOLOGICAL SOCIETY. JOURNAL. Text in English. 1966. 3/yr. INR 250, USD 50. adv. bk.rev. charts, illus, stat. index. **Document type:** *Academic/Scholarly.* **Description:** Publishes articles in all branches of anthropology including medical anthropology.
Indexed: A.I.C.P. (1966-), Anthropol.Lit., Bibl.Asian Stud. (1971-1995), Biol.Abstr., Forest.Abstr., IDA, Lang.& Lang.Behav.Abstr., Rural Devel.Abstr., SOPODA, Soc.Serv.Abstr., Sociol.Abstr.
—ingenta.
Published by: Indian Anthropological Society, 27 Jawaharlal Nehru Marg, Kolkata, West Bengal 700 016, India. Eds. A K Danda, Arabinda Basu. Circ: 700.

INDIAN JOURNAL OF PHYSICAL ANTHROPOLOGY AND HUMAN GENETICS. see *BIOLOGY—Genetics*

599.9 IDN ISSN 0216-7204
GN49
INDONESIAN JOURNAL OF BIOANTHROPOLOGY/ BERKALA BIOANTHROPOLOGI INDONESIA. Text and summaries in English, Indonesian. 1980. irreg., latest vol.4, no.3, 1984. IDR 7,500, USD 20. adv. bk.rev. charts, illus, stat. back issues avail.
—CCC.
Published by: Gadjah Mada University, College of Medicine/Universitas Gadjah Mada, Fakultas Kedokteran, Department of Physical Anthropology, Sekip, Yogyakarta, Indonesia. Ed. Teuku Jacob. Circ: 1,000.

INTERNATIONAL ASSOCIATION FOR CROSS-CULTURAL PSYCHOLOGY. INTERNATIONAL CONFERENCE. SELECTED PAPERS. see *PSYCHOLOGY*

INTERNATIONAL CONFERENCE ON THE STUDY OF SHAMANISM AND ALTERNATIVE MODES OF HEALING. PROCEEDINGS. see *ALTERNATIVE MEDICINE*

JOURNAL OF CROSS-CULTURAL GERONTOLOGY. see *GERONTOLOGY AND GERIATRICS*

JOURNAL OF ETHNOBIOLOGY. see *BIOLOGY*

▼ **JOURNAL OF MUNDANE BEHAVIOR.** see *SOCIOLOGY*

301 JPN ISSN 0286-4568
KYOTO DAIGAKU. REICHORUI KENKYUJO NENPO/KYOTO UNIVERSITY. PRIMATE RESEARCH INSTITUTE. ANNUAL REPORTS. Text in Japanese. 1971. a. free per issue. back issues avail. **Document type:** *Academic/Scholarly.*
Indexed: Jap.Per.Ind.
Published by: Kyoto University, Primate Research Institute/Kyoto Daigaku Reichorui Kenkyujo, Kanrin, Inuyama-shi, Aichi-ken 484-8506, Japan. TEL 81-568-63-0567, FAX 81-568-63-0085, shomu@pri.kyoto-u.ac.jp, Shomu@smtp.pri.kyoto-u.ac.jp, http://www.pri.kyoto-u.ac.jp/. Circ: 1,000.

A

306.4 USA ISSN 0025-2344
GN1 CODEN: MKQUA4
MANKIND QUARTERLY; an international quarterly journal dealing with both physical and cultural anthropology including related subjects such as psychology, demography, genetics, linguistics and mythology. Text in English. 1960. q. USD 37.50 domestic to individuals; USD 45.50 foreign to individuals; USD 80 domestic to libraries; USD 88 foreign to libraries (effective 1999). adv. bk.rev. charts, illus. index. reprints avail. *Refereed.* **Document type:** *Academic/Scholarly.* **Description:** Articles on anthropology, anthropological linguistics, mythology and religion, psychology, demography and genetics.
Related titles: Online - full text ed.: (from Northern Light Technology, Inc., ProQuest Information & Learning, Institute for Scientific Information).
Indexed: A.I.C.P., ASCA, ASSIA, Abstr.Anthropol., Anthropol.Lit. (coverage dropped), Arts & Hum.Cit.Ind. (coverage dropped), Bibl.Asian Stud. (1972-1991), Bibl.Ling., Biol.Abstr., Curr.Cont., E.I., Fam.Ind., Hist.Abstr. (1972-1977, dropped), IBR, IBZ, Intl.Bibl.Soc.Sci., Lang.& Lang.Behav.Abstr., M.L.A., MLA Intl.Bibl., Mid.East: Abstr.& Ind., P.A.I.S., Polit.Sci.Abstr., Psychol.Abstr., Rel.Ind.One, Rel.Ind.Two, Russ.Acad.Sci.Bibl., SOPODA, SSCI, Soc.Serv.Abstr., Sociol.Abstr., e-psyche.
—BLDSC (5360.900000), IDS, ingenta.
Published by: Scott - Townsend Publishers, PO Box 34070, N W, Washington, DC 20043. TEL 202-371-2700, FAX 202-371-1523, socecon@aol.com, http://www.mankind.org/mqartlst.htm. Ed. Richard Lynn. R&P, Adv. contact James Johnson. Circ: 1,025.

301 DNK ISSN 0106-1062
E99.E7
MEDDELELSER OM GROENLAND. MAN & SOCIETY. Variant title: Greenland Man and Society. Text in Danish. 1878. irreg., latest vol.25, 2001. price varies. charts, illus. **Document type:** *Academic/Scholarly.*
Supersedes in part (in 1979): Meddelelser om Groenland (0025-6676)
Indexed: Biol.Abstr., Zoo.Rec.
—BLDSC (5487.300000), CISTI, Linda Hall.
Published by: Danish Polar Center, Strandgade 100 H, Copenhagen K 1401, Denmark. TEL 45-32-88-01-00, FAX 45-32-88-01-01. Ed. Hans Christian Gulloev.

306.461 CHE ISSN 0145-9740
GN296 CODEN: MDANES
MEDICAL ANTHROPOLOGY; cross-cultural studies in health and illness. Text in English. 1977. q. GBP 77, USD 92, EUR 102 to individuals; GBP 358, USD 437, EUR 446 to institutions; GBP 514, USD 674, EUR 654 to corporations (effective 2002). cum.index. reprint service avail. from PQC,SCH,PSC,ISI. *Refereed.* **Document type:** *Academic/Scholarly.*
Related titles: Microform ed.
Indexed: A.I.C.P., Abstr.Anthropol., Anthropol.Lit., Behav.Med.Abstr., Chic.Per.Ind., IBZ, Ind.Med. (1977-), Indian Psychol.Abstr., Intl.Bibl.Soc.Sci., PsycInfo, Psychol.Abstr. (1985-), So.Pac.Per.Ind., e-psyche.
—BLDSC (5526.220000), GNLM, Infotrieve, ingenta. **CCC.**
Published by: Gordon and Breach - Harwood Academic (Subsidiary of: Taylor & Francis Group), PO Box 531, Lausanne 1000, Switzerland. Ed. Stacy Leigh Pigg. **Subscr. addr. in US:** International Publishers Direct, PO Box 32160, Newark, NJ 07102. FAX 215-750-6343.

306.461 USA ISSN 0745-5194
GN296 CODEN: MAQUD5
MEDICAL ANTHROPOLOGY QUARTERLY; international journal for the cultural and social analysis of health. Text in English. 1970. q. USD 75 to individuals; USD 80 to institutions (effective 1999). adv. bk.rev. illus. reprint service avail. from PQC,ISI. *Refereed.* **Document type:** *Academic/Scholarly.* **Description:** Review articles and brief research reports on health, disease and illness from a biological, cultural, linguistic, and historical perspective.
Former titles: Medical Anthropology Newsletter (0543-2499); Medical Anthropology
Related titles: Online - full text ed.: (from H. W. Wilson, Gale Group, Institute for Scientific Information).
Indexed: A.I.C.P. (1968-), ASCA, Abstr.Anthropol., AgeLine, Anthropol.Lit., Arts & Hum.Cit.Ind. (coverage dropped), Chic.Per.Ind., Curr.Cont., E.I., Fam.Ind., Ind.Med. (1983-), Int.Nurs.Ind., Intl.Bibl.Soc.Sci., Lang.& Lang.Behav.Abstr., SOPODA, SSCI, So.Pac.Per.Ind., Soc.Sci.Ind. (Jul.1999-), Soc.Serv.Abstr., Sociol.Abstr.
—BLDSC (5526.231000), GNLM, ingenta.
Published by: (Society for Medical Anthropology), American Anthropological Association, 4350 N Fairfax Dr, Ste 640, Arlington, VA 22203-1620. TEL 703-528-1902, http://www.ameranthassn.org/smapubs.htm. Ed. Mac Marshall. R&P, Adv. contact Terry Clifford. page USD 275; trim 9 x 6. Circ: 2,000.

MENTAL HEALTH, RELIGION & CULTURE. see *PSYCHOLOGY*

301 GUM ISSN 0026-279X
QH198.M48 CODEN: MCNSBU
MICRONESICA; a journal of the University of Guam. Text and summaries in English. 1964. s-a. USD 40 (effective 1999). bk.rev. charts, illus, maps. index. Supplement avail.; back issues avail. *Refereed.* **Document type:** *Magazine, Academic/Scholarly.* **Description:** Original research on anthropology, biology and related fields of the tropical Pacific.
Indexed: A.I.C.P. (1964-), Abstr.Anthropol., Aqua.Sci.& Fish.Abstr., Aquacult.Abstr., Biol.Abstr., Deep Sea Res.& Oceanogr.Abstr., Environ.Sci.Poll.Mgmt., GeoRef, MLA Intl.Bibl., So.Pac.Per.Ind., Sport Fish.Abstr., Wild.Rev., Zoo.Rec.
—BLDSC (5759.340000), ingenta.
Published by: (University of Guam USA, Graduate School and Research USA), University of Guam Press, UOG Sta, Mangilao, GU 96923. TEL 671-735-2787, 671-735-2171, FAX 671-734-1299, 671-734-2296, 671-734-4582, http://www.uog.edu/up/micronesica/. Ed. Dr. C S Lobban. R&P Dr. C.S. Lobban. Circ: 350.

301 613.2 USA
NUTRITIONAL ANTHROPOLOGY. Text in English. s-a. USD 6 (effective 1999). bk.rev. **Document type:** *Academic/Scholarly.* **Description:** Publishes notices and reports of domestic and international meetings, curriculum guides, and other information for professionals in academic and applied careers with interests in anthropological study of food and nutrition.
Formerly (until 1998): Communicator (Washington) (1062-1938)
Published by: American Anthropological Association, 4350 N Fairfax Dr, Ste 640, Arlington, VA 22203-1620. TEL 703-528-1902, FAX 703-528-3546. Ed. Gretel Pelto. R&P Terry Clifford.

PERSPECTIVES IN HUMAN BIOLOGY. see *BIOLOGY*

301 599.8 GBR ISSN 0305-8417
PRIMATE EYE. Text in English. 1967. 3/yr. GBP 15 (effective 1999). **Document type:** *Newsletter, Proceedings, Academic/Scholarly.*
—BLDSC (6612.917000).
Published by: Primate Society of Great Britain, c/o Institute of Biology, 20-22 Queensbury Pl, London SW7 2DZ, United Kingdom. TEL 44-1316-503110, FAX 44-1316-506545, bill.sellers@ed.ac.uk, http://www.ana.ed.uk/PSGB. Ed. Bill Sellers. Circ: 2,400.

PRIMATES; journal of primatology. see *BIOLOGY—Zoology*

SHAMAN; journal of the international society for shamanistic research. see *ALTERNATIVE MEDICINE*

291.22 USA ISSN 0887-8897
BL2370.S5
SHAMAN'S DRUM; a journal of experiential Shamanism. Text in English. 1985. q. USD 18 domestic; USD 22 in Canada & Mexico; USD 34 elsewhere (effective 2000). adv. bk.rev. **Document type:** *Consumer.* **Description:** Discusses cross-cultural shamanism, Native American healing and ethnic spirituality.
Published by: Cross-Cultural Shamanism Network, Shaman's Drum, 3600 Cedar Flat Rd no A, Williams, OR 97544. TEL 541-846-1313, FAX 541-846-1204. Ed. Timothy White. R&P Roberta Louis. Adv. contact Judy Wells. Circ: 14,000 (paid).

SIGN LANGUAGE STUDIES. see *LINGUISTICS*

SOCIETY FOR THE STUDY OF HUMAN BIOLOGY. SYMPOSIUM SERIES. see *BIOLOGY—Physiology*

SOUTH AFRICAN MUSEUM. ANNALS/SUID-AFRIKAANSE MUSEUM. ANNALE. see *BIOLOGY*

301 ITA ISSN 0392-6788
STUDI PER L'ECOLOGIA DEL QUATERNARIO. Text in Italian. 1979. a. ITL 45,000 (effective 1994). bk.rev. **Document type:** *Academic/Scholarly.* **Description:** Contains previously unpublished works concerning ecology of the Quaternary era, prehistoric ecology, palaeoethnology, Quaternary geology, human paleontology and anthropology.
Indexed: Anthropol.Lit., GeoRef.
Published by: Laboratorio di Ecologia del Quaternario, Via Del Proconsolo, 12, Florence, FI 50122, Italy. TEL 055-293028, FAX 055-293028. Ed. E Borzatti von Loewenstern. Circ: 800.

TRANSCULTURAL PSYCHIATRY. see *MEDICAL SCIENCES—Psychiatry And Neurology*

599.9 DEU ISSN 0044-314X
QM1 CODEN: ZMOAAN
ZEITSCHRIFT FUER MORPHOLOGIE UND ANTHROPOLOGIE. Text in English, French, German. 1899. irreg. USD 70 per issue domestic; USD 71 per issue foreign (effective 2001). **Document type:** *Journal, Academic/Scholarly.*
Indexed: A.I.C.P., Anthropol.Lit., Bibl.Asian Stud. (1971-1975), Biol.Abstr., GeoRef, IBR, Ind.Med. (1899-), P C I, Russ.Acad.Sci.Bibl., Zoo.Rec.
—BLDSC (9473.250000), CISTI, GNLM. **CCC.**
Published by: E. Schweizerbart'sche Verlagsbuchhandlung, Johannesstr 3A, Stuttgart 70176, Germany. TEL 49-711-625001, FAX 49-711-625005, mail@schweizerbart.de, schweizerbart@schweizerbart.de, http://www.schweizerbart.de. Ed. H W Juergens.

ANTHROPOLOGY—Abstracting, Bibliographies, Statistics

REFERATIVNYI ZHURNAL. MORFOLOGIYA CHELOVEKA I ZHIVOTNYKH. ANTROPOLOGIYA. see *BIOLOGY—Abstracting, Bibliographies, Statistics*

ANTIQUES

see also ART

ARCHAEOLOGY

see also ANTHROPOLOGY; ART; HISTORY; PALEONTOLOGY

FLORIDA MUSEUM OF NATURAL HISTORY. BULLETIN. see *BIOLOGY*

GUNNERIA. see *BIOLOGY*

ILLINOIS. STATE MUSEUM. SCIENTIFIC PAPERS SERIES. see *SCIENCES: COMPREHENSIVE WORKS*

JOURNAL OF ETHNOBIOLOGY. see *BIOLOGY*

NATUR UND MENSCH: JAHRESMITTEILUNGEN DER NATURHISTORISCHEN GESELLSCHAFT NUERNBERG. see *BIOLOGY*

SOUTH AFRICAN MUSEUM. ANNALS/SUID-AFRIKAANSE MUSEUM. ANNALE. see *BIOLOGY*

ARCHITECTURE

see also BUILDING AND CONSTRUCTION; ENGINEERING—Civil Engineering; HOUSING AND URBAN PLANNING; REAL ESTATE

ARCHITECTURAL PSYCHOLOGY NEWSLETTER. see *PSYCHOLOGY*

720 CHE ISSN 0379-8585
NA2542.4
ARCHITECTURE & BEHAVIOUR/ARCHITECTURE ET COMPORTEMENT. Text in English, French. 1980. q. CHF 70 to individuals; CHF 150 to institutions. adv. bk.rev. **Document type:** *Academic/Scholarly.*
Indexed: Avery Ind.Archit.Per., Geo.Abstr.H.G., IDA, Psychol.Abstr. (1980-), e-psyche.
—ingenta.
Published by: Swiss Federal Institute of Technology, Department of Architecture, Case Postale 555, Lausanne 1001, Switzerland. FAX 021-6176317. Ed. Kaj Noschis. Circ: 1,000.

363.7 DEU ISSN 0176-0513
WOHNUNG & GESUNDHEIT; Fachzeitschrift fuer oekologisches Bauen & Leben. Text in German. 1979. q. DEM 60, USD 45 (effective 2000 & 2001). adv. bk.rev. bibl. Supplement avail.; back issues avail. **Document type:** *Journal, Trade.*
Indexed: IBZ, INIS Atomind., Ref.Zh.
—CISTI.
Published by: Institut fuer Baubiologie und Oekologie, Holzham 25, Neubeuern 83115, Germany. TEL 49-8035-2039, FAX 49-8035-8164, institut@baubiologie.ibn.de. Ed. Anton Schneider. Circ: 7,500.

ART

see also ADVERTISING AND PUBLIC RELATIONS HOBBIES; MUSEUMS AND ART GALLERIES

615.85156 USA
A A T A NEWSLETTER. Text in English. q. USD 26 domestic; USD 38 foreign (effective 2000). adv. **Document type:** *Newsletter.*
Former titles: Inklinks (Mundelin); American Art Therapy Association Newsletter (1066-4076)
Published by: American Art Therapy Association, Inc., 1202 Allanson Rd., Mundelin, IL 60060. TEL 847-949-6064, FAX 847-566-4580. Ed. Deborah Mickelsen. Adv. contact Karen Savage. Circ: 5,000.

A & U; America's AIDS magazine. (Art & Understanding) see *LITERATURE*

700 620 IRL ISSN 0743-0884
AMERICAN INTERNATIONAL JOURNAL OF ARTS, SCIENCES, ENGINEERING AND MEDICINE. Text in English. 1984. q. USD 100. adv. bk.rev. **Document type:** *Academic/Scholarly.* **Description:** Aimed at providing a link between research and practice for professors, consultants and researchers in various specializations.
Published by: Royal University, Ltd., 6 Lower Hatch St., Dublin 2, Ireland. FAX 353-1-6686632. Ed. C V Ramasastry.

AMERICAN JOURNAL OF ART THERAPY; art in psychotherapy, education, and rehabilitation. see *MEDICAL SCIENCES—Physical Medicine And Rehabilitation*

ART HAZARDS NEWS. see *OCCUPATIONAL HEALTH AND SAFETY*

ART THERAPY. see *MEDICAL SCIENCES—Physical Medicine And Rehabilitation*

ARTS ACCESS NEWS. see *HANDICAPPED*

THE ARTS IN PSYCHOTHERAPY; an international journal. see *PSYCHOLOGY*

▼ **ARTS THERAPIES RESEARCH LIBRARY.** see *MEDICAL SCIENCES*

COMPOSITE ART MANUAL. see *MEDICAL SCIENCES—Forensic Sciences*

CONSTRUCTIVE CRITICISM; a journal of construct psychology and the arts. see *PSYCHOLOGY*

700 150.19 ARG
EOS; revista Argentina de arte y psicoanalisis. Text in Spanish. 1991. a.?.
Published by: Fundacion Banco Credito Argentino, 11 De Septiembre, 1990, Capital Federal, Buenos Aires 1428, Argentina. TEL 54-114-7833819.

INTERNATIONAL JOURNAL OF ARTS MEDICINE. see *MEDICAL SCIENCES*

700 616.89 JPN ISSN 0916-6688
JAPANESE BULLETIN OF ARTS THERAPY. Text in Japanese, Multiple languages. 1969. s-a. JPY 10,000 (effective 2001). adv. bk.rev. bibl, charts, illus, stat. back issues avail. *Refereed.* **Document type:** *Bulletin, Academic/Scholarly.*
Indexed: e-psyche.
Published by: Societe Japonaise de Psychopathologie de l'Expression, c/o Neuropsychiatric Research Institute, 91 Bentencho, Shin Juku-ku, Tokyo 162-0851, Japan. TEL 81-3-3260-5598, FAX 81-3-3260-5598. Ed. Dr. Makio Iimori.

KALEIDOSCOPE (AKRON); exploring the experience of disability through literature and the fine arts. see *HANDICAPPED*

701 ITA ISSN 0393-9898
RIVISTA DI PSICOLOGIA DELL'ARTE. Text in Italian. 1979. a. ITL 30,000 domestic; USD 30 foreign (effective 1999). adv. bk.rev. back issues avail. **Document type:** *Academic/Scholarly.* **Description:** Publishes experimental and theoretical studies in the field of psychology of art and empirical aesthetics.
Indexed: Artbibl.Mod., Psychol.Abstr., e-psyche.
Published by: Jartrakor, Via Dei Pianellari, 20, Rome, RM 00186, Italy. TEL 39-06-68307590, FAX 39-06-6867824, sergio.lombardo@iol.it. Ed., R&P Sergio Lombardo. Circ: 3,000.

UOMINI E IDEE. see *LITERATURE*

ARTIFICIAL INTELLIGENCE

see COMPUTERS—Artificial Intelligence

ARTS AND HANDICRAFTS

see also HOBBIES

EESTI NAINE; a magazine for women. see *WOMEN'S INTERESTS*

ASTROLOGY

see also NEW AGE PUBLICATIONS

133.5 615.89 ITA
INCANTESIMO. Text in Italian. 1992. m. adv.
Published by: Editrice Marduk, Via Samminiatese, 64, San Miniato, PI 56027, Italy. TEL 39-571-43421. Ed. Massimo Benedetti. Adv. contact Lino Ieva.

613.262 USA
VEGETARIAN ASTROLOGER. Text in English. irreg.
Address: 4216 Tod Ave, East Chicago, IN 46312. TEL 219-397-9297. Ed. Ted Pandeva.

ASTRONOMY

▼ **ASTROBIOLOGY.** see *BIOLOGY*

AUTOMATION

see COMPUTERS—Automation

AUTOMOBILES

see TRANSPORTATION—Automobiles

BAKERS AND CONFECTIONERS

see FOOD AND FOOD INDUSTRIES—Bakers And Confectioners

BALL GAMES

see SPORTS AND GAMES—Ball Games

BANKING AND FINANCE

see BUSINESS AND ECONOMICS—Banking And Finance

BEAUTY CULTURE

see also BEAUTY CULTURE—Perfumes And Cosmetics

BOOTS HEALTH & BEAUTY. see *WOMEN'S INTERESTS*

CHIMICA OGGI/CHEMISTRY TODAY. see *CHEMISTRY*

ELECTROLYSIS WORLD. see *MEDICAL SCIENCES—Dermatology And Venereology*

NATIONAL ALOPECIA AREATA FOUNDATION NEWSLETTER. see *MEDICAL SCIENCES—Dermatology And Venereology*

▼ **SHINE**; for a happier, healthier, sexier you. see *WOMEN'S HEALTH*

VIVERSANI E BELLI; settimanale di salute e belleza. see *PHYSICAL FITNESS AND HYGIENE*

606.7 658.8 GBR
THE WORLD MARKET FOR ORAL HYGIENE. Text in English. irreg., latest 1998. GBP 3,950, USD 7,900. **Document type:** *Trade.* **Description:** Provides a comprehensive and strategic review of the oral hygiene market worldwide.
Published by: Euromonitor, 60-61 Britton St, London EC1M 5UX, United Kingdom. TEL 44-20-7251-8024, info@euromonitor.com, http://www.euromonitor.com.

646.72 658.8 GBR
THE WORLD MARKET FOR SKIN CARE AND SUN CARE. Text in English. irreg., latest 1998. GBP 3,500, USD 7,000. **Document type:** *Trade.* **Description:** Provides a comprehensive and strategic review of the skin and sun care products market worldwide.
Published by: Euromonitor, 60-61 Britton St, London EC1M 5UX, United Kingdom. TEL 44-20-7251-8024, info@euromonitor.com, http://www.euromonitor.com.

646.72 USA
ZDROWIE, URODA I ZYCIE. Text in Polish. 1988. m. USD 25. adv. back issues avail. **Document type:** *Consumer.* **Description:** Provides health, fitness and beauty tips.
Published by: Back to Nature, Inc., 5627 N Milwaukee, Chicago, IL 60646. TEL 312-585-0402. Ed., Adv. contact Barbara Radlinski. Pub., R&P Marcin Hencz. page USD 325. Circ: 15,000.

ZEST; the health and beauty magazine. see *WOMEN'S INTERESTS*

BEAUTY CULTURE—Abstracting, Bibliographies, Statistics

016.66854 USA ISSN 0275-7044
CODEN: CACCD9
C A SELECTS. COSMETIC CHEMICALS. Text in English. s-w. USD 275 (effective 2001). **Document type:** *Abstract/Index.* **Description:** Covers the synthesis or manufacture of chemical substances of use in cosmetics; formulation of cosmetic preparations.
Published by: Chemical Abstracts Service (Subsidiary of: American Chemical Society), 2540 Olentangy River Rd, Box 3012, Columbus, OH 43210-0012. TEL 714-447-3600, 800-753-4227, FAX 614-447-3751.

BEAUTY CULTURE—Perfumes And Cosmetics

AERZTLICHE PRAXIS. DERMATOLOGIE. see *MEDICAL SCIENCES—Dermatology And Venereology*

668.5 USA ISSN 1098-044X
AROMA-CHOLOGY REVIEW. Text in English. 1987. biennial. USD 40 domestic; USD 50 foreign (effective 2000). **Document type:** *Newsletter.* **Description:** Reports on the latest research in olfaction.
Formerly (until 1992): Focus on Fragrance
Related titles: Online - full content ed.
Indexed: e-psyche.
Published by: Sense of Smell Institute, 145 E 32nd St, New York, NY 10016. TEL 212-725-2755, FAX 212-779-9072, www.senseofsmell.org. Ed. Annette Green.

C A SELECTS. COSMETIC CHEMICALS. see *BEAUTY CULTURE—Abstracting, Bibliographies, Statistics*

668.5 USA ISSN 1086-119X
CATEGORY REPORT - HEALTH & BEAUTY AIDS. Text in English. m. USD 1,100 (effective 2000). **Document type:** *Newsletter.* **Description:** Contains detailed product and packaging description and analysis of new foreign and domestic consumer packaged goods.
Published by: Marketing Intelligence Service Ltd., 6473D Route 64, Naples, NY 14512-9726. TEL 716-374-6326, FAX 716-374-5217, mi@productscan.com, http://www.productscan.com. Eds. Daniel Smith, Thomas Vierhile. Pub., R&P Daniel Smith.

668.5 USA ISSN 1086-1203
CATEGORY REPORT - HOUSEHOLD, PET & MISCELLANEOUS PRODUCTS. Text in English. m. USD 1,100 (effective 2000). back issues avail. **Document type:** *Newsletter.* **Description:** Contains detailed product and packaging description and analysis of new foreign and domestic consumer packaged goods.
Published by: Marketing Intelligence Service Ltd., 6473D Route 64, Naples, NY 14512-9726. TEL 716-374-6326, FAX 716-374-5217, mi@productscan.com, http://www.productscan.com. Eds. Daniel Smith, Thomas Vierhile. Pub., R&P Daniel Smith.

COSMETIC SCIENCE AND TECHNOLOGY SERIES. see *MEDICAL SCIENCES*

668.55 GBR
COSMETIC SCIENCE MONOGRAPHS. Text in English. 1997. irreg., latest vol.2, 1998. **Document type:** *Monographic series.*
—BLDSC (3477.175770).
Published by: Micelle Press, 10-12 Ullswater Cres., Weymouth, Dorset DT3 5HE, United Kingdom. TEL 44-1305-781574, http://www.wdi.co.uk. **Dist. in US and Canada by:** Scholuim International Inc., 14 Vanderventer Ave, PO Box 1519, Port Washington, NY 11050-0306. TEL 516-767-7171.

D C A T DIGEST. see *PHARMACY AND PHARMACOLOGY*

D W: DROGISTEN WEEKBLAD; onafhankelijk vakblad voor drogisterij, parfumerie, reformzaak. see *PHARMACY AND PHARMACOLOGY*

DERMATOLOGIE PRATIQUE. see *MEDICAL SCIENCES—Dermatology And Venereology*

FARMACIA DISTRIBUICAO. see *PHARMACY AND PHARMACOLOGY*

FOOD, DRUG, COSMETIC, AND MEDICAL DEVICE LAW DIGEST. see *LAW*

668.55 USA ISSN 1523-9470
RS1 CODEN: DCINAQ
GLOBAL COSMETIC INDUSTRY. Text in English. 1914. 13/yr., latest vol.166. USD 43 United States & Possessions; USD 59 in Canada & Mexico; USD 99 elsewhere; USD 5 newsstand/cover United States & Possessions (effective 2001). adv. bk.rev. abstr, illus, mkt, pat, tr.mk. index. reprints avail. **Document type:** *Magazine, Trade.* **Description:** Formulation, raw material procurement, production and packaging for marketers and manufacturers of cosmetics, personal products and OTC pharmaceuticals.
Former titles (until 1999): D C I (1096-4819); Drug and Cosmetic Industry (0012-6527); Which incorporated (1931-1997): Drug and Cosmetic Catalog (0732-0760)
Related titles: Microform ed.: (from PMC,PQC); Online - full text ed.: (from The Dialog Corporation, Gale Group, ProQuest Information & Learning, Northern Light Technology, Inc., H. W. Wilson, Factiva).
Indexed: ABI Inform. (Jan.1991-), Agri.& Environ.Biotech.Abstr. (coverage dropped), B.P.I. (Jan.1999-), Biol.Abstr., Bus.& Indus. (Jan.1994-), Bus.Ind., CBNB (1989-), Cadscan, Chem.Abstr., Chem.Indus.Notes, Chem.Titles, Curr.Cont. (coverage dropped), Curr.Pack.Abstr., Environ.Sci.Poll.Mgmt., Hlth.Ind., INIS Atomind., I.P.A., Int.Packag.Abstr., Lead Abstr., PROMT, Pollut.Abstr., Ref.Zh., Risk Abstr., Saf.Sci.Abstr., Tox.Abstr., Tr.& Indus.Ind., Zincscan.
—BLDSC (4195.384850), CASDDS, CISTI, GNLM, Infotrieve, ingenta, Linda Hall. **CCC.**
Published by: Advanstar Communications Inc., One Park Ave 2nd Fl, New York, NY 10016. TEL 440-243-8102, FAX 212-951-6623, http://www.cosmeticindex.com; http://www.globalcosmetic.com. Ed. Joyceann Conney-Curran. Pub. Glen Stout. Circ: 14,145.

668.5 GBR ISSN 0142-5463
TP983 CODEN: IJCMDW
INTERNATIONAL JOURNAL OF COSMETIC SCIENCE. Text in English, French. bi-m., latest vol.6, 2002. GBP 481 in Europe; USD 764 in North America; GBP 530 elsewhere (effective 2002). adv. back issues avail.; reprint service avail. from ISI. *Refereed.* **Document type:** *Academic/Scholarly.* **Description:** Provides a current presentation of pure and applied scientific research in cosmetics, toiletries, perfumery, and allied fields.
Related titles: Online - full text ed.: ISSN 1468-2494. GBP 433 in Europe; USD 688 in North America; GBP 433 elsewhere (effective 2002) (from EBSCO Publishing, O C L C Online Computer Library Center, Inc., RoweCom Information Quest, ingenta, Munksgaard & Blackwell Science's Synergy, Swets Blackwell).
Indexed: ASCA, Agri.& Environ.Biotech.Abstr. (coverage dropped), Biol.Abstr., C.I.S. Abstr., Chem.Abstr., Chem.Indus.Notes, Chem.Titles, Curr.Adv.Ecol.Sci., Curr.Cont. (coverage dropped), Derwent Biotech.Abstr., Eng.Ind., Environ.Sci.Poll.Mgmt., Excerp.Med., I.P.A., Ind.Med. (coverage dropped), Ind.Sci.Rev., Pollut.Abstr., Risk Abstr., Saf.Sci.Abstr., Sci.Cit.Ind. (coverage dropped).
—BLDSC (4542.178400), ADONIS, CASDDS, CISTI, Ei, GNLM, Infotrieve. **CCC.**
Published by: (Society of Cosmetic Chemists NLD, Societe Francaise de Cosmetologie FRA), Blackwell Science Ltd., PO Box 88, Oxford OX2 0NE, United Kingdom. TEL 44-1865-206180, 44-1865-206002, FAX 44-1865-206219, journals.cs@blacksci.co.uk, jnl.orders@blacksci.co.uk, http://www.blackwell-science.com/ics, http://www.blackwellpublishing.com. Eds. D Saint-Leger, D Williams. Pub. Elaine Stott. R&P Lindsay Doyle. Adv. contact Martine Cariou Keen. Circ: 2,750.

INTERNATIONAL PHARMACEUTICAL REGULATORY MONITOR; a legal, medical & scientific information series for the pharmaceutical and biotech industry. see *PHARMACY AND PHARMACOLOGY*

668.5 USA ISSN 0740-3852
LOOKOUT - NONFOODS. Text in English. 1978. s-m. USD 700 (effective 2000). **Document type:** *Newsletter.* **Description:** Reviews the most innovative and influential new product entries, complete with analyses and illustrations.
Supersedes in part: Lookout (Naples)
Related titles: Online - full text ed.: (from Gale Group, Factiva).
Indexed: Bus.& Indus. (Jan.1994-).
—CCC.
Published by: Marketing Intelligence Service Ltd., 6473D Route 64, Naples, NY 14512-9726. TEL 716-374-6326, FAX 716-374-5217, mi@productscan.com, http://www.productscan.com. Eds. Daniel Smith, Thomas Vierhile. Pub., R&P Daniel Smith.

NIEUWE DROGIST. see *PHARMACY AND PHARMACOLOGY*

668.55 ZAF ISSN 1015-4760
CODEN: PCRVDQ
PHARMACEUTICAL & COSMETIC REVIEW; devoted to the manufacture & marketing of medicines, toiletries, soaps, detergents in South Africa. Text in English. 1974. bi-m. ZAR 191.84 (effective 1999). adv. illus. **Document type:** *Trade.* **Description:** Reports on new equipment, ingredients, processes, packaging materials, legislative and marketing trends and overseas developments for manufacturers, packers and distributors of pharmaceutical, cosmetic and related products.
Formerly: South African Pharmaceutical and Cosmetic Review (0257-2028)
Indexed: INIS Atomind., I.P.A., Ind.S.A.Per.
—BLDSC (6442.750000).
Published by: National Publishing (Pty) Ltd., PO Box 2271, Clareinch 7740, South Africa. TEL 27-21-611140, FAX 27-21-611389, accirc@natpub.co.za. Ed. Lindy Hughson. Circ: 2,000. **Co-sponsors:** Aerosol Manufacturers' Association; Society of Cosmetic Chemists; South African Association of Industrial Flavor and Fragrance Manufacturers.

PHARMACEUTICAL FORMULATION & QUALITY BUYERS' GUIDE. see *PHARMACY AND PHARMACOLOGY*

PRODUCT ALERT. see *FOOD AND FOOD INDUSTRIES*

SKIN INC.; business and science for skin care professionals. see *MEDICAL SCIENCES—Dermatology And Venereology*

SO YOUNG!; dedicated to a youthful body, mind and spirit. see *PHYSICAL FITNESS AND HYGIENE*

668.5 USA ISSN 0279-1110
TOILETRIES, FRAGRANCES AND SKIN CARE: THE ROSE SHEET. Text in English. 1980. w. USD 775 domestic; USD 900 foreign (effective 2001). back issues avail.; reprints avail. **Document type:** *Newsletter, Trade.* **Description:** Provides executives in the toiletries, fragrances, skin care and related industries with specialized regulatory, legislative, scientific, financial and legal news.
Related titles: Online - full text ed.: (from Data-Star, The Dialog Corporation).
Indexed: P.N.I.
—Infotrieve. **CCC.**
Published by: F-D-C Reports, Inc., 5550 Friendship Blvd, Ste One, Chevy Chase, MD 20815-7278. TEL 800-332-2181, FAX 301-664-7238, http://www.fdcreports.com. Ed. Kate Rawson. R&P Michael Keville.

646.72 CHN
ZHONGHUA YIXUE MEIRONG ZAZHI/CHINESE JOURNAL OF MEDICAL AETHETICS AND COSMETOLOGY. Text in Chinese. bi-m. USD 17.40; USD 2.90 newsstand/cover (effective 2001). **Document type:** *Academic/Scholarly.*
Published by: Zhonghua Yixuehui Zazhishe, 42 Dongsi Xidajie, Beijing 100710, China. **Dist. by:** China International Book Trading Corp, 35, Chegongzhuang Xilu, Haidian District, Beijing 100044, China. TEL 86-1-68413849, FAX 86-1-68412048, cibtc@mail.cibtc.com.cn, http://www.cibtc.com.cn.

BEVERAGES

see also FOOD AND FOOD INDUSTRIES; PACKAGING

663 616.861 USA ISSN 1067-3105
ALCOHOL ISSUES INSIGHTS. Text in English. 1983. m. USD 270 (effective 1999). back issues avail. **Document type:** *Newsletter.* **Description:** Covers alcohol policy issues, including excise tax, drunk driving laws, advertising and availability restrictions, and alcohol and health.
Published by: Beer Marketer's Insights, Inc., PO Box 264, West Nyack, NY 10994. TEL 845-624-2337. Ed. Eric Shepard. R&P Jim Sullivan.

PODRAVKA; znanstveno-strucni casopis. see *AGRICULTURE*

PRODUCT ALERT. see *FOOD AND FOOD INDUSTRIES*

BIBLIOGRAPHIES

see also ABSTRACTING AND INDEXING SERVICES; LIBRARY AND INFORMATION SCIENCES; PUBLISHING AND BOOK TRADE; and also Abstracting, Bibliographies, Statistics subheadings under specific subjects

50 TITRES SUR... see *POPULATION STUDIES—Abstracting, Bibliographies, Statistics*

AEROSPACE MEDICINE AND BIOLOGY; a continuing bibliography. see *MEDICAL SCIENCES—Abstracting, Bibliographies, Statistics*

AIDS LEGAL BIBLIOGRAPHY. (Acquired Immune Deficiency Syndrome) see *LAW—Abstracting, Bibliographies, Statistics*

ASSOCIATION FOR GERONTOLOGY IN HIGHER EDUCATION. BRIEF BIBLIOGRAPHY. see *GERONTOLOGY AND GERIATRICS—Abstracting, Bibliographies, Statistics*

BIBLIOGRAFIA BRASILEIRA DE ODONTOLOGIA. see *MEDICAL SCIENCES—Abstracting, Bibliographies, Statistics*

BIBLIOGRAFIA DO IDOSO. see *GERONTOLOGY AND GERIATRICS—Abstracting, Bibliographies, Statistics*

BIBLIOGRAFIJA JUGOSLAVIJE. CLANCI I PRILOZI U SERIJSKIM PUBLIKACIJAMA. SERIJA B: PRIRODNE, PRIMENJENE, MEDICINSKE I TEHNICKE NAUKE. see *SCIENCES: COMPREHENSIVE WORKS—Abstracting, Bibliographies, Statistics*

BIBLIOGRAPHIA MEDICA CECHOSLOVACA. see *MEDICAL SCIENCES—Abstracting, Bibliographies, Statistics*

BIBLIOGRAPHIC GUIDE TO PSYCHOLOGY. see *PSYCHOLOGY—Abstracting, Bibliographies, Statistics*

BIBLIOGRAPHIE PSYCHOLOGISCHER LITERATUR AUS DEN DEUTSCHSPRACHIGEN LAENDERN. see *PSYCHOLOGY—Abstracting, Bibliographies, Statistics*

BIBLIOGRAPHY OF THE HISTORY OF MEDICINE. see *MEDICAL SCIENCES—Abstracting, Bibliographies, Statistics*

BIBLIOGRAPHY ON COLD REGIONS SCIENCE & TECHNOLOGY. see *ENGINEERING—Abstracting, Bibliographies, Statistics*

011 USA ISSN 0951-838X
Z7164.C81 CODEN: BPONER
BOOKS & PERIODICALS ONLINE. Text in English. 1987. a. USD 379 (effective 2001). **Document type:** *Directory, Bibliography.* **Description:** Lists 97,000 newspapers, periodicals, wire services, newsletters and reference works available online.

Incorporates (1985-1991): Directory of Periodicals Online - Law and Business (0884-089X); (1989-1994): Directory of Periodicals Online - Science and Technology (0884-0911); (in 1991): Directory of Periodicals Online - Medical and Humanities
Published by: Library Technology Alliance, Ltd., 264 Lexington Ave 4FL, PO Box 77232, New York, NY 10016-4182. TEL 212-686-8816, LTA@bellatlantic.net, http://www.periodicals.net. Ed., Pub., R&P Nuchine Nobari. Circ: 1,050.

BRITISH INSTITUTE OF LEARNING DISABILITIES. CURRENT AWARENESS SERVICE. see *EDUCATION—Abstracting, Bibliographies, Statistics*

CAB INTERNATIONAL. BUREAU OF NUTRITION. ANNOTATED BIBLIOGRAPHIES. see *NUTRITION AND DIETETICS—Abstracting, Bibliographies, Statistics*

CATALOG OF CAPTIONED FILMS FOR THE DEAF. see *MOTION PICTURES—Abstracting, Bibliographies, Statistics*

011 USA
CHICOREL INDEX SERIES. Text in English. 1970. irreg., latest vol.26, 1986. USD 125 per vol. (effective 2000). bk.rev. **Document type:** *Directory, Abstract/Index.* **Description:** Comprises series of subject guides to various fields in the humanities and social sciences, such as indexes to plays, poetry and short stories in anthologies, on audio and video. Abstracting services for reading and learning disabilities, and the mental health fields.
Related titles: Microform ed.: (from PQC).
Published by: American Library Publishing Co., PO Box 4272, Sedona, AZ 86340-4272. TEL 520-282-4922. Ed., R&P Marietta S Chicorel.

COLEGIO OFICIAL DE PSICOLOGOS DE MADRID. DOCUMENTACION PSICOLOGICA. see *PSYCHOLOGY—Abstracting, Bibliographies, Statistics*

THE COMPLETE DIRECTORY OF LARGE PRINT BOOKS AND SERIALS. see *HANDICAPPED—Abstracting, Bibliographies, Statistics*

CURRENT BIBLIOGRAPHY ON SCIENCE AND TECHNOLOGY: LIFE SCIENCES/KAGAKU GIJUTSU BUNKEN SOKUHO. RAIFUSAIENSU HEN. see *BIOLOGY—Abstracting, Bibliographies, Statistics*

CURRENT WORK IN THE HISTORY OF MEDICINE; an international bibliography. see *MEDICAL SCIENCES—Abstracting, Bibliographies, Statistics*

ERGA. see *OCCUPATIONAL HEALTH AND SAFETY—Abstracting, Bibliographies, Statistics*

FACHBUCHVERZEICHNIS MEDIZIN. see *MEDICAL SCIENCES—Abstracting, Bibliographies, Statistics*

016 614 FRA ISSN 0992-8235
FRANCE. MINISTERE DE LA SOLIDARITE, DE LA SANTE ET DE LA PROTECTION SOCIALE. BULLETIN OFFICIEL. Text in French. 1957. w. FRF 396. bk.rev.
Former titles: France. Ministere des Affaires Sociales et Solidarite National. Bulletin Officiel; France. Ministere de la Sante et de la Famille. Bulletin Officiel; France. Ministere de la Sante et de la Securite Sociale. Bulletin Officiel
Published by: Ministere des Affaires Sociales et de la Solidarite Nationale, Service de l'Information et de la Communication, 1 place de Fontenoy, Paris 75700, France. TEL 33-1-40566000. Circ: 13,500. **Subscr. to:** Journaux Officiels, 26 rue Desaix, Paris 75015, France. **Co-sponsor:** France. Ministere du Travail et de la Participation.

HEALTH INDUSTRY QUICKSOURCE; a complete descriptive reference to healthcare information resources. see *MEDICAL SCIENCES—Abstracting, Bibliographies, Statistics*

L I L A C S - CD-ROM. (Literatura Latinoamericana y del Caribe en Ciencias de la Salud) see *MEDICAL SCIENCES—Abstracting, Bibliographies, Statistics*

LETTERA; percorsi bibliografici in psichiatria. see *PSYCHOLOGY—Abstracting, Bibliographies, Statistics*

LIFE SCIENCE BOOK REVIEW. see *BIOLOGY—Abstracting, Bibliographies, Statistics*

MAGAZINES IN SPECIAL MEDIA. see *HANDICAPPED—Abstracting, Bibliographies, Statistics*

MEDICAL AND HEALTH CARE BOOKS AND SERIALS IN PRINT; an index to literature in health sciences. see *MEDICAL SCIENCES—Abstracting, Bibliographies, Statistics*

NEW LITERATURE ON OLD AGE. see *GERONTOLOGY AND GERIATRICS—Abstracting, Bibliographies, Statistics*

NEW LITERATURE ON VISUAL IMPAIRMENT. see *HANDICAPPED—Abstracting, Bibliographies, Statistics*

NOVINKY LITERATURY. ZDRAVOTNICTVI-PRIRUSTKY FONDU NARODNI LEKARSKE KNIHOVNY. see *MEDICAL SCIENCES—Abstracting, Bibliographies, Statistics*

ONLINE JOURNAL OF CLINICAL INNOVATIONS. see *MEDICAL SCIENCES—Nurses And Nursing*

610 016 MEX ISSN 0304-1840
REMEDIA. Variant title: Referencias Medicas de Informacion Actualizada. Text in Spanish. 1974. bi-m.
Published by: Instituto Mexicano del Seguro Social, Division de Bibliotecas y Documentacion Biomedica, Apdo. Postal 12976, Mexico City, DF 03001, Mexico. Circ: 2,000.

REPERTOIRE INTERNATIONAL DES BANQUES DE DONNEES BIOMEDICALES. see *MEDICAL SCIENCES—Computer Applications*

011 300 600 USA ISSN 0196-6006
SCITECH BOOK NEWS; an annotated bibliography of new books in science, technology, & medicine. Text in English. 1977. q. USD 130 domestic to individuals; USD 180 foreign to individuals; USD 175 domestic to institutions; USD 225 foreign to institutions (effective 2001). adv. bk.rev. abstr, bibl. back issues avail. **Document type:** *Bibliography.* **Description:** Presents concise reviews of newhigh-level books in science, technology, medicine, agriculture and engineering. Over 1,500 reviews in each issue.
Related titles: Online - full text ed.: (from Institute for Scientific Information).
Indexed: Bk.Rev.Ind. (1984-), Child.Bk.Rev.Ind. (1984-). —Linda Hall.
Published by: Book News, Inc. (Portland), 5739 N E Sumner St, Portland, OR 97218. TEL 503-281-9230, FAX 503-287-4485, http://www.booknews.com. Ed., Adv. contact Jane Erskine. Circ: 2,400.

SELECTED BIBLIOGRAPHIES ON AGEING. see *GERONTOLOGY AND GERIATRICS—Abstracting, Bibliographies, Statistics*

TOKYO SHIKA DAIGAKU SEIRIGAKU KYOSHITSU GYOSEKISHU/TOKYO DENTAL COLLEGE. DEPARTMENT OF PHYSIOLOGY. BIBLIOGRAPHY. see *BIOLOGY—Abstracting, Bibliographies, Statistics*

UTANO - ZIMBABWE; an annotated health information bibliography. see *MEDICAL SCIENCES—Abstracting, Bibliographies, Statistics*

WELLCOME UNIT FOR THE HISTORY OF MEDICINE. RESEARCH PUBLICATIONS. see *MEDICAL SCIENCES*

ZEITSCHRIFTENBIBLIOGRAPHIE GERONTOLOGIE. see *GERONTOLOGY AND GERIATRICS—Abstracting, Bibliographies, Statistics*

BICYCLES AND MOTORCYCLES

see SPORTS AND GAMES—Bicycles And Motorcycles

BIOENGINEERING

see BIOLOGY—Bioengineering

BIOGRAPHY

A B M S MEDICAL SPECIALIST PLUS. see *MEDICAL SCIENCES*

150 920 USA ISSN 0196-6545
BF11
AMERICAN PSYCHOLOGICAL ASSOCIATION. DIRECTORY. Text in English. 1916. quadrennial. USD 70 to non-members; USD 50 to members (effective 1999). adv. **Document type:** *Directory.*
Formerly: American Psychological Association. Biographical Directory (0090-9076)
Published by: American Psychological Association, 211 E 70th St, New York, NY 10021. TEL 202-336-5500, FAX 202-336-5633. Eds. Ed Diener, Mitch Finegold. Circ: 4,000.

CHI E CHI SANITA E SALUTE. see *PHARMACY AND PHARMACOLOGY*

CHIROPRACTIC HISTORY. see *MEDICAL SCIENCES—Chiropractic, Homeopathy, Osteopathy*

920 610 GBR ISSN 0967-7720
R134
JOURNAL OF MEDICAL BIOGRAPHY. Text in English. 1993. q. GBP 54 in Europe to individuals; USD 98 in United States to individuals; GBP 58 elsewhere to individuals; GBP 91 in Europe to institutions; USD 155 in United States to institutions; GBP 95 elsewhere to institutions (effective 2002). *Refereed.* **Document type:** *Journal, Academic/Scholarly.* **Description:** Aimed at a wide audience among both the medical and non-medical community, including clinicians, scientists, historians, archivists, librarians, and others with an interest in biographical aspects of medical history. It focuses on the lives of those in and associated with medicine and their significance in various contexts.
Indexed: Amer.Hist.& Life, Hist.Abstr. (1993-), Ind.Med. —BLDSC (5017.049000), GNLM, Infotrieve. **CCC.**
Published by: Royal Society of Medicine Press Ltd, 1 Wimpole St, London W1M 8AE, United Kingdom. TEL 44-20-7290-2921, FAX 44-20-7290-2929, rsmjournals@rsm.ac.uk, http://www.roysocmed.ac.uk/pub/jmb.htm. Ed. J M H Moll. R&P Caroline McLaughlin.

OFFICIAL A B M S DIRECTORY OF BOARD CERTIFIED MEDICAL SPECIALISTS. see *MEDICAL SCIENCES*

920 362.4 USA
RESOURCE DIRECTORY OF SCIENTISTS AND ENGINEERS WITH DISABILITIES. Text in English. 1982. irreg., latest vol.3, 1995. USD 20. **Description:** Source of role models for disabled youth and mid-career scientists and engineers. Lists 950 scientists and engineers with an address, phone number, discipline and degree(s), position, nature of and age of disability.
Published by: American Association for the Advancement of Science, Project on Science, Technology and Disability, 1200 New York Ave, N W, Washington, DC 20005. TEL 202-326-6649, FAX 202-371-9849, 1summers@aaas.org. Eds. Laureen Summers, Virginia W Stern.

SLOWNIK BIOGRAFICZNY POLSKICH NAUK MEDYCZNYCH XXX WIEKU. see *MEDICAL SCIENCES*

WHO'S WHO IN AMERICAN NURSING. see *MEDICAL SCIENCES—Nurses And Nursing*

WHO'S WHO IN MEDICINE AND HEALTHCARE. see *MEDICAL SCIENCES*

BIOCHEMISTRY

see BIOLOGY—Biochemistry

BABRAHAM INSTITUTE. CORPORATE PLAN. see *BIOLOGY—Physiology*

BABRAHAM INSTITUTE. REPORT. see *BIOLOGY—Physiology*

CELLULAR & MOLECULAR BIOLOGY LETTERS; an international journal. see *BIOLOGY*

BIOLOGY

see also BIOLOGY—Biochemistry; BIOLOGY—Bioengineering; BIOLOGY—Biophysics; BIOLOGY—Biotechnology; BIOLOGY—Botany; BIOLOGY—Computer Applications; BIOLOGY—Cytology And Histology; BIOLOGY—Entomology; BIOLOGY—Genetics; BIOLOGY—Microbiology; BIOLOGY—Microscopy; BIOLOGY—Ornithology; BIOLOGY—Physiology; BIOLOGY—Zoology; MEDICAL SCIENCES; PHARMACY AND PHARMACOLOGY

B

571.9 610 DNK ISSN 0903-4641
CODEN: APMSEL

A P M I S. (Acta Pathologica Microbiologica et Immunologica Scandinavica) Text and summaries in English. 1926. m. GBP 335 combined subscription print & online eds. combined (effective 2002). bk.rev. Supplement avail.; reprint service avail. from ISI. *Refereed.* **Document type:** *Journal, Academic/Scholarly.*

Formed by the 1988 merger of: Acta Pathologica, Microbiologica et Immunologica Scandinavica. Section A. Pathology (0108-0164); Which was formerly (1970-1982): Acta Pathologica et Microbiologica Scandinavica. Section A. Pathology (0365-4184); Acta Pathologica, Microbiologica et Immunologica Scandinavic. Section B. Microbiology (0108-0180); Which was formerly (1975-1982): Acta Pathologica et Microbiologica Scandinavica. Section B. Microbiology (0304-131X); Acta Pathologica, Microbiologica et Immunologica Scandinavic. Section C. Immunology (0108-0202); Which was formerly (1975-1982): Acta Pathologica et Microbiologica Scandinavica. Section C. Immunology (0304-1328); Section B & C superseded in part (1970-1975): Acta Pathologica et Microbiologica Scandinavica. Section B. Microbiology and Immunology (0365-5563); Section A & B superseded in part (1924-1970): Acta Pathologica et Microbiologica Scandinavica (0365-5555)

Related titles: Online - full text ed.: ISSN 1600-0463. GBP 300 (effective 2002) (from Ovid Technologies, Inc., ingenta, Swets Blackwell, Institute for Scientific Information).

Indexed: ASCA, Abstr.Hyg., AgBiotech, Agri.& Environ.Biotech.Abstr. (coverage dropped), Biol.Abstr., Chem.Abstr., Curr.Adv.Ecol.Sci., Curr.Adv.Gen.& Molec.Biol., Curr.Cont., Dairy Sci.Abstr., Dent.Ind., Derwent Biotech.Abstr., Environ.Sci.Poll.Mgmt., Excerp.Med., Helminthol.Abstr., INIS Atomind., Ind.Med. (1988-), Ind.Sci.Rev., Ind.Vet., Inpharma, Int.Abstr.Biol.Sci., Med.& Surg.Dermat., Microbiol.Abstr., NRN, Nutr.Abstr., Pig News & Info., Protozool.Abstr., Reac., Rev.Appl.Entomol., Rev.Arom.& Med.Plants, Rev.Med.& Vet.Mycol., Rev.Plant Path., Sci.Cit.Ind., Small Anim.Abstr., Trop.Dis.Bull., Vet.Bull., Wild.Rev.

—BLDSC (1568.740000), ADONIS, CASDDS, CISTI, GNLM, IDS, ingenta, KNAW. **CCC.**

Published by: Blackwell Munksgaard, Noerre Soegade 35, PO Box 2148, Copenhagen K 1016, Denmark. TEL 45-77-33-33-33, FAX 45-77-33-33-77, customerservice@munksgaard.dk, http://www.munksgaard.dk/apmis. Ed. Joergen Rygaard. Adv. contact Eric Rozario TEL 45-77-33-33-01. Circ: 800.

610 576 DNK ISSN 0903-465X
R81 CODEN: AISSE2

A P M I S SUPPLEMENTUM. Text in Danish. 1926. irreg. Free to subscribers of APMIS. reprint service avail. from ISI. **Document type:** *Academic/Scholarly.*

Formed by the 1988 merger of: Acta Pathologica, Microbiologica et Immunologica Scandinavica. Section A. Supplement (0108-0172); Which was formerly (until 1982): Acta Pathologica et Microbiologica Scandinavica. Section A. Supplement (0365-5571); Acta Pathologica, Microbiologica et Immunologica Scandinavica. Section C. Supplement (0108-0210); Which was formerly (until 1981): Acta Pathologica et Microbiologica Scandinavica. Section C. Supplement (0105-8703); Superseded in part (in 1970): Acta Pathologica et Microbiologica Scandinavica. Supplementum (0065-1486)

Related titles: Microfilm ed.: (from PMC); Online - full text ed.: ISSN 1600-5503 (from Ovid Technologies, Inc.).

Indexed: Biol.Abstr., Chem.Abstr., Curr.Cont. (coverage dropped), Dent.Ind., Helminthol.Abstr., INIS Atomind., Ind.Med. (1988-), Ind.Sci.Rev., Int.Abstr.Biol.Sci., Trop.Dis.Bull.

—BLDSC (1568.750000), ADONIS, CASDDS, CISTI, EMDOCS, ingenta, KNAW. **CCC.**

Published by: Blackwell Munksgaard, Noerre Soegade 35, PO Box 2148, Copenhagen K 1016, Denmark. TEL 45-77-33-33-33, FAX 45-77-33-33-77, customerservice@munksgaard.dk, http://www.munksgaard.dk/apmis. Ed. Joergen Rygaard. Adv. contact Eric Rozario TEL 45-77-33-33-01.

570 USA ISSN 0001-2386

A S B BULLETIN. Text in English. 1953. q. USD 20 (effective 2000). bk.rev. abstr, charts, illus, stat. reprint service avail. from PQC. **Document type:** *Bulletin, Academic/Scholarly.*

Related titles: Microform ed.: (from PQC).

Indexed: Biol.Abstr., Deep Sea Res.& Oceanogr.Abstr., Sport Fish.Abstr., Zoo.Rec.

—CISTI, Linda Hall.

Published by: Association of Southeastern Biologists, Inc., University of Tennessee, Department of Botony, Knoxville, TN 37996-1100. TEL 865-974-6219, FAX 865-974-2258, jcaponet@utk.edu, http://www.asb.appstate.edu/. Ed. James D Caponetti. Circ: 1,300.

570.752 USA

A T C C PRESERVATION METHODS: FREEZING & FREEZE-DRYING. Text in English. 1991. irreg. USD 45; USD 50 foreign.

Published by: American Type Culture Collection, 10801 University Blvd, Manassas, VA 20110. TEL 800-638-6597, FAX 301-816-4361. Eds. E M Brown, F P Simione.

ACADEMIE SERBE DES SCIENCES ET DES ARTS. CLASSE DES SCIENCES MATHEMATIQUES ET NATURELLES. BULLETIN SCIENCES NATURELLES. see *SCIENCES: COMPREHENSIVE WORKS*

571.3 JPN ISSN 0022-7722
CODEN: KAIZAN

ACTA ANATOMICA NIPPONICA/KAIBOGAKU ZASSHI. Text in English, Japanese; Summaries in English, German. 1893. bi-m. JPY 15,000. adv. bk.rev. abstr, bibl. index. **Document type:** *Academic/Scholarly.*

Indexed: Biol.Abstr., Chem.Abstr., Dent.Ind., Excerp.Med., INIS Atomind., Ind.Med. (1928-), Ind.Vet., Sport Fish.Abstr., Vet.Bull., Zoo.Rec.

—BLDSC (0595.200000), CISTI, GNLM, Infotrieve. **CCC.**

Published by: (Japanese Association of Anatomists), Business Center for Academic Societies Japan/Nihon Gakkai Jimu Senta, 5-16-9 Honkomagome, Bunkyo-ku, Tokyo 113-0021, Japan. TEL 81-3-5814-5811, FAX 81-3-5814-5822. Circ: 1,950.

570 HRV ISSN 0448-0147
QH178.Y8 CODEN: ACBLDN

ACTA BIOLOGICA. Text and summaries in Croatian, English, French, German, Russian. 1913. biennial. USD 10. back issues avail. **Document type:** *Academic/Scholarly.*

Indexed: Biol.Abstr., Zoo.Rec.

—KNAW, Linda Hall.

Published by: Hrvatska Akademija Znanosti i Umjetnosti/Croatian Academy of Sciences and Arts, Zrinski trg 11, Zagreb 41000, Croatia. TEL 385-1-4819982, FAX 385-1-4819979. Ed. Zvonimir Devide. Circ: 800.

615.532 DEU ISSN 0722-4192

ACTA BIOLOGICA; Zeitschrift fuer angewandte Homoeo-Phytotherapie, Ganzheitsbehandlungen und Sondermethoden der Medizin. Text in German. 1962. s-a. **Document type:** *Academic/Scholarly.*

—GNLM.

Published by: Pascoe Pharmazeutische Praeparate GmbH, Schiffenberger Weg 55, Giessen 35394, Germany. TEL 0641-7960-0, FAX 0641-77333. Circ: 7,500.

570 HUN ISSN 0567-7327
CODEN: ABIDAO

ACTA BIOLOGICA DEBRECINA✱. Text in English, German, Hungarian, Russian. 1962. irreg. bibl, illus. **Document type:** *Academic/Scholarly.*

Indexed: Biol.Abstr., Chem.Abstr., GeoRef.

—CASDDS, Linda Hall.

Published by: Kossuth Lajos Tudomanyegyetem, Novenytani Tanszek, PF 37, Debrecen 4010, Hungary. Circ: 450.

570 610 POL ISSN 0065-1087
QH301 CODEN: ACBMAN

ACTA BIOLOGICA ET MEDICA. Text in Polish. 1957. irreg.

Indexed: AgroLibrex.

—CISTI, GNLM.

Published by: Gdanskie Towarzystwo Naukowe/Gdansk Scientific Society, Ul Grodzka 12, Gdansk 80-841, Poland. TEL 48-58-312124, FAX 48-58-312124.

570 YUG ISSN 0514-6658
S590 CODEN: ZMBLAP

ACTA BIOLOGICA IUGOSLAVICA. SERIJA A: ZEMLJISTE I BILJKA✱. Text in Serbo-Croatian. 1952. 3/yr. USD 78. **Document type:** *Academic/Scholarly.*

Indexed: Field Crop Abstr., Herb.Abstr., Plant Grow.Reg.Abstr., Soils & Fert.

—CASDDS, CISTI.

Published by: Unija Bioloskih Naucnih Drustava Jugoslavije/Yugoslav Union of Biological Sciences, Kneza Milosa 101-111, Belgrade 11000, Yugoslavia. TEL 381-11-615315, pedja@bf.bio.bf.ac.yu. Ed. Dr. Vitko Soric.

570 615 YUG ISSN 0021-3225
QP509 CODEN: IPPABX

ACTA BIOLOGICA IUGOSLAVICA. SERIJA C: IUGOSLAVICA PHYSIOLOGICA ET PHARMACOLOGICA ACTA✱. Key Title: Iugoslavica Physiologica et Pharmacologica Acta. Text in English; Summaries in Serbo-Croatian. 1965. 3/yr. price varies. index. **Document type:** *Academic/Scholarly.*

Indexed: Biol.Abstr., Chem.Abstr., Chem.Indus.Notes, Chem.Titles, Curr.Cont. (coverage dropped), Dairy Sci.Abstr., Excerp.Med., INIS Atomind., Ind.Sci.Rev., Sci.Cit.Ind. (coverage dropped).

—CASDDS, CISTI, GNLM, Linda Hall.

Published by: Unija Bioloskih Naucnih Drustava Jugoslavije/Yugoslav Union of Biological Sciences, Kneza Milosa 101-111, Belgrade 11000, Yugoslavia. TEL 381-11-615315, pedja@bf.bio.bg.ac.yu. Ed. Dr. Vitko Soric. Circ: 1,000.

577 YUG ISSN 0531-9110

ACTA BIOLOGICA IUGOSLAVICA. SERIJA D: EKOLOGIJA✱. Key Title: Ekologija. Text in Serbo-Croatian. 1966. s-a. price varies. **Document type:** *Academic/Scholarly.* **Description:** Focuses on ecological issues.

—Linda Hall.

Published by: Unija Bioloskih Naucnih Drustava Jugoslavije/Yugoslav Union of Biological Sciences, Kneza Milosa 101-111, Belgrade 11000, Yugoslavia. TEL 381-11-615315, pedja@bf.bio.bg.ac.yu, pedja@bf.bio.bf.ac.yu. Ed. Dr. Vitko Soric.

570 BRA ISSN 0101-5354
QH301 CODEN: ABLEEC

ACTA BIOLOGICA LEOPOLDENSIA. Text in Portuguese. 1979. s-a. USD 24; or exchange basis. bibl, charts, illus. **Document type:** *Academic/Scholarly.*

Indexed: Zoo.Rec.

—CISTI.

Published by: (Universidade do Vale do Rio dos Sinos), Unisinos, Av Unisinos, 950, Sao Leopoldo, RS 93022-000, Brazil. TEL 55-51-590-8239, ext. 1951, FAX 55-51-592-8238. Ed. Elena Diehl.

570 VEN ISSN 0001-5326
QH7 CODEN: ABVEAO

ACTA BIOLOGICA VENEZUELICA. Text in English, Portuguese, Spanish. 1951. s-a. USD 10 per issue (effective (No. 2001). bk.rev. bibl, charts, illus. index. *Refereed.* **Document type:** *Academic/Scholarly.* **Description:** Publishes original contributions to systematics, ecology, physiology, parasitology and related biological disciplines. Includes short notes on methodological innovations and recent advances. Aimed at upper undergraduate, graduate students and professional staff.

Indexed: Aqua.Sci.& Fish.Abstr., Aquacult.Abstr., Biol.Abstr., Chem.Abstr., Deep Sea Res.& Oceanogr.Abstr., Forest.Abstr., Rev.Appl.Entomol., Seed Abstr., Soils & Fert., Sport Fish.Abstr., Weed Abstr., Wild.Rev., Zoo.Rec.

—Linda Hall.

Published by: Universidad Central de Venezuela, Instituto de Zoologia Tropical, Facultad de Ciencias-UCV, Apartado 47058, Caracas, DF 1041-A, Venezuela. FAX 58-2-6052136, TELEX 29452 UCVFCVC, amachado@strix.ciens.ucv.ve, imorales@strix.ciens.ucv.ve. Ed., R&P Dr. Antonio Machado. Circ: 700 (controlled).

570 NLD ISSN 0001-5342
QH301 CODEN: ABIOAN

ACTA BIOTHEORETICA. Text in English. 1935. q. EUR 294, USD 294 to institutions for print or online ed.; EUR 352.80, USD 352.80 to institutions for print & online eds. combined (effective 2002). bibl, charts, illus. back issues avail. *Refereed.* **Document type:** *Journal, Academic/Scholarly.* **Description:** Promotes theoretical biology and publishes papers on the subject, including the philosophy of biology and biomathematics.

Related titles: Microform ed.: (from PQC); Online - full text ed.: (from EBSCO Publishing, O C L C Online Computer Library Center, Inc., RoweCom Information Quest, Swets Blackwell, Kluwer Online, Institute for Scientific Information).

Indexed: ASCA, Anim.Breed.Abstr., Arts & Hum.Cit.Ind. (coverage dropped), Biol.Abstr., Chem.Abstr., Crop Physiol.Abstr., Curr.Adv.Ecol.Sci., Curr.Cont., Deep Sea Res.& Oceanogr.Abstr., Ecol.Abstr., Excerp.Med., Field Crop Abstr., Hort.Abstr., INIS Atomind., Ind.Med. (1935-), Ind.Sci.Rev., Ind.Vet., Int.Abstr.Biol.Sci., Ornam.Hort., Plant Breed.Abstr., Plant Gen.Res.Abstr., Ref.Zh., Rev.Appl.Entomol., Sci.Cit.Ind., Zoo.Rec.

—BLDSC (0604.000000), CASDDS, CISTI, EMDOCS, IDS, Infotrieve, ingenta, Linda Hall. **CCC.**

Published by: (Prof. Dr. Jan van der Hoeven Foundation for Theoretical Biology), Kluwer Academic Publishers Group (Subsidiary of: Wolters Kluwer N.V.), Spuiboulevard 50, PO Box 17, Dordrecht 3300 AA, Netherlands. TEL 31-78-639-2392, FAX 31-78-654-2254, services@wkap.nl, http://www.wkap.nl/journalhome.htm/0001-5342. Eds. A Stevens, J Demongeot, L Hemerik, U an der Heiden. **Subscr. in N America to:** Kluwer Academic - Plenum Publishers, 233 Spring St, New York, NY 10013-1578. TEL 212-620-8468, FAX 212-807-1047; **Subscr. to:** Journals Department, PO Box 322, Dordrecht 3300 AH, Netherlands. TEL 31-78-639-2392, FAX 31-78-654-6474.

571.9 DEU ISSN 1437-9546
ACTA ETHOLOGICA ONLINE. Text in English. 2/yr. *Refereed.* **Document type:** *Journal, Academic/Scholarly.*
Media: Online - full text (from EBSCO Publishing, RoweCom Information Quest, Swets Blackwell, Springer LINK). **Related titles:** Microform ed.; ♦ Print ed.: Acta Ethologica. ISSN 0873-9749.
Published by: (Instituto Superior de Psicologia Aplicada PRT), Springer-Verlag (Subsidiary of: BertelsmannSpringer), Haber Str 7, Heidelberg 69126, Germany. TEL 49-30-82787-0, FAX 49-30-82787301, service@springer.de, http://link.springer.de, http://www.springer.de.

ACTA FACULTATIS MEDICAE UNIVERSITATIS BRUNENSIS. see *MEDICAL SCIENCES*

570 POL ISSN 0065-132X
QH301.P63 CODEN: AHBPAX
ACTA HYDROBIOLOGICA. Text in English; Abstracts in Polish. 1959. q. USD 150 foreign (effective 2001). illus. *Refereed.* **Document type:** *Academic/Scholarly.* **Description:** Devoted to the study of biology of inland waters. The scope includes ecology, physiology, taxonomy and methodology.
Indexed: AgroAgen, AgroLibrex, Aqua.Sci.& Fish.Abstr., Biol.Abstr., Chem.Abstr., Chem.Indus.Notes, Chem.Titles, Curr.Adv.Ecol.Sci., Deep Sea Res.& Oceanogr.Abstr., Ecol.Abstr., Environ.Sci.Poll.Mgmt., Geo.Abstr.P.G., GeoRef, Geol.Abstr., IBR, INIS Atomind., Pollut.Abstr., Sel.J.Water, Sel.Water Res.Abstr., Sport Fish.Abstr., Vet.Bull., Wild.Rev., Zoo.Rec.
—BLDSC (0624.485000), CASDDS, CISTI, ingenta.
Published by: Polska Akademia Nauk, Zaklad Biologii Wod im. Karola Starmacha/Polish Academy of Sciences, Karol Starmach Institute of Freshwater Biology, Ul Slawkowska 17, Krakow 31016, Poland. TEL 48-12-4215082, FAX 48-12-4222115, office@zbw.pan.krakow.pl, http://www.zbw.pan.krakow.pl. Ed. Antoni Amirowicz. R&P Janusz Starmach. Circ: 650.

ACTA MEDICA ET BIOLOGICA/IGAKU SEIBUTSUGAKU KENKYU KIYO. see *MEDICAL SCIENCES*

ACTA MEDICA ROMANA. see *MEDICAL SCIENCES*

570 POL ISSN 0065-1400
QP351 CODEN: ANEXAC
ACTA NEUROBIOLOGIAE EXPERIMENTALIS. Text in English. 1928. q. USD 130 to individuals; USD 200 to institutions (effective 2002). index. reprint service avail. from ISI. *Refereed.* **Document type:** *Journal, Academic/Scholarly.*
Formerly: Acta Biologiae Experimentalis
Related titles: Online - full text ed.: (from Institute for Scientific Information).
Indexed: ASCA, AgroAgen, AgroLibrex, Anim.Behav.Abstr., Aqua.Sci.& Fish.Abstr., Biol.Abstr., Chem.Abstr., Curr.Adv.Ecol.Sci., Curr.Cont., Dent.Ind., Excerp.Med., INIS Atomind., Ind.Med. (1970-), Ind.Sci.Rev., Inpharma, Neurosci.Abstr., Neurosci.Cit.Ind., PsycInfo, Psychol.Abstr. (1952-), Reac., Ref.Zh., Rev.Plant Path., SSCI (coverage dropped), Sci.Cit.Ind. (coverage dropped), Zoo.Rec., e-psyche.
—BLDSC (0639.800000), CASDDS, CISTI, EMDOCS, GNLM, IDS, ingenta, KNAW.
Published by: Polska Akademia Nauk, Instytut Biologii Doswiadczalnej im. M. Nenckiego/Polish Academy of Sciences, M. Nencki Institute of Experimental Biology, Ul Pasteura 3, Warsaw 02093, Poland. TEL 48-22-659-8571, FAX 48-22-8225342, wrobel@nencki.gov.pl, http://www.nenckil.gov.pl/public.htm. Ed., R&P Andrzej Wrobel. **Dist. by:** Ars Polona, Krakowskie Przedmiescie 7, Warsaw, Poland.

570 610 SWE ISSN 1101-8429
ACTA REGIAE SOCIETATIS SCIENTIARUM ET LITTERARUM GOTHOBURGENSIS. BIOMEDICA. Text in English. 1991. irreg. SEK 100 (effective 2000). **Document type:** *Monographic series, Academic/Scholarly.*
Published by: Kungliga Vetenskaps- och Vitterhets-Samhaelle, c/o Goeteborgs Universitetsbibliotek, Fack 222, Goeteborg 40530, Sweden.

570 CZE ISSN 0001-7124
CODEN: ACBIBC
ACTA UNIVERSITATIS CAROLINAE: BIOLOGICA. Text in English. 1954. q. USD 80 (effective 1999). bk.rev. bibl, charts, illus, stat. index. **Document type:** *Academic/Scholarly.* **Description:** Covers cooperative research projects in the field of zoology, anthropology and botany.
Indexed: Apic.Abstr., Aqua.Sci.& Fish.Abstr., Biol.Abstr., Curr.Adv.Ecol.Sci., Entomol.Abstr., Excerp.Med., Plant Breed.Abstr., Soils & Fert., Sport Fish.Abstr., VITIS, Wild.Rev., Zoo.Rec.
—BLDSC (0584.500000), CASDDS, CISTI, Linda Hall.
Published by: (Univerzita Karlova, Prirodovedecka Fakulta), Vydavatelstvi Karolinum, Ovocny trh 3, Prague 116 36, Czech Republic. TEL 420-2-24491111, FAX 420-2-24212041, edice@cuni.cz; kinkorov@mail.natur.cuni. Ed. Milan Chvala. Circ: 650. **Subscr. to:** Vinicna 7, Prague 128 44, Czech Republic.

570 HUN ISSN 0563-0592
QH7 CODEN: AUSGAC
ACTA UNIVERSITATIS DE ATTILA JOZSEF NOMINATAE. ACTA BIOLOGICA. Text in English. 1947; N.S. 1955. a. per issue exchange basis. **Document type:** *Academic/Scholarly.* **Description:** Journal of animal and plant taxonomy and physiology, physical anthropology and ecology.
Indexed: Anthropol.Lit. (coverage dropped), GeoRef.
—CASDDS, CISTI, Linda Hall.
Published by: Attila Jozsef University, Faculty of Sciences, c/o E. Szabo, Exchange Librarian, Dugonics ter 13, PO Box 393, Szeged 6701, Hungary. Ed. Gyula Farkas. Circ: 400.

570 POL ISSN 0208-4449
ACTA UNIVERSITATIS NICOLAI COPERNICI. BIOLOGIA. Text in Polish. 1956. irreg. price varies. **Document type:** *Academic/Scholarly.*
Formerly: Uniwersytet Mikolaja Kopernika, Torun. Nauki Matematyczno-Przyrodnicze. Biologia (0083-4521)
Indexed: AgroAgen, AgroLibrex, Biol.Abstr., Curr.Adv.Ecol.Sci., Ref.Zh., Zoo.Rec.
Published by: Uniwersytet Mikolaja Kopernika, Wydawnictwo, Ul Gagarina 11, Torun 87100, Poland. TEL 48-56-14295. **Dist. by:** Osrodek Rozpowszechniania Wydawnictw Naukowych PAN, Palac Kultury i Nauki, Warsaw 00901, Poland.

570 COL ISSN 0304-3584
QH301 CODEN: ACBIEF
ACTUALIDADES BIOLOGICAS. Text in English, Portuguese, Spanish; Summaries in English, Spanish. 1972-1987; resumed 1988 (vol.20, no.68). s-a. COP 20,000 domestic; USD 25 in the Americas; USD 30 elsewhere (effective 2000). bk.rev. illus. back issues avail. *Refereed.* **Document type:** *Journal, Academic/Scholarly.* **Description:** Presents results of investigations in all fields of biology, most of which take place in Colombia.
Indexed: Aqua.Sci.& Fish.Abstr., Aquacult.Abstr., Biol.Abstr., Chem.Abstr., Environ.Sci.Poll.Mgmt., Zoo.Rec.
—CASDDS, CISTI.
Published by: Universidad de Antioquia, Departamento de Biologia, Apdo Aereo 1226, Medellin, Colombia. TEL 57-4-210-5622, FAX 57-4-233-0120, actubiol@matematicas.udea.edu.co, http://matematicas.udea.edu.co/cen/revista/actbiol.html. Eds. Daniel Aldana, Gabriel Roldan Perez. Circ: 700.

570 FRA ISSN 0753-3918
ACTUALITES BIOLOGIQUES. Text in French. m. FRF 950 (effective 1999). adv. **Document type:** *Trade.* **Description:** For professionals and administrators of biological analysis laboratories.
Published by: Centre National des Biologistes, 80 av. du Maine, Paris 75014, France. TEL 33-1-43229770, FAX 33-1-43217312. Pub. Jean Benoit. Adv. contact Jeanne Berga.

ADVANCED DRUG DELIVERY REVIEWS. see *PHARMACY AND PHARMACOLOGY*

570 USA ISSN 0301-5556
QL801
ADVANCES IN ANATOMY, EMBRYOLOGY AND CELL BIOLOGY. Text in English. 1966. irreg., latest vol.118, 1990. reprint service avail. from ISI. *Refereed.* **Document type:** *Monographic series.*
Related titles: Online - full text ed.: (from Institute for Scientific Information).
Indexed: ASCA, Biol.Abstr., GeoRef, Ind.Med. (1973-), Ind.Sci.Rev., Ind.Vet., Sci.Cit.Ind., Vet.Bull., Zoo.Rec.
—BLDSC (0698.800000), CISTI, GNLM, ingenta, KNAW. **CCC.**
Published by: Springer-Verlag, Journals (Subsidiary of: BertelsmannSpringer), 175 Fifth Ave, New York, NY 10010. TEL 212-460-1500, FAX 212-473-6272.

ADVANCES IN BEHAVIORAL BIOLOGY. see *PSYCHOLOGY*

ADVANCES IN BIOETHICS. see *PHILOSOPHY*

ADVANCES IN COLLOID AND INTERFACE SCIENCE. see *CHEMISTRY—Physical Chemistry*

570 USA
ADVANCES IN DEVELOPMENTAL BIOLOGY. Text in English. irreg. USD 128.50 per vol.. back issues avail.
Indexed: Chem.Abstr., Chem.Indus.Notes, Chem.Titles.
—BLDSC (0704.243800).
Published by: J A I Press Inc., 100 Prospect St, Box 811, Stamford, CT 06904-0811. TEL 203-323-9606, FAX 203-357-8446, jai@jaipress.com. Ed. Paul M Wassarman.

570 619 USA ISSN 0065-2598
CODEN: AEMBAP
ADVANCES IN EXPERIMENTAL MEDICINE AND BIOLOGY. Text in English. 1967. irreg., latest vol.477, 2000. price varies. *Refereed.* **Document type:** *Monographic series.*
Related titles: Online - full text ed.: (from Institute for Scientific Information).
Indexed: ASCA, Aqua.Sci.& Fish.Abstr., Bibl.Agri., Biol.Abstr., Chem.Abstr., Chem.Indus.Notes, Chem.Titles, Curr.Adv.Ecol.Sci., Dent.Ind., Environ.Sci.Poll.Mgmt., Excerp.Med., Hum.Gen.Abstr., INIS Atomind., Ind.Med. (1967-), Ind.Sci.Rev., Mass Spectr.Bull., Oncog.G.F.Abstr. (coverage dropped), Pollut.Abstr., Sci.Cit.Ind. (coverage dropped).
—BLDSC (0706.050000), ADONIS, CASDDS, CISTI, GNLM, IDS, ingenta, KNAW. **CCC.**
Published by: Kluwer Academic - Plenum Publishers (Subsidiary of: Wolters Kluwer N.V.), 233 Spring St, New York, NY 10013-1578. TEL 212-620-8000, 800-221-9369, FAX 212-463-0742, info@plenum.com, http://www.plenum.com.

570 CHE
ADVANCES IN LIFE SCIENCES. Text in English. irreg. price varies. **Document type:** *Monographic series, Academic/Scholarly.*
Published by: Birkhaeuser Verlag AG (Subsidiary of: BertelsmannSpringer), Klosterberg, Postfach 133, Basel 4010, Switzerland. TEL 41-61-2050707, FAX 41-61-2050792, orders@birkhauser.ch, http://www.birkhauser.ch.

578.77 USA ISSN 0065-2881
QH91.A1 CODEN: AMBYAR
ADVANCES IN MARINE BIOLOGY. Text in English. 1963. irreg., latest vol.32, 1997. index. reprint service avail. from ISI. *Refereed.* **Document type:** *Monographic series.*
Related titles: Online - full text ed.: (from Institute for Scientific Information).
Indexed: ASCA, Anim.Behav.Abstr. (coverage dropped), Appl.Ecol.Abstr. (coverage dropped), Aqua.Sci.& Fish.Abstr., Biol.& Agr.Ind. (Jan.1984-), Biol.Abstr., Chem.Abstr., Curr.Adv.Ecol.Sci., Deep Sea Res.& Oceanogr.Abstr., GeoRef, Helminthol.Abstr., Ind.Sci.Rev., Ocean.Abstr., Sci.Cit.Ind., Sport Fish.Abstr., Wild.Rev., Zoo.Rec.
—BLDSC (0709.340000), CASDDS, CISTI, Infotrieve, ingenta, KNAW, Linda Hall. **CCC.**
Published by: Academic Press, Inc., Journal Division (Subsidiary of: Harcourt Brace & Company), 525 B St, Ste 1900, San Diego, CA 92101-4495. TEL 619-231-0926, FAX 619-699-6715. Eds. F S Russell, J H S Blaxter. **Subscr. to:** Order Dept., 6277 Sea Harbor Dr, 4th Fl, Orlando, FL 32887. TEL 800-321-5068.

571.6 USA ISSN 1053-9506
CODEN: ARCGEH
ADVANCES IN REGULATION OF CELL GROWTH SERIES. Text in English. 1989. irreg. price varies. reprint service avail. from PQC. *Refereed.* **Document type:** *Monographic series.*

Indexed: Chem.Abstr., Chem.Indus.Notes, Chem.Titles.
—CASDDS.
Published by: Lippincott Williams & Wilkins (Philadelphia) (Subsidiary of: Wolters Kluwer N.V.), 530 Walnut St, Philadelphia, PA 19106-3621. TEL 301-223-2300, 800-638-3030, FAX 301-223-2400.

AEROSPACE MEDICINE AND BIOLOGY; a continuing bibliography. see *MEDICAL SCIENCES—Abstracting, Bibliographies, Statistics*

AFRICAN JOURNAL OF TROPICAL HYDROBIOLOGY AND FISHERIES. see *FISH AND FISHERIES*

AGRICULTURAL AND BIOLOGICAL RESEARCH. see *AGRICULTURE*

AIDS WEEKLY PLUS. see *MEDICAL SCIENCES—Communicable Diseases*

577 ITA
AIRONE. Text in Italian. 1981. m. ITL 70,000; ITL 160,000 foreign (effective 1997). adv. bk.rev. charts, illus. **Description:** Features items on ecology, nature and civilization.
Published by: Editoriale Giorgio Mondadori S.p.A., Via Andrea Ponti, 10, Milan, MI 20143, Italy. TEL 39-02-891661, FAX 39-02-8912-5888. Ed. Nicoletta Salvatori. Circ: 100,000.

570 GEO
AKADEMIYA NAUK GRUZINSKOI S.S.R. IZVESTIYA. SERIYA BIOLOGICHESKAYA. Text in Georgian, Russian. bi-m.
Indexed: Biol.Abstr., Chem.Abstr., Field Crop Abstr., INIS Atomind., Maize Abstr., Numis.Lit., Russ.Acad.Sci.Bibl., Triticale Abstr.
Published by: Akademiya Nauk Gruzinskoi S.S.R., Ul Dzerzhinskogo 8, Tbilisi, Georgia.

570 KAZ
QH301 CODEN: IKABAR
AKADEMIYA NAUK KAZAKHSTANA. IZVESTIYA. SERIYA BIOLOGICHESKAYA. Text in Russian. 1955. bi-m. charts, illus. index. **Document type:** *Academic/Scholarly.*
Formerly (until 1992): Akademiya Nauk Kazakhskoi S.S.R. Izvestiya. Seriya Biologicheskaya (0002-3183)
Indexed: Alloys Ind., Anim.Breed.Abstr., Biol.Abstr., Chem.Abstr., Crop Physiol.Abstr., Dairy Sci.Abstr., Field Crop Abstr., GeoRef, Helminthol.Abstr., Herb.Abstr., Hort.Abstr., INIS Atomind., Ind.Vet., Met.Abstr., Met.Abstr.Ind., Nonfer.Met.Alert, PCC Alert, Plant Breed.Abstr., Protozool.Abstr., Rev.Plant Path., Seed Abstr., Sel.Water Res.Abstr., Soils & Fert., Steels Alert, Triticale Abstr., Vet.Bull., Weed Abstr.
—CASDDS, CISTI, KNAW, Linda Hall.
Published by: (Akademiya Nauk Kazakhstana), Gylym, Ul Pushkina 111-113, Alma Ata 480100, Kazakstan. TEL 3272-611877. Ed. K T Tashenov. **Subscr. to:** G.R. Kondubayeva, Ul Shevchenko 28, Almaty 480021, Kazakstan.

570 TKM
CODEN: ITUBAK
AKADEMIYA NAUK TURKMENISTANA. IZVESTIYA. SERIYA BIOLOGICHESKIKH NAUK. Text in Russian. 1960. bi-m. charts, illus. index.
Formerly (until 1992): Akademiya Nauk Turkmenskoi S.S.R. Izvestiya. Seriya Biologicheskikh Nauk (0321-1746)
Indexed: Bio-Contr.News & Info., Biol.Abstr., Chem.Abstr., Helminthol.Abstr., Hort.Abstr., Ornam.Hort., Vet.Bull., Weed Abstr., Zoo.Rec.
—CASDDS, CISTI, Infotrieve. **CCC.**
Published by: Akademiya Nauk Turkmenistana, Gogolya ul 15, Ashkhabad 744000, Turkmenistan. Circ: 500.

579.8 DEU ISSN 0342-1120
QK564
ALGOLOGICAL STUDIES; Archiv fuer Hydrobiologie, Supplementbaende. Text in English, French, German. 1970. irreg. USD 78.10 per vol. domestic; USD 79.20 per vol. foreign (effective 2001). bk.rev. **Document type:** *Monographic series, Academic/Scholarly.*
Related titles: ♦ Supplement to: Archiv fuer Hydrobiologie. ISSN 0003-9136.
Indexed: Aqua.Sci.& Fish.Abstr., Aquacult.Abstr., Biol.Abstr., Environ.Sci.Poll.Mgmt., GeoRef, Int.Abstr.Biol.Sci., Sport Fish.Abstr., Wild.Rev., Zoo.Rec.
—CISTI, Infotrieve, ingenta, Linda Hall. **CCC.**
Published by: E. Schweizerbart'sche Verlagsbuchhandlung, Johannesstr 3A, Stuttgart 70176, Germany. TEL 49-711-625001, FAX 49-711-625005, mail@schweizerbart.de, schweizerbart@schweizerbart.de, http://www.schweizerbart.de. Ed. O Lhotsky.

570 ISR ISSN 0333-9815
ALON LEMOREH HABIOLOGIA/PAMPHLET FOR BIOLOGY TEACHERS. Text in Hebrew. 1969. q. USD 20. bk.rev. index. back issues avail. **Document type:** *Trade.* **Description:** Provides biology teachers with ideas and activities for classroom enrichment. Discusses current information in the biological sciences and problems and issues in biology education.
Indexed: Ind.Heb.Per. (1983-).
Published by: Hebrew University of Jerusalem, Amos De Shalit Science Teaching Centre, Jerusalem, Israel. TEL 972-2-585365. Ed. Talmona Oryan. Circ: 700.

570 551 560 DEU ISSN 0232-5381
ALTENBURGER NATURWISSENSCHAFTLICHE FORSCHUNGEN. Text in German; Summaries in English, German. 1981. a. bk.rev. back issues avail. **Document type:** *Academic/Scholarly.*
Indexed: GeoRef, Ref.Zh., Zoo.Rec.
—Linda Hall.
Published by: Naturkundliches Museum Mauritianum, Postfach 1644, Altenburg 04590, Germany. TEL 49-3447-2589, FAX 49-3447-2589. Ed. Norbert Hoeser. Circ: 1,200.

570 JPN ISSN 0065-6682
QH91.AI CODEN: ARJPB8
AMAKUSA MARINE BIOLOGICAL LABORATORY. PUBLICATIONS. Text and summaries in English. 1966. a. per issue exchange basis. **Document type:** *Academic/Scholarly.* **Description:** Publishes mainly achievements of laboratory staff and visiting scientists. Also contains ecological and taxonomic studies of benthic invertebrates in the littoral and shallow sea.
Indexed: Aqua.Sci.& Fish.Abstr., Aquacult.Abstr., Biol.Abstr., Curr.Adv.Ecol.Sci., Ecol.Abstr., Environ.Sci.Poll.Mgmt., Sport Fish.Abstr., Zoo.Rec.
—Linda Hall.
Published by: Kyushu University, Amakusa Marine Biological Laboratory/Kyushu Daigaku Rigakubu Fuzoku Amakusa Rinkai Jikkensho, 2231 Tomioka, Amakusa-gun, Reihoku Cho, Kumamoto ken 8632507, Japan. TEL 81-969-35-0003, FAX 81-969-35-2413. R&P Taiji Kikuchi. Circ: 450.

577 DEU ISSN 0065-6755
QH117 CODEN: AMAZAP
AMAZONIANA. Text in Multiple languages. 1965. a. (2 nos./vol.). DEM 88. *Refereed.* **Document type:** *Academic/Scholarly.*
Related titles: Online - full text ed.: (from Institute for Scientific Information).
Indexed: ASCA, Appl.Ecol.Abstr., Aqua.Sci.& Fish.Abstr., Aquacult.Abstr., Biol.Abstr., Curr.Adv.Ecol.Sci., Curr.Cont., Ecol.Abstr., Entomol.Abstr., Environ.Sci.Poll.Mgmt., Forest Prod.Abstr., Forest.Abstr., Geo.Abstr.H.G., Geo.Abstr.P.G., GeoRef, Geol.Abstr., Pollut.Abstr., Ref.Zh., Rev.Appl.Entomol., Sel.Water Res.Abstr., Soils & Fert., Zoo.Rec.
—IDS, ingenta.
Published by: Universitaetsbuchhandlung Muehlau, Holtenauer Str 116, Kiel 24100, Germany. TEL 49-431-8009-0, FAX 49-431-800950. Eds. Djalma Batista, Harald Sioli.

572.8 610 USA
AMERICAN BLOOD RESOURCES ASSOCIATION. JOURNAL* . Text in English. 1979. q. USD 90; USD 110 foreign. adv. tr.lit. back issues avail. **Document type:** *Trade.*
Former titles (until 1992): Plasmapheresis (0894-6779); (until 1987): Plasma Quarterly (0739-8751)
Published by: American Blood Resources Association, 147 Old Solomons Island Rd Ste 100, Annapolis, MD 21401-3822. TEL 410-263-8296, FAX 410-263-2298, 463.3276@compuserve.com. Ed. James P Reilly. R&P, Adv. contact Catherine Izzi. Circ: 4,000.

AMERICAN JOURNAL OF CLINICAL PATHOLOGY. see *MEDICAL SCIENCES*

570 USA ISSN 1042-0533
QP1 CODEN: AJHUES
AMERICAN JOURNAL OF HUMAN BIOLOGY. Text in English. 1989. bi-m. USD 830 in United States; USD 890 in Canada & Mexico; USD 941 elsewhere; USD 872 combined subscription in United States for print and online eds.; USD 932 combined subscription in Canada & Mexico for print and online eds.; USD 983 combined subscription elsewhere for print and online eds. (effective 2002). adv. back issues avail. *Refereed.* **Document type:** *Academic/Scholarly.* **Description:** Provides a forum for research in human biology. For scientists and professionals interested in understanding individual and population variations in health and disease. Covers a wide range of topics in such areas as genetic variation, anatomy and physiology, growth and aging, physical performance and evolution.
Formerly: Human Biology (New York)
Related titles: Microform ed.: (from PQC); Online - full text ed.: ISSN 1520-6300. USD 830 in United States; USD 830 in Canada & Mexico; USD 830 elsewhere (effective 2002) (from EBSCO Publishing, Gale Group, Wiley InterScience, Institute for Scientific Information).
Indexed: A.I.C.P., ASCA, AgeLine, Anthropol.Lit., Arts & Hum.Cit.Ind. (coverage dropped), Biol.Dig., Cal.Tiss.Abstr., Curr.Cont., Curr.Ind.Stat., Environ.Sci.Poll.Mgmt., Fam.Ind., Gen.Sci.Ind. (Jul.1997-), Inpharma, NRN, Nutr.Abstr., Pharm.&Out.News, Pollut.Abstr., Popul.Ind., Protozool.Abstr., Reac., Ref.Zh., Rev.Appl.Entomol., Risk Abstr., SSCI, Saf.Sci.Abstr.
—BLDSC (0824.900000), CISTI, GNLM, IDS, Infotrieve, ingenta, KNAW. **CCC.**
Published by: (Human Biology Council), John Wiley & Sons, Inc., Journals (Subsidiary of: Wiley InterScience), 605 Third Ave, New York, NY 10158. TEL 212-850-6645, FAX 212-850-6021, subinfo@jwiley.com, uscs-wis@wiley.com, http://www.wiley.co.uk, http://www.wiley.com. Ed. Robert M Malina. adv.: B&W page GBP 640, color page GBP 1,515; trim 174 x 254. Circ: 800. **Subscr. outside the Americas to:** John Wiley & Sons Ltd., Baffins Ln, Chichester, Sussex PO19 IUD, United Kingdom. TEL 44-1243-779777, FAX 44-1243-843232, cs-journals@wiley.co.uk, http://www.wiley.co.uk.

570 USA ISSN 0003-0147
QH1 CODEN: AMNTA4
THE AMERICAN NATURALIST; devoted to the advancement and correlation of the biological sciences. Text in English. 1867. m., latest vol.157, 2001, Jan. USD 71 in United States to individuals; USD 93.97 in Canada to individuals; USD 89 elsewhere to individuals; USD 328 in United States to institutions; USD 368.96 in Canada to institutions; USD 346 elsewhere to institutions; USD 49 in United States to students; USD 70.43 in Canada to students; USD 67 elsewhere to students; USD 31.35 newsstand/cover elsewhere to individuals; USD 9.90 newsstand/cover to institutions; USD 76 in United States family; USD 94 in Canada family; USD 99.32 elsewhere family (effective Sep. 2002); Prices for both print and online eds. combined. adv. bk.rev. illus. index. reprints avail. *Refereed.* **Document type:** *Academic/Scholarly.* **Description:** Addresses ecology and evolutionary biology; devoted to the conceptual unification of the biological sciences.
Related titles: Microfiche ed.: (from IDC); Microform ed.: (from PQC,PMC); Online - full text ed.: USD 47 to individuals; USD 25 to students (2001) (from EBSCO Publishing, JSTOR (Web-based Journal Archive), Gale Group, Factiva, Institute for Scientific Information).
Indexed: ASCA, Acid Pre.Dig., Agri.Eng.Abstr., Anim.Behav.Abstr., Anim.Breed.Abstr., Apic.Abstr., Appl.Ecol.Abstr., Aqua.Sci.& Fish.Abstr., Bio-Contr.News & Info., Biol.& Agr.Ind. (Nov.1982-), Biol.Abstr., Chem.Abstr., Crop Physiol.Abstr., Curr.Adv.Ecol.Sci., Curr.Adv.Gen.& Molec.Biol., Curr.Adv.Plant Sci., Curr.Cont., Curr.Ind.Stat., Curr.Ref.Fish Res., Dairy Sci.Abstr., Deep Sea Res.& Oceanogr.Abstr., Ecol.Abstr., Eng.Ind., Entomol.Abstr., Environ.Per.Bibl. (1973-), Environ.Sci.Poll.Mgmt., Field Crop Abstr., Forest.Abstr., Gen.Sci.Ind. (Jun.1984-), GeoRef, Geol.Abstr., Helminthol.Abstr., Herb.Abstr., Hort.Abstr., INIS Atomind., Ind.Sci.Rev., Ind.Vet., Int.Abstr.Biol.Sci., Int.Abstr.Oper.Res., Key Word Ind.Wildl.Res., Math.R., Nutr.Abstr., Ocean.Abstr., Ornam.Hort., Plant Breed.Abstr., Plant Gen.Res.Abstr., Plant Sci., Postharvest, Protozool.Abstr., Ref.Zh., Rev.Appl.Entomol., Rev.Med.& Vet.Mycol., Rev.Plant Path., Rice Abstr., Risk Abstr., Russ.Acad.Sci.Bibl., SSCI (coverage dropped), Sci.Cit.Ind., Seed Abstr., Sel.Water Res.Abstr., Soils & Fert., Sport Fish.Abstr., Weed Abstr., Wild.Rev., Zoo.Rec.
—BLDSC (0846.000000), ADONIS, CASDDS, CISTI, Ei, EMDOCS, IDS, ingenta, Linda Hall. **CCC.**

Published by: (American Society of Naturalists), University of Chicago Press, Journals Division, PO Box 37005, Chicago, IL 60637. TEL 773-753-3347, FAX 773-753-0811, subscriptions@journals.uchicago.edu, orders@press.uchicago.edu, http://www.journals.uchicago.edu/AN/home.html. Ed. Joseph Travis. adv.: page USD 445; trim 9.5 x 6.63. Circ: 3,300 (paid).

571.3 611 USA ISSN 0003-276X
QL801

THE ANATOMICAL RECORD. Text in English. 1906. 18/yr. USD 4,250 in United States; USD 4,430 in Canada & Mexico; USD 4,583 elsewhere; USD 4,463 combined subscription in United States for print and online eds.; USD 4,643 combined subscription in Canada & Mexico for print and online eds.; USD 4,796 combined subscription elsewhere for print and online eds. (effective 2002). adv. bk.rev. abstr, bibl, charts, illus. index. back issues avail.; reprint service avail. from SWZ. *Refereed.* **Document type:** *Academic/Scholarly.*

Related titles: Microfilm ed.: (from PMC); Microform ed.: (from PQC); Online - full text ed.: ISSN 1097-0185. USD 4,250 in United States; USD 4,250 in Canada & Mexico; USD 4,250 elsewhere (effective 2002) (from EBSCO Publishing, Wiley InterScience, Institute for Scientific Information).

Indexed: ASCA, Abstr.Anthropol., Anim.Breed.Abstr., Aqua.Sci.& Fish.Abstr., Biol.& Agr.Ind. (Jan.1990-), Biol.Abstr., Cal.Tiss.Abstr. (coverage dropped), Chem.Abstr., Chem.Indus.Notes, Chem.Titles, Curr.Adv.Cell & Devel.Biol., Curr.Adv.Ecol.Sci., Curr.Cont., Curr.Tit.Dent., Dent.Ind., Excerp.Med., Focus on: Vet.Sci.& Med., INIS Atomind., Ind.Med. (1906-), Ind.Sci.Rev., Ind.Vet., Inpharma, Int.Abstr.Biol.Sci., Neurosci.Cit.Ind., Nutr.Abstr., Pharm.&Out.News, Reac., Ref.Zh., Sci.Cit.Ind., Sport Fish.Abstr., THA, Tox.Abstr. (coverage dropped), Vet.Bull., Wild.Rev., Zoo.Rec.

—BLDSC (0898.000000), CASDDS, CISTI, EMDOCS, GNLM, IDS, ingenta, KNAW, Linda Hall. **CCC.**

Published by: (American Association of Anatomists), John Wiley & Sons, Inc., Journals (Subsidiary of: Wiley InterScience), 605 Third Ave, New York, NY 10158. TEL 212-850-6645, FAX 212-850-6021, SUBINFO@JWILEY.COM, uscs-wis@wiley.com, http://www.wiley.com. Ed. Aaron J Ladman. adv.: B&W page USD 640, color page USD 1,515; trim 210 x 279. Circ: 1,200. **Subscr. outside the Americas to:** John Wiley & Sons Ltd., Baffins Ln, Chichester, Sussex PO19 IUD, United Kingdom. TEL 44-1243-779777, FAX 44-1243-843232, cs-journals@wiley.co.uk, http://www.wiley.co.uk.

571.86 ITA ISSN 1121-1431
QL1 CODEN: AIBOE7

ANIMAL BIOLOGY. Text and summaries in English. 1980. 3/yr. ITL 150,000; ITL 200,000 foreign (effective 1996). index. reprint service avail. from ISI.

Former titles (until 1991): Acta Embryologiae et Morphologiae Experimentalis (0391-9706); (until 1980): Acta Embryologiae Experimentalis (0065-1184); (until 1968): Acta Embryologiae et Morphologiae Experimentalis (0567-7416)

Indexed: Biol.Abstr., Curr.Adv.Ecol.Sci., Curr.Cont. (coverage dropped), Excerp.Med., Helminthol.Abstr., Ind.Med. (coverage dropped), Zoo.Rec.

—CASDDS, CISTI, GNLM, ingenta, Linda Hall.

Published by: Halocynthia Association, Istituto di Zoologia Universita di Palermo, Via Archirafi, 18, Palermo, PA 90123, Italy. TEL 39-91-6621020, FAX 39-91-6172009. Ed. Giacomo De Leo. Circ: 400.

570 610 FRA ISSN 0003-3898
RB1 CODEN: ABCLAI

ANNALES DE BIOLOGIE CLINIQUE. Text in English, French; Summaries in English, French. 1943. 6/yr. FRF 750 domestic to individuals; EUR 127 in Europe to individuals; FRF 870 elsewhere to individuals; FRF 1,550 domestic to institutions; EUR 248 in Europe to institutions; FRF 1,670 elsewhere to institutions; FRF 250 newsstand/cover (effective 2001). adv. bk.rev. charts, illus. index. *Refereed.* **Document type:** *Academic/Scholarly.* **Description:** Covers all aspects of clinical biology, from instrumentation and methodology to laboratory applications, clinical investigations, animal experimentation, human pathology and evaluations of apparatus or reagents.

Related titles: Online - full text ed.: FRF 750 to individuals; FRF 1,550 to institutions (effective 2001) (from ingenta, Institute for Scientific Information).

Indexed: ASCA, Biol.Abstr., C.I.S. Abstr., Chem.Abstr., Chem.Cit.Ind., Chem.Indus.Notes, Chem.Titles, Curr.Adv.Ecol.Sci., Curr.Cont. (coverage dropped), Excerp.Med., Food Sci.& Tech.Abstr., Helminthol.Abstr., INIS Atomind., Ind.Med. (1943-), Ind.Sci.Rev., Ind.Vet., Int.Abstr.Biol.Sci., Int.Nurs.Ind., Mass Spectr.Bull., Nutr.Abstr., Pig News & Info., Protozool.Abstr., Rev.Med.& Vet.Mycol., Sci.Cit.Ind. (coverage dropped), Vet.Bull.

—BLDSC (0967.730000), CASDDS, CISTI, EMDOCS, GNLM, IDS, Infotrieve, KNAW. **CCC.**

Published by: (Societe Francaise de Biologie Clinique), John Libbey Eurotext, 127 av. de la Republique, Montrouge 92120, France. TEL 33-01-46730660, FAX 33-01-40840999, marketing@jle.com, http://www.john-libbey-eurotext.fr/. Ed. Jean Louis Dhondt. Circ: 3,000. **Subscr. to:** A T E I, 3 av. Pierre Kerautret, Romainville 92230, France. TEL 33-1-48408686, FAX 33-1-48400731, atei@club-internet.fr.

571.9 616.07 FRA ISSN 0242-6498
CODEN: ASPAD2

ANNALES DE PATHOLOGIE. Text in French; Summaries in English, French. 1924. 6/yr. FRF 1,449; FRF 1,742 foreign (effective 2000). bk.rev. bibl, illus. index. reprint service avail. from ISI. *Refereed.* **Document type:** *Academic/Scholarly.* **Description:** Publishes observations and works of a morphological order, reflecting the achievements of French-speaking anatomopathologists.

Formerly (until 1981): Annales d'Anatomie Pathologique (0003-3871)

Related titles: Microform ed.: (from PQC); Online - full text ed.: (from Institute for Scientific Information, RoweCom Information Quest).

Indexed: ASCA, Aqua.Sci.& Fish.Abstr., Biol.Abstr., Chem.Abstr., Curr.Adv.Cancer Res., Curr.Adv.Ecol.Sci., Curr.Cont., Dent.Ind., Environ.Sci.Poll.Mgmt., Excerp.Med., Ind.Med. (1981-), Ind.Sci.Rev., Inpharma, Pharm.&Out.News, Reac., Rev.Med.& Vet.Mycol., Sci.Cit.Ind.

—BLDSC (0991.300000), CASDDS, CISTI, EMDOCS, GNLM, IDS, Infotrieve, KNAW. **CCC.**

Published by: (Societe Francaise de Pathologie), Masson - Periodiques, 120 bd. St. Germain, Paris 75006, France. TEL 33-1-40466200, FAX 33-1-404662011. Ed. D Henin. Circ: 1,400. **Subscr. to:** Societe de Periodiques Specialises, BP 22, Vineuil Cedex 41354, France. TEL 33-2-54504612, FAX 33-2-54504611.

570 POL ISSN 0066-2232
QH301.L8 CODEN: AUCBAJ

ANNALES UNIVERSITATIS MARIAE CURIE-SKLODOWSKA. SECTIO C. BIOLOGIA. Text in English, Polish; Summaries in English, French, German. 1946. a. price varies. **Document type:** *Academic/Scholarly.*

Indexed: A.I.C.P., AgroLibrex, Biol.Abstr., Chem.Abstr., Curr.Adv.Ecol.Sci., Field Crop Abstr., Forest Prod.Abstr., Forest.Abstr., GeoRef, Herb.Abstr., Hort.Abstr., INIS Atomind., Int.Abstr.Biol.Sci., Plant Breed.Abstr., Rev.Appl.Entomol., Zoo.Rec.

—CASDDS, CISTI, Linda Hall.

Published by: Uniwersytet Marii Curie-Sklodowskiej, Wydawnictwo, Pl M Curie Sklodowskiej 5, Lublin 20031, Poland. TEL 48-31-375304, FAX 48-81-336699, TELEX 0643223. Ed. Zbigniew Lorkiewicz. Circ: 950.

ANNALS OF ANATOMY. see *MEDICAL SCIENCES*

570 GBR ISSN 0003-4746
QH301 CODEN: AABIAV

ANNALS OF APPLIED BIOLOGY. Text in English. 1914. bi-m. (in 2 vols.). GBP 217.50, USD 445 (effective 1999). adv. illus. cum.index: 1914-1978, 1979-1985. *Refereed.* **Document type:** *Academic/Scholarly.*

Related titles: Online - full text ed.: (from ingenta, Institute for Scientific Information); ♦ Supplement: Tests of Agrochemicals and Cultivars. ISSN 0951-4309.

Indexed: ASCA, AgBiotech, Agri.& Environ.Biotech.Abstr. (coverage dropped), Agri.Eng.Abstr., Agricola, Agroforest.Abstr., Aqua.Sci.& Fish.Abstr., Bio-Contr.News & Info., Biodet.Abstr., Biol.& Agr.Ind. (Feb.1983-), Biol.Abstr., Chem.Abstr., Chem.Indus.Notes, Chem.Titles, Crop Physiol.Abstr., Curr.Adv.Ecol.Sci., Curr.Adv.Plant Sci., Curr.Biotech.Abstr., Curr.Cont., Derwent Biotech.Abstr., Ecol.Abstr., Entomol.Abstr., Environ.Sci.Poll.Mgmt., Excerp.Med., Fababean Abstr., Field Crop Abstr., Food Sci.& Tech.Abstr., Forest Prod.Abstr., Forest.Abstr., Genet.Abstr. (coverage dropped), Helminthol.Abstr., Herb.Abstr., Hort.Abstr., Hum.Gen.Abstr., IDA, INIS Atomind., Ind.Med. (coverage dropped), Ind.Sci.Rev., Ind.Vet., Int.Abstr.Biol.Sci., Irr.& Drain.Abstr., Maize Abstr., Microbiol.Abstr., Nutr.Abstr., Ornam.Hort., Plant Breed.Abstr., Plant Gen.Res.Abstr., Plant Grow.Reg.Abstr., Plant Sci., Postharvest, Potato Abstr., Ref.Zh., Rev.Appl.Entomol., Rev.Arom.& Med.Plants, Rev.Plant Path., Rice Abstr., Sci.Cit.Ind., Seed Abstr., Soils & Fert., Sorghum & Millets Abstr., Soyabean Abstr., Sport Fish.Abstr., Triticale Abstr., Trop.Oil Seeds Abstr., Weed Abstr., Wild.Rev., Zoo.Rec.

—BLDSC (1038.000000), CASDDS, CISTI, EMDOCS, GNLM, ingenta, Linda Hall.

Published by: Association of Applied Biologists, Horticultural Research International, Horticulture Research International, Wellesbourne, Warwick CV35 9EF, United Kingdom. FAX 44-1789-470234, chris.aab@hri.ac.uk; carol.aab@hri.ac.uk, http://www.hri.ac.uk/aab/. Ed. M Parry. R&P, Adv. contact Carol Millman TEL 44-1789-470382. Circ: 1,000.

B

570 IND ISSN 0970-0153
CODEN: ANBIEO

ANNALS OF BIOLOGY; an international journal of basic and applied biology. Text in English. 1985. s-a. INR 500, USD 60 (effective 1999 & 2000). adv. bk.rev. **Document type:** *Academic/Scholarly.*

Indexed: AgBiotech, Agri.Eng.Abstr., Agrindex, Agroforest.Abstr., Anim.Breed.Abstr., Aqua.Sci.& Fish.Abstr., Bio-Contr.News & Info., Biol.Abstr., Crop Physiol.Abstr., Curr.Adv.Ecol.Sci., Dairy Sci.Abstr., Ecol.Abstr., Entomol.Abstr., Environ.Sci.Poll.Mgmt., Field Crop Abstr., Food Sci.& Tech.Abstr., Forest.Abstr., Geo.Abstr.P.G., Helminthol.Abstr., Herb.Abstr., Hort.Abstr., IDA, Ind.Vet., Indian Sci.Abstr., Irr.& Drain.Abstr., Maize Abstr., Microbiol.Abstr., Nutr.Abstr., Ocean.Abstr., Plant Breed.Abstr., Plant Gen.Res.Abstr., Plant Grow.Reg.Abstr., Pollut.Abstr., Poult.Abstr., Rev.Appl.Entomol., Rev.Arom.& Med.Plants, Rev.Med.& Vet.Mycol., Rev.Plant Path., Rice Abstr., Rural Devel.Abstr., Seed Abstr., Sel.Water Res.Abstr., Soils & Fert., Sorghum & Millets Abstr., Soyabean Abstr., Sugar Ind.Abstr., Triticale Abstr., Trop.Oil Seeds Abstr., Weed Abstr., World Ag.Econ.& Rur.Soc.Abstr., Zoo.Rec.

—BLDSC (1039.300000), CASDDS, CISTI.

Published by: Agri Bio Research Publishers, 121 Mohalla Chaudharian, Hisar 125 001, India. TEL 91-1662-37530, bajdasch@nde.vsnl.com. Eds. Dr. Manjit S Dhindsa, Dr. R K Behl. Circ: 500.

ANNALS OF CONTEMPORARY DIAGNOSTIC PATHOLOGY. see *MEDICAL SCIENCES*

ANNALS OF DIAGNOSTIC PATHOLOGY. see *MEDICAL SCIENCES*

570 GBR ISSN 0301-4460
QP34.5 CODEN: AHUBBJ

ANNALS OF HUMAN BIOLOGY. Text in English; Summaries in French, German. 1974. bi-m. GBP 514, USD 848 to institutions (effective 2002). bk.rev. bibl, charts, stat. index. *Refereed.* **Document type:** *Academic/Scholarly.* **Description:** Publishes papers concerning research into biological aspects of human populations with regard to their ecology, demography, genetics, evolution, and the growth, physiology, disease patterns and behavior of the individuals composing them.

Related titles: Microform ed.: 1974; Online - full text ed.: ISSN 1464-5033. 1974 (from CatchWord Ltd., EBSCO Publishing, O C L C Online Computer Library Center, Inc., RoweCom Information Quest, Swets Blackwell, Institute for Scientific Information).

Indexed: A.I.C.P., ASCA, Abstr.Anthropol., Abstr.Hyg., Anthropol.Lit., Bibl.Dev.Med.& Child Neur., Biol.Abstr., Chem.Abstr., Curr.Adv.Ecol.Sci., Curr.Adv.Gen.& Molec.Biol., Curr.Cont., Dairy Sci.Abstr., Dent.Ind., Ergon.Abstr., Excerp.Med., Geo.Abstr.H.G., IDA, Ind.Med. (1974-), Ind.Sci.Rev., Inpharma, Intl.Bibl.Soc.Sci., NRN, Nutr.Abstr., Popul.Ind., Protozool.Abstr., Reac., Risk Abstr., SSCI (coverage dropped), Sci.Cit.Ind., Trop.Dis.Bull.

—BLDSC (1040.900000), CASDDS, CatchWord, CISTI, GNLM, IDS, ingenta, Linda Hall. **CCC.**

Published by: (Society for the Study of Human Biology), Taylor & Francis Group, Taylor & Francis Ltd., 11 New Fetter Ln, London EC4P 4EE, United Kingdom. TEL 44-20-7583-9855, FAX 44-20-7842-2298, info@tandf.co.uk, http://www.tandf.co.uk. Eds. A H Bittles, N G Norgan, R Hauspie. **Subscr. in N american to:** Taylor & Francis Ltd., 325 Chestnut St, Suite 800, Philadelphia, PA 19016. TEL 800-354-1420, FAX 215-625-8914, info@taylorandfrancis.com, http://www.taylorandfrancis.com/.

570 FRA ISSN 0003-5017
QH3 CODEN: ANBLAT

L'ANNEE BIOLOGIQUE. Text in French. 1895. q. FRF 1,417 domestic to institutions; EUR 216.02 in Europe to institutions; USD 262 in the Americas to institutions; FRF 1,561 elsewhere to institutions (effective 2001). adv. bk.rev. bibl, charts, illus. index. back issues avail.; reprint service avail. from ISI. *Refereed.* **Document type:** *Academic/Scholarly.* **Description:** Contains articles on all topics: general biology, biochemistry, molecular biology, zoology, botany, ecology, animal and vegetal physiology, psychophysiology, and paleontology.
Related titles: Online - full text ed.: (from ingenta, ScienceDirect, Swets Blackwell).
Indexed: ASCA, AgBiotech, Aqua.Sci.& Fish.Abstr., Aquacult.Abstr., Biol.Abstr., Chem.Abstr., Chem.Indus.Notes, Chem.Titles, Curr.Adv.Ecol.Sci., Curr.Cont. (coverage dropped), Curr.Ref.Fish Res., Deep Sea Res.& Oceanogr.Abstr., Environ.Sci.Poll.Mgmt., GeoRef, Helminthol.Abstr., Ind.Med. (coverage dropped), Ind.Sci.Rev., Rev.Appl.Entomol., Sci.Cit.Ind. (coverage dropped), Sport Fish.Abstr., Zoo.Rec.
—BLDSC (1048.000000), CASDDS, CISTI, IDS, Infotrieve, Linda Hall. **CCC.**
Published by: Elsevier Paris, Editions Scientifiques et Medicales (Subsidiary of: Reed Elsevier plc. group), 23 rue Linois, Paris 75015, France. TEL 33-1-45589110, FAX 33-1-45589419, academic@elsevier-fr.com, http://www.elsevier.nl/inca/publications/store/6/0/0/7/8/5/. Eds. P Cassier, P Mazliak. Circ: 1,000.

610 FRA ISSN 1157-4135

ANNUAIRE DE LA RECHERCHE BIO-MEDICALE. Short title: A R B M. Text in French. 1989. a., latest vol.5, 1995. USD 149. **Document type:** *Directory.* **Description:** Covers all public and semi-public biomedical research centers in France, including INSERM, CEA, CNRS, ORSTOM, medical schools, science faculties, Pasteur Institutes, and centers for cancer research.
Published by: Editions Scientifiques et Medicales Elsevier, 141 rue de Javel, Paris Cedex 15 75747, France. TEL 33-1-45589022, FAX 33-1-45589421, http://www.elsevier.nl/. **Subscr. in U.S. and Canada to:** Elsevier Science, PO Box 945, New York, NY 10159-0945. TEL 212-633-3730, FAX 212-633-3680, http://www.elsevier.com.

573.6 306.7 USA

ANNUAL EDITIONS: HUMAN SEXUALITY. Text in English. 1975. a. USD 12.25. illus. *Refereed.* **Document type:** *Academic/Scholarly.*
Former titles: Annual Editions: Readings in Human Sexuality (0163-836X); Focus: Human Sexuality (0147-0655)
Indexed: e-psyche.
Published by: Dushkin - McGraw-Hill, Sluice Dock, Guilford, CT 06437-9989. TEL 203-453-4351, FAX 203-453-6000. Ed. Susan Bunting. Pub. Ian Nielsen. R&P Cheryl Greenleaf.

570 USA

ANNUAL EDITIONS: LIFE MANAGEMENT. Text in English. 1992. a. USD 12.95. illus. **Document type:** *Academic/Scholarly.*
Published by: Dushkin - McGraw-Hill, Sluice Dock, Guilford, CT 06437-9989. TEL 203-453-4351, FAX 203-453-6000. Ed. Ann Daluiso. Pub. Ian Nielsen. R&P Cheryl Greenleaf.

559.89 570 GBR ISSN 0954-1020
Q127.A48 CODEN: ANTSE8

ANTARCTIC SCIENCE. Text in English. q. GBP 136 to individuals; USD 364 to institutions (effective 2002). adv. bk.rev. illus. index. back issues avail. *Refereed.* **Document type:** *Academic/Scholarly.* **Description:** Contains both review and data papers, short notes on technical developments and recent discoveries, reports on key Antarctic meetings, book reviews, and a diary of forthcoming events.
Related titles: Microform ed.: (from PQC); Online - full text ed.: (from EBSCO Publishing, Institute for Scientific Information).
Indexed: ASCA, Aqua.Sci.& Fish.Abstr., Aquacult.Abstr., Cal.Tiss.Abstr., Chemorec.Abstr., Curr.Cont., Ecol.Abstr., Eng.Ind., Environ.Abstr., Environ.Per.Bibl. (1990-), Environ.Sci.Poll.Mgmt., Geo.Abstr.P.G., GeoRef, Geol.Abstr., INIS Atomind., Ind.Sci.Rev., Int.Abstr.Biol.Sci., Meteor.& Geoastrophys.Abstr., Microbiol.Abstr., Mineral.Abstr., Neurosci.Abstr. (coverage dropped), Ocean.Abstr. (coverage dropped), Pollut.Abstr., Ref.Zh., Sci.Cit.Ind., Sel.Water Res.Abstr., Sport Fish.Abstr., Wild.Rev., Zoo.Rec.
—BLDSC (1542.130500), CISTI, Ei, EMDOCS, IDS, Infotrieve, ingenta, Linda Hall. **CCC.**
Published by: (British Antarctic Survey), Cambridge University Press, Edinburgh Bldg, Shaftesbury Rd, Cambridge CB2 2RU, United Kingdom. FAX 44-1223-315052, information@cup.cam.ac.uk, information@cambridge.org, http://www.cup.cam.ac.uk, http://www.uk.cambridge.org/journals/pmu. Eds. Alan P.M. Vaughan, David W.H. Walton, Stephen D. Mobbs. Adv. contact Martine Cariou Keen. Circ: 455.

APOPTOSIS. see *BIOLOGY—Abstracting, Bibliographies, Statistics*

570 NLD ISSN 1386-2588
QH90.A1 CODEN: AQECF9

AQUATIC ECOLOGY; a multidisciplinary journal relating to processes and structures at different organizational levels. Text in English. 1975 (vol.9). q. EUR 268, USD 268 to institutions for print or online ed.; EUR 321.60, USD 321.60 to institutions for print & online edition (effective 2002). adv. bk.rev. *Refereed.* **Document type:** *Academic/Scholarly.* **Description:** Publishes fundamental and applied research on the ecology of fresh, brackish, estuarine, and marine environments.
Former titles (until 1997): Netherlands Journal of Aquatic Ecology (1380-8427); (until 1992): Hydrobiological Bulletin (0165-1404); (until 1973): Hydrobiologische Vereniging. Mededelingen
Related titles: Online - full text ed.: NLG 542, EUR 246 to institutions; NLG 650.40, EUR 295.20 to institutions for online & print edition (effective 2001) (from EBSCO Publishing, O C L C Online Computer Library Center, Inc., RoweCom Information Quest, Swets Blackwell, Kluwer Online).
Indexed: Appl.Ecol.Abstr., Aqua.Sci.& Fish.Abstr., Biol.Abstr., Chem.Abstr., Chem.Indus.Notes, Chem.Titles, Curr.Adv.Ecol.Sci., Ecol.Abstr., Environ.Sci.Poll.Mgmt., Excerp.Med., Genet.Abstr., Geo.Abstr.H.G., Geo.Abstr.P.G., Geol.Abstr., Hum.Gen.Abstr., Ocean.Abstr., Pollut.Abstr., Sel.Water Res.Abstr., Sport Fish.Abstr., W.R.C.Inf., Zoo.Rec.
—BLDSC (1582.372500), CASDDS, CISTI, EMDOCS, Infotrieve, ingenta, Linda Hall. **CCC.**
Published by: (Nederlandse Vereniging voor Aquatische Ecologie), Kluwer Academic Publishers Group (Subsidiary of: Wolters Kluwer N.V.), Spuiboulevard 50, PO Box 17, Dordrecht 3300 AA, Netherlands. TEL 31-78-639-2392, FAX 31-78-654-2254, services@wkap.nl, http://www.wkap.nl/journalhome.htm/1386-2588. Ed. Ramesh D Gulati. Pub. D J Larner. R&P Rene Mijs. **Subscr. in the Americas:** Kluwer Academic - Plenum Publishers, 233 Spring St, New York, NY 10013-1578. TEL 212-620-8468, FAX 212-807-1047; **Subscr. to:** Journals Department, PO Box 322, Dordrecht 3300 AH, Netherlands. TEL 31-78-639-2392, FAX 31-78-654-6474.

578.77 DEU ISSN 0003-9136
QH301 CODEN: AHYBA4

ARCHIV FUER HYDROBIOLOGIE. Text in English, French, German. 1906. m. (in 3 vols., 4 nos./vol.). USD 92 per issue domestic; USD 93.10 per issue foreign (effective 2002). adv. bk.rev. bibl, charts, illus. reprint service avail. from SWZ. *Refereed.* **Document type:** *Monographic series, Academic/Scholarly.*
Related titles: Online - full text ed.: (from Institute for Scientific Information); ♦ Supplement: Algological Studies. ISSN 0342-1120; ♦ Advances in Limnology. ISSN 0071-1128; ♦ Archiv fuer Hydrobiologie. Supplement-Band: Arbeiten aus dem Limnologischen Institut der Universitaet Konstanz. ISSN 0930-4681; ♦ Archiv fuer Hydrobiologie. Supplement-Band: Large Rivers. ISSN 0945-3784; ♦ Archiv fuer Hydrobiologie. Supplement-Band: Untersuchungen des Elbe-Aestuars. ISSN 0342-1066.
Indexed: ASCA, Anim.Behav.Abstr. (coverage dropped), Appl.Ecol.Abstr., Aqua.Sci.& Fish.Abstr., Aquacult.Abstr., Biol.Abstr., Chem.Abstr., Chem.Indus.Notes, Chem.Titles, Curr.Adv.Ecol.Sci., Curr.Adv.Gen.& Molec.Biol., Curr.Cont., Deep Sea Res.& Oceanogr.Abstr., Ecol.Abstr., Entomol.Abstr., Environ.Sci.Poll.Mgmt., Excerp.Med., Geo.Abstr.P.G., GeoRef, Geol.Abstr., Helminthol.Abstr., IBR, INIS Atomind., Ind.Sci.Rev., Irr.& Drain.Abstr., Nutr.Abstr., Pollut.Abstr., Rev.Appl.Entomol., Rev.Med.& Vet.Mycol., Rice Abstr., SSCI (coverage dropped), Sci.Cit.Ind., Sel.Water Res.Abstr., So.Pac.Per.Ind., Soils & Fert., Sport Fish.Abstr., W.R.C.Inf., Weed Abstr., Wild.Rev., Zoo.Rec.
—BLDSC (1613.000000), CASDDS, CISTI, EMDOCS, IDS, Infotrieve, ingenta, Linda Hall. **CCC.**
Published by: (International Association for Theoretical and Applied Limnology), E. Schweizerbart'sche Verlagsbuchhandlung, Johannesstr 3A, Stuttgart 70176, Germany. TEL 49-711-625001, FAX 49-711-625005, schweizerbart@schweizerbart.de, http://www.schweizerbart.de. Ed. W Lampert.

578.77 DEU ISSN 0930-4681

ARCHIV FUER HYDROBIOLOGIE. SUPPLEMENT-BAND: ARBEITEN AUS DEM LIMNOLOGISCHEN INSTITUT DER UNIVERSITAET KONSTANZ. Text in German. irreg. price varies. **Document type:** *Monographic series, Academic/Scholarly.*
Former titles (until 1980): Archiv fuer Hydrobiologie. Supplement-Band: Arbeiten aus dem Limnologischen Institut der Universitaet Freiburg (0342-1112); (until 1961): Archiv fuer Hydrobiologie. Supplement-Band: Schriften der Hydrobiologische Station Falkau - Schwarzwald (0425-6581)
Related titles: ♦ Supplement to: Archiv fuer Hydrobiologie. ISSN 0003-9136.
Indexed: Aqua.Sci.& Fish.Abstr., Aquacult.Abstr., Environ.Sci.Poll.Mgmt.
Published by: (Universitaet Konstanz, Limnologische Institut), E. Schweizerbart'sche Verlagsbuchhandlung, Johannesstr 3A, Stuttgart 70176, Germany. TEL 49-711-625001, FAX 49-711-625005, mail@schweizerbart.de, schweizerbart@schweizerbart.de, http://www.schweizerbart.de.

578.77 DEU ISSN 0945-3784

ARCHIV FUER HYDROBIOLOGIE. SUPPLEMENT-BAND: LARGE RIVERS. Text in German. irreg. USD 78 per issue domestic; USD 79 per issue foreign (effective 2001). **Document type:** *Monographic series, Academic/Scholarly.*
Related titles: ♦ Supplement to: Archiv fuer Hydrobiologie. ISSN 0003-9136.
Indexed: Aqua.Sci.& Fish.Abstr., Aquacult.Abstr., Environ.Sci.Poll.Mgmt.
Published by: E. Schweizerbart'sche Verlagsbuchhandlung, Johannesstr 3A, Stuttgart 70176, Germany. TEL 49-711-625001, FAX 49-711-625005, mail@schweizerbart.de, schweizerbart@schweizerbart.de, http://www.schweizerbart.de.

578.77 DEU ISSN 0342-1066

ARCHIV FUER HYDROBIOLOGIE. SUPPLEMENT-BAND: UNTERSUCHUNGEN DES ELBE-AESTUARS. Text in German. 1961. irreg. USD 78.20 per issue domestic; USD 79.20 per issue foreign (effective 2001). **Document type:** *Monographic series, Academic/Scholarly.*
Related titles: ♦ Supplement to: Archiv fuer Hydrobiologie. ISSN 0003-9136.
Indexed: Aqua.Sci.& Fish.Abstr., Aquacult.Abstr., Environ.Sci.Poll.Mgmt., GeoRef.
Published by: E. Schweizerbart'sche Verlagsbuchhandlung, Johannesstr 3A, Stuttgart 70176, Germany. TEL 49-711-625001, FAX 49-711-625005, mail@schweizerbart.de, schweizerbart@schweizerbart.de, http://www.schweizerbart.de.

578.77 DEU ISSN 1435-6406
QH301 CODEN: AHBSA8

ARCHIV FUER HYDROBIOLOGIE. SUPPLEMENT VOLUMES, MONOGRAPHIC STUDIES. Text in German. 1911. irreg. USD 83 per issue domestic; USD 84 per issue foreign (effective 2001). **Document type:** *Monographic series, Academic/Scholarly.*
Former titles (until 1995): Archiv fuer Hydrobiologie. Supplement-Band, Monographische Beitrage (0341-2881); (until 1967): Archiv fuer Hydrobiologie. Supplement-Band (0365-284X); Archiv fuer Hydrobiologie und Planktonkunde. Supplement-Band (0931-6256)
Indexed: Aqua.Sci.& Fish.Abstr., Aquacult.Abstr., Environ.Sci.Poll.Mgmt., GeoRef, Zoo.Rec.
—CASDDS, CISTI, Infotrieve, ingenta. **CCC.**

Published by: E. Schweizerbart'sche Verlagsbuchhandlung, Johannesstr 3A, Stuttgart 70176, Germany. TEL 49-711-625001, FAX 49-711-625005, mail@schweizerbart.de, schweizerbart@schweizerbart.de, http://www.schweizerbart.de.

570 YUG ISSN 0354-4664
ARCHIVES OF BIOLOGICAL SCIENCES. Text in English. 1949. q.?.
Formerly: Arhiv Bioloskih Nauka (0375-8575)
Indexed: GeoRef, INIS Atomind.
—CISTI.
Published by: Srpsko Biolosko Drustvo, Institut za Bioloska Istrazivanja "Sinisa Stankovic", Kneza Milosa 10/111, Belgrade 11000, Yugoslavia. Ed. Maksim Todorovic.

570 611 ITA ISSN 0004-0223
CODEN: AIAEA2
ARCHIVIO ITALIANO DI ANATOMIA E DI EMBRIOLOGIA/ITALIAN JOURNAL OF ANATOMY AND EMBRYOLOGY. Text in Italian; Summaries in English, French, German. 1902. q. ITL 150,000; ITL 200,000 foreign. adv. bk.rev. charts, illus. index.
Indexed: Biol.Abstr., Chem.Abstr., Curr.Adv.Ecol.Sci., Dent.Ind., Excerp.Med., Ind.Med. (coverage dropped), Ind.Vet., Vet.Bull.
—BLDSC (4588.339500), CASDDS, GNLM, KNAW.
Published by: Editrice Sedicesimo, Via Mannelli, 29 r, Florence, FI 50136, Italy. TEL 055-2476781, FAX 055-2478568. Ed. Enzo Brizzi. Circ: 600.

570 ARG ISSN 0004-0401
ARCHIVO DE CIENCIAS BIOLOGICAS Y NATURALES, TEORICAS Y APLICADAS* . Text in Spanish. 1956. 2/yr. USD 1.
—Linda Hall.
Published by: Librart s.r.l., Casilla Correo 5047, Buenos Aires, Argentina. Ed. A Silvia Colla.

571.3 ESP ISSN 0004-0436
ARCHIVO ESPANOL DE MORFOLOGIA. Text in English, Spanish. 1941, N.S. 1996. 3/yr. ESP 12,000 to individuals; ESP 18,000 to institutions (effective 2000). **Document type:** *Monographic series.*
—GNLM.
Published by: Morphos Ediciones S.L., C PASOS, 3, Alcantarilla, Murcia 30820, Spain. FAX 34-968-8953912, morphos@distrito.com. Ed. Andres Martinez Almagro.

570 PER ISSN 0250-5037
QP82.2.A4 CODEN: ABANDH
ARCHIVOS DE BIOLOGIA ANDINA. Text in Spanish; Text occasionally in English; Summaries in English. 1965. s-a. free per issue. abstr, bibl, charts, stat.
Formerly (until 1977): Universidad Nacional Mayor de San Marcos. Instituto de Biologia Andina. Archivos (0020-3750)
Indexed: A.I.C.P., Biol.Abstr., Chem.Abstr., Ind.Med. (coverage dropped), Rev.Plant Path., Sci.Cit.Ind. (coverage dropped).
—CASDDS.
Published by: Universidad Nacional Mayor de San Marcos, Instituto de Biologia Andina, c/o Centro de Investigacion, Apdo. 5073, Lima, Peru. Ed. Dr. E Picon Reategui. Circ: 1,000.

ARCTIC, ANTARCTIC AND ALPINE RESEARCH. see *SCIENCES: COMPREHENSIVE WORKS*

570.72 ZWE ISSN 0250-6386
AS622 CODEN: AZIMDI
ARNOLDIA ZIMBABWE. Text in English. 1964. irreg. price varies. illus. index. **Document type:** *Academic/Scholarly.* **Description:** Results of research in the natural sciences in southern Africa.
Former titles: Arnoldia Zimbabwe Rhodesia; Arnoldia Rhodesia (0066-7781)
Indexed: Aqua.Sci.& Fish.Abstr., Aquacult.Abstr., Biol.Abstr., Environ.Sci.Poll.Mgmt., GeoRef, P.L.E.S.A. (1990-), Rev.Appl.Entomol., Sport Fish.Abstr., Wild.Rev., Zoo.Rec.
—BLDSC (1684.105000).
Published by: National Museums and Monuments of Zimbabwe, PO Box 240, Bulawayo, Zimbabwe. TEL 60045. Ed. A Kumirai. Circ: 400.

570 DEU ISSN 0171-4090
ARTICULATA; Zeitschrift fuer Biologie, Systematik und Neubeschreibung von Orthopteren. Text in English, French, German. 1975. s-a. EUR 25 (effective 2001). bk.rev. index. back issues avail. *Refereed.* **Document type:** *Magazine, Academic/Scholarly.*
Indexed: Entomol.Abstr. (coverage dropped), Ref.Zh., Zoo.Rec.
Published by: Deutsche Gesellschaft fuer Orthopterologie e.V., c/o Dr. Peter Detzel, Ed., Turnierstr 9, Stuttgart 70599, Germany. TEL 49-711-4569428, FAX 49-711-4569632, articulata@goeg.de. Ed., Adv. contact Dr. Peter Detzel. Circ: 650.

ARTIFICIAL LIFE. see *COMPUTERS—Artificial Intelligence*

ASSOCIATION OF MARINE LABORATORIES OF THE CARIBBEAN. PROCEEDINGS. see *EARTH SCIENCES—Oceanography*

570 USA ISSN 1531-1074
▼ **ASTROBIOLOGY.** Text in English. 2001. q. USD 138 domestic to individuals; USD 169 foreign to individuals; USD 219 domestic to libraries; USD 259 foreign to libraries; USD 166 domestic to individuals print and online eds. combined; USD 197 foreign to individuals print and online eds. combined; USD 263 domestic to libraries print and online eds. combined; USD 303 foreign to institutions print and online eds. combined (effective 2002). adv. *Refereed.* **Document type:** *Journal, Academic/Scholarly.* **Description:** Provides a forum for scientists who define the future of astrobiology, including meteoritics, cosmochemistry, gravitational biology, and planetary geology.
Related titles: Online - full text ed.: USD 138 worldwide to individuals; USD 219 worldwide to institutions (2002) (from CatchWord Ltd., RoweCom Information Quest).
Published by: Mary Ann Liebert, Inc. Publishers, 2 Madison Ave, Larchmont, NY 10538. TEL 914—834-3100, FAX 914-834-1388, info@liebertpub.com, http://www.liebertpub.com/ast. Ed. Sherry Cady. R&P Esther Bicovany. Adv. contact Harriet Matysko.

ATENEO PARMENSE. ACTA BIO-MEDICA. see *MEDICAL SCIENCES*

577 AUS ISSN 1442-9985
QH197 CODEN: AJECDQ
AUSTRAL ECOLOGY; a journal of ecology in the Southern Hemisphere. Text in English. 1976. bi-m. AUD 165 domestic to individuals; AUD 150 in New Zealand to individuals; USD 135 elsewhere to individuals; AUD 704 domestic to institutions; AUD 640 in New Zealand to institutions; USD 695 elsewhere to institutions; AUD 182 domestic to individuals paper & online eds. combined; AUD 165 in New Zealand to individuals paper & online eds. combined; USD 149 elsewhere to individuals paper & online eds. combined; AUD 775 domestic to institutions paper & online eds. combined; AUD 704 in New Zealand to institutions paper & online eds. combined; USD 765 elsewhere to institutions paper & online eds. combined (effective 2001). adv. bk.rev. index. back issues avail.; reprint service avail. from PQC. **Document type:** *Academic/Scholarly.* **Description:** Publishes original papers describing experimental, comprehensive, observational or theoretical studies on terrestrial, marine or freshwater systems.
Formerly (until 2000): Australian Journal of Ecology (0307-692X)
Related titles: Online - full text ed.: ISSN 1442-9993. AUD 149 domestic to individuals; AUD 135 in New Zealand to individuals; USD 122 elsewhere to individuals; AUD 634 domestic to institutions; AUD 576 in New Zealand to institutions; USD 626 elsewhere to institutions (effective 2001) (from EBSCO Publishing, O C L C Online Computer Library Center, Inc., RoweCom Information Quest, ingenta, Munksgaard & Blackwell Science's Synergy, Swets Blackwell, Institute for Scientific Information).
Indexed: AESIS, ASCA, Abstr.Anthropol., Agricola, Agroforest.Abstr., Anim.Behav.Abstr., Apic.Abstr., Appl.Ecol.Abstr., Aqua.Sci.& Fish.Abstr., Aquacult.Abstr., Bibl.Agri., Bio-Contr.News & Info., Biol.Abstr., Chem.Abstr., Crop Physiol.Abstr., Curr.Adv.Ecol.Sci., Curr.Adv.Plant Sci., Curr.Cont., Curr.Ref.Fish Res., Deep Sea Res.& Oceanogr.Abstr., Ecol.Abstr., Eng.Ind., Entomol.Abstr., Environ.Per.Bibl. (1981-), Environ.Sci.Poll.Mgmt., Field Crop Abstr., Forest Prod.Abstr., Forest.Abstr., Geo.Abstr.H.G., Geo.Abstr.P.G., Helminthol.Abstr., Herb.Abstr., INIS Atomind., Ind.Sci.Rev., Ind.Vet., Irr.& Drain.Abstr., Key Word Ind.Wildl.Res., Meteor.& Geoastrophys.Abstr., Ocean.Abstr., Plant Sci., Pollut.Abstr., Rev.Appl.Entomol., Rev.Med.& Vet.Mycol., SSCI (coverage dropped), Sci.Cit.Ind., Seed Abstr., Sel.Water Res.Abstr., Soils & Fert., Sport Fish.Abstr., Weed Abstr., Zoo.Rec.
—BLDSC (1793.105000), CASDDS, CISTI, Ei, EMDOCS, IDS, Infotrieve, ingenta, Linda Hall. **CCC.**
Published by: (Ecological Society of Australia, Flinders University of South Australia, School of Biological Sciences), Blackwell Science Asia Pty Ltd, PO Box 378, Carlton South, VIC 3053, Australia. TEL 61-3-9347-0300, FAX 61-3-9347-5001, info@blacksci-asia.com.au; michael.bull@cc.flinders.edu.au, http://www.blacksci.co.uk. Ed. Michael Bull. Adv. contact Kathryn O'Brien. B&W page AUD 935, color page AUD 1,950; trim 210 x 275. Circ: 1,650.

B B A - BIOENERGETICS. (Biochimica et Biophysica Acta) see *BIOLOGY—Botany*

570 DEU ISSN 0067-2858
BADISCHER LANDESVEREIN FUER NATURKUNDE UND NATURSCHUTZ, FREIBURG. MITTEILUNGEN. NEUE FOLGE. Text in German. 1919. a. DEM 50 (effective 2000). bk.rev. **Document type:** *Academic/Scholarly.* **Description:** Publications on biology, geology and mineralogy.
Indexed: Biol.Abstr., Zoo.Rec.
Published by: Badischer Landesverein fuer Naturkunde und Naturschutz e.V., Gerberau 32, Freiburg Im Breisgau 79098, Germany. TEL 49-761-2012561, FAX 49-761-2012563. Ed. H Koerner. Circ: 2,500.

570 USA ISSN 0198-0068
CODEN: BANRDU
BANBURY REPORTS. Variant title: Banbury Reports Series. Text in English. 1979. irreg., latest vol.35, 1991. price varies. **Document type:** *Monographic series, Academic/Scholarly.* **Description:** Devoted to risk assessments including topics pertaining to human diseases.
Indexed: Biol.Abstr., Chem.Abstr.
—CASDDS, CISTI. **CCC.**
Published by: Cold Spring Harbor Laboratory Press, Publications Department, 10 Skyline Dr, Plainview, NY 11803. TEL 800-843-4388, FAX 516-349-1946, cshpress@cshl.org, http://www.cshl.org. Ed. John Inglis.

570 630 BGD ISSN 1016-4057
BANGLADESH JOURNAL OF BIOLOGICAL SCIENCES. Text in English. 1955. s-a. BDT 30, USD 5. bk.rev. back issues avail.
Former titles: Bangladesh Journal of Biological and Agricultural Sciences (0045-1428); Pakistan Journal of Biological and Agricultural Sciences (0078-8244)
Indexed: Biol.Abstr., Chem.Abstr., Dairy Sci.Abstr., Field Crop Abstr., Herb.Abstr., Plant Breed.Abstr., Zoo.Rec.
—CISTI, Linda Hall.
Published by: Bangladesh Society for Biological and Agricultural Sciences, Dept. of Biochemistry, University of Dhaka, Ramna, Dhaka 2, Bangladesh. Ed. Kamaluddin Ahmad. Circ: 500.

611.018 ITA ISSN 1120-9992
BASIC AND APPLIED MYOLOGY. Short title: B A M. Text in Italian. 1991. bi-m. ITL 15,000, USD 150 (effective 1996). back issues avail. *Refereed.* **Document type:** *Academic/Scholarly.*
—BLDSC (1861.468000), GNLM, IDS.
Published by: (Universita di Padua, Department of Biomedical Sciences), Unipress s.a.s., Via Cesare Battisti, 231, Padua, PD 35121, Italy. FAX 39-49-8752542. Ed. Ugo Carraro. Circ: 100.

570 USA ISSN 0090-5542
CODEN: BLFSBY
BASIC LIFE SCIENCES. Text in English. 1973. irreg., latest vol.66, 1999. price varies. *Refereed.* **Document type:** *Monographic series.*
Indexed: Biol.Abstr., Chem.Abstr., Chem.Indus.Notes, Chem.Titles, Derwent Biotech.Abstr., INIS Atomind., Ind.Med. (1973-).
—BLDSC (1863.980000), CASDDS, CISTI, GNLM, Infotrieve, KNAW. **CCC.**
Published by: Kluwer Academic - Plenum Publishers (Subsidiary of: Wolters Kluwer N.V.), 233 Spring St, New York, NY 10013-1578. TEL 212-620-8000, 800-221-9369, FAX 212-463-0742, info@plenum.com, http://www.plenum.com. Ed. Ernest H Y Chu.

BASLER VEROEFFENTLICHUNGEN ZUR GESCHICHTE DER MEDIZIN UND DER BIOLOGIE. NEUE FOLGE. see *MEDICAL SCIENCES*

338 USA
BAYER ALKALIZER. Text in English. 1936. q. free per issue. back issues avail. **Description:** Employee news of research-based healthcare products manufacturer.
Former titles: Miles Alkalizer; (until 1989): Alkalizer

B

Published by: Bayer Corp., 1884 Miles Ave, Elkhart, IN 46514. TEL 219-264-8111, FAX 219-262-7209, http://www.bayerus.com. Ed. Catherine Wells Bentz. Circ: 6,500 (controlled).

BEHAVIORAL AND BRAIN SCIENCES; an international journal of current research and theory with open peer commentary. see *PSYCHOLOGY*

591.7 USA ISSN 1045-2249
QL750 CODEN: BEECE3
BEHAVIORAL ECOLOGY. Text in English. 1990. bi-m. GBP 41, USD 65 to individuals; GBP 250, USD 400 to institutions (effective 2002). adv. back issues avail. *Refereed.* **Document type:** *Journal, Academic/Scholarly.* **Description:** Publishes research on environmental influences on the evolution and adaptation of animal behavior.
Related titles: Online - full text ed.: ISSN 1465-7279. GBP 225, USD 360 to institutions Online only (effective 2002) (from HighWire Pr., EBSCO Publishing, O C L C Online Computer Library Center, Inc., RoweCom Information Quest, ingenta, Swets Blackwell, Institute for Scientific Information).
Indexed: ASCA, Anim.Behav.Abstr., Anim.Breed.Abstr., Apic.Abstr., Appl.Ecol.Abstr., Aqua.Sci.& Fish.Abstr., Bio-Contr.News & Info., Biotech.& Bioeng.Abstr., Curr.Cont., Ecol.Abstr., Entomol.Abstr., Environ.Per.Bibl. (1993-), Environ.Sci.Poll.Mgmt., Forest.Abstr., Genet.Abstr., Hum.Gen.Abstr., Ind.Vet., Int.Abstr.Biol.Sci., Key Word Ind.Wildl.Res., Rev.Appl.Entomol., Rev.Med.& Vet.Mycol., Sci.Cit.Ind., Seed Abstr., Sport Fish.Abstr., Wild.Rev., Zoo.Rec.
—BLDSC (1877.390000), EMDOCS, IDS, Infotrieve, ingenta. **CCC.**
Published by: (International Society for Behavioral Ecology), Oxford University Press, Academic Division, Great Clarendon St, Oxford OX2 6DP, United Kingdom. TEL 44-1865-267907, FAX 44-1865-267835, jnlorders@oup-usa.org, jnl.info@oup.co.uk, http://beheco.oupjournals.org/, http://www.oup.co.uk/journals. Eds. Dr. Andrew Bourke, David F Westneat, Dr. Innes Cuthill. Pub. David Prosser. adv.: B&W page GBP 315, B&W page USD 565; trim 190 x 245. Circ: 1,366. **Subscr. outside N. America to:** Journals Marketing, Great Clarendon St, Oxford OX2 6DP, United Kingdom.

BEHAVIORAL ECOLOGY AND SOCIOBIOLOGY. see *ENVIRONMENTAL STUDIES*

570 DEU ISSN 0721-3468
BEITRAEGE ZUR NATURKUNDE DER WETTERAU✶. Text in German; Summaries in English, German. 1981. a. DEM 12. adv. bk.rev. back issues avail.
Related titles: Microfiche ed.: 1981.
Published by: Naturkundlicher Arbeitskreis Wetterau, Fuhrstr 5, Rosbach 61191, Germany. Circ: 800.

570 550 DEU ISSN 0342-5452
BEITRAEGE ZUR NATURKUNDE IN OSTHESSEN. Text in German. 1969. irreg., latest vol.34, 1998. DEM 30. bk.rev. **Document type:** *Monographic series.*
Indexed: GeoRef, Zoo.Rec.
Published by: (Verein fuer Naturkunde in Osthessen e.V.), Verlag Parzeller GmbH & Co. KG, Postfach 409, Fulda 36004, Germany. TEL 49-661-280-0, FAX 49-661-280-285, verlag@parzeller.de. Circ: 500.

500.9 DEU ISSN 0340-4277
QH5 CODEN: BNNIDQ
BEITRAEGE ZUR NATURKUNDE NIEDERSACHSENS. Text in German. 1948. q. DEM 45 (effective 2000). adv. bk.rev. abstr, charts, illus, stat. index. **Document type:** *Academic/Scholarly.* **Description:** Covers general biology as related to the federal state of Lower Saxony and Bremen in Germany.
Formerly (1965-1971): Natur, Kultur und Jagd (0028-0577)
Indexed: Biol.Abstr., Forest.Abstr., Key Word Ind.Wildl.Res., Zoo.Rec.
Address: Kastanienallee 13, Peine 31224, Germany. TEL 49-5171-12233, FAX 49-5171-48283, 0517112233@t-online.de. Ed., Pub. Dr. Hans Oelke. Circ: 700. **Subscr. to:** J. Streichert, Bergweg 6, Ilsede 31241, Germany.

570 580 JPN ISSN 0286-9306
QR171.I6 CODEN: BIMIDK
BIFIDOBACTERIA AND MICROFLORA. Text in Japanese. s-a. USD 65.
Indexed: Aqua.Sci.& Fish.Abstr., Environ.Sci.Poll.Mgmt., Microbiol.Abstr., Pollut.Abstr., Sugar Ind.Abstr.
—CASDDS, CISTI, GNLM.
Published by: (Japan Bifidus Foundation), Business Center for Academic Societies Japan/Nihon Gakkai Jimu Senta, 5-16-9 Honkomagome, Bunkyo-ku, Tokyo 113-0021, Japan. TEL 81-3-5814-5811, FAX 81-3-5814-5822, TELEX 2722268 BCJSP J.

570 580 JPN ISSN 0914-2509
Z5185.B53
BIFIZUSU/BIFIDUS FLORES, FRUCTUS ET SEMINA. Text in Japanese. 1987. s-a. JPY 5,150. **Document type:** *Academic/Scholarly.*
Formed by the merger of (1981-1987): Bifidus: Bibliography of Bifidobacteria and Microflora (0285-7006); (1985-1987): Bifidus, Fructus et Semina (0911-7636); (1984-1987): Nihon Bifizusukin Senta Nyusu (0914-3262)
—CISTI.
Published by: (Nihon Bifizusukin Senta/Japan Bifidus Foundation), Business Center for Academic Societies Japan/Nihon Gakkai Jimu Senta, 5-16-9 Honkomagome, Bunkyo-ku, Tokyo 113-0021, Japan. TEL 81-3-5814-5811, FAX 81-3-5814-5822, TELEX 2722268 BCJSP J.

DIE BINNENGEWAESSER; Einzeldarstellungen aus der Limnologie und ihren Grenzgebieten. see *EARTH SCIENCES—Hydrology*

BIO MED. see *MEDICAL SCIENCES*

570 IND ISSN 0970-0889
CODEN: BSRB
BIO-SCIENCE RESEARCH BULLETIN. Text in English. 1985. 2/yr. (in 18 vols.). INR 300, USD 50, GBP 30 (effective 2001). adv. bk.rev. 110 p./no. 1 cols./p. back issues avail.; reprints avail. *Refereed.* **Document type:** *Bulletin, Journal, Academic/Scholarly.* **Description:** Research papers related with Biological Science and Life Science.
Media: Large Type (11 pt.).
Indexed: Zoo.Rec.
—CCC.
Published by: A.K. Sharma, Ed. & Pub., 19-A, D D A Flats, Mansarover Park, Shahdara, New Delhi 110 032, India. TEL 91-11-2117408, bulletin@mantraonline.com;bulletin@satyam.net.in. R&P, Adv. contact A K Sharma. B&W page INR 1,000, B&W page USD 50, color page INR 2,000, color page USD 100. Circ: 600.

BIODEGRADATION. see *ENVIRONMENTAL STUDIES—Waste Management*

570 GBR ISSN 0265-9247
QH506 CODEN: BIOEEJ
BIOESSAYS; advances in molecular, cellular and developmental biology. Text in English. 1984. m. USD 685 in United States; USD 685 in Canada & Mexico; USD 745 elsewhere; USD 720 combined subscription in United States for print and online eds.; USD 720 combined subscription in Canada & Mexico for print and online eds.; USD 780 combined subscription elsewhere for print and online eds. (effective 2002). adv. reprint service avail. from SWZ. *Refereed.* **Document type:** *Academic/Scholarly.* **Description:** Current-awareness journal reviewing advances in molecular, cellular and developmental biology.
Related titles: Online - full text ed.: ISSN 1521-1878. USD 685 in United States; USD 685 in Canada & Mexico; USD 685 elsewhere (effective 2002) (from EBSCO Publishing, Gale Group, Wiley InterScience, Institute for Scientific Information).
Indexed: ASCA, AgBiotech, Anim.Breed.Abstr., Aqua.Sci.& Fish.Abstr., BBCI, CEABA, Chem.Abstr., Chem.Indus.Notes, Chem.Titles, Crop Physiol.Abstr., Curr.Adv.Biochem., Curr.Adv.Cancer Res., Curr.Adv.Cell & Devel.Biol., Curr.Adv.Ecol.Sci., Curr.Adv.Gen.& Molec.Biol., Curr.Biotech.Abstr., Curr.Cont., Environ.Sci.Poll.Mgmt., Genet.Abstr., Helminthol.Abstr., Hort.Abstr., Hum.Gen.Abstr., Ind.Med. (1984-), Ind.Sci.Rev., Inpharma, Int.Abstr.Biol.Sci., Maize Abstr., Neurosci.Abstr., Neurosci.Cit.Ind., Nuc.Acids Abstr., Nutr.Abstr., Plant Breed.Abstr., Potato Abstr., Protozool.Abstr., Reac., Ref.Zh., Rev.Appl.Entomol., Rev.Plant Path., Sci.Cit.Ind., Soyabean Abstr., Sport Fish.Abstr., Telegen, Triticale Abstr., Weed Abstr., Wild.Rev., Zoo.Rec.
—BLDSC (2072.118000), CASDDS, CISTI, EMDOCS, GNLM, ingenta, Linda Hall.
Published by: Wiley Europe Ltd., Baffins Ln, Chichester, W Sussex PO19 1UD, United Kingdom. TEL 44-1243-779777, FAX 44-1243-775878, subinfo@jwiley.com, customer@wiley.co.uk, http://www.interscience.wiley.com/jpages/0265-9247/, http://www.wiley.co.uk. Ed. Adam S Wilkins. R&P Chris Sheridan. Adv. contact Susan Levey. **Subscr. outside the Americas to:** John Wiley & Sons, Inc., Journals, 605 Third Ave, New York, NY 10158. TEL 212-850-6021, 212-850-6645, subinfo@jwiley.com.

BIOETHICS. see *PHILOSOPHY*

570 USA ISSN 1060-2488
BIOFEEDBACK (CINCINNATI). Text in English. q. USD 105 with S.L.A. membership. adv. bk.rev. bibl. **Document type:** *Newsletter.* **Description:** Contains Division news, announcements, and information of interest to biological science librarians.
Published by: Special Libraries Association, Biological Sciences Division, c/o John Tebo, Ed, Chemistry Biology Lab, University of Cincinnati, 503 Rieveschel Hall, Mail Location 0151, Cincinnati, OH 45221-0151. TEL 513-556-1494, FAX 513-556-1103, tebo@ucbeh.san.uc.edu. R&P Adam Schiff. Adv. contact Lawrence Kelland. Circ: 600 (paid).

572.8 579 DEU ISSN 0940-0079
CODEN: BFRME3
BIOFORUM. Text in German. 1978. 10/yr. EUR 82 (effective 2001). adv. **Document type:** *Magazine, Trade.*
Formerly: Forum Mikrobiologie
Indexed: CEABA, Chem.Abstr., Chem.Indus.Notes, Chem.Titles, VITIS.
—CASDDS, GNLM.
Published by: G I T Verlag GmbH, Roesslerstr 90, Darmstadt 64293, Germany. TEL 49-6151-8090-0, FAX 49-6151-8090144, gitverlaggmbh@gitverlag.com, http://www.gitverlag.com. Ed. J P Matthes. Adv. contact Elke Stoehr TEL 49-6151-8090197. B&W page XEU 3,780, color page XEU 5,260; trim 185 x 260. Circ: 10,000.

572.8 DEU
BIOFORUM INTERNATIONAL. Text in English. 1997. 6/yr. adv. **Document type:** *Magazine, Trade.*
Published by: G I T Verlag GmbH, Roesslerstr 90, Darmstadt 64293, Germany. TEL 49-6151-8090-0, FAX 49-6151-8090144, gitverlaggmbh@gitverlag.com, http://www.gitverlag.com. Ed. Joerg Peter Matthes. Adv. contact Hubert Schulz TEL 49-6151-8090116. B&W page XEU 4,420, color page XEU 5,900; trim 185 x 260. Circ: 27,000 (paid).

570 FRA ISSN 1165-6638
BIOGEOGRAPHICA. Text in English, French, Spanish. 1924. q. FRF 330 domestic to non-members; FRF 375 foreign to non-members; FRF 260 domestic to members; FRF 290 foreign to members (effective 1999). bk.rev. charts, illus. **Document type:** *Bulletin.*
Former titles (until 1992): Societe de Biogeographe. Compte Rendu des Seances (0037-9018); (until 1969): Societe de Biogeographie. Compte-Rendu Sommaire des Seances (1153-320X)
Indexed: Aqua.Sci.& Fish.Abstr., Aquacult.Abstr., Biol.Abstr., Deep Sea Res.& Oceanogr.Abstr., Environ.Sci.Poll.Mgmt., GeoRef, Ind.Med. (coverage dropped), Zoo.Rec.
—BLDSC (2072.169000).
Published by: Societe de Biogeographie, 57 rue Cuvier, Paris Cedex 5 75231, France. Ed. W R Lourenco. Circ: 550.

570.9 JPN ISSN 0067-8716
BIOGEOGRAPHICAL SOCIETY OF JAPAN. BULLETIN/NIHON SEIBUTSU CHIRI GAKKAI KAIHO. Text in English, Japanese; Summaries in English. 1928. a. JPY 6,000, USD 47 (effective 1999). index. **Document type:** *Bulletin, Directory, Proceedings.*
Indexed: Apic.Abstr., Biol.Abstr., Zoo.Rec.
—CCC.
Published by: Biogeographical Society of Japan/Nippon Seibutsu Chiri Gakkai, 2-26-12 Sendagi, Bunkyo-ku, Tokyo 113-0022, Japan. TEL 81-3-3828-0445. Ed. Seiroku Sakai.

▼ **BIOGERONTOLOGY.** see *GERONTOLOGY AND GERIATRICS*

570 ITA ISSN 0392-2510
BIOLOGI ITALIANI. Text in Italian. 1971. m. ITL 30,000, USD 14.98 to non-members. adv. bk.rev. *Refereed.* **Document type:** *Academic/Scholarly.* **Description:** Covers clinical biology, environment, biotechnology, didactic of biology.

Indexed: Helminthol.Abstr., Protozool.Abstr., Ref.Zh., Weed Abstr.
—BLDSC (2072.680000).
Published by: Ordine Nazionale dei Biologi, Via Icilio, 7, Rome, RM 00153, Italy. TEL 39-06-571061, FAX 39-06-57106235. Ed. Ernesto Landi. R&P Federico Santini. Adv. contact Federico Santico. B&W page ITL 1,850,000, color page ITL 2,400,000. Circ: 40,000.

570 MEX ISSN 0185-2000
BIOLOGIA. Text in Spanish. 1970. q. price varies. adv. bk.rev. charts, bibl, illus. cum.index: 1970-1975.
Published by: Consejo Nacional para la Ensenanza de la Biologia, Calejon de Pino 18, Chimalistac San Angel, C.P. 01070, Mexico City, DF, Mexico. Ed. Lopez de la Rosa. Circ: 1,500.

570 ITA
BIOLOGIA E ETOLOGIA. Text in Italian. 1986. irreg., latest vol.4, 1992. price varies. adv. **Document type:** *Monographic series.*
Published by: Liguori Editore srl, Via Posillipo, 394, Naples, NA 80123, Italy. TEL 39-81-7206111, FAX 39-81-7206244, http://www.liguori.it. Ed. Bruno D'Udine. Pub. Guido Liguori. Adv. contact Maria Liguori.

570 POL ISSN 0137-8031
BIOLOGIA W SZKOLE. Text in Polish. 1948. q. PLZ 34 (effective 2002). bk.rev., software rev., Website rev. bibl, illus. 64 p./no. back issues avail. **Document type:** *Journal, Academic/Scholarly.* **Description:** For biology teachers at all levels and for students in teacher training colleges and universities. Discusses developments in the biological sciences and recent achievements in the methodology of teaching biology, with articles to improve teachers' knowledge, and comments on teaching syllabi and school textbooks.
Indexed: AgroLibrex.
Published by: (Poland. Ministerstwo Edukacji Narodowej), Wydawnictwa Szkolne i Pedagogiczne, Pl Dabrowskiego 8, Warsaw 00950, Poland. FAX 48-22-8265451. Ed. Krzystof Spalik. Adv. contact Maria Podstolska. **Dist. by:** Ars Polona, Krakowskie Przedmiescie 7, Warsaw, Poland**; Dist. by:** RUCH S.A., ul Jana Kazimierza 31/33, Warsaw 00958, Poland.

BIOLOGICAL ABSTRACTS; references, abstracts, and indexes to the world's life sciences research literature. see *BIOLOGY—Abstracting, Bibliographies, Statistics*

BIOLOGICAL ABSTRACTS CUMULATIVE INDEXES. see *BIOLOGY—Abstracting, Bibliographies, Statistics*

BIOLOGICAL ABSTRACTS - R R M; references and indexes to the world's life science reports, reviews, and meeting literature. (Reports, Reviews, Meetings) see *BIOLOGY—Abstracting, Bibliographies, Statistics*

BIOLOGICAL ABSTRACTS - R R M CUMULATIVE INDEX. (Reports, Reviews, and Meetings) see *BIOLOGY—Abstracting, Bibliographies, Statistics*

570 USA ISSN 0006-3185
Microfilm 02244 CODEN: BIBUBX
BIOLOGICAL BULLETIN. Text in English. 1897. bi-m. (2 vols./yr.). USD 95 to individuals; USD 235 to institutions; USD 20 newsstand/cover to individuals; USD 40 newsstand/cover to institutions (effective 2001). adv. illus. s-a. index, cum.index (approx. every 10 yrs.). back issues avail.; reprints avail. *Refereed.* **Document type:** *Journal, Trade.* **Description:** Publishes original research reports of general interest to biologists worldwide.
Related titles: E-mail ed.; Microfilm ed.: (from PQC,PMC); Online - full text ed.: (from Gale Group, ProQuest Information & Learning, Northern Light Technology, Inc., Factiva, Institute for Scientific Information).
Indexed: Anim.Behav.Abstr. (coverage dropped), Anim.Breed.Abstr., Appl.Ecol.Abstr., Aqua.Sci.& Fish.Abstr., Biol.& Agr.Ind. (Feb.1983-), Biol.Abstr., Chem.Abstr., Curr.Adv.Ecol.Sci., Curr.Cont., Deep Sea Res.& Oceanogr.Abstr., Ecol.Abstr., Environ.Sci.Poll.Mgmt., Gen.Sci.Ind. (Apr.1984-), Genet.Abstr., GeoRef, Helminthol.Abstr., Hum.Gen.Abstr., INIS Atomind., Ind.Med. (1899-), Ind.Sci.Rev., Ind.Vet., Inpharma, Int.Abstr.Biol.Sci., Int.Aerosp.Abstr., Irr.& Drain.Abstr., Neurosci.Abstr. (coverage dropped), Neurosci.Cit.Ind., Nutr.Abstr., Ocean.Abstr., Pollut.Abstr., Protozool.Abstr., Psychol.Abstr., Reac., Rev.Appl.Entomol., Sci.Cit.Ind., Sel.Water Res.Abstr., Soils & Fert., Sport Fish.Abstr., Vet.Bull., Wild.Rev., Zoo.Rec.
—BLDSC (2075.000000), CASDDS, CISTI, IDS, ingenta, Linda Hall.
Published by: Marine Biological Laboratory, 7 MBL St, Woods Hole, MA 02543-1015. TEL 508-289-7402, subscriptions@mbl.edu; cmarrama@mbl.edu, http://www.biolbull.org/, http://hermes.mbl.edu/BiologicalBulletin/index.html. Ed. Michael J Greenberg. R&P Carol Schachinger. Adv. contact Patty Burns. Circ: 1,850. **Subscr. to:** Patty Burns. TEL 504-289-7402, FAX 508-289-7922.

570 POL ISSN 1426-5656
QH301 CODEN: BSPDAJ
BIOLOGICAL BULLETIN OF POZNAN. Text in English, French, German. 1960. a. price varies. bibl, charts, illus. **Document type:** *Bulletin.*
Formerly (until 1994): Societe des Amis des Sciences et des Lettres de Panan. Bulletin. Serie D: Sciences Biologiques (0079-4570)
Indexed: AgroAgen, Biol.Abstr., Chem.Abstr., Chem.Indus.Notes, Chem.Titles, GeoRef, INIS Atomind., Zoo.Rec.
—CASDDS, CISTI.
Published by: Poznanskie Towarzystwo Przyjaciol Nauk, Ul Sew Mielzynskiego 27-29, Poznan 61725, Poland. TEL 48-61-522205. Ed. Jozef Bielawski. **Dist. by:** Ars Polona, Krakowskie Przedmiescie 7, Warsaw, Poland.

570 USA ISSN 1049-9644
SB925 CODEN: BCIOEB
BIOLOGICAL CONTROL; theory and application in pest management. Text in English. 1991. 9/yr. USD 415 in US & Canada to institutions; USD 465 elsewhere to institutions (effective 2001). *Refereed.* **Document type:** *Academic/Scholarly.* **Description:** Promotes the science and technology of biological control and includes articles on entomology, plant pathology, nematology, and weed science.
Related titles: Online - full text ed.: (from EBSCO Publishing, O C L C Online Computer Library Center, Inc., RoweCom Information Quest, ingenta, Swets Blackwell, IDEAL Online Library, Institute for Scientific Information).
Indexed: ASCA, Agricola, Bibl.Agri., Bio-Contr.News & Info., Biotech.Cit.Ind., Crop Physiol.Abstr., Curr.Adv.Plant Sci., Curr.Cont., Derwent Biotech.Abstr., Field Crop Abstr., Food Sci.& Tech.Abstr., Forest.Abstr., Helminthol.Abstr., Herb.Abstr., Hort.Abstr., Ind.Sci.Rev., Ind.Vet., Int.Abstr.Biol.Sci., Maize Abstr., Ornam.Hort., Plant Breed.Abstr., Plant Sci., Postharvest, Potato Abstr., Poult.Abstr., Protozool.Abstr., Rev.Appl.Entomol., Rev.Med.& Vet.Mycol., Rev.Plant Path., Sci.Cit.Ind., Seed Abstr., Soyabean Abstr., Triticale Abstr., Vet.Bull., Weed Abstr., Wild.Rev., Zoo.Rec.
—BLDSC (2075.130000), ADONIS, CISTI, EMDOCS, IDS, ingenta. **CCC.**
Published by: Academic Press, Inc., Journal Division (Subsidiary of: Harcourt Brace & Company), 525 B St, Ste 1900, San Diego, CA 92101-4495. TEL 619-230-1840, FAX 619-699-6800, apsubs@acad.com, http://www.academicpress.com/biocon.

BIOLOGICAL PSYCHIATRY; a journal of psychiatric research. see *MEDICAL SCIENCES—Psychiatry And Neurology*

BIOLOGICAL PSYCHOLOGY. see *PSYCHOLOGY*

570 619 CHL ISSN 0716-9760
QH301 CODEN: ABMXA2
BIOLOGICAL RESEARCH. Text in English. 1964. q. USD 100 (effective 2000). adv. bk.rev. *Refereed.* **Document type:** *Academic/Scholarly.* **Description:** Publishes original works in the different fields of the biological sciences.
Formerly (until 1992): Archivos de Biologia y Medicina Experimentales (0004-0533)
Related titles: Microfiche ed.: (from PQC); Online - full text ed.: (from SciELO, Institute for Scientific Information).
Indexed: Aqua.Sci.& Fish.Abstr., Aquacult.Abstr., Biol.Abstr., Chem.Abstr., Chem.Indus.Notes, Chem.Titles, Curr.Adv.Ecol.Sci., Curr.Cont. (coverage dropped), Environ.Sci.Poll.Mgmt., Excerp.Med., Helminthol.Abstr., INIS Atomind., Ind.Med. (1992-), Ind.Sci.Rev., Int.Abstr.Biol.Sci., Sci.Cit.Ind. (coverage dropped), Sport Fish.Abstr., Zoo.Rec.
—BLDSC (2077.675000), CASDDS, EMDOCS, GNLM, IDS, KNAW, Linda Hall.
Published by: Sociedad de Biologia de Chile, Casilla 16164, Santiago 9, Chile. TEL 56-2-6862850, FAX 56-2-2225515, pzapata@genes.bio.puc.cl. Ed. Patricio Zapata. Circ: 1,250.

570 FIN ISSN 0356-1062
QH301
BIOLOGICAL RESEARCH REPORTS FROM THE UNIVERSITY OF JYVASKYLA. Text in Finnish. 1975. irreg. per issue exchange basis. **Document type:** *Monographic series.*
Indexed: Zoo.Rec.
Published by: Jyvaskylan Yliopisto/University of Jyvaskyla, Publications Center, PL 35, Jyvaeskylae 40100, Finland. TEL 941-601-211, FAX 603-371. Eds. Jukka Saerkkae, Markku Kuitunen. Circ: 450.

570 GBR ISSN 1464-7931
QH301 CODEN: BRCPAH
BIOLOGICAL REVIEWS. Text in English. 1923. q. GBP 186 to individuals; USD 198 to institutions (effective 2002). bibl, charts, illus. index. back issues avail.; reprint service avail. from SCH,PSC. *Refereed.* **Document type:** *Monographic series.* **Description:** Covers all aspects of biological science. Although scholarly and with extensive bibliographies, the articles are aimed at non-specialist biologists as well as researchers in the field.
Former titles (until 1997): Cambridge Philosophical Society. Biological Reviews (0006-3231); (until 1937): Cambridge Philosophical Society. Biological Reviews and Biological Proceedings (0301-7699); (until 1926): Cambridge Philosophical Society. Proceedings. Biological Sciences
Related titles: Microfiche ed.: (from IDC); Microform ed.: (from PQC); Online - full text ed.: (from EBSCO Publishing, O C L C Online Computer Library Center, Inc., RoweCom Information Quest, Gale Group, Swets Blackwell, Factiva, Institute for Scientific Information).
Indexed: ASCA, Anim.Behav.Abstr., Anim.Breed.Abstr., Appl.Ecol.Abstr., Aqua.Sci.& Fish.Abstr., Bio-Contr.News & Info., Biol.& Agr.Ind. (May 1983-), Biol.Abstr., Chem.Abstr., Curr.Adv.Ecol.Sci., Curr.Cont., Ecol.Abstr., Entomol.Abstr., Environ.Sci.Poll.Mgmt., Excerp.Med., Field Crop Abstr., Gen.Sci.Ind. (Aug.1984-), GeoRef, Geol.Abstr., Helminthol.Abstr., Herb.Abstr., Hort.Abstr., INIS Atomind., Ind.Med. (1935-), Ind.Sci.Rev., Ind.Vet., Inpharma, Int.Abstr.Biol.Sci., Nutr.Abstr., Pollut.Abstr., Protozool.Abstr., Reac., Ref.Zh., Rev.Appl.Entomol., Rev.Med.& Vet.Mycol., Rev.Plant Path., Russ.Acad.Sci.Bibl., SSCI (coverage dropped), Sci.Cit.Ind., Seed Abstr., Soils & Fert., Sport Fish.Abstr., Vet.Bull., Weed Abstr., Wild.Rev., Zoo.Rec.
—BLDSC (2079.000000), CASDDS, CISTI, EMDOCS, IDS, ingenta, Linda Hall. **CCC.**
Published by: (Cambridge Philosophical Society), Cambridge University Press, Edinburgh Bldg, Shaftesbury Rd, Cambridge CB2 2RU, United Kingdom. FAX 44-1223-315052, information@cup.cam.ac.uk, information@cambridge.org, http://www.cup.org/journals/CUPJNS.html. Ed. W A Foster. R&P Linda Nicol.

570 JPN ISSN 0045-2033
CODEN: SBTKAQ
BIOLOGICAL SCIENCE/SEIBUTSU KAGAKU. Text in Japanese. 1949. q. JPY 950 per issue.
Indexed: Chem.Abstr., GeoRef, INIS Atomind., Jap.Per.Ind., Zoo.Rec.
—Linda Hall.
Published by: (Japanese Society of Biological Scientists/Nihon Seibutsu Kagakusha Kyokai), Iwanami Shoten Publishers, 2-5-5 Hitotsubashi, Chiyoda-ku, Tokyo 101-0003, Japan. FAX 03-239-9618. Ed. K Nagano. **Dist. overseas by:** Japan Publications Trading Co., Ltd., PO Box 5030, Tokyo International, Tokyo 100-31, Japan.

570 GBR ISSN 0953-5365
BIOLOGICAL SCIENCES REVIEW. Text in English. 4/yr. GBP 19.95 in United Kingdom; GBP 26 in Europe; GBP 31 elsewhere (effective Sep. 2001). adv. illus. back issues avail. *Refereed.* **Document type:** *Magazine, Academic/Scholarly.*
—BLDSC (2080.455000).
Published by: (School of Biology, University of Manchester), Philip Allan Updates, Market Pl, Deddington, Banbury, Oxon OX15 0SE, United Kingdom. TEL 44-1869-338652, FAX 44-1869-338803, sales@philipallan.co.uk, http://www.philipallan.co.uk. Ed. Patrick Fox. Circ: 24,000.

570 USA ISSN 0006-324X
QH1 CODEN: PBSWAO
BIOLOGICAL SOCIETY OF WASHINGTON. PROCEEDINGS. Text in English. 1880. q. USD 40 (effective 2001). charts, illus. index, cum.index: 1881-1922, 1923-1961. back issues avail. *Refereed.* **Document type:** *Academic/Scholarly.* **Description:** Journal of international scope for publication of papers bearing on systematics in the biological sciences (both botany and zoology, including paleontology).
Related titles: Online - full text ed.: (from Institute for Scientific Information).

B

Indexed: ASCA, Aqua.Sci.& Fish.Abstr., Art & Archaeol.Tech.Abstr., Biol.Abstr., Curr.Adv.Ecol.Sci., Curr.Cont., Deep Sea Res.& Oceanogr.Abstr., Ecol.Abstr., Entomol.Abstr., Environ.Sci.Poll.Mgmt., GeoRef, Geol.Abstr., Ind.Sci.Rev., Ocean.Abstr., Rev.Appl.Entomol., Rev.Med.& Vet.Mycol., Sci.Cit.Ind., So.Pac.Per.Ind., Sport Fish.Abstr., Wild.Rev., Zoo.Rec.
—BLDSC (6661.000000), CISTI, IDS, ingenta, Linda Hall.
Published by: Biological Society of Washington, National Museum of Natural History, Smithsonian Institution, Washington, DC 20560. TEL 202-786-2550, pbsw@allenpress.com, http://www.allenpress.com. Ed. Brian Robbins. Circ: 900. **Subscr. to:** Allen Press Inc., PO Box 1897, Lawrence, KS 66044-8897.

570 GBR ISSN 1045-1056
RA401.A1 CODEN: BILSEC
BIOLOGICALS. Text in English. 1973. q. GBP 215 to institutions (effective 2001). adv. reprint service avail. from SWZ. *Refereed.* **Document type:** *Academic/Scholarly.* **Description:** Devoted to the timely publication of broad ranging reports relevant to the development, preparation, and quality control of biologicals used in human and veterinary medicine.
Formerly: Journal of Biological Standardization (0092-1157)
Related titles: Online - full text ed.: (from EBSCO Publishing, O C L C Online Computer Library Center, Inc., RoweCom Information Quest, ingenta, Swets Blackwell, IDEAL Online Library, Institute for Scientific Information).
Indexed: ASCA, Abstr.Hyg., Agri.& Environ.Biotech.Abstr. (coverage dropped), Agricola, Aqua.Sci.& Fish.Abstr., Biol.Abstr., Cal.Tiss.Abstr., Chem.Abstr., Chem.Indus.Notes, Chem.Titles, Chemorec.Abstr., Curr.Cont., Derwent Biotech.Abstr., Diar.Dis.Res., Dok.Arbeitsmed., Environ.Sci.Poll.Mgmt., Excerp.Med., Helminthol.Abstr., INIS Atomind., Ind.Med. (1990-), Ind.Sci.Rev., Ind.Vet., Inpharma, Int.Abstr.Biol.Sci., Med.& Pharm.Biotech.Abstr., Microbiol.Abstr., Neurosci.Abstr. (coverage dropped), Pharm.&Out.News, Poult.Abstr., Protozool.Abstr., Reac., Rev.Appl.Entomol., Rev.Med.& Vet.Mycol., Sci.Cit.Ind., Trop.Dis.Bull., Vet.Bull.
—BLDSC (2081.670000), ADONIS, CASDDS, CISTI, EMDOCS, GNLM, IDS, Infotrieve, ingenta, KNAW, Linda Hall. **CCC.**
Published by: (International Association for Biologicals CHE), Academic Press (Subsidiary of: Harcourt Publishers Ltd.), 24 Oval Rd, London NW1 7DX, United Kingdom. TEL 44-20-7267-4466, FAX 44-20-7482-2293, apsubs@acad.com, http://www.academicpress.com/biologicals. Eds. Elwyn Griffiths, F Horaud. R&P Catherine John. Adv. contact Nik Screen. **Subscr. to:** Harcourt Publishers Ltd., Foots Cray High St, Sidcup, Kent DA14 5HP, United Kingdom. TEL 44-20-300-3322, FAX 44-20-8309-0807.

570 DEU ISSN 0045-205X
CODEN: BLUZAR
BIOLOGIE IN UNSERER ZEIT. Abbreviated title: B I U Z. Text in German. 1971. bi-m. EUR 148 in Europe; CHF 238 in Switzerland & Liechtenstein; USD 178 elsewhere; EUR 156 in Europe for print and online eds.; CHF 250 in Switzerland & Liechtenstein, for print and online eds.; USD 187 elsewhere for print and online eds. (effective 2002). adv. bk.rev., software rev., Website rev. charts, illus, maps. index. reprint service avail. from ISI. **Document type:** *Journal, Academic/Scholarly.* **Description:** Presents current developments in all areas of biology.
Related titles: Online - full text ed.: ISSN 1521-415X. EUR 148 in Europe; CHF 238 in Switzerland & Liechtenstein; USD 178 elsewhere (effective 2002) (from EBSCO Publishing, Wiley InterScience).
Indexed: Biol.Abstr., Chem.Abstr., Chem.Indus.Notes, Chem.Titles, Excerp.Med., INIS Atomind., Zoo.Rec.
—CASDDS, CISTI, Infotrieve, Linda Hall. **CCC.**
Published by: Wiley - V C H, Postfach 101161, Weinheim 69451, Germany. TEL 49-6201-606-147, FAX 49-6201-606-117, subservice@wiley-vch.de, http://www.wiley-vch.de/home/biuz. Ed. C Von See. R&P Claudia Rutz. Adv. contact Marion Schulz. Circ: 9,610. **Subscr. in the Americas to:** John Wiley & Sons, Inc., Journals. TEL 44-1243-779777, 212-850-6645, FAX 212-850-6021; **Subscr. outside Germany, Austria & Switzerland to:** John Wiley & Sons Ltd., Baffins Ln, Chichester, Sussex PO19 IUD, United Kingdom. TEL 44-1243-779777, FAX 44-1243-843232.

BIOLOGISCHE TIERMEDIZIN. see *VETERINARY SCIENCE*

570 GBR ISSN 0006-3347
QH1 CODEN: BLGTB8
BIOLOGIST. Text in English. 1953. 5/yr. GBP 33 in British Isles; GBP 42 overseas (effective 2000). adv. bk.rev., software rev. illus. **Document type:** *Academic/Scholarly.* **Description:** Overview articles, news, reviews for professional biologists in the areas of biomedical, environmental, agricultural, and educational biology.
Indexed: AgBiotech, Aqua.Sci.& Fish.Abstr., Bio-Contr.News & Info., Br.Archaeol.Abstr., Cont.Pg.Educ., Curr.Adv.Ecol.Sci., Dairy Sci.Abstr., Ecol.Abstr., Environ.Abstr., Environ.Sci.Poll.Mgmt., Field Crop Abstr., Food Sci.& Tech.Abstr., Forest Prod.Abstr., Forest.Abstr., Geo.Abstr.H.G., Helminthol.Abstr., IDA, INIS Atomind., Ind.Med., Ind.Vet., Nutr.Abstr., Ornam.Hort., Plant Breed.Abstr., Rev.Appl.Entomol., Rev.Arom.& Med.Plants, Rev.Plant Path., Rural Devel.Abstr., Seed Abstr., Sel.Water Res.Abstr., Soils & Fert., Sport Fish.Abstr., Triticale Abstr., Vet.Bull., Weed Abstr., Wild.Rev., World Ag.Econ.& Rur.Soc.Abstr., Zoo.Rec.
—BLDSC (2086.200000), CASDDS, CISTI, ingenta, Linda Hall. **CCC.**
Published by: Institute of Biology, 20-22 Queensberry Pl, London SW7 2DZ, United Kingdom. TEL 44-20-7581-8333, FAX 44-20-7823-9409, info@job.primex.co.uk, http://www.iob.org. Ed. Dr. S Silver. Circ: 15,500.

578.77 551.46 RUS ISSN 0134-3475
QH91.A1 CODEN: BIMOD4
BIOLOGIYA MORYA/MARINE BIOLOGY. Text in Russian. 1975. bi-m. illus. **Document type:** *Academic/Scholarly.* **Description:** Publishes papers on marine organisms and their activities, various biological studies conducted on marine objects; practical problems of preservation, rational utilization of biological resources of the sea and limitation of activity of some harmful sea organisms.
Related titles: ♦ English Translation: Russian Journal of Marine Biology. ISSN 1063-0740.
Indexed: Anim.Breed.Abstr., Aqua.Sci.& Fish.Abstr., Aquacult.Abstr., Biol.Abstr., Chem.Abstr., Chem.Indus.Notes, Chem.Titles, Curr.Cont. (coverage dropped), Deep Sea Res.& Oceanogr.Abstr., Ecol.Abstr., Environ.Sci.Poll.Mgmt., Food Sci.& Tech.Abstr., Geol.Abstr., Helminthol.Abstr., Ind.Sci.Rev., Ocean.Abstr. (coverage dropped), Ref.Zh., Sci.Cit.Ind. (coverage dropped), Sel.Water Res.Abstr., Sport Fish.Abstr., Wild.Rev., Zoo.Rec.
—CASDDS, CISTI, East View, Infotrieve, KNAW, Linda Hall. **CCC.**
Published by: (Otdelenie Obshchei Biologii, Rossiiskaya Akademiya Nauk/Russian Academy of Sciences), M A I K Nauka - Interperiodica, Mezhdunarodnyi Otdel, Profsoyuznaya ul 90, Moscow 117864, Russian Federation. TEL 7-095-336-1600, FAX 7-095-336-0666, compmg@maik.ru, http://www.maik.rssi.ru/. Ed. Dr. Vladimir L Kasyanov. Circ: 1,200. **US dist. addr.:** Kluwer Academic Publishers, PO Box 17, Dordrecht 3300 AH, Netherlands. TEL 31-78-639-2392, FAX 31-78-654-6474, http://www.wkap.nl. **Co-sponsor:** Rossiiskaya Akademiya Nauk, Dal'nevostochnyi Nauchnyi Tsentr.

570 IRL ISSN 0791-7945
QH301 CODEN: BENVE3
BIOLOGY AND ENVIRONMENT; proceedings of the Royal Irish Academy. Text in English. 1836. 3/yr. IEP 25 to individuals; IEP 90 to institutions (effective 2000). charts, illus. index, cum.index. *Refereed.* **Document type:** *Proceedings, Academic/Scholarly.*
Formerly (until 1993): Royal Irish Academy. Proceedings. Section B: Biological, Geological and Chemical Sciences (0035-8983)
Related titles: Microform ed.: (from PMC); Online - full text ed.: (from Institute for Scientific Information).
Indexed: ASCA, Aqua.Sci.& Fish.Abstr., Aquacult.Abstr., BHA, Biol.Abstr., Br.Geol.Lit., Chem.Abstr., Curr.Adv.Ecol.Sci., Curr.Cont., Deep Sea Res.& Oceanogr.Abstr., Environ.Abstr., Environ.Sci.Poll.Mgmt., Excerp.Med., Forest.Abstr., GeoRef, Geol.Abstr., Helminthol.Abstr., Herb.Abstr., INIS Atomind., INSPEC (coverage dropped), Ind.Med. (coverage dropped), Ind.Vet., Phys.Ber., Rev.Appl.Entomol., Rev.Plant Path., Sci.Cit.Ind., Soils & Fert., Vet.Bull.
—BLDSC (2086.996500), CASDDS, CISTI, GNLM, KNAW, Linda Hall. **CCC.**
Published by: Royal Irish Academy, 19 Dawson St., Dublin 2, Ireland. TEL 353-1-676-2570, FAX 353-1-676-2346, http://www.ria.ie. Eds. Martin Steer, Paul Giller. Circ: 600.

BIOLOGY AND FERTILITY OF SOILS. see *AGRICULTURE—Crop Production And Soil*

BIOLOGY DIGEST. see *BIOLOGY—Abstracting, Bibliographies, Statistics*

570 FRA ISSN 0253-2069
QH301 CODEN: BYILDJ
BIOLOGY INTERNATIONAL: I U B S NEWSMAGAZINE. Text in French. s-a. USD 40. **Document type:** *Newsletter, Academic/Scholarly.*
Former titles: I U B S Newsmagazine; I U B S Newsletter
Indexed: Biol.Abstr., Sport Fish.Abstr.
—CASDDS, CISTI. **CCC.**
Published by: International Union of Biological Sciences, 51 bd. de Montmorency, Paris 75016, France. TEL 45-25-00-09.

573.6 USA ISSN 0006-3363
QP251.A1 CODEN: BIREBV
BIOLOGY OF REPRODUCTION. Text in English. 1969. m. (in 2 vols.). USD 400; USD 435 foreign; USD 500 both eds.; USD 535 foreign both eds. (effective 2000). adv. abstr, bibl, charts, illus. s-a. index. back issues avail. *Refereed.* **Document type:** *Academic/Scholarly.* **Description:** Publishes original research on a variety of topics in the field of reproductive biology, as well as review articles on topics of importance or controversy.
Related titles: Microform ed.: (from PQC); Online - full text ed.: (from HighWire Pr., EBSCO Publishing, Institute for Scientific Information); ♦ Supplement: Biology of Reproduction. Supplement. ISSN 0523-6754.
Indexed: ASCA, Abstr.Anthropol., AgBiotech, Agricola, Anim.Breed.Abstr., Aqua.Sci.& Fish.Abstr., Bibl.Agri., Biol.Abstr., Chem.Abstr., Chem.Indus.Notes, Chem.Titles, Curr.Adv.Ecol.Sci., Curr.Cont., Dairy Sci.Abstr., Environ.Sci.Poll.Mgmt., Excerp.Med., Focus on: Vet.Sci.& Med., Genet.Abstr., Helminthol.Abstr., Hum.Gen.Abstr., INIS Atomind., Ind.Med. (1969-), Ind.Sci.Rev., Ind.Vet., Inpharma, Int.Abstr.Biol.Sci., Neurosci.Cit.Ind., Nuc.Acids Abstr., Nutr.Abstr., Pharm.&Out.News, Pig News & Info., Pollut.Abstr., Poult.Abstr., Reac., Rev.Med.& Vet.Mycol., Risk Abstr., Saf.Sci.Abstr., Sci.Cit.Ind., Small Anim.Abstr., Soyabean Abstr., Sport Fish.Abstr., Vet.Bull., Wild.Rev., Zoo.Rec.
—BLDSC (2087.220000), CASDDS, CISTI, EMDOCS, GNLM, IDS, ingenta, Linda Hall. **CCC.**
Published by: Society for the Study of Reproduction, 1603 Monroe St, Madison, WI 53711-2021. TEL 608-256-2777, FAX 608-256-4610, ssr@ssr.org; orders@allenpress.com, http://www.biolreprod.org/. Ed. Virendra B Mahesh. R&P, Adv. contact Judith Jansen. Circ: 3,700 (paid). **Subscr. to:** Allen Press Inc., PO Box 1897, Lawrence, KS 66044-8897.

BIOLOGY OF THE NEONATE; foetal and neonatal research. see *MEDICAL SCIENCES—Obstetrics And Gynecology*

BIOMARKERS. see *MEDICAL SCIENCES*

570 USA ISSN 0067-8821
CODEN: BMATBJ
BIOMATHEMATICS. Text in English. 1970. irreg. price varies. reprint service avail. from ISI. **Document type:** *Academic/Scholarly.*
Indexed: Math.R., Sci.Cit.Ind. (coverage dropped), Zent.Math.
—CISTI, Infotrieve. **CCC.**
Published by: Springer-Verlag, Journals (Subsidiary of: BertelsmannSpringer), 175 Fifth Ave, New York, NY 10010. TEL 212-460-1500, FAX 212-473-6272.

570 GBR ISSN 0961-088X
QR1 CODEN: BILEE4
BIOMEDICAL LETTERS; a prestige international biomedical journal for the rapid publication of biomedical communications. Text in English. 1976. GBP 150. adv. bk.rev. abstr, bibl, charts, illus. index. *Refereed.* **Description:** Explores chemical microbiology, cellular pharmacology, virology, bacteriology, biochemistry, immunology, hematology, molecular biology, biochemical genetics and biophysics, radiation biology and cancer research.
Formerly: Microbios Letters (0307-5494)
Related titles: Online - full text ed.: (from Institute for Scientific Information).
Indexed: ASCA, Aqua.Sci.& Fish.Abstr., Biol.Dig., Chem.Abstr., Chem.Indus.Notes, Chem.Titles, Curr.Adv.Ecol.Sci., Curr.Biotech.Abstr., Curr.Cont. (coverage dropped), Excerp.Med., Ind.Vet., Microbiol.Abstr., Nutr.Abstr., Protozool.Abstr., Ref.Zh., Rev.Appl.Entomol., Rev.Arom.& Med.Plants, Rev.Med.& Vet.Mycol., Rev.Plant Path., Sugar Ind.Abstr., Vet.Bull.
—CASDDS, CISTI, GNLM, Infotrieve, KNAW. **CCC.**
Published by: Faculty Press, 88 Regent St, Cambridge CB2 1DP, United Kingdom.

BIOMEDICAL MEETINGS INDEX. see *MEETINGS AND CONGRESSES*

BIOMEDICAL PERSPECTIVES. see *MEDICAL SCIENCES*

B

BIOMEDICAL RESEARCH. see *MEDICAL SCIENCES*

▼ BIOMEDICAL RESEARCH; an interdisciplinary journal for the biomedical sciences. see *MEDICAL SCIENCES*

BIOMEDICAL TECHNOLOGY RESEARCH RESOURCES; a research resources directory. see *MEDICAL SCIENCES*

570 MEX ISSN 1607-6788
BIOMEDICAS. Variant title: Gaceta Biomedicas. Text in Spanish. 1996. m. **Document type:** *Academic/Scholarly.*
Formerly: Instituto de Investigaciones Biomedicas. Informe (0076-7220)
Related titles: Online - full text ed.: ISSN 1606-8378.
Published by: Universidad Nacional Autonoma de Mexico, Instituto de Investigaciones Biomedicas, Circuito Interior, Ciudad Universitaria, Mexico D.F. 04510 , Mexico. TEL 52-5-6226807, FAX 52-5-6650951, namihira@servidor.unam.mx, http://www.biomedicas.unam.mx/gaceta.asp. Ed. Rosalba Namihira. Circ: 2,000.

BIOMETEOROLOGY; proceedings of the International Congress of Biometeorology. see *METEOROLOGY*

BIOMETEOROLOGY BULLETIN. see *METEOROLOGY*

BIOMETRIC BULLETIN. see *STATISTICS*

570 DEU ISSN 0323-3847
QH323.5 CODEN: BIJODN
BIOMETRICAL JOURNAL; journal of mathematical methods in biosciences. Text in English. 1959. 8/yr. EUR 868 in Europe; CHF 1,468 in Switzerland & Liechtenstein; USD 1,148 elsewhere; EUR 912 in Europe for print and online eds.; CHF 1,542 in Switzerland & Liechtenstein, for print and online eds.; USD 1,206 elsewhere for print and online eds. (effective 2002). adv. bk.rev. abstr, bibl, charts, illus, stat. index. back issues avail.; reprints avail. *Refereed.* **Document type:** *Journal, Academic/Scholarly.* **Description:** Promotes new contributions to the mathematical and statistical theory as well as interesting and original applications of known theoretical methods in the field of biosciences.
Formerly: Biometrische Zeitschrift
Related titles: Online - full text ed.: ISSN 1521-4036. EUR 868 in Europe; CHF 1,468 in Switzerland & Liechtenstein; USD 1,148 elsewhere (effective 2002) (from EBSCO Publishing, Wiley InterScience, Institute for Scientific Information).
Indexed: ASCA, Anim.Breed.Abstr., Biol.Abstr., Biostat., C.C.M.J., Compumath, Curr.Cont. (1973-, dropped), Curr.Ind.Stat., Excerp.Med., GeoRef, INIS Atomind., J.Cont.Quant.Meth., Math.R., Oper.Res.Manage.Sci., Plant Breed.Abstr., Qual.Contr.Appl.Stat., Rice Abstr., SSCI (coverage dropped), Sport Fish.Abstr., Stat.Theor.Meth.Abstr. (1973-), VITIS, Wild.Rev., Zent.Math., Zoo.Rec.
—BLDSC (2087.990000), CISTI, IDS, ingenta, Linda Hall. **CCC.**
Published by: Wiley - V C H, Postfach 101161, Weinheim 69451, Germany. FAX 49-6201-606-117, subservice@wiley-vch.de, http://www.interscience.wiley.com/biometricaljournal, http://www.wiley-vch.de. Ed. Peter Bauer. R&P Claudia Rutz. **Subscr. in the Americas to:** John Wiley & Sons, Inc., Journals. TEL 44-1243-779777, 212-850-6645, FAX 212-850-6021; **Subscr. outside Germany, Austria & Switzerland to:** John Wiley & Sons Ltd., Baffins Ln, Chichester, Sussex PO19 IUD, United Kingdom. TEL 44-1243-779777, FAX 44-1243-843232.

BIOMETRICS. see *STATISTICS*

BIOMETRIKA. see *BIOLOGY—Abstracting, Bibliographies, Statistics*

570 NLD ISSN 0924-7734
QH301
BIONIEUWS. Text in Dutch. 1919-1993; resumed. 20/yr. NLG 130, EUR 58.99 (effective 2001). adv. bk.rev. illus. index. 8 p./no. **Document type:** *Trade.* **Description:** Covers developments in biology and labor conditions affecting the biologist, including scientific policy, education, economic, ethical and environmental topics.
Former titles (until 1992): Biovisie (0921-9234); (until 1989): Biovisie Magazine (0921-9242); Vakblad voor Biologen (0042-2215)
Indexed: Biol.Abstr., Excerp.Med., GeoRef, Leg.Per. (coverage dropped), Sport Fish.Abstr., Zoo.Rec.
—CISTI.
Published by: Nederlands Instituut voor Biologie, Postbus 8616, Utrecht 3503 RP, Netherlands. TEL 31-30-2369244, FAX 31-30-2332877, nibi@nibi.nl, http://www.nibi.nl/bionieuws. Ed. G van Caulil. adv.: B&W page NLG 5,000, color page NLG 6,000; trim 26 x 380. Circ: 9,447.

577 DNK ISSN 0107-4415
BIONYT/BIO-NEWS; populaer forskning. Text in Danish. 1981. irreg. (4-6/yr.). DKK 285 domestic; DKK 345 in Scandinavia; DKK 415 in Europe; DKK 455 rest of world (effective 2000). bk.rev. index, cum index: 1981-1993. back issues avail. **Document type:** *Newsletter.* **Description:** Contains popular reviews and news of international research in biology, medicine and environment with literature references and list of new books in Danish categorized according to subject.
Published by: Foreningen af Yngre Biologer, Falkonergaardsvej 4, Frederiksberg C 1959, Denmark. TEL 45-35-37-64-08, FAX 45-35-37-12-55, bio@forskning.dk. Ed. Ole Terney. Circ: 1,000.

570 600 USA
CODEN: BPTEEP
BIOPHARMACEUTICAL PROCESS VALIDATION. Text in English. 1986. irreg., latest vol.23, 1996. price varies. adv. *Refereed.*
Formerly: Bioprocess Technology Series (0888-7470)
Indexed: Chem.Abstr., Chem.Indus.Notes, Chem.Titles, Eng.Ind.
—BLDSC (2089.860305), CASDDS, CISTI, Ei, KNAW. **CCC.**
Published by: Marcel Dekker, Inc., Attn: Eridania Perrez, 270 Madison Ave, New York, NY 10016-0602. TEL 212-696-9000, 800-228-1160, FAX 212-685-4540, marketing@dekker.com, http://www.dekker.com. Pub. Russell Dekker. R&P Julia Mulligan. Adv. contact Eridania Perez.

BIOPHOENIX DATABASE ON CD-ROM. see *MEDICAL SCIENCES*

570 USA ISSN 0006-3568
QH1 CODEN: BISNAS
BIOSCIENCE. Text in English. 1951. m. USD 242 domestic Print & online eds.; USD 288 foreign Print & online eds. (effective 2001). adv. bk.rev. bibl, illus. index. back issues avail.; reprint service avail. from PQC. *Refereed.* **Document type:** *Journal, Academic/Scholarly.* **Description:** Contains articles from all areas of biological sciences, including animals, humans, plants, and the environment.
Related titles: Microform ed.: (from PQC); Online - full text ed.: ISSN 1525-3244. USD 218 (effective 2001) (from ProQuest Information & Learning, CatchWord Ltd., Gale Group, Ovid Technologies, Inc., BioOne, Northern Light Technology, Inc., EBSCO Publishing, H. W. Wilson, Factiva, Institute for Scientific Information).
Indexed: Abstr.Bull.Inst.Pap.Chem., Acad.Ind., Acid Pre.Dig., AgBiotech, Agri.Eng.Abstr., Agricola, Agroforest.Abstr., Anim.Behav.Abstr., Anim.Breed.Abstr., Appl.Ecol.Abstr., Aqua.Sci.& Fish.Abstr., Bibl.Agri., Bio-Contr.News & Info., Biol.& Agr.Ind. (Jun.1983-), Biol.Abstr., Biol.Dig., Bk.Rev.Ind. (1991-), CEABA, C.I.J.E., Chem.Abstr., Child.Bk.Rev.Ind. (1991-), Crop Physiol.Abstr., Curr.Adv.Ecol.Sci., Curr.Adv.Plant Sci., Curr.Biotech.Abstr., Curr.Cont., Curr.Lit.Fam.Plan., Curr.Tit.Ocean, Cyb.Abstr., Dairy Sci.Abstr., Deep Sea Res.& Oceanogr.Abstr., Entomol.Abstr., Environ.Abstr., Environ.Ind., Environ.Per.Bibl. (1973-), Environ.Sci.Poll.Mgmt., Field Crop Abstr., Forest.Abstr., Fut.Surv., Gard.Lit. (1992-1994), Gen.Sci.Ind. (Apr.1984-), GeoRef, Helminthol.Abstr., Herb.Abstr., Hlth.Ind., Hort.Abstr., INIS Atomind., Ind.Sci.Rev., Ind.Vet., Int.Abstr.Biol.Sci., Irr.& Drain.Abstr., Key Word Ind.Wildl.Res., Mag.Ind., Microbiol.Abstr., Ocean.Abstr. (coverage dropped), PMR, Plant Breed.Abstr., Plant Gen.Res.Abstr., Plant Sci., Pollut.Abstr., R.G. (Jan.1983-), R.G.Abstr. (Jan.1983-), Ref.Sour., Ref.Zh., Rev.Appl.Entomol., Rev.Arom.& Med.Plants, Rev.Med.& Vet.Mycol., Rev.Plant Path., Risk Abstr., SSCI (coverage dropped), Sci.Cit.Ind., Seed Abstr., Sel.Water Res.Abstr., Small Anim.Abstr., Soils & Fert., Sport Fish.Abstr., Telegen, Triticale Abstr., WMB, Weed Abstr., Wild.Rev., World Ag.Econ.& Rur.Soc.Abstr., Zoo.Rec.
—BLDSC (2089.611400), CASDDS, CIS, CISTI, EMDOCS, GNLM, IDS, ingenta, Linda Hall. **CCC.**
Published by: American Institute of Biological Sciences, 1313 Dolley Madison Blvd., Ste 402, McLean, VA 22101. TEL 703-790-1745, FAX 703-790-2672, bioscience@aibs.org, http://www.catchword.com, http://www.aibs.org. Ed. Rebecca Chasan. Pub. Richard T O'Grady. R&P Jill Scott. Adv. contact Caroline Jacobson. Circ: 9,000.

570 575.1 FRA ISSN 1158-467X
CODEN: BIOSER
BIOSCIENCES. Variant title: Biosciences Appliquees. Text and summaries in English, French. 1982. q. FRF 450, USD 50. adv. bk.rev. index. **Document type:** *Academic/Scholarly.*
Formerly (until 1990): Bio-Sciences (Chateaufort) (0292-8418)
Indexed: Apic.Abstr., Biodet.Abstr., Curr.Biotech.Abstr. —CASDDS, CISTI.
Published by: Dunod, 5 rue Laromiguiere, Paris 75005, France. TEL 33-1-40466200, FAX 33-1-40466201, http://www.gauthier-villars.fr. Ed. Christian Doinel. Circ: 1,000.

BIOSIS EVOLUTIONS. see *BIOLOGY—Abstracting, Bibliographies, Statistics*

BIOSIS SEARCH GUIDE (YEAR). see *BIOLOGY—Abstracting, Bibliographies, Statistics*

BIOSIS SERIAL SOURCES. see *BIOLOGY—Abstracting, Bibliographies, Statistics*

570 IRL ISSN 0303-2647
QH301 CODEN: BSYMBO
BIOSYSTEMS. Text in English. 1967. 18/yr. EUR 95 in Europe to qualified personnel (effective 2001); JPY 12,600 in Japan to qualified personnel; USD 106 elsewhere to qualified personnel; EUR 1,634 in Europe to institutions; JPY 217,200 in Japan to institutions; USD 1,828 elsewhere to institutions (effective 2002). charts, illus. index. back issues avail. *Refereed.* **Document type:** *Academic/Scholarly.* **Description:** Devoted to achieving an improved understanding of biological origins and evolution by means of the analysis and modeling of complex biological systems.
Formerly (until 1974): Currents in Modern Biology (0011-4014)
Related titles: Microform ed.: (from PQC); Online - full text ed.: (from ingenta, Swets Blackwell, ScienceDirect, Institute for Scientific Information).
Indexed: ASCA, Anim.Breed.Abstr., Aqua.Sci.& Fish.Abstr., Biol.Abstr., Chem.Abstr., Chem.Indus.Notes, Chem.Titles, Compumath, Crop Physiol.Abstr., Curr.Adv.Ecol.Sci., Curr.Cont., Dairy Sci.Abstr., Ecol.Abstr., Environ.Sci.Poll.Mgmt., Excerp.Med., Field Crop Abstr., GeoRef, INIS Atomind., Ind.Med. (1974-), Ind.Sci.Rev., Inpharma, Int.Abstr.Biol.Sci., Nutr.Abstr., Plant Breed.Abstr., Pollut.Abstr., Protozool.Abstr., Reac., Rev.Appl.Entomol., Rev.Med.& Vet.Mycol., Sci.Cit.Ind., Sport Fish.Abstr., Wild.Rev., Zoo.Rec.
—BLDSC (2089.670000), CASDDS, CISTI, EMDOCS, GNLM, IDS, ingenta, Linda Hall. **CCC.**
Published by: Elsevier Science Ireland Ltd, Elsevier House, Brookvale Plaza, E. Park, Shannon, Co. Clare, Ireland. TEL 353-61-709600, FAX 353-61-709100, http://www.elsevier.com/locate/biosystems. Eds. David B Fogel, Michael Conrad. R&P Annette Moloney. **Subscr. in Australasia and the Far East to:** Elsevier Science (Singapore) Pte Ltd, No.1 Temasek Ave, 17-01 Millenia Tower, Singapore 039192, Singapore. TEL 65-434-3727, FAX 65-337-2230, asiainfo@elsevier.com.sg; **Subscr. in the Americas to:** Elsevier Science, PO Box 945, New York, NY 10159-0945. TEL 212-633-3730, FAX 212-633-3680, usinfo-f@elsevier.com; **Subscr. to:** Elsevier Science Inc - Japan Regional Office, 9-15 Higashi-Azabu 1-chome, Minato-ku, Tokyo 106-0044, Japan. TEL 81-3-5561-5033, FAX 81-3-5561-5047, info@elsevier.co.jp. **Subscr. to:** Elsevier Science BV, PO Box 211, Amsterdam 1000 AE, Netherlands. TEL 31-20-485-3757, FAX 31-20-485-3432, nlinfo-f@elsevier.nl.

BIOTECHNOLOGY GUIDE U.S.A. see *BIOLOGY—Biotechnology*

660.6 570 USA
BIOTECHNOLOGY INDUSTRY GUIDE. Text in English. 1996. biennial. USD 49.99; USD 59.95 foreign (effective 1998). **Document type:** *Academic/Scholarly, Trade.* **Description:** Contains contact information for over 950 companies throughout the United States, including biotechnology firms from all sectors of the industry and other large corporations active in pharmaceuticals, diagnostics and agriculture.
Published by: Institute for Biotechnology Information, c/o Mark Dibner, Pres., Box 14569, Research Triangle Park, NC 27709-4569. TEL 919-544-5111, FAX 919-544-5401, ibi@mindspring.com, http://www.bitechinfo.com.

571.3 GBR ISSN 1352-2396
BIOTRANSFORMATIONS (CAMBRIDGE); a survey of the biotransformations of drugs and chemicals in animals. Text in English. 1989. irreg., latest vol.7, 1996. GBP 155 per vol. (effective 2002). 486 p./no. back issues avail. **Document type:** *Monographic series.* **Description:** Surveys the literature on biotransformations in animals.
—GNLM.
Published by: Royal Society of Chemistry, Thomas Graham House, Science Park, Milton Rd, Cambridge CB4 4WF, United Kingdom. TEL 44-1223-420066, FAX 44-1223-423429, sales@rsc.org, http://www.rsc.org/. Ed. D R Hawkins. **Dist. by:** Turpin Distribution Services Ltd., Blackhorse Rd, Letchworth, Herts SG6 1HN, United Kingdom. FAX 44-1462-480947.

570 GBR ISSN 1359-2963
BIOTRANSFORMATIONS (LONDON). Text in English. 1996. s-a. GBP 4,000; GBP 800 renewals. **Description:** Provides data on new and established methods for preparative biosynthetic reactions. Contains both archival and current material from Professor Dr. Klaus Kieslich's Databank of Biotransformations and the Warwick Biotransformation Club.
Media: CD-ROM.
Published by: Chapman & Hall, Electronic Publishing Division, Chapman & Hall, 2-6 Boundary Row, London SE1 8HN, United Kingdom. TEL 44-20-7865-0066, FAX 44-20-7522-0101, cust.serv@chall.co.uk, http://epd.chapmanhall.com. **Dist. by:** Cheriton House, North Way, Andover, Hamps SP10 5BE, United Kingdom. TEL 44-1264-332424, FAX 44-1264-342787.

BIOTRONICS; environment control and environmental biology. see *ENVIRONMENTAL STUDIES*

578.0913 USA ISSN 0006-3606
QH1 CODEN: BTROAZ
BIOTROPICA. Text in English. 1969. q. USD 120 to institutions (effective 2001). adv. back issues avail.; reprint service avail. from PQC. *Refereed.* **Document type:** *Academic/Scholarly.* **Description:** Publishes articles dealing with any phase of tropical biology with related subjects, as long as the primary emphasis is tropical and biological.
Formerly: Association for Tropical Biology. Bulletin
Related titles: Microfilm ed.: (from PQC); Online - full text ed.: (from JSTOR (Web-based Journal Archive), Institute for Scientific Information).
Indexed: ASCA, Agricola, Agroforest.Abstr., Anim.Behav.Abstr., Apic.Abstr., Appl.Ecol.Abstr., Aqua.Sci.& Fish.Abstr., Bio-Contr.News & Info., Biol.Abstr., Chemorec.Abstr., Curr.Adv.Ecol.Sci., Curr.Cont., Deep Sea Res.& Oceanogr.Abstr., Ecol.Abstr., Entomol.Abstr., Environ.Sci.Poll.Mgmt., Excerp.Med., Field Crop Abstr., Forest Prod.Abstr., Forest.Abstr., Geo.Abstr.P.G., Geol.Abstr., Helminthol.Abstr., Hort.Abstr., IDA, Ind.Sci.Rev., Key Word Ind.Wildl.Res., Maize Abstr., Microbiol.Abstr., Ornam.Hort., Plant Breed.Abstr., Protozool.Abstr., Rev.Appl.Entomol., Rev.Arom.& Med.Plants, Rev.Plant Path., Sci.Cit.Ind., Seed Abstr., Sel.Water Res.Abstr., So.Pac.Per.Ind., Soils & Fert., Sport Fish.Abstr., Weed Abstr., Wild.Rev., Zoo.Rec.
—BLDSC (2089.900000), CISTI, IDS, ingenta, Linda Hall.
Published by: Association for Tropical Biology, Inc., The Botanical Review, the New York Botanical Garden Press, Bonx, NY 10458-5126. TEL 202-357-3392, FAX 202-786-2563, atb@allenpress.com, biotropica@umsl.edu; orders@allenpress.com, http://www.allenpress.com. Ed. Robert Marquis. R&P W John Kress TEL 202-357-2534. Circ: 1,600 (paid). **Subscr. to:** Allen Press Inc., PO Box 1897, Lawrence, KS 66044-8897.

570 USA
BIOWORLD INTERNATIONAL. Text in English. w. USD 997 for fax or online eds.; USD 38 newsstand/cover for fax or online eds. (effective 2001). **Document type:** *Newsletter.*
Media: Fax. **Related titles:** Online - full text ed.
Published by: American Health Consultants, BioWorld Publishing Group (Subsidiary of: Medical Economics), PO Box 740021, Atlanta, GA 30374. TEL 404-262-7436, 800-688-2421, FAX 404-814-0759, custserv@ahcpub.com, http://www.ahcpub.com. Pub. Donald R Johnston.

570 USA
BIOWORLD TODAY. Text in English. d. USD 1,897, USD 1,927 for print or fax or online eds.; USD 15 newsstand/cover for print or fax or online eds. (effective 2001). **Document type:** *Newsletter.*
Related titles: Fax ed.; Online - full text ed.
Indexed: Inpharma, Reac.
Published by: American Health Consultants, BioWorld Publishing Group (Subsidiary of: Medical Economics), PO Box 740021, Atlanta, GA 30374. TEL 404-262-7436, 800-688-2421, FAX 404-814-0759, custserv@ahcpub.com, http://www.ahcpub.com. Pub. Donald R Johnston.

BIOWORLD TODAY INDEX. see *BIOLOGY—Abstracting, Bibliographies, Statistics*

577 USA
BIOWORLD WEEK. Text in English. w. USD 747 domestic for print or fax eds.; USD 777 foreign for print or fax eds.; USD 29 newsstand/cover for print or fax eds. (effective 2001). **Document type:** *Newsletter.*
Related titles: Fax ed.
Published by: American Health Consultants, BioWorld Publishing Group (Subsidiary of: Medical Economics), PO Box 740021, Atlanta, GA 30374. TEL 404-262-7436, 800-688-2421, FAX 404-814-0759, 404 262-7837, 800 284-3291, custserv@ahcpub.com, http://www.ahcpub.com. Pub. Donald R Johnston.

BOLETIN DE AGRICULTURA BIOLOGICO-DINAMICA. see *AGRICULTURE*

BOTANISCHER VEREIN VON BERLIN UND BRANDENBURG. VERHANDLUNGEN. see *BIOLOGY—Botany*

BRAGANTIA. see *AGRICULTURE*

570 BRA ISSN 1519-6984
QH301 CODEN: RBBIAL
BRAZILIAN JOURNAL OF BIOLOGY/REVISTA BRASILEIRA DE BIOLOGIA. Text in English, French, German, Italian, Portuguese, Spanish. 1941. q. USD 45. bk.rev. bibl, charts, illus. index.
Formerly: Revista Brasileira de Biologia (0034-7108)
Related titles: Online - full text ed.: (from SciELO).
Indexed: AgBiotech, Anim.Behav.Abstr., Anim.Breed.Abstr., Appl.Ecol.Abstr., Aqua.Sci.& Fish.Abstr., Bio-Contr.News & Info., Biol.Abstr., Chem.Abstr., Crop Physiol.Abstr., Curr.Adv.Biochem., Curr.Adv.Cell & Devel.Biol., Dent.Ind., Entomol.Abstr., Environ.Sci.Poll.Mgmt., Forest.Abstr., GeoRef, Helminthol.Abstr., Herb.Abstr., INIS Atomind., Ind.Med. (1941-), Ind.Vet., Irr.& Drain.Abstr., Nutr.Abstr., Ocean.Abstr., Ornam.Hort., Plant Breed.Abstr., Postharvest, Poult.Abstr., Protozool.Abstr., Rev.Appl.Entomol., Rev.Med.& Vet.Mycol., Rev.Plant Path., Rice Abstr., Rural Devel.Abstr., Seed Abstr., Sel.Water Res.Abstr., Soils & Fert., Sport Fish.Abstr., Triticale Abstr., Vet.Bull., Weed Abstr., Zoo.Rec.
—BLDSC (2277.401300), CASDDS, GNLM, ingenta, Linda Hall.
Published by: Instituto Internacional de Ecologia/International Institute of Ecology, Rua Bento Carlos, 759, Centro, Sao Carlos, SP 13560-660, Brazil. iie@iie.com.br. Ed. Dr. Takako Matsumura Tundisi.

BRAZILIAN JOURNAL OF MEDICAL AND BIOLOGICAL RESEARCH. see *MEDICAL SCIENCES*

570 USA ISSN 0068-2799
CODEN: BSBIAW
BROOKHAVEN SYMPOSIA IN BIOLOGY. Text in English. irreg., latest vol.36, 1991. *Refereed.* **Document type:** *Proceedings.*
Indexed: Anim.Breed.Abstr., Biol.Abstr., Dairy Sci.Abstr., Deep Sea Res.& Oceanogr.Abstr., Excerp.Med., Helminthol.Abstr., Ind.Med. (coverage dropped), Plant Breed.Abstr.
—CASDDS, CISTI.
Published by: (Brookhaven National Laboratory), Kluwer Academic - Plenum Publishers (Subsidiary of: Wolters Kluwer N.V.), 233 Spring St, New York, NY 10013-1578. TEL 212-620-8000, 800-221-9369, FAX 212-463-0742, info@plenum.com, http://www.plenum.com. **Dist. by:** National Technical Information Service, Government Research Center.

570 610 NLD ISSN 0007-4888
R850 CODEN: BEXBAN
BULLETIN OF EXPERIMENTAL BIOLOGY AND MEDICINE. Text in English. 1956. m. EUR 2,753, USD 2,758 to institutions for print or online ed.; EUR 3,303.60, USD 3,309.60 to institutions for print & online eds. combined (effective 2002). back issues avail. *Refereed.* **Document type:** *Journal, Academic/Scholarly.* **Description:** Presents the latest experimental research on key issues in modern biology and medicine, translated from the Russian.
Related titles: Microfilm ed.: (from PQC); Online - full text ed.: (from Swets Blackwell, Kluwer Online, Institute for Scientific Information, RoweCom Information Quest); ♦ Translation of: Byulleten' Eksperimental'noi Biologii i Meditsiny. ISSN 0365-9615.
Indexed: ASCA, Biol.Abstr., Chem.Titles, Curr.Adv.Biochem., Curr.Adv.Ecol.Sci., Curr.Adv.Gen.& Molec.Biol., Curr.Cont. (coverage dropped), Excerp.Med., INIS Atomind., Ind.Med. (1956-), Ind.Sci.Rev., Int.Abstr.Biol.Sci., Neurosci.Cit.Ind., SSCI (coverage dropped), Sci.Cit.Ind.
—BLDSC (0409.500000), CASDDS, CISTI, IDS, ingenta. **CCC.**
Published by: (Rossiiskaya Akademiya Meditsinskikh Nauk RUS), Kluwer Academic Publishers Group (Subsidiary of: Wolters Kluwer N.V.), Spuiboulevard 50, PO Box 17, Dordrecht 3300 AA, Netherlands. TEL 31-78-639-2392, FAX 31-78-654-2254, services@wkap.nl, http://www.wkap.nl/journalhome.htm/0007-4888. Ed. Vladimir N Yarigin. **Subscr. in N America to:** Kluwer Academic - Plenum Publishers, 233 Spring St, New York, NY 10013-1578. TEL 212-620-8468, FAX 212-807-1047; **Subscr. to:** Journals Department, PO Box 322, Dordrecht 3300 AH, Netherlands. TEL 31-78-639-2392, FAX 31-78-654-6474.

570 GBR ISSN 0092-8240
QH505.A1 CODEN: BMTBAP
BULLETIN OF MATHEMATICAL BIOLOGY. Text in English. 1939. bi-m. GBP 508 to institutions (effective 2001). adv. bk.rev., software rev. reprint service avail. from SWZ. *Refereed.* **Document type:** *Bulletin, Academic/Scholarly.* **Description:** Devoted to research at the junction of computational, theoretical and experimental biology.
Formerly: Bulletin of Mathematical Biophysics (0007-4985)
Related titles: Microfilm ed.: (from PQC); Online - full text ed.: (from EBSCO Publishing, O C L C Online Computer Library Center, Inc., RoweCom Information Quest, ingenta, Swets Blackwell, IDEAL Online Library, Institute for Scientific Information).
Indexed: ASCA, Acoust.Abstr., Anim.Breed.Abstr., Appl.Mech.Rev., Aqua.Sci.& Fish.Abstr., Bibl.Agri., Bio-Contr.News & Info., Biol.Abstr., Biostat., Chem.Abstr., Chem.Indus.Notes, Chem.Titles, Compumath, Curr.Adv.Ecol.Sci., Curr.Cont., Curr.Ind.Stat., Deep Sea Res.& Oceanogr.Abstr., Excerp.Med., Helminthol.Abstr., INIS Atomind., INSPEC (Feb.1974-1985, dropped), Ind.Med. (1973-), Ind.Sci.Rev., Ind.Vet., Inpharma, Int.Abstr.Biol.Sci., Math.R., Pharm.&Out.News, Plant Breed.Abstr., Postharvest, Protozool.Abstr., Reac., Rev.Appl.Entomol., Rev.Plant Path., Risk Abstr., Sci.Cit.Ind., Sport Fish.Abstr., Vet.Bull., Weed Abstr., Wild.Rev., Zent.Math., Zoo.Rec.
—BLDSC (2867.970000), CASDDS, CISTI, EMDOCS, GNLM, IDS, ingenta, Linda Hall. **CCC.**
Published by: (Society for Mathematical Biology), Academic Press (Subsidiary of: Harcourt Publishers Ltd.), 24-48 Oval Rd, London NW1 7DX, United Kingdom. TEL 44-20-7267-4466, FAX 44-20-7482-2293, apsubs@acad.com, http://www.academicpress.com/bmb. Ed. Lee A Segel. Circ: 1,250. **Subscr. to:** Harcourt Publishers Ltd., Foots Cray High St, Sidcup, Kent DA14 5HP, United Kingdom. TEL 44-20-8300-3322, FAX 44-20-8309-0807.

611.01816 ITA ISSN 0391-481X
CODEN: BMBMD5
BULLETIN OF MOLECULAR BIOLOGY AND MEDICINE; a journal for the rapid publication of reports in the field of biochemical sciences. Text in English. 1975. q. ITL 90,000, USD 150 (effective 1999). abstr, charts, stat. **Description:** Contains topics about molecular biology and medicine.
Indexed: Chem.Abstr., Chem.Indus.Notes, Chem.Titles, Derwent Biotech.Abstr., Excerp.Med. (1994-).
—BLDSC (2881.370000), CASDDS, CISTI, EMDOCS, GNLM.
Published by: (Dipartimento Biochimica e Biologia Molecolare, Bari and Dipartimento Biochimica e Biotecnologie Mediche, Napoli, Universita degli Studi), Casa Editrice Idelson, Via Annibale De Gasperis, 55, Naples, NA 80137, Italy. TEL 39-81-5524733, FAX 39-81-5518295, idelgno@tin.it, http://www.idelson-gnocchi.com. Eds. Ernesto Quagliariello, Francesco Salvatore.

BUNDESAMT FUER SERA UND IMPFSTOFFE. PAUL-EHRLICH-INSTITUT. ARBEITEN. see *MEDICAL SCIENCES*

570 610 RUS ISSN 0365-9615 CODEN: BEBMAE
BYULLETEN' EKSPERIMENTAL'NOI BIOLOGII I MEDITSINY. Text in Russian. 1936. m. USD 349.95. adv. **Document type:** *Academic/Scholarly.* **Description:** Publishes brief accounts of original experimental research devoted to urgent problems of biology and medicine by members of the Academy of Medical Sciences in their particular fields.
Related titles: ♦ English Translation: Bulletin of Experimental Biology and Medicine. ISSN 0007-4888.
Indexed: Agri.& Environ.Biotech.Abstr. (coverage dropped), Anim.Breed.Abstr., Aqua.Sci.& Fish.Abstr., Aquacult.Abstr., Chem.Abstr., Chem.Indus.Notes, Chem.Titles, Dairy Sci.Abstr., Dent.Ind., Derwent Biotech.Abstr., Environ.Sci.Poll.Mgmt., Excerp.Med., Helminthol.Abstr., INIS Atomind., Ind.Med. (coverage dropped), Ref.Zh., Rev.Med.& Vet.Mycol.
—BLDSC (0025.000000), CASDDS, CISTI, East View, EMDOCS, GNLM, Infotrieve. **CCC.**
Published by: Rossiiskaya Akademiya Meditsinskikh Nauk, Solyanka ul 14, Moscow 109801, Russian Federation. TEL 7-095-9248785, FAX 7-095-9286003. Ed. D S Sarkisov. Adv. contact K V Movsesyan. **Dist. by:** Mezhdunarodnaya Kniga, B Yakimanka 39, Moscow 117049, Russian Federation. TEL 7-095-2384967, FAX 7-095-2384634; **US dist. addr.:** East View Publications, 3020 Harbor Ln N, Minneapolis, MN 55447. TEL 612-550-0961.

C A L M SCIENCE. (Conservation and Land Management) see *CONSERVATION*

C A P TODAY. see *MEDICAL SCIENCES*

C A SELECTS. PSYCHOBIOCHEMISTRY. see *BIOLOGY—Abstracting, Bibliographies, Statistics*

C B E VIEWS. see *PUBLISHING AND BOOK TRADE*

C M A S BULLETIN D'INFORMATION/C M A S NEWSLETTER. (Confederation Mondiale des Activites) see *EARTH SCIENCES—Oceanography*

578.77 FRA ISSN 0007-9723
QH90 CODEN: CBIMA5
CAHIERS DE BIOLOGIE MARINE. Text in English, French. 1960. q. FRF 1,174.15; FRF 1,150 foreign (effective 1999). adv. bk.rev. bibl, charts, illus. back issues avail. *Refereed.* **Document type:** *Academic/Scholarly.* **Description:** Contains papers and short notes concerning marine biology, reproduction, life cycles, developmental biology, morphogenesis, genetics, population dynamics, ecophysiology, plankton, benthos and algology.
Related titles: Online - full text ed.: (from Institute for Scientific Information).
Indexed: ASCA, Aqua.Sci.& Fish.Abstr., Aquacult.Abstr., Biol.Abstr., Chem.Abstr., Curr.Adv.Ecol.Sci., Curr.Adv.Gen.& Molec.Biol., Curr.Cont., Deep Sea Res.& Oceanogr.Abstr., Ecol.Abstr., Environ.Sci.Poll.Mgmt., Geo.Abstr.P.G., GeoRef, Helminthol.Abstr., INIS Atomind., Ind.Sci.Rev., Ocean.Abstr., Pollut.Abstr., Rev.Appl.Entomol., Sci.Cit.Ind. (coverage dropped), Sel.Water Res.Abstr., Soils & Fert., Sport Fish.Abstr., Wild.Rev., Zoo.Rec.
—BLDSC (2948.650000), CASDDS, CISTI, IDS, ingenta, Linda Hall.
Published by: Station Biologique de Roscoff, B.P. 74, Roscoff Cedex 29682, France. TEL 33-2-98292302, FAX 33-2-98292380, jouin@sb-roscoff.fr, http://www.sb-roscoff.fr/services.html. Ed. Claude Jouin Toulmond. Pub. Andre Toulmond. Circ: 400.

570 USA ISSN 0885-4629
Q11 CODEN: CFAMBS
CALIFORNIA ACADEMY OF SCIENCES. MEMOIRS. Text in English. 1868. irreg., latest vol.25. price varies. back issues avail. *Refereed.* **Document type:** *Monographic series.* **Description:** Produces two series of publications containing the results of original research conducted by the scientific staff and research associates of the institution and others.
Indexed: GeoRef, Zoo.Rec.
—BLDSC (5580.300000), Linda Hall.
Published by: California Academy of Sciences, Golden Gate Park, San Francisco, CA 94118. TEL 415-750-7243, FAX 415-750-7090, scipubs@cas.calacademy.org, orders@allenpress.com, www.calacademy.org, http://www.allenpress.com. Ed. Alan E Leviton. R&P Katie Martin. **Subscr. to:** Allen Press Inc., PO Box 1897, Lawrence, KS 66044-8897.

570 510 GBR ISSN 0263-9424 CODEN: CSMBDC
CAMBRIDGE STUDIES IN MATHEMATICAL BIOLOGY. Text in English. 1980. irreg. price varies. **Document type:** *Monographic series.*
Indexed: Biol.Abstr., C.C.M.J., Math.R., Zent.Math., Zoo.Rec.
—BLDSC (3015.994600), CISTI.
Published by: Cambridge University Press, Edinburgh Bldg, Shaftesbury Rd, Cambridge CB2 2RU, United Kingdom. FAX 44-1223-315052, information@cup.cam.ac.uk, information@cambridge.org, http://www.cup.cam.ac.uk, http://www.uk.cambridge.org/journals/pmu. R&P Linda Nicol.

CANADIAN BULLETIN OF FISHERIES AND AQUATIC SCIENCES. see *FISH AND FISHERIES*

570 CAN ISSN 0845-5066
QH301.C246
CANADIAN FEDERATION OF BIOLOGICAL SOCIETIES. ANNUAL MEETING. PROGRAMME, PROCEEDINGS. Text in English. 1987. a. USD 10. adv. author index. **Document type:** *Proceedings.* **Description:** Contains summaries and descriptions of papers, posters and symposia presented at the annual meeting of the federation.
Formed by the 1987 merger of: Programme - Canadian Federation of Biological Societies. Annual Meeting (0845-5058); Canadian Federation of Biological Societies. Annual Meeting. Proceedings (0714-8577); Which continues in part: Canadian Federation of Biological Societies. Programme and Proceedings of the Annual Meeting (0709-1265); Which was formed by the merger of: Canadian Federation of Biological Societies. Programme of the Annual Meeting (0068-8703); Canadian Federation of Biological Societies. Annual Meeting. Proceedings (0068-869X)
Indexed: Biol.Abstr.
—BLDSC (1087.691500).
Published by: Canadian Federation of Biological Societies, 104 1750 Courtwood Cres, Ottawa, ON K2C 2B5, Canada. TEL 613-225-8889, FAX 613-225-9621. R&P Paul Hough. Adv. contact Natalie Lamarche.

570 CAN ISSN 0068-8681
CANADIAN FEDERATION OF BIOLOGICAL SOCIETIES. NEWSLETTER. Text in English, French. 1959. s-a. adv. **Document type:** *Newspaper.* **Description:** Reports about science projects, funding, and new developments in biological sciences.
Related titles: Online - full text ed.
Published by: Canadian Federation of Biological Societies, 104 1750 Courtwood Cres, Ottawa, ON K2C 2B5, Canada. TEL 613-225-8889, FAX 613-225-9621, http://www.fermentas.com/cfbs. R&P Paul Hough. Adv. contact Natalie Lamarche.

570 PRI ISSN 0008-6452
Q1 CODEN: CRJSA4
CARIBBEAN JOURNAL OF SCIENCE. Text in English. 1961. s-a. USD 25 to individuals; USD 45 to institutions; USD 20 to students (effective 2001). bk.rev. cum.index: vol.1-15, vol.16-27. *Refereed.* **Document type:** *Academic/Scholarly.* **Description:** Contains natural history papers pertinent to the Caribbean. Papers are technical, most in the area of botany, zoology, ecology and geology.
Related titles: Online - full text ed.: (from Institute for Scientific Information).
Indexed: Anim.Behav.Abstr., Appl.Ecol.Abstr., Aqua.Sci.& Fish.Abstr., Bio-Contr.News & Info., Biol.Abstr., Curr.Cont., Deep Sea Res.& Oceanogr.Abstr., Ecol.Abstr., Entomol.Abstr., Environ.Sci.Poll.Mgmt., Forest.Abstr., Geo.Abstr.P.G., GeoRef, Geol.Abstr., Hort.Abstr., Ind.Vet., Irr.& Drain.Abstr., Meteor.& Geoastrophys.Abstr., Ocean.Abstr., Pollut.Abstr., Protozool.Abstr., Seed Abstr., Soils & Fert., Sport Fish.Abstr., Wild.Rev., Zoo.Rec.
—BLDSC (3053.100000), CISTI, ingenta, Linda Hall.
Published by: University of Puerto Rico, College of Arts and Sciences, PO Box 9280, Mayaguez, PR 00681-9280. TEL 809-832-4040, ext. 3345, FAX 603-250-7332, j_mari@rumac.upr.clu.edu, http://www.caribjcsi.org, http://mayaweb.upr.clu.edu/artssciences/cjs. Ed. Jose A. Mari Mutt. Circ: 500 (paid).

CARIBBEAN RESEARCH INSTITUTE. REPORT. see *HISTORY—History Of North And South America*

CARNEGIE MUSEUM OF NATURAL HISTORY. ANNALS. see *SCIENCES: COMPREHENSIVE WORKS*

CARNEGIE MUSEUM OF NATURAL HISTORY. BULLETIN. see *SCIENCES: COMPREHENSIVE WORKS*

570.71 USA ISSN 0045-5865
CAROLINA TIPS. Text in English. 1938. 4/yr. free per issue to qualified personnel. adv. bk.rev. illus. index. **Document type:** *Newsletter, Academic/Scholarly.*
Media: Duplicated (not offset). **Related titles:** Online - full text ed.
Indexed: Biol.Abstr.
Published by: Carolina Biological Supply Co., 2700 York Rd, Burlington, NC 27215. TEL 336-584-0381, FAX 336-584-3399, tips@carolina.com. R&P Gwen W Oakley TEL 336-538-6233. Adv. contact Harry Shoffner TEL 336-222-6438. Circ: 100,000.

570 CHE ISSN 1061-5385 CODEN: CADCEF
CELL ADHESION AND COMMUNICATION. Text in English. 1993. 6/yr. GBP 143, USD 173, EUR 190 to individuals; GBP 540, USD 759, EUR 761 to institutions; GBP 828, USD 1,188, EUR 1,194 to corporations (effective 2002). *Refereed.* **Document type:** *Academic/Scholarly.* **Description:** Presents research, short communications, and reviews on all families of adhesion receptors and counterreceptors from diverse biological systems.
Related titles: CD-ROM ed.; Microform ed.; Online - full text ed.: (from EBSCO Publishing, RoweCom Information Quest, Institute for Scientific Information).
Indexed: ASCA, Aqua.Sci.& Fish.Abstr., BBCI, Curr.Cont., Excerp.Med. (1994-), Ind.Med. (1993-), Ind.Sci.Rev., Inpharma, Int.Abstr.Biol.Sci., Protozool.Abstr., Reac., Sci.Cit.Ind.
—BLDSC (3097.655000), CISTI, EMDOCS, GNLM, Infotrieve. **CCC.**
Published by: Gordon and Breach - Harwood Academic (Subsidiary of: Taylor & Francis Group), PO Box 531, Lausanne 1000, Switzerland. http://www.gbhap.com/Cell_Adhesion_Communication/. Ed. Bruce J Nicholson. **Subscr. addr. in US:** International Publishers Direct, PO Box 32160, Newark, NJ 07102. FAX 215-750-6343.

570 USA ISSN 0740-784X
QH601 CODEN: CEMBDG
CELL MEMBRANES, METHODS AND REVIEWS. Text in English. 1974. irreg., latest vol.3, 1987. price varies. *Refereed.* **Document type:** *Monographic series.*
Supersedes (in 1983): Methods in Membrane Biology (0093-4771)
Related titles: Online - full text ed.: (from Institute for Scientific Information).
Indexed: ASCA, BBCI, Biol.Abstr., Chem.Abstr., Excerp.Med., Ind.Sci.Rev., Sci.Cit.Ind.
—CASDDS, CISTI, GNLM, Linda Hall.
Published by: Kluwer Academic - Plenum Publishers (Subsidiary of: Wolters Kluwer N.V.), 233 Spring St, New York, NY 10013-1578. TEL 212-620-8000, 800-221-9369, FAX 212-463-0742, info@plenum.com, http://www.plenum.com.

570 CHN ISSN 1001-0602
CELL RESEARCH/XIBAO YANJIU. Text in English. 1990. q. USD 125 (effective 2000). 104 p./no. *Refereed.* **Document type:** *Academic/Scholarly.* **Description:** Features research work in the field of animal and plant cell biology.
Related titles: Online - full text ed.: (from Institute for Scientific Information).
Indexed: Ind.Med. (1990-).
—BLDSC (3097.858000).
Published by: (Shanghai Xibao Shengwusuo), Kexue Chubanshe/Science Press, 16 Donghuang Cheng Genbei Jie, Beijing 100717, China. Ed. Zheng Yao.

CELL STRESS & CHAPERONES. see *MEDICAL SCIENCES*

572.8 FRA ISSN 0145-5680
QH611 CODEN: CMBID4
CELLULAR AND MOLECULAR BIOLOGY. Text in English; Summaries in English. 1977. 8/yr., latest vol.47, 2001. FRF 3,200, USD 485.71 (effective 2002). adv. bk.rev. index. 150 p./no. Supplement avail.; back issues avail. *Refereed.* **Document type:** *Journal, Academic/Scholarly.* **Description:** Covers all relevant areas of the life sciences. Analyzes the relationship between structure and chemical and/or physical content.
Formerly (until 1977): Annales d'Histochimie (0003-4355); Incorporates: Cyto-Enzymology
Related titles: Online - full content ed.: ISSN 1165-158X. EUR 228.67, USD 242.85 domestic (effective 2002); Online - full text ed.: (from Institute for Scientific Information).
Indexed: ASCA, Aqua.Sci.& Fish.Abstr., BBCI, Bio-Contr.News & Info., Biol.Abstr., Biotech.Cit.Ind., Chem.Abstr., Chem.Indus.Notes, Chem.Titles, Crop Physiol.Abstr., Curr.Cont., Excerp.Med., Hort.Abstr., INIS Atomind., Immun.Abstr. (coverage dropped), Ind.Med. (1992-), Ind.Sci.Rev., Ind.Vet., Inpharma, Maize Abstr., Neurosci.Abstr., Nuc.Acids Abstr., Nutr.Abstr., Pharm.&Out.News, Plant Breed.Abstr., Poult.Abstr., Protozool.Abstr., Reac., Rev.Appl.Entomol., Rev.Arom.& Med.Plants, Rev.Med.& Vet.Mycol., Rev.Plant Path., Rice Abstr., Sci.Cit.Ind., Seed Abstr., Soils & Fert., Soyabean Abstr., Vet.Bull., Virol.Abstr. (coverage dropped).
—BLDSC (3097.921000), CASDDS, CISTI, GNLM, Infotrieve, ingenta, KNAW, Linda Hall. **CCC.**
Published by: C M B Association, 1bis av. du Pave Neuf, Noisy le Grand 93160, France. TEL 33-1-45923719, FAX 33-1-43042030, cmb-ass@wanadoo.fr, http://www.cmb-ass. Ed. Karl-Jurgen Halbhuber. R&P Raymond Wegmann. Adv. contact Mieke Wegmann. B&W page FRF 3,000, color page FRF 5,000; 17.5 x 23. Circ: 750.

571 POL ISSN 1425-8153
CELLULAR & MOLECULAR BIOLOGY LETTERS; an international journal. Text in English. 1996. q., latest vol.6, 2001. PLZ 60 domestic to individuals; DEM 80 in Europe to individuals; USD 60 elsewhere to individuals; PLZ 150 domestic to institutions; DEM 130 in Europe to institutions; USD 100 elsewhere to institutions (effective 2002). back issues avail. *Refereed.* **Document type:** *Academic/Scholarly.* **Description:** Publishes accelerated papers on biochemistry, molecular biology, cellural biology, physiology and biophysics as well as general and applied biotechnology.
Related titles: E-mail ed.; Online - full text ed.: (from Institute for Scientific Information).
Indexed: AgroAgen, BBCI, Biotech.& Bioeng.Abstr., Chem.Abstr., Excerp.Med., Genet.Abstr., Int.Abstr.Biol.Sci., Nuc.Acids Abstr., Ref.Zh., Sci.Cit.Ind. (coverage dropped).
—BLDSC (3097.921500).
Published by: (Polskie Towarzystwo Biologii Komorki/Polish Society for Cell Biology), Uniwersytet Wroclawski, Instytut Biochemii, Zaklad Biochemii Genetycznej/University of Wroclaw, Institute of Biochemistry, Department of Genetic Biochemistry, ul Przybyszewskiego 63-77, Wroclaw 51-148, Poland. http://www.microb.uni.wroc.pl/biochem/cmbl.htm. Eds. Aleksander F Sikorski, Arkadiusz Kozubek, Jan Szopa.

509 CHE ISSN 1420-682X
Q1.A1 CODEN: CMLSFI
CELLULAR AND MOLECULAR LIFE SCIENCES. Text in English. 1945. 12/yr. CHF 2,150, USD 1,522; CHF 215, USD 129.06 newsstand/cover (effective 2002). adv. charts, illus. index. back issues avail. *Refereed.* **Document type:** *Journal, Academic/Scholarly.* **Description:** Contains research articles covering the latest aspects of biological and biomedical research with contributions focusing on molecular and cellular aspects of biomedicine, cell biology, immunology, molecular genetics, neuroscience, biochemistry, pharmacology and physiology related to pharmacology.
Formerly (until 1997): Experientia (0014-4754)
Related titles: Online - full text ed.: ISSN 1420-9071 (from EBSCO Publishing, Swets Blackwell, Springer LINK, Institute for Scientific Information).
Indexed: ASCA, Abstr.Hyg., AgBiotech, Agri.& Environ.Biotech.Abstr. (coverage dropped), Agricola, Anim.Behav.Abstr., Anim.Breed.Abstr., Apic.Abstr., Aqua.Sci.& Fish.Abstr., Aquacult.Abstr., Arts & Hum.Cit.Ind. (coverage dropped), Bio-Contr.News & Info., Biodet.Abstr., Biol.Abstr., Cal.Tiss.Abstr., Chem.Abstr., Chem.Cit.Ind., Chem.Infd., Chemorec.Abstr., Cott.& Trop.Fibr.Abstr., Crop Physiol.Abstr., Curr.Adv.Biochem., Curr.Adv.Cancer Res., Curr.Adv.Cell & Devel.Biol., Curr.Adv.Ecol.Sci., Curr.Chem.React., Curr.Cont., Dairy Sci.Abstr., Deep Sea Res.& Oceanogr.Abstr., Dent.Ind., Derwent Biotech.Abstr., Dok.Arbeitsmed., Entomol.Abstr., Environ.Sci.Poll.Mgmt., Excerp.Med., Field Crop Abstr., Food Sci.& Tech.Abstr., Forest Prod.Abstr., Forest.Abstr., GeoRef, Helminthol.Abstr., Herb.Abstr., Hort.Abstr., INIS Atomind., INSPEC (coverage dropped), Ind.Chem., Ind.Med. (1997-), Ind.Sci.Rev., Ind.Vet., Int.Abstr.Biol.Sci., Irr.& Drain.Abstr., Lab.Haz.Bull., Maize Abstr., Mass Spectr.Bull., Met.Abstr., Microbiol.Abstr., NPU, NRN, Neurosci.Abstr., Neurosci.Cit.Ind., Nutr.Abstr., Ocean.Abstr. (coverage dropped), Pig News & Info., Plant Breed.Abstr., Plant Grow.Reg.Abstr., Pollut.Abstr., Poult.Abstr., Protozool.Abstr., Psychol.Abstr., RCI, Rev.Appl.Entomol., Rev.Arom.& Med.Plants, Rev.Med.& Vet.Mycol., Rev.Plant Path., Risk Abstr., SSCI (coverage dropped), Saf.Sci.Abstr., Sci.Cit.Ind., Seed Abstr., Sel.Water Res.Abstr., Soils & Fert., Soyabean Abstr., Sport Fish.Abstr., Sugar Ind.Abstr., THA, Tox.Abstr., Triticale Abstr., VITIS, Vet.Bull., W.R.C.Inf., Weed Abstr., Wild.Rev., Zoo.Rec.
—BLDSC (3097.923800), ADONIS, CASDDS, CINDOC, CISTI, EMDOCS, GNLM, IDS, ingenta, Linda Hall. **CCC.**
Published by: Birkhaeuser Verlag AG (Subsidiary of: BertelsmannSpringer), Klosterberg, Postfach 133, Basel 4010, Switzerland. TEL 41-61-2050730, FAX 41-61-2050792, cmls@birkhauser.ch, http://link.springer.de/link/service/journals/00018/index.htm, http://www.birkhauser.ch/journals. Ed. P Jolles. **Dist. in N.America by:** Springer-Verlag, 333 Meadowlands Parkway, Secaucus, NJ 07094. TEL 800-777-4643, FAX 201-348-4505.

617.22 570.22 USA ISSN 1052-5882
CODEN: CMMIEQ
CELLULAR AND MOLECULAR MECHANISMS OF INFLAMMATION; receptors of inflammatory cells: structure-function relationships. Text in English. 1990. irreg., latest vol.5, 1999.
Indexed: Chem.Abstr., Chem.Indus.Notes, Chem.Titles.
—CASDDS, CISTI, GNLM, Infotrieve, KNAW. **CCC.**
Published by: Academic Press, Inc., Journal Division (Subsidiary of: Harcourt Brace & Company), 525 B St, Ste 1900, San Diego, CA 92101-4495. TEL 619-231-0926, FAX 619-699-6715. Eds. Charles G Cochrane, Michael A Gimbrone Jr. **Subscr. to:** Order Dept., 6277 Sea Harbor Dr, 4th Fl, Orlando, FL 32887. TEL 800-321-5068.

570 MDG
CENTRE D'INFORMATION ET DE DOCUMENTATION SCIENTIFIQUE ET TECHNIQUE. RECHERCHES POUR LE DEVELOPPEMENT. SERIE SCIENCES BIOLOGIQUE. Text in French; Summaries in English, French. 1985. s-a. MGF 60, USD 10. abstr, bibl, charts, illus, stat. back issues avail.
Indexed: Zoo.Rec.
Published by: Centre d'Information et de Documentation Scientifique et Technique, BP 6224, Antananarivo 101, Madagascar. TEL 261-2-33288. Circ: 1,000.

616.96 CZE
CESKA PARAZITOLOGICKA SPOLECNOST. ZPRAVY/CZECH PARASITOLOGY SOCIETY. REPORTS. Text in Czech. q. bk.rev. **Document type:** *Academic/Scholarly.* **Description:** Contains news of recent society activities and a calendar of related events within the Czech Republic and abroad.
Published by: Ceska Akademie Ved, Parazitologicky Ustav, Branisovska 31, Ceske Budejovice 37005, Czech Republic. oleg@paru.cas.cz, http://www.paru.cas.cz. Ed. Oleg Ditrich.

578.77 CZE
CESKE AKADEMIE VED. HYDROBIOLOGICKY USTAV. ANNUAL REPORT. Text in English. 1960. a. per issue exchange basis only. back issues avail. **Document type:** *Academic/Scholarly.* **Description:** Contains brief description of scientific results and other activities of the institute during a given year.
Former titles: Academy of Sciences of the Czech Republic. Hydrobiological Institute. Annual Report (1210-9649); (until 1991): Czechoslovak Academy of Sciences. Institute of Landscape Ecology. Section of Hydrobiology. Annual Report (0232-0533); (until 1983): Czechoslovak Academy of Sciences. Institute of Landscape Ecology. Hydrobiological Laboratory. Annual Report (1210-1338); (until 1980): Czechoslovak Academy of Sciences. Hydrobiological Laboratory. Annual Report (0139-8024)
Related titles: Online - full text ed.
Indexed: Biol.Abstr.
Published by: Ceska Akademie Ved, Hydrobiologicky Ustav, Na Sadkach 7, Ceske Budejovice 37005, Czech Republic. TEL 420-38-7775819, FAX 420-38-45718, TELEX 144 406 CSAC C, hbu@hbu.cas.cz, http://www.jcu.cz/~hbu. Ed. V Straskrabova. Circ: 750.

CESKO-SLOVENSKA PATOLOGIE A SOUDNI LEKARSTVI. see *MEDICAL SCIENCES*

570 LKA ISSN 0069-2379
CODEN: CYJBA2
CEYLON JOURNAL OF SCIENCE. BIOLOGICAL SCIENCES. Text in English. 1957. a., latest vol.27. LKR 150, USD 16 (effective 2000 - 2001). bk.rev. charts, illus. 70 p./no. back issues avail.; reprints avail. *Refereed.* **Document type:** *Journal, Academic/Scholarly.*
Media: Large Type.
Indexed: Aqua.Sci.& Fish.Abstr., Bio-Contr.News & Info., Biol.Abstr., Curr.Adv.Ecol.Sci., GeoRef, Helminthol.Abstr., Herb.Abstr., Hort.Abstr., IBR, INIS Atomind., Ind.Vet., MLA Intl.Bibl., Maize Abstr., Nutr.Abstr., Ornam.Hort., Plant Breed.Abstr., Postharvest, Protozool.Abstr., Rev.Appl.Entomol., Rev.Med.& Vet.Mycol., Rev.Plant Path., Soyabean Abstr., Sri Lanka Sci.Ind., Triticale Abstr., Vet.Bull., Weed Abstr., Zoo.Rec.
—CISTI, ingenta, Linda Hall.
Published by: University of Peradeniya, P.O. Box 35, Peradeniya, Sri Lanka. TEL 94-8-88678, FAX 94-8-88018, cjs@botany.pdn.ac.lk. Ed. N K B Adikaram. Circ: 300.

CHEMICO-BIOLOGICAL INTERACTIONS; a journal of molecular and biochemical toxicology. see *ENVIRONMENTAL STUDIES—Toxicology And Environmental Safety*

CHEMISTRY & BIOLOGY. see *CHEMISTRY*

CHEMISTRY AND ECOLOGY. see *CHEMISTRY*

CHEMOECOLOGY; evolutionary, mechanistic and environmental approaches to chemically-mediated interactions. see *CHEMISTRY—Organic Chemistry*

CHIHUAHUAN DESERT DISCOVERY. see *EARTH SCIENCES*

CHIHUAHUAN DESERT NEWSBRIEFS. see *EARTH SCIENCES*

CHINESE MEDICAL SCIENCES JOURNAL. see *MEDICAL SCIENCES*

570 ITA ISSN 0390-0037
QP84.6 CODEN: CBLGA2
CHRONOBIOLOGIA. Text in English. 1974. q. ITL 250,000, USD 180. bk.rev. abstr, bibl, illus. index.
Related titles: Microfiche ed.: (from PQC).
Indexed: Apic.Abstr., Aqua.Sci.& Fish.Abstr., Biol.Abstr., Chem.Abstr., Chem.Indus.Notes, Chem.Titles, Curr.Adv.Ecol.Sci., Curr.Cont. (coverage dropped), Excerp.Med., Genet.Abstr., Hum.Gen.Abstr., Ind.Med. (coverage dropped), Psychol.Abstr. (1977-).
—CASDDS, EMDOCS, GNLM, ingenta, KNAW.
Published by: (International Society for Chronobiology USA), Casa Editrice Il Ponte, Casella Postale 1071, Milan, MI 20100, Italy. TEL (0039)-2 31072676. Circ: 6,000.

570 USA ISSN 0742-0528
CODEN: CHBIE4
CHRONOBIOLOGY INTERNATIONAL; The Journal of Biological and Medical Rhythm Research. Text in English. 1984. bi-m. USD 145 to individuals print & online eds.; USD 695 to institutions print only (effective 2002). adv. charts, illus. reprint service avail. from PQC. *Refereed.* **Document type:** *Academic/Scholarly.* **Description:** Publishes original research investigations, short communications, and commentaries in chronobiology and related disciplines.
Incorporates: Annual Review of Chronopharmacology (0743-9539)
Related titles: Online - full text ed.: (from EBSCO Publishing, O C L C Online Computer Library Center, Inc., RoweCom Information Quest, Swets Blackwell, Institute for Scientific Information).
Indexed: ASCA, Anim.Behav.Abstr., Aqua.Sci.& Fish.Abstr., Chem.Abstr., Chem.Indus.Notes, Chem.Titles, Curr.Adv.Cancer Res., Curr.Adv.Ecol.Sci., Curr.Cont., Derwent Biotech.Abstr., Excerp.Med., Ind.Med. (1984-), Ind.Sci.Rev., Inpharma, Int.Abstr.Biol.Sci., Neurosci.Abstr., Pharm.&Out.News, Psychol.Abstr. (1984-), Reac., Ref.Zh., SSCI (coverage dropped), Sci.Cit.Ind.
—BLDSC (3188.320000), CASDDS, CISTI, EMDOCS, GNLM, IDS, Infotrieve, KNAW. **CCC.**
Published by: (International Society for Chronobiology), Marcel Dekker Inc., 270 Madison Ave, New York, NY 10016. TEL 212-696-9000, 800-228-1160, FAX 212-685-4540, http://www.dekker.com/servlet/product/productid/CBI. Eds. Ludger Rensing, Michael Smolensky. R&P Julia Mulligan. Adv. contact Anne Mullins. Circ: 650. **Subscr. to:** PO Box 5005, Monticello, NY 12701. jrnlorders@dekker.com.

578.77 ITA
CIVICA STAZIONE IDROBIOLOGICA DI MILANO. QUADERNI. Text in Italian; Summaries in English. 1970. irreg. free to researchers. bibl, charts, illus. **Document type:** *Academic/Scholarly.*
Indexed: Sport Fish.Abstr., Zoo.Rec.
Published by: Civica Stazione Idrobiologica di Milano, Via Gerolamo Gadio, 2, Milan, MI 20121, Italy. TEL 39-2-86462051, FAX 39-2-8690719, IATOMI@tin.it. Ed. Mauro Mariani. R&P Cristina Gilardi.

570 GBR ISSN 0748-3007
QH83 CODEN: CLADEC
CLADISTICS; the international journal of the Willi Hennig Society. Text in English. 1986. q. GBP 198 to institutions (effective 2001). adv. reprint service avail. from SWZ. *Refereed.* **Document type:** *Academic/Scholarly.* **Description:** Covers theory, method, the philosophical aspects of systematics, and the role of systematic and evolutionary studies in the investigation of biogeographical and other general biological phenomena.
Related titles: Online - full text ed.: (from EBSCO Publishing, O C L C Online Computer Library Center, Inc., RoweCom Information Quest, ingenta, Swets Blackwell, IDEAL Online Library, Institute for Scientific Information).
Indexed: ASCA, Agricola, Curr.Cont., Ecol.Abstr., GeoRef, Geol.Abstr., Ind.Sci.Rev., Rev.Appl.Entomol., Sci.Cit.Ind., Sport Fish.Abstr., Zoo.Rec.
—BLDSC (3274.292500), CISTI, IDS, ingenta, Linda Hall. **CCC.**
Published by: (Willi Hennig Society), Academic Press (Subsidiary of: Harcourt Publishers Ltd.), 24 Oval Rd, London NW1 7DX, United Kingdom. TEL 44-20-7267-4466, FAX 44-20-7482-2293, apsubs@acad.com, http://www.academicpress.com/cladistics; http://www.europe.idealibrary.com/. Eds. C J Humphries, D Upscomb. R&P Catherine John. Adv. contact Nik Screen. Circ: 800. **Subscr. to:** Harcourt Publishers Ltd., Foots Cray High St, Sidcup, Kent DA14 5HP, United Kingdom. TEL 44-20-8300-3322, FAX 44-20-8309-0807.

CLINICAL ANATOMY. see *MEDICAL SCIENCES*

571.3 USA ISSN 0962-8827
CODEN: CDYSEJ
CLINICAL DYSMORPHOLOGY. Text in English. 1992. q. USD 159 domestic to individuals; USD 159 foreign to individuals; USD 507 per issue domestic to institutions; USD 507 per issue foreign to institutions; USD 116 newsstand/cover (effective 2002). adv. bk.rev. illus. reprints avail. *Refereed.* **Document type:** *Academic/Scholarly.* **Description:** Devoted to publishing reports of multiple congenital anomaly syndromes, original studies and review articles on etiology, clinical delineation, genetic mapping, and molecular embryology of birth defects.
Related titles: Online - full text ed.: USD 659.10 domestic academic site license; USD 659.10 foreign academic site license; USD 735.15 domestic corporate site license; USD 735.15 foreign corporate site license (2002) (from EBSCO Publishing, Institute for Scientific Information).
Indexed: ASCA, Biotech.Cit.Ind., Curr.Cont., Excerp.Med. (1994-), Ind.Med. (1992-), Inpharma, Neurosci.Cit.Ind., Pharm.&Out.News, Reac.
—BLDSC (3286.273700), ADONIS, CISTI, EMDOCS, GNLM, IDS, KNAW.
Published by: Lippincott Williams & Wilkins (Philadelphia) (Subsidiary of: Wolters Kluwer N.V.), 530 Walnut St, Philadelphia, PA 19106-3621. TEL 215-521-8300, FAX 215-521-8902, http://www.lww.com. Eds. Dian Donnai, Michael Baraitser, Robin Winter. Circ: 296. **Subscr. to:** PO Box 1600, Hagerstown, MD 21740-1600. TEL 800-777-2295, FAX 301-824-7390.

CLINICAL INVESTIGATOR NEWS. see *PHARMACY AND PHARMACOLOGY*

CLINICAL SCIENCE. see *MEDICAL SCIENCES*

016.574 USA ISSN 0084-8824
COLD SPRING HARBOR LABORATORY. ABSTRACTS OF PAPERS PRESENTED AT MEETINGS. Text in English. irreg. (8-13/yr.). **Document type:** *Abstract/Index.*
Media: Duplicated (not offset).
—CCC.
Published by: Cold Spring Harbor Laboratory Press, Publications Department, 10 Skyline Dr, Plainview, NY 11803. TEL 800-843-4388, FAX 516-349-1946, cshpress@cshl.org, http://www.cshl.org. Circ: (controlled).

570 USA ISSN 0069-5009
COLD SPRING HARBOR LABORATORY. ANNUAL REPORT. Text in English. 1924. a. **Document type:** *Corporate.*
Indexed: Environ.Abstr.
Published by: Cold Spring Harbor Laboratory Press, Publications Department, 10 Skyline Dr, Plainview, NY 11803. TEL 800-843-4388, FAX 516-349-1946, cshpress@cshl.org, http://www.cshl.org. Circ: (controlled).

570 USA ISSN 0091-7451
QH301 CODEN: CSHSAZ
COLD SPRING HARBOR LABORATORY. SYMPOSIA ON QUANTITATIVE BIOLOGY. Text in English. 1933. a. price varies. back issues avail. *Refereed.* **Document type:** *Proceedings, Academic/Scholarly.*
Related titles: Online - full text ed.: (from Institute for Scientific Information).
Indexed: ASCA, BBCI, Biol.& Agr.Ind. (Jan.1989-), Biol.Abstr., Chem.Abstr., Chem.Indus.Notes, Chem.Titles, Curr.Cont., Dent.Ind., Excerp.Med., INIS Atomind., Ind.Med. (1933-), Ind.Sci.Rev., Inpharma, Int.Abstr.Biol.Sci., Maize Abstr., Pharm.&Out.News, Reac., Sci.Cit.Ind., Sport Fish.Abstr., Zoo.Rec.
—BLDSC (3296.000000), CASDDS, CISTI, EMDOCS, GNLM, IDS, ingenta, KNAW, Linda Hall. **CCC.**
Published by: Cold Spring Harbor Laboratory Press, Publications Department, 10 Skyline Dr, Plainview, NY 11803. TEL 800-843-4388, FAX 516-349-1946, cshpress@cshl.org, http://www.cshl.org.

570 USA ISSN 0270-1847
CODEN: CHMSDK
COLD SPRING HARBOR MONOGRAPH SERIES. Text in English. 1970. irreg. price varies. illus. index. **Document type:** *Monographic series, Academic/Scholarly.*
Indexed: Aqua.Sci.& Fish.Abstr., Biol.Abstr., Chem.Abstr., Chem.Indus.Notes, Chem.Titles, Environ.Sci.Poll.Mgmt., Pollut.Abstr., Sci.Cit.Ind. (coverage dropped).
—BLDSC (3295.855000), CASDDS, CISTI, Infotrieve, KNAW. **CCC.**
Published by: Cold Spring Harbor Laboratory Press, Publications Department, 10 Skyline Dr, Plainview, NY 11803. TEL 800-843-4388, FAX 516-349-1946, cshpress@cshl.org, http://www.cshl.org.

570 ESP
COLECCION CIENCIAS BIOLOGICAS. Text in Spanish. 1974. irreg. price varies. **Document type:** *Academic/Scholarly.*
Published by: (Universidad de Navarra, Facultad de Ciencias), Ediciones Universidad de Navarra, S.A. (EUNSA), Pza. Los Sauces, 1-2, Baranain, (Navarra) 31010, Spain. TEL 34-948-256850, FAX 34-948-256854, ensaidi@abc.ibernet.com, http://www.unav.es.

570 USA ISSN 0069-6285
COLUMBIA BIOLOGICAL SERIES. Text in English. 1910. irreg., latest vol.24, 1968. *Refereed.* **Document type:** *Monographic series.*
Published by: Columbia University Press, 61 W 62nd St, New York, NY 10023. TEL 212-666-1000. Ed. Kate Witterberg. R&P Lisa Simmars.

572.8 USA
COLUMBIA SERIES IN MOLECULAR BIOLOGY. Text in English. irreg., latest 1976. price varies. *Refereed.* **Document type:** *Monographic series.*
Published by: Columbia University Press, 61 W 62nd St, New York, NY 10023. TEL 212-666-1000. Ed. Kate Witterberg. R&P Lisa Simmars.

COMMENT; a funding first publication. see *MEDICAL SCIENCES*

570 CHE ISSN 0894-8550
QH301 CODEN: CTBIEK
COMMENTS ON THEORETICAL BIOLOGY. Text in English. 1988. 6/yr. GBP 133, USD 195, EUR 177 to individuals; GBP 371, USD 415, EUR 465 to institutions; GBP 550, USD 625, USD 705 to corporations (effective 2002). **Document type:** *Academic/Scholarly.*
Related titles: Microform ed.
Indexed: Zoo.Rec.
—BLDSC (3336.042000), CISTI. **CCC.**
Published by: Gordon and Breach - Harwood Academic (Subsidiary of: Taylor & Francis Group), PO Box 531, Lausanne 1000, Switzerland. Ed. Mair Zamir. **Subscr. addr. in US:** International Publishers Direct, PO Box 32160, Newark, NJ 07102. FAX 215-750-6343.

COMPARATIVE BRAIN RESEARCH IN MAMMALS. see *MEDICAL SCIENCES—Psychiatry And Neurology*

571.9 USA ISSN 0161-6935
CODEN: CPATDJ
COMPARATIVE PATHOBIOLOGY. Text in English. 1976. irreg. **Document type:** *Monographic series.*
—CASDDS, CISTI.
Published by: Kluwer Academic - Plenum Publishers (Subsidiary of: Wolters Kluwer N.V.), 233 Spring St, New York, NY 10013-1578. TEL 212-620-8000, 800-221-9369, FAX 212-463-0742, info@plenum.com, http://www.plenum.com.

CONSERVATION BIOLOGY. see *CONSERVATION*

CONTEMPORARY TOPICS IN IMMUNOBIOLOGY. see *MEDICAL SCIENCES—Allergology And Immunology*

551.46 USA ISSN 0082-3449
CODEN: CMSCAY
CONTRIBUTIONS IN MARINE SCIENCE. Text in English. 1945. a. USD 30 to individuals; USD 80 to libraries (effective 2000). back issues avail. *Refereed.* **Document type:** *Monographic series.* **Description:** Focuses on monographs, reviews, and lengthy taxonomic keys relevant to the Gulf of Mexico. These lengthy documents are often difficult to publish but serve a valuable scientific role. A unique publication for the Gulf of Mexico and Southern United States.
Formerly (until 1967): University of Texas. Institute of Marine Science. Publications (0096-431X)
Indexed: Appl.Ecol.Abstr. (coverage dropped), Aqua.Sci.& Fish.Abstr., Biol.& Agr.Ind. (coverage dropped), Biol.Abstr., Chem.Abstr., Curr.Adv.Ecol.Sci., Deep Sea Res.& Oceanogr.Abstr., Ecol.Abstr., Environ.Sci.Poll.Mgmt., Excerp.Med., GeoRef, Geol.Abstr., Ind.Sci.Rev., Meteor.& Geoastrophys.Abstr., Nutr.Abstr., Ocean.Abstr., Sci.Cit.Ind. (coverage dropped), Sport Fish.Abstr., Wild.Rev., Zoo.Rec.
—CASDDS, CISTI, ingenta, Linda Hall.
Published by: University of Texas at Austin, Marine Science Institute, 750 Channelview Dr, Port Aransas, TX 78373. TEL 361-749-6732, FAX 361-749-6777, cms@utmsi.utexas.edu, http://www.utmsi.utexas.edu. Eds. Barbara Dorf, Tracy Villareal. Circ: 1,200 (controlled).

CORNELL FOCUS. see *AGRICULTURE*

CORNELL UNIVERSITY. NEW YORK STATE COLLEGE OF AGRICULTURE AND LIFE SCIENCES. BIOMETRICS UNIT. ANNUAL REPORT. see *BIOLOGY—Abstracting, Bibliographies, Statistics*

CRITICAL REVIEWS IN NEUROBIOLOGY. see *MEDICAL SCIENCES—Psychiatry And Neurology*

CURRENT AWARENESS IN BIOLOGICAL SCIENCES. see *BIOLOGY—Abstracting, Bibliographies, Statistics*

B

CURRENT AWARENESS. S D I SERVICE. see *MEDICAL SCIENCES*

CURRENT BIBLIOGRAPHIES ON SCIENCE AND TECHNOLOGY: BIOLOGY, PHARMACY AND FOOD SCIENCE. see *BIOLOGY—Abstracting, Bibliographies, Statistics*

CURRENT BIBLIOGRAPHY ON SCIENCE AND TECHNOLOGY: LIFE SCIENCES/KAGAKU GIJUTSU BUNKEN SOKUHO. RAIFUSAIENSU HEN. see *BIOLOGY—Abstracting, Bibliographies, Statistics*

CURRENT BIOLOGY. see *BIOLOGY—Abstracting, Bibliographies, Statistics*

CURRENT COMMENTS; the newsletter of discovery and innovation. see *MEDICAL SCIENCES—Experimental Medicine, Laboratory Technique*

CURRENT CONTENTS: LIFE SCIENCES. see *BIOLOGY—Abstracting, Bibliographies, Statistics*

572.8 USA

CURRENT PROTOCOLS IN MOLECULAR BIOLOGY. Text in English. 4 base vols. plus q. updates. USD 695 (effective 2001); USD 730 combined subscription for base vol. & update; USD 390 updates for base vol. & update (effective 2002). **Document type:** *Academic/Scholarly.*
Related titles: CD-ROM ed.: USD 675 (effective 2001); USD 705 combined subscription for base vol. & update; USD 375 renewals for base vol. & update (effective 2002).
—BLDSC (3501.540000).
Published by: John Wiley & Sons, Inc., Journals (Subsidiary of: Wiley InterScience), 605 Third Ave, New York, NY 10158. TEL 212-850-6645, FAX 212-850-6021, uscs-wis@wiley.com, http://www.wiley.com. **Subscr. to:** John Wiley & Sons Ltd., Baffins Ln, Chichester, Sussex PO19 IUD, United Kingdom. TEL 44-1243-779777, FAX 44-1243-843232, cs-journals@wiley.co.uk.

570 USA ISSN 0070-2137
QH573 CODEN: CTCRAE

CURRENT TOPICS IN CELLULAR REGULATION. Text in English. 1969. irreg., latest vol.35, 1997. reprint service avail. from ISI. *Refereed.*
Related titles: Online - full text ed.: (from Institute for Scientific Information).
Indexed: ASCA, Biol.Abstr., Chem.Abstr., Chem.Indus.Notes, Chem.Titles, Curr.Adv.Ecol.Sci., Ind.Med. (1969-), Ind.Sci.Rev., Sci.Cit.Ind.
—BLDSC (3504.875000), CASDDS, CISTI, GNLM, ingenta, Linda Hall. **CCC.**
Published by: Academic Press, Inc., Journal Division (Subsidiary of: Harcourt Brace & Company), 525 B St, Ste 1900, San Diego, CA 92101-4495. TEL 619-231-0926, FAX 619-699-6715. Eds. Bernard L Horecker, Earl R Stadtman. **Subscr. to:** Order Dept., 6277 Sea Harbor Dr, 4th Fl, Orlando, FL 32887. TEL 800-321-5068.

570 CHE ISSN 0732-4413
QH301 CODEN: CDBID9

CURRENT TOPICS IN CHINESE SCIENCE. SECTION D: BIOLOGY. Text in English. 1982. irreg., latest vol.3, 1985. *Refereed.* **Document type:** *Monographic series.*
—**CCC.**
Published by: Gordon and Breach - Harwood Academic (Subsidiary of: Taylor & Francis Group), PO Box 531, Lausanne 1000, Switzerland. **Subscr. addr. in US:** International Publishers Direct, PO Box 32160, Newark, NJ 07102. FAX 215-750-6343.

570 USA ISSN 0070-2153
QL951 CODEN: CTDBA5

CURRENT TOPICS IN DEVELOPMENTAL BIOLOGY. Text in English. 1966. irreg., latest vol.39, 1998. reprint service avail. from ISI. *Refereed.* **Document type:** *Monographic series.*
Related titles: Online - full text ed.: (from Institute for Scientific Information).
Indexed: ASCA, Anim.Breed.Abstr., Aqua.Sci.& Fish.Abstr., Aquacult.Abstr., BBCI (coverage dropped), Biol.Abstr., Chem.Abstr., Chem.Indus.Notes, Chem.Titles, Crop Physiol.Abstr., Curr.Adv.Ecol.Sci., Environ.Sci.Poll.Mgmt., Ind.Med. (1966-), Ind.Sci.Rev., Nutr.Abstr., Plant Breed.Abstr., Poult.Abstr., Sci.Cit.Ind., Seed Abstr., Sport Fish.Abstr., Wild.Rev., Zoo.Rec.
—BLDSC (3504.880000), CASDDS, CISTI, GNLM, ingenta, Linda Hall. **CCC.**
Published by: Academic Press, Inc., Journal Division (Subsidiary of: Harcourt Brace & Company), 525 B St, Ste 1900, San Diego, CA 92101-4495. TEL 619-231-0926, FAX 619-699-6715. Ed. A A Moscona. **Subscr. to:** Order Dept., 6277 Sea Harbor Dr, 4th Fl, Orlando, FL 32887. TEL 800-321-5068.

CURRENT TOPICS IN PATHOLOGY. see *MEDICAL SCIENCES*

570 IND ISSN 0378-7540
CODEN: CTSCDI

CURRENT TRENDS IN LIFE SCIENCES; recent researches in cold water fisheries. Text in English. irreg., latest vol.21, 1996. price varies. **Document type:** *Monographic series.*
Indexed: Biol.Abstr., Chem.Abstr., Chem.Indus.Notes, Chem.Titles, Curr.Adv.Ecol.Sci., Curr.Cont. (coverage dropped), Zoo.Rec.
—BLDSC (3504.945000), CASDDS, CISTI, Infotrieve. **CCC.**
Published by: Today and Tomorrow's Printers & Publishers, 24 B-5 Desh Bandhu Gupta Rd., Karol Bagh, New Delhi 110 005, India. TEL 5721928. Ed. K L Sehgal. **Dist. in U.S. by:** Scholarly Publications, 2825 Wilcrest Dr, Ste 255, Houston, TX 77042. TEL 713-781-0070.

570 USA ISSN 0340-8132
CODEN: LSRPD8

DAHLEM WORKSHOP REPORTS. LIFE SCIENCES RESEARCH REPORT. Text in English. 1976. irreg., latest vol.36, 1986. price varies. **Document type:** *Monographic series.*
Indexed: GeoRef.
—CASDDS, CISTI, KNAW. **CCC.**
Published by: Springer-Verlag, Journals (Subsidiary of: BertelsmannSpringer), 175 Fifth Ave, New York, NY 10010. TEL 212-460-1500, FAX 212-473-6272.

DANMARKS FISKERIUNDERSOEGELSER. AARSBERETNING. see *FISH AND FISHERIES*

570 550 DEU ISSN 0416-833X
CODEN: DEBEAC

DECHENIANA-BEIHEFTE (BONN). Text in German; Summaries in English. 1955. irreg., latest vol.38, 1999. price varies. back issues avail. **Document type:** *Monographic series, Academic/Scholarly.*
Indexed: Aqua.Sci.& Fish.Abstr., Aquacult.Abstr., Curr.Adv.Ecol.Sci., Environ.Sci.Poll.Mgmt., GeoRef, Zoo.Rec.
—CISTI, Linda Hall.
Published by: Naturhistorischer Verein, Nussallee 15A, Bonn 53115, Germany. TEL 49-228-735525. Ed., R&P Bodo Moeseler.

570 ITA ISSN 0416-928X
CODEN: DLPNAM

DELPINOA. Text in Italian; Summaries in English. 1959. irreg. per issue exchange basis. bibl, charts, illus.
Indexed: Biol.Abstr.
Published by: Universita degli Studi di Napoli, Dipartimento di Biologia Vegetale, Via Foria, 223, Naples, NA 80139, Italy. Ed. Giuseppe Caputo. Circ: 650.

DEUTSCHE GESELLSCHAFT FUER PATHOLOGIE. VERHANDLUNGEN. see *MEDICAL SCIENCES*

571.3 GBR ISSN 0950-1991
QL951 CODEN: DEVPED

DEVELOPMENT (CAMBRIDGE). Text in English. 1953. s-m. GBP 256 domestic to individuals print ed.; GBP 74 domestic to individuals online ed.; GBP 277 domestic to individuals print & online eds.; USD 430 in North America to individuals print ed.; USD 125 in North America to individuals online ed.; USD 465 in North America to individuals print & online eds. (effective 2001). adv. abstr, bibl, illus. index. back issues avail.; reprints avail. *Refereed.* **Document type:** *Journal, Academic/Scholarly.* **Description:** Focuses on experimental studies of genetic, molecular and cellular aspects of animal and plant development.
Formerly: Journal of Embryology and Experimental Morphology (0022-0752)
Related titles: Online - full text ed.: (from EBSCO Publishing, RoweCom Information Quest, Swets Blackwell, Institute for Scientific Information).
Indexed: AgBiotech, Anim.Breed.Abstr., Aqua.Sci.& Fish.Abstr., Biol.& Agr.Ind. (Jan.1990-), Biol.Abstr., Cal.Tiss.Abstr. (coverage dropped), Chem.Abstr., Chem.Indus.Notes, Chem.Titles, Chemorec.Abstr., Curr.Cont., Dairy Sci.Abstr., Dent.Ind., Entomol.Abstr. (coverage dropped), Excerp.Med., Genet.Abstr., Geo.Abstr.H.G., Helminthol.Abstr., Hum.Gen.Abstr., INIS Atomind., Ind.Med. (1987-), Ind.Sci.Rev., Ind.Vet., Int.Abstr.Biol.Sci., Maize Abstr., Neurosci.Abstr., Nuc.Acids Abstr., Plant Breed.Abstr., Plant Grow.Reg.Abstr., Rev.Appl.Entomol., Sci.Cit.Ind., Seed Abstr., Sport Fish.Abstr., Tox.Abstr. (coverage dropped), Vet.Bull., Wild.Rev., Zoo.Rec.
—BLDSC (3578.598000), CASDDS, CISTI, EMDOCS, GNLM, ingenta, Linda Hall.
Published by: Company of Biologists Ltd., Bidder Bldg, Bidder Building, 140 Cowley Rd, Cambridge CB4 4DL, United Kingdom. TEL 44-1223-426164, FAX 44-1223-423353, sales@biologists.com, http://dev.biologists.org, http://www.biologists.com/development. Ed. Chris Wylie. R&P R Skaer TEL 44-1223-420482. Adv. contact Amanda Sheppardson. Circ: 2,700.

571.3 DEU ISSN 0949-944X
QL951 CODEN: DGEVFT

DEVELOPMENT, GENES AND EVOLUTION. Text in English. 1894. 12/yr. EUR 644.90 domestic; EUR 625.70 in Germany; EUR 59.90 newsstand/cover foreign (effective 2002). adv. bibl, charts, illus. index. back issues avail.; reprint service avail. from ISI. *Refereed.* **Document type:** *Journal, Academic/Scholarly.* **Description:** Reports on experimental work at the systemic, cellular and molecular levels in the field of animal and plant systems.
Former titles: Roux's Archives of Developmental Biology (0930-035X); (until 1986): Wilhelm Roux's Archives of Developmental Biology (0340-0794); Roux' Archiv fuer Entwicklungsmechanik der Organismen (0043-5546)
Related titles: Microform ed.: (from PQC); Online - full text ed.: ISSN 1432-041X (from EBSCO Publishing, RoweCom Information Quest, Swets Blackwell, Springer LINK, Institute for Scientific Information).
Indexed: ASCA, AgBiotech, Anim.Breed.Abstr., Aqua.Sci.& Fish.Abstr., Aquacult.Abstr., Bio-Contr.News & Info., Biol.Abstr., Biotech.& Bioeng.Abstr., Cal.Tiss.Abstr., Chem.Abstr., Chem.Indus.Notes, Chem.Titles, Curr.Adv.Ecol.Sci., Curr.Cont., Environ.Sci.Poll.Mgmt., Excerp.Med., Genet.Abstr., GeoRef, Helminthol.Abstr., Hum.Gen.Abstr., INIS Atomind., Ind.Med. (1996-), Ind.Sci.Rev., Inpharma, Maize Abstr., Microbiol.Abstr., Neurosci.Cit.Ind., Plant Breed.Abstr., Postharvest, Poult.Abstr., Reac., Rev.Appl.Entomol., Sci.Cit.Ind., Seed Abstr., Sport Fish.Abstr., Wild.Rev., Zoo.Rec.
—BLDSC (3579.034000), CASDDS, CISTI, EMDOCS, GNLM, IDS, Infotrieve, ingenta, Linda Hall. **CCC.**
Published by: (European Developmental Biology Organization, Executive Board), Springer-Verlag (Subsidiary of: BertelsmannSpringer), Tiergartenstr 17, Heidelberg 69121, Germany. TEL 49-6221-345-0, FAX 49-6221-345229, subscriptions@springer.de, http://link.springer.de/link/service/journals/00427/index.html, http://www.springer.de. Ed. D Tautz. Adv. contact Edda Lueckermann. **Subscr. in N. America to:** Springer-Verlag New York Inc., PO Box 2485, Secaucus, NJ 07096-2485. TEL 212-460-1500, FAX 212-473-6272.

570 AUS ISSN 0012-1592
CODEN: DGDFA5

DEVELOPMENT, GROWTH AND DIFFERENTIATION/HASSEI, SEICHO, BUNKA. Text in English. 1950. bi-m. AUD 207 domestic to individuals; AUD 189 in New Zealand to individuals; USD 185 elsewhere to individuals; AUD 739 domestic to institutions; AUD 672 in New Zealand to institutions; JPY 76,350 in Japan to institutions; USD 625 elsewhere to institutions; AUD 228 domestic to individuals paper & online eds. combined; AUD 208 in New Zealand to individuals paper & online eds. combined; USD 204 elsewhere to individuals paper & online eds. combined; AUD 813 domestic to institutions paper & online eds. combined; AUD 740 in New Zealand to institutions paper & online eds. combined; JPY 83,985 in Japan to institutions paper & online eds. combined; USD 688 elsewhere to institutions paper & online eds. combined (effective 2001). adv. bibl, charts, illus. back issues avail. *Refereed.* **Document type:** *Academic/Scholarly.* **Description:** Covers developmental phenomena for all types of organisms, including plants and microorganisms. Focus is biochemical and analytical.
Formerly (until 1959): Embryologia

Related titles: Online - full text ed.: ISSN 1440-169X. AUD 187 domestic to individuals; AUD 171 in New Zealand to individuals; USD 167 elsewhere to individuals; AUD 606 domestic to institutions; AUD 605 in New Zealand to institutions; JPY 68,175 in Japan to institutions; USD 563 elsewhere to institutions (effective 2001) (from EBSCO Publishing, O C L C Online Computer Library Center, Inc., RoweCom Information Quest, ingenta, Munksgaard & Blackwell Science's Synergy, Swets Blackwell, Institute for Scientific Information).

Indexed: ASCA, AgBiotech, Anim.Breed.Abstr., Aqua.Sci.& Fish.Abstr., Biol.Abstr., Chem.Abstr., Chem.Indus.Notes, Chem.Titles, Curr.Adv.Ecol.Sci., Curr.Cont., Dairy Sci.Abstr., Excerp.Med., Genet.Abstr., Hum.Gen.Abstr., INIS Atomind., Ind.Med. (1969-), Ind.Sci.Rev., Inpharma, Neurosci.Abstr., Nuc.Acids Abstr., Pharm.&Out.News, Poult.Abstr., Reac., Ref.Zh., Rev.Appl.Entomol., Sci.Cit.Ind., Sport Fish.Abstr., Zoo.Rec.

—BLDSC (3579.035000), ADONIS, CASDDS, CISTI, GNLM, IDS, ingenta, Linda Hall. **CCC.**

Published by: (Japanese Society of Developmental Biologists JPN), Blackwell Science Asia Pty Ltd, PO Box 378, Carlton South, VIC 3053, Australia. TEL 61-3-9347-0300, FAX 61-3-9347-5001, info@blacksci-asia.com.au; dgdedit@ipc.hiroshima-u.ac.jp, http://www.blacksci.co.uk. Ed. Makoto Asashima. Adv. contact Kathryn O'Brien. B&W page AUD 1,243, color page AUD 2,497; 210 x 275. Circ: 1,850.

570 USA ISSN 0012-1606
QL951 CODEN: DEBIAO

DEVELOPMENTAL BIOLOGY; an international journal. Text in English. 1959. 24/yr. USD 4,100 in US & Canada to institutions; USD 4,675 elsewhere to institutions (effective 2001). adv. charts, illus. index every 6 mos. back issues avail.; reprints avail. *Refereed.* **Document type:** *Academic/Scholarly.* **Description:** Publishes original analytical research on mechanisms of development, differentiation, growth, regulation, and tissue repair in plants and animals at the molecular, cellular, and genetic levels.

Related titles: Online - full text ed.: (from EBSCO Publishing, O C L C Online Computer Library Center, Inc., RoweCom Information Quest, ingenta, Gale Group, Swets Blackwell, IDEAL Online Library, Institute for Scientific Information).

Indexed: ASCA, AgBiotech, Agricola, Anim.Breed.Abstr., Aqua.Sci.& Fish.Abstr., Bibl.Agri., Biol.& Agr.Ind. (Mar.1983-), Biol.Abstr., Biotech.& Bioeng.Abstr., Cal.Tiss.Abstr. (coverage dropped), Chem.Abstr., Chem.Indus.Notes, Chem.Titles, Chemorec.Abstr., Crop Physiol.Abstr., Curr.Adv.Biochem., Curr.Adv.Cell & Devel.Biol., Curr.Adv.Ecol.Sci., Curr.Adv.Gen.& Molec.Biol., Curr.Cont., Dairy Sci.Abstr., Dent.Ind., Entomol.Abstr. (coverage dropped), Excerp.Med., Field Crop Abstr., Gen.Sci.Ind. (Jun.1992-), Genet.Abstr., Helminthol.Abstr., Hort.Abstr., Hum.Gen.Abstr., INIS Atomind., Ind.Med. (1959-), Ind.Sci.Rev., Ind.Vet., Inpharma, Int.Abstr.Biol.Sci., Maize Abstr., Microbiol.Abstr., Neurosci.Abstr. (coverage dropped), Neurosci.Cit.Ind., Nuc.Acids Abstr., Nutr.Abstr., Ornam.Hort., Pig News & Info., Plant Breed.Abstr., Plant Grow.Reg.Abstr., Poult.Abstr., Reac., Ref.Zh., Rev.Appl.Entomol., Rev.Med.& Vet.Mycol., Rice Abstr., Sci.Cit.Ind., Seed Abstr., Sport Fish.Abstr., Tox.Abstr. (coverage dropped), Weed Abstr., Wild.Rev., Zoo.Rec.

—BLDSC (3579.051900), ADONIS, CASDDS, CISTI, GNLM, IDS, ingenta, Linda Hall. **CCC.**

Published by: Academic Press, Inc., Journal Division (Subsidiary of: Harcourt Brace & Company), 525 B St, Ste 1900, San Diego, CA 92101-4495. TEL 619-230-1840, FAX 619-699-6800, apsubs@acad.com, http://www.academicpress.com/db. Ed. Eric N Olson.

571.8 611 USA ISSN 1058-8388
QL801 CODEN: DEDYEI

DEVELOPMENTAL DYNAMICS. Text in English. 1901. m. USD 2,815 in United States; USD 2,935 in Canada & Mexico; USD 3,037 elsewhere; USD 2,956 combined subscription in United States for print and online eds.; USD 3,076 combined subscription in Canada & Mexico for print and online eds.; USD 3,178 combined subscription elsewhere for print and online eds. (effective 2002). adv. bk.rev. abstr, bibl, charts, illus. back issues avail.; reprint service avail. from SWZ. *Refereed.* **Document type:** *Academic/Scholarly.* **Description:** Provides a focus for communication among developmental biologists who study the emergence of form during animal development.

Formerly: American Journal of Anatomy (0002-9106)

Related titles: Microfiche ed.: (from IDC); Microform ed.: (from PMC,PQC,SWZ); Online - full text ed.: ISSN 1097-0177. USD 2,815 in United States; USD 2,815 in Canada & Mexico; USD 2,815 elsewhere (effective 2002) (from EBSCO Publishing, Wiley InterScience, Institute for Scientific Information).

Indexed: ASCA, Abstr.Anthropol., Anim.Breed.Abstr., Biol.Abstr., Chem.Abstr., Chem.Indus.Notes, Chem.Titles, Curr.Adv.Ecol.Sci., Curr.Cont., Dent.Ind., Excerp.Med., Focus on: Vet.Sci.& Med., INIS Atomind., Ind.Med. (1992-), Ind.Sci.Rev., Ind.Vet., Inpharma, Int.Abstr.Biol.Sci., Neurosci.Cit.Ind., Nutr.Abstr., Poult.Abstr., Reac., Ref.Zh., Sci.Cit.Ind., Small Anim.Abstr., Sport Fish.Abstr., Vet.Bull., Wild.Rev., Zoo.Rec.

—BLDSC (3579.054470), CASDDS, CISTI, EMDOCS, GNLM, IDS, ingenta, Linda Hall. **CCC.**

Published by: John Wiley & Sons, Inc., Journals (Subsidiary of: Wiley InterScience), 605 Third Ave, New York, NY 10158. TEL 212-850-6645, FAX 212-850-6021, subinfo@wiley.com, uscs-wis@wiley.com, http://www.wiley.com. Ed. Paul F Goetinck. adv.: B&W page GBP 640, color page GBP 1,515; trim 210 x 279. Circ: 1,250. **Subscr. outside N. America to:** John Wiley & Sons Ltd., Baffins Ln, Chichester, Sussex PO19 IUD, United Kingdom. TEL 44-1243-779777, FAX 44-1243-843232, cs-journals@wiley.co.uk, http://www.wiley.co.uk.

573.8 612.8 USA ISSN 0012-1630
QL750 CODEN: DEPBA5

DEVELOPMENTAL PSYCHOBIOLOGY. Text in English. 1967. 8/yr. USD 1,395 in United States; USD 1,475 in Canada & Mexico; USD 1,543 elsewhere; USD 1,465 combined subscription in United States for print and online eds.; USD 1,545 combined subscription in Canada & Mexico for print and online eds.; USD 1,613 combined subscription elsewhere for print and online eds. (effective 2002). adv. bk.rev. index. back issues avail.; reprint service avail. from PQC,PSC,SCH. *Refereed.* **Document type:** *Academic/Scholarly.* **Description:** Presents original research reports that contribute to the understanding of behaviorally related processes, whether in the embryo, fetus, neonate, or juvenile.

Related titles: Microform ed.: (from PQC); Online - full text ed.: ISSN 1098-2302. USD 1,395 in United States; USD 1,395 in Canada & Mexico; USD 1,395 elsewhere (effective 2002) (from EBSCO Publishing, Wiley InterScience, Institute for Scientific Information).

Indexed: ASCA, Abstr.Anthropol., Biol.Abstr., Chem.Abstr., Chem.Indus.Notes, Chem.Titles, Child Devel.Abstr., Curr.Adv.Ecol.Sci., Curr.Cont., Dairy Sci.Abstr., Excerp.Med., Fam.Ind., INIS Atomind., Ind.Med. (1968-), Ind.Sci.Rev., Ind.Vet., Inpharma, Neurosci.Abstr. (coverage dropped), Neurosci.Cit.Ind., Nutr.Abstr., Pharm.&Out.News, PsycInfo, Psychol.Abstr. (1969-), Psychol.R.G., Reac., SSCI (coverage dropped), Sci.Cit.Ind., e-psyche.

—BLDSC (3579.058000), CASDDS, CISTI, GNLM, IDS, ingenta. **CCC.**

Published by: (International Society for Developmental Psychology), John Wiley & Sons, Inc., Journals (Subsidiary of: Wiley InterScience), 605 Third Ave, New York, NY 10158. TEL 212-850-6645, FAX 212-850-6021, subinfo@wiley.com, uscs-wis@wiley.com, http://www.wiley.com. Ed. William P Smotherman. adv.: B&W page GBP 640, color page GBP 1,515; trim 165 x 254. Circ: 800. **Subscr. outside the Americas to:** John Wiley & Sons Ltd., Baffins Ln, Chichester, Sussex PO19 IUD, United Kingdom. TEL 44-1243-779777, FAX 44-1243-843232, cs-journals@wiley.co.uk, http://www.wiley.co.uk.

DEVELOPMENTS IN BIOLOGICALS. see *METROLOGY AND STANDARDIZATION*

578.77 551.4 NLD ISSN 0167-8418
CODEN: DHIMDR

DEVELOPMENTS IN HYDROBIOLOGY. Text in English. 1981. irreg., latest vol.86, 1993. price varies. *Refereed.* **Document type:** *Monographic series.*

Indexed: Anim.Behav.Abstr. (coverage dropped), Appl.Ecol.Abstr. (coverage dropped), Aqua.Sci.& Fish.Abstr., Aquacult.Abstr., Biol.Abstr., Chem.Abstr., Entomol.Abstr. (coverage dropped), Environ.Sci.Poll.Mgmt., GeoRef, Meteor.& Geoastrophys.Abstr., Microbiol.Abstr., Ocean.Abstr., Pollut.Abstr., Sel.Water Res.Abstr., Zoo.Rec.

—CASDDS, CISTI.

Published by: Kluwer Academic Publishers Group (Subsidiary of: Wolters Kluwer N.V.), Spuiboulevard 50, PO Box 17, Dordrecht 3300 AA, Netherlands. FAX 31-78-639-2254, services@wkap.nl, http://www.wkap.nl. Ed. H J Dumont. **Dist. by:** Journals Department, PO Box 322, Dordrecht 3300 AH, Netherlands. FAX 31-78-654-6474.

570 DEU ISSN 0301-4681
QH573 CODEN: DFFNAW

DIFFERENTIATION; ontogeny, neoplasia and differentiation therapy. Text in English. 1973. 10/yr. DEM 2,038, EUR 1,042.02 in Europe; DEM 2,043, EUR 1,044.57 elsewhere; DEM 2,176, EUR 1,112.57 print & online eds. combined (effective 2001). adv. back issues avail.; reprint service avail. from ISI. *Refereed.* **Document type:** *Journal, Academic/Scholarly.* **Description:** Reports on the most up-to-date research results on problems of biological diversification in plants and animals.

Related titles: Online - full text ed.: ISSN 1432-0436. DEM 1,780, EUR 910 (effective 2001) (from EBSCO Publishing, RoweCom Information Quest, Munksgaard & Blackwell Science's Synergy, Swets Blackwell, Institute for Scientific Information).

Indexed: ASCA, Aqua.Sci.& Fish.Abstr., Biol.Abstr., Biotech.& Bioeng.Abstr., Chem.Abstr., Chem.Indus.Notes, Chem.Titles, Curr.Adv.Cell & Devel.Biol., Curr.Cont., Dairy Sci.Abstr., Dent.Ind., Entomol.Abstr., Excerp.Med., Genet.Abstr., Helminthol.Abstr., INIS Atomind., Ind.Med. (1973-), Ind.Sci.Rev., Inpharma, Int.Abstr.Biol.Sci., Plant Grow.Reg.Abstr., Reac., Sci.Cit.Ind.

—BLDSC (3584.240000), ADONIS, CASDDS, CISTI, EMDOCS, GNLM, IDS, ingenta, Linda Hall. **CCC.**

Published by: (International Society of Differentiation), Blackwell Wissenschafts Verlag GmbH, Kurfuerstendamm 57, Berlin 10707, Germany. TEL 49-30-32790624, FAX 49-30-32790610, abo@blackwis.de, anzeigen@blackwis.de, http://www.blackwell.de/dif.htm. Ed. Laurence Etkin. Adv. contact Manfred Otawa. B&W page DEM 1,700, color page DEM 2,750; trim 175 x 235.

DIRASAT. MEDICAL AND BIOLOGICAL SCIENCES. see *MEDICAL SCIENCES*

DIRECTORY OF BIOTECHNOLOGY CENTERS. see *BIOLOGY—Biotechnology*

DIRECTORY OF PATHOLOGY TRAINING PROGRAMS (YEAR). see *EDUCATION—Higher Education*

570 028.5 ITA

DO DO. Text in Italian. 1990. m. ITL 60,000; ITL 90,000 foreign (effective 1997).

Formerly: Airone Junio

Published by: Editoriale Giorgio Mondadori S.p.A., Via Andrea Ponti, 10, Milan, MI 20143, Italy. TEL 02-891661, FAX 02-89125888. Ed. Nicoletta Salvaroti. adv.: B&W page ITL 8,150,000, color page ITL 12,500,000. Circ: 75,000.

595 RUS ISSN 0012-4966
QH505 CODEN: DKBSAS

DOKLADY BIOLOGICAL SCIENCES. Text in English. 1933. bi-m. EUR 2,171, USD 1,929 to institutions for print or online ed.; EUR 2,605.20 to institutions for print & online eds.combined; USD 2,314.80 to institutions for print & online eds. combined (effective 2002). index. back issues avail. *Refereed.* **Document type:** *Academic/Scholarly.* **Description:** Disseminates the most noteworthy research in the biological sciences, translated from the Russian into English.

Incorporates (1964-2001): Doklady Botanical Sciences (0012-4982)

Related titles: Microfilm ed.: (from PQC); Online - full content ed.: ISSN 1608-3105 (from Swets Blackwell); Online - full text ed.: (from RoweCom Information Quest); ♦ Partial translation of: Rossiiskaya Akademiya Nauk. Doklady. ISSN 0869-5652.

Indexed: AgBiotech, Anim.Breed.Abstr., Bio-Contr.News & Info., Biol.Abstr., Chem.Titles, Crop Physiol.Abstr., Curr.Adv.Ecol.Sci., Deep Sea Res.& Oceanogr.Abstr., Energy Res.Abstr., Excerp.Med., Field Crop Abstr., Forest.Abstr., Helminthol.Abstr., Hort.Abstr., INIS Atomind., Ind.Med. (1992-), Ind.Vet., Int.Abstr.Biol.Sci., Nutr.Abstr., Pig News & Info., Plant Breed.Abstr., Plant Grow.Reg.Abstr., Potato Abstr., Protozool.Abstr., Rev.Appl.Entomol., Rev.Arom.& Med.Plants, Rev.Med.& Vet.Mycol., Rev.Plant Path., Rice Abstr., Seed Abstr., Sel.Water Res.Abstr., Soils & Fert., Sport Fish.Abstr., Triticale Abstr., Weed Abstr., Wild.Rev., Zoo.Rec.

—BLDSC (0411.200000), CISTI, Infotrieve, ingenta. **CCC.**

B

Published by: (Rossiiskaya Akademiya Nauk/Russian Academy of Sciences), M A I K Nauka - Interperiodica, Mezhdunarodnyi Otdel, Profsoyuznaya ul 90, Moscow 117864, Russian Federation. TEL 7-095-336-1600, FAX 7-095-3360066, compmg@maik.rssi.ru; info@plenum.com, http://www.wkap.nl/journalhome.htm/0012-4966, http://www.maik.rssi.ru/journals/danbio.htm; http://www.plenum.com. Ed. Victor A. Kabanov. **Dist. by:** Kluwer Academic Publishers Group, Journals Department, PO Box 322, Dordrecht 3300 AH, Netherlands. TEL 31-78-639-23-92, FAX 31-78-654-64-74, services@wkap.nl, http://www.wkap.nl/.

577 550 DEU ISSN 0340-3947
DORTMUNDER BEITRAEGE ZUR LANDESKUNDE. Text in English, German. 1967. a. DEM 15 (effective 2001). bk.rev. back issues avail. **Document type:** *Journal, Academic/Scholarly.*
Indexed: GeoRef, Zoo.Rec.
Published by: Museum fuer Naturkunde, Muensterstr 271, Dortmund 44122, Germany. TEL 49-231-5024850, FAX 49-231-5024852, naturkundemuseum@stadtdortmund.de, http://www.museendortmund.de. Circ: 600.

ECOGRAPHY; pattern and diversity in ecology. see *ENVIRONMENTAL STUDIES*

577 ESP ISSN 0214-0896
QH171 CODEN: ECOLEV
ECOLOGIA. Text in English, Spanish; Summaries in English. 1972. a., latest vol.4, 2000. ESP 1,500 domestic; ESP 2,000 foreign (effective 2000). bk.rev. bibl, charts, illus, stat. back issues avail. *Refereed.* **Document type:** *Yearbook, Academic/Scholarly.* **Description:** Provides original papers relating to the various aspects of environmental science.
Formerly (until 1987): Estacion Central de Ecologia. Boletin (0210-2536)
Indexed: Anim.Breed.Abstr., Aqua.Sci.& Fish.Abstr., Bio-Contr.News & Info., Biol.Abstr., Chem.Abstr., Curr.Adv.Ecol.Sci., Curr.Cont. (coverage dropped), Forest Prod.Abstr., Forest.Abstr., GeoRef, Herb.Abstr., Ind.SST, Ind.Vet., Rev.Appl.Entomol., Rev.Plant Path., Seed Abstr., Soils & Fert., Sport Fish.Abstr., Weed Abstr., Wild Life Rev., Wild.Rev., Zoo.Rec.
—CINDOC.
Published by: Direccion General de Conservacion de la Naturaleza, Gran Via de San Francisco, 4, Madrid 28005, Spain. TEL 34-91-59755639, FAX 34-91-5975566, beninigno.asensio@gvsf.mma.es, http://www.mma.es/. Ed. Benigno Asensio. Circ: 3,000.

577 550 BOL
CODEN: ECBOE9
ECOLOGIA EN BOLIVIA. Text in Spanish; Abstracts in English, German. 1982. 3/yr. USD 30 (effective 1998 & 1999). bk.rev. back issues avail. *Refereed.* **Document type:** *Bulletin, Academic/Scholarly.* **Description:** Publishes scientific work on ecology and biodiversity in Bolivia.
Indexed: Crop Physiol.Abstr., Curr.Adv.Ecol.Sci., Forest Prod.Abstr., Forest.Abstr., Herb.Abstr., Hort.Abstr., Nutr.Abstr., Rev.Appl.Entomol., Rev.Arom.& Med.Plants, Seed Abstr., Soils & Fert., Sport Fish.Abstr., Weed Abstr., Wild.Rev., Zoo.Rec.
Published by: Instituto de Ecologia, Casilla 10077, La Paz, Bolivia. TEL 591-2-792582, FAX 591-2-797511, insteco@ie.rds.org.bo. Ed., R&P Cecile de Morales. Circ: 1,000.

ECOLOGICAL APPLICATIONS. see *ENVIRONMENTAL STUDIES*

ECOLOGICAL MONOGRAPHS. see *ENVIRONMENTAL STUDIES*

ECOLOGICAL SOCIETY OF AMERICA. BULLETIN. see *ENVIRONMENTAL STUDIES*

577 USA ISSN 0070-8356
CODEN: ESASAM
ECOLOGICAL STUDIES: ANALYSIS AND SYNTHESIS. Text in English. 1970. irreg., latest vol.119, 1996. price varies. reprint service avail. from ISI. **Document type:** *Monographic series.*
Indexed: Aqua.Sci.& Fish.Abstr., Aquacult.Abstr., Bibl.Agri., Biol.Abstr., Chem.Abstr., Eng.Ind., Environ.Sci.Poll.Mgmt., Forest.Abstr., GeoRef, Meteor.& Geoastrophys.Abstr., Zoo.Rec.
—BLDSC (3649.300000), CASDDS, CISTI, Ei, ingenta. **CCC.**
Published by: Springer-Verlag, Journals (Subsidiary of: BertelsmannSpringer), 175 Fifth Ave, New York, NY 10010. TEL 212-460-1500, FAX 212-473-6272.

577 IND
THE ECOLOGISTS. Text in English. bi-m. USD 40 (effective 2000). **Document type:** *Academic/Scholarly.*
Published by: H P C Publishers Distributors Pvt. Ltd., 1st Fl., Flats 1 & 2, Darya Ganj, 4805-24 Bharat Ram Rd., New Delhi 110 002, India. TEL 91-11-3254401, FAX 91-11-619-3511, hpcpd@nda.vsnl.net.in, hpcpd@hpc.cc, http://www.hpc.cc, http://www.bizdelhi.com/publisher/hpc. **Co-publisher:** The Ecologist Asia.

ECOLOGY. see *ENVIRONMENTAL STUDIES*

ECOLOGY U S A. see *ENVIRONMENTAL STUDIES*

570 610 USA ISSN 0724-6706
CODEN: EQJMD4
THE EINSTEIN QUARTERLY; journal of biology and medicine. Text in English. 1982. q. (in 1 vol., 4 nos./vol.). USD 172.60 in Germany; USD 173 elsewhere; USD 63.40 newsstand/cover in Germany; USD 63.80 newsstand/cover elsewhere (effective 2001). adv. reprint service avail. from ISI. *Refereed.* **Document type:** *Academic/Scholarly.* **Description:** Provides a forum for the discussion of the interface of medicine and the social sciences.
Related titles: Microform ed.: (from PQC); Online - full text ed.: (from Springer LINK).
Indexed: Chem.Abstr., Chem.Indus.Notes, Chem.Titles, Excerp.Med.
—BLDSC (3665.635000), CASDDS, CISTI, GNLM, Infotrieve. **CCC.**
Published by: (Albert Einstein College of Medicine), Springer-Verlag, Journals (Subsidiary of: BertelsmannSpringer), 175 Fifth Ave, New York, NY 10010. TEL 212-460-1500, FAX 212-473-6272, orders@springer-ny.com, http://www.springer-ny.com. Ed. Julie L Choderker. R&P Ian Gross. Adv. contact Jay Feinman. **N. American subscr. to:** Journal Fulfillment Services, PO Box 2485, Secaucus, NJ 07096-2485. TEL 800-777-4643, FAX 201-348-4505.

577 UKR ISSN 0203-4646
QH541.5.S3 CODEN: EKMODH
EKOLOGIYA MORYA; respublikanskii mezhvedomstvennyi sbornik nauchnykh trudov. Text in Russian; Summaries in English, Russian. 1980. q. **Document type:** *Academic/Scholarly.*
Formerly: Biologiya Morya (0320-9695)
Indexed: Aqua.Sci.& Fish.Abstr., Aquacult.Abstr., Chem.Abstr., Curr.Adv.Ecol.Sci., Deep Sea Res.& Oceanogr.Abstr., Environ.Sci.Poll.Mgmt., GeoRef, Helminthol.Abstr., Sel.Water Res.Abstr., So.Pac.Per.Ind.
—CASDDS, CISTI, Infotrieve, Linda Hall. **CCC.**
Published by: Natsional'na Akademiya Nauk Ukrainy, Institut Biologii Yuzhnykh Morei im. A.O. Kovalevskogo, Vul Tereshchenkivska 3, Kiev 252601, Ukraine. TEL 380-44-224-4068, FAX 380-44-224-7060. **Dist. by:** Mezhdunarodnaya Kniga, B Yakimanka 39, Moscow 117049, Russian Federation.

570 FRA
ELECTRICITE DE FRANCE. DIRECTION DES ETUDES ET RECHERCHES. COLLECTION DE NOTES INTERNES. BIOLOGIE, SCIENCES DE LA TERRE ET ENVIRONNEMENT. Text in French. 1992. irreg. FRF 1,500.
Indexed: Chem.Abstr., Chem.Indus.Notes, Chem.Titles.
Published by: Electricite de France, Direction des Etudes et Recherches, 1 av. du General de Gaulle, Clamart Cedex 92141, France. TEL 1-47-65-43-21, FAX 1-47-65-31-24.

570 CHE ISSN 1062-3329
QP88.45 CODEN: ENDTE9
ENDOTHELIUM. Text in English. 1993. 6/yr. GBP 105, USD 127, EUR 140 to individuals (effective 2002); GBP 387, USD 536, EUR 467 to institutions; GBP 604, USD 831, EUR 893 to corporations (effective 2000). back issues avail. *Refereed.* **Document type:** *Academic/Scholarly.* **Description:** Dedicated to the rapid turnaround of significant basic and clinical research on the endothelium, including endothelial-derived biologically active factors involved in the regulation of vascular tone and structure in haemostasis, fibrinolysis, inflamation and immune responses.
Related titles: CD-ROM ed.; Microform ed.; Online - full text ed.: (from EBSCO Publishing, RoweCom Information Quest, Institute for Scientific Information).
Indexed: BBCI, Curr.Cont., Excerp.Med. (1994-), Ind.Med. (1993-), Int.Abstr.Biol.Sci., Sci.Cit.Ind.
—BLDSC (3743.651000), CISTI, EMDOCS, GNLM, Infotrieve, KNAW. **CCC.**
Published by: Gordon and Breach - Harwood Academic (Subsidiary of: Taylor & Francis Group), PO Box 531, Lausanne 1000, Switzerland. http://www.gbhap.com/Endothelium; http://biomednet.com/library/391. Ed. Peter I Lelkes. **Subscr. addr. in US:** International Publishers Direct, PO Box 32160, Newark, NJ 07102. FAX 215-750-6343.

ENVIROFICHE. see *BIOLOGY—Abstracting, Bibliographies, Statistics*

ENVIRONMENTAL BIOLOGY. see *ENVIRONMENTAL STUDIES*

ESCUELA TECNICA SUPERIOR DE INGENIEROS DE MONTES. BIBLIOTECA. BOLETIN BIBLIOGRAFICO Y DOCUMENTAL. INFORMACION FORESTAL. SERIE A: MONOGRAFIAS. see *FORESTS AND FORESTRY—Abstracting, Bibliographies, Statistics*

ESCUELA TECNICA SUPERIOR DE INGENIEROS DE MONTES. BIBLIOTECA. BOLETIN BIBLIOGRAFICO Y DOCUMENTAL. INFORMACION FORESTAL. SERIE B: PUBLICACIONES PERIODICAS. see *FORESTS AND FORESTRY—Abstracting, Bibliographies, Statistics*

577 EST ISSN 1406-0914
QH301 CODEN: EATBEC
ESTONIAN ACADEMY OF SCIENCES. PROCEEDINGS. BIOLOGY - ECOLOGY/EESTI TEADUSTE AKADEEMIA. TOIMETISED. BIOLOOGIA. OKOLOOGIA. Text in English; Summaries in English, Estonian. 1997. q., latest vol.50, no.2. USD 85 foreign (effective 2002). adv. illus, abstr, charts, maps. 80 p./no. back issues avail. *Refereed.* **Document type:** *Journal, Academic/Scholarly.*
Formed by the merger of (1991-1997): Eesti Teaduste Akadeemia. Toimetised. Okoloogia (0868-5894); (1990-1997): Eesti Teaduste Akadeemia. Toimetised. Bioloogia (1018-7642); Which was formerly (1956-1990): Akademiya Nauk Estonskoi S.S.R. Izvestiya. Biologiya (0013-2144)
Indexed: Anim.Breed.Abstr., Appl.Ecol.Abstr., Aqua.Sci.& Fish.Abstr., Aquacult.Abstr., Biol.Abstr., Chem.Abstr., Chem.Indus.Notes, Chem.Titles, Crop Physiol.Abstr., Dairy Sci.Abstr., Entomol.Abstr., Environ.Sci.Poll.Mgmt., Field Crop Abstr., Forest.Abstr., GeoRef, Helminthol.Abstr., Herb.Abstr., Hort.Abstr., INIS Atomind., Ind.Vet., Int.Aerosp.Abstr., Irr.& Drain.Abstr., NAA, Nutr.Abstr., Ornam.Hort., Plant Breed.Abstr., Pollut.Abstr., Potato Abstr., Rev.Appl.Entomol., Rev.Plant Path., Sel.Water Res.Abstr., Soils & Fert., Vet.Bull., Weed Abstr., Zoo.Rec.
—CASDDS, CISTI, Infotrieve, KNAW, Linda Hall. **CCC.**
Published by: (Eesti Teaduste Akadeemia), Teaduste Akadeemia Kirjastus/Estonian Academy Publishers, Estonia pst 7, Tallinn 10143, Estonia. TEL 372-6-454504, FAX 372-6-466026, niine@kirj.ee, asta@kirj.ee, http://www.kirj.ee. Ed. Hillar Aben. Pub. Ulo Niine. Adv. contact Asta Tikerpae. Circ: 550.

551.4609 USA ISSN 0160-8347
S932.C47 CODEN: ESTUDO
ESTUARIES; a journal of research on any aspect of natural science and management applied to estuaries. Text in English. 1978. bi-m. USD 360 in North America; USD 375 elsewhere (effective 2001). adv. bk.rev. abstr, bibl, charts, illus, maps, stat. index. back issues avail.; reprint service avail. from PQC. *Refereed.* **Document type:** *Journal, Academic/Scholarly.* **Description:** It is devoted to publishing original papers based on research in any aspect of natural science or management of estuaries and the coastal zone, including selected interpretive review papers that lead to new and important generalizations.
Formerly: Chesapeake Science (0009-3262)
Related titles: Microform ed.: (from MIM,PQC,PMC); Online - full text ed.: (from Institute for Scientific Information).
Indexed: ASCA, Abstr.Bull.Inst.Pap.Chem., Appl.Ecol.Abstr., Aqua.Sci.& Fish.Abstr., Biodet.Abstr., Biol.Abstr., Chem.Abstr., Chem.Indus.Notes, Chem.Titles, Curr.Adv.Ecol.Sci., Curr.Cont., Curr.Tit.Ocean, Deep Sea Res.& Oceanogr.Abstr., Ecol.Abstr., Entomol.Abstr., Environ.Per.Bibl. (1996-), Environ.Sci.Poll.Mgmt., Excerp.Med., Forest.Abstr., Geo.Abstr.H.G., Geo.Abstr.P.G., GeoRef, Geol.Abstr., Helminthol.Abstr., Herb.Abstr., INIS Atomind., Ind.Sci.Rev., Int.Abstr.Biol.Sci., Meteor.& Geoastrophys.Abstr., Ocean.Abstr., Pollut.Abstr., Ref.Zh., Rev.Appl.Entomol., Sci.Cit.Ind., Seed Abstr., Sel.Water Res.Abstr., Soils & Fert., Sport Fish.Abstr., W.R.C.Inf., Weed Abstr., Wild.Rev., Zoo.Rec.
—BLDSC (3812.593700), CASDDS, CISTI, EMDOCS, IDS, ingenta, Linda Hall. **CCC.**

Published by: Estuarine Research Federation, 2018 Daffodil, PO Box 510, Port Republic, MD 20676. TEL 410-586-0997, FAX 410-586-9226, stt@estuaries-olemiss.edu, http://erf.org/journal/journal.html, http://erf.org/journal.html. R&P Harold Stevenson. Adv. contact Joy Bartholonnew. Circ: 1,800. **Subscr. to:** Allen Press Inc., PO Box 1897, Lawrence, KS 66044-8897. TEL 785-843-1235, FAX 785-843-1274, estuaries@allenpress.com.

ESTUDIOS DE ANTROPOLOGIA BIOLOGICA. see *ANTHROPOLOGY*

570 CHE ISSN 0896-4343
CODEN: EMLSE5
ETTORE MAJORANA INTERNATIONAL SCIENCE SERIES. LIFE SCIENCES. Text in English. irreg., latest vol.14. price varies. bibl. index. **Document type:** *Monographic series.*
Indexed: Chem.Abstr., INSPEC (coverage dropped), Zoo.Rec.
—CISTI.
Published by: Gordon and Breach - Harwood Academic (Subsidiary of: Taylor & Francis Group), PO Box 531, Lausanne 1000, Switzerland. Ed. Antonino Zichichi. **Subscr. addr. in US:** International Publishers Direct, PO Box 32160, Newark, NJ 07102. FAX 215-750-6343.

174.957 JPN ISSN 1173-2571
EUBIOS JOURNAL OF ASIAN AND INTERNATIONAL BIOETHICS. Text in English. 1991. bi-m. JPY 3,500, USD 35, NZD 50 (effective 2001 & 2002). adv. bk.rev. 32 p./no. back issues avail. *Refereed.* **Document type:** *Journal, Academic/Scholarly, Bibliography.* **Description:** Aims to review and update news and trends in bioethics from around the world.
Formerly (until 1995): Eubios Ethics Institute Newsletter (1170-5485)
Related titles: Online - full text ed.
Published by: Eubios Ethics Institute, PO Box 125, Tsukuba Science City 305-8591, Japan. TEL 81-298-534662, FAX 81-298-536614, macer@sakura.cc.tsukuba.ac.jp, http://www.biol.tsukuba.ac.jp/~macer/EJAIB.html. Ed., R&P, Adv. contact Darryl Macer. Circ: 500 (paid and controlled). **Co-sponsor:** Eubios Ethics Institute.

570 FRA ISSN 0999-5749
RB37.A1 CODEN: BIOLE6
EUROBIOLOGISTE. Text in French. 1955. bi-m. FRF 800 (effective 1999). adv. bk.rev. *Refereed.* **Document type:** *Academic/Scholarly.* **Description:** Scholarly articles focusing on research findings in the biological sciences.
Former titles: Biologiste (0981-6003); Pharmacien Biologiste (0553-9323)
Related titles: Online - full text ed.
Indexed: Biol.Abstr., Chem.Abstr., Excerp.Med., INIS Atomind., I.P.A., Ref.Zh.
—CASDDS, Linda Hall. **CCC.**
Published by: Centre National des Biologistes, 80 av. du Maine, Paris 75014, France. TEL 33-1-43229770, FAX 33-1-43217312. Pub. Jean Benoit. Adv. contact Jeanne Berga. Circ: 3,200.

571.3 NLD ISSN 0924-3860
QL799 CODEN: EJMOEB
EUROPEAN JOURNAL OF MORPHOLOGY; incorporating european archives & biology. Text in English. 1938. 5/yr., latest vol.39, 2001. NLG 444, USD 247 to individuals; NLG 998, USD 512 to institutions (effective 2001). adv. bk.rev. bibl. charts. index. back issues avail.; reprint service avail. from SWZ. *Refereed.* **Document type:** *Journal, Academic/Scholarly.* **Description:** Publishes research and commentary in all areas of vertabrate morphology, especially human embryology and anatomy.
Incorporates (in 1995): European Archives of Biology (0777-0553); Which was formerly (1886-1989): Archives de Biologie (0003-9624); Former titles (until 1989): Acta Morphologica Neerlando-Scandinavica (0001-6225); (until 1956): Acta Neerlandica Morphologiae Narmalis et Pathologicae (0365-4907)
Related titles: Microfiche ed.: (from BHP); Online - full text ed.: (from EBSCO Publishing, O C L C Online Computer Library Center, Inc., RoweCom Information Quest, Swets Blackwell, Institute for Scientific Information).
Indexed: ASCA, Anim.Breed.Abstr., Aqua.Sci.& Fish.Abstr., Aquacult.Abstr., Biol.Abstr., Chem.Abstr., Curr.Adv.Ecol.Sci., Curr.Cont., Dent.Ind., Environ.Sci.Poll.Mgmt., Excerp.Med., GeoRef, Helminthol.Abstr., INIS Atomind., Ind.Med. (1990-), Ind.Sci.Rev., Ind.Vet., Inpharma, Int.Abstr.Biol.Sci., Pharm.&Out.News, Pollut.Abstr., Poult.Abstr., Reac., Ref.Zh., Sci.Cit.Ind., Sport Fish.Abstr., Vet.Bull., Wild.Rev., Zoo.Rec.
—BLDSC (3829.731660), ADONIS, CASDDS, CISTI, EMDOCS, GNLM, IDS, ingenta, Linda Hall. **CCC.**
Published by: Swets & Zeitlinger BV, PO Box 825, Lisse 2160 SZ, Netherlands. TEL 31-252-435111, FAX 31-252-415888, orders@swets.nl, http://www.swets.nl/sps/journals/ejm/html. Eds. Benjamin M, Hillen B. R&P J van der Valk. Adv. contact Patrick Kliean. Circ: 600. **Dist. in N. America by:** Swets & Zeitlinger, PO Box 582, Downingtown, PA 19335-998. TEL 800-477-9387, FAX 610-524-5366.

577 FRA ISSN 1164-5563
QH84.8 CODEN: EJSBE2
EUROPEAN JOURNAL OF SOIL BIOLOGY. Text in English; Summaries in French, English. 1964. q. EUR 216 in Europe to institutions; JPY 28,700 in Japan to institutions; USD 242 elsewhere to institutions (effective 2002). adv. bk.rev. bibl, charts, illus. index. back issues avail. *Refereed.* **Document type:** *Academic/Scholarly.* **Description:** Examines biology and ecology of the soil. Also focuses on interactions of soil organisms and the ecosystem balance.
Formerly: Revue d'Ecologie et de Biologie du Sol (0035-1822)
Related titles: Microform ed.: (from PQC); Online - full text ed.: (from ingenta, Swets Blackwell, ScienceDirect, Institute for Scientific Information).
Indexed: ASCA, Appl.Ecol.Abstr. (coverage dropped), Bio-Contr.News & Info., Biol.Abstr., Chem.Abstr., Chem.Indus.Notes, Chem.Titles, Curr.Adv.Ecol.Sci., Curr.Adv.Plant Sci., Curr.Cont., Ecol.Abstr., Energy Ind., Energy Info.Abstr., Eng.Ind., Entomol.Abstr. (coverage dropped), Environ.Sci.Poll.Mgmt., Excerp.Med., Field Crop Abstr., Forest Prod.Abstr., Forest.Abstr., GeoRef, Helminthol.Abstr., Herb.Abstr., INIS Atomind., Plant Sci., Pollut.Abstr., Rev.Appl.Entomol., Rev.Plant Path., Rice Abstr., Sci.Cit.Ind. (coverage dropped), Soils & Fert., Sport Fish.Abstr., Weed Abstr., Wild.Rev., Zoo.Rec.
—BLDSC (3829.741000), CASDDS, CISTI, Ei, IDS, Infotrieve, ingenta, Linda Hall. **CCC.**
Published by: Elsevier Paris, Editions Scientifiques et Medicales (Subsidiary of: Reed Elsevier plc. group), 23 rue Linois, Paris 75015, France. TEL 33-1-45589110, FAX 33-1-45589419, academic@elsevier-fr.com, http://www.elsevier.com/locate/sbpar. Ed. Y Frenot. Circ: 1,000.

EUROPEAN JOURNAL OF ULTRASOUND. see *MEDICAL SCIENCES—Radiology And Nuclear Medicine*

EVOLUTION AND COGNITION. see *PSYCHOLOGY*

571.3 USA ISSN 1520-541X
QH359 CODEN: ELDMF9
▼ **EVOLUTION & DEVELOPMENT.** Text in English. 1999. bi-m. USD 85 domestic to individuals; USD 95 in Canada & Mexico to individuals; USD 105 overseas to individuals; USD 210 domestic to institutions; USD 220 in Canada & Mexico to institutions; USD 230 overseas to institutions; USD 93.50 to individuals print & online eds. combined; USD 231 to institutions print & online eds. combined (effective 2001). adv. bk.rev. reprints avail. *Refereed.* **Document type:** *Academic/Scholarly.* **Description:** Publishes research papers and review articles reflecting the rapid growth in research where the fields of evolutionary and developmental biology have, after some 50 years, become reintegrated.
Related titles: ♦ Online - full text ed.: Evolution & Development Online. ISSN 1525-142X.
Indexed: Curr.Cont., Zoo.Rec.
—BLDSC (3834.215000). **CCC.**
Published by: Blackwell Science Inc., Commerce Pl, 350 Main St, Malden, MA 02148-5018. TEL 781-388-8250, 800-759-6102, FAX 781-388-8255, journals@blacksci.com, http://www.blackwell-science.com. Ed. Rudolf A Raff. R&P Tracey Davies. Adv. contact Jenny Applin.

571.3 USA ISSN 1525-142X
EVOLUTION & DEVELOPMENT ONLINE. Text in English. bi-m. USD 77 to individuals; USD 189 to institutions (effective 2001). **Document type:** *Academic/Scholarly.*
Media: Online - full text (from EBSCO Publishing, O C L C Online Computer Library Center, Inc., RoweCom Information Quest, ingenta, Munksgaard & Blackwell Science's Synergy, Swets Blackwell, Institute for Scientific Information). **Related titles:** ♦ Print ed.: Evolution & Development. ISSN 1520-541X.
Published by: Blackwell Science Inc., Commerce Pl, 350 Main St, Malden, MA 02148-5018. TEL 781-388-8250, 800-759-6102, FAX 781-388-8255, website@blacksci.com, journals@blacksci.com, http://www.blackwell-science.com/~cgilib/bsinc.bin?Journal=geoscience.

599.9 USA ISSN 0272-0809
EVOLUTIONARY MONOGRAPHS. Text in English. 1979. irreg. price varies. *Refereed.* **Document type:** *Monographic series, Academic/Scholarly.* **Description:** Publishes long papers and other nonstandard items in the evolutionary half of biology and historical geology.
Indexed: Biol.Abstr., Deep Sea Res.& Oceanogr.Abstr., GeoRef.
—BLDSC (3834.452000).
Published by: University of Chicago, Department of Ecology and Evolution, 1101 E 57th St, Chicago, IL 60637. TEL 312-702-9475. Ed. Leigh M Van Valen. Circ: 200 (paid).

570 USA ISSN 0093-4755
QH359 CODEN: EVTHB4
EVOLUTIONARY THEORY; an international journal of fact and interpretation. Text in English. 1973. irreg. USD 28. bk.rev. *Refereed.* **Document type:** *Academic/Scholarly.* **Description:** Publishes factual and theoretical papers and reviews on topics in evolutionary biology.
Indexed: Anim.Breed.Abstr., Biol.Abstr., Biostat., Curr.Adv.Ecol.Sci., Curr.Cont. (coverage dropped), Curr.Ind.Stat., Deep Sea Res.& Oceanogr.Abstr., GeoRef, Sport Fish.Abstr., Zoo.Rec.
—ingenta, Linda Hall.
Published by: University of Chicago, Department of Ecology and Evolution, 1101 E 57th St, Chicago, IL 60637. TEL 312-702-9475. Eds. Leigh M Van Valen, Virginia C Maiorana. Circ: 650 (paid).

B

EXCERPTA MEDICA. SECTION 5: GENERAL PATHOLOGY AND PATHOLOGICAL ANATOMY. see *BIOLOGY—Abstracting, Bibliographies, Statistics*

570 610 USA
QP1 CODEN: PSEBAA
EXPERIMENTAL BIOLOGY AND MEDICINE (MAYWOOD). Text in English. 1903. 11/yr. membership dues include a subscription to print & online eds. adv. abstr, bibl, illus. index. back issues avail.; reprints avail. *Refereed.* **Document type:** *Academic/Scholarly.* **Description:** Attempts to promote investigation in the biomedical sciences by encouraging and facilitating the interchange of scientific information among disciplines. Presents original articles, minireviews, and symposia.
Formerly: Society for Experimental Biology and Medicine. Proceedings (0037-9727)
Related titles: Microfilm ed.: (from PMC,WWS); Online - full text ed.: ISSN 1525-1373 (from Ovid Technologies, Inc., HighWire Pr., EBSCO Publishing, O C L C Online Computer Library Center, Inc., RoweCom Information Quest, ingenta, Swets Blackwell, Institute for Scientific Information).
Indexed: ASCA, Abstr.Hyg., AgBiotech, Agri.& Environ.Biotech.Abstr. (coverage dropped), Agricola, Anim.Breed.Abstr., Aqua.Sci.& Fish.Abstr., BBCI, Bibl.Agri., Biol.Abstr., Cal.Tiss.Abstr. (coverage dropped), Chem.Abstr., Chem.Titles, Curr.Adv.Biochem., Curr.Adv.Cell & Devel.Biol., Curr.Adv.Ecol.Sci., Curr.Cont., Dairy Sci.Abstr., Dent.Ind., Derwent Biotech.Abstr., Excerp.Med., Food Sci.& Tech.Abstr., Helminthol.Abstr., INIS Atomind., Ind.Med. (1903-), Ind.Sci.Rev., Ind.Vet., Inpharma, Int.Abstr.Biol.Sci., Neurosci.Abstr. (coverage dropped), Nutr.Abstr., Pharm.&Out.News, Pig News & Info., Postharvest, Poult.Abstr., Protozool.Abstr., Reac., Rev.Appl.Entomol., Rev.Arom.& Med.Plants, Rev.Med.& Vet.Mycol., Rev.Plant Path., Sci.Cit.Ind., Small Anim.Abstr., Soyabean Abstr., Sport Fish.Abstr., THA, Tox.Abstr. (coverage dropped), Triticale Abstr., Trop.Dis.Bull., Vet.Bull., W.R.C.Inf., Weed Abstr., Wild.Rev., Zoo.Rec.
—CASDDS, CISTI, GNLM, IDS, ingenta, KNAW, Linda Hall.
Published by: Society for Experimental Biology and Medicine, 195 W. Spring Valley Ave., Maywood, NJ 07607-1727. TEL 201-291-9080, FAX 201-291-2988, sebm@inch.com, http://www.sebm.org/. Ed. Andrzej Bartke. Circ: 3,200.

570 DEU ISSN 1430-3418
EXPERIMENTAL BIOLOGY ONLINE. Text in German. 1996. irreg. DEM 238 (effective 2001). *Refereed.* **Document type:** *Academic/Scholarly.* **Description:** Specializes in short, topical research papers in experimental biology organized in three sections: animal biology, plant biology, and cell biology.
Media: Online - full content (from EBSCO Publishing, Swets Blackwell). **Related titles:** CD-ROM ed.; Online - full text ed.: (from Springer LINK, RoweCom Information Quest); Print ed.: ISSN 1435-3237.
Indexed: Chem.Abstr., Chem.Indus.Notes, Chem.Titles, Zoo.Rec.
—**CCC.**

Published by: (Society for Experimental Biology GBR), Springer-Verlag (Subsidiary of: BertelsmannSpringer), Tiergartenstr 17, Heidelberg 69121, Germany. TEL 49-6221-345-0, FAX 49-6221-345229, subscriptions@springer.de, http://link.springer.de/link/service/journals/10136/index.htm, http://www.springer.de. Eds. A Curtis, C R Bridges.

EXPERIMENTAL PARASITOLOGY. see *MEDICAL SCIENCES—Communicable Diseases*

EXPRESS BULLETINS; a series of current awareness bulletins for researchers in biology and medicine. see *BIOLOGY—Abstracting, Bibliographies, Statistics*

570 USA ISSN 0892-6638
QH301 CODEN: FAJOEC

THE F A S E B JOURNAL. Text in English. 1987. m. USD 90 domestic to members Print & online eds.; USD 110 in Canada & Mexico to members Print & online eds.; USD 142 elsewhere to members Print & online eds.; USD 154 domestic to non-members Print & online eds.; USD 174 in Canada & Mexico to non-members Print & online eds.; USD 206 elsewhere to non-members Print & online eds.; USD 540 domestic to institutions Print & online eds.; USD 560 in Canada & Mexico to institutions Print & online eds.; USD 592 elsewhere to institutions Print & online eds.; USD 45 domestic to students Print & online eds. (effective 2001). adv. abstr, charts, illus. index. back issues avail.; reprint service avail. from PQC. *Refereed.* **Document type:** *Academic/Scholarly.* **Description:** Presents scholarly papers and reviews of research in experimental biology, encompassing physiology, biological chemistry, pharmacology, experimental therapeutics, immunology, nutrition, and cell biology.

Supersedes: Federation of American Societies for Experimental Biology. Federation Proceedings (0014-9446)

Related titles: Microform ed.; Online - full text ed.: USD 540 (effective 2001) (from HighWire Pr., EBSCO Publishing, RoweCom Information Quest, Institute for Scientific Information); Supplement: Experimental Biology (Year) Abstracts.

Indexed: ASCA, AgBiotech, Agri.& Environ.Biotech.Abstr. (coverage dropped), Agricola, Anim.Breed.Abstr., Aqua.Sci.& Fish.Abstr., Bibl.Agri., Biol.& Agr.Ind. (Jan.1983-Jun.1987), Biol.Abstr., Cal.Tiss.Abstr. (coverage dropped), Chem.Abstr., Chem.Cit.Ind., Chem.Indus.Notes, Chem.Titles, Crop Physiol.Abstr., Curr.Adv.Cancer Res., Curr.Adv.Ecol.Sci., Curr.Cont., Dairy Sci.Abstr., Derwent Biotech.Abstr., Excerp.Med., Field Crop Abstr., Food Sci.& Tech.Abstr., Genet.Abstr., Helminthol.Abstr., Hum.Gen.Abstr., INIS Atomind., Immun.Abstr. (coverage dropped), Ind.Med. (1987-), Ind.Vet., Inpharma, Int.Abstr.Biol.Sci., Med.& Surg.Dermat., NRN, Neurosci.Abstr., Nuc.Acids Abstr., Nutr.Abstr., Pharm.&Out.News, Pig News & Info., Plant Breed.Abstr., Poult.Abstr., Protozool.Abstr., Reac., Rev.Appl.Entomol., Rev.Plant Path., SSCI (coverage dropped), Sci.Cit.Ind., Sport Fish.Abstr., THA, Tox.Abstr. (coverage dropped), Trop.Dis.Bull., Vet.Bull., Weed Abstr., Wild.Rev., Zoo.Rec.

—BLDSC (3896.579700), CASDDS, CISTI, EMDOCS, GNLM, IDS, ingenta, Linda Hall. **CCC.**

Published by: Federation of American Societies for Experimental Biology, 9650 Rockville Pike, Bethesda, MD 20814-3998. TEL 301-530-7100, FAX 301-571-1855, http://www.fasebj.org. Ed. Vincent T Marchesi. R&P S Jacobson. Adv. contacts Marsha Bell, Susan Mergenhagen. B&W page USD 1,765, color page USD 2,860. Circ: 6,000 (paid).

FACULTAD NACIONAL DE AGRONOMIA MEDELLIN. REVISTA. see *AGRICULTURE*

570 FRA ISSN 0428-2779
CODEN: FBIOAA

FEUILLETS DE BIOLOGIE; le repertoire medical pratique. Text in French. 1960. bi-m. FRF 740 (effective 1997). adv. bk.rev. bibl, charts, illus.

Indexed: Biol.Abstr., Chem.Abstr., Excerp.Med., INIS Atomind., Int.Abstr.Biol.Sci., Rev.Med.& Vet.Mycol.

—BLDSC (3913.600000), CASDDS, EMDOCS, GNLM.

Published by: Editions Orion, 9 av. du Bel Air, Bezons 95870, France. TEL 33-1-39472260, FAX 33-1-30762212. Ed. Dr. Bernard Bousquet. Circ: 4,000.

578.77 GBR ISSN 1050-4648
QL638.97 CODEN: FSIMEP

FISH AND SHELLFISH IMMUNOLOGY. Text in English. 1991. 8/yr. GBP 350 to institutions (effective 2001). adv. illus. Index. reprint service avail. from SWZ. *Refereed.* **Document type:** *Academic/Scholarly.* **Description:** Presents studies on the basic mechanisms of both the specific and nonspecific defense systems, the cells, tissues, and hormonal factors involved, their dependence on environmental and intrinsic factors, response to pathogens, response to vaccination, and applied studies on the development of specific vaccines for use in the aquaculture industry.

Related titles: Online - full text ed.: (from EBSCO Publishing, O C L C Online Computer Library Center, Inc., RoweCom Information Quest, ingenta, Swets Blackwell, IDEAL Online Library, Institute for Scientific Information).

Indexed: AIDS & Cancer Res., ASCA, AgBiotech, Anim.Breed.Abstr., Aqua.Sci.& Fish.Abstr., Aquacult.Abstr., Curr.Cont., Environ.Sci.Poll.Mgmt., Focus on: Vet.Sci.& Med., Helminthol.Abstr., Immun.Abstr., Ind.Med., Ind.Vet., Nutr.Abstr., Ocean.Abstr., Protozool.Abstr., Rev.Med.& Vet.Mycol., Sci.Cit.Ind., Sport Fish.Abstr., Vet.Bull., Wild.Rev., Zoo.Rec.

—BLDSC (3934.880000), CINDOC, CISTI, IDS, Infotrieve, ingenta. **CCC.**

Published by: Academic Press (Subsidiary of: Harcourt Publishers Ltd.), 24 Oval Rd, London NW1 7DX, United Kingdom. TEL 44-20-7267-4466, FAX 44-20-7482-2293, apsubs@acad.com, http://www.academicpress.com/fsi; http://www.europe.idealibrary.com/. Eds. A E Ellis, C Secombes. R&P Catherine John. Adv. contact Nik Screen. **Subscr. to:** Harcourt Publishers Ltd., Foots Cray High St, Sidcup, Kent DA14 5HP, United Kingdom. TEL 44-20-8300-3322, FAX 44-180-309-0807.

578.77 USA

FISHES OF THE WESTERN NORTH ATLANTIC. MEMOIRS. Text in English. 1948. irreg., latest vol.1, 1989, part 9. price varies. back issues avail. **Document type:** *Monographic series.*

Indexed: Deep Sea Res.& Oceanogr.Abstr.

Published by: Sears Foundation for Marine Research, Kline Geology Laboratory, Yale University, Box 208109, New Haven, CT 06520-8109. TEL 203-432-3760. Ed. Dr. Leo Buss.

578.77 USA ISSN 0095-0157
CODEN: FMPUA4

FLORIDA MARINE RESEARCH PUBLICATIONS. Text in English. 1973. irreg. per issue exchange basis. charts, illus. **Document type:** *Academic/Scholarly.*

Formed by the merger of: Florida Marine Research Institute. Educational Series (0094-2693); Florida Marine Research Institute. Leaflet Series; Florida Marine Research Institute. Professional Papers Series (0160-4473); Florida Marine Research Institute. Saltwater Fishery Leaflets; Florida Marine Research Institute. Special Scientific Report; Florida Marine Research Institute. Technical Series (0149-4015)

Indexed: Aqua.Sci.& Fish.Abstr., Aquacult.Abstr., Biol.Abstr., Curr.Adv.Ecol.Sci., Deep Sea Res.& Oceanogr.Abstr., Environ.Sci.Poll.Mgmt., GeoRef, Ocean.Abstr., Sport Fish.Abstr., Wild.Rev., Zoo.Rec.

—CISTI, Linda Hall.

Published by: Florida Marine Research Institute, Department of Environmental Protection, 100 8th Ave. S.E., St. Petersburg, FL 33701. FAX 813-823-0166. Ed. K A Steidinger. Circ: 1,000.

508 USA
QH1 CODEN: BFMSEU

FLORIDA MUSEUM OF NATURAL HISTORY. BULLETIN. Summaries in English, Spanish. 1956. irreg. price varies. cum.index. *Refereed.* **Document type:** *Bulletin, Academic/Scholarly.* **Description:** Presents the results of research in the natural sciences, emphasizing the circum-Caribbean region.

Former titles: Florida Museum of Natural History. Bulletin. Biological Sciences (1052-3669); (until 1990): Florida State Museum. Bulletin. Biological Sciences (0071-6154)

Indexed: Appl.Ecol.Abstr., Aqua.Sci.& Fish.Abstr., Aquacult.Abstr., Biol.Abstr., Curr.Adv.Ecol.Sci., Deep Sea Res.& Oceanogr.Abstr., Entomol.Abstr. (coverage dropped), Environ.Sci.Poll.Mgmt., GeoRef, Sport Fish.Abstr., Wild.Rev., Zoo.Rec.

—CISTI, Linda Hall.

Published by: Florida Museum of Natural History, University of Florida, Box 117800, Gainesville, FL 32611-7800. TEL 352-392-1721, FAX 352-846-0287, mjoyner@flmnh.ufl.edu, http://www.flmnh.edu/admin/bulletin.htm. Eds. John F Eisenberg, Richard Franz. R&P Margaret J Joyner. Circ: 700.

570 USA ISSN 0533-1242

FOCUS (ROCKVILLE). Text in English. 1979. q. free per issue. index, cum.index: vols.1-21. back issues avail. *Refereed.* **Document type:** *Newsletter.* **Description:** Describes novel techniques, improvements of common techniques, simplified protocols, and trouble shooting of life science techniques.

Related titles: Online - full text ed.

Indexed: Aqua.Sci.& Fish.Abstr., Environ.Sci.Poll.Mgmt., Pollut.Abstr., Risk Abstr., Saf.Sci.Abstr.

Published by: Life Technologies, Inc., PO Box 6482, Rockville, MD 20849-6482. TEL 301-610-8000, http://www.lifetech.com. Ed., R&P Doreen Cupo. Circ: 40,000.

FOLIA BIOCHIMICA ET BIOLOGICA GRAECA. see *BIOLOGY—Biochemistry*

570 CZE ISSN 0015-5500
QH301 CODEN: FOBLAN

FOLIA BIOLOGICA. Text and summaries in English. 1955. bi-m. GBP 136 foreign (effective 2000). adv. bk.rev. abstr, charts, illus. index. *Refereed.* **Document type:** *Academic/Scholarly.* **Description:** Publishes reports on the results of original research in the field of molecular and cellular biology.

Related titles: Online - full text ed.: (from Institute for Scientific Information).

Indexed: AgBiotech, AgroLibrex, Anim.Breed.Abstr., Aqua.Sci.& Fish.Abstr., Biol.Abstr., C.I.S. Abstr., Chem.Abstr., Chem.Indus.Notes, Chem.Titles, Curr.Adv.Cancer Res., Curr.Adv.Ecol.Sci., Curr.Cont., Dairy Sci.Abstr., Excerp.Med., Helminthol.Abstr., INIS Atomind., Ind.Med. (1955-), Ind.Sci.Rev., Ind.Vet., Inpharma, Int.Abstr.Biol.Sci., Nutr.Abstr., Pig News & Info., Poult.Abstr., Reac., Rev.Med.& Vet.Mycol., Sci.Cit.Ind., Vet.Bull.

—BLDSC (3967.000000), CASDDS, CISTI, GNLM, IDS, ingenta, Linda Hall. **CCC.**

Published by: Ceska Akademie Ved, Ustav Molekularni Genetiky, Flemingovo nam 2, Prague 16637, Czech Republic. TEL 42-2-24310234, FAX 42-2-24310955, TELEX 25775 ACPRES G, folia@img.cas.cz, http://www.img.cas.cz/. Ed. J Svoboda. R&P Catherine John. Adv. contact Nik Screen. Circ: 950. **Dist. by:** Harcourt Publishers Ltd.

570 POL ISSN 0015-5497
CODEN: FOBGA8

FOLIA BIOLOGICA; international journal of biological research. Text and summaries in English. 1953. q. PLZ 50 domestic; USD 40 foreign (effective 2000). adv. bk.rev. abstr, bibl, charts, illus. index. back issues avail. *Refereed.* **Document type:** *Academic/Scholarly.* **Description:** Publishes papers concerning various aspects of experimental zoology, nuclear and chromosome research and ultrastructural studies.

Related titles: E-mail ed.; Fax ed.; Online - full text ed.: (from Institute for Scientific Information).

Indexed: AgroAgen, Anim.Breed.Abstr., Biol.Abstr., Chem.Abstr., Chem.Indus.Notes, Chem.Titles, Curr.Adv.Ecol.Sci., Curr.Cont., Dent.Ind., Excerp.Med., INIS Atomind., Ind.Med. (1953-), Ind.Sci.Rev., Int.Abstr.Biol.Sci., Plant Breed.Abstr., Zoo.Rec.

—BLDSC (3966.900000), CASDDS, CISTI, GNLM, IDS, Linda Hall.

Published by: Polska Akademia Nauk, Instytut Systematyki i Ewolucji Zwierzat/Polish Academy of Sciences, Institute of Systematics and Evolution of Animals, Ul Slawkowska 17, Krakow 31016, Poland. TEL 48-12-4227006, FAX 48-12-4224294, TELEX 0322414 PAN PL, folia@isez.pan.krakow.pl, http://www.isez.pan.krakow.pl. Ed., R&P Halina Kosciuszko. Adv. contact Ewa Zychowska. Circ: 350.

FOLIA DENDROLOGICA. see *FORESTS AND FORESTRY*

570 CZE
CODEN: FFUBAP

FOLIA FACULTATIS SCIENTIARUM NATURALIUM UNIVERSITATIS MASARYKIANAE BRUNENSIS: BIOLOGIA. Text in Czech. a. price varies. **Document type:** *Monographic series, Academic/Scholarly.*

Formerly: Folia Facultatis Scientiarum Naturalium Universitatis Purkynianae Brunensis: Biologia (0323-0082)

Indexed: Biol.Abstr., Chem.Abstr., Helminthol.Abstr., Ref.Zh., Zoo.Rec.

—CASDDS, CISTI, Linda Hall.

Published by: Masarykova Universita, Prirodovedecka Fakulta/Masaryk University, Faculty of Sciences, Kotlarska 2, Brno 61137, Czech Republic. Ed. Jaromir Vanhara.

616.079 GBR ISSN 0954-0105
CODEN: FAIMEZ
FOOD AND AGRICULTURAL IMMUNOLOGY. Text in English. 1989. q. GBP 189, USD 312 to individuals; GBP 565, USD 927 to institutions (effective 2002). *Refereed.* **Document type:** *Academic/Scholarly.* **Description:** Features original immunological research with food, agricultural, environmental and veterinary applications.
Related titles: Online - full text ed.: ISSN 1465-3443 (from CatchWord Ltd., EBSCO Publishing, O C L C Online Computer Library Center, Inc., RoweCom Information Quest, ProQuest Information & Learning, Swets Blackwell, Institute for Scientific Information).
Indexed: AIDS & Cancer Res., ASCA, AgBiotech, Agri.& Environ.Biotech.Abstr., Agricola, Anal.Abstr., Aqua.Sci.& Fish.Abstr., Aquacult.Abstr., Biodet.Abstr., Chem.Abstr., Chem.Indus.Notes, Chem.Titles, Curr.Cont., Dairy Sci.Abstr., Environ.Sci.Poll.Mgmt., Food Sci.& Tech.Abstr., Herb.Abstr., Hort.Abstr., Immun.Abstr., Ind.Vet., Int.Abstr.Biol.Sci., Maize Abstr., Microbiol.Abstr., Nutr.Abstr., Pig News & Info., Postharvest, Rev.Appl.Entomol., Rev.Med.& Vet.Mycol., Rev.Plant Path., Rice Abstr., Soils & Fert., Soyabean Abstr., Triticale Abstr., Vet.Bull., Weed Abstr.
—BLDSC (3977.004500), CASDDS, CatchWord, CISTI, EMDOCS, IDS, Infotrieve. **CCC.**
Published by: Carfax Publishing Limited (Subsidiary of: Taylor & Francis Group), PO Box 25, Abingdon, Oxon OX14 3UE, United Kingdom. TEL 44-1235-401000, FAX 44-1235-401550, enquiries@carfax.co.uk, enquiry@tandf.co.uk, http://www.carfax.co.uk. Ed. M R A Morgan.

571.3 JPN ISSN 0911-6036
FORMA. Text in English. 1989. 4/yr. USD 120. *Refereed.* **Document type:** *Academic/Scholarly.*
Indexed: C.C.M.J.
—BLDSC (4008.314600).
Published by: Society for Science on Form Japan/Katachi no Kagakkai, Tokyo University of Agriculture & Technology, Dept of Mechanical Systems Engineering, 24-16 Naka-cho 2-chome, Koganei-shi, Tokyo-to 184-0012, Japan. TEL 81-423-88-7224, FAX 81-423-85-7204, takaki@cc.tuat.ac.jp, http://www.tuat.ac.jp/~takaki/index.html. Ed., R&P Ryuji Takaki. Circ: 400.

570 550 NLD ISSN 1381-2491
QH7
FOUNDATION FOR SCIENTIFIC RESEARCH IN THE CARIBBEAN REGION. PUBLICATION. Text in English. 1946. irreg., latest vol.137, 1996. price varies. back issues avail. **Document type:** *Monographic series.*
Formerly (until 1990): Natuurwetenschappelijke Studiekring voor Suriname en de Nederlandse Antillen. Uitgaven (0300-5534)
Indexed: Biol.Abstr., GeoRef.
Published by: Foundation for Scientific Research in the Caribbean Region/Natuurwetenschappelijke Studiekring voor het Caraibische Gebied, Instituut voor Taxonomische Zoologie, Plantage Middenlaan 45, Amsterdam 1018 DC, Netherlands. TEL 31-20-5255926, FAX 31-20-5256612. Ed. Louise J van der Steen. R&P Louise J Westermann.

570 USA ISSN 0891-5849
QP527 CODEN: FRBMEH
FREE RADICAL BIOLOGY & MEDICINE. Text in English. 1985. s-m. EUR 429 in Europe to qualified personnel; JPY 57,000 in Japan to qualified personnel; USD 480 elsewhere to qualified personnel; EUR 2,045 in Europe to institutions; JPY 271,600 in Japan to institutions; USD 2,288 elsewhere to institutions (effective 2002). back issues avail. *Refereed.* **Document type:** *Academic/Scholarly.* **Description:** Encompasses chemical, biochemical, physiological, pathological, pharmacological, toxicological and medical approaches to free-radical research.
Formed by the merger of: Advances in Free Radical Biology and Medicine (8755-9668); Journal of Free Radicals in Biology and Medicine; Which was formerly: Journal of Free Radicals in Biology (0748-5514)
Related titles: Microfilm ed.: (from PQC); Online - full text ed.: (from EBSCO Publishing, ingenta, Swets Blackwell, ScienceDirect, Institute for Scientific Information).
Indexed: ASCA, BBCI, Biotech.& Bioeng.Abstr., Chem.Abstr., Chem.Cit.Ind., Chem.Indus.Notes, Chem.Titles, Curr.Adv.Biochem., Curr.Adv.Cell & Devel.Biol., Curr.Adv.Ecol.Sci., Curr.Cont., Environ.Sci.Poll.Mgmt., Excerp.Med., Genet.Abstr., Hum.Gen.Abstr., INIS Atomind., Ind.Med. (1987-), Ind.Sci.Rev., Inpharma, Int.Abstr.Biol.Sci., Mass Spectr.Bull., NRN, Neurosci.Cit.Ind., Nuc.Acids Abstr., Pharm.&Out.News, Pollut.Abstr., Reac., Risk Abstr., Sci.Cit.Ind., THA, Tox.Abstr.
—BLDSC (4033.326480), ADONIS, CASDDS, CISTI, EMDOCS, GNLM, IDS, ingenta, KNAW. **CCC.**
Published by: (Oxygen Society), Elsevier Science, PO Box 945, New York, NY 10159-0945. TEL 212-989-5800, FAX 212-633-3990, http://www.elsevier.com/locate/freeradbiomed. Eds. K J A Davies, W A Pryor. **Subscr. in Australasia and the Far East to:** Elsevier Science (Singapore) Pte Ltd, No.1 Temasek Ave, 17-01 Millenia Tower, Singapore 039192, Singapore. TEL 65-434-3727, FAX 65-337-2230; **Subscr. in Japan to:** Elsevier Science Inc - Japan Regional Office, 9-15 Higashi-Azabu 1-chome, Minato-ku, Tokyo 106-0044, Japan. TEL 81-3-5561-5033; **Subscr. outside the Americas to:** Elsevier Science BV, PO Box 211, Amsterdam 1000 AE, Netherlands. TEL 31-20-485-3757, nlinfo-f@elsevier.nl.

578.77 GBR ISSN 0308-6739
CODEN: OPFAEI
FRESHWATER BIOLOGICAL ASSOCIATION. OCCASIONAL PUBLICATIONS. Text in English. 1976. irreg. price varies. back issues avail. **Document type:** *Monographic series, Academic/Scholarly.*
Related titles: Microfiche ed.
Indexed: Aqua.Sci.& Fish.Abstr., Aquacult.Abstr., Curr.Adv.Ecol.Sci., Environ.Sci.Poll.Mgmt., Forest.Abstr., GeoRef, Math.R., Soils & Fert., Zoo.Rec.
—BLDSC (6225.650000), Linda Hall.
Published by: Freshwater Biological Association, The Ferry House, Ambleside, Cumbria LA22 0LP, United Kingdom. TEL 44-1539-442468, FAX 44-1539-446914, chiefexec@fba.org.uk, http://www.fba.org.uk. Ed. D W Sutcliffe. Circ: 400.

578.77 GBR ISSN 0367-1887
QH96.A1 CODEN: FBSPAT
FRESHWATER BIOLOGICAL ASSOCIATION. SCIENTIFIC PUBLICATIONS. Text in English. a. price varies. back issues avail. **Document type:** *Academic/Scholarly.*
Related titles: Microfiche ed.
Indexed: Aqua.Sci.& Fish.Abstr., Aquacult.Abstr., Biol.Abstr., Curr.Adv.Ecol.Sci., Deep Sea Res.& Oceanogr.Abstr., Environ.Sci.Poll.Mgmt., Sport Fish.Abstr., Wild.Rev., Zoo.Rec.
—BLDSC (8191.000000), CISTI.
Published by: Freshwater Biological Association, The Ferry House, Ambleside, Cumbria LA22 0LP, United Kingdom. TEL 44-1539-442468, FAX 44-1539-446914, chiefexec@fba.org.uk, http://www.fba.org.uk. Eds. D W Sutcliffe, J M Elliott. Circ: 2,500.

578.77 GBR ISSN 0046-5070
QH96.A1 CODEN: FWBLAB
FRESHWATER BIOLOGY. Text in English. 1971. 12/yr. (in 3 vols.), latest vol.47, 2002. GBP 115 in Europe to individuals; USD 183 in North America to individuals; GBP 127 elsewhere to individuals; GBP 1,370 in Europe to institutions; USD 2,171 in North America to institutions; GBP 1,507 elsewhere to institutions (effective 2002). adv. bk.rev. abstr, charts, illus, stat. index. back issues avail.; reprint service avail. from ISI. *Refereed.* **Document type:** *Journal, Academic/Scholarly.*
Related titles: Microform ed.: (from PQC); ♦ Online - full text ed.: Freshwater Biology Online. ISSN 1365-2427.
Indexed: ASCA, Abstr.Bull.Inst.Pap.Chem., Acid Pre.Dig., Appl.Ecol.Abstr., Aqua.Sci.& Fish.Abstr., Aquacult.Abstr., Bio-Contr.News & Info., Biol.& Agr.Ind. (Jun.1989-), Biol.Abstr., Chem.Abstr., Chem.Indus.Notes, Chem.Titles, Curr.Adv.Ecol.Sci., Curr.Adv.Plant Sci., Curr.Cont., Curr.Ref.Fish Res., Deep Sea Res.& Oceanogr.Abstr., Ecol.Abstr., Entomol.Abstr., Environ.Abstr., Environ.Per.Bibl. (1990-), Environ.Sci.Poll.Mgmt., Excerp.Med., Forest.Abstr., Geo.Abstr.H.G., Geo.Abstr.P.G., GeoRef, Geol.Abstr., Helminthol.Abstr., INIS Atomind., Ind.Sci.Rev., Int.Abstr.Biol.Sci., Irr.& Drain.Abstr., Microbiol.Abstr., Nutr.Abstr., Plant Sci., Pollut.Abstr., Ref.Zh., Rev.Appl.Entomol., Rev.Med.& Vet.Mycol., Rural Recreat.Tour.Abstr., Sci.Cit.Ind., Sel.J.Water, Soils & Fert., Sport Fish.Abstr., W.R.C.Inf., Weed Abstr., Wild.Rev., Zoo.Rec.
—BLDSC (4037.200000), CASDDS, CISTI, EMDOCS, IDS, ingenta, Linda Hall. **CCC.**
Published by: Blackwell Science Ltd., PO Box 88, Oxford OX2 0NE, United Kingdom. TEL 44-1865-206180, 44-1865-206002, FAX 44-1865-206219, fwb@blacksci.co.uk, jnl.orders@blacksci.co.uk, http://www.blackwell-science.com/fwb, http://www.blackwellpublishing.com. Eds. Dr. Alan G. Hildrew, Dr. Colin R. Townsend. Pub. Sue Hewitt. R&P Sophie Savage. Adv. contact Jenny Applin. Circ: 840.

578.77 GBR ISSN 1365-2427
FRESHWATER BIOLOGY ONLINE. Text in English. 1998. m. GBP 104 in Europe to individuals; USD 165 in North America to individuals; GBP 104 elsewhere to individuals; GBP 1,233 in Europe to institutions; USD 1,954 in North America to institutions; GBP 1,233 elsewhere to institutions (effective 2002). *Refereed.* **Document type:** *Academic/Scholarly.*
Media: Online - full text (from EBSCO Publishing, Munksgaard & Blackwell Science's Synergy, O C L C Online Computer Library Center, Inc., RoweCom Information Quest, ingenta, Swets Blackwell, Institute for Scientific Information). **Related titles:** Microform ed.: (from PQC); ♦ Print ed.: Freshwater Biology. ISSN 0046-5070.
Published by: Blackwell Science Ltd., Osney Mead, Oxford OX2 0EL, United Kingdom. TEL 44-1685-206206, FAX 44-1685-721205, website@blacksci.com, journals.cs@blacksci.co.uk, http://www.blackwell-science.com.

FRONTIERS IN BIOSCIENCE. see *MEDICAL SCIENCES*

573.6 USA ISSN 0895-1942
QK623.S73 CODEN: FGNEEA
FUNGAL GENETICS NEWSLETTER. Text in English. 1962. a. USD 15. back issues avail. **Document type:** *Newsletter.* **Description:** Publishes articles, bibliographies and addresses for researches in fungal genetics.
Formerly: Neurospora Newsletter (0028-3975)
Related titles: Online - full text ed.
Indexed: Biol.Abstr., INIS Atomind., Rev.Plant Path.
—BLDSC (4056.650000), CISTI.
Published by: Fungal Genetics Stock Center, University of Kansas Medical School, Department of Microbiology, Kansas City, KS 66160-7420. TEL 913-588-7044, FAX 913-588-7295, fgsc@kuhub.cc.ukans.edu, http://www.fgsc.net/newslet.html. Ed. Peter J Russell. R&P Kevin McCluskey. Circ: 1,000.

GARCIA DE ORTA: SERIE DE ANTROPOBIOLOGIA. see *ANTHROPOLOGY*

570 550 IND ISSN 0251-1223
QH301 CODEN: GBOSBU
GEOBIOS; an international journal of life sciences on earth. Text in English. 1974. q. INR 200 to individuals; INR 600 to institutions (effective 2002). adv. bk.rev. 64 p./no. 2 cols./p. back issues avail.; reprints avail. *Refereed.* **Document type:** *Journal, Academic/Scholarly.*
Indexed: Biol.Abstr., Br.Geol.Lit., Chem.Abstr., Chem.Indus.Notes, Chem.Titles, Curr.Adv.Ecol.Sci., Excerp.Med., Geo.Abstr.P.G., Geol.Abstr., Hort.Abstr., INIS Atomind., Zoo.Rec.
—BLDSC (4116.901500), CASDDS, CISTI, Linda Hall.
Published by: Geobios Zion, Zion, 41B B-1-A, P.W.D. Colony, P O Box 14, Jodhpur, Rajasthan 342 001, India. TEL 91-291-431726. Ed. David Navin Sen.

570 550 IND ISSN 0253-3340
QH301
GEOBIOS NEW REPORTS; biannual journal of life sciences. Text in English. 1982. biennial. INR 100, USD 35 to individuals; INR 350, USD 70 to institutions (effective 1999). bk.rev. reprints avail. **Document type:** *Academic/Scholarly.* **Description:** Publishes research reports in the life sciences.
Indexed: Curr.Adv.Ecol.Sci., Zoo.Rec.
—Linda Hall.
Published by: Geobios Zion, Zion, 41B B-1-A, P.W.D. Colony, P O Box 14, Jodhpur, Rajasthan 342 001, India. TEL 91-291-431726. Ed. David Navin Sen.

GEORGIAN MEDICAL NEWS; monthly scientific bulletin. see *MEDICAL SCIENCES*

570 DEU ISSN 0368-2307
QH5 CODEN: JGNWA2
GESELLSCHAFT FUER NATURKUNDE IN WUERTTEMBERG. JAHRESHEFTE. Text in German. 1845. a. DEM 35 (effective 1999). **Document type:** *Proceedings.*
Formerly: Verein fuer Vaterlaendische Naturkunde in Wuerttemberg. Jahresheft
Indexed: Biol.Abstr., GeoRef, Ref.Zh., Zoo.Rec.
—Linda Hall.
Published by: Gesellschaft fuer Naturkunde in Wuerttemberg e.V., Rosensteinstr 1, Stuttgart 70191, Germany. TEL 49-711-89360. Ed. Siegmund Seybold. Circ: 1,100.

B

570 UKR ISSN 0375-8990
CODEN: GBZUAM

GIDROBIOLOGICHESKII ZHURNAL; nauchnyi zhurnal. Text in Russian; Summaries in English. 1965. bi-m. USD 410 (effective 1998). **Document type:** *Academic/Scholarly.*
Related titles: ♦ English Translation: Hydrobiological Journal. ISSN 0018-8166.
Indexed: Aqua.Sci.& Fish.Abstr., Aquacult.Abstr., Biol.Abstr., Chem.Abstr., Chem.Indus.Notes, Chem.Titles, Deep Sea Res.& Oceanogr.Abstr., Environ.Sci.Poll.Mgmt., GeoRef, Helminthol.Abstr., INIS Atomind., Ocean.Abstr. (coverage dropped), Pollut.Abstr., Protozool.Abstr., Sel.Water Res.Abstr., Sport Fish.Abstr., Wild.Rev., Zoo.Rec.
—CASDDS, CISTI, East View, Infotrieve, KNAW, Linda Hall. **CCC.**
Published by: Natsional'na Akademiya Nauk Ukrainy, Otdelenie Obshchei Biologii, Vul Tereshchenkivska 3, Kiev 252601, Ukraine. TEL 380-44-224-4068, FAX 380-44-224-7060. **Subscr. to:** Mezhdunarodnaya Kniga, B Yakimanka 39, Moscow 117049, Russian Federation.

570 500 GBR ISSN 0373-241X
CODEN: GGNTAS

GLASGOW NATURALIST. Text in English. 1908. a. GBP 3 domestic; GBP 6 foreign (effective 2001). adv. bk.rev. charts, illus. cum.index every 5 yrs. *Refereed.* **Document type:** *Academic/Scholarly.* **Description:** Contains general articles, papers, and short notes on natural history of Scotland.
Related titles: Microfilm ed.: (from PMC).
Indexed: Biol.Abstr., Curr.Adv.Ecol.Sci., Deep Sea Res.& Oceanogr.Abstr., GeoRef, Sport Fish.Abstr., Zoo.Rec.
—BLDSC (4184.000000).
Published by: Glasgow Natural History Society, c/o Dr. J.R. Downie, Ed, Graham Kerr (Zoology) Bldg, University of Glasgow, Glasgow, Lanarkshire G12 8QQ, United Kingdom. TEL 44-141-330-5157, FAX 44-141-330-5971, j.r.downie@bio.gla.ac.uk. Ed., R&P J R Downie. Circ: 500.

570 170 ITA ISSN 1128-7462

GLOBAL BIOETHICS. Text in English. 1992. q. USD 90 to individuals; USD 115 to institutions (effective 2000). bk.rev. abstr. back issues avail. **Document type:** *Academic/Scholarly.* **Description:** Forum for reflection and debate on all questions inherent in the generally-defined boundaries of bio-ethics, medical ethics and environmental ethics.
Formerly (until 1991): Problemi di Bioetica
Related titles: Online - full text ed.: ISSN 1591-7398. 2001.
—BLDSC (4195.351750).
Published by: (International Institute for the Study of Man), Angelo Pontecorboli Editore, c/o Inst.d'Antropologia, Universita di Firenze, Via Del Proconsolo, 12, Florence, FI 50122, Italy. TEL 39-55-2398065, FAX 39-55-283358, antropos@cesit1.unifi.it, http://www.digital.casalini.it/fup/periodicals.htm, http://www.unifi.it/unifi/antrop/. Ed. A B Chiarelli. Circ: 400.

GLOBAL CONNECTIONS (ROCHESTER). see *LIBRARY AND INFORMATION SCIENCES*

GORTANIA; atti del Museo Friulano di Storia Naturale. see *SCIENCES: COMPREHENSIVE WORKS*

570 590 ESP ISSN 0367-5041
QL461 CODEN: GRAEAT

GRAELLSIA; revista de zoologia. Text and summaries in English, Spanish. 1943. a. ESP 4,000 domestic to individuals; ESP 5,500 foreign to individuals; ESP 8,000 domestic to institutions; ESP 11,000 foreign to institutions. bk.rev. Supplement avail.; back issues avail. *Refereed.* **Document type:** *Newspaper, Monographic series.* **Description:** Covers contributions to the advancement of knowledge in zoological biodiversity, including taxonomy, fauna, biogeography and evolution and conservation studies.
Indexed: Entomol.Abstr. (coverage dropped), Ind.SST, Rev.Appl.Entomol., Zoo.Rec.
—CINDOC.
Published by: Museo Nacional de Ciencias Naturales, Jose Gutierrez Abascal, 2, Madrid 28006, Spain. TEL 34-1-4111328, FAX 34-1-5645078, graellsia@mncn.csic.es. Eds. Ana I Camacho, M Angeles Ramos. Circ: 400.

612.67 USA ISSN 1041-1232
QH511.A1 CODEN: GDAGE9

GROWTH, DEVELOPMENT & AGING. Text in English. 1937. q. USD 90 domestic to non-members; USD 110 foreign to non-members; USD 40 domestic to members; USD 50 foreign to members (effective 2000). adv. bk.rev. bibl, charts, illus. index. reprint service avail. from PQC,ISI. *Refereed.* **Document type:** *Journal, Academic/Scholarly.* **Description:** Devoted to problems of normal and abnormal growth patterns; relationship among growth, development and aging; and mathematical models related to these areas.
Formerly (until 1987): Growth (0017-4793)
Related titles: Microform ed.: (from PQC,PMC); Online - full text ed.: (from H. W. Wilson, Institute for Scientific Information).
Indexed: ASCA, Abstr.Anthropol., Agricola, Anim.Breed.Abstr., Aqua.Sci.& Fish.Abstr., Biol.& Agr.Ind. (Mar.1988-), Biol.Abstr., Chem.Abstr., Chem.Indus.Notes, Chem.Titles, Curr.Adv.Ecol.Sci., Curr.Cont., Dairy Sci.Abstr., Dent.Ind., Excerp.Med., INIS Atomind., Ind.Med. (1988-), Ind.Sci.Rev., Ind.Vet., Inpharma, Int.Abstr.Biol.Sci., Mid.East: Abstr.& Ind., NRN, Nutr.Abstr., Pharm.&Out.News, Pig News & Info., Poult.Abstr., Reac., Ref.Zh., Sci.Cit.Ind., THA, Vet.Bull., W.R.C.Inf., Zoo.Rec.
—BLDSC (4223.032500), CASDDS, CISTI, GNLM, IDS, ingenta, Linda Hall.
Published by: Growth Publishing Co., Inc., PO Box 205, Hulls Cove, ME 04644-0205. FAX 207-288-6079, deh@jax.org, http://www.growthdevelaging.org. Ed., R&P Dr. David E Harrison TEL 207-288-6357. Circ: 625.

570 NOR ISSN 0332-8554
QH168 CODEN: KNVGDN

GUNNERIA. Text and summaries in English, German, Norwegian. 1971. irreg., latest vol.76, 1999. *Refereed.* **Document type:** *Academic/Scholarly.*
Formerly (until no.26, 1977): Kongelige Norske Videnskabers Selskab. Museet. Miscellanea (0332-8430)
Indexed: Aqua.Sci.& Fish.Abstr., Aquacult.Abstr., Biol.Abstr., Chem.Abstr., Curr.Adv.Ecol.Sci., Deep Sea Res.& Oceanogr.Abstr., GeoRef, Herb.Abstr., NAA, Plant Gen.Res.Abstr., Zoo.Rec.
—**CCC.**
Published by: Norges Teknisk-Naturvitenskapelige Universitet, Vitenskapmuseet/Norwegian University of Science and Technology, Museum of Natural History and Archaeology, Trondheim 7491, Norway. TEL 47-73-59-21-45, FAX 47-73-59-22-23, ase.vanvik@vm.ntnu.no. Ed. Astrid Langvath. Circ: 500.

570 GBR

H M S BEAGLE. (Her Majesty's Ship) Text in English. bi-w. adv. back issues avail. **Document type:** *Newsletter, Bulletin.* **Description:** Provides a forum for researchers in the biomedical sciences to exchange Web-based resources and other ideas.
Media: Online - full text.
Published by: BioMedNet Ltd. (Subsidiary of: Elsevier Science), Flat 34, Middlesex House, 34-42 Cleveland St, London W1P 6LE, United Kingdom. TEL 44-171-323-5348, FAX 44-171-631-0819, info@biomed.net, http://www.biomednet.com/hmsbeagle. Ed. Lois Wingerson. Pub. Berlinda Kerkhof. Adv. contact Stacy Barrett.

HANDBOOK OF BEHAVIORAL NEUROBIOLOGY. see *MEDICAL SCIENCES—Psychiatry And Neurology*

HASTINGS CENTER REPORT. see *MEDICAL SCIENCES*

570 USA ISSN 0073-1331
QH91.A1

HAWAII INSTITUTE OF MARINE BIOLOGY. TECHNICAL REPORTS. Text in English. 1964. irreg., latest vol.39, 1988. price varies. *Refereed.* **Document type:** *Academic/Scholarly.*
Indexed: Deep Sea Res.& Oceanogr.Abstr., Ocean.Abstr. (coverage dropped).
Published by: Hawaii Institute of Marine Biology, PO Box 1346, Kaneohe, HI 96744. TEL 808-237-7401, FAX 808-247-6634. Ed. Philip Helfrich. Circ: 200.

570 ARM ISSN 0002-2918
QH301 CODEN: BZARAZ

HAYASTANY KENSABANAKAN ANDES/ BIOLOGICHESKII ZHURNAL ARMENII. Text in Armenian, Russian; Summaries in English. 1948. q. AMD 400. abstr, illus. **Document type:** *Academic/Scholarly.*
Indexed: Anim.Breed.Abstr., Biodet.Abstr., Biol.Abstr., Chem.Abstr., Chem.Indus.Notes, Chem.Titles, Crop Physiol.Abstr., Dairy Sci.Abstr., Field Crop Abstr., Food Sci.& Tech.Abstr., Forest.Abstr., Herb.Abstr., Hort.Abstr., INIS Atomind., Maize Abstr., Plant Breed.Abstr., Poult.Abstr., Rev.Plant Path., Seed Abstr., Sel.Water Res.Abstr., Soils & Fert., Triticale Abstr., VITIS, Vet.Bull.
—CISTI, Linda Hall.
Published by: Akademiya Nauk Armenii, Pr Marshala Bagramayana 24, Erevan 375019, Armenia. TEL 78852-524580, TELEX 243344. Ed. G G Batikian.

HELICOBACTER. see *BIOLOGY—Abstracting, Bibliographies, Statistics*

▼ **HIGH ALTITUDE MEDICINE AND BIOLOGY.** see *MEDICAL SCIENCES*

HIROSAKI IGAKU/HIROSAKI MEDICAL JOURNAL. see *MEDICAL SCIENCES*

HISTORICAL BIOLOGY; an international journal of paleobiology. see *PALEONTOLOGY*

570 GBR ISSN 0391-9714
QH305 CODEN: HPLSDO

HISTORY AND PHILOSOPHY OF THE LIFE SCIENCES. Text in English. 1916. 4/yr. GBP 108, USD 178 to individuals; GBP 209, USD 346 to institutions (effective 2002). adv. bk.rev. back issues avail. *Refereed.* **Document type:** *Academic/Scholarly.* **Description:** Explores the historical development of the life sciences and the social and epistemological implications.
Supersedes in part (in 1979): Stazione Zoologica di Napoli. Pubblicazioni (0039-081X)
Related titles: Online - full text ed.: (from Institute for Scientific Information).
Indexed: ASCA, Arts & Hum.Cit.Ind., Curr.Cont., GeoRef, Hist.Abstr. (1983-1994, dropped), Ind.Med. (1979-), Phil.Ind., Russ.Acad.Sci.Bibl., SSCI, Zoo.Rec.
—BLDSC (4317.820000), CISTI, IDS, ingenta, Linda Hall. **CCC.**
Published by: (Stazione Zoologica di Napoli ITA), Taylor & Francis Group, Taylor & Francis Ltd., 11 New Fetter Ln, London EC4P 4EE, United Kingdom. TEL 44-20-7583-9855, FAX 44-20-7842-2298, info@tandf.co.uk, http://www.tandf.co.uk. Ed. Bernardino Fantini. **Subscr. in N. America to:** Taylor & Francis Ltd., 325 Chestnut St, Suite 800, Philadelphia, PA 19016. TEL 800-354-1420, FAX 215-625-8914, info@taylorandfrancis.com, http://www.taylorandfrancis.com/.

570 JPN ISSN 0018-3393
QH301 CODEN: HKDSBF

HOKKAIDO KYOIKU DAIGAKU KIYO. DAI-2-BU, B. SEIBUTSUGAKU, CHIGAKU, NOGAKU-HEN/ HOKKAIDO UNIVERSITY OF EDUCATION. JOURNAL. SECTION 2 B. BIOLOGY, GEOLOGY, AND AGRICULTURE. Text in English, French, Japanese; Summaries in English. 1982 (vol.32). s-a. per issue exchange basis. **Document type:** *Bulletin.*
Indexed: Biol.Abstr., Chem.Abstr., GeoRef, Zoo.Rec.
Published by: Hokkaido University of Education/Hokkaido Kyoiku Daigaku, Ainosato 5-jo, 3-chome, Kita-ku, Sapporo-shi, Hokkaido 002, Japan. Circ: 500.

570 HRV

HRVATSKA AKADEMIJA ZNANOSTI I UMJETNOSTI. RAZRED ZA PRIRODNE ZNANOSTI. RAD. Text and summaries in Croatian, English, French, German. 1866. a. USD 30. **Document type:** *Academic/Scholarly.*
Formerly: Jugoslavenska Akademija Znanosti i Umjetnosti. Razred za Prirodne Znanosti. Rad. (0351-3297)
Indexed: Biol.Abstr., Concr.Abstr., GeoRef.
Published by: Hrvatska Akademija Znanosti i Umjetnosti, Razred za Prirodne Znanosti, Zrinski trg 11, Zagreb 10000, Croatia. TEL 385-1-4813344, FAX 385-1-4819979.

HUAXI YIKE DAXUE XUEBAO/WEST CHINA UNIVERSITY OF MEDICAL SCIENCES. JOURNAL. see *MEDICAL SCIENCES*

570 USA ISSN 0018-7143
GN1 CODEN: HUBIAA
HUMAN BIOLOGY (DETROIT). Text in English. 1929. bi-m. USD 85 domestic to individuals; USD 109 foreign to individuals; USD 160 domestic to institutions; USD 184 foreign to institutions (effective 2000). adv. bk.rev. charts, illus. index. back issues avail.; reprint service avail. from PSC,PQC. *Refereed.* **Document type:** *Academic/Scholarly.* **Description:** Focuses on genetics areas, including population genetics, evolutionary and genetic demography, quantitative genetics, genetic epidemiology, behavioral genetics, molecular genetics; also growth and physiological parameters of genetic and environmental interactions.
Related titles: Microform ed.: (from PQC); Online - full text ed.: (from Gale Group, ProQuest Information & Learning, H. W. Wilson, Swets Blackwell, Factiva, Institute for Scientific Information).
Indexed: A.I.C.P. (1929-), Abstr.Anthropol., AgeLine, Amer.Bibl.Slavic & E.Eur.Stud., Anthropol.Lit., Art & Archaeol.Tech.Abstr., Behav.Med.Abstr., Bibl.Asian Stud. (1970-1971, 1998), Bibl.Dev.Med.& Child Neur., Biol.& Agr.Ind. (Feb.1983-), Biol.Abstr., Biol.Dig., Chem.Abstr., Curr.Adv.Ecol.Sci., Curr.Cont., Curr.Ind.Stat., Dairy Sci.Abstr., Dok.Arbeitsmed., Excerp.Med., Gen.Sci.Ind. (Feb.1984-), Helminthol.Abstr., INIS Atomind., Ind.Med. (1929-), Ind.Sci.Rev., Inpharma, Int.Abstr.Biol.Sci., Lang.& Lang.Behav.Abstr., Mid.East: Abstr.& Ind., Nutr.Abstr., P C I, Pharm.&Out.News, Popul.Ind., Psychol.Abstr., Reac., Russ.Acad.Sci.Bibl., SOPODA, SSCI (coverage dropped), Sci.Cit.Ind., So.Pac.Per.Ind., Soc.Serv.Abstr., Sociol.Abstr., Sp.Ed.Needs Abstr., Trop.Dis.Bull.
—BLDSC (4336.000000), CASDDS, CISTI, EMDOCS, GNLM, IDS, ingenta, KNAW, Linda Hall. **CCC.**
Published by: Wayne State University Press, The Leonard N. Simons Bldg, 4809 Woodward Ave, Detroit, MI 48201-1309. TEL 313-577-6120, 313-577-6119, FAX 313-577-6131, ac3707@wayne.edu, http://www.libraries.wayne.edu/wsupress/, http://www.lark.cc.ukans.edu/~humanbio. Ed. Michael Crawford. R&P, Adv. contact Georgia Shurn. Circ: 1,654.

HUMAN ETHOLOGY BULLETIN. see *PSYCHOLOGY*

HUMAN EVOLUTION; international journal. see *ANTHROPOLOGY*

HUMAN NATURE; an interdisciplinary biosocial perspective. see *SOCIAL SCIENCES: COMPREHENSIVE WORKS*

599.9 573.6 170 GBR ISSN 1028-7825
HUMAN REPRODUCTION AND GENETIC ETHICS; an international journal. Text in English. 1995. s-a. GBP 12, USD 27 to individuals; GBP 20, USD 40 to institutions (effective 2001). adv. bk.rev. *Refereed.* **Document type:** *Academic/Scholarly.* **Description:** Publishes contributions on ethical perspectives of genetics and human reproduction across all disciplines. Themes include human genome analysis, artificial fecundation and reproduction, sex selection, privacy of genetic data and screening, human gene therapy, eugenics, biotechnology, and cloning.
Formerly (until 1998): European Journal of Genetics in Society (1023-9022)
—BLDSC (4336.431200), GNLM. **CCC.**
Published by: European Bioethical Research, 191 Leith Walk, Edinburgh, Midlothian EH6 8NX, United Kingdom. bioethics@europe.com. Ed., R&P Dr. Calum MacKellar TEL 44-131-554-8869.

578.77 NLD ISSN 0018-8158
QH90 CODEN: HYDRB8
HYDROBIOLOGIA; the international journal on limnology and marine sciences. Text in English. 1948. 23/yr. EUR 7,204, USD 7,216 to institutions for print or online ed.; EUR 8,644.80, USD 8,659.20 to institutions for print & online eds. combined (effective 2002). adv. bk.rev. bibl. reprint service avail. from SWZ. *Refereed.* **Document type:** *Journal, Academic/Scholarly.* **Description:** Publishes original articles in the fields of fundamental limnology and marine biology.
Incorporates (1992-2000): International Journal of Salt Lake Research (1037-0544)
Related titles: Microform ed.: (from PQC); Online - full text ed.: (from EBSCO Publishing, O C L C Online Computer Library Center, Inc., RoweCom Information Quest, Swets Blackwell, Kluwer Online, Institute for Scientific Information); ♦ Supplement: Journal of Applied Phycology. ISSN 0921-8971.
Indexed: ASCA, Acid Pre.Dig., AgBiotech, Agri.Eng.Abstr., Anim.Behav.Abstr., Anim.Breed.Abstr., Appl.Ecol.Abstr., Aqua.Sci.& Fish.Abstr., Bio-Contr.News & Info., Biol.Abstr., Cadscan, Chem.Abstr., Chem.Cit.Ind., Chem.Indus.Notes, Chem.Titles, Curr.Adv.Ecol.Sci., Curr.Cont., Curr.Ref.Fish Res., Deep Sea Res.& Oceanogr.Abstr., Ecol.Abstr., Eng.Ind., Entomol.Abstr., Environ.Abstr., Environ.Ind., Environ.Per.Bibl. (1993-), Environ.Sci.Poll.Mgmt., Excerp.Med., Food Sci.& Tech.Abstr., Forest Prod.Abstr., Forest.Abstr., Genet.Abstr., Geo.Abstr.H.G., Geo.Abstr.P.G., GeoRef, Geol.Abstr., Helminthol.Abstr., Herb.Abstr., Hort.Abstr., Hum.Gen.Abstr., IDA, INIS Atomind., Ind.Sci.Rev., Ind.Vet., Int.Abstr.Biol.Sci., Irr.& Drain.Abstr., Lead Abstr., Mass Spectr.Bull., Microbiol.Abstr., Nutr.Abstr., Ocean.Abstr., Plant Breed.Abstr., Plant Grow.Reg.Abstr., Pollut.Abstr., Rev.Appl.Entomol., Rev.Med.& Vet.Mycol., Rev.Plant Path., Rice Abstr., SSCI (coverage dropped), Sci.Cit.Ind., Seed Abstr., Sel.J.Water, Sel.Water Res.Abstr., So.Pac.Per.Ind., Soils & Fert., Sport Fish.Abstr., Sugar Ind.Abstr., Tox.Abstr. (coverage dropped), Triticale Abstr., Vet.Bull., W.R.C.Inf., Weed Abstr., Wild.Rev., World Ag.Econ.& Rur.Soc.Abstr., Zincscan, Zoo.Rec.
—BLDSC (4343.000000), CASDDS, CINDOC, CIS, CISTI, Ei, EMDOCS, IDS, ingenta, Linda Hall. **CCC.**
Published by: Kluwer Academic Publishers Group (Subsidiary of: Wolters Kluwer N.V.), Spuiboulevard 50, PO Box 17, Dordrecht 3300 AA, Netherlands. TEL 31-78-639-2392, FAX 31-78-654-2254, services@wkap.nl, http://www.wkap.nl/journalhome.htm/0018-8158. Ed. H J Dumont. Circ: 1,000. **Subscr. in the Americas to:** Kluwer Academic - Plenum Publishers, 233 Spring St, New York, NY 10013-1578. TEL 212-620-8468, FAX 212-807-1047; **Subscr. to:** Journals Department, PO Box 322, Dordrecht 3300 AH, Netherlands. TEL 31-78-639-2392, FAX 31-78-654-6474.

578.77 551.48 USA ISSN 0018-8166
QH91.A1 CODEN: HYBJA
HYDROBIOLOGICAL JOURNAL. Text in English. 1970. 7/yr. USD 1,323 domestic; USD 1,378 foreign (effective 2000). adv. bk.rev. charts, illus. index. **Document type:** *Academic/Scholarly.* **Description:** Focuses on freshwater and marine biology.
Related titles: Microform ed.: (from PQC); ♦ Translation of: Gidrobiologicheskii Zhurnal. ISSN 0375-8990.
Indexed: Anim.Behav.Abstr. (coverage dropped), Appl.Ecol.Abstr. (coverage dropped), Aqua.Sci.& Fish.Abstr., Biol.Abstr., Curr.Adv.Ecol.Sci., Curr.Tit.Ocean, Deep Sea Res.& Oceanogr.Abstr., Ecol.Abstr., Eng.Ind., Environ.Sci.Poll.Mgmt., Excerp.Med., Fuel & Energy Abstr., Geo.Abstr.P.G., GeoRef, Geol.Abstr., INIS Atomind., Microbiol.Abstr., Ocean.Abstr. (coverage dropped), Pollut.Abstr., Sel.J.Water, Sel.Water Res.Abstr., Soils & Fert., Sport Fish.Abstr., W.R.C.Inf., Weed Abstr., Wild.Rev., Zoo.Rec.
—BLDSC (0412.088600), CISTI, Ei, ingenta. **CCC.**
Published by: Begell House Inc., 79 Madison Ave, Ste 1205, New York, NY 10016-7892. TEL 212-725-1999, FAX 212-213-8368, begellhouse@worldnet.att.net, orders@begellhouse.com. Ed. Robert J Behnke. Circ: 325. **Co-sponsors:** Ukrainian Academy of Science; Rossiiskaya Akademiya Nauk/Russian Academy of Sciences.

578.77 BGR ISSN 0324-0924
QH90.A1 CODEN: KHIDD9
HYDROBIOLOGY. Text in Bulgarian, English, French, Russian. 1975. irreg. BGL 1.32 per issue. bibl, illus. reprint service avail. from IRC.
Indexed: Environ.Eng.Abstr., GeoRef, Sel.Water Res.Abstr.
—CASDDS, CISTI, KNAW, Linda Hall.
Published by: (Bulgarska Akademiia na Naukite/Bulgarian Academy of Sciences), Publishing House of the Bulgarian Academy of Sciences, Akad G Bonchev 6, Sofia 1113, Bulgaria. Circ: 430. **Dist. by:** Hemus, 6 Rouski blvd, Sofia 1000, Bulgaria.

570 JPN ISSN 0915-8987
HYUMAN SAIENSU* /HUMAN SCIENCE. Text in Japanese. 1990. bi-m. JPY 800 per issue.
Published by: Hyuman Saiensu Shinko Zaidan/Japan Health Science Foundation, c/o Japan Public Health Association, Koei Bldg, 29-8 Shinjuku 1-chome, Shinjuku-ku, Tokyo 160-0022, Japan.

I-BUNPI KENKYUKAISHI/JAPANESE SOCIETY OF GASTRIC SECRETION RESEARCH. PROCEEDINGS. see *MEDICAL SCIENCES—Endocrinology*

I E E E - E M B S CONFERENCE ON INFORMATION TECHNOLOGY APPLICATIONS IN BIOMEDICINE. PROCEEDINGS. see *COMPUTERS*

I M A JOURNAL OF MATHEMATICS APPLIED IN MEDICINE & BIOLOGY. see *MATHEMATICS*

I M S NEWSLETTER. (International Marine Science) see *EARTH SCIENCES—Oceanography*

IGAKU TO SEIBUTSUGAKU/MEDICINE AND BIOLOGY. see *MEDICAL SCIENCES*

570 USA ISSN 0073-4748
CODEN: ILBMA4
ILLINOIS BIOLOGICAL MONOGRAPHS SERIES. Text in English. 1914. irreg. reprint service avail. from PQC. *Refereed.* **Document type:** *Monographic series.*
Related titles: Microform ed.: (from PQC).
Indexed: Aqua.Sci.& Fish.Abstr., Aquacult.Abstr., Biol.Abstr., Environ.Sci.Poll.Mgmt., Rev.Appl.Entomol., Sport Fish.Abstr., Zoo.Rec.
—BLDSC (4365.000000), CISTI, Infotrieve, Linda Hall. **CCC.**
Published by: University of Illinois Press, 1325 S Oak St, Champaign, IL 61820. TEL 217-333-0950, FAX 217-244-8082.

570 USA ISSN 0073-490X
QH9 CODEN: INHNAH
ILLINOIS. NATURAL HISTORY SURVEY. BIOLOGICAL NOTES. Text in English. 1933. irreg., latest vol.140, 1997. USD 4 per issue (effective 2000). back issues avail. *Refereed.* **Document type:** *Government.* **Description:** Reports of research results and techniques; faunistic surveys with emphasis on Illinois species.
Indexed: Aqua.Sci.& Fish.Abstr., Biol.Abstr., Environ.Sci.Poll.Mgmt., Pollut.Abstr., Rev.Plant Path., Sport Fish.Abstr., Wild Life Rev., Wild.Rev., Zoo.Rec.
—CISTI, Linda Hall.
Published by: Department of Natural Resources, Natural History Survey, Natural Resources Bldg, 607 E Peabody Dr, Champaign, IL 61820. TEL 217-244-2115, FAX 217-333-4949. Ed. Charles Warwick. Circ: 1,500.

570 USA ISSN 0073-4918
QH1 CODEN: INHBAF
ILLINOIS. NATURAL HISTORY SURVEY. BULLETIN. Text in English. 1876. irreg., latest vol.35, no.4, 1997. USD 10 per issue (effective 2000). bibl, illus. *Refereed.* **Document type:** *Academic/Scholarly.* **Description:** Reports of research results and biological data with emphasis on Illinois.
Indexed: Biol.Abstr., Poult.Abstr., Ref.Zh., Rev.Plant Path., Sport Fish.Abstr., Wild Life Rev., Wild.Rev., Zoo.Rec.
—BLDSC (2558.000000), CISTI, ingenta, Linda Hall.
Published by: Department of Natural Resources, Natural History Survey, Natural Resources Bldg, 607 E Peabody Dr, Champaign, IL 61820. TEL 217-244-2115, FAX 217-333-4949. Ed. Charles Warwick.

ILLINOIS. STATE MUSEUM. SCIENTIFIC PAPERS SERIES. see *SCIENCES: COMPREHENSIVE WORKS*

570 510 SVN ISSN 1580-3139
CODEN: ASTLDL
IMAGE ANALYSIS AND STEREOLOGY. Text in English. 1982. 3/yr. SIT 11,000 domestic; USD 60 foreign (effective 2000). adv. bk.rev. index. *Refereed.* **Document type:** *Proceedings.* **Description:** Promotes the exchange of scientific, technical, organizational and other information among scientists interested in the quantitative analysis of populations having a geometrical structure. Includes stereology, image analysis, image processing, mathematical morphology, stochastic geometry, pattern recognition, and related topics.
Formerly (until 2000): Acta Stereologica (0351-580X)
Indexed: Alloys Ind. (1982-), Biol.Abstr., Chem.Abstr., Chem.Indus.Notes, Chem.Titles, Eng.Mat.Abstr., Excerp.Med., METADEX, Met.Abstr. (1982-), Met.Abstr.Ind. (1982-), Nonfer.Met.Alert (1982-), PCC Alert (1982-), Ref.Zh., Steels Alert (1982-), World Alum.Abstr., Zent.Math.
—BLDSC (4368.991220), CASDDS, CISTI, Linda Hall.
Published by: Slovenian Society for Stereology and Quantitative Image Analysis, Medical Faculty, Institute of Anatomy, Korytkova 2, Ljubljana 61105, Slovenia. TEL 386-1-5437300, FAX 386-1-5437301, tatjana.praprotnik@mf.uni-lj.si. Ed. Ida Erzen. adv.: page SIT 110,000, page USD 600. Circ: 500. **Co-sponsors:** International Society for Stereology; Ministrstvo za Solstvo, Znanost in Sport/Ministry of Education, Science and Sport of the Republic of Slovenia.

B

571.974 FRA ISSN 0923-2532
CODEN: IBSPE

IMMUNOANALYSE ET BIOLOGIE SPECIALISEE. Abbreviated title: I B S. Text in French. 1986. bi-m. EUR 239 in Europe to institutions; USD 304 elsewhere to institutions (effective 2002). adv. bk.rev. *Refereed.* **Document type:** *Academic/Scholarly.* **Description:** Covers research and application of clinical biology as in immunology, molecular biology, cell biology, analyses involving probes and receptors.

Formerly (until 1989): Trait-d'Union (0980-9090)

Related titles: Online - full text ed.: (from ingenta, Swets Blackwell).

Indexed: Excerp.Med., Int.Abstr.Biol.Sci.

—BLDSC (4369.654800), CISTI, EMDOCS, GNLM, Infotrieve. **CCC.**

Published by: (Societe Francaise de Biophysique et de Medecine Nucleaire), Elsevier Paris, Editions Scientifiques et Medicales (Subsidiary of: Reed Elsevier plc. group), 23 rue Linois, Paris 75015, France. TEL 33-1-45589110, FAX 33-1-45589419, labm@elsevier-fr.com; academic@elsevier-fr.com, http://www.elsevier.nl/inca/publications/store/6/2/0/7/3/7/. Ed. J Ingrand. Circ: 2,000.

IMMUNOLOGY AND CELL BIOLOGY. see *MEDICAL SCIENCES—Allergology And Immunology*

570 GBR

INDEX FILICUM. Text in English. 1906. irreg. price varies. **Document type:** *Academic/Scholarly.*

Published by: Royal Botanic Gardens, Kew, The Royal Botanic Gardens, Kew, Richmond, Surrey TW9 3AB, United Kingdom. TEL 44-20-8332-5000, jnlorders@oup.co.uk, info@rbgkew.org.uk, http://www.oup.co.uk. Ed. B S Parris. **Subscr. in N. America to:** Oxford University Press, Journals. TEL 919-677-0977, FAX 919-677-1714, http://www.oup.co.uk.

570 GBR

INDEX KEWENSIS. Text in English. 1896. every 5 yrs. price varies. **Document type:** *Academic/Scholarly.*

Related titles: Microfilm ed.: (from BHP).

Published by: (Royal Botanic Gardens, Kew), Oxford University Press, Oxford Journals, Walton St, Oxford OX2 6DP, United Kingdom. FAX 44-1865-267773, jnl.orders@oup.co.uk, http://www.oup.co.uk. **Subscr. in N. America to:** Oxford University Press, Journals, 2001 Evans Rd, Cary, NC 27513. TEL 919-677-0977, FAX 919-677-1714.

570 IND ISSN 0302-7554
QH301 CODEN: INBID9

INDIAN BIOLOGIST. Text in English. 1968. s-a. USD 30 (effective 1999). adv. bk.rev.

Indexed: Biol.Abstr., Chem.Abstr., Chem.Indus.Notes, Chem.Titles, Curr.Cont. (coverage dropped), Excerp.Med., INIS Atomind., Zoo.Rec.

—CASDDS, CISTI, ingenta, Linda Hall.

Published by: Indian Association of Biological Sciences, c/o Life Science Centre, University of Calcutta, 35 Ballygunge Circular Rd., Calcutta, West Bengal 700 019, India. Ed. T M Das. Circ: 1,000.

570 IND ISSN 0019-5189
QH301 CODEN: IJEBA6

INDIAN JOURNAL OF EXPERIMENTAL BIOLOGY. Text in English. 1963. m. INR 500, USD 300 (effective 2001). bk.rev. bibl, charts, illus. index. back issues avail. **Document type:** *Academic/Scholarly.* **Description:** Covers research in the fields of experimental botany, zoology, micrology, pharmacology and nutrition.

Indexed: Abstr.Anthropol., Abstr.Hyg., AgBiotech, Agri.& Environ.Biotech.Abstr. (coverage dropped), Agroforest.Abstr., Anal.Abstr., Anim.Breed.Abstr., Aqua.Sci.& Fish.Abstr., Aquacult.Abstr., Bio-Contr.News & Info., Biol.Abstr., Cal.Tiss.Abstr., Chem.Abstr., Chem.Indus.Notes, Chem.Titles, Crop Physiol.Abstr., Curr.Adv.Ecol.Sci., Curr.Cont. (coverage dropped), Curr.Leather Lit., Dairy Sci.Abstr., Derwent Biotech.Abstr., Diar.Dis.Res., Eng.Ind., Entomol.Abstr. (coverage dropped), Environ.Sci.Poll.Mgmt., Excerp.Med., Field Crop Abstr., Food Sci.& Tech.Abstr., Forest.Abstr., Helminthol.Abstr., Herb.Abstr., Hort.Abstr., INIS Atomind., INSPEC (coverage dropped), Ind.Med. (1963-), Ind.Sci.Rev., Ind.Vet., Irr.& Drain.Abstr., Maize Abstr., Nutr.Abstr., Ornam.Hort., Pig News & Info., Plant Breed.Abstr., Plant Gen.Res.Abstr., Plant Grow.Reg.Abstr., Postharvest, Potato Abstr., Poult.Abstr., Protozool.Abstr., Ref.Zh., Rev.Appl.Entomol., Rev.Arom.& Med.Plants, Rev.Med.& Vet.Mycol., Rev.Plant Path., Rice Abstr., Sci.Cit.Ind. (coverage dropped), Seed Abstr., Soils & Fert., Soyabean Abstr., Sport Fish.Abstr., Sugar Ind.Abstr., Text.Tech.Dig. (1963-1978), Triticale Abstr., Trop.Dis.Bull., Vet.Bull., Weed Abstr., Wild.Rev., Zoo.Rec.

—BLDSC (4412.200000), CASDDS, CISTI, Ei, GNLM, IDS, ingenta, KNAW, Linda Hall.

Published by: (India. Council of Scientific and Industrial Research, India. Publications & Information Directorate), Scientific Publishers, 5-A New Pali Rd., P O Box 91, Jodhpur, Rajasthan 342 001, India. TEL 91-291-433323, FAX 91-291-512580, scienti@sancharnet.in, http://www.scientificpub.com. Ed. K Satayanarayana. Circ: 1,200.

INDIAN JOURNAL OF MEDICAL PHOTOGRAPHY. see *PHOTOGRAPHY*

THE INDIAN JOURNAL OF MEDICAL RESEARCH. see *MEDICAL SCIENCES*

INDONESIAN BIOLOGICAL AND AGRICULTURAL INDEX/INDEKS BIOLOGI DAN PERTANIAN DE INDONESIA. see *AGRICULTURE—Abstracting, Bibliographies, Statistics*

INDONESIAN JOURNAL OF BIOANTHROPOLOGY/ BERKALA BIOANTHROPOLOGI INDONESIA. see *ANTHROPOLOGY*

INFORMATIK, BIOMETRIE UND EPIDEMIOLOGIE; in Medizin und Biologie. see *MEDICAL SCIENCES*

INFORMATION DU TECHNICIEN BIOLOGISTE. see *MEDICAL SCIENCES—Experimental Medicine, Laboratory Technique*

INSTITUT PASTEUR DE TUNIS. ARCHIVES. see *MEDICAL SCIENCES*

INSTITUTE OF ENVIRONMENTAL SCIENCES AND TECHNOLOGY. ANNUAL TECHNICAL MEETING. PROCEEDINGS. see *ENVIRONMENTAL STUDIES*

INSTITUTE OF ENVIRONMENTAL SCIENCES. TUTORIAL SERIES. see *ENVIRONMENTAL STUDIES*

570 BRA ISSN 0020-3661
CODEN: BBIBAT

INSTITUTO BIOLOGICO DA BAHIA. BOLETIM. Summaries in English, Portuguese. 1954. irreg. bibl, charts, illus.

Indexed: Biol.Abstr., Chem.Abstr.

—CASDDS.

Published by: Instituto Biologico da Bahia, Ave. ADHEMAR DE BARROS-ONDINA, Comercio, Caixa Postal 553, Salvador, BA 40001-970, Brazil. Ed. Antonio A J da Silva.

578.0913 PRT ISSN 0871-1755

INSTITUTO DE INVESTIGACAO CIENTIFICA TROPICAL. COMUNICACOES. SERIE DE CIENCIAS BIOLOGICAS. Text in Portuguese. 1989. irreg. price varies. back issues avail. **Document type:** *Monographic series.*

Published by: Instituto de Investigacao Cientifica Tropical, Rua da Junqueira, 30, Lisbon 1349-007, Portugal. TEL 351-21-3622621, FAX 351-21-3631460, iict@iict.pt. Circ: 1,000. **Subscr. to:** Centro de Documentacao e Informacao, Rua de Jau, 47, Lisbon 1300, Portugal. TEL 351-21-3644846, FAX 351-21-3628218.

INSTITUTO DE LA PATAGONIA. ANALES. CIENCIAS SOCIALES. see *HISTORY—History Of North And South America*

570 610 BRA ISSN 0074-0276
CODEN: MIOCAS

INSTITUTO OSWALDO CRUZ, RIO DE JANEIRO. MEMORIAS. Text in English. 1909. bi-m. BRL 35 domestic to individuals; BRL 45 in South America to individuals; BRL 60 elsewhere to individuals; BRL 70 domestic to institutions; BRL 80 in South America to institutions; BRL 120 elsewhere to institutions (effective 1999). adv. bk.rev. back issues avail. *Refereed.* **Document type:** *Academic/Scholarly.*

Related titles: Microform ed.: (from PMC); Online - full text ed.: (from SciELO, Institute for Scientific Information).

Indexed: ASCA, Abstr.Hyg., Anim.Behav.Abstr. (coverage dropped), Appl.Ecol.Abstr. (coverage dropped), Aqua.Sci.& Fish.Abstr., Bio-Contr.News & Info., Biol.Abstr., Curr.Cont., Dairy Sci.Abstr., Entomol.Abstr., Environ.Sci.Poll.Mgmt., GeoRef, Helminthol.Abstr., INIS Atomind., Ind.Med. (1909-), Ind.Sci.Rev., Ind.Vet., Inpharma, Microbiol.Abstr., Nutr.Abstr., Ocean.Abstr. (coverage dropped), Pharm.&Out.News, Pig News & Info., Plant Gen.Res.Abstr., Pollut.Abstr., Poult.Abstr., Protozool.Abstr., Reac., Rev.Appl.Entomol., Rev.Arom.& Med.Plants, Rev.Med.& Vet.Mycol., Rev.Plant Path., Rice Abstr., Risk Abstr., Saf.Sci.Abstr., Sci.Cit.Ind., Sel.Water Res.Abstr., Sport Fish.Abstr., Trop.Dis.Bull., Vet.Bull., Wild.Rev., Zoo.Rec.

—BLDSC (5661.000000), CISTI, GNLM, IDS, ingenta, KNAW, Linda Hall. **CCC.**

Published by: Fundacao Oswaldo Cruz, Avda. Brasil 4365, Rio De Janeiro, RJ 21045-900, Brazil. TEL 55-21-5984335, FAX 55-21-2805048, memorias@pobox.com, http://www.scielo.com/. Ed. Hooman Momen. Adv. contact Luciane Dec B Soares. Circ: 1,400.

570 MEX ISSN 0365-1932
QH301 CODEN: AENBAU

INSTITUTO POLITECNICO NACIONAL. ESCUELA NACIONAL DE CIENCIAS BIOLOGICAS. ANALES. Key Title: Anales de la Escuela Nacional de Ciencias Biologicas (Mexico). Text in Spanish; Summaries in English, Spanish. 1938. a. MXP 150, USD 50 (effective 1997). charts, illus, stat. *Refereed.* **Document type:** *Academic/Scholarly.* **Description:** Presents original research in the biological sciences: zoology, botany, morphology, ecology.

Indexed: GeoRef, Sport Fish.Abstr., VITIS, Wild.Rev., Zoo.Rec.

—CISTI, Linda Hall.

Published by: Instituto Politecnico Nacional, Escuela Nacional de Ciencias Biologicas, Carpio y Plan de Ayala,, Col Santa Tomas, Apartado Postal 42 186, Mexico City, DF 11340, Mexico. FAX 52-5-3963503. Ed. Dr. Fernando de la Jara Alcocer. Pub. Paul Vallejo de Aquino. Circ: 1,000 (controlled).

570 ROM

INSTITUTUL DE SUBINGINERI ORADEA. LUCRARI STIINTIFICE: SERIA BIOLOGIC. Text in Romanian; Text occasionally in English, French; Summaries in English, French, German, Romanian. 1967. a. **Document type:** *Journal, Abstract/Index.*

Formerly: Institutul Pedagogic Oradea. Lucrari Stiintifice Seria Biologic; Which superseded in part (in 1973): Institutul Pedagogic Oradea. Lucrari Stiintifice: Seria Educatie Fizica, Biologie, Stiinte Medicale; Which superseded in part (in 1971): Institutul Pedagogic Oradea. Lucraria Stiintifice: Seria A and Seria B; Which was formerly (until 1969): Institutul Pedagogic Oradea. Lucrari Stiintifice

Published by: Institutul de Subingineri Oradea, Calea Armatei Rosii 5, Oradea 3700, Romania.

570 GBR ISSN 0962-5968

INTERNATIONAL BIOLOGICAL PROGRAMME SERIES. Text in English. 1975. irreg., latest vol.26, 1981. price varies. **Document type:** *Monographic series.*

Indexed: Biol.Abstr.

—CISTI.

Published by: Cambridge University Press, Edinburgh Bldg, Shaftesbury Rd, Cambridge CB2 2RU, United Kingdom. FAX 44-1223-315052, information@cup.cam.ac.uk, information@cambridge.org, http://www.cup.cam.ac.uk, http://www.uk.cambridge.org/journals/pmu. R&P Linda Nicol.

616 ITA ISSN 0393-6155 CODEN: IBMAEP
INTERNATIONAL JOURNAL OF BIOLOGICAL MARKERS. Text in English. 1986. q. EUR 173 in Europe to individuals; USD 190 elsewhere to individuals; EUR 227 in Europe to institutions; USD 240 elsewhere to institutions (effective 2001). adv. abstr, bibl, charts, illus. Index. 64 p./no. back issues avail.; reprints avail. *Refereed.* **Document type:** *Journal, Academic/Scholarly.*
Related titles: Online - full text ed.: (from Institute for Scientific Information).
Indexed: ASCA, BBCI, Chem.Abstr., Chem.Indus.Notes, Chem.Titles, Curr.Cont., Ind.Med. (1986-), Inpharma, Pharm.&Out.News, Reac., Ref.Zh.
—BLDSC (4542.151100), CASDDS, CISTI, EMDOCS, GNLM, IDS, ingenta, KNAW. **CCC.**
Published by: Wichtig Editore s.r.l., Via Friuli, 72, Milan, MI 20135, Italy. TEL 39-02-55195443, FAX 39-02-55195971, info@wichtig-publisher.com, http://www.biological-markers.com. Ed. Dr. Massimo Gion. Pub. Dr. Diego Brancaccio. R&P, Adv. contact Lucia Steele. color page USD 1,350; trim 21 x 28. Circ: 1,500 (controlled).

INTERNATIONAL JOURNAL OF BIOMETEOROLOGY; the description, causes, and implications of climatic change. see *METEOROLOGY*

570 340 GBR ISSN 1353-274X
INTERNATIONAL JOURNAL OF BIOSCIENCES AND THE LAW. Text in English. 1996. 4/yr. GBP 99, USD 189 (effective 2001). bk.rev. back issues avail. **Document type:** *Academic/Scholarly.* **Description:** Provides analyses of both legal and scientific issues related to the environment; the regulation of medical, agricultural and environmental biotechnology; public health; agriculture and fisheries; food and water quality and safety. Emphasis is on furthering understanding and communication between lawyers and scientists.
Indexed: AIDS & Cancer Res., Aqua.Sci.& Fish.Abstr., Environ.Sci.Poll.Mgmt., Pollut.Abstr., Risk Abstr., Saf.Sci.Abstr., Tox.Abstr., Virol.Abstr.
—BLDSC (4542.155030).
Published by: A B Academic Publishers, PO Box 42, Bicester, Oxon OX26 6NW, United Kingdom. jrnls@abapubl.demon.co.uk.

570 ESP ISSN 0214-6282
QH491 CODEN: IJDBE5
INTERNATIONAL JOURNAL OF DEVELOPMENTAL BIOLOGY. Text in English. 1960. 8/yr. ESP 19,500 in Europe to individuals; USD 150 in United States to individuals; ESP 27,950 elsewhere to individuals; ESP 39,650 in Europe to institutions; USD 395 in United States to institutions; ESP 51,350 elsewhere to institutions (effective 2000). adv. bk.rev. Index. back issues avail. *Refereed.* **Document type:** *Academic/Scholarly.* **Description:** Reports substantial and original findings in biological development. Covers all animal or vegetable organisms.
Formerly (until 1989): Anales del Desarrollo (0569-9908)
Related titles: Online - full text ed.: (from EBSCO Publishing, Institute for Scientific Information).
Indexed: ASCA, Aqua.Sci.& Fish.Abstr., Aquacult.Abstr., Biol.Abstr., Cal.Tiss.Abstr. (coverage dropped), Chem.Abstr., Chem.Titles, Curr.Cont., Environ.Sci.Poll.Mgmt., Excerp.Med., Genet.Abstr., Hum.Gen.Abstr., Ind.Med. (1989-), Ind.Med.Esp., Ind.SST, Ind.Sci.Rev., Inpharma, Int.Abstr.Biol.Sci., Neurosci.Abstr. (coverage dropped), Nuc.Acids Abstr., Reac., Sci.Cit.Ind., Tox.Abstr. (coverage dropped), Zoo.Rec.
—BLDSC (4542.185090), CASDDS, CINDOC, EMDOCS, GNLM, IDS, ingenta, KNAW. **CCC.**
Published by: (Facultad de Medicina, Universidad del Pais Vasco), U B C Press, Apartado 1397, Bilbao, Vizcaya 48080, Spain. TEL 34-94-6012884, FAX 34-94-480-1314, gcparmaj@lg.ehu.es, http://www.ijdb.ehu.es/, http://www.lg.ehu.es/ijdb. Ed., Adv. contact Juan Arechaga. R&P Juan J Rodriguez. B&W page ESP 75,000, color page ESP 150,000. Circ: 1,000.

INTERNATIONAL JOURNAL OF FERTILITY AND WOMEN'S MEDICINE. see *MEDICAL SCIENCES*

570 USA ISSN 1094-2912
INTERNATIONAL JOURNAL OF FOOD PROPERTIES. Text in English. 1998. 3/yr. USD 85 to individuals print & online eds.; USD 350 to institutions print only (effective 2002). adv. **Document type:** *Academic/Scholarly.* **Description:** Publishes original research papers devoted to all scientific and applied aspects of food properties, with an emphasis on measurement methods, development of standard materials, and data on food properties, predictions, and applications.
Related titles: Online - full text ed.: (from Institute for Scientific Information, RoweCom Information Quest).
Indexed: Agricola, Aqua.Sci.& Fish.Abstr., Biotech.& Bioeng.Abstr., Chemorec.Abstr., Curr.Cont., Eng.Ind., Food Sci.& Tech.Abstr., Ref.Zh.
—BLDSC (4542.253100), Infotrieve. **CCC.**
Published by: Marcel Dekker Inc., 270 Madison Ave, New York, NY 10016. TEL 212-696-9000, 800-228-1160, FAX 212-685-4540, http://www.dekker.com/servlet/product/productid/JFP. Ed. Shafiur Rahman. R&P Julia Mulligan. Adv. contact Diane Saulon. B&W page USD 800. Circ: 250.

INTERNATIONAL JOURNAL OF MEDICAL AND BIOLOGICAL FRONTIERS. see *MEDICAL SCIENCES*

578.77 DEU ISSN 1434-2944
QH301 CODEN: IRHYFF
INTERNATIONAL REVIEW OF HYDROBIOLOGY; a journal covering all aspects of limnology and marine biology. Text in English, French, German. 1908. bi-m. EUR 698 in Europe; CHF 1,228 in Switzerland & Liechtenstein; USD 968 elsewhere; EUR 733 combined subscription in Europe for print and online eds.; CHF 1,290 combined subscription in Switzerland & Liechtenstein, for print and online eds.; USD 1,017 combined subscription elsewhere for print and online eds. (effective 2002). adv. charts, illus. index. *Refereed.* **Document type:** *Journal, Academic/Scholarly.* **Description:** Covers the analysis and assessment of biological structures in water in their interconnection with the internal and external cycle of materials.
Formerly: Internationale Revue der Gesamten Hydrobiologie (0020-9309)
Related titles: Online - full text ed.: ISSN 1522-2632. EUR 698 in Europe; CHF 1,228 in Switzerland & Liechtenstein; USD 968 elsewhere (effective 2002) (from EBSCO Publishing, Wiley InterScience, Institute for Scientific Information).
Indexed: ASCA, Appl.Ecol.Abstr., Aqua.Sci.& Fish.Abstr., Aquacult.Abstr., Biol.Abstr., Cal.Tiss.Abstr., Chem.Abstr., Chem.Indus.Notes, Chem.Titles, Chemorec.Abstr., Curr.Adv.Ecol.Sci., Curr.Cont., Ecol.Abstr., Entomol.Abstr., Environ.Sci.Poll.Mgmt., Excerp.Med., Geo.Abstr.P.G., GeoRef, Helminthol.Abstr., Herb.Abstr., INIS Atomind., Ind.Sci.Rev., Int.Abstr.Biol.Sci., Neurosci.Abstr. (coverage dropped), Ocean.Abstr. (coverage dropped), Pollut.Abstr., Rev.Med.& Vet.Mycol., Sci.Cit.Ind., Sel.Water Res.Abstr., Sport Fish.Abstr., W.R.C.Inf., Zoo.Rec.
—BLDSC (4547.300000), CASDDS, EMDOCS, IDS, Infotrieve, ingenta, Linda Hall. **CCC.**
Published by: Wiley - V C H, Postfach 101161, Weinheim 69451, Germany. FAX 49-6201-606-117, subservice@wiley-vch.de, http://www.wiley-vch.de. Ed. U Walz. R&P Claudia Rutz. Adv. contact Aenne Anders TEL 49-6201-606552. **Subscr. in the Americas to:** John Wiley & Sons, Inc., Journals. TEL 44-1243-779777, 212-850-6645, FAX 212-850-6021; **Subscr. outside Germany, Austria & Switzerland to:** John Wiley & Sons Ltd., Baffins Ln, Chichester, Sussex PO19 IUD, United Kingdom. TEL 44-1243-779777, FAX 44-1243-843232.

570 FRA ISSN 0445-1333
INTERNATIONAL UNION OF BIOLOGICAL SCIENCES. GENERAL ASSEMBLIES. PROCEEDINGS. Text in French. triennial. **Document type:** *Proceedings.*
Formerly: International Union of Biological Sciences. Reports of General Assemblies (0074-9362)
Published by: International Union of Biological Sciences, 51 bd. de Montmorency, Paris 75016, France. TEL 45-25-00-09.

570 ISR
ISRAEL INSTITUTE FOR BIOLOGICAL RESEARCH. PUBLICATIONS. Text in English. 1970. a. free per issue. **Document type:** *Bibliography.*
Formerly (until 1993): Israel Institute for Biological Research. Scientific Activities
Published by: Israel Institute for Biological Research, P O Box 19, Ness-ziona 74100, Israel. TEL 972-8-9381595, FAX 972-8-9401404, mambi@iibr.gov.il.

572.8 RUS ISSN 0202-7070
QH506 CODEN: ITMBCG
ITOGI NAUKI I TEKHNIKI. MOLEKULYARNAYA BIOLOGIYA. Text in Russian. irreg., latest 1989, vols. 27-28.
Indexed: Chem.Abstr.
—Linda Hall.
Published by: Vserossiiskii Institut Nauchnoi i Tekhnicheskoi Informatsii (VINITI), Usievicha ul 20-a, Moscow 125315, Russian Federation. TEL 7-095-1526441. **Dist. by:** Mezhdunarodnaya Kniga, B Yakimanka 39, Moscow 117049, Russian Federation. TEL 7-095-2384967, FAX 7-095-2384634.

570 RUS
ITOGI NAUKI I TEKHNIKI. MORFOLOGIYA CHELOVEKA I ZHIVOTNYKH. Text in Russian. irreg. **Document type:** *Academic/Scholarly.*
Published by: Vserossiiskii Institut Nauchnoi i Tekhnicheskoi Informatsii (VINITI), Usievicha ul 20-a, Moscow 125315, Russian Federation. TEL 7-095-1526441, FAX 7-095-943-0060. **US dist. addr.:** East View Publications, 3020 Harbor Ln N, Minneapolis, MN 55447. TEL 612-550-0961.

570 RUS ISSN 0203-5405
QH301
ITOGI NAUKI I TEKHNIKI. OBSHCHIE PROBLEMY BIOLOGII. Text in Russian. 1982. irreg., latest vol.6, 1987. price varies.
—Linda Hall.
Published by: Vserossiiskii Institut Nauchnoi i Tekhnicheskoi Informatsii (VINITI), Usievicha ul 20-a, Moscow 125315, Russian Federation. TEL 7-095-1526441. **Dist. by:** Mezhdunarodnaya Kniga, B Yakimanka 39, Moscow 117049, Russian Federation. TEL 7-095-2384967, FAX 7-095-2384634.

ITOGI NAUKI I TEKHNIKI. ONKOLOGIYA. see *MEDICAL SCIENCES—Oncology*

570 DEU ISSN 0944-3266
QH305
JAHRBUCH FUER GESCHICHTE UND THEORIE DER BIOLOGIE. Text in German. a. EUR 20 (effective 2001 & 2002). back issues avail. **Document type:** *Journal, Academic/Scholarly.* **Description:** Presents articles about various themes of the history of biology.
Indexed: IBZ.
Published by: (Deutsche Gesellschaft fuer Geschichte und Theorie der Biologie), V W B - Verlag fuer Wissenschaft und Bildung, Zossener Str 55, Berlin 10961, Germany. TEL 49-30-2510415, FAX 49-30-2511136, 100615.1565@compuserve.com, http://www.vwb-verlag.com. Eds. Hans Joerg Rheinberger, Michael Weingarten.

JAPAN MATRIX (COLLAGEN) CLUB. PROCEEDINGS OF THE ANNUAL MEETING OF JAPAN MARIX CLUB. see *MEDICAL SCIENCES*

JAPAN SOCIETY FOR COMPARATIVE ENDOCRINOLOGY. PROCEEDINGS. see *MEDICAL SCIENCES—Endocrinology*

JAPANESE JOURNAL OF ECOLOGY/NIPPON SEITAI GAKKAISHI. see *ENVIRONMENTAL STUDIES*

615 577 JPN ISSN 0368-9395
JAPANESE JOURNAL OF HEALTH AND HUMAN ECOLOGY. Text and summaries in English, Japanese. 1935. bi-m. JPY 17,000. **Document type:** *Academic/Scholarly.*
Published by: Kyorin Shoin, 4-2-1 Yushima, Bunkyo-ku, Tokyo 113-0034, Japan. TEL 81-3-811-4887. Ed. M Uematsu.

JAPANESE JOURNAL OF INFECTIOUS DISEASES. see *MEDICAL SCIENCES*

570 CHN ISSN 1001-1633
JIEPOUXUE ZAZHI/JOURNAL OF ANATOMY. Text in Chinese. q.
Published by: Di 2 Junyi Daxue/No.2 Military University of Medical Science, 594 Xiangyin Lu, Shanghai 200433, China. TEL 488706. Ed. Huang Ying. **Co-sponsor:** Chinese Society of Anatomy.

570 IND
JOURNAL OF ADVANCES IN BIOSCIENCE. Text in English. s-a. USD 35 (effective 2000). **Document type:** *Academic/Scholarly.*
Published by: H P C Publishers Distributors Pvt. Ltd., 1st Fl. Flats 1 & 2, Darya Ganj, 48-5-24 Bharat Ram Rd., New Delhi 110 002, India. TEL 91-11-3254401, FAX 91-11-619-3511, hpcpd@nda.vsnl.net.in, hpcpd@hpc.cc, http://www.bizdelhi.com/publisher/hpc, http://www.hpc.cc. **Co-publisher:** Society of Bio-Sciences.

B

571.3 611 GBR ISSN 0021-8782
QL801 CODEN: JOANAY
JOURNAL OF ANATOMY; molecular, cellular and experimental morphology. Text in English. m., latest vol.200, 2002. GBP 128 in Europe to individuals; USD 204 in North America to individuals; GBP 141 elsewhere to individuals; GBP 596 in Europe to institutions; USD 945 in North America to institutions; GBP 656 elsewhere to institutions (effective 2002). adv. bk.rev. bibl, charts, illus. index. cum.index: 1866-1966. back issues avail.; reprint service avail. from SWZ. *Refereed.* **Document type:** *Academic/Scholarly.*
Description: Presents articles and reviews covering normal human and comparative anatomy, including applied anatomy, physical anthropology, neurology, endocrinology, embryology.
Related titles: Microfilm ed.: (from BHP); Microform ed.: (from PQC); Online - full text ed.: GBP 116 in Europe to individuals; USD 184 in North America to individuals; GBP 116 elsewhere to individuals; GBP 537 in Europe to institutions; USD 851 in North America to institutions; GBP 537 elsewhere to institutions (effective 2002) (from EBSCO Publishing, O C L C Online Computer Library Center, Inc., RoweCom Information Quest, Swets Blackwell, Institute for Scientific Information).
Indexed: ASCA, Abstr.Anthropol., AgBiotech, Anim.Breed.Abstr., Biol.Abstr., Chem.Abstr., Chem.Indus.Notes, Chem.Titles, Curr.Cont., Dairy Sci.Abstr., Dent.Ind., Excerp.Med., GeoRef, INIS Atomind., Ind.Med. (1916-), Ind.Sci.Rev., Ind.Vet., Inpharma, Int.Abstr.Biol.Sci., Neurosci.Cit.Ind., Nutr.Abstr., Pig News & Info., Poult.Abstr., Reac., Ref.Zh., Sci.Cit.Ind., Sport Fish.Abstr., Vet.Bull., Wild.Rev., Zoo.Rec.
—BLDSC (4929.000000), CASDDS, CISTI, GNLM, IDS, ingenta, KNAW, Linda Hall. **CCC.**
Published by: (Anatomical Society of Great Britain and Ireland), Blackwell Science Ltd., PO Box 88, Oxford OX2 0NE, United Kingdom. TEL 44-1865-206180, 44-1865-206002, FAX 44-1865-206219, jnl.orders@blacksci.co.uk, http://www.blackwell-science.com/~cgilib/jnlpage.asp?Journal=joa&File=joa, http://www.blackwellpublishing.com. R&P Sophie Savage. Adv. contact Jenny Applin.

591.7 GBR ISSN 0021-8790
QL750
JOURNAL OF ANIMAL ECOLOGY. Text in English. 1932. bi-m., latest vol.71, 2002. GBP 350 in Europe; USD 555 in North America; GBP 385 elsewhere (effective 2002). adv. bk.rev. bibl, illus. index. back issues avail.; reprint service avail. from ISI. *Refereed.* **Document type:** *Academic/Scholarly.* **Description:** Publishes original research papers on most aspects of animal ecology, plus reviews that shed light on subjects central to animal ecology, including theoretical analyses of specific topics.
Related titles: Microform ed.: (from PQC); Online - full text ed.: ISSN 1365-2656. GBP 315 in Europe; USD 550 in North America; GBP 315 elsewhere (effective 2002) (from JSTOR (Web-based Journal Archive), EBSCO Publishing, O C L C Online Computer Library Center, Inc., RoweCom Information Quest, ingenta, Munksgaard & Blackwell Science's Synergy, Swets Blackwell, Institute for Scientific Information).
Indexed: ASCA, Abstr.Anthropol., Abstr.Hyg., Anim.Behav.Abstr., Anim.Breed.Abstr., Appl.Ecol.Abstr., Aqua.Sci.& Fish.Abstr., Bio-Contr.News & Info., Biol.& Agr.Ind. (Jun.1983-), Biol.Abstr., Chem.Abstr., Curr.Cont., Curr.Ind.Stat., Curr.Ref.Fish Res., Deep Sea Res.& Oceanogr.Abstr., Ecol.Abstr., Entomol.Abstr., Environ.Per.Bibl. (1974-), Environ.Sci.Poll.Mgmt., Field Crop Abstr., Food Sci.& Tech.Abstr., Forest.Abstr., Genet.Abstr., Geo.Abstr.P.G., GeoRef, Helminthol.Abstr., Herb.Abstr., Hum.Gen.Abstr., Ind.Sci.Rev., Ind.Vet., Int.Abstr.Biol.Sci., Key Word Ind.Wildl.Res., Math.R., Nutr.Abstr., P C I, Postharvest, Poult.Abstr., Protozool.Abstr., Ref.Zh., Rev.Appl.Entomol., Rev.Med.& Vet.Mycol., Sci.Cit.Ind., Seed Abstr., Sel.Water Res.Abstr., Soils & Fert., Sport Fish.Abstr., Triticale Abstr., Trop.Dis.Bull., Vet.Bull., W.R.C.Inf., Weed Abstr., Wild.Rev., Zoo.Rec.
—BLDSC (4936.000000), CISTI, EMDOCS, IDS, ingenta, Linda Hall. **CCC.**
Published by: (British Ecological Society), Blackwell Science Ltd., PO Box 88, Oxford OX2 0NE, United Kingdom. TEL 44-1865-206180, 44-1865-206002, FAX 44-1865-206219, jnl.orders@blacksci.co.uk, http://www.blackwell-science.com/~cgilib/jnlpage.asp?Journal=janim&File=janim, http://www.blackwellpublishing.com. Eds. D Raffaelli, S Albon. Pub. Sue Hewitt. R&P Sophie Savage. Adv. contact Jenny Applin. Circ: 2,715.

571.3 IND ISSN 0021-8804
QL801 CODEN: JAMPA2
JOURNAL OF ANIMAL MORPHOLOGY AND PHYSIOLOGY. Text in English. 1954. s-a. INR 125; USD 35 foreign. adv. bk.rev. charts, illus. index. **Document type:** *Academic/Scholarly.*
Indexed: Anim.Breed.Abstr., Aqua.Sci.& Fish.Abstr., Biol.Abstr., Chem.Abstr., Chem.Indus.Notes, Chem.Titles, Entomol.Abstr., Excerp.Med., Genet.Abstr., Hum.Gen.Abstr., INIS Atomind., Ind.Vet., Vet.Bull., Zoo.Rec.
—CASDDS, CISTI, Linda Hall.
Published by: Society of Animal Morphologists & Physiologists, c/o Maharaja Sayajirao University of Baroda, Dept. of Zoology, Faculty of Science, Baroda, Gujarat 390 002, India. TEL 91-265-336492. Ed., Adv. contact Bonny Pilo. Circ: 300.

577 GBR ISSN 0021-8901
S3 CODEN: JAPEAI
JOURNAL OF APPLIED ECOLOGY. Text in English. 1964. 6/yr., latest vol.39, 2002. GBP 350 in Europe; USD 555 in North America; GBP 385 elsewhere (effective 2002). adv. bk.rev. bibl, charts, illus. index. back issues avail.; reprint service avail. from ISI. *Refereed.* **Document type:** *Academic/Scholarly.* **Description:** Publishes papers that discuss the application of ecological ideas, theories, and methods to the use of biological resources in the widest sense.
Related titles: Microform ed.: (from PQC); ♦ Online - full text ed.: Journal of Applied Ecology Online. ISSN 1365-2664.
Indexed: AESIS, ASCA, AgBiotech, Agri.& Environ.Biotech.Abstr. (coverage dropped), Agricola, Agroforest.Abstr., Anim.Behav.Abstr., Anim.Breed.Abstr., Appl.Ecol.Abstr., Aqua.Sci.& Fish.Abstr., Bio-Contr.News & Info., Biol.& Agr.Ind. (Aug.1983-), Biol.Abstr., Biostat., Biotech.& Bioeng.Abstr., Chem.Abstr., Chem.Indus.Notes, Chem.Titles, Cott.& Trop.Fibr.Abstr., Crop Physiol.Abstr., Curr.Cont., Curr.Ind.Stat., Deep Sea Res.& Oceanogr.Abstr., Derwent Biotech.Abstr., Ecol.Abstr., Energy Ind., Energy Info.Abstr., Eng.Ind., Entomol.Abstr., Environ.Abstr., Environ.Per.Bibl. (1989-), Environ.Sci.Poll.Mgmt., Excerp.Med., Field Crop Abstr., Forest Prod.Abstr., Forest.Abstr., Genet.Abstr., Geo.Abstr.H.G., Geo.Abstr.P.G., GeoRef, Geomech.Abstr., Helminthol.Abstr., Herb.Abstr., Hort.Abstr., Hum.Gen.Abstr., IDA, INIS Atomind., Ind.Sci.Rev., Ind.Vet., Int.Abstr.Biol.Sci., Irr.& Drain.Abstr., Key Word Ind.Wildl.Res., Maize Abstr., Nutr.Abstr., Ocean.Abstr. (coverage dropped), Ornam.Hort., Pig News & Info., Plant Breed.Abstr., Plant Gen.Res.Abstr., Pollut.Abstr., Potato Abstr., Poult.Abstr., Protozool.Abstr., Ref.Zh., Rev.Appl.Entomol., Rev.Med.& Vet.Mycol., Rev.Plant Path., Rice Abstr., Rural Devel.Abstr., Rural Recreat.Tour.Abstr., Sci.Cit.Ind., Seed Abstr., Sel.Water Res.Abstr., Small Anim.Abstr., Soils & Fert., Sport Fish.Abstr., Tox.Abstr., Triticale Abstr., Vet.Bull., W.R.C.Inf., Weed Abstr., Wild.Rev., World Ag.Econ.& Rur.Soc.Abstr., Zoo.Rec.
—BLDSC (4942.500000), CASDDS, CISTI, Ei, EMDOCS, IDS, ingenta, Linda Hall. **CCC.**
Published by: (British Ecological Society), Blackwell Science Ltd., PO Box 88, Oxford OX2 0NE, United Kingdom. TEL 44-1865-206180, 44-1865-206002, FAX 44-1865-206219, jnl.orders@blacksci.co.uk, http://www.blackwell-science.com/~cgilib/jnlpage.asp?Journal=jappl&File=jappl, http://www.blackwellpublishing.com. Eds. Andrew Watkinson, Jon Marshall, Nigel Barlow. Pub. Sue Hewitt. Circ: 2,690.

578.77 333.91 USA ISSN 0733-2076
SH151 CODEN: JAQSDY
JOURNAL OF AQUARICULTURE AND AQUATIC SCIENCES. Text in English. 1980. irreg. USD 70 in North America to individuals; USD 85 elsewhere to individuals; USD 140 in North America to libraries; USD 170 elsewhere to libraries. adv. bk.rev. abstr, bibl, charts, illus. index. back issues avail.; reprints avail. *Refereed.* **Document type:** *Academic/Scholarly.*
Description: Publishes original scientific research and correspondence pertaining to aquariculture, the art or science of cultivating living aquatic animals in artificial ponds or tanks. Also covers related aquatic sciences.
Formerly (until 1982): Journal of Aquariculture
Related titles: Online - full text ed.: (from CompuServe, Inc.).
Indexed: Aqua.Sci.& Fish.Abstr., Aquacult.Abstr., Biol.Abstr., Biotech.& Bioeng.Abstr., Curr.Cont. (coverage dropped), Deep Sea Res.& Oceanogr.Abstr., Environ.Sci.Poll.Mgmt., Microbiol.Abstr., Ocean.Abstr. (coverage dropped), Pollut.Abstr., Sel.Water Res.Abstr., Sport Fish.Abstr., Wild.Rev., Zoo.Rec.
—CASDDS, Infotrieve, Linda Hall. **CCC.**
Published by: The Written Word, 7601 E. Forest Lake Dr., N.W., Parkville, MO 64152. TEL 816-891-6671, FAX 816-474-6486, JFK@compuserve.com, http://petsforum.com/aquascience/. Ed., Pub. John Farrell Kuhns. Adv. contact Carol L Kuhns. Circ: 800 (paid).

570 GBR ISSN 0021-9266
QH315 CODEN: JBIEAO
JOURNAL OF BIOLOGICAL EDUCATION. Text in English. 1966. 3/yr. GBP 48 in British Isles to individuals; GBP 84 in British Isles to institutions; GBP 60 overseas to individuals; GBP 100 overseas to institutions (effective 2000). adv. bk.rev. illus. index. back issues avail.; reprint service avail. from SCH,PSC. *Refereed.* **Document type:** *Academic/Scholarly.* **Description:** Presents articles on practical work, curricular matters, and teaching methods in biology.
Related titles: Online - full text ed.: (from H. W. Wilson, Institute for Scientific Information).
Indexed: ASCA, Aqua.Sci.& Fish.Abstr., Aquacult.Abstr., Biol.Abstr., Br.Educ.Ind., C.I.J.E., Chem.Abstr., Cont.Pg.Educ., Curr.Cont., Dairy Sci.Abstr., ERA, Ecol.Abstr., Educ.Ind. (Jan.1983-), Educ.Tech.Abstr., Environ.Abstr., Environ.Sci.Poll.Mgmt., High.Educ.Curr.Aware.Bull., IBR, IBZ, Media Rev.Dig. (Jan.1989-), Mult.Ed.Abstr., Plant Breed.Abstr., Ref.Zh., Res.High.Educ.Abstr., Rural Recreat.Tour.Abstr., Russ.Acad.Sci.Bibl., SSCI (coverage dropped), Tech.Educ.Abstr., Telegen, World Ag.Econ.& Rur.Soc.Abstr., Zoo.Rec.
—BLDSC (4953.100000), CIS, CISTI, IDS, ingenta, Linda Hall. **CCC.**
Published by: Institute of Biology, 20-22 Queensberry Pl, London SW7 2DZ, United Kingdom. TEL 44-20-7581-8333, FAX 44-20-7823-9409, info@iob.primex.co.uk, http://www.iob.org. Ed. Clare Chatham. Adv. contact Clare P Chatham. Circ: 2,300 (paid).

570 ITA ISSN 0393-974X
CODEN: JBRAER
JOURNAL OF BIOLOGICAL REGULATORS AND HOMEOSTATIC AGENTS. Text in English. 1987. q. EUR 173 in Europe to individuals; USD 190 elsewhere to individuals; EUR 227 in Europe to institutions; USD 240 elsewhere to institutions (effective 2001). adv. abstr, bibl, charts. 64 p./no. back issues avail.; reprints avail. *Refereed.* **Document type:** *Journal, Academic/Scholarly.*
Related titles: Online - full text ed.: (from Institute for Scientific Information).
Indexed: ASCA, Chem.Abstr., Chem.Indus.Notes, Chem.Titles, Curr.Cont., Derwent Biotech.Abstr., Ind.Med. (1987-), Inpharma, Int.Abstr.Biol.Sci., Pharm.&Out.News, Reac., Rev.Med.& Vet.Mycol.
—BLDSC (4953.220000), CASDDS, CISTI, EMDOCS, GNLM, IDS, ingenta, KNAW. **CCC.**
Published by: Wichtig Editore s.r.l., Via Friuli, 72, Milan, MI 20135, Italy. TEL 39-02-55195443, FAX 39-02-55195971, info@wichtig-publisher.com. Eds. F Dianzani, F Mandelli. Pub. Dr. Diego Brancaccio. R&P, Adv. contact Lucia Steele. color page AED 1,450; trim 21 x 28. Circ: 1,500 (controlled).

570 IND ISSN 0021-9282
QH1 CODEN: JBSBAV
JOURNAL OF BIOLOGICAL SCIENCES. Text in English. 1958. s-a. INR 30, USD 8. adv. bk.rev. charts, illus. index. reprint service avail. from PQC.
Related titles: Microfilm ed.: (from PQC).
Indexed: Biol.Abstr., Chem.Abstr., Indian Sci.Abstr., Seed Abstr., Vet.Bull.
—CASDDS, CISTI, Linda Hall.
Published by: Bombay Biological Association, c/o Biology Dept., R. J. College, Ghatkopar, Mumbai, Maharashtra 400 086, India. Eds. K P Dhage, S M Karmarkar. Circ: 250.

570 SGP ISSN 0218-3390
JOURNAL OF BIOLOGICAL SYSTEMS. Text in English. 1993. q. SGD 185, USD 110 to individuals; SGD 521, USD 308 to institutions; SGD 316, USD 187 in developing nations to institutions (effective 2001); SGD 217 to individuals Asia Pacific & Australasia except Hong Kong and China; USD 121 elsewhere to individuals; SGD 599 to institutions Asia Pacific & Australasia except Hong Kong and China; USD 333 elsewhere to institutions; SGD 364 in developing nations to institutions Asia Pacific & Australasia except Hong Kong and China; USD 202 in developing nations to institutions (effective 2002). **Document type:** *Academic/Scholarly.* **Description:** Promotes interdisciplinary approaches in biology and in medicine, including mathematical methods and general systems theory as they contribute to the study of biological situations.

B

Related titles: Online - full text ed.: (from Swets Blackwell, ScienceDirect, Institute for Scientific Information).
Indexed: Aqua.Sci.& Fish.Abstr., Environ.Sci.Poll.Mgmt., Pollut.Abstr., Zoo.Rec.
—BLDSC (4953.420000), CISTI.
Published by: World Scientific Publishing Co Pte Ltd, Farrer Rd, PO Box 128, Singapore 912805, Singapore. wspc@wspc.com.sg, http://www.worldscientific.com. Eds. P M Auger, R V Jean.

JOURNAL OF BIOMEDICAL OPTICS. see *PHYSICS—Optics*

JOURNAL OF BIOMEDICAL SCIENCE. see *MEDICAL SCIENCES*

570 IND ISSN 0250-5991
CODEN: JOBSDN
JOURNAL OF BIOSCIENCES. Text in English. 1979. irreg., latest vol.24, 2000 (4-6/yr.). INR 200, USD 100 (effective 2001). 120 p./no. 2 cols./p. back issues avail.; reprint service avail. from ISI. *Refereed.* **Document type:** *Journal, Academic/Scholarly.*
Incorporates (1934-1991): Indian Academy of Sciences. Proceedings. Animal Sciences (0253-4118); Indian Academy of Sciences. Proceedings. Plant Sciences (0253-410X)
Related titles: Online - full text ed.: (from Institute for Scientific Information).
Indexed: ASCA, AgBiotech, Agroforest.Abstr., Anim.Breed.Abstr., Apic.Abstr., Aqua.Sci.& Fish.Abstr., Aquacult.Abstr., Bio-Contr.News & Info., Biotech.& Bioeng.Abstr. (coverage dropped), Chem.Abstr., Chem.Indus.Notes, Chem.Titles, Crop Physiol.Abstr., Curr.Cont., Dairy Sci.Abstr., Ecol.Abstr., Environ.Abstr., Environ.Sci.Poll.Mgmt., Excerp.Med., Field Crop Abstr., Forest.Abstr., GeoRef, Helminthol.Abstr., Herb.Abstr., Hort.Abstr., IDA, INIS Atomind., Ind.Med. (1979-), Ind.Sci.Rev., Ind.Vet., Inpharma, Int.Abstr.Biol.Sci., Neurosci.Abstr. (coverage dropped), Ornam.Hort., Plant Breed.Abstr., Plant Grow.Reg.Abstr., Postharvest, Protozool.Abstr., Reac., Ref.Zh., Rev.Appl.Entomol., Rev.Arom.& Med.Plants, Rev.Med.& Vet.Mycol., Rev.Plant Path., Rice Abstr., Sci.Cit.Ind., Seed Abstr., Sel.Water Res.Abstr., Soils & Fert., Sorghum & Millets Abstr., Sport Fish.Abstr., Sugar Ind.Abstr., Telegen, Trop.Oil Seeds Abstr., VITIS, Vet.Bull., Weed Abstr., World Ag.Econ.& Rur.Soc.Abstr., Zoo.Rec.
—BLDSC (4954.070000), CASDDS, CIS, CISTI, EMDOCS, GNLM, IDS, ingenta, KNAW, Linda Hall.
Published by: Indian Academy of Sciences, C.V. Raman Ave., P O Box 8005, Sadashivanagar, Bangalore, Karnataka 560 080, India. TEL 91-80-3342546, FAX 91-80-3346094, jbiosci@ias.ernet.in, http://www.ias.ac.in/jbiosci, http://www.ias.ac.in/pramana. Eds. V Nanjundiah, V K Guar. Circ: 1,500.

616.079 571.9 GBR ISSN 0021-9975
CODEN: JCVPAR
JOURNAL OF COMPARATIVE PATHOLOGY. Text in English. 1888. 8/yr. (in 2 vols.). GBP 219 to individuals; GBP 439 to institutions (effective 2002). adv. bibl, charts, illus. index. reprint service avail. from PSC,SWZ. *Refereed.* **Document type:** *Academic/Scholarly.* **Description:** Directed to workers in veterinary and medical science who investigate diseases of all vertebrate animals, including domesticated zoo, wild and marine species, and man.
Related titles: Online - full text ed.: (from EBSCO Publishing, RoweCom Information Quest, Swets Blackwell, IDEAL Online Library, Institute for Scientific Information).
Indexed: ASCA, AgBiotech, Agri.& Environ.Biotech.Abstr. (coverage dropped), Agricola, Anim.Breed.Abstr., Biol.Abstr., Chem.Abstr., Chem.Indus.Notes, Chem.Titles, Curr.Cont., Curr.Ref.Fish Res., Dairy Sci.Abstr., Dent.Ind., Derwent Biotech.Abstr., Excerp.Med., Focus on: Vet.Sci.& Med., Helminthol.Abstr., INIS Atomind., Ind.Med. (1965-), Ind.Sci.Rev., Ind.Vet., Inpharma, Neurosci.Cit.Ind., Nutr.Abstr., Pig News & Info., Poult.Abstr., Protozool.Abstr., Reac., Rev.Appl.Entomol., Rev.Med.& Vet.Mycol., Rev.Plant Path., Sci.Cit.Ind., Small Anim.Abstr., Soyabean Abstr., Sport Fish.Abstr., Vet.Bull., Wild.Rev., Zoo.Rec.
—BLDSC (4962.800000), CASDDS, CISTI, GNLM, IDS, ingenta, KNAW. **CCC.**
Published by: W.B. Saunders Co. Ltd. (Subsidiary of: Harcourt Publishers Ltd.), 24-28 Oval Rd, London NW1 7DX, United Kingdom. TEL 44-20-7424-4200, FAX 44-20-7424-4515, cservice@harcourt.com, http://www.harcourt-international.com/journals/jcpa. Ed. E G R Smith. **Subsr. to:** Harcourt Publishers Ltd., Foots Cray High St, Sidcup, Kent DA14 5HP, United Kingdom. TEL 44-20-8308-5700, FAX 44-20-8309-0807.

577 GBR ISSN 0022-0477
QH540 CODEN: JECOAB
JOURNAL OF ECOLOGY. Text in English. 1913. bi-m., latest vol.90, 2002. GBP 350 in Europe; USD 555 in North America; GBP 385 elsewhere (effective 2002). adv. bk.rev. abstr, bibl, charts, illus, maps. index, cum.index: vols.1-20 (1913-1932), vols.21-50 (1933-1982). back issues avail.; reprint service avail. from ISI. *Refereed.* **Document type:** *Academic/Scholarly.*
Related titles: Microform ed.: (from PQC); Online - full text ed.: ISSN 1365-2745. GBP 315 in Europe; USD 500 in North America; GBP 315 elsewhere (effective 2002) (from JSTOR (Web-based Journal Archive), EBSCO Publishing, O C L C Online Computer Library Center, Inc., RoweCom Information Quest, ingenta, Gale Group, Munksgaard & Blackwell Science's Synergy, Swets Blackwell, Factiva, Institute for Scientific Information).
Indexed: ASCA, Agricola, Agroforest.Abstr., Anim.Behav.Abstr., Appl.Ecol.Abstr., Aqua.Sci.& Fish.Abstr., Bibl.Agri., Bio-Contr.News & Info., Biol.& Agr.Ind. (Jul.1983-), Biol.Abstr., Biostat., Br.Archaeol.Abstr., Br.Geol.Lit., Chem.Abstr., Chem.Indus.Notes, Chem.Titles, Crop Physiol.Abstr., Curr.Adv.Plant Sci., Curr.Cont., Curr.Ind.Stat., Curr.Ref.Fish Res., Deep Sea Res.& Oceanogr.Abstr., Ecol.Abstr., Energy Rev., Entomol.Abstr., Environ.Abstr., Environ.Per.Bibl. (1982-), Environ.Sci.Poll.Mgmt., Excerp.Med., Field Crop Abstr., Forest Prod.Abstr., Forest.Abstr., Gen.Sci.Ind. (Jul.1984-), Genet.Abstr., Geo.Abstr.H.G., Geo.Abstr.P.G., GeoRef, Geol.Abstr., Helminthol.Abstr., Herb.Abstr., Hort.Abstr., Hum.Gen.Abstr., IBR, Ind.Sci.Rev., Int.Abstr.Biol.Sci., Irr.& Drain.Abstr., Key Word Ind.Wildl.Res., Microbiol.Abstr., Ocean.Abstr., Ornam.Hort., P C I, Plant Breed.Abstr., Plant Gen.Res.Abstr., Plant Sci., Ref.Zh., Rev.Appl.Entomol., Rev.Plant Path., Sci.Cit.Ind., Seed Abstr., Sel.Water Res.Abstr., Soils & Fert., Sport Fish.Abstr., Triticale Abstr., W.R.C.Inf., Weed Abstr., Wild.Rev., Zoo.Rec.
—BLDSC (4972.000000), CASDDS, CISTI, EMDOCS, IDS, ingenta, Linda Hall. **CCC.**
Published by: (British Ecological Society), Blackwell Science Ltd., PO Box 88, Oxford OX2 0NE, United Kingdom. TEL 44-1865-206180, 44-1865-206002, FAX 44-1865-206219, jnl.orders@blacksci.co.uk, http://www.blackwell-science.com/~cgilib/jnlpage.asp?Journal=jecol&File=jecol, http://www.blackwellpublishing.com. Eds. A Davy, M Hutchings. Pub. Sue Hewitt. R&P Sophie Savage. Adv. contact Jenny Applin. Circ: 3,190.

573.6 IND
CODEN: JRBED2
JOURNAL OF ENDOCRINOLOGY & REPRODUCTION. Text in English. 1981. s-a., latest vol.4, 2000. USD 60 (effective 2000). **Document type:** *Academic/Scholarly.*
Formerly: Journal of Reproductive Biology and Comparative Endocrinology (0254-3583)
Indexed: Chem.Abstr., Chem.Indus.Notes, Chem.Titles.
—CASDDS, CISTI.
Published by: (Society for Reproductive Biology and Comparative Endocrinology), H P C Publishers Distributors Pvt. Ltd., 1st Fl., Flats 1 & 2, Darya Ganj, 4805-24 Bharat Ram Rd., New Delhi 110 002, India. TEL 91-11-3254401, FAX 91-11-619-3511, hpcpd@nda.vsnl.net.in, hpcpd@hpc.cc, http://www.hpc.cc, http://www.bizdelhi.com/publisher/hpc.

JOURNAL OF ENVIRONMENTAL BIOLOGY; an international research journal of environmental sciences & toxicology. see *ENVIRONMENTAL STUDIES*

JOURNAL OF EPIDEMIOLOGY AND BIOSTATISTICS. see *PUBLIC HEALTH AND SAFETY*

599.9 USA ISSN 0278-0771
GN476.7 CODEN: JOUEE9
JOURNAL OF ETHNOBIOLOGY. Abstracts in English, French, Spanish. 1981. s-a. USD 35; to individuals in N. America (Mexico $25; elsewhere 45); institutions $60 (outside N. America & Mexico $70) (effective 1999) (includes membership). adv. bk.rev. back issues avail. *Refereed.* **Document type:** *Academic/Scholarly.* **Description:** Features articles about the uses of plants and animals by native peoples worldwide, both prehistorically and historically. Covers ethnozoology, paleoethnobotany, paleozoology, and ethnobotany.
Indexed: A.I.C.P. (1981-), Abstr.Anthropol., Anthropol.Lit., Bibl.Asian Stud. (1987-1988), Biol.Abstr., Br.Archaeol.Abstr., Intl.Bibl.Soc.Sci., Numis.Lit., Sport Fish.Abstr., Wild.Rev., Zoo.Rec.
—BLDSC (4979.602350), CISTI, ingenta.
Published by: Society of Ethnobiology, c/o Gayle Fritz, Dept of Anthropology CB 1114, Washington, MO 63130-4899. TEL 314-935-8588, FAX 314-935-8535, hunn@u.washington.edu. Ed. Eugene Hunn. Circ: 400.

570 GBR ISSN 0022-0949
CODEN: BJEBAV
JOURNAL OF EXPERIMENTAL BIOLOGY. Text in English. 1923. m. GBP 192 domestic to individuals print ed.; USD 323 in North America to individuals print ed.; GBP 51 domestic to individuals online ed.; USD 86 in North America to individuals online ed.; GBP 213 domestic to individuals print & online eds.; USD 358 in North America to individuals print & online eds. (effective 2001). adv. charts, illus. index; cum.index. back issues avail.; reprints avail. *Refereed.* **Document type:** *Journal, Academic/Scholarly.* **Description:** Covers integrative biology from the molecular and sub-cellular to the whole animal.
Formerly (until 1925): British Journal of Experimental Biology (0366-0788)
Related titles: Online - full text ed.: (from EBSCO Publishing, RoweCom Information Quest, Gale Group, Swets Blackwell, Institute for Scientific Information).
Indexed: ASCA, AgBiotech, Agri.Eng.Abstr., Anim.Behav.Abstr., Anim.Breed.Abstr., Apic.Abstr., Aqua.Sci.& Fish.Abstr., BBCI, Bio-Contr.News & Info., Biol.& Agr.Ind. (Mar.1983-), Biol.Abstr., Chem.Abstr., Chem.Cit.Ind., Chem.Indus.Notes, Chem.Titles, Curr.Adv.Cell & Devel.Biol., Curr.Cont., Curr.Ref.Fish Res., Dairy Sci.Abstr., Deep Sea Res.& Oceanogr.Abstr., Dent.Ind., Entomol.Abstr., Environ.Sci.Poll.Mgmt., Excerp.Med., Forest.Abstr., Gen.Sci.Ind. (Jul.1984-), Helminthol.Abstr., Hort.Abstr., Ind.Med. (1930-), Ind.Sci.Rev., Ind.Vet., Inpharma, Int.Abstr.Biol.Sci., Key Word Ind.Wildl.Res., Med.& Surg.Dermat., Neurosci.Cit.Ind., Nutr.Abstr., Ocean.Abstr. (coverage dropped), Pollut.Abstr., Poult.Abstr., Protozool.Abstr., Psychol.Abstr., Reac., Ref.Zh., Rev.Appl.Entomol., Rev.Med.& Vet.Mycol., SSCI (coverage dropped), Sci.Cit.Ind., Soils & Fert., Sport Fish.Abstr., Tox.Abstr., Trop.Dis.Bull., Vet.Bull., W.R.C.Inf., Weed Abstr., Wild.Rev., Zoo.Rec.
—BLDSC (4980.000000), CASDDS, CISTI, EMDOCS, GNLM, ingenta, Linda Hall.
Published by: Company of Biologists Ltd., Bidder Bldg, Bidder Building, 140 Cowley Rd, Cambridge CB4 4DL, United Kingdom. TEL 44-1223-426164, FAX 44-1223-423353, sales@thecob.demon.co.uk, http://jeb.biologists.org, http://www.biologists.com. Ed. R G Boutilier. R&P R Skaer TEL 44-1223-420482. Adv. contact Amanda Sheppardson. Circ: 1,250.

578.77 NLD ISSN 0022-0981
QH91.A1 CODEN: JEMBAM
JOURNAL OF EXPERIMENTAL MARINE BIOLOGY AND ECOLOGY. Text in Dutch. 1967. 28/yr. EUR 3,333 in Europe to institutions; JPY 442,400 in Japan to institutions; USD 3,729 elsewhere to institutions (effective 2002). adv. bk.rev. illus. Index. back issues avail.; reprint service avail. from SWZ,ISI. *Refereed.* **Document type:** *Academic/Scholarly.* **Description:** Provides a forum for work in the biochemistry, physiology, behavior, and genetics of marine plants and animals in relation to their ecology.
Related titles: Microform ed.: (from PQC); Online - full text ed.: (from EBSCO Publishing, ingenta, ScienceDirect, Swets Blackwell, Institute for Scientific Information).
Indexed: ASCA, AgBiotech, Anim.Behav.Abstr. (coverage dropped), Anim.Breed.Abstr., Appl.Ecol.Abstr., Aqua.Sci.& Fish.Abstr., Aquacult.Abstr., Biol.& Agr.Ind. (coverage dropped), Biol.Abstr., Chem.Abstr., Chem.Indus.Notes, Chem.Titles, Chemorec.Abstr., Curr.Adv.Plant Sci., Curr.Cont., Curr.Ref.Fish Res., Deep Sea Res.& Oceanogr.Abstr., Ecol.Abstr., Energy Ind., Energy Info.Abstr., Environ.Abstr., Environ.Per.Bibl (1990-1993), Environ.Sci.Poll.Mgmt., Excerp.Med., Forest.Abstr., Genet.Abstr., Geo.Abstr.H.G., GeoRef, Helminthol.Abstr., Hum.Gen.Abstr., INIS Atomind., Ind.Sci.Rev., Ind.Vet., Int.Abstr.Biol.Sci., Mar.Sci.Cont.Tab., Microbiol.Abstr., Nutr.Abstr., Ocean.Abstr., Plant Sci., Pollut.Abstr., Protozool.Abstr., Rev.Med.& Vet.Mycol., SSCI (coverage dropped), Sci.Cit.Ind., Sel.Water Res.Abstr., Sport Fish.Abstr., W.R.C.Inf., Weed Abstr., Wild.Rev., Zoo.Rec.
—BLDSC (4981.600000), CASDDS, CISTI, EMDOCS, IDS, ingenta, Linda Hall. **CCC.**
Published by: Elsevier Science BV, PO Box 211, Amsterdam 1000 AE, Netherlands. TEL 31-20-485-3757, FAX 31-20-485-3432, TELEX 18582 ESPA NL, http://www.elsevier.com/locate/jembe, http://www.elsevier.nl. Eds. R Warwick, S Shumway. **Subscr. in Australasia and the Far East to:** Elsevier Science (Singapore) Pte Ltd, No.1 Temasek Ave, 17-01 Millenia Tower, Singapore 039192, Singapore. TEL 65-434-3727, FAX 65-337-2230; **Subscr. in Japan to:** Elsevier Science Inc - Japan Regional Office, 9-15 Higashi-Azabu 1-chome, Minato-ku, Tokyo 106-0044, Japan. FAX 81-3-5561-5047; **Subscr. in the Americas to:** Elsevier Science, PO Box 945, New York, NY 10159-0945. TEL 212-633-3730, FAX 212-633-3680, usinfo-f@elsevier.com.

B

578.7 IND ISSN 0970-3594
QH90.A1 CODEN: JOHYE4
JOURNAL OF HYDROBIOLOGY. Text in English. 1985. s-a. INR 750, USD 20. adv. bk.rev.
Indexed: Biol.Abstr., Zoo.Rec.
—CISTI, ingenta.
Published by: Vikram University, School of Studies in Zoology, P O Box 233, Ujjain 456 010, India. Ed. K S Rao.

570 USA ISSN 0883-1394
CODEN: JIDBE9
JOURNAL OF INFERENTIAL AND DEDUCTIVE BIOLOGY✱. Text in English. 1985. irreg. USD 188. adv. bk.rev.
—CASDDS.
Published by: Danielli Associates, c/o Richard F. Danielli, 667 Washington St Apt 223, Auburn, MA 01501-2789. Eds. Alejandro B Engel, Roger V Jean.

570 USA ISSN 0741-5400
QP185 CODEN: JLBIE7
JOURNAL OF LEUKOCYTE BIOLOGY. Text in English. 1967. m. (2 vols./yr.). USD 105 in North America to individuals; USD 153 elsewhere to individuals; USD 696 in North America to institutions; USD 716 elsewhere to institutions; USD 80 in North America to members; USD 125 elsewhere to members (effective 2000). adv. charts, illus. index. back issues avail. *Refereed.* **Document type:** *Academic/Scholarly.* **Description:** Presents manuscripts of original investigations on the origins, developmental biology, and functions of granulocytes, lymphocytes, and mononuclear phagocytes.
Formerly (until 1984): R E S. Reticuloendothelial Society. Journal (0033-6890)
Related titles: Online - full text ed.: (from EBSCO Publishing, Institute for Scientific Information).
Indexed: AIDS & Cancer Res., ASCA, Biol.Abstr., Chem.Abstr., Chem.Titles, Chemorec.Abstr., Curr.Adv.Cancer Res., Curr.Adv.Cell & Devel.Biol., Curr.Adv.Ecol.Sci., Curr.Cont., Dairy Sci.Abstr., Dent.Ind., Excerp.Med., INIS Atomind., Immun.Abstr., Ind.Med. (1984-), Ind.Sci.Rev., Ind.Vet., Inpharma, Int.Aerosp.Abstr., Neurosci.Cit.Ind., Pharm.&Out.News, Pig News & Info., Reac., Rev.Med.& Vet.Mycol., SSCI (coverage dropped), Sci.Cit.Ind., Small Anim.Abstr., Vet.Bull., Virol.Abstr. (coverage dropped).
—BLDSC (5010.305000), CASDDS, CISTI, EMDOCS, GNLM, IDS, ingenta, KNAW.
Published by: (Society for Leukocyte Biology), Federation of American Societies for Experimental Biology, 9650 Rockville Pike, Bethesda, MD 20814-3998. TEL 301-530-7100, FAX 301-571-1855, http://www.jleukbio.org/. Ed. Joost J Oppenheim. R&P S Jacobson. Adv. contact Susan Mergenhagen.

578.77 ITA ISSN 1129-5767
QH96 CODEN: MIIMAS
JOURNAL OF LIMNOLOGY. Text in English. 1942. s-a. per issue exchange basis. **Document type:** *Academic/Scholarly.* **Description:** Publishes peer-reviewed original papers, review papers, and notes in the field of limnology, including hydrochemistry, lake physics, methodology, taxonomy, all aspects of ecology, biogeography and pollution.
Formerly (until 1999): Istituto Italiano di Idrobiologia. Memorie (0374-9118)
Related titles: Online - full content ed.
Indexed: Aqua.Sci.& Fish.Abstr., Aquacult.Abstr., Biol.Abstr., Curr.Adv.Ecol.Sci., Deep Sea Res.& Oceanogr.Abstr., Ecol.Abstr., Environ.Sci.Poll.Mgmt., Geo.Abstr.H.G., Geo.Abstr.P.G., GeoRef, Ref.Zh., Sport Fish.Abstr., Water Resour.Abstr., Wild.Rev., Zoo.Rec.
—BLDSC (5010.474600), CASDDS, CISTI, EMDOCS, ingenta, Linda Hall.
Published by: Istituto Italiano di Idrobiologia, L.go V. Tonolli, 50, Verbania Pallanza, VB 28922, Italy. FAX 39-323-556513, g.giussani@iii.to.cnr.it, http://www.iii.to.cnr.it. Ed. Riccardo de Bernardi. Circ: 800.

570 DEU ISSN 0303-6812
QH323.5 CODEN: JMBLAJ
JOURNAL OF MATHEMATICAL BIOLOGY. Text in English. m. DEM 1,737.20 domestic; DEM 1,748 foreign (effective 2001). reprint service avail. from ISI. *Refereed.* **Document type:** *Journal, Academic/Scholarly.* **Description:** Includes the fields of genetics, demography, ecology, neurobiology, epidemiology, morphogenesis, and cell biology.
Related titles: Microform ed.: (from PQC); Online - full text ed.: ISSN 1432-1416 (from EBSCO Publishing, RoweCom Information Quest, Swets Blackwell, Springer LINK, Institute for Scientific Information).
Indexed: ASCA, Anim.Breed.Abstr., Appl.Ecol.Abstr. (coverage dropped), Aqua.Sci.& Fish.Abstr., Biostat., C.C.M.J., Compumath, Comput.Abstr., Curr.Adv.Biochem., Curr.Adv.Ecol.Sci., Curr.Adv.Gen.& Molec.Biol., Curr.Cont. (1990-), Curr.Ind.Stat., Deep Sea Res.& Oceanogr.Abstr., Environ.Sci.Poll.Mgmt., Excerp.Med., Helminthol.Abstr., INSPEC (1977-1997, dropped), Ind.Med. (1974-), Ind.Sci.Rev., Inpharma, Math.R., Plant Breed.Abstr., Reac., Sci.Cit.Ind., Sport Fish.Abstr., Stat.Theor.Meth.Abstr. (1990-), Wild.Rev., Zent.Math., Zoo.Rec.
—BLDSC (5012.375000), AskIEEE, CISTI, GNLM, IDS, ingenta, Linda Hall. **CCC.**
Published by: Springer-Verlag (Subsidiary of: BertelsmannSpringer), Tiergartenstr 17, Heidelberg 69121, Germany. TEL 49-6221-345-0, FAX 49-6221-345229, subscriptions@springer.de, http://link.springer.de/link/service/journals/00285/index.htm, http://www.springer.de. Eds. K P Hadeler, O Diekmann. **Subscr. in N. America to:** Springer-Verlag New York Inc., PO Box 2485, Secaucus, NJ 07096-2485. TEL 212-460-1500, FAX 212-473-6272.

570 610 SGP ISSN 0219-5194
▼ **JOURNAL OF MECHANICS IN MEDICINE AND BIOLOGY.** Text in English. 2001. q. SGD 162, USD 92 to individuals; SGD 406, USD 240 to institutions; SGD 243, USD 144 in developing nations to institutions (effective 2001); SGD 173 to individuals Asia Pacific & Australasia except Hong Kong and China; USD 96 elsewhere to individuals; SGD 432 to institutions Asia Pacific & Australasia except Hong Kong and China; USD 240 elsewhere to institutions; SGD 259 in developing nations to institutions Asia Pacific & Australasia except Hong Kong and China; USD 144 in developing nations to institutions (effective 2002). **Document type:** *Academic/Scholarly.* **Description:** Publishes original papers covering biomedical science subjects ranging from nano to macro scale, and the applied technology of the methods and techniques of medical and clinical treatment.
Published by: World Scientific Publishing Co Pte Ltd, 5 Toh Tuck Link, Singapore 596224, Singapore. http://www.worldscientific.com. Ed. Wen-Jei Yang TEL 734-764-9910. **Subscr. in N. America to:** 1060 Main St, River Edge, NJ 07661. TEL 888-977-2665, 800-227-7562, sales@wspc.com.

571.3 USA ISSN 0362-2525
QL801 CODEN: JOMOAT
JOURNAL OF MORPHOLOGY. Text in English. 1887. m. USD 3,175 in United States; USD 3,295 in Canada & Mexico; USD 3,397 elsewhere; USD 3,334 combined subscription in United States for print and online eds.; USD 3,454 combined subscription in Canada & Mexico for print and online eds.; USD 3,556 combined subscription elsewhere for print and online eds. (effective 2002). adv. abstr, bibl, charts, illus. index. back issues avail.; reprint service avail. from SWZ. *Refereed.* **Document type:** *Academic/Scholarly.* **Description:** Publishes original research in morphology including cytology, protozoology, developmental biology, and general and functional morphology.
Former titles (until 1930): Journal of Morphology and Physiology (0095-9626); (until 1923): Journal of Morphology (0022-2887)
Related titles: Microform ed.: (from PMC,PQC,SWZ); Online - full text ed.: ISSN 1097-4687. USD 3,175 in United States; USD 3,175 in Canada & Mexico; USD 3,175 elsewhere (effective 2002) (from EBSCO Publishing, Wiley InterScience, Institute for Scientific Information).
Indexed: ASCA, Agricola, Anim.Breed.Abstr., Aqua.Sci.& Fish.Abstr., Biol.Abstr., Chem.Abstr., Chem.Indus.Notes, Chem.Titles, Curr.Adv.Cell & Devel.Biol., Curr.Adv.Ecol.Sci., Curr.Cont., Deep Sea Res.& Oceanogr.Abstr., Dent.Ind., Entomol.Abstr., Environ.Sci.Poll.Mgmt., Excerp.Med., GeoRef, Helminthol.Abstr., INIS Atomind., Ind.Med. (1887-), Ind.Sci.Rev., Ind.Vet., Inpharma, Int.Abstr.Biol.Sci., Neurosci.Cit.Ind., Pollut.Abstr., Poult.Abstr., Reac., Ref.Zh., Rev.Appl.Entomol., SSCI (coverage dropped), Sci.Cit.Ind., Sport Fish.Abstr., Vet.Bull., Wild.Rev., Zoo.Rec.
—BLDSC (5021.000000), CASDDS, CISTI, EMDOCS, GNLM, IDS, ingenta, Linda Hall. **CCC.**
Published by: John Wiley & Sons, Inc., Journals (Subsidiary of: Wiley InterScience), 605 Third Ave, New York, NY 10158. TEL 212-850-6645, FAX 212-850-6021, subinfo@wiley.com, uscs-wis@wiley.com, http://www.wiley.com. Ed. Frederick W Harrison. adv.: B&W page GBP 640, color page GBP 1,515; trim 174 x 254. Circ: 900. **Subscr. outside the Americas to:** John Wiley & Sons Ltd., Baffins Ln, Chichester, Sussex PO19 IUD, United Kingdom. TEL 44-1243-779777, FAX 44-1243-843232, cs-journals@wiley.co.uk.

570 GBR ISSN 0022-2933
QH1 CODEN: JNAHA9
JOURNAL OF NATURAL HISTORY. Text in English. 1841. 18/yr. GBP 1,650, USD 2,722 to institutions (effective 2002). adv. bk.rev. *Refereed.* **Document type:** *Academic/Scholarly.* **Description:** Contains original research and reviews in systematics and evolutionary and general biology.
Formerly (until 1967): Annals and Magazine of Natural History
Related titles: Microform ed.; Online - full text ed.: ISSN 1464-5262. 199? (from CatchWord Ltd., EBSCO Publishing, O C L C Online Computer Library Center, Inc., RoweCom Information Quest, Swets Blackwell, Institute for Scientific Information).
Indexed: ASCA, Agroforest.Abstr., Anim.Behav.Abstr., Anim.Breed.Abstr., Apic.Abstr., Appl.Ecol.Abstr., Aqua.Sci.& Fish.Abstr., Bio-Contr.News & Info., Biol.Abstr., Curr.Adv.Ecol.Sci., Curr.Cont., Curr.Ref.Fish Res., Curr.Tit.Ocean, Deep Sea Res.& Oceanogr.Abstr., Ecol.Abstr., Entomol.Abstr., Environ.Per.Bibl. (1991-), Environ.Sci.Poll.Mgmt., Forest.Abstr., GeoRef, Geol.Abstr., Helminthol.Abstr., IBR, Ind.Sci.Rev., Ind.Vet., Int.Abstr.Biol.Sci., Protozool.Abstr., Ref.Sour., Rev.Appl.Entomol., Rev.Med.& Vet.Mycol., Sci.Cit.Ind., Seed Abstr., So.Pac.Per.Ind., Soils & Fert., Sport Fish.Abstr., Triticale Abstr., Weed Abstr., Wild.Rev., Zoo.Rec.
—BLDSC (5021.200000), CatchWord, CISTI, EMDOCS, IDS, Infotrieve, ingenta, Linda Hall. **CCC.**
Published by: Taylor & Francis Group, Taylor & Francis Ltd., 11 New Fetter Ln, London EC4P 4EE, United Kingdom. TEL 44-20-7583-9855, FAX 44-20-7842-2298, info@tandf.co.uk, http://www.tandf.co.uk/. Eds. A Polaszek, P Je Hayward. **Subscr. in N. America to:** Taylor & Francis Ltd., 325 Chestnut St, Suite 800, Philadelphia, PA 19016. TEL 800-354-1420, FAX 215-625-8914, info@taylorandfrancis.com, http://www.taylorandfrancis.com/.

JOURNAL OF NUCLEAR AGRICULTURE AND BIOLOGY. see *AGRICULTURE—Crop Production And Soil*

578.77 GBR ISSN 0142-7873
QH90.8.P5 CODEN: JPLRD9
JOURNAL OF PLANKTON RESEARCH. Text in English. 1979. m. GBP 160, USD 258 to individuals; GBP 380, USD 645 to institutions (effective 2002). adv. bk.rev. illus. index. back issues avail.; reprint service avail. from SWZ. *Refereed.* **Document type:** *Academic/Scholarly.* **Description:** A forum for international papers covering zooplankton and phytoplankton in three main areas: ecology (including model studies); physiology; distribution, life and taxonomy.
Related titles: Online - full text ed.: ISSN 1464-3774. GBP 342, USD 580 to institutions Online only (effective 2002) (from HighWire Pr., EBSCO Publishing, O C L C Online Computer Library Center, Inc., RoweCom Information Quest, ingenta, Swets Blackwell, Institute for Scientific Information).
Indexed: ASCA, Anim.Behav.Abstr., Appl.Ecol.Abstr., Aqua.Sci.& Fish.Abstr., Arts & Hum.Cit.Ind. (coverage dropped), Biotech.& Bioeng.Abstr., Chem.Abstr., Chem.Indus.Notes, Chem.Titles, Curr.Adv.Ecol.Sci., Curr.Adv.Plant Sci., Curr.Cont., Deep Sea Res.& Oceanogr.Abstr., Ecol.Abstr., Environ.Sci.Poll.Mgmt., Geo.Abstr.H.G., GeoRef, Geol.Abstr., Ind.Vet., Int.Abstr.Biol.Sci., Microbiol.Abstr., Ocean.Abstr., Plant Sci., Pollut.Abstr., Rev.Appl.Entomol., Sci.Cit.Ind., Sel.Water Res.Abstr., Sport Fish.Abstr., W.R.C.Inf., Zoo.Rec.
—BLDSC (5040.350000), CASDDS, CINDOC, CISTI, EMDOCS, IDS, Infotrieve, ingenta, Linda Hall. **CCC.**
Published by: Oxford University Press, Academic Division, Great Clarendon St, Oxford OX2 6DP, United Kingdom. TEL 44-1865-267907, FAX 44-1865-267835, jnl.info@oup.co.uk, http://plankt.oupjournals.org/, http://www.oup.co.uk/journals. Ed. D H Cushing. Pub. Cathy Kennedy. R&P Fiona Willis. adv.: B&W page GBP 230, B&W page USD 415; trim 195 x 125. Circ: 850. **U.S. subscr. to:** Oxford University Press, Journals, 2001 Evans Rd, Cary, NC 27513. TEL 800-852-7323, FAX 919-677-1714, jnlorders@oup-usa.org.

636.0845 USA ISSN 0022-409X
SF85 CODEN: JRMGAQ

JOURNAL OF RANGE MANAGEMENT; covering the study, management, and use of rangeland ecosystems and range resources. Text in English. 1948. bi-m. USD 95 domestic to institutions; USD 112 foreign to institutions; USD 158 foreign to institutions with Rangelands (effective 2001). adv. bk.rev. bibl, charts, illus. index. back issues avail.; reprint service avail. from PQC,PSC,SCH. *Refereed.* **Document type:** *Journal, Academic/Scholarly.* **Description:** Offers a forum of technical articles about research in range science and range management.

Related titles: Microfilm ed.: (from PQC); Online - full text ed.: (from Institute for Scientific Information); Supplement: Trail Boss News.

Indexed: ASCA, Agri.& Environ.Biotech.Abstr. (coverage dropped), Agri.Eng.Abstr., Agricola, Agroforest.Abstr., Bibl.Agri., Bio-Contr.News & Info., Biol.& Agr.Ind. (Jan.1983-), Biol.Abstr., Biol.Dig., Chem.Abstr., Crop Physiol.Abstr., Curr.Adv.Ecol.Sci., Curr.Adv.Plant Sci., Curr.Cont., Curr.Ind.Stat., Dairy Sci.Abstr., Derwent Biotech.Abstr., Ecol.Abstr., Energy Ind., Energy Info.Abstr., Environ.Per.Bibl. (1972-), Farm & Garden Ind., Field Crop Abstr., Forest Prod.Abstr., Forest.Abstr., Geo.Abstr.H.G., Geo.Abstr.P.G., GeoRef, Herb.Abstr., IDA, INIS Atomind., Ind.Sci.Rev., Ind.Vet., Int.Abstr.Biol.Sci., Int.Abstr.Oper.Res., Irr.& Drain.Abstr., Maize Abstr., Nutr.Abstr., Plant Breed.Abstr., Plant Gen.Res.Abstr., Plant Grow.Reg.Abstr., Plant Sci., Protozool.Abstr., Rev.Appl.Entomol., Rev.Plant Path., SSCI (coverage dropped), Sci.Cit.Ind., Seed Abstr., Soils & Fert., Sport Fish.Abstr., Sugar Ind.Abstr., Triticale Abstr., Vet.Bull., Weed Abstr., Wild.Rev., World Ag.Econ.& Rur.Soc.Abstr., Zoo.Rec.

—BLDSC (5046.000000), CASDDS, CISTI, EMDOCS, IDS, ingenta, Linda Hall.

Published by: Society for Range Management, 445 Union Blvd, Ste 230, Lakewood, CO 80228-1259. TEL 303-986-3309, FAX 303-986-3892, srmden@ix.netcom.com, http://uvalde.tamu.edu/jrm/jrmhome.htm, http://srm.org. Eds. Gary Frasier, Patty Rich. Circ: 3,000 (paid).

570 USA ISSN 1079-9893
QH603.C43 CODEN: JRETET

JOURNAL OF RECEPTOR AND SIGNAL TRANSDUCTION RESEARCH. Text in English. 1981. q. USD 115 to individuals print & online eds.; USD 975 to institutions print only (effective 2002). adv. bk.rev. charts, illus. index. back issues avail. *Refereed.* **Document type:** *Academic/Scholarly.* **Description:** Presents a forum for the rapid publication of laboratory and clinical research on biological receptors and associated signal transduction pathways for hormones, growth factors, drugs, and ligands involved in the immune response.

Formed by the merger of (1980-1995): Journal of Receptor Research (0197-5110); Second Messengers and Phosphoproteins (0895-7479); Which was formerly titled (until 1988): Journal of Cyclic Nucleotide and Protein Phosphorylation Research; Journal of Cyclic Nucleotide Research (0095-1544)

Related titles: Microform ed.: (from RPI); Online - full content ed.; Online - full text ed.: (from Institute for Scientific Information, RoweCom Information Quest).

Indexed: ASCA, BBCI, Biol.Abstr., Cal.Tiss.Abstr., Chem.Abstr., Chem.Indus.Notes, Chem.Titles, Curr.Adv.Biochem., Curr.Adv.Cell & Devel.Biol., Curr.Adv.Ecol.Sci., Curr.Cont., Dairy Sci.Abstr., Derwent Biotech.Abstr., Excerp.Med., INIS Atomind., Ind.Med. (1995-), Ind.Sci.Rev., Inpharma, Int.Abstr.Biol.Sci., Mass Spectr.Bull., Neurosci.Abstr., Protozool.Abstr., Reac., Ref.Zh., Sci.Cit.Ind.

—BLDSC (5047.849000), CASDDS, CISTI, EMDOCS, GNLM, IDS, Infotrieve, ingenta, Linda Hall. **CCC.**

Published by: Marcel Dekker Inc., 270 Madison Ave, New York, NY 10016. TEL 212-696-9000, 800-228-1160, FAX 212-685-4540, http://www.dekker.com/servlet/product/productid/RRS. Ed. Alex N Eberle. R&P Julia Mulligan. Adv. contact Diane Saulon. Circ: 525 (paid).

612 573.6 IND

JOURNAL OF REPRODUCTION AND FERTILITY. Text in English. q.

Related titles: Microfilm ed.: (from PMC).

Indexed: Biol.& Agr.Ind. (coverage dropped), Biol.Abstr., Chem.Abstr., Chem.Indus.Notes, Chem.Titles, Curr.Cont. (coverage dropped), Dairy Sci.Abstr., Small Anim.Abstr., Vet.Bull.

Published by: Indian Society for the Study of Reproduction and Endocrinology, c/o Department of Zoology, University of Delhi, New Delhi 110 007, India.

JOURNAL OF SOCIAL AND EVOLUTIONARY SYSTEMS. see *PSYCHOLOGY*

570 USA ISSN 1047-8477
QH573 CODEN: JSBIEM

JOURNAL OF STRUCTURAL BIOLOGY. Text in Multiple languages. 1957. m. USD 770 in US & Canada to institutions; USD 880 elsewhere to institutions (effective 2001). adv. bibl, charts, illus. index. *Refereed.* **Document type:** *Academic/Scholarly.* **Description:** Deals with the structural analysis of biological matter at all levels of organization by means of light and electron microscopy, x-ray diffraction, nuclear magnetic resonance, as well as other imaging, diffraction, spectroscopic, or scanning probe techniques yielding structural information.

Former titles: Journal of Ultrastructure and Molecular Structure Research (0889-1605); Journal of Ultrastructure Research (0022-5320)

Related titles: Online - full text ed.: (from EBSCO Publishing, O C L C Online Computer Library Center, Inc., RoweCom Information Quest, ingenta, Swets Blackwell, IDEAL Online Library, Institute for Scientific Information).

Indexed: ASCA, Abstr.Bull.Inst.Pap.Chem., Abstr.Hyg., Agricola, Anim.Breed.Abstr., Aqua.Sci.& Fish.Abstr., Aquacult.Abstr., BBCI, Bibl.Agri., Biol.Abstr., Chem.Abstr., Chem.Indus.Notes, Chem.Titles, Curr.Adv.Ecol.Sci., Curr.Cont., Dairy Sci.Abstr., Environ.Sci.Poll.Mgmt., Excerp.Med., Field Crop Abstr., GeoRef, Helminthol.Abstr., Herb.Abstr., INIS Atomind., Ind.Med. (1990-), Ind.Sci.Rev., Ind.Vet., Inpharma, Nutr.Abstr., Pig News & Info., Poult.Abstr., Protozool.Abstr., Reac., Rev.Plant Path., Sci.Cit.Ind., Soils & Fert., Sport Fish.Abstr., Trop.Dis.Bull., Vet.Bull., Wild.Rev., Zoo.Rec.

—BLDSC (5066.874500), ADONIS, CASDDS, CISTI, EMDOCS, GNLM, IDS, ingenta, Linda Hall. **CCC.**

Published by: Academic Press, Inc., Journal Division (Subsidiary of: Harcourt Brace & Company), 525 B St, Ste 1900, San Diego, CA 92101-4495. TEL 619-230-1840, FAX 619-699-6859, apsubs@acad.com, http://www.academicpress.com/jsb; http://www.idealibrary.com/. Ed. Alasdair C Steven.

571.3 611 IND
QM1 CODEN: JAINAA

JOURNAL OF THE ANATOMICAL SOCIETY OF INDIA. Text in English. 1951. s-a. INR 275, USD 45 (effective 2001). adv. bk.rev. charts, illus, abstr. index. 100 p./no. 2 cols./p. back issues avail. *Refereed.* **Document type:** *Journal, Academic/Scholarly.* **Description:** Covers anatomy, anthropology, cytology, histology, genetics and clinical applied medicine.

Formerly: Anatomical Society of India. Journal (0003-2778)

Related titles: Online - full text ed.

Indexed: Biol.Abstr., Chem.Abstr., Excerp.Med., Ind.Vet., Nutr.Abstr., Vet.Bull.

—CASDDS, CISTI.

Published by: Anatomical Society of India, Department of Anatomy, M.L.B. Medical College, Jhansi, Uttar Pradesh 284 128, India. TEL 0517-320032, editorjasi@rediffmail.com, secasi@yahoo.com. Ed. GopiChand V.V. Patnaik. adv.: page INR 1,200. Circ: 550.

570 NLD ISSN 0022-5010
QH305 CODEN: JHBIA9

JOURNAL OF THE HISTORY OF BIOLOGY. Text in English. 1968. 3/yr. EUR 293, USD 294 to institutions for print or online ed..; EUR 351.60, USD 352.80 to institutions for print & online eds.combined (effective 2002). adv. bk.rev. charts, illus. index. reprint service avail. from SWZ. *Refereed.* **Document type:** *Journal, Academic/Scholarly.* **Description:** Publishes research on the history of the biological sciences, with particular emphasis on developments of the 19th and 20th centuries, including philosophical issues.

Related titles: Microform ed.: (from PQC); Online - full text ed.: (from EBSCO Publishing, O C L C Online Computer Library Center, Inc., RoweCom Information Quest, Swets Blackwell, Kluwer Online, Institute for Scientific Information); ♦ French ed.: Revue de l'Histoire de Biologie.

Indexed: ASCA, Amer.Bibl.Slavic & E.Eur.Stud., Amer.Hist.& Life, Arts & Hum.Cit.Ind., Biol.& Agr.Ind. (Apr.1983-Mar.1989), Biol.Abstr., Curr.Adv.Ecol.Sci., Curr.Cont., Deep Sea Res.& Oceanogr.Abstr., GeoRef, Hist.Abstr. (1968-), IBR, IBZ, Ind.Med. (coverage dropped), Ind.Sci.Rev., Maize Abstr., Phil.Ind., Plant Breed.Abstr., Plant Grow.Reg.Abstr., Ref.Zh., Rev.Med.& Vet.Mycol., Russ.Acad.Sci.Bibl., SSCI, Sci.Cit.Ind., Sport Fish.Abstr., Zoo.Rec.

—BLDSC (5000.700000), CISTI, IDS, ingenta, Linda Hall. **CCC.**

Published by: Kluwer Academic Publishers Group (Subsidiary of: Wolters Kluwer N.V.), Spuiboulevard 50, PO Box 17, Dordrecht 3300 AA, Netherlands. TEL 31-78-639-2392, FAX 31-78-654-2254, services@wkap.nl, http://www.wkap.nl/journalhome.htm/0022-5010. Eds. Garland E Allen, Jane Maienschein. **Subscr. in the Americas to:** Kluwer Academic - Plenum Publishers, 233 Spring St, New York, NY 10013-1578. TEL 212-620-8468, FAX 212-807-1047; **Subscr. to:** Journals Department, PO Box 322, Dordrecht 3300 AH, Netherlands. TEL 31-78-639-2392, FAX 31-78-654-6474.

JOURNAL OF THE PERIPHERAL NERVOUS SYSTEM. see *MEDICAL SCIENCES—Psychiatry And Neurology*

JOURNAL OF THE PERIPHERAL NERVOUS SYSTEM ONLINE. see *MEDICAL SCIENCES—Psychiatry And Neurology*

B

570 GBR ISSN 0022-5193
QH301 CODEN: JTBIAP

JOURNAL OF THEORETICAL BIOLOGY; an international multidisciplinary journal. Text in English. 1961. 24/yr. GBP 2,100 to institutions (effective 2001). adv. bibl, charts, illus. index. reprint service avail. from SWZ. *Refereed.* **Document type:** *Academic/Scholarly.* **Description:** Provides a forum for theoretical papers that give insight into biological processes.

Related titles: Online - full text ed.: (from EBSCO Publishing, O C L C Online Computer Library Center, Inc., RoweCom Information Quest, ingenta, Swets Blackwell, IDEAL Online Library, Institute for Scientific Information).

Indexed: ASCA, Abstr.Anthropol., Agricola, Anim.Behav.Abstr., Apic.Abstr., Appl.Ecol.Abstr., Aqua.Sci.& Fish.Abstr., Bibl.Agri., Biol.Abstr., Biostat., Chem.Abstr., Chem.Cit.Ind., Chem.Indus.Notes, Chem.Titles, Compumath, Curr.Adv.Biochem., Curr.Adv.Cell & Devel.Biol., Curr.Adv.Ecol.Sci., Curr.Adv.Gen.& Molec.Biol., Curr.Cont., Curr.Ind.Stat., Dairy Sci.Abstr., Deep Sea Res.& Oceanogr.Abstr., Dent.Ind., Ecol.Abstr., Entomol.Abstr., Environ.Sci.Poll.Mgmt., Excerp.Med., Field Crop Abstr., Fluidex, Genet.Abstr., Geo.Abstr.H.G., GeoRef, Geol.Abstr., Helminthol.Abstr., Herb.Abstr., Hum.Gen.Abstr., INIS Atomind., Ind.Med. (1961-), Ind.Sci.Rev., Ind.Vet., Inpharma, Int.Abstr.Biol.Sci., Int.Aerosp.Abstr., Key Word Ind.Wildl.Res., Math.R., Microbiol.Abstr., Neurosci.Cit.Ind., Nuc.Acids Abstr., Nutr.Abstr., Protozool.Abstr., Reac., Ref.Zh., Risk Abstr., SSCI (coverage dropped), Sci.Cit.Ind., Sport Fish.Abstr., Vet.Bull., Weed Abstr., Wild.Rev., Zoo.Rec.

—BLDSC (5069.075000), ADONIS, CASDDS, CISTI, EMDOCS, GNLM, IDS, ingenta, Linda Hall. **CCC.**

Published by: Academic Press (Subsidiary of: Harcourt Publishers Ltd.), 24 Oval Rd, London NW1 7DX, United Kingdom. TEL 44-20-7267-4466, FAX 44-20-7482-2293, apsubs@acad.com, http://www.academicpress.com/jtb; http://www.europe.idealibrary.com/. Eds. J Tyson, L Wolpert. R&P Catherine John. Adv. contact Nik Screen. **Subscr. to:** Harcourt Publishers Ltd., Foots Cray High St, Sidcup, Kent DA14 5HP, United Kingdom. TEL 44-20-8300-3322, FAX 44-20-8309-0807.

JOURNAL OF TOXICOLOGY AND PUBLIC HEALTH. see *ENVIRONMENTAL STUDIES*

THE JOURNAL OF TRACE ELEMENTS IN EXPERIMENTAL MEDICINE. see *MEDICAL SCIENCES—Experimental Medicine, Laboratory Technique*

570 DEU ISSN 0946-672X
CODEN: JTEBFO

JOURNAL OF TRACE ELEMENTS IN MEDICINE AND BIOLOGY. Text in English. 1987. q. EUR 364, GBP 293 (effective 2002). index. back issues avail. *Refereed.* **Document type:** *Journal, Academic/Scholarly.* **Description:** Contains research papers and articles on theoretical and applied aspects of trace elements in medicine and biology.

Formerly (until 1994): Journal of Trace Elements and Electrolytes in Health and Disease (0931-2838)

Related titles: Online - full text ed.: (from Institute for Scientific Information).

Indexed: ASCA, Anal.Abstr., BBCI, Chem.Abstr., Chem.Titles, Curr.Cont., Dairy Sci.Abstr., Excerp.Med., Ind.Med. (1995-), Inpharma, Mass Spectr.Bull., Nutr.Abstr., Pharm.&Out.News, Reac., Sci.Cit.Ind., Triticale Abstr.

—BLDSC (5069.744400), CASDDS, CISTI, EMDOCS, GNLM, IDS, Infotrieve, ingenta. **CCC.**

Published by: (Society for Minerals and Trace Elements), Urban & Fischer Verlag, Loebdergraben 14a, Jena 07743, Germany. TEL 49-3641-626444, FAX 49-3641-626421, marketing.journals@urbanfischer.de, http://www.urbanfischer.de/journals. Ed. V Negretti de Bratter. R&P Kerstin Schumann TEL 49-3641-626444. **Subscr. to:** Nature Publishing Group, Brunel Rd, Basingstoke RG21 6XS, United Kingdom. TEL 44-1256-302629, FAX 44-1256-463570, j.stephens@macmillan.com.

571.986 USA ISSN 1081-1710
RA639 CODEN: BSVEDL
JOURNAL OF VECTOR ECOLOGY. Text in English. 1974. s-a. USD 50 (effective 2000). adv. bk.rev. *Refereed.* **Document type:** *Proceedings, Academic/Scholarly.* **Description:** Contains public health related research papers and proceedings from national and international conferences. Also provides members and selected nonmembers worldwide with updated information regarding disease vector-control information.
Former titles (until Jun. 1995): Society for Vector Ecology. Bulletin; Society of Vector Ecologists. Bulletin (0146-6429)
Related titles: Online - full text ed.: (from Institute for Scientific Information).
Indexed: ASCA, Abstr.Hyg., Bio-Contr.News & Info., Biol.Abstr., Chem.Abstr., Curr.Cont., Forest.Abstr., Helminthol.Abstr., Ind.Med. (1995-), Ind.Vet., Poult.Abstr., Protozool.Abstr., Rev.Appl.Entomol., Rev.Med.& Vet.Mycol., Rice Abstr., Sci.Cit.Ind., Trop.Dis.Bull., Vet.Bull., Zoo.Rec.
—BLDSC (5072.273000), CASDDS, CISTI, IDS, KNAW. **CCC.**
Published by: Society for Vector Ecology, 1966 Compton Ave, Corona, CA 91719. TEL 714-971-2421, FAX 714-971-3940, mklowden@marvin.ag.uidaho.edu. Ed. Marc J Klowden. R&P Major S Dhillon TEL 909-340-9792. Adv. contact Dan Abiaz. page USD 150; trim 11 x 8.5. Circ: 860 (paid).

KARUSHUMU SHINPOJUMU KOEN YOSHI/ABSTRACTS OF CALCIUM SYMPOSIUM. see *BIOLOGY—Abstracting, Bibliographies, Statistics*

570 IND ISSN 0374-860X
KERALA ACADEMY OF BIOLOGY. JOURNAL* . Text in Malayalam; Summaries in English. s-a. INR 15.
Indexed: Biol.Abstr.
Published by: Kerala Academy of Biology, Thiruvananthapuram, Kerala, India.

570 FIN ISSN 0453-7831
AS262.T84
KEVO SUBARCTIC RESEARCH INSTITUTE. REPORTS. Text in English, German; Summaries in English. 1964. irreg., latest vol.22, 1998. price varies. bk.rev. back issues avail.; reprints avail. *Refereed.* **Document type:** *Journal, Academic/Scholarly.* **Description:** Studies on the nature of subarctic areas.
Indexed: Bio-Contr.News & Info., Biol.Abstr., Curr.Adv.Ecol.Sci., Curr.Adv.Plant Sci., Curr.Cont. (coverage dropped), Entomol.Abstr. (coverage dropped), Forest.Abstr., Rev.Appl.Entomol., Rev.Plant Path., Zoo.Rec.
—CISTI.
Published by: University of Turku, Kevo Subarctic Research Institute, Turku 20014, Finland. TEL 358-2-333-5913, FAX 358-2-333-5960, http://www.utu.fi/erill/kevo/. Ed. Seppo Neuvonen TEL 358-2-333-5930. Circ: 400.

578.77 SAU ISSN 1012-8840
GC1 CODEN: JFMSDF
KING ABDUL AZIZ UNIVERSITY. FACULTY OF MARINE SCIENCE. JOURNAL. Text in Arabic, English. 1981. a. USD 5. illus. **Description:** Promotes research in the field of marine science.
Indexed: Aquacult.Abstr., Deep Sea Res.& Oceanogr.Abstr., Environ.Sci.Poll.Mgmt.
Published by: King Abdul Aziz University, Faculty of Marine Science, P O Box 1540, Jeddah 21441, Saudi Arabia. TEL 6952386, FAX 6952381, TELEX 601141 KAUNI SJ. Ed. A K Behairy.

KOBE UNIVERSITY. FACULTY OF AGRICULTURE. SCIENCE REPORTS. see *AGRICULTURE*

KOCHI DAIGAKU GAKUJUTSU KENKYU HOKOKU. NOGAKU/KOCHI UNIVERSITY. AGRICULTURAL SCIENCE. RESEARCH REPORTS. see *AGRICULTURE*

570 AUT ISSN 0075-6547
QL571 CODEN: KLRUAS
KOLEOPTEROLOGISCHE RUNDSCHAU. Text in German. 1912. a. ATS 400; ATS 700 foreign (effective 2000). **Document type:** *Academic/Scholarly.*
Indexed: Aqua.Sci.& Fish.Abstr., Biol.Abstr., IBR, Ref.Zh., Rev.Appl.Entomol., Zoo.Rec.
—Linda Hall.
Published by: Zoologisch-Botanische Gesellschaft in Oesterreich, Althanstrasse 14, Postfach 287, Vienna, W 1091, Austria. TEL 43-1-313361416, FAX 43-1-31336776, wolfgang.punz@univie.ac.at. Circ: 180.

570 DNK ISSN 0366-3612
QH7 CODEN: BSVSAQ
KONGELIGE DANSKE VIDENSKABERNES SELSKAB. BIOLOGISKE SKRIFTER. Text mainly in English. 1941. irreg., latest vol.51, 1998. price varies. bibl, illus. **Document type:** *Monographic series, Academic/Scholarly.*
Indexed: Aqua.Sci.& Fish.Abstr., Aquacult.Abstr., Biol.Abstr., Curr.Adv.Ecol.Sci., GeoRef, Seed Abstr., Zoo.Rec.
—CISTI, KNAW, Linda Hall.
Published by: Kongelige Danske Videnskabernes Selskab/Royal Danish Academy of Sciences and Letters, H C Andersens Blvd 35, Copenhagen V 1553, Denmark. TEL 45-33-43-5300, FAX 45-33-43-5301, pg@royalacademy.dk. Ed. Flemming Lundgreen Nielsen. **Subscr. to:** Reitzels Boghandel og Forlag, Norregade 20, Copenhagen K 1165, Denmark. TEL 45-33-12-2400, FAX 45-33-14-0270.

KYOTO DAIGAKU. REICHORUI KENKYUJO NENPO/KYOTO UNIVERSITY. PRIMATE RESEARCH INSTITUTE. ANNUAL REPORTS. see *ANTHROPOLOGY*

570 JPN ISSN 0454-7802
QH301 CODEN: MFKBBJ
KYOTO UNIVERSITY. FACULTY OF SCIENCE. MEMOIRS. SERIES OF BIOLOGY. Text in English. 1924; N.S. 1967. s-a. per issue exchange basis. back issues avail.
Indexed: Biol.Abstr., Chem.Abstr., Curr.Adv.Ecol.Sci., Deep Sea Res.& Oceanogr.Abstr., Field Crop Abstr., GeoRef, Herb.Abstr., INIS Atomind., Zoo.Rec.
—CISTI, KNAW, Linda Hall.
Published by: Kyoto University, Faculty of Science/Kyoto Daigaku Rigakubu, Kita-Shirakawaoiwake-cho, Sakyo-ku, Kyoto-shi 606-8224, Japan.

574 347 FRA ISSN 1166-0856
L A B M JURIDIQUE. Text in French. 199?. q. FRF 485 domestic to institutions; EUR 73.94 in Europe to institutions; USD 92 in the Americas to institutions; FRF 538 elsewhere to institutions (effective 2001). back issues avail.; reprints avail. *Refereed.* **Document type:** *Academic/Scholarly.*
Related titles: Online - full text ed.
Published by: (Laboratoire de Biologie Medicale), Elsevier Paris, Editions Scientifiques et Medicales (Subsidiary of: Reed Elsevier plc. group), 23 rue Linois, Paris 75015, France. TEL 33-1-45589110, FAX 33-1-45589419, academic@elsevier-fr.com, http://www.elsevier.com/locate/labmju.

LABORATORY TECHNIQUES IN BIOCHEMISTRY AND MOLECULAR BIOLOGY. see *BIOLOGY—Biochemistry*

LASERS IN THE LIFE SCIENCES. see *PHYSICS—Optics*

LATVIJAS ZINATNU AKADEMIJAS VETIS. B DALA. DABASZINATNES/LATVIAN ACADEMY OF SCIENCES. SECTION B. NATURAL SCIENCES. PROCEEDINGS. see *SCIENCES: COMPREHENSIVE WORKS*

LEBENDIGE ERDE; Zeitschrift fuer Biologisch-Dynamische Wirtschaftsweise. see *AGRICULTURE*

LECTURE NOTES IN BIOMATHEMATICS. see *MATHEMATICS*

LECTURES ON MATHEMATICS IN THE LIFE SCIENCES. see *MATHEMATICS*

580 590 LIE
LIECHTENSTEIN. BOTANISCH-ZOOLOGISCHE GESELLSCHAFT LIECHTENSTEIN SARGANS-WERDENBERG. BERICHT. Text in German. 1972. a. USD 30 (effective 2000). adv. bk.rev. bibl, illus. **Document type:** *Proceedings, Academic/Scholarly.*
Indexed: Zoo.Rec.
Published by: Botanisch-Zoologische Gesellschaft Liechtenstein-Sargans-Werdenberg, Im Bretscha 22, Schaan 9494, Liechtenstein. Ed. Mario Broggi. R&P F Flueck Wirth. Circ: 1,000.

577 LTU ISSN 0235-7224
CODEN: EKOLEJ
LIETUVOS MOKSLU AKADEMIJA. EKOLOGIJA. Text in English, Lithuanian, Russian; Summaries in Lithuanian, Russian. 1955. q. USD 80 foreign (effective 1999). adv. **Document type:** *Academic/Scholarly.*
Supersedes in part (in 1990): Lietuvos T.S.R. Mokslu Akademijos Darbai. C Serija. Biologijos Mokslai (0131-3851)
Indexed: Aqua.Sci.& Fish.Abstr., Aquacult.Abstr., Chem.Abstr., Environ.Sci.Poll.Mgmt., Forest Prod.Abstr., Forest.Abstr., GeoRef, Helminthol.Abstr., Herb.Abstr., Hort.Abstr., INIS Atomind., Vet.Bull., Zoo.Rec.
—BLDSC (0397.597950), CASDDS, CISTI, KNAW.
Published by: (Lietuvos Mokslu Akademija), Leidykla Academia, A Gostauto 12, Vilnius 2000, Lithuania. TEL 370-2-626851. Ed. T Eitminaviciute. R&P A Garliauskas. Adv. contact A. Garliauskas. Circ: 680.

LIFE SCIENCE BOOK REVIEW. see *BIOLOGY—Abstracting, Bibliographies, Statistics*

570 GBR ISSN 0024-4066
QH1 CODEN: BJLSBG
LINNEAN SOCIETY. BIOLOGICAL JOURNAL; a journal of evolution. Text in English. 1791. m., latest vol.75, 2002. GBP 1,241 in Europe; USD 1,968 in North America; GBP 1,366 elsewhere (effective 2002). adv. bk.rev. bibl, illus. index per vol. reprint service avail. from SWZ. *Refereed.* **Document type:** *Journal, Academic/Scholarly.* **Description:** Examines the process of organic evolution, with particular emphasis on theoretical and empirical contributions illustrating unifying concepts of evolutionary biology.
Formerly (until 1969): Linnean Society of London. Proceedings
Related titles: Microfilm ed.: (from BHP); Online - full text ed.: ISSN 1095-8312. GBP 1,117 in Europe; USD 1,772 in North America; GBP 1,117 elsewhere (effective 2002) (from EBSCO Publishing, O C L C Online Computer Library Center, Inc., RoweCom Information Quest, ingenta, Swets Blackwell, IDEAL Online Library, Institute for Scientific Information).
Indexed: ASCA, AgBiotech, Agricola, Anim.Behav.Abstr., Anim.Breed.Abstr., Apic.Abstr., Appl.Ecol.Abstr., Aqua.Sci.& Fish.Abstr., Bibl.Agri., Bio-Contr.News & Info., Biol.Abstr., Curr.Adv.Gen.& Molec.Biol., Curr.Adv.Plant Sci., Curr.Cont., Deep Sea Res.& Oceanogr.Abstr., Ecol.Abstr., Entomol.Abstr., Environ.Sci.Poll.Mgmt., Field Crop Abstr., Forest.Abstr., Genet.Abstr., GeoRef, Geol.Abstr., Helminthol.Abstr., Herb.Abstr., Ind.Sci.Rev., Ind.Vet., Int.Abstr.Biol.Sci., Key Word Ind.Wildl.Res., Nutr.Abstr., Plant Breed.Abstr., Plant Gen.Res.Abstr., Plant Sci., Potato Abstr., Protozool.Abstr., Rev.Appl.Entomol., Rev.Med.& Vet.Mycol., Rev.Plant Path., Sci.Cit.Ind., Seed Abstr., Sel.Water Res.Abstr., Soils & Fert., Sport Fish.Abstr., Weed Abstr., Wild.Rev., Zoo.Rec.
—BLDSC (2075.460000), CISTI, EMDOCS, IDS, ingenta, Linda Hall. **CCC.**
Published by: (Linnean Society of London), Blackwell Science Ltd., PO Box 88, Oxford OX2 0NE, United Kingdom. TEL 44-1865-206180, 44-1865-206002, FAX 44-1865-206219, apsubs@acad.com, jnl.orders@blacksci.co.uk, http://www.blackwell-science.com/~cgilib/jnlpage.asp?Journal=bij&File=bij, http://www.blackwellpublishing.com. R&Ps Catherine John, Sophie Savage. Adv. contacts Jenny Applin, Nik Screen. **Subscr. to:** Harcourt Publishers Ltd., Foots Cray High St, Sidcup, Kent DA14 5HP, United Kingdom.

570 USA ISSN 0161-6366
CODEN: LSSSDM
LINNEAN SOCIETY. SYMPOSIA SERIES. Text in English. 1976. irreg., latest vol.18, 1996. price varies. back issues avail.; reprint service avail. from ISI. **Document type:** *Proceedings.* **Description:** Publishes scholarly papers read at the Linnean Society's symposia but not included in one of its three journals.
Indexed: Biol.Abstr., Chem.Abstr., Chem.Indus.Notes, Chem.Titles, GeoRef, Zoo.Rec.
—BLDSC (5221.493000), CASDDS, CISTI. **CCC.**
Published by: (Linnaean Society of London), Academic Press, Inc., Journal Division (Subsidiary of: Harcourt Brace & Company), 525 B St, Ste 1900, San Diego, CA 92101-4495. TEL 619-231-0926, FAX 619-699-6715, john@linnean.org, http://www.linnean.org/html/publications/publications_symposia.htm. **Subscr. to:** Order Dept., 6277 Sea Harbor Dr, 4th Fl, Orlando, FL 32887. TEL 800-321-5068.

570.15195 POL ISSN 0458-0036
LISTY BIOMETRYCZNE/BIOMETRICAL LETTERS. Text and summaries in English, Polish. 1964. 2/yr. USD 10 (effective 1999). adv. bk.rev. back issues avail. *Refereed.* **Document type:** *Academic/Scholarly.* **Description:** Publishes papers concerned with different aspects of the analysis and interpretation of results obtained from biometrical experiments, using statistical methods.
Indexed: Curr.Ind.Stat.
Published by: Polskie Towarzystwo Biometryczne/Polish Biometric Society, c/o Akademia Rolnicza w Poznaniu, Dept. Metod Matematyczno-Statystycznych, Wojska Polskiego 28, Poznan 60637, Poland. TEL 48-61-8487140, FAX 48-61-8487146, smejza@au.poznan.pl; pkra@igr.poznan.pl, http://www.igr.poznan.pl. Ed. Zygmunt Kaczmarek. Pub. Stanisław Mejza. R&P, Adv. contact Pawel Krajewski TEL 48-61-233511. Circ: 100 (paid); 300 (controlled).

910 SWE ISSN 1400-1144
GF1
LUND STUDIES IN GEOGRAPHY. Text in English. 1949. irreg. price varies. index. cum.index every 4 yrs. **Document type:** *Monographic series, Academic/Scholarly.*
Formerly (until 1994): Lund Studies in Geography. Series B. Human Geography (0076-1478)
Indexed: Geo.Abstr.P.G., IDA.
—CISTI.
Published by: University of Lund, Department of Social and Economic Geography, Soelvegatan 13, Lund 22362, Sweden. TEL 46-46-2220000, FAX 46-46-2228401, kulekgeo@kulekgeo.lu.se, http://www1.ldc.lu.se/kulekgeo.

570 FIN ISSN 0024-7383
QH7 CODEN: LUTUAA
LUONNON TUTKIJA. Text in Finnish. 1897. 5/yr. FIM 150 (effective 2000). adv. bk.rev. charts, illus. index, cum.index. **Document type:** *Academic/Scholarly.*
Indexed: Biol.Abstr., Curr.Adv.Ecol.Sci., Deep Sea Res.& Oceanogr.Abstr., GeoRef, Ref.Zh.
—BLDSC (5307.350000).
Published by: Societas Biologica Fennica Vanamo, c/o Dept of Ecology and Systematics, PL 7, Helsinki 00014, Finland. TEL 358-9-191-24420, FAX 358-9-191-24456, jmanttari@fimug.fi; junani.manttari@helsinki.fi. Ed. Juhani Manttari. Circ: 2,200.

M B I. (Medico-Biologic Information) see *MEDICAL SCIENCES*

570 USA ISSN 0275-8679
CODEN: MLBID5
M B L LECTURES IN BIOLOGY. Text in English. 1981. irreg., latest vol.10, 1990. price varies.
Indexed: Biol.Abstr., Chem.Abstr., Chem.Indus.Notes, Chem.Titles.
—BLDSC (5413.408000), CASDDS, CISTI, KNAW.
Published by: (Marine Biological Laboratory), John Wiley & Sons, Inc., Journals (Subsidiary of: Wiley InterScience), 605 Third Ave, New York, NY 10158. TEL 212-475-7700. Eds. Harlyn O Halvorson, K E van Holde.

570 610 MKD ISSN 0351-3254
R91 CODEN: PANND2
MAKEDONSKA AKADEMIJA NA NAUKITE I UMETNOSTITE. ODDELENIE ZA BIOLOSKI I MEDICINSKI NAUKI. PRILOZI/MACEDONIAN ACADEMY OF SCIENCES AND ARTS. SECTION OF BIOLOGICAL AND MEDICAL SCIENCES. CONTRIBUTIONS. Text in Macedonian. 1980. s-a. **Description:** Presents research reports in botany, zoology, biochemistry, medicine and pharmacology, genetics, and agriculture.
Indexed: Chem.Abstr., INIS Atomind., Zoo.Rec.
—CASDDS, KNAW, Linda Hall.
Published by: Makedonska Akademija na Naukite i Umetnostite, Oddelenie za Bioloski i Medicinski Nauki, Bulevar Krste Misirkov 2, PO Box 428, Skopje 91000, Macedonia. TEL 398-02-114200, FAX 389-02-115903, makakad@manu.edu.mk, http://www.manu.edu.mk. Ed. Georgi Efremov.

MANAB MON; a journal depicting the modern trends in psychology, biology, and sociology. see *PSYCHOLOGY*

MANUAL OF BIOLOGICAL MARKERS OF DISEASE. see *MEDICAL SCIENCES—Allergology And Immunology*

578.77 IND ISSN 0025-3146
CODEN: JMBIAA
MARINE BIOLOGICAL ASSOCIATION OF INDIA. JOURNAL. Text mainly in English; Text occasionally in French, German, Spanish. 1959. a., latest vol.43, no.2, 2001. USD 90 (effective 2001). adv. bk.rev. charts, illus. index. **Description:** Contains original contributions about marine biology. Covers plankton, coral, ecosystems, population dynamics, propagation of cultivable species, biology of fishes, marine reptiles, sea birds, mammals and pollution.
Indexed: Aqua.Sci.& Fish.Abstr., Aquacult.Abstr., Biol.Abstr., Curr.Adv.Ecol.Sci., Deep Sea Res.& Oceanogr.Abstr., Environ.Sci.Poll.Mgmt., GeoRef, Helminthol.Abstr., INIS Atomind., Ocean.Abstr. (coverage dropped), Soils & Fert., Sport Fish.Abstr., W.R.C.Inf., Zoo.Rec.
—CASDDS, CISTI, ingenta.
Published by: (Marine Biological Association of India), Scientific Publishers, 5-A New Pali Rd., P O Box 91, Jodhpur, Rajasthan 342 001, India. TEL 91-291-433323, FAX 91-291-512580, scienti@sancharnet.in, http://www.scientificpub.com. Ed. K Rengarajan. Circ: 700.

578.77 GBR ISSN 0025-3154
QH301 CODEN: JMBAAK
MARINE BIOLOGICAL ASSOCIATION OF THE UNITED KINGDOM. JOURNAL. Key Title: Journal of the Marine Biological Association of the United Kingdom. Short title: J M B A. Text in English. 1887. bi-m. USD 535 to institutions (effective 2002). adv. bk.rev. illus. Index. back issues avail.; reprint service avail. from SWZ. *Refereed.* **Document type:** *Academic/Scholarly.* **Description:** Publishes original research on all aspects of marine biology.
Related titles: Microfilm ed.: (from BHP); Microform ed.: (from PQC); Online - full text ed.: (from EBSCO Publishing, O C L C Online Computer Library Center, Inc., RoweCom Information Quest, Swets Blackwell, Institute for Scientific Information).
Indexed: ASCA, Anim.Breed.Abstr., Aqua.Sci.& Fish.Abstr., Aquacult.Abstr., Biol.& Agr.Ind. (May 1983-Feb.1989), Biol.Abstr., Cadscan, Chem.Abstr., Chem.Indus.Notes, Chem.Titles, Curr.Adv.Ecol.Sci., Curr.Cont., Curr.Tit.Ocean, Deep Sea Res.& Oceanogr.Abstr., Ecol.Abstr., Environ.Per.Bibl. (1990-1994), Environ.Sci.Poll.Mgmt., GeoRef, Helminthol.Abstr., INIS Atomind., Int.Abstr.Biol.Sci., Lead Abstr., Nutr.Abstr., Ocean.Abstr. (coverage dropped), Protozool.Abstr., Ref.Zh., Rev.Appl.Entomol., Rev.Med.& Vet.Mycol., Sci.Cit.Ind., Sel.Water Res.Abstr., Sport Fish.Abstr., W.R.C.Inf., Wild.Rev., Zincscan, Zoo.Rec.
—BLDSC (4821.000000), CASDDS, CISTI, EMDOCS, IDS, ingenta, Linda Hall. **CCC.**
Published by: (Marine Biological Association of the United Kingdom), Cambridge University Press, Edinburgh Bldg, Shaftesbury Rd, Cambridge CB2 2RU, United Kingdom. FAX 44-1223-315052, information@cup.cam.ac.uk, information@cambridge.org, http://www.cup.cam.ac.uk, http://www.uk.cambridge.org/journals/pmu. Eds. Ann Pulsford, John A Raven, Michael Whitfield, P.A. Tyler, P.E. Gibbs, R. Seed. R&P Linda Nicol. Adv. contact Rebecca Symons.

578.77 GBR ISSN 0260-2784
MARINE BIOLOGICAL ASSOCIATION OF THE UNITED KINGDOM. OCCASIONAL PUBLICATIONS. Text in English. 1980. irreg. price varies. bk.rev. *Refereed.* **Document type:** *Monographic series, Academic/Scholarly.*
Indexed: Aqua.Sci.& Fish.Abstr., Aquacult.Abstr., Deep Sea Res.& Oceanogr.Abstr., Environ.Sci.Poll.Mgmt., GeoRef.
—CISTI.
Published by: Marine Biological Association of the United Kingdom, Citadel Hill, Plymouth PL1 2PB, United Kingdom. TEL 44-1752-633334, FAX 44-1752-633102. Ed. Ann Pulsford. Circ: 500.

578.77 DEU ISSN 0025-3162
QH91.A1 CODEN: MBIOAJ
MARINE BIOLOGY; international journal on life in oceans and coastal waters. Text in English. 1967. m. EUR 3,645.90 domestic; EUR 3,626.70 in Germany; EUR 360 newsstand/cover foreign (effective 2002). adv. charts, illus. back issues avail.; reprint service avail. from ISI. *Refereed.* **Document type:** *Journal, Academic/Scholarly.* **Description:** Reports on plankton research, theoretical biology related to the marine environment, apparatus and techniques, and underwater exploration and experimentation.
Related titles: Microform ed.: (from PQC); Online - full text ed.: ISSN 1432-1793 (from EBSCO Publishing, RoweCom Information Quest, Gale Group, Swets Blackwell, Springer LINK, Factiva, Institute for Scientific Information).
Indexed: AESIS, Anim.Behav.Abstr., Appl.Ecol.Abstr., Aqua.Sci.& Fish.Abstr., Aquacult.Abstr., Biol.& Agr.Ind. (Feb.1983-), Biol.Abstr., Cadscan, Chem.Abstr., Chem.Titles, Chemorec.Abstr., Curr.Adv.Biochem., Curr.Adv.Cell & Devel.Biol., Curr.Adv.Ecol.Sci., Curr.Adv.Plant Sci., Curr.Cont., Curr.Ref.Fish Res., Deep Sea Res.& Oceanogr.Abstr., Ecol.Abstr., Environ.Abstr., Environ.Per.Bibl. (1974-), Environ.Sci.Poll.Mgmt., Excerp.Med., Food Sci.& Tech.Abstr., Forest.Abstr., Fuel & Energy Abstr., Genet.Abstr., Geo.Abstr.H.G., Geol.Abstr., Helminthol.Abstr., Hum.Gen.Abstr., IBR, INIS Atomind., Ind.Sci.Rev., Int.Abstr.Biol.Sci., Lead Abstr., Microbiol.Abstr., Nutr.Abstr., Ocean.Abstr., Plant Breed.Abstr., Plant Sci., Pollut.Abstr., Ref.Zh., Sci.Cit.Ind., Sel.Water Res.Abstr., Soils & Fert., Sport Fish.Abstr., W.R.C.Inf., Zincscan, Zoo.Rec.
—BLDSC (5373.700000), CASDDS, CINDOC, CISTI, EMDOCS, IDS, ingenta, Linda Hall. **CCC.**
Published by: Springer-Verlag (Subsidiary of: BertelsmannSpringer), Tiergartenstr 17, Heidelberg 69121, Germany. TEL 49-6221-345-0, FAX 49-6221-345229, subscriptions@springer.de, http://link.springer.de/link/service/journals/00227/index.htm, http://www.springer.de. Ed. O Kinne. **Subscr. in N. America to:** Springer-Verlag New York Inc., PO Box 2485, Secaucus, NJ 07096-2485. TEL 212-460-1500, FAX 212-473-6272.

578.77 GBR ISSN 0268-7666
MARINE CONSERVATION. Text in English. q. GBP 20 domestic; GBP 30 foreign (effective 2001). adv. **Document type:** *Newsletter, Consumer.* **Description:** Provides current information and articles on marine biology and conservation.
Formerly (until 1985): Sea
Indexed: Sport Fish.Abstr.
Published by: Marine Conservation Society, 9 Gloucester Rd, Ross-on-Wye, Herefordshire HR9 5BU, United Kingdom. TEL 44-1989-566017, FAX 44-1989-567815, http://www.mcsuk.org. Ed., R&P Richard Harrington. Circ: 6,000 (paid).

577.7 DEU ISSN 0173-9565
CODEN: MAECDR
MARINE ECOLOGY. Text in English. 1916. 4/yr. DEM 827.32 in Europe; DEM 848.83 elsewhere; DEM 910.05 in Europe print & online eds. combined; DEM 933.71 elsewhere print & online eds. combined (effective 2001). adv. *Refereed.* **Document type:** *Journal, Academic/Scholarly.* **Description:** Covers biological and ecological topics regarding the Mediterranean and other seas.
Supersedes in part (in 1979): Stazione Zoologica di Napoli. Pubblicazioni (0039-081X)
Related titles: ♦ Online - full text ed.: Marine Ecology Online. ISSN 1439-0485.
Indexed: Appl.Ecol.Abstr., Aqua.Sci.& Fish.Abstr., Aquacult.Abstr., Biol.Abstr., Chem.Abstr., Chem.Titles, Curr.Adv.Ecol.Sci., Curr.Cont., Curr.Tit.Ocean, Ecol.Abstr., Environ.Per.Bibl. (1972-), Environ.Sci.Poll.Mgmt., Genet.Abstr., Geo.Abstr.H.G., GeoRef, Hum.Gen.Abstr., IBR, Ocean.Abstr., Pollut.Abstr., Ref.Zh., Sci.Cit.Ind., Sel.Water Res.Abstr., Sport Fish.Abstr., Wild.Rev., Zoo.Rec.
—BLDSC (5373.850000), CASDDS, CISTI, IDS, Infotrieve, ingenta, Linda Hall. **CCC.**
Published by: (Stazione Zoologica di Napoli ITA), Blackwell Wissenschafts Verlag GmbH, Kurfuerstendamm 57, Berlin 10707, Germany. TEL 49-30-32790679, FAX 49-30-32790610, abo@blackwis.de, http://www.blackwell.de. Eds. D Marino, J Ott. adv.: B&W page DEM 560; trim 122 x 196. Circ: 560.

577.7 DEU ISSN 1439-0485
MARINE ECOLOGY ONLINE. Text in English. 4/yr. DEM 745 (effective 2001). **Document type:** *Academic/Scholarly.*
Media: Online - full text (from EBSCO Publishing, ingenta, Munksgaard & Blackwell Science's Synergy, Swets Blackwell, Institute for Scientific Information). **Related titles:** ♦ Print ed.: Marine Ecology. ISSN 0173-9565.
Published by: Blackwell Wissenschafts Verlag GmbH, Kurfuerstendamm 57, Berlin 10707, Germany. TEL 49-30-32790679, FAX 49-30-32790610, abo@blackwis.de, http://www.blackwell-science.com/~cgilib/jnlpage.bin?Journal=XMECO&File=XMECO&Page=aims, http://www.blackwell.de.

B

577.78 DEU ISSN 0171-8630
QH541.5.S3 CODEN: MESEDT
MARINE ECOLOGY - PROGRESS SERIES. Text in English. 1979. 20/yr. EUR 3,517 domestic; EUR 3,588 Sat. foreign (effective 2002). adv. illus. Index. back issues avail.; reprints avail. *Refereed.* **Document type:** *Journal, Academic/Scholarly.* **Description:** Presents original papers, short notes and reviews in environmental factors, physiological mechanisms, cultivation, dynamics and ocean management.
Related titles: ♦ Online - full text ed.: Marine Ecology - Progress Series Online. ISSN 1616-1599.
Indexed: ASCA, Anim.Behav.Abstr. (coverage dropped), Appl.Ecol.Abstr., Aqua.Sci.& Fish.Abstr., Aquacult.Abstr., Biol.Abstr., Cadscan, Chem.Abstr., Chem.Indus.Notes, Chem.Titles, Curr.Adv.Ecol.Sci., Curr.Cont., Dairy Sci.Abstr., Ecol.Abstr., Environ.Sci.Poll.Mgmt., Forest.Abstr., Geo.Abstr.H.G., Geo.Abstr.P.G., GeoRef, Geol.Abstr., Helminthol.Abstr., Hum.Gen.Abstr., IBR, INIS Atomind., Ind.Sci.Rev., Int.Abstr.Biol.Sci., Lead Abstr., Microbiol.Abstr., Nutr.Abstr., Ocean.Abstr., Pollut.Abstr., Rev.Med.& Vet.Mycol., Saf.Sci.Abstr., Sci.Cit.Ind., Sel.Water Res.Abstr., Soils & Fert., Sport Fish.Abstr., Trop.Dis.Bull., Wild.Rev., Zincscan, Zoo.Rec.
—BLDSC (5373.904000), CASDDS, CISTI, EMDOCS, ingenta, Linda Hall.
Published by: Inter-Research, Nordbuente 23, Oldendorf 21385, Germany. TEL 49-4132-7127, FAX 49-4132-8883, marita@int-res.com, http://www.int-res.com. Ed. O Kinne. Adv. contact H Witt. Circ: 1,000.

577.78 DEU ISSN 1616-1599
MARINE ECOLOGY - PROGRESS SERIES ONLINE. Text in English. 18/yr. EUR 3,170 (effective 2002). *Refereed.* **Document type:** *Academic/Scholarly.*
Media: Online - full text (from Institute for Scientific Information). **Related titles:** ♦ Print ed.: Marine Ecology - Progress Series. ISSN 0171-8630.
Published by: Inter-Research, Nordbuente 23, Oldendorf 21385, Germany. TEL 49-4132-7127, FAX 49-4132-8883, webmaster@int-res.com, marita@int-res.com, http://www.int-res.com/journals/meps/index.html.

MARINE ENVIRONMENTAL RESEARCH. see *ENVIRONMENTAL STUDIES—Pollution*

570 CZE
MASARYK UNIVERSITY. FACULTY OF SCIENCES. SCRIPTA BIOLOGIA/SCRIPTA FACULTATIS SCIENTIARUM NATURALIUM UNIVERSITATIS MASARYKIANAE BRUNENSIS. BIOLOGIA. Text in English, French, Russian. a. price varies. bibl. **Document type:** *Academic/Scholarly.*
Former titles: Scripta Facultatis Scientiarum Naturalium Universitatis Purkynianae Brunensis. Biologia (0231-5777); Supersedes in part (in 1970): Universita J.E. Purkyne. Prirodovedecka Fakulta. Spisy
Indexed: Biol.Abstr., Chem.Abstr., Chem.Indus.Notes, Chem.Titles, Field Crop Abstr., GeoRef, Herb.Abstr., Plant Grow.Reg.Abstr., Ref.Zh.
—CISTI.
Published by: Masarykova Universita, Prirodovedecka Fakulta/Masaryk University, Faculty of Sciences, Kotlarska 2, Brno 61137, Czech Republic. Ed. Jiri Gaisler.

MATHEMATICAL BIOSCIENCES; an international journal. see *MATHEMATICS*

400 617.6 JPN ISSN 0385-1613
CODEN: MATSDE
MATSUMOTO SHIGAKU/MATSUMOTO DENTAL UNIVERSITY SOCIETY. JOURNAL. Text in Japanese; Summaries in English. 1975. 3/yr. JPY 3,500 domestic; USD 30 foreign (effective 2000). adv. back issues avail. *Refereed.* **Document type:** *Academic/Scholarly.*
Related titles: CD-ROM ed.; Fax ed.
Indexed: Chem.Abstr., Chem.Titles.
—BLDSC (5413.245000), CASDDS.
Published by: Matsumoto Dental University Society/Matsumoto Shika Daigaku Gakkai, 1780 Gobara-Hiroka, shiojiri-shi, Nagano-ken 399-0700, Japan. TEL 81-263-523100, FAX 81-263-533456, yamaoka@po.mdu.ac.jp. Ed. Takurou Wada. R&P, Adv. contact Minoru Yamaoka TEL 81-263-51-2075. B&W page JPY 90,000; trim 232 x 160. Circ: 1,800.

570 DNK ISSN 0106-1054
QH132.G73
MEDDELELSER OM GROENLAND, BIOSCIENCE. Variant title: Greenland Bioscience. Text in Danish. 1878. irreg., latest vol.52, 2000. price varies. charts, illus. **Document type:** *Monographic series, Academic/Scholarly.*
Supersedes in part (in 1979): Meddelelser om Groenland (0025-6676)
Indexed: Biol.Abstr., Chem.Abstr., Curr.Adv.Ecol.Sci., GeoRef, Zoo.Rec.
—CISTI, Linda Hall.
Published by: Danish Polar Center, Strandgade 100 H, Copenhagen K 1401, Denmark. TEL 45-32-88-01-00, FAX 45-32-88-01-01. Eds. G Hoepner Petersen, Gert Steen Mogensen.

MEDICINAL CHEMISTRY RESEARCH; an international journal for rapid communications on design and mechanisms of action of biologically active agents. see *MEDICAL SCIENCES*

MEDICINSKI RAZGLEDI. see *MEDICAL SCIENCES*

551.46 USA ISSN 0085-0683
QH92.3 CODEN: MHGCBG
MEMOIRS OF THE HOURGLASS CRUISES. Text in English. 1969. irreg. per issue exchange basis. charts, illus. back issues avail.
Indexed: Aqua.Sci.& Fish.Abstr., Biol.Abstr., Deep Sea Res.& Oceanogr.Abstr., Ocean.Abstr., Sport Fish.Abstr., Wild.Rev., Zoo.Rec.
—Linda Hall.
Published by: Florida Marine Research Institute, Department of Environmental Protection, 100 8th Ave. S.E., St. Petersburg, FL 33701. FAX 813-823-0166. Ed. K A Steidinger. Circ: 1,000.

MEMORIE DI BIOLOGIA MARINA E DI OCEANOGRAFIA. see *EARTH SCIENCES—Oceanography*

METABOLISM: CLINICAL AND EXPERIMENTAL. see *MEDICAL SCIENCES—Endocrinology*

572.8 USA ISSN 1064-3745
CODEN: MMBIED
METHODS IN MOLECULAR BIOLOGY. Text in English. 1984. irreg., latest vol.135, 1999. price varies. back issues avail. **Document type:** *Journal, Academic/Scholarly.* **Description:** Offers the latest molecular biology and biochemistry laboratory methods and protocols.
Indexed: Chem.Abstr., Chem.Indus.Notes, Chem.Titles, Ind.Med. (1984-), Mass Spectr.Bull.
—BLDSC (5748.201800), CASDDS, CISTI, Infotrieve. **CCC.**
Published by: Humana Press Inc., 999 Riverview Dr, Ste 208, Totowa, NJ 07512. TEL 973-256-1699, FAX 973-256-8341, humana@humanapr.com, http://humanapress.com. Ed. John Walker. R&P Richard Hruska.

570 USA ISSN 0076-8227
QH1 CODEN: PMUBAE
MICHIGAN STATE UNIVERSITY. MUSEUM PUBLICATIONS. BIOLOGICAL SERIES. Text in English; Abstracts occasionally in German. 1957. irreg. (approx. 1-2/yr.). price varies. **Document type:** *Monographic series, Academic/Scholarly.*
Indexed: Biol.Abstr., GeoRef.
—CISTI, Linda Hall.
Published by: Michigan State University, Museum, MSU Library, East Lansing, MI 48824. TEL 517-355-2370. Circ: 1,850.

MICRONESICA; a journal of the University of Guam. see *ANTHROPOLOGY*

MIDWEST BIOLOGICAL CONTROL NEWS. see *AGRICULTURE—Crop Production And Soil*

570 JPN ISSN 0910-2523
MITSUBISHI KASEI INSTITUTE OF LIFE SCIENCES. ANNUAL REPORT. Text in English. 1971. a. adv. *Refereed.* **Document type:** *Yearbook, Academic/Scholarly.* **Description:** Outlines the scientific achievements of the Institute's research activities in neuroscience, immunology, development-gerontology, and other major fields in the life sciences.
—CISTI, GNLM, KNAW.
Published by: Mitsubishi Kasei Institute of Life Sciences/Mitsubishi Kagaku Seimei Kagaku Kenkyujo, 11 Minami-Oya, Machida-shi, Tokyo-to 194-0031, Japan. TEL 81-427-24-6202, FAX 81-427-29-1252, mats@libra.ls.m-kagaku.co.jp. Ed., Adv. contact Tetsuo Jikihara. Circ: 1,000.

570 USA
MODERN BIOLOGY SERIES. Text in English. irreg. price varies. *Refereed.*
Published by: Holt, Rinehart and Winston, Inc., c/o Harcourt Brace Jovanovich, 6277 Sea Harbor Dr, Orlando, FL 32887. TEL 407-345-2500. Ed. Bob Todd.

MODERN DRUG DISCOVERY; chemical and biological perspectives. see *PHARMACY AND PHARMACOLOGY*

MODERN PATHOLOGY. see *MEDICAL SCIENCES*

572.8 USA ISSN 0737-4038
QH506 CODEN: MBEVEO
MOLECULAR BIOLOGY AND EVOLUTION. Text in English. 1983. m. USD 425 Print & online eds. (effective 2001). adv. illus. Index. reprint service avail. from PQC,ISI. *Refereed.* **Document type:** *Academic/Scholarly.* **Description:** Includes research at the interface between molecular and evolutionary biology. This includes: investigations of molecular evolutionary patterns and processes; test of evolutionary hypotheses that use molecular data.
Related titles: Microform ed.: (from PQC,PMC); Online - full text ed.: USD 335 (effective 2001) (from HighWire Pr., EBSCO Publishing, Institute for Scientific Information).
Indexed: ASCA, Abstr.Anthropol., Abstr.Hyg., AgBiotech, Anim.Breed.Abstr., Aqua.Sci.& Fish.Abstr., BBCI, Bio-Contr.News & Info., Biol.Abstr., Biotech.Cit.Ind., Chem.Abstr., Chem.Indus.Notes, Chem.Titles, Curr.Adv.Biochem., Curr.Adv.Cell & Devel.Biol., Curr.Adv.Ecol.Sci., Curr.Adv.Gen.& Molec.Biol., Curr.Cont., Curr.Ind.Stat., Dairy Sci.Abstr., Entomol.Abstr., Excerp.Med., Forest.Abstr., Genet.Abstr., GeoRef, Helminthol.Abstr., Hum.Gen.Abstr., Ind.Med. (1983-), Ind.Sci.Rev., Inpharma, Int.Abstr.Biol.Sci., Maize Abstr., Nuc.Acids Abstr., Oncog.G.F.Abstr. (coverage dropped), Plant Breed.Abstr., Plant Gen.Res.Abstr., Poult.Abstr., Protozool.Abstr., Reac., Rev.Appl.Entomol., Rev.Med.& Vet.Mycol., Rev.Plant Path., Rice Abstr., Sci.Cit.Ind., Seed Abstr., Soyabean Abstr., Sport Fish.Abstr., Triticale Abstr., Trop.Dis.Bull., Weed Abstr., Wild.Rev., Zoo.Rec.
—BLDSC (5900.782000), CASDDS, CISTI, EMDOCS, GNLM, IDS, ingenta, KNAW, Linda Hall. **CCC.**
Published by: Allen Press Inc., PO BOx 1897, Lawrence, KS 66044. TEL 785-843-1235, FAX 785-843-1274, bhall@bgh.biology.rochester.edu; smbe@allen-press.com, http://www.molbiolevol.org/. Ed. Barry G Hall. Circ: 1,000.

MOLECULAR BRAIN RESEARCH. see *MEDICAL SCIENCES—Psychiatry And Neurology*

MOLECULAR DIAGNOSIS; a journal devoted to the understanding of human disease through the clinical application of molecular biology. see *MEDICAL SCIENCES*

MOLECULAR HUMAN REPRODUCTION. see *MEDICAL SCIENCES—Obstetrics And Gynecology*

MOLECULAR PSYCHIATRY. see *MEDICAL SCIENCES—Psychiatry And Neurology*

570 ARG ISSN 0328-1620
MONOGRAFIAS DE L.O.L.A. (Literature of Latin America) Text in English, Spanish. 1994. irreg. price varies. adv. illus. back issues avail. *Refereed.* **Document type:** *Monographic series.* **Description:** Includes articles on biology.
Indexed: Zoo.Rec.
Address: Pena Rodriguez, 115 2o, Capital Federal, Buenos Aires 1020, Argentina. TEL 54-114-3720518, FAX 54-114-3722787, csharp@ba.net, http://www.thebookplace.com/lola. Ed. Colin Sharp.

570.9 NLD ISSN 0077-0639
QH301 CODEN: MOBIAN
MONOGRAPHIAE BIOLOGICAE. Text in English. 1957. irreg., latest vol.73, 1995. price varies. *Refereed.* **Document type:** *Monographic series.*
Indexed: Aqua.Sci.& Fish.Abstr., Aquacult.Abstr., Biol.Abstr., Deep Sea Res.& Oceanogr.Abstr., Environ.Sci.Poll.Mgmt., GeoRef, Meteor.& Geoastrophys.Abstr., Sport Fish.Abstr., Wild.Rev., Zoo.Rec.
—BLDSC (5917.783000), CASDDS, CISTI.
Published by: Kluwer Academic Publishers Group (Subsidiary of: Wolters Kluwer N.V.), Spuiboulevard 50, PO Box 17, Dordrecht 3300 AA, Netherlands. FAX 31-78-639-2254, services@wkap.nl, http://www.wkap.nl. Ed. M Dumont. **Dist. by:** Journals Department, PO Box 322, Dordrecht 3300 AH, Netherlands. FAX 31-78-654-6474.

MONOGRAPHS IN EPIDEMIOLOGY AND BIOSTATISTICS. see *PUBLIC HEALTH AND SAFETY*

MONOGRAPHS IN PSYCHOBIOLOGY. see *PSYCHOLOGY*

571.3 611 RUS ISSN 1026-3543 CODEN: AAGEAA
MORFOLOGIYA. Text in Russian; Summaries in English, Russian. 1916. bi-m. RUR 60, USD 10 (effective 1999). bk.rev. bibl. index. back issues avail. *Refereed.* **Document type:** *Academic/Scholarly.* **Description:** Carries original investigations; reviews and discussion of papers on cytology, histology, embryology (normal and topographic), and comparative anatomy and anthropology; methods of morphological investigation; history of morphology; reports on the latest achievements in morphological sciences.
Formerly (until 1992): Arkhiv Anatomii, Gistologii i Embriologii (0004-1947)
Related titles: E-mail ed.; Fax ed.; Online - full text ed.
Indexed: Aqua.Sci.& Fish.Abstr., Aquacult.Abstr., Biol.Abstr., Chem.Abstr., Chem.Indus.Notes, Chem.Titles, Dent.Ind., Environ.Sci.Poll.Mgmt., INIS Atomind., Ind.Med. (1992-), Ref.Zh., Zoo.Rec.
—BLDSC (0118.230000), CASDDS, CISTI, GNLM.
Published by: (Rossiiskaya Akademiya Meditsinskikh Nauk), Morfologiya, B Zelem'na 43-A, St Petersburg 197110, Russian Federation. TEL 7-812-235-3009, FAX 7-812-235-0986, aeseulap@mail.wplus.net, http://www.aeseulap.net. Ed. F V Sudzilovskii. adv.: B&W page USD 600, color page USD 2,000; trim 295 x 210. Circ: 1,000 (paid). **US dist. addr.:** East View Publications, 3020 Harbor Ln N, Minneapolis, MN 55447. TEL 612-550-0961. **Co-sponsor:** Vsesoyuznoe Nauchnoe Obshchestvo Anatomov, Gistologov i Embriologov.

MORPHOLOGIE. see *MEDICAL SCIENCES*

570 USA ISSN 0096-3925
QH301 CODEN: MUBBDD
MOSCOW STATE UNIVERSITY BIOLOGICAL SCIENCES BULLETIN. Text in English. 1974. q. USD 1,365 in US & Canada; USD 1,540 elsewhere (effective 2002). bibl, charts, illus. index. back issues avail. *Refereed.* **Document type:** *Journal, Academic/Scholarly.* **Description:** Covers human, animal and plant physiology, genetics, flora and fauna, biochemistry and biophysics, and cell physiology.
Related titles: ♦ Russian ed.: Moskovskii Gosudarstvennyi Universitet. Vestnik. Seriya 16: Biologiya. ISSN 0137-0952; ♦ Translation of: Vestnik Moskovskogo Universiteta. Seriya 17: Pochvovedenie. ISSN 0137-0944; ♦ Partial translation of: Moskovskii Gosudarstvennyi Universitet. Vestnik. Seriya 16: Biologiya. ISSN 0137-0952.
Indexed: Biol.Abstr., Crop Physiol.Abstr., Excerp.Med., Field Crop Abstr., Forest.Abstr., GeoRef, Herb.Abstr., Hort.Abstr., Ornam.Hort., Rev.Appl.Entomol., Rev.Plant Path., Soils & Fert., Sport Fish.Abstr., Weed Abstr., Wild.Rev., Zoo.Rec.
—BLDSC (0416.237000), CISTI, Infotrieve, ingenta. **CCC.**
Published by: (Moskovskii Gosudarstvennyi Universitet RUS), Allerton Press, Inc., 18 W 27th St, New York, NY 10001. TEL 646-424-9686, FAX 646-424-9695, journals@allertonpress.com, http://www.allertonpress.com/. Ed. M V Gusev.

570 RUS ISSN 0137-0952
QH301 CODEN: VMUBDF
MOSKOVSKII GOSUDARSTVENNYI UNIVERSITET. VESTNIK. SERIYA 16: BIOLOGIYA. Text in Russian; Contents page in English. 1960. irreg. USD 85. bk.rev. bibl. index.
Formerly (until 1977): Moskovskii Gosudarstvennyi Universitet. Vestnik. Seriya 6: Biologiya, Pochvovedenie (0579-9422)
Related titles: ♦ English ed.: Moscow State University Biological Sciences Bulletin. ISSN 0096-3925; ♦ English Translation: Moscow State University Soil Science Bulletin. ISSN 0147-6874; ♦ Partial English Translation: Moscow State University Biological Sciences Bulletin. ISSN 0096-3925.
Indexed: Aqua.Sci.& Fish.Abstr., Aquacult.Abstr., Biol.Abstr., Chem.Abstr., Chem.Indus.Notes, Environ.Sci.Poll.Mgmt., Field Crop Abstr., GeoRef, Plant Grow.Reg.Abstr., Ref.Zh., Russ.Acad.Sci.Bibl.
—CASDDS, CISTI, East View, Infotrieve, Linda Hall. **CCC.**
Published by: (Moskovskii Gosudarstvennyi Universitet), Izdatel'stvo Moskovskogo Gosudarstvennogo Universiteta, B Nikitskaya 5-7, Moscow 103009, Russian Federation. TEL 7-095-2033128. **Dist. by:** Mezhdunarodnaya Kniga, B Yakimanka 39, Moscow 117049, Russian Federation. TEL 7-095-2384967, FAX 7-095-2384634; **US dist. addr.:** East View Publications, 3020 Harbor Ln N, Minneapolis, MN 55447. TEL 612-550-0961.

570 RUS ISSN 0027-1403
Q60 CODEN: BYMOAB
MOSKOVSKOE OBSHCHESTVO ISPYTATELEI PRIRODA. BIOLOGICHESKII OTDEL. BYULLETEN/MOSCOW SOCIETY OF NATURALISTS. BIOLOGICAL SERIES. BULLETIN. Text in Russian; Summaries in English. 1829. bi-m. USD 104. bk.rev. abstr, bibl, charts, illus. **Document type:** *Bulletin, Academic/Scholarly.*
Formerly (1829-1917): Moskovskoe Obshchestvo Ispytatelei Priroda. Byulleten (0007-7682)
Related titles: Microfiche ed.: (from IDC).
Indexed: Aqua.Sci.& Fish.Abstr., Aquacult.Abstr., Bio-Contr.News & Info., Biol.Abstr., Deep Sea Res.& Oceanogr.Abstr., Environ.Sci.Poll.Mgmt., Forest.Abstr., GeoRef, Herb.Abstr., INIS Atomind., Key Word Ind.Wildl.Res., Ref.Zh., Rev.Appl.Entomol., Russ.Acad.Sci.Bibl., Sport Fish.Abstr., Triticale Abstr., Zoo.Rec.
—BLDSC (0022.000000), CISTI, East View, KNAW, Linda Hall.
Published by: (Moskovskoe Obshchestvo Ispytatelei Priroda, Biologicheskii Otdel), Izdatel'stvo Moskovskogo Gosudarstvennogo Universiteta, B Nikitskaya 5-7, Moscow 103009, Russian Federation. TEL 7-095-2295091. Ed. T A Rabotnov. Circ: 1,635. **Dist. by:** Mezhdunarodnaya Kniga, B Yakimanka 39, Moscow 117049, Russian Federation. TEL 7-095-2384967, FAX 7-095-2384634; **US dist. addr.:** East View Publications, 3020 Harbor Ln N, Minneapolis, MN 55447. TEL 612-550-0961.

570 USA ISSN 0097-0883
QH323 CODEN: BMDIAY
MOUNT DESERT ISLAND BIOLOGICAL LABORATORY. BULLETIN. Text in English. 1960. a. USD 10 to non-members (effective 2000). charts, illus. index. *Refereed.* **Document type:** *Bulletin, Academic/Scholarly.*
Indexed: Aqua.Sci.& Fish.Abstr., Biol.Abstr., Curr.Cont. (coverage dropped), Deep Sea Res.& Oceanogr.Abstr., Environ.Sci.Poll.Mgmt., Pollut.Abstr., Sport Fish.Abstr., Wild.Rev., Zoo.Rec.
—BLDSC (2622.000000), Linda Hall.
Published by: Mount Desert Island Biological Laboratory, Salsbury Cove, ME 04672. TEL 207-288-3605, mmckernan@mdibl.org, http://www.mdibl.org. Ed. David Miller. Circ: 1,000.

570 JPN ISSN 0910-0903
MUKIN SEIBUTSU/JOURNAL OF GERMFREE LIFE AND GNOTOBIOLOGY. Text in English, Japanese. 1971. s-a.
Published by: Nihon Mukin Seibutsu Noto Baioroji Gakkai/Japanese Association of Germfree Life and Gnotobiology, c/o Ms. Kazuko Adachi, Kobe Gakuin Daigaku Eiyogakubu, Arise, Ikawadanicho, Nishi-ku, Kobe-shi, Hyogo-ken 673, Japan.

570 ARG ISSN 0524-9481 CODEN: RANCEQ
MUSEO ARGENTINO DE CIENCIAS NATURALES "BERNARDINO RIVADAVIA." INSTITUTO NACIONAL DE INVESTIGACION DE LAS CIENCIAS NATURALES. REVISTA. ECOLOGIA. Text in Spanish. 1963. irreg., latest vol.3, no.4, 1991. **Document type:** *Academic/Scholarly.*
Indexed: Aqua.Sci.& Fish.Abstr., Aquacult.Abstr., Environ.Sci.Poll.Mgmt., GeoRef, Zoo.Rec.
—CISTI, Linda Hall.
Published by: Museo Argentino de Ciencias Naturales "Bernardino Rivadavia", Instituto Nacional de Investigacion de las Ciencias Naturales, Avda. Angel Gallardo 470, Casilla de Correo 220-Sucursal 5, Buenos Aires, Argentina.

578.77 ARG ISSN 0524-9503
QH91.A1 CODEN: RNBHD3
MUSEO ARGENTINO DE CIENCIAS NATURALES "BERNARDINO RIVADAVIA." INSTITUTO NACIONAL DE INVESTIGACION DE LAS CIENCIAS NATURALES. REVISTA. HIDROBIOLOGIA. Text in Spanish. 1963. irreg., latest vol.6, no.9, 1987.
Indexed: Aqua.Sci.& Fish.Abstr., Aquacult.Abstr., BSL Biol., Environ.Sci.Poll.Mgmt., GeoRef.
—CISTI, Linda Hall.
Published by: Museo Argentino de Ciencias Naturales "Bernardino Rivadavia", Instituto Nacional de Investigacion de las Ciencias Naturales, Avda. Angel Gallardo 470, Casilla de Correo 220-Sucursal 5, Buenos Aires, Argentina.

570 ITA ISSN 0392-758X
MUSEO REGIONALE DI SCIENZE NATURALI, TORINO. BOLLETTINO. Text in English, French, Italian, Spanish; Summaries in English. 1983. s-a. ITL 75,000 (effective 2000 - 2001). back issues avail. **Document type:** *Bulletin, Academic/Scholarly.* **Description:** Features readings on natural sciences, including paleontology, botany, mineralogy, geology and zoology.
Indexed: GeoRef, Zoo.Rec.
—BLDSC (2227.600000).
Published by: Museo Regionale di Scienze Naturali Torino, Redazione, Via Giovanni Giolitti, 36, Turin, TO 10123, Italy. TEL 39-011-4323063, FAX 39-011-4323331, TELEX 220685 REGPIE I, redazione.mrsn@regione.piemonte.it. Ed. Paolo Sibille. Adv. contact Olindo Bortesi. Circ: 700.

MUSEU MUNICIPAL DO FUNCHAL. BOLETIM. see *BIOLOGY—Zoology*

570.74 ROM
QH1 CODEN: TMNAAK
MUSEUM NATIONAL D'HISTOIRE NATURELLE "GRIGORE ANTIPA". TRAVAUX/MUZEUL NATIONAL DE ISTORIE NATURALA "GRIGORE ANTIPA". TRAVAUX. Text in English, French, German; Summaries in Romanian; Abstracts in English, French. 1957. a. price varies. adv. bk.rev. index. back issues avail. **Document type:** *Bulletin, Academic/Scholarly.*
Formerly: Museum d'Histoire Naturelle "Grigore Antipa." Travaux (0068-3078)
Indexed: GeoRef, Ocean.Abstr. (coverage dropped), Rev.Appl.Entomol., Sport Fish.Abstr., Zoo.Rec.
—BLDSC (9039.500000), CISTI, Linda Hall.
Published by: Muzeul National de Istorie Naturala "Grigore Antipa", Sos. Kiseleff 1, Bucharest 79744, Romania. TEL 40-1-3128826, FAX 40-1-3128886, dmurariu@antipa.ro. Ed., R&P Dumitru Murariu TEL 40-1-6505250. Adv. contact Elena Cursaru. Circ: 900.

570 POL ISSN 0068-466X CODEN: ASMHE9
MUZEUM GORNOSLASKIE W BYTOMIU. ROCZNIK. SERIA PRZYRODA. Text and summaries in English, Polish. 1962. irreg. USD 15. **Document type:** *Proceedings.*
Indexed: AgroLibrex, Aqua.Sci.& Fish.Abstr., Aquacult.Abstr., Environ.Sci.Poll.Mgmt.
Published by: Muzeum Gornoslaskie w Bytomiu, Pl Jana III Sobieskiego 2, Bytom 41902, Poland. TEL 48-32-2813401, FAX 48-32-2813401, dobosz@us.edu.pl.

N B I A NEWSLETTER. see *AGRICULTURE*

N C R R REPORTER. (National Center for Research Resources) see *MEDICAL SCIENCES*

NAPRALERT ON CD-ROM. see *PHARMACY AND PHARMACOLOGY*

570 IND ISSN 0369-8211
Q73 CODEN: PAIBA6
NATIONAL ACADEMY OF SCIENCES, INDIA. PROCEEDINGS. SECTION B. BIOLOGICAL SCIENCES. Text in English. 1930. q. INR 250, USD 100; USD 200 Includes Section A & B (effective 2000). bk.rev. bibl, charts, illus, stat. **Document type:** *Proceedings.*
Indexed: AgBiotech, Anim.Breed.Abstr., Aqua.Sci.& Fish.Abstr., Aquacult.Abstr., Bio-Contr.News & Info., Biol.Abstr., C.C.M.J., Chem.Abstr., Chem.Indus.Notes, Chem.Titles, Crop Physiol.Abstr., Curr.Adv.Ecol.Sci., Curr.Cont. (coverage dropped), Environ.Sci.Poll.Mgmt., Field Crop Abstr., Food Sci.& Tech.Abstr., GeoRef, Helminthol.Abstr., Hort.Abstr., INIS Atomind., INSPEC (pre-1969-), Plant Breed.Abstr., Plant Grow.Reg.Abstr., Postharvest, Protozool.Abstr., Ref.Zh., Rev.Appl.Entomol., Rev.Arom.& Med.Plants, Rev.Med.& Vet.Mycol., Rev.Plant Path., Soils & Fert., Sorghum & Millets Abstr., Weed Abstr., Zoo.Rec.
—BLDSC (6761.901000), CASDDS, CISTI, Linda Hall.
Published by: National Academy of Sciences, 5 Lajpatrai Rd., Allahabad, Uttar Pradesh 211 002, India. TEL 91-532-640224, FAX 91-532-641183, nasi@nde.vsnl.net.in. Ed. K Swarup. Circ: 500.

NATIONAL INSTITUTE OF AGRO-ENVIRONMENTAL SCIENCES. ANNUAL REPORT. see *AGRICULTURE*

570 610 JPN ISSN 0386-5541
NATIONAL INSTITUTE OF POLAR RESEARCH. MEMOIRS. SERIES E: BIOLOGY AND MEDICAL SCIENCE. Text and summaries in English. 1959. irreg., latest vol.39, 1996. per issue exchange basis. *Refereed.* **Document type:** *Monographic series.*

Supersedes: Japanese Antarctic Research Expedition, 1956-1962. Scientific Reports. Series E. Biology (0075-3394)
Indexed: Aqua.Sci.& Fish.Abstr., Aquacult.Abstr., Biol.Abstr., Sport Fish.Abstr., Zoo.Rec.
—BLDSC (5626.812000), Linda Hall.
Published by: National Institute of Polar Research/Kokuritsu Kyokuchi Kenkyujo, Publications, 9-10, Kiga 1-chome, Itabashi-ku, Tokyo 173, Japan. TEL 81-3-3962-2214, FAX 81-3-3962-2225, TELEX 272-2515 POLRSCJ, publication@nipr.ac.jp. Ed. Okitsugu Watanabe. Circ: 1,000.

570 BLR CODEN: VABBA3
NATSIONALNAYA AKADEMIYA NAVUK BELARUSI. VESTSI. SERIYA BIOLOGICHNYKH NAVUK/NATIONAL ACADEMY OF SCIENCES OF BELARUS. PROCEEDINGS. BIOLOGICAL SERIES. Text in Belorussian, Russian; Summaries in English. 1956. q. BYB 120,000, USD 129 (effective 1999). bibl, charts, illus. index. **Document type:** *Academic/Scholarly.* **Description:** Presents results of experimental research on a wide range of biological sciences from biomolecules to biosphere. Analytical reviews of the advances in science and technology.
Formerly (until 1992): Akademiya Navuk Belarusskai S.S.R. Vestsi. Seriya Biologichnykh Navuk (0002-3558)
Indexed: Biol.Abstr., Crop Physiol.Abstr., Dairy Sci.Abstr., Field Crop Abstr., Forest.Abstr., Herb.Abstr., Hort.Abstr., INIS Atomind., Nutr.Abstr., Ornam.Hort., Plant Breed.Abstr., Plant Grow.Reg.Abstr., Postharvest, Potato Abstr., Rev.Appl.Entomol., Rev.Arom.& Med.Plants, Rev.Med.& Vet.Mycol., Rev.Plant Path., Seed Abstr., Soils & Fert., Triticale Abstr., Zoo.Rec.
—CASDDS, CISTI, KNAW, Linda Hall.
Published by: (Natsionalnaya Akademiya Navuk Belarusi/National Academy of Sciences of Belarus), Vydavetstvo Belaruskaya Navuka, Kuprevicha 18, Minsk 220141, Belarus. TEL 375-172-284-2821, FAX 375-172-284-2821. Ed. A G Lobanok. Circ: 300. **Dist. by:** Mezhdunarodnaya Kniga, B Yakimanka 39, Moscow 117049, Russian Federation. TEL 7-095-2384967, FAX 7-095-2384634.

NATUR UND KOSMOS. see *ENVIRONMENTAL STUDIES*

570 930 DEU ISSN 0077-6025
NATUR UND MENSCH: JAHRESMITTEILUNGEN DER NATURHISTORISCHEN GESELLSCHAFT NUERNBERG. Text in German. 1965. a. price varies. **Document type:** *Yearbook, Academic/Scholarly.*
Formerly (until 1969): Naturhistorische Gesellschaft Nuernberg. Mitteilungen und Jahresbericht
Indexed: Biol.Abstr., GeoRef, Key Word Ind.Wildl.Res., Ref.Zh., Zoo.Rec.
Published by: Naturhistorische Gesellschaft Nuernberg e.V., Norishalle, Marientorgraben 8, Nuernberg 90402, Germany. TEL 49-911-227970, FAX 49-911-2447441, http://www.nhg-nuernberg.de. Circ: 2,500.

570 BRA
NATURA. Text in Portuguese. 1975. s-a. free per issue.
Published by: Universidade Federal da Bahia, Instituto de Biologia, Rua Barao de Geremoabo-Ondina, Salvador, Bahia 40000, Brazil. Ed. Antonio Pedreira. Circ: 1,500. **Co-sponsor:** Instituto de Ciencias da Saude.

570 DNK ISSN 0077-6033
QH7 CODEN: NAJUAC
NATURA JUTLANDICA. Text in English. 1947. irreg. DKK 100, USD 17. illus. **Document type:** *Academic/Scholarly.*
Indexed: Aqua.Sci.& Fish.Abstr., Biol.Abstr., Curr.Adv.Ecol.Sci., Ecol.Abstr., GeoRef, Key Word Ind.Wildl.Res., Sport Fish.Abstr., Wild.Rev., Zoo.Rec.
—Linda Hall.
Published by: Naturhistorisk Museum, Universitetsparken, Bygning 210, Aarhus C 8000, Denmark. TEL 86-12-97-77, FAX 86-13-08-82, nm@nathist.aau.dk, http://www.naturhistoriskmuseum.dk. Ed. Thomas Secher Jensen. Circ: 1,000.

570 BRA ISSN 0101-1944
QH7 CODEN: NTRLDP
NATURALIA. Text in Portuguese; Summaries in English, Portuguese. 1975-1979; N.S. 1980. a., latest vol.24, 1999. USD 30 (effective 2001); or exchange basis. charts, illus, stat, abstr, bibl. back issues avail. *Refereed.* **Document type:** *Journal, Academic/Scholarly.* **Description:** Publishes original contributions on biological sciences.
Indexed: Abstr.Anthropol., Apic.Abstr., Aqua.Sci.& Fish.Abstr., Aquacult.Abstr., Bio-Contr.News & Info., Biol.Abstr., Curr.Adv.Cell & Devel.Biol., Curr.Adv.Ecol.Sci., Curr.Adv.Gen.& Molec.Biol., Entomol.Abstr., Forest.Abstr., GeoRef, Helminthol.Abstr., Herb.Abstr., Hort.Abstr., INIS Atomind., Math.R., Plant Breed.Abstr., Pollut.Abstr., Rev.Appl.Entomol., Rev.Med.& Vet.Mycol., Rev.Plant Path., Seed Abstr., Sociol.Abstr., Weed Abstr., Zoo.Rec.
—BLDSC (6041.910000), CASDDS, CISTI, KNAW, Linda Hall.
Published by: Universidade Estadual Paulista, Ave. VICENTE FERREIRA, 1278, Centro, Caixa Postal 71, Marilia, SP 17515-901, Brazil. TEL 55-144-222504, FAX 55-144-222504, cgb@marilia.unesp.br. Ed. Flavio Henrique Caetano. Circ: 1,000.

570 508 GBR ISSN 0028-0771
QH1 CODEN: NTRLAM
THE NATURALIST. Text in English. 1875. q. GBP 20 (effective 2001). adv. bk.rev. index. reprint service avail. from PQC. *Refereed.* **Document type:** *Academic/Scholarly.*
Related titles: Microfilm ed.: (from PQC).
Indexed: Aqua.Sci.& Fish.Abstr., Aquacult.Abstr., Biol.Abstr., Chem.Abstr., Curr.Adv.Ecol.Sci., Environ.Per.Bibl. (1991-), GeoRef, IBR, IBZ, Rev.Plant Path.
—BLDSC (6042.000000). **CCC.**
Published by: Yorkshire Naturalists' Union, University of Bradford, Bradford, W Yorks BD7 1DP, United Kingdom. TEL 44-1274-234212, FAX 44-1274-234231, m.r.d.seaward@bradford.ac.uk. Ed. M R D Seaward. Circ: 3,600.

NATURE MEDICINE. see *MEDICAL SCIENCES*

570 USA ISSN 1072-8368
QH506 CODEN: NSBIEW
NATURE STRUCTURAL BIOLOGY. Text in English. 1994. m. USD 199 in United States to individuals; GBP 170 elsewhere to individuals; USD 975 in United States to institutions; GBP 520 elsewhere to institutions (effective 2001). adv. illus. index. back issues avail. *Refereed.* **Document type:** *Academic/Scholarly.* **Description:** Publishes biomedical research results in structural biology, including applications of new technologies and techniques.
Related titles: Online - full text ed.: (from EBSCO Publishing, ingenta, Institute for Scientific Information).
Indexed: AIDS & Cancer Res., ASCA, Agri.& Environ.Biotech.Abstr., Anim.Behav.Abstr. (coverage dropped), Aqua.Sci.& Fish.Abstr., Aquacult.Abstr., BBCI, Bio-Contr.News & Info., Cal.Tiss.Abstr., Chem.Abstr., Chem.Indus.Notes, Chem.Titles, Chemorec.Abstr., Curr.Cont., Dairy Sci.Abstr., Entomol.Abstr., Environ.Sci.Poll.Mgmt., Excerp.Med. (1995-), Field Crop Abstr., Food Sci.& Tech.Abstr., Genet.Abstr., Hort.Abstr., Hum.Gen.Abstr., Immun.Abstr., Ind.Med. (1994-), Ind.Sci.Rev., Ind.Vet., Inpharma, Int.Abstr.Biol.Sci., Med.& Pharm.Biotech.Abstr., Microbiol.Abstr., Neurosci.Abstr., Nuc.Acids Abstr., Ocean.Abstr. (coverage dropped), Oncog.G.F.Abstr., Ornam.Hort., Pollut.Abstr., Protozool.Abstr., Reac., Ref.Zh., Rev.Appl.Entomol., Rev.Arom.& Med.Plants, Rev.Med.& Vet.Mycol., Rev.Plant Path., Risk Abstr., Saf.Sci.Abstr., Sci.Cit.Ind., Sugar Ind.Abstr., Virol.Abstr. (coverage dropped).
—BLDSC (6047.375000), CASDDS, CISTI, GNLM, IDS, ingenta. **CCC.**
Published by: Macmillan Magazines Ltd. (Subsidiary of: Macmillan Publishers Ltd.), 1234 National Press Bldg, Washington, DC 20045. TEL 202-626-2513, orders@allenpress.com, http://www.structbio.nature.com. Ed. Guy Riddihough. **Subscr. to:** Allen Press Inc., PO Box 1897, Lawrence, KS 66044-8897. TEL 800-524-0384, FAX 615-377-0525; Nature, 345 Park Ave S, New York, NY 10160-1743. TEL 212-726-9244.

570 610 AUT ISSN 0379-1416
NATURWISSENSCHAFTLICH - MEDIZINISCHEN VEREINS IN INNSBRUCK. BERICHTE. Text in English, German; Summaries in English, French, German, Italian. 1870. a. ATS 500 domestic; EUR 36.50 foreign. bk.rev. abstr. back issues avail. *Refereed.* **Document type:** *Abstract/Index, Academic/Scholarly.* **Description:** Covers biological, faunistic, floristic, environmental and medical sciences. Accentuates the problems of the Alps, other high mountain groups and the Mediterranean basin.
Indexed: Aqua.Sci.& Fish.Abstr., Biol.Abstr., Entomol.Abstr., Environ.Sci.Poll.Mgmt., Pollut.Abstr., Ref.Zh., Zoo.Rec.
—BLDSC (1923.300000).
Published by: Naturwissenschaftlich - Medizinischer Verein in Innsbruck, Technikerstrasse 25, Innsbruck, T 6020, Austria. TEL 43-512-5076142, FAX 43-512-5072930, erwin.meyer@uibk.ac.at. Ed. Dr. Erwin Meyer. Circ: 500. **Distr. by:** Dr. Wolfgang Schede, Technikerstrasse 25, Innsbruck, T 6020, Austria. TEL 0512-507-6143, FAX 0512-507-2930.

570 550 DEU ISSN 0932-9447
NATURWISSENSCHAFTLICHE ZEITSCHRIFT FUER NIEDERBAYERN. Text in German. 1864. triennial. DEM 20 (effective 2001). adv. bk.rev. **Document type:** *Proceedings, Academic/Scholarly.*
Published by: Naturwissenschaftlicher Verein fuer Niederbayern, Bachstrasse 51 (Stadtarchiv), Landshut 84036, Germany. TEL 49-871-881218, FAX 49-871-881218. Ed., R&P, Adv. contact Georg Spitzlberger TEL 0871-42266.

570 DEU ISSN 0720-3705
NATURWISSENSCHAFTLICHER VEREIN FUER SCHWABEN. BERICHTE. Text in German. 1848. a. EUR 25 (effective 2001). bk.rev. 112 p./no. back issues avail. **Document type:** *Yearbook, Academic/Scholarly.*
Formerly (until 1885): Naturhistorischer Verein Augsburg. Bericht (0340-3734)
Indexed: GeoRef, IBR, Zoo.Rec.
Published by: Naturwissenschaftlicher Verein fuer Schwaben e.V., Im Thaele 3, Augsburg 86152, Germany. TEL 49-821-3246730, FAX 49-821-3246741. Eds. Hermann Oblinger, Otto Mair. Circ: 1,000.

370 550 DEU ISSN 0340-3718
NATURWISSENSCHAFTLICHER VEREIN ZU BREMEN. ABHANDLUNGEN. Text in German. 1886. irreg., latest vol.44, 1999. DEM 80 newsstand/cover. *Refereed.* **Document type:** *Journal, Academic/Scholarly.* **Description:** Presents articles and research concerning all fields of the natural sciences.
Indexed: Aqua.Sci.& Fish.Abstr., Aquacult.Abstr., GeoRef, IBZ, Ref.Zh.
—Linda Hall.
Published by: Naturwissenschaftlicher Verein zu Bremen, Bahnhofsplatz 13, Bremen 28195, Germany. TEL 49-421-36111998, nwv.bremen@lycosmail.com, http://www.bremen.de/info/nwv/publikat.htm.

570 560 NLD ISSN 0374-955X
NATUURHISTORISCH GENOOTSCHAP IN LIMBURG. PUBLICATIES. Text in Dutch, English; Summaries in English. 1948. irreg., latest vol.42, 1999 (1-2/yr.). price varies. back issues avail. **Document type:** *Monographic series, Academic/Scholarly.* **Description:** Covers the biological, geological, and paleontological research of Limburg.
Indexed: Biol.Abstr., GeoRef, Rev.Appl.Entomol., Zoo.Rec.
—CISTI.
Published by: (Natuurhistorisch Genootschap in Limburg), Publicatie Bureau N H G, Groenstraat 106, Melick 6074 EL, Netherlands. TEL 31-475-537095. R&P A Lenders. Circ: 1,000.

NAUKOVE TOVARYSTVO IMENI SHEVCHENKA. PROCEEDINGS OF THE SECTION OF CHEMISTRY, BIOLOGY AND MEDICINE. see *CHEMISTRY*

NEUROBIOLOGICAL RESEARCH. see *MEDICAL SCIENCES—Psychiatry And Neurology*

NEUROBIOLOGY OF LEARNING AND MEMORY. see *MEDICAL SCIENCES—Psychiatry And Neurology*

NEURON. see *MEDICAL SCIENCES—Psychiatry And Neurology*

NEUROSCIENCE NEWS. see *MEDICAL SCIENCES—Psychiatry And Neurology*

NEW DEVELOPMENTS IN BIOSCIENCES. see *MEDICAL SCIENCES*

577 NZL ISSN 0110-6465
QH540 CODEN: NZJED6
NEW ZEALAND JOURNAL OF ECOLOGY. Text in English. 1953. 2/yr. NZD 120 domestic; NZD 130 in Australia & Asia Pacific; USD 80 elsewhere (effective 2000). adv. bk.rev. 21 year cum.index. back issues avail. *Refereed.* **Document type:** *Academic/Scholarly.* **Description:** Publishes scientific studies of ecology in, or relevant to, New Zealand.
Formerly: New Zealand Ecological Society. Proceedings (0077-9946)
Related titles: Microfiche ed.: (from IDC); Online - full text ed.: (from Institute for Scientific Information).

Indexed: ASCA, Apic.Abstr., Appl.Ecol.Abstr., Aqua.Sci.& Fish.Abstr., Bio-Contr.News & Info., Biol.Abstr., Chem.Abstr., Curr.Adv.Ecol.Sci., Curr.Cont., Curr.Ref.Fish Res., Ecol.Abstr., Entomol.Abstr., Environ.Sci.Poll.Mgmt., Excerp.Med., Field Crop Abstr., Forest Prod.Abstr., Forest.Abstr., Genet.Abstr., Geo.Abstr.P.G., GeoRef, Helminthol.Abstr., Herb.Abstr., Hum.Gen.Abstr., Ind.Sci.Rev., Ind.Vet., Pollut.Abstr., Rev.Appl.Entomol., Rev.Plant Path., Sci.Cit.Ind., Seed Abstr., Sel.Water Res.Abstr., Soils & Fert., Sport Fish.Abstr., Vet.Bull., Weed Abstr., Wild.Rev., Zoo.Rec.
—BLDSC (6093.530000), CASDDS, CISTI, IDS, Infotrieve, Linda Hall. **CCC.**
Published by: New Zealand Ecological Society, Inc., P.O. Box 25178, Christchurch, New Zealand. TEL 64-3-384-2432, FAX 64-3-384-2432, sheppars@ihug.co.nz. Ed. David Wardle. Adv. contact Gabor Lovei. page NZD 200. Circ: 700.

570 NZL ISSN 0113-7492
CODEN: NZNSEZ
NEW ZEALAND NATURAL SCIENCES. Text in English. 1973. a. NZD 18 to individuals; NZD 25 to libraries; NZD 20 foreign (effective 2000). bk.rev. *Refereed.* **Document type:** *Academic/Scholarly.* **Description:** Documents scientific research in the earth, life and environmental sciences relevant to New Zealand or Antarctica.
Formerly (until 1988): Mauri Ora (0302-086X)
Indexed: Biol.Abstr., Curr.Adv.Ecol.Sci., Ecol.Abstr., Excerp.Med., GeoRef, Geol.Abstr., Mineral.Abstr., Sport Fish.Abstr., Wild.Rev., Zoo.Rec.
—BLDSC (6096.315000), CASDDS, CISTI, Infotrieve, Linda Hall. **CCC.**
Published by: University of Canterbury, Zoology Department, Private Bag 4800, Christchurch, 1, New Zealand. TEL 64-3-364-2860, FAX 64-3-364-2024, nzns@zool.canterbury.ac.nz. Ed., R&P Norman Ragg. Circ: 260.

570 JPN ISSN 0387-8236
CODEN: NDRHE4
NIIGATA DAIGAKU RIGAKUBU FUZOKU SADO RINKAI JIKKENJO TOKUBETSU HOKOKU/NIIGATA UNIVERSITY. SADO MARINE BIOLOGICAL STATION. SPECIAL PUBLICATION. Text in Japanese; Summaries in English, Japanese. 1978. irreg.
Indexed: Aqua.Sci.& Fish.Abstr., Aquacult.Abstr., Environ.Sci.Poll.Mgmt., Sport Fish.Abstr.
Published by: Niigata Daigaku, Rigakubu/Niigata University, Faculty of Science, Fuzoku Sado Rinkai Jikkenjo, 8050 Igarashi Nino-cho, Niigata-shi, Nigata-ken 950-21, Japan.

570 JPN ISSN 0029-0750
NISSEIKEN TAYORI/NIPPON INSTITUTE FOR BIOLOGICAL SCIENCE. JOURNAL. Text in Japanese. 1955. m. free per issue. bk.rev. charts, illus. cum.index. **Document type:** *Newsletter.* **Description:** Summary of research activities in the institute; articles for technical extension; and records of the semi-annual seminar held by the Pathology Division of the Japanese Society for Veterinary Science.
Published by: Nippon Seibutsu Kagaku Kenkyujo/Nippon Institute for Biological Science, 2221-1 Shin-Machi, Ome-shi, Tokyo-to 198-0024, Japan. TEL 81-428-33-1001, FAX 81-429-31-6166, nibs@group.lin.go.jp, http://group.lin.go.jp/nibs/. Ed. Hiromasa Tanaka. Circ: 1,600.

NOGYO KANKYO GIJUTSU KENKYUSHO HOKOKU/NATIONAL INSTITUTE OF AGRO-ENVIRONMENTAL SCIENCES. BULLETIN. see *AGRICULTURE*

570 JPN ISSN 0911-6575
CODEN: NSSHEC
NOGYO SEIBUTSU SHIGEN KENKYUJO KENKYU HOKOKU/NATIONAL INSTITUTE OF AGROBIOLOGICAL RESOURCES. BULLETIN. Text in English, Japanese. 1985. a. per issue exchange basis. **Document type:** *Bulletin.*
Indexed: Agrindex, Biol.Abstr., Chem.Abstr., Chem.Indus.Notes, Chem.Titles, Crop Physiol.Abstr., Fababean Abstr., Field Crop Abstr., Poult.Abstr., Ref.Zh., Rev.Appl.Entomol., Rev.Plant Path., Rice Abstr., Seed Abstr., Soyabean Abstr., VITIS.
—BLDSC (2640.010000), CASDDS, CISTI, Linda Hall.
Published by: Norin Suisansho, Nogyo Seibutsu Shigen Kenkyujo/Ministry of Agriculture, Forestry and Fisheries, National Institute of Agrobiological Resources, 2-1-2 Kannondai, Tsukuba-shi, Ibaraki-ken 305-0856, Japan. TEL 0298-38-7004, FAX 0298-38-7408. Ed. Kenji Takayanagi.

NONLINEAR DYNAMICS, PSYCHOLOGY, AND LIFE SCIENCES. see *PSYCHOLOGY*

570 AUS ISSN 0078-1630
CODEN: NQNAAG
NORTH QUEENSLAND NATURALIST. Text in English. 1932. irreg., latest vol.189, 1989. AUD 10 to membership. bk.rev.
Indexed: Biol.Abstr.
Published by: North Queensland Naturalists Club, PO Box 991, Cairns, QLD 4870, Australia. Circ: 220.

NOTICIAS DE GALAPAGOS. see *SCIENCES: COMPREHENSIVE WORKS*

570 CUB
NOTICIERO CIENTIFICO. SERIE: BIOLOGIA. Text in Spanish. fortn.
Published by: Academia de Ciencias, Instituto de Documentacion e Informacion Cientifico-Tecnica (I D I C T), Capitolio Nacional, Prado y San Jose, Habana 2, Cuba.

570 NLD ISSN 0166-6584
QL520 CODEN: NOODDJ
NOTULAE ODONATOLOGICAE. Text in English, French, German, Italian, Spanish. 1978. s-a. NLG 40. bk.rev. charts. **Document type:** *Bulletin.*
Indexed: Aqua.Sci.& Fish.Abstr., Biol.Abstr., Entomol.Abstr. (coverage dropped), Genet.Abstr. (coverage dropped), Zoo.Rec.
—BLDSC (6176.010000).
Published by: Societas Internationalis Odonatologica, SIO Central Office, PO Box 256, Bilthoven 3720 AG, Netherlands. Circ: 500.

570 FRA ISSN 0181-3684
NOUVEAU BIOLOGISTE*. Text in French. 10/yr. FRF 550.
Address: c/o Societe de Biologie, College de France, Paris Cedex 5 75231, France. TEL 42-65-15-97, FAX 42-65-58-05. Ed. A Bedossa. Circ: 3,500.

NUCLEAR MEDICINE AND BIOLOGY. see *MEDICAL SCIENCES—Radiology And Nuclear Medicine*

NUKADA INSTITUTE FOR MEDICAL AND BIOLOGICAL RESEARCH. REPORTS. see *MEDICAL SCIENCES*

NUTRITION AND THE BRAIN. see *NUTRITION AND DIETETICS*

571.9 BGR ISSN 0324-1998
CODEN: OSPADK
OBSTA I SRAVNITELNA PATOLOGIIA. Text in Multiple languages. 1976. s-a. price varies. reprint service avail. from IRC.
Indexed: Abstr.Bulg.Sci.Med.Lit., BSL Biol., Biol.Abstr., Chem.Abstr., Excerp.Med., Ind.Vet., Poult.Abstr., Vet.Bull.
—CASDDS, GNLM, Infotrieve, KNAW. **CCC.**
Published by: (Bulgarska Akademiia na Naukite/Bulgarian Academy of Sciences), Publishing House of the Bulgarian Academy of Sciences, Akad G Bonchev 6, Sofia 1113, Bulgaria. Circ: 500.

OCEANOGRAPHY AND MARINE BIOLOGY: AN ANNUAL REVIEW. see *EARTH SCIENCES—Oceanography*

OCROTIREA NATURII SI A MEDIULUI INCONJURATOR. see *SCIENCES: COMPREHENSIVE WORKS*

570 NLD ISSN 0375-0183
QL520 CODEN: ODTGAI
ODONATOLOGICA. Text in English, French, German. 1972. q. NLG 220. bk.rev. charts. **Document type:** *Academic/Scholarly, Abstract/Index.*
Related titles: Online - full text ed.: (from Institute for Scientific Information).
Indexed: Anim.Behav.Abstr., Appl.Ecol.Abstr. (coverage dropped), Aqua.Sci.& Fish.Abstr., Biol.Abstr., Curr.Cont., Ecol.Abstr., Entomol.Abstr., Environ.Sci.Poll.Mgmt., Genet.Abstr. (coverage dropped), Zoo.Rec.
—ingenta.
Published by: Societas Internationalis Odonatologica, SIO Central Office, PO Box 256, Bilthoven 3720 AG, Netherlands. Circ: 500.

577 DEU ISSN 0029-8549
QH540 CODEN: OECOBX
OECOLOGIA. Text in English. 1924. 16/yr. EUR 3,161.10 domestic; EUR 1,335.60 in Germany; EUR 232.50 newsstand/cover foreign (effective 2002). adv. bibl, illus. index. back issues avail.; reprint service avail. from ISI. *Refereed.* **Document type:** *Journal, Academic/Scholarly.* **Description:** Presents articles on research developments in the functional relationships between plant and animal organisms and their environment.
Formerly: Zeitschrift fuer Morphologie und Oekologie der Tiere
Related titles: Microform ed.: (from PQC); Online - full text ed.: ISSN 1432-1939 (from EBSCO Publishing, RoweCom Information Quest, Swets Blackwell, Springer LINK, Institute for Scientific Information).
Indexed: ASCA, AgBiotech, Agricola, Agroforest.Abstr., Anim.Behav.Abstr., Apic.Abstr., Appl.Ecol.Abstr., Aqua.Sci.& Fish.Abstr., Bibl.Agri., Bio-Contr.News & Info., Biol.& Agr.Ind. (Jan.1996-), Biol.Abstr., Chemorec.Abstr., Crop Physiol.Abstr., Curr.Adv.Ecol.Sci., Curr.Adv.Plant Sci., Curr.Cont., Curr.Ref.Fish Res., Deep Sea Res.& Oceanogr.Abstr., Ecol.Abstr., Entomol.Abstr., Environ.Sci.Poll.Mgmt., Excerp.Med., Field Crop Abstr., Forest Prod.Abstr., Forest.Abstr., Genet.Abstr., Geo.Abstr.H.G., Geo.Abstr.P.G., GeoRef, Helminthol.Abstr., Herb.Abstr., Hort.Abstr., Hum.Gen.Abstr., INIS Atomind., Ind.Sci.Rev., Ind.Vet., Int.Abstr.Biol.Sci., Irr.& Drain.Abstr., Key Word Ind.Wildl.Res., Maize Abstr., Meteor.& Geoastrophys.Abstr., Microbiol.Abstr., Nutr.Abstr., Ocean.Abstr., Ornam.Hort., Plant Breed.Abstr., Plant Gen.Res.Abstr., Plant Grow.Reg.Abstr., Plant Sci., Pollut.Abstr., Poult.Abstr., Ref.Zh., Rev.Appl.Entomol., Rev.Arom.& Med.Plants, Rev.Med.& Vet.Mycol., Rev.Plant Path., Rice Abstr., Sci.Cit.Ind., Seed Abstr., Sel.Water Res.Abstr., Soils & Fert., Soyabean Abstr., Sport Fish.Abstr., Sugar Ind.Abstr., Triticale Abstr., Weed Abstr., Wild.Rev., Zoo.Rec.
—BLDSC (6235.262600), CISTI, EMDOCS, IDS, ingenta, Linda Hall. **CCC.**
Published by: (International Association for Ecology, (Intecol) NLD), Springer-Verlag (Subsidiary of: BertelsmannSpringer), Tiergartenstr 17, Heidelberg 69121, Germany. TEL 49-6221-345-0, FAX 49-6221-345229, subscriptions@springer.de, http://link.springer.de/link/service/journals/00442/index.htm, http://www.springer.de. Eds. J R Ehleringer, M Schaefer. **Subscr. in N. America to:** Springer-Verlag New York Inc., PO Box 2485, Secaucus, NJ 07096-2485. TEL 212-460-1500, FAX 212-473-6272.

570 USA ISSN 0078-3994
QH105.O3 CODEN: BOBNAJ
OHIO BIOLOGICAL SURVEY. BULLETIN. NEW SERIES. Text in English. 1913; N.S. 1959. irreg., latest vol.13, no.1, 1998. price varies. *Refereed.* **Document type:** *Monographic series.*
Indexed: Biol.Abstr., GeoRef, Sport Fish.Abstr., Wild.Rev., Zoo.Rec.
—CISTI, Linda Hall.
Published by: Ohio Biological Survey, 1315 Kinnear Rd, Columbus, OH 43212. TEL 614-292-9645, FAX 614-688-4322. Ed. Veda M Cafazzo. Circ: 1,000.

570 JPN ISSN 0916-930X
QH301 CODEN: OSSHEN
OKAYAMA DAIGAKU SHIGEN SEIBUTSU KAGAKU KENKYUJO HOKOKU/OKAYAMA UNIVERSITY. RESEARCH INSTITUTE FOR BIORESOURCES. BULLETIN. Text in English, Japanese. 1990. q. per issue exchange basis.
Formed by the merger of (1916-1990): Okayama Universitaet. Berichte des Ohara Instituts fuer Landwirtschaftliche Biologie (0365-9860); Which was formerly (until 1954): Okayama Universitaet. Berichte des Ohara Instituts fuer Landwirtschaftliche Forschungen (0365-9879); (1924-1990): Nogaku Kenkyu - Ohara Institute for Agricultural Biology. Report (0029-0874); Which was formerly: Nogaku Koenshu
Indexed: Biol.Abstr., Chem.Abstr., Chem.Indus.Notes, Chem.Titles, Crop Physiol.Abstr., Field Crop Abstr., GeoRef, Hort.Abstr., INIS Atomind., Maize Abstr., Plant Breed.Abstr., Ref.Zh., Rev.Appl.Entomol., Rev.Plant Path., Rice Abstr., Seed Abstr., Triticale Abstr.
—CASDDS, CISTI, ingenta, Linda Hall.
Published by: Okayama Daigaku, Shigen Seibutsu Kagaku Kenkyujo/Okayama University, Research Institute for Bioresources, 20-1 Chuo 2-chome, Kurashiki-shi, Okayama-ken 710-0046, Japan. Ed. Isao Aoyama. Circ: 875.

570 RUS ISSN 0475-1450
CODEN: ONGZAC
ONTOGENEZ. Text in Russian. 1970. bi-m. RUR 275 for 2 mos. (effective 2001). back issues avail. *Refereed.* **Document type:** *Academic/Scholarly.* **Description:** Publishes fundamental and applied research papers and reviews on development, regeneration, and carcinogenesis at the molecular, cellular, and organismic levels.
Related titles: Microfilm ed.: (from PQC); Online - full text ed.; ♦ English Translation: Russian Journal of Developmental Biology. ISSN 1062-3604.
Indexed: Chem.Abstr., Chem.Titles, GeoRef, INIS Atomind., Ind.Med. (1970-), Ref.Zh., Zoo.Rec.

B

—BLDSC (0127.452000), CASDDS, CISTI, East View, GNLM, KNAW, Linda Hall. **CCC.**

Published by: (Rossiiskaya Akademiya Nauk/Russian Academy of Sciences), M A I K Nauka - Interperiodica, Mezhdunarodnyi Otdel, Profsoyuznaya ul 90, Moscow 117864, Russian Federation. TEL 7-095-336-1600, FAX 7-095-336-0666, compmg@maik.ru, http://www.maik.rssi.ru/journals/devbio.htm. Ed. Sergei G Vassetzky. **US dist. addr.:** Kluwer Academic Publishers, PO Box 17, Dordrecht 3300 AH, Netherlands. TEL 31-78-639-2392, FAX 31-78-654-6474, http://www.wkap.nl.

578.77 DNK ISSN 0078-5326
QH91.A1 CODEN: OPHLAN

OPHELIA; an international journal of marine biology. Text in English. 1964. 6/yr. DKK 1,430 (effective 2001). adv. illus. Index. back issues avail.; reprints avail. *Refereed.* **Document type:** *Journal, Academic/Scholarly.*

Related titles: Online - full text ed.: (from Institute for Scientific Information); ♦ Supplement: Ophelia. Supplementum. ISSN 0107-5896.

Indexed: ASCA, Appl.Ecol.Abstr. (coverage dropped), Aqua.Sci.& Fish.Abstr., Bibl.Agri., Biol.Abstr., Chem.Abstr., Curr.Adv.Biochem., Curr.Adv.Cell & Devel.Biol., Curr.Adv.Ecol.Sci., Curr.Cont., Deep Sea Res.& Oceanogr.Abstr., Ecol.Abstr., Environ.Sci.Poll.Mgmt., GeoRef, Helminthol.Abstr., IBR, Ind.Sci.Rev., Int.Abstr.Biol.Sci., Mar.Sci.Cont.Tab., Nutr.Abstr., Ocean.Abstr., Pollut.Abstr., Sci.Cit.Ind., Sel.Water Res.Abstr., Sport Fish.Abstr., Wild.Rev., Zoo.Rec.

—BLDSC (6270.800000), CISTI, EMDOCS, ingenta, Linda Hall.

Published by: (Marine Biological Laboratory), Apollo Books Aps, Kirkeby Sand 19, Stenstrup 5771, Denmark. TEL 45-62-26-37-37, FAX 45-62-26-37-80, apollobooks@vip.cybercity.dk, http://www.apollobooks.com. Ed. T. Fenchel. Circ: 600.

570 610 FRA ISSN 0992-5945

OPTION - BIO; le journal de l'analyse medicale et de la biologie clinique. Text in French. 1989. 22/yr. FRF 977 domestic to institutions; EUR 148.94 in Europe to institutions; USD 183 in the Americas to institutions; FRF 1,076, EUR 164.04 elsewhere to institutions (effective 2001). adv. back issues avail. *Refereed.* **Document type:** *Academic/Scholarly.* **Description:** Provides day-to-day news, scientific information in the medical and biological areas, diagnostic approaches and technical viewpoints.

Related titles: Online - full text ed.: (from ingenta, ScienceDirect, Swets Blackwell).

—CCC.

Published by: Elsevier Paris, Editions Scientifiques et Medicales (Subsidiary of: Reed Elsevier plc. group), 23 rue Linois, Paris 75015, France. TEL 33-1-45589110, FAX 33-1-45589419, labm@elsevier.com.fr, http://www.elsevier.nl/inca/publications/store/5/0/5/8/1/9/. Ed. F Mauriat. Circ: 6,800.

571.3 DEU ISSN 1439-6092

▼ **ORGANISMS DIVERSITY AND EVOLUTION.** Text in English. 2000. 4/yr. EUR 255, GBP 188 (effective 2002). adv. *Refereed.* **Document type:** *Journal, Academic/Scholarly.* **Description:** Devoted to the understanding of organismal diversity.

Related titles: Online - full text ed.: (from Swets Blackwell).

Indexed: Appl.Ecol.Abstr., Biotech.& Bioeng.Abstr., Entomol.Abstr., Genet.Abstr.

Published by: (Gesellschaft fuer Biologische Systematik), Urban & Fischer Verlag, Loebdergraben 14a, Jena 07743, Germany. TEL 49-3641-626430, FAX 49-3641-626421, info@urbanfischer.de, http://www.urbanfischer.de/journals. Ed. Gerhard Haszprunar. R&P Martin Huber TEL 49-3641-626430. Adv. contact Sabine Schroeter.

570 USA ISSN 0553-0342

ORGANIZATION OF AMERICAN STATES. DEPARTMENT OF SCIENTIFIC AFFAIRS. SERIE DE BIOLOGIA: MONOGRAFIAS. Text in Spanish. 1965. irreg., latest vol.20, 1978. USD 3.50 per issue. **Document type:** *Monographic series.*

Published by: Organization of American States, Department of Publications, 1889 F St, N W, Washington, DC 20006. TEL 703-941-1617. Circ: 3,000.

572.38 578 NLD ISSN 0169-6149
QH325

ORIGINS OF LIFE AND EVOLUTION OF THE BIOSPHERE. Text in Dutch. 1968. bi-m. EUR 461 to institutions for print or online ed.; EUR 553.20 to institutions print & online eds.combined (effective 2002). adv. bk.rev. bibl, illus. reprint service avail. from SWZ. *Refereed.* **Document type:** *Academic/Scholarly.* **Description:** Publishes experimental and theoretical studies of chemical evolution, including evolution of planetary atmospheres, prebiotic chemistry and biochemical evolution.

Former titles: Origins of Life (0302-1688); (until 1974): Space Life Sciences (0038-6286)

Related titles: Microform ed.: (from PQC); Online - full text ed.: (from EBSCO Publishing, O C L C Online Computer Library Center, Inc., RoweCom Information Quest, Swets Blackwell, Kluwer Online, Institute for Scientific Information).

Indexed: ASCA, Appl.Mech.Rev., Astron.& Astrophys.Abstr., Biol.Abstr., Chem.Abstr., Chem.Titles, Curr.Adv.Ecol.Sci., Curr.Cont., Deep Sea Res.& Oceanogr.Abstr., Environ.Per.Bibl. (1985-1995), Excerp.Med., GeoRef, Geol.Abstr., IBR, IBZ, INIS Atomind., INSPEC (May 1970-Dec.1973, Jan.1974-), Ind.Med. (1984-), Ind.Sci.Rev., Inpharma, Int.Aerosp.Abstr., Mass Spectr.Bull., Meteor.& Geoastrophys.Abstr., Phys.Ber., Reac., Ref.Zh., Sci.Cit.Ind.

—BLDSC (6291.265100), AskIEEE, CASDDS, CISTI, GNLM, IDS, Infotrieve, ingenta, Linda Hall. **CCC.**

Published by: (International Society for the Study of the Origins of Life), Kluwer Academic Publishers Group (Subsidiary of: Wolters Kluwer N.V.), Spuiboulevard 50, PO Box 17, Dordrecht 3300 AA, Netherlands. FAX 31-78-639-2254, services@wkap.nl, http://www.wkap.nl/journalhome.htm/0169-6149. Ed. James P Ferris. **Dist. by:** Journals Department, PO Box 322, Dordrecht 3300 AH, Netherlands. TEL 781-871-6600, FAX 31-78-654-6474.

570 JPN ISSN 0389-9047

OSAKA-SHIRITSU SHIZENSHI HAKUBUTSUKAN SHUZO SHIRYO MOKUROKU/OSAKA MUSEUM OF NATURAL HISTORY. SPECIAL PUBLICATIONS. Text in Japanese. 1969. a. price varies; also avail. on exchange basis. **Document type:** *Catalog.*

Indexed: GeoRef, Zoo.Rec.

—BLDSC (8379.670000).

Published by: Osaka-shiritsu Shizenshi Hakubutsukan/Osaka Museum of Natural History, 1-23 Nagaikoen, Higashisumiyoshi-ku, Osaka-shi 546-0034, Japan. TEL 81-6-6697-6221, FAX 81-6-6697-6225, library@mus-nh.city.osaka.jp, http://www.mus-nh.city.osaka.jp. Ed. Takayoshi Nasu. Circ: 1,000.

PARASITE IMMUNOLOGY. see *MEDICAL SCIENCES—Communicable Diseases*

577 595.7 BEL ISSN 0031-1812
SB599 CODEN: PARGAW

PARASITICA. Text in Dutch, English, French, German. 1945. q. BEF 4,755 domestic; BEF 8,100 foreign (effective 2000). adv. bk.rev. charts, illus. index. back issues avail. *Refereed.* **Document type:** *Bulletin, Academic/Scholarly.*

Related titles: Microform ed.: (from PMC).

Indexed: Agri.& Environ.Biotech.Abstr. (coverage dropped), Aqua.Sci.& Fish.Abstr., Bio-Contr.News & Info., Biol.Abstr., Chem.Abstr., Curr.Adv.Ecol.Sci., Curr.Cont. (coverage dropped), Derwent Biotech.Abstr., Entomol.Abstr., Forest.Abstr., Helminthol.Abstr., Hort.Abstr., Microbiol.Abstr., Ornam.Hort., Plant Breed.Abstr., Postharvest, Potato Abstr., Rev.Appl.Entomol., Rev.Plant Path., Rice Abstr., Seed Abstr., Soils & Fert., Triticale Abstr., Weed Abstr., Zoo.Rec.

—CASDDS, CISTI, Linda Hall.

Published by: Association pour les Etudes et Recherches de Zoologie Appliquee et de Phytopathologie, Rue du Bordia 11, Gembloux 5030, Belgium. TEL 32-81-625262, FAX 32-81-625272. Ed. R Moens. R&P R. Moens TEL 32-81-625272. Adv. contact M Galoux. page BEF 7,430. Circ: 550.

PATHOLOGIE ET BIOLOGIE. see *MEDICAL SCIENCES*

PATHOLOGY. see *MEDICAL SCIENCES*

PATHOLOGY PATTERNS. see *MEDICAL SCIENCES*

571.9 MEX ISSN 0185-4305

PATOLOGIA; revista latinoamericana. Text in Spanish; Summaries in English, Portuguese. 1992. q. MXP 300, USD 70 (effective 1996 & 1997). adv. bk.rev. charts, illus. index. back issues avail. *Refereed.* **Document type:** *Academic/Scholarly.* **Description:** Contains original articles, research reports, review articles, clinical cases and notices related to anatomical pathology.

Formerly (until 1970): Asociacion Mexicana de Patologos. Boletin

Related titles: CD-ROM ed.

Indexed: Biol.Abstr., Curr.Cont. (coverage dropped), Excerp.Med., Helminthol.Abstr., Sci.Cit.Ind. (coverage dropped).

Published by: (Asociacion Latinoamericana de Patologia), Obsidiana Editores S.A., CZDA DE TLALPAN 2365, Col Ciudad Jardin, Mexico City, DF 04370, Mexico. TEL 52-5-689-9133. Ed. Dr. Luis Benitez Bribiesca. Pub. Jorge Godoy-Gutierrez. Circ: 630 (paid); 1,370 (controlled). **Dist. by:** Distribuidora Editorial de Mexico SA de CV, P.O. Box 76-026, Mexico City, DF 04201, Mexico. TEL 52-5-544-7953, FAX 52-5-689-6545. **Co-sponsor:** Asociacion Mexicana de Patologos.

PATOLOGICHESKAYA FIZIOLOGIYA I EKSPERIMENTAL'NAYA TERAPIYA/PATHOLOGICAL PHYSIOLOGY AND EXPERIMENTAL THERAPY. see *MEDICAL SCIENCES*

PEDOBIOLOGIA. see *AGRICULTURE—Crop Production And Soil*

PELAGOS. see *EARTH SCIENCES—Oceanography*

PENNSYLVANIA ACADEMY OF SCIENCE. JOURNAL. see *SCIENCES: COMPREHENSIVE WORKS*

570 610 HRV ISSN 0031-5362
QH301 CODEN: PDBIAD

PERIODICUM BIOLOGORUM. Text in English; Summaries in Croatian, English. 1886. q. USD 25. bk.rev. index. back issues avail. **Document type:** *Academic/Scholarly.*

Related titles: Online - full text ed.: (from Institute for Scientific Information).

Indexed: Abstr.Hyg., AgBiotech, Agroforest.Abstr., Anim.Breed.Abstr., Biol.Abstr., Chem.Abstr., Chem.Indus.Notes, Chem.Titles, Crop Physiol.Abstr., Curr.Adv.Biochem., Curr.Adv.Cell & Devel.Biol., Curr.Adv.Ecol.Sci., Curr.Adv.Gen.& Molec.Biol., Curr.Cont. (coverage dropped), Dairy Sci.Abstr., Excerp.Med., Field Crop Abstr., Forest.Abstr., Helminthol.Abstr., Herb.Abstr., INIS Atomind., Ind.Vet., Int.Abstr.Biol.Sci., Maize Abstr., Nutr.Abstr., Plant Breed.Abstr., Plant Gen.Res.Abstr., Poult.Abstr., Rev.Appl.Entomol., Rev.Med.& Vet.Mycol., Rev.Plant Path., Sci.Cit.Ind. (coverage dropped), Soils & Fert., Sport Fish.Abstr., Vet.Bull., Weed Abstr., Wild.Rev., Zoo.Rec.

—BLDSC (6426.240000), CASDDS, CISTI, GNLM, IDS, ingenta, KNAW, Linda Hall.

Published by: Hrvatsko Prirodoslovno Drustvo/Croatian Society of Natural Sciences, Ilica 16-3, Zagreb 41000, Croatia. TEL 041-425-288, FAX 041-425-288. Ed. Vlatko Silobrcic. Circ: 900.

PERSPECTIVES IN BIOLOGY AND MEDICINE. see *MEDICAL SCIENCES*

571.43 CHE ISSN 0272-6327

PERSPECTIVES IN BIOMECHANICS. Text in English. irreg. *Refereed.* **Document type:** *Monographic series.*

Published by: Gordon and Breach - Harwood Academic (Subsidiary of: Taylor & Francis Group), PO Box 531, Lausanne 1000, Switzerland. Ed. D N Ghista. **Subscr. addr. in US:** International Publishers Direct, PO Box 32160, Newark, NJ 07102. FAX 215-750-6343.

599.9 AUS ISSN 1038-5762
QP34.5

PERSPECTIVES IN HUMAN BIOLOGY. Text in English. 1992. a. AUD 30, USD 24 (effective 1997). bk.rev. *Refereed.* **Document type:** *Academic/Scholarly.* **Description:** Publishes research papers and reviews which foster a primarily biological understanding of humans, with emphasis on the integration of the constituent disciplines.

Indexed: A.I.C.P. (1994-).

—BLDSC (6428.143180).

Published by: Centre for Human Biology, Dept. of Anatomy & Human Biology, Univ of Western, Nedlands, W.A. 6907, Australia. TEL 61-8-93803290, FAX 61-8-93801051, adminsec@anhb.uwa.edu.au, http://www.anhb.uwa.edu.au. Ed. Charles Oxnard. Circ: 200.

PETERSON'S GRADUATE AND PROFESSIONAL PROGRAMS: THE BIOLOGICAL SCIENCES (YEAR) (BOOK 3). see *EDUCATION—Guides To Schools And Colleges*

PHOTOCHEMICAL & PHOTOBIOLOGICAL REVIEWS. see *CHEMISTRY*

PHOTOCHEMISTRY AND PHOTOBIOLOGY. see *CHEMISTRY*

578.77 THA ISSN 0858-1088
QH193.T46 CODEN: RBPCE9
PHUKET MARINE BIOLOGICAL CENTER. RESEARCH BULLETIN. Text in English. 1973. irreg. (1-2/yr.). USD 10 (effective 1993). illus. back issues avail. *Refereed.* **Document type:** *Bulletin.* **Description:** Examines research results carried out at the center; in cooperation with the center; or independent research performed in Thailand and adjacent areas.
Indexed: Aqua.Sci.& Fish.Abstr., Aquacult.Abstr., Environ.Sci.Poll.Mgmt., Sport Fish.Abstr., Zoo.Rec.
Published by: Phuket Marine Biological Center, PO Box 60, Phuket 83000, Thailand. TEL 076-391128, FAX 076-391127. Ed. Samsak Chullasorn. Circ: 500.

573.4 616.48 IND
PINEAL GLAND: ITS MOLECULAR SIGNALS. Text in English. 1996. irreg. USD 30 per issue (effective 2000). **Document type:** *Monographic series.*
Published by: Hindustan Publishing Corporation (India), 4805-24 Bharat Ram Rd., Ist Fl., Darya Ganj, New Delhi 110 002, India. TEL 91-11-325-4401, FAX 91-11-6193511, hpcpd@nda.vsnl.net.in, hpcpd@hpc.cc, http://www.hpc.cc, http://www.bizdelhi.com/publisher/hpc. Ed. Chandana Haldar.

578.77 JPN ISSN 1343-0874
QH90.8.P5
PLANKTON BIOLOGY AND ECOLOGY. Text in English. s-a. JPY 12,000 (effective 2000). *Refereed.* **Document type:** *Academic/Scholarly.* **Description:** Publishes papers, reviews, and notes dealing with all aspects of biology; ecology of marine; freshwater plankton; and their interactions with the environments in any aquatic systems.
Indexed: Aqua.Sci.& Fish.Abstr., Biotech.& Bioeng.Abstr., Ecol.Abstr., Environ.Sci.Poll.Mgmt., Microbiol.Abstr., Ocean.Abstr., Pollut.Abstr., Risk Abstr., Saf.Sci.Abstr., Zoo.Rec.
Published by: Plankton Society of Japan/Nihon Purankuton Gakkai, c/o tokyo University of Fisheries, 4-5-7 Kounan, Minato-ku, Tokyo 108-8477, Japan. TEL 81-3-5463-0539, FAX 81-3-5463-0539, plankton@tokyo-u-fish.ac.jp, http://www2.ori.u-tokyo.ac.jp/plankton/soc/PlanktonSocJ.html. Ed. Shuhei Nishida. R&P Haruto Jshii. Circ: 700.

578.77 JPN ISSN 0387-8961
THE PLANKTON SOCIETY OF JAPAN. BULLETIN/NIHON PURANKUTON GAKKAIHO. Text in Japanese. 1953. s-a. JPY 10,000 (effective 2000). adv. bk.rev. **Document type:** *Bulletin, Academic/Scholarly.* **Description:** Covers all aspects of zoo- and phytoplankton in marine, freshwater, brackish and airborne environments.
Indexed: Agrindex, Appl.Ecol.Abstr. (coverage dropped), Aqua.Sci.& Fish.Abstr., Aquacult.Abstr., Biol.Abstr., Curr.Adv.Ecol.Sci., Deep Sea Res.& Oceanogr.Abstr., Environ.Sci.Poll.Mgmt., Jap.Per.Ind., Ocean.Abstr. (coverage dropped), Sel.Water Res.Abstr., Zoo.Rec.
—CISTI.
Published by: Plankton Society of Japan/Nihon Purankuton Gakkai, c/o tokyo University of Fisheries, 4-5-7 Kounan, Minato-ku, Tokyo 108-8477, Japan. TEL 81-3-5463-0539, FAX 81-3-5463-0539, plankton@tokyo-u-fish.ac.jp, http://www2.ori.u-tokyo.ac.jp/plankton/soc/PlanktonSocJ.html. Ed. Naonobu Shiga. R&P, Adv. contact Haruto Jshii. Circ: 700.

581.7 GBR ISSN 0140-7791
CODEN: PLCEDV
PLANT, CELL AND ENVIRONMENT. Text in English. 1978. m., latest vol.25, 2002. GBP 99 in Europe to individuals; USD 157 in North America to individuals; GBP 109 elsewhere to individuals; GBP 1,131 in Europe to institutions; USD 1,793 in North America to institutions; GBP 1,245 elsewhere to institutions (effective 2002). adv. bk.rev. bibl. illus. index. reprint service avail. from ISI. *Refereed.* **Document type:** *Academic/Scholarly.* **Description:** Publishes original research, either theoretical or experimental, in any field of the physiology of green plants.
Related titles: Microform ed.: (from PQC); Online - full text ed.: Plant, Cell and Environment Online. ISSN 1365-3040. 1998. GBP 90 in Europe to individuals; USD 142 in North America to individuals; GBP 90 elsewhere to individuals; GBP 1,018 in Europe to institutions; USD 1,614 in North America to institutions; GBP 1,018 elsewhere to institutions (effective 2002) (from EBSCO Publishing, O C L C Online Computer Library Center, Inc., RoweCom Information Quest, ingenta, Munksgaard & Blackwell Science's Synergy, Swets Blackwell, Institute for Scientific Information).
Indexed: ASCA, AgBiotech, Agri.& Environ.Biotech.Abstr. (coverage dropped), Agri.Eng.Abstr., Agricola, Agroforest.Abstr., Aqua.Sci.& Fish.Abstr., Aquacult.Abstr., Bibl.Agri., Biol.Abstr., Chem.Abstr., Chem.Cit.Ind., Chem.Indus.Notes, Chem.Titles, Cott.& Trop.Fibr.Abstr., Crop Physiol.Abstr., Curr.Adv.Ecol.Sci., Curr.Adv.Plant Sci., Curr.Cont., Derwent Biotech.Abstr., Ecol.Abstr., Environ.Abstr., Environ.Per.Bibl. (1989-), Environ.Sci.Poll.Mgmt., Excerp.Med., Fababean Abstr., Field Crop Abstr., Forest Prod.Abstr., Forest.Abstr., Geo.Abstr.P.G., Herb.Abstr., Hort.Abstr., IBR, Ind.Sci.Rev., Int.Abstr.Biol.Sci., Irr.& Drain.Abstr., Maize Abstr., Mass Spectr.Bull., Meteor.& Geoastrophys.Abstr., Nutr.Abstr., Ornam.Hort., Plant Breed.Abstr., Plant Gen.Res.Abstr., Plant Grow.Reg.Abstr., Plant Sci., Pollut.Abstr., Postharvest, Potato Abstr., Rev.Appl.Entomol., Rev.Plant Path., Rice Abstr., Sci.Cit.Ind., Seed Abstr., Sel.Water Res.Abstr., Soils & Fert., Soyabean Abstr., Triticale Abstr., VITIS, Weed Abstr.
—BLDSC (6514.200000), CASDDS, CISTI, EMDOCS, IDS, ingenta, Linda Hall. **CCC.**
Published by: Blackwell Science Ltd., Osney Mead, Oxford OX2 0EL, United Kingdom. TEL 44-1865-206206, FAX 44-1865-721205, journals.cs@blacksci.co.uk, http://www.blackwell-science.com. Ed. Harry Smith. Pub. Sue Hewitt. R&P Sophie Savage. Adv. contact Jenny Applin. Circ: 760.

572.8 NLD ISSN 0167-4412
CODEN: PMBIDB
PLANT MOLECULAR BIOLOGY; an international journal on molecular biology, biochemistry and genetic engineering. Text in English. 1981. 18/yr. EUR 2,304 to institutions for print or online ed.; EUR 2,764.80 to institutions print & online eds.combined (effective 2002). adv. bk.rev. illus. Index. back issues avail.; reprint service avail. from SWZ. *Refereed.* **Document type:** *Academic/Scholarly.* **Description:** Publishes research concerned with plant molecular biology, biochemistry and plant molecular genetics, including cyanobacteria and algae.
Related titles: Microform ed.: (from PQC); Online - full text ed.: (from EBSCO Publishing, O C L C Online Computer Library Center, Inc., RoweCom Information Quest, Swets Blackwell, Kluwer Online, Institute for Scientific Information).
Indexed: ASCA, AgBiotech, Agri.& Environ.Biotech.Abstr., Agricola, Agroforest.Abstr., Aqua.Sci.& Fish.Abstr., BBCI, Bibl.Agri., Biol.Abstr., Biotech.Cit.Ind., Chem.Abstr., Chem.Titles, Cott.& Trop.Fibr.Abstr., Crop Physiol.Abstr., Curr.Adv.Biochem., Curr.Adv.Ecol.Sci., Curr.Adv.Gen.& Molec.Biol., Curr.Adv.Plant Sci., Curr.Biotech.Abstr., Curr.Cont., Derwent Biotech.Abstr., Eng.Ind., Environ.Sci.Poll.Mgmt., Fababean Abstr., Field Crop Abstr., Food Sci.& Tech.Abstr., Forest.Abstr., Genet.Abstr., Helminthol.Abstr., Hort.Abstr., Hum.Gen.Abstr., Ind.Med. (1981-), Ind.Sci.Rev., Int.Abstr.Biol.Sci., Maize Abstr., Microbiol.Abstr., NPU, Nuc.Acids Abstr., Oncog.G.F.Abstr. (coverage dropped), Ornam.Hort., Plant Breed.Abstr., Plant Gen.Res.Abstr., Plant Grow.Reg.Abstr., Plant Sci., Postharvest, Potato Abstr., Ref.Zh., Rev.Appl.Entomol., Rev.Arom.& Med.Plants, Rev.Plant Path., Rice Abstr., Sci.Cit.Ind., Seed Abstr., Soyabean Abstr., Telegen, Triticale Abstr., VITIS, Weed Abstr.
—BLDSC (6520.350000), CASDDS, CISTI, EMDOCS, GNLM, IDS, ingenta, Linda Hall. **CCC.**
Published by: (International Society for Plant Molecular Biology), Kluwer Academic Publishers Group (Subsidiary of: Wolters Kluwer N.V.), Spuiboulevard 50, PO Box 17, Dordrecht 3300 AA, Netherlands. FAX 31-78-639-2254, services@wkap.nl, http://www.wkap.nl. Ed. Stephen H Howell. **Dist. by:** Kluwer Academic Publishing Group, PO Box 332, Dordrecht 3300 AH, Netherlands. TEL 31-78-639-2392, FAX 31-78-654-6474.

571.3 GBR ISSN 0953-7104
CODEN: PLTEEF
PLATELETS (ABINGDON). Text in English. 1990. 8/yr. GBP 155, USD 259 to individuals; GBP 504, USD 829 to institutions (effective 2002). *Refereed.* **Document type:** *Academic/Scholarly.* **Description:** Covers all aspects of platelet-related research, including vascular disease, cerebral and myocardial ischaemia, asthma, inflammation, growth factors, pathology and morphology of platelets, and comparison with other cells and clinical trials of anti-platelet agents.
Related titles: Online - full text ed.: ISSN 1369-1635 (from CatchWord Ltd., EBSCO Publishing, O C L C Online Computer Library Center, Inc., RoweCom Information Quest, Swets Blackwell, Institute for Scientific Information).
Indexed: Curr.Cont., Ind.Med., Ind.Sci.Rev., Ref.Zh., Sci.Cit.Ind.
—BLDSC (6537.844500), ADONIS, CASDDS, CatchWord, CISTI, EMDOCS, GNLM, IDS, Infotrieve, KNAW. **CCC.**
Published by: Carfax Publishing Limited (Subsidiary of: Taylor & Francis Group), Carfax Publishing Co, PO Box 24, Abingdon, Oxon OX14 3UE, United Kingdom. FAX 44-1235-401550, enquiries@carfax.co.uk, enquiries@carfax.co.uk/, http://www.carfax.co.uk. Ed. S Heptinstall. Circ: 200.

570 DEU ISSN 0722-4060
QL104 CODEN: POBIDP
POLAR BIOLOGY. Text in English. 1982. m. EUR 1,581.10 domestic; EUR 1,570.70 in Germany; EUR 155 newsstand/cover foreign (effective 2002). reprint service avail. from ISI. *Refereed.* **Document type:** *Journal, Academic/Scholarly.* **Description:** Presents results of all kinds of studies in plants, animals, and microorganisms of marine, limnic and terrestrial habitats of Arctic and Antarctic regions.
Related titles: Microfiche ed.: (from PQC); Online - full text ed.: ISSN 1432-2056 (from EBSCO Publishing, RoweCom Information Quest, Swets Blackwell, Springer LINK, Institute for Scientific Information).
Indexed: ASCA, Appl.Ecol.Abstr., Aqua.Sci.& Fish.Abstr., Aquacult.Abstr., Chem.Abstr., Curr.Adv.Ecol.Sci., Curr.Cont., Deep Sea Res.& Oceanogr.Abstr., Ecol.Abstr., Entomol.Abstr., Environ.Sci.Poll.Mgmt., Geo.Abstr.H.G., Geo.Abstr.P.G., GeoRef, Geol.Abstr., Helminthol.Abstr., INIS Atomind., Ind.Sci.Rev., Int.Abstr.Biol.Sci., Irr.& Drain.Abstr., Meteor.& Geoastrophys.Abstr., Ocean.Abstr., Plant Breed.Abstr., Plant Gen.Res.Abstr., Rev.Appl.Entomol., Rev.Med.& Vet.Mycol., Rev.Plant Path., Sci.Cit.Ind., Soils & Fert., Sport Fish.Abstr., Zoo.Rec.
—BLDSC (6541.936500), CASDDS, CISTI, EMDOCS, IDS, Infotrieve, ingenta, Linda Hall. **CCC.**
Published by: Springer-Verlag (Subsidiary of: BertelsmannSpringer), Tiergartenstr 17, Heidelberg 69121, Germany. TEL 49-6221-345-0, FAX 49-6221-345229, subscriptions@springer.de, http://link.springer.de/link/service/journals/00300/index.htm, http://www.springer.de. Ed. G Hempel. **Subscr. in N. America to:** Springer-Verlag New York Inc., PO Box 2485, Secaucus, NJ 07096-2485. TEL 212-460-1500, FAX 212-473-6272.

570.11 JPN ISSN 1344-6231
QH95.58 CODEN: PNSBEF
POLAR BIOSCIENCE. Text in English. 1967. a., latest vol.14, 2001. per issue exchange basis. *Refereed.* **Document type:** *Academic/Scholarly.*
Formerly (until 1998): N I P R Symposium on Polar Biology. Proceedings (0914-563X); Supersedes in part (in 1987): National Institute of Polar Research. Memoirs. Special Issue (0386-0744); Which was formerly (until 1972): Japanese Antarctic Research Expedition Scientific Reports. Special Issue (0386-5452)
Indexed: Aqua.Sci.& Fish.Abstr., Aquacult.Abstr., Environ.Sci.Poll.Mgmt., GeoRef, Meteor.& Geoastrophys.Abstr., Sport Fish.Abstr., Wild.Rev., Zoo.Rec.
—BLDSC (6541.936600), CASDDS, CISTI, ingenta, KNAW.
Published by: National Institute of Polar Research/Kokuritsu Kyokuchi Kenkyujo, Publications, 9-10, Kiga 1-chome, Itabashi-ku, Tokyo 173, Japan. TEL 81-3-3962-2214, FAX 81-3-3962-2225, publication@nipr.ac.jp. Ed. Okitsugu Watanabe. Circ: 1,000.

570 POL ISSN 0867-1656
QH301 CODEN: BPABEN
POLISH ACADEMY OF SCIENCES. BULLETIN. BIOLOGICAL SCIENCES. Text in English. 1953. q. PLZ 156 domestic; USD 116 foreign; PLZ 39 newsstand/cover domestic; USD 29 newsstand/cover foreign (effective 2001). adv. bibl, charts, illus. *Refereed.* **Document type:** *Bulletin, Academic/Scholarly.*
Formerly (until 1983): Academie Polonaise des Sciences. Bulletin. Serie des Sciences Biologiques (0001-4087)

Indexed: Abstr.Hyg., AgroAgen, AgroLibrex, Anim.Breed.Abstr., Biol.Abstr., Chem.Abstr., Chem.Indus.Notes, Chem.Titles, Curr.Adv.Ecol.Sci., Dairy Sci.Abstr., Deep Sea Res.& Oceanogr.Abstr., Excerp.Med., Fababean Abstr., Field Crop Abstr., Food Sci.& Tech.Abstr., GeoRef, Helminthol.Abstr., Herb.Abstr., Hort.Abstr., INIS Atomind., Ind.Med. (coverage dropped), Ind.Vet., Nutr.Abstr., Ornam.Hort., Plant Breed.Abstr., Sci.Cit.Ind. (coverage dropped), Seed Abstr., Soils & Fert., Sport Fish.Abstr., Trop.Dis.Bull., Vet.Bull., Weed Abstr., Wild.Rev., Zoo.Rec.
—CASDDS, CISTI, GNLM, Linda Hall.
Published by: Polska Akademia Nauk, Centrum Upowszechniania Nauki, Palac Kultury i Nauki, Pietro XXIII, pok 23-10, Warsaw 00901, Poland. TEL 48-22-6204900, FAX 48-22-8272768, ceunpan@warman.com.pl, ceunpan@pan.com.pl, http://www.pan.pl/bulletin/. Ed. Janusz Jeliaszewicz. R&P, Adv. contact Andrzej Kostkowski. B&W page USD 700, color page USD 1,000. Circ: 180. **Dist. by:** Ars Polona, Krakowskie Przedmiescie 7, Warsaw, Poland.

B

577 POL ISSN 1505-2249
QH162 CODEN: PJECFN
POLISH JOURNAL OF ECOLOGY. Text and summaries in English, Polish. 1953. q. USD 105 foreign (effective 2000). bk.rev. bibl, illus. **Document type:** *Academic/Scholarly.* **Description:** Original scientific papers dealing with all aspects of ecology: both fundamental and applied, physiological ecology, ecology of population, community, ecosystem, landscape as well as global ecology.
Former titles (until vol.45, no.3-4, 1997): Ekologia Polska (0420-9036); (until 1970): Ekologia Polska. Seria A (0070-9557); (until 1955): Ekologia Polska
Indexed: AgroAgen, AgroLibrex, Appl.Ecol.Abstr., Aqua.Sci.& Fish.Abstr., Bio-Contr.News & Info., Biol.Abstr., Chem.Abstr., Curr.Adv.Ecol.Sci., Curr.Cont. (coverage dropped), Curr.Ref.Fish Res., Deep Sea Res.& Oceanogr.Abstr., Ecol.Abstr., Entomol.Abstr., Environ.Sci.Poll.Mgmt., Excerp.Med., Field Crop Abstr., Forest Prod.Abstr., Forest.Abstr., Geo.Abstr.P.G., GeoRef, Herb.Abstr., Hort.Abstr., INIS Atomind., Key Word Ind.Wildl.Res., Microbiol.Abstr., Plant Breed.Abstr., Pollut.Abstr., Rev.Appl.Entomol., Sel.Water Res.Abstr., Soils & Fert., Sport Fish.Abstr., Triticale Abstr., Wild.Rev., Zoo.Rec.
—BLDSC (6543.668000), CASDDS, CISTI, ingenta, Linda Hall.
Published by: Polska Akademia Nauk, Instytut Ekologii, Dziekanow Lesny k-Warszawy, Lomianki, Poland. TEL 48-22-7513046, FAX 48-22-7513100. Ed. Leszek Grum. R&P Anna Hillbricht Ilkowska. Circ: 980. **Dist. by:** Ars Polona, Krakowskie Przedmiescie 7, Warsaw, Poland.

571.9 POL ISSN 1233-9687
CODEN: PAPOAC
POLISH JOURNAL OF PATHOLOGY. Text in Polish. 1950. q. USD 60 foreign (effective 2000). adv. bk.rev. illus. index. *Refereed.* **Document type:** *Academic/Scholarly.* **Description:** Contains papers reporting experimental research in pathology.
Formerly (until 1993): Patologia Polska (0031-3114)
Indexed: Biol.Abstr., Chem.Abstr., Chem.Indus.Notes, Chem.Titles, Excerp.Med., INIS Atomind., Ind.Med. (1994-).
—CASDDS, CISTI, GNLM.
Published by: Polskie Towarzystwo Patologow/Polish Society of Pathologists, Ul Grzegorzecka 16, Krakow 31531, Poland. TEL 48-12-4211564, FAX 48-12-4215210, mpstachu@cyf-kr.edu.pl; jszymas@ampat.amu.edu.pl, http://www.bj.uj.edu.pl/cm/pato. Ed. Jerzy Stachura. Adv. contact Wojciech Dabros. Circ: 700. **Co-sponsor:** International Academy of Pathology, Polish Division.

POLLICHIA. MITTEILUNGEN. see *EARTH SCIENCES*

570 POL ISSN 0079-4619
QH7 CODEN: PTPRAI
POZNANSKIE TOWARZYSTWO PRZYJACIOL NAUK. KOMISJA BIOLOGICZNA. PRACE. Text in English, Polish; Summaries in English. 1921. irreg., latest vol.74, 1994. price varies. **Document type:** *Academic/Scholarly.*
Indexed: Biol.Abstr., Chem.Abstr., GeoRef.
—Linda Hall.
Published by: (Komisja Biologiczna), Poznanskie Towarzystwo Przyjaciol Nauk, Ul Sew Mielzynskiego 27-29, Poznan 61725, Poland. **Dist. by:** Ars Polona, Krakowskie Przedmiescie 7, Warsaw, Poland.

DER PRAEPARATOR. see *CONSERVATION*

570 HRV ISSN 0351-0662
QH7
PRIRODA. Text in Croatian. 1911. 10/yr.
—BLDSC (6615.800000).
Published by: (Hrvatsko Prirodsovno Drustvo), Vjesnik, Avenija Bratstva i Jedinstva 4, Zagreb 41000, Croatia. TEL 041-515-555. Ed. Tomislav Krcmar. Circ: 10,000.

573.6 RUS ISSN 1025-7217
PROBLEMY REPRODUKTSII. Text in English, Russian. 1995. bi-m. RUR 288 for 6 mos. to individuals; RUR 360 for 6 mos. to institutions (effective 2002). **Document type:** *Academic/Scholarly.*
Indexed: Ref.Zh.
—BLDSC (0133.627000).
Published by: Media Sfera, Dmitrovskoe shosse 46, korp 2, etazh 4, P.O. Box 54, Moscow 127238, Russian Federation. TEL 7-095-4820604, 7-095-4884118, FAX 7-095-2676142, mediashp@mediasphera.ru. Ed. M B Anshina. **US dist. addr.:** East View Publications, 3020 Harbor Ln N, Minneapolis, MN 55447. TEL 612-550-0961.

570 USA ISSN 0172-6625
CODEN: PRLSEP
PROCEEDINGS IN LIFE SCIENCES. Text in English. 1976. irreg. price varies. **Document type:** *Proceedings.*
—CCC.
Published by: Springer-Verlag, Journals (Subsidiary of: BertelsmannSpringer), 175 Fifth Ave, New York, NY 10010. TEL 212-460-1500, FAX 212-473-6272. Eds. A Gorio, D G Weiss.

PROGRESS IN CLINICAL AND BIOLOGICAL RESEARCH. see *MEDICAL SCIENCES*

578.77 USA ISSN 0079-6603
QP551 CODEN: PNMBAF
PROGRESS IN NUCLEIC ACID RESEARCH AND MOLECULAR BIOLOGY. Text in English. 1963. irreg., latest vol.60, 1998. reprint service avail. from ISI. *Refereed.*
Formerly (until vol.2): Progress in Nucleic Acid Research
Related titles: Online - full text ed.: (from Institute for Scientific Information).
Indexed: ASCA, AgBiotech, Agricola, Anim.Breed.Abstr., Aqua.Sci.& Fish.Abstr., BBCI, Biol.Abstr., Biotech.Cit.Ind., Chem.Abstr., Chem.Cit.Ind., Chem.Titles, Curr.Adv.Ecol.Sci., Dok.Arbeitsmed., Genet.Abstr., Hum.Gen.Abstr., INIS Atomind., Ind.Med. (1964-), Ind.Sci.Rev., Nuc.Acids Abstr., Nutr.Abstr., Oncog.G.F.Abstr. (coverage dropped), Sci.Cit.Ind.
—BLDSC (6871.210000), CASDDS, CISTI, GNLM, ingenta, Linda Hall. **CCC.**
Published by: Academic Press, Inc., Journal Division (Subsidiary of: Harcourt Brace & Company), 525 B St, Ste 1900, San Diego, CA 92101-4495. TEL 619-231-0926, FAX 619-699-6715. Eds. J N Davidson, Waldo E Cohn. **Subscr. to:** Order Dept., 6277 Sea Harbor Dr, 4th Fl, Orlando, FL 32887. TEL 800-321-5068.

570 DEU ISSN 1434-4610
QL366 CODEN: PROTFA
PROTIST. Text in English. 1902. 4/yr. DEM 153, GBP 110 to individuals; EUR 368, GBP 298 to institutions (effective 2002). adv. bk.rev. bibl, charts, illus. index. cum.index: vols.1-50, 1902-1918 (in 2 vols.). reprint service avail. from ISI. *Refereed.* **Document type:** *Journal, Academic/Scholarly.* **Description:** Publishes original papers, short historical perspectives, and news and views in all areas of research on protists.
Formerly (until 1998): Archiv fuer Protistenkunde (0003-9365)
Related titles: Microfilm ed.: (from BHP); Online - full text ed.: (from EBSCO Publishing, ingenta, Swets Blackwell, Institute for Scientific Information).
Indexed: ASCA, Abstr.Hyg., Aqua.Sci.& Fish.Abstr., Bio-Contr.News & Info., Biol.Abstr., Chem.Abstr., Curr.Adv.Ecol.Sci., Curr.Adv.Plant Sci., Curr.Cont., Deep Sea Res.& Oceanogr.Abstr., Environ.Sci.Poll.Mgmt., Excerp.Med., GeoRef, Helminthol.Abstr., INIS Atomind., Ind.Med. (1998-), Ind.Sci.Rev., Ind.Vet., Int.Abstr.Biol.Sci., Microbiol.Abstr., Plant Sci., Protozool.Abstr., Sci.Cit.Ind., Soils & Fert., Trop.Dis.Bull., Vet.Bull., Zoo.Rec.
—BLDSC (6936.450000), CISTI, IDS, Infotrieve, ingenta, Linda Hall. **CCC.**
Published by: Urban & Fischer Verlag, Loebdergraben 14A, Jena 07743, Germany. TEL 49-3641-626444, FAX 49-3641-626500, info@urbanfischer.de, http://www.urbanfischer.de. Ed. Michael Melkonian. Adv. contact Sabine Schroeter. page DEM 550; trim 21.08 x 280. Circ: 350.

PSIQUIATRIA BIOLOGICA. see *MEDICAL SCIENCES—Psychiatry And Neurology*

PUERTO RICO HEALTH SCIENCES JOURNAL. see *MEDICAL SCIENCES*

THE QUARTERLY JOURNAL OF NUCLEAR MEDICINE. see *MEDICAL SCIENCES—Radiology And Nuclear Medicine*

570 USA ISSN 0033-5770
QH301 CODEN: QRBIAK
QUARTERLY REVIEW OF BIOLOGY. Text in English. 1926. q., latest vol.76, 2001, March. USD 38 in United States to individuals; USD 45.66 in Canada to individuals; USD 43 elsewhere to individuals; USD 175 in United States to institutions; USD 192.25 in Canada to institutions; USD 180 elsewhere to institutions; USD 26 in United States Retired persons; USD 32.82 in Canada Retired persons; USD 31 elsewhere Retired persons; USD 26 in United States to students; USD 32.82 in Canada to students; USD 31 elsewhere to students; USD 13.50 newsstand/cover to individuals; USD 47.75 newsstand/cover to institutions (effective 2002). adv. bk.rev., software rev. bibl, charts, illus. index. reprints avail. *Refereed.* **Document type:** *Academic/Scholarly.* **Description:** Features recent research and software reviews in the various fields of the biological sciences.
Related titles: Microform ed.: (from NRP,PQC); Online - full text ed.: (from JSTOR (Web-based Journal Archive), Gale Group, Factiva, Institute for Scientific Information).
Indexed: ASCA, Abstr.Anthropol., Acad.Ind., Anim.Behav.Abstr., Anim.Breed.Abstr., Appl.Ecol.Abstr., Aqua.Sci.& Fish.Abstr., Bio-Contr.News & Info., Biol.& Agr.Ind. (Mar.1983-), Biol.Abstr., Biol.Dig., Bk.Rev.Ind. (1989-), Chem.Abstr., Chem.Indus.Notes, Chem.Titles, Child.Bk.Rev.Ind. (1989-), Curr.Adv.Ecol.Sci., Curr.Cont., Deep Sea Res.& Oceanogr.Abstr., Ecol.Abstr., Entomol.Abstr., Environ.Sci.Poll.Mgmt., Excerp.Med., Gen.Sci.Ind. (Jun.1984-), Geo.Abstr.H.G., GeoRef, Geol.Abstr., Helminthol.Abstr., Hort.Abstr., INIS Atomind., Ind.Med. (1926-), Ind.Sci.Rev., Ind.Vet., Key Word Ind.Wildl.Res., Microbiol.Abstr., NRN, Nutr.Abstr., Plant Breed.Abstr., Protozool.Abstr., Ref.Sour., Ref.Zh., Rev.Appl.Entomol., Rev.Arom.& Med.Plants, Rev.Plant Path., Sci.Cit.Ind., Sel.Water Res.Abstr., Sport Fish.Abstr., Weed Abstr., Wild.Rev., Zoo.Rec.
—BLDSC (7206.000000), ADONIS, CASDDS, CISTI, IDS, ingenta, Linda Hall. **CCC.**
Published by: University of Chicago Press, Journals Division, PO Box 37005, Chicago, IL 60637. TEL 773-753-3347, FAX 773-753-0811, subscriptions@journals.uchicago.edu, orders@press.uchicago.edu, http://www.journals.uchicago.edu/QRB/home.html. Eds. Albert D Carlson, James D Thomson. Adv. contact Timothy Hill. page USD 510; trim 10 x 6.75. Circ: 3,200 (paid and controlled).

QUARTERLY REVIEWS OF BIOPHYSICS. see *BIOLOGY—Biophysics*

578.77 CAN
QUEBEC (PROVINCE). DIRECTION DE L'INNOVATION ET DES TECHNOLOGIES. ACTIVITES (YEAR). Text in French. 1953-1979; N.S. 1988. a. free per issue. **Document type:** *Government.*
Formerly (until 1996): Quebec (Province). Direction de la Recherche Scientifique et Technique. Activites (Year); Supersedes (in 1988): Quebec (Province). Direction Generale des Peches Maritimes. Direction de la Recherche. Rapport Annuel (0318-8779); (in 1969): Quebec (Province). Marine Biological Station, Grande-Riviere. Rapport (0079-8754)
Indexed: Aqua.Sci.& Fish.Abstr., Biol.Abstr., Ocean.Abstr. (coverage dropped).
—CISTI.
Published by: Ministere de l'Agriculture, des Pecheries et de l'Alimentation, 96 Montee de Sandy Beach, bur. 205, Gaspe, PQ G4X 2V6, Canada. TEL 418-368-7615, FAX 418-360-8211, pcarrier@agr.gouv.qc.ca.

509 AUS ISSN 0079-8843
CODEN: QLNAAE
QUEENSLAND NATURALIST. Text in English. 1908. s-a. AUD 12. *Refereed.* **Document type:** *Academic/Scholarly.* **Description:** Covers natural history and natural science.
Indexed: Aqua.Sci.& Fish.Abstr., Biol.Abstr., Environ.Sci.Poll.Mgmt., GeoRef, Ocean.Abstr., Pollut.Abstr., Sport Fish.Abstr., Wild.Rev., Zoo.Rec.
—CISTI, ingenta, Linda Hall.
Published by: Queensland Naturalists' Club Inc., Brisbane, GPO Box 5663, West End, QLD 4101, Australia. TEL 61-7-33652300, FAX 61-7-33651355, p.woodall@mailbox.uq.edu.au. Ed. Peter Woodall. Circ: 600.

570 ESP ISSN 0583-7499
REAL SOCIEDAD ESPANOLA DE HISTORIA NATURAL. BOLETIN. ACTAS. Text in Spanish; Summaries in English, French. 1872. a. ESP 7,000 to individual members; ESP 10,000 to institutional members. bk.rev. reprint service avail. from SCH,PSC. **Document type:** *Bulletin, Academic/Scholarly.*
Supersedes in part (in 1950): Real Sociedad Espanola de Historia Natural. Boletin (0365-9755); Which superseded in part (in 1901): Sociedad Espanola de Historia Natural. Anales (0210-5160)
Indexed: Biol.Abstr., Curr.Adv.Ecol.Sci., Deep Sea Res.& Oceanogr.Abstr., GeoRef, Helminthol.Abstr., Ind.SST, Rev.Appl.Entomol.
—CINDOC, CISTI.
Published by: Real Sociedad Espanola de Historia Natural, Facultades de Biologia y Geologia, Ciudad Universitaria, Madrid 28040, Spain. TEL 34-1-3945000, FAX 34-1-3945000, rsehno@eucmax.sim.ucm.es, http://www.ucm.es/info/rsehn/. Ed. Antonio Perejon Rincon. Circ: 900.

RECENT ADVANCES IN HISTOPATHOLOGY. see *MEDICAL SCIENCES*

577 IND ISSN 0971-1708
CODEN: PGECDY
RECENT RESEARCHES IN ECOLOGY, ENVIRONMENT AND POLLUTION. Text in English. 1988. irreg., latest vol.10, 1993. price varies. **Document type:** *Monographic series.*
Formerly (until 1988): Progress in Ecology (0253-665X)
Indexed: Biol.Abstr., Chem.Abstr., Curr.Cont. (coverage dropped), Zoo.Rec.
—BLDSC (7305.087900), CASDDS, CISTI, Infotrieve. **CCC.**
Published by: Today and Tomorrow's Printers & Publishers, 24 B-5 Desh Bandhu Gupta Rd., Karol Bagh, New Delhi 110 005, India. TEL 5721928. Ed. Malabika Ray. **Dist. in U.S. by:** Scholarly Publications, 2825 Wilcrest Dr, Ste 255, Houston, TX 77042. TEL 713-781-0070.

REFERATIVNYI ZHURNAL. BIOLOGIYA. see *BIOLOGY—Abstracting, Bibliographies, Statistics*

REFERATIVNYI ZHURNAL. BIOLOGIYA SEL'SKOKHOZYAISTVENNYKH ZHIVOTNYKH. see *BIOLOGY—Abstracting, Bibliographies, Statistics*

REFERATIVNYI ZHURNAL. EKOLOGIYA CHELOVEKA. see *BIOLOGY—Abstracting, Bibliographies, Statistics*

REFERATIVNYI ZHURNAL. OBSHCHIE VOPROSY PATOLOGICHESKOI ANATOMII. see *BIOLOGY—Abstracting, Bibliographies, Statistics*

REFERATIVNYI ZHURNAL. RASTENIEVODSTVO (BIOLOGICHESKIE OSNOVY). see *BIOLOGY—Abstracting, Bibliographies, Statistics*

573.6 GBR ISSN 1470-1626
▼ **REPRODUCTION.** Text in English. 2001 (Jan). m. GBP 350, EUR 560, USD 595 (effective 2001); GBP 395, EUR 633, USD 670 (effective 2002). adv. 180 p./no. 2 cols./p. back issues avail. **Document type:** *Journal, Academic/Scholarly.* **Description:** Publishes topical reviews on basic mechanisms, recent developments and new hypotheses in the field of reproductive biology.
Formed by the merger of (1996-2000): Reviews of Reproduction (1359-6004); (1960-2000): Journal of Reproduction and Fertility (0022-4251); Which was formerly (1949-1958): Society for the Study of Fertility. Proceedings (0562-4142)
Related titles: Online - full text ed.: Avail. only as part of subscr. to hard copy edition (from Institute for Scientific Information).
Indexed: Biol.& Agr.Ind. (Jan.2001-), Curr.Cont., Focus on: Vet.Sci.& Med., Ind.Med.
—BLDSC (7713.597800).
Published by: Journals of Reproduction & Fertility Ltd, 22 Newmarket Rd, Cambridge CB5 8DT, United Kingdom. TEL 44-1223-351809, FAX 44-1223-359754, jrf@journals-of-reproduction.org.uk, http://www.journals-of-reproduction.org.uk. Ed. Prof R Webb. Adv. contact Mrs. C H Clarke. **Dist. by:** Portland Press Ltd., PO Box 32, Commerce Way, Colchester, Essex C02 8HP, United Kingdom.

570 AUS ISSN 1031-3613
QH251 CODEN: RFDEEH
REPRODUCTION, FERTILITY AND DEVELOPMENT. Text in English. 1989. 8/yr. AUD 625 combined subscription domestic for print & online eds.; USD 550 combined subscription foreign for print & online eds. (effective 2002). adv. charts, illus. index. back issues avail. *Refereed.* **Document type:** *Journal, Academic/Scholarly.* **Description:** Covers reproductive biology, reproductive endocrinology and developmental biology.
Formed by the merger of (1982-1989): Clinical Reproduction and Fertility (0725-556X); (1948-1989): Australian Journal of Biological Sciences (0004-9417)
Related titles: Microform ed.: (from PQC); Online - full content ed.: AUD 555, USD 470 (effective 2002) (from EBSCO Publishing, Swets Blackwell); Online - full text ed.: (from Institute for Scientific Information).
Indexed: ASCA, Abstr.Hyg., AgBiotech, Agri.& Environ.Biotech.Abstr. (coverage dropped), Agricola, Anim.Breed.Abstr., Aqua.Sci.& Fish.Abstr., Biol.& Agr.Ind. (Jan.1983-Dec.1988), Biol.Abstr., Chem.Abstr., Chem.Indus.Notes, Chem.Titles, Curr.Adv.Ecol.Sci., Curr.Biotech.Abstr., Curr.Cont., Curr.Leather Lit., Curr.Ref.Fish Res., Dairy Sci.Abstr., Deep Sea Res.& Oceanogr.Abstr., Environ.Per.Bibl., Excerp.Med., Field Crop Abstr., Food Sci.& Tech.Abstr., Forest Prod.Abstr., Forest.Abstr., GeoRef, Helminthol.Abstr., Hort.Abstr., INIS Atomind., Ind.Med. (1989-), Ind.Sci.Rev., Ind.Vet., Inpharma, Int.Abstr.Biol.Sci., Nutr.Abstr., Ocean.Abstr., Pharm.&Out.News, Pig News & Info., Plant Breed.Abstr., Poult.Abstr., Reac., Rev.Appl.Entomol., Rev.Med.& Vet.Mycol., Rev.Plant Path., Russ.Acad.Sci.Bibl., SSCI (coverage dropped), Sci.Cit.Ind., Soils & Fert., Soyabean Abstr., Sport Fish.Abstr., Triticale Abstr., Trop.Dis.Bull., Vet.Bull., Weed Abstr., Wild.Rev., Zoo.Rec.
—BLDSC (7713.603000), CASDDS, CISTI, EMDOCS, GNLM, IDS, Infotrieve, ingenta, Linda Hall. **CCC.**
Published by: (C S I R O Australia), C S I R O Publishing, 150 Oxford St, Collingwood, VIC 3066, Australia. TEL 61-3-96627629, FAX 61-3-9662-7611, camilla.myers@publish.csiro.au, publishing@csiro.au, http://www.publish.csiro.au/journals/rfd. Ed. Camilla Myers. Circ: 600.

573.6 FRA ISSN 0926-5287
SF768 CODEN: RNDEE5
REPRODUCTION, NUTRITION, DEVELOPMENT. Text in English; Abstracts in English. 1961. bi-m. FRF 2,293 domestic; EUR 406 in the European Union; EUR 428 elsewhere (effective 2001). adv. charts, illus. index. *Refereed.* **Document type:** *Academic/Scholarly.* **Description:** Presents papers about reproduction, development and nutrition in animals.
Former titles (until 1989): Reproduction, Nutrition, Developpement (0181-1916); (until 1980): Annales de Biologie Animale, Biochimie, Biophysique (0003-388X)
Related titles: Online - full text ed.: ISSN 1297-9708 (from EBSCO Publishing, ingenta, Swets Blackwell, Institute for Scientific Information, RoweCom Information Quest).
Indexed: ASCA, AgBiotech, Agri.& Environ.Biotech.Abstr. (coverage dropped), Anal.Abstr., Anim.Breed.Abstr., Biol.Abstr., Chem.Abstr., Chem.Indus.Notes, Chem.Titles, Curr.Adv.Cell & Devel.Biol., Curr.Adv.Ecol.Sci., Curr.Adv.Gen.& Molec.Biol., Curr.Cont., Dairy Sci.Abstr., Deep Sea Res.& Oceanogr.Abstr., Dent.Ind., Derwent Biotech.Abstr., Excerp.Med., Field Crop Abstr., Focus on: Vet.Sci.& Med., Food Sci.& Tech.Abstr., Genet.Abstr. (coverage dropped), Helminthol.Abstr., Herb.Abstr., INIS Atomind., Ind.Med. (1989-), Ind.Sci.Rev., Ind.Vet., Inpharma, Int.Abstr.Biol.Sci., Maize Abstr., Nutr.Abstr., Pig News & Info., Poult.Abstr., Protozool.Abstr., Reac., Rev.Arom.& Med.Plants, Sci.Cit.Ind., Soyabean Abstr., Sport Fish.Abstr., Sugar Ind.Abstr., Triticale Abstr., Vet.Bull.
—BLDSC (7713.630000), CASDDS, CISTI, EMDOCS, GNLM, IDS, Infotrieve, ingenta, Linda Hall. **CCC.**
Published by: (France. Institut National de la Recherche Agronomique), E D P Sciences, 7 av. du Hoggar, B.P. 112, P.A. de Courtaboeuf, Les Ulis Cedex A 91944, France. TEL 33-1-69187575, FAX 33-1-69288491, subscribers@edpsciences.org, http:// www.edpsciences.org. Circ: 2,000.

573.6 PHL
REPRODUCTIONS. Text in English. 1970. irreg. (15-20/yr.). PHP 5, USD 4. bk.rev.
Published by: (University of Santo Tomas), University of Santo Tomas, Institute for the Study of Human Reproduction (Subsidiary of: University of Santo Tomas), Faculty of Medicine, Espana St, Sampaloc, Manila, Philippines. Ed. Dr. Vicente J A Rosales. Circ: 5,000.

REPUBLIC OF CHINA. NATIONAL SCIENCE COUNCIL. PROCEEDINGS. PART B: LIFE SCIENCES. see *MEDICAL SCIENCES*

RESONANCE (SUMTERVILLE). see *PHYSICS*

570 CUB ISSN 0864-3490
QH301
REVISTA BIOLOGIA. Text in Spanish, English. 1987. s-a. CUP 30 domestic; USD 30 foreign (effective 2000). back issues avail. *Refereed.* **Document type:** *Academic/Scholarly.* **Description:** Includes research in the field of biology and related issues.
Indexed: Bio-Contr.News & Info., Field Crop Abstr., Hort.Abstr., Nutr.Abstr., Ornam.Hort., Plant Breed.Abstr., Plant Gen.Res.Abstr., Ref.Zh., Rev.Appl.Entomol., Rev.Plant Path., Soils & Fert., Sugar Ind.Abstr., Zoo.Rec.
Published by: Universidad de La Habana, Facultad de Biologia, Calle 25 y J Vedado, Havana, Cuba. TEL 53-537-321321, FAX 53-537-321321, marthap@fbio.oc.uh.cu. Ed. Martha Perez. Pub. Miguel Valdes. Circ: 200 (paid); 100 (controlled).

REVISTA BRASILEIRA DE PARASITOLOGIA VETERINARIA/BRAZILIAN JOURNAL OF VETERINARY PARASITOLOGY. see *VETERINARY SCIENCE*

REVISTA CHILENA DE ANATOMIA. see *MEDICAL SCIENCES*

611.01816 610 CUB ISSN 0864-0300
REVISTA CUBANA DE INVESTIGACIONES BIOMEDICAS. Text in Spanish; Summaries in English, Spanish. s-a. USD 36 in the Americas; USD 44 in Europe; USD 52 elsewhere. bibl, charts, illus. index.
Indexed: I.P.A.
—EMDOCS.
Published by: (Cuba. Ministerio de Salud Publica, Centro Nacional de Informacion de Ciencias Medicas), Editorial de Ciencias Medicas, O'Reilly No. 4, Habana, Cuba. TEL 809-62-8091. Ed. Maura Diaz. Circ: 1,300.
Co-sponsors: Sociedad Cubana de Ciencias Fisiologicas; Instituto Superior de Ciencias Medicales de La Habana.

573.6 CUB ISSN 0138-6700
REVISTA CUBANA DE REPRODUCCION ANIMAL. Abstracts and contents page in English. 1975. 2/yr. USD 14 in North America; USD 15 in South America; USD 19 in Europe. bibl, charts, illus.
Indexed: Agrindex, Anim.Breed.Abstr., Biol.Abstr., Ind.Vet., Poult.Abstr.
—CINDOC.
Published by: Centro de Informacion y Documentacion Agropecuario, Gaveta Postal 4149, Havana 4, Cuba. Ed. J R Morales. **Dist. by:** Ediciones Cubanas, Obispo No. 527, Apdo. 605, Havana, Cuba.

570 PRT ISSN 0034-7736
QH301 CODEN: RVBIAP
REVISTA DE BIOLOGIA. Text in English, French, German, Portuguese. 1957. irreg. price varies. adv. bk.rev. charts, illus. reprint service avail. from PQC. **Document type:** *Academic/Scholarly.*
Related titles: Microform ed.: (from PQC).
Indexed: AgBiotech, Aqua.Sci.& Fish.Abstr., Biol.Abstr., Chem.Abstr., Crop Physiol.Abstr., Curr.Adv.Ecol.Sci., Field Crop Abstr., Forest.Abstr., Herb.Abstr., Hort.Abstr., Ind.Vet., Irr.& Drain.Abstr., Ocean.Abstr., Plant Breed.Abstr., Plant Grow.Reg.Abstr., Ref.Zh., Rev.Appl.Entomol., Rev.Plant Path., Seed Abstr., Soils & Fert., Triticale Abstr., W.R.C.Inf., Weed Abstr., World Ag.Econ.& Rur.Soc.Abstr., Zoo.Rec.
—BLDSC (7842.750000), CASDDS, CISTI.
Published by: Universidade de Lisboa, Museu, Laboratorio e Jardim Botanico, Rua da Escola Politecnica, 58, Lisboa 1250-102, Portugal. TEL 351-21-3921801, FAX 351-21-3970882, jbbiblio@fc.ul.pt, http://wwwjb.ul.pt/. Ed. F M Catarino TEL 351-21-3921890. R&P F.M. Catarino TEL 351-21-3921890. Adv. contact Manuel Dos Santos Lopes. Circ: 250.

570 URY ISSN 0304-971X
QH305.2.U8 CODEN: RBURDA
REVISTA DE BIOLOGIA DEL URUGUAY. Text in Spanish; Summaries in English. 1973. a. USD 20. illus. index. back issues avail. **Document type:** *Academic/Scholarly.*
Indexed: Biol.Abstr., Deep Sea Res.& Oceanogr.Abstr.
—CISTI, Linda Hall.
Published by: Fernando Mane-Garzon, Ed. & Pub., Casilla de Correo 157, Montevideo, Uruguay. Circ: 1,500.

578.77 CHL ISSN 0717-3326
QH91.A1 CODEN: RBIMAY
REVISTA DE BIOLOGIA MARINA Y OCEANOGRAFIA. Text in English, Spanish; Summaries in English, Spanish. 1948. s-a. USD 20 domestic; USD 50 foreign (effective 2000); or exchange basis. cum.index. *Refereed.* **Document type:** *Academic/Scholarly.* **Description:** Presents papers on marine biology, ecology, physical, chemical and biological oceanography, marine geology, and estuarine environment.
Formerly (until 1997): Revista de Biologia Marina (0080-2115)
Indexed: Aqua.Sci.& Fish.Abstr., Aquacult.Abstr., Biol.Abstr., Curr.Adv.Ecol.Sci., Curr.Adv.Plant Sci., Deep Sea Res.& Oceanogr.Abstr., Ecol.Abstr., Environ.Sci.Poll.Mgmt., Geo.Abstr.H.G., GeoRef, Helminthol.Abstr., Mar.Sci.Cont.Tab., Ocean.Abstr. (coverage dropped), Sel.Water Res.Abstr., Sport Fish.Abstr., Wild.Rev., Zoo.Rec.
—BLDSC (7843.100000), CINDOC, CISTI.
Published by: Universidad de Valparaiso, Instituto de Oceanologia, Casilla 13-D, Vina Del Mar, Valparaiso, Chile. FAX 56-32-833214, fbalbon@uv.cl, http://www.uv.cl/FAC/novedad/med/oce/rbiol.htm. Ed., R&P Fernando Balbontin TEL 56-32-832702. Circ: 400.

B

570.909 CRI ISSN 0034-7744
RC960 CODEN: RBTCAP
REVISTA DE BIOLOGIA TROPICAL. Text in English, Spanish. 1953. 4/yr. USD 40 (effective 2000). charts, illus. index. back issues avail.; reprint service avail. from PQC. *Refereed.* **Document type:** *Academic/Scholarly.*
Related titles: Microfilm ed.: (from OMN); Microform ed.: (from PQC); Online - full text ed.: (from Institute for Scientific Information).
Indexed: ASCA, Abstr.Hyg., Agroforest.Abstr., Anim.Breed.Abstr., Apic.Abstr., Aqua.Sci.& Fish.Abstr., Aquacult.Abstr., Bio-Contr.News & Info., Biol.Abstr., Chem.Abstr., Crop Physiol.Abstr., Curr.Adv.Ecol.Sci., Curr.Cont., Dairy Sci.Abstr., Deep Sea Res.& Oceanogr.Abstr., Ecol.Abstr., Entomol.Abstr. (coverage dropped), Environ.Sci.Poll.Mgmt., Field Crop Abstr., Forest.Abstr., GeoRef, Helminthol.Abstr., Herb.Abstr., Hort.Abstr., INIS Atomind., Ind.Med. (1953-), Ind.Vet., Microbiol.Abstr., Nutr.Abstr., Plant Breed.Abstr., Poult.Abstr., Protozool.Abstr., Rev.Appl.Entomol., Rev.Arom.& Med.Plants, Rev.Med.& Vet.Mycol., Rev.Plant Path., Seed Abstr., Sel.Water Res.Abstr., Soils & Fert., Sport Fish.Abstr., Triticale Abstr., Vet.Bull., Weed Abstr., Wild.Rev., Zoo.Rec.
—BLDSC (7843.200000), CASDDS, CINDOC, CISTI, IDS, ingenta, Linda Hall.
Published by: Editorial de la Universidad de Costa Rica, Apdo. 75-2060, Ciudad Univ. R. Facio, San Pedro de Montes de Oca, San Jose 2050, Costa Rica. TEL 506-2075957, FAX 506-2249367, cmmoreno@cariari.ucr.ac.cr. Ed. Julian Monge Najera. R&P Mario Murillo TEL 506-2075003. Circ: 1,000.

578.77 CUB ISSN 0252-1962
QH109.C9 CODEN: RIMAD2
REVISTA DE INVESTIGACIONES MARINAS. Text in Spanish; Summaries in English, Spanish. 1980. 3/yr. CUP 4.50 domestic; USD 24 in North America; USD 25 in South America; USD 26 in Europe.
Indexed: Aqua.Sci.& Fish.Abstr., Aquacult.Abstr., Deep Sea Res.& Oceanogr.Abstr., Environ.Sci.Poll.Mgmt., GeoRef, Ocean.Abstr. (coverage dropped), Zoo.Rec.
—CINDOC, CISTI, KNAW, Linda Hall.
Published by: (Universidad de La Habana, Direccion de Informacion Cientifico- Tecnica), Ediciones Cubanas, Obispo No. 527, Apdo. 605, Havana, Cuba.

REVISTA ECUATORIANA DE MEDICINA Y CIENCIAS BIOLOGICAS. see *MEDICAL SCIENCES*

570 NLD
▼ **REVUE DE L'HISTOIRE DE BIOLOGIE.** Text in French. 1999. s-a. NLG 280, EUR 127 to institutions for print or online ed.; NLG 336, EUR 152.40 to institutions print & online eds.combined (effective 2001). adv. bk.rev. charts, illus. index. reprint service avail. from SWZ. *Refereed.* **Document type:** *Academic/Scholarly.* **Description:** Publishes research on the history of the biological sciences, with emphasis on research on developments of the 19th and 20th centuries, with philosophical issues.
Related titles: Microform ed.: (from PQC); Online - full text ed.: (from O C L C Online Computer Library Center, Inc.); ♦ English ed.: Journal of the History of Biology. ISSN 0022-5010.
—CISTI, ingenta, Linda Hall.
Published by: Kluwer Academic Publishers Group (Subsidiary of: Wolters Kluwer N.V.), Spuiboulevard 50, PO Box 17, Dordrecht 3300 AA, Netherlands. FAX 31-78-639-2254. **Dist. by:** Journals Department, PO Box 322, Dordrecht 3300 AH, Netherlands. TEL 781-871-6600, FAX 31-78-639-6474.

577 FRA ISSN 1166-9632
QH541.5.M66 CODEN: REALEG
REVUE D'ECOLOGIE ALPINE. Text in English, French, German, Italian. 1963. irreg. FRF 200, USD 15. adv. bk.rev. illus, maps. back issues avail. **Document type:** *Academic/Scholarly.* **Description:** Features original articles addressing methods in map-making and applications in ecological studies.
Former titles (until 1988): Documents de Cartographie Ecologique (0335-5330); Documents pour la Carte de la Vegetation des Alpes (0419-5728)
Indexed: Bibl.Cart., Biol.Abstr., GeoRef, Zoo.Rec.
—BLDSC (7898.720000), CISTI.
Published by: Universite de Grenoble I (Universite Scientifique et Medicale de Grenoble), Centre de Biologie Alpine, Universite Joseph Fourier, B.P. 53X, Grenoble Cedex 1 38041, France. Ed. B Souchier. Circ: 900.

570 FRA ISSN 0373-2851
CODEN: RSNAA6
REVUE DES SCIENCES NATURELLES D'AUVERGNE. Text in French. 1921. a. FRF 70. back issues avail.
Indexed: GeoRef, Ref.Zh., Zoo.Rec.
Published by: Societe d'Histoire Naturelle d'Auvergne, Faculte de Botanique, 2 rue Ledru, Clermont-Ferrand 63000, France.

570 FRA ISSN 0338-9898
REVUE FRANCAISE DES LABORATOIRES. Text in French. 1972. 10/yr. EUR 173 in Europe to institutions; USD 216 elsewhere to institutions (effective 2002). adv. *Refereed.* **Document type:** *Academic/Scholarly.* **Description:** Offers articles concentrating on breaking scientific news - both biological and economical - along with developments in research in the diagnostic fields.
Formerly (until 1975): Revue Francaise des Fournisseurs de Laboratoires (0338-988X)
Related titles: Online - full text ed.: (from ScienceDirect).
Indexed: Ref.Zh.
Published by: (Labo-France), Elsevier Paris, Editions Scientifiques et Medicales (Subsidiary of: Reed Elsevier plc. group), 23 rue Linois, Paris 75015, France. TEL 33-1-45589110, FAX 33-1-45589419, http://www.elsevier.com/locate/revfra. Ed. P Lafargue. Circ: 7,000.

570 ITA ISSN 0035-6050
QH301 CODEN: RBILAV
RIVISTA DI BIOLOGIA/BIOLOGY FORUM. Text in English, Italian. 1919. 3/yr. ITL 86,000 domestic; ITL 125,000 foreign; ITL 33,000 newsstand/cover domestic; ITL 48,000 newsstand/cover foreign (effective 2000). index. reprint service avail. from PQC. *Refereed.* **Document type:** *Journal, Academic/Scholarly.* **Description:** Features essays, reviews, critiques and comments on biological topics.
Related titles: Online - full text ed.: (from Institute for Scientific Information).
Indexed: ASCA, Aqua.Sci.& Fish.Abstr., Arts & Hum.Cit.Ind. (coverage dropped), Biol.Abstr., Cal.Tiss.Abstr., Chem.Abstr., Chemorec.Abstr., Curr.Adv.Ecol.Sci., Curr.Cont., Deep Sea Res.& Oceanogr.Abstr., Environ.Per.Bibl. (1989-1994), Excerp.Med., INSPEC (coverage dropped), Ind.Med. (1919-), Nutr.Abstr., Plant Breed.Abstr., Rev.Appl.Entomol., Rev.Plant Path., Sport Fish.Abstr., Zoo.Rec.
—BLDSC (7982.100000), CASDDS, CISTI, GNLM, IDS, Linda Hall.
Published by: (Universita degli Studi di Perugia), Tilgher-Genova s.a.s., Via Assarotti 31, Genoa, MI 16122, Italy. TEL 39-10-8391140, FAX 39-10-870653, tilgher@tilgher.it, http://www.tilgher.it/biologiae.html. R&P Lucio Bozzi. Circ: 750.

571.9 ITA ISSN 0391-1551
CODEN: RBNPD3
RIVISTA DI BIOLOGIA NORMALE E PATOLOGICA. Text and summaries in English, Italian. 1975. bi-m. ITL 10,000. bk.rev. back issues avail.
Indexed: Abstr.Hyg., Biol.Abstr., Chem.Abstr., Excerp.Med., Ind.Vet., Vet.Bull.
—CASDDS. **CCC.**
Published by: Universita degli Studi di Messina, Centro Universitario di Ricerca sui Tumori, Via Giacomo Venezian, Messina, ME 98122, Italy. Ed. Carmelo Cavallaro. Circ: 300.

578.77 ITA ISSN 0048-8399
QH96.25.I8 CODEN: RIIDBN
RIVISTA DI IDROBIOLOGIA. Text in Italian; Summaries in English. 1960. q. per issue exchange basis. bk.rev. illus. cum.index. **Document type:** *Monographic series.*
Indexed: Aqua.Sci.& Fish.Abstr., Aquacult.Abstr., Biol.Abstr., Chem.Abstr., Environ.Sci.Poll.Mgmt., Forest.Abstr., Herb.Abstr., Nutr.Abstr., Sel.Water Res.Abstr., Zoo.Rec.
—BLDSC (7986.650000), CASDDS, CISTI.
Published by: Universita degli Studi di Perugia, Istituto di Idrobiologia, Via Elce Di Sotto, Perugia, PG 06123, Italy. TEL 39-75-5855705, FAX 39-75-5855709. Ed. Giampaolo Moretti. Circ: 300.

RIVISTA DI NEUROBIOLOGIA. see *MEDICAL SCIENCES—Psychiatry And Neurology*

RIVISTA ITALIANA DI BIOLOGIA E MEDICINA. see *MEDICAL SCIENCES*

570 BRA ISSN 0370-6583
QH301 CODEN: RODRAD
RODRIGUESIA; revista do Jardim Botanico do Rio de Janeiro. Text in Portuguese. 1935; N.S. 1939 (Sep.). irreg., latest vol.51. USD 36 (effective 1997). bk.rev. abstr, bibl. **Document type:** *Magazine, Abstract/Index, Bibliography.*
Indexed: Biol.Abstr., Forest Prod.Abstr., Forest.Abstr., INIS Atomind., Rev.Plant Path.
—CISTI, Linda Hall.
Published by: Ministerio do Meio Ambiente dos Recursos Hidricos e da Amazonia Legal, Jardim Botanico do Rio de Janeiro, Biblioteca Barbosa Rodrigues, Rua Jardim Botanico, 1008, Jd Botanico, Gavea, RJ 22460-000, Brazil. TEL 55-21-2748246, FAX 55-21-2744897, bibiiot@jbrj.gov.br, http://www.jardimbotanico.gov.br.

571.86 612.64 ROM ISSN 1220-0522
CODEN: RRMEEA
ROMANIAN JOURNAL OF MORPHOLOGY AND EMBRYOLOGY/REVUE ROUMAINE DE MORPHOLOGIE ET EMBRYOLOGIE. Text in English, French, German, Russian, Spanish. 1964. q. bk.rev. charts, illus. index. **Document type:** *Academic/Scholarly.*
Formerly (until 1990): Morphologie et Embryologie (0377-5038); Which supersedes in part (in 1975): Revue Roumaine de Morphologie et de Physiologie (0377-4953); Which was formed by the 1974 merger of: Revue Roumaine de Physiologie (0035-399X); Revue Roumaine de Morphologie et d'Embryologie (0377-4945); Which was formed by the 1973 merger of: Morfologia Normala si Patologica (0027-1063); Revue Roumaine d'Embryologie et de Cytologie. Serie de Cytologie (0556-8056); Revue Roumaine d'Embryologie (0300-063X); Which was formerly (1964-1972): Revue Roumaine d'Embryologie et de Cytologie. Serie d'Embryologie (0035-4007)
Indexed: Biol.Abstr., Chem.Abstr., Chem.Indus.Notes, Chem.Titles, Curr.Adv.Cancer Res., Curr.Adv.Ecol.Sci., Excerp.Med., Ind.Med. (1990-), Nutr.Abstr.
—BLDSC (8019.636500), CASDDS, CISTI, GNLM, KNAW, Linda Hall.
Published by: (Academia de Stiinte Medicale), Editura Academiei Romane, Calea 13 Septembrie 13, Bucharest 76117, Romania. Ed. V D Marza. **Dist. by:** Rodipet S.A.. TEL 401-618-5103, FAX 401-226407.

570 RUS
CODEN: IANBAM
ROSSIISKAYA AKADEMIYA NAUK. IZVESTIYA. SERIYA BIOLOGICHESKAYA. Text in Russian; Summaries in English. 1936. bi-m. bk.rev. index. **Document type:** *Academic/Scholarly.* **Description:** Focuses on fundamental studies in the fields of cell biology, biochemistry, zoology, botany, physiology, and ecology.
Formerly: Akademiya Nauk S.S.S.R. Izvestiya. Seriya Biologicheskaya (0002-3329)
Related titles: Online - full text ed.: (from Institute for Scientific Information); ♦ English Translation: Russian Academy of Sciences. Biology Bulletin. ISSN 1062-3590.
Indexed: Aqua.Sci.& Fish.Abstr., Aquacult.Abstr., Biol.Abstr., Chem.Abstr., Crop Physiol.Abstr., Curr.Cont., Deep Sea Res.& Oceanogr.Abstr., Environ.Sci.Poll.Mgmt., Field Crop Abstr., Forest Prod.Abstr., Forest.Abstr., GeoRef, Helminthol.Abstr., INIS Atomind., Ind.Med. (coverage dropped), Ind.Sci.Rev., Int.Aerosp.Abstr., Ocean.Abstr. (coverage dropped), Plant Breed.Abstr., Plant Grow.Reg.Abstr., Protozool.Abstr., Ref.Zh., Rev.Appl.Entomol., Rev.Plant Path., Rice Abstr., Sci.Cit.Ind. (coverage dropped), Soils & Fert., Soyabean Abstr., Triticale Abstr., Zoo.Rec.
—BLDSC (0082.301000), CASDDS, CISTI, East View, GNLM, IDS, Linda Hall. **CCC.**

Published by: (Rossiiskaya Akademiya Nauk/Russian Academy of Sciences), M A I K Nauka - Interperiodica, Mezhdunarodnyi Otdel, Profsoyuznaya ul 90, Moscow 117864, Russian Federation. TEL 7-095-336-1600, FAX 7-095-336-0666, compmg@maik.rssi.ru, http://www.maik.rssi.ru/journals/biobull.htm, http://hea.iki.rssi.ru/pazh. Ed. Nikolai G Khrushchev. **Dist. by:** Mezhdunarodnaya Kniga; **US dist. addr.:** East View Publications, 3020 Harbor Ln N, Minneapolis, MN 55447.

570 610 GBR ISSN 0962-8436
QH301 CODEN: PTRBAE

ROYAL SOCIETY OF LONDON. PHILOSOPHICAL TRANSACTIONS. BIOLOGICAL SCIENCES. Text in English. m. USD 1,025 in Europe printed and electronic access; GBP 1,060 in US & Canada printed and electronic access; GBP 1,105 elsewhere printed and electronic access (effective 2001). back issues avail.; reprint service avail. from PQC,PSC,SCH. *Refereed.* **Document type:** *Proceedings, Academic/Scholarly.* **Description:** Contains full reports of the Society discussion meetings, topical themes and reviews on specific subjects.

Related titles: Microfiche ed.: (from IDC); Microform ed.: (from PMC); Online - full text ed.: ISSN 1471-2970 (from JSTOR (Web-based Journal Archive), CatchWord Ltd., O C L C Online Computer Library Center, Inc., RoweCom Information Quest, Swets Blackwell, Institute for Scientific Information).

Indexed: AESIS, ASCA, Agroforest.Abstr., Anim.Behav.Abstr. (coverage dropped), Anim.Breed.Abstr., Apic.Abstr., Appl.Ecol.Abstr. (coverage dropped), Aqua.Sci.& Fish.Abstr., Aquacult.Abstr., Bio-Contr.News & Info., Biol.Abstr., Br.Archaeol.Abstr., Br.Geol.Lit., Chem.Abstr., Chem.Titles, Compumath, Curr.Adv.Ecol.Sci., Curr.Adv.Plant Sci., Curr.Biotech.Abstr., Curr.Cont., Dairy Sci.Abstr., Dent.Ind., Ecol.Abstr., Environ.Abstr., Environ.Ind., Environ.Sci.Poll.Mgmt., Excerp.Med., Field Crop Abstr., Forest Prod.Abstr., Forest.Abstr., Geo.Abstr.H.G., GeoRef, Geol.Abstr., Helminthol.Abstr., Herb.Abstr., IDA, Ind.Med. (1887-), Ind.Sci.Rev., Ind.Vet., Inpharma, Int.Abstr.Biol.Sci., Maize Abstr., Meteor.& Geoastrophys.Abstr., Nutr.Abstr., Ocean.Abstr. (coverage dropped), Petrol.Abstr. (coverage dropped), Plant Breed.Abstr., Plant Sci., Poult.Abstr., Protozool.Abstr., Reac., Rev.Appl.Entomol., Rev.Med.& Vet.Mycol., Rev.Plant Path., Sci.Cit.Ind., Seed Abstr., So.Pac.Per.Ind., Soils & Fert., Sorghum & Millets Abstr., Soyabean Abstr., Sport Fish.Abstr., Triticale Abstr., Vet.Bull., Weed Abstr., Wild.Rev., Zoo.Rec.

—BLDSC (6464.000000), ADONIS, CASDDS, CatchWord, CISTI, EMDOCS, IDS, Linda Hall. **CCC.**

Published by: Royal Society of London, 6 Carlton House Terr, London SW1Y 5AG, United Kingdom. TEL 44-207-839-5561, FAX 44-207-976-1837, sales@royalsoc.ac.uk, http://www.pubs.royalsoc.ac.uk, http://www.royalsoc.ac.uk. Ed. Semir Zeki FRS. R&P Phil Hurst. Circ: 649.

570 GBR ISSN 0962-8452
QH301

ROYAL SOCIETY OF LONDON. PROCEEDINGS. BIOLOGICAL SCIENCES. Text in English. 1832. bi-m. USD 925 in Europe includes online acces; USD 965 in US & Canada includes online access; USD 990 elsewhere includes online acces (effective 2001). back issues avail.; reprint service avail. from ISI. *Refereed.* **Document type:** *Proceedings, Journal, Academic/Scholarly.* **Description:** Publishes original papers on all aspects of the biological sciences. Including the latest research.

Related titles: Microform ed.: (from PMC); Online - full text ed.: ISSN 1471-2954 (from JSTOR (Web-based Journal Archive), CatchWord Ltd., EBSCO Publishing, O C L C Online Computer Library Center, Inc., RoweCom Information Quest, Swets Blackwell, Institute for Scientific Information).

Indexed: ASCA, AgBiotech, Anim.Behav.Abstr., Anim.Breed.Abstr., Appl.Ecol.Abstr. (coverage dropped), Aqua.Sci.& Fish.Abstr., Bibl.Agri., Bio-Contr.News & Info., Biol.Abstr., Br.Archaeol.Abstr., Br.Geol.Lit., Chem.Abstr., Chem.Titles, Compumath, Comput.Abstr., Crop Physiol.Abstr., Curr.Adv.Ecol.Sci., Curr.Cont., Dairy Sci.Abstr., Deep Sea Res.& Oceanogr.Abstr., Dent.Ind., Ecol.Abstr., Eng.Ind., Entomol.Abstr., Environ.Sci.Poll.Mgmt., Excerp.Med., Field Crop Abstr., Food Sci.& Tech.Abstr., Forest.Abstr., Genet.Abstr., Geo.Abstr.H.G., GeoRef, Geol.Abstr., Helminthol.Abstr., Herb.Abstr., Hum.Gen.Abstr., Ind.Med. (coverage dropped), Ind.Sci.Rev., Ind.Vet., Inpharma, Int.Abstr.Biol.Sci., NRN, Nutr.Abstr., Ocean.Abstr., Pharm.&Out.News, Plant Breed.Abstr., Plant Gen.Res.Abstr., Postharvest, Poult.Abstr., Protozool.Abstr., Reac., Rev.Appl.Entomol., Rev.Med.& Vet.Mycol., Rev.Plant Path., Rice Abstr., SSCI (coverage dropped), Sci.Cit.Ind., Seed Abstr., Soils & Fert., Sport Fish.Abstr., Triticale Abstr., Vet.Bull., Weed Abstr., Wild.Rev., Zoo.Rec.

—BLDSC (6804.600000), ADONIS, CASDDS, CatchWord, CISTI, EMDOCS, IDS, Linda Hall. **CCC.**

Published by: Royal Society of London, 6 Carlton House Terr, London SW1Y 5AG, United Kingdom. TEL 44-207-839-5561, FAX 44-207-976-1837, sales@royalsoc.ac.uk, http://www.pubs.royalsoc.ac.uk. Ed. R M Alexander FRS. R&P Phil Hurst. Circ: 1,064.

570 RUS ISSN 1062-3590
QH301 CODEN: BRASEK

RUSSIAN ACADEMY OF SCIENCES. BIOLOGY BULLETIN. Key Title: Biology Bulletin of the Russian Academy of Sciences. Text in English. 1936. bi-m. NLG 4,147, EUR 1,882, USD 1,720 to institutions for print or online ed.; NLG 4,976.40, EUR 2,258.40, USD 2,064 to institutions print & online eds.combined (effective 2001). bibl, charts, illus. index. back issues avail. *Refereed.* **Document type:** *Academic/Scholarly.* **Description:** Publishes current experimental studies and surveys of recent scientific problems in general biology, as well as information on scientific conferences and reviews of new books in the fields of general biology.

Formerly (until 1992): Academy of Sciences of the U S S R. Biology Bulletin (0098-2164)

Related titles: Online - full text ed.: ISSN 1608-3059 (from Swets Blackwell, RoweCom Information Quest); ♦ Translation of: Rossiiskaya Akademiya Nauk. Izvestiya. Seriya Biologicheskaya.

Indexed: AgBiotech, Anim.Breed.Abstr., Aqua.Sci.& Fish.Abstr., Bio-Contr.News & Info., Biodet.Abstr., Biol.Abstr., Biotech.& Bioeng.Abstr., Chem.Titles, Crop Physiol.Abstr., Curr.Adv.Ecol.Sci., Curr.Ref.Fish Res., Environ.Sci.Poll.Mgmt., Excerp.Med., Field Crop Abstr., Forest.Abstr., Herb.Abstr., Hort.Abstr., INIS Atomind., Ind.Med. (coverage dropped), Ind.Vet., Int.Abstr.Biol.Sci., Maize Abstr., Nutr.Abstr., Ornam.Hort., Plant Breed.Abstr., Plant Gen.Res.Abstr., Plant Grow.Reg.Abstr., Postharvest, Poult.Abstr., Rev.Appl.Entomol., Rev.Arom.& Med.Plants, Rev.Med.& Vet.Mycol., Rev.Plant Path., Rice Abstr., Seed Abstr., Soils & Fert., Triticale Abstr., Weed Abstr.

—BLDSC (0406.045000), CISTI, GNLM, Infotrieve, ingenta. **CCC.**

Published by: (Rossiiskaya Akademiya Nauk/Russian Academy of Sciences), M A I K Nauka - Interperiodica, Mezhdunarodnyi Otdel, Profsoyuznaya ul 90, Moscow 117864, Russian Federation. TEL 7-095-336-1600, FAX 7-095-336-0666, compmg@maik.rssi.ru, http://www.maik.rssi.ru/journals/biobull.htm, http://hea.iki.rssi.ru/pazh. Ed. Sergei G Vassetzky. **Subscr. in N America to:** Kluwer Academic - Plenum Publishers, 233 Spring St, New York, NY 10013-1578. TEL 212-620-8468, 800-221-9369, FAX 212-807-1047. **Dist. by:** Kluwer Academic Publishers Group, Journals Department, PO Box 322, Dordrecht 3300 AH, Netherlands. TEL 31-78-6546392, 31-78-654-6474, services@wkap.nl, http://www.wkap.nl, http://www.wkap.nl/journalhome.htm/1062-3590.

570 RUS ISSN 1062-3604
QL951 CODEN: RJDBE2

RUSSIAN JOURNAL OF DEVELOPMENTAL BIOLOGY. Text in English. 1970. bi-m. EUR 2,111 for print or online ed.; EUR 2,533.20 print & online eds.combined (effective 2002). back issues avail. *Refereed.* **Document type:** *Academic/Scholarly.* **Description:** Publishes fundamental and applied research papers and reviews on development, regeneration, and carcinogenesis at the molecular, cellular, and organismic levels.

Formerly (until 1993): Soviet Journal of Developmental Biology (0049-173X)

Related titles: Microfilm ed.: (from PQC); Online - full text ed.: ISSN 1608-3326 (from Swets Blackwell, Kluwer Online); ♦ Translation of: Ontogenez. ISSN 0475-1450.

Indexed: Biol.Abstr., Curr.Adv.Ecol.Sci., GeoRef, INIS Atomind., Ind.Med. (coverage dropped), Psychol.Abstr.

—BLDSC (0420.760900), CASDDS, CISTI, GNLM, ingenta. **CCC.**

Published by: (Rossiiskaya Akademiya Nauk/Russian Academy of Sciences), M A I K Nauka - Interperiodica, Mezhdunarodnyi Otdel, Profsoyuznaya ul 90, Moscow 117864, Russian Federation. TEL 7-095-336-1600, FAX 7-095-336-0666, compmg@maik.ru, http://www.maik.rssi.ru/journals/devbio.htm. Ed. Sergei G Vassetzky. **Dist. by:** Kluwer Academic Publishers, PO Box 17, Dordrecht 3300 AH, Netherlands. TEL 31-78-639-2392, FAX 31-78-654-6474, http://www.wkap.nl.

578.77 RUS ISSN 1063-0740
QH91.A1 CODEN: RJMBED

RUSSIAN JOURNAL OF MARINE BIOLOGY. Text in English. 1975. bi-m. EUR 1,581 to institutions for print or online ed.; EUR 1,897.20 to institutions print & online eds.combined (effective 2002). back issues avail. *Refereed.* **Document type:** *Academic/Scholarly.* **Description:** Covers a range of topics in marine biology and related studies of marine biota and the environment.

Formerly (until 1993): Soviet Journal of Marine Biology (0145-1456)

Related titles: Microfilm ed.: (from PQC); Online - full text ed.: ISSN 1608-3377 (from Swets Blackwell, Kluwer Online, RoweCom Information Quest); ♦ Translation of: Biologiya Morya. ISSN 0134-3475.

Indexed: Aqua.Sci.& Fish.Abstr., Biol.Abstr., Curr.Adv.Ecol.Sci., Curr.Cont. (coverage dropped), Deep Sea Res.& Oceanogr.Abstr., Environ.Sci.Poll.Mgmt., GeoRef, Int.Abstr.Biol.Sci., Ocean.Abstr., Pollut.Abstr., Sport Fish.Abstr.

—BLDSC (0420.761500), CISTI, Infotrieve, ingenta. **CCC.**

Published by: (Rossiiskaya Akademiya Nauk/Russian Academy of Sciences), M A I K Nauka - Interperiodica, Mezhdunarodnyi Otdel, Profsoyuznaya ul 90, Moscow 117864, Russian Federation. TEL 7-095-336-1600, FAX 7-095-336-0666, http://www.maik.rssi.ru/. Ed. Vladimir L Kas'yanov. **Dist. by:** Kluwer Academic Publishers, PO Box 17, Dordrecht 3300 AH, Netherlands. TEL 31-78-639-2392, FAX 31-78-654-6474, http://www.wkap.nl.

570 FRA ISSN 1260-0199

RYTHMES. Text in French. 1969. q. FRF 150, EUR 22.87 (effective 2000 - 2001). adv. *Refereed.* **Document type:** *Bulletin.*

Formerly (until 1995): Groupe d'Etude des Rythmes Biologiques. Bulletin (0154-0238)

Published by: Societe Francophone de Chronobiologie, c/o Laboratoire de Biologie Animale et Appliquee, Faculte des Sciences et Techniques, 23 rue Paul Michelon, Saint-Etienne Cedex 2 42023, France. TEL 33-4-77481517, FAX 33-4-77481520. Ed. Bernard Millet. Pub. Bernard Canguilhem. R&P Alain Blanc. Adv. contact Bernard Buisson.

570 JPN ISSN 0289-6389
QH91.A1 CODEN: NRFHE8

SADO MARINE BIOLOGICAL STATION. REPORT/NIIGATA DAIGAKU RIGAKUBU FUZOKU SADO RINKAI JIKKENJO KENKYU HOKOKU. Text and summaries in English. 1971. a. per issue exchange basis. bibl. *Refereed.* **Document type:** *Academic/Scholarly.*

Formerly: Sado Marine Biological Station. Annual Report (0388-0117)

Related titles: CD-ROM ed.; Online - full text ed.

Indexed: Aqua.Sci.& Fish.Abstr., Aquacult.Abstr., Biol.Abstr., Environ.Sci.Poll.Mgmt., Sport Fish.Abstr., Zoo.Rec.

Published by: Niigata Daigaku, Rigakubu Fuzoku Sado Rinkai Jikkenjo/Niigata University, Sado Marine Biological Station, 2-8050 Igarashi, Niigata 950-21, Japan. TEL 0259-75-2012, FAX 0259-75-2012. Ed. Yoshiharu Honma. Circ: 600 (controlled).

SALUSVITA; revista da area de ciencias biologicas e da saude. see *MEDICAL SCIENCES*

570 RUS
AS262 CODEN: VLUBB6
SANKT-PETERBURGSKII UNIVERSITET. VESTNIK. SERIYA BIOLOGIYA. Text in Russian; Abstracts and contents page in English. 1946. q. bk.rev. charts, illus. index. **Document type:** *Academic/Scholarly.*
Formerly (until 1992): Leningradskii Universitet. Vestnik. Seriya Biologiya (0321-186X)
Related titles: Microform ed.: (from EVP).
Indexed: Aqua.Sci.& Fish.Abstr., Aquacult.Abstr., Bio-Contr.News & Info., Biol.Abstr., Chem.Abstr., Chem.Indus.Notes, Chem.Titles, Crop Physiol.Abstr., Environ.Sci.Poll.Mgmt., Field Crop Abstr., Forest.Abstr., GeoRef, Helminthol.Abstr., Herb.Abstr., Hort.Abstr., Int.Aerosp.Abstr., Plant Breed.Abstr., Plant Grow.Reg.Abstr., Ref.Zh., Russ.Acad.Sci.Bibl., Zoo.Rec.
—BLDSC (0032.757100), CASDDS, CISTI, GNLM, Infotrieve, Linda Hall. **CCC.**
Published by: Sankt-Peterburgskii Universitet, Universitetskaya nab 7-9, St Petersburg 199034, Russian Federation. TEL 812-2189784. Ed. S P Merkur'ev. Circ: 1,330. **Subscr. to:** Mezhdunarodnaya Kniga, B Yakimanka 39, Moscow 117049, Russian Federation. **US dist. addr.:** East View Publications, 3020 Harbor Ln N, Minneapolis, MN 55447. TEL 612-550-0961.

570 615.8 531.6 FRA ISSN 0767-6891
SCIENCES ORGONOMIQUES; revue des lois de la vie. Text in French. 1986. q. FRF 150; FRF 308 foreign. illus. back issues avail. **Description:** Deals with biology, physics and medicine from an energetic or orgonomic perspective; discusses applications of the theories and works of Wilhelm Reich.
Published by: Societe d'Edition pour la Diffusion de l'Orgonomie (S.E.DIF.OR.), Allee du Chene Vert-Parc Liserb, Nice 06000, France. Circ: 1,800.

570 GBR ISSN 0268-3385
THE SCOTTISH NATURALIST. Text in English. 1871. 3/yr. GBP 35 (effective 1999). bk.rev. charts, illus, maps. back issues avail. **Document type:** *Academic/Scholarly.* **Description:** Covers all aspects of Scottish natural history.
Former titles (until 1982): Western Naturalist (0141-5247); Scottish Naturalist
Indexed: Zoo.Rec.
—BLDSC (8211.000000).
Published by: Scottish Natural History Library, Foremount House, Easwald Bank, Milliken Park, Johnstone, Kilbarchan, Renfrewshire PA10 2EZ, United Kingdom. TEL 44-1505-702419. Ed. J A Gibson. Circ: 1,000.

570 JPN ISSN 0385-5996
SEIBUTSU KAGAKU NYUSU/BIOLOGICAL SCIENCE NEWS. Text in Japanese. 1971. m. **Document type:** *Newsletter.*
Published by: Zoological Society of Japan/Nihon Dobutsu Gakkai, Toshin Bldg 2F, 2-27-2 Hongo, Bunkyo-ku, Tokyo 113-0033, Japan. TEL 81-3-3814-5461, FAX 81-3-3814-5352.

570 JPN ISSN 0370-9531
CODEN: SEKAA6
SEITAI NO KAGAKU/LIFE SCIENCE. Text in Japanese. 1949. bi-m. JPY 14,210, USD 109 (effective 2001). bk.rev. 90 p./no. back issues avail. *Refereed.* **Document type:** *Journal, Academic/Scholarly.*
Indexed: Chem.Abstr., Chem.Indus.Notes, Chem.Titles, INIS Atomind.
—CASDDS, CISTI.
Published by: (Ichiro kanehara Foundation), Igaku-Shoin Ltd., Akamon Royal Heights 1003, 5-29-12 Hongo, Bunkyo-ku, Tokyo 113-0033, Japan. TEL 81-3-3815-7801, FAX 81-3-5800-2722, http://www.igaku-shoin.co.jp. Eds. Dr. A Wonomura, Dr. H Ishikawa, Dr. M Fieyita, Dr. M Ito. R&P Hideho Nakamura TEL 81-3-3817-5616. Circ: 3,000.

SENCKENBERGIANA MARITIMA. see *EARTH SCIENCES—Oceanography*

570 551 DEU ISSN 0365-7000
QH5 CODEN: ASNGA7
SENCKENBERGISCHE NATURFORSCHENDE GESELLSCHAFT. ABHANDLUNGEN. Text in German, English. 1884. irreg., latest vol.554, 2001. USD 61.70 per vol. domestic; USD 61.90 per vol. foreign (effective 2002). back issues avail. **Document type:** *Monographic series, Academic/Scholarly.* **Description:** Contains extensive papers on zoology, geology, paleontology and botany.
Indexed: Biol.Abstr., Deep Sea Res.& Oceanogr.Abstr., GeoRef, Ref.Zh., Sport Fish.Abstr., Wild.Rev.
—CISTI, Linda Hall. **CCC.**
Published by: (Senckenbergische Naturforschende Gesellschaft), E. Schweizerbart'sche Verlagsbuchhandlung, Johannesstr 3A, Stuttgart 70176, Germany. TEL 49-711-625001, FAX 49-711-625005, schweizerbart@schweizerbart.de. Ed. Fritz F Steininger. Circ: 550 (paid).

SENEGAL. CENTRE DE RECHERCHE OCEANOGRAPHIQUE. DOCUMENT SCIENTIFIQUE. see *EARTH SCIENCES—Oceanography*

SENSORY SYSTEMS. see *PSYCHOLOGY*

570 KOR ISSN 0377-5232
QH301 CODEN: SNBAAO
SEOUL NATIONAL UNIVERSITY. FACULTY PAPERS. BIOLOGY AND AGRICULTURE SERIES. Text in English. 1971. a. **Document type:** *Monographic series.*
Indexed: Excerp.Med.
—GNLM.
Published by: Seoul National University, San 56-1 Sinlim-dong, Kwanak-ku, Seoul 151742, Korea, S..

578.77 JPN ISSN 0037-2870
QH91.A1 CODEN: PSMBAG
SETO MARINE BIOLOGICAL LABORATORY. PUBLICATIONS/SETO RINKAI JIKKENJO KIYO. Text in English. 1949. s-a. per issue exchange basis. charts, illus. index. *Refereed.* **Document type:** *Academic/Scholarly.* **Description:** Publishes scientific papers on marine biology related to Japanese and Indo-Pacific waters, especially those on taxonomy, morphology and biology.
Indexed: Aqua.Sci.& Fish.Abstr., Aquacult.Abstr., Curr.Adv.Ecol.Sci., Deep Sea Res.& Oceanogr.Abstr., GeoRef, Ocean.Abstr., Sel.Water Res.Abstr., Sport Fish.Abstr., Zoo.Rec.
—BLDSC (7112.000000).
Published by: Kyoto University, Graduate School of Science, Seto Marine Biological Laboratory/Kyoto Daigaku, Daigakuin Rigaku Kenkyuka Fuzoku Seto Rinkai Jikkenjo, Nishimuro-gun, shirahama-cho, Wakayama-ken 649-2211, Japan. TEL 81-739-42-3515, FAX 81-739-42-4518, http://www.seto.kyoto-u.ac.jp, http://www.seto.kyoto.u.ac.jp. Ed. Yoshihisa Shirayama. Circ: 460.

578.77 JPN ISSN 0389-6609
SETO MARINE BIOLOGICAL LABORATORY. SPECIAL PUBLICATION SERIES. Text in English. 1959. irreg. per issue exchange basis. *Refereed.* **Document type:** *Monographic series, Academic/Scholarly.*
Formerly: Seto Marine Biological Laboratory. Special Publications (0080-9098)
Indexed: Aqua.Sci.& Fish.Abstr., Aquacult.Abstr., Biol.Abstr., Deep Sea Res.& Oceanogr.Abstr., Environ.Sci.Poll.Mgmt.
Published by: Kyoto University, Graduate School of Science, Seto Marine Biological Laboratory/Kyoto Daigaku, Daigakuin Rigaku Kenkyuka Fuzoku Seto Rinkai Jikkenjo, Nishimuro-gun, shirahama-cho, Wakayama-ken 649-2211, Japan. TEL 81-739-42-3515, FAX 81-739-42-4518, http://www.seto.kyoto.u.ac.jp. Ed. Yoshihisa Shirayama. Circ: 460.

SHANXI YIYAO ZAZHI/SHANXI MEDICAL JOURNAL. see *PHARMACY AND PHARMACOLOGY*

570 CHN ISSN 0006-3193
QH301 CODEN: SWHTA4
SHENGWUXUE TONGBAO/BULLETIN OF BIOLOGY. Text in Chinese, English. bi-m. charts, illus. *Refereed.*
Indexed: Chem.Abstr., Chem.Indus.Notes, Chem.Titles.
—CASDDS, Linda Hall.
Published by: (Chinese Society of Zoology), Kexue Chubanshe/Science Press, 16 Donghuang Cheng Genbei Jie, Beijing 100717, China. TELEX 210247-SPBJ-CN. **Co-sponsor:** Chinese Botanical Society.

578.77 JPN ISSN 0385-1109
SHIMA MARINELAND. SCIENCE REPORT. Text in English, Japanese. 1972. irreg. per issue exchange basis. adv. **Document type:** *Academic/Scholarly.*
Indexed: Biol.Abstr., Deep Sea Res.& Oceanogr.Abstr., Sport Fish.Abstr.
Published by: Shima Marineland Foundation, Kashikojima, Shima-gun, Ago-cho, Mie 517-05, Japan. TEL 81-5994-3-1225, FAX 81-5994-3-1224. Ed. T Tsujii. R&P Tadashi Tsujii. Adv. contact Shuzo Okubo. Circ: 1,500.

570 CHN ISSN 1000-3207
CODEN: SSXUET
SHUISHENG SHENGWU XUEBAO/ACTA HYDROBIOLOGICA SINICA. Text in Chinese; Summaries in English. 1955. q. USD 72 (effective 2000). adv. *Refereed.* **Document type:** *Academic/Scholarly.* **Description:** Directed to college instructors, students, and researchers; contains research articles, brief reports and reviews about taxonomy, ecology, physiology, pathology, toxicology, disease prevention; genetics and breeding of freshwater fish, algae, and other organisms.
Indexed: AgBiotech, Anim.Breed.Abstr., Aqua.Sci.& Fish.Abstr., Aquacult.Abstr., Bio-Contr.News & Info., Environ.Sci.Poll.Mgmt., GeoRef, Helminthol.Abstr., Ind.Vet., Irr.& Drain.Abstr., Nutr.Abstr., Plant Breed.Abstr., Plant Grow.Reg.Abstr., Poult.Abstr., Protozool.Abstr., Rev.Appl.Entomol., Rev.Med.& Vet.Mycol., Seed Abstr., Soils & Fert., Sport Fish.Abstr., Triticale Abstr., Vet.Bull., Weed Abstr., Zoo.Rec.
—BLDSC (0624.500000), CASDDS, CISTI.
Published by: (Chinese Academy of Sciences/Zhongguo Kexueyuan), Kexue Chubanshe/Science Press, 16 Donghuang Cheng Genbei Jie, Beijing 100717, China. Circ: 6,000.

570 JPN ISSN 0559-9822
CODEN: SIEBA7
SIEBOLDIA ACTA BIOLOGICA/SHIBORUDIA. Text in English, Japanese. 1952. irreg. per issue exchange basis. reprint service avail. from PQC.
Indexed: Biol.Abstr.
—CASDDS.
Published by: (Biological Laboratory), Kyushu University, College of General Education, 4-2-1 Ropponmatsu, Chuo-ku, Fukuoka-shi 810-0044, Japan. TEL 81-92-731-8745, FAX 81-92-771-4161.

570 SVK ISSN 0037-6930
QH7 CODEN: BLGPAT
SLOVENSKA AKADEMIA VIED. BIOLOGICKE PRACE/SLOVAK ACADEMY OF SCIENCES. TREATISES ON BIOLOGY. Text in English, Slovak; Summaries in English, German, Russian. 1955. irreg. USD 5. charts, illus.
Indexed: Biol.Abstr.
—CISTI, Linda Hall.
Published by: (Slovenska Akademia Vied/Slovak Academy of Sciences), Veda Publishing House of the Slovak Academy of Sciences, Bradacova 7, Bratislava 85286, Slovakia. Circ: 500. **Dist. by:** Slovart, Nam Slobody 6, Bratislava 81764, Slovakia.

570 BOL
SOCIEDAD BOLIVIANA DE HISTORIA NATURAL. REVISTA. Text in Spanish; Abstracts occasionally in English. 1974. irreg. illus.
Indexed: Biol.Abstr.
Published by: Sociedad Boliviana de Historia Natural, Casilla de Correos 538, Cochabamba, Bolivia.

570 CHL ISSN 0037-850X
QH301 CODEN: BOBCAK
SOCIEDAD DE BIOLOGIA DE CONCEPCION. BOLETIN. Summaries in Spanish, English. 1927. s-a. per issue exchange basis. charts, illus. index. back issues avail. **Document type:** *Bulletin, Academic/Scholarly.*
Indexed: Aqua.Sci.& Fish.Abstr., Aquacult.Abstr., Biol.Abstr., Chem.Abstr., Deep Sea Res.& Oceanogr.Abstr., Entomol.Abstr., Environ.Sci.Poll.Mgmt., GeoRef, Sport Fish.Abstr., Zoo.Rec.
—GNLM, Linda Hall.
Published by: Sociedad de Biologia de Concepcion, Casilla 4006, Concepcion, Chile. Ed. Hugo I Moyano. Circ: 500.

570 ITA ISSN 0366-2047
CODEN: BONNAB
SOCIETA DEI NATURALISTI IN NAPOLI. BOLLETTINO. Text in Italian; Summaries in English. 1887. a. **Document type:** *Bulletin, Academic/Scholarly.*
Indexed: Biol.Abstr., Chem.Abstr., Deep Sea Res.& Oceanogr.Abstr., GeoRef.
—CASDDS.
Published by: (Societa dei Naturalisti in Napoli), Giannini Editore, Via Cisterna dell'Olio, Naples, NA 80134, Italy. TEL 39-81-5513928.

B

570 ITA ISSN 0037-8771
QH301 CODEN: BSIBAC
SOCIETA ITALIANA DI BIOLOGIA SPERIMENTALE. BOLLETTINO/JOURNAL OF BIOLOGICAL RESEARCH. Text in English, Italian. 1924. bi-m. ITL 130,000, USD 200 (effective 1999). adv. charts, illus, stat. index. **Description:** Features articles and research papers covering a wide variety of topics in experimental biology; includes anatomy, molecular biology, botany, cardiology and clinical chemistry.
Related titles: Microform ed.: (from PMC).
Indexed: Agri.& Environ.Biotech.Abstr. (coverage dropped), Anal.Abstr., Anim.Breed.Abstr., Biol.Abstr., Chem.Abstr., Chem.Indus.Notes, Chem.Titles, Curr.Adv.Ecol.Sci., Dairy Sci.Abstr., Deep Sea Res.& Oceanogr.Abstr., Dent.Ind., Derwent Biotech.Abstr., Excerp.Med., INIS Atomind., Ind.Med. (1925-), Ind.Vet., Nutr.Abstr., Poult.Abstr., Vet.Bull.
—BLDSC (2231.000000), CASDDS, CISTI, GNLM, KNAW, Linda Hall.
Published by: Casa Editrice Idelson, Via Annibale De Gasperis, 55, Naples, NA 80137, Italy. TEL 39-81-5524733, FAX 39-81-5518295, idelgno@tin.it, http://www.idelson-gnocchi.com. Ed. Pietro de Franciscis.

570 NLD ISSN 0926-3551
SOCIETAS INTERNATIONALIS ODONATOLOGICA. RAPID COMMUNICATIONS. Text in Dutch. 1980. irreg. price varies. bk.rev. charts. **Document type:** *Academic/Scholarly.*
Indexed: Biol.Abstr., Entomol.Abstr. (coverage dropped), Genet.Abstr. (coverage dropped), Zoo.Rec.
Published by: Societas Internationalis Odonatologica, SIO Central Office, PO Box 256, Bilthoven 3720 AG, Netherlands. Circ: 500.

581 591 FIN ISSN 0373-6873
QH7 CODEN: MSFFAS
SOCIETAS PRO FAUNA ET FLORA FENNICA. MEMORANDA. Text in English, Finnish, German, Swedish; Summaries in English. 1927. 2/yr. FIM 80. adv. bk.rev. back issues avail. *Refereed.* **Document type:** *Academic/Scholarly.*
Indexed: Biol.Abstr., Ecol.Abstr., GeoRef, IBR, Ref.Zh., Rev.Appl.Entomol., Sport Fish.Abstr., Weed Abstr., Wild.Rev., Zoo.Rec.
—BLDSC (5645.000000), CISTI, ingenta, KNAW, Linda Hall.
Published by: Societas pro Fauna et Flora Fennica, University of Helsinki, PL 17, Helsinki 00014, Finland. Ed. Olof Bistroem. Circ: 1,550.

570 FRA ISSN 1295-0661
CODEN: CRSBAW
SOCIETE DE BIOLOGIE. JOURNAL. Text in French. 1849. bi-m. FRF 960; FRF 1,066 foreign (effective 1997). adv. index. reprint service avail. from ISI. **Document type:** *Academic/Scholarly.* **Description:** Accounts of meetings of the society and its branches.
Formerly (until 1999): Societe de Biologie et de Ses Filiales. Comptes Rendus des Seances (0037-9026)
Related titles: Microform ed.: (from PMC).
Indexed: Agri.& Environ.Biotech.Abstr. (coverage dropped), Anim.Breed.Abstr., Apic.Abstr., Aqua.Sci.& Fish.Abstr., Aquacult.Abstr., Bio-Contr.News & Info., Biol.Abstr., Chem.Abstr., Chem.Indus.Notes, Chem.Titles, Crop Physiol.Abstr., Curr.Adv.Biochem., Curr.Adv.Cell & Devel.Biol., Curr.Adv.Gen.& Molec.Biol., Dairy Sci.Abstr., Deep Sea Res.& Oceanogr.Abstr., Derwent Biotech.Abstr., Environ.Sci.Poll.Mgmt., Excerp.Med., Field Crop Abstr., Food Sci.& Tech.Abstr., Forest Prod.Abstr., Forest.Abstr., Helminthol.Abstr., Herb.Abstr., Hort.Abstr., INIS Atomind., Ind.Med. (coverage dropped), Ind.Vet., Maize Abstr., Nutr.Abstr., Ornam.Hort., Poult.Abstr., Protozool.Abstr., Ref.Zh., Rev.Appl.Entomol., Rev.Arom.& Med.Plants, Rev.Plant Path., Seed Abstr., Sport Fish.Abstr., Trop.Dis.Bull., Vet.Bull., Wild.Rev., Zoo.Rec.
—BLDSC (4876.800000), CASDDS, CISTI, GNLM, IDS, Infotrieve, ingenta, KNAW. **CCC.**
Published by: (Societe de Biologie et de Ses Filiales), Masson - Periodiques, 120 bd. St. Germain, Paris 75006, France. TEL 33-1-40466200, FAX 33-1-40466201. Ed. Miss Faibie. Circ: 1,300. **Subscr. to:** Societe de Periodiques Specialises, BP 22, Vineuil Cedex 41354, France. TEL 33-2-54504612, FAX 33-2-54504611.

570 550 LUX ISSN 0304-9620
CODEN: BNLXAO
SOCIETE DES NATURALISTES LUXEMBOURGEOIS. BULLETIN. Text and summaries in English, French, German. 1890. a. LUF 500, USD 8. bk.rev. back issues avail. **Document type:** *Bulletin.*
Indexed: GeoRef, Zoo.Rec.
—BLDSC (2747.000000), Linda Hall.
Published by: Societe des Naturalistes Luxembourgeois, B.P. 327, Luxembourg L-2013, Luxembourg. FAX 352-31-38-19. Ed. Paul Diederich. Circ: 850.

570 FRA ISSN 0366-1326
CODEN: BMSLAG
SOCIETE LINNEENNE DE LYON. BULLETIN MENSUEL. Text in French; Summaries in English. 1822. 10/yr. FRF 250 (effective 2001). adv. bk.rev. index. back issues avail. **Document type:** *Bulletin.*
Indexed: A.I.C.P., Aqua.Sci.& Fish.Abstr., Aquacult.Abstr., Biol.Abstr., Environ.Sci.Poll.Mgmt., GeoRef, Ref.Zh., Rev.Plant Path., Zoo.Rec.
—BLDSC (2875.300000), Linda Hall.
Published by: Societe Linneenne de Lyon, 33 rue Bossuet, Lyon 69006, France. societe.linneenne.lyon@wanadoo.fr, http://www.linneenne-lyon.org. Ed. Paul Berthet. Circ: 1,600.

571.4645 USA ISSN 1069-3610
SOCIETY FOR CRYOBIOLOGY. NEWS NOTES. Text in English. 1979. q. membership only. bk.rev. **Document type:** *Newsletter.* **Description:** News of interest about the society.
Published by: Society for Cryobiology, 8650 Rockville Pike, Bethesda, MD 20814. TEL 706-721-4173, FAX 706-721-2347. Ed. A M Karow. Circ: 500.

570 USA ISSN 0583-9009
QH511 CODEN: SBSYAT
SOCIETY FOR DEVELOPMENTAL BIOLOGY. SYMPOSIUM. Text in English. 1981 (no.39). irreg., latest vol.47, 1989. price varies.
Indexed: Biol.Abstr., Chem.Abstr., Chem.Indus.Notes, Chem.Titles, Ind.Med. (coverage dropped).
—CASDDS, GNLM.
Published by: John Wiley & Sons, Inc., Journals (Subsidiary of: Wiley InterScience), 605 Third Ave, New York, NY 10158. TEL 212-475-7700.

570 GBR ISSN 0309-6831
CODEN: SEBSDI
SOCIETY FOR EXPERIMENTAL BIOLOGY. SEMINAR SERIES. Text in English. 197?. irreg. price varies. index. **Document type:** *Proceedings.*
Indexed: Aqua.Sci.& Fish.Abstr., Biol.Abstr., Chem.Abstr., Chem.Indus.Notes, Chem.Titles, GeoRef, Zoo.Rec.
—CASDDS, CISTI, KNAW.
Published by: (Society for Experimental Biology), Cambridge University Press, Edinburgh Bldg, Shaftesbury Rd, Cambridge CB2 2RU, United Kingdom. FAX 44-1223-315052, information@cup.cam.ac.uk, information@cambridge.org, http://www.cup.cam.ac.uk, http://www.uk.cambridge.org/journals/pmu. R&P Linda Nicol.

570 GBR ISSN 0081-1386
QH302 CODEN: SSEBA9
SOCIETY FOR EXPERIMENTAL BIOLOGY. SYMPOSIA. Text in English. 1947. irreg., latest vol.51, 1998. GBP 70, USD 115. **Document type:** *Proceedings.*
Indexed: ASCA, Biol.Abstr., Chem.Abstr., Chem.Indus.Notes, Chem.Titles, Curr.Adv.Ecol.Sci., Ind.Med. (1947-), Rev.Plant Path., Seed Abstr., Sport Fish.Abstr., Weed Abstr., Zoo.Rec.
—BLDSC (8585.000000), CASDDS, CISTI, Infotrieve, ingenta, KNAW. **CCC.**
Published by: Society for Experimental Biology, Burlington House, Piccadilly, London W1V 0LQ, United Kingdom. TEL 44-20-7439-8732, FAX 44-20-7287-4786, seb@sebiol.demon.co.uk, http://www.demon.co.uk/SEB/. **Subscr. to:** Portland Press Ltd., Commerce Way, Colchester, Essex CO2 8HP, United Kingdom. TEL 44-1206-796351, FAX 44-1206-779331.

570 USA ISSN 0361-6525
QH301 CODEN: SOCIDT
SOCIOBIOLOGY. Text in English. 1976. irreg. (approx. a.). USD 100 (effective 2000 - 2001). bk.rev. illus. index. back issues avail. *Refereed.* **Document type:** *Academic/Scholarly.* **Description:** Provides research articles and translations of classic papers on various aspects of the biology of social animals.
Related titles: Online - full text ed.: (from Institute for Scientific Information).
Indexed: ASCA, Agricola, Anim.Behav.Abstr., Appl.Ecol.Abstr., Aqua.Sci.& Fish.Abstr., Bibl.Agri., Bio-Contr.News & Info., Biol.Abstr., Biotech.& Bioeng.Abstr., Curr.Adv.Ecol.Sci., Curr.Cont., Entomol.Abstr., Environ.Sci.Poll.Mgmt., Forest Prod.Abstr., Forest.Abstr., Genet.Abstr., Herb.Abstr., Hum.Gen.Abstr., Maize Abstr., Rev.Appl.Entomol., Rev.Med.& Vet.Mycol., Sci.Cit.Ind., Seed Abstr., Soils & Fert., Sport Fish.Abstr., Wild.Rev., Zoo.Rec.
—BLDSC (8319.562000), CISTI, IDS, Infotrieve, ingenta, Linda Hall. **CCC.**

Published by: California State University, Chico, Department of Biological Sciences, Chico, CA 95926. TEL 530-898-5116, FAX 530-898-4363, dkistner@csuchico.edu. Ed., R&P David H Kistner. Circ: 400.

570 BGR ISSN 0081-1823
SOFIISKI UNIVERSITET. BIOLOGICHESKI FAKULTET. GODISHNIK. Text in Bulgarian. irreg., latest vol.71, 1977. price varies. reprint service avail. from IRC.
Indexed: Biol.Abstr., Chem.Abstr., Field Crop Abstr., INIS Atomind.
Published by: (Biologicheski Fakultet, Sofiiski Universitet), Publishing House of the Bulgarian Academy of Sciences, Akad G Bonchev 6, Sofia 1113, Bulgaria. Ed. I Penev. Circ: 550.

SOUTH AFRICAN INSTITUTE FOR MEDICAL RESEARCH. PUBLICATION. see *MEDICAL SCIENCES*

301 ZAF ISSN 0303-2515
QH1 CODEN: ASAMAS
SOUTH AFRICAN MUSEUM. ANNALS/SUID-AFRIKAANSE MUSEUM. ANNALE. Text in English. 1898. irreg. price varies. illus. back issues avail. *Refereed.* **Document type:** *Monographic series, Academic/Scholarly.* **Description:** Publishes research and review articles in the fields of anthropology, archeology, geology, paleontology, entomology, and vertebrate and invertebrate zoology.
Indexed: Abstr.Anthropol., Aqua.Sci.& Fish.Abstr., Biol.Abstr., Deep Sea Res.& Oceanogr.Abstr., Environ.Sci.Poll.Mgmt., GeoRef, Ind.S.A.Per., Ocean.Abstr., Pollut.Abstr., Ref.Zh., Sel.Water Res.Abstr., Sport Fish.Abstr., Wild.Rev., Zoo.Rec.
—BLDSC (1032.000000), CISTI, ingenta.
Published by: South African Museum, PO Box 61, Cape Town 8000, South Africa. TEL 27-21-4243330, FAX 27-21-4246716, elouw@samuseum. ac.za. Ed. Elizabeth Louw. R&P E Louw. Circ: 450 (controlled).

570 610 FRA ISSN 0295-1967
CODEN: SPEBEQ
SPECTRA BIOLOGIE. Text in French. 1982. 7/yr. FRF 430; FRF 580 foreign. adv. bk.rev. **Document type:** *Academic/Scholarly.* **Description:** Focuses on analytical techniques and instruments routinely used in clinical laboratories. Disseminates information on the growth of the profession and on new concepts, which are expected to greatly affect clinical laboratory practice.
Indexed: Chem.Abstr., Chem.Indus.Notes, Chem.Titles.
—BLDSC (8408.690000), CASDDS, CISTI.
Published by: P C I, 176 rue du Temple, Paris 75003, France. TEL 33-1-44593838, FAX 33-1-44593839. Ed. Monique Chevalier. Adv. contact Catherine Leclerq Bourdon. Circ: 4,500.

SPEZIELLE PATHOLOGISCHE ANATOMIE. see *MEDICAL SCIENCES*

572.8 USA ISSN 1066-5099
QH442.2 CODEN: STCEEJ
STEM CELLS; reporting on clinical and experimental research in the field of progenitor cell differentiation and proliferation. Text in English. 1983. bi-m. USD 130 domestic to individuals; USD 145 in Canada to individuals; USD 160 elsewhere to individuals; USD 195 domestic to institutions; USD 210 in Canada to institutions; USD 225 elsewhere to institutions (effective 2001). adv. bk.rev. back issues avail. *Refereed.* **Document type:** *Academic/Scholarly.* **Description:** Publishes investigative papers and concise reviews with significant new information on normal and neoplastic stem and progenitor cell biology and molecular biology, clinical applications of gene manipulation, growth factors and cytokines, peripheral blood sten cell mobilization and transplantation and tumor cell purging.
Formerly (until 1992): International Journal of Cell Cloning (0737-1454)
Related titles: Online - full text ed.: (from HighWire Pr., EBSCO Publishing, Institute for Scientific Information).

Indexed: ASCA, Biol.Dig., Biotech.Cit.Ind., Chem.Abstr., Chem.Indus.Notes, Chem.Titles, Curr.Adv.Cancer Res., Curr.Adv.Cell & Devel.Biol., Curr.Adv.Ecol.Sci., Curr.Cont., Excerp.Med., INIS Atomind., Ind.Med. (1993-), Ind.Sci.Rev., Inpharma, Int.Abstr.Biol.Sci., Pharm.&Out.News, Reac., Sci.Cit.Ind., Telegen.
—BLDSC (8464.133510), CASDDS, CISTI, EMDOCS, GNLM, IDS, ingenta, KNAW, Linda Hall. **CCC.**
Published by: AlphaMed Press, Inc., One Prestige Pl, Ste 290, Miamisburg, OH 45342-3758. TEL 937-291-2355, FAX 937-291-4229, stemcells@alphamedpress.com, alphamedpress@alphamedpress.com; subscribers@alphamedpress.com, http://www.stemcells.com. Ed. Curt I. Civin. R&P Tim Sparling. Adv. contact Ann Murphy. B&W page USD 900, color page USD 1,550. Circ: 2,050.
Stem Cells provides a premier, peer-reviewed international forum for the publication of original papers and concise reviews describing basic laboratory investigations of stem cells and the translation of clinical aspects of its characterization and manipulation from the bench to patient care, and provocative proposals from Young Turks for new research directions. *Publisher provided annotation.*

577.7 USA ISSN 0969-2126
QH506 CODEN: STRUE6
STRUCTURE. Cover title: Structure with Folding & Design. Text in English. 1993. m. NLG 578, EUR 262.28 in Europe to individuals; JPY 38,100 in Japan to individuals; USD 293 elsewhere to individuals; NLG 2,262, EUR 1,026.45 in Europe to institutions; JPY 142,400 in Japan to institutions; USD 1,148 elsewhere to institutions (effective 2001). adv. reprints avail. *Refereed.* **Document type:** *Academic/Scholarly.* **Description:** Directed toward researchers, educators and students of biology. Features original research and reviews.
Incorporates (1995-1998): Folding and Design (1359-0278)
Related titles: Online - full text ed.: (from EBSCO Publishing, ingenta, Swets Blackwell, Institute for Scientific Information, ScienceDirect).
Indexed: BBCI, Chem.Abstr., Chem.Indus.Notes, Chem.Titles, Curr.Cont., Dairy Sci.Abstr., Food Sci.& Tech.Abstr., Ind.Med. (1999-), Mass Spectr.Bull., Sci.Cit.Ind.
—BLDSC (8478.955000), ADONIS, CASDDS, CISTI, EMDOCS, GNLM, IDS, Infotrieve, ingenta, KNAW. **CCC.**
Published by: Cell Press (Subsidiary of: Reed Elsevier plc), 1100 Massachusetts Ave, Cambridge, MA 02138. TEL 617-661-7057, FAX 617-661-7061, structure@cell.com, http://www.structure.org/, http://www.cellpress.com/. R&P Diana McKinney. adv.: B&W page USD 660, color page USD 1,510; trim 11 x 8.5. Circ: 600. **Subscr. to:** Quadrant Subscription Services. **Dist. by:** Turpin Distribution Services Ltd.

570 ROM ISSN 1221-8103
QH301 CODEN: SUBBA8
STUDIA UNIVERSITATIS "BABES-BOLYAI". BIOLOGIA. Text in English, French, German, Romanian. 1958. s-a. per issue exchange basis. bk.rev. abstr, charts, illus. **Document type:** *Academic/Scholarly.*
Indexed: Biol.Abstr., Chem.Abstr., Excerp.Med., Field Crop Abstr., Forest.Abstr., GeoRef, Herb.Abstr., Maize Abstr., Rev.Plant Path., Soils & Fert., VITIS, Zoo.Rec.
Published by: Universitatea "Babes-Bolyai", Biblioteca Centrala Universitara, Str. Gh. Bilascu 24, Cluj-Napoca 3400, Romania. TEL 36-64-194315, FAX 36-64-191906, puc@hera.ubbcluj.ro. Ed. A Marga.

STUDIES IN FERTILITY AND STERILITY. see *MEDICAL SCIENCES*

570 SGP
STUDIES OF NONLINEAR PHENOMENA IN LIFE SCIENCE. Text in English. 1990. irreg., latest vol.8, 1999, May. USD 68, GBP 43 per vol. for vol. 8 (effective 2002); price varies with each vol.. **Document type:** *Monographic series.*
Indexed: C.C.M.J., Zent.Math.
—BLDSC.
Published by: World Scientific Publishing Co Pte Ltd, Farrer Rd, PO Box 128, Singapore 912805, Singapore. TEL 65-3825663, FAX 65-3825919, wspcl@singnet.com.sg; sales@wspc2.demon.co.uk; wspc@wspc.com, http://www.singnet.com.sg/~wspclib/. Ed. B J West.

STUDII SI CERCETARI DE BIOLOGIE. SERIA BIOLOGIE ANIMALA. see *BIOLOGY—Zoology*

SURFACTANT SCIENCE SERIES. see *CHEMISTRY*

577.85 ISR ISSN 0334-5114
CODEN: SYMBER
SYMBIOSIS. Text in English. 1985. bi-m. USD 410 (effective 2002). reprint service avail. from PQC. *Refereed.* **Document type:** *Academic/Scholarly.* **Description:** Contains original research in symbiotic interactions at the molecular, cellular and organismic levels.
Related titles: Online - full text ed.: (from Institute for Scientific Information).
Indexed: ASCA, AgBiotech, Agricola, Agroforest.Abstr., Appl.Ecol.Abstr., Aqua.Sci.& Fish.Abstr., Bio-Contr.News & Info., Chem.Abstr., Chem.Indus.Notes, Chem.Titles, Crop Physiol.Abstr., Curr.Adv.Plant Sci., Curr.Cont., Ecol.Abstr., Environ.Sci.Poll.Mgmt., Fababean Abstr., Field Crop Abstr., Food Sci.& Tech.Abstr., Forest Prod.Abstr., Forest.Abstr., Geo.Abstr.P.G., Helminthol.Abstr., Herb.Abstr., Hort.Abstr., Ind.Sci.Rev., Int.Abstr.Biol.Sci., Maize Abstr., Microbiol.Abstr., Ocean.Abstr., Plant Breed.Abstr., Plant Grow.Reg.Abstr., Plant Sci., Potato Abstr., Rev.Appl.Entomol., Rev.Arom.& Med.Plants, Rev.Med.& Vet.Mycol., Rev.Plant Path., Rice Abstr., Sci.Cit.Ind., Seed Abstr., Soils & Fert., Soyabean Abstr., Sport Fish.Abstr., Triticale Abstr., Weed Abstr., Zoo.Rec.
—BLDSC (8581.640000), CASDDS, CISTI, EMDOCS, IDS, ingenta, Linda Hall.
Published by: Balaban Publishers, International Science Services, P O Box 2039, Rehovot 76100, Israel. TEL 972-8-9476216, FAX 972-8-9467632. Ed. Margalith Galun.

570 NLD ISSN 0165-5752
QL757 CODEN: SYPAD4
SYSTEMATIC PARASITOLOGY. Text in English. 1979. 9/yr. EUR 924 to institutions for print or online ed.; EUR 1,108.80 to institutions print & online eds.combined (effective 2002). adv. illus. Index. back issues avail.; reprint service avail. from SWZ. *Refereed.* **Document type:** *Academic/Scholarly.* **Description:** Publishes original papers on the systematics, taxonomy and nomenclature of parasites, including nematodes, arthropods, and other parasitic groups.
Related titles: Microform ed.: (from PQC); Online - full text ed.: (from EBSCO Publishing, O C L C Online Computer Library Center, Inc., RoweCom Information Quest, Swets Blackwell, Kluwer Online, Institute for Scientific Information).
Indexed: ASCA, Abstr.Hyg., Agricola, Aqua.Sci.& Fish.Abstr., Bio-Contr.News & Info., Biol.Abstr., Curr.Adv.Ecol.Sci., Curr.Cont., Entomol.Abstr., Environ.Sci.Poll.Mgmt., Helminthol.Abstr., Ind.Med. (1979-), Ind.Sci.Rev., Ind.Vet., Int.Abstr.Biol.Sci., Microbiol.Abstr., Protozool.Abstr., Rev.Appl.Entomol., Rev.Med.& Vet.Mycol., Sci.Cit.Ind., Soils & Fert., Sport Fish.Abstr., Trop.Dis.Bull., Vet.Bull., Zoo.Rec.
—BLDSC (8589.188000), CISTI, EMDOCS, IDS, Infotrieve, ingenta, Linda Hall. **CCC.**
Published by: Kluwer Academic Publishers Group (Subsidiary of: Wolters Kluwer N.V.), Spuiboulevard 50, PO Box 17, Dordrecht 3300 AA, Netherlands. FAX 31-78-639-2254, services@wkap.nl, http://www.wkap.nl/journalhome.htm/0165-5752. Ed. D I Gibson. **Dist. by:** Journals Department, PO Box 322, Dordrecht 3300 AH, Netherlands. TEL 781-871-6600, FAX 31-78-654-6474.

570 540 JPN ISSN 0371-5167
CODEN: TAKHAA
TAKEDA RESEARCH LABORATORIES. JOURNAL. Text in Japanese, English; Summaries in English. 1936. a., latest vol.57, 1998. JPY 2,000 (effective 1999). back issues avail. **Document type:** *Academic/Scholarly.*
Indexed: Biol.Abstr., CEABA, Chem.Abstr., Excerp.Med., INIS Atomind., Ref.Zh.
—CASDDS, EMDOCS, GNLM, Linda Hall.
Published by: Takeda Chemical Industries Ltd., Pharmaceutical Research Division, 17-85 Juso-Hon-Machi 2-chome, Yodogawa-ku, Osaka-shi 532-0024, Japan. Ed. Kanji Meguro. Circ: 1,500.

570 AUS ISSN 0819-6826
TASMANIAN NATURALIST. Text in English. 1904. a. AUD 15 domestic to individuals; AUD 20 domestic to libraries; AUD 25 foreign (effective 2001). bk.rev. bibl, illus, maps. 56 p./no. back issues avail. *Refereed.* **Document type:** *Journal, Academic/Scholarly.* **Description:** Covers natural history of Tasmania, including views on management of natural areas and values.
Indexed: Zoo.Rec.
Published by: Tasmanian Field Naturalist Club Inc., GPO Box 68, Hobart, TAS 7001, Australia. TEL 61-3-6233-4914, julia.jp.scott@centrelink.gov.au, http://www.tased.edu.au/tasonline/tasfield/tasfield.htm. Ed. Owen Seeman. R&P G Gates TEL 61-3-6227-8638. Circ: 200 (paid).

TAUCHEN; internationales Unterwasser-Magazin. see *SPORTS AND GAMES*

TECHNIQUE ET BIOLOGIE; revue de documentation scientifique et d'information professionnelle. see *MEDICAL SCIENCES—Experimental Medicine, Laboratory Technique*

TECHNIQUES IN DIAGNOSTIC PATHOLOGY. see *MEDICAL SCIENCES*

571.976 USA ISSN 0040-3709
QM691 CODEN: TJADAB
TERATOLOGY; the international journal of abnormal development. Text in English. 1968. m. USD 2,660 in United States; USD 2,780 in Canada & Mexico; USD 2,882 elsewhere; USD 2,793 combined subscription in United States for print and online eds.; USD 2,913 combined subscription in Canada & Mexico for print and online eds.; USD 3,015 combined subscription elsewhere for print and online eds. (effective 2002). adv. bk.rev. bibl, charts, illus. index. back issues avail.; reprint service avail. from SWZ. *Refereed.* **Document type:** *Academic/Scholarly.* **Description:** Investigates abnormal fetal development in humans and in experimental animal models.
Related titles: Microform ed.: (from PQC,SWZ); Online - full text ed.: ISSN 1096-9926. 1996. USD 2,660 in United States; USD 2,660 in Canada & Mexico; USD 2,660 elsewhere (effective 2002) (from EBSCO Publishing, Wiley InterScience, Institute for Scientific Information).
Indexed: ASCA, Agri.& Environ.Biotech.Abstr. (coverage dropped), Anim.Breed.Abstr., Art & Archaeol.Tech.Abstr., Bibl.Dev.Med.& Child Neur., Biol.Abstr., Chem.Abstr., Chem.Indus.Notes, Chem.Titles, Curr.Adv.Cell & Devel.Biol., Curr.Adv.Ecol.Sci., Curr.Adv.Gen.& Molec.Biol., Curr.Cont., Dent.Ind., Derwent Biotech.Abstr., Excerp.Med., Helminthol.Abstr., INIS Atomind., I.P.A., Ind.Med. (1968-), Ind.Sci.Rev., Ind.Vet., Inpharma, NRN, Neurosci.Cit.Ind., Nutr.Abstr., Pharm.&Out.News, Poult.Abstr., Reac., Rev.Med.& Vet.Mycol., Sci.Cit.Ind., Sport Fish.Abstr., THA, Vet.Bull., Wild.Rev., Zoo.Rec.
—BLDSC (8792.180000), CASDDS, CISTI, GNLM, IDS, ingenta, KNAW, Linda Hall. **CCC.**
Published by: (Teratology Society), John Wiley & Sons, Inc., Journals (Subsidiary of: Wiley InterScience), 605 Third Ave, New York, NY 10158. TEL 212-850-6645, FAX 212-850-6021, subinfo@wiley.com, uscs-wis@wiley.com, http://www.wiley.com. Ed. Thomas W Sadler. adv.: B&W page GBP 640, color page GBP 1,515; trim 210 x 279. Circ: 1,600. **Subscr. outside the Americas to:** John Wiley & Sons Ltd., Baffins Ln, Chichester, Sussex PO19 IUD, United Kingdom. TEL 44-1243-779777, FAX 44-1243-843232, cs-journals@wiley.co.uk.

572.8 GBR ISSN 1472-9288
▼ **THALAMUS AND RELATED SYSTEMS.** Text in English. 2001. q. EUR 194 in Europe to institutions; JPY 25,800 in Japan to institutions; USD 217 elsewhere to institutions (effective 2002). abstr. **Description:** Publishes papers on the structure, organization and chemistry of thalamic neurons, including the development, single-cell electrophysiology and synaptic interactions, molecular biology and genetics, neuropsychology, computational neurobiology, and pathology of the thalamus.
Related titles: Online - full text ed.
—BLDSC (8814.142000).

Published by: Elsevier Science BV, PO Box 211, Amsterdam 1000 AE, Netherlands. TEL 31-20-485-2911, FAX 31-20-485-2457, nlinfo-f@elsevier.nl, http://www.elsevier.nl/inca/publications/store/6/2/1/9/2/1/. Eds. Edward G Jones, Mircea Steriade.

570 551.46 ESP ISSN 0212-5919
CODEN: THALEP
THALASSAS; revista de ciencias del mar. Text and summaries in English, Spanish. 1983. a. ESP 3,500 (effective 1998 & 1999). charts, illus. back issues avail. *Refereed.* **Document type:** *Academic/Scholarly.* **Description:** Covers marine geology, biology, chemistry and oceanography.
Indexed: Aqua.Sci.& Fish.Abstr., Aquacult.Abstr., Environ.Sci.Poll.Mgmt., GeoRef, Ind.SST, Sport Fish.Abstr., Wild.Rev., Zoo.Rec.
—**CCC.**
Published by: Universidad de Vigo, Servicio de Publicacion, Campus Lagoas-Marcosende, Vigo 36200, Spain. TEL 34-986-812235, FAX 34-986-812180, sep@uvigo.es. Ed. Federico Vilas Martin. Pub., R&P Manuel Vazquez Vazquez. Circ: 500.

570 HRV ISSN 0495-4025
QL1 CODEN: THJUAP
THALASSIA JUGOSLAVICA. Text in Croatian. 1956. q. per issue exchange basis. illus. **Document type:** *Academic/Scholarly.*
Indexed: Aqua.Sci.& Fish.Abstr., Deep Sea Res.& Oceanogr.Abstr.
—CASDDS.
Published by: Rudier Boskovic Institute, Center for Marine Research, PO Box 1016, Zagreb 41001, Croatia. Ed. Tomo Gamulin.

570 USA ISSN 0082-3945
THEORETICAL AND EXPERIMENTAL BIOLOGY; an international series of monographs. Text in English. 1961. irreg., latest vol.6, 1967. reprint service avail. from ISI. *Refereed.* **Document type:** *Monographic series.*
Indexed: Biol.Abstr.
—CISTI, GNLM.
Published by: Academic Press, Inc., Journal Division (Subsidiary of: Harcourt Brace & Company), 525 B St, Ste 1900, San Diego, CA 92101-4495. TEL 619-231-0962, FAX 619-699-6715. Ed. J F Danielli. **Subscr. to:** Order Dept., 6277 Sea Harbor Dr, 4th Fl, Orlando, FL 32887. TEL 800-321-5068.

570 USA ISSN 0040-5809
QH301 CODEN: TLPBAQ
THEORETICAL POPULATION BIOLOGY; an international journal. Text in English. 1970. 8/yr. USD 770 in US & Canada to institutions; USD 885 elsewhere to institutions (effective 2001). *Refereed.* **Document type:** *Academic/Scholarly.* **Description:** Covers the theoretical aspects of the biology of populations, particularly in the areas of ecology, genetics, demography, and epidemiology.
Related titles: Online - full text ed.: (from EBSCO Publishing, O C L C Online Computer Library Center, Inc., RoweCom Information Quest, ingenta, Swets Blackwell, IDEAL Online Library, Institute for Scientific Information).
Indexed: ASCA, Abstr.Hyg., AgBiotech, Anim.Breed.Abstr., Appl.Ecol.Abstr., Aqua.Sci.& Fish.Abstr., Bio-Contr.News & Info., Biol.Abstr., Biotech.& Bioeng.Abstr., Curr.Adv.Ecol.Sci., Curr.Adv.Gen.& Molec.Biol., Curr.Cont., Curr.Ind.Stat., Dairy Sci.Abstr., Deep Sea Res.& Oceanogr.Abstr., Ecol.Abstr., Entomol.Abstr., Environ.Per.Bibl., Environ.Sci.Poll.Mgmt., Forest.Abstr., Genet.Abstr., Helminthol.Abstr., Hum.Gen.Abstr., Ind.Med. (1970-), Ind.Sci.Rev., Ind.Vet., Inpharma, Int.Abstr.Biol.Sci., Math.R., Plant Breed.Abstr., Popul.Ind., Protozool.Abstr., Reac., Rev.Appl.Entomol., Rev.Plant Path., Sci.Cit.Ind., Seed Abstr., Soils & Fert., Sport Fish.Abstr., Wild.Rev., Zent.Math., Zoo.Rec.
—BLDSC (8814.566000), CISTI, EMDOCS, GNLM, IDS, ingenta, Linda Hall. **CCC.**
Published by: Academic Press, Inc., Journal Division (Subsidiary of: Harcourt Brace & Company), 525 B St, Ste 1900, San Diego, CA 92101-4495. TEL 619-230-1840, FAX 619-699-6800, http://www.academicpress.com/tpb.

570 DEU ISSN 1431-7613
QH301 CODEN: THBIFM
THEORY IN BIOSCIENCES/THEORIE IN DEN BIOWISSENSCHAFTEN. Text and summaries in English, German. 1881. 4/yr. EUR 218, GBP 180 (effective 2002). adv. bk.rev. charts, illus. reprint service avail. from PQC. *Refereed.* **Document type:** *Journal, Academic/Scholarly.*
Formerly (until 1997): Biologisches Zentralblatt (0006-3304)
Related titles: Microform ed.: (from PQC,PMC); Online - full text ed.: (from EBSCO Publishing, O C L C Online Computer Library Center, Inc., ingenta, Swets Blackwell, Institute for Scientific Information).
Indexed: ASCA, Anim.Breed.Abstr., Aqua.Sci.& Fish.Abstr., Biol.Abstr., Chem.Abstr., Chem.Indus.Notes, Chem.Titles, Curr.Adv.Ecol.Sci., Curr.Cont., Deep Sea Res.& Oceanogr.Abstr., Ecol.Abstr., Excerp.Med., Fababean Abstr., Field Crop Abstr., Helminthol.Abstr., Herb.Abstr., Hort.Abstr., INIS Atomind., Ind.Sci.Rev., Ind.Vet., Int.Abstr.Biol.Sci., Key Word Ind.Wildl.Res., Plant Breed.Abstr., Plant Grow.Reg.Abstr., Rev.Appl.Entomol., Rev.Med.& Vet.Mycol., Rev.Plant Path., Rice Abstr., SSCI (coverage dropped), Sci.Cit.Ind., Seed Abstr., Vet.Bull., Weed Abstr., Wild.Rev., Zoo.Rec.
—BLDSC (8814.630200), CASDDS, CISTI, EMDOCS, IDS, Infotrieve, ingenta, Linda Hall. **CCC.**
Published by: Urban & Fischer Verlag, Loebdergraben 14A, Jena 07743, Germany. TEL 49-3641-626444, FAX 49-3641-626500, info@urbanfischer.de, http://www.urbanfischer.de. Eds. M Weingarten, O Breidbach. R&P Martin Huber TEL 49-3641-626430. Adv. contact Sabine Schroeter. page DEM 600; trim 240 x 170. Circ: 300.

577 HUN ISSN 0563-587X
QH178.H8 CODEN: TSCAB8
TISCIA; an ecological journal. Text in English. 1965. a. per issue exchange basis. charts, illus. **Document type:** *Academic/Scholarly.* **Description:** Covers the biology and ecology of ecosystems and the pollution of the environment in and around the Tisza River.
Indexed: Aqua.Sci.& Fish.Abstr., Biol.Abstr., Chem.Abstr., Chem.Titles, Entomol.Abstr. (coverage dropped), GeoRef, Microbiol.Abstr., Russ.Acad.Sci.Bibl., Sel.Water Res.Abstr., Zoo.Rec.
—CASDDS.
Published by: Attila Jozsef University, Department of Ecology, c/o Laszlo Kormoczy, PO Box 659, Szeged 6701, Hungary. kormoczy@sol.cc.u-sezeged.hu. Ed. Laszlo Galle. Circ: 300. **Co-sponsor:** Tisza Kutato Bizottsag.

TISSUE ANTIGENS. see *MEDICAL SCIENCES*

570 JPN ISSN 0040-8786
CODEN: STUBAS
TOHOKU UNIVERSITY. SCIENCE REPORTS. SERIES 4: BIOLOGY/TOHOKU DAIGAKU RIKA HOKOKU. DAI-4-SHU, SEIBUTSUGAKU. Text in English. 1924. a. per issue exchange basis. bibl, charts, illus. index.
Related titles: Microform ed.: (from PMC).
Indexed: Agrindex, Aqua.Sci.& Fish.Abstr., Aquacult.Abstr., Biol.Abstr., Chem.Abstr., Deep Sea Res.& Oceanogr.Abstr., Environ.Sci.Poll.Mgmt., Excerp.Med., GeoRef, Met.Abstr., Zoo.Rec.
—CASDDS, CISTI.
Published by: Tohoku Daigaku, Rigakubu/Tohoku University, Faculty of Science, Laboratory of Nuclear Science, Aramaki, Aoba-ku, Sendai-shi, Miyagi-ken 981-0945, Japan. Ed. Dr. K Sohma. Circ: 700.

TOPICS IN GEOBIOLOGY. see *EARTH SCIENCES—Geology*

570 CAN ISSN 0820-683X
TORONTO FIELD NATURALIST. Text in English. 1938. 8/yr. CND 25. bk.rev. **Document type:** *Newsletter.* **Description:** Stimulates public interest in natural history and encourages the preservation of Canada's natural heritage through conservation.
Address: 2 Carlton St No 1519, Toronto, ON M5B 1J3, Canada. TEL 416-593-2656. Ed. Helen Juhola. Circ: 1,500 (paid).

TRANSYLVANIA UNIVERSITY OF BRASOV. BULLETIN. SERIES B; mathematics, economical sciences, philology, medicine, physics, chemistry, sports. see *MATHEMATICS*

577 GBR ISSN 0169-5347
QH540 CODEN: TREEEQ
TRENDS IN ECOLOGY AND EVOLUTION. Text in English. 1986. m. GBP 92 in Europe to individuals; EUR 115 in Europe to individuals Print & online eds. combined; JPY 14,000 in Japan to individuals; USD 126 elsewhere to individuals; EUR 908 in Europe to institutions; JPY 125,900 in Japan to institutions; USD 1,015 elsewhere to institutions; GBP 47 in Europe to students; JPY 10,100 in Japan to students; USD 78 elsewhere to students; USD 1,308 to institutions Print & online eds. combined; EUR 144, JPY 17,500 in Europe to qualified personnel; USD 157 elsewhere to qualified personnel (effective 2002). adv. bk.rev., software rev. charts, illus. index. back issues avail.; reprints avail. *Refereed.* **Document type:** *Academic/Scholarly.* **Description:** Contains reviews, commentaries, discussions and letters in all areas of ecology and evolutionary science.
Related titles: Online - full text ed.: (from ingenta, Swets Blackwell, Institute for Scientific Information, ScienceDirect).
Indexed: ASCA, AgBiotech, Anim.Behav.Abstr., Anim.Breed.Abstr., Apic.Abstr., Appl.Ecol.Abstr., Aqua.Sci.& Fish.Abstr., Arts & Hum.Cit.Ind. (coverage dropped), Bio-Contr.News & Info., Biol.Abstr., Biol.Dig., Chemorec.Abstr., Crop Physiol.Abstr., Curr.Cont., Ecol.Abstr., Entomol.Abstr., Environ.Abstr., Environ.Per.Bibl. (1989-), Environ.Sci.Poll.Mgmt., Food Sci.& Tech.Abstr., Forest.Abstr., Genet.Abstr., Geo.Abstr.H.G., Geo.Abstr.P.G., GeoRef, Geol.Abstr., Helminthol.Abstr., Herb.Abstr., Hort.Abstr., Hum.Gen.Abstr., IBR, INIS Atomind., Ind.Sci.Rev., Int.Abstr.Biol.Sci., Nuc.Acids Abstr., Plant Breed.Abstr., Poult.Abstr., Protozool.Abstr., Rev.Appl.Entomol., Rev.Med.& Vet.Mycol., Rev.Plant Path., SSCI (coverage dropped), Saf.Sci.Abstr., Sci.Cit.Ind., Seed Abstr., Soils & Fert., Sport Fish.Abstr., Weed Abstr., Wild.Rev., World Ag.Econ.& Rur.Soc.Abstr., Zoo.Rec.
—BLDSC (9049.569000), ADONIS, CISTI, IDS, ingenta, Linda Hall. **CCC.**
Published by: Elsevier Science Ltd., Elsevier Trends Journals, 68 Hills Rd, Cambridge CB2 1LA, United Kingdom. TEL 44-1865-315961, FAX 44-1233-464430, tree@elsevier.co.uk, TREE@elsevier.co.uk, http://www.elsevier.com/locate/issn/01695347. Eds. Andrew M Sugden, C MacCallum, H Carroll. Adv. contact Thelma Reid. Circ: 1,649. **Subscr. in Australasia and the Far East to:** Elsevier Science (Singapore) Pte Ltd, No.1 Temasek Ave, 17-01 Millenia Tower, Singapore 039192, Singapore. TEL 65-434-3727, FAX 65-337-2230**; Subscr. in the Americas to:** Elsevier Science, PO Box 945, New York, NY 10159-0945. TEL 212-633-3730, FAX 212-633-3680, http://www.elsevier.com**; Subscr. to:** Elsevier Current Trends Subscriptions, PO Box 331, Haywards Heath, W Sussex RH16 3FG, United Kingdom. TEL 44-1444-475650, FAX 44-1444-445423.

570 TUR ISSN 1300-0152
QH301 CODEN: TJBIEZ
TURKISH JOURNAL OF BIOLOGY/TURK BIYOLOJI DERGISI. Text in English, Turkish. 1976. 4/yr. USD 100 (effective 1999). *Refereed.* **Document type:** *Journal, Academic/Scholarly.*
Formerly (until 1994): Doga Turkish Journal of Biology - Doga Turk Biyoloji Dergisi (1010-7576)
Related titles: Online - full text ed.
Indexed: Abstr.Hyg., AgBiotech, Anim.Breed.Abstr., Apic.Abstr., Bio-Contr.News & Info., Biol.Abstr., Chem.Abstr., Crop Physiol.Abstr., Dairy Sci.Abstr., Field Crop Abstr., Food Sci.& Tech.Abstr., Forest Prod.Abstr., Herb.Abstr., Hort.Abstr., Ind.Vet., Maize Abstr., Nutr.Abstr., Ornam.Hort., Plant Breed.Abstr., Plant Grow.Reg.Abstr., Postharvest, Poult.Abstr., Rev.Appl.Entomol., Rev.Arom.& Med.Plants, Rev.Med.& Vet.Mycol., Rev.Plant Path., Rice Abstr., Seed Abstr., Soils & Fert., Soyabean Abstr., Triticale Abstr., Trop.Dis.Bull., Weed Abstr., Zoo.Rec.
—BLDSC, CASDDS, Linda Hall.
Published by: Scientific and Technical Research Council of Turkey - TUBITAK/Turkiye Bilimsel ve Teknik Arastirma Kurumu, Ataturk Bulvari No. 221, Kavaklidere, Ankara 06100, Turkey. TEL 90-312-468-5300, FAX 90-312-426-8073, bdym@tubitak.gov.tr, http://www.tubitak.gov.tr/journals/biology/. Ed. Dr. Ahmet Noyan.

TURKISH JOURNAL OF MEDICAL & BIOLOGICAL RESEARCH. see *MEDICAL SCIENCES*

570 FIN ISSN 0082-6979
CODEN: ATYBAK
TURUN YLIOPISTO. JULKAISUJA. SARJA A. II. BIOLOGICA - GEOGRAPHICA - GEOLOGICA/ ANNALES UNIVERSITATIS TURKUENSIS. Text in English, Finnish, French, German. 1957. irreg. price varies. **Document type:** *Monographic series, Academic/Scholarly.* **Description:** Studies biology, genetics, geography and geology.
Indexed: GeoRef, INIS Atomind.
—CASDDS, CISTI, EMDOCS, Linda Hall.
Published by: Turun Yliopiston Kirjasto/University of Turku, Turku 20500, Finland. FAX 358-2-3335050, annales@utu.fi, http://www.utu.fi/kirjasto.

U.S. CENTERS FOR DISEASE CONTROL. CONGENITAL MALFORMATIONS SURVEILLANCE. see *BIOLOGY—Abstracting, Bibliographies, Statistics*

570 USA ISSN 0301-5629
RM862.7 CODEN: USMBA3
ULTRASOUND IN MEDICINE & BIOLOGY. Text in English. 1974. 12/yr. EUR 1,023 in Europe to institutions; JPY 136,000 in Japan to institutions; USD 1,145 elsewhere to institutions; EUR 89 in Europe in Residence; JPY 11,800 in Japan in Residence; USD 100 elsewhere in Residence (effective 2002). adv. charts, illus. index. back issues avail. *Refereed.* **Document type:** *Academic/Scholarly.* **Description:** Publishes original contributions on significant advances in clinical diagnostic, interventional and therapeutic applications, new and improved clinical techniques, the physics, engineering and technology of ultrasound in medicine and biology, and the interactions between ultrasound and biological materials.
Related titles: Microfilm ed.: (from PQC); Online - full text ed.: (from ingenta, Swets Blackwell, Institute for Scientific Information, ScienceDirect).
Indexed: ASCA, Acoust.Abstr., Appl.Mech.Rev., Aqua.Sci.& Fish.Abstr., Bioeng.Abstr., Biol.Abstr., Cal.Tiss.Abstr., Comput.& Info.Sys., Curr.Adv.Ecol.Sci., Curr.Cont., Dent.Ind., Electron.& Communic.Abstr.J., Eng.Ind., Environ.Sci.Poll.Mgmt., Excerp.Med., INSPEC (Sep.1973-), ISMEC, Ind.Imag.Lit., Ind.Med. (1973-), Ind.Sci.Rev., Inpharma, Pharm.&Out.News, Pollut.Abstr., Reac., Risk Abstr., Saf.Sci.Abstr., Sci.Cit.Ind.
—BLDSC (9082.815000), AskIEEE, CISTI, Ei, EMDOCS, GNLM, IDS, ingenta, KNAW, Linda Hall. **CCC.**
Published by: (World Federation for Ultrasound in Medicine and Biology), Elsevier Science, 655 Ave of the Americas, New York, NY 10010. TEL 212-989-5800, FAX 212-633-3990, usinfo-f@elsevier.com, http://www.elsevier.nl/locate/issn/03015629. Eds. Dennis N White, P N T Wells. Adv. contact Tino DeCarlo. B&W page USD 985, color page USD 1,175. Circ: 1,500 (paid). **Subscr. in Australasia and the Far East to:** Elsevier Science (Singapore) Pte Ltd, No.1 Temasek Ave, 17-01 Millenia Tower, Singapore 039192, Singapore. TEL 65-434-3727, FAX 65-337-2230; **Subscr. in Japan to:** Elsevier Science Inc - Japan Regional Office, 9-15 Higashi-Azabu 1-chome, Minato-ku, Tokyo 106-0044, Japan. TEL 81-3-5561-5033; **Subscr. outside the Americas to:** Elsevier Science BV, PO Box 211, Amsterdam 1000 AE, Netherlands. TEL 31-20-485-3757.

570 COL ISSN 0120-8063
UNIVERSIDAD DE BOGOTA JORGE TADEO LOZANO. MUSEO DEL MAR. INFORME. Text in Spanish; Summaries in English. 1971. irreg. price varies. bibl. **Document type:** *Monographic series.*
Indexed: Aqua.Sci.& Fish.Abstr., Aquacult.Abstr., Environ.Sci.Poll.Mgmt.
Published by: Universidad de Bogota Jorge Tadeo Lozano, Museo del Mar, Carrera 4 No. 22-61, Bogota, CUND, Colombia. TEL 57-1-3426581, FAX 57-1-2826197. Ed. Elvira Maria Alvarado Chacon.

570 URY ISSN 0250-653X
QH301
UNIVERSIDAD DE LA REPUBLICA. FACULTAD DE HUMANIDADES Y CIENCIAS. REVISTA. SERIE CIENCIAS BIOLOGICAS. Text in Spanish. N.S. 1978. irreg. per issue exchange basis.
Formerly: Universidad de la Republica. Facultad de Humanidades y Ciencias. Revista. Serie Ciencias; Supersedes in part: Universidad de la Republica. Facultad de Humanidades y Ciencias. Revista
Published by: Universidad de la Republica, Facultad de Humanidades y Ciencias, c/o Seccion Revista, Dr. Tristan Narvaja, 1674, Montevideo 11205, Uruguay. Ed. Beatriz Martinez Osorio.

570 ESP
UNIVERSIDAD DE MURCIA. ANALES DE BIOLOGIA. Text mainly in English, Spanish. 1984. a., latest vol.22, 1999, for the year 1997. ESP 2,000 (effective 2001). bk.rev. back issues avail. **Document type:** *Academic/Scholarly.* **Description:** Contains original advances in the field of the biological sciences.
Indexed: Entomol.Abstr. (coverage dropped), Ind.SST, Rev.Med.& Vet.Mycol.
Published by: Universidad de Murcia, Servicio de Publicaciones, C Actor Isidoro Maiquez 9, Murcia 30007, Spain. TEL 34-68-363014, FAX 34-68-363414, vgm@um.es, http://www.um.es/spumweb. Ed. Diego Jose Rivera Nunez TEL 34-968-364958. Circ: 606.

577 ESP ISSN 0213-4004
QH540 CODEN: ABSAEZ
UNIVERSIDAD DE MURCIA. ANALES DE BIOLOGIA. SECCION BIOLOGIA AMBIENTAL. Text mainly in English, Spanish. 1984. a., latest vol.22, 1999, for the year 1997. ESP 2,000 (effective 2001). bk.rev. back issues avail. **Document type:** *Academic/Scholarly.*
Indexed: Ind.SST.
—CISTI.
Published by: Universidad de Murcia, Servicio de Publicaciones, C Actor Isidoro Maiquez 9, Murcia 30007, Spain. TEL 34-68-363014, FAX 34-68-363414, vgm@um.es, http://www.um.es/spumweb. Ed. Diego Jose Rivera Nunez TEL 34-968-364958. Circ: 606.

572.8 ESP
UNIVERSIDAD DE MURCIA. ANALES DE BIOLOGIA. SECCION BIOLOGIA MOLECULAR Y MICROBIANA. Text mainly in English, Spanish. 1984. irreg., latest vol.22, 1999, for the year 1997. ESP 2,000 (effective 1997). bk.rev. back issues avail. **Document type:** *Academic/Scholarly.*
Formerly: Universidad de Murcia. Anales de Biologia. Seccion Biologia General (0213-5442)
Indexed: Field Crop Abstr., Herb.Abstr., Plant Grow.Reg.Abstr.
—CISTI.
Published by: Universidad de Murcia, Servicio de Publicaciones, C Actor Isidoro Maiquez 9, Murcia 30007, Spain. TEL 34-68-363014, FAX 34-68-363414, vgm@um.es, http://www.um.es/spumweb. Ed. Diego Jose Rivera Nunez TEL 34-968-364958. Circ: 500.

570 ESP ISSN 0212-8977
CODEN: RBUOE2
UNIVERSIDAD DE OVIEDO. REVISTA DE BIOLOGIA. Text in Spanish; Abstracts in English, Spanish. 1942. a. ESP 2,500. **Document type:** *Academic/Scholarly.*
Formerly (until 1981): Universidad de Oviedo. Facultad de Ciencias, Revista. Serie Biologia (0473-6303)
Related titles: ♦ Supplement: Biodatos Basicos.
Indexed: Aquacult.Abstr., Biol.Abstr., Curr.Adv.Ecol.Sci., GeoRef, Ind.SST, Sport Fish.Abstr.
—CASDDS, CISTI.
Published by: Universidad de Oviedo, Facultad de Biologia, c/o Carlos Lastra, Redactor, Departamento de Zoologia, Oviedo 33071, Spain. Circ: 750. **Subscr. to:** Servicio de Publicaciones, Arguelles, 19, Oviedo 33003, Spain. TEL 34-85-104486, FAX 34-85-104488.

578.77 551.46 BRA ISSN 0374-0412
QH91.A1 CODEN: URTBAV
UNIVERSIDADE FEDERAL DE PERNAMBUCO. DEPARTAMENTO DE OCEANOGRAFIA. CENTRO DE TECNOLOGIA. TRABALHOS OCEANOGRAFICOS. Text in Spanish, Portuguese, English. 1960. a. BRL 20 domestic; USD 20 foreign (effective 2000). adv. bk.rev. abstr. back issues avail. *Refereed.* **Document type:** *Bulletin.* **Description:** Informs about estuarine, coastal and oceanic oceanography research, mainly in tropical areas.
Former titles (until 1966): Universidade Federal de Pernambuco. Instituto Oceanografico. Trabalhos (0080-0236); (until 1963): Universidade do Recife. Instituto Oceanografico. Trabalhos; (until 1960): Instituto de Biologia Marinha e Oceanografia. Trabalhos
Related titles: Fax ed.
Indexed: Aqua.Sci.& Fish.Abstr., Aquacult.Abstr., Biol.Abstr., Deep Sea Res.& Oceanogr.Abstr., Environ.Sci.Poll.Mgmt., GeoRef, Sport Fish.Abstr.
Published by: Editoria Universitaria U F P E, Departamento de Oceanografia, Centro de Tecnologia, Campus Universitario, C D U, Recife, PE 50670901, Brazil. TEL 55-81-2718397, FAX 55-81-2718395, TELEX 811267, oceano@npd.ufpe.br. Ed., R&P Sigrid Neumann Leitao TEL 55-81-2718225. adv.: B&W page USD 15, color page USD 30; trim 140 x 200. Circ: 250.

570 ITA ISSN 0085-0950
UNIVERSITA DEGLI STUDI DI GENOVA. MUSEI E ISTITUTI BIOLOGICI. BOLLETTINO. Key Title: Bollettino dei Musei e degli Istituti Biologici dell'Universita di Genova. Text in English, Italian; Summaries in English. 1891. a. per issue exchange basis. **Document type:** *Academic/Scholarly.*
Indexed: Biol.Abstr., Deep Sea Res.& Oceanogr.Abstr., Zoo.Rec.
Published by: Universita degli Studi di Genova, Istituto di Zoologia, Via Balbi 5, Genoa 16126, Italy. TEL 39-010-2099454, FAX 39-010-2099323, zoologia@unige.it. Ed. Silvio Spano. Circ: 500.

571.9 640 ITA ISSN 1125-0720
UNIVERSITA DI FERRARA. ANNALI. SEZIONE 2: PATOLOGIA CHIRURGICA. Text in Italian. 1952. a.
Published by: (Universita di Ferrara), Casa Editrice Leo S. Olschki, Viuzzo Del Pozzetto, Florence, FI 50126, Italy. TEL 39-55-6530684, FAX 39-55-6530214.

571.86 ITA ISSN 0373-5907
UNIVERSITA DI FERRARA. ANNALI. SEZIONE 3: BIOLOGIA ANIMALE. Text in Italian. 1951. irreg.
Published by: (Universita di Ferrara), Casa Editrice Leo S. Olschki, Viuzzo Del Pozzetto, Florence, FI 50126, Italy. TEL 39-55-6530684, FAX 39-55-6530214.

570 AUT ISSN 0587-484X
UNIVERSITAET INNSBRUCK. ALPIN-BIOLOGISCHE STUDIEN* . Text in German. 1970. irreg., latest vol.6, 1974. price varies.
Published by: (Universitaet Innsbruck), Oesterreichische Kommissionsbuchhandlung, Glasmalereistr 6, Innsbruck, T 6020, Austria. TEL 43-512-587039, FAX 43-512-5870394, oekobuch@aon.at, http://www.oekobuch.com. Ed. Heinz Janetschek.

570 ROM ISSN 0041-9133
QH301 CODEN: AUIBAF
UNIVERSITATEA "AL. I. CUZA" DIN IASI. ANALELE STIINTIFICE. SECTIUNEA 2A: BIOLOGIE. Text in French, German, Romanian, Russian. 1955. a. ROL 35. bk.rev. abstr. charts, illus. **Description:** Contains information on genetics, microbiology, plant anatomy, vegetal taxonomy, entomology, ecology and cellular biology.
Indexed: Biol.Abstr., Chem.Abstr., Chem.Indus.Notes, Chem.Titles, Hort.Abstr., Math.R., Ornam.Hort., Ref.Zh., Rev.Plant Path., Seed Abstr.
—CASDDS, CISTI, Linda Hall.
Published by: Universitatea "Al. I. Cuza" din Iasi, Calea M. Eminescu 11, Jassy, Romania. Ed. C Toma. Circ: 550. **Subscr. to:** ILEXIM, Str. 13 Decembrie 3, PO Box 136-137, Bucharest 70116, Romania.

570 630 ROM ISSN 0254-7236
CODEN: AUCHD6
UNIVERSITATEA DIN CRAIOVA. ANALE. SERIA: BIOLOGIE, AGRONOMIE, HORTICULTURA. Text in Romanian; Summaries in English, French, German. 1972. a. ROL 80, USD 15.
—CASDDS.
Published by: Universitatea din Craiova, Str. A.I. Cuza 13, Craiova 1100, Romania. Circ: 300.

570 TGO ISSN 1016-9210
UNIVERSITE DU BENIN. ANNALES. SERIE SCIENCE. Text in French; Summaries in English, French. 1975. a. FRF 15,000 (effective Jun. 2000); USD 25 (effective 2000). bk.rev. **Document type:** *Academic/Scholarly.*
Published by: Universite du Benin, BP 1515, Lome, Togo. TEL 25-48-44, FAX 25-87-84, TELEX 52-58 UBTO, gbesson@syfed.tg.refer.org. Ed. Messanvi Gbeassor.

570 USA ISSN 0568-8604
QH1
UNIVERSITY OF ALASKA. BIOLOGICAL PAPERS. Text in English. 1955. irreg., latest vol.25, 1996. USD 30. bibl, illus. back issues avail. *Refereed.* **Document type:** *Monographic series.*
Indexed: Biol.Abstr., GeoRef, Sport Fish.Abstr., Wild.Rev., Zoo.Rec.
—CISTI, Linda Hall.
Published by: (Library), University of Alaska at Fairbanks, Institute of Arctic Biology, 308 Irving I, PO Box 757000, Fairbanks, AK 99775-7000. TEL 907-474-7658, FAX 907-474-7666. Ed., R&P Jean James. Circ: 500.

570 USA ISSN 0161-3243
CODEN: BPURDY
UNIVERSITY OF ALASKA. BIOLOGICAL PAPERS. SPECIAL REPORTS. Text in English. 1975. irreg., latest vol.5, 1992. USD 30. **Document type:** *Monographic series.*
Indexed: Zoo.Rec.

—CASDDS, CISTI.
Published by: (Library), University of Alaska at Fairbanks, Institute of Arctic Biology, 308 Irving I, PO Box 757000, Fairbanks, AK 99775-7000. TEL 907-474-7658, FAX 907-474-7666. Ed. Jean James.

570 USA ISSN 0272-9075
UNIVERSITY OF CALIFORNIA. LAWRENCE BERKELEY LABORATORY. BIOLOGY AND MEDICINE DIVISION. ANNUAL REPORT. Text in English. a.
Published by: (Lawrence Berkeley Laboratory, University of California, Biology and Medicine Division), U.S. National Technical Information Service, 5285 Port Royal Rd, Springfield, VA 22161. TEL 703-605-6060.

570 500.9 USA ISSN 0272-2658
UNIVERSITY OF KANSAS. MUSEUM OF NATURAL HISTORY. PUBLIC EDUCATION SERIES. Text in English. 1974. irreg., latest vol.12, 1992. price varies. reprints avail.
—Linda Hall.
Published by: University of Kansas, Museum of Natural History, 602 Dyche Hall, Lawrence, KS 66044-2454. Ed. Joseph T Collins.

570 500.9 USA ISSN 0193-7766
UNIVERSITY OF KANSAS. MUSEUM OF NATURAL HISTORY. SPECIAL PUBLICATIONS. Text in English. irreg., latest vol.19, 1991. price varies. reprints avail. *Refereed.* **Document type:** *Academic/Scholarly.*
Indexed: GeoRef, Zoo.Rec.
—Linda Hall.
Published by: University of Kansas, Museum of Natural History, 602 Dyche Hall, Lawrence, KS 66044-2454. TEL 785-654-4450, FAX 785-864-5335, kunhm@ukans.edu, http://www.nhm.ukans.edu. Ed. William E Duellman.

578.77 SDN ISSN 0379-9611
CODEN: AUKUDH
UNIVERSITY OF KHARTOUM. HYDROBIOLOGICAL RESEARCH UNIT. ANNUAL REPORT. Text in English. a.
Published by: University of Khartoum, Hydrobiological Research Unit, P O Box 321, Khartoum, Sudan.

UNIVERSITY OF OSAKA PREFECTURE. COLLEGE OF AGRICULTURE. SCIENTIFIC REPORT. see *AGRICULTURE*

UNIVERSITY OF SANTO TOMAS. GRADUATE SCHOOL. JOURNAL OF GRADUATE RESEARCH. see *SOCIAL SCIENCES: COMPREHENSIVE WORKS*

611.01816 USA
UNIVERSITY OF SOUTH FLORIDA. INTERNATIONAL BIOMEDICAL SYMPOSIA SERIES. Text in English. 1986. irreg., latest vol.3, 1987. price varies. charts, illus. *Refereed.* **Document type:** *Proceedings.*
Published by: (University of South Florida), Kluwer Academic - Plenum Publishers (Subsidiary of: Wolters Kluwer N.V.), 233 Spring St, New York, NY 10013-1578. TEL 212-620-8000, 800-221-9369, FAX 212-463-0742, info@plenum.com, http://www.plenum.com. Ed. Andor Szentivanyi.

UNIVERSITY OF WAIKATO. ANTARCTIC RESEARCH UNIT. REPORT. see *EARTH SCIENCES—Geology*

570 CAN ISSN 0317-3348
UNIVERSITY OF WATERLOO BIOLOGY SERIES. Text in English. 1971. irreg. price varies. **Document type:** *Academic/Scholarly.*
—CISTI.
Published by: University of Waterloo, Department of Biology, Waterloo, ON N2L 3G1, Canada. TEL 519-885-1211, FAX 519-746-0614. Ed. J C Semple.

570 550 USA
UNIVERSITY OF WISCONSIN-MILWAUKEE. FIELD STATION BULLETIN. Text in English. 1968. s-a. free per issue. back issues avail. **Document type:** *Bulletin.*
Indexed: Biol.Abstr., Zoo.Rec.
Published by: University of Wisconsin-Milwaukee, Field Station, 3095 Blue Goose Rd, Saukville, WI 53080. TEL 414-675-6844, FAX 414-675-0337, jimr@csd.uwm.edu. Ed., R&P James A Reinartz. Circ: 400.

570 POL ISSN 0554-811X
UNIWERSYTET IM. ADAMA MICKIEWICZA. BIOLOGIA. Text in Polish; Summaries in English. 1961. irreg., latest vol.57, 1996. price varies. **Document type:** *Monographic series, Academic/Scholarly.* **Description:** Contains current research results of the university's biologists, their Ph.D. works, monographs and other scientific works. Each volume is devoted to the work of one author.
Formerly: Uniwersytet im. Adama Mickiewicza w Poznaniu. Wydzial Biologii i Nauk o Ziemi. Seria Biologia
Indexed: AgroLibrex, Zoo.Rec.
—CISTI, Linda Hall.
Published by: (Uniwersytet im. Adama Mickiewicza), Adam Mickiewicz University Press, Nowowiejskiego 55, Poznan 61734, Poland. TEL 48-61-527380, FAX 48-61-527701. Pub. Maria Jankowska. R&P Malgorzata Bis. Circ: 400.

570 POL ISSN 0860-2441
UNIWERSYTET SLASKI W KATOWICACH. PRACE NAUKOWE. ACTA BIOLOGICA SILESIANA. Text in English, Polish; Summaries in English, Polish, Russian. 1975. irreg. price varies. **Document type:** *Academic/Scholarly.* **Description:** Covers biochemistry, botany, histology, microbiology, physiology, zoology, morphology, systematics, environmental protection.
Formerly (until 1985): Acta Biologica (0208-5046)
Indexed: AgroLibrex, Triticale Abstr., Zoo.Rec.
Published by: (Uniwersytet Slaski w Katowicach), Wydawnictwa Szkolne i Pedagogiczne, Ul Bankowa 12 B, Katowice 40007, Poland. TEL 48-32-596915, FAX 48-32-599-605, wydawus@us.edu.pl, http://www.us.edu.pl/uniwersytet/jednostki/ogolne. R&P Barbara Woznica. **Dist. by:** CHZ Ars Polona, Biblioteka PAN w Warszawie, PO Box 1001, Warsaw 00950, Poland.

570.71 DEU ISSN 0341-5260
UNTERRICHT BIOLOGIE; Beitraege zu seiner Gestaltung. Text in German. 1965. 10/yr. DEM 158.60 domestic; DEM 168.60 foreign; DEM 18.80 newsstand/cover (effective 2001). abstr. cum.index. **Document type:** *Journal, Academic/Scholarly.*
Incorporates: Naturwissenschaften im Unterricht Biologie (0342-5487); Formerly: Biologieunterricht (0006-3274)
Indexed: Biol.Abstr., IBR.
—CISTI. **CCC.**
Published by: Erhard Friedrich Verlag GmbH, Im Brande 17, Seelze 30926, Germany. TEL 49-511-40004-0, FAX 49-511-40004119, info@friedrich-verlag.de, http://www.friedrich-verlag.de. Ed. Barbara Dulitz. Circ: 15,000.

572.8 BGR ISSN 0205-0625
QH506 CODEN: UMBIEX
USPEHI NA MOLECULIARNATA BIOLOGIA/ADVANCES IN MOLECULAR BIOLOGY. Text in Bulgarian. 1975. s-a. BGL 1.36 per issue. reprint service avail. from IRC.
Supersedes: Molekulna Biologiia
—CASDDS, Linda Hall.
Published by: (Bulgarska Akademiia na Naukite/Bulgarian Academy of Sciences), Publishing House of the Bulgarian Academy of Sciences, Akad G Bonchev 6, Sofia 1113, Bulgaria. Circ: 450.

570 RUS ISSN 0042-1324
QH301 CODEN: USBIA3
USPEKHI SOVREMENNOI BIOLOGII. Text in Russian. 1932. bi-m. USD 143.75. bk.rev.
Indexed: AgBiotech, Anim.Breed.Abstr., Aqua.Sci.& Fish.Abstr., Aquacult.Abstr., Bio-Contr.News & Info., Biol.Abstr., Chem.Abstr., Chem.Indus.Notes, Crop Physiol.Abstr., Deep Sea Res.& Oceanogr.Abstr., Environ.Sci.Poll.Mgmt., Field Crop Abstr., Helminthol.Abstr., Herb.Abstr., Hort.Abstr., INIS Atomind., Ind.Med. (coverage dropped), Ind.Vet., Int.Aerosp.Abstr., Maize Abstr., Nutr.Abstr., Plant Breed.Abstr., Plant Grow.Reg.Abstr., Poult.Abstr., Protozool.Abstr., Ref.Zh., Rev.Appl.Entomol., Rev.Med.& Vet.Mycol., Rev.Plant Path., Russ.Acad.Sci.Bibl., Seed Abstr., Triticale Abstr., Trop.Oil Seeds Abstr., Weed Abstr., Zoo.Rec.
—CASDDS, CISTI, East View, GNLM, KNAW, Linda Hall.
Published by: (Rossiiskaya Akademiya Nauk/Russian Academy of Sciences), M A I K Nauka - Interperiodica, Mezhdunarodnyi Otdel, Profsoyuznaya ul 90, Moscow 117864, Russian Federation. TEL 7-095-3360266, FAX 7-095-420-2220. Ed. Yu I Chernov. **US dist. addr.:** East View Publications, 3020 Harbor Ln N, Minneapolis, MN 55447. TEL 612-550-0961.

570 UZB ISSN 0042-1685
QH301.A3652 CODEN: UZBZAZ
UZBEKSKII BIOLOGICHESKII ZHURNAL. Text in Russian. 1957. bi-m. charts, illus.
Indexed: Bio-Contr.News & Info., Biol.Abstr., Chem.Abstr., Crop Physiol.Abstr., Dairy Sci.Abstr., Field Crop Abstr., GeoRef, Helminthol.Abstr., Herb.Abstr., Hort.Abstr., INIS Atomind., Ind.Vet., Pig News & Info., Plant Grow.Reg.Abstr., Rev.Plant Path., Sorghum & Millets Abstr., Vet.Bull., Weed Abstr., Zoo.Rec.
—CASDDS, CISTI, Infotrieve, Linda Hall. **CCC.**
Published by: (Akademiya Nauk Uzbekistana), Izdatel'stvo Fan, Ya Gulyamov ul 70, k 105, Tashkent 700047, Uzbekistan.

577 FRA ISSN 0240-8759
CODEN: VIMID2
VIE ET MILIEU/LIFE AND ENVIRONMENT; periodique d'ecologie generale. Text in English, French. 1950. q. FRF 950 domestic to individuals; FRF 1,050 foreign to individuals (effective 1999). adv. bk.rev. charts, illus. index. back issues avail. *Refereed.* **Document type:** *Academic/Scholarly.* **Description:** Journal of general ecology: Organisms, communities and ecosystems biology and ecology; trophic webs, energetics; benthic ecology; pollution; numerical ecology, modelings; evolutionary biology and phylogeny, with emphasis on marine, lagoonar and terrestrial milieus. Includes one special topic issue each year.
Related titles: Online - full text ed.: (from Institute for Scientific Information).
Indexed: Agroforest.Abstr., Anim.Behav.Abstr., Appl.Ecol.Abstr., Aqua.Sci.& Fish.Abstr., Aquacult.Abstr., Biol.& Agr.Ind. (coverage dropped), Biol.Abstr., Curr.Adv.Ecol.Sci., Curr.Cont., Deep Sea Res.& Oceanogr.Abstr., Ecol.Abstr., Entomol.Abstr., Environ.Sci.Poll.Mgmt., Excerp.Med., Forest.Abstr., Geo.Abstr.H.G., GeoRef, Geol.Abstr., Helminthol.Abstr., Ind.Vet., Ocean.Abstr. (coverage dropped), Pollut.Abstr., Rev.Appl.Entomol., Rev.Med.& Vet.Mycol., Sci.Cit.Ind., Sel.Water Res.Abstr., Soils & Fert., Sport Fish.Abstr., Wild.Rev., Zoo.Rec.
—BLDSC (9235.000000), CISTI, IDS, ingenta, Linda Hall.
Published by: Universite de Paris VI (Pierre et Marie Curie), Laboratoire Arago, Banyuls Sur Mer 66650, France. TEL 33-4-68887327, FAX 33-4-68881699, vimilieu@arago.obs-banyuls.fr. Ed. Alain Guille. R&P, Adv. contact Nicole Coineau.

571.9 616.07 DEU ISSN 0945-6317
RB1 CODEN: VARCEM
VIRCHOWS ARCHIV; an international journal of pathology. Text in English. 1847. m. EUR 1,155.90 domestic; EUR 1,136.70 in Germany; EUR 111 newsstand/cover foreign (effective 2002). adv. bibl, charts, illus. index, cum.index: vols.301-325, vols.326-343. back issues avail.; reprint service avail. from ISI. *Refereed.* **Document type:** *Journal, Academic/Scholarly.* **Description:** Provides fundamental research on disease and on human pathological anatomy and histology in particular.
Formed by the 1994 merger of: Virchows Archiv. Section B: Cell Pathology (0340-6075); Virchows Archiv. Section A: Pathological Anatomy and Histopathology (0174-7398); Which was formerly: Virchows Archiv. Section A: Pathological Anatomy and Histology. (0340-1227); Virchows Archiv. Abteilung A: Pathologische Anatomie (0042-6423)
Related titles: Microform ed.: (from PQC,PMC); Online - full text ed.: ISSN 1432-2307 (from EBSCO Publishing, RoweCom Information Quest, Swets Blackwell, Springer LINK, Institute for Scientific Information).
Indexed: ASCA, Biol.Abstr., Chem.Abstr., Chem.Indus.Notes, Curr.Adv.Cancer Res., Curr.Adv.Cell & Devel.Biol., Curr.Adv.Ecol.Sci., Curr.Adv.Gen.& Molec.Biol., Curr.Cont., Dairy Sci.Abstr., Dent.Ind., Excerp.Med., Helminthol.Abstr., INIS Atomind., Ind.Med. (1994-), Ind.Sci.Rev., Ind.Vet., Inpharma, Int.Abstr.Biol.Sci., Med.& Surg.Dermat., Neurosci.Cit.Ind., Nutr.Abstr., Pharm.&Out.News, Protozool.Abstr., Reac., Rev.Med.& Vet.Mycol., Sci.Cit.Ind., Vet.Bull.
—BLDSC (9238.000000), ADONIS, CASDDS, CISTI, EMDOCS, GNLM, IDS, ingenta, KNAW. **CCC.**
Published by: (European Society of Pathologists), Springer-Verlag (Subsidiary of: BertelsmannSpringer), Tiergartenstr 17, Heidelberg 69121, Germany. TEL 49-6221-345-0, FAX 49-6221-345229, subscriptions@springer.de, http://link.springer.de/link/service/journals/00428/index.htm, http://www.springer.de. Eds. C L Berry, M Dietel. **Subscr. in N. America to:** Springer-Verlag New York Inc., PO Box 2485, Secaucus, NJ 07096-2485. TEL 212-460-1500, FAX 212-473-6272.

578.77 USA ISSN 0083-6427
VIRGINIA INSTITUTE OF MARINE SCIENCE, GLOUCESTER POINT. EDUCATIONAL SERIES. Text in English. 1943. irreg., latest 1994. price varies. **Document type:** *Monographic series.*

Published by: Virginia Institute of Marine Science, PO Box 1346, Gloucester, VA 23062. TEL 804-684-7170, FAX 804-684-7161, http://www.vims.edu. Ed., R&P Lee Larkin TEL 804-684-7000.

578.77 USA ISSN 0083-6435
VIRGINIA INSTITUTE OF MARINE SCIENCE, GLOUCESTER POINT. MARINE RESOURCES ADVISORY SERIES. Text in English. 1970. irreg., latest 1998. price varies. **Document type:** *Monographic series.*
Published by: Virginia Institute of Marine Science, PO Box 1346, Gloucester, VA 23062. TEL 804-684-7170, FAX 804-684-7161, http://www.vims.edu.

578.77 USA ISSN 0083-6443
VIRGINIA INSTITUTE OF MARINE SCIENCE, GLOUCESTER POINT. SPECIAL SCIENTIFIC REPORT. Text in English. 1948. irreg., latest vol.136, 1998. price varies.
Related titles: Microfiche ed.
Indexed: Biol.Abstr., GeoRef, Ocean.Abstr. (coverage dropped).
Published by: Virginia Institute of Marine Science, PO Box 1346, Gloucester, VA 23062. TEL 804-684-7116, FAX 804-684-7113, http://www.vims.edu. R&P Eugene Burreson TEL 804-684-7000.

B

570 610 RUS
VOPROSY BIOLOGICHESKOI, MEDITSINSKOI, I FARMATSEVTICHESKOI KHIMII/PROBLEMS OF BIOLOGICAL, MEDICAL AND PHARMACOLOGICAL. Text in Russian. 1998. q. USD 180 foreign (effective 2000). adv. bk.rev., Website rev. **Document type:** *Journal, Academic/Scholarly.* **Description:** Deals with problems of biological, medical, and pharmocological chemistry.
Indexed: Ref.Zh.
Published by: Izdatel'stvo Meditsina, Petroverigskii per 6-8, Moscow 101000, Russian Federation. TEL 7-095-9248785, 7-095-928-86-48, FAX 7-095-9211355, 7-095-9286003, http://www.medit.ru. Ed. E.V. Severin. Pub. A M Stochik. R&P E V Severin. Adv. contact O A Fadeeva TEL 7-095-923-51-40. Circ: 200. **Dist. by:** Mezhdunarodnaya Kniga, B Yakimanka 39, Moscow 117049, Russian Federation. TEL 7-095-2384967, FAX 7-095-2384634; **US dist. addr.:** East View Publications, 3020 Harbor Ln N, Minneapolis, MN 55447. TEL 612-550-0961.

VOPROSY RADIOBIOLOGII I BIOLOGICHESKOGO DEISTVIYA TSITOSTATICHESKIKH PREPARATOV. see *MEDICAL SCIENCES—Radiology And Nuclear Medicine*

570 550 JPN ISSN 0913-0187
WASEDA DAIGAKU KYOIKUGAKUBU GAKUJUTSU KENKYU. SEIBUTSUGAKU, CHIGAKU HEN/WASEDA UNIVERSITY. SCHOOL OF EDUCATION. SCIENTIFIC RESEARCHES: BIOLOGY, GEOLOGY. Text and summaries in English, Japanese. 1952. a. membership.
Indexed: Jap.Per.Ind.
Published by: Waseda Daigaku, Kyoikugakubu/Waseda University, School of Education, Shinjuku-ku, Tokyo 169-50, Japan. TEL 03-3203-4141, FAX 03-3208-1032.

570 USA ISSN 0043-0927
QH1 CODEN: WMJBA2
WASMANN JOURNAL OF BIOLOGY. Text in English. 1937. s-a. USD 6.50. abstr, bibl, charts, illus. index. *Refereed.* **Document type:** *Academic/Scholarly.*
Indexed: Biol.Abstr., Biol.Dig., Chem.Abstr., Curr.Adv.Ecol.Sci., Deep Sea Res.& Oceanogr.Abstr., Ecol.Abstr., Nutr.Abstr., Soils & Fert., Sport Fish.Abstr., Wild.Rev., Zoo.Rec.
—CISTI, ingenta, Linda Hall.
Published by: University of San Francisco, Biology Department, San Francisco, CA 94117. TEL 415-666-6381. Ed. Gary L Stevens. Circ: 400.

WENNER GREN CENTER INTERNATIONAL SYMPOSIUM SERIES. see *SCIENCES: COMPREHENSIVE WORKS*

WHALEWATCHER. see *CONSERVATION*

577 POL ISSN 0013-2969
CODEN: WEKLAF
WIADOMOSCI EKOLOGICZNE. Text in Polish; Summaries in English. 1955. q. USD 35 foreign (effective 2002). adv. bk.rev. bibl. 100 p./no. 1 cols./p. back issues avail. **Document type:** *Academic/Scholarly.* **Description:** Publishes various articles, reports from conferences as well as information on activities of ecological institutions in Poland and other countries.
Formerly: Ekologia Polska. Seria B
Indexed: AgroLibrex, Biol.Abstr., Field Crop Abstr., GeoRef, Herb.Abstr., INIS Atomind., Russ.Acad.Sci.Bibl., Sel.Water Res.Abstr., Zoo.Rec.
—BLDSC (9313.100000).
Published by: Polska Akademia Nauk, Instytut Ekologii, Dziekanow Lesny, Lomianki 05092, Poland. TEL 48-22-7513046, FAX 48-22-7513100. Ed., R&P, Adv. contact Eligiusz Pieczynski. Circ: 860. **Dist. by:** Ars Polona, Krakowskie Przedmiescie 7, Warsaw, Poland.

616.96 POL ISSN 0043-5163
CODEN: WIPAAZ
WIADOMOSCI PARAZYTOLOGICZNE. Text in Polish, English. 1955. bi-m. USD 33. bk.rev. bibl, charts, illus, tr.lit. index.
Related titles: ♦ Includes: International Commission on Trichinellosis. Proceedings. ISSN 0074-3356.
Indexed: Abstr.Hyg., AgroAgen, AgroLibrex, Apic.Abstr., Biol.Abstr., Chem.Abstr., Curr.Adv.Ecol.Sci., Excerp.Med., Helminthol.Abstr., INIS Atomind., Ind.Med. (1955-), Ind.Vet., Pig News & Info., Poult.Abstr., Protozool.Abstr., Rev.Appl.Entomol., Rev.Med.& Vet.Mycol., Rev.Plant Path., Trop.Dis.Bull., Vet.Bull., Zoo.Rec.
—CASDDS, CISTI, GNLM.
Published by: Polskie Towarzystwo Parazytologiczne/ Polish Parasitological Society, Ul Grochowska 272, Warsaw 03849, Poland. bielecki@matman.wsp.olsztyn.pl. Ed. Aleksander Bielecki. Circ: 1,150.

577 USA ISSN 0084-0122
WILDLIFE BEHAVIOR AND ECOLOGY. Text in English. 1971. irreg., latest 1995. price varies. reprint service avail. from PQC,ISI. *Refereed.*
Published by: University of Chicago Press, 5801 S Ellis Ave, Chicago, IL 60637. TEL 773-702-7899, sales@press.uchicago.edu, http://www.press.uchicago.edu. Ed. George B Schaller.

WOHNUNG & GESUNDHEIT; Fachzeitschrift fuer oekologisches Bauen & Leben. see *ARCHITECTURE*

571.864 FRA ISSN 0084-1641
RC889
WORLD CONGRESS ON FERTILITY AND STERILITY. PROCEEDINGS. Text in English. 1953. triennial, latest 1995, 15th, Montpellier. **Document type:** *Proceedings.*
Indexed: Anim.Breed.Abstr., Biol.Abstr.
Published by: International Federation of Fertility Societies, CSI c/o Prof. Bernard Hedon, 337 rue de la Combe Caude, Montpellier 34090, France. TEL 33-4-67635340, FAX 33-4-67419427, algcsi@mnet.fr; bhiffs@mnet.fr. R&P B Hedon. Circ: 3,000.

570 USA
THE WORLD WIDE WEB JOURNAL OF BIOLOGY. Text in English. 1995. a., latest vol.4, 1999. back issues avail. **Document type:** *Journal, Academic/Scholarly.*
Media: Online - full text. **Related titles:** CD-ROM ed.
Indexed: Zoo.Rec.
Published by: Epress Inc, 130 Union Terrace Ln, Plymouth, MN 55441. http://epress.com/w3jbio/wjbhome.htm. Ed. Lester F Harris.

570.71 POL
WYZSZA SZKOLA PEDAGOGICZNA IM. KOMISJI EDUKACJI NARODOWEJ W KRAKOWIE. ROCZNIK NAUKOWO-DYDAKTYCZNY. PRACE Z DYDAKTYKI BIOLOGII. Text in Polish. 1964. irreg., latest vol.4, 1990. price varies.
Published by: (Wyzsza Szkola Pedagogiczna im. Komisji Edukacji Narodowej w Krakowie), Wydawnictwo Naukowe W S P, Ul Karmelicka 41, Krakow 31128, Poland. TEL 33-78-20. **Co-sponsor:** Ministerstwo Edukacji Narodowej.

YALE JOURNAL OF BIOLOGY AND MEDICINE. see *MEDICAL SCIENCES*

YANBIAN - JIBIAN - TUBIAN/CARCINOGENSIS, TERATOGENSIS AND MUTAGENESIS. see *MEDICAL SCIENCES—Oncology*

YOKOHAMA MEDICAL JOURNAL. see *MEDICAL SCIENCES*

570 JPN
YOKOHAMA NATIONAL UNIVERSITY. SCIENCE REPORTS. SECTION 2: BIOLOGICAL AND GEOLOGICAL SCIENCES/YOKOHAMA KOKURITSU DAIGAKU RIKA KIYO. DAI-2-RUI. SEIBUTSUGAKU, CHIGAKU. Text in Multiple languages, Japanese. 1952. a. per issue exchange basis only. illus. **Document type:** *Academic/Scholarly.*
Formerly: Yokohama National University. Science Reports. Section 2: Biological Sciences (0513-5613)
Indexed: Biol.Abstr., Forest Prod.Abstr., Forest.Abstr., GeoRef, JTA, Jap.Per.Ind., Rev.Plant Path.
—Linda Hall.
Published by: Yokohama Kokuritsu Daigaku, Kyoikugakubu/Yokohama National University, Faculty of Education, 156 Tokiwa-Dai, Hodogaya-ku, Yokohama-shi, Kanagawa-ken 240-0067, Japan.

YUNYI NATURALIST. see *CHILDREN AND YOUTH—For*

570 910.02 DEU
ZEITSCHRIFT FUER ANGEWANDTE GEWASSEROEKOLOGIE. Text in German. 1995. biennial. back issues avail. **Document type:** *Magazine, Academic/Scholarly.*
Related titles: E-mail ed.; Fax ed.
Published by: (Institut zur Angewandte Gewasseroekologie), Natur und Text in Brandenburg GmbH, Friedensallee 21, Rangsdorf 15834, Germany. TEL 49-708-20432, FAX 49-708-20433, nut-brandenburg@t-online.de. Ed. Jens Meisel.

ZEITSCHRIFT FUER MORPHOLOGIE UND ANTHROPOLOGIE. see *ANTHROPOLOGY*

570 DEU ISSN 0939-5075
QH301 CODEN: ZNCBDA
ZEITSCHRIFT FUER NATURFORSCHUNG. SECTION C: A JOURNAL OF BIOSCIENCES. Text in English. 1946. bi-m. DEM 740 (effective 2001). bk.rev. bibl, charts, illus. index. *Refereed.* **Document type:** *Journal, Academic/Scholarly.*
Formerly (until 1986): Zeitschrift fuer Naturforschung. Section C: Biosciences (0341-0382)
Related titles: Online - full text ed.: (from Institute for Scientific Information).
Indexed: ASCA, Abstr.Hyg., AgBiotech, Agri.& Environ.Biotech.Abstr. (coverage dropped), Agroforest.Abstr., Apic.Abstr., Aqua.Sci.& Fish.Abstr., Aquacult.Abstr., BBCI, Biol.Abstr., Chem.Abstr., Chem.Cit.Ind., Chem.Indus.Notes, Chem.Titles, Crop Physiol.Abstr., Curr.Adv.Ecol.Sci., Curr.Adv.Plant Sci., Curr.Cont., Dairy Sci.Abstr., Deep Sea Res.& Oceanogr.Abstr., Dent.Ind., Derwent Biotech.Abstr., Entomol.Abstr. (coverage dropped), Environ.Sci.Poll.Mgmt., Excerp.Med., Fababean Abstr., Field Crop Abstr., Forest Prod.Abstr., Forest.Abstr., Helminthol.Abstr., Herb.Abstr., Hort.Abstr., INIS Atomind., Ind.Med. (1986-), Ind.Sci.Rev., Ind.Vet., Inpharma, Int.Abstr.Biol.Sci., Irr.& Drain.Abstr., Maize Abstr., Mass Spectr.Bull., NPU, Nutr.Abstr., Ornam.Hort., Pharm.&Out.News, Plant Breed.Abstr., Plant Gen.Res.Abstr., Plant Grow.Reg.Abstr., Plant Sci., Potato Abstr., Poult.Abstr., Protozool.Abstr., Reac., Rev.Appl.Entomol., Rev.Arom.& Med.Plants, Rev.Med.& Vet.Mycol., Rev.Plant Path., Rice Abstr., Sci.Cit.Ind., Seed Abstr., Soils & Fert., Soyabean Abstr., Sport Fish.Abstr., Sugar Ind.Abstr., Triticale Abstr., Trop.Dis.Bull., VITIS, Vet.Bull., Weed Abstr., Wild.Rev., Zoo.Rec.
—BLDSC (9475.010000), CASDDS, CINDOC, CISTI, EMDOCS, GNLM, IDS, ingenta, Linda Hall. **CCC.**
Published by: Verlag der Zeitschrift fuer Naturforschung, Postfach 2645, Tuebingen 72016, Germany. TEL 49-7071-31555, FAX 49-7071-360571, mail@znaturforsch.com, http://www.znaturforsch.com. Eds. H Hausen, P. Boeger. R&P Tamina Greifeld.

ZHONGGUO HAIYANG YAOWU ZAZHI/CHINESE JOURNAL OF MARINE DRUGS. see *PHARMACY AND PHARMACOLOGY*

ZHONGGUO JISHENGCHONG YU JISHENGCHONGBING ZAZHI/CHINESE JOURNAL OF PARASITOLOGY AND PARASITIC DISEASES. see *MEDICAL SCIENCES—Communicable Diseases*

ZHONGGUO JISHENGCHONGBING FANGZHI ZAZHI/CHINESE JOURNAL OF PARASITIC DISEASE CONTROL. see *MEDICAL SCIENCES—Communicable Diseases*

ZHONGHUA FENGSHIBINGXUE ZAZHI/CHINESE JOURNAL OF RHEUMATOLOGY. see *MEDICAL SCIENCES—Rheumatology*

570 RUS ISSN 0044-4596
CODEN: ZOBIAU
ZHURNAL OBSHCHEI BIOLOGII. Text in Russian; Summaries in English. 1940. bi-m. USD 223.75. index. *Refereed.*
Related titles: Online - full text ed.: (from Institute for Scientific Information).

Indexed: ASCA, Abstr.Hyg., Anim.Breed.Abstr., Aqua.Sci.& Fish.Abstr., Aquacult.Abstr., Bio-Contr.News & Info., Biol.Abstr., Chem.Abstr., Chem.Indus.Notes, Chem.Titles, Crop Physiol.Abstr., Curr.Adv.Ecol.Sci., Curr.Cont., Dairy Sci.Abstr., Deep Sea Res.& Oceanogr.Abstr., Environ.Sci.Poll.Mgmt., Excerp.Med., Field Crop Abstr., Forest.Abstr., GeoRef, Helminthol.Abstr., Herb.Abstr., INIS Atomind., Ind.Med. (1940-), Ind.Sci.Rev., Ind.Vet., Int.Aerosp.Abstr., Plant Breed.Abstr., Plant Grow.Reg.Abstr., Protozool.Abstr., Ref.Zh., Rev.Appl.Entomol., Russ.Acad.Sci.Bibl., Sci.Cit.Ind., Soils & Fert., Triticale Abstr., Trop.Dis.Bull., Vet.Bull., Weed Abstr., Zoo.Rec.
—CASDDS, CISTI, East View, GNLM, IDS, Infotrieve, KNAW, Linda Hall. **CCC.**
Published by: (Otdelenie Obshchei Biologii, Rossiiskaya Akademiya Nauk/Russian Academy of Sciences), M A I K Nauka - Interperiodica, Mezhdunarodnyi Otdel, Profsoyuznaya ul 90, Moscow 117864, Russian Federation. TEL 7-095-3360266, FAX 7-095-420-2220. Ed. L N Andreev. **Dist. in U.S. by:** Victor Kamkin Inc., 4956 Boiling Brook Pkwy, Rockville, MD 20852.

571.3 DEU ISSN 0720-213X
QL1 CODEN: ZMPHDI
ZOOMORPHOLOGY; an international journal of comparative and functional morphology. Text in English. 1924. q. EUR 1,008.30 domestic; EUR 1,004.90 in Germany; EUR 299.40 newsstand/cover foreign (effective 2002). adv. bibl, illus. back issues avail.; reprint service avail. from ISI. *Refereed.* **Document type:** *Journal, Academic/Scholarly.* **Description:** Reviews research on animal morphology at all levels of ontogeny and organization, including ultrastructure of invertebrates and vertebrates.
Former titles: Zoomorphologie (0340-6725); Zeitschrift fuer Morphologie der Tiere (0044-3131)
Related titles: Microform ed.: (from PQC); Online - full text ed.: ISSN 1432-234X (from EBSCO Publishing, RoweCom Information Quest, Swets Blackwell, Springer LINK, Institute for Scientific Information).
Indexed: ASCA, Aqua.Sci.& Fish.Abstr., Bio-Contr.News & Info., Biol.Abstr., Curr.Adv.Ecol.Sci., Curr.Cont., Curr.Ref.Fish Res., Deep Sea Res.& Oceanogr.Abstr., Entomol.Abstr., Helminthol.Abstr., INIS Atomind., Ind.Sci.Rev., Ref.Zh., Rev.Appl.Entomol., Rev.Med.& Vet.Mycol., Sci.Cit.Ind., Sport Fish.Abstr., Wild.Rev., Zoo.Rec.
—BLDSC (9530.310000), ADONIS, CISTI, IDS, Infotrieve, ingenta, Linda Hall. **CCC.**
Published by: Springer-Verlag (Subsidiary of: BertelsmannSpringer), Tiergartenstr 17, Heidelberg 69121, Germany. TEL 49-6221-345-0, FAX 49-6221-345229, subscriptions@springer.de, http://link.springer.de/link/service/journals/00435/index.htm, http://www.springer.de. Ed. O Kraus. **Subscr. in N. America to:** Springer-Verlag New York Inc., PO Box 2485, Secaucus, NJ 07096-2485. TEL 212-460-1500, FAX 212-473-6272.

577 USA ISSN 0720-1842
CODEN: ZOOPDH
ZOOPHYSIOLOGY. Text in English. 1971. irreg., latest vol.33, 1995. price varies. reprint service avail. from ISI. **Document type:** *Monographic series.*
Formerly (until 1977): Zoophysiology and Ecology (0084-5663)
Indexed: Aqua.Sci.& Fish.Abstr., Aquacult.Abstr., Biol.Abstr., Environ.Sci.Poll.Mgmt., Zoo.Rec.
—BLDSC (9531.259000), CISTI, KNAW.
Published by: Springer-Verlag, Journals (Subsidiary of: BertelsmannSpringer), 175 Fifth Ave, New York, NY 10010. TEL 212-460-1500, FAX 212-473-6272. Ed. D S Farne.

BIOLOGY—Abstracting, Bibliographies, Statistics

016.58 BEL ISSN 0066-9784
A E T F A T INDEX; releve des travaux de phanerogamie systematique et des taxons nouveaux concernant l'Afrique au sud du Sahara et Madagascar. Text in English, French. 1953. a. USD 8.50. cum.index: 1953-1985.
Published by: Association pour l'Etude Taxonomique de la Flore d'Afrique Tropicale, Rue de la Hulpe 136, Rosieres 1331, Belgium. Ed. J Lejoly.

016.6606 USA ISSN 1043-8971
TP248.27.M37
A S F A MARINE BIOTECHNOLOGY ABSTRACTS. (Aquatic Sciences & Fisheries Abstracts) Text in English. 1989. q. USD 465 print & online eds. (effective 2002). abstr. index. back issues avail. **Document type:** *Abstract/Index.* **Description:** Covers the application of molecular biology and genetics to marine and aquatic organisms.
Formerly: Marine Biotechnology Abstracts
Related titles: Online - full text ed.: USD 350 (effective 2002) (from CSA, CISTI).
—BLDSC (1740.620000).
Published by: Cambridge Scientific Abstracts, 7200 Wisconsin Ave., Suite 601, Bethesda, MD 20814. TEL 301-961-6798, FAX 301-961-6799, journals@csa.com, http://www.csa.com/journals. Ed. Deborah Whitman. Pub. Ted Caris.

016.612015 GBR ISSN 0261-4553
A T PASES. (Adenosine Triphosphatases) Text in English. s-m. GBP 96 for print ed. or e-mail (effective 2001). adv. back issues avail. **Document type:** *Abstract/Index.* **Description:** Provides a current-awareness service for researchers in clinical and life sciences.
Related titles: E-mail ed.; Online - full text ed.: GBP 108 to individuals (effective 2001).
—CCC.
Published by: S U B I S (Subsidiary of: Sheffield Academic Press Ltd), Mansion House, 19 Kingfield Rd, Sheffield, S Yorks S11 9AS, United Kingdom. TEL 44-114-255-4433, FAX 44-114-255-4626, subis@sheffac.demon.co.uk, http://www.shef-ac-press.co.uk/subis. Ed. S Huntridge. Adv. contact C Evans.

016.597 USA ISSN 0001-3579
Z5856 CODEN: AEMYA
ABSTRACTS OF ENTOMOLOGY. Text in English. 1970. m. USD 630 (effective 2001); includes cumulative index. bk.rev. abstr, bibl. index, cum.index. **Document type:** *Abstract/Index.* **Description:** Current awareness journal containing abstracts and content summaries in English of pure and applied research involving insects, arachnids and insecticides.
Indexed: Rev.Appl.Entomol.
—BLDSC (0564.230000), CISTI.
Published by: BIOSIS, 2001 Market Street, Suite 700, Philadelphia, PA 19103-7095. TEL 215-587-4800, FAX 215-587-2016, info@mail.biosis.org, http://www.biosis.org.

016.5795 USA ISSN 0001-3617
QK600 CODEN: ABMYA5
ABSTRACTS OF MYCOLOGY. Text in English. 1967. m. USD 630 (effective 2001); includes cumulative index. bk.rev. abstr, bibl. index, cum.index. **Document type:** *Abstract/Index.* **Description:** Contains abstracts in English about research involving fungi, lichens, and fungicides.
—BLDSC (0565.430000), CASDDS, CISTI.
Published by: BIOSIS, 2001 Market Street, Suite 700, Philadelphia, PA 19103-7095. TEL 215-587-4800, FAX 215-587-2016, info@mial.biosis.org, http://www.biosis.org.

016.63 GBR ISSN 0954-9897
S494.5.B563
AGBIOTECH NEWS AND INFORMATION. Text in English. 1989. m. GBP 765, USD 1,340 (effective 2001). back issues avail. **Document type:** *Abstract/Index.* **Description:** Contains a comprehensive selection of abstracts of the world's literature on agricultural biotechnology and some human applications of biotechnology. Focuses on the impact of biotechnology in agriculture and policy issues, as well as the purely scientific ones.
Related titles: Online - full text ed.: (from DIMDI, The Dialog Corporation, S T N International).
Indexed: Food Sci.& Tech.Abstr., Hort.Abstr., Rev.Appl.Entomol., Rev.Arom.& Med.Plants, Rev.Plant Path., Seed Abstr., Weed Abstr.
—BLDSC (0736.034000), CISTI, Infotrieve. **CCC.**
Published by: CABI Publishing, Wallingford, Oxon OX10 8DE, United Kingdom. TEL 44-1491-832111, FAX 44-1491-829198, publishing@cabi.org, http://www.agbiotechnet.com. Ed. David Hemming. **US subscr. to:** 10 E 40th St, Ste 3203, New York, NY 10016. TEL 212-481-7018, 800-528-4841, FAX 212-686-7993, cabi-nao@cabi.org.

016.5736 GBR ISSN 0268-1544
AGING. Text in English. s-m. GBP 120 (effective 2001). adv. back issues avail. **Document type:** *Abstract/Index.* **Description:** Current awareness service for researchers in the clinical and life sciences.
Related titles: E-mail ed.: GBP 120 (effective 2001); Online - full text ed.: GBP 108 (effective 2001) (from Northern Light Technology, Inc.).
Indexed: AgeLine, Environ.Sci.Poll.Mgmt., Int.Nurs.Ind., Pollut.Abstr., Risk Abstr., Saf.Sci.Abstr.
—Infotrieve. **CCC.**
Published by: S U B I S (Subsidiary of: Sheffield Academic Press Ltd), Mansion House, 19 Kingfield Rd, Sheffield, S Yorks S11 9AS, United Kingdom. TEL 44-114-255-4433, FAX 44-114-255-4626, subis@sheffac.demon.co.uk, http://www.shef-ac-press.co.uk/subis. Ed. S Huntridge. Adv. contact C Evans.

016.579 USA ISSN 1060-2011
QR1
AMERICAN SOCIETY FOR MICROBIOLOGY. ABSTRACTS OF THE GENERAL MEETING. Text in English. 1948. a. USD 25. index. reprint service avail. from PQC. **Document type:** *Proceedings.*
Former titles: American Society for Microbiology. Abstracts of the Annual Meeting (0094-8519); Bacteriological Proceedings (0067-2777)
Indexed: Biol.Abstr., Dairy Sci.Abstr., Derwent Biotech.Abstr., Food Sci.& Tech.Abstr., INIS Atomind., Ind.Vet., Nutr.Abstr., Soils & Fert., Vet.Bull., Weed Abstr.
—BLDSC (0564.255000), CISTI, GNLM, Linda Hall. **CCC.**
Published by: American Society for Microbiology, 1325 Massachusetts Ave, N W, Washington, DC 20005-4171. TEL 202-737-3600. Circ: 10,000.

016.5915 USA ISSN 0301-8695
QL750
ANIMAL BEHAVIOR ABSTRACTS. Text in English. 1972. q. USD 850 print & online eds. (effective 2002). bk.rev. abstr. index. back issues avail. **Document type:** *Abstract/Index.* **Description:** Covers field and laboratory studies of all aspects of animal behavior.
Formerly: Behavioural Biology Abstracts, Section A: Animal Behaviour (0300-5852)
Related titles: Online - full text ed.: USD 640 (effective 2002) (from The Dialog Corporation, S T N International, EBSCO Publishing, CSA).
Indexed: Russ.Acad.Sci.Bibl.
—BLDSC (0902.960000), CISTI.
Published by: Cambridge Scientific Abstracts, 7200 Wisconsin Ave., Suite 601, Bethesda, MD 20814. TEL 301-961-6798, FAX 301-961-6799, journals@csa.com, http://www.csa.com/journals. Ed. R Hilton. Pub. Ted Caris.

016.57 GBR ISSN 1350-4541
APOPTOSIS. Text in English. 1993. s-m. GBP 96 for print ed. or e-mail (effective 2001). adv. **Document type:** *Abstract/Index.* **Description:** Provides current awareness service for researchers in clinical and life sciences.
Related titles: E-mail ed.; Online - full text ed.: GBP 108 to individuals (effective 2001) (from Kluwer Online).
Indexed: Inpharma, Reac.
—CCC.
Published by: S U B I S (Subsidiary of: Sheffield Academic Press Ltd), Mansion House, 19 Kingfield Rd, Sheffield, S Yorks S11 9AS, United Kingdom. TEL 44-114-255-4433, FAX 44-114-255-4626, subis@sheffac.demon.co.uk, http://www.shef-ac-press.co.uk/subis. Ed. S Huntridge. Adv. contact C Evans.

016.571 612 USA ISSN 1080-4757
APSTRACTS. Text in English. w. free. **Description:** Features current articles that are accepted and scheduled to be published in the journals of the American Physiological Society.
Media: Online - full text.
Published by: American Physiological Society, 9650 Rockville Pike, Bethesda, MD 20814-3991. TEL 301-530-7164, FAX 301-571-8305, info@aps.faseb.org, info@the-aps.org, http://www.uth.tmc.edu/apstracts. Ed. M Frank.

016.57877 ZAF ISSN 1083-883X
AQUATIC BIOLOGY, AQUACULTURE & FISHERIES RESOURCES. Text in English. 1995. q. ZAR 27,420. **Document type:** *Abstract/Index.* **Description:** Provides access to comprehensive information on the science and management of aquatic organisms and environments.
Media: Online - full content. **Related titles:** CD-ROM ed.: (from National Information Services Corp. (NISC)).
Published by: (National Inquiry Services Centre (Pty) Ltd), N I S C South Africa, 22 Somerset St, Grahamstown 6139, South Africa. FAX 27-46-622-9550, 27-46-622-9550, nisc@ru.ac.za, info@nisc.co.za, http://education.nation.co.za/nisc/aquatic.html, http://www.nisc.co.za.

016.5765 AUS

AUSTRALIAN AND NEW ZEALAND DIRECTORY OF GENETICS SUPPORT GROUPS, SERVICES AND INFORMATION. Text in English. 1992. biennial. AUD 35 (effective 1999). *Refereed.* **Document type:** *Directory.* **Description:** Provides information about genetic support groups and services for the health professionals, students, teachers, and the general community.

Published by: New South Wales Genetics Education Program, PO Box 317, St Leonards, NSW 2065, Australia. FAX 61-2-9906-7529, gethi@blackburn.med.usyd.edu.au, http://www.genetics.com.au. Ed., R&P Kristine Barlow-Stewart TEL 61-2-9926-7324. Pub. Kristine Barlow Stewart. Circ: 1,500.

016.5714 GBR ISSN 0952-0384

BIO-ELECTRONICS AND BIOSENSORS. Text in English. 1986. s-m. GBP 120 (effective 2001). adv. **Document type:** *Abstract/Index.* **Description:** Current awareness service for researchers in clinical and life sciences. Covers bioelectricity, biochips, enzyme electrodes and in vivo NMR.

Formerly (until 1987): Bio-electronics (0268-1633)

Related titles: E-mail ed.: GBP 120 (effective 2001); Online - full text ed.: GBP 108 (effective 2001).

Indexed: Nutr.Abstr.

—Infotrieve. **CCC.**

Published by: S U B I S (Subsidiary of: Sheffield Academic Press Ltd), Mansion House, 19 Kingfield Rd, Sheffield, S Yorks S11 9AS, United Kingdom. TEL 44-114-255-4433, FAX 44-114-255-4626, subis@sheffac.demon.co.uk, http://www.shef-ac-press.co.uk/subis. Ed. S Huntridge. Adv. contact C Evans.

016.572 USA ISSN 1065-7509

BIOCHEMISTRY AND BIOPHYSICS CITATION INDEX. Text in English. bi-m. USD 1,170 for CD-ROM. **Document type:** *Academic/Scholarly, Bibliography.* **Description:** Provides bibliographic data, cited references, related records and English-language author abstracts for international scholarly research journals and conference proceedings.

Related titles: CD-ROM ed.: (from Institute for Scientific Information); Magnetic Tape ed.

Published by: Institute for Scientific Information, 3501 Market St., Philadelphia, PA 19104. TEL 215-386-0100, FAX 215-386-2911.

016.57 USA ISSN 0006-3169
QH301 CODEN: BIABA4

BIOLOGICAL ABSTRACTS; references, abstracts, and indexes to the world's life sciences research literature. Text in English. 1926. s-m. USD 8,330 to institutions; USD 9,160 foreign to institutions; USD 7,370 to libraries; USD 8,200 foreign to libraries (effective 1999). abstr, illus. index, cum.index. reprint service avail. from SCH,PSC. **Document type:** *Abstract/Index.*

Formed by the 1926 merger of: Abstracts of Bacteriology (0096-5340); Botanical Abstracts (0096-526X)

Related titles: CD-ROM ed.: ISSN 1058-4129 (from SilverPlatter Information, Inc.); Microfilm ed.: USD 9,200 (effective 2000) (from BIO); Online - full text ed.: (from DIMDI, Data-Star, The Dialog Corporation, S T N International).

Indexed: Popul.Ind.

—BLDSC (2074.000000), CASDDS, CISTI, Linda Hall.

Published by: BIOSIS, 2001 Market Street, Suite 700, Philadelphia, PA 19103-7095. TEL 215-523-4806, 215-587-4800, FAX 215-587-2016, info@mail.biosis.org, http://www.biosis.org.

016.57 USA

BIOLOGICAL ABSTRACTS CUMULATIVE INDEXES. Text in English. 1927. s-a. USD 3,350 to institutions; USD 3,620 foreign to institutions; USD 3,210 to libraries; USD 3,450 foreign to libraries (effective 1999). **Document type:** *Abstract/Index.*

Related titles: Microform ed.: (from BIO).

—Linda Hall.

Published by: BIOSIS, 2001 Market Street, Suite 700, Philadelphia, PA 19103-7095. TEL 215-587-4800, FAX 215-587-2016, info@mail.biosis.org, http://www.biosis.org.

016.57 USA ISSN 0192-6985
Z5321 CODEN: BARRDG

BIOLOGICAL ABSTRACTS - R R M; references and indexes to the world's life science reports, reviews, and meeting literature. (Reports, Reviews, Meetings) Text in English. 1965. s-m. USD 4,160 to institutions; USD 4,520 foreign to institutions; USD 3,690 to libraries; USD 4,100 foreign to libraries (effective 1999). bk.rev. bibl. index. **Document type:** *Abstract/Index.* **Description:** Provides indexed and classified bibliographic entries for research reports, reviews; books on biology and biomedicine; conference literature.

Formerly (until 1980): BioResearch Index (0006-3541)

Related titles: CD-ROM ed.: ISSN 1058-4137 (from SilverPlatter Information, Inc.); Microfiche ed.; Online - full text ed.: (from DIMDI, Data-Star, The Dialog Corporation, S T N International).

—BLDSC (2074.100000), CASDDS, CISTI, Linda Hall.

Published by: BIOSIS, 2001 Market Street, Suite 700, Philadelphia, PA 19103-7095. TEL 215-587-4800, FAX 215-587-2016, info@mail.biosis.org, http://www.biosis.org/.

016.57 USA

BIOLOGICAL ABSTRACTS - R R M CUMULATIVE INDEX. (Reports, Reviews, and Meetings) Text in English. 1970. s-a. USD 1,665 domestic to institutions; USD 1,845 foreign to institutions; USD 1,630 domestic to libraries; USD 1,715 foreign to libraries (effective 1999). bk.rev. **Document type:** *Abstract/Index.*

Former titles: Cumulative Index to Biological Abstracts R R M; Cumulative Index to Bioresearch Index; Annual Cumulative Index to Bioresearch Index

Related titles: Microfiche ed.: (from BIO).

Published by: BIOSIS, 2001 Market Street, Suite 700, Philadelphia, PA 19103-7095. TEL 215-587-4800, FAX 215-587-2016, info@mail.biosis.org, http://www.biosis.org.

016.57 USA ISSN 0006-3177
Z5073

BIOLOGICAL & AGRICULTURAL INDEX. Text in English. 1964. m. (except Aug.). **Document type:** *Abstract/Index.* **Description:** Provides a cumulative subject index to periodicals in the fields of biology, agriculture and related sciences.

Formerly: Agricultural Index

Related titles: CD-ROM ed.: ISSN 1076-7037 (from SilverPlatter Information, Inc., H. W. Wilson); Magnetic Tape ed.; Online - full text ed.; Cumulative ed.

—CISTI, Linda Hall.

Published by: H.W. Wilson Co., 950 University Ave, Bronx, NY 10452-4224. TEL 718-588-8400, 800-367-6770, FAX 718-590-1617, custserv@hwwilson.com, http://www.hwwilson.com. Ed. Syed Shah.

016.57 GBR ISSN 0142-8004

BIOLOGICAL RHYTHMS. Text in English. 1970. s-m. GBP 120 (effective 2001). adv. **Document type:** *Abstract/Index.* **Description:** Current awareness service for researchers in clinical and life sciences.

Formerly: Circadian Rhythms

Related titles: E-mail ed.: GBP 120 (effective 2001); Online - full text ed.: GBP 108 (effective 2001).

—CCC.

Published by: S U B I S (Subsidiary of: Sheffield Academic Press Ltd), Mansion House, 19 Kingfield Rd, Sheffield, S Yorks S11 9AS, United Kingdom. TEL 44-114-255-4433, FAX 44-114-255-4626, subis@sheffac.demon.co.uk, http://www.shef-ac-press.co.uk/subis. Ed. S Huntridge. Adv. contact C Evans.

016.57 USA ISSN 0095-2958
QH301

BIOLOGY DIGEST. Text in English. 1974. m., latest vol.28 (Sep.-May). USD 139 (effective 2001). bk.rev. abstr, bibl, illus. cum.index. 140 p./no. back issues avail.; reprints avail. **Document type:** *Journal, Abstract/Index.* **Description:** Contains abstracts of current life science articles and research reports for high school and college students.

Incorporates: Environmental Quality Abstracts (0095-0149)

Related titles: CD-ROM ed.; Microfiche ed.: (from PQC); Online - full text ed.

—BLDSC (2087.058000).

Published by: Plexus Publishing, Inc., 143 Old Marlton Pike, Medford, NJ 08055. TEL 609-654-6500, FAX 609-654-4309, info@plexuspublishing.com, http://www.plexuspublishing.com. Ed. Thomas H Hogan. Circ: 2,000 (paid). **Subscr. to:** Information Today, Inc.

570.15195 GBR ISSN 0006-3444
QH301

BIOMETRIKA. Text in English. 1901. q. GBP 31, USD 52 to individuals; GBP 88, USD 150 to institutions (effective Mar. 2002). charts, illus. author index: vols.1-78, 1901-1991; subject index: vols.1-37, 1901-1950. back issues avail.; reprint service avail. from PQC. *Refereed.* **Document type:** *Journal, Academic/Scholarly.* **Description:** Contains statistics with theoretical papers of direct or potential value in applications.

Related titles: Microform ed.: (from PQC,PMC); Online - full text ed.: ISSN 1464-3510. 199? (from JSTOR (Web-based Journal Archive), EBSCO Publishing, O C L C Online Computer Library Center, Inc., RoweCom Information Quest, ingenta, Swets Blackwell, Institute for Scientific Information).

Indexed: A.S.& T.Ind. (Jan.2001-), ASCA, Anim.Breed.Abstr., Aqua.Sci.& Fish.Abstr., Aquacult.Abstr., Biol.& Agr.Ind. (Aug.1983-Mar.1989), Biol.Abstr., Biostat., C.C.M.J., C.I.S. Abstr., Chem.Abstr., Compumath, Curr.Adv.Ecol.Sci., Curr.Cont. (1964-), Curr.Ind.Stat., Dairy Sci.Abstr., Environ.Sci.Poll.Mgmt., Excerp.Med., Helminthol.Abstr., Hort.Abstr., INSPEC (Apr.1977-Dec.1986, dropped), Ind.Sci.Rev., Inpharma, J.Cont.Quant.Meth., Math.R., Nutr.Abstr., Oper.Res.Manage.Sci., Plant Breed.Abstr., Qual.Contr.Appl.Stat., Reac., Ref.Zh., Risk Abstr., Russ.Acad.Sci.Bibl., SSCI (coverage dropped), Sci.Cit.Ind., Sport Fish.Abstr., Stat.Theor.Meth.Abstr. (1964-), W.R.C.Inf., Wild.Rev., Zent.Math., Zoo.Rec.

—BLDSC (2089.000000), CISTI, GNLM, ingenta, Linda Hall. **CCC.**

Published by: (Biometrika Trust), Oxford University Press, Academic Division, Great Clarendon St, Oxford OX2 6DP, United Kingdom. TEL 44-1865-267907, FAX 44-1865-267835, jnl.info@oup.co.uk, http://www.biomet.oupjournals.org, http://www.oup.co.uk/journals, http://www3.oup.co.uk/biomet/. Ed. D M Titterington. Pub. Ian McIntosh. R&P Fionna Willis. Circ: 3,700. **Subscr. in U.S. to:** Oxford University Press, Journals, 2001 Evans Rd, Cary, NC 27513. TEL 919-677-0977, 800-852-7323, FAX 919-677-1714, jnlorders@oup-usa.org, http://www.oup-usa.org; **Subscr. to:** Journals Marketing, Great Clarendon St, Oxford OX2 6DP, United Kingdom.

016.5714 USA ISSN 0523-6800
QH505.A1

BIOPHYSICAL SOCIETY. ANNUAL MEETING. ABSTRACTS. Text in English. 1958. a. USD 775 domestic includes Biophysical Journal; USD 825 foreign includes Biophysical Journal (effective 2000). adv. *Refereed.* **Document type:** *Proceedings, Academic/Scholarly, Abstract/Index.*

Formerly: Biophysical Society. Abstracts (0067-8910); Supersedes: Biophysical Society. Symposium Proceedings (0520-1985)

Related titles: ♦ Supplement to: Biophysical Journal. ISSN 0006-3495.

Indexed: Biol.Abstr.

—CISTI.

Published by: Biophysical Society, 9650 Rockville Pike, Bethesda, MD 20814. TEL 301-530-7199, FAX 301-530-7133, http://www.biophysics.org/biophys. Ed. Peter Moore. R&P Cathy Kenney. Adv. contact Jeanne Brooksbank.

016.57 USA ISSN 1081-8669
CODEN: BISCDW

BIOSIS EVOLUTIONS. Text in English. 1994. bi-m., latest vol.8, 2001. free. back issues avail. **Document type:** *Newsletter.* **Description:** Reports information on BIOSIS's products and services, as well as items of current interest to the users of biological and biomedical information.

Formed by the merger of (1970-1994): BioScene (0090-3337); (1983-1994): BioSearch (1041-8946)

Related titles: Online - full text ed.

Indexed: Biol.Dig., C.I.J.E.

—CISTI, Linda Hall.

Published by: BIOSIS, Marketing, Sales, and Product Development, 2001 Market St. suite 700, Philadelphia, PA 19103-7095. TEL 800-523-4806, FAX 215-587-2016, info@mail.biosis.org, http://www.biosis.org/evol/index.html, http://www.biosis.org/htmls/evol. Eds. Christopher D'Lauro Christopher D'Lauro, Robert Connor. R&P John Anderson TEL 215-587-4800. Circ: 10,000.

016.57 USA
Z695.1.B5

BIOSIS SEARCH GUIDE (YEAR). Text in English. 1977. biennial. USD 175 (effective 2000). **Document type:** *Abstract/Index.*

Former titles: BIOSIS Previews Search Guide (Year) (0898-2414); BIOSIS Search Guide

Published by: BIOSIS, 2001 Market Street, Suite 700, Philadelphia, PA 19103-7095. TEL 215-587-4800, FAX 215-587-2016, info@mail.biosis.org, http://www.biosis.org.

016.57 USA ISSN 1086-2951
Z5321 CODEN: SSBDE4
BIOSIS SERIAL SOURCES. Text in English. 1938. a. USD 140 (effective 2001). **Document type:** *Abstract/Index.*
Former titles (until 1996): Serial Sources for the BIOSIS Previers Database (1044-4297); (until 1989): Serial Sources for the BIOSIS Database (0162-2048); (until 1978): BIOSIS: List of Serials with Coden, Title Abbreviations, New, Changed and Ceased Titles (0067-8937); (until 1969): Biological Abstracts List of Serials with Title Abbreviations (0523-6568)
Related titles: CD-ROM ed.
—BLDSC (2089.612600), CASDDS, CISTI, Linda Hall.
Published by: BIOSIS, 2001 Market Street, Suite 700, Philadelphia, PA 19103-7095. TEL 215-231-7532, FAX 215-587-2016, info@mail.biosis.org, http://www.biosis.org. **Affiliate:** BIOSIS UK.

570.15195 USA ISSN 1041-7648
QH323.5
BIOSTATISTICA. Text in English. 1989. q., latest vol.12. USD 150; USD 165 foreign (effective 2002). bk.rev. stat, abstr. annual. 96 p./no. back issues avail. **Document type:** *Abstract/Index.* **Description:** Includes mathematical biological abstracts, current book contents, and an annual index.
Published by: Executive Sciences Institute, 1005 Mississippi Ave, Davenport, IA 52803. TEL 319-324-4463, FAX 319-327-3725, greta.lane@usa.net. Ed., R&P Bruce Brocka. Circ: 300 (paid).

016.6606 GBR ISSN 0262-5318
TP248.13
BIOTECHNOLOGY ABSTRACTS. Key Title: Derwent Biotechnology Abstracts. Text in English. 1982. fortn. USD 2,142. **Document type:** *Abstract/Index.* **Description:** Covers a broad range of technical aspects of biotechnology, from genetic manipulation and biochemical engineering to fermentation and downstream processing.
Related titles: CD-ROM ed.: ISSN 1358-6009 (from National Information Services Corp. (NISC)); Online - full text ed.: (from The Dialog Corporation, Questel Orbit Inc., NISC).
Published by: Derwent Information Ltd., 14 Great Queen St, London WC2B 5DF, United Kingdom. TEL 44-171-3442800. **US subscr. to:** Derwent Information, 1725 Duke St, Ste 250, Alexandria, VA 22314. TEL 703-706-4220.

016.6606 HUN ISSN 0237-0115
BIOTECHNOLOGY INFORMATION. Variant title: Biotech-Info. Text in Hungarian. 1984. m. HUF 3,600. abstr.
Published by: Orszagos Muszaki Informacios Kozpont es Konyvtar/National Technical Information Centre and Library, Muzeum utca 17, PO Box 12, Budapest 1428, Hungary. Ed. Fazekasne Zsuzsanna Horvath. Circ: 420.

016.57 USA
BIOWORLD TODAY INDEX. Text in English. 1994. q. USD 251; USD 281 foreign (effective 1997). **Document type:** *Abstract/Index, Trade.*
Media: Diskette.
Published by: American Health Consultants, BioWorld Publishing Group (Subsidiary of: Medical Economics), PO Box 95278, Chicago, IL 60694-5278. TEL 404-262-7436, FAX 404-814-0759, custserv@ahcpub.com, http://www.ahcpub.com. Pub. Donald Johnston.

016.58 DNK ISSN 0900-2367
BOTANISK CENTRALBIBLIOTEK. FORTEGNELSE OVER LOEBENDE PERIODICA VED BOTANISK CENTRALBIBLITEK. Text in Danish. 1977. irreg., latest 1998. free per issue. **Document type:** *Catalog.*
Published by: Botanisk Centralbibliotek, OPG S, Soelvgade 83, Copenhagen K 1307, Denmark. bcb@bot.ku.dk. Ed. Annelise Hartmann.

016.572 USA ISSN 0895-6626
CODEN: CBUREG
C A S BIOTECH UPDATES. BIOCHEMICAL IMMOBILIZATION & BIOCATALYTIC REACTORS. Text in English. s-w. USD 270 (effective 2001). **Document type:** *Abstract/Index.* **Description:** Preparation and use of biological reactors and of immobilized microorganisms, plant and animal cells, enzymes, and other biological molecules; fermentors, biological electrodes, affinity chromatography, and enzyme immunoassay.
Published by: Chemical Abstracts Service (Subsidiary of: American Chemical Society), 2540 Olentangy River Rd, Box 3012, Columbus, OH 43210-0012. TEL 614-447-3600, FAX 800-753-4227.

016.572 USA ISSN 0884-7479
CODEN: CBUBE2
C A S BIOTECH UPDATES. BIOSENSORS. Text in English. s-w. USD 270 (effective 2001). **Document type:** *Abstract/Index.* **Description:** Covers use of immobilized enzymes, immunological components, and cell fractions or whole cells for biochemical analysis, body fluid monitoring, and diagnostics; electrodes, thermistors, transistors, and light-detection-type biosensors in the detection and determination of sample components.
Published by: Chemical Abstracts Service (Subsidiary of: American Chemical Society), 2540 Olentangy River Rd, Box 3012, Columbus, OH 43210-0012. TEL 614-447-3600, 800-753-4227, FAX 614-447-3751.

016.5716 USA ISSN 1040-709X
CODEN: CUCCEE
C A S BIOTECH UPDATES. CELL & TISSUE CULTURE. Text in English. s-w. USD 270 (effective 2001). **Document type:** *Abstract/Index.* **Description:** Covers methods and applications of culturing animal and plant cells; studies of organism metabolism and physiology as well as processes for the laboratory or commercial-scale production of cell metabolites.
Published by: Chemical Abstracts Service (Subsidiary of: American Chemical Society), 2540 Olentangy River Rd, Box 3012, Columbus, OH 43210-0012. TEL 614-447-3600, 800-753-4227, FAX 614-447-3751.

016.572 USA ISSN 1045-8565
CODEN: CBUFEE
C A S BIOTECH UPDATES. COMMERCIAL FERMENTATION. Text in English. s-w. USD 270 (effective 2001). **Document type:** *Abstract/Index.* **Description:** Covers processes, products, and equipment of industry-scale production using microorganisms or enzymes; organism strain selection, culturing, fermentation, culture enhancement, immobilization, assays, and product recovery.
Published by: Chemical Abstracts Service (Subsidiary of: American Chemical Society), 2540 Olentangy River Rd, Box 3012, Columbus, OH 43210-0012. TEL 614-447-3600, 800-753-4227, FAX 614-447-3751.

016.57286 USA ISSN 1045-8581
CODEN: CBDPER
C A S BIOTECH UPDATES. D N A & R N A PROBES. Text in English. s-w. USD 270 (effective 2001). **Document type:** *Abstract/Index.* **Description:** Covers DNA and RNA probes and their applications - such as detection of biological species or strains; taxonomy; clinical diagnosis of microbial infections and genetic diseases.
Published by: Chemical Abstracts Service (Subsidiary of: American Chemical Society), 2540 Olentangy River Rd, Box 3012, Columbus, OH 43210-0012. TEL 614-447-3600, 800-753-4227, FAX 614-447-3751.

016.57286 USA ISSN 0895-6618
CODEN: CUDREU
C A S BIOTECH UPDATES. D N A FORMATION & REPAIR. Text in English. s-w. USD 270 (effective 2001). **Document type:** *Abstract/Index.* **Description:** Covers aspects of the biosynthesis and repair of DNA; enzyme studies of the various DNA polymerases and factors involved in DNA formation.
Published by: Chemical Abstracts Service (Subsidiary of: American Chemical Society), 2540 Olentangy River Rd, Box 3012, Columbus, OH 43210-0012. TEL 614-447-3600, 800-753-4227, FAX 614-447-3751.

016.572 USA ISSN 1040-7081
CODEN: CUEBEL
C A S BIOTECH UPDATES. ENZYMES IN BIOTECHNOLOGY. Text in English. s-w. USD 270 (effective 2001). **Document type:** *Abstract/Index.* **Description:** Covers laboratory, commercial, and industrial uses as well as applications of enzymes in genetics, medicine, organic synthesis, electrochemistry, and clinical and medical analysis.
Published by: Chemical Abstracts Service (Subsidiary of: American Chemical Society), 2540 Olentangy River Rd, Box 3012, Columbus, OH 43210-0012. TEL 614-447-3600, 800-753-4227, FAX 614-447-3751.

016.5765 USA ISSN 0884-7460
CODEN: CBUEEB
C A S BIOTECH UPDATES. GENETIC ENGINEERING. Text in English. s-w. USD 270 (effective 2001). **Document type:** *Abstract/Index.* **Description:** Covers various aspects of genetic manipulation and genetic engineering in animals, plants, microorganisms, and viruses; recombinant DNA technology, gene splicing, molecular cloning, and plasmid and cosmid vector methodology.
Published by: Chemical Abstracts Service (Subsidiary of: American Chemical Society), 2540 Olentangy River Rd, Box 3012, Columbus, OH 43210-0012. TEL 614-447-3600, 800-753-4227, FAX 614-447-3751.

016.57286 USA ISSN 1045-859X
CODEN: CBNSEI
C A S BIOTECH UPDATES. NUCLEIC ACID & PROTEIN SEQUENCES. Text in English. s-w. USD 270 (effective 2001). **Document type:** *Abstract/Index.* **Description:** Covers newly determined biopolymer sequences, including the nucleotide sequences of DNA and RNA and the amino acid sequences of proteins (enzymes, hormones); partial and complete sequences; database management and computerized manipulation of sequence information.
Formerly (until Jan. 1990): Biopolymer Sequences
Published by: Chemical Abstracts Service (Subsidiary of: American Chemical Society), 2540 Olentangy River Rd, Box 3012, Columbus, OH 43210-0012. TEL 614-447-3600, 800-753-4227, FAX 614-447-3751.

016.579 USA ISSN 0884-7487
CODEN: CBUAEX
C A S BIOTECH UPDATES. PHARMACEUTICAL APPLICATIONS. Text in English. s-w. USD 270 (effective 2001). **Document type:** *Abstract/Index.* **Description:** Covers the production of pharmaceuticals by microorganisms and nonmicrobial tissue cultures, bioreactors and enzymes, and genetic engineering; antibiotics, hormones, immunological substances (interferon, antibodies), vaccines, blood factors and related products, and other pharmaceuticals.
Published by: Chemical Abstracts Service (Subsidiary of: American Chemical Society), 2540 Olentangy River Rd, Box 3012, Columbus, OH 43210-0012. TEL 614-447-3600, 800-753-4227, FAX 614-447-3751.

016.59 USA ISSN 0162-7694
CODEN: CSLAD4
C A SELECTS. ANIMAL LONGEVITY AND AGING. Text in English. s-w. USD 275 (effective 2001). **Document type:** *Abstract/Index.* **Description:** Covers animal longevity and senescence, senility, limb regeneration, geriatrics, and gerontology.
Published by: Chemical Abstracts Service (Subsidiary of: American Chemical Society), 2540 Olentangy River Rd, Box 3012, Columbus, OH 43210-0012. TEL 614-447-3600, 800-753-4227, FAX 614-447-3751.

016.579 USA ISSN 1047-8167
CODEN: CSATE7
C A SELECTS. ANTIFUNGAL & ANTIMYCOTIC AGENTS. Text in English. 1988. s-w. USD 275 (effective 2001). **Document type:** *Abstract/Index.* **Description:** Covers the antifungal and antimycotic activities of both established and developmental drugs. Includes synthesis, mechanism(s) of action, formulation, and structure-activity relationships.
Formerly (until 1989): BIOSIS CAS Selects: Antifungal Agents
Published by: Chemical Abstracts Service (Subsidiary of: American Chemical Society), 2540 Olentangy River Rd, Box 3012, Columbus, OH 43210-0012. TEL 614-447-3600, 800-753-4227, FAX 614-447-3751.

016.572 USA ISSN 0895-5905
CODEN: CAFRE2
C A SELECTS. FREE RADICALS (BIOCHEMICAL ASPECTS). Text in English. 1988. s-w. USD 275 (effective 2001). **Document type:** *Abstract/Index.* **Description:** Covers reactions and interactions of free radicals, including activated oxygen species in biological systems; formation, metabolic aspects, and toxicity of free radicals in intact organisms, isolated organs, tissues, cells, and subcellular systems, as well as in model biological systems.
Published by: Chemical Abstracts Service (Subsidiary of: American Chemical Society), 2540 Olentangy River Rd, Box 3012, Columbus, OH 43210-0012. TEL 614-447-3600, 800-753-4227, FAX 614-447-3751.

B

016.61601 USA ISSN 1047-8094 CODEN: CMOAEC
C A SELECTS. MONOCLONAL ANTIBODIES. Text in English. 1984. s-w. USD 275 (effective 2001). **Document type:** *Abstract/Index.* **Description:** Covers the preparation, characterization, and use of monoclonal antibodies and monoclonal antibody conjugates. Includes pathophysiology and hybridoma technology.
Formerly (until 1989): BIOSIS CAS Selects: Monoclonal Antibodies
Published by: Chemical Abstracts Service (Subsidiary of: American Chemical Society), 2540 Olentangy River Rd, Box 3012, Columbus, OH 43210-0012. TEL 614-447-3600, 800-753-4227, FAX 614-447-3751.

016.57265 USA ISSN 1083-2750 CODEN: CSPPF3
C A SELECTS PLUS. AMINO ACIDS, PEPTIDES AND PROTEINS. Text in English. s-w. USD 275 (effective 2001). **Document type:** *Abstract/Index.* **Description:** Covers chemistry and synthesis of amino acids, peptides, and proteins.
Formerly: C A Selects. Amino Acids, Peptides and Proteins (0275-701X)
Published by: Chemical Abstracts Service (Subsidiary of: American Chemical Society), 2540 Olentangy River Rd, Box 3012, Columbus, OH 43210-0012. TEL 614-447-3600, 800-753-4227, FAX 614-447-3751.

016.5719 USA ISSN 0362-9848 CODEN: CASPDQ
C A SELECTS. PSYCHOBIOCHEMISTRY. Text in English. s-w. USD 275 (effective 2001). **Document type:** *Abstract/Index.* **Description:** Covers the pathological and pharmacological aspects of mental function, including human and animal behavior, and emotions.
Published by: Chemical Abstracts Service (Subsidiary of: American Chemical Society), 2540 Olentangy River Rd, Box 3012, Columbus, OH 43210-0012. TEL 614-447-3600, 800-753-4227, FAX 614-447-3751.

016.572 USA ISSN 0160-9173 CODEN: CSBSDB
C A SELECTS. STEROIDS (BIOCHEMICAL ASPECTS). Text in English. s-w. USD 275 (effective 2001). **Document type:** *Abstract/Index.* **Description:** Covers pharmacology, toxicology, general biochemistry, and nutritional uses of steroids.
Published by: Chemical Abstracts Service (Subsidiary of: American Chemical Society), 2540 Olentangy River Rd, Box 3012, Columbus, OH 43210-0012. TEL 614-447-3600, 800-753-4227, FAX 614-447-3751.

016.5792 USA ISSN 1047-8078 CODEN: CSVVEG
C A SELECTS. VIRUCIDES & VIRUSTATS. Text in English. 1986. s-w. USD 275 (effective 2001). **Document type:** *Abstract/Index.* **Description:** Covers the antiviral activity of both established and developmental drugs; includes synthesis, mechanism of action, formulation and structure-activity relationships.
Formerly (until 1989): BIOSIS CAS Selects: Antiviral Agents (0885-6990)
Indexed: Chem.Abstr.
Published by: Chemical Abstracts Service (Subsidiary of: American Chemical Society), 2540 Olentangy River Rd, Box 3012, Columbus, OH 43210-0012. TEL 614-447-3600, 800-753-4227, FAX 614-447-3751.

016.5715 USA ISSN 1069-5540
QP88.2
CALCIUM AND CALCIFIED TISSUE ABSTRACTS. Text in English. 1969. q. USD 840 print & online eds. (effective 2002). adv. bk.rev. abstr. index. back issues avail. **Document type:** *Abstract/Index.* **Description:** Covers the role of calcium metabolism in maintaining body function, including bone structure and diseases.
Formerly (until 1994): Calcified Tissue Abstracts (0008-0586)
Related titles: Online - full text ed.: USD 630 (effective 2002) (from The Dialog Corporation, S T N International, EBSCO Publishing, CSA).
—GNLM.
Published by: Cambridge Scientific Abstracts, 7200 Wisconsin Ave., Suite 601, Bethesda, MD 20814. TEL 301-961-6798, FAX 301-961-6799, journals@csa.com, http://www.csa.com/journals. Ed. Janet Padgett. Pub. Ted Caris.

016.5728 GBR ISSN 0142-8020
CELL CALCIUM (SHEFFIELD). Text in English. 1976. s-m. GBP 120 for print or e-mail eds. (effective 2001). adv. **Document type:** *Abstract/Index.* **Description:** Current awareness service for researchers in clinical and life sciences. Covers calcium in signal transduction, calcium transport, calcium-binding proteins, muscle and nerve cell calcium.
Related titles: E-mail ed.; Online - full text ed.: GBP 108 (effective 2001).
Indexed: Curr.Adv.Biochem., Curr.Adv.Cell & Devel.Biol., Curr.Adv.Ecol.Sci., Vet.Bull.
—CCC.
Published by: S U B I S (Subsidiary of: Sheffield Academic Press Ltd), Mansion House, 19 Kingfield Rd, Sheffield, S Yorks S11 9AS, United Kingdom. TEL 44-114-255-4433, FAX 44-114-255-4626, subis@sheffac.demon.co.uk, http://www.shef-ac-press.co.uk/subis. Ed. S Huntridge. Adv. contact C Evans.

016.5716 GBR ISSN 0263-726X
CELL DIFFERENTIATION. Text in English. 1983. s-m. GBP 96 for print ed. or e-mail (effective 2001). adv. back issues avail. **Document type:** *Abstract/Index.* **Description:** Current awareness service for researchers in clinical and life sciences.
Related titles: E-mail ed.; Online - full text ed.: GBP 108 to individuals (effective 2001).
—CCC.
Published by: S U B I S (Subsidiary of: Sheffield Academic Press Ltd), Mansion House, 19 Kingfield Rd, Sheffield, S Yorks S11 9AS, United Kingdom. TEL 44-114-255-4433, FAX 44-114-255-4626, subis@sheffac.demon.co.uk, http://www.shef-ac-press.co.uk/subis. Ed. S Huntridge. Adv. contact C Evans.

016.572 GBR ISSN 0142-8047
CELL MEMBRANES. Text in English. 1970. s-m. GBP 120 for print or e-mail eds. (effective 2001). adv. **Document type:** *Abstract/Index.* **Description:** Current awareness service for researchers in clinical and life sciences. Covers membrane transport, protein transport, channels, electrical properties, lipids and model systems.
Related titles: E-mail ed.; Online - full text ed.: GBP 108 (effective 2001).
Indexed: Chem.Abstr., Chem.Indus.Notes, Chem.Titles, Sci.Cit.Ind. (coverage dropped).
—CCC.
Published by: S U B I S (Subsidiary of: Sheffield Academic Press Ltd), Mansion House, 19 Kingfield Rd, Sheffield, S Yorks S11 9AS, United Kingdom. TEL 44-114-255-4433, FAX 44-114-255-4626, subis@sheffac.demon.co.uk, http://www.shef-ac-press.co.uk/subis. Ed. S Huntridge. Adv. contact C Evans.

016.5954 FRA ISSN 0295-060X
CENTRE INTERNATIONAL DE DOCUMENTATION ARACHNOLOGIQUE. LISTE DES TRAVAUX ARACHNOLOGIQUES. Text in French. 1968. a. FRF 100. adv. bibl. index. **Description:** Presents a listing of publications covering arachnology. Includes author's name, title of work, and year first published.
Related titles: Record ed.
Indexed: Zoo.Rec.
Published by: Centre International de Documentation Arachnologique, 61 rue de Buffon, Paris 75005, France. FAX 40-79-38-63, arachne@mnhn.fr. Ed. Jacqueline Heurtault.

016.572 USA ISSN 0009-2304 CODEN: CABSBG
CHEMICAL ABSTRACTS - BIOCHEMISTRY SECTIONS. Abbreviated title: C A B S. Text in English. 1963. s-w. USD 2,525 to CA subscribers; USD 2,795 others; USD 559 to members (effective 2001). charts, pat, stat. index. **Document type:** *Abstract/Index.*
Related titles: Online - full text ed.: (from S T N International).
Indexed: Dairy Sci.Abstr., VITIS.
—CASDDS, CISTI.
Published by: Chemical Abstracts Service (Subsidiary of: American Chemical Society), 2540 Olentangy River Rd, Box 3012, Columbus, OH 43210-0012. TEL 614-447-3600, 800-753-4227, FAX 614-447-3751. Ed. David W Weisgerber.

016.5716592 GBR ISSN 0264-9640
CHLOROPLASTS. Text in English. 1984. s-m. GBP 96 for print ed. or e-mail (effective 2001). adv. back issues avail. **Document type:** *Abstract/Index.* **Description:** Current awareness service for researchers in life sciences.
Related titles: E-mail ed.; Online - full text ed.: GBP 108 to individuals (effective 2001).
—CCC.
Published by: S U B I S (Subsidiary of: Sheffield Academic Press Ltd), Mansion House, 19 Kingfield Rd, Sheffield, S Yorks S11 9AS, United Kingdom. TEL 44-114-255-4433, FAX 44-114-255-4626, subis@sheffac.demon.co.uk, http://www.shef-ac-press.co.uk/subis. Ed. S Huntridge. Adv. contact C Evans.

016.57257 GBR ISSN 0964-7597
CHOLESTEROL & LIPOPROTEINS. Text in English. 1992. s-m. GBP 96 for print ed. or e-mail (effective 2001). adv. **Document type:** *Abstract/Index.* **Description:** Current awareness service for researchers in life sciences.
Related titles: E-mail ed.; Online - full text ed.: GBP 108 to individuals (effective 2001).
Published by: S U B I S (Subsidiary of: Sheffield Academic Press Ltd), Mansion House, 19 Kingfield Rd, Sheffield, S Yorks S11 9AS, United Kingdom. TEL 44-114-255-4433, FAX 44-114-255-4626, subis@sheffac.demon.co.uk, http://www.shef-ac-press.co.uk/subis. Ed. S Huntridge. Adv. contact C Evans.

016.5765 GBR ISSN 0260-5872
CLINICAL CYTOGENETICS. Text in English. 1981. s-m. GBP 120 for print or e-mail eds. (effective 2001). adv. **Document type:** *Abstract/Index.* **Description:** Current awareness service for researchers. Covers chromosomal birth defects, banding techniques, DNA cytometry, DNA probes and gene mapping, leukemias and lymphomas, solid tumors, genetic amniocentesis.
Related titles: E-mail ed.; Online - full text ed.: GBP 108 (effective 2001).
—CCC.
Published by: S U B I S (Subsidiary of: Sheffield Academic Press Ltd), Mansion House, 19 Kingfield Rd, Sheffield, S Yorks S11 9AS, United Kingdom. TEL 44-114-255-4433, FAX 44-114-255-4626, subis@sheffac.demon.co.uk, http://www.shef-ac-press.co.uk/subis. Ed. S Huntridge. Adv. contact C Evans.

570.15195 USA
CORNELL UNIVERSITY. NEW YORK STATE COLLEGE OF AGRICULTURE AND LIFE SCIENCES. BIOMETRICS UNIT. ANNUAL REPORT. Text in English. 1949. a. free per issue. bk.rev. **Document type:** *Corporate.*
Published by: New York State College of Agriculture and Life Sciences, Department of Plant Breeding and Biometry, Cornell University, 436 Warren Hall, Ithaca, NY 14853. TEL 607-255-5488, FAX 607-255-4698, biometrics@cornell.edu. Ed. Janet L Breslin. Circ: (controlled).

016.579 GBR ISSN 0964-8712
Z5180
CURRENT ADVANCES IN APPLIED MICROBIOLOGY & BIOTECHNOLOGY. Text in English. 1984. m. EUR 120 in Europe to qualified personnel; JPY 16,275 in Japan to individuals; USD 135 elsewhere to qualified personnel; EUR 1,384 in Europe to qualified personnel; JPY 183,484 in Japan to qualified personnel; USD 1,548 elsewhere to qualified personnel (effective 2002). adv. back issues avail. **Document type:** *Abstract/Index.* **Description:** Provides current awareness service in the sphere of applied microbiology and biotechnology. Gives listings of titles of microbiological papers published throughout the world classified into 149 main areas and provides a comprehensive listing of review articles.
Formerly (until 1992): Current Advances in Microbiology (0741-1669)
Related titles: Diskette ed.; Microfilm ed.: (from PQC); Online - full text ed.
—BLDSC (3494.060900), Infotrieve. **CCC.**
Published by: Elsevier Science BV, PO Box 211, Amsterdam 1000 AE, Netherlands. TEL 31-20-485-2911, FAX 31-20-485-2457, http://www.elsevier.com/locate/camicrobio, http://www.elsevier.nl. **Subscr. in Australasia and the Far East to:** Elsevier Science (Singapore) Pte Ltd, No.1 Temasek Ave, 17-01 Millenia Tower, Singapore 039192, Singapore. TEL 65-434-3727, FAX 65-337-2230; **Subscr. in Japan to:** Elsevier Science Inc - Japan Regional Office, 9-15 Higashi-Azabu 1-chome, Minato-ku, Tokyo 106-0044, Japan. TEL 81-3-5561-5033; **Subscr. in the Americas to:** Elsevier Science, PO Box 945, New York, NY 10159-0945. TEL 212-633-3730, FAX 212-633-3680, usinfo-f@elsevier.com.

016.5716 GBR ISSN 0741-1626
Z5322.C3

CURRENT ADVANCES IN CELL & DEVELOPMENTAL BIOLOGY. Text in English. 1984. m. EUR 120 in Europe to qualified personnel; JPY 16,275 in Japan to qualified personnel; USD 135 elsewhere to qualified personnel; EUR 1,467 in Europe to institutions; JPY 194,436 in Japan to institutions; USD 1,641 elsewhere to institutions (effective 2002). **Document type:** *Abstract/Index.* **Description:** Provides a current awareness service in the sphere of cell and developmental biology. Gives listings of titles of cell and developmental biology papers published throughout the world classified into 76 main areas and provides a comprehensive listing of review articles.

Related titles: Diskette ed.; Microfilm ed.: (from PQC); Online - full text ed.

—BLDSC (3494.062000), Infotrieve. **CCC.**

Published by: Elsevier Science BV, PO Box 211, Amsterdam 1000 AE, Netherlands. TEL 31-20-485-2911, FAX 31-20-485-2457, http://www.elsevier.com/locate/cacell. **Subscr. in Australasia and the Far East to:** Elsevier Science (Singapore) Pte Ltd, No.1 Temasek Ave, 17-01 Millenia Tower, Singapore 039192, Singapore. TEL 65-434-3727, FAX 65-337-2230; **Subscr. in Japan to:** Elsevier Science Inc - Japan Regional Office, 9-15 Higashi-Azabu 1-chome, Minato-ku, Tokyo 106-0044, Japan. TEL 81-3-5561-5033; **Subscr. in the Americas to:** Elsevier Science, PO Box 945, New York, NY 10159-0945. TEL 212-633-3730, FAX 212-633-3680, usinfo-f@elsevier.com.

016.579 GBR ISSN 0741-1642
Z5322.G4

CURRENT ADVANCES IN GENETICS AND MOLECULAR BIOLOGY. Text in English. 1984. m. EUR 120 in Europe to qualified personnel; JPY 16,275 in Japan to qualified personnel; USD 135 elsewhere to qualified personnel; EUR 2,183 in Europe to institutions; JPY 289,390 in Japan to institutions; USD 2,442 elsewhere to institutions (effective 2002). adv. **Document type:** *Abstract/Index.* **Description:** Provides current awareness service for biologists, ecologists and environmental scientists. Gives listings of titles of ecological papers published throughout the world classified into 61 main areas and provides a comprehensive listing of review articles.

Related titles: Diskette ed.; Microfilm ed.: (from PQC); Online - full text ed.

—BLDSC (3494.064100), Infotrieve. **CCC.**

Published by: Elsevier Science BV, PO Box 211, Amsterdam 1000 AE, Netherlands. TEL 31-20-485-2911, FAX 31-20-485-2457, nlinfo-f@elsevier.nl; usinfo-f@elsevier.com; forinfo-kyf04035@niftyserve.or.jp, http://www.elsevier.nl/inca/publications/store/7/3/5/. **Subscr. in Australasia and the Far East to:** Elsevier Science (Singapore) Pte Ltd, No.1 Temasek Ave, 17-01 Millenia Tower, Singapore 039192, Singapore. TEL 65-434-3727, FAX 65-337-2230; **Subscr. in Japan to:** Elsevier Science Inc - Japan Regional Office, 9-15 Higashi-Azabu 1-chome, Minato-ku, Tokyo 106-0044, Japan. TEL 81-3-5561-5033; **Subscr. in the Americas to:** Elsevier Science, PO Box 945, New York, NY 10159-0945. TEL 212-633-3730, FAX 212-633-3680.

016.572 GBR ISSN 0965-0504
Z5524.B54

CURRENT ADVANCES IN PROTEIN BIOCHEMISTRY. Text in English. 1984. m. EUR 120 in Europe to qualified personnel; JPY 16,275 in Japan to qualified personnel; USD 135 elsewhere to qualified personnel; EUR 1,226 in Europe to institutions; JPY 162,500 in Japan to institutions; USD 1,371 elsewhere to institutions (effective 2002). adv. **Document type:** *Abstract/Index.* **Description:** Lists titles of protein biochemistry papers published throughout the world classified into 141 main areas; and provides a comprehensive listing of review articles.

Formerly (until 1992): Current Advances in Biochemistry (0741-1618)

Related titles: Diskette ed.; Microform ed.: (from PQC); Online - full text ed.

—BLDSC (3494.067000), Infotrieve. **CCC.**

Published by: Elsevier Science BV, PO Box 211, Amsterdam 1000 AE, Netherlands. TEL 31-20-485-2911, FAX 31-20-485-2457, http://www.elsevier.com/locate/caprobio, http://www.elsevier.nl. **Subscr. in Australasia and the Far East to:** Elsevier Science (Singapore) Pte Ltd, No.1 Temasek Ave, 17-01 Millenia Tower, Singapore 039192, Singapore. TEL 65-434-3727, FAX 65-337-2230; **Subscr. in Japan to:** Elsevier Science Inc - Japan Regional Office, 9-15 Higashi-Azabu 1-chome, Minato-ku, Tokyo 106-0044, Japan. TEL 81-3-5561-5033; **Subscr. in the Americas to:** Elsevier Science, PO Box 945, New York, NY 10159-0945. TEL 212-633-3730, FAX 212-633-3680, usinfo-f@elsevier.com.

016.57 NLD ISSN 0733-4443
QH301

CURRENT AWARENESS IN BIOLOGICAL SCIENCES. (Consists of 12 sections, Current Advances in: Applied Microbiology & Biotechnology; Cancer Research; Cell & Developmental Biology; Clinical Chemistry; Ecological & Environmental Sciences; Endocrinology & Metabolism; Genetics & Molecular Biology; Immunology & Infectious Diseases; Neuroscience; Plant Science; Protein Biochemistry; Toxicology) Text in Dutch. 1954. 144/yr. EUR 7,623.51 in Europe all 12 sections; JPY 1,033,400 in Japan all 12 sections; USD 8,528 elsewhere all 12 sections (effective 2001). adv. back issues avail. **Document type:** *Abstract/Index.* **Description:** Provides comprehensive coverage of recent publications in the entire spectrum of biological sciences, including relevant work in toxicology and the biomedical and environmental sciences.

Formerly (until 1983): International Abstracts of Biological Sciences (0020-5818)

Related titles: Microfilm ed.: (from PQC); Online - full text ed.

—CISTI, GNLM, Infotrieve, Linda Hall. **CCC.**

Published by: Elsevier Science BV, PO Box 211, Amsterdam 1000 AE, Netherlands. http://www.elsevier.nl/locate/cabs. Circ: 1,000. **Subscr. in Australasia and the Far East to:** Elsevier Science (Singapore) Pte Ltd, No.1 Temasek Ave, 17-01 Millenia Tower, Singapore 039192, Singapore. TEL 65-434-3727, FAX 65-337-2230; **Subscr. in Japan to:** Elsevier Science Inc - Japan Regional Office, 9-15 Higashi-Azabu 1-chome, Minato-ku, Tokyo 106-0044, Japan. TEL 81-3-5561-5033; **Subscr. in the Americas to:** Elsevier Science, PO Box 945, New York, NY 10159-0945. TEL 212-633-3730, FAX 212-633-3680, usinfo-f@elsevier.com, http://www.elsevier.com.

016.57 KOR

CURRENT BIBLIOGRAPHIES ON SCIENCE AND TECHNOLOGY: BIOLOGY, PHARMACY AND FOOD SCIENCE. Text in Korean. 1962. m. USD 107. reprint service avail. from PQC.

Formerly: Current Index to Journals in Science and Technology: Biology, Agriculture, Pharmacy; Which superseded in part: Current Bibliography on Science and Technology

Published by: Korea Institute for Economics and Technology, 206-9 Cheongryangri-Dong, Dongdaimun-Ku, P.O. Box 205, Seoul, Korea, S.. Circ: 300.

016.57 JPN ISSN 0285-5100

CURRENT BIBLIOGRAPHY ON SCIENCE AND TECHNOLOGY: LIFE SCIENCES/KAGAKU GIJUTSU BUNKEN SOKUHO. RAIFUSAIENSU HEN. Text in Japanese. 1981. 3/m. USD 2,500. index. **Document type:** *Bibliography.*

Related titles: CD-ROM ed.; Online - full text ed.: (from JICST).

Published by: Japan Science and Technology Corporation, Information Center for Science and Technology/Kagaku Gijutsu Shinko Jigyodan, 5-3 Yonban-cho, Chiyoda-ku, Tokyo 102-0081, Japan. TEL 81-3-5214-8413, FAX 81-3-5214-8410. Circ: 600.

016.57 USA ISSN 0960-9822
QH301 CODEN: CUBLE2

CURRENT BIOLOGY. Text in English. 1991. s-m. NLG 350, EUR 158.82 in Europe to individuals; JPY 23,100 in Japan to individuals; USD 178 elsewhere to individuals; NLG 1,665, EUR 755.54 in Europe to institutions; JPY 104,800 in Japan to institutions; USD 845 elsewhere to institutions (effective 2001). adv. illus. back issues avail.; reprints avail. *Refereed.* **Document type:** *Academic/Scholarly.* **Description:** Directed toward researchers, educators and students of biology. Features original research and reviews of the latest developments in the different specializations within the field.

Related titles: Online - full text ed.: (from EBSCO Publishing, ingenta, ScienceDirect, Institute for Scientific Information).

Indexed: AIDS & Cancer Res., ASCA, AgBiotech, Agri.& Environ.Biotech.Abstr. (coverage dropped), Anim.Behav.Abstr., Anim.Breed.Abstr., Aqua.Sci.& Fish.Abstr., BBCI, Biol.Dig., Cal.Tiss.Abstr., Chem.Indus.Notes, Chem.Titles, Crop Physiol.Abstr., Curr.Cont., Entomol.Abstr., Environ.Sci.Poll.Mgmt., Field Crop Abstr., Genet.Abstr., Helminthol.Abstr., Hort.Abstr., Hum.Gen.Abstr., Immun.Abstr. (coverage dropped), Ind.Med. (1991-), Ind.Vet., Inpharma, Int.Abstr.Biol.Sci., Med.& Pharm.Biotech.Abstr. (coverage dropped), Neurosci.Abstr., Neurosci.Cit.Ind., Nuc.Acids Abstr., Nutr.Abstr., Oncog.G.F.Abstr. (coverage dropped), Plant Breed.Abstr., Plant Gen.Res.Abstr., Plant Grow.Reg.Abstr., Postharvest, Poult.Abstr., Protozool.Abstr., PsycInfo, Reac., Rev.Appl.Entomol., Rev.Med.& Vet.Mycol., Rev.Plant Path., Rice Abstr., SSCI (coverage dropped), Seed Abstr., Soils & Fert., Sport Fish.Abstr., Triticale Abstr., Weed Abstr., Wild.Rev., Zoo.Rec., e-psyche.

—BLDSC (3494.651300), ADONIS, CASDDS, CISTI, EMDOCS, GNLM, IDS, ingenta. **CCC.**

Published by: Cell Press (Subsidiary of: Reed Elsevier plc), 1100 Massachusetts Ave, Cambridge, MA 02138. TEL 617-661-7057, FAX 617-661-7061, cbiol@current-biology.com, http://www.current-biology.com/, http://www.cellpress.com/. Ed. Geoffrey North. adv.: B&W page USD 1,125, color page USD 2,400; trim 11 x 8.5. Circ: 9,100. **Subscr. to:** Quadrant Subscription Services. **Dist. by:** Turpin Distribution Services Ltd.

B

016.6606 DEU ISSN 0960-5037
TP248.2 CODEN: CUBIER

CURRENT BIOTECHNOLOGY. Text in English. 1983. m. DEM 1,683 in Germany; USD 1,229 in United States; GBP 727 elsewhere (effective 2000). adv. **Document type:** *Bulletin, Abstract/Index.* **Description:** Reports on the latest scientific, technical and techno-commercial advances in the broad field of biotechnology.

Incorporates (in 2000): Biotechnology: Apparatus, Plant, and Equipment (0938-5584); Formerly (until 1990): Current Biotechnology Abstracts (0264-3391)

Related titles: CD-ROM ed.: (from The Dialog Corporation); Online - full text ed.: (from Data-Star, The Dialog Corporation).

Published by: DECHEMA e.V., Postfach 150104, Frankfurt Am Main D-60061, Germany. TEL 49-69-7564-349, FAX 49-69-7564-201, forsyth@dechema.de, http://www.dechema.de. Ed. John Taylor. **Subscr. to:** Turpin Distribution Services Ltd., Blackhorse Rd, Letchworth, Herts SG6 1HN, United Kingdom. TEL 44-1462-672555.

016.57 USA ISSN 0011-3409
Z5321 CODEN: CCLSBC

CURRENT CONTENTS: LIFE SCIENCES. Short title: C C: L S. Text in English. 1958. w. USD 1,015. Index. **Document type:** *Academic/Scholarly, Bibliography.* **Description:** Lists the tables of contents of the world's leading scientific publications in life sciences including biochemistry, biomedical research, experimental medicine, immunology, microbiology, neuroscience, physiology and toxicology.

Formerly: Current Contents, Chemical, Pharmaco-Medical and Life Sciences

Related titles: CD-ROM ed.: (from Institute for Scientific Information); Diskette ed.; Magnetic Tape ed.; Online - full text ed.: (from The Dialog Corporation).

Indexed: Inpharma, Pharm.&Out.News, Reac., Russ.Acad.Sci.Bibl.

—BLDSC (3496.170000), CASDDS, GNLM.

Published by: Institute for Scientific Information, 3501 Market St., Philadelphia, PA 19104. TEL 215-386-0100, FAX 215-386-2911.

016.5716 GBR ISSN 0268-1625

CYTOSKELETON. Text in English. s-m. GBP 120 for print or e-mail eds. (effective 2001). adv. **Document type:** *Abstract/Index.* **Description:** Current awareness service for researchers. Covers tubulin, microtubules, microfilaments, neurofilaments, cell motility, cilia and flagella.

Formerly: Microfilaments and Microtubules (0142-8209)

Related titles: E-mail ed.; Online - full text ed.: GBP 108 (effective 2001).

—Infotrieve. **CCC.**

Published by: S U B I S (Subsidiary of: Sheffield Academic Press Ltd), Mansion House, 19 Kingfield Rd, Sheffield, S Yorks S11 9AS, United Kingdom. TEL 44-114-255-4433, FAX 44-114-255-4626, subis@sheffac.demon.co.uk, http://www.shef-ac-press.co.uk/subis. Ed. S Huntridge. Adv. contact C Evans.

016.57286 GBR ISSN 0266-6308

D N A PROBES. Text in English. 1985. s-m. GBP 120 for print or e-mail eds. (effective 2001). adv. **Document type:** *Abstract/Index.* **Description:** Covers probes for all organisms: RFLPs, DNA fingerprinting, and polymerase chain reaction.

Related titles: E-mail ed.; Online - full text ed.: GBP 108 (effective 2001).

—CCC.

Published by: S U B I S (Subsidiary of: Sheffield Academic Press Ltd), Mansion House, 19 Kingfield Rd, Sheffield, S Yorks S11 9AS, United Kingdom. TEL 44-114-255-4433, FAX 44-114-255-4626, subis@sheffac.demon.co.uk, http://www.shef-ac-press.co.uk/subis. Ed. S Huntridge. Adv. contact C Evans.

016.57155 GBR ISSN 0957-3518

ENDOTHELIUM. Text in English. 1990. s-m. GBP 120 for print ed. or e-mail (effective 2001). adv. **Document type:** *Abstract/Index.* **Description:** Current awareness service for researchers. Covers all aspects of endothelial structure and function, including endothelins and EDRF.

Related titles: E-mail ed.; Online - full text ed.: GBP 108 (effective 2001).

Published by: S U B I S (Subsidiary of: Sheffield Academic Press Ltd), Mansion House, 19 Kingfield Rd, Sheffield, S Yorks S11 9AS, United Kingdom. TEL 44-114-255-4433, FAX 44-114-255-4626, subis@sheffac.demon.co.uk, http://www.shef-ac-press.co.uk/subis. Ed. S Huntridge. Adv. contact C Evans.

016.5957 USA ISSN 0013-8924
QL461

ENTOMOLOGY ABSTRACTS. Text in English. 1969. m. USD 420 for print & online combined (effective 2002). a. index on CD-ROM. back issues avail. **Document type:** *Abstract/Index.* **Description:** Covers insects, arachnids, myriapods, onychophorans, and terrestrial isopods.

Related titles: Online - full text ed.: USD 1,065 (effective 2002) (from The Dialog Corporation, NISC, S T N International, EBSCO Publishing, CSA).

Published by: Cambridge Scientific Abstracts, 7200 Wisconsin Ave., Suite 601, Bethesda, MD 20814. TEL 301-961-6798, FAX 301-961-6799, journals@csa.com, http://www.csa.com/journals. Ed. Robert Hilton. Pub. Ted Caris.

016.572 576.5 USA ISSN 1078-7712
QP625.N89

ENTREZ DOCUMENT RETRIEVAL SYSTEM. Text in English. bi-m. **Document type:** *Abstract/Index, Government.* **Description:** Cites and abstracts papers with molecular sequence data from MEDLINE, as well as nucleotide sequences from GenBank, EMBL, DDBJ, and dbEST and protein sequences from PIR, Swiss-Prot, PDB, and PRF. DNA, protein, and bibliographic records are linked.

Formed by the merger of (1992-1995): Entrez: Sequences (1065-707X); (1992-1995): Entrez: References (1072-3072); Incorporates (in 1995): N C B I - Sequences (1080-7438)

Media: Online - full text.

Published by: U.S. National Center for Biotechnology Information, National Library of Medicine, Bldg 38A, Rm 8N 803, 8600 Rockville Pike, Bethesda, MD 20894. TEL 301-496-2475, FAX 301-480-9241, info@ncbi.nlm.nih.gov, http://www.ncbi.nlm.nih.gov.

016.577 USA

ENVIROFICHE. Text in English. m. price varies. back issues avail. **Document type:** *Abstract/Index.* **Description:** Full text of the vast majority of abstracted articles and proceedings in Environment Abstracts. Items on microfiche are linked to the print and electronic services through the unique accession number.

Media: Microfiche.

Published by: Congressional Information Service, Inc. (Subsidiary of: LexisNexis), 4520 East West Hwy, Bethesda, MD 20814. TEL 301-654-1550, 800-638-8380, FAX 301-654-4033, cisinfo@lexis-nexis.com, http://www.cispubs.com. Ed. Larry Sheridan. R&P Tim Fusco.

016.57965 NLD ISSN 0921-822X

EXCERPTA MEDICA. ABSTRACT JOURNALS. (Consists of 41 Sections) Text in English. 1947. 12/yr. (each section). USD 49,812 for the full set series (effective 2001). illus. index, cum.index. back issues avail.; reprints avail. **Document type:** *Abstract/Index, Academic/Scholarly.*

Related titles: CD-ROM ed.: (from SilverPlatter Information, Inc.); Online - full text ed.: (from DIMDI, Data-Star, The Dialog Corporation, JICST).

—Linda Hall.

Published by: Excerpta Medica Medical Communications BV (Subsidiary of: Reed Elsevier plc), Rooseveltweg 15, Almere-Stad 1314 SJ, Netherlands. TEL 31-36-538-5600, FAX 31-36-538-5650, nlinfo-f@elsevier.nl, http://www.elsevier.com/locate/emset, http://www.excerptamedica.com. **Subscr. in Australasia and the Far East to:** Elsevier Science (Singapore) Pte Ltd, No.1 Temasek Ave, 17-01 Millenia Tower, Singapore 039192, Singapore. TEL 65-434-3727, FAX 65-337-2230, asiainfo@elsevier.com.sg; **Subscr. in Japan to:** Elsevier Science Inc - Japan Regional Office, 9-15 Higashi-Azabu 1-chome, Minato-ku, Tokyo 106-0044, Japan. TEL 81-3-5561-5033, FAX 81-3-5561-5047, info@elsevier.co.jp; **Subscr. in the Americas to:** Elsevier Science, PO Box 945, New York, NY 10159-0945. TEL 212-633-3730, 888-437-4636, FAX 212-633-3680. **Dist. by:** Elsevier Science (Brazil).; Elsevier Science BV, PO Box 211, Amsterdam 1000 AE, Netherlands. TEL 31-20-485-3757, FAX 31-20-485-3432, nlinfo-f@elsevier.nl, http://www.elsevier.nl.

016.61 NLD ISSN 0014-4053
CODEN: AAEHA9

EXCERPTA MEDICA. SECTION 1: ANATOMY, ANTHROPOLOGY, EMBRYOLOGY & HISTOLOGY. Text in English. 1947. m. EUR 1,581 in Europe to institutions; JPY 209,583 in Japan to institutions; USD 1,769 elsewhere to institutions (effective 2002). adv. index, cum.index. **Document type:** *Abstract/Index, Academic/Scholarly.* **Description:** Provides a comprehensive current-awareness service for academic and trade articles in the fields of anatomy, anthropology, embryology, and histology.

Related titles: CD-ROM ed.: (from SilverPlatter Information, Inc.); Online - full text ed.: (from DIMDI, Data-Star, The Dialog Corporation, JICST).

—GNLM. **CCC.**

Published by: Excerpta Medica Medical Communications BV (Subsidiary of: Reed Elsevier plc), Rooseveltweg 15, Almere-Stad 1314 SJ, Netherlands. TEL 31-36-538-5600, FAX 31-36-538-5650, http://www.elsevier.com/locate/anatomy, http://www.excerptamedica.com. **Subscr. in Australasia and the Far East to:** Elsevier Science (Singapore) Pte Ltd, No.1 Temasek Ave, 17-01 Millenia Tower, Singapore 039192, Singapore. TEL 65-434-3727, FAX 65-337-2230, asiainfo@elsevier.com.sg; **Subscr. in Japan to:** Elsevier Science Inc - Japan Regional Office, 9-15 Higashi-Azabu 1-chome, Minato-ku, Tokyo 106-0044, Japan. TEL 81-3-5561-5033, FAX 81-3-5561-5047, info@elsevier.co.jp; **Subscr. in the Americas to:** Elsevier Science, PO Box 945, New York, NY 10159-0945. TEL 212-633-3730, 888-437-4636, FAX 212-633-3680, usinfo-f@elsevier.com, http://www.elsevier.com. **Dist. by:** Elsevier Science (Brazil).; Elsevier Science BV, PO Box 211, Amsterdam 1000 AE, Netherlands. TEL 31-20-485-3757, FAX 31-20-485-3432, nlinfo-f@elsevier.nl, http://www.elsevier.nl.

EXCERPTA MEDICA. SECTION 2: PHYSIOLOGY. see *MEDICAL SCIENCES—Abstracting, Bibliographies, Statistics*

016.612 NLD ISSN 0014-4258
CODEN: DBITA

EXCERPTA MEDICA. SECTION 21: DEVELOPMENTAL BIOLOGY AND TERATOLOGY. Text in English. 1961. m. NLG 3,879, EUR 1,760.21 in Europe to institutions; JPY 238,600 in Japan to institutions; USD 1,970 elsewhere to institutions (effective 2001). adv. index, cum.index. back issues avail. **Document type:** *Abstract/Index, Academic/Scholarly.* **Description:** Provides a comprehensive current-awareness service of trade and academic articles covering both the experimental and clinical aspects of embryology and fetal, neonatal development.

Related titles: CD-ROM ed.: (from SilverPlatter Information, Inc.); Online - full text ed.: (from DIMDI, Data-Star, The Dialog Corporation, JICST).

—GNLM, Infotrieve, Linda Hall. **CCC.**

Published by: Excerpta Medica Medical Communications BV (Subsidiary of: Reed Elsevier plc), Rooseveltweg 15, Almere-Stad 1314 SJ, Netherlands. TEL 31-36-538-5600, FAX 31-36-538-5650, http://www.elsevier.com/locate/devbioter, http://www.excerptamedica.com. **Subscr. in Australasia and the Far East to:** Elsevier Science (Singapore) Pte Ltd, No.1 Temasek Ave, 17-01 Millenia Tower, Singapore 039192, Singapore. TEL 65-434-3727, FAX 65-337-2230; **Subscr. in Japan to:** Elsevier Science Inc - Japan Regional Office, 9-15 Higashi-Azabu 1-chome, Minato-ku, Tokyo 106-0044, Japan. TEL 81-3-5561-5033, FAX 81-3-5561-5047; **Subscr. in the Americas to:** Elsevier Science, PO Box 945, New York, NY 10159-0945. TEL 212-633-3730, 888-437-4636, FAX 212-633-3680, usinfo-f@elsevier.com, http://www.elsevier.com. **Dist. by:** Elsevier Science (Brazil).; Elsevier Science BV, PO Box 211, Amsterdam 1000 AE, Netherlands. TEL 31-20-485-3757, FAX 31-20-485-3432.

016.5999 NLD ISSN 0014-4266
QH431 CODEN: HUGEA

EXCERPTA MEDICA. SECTION 22: HUMAN GENETICS. Text in English. 1963. s-m. EUR 335 in Europe to qualified personnel; JPY 45,360 in Japan to qualified personnel; USD 374 elsewhere to qualified personnel; EUR 3,115 in Europe to institutions; JPY 412,937 in Japan to institutions; USD 3,484 elsewhere to institutions (effective 2002). adv. index, cum.index. **Document type:** *Abstract/Index, Academic/Scholarly.* **Description:** Provides a comprehensive current-awareness service of trade and academic articles covering both the clinical and experimental aspects of human genetics; includes genetics of lower animals when potentially relevant to human medicine; congenital defects and malformations; basic genetics such as DNA synthesis, gene structure and regulation, genetics recombination and mutagenesis.

Related titles: CD-ROM ed.: (from SilverPlatter Information, Inc.); Online - full text ed.: (from DIMDI, Data-Star, The Dialog Corporation, JICST).

—GNLM, Infotrieve, Linda Hall. **CCC.**

Published by: Excerpta Medica Medical Communications BV (Subsidiary of: Reed Elsevier plc), Rooseveltweg 15, Almere-Stad 1314 SJ, Netherlands. TEL 31-36-538-5600, FAX 31-36-538-5650, http://www.elsevier.com/locate/humgene, http://www.excerptamedica.com. **Subscr. in Australasia and the Far East to:** Elsevier Science (Singapore) Pte Ltd, No.1 Temasek Ave, 17-01 Millenia Tower, Singapore 039192, Singapore. TEL 65-434-3727, FAX 65-337-2230; **Subscr. in Japan to:** Elsevier Science Inc - Japan Regional Office, 9-15 Higashi-Azabu 1-chome, Minato-ku, Tokyo 106-0044, Japan. TEL 81-3-5561-5033, FAX 81-3-5561-5047; **Subscr. in the Americas to:** Elsevier Science, PO Box 945, New York, NY 10159-0945. TEL 212-633-3730, 888-437-4636, FAX 212-633-3680, usinfo-f@elsevier.com, http://www.elsevier.com. **Dist. by:** Elsevier Science (Brazil).; Elsevier Science BV, PO Box 211, Amsterdam 1000 AE, Netherlands. TEL 31-20-485-3757, FAX 31-20-485-3432.

016.57145 NLD ISSN 0014-4312 CODEN: BBMIA

EXCERPTA MEDICA. SECTION 27: BIOPHYSICS, BIO-ENGINEERING AND MEDICAL INSTRUMENTATION. Text in English. 1967. 16/yr. EUR 2,151 in Europe to institutions; JPY 285,129 in Japan to institutions; USD 2,406 elsewhere to institutions (effective 2002). adv. index, cum.index. **Document type:** *Abstract/Index, Academic/Scholarly.* **Description:** Provides a comprehensive current-awareness service for articles that cover the application of biophysical principles to the development of instrumentation, the use of automation in biomedicine, biomechanics, and bioengineering.

Related titles: CD-ROM ed.: (from SilverPlatter Information, Inc.); Online - full text ed.: (from DIMDI, Data-Star, The Dialog Corporation, JICST).

—GNLM, Infotrieve, Linda Hall. **CCC.**

Published by: Excerpta Medica Medical Communications BV (Subsidiary of: Reed Elsevier plc), Rooseveltweg 15, Almere-Stad 1314 SJ, Netherlands. TEL 31-36-538-5600, FAX 31-36-538-5650, http://www.elsevier.nl/locate/biomedinstr, http://www.excerptamedica.com. **Subscr. in Australasia and the Far East to:** Elsevier Science (Singapore) Pte Ltd, No.1 Temasek Ave, 17-01 Millenia Tower, Singapore 039192, Singapore. TEL 65-434-3727, FAX 65-337-2230, asiainfo@elsevier.com.sg; **Subscr. in Japan to:** Elsevier Science Inc - Japan Regional Office, 9-15 Higashi-Azabu 1-chome, Minato-ku, Tokyo 106-0044, Japan. TEL 81-3-5561-5033, FAX 81-3-5561-5047, info@elsevier.co.jp; **Subscr. in the Americas to:** Elsevier Science. **Dist. by:** Elsevier Science (Brazil).; Elsevier Science BV, PO Box 211, Amsterdam 1000 AE, Netherlands. TEL 31-20-485-3757, FAX 31-20-485-3432, nlinfo-f@elsevier.nl, http://www.elsevier.nl.

016.572 NLD ISSN 0927-278X

EXCERPTA MEDICA. SECTION 29: CLINICAL AND EXPERIMENTAL BIOCHEMISTRY. Text in English. 1948. 40/yr. NLG 7,621, EUR 3,770 in Europe to institutions; JPY 499,761 in Japan to institutions; USD 4,217 elsewhere to institutions (effective 2002). adv. bk.rev. charts. index, cum.index. **Document type:** *Abstract/Index, Academic/Scholarly.* **Description:** Provides a current-awareness service for articles covering both clinical chemistry and general biochemistry and includes analytical methods, chemical function tests, enzyme assay, enzyme mode of action studies, biochemical roles in disease, metabolic biochemistry, nutritional analysis, and molecular transport.

Former titles (until 1992): Excerpta Medica. Section 29. Clinical Biochemistry (0300-5372); Excerpta Medica. Section 29: Biochemistry (0014-4339); Which supersedes in part (in 1964): Excerpta Medica. Section 2: Physiology, Biochemistry and Pharmacology (0014-4061)

Related titles: CD-ROM ed.: (from SilverPlatter Information, Inc.); Online - full text ed.: (from DIMDI, Data-Star, The Dialog Corporation, JICST).

—GNLM, Infotrieve, Linda Hall. **CCC.**

Published by: Excerpta Medica Medical Communications BV (Subsidiary of: Reed Elsevier plc), Rooseveltweg 15, Almere-Stad 1314 SJ, Netherlands. TEL 31-36-538-5600, FAX 31-36-538-5650, http://www.elsevier.com/locate/clinexpbio, http://www.excerptamedica.com. **Subscr. in Australasia and the Far East to:** Elsevier Science (Singapore) Pte Ltd, No.1 Temasek Ave, 17-01 Millenia Tower, Singapore 039192, Singapore. TEL 65-434-3727, FAX 65-337-2230, asiainfo@elsevier.com.sg; **Subscr. in Japan to:** Elsevier Science Inc - Japan Regional Office, 9-15 Higashi-Azabu 1-chome, Minato-ku, Tokyo 106-0044, Japan. TEL 81-3-5561-5033, FAX 81-3-5561-5047, info@elsevier.co.jp; **Subscr. in the Americas to:** Elsevier Science, PO Box 945, New York, NY 10159-0945. TEL 212-633-3730, 888-437-4636, FAX 212-633-3680, usinfo-f@elsevier.com, http://www.elsevier.com. **Dist. by:** Elsevier Science (Brazil).; Elsevier Science BV, PO Box 211, Amsterdam 1000 AE, Netherlands. TEL 31-20-485-3757, FAX 31-20-485-3432, nlinfo-f@elsevier.nl, http://www.elsevier.nl.

016.579 NLD ISSN 0927-2771

EXCERPTA MEDICA. SECTION 4: MICROBIOLOGY: BACTERIOLOGY, MYCOLOGY, PARASITOLOGY AND VIROLOGY. Text in English. 1948. 40/yr. EUR 4,793 in Europe to institutions; JPY 635,374 in Japan to institutions; USD 5,361 elsewhere to institutions (effective 2002). adv. index, cum.index. back issues avail. **Document type:** *Abstract/Index, Academic/Scholarly.* **Description:** Covers general aspects of infectious diseases, diagnosis, treatment, epidemiology and prevention of diseases. Includes bacteriology, parasitology, mycology, algae and sexually transmitted diseases.

Incorporates (1971-1991): Excerpta Medica. Section 47: Virology (0031-6520); Former titles (until 1992): Excerpta Medica. Section 4: Microbiology (0167-4285); Excerpta Medica. Section 4: Microbiology: Bacteriology, Mycology and Parasitology (0376-6314)

Related titles: CD-ROM ed.: (from SilverPlatter Information, Inc.); Online - full text ed.: (from DIMDI, Data-Star, The Dialog Corporation, JICST).

—GNLM, Infotrieve. **CCC.**

Published by: Excerpta Medica Medical Communications BV (Subsidiary of: Reed Elsevier plc), Rooseveltweg 15, Almere-Stad 1314 SJ, Netherlands. TEL 31-36-538-5600, FAX 31-36-538-5650, http://www.elsevier.nl/locate/mbmpv, http://www.excerptamedica.com. **Subscr. to:** Elsevier Science (Singapore) Pte Ltd; Elsevier Science Inc - Japan Regional Office, 9-15 Higashi-Azabu 1-chome, Minato-ku, Tokyo 106-0044, Japan. TEL 81-3-5561-5033, FAX 81-3-5561-5047; Elsevier Science, PO Box 945, New York, NY 10159-0945. TEL 212-633-3730, 888-437-4636, FAX 212-633-3680, usinfo-f@elsevier.com, http://www.elsevier.com. **Dist. by:** Elsevier Science (Brazil).; Elsevier Science BV, PO Box 211, Amsterdam 1000 AE, Netherlands. TEL 31-20-485-3757, FAX 31-20-485-3432.

016.5719 NLD ISSN 0014-4096 RB1 CODEN: GPPABB

EXCERPTA MEDICA. SECTION 5: GENERAL PATHOLOGY AND PATHOLOGICAL ANATOMY. Text in English. 1948. 30/yr. EUR 3,667 in Europe to institutions; JPY 486,187 in Japan to institutions; USD 4,103 elsewhere to institutions (effective 2002). adv. index, cum.index. back issues avail. **Document type:** *Abstract/Index, Academic/Scholarly.* **Description:** Provides users with a current-awareness service of clinical and experimental articles in general pathology.

Related titles: CD-ROM ed.: (from SilverPlatter Information, Inc.); Online - full text ed.: (from DIMDI, Data-Star, The Dialog Corporation, JICST).

—GNLM, Infotrieve. **CCC.**

Published by: Excerpta Medica Medical Communications BV (Subsidiary of: Reed Elsevier plc), Rooseveltweg 15, Almere-Stad 1314 SJ, Netherlands. TEL 31-36-538-5600, FAX 31-36-538-5650, nlinfo-f@elsevier.nl, http://www.elsevier.com/locate/genpathana, http://www.excerptamedica.com. **Subscr. to:** Elsevier Science (Singapore) Pte Ltd, No.1 Temasek Ave, 17-01 Millenia Tower, Singapore 039192, Singapore. TEL 65-434-3727, FAX 65-337-2230, asiainfo@elsevier.com.sg; Elsevier Science Inc - Japan Regional Office, 9-15 Higashi-Azabu 1-chome, Minato-ku, Tokyo 106-0044, Japan. TEL 81-3-5561-5033, FAX 81-3-5561-5047, info@elsevier.co.jp; Elsevier Science, PO Box 945, New York, NY 10159-0945. TEL 212-633-3730, 888-437-4636, FAX 212-633-3680, usinfo-f@elsevier.com, http://www.elsevier.com. **Dist. by:** Elsevier Science (Brazil).; Elsevier Science BV, PO Box 211, Amsterdam 1000 AE, Netherlands. TEL 31-20-485-3757, FAX 31-20-485-3432, nlinfo-f@elsevier.nl, http://www.elsevier.nl.

016.57 016.61 GBR

EXPRESS BULLETINS; a series of current awareness bulletins for researchers in biology and medicine. Text in English. 1967. s-m. GBP 100 (effective 1999); per title online; diskette price varies. **Document type:** *Abstract/Index.*

Media: Diskette. **Related titles:** Online - full text ed.

Published by: S U B I S (Subsidiary of: Sheffield Academic Press Ltd), Mansion House, 19 Kingfield Rd, Sheffield, S Yorks S11 9AS, United Kingdom. TEL 44-114-255-4433, FAX 44-114-255-4626, subis@sheffac.demon.co.uk.

016.5716 GBR ISSN 0268-1617

EXTRACELLULAR MATRIX. Text in English. 1986. s-m. GBP 120 for print or e-mail eds. (effective 2001). adv. **Document type:** *Abstract/Index.* **Description:** Current awareness service for researchers in clinical and life sciences.

Related titles: E-mail ed.; Online - full text ed.: GBP 108 (effective 2001).

—**CCC.**

Published by: S U B I S (Subsidiary of: Sheffield Academic Press Ltd), Mansion House, 19 Kingfield Rd, Sheffield, S Yorks S11 9AS, United Kingdom. TEL 44-114-255-4433, FAX 44-114-255-4626, subis@sheffac.demon.co.uk, http://www.shef-ac-press.co.uk/subis. Ed. S Huntridge. Adv. contact C Evans.

FOCUS ON: MOLECULAR MEDICINE. see *MEDICAL SCIENCES—Abstracting, Bibliographies, Statistics*

016.5765 GBR ISSN 1356-1308

GENE THERAPY (SHEFFIELD). Text in English. 1995. s-m. GBP 120 for print ed. or e-mail (effective 2001). adv. **Document type:** *Abstract/Index.* **Description:** Current awareness service for researchers in clinical and life sciences.

Related titles: E-mail ed.; Online - full text ed.: GBP 108 (effective 2001).

Indexed: Inpharma, Pharm.&Out.News, Reac.

Published by: S U B I S (Subsidiary of: Sheffield Academic Press Ltd), Mansion House, 19 Kingfield Rd, Sheffield, S Yorks S11 9AS, United Kingdom. TEL 44-114-255-4433, FAX 44-114-255-4626, subis@sheffac.demon.co.uk, http://www.shef-ac-press.co.uk/subis. Ed. S Huntridge. Adv. contact C Evans.

016.5765 USA ISSN 0016-674X QH431

GENETICS ABSTRACTS. Text in English. 1968. m. USD 1,450 for print & online eds. combined (effective 2002). bk.rev. abstr. index. back issues avail. **Document type:** *Abstract/Index.* **Description:** Covers all aspects of genetics in humans, animals, and plants, with emphasis on molecular genetics.

Related titles: Online - full text ed.: USD 1,090 (effective 2002) (from The Dialog Corporation, S T N International).

—BLDSC (4115.050000).

Published by: Cambridge Scientific Abstracts, 7200 Wisconsin Ave., Suite 601, Bethesda, MD 20814. TEL 301-961-6798, FAX 301-961-6799, journals@csa.com, http://www.csa.com/journals. Ed. Jennifer Phillips. Pub. Ted Caris.

016.5765 JPN

GENETICS SOCIETY OF JAPAN. ABSTRACTS OF THE ANNUAL MEETING/NIHON IDEN GAKKAI TAIKAI PUROGURAMU YOKOSHU. Text in English. a. JPY 10,000, USD 130 (effective 2000). bk.rev. *Refereed.* **Document type:** *Abstract/Index, Academic/Scholarly.*

Published by: Genetics Society of Japan/Nihon Iden Gakkai, c/o National Institute of Genetics, 1111 Yata, Mishima-shi, Shizuoka-ken 411-0801, Japan. shinagaw@biken.osaka-u.ac.jp. Ed., R&P Hideo Shinagawa. **Dist. outside Japan by:** Business Center for Academic Societies Japan, 5-16-9 Honkomagome, Bunkyo-ku, Tokyo 113-0021, Japan. TEL 81-3-5814-5811, 81-3-5814-5822, FAX 81-3-5814-5822.

016.572566 GBR ISSN 1356-1316

GLYCOBIOLOGY RESEARCH. Text in English. 1995. s-m. GBP 120 for print ed. or e-mail (effective 2001). adv. **Document type:** *Abstract/Index.* **Description:** Current awareness service for researchers in clinical and life sciences.

Related titles: E-mail ed.; Online - full text ed.: GBP 108 (effective 2001).

Published by: S U B I S (Subsidiary of: Sheffield Academic Press Ltd), Mansion House, 19 Kingfield Rd, Sheffield, S Yorks S11 9AS, United Kingdom. TEL 44-114-255-4433, FAX 44-114-255-4626, subis@sheffac.demon.co.uk, http://www.shef-ac-press.co.uk/subis. Ed. S Huntridge. Adv. contact C Evans.

016.57 GBR ISSN 1351-5284

HELICOBACTER. Text in English. 1994. s-m. GBP 96 for print or email ed. (effective 2001). adv. **Document type:** *Abstract/Index.* **Description:** Current awareness service for researchers in clinical and life sciences.

Related titles: E-mail ed.; Online - full text ed.: GBP 108 to individuals (effective 2001).

Indexed: Inpharma, Pharm.&Out.News, Reac.

B

Published by: S U B I S (Subsidiary of: Sheffield Academic Press Ltd), Mansion House, 19 Kingfield Rd, Sheffield, S Yorks S11 9AS, United Kingdom. TEL 44-114-255-4433, FAX 44-114-255-4626, subis@sheffac.demon.co.uk, http://www.shef-ac-press.co.uk/subis. Ed. S Huntridge. Adv. contact C Evans.

016.5923 GBR ISSN 0957-6789
QL392.A1 CODEN: HEABEC
HELMINTHOLOGICAL ABSTRACTS. Text in English. 1932. m. GBP 565 to institutions pjrint only; USD 990 in the Americas to institutions print only; GBP 580 to institutions print & online; USD 1,015 in the Americas to institutions print & online (effective 2002). adv. bk.rev. abstr. index, cum.index. back issues avail.; reprints avail. **Document type:** *Abstract/Index.* **Description:** Covers the literature on parasitic helminths: gastrointestinal nematodes, liver flukes, hydatid, trichinella, schistosomes, filariids, and taenia. Aspects covered include morphology, taxonomy, immunology, pathology, biochemistry, epidemiology, life history, control, and molecular biology.
Supersedes: Helminthological Abstracts. Series A: Animal and Human Helminthology (0300-8339)
Related titles: Online - full text ed.: GBP 490 to institutions online only; USD 855 in the Americas to institutions online only (effective 2002) (from DIMDI, The Dialog Corporation, S T N International).
Indexed: Ind.Vet.
—CISTI, GNLM, Linda Hall.
Published by: CABI Publishing, Wallingford, Oxon OX10 8DE, United Kingdom. TEL 44-1491-832111, FAX 44-1491-829198, publishing@cabi.org, http://www.cabi.org/Publishing/Products/Journals/Abstract/HMA/Index.asp. Adv. contact S Harris. B&W page GBP 150; 170 x 267. **US subscr. to:** 10 E 40th St, Ste 3203, New York, NY 10016. TEL 212-481-7018, 800-528-4841, FAX 212-686-7993, cabi-nao@cabi.org.

016.5737 GBR ISSN 1355-4786
QP251 CODEN: HRUPF8
HUMAN REPRODUCTION UPDATE. Text in English. 1963. bi-m. GBP 145, USD 275 to individuals; GBP 455, USD 840 to institutions (effective 2002). adv. bibl. s-a. index. back issues avail. *Refereed.* **Document type:** *Journal, Academic/Scholarly.* **Description:** Comprehensive review service of research within the field of human reproduction.
Formed by the 1995 merger of: Oxford Review of Reproductive Biology (0955-8713); Bibliography of Reproduction (0006-1565)
Related titles: Online - full text ed.: ISSN 1460-2369. GBP 130, USD 247 to individuals Online only; GBP 410, USD 755 to institutions Online only (effective 2002) (from EBSCO Publishing, O C L C Online Computer Library Center, Inc., RoweCom Information Quest, ingenta, Swets Blackwell, Institute for Scientific Information).
Indexed: Curr.Cont., Ind.Med. (1995-), Inpharma, Pharm.&Out.News, Reac., Sci.Cit.Ind.
—BLDSC (4336.431500), CASDDS, CISTI, EMDOCS, GNLM, IDS, Infotrieve, ingenta, Linda Hall. **CCC.**
Published by: (Reproduction Research Information Service Ltd.), Oxford University Press, Academic Division, Great Clarendon St, Oxford OX2 6DP, United Kingdom. TEL 44-1865-267907, FAX 44-1865-267835, jnl.info@oup.co.uk, http://www.humupd.oupjournals.org, http://www.oup.co.uk/journals. Eds. Claus Yding Andersen, H Kentenich, R G Edwards. Pub. J Boullin. R&P Fionna Willis. adv.: page GBP 315, page USD 595. Circ: 1,050. **Subscr. in the Americas to:** Oxford University Press, Journals, 2001 Evans Rd, Cary, NC 27513. TEL 800-852-7323, FAX 919-677-1714, jnlorders@oup-usa.org; **Subscr. to:** Journals Marketing, Great Clarendon St, Oxford OX2 6DP, United Kingdom.

016.5715 GBR ISSN 0142-8136
IMMUNOHISTOCHEMISTRY. Text in English. 1970. s-m. GBP 120 for print ed. or e-mail (effective 2001). adv. **Document type:** *Abstract/Index.* **Description:** Current awareness service for researchers. Covers immunocytochemistry, immunohistology and immuno-electron microscopy.
Formerly (until 1973): Ferritin
Related titles: E-mail ed.; Online - full text ed.: USD 108 (effective 2001).
—CCC.
Published by: S U B I S (Subsidiary of: Sheffield Academic Press Ltd), Mansion House, 19 Kingfield Rd, Sheffield, S Yorks S11 9AS, United Kingdom. TEL 44-114-255-4433, FAX 44-114-255-4626, subis@sheffac.demon.co.uk, http://www.shef-ac-press.co.uk/subis. Ed. S Huntridge. Adv. contact C Evans.

INDONESIAN BIOLOGICAL AND AGRICULTURAL INDEX/INDEKS BIOLOGI DAN PERTANIAN DE INDONESIA. see *AGRICULTURE—Abstracting, Bibliographies, Statistics*

016.5714 USA
INTERNATIONAL BIOPHYSICS CONGRESS. ABSTRACTS. Text in English. 1961. irreg. USD 10. **Document type:** *Proceedings.*
Published by: Massachusetts Institute of Technology, International Biophysics Congress, Cambridge, MA 02139. Ed. Walter Rosenelith.

016.5738 016.6168 GBR ISSN 0261-4952
INVERTEBRATE NEUROBIOLOGY. Text in English. 1982. s-m. GBP 120 for print ed. or e-mail (effective 2001). adv. **Document type:** *Abstract/Index.* **Description:** Current awareness service for researchers. Examines invertebrate neuroscience: development, structure, physiology, biochemistry, peptides and transmitters.
Related titles: E-mail ed.; Online - full text ed.: GBP 108 (effective 2001).
—CCC.
Published by: S U B I S (Subsidiary of: Sheffield Academic Press Ltd), Mansion House, 19 Kingfield Rd, Sheffield, S Yorks S11 9AS, United Kingdom. TEL 44-114-255-4433, FAX 44-114-255-4626, subis@sheffac.demon.co.uk, http://www.shef-ac-press.co.uk/subis. Ed. S Huntridge. Adv. contact C Evans.

016.5724 GBR ISSN 0142-8152
IRON METABOLISM. Text in English. 1992. s-m. GBP 96 for print ed. or e-mail (effective 2001). adv. back issues avail. **Document type:** *Abstract/Index.* **Description:** Current awareness service for researchers in clinical and life sciences.
Related titles: E-mail ed.; Online - full text ed.: GBP 108 to individuals (effective 2001).
—Infotrieve. **CCC.**
Published by: S U B I S (Subsidiary of: Sheffield Academic Press Ltd), Mansion House, 19 Kingfield Rd, Sheffield, S Yorks S11 9AS, United Kingdom. TEL 44-114-255-4433, FAX 44-114-255-4626, subis@sheffac.demon.co.uk, http://www.shef-ac-press.co.uk/subis. Ed. S Huntridge. Adv. contact C Evans.

016.58135 DEU ISSN 1436-8730
QK867
JOURNAL OF PLANT NUTRITION AND SOIL SCIENCE/ZEITSCHRIFT FUER PFLANZENERNAEHRUNG UND BODENKUNDE. Text in English, German. 1922. bi-m. EUR 448 in Europe; CHF 788 in Switzerland & Liechtenstein; USD 588 elsewhere; EUR 471 combined subscription in Europe for print and online eds.; CHF 828 combined subscription in Switzerland & Liechtenstein, for print and online eds.; USD 618 combined subscription elsewhere for print and online eds. (effective 2002). adv. bk.rev. abstr. charts, illus. reprint service avail. from ISI. *Refereed.* **Document type:** *Journal, Academic/Scholarly.* **Description:** Covers the entire spectrum of plant nutrition and soil science.
Former titles (until 1999): Zeitschrift fuer Pflanzenernaehrung und Bodenkunde (0044-3263); (until 1966): Zeitschrift fuer Pflanzenernaehrung, Duengung, Bodenkunde (0932-6707)
Related titles: Microfiche ed.; Online - full text ed.: ISSN 1522-2624. EUR 448 in Europe; CHF 788 in Switzerland & Liechtenstein; USD 588 elsewhere (effective 2002) (from Wiley InterScience, Institute for Scientific Information).
Indexed: ASCA, AgBiotech, Agroforest.Abstr., Aqua.Sci.& Fish.Abstr., Biol.Abstr., Chem.Abstr., Chem.Indus.Notes, Chem.Titles, Crop Physiol.Abstr., Curr.Adv.Ecol.Sci., Curr.Cont., Environ.Sci.Poll.Mgmt., Field Crop Abstr., Food Sci.& Tech.Abstr., Forest.Abstr., GeoRef, Herb.Abstr., Hort.Abstr., IBZ, INIS Atomind., Ind.Sci.Rev., Irr.& Drain.Abstr., Maize Abstr., Nutr.Abstr., Plant Breed.Abstr., Plant Grow.Reg.Abstr., Potato Abstr., Rev.Appl.Entomol., Rev.Plant Path., Rice Abstr., Sci.Cit.Ind., Seed Abstr., Sel.Water Res.Abstr., Soils & Fert., Sorghum & Millets Abstr., Triticale Abstr., VITIS, Weed Abstr.
—BLDSC (9478.500000), CASDDS, CISTI, IDS, Infotrieve, ingenta, Linda Hall. **CCC.**
Published by: (Deutsche Bodenkundliche Gesellschaft), Wiley - V C H, Postfach 101161, Weinheim 69451, Germany. FAX 49-6201-606-117, adsales@wiley-vch.de, subservice@wiley-vch.de, http://www.wiley-vch.de. Eds. H Beringer, P Leinweber. R&P Claudia Rutz. **Subscr. in the Americas to:** John Wiley & Sons, Inc., Journals. TEL 44-1243-779777, 212-850-6645, FAX 212-850-6021; **Subscr. outside Germany, Austria & Switzerland to:** John Wiley & Sons Ltd., Baffins Ln, Chichester, Sussex PO19 IUD, United Kingdom. TEL 44-1243-779777, FAX 44-1243-843232. **Co-sponsor:** Deutsche Gesellschaft fuer Pflanzenernaehrung.

016.57 JPN
KARUSHUMU SHINPOJUMU KOEN YOSHI/ABSTRACTS OF CALCIUM SYMPOSIUM. Text in Japanese. 1989. s-a. **Document type:** *Abstract/Index.*
Published by: Karushumu Shinpojumu Un'ei Iinkai/Management Committee of Calcium Symposium, Shokuseikatsu Kenkyukai, 12-19 Nishi-Hon-Machi 1-chome, Nishi-ku, Osaka-shi 550-0005, Japan.

016.5765 JPN
KIKAN KEISEI KENKYUKAI KOEN YOSHISHU/ JAPANESE SOCIETY FOR BASIC AND APPLIED ORGAN RESEARCH. ABSTRACTS OF THE MEETING. Text in Japanese. s-a.
Published by: Kikan Keisei Kenkyukai, Nagoya Daigaku Igakubu, Koku Gekagaku Kyoshitsu, 65 Tsurumai-cho, Showa-ku, Nagoya-shi, Aichi-ken 466-0065, Japan.

016.612015 GBR ISSN 0143-4217
LECTINS. Text in English. 1992. s-m. GBP 96 for print ed. or e-mail (effective 2001). adv. back issues avail. **Document type:** *Abstract/Index.* **Description:** Current awareness service for researchers in clinical and life sciences.
Related titles: E-mail ed.; Online - full text ed.: GBP 108 to individuals (effective 2001).
—CCC.
Published by: S U B I S (Subsidiary of: Sheffield Academic Press Ltd), Mansion House, 19 Kingfield Rd, Sheffield, S Yorks S11 9AS, United Kingdom. TEL 44-114-255-4433, FAX 44-114-255-4626, subis@sheffac.demon.co.uk, http://www.shef-ac-press.co.uk/subis. Ed. S Huntridge. Adv. contact C Evans.

LEUCOCYTES. see *MEDICAL SCIENCES—Abstracting, Bibliographies, Statistics*

016.57 USA
LIFE SCIENCE BOOK REVIEW. Text in English. 1991. bi-m. USD 24. **Description:** Covers all areas of the life sciences.
Published by: Carolina Press, PO Box 24906, Winston Salem, NC 27114. TEL 919-768-9180. Ed. Andrew Goliszek.

016.57257 GBR ISSN 0264-9659
LIPOSOMES. Text in English. 1984. s-m. GBP 120 for print ed. or e-mail (effective 2001). adv. **Document type:** *Abstract/Index.* **Description:** Current awareness service for researchers. Offers information on the structure and pharmacology of liposomes and natural membrane vesicles.
Related titles: E-mail ed.; Online - full text ed.: GBP 108 (effective 2001).
—CCC.
Published by: S U B I S (Subsidiary of: Sheffield Academic Press Ltd), Mansion House, 19 Kingfield Rd, Sheffield, S Yorks S11 9AS, United Kingdom. TEL 44-114-255-4433, FAX 44-114-255-4626, subis@sheffac.demon.co.uk, http://www.shef-ac-press.co.uk/subis. Ed. S Huntridge. Adv. contact C Evans.

016.571655 GBR ISSN 1351-5322
LYSOSOMES AND ENDOCYTOSIS. Text in English. 1994. s-m. GBP 96 fo rprint ed. or e-mail (effective 2001). adv. back issues avail. **Document type:** *Abstract/Index.* **Description:** Current awareness service for researchers in clinical and life sciences.
Formerly (until 1993): Lysosomes (0142-8187)
Related titles: E-mail ed.; Online - full text ed.: GBP 108 to individuals (effective 2001).
—CCC.
Published by: S U B I S (Subsidiary of: Sheffield Academic Press Ltd), Mansion House, 19 Kingfield Rd, Sheffield, S Yorks S11 9AS, United Kingdom. TEL 44-114-255-4433, FAX 44-114-255-4626, subis@sheffac.demon.co.uk, http://www.shef-ac-press.co.uk/subis. Ed. S Huntridge. Adv. contact C Evans.

MACROPHAGES. see *MEDICAL SCIENCES—Abstracting, Bibliographies, Statistics*

016.573679 016.6181 GBR ISSN 0964-7600
MAMMARY GLAND. Text in English. 1992. s-m. GBP 96 for print ed. or e-mail ed. (effective 2001). adv. **Document type:** *Abstract/Index.* **Description:** Current awareness service for researchers. Covers all aspects of the mammary gland.
Related titles: E-mail ed.; Online - full text ed.: GBP 108 to individuals (effective 2001).
Published by: S U B I S (Subsidiary of: Sheffield Academic Press Ltd), Mansion House, 19 Kingfield Rd, Sheffield, S Yorks S11 9AS, United Kingdom. TEL 44-114-255-4433, FAX 44-114-255-4626, subis@sheffac.demon.co.uk, http://www.shef-ac-press.co.uk/subis. Ed. S Huntridge. Adv. contact C Evans.

016.579 USA ISSN 0300-838X
QR53
MICROBIOLOGY ABSTRACTS: SECTION A. INDUSTRIAL & APPLIED MICROBIOLOGY. Text in English. 1965. m. USD 1,440 for print & online combined (effective 2002). bk.rev. back issues avail. **Document type:** *Abstract/Index.* **Description:** Covers scientific research and practical applications in pharmaceuticals, foods, and agriculture.
Related titles: Online - full text ed.: USD 1,080 (effective 2002) (from The Dialog Corporation, S T N International).
—BLDSC (5757.770000), GNLM.
Published by: Cambridge Scientific Abstracts, 7200 Wisconsin Ave., Suite 601, Bethesda, MD 20814. TEL 301-961-6798, FAX 301-961-6799, journals@csa.com, http://www.csa.com/journals. Ed. Roberta Gardner. Pub. Ted Caris.

016.5793 USA ISSN 0300-8398
QR1
MICROBIOLOGY ABSTRACTS: SECTION B. BACTERIOLOGY. Text in English. 1966. m. USD 1,435 for print & online combined (effective 2002). adv. bk.rev. abstr. back issues avail. **Document type:** *Abstract/Index.* **Description:** Covers clinical applications and pure research in all aspects of bacteriology.
Related titles: Online - full text ed.: USD 1,075 (effective 2002) (from The Dialog Corporation, S T N International, CSA).
Published by: Cambridge Scientific Abstracts, 7200 Wisconsin Ave., Suite 601, Bethesda, MD 20814. TEL 301-961-6798, FAX 301-961-6799, journals@csa.com, http://www.csa.com/journals. Ed. Roberta Gardner. Pub. Ted Caris.

016.579 USA ISSN 0301-2328
QK564
MICROBIOLOGY ABSTRACTS: SECTION C. ALGOLOGY, MYCOLOGY AND PROTOZOOLOGY. Text in English. 1972. m. USD 1,360 for print & online combined (effective 2002). bk.rev. abstr. back issues avail. **Document type:** *Abstract/Index.* **Description:** Covers life cycles of algae, fungi, and protozoa, and their interactions with animals and plants.
Related titles: Online - full text ed.: USD 1,020 (effective 2002) (from The Dialog Corporation, S T N International, CSA).
Published by: Cambridge Scientific Abstracts, 7200 Wisconsin Ave., Suite 601, Bethesda, MD 20814. TEL 301-961-6798, FAX 301-961-6799, journals@csa.com, http://www.csa.com/journals. Ed. Roberta Gardner. Pub. Ted Caris.

016.571657 GBR ISSN 0142-8217
Z5322.C3
MITOCHONDRIA. Text in English. 1978. s-m. GBP 120 for print ed. or e-mail (effective 2001). adv. **Document type:** *Abstract/Index.* **Description:** Current awareness service for researchers. Covers electron transport, cytochromes, oxidative phosphorylation, TCA cycle, pathology.
Related titles: E-mail ed.; Online - full text ed.: GBP 108 (effective 2001).
—CCC.
Published by: S U B I S (Subsidiary of: Sheffield Academic Press Ltd), Mansion House, 19 Kingfield Rd, Sheffield, S Yorks S11 9AS, United Kingdom. TEL 44-114-255-4433, FAX 44-114-255-4626, subis@sheffac.demon.co.uk, http://www.shef-ac-press.co.uk/subis. Ed. S Huntridge. Adv. contact C Evans.

016.5728 GBR ISSN 1356-1324
MOLECULAR BIOLOGY TECHNIQUES. Text in English. 1995. s-m. GBP 120 for print ed. or e-mail (effective 2001). adv. **Document type:** *Abstract/Index.* **Description:** Current awareness service for researchers in clinical and life sciences. Covers all aspects of investigations in the field of molecular biology.
Related titles: E-mail ed.; Online - full text ed.: GBP 108 (effective 2001).
Published by: S U B I S (Subsidiary of: Sheffield Academic Press Ltd), Mansion House, 19 Kingfield Rd, Sheffield, S Yorks S11 9AS, United Kingdom. TEL 44-114-255-4433, FAX 44-114-255-4626, subis@sheffac.demon.co.uk, http://www.shef-ac-press.co.uk/subis. Ed. S Huntridge. Adv. contact C Evans.

016.61697 GBR ISSN 0261-4960
MONOCLONAL ANTIBODIES. Text in English. 1981. s-m. GBP 120 for print ed. or e-mail (effective 2001). adv. bk.rev. **Document type:** *Abstract/Index.* **Description:** Current awareness service for researchers. Covers antibodies, molecules and cell types. Includes information on assays and separation techniques using MABs.
Related titles: E-mail ed.; Online - full text ed.: GBP 108 (effective 2001).
—CCC.
Published by: S U B I S (Subsidiary of: Sheffield Academic Press Ltd), Mansion House, 19 Kingfield Rd, Sheffield, S Yorks S11 9AS, United Kingdom. TEL 44-114-255-4433, FAX 44-114-255-4626, subis@sheffac.demon.co.uk, http://www.shef-ac-press.co.uk/subis. Ed. S Huntridge. Adv. contact C Evans.

016.5793 GBR ISSN 1351-5292
MYCOBACTERIA. Text in English. 1994. s-m. GBP 96 for print or email ed. (effective 2001). adv. **Document type:** *Abstract/Index.* **Description:** Current awareness service for researchers in clinical and life sciences.
Related titles: E-mail ed.; Online - full text ed.: GBP 108 to individuals (effective 2001).
Indexed: Abstr.Hyg.
Published by: S U B I S (Subsidiary of: Sheffield Academic Press Ltd), Mansion House, 19 Kingfield Rd, Sheffield, S Yorks S11 9AS, United Kingdom. TEL 44-114-255-4433, FAX 44-114-255-4626, subis@sheffac.demon.co.uk, http://www.shef-ac-press.co.uk/subis. Ed. S Huntridge. Adv. contact C Evans.

016.59257 GBR ISSN 0957-6797
SB998.N4 CODEN: NEABEA
NEMATOLOGICAL ABSTRACTS. Text in English. 1932. q. GBP 250 Includes single site Internet access; USD 435 in the Americas Includes single site Internet access; GBP 260 For Internet only (effective 2001); USD 455 For Internet only (effective 2000). adv. bk.rev. back issues avail.; reprints avail. **Document type:** *Abstract/Index.* **Description:** Contains abstracts of the world literature on: nematodes parasitic on plants, free-living and marine nematodes, and nematodes parasitic on insects or other invertebrates.
Supersedes: Helminthological Abstracts. Series B: Plant Nematology (0300-8320)
Related titles: Online - full text ed.: (from DIMDI, The Dialog Corporation, S T N International).
Indexed: Rev.Appl.Entomol.
—CISTI, Linda Hall.
Published by: CABI Publishing, Wallingford, Oxon OX10 8DE, United Kingdom. TEL 44-1491-832111, FAX 44-1491-829198, publishing@cabi.org, http://www.cabi.org. **U.S. subscr. to:** 10 E 40th St, Ste 3203, New York, NY 10016. TEL 212-481-7018, 800-528-4841, FAX 212-686-7993, cabi-nao@cabi.org.

016.5716 016.6168 GBR ISSN 0142-8225
NERVE CELL BIOLOGY. Text in English. 1972. s-m. GBP 120 for print ed. or e-mail (effective 2001). adv. **Document type:** *Abstract/Index.* **Description:** Current awareness service for researchers. Covers nerve cell biology: development, regeneration, structure, tissue culture, pharmacology, immunology, membranes and sensory receptors.
Related titles: E-mail ed.; Online - full text ed.: GBP 108 (effective 2001).
—CCC.
Published by: S U B I S (Subsidiary of: Sheffield Academic Press Ltd), Mansion House, 19 Kingfield Rd, Sheffield, S Yorks S11 9AS, United Kingdom. TEL 44-114-255-4433, FAX 44-114-255-4626, subis@sheffac.demon.co.uk, http://www.shef-ac-press.co.uk/subis. Ed. S Huntridge. Adv. contact C Evans.

016.572 GBR ISSN 0142-8233
NEUROPEPTIDES (SHEFFIELD). Text in English. 1979. s-m. GBP 120 for print ed. or e-mail (effective 2001). adv. **Document type:** *Abstract/Index.* **Description:** Current awareness service for researchers. Covers opioids, endorphins, neurotensin, cholecystokinin, TRH, VIP, neuropeptide Y, and invertebrate peptides.
Related titles: E-mail ed.; Online - full text ed.: GBP 108 (effective 2001).
Indexed: Chem.Abstr., Curr.Adv.Ecol.Sci., Excerp.Med., Ind.Sci.Rev., Sci.Cit.Ind. (coverage dropped).
—CCC.
Published by: S U B I S (Subsidiary of: Sheffield Academic Press Ltd), Mansion House, 19 Kingfield Rd, Sheffield, S Yorks S11 9AS, United Kingdom. TEL 44-114-255-4433, FAX 44-114-255-4626, subis@sheffac.demon.co.uk, http://www.shef-ac-press.co.uk/subis. Ed. S Huntridge. Adv. contact C Evans.

016.5738 016.6168 GBR ISSN 0142-8241
NEUROPHYSIOLOGY. Text in English. 1972. s-m. GBP 120 for print ed. or e-mail (effective 2001). adv. **Document type:** *Abstract/Index.* **Description:** Current awareness service for researchers. Covers the electrophysiology and pharmacology of the vertebrate central, autonomic and peripheral nervous systems.
Related titles: E-mail ed.; Online - full text ed.: GBP 108 (effective 2001) (from Kluwer Online).
Indexed: Biol.Abstr., Chem.Abstr., Curr.Adv.Ecol.Sci., Excerp.Med., Ind.Sci.Rev., Psychol.Abstr., Sci.Cit.Ind. (coverage dropped), e-psyche.
—Infotrieve. **CCC.**
Published by: S U B I S (Subsidiary of: Sheffield Academic Press Ltd), Mansion House, 19 Kingfield Rd, Sheffield, S Yorks S11 9AS, United Kingdom. TEL 44-114-255-4433, FAX 44-114-255-4626, subis@sheffac.demon.co.uk, http://www.shef-ac-press.co.uk/subis. Ed. S Huntridge. Adv. contact C Evans.

016.579321 JPN
NIHON BOKIN BOBAI GAKKAI. NENJI TAIKAI YOSHISHU/SOCIETY FOR ANTIBACTERIAL AND ANTIFUNGAL AGENTS, JAPAN. ABSTRACTS OF THE MEETING. Text in Japanese. a. JPY 3,000 (effective 2000). adv. **Document type:** *Academic/Scholarly, Abstract/Index.*
Published by: Nihon Bokin Bobai Gakkai/Society for Antibacterial and Antifungal Agents, Japan, 9th Fl, Shin-Kousan Bldg, 13-38, Nishimotocho 1-chome, Nishi-ku, Osaka-shi 550-0005, Japan. Ed. Tetsuaki Tsuchido. R&P K Arai TEL 81-6-6538-2166. Adv. contact Iwao Yamamoto.

016.590724 JPN
NIHON JIKKEN DOBUTSU GAKKAI SOKAI KOEN YOSHISHU/JAPANESE ASSOCIATION FOR LABORATORY ANIMAL SCIENCE. ABSTRACTS OF GENERAL MEETING. Text in Japanese. a. **Document type:** *Abstract/Index.*
Published by: Japanese Association for Laboratory Animal Science/Nihon Jikken Dobutsu Gakkai, Akamon Royal Heights, Rm 1103, 5-29-12 Hongo, Bunkyo-ku, Tokyo 113-0033, Japan. TEL 81-3-3814-8276, FAX 81-3-3814-3990, http://www.jalas.or.jp/.

016.5999 JPN
NIHON JINRUI IDEN GAKKAI TAIKAI SHOROKUSHU/ JAPAN SOCIETY OF HUMAN GENETICS. ABSTRACTS OF THE ANNUAL MEETING. Text in English, Japanese. a. **Document type:** *Abstract/Index.*
Published by: Nihon Jinrui Iden Gakkai/Japan Society of Human Genetics, Ika Shika Daigaku Jinrui Idengaku Kenkyushitsu, 5-45 Yushima 1-chome, Bunkyo-ku, Tokyo 113-0034, Japan.

016.571 JPN
NIHON SEIRI JINRUI GAKKAI TAIKAI SHOROKUSHU/JAPAN SOCIETY OF PHYSIOLOGICAL ANTHROPOLOGY. ABSTRACTS OF THE MEETING. Text in Japanese. a. **Document type:** *Abstract/Index.*
Published by: Nihon Seiri Jinrui Gakkai, c/o Business Center for Academic Societies Japan, 5-16-9 Honkomagome, Bunkyo-ku, Tokyo 113-0021, Japan. TEL 81-3-5814—5801, FAX 81-3-5814-5820, iwanaga@design.ti.chiba-u.ac.jp.

016.57287 JPN
NIHON SENSHOKUTAI KENSA GAKKAI SHOROKUSHU/JAPANESE ASSOCIATION FOR CHROMOSOME ANALYSIS. ABSTRACT OF ANNUAL MEETING. Text in English, Japanese. 1988. a. **Document type:** *Abstract/Index.*

Published by: Nihon Senshokutai Kensa Gakkai, c/o Nihon Gene Research Lab's Inc., 3-36 Ogi-Machi 2-chome, Miyagino-ku, Sendai-shi, Miyagi-ken 983-0034, Japan. TEL 81-22-238-070, kgg0250@niftyserve.or.jp.

016.5738 GBR ISSN 1351-525X
NITRIC OXIDE. Text in English. 1994. s-m. GBP 120 for print ed. or e-mail (effective 2001). adv. **Document type:** *Abstract/Index.* **Description:** Current awareness service for researchers in clinical and life sciences.
Related titles: E-mail ed.; Online - full text ed.: GBP 108 (effective 2001).
Indexed: Ind.Med. (coverage dropped).
Published by: S U B I S (Subsidiary of: Sheffield Academic Press Ltd), Mansion House, 19 Kingfield Rd, Sheffield, S Yorks S11 9AS, United Kingdom. TEL 44-114-255-4433, FAX 44-114-255-4626, subis@sheffac.demon.co.uk, http://www.shef-ac-press.co.uk/subis. Ed. S Huntridge. Adv. contact C Evans.

016.5738 JPN
NO NO IGAKU SEIBUTSUGAKU KONWAKAI SHOROKU/ABSTRACTS OF CONFERENCE ON MEDICINE AND BIOLOGY OF THE BRAIN. Text in Japanese. 1986. s-a. **Document type:** *Abstract/Index.*
Published by: No no Igaku Seibutsugaku Konwakai, Fujita Gakuen Hoken Eisei Daigaku, Igakubu Seirigaku Kyoshitsu, 1-98 Dengakugakubo-kutsukakecho, Toyoake-shi, Aichi-ken 470-1100, Japan.

016.572 USA ISSN 1070-2466
QP551
NUCLEIC ACIDS ABSTRACTS. Text in English. 1971. m. USD 1,280 for print & online combined (effective 2002). bk.rev. abstr. index. **Document type:** *Abstract/Index.* **Description:** Covers physical, chemical, and biological aspects of nucleic acids and nucleoproteins.
Former titles (until 1994): Cambridge Scientific Biochemistry Abstracts: Part 2. Nucleic Acids (8756-7512); Biochemistry Abstracts: Part 2. Nucleic Acids (0143-3318); Nucleic Acids Abstracts (0048-1041)
Related titles: Online - full text ed.: USD 960 (effective 2002) (from The Dialog Corporation, S T N International, CSA).
—GNLM.
Published by: Cambridge Scientific Abstracts, 7200 Wisconsin Ave., Suite 601, Bethesda, MD 20814. TEL 301-961-6798, FAX 301-961-6799, journals@csa.com, http://www.csa.com/journals. Ed. Jennifer Phillips. Pub. Ted Caris.

016.572 GBR ISSN 0950-057X
OXYGEN RADICALS. Text in English. 1988. s-m. GBP 120 for print ed. or email (effective 2001). adv. bk.rev. back issues avail. **Document type:** *Abstract/Index.* **Description:** Current awareness service for researchers in clinical and life sciences.
Related titles: E-mail ed.; Online - full text ed.: GBP 108 (effective 2001).
—CCC.
Published by: S U B I S (Subsidiary of: Sheffield Academic Press Ltd), Mansion House, 19 Kingfield Rd, Sheffield, S Yorks S11 9AS, United Kingdom. TEL 44-114-255-4433, FAX 44-114-255-4626, subis@sheffac.demon.co.uk, http://www.shef-ac-press.co.uk/subis. Ed. S Huntridge. Adv. contact C Evans.

016.579 GBR ISSN 0267-6850
P H L S LIBRARY BULLETIN. Text in English. ceased; resumed 1948. w. GBP 65 in United Kingdom; GBP 110 in Europe; GBP 160 elsewhere (effective 2000). **Document type:** *Bibliography.* **Description:** Provides compiled information specifically deals with the public health and medical laboratory microbiologist in mind. Lists authors and titles of 350 relevant papers each week.
Published by: Public Health Laboratory Service, 61 Colindale Ave, London NW9 5HT, United Kingdom. TEL 44-20-8200-4400, FAX 44-20-8200-7875. Ed. Margaret Clennett. Circ: 600.

016.5734 GBR ISSN 0142-825X
PANCREATIC AND SALIVARY SECRETION. Text in English. 1979. s-m. GBP 120 for print ed. or email (effective 2001). adv. **Document type:** *Abstract/Index.* **Description:** Provides a current-awareness service for researchers. Covers the pharmacology, structure and function of the pancreatic and salivary glands.
Related titles: E-mail ed.; Online - full text ed.: GBP 108 (effective 2001).
—CCC.
Published by: S U B I S (Subsidiary of: Sheffield Academic Press Ltd), Mansion House, 19 Kingfield Rd, Sheffield, S Yorks S11 9AS, United Kingdom. TEL 44-114-255-4433, FAX 44-114-255-4626, subis@sheffac.demon.co.uk, http://www.shef-ac-press.co.uk/subis. Ed. S Huntridge. Adv. contact C Evans.

016.57965 GBR ISSN 0964-7570
PARASITOLOGY (SHEFFIELD). Text in English. 1992. s-m. GBP 120 for print ed. or email (effective 2001). adv. **Document type:** *Abstract/Index.* **Description:** Current awareness service for researchers investigating all aspects of parasitology.
Related titles: E-mail ed.; Online - full text ed.: GBP 108 (effective 2001).
Indexed: Curr.Cont. (coverage dropped), Ind.Sci.Rev., Nuc.Acids Abstr.
Published by: S U B I S (Subsidiary of: Sheffield Academic Press Ltd), Mansion House, 19 Kingfield Rd, Sheffield, S Yorks S11 9AS, United Kingdom. TEL 44-114-255-4433, FAX 44-114-255-4626, subis@sheffac.demon.co.uk, http://www.shef-ac-press.co.uk/subis. Ed. S Huntridge. Adv. contact C Evans.

016.58 660 GBR ISSN 0260-5902
PLANT BIOTECHNOLOGY. Text in English. 1981. s-m. GBP 120 for print ed. or e-mail (effective 2001). adv. bk.rev. **Document type:** *Abstract/Index.* **Description:** Current awareness service for researchers. Covers plant tissue culture, protoplasts, recombinant work, chemostat technology, immobilized enzymes and cells, biomass production and production of primary and secondary products.
Related titles: E-mail ed.; Online - full text ed.: GBP 108 (effective 2001).
Indexed: Abstr.Bull.Inst.Pap.Chem., Chem.Abstr., Chem.Indus.Notes, Chem.Titles, Food Sci.& Tech.Abstr.
—BLDSC (6513.770000). **CCC.**
Published by: S U B I S (Subsidiary of: Sheffield Academic Press Ltd), Mansion House, 19 Kingfield Rd, Sheffield, S Yorks S11 9AS, United Kingdom. TEL 44-114-255-4433, FAX 44-114-255-4626, subis@sheffac.demon.co.uk, http://www.shef-ac-press.co.uk/subis. Ed. S Huntridge. Adv. contact C Evans.

016.573159 GBR ISSN 0142-8268
PLATELETS (SHEFFIELD). Text in English. 1976. s-m. GBP 120 for print ed. or e-mail (effective 2001). adv. **Document type:** *Abstract/Index.* **Description:** Current awareness service for researchers. Covers thrombocytopoiesis, pharmacology, aggregation, structure, biochemistry and functions of platelets.
Related titles: E-mail ed.; Online - full text ed.: GBP 108 (effective 2001).
Indexed: Sci.Cit.Ind. (coverage dropped).
—Infotrieve. **CCC.**
Published by: S U B I S (Subsidiary of: Sheffield Academic Press Ltd), Mansion House, 19 Kingfield Rd, Sheffield, S Yorks S11 9AS, United Kingdom. TEL 44-114-255-4433, FAX 44-114-255-4626, subis@sheffac.demon.co.uk, http://www.shef-ac-press.co.uk/subis. Ed. S Huntridge. Adv. contact C Evans.

016.572 GBR ISSN 0952-0406
PROTEINS: POST-TRANSLATIONAL PROCESSING. Text in English. 1976. s-m. GBP 120 for print ed. or e-mail (effective 2001). adv. **Document type:** *Abstract/Index.* **Description:** Current awareness service for researchers. Covers phosphorylation, methylation, acetylation, amidation, sulphation, hydroxylation and glycoslation as well as transport of proteins.
Formerly (until 1987): Protein Phosphorylation (0142-8292)
Related titles: E-mail ed.; Online - full text ed.: GBP 108 (effective 2001).
—CCC.
Published by: S U B I S (Subsidiary of: Sheffield Academic Press Ltd), Mansion House, 19 Kingfield Rd, Sheffield, S Yorks S11 9AS, United Kingdom. TEL 44-114-255-4433, FAX 44-114-255-4626, subis@sheffac.demon.co.uk, http://www.shef-ac-press.co.uk/subis. Ed. S Huntridge. Adv. contact C Evans.

016.59 GBR ISSN 0309-1287
PROTOZOOLOGICAL ABSTRACTS. Text in English. 1977. m. GBP 635 to institutions; USD 1,085 in the Americas to institutions; GBP 650 to institutions Includes single site online access; USD 1,115 in the Americas to institutions Includes single site online access (effective 2002). adv. back issues avail. **Document type:** *Abstract/Index.* **Description:** Covers all protozoan diseases, many endemic to the tropics, affecting humans and animals.
Related titles: Online - full text ed.: GBP 550, USD 960 to institutions (effective 2002) (from DIMDI, The Dialog Corporation, S T N International).
—CISTI, Linda Hall.
Published by: CABI Publishing, Wallingford, Oxon OX10 8DE, United Kingdom. TEL 44-1491-832111, FAX 44-1491-829198, publishing@cabi.org, http://www.cabi.org/Publishing/Products/Journals/Abstract/PZA/Index.asp. Adv. contact S Harris. B&W page GBP 75; 170 x 267. **U.S. subscr. to:** 10 E 40th St, Ste 3203, New York, NY 10016. TEL 212-481-7018, 800-528-4841, FAX 212-686-7993, cabi-nao@cabi.org.

016.57 RUS ISSN 0034-2300
QH7 CODEN: RZBLAS
REFERATIVNYI ZHURNAL. BIOLOGIYA. Text in Russian. 1953. m. abstr, bibl. index. **Document type:** *Abstract/Index.*
Formerly: Referativnyi Zhurnal. Biologicheskaya Khimiya (0486-2260)
Indexed: Apic.Abstr., Biol.Abstr., Chem.Abstr., Helminthol.Abstr.
—CASDDS, East View, Linda Hall.
Published by: Vserossiiskii Institut Nauchnoi i Tekhnicheskoi Informatsii (VINITI), Usievicha ul 20-a, Moscow 125315, Russian Federation. TEL 7-095-1526441. Ed. Rem Petrov. Circ: 2,930. **Dist. by:** Mezhdunarodnaya Kniga, B Yakimanka 39, Moscow 117049, Russian Federation. TEL 7-095-2384967, FAX 7-095-2384634; **US dist. addr.:** East View Publications, 3020 Harbor Ln N, Minneapolis, MN 55447. TEL 612-550-0961.

016.57 RUS ISSN 0235-3105
REFERATIVNYI ZHURNAL. BIOLOGIYA SEL'SKOKHOZYAISTVENNYKH ZHIVOTNYKH. Text in Russian. 1959. m. USD 396. **Document type:** *Abstract/Index.*
Formerly: Referativnyi Zhurnal. Zhivotnovodstvo (0206-5533)
Indexed: Chem.Abstr.
—East View.
Published by: Vserossiiskii Institut Nauchnoi i Tekhnicheskoi Informatsii (VINITI), Usievicha ul 20-a, Moscow 125315, Russian Federation. TEL 7-095-1526441. **Dist. by:** Mezhdunarodnaya Kniga, B Yakimanka 39, Moscow 117049, Russian Federation. TEL 7-095-2384967, FAX 7-095-2384634; **US dist. addr.:** East View Publications, 3020 Harbor Ln N, Minneapolis, MN 55447. TEL 612-550-0961.

016.5714 RUS ISSN 0202-912X
REFERATIVNYI ZHURNAL. BIONIKA. BIOKIBERNETIKA. BIOINZHENERIYA. Text in Russian. 1975. m. USD 279. **Document type:** *Abstract/Index.*
Published by: Vserossiiskii Institut Nauchnoi i Tekhnicheskoi Informatsii (VINITI), Usievicha ul 20-a, Moscow 125315, Russian Federation. TEL 7-095-1526441. **Dist. by:** Mezhdunarodnaya Kniga, B Yakimanka 39, Moscow 117049, Russian Federation. TEL 7-095-2384967, FAX 7-095-2384634.

016.577 RUS ISSN 0868-4588
REFERATIVNYI ZHURNAL. EKOLOGIYA CHELOVEKA. Text in Russian. 1987. m. USD 320.
Formerly: Referativnyi Sbornik. Ekologiya Cheloveka (0202-5140)
Indexed: Ref.Zh.
Published by: Vserossiiskii Institut Nauchnoi i Tekhnicheskoi Informatsii (VINITI), Usievicha ul 20-a, Moscow 125315, Russian Federation. TEL 7-095-1526441. **Dist. by:** Mezhdunarodnaya Kniga, B Yakimanka 39, Moscow 117049, Russian Federation. TEL 7-095-2384967, FAX 7-095-2384634; **US dist. addr.:** East View Publications, 3020 Harbor Ln N, Minneapolis, MN 55447. TEL 612-550-0961, FAX 612-559-2931.

016.58 RUS ISSN 0202-9235
REFERATIVNYI ZHURNAL. FITOPATOLOGIYA. Text in Russian. 1978. m. USD 171. **Document type:** *Abstract/Index.*
Published by: Vserossiiskii Institut Nauchnoi i Tekhnicheskoi Informatsii (VINITI), Usievicha ul 20-a, Moscow 125315, Russian Federation. TEL 7-095-1526441. **Dist. by:** Mezhdunarodnaya Kniga, B Yakimanka 39, Moscow 117049, Russian Federation. TEL 7-095-2384967, FAX 7-095-2384634.

016.571 RUS ISSN 0207-141X
REFERATIVNYI ZHURNAL. FIZIOLOGIYA I MORFOLOGIYA CHELOVEKA I ZHIVOTNYKH. Text in Russian. 1959. m. USD 2,168. **Document type:** *Abstract/Index.*

Published by: Vserossiiskii Institut Nauchnoi i Tekhnicheskoi Informatsii (VINITI), Usievicha ul 20-a, Moscow 125315, Russian Federation. TEL 7-095-1526441. **Dist. by:** Mezhdunarodnaya Kniga, B Yakimanka 39, Moscow 117049, Russian Federation. TEL 7-095-2384967, FAX 7-095-2384634.

016.5765 RUS ISSN 0202-9146
REFERATIVNYI ZHURNAL. GENETIKA CHELOVEKA. Text in Russian. 1969. m. USD 462. **Document type:** *Abstract/Index.*
—East View.
Published by: Vserossiiskii Institut Nauchnoi i Tekhnicheskoi Informatsii (VINITI), Usievicha ul 20-a, Moscow 125315, Russian Federation. TEL 7-095-1526441, FAX 7-095-943-0060. **Dist. by:** Mezhdunarodnaya Kniga, B Yakimanka 39, Moscow 117049, Russian Federation. TEL 7-095-2384967, FAX 7-095-2384634; **US dist. addr.:** East View Publications, 3020 Harbor Ln N, Minneapolis, MN 55447. TEL 612-550-0961.

016.5999 RUS ISSN 0235-8913
REFERATIVNYI ZHURNAL. GENETIKA I SELEKTSIYA MIKROORGANIZMOV. Text in Russian. 1991. m. USD 525 in United States. **Document type:** *Abstract/Index.*
—East View.
Published by: Vserossiiskii Institut Nauchnoi i Tekhnicheskoi Informatsii (VINITI), Usievicha ul 20-a, Moscow 125315, Russian Federation. TEL 7-095-1526441, FAX 7-095-943-0060. **US dist. addr.:** East View Publications, 3020 Harbor Ln N, Minneapolis, MN 55447. TEL 612-550-0961.

016.5999 RUS ISSN 0235-8921
REFERATIVNYI ZHURNAL. GENETIKA I SELEKTSIYA SEL'SKOKHOZYAISTVENNYKH ZHIVOTNYKH. Text in Russian. 1990. m. USD 295 in United States. **Document type:** *Abstract/Index.*
—East View.
Published by: Vserossiiskii Institut Nauchnoi i Tekhnicheskoi Informatsii (VINITI), Usievicha ul 20-a, Moscow 125315, Russian Federation. TEL 7-095-1526441, FAX 7-095-943-0060. **US dist. addr.:** East View Publications, 3020 Harbor Ln N, Minneapolis, MN 55447. TEL 612-550-0961.

016.5765 RUS ISSN 0202-9138
REFERATIVNYI ZHURNAL. GENETIKA I SELEKTSIYA VOZDELYVAEMYKH RASTENII. Text in Russian. 1978. m. USD 261. **Document type:** *Abstract/Index.*
—East View.
Published by: Vserossiiskii Institut Nauchnoi i Tekhnicheskoi Informatsii (VINITI), Usievicha ul 20-a, Moscow 125315, Russian Federation. TEL 7-095-1526441, FAX 7-095-943-0060. **Dist. by:** Mezhdunarodnaya Kniga, B Yakimanka 39, Moscow 117049, Russian Federation. TEL 7-095-2384967, FAX 7-095-2384634; **US dist. addr.:** East View Publications, 3020 Harbor Ln N, Minneapolis, MN 55447. TEL 612-550-0961.

016.5999 RUS ISSN 0869-4060
REFERATIVNYI ZHURNAL. GENETIKA: TSITOLOGIYA. Text in Russian. m. USD 2,100 in United States. **Document type:** *Abstract/Index.*
—East View.
Published by: Vserossiiskii Institut Nauchnoi i Tekhnicheskoi Informatsii (VINITI), Usievicha ul 20-a, Moscow 125315, Russian Federation. TEL 7-095-1526441, FAX 7-095-943-0060. **US dist. addr.:** East View Publications, 3020 Harbor Ln N, Minneapolis, MN 55447. TEL 612-550-0961.

016.579 RUS ISSN 0206-5517
REFERATIVNYI ZHURNAL. MIKROBIOLOGIYA SANITARNAYA I MEDITSINSKAYA. Text in Russian. m. USD 645 in United States. **Document type:** *Abstract/Index.*
—East View.
Published by: Vserossiiskii Institut Nauchnoi i Tekhnicheskoi Informatsii (VINITI), Usievicha ul 20-a, Moscow 125315, Russian Federation. TEL 7-095-1526441, FAX 7-095-943-0060. **US dist. addr.:** East View Publications, 3020 Harbor Ln N, Minneapolis, MN 55447. TEL 612-550-0961.

016.5728 RUS ISSN 0207-8619
REFERATIVNYI ZHURNAL. MOLEKULYARNAYA BIOLOGIYA. Text in Russian. m. USD 275 in United States. **Document type:** *Abstract/Index.*
—East View.
Published by: Vserossiiskii Institut Nauchnoi i Tekhnicheskoi Informatsii (VINITI), Usievicha ul 20-a, Moscow 125315, Russian Federation. TEL 7-095-1526441, FAX 7-095-943-0060. **US dist. addr.:** East View Publications, 3020 Harbor Ln N, Minneapolis, MN 55447. TEL 612-550-0961.

016.57 016.61 016.301 RUS ISSN 0207-1428
REFERATIVNYI ZHURNAL. MORFOLOGIYA CHELOVEKA I ZHIVOTNYKH. ANTROPOLOGIYA. Text in Russian. 1958. m. USD 895 in United States. **Document type:** *Abstract/Index.*
—East View.
Published by: Vserossiiskii Institut Nauchnoi i Tekhnicheskoi Informatsii (VINITI), Usievicha ul 20-a, Moscow 125315, Russian Federation. TEL 7-095-1526441, FAX 7-095-943-0060. **US dist. addr.:** East View Publications, 3020 Harbor Ln N, Minneapolis, MN 55447. TEL 612-550-0961.

016.5765 RUS
REFERATIVNYI ZHURNAL. OBSHCHAYA GENETIKA. Text in Russian. 1964. m. USD 795 in United States. **Document type:** *Abstract/Index.*
Published by: Vserossiiskii Institut Nauchnoi i Tekhnicheskoi Informatsii (VINITI), Usievicha ul 20-a, Moscow 125315, Russian Federation. TEL 7-095-1526441, FAX 7-095-943-0060. **US dist. addr.:** East View Publications, 3020 Harbor Ln N, Minneapolis, MN 55447. TEL 612-550-0961.

016.5719 RUS
REFERATIVNYI ZHURNAL. OBSHCHIE VOPROSY PATOLOGICHESKOI ANATOMII. Text in Russian. 1976. m. USD 396. **Document type:** *Abstract/Index.*
Formerly: Referativnyi Zhurnal. Obshchie Voprosy Patologii (0202-9189)
Published by: Vserossiiskii Institut Nauchnoi i Tekhnicheskoi Informatsii (VINITI), Usievicha ul 20-a, Moscow 125315, Russian Federation. TEL 7-095-1526441, FAX 7-095-943-0060. **Dist. by:** Mezhdunarodnaya Kniga, B Yakimanka 39, Moscow 117049, Russian Federation. TEL 7-095-2384967, FAX 7-095-2384634; **US dist. addr.:** East View Publications, 3020 Harbor Ln N, Minneapolis, MN 55447. TEL 612-550-0961.

016.5714 RUS ISSN 0131-355X
QH652.A1 CODEN: RZRBDD
REFERATIVNYI ZHURNAL. RADIATSIONNAYA BIOLOGIYA. Text in Russian. 1973. m. USD 453. **Document type:** *Abstract/Index.*
Indexed: Chem.Abstr.
—CASDDS, East View, Linda Hall.
Published by: Vserossiiskii Institut Nauchnoi i Tekhnicheskoi Informatsii (VINITI), Usievicha ul 20-a, Moscow 125315, Russian Federation. TEL 7-095-1526441, FAX 7-095-943-0060. **Dist. by:** Mezhdunarodnaya Kniga, B Yakimanka 39, Moscow 117049, Russian Federation. TEL 7-095-2384967, FAX 7-095-2384634; **US dist. addr.:** East View Publications, 3020 Harbor Ln N, Minneapolis, MN 55447. TEL 612-550-0961.

016.57 RUS ISSN 0202-9200
CODEN: RZRAA7
REFERATIVNYI ZHURNAL. RASTENIEVODSTVO (BIOLOGICHESKIE OSNOVY). Text in Russian. 1961. m. USD 396. **Document type:** *Abstract/Index.*
Indexed: Chem.Abstr.
Published by: Vserossiiskii Institut Nauchnoi i Tekhnicheskoi Informatsii (VINITI), Usievicha ul 20-a, Moscow 125315, Russian Federation. TEL 7-095-1526441, FAX 7-095-943-0060. **Dist. by:** Mezhdunarodnaya Kniga, B Yakimanka 39, Moscow 117049, Russian Federation. TEL 7-095-2384967, FAX 7-095-2384634; **US dist. addr.:** East View Publications, 3020 Harbor Ln N, Minneapolis, MN 55447. TEL 612-550-0961.

016.5716 RUS ISSN 0202-9103
REFERATIVNYI ZHURNAL. TSITOLOGIYA. Text in Russian. m. **Document type:** *Abstract/Index.*
—East View.
Published by: Vserossiiskii Institut Nauchnoi i Tekhnicheskoi Informatsii (VINITI), Usievicha ul 20-a, Moscow 125315, Russian Federation. TEL 7-095-1526441, FAX 7-095-943-0060. **US dist. addr.:** East View Publications, 3020 Harbor Ln N, Minneapolis, MN 55447. TEL 612-550-0961.

016.579 RUS
REFERATIVNYI ZHURNAL. VIRUSOLOGIYA. Text in Russian. 1959. m. **Document type:** *Abstract/Index.*
Published by: Vserossiiskii Institut Nauchnoi i Tekhnicheskoi Informatsii (VINITI), Usievicha ul 20-a, Moscow 125315, Russian Federation. TEL 7-095-1526441, FAX 7-095-943-0060. **Dist. by:** Mezhdunarodnaya Kniga, B Yakimanka 39, Moscow 117049, Russian Federation. TEL 7-095-2384967, FAX 7-095-2384634.

016.5792 RUS ISSN 0201-5226
REFERATIVNYI ZHURNAL. VIRUSOLOGIYA. MIKROBIOLOGIYA. Text in Russian. 1959. m. USD 1,525 in United States.
Published by: Vserossiiskii Institut Nauchnoi i Tekhnicheskoi Informatsii (VINITI), Usievicha ul 20-a, Moscow 125315, Russian Federation. TEL 7-095-1526441, FAX 7-095-943-0060. **US dist. addr.:** East View Publications, 3020 Harbor Ln N, Minneapolis, MN 55447. TEL 612-550-0961.

016.5734 016.6163 GBR ISSN 0300-3434
RENAL PHYSIOLOGY. Text in English. 1970. s-m. GBP 120 for print Ed. or e-mail (effective 2001). adv. **Document type:** *Abstract/Index.* **Description:** Current awareness service for researchers. Covers the structure and function of kidneys, immunology, toxicology, pharmacology.
Related titles: E-mail ed.; Online - full text ed.: GBP 108 to individuals (effective 2001).
Indexed: Biol.Abstr., Chem.Abstr., Ind.Med. (coverage dropped).
—Infotrieve. **CCC.**
Published by: S U B I S (Subsidiary of: Sheffield Academic Press Ltd), Mansion House, 19 Kingfield Rd, Sheffield, S Yorks S11 9AS, United Kingdom. TEL 44-114-255-4433, FAX 44-114-255-4626, subis@sheffac.demon.co.uk, http://www.shef-ac-press.co.uk/subis. Ed. S Huntridge. Adv. contact C Evans.

016.5734 016.6164 GBR ISSN 0143-4284
RENIN, ANGIOTENSIN & KININS. Text in English. 1980. s-m. GBP 120 for print Ed. or e-mail (effective 2001). adv. **Document type:** *Abstract/Index.* **Description:** Current awareness service for researchers.
Related titles: E-mail ed.; Online - full text ed.: GBP 108 to individuals (effective 2001).
—Infotrieve. **CCC.**
Published by: S U B I S (Subsidiary of: Sheffield Academic Press Ltd), Mansion House, 19 Kingfield Rd, Sheffield, S Yorks S11 9AS, United Kingdom. TEL 44-114-255-4433, FAX 44-114-255-4626, subis@sheffac.demon.co.uk, http://www.shef-ac-press.co.uk/subis. Ed. S Huntridge. Adv. contact C Evans.

016.5736 GBR
QP251
REPRODUCTION. ABSTRACT SERIES. Text in English. 1988. irreg., latest vol.27. price varies. adv. back issues avail. **Document type:** *Proceedings.*
Formerly (until 2001): Journal of Reproduction and Fertility. Abstract Series (0954-0725)
Related titles: ♦ Supplement to: Journal of Reproduction and Fertility. ISSN 0022-4251.
Indexed: AgBiotech, Anim.Breed.Abstr., Ind.Med. (1988-), Ind.Vet., Poult.Abstr., Sport Fish.Abstr., Vet.Bull., Wild.Rev.
—BLDSC (5049.600500), CISTI, Infotrieve, KNAW, Linda Hall. **CCC.**
Published by: Journals of Reproduction & Fertility Ltd, 22 Newmarket Rd, Cambridge CB5 8DT, United Kingdom. TEL 44-1223-351809, FAX 44-1223-359754, office@ssf.org.uk, jrf@journals-of-reproduction.org.uk, http://www.journals-of-reproduction.org.uk. Ed. Dr. C A Doberska. Adv. contact Mrs. C H Clarke. **Dist. by:** Portland Press Ltd., PO Box 32, Commerce Way, Colchester, Essex C02 8HP, United Kingdom.

016.581634 GBR ISSN 1356-1421
REVIEW OF AROMATIC AND MEDICINAL PLANTS. Text in English. 1995. bi-m. GBP 225 Includes single site Internet access; USD 395 in the Americas Includes single site Internet access; GBP 235, USD 410 For Internet Access only (effective 2001). back issues avail. **Document type:** *Abstract/Index.* **Description:** Series of annotated bibliographies covering medicinal, aromatic and pesticidal plants.
Related titles: Online - full text ed.
Published by: CABI Publishing, Wallingford, Oxon OX10 8DE, United Kingdom. TEL 44-1491-832111, FAX 44-1491-829198, publishing@cabi.org, http://www.cabi.org. Adv. contact S Harris. **U.S. subscr. to:** 10 E 40th St, Ste 3203, New York, NY 10016. TEL 212-481-7018, 800-528-4841, FAX 212-686-7993, cabi-nao@cabi.org.

B

REVIEW OF MEDICAL AND VETERINARY ENTOMOLOGY. see *MEDICAL SCIENCES—Abstracting, Bibliographies, Statistics*

016.5795 GBR ISSN 0034-6624
REVIEW OF MEDICAL AND VETERINARY MYCOLOGY. Text in English. 1943. q. GBP 375 to institutions; USD 630 in the Americas to institutions; GBP 385 to institutions Includes single site online access; USD 650 in the Americas to institutions Includes single site online access (effective 2002). adv. **Document type:** *Academic/Scholarly, Abstract/Index.* **Description:** Covers mycoses of man and domestic, farm, and wild animals, along with allergic disorders associated with fungi and poisoning by fungi or mold-contaminated foods.
Related titles: Online - full text ed.: GBP 295, USD 560 to institutions (effective 2002) (from DIMDI, The Dialog Corporation, S T N International).
—CISTI, GNLM. **CCC.**
Published by: CABI Publishing, Wallingford, Oxon OX10 8DE, United Kingdom. TEL 44-1491-832111, FAX 44-1491-829198, publishing@cabi.org, http://www.cabi.org/Publishing/Products/Journals/Abstract/RMVM/Index.asp. Adv. contact S Harris. B&W page GBP 75; 170 x 267. **US subscr. to:** 10 E 40th St, Ste 3203, New York, NY 10016. TEL 212-481-7018, 800-528-4841, FAX 212-686-7993, cabi-nao@cabi.org.

016.57192 GBR
SB599
REVIEW OF PLANT PATHOLOGY; consisting of abstracts and reviews of current literature on plant pathology. Text in English. 1922. m. GBP 720 Includes single site Internet access; USD 1,260 in the Americas Includes single site Internet access; GBP 745, USD 1,260 For Internet access only (effective 2001). adv. bk.rev. abstr. index. **Document type:** *Academic/Scholarly, Abstract/Index.* **Description:** Covers diseases of crop plants, ornamental plants and forest trees caused by fungi, bacteria, viruses, mycoplasma-like organisms, and nonparasitic factors and their control.
Formerly: Review of Applied Mycology
Related titles: Online - full text ed.: (from DIMDI, The Dialog Corporation, S T N International, EBSCO Publishing).
—CISTI, Linda Hall.
Published by: CABI Publishing, Wallingford, Oxon OX10 8DE, United Kingdom. TEL 44-1491-832111, FAX 44-1491-829198, publishing@cabi.org, http://www.cabi.org. Ed. S Harris. **US subscr. to:** 10 E 40th St, Ste 3203, New York, NY 10016. TEL 212-481-7018, 800-528-4841, FAX 212-686-7993, cabi-nao@cabi.org.

016.571658 GBR ISSN 0952-0414
RIBOSOMES AND TRANSLATION. Text in English. 1970. s-m. GBP 96 for print ed. or email (effective 2001). adv. **Document type:** *Abstract/Index.* **Description:** Current awareness service for researchers in clinical and life sciences.
Formerly (until 1987): Ribosomes (0142-8322)
Related titles: E-mail ed.; Online - full text ed.: GBP 108 to individuals (effective 2001).
—CCC.
Published by: S U B I S (Subsidiary of: Sheffield Academic Press Ltd), Mansion House, 19 Kingfield Rd, Sheffield, S Yorks S11 9AS, United Kingdom. TEL 44-114-255-4433, FAX 44-114-255-4626, subis@sheffac.demon.co.uk, http://www.shef-ac-press.co.uk/subis. Ed. S Huntridge. Adv. contact C Evans.

016.597079 USA ISSN 0887-4220
SEA GRANT ABSTRACTS; publications from the nation's Sea Grant programs. Text in English. 1985. q. free per issue to qualified personnel. bk.rev. back issues avail. **Document type:** *Abstract/Index.* **Description:** Documents and facilitates the acquisition of publications originating from the program.
Related titles: CD-ROM ed.: (from National Information Services Corp. (NISC)).
Published by: (National Sea Grant Depository), Woods Hole Data Base, Inc., PO Box 712, Woods Hole, MA 02543. TEL 508-548-2743. Eds. Cynthia Murray, Frank Shephard. Circ: 6,000. **Subscr. to:** PO Box 84, Woods Hole, MA 02543.

016.572 GBR ISSN 0964-7589
SIGNAL TRANSDUCTION & CYCLIC NUCLEOTIDES. Text in English. 1970. s-m. GBP 120 for print ed. or e-mail (effective 2001). adv. **Document type:** *Abstract/Index.* **Description:** Current awareness service for researchers in clinical and life sciences.
Supersedes: Signal Transduction (0952-0392); Cyclic A M P (0142-8055)
Related titles: E-mail ed.; Online - full text ed.: GBP 108 to individuals (effective 2001).
—CCC.
Published by: S U B I S (Subsidiary of: Sheffield Academic Press Ltd), Mansion House, 19 Kingfield Rd, Sheffield, S Yorks S11 9AS, United Kingdom. TEL 44-114-255-4433, FAX 44-114-255-4626, subis@sheffac.demon.co.uk, http://www.shef-ac-press.co.uk/subis. Ed. S Huntridge. Adv. contact C Evans.

016.5713 RUS ISSN 0233-6618
SIGNAL'NAYA INFORMATSIYA. FIZIOLOGIYA I MORFOLOGIYA CHELOVEKA I ZHIVOTNYKH: KROV' I LIMFA. Text in Russian. 1985. m. **Document type:** *Abstract/Index.*
Formerly: Signal'naya Informatsiya. Fiziologiya Cheloveka i Zhivotnykh: Krov' i Limfa (0131-6559)
Published by: Vserossiiskii Institut Nauchnoi i Tekhnicheskoi Informatsii (VINITI), Usievicha ul 20-a, Moscow 125315, Russian Federation. TEL 7-095-1526441. **Dist. by:** Mezhdunarodnaya Kniga, B Yakimanka 39, Moscow 117049, Russian Federation. TEL 7-095-2384967, FAX 7-095-2384634.

016.5716 GBR ISSN 0142-8810
TISSUE CULTURE. Text in English. 1981. s-m. GBP 120 for print ed. or e-mail (effective 2001). adv. **Document type:** *Abstract/Index.* **Description:** Current awareness service for researchers. Focuses on animal cells, especially growth factors tested in vitro, cell growth in vitro, organ culture.
Related titles: E-mail ed.; Online - full text ed.: GBP 108 to individuals (effective 2001).
—Infotrieve. **CCC.**
Published by: S U B I S (Subsidiary of: Sheffield Academic Press Ltd), Mansion House, 19 Kingfield Rd, Sheffield, S Yorks S11 9AS, United Kingdom. TEL 44-114-255-4433, FAX 44-114-255-4626, subis@sheffac.demon.co.uk, http://www.shef-ac-press.co.uk/subis. Ed. S Huntridge. Adv. contact C Evans.

016.571 JPN
TOKYO SHIKA DAIGAKU SEIRIGAKU KYOSHITSU GYOSEKISHU/TOKYO DENTAL COLLEGE. DEPARTMENT OF PHYSIOLOGY. BIBLIOGRAPHY. Text in English, Japanese. 1964. irreg. **Document type:** *Bibliography.*
Published by: Tokyo Shika Daigaku/Tokyo Dental College, Seirigaku Kyoshitsu, 1-2-2 Masago, Mihama-ku, Chiba-shi 261-0011, Japan.

016.57179 USA ISSN 0092-5594
RG627
U.S. CENTERS FOR DISEASE CONTROL. CONGENITAL MALFORMATIONS SURVEILLANCE. Key Title: Congenital Malformations Surveillance. Text in English. q. stat. **Document type:** *Government.*
Indexed: Curr.Lit.Fam.Plan.
Published by: U.S. Centers for Disease Control, 1600 Clifton Rd, Atlanta, GA 30333. TEL 404-639-3311.

016.579 JPN ISSN 0082-481X
QR1
UNIVERSITY OF TOKYO. INSTITUTE OF APPLIED MICROBIOLOGY. REPORTS. Text in English. 1961. a. free per issue. author index. **Description:** Contains abstracts of original papers.
Indexed: JTA.
—CISTI.
Published by: University of Tokyo, Institute of Applied Microbiology/Tokyo Daigaku Oyo Biseibutsu Kenkyujo, 1-1-1 Yayoi, Bunkyo-ku, Tokyo 113-0032, Japan. Ed. Shoji Mizushima. Circ: (controlled).

016.5792 USA ISSN 0896-5919
QR360
VIROLOGY AND AIDS ABSTRACTS. Text in English. 1967. m. USD 1,340 for print & online combined (effective 2002). bk.rev. abstr. index. back issues avail. **Document type:** *Abstract/Index.* **Description:** Covers viruses of humans, animals and plants, with emphasis on AIDS.
Formerly: Virology Abstracts (0042-6830)
Related titles: Online - full text ed.: USD 1,005 (effective 2002) (from The Dialog Corporation, S T N International).
Published by: Cambridge Scientific Abstracts, 7200 Wisconsin Ave., Suite 601, Bethesda, MD 20814. TEL 301-961-6798, FAX 301-961-6799, journals@csa.com, http://www.csa.com/journals. Ed. Christine Hong. Pub. Ted Caris.

016.59 USA ISSN 0144-3607
Z7991 CODEN: ZOREAU
ZOOLOGICAL RECORD. (Consists of 27 sections and subsections avail. separately) Text in English. 1864. a. USD 4,300 to institutions (effective 2001). illus. index. back issues avail.; reprints avail. **Document type:** *Abstract/Index, Academic/Scholarly.* **Description:** A comprehensive index to worldwide publications covering all areas of zoology and animal science including anatomy, behavior, conservation, distribution, ecology & environment, evolution, nutrition, systematics, veterinary science. Includes author, subject, geographical, palaeontological and systematic indexes.
Related titles: CD-ROM ed.: (from SilverPlatter Information, Inc.); Microfiche ed.: (from BHP); Microfilm ed.: (from PQC); Online - full text ed.: (from The Dialog Corporation).
Indexed: GeoRef.
—BLDSC (9520.000000), CISTI, Linda Hall.
Published by: BIOSIS, 2100 Arch St, Philadelphia, PA 19103-1399. TEL 215-587-2016, 215-523-4806, 215-587-4800, FAX 215-587-2016, zoorec@york.biosis.org, info@mail.biosis.org, http://www.biosis.org. Ed. Marcia Edwards. **Affiliate:** BIOSIS UK. **Co-publisher:** Zoological Society of London, UK.

BIOLOGY—Bioengineering

A I U M REPORTER. see *MEDICAL SCIENCES—Radiology And Nuclear Medicine*

574.28 610.28 POL ISSN 1509-409X
▼ **ACTA OF BIOENGINEERING AND BIOMECHANICS.** Text and summaries in English. 1999. 2/yr. price varies. bk.rev. back issues avail. *Refereed.* **Document type:** *Academic/Scholarly.*
Published by: (Politechnika Wroclawska), Oficyna Wydawnicza Politechniki Wroclawskiej, Wybrzeze Wyspianskiego 27, Wroclaw 50370, Poland. TEL 48-71-3282940, FAX 48-71-3282940, oficwyd@pwr.wroc.pl. Ed. Romuald Bedzinski. R&P Halina Dudek. **Dist. by:** Ars Polona, Krakowskie Przedmiescie 7, Warsaw, Poland.

ADVANCES IN BIOCHEMICAL ENGINEERING - BIOTECHNOLOGY. see *BIOLOGY—Biotechnology*

571.43 USA ISSN 0360-9960
R856.A1 CODEN: ADBIDL
ADVANCES IN BIOENGINEERING. Text in English. a. USD 40 to non-members; USD 20 to members. illus. *Refereed.*
Indexed: Biol.Abstr., Chem.Abstr.
—Linda Hall. **CCC.**
Published by: A S M E International, 22 Law Dr, PO Box 2900, Fairfield, NJ 07007-2900. Ed. L Thibault.

571.43 GBR
▼ **ADVANCES IN BIOENGINEERING SERIES.** Text in English. 1999. irreg., latest vol.4, 2000. **Document type:** *Monographic series, Academic/Scholarly.* **Description:** Covers areas of current interest on active research in the application of computing to analyze numerically biomedical processes and medical data.
Published by: WIT Press, Ashurst Lodge, Lyndhurst Rd, Ashurst, Southampton, Hants SO40 7AA, United Kingdom. TEL 44-238-0293223, FAX 44-238-0292853, marketing@witpress.com, http://www.witpress.com/advbiser.html. **Dist. by:** Computational Mechanics Inc.. TEL 978-667-5841, FAX 978-667-7582, marketing@compmech.com, http://www.compmech.com/witpress.

610.28 GBR ISSN 1465-3222
ADVANCES IN COMPUTATIONAL BIOENGINEERING. Text in English. irreg., latest vol.5, 2001. *Refereed.* **Document type:** *Monographic series, Academic/Scholarly.* **Description:** Covers state-of-the-art advances in the field of biomedical engineering. Contains papers from leading researchers in bioengineering. Each volume covers areas of current interest or active research.
Formerly (until 1999): Advances in Bioengineering
Published by: WIT Press, Ashurst Lodge, Lyndhurst Rd, Ashurst, Southampton, Hants SO40 7AA, United Kingdom. TEL 44-238-0293223, FAX 44-238-0292853, marketing@witpress.com, http://www.witpress.com/advbiser.html. **Dist. by:** Computational Mechanics Inc., 25 Bridge St, Billerica, MA 01821-1007. TEL 978-667-5841, FAX 978-667-7582, marketing@compmech.com, http://www.compmech.com/witpress.

ANNALS OF BIOMEDICAL ENGINEERING. see *MEDICAL SCIENCES*

610.28 JPN
BAIOENJINIARINGU SHINPOJUMU RONBUNJU/ BIOENGINEERING SYMPOSIUM. Text in Japanese; Summaries in English. 1989. a. JPY 5,000.
Published by: Nihon Kikai Gakkai/Japan Society of Mechanical Engineers, 4-9 Yoyogi 2-chome, Shibuya-ku, Tokyo 151-0053, Japan.

610.28 JPN ISSN 0913-7556
CODEN: BMEEEV
BIO MEDICAL ENGINEERING. Short title: B M E. Text in Japanese. 1987. m. JPY 1,500 per issue.
Indexed: Chem.Abstr., Chem.Indus.Notes, Chem.Titles, INSPEC (1968-1977, dropped).
—CASDDS, CISTI, GNLM.
Published by: Nihon M E Gakkai/Japan Society of Medical Electronics and Biological Engineering, c/o Nihon Gakkai Jimu Senta, 16-0 Honkomagome 5-chome, Bunkyo-ku, Tokyo 113-0021, Japan.

610.28 574 NLD ISSN 0959-2989
R857.M3 CODEN: BMENEO
BIO-MEDICAL MATERIALS AND ENGINEERING; an international journal. Text in English. 1991. quadrennial. EUR 464, USD 422 to institutions (effective 2002). back issues avail. *Refereed.* **Document type:** *Journal, Academic/Scholarly.* **Description:** Covers materials and engineering for biological and medical systems.
Related titles: Microform ed.: (from PQC); Online - full text ed.: (from EBSCO Publishing, O C L C Online Computer Library Center, Inc., Swets Blackwell, Institute for Scientific Information, RoweCom Information Quest).
Indexed: ASCA, Alloys Ind. (1991-), Appl.Mech.Rev., Biol.Abstr., Biotech.& Bioeng.Abstr., Cal.Tiss.Abstr., Chem.Abstr., Chem.Indus.Notes, Chem.Titles, Eng.Mat.Abstr., Environ.Sci.Poll.Mgmt., Excerp.Med., Ind.Med. (1991-), Mat.Sci.Cit.Ind., Med.& Pharm.Biotech.Abstr., Met.Abstr. (1991-), Met.Abstr.Ind. (1991-), Nonfer.Met.Alert (1991-), PCC Alert (1991-), Pollut.Abstr., Risk Abstr., Saf.Sci.Abstr., Steels Alert (1991-), World Alum.Abstr.
—BLDSC (2087.839000), CASDDS, CISTI, GNLM, IDS, Infotrieve. **CCC.**
Published by: I O S Press, Nieuwe Hemweg 6B, Amsterdam 1013 BG, Netherlands. TEL 31-20-688-3355, FAX 31-20-620-3419, market@iospress.nl, http://www.iospress.nl. Ed. Takeo Yokobori. **Subscr. to:** I O S Press, Inc, 5795-G Burke Centre Pkwy, Burke, VA 22015. TEL 703-323-5554, FAX 703-323-3668, iosbooks@iospress.com; Kinokuniya Company Ltd, Shinjuku 3-chome, Shinjuku-ku, Tokyo 160-0022, Japan. FAX 81-3-3439-1094, journal@kinokuniya.co.jp, http://www.kinokuniya.co.jp; Globe Publication Pvt. Ltd., C-62 Inderpuri, New Delhi 100 012, India. TEL 91-11-579-3211, 91-11-579-3212, FAX 91-11-579-8876, custserve@globepub.com, http://www.globepub.com.

610.28 POL ISSN 0208-5216
BIOCYBERNETICS AND BIOMEDICAL ENGINEERING. Text in English; Summaries in Polish. 1981. irreg., latest vol.19, 1999. price varies. bibl, illus. **Description:** Publishes original papers on biocybernetics and biomedical engineering.
—BLDSC (2071.215000), GNLM.
Published by: (Polska Akademia Nauk/Polish Academy of Sciences, Instytut Biocybernetyki i Inzynierii Biomedycznej), Wydawnictwo Naukowe P W Nowe, Ul Miodowa 10, Warsaw 00251, Poland. TEL 48-22-6954321, FAX 48-22-6954288. Ed. Maciej Nalecz. Circ: 300. **Dist. by:** Ars Polona, Krakowskie Przedmiescie 7, Warsaw, Poland.

344 610.28 174 USA
BIOLAW: A LEGAL AND ETHICAL REPORTER ON MEDICINE, HEALTH CARE, AND BIOENGINEERING. Text in English. base vol. plus m. updates. USD 495 (effective 1999); for Resource Manual, Monthly Updates, & Special Sections. back issues avail. **Document type:** *Academic/Scholarly.* **Description:** Covers the most recent developments in case law concerning bioethics.
Incorporates (in 1986): Bioethics Reporter
Related titles: Microfiche ed.
Published by: University Publications of America (Subsidiary of: Congressional Information Service Inc.), 4520 East West Hwy Ste 800, Bethesda, MD 20814-3389. TEL 301-654-1550, 800-638-8380, FAX 301-657-3203, cisinfor@lexis-nexis.com, http://www.cispubs.com.

BIOTECHNOLOGY ADVANCES; research reviews and patent abstracts. see *BIOLOGY—Biotechnology*

BIOTECHNOLOGY AND BIOENGINEERING. see *BIOLOGY—Biotechnology*

BIOTECHNOLOGY AND BIOTECHNOLOGICAL EQUIPMENT; international scientific-theoretical and applied publication. see *BIOLOGY—Biotechnology*

BIOTECHNOLOGY AND GENETIC ENGINEERING REVIEWS. see *BIOLOGY—Biotechnology*

BIOTEKHNOLOGIYA. see *BIOLOGY—Biotechnology*

610.28 USA
C R I S P: BIOMEDICAL RESEARCH INFORMATION ON CD-ROM. Text in English. 1972. q. USD 74 domestic; USD 92.50 foreign (effective 2000). back issues avail. **Document type:** *Government.* **Description:** Contains information on research programs supported by PHS. Includes research on extramural projects such as grants, contracts, and agreements conducted primarily by universities, hospitals, and other research institutions.
Formerly (until 1980): CRISP: Biomedical Research Information
Media: CD-ROM.
Published by: U.S. Department of Health and Human Services, Hubert H. Humphrey Bldg., 200 Independence Ave., S.W., Washington, DC 20201. **Subscr. to:** U.S. Government Printing Office, Superintendent of Documents, PO Box 371954, Pittsburgh, PA 15250-7954. TEL 202-512-1800, FAX 202-512-2250, orders@gpo.gov, http://www.access.gpo.gov.

610.28 USA
R856.A1 CODEN: CRBEDR
CRITICAL REVIEWS IN BIOMEDICAL ENGINEERING. Text in English. 1974. bi-m. USD 105 to individuals; USD 567 to institutions (effective 2000). adv. bibl, charts, illus. back issues avail.; reprints avail. *Refereed.* **Document type:** *Academic/Scholarly.* **Description:** Critically surveys the wide range of research and applied activities in this field.
Former titles: C R C Critical Reviews in Biomedical Engineering (0278-940X); Critical Reviews in Bioengineering (0731-6984); C R C Critical Reviews in Bioengineering (0045-642X)
Related titles: Online - full text ed.: (from Institute for Scientific Information).
Indexed: ASCA, Appl.Mech.Rev., Bioeng.Abstr., Biol.Abstr., Biotech.& Bioeng.Abstr., Curr.Adv.Ecol.Sci., Curr.Cont., Eng.Ind., Excerp.Med., INIS Atomind., INSPEC (1978-, dropped), Ind.Med. (1981-), Ind.Sci.Rev., Inpharma, Int.Abstr.Biol.Sci., Pharm.&Out.News, Reac., Sci.Cit.Ind.
—BLDSC (3487.472300), AskIEEE, CISTI, EMDOCS, GNLM, IDS, Infotrieve, ingenta, Linda Hall. **CCC.**
Published by: Begell House Inc., 79 Madison Ave, Ste 1205, New York, NY 10016-7892. TEL 212-725-1999, FAX 212-213-8368, begellhouse@worldnet.att.net, orders@begellhouse.com, http://www.begellhouse.com. Ed. John R Bourne. R&P Jim Kelly. Adv. contact Jm Kelly. Circ: 680.

CRITICAL REVIEWS IN CLINICAL LABORATORY SCIENCES. see *MEDICAL SCIENCES*

E S E M NEWS. see *MEDICAL SCIENCES*

EUROPEAN BIOPHARMACEUTICAL REVIEW. see *PHARMACY AND PHARMACOLOGY*

EUROPEAN SYMPOSIUM ON BIOCHEMICAL ENGINEERING SCIENCE. PROCEEDINGS. see *ENGINEERING—Chemical Engineering*

FOLIA MICROBIOLOGICA. see *BIOLOGY—Biochemistry*

610.28 USA
FOUNDATION FOR BIOMEDICAL RESEARCH. NEWS. Text in English. 1984. bi-m. USD 25. back issues avail. **Document type:** *Newsletter.*
Formerly (until May 1993): Foundation for Biomedical Research. Newsletter
Published by: Foundation for Biomedical Research, 818 Connecticut Ave N W, 3rd Fl, Washington, DC 20006. TEL 202-457-0654, FAX 202-457-0659. Circ: 1,800.

610.28 NLD ISSN 0921-3775
CODEN: FMBEEQ
FRONTIERS OF MEDICAL AND BIOLOGICAL ENGINEERING. Text in English. 1988. q. EUR 460, USD 533 includes online ed. (effective 2002). back issues avail. *Refereed.* **Document type:** *Journal, Academic/Scholarly.* **Description:** Covers the field of medical and biological engineering in the broadest sense, including clinical, industrial and technical data and applications.
Related titles: Online - full content ed.: 2000 (from EBSCO Publishing, Swets Blackwell); Online - full text ed.: (from CatchWord Ltd.).
Indexed: INSPEC (1999-), Ind.Med. (1988-).
—BLDSC (4042.037000), GNLM, KNAW.
Published by: (Japan Society of Medical Electronics and Biological Engineering/Nihon me Gakkai JPN), V S P (Subsidiary of: Brill Academic Publishers), PO Box 346, Zeist 3700 AH, Netherlands. TEL 31-30-692-5790, FAX 31-30-693-2081, vsppub@compuserve.com, http://www.vsppub.com/journals/jn-FroMedBioEng.html. Ed. K Yamamoto.

GENEWATCH. see *BIOLOGY—Genetics*

574.28 CHN ISSN 1001-1110
GUOWAI YIXUE (SHENGWU YIXUE GONGCHENG FENCE)/FOREIGN MEDICAL SCIENCES (BIOMEDICAL ENGINEERING). Text in Chinese. 1978. bi-m. USD 25.20; USD 4.20 newsstand/cover (effective 2001). **Document type:** *Academic/Scholarly.*
Published by: China International Book Trading Corp/Zhongguo Guoji Tushu Maoyi Zonggongsi cibtc@mail.cibtc.com.cn, http://www.cibtc.com.cn. **Dist. by:** 35, Chegongzhuang Xilu, Haidian District, Beijing 100044, China.

B

610.28 600 USA ISSN 0739-5175
R856.A1 CODEN: IEMBDE
I E E E ENGINEERING IN MEDICINE AND BIOLOGY MAGAZINE. Text in English. bi-m. USD 195 in North America for print or online ed.; USD 220 elsewhere for print or online ed. (effective 2002). adv. bk.rev. charts, illus, pat. index. back issues avail. *Refereed.* **Description:** Technical, short items on current technologies and methods used in biomedical and clinical engineering. Includes news items and correspondence.
Formerly (until June 1982): Engineering in Medicine and Biology; Supersedes (1962-19??): I E E E - E M B S Newsletter
Related titles: CD-ROM ed.; Microfiche ed.; Online - full text ed.: (from EBSCO Publishing, Institute for Scientific Information).
Indexed: AMED, A.S.& T.Ind. (Jan.2001-), Bioeng.Abstr., Biotech.& Bioeng.Abstr., Curr.Cont., Eng.Ind., Excerp.Med., INSPEC (Jun.1982-), Ind.Med. (1982-), Inpharma, Reac., SSCI (coverage dropped).
—BLDSC (4362.927800), AskIEEE, CISTI, Ei, EMDOCS, GNLM, IDS, Infotrieve, ingenta, Linda Hall. **CCC.**
Published by: Institute of Electrical and Electronics Engineers, Inc. TEL 800-701-4333, customer.service@ieee.org, subscription-service@ieee.org, http://www.ieee.org. Ed. Dr. Alvin S Wald. **Subscr. to:** Maruzen Co. Ltd., 3-10 Nihonbashi 2-chome, Chuo-ku, Tokyo 103-0027, Japan. FAX 81-3-3275-0657; Universal Subscription Agency, Pvt. Ltd., 877, Udyog Vihar, V, Gurgoan 122001, India. TEL 91-124-347261, FAX 91-124-342496. **Co-sponsor:** Engineering in Medicine and Biology Society.

610.28 USA ISSN 0018-9294
R895.A1 CODEN: IEBEAX
I E E E TRANSACTIONS ON BIOMEDICAL ENGINEERING. Text in English. 1953. m. USD 615 in North America for print or online ed.; USD 640 elsewhere for print or online ed. (effective 2002). bk.rev. abstr, illus. index. *Refereed.* **Description:** Focuses on concepts and methods of the physical and engineering sciences applied in biology and medicine.
Former titles (until 1963): I E E E Transactions on Bio-Medical Electronics; (until 1962): I R E Transactions on Bio-Medical Electronics; (until 1960): I R E Transactions on Medical Electronics; (until 1955): Professional Group on Medical Electronics. Transactions
Related titles: Microform ed.; Online - full text ed.: (from EBSCO Publishing, Gale Group, Institute for Scientific Information).
Indexed: A.S.& T.Ind. (Jan.1991-), ASCA, Appl.Mech.Rev., Bioeng.Abstr., Biol.Abstr., Biostat., Chem.Abstr., Compumath, Comput.& Info.Sys., Curr.Adv.Ecol.Sci., Curr.Cont., Deep Sea Res.& Oceanogr.Abstr., Dent.Ind., Electron.& Communic.Abstr.J., Eng.Ind., Environ.Sci.Poll.Mgmt., Ergon.Abstr., Excerp.Med., INIS Atomind., INSPEC (pre-1969-), ISMEC, Ind.Med. (1964-), Ind.Sci.Rev., Inpharma, Int.Aerosp.Abstr., Math.R., Neurosci.Abstr. (coverage dropped), Neurosci.Cit.Ind., Pollut.Abstr., Psychol.Abstr., Reac., Ref.Zh., Risk Abstr., SSCI (coverage dropped), Saf.Sci.Abstr., Sci.Cit.Ind., Solid St.Abstr.
—BLDSC (4363.152000), AskIEEE, CASDDS, CISTI, Ei, GNLM, IDS, ingenta, Linda Hall. **CCC.**

Published by: Institute of Electrical and Electronics Engineers, Inc. TEL 800-701-4333, customer.service@ieee.org, subscription-service@ieee.org, http://www.ieee.org. Ed. Dr. John Louis Coatrieux. **Subscr. to:** Maruzen Co. Ltd., 3-10 Nihonbashi 2-chome, Chuo-ku, Tokyo 103-0027, Japan. FAX 81-3-3275-0657; Universal Subscription Agency, Pvt. Ltd., 877, Udyog Vihar, V, Gurgoan 122001, India. TEL 91-124-347261, FAX 91-124-342496. **Co-sponsor:** Engineering in Medicine and Biology Society.

572.43 USA ISSN 1534-4320
RM950 CODEN: IEEREN

I E E E TRANSACTIONS ON NEURAL SYSTEMS AND REHABILITATION ENGINEERING. Text in English. 1993. q. USD 265 in North America; USD 290 elsewhere (effective 2001). adv. **Description:** Covers human performance measurement and analysis, nerve stimulation, motor control and simulation, biomechanics, signal processing, hardware and software for rehabilitation engineering applications.
Formerly (until 2000): I E E E Transactions on Rehabilitation Engineering (1063-6528)
Related titles: CD-ROM ed.; Microfiche ed.; Online - full text ed.: (from EBSCO Publishing, Institute for Scientific Information).
Indexed: AMED, A.S.& T.Ind. (Jan.1997-), ASCA, Bioeng.Abstr., Biotech.& Bioeng.Abstr., Curr.Cont., Eng.Ind., Excerp.Med. (1996-), INSPEC (Mar.1993-, dropped), Ind.Med. (1993-), Ref.Zh.
—BLDSC (4363.218500), AskIEEE, CISTI, Ei, GNLM, IDS, ingenta, Linda Hall. **CCC.**
Published by: Institute of Electrical and Electronics Engineers, Inc., 3 Park Ave, 17th Fl, New York, NY 10017. TEL 908-981-0060, 800-701-4333, FAX 908-981-9667, subscription-service@ieee.org, http://www.ieee.org. Ed. Charles J Robinson. **Subscr. to:** Maruzen Co. Ltd., 3-10 Nihonbashi 2-chome, Chuo-ku, Tokyo 103-0027, Japan; Universal Subscription Agency, Pvt. Ltd., 877, Udyog Vihar, V, Gurgoan 122001, India. TEL 91-124-347261, FAX 91-124-342496.

570.285 GBR ISSN 1359-0944

I F M B E NEWS. (International Federation for Medical & Biological Engineering) Text in English. 1977. bi-m. **Document type:** *Newsletter, Academic/Scholarly.*
Formerly (until 1995): M B E C News (0140-0134)
Related titles: ♦ Supplement to: Medical & Biological Engineering & Computing. ISSN 0140-0118.
—BLDSC (4363.315950).
Published by: INSPEC, I.E.E., Michael Faraday House, Six Hills Way, Stevenage, Herts SG1 2AY, United Kingdom. TEL 44-1438-767266, FAX 44-1438-742849, inspec@iee.org.uk, http://ifmbe-news.iee.org, http://www.iee.org.uk. Ed. Peter Rolfe.

610.28 GBR ISSN 0954-4119
R856.A1 CODEN: PIHMEQ

INSTITUTION OF MECHANICAL ENGINEERS. PROCEEDINGS. PART H: JOURNAL OF ENGINEERING IN MEDICINE. Text in English. 1971. bi-m. USD 824 in the Americas; GBP 514 elsewhere (effective 2002). adv. illus. back issues avail.; reprint service avail. from PQC. *Refereed.* **Document type:** *Journal, Academic/Scholarly.* **Description:** Publishes scholarly research articles on theoretical and experimental application in joint and bone replacement prosthetics, mechanical coupling, and ambulatory design; with reviews of supplies and medical equipment; and announcements of conferences, seminars, and exhibitions.
Formerly (until 1989): Engineering in Medicine (0046-2039)
Related titles: Microform ed.: (from PQC); Online - full text ed.: (from EBSCO Publishing, O C L C Online Computer Library Center, Inc., RoweCom Information Quest, ingenta, CatchWord Ltd., Swets Blackwell, Institute for Scientific Information).
Indexed: AMED, A.S.& T.Ind. (Jan.2001-), ASCA, Alloys Ind., Appl.Mech.Rev., Bioeng.Abstr., Biotech.& Bioeng.Abstr., Br.Tech.Ind., Comput.& Info.Sys., Curr.Cont., Dent.Ind., Eng.Ind., Eng.Mat.Abstr., Excerp.Med., Fluidex, INSPEC (Apr.1973-Oct.1988, 1989-), ISMEC, Ind.Med. (1989-), Met.Abstr., Met.Abstr.Ind., Nonfer.Met.Alert, PCC Alert, Sci.Cit.Ind., Steels Alert, World Alum.Abstr.
—BLDSC (6724.900900), AskIEEE, CISTI, Ei, EMDOCS, GNLM, IDS, Infotrieve, ingenta, Linda Hall. **CCC.**
Published by: (Institution of Mechanical Engineers), Professional Engineering Publishing, Northgate Ave, Bury St Edmunds, Suffolk IP32 6BW, United Kingdom. TEL 44-1284-763277, FAX 44-1284-718692, orders@pepublishing.com, http://www.pepublishing.com. Ed. A Unsworth. Pub. Rosie Grimes. Circ: 800. **Subscr. to:** PO Box 361, Birmingham, AL 35201-0361. TEL 800-633-4931, FAX 205-995-1588.

610.28 JPN ISSN 0910-1705

IYO KOGAKU KENKYU SHISETSU HOKOKU/TOKYO WOMEN'S MEDICAL COLLEGE. INSTITUTE OF BIOMEDICAL ENGINEERING. REPORTS. Text in English, Japanese. 1976. a.
—BLDSC (7520.276000).
Published by: Tokyo Joshi Ika Daigaku, Iyo Kogaku Kenkyu Shisetsu, 10 Kawada-cho, Shinjuku-ku, Tokyo 162-0054, Japan.

THE JOURNAL OF BIOMECHANICS. see *MEDICAL SCIENCES*

660 JPN ISSN 1389-1723
QH301 CODEN: JBBIF6

JOURNAL OF BIOSCIENCE AND BIOENGINEERING. Text in English. 1923. m. EUR 1,063 in Europe to institutions; USD 1,189 elsewhere to institutions (effective 2002). adv. index. back issues avail. *Refereed.* **Document type:** *Academic/Scholarly.* **Description:** Publishes original research papers, review articles and letters concerning fermentation technology, biochemical technology, food technology and microbiology.
Former titles: Journal of Fermentation and Bioengineering (0922-338X); Journal of Fermentation Technology (0385-6380)
Related titles: Online - full text ed.: (from ingenta, Institute for Scientific Information).
Indexed: ASCA, AgBiotech, Agri.& Environ.Biotech.Abstr., Aqua.Sci.& Fish.Abstr., BBCI, Bio-Contr.News & Info., Bioeng.Abstr., Biol.Abstr., Biotech.Cit.Ind., CEABA, Chem.Abstr., Chem.Cit.Ind., Chem.Indus.Notes, Chem.Titles, Compumath, Comput.& Info.Sys., Crop Physiol.Abstr., Curr.Adv.Biochem., Curr.Adv.Gen.& Molec.Biol., Curr.Biotech.Abstr., Curr.Cont., Dairy Sci.Abstr., Derwent Biotech.Abstr., Electron.& Communic.Abstr.J., Energy Ind., Energy Info.Abstr., Eng.Ind., Environ.Sci.Poll.Mgmt., Excerp.Med., Field Crop Abstr., Food Sci.& Tech.Abstr., Hort.Abstr., INIS Atomind., ISMEC, Ind.Sci.Rev., Inpharma, Int.Abstr.Biol.Sci., JTA, Microbiol.Abstr., Plant Breed.Abstr., Plant Grow.Reg.Abstr., Pollut.Abstr., Potato Abstr., Reac., Rev.Appl.Entomol., Rev.Arom.& Med.Plants, Rev.Med.& Vet.Mycol., Rev.Plant Path., Rice Abstr., Sci.Cit.Ind., Sel.Water Res.Abstr., Soils & Fert., Soyabean Abstr., Sugar Ind.Abstr., Weed Abstr.
—BLDSC (4954.067000), ADONIS, CASDDS, CISTI, Ei, EMDOCS, IDS, Infotrieve, ingenta, Linda Hall. **CCC.**
Published by: The Society for Fermentation and Bioengineering Japa/Seibutsu Kogakkai, Business office c/o Faculty of Engineering Osaka University, 2-1 Yamada-Oka, Suita-shi, Osaka-fu 565-0871, Japan. TEL 81-6-877-5111, FAX 81-6-879-2034, sfbj@ijnet.or.jp, http://www.elsevier.nl/locate/jfermbio. Ed. Itaru Urabe. Pub. Shiro Nagai. Adv. contact Takekuma Kuroki. **Subscr. in U.S. and Canada to:** Elsevier Science, 655 Ave of the Americas, New York, NY 10010. TEL 212-633-3730. **Dist. outside Japan by:** Elsevier Science BV, PO Box 2227, Amsterdam 1000 CE, Netherlands. TEL 31-20-4853642, FAX 31-20-4853598.

610.28 USA ISSN 0363-8855
R856.A1 CODEN: JCEND7

JOURNAL OF CLINICAL ENGINEERING. Text in English. 1976. bi-m. USD 239 domestic; USD 248 foreign (effective 2000);). adv. bk.rev. charts, illus, tr.lit. index. back issues avail. *Refereed.* **Document type:** *Newsletter, Academic/Scholarly.* **Description:** Publishes professional papers covering advances in, and practical aspects of, clinical and biomedical engineering.
Related titles: Microform ed.: 1976 (from PQC); Online - full text ed.: 1976.
Indexed: Abstr.Health Care Manage.Stud., Bioeng.Abstr., Biol.Abstr., Comput.& Info.Sys., Eng.Ind., Excerp.Med., Hosp.Lit.Ind., INSPEC (Jan.1979-).
—BLDSC (4958.420000), AskIEEE, CISTI, Ei, EMDOCS, GNLM, ingenta, Linda Hall. **CCC.**
Published by: Aspen Publishers, Inc., 200 Orchard Ridge Dr, Ste 200, Gaithersburg, MD 20878. TEL 301-417-7500, FAX 301-695-7931, http://www.aspenpublishers.com. adv.: B&W page USD 890, color page USD 1,865. Circ: 2,526.

▼ **JOURNAL OF MICROMECHATRONICS.** see *ENGINEERING—Electrical Engineering*

MEDICAL AND BIOMEDICAL ENGINEERING REPORTS. see *ENGINEERING*

572.4 USA ISSN 1096-7176
CODEN: MEENFM

METABOLIC ENGINEERING. Text in English. 1998. q. USD 195 in US & Canada to institutions; USD 230 rest of world to institutions (effective 2001). adv. **Document type:** *Academic/Scholarly.* **Description:** Publishes original research on the targeted improvement of cellular properties or metabolite production via manipulation of specific metabolic or signal transduction pathways.
Related titles: Online - full text ed.: (from EBSCO Publishing, O C L C Online Computer Library Center, Inc., ingenta, Swets Blackwell, IDEAL Online Library).
Indexed: Ind.Med. (1999-).
—BLDSC (5683.269000), ADONIS.
Published by: Academic Press, Inc., Journal Division (Subsidiary of: Harcourt Brace & Company), 525 B St, Ste 1900, San Diego, CA 92101-4495. http://www.apnet.com/mbe, http://www.academicpress.com/mbe. **Subscr. to:** Order Dept., 6277 Sea Harbor Dr, 4th Fl, Orlando, FL 32887. TEL 800-321-5068.

METHODS IN BIOTECHNOLOGY. see *BIOLOGY—Biotechnology*

610.28 USA ISSN 0277-1063
CODEN: BENYDB

NORTHEAST BIOENGINEERING CONFERENCE. PROCEEDINGS. Key Title: Bioengineering. (Conferences prior to 1982 published by Pergamon Press plc; conferences not held 1983-1984) Text in English. 1973. a. USD 128 to institutions (effective 2001). **Description:** Forum for the exchange of technical and scientific information among engineers, physicians and other scientists interested in research, development and education.
Former titles (until 1979): New England (Northeast) Bioengineering Conference. Proceedings (0270-1820); (until 1978): New England Bioengineering Conference. Proceedings (0163-1896)
Related titles: CD-ROM ed.; Microfiche ed.
Indexed: ASCA.
—BLDSC (6842.154400), CASDDS, Infotrieve. **CCC.**
Published by: Institute of Electrical and Electronics Engineers, Inc., 3 Park Ave, 17th Fl, New York, NY 10017. TEL 800-678-4333, customer.service@ieee.org, http://www.ieee.org.

OF VALUE. see *PHILOSOPHY*

610.28 DEU ISSN 1431-8202

PROGRESS IN BIOMEDICAL RESEARCH. Text in English. 1996. bi-m.
—BLDSC (6865.992500).
Published by: Friedrich-Alexander University Erlangen-Nuremberg, Department of Biomedical Engineering, Turnstrabe 5, Erlangen D-91054, Germany. TEL 49-9131-852-2407, FAX 49-9131-27196. Ed. Dr. M Schaldach.

610.28 JPN

RAIOENJINIARINGU BUMON GAKUJUTSU KOENKAI KOEN RONBUNSHU/JAPANESE SOCIETY OF MECHANICAL ENGINEERS. BIOENGINEERING DIVISION CONFERENCE. Text in Japanese; Summaries in English. 1989. a. JPY 6,000.
Published by: Nihon Kikai Gakkai/Japan Society of Mechanical Engineers, 4-9 Yoyogi 2-chome, Shibuya-ku, Tokyo 151-0053, Japan.

SCHERING ANNUAL REPORT (YEAR). see *PHARMACY AND PHARMACOLOGY*

TECHNOLOGY AND HEALTH CARE. see *MEDICAL SCIENCES*

TISSUE ENGINEERING. see *BIOLOGY—Cytology And Histology*

TRANSGENIC RESEARCH. see *BIOLOGY—Genetics*

660.6 IND ISSN 0971-5622

V A T I S UPDATE. BIOTECHNOLOGY. (Value Added Technology Information Service) Text in English. 1993. bi-m. INR 1,000, USD 100; USD 17 newsstand/cover (effective 2000). adv. bk.rev. bibl, charts, illus, mkt, pat, tr.lit. 20 p./no. 2 cols./p. back issues avail. *Refereed.* **Document type:** *Bulletin, Newsletter, Trade.* **Description:** Keeps readers up-to-date with the latest technological developments and events in the field of biotechnology. Designed for policy makers, industries and technology transfer intermediaries.

B

Published by: Asian and Pacific Centre for Transfer of Technology, Qutab Institutional Area, Off New Mehrauli Rd., P O Box 4575, New Delhi 110 016, India. TEL 91-11-6856276, 91-11-6966509, FAX 91-11-6856274, TELEX 31-73271 APCT IN, postmaster@apctt.org, http://www.apctt.org. Ed., R&P, Adv. contact N Srinivasan. page INR 3,750, page USD 105; 220 x 280. Circ: 700. **Co-sponsor:** Biotech Consortium India Ltd.

ZHONGGUO SHENGWU YIXUE GONGCHENG XUEBAO/CHINESE JOURNAL OF BIOMEDICAL ENGINEERING. see *MEDICAL SCIENCES*

BIOLOGY—Biochemistry

572.06 GBR ISSN 0959-860X
A C B NATIONAL MEETING HANDBOOK. Text in English. 1985. a. adv. back issues avail. **Document type:** *Bulletin.*
—CCC.
Published by: (Association of Clinical Biochemists), P R C Associates, The Annexe, Fitznells Manor, Chessington Rd, Ewell Village, Epsom, Surrey KT17 1TF, United Kingdom. TEL 44-20-8786-7376, FAX 44-20-8786-7262. Ed. J D Berg. Circ: 4,500.

572.06 GBR ISSN 0959-9029
A C B NATIONAL MEETING PROCEEDINGS. Text in English. 1987. a. GBP 10 in Europe; USD 20 elsewhere. adv. back issues avail. **Document type:** *Bulletin, Proceedings.*
—CCC.
Published by: (Association of Clinical Biochemists), P R C Associates, The Annexe, Fitznells Manor, Chessington Rd, Ewell Village, Epsom, Surrey KT17 1TF, United Kingdom. TEL 44-20-8786-7376, FAX 44-20-8786-7262. Ed. S P Halloran. Circ: 2,500.

A D C NEWS. see *MEDICAL SCIENCES—Oncology*

572.86 USA
A T C C CATALOGUE OF RECOMBINANT D N A MATERIALS. Text in English. irreg., latest vol.3, 1993. USD 5. **Document type:** *Catalog.*
Formerly: American Type Culture Collection. Catalogue of Recombinant D N A Collections; Supersedes in part: American Type Culture Collection. Catalogue of Bacteria, Phages, and D N A Vectors; American Type Culture Collection. Catalogue of Strains 1: Algae, Bacteria, Bacteriophages, Plasmids, Fungi, Plant Viruses and Antisera and Protozoa; Former titles: American Type Culture Collection. Catalogue of Strains 1: Algae, Bacteria, Bacteriophages, Fungi, Plant Viruses and Antisera and Protozoa; American Type Culture Collection. Catalogue of Strains: Algae, Bacteria, Bacteriophages, Fungi and Protozoa (0363-2970)
—CISTI. **CCC.**
Published by: American Type Culture Collection, 10801 University Blvd, Manassas, VA 20110. TEL 800-638-6597, FAX 301-816-4361, sales@atcc.org. Eds. D R Maglott, W C Nierman.

A T PASES. (Adenosine Triphosphatases) see *BIOLOGY—Abstracting, Bibliographies, Statistics*

ACTA BIOPHYSICS SINICA. see *BIOLOGY—Biophysics*

572 ARG ISSN 0325-2957
CODEN: ABCLDL
ACTA BIOQUIMICA CLINICA LATINOAMERICANA. Text in Spanish; Summaries in English, Spanish. 1966. q. USD 70. adv. bk.rev. abstr, bibl, charts, illus. index. *Refereed.*
Formerly: Bioquimica Clinica (0006-3533)
Related titles: Online - full text ed.: (from Institute for Scientific Information).
Indexed: ASCA, BBCI, Biol.Abstr., Chem.Abstr., Chem.Indus.Notes, Chem.Titles, Curr.Adv.Ecol.Sci., Excerp.Med., INIS Atomind., Ind.Med. (coverage dropped).
—BLDSC (0603.500000), CASDDS, CISTI, IDS, KNAW.
Published by: Federacion Bioquimica de la Provincia de Buenos Aires, Calle 6, 1344, La Plata, Buenos Aires 1900, Argentina. TEL 54-114-3882142797, FAX 54-114-254224. Ed. Juan M Castagnino. Circ: 3,000 (controlled).

572 DEU ISSN 0065-1281
CODEN: AHISA9
ACTA HISTOCHEMICA; journal of structural biochemistry. Text in English. 1954. 4/yr. EUR 490, GBP 359 to institutions (effective 2002). adv. bk.rev. bibl, charts, illus. index. reprint service avail. from ISI. *Refereed.* **Document type:** *Journal, Academic/Scholarly.*
Related titles: Microform ed.: (from PMC,SWZ); Online - full text ed.: (from Swets Blackwell, Institute for Scientific Information).
Indexed: ASCA, BBCI, Biol.Abstr., Chem.Abstr., Chem.Indus.Notes, Chem.Titles, Curr.Adv.Ecol.Sci., Curr.Cont., Dairy Sci.Abstr., Dent.Ind., Eng.Ind., Excerp.Med., Helminthol.Abstr., INIS Atomind., Ind.Med. (1954-), Ind.Sci.Rev., Ind.Vet., Inpharma, Neurosci.Cit.Ind., Nutr.Abstr., Reac., Rev.Arom.& Med.Plants, Sci.Cit.Ind., Sport Fish.Abstr., Vet.Bull., Wild.Rev., Zoo.Rec.
—BLDSC (0624.000000), CASDDS, CISTI, Ei, EMDOCS, GNLM, IDS, ingenta, KNAW, Linda Hall. **CCC.**
Published by: Urban & Fischer Verlag, Loebdergraben 14a, Jena 07743, Germany. TEL 49-3641-626444, FAX 49-3641-626500, journals@urbanfischer.de, http://www.urbanfischer.de/journals. Eds. C J F van Noorden, R Gossrau. R&P Martin Huber TEL 49-3641-626430. Adv. contact Sabine Schroeter. page DEM 600; trim 200 x 135. Circ: 400. **Dist. by:** Nature Publishing Group, Brunel Rd, Basingstoke RG21 6XS, United Kingdom. TEL 44-1256-302629, FAX 44-1256-463570, j.stephens@macmillan.com.

ACTA HISTOCHEMICA ET CYTOCHEMICA/NIHON SOSHIKI SAIBO KAGAKKAI GAKKAISHI. see *BIOLOGY—Cytology And Histology*

572 POL ISSN 0208-614X
QP501 CODEN: AUFBD3
ACTA UNIVERSITATIS LODZIENSIS: FOLIA BIOCHIMICA ET BIOPHYSICA. Text in Polish; Summaries in Multiple languages. 1955; N.S. 1981. irreg. **Document type:** *Academic/Scholarly.* **Description:** Publishes articles devoted to the studies on biochemistry and biophysics.
Supersedes in part: Uniwersytet Lodzki. Zeszyty Naukowe. Seria 2: Nauki Matematyczno-Przyrodnicze (0076-0366)
Indexed: AgroLibrex, Chem.Abstr., Chem.Indus.Notes, Chem.Titles, INIS Atomind., Ref.Zh., Zoo.Rec.
—CASDDS, CISTI, KNAW, Linda Hall.
Published by: Wydawnictwo Uniwersytetu Lodzkiego, Ul. Jaracza 34, Lodz, Poland. TEL 331671. **Dist. by:** Ars Polona, Krakowskie Przedmiescie 7, Warsaw, Poland.

572.65 USA
ADVANCES IN AMINO ACID MIMETICS AND PEPTIDOMIMETICS. Text in English. 1998. irreg. USD 109.50. **Document type:** *Monographic series, Academic/Scholarly.*
—BLDSC (0698.630000).
Published by: J A I Press Inc., 100 Prospect St, Box 811, Stamford, CT 06904-0811. TEL 203-323-9606, FAX 203-357-8446, jai@jaipress.com. Ed. Andrew Abell.

ADVANCES IN ANTIVIRAL DRUG DESIGN. see *PHARMACY AND PHARMACOLOGY*

572.57 USA
ADVANCES IN APPLIED LIPID RESEARCH. Text in English. 1992. irreg., latest vol.3. USD 109.50. **Document type:** *Monographic series, Academic/Scholarly.*
Indexed: Chem.Abstr., Chem.Indus.Notes, Chem.Titles.
Published by: J A I Press Inc., 100 Prospect St, Box 811, Stamford, CT 06904-0811. TEL 203-323-9606, FAX 203-357-8446, jai@jaipress.com. Ed. Fred Padley.

ADVANCES IN BIOCHEMICAL ENGINEERING - BIOTECHNOLOGY. see *BIOLOGY—Biotechnology*

572 NLD ISSN 0272-3840
CODEN: ABIODQ
ADVANCES IN BIOMATERIALS. Text in Dutch. 1983. irreg., latest vol.10, 1992. price varies. *Refereed.* **Document type:** *Monographic series, Academic/Scholarly.* **Description:** Chronicles research and development in the field of biomaterials.
Indexed: Chem.Abstr., Chem.Indus.Notes, Chem.Titles.
—CASDDS, CISTI, KNAW. **CCC.**
Published by: (European Society for Biomaterials GBR), Elsevier Science BV, PO Box 211, Amsterdam 1000 AE, Netherlands. TEL 31-20-485-3757, 31-20-485-3911, FAX 31-20-485-3432, 31-20-485-3598, nlinfo-f@elsevier.nl; usinfo-f@elsevier.com; forinfo-kyf04035@niftyserve.or.jp, http://www.elsevier.nl/. **Subscr. in Australasia and the Far East to:** Elsevier Science (Singapore) Pte Ltd, No.1 Temasek Ave, 17-01 Millenia Tower, Singapore 039192, Singapore. TEL 65-434-3727, FAX 65-337-2230, asiainfo@elsevier.com.sg; **Subscr. in Japan to:** Elsevier Science Inc - Japan Regional Office, 9-15 Higashi-Azabu 1-chome, Minato-ku, Tokyo 106-0044, Japan. TEL 81-3-5561-5033, FAX 81-3-5561-5047, info@elsevier.co.jp; **Subscr. in the Americas to:** Elsevier Science, PO Box 945, New York, NY 10159-0945. TEL 212-633-3730, 888-437-4636, FAX 212-633-3680, usinfo-f@elsevier.com, http://www.elsevier.com

ADVANCES IN BIOPHYSICAL CHEMISTRY. see *CHEMISTRY—Physical Chemistry*

ADVANCES IN CARBOHYDRATE CHEMISTRY AND BIOCHEMISTRY. see *MEDICAL SCIENCES*

572 USA ISSN 0065-2423
RB1
ADVANCES IN CLINICAL CHEMISTRY. Text in English. 1958. irreg., latest vol.32, 1996. index, cum.index: vols.1-5 (1958-1962). reprint service avail. from ISI. *Refereed.*
Related titles: Online - full text ed.: (from Institute for Scientific Information).
Indexed: ASCA, BBCI, Biol.Abstr., Chem.Abstr., Chem.Indus.Notes, Chem.Titles, Curr.Adv.Ecol.Sci., Diar.Dis.Res., Ind.Med. (1958-), Ind.Sci.Rev., Sci.Cit.Ind.
—BLDSC (0703.900000), CASDDS, CISTI, GNLM, Linda Hall. **CCC.**
Published by: Academic Press, Inc., Journal Division (Subsidiary of: Harcourt Brace & Company), 525 B St, Ste 1900, San Diego, CA 92101-4495. TEL 619-231-0926, FAX 619-699-6715. Ed. Herbert E Spiegel. **Subscr. to:** Order Dept., 6277 Sea Harbor Dr, 4th Fl, Orlando, FL 32887. TEL 800-321-5068.

572.7 GBR ISSN 0065-2571
QP601.A1 CODEN: AEZRA2
ADVANCES IN ENZYME REGULATION. Text in English. 1963. a. EUR 703 in Europe to institutions; JPY 93,300 in Japan to institutions; USD 786 elsewhere to institutions (effective 2002). adv. back issues avail. *Refereed.* **Document type:** *Proceedings, Academic/Scholarly.* **Description:** Evaluates topics including metabolic regulation, inborn errors of metabolism, metabolic diseases, diabetes, and cancer in the light of new research results.
Related titles: Microform ed.: (from PQC); Online - full text ed.: (from ingenta, Swets Blackwell, ScienceDirect, Institute for Scientific Information).
Indexed: ASCA, BBCI, Biol.Abstr., Chem.Abstr., Chem.Indus.Notes, Chem.Titles, Curr.Adv.Ecol.Sci., Curr.Cont. (coverage dropped), Ind.Med. (1963-), Ind.Sci.Rev., Int.Abstr.Biol.Sci., Sci.Cit.Ind.
—BLDSC (0705.950000), CASDDS, CISTI, EMDOCS, GNLM, IDS, ingenta. **CCC.**
Published by: Pergamon (Subsidiary of: Elsevier Science), The Boulevard, Langford Ln, East Park, Kidlington, Oxford OXB 1GB, United Kingdom. FAX 44-1865-843010, nlinfo-f@elsevier/nl; usinfo-f@elsevier.com; forinfo-kyf04035@niftyserve.or.jp, http://www.elsevier.com/locate/advenzreg. Ed. George Weber. **Subscr. in Australasia and the Far East to:** Elsevier Science (Singapore) Pte Ltd, No.1 Temasek Ave, 17-01 Millenia Tower, Singapore 039192, Singapore. TEL 65-434-3727, FAX 65-337-2230; **Subscr. in the Americas to:** Elsevier Science, PO Box 945, New York, NY 10159-0945. TEL 212-633-3730, FAX 212-633-3680, usinfo-f@elsevier.com; **Subscr. to:** Elsevier Science BV, PO Box 211, Amsterdam 1000 AE, Netherlands. TEL 31-20-485-3757, FAX 31-20-485-3432, nlinfo-f@elsevier.nl.

572.7 GBR ISSN 0065-258X
QP601.A1 CODEN: AERAAD
ADVANCES IN ENZYMOLOGY AND RELATED AREAS OF MOLECULAR BIOLOGY. Text in English. 1942. irreg., latest vol.72, 1998. GBP 100. *Refereed.* **Document type:** *Academic/Scholarly.*
Formerly: Advances in Enzymology and Related Subjects of Biochemistry
Related titles: Online - full text ed.: (from Institute for Scientific Information).
Indexed: ASCA, Agricola, BBCI, Biol.Abstr., Biotech.Cit.Ind., Chem.Abstr., Chem.Indus.Notes, Chem.Titles, Curr.Adv.Ecol.Sci., Curr.Biotech.Abstr., Dairy Sci.Abstr., Derwent Biotech.Abstr., Ind.Med. (1967-), Ind.Sci.Rev., Sci.Cit.Ind., Trop.Dis.Bull.

—BLDSC (0705.970000), CASDDS, CISTI, GNLM, IDS, ingenta, Linda Hall. **CCC.**
Published by: Wiley Europe Ltd., Baffins Ln, Chichester, W Sussex PO19 1UD, United Kingdom. TEL 44-1243-779777, FAX 44-1243-775878, info-assests@wiley.co.uk, customer@wiley.co.uk, http://www.wiley.co.uk. Ed. Daniel Purich.

ADVANCES IN GENOME BIOLOGY. see *BIOLOGY—Genetics*

572 USA ISSN 0941-3472
ADVANCES IN LECTIN RESEARCH. Text in English. 1988. irreg. **Document type:** *Monographic series.*
—GNLM.
Published by: Springer-Verlag, Journals (Subsidiary of: BertelsmannSpringer), 175 Fifth Ave, New York, NY 10010. TEL 212-460-1500, FAX 212-473-6272.

572.757 USA
ADVANCES IN LIPOBIOLOGY. Text in English. 1996. irreg., latest vol.2, 1996. USD 128.50. **Document type:** *Monographic series, Academic/Scholarly.*
Indexed: Chem.Abstr., Chem.Indus.Notes, Chem.Titles.
Published by: J A I Press Inc., 100 Prospect St, Box 811, Stamford, CT 06904-0811. TEL 203-323-9606, FAX 203-357-8446, jai@jaipress.com. Ed. Richard Gross.

573.84 USA ISSN 0098-6089
QP356.3 CODEN: ADNEDZ
ADVANCES IN NEUROCHEMISTRY. Text in English. 1975. irreg., latest vol.9. price varies. *Refereed.* **Document type:** *Monographic series.*
Indexed: Biol.Abstr., Chem.Abstr., Chem.Indus.Notes, Curr.Adv.Ecol.Sci., e-psyche.
—CASDDS, CISTI, GNLM, KNAW. **CCC.**
Published by: Kluwer Academic - Plenum Publishers (Subsidiary of: Wolters Kluwer N.V.), 233 Spring St, New York, NY 10013-1578. TEL 212-620-8000, 800-221-9369, FAX 212-463-0742, info@plenum.com, http://www.plenum.com. Eds. B W Agranoff, K Suzuki.

572.6 USA ISSN 0065-3233
QD431 CODEN: APCHA2
ADVANCES IN PROTEIN CHEMISTRY. Text in English. 1944. irreg., latest vol.51, 1998. reprint service avail. from ISI. *Refereed.* **Document type:** *Monographic series.*
Related titles: Online - full text ed.: (from Institute for Scientific Information).
Indexed: ASCA, Abstr.Hyg., BBCI, Biol.Abstr., Chem.Abstr., Chem.Cit.Ind., Chem.Indus.Notes, Chem.Titles, Curr.Adv.Ecol.Sci., Dairy Sci.Abstr., Excerp.Med., Food Sci.& Tech.Abstr., Ind.Med. (1944-), Ind.Sci.Rev., Int.Abstr.Biol.Sci., Nutr.Abstr., Sci.Cit.Ind., Trop.Dis.Bull.
—BLDSC (0711.000000), CASDDS, CISTI, EMDOCS, GNLM, ingenta, KNAW, Linda Hall. **CCC.**
Published by: Academic Press, Inc., Journal Division (Subsidiary of: Harcourt Brace & Company), 525 B St, Ste 1900, San Diego, CA 92101-4495. TEL 619-231-0926, FAX 619-699-6715. Eds. John T Edsall, M L Anson. **Subscr. to:** Order Dept., 6277 Sea Harbor Dr, 4th Fl, Orlando, FL 32887. TEL 800-321-5068.

572 USA ISSN 1040-7952
QP625.N89 CODEN: ACNREY
ADVANCES IN SECOND MESSENGER AND PHOSPHOPROTEIN RESEARCH. Text in English. 1972. irreg. price varies. reprint service avail. from PQC. *Refereed.* **Document type:** *Proceedings.*
Former titles (until 1988): Advances in Cyclic Nucleotide Research and Protein Phosphorylation Research (0747-7767); (until 1984): Advances in Cyclic Nucleotide Research (0084-5930)
Related titles: Online - full text ed.: (from Institute for Scientific Information).
Indexed: ASCA, BBCI, Biol.Abstr., Chem.Abstr., Chem.Indus.Notes, Chem.Titles, Curr.Adv.Ecol.Sci., Curr.Cont. (coverage dropped), Ind.Med. (1988-), Ind.Sci.Rev., Sci.Cit.Ind.
—BLDSC (0711.383350), CASDDS, CISTI, GNLM, ingenta, Linda Hall.
Published by: Lippincott Williams & Wilkins (Philadelphia) (Subsidiary of: Wolters Kluwer N.V.), 530 Walnut St, Philadelphia, PA 19106-3621. TEL 301-223-2300, 800-638-3030, FAX 301-223-2400.

▼ **AMERICAN JOURNAL OF PHARMACOGENOMICS.** see *BIOLOGY—Genetics*

AMERICAN JOURNAL OF PHYSIOLOGY: LUNG CELLULAR AND MOLECULAR PHYSIOLOGY. see *BIOLOGY—Physiology*

AMERICAN SOCIETY FOR NEUROCHEMISTRY. TRANSACTIONS. see *MEDICAL SCIENCES—Psychiatry And Neurology*

572.65 AUT ISSN 0939-4451
QD431.A1 CODEN: AACIE6
AMINO ACIDS. Text in English. 1991. 8/yr. EUR 840 foreign; EUR 833.60 per issue in Germany; EUR 122 newsstand/cover foreign (effective 2002). adv. abstr. back issues avail.; reprints avail. *Refereed.* **Document type:** *Journal, Academic/Scholarly.* **Description:** Publishes contributions from all fields of amino acids research.
Related titles: Online - full text ed.: ISSN 1438-2199 (from EBSCO Publishing, RoweCom Information Quest, Swets Blackwell, Springer LINK, Institute for Scientific Information).
Indexed: ASCA, Agricola, Aqua.Sci.& Fish.Abstr., BBCI, Chem.Abstr., Chem.Cit.Ind., Chem.Indus.Notes, Chem.Titles, Compumath, Curr.Cont., Excerp.Med. (1993-), Helminthol.Abstr., Ind.Med. (1991-), Ind.Sci.Rev., Inpharma, Int.Abstr.Biol.Sci., Mass Spectr.Bull., Neurosci.Abstr. (coverage dropped), Nutr.Abstr., Pharm.&Out.News, Pig News & Info., Protozool.Abstr., Reac., Rev.Plant Path., Sci.Cit.Ind., Weed Abstr.
—BLDSC (0859.152000), ADONIS, CASDDS, CISTI, EMDOCS, GNLM, IDS, Infotrieve, KNAW. **CCC.**
Published by: Springer-Verlag Wien (Subsidiary of: BertelsmannSpringer), Sachsenplatz 4-6, PO Box 89, Vienna, W 1201, Austria. TEL 43-1-3302415-0, FAX 43-1-330242665, journals@springer.at, http://www.springer.at/amino_acids. Eds. C L McLeod, G Lubec, M Herrera-Marschitz. R&P Angela Foessl TEL 43-1-3302415517. Adv. contact Michael Katzenberger TEL 43-1-3302415220. B&W page XEU 1,000; 170 x 230. **Subscr. in N. America to:** Springer-Verlag, Journals, 175 Fifth Ave, New York, NY 10010. TEL 212-460-1500, FAX 212-473-6272, orders@springer-ny.com, http://www.springer-ny.com.

572.65 GBR ISSN 1361-5904
QD431.A1 CODEN: AACPER
AMINO ACIDS, PEPTIDES AND PROTEINS. Text in English. 1968. a. GBP 189.50, USD 314 (effective 2002). charts, illus. index. back issues avail. **Document type:** *Academic/Scholarly.*
Former titles (until 1994): Amino Acids and Peptides (0269-7521); (until 1985): Amino Acids, Peptides and Proteins (0306-0004)
Indexed: Chem.Abstr., Chem.Indus.Notes, Chem.Titles, Food Sci.& Tech.Abstr.
—BLDSC (0859.155000), CASDDS, CISTI, GNLM, Infotrieve, Linda Hall. **CCC.**
Published by: Royal Society of Chemistry, Thomas Graham House, Science Park, Milton Rd, Cambridge CB4 4WF, United Kingdom. TEL 44-1223-420066, FAX 44-1223-423429, sales@rsc.org, http://www.rsc.org/spr. Ed. J S Davies. **Subscr. to:** Turpin Distribution Services Ltd., Blackhorse Rd, Letchworth, Herts SG6 1HN, United Kingdom. TEL 44-1462-672555.

572.579 USA
▼ **ANABOLIC INSIDER.** Text in English. 2001. bi-m. USD 29.99 for 12 nos.; USD 3.99 newsstand/cover for 12 nos. (effective 2001). adv. **Document type:** *Magazine, Consumer.* **Description:** Openly and honestly discusses all the facets of anabolic compounds and their use, including pharmaceutical resources, what's out there, counterfeits, how much, how often, what compounds to stack together and which ones not to, new anabolics, new evaluations of old anabolics, and much more.
Address: 1155 South Havana, Ste 11-392, Aurora, CO 80012. TEL 303-750-8844, 888-577-4464, http://www.anabolicinsider.com.

572 USA ISSN 0003-2697
QP501 CODEN: ANBCA2
ANALYTICAL BIOCHEMISTRY; methods in the biological sciences. Text in English. 1960. 24/yr. GBP 225 to institutions (effective 2001). adv. bk.rev. charts, illus. index. back issues avail.; reprints avail. *Refereed.* **Document type:** *Academic/Scholarly.* **Description:** Emphasizes methods in the biological and biochemical sciences and all related fields.
Related titles: Online - full text ed.: (from EBSCO Publishing, O C L C Online Computer Library Center, Inc., RoweCom Information Quest, ingenta, Swets Blackwell, IDEAL Online Library, Institute for Scientific Information).
Indexed: AESIS, ASCA, Abstr.Bull.Inst.Pap.Chem., AgBiotech, Agri.& Environ.Biotech.Abstr. (coverage dropped), Anal.Abstr., Anim.Breed.Abstr., Apic.Abstr., Aqua.Sci.& Fish.Abstr., BBCI, Biol.Abstr., Chem.Abstr., Chem.Cit.Ind., Chem.Indus.Notes, Chem.Titles, Chromat.Abstr., Crop Physiol.Abstr., Curr.Adv.Biochem., Curr.Adv.Cell & Devel.Biol., Curr.Adv.Gen.& Molec.Biol., Curr.Cont., Curr.Leather Lit., Dairy Sci.Abstr., Deep Sea Res.& Oceanogr.Abstr., Dent.Ind., Derwent Biotech.Abstr., Excerp.Med., Field Crop Abstr., Food Sci.& Tech.Abstr., Genet.Abstr. (coverage dropped), Helminthol.Abstr., Herb.Abstr., Hort.Abstr., Hum.Gen.Abstr., INIS Atomind., Ind.Med. (1960-), Ind.Sci.Rev., Ind.Vet., Inpharma, Int.Abstr.Biol.Sci., Maize Abstr., Mass Spectr.Bull., Neurosci.Cit.Ind., Nuc.Acids Abstr., Nutr.Abstr., Plant Breed.Abstr., Protozool.Abstr., Reac., Ref.Zh., Rev.Appl.Entomol., Rev.Med.& Vet.Mycol., Sci.Cit.Ind., Soils & Fert., Sport Fish.Abstr., Sugar Ind.Abstr., THA, Vet.Bull.
—BLDSC (0896.500000), ADONIS, CASDDS, CINDOC, CISTI, EMDOCS, GNLM, IDS, ingenta, Linda Hall. **CCC.**
Published by: Academic Press, Inc., Journal Division (Subsidiary of: Harcourt Brace & Company), 525 B St, Ste 1900, San Diego, CA 92101-4495. TEL 619-230-1840, FAX 619-699-6800, apsubs@acad.com, http://www.academicpress.com/ab. Ed. William B Jakoby.

612.015 GBR ISSN 0004-5632
CODEN: ACBOBU
ANNALS OF CLINICAL BIOCHEMISTRY. Text in English. 1960. bi-m. GBP 136 in Europe; USD 234 in United States; GBP 142 elsewhere (effective 2002). adv. bk.rev. illus. index. back issues avail. *Refereed.* **Document type:** *Journal, Academic/Scholarly.* **Description:** Presents international papers about clinical biochemistry, especially for the understanding, diagnosis and treatment of human disease.
Formerly (until 1969): Association of Clinical Biochemists. Proceedings (0369-8564)
Related titles: Online - full text ed.: (from CatchWord Ltd., Institute for Scientific Information).
Indexed: ASCA, Anal.Abstr., BBCI, Biol.Abstr., Chem.Abstr., Chem.Indus.Notes, Chem.Titles, Curr.Adv.Ecol.Sci., Curr.Cont., Dent.Ind., Excerp.Med., INIS Atomind., Ind.Med. (1969-), Ind.Sci.Rev., Inpharma, Int.Abstr.Biol.Sci., Int.Nurs.Ind., Kidney, Mass Spectr.Bull., Nutr.Abstr., Pharm.&Out.News, Reac., Ref.Zh., Rev.Med.& Vet.Mycol., SSCI (coverage dropped), Sci.Cit.Ind., THA, Vet.Bull.
—BLDSC (1040.230000), ADONIS, CASDDS, CISTI, EMDOCS, GNLM, IDS, ingenta, KNAW. **CCC.**
Published by: (Association of Clinical Biochemists), Royal Society of Medicine Press Ltd, 1 Wimpole St, London W1M 8AE, United Kingdom. TEL 44-20-7290-2921, FAX 44-20-7290-2929, http://www.roysocmed.ac.uk/pub/acb.htm. Ed. Stephen P Halloran. Pub. Delia Siedle. R&P Caroline McLaughlin. Circ: 3,650.

572 USA ISSN 0066-4154
QP501 CODEN: ARBOAW
ANNUAL REVIEW OF BIOCHEMISTRY. Text in English. 1932. a. USD 68 domestic to individuals; USD 74 foreign to individuals; USD 136 domestic to institutions; USD 148 foreign to institutions (effective 1999). adv. bibl, charts. index, cum.index. back issues avail.; reprints avail. *Refereed.* **Document type:** *Academic/Scholarly.* **Description:** Original critical reviews of the significant primary literature and current developments in biochemistry.
Related titles: Microfilm ed.: (from PQC); Online - full text ed.: (from HighWire Pr., EBSCO Publishing, H. W. Wilson, Gale Group, Institute for Scientific Information).
Indexed: ASCA, Abstr.Bull.Inst.Pap.Chem., Agri.& Environ.Biotech.Abstr. (coverage dropped), Anim.Breed.Abstr., Aqua.Sci.& Fish.Abstr., BBCI, Biol.& Agr.Ind. (Jan.1983-), Biol.Abstr., Chem.Abstr., Chem.Cit.Ind., Chem.Indus.Notes, Chem.Titles, Curr.Adv.Ecol.Sci., Curr.Cont., Dairy Sci.Abstr., Diar.Dis.Res., Excerp.Med., Field Crop Abstr., Food Sci.& Tech.Abstr., Gen.Sci.Ind. (Jul.1997-), Genet.Abstr., Helminthol.Abstr., Hort.Abstr., Hum.Gen.Abstr., INIS Atomind., Ind.Med. (1932-), Ind.Sci.Rev., Inpharma, Int.Abstr.Biol.Sci., Media Rev.Dig., Neurosci.Abstr., Nuc.Acids Abstr., Nutr.Abstr., Pharm.&Out.News, Plant Breed.Abstr., Reac., SSCI (coverage dropped), Sci.Cit.Ind., Soils & Fert., THA, Trop.Dis.Bull., VITIS, Weed Abstr.
—BLDSC (1522.000000), ADONIS, CASDDS, CINDOC, CISTI, EMDOCS, GNLM, IDS, ingenta, KNAW, Linda Hall. **CCC.**

Published by: Annual Reviews Inc., 4139 El Camino Way, Box 10139, Palo Alto, CA 94303-0139. TEL 650-493-4400, 800-523-8635, FAX 650-424-0910, service@annurev.org; orders@allenpress.com, http://www.annualreviews.org; www.allenpress.com. Ed. Samuel Gubins. R&P, Adv. contact Swati Aneja TEL 650-843-6634. **Subscr. to:** Allen Press Inc., PO Box 1897, Lawrence, KS 66044-8897.

ANNUAL REVIEW OF BIOPHYSICS AND BIOMOLECULAR STRUCTURE. see *BIOLOGY—Biophysics*

ANTI-CANCER DRUG DESIGN. see *MEDICAL SCIENCES—Oncology*

▼ **ANTIOXIDANTS & REDOX SIGNALING.** see *MEDICAL SCIENCES*

ANTISENSE AND NUCLEIC ACID DRUG DEVELOPMENT. see *BIOLOGY—Genetics*

572 615 616.9 GBR ISSN 0956-3202
CODEN: ACCHEH

ANTIVIRAL CHEMISTRY AND CHEMOTHERAPY. Text in English. 1990. bi-m. GBP 65 domestic to individuals; USD 105 foreign to individuals; GBP 259 domestic to institutions; USD 419 foreign to institutions (effective 2000). bk.rev. illus. index. back issues avail. *Refereed.* **Document type:** *Academic/Scholarly.* **Description:** Contains original research and reviews of the biochemistry, mode of action, chemistry, pharmacology and virology of antiviral compounds.

Related titles: Microform ed.: (from PQC); Online - full text ed.: (from Institute for Scientific Information).

Indexed: AIDS & Cancer Res., AIDS Abstr., ASCA, Abstr.Hyg., Biotech.& Bioeng.Abstr., Chem.Abstr., Chem.Cit.Ind., Chem.Indus.Notes, Chem.Titles, Curr.Cont., Derwent Biotech.Abstr., Eng.Ind., Environ.Sci.Poll.Mgmt., Excerp.Med., Ind.Med. (1990-), Ind.Sci.Rev., Ind.Vet., Inpharma, Med.& Pharm.Biotech.Abstr., Microbiol.Abstr., Pharm.&Out.News, Reac., Rev.Appl.Entomol., Rev.Arom.& Med.Plants, Sci.Cit.Ind., Virol.Abstr.

—BLDSC (1552.828000), CASDDS, CISTI, Ei, EMDOCS, GNLM, IDS, Infotrieve, KNAW. **CCC.**

Published by: (International Society for Antiviral Research NLD), International Medical Press, 125 High Holborn, London WC1V 6QA, United Kingdom. TEL 44-20-7831-3106, FAX 44-20-7831-0036, imp@intmedpress.com, http://www.intmedpress.com. Ed. Graham K Darby. Pub. Stephen Cameron. R&P Colin Drummond. Circ: 285.

ANTIVIRAL THERAPY. see *MEDICAL SCIENCES—Communicable Diseases*

572 USA ISSN 0273-2289
TP248.3 CODEN: ABIBDL

APPLIED BIOCHEMISTRY AND BIOTECHNOLOGY. Text in English. 1976. 21/yr. USD 1,025 domestic; USD 1,080 foreign (effective 2000). adv. bk.rev. bibl, charts, illus. *Refereed.* **Document type:** *Journal, Academic/Scholarly.* **Description:** Presents innovative, practically oriented research articles in the applications of biotechnology covering genetic engineering, enzyme engineering, fermentation technology, proteins and nucleic acids.

Formerly (until vol.5, 1980): Journal of Solid-Phase Biochemistry (0146-0641)

Related titles: Online - full text ed.: (from O C L C Online Computer Library Center, Inc., Institute for Scientific Information).

Indexed: AESIS, ASCA, Agri.& Environ.Biotech.Abstr., Agricola, Aqua.Sci.& Fish.Abstr., BBCI, Biodet.Abstr., Biol.Abstr., Biotech.Cit.Ind., CEABA, Chem.Abstr., Chem.Cit.Ind., Chem.Indus.Notes, Chem.Titles, Curr.Adv.Ecol.Sci., Curr.Biotech.Abstr., Curr.Cont., Dairy Sci.Abstr., Derwent Biotech.Abstr., Eng.Ind., Environ.Sci.Poll.Mgmt., Excerp.Med., Field Crop Abstr., Food Sci.& Tech.Abstr., INIS Atomind., Ind.Med. (1981-), Ind.Sci.Rev., Inpharma, Maize Abstr., Mat.Sci.Cit.Ind. (coverage dropped), Med.& Pharm.Biotech.Abstr., Microbiol.Abstr., Nutr.Abstr., Pharm.&Out.News, Poult.Abstr., Reac., Rev.Appl.Entomol., Rice Abstr., SSCI (coverage dropped), Sci.Cit.Ind., Soils & Fert., Sugar Ind.Abstr., Telegen, Triticale Abstr., Weed Abstr., World Ag.Econ.& Rur.Soc.Abstr.

—BLDSC (1571.880000), ADONIS, CASDDS, CISTI, Ei, GNLM, IDS, ingenta, Linda Hall. **CCC.**

Published by: Humana Press Inc., 999 Riverview Dr, Ste 208, Totowa, NJ 07512. TEL 973-256-1699, FAX 973-256-8341, humana@humanapr.com, http://humanapress.com. Eds. David R. Walt, John M. Walker. R&P Richard Hruska. Adv. contact Thomas B Lanigan Jr. **Dist. in Japan by:** Maruzen Co., Ltd., International Division, Export Dept, P.O. Box 5050, Tokyo International 100-3191, Japan. TEL 81-3-3275-8591.

572 RUS ISSN 0003-6838
QH345 CODEN: APBMAC

APPLIED BIOCHEMISTRY AND MICROBIOLOGY. Text in English. 1965. bi-m. EUR 2,552, USD 2,284 to institutions for print or online ed.; EUR 3,062.40, USD 2,740.80 to institutions print & online eds.combined (effective 2002). back issues avail. *Refereed.* **Document type:** *Academic/Scholarly.* **Description:** Offers original accounts and reviews of the latest theoretical, experimental, and applied research in the fields of biochemistry, microbiology, and biotechnology.

Related titles: Microfilm ed.: (from PQC); Online - full text ed.: ISSN 1608-3024 (from Swets Blackwell, Kluwer Online, Institute for Scientific Information, RoweCom Information Quest); ♦ Translation of: Prikladnaya Biokhimiya i Mikrobiologiya. ISSN 0555-1099.

Indexed: ASCA, Agri.& Environ.Biotech.Abstr., Aqua.Sci.& Fish.Abstr., BBCI, Biol.Abstr., Biotech.Cit.Ind., Chem.Cit.Ind., Chem.Titles, Curr.Biotech.Abstr., Environ.Sci.Poll.Mgmt., Excerp.Med., Food Sci.& Tech.Abstr., Forest Prod.Abstr., GeoRef, INIS Atomind., Ind.Med. (coverage dropped), Med.& Pharm.Biotech.Abstr., Microbiol.Abstr., Pollut.Abstr.

—BLDSC (0404.670000), CISTI, IDS, Infotrieve, ingenta. **CCC.**

Published by: (Rossiiskaya Akademiya Nauk/Russian Academy of Sciences), M A I K Nauka - Interperiodica, Mezhdunarodnyi Otdel, Profsoyuznaya ul 90, Moscow 117864, Russian Federation. TEL 7-095-3360666, FAX 7-095-3361600, compmg@maik.rssi.ru; kluwer@wkap.com; services@wkap.nl, http://www.wkap.nl/journalhome.htm/0003-6838, http://www.maik.rssi.ru/. Ed. B F Poglazov. **Dist. by:** Kluwer Academic Publishers, PO Box 17, Dordrecht 3300 AH, Netherlands.

AQUATIC TOXICOLOGY. see *ENVIRONMENTAL STUDIES—Toxicology And Environmental Safety*

572 USA ISSN 0003-9861
QP501 CODEN: ABBIA4

ARCHIVES OF BIOCHEMISTRY AND BIOPHYSICS. Text in English. 1942. 24/yr. USD 3,845 in US & Canada to institutions; USD 4,422 elsewhere to institutions (effective 2001). adv. bibl, illus. index. back issues avail. *Refereed.* **Document type:** *Academic/Scholarly.* **Description:** Presents articles in the areas of biochemistry and biophysics, especially those related to molecular biology, cell biology, and developmental biology.

Related titles: Online - full text ed.: (from EBSCO Publishing, O C L C Online Computer Library Center, Inc., RoweCom Information Quest, ingenta, Swets Blackwell, IDEAL Online Library, Institute for Scientific Information).

Indexed: AIDS Abstr., ASCA, Abstr.Bull.Inst.Pap.Chem., Agri.& Environ.Biotech.Abstr. (coverage dropped), Agricola, Anim.Breed.Abstr., Aqua.Sci.& Fish.Abstr., BBCI, Bibl.Agri., Biodet.Abstr., Biol.Abstr., C.I.S. Abstr., Chem.Abstr., Chem.Cit.Ind., Chem.Indus.Notes, Chem.Titles, Crop Physiol.Abstr., Curr.Adv.Biochem., Curr.Adv.Cell & Devel.Biol., Curr.Adv.Ecol.Sci., Curr.Adv.Gen.& Molec.Biol., Curr.Cont., Dairy Sci.Abstr., Deep Sea Res.& Oceanogr.Abstr., Dent.Ind., Derwent Biotech.Abstr., Eng.Ind., Environ.Abstr., Environ.Sci.Poll.Mgmt., Excerp.Med., Field Crop Abstr., Food Sci.& Tech.Abstr., GeoRef, Helminthol.Abstr., Herb.Abstr., Hort.Abstr., INIS Atomind., Ind.Med. (1951-), Ind.Sci.Rev., Ind.Vet., Inpharma, Int.Abstr.Biol.Sci., Maize Abstr., Mass Spectr.Bull., Microbiol.Abstr., NRN, Neurosci.Cit.Ind., Nuc.Acids Abstr., Nutr.Abstr., Ornam.Hort., Pharm.&Out.News, Pig News & Info., Plant Breed.Abstr., Potato Abstr., Protozool.Abstr., Reac., Ref.Zh., Rev.Appl.Entomol., Rev.Arom.& Med.Plants, Rev.Med.& Vet.Mycol., Rev.Plant Path., Sci.Cit.Ind., Seed Abstr., Soils & Fert., Sorghum & Millets Abstr., Soyabean Abstr., Sport Fish.Abstr., Sugar Ind.Abstr., Triticale Abstr., Trop.Dis.Bull., Trop.Oil Seeds Abstr., Vet.Bull., Weed Abstr., Wild.Rev., Zoo.Rec.

—BLDSC (1633.000000), ADONIS, CASDDS, CINDOC, CISTI, Ei, EMDOCS, GNLM, IDS, ingenta, Linda Hall. **CCC.**

Published by: Academic Press, Inc., Journal Division (Subsidiary of: Harcourt Brace & Company), 525 B St, Ste 1900, San Diego, CA 92101-4495. TEL 619-230-1840, FAX 619-699-6800, apsubs@acad.com, http://www.academicpress.com/abb. Ed. J Thomas August.

ARCHIVES OF MICROBIOLOGY. see *BIOLOGY—Microbiology*

ARCHIVES OF PHYSIOLOGY AND BIOCHEMISTRY. see *BIOLOGY—Physiology*

572 ARG ISSN 0004-4768
QP501 CODEN: RABAAO

ASOCIACION BIOQUIMICA ARGENTINA. REVISTA. Text in Spanish. 1934. q. USD 60. adv. bk.rev. abstr, charts, illus. index.

Indexed: Biol.Abstr., Chem.Abstr.

—CASDDS, CISTI, Linda Hall.

Published by: Asociacion Bioquimica Argentina, Venezuela, 1823-Piso 3, Capital Federal, Buenos Aires 1096, Argentina. Ed. Raul G Coronato. Circ: 3,000.

572.06 GBR ISSN 0141-8912

ASSOCIATION OF CLINICAL BIOCHEMISTS. NEWS SHEET. Key Title: News Sheet - Association of Biochemists Limited. Cover title: A C B News Sheet. Text in English. 1951. m. membership. adv. bk.rev. **Description:** Focuses on information about developments in laboratory health care in the U.K. and abroad.

—**CCC.**

Published by: Association of Clinical Biochemists, c/o Dr. Jonathan D. Berg, Ed, Department of Clinical Biochemistry, Sandwell District General Hospital, West Bromwich, W Mids B71 4HJ, United Kingdom. TEL 44-1836-635771, FAX 44-121-745-7929. Pub. Peter Carpenter. Circ: 3,600.

572.06094 AUS ISSN 0067-1703
QD415.A1 CODEN: ABIPBR

AUSTRALIAN BIOCHEMICAL SOCIETY. PROCEEDINGS. Text in English. 1968. a. AUD 17.25. adv. **Document type:** *Monographic series.*

Formerly: Australian Biochemical Society. Programme and Abstracts

Indexed: Biol.Abstr., Curr.Adv.Ecol.Sci., Curr.Cont. (coverage dropped), Dairy Sci.Abstr., Helminthol.Abstr., INIS Atomind., Nutr.Abstr.

—CASDDS, CISTI, GNLM, Linda Hall.

Published by: (Australian Biochemical Society), D A Information Services, 648 Whitehorse Rd, Mitcham, VIC 3132, Australia. TEL 61-3-92107777, FAX 61-3-92107788, service@dadirect.com.au, http://www.dadirect.com.au. Ed. M G Clark. Circ: 1,400. **Co-sponsor:** C S I R O, Division of Human Nutrition.

AUTOIMMUNE DISEASES. see *MEDICAL SCIENCES—Abstracting, Bibliographies, Statistics*

572 NLD ISSN 0304-4165

B B A - GENERAL SUBJECTS. Text in Dutch. 1947. 18/yr. EUR 1,952 in Europe to institutions; JPY 259,200 in Japan to institutions; USD 2,182 elsewhere to institutions (effective 2002). *Refereed.* **Document type:** *Academic/Scholarly.* **Description:** Contains a collection of diverse, authoritative papers which complete BBA's comprehensive coverage of the fields of biochemistry and biophysics.

Related titles: Microform ed.: (from PQC); Online - full text ed.: (from EBSCO Publishing, ingenta, Swets Blackwell, ScienceDirect, Institute for Scientific Information).

Indexed: ASCA, BBCI, Biodet.Abstr., Curr.Cont., Curr.Leather Lit., Dairy Sci.Abstr., Derwent Biotech.Abstr., Field Crop Abstr., Hort.Abstr., INIS Atomind., Ind.Vet., Inpharma, Int.Abstr.Biol.Sci., Nutr.Abstr., Ornam.Hort., Phys.Ber., Pig News & Info., Protozool.Abstr., Reac., Ref.Zh., Rev.Appl.Entomol., Rev.Plant Path., Sci.Cit.Ind., Seed Abstr., Soils & Fert., Triticale Abstr.

—ADONIS, CISTI, EMDOCS, IDS, Infotrieve, ingenta. **CCC.**

B

Published by: Elsevier Science BV, PO Box 211, Amsterdam 1000 AE, Netherlands. TEL 31-20-485-2911, FAX 31-20-485-2457, nlinfo-f@elsevier.nl, http://www.elsevier.com/locate/bbagen, http://www.elsevier.nl. Eds. C G Gahmberg, M Fukuda. **Subscr. in Australasia and the Far East to:** Elsevier Science (Singapore) Pte Ltd, No.1 Temasek Ave, 17-01 Millenia Tower, Singapore 039192, Singapore. TEL 65-434-3727, FAX 65-337-2230; **Subscr. in Japan to:** Elsevier Science Inc - Japan Regional Office, 9-15 Higashi-Azabu 1-chome, Minato-ku, Tokyo 106-0044, Japan. TEL 81-3-5561-5033, FAX 81-3-5561-5047; **Subscr. in the Americas to:** Elsevier Science, PO Box 945, New York, NY 10159-0945. TEL 212-633-3730, FAX 212-633-3680, usinfo-f@elsevier.com, http://www.elsevier.com.

572.57 NLD ISSN 1388-1981
QD1
B B A - MOLECULAR AND CELL BIOLOGY OF LIPIDS. (Biochimica and Biophysica Acta) Text in Dutch. 18/yr. EUR 2,083 in Europe to institutions; JPY 276,600 in Japan to institutions; USD 2,330 elsewhere to institutions (effective 2002). *Refereed.* **Document type:** *Academic/Scholarly.* **Description:** Focuses on lipid isolation and characterization, lipid biosynthesis and metabolism, phospholipids and phospholipases, glycolipids, fatty acid metabolism, prostaglandins and related substances, sterols and bile acids, functions of lipids in health and disease.
Former titles (until 1999): B B A - Lipids and Lipid Metabolism (0005-2760); (until 1965): Biochimica et Biophysica Acta. Lipids and Related Subjects (0926-6542)
Related titles: Microform ed.: (from PQC); Online - full text ed.: (from EBSCO Publishing, ingenta, Swets Blackwell, ScienceDirect, Institute for Scientific Information).
Indexed: ASCA, BBCI, Crop Physiol.Abstr., Curr.Adv.Ecol.Sci., Curr.Cont., Derwent Biotech.Abstr., Excerp.Med., Field Crop Abstr., Helminthol.Abstr., Hort.Abstr., INIS Atomind., Ind.Vet., Inpharma, Maize Abstr., Nutr.Abstr., Poult.Abstr., Protozool.Abstr., Reac., Ref.Zh., Rev.Appl.Entomol., Rev.Med.& Vet.Mycol., Rev.Plant Path., Sci.Cit.Ind., Seed Abstr.
—ADONIS, CISTI, EMDOCS, GNLM, IDS, Infotrieve, ingenta, Linda Hall. **CCC.**
Published by: Elsevier Science BV, PO Box 211, Amsterdam 1000 AE, Netherlands. TEL 31-20-485-3757, FAX 31-20-485-3432, TELEX 18582 ESPA NL, nlinfo-f@elsevier.nl, http://www.elsevier.com/locate/bbalip, http://www.elsevier.nl. Eds. D E Vance, F Spener. **Subscr. in Australasia and the Far East to:** Elsevier Science (Singapore) Pte Ltd, No.1 Temasek Ave, 17-01 Millenia Tower, Singapore 039192, Singapore. TEL 65-434-3727, FAX 65-337-2230, asiainfo@elsevier.com.sg; **Subscr. in Japan to:** Elsevier Science Inc - Japan Regional Office, 9-15 Higashi-Azabu 1-chome, Minato-ku, Tokyo 106-0044, Japan. TEL 81-3-5561-5033, FAX 81-3-5561-5047, info@elsevier.co.jp; **Subscr. in the Americas to:** Elsevier Science, PO Box 945, New York, NY 10159-0945. TEL 212-633-3730, FAX 212-633-3680, usinfo-f@elsevier.com, http://www.elsevier.com.

B B A - MOLECULAR BASIS OF DISEASE. see *BIOLOGY—Genetics*

572 NLD ISSN 0167-4838
QD1
B B A - PROTEIN STRUCTURE AND MOLECULAR ENZYMOLOGY. Text in Dutch. 1967. 16/yr. EUR 22,430 in Europe to institutions; JPY 322,400 in Japan to institutions; USD 2,718 elsewhere to institutions (effective 2002). back issues avail. *Refereed.* **Document type:** *Academic/Scholarly.* **Description:** Focuses on protein structure, protein conformation, metalloproteins. protein spectroscopy, structure in solution, and protein dynamics.
Formerly (until 1982): B B A - Protein Structure (0005-2795)
Related titles: Microform ed.: (from PQC); Online - full text ed.: (from EBSCO Publishing, ingenta, Swets Blackwell, ScienceDirect, Institute for Scientific Information).
Indexed: ASCA, AgBiotech, Anim.Breed.Abstr., Aqua.Sci.& Fish.Abstr., BBCI, Biol.Abstr., Chem.Abstr., Crop Physiol.Abstr., Curr.Adv.Ecol.Sci., Curr.Cont., Dairy Sci.Abstr., Derwent Biotech.Abstr., Excerp.Med., Field Crop Abstr., GeoRef, Helminthol.Abstr., Hort.Abstr., INIS Atomind., Ind.Chem. (coverage dropped), Inpharma, Int.Abstr.Biol.Sci., Nutr.Abstr., Pig News & Info., Plant Breed.Abstr., Protozool.Abstr., Reac., Ref.Zh., Rev.Appl.Entomol., Rev.Arom.& Med.Plants, Rev.Med.& Vet.Mycol., Rev.Plant Path., Sci.Cit.Ind., Seed Abstr., Soils & Fert., Soyabean Abstr., Triticale Abstr., Trop.Dis.Bull., Vet.Bull.
—ADONIS, CISTI, GNLM, IDS. **CCC.**
Published by: Elsevier Science BV, PO Box 211, Amsterdam 1000 AE, Netherlands. TEL 31-20-485-3757, FAX 31-20-485-3432, TELEX 18582 ESPA NL, nlinfo-f@elsevier.nl, http://www.elsevier.com/locate/bbapro, http://www.elsevier.nl. Eds. A Fink, Y Lindqvist. **Subscr. in Australasia and the Far East to:** Elsevier Science (Singapore) Pte Ltd, No.1 Temasek Ave, 17-01 Millenia Tower, Singapore 039192, Singapore. TEL 65-434-3727, FAX 65-337-2230, asiainfo@elsevier.com.sg; **Subscr. in Japan to:** Elsevier Science Inc - Japan Regional Office, 9-15 Higashi-Azabu 1-chome, Minato-ku, Tokyo 106-0044, Japan. TEL 81-3-5561-5033, FAX 81-3-5561-5047, info@elsevier.co.jp; **Subscr. in the Americas to:** Elsevier Science, PO Box 945, New York, NY 10159-0945. TEL 212-633-3730, FAX 212-633-3680, usinfo-f@elsevier.com, http://www.elsevier.com.

572 BEL
BELGIUM. STATION DE RECHERCHES FORESTIERES ET HYDROBIOLOGIQUES. TRAVAUX. SERIE D. HYDROBIOLOGIE. Text in Dutch, French. 1941. irreg.
Formerly: Belgium. Administration des Eaux et Forets. Station de Recherche des Eaux et Forets. Travaux. Serie D. Hydrobiologie (0067-5369)
Indexed: Aqua.Sci.& Fish.Abstr., Aquacult.Abstr., Environ.Sci.Poll.Mgmt.
Published by: Station de Recherches Forestieres et Hydrobiologiques, Groenendaal, Duboislaan 14, Hoeilaart 1560, Belgium.

BIOCATALYSIS AND BIOTRANSFORMATION. see *BIOLOGY—Biotechnology*

572 DEU ISSN 0946-1310
CODEN: BIOCFE
BIOCHEMICA. Text in English. 1994. q. free per issue. **Document type:** *Academic/Scholarly.* **Description:** Disseminates information of interest to the research community.
Formed by the merger of (1993-1994): Colloquium (0945-1110); (1993-1994): Biochemica - Information (Internationale Ausgabe) (0945-1102)
Indexed: Chem.Abstr., Chem.Indus.Notes, Chem.Titles.
—BLDSC (2066.821000), CASDDS.
Published by: Roche Molecular Biochemicals, Sandhofer Str 116, Mannheim 68305, Germany. TEL 49-621-759-8555, FAX 49-621-759-8830, burkhard_ziebolz@bmg.boehringer-mannheim.com, burkhard.ziebolz@roche.com, http://biochem.boehringer-mannheim.com, http://biochem.roche.com. Ed. Dr. Burkhard Ziebolz.

572 USA ISSN 0006-291X
QH301 CODEN: BBRCA9
BIOCHEMICAL AND BIOPHYSICAL RESEARCH COMMUNICATIONS. Text in English. 1959. 50/yr. USD 3,999 in US & Canada to institutions; USD 4,350 elsewhere to institutions (effective 2001). adv. bibl, charts, illus. index. cum.index. back issues avail.; reprints avail. *Refereed.* **Document type:** *Academic/Scholarly.* **Description:** Devoted to the rapid dissemination of timely and significant experimental results in the diverse fields of modern biology.
Related titles: Online - full text ed.: (from EBSCO Publishing, O C L C Online Computer Library Center, Inc., RoweCom Information Quest, ingenta, Swets Blackwell, IDEAL Online Library, Institute for Scientific Information).
Indexed: AIDS Abstr., ASCA, Abstr.Bull.Inst.Pap.Chem., Abstr.Hyg., AgBiotech, Agri.& Environ.Biotech.Abstr. (coverage dropped), Agricola, Anim.Breed.Abstr., Apic.Abstr., Aqua.Sci.& Fish.Abstr., BBCI, Bibl.Agri., Bio-Contr.News & Info., Biodet.Abstr., Biol.Abstr., Chem.Abstr., Chem.Cit.Ind., Chem.Indus.Notes, Chem.Titles, Chemorec.Abstr., Crop Physiol.Abstr., Curr.Adv.Biochem., Curr.Adv.Cancer Res., Curr.Adv.Cell & Devel.Biol., Curr.Adv.Ecol.Sci., Curr.Adv.Gen.& Molec.Biol., Curr.Cont., Dairy Sci.Abstr., Dent.Ind., Derwent Biotech.Abstr., Environ.Sci.Poll.Mgmt., Excerp.Med., Field Crop Abstr., Food Sci.& Tech.Abstr., Forest Prod.Abstr., Forest.Abstr., Genet.Abstr., Helminthol.Abstr., Herb.Abstr., Hort.Abstr., Hum.Gen.Abstr., INIS Atomind., Ind.Med. (1959-), Ind.Sci.Rev., Ind.Vet., Inpharma, Int.Abstr.Biol.Sci., Mass Spectr.Bull., Microbiol.Abstr., Neurosci.Abstr. (coverage dropped), Neurosci.Cit.Ind., Nuc.Acids Abstr., Nutr.Abstr., Pharm.&Out.News, Pig News & Info., Plant Breed.Abstr., Plant Gen.Res.Abstr., Plant Grow.Reg.Abstr., Potato Abstr., Poult.Abstr., Protozool.Abstr., RCI, Reac., Ref.Zh., Rev.Appl.Entomol., Rev.Med.& Vet.Mycol., Rev.Plant Path., Rice Abstr., Sci.Cit.Ind., Seed Abstr., Soils & Fert., Soyabean Abstr., Sport Fish.Abstr., Sugar Ind.Abstr., THA, Trop.Dis.Bull., Virol.Abstr. (coverage dropped), Weed Abstr., Wild.Rev., Zoo.Rec.
—BLDSC (2066.900000), ADONIS, CASDDS, CINDOC, CISTI, EMDOCS, GNLM, IDS, ingenta, Linda Hall. **CCC.**
Published by: Academic Press, Inc., Journal Division (Subsidiary of: Harcourt Brace & Company), 525 B St, Ste 1900, San Diego, CA 92101-4495. TEL 619-230-1840, FAX 619-699-6800, apsubs@acad.com, http://www.academicpress.com/bbrc.

BIOCHEMICAL GENETICS. see *BIOLOGY—Genetics*

572 GBR ISSN 0264-6021
QP501 CODEN: BIJOAK
BIOCHEMICAL JOURNAL. Text in English. 1906. s-m. (in 8 vols., 3 nos./vol.). USD 2,189 in US & Canada Print & online eds.; GBP 1,245 elsewhere Print & online eds. (effective 2002). adv. bk.rev. illus. index. back issues avail.; reprints avail. *Refereed.* **Document type:** *Journal, Academic/Scholarly.* **Description:** Contains original refereed papers about all aspects of biochemistry.
Formed by the merger of: Biochemical Journal. Part 1: Cellular Aspects (0306-3283); Biochemical Journal. Part 2: Molecular Aspects (0306-3275)
Related titles: Microfiche ed.; Microfilm ed.: (from PQC,PMC); Online - full text ed.: ISSN 1470-8728. USD 2,048 in US & Canada; GBP 1,165 elsewhere (effective 2002) (from EBSCO Publishing, RoweCom Information Quest, ingenta, Swets Blackwell, Institute for Scientific Information).
Indexed: ASCA, Abstr.Bull.Inst.Pap.Chem., Abstr.Hyg., AgBiotech, Agri.& Environ.Biotech.Abstr. (coverage dropped), Agricola, Anal.Abstr., Anim.Breed.Abstr., Aqua.Sci.& Fish.Abstr., BBCI, Bibl.Agri., Bio-Contr.News & Info., Biol.Abstr., C.I.S. Abstr., Cal.Tiss.Abstr., Chem.Abstr., Chem.Cit.Ind., Chem.Indus.Notes, Chem.Titles, Chemorec.Abstr., Crop Physiol.Abstr., Curr.Adv.Biochem., Curr.Adv.Cancer Res., Curr.Adv.Ecol.Sci., Curr.Adv.Gen.& Molec.Biol., Curr.Cont., Dairy Sci.Abstr., Dent.Ind., Derwent Biotech.Abstr., Eng.Ind., Excerp.Med., Fababean Abstr., Field Crop Abstr., Food Sci.& Tech.Abstr., Genet.Abstr., Helminthol.Abstr., Herb.Abstr., Hort.Abstr., Hum.Gen.Abstr., INIS Atomind., Ind.Med. (1906-), Ind.Sci.Rev., Ind.Vet., Inpharma, Int.Abstr.Biol.Sci., Maize Abstr., Mass Spectr.Bull., Microbiol.Abstr., Neurosci.Cit.Ind., Nuc.Acids Abstr., Nutr.Abstr., Ornam.Hort., Pharm.&Out.News, Pig News & Info., Plant Breed.Abstr., Plant Grow.Reg.Abstr., Potato Abstr., Poult.Abstr., Protozool.Abstr., Reac., Ref.Zh., Rev.Appl.Entomol., Rev.Arom.& Med.Plants, Rev.Med.& Vet.Mycol., Rev.Plant Path., Rice Abstr., Sci.Cit.Ind., Seed Abstr., Small Anim.Abstr., So.Pac.Per.Ind., Soils & Fert., Soyabean Abstr., Sport Fish.Abstr., Sugar Ind.Abstr., Tox.Abstr. (coverage dropped), Triticale Abstr., Trop.Dis.Bull., Vet.Bull., Weed Abstr.
—BLDSC (2067.000000), ADONIS, CASDDS, CINDOC, CISTI, EMDOCS, GNLM, IDS, Infotrieve, ingenta, Linda Hall. **CCC.**
Published by: (Biochemical Society), Portland Press Ltd., 59 Portland Pl, London W1N 3AJ, United Kingdom. TEL 44-20-7580-5530, FAX 44-20-7323-1136, sales@portland-service.com, editl@portlandpress.com, http://www.BiochemJ.org, http://www.biochemj.org, http://www.portlandpress.com/. Ed. P J Parker. Pub. Rhonda Oliver. R&P Adam Marshall. Adv. contact Sarah Laflin. Circ: 2,300. **Subscr. to:** Commerce Way, Colchester, Essex CO2 8HP, United Kingdom. TEL 44-1206-796351, FAX 44-1206-799331, sales@portland-services.com.

BIOCHEMICAL PHARMACOLOGY. see *PHARMACY AND PHARMACOLOGY*

572 IND ISSN 0365-9429
QP501 CODEN: BCRVA5
BIOCHEMICAL REVIEWS. Text in English. 1972 (vol.43). a.
Indexed: Biol.Abstr., Chem.Abstr.
—CASDDS, CISTI, Linda Hall.
Published by: Society of Biological Chemists, Department of Biochemistry, Indian Institute of Science, Bangalore, Karnataka 560 012, India.

572 GBR ISSN 0067-8694
QH345 CODEN: BSSYAT
BIOCHEMICAL SOCIETY SYMPOSIUM. Text in English. 1948. a. GBP 65, EUR 285, USD 110.50; GBP 48, EUR 77, USD 80 newsstand/cover (effective 2002). back issues avail. *Refereed.* **Document type:** *Proceedings.*
Related titles: Online - full text ed.: (from Institute for Scientific Information).
Indexed: ASCA, BBCI, Ind.Med. (1948-), Sci.Cit.Ind.
—BLDSC (2068.150000), CASDDS, CISTI, GNLM, IDS, KNAW, Linda Hall. **CCC.**

Published by: (Biochemical Society), Portland Press Ltd., 59 Portland Pl, London W1N 3AJ, United Kingdom. TEL 44-20-7580-5530, FAX 44-20-7323-1136, sales@portland-service.com, http://www.portlandpress.com/bst/default.htm. R&P Adam Marshall. **Subscr. to:** Commerce Way, Colchester, Essex CO2 8HP, United Kingdom. TEL 44-1206-796351, FAX 44-1206-799331.

572 GBR ISSN 0300-5127
QH345 CODEN: BCSTBS
BIOCHEMICAL SOCIETY TRANSACTIONS. Text in English. 1973. bi-m. USD 338 in United States Print & online eds.; GBP 198 elsewhere Print & online eds. (effective 2002). adv. bk.rev. abstr, bibl, charts. index. back issues avail. *Refereed.* **Document type:** *Journal, Academic/Scholarly.* **Description:** Contains short reviews from colloquia sponsored by the society.
Related titles: Online - full text ed.: ISSN 1470-8752. USD 317 in United States; GBP 185.50 elsewhere (effective 2002) (from Swets Blackwell, Institute for Scientific Information).
Indexed: ASCA, Abstr.Hyg., AgBiotech, Agricola, Anal.Abstr., Anim.Breed.Abstr., Apic.Abstr., Aqua.Sci.& Fish.Abstr., BBCI, Bio-Contr.News & Info., Biol.Abstr., Chem.Abstr., Chem.Cit.Ind., Chem.Indus.Notes, Chem.Titles, Crop Physiol.Abstr., Curr.Adv.Biochem., Curr.Adv.Cell & Devel.Biol., Curr.Adv.Ecol.Sci., Curr.Adv.Gen.& Molec.Biol., Curr.Cont., Dairy Sci.Abstr., Derwent Biotech.Abstr., Diar.Dis.Res., Environ.Sci.Poll.Mgmt., Excerp.Med., Field Crop Abstr., Food Sci.& Tech.Abstr., Helminthol.Abstr., Herb.Abstr., Hort.Abstr., INIS Atomind., Ind.Med. (1973-), Ind.Sci.Rev., Ind.Vet., Inpharma, Int.Abstr.Biol.Sci., Maize Abstr., Mass Spectr.Bull., Neurosci.Cit.Ind., Nutr.Abstr., Ornam.Hort., Pharm.&Out.News, Plant Breed.Abstr., Plant Grow.Reg.Abstr., Pollut.Abstr., Poult.Abstr., Protozool.Abstr., Reac., Ref.Zh., Rev.Appl.Entomol., Rev.Med.& Vet.Mycol., Rev.Plant Path., Rice Abstr., Sci.Cit.Ind., Seed Abstr., Sel.Water Res.Abstr., Soils & Fert., Triticale Abstr., Trop.Dis.Bull., Vet.Bull., Weed Abstr., Zoo.Rec.
—BLDSC (2068.155000), ADONIS, CASDDS, CISTI, EMDOCS, GNLM, IDS, ingenta, Linda Hall. **CCC.**
Published by: (Biochemical Society), Portland Press Ltd., 59 Portland Pl, London W1N 3AJ, United Kingdom. TEL 44-20-7580-5530, FAX 44-20-7323-1136, sales@portland-service.com, http://www.portlandpress.com/bst/default.htm. Ed. N Ryan. Adv. contact Sarah Laflin. Circ: 1,200. **Subscr. to:** Commerce Way, Colchester, Essex CO2 8HP, United Kingdom. TEL 44-1206-796351, FAX 44-1206-799331.

572 GBR ISSN 0305-1978
QH83 CODEN: BSECBU
BIOCHEMICAL SYSTEMATICS AND ECOLOGY. Text in English. 1973. 11/yr. EUR 136 in Europe to qualified personnel; JPY 18,000 in Japan to qualified personnel; USD 151 elsewhere to qualified personnel; EUR 1,180 in Europe to institutions; JPY 156,700 in Japan to institutions; USD 1,321 elsewhere to institutions (effective 2002). adv. bk.rev. abstr. back issues avail. *Refereed.* **Document type:** *Academic/Scholarly.* **Description:** Publishes papers on the application of biochemistry and chemistry to systematic problems in biology, and on the role of biochemistry in interactions between organisms or between organisms and their environments.
Formerly (until 1974): Biochemical Systematics (0045-2025)
Related titles: Microfilm ed.: (from PQC); Online - full text ed.: (from ingenta, Swets Blackwell, ScienceDirect, Institute for Scientific Information).
Indexed: ASCA, AgBiotech, Agricola, Agroforest.Abstr., Anim.Breed.Abstr., Apic.Abstr., Appl.Ecol.Abstr., Aqua.Sci.& Fish.Abstr., BBCI, Bibl.Agri., Bio-Contr.News & Info., Biodet.Abstr., Biol.Abstr., Chem.Abstr., Chem.Indus.Notes, Chem.Titles, Chemorec.Abstr., Crop Physiol.Abstr., Curr.Adv.Biochem., Curr.Adv.Ecol.Sci., Curr.Adv.Plant Sci., Curr.Cont., Deep Sea Res.& Oceanogr.Abstr., Ecol.Abstr., Entomol.Abstr., Environ.Sci.Poll.Mgmt., Excerp.Med., Fababean Abstr., Field Crop Abstr., Food Sci.& Tech.Abstr., Forest Prod.Abstr., Forest.Abstr., Genet.Abstr., Helminthol.Abstr., Herb.Abstr., Hort.Abstr., Hum.Gen.Abstr., Ind.Sci.Rev., Int.Abstr.Biol.Sci., Maize Abstr., Ocean.Abstr. (coverage dropped), Ornam.Hort., Plant Breed.Abstr., Plant Gen.Res.Abstr., Plant Grow.Reg.Abstr., Plant Sci., Rev.Appl.Entomol., Rev.Arom.& Med.Plants, Rev.Med.& Vet.Mycol., Rev.Plant Path., Sci.Cit.Ind., Seed Abstr., Sel.Water Res.Abstr., Soils & Fert., Sorghum & Millets Abstr., Soyabean Abstr., Sport Fish.Abstr., Triticale Abstr., Weed Abstr., Wild.Rev., Zoo.Rec.
—BLDSC (2068.162000), CASDDS, CISTI, EMDOCS, IDS, ingenta, Linda Hall. **CCC.**
Published by: Pergamon (Subsidiary of: Elsevier Science), The Boulevard, Langford Ln, East Park, Kidlington, Oxford OXB 1GB, United Kingdom. FAX 44-1865-843010, nlinfo-f@elsevier/nl; usinfo-f@elsevier.com; forinfo-kyf04035@niftyserve.or.jp, http://www.elsevier.com/locate/biochemsyseco, http://www.elsevier.nl/. Eds. L Maxson, Peter Waterman. Circ: 1,000. **Subscr. in Australasia and the Far East to:** Elsevier Science (Singapore) Pte Ltd, No.1 Temasek Ave, 17-01 Millenia Tower, Singapore 039192, Singapore. TEL 65-434-3727, FAX 65-337-2230; **Subscr. in the Americas to:** Elsevier Science, PO Box 945, New York, NY 10159-0945. TEL 212-633-3730, FAX 212-633-3680, usinfo-f@elsevier.com, http://www.elsevier.com; **Subscr. to:** Elsevier Science BV, PO Box 211, Amsterdam 1000 AE, Netherlands. TEL 31-20-485-3757, nlinfo-f@elsevier.nl, http://www.elsevier.nl.

572 USA ISSN 0006-2960
QP501 CODEN: BICHAW
BIOCHEMISTRY. Text in English. 1962. 51/yr. USD 2,660 in North America to institutions; USD 3,104 elsewhere to institutions; USD 3,192 in North America to institutions Print & online eds.; USD 3,636 elsewhere to institutions Print & online eds. (effective 2002); for additional pricing options for print and web editions contact inside sales specialist, Ms. Chako Dickinson, at 202-872-4063. adv. charts, illus. index. back issues avail.; reprints avail. *Refereed.* **Document type:** *Journal, Academic/Scholarly.* **Description:** Contains papers on the most current results of original research in all areas of biochemistry. Emphasis is given to the close relationship of chemistry, biochemistry, molecular and cell biology.
Related titles: CD-ROM ed.; Microfiche ed.: USD 2,660 in North America; USD 2,737 elsewhere (effective 2002); Microfilm ed.: USD 2,660 in North America; USD 2,710 elsewhere (effective 2002); Online - full text ed.: ISSN 1520-4995. USD 2,793 (effective 2002) (from EBSCO Publishing, Gale Group, Institute for Scientific Information).
Indexed: AIDS & Cancer Res., AIDS Abstr., ASCA, Abstr.Bull.Inst.Pap.Chem., Abstr.Hyg., Agri.& Environ.Biotech.Abstr. (coverage dropped), Agricola, Anim.Breed.Abstr., Aqua.Sci.& Fish.Abstr., BBCI, Bibl.Agri., Bio-Contr.News & Info., Biol.& Agr.Ind. (Jan.1983-), Biol.Abstr., Biwk.Pap.Rad.Chem.& Photochem., Cal.Tiss.Abstr., Chem.Abstr., Chem.Cit.Ind., Chemorec.Abstr., Crop Physiol.Abstr., Curr.Adv.Biochem., Curr.Adv.Cancer Res., Curr.Adv.Cell & Devel.Biol., Curr.Adv.Ecol.Sci., Curr.Adv.Gen.& Molec.Biol., Curr.Cont., Curr.Leather Lit., Dairy Sci.Abstr., Deep Sea Res.& Oceanogr.Abstr., Dent.Ind., Derwent Biotech.Abstr., Eng.Ind., Environ.Abstr., Environ.Sci.Poll.Mgmt., Excerp.Med., Field Crop Abstr., Food Sci.& Tech.Abstr., Forest.Abstr., Gen.Sci.Ind. (Mar.1984-), Genet.Abstr., Helminthol.Abstr., Hort.Abstr., Hum.Gen.Abstr., INIS Atomind., Immun.Abstr. (coverage dropped), Ind.Med. (1962-), Ind.Sci.Rev., Ind.Vet., Int.Abstr.Biol.Sci., Maize Abstr., Mass Spectr.Bull., Mat.Sci.Cit.Ind. (coverage dropped), Microbiol.Abstr., Neurosci.Abstr., Neurosci.Cit.Ind., Nuc.Acids Abstr., Nutr.Abstr., Potato Abstr., Protozool.Abstr., Ref.Zh., Rev.Appl.Entomol., Rev.Arom.& Med.Plants, Rev.Med.& Vet.Mycol., Rev.Plant Path., Saf.Sci.Abstr., Sci.Cit.Ind., Soils & Fert., Sport Fish.Abstr., Telegen, Tox.Abstr., Trop.Dis.Bull., Vet.Bull., Virol.Abstr., Weed Abstr., Wild.Rev., Zoo.Rec.
—BLDSC (2069.200000), CASDDS, CISTI, EMDOCS, GNLM, IDS, ingenta, Linda Hall. **CCC.**
Published by: American Chemical Society, 1155 16th St, N W, Washington, DC 20036. TEL 202-332-5544, 800-333-9511, FAX 202-332-4559, service@acs.org, http://pubs.acs.org/biochemistry. Ed. Dr. Gordon G Hammes. Circ: 6,200. **Subscr. to:** American Chemical Society, Member and Subscriber Services, PO Box 3337, Columbus, OH 43210. TEL 614-447-3674, FAX 614-447-3671.

BIOCHEMISTRY AND BIOPHYSICS CITATION INDEX.
see *BIOLOGY—Abstracting, Bibliographies, Statistics*

572 CAN ISSN 0829-8211
QP501 CODEN: BCBIEQ
BIOCHEMISTRY AND CELL BIOLOGY/BIOCHIMIE ET BIOLOGIE CELLULAIRE. Text in English; Text occasionally in French. 1929. bi-m. CND 116 domestic to individuals; USD 116 foreign to individuals; CND 350 domestic to institutions; USD 350 foreign to institutions (effective 1999). adv. bibl, illus. index. reprint service avail. from PQC. *Refereed.* **Document type:** *Academic/Scholarly.*
Former titles (until 1986): Canadian Journal of Biochemistry and Cell Biology - Revue Canadien de Biochimie et Biologie Cellulaire (0714-7511); (until 1983): Canadian Journal of Biochemistry (0008-4018); Which supersedes in part (in 1963): Canadian Journal of Biochemistry and Physiology (0576-5544); Which was formerly (until 1954): Canadian Journal of Medical Sciences (0316-4403); (until 1950): Canadian Journal of Research. Section E: Medical Sciences (0366-743X)
Related titles: Microfiche ed.: (from MML); Microform ed.: (from PQC,PMC,MML); Online - full text ed.: ISSN 1208-6002 (from EBSCO Publishing, O C L C Online Computer Library Center, Inc., RoweCom Information Quest, ProQuest Information & Learning, CISTI, Swets Blackwell, Institute for Scientific Information).
Indexed: ASCA, Abstr.Bull.Inst.Pap.Chem., Abstr.Hyg., AgBiotech, Agri.& Environ.Biotech.Abstr. (coverage dropped), Agricola, Anal.Abstr., Anim.Breed.Abstr., Apic.Abstr., Aqua.Sci.& Fish.Abstr., BBCI, Bibl.Agri., Biol.& Agr.Ind. (May 1983-Dec.1985), Biol.Abstr., CBCA Ref., Chem.Abstr., Chem.Indus.Notes, Chem.Titles, Crop Physiol.Abstr., Curr.Adv.Ecol.Sci., Curr.Cont., Dairy Sci.Abstr., Dent.Ind., Derwent Biotech.Abstr., Eng.Ind., Excerp.Med., Field Crop Abstr., Food Sci.& Tech.Abstr., Genet.Abstr., Helminthol.Abstr., Herb.Abstr., Hort.Abstr., Hum.Gen.Abstr., INIS Atomind., Ind.Med. (1986-), Ind.Sci.Rev., Ind.Vet., Inpharma, Int.Abstr.Biol.Sci., Maize Abstr., Nuc.Acids Abstr., Nutr.Abstr., Ornam.Hort., Pig News & Info., Plant Breed.Abstr., Poult.Abstr., Reac., Rev.Arom.& Med.Plants, Rev.Med.& Vet.Mycol., Sci.Cit.Ind., Seed Abstr., Soils & Fert., Soyabean Abstr., Sport Fish.Abstr., Triticale Abstr., Trop.Dis.Bull., Vet.Bull., Weed Abstr., Wild.Rev., World Text.Abstr., Zoo.Rec.
—BLDSC (2069.474000), ADONIS, CASDDS, CINDOC, CISTI, GNLM, IDS, ingenta, KNAW, Linda Hall. **CCC.**
Published by: N R C Research Press, Building M 55, Ottawa, ON K1A 0R6, Canada. TEL 613-993-9084, FAX 613-952-7656, research.journal@nrc.ca, http://www.nrc.ca/cisti/journals/. Eds. Dr. David L Brown, Martin Tenniswood. Adv. contact Judy Heyman. B&W page CND 675; trim 11 x 8.5. Circ: 913.

572.3071 GBR ISSN 1470-8175
QP518 CODEN: BIEDDX
BIOCHEMISTRY AND MOLECULAR BIOLOGY EDUCATION. Text in English. 1972. bi-m. NLG 210, EUR 95.29 in Europe to individuals; JPY 13,200 in Japan to individuals; USD 107 elsewhere to individuals; NLG 608, EUR 275.90 in Europe to institutions; JPY 38,200 in Japan to institutions; USD 308 elsewhere to institutions (effective 2001). adv. bk.rev. abstr. back issues avail.; reprint service avail. from PQC. *Refereed.* **Document type:** *Academic/Scholarly.* **Description:** Assists in the teaching of biochemistry to science and medical students throughout the world.
Formerly (until 2000): Biochemical Education (0307-4412)
Related titles: Microfilm ed.: (from PQC); Online - full text ed.: (from ingenta, Swets Blackwell, ScienceDirect, Institute for Scientific Information).
Indexed: ASCA, BBCI, C.I.J.E., Chem.Abstr., Chem.Indus.Notes, Chem.Titles, Cont.Pg.Educ., Curr.Adv.Ecol.Sci., ERA, Educ.Ind. (Oct.2000-), Educ.Tech.Abstr., Excerp.Med., Ind.Sci.Rev., Res.High.Educ.Abstr., SSCI (coverage dropped).
—BLDSC (2069.510000), CASDDS, CISTI, IDS, Infotrieve, ingenta. **CCC.**
Published by: (International Union of Biochemistry USA), Pergamon (Subsidiary of: Elsevier Science), The Boulevard, Langford Ln, East Park, Kidlington, Oxford OXB 1GB, United Kingdom. TEL 44-1865-843565, FAX 44-1865-843976, voet@sas.upenn.edu, http://www.elsevier.com/locate/bambed, http://www.elsevier.nl. Eds. Donald Voet, G Parslow, J G Voet. Circ: 5,000. **Subscr. in Australasia and the Far East to:** Elsevier Science (Singapore) Pte Ltd, No.1 Temasek Ave, 17-01 Millenia Tower, Singapore 039192, Singapore. TEL 65-434-3727, FAX 65-337-2230, asiainfo@elsevier.com.sg; **Subscr. in the Americas to:** Elsevier Science, PO Box 945, New York, NY 10159-0945. TEL 212-633-3730, 888-437-4636, FAX 212-633-3680, usinfo-f@elsevier.com, http://www.elsevier.com; **Subscr. to:** Elsevier Science Inc - Japan Regional Office, 9-15 Higashi-Azabu 1-chome, Minato-ku, Tokyo 106-0044, Japan. TEL 81-3-5561-5033, FAX 81-3-5561-5047, info@elsevier.co.jp. **Subscr. to:** Elsevier Science BV, PO Box 211, Amsterdam 1000 AE, Netherlands. TEL 31-20-485-3757, FAX 31-20-485-3432, nlinfo-f@elsevier.nl, http://www.elsevier.nl.; **Dist. by:** Elsevier Science (Brazil).

B

572 RUS ISSN 0006-2979
QH301 CODEN: BIORAK

BIOCHEMISTRY (MOSCOW). Text in English. 1956. m. USD 2,812, EUR 3,145 to institutions for print or online ed.; USD 3,374.40, EUR 3,774 to institutions print & online eds.combined (effective 2002). bk.rev. back issues avail. *Refereed.* **Document type:** *Academic/Scholarly.* **Description:** Publishes important research in biochemistry, as well as the related fields of molecular biology, bioorganic chemistry, microbiology, immunology, physiology, and the biological sciences, translated into English from the Russian journal Biokhimiya.

Related titles: Online - full text ed.: ISSN 1608-3040 (from Swets Blackwell, Kluwer Online, Institute for Scientific Information, RoweCom Information Quest); ♦ Translation of: Biokhimiya. ISSN 0320-9725.

Indexed: Apic.Abstr., Aqua.Sci.& Fish.Abstr., BBCI, Biol.Abstr., Chem.Abstr., Chem.Indus.Notes, Chem.Titles, Crop Physiol.Abstr., Curr.Adv.Biochem., Curr.Adv.Cancer Res., Curr.Adv.Cell & Devel.Biol., Curr.Adv.Ecol.Sci., Curr.Adv.Gen.& Molec.Biol., Curr.Cont., Curr.Leather Lit., Dairy Sci.Abstr., Excerp.Med., Food Sci.& Tech.Abstr., Hort.Abstr., INIS Atomind., Ind.Med. (1956-), Ind.Sci.Rev., Int.Abstr.Biol.Sci., Mass Spectr.Bull., Nutr.Abstr., Potato Abstr., Protozool.Abstr., Rev.Med.& Vet.Mycol., Rev.Plant Path., Sci.Cit.Ind., Soyabean Abstr., Triticale Abstr., Weed Abstr.

—BLDSC (0406.000000), CASDDS, CISTI, GNLM, IDS, ingenta, Linda Hall. **CCC.**

Published by: (Rossiiskaya Akademiya Nauk/Russian Academy of Sciences), M A I K Nauka - Interperiodica, Mezhdunarodnyi Otdel, Podsosenskii per 21, room 31, Moscow 103062, Russian Federation. ozrina@jnlbioch.bio.msu.su, compmg@maik.ru, http://www.protein.bio.msu.su/biokhimiya, http://www.maik.rssi.ru/. Ed. V P Skulachev. **Dist. by:** Kluwer Academic Publishers, PO Box 17, Dordrecht 3300 AH, Netherlands. TEL 31-78-6392392, FAX 31-78-546474.

572 USA ISSN 0887-6495
CODEN: BIELEO

BIOCHEMISTRY OF THE ELEMENTS. Text in English. 1980. irreg., latest vol.13-II. price varies. back issues avail. *Refereed.* **Document type:** *Monographic series.*

Indexed: Chem.Abstr., Chem.Indus.Notes, Chem.Titles.

—BLDSC (2069.720000), CASDDS, CISTI, KNAW.

Published by: Kluwer Academic - Plenum Publishers (Subsidiary of: Wolters Kluwer N.V.), 233 Spring St, New York, NY 10013-1578. TEL 212-620-8000, 800-221-9369, FAX 212-463-0742, info@plenum.com, http://www.plenum.com. Ed. Earl Frieden.

572 USA ISSN 0194-0538

BIOCHEMISTRY: SERIES OF MONOGRAPHS. Text in English. 1980. irreg., latest 1985. price varies. *Refereed.*

—CISTI, Infotrieve. **CCC.**

Published by: John Wiley & Sons, Inc., Journals (Subsidiary of: Wiley InterScience), 605 Third Ave, New York, NY 10158. TEL 212-850-6000. Ed. Alton Meister.

572 NLD ISSN 0006-3002
QD1 CODEN: BBACAQ

BIOCHIMICA ET BIOPHYSICA ACTA; international journal of biochemistry and biophysics. Short title: B B A. Text in English. 1947. 132/yr. USD 12,127 subscription to all 10 sections (effective 2001). adv. charts, illus. index, cum.index. back issues avail.; reprints avail. *Refereed.* **Document type:** *Academic/Scholarly.*

Related titles: Microform ed.: (from PQC); Online - full text ed.: (from EBSCO Publishing).

Indexed: AESIS, Agricola, Anal.Abstr., Anim.Breed.Abstr., Apic.Abstr., Aqua.Sci.& Fish.Abstr., Aquacult.Abstr., Bibl.Agri., Bio-Contr.News & Info., Biol.Abstr., Biwk.Pap.Rad.Chem.& Photochem., Chem.Abstr., Chem.Cit.Ind., Crop Physiol.Abstr., Curr.Adv.Biochem., Curr.Adv.Cancer Res., Curr.Adv.Gen.& Molec.Biol., Curr.Cont. (coverage dropped), Dent.Ind., Entomol.Abstr. (coverage dropped), Environ.Sci.Poll.Mgmt., Excerp.Med., Fababean Abstr., Field Crop Abstr., Food Sci.& Tech.Abstr., GeoRef, Helminthol.Abstr., Herb.Abstr., INIS Atomind., Ind.Med. (1947-), Inpharma, Kidney, Maize Abstr., Mass Spectr.Bull., Mat.Sci.Cit.Ind. (coverage dropped), Microbiol.Abstr., Neurosci.Cit.Ind., Nuc.Acids Abstr., Nutr.Abstr., Plant Grow.Reg.Abstr., Reac., Rev.Appl.Entomol., Rev.Plant Path., Seed Abstr., Soyabean Abstr., Telegen, Vet.Bull., Weed Abstr., Wild.Rev.

—BLDSC (2070.000000), CASDDS, CINDOC, CISTI, GNLM, IDS, ingenta, Linda Hall. **CCC.**

Published by: Elsevier Science BV, PO Box 211, Amsterdam 1000 AE, Netherlands. TEL 31-20-485-3757, FAX 31-20-485-3432, TELEX 18582 ESPA NL, http://www.elsevier.com/locate/bba. Circ: 4,500. **Subscr. in Australasia and the Far East to:** Elsevier Science (Singapore) Pte Ltd, No.1 Temasek Ave, 17-01 Millenia Tower, Singapore 039192, Singapore. TEL 65-434-3727, FAX 65-337-2230; **Subscr. in Japan to:** Elsevier Science Inc - Japan Regional Office, 9-15 Higashi-Azabu 1-chome, Minato-ku, Tokyo 106-0044, Japan. TEL 81-3-5561-5033, FAX 81-3-5561-5047; **Subscr. in the Americas to:** Elsevier Science, PO Box 945, New York, NY 10159-0945. TEL 212-633-3730, FAX 212-633-3680, usinfo-f@elsevier.com, http://www.elsevier.com.

572 FRA ISSN 0300-9084
QP501 CODEN: BICMBE

BIOCHIMIE. Text and summaries in English. 1914. m. EUR 716 in Europe to institutions; JPY 94,900 in Japan to institutions; USD 801 elsewhere to institutions (effective 2002). adv. bk.rev. bibl, charts, illus. reprint service avail. from ISI. *Refereed.* **Document type:** *Academic/Scholarly.* **Description:** Publishes original work, review articles and mini-reviews in enzymology, genetics, immunology, microbiology, structure of macromolecules.

Formerly (until 1971): Societe de Chimie Biologique. Bulletin (0037-9042)

Related titles: Microform ed.: (from PQC); Online - full text ed.: (from ingenta, Swets Blackwell, ScienceDirect, Institute for Scientific Information).

Indexed: ASCA, AgBiotech, Agri.& Environ.Biotech.Abstr. (coverage dropped), Anal.Abstr., Aqua.Sci.& Fish.Abstr., Aquacult.Abstr., BBCI, Biol.Abstr., Chem.Abstr., Chem.Cit.Ind., Chem.Indus.Notes, Chem.Titles, Crop Physiol.Abstr., Curr.Adv.Ecol.Sci., Curr.Cont., Dairy Sci.Abstr., Derwent Biotech.Abstr., Environ.Sci.Poll.Mgmt., Excerp.Med., Field Crop Abstr., Food Sci.& Tech.Abstr., Helminthol.Abstr., INIS Atomind., Ind.Med. (1971-), Ind.Sci.Rev., Ind.Vet., Inpharma, Int.Abstr.Biol.Sci., Mass Spectr.Bull., Microbiol.Abstr., Nuc.Acids Abstr., Nutr.Abstr., Pharm.&Out.News, Plant Breed.Abstr., Protozool.Abstr., Reac., Ref.Zh., Rev.Med.& Vet.Mycol., Rev.Plant Path., Sci.Cit.Ind., Sport Fish.Abstr., Sugar Ind.Abstr., Triticale Abstr., Trop.Dis.Bull., Vet.Bull., Weed Abstr.

—BLDSC (2070.500000), CASDDS, CISTI, EMDOCS, GNLM, IDS, ingenta, Linda Hall. **CCC.**

Published by: (Societe Francaise de Biochimie et Biologie Moleculaire, Centre Universitaire des Saints-Peres), Elsevier Paris, Editions Scientifiques et Medicales (Subsidiary of: Reed Elsevier plc. group), 23 rue Linois, Paris 75015, France. TEL 33-1-45589110, FAX 33-1-45589419, academic@elsevier-fr.com, http://www.elsevier.com/locate/biochi. Eds. M Grunberg-Manago, R H Buckingham. Circ: 3,000.

572 USA ISSN 1043-1802
QP517.B49 CODEN: BCCHES

BIOCONJUGATE CHEMISTRY. Text in English. 1990. bi-m. USD 648 in North America to institutions; USD 706 elsewhere to institutions; USD 778 in North America to institutions Print & online eds.; USD 836 elsewhere to institutions Print online eds. (effective 2002); for additional pricing options for print and web editions contact inside sales specialist, Ms. Chako Dickinson, at 202-872-4063. back issues avail. *Refereed.* **Document type:** *Journal, Academic/Scholarly.* **Description:** Emphasizes the joining of two different molecular functions by chemical or biological means.

Related titles: Microform ed.; Online - full text ed.: ISSN 1520-4812. USD 680 (effective 2002) (from EBSCO Publishing, Institute for Scientific Information).

Indexed: ASCA, BBCI, Biotech.Cit.Ind., Chem.Abstr., Chem.Cit.Ind., Chem.Indus.Notes, Chem.Titles, Curr.Cont., INIS Atomind., Ind.Med. (1990-), Ind.Sci.Rev., Inpharma, Int.Abstr.Biol.Sci., Mat.Sci.Cit.Ind. (coverage dropped), Pharm.&Out.News, Reac., Sci.Cit.Ind.

—BLDSC (2071.080000), CASDDS, CISTI, EMDOCS, GNLM, IDS, ingenta, Linda Hall. **CCC.**

Published by: American Chemical Society, 1155 16th St, N W, Washington, DC 20036. TEL 202-332-5544, 800-333-9511, FAX 202-332-4559, service@acs.org, http://pubs.acs.org/bc. Ed. Claude F Meares. Circ: 1,100. **Subscr. to:** American Chemical Society, Member and Subscriber Services, PO Box 3337, Columbus, OH 43210. TEL 614-447-3674, FAX 614-447-3671.

572 CHE ISSN 1422-4208
QP341 CODEN: BEBEBP

BIOELECTROCHEMISTRY; an international journal devoted to electrochemical aspects of biology and biological aspects of electrochemistry. Text in English. 1974. bi-m. EUR 1,484 in Europe to institutions; JPY 197,100 in Japan to institutions; USD 1,659 elsewhere to institutions (effective 2002). adv. bk.rev. back issues avail. *Refereed.* **Document type:** *Academic/Scholarly.* **Description:** Publishes papers on electrochemical aspects of biology and biological aspects of electrochemistry.

Formerly (until 1995): Bioelectrochemistry and Bioenergetics (0302-4598)

Related titles: Microform ed.: (from PQC); Online - full text ed.: (from ingenta, Swets Blackwell, ScienceDirect, Institute for Scientific Information).

Indexed: ASCA, Alloys Ind. (1983-1994), Anal.Abstr., Aqua.Sci.& Fish.Abstr., BBCI, Biol.Abstr., CEABA, Chem.Abstr., Chem.Cit.Ind., Chem.Indus.Notes, Chem.Titles, Curr.Adv.Ecol.Sci., Curr.Cont., Curr.Tit.Electrochem., Eng.Ind., Excerp.Med., Ind.Med. (coverage dropped), Ind.Sci.Rev., Inpharma, Int.Abstr.Biol.Sci., Met.Abstr. (1983-1994), Met.Abstr.Ind. (1983-1994), Nonfer.Met.Alert (1983-1994), PCC Alert (1983-1994), Pharm.&Out.News, Poult.Abstr., Reac., Ref.Zh., Sci.Cit.Ind., Steels Alert (1983-1994).

—BLDSC (2072.008000), CASDDS, CISTI, Ei, EMDOCS, GNLM, IDS, ingenta, Linda Hall. **CCC.**

Published by: Elsevier Science S.A., PO Box 564, Lausanne, 1 1001, Switzerland. TEL 41-21-3207381, FAX 41-21-3235444, http://www.elsevier.com/locate/bioelechem. Eds. D Walz, R Guidelli. **Subscr. in Australasia to:** Elsevier Science (Singapore) Pte Ltd, No.1 Temasek Ave, 17-01 Millenia Tower, Singapore 039192, Singapore. TEL 65-434-3727, FAX 65-337-2230; **Subscr. in the Americas to:** Elsevier Science, PO Box 945, New York, NY 10159-0945. TEL 212-633-3730, FAX 212-633-3680; **Subscr. to:** Elsevier Science BV, PO Box 211, Amsterdam 1000 AE, Netherlands. TEL 31-20-485-3757.

572 CHE

BIOELECTROCHEMISTRY: PRINCIPLES AND PRACTICE. Text in English. 1994. irreg. price varies. **Document type:** *Monographic series, Academic/Scholarly.* **Description:** Compiles information on all the physiochemical aspects of the different biochemical and physiological processes.

Indexed: Chem.Abstr., Chem.Indus.Notes, Chem.Titles.

Published by: Birkhaeuser Verlag AG (Subsidiary of: BertelsmannSpringer), Klosterberg, Postfach 133, Basel 4010, Switzerland. TEL 41-61-2050707, FAX 41-61-2050792, orders@birkhauser.ch, http://www.birkhauser.ch.

572 NLD ISSN 0951-6433
QP771 CODEN: BIFAEU

BIOFACTORS; vitamins - autoregulatory substances - trace elements - growth factors. Text in English. 1988. m. (in 3 vols). EUR 829, USD 786 to institutions (effective 2002). index. back issues avail.; reprint service avail. from SWZ. *Refereed.* **Document type:** *Journal, Academic/Scholarly.* **Description:** Contains papers and short communications aimed at identifying and investigating effects and roles of trace substances required by organisms.

Related titles: Online - full text ed.: (from EBSCO Publishing, O C L C Online Computer Library Center, Inc., Swets Blackwell, Institute for Scientific Information, RoweCom Information Quest).

Indexed: Anim.Breed.Abstr., Aqua.Sci.& Fish.Abstr., BBCI, Biol.Abstr., Chem.Abstr., Chem.Indus.Notes, Chem.Titles, Curr.Adv.Biochem., Curr.Adv.Cell & Devel.Biol., Curr.Adv.Gen.& Molec.Biol., Curr.Cont. (coverage dropped), Dairy Sci.Abstr., Environ.Sci.Poll.Mgmt., Excerp.Med. (1988-1993, 1996-), Immun.Abstr. (coverage dropped), Ind.Med. (1988-), Int.Abstr.Biol.Sci., Mat.Sci.Cit.Ind. (coverage dropped), Nutr.Abstr., Pollut.Abstr., Sci.Cit.Ind. (coverage dropped), Weed Abstr.

—BLDSC (2072.123000), ADONIS, CASDDS, CISTI, EMDOCS, GNLM, IDS, Infotrieve, ingenta, Linda Hall. **CCC.**

Published by: (International Union of Biochemistry and Molecular Biology AUS), I O S Press, Nieuwe Hemweg 6B, Amsterdam 1013 BG, Netherlands. TEL 31-20-688-3355, FAX 31-20-620-3419, nikie@cc.utsunomiya-u.ac.jp, market@iospress.nl, http://www.iospress.nl. Eds. L Flohe TEL 49-531-6181-599, W J Whelan. **Subscr. to:** I O S Press, Inc, 5795-G Burke Centre Pkwy, Burke, VA 22015. TEL 703-323-5554, FAX 703-323-3668, iosbooks@iospress.com; Globe Publication Pvt. Ltd., C-62 Inderpuri, New Delhi 100 012, India. TEL 91-11-579-3211, 91-11-579-3212, FAX 91-11-579-8876, custserve@globepub.com, http://www.globepub.com; Kinokuniya Company Ltd, Shinjuku 3-chome, Shinjuku-ku, Tokyo 160-0022, Japan. FAX 81-3-3439-1094, journal@kinokuniya.co.jp, http://www.kinokuniya.co.jp.

572.65 NLD ISSN 0168-8561
QP801.B66 CODEN: BIAME7
BIOGENIC AMINES. Text in English. 1984. bi-m. EUR 358, USD 415 (effective 2002). back issues avail. *Refereed.* **Document type:** *Journal, Academic/Scholarly.* **Description:** Publishes research on all aspects of biogenic amines and amino acid transmitters, related compounds, and interactions.
Related titles: Online - full text ed.: (from Institute for Scientific Information).
Indexed: ASCA, BBCI, Chem.Abstr., Chem.Indus.Notes, Chem.Titles, Curr.Cont., Excerp.Med., Ind.Sci.Rev., Inpharma, Neurosci.Cit.Ind., Pharm.&Out.News, Reac., Sci.Cit.Ind.
—BLDSC (2072.149000), CASDDS, CISTI, GNLM, Infotrieve. **CCC.**
Published by: V S P (Subsidiary of: Brill Academic Publishers), PO Box 346, Zeist 3700 AH, Netherlands. TEL 31-30-692-5790, FAX 31-30-693-2081, vsppub@compuserve.com, http://www.vsppub.com/journals/jn-BioAmi.html. Eds. S H Parvez, T Nagatsu.

572 NLD ISSN 0168-2563
QH343.7 CODEN: BIOGEP
BIOGEOCHEMISTRY; an international journal. Text and summaries in English. 1984. m. NLG 2,880, EUR 1,307, USD 1,309 to institutions for print or online ed.; NLG 3,456, EUR 1,568.40, USD 1,570.80 to institutions for print & online eds. combined (effective 2001). adv. bk.rev. reprint service avail. from SWZ. *Refereed.* **Document type:** *Academic/Scholarly.* **Description:** Publishes original papers dealing with biotic controls on the chemistry of the environment or the geochemical control of the structure and function of ecosystems.
Related titles: Microform ed.: (from PQC); Online - full text ed.: (from EBSCO Publishing, O C L C Online Computer Library Center, Inc., RoweCom Information Quest, Swets Blackwell, Kluwer Online, Institute for Scientific Information).
Indexed: AESIS, ASCA, Agricola, Agroforest.Abstr., Aqua.Sci.& Fish.Abstr., Bibl.Agri., Biol.Abstr., Chem.Abstr., Chem.Indus.Notes, Chem.Titles, Curr.Adv.Ecol.Sci., Curr.Adv.Plant Sci., Curr.Cont., Deep Sea Res.& Oceanogr.Abstr., Ecol.Abstr., Environ.Per.Bibl. (1993-), Environ.Sci.Poll.Mgmt., Excerp.Med. (until 19??), Field Crop Abstr., Forest.Abstr., Geo.Abstr.H.G., Geo.Abstr.P.G., GeoRef, Geol.Abstr., Herb.Abstr., Hort.Abstr., INIS Atomind., Ind.Sci.Rev., Int.Abstr.Biol.Sci., Irr.& Drain.Abstr., Microbiol.Abstr., Plant Sci., Pollut.Abstr., Rev.Plant Path., Rice Abstr., Sci.Cit.Ind., Sel.Water Res.Abstr., Soils & Fert.
—BLDSC (2072.163000), CASDDS, CISTI, EMDOCS, IDS, Infotrieve, ingenta, Linda Hall. **CCC.**
Published by: Kluwer Academic Publishers Group (Subsidiary of: Wolters Kluwer N.V.), Spuiboulevard 50, PO Box 17, Dordrecht 3300 AA, Netherlands. TEL 31-78-639-2392, FAX 31-78-654-2254, services@wkap.nl, http://www.wkap.nl/journalhome.htm/0168-2563. Ed. Robert W Howarth. **Subscr. in N America to:** Kluwer Academic - Plenum Publishers, 233 Spring St, New York, NY 10013-1578. TEL 212-620-8468, 800-221-9369, FAX 212-807-1047; **Subscr. to:** Journals Department, PO Box 322, Dordrecht 3300 AH, Netherlands. TEL 31-78-639-2392, FAX 31-78-654-6474.

572 RUS ISSN 0320-9725
QH301 CODEN: BIOHAO
BIOKHIMIYA. Text in Russian; Summaries in English. 1936. m. RUR 310 per month (effective 2001). adv. bk.rev. illus. index, cum.index: 1946-1955.
Related titles: Online - full text ed.; ♦ English Translation: Biochemistry (Moscow). ISSN 0006-2979.
Indexed: Abstr.Bull.Inst.Pap.Chem., Agri.& Environ.Biotech.Abstr. (coverage dropped), Anal.Abstr., Aqua.Sci.& Fish.Abstr., Aquacult.Abstr., Biol.Abstr., Chem.Abstr., Curr.Cont. (coverage dropped), Dairy Sci.Abstr., Derwent Biotech.Abstr., Eng.Ind., Environ.Sci.Poll.Mgmt., Excerp.Med., Food Sci.& Tech.Abstr., Helminthol.Abstr., INIS Atomind., Ind.Med. (coverage dropped), Inpharma, Nutr.Abstr., Reac., Ref.Zh., Soils & Fert., Zoo.Rec.
—BLDSC (0018.100000), CASDDS, CINDOC, CISTI, East View, GNLM, KNAW, Linda Hall. **CCC.**
Published by: (Rossiiskaya Akademiya Nauk/Russian Academy of Sciences), M A I K Nauka - Interperiodica, Mezhdunarodnyi Otdel, Podsosenskii per 21, room 31, Moscow 103062, Russian Federation. ozrina@jnlbioch.bio.msu.su/biokhimiya, compmg@maik.rssi.ru, http://www.protein.bio.msu.su/biokhimiya, http://www.maik.rssi.ru/. Ed. V P Skulachev. Circ: 4,230. **US dist. addr.:** Kluwer Academic Publishers, PO Box 17, Dordrecht 3300 AH, Netherlands. TEL 31-78-392392.

572 UKR ISSN 0136-9377
QP1 CODEN: BZCHDI
BIOKHIMIYA ZHIVOTNYKH I CHELOVEKA; respublikanskii mezhvedomstvennyi sbornik nauchnykh trudov. Text in Russian. 1977. a.
Indexed: Chem.Abstr., Chem.Indus.Notes, Chem.Titles.
—CASDDS, Linda Hall.
Published by: Natsional'na Akademiya Nauk Ukrainy, Institut Biokhimii im. A.V. Palladina, Vul Tereshchenkivska 3, Kiev 252601, Ukraine. TEL 044-224-4060, FAX 044-224-7060, oficer@biochem.freenet.Kiev.ua. **Dist. by:** Mezhdunarodnaya Kniga, B Yakimanka 39, Moscow 117049, Russian Federation.

572.8 SVK ISSN 1335-6399
CODEN: BLOAAO
BIOLOGIA. SECTION: CELLULAR AND MOLECULAR BIOLOGY. Text in English. 1946. s-a. USD 168 for 3 sections (effective 2001). adv. bk.rev. charts, illus. index. **Document type:** *Academic/Scholarly.* **Description:** Covers original experimental and theoretical works in basic biological research from molecular and cell biology and biochemistry.
Formerly (until 1994): Biologia. D: Biochemia a Molekularna Biologia (0862-1152); Supersedes in part (in 1969): Biologia (0006-3088)
Indexed: Biodet.Abstr., Biol.Abstr., Chem.Abstr., Curr.Cont. (coverage dropped), INIS Atomind., Ind.Med. (coverage dropped), Soyabean Abstr., Sport Fish.Abstr., Triticale Abstr., Wild.Rev., Zoo.Rec.
—BLDSC (2072.700000), CASDDS, CISTI, GNLM, IDS, KNAW, Linda Hall.
Published by: Slovak Academy of Sciences, Institute of Microbiology, Stefanikova 3, Bratislava 81434, Slovakia. TEL 421-7-394845, FAX 421-7-393824, sjanecek@ue.savba.sk. Ed. Stefan Janecek. **Dist. by:** Slovak Academic Press Ltd.

BIOLOGICAL & PHARMACEUTICAL BULLETIN. see *PHARMACY AND PHARMACOLOGY*

572 DEU ISSN 1431-6730
QP501 CODEN: BICHF3
BIOLOGICAL CHEMISTRY. Text and summaries in English, German. 1877. m. EUR 210.30 domestic to individuals; EUR 219.50 foreign to individuals; EUR 910.30 domestic to institutions; EUR 919.50 foreign to institutions; EUR 848 online ed. only (effective 2002). adv. abstr, bibl, charts, illus, stat. index. *Refereed.* **Document type:** *Journal, Academic/Scholarly.*
Former titles: Biological Chemistry Hoppe-Seyler (0177-3593); Hoppe-Seyler's Zeitschrift fuer Physiologische Chemie (0018-4888)
Related titles: Microform ed.: (from PQC,PMC); Online - full text ed.: (from EBSCO Publishing, O C L C Online Computer Library Center, Inc., Swets Blackwell, Institute for Scientific Information).
Indexed: ASCA, Agri.& Environ.Biotech.Abstr. (coverage dropped), Agricola, Anim.Breed.Abstr., Aqua.Sci.& Fish.Abstr., Aquacult.Abstr., BBCI, Bibl.Agri., Biodet.Abstr., Biol.Abstr., Chem.Abstr., Chem.Cit.Ind., Chem.Indus.Notes, Chem.Infd., Chem.Titles, Curr.Adv.Biochem., Curr.Adv.Cancer Res., Curr.Adv.Cell & Devel.Biol., Curr.Adv.Ecol.Sci., Curr.Adv.Gen.& Molec.Biol., Curr.Cont., Dairy Sci.Abstr., Dent.Ind., Derwent Biotech.Abstr., Environ.Sci.Poll.Mgmt., Excerp.Med., Food Sci.& Tech.Abstr., INIS Atomind., Ind.Med. (1996-), Ind.Sci.Rev., Ind.Vet., Inpharma, Int.Abstr.Biol.Sci., Mass Spectr.Bull., Nutr.Abstr., Pharm.&Out.News, Plant Gen.Res.Abstr., Protozool.Abstr., RCI, Reac., Rev.Appl.Entomol., Rev.Plant Path., Sci.Cit.Ind., Sport Fish.Abstr., THA, Vet.Bull., Wild.Rev., Zoo.Rec.
—BLDSC (2075.070000), CASDDS, CINDOC, CISTI, EMDOCS, GNLM, IDS, ingenta, Linda Hall. **CCC.**
Published by: Walter de Gruyter und Co., Genthiner Str 13, Berlin 10785, Germany. TEL 49-30-26005-0, FAX 49-30-26005-251, wdg-info@degruyter.de, http://www.degruyter.de. Ed. Walter Schaffner. adv.: B&W page DEM 2,300; trim 210 x 297. Circ: 6,000 (paid).

BIOLOGICAL PSYCHIATRY; a journal of psychiatric research. see *MEDICAL SCIENCES—Psychiatry And Neurology*

572 USA ISSN 0271-9355
CODEN: BRDEDQ
BIOLOGICAL REGULATION & DEVELOPMENT. Text in English. 1979. irreg., latest vol.3, 1984. price varies. *Refereed.* **Document type:** *Monographic series.*
Indexed: Chem.Abstr.
—CASDDS, CISTI.
Published by: Kluwer Academic - Plenum Publishers (Subsidiary of: Wolters Kluwer N.V.), 233 Spring St, New York, NY 10013-1578. TEL 212-620-8000, 800-221-9369, FAX 212-463-0742, info@plenum.com, http://www.plenum.com. Ed. Robert F Goldberger.

572 USA ISSN 0163-4984
QP534 CODEN: BTERDG
BIOLOGICAL TRACE ELEMENT RESEARCH. Text in English. 1979. 18/yr. USD 965 domestic; USD 995 foreign (effective 2000). adv. bk.rev. bibl, charts, illus. *Refereed.* **Document type:** *Journal, Academic/Scholarly.* **Description:** Forum for original papers in biological, environmental and biomedical research on trace elements. Stresses the integrative aspects of trace element research in all relevant fields, especially focusing on nutritional studies in humans and in animals models.
Related titles: Online - full text ed.: (from Institute for Scientific Information).
Indexed: ASCA, Agricola, Agroforest.Abstr., Aqua.Sci.& Fish.Abstr., BBCI, Biol.Abstr., Cal.Tiss.Abstr., Chem.Abstr., Chem.Cit.Ind., Chem.Indus.Notes, Chem.Titles, Crop Physiol.Abstr., Curr.Adv.Ecol.Sci., Curr.Cont., Dairy Sci.Abstr., Environ.Sci.Poll.Mgmt., Excerp.Med., Field Crop Abstr., GeoRef, Hort.Abstr., INIS Atomind., Ind.Med. (1979-), Ind.Sci.Rev., Ind.Vet., Inpharma, Irr.& Drain.Abstr., Lab.Haz.Bull., Mass Spectr.Bull., Nutr.Abstr., Pharm.&Out.News, Pig News & Info., Pollut.Abstr., Poult.Abstr., Protozool.Abstr., Reac., Rev.Appl.Entomol., Rev.Arom.& Med.Plants, Rice Abstr., Risk Abstr., Saf.Sci.Abstr., Sci.Cit.Ind., Seed Abstr., Sel.Water Res.Abstr., Soils & Fert., Soyabean Abstr., Sport Fish.Abstr., Tox.Abstr., Triticale Abstr., Vet.Bull., Weed Abstr., Wild.Rev.
—BLDSC (2081.600000), ADONIS, CASDDS, CISTI, EMDOCS, GNLM, IDS, ingenta, Linda Hall. **CCC.**
Published by: (International Association of Bioinorganic Scientists), Humana Press Inc., 999 Riverview Dr, Ste 208, Totowa, NJ 07512. TEL 973-256-1699, FAX 973-256-8341, humana@humanapr.com, http://humanapress.com. Ed. Gerhard N Schrauzer. R&P Richard Hruska. Adv. contact Thomas B Lanigan Jr. **Dist. in Japan by:** Maruzen Co., Ltd., International Division, Export Dept, P.O. Box 5050, Tokyo International 100-3191, Japan. TEL 81-3-3278-1937, 81-3-3275-8591.

BIOMATERIALS. see *MEDICAL SCIENCES*

572 JPN ISSN 0916-717X
CODEN: BRTEE5
BIOMEDICAL RESEARCH ON TRACE ELEMENTS. Text in English, Japanese; Summaries in English. 1990. irreg. JPY 75,000. **Document type:** *Academic/Scholarly.*
Indexed: Chem.Abstr., Chem.Indus.Notes, Chem.Titles.
—BLDSC (2087.875000), CASDDS, GNLM.
Published by: Japan Society for Biomedical Research on Trace Elements/Nihon Biryo Genso Gakkai, Nihon Daigaku Igakubu Kagaku Kyoshitsu, 30-1, Oyaguchi Kamicho, Itabashi-ku, Tokyo 173, Japan. TEL 03-3972-8111, FAX 03-5995-6956. Ed. Yasuyuki Arakawa.

BIOORGANICHESKAYA KHIMIYA. see *CHEMISTRY—Organic Chemistry*

BIOPHYSICAL CHEMISTRY; an international journal devoted to the physics and chemistry of biological phenomena. see *BIOLOGY—Biophysics*

BIOSCIENCE, BIOTECHNOLOGY, AND BIOCHEMISTRY. see *BIOLOGY—Biotechnology*

BIOSCIENCE REPORTS; molecular and cellular biology of the cell surface. see *BIOLOGY—Cytology And Histology*

B

BIOTECHNOLOGY AND APPLIED BIOCHEMISTRY. see *BIOLOGY—Biotechnology*

BIOTECHNOLOGY AND BIOENGINEERING. see *BIOLOGY—Biotechnology*

572.8 TUR ISSN 0250-4685
BIYOKIMYA DERGISI. Text in Turkish, English. 3/yr. *Refereed.* **Document type:** *Journal, Academic/Scholarly.* **Description:** Publishes research in the field of biochemistry.
Published by: Turk Biyokimya Dernegi'nin Yayin Organidir/Turkish Biochemical Society, PK 407, Yenisehir, Ankara 06444, Turkey. FAX 90-312-311-6616.

BLOOD. see *MEDICAL SCIENCES—Hematology*

612.015 USA ISSN 1078-0491
BLOOD CELL BIOCHEMISTRY. Text in English. 1990. irreg., latest vol.8, 1999. price varies. **Document type:** *Monographic series, Academic/Scholarly.*
Supersedes in part (in 1990): SubCellular Biochemistry (0306-0225)
—BLDSC (2112.180000).
Published by: Kluwer Academic - Plenum Publishers (Subsidiary of: Wolters Kluwer N.V.), 233 Spring St, New York, NY 10013-1578. http://www.wkap.nl/series.htm/BLBI. **Subscr. elsewhere to:** Kluwer Academic Publishers, PO Box 17, Dordrecht 3300 AH, Netherlands. TEL 31-78-639-2392, FAX 31-78-654-6474; **Subscr. in the Americas to:** Kluwer Academic Publishers, Accord Station, PO Box358, Hingham, MA 02018-0358. TEL 781-871-6600, FAX 781-871-6528.

C A S BIOTECH UPDATES. BIOCHEMICAL IMMOBILIZATION & BIOCATALYTIC REACTORS. see *BIOLOGY—Abstracting, Bibliographies, Statistics*

C A S BIOTECH UPDATES. BIOSENSORS. see *BIOLOGY—Abstracting, Bibliographies, Statistics*

C A S BIOTECH UPDATES. COMMERCIAL FERMENTATION. see *BIOLOGY—Abstracting, Bibliographies, Statistics*

C A S BIOTECH UPDATES. D N A & R N A PROBES. see *BIOLOGY—Abstracting, Bibliographies, Statistics*

C A S BIOTECH UPDATES. D N A FORMATION & REPAIR. see *BIOLOGY—Abstracting, Bibliographies, Statistics*

C A S BIOTECH UPDATES. ENZYMES IN BIOTECHNOLOGY. see *BIOLOGY—Abstracting, Bibliographies, Statistics*

C A S BIOTECH UPDATES. NUCLEIC ACID & PROTEIN SEQUENCES. see *BIOLOGY—Abstracting, Bibliographies, Statistics*

C A SELECTS. FREE RADICALS (BIOCHEMICAL ASPECTS). see *BIOLOGY—Abstracting, Bibliographies, Statistics*

C A SELECTS. PHOTOBIOCHEMISTRY. see *CHEMISTRY—Abstracting, Bibliographies, Statistics*

C A SELECTS PLUS. AMINO ACIDS, PEPTIDES AND PROTEINS. see *BIOLOGY—Abstracting, Bibliographies, Statistics*

C A SELECTS. STEROIDS (BIOCHEMICAL ASPECTS). see *BIOLOGY—Abstracting, Bibliographies, Statistics*

572.8 CAN CODEN: CBCBBB
CANADIAN SOCIETY OF BIOCHEMISTRY, MOLECULAR AND CELLULAR BIOLOGY. BULLETIN. Text mainly in English; Text occasionally in French. s-a. CND 10, USD 10. adv. bk.rev. **Document type:** *Bulletin.* **Description:** Covers news and meetings in Canada's biochemistry field.
Former titles: Canadian Society of Biochemistry and Molecular Biology. Bulletin; Canadian Biochemical Society. Bulletin (0008-302X)
Indexed: Ref.Zh.
—CASDDS, CISTI.
Published by: Canadian Society of Biochemistry, Molecular and Cellular Biology, c/o Dr E R Tustanoff, Sec, Dept of Biochemistry, University of Western Ontario, London, ON N6A 5C1, Canada. TEL 519-471-1961, FAX 519-661-3175. Ed. David Tinker. Circ: 750.

CANCER BIOCHEMISTRY BIOPHYSICS. see *MEDICAL SCIENCES—Oncology*

572 CHE ISSN 1073-5070 CODEN: CLETEC
CARBOHYDRATE LETTERS. Text in English. 1994. 12/yr. (in 2 vols., 6 nos./vol.). EUR 470 to institutions; EUR 728 to corporations (effective 2000). back issues avail. *Refereed.* **Document type:** *Academic/Scholarly.* **Description:** Promotes the understanding of the precise biological role of sugars, as defined through developments in the chemistry of carbohydrates.
Related titles: CD-ROM ed.; Online - full text ed.: (from EBSCO Publishing, RoweCom Information Quest).
Indexed: Food Sci.& Tech.Abstr., Int.Abstr.Biol.Sci.
—BLDSC (3050.990150), EMDOCS, Infotrieve. **CCC.**
Published by: Gordon and Breach - Harwood Academic (Subsidiary of: Taylor & Francis Group), PO Box 531, Lausanne 1000, Switzerland. http://www.gbhap.com/Carbohydrate_Letters/. Ed. Pierre G Sinay. **Subscr. addr. in US:** International Publishers Direct, PO Box 32160, Newark, NJ 07102. FAX 215-750-6343.

572 USA ISSN 0069-0732
CAROTENOIDS OTHER THAN VITAMIN A. Text in English. 1967. irreg., latest 1972, 3rd, Cluj, Rumania. price varies. **Document type:** *Monographic series, Proceedings.*
Published by: (International Union of Pure and Applied Chemistry), C R C Press, LLC, 2000 Corporate Blvd, N W, Boca Raton, FL 33431. TEL 561-994-0555, 800-272-7737, FAX 561-998-9784.

CELL BIOCHEMISTRY AND BIOPHYSICS. see *BIOLOGY—Cytology And Histology*

571.6 GBR ISSN 0263-6484
QH611 CODEN: CBFUDH
CELL BIOCHEMISTRY AND FUNCTION. Text in English. 1983. q. USD 1,425 in United States; USD 1,425 in Canada & Mexico; USD 1,425 elsewhere; USD 1,497 combined subscription in United States for print and online eds.; USD 1,497 combined subscription in Canada & Mexico for print and online eds.; USD 1,497 combined subscription elsewhere for print and online eds. (effective 2002). adv. bk.rev. abstr, illus. index. back issues avail.; reprint service avail. from SWZ. *Refereed.* **Document type:** *Academic/Scholarly.* **Description:** Provides a forum for reporting and discussing the biochemistry of whole cells and of the link between the biochemistry and the functioning of cells in isolation, in assemblies, and in tissues.
Related titles: Microform ed.: (from PQC); Online - full text ed.: ISSN 1099-0844. USD 1,425 in United States; USD 1,425 in Canada & Mexico; USD 1,425 elsewhere (effective 2002) (from EBSCO Publishing, Wiley InterScience, Institute for Scientific Information).
Indexed: Aqua.Sci.& Fish.Abstr., BBCI, Chem.Abstr., Chem.Indus.Notes, Chem.Titles, Curr.Adv.Ecol.Sci., Curr.Cont., Environ.Sci.Poll.Mgmt., Excerp.Med., Ind.Med. (1983-), Ind.Sci.Rev., Inpharma, Int.Abstr.Biol.Sci., Nutr.Abstr., Pharm.&Out.News, Reac., Sci.Cit.Ind., Soyabean Abstr.
—BLDSC (3097.702000), CASDDS, CISTI, EMDOCS, GNLM, IDS, ingenta, KNAW. **CCC.**
Published by: Wiley Europe Ltd., Baffins Ln, Chichester, W Sussex PO19 1UD, United Kingdom. TEL 44-1243-779777, FAX 44-1243-775878, customer@wiley.co.uk, http://www.interscience.wiley.com/jpages/0263-6484/, http://www.wiley.co.uk. adv.: B&W page GBP 650, color page GBP 1,550; trim 200 x 260. Circ: 300. **Subscr. to:** John Wiley & Sons, Inc., Journals, 605 Third Ave, New York, NY 10158. TEL 212-850-6021, 212-850-6645, subinfo@jwiley.com.

CELL CALCIUM (SHEFFIELD). see *BIOLOGY—Abstracting, Bibliographies, Statistics*

CELL MEMBRANES. see *BIOLOGY—Abstracting, Bibliographies, Statistics*

CELLULAR PHYSIOLOGY AND BIOCHEMISTRY; international journal of experimental cellular physiology, biochemistry and pharmacology. see *BIOLOGY—Cytology And Histology*

CHEMICAL ABSTRACTS - BIOCHEMISTRY SECTIONS. see *BIOLOGY—Abstracting, Bibliographies, Statistics*

572 USA ISSN 0093-6855 CODEN: CMMUAO
CHEMICAL MUTAGENS. Text in English. 1971. irreg., latest vol.10, 1986. **Document type:** *Monographic series.*
Related titles: Online - full text ed.: (from Institute for Scientific Information).
Indexed: BBCI, Sci.Cit.Ind.
—CASDDS, CISTI, GNLM, Infotrieve. **CCC.**
Published by: Kluwer Academic - Plenum Publishers (Subsidiary of: Wolters Kluwer N.V.), 233 Spring St, New York, NY 10013-1578. TEL 212-620-8000, 800-221-9369, FAX 212-463-0742, info@plenum.com, http://www.plenum.com.

CHEMICAL SENSES. see *BIOLOGY—Physiology*

CHEMICO-BIOLOGICAL INTERACTIONS; a journal of molecular and biochemical toxicology. see *ENVIRONMENTAL STUDIES—Toxicology And Environmental Safety*

CHEMISTRY AND ECOLOGY. see *CHEMISTRY*

572.57 IRL ISSN 0009-3084 CODEN: CPLIA4
CHEMISTRY AND PHYSICS OF LIPIDS. Text in English. 1967. m. EUR 2,208 in Europe to institutions; JPY 293,400 in Japan to institutions; USD 2,470 elsewhere to institutions (effective 2002). illus. index. back issues avail. *Refereed.* **Document type:** *Academic/Scholarly.* **Description:** Publishes papers and review articles in the field of molecular biology which emphasize chemical and biophysical aspects of lipids.
Related titles: Microform ed.: (from PQC); Online - full text ed.: (from ingenta, Swets Blackwell, ScienceDirect, Institute for Scientific Information).
Indexed: ASCA, Apic.Abstr., BBCI, Biol.Abstr., Chem.Abstr., Chem.Cit.Ind., Chem.Indus.Notes, Chem.Titles, Curr.Adv.Biochem., Curr.Adv.Cell & Devel.Biol., Curr.Adv.Ecol.Sci., Curr.Cont., Eng.Ind., Excerp.Med., INIS Atomind., Ind.Med. (1966-), Ind.Sci.Rev., Inpharma, Int.Abstr.Biol.Sci., Mass Spectr.Bull., Nutr.Abstr., Pharm.&Out.News, Reac., Rev.Appl.Entomol., Rev.Med.& Vet.Mycol., Sci.Cit.Ind.
—BLDSC (3170.100000), ADONIS, CASDDS, CISTI, Ei, EMDOCS, GNLM, IDS, ingenta, Linda Hall. **CCC.**
Published by: Elsevier Science Ireland Ltd, Elsevier House, Brookvale Plaza, E. Park, Shannon, Co. Clare, Ireland. TEL 353-61-709600, FAX 353-61-709100, http://www.elsevier.com/locate/chemphyslip, http://www.elsevier.nl. Eds. F Paltauf, H H O Schmid. R&P Annette Moloney. **Subscr. in Australasia and the Far East to:** Elsevier Science (Singapore) Pte Ltd, No.1 Temasek Ave, 17-01 Millenia Tower, Singapore 039192, Singapore. TEL 65-434-3727, FAX 65-337-2230, asiainfo@elsevier.com.sg; **Subscr. in the Americas to:** Elsevier Science, PO Box 945, New York, NY 10159-0945. TEL 212-633-3730, FAX 212-633-3680, usinfo-f@elsevier.com; **Subscr. to:** Elsevier Science Inc - Japan Regional Office, 9-15 Higashi-Azabu 1-chome, Minato-ku, Tokyo 106-0044, Japan. TEL 81-3-5561-5033, FAX 81-3-5561-5047, info@elsevier.co.jp. **Subscr. to:** Elsevier Science BV, PO Box 211, Amsterdam 1000 AE, Netherlands. TEL 31-20-485-3757, FAX 31-20-485-3432, nlinfo-f@elsevier.nl.

572 AUT ISSN 1608-2265
▼ **CHEMOTAXIS AND MIGRATION.** Text in English. 2000. q. USD 75 domestic; USD 115 foreign; USD 35 newsstand/cover (effective 2001). adv. back issues avail. *Refereed.* **Document type:** *Journal, Academic/Scholarly.* **Description:** Publishes articles, case reports, reviews, and letters on improving communications in understanding the multidisciplinary fields of chemotaxis, cell locomotion, and migration.
Related titles: Online - full text ed.
Published by: V I C E R Publishing, PO Box 14, Vienna A-1097, Austria. TEL 43-676-9568085, FAX 43-676-9568086, vicer@vicer.org, http://www.vicer.org. Ed., R&P Roland Hofbauer. adv.: B&W page USD 1,700, color page USD 2,200. Circ: 1,000 (paid and controlled).

572.8 USA ISSN 0899-0042
QP517.C57 CODEN: CHRLEP
CHIRALITY; the pharmacological, biological, and chemical consequences of molecular asymmetry. Text in English. 1989. 9/yr. USD 1,545 in United States; USD 1,645 in Canada & Mexico; USD 1,730 elsewhere; USD 1,623 combined subscription in United States for print and online eds.; USD 1,723 combined subscription in Canada & Mexico for print and online eds.; USD 1,808 combined subscription elsewhere for print and online eds. (effective 2002). adv. bk.rev. back issues avail. *Refereed.* **Document type:** *Academic/Scholarly.* **Description:** Devoted to molecular asymmetry and its relevance in biological or chemical processes.
Related titles: Microform ed.: (from PQC); Online - full text ed.: ISSN 1520-636X. USD 1,545 in United States; USD 1,545 in Canada & Mexico; USD 1,545 elsewhere (effective 2002) (from EBSCO Publishing, Wiley InterScience, Institute for Scientific Information).

Indexed: ASCA, Anal.Abstr., Aqua.Sci.& Fish.Abstr., Chem.Abstr., Chem.Cit.Ind., Chem.Indus.Notes, Chem.Titles, Chromat.Abstr., Curr.Cont., Environ.Sci.Poll.Mgmt., INIS Atomind., Ind.Med. (1989-), Inpharma, Mass Spectr.Bull., Pharm.&Out.News, Pollut.Abstr., RCI, Reac., Ref.Zh., Sci.Cit.Ind., Sugar Ind.Abstr., Tox.Abstr.
—BLDSC (3181.124450), CASDDS, CISTI, EMDOCS, GNLM, IDS, ingenta. **CCC.**
Published by: John Wiley & Sons, Inc., Journals (Subsidiary of: Wiley InterScience), 605 Third Ave, New York, NY 10158. TEL 212-850-6645, FAX 212-850-6021, subinfo@wiley.com, uscs-wis@wiley.com, http://www.interscience.wiley.com/jpages/0899-0042/, http://www.wiley.com. Eds. Daniel W Armstrong, William F Trager. adv.: B&W page GBP 640, color page GBP 1,515; trim 210 x 279. Circ: 550. **Subscr. outside the Americas to:** John Wiley & Sons Ltd., Baffins Ln, Chichester, Sussex PO19 IUD, United Kingdom. TEL 44-1243-779777, FAX 44-1243-843232, cs-journals@wiley.co.uk, http://www.wiley.co.uk.

CHOLESTEROL & LIPOPROTEINS. see *BIOLOGY—Abstracting, Bibliographies, Statistics*

572 USA ISSN 0009-9120
RB112.5 CODEN: CLBIAS
CLINICAL BIOCHEMISTRY. Text in English, French. 1967. 8/yr. EUR 420 in Europe to institutions; JPY 55,700 in Japan to institutions; USD 470 elsewhere to institutions (effective 2002). adv. charts, illus, stat. back issues avail. *Refereed.* **Document type:** *Journal, Academic/Scholarly.* **Description:** Publishes articles relating to the applications of molecular biology, biochemistry, chemistry and immunology to clinical investigation and to the diagnosis, therapy, and monitoring of human diseases.
Related titles: Microfilm ed.: (from PQC); Online - full text ed.: (from ingenta, Swets Blackwell, ScienceDirect, Institute for Scientific Information).
Indexed: Agri.& Environ.Biotech.Abstr. (coverage dropped), Anal.Abstr., BBCI, Biol.Abstr., Chem.Abstr., Chem.Indus.Notes, Chem.Titles, Compumath, Curr.Adv.Biochem., Curr.Cont., Dairy Sci.Abstr., Derwent Biotech.Abstr., Excerp.Med., Helminthol.Abstr., INIS Atomind., Ind.Med. (1967-), Ind.Sci.Rev., Inpharma, Int.Abstr.Biol.Sci., Mass Spectr.Bull., Nutr.Abstr., Pharm.&Out.News, Reac., Rev.Plant Path., Sci.Cit.Ind., Sugar Ind.Abstr.
—BLDSC (3286.262000), ADONIS, CASDDS, CISTI, EMDOCS, GNLM, IDS, ingenta, KNAW, Linda Hall. **CCC.**
Published by: (Canadian Society of Clinical Chemists CAN), Elsevier Science, Box 945, New York, NY 10159-0945. TEL 212-989-5800, FAX 212-633-3990, usinfo-f@elsevier.com, http://www.elsevier.nl/locate/clinbiochem, http://www.elsevier.com. Eds. Khosrow Adeli, M Oellerich. Circ: 1,500. **Subscr. in Australasia and the Far East to:** Elsevier Science (Singapore) Pte Ltd, No.1 Temasek Ave, 17-01 Millenia Tower, Singapore 039192, Singapore. TEL 65-434-3727, FAX 65-337-2230; **Subscr. in Japan to:** Elsevier Science Inc - Japan Regional Office, 9-15 Higashi-Azabu 1-chome, Minato-ku, Tokyo 106-0044, Japan. TEL 81-3-5561-5033, FAX 81-3-5561-5047; **Subscr. outside the Americas to:** Elsevier Science BV, PO Box 211, Amsterdam 1000 AE, Netherlands. TEL 31-20-485-3757, FAX 31-20-485-3432. **Co-sponsor:** National Academy of Biochemistry.

572.7 CHE ISSN 0892-2187
CODEN: CCECEY
CLINICAL CHEMISTRY AND ENZYMOLOGY COMMUNICATIONS. Text in English. 1988. 6/yr. USD 590 to institutions; USD 920 to corporations (effective 1999). *Refereed.* **Document type:** *Academic/Scholarly.*
Related titles: CD-ROM ed.; Microform ed.; Online - full text ed.
Indexed: Eng.Ind., Environ.Sci.Poll.Mgmt., Int.Abstr.Biol.Sci., Pollut.Abstr.
—CISTI, Ei, EMDOCS, GNLM, ingenta. **CCC.**
Published by: Gordon and Breach - Harwood Academic (Subsidiary of: Taylor & Francis Group), PO Box 531, Lausanne 1000, Switzerland. http://www.gbhap.com/Clinical_Chemistry_Enzymology_Communications/. Ed. Giorgio Federici. **Subscr. addr. in US:** International Publishers Direct, PO Box 32160, Newark, NJ 07102. FAX 215-750-6343.

572 DEU ISSN 1434-6621
RB40.A1 CODEN: CCLMFW
CLINICAL CHEMISTRY AND LABORATORY MEDICINE. Text in English, French, German. 1963. m. EUR 814.85 domestic; EUR 821 foreign; EUR 748 online ed. only (effective 2002). adv. bk.rev. charts, illus. index. *Refereed.* **Document type:** *Journal, Academic/Scholarly.*
Former titles (until 1998): European Journal of Clinical Chemistry and Clinical Biochemistry (0939-4974); (until 1991): Journal of Clinical Chemistry and Clinical Biochemistry (0340-076X); Zeitschrift fuer Klinische Chemie und Klinische Biochemie (0044-2933)
Related titles: Online - full text ed.: (from EBSCO Publishing, O C L C Online Computer Library Center, Inc., Swets Blackwell, Institute for Scientific Information).
Indexed: ASCA, Anal.Abstr., BBCI, Biol.Abstr., Chem.Abstr., Curr.Adv.Biochem., Curr.Cont., Dairy Sci.Abstr., Dent.Ind., Excerp.Med., Helminthol.Abstr., INIS Atomind., Ind.Med. (1998-), Ind.Sci.Rev., Ind.Vet., Inpharma, Int.Abstr.Biol.Sci., Nutr.Abstr., Protozool.Abstr., Reac., Rev.Med.& Vet.Mycol., Sci.Cit.Ind.
—BLDSC (3286.268100), CASDDS, CINDOC, CISTI, EMDOCS, GNLM, IDS, Infotrieve, ingenta, KNAW, Linda Hall. **CCC.**
Published by: (Deutsche Gesellschaft fuer Klinische Chemie), Walter de Gruyter und Co., Genthiner Str 13, Berlin 10785, Germany. TEL 49-30-26005-0, FAX 49-30-26005-251, wdg-info@degruyter.de, http://www.degruyter.de. Ed. Gerard Siest. adv.: B&W page DEM 1,290; trim 180 x 264. Circ: 2,000 (paid and controlled).

573.84 GBR ISSN 0885-7431
CLINICAL NEUROCHEMISTRY. Text in English. 1986. irreg. **Document type:** *Monographic series, Academic/Scholarly.*
—CISTI.
Published by: Academic Press (Subsidiary of: Harcourt Publishers Ltd.), 24 Oval Rd, London NW1 7DX, United Kingdom. TEL 44-20-7267-4466, FAX 44-20-7482-2293.

572 USA ISSN 0366-5887
CODEN: CGBCA9
COLLOQUIUM MOSBACH. Variant title: Gesellschaft fuer Biologische Chemie, Mosbach. Colloquium. Text in English, French, German. 1951. irreg., latest vol.45, 1995. price varies. reprint service avail. from ISI. **Document type:** *Academic/Scholarly.*
Formerly: Gesellschaft fuer Physiologische Chemie, Mosbach. Colloquium (0072-4246)
Indexed: Biol.Abstr.
—CASDDS, GNLM, Infotrieve, KNAW. **CCC.**
Published by: Springer-Verlag, Journals (Subsidiary of: BertelsmannSpringer), 175 Fifth Ave, New York, NY 10010. TEL 212-460-1500, FAX 212-473-6272.

COMPARATIVE BIOCHEMISTRY AND PHYSIOLOGY. PART A: MOLECULAR & INTEGRATIVE PHYSIOLOGY. see *BIOLOGY—Physiology*

572 USA ISSN 1096-4959
QP33 CODEN: CBPBB8
COMPARATIVE BIOCHEMISTRY AND PHYSIOLOGY. PART B: BIOCHEMISTRY & MOLECULAR BIOLOGY. Text and summaries in English, French, German. 1961. m. EUR 3,811 in Europe to institutions; JPY 506,100 in Japan to institutions; USD 4,262 elsewhere to institutions (effective 2002). adv. bk.rev. bibl, charts, illus. back issues avail. *Refereed.* **Document type:** *Journal, Academic/Scholarly.* **Description:** Original research on the biochemistry and physiology of animals.
Formerly (until 1994): Comparative Biochemistry and Physiology. Part B: Comparative Biochemistry (0305-0491)
Related titles: Microfiche ed.: (from MIM); Microfilm ed.: (from PQC); Online - full text ed.: (from ingenta, Swets Blackwell, ScienceDirect, Institute for Scientific Information).
Indexed: ASCA, AgBiotech, Agricola, Anim.Behav.Abstr., Anim.Breed.Abstr., Apic.Abstr., Aqua.Sci.& Fish.Abstr., Aquacult.Abstr., BBCI, Bio-Contr.News & Info., Biodet.Abstr., Biol.Abstr., Cal.Tiss.Abstr., Chem.Abstr., Chem.Cit.Ind., Chemorec.Abstr., Curr.Adv.Biochem., Curr.Adv.Cell & Devel.Biol., Curr.Adv.Ecol.Sci., Curr.Adv.Gen.& Molec.Biol., Curr.Cont., Dairy Sci.Abstr., Deep Sea Res.& Oceanogr.Abstr., Dent.Ind., Entomol.Abstr., Environ.Sci.Poll.Mgmt., Excerp.Med., Genet.Abstr., GeoRef, Helminthol.Abstr., Hort.Abstr., Hum.Gen.Abstr., INIS Atomind., Ind.Med. (1994-), Ind.Sci.Rev., Ind.Vet., Int.Abstr.Biol.Sci., Maize Abstr., Mass Spectr.Bull., Neurosci.Abstr. (coverage dropped), Neurosci.Cit.Ind., Nuc.Acids Abstr., Nutr.Abstr., Ocean.Abstr., Pig News & Info., Pollut.Abstr., Postharvest, Poult.Abstr., Protozool.Abstr., Rev.Appl.Entomol., Rev.Arom.& Med.Plants, Rev.Med.& Vet.Mycol., Rev.Plant Path., SSCI (coverage dropped), Sci.Cit.Ind., Small Anim.Abstr., Soils & Fert., Soyabean Abstr., Sport Fish.Abstr., Vet.Bull., Weed Abstr., Wild.Rev., Zoo.Rec.
—BLDSC (3363.752000), ADONIS, CASDDS, CISTI, EMDOCS, IDS, ingenta. **CCC.**
Published by: Elsevier Science, Box 945, New York, NY 10159-0945. TEL 212-989-5800, FAX 212-633-3990, usinfo-f@elsevier.com, http://www.elsevier.com/locate/cbpb. Eds. Peter W Hochachka, Thomas P Mommsen. adv.: B&W page USD 550, color page USD 1,350. Circ: 2,000. **Subscr. in Australasia and the Far East to:** Elsevier Science (Singapore) Pte Ltd, No.1 Temasek Ave, 17-01 Millenia Tower, Singapore 039192, Singapore. TEL 65-434-3727, FAX 65-337-2230; **Subscr. in Japan to:** Elsevier Science Inc - Japan Regional Office, 9-15 Higashi-Azabu 1-chome, Minato-ku, Tokyo 106-0044, Japan. TEL 81-3-5561-5033, FAX 81-3-5561-5047; **Subscr. outside the Americas to:** Elsevier Science BV, PO Box 211, Amsterdam 1000 AE, Netherlands. TEL 31-20-485-3757, FAX 31-20-485-3432.

615.1 USA ISSN 1532-0456
QP33 CODEN: CBPCEE
COMPARATIVE BIOCHEMISTRY AND PHYSIOLOGY. TOXICOLOGY & PHARMACOLOGY. Text in English, French. 1975. m. EUR 2,776 in Europe to institutions; JPY 368,700 in Japan to institutions; USD 3,105 elsewhere to institutions (effective 2002). adv. bk.rev. abstr, charts, illus. index. back issues avail. *Refereed.* **Document type:** *Academic/Scholarly.* **Description:** Publishes research studying the actions of drugs and chemicals on cells, tissues, and whole animals.
Former titles (until 2000): Comparative Biochemistry and Physiology. Part C: Pharmacology, Toxicology & Endocrinology (1367-8280); (until 1994): Comparative Biochemistry and Physiology. Part C: Comparative Pharmacology & Toxicology (0742-8413); (until 1993): Comparative Biochemistry and Physiology. Part C: Comparative Pharmacology (0306-4492); Supersedes in part: Comparative Biochemistry and Physiology (0010-406X)
Related titles: Microfiche ed.: (from MIM); Microfilm ed.: (from PQC); Online - full text ed.: (from ingenta, Swets Blackwell, ScienceDirect, Institute for Scientific Information).
Indexed: ASCA, AgBiotech, Anim.Behav.Abstr., Anim.Breed.Abstr., Apic.Abstr., Aqua.Sci.& Fish.Abstr., BBCI, Biol.Abstr., Cal.Tiss.Abstr., Chem.Abstr., Chemorec.Abstr., Curr.Adv.Ecol.Sci., Curr.Cont., Dairy Sci.Abstr., Deep Sea Res.& Oceanogr.Abstr., Entomol.Abstr., Environ.Sci.Poll.Mgmt., Excerp.Med., Helminthol.Abstr., INIS Atomind., Ind.Med. (coverage dropped), Ind.Sci.Rev., Ind.Vet., Int.Abstr.Biol.Sci., Neurosci.Abstr. (coverage dropped), Neurosci.Cit.Ind., Nutr.Abstr., Ocean.Abstr., Pig News & Info., Poult.Abstr., Protozool.Abstr., Rev.Appl.Entomol., Rev.Arom.& Med.Plants, Rev.Med.& Vet.Mycol., Rev.Plant Path., Sci.Cit.Ind., Sel.Water Res.Abstr., Soils & Fert., Soyabean Abstr., Sport Fish.Abstr., Sugar Ind.Abstr., Trop.Dis.Bull., Vet.Bull., Weed Abstr., Wild.Rev., Zoo.Rec.
—BLDSC (3363.752500), ADONIS, CASDDS, CISTI, EMDOCS, IDS, ingenta, Linda Hall. **CCC.**
Published by: Elsevier Science, 655 Ave of the Americas, New York, NY 10010. TEL 212-989-5800, FAX 212-633-3990, usinfo-f@elsevier.com, http://www.elsevier.com/locate/cbpc. Eds. Peter W Hochachka, Thomas P Mommsen. adv.: B&W page USD 550, color page USD 1,350. Circ: 1,500. **Subscr. in Australasia and the Far East to:** Elsevier Science (Singapore) Pte Ltd, No.1 Temasek Ave, 17-01 Millenia Tower, Singapore 039192, Singapore. TEL 65-434-3727; **Subscr. outside the Americas to:** Elsevier Science BV, PO Box 211, Amsterdam 1000 AE, Netherlands. TEL 31-20-485-3757.

572 NLD ISSN 0069-8032
COMPREHENSIVE BIOCHEMISTRY. Text in Dutch. 1962. irreg., latest vol.37, 1990. price varies. *Refereed.* **Document type:** *Monographic series.*
Indexed: Ind.Sci.Rev., Sci.Cit.Ind. (coverage dropped).
—BLDSC (3366.300000), Infotrieve. **CCC.**
Published by: Elsevier Science BV, PO Box 211, Amsterdam 1000 AE, Netherlands. TEL 31-20-485-3757, 31-20-485-3911, FAX 31-20-485-3432, 31-20-485-3598, nlinfo-f@elsevier.nl; usinfo-f@elsevier.com; forinfo-kyf04035@niftyserve.or.jp, http://www.elsevier.nl/. Eds. E H Stotz, M Florkin. **Subscr. in Australasia and the Far East to:** Elsevier Science (Singapore) Pte Ltd, No.1 Temasek Ave, 17-01 Millenia Tower, Singapore 039192, Singapore. TEL 65-434-3727, FAX 65-337-2230, asiainfo@elsevier.com.sg; **Subscr. in Japan to:** Elsevier Science Inc - Japan Regional Office, 9-15 Higashi-Azabu 1-chome, Minato-ku, Tokyo 106-0044, Japan. TEL 81-3-5561-5033, FAX 81-3-5561-5047, info@elsevier.co.jp; **Subscr. in the Americas to:** Elsevier Science, PO Box 945, New York, NY 10159-0945. TEL 212-633-3730, 888-437-4636, FAX 212-633-3680, usinfo-f@elsevier.com, http://www.elsevier.com

B

572 CHL ISSN 0069-8784
CONFERENCIAS DE BIOQUIMICA*. Text in Spanish. 1967. a. **Document type:** *Proceedings, Academic/Scholarly.*
Published by: Universidad de Chile, Instituto de Quimica Fisiologica y Patologica, Diag. Paraguay, 265, Torre 15, Santiago, Chile.

612.015 572.8 USA
CONTEMPORARY BIOMEDICINE. Text in English. 1979. irreg., latest 1997. price varies. illus. back issues avail. *Refereed.* **Document type:** *Monographic series, Academic/Scholarly.* **Description:** Discusses scientific and medical research in biological chemistry.
Formerly (until 1995): Contemporary Issues in Biomedicine, Ethics, and Society
Published by: Humana Press Inc., 999 Riverview Dr, Ste 208, Totowa, NJ 07512. TEL 973-256-1699, FAX 973-256-8431, humana@humanapr.com, http://humanapress.com. R&P Richard Hruska.

CONTEMPORARY NEUROSCIENCE. see *MEDICAL SCIENCES—Psychiatry And Neurology*

572 USA ISSN 1040-9238
QP501 CODEN: CRBBEJ
CRITICAL REVIEWS IN BIOCHEMISTRY AND MOLECULAR BIOLOGY. Text in English. 1971. bi-m. USD 495 (effective 1998). bibl, charts, illus. back issues avail. *Refereed.* **Document type:** *Academic/Scholarly.* **Description:** Includes, in each issue, several critical surveys on specific topics of current interest.
Formerly: C R C Critical Reviews in Biochemistry (0045-6411)
Related titles: Online - full text ed.: (from O C L C Online Computer Library Center, Inc., Swets Blackwell, ScienceDirect, Institute for Scientific Information).
Indexed: ASCA, Agricola, Aqua.Sci.& Fish.Abstr., BBCI, Biol.Abstr., Chem.Abstr., Chem.Indus.Notes, Chem.Titles, Curr.Adv.Ecol.Sci., Curr.Cont., Derwent Biotech.Abstr., Food Sci.& Tech.Abstr., Genet.Abstr., Helminthol.Abstr., Hum.Gen.Abstr., INIS Atomind., Ind.Med. (1989-), Ind.Sci.Rev., Inpharma, Int.Abstr.Biol.Sci., Neurosci.Abstr., Nuc.Acids Abstr., Nutr.Abstr., Reac., Sci.Cit.Ind.
—BLDSC (3487.471500), ADONIS, CASDDS, CISTI, EMDOCS, GNLM, IDS, ingenta, Linda Hall. **CCC.**
Published by: C R C Press, LLC, 2000 Corporate Blvd, N W, Boca Raton, FL 33431. TEL 561-994-0555, 800-272-7737, FAX 561-998-9784. Ed. Gerald D Fasman. Circ: 570.

CURRENT ADVANCES IN ENDOCRINOLOGY & METABOLISM. see *MEDICAL SCIENCES—Endocrinology*

CURRENT ADVANCES IN GENETICS AND MOLECULAR BIOLOGY. see *BIOLOGY—Abstracting, Bibliographies, Statistics*

CURRENT ADVANCES IN PROTEIN BIOCHEMISTRY. see *BIOLOGY—Abstracting, Bibliographies, Statistics*

572.8 USA ISSN 1063-8806
CODEN: CCCBEL
CURRENT COMMUNICATIONS IN CELL AND MOLECULAR BIOLOGY SERIES. Text in English. 1983. irreg. price varies. reprints avail. **Document type:** *Monographic series.* **Description:** Examines topics on which the impact of the techniques and concepts of molecular and cell biology is particularly evident.
Formerly (until 1990): Current Communications in Molecular Biology
Indexed: Chem.Abstr., Chem.Indus.Notes, Chem.Titles.
—CASDDS, CISTI, KNAW. **CCC.**
Published by: Cold Spring Harbor Laboratory Press, Publications Department, 10 Skyline Dr, Plainview, NY 11803. TEL 800-843-4388, FAX 516-349-1946, cshpress@cshl.org, http://www.cshl.org. Eds. Jan Witkowski, John Inglis.

572 GBR ISSN 1467-3037
CURRENT ISSUES IN MOLECULAR BIOLOGY. (Online edition available from January 2002.) Text in English. 1998. q. GBP 75, USD 150 to individuals; GBP 130, USD 260 to institutions (effective 2002). back issues avail. *Refereed.* **Document type:** *Academic/Scholarly.*
Related titles: Online - full content ed.: ISSN 1467-3045. 2002. GBP 40, USD 80 to individuals; GBP 80, USD 160 to institutions (effective 2002).
Indexed: AgBiotech, Agri.& Environ.Biotech.Abstr., Aqua.Sci.& Fish.Abstr., Biotech.& Bioeng.Abstr., Dairy Sci.Abstr., Environ.Sci.Poll.Mgmt., Genet.Abstr., Ind.Vet., Med.& Pharm.Biotech.Abstr., Plant Breed.Abstr., Rev.Plant Path., Vet.Bull., Virol.Abstr.
—BLDSC (3499.075250).
Published by: Caister Academic Press, 32 Hewitts Ln, Wymondham, Norfolk NR18 0JA, United Kingdom. TEL 44-870-321-3681, FAX 44-870-321-3692, mail@caister.com, http://www.cimb.org/, http://www.horizonpress.com/.

572 GBR ISSN 0959-440X
QH506 CODEN: COSBEF
CURRENT OPINION IN STRUCTURAL BIOLOGY. Text in English. 1991. bi-m. EUR 170 in Europe to individuals; JPY 20,600 in Japan to individuals; USD 184 elsewhere to individuals; EUR 213 in Europe to qualified personnel; JPY 25,700 in Japan to qualified personnel; USD 230 domestic to qualified personnel; EUR 1,015 in Europe to institutions; JPY 140,800 in Japan to institutions; USD 1,135 elsewhere to institutions (effective 2002). adv. bibl, illus. back issues avail. *Refereed.* **Document type:** *Academic/Scholarly.* **Description:** Presents review articles, followed by annotated bibliographies of references consulted; includes a "Paper Alert" section, giving brief summaries of relevant papers recently published in other journals.
Related titles: CD-ROM ed.; Online - full text ed.: USD 227 in North America to individuals; USD 90 in North America to students (effective 1999 & 2000) (from EBSCO Publishing, ingenta, Swets Blackwell, ScienceDirect, Institute for Scientific Information).
Indexed: ASCA, Aqua.Sci.& Fish.Abstr., BBCI, Chem.Abstr., Chem.Cit.Ind., Chem.Indus.Notes, Chem.Titles, Curr.Cont., Environ.Sci.Poll.Mgmt., Excerp.Med. (1993-), Food Sci.& Tech.Abstr., Ind.Med. (1991-), Ind.Sci.Rev., Inpharma, Int.Abstr.Biol.Sci., Mass Spectr.Bull., Neurosci.Abstr., Nuc.Acids Abstr., Reac., Saf.Sci.Abstr., Sci.Cit.Ind.
—BLDSC (3500.779000), ADONIS, CASDDS, CISTI, EMDOCS, GNLM, IDS, Infotrieve, ingenta. **CCC.**
Published by: Elsevier Science Ltd., Elsevier Trends Journals, 68 Hills Rd, Cambridge CB2 1LA, United Kingdom. TEL 44-20-7611-4400, FAX 44-20-7611-4468, info@current-opinion.com, http://www.current-opinion.com, http://www.elsevier.nl. Eds. Andrew M Sugden, Rachel Page. Circ: 1,800. **Subscr. to:** TEL 44-1444-475650, FAX 44-1444-445423.

572 USA ISSN 1389-2037
▼ **CURRENT PROTEIN AND PEPTIDE SCIENCE.** Text in English. 2000 (Jun.). q. USD 110, USD 600 to institutions (effective 2000). adv. *Refereed.* **Document type:** *Academic/Scholarly.* **Description:** Features reviews in protein and peptide science and related areas.
Related titles: Online - full text ed.: (from Swets Blackwell).
Indexed: Med.& Pharm.Biotech.Abstr.
—BLDSC (3501.531000).
Published by: Bentham Science Publishers, 102 N.E. 2nd St, Mail Box 135, Boca Raton, FL 33432. FAX 561-393-7229, m.bentham@inter.nl.net. Ed. Ben M Dunn. Adv. contact Tom Lucas.

572 USA
CURRENT PROTOCOLS IN PROTEIN SCIENCE. Text in English. a., 2 base vols. plus q. updates (plus q. updates). USD 575 (effective 2001); USD 610 combined subscription for base vol. & update; USD 330 updates (effective 2002). **Document type:** *Monographic series, Academic/Scholarly.* **Description:** Covers both basic and advanced methods used in protein purification, characterization, and analysis.
Related titles: CD-ROM ed.: USD 565 (effective 2001); USD 595 combined subscription for base vol. & update; USD 325 renewals (effective 2002).
Published by: John Wiley & Sons, Inc., Journals (Subsidiary of: Wiley InterScience), 605 Third Ave, New York, NY 10158. TEL 212-850-6645, FAX 212-850-6021, subinfo@jwiley.com, uscs-wis@wiley.com, http://www.wiley.com. **Subscr. to:** John Wiley & Sons Ltd., Baffins Ln, Chichester, Sussex PO19 IUD, United Kingdom. TEL 44-1243-779777, FAX 44-1243-843232, cs-journals@wiley.co.uk.

572.65 GBR ISSN 1359-6101
QP552.G76 CODEN: CGFRFB
CYTOKINE AND GROWTH FACTOR REVIEWS. Text in English. 1989. q. EUR 106 in Europe to individuals (effective 2001); JPY 14,100 in Japan to individuals; USD 119 elsewhere to individuals; EUR 497 in Europe to institutions; JPY 65,900 in Japan to institutions; USD 555 elsewhere to institutions (effective 2002). abstr. back issues avail. *Refereed.* **Document type:** *Academic/Scholarly.* **Description:** Features reviews of current research and applications on cytokines, growth factors and related regulatory peptides.
Formerly (until vol.7): Progress in Growth Factor Research (0955-2235)
Related titles: Microfilm ed.: (from PQC); Online - full text ed.: (from ingenta, Swets Blackwell, ScienceDirect, Institute for Scientific Information).
Indexed: AIDS & Cancer Res., BBCI, Cal.Tiss.Abstr., Chem.Abstr., Chem.Indus.Notes, Chem.Titles, Chemorec.Abstr., Immun.Abstr., Ind.Med. (1996-), Int.Abstr.Biol.Sci., Neurosci.Abstr. (coverage dropped), Nuc.Acids Abstr., Oncog.G.F.Abstr.
—BLDSC (3506.778500), CASDDS, CISTI, GNLM, IDS, Infotrieve, ingenta, KNAW. **CCC.**
Published by: Pergamon (Subsidiary of: Elsevier Science), The Boulevard, Langford Ln, East Park, Kidlington, Oxford OXB 1GB, United Kingdom. FAX 44-1865-843010, http://www.elsevier.com/locate/cytogfr. Eds. J VilCaccaron, M Sporn. **Subscr. in Australasia and the Far East to:** Elsevier Science (Singapore) Pte Ltd, No.1 Temasek Ave, 17-01 Millenia Tower, Singapore 039192, Singapore. TEL 65-434-3727, FAX 65-337-2230; **Subscr. in the Americas to:** Elsevier Science, PO Box 945, New York, NY 10159-0945. TEL 212-633-3730, FAX 212-633-3680, usinfo-f@elsevier.com; **Subscr. to:** Elsevier Science BV, PO Box 211, Amsterdam 1000 AE, Netherlands. TEL 31-20-485-3757.

572.86 USA ISSN 1044-5498
QH442 CODEN: DCEBE8
D N A AND CELL BIOLOGY. Text in English. 1981. m. USD 299 domestic to individuals; USD 483 foreign to individuals; USD 359 domestic to individuals print and online eds. combined; USD 543 foreign to individuals print and online eds. combined; USD 1,137 domestic to institutions; USD 1,256 foreign to institutions; USD 1,364 domestic to institutions print and online eds. combined; USD 1,484 foreign to institutions print and online eds. combined (effective 2002). back issues avail.; reprints avail. *Refereed.* **Document type:** *Journal, Academic/Scholarly.* **Description:** Covers molecular immunology, molecular medicine, gene structure and function, genetic vaccines, cell cycle and apoptosis. Publishes papers relating to all aspects of biochemistry, cell and molecular biology, structural and disease related molecular science.
Former titles: D N A (0198-0238); Recombinant D N A
Related titles: Online - full text ed.: USD 299 to individuals; USD 1,137 to institutions (effective 2002) (from CatchWord Ltd., EBSCO Publishing, O C L C Online Computer Library Center, Inc., RoweCom Information Quest, Swets Blackwell, Institute for Scientific Information).
Indexed: AIDS & Cancer Res., ASCA, Abstr.Anthropol., AgBiotech, Agri.& Environ.Biotech.Abstr., Anim.Breed.Abstr., Aqua.Sci.& Fish.Abstr., BBCI, Biol.Abstr., Biotech.Cit.Ind., Chem.Abstr., Chem.Indus.Notes, Chem.Titles, Curr.Adv.Biochem., Curr.Adv.Ecol.Sci., Curr.Adv.Gen.& Molec.Biol., Curr.Biotech.Abstr., Curr.Cont., Dairy Sci.Abstr., Derwent Biotech.Abstr., Environ.Sci.Poll.Mgmt., Excerp.Med., Food Sci.& Tech.Abstr., Genet.Abstr., Helminthol.Abstr., Hum.Gen.Abstr., INIS Atomind., Immun.Abstr., Ind.Med. (1990-), Ind.Sci.Rev., Ind.Vet., Inpharma, Int.Abstr.Biol.Sci., Med.& Pharm.Biotech.Abstr., Microbiol.Abstr., Nuc.Acids Abstr., Oncog.G.F.Abstr., Reac., Sci.Cit.Ind., Telegen.
—BLDSC (3605.721420), ADONIS, CASDDS, CatchWord, CISTI, EMDOCS, GNLM, IDS, ingenta. **CCC.**
Published by: Mary Ann Liebert, Inc. Publishers, 2 Madison Ave, Larchmont, NY 10538. TEL 914—834-3100, FAX 914-834-1388, info@liebertpub.com, www.liebertpub.com/dna, http://www.liebertpub.com. Ed. Mark I Greene.

D N A PROBES. see *BIOLOGY—Abstracting, Bibliographies, Statistics*

572.86 CHE ISSN 1042-5179
QP624 CODEN: DNSEES
D N A SEQUENCE; the journal of DNA sequencing and mapping. Text in English. 1990. bi-m. GBP 116, USD 140, EUR 154 to individuals; GBP 475, USD 616, EUR 632 to institutions; GBP 777, USD 1,008, EUR 1,037 to corporations (effective 2002). *Refereed.* **Document type:** *Journal, Academic/Scholarly.* **Description:** Covers mapping data, full DNA sequences and their analyses, new sequencing procedures, computer methods to analyze sequences, and compilations of DNA and protein motifs.
Related titles: CD-ROM ed.; Microform ed.; Online - full text ed.: (from EBSCO Publishing, ingenta, Institute for Scientific Information, RoweCom Information Quest).
Indexed: ASCA, AgBiotech, Anim.Breed.Abstr., Bibl.Agri., Biotech.Cit.Ind., Curr.Cont., Dairy Sci.Abstr., Food Sci.& Tech.Abstr., Forest.Abstr., Helminthol.Abstr., Ind.Med. (1990-), Ind.Vet., Inpharma, Int.Abstr.Biol.Sci., Nutr.Abstr., Plant Breed.Abstr., Plant Grow.Reg.Abstr., Postharvest, Poult.Abstr., Protozool.Abstr., Reac., Rev.Appl.Entomol., Rev.Med.& Vet.Mycol., Rev.Plant Path., Rice Abstr., Sci.Cit.Ind., Vet.Bull., Weed Abstr.
—BLDSC (3605.723500), CISTI, EMDOCS, GNLM, Infotrieve, KNAW. **CCC.**

Published by: Gordon and Breach - Harwood Academic (Subsidiary of: Taylor & Francis Group), PO Box 531, Lausanne 1000, Switzerland. TEL 41-21-6411280, FAX 41-21-6411281, info@gbhap.com, http://www.gbhap.com/DNA_Sequence/. Ed. Bart Barrell. **Subscr. addr. in US:** International Publishers Direct, PO Box 32160, Newark, NJ 07102. FAX 215-750-6343.

572 NLD ISSN 0167-4978
CODEN: DLCBDQ
DEVELOPMENTS IN CLINICAL BIOCHEMISTRY. Text in English. 1980. irreg. price varies. *Refereed.* **Document type:** *Monographic series.*
—CASDDS, CISTI.
Published by: (Commission of the European Communities BEL), Kluwer Academic Publishers Group (Subsidiary of: Wolters Kluwer N.V.), Spuiboulevard 50, PO Box 17, Dordrecht 3300 AA, Netherlands. FAX 31-78-639-2254, services@wkap.nl, http://www.wkap.nl. **Dist. by:** Journals Department, PO Box 322, Dordrecht 3300 AH, Netherlands. FAX 31-78-654-6474.

572.8 NLD ISSN 0167-9023
CODEN: DMCBDX
DEVELOPMENTS IN MOLECULAR AND CELLULAR BIOCHEMISTRY. Text in English. 1981. irreg., latest vol.11, 1993. price varies. *Refereed.* **Document type:** *Monographic series.*
Indexed: Agri.& Environ.Biotech.Abstr. (coverage dropped), Biol.Abstr., Curr.Adv.Cancer Res., Protozool.Abstr.
—CISTI. **CCC.**
Published by: Kluwer Academic Publishers Group (Subsidiary of: Wolters Kluwer N.V.), Spuiboulevard 50, PO Box 17, Dordrecht 3300 AA, Netherlands. FAX 31-78-639-2254, services@wkap.nl, http://www.wkap.nl. **Dist. by:** Journals Department, PO Box 322, Dordrecht 3300 AH, Netherlands. FAX 31-78-654-6474.

572.014 MEX
DICCIONARIO DE ESPECIALIDADES BIOQUIMICAS. Text in Spanish. 1984. a. MXP 200, USD 100. adv. bk.rev.
Published by: Ediciones P L M S.A. de C.V., San BERNADINO 17, Col del Valle, Mexico City, DF 03100, Mexico. TEL 52-5-6871766, FAX 52-5-5365027. Ed. Federico Garcia Ortega. Circ: 6,000.

DOJIN NYUSU/DOJIN NEWS. see *CHEMISTRY—Analytical Chemistry*

DRUG TARGETING. see *PHARMACY AND PHARMACOLOGY—Abstracting, Bibliographies, Statistics*

572 GBR ISSN 0261-4189
QH506 CODEN: EMJODG
THE E M B O JOURNAL. Text in English. 1982. s-m. GBP 140, USD 240 to individuals; GBP 820, USD 1,330 to institutions (effective 2002). adv. bk.rev. illus. index. back issues avail.; reprint service avail. from SWZ. *Refereed.* **Document type:** *Journal, Academic/Scholarly.* **Description:** Covers all areas of molecular biology, including immunology, cell biology, molecular genetics, expression, neurobiology, virology, and plant science.
Related titles: Online - full text ed.: ISSN 1460-2075. GBP 126, USD 216 to individuals Online only; GBP 738, USD 1,197 to institutions Online only (effective 2002) (from HighWire Pr., Ovid Technologies, Inc., EBSCO Publishing, O C L C Online Computer Library Center, Inc., RoweCom Information Quest, ingenta, Swets Blackwell, Institute for Scientific Information).
Indexed: AIDS & Cancer Res., ASCA, AgBiotech, Agri.& Environ.Biotech.Abstr., Agricola, Anim.Breed.Abstr., Aqua.Sci.& Fish.Abstr., BBCI, Bibl.Agri., Biol.& Agr.Ind. (Jan.1990-), Biotech.Cit.Ind., Cal.Tiss.Abstr. (coverage dropped), Chem.Abstr., Chem.Cit.Ind., Chem.Indus.Notes, Chem.Titles, Chemorec.Abstr., Crop Physiol.Abstr., Curr.Adv.Biochem., Curr.Adv.Cancer Res., Curr.Adv.Cell & Devel.Biol., Curr.Adv.Ecol.Sci., Curr.Adv.Gen.& Molec.Biol., Curr.Biotech.Abstr., Curr.Cont., Dairy Sci.Abstr., Derwent Biotech.Abstr., Entomol.Abstr. (coverage dropped), Environ.Sci.Poll.Mgmt., Field Crop Abstr., Food Sci.& Tech.Abstr., Genet.Abstr., Helminthol.Abstr., Hort.Abstr., Hum.Gen.Abstr., INIS Atomind., Immun.Abstr., Ind.Med. (1982-), Ind.Vet., Inpharma, Int.Abstr.Biol.Sci., Maize Abstr., Med.& Pharm.Biotech.Abstr., Microbiol.Abstr., Neurosci.Abstr., Neurosci.Cit.Ind., Nuc.Acids Abstr., Nutr.Abstr., Oncog.G.F.Abstr., Plant Breed.Abstr., Plant Grow.Reg.Abstr., Potato Abstr., Poult.Abstr., Protozool.Abstr., Reac., Ref.Zh., Rev.Appl.Entomol., Rev.Med.& Vet.Mycol., Rev.Plant Path., Rice Abstr., Sci.Cit.Ind., Seed Abstr., Soils & Fert., Soyabean Abstr., Telegen, Tox.Abstr. (coverage dropped), Triticale Abstr., Vet.Bull., Virol.Abstr. (coverage dropped), Weed Abstr., Zoo.Rec.
—BLDSC (3733.085000), CASDDS, CISTI, EMDOCS, GNLM, IDS, ingenta, Linda Hall. **CCC.**
Published by: (European Molecular Biology Organization), Oxford University Press, Academic Division, Great Clarendon St, Oxford OX2 6DP, United Kingdom. TEL 44-1865-267907, FAX 44-1865-267835, jnl.info@oup.co.uk, http://www.emboj.org/, http://www.oup.co.uk/journals. Eds. Dr. Astrid Lunkes, Herbert Jackle. Pub. David Prosser. R&P Fionna Willis. adv.: page GBP 550, page USD 990. Circ: 4,200. **U.S. subscr. to:** Oxford University Press, Journals, 2001 Evans Rd, Cary, NC 27513. TEL 800-852-7323, FAX 919-677-1714, jnlorders@oup-usa.org; **Subscr. to:** Journals Marketing, Great Clarendon St, Oxford OX2 6DP, United Kingdom.

ELECTRONIC JOURNAL OF BIOTECHNOLOGY. see *BIOLOGY—Biotechnology*

572 CHE
EMERGING BIOCHEMICAL AND BIOPHYSICAL TECHNIQUES. Text in English. 1994. irreg. CHF 188 (effective 2000). **Document type:** *Monographic series, Academic/Scholarly.*
Published by: Birkhaeuser Verlag AG (Subsidiary of: BertelsmannSpringer), Klosterberg, Postfach 133, Basel 4010, Switzerland. TEL 41-61-2050707, FAX 41-61-2050792, orders@birkhauser.ch, http://www.birkhauser.ch. Eds. T M Laue, T M Schuster.

572.43 DEU ISSN 0013-7472
ENERGY AND CHARACTER* ; journal of bio-energetic research. Text in German. 1970. 3/yr. adv. bk.rev. index.
Related titles: Microfiche ed.: 1970.
Indexed: Psychol.Abstr., e-psyche.
—BLDSC (3747.500000).
Published by: Deutsches Institut fuer Biosynthese, Hakenweg 17, Jaderberg 26349, Germany. Ed. Andreas Wehowsky. Circ: 1,000.

ENTREZ DOCUMENT RETRIEVAL SYSTEM. see *BIOLOGY—Abstracting, Bibliographies, Statistics*

ENVIRONMENTAL AND MOLECULAR MUTAGENESIS. SUPPLEMENT. see *BIOLOGY—Genetics*

ENVIRONMENTAL TOXICOLOGY AND CHEMISTRY. see *ENVIRONMENTAL STUDIES—Toxicology And Environmental Safety*

572.7 USA ISSN 0094-8500
TP248.E5 CODEN: ENENDT
ENZYME ENGINEERING. Text in English. irreg., latest vol.13, 1996. *Refereed.*
Indexed: Curr.Biotech.Abstr.
—CASDDS, CISTI, Infotrieve. **CCC.**
Published by: New York Academy of Sciences, 2 E 63rd St, New York, NY 10021. TEL 212-838-0230.

572 GBR ISSN 0071-1365
QH345 CODEN: ESBIAV
ESSAYS IN BIOCHEMISTRY. Text in English. 1965. a. GBP 19, USD 29.95 (effective 2002). reprint service avail. from ISI. *Refereed.* **Document type:** *Academic/Scholarly.*
Related titles: Online - full text ed.: (from Institute for Scientific Information).
Indexed: ASCA, Anim.Breed.Abstr., BBCI, Biol.Abstr., Chem.Abstr., Chem.Indus.Notes, Chem.Titles, Curr.Adv.Ecol.Sci., Ind.Med. (1965-), Ind.Sci.Rev., Nutr.Abstr., Sci.Cit.Ind.
—BLDSC (3811.676000), CASDDS, CISTI, GNLM, ingenta, Linda Hall. **CCC.**
Published by: (Biochemical Society), Portland Press Ltd., 59 Portland Pl, London W1N 3AJ, United Kingdom. TEL 44-20-7580-5530, FAX 44-20-7323-1136, sales@portland-service.com, http://www.portlsndpress.com/bst/default.htm, http://www.portlandpress.com/bst/default.htm. Ed. S J Higgins. R&P Adam Marshall. **Subscr. to:** Commerce Way, Colchester, Essex CO2 8HP, United Kingdom. TEL 44-1206-796351, FAX 44-1206-799331.

EUROPEAN BIOPHARMACEUTICAL REVIEW. see *PHARMACY AND PHARMACOLOGY*

572 GBR ISSN 0014-2956
QP501 CODEN: EJBCAI
EUROPEAN JOURNAL OF BIOCHEMISTRY; the FEBS journal. Text in English. 1967. fortn., latest vol.269, 2002. GBP 1,617 in Europe; USD 2,562 in North America; GBP 1,779 elsewhere (effective 2002). adv. bibl, charts, illus. index. back issues avail.; reprint service avail. from ISI. *Refereed.* **Document type:** *Academic/Scholarly.* **Description:** Covers the entire basic biomedical sciences community, including molecular genetics, enzymology, physical and inorganic chemistry, metabolic regulation, molecular neurobiology, and developmental biochemistry and immunology.
Related titles: Microform ed.: (from PQC); Online - full text ed.: ISSN 1432-1033. GBP 1,456 in Europe; USD 2,306 in North America; GBP 1,456 elsewhere (effective 2002) (from HighWire Pr., EBSCO Publishing, O C L C Online Computer Library Center, Inc., RoweCom Information Quest, ingenta, Munksgaard & Blackwell Science's Synergy, Swets Blackwell, Institute for Scientific Information).
Indexed: ASCA, AgBiotech, Agri.& Environ.Biotech.Abstr. (coverage dropped), Agricola, Anim.Breed.Abstr., Apic.Abstr., Aqua.Sci.& Fish.Abstr., BBCI, Bibl.Agri., Biol.& Agr.Ind. (Jan.1996-), Biol.Abstr., Cal.Tiss.Abstr. (coverage dropped), Chem.Abstr., Chem.Cit.Ind., Chem.Indus.Notes, Chem.Titles, Chemorec.Abstr., Crop Physiol.Abstr., Curr.Adv.Biochem., Curr.Adv.Cancer Res., Curr.Adv.Cell & Devel.Biol., Curr.Adv.Ecol.Sci., Curr.Adv.Gen.& Molec.Biol., Curr.Cont., Curr.Ref.Fish Res., Dairy Sci.Abstr., Dent.Ind., Derwent Biotech.Abstr., Eng.Ind., Excerp.Med., Field Crop Abstr., Food Sci.& Tech.Abstr., Forest.Abstr., Genet.Abstr., Helminthol.Abstr., Herb.Abstr., Hort.Abstr., Hum.Gen.Abstr., INIS Atomind., Immun.Abstr. (coverage dropped), Ind.Med. (1967-), Ind.Sci.Rev., Ind.Vet., Inpharma, Int.Abstr.Biol.Sci., Maize Abstr., Mass Spectr.Bull., Microbiol.Abstr., NPU, Neurosci.Abstr. (coverage dropped), Neurosci.Cit.Ind., Nuc.Acids Abstr., Nutr.Abstr., Pharm.&Out.News, Pig News & Info., Plant Breed.Abstr., Plant Grow.Reg.Abstr., Postharvest, Potato Abstr., Poult.Abstr., Protozool.Abstr., Reac., Ref.Zh., Rev.Appl.Entomol., Rev.Arom.& Med.Plants, Rev.Med.& Vet.Mycol., Rev.Plant Path., Rice Abstr., Sci.Cit.Ind., Seed Abstr., Soils & Fert., Soyabean Abstr., Sugar Ind.Abstr., Tox.Abstr. (coverage dropped), Triticale Abstr., Trop.Dis.Bull., Vet.Bull., Weed Abstr., Wild.Rev., Zoo.Rec.
—BLDSC (3829.723000), ADONIS, CASDDS, CINDOC, CISTI, Ei, GNLM, IDS, ingenta, KNAW, Linda Hall. **CCC.**
Published by: (Federation of European Biochemical Societies NLD), Blackwell Science Ltd., PO Box 88, Oxford OX2 0NE, United Kingdom. TEL 44-1865-206180, 44-1865-206002, FAX 44-1865-206219, jnl.orders@blacksci.co.uk, http://www.blackwell-science.com/~cgilib/jnlpage.asp?Journal=ejb&File=ejb, http://www.blackwellpublishing.com. Ed. Federick Sanger. Pub. Amanda McLean Inglis. R&P Sophie Savage. Adv. contact Jenny Applin. Circ: 1,950.

572 ITA ISSN 1121-760X
CODEN: EJHIE2
EUROPEAN JOURNAL OF HISTOCHEMISTRY. Cover title: E J H. Text in English. 1954. q. USD 200. adv. bk.rev. *Refereed.* **Document type:** *Academic/Scholarly.*
Former titles (until 1991): European Journal of Basic and Applied Histochemistry (1121-4201); (until 1990): Basic and Applied Histochemistry (0391-7258); (until 1979): Rivista di Istochimica Normale e Patologica (0485-2400)
Related titles: Online - full text ed.: (from Institute for Scientific Information).
Indexed: ASCA, BBCI, Chem.Abstr., Chem.Indus.Notes, Chem.Titles, Curr.Adv.Cell & Devel.Biol., Curr.Adv.Ecol.Sci., Curr.Cont., Dairy Sci.Abstr., Excerp.Med., Ind.Med. (1992-), Ind.Sci.Rev., Ind.Vet., Inpharma, Int.Abstr.Biol.Sci., Neurosci.Abstr. (coverage dropped), Neurosci.Cit.Ind., Reac., Ref.Zh., Risk Abstr., Sci.Cit.Ind., Vet.Bull., Zoo.Rec.
—BLDSC (3829.729900), CASDDS, CISTI, EMDOCS, GNLM, IDS, KNAW.
Published by: (Societa Italiana di Istochimica), Luigi Ponzio e Figlio Editori, Via D da Catalogna, 1-3, Pavia, PV 27100, Italy. TEL 382-35000, FAX 382-304435. Ed. Maria G M Romanini. Circ: 500.

B

B

615 FRA ISSN 0223-5234
CODEN: EJMCA5

EUROPEAN JOURNAL OF MEDICINAL CHEMISTRY. Text and summaries in English. 1965. m. EUR 627 in Europe to institutions; JPY 83,300 in Japan to institutions; USD 702 elsewhere to institutions (effective 2002). adv. bk.rev. bibl, charts. index. back issues avail. *Refereed.* **Document type:** *Academic/Scholarly.* **Description:** Publishes original papers, laboratory notes, short or preliminary communications, and descriptions of new products involving all aspects of medicinal chemistry.
Formerly (until 1973): Chimica Therapeutica (0009-4374)
Related titles: Microform ed.: (from PQC); Online - full text ed.: (from ingenta, Swets Blackwell, ScienceDirect, Institute for Scientific Information).
Indexed: ASCA, Agri.& Environ.Biotech.Abstr. (coverage dropped), BBCI, Biol.Abstr., Chem.Abstr., Chem.Cit.Ind., Chem.Indus.Notes, Chem.Titles, Curr.Adv.Ecol.Sci., Curr.Chem.React., Curr.Cont., Derwent Biotech.Abstr., Excerp.Med., Helminthol.Abstr., INIS Atomind., I.P.A., Ind.Chem., Ind.Med. (1974-), Ind.Sci.Rev., Inpharma, Neurosci.Cit.Ind., Pharm.&Out.News, Protozool.Abstr., RCI, Reac., Ref.Zh., Rev.Med.& Vet.Mycol., Sci.Cit.Ind.
—BLDSC (3829.731500), ADONIS, CASDDS, CISTI, EMDOCS, GNLM, IDS, Infotrieve, KNAW, Linda Hall. **CCC.**
Published by: (Societe Francaise de Chimie Therapeutique), Elsevier Paris, Editions Scientifiques et Medicales (Subsidiary of: Reed Elsevier plc. group), 23 rue Linois, Paris 75015, France. TEL 33-1-45589110, FAX 33-1-45589419, academic@elsevier-fr.com, http://www.elsevier.com/locate/ejmech. Eds. C Combet Farnoux, O Lafont. Circ: 3,000. **Co-sponsor:** European Federation of Medicinal Chemistry.

EUROPEAN JOURNAL OF NEUROSCIENCE. see *MEDICAL SCIENCES—Psychiatry And Neurology*

EXCERPTA MEDICA. SECTION 29: CLINICAL AND EXPERIMENTAL BIOCHEMISTRY. see *BIOLOGY—Abstracting, Bibliographies, Statistics*

572 KOR ISSN 1226-3613
CODEN: KJBID3

EXPERIMENTAL AND MOLECULAR MEDICINE. Text and summaries in English. 1964. q. KRW 30,000 domestic to individuals; USD 40 foreign to individuals; KRW 100,000 domestic to institutions; USD 130 foreign to institutions; KRW 15,000 domestic to students; USD 20 foreign to students (effective 2001). adv. bk.rev. *Refereed.* **Document type:** *Academic/Scholarly.* **Description:** Publishes research papers and mini-reviews in the fields of basic and applied molecular biology, and experimental biochemistry in medicine.
Formerly (until 1996): Korean Journal of Biochemistry (0378-8512)
Related titles: Online - full text ed.: (from Institute for Scientific Information).
Indexed: ASCA, BBCI, Biol.Abstr., Chem.Abstr., Chem.Indus.Notes, Chem.Titles, Excerp.Med., Ind.Med. (1996-).
—BLDSC (3838.690000), CASDDS, CISTI, GNLM, IDS.
Published by: Korean Society of Medical Biochemistry and Molecular Biology, #812 KSTC, 635-4 Yoksam-dong Kangnam-gu, Seoul 135-703, Korea, S.. TEL 82-2-565-1621, FAX 82-2-565-1622, ksmbmb@ksmbmb.or.kr, http://www.ksmbmb.or.kr. Ed., R&P Soo Il Chung. Adv. contact So Young Kang. Circ: 1,500. **Subscr. to:** #812 KOFST, 635-4 Yoksam-dong Kangnam-gu, Seoul 135-703, Korea, S. **Co-sponsor:** Korean Federation of Science and Technology Societies.

EXPERIMENTAL BIOLOGY AND MEDICINE (TOTOWA). see *MEDICAL SCIENCES—Experimental Medicine, Laboratory Technique*

▼ **EXPERT OPINION ON BIOLOGICAL THERAPY.** see *MEDICAL SCIENCES*

572 NLD ISSN 0014-5793
QP501 CODEN: FEBLAL

F E B S LETTERS. Text in English, French, German; Summaries in English. 1968. 69/yr. EUR 528 in Europe to individuals; JPY 69,000 in Japan to individuals; USD 590 elsewhere to individuals; EUR 3,600 in Europe to institutions; JPY 514,000 in Japan to institutions; USD 4,027 elsewhere to institutions (effective 2002). adv. bk.rev. charts, illus, stat. cum.index. reprint service avail. from ISI. *Refereed.* **Document type:** *Academic/Scholarly.* **Description:** Publishes short reports of immediate importance to investigators in biochemistry, biophysics and molecular biology.
Related titles: Microform ed.: (from PQC); Online - full text ed.: (from EBSCO Publishing, ingenta, Swets Blackwell, ScienceDirect, Institute for Scientific Information).
Indexed: AIDS Abstr., ASCA, AgBiotech, Agri.& Environ.Biotech.Abstr. (coverage dropped), Anim.Breed.Abstr., Apic.Abstr., Aqua.Sci.& Fish.Abstr., BBCI, Bio-Contr.News & Info., Biol.Abstr., Biwk.Pap.Rad.Chem.& Photochem., Cal.Tiss.Abstr. (coverage dropped), Chem.Abstr., Chem.Cit.Ind., Chem.Indus.Notes, Chem.Titles, Chemorec.Abstr., Crop Physiol.Abstr., Curr.Adv.Biochem., Curr.Adv.Cancer Res., Curr.Adv.Cell & Devel.Biol., Curr.Adv.Ecol.Sci., Curr.Adv.Gen.& Molec.Biol., Curr.Cont., Dairy Sci.Abstr., Dent.Ind., Derwent Biotech.Abstr., Environ.Abstr., Excerp.Med., Field Crop Abstr., Food Sci.& Tech.Abstr., Forest.Abstr., Genet.Abstr., GeoRef, Helminthol.Abstr., Herb.Abstr., Hort.Abstr., Hum.Gen.Abstr., INIS Atomind., Ind.Med. (1968-), Ind.Sci.Rev., Ind.Vet., Inpharma, Int.Abstr.Biol.Sci., Maize Abstr., Mass Spectr.Bull., Microbiol.Abstr., Neurosci.Abstr. (coverage dropped), Neurosci.Cit.Ind., Nuc.Acids Abstr., Nutr.Abstr., Ornam.Hort., Pharm.&Out.News, Pig News & Info., Plant Breed.Abstr., Plant Grow.Reg.Abstr., Postharvest, Potato Abstr., Poult.Abstr., Protozool.Abstr., RCI, Reac., Ref.Zh., Rev.Appl.Entomol., Rev.Arom.& Med.Plants, Rev.Med.& Vet.Mycol., Rev.Plant Path., Rice Abstr., Sci.Cit.Ind., Seed Abstr., Soils & Fert., Sorghum & Millets Abstr., Soyabean Abstr., Sport Fish.Abstr., Sugar Ind.Abstr., THA, Telegen, Tox.Abstr. (coverage dropped), Triticale Abstr., Trop.Dis.Bull., Trop.Oil Seeds Abstr., Vet.Bull., Virol.Abstr. (coverage dropped), Weed Abstr.
—BLDSC (3901.600000), ADONIS, CASDDS, CISTI, GNLM, IDS, ingenta, Linda Hall. **CCC.**
Published by: (Federation of European Biochemical Societies), Elsevier Science BV, PO Box 211, Amsterdam 1000 AE, Netherlands. TEL 31-20-485-3757, FAX 31-20-485-3432, nlinfo-f@elsevier.nl, http://www.elsevier.com/locate/febslet, http://www.elsevier.nl. Ed. M Saraste. Circ: (controlled). **Subscr. in Australasia and the Far East to:** Elsevier Science (Singapore) Pte Ltd, No.1 Temasek Ave, 17-01 Millenia Tower, Singapore 039192, Singapore. TEL 65-434-3727, FAX 65-337-2230, asiainfo@elsevier.com.sg; **Subscr. in Japan to:** Elsevier Science Inc - Japan Regional Office, 9-15 Higashi-Azabu 1-chome, Minato-ku, Tokyo 106-0044, Japan. TEL 81-3-5561-5033, FAX 81-3-5561-5047, info@elsevier.co.jp; **Subscr. in the Americas to:** Elsevier Science, PO Box 945, New York, NY 10159-0945. TEL 212-633-3730, 888-437-4636, FAX 212-633-3680, usinfo-f@elsevier.com, http://www.elsevier.com. **Dist. by:** Elsevier Science (Brazil).

FIZIOLOGIYA I BIOKHIMIYA KUL'TURNYKH RASTENII/PHYSIOLOGY AND BIOCHEMISTRY OF CULTIVATED PLANTS; nauchno-teoreticheskii zhurnal. see *BIOLOGY—Physiology*

572 GRC ISSN 0015-5489
CODEN: FBBGAJ

FOLIA BIOCHIMICA ET BIOLOGICA GRAECA. Text in English, French, German, Greek. 1964. irreg. (3-4/yr.). per issue exchange basis.
Indexed: Biol.Abstr., Chem.Abstr., Excerp.Med., GeoRef.
—CASDDS, CISTI.
Published by: (Hellenic Society of Marine Molecular Biology), Institute of Marine Molecular Biology, 2 Lampsakou St, Athens 611, Greece. Ed. A Christomanos.

579 GBR ISSN 0015-5632
CODEN: FOMIAZ

FOLIA MICROBIOLOGICA. Text and summaries in English. 1956. bi-m. GBP 169 domestic; GBP 190 foreign (effective 2000). adv. bk.rev. abstr, charts, illus, mkt. index. *Refereed.* **Document type:** *Academic/Scholarly.* **Description:** A forum for microbiologists and immunologists all over the world. Includes papers and reports from meetings of international nomenclature committees in microbiology and biochemistry.
Formerly (until 1958): Ceskoslovenska Mikrobiologie
Related titles: Online - full text ed.: (from Institute for Scientific Information).
Indexed: ASCA, Abstr.Hyg., Agri.& Environ.Biotech.Abstr. (coverage dropped), Agri.Eng.Abstr., Agroforest.Abstr., Aqua.Sci.& Fish.Abstr., Bio-Contr.News & Info., Biol.Abstr., Biotech.Cit.Ind., Chem.Abstr., Chem.Indus.Notes, Chem.Titles, Crop Physiol.Abstr., Curr.Adv.Ecol.Sci., Curr.Biotech.Abstr., Curr.Cont., Dairy Sci.Abstr., Deep Sea Res.& Oceanogr.Abstr., Derwent Biotech.Abstr., Environ.Sci.Poll.Mgmt., Excerp.Med., Field Crop Abstr., Food Sci.& Tech.Abstr., Forest Prod.Abstr., Helminthol.Abstr., Hort.Abstr., INIS Atomind., Ind.Med. (1959-), Ind.Sci.Rev., Ind.Vet., Inpharma, Maize Abstr., Microbiol.Abstr., Nutr.Abstr., Pharm.&Out.News, Plant Grow.Reg.Abstr., Postharvest, Poult.Abstr., Protozool.Abstr., Reac., Rev.Appl.Entomol., Rev.Med.& Vet.Mycol., Rev.Plant Path., Sci.Cit.Ind., Seed Abstr., Soils & Fert., Soyabean Abstr., Sugar Ind.Abstr., Triticale Abstr., Trop.Dis.Bull., Vet.Bull., W.R.C.Inf., Weed Abstr.
—BLDSC (3971.500000), CASDDS, CISTI, GNLM, IDS, ingenta, Linda Hall. **CCC.**
Published by: Academy of Sciences of the Czech Republic, Institute of Microbiology/Czech Academy of Sciences, Institute of Microbiology, Videnska 1083, 142 20 Prague 4, Prague 142 20, Czech Republic. FAX 420-2-4447-2278, 420-2-4447-1286, folia.micro@usa.net, http://www.biomed.cas.cz/mbu/folia/index.html. Ed., R&P J Cudlin. Circ: 1,200. **Subscr. to:** Harcourt Publishers Ltd., Foots Cray High St, Sidcup, Kent DA14 5HP, United Kingdom. TEL 44-20-8300-3322. **Co-sponsor:** Ceskoslovenska Spolecnost Mikrobiologicka.

572 GBR ISSN 1353-6516

FRONTIERS IN METABOLISM. Text in English. 1996. irreg. GBP 18.95, USD 40 (effective 2002). *Refereed.* **Document type:** *Monographic series.*
Published by: Portland Press Ltd., 59 Portland Pl, London W1N 3AJ, United Kingdom. TEL 44-20-7580-5530, FAX 44-20-7323-1136, sales@portland-service.com, http://www.portlandpress.com/bst/default.htm. Ed. K Snell. R&P Adam Marshall. **Subscr. to:** Commerce Way, Colchester, Essex CO2 8HP, United Kingdom. TEL 44-1206-796351, FAX 44-1206-799331.

572 USA

G W U M C. DEPARTMENT OF BIOCHEMISTRY. ANNUAL SPRING SYMPOSIA SERIES. Text in English. 1982. irreg., latest 1996. price varies. *Refereed.* **Document type:** *Proceedings.*
—BLDSC (1531.702000).
Published by: (George Washington University Medical Center), Kluwer Academic - Plenum Publishers (Subsidiary of: Wolters Kluwer N.V.), 233 Spring St, New York, NY 10013-1578. TEL 212-620-8000, 800-221-9369, FAX 212-463-0742, info@plenum.com, http://www.plenum.com.

572.86 USA ISSN 1080-742X

GENBANK. Text in English. 1992. bi-m. USD 192; USD 240 foreign (effective 1999). **Document type:** *Academic/Scholarly, Government.* **Description:** Provides DNA sequence data in the traditional GenBank flat file format, including annotation and conceptual translations.
Formerly (until 1993): N C B I - GenBank, Genetic Sequence Databank (Flat File) (1080-7411)
Media: Online - full text.
Published by: U.S. National Library of Medicine, U.S. National Center for Biotechnology Information, Bldg 38A, Rm 8N 803, 8600 Rockville Pike, Bethesda, MD 20894. TEL 301-435-5946, FAX 301-480-2233, info@ncbi.nlm.nih.gov, http://www.ncbi.nlm.nih.gov.

GENE EXPRESSION; international journal of molecular and cellular science. see *BIOLOGY—Genetics*

572.7 GBR
CODEN: ISBLEK

GENE FAMILIES AND ISOZYMES BULLETIN. Text in English. 1967. a. adv. bk.rev. **Document type:** *Bulletin.*
Supersedes (in 1998): Isozyme (0197-887X)
Indexed: Sport Fish.Abstr., Wild.Rev., Zoo.Rec.
—BLDSC (4096.402460), CISTI.
Address: c/o W.R. Chegwidden Ed, Hallam University, Sheffield, City Campus, Pond St, Sheffield, S Yorks S1 1WB, United Kingdom. TEL 44-114-253-3042, FAX 44-114-253-2020, w.r.chegwidden@shu.ac.uk. Circ: 150 (paid).

GENOME RESEARCH. see *BIOLOGY—Genetics*

GENOMICS; international journal for analysis of the human and other genomes. see *BIOLOGY—Genetics*

572.86 GBR
▼ **GENOMIKA.** Text in English. 1999 (Dec.). 22/yr. GBP 325 in Europe; USD 585 in US & Canada; JPY 80,600 in Japan; GBP 360 rest of world (effective 2001). 8 p./no. 3 cols./p. back issues avail.; reprints avail. **Document type:** *Newsletter.* **Description:** Provides the latest market and business information on the fast-expanding field of DNA, RNA and protein analysis.
Related titles: E-mail ed.; Online - full text ed.: (from The Dialog Corporation, S T N International, Ovid Technologies, Inc., Data-Star).
Published by: P J B Publications Ltd., 18-20 Hill Rise, Richmond, Surrey TW10 6UA, United Kingdom. TEL 44-20-8948-3262, FAX 44-20-8332-8990, genomika@pjbpubs.com, info@pjbpubs.com, http://www.genomika.com/, http://www.pjbpubs.com. Ed. Philip Greenfield. Pub. Philip Brown. R&P Annette Watts TEL 44-20-8332-8961. **Subscr. addr. in N America:** Pharmabooks Ltd., 1775 Broadway, Ste 511, New York, NY 10019. TEL 212-262-8230, FAX 212-262-8234.

GEOMICROBIOLOGY JOURNAL; an international journal of geomicrobiology and microbial biogeochemistry. see *BIOLOGY—Microbiology*

572.566 USA ISSN 0959-6658
QP552.G59 CODEN: GLYCE3
GLYCOBIOLOGY. Text in English. 1991. m. GBP 178, USD 285 to individuals; GBP 495, USD 795 to institutions (effective 2002). adv. bk.rev. back issues avail.; reprint service avail. from SWZ. *Refereed.* **Document type:** *Journal, Academic/Scholarly.* **Description:** Provides a forum for the publication of original research papers on any aspect of the structure and functions of glycobiology or any aspect of proteins that specifically interact with saccharides.
Related titles: Online - full text ed.: ISSN 1460-2423. GBP 445, USD 715 to institutions Online only (effective 2002) (from HighWire Pr., EBSCO Publishing, O C L C Online Computer Library Center, Inc., RoweCom Information Quest, ingenta, Swets Blackwell, Institute for Scientific Information).
Indexed: ASCA, AgBiotech, Agricola, BBCI, Bibl.Agri., Chem.Abstr., Chem.Indus.Notes, Chem.Titles, Curr.Cont., Helminthol.Abstr., Ind.Med. (1990-), Ind.Sci.Rev., Inpharma, Int.Abstr.Biol.Sci., Mass Spectr.Bull., Plant Breed.Abstr., Protozool.Abstr., Reac., Rev.Appl.Entomol., Rev.Med.& Vet.Mycol., Sci.Cit.Ind.
—BLDSC (4196.303000), CASDDS, CISTI, EMDOCS, GNLM, IDS, ingenta, KNAW, Linda Hall. **CCC.**
Published by: Oxford University Press, Academic Division, Great Clarendon St, Oxford OX2 6DP, United Kingdom. TEL 44-1865-267907, FAX 44-1865-267835, jnlorders@oup-usa.org, jnl.info@oup.co.uk, http://glycob.oupjournals.org/, http://www.oup.co.uk/journals. Eds. Akira Kobata, Anne Dell, Gerald W Hart. Pub. Janet Fox. R&P Fionna Willis. adv.: page GBP 380, page USD 685. Circ: 1,200. **Subscr. outside the Americas to:** Journals Marketing, Great Clarendon St, Oxford OX2 6DP, United Kingdom.

GLYCOBIOLOGY RESEARCH. see *BIOLOGY—Abstracting, Bibliographies, Statistics*

572 USA ISSN 0282-0080
CODEN: GLJOEW
GLYCOCONJUGATE JOURNAL. Text in English. 1984. 9/yr. USD 1,011, EUR 1,009.50 to institutions for print or online ed.; USD 1,213.20, EUR 1,211.40 to institutions for print & online eds. combined (effective 2002). adv. back issues avail.; reprints avail. *Refereed.* **Document type:** *Journal, Academic/Scholarly.* **Description:** Publishes articles and reviews on all areas concerned with the composition, degradation, function, interactions, structure, and synthesis of glycoconjugates (glycoproteins, glycolipids, oligosaccharides, polysaccharides, Proteoglycans), including those aspects that are related to disease processes (eg, immunological, inflammatory, and arthritic diseases, infections, metabolic disorders, Malignancy, neurological disorders).
Incorporates (1994-1996): Glycosylation and Disease (0969-3653)
Related titles: Online - full text ed.: (from EBSCO Publishing, O C L C Online Computer Library Center, Inc., RoweCom Information Quest, Swets Blackwell, Kluwer Online, Institute for Scientific Information).
Indexed: ASCA, BBCI, Chem.Abstr., Chem.Cit.Ind., Chem.Indus.Notes, Chem.Titles, Curr.Adv.Biochem., Curr.Adv.Cancer Res., Curr.Adv.Ecol.Sci., Curr.Cont., Excerp.Med., Hort.Abstr., Ind.Med. (1984-), Ind.Sci.Rev., Ind.Vet., Inpharma, Int.Abstr.Biol.Sci., Neurosci.Cit.Ind., Pharm.&Out.News, Protozool.Abstr., RCI, Reac., Rev.Appl.Entomol., Sci.Cit.Ind.
—BLDSC (4196.305000), ADONIS, CASDDS, CISTI, EMDOCS, GNLM, IDS, Infotrieve, KNAW. **CCC.**
Published by: (International Glyconjugate Organization), Kluwer Academic Publishers Boston, 101 Philip Dr, Assinippi Park, Norwell, MA 02061. TEL 781-871-6600, FAX 781-871-9045, services@wkap.nl, http://www.wkap.nl/journalhome.htm/0282-0080. Ed. Graham A Turner. R&P Rose Luongo TEL 781-871-6311. Adv. contact Gemma Heiser TEL 781-871-6600. **Subscr. outside the Americas to:** Kluwer Academic Publishers Group, Journals Department, PO Box 322, Dordrecht 3300 AH, Netherlands. TEL 31-78-639-2392, FAX 31-78-654-6474; **Subscr. to:** Kluwer Academic - Plenum Publishers, 233 Spring St, New York, NY 10013-1578. TEL 212-620-8468, FAX 212-807-1047.

572 USA ISSN 1043-9811
QP514
HARPER'S BIOCHEMISTRY*. Text in English. 1939. biennial. USD 36.95 (effective 1998). bk.rev. **Document type:** *Academic/Scholarly.*
Former titles (until 1988): Harper's Review of Biochemistry (0734-9866); (until 1979): Review of Physiological Chemistry (0080-1976)
—BLDSC (4264.885500), CISTI, Infotrieve. **CCC.**
Published by: Appleton & Lange, Journal Division (Subsidiary of: Simon & Schuster Company), 11 W 19th St, New York, CT 10011-4209. TEL 203-406-4500, FAX 203-406-4600.

THE HISTOCHEMICAL JOURNAL; a journal of cell and tissue biochemistry. see *BIOLOGY—Cytology And Histology*

HISTOCHEMISTRY AND CELL BIOLOGY. see *BIOLOGY—Cytology And Histology*

572.8 USA ISSN 0272-457X
QR185.8.H93 CODEN: HYBRDY
HYBRIDOMA; a journal of molecular immunology and experimental and clinical immunotherapy. Text in English. 1981. bi-m. USD 278 domestic to individuals; USD 399 foreign to individuals; USD 334 domestic to individuals print and online eds. combined; USD 454 foreign to individuals print and online eds. combined; USD 635 domestic to institutions; USD 788 foreign to institutions; USD 762 domestic to institutions print and online eds. combined; USD 915 foreign to institutions print and online eds. combined (effective 2002). adv. back issues avail.; reprints avail. *Refereed.* **Document type:** *Journal, Academic/Scholarly.* **Description:** Publishes research in molecular immunology and experimental and clinical immunotherapy. Includes papers on the application of monoclonal antibodies for diagnostics and therapy, and original articles on various aspects of hybridoma research.
Incorporates (in 1990): Monoclonal Antibodies (1047-871X); Formerly (until 1990): Monoclonal Antibody News (0272-4588)
Related titles: Online - full text ed.: USD 278 to individuals; USD 635 to institutions (effective 2002) (from EBSCO Publishing, O C L C Online Computer Library Center, Inc., RoweCom Information Quest, Swets Blackwell, Institute for Scientific Information).
Indexed: AIDS & Cancer Res., ASCA, Agri.& Environ.Biotech.Abstr. (coverage dropped), Biol.Abstr., Biotech.Cit.Ind., Chem.Abstr., Chem.Indus.Notes, Chem.Titles, Curr.Adv.Cancer Res., Curr.Adv.Ecol.Sci., Curr.Biotech.Abstr., Curr.Cont., Dairy Sci.Abstr., Derwent Biotech.Abstr., Excerp.Med., Genet.Abstr. (coverage dropped), Helminthol.Abstr., INIS Atomind., Immun.Abstr., Ind.Med. (1981-), Ind.Sci.Rev., Ind.Vet., Inpharma, Int.Abstr.Biol.Sci., Med.& Pharm.Biotech.Abstr., Pharm.&Out.News, Poult.Abstr., Reac., Ref.Zh., Rev.Med.& Vet.Mycol., Sci.Cit.Ind., Sugar Ind.Abstr., Telegen, Vet.Bull., Weed Abstr.
—BLDSC (4340.385000), ADONIS, CASDDS, CatchWord, CISTI, EMDOCS, GNLM, IDS, ingenta. **CCC.**
Published by: Mary Ann Liebert, Inc. Publishers, 2 Madison Ave, Larchmont, NY 10538. TEL 914–834-3100, FAX 914-834-1388, info@liebertpub.com, www.liebertpub.com/hyb, http://www.liebertpub.com. Ed. Dr. Zenon Steplewski.

572 GBR ISSN 1521-6543
QP501 CODEN: IULIF8
I U B M B LIFE. Text in English. 1980. 12/yr. GBP 153, USD 253 to individuals; GBP 589, USD 972 to institutions (effective 2002). *Refereed.* **Document type:** *Academic/Scholarly.* **Description:** Devoted to the dissemination of original research findings among the scientific communities of the forty nations represented by the International Union of Biochemistry.
Former titles (until 1999): Biochemistry and Molecular Biology International (1039-9712); (until 1993): Biochemistry International (0158-5231)
Related titles: Online - full text ed.: ISSN 1521-6551 (from O C L C Online Computer Library Center, Inc., RoweCom Information Quest, CatchWord Ltd., Swets Blackwell, Institute for Scientific Information).
Indexed: ASCA, Abstr.Hyg., AgBiotech, Agri.& Environ.Biotech.Abstr. (coverage dropped), Agricola, Anim.Breed.Abstr., Aqua.Sci.& Fish.Abstr., BBCI, Bibl.Agri., Chem.Abstr., Chem.Cit.Ind., Chem.Indus.Notes, Chem.Titles, Crop Physiol.Abstr., Curr.Adv.Biochem., Curr.Adv.Cancer Res., Curr.Adv.Cell & Devel.Biol., Curr.Adv.Ecol.Sci., Curr.Adv.Gen.& Molec.Biol., Curr.Cont., Dairy Sci.Abstr., Excerp.Med., Field Crop Abstr., Helminthol.Abstr., Hort.Abstr., Ind.Med. (1999-), Ind.Sci.Rev., Ind.Vet., Inpharma, Int.Abstr.Biol.Sci., Maize Abstr., Neurosci.Cit.Ind., Nutr.Abstr., Pharm.&Out.News, Pig News & Info., Plant Breed.Abstr., Plant Gen.Res.Abstr., Plant Grow.Reg.Abstr., Postharvest, Poult.Abstr., Protozool.Abstr., Reac., Rev.Appl.Entomol., Rev.Arom.& Med.Plants, Rev.Med.& Vet.Mycol., Rev.Plant Path., Rice Abstr., Sci.Cit.Ind., Seed Abstr., Soils & Fert., Sport Fish.Abstr., Sugar Ind.Abstr., Triticale Abstr., Trop.Dis.Bull., Vet.Bull., Weed Abstr., Wild.Rev., Zoo.Rec.
—BLDSC (4588.826000), CASDDS, CatchWord, CISTI, EMDOCS, GNLM, IDS, ingenta, Linda Hall.
Published by: (International Union of Biochemistry and Molecular Biology AUS), Taylor & Francis Ltd. (Subsidiary of: Taylor & Francis Group), 11 New Fetter Ln, London EC4P 4EE, United Kingdom. TEL 44-20-7842-2346, FAX 44-20-7583-0701, info@tandf.co.uk, http://www.tandf.co.uk. Ed. Kelvin J A Davies. Circ: 1,000.

IMMUNOHISTOCHEMISTRY. see *BIOLOGY—Abstracting, Bibliographies, Statistics*

572 IND ISSN 0301-1208
QP501 CODEN: IJBBBQ
INDIAN JOURNAL OF BIOCHEMISTRY AND BIOPHYSICS. Text in English. 1963. bi-m. (in 2 vols.). INR 400, USD 150 (effective 2001). adv. back issues avail. *Refereed.* **Document type:** *Academic/Scholarly.* **Description:** Provides original research in biochemistry and biophysics.
Formerly (until 1971): Indian Journal of Biochemistry (0019-5081)
Related titles: Online - full text ed.: (from Institute for Scientific Information).
Indexed: ASCA, Abstr.Hyg., AgBiotech, Agri.& Environ.Biotech.Abstr. (coverage dropped), Anal.Abstr., Anim.Breed.Abstr., Aqua.Sci.& Fish.Abstr., Aquacult.Abstr., BBCI, Biol.Abstr., Chem.Abstr., Chem.Indus.Notes, Chem.Titles, Crop Physiol.Abstr., Curr.Adv.Ecol.Sci., Curr.Cont., Dairy Sci.Abstr., Dent.Ind., Derwent Biotech.Abstr., Eng.Ind., Environ.Sci.Poll.Mgmt., Field Crop Abstr., Food Sci.& Tech.Abstr., Helminthol.Abstr., Hort.Abstr., INIS Atomind., Ind.Med. (1971-), Ind.Sci.Rev., Ind.Vet., Inpharma, NPU, Nutr.Abstr., Ornam.Hort., Pharm.&Out.News, Plant Breed.Abstr., Plant Grow.Reg.Abstr., Potato Abstr., Protozool.Abstr., Reac., Ref.Zh., Rev.Appl.Entomol., Rev.Arom.& Med.Plants, Rev.Med.& Vet.Mycol., Rev.Plant Path., SSCI (coverage dropped), Sci.Cit.Ind. (coverage dropped), Seed Abstr., Sport Fish.Abstr., Triticale Abstr., Trop.Dis.Bull., Vet.Bull., Weed Abstr.
—BLDSC (4410.420000), CASDDS, CISTI, Ei, GNLM, IDS, ingenta, Linda Hall.
Published by: (India. Council of Scientific and Industrial Research, India. Publications and Information Directorate), Scientific Publishers, 5-A New Pali Rd., P O Box 91, Jodhpur, Rajasthan 342 001, India. TEL 91-291-433323, FAX 91-291-512580, scienti@sancharnet.in, http://www.scientificpub.com. Ed. B S Janqi. Circ: 1,000. **Co-sponsor:** Society of Biological Chemists.

INSTITUT PASTEUR. ANNALES. ACTUALITES. see *BIOLOGY—Microbiology*

INTERNATIONAL ANTIVIRAL NEWS. see *MEDICAL SCIENCES—Communicable Diseases*

572 FIN ISSN 0074-3690
INTERNATIONAL CONGRESS OF HISTOCHEMISTRY AND CYTOCHEMISTRY. PROCEEDINGS. (Proceedings published in host country) Text in Finnish. 1960. quadrennial, latest 1984 (Helsinki). price varies. adv. **Document type:** *Proceedings.*
—CISTI.
Published by: University of Helsinki, Department of Anatomy, c/o Dr Pertti Panula, Siltavuorenpenger 20 A, Helsinki 00170, Finland. Circ: 1,000.

572 GBR ISSN 1357-2725
QP501 CODEN: IJBBFU
INTERNATIONAL JOURNAL OF BIOCHEMISTRY & CELL BIOLOGY. Text in English. 1970. m. EUR 2,243 in Europe to institutions; JPY 297,800 in Japan to institutions; USD 2,509 elsewhere to institutions (effective 2002). adv. charts, illus, stat. index. back issues avail.; reprint service avail. from PQC. *Refereed.* **Document type:** *Academic/Scholarly.* **Description:** Provides comprehensive coverage of new research in growth areas of biochemistry.
Formerly (until 1995): International Journal of Biochemistry (0020-711X)
Related titles: Microfilm ed.: (from PQC); Online - full text ed.: (from EBSCO Publishing, ingenta, Swets Blackwell, ScienceDirect, Institute for Scientific Information).
Indexed: ASCA, AgBiotech, Agricola, Anim.Breed.Abstr., BBCI, Biol.Abstr., Chem.Abstr., Chem.Cit.Ind., Chem.Indus.Notes, Chem.Titles, Curr.Adv.Biochem., Curr.Adv.Cancer Res., Curr.Adv.Ecol.Sci., Curr.Adv.Gen.& Molec.Biol., Curr.Cont., Dairy Sci.Abstr., Dent.Ind., Derwent Biotech.Abstr., Eng.Ind., Excerp.Med., Helminthol.Abstr., Hort.Abstr., Ind.Med. (1995-), Ind.Sci.Rev., Ind.Vet., Inpharma, Int.Abstr.Biol.Sci., Neurosci.Cit.Ind., Nutr.Abstr., Pharm.&Out.News, Poult.Abstr., Protozool.Abstr., Reac., Ref.Zh., Rev.Appl.Entomol., Rev.Arom.& Med.Plants, Rev.Med.& Vet.Mycol., SSCI (coverage dropped), Sci.Cit.Ind., Seed Abstr., Sport Fish.Abstr., Trop.Dis.Bull., Vet.Bull., Wild.Rev., Zoo.Rec.
—BLDSC (4542.135000), ADONIS, CASDDS, CISTI, Ei, GNLM, IDS, ingenta, Linda Hall. **CCC.**
Published by: Pergamon (Subsidiary of: Elsevier Science), The Boulevard, Langford Ln, East Park, Kidlington, Oxford OXB 1GB, United Kingdom. FAX 44-1865-843010, http://www.elsevier.com/locate/biocel. Eds. Geoffrey J Laurent, Robert P Mecham. Circ: 1,000. **Subscr. in Australasia and the Far East to:** Elsevier Science (Singapore) Pte Ltd, No.1 Temasek Ave, 17-01 Millenia Tower, Singapore 039192, Singapore. TEL 65-434-3727, FAX 65-337-2230; **Subscr. in the Americas to:** Elsevier Science, PO Box 945, New York, NY 10159-0945. TEL 212-633-3730, FAX 212-633-3680, usinfo-f@elsevier.com; **Subscr. to:** Elsevier Science BV, PO Box 211, Amsterdam 1000 AE, Netherlands. TEL 31-20-485-3757.

572.8 NLD ISSN 0141-8130
QP801.P64 CODEN: IJBMDR
INTERNATIONAL JOURNAL OF BIOLOGICAL MACROMOLECULES; structure, function and interactions. Text in English. 1979. 10/yr. EUR 158 in Europe to qualified personnel; JPY 21,000 in Japan to qualified personnel; USD 177 elsewhere to qualified personnel; EUR 1,348 in Europe to institutions; JPY 179,000 in Japan to institutions; USD 1,507 elsewhere to institutions (effective 2002). adv. bk.rev. abstr, illus. index. back issues avail. *Refereed.* **Document type:** *Academic/Scholarly.* **Description:** Reports research into the structure of natural macromolecules: proteins, carbohydrates, nucleic acids, viruses and membranes.
Related titles: Microform ed.: (from PQC); Online - full text ed.: (from ingenta, Swets Blackwell, ScienceDirect, Institute for Scientific Information).
Indexed: ASCA, Abstr.Bull.Inst.Pap.Chem., BBCI, Biol.Abstr., Chem.Abstr., Chem.Cit.Ind., Chem.Indus.Notes, Chem.Titles, Curr.Adv.Biochem., Curr.Adv.Cell & Devel.Biol., Curr.Adv.Gen.& Molec.Biol., Curr.Cont., Dairy Sci.Abstr., Excerp.Med., Food Sci.& Tech.Abstr., Ind.Med. (1979-), Ind.Sci.Rev., Inpharma, Int.Abstr.Biol.Sci., Maize Abstr., Mat.Sci.Cit.Ind. (coverage dropped), Pharm.&Out.News, Reac., Rev.Arom.& Med.Plants, Sci.Cit.Ind., Seed Abstr., Telegen.
—BLDSC (4542.151000), CASDDS, CISTI, GNLM, IDS, Infotrieve, ingenta, Linda Hall. **CCC.**
Published by: Elsevier Science BV, PO Box 211, Amsterdam 1000 AE, Netherlands. TEL 31-20-485-3757, FAX 31-20-485-3432, TELEX 18582 ESPA NL, http://www.elsevier.com/locate/ijbiomac. Ed. Steven T Case. **Subscr. in Australasia and the Far East to:** Elsevier Science (Singapore) Pte Ltd, No.1 Temasek Ave, 17-01 Millenia Tower, Singapore 039192, Singapore. TEL 65-434-3727, FAX 65-337-2230; **Subscr. in Japan to:** Elsevier Science Inc - Japan Regional Office, 9-15 Higashi-Azabu 1-chome, Minato-ku, Tokyo 106-0044, Japan. TEL 81-3-5561-5033, FAX 81-3-5561-5047; **Subscr. in the Americas to:** Elsevier Science, PO Box 945, New York, NY 10159-0945. TEL 212-633-3730, 888-437-4636, FAX 212-633-3680, usinfo-f@elsevier.com, http://www.elsevier.com. **Dist. by:** Elsevier Science (Brazil).

INTERNATIONAL JOURNAL OF NEUROSCIENCE. see *MEDICAL SCIENCES—Psychiatry And Neurology*

INTERNATIONAL REINHARDSBRUNN SYMPOSIUM PROCEEDINGS. see *BIOLOGY—Botany*

572 GBR ISSN 1462-2149
INTERNET JOURNAL OF SCIENCE - BIOLOGICAL CHEMISTRY. Text in English. 1997. irreg. back issues avail. **Document type:** *Journal, Academic/Scholarly.* **Description:** Includes all aspects of chemistry, but with particular emphasis on studies of biologically important molecules.
Media: Online - full text.
Published by: Emedia Science Ltd, P O Box 92, New Ferry CH63 9WA, United Kingdom. TEL 44-151-647-0008, FAX 44-702-095-9300, sales@emedia-science.co.uk, http://www.netsci-journal.com/, http://www.emedia-science.co.uk. Ed. Dr. Paul Heelis.

IRON METABOLISM. see *BIOLOGY—Abstracting, Bibliographies, Statistics*

572 ITA ISSN 0021-2938
CODEN: IJBIAC
ITALIAN JOURNAL OF BIOCHEMISTRY. Text in English. 1955-1995 (Dec.); resumed. bi-m. ITL 379,500, USD 230 (effective 1995). adv. bk.rev. charts, illus. index. reprint service avail. from ISI. *Refereed.* **Document type:** *Academic/Scholarly.*
Related titles: Online - full text ed.: (from Institute for Scientific Information).
Indexed: ASCA, Agri.& Environ.Biotech.Abstr. (coverage dropped), Anal.Abstr., Aqua.Sci.& Fish.Abstr., Biol.Abstr., Chem.Abstr., Chem.Indus.Notes, Chem.Titles, Curr.Adv.Biochem., Curr.Adv.Gen.& Molec.Biol., Curr.Cont. (coverage dropped), Dairy Sci.Abstr., Excerp.Med., Ind.Med. (1957-), Ind.Sci.Rev., NPU, Neurosci.Cit.Ind., Nutr.Abstr., Poult.Abstr., Sci.Cit.Ind. (coverage dropped).
—BLDSC (4588.340000), CASDDS, CISTI, GNLM, ingenta, Linda Hall.
Published by: Biomedia s.r.l., Via Carlo Farini, 70, Milan, MI 20159, Italy. TEL 39-2-69001316, FAX 39-2-69001311. Circ: 600.

572.4 ITA ISSN 1121-1709
CODEN: IMEME
ITALIAN JOURNAL OF MINERAL & ELECTROLYTE METABOLISM. Text in English. 1987. q. USD 110 to individuals; USD 160 to institutions (effective 1999). adv. *Refereed.* **Document type:** *Academic/Scholarly.* **Description:** Deals with mineral and electrolyte metabolism and with calcified tissue.
Formerly (until 1990): Giornale Italiano di Metabolismo Minerale ed Elettrolitico (0394-1566)
Related titles: Online - full text ed.: (from Institute for Scientific Information).
Indexed: ASSIA, BBCI, Chem.Abstr., Chem.Indus.Notes, Chem.Titles, Excerp.Med. (1994-), Int.Abstr.Biol.Sci.
—BLDSC (4588.340640), CASDDS, EMDOCS, GNLM, IDS.
Published by: (Italian Society of Mineral and Electrolyte Metabolism), Edizioni Minerva Medica, Corso Bramante, 83-85, Turin, TO 10126, Italy. TEL 39-11-678282, FAX 39-11-674502. Ed. Giorgio Coen. Pub. Alberto Oliaro. Adv. contact F Filippo. B&W page USD 1,200, color page USD 2,000; trim 280 x 215. Circ: 2,000 (paid).

572 RUS ISSN 0202-795X
QP501 CODEN: INBKBD
ITOGI NAUKI I TEKHNIKI. BIOLOGICHESKAYA KHIMIYA. Text in Russian. irreg., latest vol.32, 1989.
Indexed: Chem.Abstr., Chem.Indus.Notes, Chem.Titles.
—CASDDS, Linda Hall.
Published by: Vserossiiskii Institut Nauchnoi i Tekhnicheskoi Informatsii (VINITI), Usievicha ul 20-a, Moscow 125315, Russian Federation. TEL 7-095-1526441. **Dist. by:** Mezhdunarodnaya Kniga, B Yakimanka 39, Moscow 117049, Russian Federation. TEL 7-095-2384967, FAX 7-095-2384634; **US dist. addr.:** East View Publications, 3020 Harbor Ln N, Minneapolis, MN 55447. TEL 612-550-0961.

572 571.4 RUS ISSN 0233-6715
CODEN: ISOBEL
ITOGI NAUKI I TEKHNIKI. OBSHCHIE PROBLEMY FIZIKO-KHIMICHESKOI BIOLOGII. Text in Russian. irreg. **Document type:** *Academic/Scholarly.*
—CASDDS, Linda Hall.
Published by: Vserossiiskii Institut Nauchnoi i Tekhnicheskoi Informatsii (VINITI), Usievicha ul 20-a, Moscow 125315, Russian Federation. TEL 7-095-1526441, FAX 7-095-943-0060. **US dist. addr.:** East View Publications, 3020 Harbor Ln N, Minneapolis, MN 55447. TEL 612-550-0961.

IYAKU ANZENSEI KENKYUKAI KAIHO/JAPANESE SOCIETY FOR BIOPHARMACEUTICAL STATISTICS. BULLETIN. see *PHARMACY AND PHARMACOLOGY*

IYAKU ANZENSEI KENKYUKAI TEIREIKAI SHIRYO/PROCEEDINGS OF REGULAR MEETINGS ON BIOPHARMACEUTICAL STATISTICS. see *PHARMACY AND PHARMACOLOGY*

612.015 616.4 AUT ISSN 1023-7763
JOURNAL FUER MINERALSTOFFWECHSEL; Zeitschrift fuer Physiologie, Pathophysiologie und Klinik des Mineralstoffwechsels. Text in German. 1994. q. ATS 400 (effective 2001). adv. abstr, bibl. back issues avail. *Refereed.* **Document type:** *Journal, Academic/Scholarly.* **Description:** Presents available scientific information on safety and efficacy issues related to osteoporosis and the intake of calcium and vitamin D.
—BLDSC (5020.144500).
Published by: Krause & Pachernegg GmbH, Mozartgasse 10, Gablitz 3003, Austria. TEL 43-2231-61258-0, FAX 43-2231-6125810, k_u_p@eunet.at, http://members.eunet.at/k_u_p/min.htm, http://members.eunet.at/k_u_p/verlag.htm. Ed. Dr. Peter Bernecker.

JOURNAL OF BASIC MICROBIOLOGY; an international journal on biochemistry, physiology, genetics, morphology and ecology of microorganisms. see *BIOLOGY—Microbiology*

572.33 USA ISSN 0883-9115
CODEN: JBCPEV
JOURNAL OF BIOACTIVE AND COMPATIBLE POLYMERS. Text in English. 1986. bi-m. USD 665 for print or electronic eds.; USD 765 for print and electronic eds. (effective 2001). back issues avail.; reprints avail. *Refereed.* **Document type:** *Journal, Academic/Scholarly.* **Description:** Provides a forum for both biological scientists and polymer chemists to publish refereed research papers and short communications in an area that is of common interest.
Related titles: E-mail ed.; Online - full content ed.; Online - full text ed.: (from Institute for Scientific Information).
Indexed: ASCA, Alloys Ind., Bioeng.Abstr., Biotech.& Bioeng.Abstr., Chem.Abstr., Chem.Cit.Ind., Chem.Indus.Notes, Chem.Titles, Curr.Cont., Eng.Ind., Eng.Mat.Abstr., Excerp.Med., Intl.Polym.Sci.& Tech., METADEX, Mat.Sci.Cit.Ind., Met.Abstr., Met.Abstr.Ind., Nonfer.Met.Alert, PCC Alert, RAPRA (1989-), Sci.Cit.Ind., Solid St.Abstr., Steels Alert, World Alum.Abstr.
—BLDSC (4951.567000), CASDDS, CISTI, Ei, EMDOCS, GNLM, IDS, Infotrieve, Linda Hall. **CCC.**
Published by: Sage Publications, Inc., 2111 W Hillcrest Dr, Thousand Oaks, CA 91320. Circ: 185 (paid).

572 NLD ISSN 0165-022X
QP519.7 CODEN: JBBMDG
JOURNAL OF BIOCHEMICAL AND BIOPHYSICAL METHODS. Text in Dutch. 1979. 9/yr. EUR 1,167 in Europe to institutions; JPY 154,800 in Japan to institutions; USD 1,303 elsewhere to institutions (effective 2002). adv. bk.rev. back issues avail.; reprint service avail. from SWZ,ISI. *Refereed.* **Document type:** *Academic/Scholarly.* **Description:** Publishes research papers dealing with the development of new methods or the significant modification of existing techniques to solve biological problems.
Related titles: Microform ed.: (from PQC); Online - full text ed.: (from ingenta, Swets Blackwell, ScienceDirect, Institute for Scientific Information).
Indexed: ASCA, BBCI, Biol.Abstr., CEABA, Chem.Abstr., Chem.Cit.Ind., Chem.Indus.Notes, Chem.Titles, Curr.Adv.Biochem., Curr.Adv.Cell & Devel.Biol., Curr.Adv.Gen.& Molec.Biol., Curr.Cont., Dairy Sci.Abstr., Eng.Ind., Excerp.Med., Food Sci.& Tech.Abstr., INIS Atomind., INSPEC (May 1979-), Ind.Med. (1979-), Ind.Sci.Rev., Inpharma, Mass Spectr.Bull., Reac., Ref.Zh., Sci.Cit.Ind., Sugar Ind.Abstr., VITIS.
—ADONIS, AskIEEE, CASDDS, CISTI, GNLM, IDS, ingenta, Linda Hall. **CCC.**
Published by: Elsevier Science BV, PO Box 211, Amsterdam 1000 AE, Netherlands. TEL 31-20-485-2911, FAX 31-20-485-2457, http://www.elsevier.nl/locate/jbbm. Eds. C F Chignell, S Hjerten. **Subscr. in Australasia and the Far East to:** Elsevier Science (Singapore) Pte Ltd, No.1 Temasek Ave, 17-01 Millenia Tower, Singapore 039192, Singapore. TEL 65-434-3727, FAX 65-337-2230; **Subscr. in U.S. and Canada to:** Elsevier Science, PO Box 882, New York, NY 10159-0882. TEL 212-633-3730, FAX 212-633-3680, usinfo-f@elsevier.com.

572 JPN ISSN 0021-924X
QP501 CODEN: JOBIAO
JOURNAL OF BIOCHEMISTRY. Text in English. 1922. m. USD 240. adv. abstr, bibl, charts, illus, stat. index. back issues avail.; reprints avail. *Refereed.* **Description:** Publishes original papers in the fields of biochemistry, molecular biology, cell, and biotechnology.
Related titles: Microfilm ed.: (from PMC); Online - full text ed.: (from Institute for Scientific Information).
Indexed: ASCA, AgBiotech, Agricola, Agroforest.Abstr., Anim.Breed.Abstr., Apic.Abstr., Aqua.Sci.& Fish.Abstr., BBCI, Bibl.Agri., Biol.Abstr., Cal.Tiss.Abstr. (coverage dropped), Chem.Abstr., Chem.Cit.Ind., Chem.Indus.Notes, Chem.Titles, Crop Physiol.Abstr., Curr.Adv.Biochem., Curr.Adv.Cancer Res., Curr.Adv.Cell & Devel.Biol., Curr.Adv.Gen.& Molec.Biol., Curr.Cont., Curr.Ref.Fish Res., Dairy Sci.Abstr., Deep Sea Res.& Oceanogr.Abstr., Dent.Ind., Derwent Biotech.Abstr., Eng.Ind., Environ.Sci.Poll.Mgmt., Excerp.Med., Field Crop Abstr., Food Sci.& Tech.Abstr., Forest.Abstr., Genet.Abstr., Helminthol.Abstr., Hort.Abstr., Hum.Gen.Abstr., INIS Atomind., Ind.Med. (1922-), Ind.Sci.Rev., Ind.Vet., Inpharma, Int.Abstr.Biol.Sci., Mass Spectr.Bull., Microbiol.Abstr., NPU, Neurosci.Cit.Ind., Nuc.Acids Abstr., Nutr.Abstr., Ornam.Hort., Pharm.&Out.News, Pig News & Info., Plant Breed.Abstr., Postharvest, Poult.Abstr., Protozool.Abstr., Reac., Ref.Zh., Rev.Appl.Entomol., Rev.Arom.& Med.Plants, Rev.Med.& Vet.Mycol., Rev.Plant Path., Rice Abstr., Sci.Cit.Ind., Seed Abstr., Soils & Fert., Soyabean Abstr., Sugar Ind.Abstr., Tox.Abstr. (coverage dropped), Triticale Abstr., Trop.Dis.Bull., Vet.Bull.
—BLDSC (4952.000000), CASDDS, CINDOC, CISTI, Ei, GNLM, IDS, ingenta, KNAW, Linda Hall. **CCC.**
Published by: Japanese Biochemical Society/Nihon Seikagakkai, 26-16 Hongo 5-chome, Bunkyo-ku, Tokyo 113-0033, Japan. TEL 81-3-38151913, FAX 81-3-38151934, TELEX 2722268 BCJSP J, jbs-ho@bcasj.or.jp, http://jb.bcasj.or.jp/. Circ: 2,650. **Dist. by:** Business Center for Academic Societies Japan, 5-16-9 Honkomagome, Bunkyo-ku, Tokyo 113-0021, Japan. TEL 5814-5811.

572 HKG ISSN 1225-8687
QD415.A1 CODEN: JBMBE5
JOURNAL OF BIOCHEMISTRY AND MOLECULAR BIOLOGY. Text in English. 1968. bi-m. USD 403.40 domestic; USD 397.10 in Germany; USD 74 newsstand/cover foreign (effective 2002). 100 p./no. *Refereed.* **Document type:** *Journal, Academic/Scholarly.*
Formerly (until 1995): Korean Biochemical Journal (0368-4881)
Related titles: ♦ Online - full content ed.: Journal of Biochemistry and Molecular Biology Online. ISSN 0219-1024; Online - full text ed.: (from Springer LINK, Institute for Scientific Information, RoweCom Information Quest).
Indexed: BBCI, Chem.Abstr., Chem.Indus.Notes, Chem.Titles, Food Sci.& Tech.Abstr., INIS Atomind., Sugar Ind.Abstr., Zoo.Rec.
—BLDSC (4952.110000), CASDDS, GNLM, IDS.
Published by: (Biochemical Society of the Republic of Korea SGP), Springer-Verlag Hong Kong Ltd. (Subsidiary of: BertelsmannSpringer), Unit 1702, Tower 1, Enterprise Square, 9 Sheung Yuet Rd, Kowloon Bay, Kowloon, Hong Kong. TEL 852-2723-9698, FAX 852-2724-2366, springer@springer.com.hk, http://link.springer.de/link/service/journals/10060/index.htm. Ed. Doe Sun Na.

572 HKG ISSN 0219-1024
JOURNAL OF BIOCHEMISTRY AND MOLECULAR BIOLOGY ONLINE. Text in English. bi-m. **Document type:** *Academic/Scholarly.*
Media: Online - full content (from EBSCO Publishing, Swets Blackwell). **Related titles:** Online - full text ed.: (from Springer LINK, Institute for Scientific Information, RoweCom Information Quest); ♦ Print ed.: Journal of Biochemistry and Molecular Biology. ISSN 1225-8687.
Published by: Springer-Verlag Hong Kong Ltd. (Subsidiary of: BertelsmannSpringer), Unit 1702, Tower 1, Enterprise Square, 9 Sheung Yuet Rd, Kowloon Bay, Kowloon, Hong Kong. TEL 852-723-9698, FAX 852-724-2366, springer@springer.com.hk, http://link.springer.de/link/service/journals/10060/index.htm.

572 CHE ISSN 1025-8140
JOURNAL OF BIOCHEMISTRY, MOLECULAR BIOLOGY AND BIOPHYSICS. Text in English. 1997. 6/yr. GBP 66, USD 80, EUR 88 to individuals; GBP 264, USD 340, EUR 357 to institutions; GBP 403, USD 508, EUR 542 to corporations (effective 2002). **Document type:** *Journal, Academic/Scholarly.* **Description:** Dedicated to the rapid publication of reviews and stories from the world's scientific community.
Related titles: CD-ROM ed.; Microfilm ed.; Online - full text ed.: (from EBSCO Publishing, RoweCom Information Quest).
Indexed: ASCA, Aqua.Sci.& Fish.Abstr., Crop Physiol.Abstr., Environ.Sci.Poll.Mgmt., Genet.Abstr., Hort.Abstr., Hum.Gen.Abstr., Microbiol.Abstr., Nuc.Acids Abstr., Plant Breed.Abstr., Postharvest, Rev.Plant Path., Tox.Abstr.
—CISTI, Infotrieve. **CCC.**
Published by: (Federation of Asian and Oceanian Biochemists and Molecular Biologists), Gordon and Breach - Harwood Academic (Subsidiary of: Taylor & Francis Group), PO Box 531, Lausanne 1000, Switzerland. TEL 41-21-6411280, FAX 41-21-6411281, info@gbhap.com, http://www.gbhap.com. Eds. Ikuo Yamashima, Richard John Guillory. **Subscr. addr. in US:** International Publishers Direct, PO Box 32160, Newark, NJ 07102. FAX 215-750-6343.

572.43 USA ISSN 0145-479X
QH511.A1 CODEN: JBBID4
JOURNAL OF BIOENERGETICS AND BIOMEMBRANES. Text in English. 1970. bi-m. USD 627, EUR 626 to institutions for print or online ed.; USD 752.40, EUR 751.20 to institutions for print & online eds. combined (effective 2002). adv. bibl, charts, illus. back issues avail. *Refereed.* **Document type:** *Journal, Academic/Scholarly.* **Description:** Publishes original research contributions in the areas of bioenergetics, biomembranes and transport, including muscle contraction, electron transport, ATP synthesis, and membrane transport.
Formerly (until 1976): Journal of Bioenergetics (0449-5705)
Related titles: Microfilm ed.: (from PQC); Online - full text ed.: (from Ovid Technologies, Inc., EBSCO Publishing, O C L C Online Computer Library Center, Inc., RoweCom Information Quest, Swets Blackwell, Kluwer Online, Institute for Scientific Information).
Indexed: ASCA, Abstr.Bull.Inst.Pap.Chem., Aqua.Sci.& Fish.Abstr., BBCI, Biol.Abstr., Chem.Abstr., Chem.Cit.Ind., Chem.Indus.Notes, Chem.Titles, Curr.Adv.Biochem., Curr.Cont., Excerp.Med., INIS Atomind., INSPEC (Jan.1973-Aug.1976, Oct.1976-), Ind.Med. (1976-), Ind.Sci.Rev., Inpharma, Int.Abstr.Biol.Sci., Pharm.&Out.News, Reac., Ref.Zh., Sci.Cit.Ind.
—BLDSC (4952.820000), AskIEEE, CASDDS, CISTI, GNLM, IDS, Infotrieve, ingenta, Linda Hall. **CCC.**
Published by: Kluwer Academic - Plenum Publishers (Subsidiary of: Wolters Kluwer N.V.), 233 Spring St, New York, NY 10013-1578. TEL 212-620-8000, 800-221-9369, FAX 212-463-0742, info@plenum.com, http://www.wkap.nl/journalhome.htm/0145-479X. Ed. Peter L Pedersen. R&P Rose Luongo TEL 781-871-6311. **Subscr. outside the Americas to:** Kluwer Academic Publishers Group, Journals Department, PO Box 322, Dordrecht 3300 AH, Netherlands. TEL 31-78-639-2392, FAX 31-78-654-6474.

572 USA ISSN 0021-9258
QP501 CODEN: JBCHA3
JOURNAL OF BIOLOGICAL CHEMISTRY. Text in English. 1905. w. USD 1,600; USD 1,962 in Canada; USD 1,850 elsewhere (effective 2000). adv. illus. index. reprint service avail. from PQC. *Refereed.* **Document type:** *Academic/Scholarly.*
Related titles: CD-ROM ed.: ISSN 1067-8816. 1992; Microform ed.: (from PQC,PMC); Online - full text ed.: ISSN 1083-351X. USD 1,100 (effective 2000) (from HighWire Pr., EBSCO Publishing, RoweCom Information Quest, Institute for Scientific Information).
Indexed: AIDS Abstr., ASCA, Abstr.Bull.Inst.Pap.Chem., AgBiotech, Agri.& Environ.Biotech.Abstr. (coverage dropped), Agricola, Anim.Breed.Abstr., Aqua.Sci.& Fish.Abstr., BBCI, Bibl.Agri., Bio-Contr.News & Info., Biol.& Agr.Ind. (Jan.1983-), Biol.Abstr., Biwk.Pap.Rad.Chem.& Photochem., Cal.Tiss.Abstr. (coverage dropped), Chem.Abstr., Chem.Cit.Ind., Chem.Indus.Notes, Chem.Titles, Chemorec.Abstr., Crop Physiol.Abstr., Curr.Adv.Biochem., Curr.Adv.Cancer Res., Curr.Adv.Cell & Devel.Biol., Curr.Adv.Gen.& Molec.Biol., Curr.Cont., Curr.Ref.Fish Res., Dairy Sci.Abstr., Deep Sea Res.& Oceanogr.Abstr., Dent.Ind., Derwent Biotech.Abstr., Eng.Ind., Entomol.Abstr. (coverage dropped), Environ.Sci.Poll.Mgmt., Excerp.Med., Field Crop Abstr., Food Sci.& Tech.Abstr., Forest Prod.Abstr., Forest.Abstr., Genet.Abstr., Helminthol.Abstr., Herb.Abstr., Hort.Abstr., Hum.Gen.Abstr., INIS Atomind., Immun.Abstr. (coverage dropped), Ind.Med. (1905-), Ind.Sci.Rev., Ind.Vet., Inpharma, Int.Abstr.Biol.Sci., Maize Abstr., Mass Spectr.Bull., Microbiol.Abstr., Neurosci.Abstr., Neurosci.Cit.Ind., Nuc.Acids Abstr., Nutr.Abstr., Ornam.Hort., Pharm.&Out.News, Pig News & Info., Plant Breed.Abstr., Plant Gen.Res.Abstr., Plant Grow.Reg.Abstr., Potato Abstr., Poult.Abstr., Protozool.Abstr., Reac., Ref.Zh., Rev.Appl.Entomol., Rev.Arom.& Med.Plants, Rev.Med.& Vet.Mycol., Rev.Plant Path., Rice Abstr., Sci.Cit.Ind., Seed Abstr., Soils & Fert., Soyabean Abstr., Sport Fish.Abstr., Sugar Ind.Abstr., Telegen, Tox.Abstr. (coverage dropped), Triticale Abstr., Trop.Dis.Bull., Vet.Bull., Virol.Abstr. (coverage dropped), Weed Abstr., Wild.Rev., Zoo.Rec.
—BLDSC (4953.000000), CASDDS, CINDOC, CISTI, GNLM, IDS, ingenta, Linda Hall. **CCC.**
Published by: American Society for Biochemistry and Molecular Biology, Inc., 9650 Rockville Pike, Bethesda, MD 20814. asbmb@asbmb.faseb.org, http://www.jbc.org. Ed. Herbert Tabor. Circ: 6,000.

572.8 USA ISSN 1087-0571
RS189 CODEN: JBISF3
JOURNAL OF BIOMOLECULAR SCREENING. Text in English. 1996. bi-m. USD 319 domestic to individuals; USD 369 foreign to individuals; USD 383 domestic to individuals print and online eds. combined; USD 433 foreign to individuals print and online eds. combined; USD 443 domestic to institutions; USD 576 foreign to institutions; USD 532 domestic to institutions print and online eds. combined; USD 664 foreign to institutions print and online eds. combined (effective 2002). back issues avail.; reprints avail. *Refereed.* **Document type:** *Journal, Academic/Scholarly.* **Description:** Covers chemistry, biology, automation and information management, including all aspects of the discovery process, from basic research through the early stages of product development.
Related titles: Online - full content ed.: USD 319 to individuals; USD 443 to institutions (effective 2002) (from Swets Blackwell); Online - full text ed.: (from CatchWord Ltd., Institute for Scientific Information, RoweCom Information Quest).
Indexed: Biotech.Cit.Ind., Chem.Abstr., Chem.Indus.Notes, Chem.Titles, Curr.Cont., Excerp.Med., Ind.Med., Mass Spectr.Bull.
—BLDSC (4953.845000), CASDDS, CatchWord, CISTI, GNLM, IDS, Infotrieve. **CCC.**
Published by: (Society for Biomolecular Screening), Mary Ann Liebert, Inc. Publishers, 2 Madison Ave, Larchmont, NY 10538. TEL 914—834-3100, FAX 914-834-1388, info@liebertpub.com, http://www.liebertpub.com/bsc. Ed. Larry Walker.

JOURNAL OF BRAIN SCIENCE. see *MEDICAL SCIENCES—Psychiatry And Neurology*

B

572 USA ISSN 0730-2312
QH506 CODEN: JCEBD5

JOURNAL OF CELLULAR BIOCHEMISTRY. Text in English. 1972. 18/yr. (in 4 vols., 3 nos./vol.). USD 4,995 in United States; USD 5,175 in Canada & Mexico; USD 5,328 elsewhere; USD 5,245 combined subscription in United States for print and online eds.; USD 5,425 combined subscription in Canada & Mexico for print and online eds.; USD 5,578 combined subscription elsewhere for print and online eds. (effective 2002). adv. bk.rev. charts, illus, stat. back issues avail.; reprint service avail. from ISI. *Refereed.* **Document type:** *Academic/Scholarly.* **Description:** Publishes timely reviews, commentaries, and descriptions of original research in areas where complex cellular, photogenic, clinical, or animal model systems are studied by biochemical, genetic or quantitative ultrastructural approaches.

Former titles (until 1982): Journal of Supramolecular Structure and Cellular Biochemistry (0275-3723); (until 1981): Journal of Supramolecular Structure (0091-7419)

Related titles: Microform ed.: (from PQC); Online - full text ed.: ISSN 1097-4644. 1996. USD 4,995 in United States; USD 4,995 in Canada & Mexico; USD 4,995 elsewhere (effective 2002) (from EBSCO Publishing, Wiley InterScience, Institute for Scientific Information); ♦ Supplement: Journal of Cellular Biochemistry. Supplement. ISSN 0733-1959.

Indexed: ASCA, Abstr.Anthropol., Agri.& Environ.Biotech.Abstr. (coverage dropped), BBCI, Biol.Abstr., Chem.Abstr., Chem.Indus.Notes, Chem.Titles, Curr.Adv.Biochem., Curr.Adv.Cell & Devel.Biol., Curr.Adv.Ecol.Sci., Curr.Adv.Gen.& Molec.Biol., Curr.Cont., Derwent Biotech.Abstr., Excerp.Med., INIS Atomind., Ind.Med. (1982-), Ind.Sci.Rev., Inpharma, Mat.Sci.Cit.Ind. (coverage dropped), Neurosci.Cit.Ind., Nutr.Abstr., Protozool.Abstr., Reac., Ref.Zh., Rev.Med.& Vet.Mycol., SSCI (coverage dropped), Sci.Cit.Ind., Sport Fish.Abstr., Wild.Rev., Zoo.Rec.

—BLDSC (4955.010000), CASDDS, CISTI, EMDOCS, GNLM, IDS, Infotrieve, ingenta, Linda Hall. **CCC.**

Published by: John Wiley & Sons, Inc., Journals (Subsidiary of: Wiley InterScience), 605 Third Ave, New York, NY 10158. TEL 212-850-6645, FAX 212-850-6021, subinfo@wiley.com, uscs-wis@wiley.com, http://www.wiley.com. adv.: B&W page GBP 640, color page GBP 1,515; trim 174 x 254. Circ: 850. **Subscr. outside the Americas to:** John Wiley & Sons Ltd., Baffins Ln, Chichester, Sussex PO19 IUD, United Kingdom. TEL 44-1243-779777, FAX 44-1243-843232, cs-journals@wiley.co.uk, http://www.wiley.co.uk.

JOURNAL OF CEREBRAL BLOOD FLOW AND METABOLISM. see *MEDICAL SCIENCES—Psychiatry And Neurology*

JOURNAL OF CHEMICAL AND BIOCHEMICAL KINETICS. see *CHEMISTRY*

JOURNAL OF CHEMICAL NEUROANATOMY. see *MEDICAL SCIENCES—Psychiatry And Neurology*

JOURNAL OF CHROMATOGRAPHY. B, BIOMEDICAL SCIENCES AND APPLICATIONS. see *CHEMISTRY*

572 613.2 JPN ISSN 0912-0009

JOURNAL OF CLINICAL BIOCHEMICAL AND NUTRITION. Text in English. 1986. bi-m. *Refereed.* **Document type:** *Academic/Scholarly.*

Related titles: Online - full text ed.: (from Institute for Scientific Information).

Indexed: BBCI, Dairy Sci.Abstr., Ind.Vet., Int.Abstr.Biol.Sci., Nutr.Abstr., Protozool.Abstr.

—BLDSC (4958.381850).

Published by: Institute of Applied Biochemistry, 1-1-1 Tennodai, Tsukuba, Ibaraki 305-8572, Japan. TEL 81-298-53-4936, FAX 81-298-53-4605, abc@agbi.tsukuba.ac.jp, http://www.agbi.tsukuba.ac.jp/~abc/.

JOURNAL OF COMPARATIVE PHYSIOLOGY. B: BIOCHEMICAL, SYSTEMIC, AND ENVIRONMENTAL PHYSIOLOGY. see *BIOLOGY—Physiology*

572.7 CHE ISSN 8755-5093
CODEN: ENINEG

JOURNAL OF ENZYME INHIBITION. Text in English. 6/yr. GBP 167, USD 203, EUR 223 to individuals; GBP 713, USD 900, EUR 950 to institutions; GBP 1,201, USD 1,474, EUR 1,601 to corporations (effective 2002). *Refereed.* **Document type:** *Journal, Academic/Scholarly.*

Related titles: CD-ROM ed.; Microform ed.; Online - full text ed.: (from EBSCO Publishing, RoweCom Information Quest, Institute for Scientific Information).

Indexed: ASCA, BBCI, Biotech.Cit.Ind., Chem.Cit.Ind., Curr.Cont., Derwent Biotech.Abstr., Field Crop Abstr., Food Sci.& Tech.Abstr., Ind.Med. (1985-), Inpharma, Int.Abstr.Biol.Sci., Pharm.&Out.News, Protozool.Abstr., Reac., Rev.Med.& Vet.Mycol., Sci.Cit.Ind.

—BLDSC (4979.460000), CISTI, EMDOCS, GNLM, ingenta. **CCC.**

Published by: Gordon and Breach - Harwood Academic (Subsidiary of: Taylor & Francis Group), PO Box 531, Lausanne 1000, Switzerland. TEL 41-21-6411280, FAX 41-21-6411281, info@gbhap.com, http://www.gbhap.com/Enzyme_Inhibition/. Ed. H J Smith. **Subscr. addr. in US:** International Publishers Direct, PO Box 32160, Newark, NJ 07102. FAX 215-750-6343.

572 RUS ISSN 0022-0930
QP1 CODEN: JEBPA9

JOURNAL OF EVOLUTIONARY BIOCHEMISTRY AND PHYSIOLOGY. Text in English. 1965. bi-m. EUR 2,557 to institutions for print or online ed.; EUR 3,068.40 to institutions print & online eds.combined (effective 2002). back issues avail. *Refereed.* **Document type:** *Academic/Scholarly.* **Description:** Illuminates the most recent research findings on the evolution of basic forms of metabolism, comparative and developmental physiology, and biochemistry and the biochemical evolution of the animal world.

Related titles: Microfilm ed.: (from PQC); Online - full text ed.: ISSN 1608-3202 (from Swets Blackwell, Kluwer Online, Institute for Scientific Information, RoweCom Information Quest); ♦ Translation of: Zhurnal Evolyutsionnoi Biokhimii i Fiziologii. ISSN 0044-4529.

Indexed: ASCA, Aqua.Sci.& Fish.Abstr., Aquacult.Abstr., BBCI, Biol.Abstr., Environ.Sci.Poll.Mgmt., Excerp.Med., Ind.Med. (coverage dropped), Int.Abstr.Biol.Sci., Neurosci.Cit.Ind.

—BLDSC (0414.450000), CASDDS, CISTI, IDS, ingenta. **CCC.**

Published by: (Rossiiskaya Akademiya Nauk/Russian Academy of Sciences), M A I K Nauka - Interperiodica, S.-Peterburgskoe Otdelenie, Thorez Ave 44, St Petersburg 194223, Russian Federation. compmg@maik.ru, http://maik.rssi.ru/journals/evolbp.htm. Ed. Vladimir L Svidersky. **Dist. by:** Kluwer Academic Publishers, PO Box 17, Dordrecht 3300 AH, Netherlands. TEL 31-78-639-2392, FAX 31-78-654-6474, http://www.wkap.nl.

JOURNAL OF HEALTH SCIENCE/EISEI KAGAKU. see *ENVIRONMENTAL STUDIES—Toxicology And Environmental Safety*

JOURNAL OF HISTOTECHNOLOGY. see *BIOLOGY—Cytology And Histology*

572 USA ISSN 0162-0134
QP501 CODEN: JIBIDJ

JOURNAL OF INORGANIC BIOCHEMISTRY; an interdisciplinary journal. Text in English. 1971. 20/yr. EUR 1,700 in Europe to institutions; JPY 225,500 in Japan to institutions; USD 1,902 elsewhere to institutions (effective 2002). adv. bk.rev. charts, illus. index. *Refereed.* **Document type:** *Journal, Academic/Scholarly.* **Description:** Publishes research papers and short communications in all areas of inorganic biochemistry.

Formerly (until vol.10): Bioinorganic Chemistry (0006-3061)

Related titles: Microform ed.: (from PQC); Online - full text ed.: (from ingenta, ScienceDirect, Swets Blackwell, Institute for Scientific Information).

Indexed: ASCA, Agricola, Apic.Abstr., BBCI, Bibl.Agri., Biol.Abstr., CEABA, Cadscan, Chem.Abstr., Chem.Cit.Ind., Chem.Indus.Notes, Chem.Titles, Crop Physiol.Abstr., Curr.Adv.Biochem., Curr.Adv.Ecol.Sci., Curr.Cont., Excerp.Med., Hort.Abstr., INIS Atomind., Ind.Med. (1979-), Ind.Sci.Rev., Inpharma, Int.Abstr.Biol.Sci., Lead Abstr., METADEX, Mass Spectr.Bull., Nutr.Abstr., RCI, Reac., Ref.Zh., Rev.Plant Path., Sci.Cit.Ind., Zincscan.

—BLDSC (5007.150000), CASDDS, CISTI, GNLM, IDS, ingenta, Linda Hall. **CCC.**

Published by: Elsevier Science, Box 945, New York, NY 10159-0945. TEL 212-989-5800, FAX 212-633-3990, usinfo-f@elsevier.com, http://www.elsevier.com/locate/jinorgbio. Eds. J H Dawson, M Sono. **Subscr. in Australasia and the Far East to:** Elsevier Science (Singapore) Pte Ltd, No.1 Temasek Ave, 17-01 Millenia Tower, Singapore 039192, Singapore. TEL 65-434-3727, FAX 65-337-2230; **Subscr. in Japan to:** Elsevier Science Inc - Japan Regional Office, 9-15 Higashi-Azabu 1-chome, Minato-ku, Tokyo 106-0044, Japan. TEL 81-3-5561-5033; **Subscr. outside the Americas to:** Elsevier Science BV, PO Box 211, Amsterdam 1000 AE, Netherlands. TEL 31-20-485-3757.

572.57 USA ISSN 0022-2275
QP751 CODEN: JLPRAW

JOURNAL OF LIPID RESEARCH. Text in English. 1959. m. USD 110 to individuals; USD 134 in Canada & Mexico to individuals; USD 165 elsewhere to individuals; USD 366 to institutions; USD 390 in Canada & Mexico to institutions; USD 421 elsewhere to institutions (effective 1999). adv. bibl, illus. index. back issues avail. *Refereed.* **Document type:** *Academic/Scholarly.* **Description:** Publishes original articles and invited reviews on subjects involving lipids in any scientific discipline.

Related titles: Microform ed.: (from PQC); Online - full text ed.: (from HighWire Pr., EBSCO Publishing, Institute for Scientific Information).

Indexed: ASCA, AgBiotech, Agri.& Environ.Biotech.Abstr. (coverage dropped), Agricola, Anal.Abstr., Anim.Breed.Abstr., BBCI, Bibl.Agri., Biol.Abstr., Biol.Dig., Chem.Abstr., Chem.Cit.Ind., Chem.Indus.Notes, Chem.Titles, Curr.Adv.Biochem., Curr.Adv.Cell & Devel.Biol., Curr.Adv.Ecol.Sci., Curr.Adv.Gen.& Molec.Biol., Curr.Chem.React., Curr.Cont., Dairy Sci.Abstr., Dent.Ind., Derwent Biotech.Abstr., Excerp.Med., Food Sci.& Tech.Abstr., Helminthol.Abstr., INIS Atomind., Ind.Chem., Ind.Med. (1959-), Ind.Sci.Rev., Ind.Vet., Inpharma, Int.Abstr.Biol.Sci., Maize Abstr., Mass Spectr.Bull., NPU, NRN, Nutr.Abstr., Pharm.&Out.News, RCI, Reac., Ref.Zh., Rev.Appl.Entomol., Rev.Med.& Vet.Mycol., Sci.Cit.Ind., Sport Fish.Abstr., THA, Telegen, Vet.Bull., Wild.Rev., Zoo.Rec.

—BLDSC (5010.500000), CASDDS, CINDOC, CISTI, GNLM, IDS, ingenta, Linda Hall. **CCC.**

Published by: Lipid Research, Inc., 9650 Rockville Pike, Bethesda, MD 20814. TEL 301-530-7100, FAX 301-571-5723, lgidez@faseb.org, http://www.jlr.org/. Ed. Arthur A Spector. R&P Lewis I Gidez. Adv. contact Susan Mergenhagen. Circ: 1,650.

572 GBR ISSN 0022-2836
QH301 CODEN: JMOBAK

JOURNAL OF MOLECULAR BIOLOGY. Text in English. 1959. w. (50/yr.). GBP 3,200 to institutions (effective 2001). adv. bibl, charts, illus. index,cum.index. reprint service avail. from SWZ. *Refereed.* **Document type:** *Academic/Scholarly.* **Description:** Presents original scientific research concerning studies of organisms or their components at the molecular level.

Related titles: Online - full text ed.: J M B Online. ISSN 1089-8638. 199? (from EBSCO Publishing, O C L C Online Computer Library Center, Inc., RoweCom Information Quest, ingenta, Swets Blackwell, IDEAL Online Library, Institute for Scientific Information).

Indexed: ASCA, Abstr.Hyg., AgBiotech, Agri.& Environ.Biotech.Abstr. (coverage dropped), Agricola, Anim.Breed.Abstr., Aqua.Sci.& Fish.Abstr., BBCI, Bibl.Agri., Bio-Contr.News & Info., Biol.& Agr.Ind. (Dec.1989-), Biol.Abstr., Biostat., Biotech.Cit.Ind., Chem.Abstr., Chem.Cit.Ind., Chem.Titles, Compumath, Crop Physiol.Abstr., Curr.Adv.Biochem., Curr.Adv.Cancer Res., Curr.Adv.Cell & Devel.Biol., Curr.Adv.Ecol.Sci., Curr.Adv.Gen.& Molec.Biol., Curr.Cont., Dairy Sci.Abstr., Derwent Biotech.Abstr., Environ.Sci.Poll.Mgmt., Excerp.Med., Field Crop Abstr., Food Sci.& Tech.Abstr., Genet.Abstr., Helminthol.Abstr., Herb.Abstr., Hum.Gen.Abstr., INIS Atomind., Ind.Med. (1959-), Ind.Sci.Rev., Ind.Vet., Inpharma, Int.Abstr.Biol.Sci., Mass Spectr.Bull., Microbiol.Abstr., Neurosci.Abstr., Nuc.Acids Abstr., Nutr.Abstr., Oncog.G.F.Abstr. (coverage dropped), Ornam.Hort., Pig News & Info., Plant Breed.Abstr., Plant Grow.Reg.Abstr., Potato Abstr., Poult.Abstr., Protozool.Abstr., Reac., Ref.Zh., Rev.Appl.Entomol., Rev.Med.& Vet.Mycol., Rev.Plant Path., Rice Abstr., Sci.Cit.Ind., Seed Abstr., Soils & Fert., Soyabean Abstr., Sport Fish.Abstr., Sugar Ind.Abstr., Triticale Abstr., Trop.Dis.Bull., Vet.Bull., Virol.Abstr. (coverage dropped), Weed Abstr., Wild.Rev., Zoo.Rec.

—BLDSC (5020.700000), ADONIS, CASDDS, CISTI, GNLM, IDS, ingenta, Linda Hall. **CCC.**

Published by: Academic Press (Subsidiary of: Harcourt Publishers Ltd.), 24 Oval Rd, London NW1 7DX, United Kingdom. TEL 44-20-7267-4466, FAX 44-20-7482-2293, apsubs@acad.com, http://www.academicpress.com/jmb; http://www.europe.idealibrary.com/. Ed. P Wright. R&P Catherine John. Adv. contact Nik Screen. **Subscr. to:** Harcourt Publishers Ltd., Foots Cray High St, Sidcup, Kent DA14 5HP, United Kingdom. TEL 44-20-8300-3322, FAX 44-20-8309-0807.

JOURNAL OF NATURAL PRODUCTS. see *PHARMACY AND PHARMACOLOGY*

573.84 GBR ISSN 0022-3042
QP351 CODEN: JONRA9
JOURNAL OF NEUROCHEMISTRY. Text in English. 1956. m., latest vol.80, 2002. GBP 378 in Europe to individuals; USD 598 in North America to individuals; GBP 415 per issue elsewhere to individuals; GBP 1,453 per issue in Europe to institutions; USD 2,301 per issue in North America to institutions; GBP 1,599 per issue elsewhere to institutions (effective 2002). adv. bk.rev. bibl, charts, illus. index. back issues avail.; reprint service avail. from PQC. *Refereed.* **Document type:** *Journal, Academic/Scholarly.* **Description:** Provides complete coverage of the biochemical aspects of behavior and brain function.
Related titles: Microform ed.: (from PQC); Online - full text ed.: ISSN 1471-4159. GBP 341 in Europe to individuals; USD 539 in North America to individuals; GBP 341 elsewhere to individuals; GBP 1,308 in Europe to institutions; USD 2,071 in North America to institutions; GBP 1,308 elsewhere to institutions (effective 2002) (from HighWire Pr., EBSCO Publishing, Munksgaard & Blackwell Science's Synergy, Swets Blackwell, Institute for Scientific Information, RoweCom Information Quest).
Indexed: AIDS Abstr., ASCA, Agri.& Environ.Biotech.Abstr. (coverage dropped), Aqua.Sci.& Fish.Abstr., BBCI, Biol.Abstr., Cal.Tiss.Abstr. (coverage dropped), Chem.Abstr., Chem.Cit.Ind., Chem.Indus.Notes, Chem.Titles, Chemorec.Abstr., Curr.Adv.Biochem., Curr.Adv.Ecol.Sci., Curr.Cont., Dairy Sci.Abstr., Dent.Ind., Derwent Biotech.Abstr., Excerp.Med., INIS Atomind., Ind.Med. (1956-), Ind.Sci.Rev., Ind.Vet., Inpharma, Int.Abstr.Biol.Sci., Mass Spectr.Bull., Neurosci.Abstr., Neurosci.Cit.Ind., Nutr.Abstr., Pharm.&Out.News, Reac., Ref.Zh., SSCI (coverage dropped), Sci.Cit.Ind., Sport Fish.Abstr., THA, Tox.Abstr. (coverage dropped), Trop.Dis.Bull., Vet.Bull., e-psyche.
—BLDSC (5021.500000), CASDDS, CISTI, GNLM, IDS, ingenta, KNAW, Linda Hall.
Published by: (International Society for Neurochemistry USA), Blackwell Science Ltd., PO Box 88, Oxford OX2 0NE, United Kingdom. TEL 44-1865-206180, 44-1865-206002, FAX 44-1865-206219, jnl.orders@blacksci.co.uk, http://www.blackwell-science.com/~cgilib/jnlpage.asp?Journal=jnc&File=jnc, http://www.blackwellpublishing.com. Ed. Brian Collier. adv.: B&W page USD 915, color page USD 2,070. Circ: 2,189 (paid).

JOURNAL OF NUTRITIONAL BIOCHEMISTRY. see *NUTRITION AND DIETETICS*

572.65 DNK ISSN 1397-002X
CODEN: JPERFA
JOURNAL OF PEPTIDE RESEARCH. Text in English. 1997. m. USD 648 in the Americas to institutions print & online eds combined; GBP 450 elsewhere to institutions print & online eds. combined (effective 2002). adv. charts, illus. index. reprint service avail. from SWZ,ISI. *Refereed.* **Document type:** *Academic/Scholarly.*
Formed by the merger of (1968-1997): International Journal of Peptide and Protein Research (0367-8377); (1988-1997): Peptide Research (1040-5704)
Related titles: Online - full text ed.: USD 583 (2002) (from Ovid Technologies, Inc., EBSCO Publishing, O C L C Online Computer Library Center, Inc., RoweCom Information Quest, ingenta, Munksgaard & Blackwell Science's Synergy, Swets Blackwell, Institute for Scientific Information).
Indexed: ASCA, Abstr.Hyg., Agri.& Environ.Biotech.Abstr. (coverage dropped), Anim.Breed.Abstr., Aqua.Sci.& Fish.Abstr., BBCI, Biol.Abstr., Chem.Abstr., Chem.Cit.Ind., Chem.Indus.Notes, Chem.Titles, Curr.Adv.Biochem., Curr.Adv.Gen.& Molec.Biol., Curr.Chem.React., Curr.Cont., Dairy Sci.Abstr., Dent.Ind., Derwent Biotech.Abstr., Eng.Ind., INIS Atomind., Ind.Chem., Ind.Med. (1997-), Ind.Sci.Rev., Ind.Vet., Inpharma, Int.Abstr.Biol.Sci., Mass Spectr.Bull., Mat.Sci.Cit.Ind. (coverage dropped), Protozool.Abstr., RCI, Reac., Rev.Med.& Vet.Mycol., Rev.Plant Path., Sci.Cit.Ind., Trop.Dis.Bull., Vet.Bull.
—BLDSC (5030.528000), ADONIS, CASDDS, CISTI, Ei, EMDOCS, GNLM, IDS, Infotrieve, ingenta, Linda Hall. **CCC.**
Published by: (American Peptide Society USA), Blackwell Munksgaard, Noerre Soegade 35, PO Box 2148, Copenhagen K 1016, Denmark. FAX 45-77-33-33-77, fsub@munksgaard.dk, http://www.blackwellmunksgaard.com/peptideresearch. Ed. Victor J Hruby. Circ: 1,400.

JOURNAL OF PHARMACOLOGICAL AND TOXICOLOGICAL METHODS. see *ENVIRONMENTAL STUDIES—Toxicology And Environmental Safety*

572 CHE ISSN 1011-1344
QH515 CODEN: JPPBEG
JOURNAL OF PHOTOCHEMISTRY AND PHOTOBIOLOGY, B: BIOLOGY. Text in English. 1987. 18/yr. EUR 2,232 in Europe to institutions; JPY 309,100 in Japan to institutions; USD 2,497 elsewhere to institutions (effective 2002). bk.rev. back issues avail. *Refereed.* **Document type:** *Academic/Scholarly.* **Description:** Publishes papers for scientists who seek to understand light and its interactions with the processes of life. Also includes technological developments, forthcoming events, conference reports, and reports on current areas of research.
Related titles: Microform ed.: (from PQC); Online - full text ed.: (from ingenta, ScienceDirect, Swets Blackwell, Institute for Scientific Information).
Indexed: ASCA, Aqua.Sci.& Fish.Abstr., BBCI, Cal.Tiss.Abstr., Chem.Abstr., Chem.Cit.Ind., Chem.Indus.Notes, Chem.Titles, Curr.Adv.Biochem., Curr.Adv.Cancer Res., Curr.Cont., Eng.Ind., Environ.Sci.Poll.Mgmt., Excerp.Med. (1993-), Ind.Med. (1987-), Ind.Sci.Rev., Inpharma, Int.Abstr.Biol.Sci., Jrnl.Watch Derm., Met.Abstr., Meteor.& Geoastrophys.Abstr., Pharm.&Out.News, Photo.Abstr., Phys.Ber., Pollut.Abstr., Reac., Ref.Zh., Sci.Cit.Ind., Zoo.Rec.
—BLDSC (5034.850000), CASDDS, EMDOCS, GNLM, IDS, Infotrieve, ingenta, Linda Hall. **CCC.**
Published by: (European Society for Photobiology), Elsevier Science S.A., PO Box 564, Lausanne, 1 1001, Switzerland. TEL 41-21-3207381, FAX 41-21-3235444, http://www.elsevier.com/locate/jphotobiol. Eds. G Jori, T Vidoacuteczy. **Subscr. in Australasia to:** Elsevier Science (Singapore) Pte Ltd, No.1 Temasek Ave, 17-01 Millenia Tower, Singapore 039192, Singapore. TEL 65-434-3727, FAX 65-337-2230; **Subscr. in the Americas to:** Elsevier Science, PO Box 945, New York, NY 10159-0945. TEL 212-633-3730, FAX 212-633-3680; **Subscr. to:** Elsevier Science BV, PO Box 211, Amsterdam 1000 AE, Netherlands. TEL 31-20-485-3757.

572.4 USA ISSN 0277-8033
QP551 CODEN: JPCHD2
JOURNAL OF PROTEIN CHEMISTRY. Text in English. 1982. 8/yr. USD 801, EUR 800 to institutions for print or online ed.; USD 961.20, EUR 960 to institutions for print & online eds.combined (effective 2002). adv. back issues avail. *Refereed.* **Document type:** *Journal, Academic/Scholarly.* **Description:** Publishes original research investigating the molecular basis for protein function. Covers all aspects of protein activity.
Related titles: Microfilm ed.: (from PQC); Online - full text ed.: (from EBSCO Publishing, O C L C Online Computer Library Center, Inc., Swets Blackwell, Kluwer Online, Institute for Scientific Information, RoweCom Information Quest).
Indexed: ASCA, Aqua.Sci.& Fish.Abstr., BBCI, Chem.Abstr., Chem.Cit.Ind., Chem.Indus.Notes, Chem.Titles, Curr.Adv.Biochem., Curr.Adv.Cell & Devel.Biol., Curr.Cont., Eng.Ind., Hort.Abstr., INIS Atomind., Ind.Med. (1982-), Ind.Sci.Rev., Inpharma, Int.Abstr.Biol.Sci., Mass Spectr.Bull., Nutr.Abstr., Postharvest, Reac., Rev.Appl.Entomol., Rev.Med.& Vet.Mycol., Rev.Plant Path., Sci.Cit.Ind., Seed Abstr., Triticale Abstr.
—BLDSC (5042.950000), CASDDS, CISTI, Ei, EMDOCS, GNLM, IDS, ingenta, Linda Hall. **CCC.**
Published by: Kluwer Academic - Plenum Publishers (Subsidiary of: Wolters Kluwer N.V.), 233 Spring St, New York, NY 10013-1578. TEL 212-620-8000, 800-221-9369, FAX 212-463-0742, info@plenum.com, http://www.wkap.nl/journalhome.htm/0277-8033. Ed. M Zouhair Atassi. R&P Rose Luongo TEL 781-871-6311. **Subscr. outside the Americas to:** Kluwer Academic Publishers Group, Journals Department, PO Box 322, Dordrecht 3300 AH, Netherlands. TEL 31-78-639-2392, FAX 31-78-654-6474.

572 GBR ISSN 0960-0760
QP801.S6 CODEN: JSBBEZ
JOURNAL OF STEROID BIOCHEMISTRY AND MOLECULAR BIOLOGY. Text in English. 1970. 20/yr. EUR 262 in Europe to qualified personnel; JPY 34,800 in Japan to qualified personnel; USD 293 elsewhere to qualified personnel; EUR 3,369 in Europe to institutions; JPY 447,200 in Japan to institutions; USD 3,768 elsewhere to institutions (effective 2002). adv. bk.rev. abstr. back issues avail. *Refereed.* **Document type:** *Academic/Scholarly.* **Description:** Covers recent experimental and theoretical developments in disciplines related to steroids.
Formerly (until 1991): Journal of Steroid Biochemistry (0022-4731)
Related titles: Microfilm ed.: (from PQC); Online - full text ed.: (from ingenta, ScienceDirect, Swets Blackwell, Institute for Scientific Information).
Indexed: ASCA, AgBiotech, Anal.Abstr., Anim.Breed.Abstr., Aqua.Sci.& Fish.Abstr., BBCI, Biol.Abstr., Chem.Abstr., Chem.Cit.Ind., Chem.Indus.Notes, Chem.Titles, Chemorec.Abstr., Curr.Adv.Biochem., Curr.Adv.Cancer Res., Curr.Adv.Ecol.Sci., Curr.Adv.Gen.& Molec.Biol., Curr.Cont., Dairy Sci.Abstr., Excerp.Med., Genet.Abstr., Helminthol.Abstr., Hum.Gen.Abstr., INIS Atomind., Ind.Med. (1990-), Ind.Sci.Rev., Ind.Vet., Inpharma, Int.Abstr.Biol.Sci., Mass Spectr.Bull., NPU, Neurosci.Abstr. (coverage dropped), Neurosci.Cit.Ind., Nuc.Acids Abstr., Nutr.Abstr., Pharm.&Out.News, Pig News & Info., Poult.Abstr., Protozool.Abstr., Reac., Rev.Appl.Entomol., Rev.Plant Path., SSCI (coverage dropped), Sci.Cit.Ind., Sport Fish.Abstr.
—BLDSC (5066.850010), ADONIS, CASDDS, CISTI, EMDOCS, GNLM, IDS, Infotrieve, ingenta, Linda Hall. **CCC.**
Published by: Pergamon (Subsidiary of: Elsevier Science), The Boulevard, Langford Ln, East Park, Kidlington, Oxford OXB 1GB, United Kingdom. FAX 44-1865-843010, nlinfo-f@elsevier.nl, http://www.elsevier.com/locate/jsbmb. Eds. J R Pasqualini, R Scholler. Circ: 1,250. **Subscr. in Australasia and the Far East to:** Elsevier Science (Singapore) Pte Ltd, No.1 Temasek Ave, 17-01 Millenia Tower, Singapore 039192, Singapore. TEL 65-434-3727, FAX 65-337-2230; **Subscr. in the Americas to:** Elsevier Science, PO Box 945, New York, NY 10159-0945. TEL 212-633-3730, FAX 212-633-3680; **Subscr. to:** Elsevier Science BV, PO Box 211, Amsterdam 1000 AE, Netherlands. TEL 31-20-485-3757.

572 YUG ISSN 0354-3447
CODEN: JMBIFF
JUGOSLOVENSKA MEDICINSKA BIOHEMIJA. Text in English, Serbo-Croatian; Summaries in English. 1982. 4/yr. YUN 2,500, USD 50 (effective 2000). adv. bk.rev. back issues avail. *Refereed.* **Document type:** *Academic/Scholarly.* **Description:** Publishes scientific papers on clinical chemistry.
Supersedes in part (in 1992): Jugoslavenska Medicinska Biokemija (0352-1311)
Related titles: Online - full text ed.: (from Institute for Scientific Information).
Indexed: ASCA, BBCI, Chem.Abstr., Chem.Titles, Excerp.Med. (until 1993, 1994-), Int.Abstr.Biol.Sci., Ref.Zh.
—CASDDS, EMDOCS, GNLM, IDS.
Published by: Drustvo Medicinskih Biohemicara Jugoslavije/Yugoslav Society of Medical Biochemists, Vojvode Stepe 450, Postanski Fah 146, Belgrade 11221, Yugoslavia. TEL 381-11-3615631, FAX 381-11-3615631, singh@eunet.yu. Ed., Adv. contact Nada Majkic Singh. Circ: 1,000.

KISO ROKA GAKKAI SAKYURA/BIOMEDICAL GERONTOLOGY CIRCULAR. see *GERONTOLOGY AND GERIATRICS*

572 JPN ISSN 0912-8921
KISO ROKA KENKYU/BIOMEDICAL GERONTOLOGY. Text in English, Japanese. 1977. s-a.
Published by: Nihon Kiso Roka Gakkai/Japan Society for Biomedical Gerontology, Tokyoto Rojin Sogo Kenkyujo, 35-2 Sakae-cho, Itabashi-ku, Tokyo 173-0015, Japan.

572.4 CZE ISSN 1210-7921
CODEN: KBMEF
KLINICKA BIOCHEMIE A METABOLISMUS. Text in Czech, Slovak; Summaries in Czech, English. 1972. q. EUR 60, USD 76 (effective 2001). adv. bk.rev. *Refereed.* **Document type:** *Academic/Scholarly.*
Formerly (until 1993): Biochemia Clinica Bohemoslovaca (0139-9608)
Indexed: Chem.Abstr., Chem.Titles, Curr.Adv.Ecol.Sci., Excerp.Med. (until 1992, 1996-), Int.Abstr.Biol.Sci.
—BLDSC (5099.284790), CASDDS, EMDOCS, GNLM, Infotrieve. **CCC.**
Published by: (Ceska Lekarska Spolecnost J.E. Purkyne/Czech Medical Association), Nakladatelske Stredisko C L S J.E. Purkyne, Sokolska 31, Prague 12026, Czech Republic. TEL 42-2-24911420, FAX 42-2-24911420, nts@iol.cz, http://www.clsjep.cz, http://www.medical.cz. Ed. A Kazda. adv.: B&W page CZK 21,100, color page CZK 31,600; 250 x 170. Circ: 950. **Dist. by:** Abont s.r.o., Chlumova 17, Prague, 3 130 00, Czech Republic; **Dist. in Western Countries by:** Kubon & Sagner, Hesstr 39-41, Munich 80798, Germany.

KLINISK KEMI; medlemsblad foer S F K K. see *MEDICAL SCIENCES*

KLINISK KEMI I NORDEN. see *MEDICAL SCIENCES*

B

572.8 NLD ISSN 0075-7535
QP519 CODEN: LTBBDT

LABORATORY TECHNIQUES IN BIOCHEMISTRY AND MOLECULAR BIOLOGY. Text in English. 1968. irreg., latest vol.28, 1999. price varies. back issues avail. *Refereed.* **Document type:** *Monographic series, Academic/Scholarly.* **Description:** Covers all aspects of laboratory work in biochemistry and molecular biology.

Indexed: Eng.Ind.

—BLDSC (5141.915000), CISTI, Ei, Infotrieve, KNAW. **CCC.**

Published by: Elsevier Science BV, PO Box 211, Amsterdam 1000 AE, Netherlands. TEL 31-20-485-3757, 31-20-485-3911, FAX 31-20-485-3432, 31-20-485-3598, nlinfo-f@elsevier.nl; usinfo-f@elsevier.com; forinfo-kyf04035@niftyserve.or.jp, http://www.elsevier.nl/. Eds. A J Levine, P C van der Vliet. **Subscr. in Australasia and the Far East to:** Elsevier Science (Singapore) Pte Ltd, No.1 Temasek Ave, 17-01 Millenia Tower, Singapore 039192, Singapore. TEL 65-434-3727, FAX 65-337-2230, asiainfo@elsevier.com.sg; **Subscr. in Japan to:** Elsevier Science Inc - Japan Regional Office, 9-15 Higashi-Azabu 1-chome, Minato-ku, Tokyo 106-0044, Japan. TEL 81-3-5561-5033, FAX 81-3-5561-5047, info@elsevier.co.jp; **Subscr. in the Americas to:** Elsevier Science, PO Box 945, New York, NY 10159-0945. TEL 888-437-4636, FAX 212-633-3680, http://www.elsevier.com

LE LAIT. see *BIOLOGY—Microbiology*

LECTINS. see *BIOLOGY—Abstracting, Bibliographies, Statistics*

572.57 GBR ISSN 0956-666X

LIPID TECHNOLOGY. Text in English. 1989. bi-m. GBP 175, USD 285 (effective 2002). abstr, pat, stat. cum.index: 1989-1998. back issues avail. **Document type:** *Trade.* **Description:** Contains commissioned feature articles from leading experts, news stories, and regular sections on nutrition, analysis, patent abstracts, research highlights, and market updates.

Indexed: Food Sci.& Tech.Abstr.

—BLDSC (5221.797000).

Published by: P.J. Barnes & Associates, P J Barnes & Associates, PO Box 200, Bridgwater TA7 0YZ, United Kingdom. TEL 44-1823-698973, FAX 44-1823-693971, sales@pbarnes.demon.co.uk, http://www.pbarnes.demon.co.uk. Ed. Frank D Gunstone. Pub. Peter J Barnes.

572.57 GBR ISSN 1357-7166
CODEN: LITEEI

LIPID TECHNOLOGY NEWSLETTER. Text in English. 1995. bi-m. GBP 175, USD 285 (effective 2002). back issues avail. *Refereed.* **Document type:** *Newsletter, Journal, Trade.* **Description:** Presents recent international developments in oils, fats and lipids in food technology, biotechnology, nutrition and pharmaceuticals. Contains news, stories, feature articles, research reports and market reports.

Indexed: Food Sci.& Tech.Abstr.

—BLDSC (5221.798000).

Published by: P.J. Barnes & Associates, P J Barnes & Associates, PO Box 200, Bridgwater TA7 0YZ, United Kingdom. TEL 44-1823-698973, FAX 44-1823-698971, sales@pbarnes.demon.co.uk, http://www.pbarnes.demon.co.uk. Ed. P J Barnes.

572.57 USA ISSN 0024-4201
QP501 CODEN: LPDSAP

LIPIDS. Text in English. 1966. m. USD 120 domestic to individuals; USD 130 foreign to individuals; USD 160 domestic to individuals for print & online eds.; USD 170 foreign to individuals for print & online eds; USD 283 domestic to institutions; USD 293 foreign to institutions (effective 2002). adv. charts, illus. back issues avail.; reprint service avail. from PQC. *Refereed.* **Document type:** *Journal, Academic/Scholarly.* **Description:** Contains original research on lipids, biochemistry, and related biomedical subjects.

Related titles: Microfilm ed.: (from PQC); Online - full text ed.: USD 100 domestic; USD 118 foreign (effective 2001) (from Institute for Scientific Information).

Indexed: ASCA, AgBiotech, Agricola, Anal.Abstr., Aqua.Sci.& Fish.Abstr., BBCI, Bibl.Agri., Bio-Contr.News & Info., Biol.Abstr., Chem.Abstr., Chem.Cit.Ind., Chem.Indus.Notes, Chem.Titles, Chromat.Abstr., Crop Physiol.Abstr., Curr.Adv.Biochem., Curr.Adv.Cell & Devel.Biol., Curr.Adv.Ecol.Sci., Curr.Cont., Dairy Sci.Abstr., Deep Sea Res.& Oceanogr.Abstr., Eng.Ind., Excerp.Med., Field Crop Abstr., Food Sci.& Tech.Abstr., Forest.Abstr., GeoRef, Helminthol.Abstr., Hort.Abstr., INIS Atomind., Ind.Med. (1966-), Ind.Sci.Rev., Ind.Vet., Inpharma, Int.Abstr.Biol.Sci., Maize Abstr., Mass Spectr.Bull., NPU, NRN, Neurosci.Cit.Ind., Nutr.Abstr., Ornam.Hort., Pharm.&Out.News, Pig News & Info., Plant Breed.Abstr., Postharvest, Potato Abstr., Poult.Abstr., R.G. (Jan.1999-, dropped), R.G.Abstr. (Jan.1999-), Reac., Ref.Zh., Rev.Appl.Entomol., Rev.Arom.& Med.Plants, Rev.Med.& Vet.Mycol., Rev.Plant Path., Rice Abstr., SSCI (coverage dropped), Sci.Cit.Ind., Seed Abstr., Soils & Fert., Soyabean Abstr., Sport Fish.Abstr., Sugar Ind.Abstr., THA, Trop.Oil Seeds Abstr., Vet.Bull., Weed Abstr., Wild.Rev., Zoo.Rec.

—BLDSC (5221.850000), CASDDS, CISTI, Ei, GNLM, IDS, ingenta, Linda Hall. **CCC.**

Published by: (American Oil Chemists' Society), A O C S Press, 2211 W Bradley Ave, Champaign, IL 61821. TEL 217-359-2344, FAX 217-351-8091, publications@aocs.org, http://www.aocs.org/press/lipids.htm. Ed. Howard R Knapp. Pub. Mary Lane. R&P Connie Winslow. adv.: B&W page USD 725; 8.25 x 11. Circ: 1,500 (paid).

LIPOSOMES. see *BIOLOGY—Abstracting, Bibliographies, Statistics*

LUMINESCENCE; journal of biological and chemical luminescence. see *CHEMISTRY—Physical Chemistry*

612.015 CHE ISSN 1027-0256

▼ **MEDICAL BIOCHEMISTRY.** Text in English. 1999. q. EUR 225 to institutions; EUR 364 to corporations (effective 2000). **Document type:** *Academic/Scholarly.*

Related titles: Online - full text ed.: (from EBSCO Publishing, RoweCom Information Quest).

Published by: Gordon and Breach - Harwood Academic (Subsidiary of: Taylor & Francis Group), PO Box 531, Lausanne 1000, Switzerland. http://www.gbhap.com. Ed. Peter Hayes. **Subscr. addr. in US:** International Publishers Direct, PO Box 32160, Newark, NJ 07102. FAX 215-750-6343.

MEDICAL ENGINEERING & PHYSICS. see *MEDICAL SCIENCES*

572 BGR ISSN 0204-9716

MEDITSINSKI PREGLED. KLINICHNA LABORATORIIA. Text in Bulgarian. 1970. q., latest vol.32, 2001. BGL 14 domestic; USD 48 foreign (effective 2001 - 2002). adv. bk.rev. abstr, bibl. index. 48 p./no. back issues avail. *Refereed.* **Document type:** *Journal, Academic/Scholarly, Abstract/Index, Bibliography.* **Description:** Abstracts of foreign publications in the field of medical laboratory, includes methods, techniques and equipment.

Published by: Meditsinski Universitet - Sofia, Tsentur za Informatsiia po Meditsina/Medical University - Sofia, Medical Information Center, 1 Sv Georgi Sofiiski ul, Sofia 1431, Bulgaria. TEL 359-2-9522342, FAX 359-2-9522393, mutafov@sun.medun.acad.bg, http://www.medun.acad.bg. Ed. Dr. K Tsachev. R&P, Adv. contact Dr. Christo Mutafov. B&W page USD 50, color page USD 150; 12 x 18. Circ: 200. **Dist. by:** Sofia Books, Ul Silivria 16, Sofia 1404, Bulgaria. TEL 359-2-9586257, sofiabooks@hotmail.com, http://www.sofiabooks.hit.bg.

572.7 USA ISSN 1046-2023
QR180 CODEN: IMUME8

METHODS: A COMPANION TO METHODS IN ENZYMOLOGY. Key Title: Methods (San Diego). Text in English. 1990. m. USD 315 in US & Canada to institutions; USD 365 elsewhere to institutions (effective 2001). abstr. back issues avail. *Refereed.* **Document type:** *Academic/Scholarly.* **Description:** Contains topic-oriented articles that cover new methods applicable to a number of disciplines.

Incorporates (in 1995): Methods - GenoMethods (1078-1501); (1992-1995): NeuroProtocols (1058-6741); (in 1995): Methods - Immunomethods (1078-151X); Which was formerly (1992-1994): Immunomethods (1058-6687)

Related titles: Online - full text ed.: ISSN 1095-9130 (from EBSCO Publishing, O C L C Online Computer Library Center, Inc., RoweCom Information Quest, ingenta, Swets Blackwell, IDEAL Online Library, Institute for Scientific Information).

Indexed: ASCA, BBCI, Chem.Abstr., Chem.Indus.Notes, Chem.Titles, Curr.Cont., Excerp.Med. (1994-), Ind.Med. (1990-), Neurosci.Cit.Ind., Sci.Cit.Ind.

—BLDSC (5746.575000), ADONIS, CASDDS, CINDOC, CISTI, EMDOCS, GNLM, IDS, Infotrieve, ingenta, Linda Hall. **CCC.**

Published by: Academic Press, Inc., Journal Division (Subsidiary of: Harcourt Brace & Company), 525 B St, Ste 1900, San Diego, CA 92101-4495. TEL 619-230-1840, FAX 619-699-6800, apsubs@acad.com, http://www.academicpress.com/methods. Eds. John N Abelson, Kenneth W Adolph.

572.7 USA ISSN 0076-6879
QP601 CODEN: MENZAU

METHODS IN ENZYMOLOGY. Text in English. 1955. irreg., latest vol.290, 1998. price varies. reprint service avail. from ISI. *Refereed.* **Document type:** *Monographic series.*

Related titles: Online - full text ed.: (from Institute for Scientific Information).

Indexed: ASCA, Abstr.Hyg., Aqua.Sci.& Fish.Abstr., Aquacult.Abstr., BBCI, Biol.Abstr., Biotech.Cit.Ind., Chem.Abstr., Chem.Cit.Ind., Chem.Indus.Notes, Chem.Titles, Dairy Sci.Abstr., Dent.Ind., Environ.Sci.Poll.Mgmt., Excerp.Med., INIS Atomind., Ind.Med. (1955-), Ind.Sci.Rev., Lab.Haz.Bull., Mass Spectr.Bull., Microbiol.Abstr., Nutr.Abstr., Protozool.Abstr., Rev.Appl.Entomol., Rev.Med.& Vet.Mycol., Sci.Cit.Ind., Sport Fish.Abstr., Sugar Ind.Abstr.

—BLDSC (5748.060000), CASDDS, CISTI, GNLM, ingenta, KNAW. **CCC.**

Published by: Academic Press, Inc., Journal Division (Subsidiary of: Harcourt Brace & Company), 525 B St, Ste 1900, San Diego, CA 92101-4495. TEL 619-231-0926, FAX 619-699-6715, ap@acad.com, http://www.apnet.com. Eds. N O Kaplan, S P Colowick. **Subscr. to:** Order Dept., 6277 Sea Harbor Dr, 4th Fl, Orlando, FL 32887. TEL 800-321-5068.

572 USA ISSN 0076-6941
QD271 CODEN: MBANAA

METHODS OF BIOCHEMICAL ANALYSIS. Text in English. 1954. irreg., latest vol.34, 1990. price varies. *Refereed.* **Document type:** *Monographic series.*

Related titles: Online - full text ed.: (from Institute for Scientific Information).

Indexed: ASCA, Abstr.Hyg., Agri.& Environ.Biotech.Abstr. (coverage dropped), BBCI, Biol.Abstr., Chem.Abstr., Chem.Indus.Notes, Chem.Titles, Comput.Rev., Curr.Adv.Ecol.Sci., Derwent Biotech.Abstr., INIS Atomind., Ind.Med. (1954-), Ind.Sci.Rev., Math.R., Nutr.Abstr., Sci.Cit.Ind.

—BLDSC (5747.000000), CASDDS, CISTI, GNLM, ingenta, Linda Hall. **CCC.**

Published by: John Wiley & Sons, Inc., Journals (Subsidiary of: Wiley InterScience), 605 Third Ave, New York, NY 10158. TEL 212-850-6000. Ed. David Glick.

MICROBIAL PATHOGENESIS; molecular and cellular biology of infectious disease. see *MEDICAL SCIENCES—Communicable Diseases*

MICROBIOLOGY AND MOLECULAR BIOLOGY REVIEWS. see *BIOLOGY—Microbiology*

MICROCIRCULATION, ENDOTHELIUM AND LYMPHATICS. see *MEDICAL SCIENCES—Hematology*

MITTEILUNGEN AUS DER GEBIETE DER LEBENSMITTELUNTERSUCHUNG UND HYGIENE/TRAVAUX DE CHIMIE ALIMENTAIRE ET D'HYGIENE. see *NUTRITION AND DIETETICS*

572.8 NLD ISSN 0166-6851
CODEN: MBIPDP

MOLECULAR AND BIOCHEMICAL PARASITOLOGY. Text in Dutch. 1980. 14/yr. EUR 3,187 in Europe to institutions; JPY 423,500 in Japan to institutions; USD 3,565 elsewhere to institutions (effective 2002). adv. back issues avail. *Refereed.* **Document type:** *Academic/Scholarly.* **Description:** Provides a medium for the rapid publication of investigations of the molecular biology, molecular immunology and biochemistry of parasitic protozoa and helminths and their interactions with the host.

Related titles: Microform ed.: (from PQC); Online - full text ed.: (from ingenta, ScienceDirect, Swets Blackwell, Institute for Scientific Information).

Indexed: AIDS & Cancer Res., ASCA, Abstr.Hyg., AgBiotech, Agri.& Environ.Biotech.Abstr. (coverage dropped), Aqua.Sci.& Fish.Abstr., BBCI, Bibl.Agri., Biol.Abstr., Chem.Abstr., Chem.Titles, Curr.Adv.Biochem., Curr.Adv.Cell & Devel.Biol., Curr.Adv.Ecol.Sci., Curr.Adv.Gen.& Molec.Biol., Curr.Cont., Derwent Biotech.Abstr., Entomol.Abstr. (coverage dropped), Environ.Sci.Poll.Mgmt., Excerp.Med., Genet.Abstr., Helminthol.Abstr., Hum.Gen.Abstr., Immun.Abstr., Ind.Med. (1980-), Ind.Sci.Rev., Ind.Vet., Inpharma, Int.Abstr.Biol.Sci., Microbiol.Abstr., Nuc.Acids Abstr., Protozool.Abstr., Reac., Rev.Appl.Entomol., Rev.Med.& Vet.Mycol., Sci.Cit.Ind., Trop.Dis.Bull., Vet.Bull., Zoo.Rec.

—BLDSC (5900.753000), ADONIS, CASDDS, CISTI, GNLM, IDS, ingenta. **CCC.**

Published by: Elsevier Science BV, PO Box 211, Amsterdam 1000 AE, Netherlands. TEL 31-20-485-2911, FAX 31-20-485-2457, http://www.elsevier.com/locate/molbiopara. Eds. A P Waters, C E Clayton. **Subscr. in Australasia and the Far East to:** Elsevier Science (Singapore) Pte Ltd, No.1 Temasek Ave, 17-01 Millenia Tower, Singapore 039192, Singapore. TEL 65-434-3727, FAX 65-337-2230; **Subscr. in Japan to:** Elsevier Science Inc - Japan Regional Office, 9-15 Higashi-Azabu 1-chome, Minato-ku, Tokyo 106-0044, Japan. TEL 81-3-5561-5033; **Subscr. in the Americas to:** Elsevier Science, PO Box 945, New York, NY 10159-0945. TEL 212-633-3730, FAX 212-633-3680, usinfo-f@elsevier.com.

572 USA ISSN 0300-8177
QR151 CODEN: MCBIB8

MOLECULAR AND CELLULAR BIOCHEMISTRY; an international journal for chemical biology in health and disease. Text in English. 1973. 26/yr. EUR 4,175 to institutions for print or online ed.; EUR 5,010 to institutions print & online eds.combined (effective 2002). adv. bk.rev. bibl, illus. back issues avail.; reprint service avail. from SWZ,PQC. *Refereed.* **Document type:** *Academic/Scholarly.* **Description:** Publishes original, full-length research papers and short communications in all areas of the biochemical sciences, the emphasis being on those papers which present novel findings relevant to the biochemical basis of cellular function and disease processes, as well as the mechanics of action of hormones and chemical agents.

Supersedes: Enzymologia (0013-9424)

Related titles: Microform ed.: (from PQC,PMC); Online - full text ed.: (from EBSCO Publishing, O C L C Online Computer Library Center, Inc., RoweCom Information Quest, Swets Blackwell, Kluwer Online, Institute for Scientific Information).

Indexed: ASCA, Abstr.Hyg., Agricola, Anal.Abstr., Anim.Breed.Abstr., Aqua.Sci.& Fish.Abstr., BBCI, Bibl.Agri., Biol.Abstr., Biotech.Cit.Ind., Chem.Abstr., Chem.Titles, Curr.Adv.Cancer Res., Curr.Adv.Ecol.Sci., Curr.Cont., Dairy Sci.Abstr., Dent.Ind., Derwent Biotech.Abstr., Excerp.Med., Food Sci.& Tech.Abstr., Genet.Abstr., Helminthol.Abstr., Hort.Abstr., Hum.Gen.Abstr., INIS Atomind., Ind.Med. (1973-), Ind.Sci.Rev., Ind.Vet., Inpharma, Int.Abstr.Biol.Sci., Mass Spectr.Bull., Neurosci.Abstr. (coverage dropped), Neurosci.Cit.Ind., Nuc.Acids Abstr., Nutr.Abstr., Ornam.Hort., Pharm.&Out.News, Poult.Abstr., Protozool.Abstr., Reac., Rev.Appl.Entomol., Rev.Arom.& Med.Plants, Rev.Med.& Vet.Mycol., Rev.Plant Path., Sci.Cit.Ind., Seed Abstr., Trop.Dis.Bull., Weed Abstr.

—BLDSC (5900.756000), CASDDS, CISTI, EMDOCS, GNLM, IDS, ingenta, Linda Hall. **CCC.**

Published by: Kluwer Academic Publishers Boston, 101 Philip Dr, Assinippi Park, Norwell, MA 02061. TEL 781-871-6600, FAX 781-871-9045, services@wkap.nl, http://www.wkap.nl/journalhome.htm/0300-8177. Ed. Naranjan S Dhalla. R&P Rose Luongo TEL 781-871-6311. Circ: 1,000. **Subscr. outside the Americas to:** Kluwer Academic Publishers Group, Journals Department, PO Box 322, Dordrecht 3300 AH, Netherlands. TEL 31-78-639-2392, FAX 31-78-654-6474; **Subscr. to:** Kluwer Academic - Plenum Publishers, 233 Spring St, New York, NY 10013-1578. TEL 212-620-8468, FAX 212-807-1047.

572.8 USA ISSN 0270-7306
QH506 CODEN: MCEBD4

MOLECULAR AND CELLULAR BIOLOGY. Text in English. 1981. fortn. USD 99 domestic to members; USD 644 domestic to non-members; USD 685 in Canada to non-members; USD 738 in Europe to non-members; USD 750 in Latin America to non-members; USD 778 elsewhere to non-members (effective 2001). adv. illus. Index. back issues avail.; reprint service avail. from PQC. *Refereed.* **Document type:** *Academic/Scholarly.* **Description:** Covers the molecular biology of eukaryotic cells of both microbial and higher organisms. Sections include gene expression, transcriptional regulation, cell growth and development, nucleocytoplasmic communication, cell and organelle structure and assembly, DNA dynamics and chromosome structure, and mammalian genetic models with minimal or complex phenotypes.

Related titles: CD-ROM ed.: USD 500 in North America; USD 524 elsewhere; Microform ed.: (from PQC); Online - full text ed.: ISSN 1098-5549 (from HighWire Pr., EBSCO Publishing, Institute for Scientific Information).

Indexed: AIDS & Cancer Res., ASCA, AgBiotech, Agri.& Environ.Biotech.Abstr., Anim.Breed.Abstr., Aqua.Sci.& Fish.Abstr., BBCI, Biol.& Agr.Ind. (Jan.1996-), Biol.Abstr., Biotech.& Bioeng.Abstr., Biotech.Cit.Ind., Cal.Tiss.Abstr. (coverage dropped), Chem.Abstr., Chem.Indus.Notes, Chem.Titles, Chemorec.Abstr., Curr.Adv.Biochem., Curr.Adv.Cancer Res., Curr.Adv.Cell & Devel.Biol., Curr.Adv.Ecol.Sci., Curr.Adv.Gen.& Molec.Biol., Curr.Cont., Dairy Sci.Abstr., Dent.Ind., Derwent Biotech.Abstr., Entomol.Abstr. (coverage dropped), Environ.Sci.Poll.Mgmt., Excerp.Med., Genet.Abstr., Helminthol.Abstr., Hum.Gen.Abstr., INIS Atomind., Immun.Abstr., Ind.Med. (1981-), Ind.Sci.Rev., Ind.Vet., Inpharma, Int.Abstr.Biol.Sci., Maize Abstr., Med.& Pharm.Biotech.Abstr., Microbiol.Abstr., Neurosci.Abstr., Neurosci.Cit.Ind., Nuc.Acids Abstr., Oncog.G.F.Abstr., Pharm.&Out.News, Plant Breed.Abstr., Poult.Abstr., Protozool.Abstr., Reac., Ref.Zh., Rev.Appl.Entomol., Rev.Med.& Vet.Mycol., Rev.Plant Path., Sci.Cit.Ind., Sport Fish.Abstr., Telegen, Tox.Abstr. (coverage dropped), Virol.Abstr. (coverage dropped), Weed Abstr., Zoo.Rec.

—BLDSC (5900.757000), CASDDS, CISTI, EMDOCS, GNLM, IDS, ingenta, KNAW, Linda Hall. **CCC.**

Published by: American Society for Microbiology, 1752 N St N W, Washington, DC 20036-2904. TEL 202-737-3600, 800-633-4931, subscriptions@asmusa.org, http://mcb.asm.org/, http://www.asmusa.org, http://www.journals.asm.org. Ed. James N Ihle. Circ: 4,700 (paid).

572.8 RUS ISSN 0026-8933
QH506 CODEN: MOLBBJ

MOLECULAR BIOLOGY. Text in English. 1967. bi-m. EUR 2,911 to institutions for print or online ed.; EUR 3,493.20 to institutions print & online eds.combined (effective 2002). back issues avail. *Refereed.* **Document type:** *Academic/Scholarly.* **Description:** Covers advances in the field of chemical and physical bases of principal life phenomena, including studies on the chemistry and physics of the most important biopolymers (proteins and nucleic acids), their structure, and their functions.

Related titles: Microfilm ed.: (from PQC); Online - full text ed.: (from Swets Blackwell, Kluwer Online, Institute for Scientific Information, RoweCom Information Quest); ♦ Translation of: Molekulyarnaya Biologiya. ISSN 0026-8984.

Indexed: ASCA, Anim.Breed.Abstr., Aqua.Sci.& Fish.Abstr., BBCI, Biol.& Agr.Ind. (Jan.1996-), Biol.Abstr., Biotech.Cit.Ind., Chem.Cit.Ind., Chem.Titles, Curr.Adv.Ecol.Sci., Curr.Cont., Excerp.Med., Genet.Abstr. (coverage dropped), INIS Atomind., Ind.Med. (coverage dropped), Ind.Sci.Rev., Inpharma, Int.Abstr.Biol.Sci., Neurosci.Abstr. (coverage dropped), Nuc.Acids Abstr., Pharm.&Out.News, Reac., Sci.Cit.Ind.

—BLDSC (0416.235000), CASDDS, CISTI, GNLM, IDS, Infotrieve, ingenta. **CCC.**

Published by: (Rossiiskaya Akademiya Nauk/Russian Academy of Sciences), M A I K Nauka - Interperiodica, Mezhdunarodnyi Otdel, Profsoyuznaya ul 90, Moscow 117864, Russian Federation. TEL 7-095-336-1600, FAX 7-095-336-0666, compmg@maik.ru, http://www.maik.rssi.ru/journals/molbio.htm. Ed. L L Kiselev. **Dist. by:** Kluwer Academic Publishers, PO Box 17, Dordrecht 3300 AH, Netherlands. TEL 31-78-639-2392, FAX 31-78-654-6474, http://www.wkap.nl.

572 USA ISSN 0077-0221
CODEN: MBBBAD

MOLECULAR BIOLOGY, BIOCHEMISTRY AND BIOPHYSICS. Text in English. 1967. irreg. price varies. reprint service avail. from ISI. **Document type:** *Academic/Scholarly.*

Indexed: Biol.Abstr., Chem.Abstr., Curr.Adv.Ecol.Sci., Ind.Med. (coverage dropped).

—CASDDS, CISTI, GNLM, KNAW, Linda Hall. **CCC.**

Published by: Springer-Verlag, Journals (Subsidiary of: BertelsmannSpringer), 175 Fifth Ave, New York, NY 10010. TEL 212-460-1500, FAX 212-473-6272.

572 NLD ISSN 0301-4851
QH506 CODEN: MLBRBU

MOLECULAR BIOLOGY REPORTS; an international journal on molecular and cellular biology. Text in Dutch. 1973. q. EUR 399 to institutions for print or online ed.; EUR 437.40 to institutions print & online eds.combined (effective 2002). adv. bk.rev. reprint service avail. from SWZ. *Refereed.* **Document type:** *Academic/Scholarly.* **Description:** Publishes original research papers on molecular and cellular biology, including DNA replication, protein biosynthesis and related subjects.

Related titles: Microform ed.: (from PQC); Online - full text ed.: (from EBSCO Publishing, O C L C Online Computer Library Center, Inc., RoweCom Information Quest, Swets Blackwell, Kluwer Online, Institute for Scientific Information).

Indexed: ASCA, AgBiotech, Agri.& Environ.Biotech.Abstr. (coverage dropped), Agricola, Anim.Breed.Abstr., Aqua.Sci.& Fish.Abstr., BBCI, Biol.Abstr., Biotech.& Bioeng.Abstr., Biotech.Cit.Ind., Chem.Abstr., Chem.Indus.Notes, Chem.Titles, Curr.Adv.Ecol.Sci., Curr.Cont., Derwent Biotech.Abstr., Genet.Abstr., Helminthol.Abstr., Hort.Abstr., Hum.Gen.Abstr., INIS Atomind., Ind.Med. (1973-), Ind.Sci.Rev., Ind.Vet., Inpharma, Int.Abstr.Biol.Sci., Mass Spectr.Bull., Nuc.Acids Abstr., Ornam.Hort., Plant Breed.Abstr., Reac., Rev.Plant Path., Rice Abstr., Sci.Cit.Ind., Telegen.

—BLDSC (5900.798000), CASDDS, CISTI, EMDOCS, GNLM, IDS, ingenta, Linda Hall. **CCC.**

Published by: Kluwer Academic Publishers Group (Subsidiary of: Wolters Kluwer N.V.), Spuiboulevard 50, PO Box 17, Dordrecht 3300 AA, Netherlands. FAX 31-78-639-2254, services@wkap.nl, http://www.wkap.nl. Eds. Andre J van Wijnen, Gary Stein. **Dist. by:** Journals Department, PO Box 322, Dordrecht 3300 AH, Netherlands. TEL 781-871-6600, FAX 31-78-654-6474.

MOLECULAR BIOLOGY TECHNIQUES. see *BIOLOGY—Abstracting, Bibliographies, Statistics*

MOLECULAR GENETICS AND METABOLISM; an international journal. see *MEDICAL SCIENCES*

MOLECULAR GENETICS, MICROBIOLOGY AND VIROLOGY. see *BIOLOGY—Microbiology*

572 GBR ISSN 0161-5890
QR180 CODEN: MOIMD5

MOLECULAR IMMUNOLOGY. Text in English, French, German, Spanish. 1964. 18/yr. EUR 288 in Europe to qualified personnel; JPY 38,300 in Japan to qualified personnel; USD 323 elsewhere to qualified personnel; EUR 2,358 in Europe to institutions; JPY 313,100 in Japan to institutions; USD 2,637 elsewhere to institutions (effective 2002). adv. bk.rev. charts, illus. index. back issues avail. *Refereed.* **Document type:** *Academic/Scholarly.* **Description:** Communicates immunological knowledge which can be delineated at the molecular level.

Formerly: Immunochemistry (0019-2791)

Related titles: Microfilm ed.: (from PQC); Online - full text ed.: (from ingenta, ScienceDirect, Swets Blackwell, Institute for Scientific Information).

Indexed: AIDS & Cancer Res., ASCA, Abstr.Hyg., AgBiotech, Agri.& Environ.Biotech.Abstr. (coverage dropped), Anim.Breed.Abstr., Apic.Abstr., BBCI, Biol.Abstr., Biotech.Cit.Ind., Chem.Abstr., Chem.Indus.Notes, Chem.Titles, Curr.Adv.Cancer Res., Curr.Adv.Ecol.Sci., Curr.Cont., Dairy Sci.Abstr., Dent.Ind., Derwent Biotech.Abstr., Excerp.Med., Focus on: Mol.Med., Forest.Abstr., Genet.Abstr., Helminthol.Abstr., Hum.Gen.Abstr., INIS Atomind., Immun.Abstr., Ind.Med. (1979-), Ind.Sci.Rev., Ind.Vet., Inpharma, Int.Abstr.Biol.Sci., Nuc.Acids Abstr., Nutr.Abstr., Pharm.&Out.News, Plant Breed.Abstr., Protozool.Abstr., Reac., Rev.Appl.Entomol., Rev.Med.& Vet.Mycol., Sci.Cit.Ind., Sport Fish.Abstr., Trop.Dis.Bull., Vet.Bull., Weed Abstr.

—BLDSC (5900.817700), ADONIS, CASDDS, CISTI, GNLM, IDS, ingenta, Linda Hall. **CCC.**

Published by: Pergamon (Subsidiary of: Elsevier Science), The Boulevard, Langford Ln, East Park, Kidlington, Oxford OXB 1GB, United Kingdom. FAX 44-1865-843010, http://www.elsevier.com/locate/molimm. Eds. H Ploegh, M Carroll. Circ: 2,100. **Subscr. in Australasia and the Far East to:** Elsevier Science (Singapore) Pte Ltd, No.1 Temasek Ave, 17-01 Millenia Tower, Singapore 039192, Singapore. TEL 65-434-3727, FAX 65-337-2230; **Subscr. in the Americas to:** Elsevier Science, PO Box 945, New York, NY 10159-0945. TEL 212-633-3730, FAX 212-633-3680, usinfo-f@elsevier.com; **Subscr. to:** Elsevier Science BV, PO Box 211, Amsterdam 1000 AE, Netherlands. TEL 31-20-485-3757.

572.8 GBR ISSN 0968-7688
QH601 CODEN: MMEBE7

MOLECULAR MEMBRANE BIOLOGY. Text in English. 1978. q. GBP 89, USD 147 to individuals; GBP 257, USD 424 to institutions (effective 2002). adv. abstr. index. *Refereed.* **Document type:** *Academic/Scholarly.* **Description:** Provides specialists in physiology, biochemistry, biophysics and medicine, with a forum for research in the study of membranes.

Formerly (until 1994): Membrane Biochemistry (0149-046X)

Related titles: Online - full text ed.: ISSN 1464-5203 (from CatchWord Ltd., EBSCO Publishing, O C L C Online Computer Library Center, Inc., RoweCom Information Quest, Swets Blackwell, Institute for Scientific Information).

Indexed: AgBiotech, Aqua.Sci.& Fish.Abstr., BBCI, Biol.Abstr., Chem.Abstr., Chem.Indus.Notes, Chem.Titles, Curr.Adv.Ecol.Sci., Curr.Cont., Excerp.Med., Genet.Abstr. (coverage dropped), INIS Atomind., Ind.Med. (1994-), Ind.Sci.Rev., Inpharma, Int.Abstr.Biol.Sci., Reac., Rev.Med.& Vet.Mycol., Sci.Cit.Ind.

—BLDSC (5900.817955), CASDDS, CatchWord, CISTI, GNLM, IDS, ingenta, KNAW, Linda Hall. **CCC.**

Published by: Taylor & Francis Group, Taylor & Francis Ltd., 11 New Fetter Ln, London EC4P 4EE, United Kingdom. TEL 44-20-7583-9855, FAX 44-20-7842-2298, info@tandf.co.uk, http://www.tandf.co.uk. **Subscr. in N. America to:** Taylor & Francis Ltd., 325 Chestnut St, Suite 800, Philadelphia, PA 19016. TEL 800-354-1420, FAX 215-625-8914, info@taylorandfrancis.com, http://www.taylorandfrancis.com/.

573.8 USA ISSN 0893-7648
QP365.2 CODEN: MONBEW

MOLECULAR NEUROBIOLOGY; a review journal. Text in English. 1987. bi-m. USD 490 domestic; USD 525 foreign (effective 2000). adv. bk.rev. abstr, bibl, charts, illus. index. back issues avail. *Refereed.* **Document type:** *Journal, Academic/Scholarly.* **Description:** Publishes review articles for neuroscientists needing to keep abreast of current experimental and clinical brain research at the molecular level.

Related titles: Online - full text ed.: (from Institute for Scientific Information).

Indexed: ASCA, Aqua.Sci.& Fish.Abstr., BBCI, Biol.Abstr., Chem.Abstr., Chem.Indus.Notes, Chem.Titles, Chemorec.Abstr., Curr.Cont. (coverage dropped), Excerp.Med., Ind.Med. (1987-), Ind.Sci.Rev., Inpharma, Neurosci.Abstr., Neurosci.Cit.Ind., Pharm.&Out.News, Reac., Sci.Cit.Ind., e-psyche.

—BLDSC (5900.817980), ADONIS, CASDDS, CISTI, GNLM, IDS, ingenta, KNAW. **CCC.**

Published by: Humana Press Inc., 999 Riverview Dr, Ste 208, Totowa, NJ 07512. TEL 973-256-1699, FAX 973-256-8341, humana@humanapr.com, http://humanapress.com. Eds. Jacques Mallet, Nicolas G Bazan. R&P Richard Hruska. Adv. contact Thomas B Lanigan Jr. **Dist. in Japan by:** Maruzen Co., Ltd., International Division, Export Dept, P.O. Box 5050, Tokyo International 100-3191, Japan. TEL 81-3-3275-8591.

572.8 USA ISSN 0894-0282
SB732.6 CODEN: MPMIEL

MOLECULAR PLANT - MICROBE INTERACTIONS. Text in English. 1988. m. USD 410 domestic; USD 471 foreign (effective 2001). back issues avail. *Refereed.* **Document type:** *Journal, Academic/Scholarly.* **Description:** Devoted to significant research on the molecular genetics and molecular biology of pathological, symbiotic, and associative interactions of microbes with plants or microbes that affect such interactions.

Related titles: Online - full text ed.: USD 550 domestic; USD 611 foreign (effective 2001) (from Institute for Scientific Information).

Indexed: ASCA, AgBiotech, Agricola, Aqua.Sci.& Fish.Abstr., BBCI, Bio-Contr.News & Info., Biotech.Cit.Ind., Chem.Abstr., Chem.Indus.Notes, Chem.Titles, Crop Physiol.Abstr., Curr.Adv.Gen.& Molec.Biol., Curr.Cont., Environ.Sci.Poll.Mgmt., Field Crop Abstr., Food Sci.& Tech.Abstr., Forest.Abstr., Genet.Abstr., Helminthol.Abstr., Herb.Abstr., Hort.Abstr., Ind.Med. (1988-), Ind.Sci.Rev., Int.Abstr.Biol.Sci., Maize Abstr., Microbiol.Abstr., Plant Breed.Abstr., Plant Gen.Res.Abstr., Plant Grow.Reg.Abstr., Plant Sci., Postharvest, Potato Abstr., Rev.Plant Path., Rice Abstr., Sci.Cit.Ind., Soils & Fert., Soyabean Abstr., Triticale Abstr., VITIS, Weed Abstr.

—BLDSC (5900.826000), CASDDS, CISTI, EMDOCS, GNLM, IDS, ingenta, Linda Hall.

Published by: (American Phytopathological Society), A P S Press, 3340 Pilot Knob Rd., St. Paul, MN 55121-2097. TEL 651-454-7250, 800-328-7560, FAX 651-454-0766, aps@scisoc.org, ismpmi@scisoc.org, http://www.scisoc.org/ismpmi. Ed. Herman P Spaink. Adv. contact Rhonda Wike. Circ: 1,492. **Co-sponsor:** International Society for Molecular Plant - Microbe Interactions.

572.8 USA ISSN 1040-452X
QP251 CODEN: MREDEE

MOLECULAR REPRODUCTION AND DEVELOPMENT. Text in English. 1988. 12/yr. (in 3 vols., 4 nos./vol.). USD 3,850 in United States; USD 3,970 in Canada & Mexico; USD 4,072 elsewhere; USD 4,043 combined subscription in United States for print and online eds.; USD 4,163 combined subscription in Canada & Mexico for print and online eds.; USD 4,265 combined subscription elsewhere for print and online eds. (effective 2002). adv. bk.rev. back issues avail. *Refereed.* **Document type:** *Academic/Scholarly.* **Description:** Covers molecular biology of spermatogenesis, oogenesis, and embryonic and fetal development.

Incorporates: Gamete Research

Related titles: Microform ed.: (from PQC); Online - full text ed.: ISSN 1098-2795. 1996. USD 3,850 in United States; USD 3,850 in Canada & Mexico; USD 3,850 elsewhere (effective 2002) (from EBSCO Publishing, Wiley InterScience, Institute for Scientific Information).

Indexed: ASCA, Abstr.Hyg., AgBiotech, Agricola, Anim.Breed.Abstr., Aqua.Sci.& Fish.Abstr., BBCI, Biotech.Cit.Ind., Chem.Abstr., Chem.Indus.Notes, Chem.Titles, Curr.Cont., Dairy Sci.Abstr., Genet.Abstr., Helminthol.Abstr., Hum.Gen.Abstr., INIS Atomind., Ind.Med. (1988-), Ind.Sci.Rev., Ind.Vet., Inpharma, Int.Abstr.Biol.Sci., Nuc.Acids Abstr., Nutr.Abstr., Pig News & Info., Poult.Abstr., Reac., Ref.Zh., Rev.Appl.Entomol., Sci.Cit.Ind., Vet.Bull., Zoo.Rec.

—BLDSC (5900.828000), CASDDS, CISTI, EMDOCS, GNLM, IDS, Linda Hall. **CCC.**

Published by: John Wiley & Sons, Inc., Journals (Subsidiary of: Wiley InterScience), 605 Third Ave, New York, NY 10158. TEL 212-850-6645, FAX 212-850-6021, subinfo@wiley.com, uscs-wis@wiley.com, http://www.wiley.com. Ed. Ralph B Gwatkin. adv.: B&W page GBP 640, color page GBP 1,515; trim 210 x 279. Circ: 800. **Subscr. outside the Americas to:** John Wiley & Sons Ltd., Baffins Ln, Chichester, Sussex PO19 IUD, United Kingdom. TEL 44-1243-779777, FAX 44-1243-843232, cs-journals@wiley.co.uk.

MOLECULAR THERAPY. see *MEDICAL SCIENCES—Oncology*

572.8 USA ISSN 1090-0535

MOLECULAR VISION. Text in English. 1995. irreg. abstr. back issues avail. *Refereed.* **Document type:** *Journal, Academic/Scholarly.* **Description:** Dedicated to the dissemination of research results in molecular biology, cell biology and the generics of the visual system.

Media: Online - full text (from Institute for Scientific Information).

Indexed: BBCI, Biotech.Cit.Ind., Curr.Cont., Ind.Med. (1995-), Sci.Cit.Ind., Zoo.Rec.

Address: Lab B-5500 Emory Eye Center, 1327 Clifton Rd N E, Atlanta, GA 30322. http://www.molvis.org/molvis/. Ed. Stephen M Cristol.

572.8 RUS ISSN 0026-8984
QH506 CODEN: MOBIBO

MOLEKULYARNAYA BIOLOGIYA. Text in Russian. 1967. bi-m. RUR 435 for 2 mos. (effective 2001). charts. index. **Description:** Covers advances in the field of chemical and physical bases of principal life phenomena, including studies on the chemistry and physics of the most important biopolymers (proteins and nucleic acids), their structure, and their functions.

Related titles: Online - full text ed.; ♦ English Translation: Molecular Biology. ISSN 0026-8933.

Indexed: Agri.& Environ.Biotech.Abstr. (coverage dropped), Aqua.Sci.& Fish.Abstr., Biol.Abstr., Chem.Abstr., Derwent Biotech.Abstr., Excerp.Med., INIS Atomind., Ind.Med. (1967-), Nuc.Acids Abstr., Ref.Zh., Zoo.Rec.

—BLDSC (0115.926000), CASDDS, CISTI, GNLM, KNAW, Linda Hall. **CCC.**

Published by: (Rossiiskaya Akademiya Nauk/Russian Academy of Sciences), M A I K Nauka - Interperiodica, Mezhdunarodnyi Otdel, Profsoyuznaya ul 90, Moscow 117864, Russian Federation. TEL 7-095-336-1600, FAX 7-095-336-0666, compmg@maik.ru, http://www.maik.rssi.ru/journals/molbio.htm. Ed. L L Kiselev. **US dist. addr.:** Kluwer Academic Publishers, PO Box 17, Dordrecht 3300 AH, Netherlands. TEL 31-78-639-2392, FAX 31-78-654-6474, http://www.wkap.nl.

572 POL ISSN 0077-0485
CODEN: MOBCA5

MONOGRAFIE BIOCHEMICZNE. Text in Polish. 1962. irreg., latest vol.43, 2001. price varies. bk.rev. bibl, charts, illus. 60 p./no. 1 cols./p. back issues avail. **Document type:** *Monographic series, Academic/Scholarly.*

—CASDDS.

Published by: Polskie Towarzystwo Biochemiczne, Ul Pasteura 3, Warsaw 02093, Poland. TEL 48-22-6582099, konarska@nencki.gov.pl, http://www.ptbioch.edu.pl. Ed. Liliana Konarska. **Dist by:** Ars Polona, Krakowskie Przedmiescie 7, Warsaw, Poland.

572 GBR ISSN 0309-0698

MONOGRAPHS ON PHYSICAL BIOCHEMISTRY. Text in English. 1972. irreg. price varies. *Refereed.* **Document type:** *Monographic series.*

Published by: Oxford University Press, Oxford Journals, Walton St, Oxford OX2 6DP, United Kingdom. TEL 44-1865-56767, FAX 44-1865-56646, jnlorders@oup.co.uk, jnl.orders@oup.co.uk, http://www.oup.co.uk. **Orders in N. America to:** Oxford University Press, Journals. TEL 919-677-0977, FAX 919-677-1714, http://www.oup.co.uk.

MUTAGENESIS. see *BIOLOGY—Genetics*

MUTATION RESEARCH; international journal on mutagenesis, chromosome breakage and related subjects. see *BIOLOGY—Genetics*

572.86 NLD ISSN 0921-8777
CODEN: MDRRE

MUTATION RESEARCH - D N A REPAIR. Text in Dutch. 1983. m. NLG 2,251, EUR 1,021.46 in Europe to institutions; JPY 141,400 in Japan to institutions; USD 1,143 elsewhere to institutions (effective 2001). back issues avail. *Refereed.* **Document type:** *Academic/Scholarly.* **Description:** Topics include: comparisons of cell-to-tissues systems; cloned DNA repair genes; transformation and mutagen testing.

Formerly (until 1988): Mutation Research - D N A Repair - Reports (0167-8817)

Related titles: Microform ed.: (from PQC); Online - full text ed.: (from EBSCO Publishing, ingenta, ScienceDirect, Swets Blackwell, Institute for Scientific Information); ♦ Special ed. of: Mutation Research. ISSN 0921-8262.

Indexed: ASCA, Aqua.Sci.& Fish.Abstr., BBCI, Biol.Abstr., Biotech.& Bioeng.Abstr., Biotech.Cit.Ind., Chem.Abstr., Curr.Cont., Environ.Sci.Poll.Mgmt., Excerp.Med., Genet.Abstr., Hum.Gen.Abstr., INIS Atomind., Ind.Med. (coverage dropped), Ind.Sci.Rev., Inpharma, Int.Abstr.Biol.Sci., Microbiol.Abstr., Nuc.Acids Abstr., Oncog.G.F.Abstr. (coverage dropped), Reac., Ref.Zh., Russ.Acad.Sci.Bibl., Sci.Cit.Ind.

—ADONIS, CISTI, EMDOCS, IDS. **CCC.**

Published by: Elsevier Science BV, PO Box 211, Amsterdam 1000 AE, Netherlands. TEL 31-20-485-3757, TELEX 18582 ESPA NL, usinfo-f@elsevier.com, nlinfo-f@elsevier.nl, http://www.elsevier.com/locate/mrdnarepair, http://www.elsevier.nl. **Subscr. in Australasia and the Far East to:** Elsevier Science (Singapore) Pte Ltd, No.1 Temasek Ave, 17-01 Millenia Tower, Singapore 039192, Singapore. TEL 65-434-3727, FAX 65-337-2230; **Subscr. in Japan to:** Elsevier Science Inc - Japan Regional Office, 9-15 Higashi-Azabu 1-chome, Minato-ku, Tokyo 106-0044, Japan. TEL 81-3-5561-5033, FAX 81-3-5561-5047, info@elsevier.co.jp; **Subscr. in the Americas to:** Elsevier Science, PO Box 945, New York, NY 10159-0945. TEL 212-633-3730, FAX 212-633-3680.

MUTATION RESEARCH - FUNDAMENTAL AND MOLECULAR MECHANISMS OF MUTAGENESIS. see *BIOLOGY—Genetics*

MUTATION RESEARCH - GENETIC TOXICOLOGY AND ENVIRONMENTAL MUTAGENESIS. see *BIOLOGY—Genetics*

MUTATION RESEARCH LETTERS. see *BIOLOGY—Genetics*

MUTATION RESEARCH - REVIEWS IN GENETIC TOXICOLOGY. see *BIOLOGY—Genetics*

572.65 GBR ISSN 0143-4179
Discard CODEN: NRPPDD
NEUROPEPTIDES (EDINBURGH). Text in English. 1979. bi-m. GBP 141 to individuals; GBP 771 to institutions (effective 2002). adv. bk.rev. bibl. back issues avail. *Refereed.* **Document type:** *Journal, Academic/Scholarly.* **Description:** Contains articles dealing with the structure, distribution, actions and functions of peptides in the central and peripheral nervous systems.
Related titles: Online - full text ed.: (from EBSCO Publishing, RoweCom Information Quest, Swets Blackwell, IDEAL Online Library, Institute for Scientific Information).
Indexed: Anim.Behav.Abstr., Aqua.Sci.& Fish.Abstr., BBCI, Chem.Abstr., Chem.Indus.Notes, Chem.Titles, Curr.Adv.Ecol.Sci., Curr.Cont., Ind.Med. (1980-), Ind.Sci.Rev., Int.Abstr.Biol.Sci., Neurosci.Abstr., Neurosci.Cit.Ind., Ref.Zh., Sci.Cit.Ind.
—BLDSC (6081.516000), ADONIS, CASDDS, CISTI, GNLM, IDS, ingenta, KNAW. **CCC.**
Published by: Churchill Livingstone (Subsidiary of: Harcourt Publishers Ltd.), Robert Stevenson House, 1-3 Baxter's Pl, Leith Walk, Edinburgh, Midlothian EH1 3AF, United Kingdom. TEL 44-131-556-2424, FAX 44-131-459-1177, cservice@harcourt.com, http://www.harcourt-international.com/journals/npep. Eds. J Hughes, Dr. J N Crawley. Pub. Gillian Griffith. R&P Catherine John TEL 212-424-4200. Adv. contact David Dunnachie. Circ: 390. **Subscr. to:** Harcourt Publishers Ltd., Foots Cray High St, Sidcup, Kent DA14 5HP, United Kingdom. TEL 44-20-8308-5700, FAX 44-20-8309-0807.

NEUROPEPTIDES (SHEFFIELD). see *BIOLOGY—Abstracting, Bibliographies, Statistics*

NEUROSCIENCE COMMUNICATIONS. see *MEDICAL SCIENCES—Abstracting, Bibliographies, Statistics*

572 CHE ISSN 1424-862X
CODEN: BISIEH
NEUROSIGNALS. Text in English. 1992. bi-m. CHF 809, EUR 577.80 in Europe to institutions; CHF 826.40 overseas to institutions; USD 631 elsewhere to institutions (effective 2002). adv. back issues avail. *Refereed.* **Document type:** *Journal, Academic/Scholarly.* **Description:** Provides a platform for new ideas, novel concepts, and innovative hypotheses which do not always conform to classical theories and teaching. Publishes original articles, reviews and communications in the broad field of production, transmission, processing, recognition, effects, modification and evolution of biological signals.
Former titles: Biological Signals and Receptors (1422-4933); (until 1998): Biological Signals (1016-0922)
Related titles: Microform ed.: (from PQC); Online - full text ed.: ISSN 1424-8638. CHF 58, EUR 42, USD 45 to institutions with print edition (effective 2002) (from EBSCO Publishing, O C L C Online Computer Library Center, Inc., RoweCom Information Quest, Swets Blackwell, Institute for Scientific Information).
Indexed: ASCA, BBCI, Chem.Abstr., Chem.Indus.Notes, Chem.Titles, Excerp.Med. (1993-), Ind.Med. (1998-), Int.Abstr.Biol.Sci., Mass Spectr.Bull.
—BLDSC (2080.720000), CASDDS, CISTI, EMDOCS, GNLM, IDS, Infotrieve, ingenta, KNAW. **CCC.**
Published by: S. Karger AG, Allschwilerstr 10, PO Box, Basel 4009, Switzerland. TEL 41-61-306-1111, FAX 41-61-306-1234, karger@karger.ch, http://www.online.karger.com/journals/bsi, http://www.karger.com. Eds. D P Cardinali, P A Ward, S F Pang. adv.: page USD 1,185.

572 NLD ISSN 0167-7306
CODEN: NCBIDL
NEW COMPREHENSIVE BIOCHEMISTRY. Text in English. 1979. irreg., latest vol.34, 1999. price varies. back issues avail. *Refereed.* **Document type:** *Monographic series, Academic/Scholarly.* **Description:** Informs scientists of developments in the biochemical sciences and provides them with an authoritative reference work.
Supersedes (in 1981): Comprehensive Biochemistry
Indexed: Chem.Abstr., Chem.Indus.Notes, Chem.Titles.
—BLDSC (6082.890000), CASDDS, CISTI. **CCC.**
Published by: Elsevier Science BV, PO Box 211, Amsterdam 1000 AE, Netherlands. TEL 31-20-485-3757, 31-20-485-3911, FAX 31-20-485-3432, 31-20-485-3598, nlinfo-f@elsevier.nl, http://www.elsevier.nl/. Eds. A Neuberger, L L M van Deenen. **Subscr. in Australasia and the Far East to:** Elsevier Science (Singapore) Pte Ltd, No.1 Temasek Ave, 17-01 Millenia Tower, Singapore 039192, Singapore. TEL 65-434-3727, FAX 65-337-2230, asiainfo@elsevier.com.sg; **Subscr. in Japan to:** Elsevier Science Inc - Japan Regional Office, 9-15 Higashi-Azabu 1-chome, Minato-ku, Tokyo 106-0044, Japan. TEL 81-3-5561-5033, FAX 81-3-5561-5047, info@elsevier.co.jp; **Subscr. in the Americas to:** Elsevier Science, PO Box 945, New York, NY 10159-0945. TEL 212-633-3730, 888-437-4636, FAX 212-633-3680, usinfo-f@elsevier.com, http://www.elsevier.com

572 JPN ISSN 0913-3348
CODEN: NOKKEL
NIHON OYO KOSO KYOKAISHI/JAPAN FOUNDATION FOR APPLIED ENZYMOLOGY. JOURNAL. Text in Japanese. a.
Indexed: Chem.Abstr.
—BLDSC (6112.915600), CASDDS.
Published by: Nihon Oyo Koso Kyokai/Japan Foundation of Applied Enzymology, 16-89 Kashima 3-chome, Yodogawa-ku, Osaka-shi 532-0031, Japan.

NIHON SENSHOKUTAI KENSA GAKKAI SHOROKUSHU/JAPANESE ASSOCIATION FOR CHROMOSOME ANALYSIS. ABSTRACT OF ANNUAL MEETING. see *BIOLOGY—Abstracting, Bibliographies, Statistics*

572.87 JPN ISSN 0917-8155
NIHON SENSHOKUTAI KENSA GAKKAI ZASSHI/JAPANESE ASSOCIATION FOR CHROMOSOME ANALYSIS. OFFICIAL JOURNAL. Text in English, Japanese; Summaries in English. 1983. q.
Published by: Nihon Senshokutai Kensa Gakkai, c/o Kurasuta Koa Kenkyujo Idenshi Kenkyubu, 11-18 Tsubamesawa-Higashi 3-chome, Miyagino-ku, Sendai-shi, Miyagi-ken 983-0000, Japan.

NITRIC OXIDE. see *BIOLOGY—Abstracting, Bibliographies, Statistics*

NUCLEIC ACIDS ABSTRACTS. see *BIOLOGY—Abstracting, Bibliographies, Statistics*

572.65 USA ISSN 0933-1891
QP620 CODEN: NAMBE8
NUCLEIC ACIDS AND MOLECULAR BIOLOGY. Text in English. 1987. irreg., latest vol.9. **Document type:** *Monographic series.*
Indexed: Agricola, Chem.Abstr., Chem.Titles, Derwent Biotech.Abstr.
—BLDSC (6183.745000), CASDDS, CISTI, GNLM, ingenta, KNAW. **CCC.**
Published by: Springer-Verlag, Journals (Subsidiary of: BertelsmannSpringer), 175 Fifth Ave, New York, NY 10010. TEL 212-460-1500, FAX 212-473-6272.

572.6 GBR ISSN 0305-1048
QP620 CODEN: NARHAD
NUCLEIC ACIDS RESEARCH. Text in English. 1974. 24/yr. GBP 335, USD 570 to individuals; GBP 1,250, USD 2,165 to institutions (effective 2002). adv. illus. index. 248 p./no. back issues avail.; reprint service avail. from SWZ. *Refereed.* **Document type:** *Journal, Academic/Scholarly.* **Description:** International rapid-publication journal on nucleic acids, constituents and analogues. Publishing RFLP sequence reprints, sequence data, NMR assignment data and methods.
Related titles: CD-ROM ed.; Online - full text ed.: ISSN 1362-4962. GBP 1,125, USD 1,948 to institutions Online only (effective 2002) (from HighWire Pr., EBSCO Publishing, O C L C Online Computer Library Center, Inc., RoweCom Information Quest, ingenta, Swets Blackwell, Institute for Scientific Information).
Indexed: ASCA, AgBiotech, Agricola, Anim.Breed.Abstr., Aqua.Sci.& Fish.Abstr., BBCI, Bibl.Agri., Bio-Contr.News & Info., Biotech.Cit.Ind., CEABA, Chem.Abstr., Chem.Cit.Ind., Chem.Indus.Notes, Chem.Titles, Curr.Adv.Biochem., Curr.Adv.Cell & Devel.Biol., Curr.Adv.Ecol.Sci., Curr.Adv.Gen.& Molec.Biol., Curr.Biotech.Abstr., Curr.Cont., Dairy Sci.Abstr., Derwent Biotech.Abstr., Entomol.Abstr., Environ.Sci.Poll.Mgmt., Fababean Abstr., Food Sci.& Tech.Abstr., Forest.Abstr., Genet.Abstr., Helminthol.Abstr., Hum.Gen.Abstr., INIS Atomind., Immun.Abstr. (coverage dropped), Ind.Med. (1974-), Ind.Sci.Rev., Ind.Vet., Inpharma, Int.Abstr.Biol.Sci., Maize Abstr., Mass Spectr.Bull., Med.& Pharm.Biotech.Abstr., Microbiol.Abstr., Neurosci.Abstr. (coverage dropped), Neurosci.Cit.Ind., Nuc.Acids Abstr., Nutr.Abstr., Oncog.G.F.Abstr. (coverage dropped), Plant Breed.Abstr., Plant Grow.Reg.Abstr., Potato Abstr., Poult.Abstr., Protozool.Abstr., RCI, Reac., Ref.Zh., Rev.Appl.Entomol., Rev.Med.& Vet.Mycol., Rev.Plant Path., Rice Abstr., Sci.Cit.Ind., Seed Abstr., Soils & Fert., Soyabean Abstr., Triticale Abstr., VITIS, Vet.Bull., Virol.Abstr. (coverage dropped).
—BLDSC (6183.850000), CASDDS, CISTI, EMDOCS, GNLM, IDS, ingenta, Linda Hall. **CCC.**
Published by: Oxford University Press, Academic Division, Great Clarendon St, Oxford OX2 6DP, United Kingdom. TEL 44-1865-267907, FAX 44-1865-267835, jnl.info@oup.co.uk, http://nar.oupjournals.org/, http://www.oup.co.uk/journals. Eds. Michael Gait, Richard J Roberts. Pub. David Prosser. R&P Fionna Willis. adv.: page GBP 470, page USD 845. Circ: 2,800. **Subscr. in U.S. to:** Oxford University Press, Journals, 2001 Evans Rd, Cary, NC 27513. TEL 800-852-7323, FAX 919-677-1714, jnlorders@oup-usa.org; **Subscr. to:** Journals Marketing, Great Clarendon St, Oxford OX2 6DP, United Kingdom.

O M I C S: A JOURNAL OF INTEGRATIVE BIOLOGY. see *BIOLOGY—Genetics*

572.57 GBR
THE OILY PRESS LIPID LIBRARY. Text in English. irreg. **Document type:** *Monographic series, Academic/Scholarly.*
—BLDSC (6252.622500).
Published by: P J Barnes and Associates, PO Box 200, Bridgwater TA7 0YZ, United Kingdom. TEL 44-1823-698973, FAX 44-1823-698971, sales@pbarnes.demon.co.uk, http://www.pbarnes.demon.co.uk. Ed. Michael I Gurr.

572 DEU
OLD HERBORN UNIVERSITY SEMINAR MONOGRAPHS. Text in English. irreg., latest vol.5, 1994. **Document type:** *Monographic series.*
Indexed: Chem.Abstr., Chem.Titles.
—BLDSC (6253.813500).
Published by: Institute for Microbiology and Biochemistry, Kornmarkt 34, Herborn 35745, Germany. TEL 02772-41033, FAX 02772-41039.

ONCOGENE. see *MEDICAL SCIENCES—Oncology*

572 JPN
OSAKA SHIKA DAIGAKU SEIKAGAKU KYOSHITSU GYOSEKISHU/OSAKA DENTAL UNIVERSITY. DEPARTMENT OF BIOCHEMISTRY. ACHIEVEMENT. Text in English, Japanese. 1961. irreg.
Published by: Osaka Shika Daigaku, Seirigaku Kyoshitsu, 1-47, Kyobashi, Higashi-ku, Osaka-shi 540, Japan.

572.6 JPN ISSN 0078-6705
QP551
OSAKA UNIVERSITY. INSTITUTE FOR PROTEIN RESEARCH. MEMOIRS/OSAKA DAIGAKU TANPAKUSHITSU KENKYUSHO KIYO. Text in English. 1959. a. per issue exchange basis. **Document type:** *Abstract/Index.*
Indexed: INIS Atomind., Nutr.Abstr., Ref.Zh.
—CISTI, Linda Hall.
Published by: Osaka Daigaku, Tanpakushitsu Kenkyusho/Osaka University, Institute for Protein Research, 3-2 Yamada-Oka, Suita-shi, Osaka-fu 565-0871, Japan. TEL 81-6-877-5111, FAX 81-6-876-2533. Ed. Toshio Takagi. Circ: 300.

OXYGEN RADICALS. see *BIOLOGY—Abstracting, Bibliographies, Statistics*

572 PHL ISSN 0115-6403
CODEN: BPBSDA
P B S BULLETIN. Text in English. 1978. a. PHP 50, USD 10. adv. bk.rev.
—CASDDS.

B

Published by: Philippine Biochemical Society, c/o Dept. of Biochemistry, University of the College of Medicine, PO Box 593, Manila, Philippines. FAX 63-2-50-17-06. Ed. E M T Mendoza. Circ: 200.

572 PAK
QP501 CODEN: PJBIAL
PAKISTAN JOURNAL OF BIOCHEMISTRY AND MOLECULAR BIOLOGY. Text in English. 1968. s-a. PKR 100, USD 50. adv. **Document type:** *Academic/Scholarly.*
Formerly: Pakistan Journal of Biochemistry (0300-8185)
Related titles: CD-ROM ed.
Indexed: Biol.Abstr., Chem.Abstr., Chem.Titles, Curr.Adv.Ecol.Sci., ExtraMED, INIS Atomind.
—BLDSC (6340.897500), CASDDS, CISTI, ingenta, Linda Hall.
Published by: Pakistan Society of Biochemists, Institute of Chemistry, University of Punjab, Lahore 54590, Pakistan. Ed. Nazrul S Hasnain. Circ: 400.

PAKISTAN JOURNAL OF PHARMACEUTICAL SCIENCES. see *PHARMACY AND PHARMACOLOGY*

PATHOPHYSIOLOGY. see *BIOLOGY—Physiology*

572.65 USA ISSN 0196-9781
QP552.P4 CODEN: PPTDD5
PEPTIDES; an international journal. Text in English. 1980. m. EUR 214 in Europe to individuals; JPY 28,400 in Japan to individuals; USD 240 elsewhere to individuals; EUR 2,809 in Europe to institutions; JPY 373,000 in Japan to institutions; USD 3,142 elsewhere to institutions (effective 2002). adv. illus. index. back issues avail.; reprint service avail. from PQC,ISI. *Refereed.* **Document type:** *Academic/Scholarly.* **Description:** Original contributions on the chemistry, biochemistry, endocrinology, gastroenterology, physiology and pharmacology of peptides and their neurological, psychological and behavioral effects.
Related titles: Microfilm ed.: (from PQC); Online - full text ed.: (from ingenta, ScienceDirect, Swets Blackwell, Institute for Scientific Information).
Indexed: AgBiotech, Anim.Behav.Abstr., Anim.Breed.Abstr., Aqua.Sci.& Fish.Abstr., BBCI, Biol.Abstr., Chem.Abstr., Chem.Cit.Ind., Chem.Indus.Notes, Chem.Titles, Curr.Adv.Ecol.Sci., Curr.Cont., Dairy Sci.Abstr., Dent.Ind., Environ.Sci.Poll.Mgmt., Excerp.Med., Helminthol.Abstr., INIS Atomind., Ind.Med. (1980-), Ind.Sci.Rev., Ind.Vet., Indian Psychol.Abstr., Inpharma, Int.Abstr.Biol.Sci., Mass Spectr.Bull., Neurosci.Abstr. (coverage dropped), Neurosci.Cit.Ind., Pharm.&Out.News, Poult.Abstr., Protozool.Abstr., PsycInfo, Psychol.Abstr. (1981-), Reac., Sci.Cit.Ind., Small Anim.Abstr., Trop.Dis.Bull., Vet.Bull., e-psyche.
—BLDSC (6422.954000), ADONIS, CASDDS, CISTI, GNLM, IDS, ingenta, KNAW, Linda Hall. **CCC.**
Published by: Elsevier Science, 655 Ave of the Americas, New York, NY 10010. TEL 212-989-5800, FAX 212-633-3990, usinfo-f@elsevier.com, http://www.elsevier.nl/locate/peptides. Ed. Abba J Kastin. **Subscr. in Australasia and the Far East to:** Elsevier Science (Singapore) Pte Ltd, No.1 Temasek Ave, 17-01 Millenia Tower, Singapore 039192, Singapore. TEL 65-434-3727, FAX 65-337-2230; **Subscr. in Japan to:** Elsevier Science Inc - Japan Regional Office, 9-15 Higashi-Azabu 1-chome, Minato-ku, Tokyo 106-0044, Japan. TEL 81-3-5561-5033; **Subscr. outside the Americas to:** Elsevier Science BV, PO Box 211, Amsterdam 1000 AE, Netherlands. TEL 31-20-485-3757.

PESTICIDE BIOCHEMISTRY AND PHYSIOLOGY; an international journal. see *AGRICULTURE—Crop Production And Soil*

572.43 NLD ISSN 0166-8595
CODEN: PHRSDI
PHOTOSYNTHESIS RESEARCH; an international journal. Text in English. 1980. m. EUR 1,340 to institutions for print or online ed.; EUR 1,476.60 to institutions print & online eds.combined (effective 2002). adv. bk.rev. back issues avail.; reprint service avail. from SWZ. *Refereed.* **Document type:** *Academic/Scholarly.* **Description:** Publishes papers dealing with basic and applied aspects of photosynthesis, including light absorption and emission, primary photochemistry, photorespiration, molecular biology, environmental and ecological aspects, and bacterial and algal photosynthesis.
Related titles: Microform ed.: (from PQC); Online - full text ed.: NLG 107.50, EUR 50 (effective 2001) (from EBSCO Publishing, O C L C Online Computer Library Center, Inc., RoweCom Information Quest, Swets Blackwell, Kluwer Online, Institute for Scientific Information).
Indexed: ASCA, AgBiotech, Agricola, Agroforest.Abstr., Aqua.Sci.& Fish.Abstr., BBCI, Biol.Abstr., Chem.Abstr., Chem.Cit.Ind., Chem.Indus.Notes, Chem.Titles, Crop Physiol.Abstr., Curr.Adv.Ecol.Sci., Curr.Adv.Plant Sci., Curr.Cont., Eng.Ind., Environ.Sci.Poll.Mgmt., Field Crop Abstr., Forest.Abstr., GeoRef, Herb.Abstr., Hort.Abstr., INSPEC (Jan.1988-), Ind.Sci.Rev., Inpharma, Int.Abstr.Biol.Sci., Maize Abstr., Microbiol.Abstr., Ornam.Hort., Plant Breed.Abstr., Plant Grow.Reg.Abstr., Plant Sci., Potato Abstr., Reac., Rice Abstr., Sci.Cit.Ind., Soils & Fert., Soyabean Abstr., Triticale Abstr., Weed Abstr.
—BLDSC (6474.365000), AskIEEE, CASDDS, CISTI, Ei, EMDOCS, IDS, ingenta, Linda Hall. **CCC.**
Published by: Kluwer Academic Publishers Group (Subsidiary of: Wolters Kluwer N.V.), Spuiboulevard 50, PO Box 17, Dordrecht 3300 AA, Netherlands. FAX 31-78-639-2254, services@wkap.nl, http://www.wkap.nl. Ed. R E Blankenship. **Dist. by:** Journals Department, PO Box 322, Dordrecht 3300 AH, Netherlands. TEL 781-871-6600, FAX 31-78-654-6474.

572 JPN ISSN 0031-9082
QP501 CODEN: SBBKA4
PHYSICO-CHEMICAL BIOLOGY/SEIBUTSU BUTSURI KAGAKU. Text in English, Japanese. 1951. bi-m. JPY 1,200 per issue. adv. bk.rev. illus. index.
Indexed: Biol.Abstr., Chem.Abstr., Chem.Titles, INIS Atomind.
—CASDDS, CISTI. **CCC.**
Published by: Society of Electrophoresis/Denki Eido Gakkai, Azabu Daigaku Juigakubu Kachiku Eiseigaku Kyoshitsu, 17-71 Fuchinobe 1-chome, Sagamihara-shi, Kanagawa-ken 229-0006, Japan. Ed. Toshitsugu Oda. Circ: 1,600.

PHYSIOLOGICAL CHEMISTRY AND PHYSICS AND MEDICAL N M R. (Nuclear Magnetic Resonance) see *BIOLOGY—Biophysics*

572.8 USA ISSN 1094-8341
▼ **PHYSIOLOGICAL GENOMICS.** Text in English. 1999. m. USD 135 domestic to non-members; USD 150 in Canada & Mexico to non-members; USD 165 elsewhere to non-members; USD 200 domestic to institutions; USD 215 in Canada & Mexico to institutions; USD 230 elsewhere to institutions; USD 140 domestic to non-members for both print & online eds.; USD 155 in Canada & Mexico to non-members for both print & onlne eds.; USD 170 elsewhere to non-members for both print & onlne eds.; USD 65 domestic to members for both print & online eds.; USD 80 in Canada & Mexico to members for both print & online eds.; USD 95 elsewhere to members for both print & online eds.; USD 210 domestic to institutions for both print & online eds.; USD 225 in Canada & Mexico to institutions for both print & online eds. (effective 2002); print & online eds.. bk.rev. *Refereed.* **Description:** Publishes the result of a wide variety of studies from human and from informative model systems with techniques linking genes and pathways to physiology from prokaryotes to eukaryotes.
Related titles: Online - full text ed.: 1999 (Jul.). USD 115 to individuals; USD 175 to institutions (effective 2002) (from HighWire Pr., EBSCO Publishing, Institute for Scientific Information).
Indexed: BBCI, Biotech.Cit.Ind., Curr.Cont., Ind.Med., Sci.Cit.Ind.
—BLDSC (6484.730000).
Published by: American Physiological Society, 9650 Rockville Pike, Bethesda, MD 20814-3991. TEL 301-530-7164, FAX 301-571-8305, publicat@asp.faseb.org, info@the-aps.org, http://www.physiolgenomics.org/, http://www.faseb.org/aps. Ed. Victor J Dzau.

PHYTOCHEMICAL ANALYSIS. see *BIOLOGY—Botany*

572 GBR ISSN 0197-8969
CODEN: APPEDR
PHYTOCHEMICAL SOCIETY OF EUROPE. ANNUAL PROCEEDINGS. Text in English. a. price varies. adv. **Document type:** *Proceedings.*
Indexed: Chem.Abstr., Chem.Indus.Notes, Chem.Titles, Environ.Sci.Poll.Mgmt., Sel.Water Res.Abstr.
—BLDSC (6787.560000), CISTI, Infotrieve. **CCC.**
Published by: Oxford University Press, Oxford Journals, Walton St, Oxford OX2 6DP, United Kingdom. FAX 44-1865-267773, jnlorders@oup.co.uk, jnl.orders@oup.co.uk, http://www.oup.co.uk. Ed. Peter J Lea. **Subscr. in N. America to:** Oxford University Press, Journals. TEL 919-677-0977, FAX 919-677-1714.

572 GBR ISSN 0964-5845
CODEN: PPRMEN
PORTLAND PRESS RESEARCH MONOGRAPH. Text in English. 1992. irreg., latest vol.12, 1998. back issues avail. *Refereed.* **Document type:** *Monographic series.*
Indexed: Chem.Abstr., Chem.Indus.Notes, Chem.Titles.
—BLDSC (6555.660000), CASDDS, CISTI.
Published by: Portland Press Ltd., 59 Portland Pl, London W1N 3AJ, United Kingdom. TEL 44-20-7580-5530, FAX 44-20-7323-1136, sales@portland-service.com, http://www.portlandpress.com/bst/default.htm. R&P Adam Marshall. **Subscr. to:** Commerce Way, Colchester, Essex CO2 8HP, United Kingdom. TEL 44-1206-796351, FAX 44-1206-799331.

572 POL ISSN 0032-5422
QP501 CODEN: PSTBAH
POSTEPY BIOCHEMII. Text in Polish; Summaries in English. 1953. q., latest vol.47, 2001. USD 80. bk.rev. charts, illus, bibl. index. 100 p./no. 2 cols./p. back issues avail. **Document type:** *Journal, Academic/Scholarly.*
Indexed: AgroAgen, AgroLibrex, Anim.Breed.Abstr., Biol.Abstr., Chem.Abstr., Chem.Indus.Notes, Chem.Titles, Curr.Adv.Ecol.Sci., Dairy Sci.Abstr., INIS Atomind., Ind.Med. (1955-).
—CASDDS, CISTI, GNLM, Linda Hall.
Published by: Polskie Towarzystwo Biochemiczne, Ul Pasteura 3, Warsaw 02093, Poland. TEL 48-22-6582099, postepy@nencki.gov.pl. Ed. Grazyna Palamarczyk. Circ: 1,810. **Dist. by:** Ars Polona, Krakowskie Przedmiescie 7, Warsaw, Poland.

572 USA ISSN 1082-6068
QH324 CODEN: PBBIF4
PREPARATIVE BIOCHEMISTRY AND BIOTECHNOLOGY. Text in English. 1971. q. USD 120 to individuals print & online eds.; USD 895 to institutions print only (effective 2002). adv. *Refereed.* **Document type:** *Academic/Scholarly.* **Description:** An international forum of research results dealing with all aspects of preparitive techniques in biotechnology, and other topics.
Formerly: Preparative Biochemistry (0032-7484)
Related titles: Microform ed.: (from RPI); Online - full content ed.; Online - full text ed.: (from Institute for Scientific Information, RoweCom Information Quest).
Indexed: ASCA, Agri.& Environ.Biotech.Abstr., Agricola, Aqua.Sci.& Fish.Abstr., Aquacult.Abstr., BBCI, Biol.Abstr., Chem.Abstr., Chem.Indus.Notes, Chem.Titles, Crop Physiol.Abstr., Curr.Adv.Ecol.Sci., Curr.Cont., Dairy Sci.Abstr., Derwent Biotech.Abstr., Environ.Sci.Poll.Mgmt., Excerp.Med., Field Crop Abstr., Helminthol.Abstr., INIS Atomind., Ind.Med. (1996-), Ind.Sci.Rev., Inpharma, Int.Abstr.Biol.Sci., Int.Aerosp.Abstr., Med.& Pharm.Biotech.Abstr., Microbiol.Abstr., Pollut.Abstr., Reac., Ref.Zh., Sci.Cit.Ind.
—BLDSC (6607.841000), CASDDS, CISTI, GNLM, IDS, Infotrieve, ingenta, Linda Hall. **CCC.**
Published by: Marcel Dekker Inc., 270 Madison Ave, New York, NY 10016. TEL 212-696-9000, 800-228-1160, FAX 212-685-4540, http://www.dekker.com/servlet/product/productid/PB. Ed. Jack Cazes. R&P Julia Mulligan. Adv. contact Diane Saulon. Circ: 300.

572 RUS ISSN 0555-1099
QH345 CODEN: PBMIAK
PRIKLADNAYA BIOKHIMIYA I MIKROBIOLOGIYA. Text in Russian. 1965. bi-m. RUR 370 for 2 mos. (effective 2001).
Related titles: Online - full text ed.; ♦ English Translation: Applied Biochemistry and Microbiology. ISSN 0003-6838.
Indexed: Abstr.Bull.Inst.Pap.Chem., Aqua.Sci.& Fish.Abstr., CEABA, Chem.Abstr., Chem.Indus.Notes, Chem.Titles, Crop Physiol.Abstr., Curr.Biotech.Abstr., Derwent Biotech.Abstr., Environ.Sci.Poll.Mgmt., Field Crop Abstr., Food Sci.& Tech.Abstr., GeoRef, Herb.Abstr., Hort.Abstr., INIS Atomind., Ind.Med. (1965-), Microbiol.Abstr., Ref.Zh., Seed Abstr., VITIS.
—BLDSC (0131.920000), CASDDS, CISTI, East View, GNLM, Infotrieve, KNAW, Linda Hall. **CCC.**
Published by: (Rossiiskaya Akademiya Nauk/Russian Academy of Sciences), M A I K Nauka - Interperiodica, Mezhdunarodnyi Otdel, Leninskii prospect 33, Moscow 117071, Russian Federation. compmg@maik.rssi.ru, http://www.maik.rssi.ru/. Ed. B F Poglazov. **US dist. addr.:** East View Publications, 3020 Harbor Ln N, Minneapolis, MN 55447. TEL 612-550-0961.

PROCESS BIOCHEMISTRY. see *BIOLOGY—Biotechnology*

572 USA ISSN 0177-8757
RB112.5 CODEN: PCBMEM
PROGRESS IN CLINICAL BIOCHEMISTRY AND MEDICINE. Text in English. 1984. irreg. price varies. reprint service avail. from ISI. **Document type:** *Monographic series.*
Indexed: Chem.Abstr., Chem.Titles, Curr.Adv.Ecol.Sci. —CASDDS, CISTI, Linda Hall.
Published by: Springer-Verlag, Journals (Subsidiary of: BertelsmannSpringer), 175 Fifth Ave, New York, NY 10010. TEL 212-460-1500, FAX 212-473-6272.

572 DEU ISSN 0079-6336
QH611 CODEN: PHCCAS
PROGRESS IN HISTOCHEMISTRY AND CYTOCHEMISTRY. Text in English. 1970. 4/yr. EUR 289, GBP 221 (effective 2002). *Refereed.* **Document type:** *Monographic series, Academic/Scholarly.* **Description:** Publishes comprehensive and analytical reviews within the entire field of histochemistry and cytochemistry.
Related titles: Online - full text ed.: (from Institute for Scientific Information).
Indexed: ASCA, BBCI, Biol.Abstr., Chem.Abstr., Chem.Titles, Curr.Adv.Biochem., Curr.Adv.Cancer Res., Curr.Adv.Cell & Devel.Biol., Curr.Adv.Ecol.Sci., Excerp.Med., Ind.Med. (until 1999, dropped), Ind.Sci.Rev., Sci.Cit.Ind.
—BLDSC (6868.437000), CASDDS, CISTI, EMDOCS, GNLM. **CCC.**
Published by: Urban & Fischer Verlag, Loebdergraben 14A, Jena 07743, Germany. TEL 49-3641-626444, FAX 49-3641-626443, info@urbanfischer.de, http://www.urbanfischer.de. Ed. Dr. W Graumann.

571.74 NLD
PROGRESS IN HORMONE BIOCHEMISTRY. Text in English. irreg. price varies. *Refereed.* **Document type:** *Monographic series.*
Published by: Kluwer Academic Publishers Group (Subsidiary of: Wolters Kluwer N.V.), Spuiboulevard 50, PO Box 17, Dordrecht 3300 AA, Netherlands. FAX 31-78-639-2254, services@wkap.nl, http://www.wkap.nl. **Dist. by:** Journals Department, PO Box 322, Dordrecht 3300 AH, Netherlands. FAX 31-78-654-6474.

PROGRESS IN MOLECULAR AND SUBCELLULAR BIOLOGY. see *BIOLOGY—Cytology And Histology*

PROSTAGLANDINS - BIOLOGY. see *MEDICAL SCIENCES—Abstracting, Bibliographies, Statistics*

PROSTAGLANDINS, LEUKOTRIENES AND CANCER. see *MEDICAL SCIENCES—Oncology*

572.7 616.3 615.1 USA
PROTEASE INHIBITOR REFERENCE. Text in English. 1997. a. USD 269 (effective 1999). **Document type:** *Trade.*
Published by: American Health Consultants (Subsidiary of: Medical Economics Co., Inc.), 3525 Piedmont Rd, N E, 6 Piedmont Center, Ste 400, Atlanta, GA 30305. TEL 404-262-5476, custserv@ahcpub.com, http://www.ahcpub.com.

572 GBR ISSN 0269-2139
TP248.P77 CODEN: PRENE9
PROTEIN ENGINEERING. Text in English. 1986. m. GBP 156, USD 256 to individuals; GBP 525, USD 855 to institutions (effective 2002). adv. bk.rev. illus. index. 124 p./no. back issues avail.; reprint service avail. from SWZ. *Refereed.* **Document type:** *Journal, Academic/Scholarly.* **Description:** International research results advancing the understanding of the structural and biochemical basis of protein function.
Related titles: Online - full text ed.: ISSN 1460-213X. GBP 472, USD 770 to institutions online only (effective 2002) (from HighWire Pr., EBSCO Publishing, O C L C Online Computer Library Center, Inc., RoweCom Information Quest, ingenta, Swets Blackwell, Institute for Scientific Information).
Indexed: AIDS & Cancer Res., ASCA, Agri.& Environ.Biotech.Abstr., Aqua.Sci.& Fish.Abstr., BBCI, Biol.Abstr., Biotech.Cit.Ind., Chem.Abstr., Chem.Cit.Ind., Chem.Titles, Curr.Adv.Biochem., Curr.Adv.Gen.& Molec.Biol., Curr.Biotech.Abstr., Curr.Cont., Dairy Sci.Abstr., Derwent Biotech.Abstr., Eng.Ind., Environ.Sci.Poll.Mgmt., Excerp.Med., Food Sci.& Tech.Abstr., Ind.Med. (1986-), Inpharma, Int.Abstr.Biol.Sci., Med.& Pharm.Biotech.Abstr., Microbiol.Abstr., Nuc.Acids Abstr., Protozool.Abstr., Reac., Ref.Zh., Saf.Sci.Abstr., Sci.Cit.Ind., Sugar Ind.Abstr., Telegen, Tox.Abstr., Virol.Abstr.
—BLDSC (6936.050000), CASDDS, CISTI, Ei, EMDOCS, GNLM, IDS, ingenta, Linda Hall. **CCC.**
Published by: Oxford University Press, Academic Division, Great Clarendon St, Oxford OX2 6DP, United Kingdom. TEL 44-1865-267907, FAX 44-1865-267835, jnl.info@oup.co.uk, http://www.oup.co.uk/proeng/, http://www.oup.co.uk/journals. Eds. A R Rees, G Petsko. Pub. David Prosser. R&P Fionna Willis. adv.: page GBP 300, page USD 570. Circ: 900. **U.S. subscr. to:** Oxford University Press, Journals, 2001 Evans Rd, Cary, NC 27513. TEL 800-852-7323, FAX 919-677-1714, jnlorders@oup-usa.org; **Subscr. to:** Journals Marketing, Great Clarendon St, Oxford OX2 6DP, United Kingdom.

572.8 USA ISSN 1046-5928
QP551 CODEN: PEXPEJ
PROTEIN EXPRESSION AND PURIFICATION. Text in English. 1990. 9/yr. USD 431 in US & Canada to institutions; USD 495 rest of world to institutions (effective 2001). back issues avail. *Refereed.* **Document type:** *Academic/Scholarly.* **Description:** Presents papers on protein isolations based on conventional fractionation techniques as well as those employing the variety of molecular biological procedures used in the expression of proteins.
Related titles: Online - full text ed.: (from EBSCO Publishing, O C L C Online Computer Library Center, Inc., RoweCom Information Quest, ingenta, Swets Blackwell, IDEAL Online Library, Institute for Scientific Information).
Indexed: ASCA, Aqua.Sci.& Fish.Abstr., BBCI, Biotech.Cit.Ind., Chem.Abstr., Chem.Cit.Ind., Chem.Indus.Notes, Chem.Titles, Curr.Cont., Food Sci.& Tech.Abstr., Ind.Med. (1990-), Inpharma, Int.Abstr.Biol.Sci., Mass Spectr.Bull., Reac., Sci.Cit.Ind.
—BLDSC (6936.060000), ADONIS, CASDDS, CISTI, EMDOCS, GNLM, IDS, ingenta, Linda Hall. **CCC.**
Published by: Academic Press, Inc., Journal Division (Subsidiary of: Harcourt Brace & Company), 525 B St, Ste 1900, San Diego, CA 92101-4495. TEL 619-230-1840, FAX 619-699-6800, apsubs@acad.com, http://www.academicpress.com/pep. Ed. Owen W Griffith.

572.6 GBR ISSN 1369-4804
▼ **PROTEIN PROFILE ONLINE.** Text in English. 1999. a. GBP 200, USD 320 (effective 2002); Online only. **Document type:** *Academic/Scholarly.*
Media: Online - full text (from O C L C Online Computer Library Center, Inc.).
Published by: Oxford University Press, Academic Division, Great Clarendon St, Oxford OX2 6DP, United Kingdom. TEL 44-1865-267907, FAX 44-1865-267835, jnl.info@oup.co.uk, http://www3.oup.co.uk/propro/, http://www.oup.co.uk/journals. Pub. David Prosser. **Subscr. in the Americas to:** Oxford University Press, Journals, 2001 Evans Rd, Cary, NC 27513. TEL 919-677-1714, 800-852-7323, jnlorders@oup-usa.org.

572 USA ISSN 0961-8368
QP551 CODEN: PRCIEI
PROTEIN SCIENCE. Text in English. 1992. m. USD 235 domestic to non-members; USD 291 in Canada & Mexico to non-members; USD 315 elsewhere to non-members; USD 967 domestic to institutions; USD 1,023 in Canada & Mexico to institutions; USD 1,047 elsewhere to institutions; USD 118 to members (effective 2001). adv. bk.rev. illus. back issues avail. *Refereed.* **Document type:** *Journal, Academic/Scholarly.* **Description:** Publishes papers on protein structure, function, and biochemical significance.
Related titles: Online - full text ed.: 1999 (from HighWire Pr., EBSCO Publishing, O C L C Online Computer Library Center, Inc., RoweCom Information Quest, Swets Blackwell, Institute for Scientific Information).
Indexed: ASCA, BBCI, Chem.Abstr., Chem.Cit.Ind., Chem.Indus.Notes, Chem.Titles, Curr.Cont., Dairy Sci.Abstr., Excerp.Med. (1993-), Food Sci.& Tech.Abstr., Ind.Med. (1992-), Ind.Sci.Rev., Inpharma, Int.Abstr.Biol.Sci., Mass Spectr.Bull., Reac., SSCI (coverage dropped), Sci.Cit.Ind.
—BLDSC (6936.105500), CASDDS, CISTI, EMDOCS, GNLM, IDS, ingenta, KNAW. **CCC.**
Published by: (Protein Society), Cold Spring Harbor Laboratory Press, Publications Department, 10 Skyline Dr, Plainview, NY 11803. TEL 516-349-1930, FAX 516-349-1946, cshpress@cshl.org, http:// www.proteinscience.org, http://www.cshl.org. Ed. Mark Hermodson.

PROTEINS: POST-TRANSLATIONAL PROCESSING. see *BIOLOGY—Abstracting, Bibliographies, Statistics*

572 USA ISSN 0887-3585
QP551 CODEN: PSFGEY
PROTEINS: STRUCTURE, FUNCTION, AND GENETICS. Text in English. 1987. 18/yr. (in 4 vols., 4 nos./vol.). USD 2,190 in United States; USD 2,350 in Canada & Mexico; USD 2,486 elsewhere; USD 2,300 combined subscription in United States for print and online eds.; USD 2,460 combined subscription in Canada & Mexico for print and online eds.; USD 2,596 combined subscription elsewhere for print and online eds. (effective 2002). adv. bk.rev. abstr. Supplement avail.; back issues avail. *Refereed.* **Document type:** *Academic/Scholarly.* **Description:** Concentrates on advances in all areas of biochemistry: structure, function, genetics, computation, and design.
Related titles: Microform ed.: (from PQC); Online - full text ed.: ISSN 1097-0134. USD 2,190 in United States; USD 2,190 in Canada & Mexico; USD 2,190 elsewhere (effective 2002) (from EBSCO Publishing, Wiley InterScience, Institute for Scientific Information).
Indexed: ASCA, Apic.Abstr., Aqua.Sci.& Fish.Abstr., BBCI, Biol.Abstr., Biotech.Cit.Ind., Chem.Abstr., Chem.Cit.Ind., Chem.Titles, Curr.Cont., Environ.Sci.Poll.Mgmt., Excerp.Med., Food Sci.& Tech.Abstr., Helminthol.Abstr., INIS Atomind., Ind.Med. (1986-), Ind.Sci.Rev., Inpharma, Int.Abstr.Biol.Sci., Mass Spectr.Bull., Microbiol.Abstr., Protozool.Abstr., Reac., Rev.Appl.Entomol., Rev.Med.& Vet.Mycol., Rev.Plant Path., Sci.Cit.Ind.
—BLDSC (6936.164000), CASDDS, CISTI, EMDOCS, GNLM, IDS, ingenta, Linda Hall. **CCC.**
Published by: John Wiley & Sons, Inc., Journals (Subsidiary of: Wiley InterScience), 605 Third Ave, New York, NY 10158. TEL 212-850-6645, FAX 212-850-6021, subinfo@wiley.com, uscs-wis@wiley.com, http://www.wiley.com. Ed. E E Lattman. adv.: B&W page GBP 640, color page GBP 1,515; trim 210 x 279. Circ: 1,200. **Subscr. outside the Americas to:** John Wiley & Sons Ltd., Baffins Ln, Chichester, Sussex PO19 IUD, United Kingdom. TEL 44-1243-779777, FAX 44-1243-843232, cs-journals@wiley.co.uk.

572 DEU ISSN 1615-9853
▼ **PROTEOMICS.** Text in English. 2001. m. EUR 698 in Europe; CHF 1,348 Switzerland & Liechtenstein; USD 698 elsewhere; EUR 733 combined subscription in Europe for print and online eds.; CHF 1,416 combined subscription in Switzerland & Liechtenstein, for print and online eds.; USD 733 combined subscription elsewhere for print and online eds. (effective 2002). bk.rev. abstr, bibl, charts, illus. back issues avail.; reprints avail. *Refereed.* **Document type:** *Journal, Academic/Scholarly.* **Description:** Aims to integrate the various areas of proteomics, including methodological developments in protein separation and characterization, advances in bioinformatics, and novel applications of proteomics in all areas of the life sciences and industry.
Related titles: Online - full text ed.: ISSN 1615-9861. 2001. EUR 698 in Europe; CHF 1,348 in Switzerland & Liechtenstein; USD 698 elsewhere (effective 2002) (from Wiley InterScience, Institute for Scientific Information).
Indexed: Biotech.& Bioeng.Abstr., Genet.Abstr., Med.& Pharm.Biotech.Abstr.
Published by: Wiley - V C H, Postfach 101161, Weinheim 69451, Germany. TEL 49-6201-606-0, FAX 49-6201-606-328, subservice@wiley-vch.de, http://www.wiley-vch.de. Ed. Michael J Dunn. R&P Claudia Rutz. Adv. contact Achim Kraus.

572.8 GBR ISSN 1355-8382
QP623 CODEN: RNARFU
R N A. (Ribonucleic Acid) Text in English. 1995. m. GBP 240 to individuals; USD 650 to institutions (effective 2002). adv. bk.rev. *Refereed.* **Document type:** *Academic/Scholarly.* **Description:** Surveys original research in all areas of RNA structure and function in eukaryotic, prokaryotic, and viral systems.
Related titles: Online - full text ed.: (from EBSCO Publishing, O C L C Online Computer Library Center, Inc., RoweCom Information Quest, Swets Blackwell, Institute for Scientific Information).
Indexed: ASCA, Aqua.Sci.& Fish.Abstr., BBCI, Curr.Cont., Environ.Sci.Poll.Mgmt., Genet.Abstr., Hum.Gen.Abstr., Ind.Med. (1995-), Inpharma, Int.Abstr.Biol.Sci., Nuc.Acids Abstr., Pollut.Abstr., Protozool.Abstr., Reac., Sci.Cit.Ind.
—BLDSC (7993.990800), CASDDS, GNLM, IDS. **CCC.**
Published by: (R N A Society), Cambridge University Press, Edinburgh Bldg, Shaftesbury Rd, Cambridge CB2 2RU, United Kingdom. FAX 44-1223-315052, information@cup.cam.ac.uk, information@cambridge.org, http://www.cup.cam.ac.uk, http://www.uk.cambridge.org/journals/pmu. Ed. Timothy W Nilsen. R&P Linda Nicol. Adv. contact Rebecca Symons.

B

572 GBR ISSN 0143-6767
CODEN: RACBDZ
RECENT ADVANCES IN CLINICAL BIOCHEMISTRY. Text in English. 1978. irreg., latest vol.3. **Document type:** *Monographic series, Academic/Scholarly.*
—CASDDS, GNLM.
Published by: Churchill Livingstone (Subsidiary of: Harcourt Publishers Ltd.), Robert Stevenson House, 1-3 Baxter's Pl, Leith Walk, Edinburgh, Midlothian EH1 3AF, United Kingdom. TEL 44-131-556-2424, FAX 44-131-459-1177, http://www.churchillmed.com. **US subscr. to:** Churchill Livingstone, 650 Ave of the Americas, New York, NY 10011. TEL 212-206-5000.

THE RECEPTORS. see *MEDICAL SCIENCES—Psychiatry And Neurology*

REFERATIVNYI ZHURNAL. MOLEKULYARNAYA BIOLOGIYA. see *BIOLOGY—Abstracting, Bibliographies, Statistics*

572.65 NLD ISSN 0167-0115
CODEN: REPPDY
REGULATORY PEPTIDES. Text in Dutch. 1980. 21/yr. EUR 2,321 in Europe to institutions; JPY 308,000 in Japan to institutions; USD 2,597 elsewhere to institutions (effective 2002). abstr. reprint service avail. from SWZ,ISI. *Refereed.* **Document type:** *Academic/Scholarly.* **Description:** Provides a medium for the rapid publication of interdisciplinary studies on the physiology and pathology of peptides of the gut, endocrine and nervous systems which regulate cell or tissue function.
Related titles: Microform ed.: (from PQC); Online - full text ed.: (from ingenta, Swets Blackwell, Institute for Scientific Information, ScienceDirect).
Indexed: ASCA, AgBiotech, Anim.Breed.Abstr., Aqua.Sci.& Fish.Abstr., BBCI, Biol.Abstr., Chem.Abstr., Chem.Indus.Notes, Chem.Titles, Curr.Adv.Cell & Devel.Biol., Curr.Adv.Ecol.Sci., Curr.Cont., Dairy Sci.Abstr., Excerp.Med., Ind.Med. (1980-), Ind.Sci.Rev., Inpharma, Int.Abstr.Biol.Sci., Neurosci.Cit.Ind., Nutr.Abstr., Pharm.&Out.News, Reac., Rev.Appl.Entomol., Sci.Cit.Ind., Sport Fish.Abstr.
—BLDSC (7350.030000), ADONIS, CASDDS, CISTI, GNLM, IDS, ingenta, KNAW. **CCC.**
Published by: Elsevier Science BV, PO Box 211, Amsterdam 1000 AE, Netherlands. TEL 31-20-485-2911, FAX 31-20-485-2457, http://www.elsevier.com/locate/regpep. Eds. M I Phillips, W E Schmidt. **Subscr. in Australasia and the Far East to:** Elsevier Science (Singapore) Pte Ltd, No.1 Temasek Ave, 17-01 Millenia Tower, Singapore 039192, Singapore. TEL 65-434-3727, FAX 65-337-2230; **Subscr. in Japan to:** Elsevier Science Inc - Japan Regional Office, 9-15 Higashi-Azabu 1-chome, Minato-ku, Tokyo 106-0044, Japan. TEL 81-3-5561-5033; **Subscr. in the Americas to:** Elsevier Science, PO Box 945, New York, NY 10159-0945. TEL 212-633-3730, FAX 212-633-3680, usinfo-f@elsevier.com.

RELAZIONI CLINICO SCIENTIFICHE. see *MEDICAL SCIENCES*

REPRODUCTION, NUTRITION, DEVELOPMENT. see *BIOLOGY*

REPRODUCTION. SUPPLEMENT. see *BIOLOGY—Physiology*

REPRODUCTIVE TOXICOLOGY. see *BIOLOGY—Physiology*

572.65 JPN ISSN 0387-4141
CODEN: HAMKE3
RESEARCH COMMITTEE OF ESSENTIAL AMINO ACIDS. REPORTS/HISSU AMINOSAN KENKYU. Text in Japanese. 1958. bi-m. charts. **Description:** Contains research reports focusing on nutrition and its physiological effects.
Indexed: Chem.Abstr., Chem.Indus.Notes, Chem.Titles.
—CASDDS.
Published by: Research Committee of Essential Amino Acids/Hissu Aminosan Kenkyu Iinkai, Kyoritsu Joshi Daigaku Kasei Gakubu Shokumotsu Gakka, 2-1 Hitotsubashi 2-chome, Chiyoda-ku, Tokyo 101-0003, Japan.

572.8 USA ISSN 1087-111X
CODEN: RCBBFC1
RESEARCH COMMUNICATIONS IN BIOCHEMISTRY AND CELL & MOLECULAR BIOLOGY. Text in English. 1997. q. illus. back issues avail.; reprints avail. *Refereed.* **Document type:** *Journal, Academic/Scholarly.* **Description:** Publishes laboratory and clinical research in biochemicistry and cytology, with applications in the medical and biological sciences.
Indexed: Zoo.Rec.
—BLDSC (7736.430000). **CCC.**
Published by: P J D Publications Ltd, PO Box 966, Westbury, NY 11590. TEL 516-626-0650, FAX 516-626-5546. Ed. Akira Tsugita.

573.84 USA ISSN 0096-2902
QP356.3 CODEN: RMNUBP
RESEARCH METHODS IN NEUROCHEMISTRY. Text in English. 1972. irreg., latest vol.6, 1985. price varies. *Refereed.* **Document type:** *Monographic series.*
Indexed: Biol.Abstr., Chem.Abstr., Chem.Indus.Notes, Chem.Titles, e-psyche.
—CASDDS, CISTI, GNLM, Linda Hall. **CCC.**
Published by: Kluwer Academic - Plenum Publishers (Subsidiary of: Wolters Kluwer N.V.), 233 Spring St, New York, NY 10013-1578. TEL 212-620-8000, 800-221-9369, FAX 212-463-0742, info@plenum.com, http://www.plenum.com. Eds. Neville Marks, Richard Rodnight.

REVIEWS OF PHYSIOLOGY, BIOCHEMISTRY AND PHARMACOLOGY. see *BIOLOGY—Physiology*

572 ROM ISSN 0001-4214
QP501 CODEN: RRBCAD
REVUE ROUMAINE DE BIOCHIMIE. Text and summaries in English, French, German, Russian. 1964. 4/yr. charts, illus. index.
Indexed: Agri.& Environ.Biotech.Abstr. (coverage dropped), Anal.Abstr., Biol.Abstr., Chem.Abstr., Chem.Indus.Notes, Chem.Titles, Curr.Adv.Cancer Res., Curr.Adv.Ecol.Sci., Curr.Cont. (coverage dropped), Dairy Sci.Abstr., Derwent Biotech.Abstr., Excerp.Med., INIS Atomind., NPU, Nutr.Abstr., Plant Breed.Abstr.
—BLDSC (7946.050000), CASDDS, CISTI, GNLM, KNAW, Linda Hall.
Published by: (Academia Romana), Editura Academiei Romane, Calea 13 Septembrie 13, Bucharest 76117, Romania. Ed. Mihai Serban. Circ: 1,000. **Dist. by:** Rodipet S.A.. TEL 401-618-5103, FAX 401-222-6407.

RIBOSOMES AND TRANSLATION. see *BIOLOGY—Abstracting, Bibliographies, Statistics*

ROYAL CHEMICAL SOCIETY. JOURNAL. PERKIN TRANSACTIONS 1. see *CHEMISTRY—Organic Chemistry*

RUSSIAN JOURNAL OF BIOORGANIC CHEMISTRY. see *CHEMISTRY—Organic Chemistry*

572 IND
S B C NEWSLETTER. Text in English. 3/yr.
Published by: Society of Biological Chemists, Department of Biochemistry, Indian Institute of Science, Bangalore, Karnataka 560 012, India.

572 JPN ISSN 0037-1017
CODEN: SEIKAQ
SEIKAGAKU/JAPANESE BIOCHEMICAL SOCIETY. JOURNAL. Text in Japanese. 1925. m. JPY 18,000. adv. bk.rev. charts, illus. index. *Refereed.*
Related titles: Online - full text ed.: (from Institute for Scientific Information).
Indexed: ASCA, BBCI, Biol.Abstr., Chem.Abstr., Chem.Titles, Curr.Adv.Biochem., Curr.Adv.Cancer Res., Curr.Adv.Cell & Devel.Biol., Curr.Adv.Ecol.Sci., Curr.Adv.Gen.& Molec.Biol., Curr.Cont. (coverage dropped), INIS Atomind., Ind.Med. (1948-), JTA, Ref.Zh., Sci.Cit.Ind. (coverage dropped).
—BLDSC (8219.700000), CASDDS, CISTI, GNLM, IDS, Infotrieve, ingenta, Linda Hall. **CCC.**
Published by: Nihon Seikagakkai/Japanese Biochemical Society, c/o Ishikawa Bldg 3F, 25-16 Hongo 5-chome, Bunkyo-ku, Tokyo 113-0033, Japan. FAX 03-3815-1934. Ed. Y Nagai. Circ: 20,709.

SEITAI NO KAGAKU/LIFE SCIENCE. see *BIOLOGY*

572.6 USA
SEQUENCES OF PROTEINS OF IMMUNOLOGICAL INTEREST. Text in English. irreg., latest vol.5, 1994. USD 30 in North America; USD 51 elsewhere. **Document type:** *Academic/Scholarly, Government.* **Description:** Discusses N.I.H. research in this area; includes summary distribution tables, variability plots, protein index, antibody specificity index, and general reference index.
Published by: U.S. National Center for Biotechnology Information, National Library of Medicine, Bldg 38A, Rm 8N 803, 8600 Rockville Pike, Bethesda, MD 20894. TEL 301-496-2475, FAX 301-480-9241, info@ncbi.nlm.nih.gov. **Subscr. to:** National Technical Information Service, Government Research Center. FAX 703-321-8547.

572 DEU
SERVA MAIN CATALOG (YEAR). Text in German. a. **Document type:** *Catalog.*
Published by: Serva Feinbiochemica GmbH und Co. KG, Carl-Benz-Str 7, Heidelberg 69115, Germany. TEL 06221-502-0, FAX 06221-502113.

572 CHN ISSN 1000-3282
CODEN: SHYCD4
SHENGWU HUAXUE YU SHENGWU WULI JINZHAN/PROGRESS IN BIOCHEMISTRY AND BIOPHYSICS. Text in Chinese. 1973. bi-m. USD 85 (effective 2000). adv. *Refereed.* **Document type:** *Academic/Scholarly.* **Description:** Covers the latest scientific developments in biochemistry, biophysics, molecular biology, and neuroscience. Includes review articles, research papers, short communications, and lectures on basic theories and applied knowledge.
Related titles: Online - full text ed.: (from Institute for Scientific Information).
Indexed: ASCA, BBCI, Chem.Abstr., Chem.Titles.
—BLDSC (6865.968000), CASDDS, IDS, Linda Hall.
Published by: (Chinese Academy of Sciences/Zhongguo Kexueyuan), Kexue Chubanshe/Science Press, 16 Donghuang Cheng Genbei Jie, Beijing 100717, China. Circ: 11,000.

572 CHN ISSN 0582-9879
CODEN: SHWPAU
SHENGWU HUAXUE YU SHENGWU WULI XUEBAO/ACTA BIOCHIMICA ET BIOPHYSICA SINICA. Text in Chinese, English. 1958. bi-m. USD 12 per issue (effective 2000). adv. *Refereed.* **Document type:** *Academic/Scholarly.*
Related titles: Online - full text ed.: (from Institute for Scientific Information).
Indexed: Abstr.Anthropol., BBCI, Biol.Abstr., CEABA, Chem.Abstr., Chem.Indus.Notes, Chem.Titles, Crop Physiol.Abstr., Curr.Adv.Ecol.Sci., Field Crop Abstr., Hort.Abstr., Ind.Sci.Rev., Ind.Vet., Maize Abstr., Mass Spectr.Bull., Plant Breed.Abstr., Plant Grow.Reg.Abstr., Rev.Appl.Entomol., Rev.Arom.& Med.Plants, Rev.Plant Path., Rice Abstr., Seed Abstr., Soils & Fert., Soyabean Abstr., Zoo.Rec.
—BLDSC (0600.800000), CASDDS, CISTI, Linda Hall.
Published by: (Zhongguo Kexueyuan, Shengwu Huaxue Yanjiusuo/Chinese Academy of Sciences, Shanghai Institute of Biochemistry), Shanghai Scientific and Technical Publishers, Journal Department, 450 Ruijin Er Rd, Shanghai 200020, China. TEL 86-21-6473-6055, FAX 86-21-6473-0679, abbs@sunm.shcnc.ac.cn. Ed. De Bao Wang. Pub. Xiang Yang Hou. R&P Zu Xun Gong. Adv. contact Lian Kang Shen. **Dist. overseas by:** China International Book Trading Corp, 35 Chegongzhuang Xilu, Haidian District, Beijing 100044, China.

▼ **SIGNAL TRANSDUCTION**; receptors, mediators and genes. see *BIOLOGY—Cytology And Histology*

SIGNAL TRANSDUCTION & CYCLIC NUCLEOTIDES. see *BIOLOGY—Abstracting, Bibliographies, Statistics*

SOCIETY FOR NEUROSCIENCE. ABSTRACTS. see *MEDICAL SCIENCES—Psychiatry And Neurology*

572 IND ISSN 0300-0486
CODEN: PSBCAW
SOCIETY OF BIOLOGICAL CHEMISTS. PROCEEDINGS. Text in English. a.
Indexed: Biol.Abstr.
—CISTI.
Published by: Society of Biological Chemists, Department of Biochemistry, Indian Institute of Science, Bangalore, Karnataka 560 012, India.

572 GBR ISSN 0038-0717
S590 CODEN: SBIOAH
SOIL BIOLOGY & BIOCHEMISTRY. Text in English. 1969. 15/yr. EUR 247 in Europe to qualified personnel; JPY 32,800 in Japan to qualified personnel; USD 276 elsewhere to qualified personnel; EUR 1,769 in Europe to institutions; JPY 235,000 in Japan to institutions; USD 1,979 elsewhere to institutions (effective 2002). adv. bk.rev. charts, stat, abstr. reprints avail. *Refereed.* **Document type:** *Academic/Scholarly.* **Description:** Provides a forum for research on soil organisms, their biochemical activities, and the influence on the soil environment and plant growth.
Related titles: Microfiche ed.: (from MIM); Microfilm ed.: (from PQC); Online - full text ed.: (from ingenta, Swets Blackwell, Institute for Scientific Information, ScienceDirect).
Indexed: ASCA, Agri.& Environ.Biotech.Abstr. (coverage dropped), Agricola, Agroforest.Abstr., Appl.Ecol.Abstr., Aqua.Sci.& Fish.Abstr., Bibl.Agri., Bio-Contr.News & Info., Biol.& Agr.Ind. (Jan.1983-), Biol.Abstr., Biol.Dig., Biotech.& Bioeng.Abstr., Chem.Abstr., Chem.Indus.Notes, Chem.Titles, Curr.Adv.Ecol.Sci., Curr.Adv.Plant Sci., Curr.Biotech.Abstr., Curr.Cont., Dairy Sci.Abstr., Deep Sea Res.& Oceanogr.Abstr., Derwent Biotech.Abstr., Ecol.Abstr., Energy Ind., Energy Info.Abstr., Entomol.Abstr., Environ.Per.Bibl. (1972-1994), Environ.Sci.Poll.Mgmt., Excerp.Med., Field Crop Abstr., Forest Prod.Abstr., Forest.Abstr., Geo.Abstr.H.G., Geo.Abstr.P.G., GeoRef, Helminthol.Abstr., Herb.Abstr., Hort.Abstr., IDA, INIS Atomind., Ind.Sci.Rev., Int.Abstr.Biol.Sci., Irr.& Drain.Abstr., Maize Abstr., Mass Spectr.Bull., Microbiol.Abstr., Plant Breed.Abstr., Plant Grow.Reg.Abstr., Plant Sci., Pollut.Abstr., Rev.Appl.Entomol., Rev.Plant Path., Rice Abstr., Sci.Cit.Ind., Seed Abstr., Sel.Water Res.Abstr., Soils & Fert., Sorghum & Millets Abstr., Soyabean Abstr., Sugar Ind.Abstr., Triticale Abstr., W.R.C.Inf., Weed Abstr., Zoo.Rec.
—BLDSC (8321.820100), CASDDS, CISTI, EMDOCS, IDS, Infotrieve, ingenta, Linda Hall. **CCC.**
Published by: (Council of Biological and Medical Abstracts), Pergamon (Subsidiary of: Elsevier Science), The Boulevard, Langford Ln, East Park, Kidlington, Oxford OXB 1GB, United Kingdom. FAX 44-1865-843010, http://www.elsevier.com/locate/soilbio. Ed. J S Waid. Circ: 1,250. **Subscr. in Australasia and the Far East to:** Elsevier Science (Singapore) Pte Ltd, No.1 Temasek Ave, 17-01 Millenia Tower, Singapore 039192, Singapore. TEL 65-434-3727, FAX 65-337-2230; **Subscr. in the Americas to:** Elsevier Science, PO Box 945, New York, NY 10159-0945. TEL 212-633-3730, FAX 212-633-3680, usinfo-f@elsevier.com; **Subscr. to:** Elsevier Science BV, PO Box 211, Amsterdam 1000 AE, Netherlands. TEL 31-20-485-3757.

SOSHIKI BAIYO KENKYU/TISSUE CULTURE RESEARCH COMMUNICATIONS. see *BIOLOGY—Cytology And Histology*

572.579 USA ISSN 0039-128X
QP752.S7 CODEN: STEDAM
STEROIDS. Text in English. 1963. m. EUR 1,031 in Europe to institutions; JPY 136,900 in Japan to institutions; USD 1,154 elsewhere to institutions (effective 2002). adv. bk.rev. abstr, bibl, charts. index. back issues avail.; reprints avail. *Refereed.* **Document type:** *Journal, Academic/Scholarly.* **Description:** Provides a forum for the communication of articles dealing with all aspects of steroid hormones.
Related titles: Microform ed.: (from PQC); Online - full text ed.: (from ingenta, Swets Blackwell, Institute for Scientific Information, ScienceDirect).
Indexed: ASCA, AgBiotech, Agri.& Environ.Biotech.Abstr. (coverage dropped), Anal.Abstr., Anim.Breed.Abstr., BBCI, Biol.Abstr., Chem.Abstr., Chem.Cit.Ind., Chem.Indus.Notes, Chem.Titles, Curr.Adv.Ecol.Sci., Curr.Chem.React., Curr.Cont., Dairy Sci.Abstr., Dent.Ind., Derwent Biotech.Abstr., Excerp.Med., INIS Atomind., Ind.Chem., Ind.Med. (1963-), Ind.Sci.Rev., Ind.Vet., Inpharma, Int.Abstr.Biol.Sci., Mass Spectr.Bull., NPU, Nutr.Abstr., Ocean.Abstr. (coverage dropped), Ornam.Hort., Pharm.&Out.News, Pig News & Info., Plant Grow.Reg.Abstr., Poult.Abstr., RCI, Reac., Rev.Appl.Entomol., Rev.Plant Path., Sci.Cit.Ind., Soyabean Abstr., Vet.Bull.
—BLDSC (8464.600000), CASDDS, CINDOC, CISTI, GNLM, IDS, ingenta, KNAW, Linda Hall. **CCC.**
Published by: Elsevier Science, Box 945, New York, NY 10159-0945. TEL 212-989-5800, FAX 212-633-3990, usinfo-f@elsevier.com, http://www.elsevier.nl/inca/publications/store/5/2/5/0/2/2/, http://www.elsevier.com. Eds. Richard Hochberg, William Rosner. **Subscr. in Australasia and the Far East to:** Elsevier Science (Singapore) Pte Ltd, No.1 Temasek Ave, 17-01 Millenia Tower, Singapore 039192, Singapore. TEL 65-434-3727, FAX 65-337-2230; **Subscr. in Japan to:** Elsevier Science Inc - Japan Regional Office, 9-15 Higashi-Azabu 1-chome, Minato-ku, Tokyo 106-0044, Japan. TEL 81-3-5561-5033, FAX 81-3-5561-5047; **Subscr. outside the Americas to:** Elsevier Science BV, PO Box 211, Amsterdam 1000 AE, Netherlands. TEL 31-20-485-3757, FAX 31-20-485-3432.

572 ROM ISSN 0049-2396
CODEN: SCBIA5
STUDII SI CERCETARI DE BIOCHIMIE. Text in Romanian; Summaries in English, Romanian. 1976 (vol.19). 2/yr. bk.rev. bibl, charts, illus.
Indexed: Apic.Abstr., Biol.Abstr., Chem.Abstr., Chem.Indus.Notes, Chem.Titles, Dairy Sci.Abstr., INIS Atomind.
—CASDDS, CISTI, Linda Hall.
Published by: (Institutul de Biochimie, Academia Romana), Editura Academiei Romane, Calea 13 Septembrie 13, Bucharest 76117, Romania. Ed. Mihai Serban. **Dist. by:** Rodipet S.A.. TEL 401-618-5103, FAX 401-222-6407.

572 USA ISSN 0306-0225
QH611 CODEN: SBCBAG
SUBCELLULAR BIOCHEMISTRY. Text in English. 1971. irreg., latest vol.35, 2000, Dec. price varies. adv. bk.rev. charts, illus. index. *Refereed.* **Document type:** *Monographic series.*
Supersedes (in 1975): Journal of Sub-Cellular Biochemistry
Indexed: Agricola, Biol.Abstr., Chem.Abstr., Chem.Indus.Notes, Chem.Titles, Curr.Cont. (coverage dropped), Excerp.Med., GeoRef, Ind.Med. (1971-).
—BLDSC (8501.890000), CASDDS, CISTI, GNLM, Linda Hall. **CCC.**
Published by: Kluwer Academic - Plenum Publishers (Subsidiary of: Wolters Kluwer N.V.), 233 Spring St, New York, NY 10013-1578. TEL 212-620-8000, 800-221-9369, FAX 212-463-0742, info@plenum.com, http://www.wkap.nl/series.htm/SCBI, http://www.plenum.com. Eds. B B Biswas, Herwig J Hilderson, J R Harris. **Subscr. elsewhere to:** Kluwer Academic Publishers, PO Box 17, Dordrecht 3300 AH, Netherlands; **Subscr. in the Americas to:** Kluwer Academic Publishers, Accord Station, PO Box358, Hingham, MA 02018-0358. TEL 781-871-6600, FAX 781-871-6528.

SUPPLEMENT TO THE EUROPEAN JOURNAL OF NEUROSCIENCE. see *MEDICAL SCIENCES—Psychiatry And Neurology*

572 JPN ISSN 0039-9450
QP501 CODEN: TAKKAJ
TANPAKUSHITSU KAKUSAN KOSO/PROTEIN, NUCLEIC ACID, ENZYME. Text in Japanese. 1956. m. JPY 16,200 (effective 2001). adv. bk.rev. bibl, charts, illus. s-a. index.
Indexed: Chem.Abstr., Chem.Indus.Notes, Chem.Titles, Dent.Ind., INIS Atomind., Ind.Med. (1956-), JTA, Jap.Per.Ind., Ref.Zh.
—CASDDS, CISTI, GNLM, Linda Hall.
Published by: Kyoritsu Shuppan Co. Ltd., 4-6-19 Kohinata, Bunkyo-ku, Tokyo 112-0006, Japan. TEL 81-3-3947-2511, FAX 81-3-3947-2539, kaneko@kyoritsu-pub.co.jp, http://kyoritsu-pub.co.jp. Ed. Yumiko Kita. R&P Yasuo Hirayama TEL 81-3-3947-2517. Circ: 6,000.

572 JPN
TETSU TAISHA KENKYUKAI PUROGURAMU SHOROKUSHU/CONFERENCE ON CURRENT TOPICS FOR IRON METABOLISM. PROGRAM AND ABSTRACTS. Text in Japanese. 1977. a.
Published by: Tetsu Taisha Kenkyukai/Iron Metabolism Research, Shigei Igaku Kenkyujo, 2117 Yamada, Okayama-shi 701-0202, Japan.

▼ **THALAMUS AND RELATED SYSTEMS.** see *BIOLOGY*

TOXICOLOGY IN VITRO. see *ENVIRONMENTAL STUDIES—Toxicology And Environmental Safety*

▼ **TRAFFIC**; the international journal of intracellular transport. see *BIOLOGY—Cytology And Histology*

572 GBR ISSN 0968-0004
QH345 CODEN: TBSCDB
TRENDS IN BIOCHEMICAL SCIENCES. Variant title: T i B S. Text in English. 1976. m. GBP 92, EUR 115 in Europe to individuals; JPY 14,000 in Japan to individuals; USD 126 elsewhere to individuals; EUR 908 in Europe to institutions; JPY 125,900 in Japan to institutions; USD 1,015 elsewhere to institutions; GBP 47 in Europe to students; JPY 10,100 in Japan to students; USD 78 elsewhere to students; EUR 144 in Europe to qualified personnel; JPY 17,500 in Japan to qualified personnel; USD 157 elsewhere to qualified personnel (effective 2002). adv. bk.rev. illus. index. back issues avail.; reprint service avail. from SWZ. *Refereed.* **Document type:** *Academic/Scholarly.* **Description:** Provides students and researchers with information on recent developments in a wide range of biochemically based sciences.
Related titles: Microfilm ed.: (from PQC); Online - full text ed.: (from ingenta, Swets Blackwell, Institute for Scientific Information, ScienceDirect).
Indexed: ASCA, Abstr.Hyg., AgBiotech, Agri.& Environ.Biotech.Abstr. (coverage dropped), Anim.Breed.Abstr., Aqua.Sci.& Fish.Abstr., BBCI, Biol.Abstr., Chem.Abstr., Chem.Cit.Ind., Chem.Titles, Crop Physiol.Abstr., Curr.Adv.Biochem., Curr.Adv.Cell & Devel.Biol., Curr.Adv.Ecol.Sci., Curr.Adv.Gen.& Molec.Biol., Curr.Cont., Dairy Sci.Abstr., Deep Sea Res.& Oceanogr.Abstr., Derwent Biotech.Abstr., Entomol.Abstr., Excerp.Med., Field Crop Abstr., Food Sci.& Tech.Abstr., Forest Prod.Abstr., Gen.Sci.Ind. (Jul.1997-), Genet.Abstr., Helminthol.Abstr., Hort.Abstr., Hum.Gen.Abstr., Ind.Med. (1976-), Ind.Sci.Rev., Ind.Vet., Inpharma, Int.Abstr.Biol.Sci., Neurosci.Abstr., Nuc.Acids Abstr., Nutr.Abstr., Pharm.&Out.News, Plant Breed.Abstr., Plant Grow.Reg.Abstr., Reac., Ref.Zh., Rev.Med.& Vet.Mycol., Rev.Plant Path., SSCI (coverage dropped), Sci.Cit.Ind., Soils & Fert., Sport Fish.Abstr., Wild.Rev.
—BLDSC (9049.546000), ADONIS, CASDDS, CISTI, EMDOCS, IDS. **CCC.**
Published by: (International Union of Biochemistry and Molecular Biology AUS), Elsevier Science Ltd., Elsevier Trends Journals, 68 Hills Rd, Cambridge CB2 1LA, United Kingdom. TEL 44-1223-315961, FAX 44-1223-464430, TTEC@elsevier.co.uk, http://www.elsevier.nl/locate/issn/09680004/. Eds. A Heinrichs, E K Wilson, Mary Purton. Adv. contact Thelma Reid. **Subscr. in Australasia and the Far East to:** Elsevier Science (Singapore) Pte Ltd, No.1 Temasek Ave, 17-01 Millenia Tower, Singapore 039192, Singapore. TEL 65-434-3727, FAX 65-337-2230; **Subscr. in the Americas to:** Elsevier Science, PO Box 945, New York, NY 10159-0945. TEL 212-633-3730, FAX 212-633-3680, http://www.elsevier.com; **Subscr. to:** Elsevier Current Trends Subscriptions, PO Box 331, Haywards Heath, W Sussex RH16 3FG, United Kingdom. TEL 44-1444-475650, FAX 44-1444-445423.

TRENDS IN BIOTECHNOLOGY. see *BIOLOGY—Biotechnology*

TUMOR BIOLOGY; from basic science to clinical application. see *MEDICAL SCIENCES—Oncology*

572 GBR ISSN 0968-6797
U K PRODUCT REVIEW. Text in English. 1986. bi-m. free per issue. adv. software rev. tr.lit. back issues avail. **Document type:** *Trade.*
Published by: Macmillan Magazines Ltd, 4-7 Porters South, Crinan St, London N1 9XW, United Kingdom. TEL 44-20-7833-4000, FAX 44-20-7843-4640. Ed. Charles Wenz. Adv. contact Karen O'Neill. B&W page GBP 1,170. Circ: 15,000 (controlled).

572 UKR ISSN 0201-8470
QP501 CODEN: UBZHD4
UKRAIN'SKII BIOKHIMICHESKII ZHURNAL/UKRAINIAN BIOCHEMICAL JOURNAL; nauchno-teoreticheskii zhurnal. Text in Russian; Summaries in English, Russian. 1926. bi-m. USD 110. adv. bk.rev. abstr, bibl, charts, illus. index.
Indexed: ASCA, Agri.& Environ.Biotech.Abstr. (coverage dropped), Apic.Abstr., Aqua.Sci.& Fish.Abstr., Aquacult.Abstr., Biol.Abstr., Chem.Abstr., Chem.Indus.Notes, Curr.Adv.Ecol.Sci., Dairy Sci.Abstr., Derwent Biotech.Abstr., Djerelo, Environ.Sci.Poll.Mgmt., INIS Atomind., Ind.Med. (1978-), Ind.Vet., Nutr.Abstr., Vet.Bull., Zoo.Rec.
—BLDSC (0384.180000), CASDDS, CISTI, East View, GNLM, IDS, KNAW, Linda Hall. **CCC.**
Published by: Natsional'na Akademiya Nauk Ukrainy, Institut Biokhimii im. A.V. Palladina, Ul N Leontovicha 9, Kiev, Ukraine. TEL 38-44-2241181. Ed. V K Lishko. Circ: 1,496. **US dist. addr.:** East View Publications, 3020 Harbor Ln N, Minneapolis, MN 55447. TEL 612-550-0961.

B

B

572 RUS ISSN 0042-8809
CODEN: VMDKAM
VOPROSY MEDITSINSKOI KHIMII/PROBLEMS OF MEDICAL CHEMISTRY. Text in Russian; Summaries in English. 1955. bi-m. USD 165. bk.rev. index. *Refereed.* **Description:** Publishes original experimental works covering various branches of medical chemistry.
Related titles: Online - full text ed.: (from Institute for Scientific Information).
Indexed: ASCA, Agri.& Environ.Biotech.Abstr. (coverage dropped), Aqua.Sci.& Fish.Abstr., BBCI, Biol.Abstr., Biotech.& Bioeng.Abstr. (coverage dropped), Cal.Tiss.Abstr., Chem.Abstr., Chem.Indus.Notes, Chemorec.Abstr., Curr.Adv.Ecol.Sci., Curr.Cont. (coverage dropped), Dairy Sci.Abstr., Dent.Ind., Derwent Biotech.Abstr., Excerp.Med., Helminthol.Abstr., INIS Atomind., Ind.Med. (1955-), Int.Aerosp.Abstr., Neurosci.Abstr. (coverage dropped), Nutr.Abstr., Ref.Zh., Rev.Med.& Vet.Mycol.
—CASDDS, CISTI, East View, GNLM, IDS, Infotrieve, KNAW, Linda Hall. **CCC.**
Published by: Rossiiskaya Akademiya Meditsinskikh Nauk, Pogodinskaya 10, Moscow 119832, Russian Federation. TEL 7-095-2466584. Ed. A I Archakov. Circ: 3,000. **Dist. by:** Mezhdunarodnaya Kniga, B Yakimanka 39, Moscow 117049, Russian Federation. TEL 7-095-2384967, FAX 7-095-2384634; **US dist. addr.:** East View Publications, 3020 Harbor Ln N, Minneapolis, MN 55447. TEL 612-550-0961.

WALTER AND ANDREE DE NOTTBECK FOUNDATION SCIENTIFIC REPORTS. see *BIOLOGY—Microbiology*

572 NGA ISSN 0043-2989
CODEN: WAJBAK
WEST AFRICAN JOURNAL OF BIOLOGICAL AND APPLIED CHEMISTRY. Text in English. 1957. q. NGN 40. adv. bk.rev. charts. **Document type:** *Academic/Scholarly.*
Indexed: Biol.Abstr., Chem.Abstr., Chem.Indus.Notes, Chem.Titles, Field Crop Abstr., Herb.Abstr., Nutr.Abstr.
—CASDDS, CISTI, Linda Hall.
Address: U.I. Post Office, University of Ibadan, PO Box 4021, Ibadan, Oyo, Nigeria. TEL 234-22-410247. Ed. Olumbe Bassir. Circ: 1,000.

572 GBR ISSN 0049-8254
QP909 CODEN: XENOBH
XENOBIOTICA; the fate of foreign compounds in biological systems. Text in English. 1971. m. GBP 1,014, USD 1,672 to institutions (effective 2002). adv. bk.rev. charts, stat. index. *Refereed.* **Document type:** *Academic/Scholarly.* **Description:** Covers three main areas: general xenobiochemistry, molecular toxicology, and clinical pharmacokinetics and metabolism.
Related titles: Online - full text ed.: ISSN 1366-5928 (from CatchWord Ltd., EBSCO Publishing, O C L C Online Computer Library Center, Inc., RoweCom Information Quest, Swets Blackwell, Institute for Scientific Information).
Indexed: ASCA, Agri.& Environ.Biotech.Abstr. (coverage dropped), Agricola, Aqua.Sci.& Fish.Abstr., BBCI, Bibl.Agri., Biol.Abstr., Chem.Abstr., Chem.Cit.Ind., Chem.Indus.Notes, Curr.Adv.Biochem., Curr.Adv.Ecol.Sci., Curr.Cont., Dairy Sci.Abstr., Deep Sea Res.& Oceanogr.Abstr., Dent.Ind., Derwent Biotech.Abstr., Environ.Per.Bibl. (1979-), Environ.Sci.Poll.Mgmt., Excerp.Med., Helminthol.Abstr., Ind.Med. (1971-), Ind.Sci.Rev., Ind.Vet., Inpharma, Int.Abstr.Biol.Sci., Lab.Haz.Bull., Mass Spectr.Bull., Microbiol.Abstr., Nutr.Abstr., Pharm.&Out.News, Pig News & Info., Pollut.Abstr., Poult.Abstr., Protozool.Abstr., Reac., Ref.Zh., Rev.Appl.Entomol., Rev.Med.& Vet.Mycol., Sci.Cit.Ind., Small Anim.Abstr., Tox.Abstr., Vet.Bull., Weed Abstr., Zoo.Rec.
—BLDSC (9367.020000), ADONIS, CASDDS, CatchWord, CISTI, GNLM, IDS, ingenta, Linda Hall. **CCC.**
Published by: Taylor & Francis Group, Taylor & Francis Ltd., Journals Customer Service, Rankine Rd, Basingstoke, Hants RG24 8PR, United Kingdom. Ed. G G Gibson. **Subscr. in N. America to:** Taylor & Francis Ltd., 325 Chestnut St, Suite 800, Philadelphia, PA 19016. TEL 800-354-1420, FAX 215-625-8914, info@taylorandfrancis.com, http://www.taylorandfrancis.com/.

572 CHN ISSN 1007-7626
CODEN: SHZAE4
ZHONGGUO SHENGWU HUAXUE YU FENZI SHENGWU XUEBAO/CHINESE JOURNAL OF BIOCHEMISTRY AND MOLECULAR BIOLOGY. Text in Chinese. 1985. bi-m. CNY 16 (effective (No. 2001). adv. bk.rev. *Refereed.* **Document type:** *Journal, Academic/Scholarly.* **Description:** Contains research reports and short communications on biochemistry and molecular biology.
Formerly (until vol.13, no.6, 1997): Shengwu Huaxue Zazhi/Chinese Biochemical Journal (1000-8543)
Related titles: Online - full content ed.: (from WanFang Data Corp.).
Indexed: Chem.Abstr., Chem.Titles.
—BLDSC (3180.295650), CASDDS.
Published by: Zhongguo Shengwu Huaxue yu Fenzi Shengwu Xuehui, Peking Xueyuan Lu, Peking Daxue Yixuebu, Shenghualou 331 Shi, Beijing 100083, China. shxb@mail.bjmu.edu.cn, http://www.periodicals.com.cn/gyjs.asp?ID=297609, http://www.bjmu.edu.cn/. Circ: 3,000. **Dist. outside of China by:** China International Book Trading Corp, 35 Chegongzhuang Xilu, Haidian District, Beijing 100044, China. TEL 86-10-68411769, FAX 86-10-68420340, bk@mail.cibtc.com.cn, http://www.cibtc.com.cn/.

572 RUS ISSN 0044-4529
QH345.Z5 CODEN: ZEBFAJ
ZHURNAL EVOLYUTSIONNOI BIOKHIMII I FIZIOLOGII. Text in Russian; Summaries in English. 1965. bi-m. bk.rev. charts, illus. index. **Description:** Illuminates the most recent research findings on the evolution of basic forms of metabolism, comparative and developmental physiology, and biochemistry and the biochemical evolution of the animal world.
Related titles: ♦ English Translation: Journal of Evolutionary Biochemistry and Physiology. ISSN 0022-0930.
Indexed: Anim.Breed.Abstr., Biol.Abstr., Chem.Abstr., Chem.Indus.Notes, Chem.Titles, Excerp.Med., Field Crop Abstr., Ind.Med. (1965-), Int.Aerosp.Abstr., Ref.Zh., Seed Abstr., Soyabean Abstr., Zoo.Rec.
—BLDSC (0067.700000), CASDDS, CISTI, GNLM, Infotrieve, KNAW, Linda Hall. **CCC.**
Published by: (Rossiiskaya Akademiya Nauk/Russian Academy of Sciences), M A I K Nauka - Interperiodica, S.-Peterburgskoe Otdelenie, Thorez Ave 44, St Petersburg 194223, Russian Federation. compmg@maik.ru, http://www.maik.rssi.ru/journals/evolbp.htm. Ed. Vladimir L Svidersky. **US dist. addr.:** Kluwer Academic Publishers, PO Box 17, Dordrecht 3300 AH, Netherlands. TEL 31-78-639-2392, FAX 31-78-654-6474, http://www.wkap.nl.

BIOLOGY—Biophysics

571 CHN ISSN 1000-6737
ACTA BIOPHYSICS SINICA. Text in Chinese; Summaries in English. 1985. q. CNY 200 domestic; USD 100 foreign (effective 2000). abstr, bibl, charts, illus, mkt. index. back issues avail. **Document type:** *Academic/Scholarly.* **Description:** Covers molecular biophysics, cell and membrane biophysics, neurobiophysics, bioinformatics, biocybernetics, theoretical biophysics, radiation and environmental biophysics, biomechanics, and biophysical expermental techniques.
Related titles: CD-ROM ed.
Indexed: GeoRef.
Published by: Biophysical Society of China, 15 Datun Rd, Chaoyang District, Beijing, China. TEL 86-10-6488-8458, FAX 86-10-6487-7837, acta@sun5.ibp.ac.cn. Ed. Yang Fuyu. R&P Ke-Ding Lu. Adv. contact Xue-Hong Liang. Circ: 800 (paid); 200 (controlled).

ACTA UNIVERSITATIS LODZIENSIS: FOLIA BIOCHIMICA ET BIOPHYSICA. see *BIOLOGY—Biochemistry*

571.47 USA
ADVANCES IN ELECTROMAGNETIC FIELDS IN LIVING SYSTEMS. Text in English. 1994. irreg., latest vol.2, 1997. price varies. *Refereed.* **Document type:** *Monographic series.* **Description:** Presents research on the theory, interactions and applications of electromagnetic fields in biology and medicine.
—BLDSC (0704.750000).
Published by: Kluwer Academic - Plenum Publishers (Subsidiary of: Wolters Kluwer N.V.), 233 Spring St, New York, NY 10013-1578. TEL 212-620-8000, 800-221-9369, FAX 212-463-0742, info@plenum.com, http://www.plenum.com. Ed. James C Lin.

571.45 USA ISSN 1056-8700
QH505 CODEN: ABBSE4
ANNUAL REVIEW OF BIOPHYSICS AND BIOMOLECULAR STRUCTURE. Text in English. 1972. a. USD 70 domestic to individuals; USD 75 foreign to individuals; USD 140 domestic to institutions; USD 150 foreign to institutions (effective 1999). adv. bibl. charts. index, cum.index every 5 yrs. back issues avail.; reprints avail. *Refereed.* **Document type:** *Academic/Scholarly.* **Description:** Original reviews of critical literature and current developments in biophysics and biomolecular structure.
Former titles (until vol.20, 1991): Annual Review of Biophysics and Biophysical Chemistry (0883-9182); (until vol.14, 1985): Annual Review of Biophysics and Bioengineering (0084-6589)
Related titles: Microfilm ed.: (from PQC); Online - full text ed.: (from HighWire Pr., EBSCO Publishing, Institute for Scientific Information).
Indexed: ASCA, Agri.& Environ.Biotech.Abstr., BBCI, Biol.Abstr., Chem.Abstr., Chem.Cit.Ind., Chem.Indus.Notes, Chem.Titles, Curr.Adv.Ecol.Sci., Curr.Cont., Curr.Ind.Stat., Deep Sea Res.& Oceanogr.Abstr., INIS Atomind., INSPEC (1968-, dropped), Immun.Abstr., Ind.Med. (1992-), Ind.Sci.Rev., Inpharma, Int.Abstr.Biol.Sci., Med.& Pharm.Biotech.Abstr., Neurosci.Abstr., Nuc.Acids Abstr., Oncog.G.F.Abstr., Reac., Sci.Cit.Ind.
—BLDSC (1522.060000), ADONIS, CASDDS, CISTI, EMDOCS, GNLM, IDS, ingenta, KNAW, Linda Hall. **CCC.**
Published by: Annual Reviews Inc., 4139 El Camino Way, Box 10139, Palo Alto, CA 94303-0139. TEL 650-493-4400, 800-523-8635, FAX 650-424-0910, service@annurev.org; orders@annurev.org, http://www.annurev.org; http://www.allenpress.com. Ed. Samuel Gubins. R&P, Adv. contact Swati Aneja TEL 650-843-6634. **Subscr. to:** Allen Press Inc., PO Box 1897, Lawrence, KS 66044-8897.

ARCHIVES OF BIOCHEMISTRY AND BIOPHYSICS. see *BIOLOGY—Biochemistry*

B B A - GENERAL SUBJECTS. see *BIOLOGY—Biochemistry*

B B A - MOLECULAR AND CELL BIOLOGY OF LIPIDS. (Biochimica and Biophysica Acta) see *BIOLOGY—Biochemistry*

B B A - PROTEIN STRUCTURE AND MOLECULAR ENZYMOLOGY. see *BIOLOGY—Biochemistry*

BIO-ELECTRONICS AND BIOSENSORS. see *BIOLOGY—Abstracting, Bibliographies, Statistics*

BIOCHEMICAL AND BIOPHYSICAL RESEARCH COMMUNICATIONS. see *BIOLOGY—Biochemistry*

BIOCHEMISTRY AND BIOPHYSICS CITATION INDEX. see *BIOLOGY—Abstracting, Bibliographies, Statistics*

BIOCHIMICA ET BIOPHYSICA ACTA; international journal of biochemistry and biophysics. see *BIOLOGY—Biochemistry*

BIOELECTROCHEMISTRY; an international journal devoted to electrochemical aspects of biology and biological aspects of electrochemistry. see *BIOLOGY—Biochemistry*

571.4 USA ISSN 0197-8462
QP82.2.E43 CODEN: BLCTDO
BIOELECTROMAGNETICS. Text in English. 1980. 8/yr. USD 865 in United States; USD 945 in Canada & Mexico; USD 1,013 elsewhere; USD 909 combined subscription in United States for print and online eds.; USD 989 combined subscription in Canada & Mexico for print and online eds.; USD 1,057 combined subscription elsewhere for print and online eds. (effective 2002). adv. bk.rev. bibl, charts, illus. index. back issues avail. *Refereed.* **Document type:** *Academic/Scholarly.* **Description:** Devoted to research on biological systems as they are influenced by natural or manufactured electric and-or magnetic fields at frequencies from D.C. to visible light.
Related titles: Microform ed.: ISSN 1521-186X. 1998 (from PQC); Online - full text ed.: ISSN 1521-186X. USD 865 in United States; USD 865 in Canada & Mexico; USD 865 elsewhere (effective 2002) (from EBSCO Publishing, Wiley InterScience, Institute for Scientific Information).
Indexed: ASCA, BBCI, Biol.Abstr., Chem.Abstr., Chem.Indus.Notes, Chem.Titles, Curr.Adv.Ecol.Sci., Curr.Cont., Dent.Ind., Excerp.Med., INIS Atomind., INSPEC (1982-), Ind.Med. (1980-), Ind.Sci.Rev., Inpharma, Neurosci.Cit.Ind., Nutr.Abstr., Reac., Ref.Zh., SSCI (coverage dropped), Sci.Cit.Ind.
—BLDSC (2072.009000), AskIEEE, CASDDS, CISTI, GNLM, IDS, ingenta, Linda Hall. **CCC.**

Published by: (Bioelectromagnetics Society), John Wiley & Sons, Inc., Journals (Subsidiary of: Wiley InterScience), 605 Third Ave, New York, NY 10158. TEL 212-850-6645, FAX 212-850-6021, subinfo@wiley.com, uscs-wis@wiley.com, http://www.interscience.wiley.com/jpages/0197-8462/, http://www.wiley.com. Ed. Ben Greenebaum. adv.: B&W page GBP 640, color page GBP 1,515; trim 210 x 279. Circ: 950. **Subscr. outside the Americas to:** John Wiley & Sons Ltd., Baffins Ln, Chichester, Sussex PO19 IUD, United Kingdom. TEL 44-1243-779777, FAX 44-1243-843232, cs-journals@wiley.co.uk, http://www.wiley.co.uk.

571.4 USA ISSN 0889-4191
BIOELECTROMAGNETICS SOCIETY NEWSLETTER. Text in English. 1978. 6/yr. USD 65 domestic to non-members; USD 75 foreign to non-members. bk.rev. back issues avail. **Document type:** *Newsletter.*
Published by: Bioelectromagnetics Society, 7519 Ridge Rd, Frederick, MD 21702-3519. TEL 301-663-4252, FAX 301-371-8955. Ed. Mary Ellen O'Connor. Circ: 800.

571.4 RUS ISSN 0006-3029
QH505.A1 CODEN: BIOFAI
BIOFIZIKA. Text in Russian; Summaries in English. 1956. bi-m. RUR 470 for 2 mos. (effective 2001). index. *Refereed.*
Related titles: Online - full text ed.: (from Institute for Scientific Information); ♦ English Translation: Biophysics. ISSN 0006-3509.
Indexed: ASCA, Agri.& Environ.Biotech.Abstr. (coverage dropped), Apic.Abstr., BBCI, Biol.Abstr., Chem.Abstr., Chem.Indus.Notes, Chem.Titles, Curr.Adv.Ecol.Sci., Curr.Cont., Dairy Sci.Abstr., Dent.Ind., Derwent Biotech.Abstr., Excerp.Med., INIS Atomind., INSPEC (1973-), Ind.Med. (1956-), Ind.Sci.Rev., Inpharma, Int.Aerosp.Abstr., Neurosci.Cit.Ind., Phys.Ber., Psychol.Abstr., Reac., Ref.Zh., Sci.Cit.Ind., Zoo.Rec.
—BLDSC (0018.030000), AskIEEE, CASDDS, CISTI, East View, GNLM, IDS, Linda Hall. **CCC.**
Published by: (Rossiiskaya Akademiya Nauk/Russian Academy of Sciences), M A I K Nauka - Interperiodica, Mezhdunarodnyi Otdel, Profsoyuznaya ul 90, Moscow 117864, Russian Federation. TEL 7-095-336-1600, FAX 7-095-336-0666, compmg@maik.rssi.ru, http://www.maik.rssi.ru/journals/biophys.htm, http://hea.iki.rssi.ru/pazh. Ed. Evgenii E Fesenko. **Dist. by:** Mezhdunarodnaya Kniga**; US dist. addr.:** East View Publications.

571.4 RUS ISSN 0301-2425
QH573
BIOFIZIKA ZHIVOI KLETKI/BIOPHYSICS OF LIVING CELLS. Text in Russian. 1970. irreg. USD 40. adv. bk.rev. illus. reprint service avail. from IRC. *Refereed.* **Document type:** *Academic/Scholarly.*
—Linda Hall.
Published by: (Institut Biofiziki Kletki/Institute of Cell Biophysics, Rossiiskaya Akademiya Nauk/Russian Academy of Sciences), Radical Enterprise, A-ya 84 (AB 7-67), Pushchino, Moskovskaya Oblast' 142292, Russian Federation. TEL 7-095-238-7940, vkar@ibfk.nifhi.ac.ru. Ed. V N Kharnaukhov. Adv. contact V.N. Kharnaukhov. Circ: 500.

571.4 RUS ISSN 0233-4755
QH601 CODEN: BIMEE9
BIOLOGICHESKIE MEMBRANY. Text in Russian. 1984. bi-m. RUR 1,105; USD 231 foreign (effective 2000). adv. bk.rev. index. *Refereed.* **Document type:** *Academic/Scholarly.* **Description:** Presents experimental and theoretical work on the physics, chemistry and biology of membranes at the molecular and cellular levels.
Related titles: Online - full text ed.: (from Institute for Scientific Information); Translation: Membrane and Cell Biology. ISSN 1023-6597. EUR 1338 ($1472) to academic institutions; corporations EUR 2087 ($2297) (effective 2000).
Indexed: BBCI, Chem.Abstr., Chem.Indus.Notes, Chem.Titles, Curr.Cont., Nutr.Abstr., Plant Breed.Abstr., Ref.Zh., Rev.Med.& Vet.Mycol., Sci.Cit.Ind., Triticale Abstr., Zoo.Rec.
—BLDSC (0017.845000), CASDDS, CISTI, East View, IDS, Infotrieve, Linda Hall. **CCC.**
Published by: (Rossiiskaya Akademiya Nauk/Russian Academy of Sciences), Biologicheskie Membrany, Vavilova ul 34, kom 335, Moscow 117990, Russian Federation. TEL 7-095-1359886, FAX 7-095-1359886, biomem@genome.eimb.relarn.ru. Ed. Yu A Chizmadzhev. Adv. contact Yuri Ermakov. page USD 100.

571.4 BGR ISSN 0204-7594
BIOMEKHANIKA/BIOMECHANICS. Text in Bulgarian, Russian; Summaries in English, Russian. 1974. irreg. BGL 2 per issue. bibl, illus. reprint service avail. from IRC.
Indexed: BSL Math., Biol.Abstr.
—GNLM.
Published by: (Tsentralna Laboratoriia po Biomekhanika, Bulgarska Akademiia na Naukite/Bulgarian Academy of Sciences), Publishing House of the Bulgarian Academy of Sciences, Akad G Bonchev 6, Sofia 1113, Bulgaria. Ed. G Brankov. Circ: 470. **Dist. by:** Hemus, 6 Rouski blvd, Sofia 1000, Bulgaria.

571.4 UKR ISSN 0374-6569
CODEN: BNKABJ
BIONIKA; respublikanskii mezhvedomstvennyi sbornik nauchnykh trudov. Text in Russian. 1965. a. USD 199.
Indexed: GeoRef, INSPEC (1972-1993, dropped).
—AskIEEE, CISTI, Infotrieve, Linda Hall. **CCC.**
Published by: Natsional'na Akademiya Nauk Ukrainy, Institut Gidromekhaniki, Vul Tereshchenkivska 3, Kiev 252601, Ukraine. TEL 044-224-4068, FAX 044-224-7060, vgr@ihm.Kiev.ua. **Dist. by:** Mezhdunarodnaya Kniga, B Yakimanka 39, Moscow 117049, Russian Federation.

571.4 NLD ISSN 0301-4622
QH345 CODEN: BICIAZ
BIOPHYSICAL CHEMISTRY; an international journal devoted to the physics and chemistry of biological phenomena. Text in Dutch. 1974. 15/yr. EUR 193 in Europe to qualified personnel; JPY 25,500 in Japan to qualified personnel; USD 215 elsewhere to qualified personnel; EUR 2,619 in Europe to institutions; JPY 347,500 in Japan to institutions; USD 2,930 elsewhere to institutions (effective 2002). adv. bk.rev. index. back issues avail.; reprint service avail. from SWZ,ISI. *Refereed.* **Document type:** *Academic/Scholarly.* **Description:** Devoted to the interpretation of biological phenomena in terms of the principles and methods of physics and chemistry.
Related titles: Microform ed.: (from PQC); Online - full text ed.: (from ingenta, Swets Blackwell, ScienceDirect, Institute for Scientific Information).
Indexed: ASCA, Apic.Abstr., Aqua.Sci.& Fish.Abstr., BBCI, Biol.Abstr., Chem.Abstr., Chem.Cit.Ind., Chem.Indus.Notes, Chem.Titles, Curr.Adv.Biochem., Curr.Adv.Cell & Devel.Biol., Curr.Adv.Ecol.Sci., Curr.Adv.Gen.& Molec.Biol., Curr.Cont., Dairy Sci.Abstr., Excerp.Med., INIS Atomind., Ind.Med. (1973-), Ind.Sci.Rev., Inpharma, Int.Abstr.Biol.Sci., Pharm.&Out.News, Reac., Rev.Plant Path., Sci.Cit.Ind.
—BLDSC (2089.380000), CASDDS, CISTI, EMDOCS, GNLM, IDS, ingenta, Linda Hall. **CCC.**
Published by: Elsevier Science BV, PO Box 211, Amsterdam 1000 AE, Netherlands. TEL 31-20-485-2911, FAX 31-20-485-2457, nlinfo-f@elsevier.nl, http://www.elsevier.nl/locate/bpc. Eds. A Cooper, E Di Cera. **Subscr. in Australasia and the Far East to:** Elsevier Science (Singapore) Pte Ltd, No.1 Temasek Ave, 17-01 Millenia Tower, Singapore 039192, Singapore. TEL 65-434-3727, FAX 65-337-2230**; Subscr. in Japan to:** Elsevier Science Inc - Japan Regional Office, 9-15 Higashi-Azabu 1-chome, Minato-ku, Tokyo 106-0044, Japan. TEL 81-3-5561-5033, FAX 81-3-5561-5047**; Subscr. in the Americas to:** Elsevier Science, PO Box 945, New York, NY 10159-0945. TEL 212-633-3730, FAX 212-633-3680, usinfo-f@elsevier.com, http://www.elsevier.com.

571.4 USA ISSN 0006-3495
QH505.A1 CODEN: BIOJAU
BIOPHYSICAL JOURNAL. Text in English. 1960. m. (in 2 vols., 6 nos./vol.). USD 775 domestic; USD 825 foreign (effective 2000); includes Biophysical Society. Annual Meeting. Abstracts. adv. bibl, charts, illus. index. back issues avail.; reprints avail. *Refereed.* **Document type:** *Journal, Academic/Scholarly.* **Description:** Reports on the latest theoretical and experimental developments in biophysical research.
Related titles: Microfiche ed.: (from PQC); Microfilm ed.: (from PQC); Online - full text ed.: (from HighWire Pr., Northern Light Technology, Inc., EBSCO Publishing, RoweCom Information Quest, ProQuest Information & Learning, Institute for Scientific Information); ♦ Supplement: Biophysical Society. Annual Meeting. Abstracts. ISSN 0523-6800.
Indexed: ASCA, Agricola, Anim.Breed.Abstr., Apic.Abstr., Appl.Mech.Rev., Aqua.Sci.& Fish.Abstr., BBCI, Bibl.Agri., Biol.Abstr., Biwk.Pap.Rad.Chem.& Photochem., Chem.Abstr., Chem.Cit.Ind., Chem.Indus.Notes, Chem.Titles, Curr.Adv.Biochem., Curr.Adv.Cell & Devel.Biol., Curr.Adv.Ecol.Sci., Curr.Adv.Gen.& Molec.Biol., Curr.Cont., Dairy Sci.Abstr., Deep Sea Res.& Oceanogr.Abstr., Eng.Ind., Excerp.Med., Field Crop Abstr., Food Sci.& Tech.Abstr., INIS Atomind., INSPEC (Feb.1974-), Ind.Med. (1960-), Ind.Sci.Rev., Inpharma, Int.Abstr.Biol.Sci., Mat.Sci.Cit.Ind. (coverage dropped), Neurosci.Abstr. (coverage dropped), Neurosci.Cit.Ind., Pharm.&Out.News, Phys.Ber., Protozool.Abstr., Reac., Ref.Zh., Rev.Appl.Entomol., Sci.Cit.Ind., Sport Fish.Abstr., Sugar Ind.Abstr., Triticale Abstr.
—BLDSC (2089.400000), AskIEEE, CASDDS, CISTI, Ei, EMDOCS, GNLM, IDS, ingenta, Linda Hall. **CCC.**
Published by: Biophysical Society, 9650 Rockville Pike, Bethesda, MD 20814. TEL 301-530-7199, FAX 301-530-7133, ckenney@biophysics.faseb.org, http://www.biophysics.org/. Ed. Peter Moore. Adv. contacts Jeanne Brooksbank, Jill Kooyman. B&W page USD 1,000, color page USD 1,500.

BIOPHYSICAL SOCIETY. ANNUAL MEETING. ABSTRACTS. see *BIOLOGY—Abstracting, Bibliographies, Statistics*

571.4 RUS ISSN 0006-3509
QH505.A1 CODEN: BIOPAE
BIOPHYSICS. Text in English. 1957. bi-m. USD 2,825 in North America; USD 2,943 elsewhere (effective 2001). adv. abstr, charts. index. back issues avail.; reprint service avail. from PQC. *Refereed.* **Document type:** *Journal, Academic/Scholarly.* **Description:** Covers a wide scope of problems related to the main physical mechanisms of processes taking place on different organization levels in biosystems.
Related titles: Microfilm ed.: (from PQC); Online - full text ed.: (from ingenta); ♦ Translation of: Biofizika. ISSN 0006-3029.
Indexed: Appl.Mech.Rev., Aqua.Sci.& Fish.Abstr., Biol.Abstr., Cal.Tiss.Abstr., Curr.Adv.Ecol.Sci., Excerp.Med., INIS Atomind., INSPEC (1972-), Ind.Med. (coverage dropped).
—BLDSC (0406.100000), AskIEEE, CISTI, GNLM, Infotrieve, ingenta, Linda Hall. **CCC.**
Published by: M A I K Nauka - Interperiodica, Mezhdunarodnyi Otdel, Profsoyuznaya ul 90, Moscow 117864, Russian Federation. TEL 7-095-3360666, FAX 7-095-3361600, compmg@maik.ru, http://www.maik.ru/journals/biophys.htm, http://www.maik.rssi.ru/. Ed. Evgenii E Fesenko. Circ: 1,000. **Subscr. to:** Maik Nauka - Interperiodica. **Dist. by:** East View Publications.

571.7 NLD ISSN 0006-355X
QH505 CODEN: BRHLAU
BIORHEOLOGY; an international journal. Text in English, French, German. 1962. bi-m. EUR 736, USD 673 to institutions (effective 2002). adv. bk.rev. charts, illus. back issues avail. *Refereed.* **Document type:** *Journal, Academic/Scholarly.* **Description:** Features articles on deformation and flow-related processes, in vivo and extra vivum, on biological systems under physiological and pathological conditions.
Related titles: Microfilm ed.: (from PQC); Online - full text ed.: (from EBSCO Publishing, O C L C Online Computer Library Center, Inc., ingenta, Swets Blackwell, Institute for Scientific Information, RoweCom Information Quest).
Indexed: ASCA, Agri.Eng.Abstr., Appl.Mech.Rev., BBCI, Biol.Abstr., Chem.Abstr., Chem.Indus.Notes, Chem.Titles, Crop Physiol.Abstr., Curr.Adv.Ecol.Sci., Curr.Cont., Dairy Sci.Abstr., Excerp.Med., Food Sci.& Tech.Abstr., Hort.Abstr., IBZ, INIS Atomind., INSPEC (1978-), Ind.Med. (1962-), Ind.Sci.Rev., Ind.Vet., Inpharma, Int.Abstr.Biol.Sci., Mat.Sci.Cit.Ind. (coverage dropped), Pharm.&Out.News, Reac., Ref.Zh., Sci.Cit.Ind., Sugar Ind.Abstr., Vet.Bull.
—BLDSC (2089.500000), ADONIS, AskIEEE, CASDDS, CISTI, EMDOCS, GNLM, IDS, ingenta, Linda Hall. **CCC.**
Published by: (International Society of Biorheology), I O S Press, Nieuwe Hemweg 6B, Amsterdam 1013 BG, Netherlands. TEL 31-20-688-3355, FAX 31-20-620-3419, market@iospress.nl, http://www.iospress.nl. Ed. Harry L Goldsmith. Circ: 1,150. **Subscr. to:** I O S Press, Inc, 5795-G Burke Centre Pkwy, Burke, VA 22015. TEL 703-323-5554, FAX 703-323-3668, iosbooks@iospress.com; Globe Publication Pvt. Ltd., C-62 Inderpuri, New Delhi 100 012, India; Kinokuniya Company Ltd, Shinjuku 3-chome, Shinjuku-ku, Tokyo 160-0022, Japan.

BIOSENSORS AND BIOELECTRONICS. see *BIOLOGY—Biotechnology*

B

BIOSPECTROSCOPY; an international interdisciplinary journal. see *CHEMISTRY—Analytical Chemistry*

CANCER BIOCHEMISTRY BIOPHYSICS. see *MEDICAL SCIENCES—Oncology*

CELL BIOCHEMISTRY AND BIOPHYSICS. see *BIOLOGY—Cytology And Histology*

571.4 CHE ISSN 0143-8123
QH506 CODEN: CMCBDM
COMMENTS ON MOLECULAR AND CELLULAR BIOPHYSICS. Text in French. 6/yr. USD 854 to institutions; USD 1,332 to corporations (effective 1999). bk.rev. **Document type:** *Academic/Scholarly.*
Related titles: Microform ed.
Indexed: Chem.Abstr., INSPEC (1980-1995, dropped), Phys.Ber.
—BLDSC (3336.029300), AskIEEE, CISTI, Infotrieve. **CCC.**
Published by: Gordon and Breach - Harwood Academic (Subsidiary of: Taylor & Francis Group), PO Box 531, Lausanne 1000, Switzerland. Eds. David M Jameson, Dinu Georgescauld. **Subscr. addr. in US:** International Publishers Direct, PO Box 32160, Newark, NJ 07102. FAX 215-750-6343.

571.464 USA ISSN 0011-2240
QH324 CODEN: CRYBAS
CRYOBIOLOGY; international journal of low temperature biology. Text in English. 1964. 8/yr. USD 399 in US & Canada to institutions; USD 465 elsewhere to institutions (effective 2001). adv. index. *Refereed.* **Document type:** *Academic/Scholarly.* **Description:** Publishes research articles on all aspects of low temperature biology.
Related titles: Online - full text ed.: (from EBSCO Publishing, O C L C Online Computer Library Center, Inc., RoweCom Information Quest, ingenta, Swets Blackwell, IDEAL Online Library, Institute for Scientific Information).
Indexed: ASCA, Agri.& Environ.Biotech.Abstr., Agricola, Anim.Breed.Abstr., Aqua.Sci.& Fish.Abstr., Biol.Abstr., Chem.Abstr., Chem.Indus.Notes, Chem.Titles, Crop Physiol.Abstr., Curr.Adv.Cell & Devel.Biol., Curr.Adv.Ecol.Sci., Curr.Cont., Dairy Sci.Abstr., Deep Sea Res.& Oceanogr.Abstr., Environ.Sci.Poll.Mgmt., Helminthol.Abstr., Hort.Abstr., INIS Atomind., INSPEC, Ind.Med. (1964-), Ind.Sci.Rev., Ind.Vet., Inpharma, Med.& Pharm.Biotech.Abstr., Microbiol.Abstr., Nutr.Abstr., Reac., Sci.Cit.Ind., Sport Fish.Abstr., Sugar Ind.Abstr., Vet.Bull., Wild.Rev., Zoo.Rec.
—BLDSC (3490.135000), ADONIS, CASDDS, CISTI, GNLM, IDS, ingenta, Linda Hall. **CCC.**
Published by: (Society for Cryobiology), Academic Press, Inc., Journal Division (Subsidiary of: Harcourt Brace & Company), 525 B St, Ste 1900, San Diego, CA 92101-4495. TEL 619-230-1840, FAX 619-699-6800, apsubs@acad.com, http://www.academicpress.com/cryobio. Ed. David E Pegg.

571.4 USA ISSN 0070-2129
QH511.A1 CODEN: CUTBAO
CURRENT TOPICS IN BIOENERGETICS. Text in English. 1966. irreg., latest vol.17, 1994. reprint service avail. from ISI. *Refereed.*
Related titles: Online - full text ed.: (from Institute for Scientific Information).
Indexed: ASCA, BBCI, Biol.Abstr., Chem.Abstr., Chem.Indus.Notes, Chem.Titles, Curr.Adv.Ecol.Sci., Ind.Sci.Rev., Nutr.Abstr., Sci.Cit.Ind.
—BLDSC (3504.870000), CASDDS, CISTI, Infotrieve, ingenta, Linda Hall. **CCC.**
Published by: Academic Press, Inc., Journal Division (Subsidiary of: Harcourt Brace & Company), 525 B St, Ste 1900, San Diego, CA 92101-4495. TEL 619-231-0926, FAX 619-699-6715. Ed. C P Lee. **Subscr. to:** Order Dept., 6277 Sea Harbor Dr, 4th Fl, Orlando, FL 32887. TEL 800-321-5068.

571.4 USA ISSN 1061-9526
QP341 CODEN: ELAGE9
ELECTRO- AND MAGNETOBIOLOGY. Text in English. 1982. 3/yr. USD 95 to individuals print & online eds.; USD 895 to institutions print only (effective 2002). adv. *Refereed.* **Document type:** *Academic/Scholarly.* **Description:** Examines questions concerning the role of intrinsic electromagnetism in the regulation of living systems.
Formerly: Journal of Bioelectricity (0730-823X)
Related titles: Microform ed.: (from RPI); Online - full text ed.: (from EBSCO Publishing, O C L C Online Computer Library Center, Inc., RoweCom Information Quest, Swets Blackwell, Institute for Scientific Information).
Indexed: ASCA, BBCI, Biol.Abstr., Chem.Abstr., Crop Physiol.Abstr., Curr.Cont., Excerp.Med., Field Crop Abstr., INSPEC (1982-, dropped), Ind.Sci.Rev., Inpharma, Reac., Ref.Zh., Sci.Cit.Ind., Weed Abstr.
—BLDSC (3698.187000), AskIEEE, CASDDS, CISTI, GNLM, IDS, Infotrieve, ingenta. **CCC.**
Published by: (International Society for Bioelectricity), Marcel Dekker Inc., 270 Madison Ave, New York, NY 10016. TEL 212-696-9000, 800-228-1160, FAX 212-685-4540, http://www.dekker.com/servlet/product/productid/JBC. Ed. Stephen D Smith. R&P Julia Mulligan. Adv. contact Anne Mullins. Circ: 250.

EMERGING BIOCHEMICAL AND BIOPHYSICAL TECHNIQUES. see *BIOLOGY—Biochemistry*

EURO COURSES. HEALTH PHYSICS AND RADIATION PROTECTION. see *ENERGY—Nuclear Energy*

571.4 DEU ISSN 0175-7571
QH505 CODEN: EBJOE8
EUROPEAN BIOPHYSICS JOURNAL. Text in English. 8/yr. EUR 797.80 domestic; EUR 792.80 in Germany; EUR 116.90 newsstand/cover foreign (effective 2002). adv. reprint service avail. from ISI. *Refereed.* **Document type:** *Journal, Academic/Scholarly.* **Description:** Topics covered include molecular and structural interactions, membrane and receptor biophysics, thermodynamics, and energetics of biological processes.
Former titles: European Biophysical Journal; (until 1984): Biophysics of Structure and Mechanism (0340-1057); Supersedes in part (in 1974): Biophysik (0006-3517)
Related titles: Microform ed.: (from PQC); Online - full text ed.: ISSN 1432-1017 (from EBSCO Publishing, RoweCom Information Quest, Swets Blackwell, Springer LINK, Institute for Scientific Information).
Indexed: ASCA, BBCI, Chem.Abstr., Chem.Cit.Ind., Chem.Indus.Notes, Chem.Titles, Curr.Adv.Ecol.Sci., Curr.Cont., Dairy Sci.Abstr., Eng.Ind., Excerp.Med., INIS Atomind., INSPEC (1974-), Ind.Med. (1984-), Ind.Sci.Rev., Inpharma, Int.Abstr.Biol.Sci., Phys.Ber., Reac., Ref.Zh., Rev.Appl.Entomol., SSCI (coverage dropped), Sci.Cit.Ind.
—BLDSC (3829.489400), AskIEEE, CASDDS, CISTI, Ei, GNLM, IDS, Infotrieve, ingenta, Linda Hall. **CCC.**
Published by: Springer-Verlag (Subsidiary of: BertelsmannSpringer), Tiergartenstr 17, Heidelberg 69121, Germany. TEL 49-6221-345-0, FAX 49-6221-345229, subscriptions@springer.de, http://link.springer.de/link/service/journals/00249/index.htm, http://www.springer.de. Ed. A Watts. **Subscr. in N. America to:** Springer-Verlag New York Inc., PO Box 2485, Secaucus, NJ 07096-2485. TEL 212-460-1500, FAX 212-473-6272.

EXCERPTA MEDICA. SECTION 27: BIOPHYSICS, BIO-ENGINEERING AND MEDICAL INSTRUMENTATION. see *BIOLOGY—Abstracting, Bibliographies, Statistics*

F E B S LETTERS. see *BIOLOGY—Biochemistry*

FARMACEVTSKI VESTNIK; strokovno glasilo slovenske farmacije. see *PHARMACY AND PHARMACOLOGY*

571.4 JPN ISSN 0435-1096
CODEN: GFSYAR
GAMMA FIELD SYMPOSIA. Text in English; Summaries in Japanese. 1962. a. per issue exchange basis. **Document type:** *Proceedings.*
Indexed: Chem.Abstr., INIS Atomind., Maize Abstr., Plant Breed.Abstr., Seed Abstr., Soyabean Abstr., Triticale Abstr.
—BLDSC (4069.200000), CASDDS, Linda Hall.
Published by: Institute of Radiation Breeding (NIAR, MAFF), Naka-gun, P.O. Box 3, Ohmiya-machi, Ibaraki-ken 319-22, Japan. TEL 81-2955-2-1138, FAX 81-2955-3-1075.

GENERAL PHYSIOLOGY AND BIOPHYSICS. see *BIOLOGY—Physiology*

571.4 USA ISSN 0073-0475
CODEN: HBBIAD
HARVARD BOOKS IN BIOPHYSICS. Text in English. 1965. irreg., latest vol.3, 1983. price varies. adv. *Refereed.* **Document type:** *Monographic series.*
Indexed: Biol.Abstr., Chem.Abstr.
—CASDDS.
Published by: (Harvard University Medical School, Department of Biophysics), Harvard University Press, 79 Garden St, Cambridge, MA 02138. TEL 617-495-2600, FAX 617-495-5898, http://www.hup.harvard.edu. R&P Mindy Koyanis TEL 617-495-2619. Adv. contact Denise Waddington.

571.4 JPN ISSN 0441-747X
CODEN: HSKEAT
HOSHASEN SEIBUTSU KENKYU/RADIATION BIOLOGY RESEARCH COMMUNICATION. Text in Japanese. 1965. q. JPY 3,000; USD 45 foreign. adv. bk.rev. *Refereed.* **Document type:** *Academic/Scholarly.*
Indexed: Chem.Abstr., INIS Atomind.
—BLDSC (7227.945000), CASDDS.
Published by: Hoshasen Seibutsu Kenkyukai/Society of Radiation Biology Research, c/o Research Reactor Institute, Kyoto University, Sennan-gun, Kumatori-cho, Osaka 590-04, Japan. TEL 81-724-51-2628, FAX 81-724-51-2628, akahon@rri.kyoto-u.ac.jp. Ed. Takeo Ohnishi. R&P, Adv. contact Hiroshi Utsumi.

INTERNATIONAL AGROPHYSICS; a quarterly journal on physics in agricultural and environmental sciences. see *AGRICULTURE—Crop Production And Soil*

INTERNATIONAL BIOPHYSICS CONGRESS. ABSTRACTS. see *BIOLOGY—Abstracting, Bibliographies, Statistics*

INTERNATIONAL JOURNAL OF RADIATION BIOLOGY. see *MEDICAL SCIENCES—Oncology*

ITOGI NAUKI I TEKHNIKI. OBSHCHIE PROBLEMY FIZIKO-KHIMICHESKOI BIOLOGII. see *BIOLOGY—Biochemistry*

JOURNAL OF BIOCHEMICAL AND BIOPHYSICAL METHODS. see *BIOLOGY—Biochemistry*

JOURNAL OF BIOCHEMISTRY, MOLECULAR BIOLOGY AND BIOPHYSICS. see *BIOLOGY—Biochemistry*

571.4 GBR ISSN 1050-6411
QP321 CODEN: JEKIE3
JOURNAL OF ELECTROMYOGRAPHY AND KINESIOLOGY. Text in English. 1991. bi-m. EUR 111 in Europe to individuals; JPY 14,700 in Japan to individuals; USD 124 elsewhere to individuals; EUR 443 in Europe to institutions; JPY 58,800 in Japan to institutions; USD 495 elsewhere to institutions (effective 2002). adv. charts, illus. back issues avail.; reprint service avail. from PQC. *Refereed.* **Document type:** *Academic/Scholarly.* **Description:** Presents original articles on the study of muscle interaction and motion, using both mechanical and electrical detection techniques.
Related titles: Microform ed.: (from PQC); Online - full text ed.: (from ingenta, ScienceDirect, Swets Blackwell, Institute for Scientific Information).
Indexed: AMED, ASCA, Curr.Cont., Ergon.Abstr., Excerp.Med. (1992-), Focus on: Sports Sci.& Med., Ind.Med. (1991-), Inpharma, Int.Abstr.Biol.Sci., Neurosci.Cit.Ind., Reac., SSCI (coverage dropped).
—BLDSC (4974.855000), CISTI, EMDOCS, GNLM, IDS, Infotrieve, ingenta. **CCC.**
Published by: Elsevier Science, PO Box 800, Kidlington, Oxon OX5 1XD, United Kingdom. TEL 44-1865-843000, FAX 44-1865-843010, http://www.elsevier.nl/locate/jelekin. Eds. Moshe Solomonow, Toshio Moritani. Circ: 1,000. **Subscr. in Australasia and the Far East to:** Elsevier Science (Singapore) Pte Ltd, No.1 Temasek Ave, 17-01 Millenia Tower, Singapore 039192, Singapore. TEL 65-434-3727, FAX 65-337-2230; **Subscr. in the Americas to:** Elsevier Science, PO Box 945, New York, NY 10159-0945. TEL 212-633-3730, FAX 212-633-3680, usinfo-f@elsevier.com; **Subscr. to:** Elsevier Science BV, PO Box 211, Amsterdam 1000 AE, Netherlands. TEL 31-20-485-3757, nlinfo-f@elsevier.nl.

JOURNAL OF ENVIRONMENTAL RADIOACTIVITY. see *ENVIRONMENTAL STUDIES*

JOURNAL OF LUMINESCENCE; an interdisciplinary journal of research on excited state processes in condensed matter. see *PHYSICS—Optics*

JOURNAL OF PURE AND APPLIED ULTRASONICS. see *PHYSICS—Sound*

JOURNAL OF SUBMICROSCOPIC CYTOLOGY AND PATHOLOGY. see *BIOLOGY—Cytology And Histology*

571.4 GBR ISSN 0306-4565
QH516 CODEN: JTBIDS
JOURNAL OF THERMAL BIOLOGY. Text in English. 1976. bi-m. EUR 172 in Europe to qualified personnel; JPY 22,800 in Japan to qualified personnel; USD 192 elsewhere to qualified personnel; EUR 872 in Europe to institutions; JPY 115,800 in Japan to institutions; USD 976 elsewhere to institutions (effective 2002). adv. bk.rev. illus, stat. index. back issues avail. *Refereed.* **Document type:** *Academic/Scholarly.* **Description:** Covers research into the mechanisms by which living organisms respond to temperature change.
Related titles: Microfilm ed.: (from PQC); Online - full text ed.: (from ingenta, ScienceDirect, Swets Blackwell, Institute for Scientific Information).
Indexed: ASCA, Agri.Eng.Abstr., Agricola, Anim.Behav.Abstr., Anim.Breed.Abstr., Apic.Abstr., Aqua.Sci.& Fish.Abstr., BBCI, Cal.Tiss.Abstr., Chem.Abstr., Chem.Indus.Notes, Chem.Titles, Crop Physiol.Abstr., Curr.Adv.Ecol.Sci., Curr.Cont., Curr.Ref.Fish Res., Dairy Sci.Abstr., Deep Sea Res.& Oceanogr.Abstr., Entomol.Abstr., Environ.Sci.Poll.Mgmt., Excerp.Med., Field Crop Abstr., Forest.Abstr., Helminthol.Abstr., Hort.Abstr., INSPEC (Apr.1984-), Ind.Sci.Rev., Ind.Vet., Inpharma, Int.Abstr.Biol.Sci., Maize Abstr., Nutr.Abstr., Pig News & Info., Plant Breed.Abstr., Poult.Abstr., Protozool.Abstr., Reac., Rev.Appl.Entomol., Rev.Med.& Vet.Mycol., Sci.Cit.Ind., Sport Fish.Abstr., Triticale Abstr., Vet.Bull., Wild.Rev., Zoo.Rec.
—BLDSC (5069.095000), AskIEEE, CASDDS, CISTI, EMDOCS, IDS, Infotrieve, ingenta, Linda Hall. **CCC.**
Published by: Elsevier Science Ltd., Pergamon, PO Box 800, Kidlington, Oxon 0X5 1DX, United Kingdom. TEL 44-1865-843000, FAX 44-1865-843010, http://www.elsevier.com/locate/jtherbio. Eds. James E Heath, K Bowler. Circ: 1,000. **Subscr. in Australasia and the Far East to:** Elsevier Science (Singapore) Pte Ltd, No.1 Temasek Ave, 17-01 Millenia Tower, Singapore 039192, Singapore. TEL 65-434-3727, FAX 65-337-2230**; Subscr. in the Americas to:** Elsevier Science, PO Box 945, New York, NY 10159-0945. TEL 212-633-3730, FAX 212-633-3680, usinfo-f@elsevier.com; **Subscr. to:** Elsevier Science BV, PO Box 211, Amsterdam 1000 AE, Netherlands. TEL 31-20-485-3757.

MEDECINE NUCLEAIRE; imagerie fonctionelle et metabolique. see *MEDICAL SCIENCES—Radiology And Nuclear Medicine*

MOLECULAR BIOLOGY, BIOCHEMISTRY AND BIOPHYSICS. see *BIOLOGY—Biochemistry*

571.4 RUS ISSN 0134-8485
CODEN: MFBVAX
MOLEKULYARNAYA FIZIKA I BIOFIZIKA VODNYKH SISTEM. Text in Russian. 1973. irreg. illus.
Supersedes: Struktura i Rol' Vody v Zhivom Organizme (0585-4393)
Indexed: Chem.Abstr.
—CASDDS.
Published by: Sankt-Peterburgskii Universitet, Universitetskaya nab 7-9, St Petersburg 199034, Russian Federation.

571.4 JPN ISSN 0915-0374
NIHON SEITAI JIKI GAKKAISHI/JAPAN BIOMAGNETISM AND BIOELECTROMAGNETICS SOCIETY. JOURNAL. Text in English, Japanese. 1988. s-a.
Published by: Nihon Seitai Jiki Gakkai, Daigaku Igakubu, Iyo Denshi Kenkyu Shisetsu, 3-1 Hongo 7-chome, Bunkyo-ku, Tokyo 113-0033, Japan.

PHYSICO-CHEMICAL BIOLOGY/SEIBUTSU BUTSURI KAGAKU. see *BIOLOGY—Biochemistry*

571.45 GBR ISSN 0031-9155
QH505 CODEN: PHMBA7
PHYSICS IN MEDICINE AND BIOLOGY. Text in English; Abstracts in English, French, German. 1956. m. USD 1,710 to institutions; USD 1,283 microfiche ed. (effective 2000). adv. bk.rev. bibl, charts, illus. index. back issues avail.; reprint service avail. from IRC. *Refereed.* **Document type:** *Academic/Scholarly.* **Description:** Covers the use of physical agents such as ionizing and non-ionizing radiation, electromagnetic fields and ultrasound in diagnosis, therapy and radiobiology; corresponding physical methods of dosimetry; associated hazards and protection requirements.
Related titles: Microfiche ed.: (from AIP); Microfilm ed.: (from AIP); Online - full text ed.: (from EBSCO Publishing, RoweCom Information Quest, Swets Blackwell, Institute for Scientific Information).
Indexed: ASCA, Biol.Abstr., Chem.Abstr., Chem.Titles, Curr.Adv.Ecol.Sci., Curr.Cont., Dairy Sci.Abstr., Dok.Arbeitsmed., Eng.Ind., Excerp.Med., INIS Atomind., INSPEC (pre-1969-), Ind.Med. (1956-), Ind.Sci.Rev., Inpharma, Nutr.Abstr., Reac., Sci.Cit.Ind.
—BLDSC (6478.800000), AskIEEE, CASDDS, CISTI, Ei, GNLM, IDS, ingenta, Linda Hall. **CCC.**
Published by: (Institute of Physics), I O P Publishing Ltd., Dirac House, Temple Back, Bristol BS1 6BE, United Kingdom. TEL 44-117-929-7481, FAX 44-117-929-4318, custserv@ioppublishing.co.uk, http:/www.iop.org. Ed. M O Leach. Adv. contact John Irish. Circ: 769. **US subscr. to:** American Institute of Physics, Member and Subscriber Services, 500 Sunnyside Blvd, Woodbury, NY 11797-2900. TEL 516-349-7800. **Co-sponsors:** Hospital Physicists Association, UK; International Organization for Medical Physics; European Federation of Organizations for Medical Physics.

571.4 USA ISSN 0748-6642
QP501 CODEN: PCPNER
PHYSIOLOGICAL CHEMISTRY AND PHYSICS AND MEDICAL N M R. (Nuclear Magnetic Resonance) Text in English. 1969. s-a., latest vol.32, 2000. USD 80 domestic; USD 87 foreign (effective 2001). bk.rev. index. back issues avail. *Refereed.* **Document type:** *Journal, Academic/Scholarly.* **Description:** Reviews of and reports on original research in biophysics, biochemistry, cellular physiology, nuclear magnetic resonance and related areas.
Formerly (until 1983): Physiological Chemistry and Physics (0031-9325)
Indexed: ASCA, Apic.Abstr., BBCI (coverage dropped), Biol.Abstr., Chem.Abstr., Chem.Cit.Ind., Chem.Indus.Notes, Chem.Titles, Curr.Adv.Ecol.Sci., Curr.Cont. (coverage dropped), INIS Atomind., INSPEC (1977-1981, dropped), Ind.Med. (1983-), Inpharma, Reac., Ref.Zh., Rev.Appl.Entomol., Sci.Cit.Ind. (coverage dropped).
—BLDSC (6484.710000), CASDDS, CISTI, GNLM, IDS, ingenta, Linda Hall.
Published by: Pacific Press, Inc., PO Box 1452, Melville, NY 11747. TEL 631-694-2929, FAX 631-249-3734, pacificpressny@aol.com. Ed., R&P Gilbert N Ling. Pub. Raymond V Damadian. Circ: 350 (paid).

571.46 UKR ISSN 0869-2327
CODEN: KRBIEQ
PROBLEMY KRIOBIOLOGII/PROBLEMS OF CRYOBIOLOGY. Text in Russian; Summaries in English. 1985. q. USD 105 in North America. **Description:** Provides basic information to researchers investigating the various phenomena involved in the interaction between low temperatures and living cells or tissue, as well as to clinicians who are undertaking trials of hypothermia.
Formerly: Kriobiologiya (0233-7673)
Indexed: Chem.Abstr., Chem.Indus.Notes, Chem.Titles, Zoo.Rec.
—CASDDS, East View, GNLM, Linda Hall.
Published by: Natsional'na Akademiya Nauk Ukrainy, Institut Problem Kriobiologii i Kriomeditsiny/National Ukrainian Academy of Sciences, Institute of Problems of Cryobiology and Cryomedicine, Ul Pereyaslavskaya 23, Kharkov 310015, Ukraine. TEL 721039, FAX 720084. Ed. V I Grishchenko. **US dist. addr.:** East View Publications, 3020 Harbor Ln N, Minneapolis, MN 55447. TEL 612-550-0961.

571.4 GBR ISSN 0079-6107
QH505.A1 CODEN: PBIMAC
PROGRESS IN BIOPHYSICS & MOLECULAR BIOLOGY. Text in English. 1950. 9/yr. EUR 1,549 in Europe to institutions; JPY 205,800 in Japan to institutions; USD 1,733 elsewhere to institutions (effective 2002). abstr. index. *Refereed.* **Document type:** *Academic/Scholarly.* **Description:** Integrates developments in the physical and biological sciences.
Related titles: Microfilm ed.: (from PQC); Online - full text ed.: (from ingenta, Swets Blackwell, Institute for Scientific Information, ScienceDirect).
Indexed: ASCA, Appl.Mech.Rev., BBCI, Biol.Abstr., Biotech.Cit.Ind., Chem.Abstr., Chem.Cit.Ind., Chem.Titles, Curr.Adv.Ecol.Sci., Curr.Cont., Excerp.Med., INSPEC (1975-), Ind.Med. (1963-), Ind.Sci.Rev., Inpharma, Int.Abstr.Biol.Sci., Mass Spectr.Bull., Plant Breed.Abstr., Reac., Sci.Cit.Ind.
—BLDSC (6866.100000), ADONIS, AskIEEE, CASDDS, CISTI, GNLM, IDS, ingenta, Linda Hall. **CCC.**
Published by: Pergamon (Subsidiary of: Elsevier Science), The Boulevard, Langford Ln, East Park, Kidlington, Oxford OXB 1GB, United Kingdom. FAX 44-1865-843010, http://www.elsevier.com/locate/pbiomolbio. Eds. D Noble, T L Blundell. **Subscr. in Australasia and the Far East to:** Elsevier Science (Singapore) Pte Ltd, No.1 Temasek Ave, 17-01 Millenia Tower, Singapore 039192, Singapore. TEL 65-434-3727, FAX 65-337-2230; **Subscr. in the Americas to:** Elsevier Science, PO Box 945, New York, NY 10159-0945. TEL 212-633-3730, FAX 212-633-3680, usinfo-f@elsevier.com**; Subscr. to:** Elsevier Science BV, PO Box 211, Amsterdam 1000 AE, Netherlands. TEL 31-20-485-3757.

571.4 GBR ISSN 0033-5835
QH505.A1 CODEN: QURBAW
QUARTERLY REVIEWS OF BIOPHYSICS. Text in English, French, German. 1968. q. GBP 150 to individuals; USD 340 to institutions (effective 2002). adv. bibl, charts, illus. index. back issues avail.; reprint service avail. from SWZ. *Refereed.* **Document type:** *Academic/Scholarly.* **Description:** Reviews recent progress and problems in biophysics and molecular biology.
Related titles: Microform ed.: (from PQC); Online - full text ed.: (from EBSCO Publishing, O C L C Online Computer Library Center, Inc., RoweCom Information Quest, Swets Blackwell, Institute for Scientific Information).
Indexed: ASCA, Appl.Mech.Rev., Aqua.Sci.& Fish.Abstr., BBCI, Biol.Abstr., Chem.Abstr., Chem.Indus.Notes, Chem.Titles, Crop Physiol.Abstr., Curr.Adv.Biochem., Curr.Adv.Cancer Res., Curr.Cont. (coverage dropped), Dairy Sci.Abstr., Excerp.Med., INIS Atomind., Ind.Med. (1968-), Ind.Sci.Rev., Inpharma, Int.Abstr.Biol.Sci., Mass Spectr.Bull., Reac., Sci.Cit.Ind.
—BLDSC (7206.300000), CASDDS, CISTI, GNLM, IDS, ingenta, Linda Hall. **CCC.**
Published by: (International Union for Pure and Applied Biophysics), Cambridge University Press, Edinburgh Bldg, Shaftesbury Rd, Cambridge CB2 2RU, United Kingdom. FAX 44-1223-315052, information@cup.cam.ac.uk, information@cambridge.org, http://www.cup.cam.ac.uk, http://www.uk.cambridge.org/journals/pmu. Eds. A. Graslund, Chris Miller, David Neuhaus, Donald M. Crothers, John Kuriyan, Kurt Wuthrich, Peter G. Wolynes. R&P Linda Nicol. Adv. contact Rebecca Symons.

571.4 DEU ISSN 0301-634X
QH505.A1 CODEN: REBPAT
RADIATION AND ENVIRONMENTAL BIOPHYSICS. Text in English. 1963. q. EUR 1,010.30 domestic; EUR 1,006.90 in Germany; EUR 300 newsstand/cover foreign (effective 2002). adv. charts, illus. index. back issues avail.; reprint service avail. from ISI. *Refereed.* **Document type:** *Journal, Academic/Scholarly.* **Description:** Covers the biophysics of ionizing and non-ionizing radiation. Examines the biological effects of temperature, pressure, gravitational forces, electricity, and magnetism, and the biophysical aspects of environmental and space influence.
Supersedes in part (in 1974): Biophysik (0006-3517)
Related titles: Microform ed.: (from PQC); Online - full text ed.: ISSN 1432-2099 (from EBSCO Publishing, RoweCom Information Quest, Swets Blackwell, Springer LINK, Institute for Scientific Information).
Indexed: ASCA, BBCI, Biol.Abstr., Chem.Abstr., Chem.Indus.Notes, Chem.Titles, Curr.Adv.Biochem., Curr.Adv.Cell & Devel.Biol., Curr.Adv.Ecol.Sci., Curr.Adv.Gen.& Molec.Biol., Curr.Cont., Curr.Ind.Stat., Deep Sea Res.& Oceanogr.Abstr., Excerp.Med., INIS Atomind., INSPEC (1971-, dropped), Ind.Med. (1974-), Inpharma, Plant Breed.Abstr., Reac., Risk Abstr., Sci.Cit.Ind.
—BLDSC (7227.930000), AskIEEE, CASDDS, CISTI, EMDOCS, GNLM, IDS, Infotrieve, ingenta, Linda Hall. **CCC.**
Published by: Springer-Verlag (Subsidiary of: BertelsmannSpringer), Tiergartenstr 17, Heidelberg 69121, Germany. TEL 49-6221-345-0, FAX 49-6221-345229, subscriptions@springer.de, http://link.springer.de/link/service/journals/00411/index.htm, http://www.springer.de. Eds. A Kellerer, T Roedler-Vogelsang. **Subscr. in N. America to:** Springer-Verlag New York Inc., PO Box 2485, Secaucus, NJ 07096-2485. TEL 212-460-1500, FAX 212-473-6272.

RADIATSIONNAYA BIOLOGIYA, RADIOEKOLOGIYA. see *MEDICAL SCIENCES—Radiology And Nuclear Medicine*

REFERATIVNYI ZHURNAL. BIONIKA. BIOKIBERNETIKA. BIOINZHENERIYA. see *BIOLOGY—Abstracting, Bibliographies, Statistics*

B

REFERATIVNYI ZHURNAL. RADIATSIONNAYA BIOLOGIYA. see *BIOLOGY—Abstracting, Bibliographies, Statistics*

REPRODUCTION, NUTRITION, DEVELOPMENT. see *BIOLOGY*

SEITAI NO KAGAKU/LIFE SCIENCE. see *BIOLOGY*

SHENGWU HUAXUE YU SHENGWU WULI JINZHAN/PROGRESS IN BIOCHEMISTRY AND BIOPHYSICS. see *BIOLOGY—Biochemistry*

SHENGWU HUAXUE YU SHENGWU WULI XUEBAO/ACTA BIOCHIMICA ET BIOPHYSICA SINICA. see *BIOLOGY—Biochemistry*

571.4 USA ISSN 0932-2353 CODEN: SSBIEJ
SPRINGER SERIES IN BIOPHYSICS. Text in English. 1986. irreg. price varies. reprint service avail. from ISI. **Document type:** *Monographic series.*
—CASDDS, CISTI, Infotrieve, KNAW. **CCC.**
Published by: Springer-Verlag, Journals (Subsidiary of: BertelsmannSpringer), 175 Fifth Ave, New York, NY 10010. TEL 212-460-1500, FAX 212-473-6272.

B

BIOLOGY—Biotechnology

see also ENGINEERING—Chemical Engineering

A S F A MARINE BIOTECHNOLOGY ABSTRACTS. (Aquatic Sciences & Fisheries Abstracts) see *BIOLOGY—Abstracting, Bibliographies, Statistics*

660 DEU ISSN 0138-4988
TA164 CODEN: ACBTDD
ACTA BIOTECHNOLOGICA. Text in English. 1981. q. EUR 528 in Europe; CHF 898 in Switzerland & Liechtenstein; USD 698 elsewhere; EUR 555 in Europe for print and online eds.; CHF 943 in Switzerland & Liechtenstein, for print and online eds.; USD 733 elsewhere for print and online eds. (effective 2002). bk.rev., Website rev. reprints avail. *Refereed.* **Document type:** *Journal, Academic/Scholarly.* **Description:** Interdisciplinary forum for environmental, industrial, and agricultural biotechnology.
Related titles: CD-ROM ed.; Online - full text ed.: ISSN 1521-3846. EUR 528 in Europe; CHF 898 in Switzerland & Liechtenstein; USD 698 elsewhere (effective 2002) (from Wiley InterScience, Institute for Scientific Information).
Indexed: AESIS, ASCA, Agri.& Environ.Biotech.Abstr., Aqua.Sci.& Fish.Abstr., Aquacult.Abstr., Biodet.Abstr., Biotech.Cit.Ind., Chem.Abstr., Chem.Indus.Notes, Chem.Titles, Curr.Adv.Ecol.Sci., Curr.Biotech.Abstr., Curr.Cont., Dairy Sci.Abstr., Derwent Biotech.Abstr., Ecol.Abstr., Eng.Ind., Environ.Sci.Poll.Mgmt., Excerp.Med., Food Sci.& Tech.Abstr., Geo.Abstr.P.G., Hort.Abstr., INIS Atomind., Ind.Sci.Rev., Int.Abstr.Biol.Sci., Med.& Pharm.Biotech.Abstr., Microbiol.Abstr., Nutr.Abstr., Plant Grow.Reg.Abstr., Russ.Acad.Sci.Bibl., Sci.Cit.Ind., Soils & Fert., Sugar Ind.Abstr., Telegen, Weed Abstr.
—BLDSC (0603.700000), CASDDS, CISTI, Ei, EMDOCS, GNLM, IDS, Infotrieve, ingenta, Linda Hall. **CCC.**
Published by: Wiley - V C H, Postfach 101161, Weinheim 69451, Germany. TEL 49-6201-606-0, FAX 49-6201-606-117, subservice@wiley-vch.de, http://www.wiley-vch.de. Ed. W Babel. R&P Claudia Rutz. Adv. contact Aenne Anders TEL 49-6201-606552. Circ: 300. **Subscr. in the Americas to:** John Wiley & Sons, Inc., Journals, 605 Third Ave, New York, NY 10158. TEL 44-1243-779777, 212-850-6645, FAX 212-850-6021; **Subscr. outside Germany, Austria & Switzerland to:** John Wiley & Sons Ltd., Baffins Ln, Chichester, Sussex PO19 IUD, United Kingdom. TEL 44-1243-779777, FAX 44-1243-843232.

660.63 USA ISSN 0724-6145
TP248.3 CODEN: ABEBDZ
ADVANCES IN BIOCHEMICAL ENGINEERING - BIOTECHNOLOGY. Text in English. 1972. irreg., latest vol.54, 1996. price varies. reprint service avail. from ISI. **Document type:** *Monographic series.* **Description:** Publishes new research in biochemical engineering and other areas of biotechnology.
Formerly: Advances in Biochemical Engineering (0065-2210)
Indexed: Agri.& Environ.Biotech.Abstr. (coverage dropped), Bibl.Agri., Chem.Abstr., Chem.Indus.Notes, Chem.Titles, Curr.Biotech.Abstr., Derwent Biotech.Abstr., Eng.Ind., Food Sci.& Tech.Abstr., Ind.Med. (1983-).
—BLDSC (0699.925500), CASDDS, CISTI, Ei, GNLM, Infotrieve, ingenta, KNAW, Linda Hall. **CCC.**
Published by: Springer-Verlag, Journals (Subsidiary of: BertelsmannSpringer), 175 Fifth Ave, New York, NY 10010. TEL 212-460-1500, FAX 212-473-6272, orders@springer-ny.com, http://springer-ny.com. Eds. A Fiechter, T K Ghose.

574.28 CUB ISSN 1027-2860
ADVANCES IN MODERN BIOTECHNOLOGY/AVANCES EN BIOTECNOLOGIA MODERNA. Text in English, Spanish. 1992. irreg. USD 12 domestic; USD 15 foreign (effective 2000). back issues avail. *Refereed.* **Document type:** *Proceedings.* **Description:** Presents short papers of oral and poster presentations for scientific congresses.
Published by: (Center for Genetic Engineering and Biotechnology), Elfos Scientiae, Ave. 31 entre 158 y 190, PO Box 6072, Cubanacan, La Playa, Ciudad de La Playa 10600, Cuba. TEL 53-7-33-1917, FAX 53-7-33-1917, elfos@cigb.edu.cu, http://www.cigb.edu.cu, http://www.elfosscientiae.com.cu. Ed., R&P Guillermo J Padron. Circ: 2,000. **Subscr. to:** EBSCO Mexico, SA de CV, Ensenada 91, Col. Hipodromo Condesa, Mexico, DF 06170, Mexico. TEL 52-5-2738218, FAX 52-5-2735550.

AGBIOTECH NEWS AND INFORMATION. see *BIOLOGY—Abstracting, Bibliographies, Statistics*

AGBIOTECH REPORTER; agricultural research - business. see *AGRICULTURE*

660 542 USA ISSN 0749-3223 CODEN: ABLAEY
AMERICAN BIOTECHNOLOGY LABORATORY. Text in English. 1983. 13/yr. USD 160; USD 193 foreign. adv. charts, illus, stat, tr.lit. **Document type:** *Trade.*
Related titles: Special ed.: American Biotechnology Laboratory. Buyers' Guide.
Indexed: ASCA, Chem.Abstr., Chem.Indus.Notes, Chem.Titles, Curr.Biotech.Abstr., Eng.Ind., Int.Abstr.Biol.Sci., Mass Spectr.Bull., Telegen.
—BLDSC (0810.806000), CASDDS, Ei, GNLM, IDS, KNAW.
Published by: International Scientific Communications, Inc., 30 Controls Dr, Box 870, Shelton, CT 06484-0870. TEL 203-926-9300, FAX 203-926-9310, iscpubs@iscpubs.com, http://www.iscpubs.com. Ed. Brian Howard. Pub. William Wham. R&P Patricia Ekbatani. Adv. contact Robert G Sweeney. B&W page USD 4,295, color page USD 5,915. Circ: 70,016 (controlled).

▼ **AMERICAN JOURNAL OF PHARMACOGENOMICS.** see *BIOLOGY—Genetics*

660 636 USA ISSN 1049-5398
SF140.B54 CODEN: ANBTEN
ANIMAL BIOTECHNOLOGY. Text in English. 1984. 2/yr. USD 60 to individuals print & online eds.; USD 650 to institutions print only (effective 2002). adv. *Refereed.* **Document type:** *Academic/Scholarly.* **Description:** Covers the identification and manipulation of genes and their products in domesticated animals.
Related titles: Online - full content ed.; Online - full text ed.: (from Institute for Scientific Information, RoweCom Information Quest).
Indexed: ASCA, AgBiotech, Agri.& Environ.Biotech.Abstr., Agricola, Anim.Breed.Abstr., Aqua.Sci.& Fish.Abstr., Biotech.& Bioeng.Abstr., Biotech.Cit.Ind., Chem.Abstr., Chem.Indus.Notes, Chem.Titles, Curr.Cont., Dairy Sci.Abstr., Derwent Biotech.Abstr., Eng.Ind., Environ.Per.Bibl. (1992-1993), Environ.Sci.Poll.Mgmt., Food Sci.& Tech.Abstr., Genet.Abstr., Hum.Gen.Abstr., Ind.Med. (1990-), Ind.Vet., Maize Abstr., Pig News & Info., Plant Breed.Abstr., Poult.Abstr., Ref.Zh., Sci.Cit.Ind., Vet.Bull.
—BLDSC (0902.975000), CASDDS, IDS, Infotrieve. **CCC.**
Published by: Marcel Dekker Inc., 270 Madison Ave, New York, NY 10016. TEL 212-696-9000, 800-228-1160, FAX 212-685-4540, http://www.dekker.com/servlet/product/productid/ABIO. Ed. Lawrence B Schook. R&P Julia Mulligan. Adv. contact Diane Saulon. B&W page USD 800. Circ: 300 (paid).

ANTIVIRAL AGENTS BULLETIN; antiviral drug and vaccine development information. see *PHARMACY AND PHARMACOLOGY*

660.62 NLD ISSN 0003-6072 CODEN: ALJMAO
ANTONIE VAN LEEUWENHOEK; international journal of general and molecular microbiology. Text in English. 1935. 8/yr. EUR 1,239, USD 1,240 to institutions for print or online ed.; EUR 795, USD 795 to individuals for print or online ed.; EUR 1,486.80, USD 1,488 to institutions print & onlilne eds.combined (effective 2002). charts, stat. index. reprint service avail. from SWZ. *Refereed.* **Document type:** *Academic/Scholarly.* **Description:** Publishes fundamental and applied research connected with microbiology, including food microbiology, medical microbiology and applications of microbiology in biotechnology.
Supersedes (in 1934): Nederlandsch Tijdschrift voor Hygiene, Microbiologie en Serologie (0369-3821)
Related titles: Microform ed.: (from PQC); Online - full text ed.: (from EBSCO Publishing, O C L C Online Computer Library Center, Inc., RoweCom Information Quest, Swets Blackwell, Kluwer Online, Institute for Scientific Information).
Indexed: ASCA, Abstr.Hyg., AgBiotech, Agri.& Environ.Biotech.Abstr. (coverage dropped), Aqua.Sci.& Fish.Abstr., Bio-Contr.News & Info., Biodet.Abstr., Biol.Abstr., Biotech.Cit.Ind., Chem.Abstr., Chem.Indus.Notes, Chem.Titles, Curr.Adv.Ecol.Sci., Curr.Biotech.Abstr., Curr.Cont., Dairy Sci.Abstr., Deep Sea Res.& Oceanogr.Abstr., Derwent Biotech.Abstr., Ecol.Abstr., Environ.Sci.Poll.Mgmt., Excerp.Med., Food Sci.& Tech.Abstr., Helminthol.Abstr., Herb.Abstr., Hort.Abstr., Ind.Med. (1934-), Ind.Sci.Rev., Ind.Vet., Inpharma, Int.Abstr.Biol.Sci., Microbiol.Abstr., Nutr.Abstr., Pig News & Info., Plant Breed.Abstr., Protozool.Abstr., Reac., Rev.Appl.Entomol., Rev.Arom.& Med.Plants, Rev.Med.& Vet.Mycol., Rev.Plant Path., Sci.Cit.Ind., Small Anim.Abstr., Soils & Fert., Sport Fish.Abstr., Sugar Ind.Abstr., Vet.Bull., W.R.C.Inf., Weed Abstr.
—BLDSC (1553.000000), CASDDS, CISTI, EMDOCS, GNLM, IDS, ingenta, KNAW, Linda Hall. **CCC.**
Published by: (Stichting Antonie van Leeuwenhoek), Kluwer Academic Publishers Group (Subsidiary of: Wolters Kluwer N.V.), Spuiboulevard 50, PO Box 17, Dordrecht 3300 AA, Netherlands. FAX 31-78-639-2254, services@wkap.nl, http://www.wkap.nl/journalhome.htm/0020-3157. Ed. M Goodfellow. **Dist. by:** Journals Department, PO Box 322, Dordrecht 3300 AH, Netherlands. TEL 781-871-6600, FAX 31-78-654-6474.

APPLIED AND ENVIRONMENTAL MICROBIOLOGY. see *BIOLOGY—Microbiology*

APPLIED BIOCHEMISTRY AND BIOTECHNOLOGY. see *BIOLOGY—Biochemistry*

APPLIED CYTOGENETICS. see *BIOLOGY—Genetics*

APPLIED GENETICS NEWS. see *BIOLOGY—Genetics*

660.62 DEU ISSN 0175-7598
QR53 CODEN: AMBIDG
APPLIED MICROBIOLOGY AND BIOTECHNOLOGY. Text in English. 1975. m. EUR 3,568.80 domestic; EUR 3,540.20 in Germany; EUR 233.30 newsstand/cover foreign (effective 2002). reprint service avail. from ISI. *Refereed.* **Document type:** *Journal, Academic/Scholarly.* **Description:** Publishes original papers, short communications and mini-reviews on the following aspects of applied microbiology and biotechnology: biotechnology, biochemical engineering, applied genetics and regulation, applied microbial and cell physiology, food biotechnology, and environmental biotechnology.
Former titles (until 1984): European Journal of Applied Microbiology and Biotechnology (0171-1741); European Journal of Applied Microbiology (0340-2118)

Related titles: Microform ed.: (from PQC); Online - full text ed.: ISSN 1432-0614 (from EBSCO Publishing, RoweCom Information Quest, Swets Blackwell, Springer LINK, Institute for Scientific Information).
Indexed: AESIS, A.S.& T.Ind. (Jan.1997-), ASCA, Abstr.Hyg., AgBiotech, Agri.& Environ.Biotech.Abstr., Agricola, Aqua.Sci.& Fish.Abstr., Aquacult.Abstr., BBCI, Bio-Contr.News & Info., Biodet.Abstr., Biol.& Agr.Ind. (Oct.1989-), Biotech.Cit.Ind., CEABA, Chem.Abstr., Chem.Cit.Ind., Chem.Indus.Notes, Chem.Titles, Chemorec.Abstr., Curr.Adv.Biochem., Curr.Adv.Ecol.Sci., Curr.Adv.Gen.& Molec.Biol., Curr.Biotech.Abstr., Curr.Cont., Dairy Sci.Abstr., Deep Sea Res.& Oceanogr.Abstr., Derwent Biotech.Abstr., Ecol.Abstr., Environ.Sci.Poll.Mgmt., Excerp.Med., Fluidex, Food Sci.& Tech.Abstr., Forest.Abstr., Geo.Abstr.P.G., Helminthol.Abstr., Hort.Abstr., INIS Atomind., Ind.Med. (1984-), Ind.Sci.Rev., Ind.Vet., Inpharma, Int.Abstr.Biol.Sci., Mass Spectr.Bull., Mat.Sci.Cit.Ind. (coverage dropped), Microbiol.Abstr., Nutr.Abstr., Ocean.Abstr., Pig News & Info., Plant Breed.Abstr., Pollut.Abstr., Potato Abstr., Reac., Ref.Zh., Rev.Appl.Entomol., Rev.Med.& Vet.Mycol., Rev.Plant Path., Rice Abstr., Sci.Cit.Ind., Sel.Water Res.Abstr., Soils & Fert., Sugar Ind.Abstr., Triticale Abstr., Vet.Bull., W.R.C.Inf., Weed Abstr., Wild.Rev.
—BLDSC (1576.100000), ADONIS, CASDDS, CINDOC, CISTI, EMDOCS, GNLM, IDS, Infotrieve, ingenta, Linda Hall. **CCC.**
Published by: Springer-Verlag (Subsidiary of: BertelsmannSpringer), Tiergartenstr 17, Heidelberg 69121, Germany. TEL 49-6221-345-0, FAX 49-6221-345229, subscriptions@springer.de, http://link.springer.de/link/service/journals/00253/index.htm, http://www.springer.de. Ed. A Steinbuechel. **Subscr. in N. America to:** Springer-Verlag New York Inc., PO Box 2485, Secaucus, NJ 07096-2485. TEL 212-460-1500, FAX 212-473-6272.

660 EGY ISSN 1110-6875
ARAB JOURNAL OF BIOTECHNOLOGY. Text in Arabic. 1998. s-a. (July & December). USD 25 to individuals; USD 100 to institutions (effective 2000). *Refereed.* **Document type:** *Academic/Scholarly.* **Description:** Aims at the advancement and dissemination of knowledge in agriculture, medicine, veterenary medicine, environment and pharmacology.
Related titles: CD-ROM ed.: EGP 50 per issue in Egypt; USD 30 per issue rest of world (effective 2000); Diskette ed.; E-mail ed.; Fax ed.
Published by: Arab Council for Graduate Studies & Scientific Research, Tharwat Street, Cairo Univ, Hostel, Giza 12613, Egypt. TEL 20-2-5676055, 20-2-5676048, FAX 20-2-3602658, acgssr@intouch.com, http://www.frcu.eun.eg/www/homepage/accgr/accgr.htm. Ed. Deyaa El Kadi.

ARTIFICIAL CELLS, BLOOD SUBSTITUTES, AND IMMOBILIZATION BIOTECHNOLOGY. see *MEDICAL SCIENCES—Experimental Medicine, Laboratory Technique*

ASIAN - AUSTRALASIAN JOURNAL OF ANIMAL SCIENCES. see *AGRICULTURE—Poultry And Livestock*

660 AUS ISSN 1036-7128
CODEN: AUBIE5
AUSTRALASIAN BIOTECHNOLOGY. Text in English. 1987. bi-m. AUD 90; AUD 120 foreign (effective 1999). adv. bk.rev. index. back issues avail. *Refereed.* **Document type:** *Newsletter.*
Formerly (until 1991): Australian Journal of Biotechnology (0819-3355)
Related titles: Online - full text ed.: (from Institute for Scientific Information).
Indexed: AESIS, ASCA, AgBiotech, Anim.Breed.Abstr., Arts & Hum.Cit.Ind. (coverage dropped), Bio-Contr.News & Info., Biotech.Cit.Ind., CBNB (1992-), CEABA, Chem.Abstr., Chem.Indus.Notes, Chem.Titles, Curr.Biotech.Abstr., Dairy Sci.Abstr., Derwent Biotech.Abstr., Food Sci.& Tech.Abstr., Helminthol.Abstr., Int.Abstr.Biol.Sci., Plant Breed.Abstr., Rev.Appl.Entomol., Rev.Plant Path., Sugar Ind.Abstr., World Ag.Econ.& Rur.Soc.Abstr.
—BLDSC (1793.610000), CASDDS, CISTI, EMDOCS, IDS, ingenta.
Published by: Australian Biotechnology Association Ltd., PO Box 4, Gardenvale, VIC 3185, Australia. TEL 61-3-95968879, FAX 61-3-95968874, aba@netspace.net.au, http://www.aba.asn.au/. Eds. D Tribe, M Playne. R&P Barbara Arnold. Adv. contact Gary Dolder. Circ: 1,200 (paid).

660 GBR
B B S R C BUSINESS. Text in English. 1967. q. free per issue. charts, illus. **Document type:** *Newsletter.* **Description:** Presents research in biology and biotechnology, agriculture, food, chemicals, and pharmaceuticals.
Supersedes in part (in Apr. 1994): A F R C News (0267-8489)
Indexed: Environ.Abstr.
Published by: Biotechnology and Biological Sciences Research Council, Polaris House, N Star Ave, Swindon, Wilts SN2 1UH, United Kingdom. TEL 44-1793-413200, FAX 44-1793-413201, http://www.bbsrc.ac.uk. Ed. Monica Winstanley.

660 JPN
BAIOINDASUTORI NENKAN/YEARBOOK OF BIOINDUSTRY. Text in Japanese. 1985. a. JPY 55,000.
Published by: C M C Co. Ltd., 5-4 Uchikanda 1-chome, Chiyoda-ku, Tokyo 101-0047, Japan.

660 USA
BIO NEWS; news & events from the biotechnology industry. Text in English. bi-m. adv. **Document type:** *Newsletter.*
Published by: Biotechnology Industry Organization, 1625 K St, N W, Ste 1100, Washington, DC 20006. TEL 202-857-0244, FAX 202-857-0237, info@bio.org, http://www.hol.gr/bio. Ed., R&P Megan Matthews. Adv. contact Susan Rathbone.

660 CHE ISSN 1024-2422
TP248.65.E59 CODEN: BOBOEQ
BIOCATALYSIS AND BIOTRANSFORMATION. Text in English. 6/yr. GBP 68, USD 145, EUR 159 to individuals; GBP 506, USD 660, EUR 675 to institutions; GBP 1,137, USD 1,442, EUR 1,517 to corporations (effective 2002). adv. bk.rev. back issues avail. *Refereed.* **Document type:** *Journal, Academic/Scholarly.* **Description:** International journal covering the industrial exploitation of biological catalysts for the interconversion of chemical species.
Formerly: Biocatalysis (0886-4454)
Related titles: CD-ROM ed.; Microform ed.; Online - full text ed.: (from EBSCO Publishing, RoweCom Information Quest, Institute for Scientific Information).
Indexed: ASCA, Agri.& Environ.Biotech.Abstr., Aqua.Sci.& Fish.Abstr., BBCI, Biotech.Cit.Ind., CEABA, Chem.Abstr., Chem.Cit.Ind., Curr.Cont., Derwent Biotech.Abstr., Eng.Ind., Environ.Sci.Poll.Mgmt., Food Sci.& Tech.Abstr., Inpharma, Int.Abstr.Biol.Sci., Microbiol.Abstr., Reac., Sci.Cit.Ind.
—BLDSC (2066.809100), CISTI, Ei, Infotrieve. **CCC.**
Published by: Gordon and Breach - Harwood Academic (Subsidiary of: Taylor & Francis Group), PO Box 531, Lausanne 1000, Switzerland. TEL 41-21-6411280, FAX 41-21-6411281, info@gbhap.com, http://www.gbhap.com. Ed. Dr. David Leak. **Subscr. addr. in US:** International Publishers Direct, PO Box 32160, Newark, NJ 07102. FAX 215-750-6343.

BIOCHIMIE. see *BIOLOGY—Biochemistry*

660 GBR
▼ **BIOCOMMERCE DATA'S BUSINESS PROFILE SERIES. VOLUME 1: THE U S BIOTECHNOLOGY DIRECTORY.** Text in English. 2000 (Apr.). irreg. price varies with each vol.. **Document type:** *Monographic series, Academic/Scholarly, Trade.* **Description:** Provides information such as profile, personnel, addresses & phone numbers, products & services on over 860 companies involved in biotechnology in the US.
Published by: Scrip Reports (Subsidiary of: P J B Publications Ltd.), 18/20 Hill Rise, Richmond, Surrey TW10 6UA, United Kingdom. TEL 44-20-8332-8964, FAX 44-20-8332-8992, 44-20-8948-6866, custserv@repsinfo.demon.co.uk, http://www.pjbpubs.com/scriprep/index.html.

660 GBR
▼ **BIOCOMMERCE DATA'S BUSINESS PROFILE SERIES. VOLUME 2. THE EUROPEAN BIOTECHNOLOGY DIRECTORY.** Text in English. 2000 (May). irreg. price varies with each vol.. **Document type:** *Monographic series, Academic/Scholarly, Trade.* **Description:** Contains over 650 profiles of biotechnology companies in 25 European countries, including 15 review articles and contact details for European venture capitalists, trade associations and universities. All profiles have been extensively revised and updated.
Published by: Scrip Reports (Subsidiary of: P J B Publications Ltd.), 18/20 Hill Rise, Richmond, Surrey TW10 6UA, United Kingdom. TEL 44-20-8332-8964, FAX 44-20-8332-8992, 44-20-8948-6866, custserv@repsinfo.demon.co.uk, http://www.pjbpubs.com/scriprep/index.html.

660 GBR
▼ **BIOCOMMERCE DATA'S BUSINESS PROFILE SERIES. VOLUME 3: THE INTERNATIONAL BIOTECHNOLOGY DIRECTORY.** Text in English. 2000 (Jun.). irreg. price varies with each vol.. **Document type:** *Monographic series, Academic/Scholarly, Trade.* **Description:** Provides information on 530 worldwide biotechnology companies and trade associations, giving you access to over 1,000 key industry contacts.
Published by: Scrip Reports (Subsidiary of: P J B Publications Ltd.), 18/20 Hill Rise, Richmond, Surrey TW10 6UA, United Kingdom. TEL 44-20-8332-8964, FAX 44-20-8332-8992, 44-20-8948-6866, custserv@repsinfo.demon.co.uk, http://www.pjbpubs.com/scriprep/index.html.

660 GBR
BIOCOMMERCE DATA'S BUSINESS PROFILE SERIES. VOLUME 4: THE U K BIOTECHNOLOGY DIRECTORY. Text in English. 1988. a., latest 2000, 11th Edition. GBP 195, USD 320, JPY 47,000 per vol. (effective 2000). adv. **Document type:** *Directory.* **Description:** Profiles more than 1000 U.K. organizations involved in biotechnology. Contains review articles.
Formerly: The U K Biotechnology Handbook (Year)
Related titles: Online - full text ed.
—BLDSC.
Published by: Scrip Reports (Subsidiary of: P J B Publications Ltd.), 18/20 Hill Rise, Richmond, Surrey TW10 6UA, United Kingdom. TEL 44-20-8332-8964, FAX 44-20-8332-8992, 44-20-8948-6866, custserv@repsinfo.demon.co.uk, http://www.pjbpubs.com/scriprep/index.html.

BIOFORUM INTERNATIONAL. see *BIOLOGY*

660.6 FRA ISSN 0294-3506
TP248.13 CODEN: BIOFEM
BIOFUTUR; mensuel Europeen de biotechnologie. Text mainly in French. 1982. m. (11/yr.). EUR 156 in Europe to institutions; USD 189 elsewhere to institutions except Japan; EUR 94 in Europe to individuals; USD 116 elsewhere to individuals except Japan (effective 2002). adv. bk.rev. back issues avail. *Refereed.* **Document type:** *Academic/Scholarly.* **Description:** Provides a comprehensive picture of the world of biotechnology and its application in all relevant sectors such as health, agro-food, agriculture, the environment.
Related titles: Microform ed.: (from PQC); Online - full text ed.: (from ingenta, Swets Blackwell, ScienceDirect, Institute for Scientific Information); Supplement: Technoscope.
Indexed: ASCA, AgBiotech, Agroforest.Abstr., Anim.Breed.Abstr., Biol.Abstr., Biotech.Cit.Ind., CEABA, Chem.Abstr., Crop Physiol.Abstr., Curr.Adv.Ecol.Sci., Curr.Biotech.Abstr., Curr.Cont., Dairy Sci.Abstr., Derwent Biotech.Abstr., Environ.Abstr., Excerp.Med., Field Crop Abstr., Forest Prod.Abstr., Forest.Abstr., Hort.Abstr., INIS Atomind., Ind.Med. (coverage dropped), Ind.Vet., Int.Abstr.Biol.Sci., Nonwov.Abstr., Paper & Bd.Abstr., Plant Breed.Abstr., Ref.Zh., Rev.Appl.Entomol., Rev.Plant Path., Rice Abstr., Rural Devel.Abstr., SSCI (coverage dropped), Sci.Cit.Ind. (coverage dropped), Seed Abstr., Telegen, World Ag.Econ.& Rur.Soc.Abstr.
—BLDSC (2072.147000), CASDDS, CISTI, EMDOCS, GNLM, IDS, Infotrieve. **CCC.**
Published by: Elsevier Paris, Editions Scientifiques et Medicales (Subsidiary of: Reed Elsevier plc. group), 23 rue Linois, Paris 75015, France. TEL 33-1-45589110, FAX 33-1-45589419, biofutur@elsevier-fr.com, http://www.elsevier.com/locate/biofut. Ed. Catherine Tastemain. Circ: 10,000.

BIOMATERIALS. see *MEDICAL SCIENCES*

660.6 NLD ISSN 1389-0344
CODEN: BIENFV
BIOMOLECULAR ENGINEERING. Text in Dutch. 1983. bi-m. EUR 93 in Europe to individuals; JPY 12,300 in Japan to individuals; USD 104 elsewhere to individuals; EUR 419 in Europe to institutions; JPY 55,600 in Japan to institutions; USD 469 elsewhere to institutions (effective 2002). abstr, bibl. reprint service avail. from SWZ. *Refereed.* **Document type:** *Academic/Scholarly.* **Description:** Publishes papers on new methods, materials and instruments for biomolecular engineering, molecular biology, cell biology, biochemistry, and genetics.

Former titles (until 1995): Genetic Analysis: Biomolecular Engineering - Techniques and Applications (1050-3862); (until 1990): Genetic Analysis Techniques (0735-0651)
Related titles: Microform ed.: (from PQC); Online - full text ed.: (from ingenta, Swets Blackwell, ScienceDirect, Institute for Scientific Information).
Indexed: ASCA, AgBiotech, Anim.Breed.Abstr., Aqua.Sci.& Fish.Abstr., BBCI, Biol.Abstr., Biotech.Cit.Ind., Chem.Abstr., Chem.Indus.Notes, Chem.Titles, Curr.Adv.Ecol.Sci., Curr.Cont., Dairy Sci.Abstr., Derwent Biotech.Abstr., Environ.Sci.Poll.Mgmt., Excerp.Med., Genet.Abstr., Hum.Gen.Abstr., INIS Atomind., Ind.Med. (1999-), Ind.Vet., Inpharma, Int.Abstr.Biol.Sci., Mass Spectr.Bull., Med.& Pharm.Biotech.Abstr., Microbiol.Abstr., Nuc.Acids Abstr., Nutr.Abstr., Oncog.G.F.Abstr. (coverage dropped), Pig News & Info., Plant Breed.Abstr., Reac., Rev.Appl.Entomol., Rev.Med.& Vet.Mycol., Sci.Cit.Ind., Telegen, Vet.Bull., World Ag.Econ.& Rur.Soc.Abstr.
—BLDSC (2089.255000), CASDDS, CISTI, EMDOCS, GNLM, IDS, ingenta, Linda Hall. **CCC.**
Published by: Elsevier Science BV, PO Box 211, Amsterdam 1000 AE, Netherlands. TEL 31-20-485-2911, FAX 31-20-485-2457, nlinfo-f@elsevier.nl, http://www.elsevier.com/locate/geneanabioeng, http://www.elsevier.nl. Eds. Cassandra L Smith, Changwong Kang. **Subscr. in Australasia and the Far East to:** Elsevier Science (Singapore) Pte Ltd, No.1 Temasek Ave, 17-01 Millenia Tower, Singapore 039192, Singapore. TEL 65-434-3727; **Subscr. in Japan to:** Elsevier Science Inc - Japan Regional Office, 9-15 Higashi-Azabu 1-chome, Minato-ku, Tokyo 106-0044, Japan. TEL 81-3-5561-5033; **Subscr. in the Americas to:** Elsevier Science, PO Box 945, New York, NY 10159-0945. TEL 212-633-3730, usinfo-f@elsevier.com, http://www.elsevier.com.

BIOPHOENIX DATABASE ON CD-ROM. see *MEDICAL SCIENCES*

BIOPHOTONICS INTERNATIONAL; photonic solutions for biotechnology and medicine. see *MEDICAL SCIENCES*

660.6 572 JPN ISSN 0916-8451
QH345 CODEN: BBBIEJ
BIOSCIENCE, BIOTECHNOLOGY, AND BIOCHEMISTRY. Text in English. 1924. m. USD 360 to non-members; USD 100 to members (effective 2000). adv. *Refereed.* **Document type:** *Academic/Scholarly.* **Description:** Publishes original papers and reviews in the fields of bioscience, biotechnology and biochemistry.
Formerly (until 1992): Agricultural and Biological Chemistry (0002-1369)
Related titles: Online - full text ed.: (from Institute for Scientific Information).
Indexed: ASCA, AgBiotech, Agri.& Environ.Biotech.Abstr., Agri.Eng.Abstr., Agroforest.Abstr., Anal.Abstr., Anim.Breed.Abstr., Apic.Abstr., Aqua.Sci.& Fish.Abstr., BBCI, Biodet.Abstr., Biol.& Agr.Ind. (Jan.1992-), Biol.Abstr., Biotech.Cit.Ind., CEABA, Chem.Abstr., Chem.Cit.Ind., Chem.Indus.Notes, Chem.Titles, Chemorec.Abstr., Cott.& Trop.Fibr.Abstr., Crop Physiol.Abstr., Curr.Adv.Biochem., Curr.Adv.Ecol.Sci., Curr.Adv.Gen.& Molec.Biol., Curr.Adv.Plant Sci., Curr.Biotech.Abstr., Curr.Cont., Dairy Sci.Abstr., Derwent Biotech.Abstr., Energy Ind., Energy Info.Abstr., Environ.Abstr., Environ.Sci.Poll.Mgmt., Excerp.Med., Fababean Abstr., Field Crop Abstr., Food Sci.& Tech.Abstr., Forest Prod.Abstr., Forest.Abstr., Genet.Abstr., Helminthol.Abstr., Herb.Abstr., Hort.Abstr., Hum.Gen.Abstr., INIS Atomind., Ind.Med. (1992-), Ind.Sci.Rev., Ind.Vet., Int.Abstr.Biol.Sci., Irr.& Drain.Abstr., MOS, Maize Abstr., Mass Spectr.Bull., Med.& Pharm.Biotech.Abstr., Microbiol.Abstr., NPU, Neurosci.Abstr., Neurosci.Cit.Ind., Nutr.Abstr., Ornam.Hort., Pig News & Info., Plant Breed.Abstr., Plant Grow.Reg.Abstr., Plant Sci., Pollut.Abstr., Postharvest, Potato Abstr., Poult.Abstr., Protozool.Abstr., RCI, Ref.Zh., Rev.Appl.Entomol., Rev.Arom.& Med.Plants, Rev.Med.& Vet.Mycol., Rev.Plant Path., Rice Abstr., Rural Recreat.Tour.Abstr., SSCI (coverage dropped), Sci.Cit.Ind., Seed Abstr., Sel.Water Res.Abstr., Soils & Fert., Sorghum & Millets Abstr., Soyabean Abstr., Sport Fish.Abstr., Sugar Ind.Abstr., Telegen, Triticale Abstr., VITIS, Vet.Bull., Weed Abstr., Wild.Rev., World Ag.Econ.& Rur.Soc.Abstr.
—BLDSC (2089.611470), CASDDS, CINDOC, CISTI, GNLM, IDS, Infotrieve, ingenta, KNAW, Linda Hall. **CCC.**
Published by: Japan Society for Bioscience Biotechnology and Agrochemistry/Nippon Nogeikagaku Kai, 2-4-16 Yayoi, Bunkyo-ku, Tokyo 113-0032, Japan. TEL 81-3-3811-8789, FAX 81-3-3815-1920, http://wwwsoc.nacsis.ac.jp/jsbba, http://www.jsbba.or.jp/. Ed. Shuichi Kaminogawa. Circ: 3,000.

660.6 GBR ISSN 0956-5663
R857.B54 CODEN: BBIOE4
BIOSENSORS AND BIOELECTRONICS. Text in English. 1985. m. EUR 1,060 in Europe to institutions; JPY 140,700 in Japan to institutions; USD 1,186 elsewhere to institutions (effective 2002). adv. bk.rev. charts, illus. index. back issues avail. *Refereed.* **Document type:** *Academic/Scholarly.* **Description:** Covers research, technology and applications of biosensors and the exploitation of biochemicals in electronic devices.
Formerly (until 1989): Biosensors (0265-928X)
Related titles: Online - full text ed.: (from ingenta, Swets Blackwell, ScienceDirect, Institute for Scientific Information).
Indexed: ASCA, Agri.& Environ.Biotech.Abstr. (coverage dropped), Agri.Eng.Abstr., Anal.Abstr., Anim.Breed.Abstr., Aqua.Sci.& Fish.Abstr., BBCI, Bioeng.Abstr., Biol.Abstr., Biotech.Cit.Ind., CEABA, Chem.Abstr., Chem.Cit.Ind., Chem.Indus.Notes, Chem.Titles, Chemorec.Abstr., Curr.Adv.Ecol.Sci., Curr.Biotech.Abstr., Curr.Cont., Dairy Sci.Abstr., Derwent Biotech.Abstr., Eng.Ind., Environ.Abstr., Environ.Sci.Poll.Mgmt., Excerp.Med., Helminthol.Abstr., INSPEC (1990-), Ind.Med. (1990-), Ind.Sci.Rev., Ind.Vet., Int.Abstr.Biol.Sci., Med.& Pharm.Biotech.Abstr., Nutr.Abstr., Pollut.Abstr., Ref.Zh., Rev.Appl.Entomol., Rev.Arom.& Med.Plants, Rev.Plant Path., Sci.Cit.Ind., Sugar Ind.Abstr., Telegen, W.R.C.Inf., Weed Abstr.
—BLDSC (2089.611910), ADONIS, AskIEEE, CASDDS, CISTI, Ei, EMDOCS, GNLM, IDS, ingenta, Linda Hall. **CCC.**
Published by: Pergamon (Subsidiary of: Elsevier Science), The Boulevard, Langford Ln, East Park, Kidlington, Oxford OXB 1GB, United Kingdom. FAX 44-1865-843010, nlinfo-f@elsevier.nl; usinfo-f@elsevier.com; forinfo-kyf04035@niftyserve.or.jp, http://www.elsevier.com/locate/bios, http://www.elsevier.nl/. Eds. A P F Turner, D Cullen. **Subscr. in Australasia and the Far East to:** Elsevier Science (Singapore) Pte Ltd, No.1 Temasek Ave, 17-01 Millenia Tower, Singapore 039192, Singapore. TEL 65-434-3727, FAX 65-337-2230; **Subscr. in the Americas to:** Elsevier Science, PO Box 945, New York, NY 10159-0945. TEL 212-633-3730, FAX 212-633-3680, usinfo-f@elsevier.com, http://www.elsevier.com; **Subscr. to:** Elsevier Science BV, PO Box 211, Amsterdam 1000 AE, Netherlands. TEL 31-20-485-3757, FAX 31-20-485-3432, nlinfo-f@elsevier.nl, http://www.elsevier.nl.

660 DEU ISSN 0937-2725
BIOTEC. Text in German. 1989. bi-m. EUR 33 domestic; EUR 54 foreign; EUR 6.50 newsstand/cover (effective 2002). **Document type:** *Magazine, Trade.*
Published by: Vereinigte Fachverlage GmbH, Lise-Meitner-Str 2, Mainz 55129, Germany. TEL 49-6131-992-0, FAX 49-6131-992-100, info@vfmz.de, http://www.industrie-service.de.

660.6 USA ISSN 0899-5702
BIOTECH BUSINESS. Text in English. 1988. m. USD 150 in North America; USD 165 elsewhere (effective 2001). pat. **Document type:** *Newsletter, Trade.* **Description:** Focuses on the latest fast-breaking developments in the technology and business of biotechnology. Provides news on patents, international business deals, licensing agreements, and developments in human, animal, and plant genetic engineering.
Related titles: Online - full text ed.: (from Data-Star, The Dialog Corporation, Gale Group, NewsNet, LexisNexis, ProQuest Information & Learning, Factiva).
—CCC.
Published by: Worldwide Videotex, PO Box 3273, Boynton Beach, FL 33424-3273. TEL 561-738-2276, markedit@juno.com, http://www.wvpubs.com. Ed., Pub. Mark Wright.

660 681 USA
BIOTECH EQUIPMENT UPDATE. Text in English. m. USD 150 in North Africa; USD 165 elsewhere (effective 2001). **Document type:** *Newsletter, Trade.* **Description:** Covers news and the latest information about biotechnology laboratory and manufacturing equipment and products.
Published by: Worldwide Videotex, PO Box 3273, Boynton Beach, FL 33424-3273. TEL 561-738-2276, markedit@juno.com, http://www.wvpubs.com. Ed., Pub., R&P Mark Wright.

330 660 340 USA
BIOTECH MARKET NEWS & LEGAL STRATEGIES. Text in English. 1985. m. USD 322 (effective 1998). **Document type:** *Newsletter.*
Formerly: BioTech Market News and Strategies (0740-1221)
Published by: Chandler Publishing Ltd., PO Box 11155, Ft. Lauderdale, FL 33339. TEL 954-522-4344, FAX 954-522-7750. Ed. Edward J Chandler. Circ: 15,000.

BIOTECH NAVIGATOR. see *BUSINESS AND ECONOMICS—Investments*

660 USA ISSN 1527-9162
TP248.25.A96 CODEN: BSIJF7
BIOTECH SOFTWARE AND INTERNET REPORT; the computer software journal for scientists. Text in English. 1984. bi-m. USD 99 domestic online; USD 298 foreign online (effective 2002). software rev., bk.rev. back issues avail. *Refereed.* **Document type:** *Academic/Scholarly.* **Description:** Contains news and reviews of all areas of scientific computing, including software, hardware and network products. Expanded coverage to include rapidly expanding base of Internet applications available to researchers.
Former titles (until 1999): Biotechnology Software & Internet Journal (1088-4270); (until 1996): Biotechnology Software Journal (1077-4890); (until 1994): Biotechnology Software (0749-0372)
Related titles: Online - full text ed.: USD 99 to individuals; USD 298 to institutions (effective 2002); Free with Print Edition (from CatchWord Ltd., EBSCO Publishing, O C L C Online Computer Library Center, Inc., RoweCom Information Quest, Swets Blackwell, Institute for Scientific Information).
Indexed: Biotech.Cit.Ind., Telegen.
—CASDDS, CatchWord, CISTI, IDS, Infotrieve, ingenta. **CCC.**
Published by: Mary Ann Liebert, Inc. Publishers, 2 Madison Ave, Larchmont, NY 10538. TEL 914—834-3100, FAX 914-834-1388, info@liebertpub.com, www.liebertpub.com/bsw, http://www.liebertpub.com. Eds. Darryl Nishimura, Robert H Gross.

660 BEL
BIOTECH TECH INTERNATIONAL; The European Magazine for the life sciences Industry. Variant title: B T I. Text in English. 1989. bi-m. BEF 3,000 in Europe; USD 90 in Africa; USD 95 in the Americas. adv. illus, tr.lit. **Document type:** *Magazine, Trade.* **Description:** Provides a mix of technology, research, product & industry news.
Formerly (until 1999): Biotech Products International
Published by: Elsevier Business Information - Belgium (Subsidiary of: Reed Elsevier plc), Rue des Palais 100, Brussels B-1030, Belgium. TEL 32-2-240-2611, FAX 32-2-242-7111, ebi@ebi.be, http://www.ebi.be. Ed. Tony Spit. Pub., R&P Dr. Bernard Leger. Adv. contact Astrid Wydouw. Circ: 27,003 (controlled).

660 USA
BIOTECH WATCH. Text in English. d.
Media: Online - full text.
Published by: The Bureau of National Affairs, Inc., 1231 25th St, N W, Washington, DC 20037. TEL 800-372-1033, http://www.bna.com. **Subscr. to:** 9435 Key West Ave, Rockville, MD 20850.

BIOTECHNIC AND HISTOCHEMISTRY; a journal for microtechnic and histochemistry. see *BIOLOGY—Microscopy*

660.6 USA ISSN 0736-6205
CODEN: BTNQDO
BIOTECHNIQUES; the journal of laboratory technology for bioresearch. Text in English. 1983. 12/yr. USD 110 domestic; USD 142 foreign (effective 2000). adv. bk.rev. back issues avail.; reprints avail. *Refereed.* **Document type:** *Journal, Academic/Scholarly.*
Related titles: Online - full text ed.: (from Institute for Scientific Information); Regional ed.: BioTechniques (Euro Edition).
Indexed: ASCA, AgBiotech, BBCI, Bio-Contr.News & Info., Biotech.Cit.Ind., Cal.Tiss.Abstr., Chem.Abstr., Chem.Cit.Ind., Chem.Indus.Notes, Chem.Titles, Curr.Adv.Biochem., Curr.Adv.Ecol.Sci., Curr.Adv.Gen.& Molec.Biol., Curr.Cont., Derwent Biotech.Abstr., Eng.Ind., Environ.Sci.Poll.Mgmt., Excerp.Med., Food Sci.& Tech.Abstr., Forest.Abstr., INIS Atomind., Ind.Med. (1983-), Ind.Sci.Rev., Inpharma, Int.Abstr.Biol.Sci., Plant Breed.Abstr., Protozool.Abstr., Reac., Rev.Appl.Entomol., Sci.Cit.Ind., Soils & Fert., Sport Fish.Abstr., Telegen, Triticale Abstr.
—BLDSC (2089.820000), CASDDS, CISTI, Ei, EMDOCS, GNLM, IDS, ingenta, Linda Hall. **CCC.**
Published by: Eaton Publishing Co., One Research Dr, Suite 400A, PO Box 1070, Westboro, MA 01581. TEL 508-655-8282, FAX 508-655-9910, bioeditor@biotechniques.com, http://www.biotechniques.com. Ed., R&P James Ellingboe. Pub. Frank Eaton. Adv. contact Esta Campbell. Circ: 60,000 (controlled).

BIOTECHNOLOGY ABSTRACTS. see *BIOLOGY—Abstracting, Bibliographies, Statistics*

660 610.28 USA ISSN 0734-9750
TP248.2 CODEN: BIADDD
BIOTECHNOLOGY ADVANCES; research reviews and patent abstracts. Text in English. 1983. 8/yr. EUR 1,124 in Europe to institutions; JPY 149,300 in Japan to institutions; USD 1,257 elsewhere to institutions (effective 2002). pat, abstr. back issues avail. *Refereed.* **Document type:** *Academic/Scholarly.* **Description:** Covers all aspects of biotechnology including relevant developments in related disciplines of biology, chemistry, and engineering.
Related titles: Microfilm ed.: (from PQC); Online - full text ed.: (from ingenta, Swets Blackwell, ScienceDirect, Institute for Scientific Information).
Indexed: ASCA, AgBiotech, Agri.& Environ.Biotech.Abstr., Aqua.Sci.& Fish.Abstr., Bibl.Agri., Biodet.Abstr., Bioeng.Abstr., Biotech.Cit.Ind., Chem.Abstr., Chem.Cit.Ind., Chem.Indus.Notes, Chem.Titles, Curr.Adv.Ecol.Sci., Curr.Biotech.Abstr., Curr.Cont., Dairy Sci.Abstr., Derwent Biotech.Abstr., Ecol.Abstr., Eng.Ind., Environ.Sci.Poll.Mgmt., Geo.Abstr.P.G., Hort.Abstr., Ind.Sci.Rev., Ind.Vet., Int.Abstr.Biol.Sci., Med.& Pharm.Biotech.Abstr., Microbiol.Abstr., Ornam.Hort., Paper & Bd.Abstr., Plant Breed.Abstr., Plant Grow.Reg.Abstr., Pollut.Abstr., Ref.Zh., Rev.Appl.Entomol., Rev.Arom.& Med.Plants, Rev.Plant Path., Sci.Cit.Ind., Soils & Fert., Sugar Ind.Abstr., Telegen, Trop.Dis.Bull.
—BLDSC (2089.845000), ADONIS, CASDDS, CISTI, Ei, EMDOCS, GNLM, IDS, Infotrieve, ingenta, Linda Hall. **CCC.**
Published by: Elsevier Science, PO Box 945, New York, NY 10159-0945. TEL 212-989-5800, FAX 212-633-3990, usinfo-f@elsevier.com, http://www.elsevier.nl/locate/biotechadv, http://www.elsevier.com. Ed. M Moo Young. **Subscr. in Australasia and the Far East to:** Elsevier Science (Singapore) Pte Ltd, No.1 Temasek Ave, 17-01 Millenia Tower, Singapore 039192, Singapore. TEL 65-434-3727, FAX 65-337-2230**; Subscr. in Japan to:** Elsevier Science Inc - Japan Regional Office, 9-15 Higashi-Azabu 1-chome, Minato-ku, Tokyo 106-0044, Japan. TEL 81-3-5561-5033, FAX 81-3-5561-5047**; Subscr. outside the Americas to:** Elsevier Science BV, PO Box 211, Amsterdam 1000 AE, Netherlands. TEL 31-20-485-3757, FAX 31-20-485-3432, nlinfo-f@elsevier.nl, http://www.elsevier.nl.

660 612.015 GBR ISSN 0885-4513
QP501 CODEN: BABIEC
BIOTECHNOLOGY AND APPLIED BIOCHEMISTRY. Text in English. 1979. bi-m. USD 141 in US & Canada to individuals; GBP 92.89 elsewhere to individuals; USD 292 in US & Canada Print & online eds.; GBP 168 elsewhere Print & online eds. (effective 2002). adv. index. back issues avail. *Refereed.* **Document type:** *Journal, Academic/Scholarly.* **Description:** Publication of articles concerning expression, purification, characterization and application of biological macromolecules in therapeutics and diagnostics with medical, dental and veterinary applications.
Formerly: Journal of Applied Biochemistry (0161-7354)
Related titles: CD-ROM ed.; Online - full text ed.: ISSN 1470-8744. USD 131 in US & Canada to individuals; GBP 75 elsewhere to individuals; USD 275 in US & Canada to institutions; GBP 157 elsewhere to institutions (effective 2001) (from EBSCO Publishing, RoweCom Information Quest, Swets Blackwell, Institute for Scientific Information).
Indexed: A.S.& T.Ind. (Jan.2001-), ASCA, Abstr.Bull.Inst.Pap.Chem., AgBiotech, Agri.& Environ.Biotech.Abstr., Agricola, Anim.Breed.Abstr., Aqua.Sci.& Fish.Abstr., BBCI, Bio-Contr.News & Info., Biodet.Abstr., Biotech.Cit.Ind., CEABA, Chem.Abstr., Chem.Cit.Ind., Chem.Indus.Notes, Chem.Titles, Curr.Biotech.Abstr., Curr.Cont., Curr.Leather Lit., Dairy Sci.Abstr., Derwent Biotech.Abstr., Eng.Ind., Environ.Sci.Poll.Mgmt., Excerp.Med., Food Sci.& Tech.Abstr., INIS Atomind., Ind.Med. (1986-), Ind.Vet., Inpharma, Int.Abstr.Biol.Sci., Maize Abstr., Mass Spectr.Bull., Med.& Pharm.Biotech.Abstr., Microbiol.Abstr., Ocean.Abstr. (coverage dropped), Pharm.&Out.News, Plant Breed.Abstr., Plant Grow.Reg.Abstr., Potato Abstr., Protozool.Abstr., Reac., Rev.Appl.Entomol., Rev.Med.& Vet.Mycol., Rev.Plant Path., Sci.Cit.Ind., Sugar Ind.Abstr., Vet.Bull.
—BLDSC (2089.848000), ADONIS, CASDDS, CINDOC, CISTI, Ei, EMDOCS, GNLM, IDS, ingenta, Linda Hall. **CCC.**
Published by: (International Union of Biochemistry USA), Portland Press Ltd., 59 Portland Pl, London W1N 3AJ, United Kingdom. TEL 44-20-7580-5530, FAX 44-20-7323-1136, editl@portlandpress.com, http://bab.portlandpress.com, http:// www.portlandpress.com/. Ed. R L Lundblad. Adv. contact Sarah Laflin. Circ: 575. **Subscr. to:** Commerce Way, Colchester, Essex CO2 8HP, United Kingdom. FAX 44-1206-796351, 44-1206-799331.

660.6 574.28 USA ISSN 0006-3592
QH324 CODEN: BIBIAU
BIOTECHNOLOGY AND BIOENGINEERING. Text in English. 1958. 28/yr. USD 4,125 in United States; USD 4,405 in Canada & Mexico; USD 4,643 elsewhere; USD 4,332 combined subscription in United States for print and online eds.; USD 4,612 combined subscription in Canada & Mexico for print and online eds.; USD 4,850 combined subscription elsewhere for print and online eds. (effective 2002). adv. bibl, charts, illus. index. back issues avail.; reprints avail. *Refereed.* **Document type:** *Proceedings, Academic/Scholarly.* **Description:** Presents original research on all aspects of biochemical and microbial technology.
Related titles: CD-ROM ed.: (from The Dialog Corporation); Microform ed.: (from PQC); Online - full text ed.: ISSN 1097-0290. USD 4,125 in United States; USD 4,125 in Canada & Mexico; USD 4,125 elsewhere (effective 2002) (from EBSCO Publishing, Wiley InterScience, Institute for Scientific Information).
Indexed: AESIS, ASCA, Abstr.Bull.Inst.Pap.Chem., AgBiotech, Agri.& Environ.Biotech.Abstr., Agricola, Anal.Abstr., Aqua.Sci.& Fish.Abstr., Bio-Contr.News & Info., Biodet.Abstr., Bioeng.Abstr., Biol.& Agr.Ind. (Mar.1990-), Biol.Abstr., Biotech.Cit.Ind., CEABA, Chem.Abstr., Chem.Cit.Ind., Chem.Eng.Abstr., Chem.Indus.Notes, Chem.Titles, Comput.& Info.Sys., Crop Physiol.Abstr., Curr.Adv.Biochem., Curr.Adv.Cancer Res., Curr.Adv.Cell & Devel.Biol., Curr.Adv.Ecol.Sci., Curr.Adv.Gen.& Molec.Biol., Curr.Biotech.Abstr., Curr.Cont., Dairy Sci.Abstr., Deep Sea Res.& Oceanogr.Abstr., Derwent Biotech.Abstr., Energy Ind., Energy Info.Abstr., Eng.Ind., Environ.Sci.Poll.Mgmt., Excerp.Med., Field Crop Abstr., Food Sci.& Tech.Abstr., Forest Prod.Abstr., Gas Abstr., Helminthol.Abstr., Herb.Abstr., Hort.Abstr., INIS Atomind., Ind.Med. (1962-), Ind.Sci.Rev., Ind.Vet., Inpharma, Int.Abstr.Biol.Sci., Int.Abstr.Oper.Res., Maize Abstr., Mass Spectr.Bull., Mat.Sci.Cit.Ind. (coverage dropped), Med.& Pharm.Biotech.Abstr., Microbiol.Abstr., Nutr.Abstr., Ocean.Abstr. (coverage dropped), Pig News & Info., Plant Breed.Abstr., Plant Grow.Reg.Abstr., Pollut.Abstr., Potato Abstr., Poult.Abstr., Reac., Ref.Zh., Rev.Appl.Entomol., Rev.Arom.& Med.Plants, Rev.Med.& Vet.Mycol., Rev.Plant Path., Rice Abstr., Sci.Cit.Ind., Sel.J.Water, Sel.Water Res.Abstr., Soils & Fert., Sorghum & Millets Abstr., Sugar Ind.Abstr., T.C.E.A., Triticale Abstr., Vet.Bull., W.R.C.Inf., Weed Abstr.
—BLDSC (2089.850000), CASDDS, Ei, EMDOCS, GNLM, IDS, ingenta, Linda Hall. **CCC.**
Published by: John Wiley & Sons, Inc., Journals (Subsidiary of: Wiley InterScience), 605 Third Ave, New York, NY 10158. TEL 212-850-6645, FAX 212-850-6021, subinfo@jwiley.com, uscs-wis@wiley.com, http://www.wiley.com. Ed. Douglas S Clark. adv.: B&W page GBP 640, color page GBP 1,515. Circ: 1,700. **Subscr. addr. outside the Americans:** John Wiley & Sons Ltd., Baffins Ln, Chichester, Sussex PO19 IUD, United Kingdom. TEL 44-1243-779777, FAX 44-1243-843232, cs-journals@wiley.co.uk, http://www.wiley.co.uk.

660.6 572.43 BGR ISSN 0205-2067
BIOTECHNOLOGY AND BIOTECHNOLOGICAL EQUIPMENT; international scientific-theoretical and applied publication. Text in English. 1984. s-a. BGL 120 domestic; USD 180 foreign (effective 2000). adv. abstr, illus. back issues avail. *Refereed.* **Document type:** *Magazine, Proceedings, Academic/Scholarly.*
Related titles: CD-ROM ed.; Diskette ed.; E-mail ed.; Fax ed.; Online - full text ed.: (from Institute for Scientific Information).
Indexed: Biotech.Cit.Ind.
—BLDSC.
Published by: Diagnosis Press Ltd., 5 Malusba Str, Sofia 1421, Bulgaria. diagnosis@ibn.bg, http:// www.diagnosispress.com. Ed. Atanas Atanassov. Pub. Snejana Pavlova. Circ: 250 (paid); 250 (controlled).

663.1 NLD ISSN 0924-9877
BIOTECHNOLOGY AND DEVELOPMENT MONITOR. Text in English. 1989. q. free. *Refereed.* **Document type:** *Journal, Academic/Scholarly.* **Description:** Analyzes worldwide developments in biotechnology, and trade and technology related international regulation, in the context of its socio-economic implications for developing countries.
Related titles: Online - full text ed.: (from Institute for Scientific Information).
Indexed: AgBiotech, Bio-Contr.News & Info., Biotech.Cit.Ind., Plant Breed.Abstr., Plant Gen.Res.Abstr., Potato Abstr., Rice Abstr., Rural Devel.Abstr., Seed Abstr., Weed Abstr., World Ag.Econ.& Rur.Soc.Abstr.
—BLDSC (2089.860350).
Address: Universiteit van Amsterdam, Department of Social Sciences, Oudezijds Achterburgwal 237, Amsterdam 1012 DL, Netherlands. TEL 31-20-5252177, FAX 31-20-5252086, monitor@pscw.uva.nl, http://www.pscw.uva.nl/monitor. Ed. Bert Ernste.

660 574.28 610 GBR ISSN 0264-8725
TP248.13 CODEN: BGERES
BIOTECHNOLOGY AND GENETIC ENGINEERING REVIEWS. Text in English. 1984. a. GBP 110 (effective Jun. 2001). index. back issues avail. *Refereed.* **Document type:** *Academic/Scholarly.* **Description:** Contains original major review articles covering important developments in industrial, agricultural and medical applications of biotechnology, with particular emphasis on the generic manipulation of the organisms concerned.
Related titles: Online - full text ed.: (from Institute for Scientific Information).
Indexed: ASCA, AgBiotech, Agricola, Biol.& Agr.Ind. (Jan.1996-), Biol.Abstr., Biotech.Cit.Ind., Chem.Abstr., Chem.Indus.Notes, Chem.Titles, Crop Physiol.Abstr., Curr.Adv.Ecol.Sci., Curr.Biotech.Abstr., Curr.Cont. (coverage dropped), Derwent Biotech.Abstr., Eng.Ind., Field Crop Abstr., Ind.Med. (1984-), Ind.Sci.Rev., Ind.Vet., Int.Abstr.Biol.Sci., Maize Abstr., Plant Breed.Abstr., Plant Sci., Potato Abstr., Sci.Cit.Ind., Telegen, Triticale Abstr., Vet.Bull.
—BLDSC (2089.860500), CASDDS, CISTI, Ei, GNLM, Infotrieve, ingenta, KNAW, Linda Hall. **CCC.**
Published by: Intercept Ltd, PO Box 716, Andover, Hants SP10 1YG, United Kingdom. TEL 44-1264-334748, FAX 44-1264-334058, intercept@andover.co.uk, http://www.intercept.co.uk. Ed. Stephen Harding. Circ: 300.

660 USA
BIOTECHNOLOGY AT WORK SERIES. Text in English. irreg., latest vol.10, 1992. **Document type:** *Monographic series.* **Description:** Covers the latest developments of biotechnology in the environmental, agricultural and medical fields.
Published by: Biotechnology Industry Organization, 1625 K St, N W, Ste 1100, Washington, DC 20006. TEL 202-857-0244, FAX 202-857-0237, info@bio.org, http://www.bio.org, http://www.hol.gr/bio. R&P Dan Eramian.

660.607 GBR ISSN 0955-6621
TP248.13 CODEN: BIEDEY
BIOTECHNOLOGY EDUCATION. Text in English. 1990. 4/yr. GBP 75 (effective 1993). back issues avail. *Refereed.* **Document type:** *Academic/Scholarly.* **Description:** Resource for teachers and students in the biological sciences.
Related titles: Microfilm ed.: (from PQC).
Indexed: Chem.Abstr., Chem.Indus.Notes, Chem.Titles.
—CASDDS.
Published by: Helix Publishing, 1 Howard Ct, 94-96 Blackheath Hill, Greenwich, London SE10 8AF, United Kingdom. Ed. Paul Wymer.

570 660.6 USA
BIOTECHNOLOGY GUIDE U.S.A. Text in English. 1989. a. USD 249 (effective 1998). **Document type:** *Academic/Scholarly, Trade.* **Description:** Profiles over 1,300 companies active in biotechnology, lists venture capital firms, and analyzes the biotechnology industry.
Published by: Institute for Biotechnology Information, c/o Mark Dibner, Pres., Box 14569, Research Triangle Park, NC 27709-4569. TEL 919-544-5111, FAX 919-544-5401, ibi@mindspring.com, http://www.biotechinfo.com.

660 USA ISSN 1052-6153
CODEN: BHANE3
BIOTECHNOLOGY HANDBOOKS. Text in English. 1987. irreg., latest vol.10, 1998. **Document type:** *Monographic series, Academic/Scholarly.*
Indexed: Chem.Abstr., Chem.Indus.Notes, Chem.Titles.
—BLDSC (2089.861590), CASDDS, CISTI. **CCC.**
Published by: Kluwer Academic - Plenum Publishers (Subsidiary of: Wolters Kluwer N.V.), 233 Spring St, New York, NY 10013-1578. TEL 212-620-8000, 800-221-9369, FAX 212-463-0742, info@plenum.com, http://www.plenum.com. Eds. Roger F Sherwood, Tony Atkinson.

660 630 USA ISSN 0934-943X
CODEN: BAFOEG
BIOTECHNOLOGY IN AGRICULTURE AND FORESTRY. Text in English. 1986. irreg., latest vol.34, 1995. price varies. reprint service avail. from ISI. **Document type:** *Academic/Scholarly.*
Indexed: Chem.Abstr., Chem.Indus.Notes, Chem.Titles.
—BLDSC (2089.847000), CASDDS, CISTI, Infotrieve. **CCC.**

B

Published by: Springer-Verlag, Journals (Subsidiary of: BertelsmannSpringer), 175 Fifth Ave, New York, NY 10010. TEL 212-460-1500, FAX 212-473-6272.

660.6 615.1 USA ISSN 1074-6072
BIOTECHNOLOGY IN THE U.S. PHARMACEUTICAL INDUSTRY. Text in English. 1995. a. USD 279 (effective 1998). **Document type:** *Academic/Scholarly, Trade.*
Published by: Institute for Biotechnology Information, c/o Mark Dibner, Pres., Box 14569, Research Triangle Park, NC 27709-4569. TEL 919-544-5111, FAX 919-544-5401, ibi@mindspring.com, http://www.biotechinfo.com.

BIOTECHNOLOGY INDUSTRY GUIDE. see *BIOLOGY*

BIOTECHNOLOGY INFORMATION. see *BIOLOGY—Abstracting, Bibliographies, Statistics*

B

343.0786606 USA ISSN 0730-031X
KF3827.G4 CODEN: BLREEL
BIOTECHNOLOGY LAW REPORT. Text in English. 1982. bi-m. USD 999 domestic to institutions; USD 1,145 foreign to institutions; USD 1,199 domestic to institutions Print & Online eds.; USD 1,344 foreign to institutions Print & Online eds. (effective 2002). back issues avail.; reprint service avail. from PSC,SCH. *Refereed.* **Document type:** *Journal, Academic/Scholarly.* **Description:** Includes papers by leading international experts on current biotechnology issues;up-to-date information on legal issues related to biotechnology.
Related titles: Online - full content ed.: USD 891 (effective 2001) (from EBSCO Publishing, O C L C Online Computer Library Center, Inc., Swets Blackwell); Online - full text ed.: USD 999 worldwide to institutions (effective 2002) (from CatchWord Ltd., Institute for Scientific Information, RoweCom Information Quest).
Indexed: ABC, ASCA, Arts & Hum.Cit.Ind. (coverage dropped), Biotech.Cit.Ind., Curr.Biotech.Abstr., SSCI (coverage dropped), Telegen.
—CatchWord, IDS, ingenta. **CCC.**
Published by: Mary Ann Liebert, Inc. Publishers, 20 W Third St., Ste 200, Media, PA 19063-2824. TEL 610-892-9580, FAX 610-892-9577, info@liebertpub.com, http://www.liebertpub.com/blr. Eds. Robert A Bohrerz, Gerry J Elman.

660 NLD ISSN 0141-5492
QR53 CODEN: BILED3
BIOTECHNOLOGY LETTERS. Text in Dutch. 1979. s-m. EUR 2,050, USD 2,054 to institutions for print or online ed.; EUR 2,460, USD 2,464.80 to institutions for print & online eds. combined (effective 2002). adv. abstr, bibl, charts, illus. reprints avail. *Refereed.* **Document type:** *Academic/Scholarly.* **Description:** Covers topics relating to actual or potential applications of biological reactions effected by microbial, plant, or animal cells and derived bio-catalysts.
Incorporates (1987-2000): Biotechnology Techniques (0951-208X)
Related titles: Online - full text ed.: (from EBSCO Publishing, O C L C Online Computer Library Center, Inc., RoweCom Information Quest, Swets Blackwell, Kluwer Online, Institute for Scientific Information).
Indexed: AESIS, ASCA, AgBiotech, Agri.& Environ.Biotech.Abstr., Agri.Eng.Abstr., Agricola, Aqua.Sci.& Fish.Abstr., Bibl.Agri., Bio-Contr.News & Info., Biodet.Abstr., Biol.Abstr., Biotech.Cit.Ind., CEABA, Chem.Abstr., Chem.Cit.Ind., Chem.Indus.Notes, Chem.Titles, Chemorec.Abstr., Cott.& Trop.Fibr.Abstr., Crop Physiol.Abstr., Curr.Adv.Biochem., Curr.Adv.Ecol.Sci., Curr.Adv.Gen.& Molec.Biol., Curr.Biotech.Abstr., Curr.Cont., Dairy Sci.Abstr., Derwent Biotech.Abstr., Energy Info.Abstr., Environ.Abstr., Environ.Sci.Poll.Mgmt., Excerp.Med., Field Crop Abstr., Food Sci.& Tech.Abstr., Forest Prod.Abstr., Forest.Abstr., Helminthol.Abstr., Hort.Abstr., INIS Atomind., Ind.Sci.Rev., Ind.Vet., Inpharma, Int.Abstr.Biol.Sci., Maize Abstr., Med.& Pharm.Biotech.Abstr., Microbiol.Abstr., Nutr.Abstr., Ornam.Hort., Plant Breed.Abstr., Plant Grow.Reg.Abstr., Pollut.Abstr., Potato Abstr., Reac., Rev.Appl.Entomol., Rev.Arom.& Med.Plants, Rev.Med.& Vet.Mycol., Rev.Plant Path., Rice Abstr., Saf.Sci.Abstr., Sci.Cit.Ind., Seed Abstr., Sel.Water Res.Abstr., Soils & Fert., Sport Fish.Abstr., Sugar Ind.Abstr., Telegen, Triticale Abstr., Weed Abstr.
—BLDSC (2089.863000), CASDDS, CIS, CISTI, GNLM, IDS, Infotrieve, ingenta. **CCC.**
Published by: Kluwer Academic Publishers Group (Subsidiary of: Wolters Kluwer N.V.), Spuiboulevard 50, PO Box 17, Dordrecht 3300 AA, Netherlands. TEL 31-78-639-2392, FAX 31-78-654-2254, services@wkap.nl, http://www.wkap.nl/journalhome.htm/0141-5492. Ed. Colin Ratledge TEL 44-1482-465243. Adv. contact Gemma Heiser. **Subscr. in N American to:** Kluwer Academic - Plenum Publishers, 233 Spring St, New York, NY 10013-1578. TEL 212-620-8468, FAX 212-807-1047; **Subscr. to:** Journals Department, PO Box 322, Dordrecht 3300 AH, Netherlands. TEL 31-78-639-2392, FAX 31-78-654-6474.

660 USA ISSN 0930-8938
CODEN: BIMOE5
BIOTECHNOLOGY MONOGRAPHS. Text in English. 1985. irreg., latest vol.5. **Document type:** *Monographic series, Academic/Scholarly.*
Indexed: Chem.Abstr., Chem.Indus.Notes, Chem.Titles.
—CASDDS, CISTI, KNAW.
Published by: Springer-Verlag, Journals (Subsidiary of: BertelsmannSpringer), 175 Fifth Ave, New York, NY 10010. TEL 212-460-1500, FAX 212-473-6272.

660 USA ISSN 0273-3226
CODEN: BINWEY
BIOTECHNOLOGY NEWS. Text in English. 1981. 30/yr. USD 634 in US & Canada; USD 658 elsewhere (effective 2001). bk.rev. tr.lit. index. back issues avail. **Document type:** *Newsletter.* **Description:** Written for executives in the biotechnology industry. Covers company news, regulatory changes, financial trends, technical developments, market analyses and patents.
Related titles: Supplement: Bioindustry Directory; Pharma Industry Directory.
Indexed: CEABA, Chem.Abstr., Chem.Indus.Notes, Chem.Titles, Curr.Biotech.Abstr.
—BLDSC (2089.867000), CASDDS, CISTI, Infotrieve. **CCC.**
Published by: C T B International Publishing Inc., PO Box 218, Maplewood, NJ 07040-0218. TEL 973-379-7749, FAX 973-379-1158, info@ctbintl.com, http://www.ctbintl.com. Eds. Christine Yanicek, Christopher Brogna. Pub. Oykue Brogna. R&P Christopher Brogna.

660 USA ISSN 8756-7938
TP248.13 CODEN: BIPRET
BIOTECHNOLOGY PROGRESS. Text in English. 1985. bi-m. USD 718 in North America to institutions; USD 750 elsewhere to institutions; USD 862 in North America to institutions Print & online eds.; USD 894 elsewhere to institutions Print & online eds. (effective 2002); for additional pricing options for print and web editions contact inside sales specialist, Ms. Chako Dickinson, at 202-872-4063. adv. bibl, charts, illus. index. back issues avail.; reprint service avail. from PQC. *Refereed.* **Document type:** *Journal, Trade.* **Description:** Reports developments and research results impacting the food, pharmaceutical and bioengineering fields.
Related titles: Microform ed.: (from PQC); Online - full text ed.: ISSN 1520-6033. USD 754 to institutions (effective 2002) (from EBSCO Publishing, Institute for Scientific Information).
Indexed: AESIS, A.S.& T.Ind. (Jan.1991-), ASCA, AgBiotech, Agri.& Environ.Biotech.Abstr., Agri.Eng.Abstr., Agricola, Aqua.Sci.& Fish.Abstr., Bioeng.Abstr., Biol.Abstr., Biotech.Cit.Ind., CEABA, Chem.Abstr., Chem.Cit.Ind., Chem.Indus.Notes, Chem.Titles, Curr.Adv.Ecol.Sci., Curr.Adv.Plant Sci., Curr.Biotech.Abstr., Curr.Cont., Dairy Sci.Abstr., Derwent Biotech.Abstr., Eng.Ind., Environ.Abstr., Environ.Sci.Poll.Mgmt., Food Sci.& Tech.Abstr., Forest Prod.Abstr., Forest.Abstr., Hort.Abstr., INIS Atomind., ISMEC, Ind.Med. (1985-), Ind.Sci.Rev., Ind.Vet., Inpharma, Int.Abstr.Biol.Sci., Maize Abstr., Med.& Pharm.Biotech.Abstr., Microbiol.Abstr., Nutr.Abstr., Ornam.Hort., Plant Breed.Abstr., Plant Gen.Res.Abstr., Plant Grow.Reg.Abstr., Plant Sci., Pollut.Abstr., Poult.Abstr., Reac., Ref.Zh., Rev.Appl.Entomol., Rev.Arom.& Med.Plants, Rev.Med.& Vet.Mycol., Rev.Plant Path., Sci.Cit.Ind., Seed Abstr., Sel.Water Res.Abstr., Sugar Ind.Abstr., Telegen, Vet.Bull.
—BLDSC (2089.868330), CASDDS, CINDOC, CISTI, Ei, EMDOCS, GNLM, IDS, ingenta, Linda Hall. **CCC.**
Published by: (American Institute of Chemical Engineers), American Chemical Society, 1155 16th St, N W, Washington, DC 20036. TEL 800-333-9511, jssbio@vms.cis.pitt.edu; orders@allenpress.com, http://pubs.acs.org/bp. Ed. Jerome S Schultz. Circ: 2,800. **Subscr.to:** Allen Press Inc., PO Box 1897, Lawrence, KS 66044-8897.

660.6 USA
BIOTECHNOLOGY STATE OF THE INDUSTRY REPORT. Text in English. 1993. a. USD 429 domestic; USD 459 foreign (effective 2001). **Document type:** *Trade.* **Description:** Covers market trends and technical developments in the biotechnology industry.
Published by: American Health Consultants (Subsidiary of: Medical Economics Co., Inc.), 3525 Piedmont Rd, N E, 6 Piedmont Center, Ste 400, Atlanta, GA 30305. TEL 404-262-5476, 404-262-7436, 800-688-2421, FAX 404-262-7837, 800-284-3291, custserv@ahcpub.com, http://www.ahcpub.com.

660 610.28 RUS ISSN 0234-2758
CODEN: BTKNEZ
BIOTEKHNOLOGIYA. Text in Russian; Summaries in English. 1984. bi-m. adv. cum.index: 1985-1995. back issues avail. **Document type:** *Academic/Scholarly.* **Description:** Presents papers and reviews on biotechnology and bioengineering.
Related titles: Diskette ed.; ♦ English Translation: Russian Biotechnology. ISSN 1068-3682.
Indexed: AgBiotech, Anim.Breed.Abstr., Bio-Contr.News & Info., CEABA, Chem.Abstr., Chem.Indus.Notes, Chem.Titles, Crop Physiol.Abstr., Dairy Sci.Abstr., Forest Prod.Abstr., Forest.Abstr., Herb.Abstr., Hort.Abstr., Ind.Vet., Nutr.Abstr., Ornam.Hort., Pig News & Info., Plant Breed.Abstr., Plant Gen.Res.Abstr., Plant Grow.Reg.Abstr., Potato Abstr., Ref.Zh., Rev.Appl.Entomol., Rev.Arom.& Med.Plants, Rev.Med.& Vet.Mycol., Rev.Plant Path., Soils & Fert., Sugar Ind.Abstr., Vet.Bull.
—BLDSC (0017.999000), CASDDS. **CCC.**
Published by: (State Scientific Research Institute for Genetics and Selection of Industrial Microorganisms, G N I I Genetika), M A I K Nauka - Interperiodica, Mezhdunarodnyi Otdel, Profsoyuznaya ul 90, Moscow 117864, Russian Federation. TEL 7-095-3661600, FAX 7-095-336-0666, boss@genetika.ru, compmg@maik.ru, http://www.maik.rssi.ru/. Ed. Vladimir G Debabov. adv.: page RUR 15,000, page USD 500; trim 220 x 160. Circ: 600. **US dist. addr.:** Maik Nauka - Interperiodica. **Dist. by:** Mezhdunarodnaya Kniga.

616 JPN ISSN 0914-2223
CODEN: BITPE9
BIOTHERAPY. Text in Japanese; Summaries in English. 1987. bi-m., latest vol.16. JPY 19,000 (effective 2002). adv. bk.rev. *Refereed.* **Document type:** *Journal, Academic/Scholarly.* **Description:** Covers immunology, molecular biology, cytology and gene therapy. Focuses especially on biological response modifiers. Serves as the official journal of the Society.
Related titles: Microfilm ed.
Indexed: Biol.Abstr., INIS Atomind.
—BLDSC (2089.873900), GNLM.
Published by: (Biological Response Modifiers Society), Japanese Journal of Cancer and Chemotherapy Publishers Inc., Risshu Bldg, 2-2-3 Nihonbashi, Chuo-ku, Tokyo 103-0027, Japan. TEL 81-3-3278-0052, FAX 81-3-3281-0435. Ed., Pub. Tetsuo Taguchi. Adv. contact Katsuko Watanabe. Circ: 2,000 (paid).

660 USA ISSN 0892-1903
CODEN: BIVIEW
BIOVENTURE VIEW. Text in English. 1986. m. (except July-Aug. combined). GBP 485 in Europe; USD 685 in US & Canada; JPY 120,000 in Japan; GBP 510 rest of world (effective 2001). adv. 3 cols./p. back issues avail.; reprints avail. **Document type:** *Newsletter, Magazine, Trade.* **Description:** Offers analysis of the companies, products, and events that drive the multibillion-dollar biotechnology industry.
Related titles: Online - full text ed.: (from CompuServe, Inc., Data-Star, The Dialog Corporation, Dow Jones Interactive, European Space Agency, Gale Group, Northern Light Technology, Inc., Factiva).
—BLDSC (2090.100000), Infotrieve. **CCC.**
Published by: P J B Publications Ltd., 18-20 Hill Rise, Richmond, Surrey TW10 6UA, United Kingdom. TEL 44-20-8948-3262, FAX 44-20-8332-8990, info@pjbpubs.com, http://www.pjbpubs.com/bvv/index.html. Eds. Mark Swallow TEL 44-20-8948-3262, Sukaina Virji. Pub. Philip Brown. Adv. contacts Jason Douglas TEL 212-262-8230, Peter Coltart TEL 44-20-8332-8802. B&W page USD 900; trim 11 x 8.5. Circ: 550 (paid). **Subscr. addr. in N America:** Pharmabooks Ltd., 1775 Broadway, Ste 511, New York, NY 10019. TEL 212-262-8230, FAX 212-262-8234.

660 610.28 CRI ISSN 0255-7924
BOLETIN DE BIOTECNOLOGIA. Text in Spanish. 1984. q. free per issue. bk.rev.
Published by: Consejo Nacional para Investigaciones Cientificas y Tecnologicas, Departamento de Informacion y Documentacion, Apdo. 10318, San Jose, Costa Rica. Circ: 1,500.

C A S BIOTECH UPDATES. ENVIRONMENTAL BIOTECHNOLOGY. see *ENVIRONMENTAL STUDIES—Abstracting, Bibliographies, Statistics*

C A S BIOTECH UPDATES. ENZYMES IN BIOTECHNOLOGY. see *BIOLOGY—Abstracting, Bibliographies, Statistics*

660 GBR ISSN 0957-0330
CODEN: CSBIED
CAMBRIDGE STUDIES IN BIOTECHNOLOGY. Text in English. 1985. irreg. price varies. **Document type:** *Monographic series.*
Indexed: Food Sci.& Tech.Abstr.
—BLDSC (3015.992500), CISTI.
Published by: Cambridge University Press, Edinburgh Bldg, Shaftesbury Rd, Cambridge CB2 2RU, United Kingdom. FAX 44-1223-315052, information@cup.cam.ac.uk, information@cambridge.org, http://www.cup.cam.ac.uk, http://www.uk.cambridge.org/journals/pmu. R&P Linda Nicol.

660.6 CAN ISSN 1188-455X
CANADIAN BIOTECH NEWS. Text in English. 1988. 52/yr. CND 500, USD 425 (effective 1999). adv. bk.rev. back issues avail. **Document type:** *Newsletter.* **Description:** Covers economics and finance in biotechnology. Includes information on company developments, patents and technology transfer.
Incorporates (in 1997): Intron - Canadian Molecular Biology; Formerly (until vol.4, no.10): New Biotech Business (0838-5777)
Related titles: Microfiche ed.: (from MML).
Indexed: CBCA Ref., Can.B.P.I.
Published by: Canadian Biotechnology News Service, 20 Stonepark Lane, Nepean, ON K2H 9P4, Canada. TEL 613-726-0115, FAX 613-726-7344, http://www.faxon.ca/publishers/subscripton-rates.html. Ed. Peter Winter. Adv. contact Carole Winter. Circ: 3,000.

660.6 CAN
CANADIAN BIOTECH RESEARCH. Text in English. 1996. m. CND 120, USD 180 (effective 1999). **Document type:** *Trade.* **Description:** Provides articles and news on the application of biotech research to various sections. Principle focus is the health care, but applications of biotechnology to agriculture and the environment are also covered.
Published by: Canadian Biotechnology News Service, 20 Stonepark Lane, Nepean, ON K2H 9P4, Canada. TEL 613-726-0115, FAX 613-726-7344, pwinter@netcom.ca, http://www.faxon.ca/publishers/subscription-rates.html. Ed. Peter Winter. Circ: 3,000 (controlled).

CELL TRANSPLANTATION. see *BIOLOGY—Cytology And Histology*

▼ **CLONING AND STEM CELLS.** see *BIOLOGY—Genetics*

660 USA
TP248.13 CODEN: CRBTE5
CRITICAL REVIEWS IN BIOTECHNOLOGY. Text in English. 1983. q. USD 375 (effective 1998). *Refereed.* **Document type:** *Academic/Scholarly.* **Description:** Presents state-of-the-art review articles covering the spectrum of technologies involving the use of living organisms and biological processes in a wide range of industrial, agricultural, and medical applications.
Formerly: C R C Critical Reviews in Biotechnology (0738-8551)
Related titles: Online - full text ed.: (from O C L C Online Computer Library Center, Inc., Swets Blackwell, ScienceDirect, Institute for Scientific Information).
Indexed: AESIS, ASCA, AgBiotech, Agri.& Environ.Biotech.Abstr., Agricola, Aqua.Sci.& Fish.Abstr., Bioeng.Abstr., Biotech.Cit.Ind., Chem.Abstr., Chem.Indus.Notes, Chem.Titles, Curr.Adv.Ecol.Sci., Curr.Biotech.Abstr., Curr.Cont., Derwent Biotech.Abstr., Eng.Ind., Entomol.Abstr., Environ.Sci.Poll.Mgmt., Field Crop Abstr., Food Sci.& Tech.Abstr., Helminthol.Abstr., INIS Atomind., Ind.Med. (1983-), Ind.Sci.Rev., Int.Abstr.Biol.Sci., Maize Abstr., Med.& Pharm.Biotech.Abstr., Microbiol.Abstr., Rev.Plant Path., Rice Abstr., Sci.Cit.Ind., Soils & Fert., Sport Fish.Abstr., Wild.Rev.
—BLDSC (3487.472400), ADONIS, CASDDS, CISTI, GNLM, IDS, ingenta, Linda Hall. **CCC.**
Published by: C R C Press, LLC, 2000 Corporate Blvd, N W, Boca Raton, FL 33431. TEL 561-994-0555, 800-272-7737, FAX 561-998-9784. Eds. Graham G Stewart, Inge Russell.

CURRENT ADVANCES IN APPLIED MICROBIOLOGY & BIOTECHNOLOGY. see *BIOLOGY—Abstracting, Bibliographies, Statistics*

CURRENT BIOTECHNOLOGY. see *BIOLOGY—Abstracting, Bibliographies, Statistics*

CURRENT ISSUES IN MOLECULAR BIOLOGY. see *BIOLOGY—Biochemistry*

660 GBR ISSN 0958-1669
TP248.13 CODEN: CUOBE3
CURRENT OPINION IN BIOTECHNOLOGY. Text in English. 1990. 6/yr. GBP 271 in Europe to individuals; JPY 57,900 in Japan to individuals; USD 445 elsewhere to individuals; NLG 2,453, EUR 1,113.12 in Europe to institutions; JPY 154,100 in Japan to institutions; USD 1,245 elsewhere to institutions; USD 1,681 to institutions Print & online combined (effective 2001). adv. bibl, illus. back issues avail. *Refereed.* **Document type:** *Academic/Scholarly.* **Description:** Presents review articles followed by annotated bibliographies for researchers and educators in biotechnology. Includes a "Paper Alert" section, giving brief summaries of relevant papers recently published in other journals.
Related titles: Online - full text ed.: USD 452 in North America to individuals; USD 493 in North America to individuals with online ed; GBP 250 elsewhere to individuals; GBP 300 elsewhere to individuals with online ed; USD 1,086 in North America to institutions includes online ed; GBP 660 elsewhere to institutions includes online ed (effective 1999 & 2000) (from EBSCO Publishing, ingenta, Swets Blackwell, ScienceDirect, Institute for Scientific Information).
Indexed: AESIS, ASCA, AgBiotech, Agri.& Environ.Biotech.Abstr., Anim.Breed.Abstr., Aqua.Sci.& Fish.Abstr., Bio-Contr.News & Info., Biol.Abstr., Biotech.Cit.Ind., CEABA, Chem.Abstr., Chem.Cit.Ind., Chem.Indus.Notes, Chem.Titles, Crop Physiol.Abstr., Curr.Cont., Dairy Sci.Abstr., Eng.Ind., Entomol.Abstr., Environ.Sci.Poll.Mgmt., Excerp.Med. (1993-), Field Crop Abstr., Forest Prod.Abstr., Ind.Med. (1990-), Ind.Vet., Inpharma, Int.Abstr.Biol.Sci., Maize Abstr., Mass Spectr.Bull., Med.& Pharm.Biotech.Abstr., Microbiol.Abstr., Nutr.Abstr., Pharm.&Out.News, Plant Breed.Abstr., Plant Grow.Reg.Abstr., Poult.Abstr., Reac., Rev.Appl.Entomol., Rev.Arom.& Med.Plants, Rev.Plant Path., Sci.Cit.Ind., Sel.Water Res.Abstr., Soils & Fert., Soyabean Abstr., Sugar Ind.Abstr., Weed Abstr., World Ag.Econ.& Rur.Soc.Abstr.
—BLDSC (3500.772500), ADONIS, CASDDS, CISTI, Ei, EMDOCS, GNLM, IDS, Infotrieve. **CCC.**
Published by: Elsevier Science Ltd., Elsevier Trends Journals, 84 Theobald's Rd, London WC1X 8RR, United Kingdom. TEL 44-20-7611-4400, FAX 44-20-7611-4468, http://www.elsevier.com/locate/copbio. Circ: 1,000. **Subscr. to:** Quadrant Subscription Services. FAX 44-1444-445423. **Dist. by:** Turpin Distribution Services Ltd.

660.6 338.476 USA ISSN 1389-2010
▼ **CURRENT PHARMACEUTICAL BIOTECHNOLOGY.** Text in English. 2000 (Jun.). q. USD 110, USD 600 to institutions (effective 2000). adv. *Refereed.* **Document type:** *Academic/Scholarly.* **Description:** Features reviews in pharmaceutical biotechnology and related areas.
Related titles: Online - full text ed.: (from Swets Blackwell).
Indexed: Biotech.& Bioeng.Abstr., Cal.Tiss.Abstr., Med.& Pharm.Biotech.Abstr.
—BLDSC (3501.280450).
Published by: Bentham Science Publishers, 102 N.E. 2nd St, Mail Box 135, Boca Raton, FL 33432. FAX 561-393-7229, m.bentham@inter.nl.net, http://www.bentham.org/cpb. Adv. contact Tom Lucas.

CYTOTECHNOLOGY; international journal of cell culture and biotechnology. see *BIOLOGY—Cytology And Histology*

DEVELOPMENTS IN BIOLOGICALS. see *METROLOGY AND STANDARDIZATION*

610.285 660 NLD
DEVELOPMENTS IN BIOTHERAPY. Text in Dutch. 1991. irreg. price varies. **Document type:** *Monographic series.*
Published by: Kluwer Academic Publishers Group (Subsidiary of: Wolters Kluwer N.V.), Spuiboulevard 50, PO Box 17, Dordrecht 3300 AA, Netherlands. FAX 31-78-639-2254, services@wkap.nl, http://www.wkap.nl. **Dist. by:** Journals Department, PO Box 322, Dordrecht 3300 AH, Netherlands. FAX 31-78-654-6474.

660 170 FRA
DICTIONNAIRE PERMANENT: BIOETHIQUE ET BIOTECHNOLOGIES. Text in French. 1995. base vol. plus m. updates. FRF 1,860 per vol.; FRF 400 updates. **Description:** Covers legal and business issues in bioethics and biotechnology.
Published by: Editions Legislatives, 80 av. de la Marne, Montrouge Cedex 92546, France. TEL 40-92-68-68, FAX 46-56-00-15, TELEX 632 855 F. Ed. Daniel Vigneau.

DIRECTORY OF AUSTRALIAN BIOTECHNOLOGY COMPANIES. see *BUSINESS AND ECONOMICS—Trade And Industrial Directories*

660.6025 570 USA
DIRECTORY OF BIOTECHNOLOGY CENTERS. Text in English. 1987. a. USD 79 (effective 1998). **Document type:** *Directory, Academic/Scholarly.* **Description:** Provides information on approximately 100 biotechnology centers in the United States. The directory is arranged alphabetically by state.
Published by: Institute for Biotechnology Information, c/o Mark Dibner, Pres., Box 14569, Research Triangle Park, NC 27709-4569. TEL 919-544-5111, FAX 919-544-5401, ibi@mindspring.com, http://www.biotechinfo.com.

DRUG DISCOVERY TODAY. see *PHARMACY AND PHARMACOLOGY*

660.6 CHL ISSN 0717-3458
CODEN: EEBIF6
ELECTRONIC JOURNAL OF BIOTECHNOLOGY. Short title: E J B. Text in English. 1998. q. free per issue. adv. *Refereed.* **Description:** Publishes papers from all areas of biotechnology, including molecular biology and environmental aspects, as well as computer applications in biotechnology.
Media: Online - full content (from SciELO). **Related titles:** Online - full text ed.: (from SciELO).
Indexed: Agri.& Environ.Biotech.Abstr., Biotech.& Bioeng.Abstr., Environ.Sci.Poll.Mgmt., Med.& Pharm.Biotech.Abstr.
—CASDDS.
Published by: EJB Electronic Journal of Biotechnology, Casilla 4059, Valparaiso, Chile. TEL 56-32-273000, FAX 56-32-212746, gmunoz@ucv.cl, http://www.ejb.org, http://www.ejb.ucv.cl. Ed., R&P Graciela Munoz TEL 56-32-273120. Pub. Atillo Bustos. Adv. contact Alejandra Munoz TEL 56-32-273287. **Co-sponsor:** Comision Nacional de Investigacion Cientifica y Tecnologica.

660 USA
ELECTRONICS AND BIOTECHNOLOGY ADVANCED. FORUM SERIES. Text in English. irreg., latest vol.3, 1998.
Indexed: Chem.Abstr., Chem.Indus.Notes, Chem.Titles.
—BLDSC (3703.120000).
Published by: (Electronics and Biotechnology Advanced), Kluwer Academic - Plenum Publishers (Subsidiary of: Wolters Kluwer N.V.), 233 Spring St, New York, NY 10013-1578. TEL 212-620-8000, 800-221-9369, FAX 212-463-0742, info@plenum.com, http://www.plenum.com.

591 636.089 USA ISSN 1083-4699
EMBRYO TRANSFER NEWSLETTER. Text in English. 1978. q. USD 80 to membership; USD 40 to students (effective 2000). adv. bk.rev. abstr. *Refereed.* **Document type:** *Newsletter.* **Description:** Features articles and announcements related to embryo transfer.
Related titles: Online - full text ed.
Published by: International Embryo Transfer Society, 1111 N Dunlap Ave, Savoy, IL 61874. TEL 217-356-3182, FAX 217-398-4119, iets@assochq.org, http://www.uets.org. Ed. Matt Wheeler. R&P, Adv. contact Fran Gardner. Circ: 1,100 (paid).

EMERGING TECHNOLOGY SERIES: GENETIC ENGINEERING AND BIOTECHNOLOGY. see *BIOLOGY—Genetics*

▼ **ENVIRONMENTAL MICROBIOLOGY.** see *BIOLOGY—Microbiology*

660.62 USA ISSN 0141-0229
TP248.E5 CODEN: EMTED2
ENZYME AND MICROBIAL TECHNOLOGY; biotechnology research and reviews. Text in English. 1979. 20/yr. EUR 229 in Europe to qualified personnel (effective 2001); JPY 30,400 in Japan to individuals; USD 256 elsewhere to individuals; EUR 1,862 in Europe to institutions; JPY 247,200 in Japan to institutions; USD 2,082 elsewhere to institutions (effective 2002). adv. bk.rev. illus. index. back issues avail. *Refereed.* **Document type:** *Academic/Scholarly.* **Description:** Encompasses basic and applied aspects of the use of enzymes, microbes and cells of mammalian or plant origin. Also covers economic and legal issues bearing on the 'new' biotechnology.

Related titles: Microform ed.: (from PQC); Online - full text ed.: (from ingenta, Swets Blackwell, ScienceDirect, Institute for Scientific Information).
Indexed: AESIS, ASCA, AgBiotech, Agri.& Environ.Biotech.Abstr., Anal.Abstr., Aqua.Sci.& Fish.Abstr., BBCI, Bio-Contr.News & Info., Biodet.Abstr., Biol.Abstr., Biotech.Cit.Ind., CEABA, Chem.Abstr., Chem.Cit.Ind., Chem.Indus.Notes, Chem.Titles, Cott.& Trop.Fibr.Abstr., Crop Physiol.Abstr., Curr.Adv.Biochem., Curr.Adv.Ecol.Sci., Curr.Biotech.Abstr., Curr.Cont., Dairy Sci.Abstr., Derwent Biotech.Abstr., Eng.Ind., Environ.Sci.Poll.Mgmt., Excerp.Med., Field Crop Abstr., Food Sci.& Tech.Abstr., Forest Prod.Abstr., Forest.Abstr., Helminthol.Abstr., Hort.Abstr., INIS Atomind., ISMEC, Ind.Sci.Rev., Inpharma, Int.Abstr.Biol.Sci., Maize Abstr., Mat.Sci.Cit.Ind. (coverage dropped), Microbiol.Abstr., Nonwov.Abstr., Nutr.Abstr., Paper & Bd.Abstr., Plant Grow.Reg.Abstr., Reac., Ref.Zh., Rev.Appl.Entomol., Rev.Arom.& Med.Plants, Rev.Plant Path., Risk Abstr., Sci.Cit.Ind., Soils & Fert., Sugar Ind.Abstr., Telegen, Triticale Abstr., Weed Abstr.
—BLDSC (3791.933000), ADONIS, CASDDS, CISTI, Ei, GNLM, IDS, Infotrieve, ingenta, Linda Hall. **CCC.**
Published by: Elsevier Science, 655 Ave of the Americas, New York, NY 10010. TEL 212-989-5800, FAX 212-633-3990, usinfo-f@elsevier.com, http://www.elsevier.com/locate/enzmictec. Eds. Raymond E Spier, Sheldon W May. **Subscr. in Australasia and the Far East to:** Elsevier Science (Singapore) Pte Ltd, No.1 Temasek Ave, 17-01 Millenia Tower, Singapore 039192, Singapore. TEL 65-434-3727, FAX 65-337-2230; **Subscr. in Japan to:** Elsevier Science Inc - Japan Regional Office, 9-15 Higashi-Azabu 1-chome, Minato-ku, Tokyo 106-0044, Japan. TEL 81-3-5561-5033; **Subscr. outside the Americas to:** Elsevier Science BV, PO Box 211, Amsterdam 1000 AE, Netherlands. TEL 31-20-485-3757.

B

EUROPEAN BIOPHARMACEUTICAL REVIEW. see *PHARMACY AND PHARMACOLOGY*

660 FRA ISSN 0765-2046
CODEN: EBNWEI
EUROPEAN BIOTECHNOLOGY NEWSLETTER. Text in English. 1986. 22/yr. FRF 3,500 domestic; FRF 3,574 in the European Union; FRF 3,500 elsewhere. **Document type:** *Newsletter, Academic/Scholarly.* **Description:** Publishes full-length articles and short communications on various aspects of biotechnology.
Related titles: Microform ed.: (from PQC); Online - full text ed.: (from ingenta).
Indexed: Chem.Abstr., Chem.Indus.Notes, Chem.Titles.
—CASDDS, Infotrieve. **CCC.**
Published by: Editions Scientifiques et Medicales Elsevier, 141 rue de Javel, Paris Cedex 15 75747, France. TEL 33-1-45589049, FAX 33-1-45589421, http://www.elsevier.nl/. Ed. O Revelant. **Subscr. in U.S. and Canada to:** Elsevier Science, PO Box 945, New York, NY 10159-0945. TEL 212-633-3730, FAX 212-633-3680, http://www.elsevier.com.

F E M S MICROBIOLOGY. see *BIOLOGY—Microbiology*

660.6029 GBR
F T BIOTECHNOLOGY & PHARMACEUTICAL COMPANIES DATABASE CD-ROM (YEARS). (Financial Times) Text in English. 1997. a. GBP 450 (effective 1997-98). adv. **Description:** Serves as a guide to the activities, performance and personnel of pharmaceutical and biotechnology companies worldwide.
Media: CD-ROM.
Published by: Financial Times Healthcare, Maple House, 149 Tottenham Ct Rd, London W1P 9LL, United Kingdom. TEL 44-207-896-2066, FAX 44-20-7896-2213, lizg@pearson-pro.com, http://www.fthealthcare.com. Adv. contact Liz Godden.

660 608.7 USA
FEDERAL BIO-TECHNOLOGY TRANSFER DIRECTORY. Text in English. 1994. a. adv. **Document type:** *Directory.* **Description:** Catalogs all federal government inventions and technology transfer in the biomedical and basic biotechnology fields from 1980 to present.
Published by: Biotechnology Information Institute, 1700 Rockville Pike, Ste 400, Rockville, MD 20852. TEL 301-424-0255, FAX 301-424-0257. Ed., R&P, Adv. contact Ronald A Rader.

660 FRA ISSN 0985-2662
FLASH ETATS-UNIS. Text in French. 1984. 11/yr. FRF 2,000, USD 399. back issues avail. **Document type:** *Newsletter.* **Description:** Scientific, technological and economic information about biotechnology in the U.S.
Related titles: Microform ed.: (from PQC).
—**CCC.**
Published by: Editions Scientifiques et Medicales Elsevier, 141 rue de Javel, Paris Cedex 15 75747, France. TEL 33-1-45589049. **Subscr. in U.S. and Canada to:** Elsevier Science, PO Box 945, New York, NY 10159-0945. TEL 212-633-3730, FAX 212-633-3680.

660.6 FRA ISSN 0985-2654
FLASH JAPON. Text in French. 1984. 11/yr. FRF 2,000, USD 399. **Document type:** *Newsletter.* **Description:** Scientific, economic and technological information about biotechnology in Japan.
Related titles: Microform ed.: (from PQC).
—**CCC.**
Published by: Editions Scientifiques et Medicales Elsevier, 141 rue de Javel, Paris Cedex 15 75747, France. TEL 33-1-45589049, FAX 33-1-45589421, http://www.elsevier.nl/. **Subscr. in U.S. and Canada to:** Elsevier Science, PO Box 945, New York, NY 10159-0945. TEL 212-633-3730, FAX 212-633-3680, http://www.elsevier.com.

FRONTIERS IN BIOMEDICAL POLYMER APPLICATIONS. see *PHARMACY AND PHARMACOLOGY*

660.65 NLD ISSN 0378-1119
QH442 CODEN: GENED6
GENE; an international journal focusing on gene cloning and gene structure and function. Text in Dutch. 1977. 40/yr. EUR 574 in Europe to individuals; JPY 75,600 in Japan to individuals; USD 642 elsewhere to individuals; EUR 7,086 in Europe to institutions; JPY 940,800 in Japan to institutions; USD 7,927 elsewhere to institutions (effective 2002). adv. back issues avail.; reprint service avail. from SWZ. *Refereed.* **Document type:** *Academic/Scholarly.* **Description:** Explores and analyzes gene structure, function and regulation, recombinant DNA techniques, mapping, sequencing and study of plant, animal, human and microbial genomes, as well as basic and practical applications of genetic engineering and RNA technology.
Related titles: Microform ed.: (from PQC); Online - full text ed.: Gene - C O M B I S (from EBSCO Publishing, ingenta, Swets Blackwell, ScienceDirect, Institute for Scientific Information).
Indexed: ASCA, Abstr.Anthropol., AgBiotech, Agri.& Environ.Biotech.Abstr. (coverage dropped), Agricola, Anim.Breed.Abstr., Aqua.Sci.& Fish.Abstr., BBCI, Bibl.Agri., Bio-Contr.News & Info., Biol.& Agr.Ind. (Jan.1996-), Biol.Abstr., Biotech.Cit.Ind., CEABA, Chem.Abstr., Chem.Indus.Notes, Chem.Titles, Crop Physiol.Abstr., Curr.Adv.Biochem., Curr.Adv.Cancer Res., Curr.Adv.Cell & Devel.Biol., Curr.Adv.Ecol.Sci., Curr.Adv.Gen.& Molec.Biol., Curr.Biotech.Abstr., Curr.Cont., Dairy Sci.Abstr., Derwent Biotech.Abstr., Entomol.Abstr., Environ.Sci.Poll.Mgmt., Excerp.Med., Food Sci.& Tech.Abstr., Forest Prod.Abstr., Forest.Abstr., Genet.Abstr., Helminthol.Abstr., Hort.Abstr., Hum.Gen.Abstr., INIS Atomind., Immun.Abstr. (coverage dropped), Ind.Med. (1976-), Ind.Sci.Rev., Ind.Vet., Int.Abstr.Biol.Sci., Maize Abstr., Microbiol.Abstr., Neurosci.Abstr. (coverage dropped), Neurosci.Cit.Ind., Nuc.Acids Abstr., Nutr.Abstr., Ornam.Hort., Pig News & Info., Plant Breed.Abstr., Plant Gen.Res.Abstr., Plant Grow.Reg.Abstr., Postharvest, Potato Abstr., Poult.Abstr., Protozool.Abstr., Rev.Appl.Entomol., Rev.Arom.& Med.Plants, Rev.Med.& Vet.Mycol., Rev.Plant Path., Rice Abstr., Risk Abstr., Sci.Cit.Ind., Seed Abstr., Small Anim.Abstr., Soils & Fert., Sorghum & Millets Abstr., Sport Fish.Abstr., Sugar Ind.Abstr., Telegen, Triticale Abstr., Vet.Bull., Virol.Abstr. (coverage dropped), Wild.Rev., Zoo.Rec.
—BLDSC (4096.402000), ADONIS, CASDDS, CISTI, EMDOCS, GNLM, IDS, ingenta, Linda Hall. **CCC.**
Published by: Elsevier Science BV, PO Box 211, Amsterdam 1000 AE, Netherlands. TEL 31-20-485-2911, FAX 31-20-485-2457, http://www.elsevier.com/locate/gene. Ed. G Bernardina. Pub. Nicolien Var Derlinden. **Subscr. in Australasia and the Far East to:** Elsevier Science (Singapore) Pte Ltd, No.1 Temasek Ave, 17-01 Millenia Tower, Singapore 039192, Singapore. TEL 65-434-3727, FAX 65-337-2230; **Subscr. in Japan to:** Elsevier Science Inc - Japan Regional Office, 9-15 Higashi-Azabu 1-chome, Minato-ku, Tokyo 106-0044, Japan. TEL 81-3-5561-5033; **Subscr. in the Americas to:** Elsevier Science, PO Box 945, New York, NY 10159-0945. TEL 212-633-3730, FAX 212-633-3680, usinfo-f@elsevier.com.

▼ **GENE THERAPY AND REGULATION**; an international interdisciplinary journal. see *BIOLOGY—Genetics*

660 576.5 GBR ISSN 1354-1366
GENETHICS NEWS. Text in English. 1994. bi-m. GBP 14.95 (effective 2001). adv. bk.rev. charts, illus. back issues avail. **Document type:** *Newsletter, Academic/Scholarly.* **Description:** Covers ethical, social and environmental issues related to genetics and biotechnology.
Address: 22B St Kilda's Rd, London N16 5BZ, United Kingdom. TEL 44-20-8809-4513, FAX 44-20-7502-7516, genethicsnews@compuserve.com, http://www.ink.uk.com/gen_p.htm, http://ourworld.compuserve.com/homepages/genethicsnews. Ed., Pub. Dr. David King. Circ: 500 (paid).

GENETIC ENGINEERING. see *BIOLOGY—Genetics*

660.65 576 USA ISSN 0196-3716
QH442 CODEN: GENGDC
GENETIC ENGINEERING; principles and methods. Text in English. 1979. irreg., latest vol.21, 1999. price varies. *Refereed.* **Document type:** *Monographic series.*
Indexed: Agri.& Environ.Biotech.Abstr. (coverage dropped), Agricola, Chem.Abstr., Chem.Indus.Notes, Chem.Titles, Curr.Biotech.Abstr., Derwent Biotech.Abstr., Ind.Med. (1979-).
—BLDSC (4111.847000), CASDDS, CISTI, GNLM, ingenta, KNAW. **CCC.**
Published by: Kluwer Academic - Plenum Publishers (Subsidiary of: Wolters Kluwer N.V.), 233 Spring St, New York, NY 10013-1578. TEL 212-620-8000, 800-221-9369, FAX 212-463-0742, info@plenum.com, http://www.plenum.com. Eds. A Hollaender, J K Setlow.

GENETIC ENGINEERING NEWS; the information source of the biotechnology industry. see *BIOLOGY—Genetics*

GENEWATCH. see *BIOLOGY—Genetics*

GENOMICS; international journal for analysis of the human and other genomes. see *BIOLOGY—Genetics*

660 JPN ISSN 0912-6686
I C BIOTECH. ANNUAL REPORTS. Text in English. 1978. a. **Document type:** *Academic/Scholarly.*
Formerly (until 1985): International Center of Cooperative Research and Development in Microbial Engineering. Annual Reports (0387-5377)
Published by: Osaka University, International Center for Biotechnology/Osaka Daigaku Seibutsu Kogaku Kokusai Koryu Senta, 2-1 Yamada-Oka, Suita-shi, Osaka-fu 565-0871, Japan. TEL 81-6-879-7455, FAX 81-6-879-7454, yoshida@icb.osaka-u.ac.jp, http://www.icb.osaka-u.ac.jp/. Ed. Toshiomi Yoshida.

660 619 610 USA
I E E E BIOMEDICAL ENGINEERING DAYS. Text in English. a. USD 140. **Document type:** *Proceedings.*
Published by: Institute of Electrical and Electronics Engineers, Inc., 3 Park Ave, 17th Fl, New York, NY 10017. TEL 800-678-4333, customer.service@ieee.org, http://www.ieee.org.

610.28 USA ISSN 1089-7771
R858.A1 CODEN: ITIBFX
I E E E TRANSACTIONS ON INFORMATION TECHNOLOGY IN BIOMEDICINE. Text in English. 1997. q. USD 195 in North America for print or online eds.; USD 220 elsewhere for print or online eds. (effective 2002). **Description:** Covers national and international developments in biomedical and health applications using information and computer networking.
Related titles: CD-ROM ed.; Microfiche ed.; Online - full text ed.: (from EBSCO Publishing, Institute for Scientific Information).
Indexed: A.S.& T.Ind. (Jan.2001-), Bioeng.Abstr., Biotech.& Bioeng.Abstr., Curr.Cont., Eng.Ind., INSPEC (Mar.1997-), Ind.Med. (1997-), Ref.Zh.
—BLDSC (4363.196500), CISTI, ingenta, Linda Hall.
Published by: Institute of Electrical and Electronics Engineers, Inc. TEL 800-701-4333, customer.service@ieee.org, subscription-service@ieee.org, http://www.ieee.org. Ed. Swamy Laxminarayan. **Subscr. to:** Maruzen Co. Ltd., 3-10 Nihonbashi 2-chome, Chuo-ku, Tokyo 103-0027, Japan. FAX 81-3-3275-0657; Universal Subscription Agency, Pvt. Ltd., 877, Udyog Vihar, V, Gurgoan 122001, India. TEL 91-124-347261, FAX 91-124-342496. **Co-sponsor:** Engineering in Medicine and Biology Society.

610.285 FRA ISSN 1297-9562

▼ **I T B M - R B M.** (Innovation et Technologie en Biologie et Medecine - Revue Europeenne de Biotechnologie Medicale) (In 2 sections: RBM La Revue (4 nos.); RBM News (6 nos.)) Text and summaries in English, French. 2000. m. EUR 218 in Europe to institutions; USD 264 elsewhere to institutions (effective 2002). *Refereed.* **Document type:** *Academic/Scholarly.* **Description:** Publishes objective, scientific medical and technical information on all aspects of biomedical technology involved in cardiology, radiology, NMR, surgery, intensive care and emergency medicine, resuscitation and clinical chemistry equipment.

Formed by the merger of part of (1979-2000): Revue Europeenne de Biotechnologie Medicale (0222-0776); (1980-2000): Innovation et Technologie en Biologie et Medecine (0243-7228)

Related titles: Online - full text ed.: (from ingenta, ScienceDirect).

Indexed: Excerp.Med. (1993-), INIS Atomind.

—BLDSC (4588.506700), CISTI, EMDOCS, GNLM, Infotrieve. **CCC.**

Published by: Elsevier Paris, Editions Scientifiques et Medicales (Subsidiary of: Reed Elsevier plc. group), 23 rue Linois, Paris 75015, France. TEL 33-1-45589110, FAX 33-1-45589419, rbm@elsevier.fr; academic@elsevier-fr.com, http://www.elsevire.com/locate/rbmret. Eds. B Kastler, C A Cuenod, J Rousseau. Circ: 6,000.

660 FRA ISSN 1297-9570

I T B M - R B M NEWS. (Innovation et Technologie en Biologie et Medecine - Revue Europeene de Biotechnologie Medicale) Text in English, French. 1979. bi-m. EUR 47 in Europe to institutions; USD 54 elsewhere to institutions (effective 2002).

Supersedes in part (in 2000): Revue Europeenne de Biotechnologie Medicale (0222-0776)

Related titles: Online - full text ed.: (from ingenta, Swets Blackwell, ScienceDirect).

Published by: Elsevier Paris, Editions Scientifiques et Medicales (Subsidiary of: Reed Elsevier plc. group), 23 rue Linois, Paris 75015, France. TEL 33-1-71724500, FAX 33-1-71724664, http://www.elsevier.com/locate/rbmnew. Ed. R Talec.

IMMUNOTECHNOLOGY; an international journal of immunological engineering. see *MEDICAL SCIENCES—Allergology And Immunology*

IN VITRO CELLULAR & DEVELOPMENTAL BIOLOGY - PLANT. see *BIOLOGY—Botany*

620.1 GBR
QH530.5.I56

INTERNATIONAL BIODETERIORATION SYMPOSIUM. PROCEEDINGS. Variant title: Biodeterioration and Biodegradation. Text in English. biennial (8th 1990, Windsor, Canada). GBP 135. bibl, illus. *Refereed.* **Document type:** *Proceedings.*

Published by: Pergamon (Subsidiary of: Elsevier Science), The Boulevard, Langford Ln, East Park, Kidlington, Oxford OXB 1GB, United Kingdom. FAX 44-1865-843010, nlinfo-f@elsevier.nl; usinfo-f@elsevier.com; forinfo-kyf04035@niftyserve.or.jp, nlinfo-f@elsevier/nl; usinfo-f@elsevier.com; forinfo-kyf04035@niftyserve.or.jp, http://www.elsevier.nl/. Ed. H W Rossmore. **Subscr. in Australasia and the Far East to:** Elsevier Science (Singapore) Pte Ltd, No.1 Temasek Ave, 17-01 Millenia Tower, Singapore 039192, Singapore. TEL 65-434-3727, FAX 65-337-2230; **Subscr. in the Americas to:** Elsevier Science, PO Box 945, New York, NY 10159-0945. TEL 212-633-3730, FAX 212-633-3680, usinfo-f@elsevier.com, http://www.elsevier.com; **Subscr. to:** Elsevier Science BV, PO Box 211, Amsterdam 1000 AE, Netherlands. TEL 31-20-485-3757, FAX 31-20-485-3432, nlinfo-f@elsevier.nl, http://www.elsevier.nl.

660 542 USA ISSN 0888-7225
TP248.13

INTERNATIONAL BIOTECHNOLOGY LABORATORY. Text in English. 1983. 7/yr. USD 135; USD 165 foreign. bk.rev. charts, illus, stat, tr.lit. **Document type:** *Trade.*

Related titles: Special ed.: International Biotechnology Laboratory. Buyers' Guide.

Indexed: CEABA, Curr.Adv.Ecol.Sci., Curr.Biotech.Abstr., Derwent Biotech.Abstr., INIS Atomind., Mass Spectr.Bull.

—BLDSC (4537.195100).

Published by: International Scientific Communications, Inc., 30 Controls Dr, Box 870, Shelton, CT 06484-0870. TEL 203-926-9300, FAX 203-926-9310, TELEX 964292, iscpubs@iscpubs.com, http://www.iscpubs.com. Ed. Brian Howard. Pub. William Wham. adv.: B&W page USD 4,255, color page USD 5,815. Circ: 37,000 (controlled). **U.K. subscr. to:** I.S.C. House, Progress Business Centre, Whittle Parkway, 5 Whittle Pkwy, Slough, Berks SL1 6DQ, United Kingdom. TEL 44-1628-668881.

INTERNATIONAL JOURNAL OF ANIMAL SCIENCES. see *AGRICULTURE—Poultry And Livestock*

660.2 CHE ISSN 0963-6048
TP248.13

▼ **INTERNATIONAL JOURNAL OF BIOTECHNOLOGY.** Abbreviated title: I J B T. Text in English. 1999. q., latest vol.4, 2002, six issues per volume, one vol. USD 470 in United Kingdom; USD 510 elsewhere; USD 565 combined subscription in United Kingdom print & online eds. (effective 2002); USD 605 combined subscription elsewhere print & online eds. (effective 2001). adv. *Refereed.* **Document type:** *Journal, Academic/Scholarly.* **Description:** Provides an international forum and authoritative source of information in the fields of biotechnology and biotechnics with an emphasis on the management and economics as well as the political and social issues.

Related titles: Online - full text ed.

Indexed: AgBiotech, Agri.& Environ.Biotech.Abstr., Aqua.Sci.& Fish.Abstr., Aquacult.Abstr., Biotech.& Bioeng.Abstr., Environ.Sci.Poll.Mgmt., METADEX, Med.& Pharm.Biotech.Abstr., Plant Gen.Res.Abstr., Risk Abstr., Rural Devel.Abstr., Saf.Sci.Abstr., Soils & Fert., World Ag.Econ.& Rur.Soc.Abstr.

—BLDSC (4542.155200), CISTI.

Published by: Inderscience Enterprises Ltd., World Trade Centre Bldg., 29 route de Pre Bois, Case Postale 896, Geneva, 15 1215, Switzerland. FAX 41-22-7910885, 44-1234-240515, ijbt@inderscience.com, info@inderscience.com, http://www.inderscience.com. Ed. Dr. M A Dorgham.

660 610 USA ISSN 0021-9304
R856 CODEN: JBMRBG

JOURNAL OF BIOMEDICAL MATERIALS RESEARCH. Text in English. 1966. bi-m. USD 4,495 in United States; USD 4,715 in Canada & Mexico; USD 4,902 elsewhere; USD 4,720 combined subscription in United States for print and online eds.; USD 4,940 combined subscription in Canada & Mexico for print and online eds.; USD 5,127 combined subscription elsewhere for print and online eds. (effective 2002). adv. illus. Supplement avail.; back issues avail.; reprint service avail. from PQC. *Refereed.* **Document type:** *Academic/Scholarly.* **Description:** Covers topics ranging from alloys, polymers and ceramics to surgery, dentistry and implanted devices.

Incorporates (1990-1995): Journal of Applied Biomaterials (1045-4861)

Related titles: Microform ed.: (from PQC); Online - full text ed.: ISSN 1097-4636. 1996. USD 4,495 in United States; USD 4,495 in Canada & Mexico; USD 4,495 elsewhere (effective 2002) (from EBSCO Publishing, Wiley InterScience, Institute for Scientific Information).

Indexed: A.S.& T.Ind. (Jan.2001-), ASCA, Agri.& Environ.Biotech.Abstr., Alloys Ind., Appl.Mech.Rev., Aqua.Sci.& Fish.Abstr., Bioeng.Abstr., Biol.& Agr.Ind. (coverage dropped), Biol.Abstr., Biotech.& Bioeng.Abstr., Cal.Tiss.Abstr., Chem.Abstr., Chem.Cit.Ind., Chem.Indus.Notes, Chem.Titles, Curr.Adv.Cell & Devel.Biol., Curr.Cont., Dent.Ind., Electron.& Communic.Abstr.J., Eng.Ind., Eng.Mat.Abstr., Environ.Sci.Poll.Mgmt., Excerp.Med., INIS Atomind., ISMEC, Ind.Med. (1967-), Ind.Sci.Rev., Inpharma, Intl.Polym.Sci.& Tech., METADEX, Mass Spectr.Bull., Mat.Sci.Cit.Ind., Med.& Pharm.Biotech.Abstr., Met.Abstr., Met.Abstr.Ind., Microbiol.Abstr., Nonfer.Met.Alert, PCC Alert, Pollut.Abstr., RAPRA (1974-), Reac., Risk Abstr., Saf.Sci.Abstr., Sci.Cit.Ind., Steels Alert, Tox.Abstr., World Alum.Abstr.

—BLDSC (4953.700000), CASDDS, CISTI, Ei, GNLM, IDS, ingenta, KNAW. **CCC.**

Published by: (Society for Biomaterials), John Wiley & Sons, Inc., Journals (Subsidiary of: Wiley InterScience), 605 Third Ave, New York, NY 10158. TEL 212-850-6645, FAX 212-850-6021, subinfo@wiley.com, uscs-wis@wiley.com, http://www.wiley.com. Ed. James Anderson. adv.: B&W page GBP 640, color page GBP 1,515; trim 210 x 279. Circ: 2,500. **Subscr. outside the Americas to:** John Wiley & Sons Ltd., Baffins Ln, Chichester, Sussex PO19 IUD, United Kingdom. TEL 44-1243-779777, FAX 44-1243-843232, cs-journals@wiley.co.uk, http://www.wiley.co.uk. **Co-sponsor:** European Society for Biomaterials.

▼ **JOURNAL OF BIOMEDICINE AND BIOTECHNOLOGY.** see *MEDICAL SCIENCES*

JOURNAL OF BIOSCIENCE AND BIOENGINEERING. see *BIOLOGY—Bioengineering*

660 NLD ISSN 0168-1656
CODEN: JBITD4

JOURNAL OF BIOTECHNOLOGY. Text and summaries in English. 1984. s-m. (25/yr.). NLG 587, EUR 266.37 in Europe to individuals includes Reviews in Molecular Biotechnolog; JPY 36,900 in Japan to individuals includes Reviews in Molecular Biotechnolog; USD 298 elsewhere to individuals includes Reviews in Molecular Biotechnolog; NLG 5,434, EUR 2,465.84 in Europe to institutions includes Reviews in Molecular Biotechnolog; JPY 341,400 in Japan to institutions includes Reviews in Molecular Biotechnolog; USD 2,758 elsewhere to institutions includes Reviews in Molecular Biotechnolog (effective 2001); y. adv. bk.rev. abstr. back issues avail.; reprint service avail. from SWZ,ISI. *Refereed.* **Document type:** *Academic/Scholarly.* **Description:** Provides a medium for full-length and short articles on various aspects of biotechnology.

Related titles: Microform ed.: (from PQC); Online - full text ed.: (from ingenta, Swets Blackwell, ScienceDirect, Institute for Scientific Information).

Indexed: AESIS, ASCA, AgBiotech, Agri.& Environ.Biotech.Abstr., Agri.Eng.Abstr., Agricola, Anim.Breed.Abstr., Aqua.Sci.& Fish.Abstr., Bibl.Agri., Bio-Contr.News & Info., Biodet.Abstr., Biol.& Agr.Ind. (Aug.1989-), Biotech.Cit.Ind., CEABA, Chem.Abstr., Chem.Cit.Ind., Chem.Indus.Notes, Crop Physiol.Abstr., Curr.Adv.Biochem., Curr.Adv.Cell & Devel.Biol., Curr.Biotech.Abstr., Curr.Cont., Cyb.Abstr., Dairy Sci.Abstr., Derwent Biotech.Abstr., Eng.Ind., Environ.Sci.Poll.Mgmt., Excerp.Med., Field Crop Abstr., Food Sci.& Tech.Abstr., Forest Prod.Abstr., Helminthol.Abstr., Hort.Abstr., INIS Atomind., Immun.Abstr. (coverage dropped), Ind.Med. (1984-), Ind.Sci.Rev., Ind.Vet., Inpharma, Int.Abstr.Biol.Sci., Mass Spectr.Bull., Mat.Sci.Cit.Ind. (coverage dropped), Med.& Pharm.Biotech.Abstr., Microbiol.Abstr., Nutr.Abstr., Pharm.&Out.News, Pig News & Info., Plant Breed.Abstr., Plant Grow.Reg.Abstr., Potato Abstr., Protozool.Abstr., Reac., Ref.Zh., Rev.Appl.Entomol., Rev.Arom.& Med.Plants, Rev.Plant Path., Rice Abstr., Sci.Cit.Ind., Seed Abstr., Sel.Water Res.Abstr., Soils & Fert., Sugar Ind.Abstr., Telegen, Vet.Bull., Weed Abstr., World Ag.Econ.& Rur.Soc.Abstr.

—BLDSC (4954.120000), ADONIS, CASDDS, CISTI, Ei, GNLM, IDS, ingenta, Linda Hall. **CCC.**

Published by: Elsevier Science BV, PO Box 211, Amsterdam 1000 AE, Netherlands. TEL 31-20-485-2911, FAX 31-20-485-2457, nlinfo-f@elsevier.nl, http://www.elsevier.nl/locate/biofui. Ed. A Fiechter. **Subscr. in Australasia and the Far East to:** Elsevier Science (Singapore) Pte Ltd, No.1 Temasek Ave, 17-01 Millenia Tower, Singapore 039192, Singapore. TEL 65-434-3727, FAX 65-337-2230; **Subscr. in Japan to:** Elsevier Science Inc - Japan Regional Office, 9-15 Higashi-Azabu 1-chome, Minato-ku, Tokyo 106-0044, Japan. TEL 81-3-5561-5033, FAX 81-3-5561-5047; **Subscr. in the Americas to:** Elsevier Science, PO Box 945, New York, NY 10159-0945. TEL 212-633-3730, FAX 212-633-3680, usinfo-f@elsevier.com.

660 GBR ISSN 1462-8732

JOURNAL OF COMMERCIAL BIOTECHNOLOGY. Text in English. 1994. q. GBP 90 in Europe to individuals; USD 135 in North America to individuals; GBP 105 rest of world to individuals; GBP 350 in Europe to institutions; USD 525 in North America to institutions; GBP 365 rest of world to institutions; GBP 170 in Europe to Biotech companies; USD 255 in North America to Biotech companies; GBP 185 rest of world to Biotech companies (effective 2001). bk.rev. 96 p./no. 2 cols./p. back issues avail.; reprints avail. *Refereed.* **Document type:** *Journal, Academic/Scholarly.* **Description:** Provides systematic, comprehensive coverage of business and strategic management, regulation and research.

Formerly (until 1998): Journal of Biotechnology in Healthcare (1353-3010)

Indexed: Derwent Biotech.Abstr.

—BLDSC (4961.071000), CISTI, Infotrieve. **CCC.**

Published by: Henry Stewart Publications, Russell House, 28/30 Little St, London WC1A 2HN, United Kingdom. TEL 44-20-7404-3040, gweny@henrystewart.co.uk, http://www.henrystewart.com/journals/cb/. Ed. Julie Simkins. R&P Daryn Moody. Adv. contact Lorna Titley. Circ: 600 (paid). **Subscr. addr. in US & Canada:** Henry Stewart Publications, Subscriptions Office, PO Box 10812, Birmingham, AL 35202-1588. TEL 800-633-4931, FAX 205-955-1588, hsp@ebsco.com.

JOURNAL OF FOOD MYCOLOGY. see *BIOLOGY—Microbiology*

660.62 GBR ISSN 1367-5435
QR53 CODEN: JIMBFL
JOURNAL OF INDUSTRIAL MICROBIOLOGY AND BIOTECHNOLOGY. Text in English. 1986. m., latest vol.27, 2001. EUR 667 in Europe to institutions for print or online ed.; USD 1,000 rest of world to institutions for print or online ed.; EUR 667 combined subscription rest of world to institutions for prinr & online; USD 1,000 combined subscription rest of world to institutions for print or online (effective 2002). bk.rev. illus, charts, stat. cum.index. back issues avail.; reprints avail. *Refereed.* **Document type:** *Journal, Academic/Scholarly.* **Description:** Publishes original research articles, short communications, critical reviews in the fields of biotechnology, fermentation, environmental microbiology, biodegradation, biodeterioration, quality control, and other areas of applied microbiology.
Formerly: Journal of Industrial Microbiology (0169-4146)
Related titles: Online - full text ed.: (from EBSCO Publishing, O C L C Online Computer Library Center, Inc., RoweCom Information Quest, ingenta, Swets Blackwell, Institute for Scientific Information).
Indexed: ASCA, AgBiotech, Agri.& Environ.Biotech.Abstr., Agricola, Aqua.Sci.& Fish.Abstr., Bio-Contr.News & Info., Biodet.Abstr., Biotech.Cit.Ind., CEABA, Chem.Abstr., Chem.Indus.Notes, Chem.Titles, Curr.Adv.Biochem., Curr.Adv.Ecol.Sci., Curr.Adv.Gen.& Molec.Biol., Curr.Biotech.Abstr., Curr.Cont., Dairy Sci.Abstr., Derwent Biotech.Abstr., Eng.Ind., Environ.Sci.Poll.Mgmt., Excerp.Med. (until 1993), Food Sci.& Tech.Abstr., Forest Prod.Abstr., Forest.Abstr., Helminthol.Abstr., Herb.Abstr., Hort.Abstr., INIS Atomind., Ind.Vet., Int.Abstr.Biol.Sci., Microbiol.Abstr., Nutr.Abstr., Pollut.Abstr., Postharvest, Poult.Abstr., Rev.Appl.Entomol., Rev.Med.& Vet.Mycol., Rev.Plant Path., Sci.Cit.Ind., Soils & Fert., Soyabean Abstr., Sugar Ind.Abstr., Triticale Abstr., Vet.Bull., Weed Abstr.
—BLDSC (5006.330500), ADONIS, CASDDS, CISTI, Ei, IDS, Infotrieve, ingenta, Linda Hall. **CCC.**
Published by: (Society for Industrial Microbiology USA), Nature Publishing Group Specialist Journals (Subsidiary of: Holtzbrink Publishers), Houndmills, Basingstoke, Hants RG21 6XS, United Kingdom. TEL 44-1256-329242, FAX 44-1256-328339, subscriptions@nature.com, http://www.nature.com/jim. Ed. Joseph J Cooney. Pub. Julia Schulhof. R&P Trace Noel. Adv. contact Robert Sloan TEL 44-20-8882-7199. **Affiliate:** Nature Publishing Group Specialist Journals.

660.62 HKG ISSN 1017-7825
CODEN: JOMBES
JOURNAL OF MICROBIOLOGY AND BIOTECHNOLOGY. Text in English. 1991. bi-m. USD 403.40 domestic; USD 397.10 in Germany; USD 74 newsstand/cover foreign (effective 2002). 96 p./no. *Refereed.* **Document type:** *Journal, Academic/Scholarly.* **Description:** Devoted to the advancement and dissemination of scientific knowledge concerning microbiology, biotechnology, and related academic disciplines.
Related titles: Online - full text ed.: (from Institute for Scientific Information).
Indexed: ASCA, Biotech.Cit.Ind., Chem.Abstr., Chem.Titles, Int.Abstr.Biol.Sci., Mass Spectr.Bull., Sci.Cit.Ind.
—BLDSC (5019.285900), CASDDS, CISTI, IDS.
Published by: (Korean Society for Applied Microbiology SGP), Springer-Verlag Hong Kong Ltd. (Subsidiary of: BertelsmannSpringer), Unit 1702, Tower 1, Enterprise Square, 9 Sheung Yuet Rd, Kowloon Bay, Kowloon, Hong Kong. TEL 852-2723-9698, FAX 852-2724-2366, springer@springer.com.hk. Ed. Yung Hee Koh.

660 USA ISSN 0275-3685
MCGRAW-HILL'S BIOTECHNOLOGY NEWSWATCH. Text in English. s-m. reprint service avail. from PQC.
Related titles: Online - full text ed.: (from The Dialog Corporation, Dow Jones Interactive, LexisNexis, NewsNet, Gale Group).
Indexed: CBNB (1989-), CEABA, Inpharma, L.R.I., Reac.
—BLDSC (2089.868000).
Published by: McGraw-Hill Companies, Chemical Engineering, 2 Penn Plaza, 5th Fl, New York, NY 10121. TEL 212-904-6410. Ed. Mara Bovsun.

MEDICAL AND BIOMEDICAL ENGINEERING REPORTS. see *ENGINEERING*

MEDICAL & PHARMACEUTICAL BIOTECHNOLOGY ABSTRACTS. see *MEDICAL SCIENCES—Abstracting, Bibliographies, Statistics*

660 574.28 USA
METHODS IN BIOTECHNOLOGY. Text in English. 1996. irreg., latest vol.12, 1999. price varies. illus. back issues avail. *Refereed.* **Document type:** *Monographic series, Academic/Scholarly.* **Description:** Offers the latest step-by-step laboratory methods for biotechnology and enzyme engineering.
Indexed: GeoRef, Mass Spectr.Bull.
—BLDSC (5747.050000).
Published by: Humana Press Inc., 999 Riverview Dr, Ste 208, Totowa, NJ 07512. TEL 973-256-1699, FAX 973-256-8341, humana@humanapr.com, http://humanapress.com. Ed. John M Walker. R&P Richard Hruska.

▼ **MICROSPHERES, MICROCAPSULES & LIPOSOMES.** see *PHARMACY AND PHARMACOLOGY*

660 610 USA ISSN 1073-6085
TP248.13 CODEN: MLBOEO
MOLECULAR BIOTECHNOLOGY. (Part B of Applied Biochemistry and Biotechnology (ISSN 0273-2289)) Text in English. 1994. 9/yr. USD 420 domestic; USD 455 foreign (effective 2000). adv. bk.rev., software rev. *Refereed.* **Document type:** *Journal, Academic/Scholarly.* **Description:** Provides detailed laboratory protocols and methods for molecular biology techniques, and publishes review articles and critical research results on the application of these techniques in basic and applied research in biotechnology.
Related titles: Online - full text ed.: (from O C L C Online Computer Library Center, Inc., Institute for Scientific Information).
Indexed: ASCA, AgBiotech, Agri.& Environ.Biotech.Abstr., Agricola, Anim.Breed.Abstr., Bibl.Agri., Biol.Abstr., Biotech.Cit.Ind., CEABA, Chem.Abstr., Chem.Indus.Notes, Chem.Titles, Curr.Cont. (coverage dropped), Environ.Sci.Poll.Mgmt., Excerp.Med., Food Sci.& Tech.Abstr., Ind.Med. (1994-), Mass Spectr.Bull., Med.& Pharm.Biotech.Abstr., Microbiol.Abstr., Neurosci.Abstr. (coverage dropped), Nuc.Acids Abstr., Plant Breed.Abstr.
—BLDSC (5900.798400), ADONIS, CASDDS, CISTI, GNLM, IDS, Infotrieve, Linda Hall. **CCC.**
Published by: Humana Press Inc., 999 Riverview Dr, Ste 208, Totowa, NJ 07512. TEL 973-256-1699, FAX 973-256-8341, humana@humanapr.com, http://humanapress.com. Ed. John M Walker. R&P Richard Hruska. Adv. contact Thomas B Lanigan Jr. Circ: 500. **Dist. in Japan by:** Maruzen Co., Ltd., International Division, Export Dept, P.O. Box 5050, Tokyo International 100-3191, Japan. TEL 81-3-3275-8591.

660.6 USA ISSN 1087-0156
TP248.3 CODEN: NABIF9
NATURE BIOTECHNOLOGY. Text in English. 1983. m. USD 119 domestic to individuals; GBP 89 foreign to individuals; USD 710 domestic to institutions; GBP 320 foreign to institutions (effective 2001). adv. bk.rev. charts, illus, tr.lit. back issues avail. *Refereed.* **Document type:** *Journal, Academic/Scholarly.* **Description:** It is the first source for finding reports on the increasing number of important developments in the international industrial biotechnology industries.
Formerly (until vol.14, no.3, Mar. 1996): Bio-Technology (0733-222X)
Related titles: E-mail ed.; Microfilm ed.: (from PQC); Online - full text ed.: (from EBSCO Publishing, ingenta, Gale Group, Factiva, Institute for Scientific Information).
Indexed: ASCA, Abstr.Bull.Inst.Pap.Chem., AgBiotech, Agri.& Environ.Biotech.Abstr., Agricola, Anim.Breed.Abstr., Aqua.Sci.& Fish.Abstr., Bio-Contr.News & Info., Biol.& Agr.Ind. (Mar.1996-), Biol.Dig., Biotech.& Bioeng.Abstr., Biotech.Cit.Ind., CEABA, C.I.J.E. (coverage dropped), Cal.Tiss.Abstr., Chem.Abstr., Chem.Indus.Notes, Chem.Titles, Crop Physiol.Abstr., Curr.Adv.Biochem., Curr.Adv.Cell & Devel.Biol., Curr.Adv.Ecol.Sci., Curr.Adv.Gen.& Molec.Biol., Curr.Biotech.Abstr., Curr.Cont., Dairy Sci.Abstr., Deep Sea Res.& Oceanogr.Abstr., Derwent Biotech.Abstr., Eng.Ind., Entomol.Abstr., Environ.Sci.Poll.Mgmt., Excerp.Med., Food Sci.& Tech.Abstr., Forest Prod.Abstr., Forest.Abstr., Genet.Abstr., Helminthol.Abstr., Hort.Abstr., Hum.Gen.Abstr., INIS Atomind., Immun.Abstr. (coverage dropped), Ind.Med. (1996-), Ind.Sci.Rev., Ind.Vet., Inpharma, Int.Abstr.Biol.Sci., Maize Abstr., Med.& Pharm.Biotech.Abstr., Microbiol.Abstr., NRN, Neurosci.Abstr., Nuc.Acids Abstr., Nutr.Abstr., Pharm.&Out.News, Pig News & Info., Plant Breed.Abstr., Plant Gen.Res.Abstr., Plant Grow.Reg.Abstr., Pollut.Abstr., Postharvest, Potato Abstr., Protozool.Abstr., Reac., Ref.Zh., Rev.Appl.Entomol., Rev.Med.& Vet.Mycol., Rev.Plant Path., Rice Abstr., Russ.Acad.Sci.Bibl., SSCI (coverage dropped), Sci.Cit.Ind., Seed Abstr., Soils & Fert., Soyabean Abstr., Telegen, Triticale Abstr., VITIS, Vet.Bull., Virol.Abstr., W.R.C.Inf., Weed Abstr., World Ag.Econ.& Rur.Soc.Abstr.
—BLDSC (6046.257000), CASDDS, CISTI, Ei, EMDOCS, GNLM, IDS, ingenta, Linda Hall. **CCC.**
Published by: Nature Publishing Co. (Subsidiary of: Macmillan Magazines, Ltd.), 345 Park Ave S, 10th Fl, New York, NY 10012-2467. TEL 212-726-9200, 800-524-0384, FAX 615-377-0525, subscriptions@natureny.com, http://www.nature.com/nbt, http://www.biotech.nature.com. Ed. Susan Hassler. Pub. James Skowrenski. Adv. contact Bill Moran. Circ: 15,000. **Subscr. in US to:** Allen Press Inc., PO Box 1897, Lawrence, KS 66044-8897; **Subscr. outside N. America to:** Macmillan Magazines Ltd, Brunel Rd, Basingstoke, Hants RG21 6XT, United Kingdom. **Dist. by:** PO Box 5054, Brentwood, TN 37024-5054.

660 630.24 JPN
CODEN: NNKKAA
NIPPON NOGEIKAGAKU KAISHI/JAPAN SOCIETY FOR BIOSCIENCE, BIOTECHNOLOGY, AND AGROCHEMISTRY. JOURNAL. Text in Japanese; Contents page in English. 1924. m. USD 200 to non-members; USD 80 to members. adv. bk.rev. **Document type:** *Academic/Scholarly.* **Description:** Contains original and review papers in the fields of bioscience, biotechnology and biochemistry.
Formerly: Agricultural Chemical Society of Japan. Journal (0002-1407)
Related titles: Online - full text ed.: (from Institute for Scientific Information).
Indexed: ASCA, AgBiotech, Anim.Breed.Abstr., Aqua.Sci.& Fish.Abstr., Aquacult.Abstr., Bio-Contr.News & Info., Biol.Abstr., CEABA, Chem.Abstr., Chem.Indus.Notes, Chem.Titles, Crop Physiol.Abstr., Curr.Adv.Biochem., Curr.Adv.Gen.& Molec.Biol., Curr.Biotech.Abstr., Curr.Chem.React., Curr.Cont., Dairy Sci.Abstr., Environ.Sci.Poll.Mgmt., Field Crop Abstr., Food Sci.& Tech.Abstr., Forest Prod.Abstr., GeoRef, Helminthol.Abstr., Herb.Abstr., Hort.Abstr., Ind.Chem., Ind.Vet., JTA, MOS, Maize Abstr., Mass Spectr.Bull., NPU, Nutr.Abstr., Ornam.Hort., Plant Grow.Reg.Abstr., Potato Abstr., RCI, Rev.Appl.Entomol., Rev.Arom.& Med.Plants, Rev.Med.& Vet.Mycol., Rev.Plant Path., Rice Abstr., Seed Abstr., Soyabean Abstr., Sport Fish.Abstr., Sugar Ind.Abstr., Triticale Abstr.
—BLDSC (6113.431500), CASDDS, CISTI, IDS, ingenta, Linda Hall. **CCC.**
Published by: Nippon Nogeikagaku Kai/Japan Society for Bioscience, Biotechnology and Agrochemistry, c/o Japan Academic Societies Centre Bldg, 2-4-16 Yayoi, Bunkyo-ku, Tokyo 113-0032, Japan. FAX 81-3-3815-1920, http://wwwsoc.nacsis.ac.jp/jsbba. Ed. Shuichi Kaminogawa. Circ: 13,800.

O M I C S: A JOURNAL OF INTEGRATIVE BIOLOGY. see *BIOLOGY—Genetics*

615.285 USA
PHARMACEUTICAL BIOTECHNOLOGY. Text in English. 1992. irreg., latest vol.12, 1999. price varies. back issues avail. **Document type:** *Monographic series.* **Description:** Scholarly monographs on theoretical and practical advances in the pharmaceutical sciences, focusing on biotechnology applications and developments in drug dosage design.
Indexed: Chem.Abstr., Chem.Indus.Notes, Chem.Titles, Ind.Med. (1992-).
—BLDSC (6442.770000).
Published by: Kluwer Academic - Plenum Publishers (Subsidiary of: Wolters Kluwer N.V.), 233 Spring St, New York, NY 10013-1578. TEL 212-620-8000, 800-221-9369, FAX 212-463-0742, info@plenum.com, http://www.plenum.com. Ed. Ronald T Borchardt.

PHARMACEUTICAL STRATEGIC ALLIANCES; the drug and biotech alliances reference guide. see *PHARMACY AND PHARMACOLOGY*

PLANT BIOTECHNOLOGY. see *BIOLOGY—Abstracting, Bibliographies, Statistics*

660 630 NLD ISSN 0925-5214
SB129 CODEN: PBTEED
POSTHARVEST BIOLOGY AND TECHNOLOGY. Text in English. 1991. 9/yr. EUR 814 in Europe to institutions; JPY 108,000 in Japan to institutions; USD 910 elsewhere to institutions (effective 2002). adv. bk.rev. back issues avail. *Refereed.* **Document type:** *Academic/Scholarly.* **Description:** Contains exclusive original papers and review articles on biological and technological research on postharvest handling or treatment, quality evaluation, packaging, storage and distribution - transportation of agronomic (including forage) and horticultural crops.
Related titles: Microform ed.: (from PQC); Online - full text ed.: (from ingenta, Swets Blackwell, Institute for Scientific Information, ScienceDirect).
Indexed: ASCA, Agri.Eng.Abstr., Agricola, Aqua.Sci.& Fish.Abstr., Bio-Contr.News & Info., Chem.Abstr., Chem.Indus.Notes, Chem.Titles, Crop Physiol.Abstr., Curr.Adv.Plant Sci., Curr.Cont., Entomol.Abstr., Field Crop Abstr., Food Sci.& Tech.Abstr., Hort.Abstr., Int.Abstr.Biol.Sci., Maize Abstr., Ornam.Hort., Plant Breed.Abstr., Plant Grow.Reg.Abstr., Plant Sci., Postharvest, Potato Abstr., Rev.Appl.Entomol., Rev.Arom.& Med.Plants, Rev.Plant Path., Sci.Cit.Ind., Seed Abstr., Soils & Fert., Soyabean Abstr., Sugar Ind.Abstr., Triticale Abstr., Weed Abstr.
—BLDSC (6563.921500), CASDDS, CISTI, EMDOCS, IDS, Infotrieve, ingenta. **CCC.**
Published by: Elsevier Science BV, PO Box 211, Amsterdam 1000 AE, Netherlands. TEL 31-20-485-2911, FAX 31-20-485-2457, http://www.elsevier.com/locate/postharvbio. Eds. Graeme E Hobson, I B Ferguson, R P Cavalieri. **Subscr. in Australasia and the Far East to:** Elsevier Science (Singapore) Pte Ltd, No.1 Temasek Ave, 17-01 Millenia Tower, Singapore 039192, Singapore. TEL 65-434-3727, FAX 65-337-2230; **Subscr. in Japan to:** Elsevier Science Inc - Japan Regional Office, 9-15 Higashi-Azabu 1-chome, Minato-ku, Tokyo 106-0044, Japan. TEL 81-3-5561-5033; **Subscr. in the Americas to:** Elsevier Science, PO Box 945, New York, NY 10159-0945. TEL 212-633-3730, FAX 212-633-3680, usinfo-f@elsevier.com.

PREPARATIVE BIOCHEMISTRY AND BIOTECHNOLOGY. see *BIOLOGY—Biochemistry*

660 GBR ISSN 0032-9592
TP500 CODEN: PRBCAP
PROCESS BIOCHEMISTRY. Text in English. 1966. m. EUR 899 in Europe to institutions; JPY 119,400 in Japan to institutions; USD 1,006 elsewhere to institutions (effective 2002). adv. bk.rev. charts, illus, tr.lit. index. *Refereed.* **Document type:** *Academic/Scholarly.* **Description:** Reports advances in the science and technology of the application of living organisms to processing and production methods in the food, beverage and pharmaceutical industries, and the energy, waste and water treatment industries.
Formerly (until 1991): Process Biochemistry International
Related titles: Microform ed.: (from PQC); Online - full text ed.: (from ingenta, Swets Blackwell, Institute for Scientific Information, ScienceDirect).
Indexed: ASCA, AgBiotech, Agri.& Environ.Biotech.Abstr., Agri.Eng.Abstr., Agricola, Agroforest.Abstr., Aqua.Sci.& Fish.Abstr., BBCI, Bibl.Agri., Bio-Contr.News & Info., Biol.Abstr., Biotech.Cit.Ind., Br.Tech.Ind., CEABA, Chem.Abstr., Chem.Cit.Ind., Chem.Eng.Abstr., Chem.Indus.Notes, Chem.Titles, Crop Physiol.Abstr., Curr.Adv.Ecol.Sci., Curr.Biotech.Abstr., Curr.Cont., Dairy Sci.Abstr., Derwent Biotech.Abstr., Energy Ind., Energy Info.Abstr., Eng.Ind., Environ.Sci.Poll.Mgmt., Excerp.Med., Field Crop Abstr., Food Sci.& Tech.Abstr., Forest Prod.Abstr., Hort.Abstr., INIS Atomind., Ind.Sci.Rev., Ind.Vet., Inpharma, Int.Abstr.Biol.Sci., Maize Abstr., Microbiol.Abstr., Nutr.Abstr., Plant Grow.Reg.Abstr., Postharvest, Potato Abstr., Poult.Abstr., Reac., Rev.Appl.Entomol., Rev.Arom.& Med.Plants, Rev.Plant Path., Sci.Cit.Ind., Seed Abstr., Sel.Water Res.Abstr., Soils & Fert., Soyabean Abstr., Sugar Ind.Abstr., T.C.E.A., Telegen, Vet.Bull., W.R.C.Inf.
—BLDSC (6849.983500), CASDDS, CISTI, Ei, EMDOCS, GNLM, IDS, Infotrieve, ingenta, Linda Hall. **CCC.**
Published by: Pergamon (Subsidiary of: Elsevier Science), The Boulevard, Langford Ln, East Park, Kidlington, Oxford OXB 1GB, United Kingdom. FAX 44-1865-843010, nlinfo-f@elsevier.nl; usinfo-f@elsevier.com; forinfo-kyf04035@niftyserve.or.jp, nlinfo-f@elsevier/nl; usinfo-f@elsevier.com; forinfo-kyf04035@niftyserve.or.jp, http://www.elsevier.com/locate/procbio. Ed. C M Brown. Circ: 3,750. **Subscr. in Australasia and the Far East to:** Elsevier Science (Singapore) Pte Ltd, No.1 Temasek Ave, 17-01 Millenia Tower, Singapore 039192, Singapore. TEL 65-434-3727, FAX 65-337-2230; **Subscr. in the Americas to:** Elsevier Science, PO Box 945, New York, NY 10159-0945. TEL 212-633-3730, FAX 212-633-3680, usinfo-f@elsevier.com; **Subscr. to:** Elsevier Science BV, PO Box 211, Amsterdam 1000 AE, Netherlands. TEL 31-20-485-3757, FAX 31-20-485-3432, nlinfo-f@elsevier.nl.

PROGRESS IN BIOMEDICAL RESEARCH. see *BIOLOGY—Bioengineering*

660 RUS ISSN 1068-3682
TP248.19.S65
RUSSIAN BIOTECHNOLOGY. Text in English. 1986. bi-m., latest 1999. USD 700 in United States; USD 795 elsewhere (effective 2001). **Document type:** *Academic/Scholarly.* **Description:** Covers industrial microbiology, genetic engineering, biosynthesis of antibiotics, immunomodulators and immunoassays, and monoclonal antibodies.
Formerly (until 1993): Soviet Biotechnology (0890-734X)
Related titles: ♦ Translation of: Biotekhnologiya. ISSN 0234-2758.
Indexed: Derwent Biotech.Abstr., Food Sci.& Tech.Abstr., INIS Atomind., Sugar Ind.Abstr.
—CISTI, Infotrieve. **CCC.**
Published by: (State Scientific Research Institute for Genetics and Selection of Industrial Microorganisms, G N I I Genetika), M A I K Nauka - Interperiodica, Mezhdunarodnyi Otdel, Profsoyuznaya ul 90, Moscow 117864, Russian Federation. TEL 7-095-336-1600, FAX 7-095-336-0666, compmg@maik.ru, http://www.maik.rssi.ru/. Ed. Vladimir G Debabov. **Dist. by:** Maik Nauka - Interperiodica, Subscription Office, PO Box 1831, Birmingham, AL 35201-1831. TEL 205-995-1567.

660 CHN ISSN 1003-3505
SHENGWU GONGCHENG JINZHAN/PROGRESS IN BIOTECHNOLOGY. Text in Chinese. 1976. bi-m. USD 30 (effective 2000). adv. **Document type:** *Academic/Scholarly.* **Description:** Reports the new developments in the field of biotechnology all over the world.
Related titles: CD-ROM ed.
—BLDSC (6866.170000).
Published by: Zhongguo Kexueyuan, Wenxian Qingbao Zhongxin/Chinese Academy of Sciences, Documentation and Information Center, 8 Kexueyuan Nanlu, Zhongguancun, Beijing 100080, China. TEL 86-1-6256-2548, FAX 86-1-6256-7325. Ed. Zhang Shuyong. R&P Ziyi Chen. adv.: page USD 500. Circ: 5,000.

660 CHN ISSN 1000-3061
TP248.13 CODEN: SGXUED
SHENGWU GONGCHENG XUEBAO/CHINESE JOURNAL OF BIOTECHNOLOGY. Text in Chinese; Summaries in English. 1985. q. USD 72 (effective 2000). adv. abstr. *Refereed.* **Document type:** *Academic/Scholarly.* **Description:** Contains research papers on genetic, fermentation, cell and enzyme engineering. Includes new methods for strain breeding, kinetics, regulation of biosynthesis; biochemical engineering unit operations and processes, resource development and environmental protection.
Indexed: Chem.Abstr., Chem.Indus.Notes, Chem.Titles, Ind.Med. (1985-).
—BLDSC (3180.297000), CASDDS.
Published by: (Chinese Academy of Sciences/Zhongguo Kexueyuan), Kexue Chubanshe/Science Press, 16 Donghuang Cheng Genbei Jie, Beijing 100717, China. Circ: 6,000.

618.178059 USA
SOCIETY FOR IN VITRO BIOLOGY. MONOGRAPH SERIES. Text in English. irreg. price varies. *Refereed.* **Document type:** *Monographic series.* **Description:** Covers specific topics of interest to tissue culture researchers.
Formerly: Tissue Culture Association. Monograph Series
Published by: Society for In Vitro Biology, 9315 Largo Dr. W., Ste. 255, Largo, MD 20774. TEL 301-324-5054, FAX 301-324-5057, sivb@sivb.org, http://www.sivb.org.

SOSHIKI BAIYO KENKYU/TISSUE CULTURE RESEARCH COMMUNICATIONS. see *BIOLOGY—Cytology And Histology*

660.6 GBR ISSN 0167-7799
TP248.13 CODEN: TRBIDM
TRENDS IN BIOTECHNOLOGY. Text in English. 1983. m. GBP 92 in Europe to individuals; EUR 115 in Europe to individuals Print & online eds. combined; JPY 14,000 in Japan to individuals; USD 126 elsewhere to individuals; EUR 908 in Europe to institutions; JPY 125,900 in Japan to institutions; USD 1,015 elsewhere to institutions; USD 1,308 to institutions Print & online eds. combined; GBP 47 in Europe to students; JPY 10,100 in Japan to students; USD 78 elsewhere to students; EUR 144 in Europe to qualified personnel Print & online eds. combined; JPY 1,750 in Japan to qualified personnel Print & online eds. combined; USD 157 elsewhere to qualified personnel Print & online eds. combined (effective 2002). adv. bk.rev. illus. index. back issues avail.; reprints avail. *Refereed.* **Document type:** *Academic/Scholarly.* **Description:** Covers all aspects of applied biosciences, including microbiology, molecular biology, immunology, plant and animal cell culture, agriculture and medicine.
Related titles: Online - full text ed.: (from ingenta, Swets Blackwell, Institute for Scientific Information, ScienceDirect).
Indexed: A.S.& T.Ind. (Jan.2001-), ASCA, AgBiotech, Agri.& Environ.Biotech.Abstr., Agricola, Anim.Breed.Abstr., Aqua.Sci.& Fish.Abstr., Bioeng.Abstr., Biol.Abstr., Biotech.Cit.Ind., CEABA, Chem.Abstr., Chem.Cit.Ind., Chem.Indus.Notes, Curr.Adv.Ecol.Sci., Curr.Biotech.Abstr., Curr.Cont., Dairy Sci.Abstr., Ecol.Abstr., Eng.Ind., Entomol.Abstr., Environ.Sci.Poll.Mgmt., Excerp.Med., Food Sci.& Tech.Abstr., Helminthol.Abstr., Hort.Abstr., Ind.Med. (1983-), Ind.Sci.Rev., Ind.Vet., Inpharma, Int.Abstr.Biol.Sci., Med.& Pharm.Biotech.Abstr., Microbiol.Abstr., Nutr.Abstr., Ornam.Hort., Pharm.&Out.News, Pig News & Info., Plant Breed.Abstr., Reac., Ref.Zh., Rev.Appl.Entomol., Rev.Plant Path., Rice Abstr., Sci.Cit.Ind., Soils & Fert., Soyabean Abstr., Telegen, Weed Abstr.
—BLDSC (9049.547000), ADONIS, CASDDS, CISTI, GNLM, IDS, ingenta. **CCC.**
Published by: Elsevier Science Ltd., Elsevier Trends Journals, 68 Hills Rd, Cambridge CB2 1LA, United Kingdom. TEL 44-1223-315961, FAX 44-1223-464430, TTEC@elsevier.co.uk, http://www.elsevier.nl/locate/issn/01677799. Eds. A Hinde, Meran Owen. Adv. contact Thelma Reid. **Subscr. in Australasia and the Far East to:** Elsevier Science (Singapore) Pte Ltd, No.1 Temasek Ave, 17-01 Millenia Tower, Singapore 039192, Singapore. TEL 65-434-3727, FAX 65-337-2230; **Subscr. in the Americas to:** Elsevier Science, PO Box 945, New York, NY 10159-0945. TEL 212-633-3730, FAX 212-633-3680, http://www.elsevier.com; **Subscr. to:** Elsevier Current Trends Subscriptions, PO Box 331, Haywards Heath, W Sussex RH16 3FG, United Kingdom. TEL 44-1444-475650, FAX 44-1444-445423.

660.6 ROM ISSN 1224-7774
UNIVERSITATEA DE STIINTE AGRONOMICE SI MEDICINA VETERINARA. LUCRARI STIINTIFICE. SERIA F, BIOTEHNOLOGII. Text in Romanian; Summaries in English. a. per issue exchange basis only. **Document type:** *Academic/Scholarly.*
Formerly (until 1995): Universitatea de Stiinte Agronomice. Lucrari Stiintifice. Seria F, Biotehnologii Vegetale, Biotehnologii Industriale, Biotehnologii Animale
Published by: Universitatea de Stiinte Agronomice si Medicina Veterinara, B-dul. Marasti 59, Sector 1, Bucharest 71331, Romania. TEL 40-1-2242576, FAX 40-1-2232693.

660.62 GBR ISSN 0959-3993
QR53 CODEN: WJMBEY
WORLD JOURNAL OF MICROBIOLOGY AND BIOTECHNOLOGY. Text in English. 1985. bi-m. EUR 1,500 to institutions for print or online ed.; EUR 1,800 to institutions print & online eds.combined (effective 2002). adv. bk.rev. back issues avail. *Refereed.* **Document type:** *Academic/Scholarly.* **Description:** Publishes research papers, short communications, technical communications and review articles on all aspects of applied microbiology and biotechnology, including management of culture collections, foodstuffs and biological control agents.
Formerly (until 1990): Mircen - Journal of Applied Microbiology and Biotechnology (0265-0762)
Related titles: CD-ROM ed.; Online - full text ed.: (from EBSCO Publishing, O C L C Online Computer Library Center, Inc., RoweCom Information Quest, Swets Blackwell, Kluwer Online, Institute for Scientific Information).
Indexed: AESIS, ASCA, AgBiotech, Agri.& Environ.Biotech.Abstr., Agri.Eng.Abstr., Agricola, Agroforest.Abstr., Aqua.Sci.& Fish.Abstr., Bio-Contr.News & Info., Biol.Abstr., Biotech.Cit.Ind., CEABA, Chem.Abstr., Chem.Indus.Notes, Chem.Titles, Crop Physiol.Abstr., Curr.Adv.Biochem., Curr.Adv.Plant Sci., Curr.Biotech.Abstr., Curr.Cont., Dairy Sci.Abstr., Derwent Biotech.Abstr., Diar.Dis.Res., Environ.Sci.Poll.Mgmt., Field Crop Abstr., Food Sci.& Tech.Abstr., Forest Prod.Abstr., Forest.Abstr., Helminthol.Abstr., Herb.Abstr., Hort.Abstr., INIS Atomind., Ind.Vet., Int.Abstr.Biol.Sci., Maize Abstr., Microbiol.Abstr., Nutr.Abstr., Pig News & Info., Plant Breed.Abstr., Plant Grow.Reg.Abstr., Plant Sci., Pollut.Abstr., Postharvest, Poult.Abstr., Protozool.Abstr., Rev.Appl.Entomol., Rev.Arom.& Med.Plants, Rev.Med.& Vet.Mycol., Rev.Plant Path., Rice Abstr., Seed Abstr., Soils & Fert., Soyabean Abstr., Sugar Ind.Abstr., Triticale Abstr., Trop.Oil Seeds Abstr., Vet.Bull., Weed Abstr., World Ag.Econ.& Rur.Soc.Abstr.
—BLDSC (9356.073500), ADONIS, CASDDS, CISTI, EMDOCS, IDS, Infotrieve. **CCC.**
Published by: (International Union of Microbiological Societies NLD), Kluwer Academic Publishers Group (Subsidiary of: Wolters Kluwer N.V.), Spuiboulevard 50, PO Box 17, Dordrecht 3300 AA, Netherlands. FAX 31-78-639-2254, services@wkap.nl, http://www.wkap.nl. Ed. Colin Ratledge TEL 44-1482-465243. Adv. contact Gemma Heiser. **Dist. by:** Journals Department, PO Box 322, Dordrecht 3300 AH, Netherlands. TEL 781-871-6600, FAX 31-78-654-6474.

660 615.19 USA
WORLDWIDE BIOTECH. Text in English. 1989. m. USD 150 in North America; USD 165 elsewhere (effective 2001). bk.rev. back issues avail. **Document type:** *Newsletter, Trade.* **Description:** Provides news and information on biotechnology as an international industry, reporting on the deals between US biotechnology companies and both US and international pharmaceutical corporations. Monitors the emerging EC marketplace and the growing Japanese interest.
Related titles: Online - full text ed.: (from Data-Star, The Dialog Corporation, Gale Group).
Published by: Worldwide Videotex, PO Box 3273, Boynton Beach, FL 33424-3273. TEL 561-738-2276, markedit@juno.com, http://www.wvpubs.com. Ed., Pub. Mark Wright.

BIOLOGY—Botany

see also AGRICULTURE—Crop Production And Soil FORESTS AND FORESTRY; GARDENING AND HORTICULTURE

A E T F A T INDEX; releve des travaux de phanerogamie systematique et des taxons nouveaux concernant l'Afrique au sud du Sahara et Madagascar. see *BIOLOGY—Abstracting, Bibliographies, Statistics*

571.2 USA ISSN 1535-5489
A S P B NEWS; the newsletter of the American Society of Plant Biologists. Text in English. 1974. bi-m., latest vol.28, no.3. USD 30 to non-members; USD 2 to members (effective 2000). back issues avail. **Document type:** *Newsletter, Newspaper-distributed.* **Description:** Keeps society members informed on items of professional interest.
Formerly: A S P P Newsletter (0279-9936)
Published by: American Society of Plant Biologists, 15501 Monona Dr, Rockville, MD 20855. TEL 301-251-0560, FAX 301-279-2996, nancyw@aspb.org, http://www.aspb.org. Ed., R&P, Adv. contact Nancy Winchester. Pub. John Lisack Jr. Circ: 5,100.

A T C C CATALOGUE OF PLANT VIRUSES AND ANTISERA. see *BIOLOGY—Microbiology*

579.5 USA
QK600.73.U62
A T C C FILAMENTOUS FUNGI. Text in English. 1986. irreg., latest vol.19, 1996. USD 34 in North America; USD 44 elsewhere. **Document type:** *Catalog.*
Formerly: A T C C Catalogue of Filamentous Fungi (1065-0598); Supersedes in part (in 1991): American Type Culture Collection. Catalogue of Fungi - Yeasts (1053-3370); Which superseded in part: American Type Culture Collection. Catalogue of Strains 1: Algae, Bacteria, Bacteriophages, Plasmids, Fungi, Plant Viruses and Antisera and Protozoa
—CISTI.
Published by: American Type Culture Collection, 10801 University Blvd, Manassas, VA 20110. TEL 800-638-6597, FAX 301-816-4361, sales@ATCC.org.

579.562 USA
A T C C YEASTS. Text in English. 1986. irreg., latest vol.19, 1995. USD 35 in North America; USD 47 elsewhere. **Document type:** *Catalog.*
Formerly (until 1995): A T C C Catalogue of Yeasts; Supersedes in part (in 1991): American Type Culture Collection. Catalogue of Fungi - Yeasts (1053-3370); Which supersedes in part: American Type Culture Collection. Catalogue of Strains 1
—CISTI.
Published by: American Type Culture Collection, 10801 University Blvd, Manassas, VA 20110. TEL 800-638-6597, FAX 301-816-4361. Eds. M J Edwards, S C Jong.

ABSTRACTS OF MYCOLOGY. see *BIOLOGY—Abstracting, Bibliographies, Statistics*

986.1 580 COL ISSN 0120-548X
ACTA BIOLOGICA COLOMBIANA. Text in Spanish. 1982. 2/yr. COP 6,000 (effective 1999). back issues avail. *Refereed.* **Description:** Describes many aspects of the studies done by the Department of Biology at the National University and includes data on Colombian flora and fauna.
Indexed: VITIS, Zoo.Rec.
Published by: Universidad Nacional de Colombia, Facultad de Biologia, Apartado Aereo 14490, Bogota, Colombia. TEL 57-1-368-4273, FAX 57-1-225-5192. Ed. Dr. Marcela Camacho. Circ: 500.

580 HRV ISSN 0365-0588
CODEN: ABCRA2
ACTA BOTANICA CROATICA. Text and summaries in English. 1925. 2/yr. HRK 300 domestic; USD 80 foreign (effective 2000 - 2001). adv. bk.rev. bibl, illus. index, cum.index. back issues avail. *Refereed.* **Description:** Publishes original scientific papers on various fields of botany.
Indexed: AgBiotech, Aqua.Sci.& Fish.Abstr., Biol.Abstr., Chem.Abstr., Chem.Indus.Notes, Chem.Titles, Crop Physiol.Abstr., Environ.Sci.Poll.Mgmt., Field Crop Abstr., Forest.Abstr., Herb.Abstr., Hort.Abstr., Maize Abstr., Ornam.Hort., Plant Breed.Abstr., Plant Gen.Res.Abstr., Plant Grow.Reg.Abstr., Pollut.Abstr., Potato Abstr., Rev.Med.& Vet.Mycol., Rev.Plant Path., Soils & Fert., Weed Abstr., Zoo.Rec.
—CASDDS, Linda Hall.
Published by: Sveuciliste u Zagrebu, Prirodoslovno-Matematicki Fakultet/University of Zagreb, Faculty of Science, Division of Biology, Bioloski Odjel, Rooseveltov trg 6, Zagreb 10000, Croatia. TEL 385-1-4895561, grozdana@lipa.botanic.hr, http://hirc.botanic.hr/actabot/actahome.htm. Ed. Damir Vilicic. Adv. contact Grozdana Sirotic. B&W page USD 200, color page USD 300. Circ: 400.

ALGOLOGICAL STUDIES; Archiv fuer Hydrobiologie, Supplementbaende. see *BIOLOGY*

582.14 635.955 ZWE ISSN 1016-524X
ALOE, CACTUS & SUCCULENT SOCIETY OF ZIMBABWE. INGENS BULLETIN. Text in English. 1989. 2/yr. ZAR 80, GBP 12, USD 20, DEM 40 to individuals; ZAR 120, GBP 20, USD 30, DEM 60 to institutions (effective 1999). adv. **Document type:** *Bulletin.*
Published by: Aloe Cactus and Succulent Society of Zimbabwe, PO Box CY 300, Causeway, Harare, Zimbabwe. TEL 263-4-481418. Ed. Michael J Kimberley. R&P Doreen Richards. Adv. contact Michael J Kimberly. Circ: 1,000.

580 FIN ISSN 0570-5169
CODEN: ASBOD8
AQUILO. SERIE BOTANICA. Text in English, German. 1963. s-a. price varies. back issues avail. *Refereed.* **Document type:** *Academic/Scholarly.* **Description:** Covers botany, ecology, pollution and plant physiology.
Indexed: Aqua.Sci.& Fish.Abstr., Biol.Abstr., Chem.Abstr., Curr.Adv.Ecol.Sci., Deep Sea Res.& Oceanogr.Abstr., Ecol.Abstr., Environ.Sci.Poll.Mgmt., GeoRef, Geol.Abstr., Hort.Abstr., Pollut.Abstr., Seed Abstr., Sel.Water Res.Abstr., Soils & Fert.
—CASDDS.
Published by: Societas Amicorum Naturae Ouluensis, Department of Botany, University of Oulu, Linnanmaa, Oulu 90570, Finland. TEL 358-8-553-1546, FAX 358-981-553-1500, se@abore. Ed., R&P Pekka Lahdesmaki. Circ: 305 (controlled).

ARBOR AGE. see *FORESTS AND FORESTRY*

ARCHIV FUER HYDROBIOLOGIE. see *BIOLOGY*

ARCHIV FUER HYDROBIOLOGIE. SUPPLEMENT-BAND: ARBEITEN AUS DEM LIMNOLOGISCHEN INSTITUT DER UNIVERSITAET KONSTANZ. see *BIOLOGY*

ARCHIV FUER HYDROBIOLOGIE. SUPPLEMENT-BAND: LARGE RIVERS. see *BIOLOGY*

ARCHIV FUER HYDROBIOLOGIE. SUPPLEMENT-BAND: UNTERSUCHUNGEN DES ELBE-AESTUARS. see *BIOLOGY*

ARCHIV FUER HYDROBIOLOGIE. SUPPLEMENT VOLUMES, MONOGRAPHIC STUDIES. see *BIOLOGY*

580 NLD ISSN 0005-2728
QD1
B B A - BIOENERGETICS. (Biochimica et Biophysica Acta) Text in Dutch. 1970. 15/yr. EUR 1,736 in Europe to institutions; JPY 230,500 in Japan to institutions; USD 1,942 elsewhere to institutions (effective 2002). back issues avail. *Refereed.* **Document type:** *Academic/Scholarly.* **Description:** Covers the area of biological energy transfer and conversion, focusing on the kinetics and thermodynamics of molecular mechanisms involved in photosynthesis, mitochondrial and bacterial respiration, oxidative phosphorylation, motility and transport, as well as the underlying molecular structures.
Related titles: Microform ed.: (from PQC); Online - full text ed.: (from EBSCO Publishing, ingenta, Swets Blackwell, ScienceDirect, Institute for Scientific Information).
Indexed: ASCA, AgBiotech, Agri.& Environ.Biotech.Abstr. (coverage dropped), Anim.Breed.Abstr., BBCI, Chem.Abstr., Chem.Indus.Notes, Chem.Titles, Crop Physiol.Abstr., Curr.Adv.Ecol.Sci., Curr.Cont., Dairy Sci.Abstr., Derwent Biotech.Abstr., Excerp.Med., Field Crop Abstr., Hort.Abstr., INIS Atomind., Ind.Sci.Rev., Ind.Vet., Inpharma, Int.Abstr.Biol.Sci., Nutr.Abstr., Reac., Ref.Zh., Rev.Appl.Entomol., Sci.Cit.Ind., Triticale Abstr., Weed Abstr.
—ADONIS, CISTI, EMDOCS, GNLM, IDS, ingenta. **CCC.**
Published by: Elsevier Science BV, PO Box 211, Amsterdam 1000 AE, Netherlands. TEL 31-20-485-3757, FAX 31-20-485-3432, TELEX 18582 ESPA NL, nlinfo-f@elsevier.nl, http://www.elsevier.com/locate/bbabio, http://www.elsevier.nl. Ed. P R Rich. **Subscr. in Australasia and the Far East to:** Elsevier Science (Singapore) Pte Ltd, No.1 Temasek Ave, 17-01 Millenia Tower, Singapore 039192, Singapore. TEL 65-434-3727, FAX 65-337-2230, asiainfo@elsevier.com.sg; **Subscr. in Japan to:** Elsevier Science Inc - Japan Regional Office, 9-15 Higashi-Azabu 1-chome, Minato-ku, Tokyo 106-0044, Japan. TEL 81-3-5561-5033, FAX 81-3-5561-5047, info@elsevier.co.jp; **Subscr. in the Americas to:** Elsevier Science, PO Box 945, New York, NY 10159-0945. TEL 212-633-3730, FAX 212-633-3680, usinfo-f@elsevier.com, http://www.elsevier.com.

580 BGD ISSN 0253-5416
QK358.7 CODEN: BJBTB3
BANGLADESH JOURNAL OF BOTANY. Text in English. 1972. 2/yr. BDT 599 per vol. domestic; USD 66 per issue foreign (effective 2001 & 2002). adv. bk.rev. 100 p./no. back issues avail. *Refereed.* **Document type:** *Journal, Academic/Scholarly.*
Related titles: CD-ROM ed.; Online - full text ed.: (from Institute for Scientific Information).
Indexed: ASCA, Agroforest.Abstr., Bio-Contr.News & Info., Biol.Abstr., Chem.Abstr., Crop Physiol.Abstr., Curr.Adv.Ecol.Sci., Curr.Cont., ExtraMED, Field Crop Abstr., Food Sci.& Tech.Abstr., Forest.Abstr., Herb.Abstr., Hort.Abstr., Maize Abstr., Nutr.Abstr., Ornam.Hort., Plant Breed.Abstr., Plant Grow.Reg.Abstr., Rev.Arom.& Med.Plants, Rev.Plant Path., Rice Abstr., Seed Abstr., Sel.Water Res.Abstr., Soils & Fert., Soyabean Abstr., Triticale Abstr., Weed Abstr., Zoo.Rec.
—BLDSC (1861.670000), CASDDS, CISTI, IDS, ingenta, Linda Hall.

Published by: Bangladesh Botanical Society, c/o Department of Botany, University of Dhaka, Dhaka 1000, Bangladesh. TEL 880-2-505848 ext 6048, FAX 880-2-865583, botany@du.bangla.net. Ed. M R Khan. adv.: page USD 3,000. Circ: 1,000.

580 DEU ISSN 0341-3624
BAUM-ZEITUNG; fuer Baumfreunde, Natur und Umwelt. Text in German. 1966. q. DEM 64.80 (effective 1998). adv. bk.rev. back issues avail. **Document type:** *Academic/Scholarly.*
Indexed: Avery Ind.Archit.Per., Ref.Zh.
Address: Stiftsallee 29B, Minden 32425, Germany. FAX 49-571-9460721. Ed. Klaus Scheidler. Circ: 2,500.

BIFIDOBACTERIA AND MICROFLORA. see *BIOLOGY*

BIFIZUSU/BIFIDUS FLORES, FRUCTUS ET SEMINA. see *BIOLOGY*

571.2 USA ISSN 0887-2236
SB732.6
BIOLOGICAL AND CULTURAL TESTS FOR CONTROL OF PLANT DISEASES. Short title: B and C Tests. Text in English. 1986. a. USD 38 to individuals; USD 150 to institutions (effective 2001). back issues avail. **Document type:** *Monographic series, Academic/Scholarly.* **Description:** Reviews current experiments in disease control. Also includes short guidelines on how to prepare reports and how to convert US units of measurement to the metric system.
Related titles: Online - full content ed.
—CISTI, ingenta, Linda Hall.
Published by: (American Phytopathological Society), A P S Press, 3340 Pilot Knob Rd., St. Paul, MN 55121-2097. TEL 651-454-7250, 800-328-7560, FAX 651-454-0766, aps@scisoc.org, http://www.scisoc.org. Ed. Steven C Bost. Circ: 1,453.

BIOLOGICAL SOCIETY OF WASHINGTON. PROCEEDINGS. see *BIOLOGY*

579.5 CHL ISSN 0716-114X
BOLETIN MICOLOGICO. Text in English, Spanish. 1982. a., latest vol.15. USD 20. **Description:** Publishes research papers, notes, commentaries, reviews and conference proceedings on general mycology.
Indexed: Bio-Contr.News & Info., Forest.Abstr., Ind.Vet., Maize Abstr., Nutr.Abstr., Plant Breed.Abstr., Postharvest, Rev.Appl.Entomol., Rev.Med.& Vet.Mycol., Rev.Plant Path., Sugar Ind.Abstr., Triticale Abstr., Trop.Dis.Bull., Vet.Bull.
—GNLM.
Published by: Universidad de Valparaiso, Facultad de Medicina, Casilla 92-V, Valparaiso, Chile. TEL 56-32-507370, FAX 56-32-212011, eduardo.piontelli@uv.cl. Ed., R&P Eduardo Piontelli TEL 56-32-212011.

580 ESP ISSN 0214-4565
QK329 CODEN: TDBCD8
BOTANICA COMPLUTENSIS. Text in Spanish. 1968. a. ESP 2,500, USD 30 (effective 2001). adv. bk.rev. bibl, illus. *Refereed.* **Document type:** *Academic/Scholarly.* **Description:** Covers all aspects of basic investigations and applications in the field of Botany.
Former titles (until 1986): Universidad Complutense. Departamento de Botanica. Trabajos (0212-4890); (until 1982): Universidad Complutense. Departamento de Botanica y Fisiologia Vegetal. Trabajos (0210-5179); (until 1975): Universidad Complutense. Departamento de Botanica. Trabajos (0377-8371); (until 1974): Universidad de Madrid. Departamento de Botanica y Fisiologia Vegetal. Trabajos (0580-468X)
Indexed: Biodet.Abstr., GeoRef, Ind.SST.
—CASDDS, CINDOC, CISTI.
Published by: Universidad Complutense de Madrid, Facultad de Ciencias Biologicas, Departamento de Biologia Vegetal I, Servicio de Publicaciones, C. Isaac Peral s/n, Madrid 28040, Spain. TEL 34-91-3946934, FAX 34-1-3946978, bioveg@eucmax.sim.ucm.es, http://www.ucm.es/info/extensio/publicaciones/sepindex.htm. Ed. Santiago Pajaron. Circ: 500.

580.74 570 DEU ISSN 0945-4292
BOTANISCHER VEREIN VON BERLIN UND BRANDENBURG. VERHANDLUNGEN. Text in German. 1859. a. DEM 30 (effective 2000). bk.rev. **Document type:** *Proceedings.*
Formerly: Berliner Botanischer Verein. Verhandlung (0724-3111)
Indexed: Biol.Abstr.
—Linda Hall.
Published by: Botanischer Verein von Berlin und Brandenburg e.V., Koenigin-Luise-Str 6-8, Berlin 14195, Germany. Ed. Gunther Klemm.

BOTANISK CENTRALBIBLIOTEK. FORTEGNELSE OVER LOEBENDE PERIODICA VED BOTANISK CENTRALBIBLITEK. see *BIOLOGY—Abstracting, Bibliographies, Statistics*

BRITISH JOURNAL OF PHYTOTHERAPY. see *ALTERNATIVE MEDICINE*

580 DEU ISSN 0724-0155
DIE BROMELIE. Text in German. 1980. 3/yr. DEM 55 to members (effective 2001). adv. bk.rev. back issues avail. **Document type:** *Journal, Academic/Scholarly.*
Published by: Deutsche Bromelien-Gesellschaft e.V., Burgstaller Str 21, Kirchberg 71737, Germany. TEL 49-7144-36639, roesslein-kirchberg@t-online.de. Ed. Wolfgang Tittelbach. Circ: 400.

580 DEU ISSN 0723-2470
BRYOLOGISCHE BEITRAEGE. Text in English, German. 1982. a. DEM 35. back issues avail.
Published by: I D H - Verlag, Funkenstr 13, Bad Muenstereifel 53902, Germany. Ed. Ruprecht Duell.

BULLETIN OF MEDICO-ETHNO-BOTANICAL RESEARCH. see *ALTERNATIVE MEDICINE*

CANADIAN JOURNAL OF HERBALISM. see *ALTERNATIVE MEDICINE*

632 CAN ISSN 0706-0661
CODEN: CJPPD6
CANADIAN JOURNAL OF PLANT PATHOLOGY. Text in English, French. 1979. q. CND 75; USD 85 foreign. back issues avail. *Refereed.* **Document type:** *Academic/Scholarly.* **Description:** Publication of original research in plant pathology including technology aspects of plant disease control.
Related titles: Online - full text ed.: (from Institute for Scientific Information).
Indexed: ASCA, AgBiotech, Agri.& Environ.Biotech.Abstr. (coverage dropped), Agri.Eng.Abstr., Agricola, Agroforest.Abstr., Bio-Contr.News & Info., Biodet.Abstr., Biol.& Agr.Ind. (Mar.1989-), Biol.Abstr., Chem.Abstr., Chem.Indus.Notes, Chem.Titles, Cott.& Trop.Fibr.Abstr., Curr.Adv.Ecol.Sci., Curr.Adv.Plant Sci., Curr.Cont., Derwent Biotech.Abstr., Environ.Abstr., Fababean Abstr., Field Crop Abstr., Forest Prod.Abstr., Forest.Abstr., Helminthol.Abstr., Herb.Abstr., Hort.Abstr., INIS Atomind., Int.Abstr.Biol.Sci., Irr.& Drain.Abstr., Maize Abstr., Nutr.Abstr., Ornam.Hort., Plant Breed.Abstr., Plant Sci., Postharvest, Potato Abstr., Ref.Zh., Rev.Appl.Entomol., Rev.Arom.& Med.Plants, Rev.Med.& Vet.Mycol., Rev.Plant Path., Seed Abstr., Soils & Fert., Soyabean Abstr., Triticale Abstr., Trop.Oil Seeds Abstr., Weed Abstr., World Ag.Econ.& Rur.Soc.Abstr.
—BLDSC (3034.400000), CASDDS, CISTI, IDS, Infotrieve, ingenta, Linda Hall. **CCC.**
Published by: Canadian Phytopathological Society, Dept of Environmental Biology, University of Guelph, Guelph, ON N1G 2W1, Canada. TEL 519-824-4120, FAX 519-837-0442. Ed. Dr. R P Singh. Circ: 900.

580 ITA
CENTRO MICOLOGICO FRIULANO. BOLLETTINO. Text in Italian. 1976. a.
Published by: Centro Micologico Friulano, Via Beato Odorico da Pordenone, 3, Udine, UD 33100, Italy.

CHEMISTRY OF PLANT PROTECTION SERIES. see *CHEMISTRY*

580 CHN ISSN 1001-0718
QK1 CODEN: CJBOE2
CHINESE JOURNAL OF BOTANY. Text in English. 1989. s-a. USD 49 domestic to individuals; USD 59 foreign to individuals; USD 78 domestic to institutions; USD 88 foreign to institutions (effective 1999). adv. bk.rev. 96 p./no. *Refereed.* **Document type:** *Academic/Scholarly.* **Description:** Publishes original articles on all aspects of plant sciences with emphasis on basic research. Includes reviews, notes, short communications, and institution briefs.
Related titles: ♦ Chinese ed.: Zhiwu Xuebao. ISSN 0577-7496.
Published by: (Chinese Academy of Sciences/Zhongguo Kexueyuan), Kexue Chubanshe/Science Press, 16 Donghuang Cheng Genbei Jie, Beijing 100717, China. Ed. Wang Fuxiong. Circ: 5,000. **Overseas dist. by:** Science Press New York Ltd.

580 615 CUB ISSN 0138-8037
CUBA. CENTRO DE INFORMACION Y DOCUMENTACION AGROPECUARIO. BOLETIN DE RESENAS. SERIE: PLANTAS MEDICINALES. Abstracts in English. 1983. irreg. CUP 1; or exchange basis. charts, stat.
Formerly: Cuba. Centro de Informacion y Divulgacion Agropecuario. Boletin de Resenas. Serie: Plantas Medicinales
Indexed: Agrindex.
—CISTI.
Published by: Centro de Informacion y Documentacion Agropecuario, Gaveta Postal 4149, Havana 4, Cuba. TEL 301672, TELEX 051-1007. **Dist. by:** Ediciones Cubanas, Obispo No. 461, Apdo. 605, Havana, Cuba.

CURRENT TOPICS IN MEDICAL MYCOLOGY. see *MEDICAL SCIENCES—Communicable Diseases*

CZECH JOURNAL OF GENETICS AND PLANT BREEDING. see *BIOLOGY—Genetics*

580 DOM
DOMINICAN REPUBLIC. CENTRO NACIONAL DE INVESTIGACIONES AGROPECUARIAS. LABORATORIO DE SANIDAD VEGETAL. SANIDAD VEGETAL✶ . Text in Spanish. irreg. (5-6/yr.). free per issue.
Media: Duplicated (not offset).
Published by: Centro Nacional de Investigaciones Agropecuarias, Laboratorio de Sanidad Vegetal, San Cristobal, Dominican Republic. Circ: (controlled).

580 615 IND ISSN 0971-1252
ETHNOBOTANY. Text in English. 1989. a. INR 200, USD 50 (effective 2000). adv. bk.rev. back issues avail. *Refereed.* **Document type:** *Academic/Scholarly.* **Description:** Carries original research papers, review articles, short communications on ethnobotany, ethno-medicine, ethno-chemistry, ethno-pharmacology, ethno-taxonomy, ethno-pharmacognosy.
Published by: (Society of Ethnobotanists), Deep Publications, A-3/27A DDA Flats, Paschim Vihar, New Delhi, Bihar 110 063, India. TEL 91-11-5579514, FAX 91-11-6519849. Ed. S L Kapoor. Pub., Adv. contact Vipul Jain. R&P Vikas Jain. Circ: 450.

582.14 ZWE ISSN 1022-5919
EXCELSA TAXONOMIC SERIES. Text in English. 1978. irreg., latest vol.4. adv. bibl, charts, illus. index. **Document type:** *Monographic series.*
Published by: Aloe Cactus and Succulent Society of Zimbabwe, PO Box CY 300, Causeway, Harare, Zimbabwe. TEL 263-4-481418, dorichards@zol.co.zw. Ed. Michael J Kimberley. R&P Doreen Richards. Adv. contact Michael J Kimberly. Circ: 1,000.

579.8 615 ARG ISSN 1514-0792
FITOCIENCIA REVISTA. Text in Spanish. 1997. q. USD 45. adv. bk.rev. illus. back issues avail. *Refereed.* **Document type:** *Monographic series.* **Description:** Publishes results of research on phytotherapy, phytopharmacology and phytotoxicology obtained with Latin American plant extracts.
Published by: Isis Ediciones s.r.l., Machado 637, Capital Federal, Buenos Aires 1405, Argentina. TEL 54-1-982-0980, FAX 54-1-982-0980. Ed. Angelica Prieto. Circ: 5,000.

580 HUN ISSN 1219-2155
FITOTERAPIA. Text in Hungarian; Contents page in English, Hungarian. 1995. irreg. HUF 250.
Indexed: Helminthol.Abstr., Nutr.Abstr., Protozool.Abstr.
Published by: Magyar Fitoterapias Tarsasag, Zrinyi utca 3, Budapest 1051, Hungary. TEL 1171488. Ed. Zoltan Hanko.

581.634 ITA ISSN 0367-326X
RS164 CODEN: FTRPAE
FITOTERAPIA; journal for the study of medicinal plants - rivista di studi ed applicazioni delle piante medicinali. Text in English, French, Italian; Summaries in English. 1934. 8/yr. EUR 206 in Europe to institutions; JPY 27,300 in Japan to institutions; USD 230 elsewhere to institutions (effective 2002). adv. bk.rev. back issues avail. *Refereed.* **Document type:** *Journal, Academic/Scholarly.* **Description:** Publishes articles concerning chemistry, pharmacology and the use of medicinal plants and their derivatives.
Related titles: Microform ed.: (from PQC); Online - full text ed.: (from ingenta, Swets Blackwell, ScienceDirect, Institute for Scientific Information).

B

Indexed: AIDS & Cancer Res., AgBiotech, Agri.& Environ.Biotech.Abstr. (coverage dropped), Agroforest.Abstr., Apic.Abstr., Aqua.Sci.& Fish.Abstr., BBCI, Biol.Abstr., Biotech.& Bioeng.Abstr., Chem.Abstr., Chem.Indus.Notes, Chem.Titles, Crop Physiol.Abstr., Derwent Biotech.Abstr., Environ.Sci.Poll.Mgmt., Excerp.Med., Field Crop Abstr., Forest Prod.Abstr., Forest.Abstr., Herb.Abstr., Hort.Abstr., I.P.A., Ind.Med., Ind.Vet., Irr.& Drain.Abstr., Mass Spectr.Bull., Microbiol.Abstr., NPU, Ornam.Hort., Plant Breed.Abstr., Plant Grow.Reg.Abstr., Rev.Med.& Vet.Mycol., Seed Abstr., Soils & Fert., Vet.Bull., Virol.Abstr.
—CASDDS, CISTI, EMDOCS, GNLM, IDS, KNAW, Linda Hall.
Published by: (Idena SpA), Elsevier Science BV, PO Box 211, Amsterdam 1000 AE, Netherlands. http://www.elsevier.com/locate/fitote, http://www.elsevier.nl. Ed. Romano Vitali. Circ: 4,000 (controlled).

580.09569403 ISR
FLORA PALAESTINA. Text in English. 1966. irreg., latest 1995. price varies. adv. Supplement avail. *Refereed.* **Document type:** *Monographic series.* **Description:** Illustrated compendium of the flora of the region.
Published by: Israel Academy of Sciences and Humanities, 43 Jabotinski St, P O Box 4040, Jerusalem 91040, Israel. TEL 972-2-5676233, FAX 972-2-5666059, tami@academy.ac.il, http://www.academy.ac.il. Ed. Zofia Lasman. Adv. contact Tami Korman.

571.2 AUS ISSN 1445-4408
QK710 CODEN: AJPPCH
FUCTIONAL PLANT BIOLOGY. Text in English. 1974. m. AUD 200 combined subscription to individuals for print & online eds.; USD 900 combined subscription domestic to institutions for print & online eds.; USD 965 combined subscription foreign to institutions for print & online eds. (effective 2001 & 2002). adv. index. 100 p./no. back issues avail. *Refereed.* **Document type:** *Journal, Academic/Scholarly.* **Description:** Covers all aspects of plant physiology, including biochemistry and biophysics, cell biology, genetics, plant-environment interactions, plant-microbe interactions and molecular biology.
Formerly (until Jan. 2002): Australian Journal of Plant Physiology (0310-7841)
Related titles: Microform ed.: (from PQC); Online - full text ed.: AUD 895, USD 830 (effective 2001) (from EBSCO Publishing, Swets Blackwell, Institute for Scientific Information).
Indexed: ASCA, Abstr.Bull.Inst.Pap.Chem., AgBiotech, Agri.& Environ.Biotech.Abstr. (coverage dropped), Agricola, Agroforest.Abstr., Aqua.Sci.& Fish.Abstr., BBCI, Biol.Abstr., Biotech.& Bioeng.Abstr., Chem.Abstr., Chem.Indus.Notes, Chem.Titles, Cott.& Trop.Fibr.Abstr., Crop Physiol.Abstr., Curr.Adv.Biochem., Curr.Adv.Ecol.Sci., Curr.Adv.Plant Sci., Curr.Cont., Derwent Biotech.Abstr., Ecol.Abstr., Eng.Ind., Environ.Sci.Poll.Mgmt., Excerp.Med., Field Crop Abstr., Food Sci.& Tech.Abstr., Forest Prod.Abstr., Forest.Abstr., Genet.Abstr., Geo.Abstr.P.G., Helminthol.Abstr., Herb.Abstr., Hort.Abstr., Hum.Gen.Abstr., IDA, INIS Atomind., Ind.Sci.Rev., Int.Abstr.Biol.Sci., Irr.& Drain.Abstr., Maize Abstr., Nuc.Acids Abstr., Ornam.Hort., Plant Breed.Abstr., Plant Gen.Res.Abstr., Plant Grow.Reg.Abstr., Plant Sci., Pollut.Abstr., Postharvest, Potato Abstr., Rev.Appl.Entomol., Rev.Arom.& Med.Plants, Rev.Plant Path., Rice Abstr., Sci.Cit.Ind., Seed Abstr., Sel.Water Res.Abstr., Soils & Fert., Soyabean Abstr., Triticale Abstr., Trop.Oil Seeds Abstr., VITIS, Weed Abstr.
—BLDSC (1811.120000), CASDDS, CISTI, EMDOCS, IDS, Infotrieve, ingenta, Linda Hall. **CCC.**
Published by: (C S I R O Australia), C S I R O Publishing, 150 Oxford St, Collingwood, VIC 3066, Australia. TEL 61-3-9662-7625, FAX 61-3-9662-7611, fpb@publish.csiro.au, fpb@csiro.au, http://www.publish.csiro.au/journals/fpb, http://www.publish.csiro.au/journals/ajpp. Ed., Adv. contact J S McCutchan. Pub. A Stammer. R&P L Hamiltan TEL 61-3-9662-7610. Circ: 800.

GENETIKA I SELEKTSIIA/GENETICS AND PLANT BREEDING. see *BIOLOGY—Genetics*

580 NLD ISSN 0167-2932
GRASDUINEN. Text in Dutch. 1979. m. adv. illus. **Document type:** *Magazine, Consumer.*
Published by: V N U Tijdschriften B.V., Postbus 1900, Hoofddorp 2130 JH, Netherlands. TEL 31-23-556-6770, FAX 31-23-556-6771, ServiceTeam@tijdschriften.vnu.com, http://www.vnu.nl/vnu/organisatie. Circ: 55,000.

GUNNERIA. see *BIOLOGY*

HEATHER SOCIETY. YEARBOOK. see *GARDENING AND HORTICULTURE*

580.9438 POL ISSN 0018-0599
CODEN: HPBIA9
HERBA POLONICA. Text in English, German, Polish; Summaries in English. 1955. q. USD 40 foreign (effective 2002). adv. bk.rev. bibl, charts, illus. index. *Refereed.* **Document type:** *Journal, Academic/Scholarly.*
Formerly: Instytut Roslin Leczniczny. Biuletyn
Related titles: Online - full text ed.
Indexed: AgBiotech, Agri.& Environ.Biotech.Abstr. (coverage dropped), AgroAgen, AgroLibrex, Anal.Abstr., Bibl.Agri., Biol.& Agr.Ind. (coverage dropped), Biol.Abstr., Chem.Abstr., Chem.Indus.Notes, Chem.Titles, Crop Physiol.Abstr., Curr.Adv.Ecol.Sci., Curr.Cont. (coverage dropped), Derwent Biotech.Abstr., Excerp.Med., Forest Prod.Abstr., Forest.Abstr., Hort.Abstr., INIS Atomind., I.P.A., Mass Spectr.Bull., Nutr.Abstr., Ornam.Hort., Plant Breed.Abstr., Plant Grow.Reg.Abstr., Postharvest, Rev.Appl.Entomol., Rev.Arom.& Med.Plants, Rev.Plant Path., Seed Abstr., Weed Abstr.
—CASDDS, GNLM.
Published by: Instytut Roslin i Przetworow Zielarskich/Research Institute of Medicinal Plants, Libelta 27, Poznan 61707, Poland. TEL 48-61-8525616, FAX 48-61-8527463, ak_iripz@man.poznan.pl. Ed. Jerzy Lutomski. Adv. contact Anna Krajewska Patan. Circ: 1,000. **Co-sponsor:** State Committe for Scientific Research.

581.63 615.321 USA ISSN 0899-5648
HERBALGRAM✱ ; the journal of the American botanical council & the herb research foundation. Text in English. 1983. q. USD 29 domestic; USD 36 in Canada; USD 44 elsewhere; USD 6.95 newsstand/cover (effective 2000). adv. bk.rev., software rev., video rev. stat, tr.lit, charts, illus, mkt. Index. back issues avail. *Refereed.* **Document type:** *Magazine, Trade, Consumer.* **Description:** Covers many of the facets of the Herb movement, both within the US and abroad. Covers herbs and medicinal plants, history of their use, legal and regulatory developments regarding sales and marketing.
Related titles: Online - full text ed.
Indexed: Agricola, Forest.Abstr., Gard.Lit. (1992-1994), Hort.Abstr., Nutr.Abstr., Rev.Arom.& Med.Plants, World Ag.Econ.& Rur.Soc.Abstr.
—GNLM, ingenta.
Published by: American Botanical Council, P O Box 144345, Austin, TX 78714-4345. TEL 512-926-4900, FAX 512-926-2345, abc@herbalgram.org, http://www.herbalgram.org/herbalgram/index.html. Ed., Pub. Mark Blumenthal. R&P Barbara Johnston TEL 512-451-4820. Adv. contact Debbie Jones. B&W page USD 1,892, color page USD 2,882; trim 8.625 x 11.125. Circ: 50,000 (paid).

581.3 USA ISSN 1054-5476
QK725 CODEN: IVCPEO
IN VITRO CELLULAR & DEVELOPMENTAL BIOLOGY - PLANT. Text in English. 1965. 6/yr. USD 215 in North America; USD 268 elsewhere; GBP 426 in North America Animal & Plant Parts; GBP 495 elsewhere Animal & Plant Parts (effective 2001). adv. bk.rev. index. back issues avail. *Refereed.* **Document type:** *Academic/Scholarly.* **Description:** Publishes original papers in plant cellular and developmental biology with emphasis on the developmental, molecular and cellular biology of cells, tissues, and organs.
Supersedes in part (in 1991): In Vitro Cellular and Developmental Biology (0883-8364); Which was formerly: In Vitro (0073-5655)
Related titles: Microform ed.: (from PQC); Online - full text ed.: (from EBSCO Publishing, RoweCom Information Quest, ingenta, Swets Blackwell, BioOne, Institute for Scientific Information).
Indexed: ASCA, AgBiotech, Agri.& Environ.Biotech.Abstr., Agri.Eng.Abstr., Agricola, BBCI, Biol.Abstr., Biotech.& Bioeng.Abstr., Biotech.Cit.Ind., Chem.Abstr., Chem.Indus.Notes, Chem.Titles, Crop Physiol.Abstr., Curr.Adv.Plant Sci., Curr.Cont., Derwent Biotech.Abstr., Environ.Sci.Poll.Mgmt., Field Crop Abstr., Forest.Abstr., Helminthol.Abstr., Herb.Abstr., Hort.Abstr., Ind.Med (coverage dropped), Int.Abstr.Biol.Sci., Maize Abstr., Microbiol.Abstr., Ornam.Hort., Plant Breed.Abstr., Plant Gen.Res.Abstr., Plant Grow.Reg.Abstr., Plant Sci., Rev.Appl.Entomol., Rev.Arom.& Med.Plants, Rev.Plant Path., Rice Abstr., Sci.Cit.Ind., Seed Abstr., Triticale Abstr., VITIS, Weed Abstr., World Ag.Econ.& Rur.Soc.Abstr.
—BLDSC (4372.500800), CASDDS, CISTI, EMDOCS, GNLM, IDS, ingenta, Linda Hall. **CCC.**
Published by: Society for In Vitro Biology, 9315 Largo Dr. W., Ste. 255, Largo, MD 20774. TEL 301-324-5054, FAX 301-324-5057, sivb@sivb.org, http://www.sivb.org. Ed. Trevor A Thrope. Adv. contact Denise McCall. B&W page USD 275, B&W page GBP 170; trim 7 x 9.5. Circ: 1,400. **Subscr. to:** Allen Press Inc., PO Box 1897, Lawrence, KS 66044-8897.

INDEX KEWENSIS. see *BIOLOGY*

580 ISR
INDEX SEMINUM; wild and cultivated plants. Text in English. a. free per issue.
Published by: Tel Aviv University, Department of Botany, Ramat Aviv, Tel Aviv 69978, Israel. TEL 03-420151. Ed. Yeduha Tankus.

581.35 IND ISSN 0019-5200
SB123 CODEN: IJGBAG
INDIAN JOURNAL OF GENETICS AND PLANT BREEDING. Text in English. 1960. q. INR 450, USD 75 (effective 2001). adv. bk.rev. charts, illus. index, cum.index: vols.1-20, vols.21-30. **Document type:** *Academic/Scholarly.* **Description:** Covers electrical and electronics, metallurgy, mechanical, chemical, software engineering and computer science, mining, steel, environmental technology, power and energy.
Indexed: AgBiotech, Biol.Abstr., Chem.Abstr., Chem.Indus.Notes, Chem.Titles, Cott.& Trop.Fibr.Abstr., Crop Physiol.Abstr., Curr.Cont. (coverage dropped), Entomol.Abstr. (coverage dropped), Fababean Abstr., Field Crop Abstr., Forest.Abstr., Genet.Abstr., Helminthol.Abstr., Herb.Abstr., Hort.Abstr., Hum.Gen.Abstr., INIS Atomind., Irr.& Drain.Abstr., Maize Abstr., Nuc.Acids Abstr., Ornam.Hort., Plant Breed.Abstr., Plant Gen.Res.Abstr., Plant Grow.Reg.Abstr., Postharvest, Rev.Appl.Entomol., Rev.Arom.& Med.Plants, Rev.Plant Path., Rice Abstr., Seed Abstr., Soils & Fert., Soyabean Abstr., Triticale Abstr., Trop.Oil Seeds Abstr., Weed Abstr.
—CASDDS, CISTI, ingenta, Linda Hall.
Published by: (Indian Society of Genetics and Plant Breeding, Division of Genetics), Scientific Publishers, 5-A New Pali Rd., P O Box 91, Jodhpur, Rajasthan 342 001, India. TEL 91-291-433323, FAX 91-291-512580, scienti@sancharnet.in, http://www.scientificpub.com. Ed. Mihir Sen. adv.: B&W page USD 422, color page USD 845. Circ: 9,000.

579.5 IND
CODEN: IJMPAK
INDIAN JOURNAL OF MYCOLOGY AND PLANT PATHOLOGY. Text in English. 1971. 3/yr. INR 2,000, USD 200 (effective 2001). adv. bk.rev. bibl, charts, illus. back issues avail. *Refereed.* **Document type:** *Academic/Scholarly.*
Former titles: Journal of Mycology and Plant Pathology (0971-9393); (until 1996): Indian Journal of Mycology and Plant Pathology (0303-4097)
Indexed: Agri.Eng.Abstr., Agroforest.Abstr., Aqua.Sci.& Fish.Abstr., Bibl.Agri., Bio-Contr.News & Info., Biol.Abstr., Biotech.& Bioeng.Abstr., Chem.Abstr., Chem.Indus.Notes, Cott.& Trop.Fibr.Abstr., Crop Physiol.Abstr., Environ.Sci.Poll.Mgmt., Fababean Abstr., Field Crop Abstr., Forest.Abstr., Helminthol.Abstr., Herb.Abstr., Hort.Abstr., Indian Sci.Abstr., Maize Abstr., Microbiol.Abstr., Ornam.Hort., Plant Breed.Abstr., Plant Grow.Reg.Abstr., Postharvest, Potato Abstr., Rev.Appl.Entomol., Rev.Arom.& Med.Plants, Rev.Med.& Vet.Mycol., Rev.Plant Path., Rice Abstr., Seed Abstr., Soils & Fert., Sorghum & Millets Abstr., Soyabean Abstr., Triticale Abstr., Trop.Oil Seeds Abstr., Weed Abstr.
—CASDDS, CISTI, ingenta, Linda Hall.
Published by: (Indian Society of Mycology and Plant Pathology), Scientific Publishers, 5-A New Pali Rd., P O Box 91, Jodhpur, Rajasthan 342 001, India. TEL 91-291-433323, FAX 91-291-512580, scienti@sancharnet.in, http://www.scientificpub.com. Circ: 500. **Dist. overseas by:** H P C Publishers Distributors Pvt. Ltd., 1st Fl., Flats 1 & 2, Darya Ganj, 4805-24 Bharat Ram Rd., New Delhi 110 002, India. TEL 91-11-395-4401, FAX 91-11-686-3511.

580 CUB
INFORMACION EXPRESS. SERIE: PLANTAS MEDICINALES Y FLORES. Text in Spanish. 1985. a. CUP 30 domestic; USD 3 in North America; USD 6 in Europe; USD 5 elsewhere. stat.
Indexed: Agrindex.
Published by: Centro de Informacion y Documentacion Agropecuario, Gaveta Postal 4149, Havana 4, Cuba. TEL 301672. **Dist. by:** Ediciones Cubanas, Obispo No. 527, Apdo. 605, Havana, Cuba.

589.5 USA ISSN 1067-909X
QK600
INOCULUM. Text in English. 1948. bi-m. USD 60 to members. **Document type:** *Newsletter.*
Formerly (until 1992): Mycological Society of America Newsletter (0541-4938)
Related titles: Online - full text ed.; ♦ Supplement to: Mycologia. ISSN 0027-5514.
Indexed: Rev.Med.& Vet.Mycol.
Published by: Mycological Society of America, c/o Lorelei Norvell, Ed, Pacific Northwest Mycology Service, 6720 N W Skyline Blvd, Portland, OR 97229-1309. TEL 503-297-3296, FAX 503-296-6745, lorelei@teleport.com, http://www.erin.utoronto.ca/~w3msa. Circ: 1,500.

622.331 553.21 FIN ISSN 0782-7784
CODEN: IPEJE8
INTERNATIONAL PEAT JOURNAL. Text in English. 1986. irreg., latest 1998. FIM 100, USD 20 (effective 1999). bk.rev. **Document type:** *Academic/Scholarly.*
Indexed: GeoRef, INIS Atomind.
—CASDDS, CISTI.
Published by: International Peat Society, Kuokkalantie 4, Jyvaskylva 40520, Finland. TEL 358-14-674-042, FAX 358-14-677-405. Ed. Jack Rieley.

579.5 615.9 GBR
INTERNATIONAL REINHARDSBRUNN SYMPOSIUM PROCEEDINGS. Text in English. irreg., latest 1998, 12th Symposium. price varies. *Refereed.* **Document type:** *Proceedings, Academic/Scholarly.* **Description:** Publishes research papers in biological chemistry and related areas presented at the Reinhardsbrunn Symposium.
—CCC.
Published by: (Deutsche Phytomedizinische Gesellschaft eV DEU, British Crop Protection Council), Intercept Ltd, PO Box 716, Andover, Hants SP10 1YG, United Kingdom. TEL 44-1264-334748, FAX 44-1264-334058, intercept@andover.co.uk, http://www.intercept.co.uk.

581.3 POL ISSN 1234-1983
SB123 CODEN: JAGEFC
JOURNAL OF APPLIED GENETICS; an international journal of genetics and breeding. Text and summaries in English. 1960. q. PLZ 80 domestic; USD 120 foreign (effective 2000 & 2001). adv. bk.rev. abstr, bibl, charts, illus. index. back issues avail. *Refereed.* **Document type:** *Academic/Scholarly.* **Description:** Publishes original scientific papers on plant and animal genetics and breeding, on microorganisms and human genetics.
Formerly (until 1995): Genetica Polonica (0016-6715)
Indexed: AgBiotech, AgroAgen, AgroLibrex, Anim.Breed.Abstr., Aqua.Sci.& Fish.Abstr., Biol.Abstr., Chem.Abstr., Crop Physiol.Abstr., Curr.Adv.Biochem., Curr.Adv.Cell & Devel.Biol., Curr.Adv.Ecol.Sci., Curr.Adv.Gen.& Molec.Biol., Curr.Cont. (coverage dropped), Dairy Sci.Abstr., Excerp.Med., Field Crop Abstr., Food Sci.& Tech.Abstr., Genet.Abstr., Helminthol.Abstr., Herb.Abstr., Hort.Abstr., Hum.Gen.Abstr., INIS Atomind., Ind.Sci.Rev., Ind.Vet., Maize Abstr., Nutr.Abstr., Plant Breed.Abstr., Plant Gen.Res.Abstr., Plant Grow.Reg.Abstr., Potato Abstr., Poult.Abstr., Rev.Appl.Entomol., Rev.Plant Path., Sci.Cit.Ind. (coverage dropped), Seed Abstr., Soils & Fert., Soyabean Abstr., Triticale Abstr., Vet.Bull.
—BLDSC (4942.612000), CASDDS, CISTI, Infotrieve. **CCC.**
Published by: Instytut Genetyki Roslin, Polska Akademia Nauk/Institute of Plant Genetics, Polish Academy of Sciences, Ul Strzeszynska 34, Poznan 60479, Poland. TEL 48-61-8221112, FAX 48-61-8233671, edyb@igr.poznan.pl, http://saturn.ci.uw.edu.pl/psjc/; http://ciuw.warman.net.pl/alf/psjc. Ed. Zygmunt Kaczmarek. R&P Eleonora Dybizbanska. Adv. contact Bogumila Szymanska. Circ: 350. **Subscr. to:** Ars Polona, Krakowskie Przedmiescie 7, Warsaw, Poland. TEL 48-22-8201201, FAX 44-22-8268673.

JOURNAL OF EVOLUTIONARY BIOLOGY. see *BIOLOGY—Genetics*

JOURNAL OF HERBS, SPICES & MEDICINAL PLANTS. see *GARDENING AND HORTICULTURE*

JOURNAL OF PLANT NUTRITION AND SOIL SCIENCE/ZEITSCHRIFT FUER PFLANZENERNAEHRUNG UND BODENKUNDE. see *BIOLOGY—Abstracting, Bibliographies, Statistics*

580 JPN
KINKI SHOKUBUTSU DOKOKAI KAISHI/KINKI BOTANICAL SOCIETY. BULLETIN. Text in Japanese. 1950. biennial. membership. adv. back issues avail.
Published by: Kinki Shokubutsu Dokokai/Kinki Botanical Society, c/o Mr Kozi Hirano, 36-15, Sayamadai 3-chome, Sakai-shi, Osaka 581, Japan.

LECTINS. see *BIOLOGY—Abstracting, Bibliographies, Statistics*

MEDICAL MYCOLOGY. see *MEDICAL SCIENCES—Communicable Diseases*

579.5 RUS ISSN 0026-3648
CODEN: MIFIB2
MIKOLOGIYA I FITOPATOLOGIYA. Text in Russian. 1967. bi-m. USD 131. *Refereed.*
Related titles: Online - full text ed.: (from Institute for Scientific Information).
Indexed: ASCA, Agri.& Environ.Biotech.Abstr. (coverage dropped), Aqua.Sci.& Fish.Abstr., Bio-Contr.News & Info., Biol.Abstr., Chem.Abstr., Chem.Indus.Notes, Chem.Titles, Cott.& Trop.Fibr.Abstr., Crop Physiol.Abstr., Curr.Adv.Ecol.Sci., Curr.Cont., Dairy Sci.Abstr., Derwent Biotech.Abstr., Environ.Sci.Poll.Mgmt., Forest.Abstr., Hort.Abstr., INIS Atomind., Ind.Sci.Rev., Maize Abstr., Microbiol.Abstr., Plant Grow.Reg.Abstr., Potato Abstr., Ref.Zh., Rev.Appl.Entomol., Rev.Arom.& Med.Plants, Rev.Med.& Vet.Mycol., Rev.Plant Path., Rice Abstr., Sci.Cit.Ind., Seed Abstr., Soils & Fert., Soyabean Abstr., Triticale Abstr., Weed Abstr., Zoo.Rec.
—BLDSC (0114.750000), CASDDS, CISTI, IDS, Infotrieve, Linda Hall. **CCC.**
Published by: (Rossiiskaya Akademiya Nauk/Russian Academy of Sciences), M A I K Nauka - Interperiodica, S.-Peterburgskoe Otdelenie, Mendeleevskaya liniya 1, St Petersburg 199034, Russian Federation. TEL 812-2184615. **US dist. addr.:** East View Publications, 3020 Harbor Ln N, Minneapolis, MN 55447. TEL 612-550-0961.

571.2 590 GBR ISSN 1468-5698
▼ **MOLECULAR BIOLOGY TODAY.** Text in English. 2000. 3/yr. GBP 75, USD 150 to individuals; GBP 130, USD 260 to institutions (effective 2002). *Refereed.* **Description:** Contains primary research papers, short communications, and review articles on all aspects of molecular biology, including plant and animal systems, human genetics, molecular microbiology, virology, and biotechnology. Also publishes laboratory protocols of general interest to molecular biologists.
Related titles: Online - full text ed.: ISSN 1468-568X. GBP 40, USD 80 to individuals; GBP 80, USD 160 to institutions (effective 2002).
Indexed: Biotech.& Bioeng.Abstr., Environ.Sci.Poll.Mgmt., Genet.Abstr., Med.& Pharm.Biotech.Abstr., Virol.Abstr.
—BLDSC (5900.798050).
Published by: Caister Academic Press, 32 Hewitts Ln, Wymondham, Norfolk NR18 0JA, United Kingdom. TEL 44-870-321-3681, FAX 44-870-321-3692, mail@caister.com, http://www.molbio.net, http://www.horizonpress.com/.

MOLECULAR PLANT - MICROBE INTERACTIONS. see *BIOLOGY—Biochemistry*

571 616.07 GBR ISSN 1464-6722
▼ **MOLECULAR PLANT PATHOLOGY.** Text in English. 2000. bi-m., latest vol.3, 2002. GBP 63 in Europe to individuals; USD 101 in North America to individuals; GBP 70 elsewhere to individuals; GBP 280 in Europe to institutions; USD 444 in North America to institutions; GBP 308 elsewhere to institutions (effective 2002). adv. **Document type:** *Journal.* **Description:** Features submissions from all areas of molecular plant pathology including research on diseases caused by fungi, oomycetes, viruses, nematodes, bacteria, insects, parasitic plants and other organisms.
Related titles: Online - full text ed.: ISSN 1364-3703. GBP 57 in Europe to individuals; USD 91 in North America to individuals; GBP 57 elsewhere to individuals; GBP 252 in Europe to institutions; USD 400 in North America to institutions; GBP 252 elsewhere to institutions (effective 2002) (from EBSCO Publishing, O C L C Online Computer Library Center, Inc., ingenta, Munksgaard & Blackwell Science's Synergy, Swets Blackwell, RoweCom Information Quest).
Indexed: AgBiotech, Crop Physiol.Abstr., Field Crop Abstr., Plant Breed.Abstr., Rev.Plant Path., Triticale Abstr.
—BLDSC (5900.826100).
Published by: (British Society for Plant Pathology), Blackwell Science Ltd., PO Box 88, Oxford OX2 0NE, United Kingdom. TEL 44-1865-206180, 44-1865-206002, FAX 44-1865-206219, jnl.orders@blacksci.co.uk, http://www.blackwell-science.com/~cgilib/jnlpage.asp?Journal=mpp&File=mpp, http://www.blackwellpublishing.com. Ed. G D Foster. Pub. Sue Hewitt. R&P Sophie Savage. Adv. contact Jenny Applin. B&W page GBP 400, color 1/4 page GBP 1,000.

579.5 NLD ISSN 0301-486X
QK600 CODEN: MYCPAH
MYCOPATHOLOGIA. Text in English. 1938. m. EUR 14.50 to institutions for print or online ed; EUR 1,098 to institutions print & online eds.combined (effective 2002). adv. bk.rev. illus. reprint service avail. from SWZ. *Refereed.* **Document type:** *Academic/Scholarly.* **Description:** Covers the study of the role of fungi in disease and biodeterioration. As such, the journal covers a range of topics that is unique in breadth and depth, including original articles and critical reviews in the fields of medical and veterinary mycology, plant mycology (crop protection), mycotoxicosis, mycetism, entomopathogenic fungi, environmental aeromycology, and applied industrial mycology.
Formerly: Mycopathologia et Mycologia - Applicata (0027-5530)
Related titles: Microform ed.: (from PQC); Online - full text ed.: (from EBSCO Publishing, O C L C Online Computer Library Center, Inc., RoweCom Information Quest, Swets Blackwell, Kluwer Online, Institute for Scientific Information).
Indexed: ASCA, Abstr.Hyg., Agri.& Environ.Biotech.Abstr. (coverage dropped), Agricola, Agroforest.Abstr., Apic.Abstr., Aqua.Sci.& Fish.Abstr., Bio-Contr.News & Info., Biol.Abstr., Biotech.& Bioeng.Abstr., Chem.Abstr., Chem.Indus.Notes, Chem.Titles, Crop Physiol.Abstr., Curr.Adv.Ecol.Sci., Curr.Adv.Plant Sci., Curr.Cont., Dairy Sci.Abstr., Derwent Biotech.Abstr., Environ.Sci.Poll.Mgmt., Excerp.Med., Field Crop Abstr., Food Sci.& Tech.Abstr., Forest Prod.Abstr., Forest.Abstr., Hort.Abstr., INIS Atomind., Ind.Med. (1975-), Ind.Sci.Rev., Ind.Vet., Inpharma, Int.Abstr.Biol.Sci., Maize Abstr., Microbiol.Abstr., NRN, Nutr.Abstr., Pig News & Info., Plant Sci., Postharvest, Poult.Abstr., Reac., Rev.Appl.Entomol., Rev.Arom.& Med.Plants, Rev.Med.& Vet.Mycol., Rev.Plant Path., Rice Abstr., Sci.Cit.Ind., Seed Abstr., Small Anim.Abstr., Soils & Fert., Soyabean Abstr., Sport Fish.Abstr., Triticale Abstr., Trop.Dis.Bull., Vet.Bull., Weed Abstr.
—BLDSC (5995.740000), CASDDS, CISTI, EMDOCS, GNLM, IDS, Infotrieve, ingenta, KNAW, Linda Hall. **CCC.**
Published by: (C A B International Mycological Institute GBR), Kluwer Academic Publishers Group (Subsidiary of: Wolters Kluwer N.V.), Spuiboulevard 50, PO Box 17, Dordrecht 3300 AA, Netherlands. FAX 31-78-639-2254, services@wkap.nl, http://www.wkap.nl. **Dist. by:** Journals Department, PO Box 322, Dordrecht 3300 AH, Netherlands. TEL 781-871-6600, FAX 31-78-654-6474.

580 SVK ISSN 0323-2646
NASE LIECIVE RASTLINY. Text in Slovak. bi-m. USD 27.
Indexed: Hort.Abstr., Seed Abstr., Weed Abstr.
Published by: Herba, Svabinsheho 4-a, Bratislava 85101, Slovakia.

580.74 IRL ISSN 0790-0422
NATIONAL BOTANIC GARDENS. OCCASIONAL PAPERS. Text in English. 1981. irreg., latest vol.12, 1999. per issue exchange basis. *Refereed.* **Document type:** *Academic/Scholarly, Government.*
—BLDSC (6218.200000), CISTI.
Published by: National Botanic Gardens, Glasnevin, Dublin 9, Ireland. TEL 353-1-8374388, FAX 353-1-8360080, nbg@indigo.ie. Ed. Matthew Jebb. Circ: 400.

580 615.19 NPL
NEPAL. DEPARTMENT OF MEDICINAL PLANTS. ANNUAL REPORT. Text in English. 1969. a. free per issue.
Published by: Ministry of Forests, Department of Medicinal Plants, Thapathali, Katmandu, Nepal. Circ: 500.

580.09436 AUT
NOTIZEN ZUR FLORA DER STEIERMARK. Text in German. 1974. irreg. price varies. **Document type:** *Academic/Scholarly.* **Description:** Results of research on the flora of the province of Styria.
Published by: Landesmuseum Joanneum, Referat Botanik, Raubergasse 10, Graz, St 8010, Austria. TEL 43-316-80179750, FAX 43-316-80179800, TELEX 311838-LRGGR-A, post@lmj-bot.stmk.gv.at. Eds. Arnold Zimmermann, Detlef Ernet. Circ: 400. **Co-sponsor:** Steiermaerkische Landesregierung.

OSAKA-SHIRITSU SHIZENSHI HAKUBUTSUKAN SHUZO SHIRYO MOKUROKU/OSAKA MUSEUM OF NATURAL HISTORY. SPECIAL PUBLICATIONS. see *BIOLOGY*

PHARMACOGNOSY, PHYTOCHEMISTRY, MEDICINAL PLANTS. see *PHARMACY AND PHARMACOLOGY*

580 GBR ISSN 0958-0344
QK865 CODEN: PHANEL
PHYTOCHEMICAL ANALYSIS. Text in English. 1990. bi-m. USD 1,050 in United States; USD 1,050 in Canada & Mexico; USD 1,050 elsewhere; USD 1,103 combined subscription in United States for print and online eds.; USD 1,103 combined subscription in Canada & Mexico for print and online eds.; USD 1,103 combined subscription elsewhere for print and online eds. (effective 2002). adv. back issues avail.; reprint service avail. from SWZ. *Refereed.* **Document type:** *Academic/Scholarly.* **Description:** Publishes original articles on the application of analytical methodology in the plant sciences.
Related titles: Microform ed.: (from PQC); Online - full text ed.: ISSN 1099-1565. USD 1,050 in United States; USD 1,050 in Canada & Mexico; USD 1,050 elsewhere (effective 2002) (from EBSCO Publishing, Wiley InterScience, Institute for Scientific Information).
Indexed: ASCA, AgBiotech, Agroforest.Abstr., Anal.Abstr., Aqua.Sci.& Fish.Abstr., BBCI, Bio-Contr.News & Info., Chem.Abstr., Chem.Cit.Ind., Chem.Titles, Chromat.Abstr., Crop Physiol.Abstr., Curr.Cont., Excerp.Med. (1993-), Field Crop Abstr., Forest Prod.Abstr., Forest.Abstr., Herb.Abstr., Hort.Abstr., Ind.Vet., Int.Abstr.Biol.Sci., Mass Spectr.Bull., Nutr.Abstr., Ocean.Abstr. (coverage dropped), Ornam.Hort., Plant Breed.Abstr., Plant Grow.Reg.Abstr., Protozool.Abstr., Rev.Appl.Entomol., Rev.Arom.& Med.Plants, Rev.Med.& Vet.Mycol., Rev.Plant Path., Rice Abstr., Sci.Cit.Ind., Seed Abstr., Triticale Abstr., Weed Abstr.
—BLDSC (6489.695000), CASDDS, CISTI, EMDOCS, GNLM, IDS, Infotrieve, ingenta. **CCC.**
Published by: Wiley Europe Ltd., Baffins Ln, Chichester, W Sussex PO19 1UD, United Kingdom. TEL 44-1243-779777, FAX 44-1243-775878, customer@wiley.co.uk, http://www.wiley.co.uk. R&P Diane Southern TEL 44-1243-770347. adv.: B&W page GBP 650, color page GBP 1,550; trim 210 x 297. Circ: 350. **Subscr. to:** John Wiley & Sons, Inc., Journals, 605 Third Ave, New York, NY 10158. TEL 212-850-6021, 212-850-6645, subinfo@jwiley.com.

615.53 GBR ISSN 0951-418X
CODEN: PHYREH
PHYTOTHERAPY RESEARCH; an international journal devoted to medical and scientific research on plants and plant products. Text in English. 1987. 8/yr. USD 1,430 in United States; USD 1,430 in Canada & Mexico; USD 1,430 elsewhere; USD 1,502 combined subscription in United States for print and online eds.; USD 1,502 combined subscription in Canada & Mexico for print and online eds.; USD 1,502 combined subscription elsewhere for print and online eds. (effective 2002). adv. back issues avail.; reprint service avail. from SWZ. *Refereed.* **Document type:** *Academic/Scholarly.* **Description:** Publishes original medical plant research, including biochemistry and molecular pharmacology, toxicology, pathology, and the clinical application of herbs and natural products to both human and animal medicine.
Related titles: Microform ed.: (from PQC); Online - full text ed.: ISSN 1099-1573. USD 1,430 in United States; USD 1,430 in Canada & Mexico; USD 1,430 elsewhere (effective 2002) (from EBSCO Publishing, Wiley InterScience, Institute for Scientific Information).
Indexed: AMED, ASCA, Agricola, Agroforest.Abstr., Aqua.Sci.& Fish.Abstr., Bibl.Agri., Chem.Abstr., Chem.Cit.Ind., Chem.Indus.Notes, Chem.Titles, Curr.Cont., Excerp.Med., Forest Prod.Abstr., Forest.Abstr., Helminthol.Abstr., Hort.Abstr., Ind.Med. (1987-), Ind.Sci.Rev., Ind.Vet., Inpharma, Int.Abstr.Biol.Sci., NPU, Nutr.Abstr., Ornam.Hort., Plant Breed.Abstr., Plant Grow.Reg.Abstr., Postharvest, Protozool.Abstr., Reac., Rev.Appl.Entomol., Rev.Arom.& Med.Plants, Rev.Med.& Vet.Mycol., Rev.Plant Path., SSCI (coverage dropped), Sci.Cit.Ind., Soyabean Abstr., Trop.Dis.Bull., Weed Abstr.
—BLDSC (6497.060000), CASDDS, EMDOCS, GNLM, IDS, Infotrieve, KNAW. **CCC.**
Published by: Wiley Europe Ltd., Baffins Ln, Chichester, W Sussex PO19 1UD, United Kingdom. TEL 44-1243-779777, FAX 44-1243-843232, customer@wiley.co.uk, http://www.wiley.co.uk. Ed. Fred J Evans. Pub. Janie Curtis. adv.: B&W page GBP 650, color page GBP 1,550; trim 210 x 297. Circ: 450. **Subscr. in the Americas to:** John Wiley & Sons, Inc., Journals, 605 Third Ave, New York, NY 10158. TEL 212-850-6645, FAX 212-850-6021, uscs-wis@wiley.com; **Subscr. to:** John Wiley & Sons Ltd., Baffins Ln, Chichester, Sussex PO19 IUD, United Kingdom. cs-journals@wiley.co.uk.

PLANT AND CELL PHYSIOLOGY. see *BIOLOGY—Cytology And Histology*

PLANT BIOTECHNOLOGY. see *BIOLOGY—Abstracting, Bibliographies, Statistics*

579.8 NLD ISSN 0167-8574
QK564 CODEN: PPREEX
PROGRESS IN PHYCOLOGICAL RESEARCH. Text in Dutch. 1982. irreg., latest vol.2, 1983. price varies. *Refereed.* **Document type:** *Monographic series.*
Indexed: Chem.Abstr., Chem.Titles, Zoo.Rec.
—CASDDS, CISTI, ingenta, Linda Hall.
Published by: Elsevier Science BV, Books Division, PO Box 211, Amsterdam 1000 AE, Netherlands. TEL 31-20-485-2911, nlinfo-f@elsevier.nl; usinfo-f@elsevier.com; forinfo-kyf04035@niftyserve.or.jp, http://www.elsevier.nl. Eds. D J Chapman, F E Round. **Subscr. in Australasia and the Far East to:** Elsevier Science (Singapore) Pte Ltd, No.1 Temasek Ave, 17-01 Millenia Tower, Singapore 039192, Singapore. TEL 65-434-3727, FAX 65-337-2230; **Subscr. in Japan to:** Elsevier Science Inc - Japan Regional Office, 9-15 Higashi-Azabu 1-chome, Minato-ku, Tokyo 106-0044, Japan. TEL 81-3-5561-5033, FAX 81-3-5561-5047; **Subscr. in the Americas to:** Elsevier Science, PO Box 945, New York, NY 10159-0945. TEL 212-633-3730, FAX 212-633-3680, usinfo-f@elsevier.com.

581.636 KEN ISSN 0048-6043
SB952.P9 CODEN: PYRPAN
PYRETHRUM POST. Text in English. 1948. s-a., latest vol.20. USD 40 (effective 1999). bk.rev. abstr, charts, stat. biennial index. 44 p./no. 2 cols./p. back issues avail.; reprints avail. *Refereed.* **Document type:** *Journal, Academic/Scholarly.* **Description:** Provides a vehicle to disseminate scientific research findings about pyrethrum and related products.
Related titles: CD-ROM ed.
Indexed: Agri.& Environ.Biotech.Abstr. (coverage dropped), Anal.Abstr., Biol.Abstr., Chem.Abstr., Chem.Indus.Notes, Chem.Titles, Derwent Biotech.Abstr., Excerp.Med., Hort.Abstr., Ind.Vet., Plant Breed.Abstr., Rev.Appl.Entomol., Rev.Arom.& Med.Plants, Small Anim.Abstr., Vet.Bull.
—BLDSC (7162.000000), CASDDS, CISTI, Linda Hall.
Published by: (Pyrethrum Bureau), Ketona Publishers, Pyrethrum Board of Kenya, PO Box 420, Nakuru, Kenya. TEL 254-37-211567, 43-6245-833810, FAX 254-37-45274, 43-6245-82356, TELEX 33080 PYBOARD KE, pbk@pyrethrum.co.ke. Ed. James N Kuria.

REFERATIVNYI ZHURNAL. FITOPATOLOGIYA. see *BIOLOGY—Abstracting, Bibliographies, Statistics*

REVIEW OF AROMATIC AND MEDICINAL PLANTS. see *BIOLOGY—Abstracting, Bibliographies, Statistics*

REVIEW OF MEDICAL AND VETERINARY MYCOLOGY. see *BIOLOGY—Abstracting, Bibliographies, Statistics*

REVIEW OF PLANT PATHOLOGY; consisting of abstracts and reviews of current literature on plant pathology. see *BIOLOGY—Abstracting, Bibliographies, Statistics*

579.5 MEX ISSN 0187-3180
CODEN: RMMIEL
REVISTA MEXICANA DE MICOLOGIA. Text in Spanish; Summaries in English, Spanish. 1968. a. adv. bk.rev. bibl, charts, illus. index. cum.index. reprint service avail. from PQC. *Refereed.* **Document type:** *Academic/Scholarly.*
Former titles (until 1985): Sociedad Mexicana de Micologia. Boletin (0085-6223); Sociedad Mexicana de Micologia. Boletin Informativo
Media: Duplicated (not offset). **Related titles:** Microform ed.: (from PQC).
Indexed: Biol.Abstr., Forest.Abstr., Hort.Abstr., Ind.Vet., Potato Abstr., Rev.Med.& Vet.Mycol., Rev.Plant Path., Seed Abstr., Sugar Ind.Abstr., Triticale Abstr., Vet.Bull.
Published by: Sociedad Mexicana de Micologia, Calle INSURGENTES SUR 3700, Col Insurgentes Cuicuilco, Apartado Postal 101 63, Mexico City, DF 04530, Mexico. Ed. Joachim Cifuentes. Circ: 1,000.

REVUE DES SCIENCES NATURELLES D'AUVERGNE. see *BIOLOGY*

579.7 CHE ISSN 0373-2959
CODEN: SZPLA7
SCHWEIZERISCHE ZEITSCHRIFT FUER PILZKUNDE/BOLLETTINO SVIZZERO DI MICOLOGIA/BULLETIN SUISSE DE MYCOLOGIE. Text in French, German, Italian. 1922. 10/yr. CHF 35. adv. bk.rev. illus. back issues avail. **Document type:** *Academic/Scholarly.* **Description:** Contains comprehensive information on all types of fungi, including special features on mushrooms and a fungus of the month.
Indexed: Rev.Plant Path.
Published by: Association Swiss Societies of Mycology, Rigistr 23, Obfelden 8912, Switzerland. Ed., Adv. contact Ivan Cucchi. Circ: 5,200.

580 JPN ISSN 0286-6102
SHOKUCHU SHOKUBUTSU KENKYUKAI KAISHI/INSECTIVOROUS PLANT SOCIETY. JOURNAL. Text in Japanese; Summaries in English. 1950. q. JPY 5,000, USD 48 (effective 2001). bk.rev. back issues avail. **Document type:** *Bulletin, Academic/Scholarly.*
Indexed: Ref.Zh.
Published by: Shokuchu Shokubutsu Kenkyukai/ Insectivorous Plant Society, c/o Department of Biology, Nippon Dental University, 9-20 Fujimi 1-chome, Chiyoda-ku, Tokyo 102-0071, Japan. TEL 81-3-3261-8311, FAX 81-3-3264-8399, zvbo1357@nifty.ne.jp. Ed. Shigeo Kurata. Circ: 600.

580 USA ISSN 0883-1475
SIDA: BOTANICAL MISCELLANY. Text in English. 1987. irreg., latest vol.21, 2001. price varies. Website rev. *Refereed.* **Document type:** *Monographic series, Academic/Scholarly.*
—CISTI, Linda Hall.
Published by: Botanical Research Institute of Texas, Inc., 509 Pecan St, Fort Worth, TX 76102-4060. TEL 817-332-4441, sida@brit.org. Ed. Barney L Lipscomb TEL 817-332-7432. R&P Yonie Hudson. Circ: 850.

581.3 DEU ISSN 0037-5349
CODEN: SIGEAQ
SILVAE GENETICA; Zeitschrift fuer Forstgenetik und Forstpflanzenzuechtung. Text in English, French, German. 1951. 6/yr. EUR 256.15 domestic; EUR 259.70 foreign (effective 2002). adv. bk.rev. abstr, charts, illus. index. *Refereed.* **Document type:** *Journal, Academic/Scholarly.* **Description:** Includes announcements and reports on meetings and congresses on forest tree breeding and genetics as well as other related fields.
Related titles: Online - full text ed.: (from Institute for Scientific Information).
Indexed: ASCA, Abstr.Bull.Inst.Pap.Chem., AgBiotech, Agricola, Agroforest.Abstr., Aqua.Sci.& Fish.Abstr., Biol.Abstr., Chem.Abstr., Crop Physiol.Abstr., Curr.Adv.Ecol.Sci., Curr.Adv.Plant Sci., Curr.Cont., Curr.Ind.Stat., Eng.Ind., Entomol.Abstr. (coverage dropped), Forest Prod.Abstr., Forest.Abstr., Genet.Abstr., Hort.Abstr., Hum.Gen.Abstr., INIS Atomind., Int.Abstr.Biol.Sci., Plant Breed.Abstr., Plant Gen.Res.Abstr., Plant Grow.Reg.Abstr., Plant Sci., Ref.Zh., Rev.Appl.Entomol., Rev.Arom.& Med.Plants, Rev.Plant Path., Sci.Cit.Ind., Seed Abstr., Soils & Fert., VITIS.
—BLDSC (8281.500000), CASDDS, CISTI, EMDOCS, IDS, Infotrieve, ingenta, Linda Hall. **CCC.**
Published by: J.D. Sauerlaender's Verlag, Finkenhofstr 21, Frankfurt Am Main 60322, Germany. TEL 49-69-555217, FAX 49-69-5964344, j.d.sauerlaenders.verlag@t-online.de. Ed. H J Muhs.

580 FRA ISSN 0373-0875
SOCIETE LINNEENNE DE PROVENCE. BULLETIN. Text in Esperanto, French, German, Spanish; Summaries in Catalan, English, Esperanto, French, German, Spanish. 1909. a. FRF 100 (effective 1999). adv. bk.rev. back issues avail. *Refereed.* **Document type:** *Bulletin.* **Description:** Publishes articles on botany, zoology, geology and prehistoric ecology.
Published by: Societe Linneenne de Provence, Lycee Victor Hugo, 3 bd. Desplaces, Marseille 13003, France. TEL 33-4-91632832, FAX 33-4-91632832. Ed. Claude Roux. Adv. contact Rene Thomas. Circ: 300. **Subscr. to:** Arlette Torre-Legueult, Lycee Victor Hugo, 3 bd. Desplaces, Marseille 13003, France.

SPAIN. MINISTERIO DE AGRICULTURA, PESCA Y ALIMENTACION. BOLETIN DE SANIDAD VEGETAL: PLAGAS. see *AGRICULTURE—Crop Production And Soil*

580 USA ISSN 1090-1876
TIPULARIA; a botanical magazine. Text in English. 1986. a. USD 10 (effective 2000). bk.rev. **Document type:** *Magazine, Academic/Scholarly.*
Published by: Georgia Botanical Society, c/o Sally Emory, Bus Mgr, 7575 Rico Rd, Palmetto, GA 30268. TEL 770-463-4227, dandsemory@aol.com. Eds. Eric Van de Genachte, Shan Cammack. R&P David Emory. Circ: 450.

582.16 CAN CODEN: TRPHEM
TREE PHYSIOLOGY; an international botanical journal. Text in English. 1986. 18/yr. CND 1,116 domestic; USD 848 foreign (effective 2002); includes online access. adv. bk.rev. illus. index. reprints avail. *Refereed.* **Document type:** *Academic/Scholarly.* **Description:** International journal devoted to research reports and technical reviews on all aspects of the physiology of trees.
Related titles: Online - full text ed.: (from The Dialog Corporation, Institute for Scientific Information).
Indexed: ASCA, AgBiotech, Agricola, Agroforest.Abstr., Appl.Ecol.Abstr., Bibl.Agri., Biol.Abstr., Chem.Abstr., Chem.Indus.Notes, Crop Physiol.Abstr., Curr.Adv.Plant Sci., Curr.Cont., Ecol.Abstr., Environ.Abstr., Environ.Sci.Poll.Mgmt., Field Crop Abstr., Forest Prod.Abstr., Forest.Abstr., Geo.Abstr.P.G., Herb.Abstr., Hort.Abstr., INIS Atomind., Ind.Sci.Rev., Int.Abstr.Biol.Sci., Irr.& Drain.Abstr., Ornam.Hort., Plant Breed.Abstr., Plant Gen.Res.Abstr., Plant Grow.Reg.Abstr., Plant Sci., Pollut.Abstr., Rev.Appl.Entomol., Rev.Arom.& Med.Plants, Rev.Plant Path., Sci.Cit.Ind., Seed Abstr., Sel.Water Res.Abstr., Soils & Fert., Weed Abstr.
—BLDSC (9047.625000), CASDDS, CISTI, Infotrieve, ingenta, Linda Hall. **CCC.**
Published by: Heron Publishing, 202-3994 Shelbourne St, Victoria, BC V8N 3E2, Canada. TEL 250-721-9921, FAX 250-721-9924, publisher@heronpublishing.com, http://heronpublishing.com/tphome.html. Pub., R&P Alfred Burdett.

TREEWORKER. see *FORESTS AND FORESTRY*

580 ESP ISSN 0213-5450
UNIVERSIDAD DE MURCIA. ANALES DE BIOLOGIA. SECCION BIOLOGIA VEGETAL. Text mainly in English, Spanish. 1984. a., latest vol.9, 1995. ESP 2,000 (effective 2001). bk.rev. back issues avail. **Document type:** *Academic/Scholarly.*
Indexed: Field Crop Abstr., Ind.SST.
—CISTI.
Published by: Universidad de Murcia, Servicio de Publicaciones, C Actor Isidoro Maiquez 9, Murcia 30007, Spain. TEL 34-68-363207, FAX 34-68-363414, vgm@um.es, http://www.um.es/spumweb. Ed. Diego Jose Rivera Nunez TEL 34-968-364958. Circ: 606.

UNIVERSITY OF WAIKATO. ANTARCTIC RESEARCH UNIT. REPORT. see *EARTH SCIENCES—Geology*

581.652 JPN ISSN 0372-798X CODEN: ZASKAN
WEED RESEARCH. Text in English, Japanese. 1962. q. JPY 5,000. back issues avail.
Indexed: Agroforest.Abstr., Bio-Contr.News & Info., Crop Physiol.Abstr., Curr.Cont. (coverage dropped), Derwent Biotech.Abstr., Field Crop Abstr., Herb.Abstr., Hort.Abstr., Ind.Vet., Irr.& Drain.Abstr., Maize Abstr., Plant Grow.Reg.Abstr., Rev.Appl.Entomol., Seed Abstr., Soils & Fert., Soyabean Abstr., Triticale Abstr., Trop.Oil Seeds Abstr., Weed Abstr.
—CASDDS, CISTI.
Published by: Weed Science Society of Japan, Shokucho Bldg 26-6 Taito, Taito 1-chome, Taito-ku, Tokyo 110-0016, Japan. Ed. Kozo Ishizuka. Circ: 2,000.

579.562 GBR ISSN 0749-503X CODEN: YESTE3
YEAST; a forum for yeast researchers. Text in English. 1985. 20/yr. USD 1,805 in United States; USD 1,805 in Canada & Mexico; USD 1,805 elsewhere; USD 1,896 in United States for print and online eds.; USD 1,896 in Canada & Mexico for print and online eds.; USD 1,896 elsewhere for print and online eds. (effective 2002). adv. back issues avail.; reprint service avail. from SWZ. *Refereed.* **Document type:** *Academic/Scholarly.* **Description:** Contains original research articles along with major and minor reviews and short communications on all aspects of saccharomyces and other yeast genera.
Related titles: Microform ed.: (from PQC); Online - full text ed.: ISSN 1097-0061. USD 1,805 in United States; USD 1,805 in Canada & Mexico; USD 1,805 elsewhere (effective 2002) (from EBSCO Publishing, Wiley InterScience, Institute for Scientific Information).
Indexed: BBCI, Biotech.& Bioeng.Abstr., Biotech.Cit.Ind., Chem.Abstr., Chem.Indus.Notes, Curr.Adv.Ecol.Sci., Curr.Cont., Dairy Sci.Abstr., Derwent Biotech.Abstr., Excerp.Med. (1992-), Food Sci.& Tech.Abstr., Genet.Abstr., Hum.Gen.Abstr., Ind.Med. (1985-), Ind.Sci.Rev., Inpharma, Int.Abstr.Biol.Sci., Mass Spectr.Bull., Microbiol.Abstr., Nuc.Acids Abstr., Reac., Rev.Med.& Vet.Mycol., Sci.Cit.Ind., Sugar Ind.Abstr., Telegen.
—BLDSC (9417.976000), CASDDS, CISTI, EMDOCS, GNLM, IDS, ingenta, Linda Hall. **CCC.**
Published by: Wiley Europe Ltd., Baffins Ln, Chichester, W Sussex PO19 1UD, United Kingdom. TEL 44-1243-779777, FAX 44-1243-843232, customer@wiley.co.uk, http://www.wiley.co.uk. Ed. S G Oliver. adv.: B&W page GBP 650, color page GBP 1,550; trim 200 x 260. **Subscr. in the Americas to:** John Wiley & Sons, Inc., Journals, 605 Third Ave, New York, NY 10158. TEL 212-850-6645, FAX 212-850-6021, uscs-wis@wiley.com; **Subscr. to:** John Wiley & Sons Ltd., Baffins Ln, Chichester, Sussex PO19 IUD, United Kingdom. cs-journals@wiley.co.uk.

580 CHN ISSN 0253-2700
QK1 CODEN: YCWCDP
YUNNAN ZHIWU YANJIU/ACTA BOTANICA YUNNANICA. Text in Chinese; Abstracts in English. 1979. bi-m. (q. until 2002). CNY 48 domestic; USD 60 foreign (effective 2001). adv. bk.rev. abstr. 126 p./no. *Refereed.* **Document type:** *Academic/Scholarly.* **Description:** Publishes original papers and notes on various fields of botany, including phytotaxonomy, phytogeography, phytochemistry, plant physiology, morphology, ecology and geobotany, domestication of introduced species, utilization of plant resources, and new techniques and achievements in China and abroad.
Related titles: CD-ROM ed.
Indexed: AgBiotech, Agroforest.Abstr., Chem.Abstr., Chem.Indus.Notes, Chem.Titles, Crop Physiol.Abstr., Curr.Adv.Ecol.Sci., Field Crop Abstr., Food Sci.& Tech.Abstr., Forest Prod.Abstr., Forest.Abstr., Herb.Abstr., Hort.Abstr., Maize Abstr., Ornam.Hort., Plant Breed.Abstr., Plant Gen.Res.Abstr., Plant Grow.Reg.Abstr., Ref.Zh., Rev.Appl.Entomol., Rev.Arom.& Med.Plants, Rev.Plant Path., Rice Abstr., Rural Devel.Abstr., Seed Abstr., Soils & Fert., Weed Abstr.
—BLDSC (0608.120000), CASDDS, Linda Hall.
Published by: Zhongguo Kexueyuan, Kunming Zhiwu Yanjiusuo/Chinese Academy of Sciences, Kunming Institute of Botany, Heilongtan, Kunming, Yunnan 650204, China. TEL 86-871-5223036, FAX 86-871-5150227, bianji@mail.kib.ac.cn, http://159.226.148.66. Ed. Zhengyi Wu. Adv. contact Aiqin Liu. Circ: 1,300 (paid and controlled). **Subscr. outside of China to:** Kexue Chubanshe, 16 Donghuang Cheng Gen Beijie, Beijing 100707, China.

ZEITSCHRIFT FUER PHYTOTHERAPIE. see *MEDICAL SCIENCES*

580 CHN ISSN 0577-7518 CODEN: CWPHA2
ZHIWU BAOHU XUEBAO/ACTA PHYTOPHYLACTICA SINICA. Variant title: Journal of Plant Protection. Text in Chinese; Abstracts in English. q. CNY 16 newsstand/cover domestic (effective 2000). **Document type:** *Academic/Scholarly.* **Description:** Contains research reports in this field of botany.
Related titles: Online - full content ed.: (from WanFang Data Corp.).
Indexed: AgBiotech, Agri.Eng.Abstr., Bio-Contr.News & Info., Biol.Abstr., Cott.& Trop.Fibr.Abstr., Curr.Adv.Ecol.Sci., Field Crop Abstr., Forest.Abstr., Helminthol.Abstr., Hort.Abstr., Maize Abstr., Plant Breed.Abstr., Postharvest, Potato Abstr., Rev.Appl.Entomol., Rev.Arom.& Med.Plants, Rev.Plant Path., Rice Abstr., Seed Abstr., Soyabean Abstr., Triticale Abstr., Weed Abstr., Zoo.Rec.
—BLDSC (0656.700000), CISTI, Linda Hall.
Published by: Zhongguo Zhiwu Baohu Xuehui, Department of Plant Protection, China Agricultural University, Beijing 100094, China. TEL 86-10-2582244 ext. 319, xxf@public.sti.ac.cn. Ed. Mingtsang Cheo.

580 CHN ISSN 0412-0914
QK710 CODEN: CWSPDA
ZHIWU BINGLI XUEBAO/ACTA PHYTOPATHOLOGICA SINICA. Text in Chinese. q. USD 1.80 per issue. 96 p./no. *Refereed.* **Document type:** *Academic/Scholarly.*
Indexed: AgBiotech, Bio-Contr.News & Info., Cott.& Trop.Fibr.Abstr., Crop Physiol.Abstr., Curr.Adv.Ecol.Sci., Field Crop Abstr., Food Sci.& Tech.Abstr., Forest.Abstr., Helminthol.Abstr., Hort.Abstr., Maize Abstr., Ornam.Hort., Plant Breed.Abstr., Potato Abstr., Rev.Appl.Entomol., Rev.Arom.& Med.Plants, Rev.Plant Path., Rice Abstr., Seed Abstr., Soyabean Abstr., Triticale Abstr., Weed Abstr., Zoo.Rec.
—BLDSC (0656.500000), Linda Hall.
Published by: Zhongguo Zhiwu Bingli Xuehui/China Phytopathological Society, Department of Plant Protection, Beijing University of Agriculture, Beijing 100094, China. TEL 86-10-62892364, FAX 86-10-62891025. Ed. Zeng Shimai.

571.2 CHN ISSN 0412-0922 CODEN: CHWSAX
ZHIWU SHENGLIXUE TONGXUN/PLANT PHYSIOLOGY COMMUNICATIONS. Text in Chinese. 1951. bi-m. USD 90 (effective 2000). adv. bk.rev. **Document type:** *Academic/Scholarly.* **Description:** Contains original papers, communications, and review articles on plant physiology, biochemistry, and biophysics, from the molecular level to the community level. Also contains columns on techniques and methods, teaching, and news.
Indexed: AgBiotech, Chem.Abstr., Chem.Indus.Notes, Chem.Titles, Crop Physiol.Abstr., Field Crop Abstr., Forest Prod.Abstr., Forest.Abstr., Herb.Abstr., Hort.Abstr., Irr.& Drain.Abstr., Maize Abstr., Ornam.Hort., Plant Breed.Abstr., Plant Gen.Res.Abstr., Plant Grow.Reg.Abstr., Postharvest, Potato Abstr., Rev.Plant Path., Rice Abstr., Seed Abstr., Soyabean Abstr., Triticale Abstr., Weed Abstr.
—BLDSC (6522.100000), CASDDS, CISTI.
Published by: (Chinese Society of Plant Physiology), Kexue Chubanshe/Science Press, 16 Donghuang Cheng Genbei Jie, Beijing 100717, China.

580 CHN ISSN 1005-264X
QK355
ZHIWU SHENGTAI XUEBAO/ACTA PHYTOECOLOGICA SINICA. Text in Chinese, English. 1955. bi-m. USD 90 (effective 2000). adv. bk.rev. *Refereed.* **Document type:** *Academic/Scholarly.* **Description:** Contains original research papers on plant ecology, including plant ecophysiology, population ecology, community ecology, vegetation science, landscape ecology, ecosystem ecology, and conservation.
Formerly (until 1994): Zhiwu Shengtaixue yu Diziwuxue Xuebao - Acta Phytoecologica et Geobotanica Sinica (1000-0011)
Indexed: Ref.Zh.
—Linda Hall.
Published by: (Chinese Academy of Sciences, Institute of Botany), Kexue Chubanshe/Science Press, 16 Donghuang Cheng Genbei Jie, Beijing 100717, China. Eds. Yihui Hu, Yonghong Li. R&P Yihui Hu. Adv. contact Yonghong Li. Circ: 1,300.

580 TWN ISSN 0006-8063
QK1 CODEN: BBASA6
ZHONGYANG YANJIUYUAN ZHIWUXUE HUIKAN/ACADEMIA SINICA. BOTANICAL BULLETIN. Text in English; Summaries in Chinese. 1960. q. USD 60 per vol. to individuals; USD 100 per vol. to institutions; USD 15 per issue to individuals; USD 25 per issue to institutions (effective 2001). adv. bibl, charts, illus, stat. index, cum.index. *Refereed.* **Document type:** *Academic/Scholarly.* **Description:** Publishes both original and review papers on all aspects of modern plant science from researchers around the world.
Related titles: CD-ROM ed.; Microfilm ed.; Online - full text ed.: (from Institute for Scientific Information).
Indexed: ASCA, AgBiotech, Bio-Contr.News & Info., Biol.Abstr., Cadscan, Chem.Abstr., Chem.Indus.Notes, Chem.Titles, Crop Physiol.Abstr., Curr.Adv.Plant Sci., Curr.Cont., Field Crop Abstr., Food Sci.& Tech.Abstr., Forest.Abstr., Genet.Abstr. (coverage dropped), Helminthol.Abstr., Herb.Abstr., Hort.Abstr., Lead Abstr., Maize Abstr., Nutr.Abstr., Ornam.Hort., Plant Breed.Abstr., Plant Grow.Reg.Abstr., Plant Sci., Rev.Appl.Entomol., Rev.Arom.& Med.Plants, Rev.Plant Path., Rice Abstr., Sci.Cit.Ind., Seed Abstr., Soils & Fert., Soyabean Abstr., Triticale Abstr., Virol.Abstr. (coverage dropped), Weed Abstr., Zincscan.
—BLDSC (2253.000000), CASDDS, CISTI, EMDOCS, IDS, ingenta, KNAW, Linda Hall.
Published by: Academia Sinica, Institute of Botany/Chung Yang Yen Chiu Yuan, Chih Wu Hsueh Yen Chiu So, Nankang, Taipei 11529, Taiwan. TEL 886-2-2789-9590, FAX 886-2-27827954, boyhlin@ccvax.sinica.edu.tw, http://www.ejournal.sinica.edu.tw/bbas. Ed. Yaw Huei Lin. Pub. Jei Fu Shaw. Circ: 570 (paid and controlled). **Dist. by:** Lily Journal and Book Co. & Ltd., 4F-3, No 125, Roosevelt Rd, Sec3, Taipei, Taiwan. TEL 886-2-2363-3168, FAX 886-2-2362-7448, hcling@ms4.hint.net.

BIOLOGY—Computer Applications

570.285 GBR ISSN 1462-1355
THE BIOINFORMER. Text in English. 1997. q. free per issue. **Document type:** *Newsletter.* **Description:** Focuses on bioinformatics research, services and developments at the Institute, including a list of the most worthwhile symposia and conferences on the field.
Related titles: Online - full text ed.: ISSN 1462-1363.

B

Published by: European Bioinformatics Institute, Welcome Trust Genome Campus, Hinxton, Cambs CB10 1SD, United Kingdom. TEL 44-1223-494635, FAX 44-1223-494468, pow@ebi.ac.uk;, http://bioinformer.ebi.ac.uk/. Ed. Jean Jack M Riethoven. R&P Jean Jack M Reithoven. Circ: 3,000.

570.285 CHE ISSN 1025-5842
COMPUTER METHODS IN BIOMECHANICS AND BIOMEDICAL ENGINEERING. Text in English. 1997. 6/yr. GBP 81, USD 98 to individuals; GBP 252, USD 377 to institutions (effective 2002). **Document type:** *Academic/Scholarly.* **Description:** Focuses on the importance of integrating the disciplines of engineering with medical technology and clinical expertise.
Published by: Gordon and Breach - Harwood Academic (Subsidiary of: Taylor & Francis Group), PO Box 531, Lausanne 1000, Switzerland. Eds. John Middleton, Nigel Shrive. **Subscr. addr. in US:** International Publishers Direct, PO Box 32160, Newark, NJ 07102. FAX 215-750-6343.

B

570.285 GBR ISSN 0010-4825
R858.A1 CODEN: CBMDAW
COMPUTERS IN BIOLOGY AND MEDICINE; an international journal. Text in English. 1971. 6/yr. EUR 216 in Europe to individuals; JPY 28,700 in Japan to individuals; USD 242 elsewhere to individuals (effective 2001). adv. bk.rev. back issues avail. *Refereed.* **Document type:** *Academic/Scholarly.* **Description:** Provides an international medium for the exchange of research, ideas and information on all aspects of the growing use of computers in the fields of bioscience and medicine.
Related titles: Microfilm ed.: (from PQC); Online - full text ed.: (from ingenta, Swets Blackwell, ScienceDirect, Institute for Scientific Information).
Indexed: ASCA, Anim.Breed.Abstr., Appl.Mech.Rev., Aqua.Sci.& Fish.Abstr., Bioeng.Abstr., Biol.Abstr., Biostat., Chem.Abstr., Chem.Indus.Notes, Chem.Titles, Compumath, Comput.Abstr., Comput.Cont., Comput.Dtbs., Curr.Adv.Ecol.Sci., Curr.Cont., Curr.Ind.Stat., Eng.Ind., Environ.Sci.Poll.Mgmt., Excerp.Med., INIS Atomind., INSPEC (Aug.1970-), Ind.Med. (1970-), Ind.Sci.Rev., Inpharma, Int.Abstr.Biol.Sci., Int.Nurs.Ind., LISA, Pharm.&Out.News, Pollut.Abstr., Reac., Risk Abstr., Saf.Sci.Abstr., Sci.Cit.Ind., Telegen.
—BLDSC (3394.880000), ADONIS, AskIEEE, CASDDS, CISTI, Ei, EMDOCS, GNLM, IDS, ingenta, Linda Hall. **CCC.**
Published by: Pergamon (Subsidiary of: Elsevier Science), The Boulevard, Langford Ln, East Park, Kidlington, Oxford OXB 1GB, United Kingdom. FAX 44-1865-843010, http://www.elsevier.com/locate/compbiomed. Ed. Robert S Ledley. Circ: 1,200. **Subscr. in Australasia and the Far East to:** Elsevier Science (Singapore) Pte Ltd, No.1 Temasek Ave, 17-01 Millenia Tower, Singapore 039192, Singapore. TEL 65-434-3727, FAX 65-337-2230; **Subscr. in the Americas to:** Elsevier Science, PO Box 945, New York, NY 10159-0945. TEL 212-633-3730, FAX 212-633-3680, usinfo-f@elsevier.com; **Subscr. to:** Elsevier Science BV, PO Box 211, Amsterdam 1000 AE, Netherlands. TEL 31-20-485-3757, http://www.elsevier.nl.

570.285 USA ISSN 1089-778X
QA76.87 CODEN: ITEVF5
I E E E TRANSACTIONS ON EVOLUTIONARY COMPUTATION. Text in English. 1997. bi-m. USD 360 in North America for print or online ed.; USD 385 elsewhere for print or online ed. (effective 2002). **Description:** Covers specific techniques such as evolution strategies, evolutionary programming, genetic algorithms and associated methods of genetic programming and classifier systems.
Related titles: CD-ROM ed.; Microfiche ed.; Online - full text ed.: (from EBSCO Publishing, Institute for Scientific Information).
Indexed: A.S.& T.Ind. (Jan.2001-), Comp.Com.Sec.Abstr., Compumath, Comput.Abstr., Curr.Cont., Eng.Ind., INSPEC (Apr.1997-), Ref.Zh., Sci.Cit.Ind.
—BLDSC (4363.187400), ingenta, Linda Hall.
Published by: Institute of Electrical and Electronics Engineers, Inc. TEL 800-701-4333, customer.service@ieee.org; webmaster@computer.org, subscription-service@ieee.org, http://www.ieee.org. Ed. David B Fogel. **Subscr. to:** Maruzen Co. Ltd., 3-10 Nihonbashi 2-chome, Chuo-ku, Tokyo 103-0027, Japan. FAX 81-3-3275-0657; Universal Subscription Agency, Pvt. Ltd., 877, Udyog Vihar, V, Gurgoan 122001, India. TEL 91-124-347261, FAX 91-124-342496. **Co-sponsor:** Natural Networks Council.

I F M B E NEWS. (International Federation for Medical & Biological Engineering) see *BIOLOGY—Bioengineering*

INTERNATIONAL JOURNAL OF EVOLUTIONARY OPTIMIZATION. see *BIOLOGY—Genetics*

INTERNATIONAL JOURNAL OF MEDICAL INFORMATICS. see *MEDICAL SCIENCES—Computer Applications*

JOURNAL OF MOLECULAR GRAPHICS AND MODELLING. see *CHEMISTRY—Computer Applications*

570.285 GBR ISSN 0140-0118
R895.A1 CODEN: MBECDY
MEDICAL & BIOLOGICAL ENGINEERING & COMPUTING. Text in English. 1962. bi-m. GBP 415, USD 762 (effective 2001). adv. bk.rev. abstr, bibl, charts, illus. index. *Refereed.* **Document type:** *Journal, Academic/Scholarly.* **Description:** Contains technical papers on subjects such as medical electronics, biomechanics, medical computing, patient monitoring, nuclear medicine, imaging, rehabilitation and biosensors.
Incorporates (in 1998): Cellular Engineering (1357-5481); Which superseded: Journal of Cellular Engineering (1364-4068); Former titles: Medical and Biological Engineering (0025-696X); Biological Engineering; Medical Electronics
Related titles: Microform ed.: (from PQC); Online - full text ed.: (from Institute for Scientific Information); ♦ Supplement: I F M B E News. ISSN 1359-0944.
Indexed: AMED, A.S.& T.Ind. (coverage dropped), ASCA, Appl.Mech.Rev., Bioeng.Abstr., Biol.Abstr., Biotech.& Bioeng.Abstr., Chem.Abstr., Chem.Cit.Ind., Compumath, Comput.& Info.Sys., Comput.Cont., Curr.Adv.Ecol.Sci., Curr.Cont., Curr.Ind.Stat., Cyb.Abstr., Electron.& Communic.Abstr.J., Eng.Ind., Environ.Sci.Poll.Mgmt., Ergon.Abstr., Excerp.Med., INIS Atomind., INSPEC (pre-1969-Nov.1976, Jan.1977-), Ind.Med. (1977-), Ind.Sci.Rev., Ind.Vet., Inpharma, Mass Spectr.Bull., Med.& Pharm.Biotech.Abstr., Neurosci.Cit.Ind., Reac., Rev.Appl.Entomol., SSCI (coverage dropped), Sci.Cit.Ind., Vet.Bull.
—BLDSC (5525.770000), AskIEEE, CASDDS, CISTI, Ei, GNLM, IDS, ingenta, Linda Hall. **CCC.**
Published by: I.E.E., Michael Faraday House, Six Hills Way, Stevenage, Herts SG1 2AY, United Kingdom. TEL 44-1438-767266, FAX 44-1438-742849, inspec@iee.org.uk, http://www.iee.org.uk. Ed. Peter Wolfe. Circ: 1,300. **Subscr. to:** INSPEC, I.E.E., .Box 96, Stevenage, Herts SG1 2SD, United Kingdom. TEL 44-1483-313311, FAX 44-1438-742792.

570.285 AUS ISSN 1443-2250
▼ **ONLINE JOURNAL OF BIOINFORMATICS.** Text in English. 1999. irreg. **Document type:** *Academic/Scholarly.* **Description:** Focuses on original research work either as full-text reports on short communications. Intended to meet the demand of rapid growth in the use of computer science in biology.
Media: Online - full text.
Published by: Pestsearch International Pty. Ltd., 173 Chatswood Rd, Daisy Hill, QLD 4127, Australia. http://www.uq.edu.au/~csvguerr/bioinfo.htm, http://www.cpb.uokhsc.edu/ojvr/jvet196a.htm. Ed. V H Guerrini.

570.285 SGP
PACIFIC SYMPOSIUM ON BIOCOMPUTING (YEAR). Text in English. a. USD 138, GBP 86 per issue (effective 2001). *Refereed.* **Document type:** *Proceedings, Academic/Scholarly.*
—BLDSC (6331.530000).
Published by: World Scientific Publishing Co Pte Ltd, 5 Toh Tuck Link, Singapore 596224, Singapore. http://www.worldscientific.com.sg. Ed. Dr. Russ B Altman. **Subscr. in N. Amerca to:** 1060 Main St, River Edge, NJ 07661.

BIOLOGY—Cytology And Histology

A C T INTERNATIONAL CYTOGENETICS LABORATORY DIRECTORY. see *MEDICAL SCIENCES—Experimental Medicine, Laboratory Technique*

571.6 USA
A T C C CELL LINES AND HYBRIDOMAS. Text in English. irreg., latest vol.8, 1994. USD 22 in North America; USD 32 elsewhere. **Document type:** *Catalog.*
Former titles: A T C C Catalogue of Cell Lines and Hybridomas; Supersedes in part: American Type Culture Collection. Catalogue of Strains 2: Animal Cell Lines, Animal Viruses, Bacterial Viruses, Mycoviruses, Plant Viruses, Rickettsiae, Chlamydiae; Which was formerly titled: American Type Culture Collection. Catalogue of Strains 2: Animal Cell Lines, Animal Viruses, Bacterial Viruses, Mycoviruses, Rickettsiae, Chlamydiae; American Type Culture Collection. Catalogue of Strains: 2. Animal Viruses, Rickettsiae, Chlamydiae; American Type Culture Collection. Catalogue of Viruses, Rickettsiae, Chlamydiae
Published by: American Type Culture Collection, 10801 University Blvd, Manassas, VA 20110. TEL 800-638-6597, FAX 301-816-4361, sales@ATCC.org. Ed. R Hay.

571.6 USA
A T C C QUALITY CONTROL METHODS FOR CELL LINES. Text in English. 1992. irreg. USD 40; USD 45 foreign.
Published by: American Type Culture Collection, 10801 University Blvd, Manassas, VA 20110. TEL 800-638-6597, FAX 301-816-4361, Sales@ATCC.org.

ACTA ANATOMICA NIPPONICA/KAIBOGAKU ZASSHI. see *BIOLOGY*

571.6 USA ISSN 0001-5547
RG1 CODEN: ACYTAN
ACTA CYTOLOGICA; the journal of clinical cytology and cytopathology. Text in English. 1957. bi-m. USD 178 to individuals; USD 249 to institutions (effective 2000). adv. bk.rev. abstr, bibl, illus, stat. index. back issues avail. *Refereed.* **Document type:** *Academic/Scholarly.*
Related titles: Microfilm ed.: (from WWS); Microform ed.: (from PMC); Online - full text ed.: (from Institute for Scientific Information).
Indexed: AESIS, AIDS Abstr., ASCA, Abstr.Hyg., BBCI, Biol.Abstr., Chem.Abstr., Curr.Adv.Ecol.Sci., Curr.Cont., Dairy Sci.Abstr., Dent.Ind., Excerp.Med., Helminthol.Abstr., INIS Atomind., Ind.Med. (1957-), Ind.Sci.Rev., Inpharma, Int.Abstr.Biol.Sci., Int.Nurs.Ind., Neurosci.Cit.Ind., Pharm.&Out.News, Protozool.Abstr., Reac., Ref.Zh., Rev.Med.& Vet.Mycol., Rev.Plant Path., Sci.Cit.Ind., Trop.Dis.Bull.
—BLDSC (0612.100000), CASDDS, CISTI, EMDOCS, GNLM, IDS, ingenta, KNAW. **CCC.**
Published by: (International Academy of Cytology), Science Printers and Publishers, Inc., 8342 Olive Blvd., St. Louis, MO 63132. TEL 314-991-4440, FAX 314-991-4654, editor@acta-cytol.com, http://www.acta-cytol.com. Ed. Dr. Marluce Bibbo. Pub., R&P, Adv. contact Donna Kessel. Circ: 6,080.

571.6 JPN ISSN 0044-5991
QM551 CODEN: ACHCBO
ACTA HISTOCHEMICA ET CYTOCHEMICA/NIHON SOSHIKI SAIBO KAGAKKAI GAKKAISHI. Text in English. 1960. bi-m. JPY 12,000. adv. bk.rev. abstr, bibl, charts, illus. index. reprint service avail. from PQC. *Refereed.* **Document type:** *Academic/Scholarly.* **Description:** Features original articles in all fields of histochemistry and cytochemistry. Contains proceedings of the annual meeting of the society.
Related titles: Microform ed.: (from PQC); Online - full text ed.: (from Institute for Scientific Information).
Indexed: ASCA, BBCI, Biol.Abstr., Cal.Tiss.Abstr., Chem.Abstr., Chem.Indus.Notes, Chem.Titles, Curr.Adv.Ecol.Sci., Curr.Cont., Dairy Sci.Abstr., Helminthol.Abstr., INIS Atomind., Ind.Sci.Rev., Inpharma, Int.Abstr.Biol.Sci., Nutr.Abstr., Pharm.&Out.News, Reac., Ref.Zh., Sci.Cit.Ind., Weed Abstr.
—BLDSC (0624.040000), CASDDS, CISTI, EMDOCS, GNLM, IDS, Infotrieve, ingenta, KNAW, Linda Hall. **CCC.**
Published by: Japan Society of Histochemistry and Cytochemistry, c/o Nakanishi Printing Co, Shimotachiuri-Ogawa, Kamikyo-ku, Kyoto-shi 602, Japan. TEL 81-75-415-3661, FAX 81-75-415-3662, HBE 02610@niftyserve.or.jp. Ed. Tsukasa Ashihara. Circ: 1,800. **Dist. overseas by:** Japan Publications Trading Co. Ltd., Tokyo International, PO Box 5030, Tokyo 100-31, Japan.

ADVANCES IN ANATOMY, EMBRYOLOGY AND CELL BIOLOGY. see *BIOLOGY*

AMERICAN JOURNAL OF KIDNEY DISEASES. see *MEDICAL SCIENCES—Urology And Nephrology*

AMERICAN JOURNAL OF PHYSIOLOGY: CELL PHYSIOLOGY. see *BIOLOGY—Physiology*

AMERICAN JOURNAL OF PHYSIOLOGY: LUNG CELLULAR AND MOLECULAR PHYSIOLOGY. see *BIOLOGY—Physiology*

571.5 USA ISSN 0884-6812
RB43 CODEN: AQCHED
ANALYTICAL AND QUANTITATIVE CYTOLOGY AND HISTOLOGY. Text in English. 1979. bi-m. USD 255 to individuals; USD 345 to institutions (effective 2000). adv. index. back issues avail. *Refereed.* **Document type:** *Academic/Scholarly.*
Formerly: Analytical and Quantitative Cytology (0190-0471)
Related titles: Microform ed.: (from PQC,PMC); Online - full text ed.: (from Institute for Scientific Information).
Indexed: ASCA, BBCI, Biol.Abstr., Chem.Abstr., Curr.Adv.Ecol.Sci., Curr.Adv.Gen.& Molec.Biol., Curr.Cont., Excerp.Med., INIS Atomind., Ind.Med. (1985-), Ind.Sci.Rev., Ind.Vet., Inpharma, Int.Abstr.Biol.Sci., Reac., Ref.Zh., SSCI (coverage dropped), Sci.Cit.Ind., Vet.Bull.
—BLDSC (0896.380000), CASDDS, CISTI, EMDOCS, GNLM, IDS, ingenta, KNAW, Linda Hall. **CCC.**
Published by: (International Academy of Cytology), Science Printers and Publishers, Inc., 8342 Olive Blvd., St. Louis, MO 63132. TEL 314-991-4440, FAX 314-991-4654, editor@aqch.com, http://www.aqch.com. Ed. Dr. George L Wied. Pub., R&P, Adv. contact Donna Kessel. Circ: 3,000. **Co-sponsor:** American Society of Cytology.

571.6 NLD ISSN 0921-8912
CODEN: ACPAER
ANALYTICAL CELLULAR PATHOLOGY. (Includes: Bibliographic Alerting Service) Text in English. 1989. 8/yr. (in 2 vols). EUR 566, USD 523 to institutions (effective 2002). adv. bibl, illus. index. back issues avail. *Refereed.* **Document type:** *Journal, Academic/Scholarly.* **Description:** Addresses all aspects of analytical and quantitative approaches to cytology and histology with emphasis on applications to pathology.
Related titles: Online - full text ed.: (from EBSCO Publishing, O C L C Online Computer Library Center, Inc., ingenta, Swets Blackwell, Institute for Scientific Information, RoweCom Information Quest).
Indexed: ASCA, BBCI, Biol.Abstr., Chem.Abstr., Chem.Indus.Notes, Chem.Titles, Curr.Cont., Excerp.Med., Ind.Med. (1989-), Inpharma, Int.Abstr.Biol.Sci., Reac., Sci.Cit.Ind.
—BLDSC (0896.540000), ADONIS, CASDDS, CISTI, EMDOCS, GNLM, IDS, Infotrieve. **CCC.**
Published by: (European Society for Analytical Cellular Pathology), I O S Press, Nieuwe Hemweg 6B, Amsterdam 1013 BG, Netherlands. TEL 31-20-688-3355, FAX 31-20-620-3419, areith@labmed.uio.no, market@iospress.nl, http://www.iospress.nl. Ed. Albrecht Reith TEL 47-22-934217. **Subscr. to:** I O S Press, Inc, 5795-G Burke Centre Pkwy, Burke, VA 22015. TEL 703-323-5554, FAX 703-323-3668, iosbooks@iospress.com; Globe Publication Pvt. Ltd., C-62 Inderpuri, New Delhi 100 012, India. TEL 91-11-579-3211, 91-11-579-3212, custserve@globepub.com, http://www.globepub.com; Kinokuniya Company Ltd, Shinjuku 3-chome, Shinjuku-ku, Tokyo 160-0022, Japan. FAX 81-3-3439-1094, journal@kinokuniya.co.jp, http://www.kinokuniya.co.jp.

571.6 USA ISSN 1081-0706
QH573 CODEN: ARDBF8
ANNUAL REVIEW OF CELL AND DEVELOPMENTAL BIOLOGY. Text in English. 1985. a. USD 64 domestic to individuals; USD 69 foreign to individuals; USD 128 domestic to institutions; USD 138 foreign to institutions (effective 1999). adv. illus. index, cum.index. back issues avail.; reprints avail. *Refereed.* **Document type:** *Academic/Scholarly.* **Description:** Synthesizes and filters primary research to identify the principal contributions in the fields of developmental and cell biology.
Formerly (until vol.10, 1994): Annual Review of Cell Biology (0743-4634)
Related titles: Microfilm ed.: (from PQC); Online - full text ed.: (from HighWire Pr., EBSCO Publishing, H. W. Wilson, Institute for Scientific Information).
Indexed: ASCA, Aqua.Sci.& Fish.Abstr., BBCI, Biol.& Agr.Ind. (Jan.1990-Jan.1994), Biol.Dig., Chem.Abstr., Chem.Indus.Notes, Chem.Titles, Curr.Adv.Ecol.Sci., Curr.Cont., Genet.Abstr., Hum.Gen.Abstr., Ind.Med. (1995-), Inpharma, Int.Abstr.Biol.Sci., Neurosci.Abstr., Reac., Sci.Cit.Ind.
—BLDSC (1522.108500), ADONIS, CASDDS, CISTI, EMDOCS, GNLM, IDS, ingenta, KNAW, Linda Hall. **CCC.**
Published by: Annual Reviews Inc., 4139 El Camino Way, Box 10139, Palo Alto, CA 94303-0139. TEL 650-493-4400, 800-523-8535, FAX 650-424-0910, service@annualreviews.org, http://www.annurev.org; http://www.allenpress.com. Ed. Samuel Gubins. R&P, Adv. contact Swati Aneja TEL 650-843-6634. **Subscr. to:** Allen Press Inc., PO Box 1897, Lawrence, KS 66044-8897.

571.6 JPN
ANNUAL REVIEW SAIBO SEIBUTSUGAKU/ANNUAL REVIEW OF CELL BIOLOGY. Text in Japanese. a. JPY 7,980 (effective 1998). adv. **Document type:** *Academic/Scholarly.*
Published by: Chugai Igakusha, 62 Yarai-cho, Shinjuku-ku, Tokyo 162-0805, Japan. R&P M Takahashi. Adv. contact M. Takahashi.

571.6 USA ISSN 1360-8185
CODEN: APOPFN
APOPTOSIS; an international journal on programmed cell death. Text in English. 1996. bi-m. EUR 598, USD 598 to individuals for print or online ed.; EUR 716.60, USD 598 to institutions for print or online ed.; EUR 716.60, USD 717.60 to institutions for print & online eds. (effective 2002). adv. *Refereed.* **Document type:** *Academic/Scholarly.* **Description:** Provides the rapid publication of innovative basic and clinically oriented investigations into apoptosis and programmed cell-death.
Related titles: Online - full text ed.: (from EBSCO Publishing, O C L C Online Computer Library Center, Inc., RoweCom Information Quest, Swets Blackwell, Kluwer Online, Institute for Scientific Information).
Indexed: Biotech.Cit.Ind., Chem.Abstr., Curr.Cont., Ind.Med., Sci.Cit.Ind.
—BLDSC (1568.884400), CASDDS, IDS, Infotrieve. **CCC.**
Published by: Kluwer Academic Publishers Boston, 101 Philip Dr, Assinippi Park, Norwell, MA 02061. TEL 781-871-6600, FAX 781-871-9045, services@wkap.nl, http://www.wkap.nl/journalhome.htm/1360-8185. Ed. Dr. Mels Sluyser. R&P Rose Luongo TEL 781-871-6311. **Subscr. outside the Americas to:** Kluwer Academic Publishers Group, Journals Department, PO Box 322, Dordrecht 3300 AH, Netherlands. TEL 31-78-639-2392, FAX 31-78-654-6474; **Subscr. to:** Kluwer Academic - Plenum Publishers, 233 Spring St, New York, NY 10013-1578. TEL 212-620-8468, FAX 212-807-1047.

APPLIED CYTOGENETICS. see *BIOLOGY—Genetics*

571.5 JPN ISSN 0914-9465
CODEN: AHCYEZ
ARCHIVES OF HISTOLOGY AND CYTOLOGY/SOSHIKI SAIBOGAKU KIROKU. Text in English. 1950. 5/yr. USD 250 (effective 2001). adv. bk.rev. charts, illus. index. 100 p./no. back issues avail. *Refereed.* **Document type:** *Journal, Academic/Scholarly.*
Formerly (until 1988): Archivum Histologicum Japonicum (0004-0681)
Related titles: Online - full text ed.: (from Institute for Scientific Information).
Indexed: ASCA, Abstr.Anthropol., Biol.Abstr., Chem.Abstr., Chem.Indus.Notes, Chem.Titles, Curr.Adv.Ecol.Sci., Curr.Cont., Dairy Sci.Abstr., Dent.Ind., Excerp.Med., INIS Atomind., Ind.Med. (1988-), Ind.Sci.Rev., Inpharma, Neurosci.Cit.Ind., Nutr.Abstr., Pharm.&Out.News, Reac., Sci.Cit.Ind., Zoo.Rec.
—BLDSC (1634.413000), CASDDS, CISTI, EMDOCS, GNLM, IDS, ingenta, KNAW.
Published by: International Society of Histology and Cytology/Kokusai Soshiki Saibou Gakkai, c/o Department of Anatomy, University School of Medicine, Asahima-cho, Niigata-shi 951-8122, Japan. TEL 81-25-227-2058, FAX 81-25-224-1767, fujita@fancy.ocn.ne.jp, t-ushiki@medws1.med.niigata-u.ac.jp, http://www.ishc.net. Eds. Tsuneo Fujita, Yasuo Uchiyama. Circ: 700 (controlled).

571.6 NLD ISSN 0005-2736
QD1
B B A - BIOMEMBRANES. (Biochimica et Biophysica Acta) Text in Dutch. 1947. 12/yr. EUR 3,367 in Europe to institutions; JPY 447,000 in Japan to institutions; USD 3,766 elsewhere to institutions (effective 2002). *Refereed.* **Document type:** *Academic/Scholarly.* **Description:** Focuses on research in membrane structure and organization, membrane fluidity and lipid composition, model membranes, and membrane-protein interactions.
Incorporates (1972-2002): B B A - Reviews on Biomembranes (0304-4157)
Related titles: Microform ed.: (from PQC); Online - full text ed.: (from EBSCO Publishing, ingenta, Swets Blackwell, ScienceDirect, Institute for Scientific Information).
Indexed: ASCA, AgBiotech, Agri.& Environ.Biotech.Abstr. (coverage dropped), Anim.Breed.Abstr., BBCI, Crop Physiol.Abstr., Curr.Adv.Ecol.Sci., Curr.Cont., Dairy Sci.Abstr., Derwent Biotech.Abstr., Eng.Ind., Excerp.Med., Field Crop Abstr., Helminthol.Abstr., Hort.Abstr., INIS Atomind., Ind.Sci.Rev., Ind.Vet., Inpharma, Int.Abstr.Biol.Sci., Nutr.Abstr., Pharm.&Out.News, Plant Breed.Abstr., Protozool.Abstr., Reac., Ref.Zh., Rev.Appl.Entomol., Rev.Arom.& Med.Plants, Rev.Med.& Vet.Mycol., Rev.Plant Path., Rice Abstr., Sci.Cit.Ind., Seed Abstr., Sugar Ind.Abstr., Triticale Abstr.
—ADONIS, CISTI, Ei, EMDOCS, IDS, ingenta. **CCC.**
Published by: Elsevier Science BV, PO Box 211, Amsterdam 1000 AE, Netherlands. TEL 31-20-485-3757, FAX 31-20-485-3432, TELEX 18582 ESPA NL, nlinfo-f@elsevier.nl, http://www.elsevier.com/locate/bbamem, http://www.elsevier.nl. Eds. A G Lee, P L Yeagle. **Subscr. in Australasia and the Far East to:** Elsevier Science (Singapore) Pte Ltd, No.1 Temasek Ave, 17-01 Millenia Tower, Singapore 039192, Singapore. TEL 65-434-3727, FAX 65-337-2230, asiainfo@elsevier.com.sg; **Subscr. in Japan to:** Elsevier Science Inc - Japan Regional Office, 9-15 Higashi-Azabu 1-chome, Minato-ku, Tokyo 106-0044, Japan. TEL 81-3-5561-5033, FAX 81-3-5561-5047, info@elsevier.co.jp; **Subscr. in the Americas to:** Elsevier Science, PO Box 945, New York, NY 10159-0945. TEL 212-633-3730, FAX 212-633-3680, usinfo-f@elsevier.com, http://www.elsevier.com.

571.6 NLD ISSN 0167-4889
B B A - MOLECULAR CELL RESEARCH. Text in Dutch. 1982. 15/yr. EUR 1,736 in Europe to institutions; JPY 230,500 in Japan to institutions; USD 1,942 elsewhere to institutions (effective 2002). back issues avail. *Refereed.* **Document type:** *Academic/Scholarly.* **Description:** Focuses on intact cellular studies at the molecular level. Includes hormone and neurotransmitter action, molecular endocrinology, cell regulation, as well as whole-cell and whole-tissue spectroscopy.
Related titles: Microform ed.: (from PQC); Online - full text ed.: (from EBSCO Publishing, ingenta, Swets Blackwell, ScienceDirect, Institute for Scientific Information).
Indexed: ASCA, AgBiotech, Anim.Breed.Abstr., BBCI, Biol.Abstr., Chem.Abstr., Crop Physiol.Abstr., Curr.Cont., Dairy Sci.Abstr., Derwent Biotech.Abstr., Excerp.Med., Field Crop Abstr., Ind.Chem. (coverage dropped), Ind.Med. (coverage dropped), Inpharma, Int.Abstr.Biol.Sci., Nutr.Abstr., Plant Breed.Abstr., Reac., Ref.Zh., Rev.Appl.Entomol., Sci.Cit.Ind.
—ADONIS, CISTI, IDS. **CCC.**
Published by: Elsevier Science BV, PO Box 211, Amsterdam 1000 AE, Netherlands. TEL 31-20-485-2911, FAX 31-20-485-2457, nlinfo-f@elsevier.nl, http://www.elsevier.com/locate/bbamcr, http://www.elsevier.nl. Eds. E L F Holzbauer, N Pfanner. **Subscr. in Australasia and the Far East to:** Elsevier Science (Singapore) Pte Ltd, No.1 Temasek Ave, 17-01 Millenia Tower, Singapore 039192, Singapore. TEL 65-434-3727, FAX 65-337-2230; **Subscr. in Japan to:** Elsevier Science Inc - Japan Regional Office, 9-15 Higashi-Azabu 1-chome, Minato-ku, Tokyo 106-0044, Japan. TEL 81-3-5561-5033; **Subscr. in the Americas to:** Elsevier Science, PO Box 945, New York, NY 10159-0945. TEL 212-633-3730, FAX 212-633-3680.

571.5 USA ISSN 0891-2106
BASIC HISTOLOGY* . Text in English. 1975. triennial. **Document type:** *Monographic series.*
—CISTI.
Published by: Appleton & Lange, Journal Division (Subsidiary of: Simon & Schuster Company), 11 W 19th St, New York, CT 10011-4209. TEL 203-406-4500, FAX 203-406-4600.

571.6 ARG ISSN 0327-9545
CODEN: BOCEEZ
BIOCELL. Text in English. 1972. 3/yr. (in 1 vol., 3 nos./vol.). USD 80 to individuals; USD 100 to institutions. adv. charts, illus. index. reprint service avail. from ISI. *Refereed.* **Document type:** *Academic/Scholarly.* **Description:** Covers all aspects of biological electron microscopy and cell biology, from the molecular level to cell and tissue organization.
Former titles (until 1993): Microscopia Electronica y Biologia Celular - Electronic Microscopy and Cellular Biology (0326-3142); (until 1983): Revista de Microscopia Electronica
Related titles: Online - full text ed.: (from Institute for Scientific Information).
Indexed: ASCA, AgBiotech, Anim.Breed.Abstr., Biol.Abstr., Chem.Abstr., Chem.Indus.Notes, Chem.Titles, Curr.Cont., Excerp.Med. (until 1988), Field Crop Abstr., Hort.Abstr., Ind.Med. (1994-), Ind.Sci.Rev., Inpharma, Int.Abstr.Biol.Sci., Plant Breed.Abstr., Reac., Rev.Med.& Vet.Mycol., Sci.Cit.Ind., Zoo.Rec.

B

—BLDSC (2066.809400), CASDDS, CISTI, GNLM, IDS.

Published by: (Universidad Nacional de Cuyo, Facultad de Ciencias Medicas, Instituto de Histologia y Embriologia), Centro Regional de Investigaciones Cientificas y Tecnologicas, Casilla de Correos 131, Mendoza 5500, Argentina. TEL 54-61-205020 ext. 2670, FAX 54-61-380232, biocell@fmed2.uncu.edu.ar. Eds. Mario H Burgos, Ramon S Piezzi. Adv. contact Gabriel Puebla. B&W page USD 200, color page USD 300. Circ: 300 (controlled). **Co-sponsors:** Latin American Electron Microscopy Society; Sociedad Iberoamericana de Biologia Celular.

BIOCHEMISTRY AND CELL BIOLOGY/BIOCHIMIE ET BIOLOGIE CELLULAIRE. see *BIOLOGY—Biochemistry*

BIOLOGICHESKIE MEMBRANY. see *BIOLOGY—Biophysics*

571.6 USA ISSN 0887-3224
QP88.23 CODEN: ICOTAR

BIOLOGY OF EXTRACELLULAR MATRIX. Text in English. 1963. irreg. index. **Document type:** *Monographic series.*

Formerly (until 1986): International Review of Connective Tissue Research (0074-767X)

Indexed: Biol.Abstr., Dent.Ind., Excerp.Med., INIS Atomind., Ind.Med. (coverage dropped), Ind.Sci.Rev., Nutr.Abstr., Sci.Cit.Ind. (coverage dropped).

—CASDDS, CISTI, GNLM, KNAW, Linda Hall. **CCC.**

Published by: Academic Press, Inc., Journal Division (Subsidiary of: Harcourt Brace & Company), 525 B St, Ste 1900, San Diego, CA 92101-4495. TEL 619-231-0926, FAX 619-699-6715.

571.6 FRA ISSN 0248-4900
QH212.E4 CODEN: BCELDF

BIOLOGY OF THE CELL. Text in English. 1962. 9/yr. EUR 663 in Europe to institutions; JPY 87,900 in Japan to institutions; USD 741 elsewhere to institutions (effective 2002). adv. charts, illus. index. *Refereed.* **Document type:** *Academic/Scholarly.* **Description:** Presents reports, review articles and rapid communications concerning the structure and function of cells in the context of developmental biology, genetics, immunology and physiology.

Former titles (until 1981): Biologie Cellulaire; Journal de Microscopie et Biologie Cellulaire; Journal de Microscopie

Related titles: Microform ed.: (from PQC); Online - full text ed.: (from ingenta, Swets Blackwell, ScienceDirect, Institute for Scientific Information).

Indexed: ASCA, Anim.Breed.Abstr., Aqua.Sci.& Fish.Abstr., BBCI, Biol.Abstr., Chem.Abstr., Chem.Indus.Notes, Chem.Titles, Crop Physiol.Abstr., Curr.Adv.Ecol.Sci., Curr.Cont., Dairy Sci.Abstr., Dent.Ind., Excerp.Med., Field Crop Abstr., Helminthol.Abstr., Herb.Abstr., Hort.Abstr., INIS Atomind., Ind.Med. (1981-), Ind.Sci.Rev., Ind.Vet., Inpharma, Int.Abstr.Biol.Sci., Nuc.Acids Abstr., Plant Breed.Abstr., Plant Grow.Reg.Abstr., Protozool.Abstr., Reac., Rev.Appl.Entomol., Rev.Med.& Vet.Mycol., Sci.Cit.Ind., Sport Fish.Abstr., Triticale Abstr., Zoo.Rec.

—BLDSC (2087.045000), CASDDS, CISTI, EMDOCS, GNLM, IDS, ingenta, Linda Hall. **CCC.**

Published by: (European Cell Biology Organization DEU, Universite Paris, Institute Jacques-Monod), Elsevier Paris, Editions Scientifiques et Medicales (Subsidiary of: Reed Elsevier plc. group), 23 rue Linois, Paris 75015, France. redacion-emc@elsevier.fr, http://www.elsevier.com/locate/bicell. Eds. B Maro, M Fukuda. Circ: 3,000. **Co-sponsors:** Societe Francaise de Microscopie Electronique; Societe de Biologie Cellulaire de France.

571.64 USA ISSN 0067-8864
QH601 CODEN: BOMBB5

BIOMEMBRANES. Text in English. 1971. irreg., latest vol.12, 1984. price varies. *Refereed.* **Document type:** *Monographic series.*

Indexed: Chem.Abstr., INIS Atomind., Ind.Med. (coverage dropped).

—CASDDS, CISTI, GNLM, Infotrieve, Linda Hall. **CCC.**

Published by: Kluwer Academic - Plenum Publishers (Subsidiary of: Wolters Kluwer N.V.), 233 Spring St, New York, NY 10013-1578. TEL 212-620-8000, 800-221-9369, FAX 212-463-0742, info@plenum.com, http://www.plenum.com. Ed. L A Manson.

571.6 USA ISSN 0144-8463
QH506 CODEN: BRPTDT

BIOSCIENCE REPORTS; molecular and cellular biology of the cell surface. Text in English. 1981. bi-m. EUR 691, USD 692 to institutions for print or online ed.; EUR 829.20, USD 830.40 to institutions for print & online eds. combined (effective 2002). adv. back issues avail. *Refereed.* **Document type:** *Academic/Scholarly.* **Description:** Publishes research papers in all areas of cell surface function, including biochemical genetics, development, pharmacology, endocrinology, and immunology.

Related titles: Microfilm ed.: (from PQC); Online - full text ed.: (from EBSCO Publishing, O C L C Online Computer Library Center, Inc., Swets Blackwell, Kluwer Online, Institute for Scientific Information, RoweCom Information Quest).

Indexed: ASCA, Agri.& Environ.Biotech.Abstr. (coverage dropped), Agricola, BBCI, Biol.Abstr., CEABA, Cal.Tiss.Abstr. (coverage dropped), Chem.Abstr., Chem.Indus.Notes, Chem.Titles, Crop Physiol.Abstr., Curr.Adv.Ecol.Sci., Curr.Biotech.Abstr., Curr.Cont., Dairy Sci.Abstr., Derwent Biotech.Abstr., Excerp.Med., Field Crop Abstr., INIS Atomind., Ind.Med. (1981-), Ind.Sci.Rev., Inpharma, Int.Abstr.Biol.Sci., Maize Abstr., Nutr.Abstr., Pharm.&Out.News, Plant Breed.Abstr., Poult.Abstr., Protozool.Abstr., Reac., Ref.Zh., Rev.Appl.Entomol., Sci.Cit.Ind., Soils & Fert., Sugar Ind.Abstr., Tox.Abstr. (coverage dropped), Trop.Dis.Bull., Weed Abstr.

—BLDSC (2089.611600), ADONIS, CASDDS, CISTI, EMDOCS, GNLM, IDS, ingenta, Linda Hall. **CCC.**

Published by: (Biochemical Society GBR), Kluwer Academic - Plenum Publishers (Subsidiary of: Wolters Kluwer N.V.), 233 Spring St, New York, NY 10013-1578. TEL 212-620-8000, 800-221-9369, FAX 212-463-0742, info@plenum.com, http://www.wkap.nl/jrnltoc.htm/0144-8463. Ed. Charles A Pasternak. R&P Rose Luongo TEL 781-871-6311. **Subscr outside N America to:** Kluwer Academic Publishers Group, Journals Department, PO Box 322, Dordrecht 3300 AH, Netherlands. TEL 31-78-639-2392, FAX 31-78-654-6474.

BIOTECHNIC AND HISTOCHEMISTRY; a journal for microtechnic and histochemistry. see *BIOLOGY—Microscopy*

BLOOD. see *MEDICAL SCIENCES—Hematology*

571.6 GBR

BRITISH SOCIETY FOR CELL BIOLOGY. SYMPOSIA. Text in English. 1976. irreg. price varies. **Document type:** *Proceedings.*

Indexed: Biol.Abstr.

Published by: Cambridge University Press, Edinburgh Bldg, Shaftesbury Rd, Cambridge CB2 2RU, United Kingdom. FAX 44-1223-315052, information@cup.cam.ac.uk, information@cambridge.org, http://www.cup.cam.ac.uk, http://www.uk.cambridge.org/journals/pmu. R&P Linda Nicol.

C A S BIOTECH UPDATES. CELL & TISSUE CULTURE. see *BIOLOGY—Abstracting, Bibliographies, Statistics*

CALCIUM AND CALCIFIED TISSUE ABSTRACTS. see *BIOLOGY—Abstracting, Bibliographies, Statistics*

CANADIAN JOURNAL OF PLANT PATHOLOGY. see *BIOLOGY—Botany*

571.3 ITA ISSN 0008-7114
QH1 CODEN: CARYAB

CARYOLOGIA; international journal of cytology, cytosystematics and cytogenetics. Text and summaries in English. 1948. 4/yr. ITL 170,000 (effective 1995). bibl, charts, illus. *Refereed.*

Related titles: Online - full text ed.: (from Institute for Scientific Information).

Indexed: ASCA, AgBiotech, Anim.Breed.Abstr., Aqua.Sci.& Fish.Abstr., Aquacult.Abstr., Biol.Abstr., Chem.Abstr., Curr.Adv.Ecol.Sci., Curr.Cont., Environ.Sci.Poll.Mgmt., Excerp.Med., Forest.Abstr., Herb.Abstr., Hort.Abstr., INIS Atomind., Ind.Sci.Rev., Ornam.Hort., Plant Breed.Abstr., Plant Gen.Res.Abstr., Ref.Zh., Rev.Appl.Entomol., Rev.Plant Path., Sci.Cit.Ind., Seed Abstr., Soils & Fert., Sport Fish.Abstr., Triticale Abstr., Zoo.Rec.

—BLDSC (3057.960000), CASDDS, CISTI, ingenta, Linda Hall.

Published by: Universita degli Studi di Firenze, Orto Botanico, Via Pier Antonio Micheli, 3, Florence, FI 50121, Italy. TEL 39-55-284696, FAX 39-55-2757438. Ed. Fernando Fabbri.

571.6 USA ISSN 0092-8674
QH573 CODEN: CELLB5

CELL. Text in English. 1974. bi-w. USD 115 domestic to individuals; USD 200 in Canada to individuals; USD 230 elsewhere to individuals; USD 755 domestic to institutions; USD 800 in Canada to institutions; USD 843 elsewhere to institutions; USD 30 newsstand/cover (effective 2001); Individual price includes online access. adv. bk.rev. charts, illus. Index. back issues avail.; reprint service avail. from PQC,ISI. *Refereed.* **Document type:** *Academic/Scholarly.* **Description:** Publishes research and reports on developments in molecular biology.

Related titles: Online - full text ed.: USD 99 to individuals (effective 2001) (from HighWire Pr., ingenta, Gale Group, Institute for Scientific Information).

Indexed: AIDS & Cancer Res., AIDS Abstr., ASCA, Abstr.Bull.Inst.Pap.Chem., Abstr.Hyg., AgBiotech, Agri.& Environ.Biotech.Abstr., Anim.Breed.Abstr., Aqua.Sci.& Fish.Abstr., BBCI, Biol.& Agr.Ind. (1989-), Biol.Abstr., Cal.Tiss.Abstr. (coverage dropped), Chem.Abstr., Chemorec.Abstr., Curr.Adv.Biochem., Curr.Adv.Cell & Devel.Biol., Curr.Adv.Ecol.Sci., Curr.Adv.Gen.& Molec.Biol., Curr.Cont., Dairy Sci.Abstr., Dent.Ind., Derwent Biotech.Abstr., Eng.Ind., Entomol.Abstr. (coverage dropped), Environ.Sci.Poll.Mgmt., Excerp.Med., Food Sci.& Tech.Abstr., Gen.Sci.Ind. (Jun.1992-), Genet.Abstr., Helminthol.Abstr., Hort.Abstr., Hum.Gen.Abstr., INIS Atomind., Immun.Abstr., Ind.Med. (1974-), Ind.Sci.Rev., Ind.Vet., Inpharma, Int.Abstr.Biol.Sci., Jrnl.Watch Psych., Med.& Pharm.Biotech.Abstr., Med.& Surg.Dermat., Microbiol.Abstr., Neurosci.Abstr., Neurosci.Cit.Ind., Nuc.Acids Abstr., Nutr.Abstr., Oncog.G.F.Abstr., Ornam.Hort., Pharm.&Out.News, Plant Breed.Abstr., Plant Grow.Reg.Abstr., Poult.Abstr., Protozool.Abstr., Reac., Ref.Zh., Rev.Appl.Entomol., Rev.Med.& Vet.Mycol., Rev.Plant Path., SSCI (coverage dropped), Sci.Cit.Ind., Soils & Fert., Sorghum & Millets Abstr., Telegen, Tox.Abstr. (coverage dropped), Triticale Abstr., Trop.Dis.Bull., Vet.Bull., Virol.Abstr. (coverage dropped), Weed Abstr., Zoo.Rec.

—BLDSC (3097.600000), ADONIS, CASDDS, CISTI, EMDOCS, GNLM, ingenta, Linda Hall.

Published by: Cell Press (Subsidiary of: Reed Elsevier plc), 1100 Massachusetts Ave, Cambridge, MA 02138. TEL 617-661-7057, FAX 617-661-7061, editor@cell.com, http://www.cell.com, http://www.cellpress.com. Ed. Vivian Siegel. Pub. Lynne Herndon. Circ: 15,500.

571.6 USA ISSN 0737-1233

CELL ANALYSIS. Text in English. 1982. irreg. **Document type:** *Monographic series.*

—CISTI.

Published by: Kluwer Academic - Plenum Publishers (Subsidiary of: Wolters Kluwer N.V.), 233 Spring St, New York, NY 10013-1578. TEL 212-620-8000, 800-221-9369, FAX 212-463-0742, info@plenum.com, http://www.plenum.com.

571.6 IND ISSN 0254-2935
CODEN: CCREE3

CELL AND CHROMOSOME RESEARCH JOURNAL. Text in English. 1978. 2/yr. INR 150, USD 20. bk.rev. back issues avail. *Refereed.* **Document type:** *Academic/Scholarly.*

Formerly (until 1981): Cell and Chromosome Research Association. Newsletter

Indexed: Biol.Abstr., Chem.Abstr., Chem.Indus.Notes, Chem.Titles.

—CASDDS, CISTI.

Published by: (Association for Cell and Chromosome Research), University of Calcutta, Centre of Advanced Studies in Botany, 35 Ballygunge Circular Rd., Kolkata, West Bengal 700 019, India. FAX 91-33-4754772. Ed. Sibdas Ghosh. Circ: 200.

571.5 NLD ISSN 1389-9333

▼ **CELL AND TISSUE BANKING.** Text in English. 2000. q. USD 63 in the Americas to individuals for print or online ed.; EUR 63 elsewhere to individuals for print or online ed.; USD 165 in the Americas to institutions for print or online ed.; EUR 165 elsewhere to institutions for print or online ed.; USD 198 in the Americas to institutions for print & online eds.; EUR 198 elsewhere to institutions for print & online eds. (effective 2002). *Refereed.* **Document type:** *Journal.* **Description:** Provides information to scientists and clinicians involved in the banking and transplantation of cells and tissues.

Related titles: Online - full text ed.: (from Swets Blackwell, Kluwer Online, RoweCom Information Quest).

Indexed: Biotech.& Bioeng.Abstr., Cal.Tiss.Abstr., Med.& Pharm.Biotech.Abstr.

—BLDSC (3097.678000).

Published by: Kluwer Academic Publishers Group (Subsidiary of: Wolters Kluwer N.V.), Spuiboulevard 50, PO Box 17, Dordrecht 3300 AA, Netherlands. TEL 31-78-639-2392, FAX 31-78-654-2254, services@wkap.nl, http://www.wkap.nl/journalhome.htm/1389-9333. Ed. Rudiger von Versen. **Subscr. in N America to:** Kluwer Academic - Plenum Publishers, 233 Spring St, New York, NY 10013-1578. TEL 212-620-8468, FAX 212-807-1047; **Subscr. to:** Journals Department, PO Box 322, Dordrecht 3300 AH, Netherlands. TEL 31-78-639-2392, FAX 31-78-654-6474.

571.6 DEU ISSN 0302-766X
QH301 CODEN: CTSRCS
CELL AND TISSUE RESEARCH. Text in English. m. EUR 4,245 domestic; EUR 4,206.40 in Germany; EUR 417 newsstand/cover foreign (effective 2002). adv. reprint service avail. from ISI. *Refereed.* **Document type:** *Academic/Scholarly.* **Description:** Presents significant advances encompassing the broad field of cell biology and microscopical anatomy, ranging from invertebrates to mammals, including humans.
Continues: Zeitschrift fuer Zellforschung und Mikroskopische Anatomie (0044-3794)
Related titles: Microform ed.: (from PQC); Online - full text ed.: ISSN 1432-0878 (from EBSCO Publishing, RoweCom Information Quest, Swets Blackwell, Springer LINK, Institute for Scientific Information).
Indexed: ASCA, AgBiotech, Anim.Breed.Abstr., Apic.Abstr., Aqua.Sci.& Fish.Abstr., Aquacult.Abstr., BBCI, Bio-Contr.News & Info., Biol.Abstr., Chem.Abstr., Chem.Indus.Notes, Chem.Titles, Curr.Adv.Biochem., Curr.Adv.Cell & Devel.Biol., Curr.Adv.Ecol.Sci., Curr.Cont., Dairy Sci.Abstr., Dent.Ind., Excerp.Med., Helminthol.Abstr., INIS Atomind., Ind.Med. (1974-), Ind.Sci.Rev., Ind.Vet., Inpharma, Int.Abstr.Biol.Sci., Neurosci.Cit.Ind., Nutr.Abstr., Pharm.&Out.News, Pig News & Info., Poult.Abstr., Reac., Ref.Zh., Rev.Appl.Entomol., Rev.Med.& Vet.Mycol., Sci.Cit.Ind., Soils & Fert., Sport Fish.Abstr., Vet.Bull., Wild.Rev., Zoo.Rec.
—BLDSC (3097.700000), ADONIS, CASDDS, CISTI, EMDOCS, GNLM, IDS, Infotrieve, ingenta, KNAW, Linda Hall. **CCC.**
Published by: Springer-Verlag (Subsidiary of: BertelsmannSpringer), Tiergartenstr 17, Heidelberg 69121, Germany. TEL 49-6221-345-0, FAX 49-6221-345229, subscriptions@springer.de, http://link.springer.de/link/service/journals/00441/index.htm, http://www.springer.de. Ed. K Unsicker. **Subscr. in N. America to:** Springer-Verlag New York Inc., PO Box 2485, Secaucus, NJ 07096-2485. TEL 212-460-1500, FAX 212-473-6272.

571.6 USA ISSN 1085-9195
QH573 CODEN: CBBIFV
CELL BIOCHEMISTRY AND BIOPHYSICS. Text in English. 1979. bi-m. USD 360 domestic; USD 400 foreign (effective 2000). adv. bk.rev. bibl, charts, illus. *Refereed.* **Document type:** *Journal, Academic/Scholarly.* **Description:** Publishes original papers covering experimental, methodological and theoretical investigations on cells, tissues, organelles and subfragments with emphasis on the mechanisms of cell behavior.
Formerly: Cell Biophysics (0163-4992)
Related titles: Online - full text ed.: (from Institute for Scientific Information).
Indexed: ASCA, Agri.& Environ.Biotech.Abstr. (coverage dropped), BBCI, Biol.Abstr., Chem.Abstr., Chem.Indus.Notes, Chem.Titles, Curr.Adv.Ecol.Sci., Curr.Cont. (coverage dropped), Derwent Biotech.Abstr., Excerp.Med., Ind.Med. (1996-), Ind.Sci.Rev., Sci.Cit.Ind. (coverage dropped).
—BLDSC (3097.701000), CASDDS, CISTI, GNLM, IDS, Infotrieve, ingenta, Linda Hall. **CCC.**
Published by: Humana Press Inc., 999 Riverview Dr, Ste 208, Totowa, NJ 07512. TEL 973-256-1699, FAX 973-256-8341, humana@humanapr.com, http://humanapress.com. Ed. Edward Massaro. R&P Richard Hruska. Adv. contact Thomas B Lanigan Jr. **Dist. in Japan by:** Maruzen Co., Ltd., International Division, Export Dept, P.O. Box 5050, Tokyo International 100-3191, Japan. TEL 81-3-3275-8591.

CELL BIOCHEMISTRY AND FUNCTION. see *BIOLOGY—Biochemistry*

CELL BIOLOGY AND TOXICOLOGY; an international journal devoted to research at the cellular level. see *ENVIRONMENTAL STUDIES—Toxicology And Environmental Safety*

571.6 USA ISSN 0172-4665
CODEN: CBMODY
CELL BIOLOGY MONOGRAPHS. Text in English. 1977. irreg., latest vol.12, 1985. price varies. reprint service avail. from ISI. **Document type:** *Monographic series.*
Supersedes: Protoplasmologia: Handbuch der Protoplasmaforschung (0079-7073)
Indexed: Biol.Abstr.
—CISTI.
Published by: Springer-Verlag, Journals (Subsidiary of: BertelsmannSpringer), 175 Fifth Ave, New York, NY 10010. TEL 212-460-1500, FAX 212-473-6272.

571.6 GBR ISSN 0143-4160
CODEN: CECADV
CELL CALCIUM (EDINBURGH). Text in English. 1980. m. GBP 706 to individuals (effective 2002). adv. bibl. *Refereed.* **Document type:** *Journal, Academic/Scholarly.* **Description:** Covers all fields of calcium metabolism and signalling in living systems, including all aspects of calcium in biological systems from inorganic chemistry to physiology, molecular biology and pathology.
Related titles: Microform ed.: (from PQC); Online - full text ed.: (from EBSCO Publishing, RoweCom Information Quest, Swets Blackwell, IDEAL Online Library, Institute for Scientific Information).
Indexed: AgBiotech, Anim.Breed.Abstr., Aqua.Sci.& Fish.Abstr., BBCI, Cal.Tiss.Abstr., Chem.Abstr., Chem.Indus.Notes, Chem.Titles, Curr.Adv.Biochem., Curr.Adv.Ecol.Sci., Curr.Cont., Dent.Ind., Excerp.Med., Ind.Med. (1980-), Ind.Sci.Rev., Int.Abstr.Biol.Sci., Plant Breed.Abstr., Sci.Cit.Ind., Tox.Abstr. (coverage dropped), Vet.Bull.
—BLDSC (3097.724000), CASDDS, CISTI, EMDOCS, GNLM, IDS, ingenta, KNAW. **CCC.**
Published by: Churchill Livingstone (Subsidiary of: Harcourt Publishers Ltd.), Robert Stevenson House, 1-3 Baxter's Pl, Leith Walk, Edinburgh, Midlothian EH1 3AF, United Kingdom. TEL 44-131-556-2424, FAX 44-131-459-1177, cservice@harcourt.com, http://www.harcourt-international.com/journals/ceca. Eds. Dr. A Scarpa, Dr. Alex Verkhratsky. Pub. Gillian Griffith. R&P Catherine John TEL 212-424-4200. Adv. contact Kathy Crawford. Circ: 495. **Subscr. to:** Harcourt Publishers Ltd., Foots Cray High St, Sidcup, Kent DA14 5HP, United Kingdom. TEL 44-20-8308-5700, FAX 44-20-8309-0807.

571.6 GBR ISSN 1350-9047
CODEN: CDDIEK
CELL DEATH AND DIFFERENTIATION. Text in English. 1994. m. GBP 145 in Europe to individuals print or online ed.; USD 218 elsewhere to individuals print or online ed.; GBP 160 combined subscription in Europe to individuals print & online; USD 240 combined subscription elsewhere to individuals print & online; GBP 495 in Europe to institutions print or online ed.; USD 698 elsewhere to institutions print or online ed.; GBP 512 combined subscription in Europe to institutions print & online; USD 768 combined subscription elsewhere to individuals print & online (effective 2002). adv. bk.rev. charts, illus, stat. back issues avail. *Refereed.* **Document type:** *Journal, Academic/Scholarly.* **Description:** Aims to provide a forum for high-quality papers on cell death, proliferation, differentiation, and development in various eukaryotic models.
Related titles: Online - full text ed.: (from EBSCO Publishing, O C L C Online Computer Library Center, Inc., RoweCom Information Quest, ingenta, Swets Blackwell, Institute for Scientific Information).
Indexed: ASCA, BBCI, Chem.Abstr., Chem.Indus.Notes, Chem.Titles, Curr.Cont., Entomol.Abstr., Excerp.Med (1996-), Immun.Abstr., Ind.Med. (1994-), Inpharma, Int.Abstr.Biol.Sci., Oncog.G.F.Abstr., Pharm.&Out.News, Reac., Rev.Med.& Vet.Mycol., Sci.Cit.Ind.
—BLDSC (3097.748600), CASDDS, CISTI, EMDOCS, GNLM, IDS, Infotrieve, KNAW. **CCC.**
Published by: Nature Publishing Group Specialist Journals (Subsidiary of: Holtzbrink Publishers), Houndmills, Basingstoke, Hants RG21 6XS, United Kingdom. TEL 44-1256-329242, FAX 44-1256-328339, subscriptions@nature.com, http://www.nature.com/cdd. Ed. Gerry Melino. Pub. Sue Deeley. R&P Trace Noel. Adv. contact Robert Sloan TEL 44-20-8882-7199. B&W page GBP 595, color page GBP 1,090; trim 210 x 280. Circ: 600.

CELL DIFFERENTIATION. see *BIOLOGY—Abstracting, Bibliographies, Statistics*

CELL MEMBRANES. see *BIOLOGY—Abstracting, Bibliographies, Statistics*

571.6 USA ISSN 0886-1544
QH647 CODEN: CMCYEO
CELL MOTILITY AND THE CYTOSKELETON. Text in English. 1980. m. USD 3,225 in United States; USD 3,345 in Canada & Mexico; USD 3,447 elsewhere; USD 3,387 combined subscription in United States for print and online eds.; USD 3,507 combined subscription in Canada & Mexico for print and online eds.; USD 3,609 combined subscription elsewhere for print and online eds. (effective 2002). adv. bibl, charts, illus. index. back issues avail. *Refereed.* **Document type:** *Academic/Scholarly.* **Description:** Specializes in the rapid publication of articles concerning all phenomena related to cell motility, including structural, biochemical, biophysical, and theoretical approaches.
Formerly: Cell Motility (0271-6585)
Related titles: Microform ed.: (from PQC); Online - full text ed.: ISSN 1097-0169. 1998. USD 3,225 in United States; USD 3,225 in Canada & Mexico; USD 3,225 elsewhere (effective 2002) (from EBSCO Publishing, Wiley InterScience, Institute for Scientific Information).
Indexed: ASCA, Anim.Breed.Abstr., BBCI, Biol.Abstr., Chem.Abstr., Chem.Indus.Notes, Chem.Titles, Curr.Adv.Cell & Devel.Biol., Curr.Adv.Ecol.Sci., Curr.Cont., Eng.Ind., Excerp.Med., Helminthol.Abstr., Ind.Med. (1986-), Ind.Sci.Rev., Inpharma, Int.Abstr.Biol.Sci., Neurosci.Cit.Ind., Pharm.&Out.News, Protozool.Abstr., Reac., Sci.Cit.Ind., Zoo.Rec.
—BLDSC (3097.826000), CASDDS, CISTI, Ei, EMDOCS, GNLM, IDS, ingenta, Linda Hall. **CCC.**
Published by: John Wiley & Sons, Inc., Journals (Subsidiary of: Wiley InterScience), 605 Third Ave, New York, NY 10158. TEL 212-850-6645, FAX 212-850-6021, subinfo@jwiley.com, uscs-wis@wiley.com, http://www.interscience.wiley.com/jpages/0886-1544/, http://www.wiley.com. Ed. B R Brinkley. adv.: B&W page GBP 640, color page GBP 1,515; trim 210 x 279. Circ: 700. **Subscr. outside the Americas to:** John Wiley & Sons Ltd., Baffins Ln, Chichester, Sussex PO19 IUD, United Kingdom. TEL 44-1243-779777, FAX 44-1243-843232, cs-journals@wiley.co.uk, http://www.wiley.co.uk.

571.6 GBR ISSN 0960-7722
QH631 CODEN: CPROEM
CELL PROLIFERATION. Text in English. 1968. bi-m., latest vol.35, 2002. GBP 96 in Europe to individuals; USD 157 in North America to individuals; GBP 109 elsewhere to individuals; GBP 375 in Europe to institutions; USD 594 in North America to institutions; GBP 412.50 elsewhere to institutions (effective 2002). adv. bk.rev. charts, illus. index. back issues avail.; reprint service avail. from ISI. *Refereed.* **Document type:** *Academic/Scholarly.* **Description:** Devoted to studies into all aspects of cell proliferation and differentiation in normal and abnormal states.
Formerly: Cell and Tissue Kinetics (0008-8730)
Related titles: Microform ed.: (from PQC); Online - full text ed.: ISSN 1365-2184. 1997. GBP 87 in Europe to individuals; USD 142 in North America to individuals; GBP 87 elsewhere to individuals; GBP 338 in Europe to institutions; USD 535 in North America to institutions; GBP 338 elsewhere to institutions (effective 2002) (from EBSCO Publishing, O C L C Online Computer Library Center, Inc., RoweCom Information Quest, ingenta, Munksgaard & Blackwell Science's Synergy, Swets Blackwell, Institute for Scientific Information).
Indexed: ASCA, Anim.Breed.Abstr., Biol.Abstr., Chem.Abstr., Chem.Indus.Notes, Chem.Titles, Curr.Adv.Ecol.Sci., Curr.Cont., Curr.Ind.Stat., Dairy Sci.Abstr., Dent.Ind., Excerp.Med., Helminthol.Abstr., INIS Atomind., Ind.Med. (1991-), Ind.Sci.Rev., Ind.Vet., Inpharma, Int.Abstr.Biol.Sci., Pharm.&Out.News, Reac., Ref.Zh., Sci.Cit.Ind., Vet.Bull.
—BLDSC (3097.854000), ADONIS, CASDDS, CISTI, EMDOCS, GNLM, IDS, ingenta, Linda Hall. **CCC.**
Published by: (Cell Kinetics Society), Blackwell Science Ltd., PO Box 88, Oxford OX2 0NE, United Kingdom. TEL 44-1865-206180, 44-1865-206002, FAX 44-1865-206219, jnl.orders@blacksci.co.uk, http://www.blackwell-science.com/products/journals/cpro.htm, http://www.blackwellpublishing.com. Ed. C S Potten. Pub. Elizabeth Whelan. R&P Sophie Savage. Adv. contact Jenny Applin. Circ: 465. **Co-sponsors:** European Study Group for Cell Proliferation; International Cell Cycle Society.

571.6 JPN ISSN 0915-907X
CODEN: CELSET
CELL SCIENCE. Text in English, Japanese. 1985. m. JPY 16,800.
—CASDDS.
Published by: Igaku Shuppan Senta/Medical Publication Center Inc., 25-2 Asakusa-Bashi 1-chome, Taito-ku, Tokyo 111-0053, Japan.

B

571.6 JPN ISSN 0386-7196
QH573 CODEN: CSFUDY
CELL STRUCTURE AND FUNCTION. Text in English. 1975. bi-m. USD 136 (effective 1998 & 1999). bk.rev. *Refereed.* **Document type:** *Academic/Scholarly.*
Related titles: Online - full text ed.: (from Institute for Scientific Information).
Indexed: ASCA, AgBiotech, BBCI, Biol.Abstr., Chem.Abstr., Chem.Indus.Notes, Chem.Titles, Curr.Adv.Biochem., Curr.Adv.Ecol.Sci., Curr.Cont., Excerp.Med., Helminthol.Abstr., INIS Atomind., INSPEC (coverage dropped), Ind.Med. (1975-), Ind.Sci.Rev., Ind.Vet., Inpharma, Int.Abstr.Biol.Sci., Pharm.&Out.News, Plant Breed.Abstr., Protozool.Abstr., Reac., Sci.Cit.Ind., Vet.Bull., Zoo.Rec.
—BLDSC (3097.870000), CASDDS, CISTI, EMDOCS, GNLM, IDS, ingenta, KNAW, Linda Hall. **CCC.**
Published by: Japan Society for Cell Biology/Nihon Saibo Seibutsu Gakkai, Shimodachuri Ogawa Higashi, Kamigyo-ku, Kyoto-shi 602-8048, Japan. TEL 81-75-415-3661, FAX 81-75-415-3662. Ed. Dr. N Hirokawa. Circ: 1,600.

571.6 USA ISSN 0963-6897
QP89 CODEN: CTRAE8
CELL TRANSPLANTATION. Text in English. 1992. 8/yr. USD 775 domestic; USD 825 foreign (effective 2001). index. back issues avail. *Refereed.* **Document type:** *Academic/Scholarly.* **Description:** Deals with a wide range of topics including physiological, medical, preclinical, tissue engineering, and device-oriented aspects of transplantation of nervous system, endocrine, growth factor-secreting, bone marrow, epithelial, endothelial, and genetically engineered cells.
Related titles: Microfilm ed.: (from PQC); Online - full text ed.: (from ingenta, ScienceDirect, Institute for Scientific Information).
Indexed: ASCA, Curr.Cont., Excerp.Med. (1993-), Ind.Med. (1992-), Ind.Sci.Rev., Inpharma, Int.Abstr.Biol.Sci., Neurosci.Cit.Ind., Pharm.&Out.News, Reac., Sci.Cit.Ind.
—BLDSC (3097.877000), CISTI, EMDOCS, GNLM, IDS, KNAW. **CCC.**
Published by: Cognizant Communication Corporation, 3 Hartsdale Rd, Elmsford, NY 10523-3701. TEL 914-592-7720, FAX 914-592-8981, cogcomm@aol.com, http://www.cognizantcommunication.com. Ed. Dr. Paul Sanberg.

571.6 USA ISSN 1060-9989
CODEN: CMSUEO
CELLS AND MATERIALS SUPPLEMENT. Text in English. 1991. irreg. price varies. **Document type:** *Monographic series.*
Indexed: Chem.Abstr., Chem.Indus.Notes, Chem.Titles.
—CASDDS, KNAW. **CCC.**
Published by: Scanning Microscopy International, Inc., AMF O Hare, PO Box 66507, Chicago, IL 60666-0507. TEL 708-529-6677, FAX 708-980-6698.

CELLS, TISSUES, ORGANS; in vivo, in vitro. see *MEDICAL SCIENCES*

CELLULAR IMMUNOLOGY. see *MEDICAL SCIENCES—Allergology And Immunology*

571.6 USA ISSN 0892-0346
QP351 CODEN: ADCND7
CELLULAR NEUROBIOLOGY. Text in English. 1980. irreg. back issues avail.; reprint service avail. from ISI. *Refereed.*
Formerly (until 1984): Advances in Cellular Neurobiology (0270-0794)
Indexed: Biol.Abstr., Chem.Abstr., e-psyche.
—CASDDS, CISTI, GNLM. **CCC.**
Published by: Academic Press, Inc., Journal Division (Subsidiary of: Harcourt Brace & Company), 525 B St, Ste 1900, San Diego, CA 92101-4495. TEL 619-231-0926, FAX 619-699-6715. Ed. Sergey Federoff. **Subscr. to:** Order Dept., 6277 Sea Harbor Dr, 4th Fl, Orlando, FL 32887. TEL 800-321-5068.

571.6 DEU ISSN 1015-8987
CODEN: CEPBEW
CELLULAR PHYSIOLOGY AND BIOCHEMISTRY; international journal of experimental cellular physiology, biochemistry and pharmacology. Text in English. 1991-1999; resumed 2000. bi-m. CHF 824 in Europe to institutions; CHF 841.40 overseas to institutions; EUR 588.80 in Europe to institutions; USD 642 overseas to institutions (effective 2002). adv. back issues avail. *Refereed.* **Document type:** *Journal, Academic/Scholarly.* **Description:** Covers mechanisms of intracellular transmission; cellular pharmacology; maintenance, regulation, and disturbance of cell volume; regulation of cell growth and differentiation; control of cellular metabolism; and molecular biology and function of ion carriers.
Related titles: Online - full text ed.: ISSN 1421-9778. CHF 58, EUR 42, USD 45 to institutions with print edition (effective 2002) (from EBSCO Publishing, RoweCom Information Quest, Swets Blackwell, Institute for Scientific Information).
Indexed: ASCA, BBCI, Chem.Abstr., Chem.Indus.Notes, Chem.Titles, Curr.Cont., Excerp.Med. (1993-), Ind.Med. (1991-), Inpharma, Int.Abstr.Biol.Sci., Reac.
—BLDSC (3097.934000), CASDDS, CISTI, EMDOCS, GNLM, IDS, Infotrieve, ingenta, KNAW, Linda Hall. **CCC.**
Address: c/o Dr Florian Lang, Gmelinstr 5, Tuebingen 72078, Germany. TEL 49-7071-2972194, FAX 49-7071-293073, http://www.online.karger.com/journals/cpb. Ed., Pub. Dr. Florian Lang. adv.: page USD 1,195. **Subscr. to:** S. Karger AG, Allschwilerstr 10, PO Box, Basel 4009, Switzerland.

571.6 USA ISSN 0898-6568
QH604.2 CODEN: CESIEY
CELLULAR SIGNALLING. Text in English. 1989. 12/yr. EUR 191 in Europe to individuals; JPY 25,300 in Japan to individuals; USD 213 elsewhere to individuals; EUR 1,233 in Europe to institutions; JPY 163,700 in Japan to institutions; USD 1,379 elsewhere to institutions (effective 2002). back issues avail. *Refereed.* **Document type:** *Academic/Scholarly.* **Description:** Publishes original papers on all aspects of the mechanisms, actions and structural components of cellular signalling systems, with emphasis on the production, regulation and action of second messengers, receptors, regulatory proteins, effector systems, and the effect of cellular signalling events.
Related titles: Microfilm ed.: (from PQC); Online - full text ed.: (from ingenta, Swets Blackwell, ScienceDirect, Institute for Scientific Information).
Indexed: ASCA, Aqua.Sci.& Fish.Abstr., BBCI, Cal.Tiss.Abstr., Chem.Abstr., Chem.Indus.Notes, Chem.Titles, Curr.Cont., Excerp.Med., Ind.Med. (1989-), Ind.Sci.Rev., Inpharma, Int.Abstr.Biol.Sci., Neurosci.Abstr. (coverage dropped), Neurosci.Cit.Ind., Protozool.Abstr., Reac., Sci.Cit.Ind., Tox.Abstr. (coverage dropped).
—BLDSC (3097.942000), ADONIS, CASDDS, CISTI, EMDOCS, GNLM, IDS, ingenta, KNAW, Linda Hall. **CCC.**
Published by: Elsevier Science, PO Box 945, New York, NY 10159-0945. TEL 212-989-5800, FAX 212-633-3990, usinfo-f@elsevier.com, http://www.elsevier.nl/locate/cellsig, http://www.elsevier.com. Ed. Miles D Houslay. **Subscr. in Australasia and the Far East to:** Elsevier Science (Singapore) Pte Ltd, No.1 Temasek Ave, 17-01 Millenia Tower, Singapore 039192, Singapore. TEL 65-434-3727, FAX 65-337-2230; **Subscr. in Japan to:** Elsevier Science Inc - Japan Regional Office, 9-15 Higashi-Azabu 1-chome, Minato-ku, Tokyo 106-0044, Japan. TEL 81-3-5561-5033, FAX 81-3-5561-5047; **Subscr. outside the Americas to:** Elsevier Science BV, PO Box 211, Amsterdam 1000 AE, Netherlands. TEL 31-20-485-3757, FAX 31-20-485-3432, nlinfo-f@elsevier.nl, http://www.elsevier.nl.

CHLOROPLASTS. see *BIOLOGY—Abstracting, Bibliographies, Statistics*

CLINICAL CYTOGENETICS. see *BIOLOGY—Abstracting, Bibliographies, Statistics*

571.5 CHE ISSN 0300-8207
QP88.23 CODEN: CVTRBC
CONNECTIVE TISSUE RESEARCH; an international journal. Text in English. 1972. 6/yr. GBP 259, USD 345, EUR 345 to individuals; GBP 1,166, USD 1,505, EUR 1,526 to institutions; GBP 2,577, USD 3,340, EUR 3,359 to corporations (effective 2002). adv. bk.rev. charts, illus. index. *Refereed.* **Document type:** *Journal, Academic/Scholarly.*
Related titles: Online - full text ed.: (from EBSCO Publishing, ingenta, Institute for Scientific Information, RoweCom Information Quest).
Indexed: ASCA, Aqua.Sci.& Fish.Abstr., BBCI, Biol.Abstr., Cal.Tiss.Abstr., Chem.Abstr., Curr.Adv.Ecol.Sci., Curr.Cont., Dent.Ind., Excerp.Med., Ind.Med. (1972-), Ind.Sci.Rev., Inpharma, Int.Abstr.Biol.Sci., Med.& Surg.Dermat., Nutr.Abstr., Pharm.&Out.News, Reac., Sci.Cit.Ind., Tox.Abstr. (coverage dropped).
—BLDSC (3417.665000), CISTI, EMDOCS, GNLM, ingenta. **CCC.**
Published by: Gordon and Breach - Harwood Academic (Subsidiary of: Taylor & Francis Group), PO Box 531, Lausanne 1000, Switzerland. TEL 41-21-6411280, FAX 41-21-6411281, info@gbhap.com, http://www.gbhap.com. Ed. Arthur Veis. **Subscr. addr. in US:** International Publishers Direct, PO Box 32160, Newark, NJ 07102. FAX 215-750-6343.

CURRENT ADVANCES IN CELL & DEVELOPMENTAL BIOLOGY. see *BIOLOGY—Abstracting, Bibliographies, Statistics*

CURRENT COMMUNICATIONS IN CELL AND MOLECULAR BIOLOGY SERIES. see *BIOLOGY—Biochemistry*

571.6 GBR ISSN 0955-0674
QH573 CODEN: COCBE3
CURRENT OPINION IN CELL BIOLOGY. Text in English. 1989. bi-m. EUR 170 in Europe to individuals; JPY 20,600 in Japan to individuals; USD 184 elsewhere to individuals; EUR 213 in Europe to qualified personnel; JPY 25,700 in Japan to qualified personnel; USD 230 elsewhere to qualified personnel; EUR 908 in Europe to institutions; JPY 125,900 in Japan to institutions; USD 1,015 elsewhere to institutions (effective 2002). adv. bibl, illus. back issues avail. *Refereed.* **Document type:** *Academic/Scholarly.* **Description:** Directed toward researchers, educators and students in cell biology. Presents review articles, followed by annotated bibliographies of references consulted. Includes a "Paper Alert" section, giving brief summaries of relevant papers recently published in other journals.
Related titles: CD-ROM ed.; Online - full text ed.: USD 227 in North America to individuals; USD 247 in North America to individuals with print ed; GBP 137 elsewhere to individuals; GBP 150 elsewhere to individuals with print ed; USD 822 in North America to institutions includes print ed; GBP 500 elsewhere to institutions includes print ed (effective 1999 & 2000) (from EBSCO Publishing, ingenta, Swets Blackwell, ScienceDirect, Institute for Scientific Information).
Indexed: ASCA, Aqua.Sci.& Fish.Abstr., Chem.Abstr., Chem.Indus.Notes, Chem.Titles, Curr.Cont., Excerp.Med., Genet.Abstr., Hum.Gen.Abstr., Ind.Med. (1989-), Ind.Sci.Rev., Inpharma, Int.Abstr.Biol.Sci., Neurosci.Abstr., Nuc.Acids Abstr., Pharm.&Out.News, Reac., Sci.Cit.Ind.
—BLDSC (3500.773500), ADONIS, CASDDS, CISTI, EMDOCS, GNLM, IDS. **CCC.**
Published by: Elsevier Science Ltd., Elsevier Trends Journals, 84 Theobald's Rd, London WC1X 8RR, United Kingdom. TEL 44-20-7611-4400, FAX 44-20-7611-4468, info@current-opinion.com, http://www.elsevier.com/inca/publications/store/6/0/1/2/9/6/index.htt, http://www.current-opinion.com. Eds. K Simons, M Kirschner. Circ: 3,200. **Subscr. to:** PO Box 331, Haywards Heath, West Sussex RH16 3FG, United Kingdom. TEL 44-1444-475650, FAX 44-1444-445423.

571.6 USA
CURRENT PROTOCOLS IN CYTOMETRY. Text in English. 1997. base vol. plus q. updates. USD 445 (effective 2001); USD 480 combined subscription for base vol. & update; USD 220 updates (effective 2002). **Document type:** *Monographic series, Academic/Scholarly.*
Related titles: CD-ROM ed.: USD 490 (effective 2001); USD 520 combined subscription for base vol. & update; USD 260 renewals for base vol. & update (effective 2002).
—BLDSC (3501.532000).
Published by: (International Society for Analytical Cytology), John Wiley & Sons, Inc., Journals (Subsidiary of: Wiley InterScience), 605 Third Ave, New York, NY 10158. TEL 212-850-6645, FAX 212-850-6021, subinfo@jwiley.com, uscs-wis@wiley.com, http://www.wiley.com. **Dist. in UK by:** John Wiley & Sons Ltd., Baffins Ln, Chichester, Sussex PO19 IUD, United Kingdom. TEL 44-1243-779777, FAX 44-1243-843232, cs-journals@wiley.co.uk.

571.64 USA ISSN 1063-5823
QH601 CODEN: CTMTA2
CURRENT TOPICS IN MEMBRANES. Text in English. 1970. irreg., latest vol.45, 1997. reprints avail. *Refereed.*
Formerly (until 1991): Current Topics in Membranes and Transport (0070-2161)
Related titles: Online - full text ed.: (from Institute for Scientific Information).
Indexed: BBCI, Biol.Abstr., Chem.Abstr., Curr.Adv.Biochem., Curr.Adv.Cell & Devel.Biol., Curr.Adv.Ecol.Sci., Curr.Adv.Gen.& Molec.Biol., Ind.Sci.Rev., Nutr.Abstr., Sci.Cit.Ind.
—BLDSC (3504.884980), CASDDS, CISTI, GNLM, Linda Hall. **CCC.**
Published by: Academic Press, Inc., Journal Division (Subsidiary of: Harcourt Brace & Company), 525 B St, Ste 1900, San Diego, CA 92101-4495. TEL 619-231-0926, FAX 619-699-6715. Eds. Arnest Kleinzeller, Felix Bronner.

CYTOGENETIC AND GENOME RESEARCH. see *BIOLOGY—Genetics*

571.6 JPN ISSN 0011-4545
QH301 CODEN: CYTOAN
CYTOLOGIA/KITOROGIA. Text in English. 1929. q. JPY 25,000 (effective 2001). adv. **Document type:** *Academic/Scholarly.*
Related titles: Microfilm ed.: (from PMC).
Indexed: AgBiotech, Agricola, Anim.Breed.Abstr., Aqua.Sci.& Fish.Abstr., Bio-Contr.News & Info., Biol.Abstr., Chem.Abstr., Chem.Indus.Notes, Chem.Titles, Cott.& Trop.Fibr.Abstr., Crop Physiol.Abstr., Curr.Adv.Ecol.Sci., Curr.Cont. (coverage dropped), Entomol.Abstr. (coverage dropped), Excerp.Med., Fababean Abstr., Field Crop Abstr., Forest.Abstr., Genet.Abstr., Helminthol.Abstr., Herb.Abstr., Hort.Abstr., Hum.Gen.Abstr., INIS Atomind., Ind.Sci.Rev., Int.Abstr.Biol.Sci., Maize Abstr., Nuc.Acids Abstr., Ornam.Hort., Plant Breed.Abstr., Plant Gen.Res.Abstr., Plant Grow.Reg.Abstr., Postharvest, Potato Abstr., Ref.Zh., Rev.Appl.Entomol., Rev.Arom.& Med.Plants, Rev.Med.& Vet.Mycol., Rev.Plant Path., Rice Abstr., Sci.Cit.Ind. (coverage dropped), Seed Abstr., Soils & Fert., Sorghum & Millets Abstr., Triticale Abstr., Trop.Oil Seeds Abstr., Weed Abstr., Zoo.Rec.
—BLDSC (3506.800000), CASDDS, CISTI, EMDOCS, GNLM, ingenta, Linda Hall.
Address: c/o Japan Mendel Society, Toshin Bldg., Hongo 2-27-2, Bunkyo-ku, Tokyo 113-0033, Japan. FAX 81-3-3814-5352. Ed. Tsuneyoshi Kuroiwa. Pub. Tadashi Hirano. R&P, Adv. contact Yukihiro Yoshida. Circ: 1,000.

CYTOLOGY AND GENETICS. see *BIOLOGY—Genetics*

571.6 USA ISSN 0196-4763
QH573 CODEN: CYTODQ
CYTOMETRY. Text in English. 1983. 19/yr. USD 968 in United States; USD 1,148 in Canada & Mexico; USD 1,301 elsewhere; USD 1,017 combined subscription in United States for print and online eds.; USD 1,197 combined subscription in Canada & Mexico for print and online eds.; USD 1,350 combined subscription elsewhere for print and online eds. (effective 2002). adv. bk.rev. bibl, charts, illus. index. back issues avail.; reprint service avail. from ISI. *Refereed.* **Document type:** *Academic/Scholarly.* **Description:** Embraces all aspects of cytology, including image and flow cytometry, flow sorting, and applications of quantitative analytical cytology to basic research and clinical medicine.
Incorporates (1993-1999): Bioimaging (0966-9051)
Related titles: Microfilm ed.: (from WWS); Microform ed.: (from PQC); Online - full text ed.: ISSN 1097-0320. USD 968 in United States; USD 968 in Canada & Mexico; USD 968 elsewhere (effective 2002) (from EBSCO Publishing, Wiley InterScience, Institute for Scientific Information).
Indexed: ASCA, BBCI, Biol.Abstr., Chem.Abstr., Chem.Indus.Notes, Chem.Titles, Curr.Adv.Ecol.Sci., Curr.Cont., INIS Atomind., Ind.Med. (1980-), Ind.Sci.Rev., Inpharma, Int.Abstr.Biol.Sci., Pharm.&Out.News, Protozool.Abstr., Reac., Rev.Appl.Entomol., Sci.Cit.Ind.
—BLDSC (3506.855000), CASDDS, CISTI, EMDOCS, GNLM, IDS, ingenta, KNAW. **CCC.**
Published by: (International Society for Analytical Cytology), John Wiley & Sons, Inc., Journals (Subsidiary of: Wiley InterScience), 605 Third Ave, New York, NY 10158. TEL 212-850-6645, FAX 212-850-6021, subinfo@wiley.com, uscs-wis@wiley.com, http://www.wiley.com. Ed. Dr. Brian H Mayall. adv.: B&W page GBP 640, color page GBP 1,515; trim 210 x 279. Circ: 3,300. **Subscr. outside the Americas to:** John Wiley & Sons Ltd., Baffins Ln, Chichester, Sussex PO19 IUD, United Kingdom. TEL 44-1243-779777, FAX 44-1243-843232, cs-journals@wiley.co.uk, http://www.wiley.co.uk.

571.6 GBR ISSN 0956-5507
CODEN: CYTPEU
CYTOPATHOLOGY. Text in English. 1990. bi-m., latest vol.13, 2002. GBP 265 in Europe; USD 420 in North America; GBP 291.50 elsewhere (effective 2002). adv. bk.rev. bibl, charts, illus. back issues avail. *Refereed.* **Document type:** *Academic/Scholarly.* **Description:** Contains original articles and critical reviews on all aspects of clinical cytology.
Related titles: Microform ed.: (from PQC); Online - full text ed.: ISSN 1365-2303. 1997. GBP 239 in Europe; USD 378 in North America; GBP 239 elsewhere (effective 2002) (from EBSCO Publishing, O C L C Online Computer Library Center, Inc., RoweCom Information Quest, ingenta, Munksgaard & Blackwell Science's Synergy, Swets Blackwell, Institute for Scientific Information); Supplement:.
Indexed: ASCA, Curr.Cont., Helminthol.Abstr., Ind.Med. (1990-), Ind.Sci.Rev., Inpharma, Int.Abstr.Biol.Sci., Pharm.&Out.News, Reac., Rev.Med.& Vet.Mycol., Sci.Cit.Ind.
—BLDSC (3506.856000), ADONIS, CISTI, EMDOCS, GNLM, IDS, Infotrieve, KNAW. **CCC.**
Published by: (British Society for Clinical Cytology), Blackwell Science Ltd., PO Box 88, Oxford OX2 0NE, United Kingdom. TEL 44-1865-206180, 44-1865-206002, FAX 44-1865-206219, jnl.orders@blacksci.co.uk, http://www.blackwell-science.com/products/journals/cyto.htm, http://www.blackwellpublishing.com. Ed. D V Coleman. Pub. Elizabeth Whelan. R&P Sophie Savage. Adv. contact Jenny Applin. Circ: 980.

CYTOSKELETON. see *BIOLOGY—Abstracting, Bibliographies, Statistics*

571.6 NLD ISSN 0920-9069
CODEN: CYTOER
CYTOTECHNOLOGY; international journal of cell culture and biotechnology. Text in English. 1988. 9/yr. EUR 1,100, USD 1,101 to institutions for print or online ed.; EUR 1,320, USD 1,321.20 to institutions for print & online eds.combined (effective 2002). back issues avail.; reprint service avail. from SWZ. *Refereed.* **Document type:** *Journal, Academic/Scholarly.* **Description:** Represents a central repository for information on both the infrastructure of cell technology and the applied use of cell cultures, thus providing a panoramic perspective of the many facets and disciplines needed to develop successful cell cultures.
Related titles: Microform ed.: (from PQC); Online - full text ed.: (from EBSCO Publishing, O C L C Online Computer Library Center, Inc., RoweCom Information Quest, Swets Blackwell, Kluwer Online, Institute for Scientific Information).
Indexed: ASCA, AgBiotech, Agri.& Environ.Biotech.Abstr., Agri.Eng.Abstr., Anim.Breed.Abstr., Aqua.Sci.& Fish.Abstr., Bio-Contr.News & Info., Biol.Abstr., Biotech.Cit.Ind., Curr.Cont., Dairy Sci.Abstr., Derwent Biotech.Abstr., Environ.Sci.Poll.Mgmt., Helminthol.Abstr., Ind.Vet., Int.Abstr.Biol.Sci., Mat.Sci.Cit.Ind. (coverage dropped), Med.& Pharm.Biotech.Abstr., Microbiol.Abstr., Neurosci.Cit.Ind., Nutr.Abstr., Plant Breed.Abstr., Poult.Abstr., Ref.Zh., Rev.Appl.Entomol., Rev.Arom.& Med.Plants, Vet.Bull.
—BLDSC (3506.882000), CASDDS, EMDOCS, GNLM, IDS, Infotrieve, ingenta. **CCC.**
Published by: Kluwer Academic Publishers Group (Subsidiary of: Wolters Kluwer N.V.), Spuiboulevard 50, PO Box 17, Dordrecht 3300 AA, Netherlands. TEL 31-78-639-2392, FAX 31-78-654-2254, services@wkap.nl, http://www.wkap.nl/journalhome.htm/0920-9069. **Subscr. in the Americas to:** Kluwer Academic - Plenum Publishers, 233 Spring St, New York, NY 10013-1578. TEL 212-620-8468, FAX 212-807-1047; **Subscr. to:** Journals Department, PO Box 322, Dordrecht 3300 AH, Netherlands. TEL 31-78-639-2392, FAX 31-78-654-6474.

571.6 GBR ISSN 0951-0818
CODEN: DVCBAP
DEVELOPMENTAL AND CELL BIOLOGY SERIES. Text in English. irreg. price varies. illus. **Document type:** *Monographic series.*
Formerly: Developmental and Cell Biology Monographs
Indexed: Zoo.Rec.
—BLDSC (3579.050100).
Published by: Cambridge University Press, Edinburgh Bldg, Shaftesbury Rd, Cambridge CB2 2RU, United Kingdom. FAX 44-1223-315052, information@cup.cam.ac.uk, information@cambridge.org, http://www.cup.cam.ac.uk, http://www.uk.cambridge.org/journals/pmu. R&P Linda Nicol.

571.6 USA
▼ **DEVELOPMENTAL CELL.** Text in English. 2001. m. USD 115 domestic to individuals; USD 200 in Canada to individuals; USD 230 rest of world to individuals; USD 755 domestic to institutions; USD 800 in Canada to institutions; USD 843 rest of world to institutions (effective 2001). adv. back issues avail. **Document type:** *Academic/Scholarly.* **Description:** Covers the filed of cell biology and developmental biology.
Related titles: Online - full text ed.: USD 115 to individuals (effective 2001).
Indexed: Biotech.& Bioeng.Abstr., Entomol.Abstr., Tox.Abstr., Virol.Abstr.
Published by: Cell Press (Subsidiary of: Reed Elsevier plc), 1100 Massachusetts Ave, Cambridge, MA 02138. TEL 617-661-7057, FAX 617-661-7061, devcell@cell.com, http://www.cell.com/. Ed. Vivian Siegel. adv.: B&W page USD 550, color page USD 1,450; trim 8.5 x 11.

DEVELOPMENTS IN MOLECULAR AND CELLULAR BIOCHEMISTRY. see *BIOLOGY—Biochemistry*

571.6 USA ISSN 8755-1039
CODEN: DICYE7
DIAGNOSTIC CYTOPATHOLOGY. Text in English. 1985. m. USD 1,295 in United States; USD 1,415 in Canada & Mexico; USD 1,517 elsewhere; USD 1,360 combined subscription in United States for print and online eds.; USD 1,480 combined subscription in Canada & Mexico for print and online eds.; USD 1,582 combined subscription elsewhere for print and online eds. (effective 2002). adv. bk.rev. abstr, illus. back issues avail. *Refereed.* **Document type:** *Academic/Scholarly.* **Description:** International forum for original research and review articles on clinical aspects of cytology, encompassing such areas as flow cytometry, electron microscopy, image analysis, and immunocytochemistry.
Related titles: Microform ed.: (from PQC); Online - full text ed.: ISSN 1097-0339. USD 1,295 in United States; USD 1,295 in Canada & Mexico; USD 1,295 elsewhere (effective 2002) (from EBSCO Publishing, Wiley InterScience, Institute for Scientific Information).
Indexed: ASCA, Curr.Cont., Excerp.Med. (1992-), Helminthol.Abstr., INIS Atomind., Ind.Med. (1985-), Inpharma, Pharm.&Out.News, Protozool.Abstr., Reac., Rev.Med.& Vet.Mycol.
—BLDSC (3579.656500), CISTI, EMDOCS, GNLM, IDS, Infotrieve, ingenta, KNAW. **CCC.**
Published by: John Wiley & Sons, Inc., Journals (Subsidiary of: Wiley InterScience), 605 Third Ave, New York, NY 10158. TEL 212-850-6645, FAX 212-850-6021, subinfo@wiley.com, uscs-wis@wiley.com, http://www.wiley.com. Ed. Carlos W M Bedrossian. adv.: B&W page GBP 640, color page GBP 1,515; trim 210 x 279. Circ: 1,750. **Subscr. outside the Americas to:** John Wiley & Sons Ltd., Baffins Ln, Chichester, Sussex PO19 IUD, United Kingdom. TEL 44-1243-779777, FAX 44-1243-843232, cs-journals@wiley.co.uk, http://www.wiley.co.uk.

THE E M B O JOURNAL. see *BIOLOGY—Biochemistry*

EGYPTIAN JOURNAL OF GENETICS AND CYTOLOGY. see *BIOLOGY—Genetics*

571.6 DEU ISSN 0256-1514
ENDOCYTOBIOSIS AND CELL RESEARCH. Text in English. 1984. 3/yr. DEM 135. adv. bk.rev. index. back issues avail. *Refereed.* **Document type:** *Academic/Scholarly.*
Related titles: Online - full text ed.: (from Institute for Scientific Information).
Indexed: ASCA, Curr.Cont., Ind.Sci.Rev., Sci.Cit.Ind., Zoo.Rec.
—BLDSC (3743.095000), CISTI, GNLM, IDS, Infotrieve. **CCC.**
Published by: (International Society on Endocytobiology), Tuebingen University Press, Wilhelmstr 5, Tuebingen 72074, Germany. TEL 07071-292502, FAX 07071-293287.

571.6 NLD ISSN 1384-1270
ENDOTHELIAL CELL RESEARCH SERIES. Text in English. 1996. irreg., latest vol.8, 2000. **Document type:** *Monographic series, Academic/Scholarly.* **Description:** Contains reviews of basic and clinical research related to the endothelium.
—BLDSC (3743.648000).
Published by: Gordon and Breach - Harwood Academic (Subsidiary of: Taylor & Francis Group), O P A, Alfa Piazza Business Park, Zekeringstraat, Amsterdam 1014 BM, Netherlands. Ed. Gabor Rubanyi.

571.6 DEU ISSN 0171-9335
QH573 CODEN: EJCBDN
EUROPEAN JOURNAL OF CELL BIOLOGY. Text in English. 1969. m. EUR 232, GBP 182 to individuals; EUR 1,050, GBP 832 to institutions (effective 2002). *Refereed.* **Document type:** *Journal, Academic/Scholarly.*
Formerly: Cytobiologie (0070-2463)
Related titles: Online - full text ed.: (from Swets Blackwell, Institute for Scientific Information).
Indexed: ASCA, AgBiotech, Anim.Breed.Abstr., Aqua.Sci.& Fish.Abstr., BBCI, Biol.Abstr., Chem.Abstr., Chem.Indus.Notes, Chem.Titles, Chemorec.Abstr., Curr.Adv.Ecol.Sci., Curr.Cont., Dairy Sci.Abstr., Dent.Ind., Derwent Biotech.Abstr., Excerp.Med., Helminthol.Abstr., INIS Atomind., Ind.Med. (1979-), Ind.Sci.Rev., Inpharma, Int.Abstr.Biol.Sci., Nuc.Acids Abstr., Nutr.Abstr., Pharm.&Out.News, Plant Breed.Abstr., Protozool.Abstr., Reac., Ref.Zh., Rev.Appl.Entomol., Rev.Med.& Vet.Mycol., Rev.Plant Path., Sci.Cit.Ind.
—BLDSC (3829.725700), CASDDS, CISTI, GNLM, ingenta, Linda Hall. **CCC.**

B

Published by: (European Cell Biology Organization), Urban & Fischer Verlag, Loebdergraben 14a, Jena 07743, Germany. FAX 49-3641-6264210, marketing.journals@urbanfischer.de, http://www.urbanfischer.de/journals. Eds. Hans Bloemendal, Reinhard Jahn, Sabine Werner, Spyridon Artavanis-Tsakonas. R&P Martin Huber TEL 49-3641-626430. Circ: 1,400. **Subscr. to:** Nature Publishing Group Specialist Journals. **Co-sponsors:** Deutsche Gesellschaft fuer Elektronenmikroskopie e.V.; Deutsche Gesellschaft fuer Zellbiologie e.V.

EUROPEAN JOURNAL OF HISTOCHEMISTRY. see *BIOLOGY—Biochemistry*

EXTRACELLULAR MATRIX. see *BIOLOGY—Abstracting, Bibliographies, Statistics*

571.6 POL ISSN 0239-8508
CODEN: FHCYEM

FOLIA HISTOCHEMICA ET CYTOBIOLOGICA. Text and summaries in English. 1963. q., latest vol.39, 2001. PLZ 100 domestic; USD 40 in Europe to individuals; USD 50 elsewhere to individuals; USD 50 in Europe to institutions; USD 65 elsewhere to institutions (effective 2002). bk.rev. charts, illus, abstr, bibl. index. back issues avail. *Refereed.* **Document type:** *Journal, Academic/Scholarly.* **Description:** Publishes review articles, original articles, letters to the editor, proceedings of scientific congresses/symposia. Covers development and applications of modern histochemical techniques, cell biology and pathology, cell-microenvironment interaction, tissue organization and pathology.
Formerly (until 1984): Folia Histochemica et Cytochemica (0015-5586)
Related titles: Online - full text ed.: (from Institute for Scientific Information).
Indexed: ASCA, AgroAgen, AgroLibrex, Anim.Breed.Abstr., BBCI, Biol.Abstr., Chem.Abstr., Chem.Indus.Notes, Chem.Titles, Curr.Adv.Biochem., Curr.Adv.Cell & Devel.Biol., Curr.Adv.Ecol.Sci., Curr.Cont. (coverage dropped), Excerp.Med., GeoRef, Helminthol.Abstr., INIS Atomind., Ind.Med. (1984-), Ind.Sci.Rev., Int.Abstr.Biol.Sci., Nutr.Abstr., Sci.Cit.Ind. (coverage dropped).
—BLDSC (3970.295000), CASDDS, CISTI, GNLM, IDS, Infotrieve, Linda Hall. **CCC.**
Published by: Polskie Towarzystwo Histochemikow i Cytochemikow/Polish Histochemical and Cytochemical Society, PO Box 843, Krakow 30960, Poland. TEL 48-12-4227027, FAX 48-12-4227027, mmlitwin@cyf-kr.edu.pl, http://www.cm-uj.krakow.pl/FHC. Ed. Jan A Litwin. Circ: 500.

FOLIA MICROBIOLOGICA. see *BIOLOGY—Biochemistry*

GENES TO CELLS. see *BIOLOGY—Genetics*

GENETIC RESOURCES AND CROP EVOLUTION; an international journal. see *BIOLOGY—Genetics*

GENOME. see *BIOLOGY—Genetics*

HEREDITAS; a periodical devoted to the publication of original research in all aspects of genetics and cytology. see *BIOLOGY—Genetics*

571.5 NLD ISSN 0018-2214
QH611 CODEN: HISJAE

THE HISTOCHEMICAL JOURNAL; a journal of cell and tissue biochemistry. Text in English. 1969. m. EUR 1,510, USD 1,512 to institutions for print or online ed.; EUR 1,812, USD 1,814.40 to institutions for print & online eds. combined (effective 2002). adv. bk.rev. charts, illus. index. reprint service avail. from PQC,ISI. *Refereed.* **Document type:** *Journal, Academic/Scholarly.* **Description:** Publishes original research papers in those areas of biochemistry, biophysics and cell biology concerned with the chemical composition and activities of tissues, cells and cellular components.
Related titles: Online - full text ed.: (from EBSCO Publishing, O C L C Online Computer Library Center, Inc., RoweCom Information Quest, Swets Blackwell, Kluwer Online, Institute for Scientific Information).
Indexed: ASCA, Abstr.Hyg., Agri.Eng.Abstr., Anim.Breed.Abstr., BBCI, Biol.Abstr., Chem.Abstr., Chem.Indus.Notes, Chem.Titles, Curr.Adv.Ecol.Sci., Curr.Cont., Dairy Sci.Abstr., Dent.Ind., Excerp.Med., Helminthol.Abstr., Hort.Abstr., INIS Atomind., Ind.Med. (1968-), Ind.Sci.Rev., Ind.Vet., Inpharma, Int.Abstr.Biol.Sci., Neurosci.Cit.Ind., Nutr.Abstr., Pig News & Info., Postharvest, Poult.Abstr., Protozool.Abstr., Reac., Rev.Med.& Vet.Mycol., Rev.Plant Path., Sci.Cit.Ind., Trop.Dis.Bull., Vet.Bull.
—BLDSC (4315.790000), ADONIS, CASDDS, CISTI, GNLM, IDS, ingenta, Linda Hall. **CCC.**
Published by: (Royal Microscopical Society GBR), Kluwer Academic Publishers Group (Subsidiary of: Wolters Kluwer N.V.), Spuiboulevard 50, PO Box 17, Dordrecht 3300 AA, Netherlands. TEL 31-78-639-2392, FAX 31-78-654-2254, services@wkap.nl, http://www.wkap.nl/journalhome.htm/0018-2214. Ed. P J Stoward. Adv. contact Gemma Heiser. **Subscr. in the Americas to:** Kluwer Academic - Plenum Publishers, 233 Spring St, New York, NY 10013-1578. TEL 212-620-8468, FAX 212-807-1047; **Subscr. to:** Journals Department, PO Box 322, Dordrecht 3300 AH, Netherlands. TEL 31-78-639-2392, FAX 31-78-654-6474.

571.6 DEU ISSN 0948-6143
QH611 CODEN: HCMYAL

HISTOCHEMISTRY AND CELL BIOLOGY. Text in English. 1958. m. (in 2 vols.). EUR 2,455 domestic; EUR 2,436.70 in Germany; EUR 241 newsstand/cover foreign (effective 2002). adv. charts, illus. back issues avail.; reprint service avail. from ISI. *Refereed.* **Document type:** *Journal, Academic/Scholarly.* **Description:** Contains original papers on all areas of cyto- and histochemistry, especially morphology and cell biology. Focus is on theory and methodology (including fractionation, homogenization techniques, autoradiography, polarization optics, and fluorescence microscopy).
Former titles: Histochemistry (0301-5564); Histochemie - Histochemistry - Histochimie (0018-2222)
Related titles: Microform ed.: (from PQC); Online - full text ed.: ISSN 1432-119X (from EBSCO Publishing, RoweCom Information Quest, Swets Blackwell, Springer LINK, Institute for Scientific Information).
Indexed: ASCA, BBCI, Biol.Abstr., Chem.Abstr., Chem.Indus.Notes, Chem.Titles, Curr.Adv.Cancer Res., Curr.Adv.Cell & Devel.Biol., Curr.Adv.Ecol.Sci., Curr.Cont., Dairy Sci.Abstr., Dent.Ind., Excerp.Med., Helminthol.Abstr., INIS Atomind., Ind.Med. (1995-), Ind.Sci.Rev., Ind.Vet., Inpharma, Int.Abstr.Biol.Sci., Kidney, Neurosci.Cit.Ind., Nutr.Abstr., Reac., Sci.Cit.Ind., Vet.Bull., Zoo.Rec.
—BLDSC (4316.003100), ADONIS, CASDDS, CISTI, EMDOCS, GNLM, IDS, ingenta, Linda Hall. **CCC.**
Published by: (Society for Histochemistry), Springer-Verlag (Subsidiary of: BertelsmannSpringer), Tiergartenstr 17, Heidelberg 69121, Germany. TEL 49-6221-345-0, FAX 49-6221-345229, subscriptions@springer.de, http://link.springer.de/link/service/journals/00418/ index.htm, http://www.springer.de. Eds. D Drenckhahn, J Roth. **Subscr. in N. America to:** Springer-Verlag New York Inc., PO Box 2485, Secaucus, NJ 07096-2485. TEL 212-460-1500, FAX 212-473-6272.

571.5 616.07 ESP ISSN 0213-3911
CODEN: HIHIES

HISTOLOGY AND HISTOPATHOLOGY; cellular and molecular biology. Text in English. 1986. a., latest vol.16. USD 400 (effective 2002). adv. 330 p./no. back issues avail. *Refereed.* **Document type:** *Journal, Academic/Scholarly.* **Description:** Publishes original works in anatomy, histology, histopathology and cell biology.
Related titles: Online - full text ed.: (from Institute for Scientific Information).
Indexed: ASCA, Anim.Breed.Abstr., BBCI, Chem.Abstr., Chem.Indus.Notes, Chem.Titles, Curr.Cont., Excerp.Med., Ind.Med. (1986-), Ind.Sci.Rev., Inpharma, Int.Abstr.Biol.Sci., Neurosci.Cit.Ind., Reac., Sci.Cit.Ind., Zoo.Rec.
—BLDSC (4316.023100), CASDDS, CISTI, EMDOCS, GNLM, IDS, Infotrieve, ingenta, KNAW. **CCC.**
Address: Plaza Fuensanta, 2, 7o C., Murcia 30008, Spain. FAX 34-968-364150, http://www.ehu.es/histol-histopathol/. Eds. F Hernandez, F Madrid. R&P F Madrid.

571.6 AUT ISSN 1609-5537

▼ **HOFBAUER CELLS.** Text in English. 2000. q. USD 75 domestic; USD 115 foreign; USD 35 newsstand/cover (effective 2001). adv. back issues avail.; reprints avail. *Refereed.* **Document type:** *Journal, Academic/Scholarly.* **Description:** Publishes articles, case reports, reviews, and letters that aim to improve communications in understanding the multidisciplinary fields of modern Hofbauer cell research and placenta research.
Related titles: Online - full text ed.: ISSN 1609-5545.
Published by: V I C E R Publishing, PO Box 14, Vienna A-1097, Austria. TEL 43-676-9568085, FAX 43-676-9568086, vicer@vicer.org, http://www.vicer.org. Ed., R&P Roland Hofbauer. adv.: B&W page USD 1,700, color page USD 2,200. Circ: 1,000 (paid and controlled).

HONYU DOBUTSU SHIKEN BUNKAKAI KAIHO/MAMMALIAN MUTAGENICITY STUDY GROUP COMMUNICATIONS. see *BIOLOGY—Genetics*

IMMUNOHISTOCHEMISTRY. see *BIOLOGY—Abstracting, Bibliographies, Statistics*

INSTITUTE FOR FERMENTATION, OSAKA. RESEARCH COMMUNICATIONS/HAKKO KENKYUJO HOKOKU. see *BIOLOGY—Microbiology*

571.6 GBR ISSN 0957-0799
CODEN: IINCEH

INTERCELLULAR AND INTRACELLULAR COMMUNICATIONS. Text in English. 1986. irreg. price varies. **Document type:** *Monographic series.*
Indexed: Chem.Abstr., Chem.Indus.Notes, Chem.Titles.
—CASDDS, CISTI.
Published by: Cambridge University Press, Edinburgh Bldg, Shaftesbury Rd, Cambridge CB2 2RU, United Kingdom. FAX 44-1223-315052, information@cup.cam.ac.uk, information@cambridge.org, http://www.cup.cam.ac.uk, http://www.uk.cambridge.org/journals/pmu.

INTERNATIONAL CONGRESS OF HISTOCHEMISTRY AND CYTOCHEMISTRY. PROCEEDINGS. see *BIOLOGY—Biochemistry*

INTERNATIONAL JOURNAL OF BIOCHEMISTRY & CELL BIOLOGY. see *BIOLOGY—Biochemistry*

571.6 USA ISSN 0074-7696
QH573 CODEN: IRCYAJ

INTERNATIONAL REVIEW OF CYTOLOGY. Text in English. 1952. irreg., latest vol.182, 1998. index; cum.index: 1952-1960, vols.1-9 in vol.10. reprint service avail. from ISI. *Refereed.* **Document type:** *Academic/Scholarly.*
Related titles: Online - full text ed.: (from Institute for Scientific Information).
Indexed: Abstr.Hyg., AgBiotech, Agricola, Anim.Breed.Abstr., Aqua.Sci.& Fish.Abstr., BBCI, Bibl.Agri., Biol.Abstr., Chem.Abstr., Chem.Indus.Notes, Chem.Titles, Crop Physiol.Abstr., Curr.Adv.Biochem., Excerp.Med., Genet.Abstr., Hum.Gen.Abstr., INIS Atomind., Ind.Med. (1952-), Ind.Sci.Rev., Int.Abstr.Biol.Sci., Maize Abstr., Neurosci.Cit.Ind., Nuc.Acids Abstr., Plant Breed.Abstr., Rev.Appl.Entomol., Rev.Med.& Vet.Mycol., Sci.Cit.Ind., Sport Fish.Abstr., Triticale Abstr., Trop.Dis.Bull., Wild.Rev., Zoo.Rec.
—BLDSC (4547.050000), CASDDS, CISTI, GNLM, ingenta, KNAW, Linda Hall. **CCC.**
Published by: Academic Press, Inc., Journal Division (Subsidiary of: Harcourt Brace & Company), 525 B St, Ste 1900, San Diego, CA 92101-4495. TEL 619-231-0926, FAX 619-699-6715. Eds. G H Bourne, J F Danielli. **Subscr. to:** Order Dept., 6277 Sea Harbor Dr, 4th Fl, Orlando, FL 32887. TEL 800-321-5068.

571.64 RUS ISSN 0234-2979
QH601

ITOGI NAUKI I TEKHNIKI. BIOFIZIKA MEMBRAN. Text in Russian. irreg., latest vol.6, 1989. price varies.
Formerly: Itogi Nauki i Tekhniki. Biofizika (0202-7003)
Indexed: Crop Physiol.Abstr., Field Crop Abstr., Herb.Abstr.
—Infotrieve, Linda Hall. **CCC.**
Published by: Vserossiiskii Institut Nauchnoi i Tekhnicheskoi Informatsii (VINITI), Usievicha ul 20-a, Moscow 125315, Russian Federation. TEL 7-095-1526441. **Dist. by:** Mezhdunarodnaya Kniga, B Yakimanka 39, Moscow 117049, Russian Federation. TEL 7-095-2384967, FAX 7-095-2384634; **US dist. addr.:** East View Publications, 3020 Harbor Ln N, Minneapolis, MN 55447. TEL 612-550-0961.

JOURNAL OF BIOCHEMISTRY, MOLECULAR BIOLOGY AND BIOPHYSICS. see *BIOLOGY—Biochemistry*

571.6 USA ISSN 0021-9525
QH301 CODEN: JCLBA3

JOURNAL OF CELL BIOLOGY. Text in English. 1955. bi-w. USD 940 in US & Canada to institutions print ed.; USD 1,125 elsewhere to institutions print ed.; USD 750 newsstand/cover to institutions online ed. (effective 2001). adv. charts, illus. Index. 242 p./no. 2 cols./p. back issues avail.; reprint service avail. from PQC,ISI. *Refereed.* **Document type:** *Journal, Academic/Scholarly.* **Description:** Provides a forum for articles in all branches of contemporary cell biology from the international community.
Related titles: Microform ed.: (from PQC); Online - full text ed.: (from HighWire Pr., Factiva, Institute for Scientific Information, RoweCom Information Quest).

Indexed: ASCA, Abstr.Bull.Inst.Pap.Chem., Abstr.Hyg., AgBiotech, Agri.& Environ.Biotech.Abstr. (coverage dropped), Agricola, Anim.Breed.Abstr., Aqua.Sci.& Fish.Abstr., BBCI, Bibl.Agri., Biol.& Agr.Ind. (Jan.1983-), Biol.Abstr., Cal.Tiss.Abstr. (coverage dropped), Chem.Abstr., Chem.Indus.Notes, Chem.Titles, Chemorec.Abstr., Crop Physiol.Abstr., Curr.Adv.Biochem., Curr.Adv.Cancer Res., Curr.Adv.Cell & Devel.Biol., Curr.Adv.Gen.& Molec.Biol., Curr.Cont., Dairy Sci.Abstr., Dent.Ind., Derwent Biotech.Abstr., Environ.Sci.Poll.Mgmt., Excerp.Med., Field Crop Abstr., Gen.Sci.Ind. (Jun.1992-), Genet.Abstr., Helminthol.Abstr., Herb.Abstr., Hort.Abstr., Hum.Gen.Abstr., INIS Atomind., Immun.Abstr. (coverage dropped), Ind.Med. (1962-), Ind.Sci.Rev., Ind.Vet., Inpharma, Int.Abstr.Biol.Sci., Maize Abstr., Microbiol.Abstr., Neurosci.Abstr., Neurosci.Cit.Ind., Nuc.Acids Abstr., Nutr.Abstr., Ornam.Hort., Plant Breed.Abstr., Poult.Abstr., Protozool.Abstr., Reac., Ref.Zh., Rev.Appl.Entomol., Rev.Med.& Vet.Mycol., Rev.Plant Path., Sci.Cit.Ind., Seed Abstr., Soils & Fert., Tox.Abstr. (coverage dropped), Trop.Dis.Bull., Vet.Bull., Weed Abstr., Zoo.Rec.
—BLDSC (4954.920000), CASDDS, CISTI, GNLM, IDS, ingenta, Linda Hall. **CCC.**
Published by: Rockefeller University Press, 1114 First Ave, New York, NY 10021. TEL 212-327-8572, FAX 212-327-7944, rupcd@rockefeller.edu, rupress@rockefeller.edu, http://www.jcb.org; http://www.rockefeller.edu/rupress. Ed. Ira Mellman. R&P Laura Smith TEL 212-327-8025. Adv. contact Lorna Peterson TEL 212-327-8880. color page USD 2,130, B&W page USD 730; 7.75 x 10.25. Circ: 3,931.

571.6 GBR ISSN 0021-9533
QH573 CODEN: JNCSAI
JOURNAL OF CELL SCIENCE. Text in English. 1852. s-m. GBP 193 domestic to individuals print ed.; USD 324 in North America to individuals print ed.; GBP 51 domestic to individuals online ed.; USD 86 in North America to individuals online ed.; GBP 213 domestic to individuals print & online eds.; USD 359 in North America to individuals print & online eds. (effective 2001). adv. charts, illus. index, cum.index. reprints avail. *Refereed.*
Document type: *Journal, Academic/Scholarly.*
Description: Covers all aspects of cell biology. Of interest to cell biologists, molecular biologists, geneticists, and particularly those working in the cell cycle and cell signaling fields.
Formerly (until 1966): Quarterly Journal of Microscopical Science (0370-2952)
Related titles: Microfilm ed.: (from BHP); Online - full text ed.: (from EBSCO Publishing, RoweCom Information Quest, Swets Blackwell, Institute for Scientific Information).
Indexed: ASCA, Abstr.Hyg., AgBiotech, Agricola, Anim.Breed.Abstr., Aqua.Sci.& Fish.Abstr., Aquacult.Abstr., BBCI, Bibl.Agri., Biol.& Agr.Ind. (Jan.1990-), Biol.Abstr., Chem.Abstr., Chem.Indus.Notes, Chem.Titles, Chemorec.Abstr., Curr.Adv.Biochem., Curr.Adv.Cancer Res., Curr.Adv.Cell & Devel.Biol., Curr.Adv.Gen.& Molec.Biol., Curr.Biotech.Abstr., Curr.Cont., Dairy Sci.Abstr., Dent.Ind., Environ.Sci.Poll.Mgmt., Excerp.Med., Field Crop Abstr., GeoRef, Helminthol.Abstr., Hort.Abstr., INIS Atomind., Ind.Med. (1966-), Ind.Sci.Rev., Ind.Vet., Inpharma, Int.Abstr.Biol.Sci., Maize Abstr., Microbiol.Abstr., Neurosci.Cit.Ind., Nuc.Acids Abstr., Nutr.Abstr., Ornam.Hort., Plant Breed.Abstr., Poult.Abstr., Protozool.Abstr., Reac., Ref.Zh., Rev.Appl.Entomol., Rev.Med.& Vet.Mycol., Rev.Plant Path., Sci.Cit.Ind., Soils & Fert., Soyabean Abstr., Sport Fish.Abstr., Triticale Abstr., Trop.Dis.Bull., Vet.Bull., Zoo.Rec.
—BLDSC (4954.960000), CASDDS, CISTI, GNLM, ingenta, Linda Hall.
Published by: Company of Biologists Ltd., Bidder Bldg, Bidder Building, 140 Cowley Rd, Cambridge CB4 4DL, United Kingdom. TEL 44-1223-426164, FAX 44-1223-423353, sales@thecob.demon.co.uk, http://jcs.biologists.org, http://www.biologists.com. Ed. Fiona M Watt. R&P R Skaer TEL 44-1223-420482. Adv. contact Amanda Sheppardson. Circ: 1,550.

JOURNAL OF CELLULAR BIOCHEMISTRY. see *BIOLOGY—Biochemistry*

571.6 GBR ISSN 1359-7388
RB25
JOURNAL OF CELLULAR PATHOLOGY. Text in English. 1996. q. GBP 45 to individuals; USD 72 in United States to individuals; GBP 115 to institutions; USD 185 in United States to institutions. back issues avail. *Refereed.* **Document type:** *Academic/Scholarly.*
Description: Contains articles on current and new techniques appropriate to cellular pathology in its broadest sense and relevant to hospitals and to industrial and research laboratories.
—BLDSC (4955.015000).
Published by: Greenwich Medical Media, 219 Linen Hall, Greenwich Medical Media Ltd, Flat 162, 162-168 Regent St, London W1R 5TB, United Kingdom. TEL 44-207-494-1515, FAX 44-207-494-1616, gm@greenwich-medical.co.uk, http://www.greenwich-medical.co.uk. Ed. John Bancroft. R&P Joolz Longley. **Subscr. to:** Royal Society of Medicine Press Ltd, PO Box 9002, London W1A 0ZA, United Kingdom. TEL 44-20-7290-2900, FAX 44-20-7290-2929.

JOURNAL OF CLINICAL ONCOLOGY. see *MEDICAL SCIENCES—Oncology*

THE JOURNAL OF CYTOLOGY AND GENETICS. see *BIOLOGY—Genetics*

571.5 USA ISSN 0022-1554
QP501 CODEN: JHCYAS
JOURNAL OF HISTOCHEMISTRY AND CYTOCHEMISTRY. Text in English. 1953. m. USD 550 domestic for print & online eds.; USD 585 foreign for print & online eds. (effective 2001). adv. bk.rev. bibl, charts, illus. index. back issues avail. *Refereed.*
Document type: *Journal.* **Description:** Publishes papers that report the development of new histochemical and cytochemical methods, significant modifications of existing techniques, or original research in which histochemical and cytochemical methods make a significant contribution.
Related titles: Microform ed.: 1953 (from WWS); Online - full text ed.: 1953. USD 100 to individuals for Online only; USD 330 to institutions for Online only (effective 2001) (from HighWire Pr., EBSCO Publishing, RoweCom Information Quest, Institute for Scientific Information).
Indexed: ASCA, Anim.Breed.Abstr., BBCI, Biol.Abstr., Chem.Abstr., Chem.Indus.Notes, Chem.Titles, Curr.Adv.Cell & Devel.Biol., Curr.Adv.Ecol.Sci., Curr.Cont., Dairy Sci.Abstr., Dent.Ind., Excerp.Med., Helminthol.Abstr., INIS Atomind., Ind.Med. (1953-), Ind.Sci.Rev., Ind.Vet., Inpharma, Int.Abstr.Biol.Sci., Mass Spectr.Bull., Neurosci.Cit.Ind., Nutr.Abstr., Pig News & Info., Poult.Abstr., Reac., Sci.Cit.Ind., Small Anim.Abstr., Trop.Dis.Bull., Vet.Bull.
—BLDSC (5000.000000), CASDDS, CISTI, GNLM, IDS, ingenta, KNAW, Linda Hall. **CCC.**
Published by: Histochemical Society, University Station, PO Box 85630, Seattle, WA 98145-1630. FAX 206-616-5842, johc@u.washington.edu, http://www.jhc.org/, http://intl.jhc.org. Ed. Dr. Denis G Baskin. Circ: 4,000.

571.5 USA ISSN 0147-8885
RB43 CODEN: JOHIDN
JOURNAL OF HISTOTECHNOLOGY. Text in English. 1977. q. USD 70 domestic to individuals; USD 100 foreign to individuals; USD 80 domestic to institutions; USD 110 foreign to institutions (effective 2002). adv. bk.rev. charts, illus, tr.lit. index. 89 p./no. 2 cols./p. back issues avail. *Refereed.* **Document type:** *Trade.*
Description: Publishes original articles, brief reports, notes on techniques, case studies dealing with anatomy, histochemistry, pathology, microscopy, and immunohistochemistry. Includes articles on applications and evaluations of commercially prepared kits, continuing education, and medical news.
Related titles: Online - full text ed.: (from Institute for Scientific Information).
Indexed: ASCA, BBCI, Biol.Abstr., Chem.Abstr., Chem.Indus.Notes, Chem.Titles, Curr.Cont., Excerp.Med., INIS Atomind., Ind.Sci.Rev., Inpharma, Reac., Rev.Appl.Entomol., Rev.Med.& Vet.Mycol., Sci.Cit.Ind.
—BLDSC (5002.400000), CASDDS, CISTI, GNLM, IDS, ingenta, KNAW.
Published by: National Society for Histotechnology, 4201 Northview Dr, Ste 502, Bowie, MD 20716-2604. TEL 301-262-6221, FAX 301-262-9188, histo@nsh.org, http://www.nsh.org. Ed. James Hendricks. R&P Roberta Mosedale. Circ: 5,000 (paid).

571.6 USA ISSN 0022-2631
QH601 CODEN: JMBBBO
JOURNAL OF MEMBRANE BIOLOGY; an international journal for studies on the structure, function and genesis of biomembranes. Text in English. 1969. 18/yr. (in 6 vols., 3 nos./vol.). USD 2,004.90 domestic for Print & Online Eds.; USD 1,924.90 in Germany for Print & Online Eds.; USD 122.90 newsstand/cover foreign (effective 2001). adv. back issues avail.; reprint service avail. from ISI. *Refereed.* **Document type:** *Academic/Scholarly.* **Description:** Contains articles examining the nature, structure, function, and genesis of biological membranes, and the physics and chemistry of artificial membranes as relevant to biomembranes.
Related titles: Microform ed.: (from PQC); Online - full text ed.: ISSN 1432-1424 (from EBSCO Publishing, RoweCom Information Quest, Swets Blackwell, Springer LINK, Institute for Scientific Information).
Indexed: ASCA, Agricola, Aqua.Sci.& Fish.Abstr., BBCI, Bio-Contr.News & Info., Biol.Abstr., Chem.Abstr., Chem.Indus.Notes, Chem.Titles, Chemorec.Abstr., Curr.Adv.Biochem., Curr.Adv.Cell & Devel.Biol., Curr.Adv.Ecol.Sci., Curr.Cont., Dairy Sci.Abstr., Excerp.Med., INIS Atomind., Ind.Med. (1969-), Ind.Sci.Rev., Inpharma, Int.Abstr.Biol.Sci., Neurosci.Abstr. (coverage dropped), Neurosci.Cit.Ind., Nutr.Abstr., Poult.Abstr., Protozool.Abstr., Reac., Rev.Appl.Entomol., Sci.Cit.Ind.
—BLDSC (5017.600000), ADONIS, CASDDS, CISTI, GNLM, IDS, ingenta, Linda Hall. **CCC.**
Published by: Springer-Verlag, Journals (Subsidiary of: BertelsmannSpringer), 175 Fifth Ave, New York, NY 10010. TEL 212-460-1500, FAX 212-473-6272, orders@springer-ny.com, http://www.springer-ny.com. Ed. W R Loewenstein. R&P Ian Gross. Adv. contact Brian Skepton. **N. American subscr. to:** Journal Fulfillment Services, PO Box 2485, Secaucus, NJ 07096-2485. TEL 800-777-4643, FAX 201-348-4505; **Subscr. to:** Heidelberger Platz 33, Berlin 14197, Germany. orders@springer-ny.com.

JOURNAL OF MUSCLE RESEARCH AND CELL MOTILITY. see *MEDICAL SCIENCES—Orthopedics And Traumatology*

571.6 USA ISSN 0300-4864
QP351 CODEN: JNCYA2
JOURNAL OF NEUROCYTOLOGY; a journal of cellular neurobiology. Text in English. 1972. 9/yr. USD 1,186, EUR 1,184.50 to institutions for print or online ed.; USD 1,423.20, EUR 1,422 to institutions for print & online eds.combined (effective 2002). bk.rev. bibl, illus. index. reprint service avail. from PQC,ISI. *Refereed.*
Document type: *Journal, Academic/Scholarly.*
Description: Publishes research papers (and occasionally reviews and letters) dealing the structure and function of nervous tissue. The scope of the Journal is wide: it embraces the organization and fine structure, and the associated molecular biology, biochemistry, cytochemistry, biophysics, physiology and pharmacology of neurons, receptor and glial cells, synapses and other intercellular specializations, in vertebrates and invertebrates under normal, experimental and pathological condititions.
Related titles: Online - full text ed.: (from EBSCO Publishing, O C L C Online Computer Library Center, Inc., RoweCom Information Quest, Swets Blackwell, Kluwer Online, Institute for Scientific Information).
Indexed: ASCA, Aqua.Sci.& Fish.Abstr., BBCI, Biol.Abstr., Chem.Abstr., Chem.Titles, Curr.Adv.Cell & Devel.Biol., Curr.Adv.Ecol.Sci., Curr.Cont., Dent.Ind., Excerp.Med., INIS Atomind., Ind.Med. (1972-), Ind.Sci.Rev., Inpharma, Int.Abstr.Biol.Sci., Neurosci.Abstr., Neurosci.Cit.Ind., Reac., Sci.Cit.Ind.
—BLDSC (5021.540000), ADONIS, CASDDS, CISTI, EMDOCS, GNLM, IDS, ingenta, Linda Hall. **CCC.**
Published by: Kluwer Academic Publishers Boston, 101 Philip Dr, Assinippi Park, Norwell, MA 02061. TEL 781-871-6600, FAX 781-871-9045, services@wkap.nl, http://www.wkap.nl/journalhome.htm/0300-4864. Eds. A R Lieberman, M W Brightman. **Subscr. outside the Americas to:** Kluwer Academic Publishers Group, Journals Department, PO Box 322, Dordrecht 3300 AH, Netherlands. TEL 31-78-639-2392, FAX 31-78-654-6474; **Subscr. to:** Kluwer Academic - Plenum Publishers, 233 Spring St, New York, NY 10013-1578. TEL 212-620-8468, FAX 212-807-1047.

571.6 ITA ISSN 1122-9497
CODEN: JSCPEE
JOURNAL OF SUBMICROSCOPIC CYTOLOGY AND PATHOLOGY. Text in English. 1969. q. ITL 180,000, USD 150 (effective 1998). *Refereed.* **Document type:** *Academic/Scholarly.* **Description:** Presents papers dealing with applications of electronmicroscopy, biology, physiology and experimental and diagnostic pathology.
Formerly (until 1988): Journal of Submicroscopic Cytology (0022-4782)
Indexed: ASCA, Biol.Abstr., Chem.Abstr., Chem.Indus.Notes, Chem.Titles, Curr.Cont. (coverage dropped), Excerp.Med. (1988-1992), Ind.Med. (1988-), Ind.Sci.Rev., Inpharma, Reac., Sci.Cit.Ind. (coverage dropped), Sport Fish.Abstr., Zoo.Rec.
—BLDSC (5066.930500), CASDDS, CISTI, GNLM, IDS, ingenta, KNAW, Linda Hall.
Published by: N I E Nuova Immagine Editrice, Strada di Montechiaro 56, Siena 53100, Italy. TEL 39-0577-42625, FAX 39-0577-44633. Circ: 500.

KLINICHNA I TRANSFUZIONNA HEMATOLOGIIA. see *MEDICAL SCIENCES—Hematology*

B

LEUCOCYTES. see *MEDICAL SCIENCES—Abstracting, Bibliographies, Statistics*

LYSOSOMES AND ENDOCYTOSIS. see *BIOLOGY—Abstracting, Bibliographies, Statistics*

MACROPHAGES. see *MEDICAL SCIENCES—Abstracting, Bibliographies, Statistics*

571.64 JPN ISSN 0385-1036
CODEN: MAKUD9
MAKU/MEMBRANE. Text in Japanese; Summaries in English. 1976. bi-m. JPY 2,800. adv. bk.rev. 90 p./no. back issues avail. *Refereed.* **Document type:** *Journal, Academic/Scholarly.*
Indexed: Biol.Abstr., Chem.Abstr., Chem.Titles, Excerp.Med.
—BLDSC (5548.025000), CASDDS, CISTI, Infotrieve. **CCC.**
Published by: Nihon Maku Gakkai/Membrane Society of Japan, 14-9 Hongo 4-chome, Bunkyo-ku, Tokyo 113-0033, Japan. TEL 81-3-3815-2818, FAX 81-3-3815-2818, membrane@muu.biglobe.ne.jp, http://wwwsoc.nacsis.ac.jp/membrane/index.html. Ed. Yoshinori Nozuwa. Circ: 850.

571.6 AUT ISSN 1609-5510
▼ **MAST CELLS.** Text in English. 2000. q. USD 75 domestic; USD 115 foreign; USD 35 newsstand/cover (effective 2001). adv. back issues avail. *Refereed.* **Document type:** *Journal, Academic/Scholarly.* **Description:** Publishes articles, case reports, reviews, and letters that aim to improve communications in understanding the multidisciplinary field of modern mast cell research.
Related titles: Online - full text ed.: ISSN 1609-5529.
Published by: V I C E R Publishing, PO Box 14, Vienna A-1097, Austria. TEL 43-676-9568085, FAX 43-676-9568086, vicer@vicer.org, http://www.vicer.org. Ed., R&P Roland Hofbauer. adv.: B&W page USD 1,700, color page USD 2,200. Circ: 1,000 (paid and controlled).

571.6 IRL ISSN 0925-4773
QH607 CODEN: MEDVE6
MECHANISMS OF DEVELOPMENT. Text in English. 1972. 20/yr. EUR 173 in Europe to individuals; JPY 23,000 in Japan to individuals; USD 193 elsewhere to individuals; EUR 2,712 in Europe to institutions; JPY 360,000 in Japan to institutions; USD 3,034 elsewhere to institutions (effective 2002). charts, illus. back issues avail.; reprint service avail. from SWZ. *Refereed.* **Document type:** *Academic/Scholarly.* **Description:** Disseminates research in developmental biology, with emphasis on the characterization of molecular mechanisms underlying the development processes in plants and vertebrate and non vertebrate animals.
Former titles (until 1990): Cell Differentiation and Development (0922-3371); (until 1988): Cell Differentiation (0045-6039)
Related titles: Microform ed.: (from PQC); Online - full text ed.: (from EBSCO Publishing, ingenta, ScienceDirect, Swets Blackwell, Institute for Scientific Information).
Indexed: ASCA, AgBiotech, Anim.Breed.Abstr., BBCI, Biol.Abstr., Chem.Abstr., Chem.Indus.Notes, Chem.Titles, Curr.Adv.Ecol.Sci., Curr.Cont., Excerp.Med., Helminthol.Abstr., INIS Atomind., Ind.Med. (1990-), Ind.Sci.Rev., Inpharma, Int.Abstr.Biol.Sci., Neurosci.Cit.Ind., Postharvest, Reac., Rev.Appl.Entomol., Sci.Cit.Ind., Zoo.Rec.
—BLDSC (5424.571280), CASDDS, CISTI, EMDOCS, GNLM, IDS, ingenta, Linda Hall. **CCC.**
Published by: Elsevier Science Ireland Ltd, Elsevier House, Brookvale Plaza, E. Park, Shannon, Co. Clare, Ireland. TEL 353-61-709600, FAX 353-61-709100, http://www.elsevier.nl/locate/modo. Eds. H Jaumlckle, P Gruss. **Subscr. in Australasia and the Far East to:** Elsevier Science (Singapore) Pte Ltd, No.1 Temasek Ave, 17-01 Millenia Tower, Singapore 039192, Singapore. TEL 65-434-3727, FAX 65-337-2230, asiainfo@elsevier.com.sg; **Subscr. in the Americas to:** Elsevier Science, PO Box 945, New York, NY 10159-0945. TEL 212-633-3730, FAX 212-633-3680, usinfo-f@elsevier.com; **Subscr. to:** Elsevier Science Inc - Japan Regional Office, 9-15 Higashi-Azabu 1-chome, Minato-ku, Tokyo 106-0044, Japan. TEL 81-3-5561-5033, FAX 81-3-5561-5047, info@elsevier.co.jp. **Subscr. to:** Elsevier Science BV, PO Box 211, Amsterdam 1000 AE, Netherlands. TEL 31-20-485-3757, FAX 31-20-485-3432, nlinfo-f@elsevier.nl.

571.64 NLD ISSN 0927-5193
CODEN: MSSREV
MEMBRANE SCIENCE AND TECHNOLOGY SERIES. Text in English. 1991. irreg., latest vol.5, 2000. *Refereed.* **Document type:** *Monographic series, Academic/Scholarly.* **Description:** Discusses advances in membrane science and technology.
Indexed: Chem.Abstr., Chem.Cit.Ind., Chem.Indus.Notes, Chem.Titles.
—BLDSC (5548.026350), CASDDS, CISTI. **CCC.**
Published by: Elsevier Science BV, PO Box 211, Amsterdam 1000 AE, Netherlands. TEL 31-20-485-3757, 31-20-485-3911, FAX 31-20-485-3432, 31-20-485-3598, nlinfo-f@elsevier.nl, http://www.elsevier.nl/. **Subscr. in Australasia and the Far East to:** Elsevier Science (Singapore) Pte Ltd, No.1 Temasek Ave, 17-01 Millenia Tower, Singapore 039192, Singapore. TEL 65-434-3727, FAX 65-337-2230, asiainfo@elsevier.com.sg; **Subscr. in Japan to:** Elsevier Science Inc - Japan Regional Office, 9-15 Higashi-Azabu 1-chome, Minato-ku, Tokyo 106-0044, Japan. TEL 81-3-5561-5033, FAX 81-3-5561-5047, info@elsevier.co.jp; **Subscr. in the Americas to:** Elsevier Science, PO Box 945, New York, NY 10159-0945. TEL 212-633-3730, 888-437-4636, FAX 212-633-3680, usinfo-f@elsevier.com, http://www.elsevier.com

METABOLIC ENGINEERING. see *BIOLOGY—Bioengineering*

571.6 USA ISSN 0091-679X
QH585 CODEN: MCBLAG
METHODS IN CELL BIOLOGY. Text in English. 1964. irreg., latest vol.56, 1998. illus. reprint service avail. from ISI. *Refereed.*
Formerly: Methods in Cell Physiology (0091-6579)
Related titles: Online - full text ed.: (from Institute for Scientific Information).
Indexed: ASCA, BBCI, Biol.Abstr., Chem.Abstr., Chem.Indus.Notes, Chem.Titles, Excerp.Med., INIS Atomind., Ind.Med. (1973-), Ind.Sci.Rev., Nutr.Abstr., Rev.Plant Path., Sci.Cit.Ind., Zoo.Rec.
—BLDSC (5747.250000), CASDDS, CISTI, GNLM, ingenta, KNAW. **CCC.**
Published by: Academic Press, Inc., Journal Division (Subsidiary of: Harcourt Brace & Company), 525 B St, Ste 1900, San Diego, CA 92101-4495. TEL 619-231-0926, FAX 619-699-6715. Ed. Leslie Wilson. **Subscr. to:** Order Dept., 6277 Sea Harbor Dr, 4th Fl, Orlando, FL 32887. TEL 800-321-5068.

571.6 NLD ISSN 1381-5741
QH585 CODEN: MCSCFB
METHODS IN CELL SCIENCE. Text in Dutch. 1975. q. EUR 275 to institutions for print or online ed.; USD 660, EUR 330 to institutions print & online eds.combined (effective 2002). adv. back issues avail. *Refereed.* **Document type:** *Academic/Scholarly.* **Description:** Publishes papers describing techniques developed during cell, tissue and organ culture from multicellular animals and plants. Emphasis is on detailed presentation of laboratory protocols for cell tissue and organ culture.
Former titles (until 1995): Journal of Tissue Culture Methods (0271-8057); (until 1978): T C A Manual (Tissue Culture Association) (0361-0268)
Related titles: Online - full text ed.: (from EBSCO Publishing, O C L C Online Computer Library Center, Inc., RoweCom Information Quest, Swets Blackwell, Kluwer Online).
Indexed: AgBiotech, Agri.& Environ.Biotech.Abstr., Aqua.Sci.& Fish.Abstr., Bio-Contr.News & Info., Biol.Abstr. (until 1979), Biotech.& Bioeng.Abstr. (coverage dropped), CEABA, Cal.Tiss.Abstr., Chem.Abstr., Chemorec.Abstr., Curr.Cont. (coverage dropped), Dairy Sci.Abstr., Environ.Sci.Poll.Mgmt., Excerp.Med., Forest.Abstr., Helminthol.Abstr., Ind.Med. (1995-), Ind.Vet., Int.Abstr.Biol.Sci., Med.& Pharm.Biotech.Abstr., Neurosci.Abstr. (coverage dropped), Plant Breed.Abstr., Protozool.Abstr., Rev.Appl.Entomol., Vet.Bull.
—BLDSC (5747.305000), CASDDS, CISTI, GNLM, ingenta. **CCC.**
Published by: (Society of In Vitro Biology), Kluwer Academic Publishers Group (Subsidiary of: Wolters Kluwer N.V.), Spuiboulevard 50, PO Box 17, Dordrecht 3300 AA, Netherlands. FAX 31-78-639-2254, services@wkap.nl, http://www.wkap.nl. Ed. Warren I Schaeffer. **Dist. by:** Journals Department, PO Box 322, Dordrecht 3300 AH, Netherlands. TEL 781-871-6600, FAX 31-78-654-6474.

MICROBIAL PATHOGENESIS; molecular and cellular biology of infectious disease. see *MEDICAL SCIENCES—Communicable Diseases*

MITOCHONDRIA. see *BIOLOGY—Abstracting, Bibliographies, Statistics*

▼ **MITOCHONDRION.** see *BIOLOGY—Microbiology*

571.6 USA ISSN 0745-3000
CODEN: MOCBDA
MODERN CELL BIOLOGY. Text in English. 1983. irreg., latest vol.15. **Document type:** *Monographic series.*
Indexed: Chem.Abstr., Chem.Titles, Zoo.Rec.
—BLDSC (5885.410000), CASDDS, CISTI, KNAW. **CCC.**
Published by: John Wiley & Sons, Inc., Journals (Subsidiary of: Wiley InterScience), 605 Third Ave, New York, NY 10158. **Subscr. outside the Americas to:** John Wiley & Sons Ltd., Baffins Ln, Chichester, Sussex PO19 IUD, United Kingdom. FAX 44-1243-776128.

571.6 GBR
MOLECULAR AND CELL BIOLOGY OF HUMAN DISEASES. Text in English. a., latest vol.5, 1995. **Document type:** *Monographic series.*
Indexed: Chem.Abstr., Chem.Indus.Notes, Chem.Titles, Ind.Med. (coverage dropped), Rev.Appl.Entomol.
—BLDSC (5900.755000).
Published by: Chapman & Hall Ltd. (Subsidiary of: International Thomson Publishing Group), Journals Department, Chapman & Hall, 2-6 Boundary Row, London SE1 8HN, United Kingdom. TEL 44-20-7865-0066, FAX 44-20-7522-9623.

MOLECULAR AND CELLULAR BIOCHEMISTRY; an international journal for chemical biology in health and disease. see *BIOLOGY—Biochemistry*

MOLECULAR AND CELLULAR BIOLOGY. see *BIOLOGY—Biochemistry*

571.6 USA ISSN 1065-3074
QH607 CODEN: MCDIEL
MOLECULAR & CELLULAR DIFFERENTIATION. Text in English. 1992. q. USD 80 to individuals; USD 285 to institutions. **Document type:** *Academic/Scholarly.*
Indexed: Biotech.Cit.Ind. (coverage dropped), Chem.Abstr., Chem.Titles, Curr.Cont. (coverage dropped), Sci.Cit.Ind. (coverage dropped).
—CASDDS, CISTI, EMDOCS, GNLM, IDS, Infotrieve. **CCC.**
Published by: C R C Press, LLC, 2000 Corporate Blvd, N W, Boca Raton, FL 33431. TEL 561-994-0555, 800-272-7737, FAX 561-998-9784.

MOLECULAR BIOLOGY. see *BIOLOGY—Biochemistry*

MOLECULAR BIOLOGY REPORTS; an international journal on molecular and cellular biology. see *BIOLOGY—Biochemistry*

571.6 USA ISSN 1097-2765
MOLECULAR CELL. Text in English. 1997. m. EUR 3,589 in Europe to institutions; JPY 476,400 in Japan to institutions; USD 4,014 elsewhere to institutions (effective 2002). adv. back issues avail. *Refereed.* **Document type:** *Academic/Scholarly.* **Description:** Extends coverage from structure to human diseases, concentrating on molecular analyses.
Related titles: Online - full text ed.: ISSN 1097-4164. USD 80 (effective 2001) (from HighWire Pr., ingenta, Institute for Scientific Information).
Indexed: AIDS & Cancer Res., Abstr.Bull.Inst.Pap.Chem., BBCI, Biotech.& Bioeng.Abstr., Curr.Cont., Eng.Ind., Environ.Sci.Poll.Mgmt., Genet.Abstr., Hum.Gen.Abstr. (coverage dropped), Immun.Abstr., Ind.Med. (1997-), Med.& Pharm.Biotech.Abstr., Microbiol.Abstr., Neurosci.Abstr., Nuc.Acids Abstr., Oncog.G.F.Abstr., Plant Breed.Abstr., Rev.Appl.Entomol., Rev.Plant Path., Saf.Sci.Abstr., Sci.Cit.Ind., Tox.Abstr. (coverage dropped), Virol.Abstr.
—BLDSC (5900.802750), ADONIS.
Published by: Cell Press (Subsidiary of: Reed Elsevier plc), 1100 Massachusetts Ave, Cambridge, MA 02138. TEL 617-661-7057, FAX 617-661-7061, editor@cell.com, http://www.elsevier.com/locate/molbrainres, http://www.cellpress.com. Ed. Vivian Siegel. Pub. Lynne Herndon.

571.6 USA ISSN 1522-4724
QH573 CODEN: MCBCFS
MOLECULAR CELL BIOLOGY RESEARCH COMMUNICATIONS. Abbreviated title: M C B R C. Text in English. 1998. m. USD 550 in US & Canada; USD 595 elsewhere (effective 2001). **Description:** Disseminates observations of how cells interact with their environment and how they interpret and respond to the resulting stimuli.
Related titles: Online - full text ed.: (from EBSCO Publishing, O C L C Online Computer Library Center, Inc., ingenta, Swets Blackwell, IDEAL Online Library).

Indexed: Derwent Biotech.Abstr., Ind.Med.
—BLDSC (5900.802800), CINDOC, Linda Hall.
Published by: Academic Press, Inc., Journal Division (Subsidiary of: Harcourt Brace & Company), 525 B St, Ste 1900, San Diego, CA 92101-4495. TEL 619-231-6616, FAX 619-699-6715, http://www.academicpress.com, http://www.academicpress.com/ideal-alert. **Subscr. to:** Order Dept., 6277 Sea Harbor Dr, 4th Fl, Orlando, FL 32887. TEL 800-321-5068.

MOLECULAR MEMBRANE BIOLOGY. see *BIOLOGY—Biochemistry*

MOLECULAR VISION. see *BIOLOGY—Biochemistry*

MONALDI ARCHIVES FOR CHEST DISEASE. see *MEDICAL SCIENCES—Respiratory Diseases*

MONOGRAPHS IN CLINICAL CYTOLOGY. see *MEDICAL SCIENCES*

571.6 NLD ISSN 1010-8793
CODEN: NASBE4
N A T O ADVANCED SCIENCE INSTITUTES SERIES H: CELL BIOLOGY. Text in Dutch. 1986. irreg., latest vol.2, 1986. price varies. reprint service avail. from ISI. *Refereed.* **Document type:** *Monographic series.*
Formerly: N A T O Advanced Study Institute. Series H: Cell Biology
Related titles: Online - full text ed.: (from European Space Agency).
Indexed: Chem.Abstr., Chem.Indus.Notes, Chem.Titles, Zoo.Rec.
—BLDSC (6033.648830), CASDDS, CISTI, KNAW. **CCC.**
Published by: (Scientific Affairs Division BEL, North Atlantic Treaty Organization BEL), Kluwer Academic Publishers Group (Subsidiary of: Wolters Kluwer N.V.), Spuiboulevard 50, PO Box 17, Dordrecht 3300 AA, Netherlands. FAX 31-78-639-2254, services@wkap.nl, http://www.wkap.nl. **Dist. by:** Journals Department, PO Box 322, Dordrecht 3300 AH, Netherlands. FAX 31-78-654-6474.

NERVE CELL BIOLOGY. see *BIOLOGY—Abstracting, Bibliographies, Statistics*

571.6 JPN
NIHON SOSHIKI BAIYO GAKKAI KAIIN TSUSHIN/JAPANESE TISSUE CULTURE ASSOCIATION. NEWS. Text in Japanese. 4/yr. **Document type:** *Academic/Scholarly.*
Published by: Nihon Soshiki Baiyo Gakkai/Japanese Tissue Culture Association, Kinosei Pepuchido Kenkyujo, 4-3-32 Shimo-Jo-Machi, Yamagata-shi 990-0823, Japan. TEL 81-236-46-2525, FAX 81-236-46-2526. Ed. Hiroyoshi Hoshi.

571.6 IND ISSN 0029-568X
QH573 CODEN: NULSAK
NUCLEUS; international journal of cytology and allied topics. Text in English. 1958. 4/yr. INR 600, USD 60 (effective 1999). adv. bk.rev. charts, illus. index. Supplement avail.; back issues avail. *Refereed.* **Document type:** *Academic/Scholarly.*
Indexed: Anim.Breed.Abstr., Biol.Abstr., Chem.Abstr., Chem.Indus.Notes, Chem.Titles, Curr.Adv.Ecol.Sci., Environ.Sci.Poll.Mgmt., Excerp.Med., Genet.Abstr. (coverage dropped), Hort.Abstr., INIS Atomind., Microbiol.Abstr., Ornam.Hort., Plant Breed.Abstr., Pollut.Abstr., Rev.Appl.Entomol., Zoo.Rec.
—BLDSC (6184.202000), CASDDS, CISTI, ingenta, Linda Hall.
Published by: University of Calcutta, Department of Botany, Centre for Advanced Study in Cell and Chromosome Research, 35 Ballygunj Circular Rd., Kolkata, West Bengal 700 019, India. TEL 91-33-440-5802, FAX 91-33-478-7603. Ed., Adv. contact Archana Sharma. Pub. Arun Kumar Sharma. Circ: 500.

PATHOBIOLOGY; journal of immunopathology, molecular and cellular biology. see *MEDICAL SCIENCES—Allergology And Immunology*

PERSPECTIVES IN CYTOLOGY & GENETICS; proceedings of the all India Congress of cytology and genetics. see *BIOLOGY—Genetics*

571.6 DNK ISSN 0893-5785
QL767 CODEN: PCREEA
PIGMENT CELL RESEARCH. Text in English. bi-m. USD 384 in the Americas to institutions print & online eds. combined; GBP 267 elsewhere to institutions print & online eds. combined (effective 2002). adv. charts, illus. reprints avail. *Refereed.* **Document type:** *Academic/Scholarly.*
Related titles: Online - full text ed.: USD 346 (effective 2002) (from EBSCO Publishing, ingenta, Munksgaard & Blackwell Science's Synergy, Swets Blackwell, Institute for Scientific Information).
Indexed: ASCA, BBCI, Biol.Abstr., Chem.Abstr., Chem.Titles, Curr.Cont., INIS Atomind., Ind.Med. (1987-), Inpharma, Med.& Surg.Dermat., Pharm.&Out.News, Reac., Sci.Cit.Ind., Zoo.Rec.
—BLDSC (6500.148000), CASDDS, CISTI, GNLM, IDS, Infotrieve, KNAW. **CCC.**
Published by: (International Federation of Pigment Cell Societies), Blackwell Munksgaard, Noerre Soegade 35, PO Box 2148, Copenhagen K 1016, Denmark. TEL 45-77-33-33-33, FAX 45-77-33-33-77, fsub@mail.munksgaard.dk, http://www.blackwellmunksgaard.com/pcr. Ed. Vincent Hearing. Circ: 600.

571.6 GBR ISSN 0032-0781
QK710 CODEN: PCPHA5
PLANT AND CELL PHYSIOLOGY. Text in English. 1960. m. GBP 145, USD 230 to individuals; GBP 325, USD 525 to institutions (effective 2002). adv. index. 144 p./no. back issues avail. *Refereed.* **Document type:** *Journal, Academic/Scholarly.* **Description:** Covers broad areas of plant sciences, including physiology, biochemistry, biophysics, chemistry, molecular and cell biology, as well as gene engineering of plants and microorganisms.
Related titles: Microform ed.: (from PMC); Online - full text ed.: GBP 292, USD 472 to institutions Online only (effective 2002) (from HighWire Pr., Swets Blackwell, Institute for Scientific Information).
Indexed: ASCA, Abstr.Bull.Inst.Pap.Chem., AgBiotech, Agri.& Environ.Biotech.Abstr., Agricola, Agroforest.Abstr., Aqua.Sci.& Fish.Abstr., BBCI, Bibl.Agri., Biol.& Agr.Ind. (1989-), Biol.Abstr., Cal.Tiss.Abstr., Chem.Abstr., Chem.Titles, Crop Physiol.Abstr., Curr.Adv.Plant Sci., Curr.Cont., Derwent Biotech.Abstr., Environ.Sci.Poll.Mgmt., Fababean Abstr., Field Crop Abstr., Food Sci.& Tech.Abstr., Forest Prod.Abstr., Forest.Abstr., Genet.Abstr., Herb.Abstr., Hort.Abstr., Hum.Gen.Abstr., INIS Atomind., Ind.Med. (1959-), Ind.Sci.Rev., Int.Abstr.Biol.Sci., Irr.& Drain.Abstr., Maize Abstr., Microbiol.Abstr., Ornam.Hort., Plant Breed.Abstr., Plant Grow.Reg.Abstr., Plant Sci., Postharvest, Potato Abstr., Ref.Zh., Rev.Appl.Entomol., Rev.Arom.& Med.Plants, Rev.Plant Path., Rice Abstr., Sci.Cit.Ind., Seed Abstr., Soils & Fert., Soyabean Abstr., Triticale Abstr., Weed Abstr.
—BLDSC (6512.250000), CASDDS, CISTI, EMDOCS, ingenta, Linda Hall. **CCC.**
Published by: (Japanese Society of Plant Physiologists/Nihon Shokubutsu Seiri Gakkai JPN), Oxford University Press, Academic Division, Great Clarendon St, Oxford OX2 6DP, United Kingdom. TEL 44-1865-267907, FAX 44-1865-267835, jspp@nacos.com, jnl.info@oup.co.uk, http://www.pcp.oupjournals.org/, http://www.oup.co.uk/journals. Pub. Janet Boullin. R&P Fionna Willis. Circ: 3,400. **Subscr. in the Americas to:** Oxford University Press, Journals, 2001 Evans Rd, Cary, NC 27513. TEL 800-852-7323, FAX 919-677-1714, jnlorders@oup-usa.org; **Subscr. to:** Journals Marketing, Great Clarendon St, Oxford OX2 6DP, United Kingdom.

571.5 NLD ISSN 0167-6857
CODEN: PTCEDJ
PLANT CELL, TISSUE AND ORGAN CULTURE; an international journal on in vitro culture of higher plants. Text in English. 1981. m. EUR 1,512 to institutions for print or online ed.; USD 1,814.40, EUR 1,814.40 to institutions print & online eds.combined (effective 2002). adv. bk.rev. back issues avail.; reprint service avail. from SWZ. *Refereed.* **Document type:** *Academic/Scholarly.* **Description:** Publishes original results of fundamental research on plant cells, tissues and organs, including plant genetics and biotechnology.
Related titles: Microform ed.: (from PQC); Online - full text ed.: (from EBSCO Publishing, O C L C Online Computer Library Center, Inc., RoweCom Information Quest, Swets Blackwell, Kluwer Online, Institute for Scientific Information).
Indexed: ASCA, Abstr.Bull.Inst.Pap.Chem., AgBiotech, Agricola, Agroforest.Abstr., Bibl.Agri., Bio-Contr.News & Info., Biol.Abstr., Biotech.Cit.Ind., CEABA, Chem.Abstr., Chem.Indus.Notes, Chem.Titles, Cott.& Trop.Fibr.Abstr., Crop Physiol.Abstr., Curr.Adv.Ecol.Sci., Curr.Adv.Plant Sci., Curr.Biotech.Abstr., Curr.Cont., Derwent Biotech.Abstr., Eng.Ind., Environ.Abstr., Field Crop Abstr., Food Sci.& Tech.Abstr., Forest.Abstr., Helminthol.Abstr., Herb.Abstr., Hort.Abstr., Ind.Sci.Rev., Int.Abstr.Biol.Sci., Maize Abstr., Ornam.Hort., Plant Breed.Abstr., Plant Gen.Res.Abstr., Plant Grow.Reg.Abstr., Plant Sci., Potato Abstr., Rev.Appl.Entomol., Rev.Arom.& Med.Plants, Rev.Plant Path., Rice Abstr., Sci.Cit.Ind., Seed Abstr., Soils & Fert., Soyabean Abstr., Sugar Ind.Abstr., Telegen, Triticale Abstr., VITIS, Weed Abstr.
—BLDSC (6514.300000), CASDDS, CISTI, Ei, EMDOCS, IDS, Infotrieve, ingenta, Linda Hall. **CCC.**
Published by: Kluwer Academic Publishers Group (Subsidiary of: Wolters Kluwer N.V.), Spuiboulevard 50, PO Box 17, Dordrecht 3300 AA, Netherlands. FAX 31-78-639-2254, services@wkap.nl, http://www.wkap.nl. **Dist. by:** Journals Department, PO Box 322, Dordrecht 3300 AH, Netherlands. TEL 781-871-6600, FAX 31-78-654-6474.

B

571.6 POL ISSN 0324-833X
QH573 CODEN: PBKODV
POSTEPY BIOLOGII KOMORKI/ADVANCES IN CELL BIOLOGY. Text in Polish; Summaries in English. 1974. q. PLZ 25 to individuals; PLZ 68 to institutions; USD 20 foreign (effective 2000). bk.rev. bibl, illus. *Refereed.* **Document type:** *Academic/Scholarly.*
Indexed: AgroLibrex, Biol.Abstr., Chem.Abstr., Chem.Indus.Notes, Chem.Titles, INIS Atomind., Ref.Zh.
—CASDDS.
Published by: (Polskie Towarzystwo Anatomiczne/Polish Anatomical Society), Fundacja Postepu Biologii Komorki, Ul Marymoncka 99, Warsaw 01813, Poland. TEL 48-22-8340344, FAX 48-22-8340470, jkawiak@cmkp.edu.pl, http://www.mol.uj.pl/pbk. Ed., R&P Jerzy Kawiak. Circ: 640. **Co-sponsor:** Polskie Towarzystwo Biologii Komorki/Polish Society for Cell Biology.

PROGRESS AND TOPICS IN CYTOGENETICS. see *BIOLOGY—Genetics*

571.6 USA ISSN 1087-2957
QH605 CODEN: PCCRF9
PROGRESS IN CELL CYCLE RESEARCH. Text in English. 1995. a., latest vol.4, 1999.
Indexed: Chem.Abstr., Chem.Indus.Notes, Chem.Titles, Ind.Med. (1995-).
—BLDSC (6866.750000), CASDDS, Infotrieve. **CCC.**
Published by: Kluwer Academic - Plenum Publishers (Subsidiary of: Wolters Kluwer N.V.), 233 Spring St, New York, NY 10013-1578. TEL 212-620-8000, 800-221-9369, FAX 212-463-6742, info@plenum.com, http://www.plenum.com.

PROGRESS IN HISTOCHEMISTRY AND CYTOCHEMISTRY. see *BIOLOGY—Biochemistry*

571.6 USA ISSN 0079-6484
QH506 CODEN: PMSBA4
PROGRESS IN MOLECULAR AND SUBCELLULAR BIOLOGY. Text in English. 1969. irreg., latest vol.9, 1985. price varies. reprint service avail. from ISI. *Refereed.* **Document type:** *Academic/Scholarly.*
Indexed: Agricola, Biol.Abstr., Chem.Abstr., Chem.Titles, Ind.Med. (1969-), Zoo.Rec.
—CASDDS, CISTI, GNLM, Infotrieve, ingenta, KNAW, Linda Hall. **CCC.**
Published by: Springer-Verlag, Journals (Subsidiary of: BertelsmannSpringer), 175 Fifth Ave, New York, NY 10010. TEL 212-460-1500, FAX 212-473-6272. Ed. F E Hahn.

REFERATIVNYI ZHURNAL. TSITOLOGIYA. see *BIOLOGY—Abstracting, Bibliographies, Statistics*

RESEARCH COMMUNICATIONS IN BIOCHEMISTRY AND CELL & MOLECULAR BIOLOGY. see *BIOLOGY—Biochemistry*

571.6 USA ISSN 0080-1844
QH607 CODEN: RCLDAT
RESULTS AND PROBLEMS IN CELL DIFFERENTIATION. Text in English. 1968. irreg., latest vol.20, 1994. price varies. reprint service avail. from ISI. **Document type:** *Academic/Scholarly.*
Indexed: Biol.Abstr., Chem.Abstr., Chem.Indus.Notes, Chem.Titles, Ind.Med. (1968-), Zoo.Rec.

—BLDSC (7780.220000), CASDDS, CISTI, GNLM, Infotrieve, ingenta, KNAW. **CCC.**

Published by: Springer-Verlag, Journals (Subsidiary of: BertelsmannSpringer), 175 Fifth Ave, New York, NY 10010. TEL 212-460-1500, FAX 212-473-6272.

RIBOSOMES AND TRANSLATION. see *BIOLOGY—Abstracting, Bibliographies, Statistics*

571.6 GBR ISSN 1084-9521
QH573 CODEN: SCDBFX

SEMINARS IN CELL AND DEVELOPMENTAL BIOLOGY. Text in English. 1996. bi-m. GBP 285 to institutions (effective 2001). adv. reprint service avail. from SWZ. *Refereed.* **Document type:** *Academic/Scholarly.* **Description:** Covers the latest advances in molecular cell biology and developmental biology.

Formed by the merger of (1990-1996): Seminars in Cell Biology (1043-4682); (1990-1996): Seminars in Developmental Biology (1044-5781)

Related titles: Online - full text ed.: (from EBSCO Publishing, O C L C Online Computer Library Center, Inc., RoweCom Information Quest, ingenta, Swets Blackwell, IDEAL Online Library, Institute for Scientific Information).

Indexed: ASCA, Aqua.Sci.& Fish.Abstr., Biotech.& Bioeng.Abstr., Chem.Abstr., Chem.Indus.Notes, Chem.Titles, Chemorec.Abstr., Curr.Cont., Genet.Abstr., Hum.Gen.Abstr., Ind.Med. (1996-), Ind.Sci.Rev., Inpharma, Neurosci.Abstr., Nuc.Acids Abstr., Reac., Sci.Cit.Ind., Zoo.Rec.

—BLDSC (8239.448346), ADONIS, CASDDS, CISTI, GNLM, IDS, Infotrieve, ingenta, KNAW, Linda Hall. **CCC.**

Published by: Academic Press (Subsidiary of: Harcourt Publishers Ltd.), 24 Oval Rd, London NW1 7DX, United Kingdom. TEL 44-20-7267-4466, FAX 44-20-7482-2293, apsubs@acad.com, http://www.academicpress.com/semcdb; http://www.europe.idealibrary.com/. Ed. Alan Colman. R&P Catherine John. Adv. contact Nik Screen. **Subscr. to:** Harcourt Publishers Ltd., Foots Cray High St, Sidcup, Kent DA14 5HP, United Kingdom. TEL 44-20-8300-3322, FAX 44-20-8309-0807.

SEMINARS IN HEMATOLOGY. see *MEDICAL SCIENCES—Hematology*

SEMINARS IN RESPIRATORY INFECTIONS. see *MEDICAL SCIENCES—Respiratory Diseases*

571.6 JPN ISSN 0915-3896

SHINKEI SOSHIKI NO SEICHO SAISEI ISHOKU/NEURAL GROWTH, REGENERATION AND TRANSPLANTATION. Text in Japanese. 1989. a. **Document type:** *Academic/Scholarly.*

Published by: (Shinkei Soshiki no Seicho Saisei Ishoku Kenkyukai/Japanese Society for Neural Growth, Regeneration and Transplantation), Nyuronsha, 21-19-305 Higashi-Gotanda 5-chome, Shinagawa-ku, Tokyo 141-0022, Japan.

571.6 CHN ISSN 0001-5334
QH301 CODEN: SYSWAE

SHIYAN SHENGWU XUEBAO/ACTA BIOLOGIAE EXPERIMENTALIS SINICA. Variant title: Shih Yen Sheng Wu Hsueh Pao. Text in Chinese; Summaries in English. 1936. q. CNY 12 domestic; USD 33.20 foreign (effective 1999). adv. charts, illus. back issues avail. *Refereed.* **Document type:** *Academic/Scholarly.* **Description:** Covers cell biology and publishes papers of experimental biology mainly in the fields of cell biology, developmental biology, reproductive biology, cancer biology, and immunobiology.

Indexed: Biol.Abstr., Chem.Abstr., Chem.Indus.Notes, Chem.Titles, Curr.Adv.Ecol.Sci., GeoRef, Ind.Med. (1953-), Ind.Vet., Pig News & Info., Zoo.Rec.

—BLDSC (0601.700000), CASDDS, CISTI, GNLM, Linda Hall.

Published by: (Shanghai Xibao Shengwu Yanjiusuo/Shanghai Institute of Cell Biology), Shanghai Scientific & Technical Publishers, Ruijin Er Rd, Shanghai 200020, China. TEL 86-21-64736055, FAX 86-21-64730679, edto@sunm.shcnc.ac.cn. Ed. Wang Yahui. Adv. contact Ping Luo. **Subscr. to:** China International Book Trading Corp, 35 Chegongzhuang Xilu, Haidian District, Beijing 100044, China. TEL 86-10-68411769, FAX 86-10-68420340, bk@mail.cibtc.com.cn, http://www.cibtc.com.cn/.

571.6 DEU ISSN 1615-4053

▼ **SIGNAL TRANSDUCTION**; receptors, mediators and genes. Text in English. 2001. 4/yr. EUR 358 in Europe; CHF 698 in Switzerland & Liechtenstein; USD 358 elsewhere; EUR 376 combined subscription in Europe for print and online eds.; CHF 733 combined subscription in Switzerland & Liechtenstein, for print and online eds.; USD 376 combined subscription elsewhere for print and online eds. (effective 2002). abstr. reprints avail. *Refereed.* **Document type:** *Journal, Academic/Scholarly.* **Description:** Covers all stages of signal transfer between cell surface and nucleus as well as the control of general cell physiology in normal and transformed cells.

Related titles: Online - full content ed.: ISSN 1615-4061. 2000.

Published by: Wiley - V C H, Postfach 101161, Weinheim 69451, Germany. TEL 49-6201-606-0, FAX 49-6201-606-328, signaltrans@wiley-vch.de, adsales@wiley-vch.de, subservice@wiley-vch.de, http://www.signaltrans.de, http://www.wiley-vch.de. R&P Claudia Rutz. Adv. contact Aenne Anders TEL 49-6201-606552.

SOMATIC CELL AND MOLECULAR GENETICS. see *BIOLOGY—Genetics*

571.6 JPN ISSN 0912-3636

SOSHIKI BAIYO KENKYU/TISSUE CULTURE RESEARCH COMMUNICATIONS. Text mainly in English; Text occasionally in Japanese. 1982. 4/yr. JPY 6,000. *Refereed.* **Document type:** *Academic/Scholarly.* **Description:** Covers cytology and histology, biological chemistry, biotechnology, genetics, physiology, cell biology and molecular biology.

Published by: Nihon Soshiki Baiyo Gakkai/Japanese Tissue Culture Association, Kinosei Pepuchido Kenkyujo, 4-3-32 Shimo-Jo-Machi, Yamagata-shi 990-0823, Japan. TEL 81-236-46-2525, FAX 81-236-46-2526. Ed. Hiroyoshi Hoshi. Circ: 1,200.

571.6 JPN

SOSHIKI SAIBO KAGAKU KOSHUKAI/COURSE TEXT OF HISTOCHEMISTRY AND CYTOCHEMISTRY. Text in Japanese. 1976. a. JPY 6,000.

Indexed: Chem.Abstr., Chem.Indus.Notes, Chem.Titles.

Published by: (Nihon Soshiki Saibo Kagakkai/Japan Society of Histochemistry and Cytochemistry), Gakusai Kikaku K.K., 5-24 Mejiro 2-chome, Toshima-ku, Tokyo 171-0031, Japan.

571.6 GBR ISSN 0040-8166
QH573 CODEN: TICEBI

TISSUE & CELL. Text in English. 1969. bi-m. GBP 494 to individuals (effective 2002). adv. abstr, charts, illus. index. *Refereed.* **Document type:** *Journal, Academic/Scholarly.* **Description:** Presents research papers on the organization of cells, their components and extracellular products.

Related titles: Microform ed.: (from PQC); Online - full text ed.: (from EBSCO Publishing, RoweCom Information Quest, Swets Blackwell, IDEAL Online Library, Institute for Scientific Information).

Indexed: ASCA, AgBiotech, Agroforest.Abstr., Anim.Breed.Abstr., Apic.Abstr., Aqua.Sci.& Fish.Abstr., Aquacult.Abstr., BBCI, Biol.Abstr., Biol.Dig., Cal.Tiss.Abstr., Chem.Abstr., Chem.Indus.Notes, Chem.Titles, Chemorec.Abstr., Curr.Adv.Ecol.Sci., Curr.Cont., Dairy Sci.Abstr., Entomol.Abstr., Excerp.Med., Helminthol.Abstr., INIS Atomind., Ind.Med. (1969-), Ind.Sci.Rev., Ind.Vet., Inpharma, Int.Abstr.Biol.Sci., Neurosci.Abstr. (coverage dropped), Nutr.Abstr., Plant Breed.Abstr., Plant Grow.Reg.Abstr., Poult.Abstr., Protozool.Abstr., Reac., Ref.Zh., Rev.Appl.Entomol., Rev.Med.& Vet.Mycol., Sci.Cit.Ind., Sport Fish.Abstr., Trop.Dis.Bull., Vet.Bull., Zoo.Rec.

—BLDSC (8858.680000), CASDDS, CISTI, GNLM, IDS, ingenta, KNAW, Linda Hall. **CCC.**

Published by: Churchill Livingstone (Subsidiary of: Harcourt Publishers Ltd.), Robert Stevenson House, 1-3 Baxter's Pl, Leith Walk, Edinburgh, Midlothian EH1 3AF, United Kingdom. TEL 44-131-556-2424, FAX 44-131-459-1177, cservice@harcourt.com, http://www.harcourt-international.com/journals/tice. Ed. L D Russell. Pub. Gillian Griffith. R&P Catherine John TEL 212-424-4200. Adv. contact David Dunnachie. Circ: 660. **Subscr. to:** Harcourt Publishers Ltd., Foots Cray High St, Sidcup, Kent DA14 5HP, United Kingdom. TEL 44-20-8308-5700, FAX 44-20-8309-0807.

TISSUE CULTURE. see *BIOLOGY—Abstracting, Bibliographies, Statistics*

571.5 USA ISSN 1076-3279
CODEN: TIENFP

TISSUE ENGINEERING. Text in English. 1993. bi-m. USD 159 domestic to individuals; USD 267 foreign to individuals; USD 191 domestic to individuals print and online eds. combined; USD 299 foreign to individuals print and online eds. combined; USD 394 domestic to institutions; USD 498 foreign to institutions; USD 473 domestic to institutions print and online eds combined.; USD 577 foreign to institutions print and online eds. combined (effective 2002). back issues avail.; reprints avail. *Refereed.* **Document type:** *Journal, Academic/Scholarly.* **Description:** Provides information on an interdisciplinary field dedicated to engineering new tissue that applies the principles and methods of engineering and the life sciences toward the fundamental understanding of structure-function relationships in normal and pathologic tissue and the development of biological substitutes.

Related titles: Online - full content ed.: USD 159 to individuals; USD 394 to institutions (effective 2002) (from EBSCO Publishing, O C L C Online Computer Library Center, Inc., Swets Blackwell); Online - full text ed.: (from CatchWord Ltd., Institute for Scientific Information, RoweCom Information Quest).

Indexed: Biotech.& Bioeng.Abstr., Biotech.Cit.Ind., Cal.Tiss.Abstr., Chem.Abstr., Chem.Indus.Notes, Chem.Titles, Curr.Cont., Excerp.Med., Ind.Med. (1995-), Med.& Pharm.Biotech.Abstr., Sci.Cit.Ind.

—CASDDS, CatchWord, CISTI, IDS, Infotrieve. **CCC.**

Published by: (Tissue Engineering Society), Mary Ann Liebert, Inc. Publishers, 2 Madison Ave, Larchmont, NY 10538. TEL 914—834-3100, FAX 914-834-1388, info@liebertpub.com, www.liebertpub.com/ten, http://www.liebertpub.com. Eds. Anthony G Mikos, Charles A Vacanti.

571.6 CHE ISSN 0250-0868
CODEN: IJTEDP

TISSUE REACTIONS. Text in English. q. CHF 400 (effective 2002). *Refereed.* **Document type:** *Journal, Academic/Scholarly.* **Description:** Contains the results of research on problems related to alterations of physiological origin, either experimentally induced or of a pathogenic nature, which occur at cellular or tissue levels.

Related titles: Online - full text ed.: (from Institute for Scientific Information).

Indexed: Aqua.Sci.& Fish.Abstr., Curr.Cont., Derwent Biotech.Abstr., Ind.Med. (1980-), Ref.Zh., Sci.Cit.Ind.

—BLDSC (4542.695600), CASDDS, CISTI, EMDOCS, GNLM, IDS, ingenta, KNAW. **CCC.**

Published by: Bioscience Ediprint Inc., Rue Alexandre Gavard 16, Carouge 1227, Switzerland. TEL 41-22-3003383, FAX 41-22-3002489, bioscience.smey@gkb.com. Ed. A Bertelli.

571.6 DNK ISSN 1398-9219

▼ **TRAFFIC**; the international journal of intracellular transport. Text in English. 2000. m. USD 149 in the Americas to individuals; USD 432 elsewhere to institutions (effective 2002). adv. bk.rev. index. back issues avail. *Refereed.* **Document type:** *Journal, Academic/Scholarly.* **Description:** Publishes research and review articles dealing with structural biology, cell biology, protein biochemistry, molecular biology, morphology, intracellular signalling and genetic and infectious diseases in for mammalian and non-mammalian systems.

Related titles: Online - full text ed.: 2000. USD 130 to individuals; USD 389 to institutions (effective 2002) (from EBSCO Publishing, O C L C Online Computer Library Center, Inc., ingenta, Munksgaard & Blackwell Science's Synergy, Swets Blackwell, Institute for Scientific Information).

Indexed: Curr.Cont., Ind.Med.

—BLDSC (8881.575000).

Published by: Blackwell Munksgaard, Noerre Soegade 35, PO Box 2148, Copenhagen K 1016, Denmark. TEL 45-77-33-33-33, FAX 45-77-33-33-77, customerservice@munksgaard.dk, http://www.traffic.dk, http://www.blackwellmunksgaard.com. Ed. Lisa Hannan.

TRANSPLANTATION PROCEEDINGS. see *MEDICAL SCIENCES—Surgery*

571.6 GBR ISSN 0962-8924
QH573 CODEN: TCBIEK
TRENDS IN CELL BIOLOGY. Text in English. 1991. m. GBP 92 in Europe to individuals; EUR 115 elsewhere to individuals; JPY 14,000 in Japan to individuals; USD 126 elsewhere to individuals; EUR 9,081 in Europe to institutions; JPY 125,900 in Japan to institutions; USD 1,015 elsewhere to institutions; GBP 47 in Europe to students; JPY 10,100 in Japan to students; USD 78 elsewhere to students; USD 1,308 to institutions Print & online eds. combined; EUR 144 to qualified personnel; JPY 17,500 in Japan to qualified personnel; USD 157 elsewhere to qualified personnel (effective 2002). adv. bk.rev., software rev. illus. index. back issues avail.; reprints avail. *Refereed.* **Document type:** *Academic/Scholarly.* **Description:** Provides comprehensive coverage of new research developments, methodologies, and theories in all specializations of cell biology.
Related titles: Online - full text ed.: (from ingenta, Swets Blackwell, Institute for Scientific Information, ScienceDirect).
Indexed: AIDS & Cancer Res., AIDS Abstr., ASCA, Aqua.Sci.& Fish.Abstr., BBCI, Chem.Abstr., Chem.Indus.Notes, Curr.Cont., Excerp.Med. (1992-), Genet.Abstr., Hum.Gen.Abstr., Immun.Abstr., Ind.Med. (1991-), Ind.Sci.Rev., Inpharma, Int.Abstr.Biol.Sci., Neurosci.Abstr., Nuc.Acids Abstr., Pharm.&Out.News, Reac., Ref.Zh., Sci.Cit.Ind.
—BLDSC (9049.552000), ADONIS, CASDDS, CISTI, EMDOCS, GNLM, IDS, Infotrieve, ingenta. **CCC.**
Published by: Elsevier Science Ltd., Elsevier Trends Journals, 68 Hills Rd, Cambridge CB2 1LA, United Kingdom. TEL 44-1223-315961, FAX 44-1223-464430, TCB@elsevier.co.uk, http://www.elsevier.com/locate/09628924. Eds. D Hatton, Deborah Sweet, P Carmeliet. Adv. contact Thelma Reid. **Subscr. in Australasia and the Far East to:** Elsevier Science (Singapore) Pte Ltd, No.1 Temasek Ave, 17-01 Millenia Tower, Singapore 039192, Singapore. TEL 65-434-3727, FAX 65-337-2230; **Subscr. in the Americas to:** Elsevier Science, PO Box 945, New York, NY 10159-0945. TEL 212-633-3730, FAX 212-633-3680, http://www.elsevier.com; **Subscr. to:** Elsevier Current Trends Subscriptions, PO Box 331, Haywards Heath, W Sussex RH16 3FG, United Kingdom. TEL 44-1444-475650, FAX 44-1444-445423.

TRENDS IN MICROBIOLOGY. see *BIOLOGY—Microbiology*

571.6 RUS ISSN 0041-3771
QH573 CODEN: TSITAQ
TSITOLOGIYA/CYTOLOGY. Text in Russian; Abstracts and contents page in English. 1959. m. USD 258. adv. bk.rev. charts, illus. index. *Refereed.*
Indexed: AgBiotech, Agri.& Environ.Biotech.Abstr. (coverage dropped), Anim.Breed.Abstr., Bio-Contr.News & Info., Biol.Abstr., Chem.Abstr., Crop Physiol.Abstr., Curr.Adv.Ecol.Sci., Curr.Cont. (coverage dropped), Dairy Sci.Abstr., Derwent Biotech.Abstr., Excerp.Med., Field Crop Abstr., Forest.Abstr., Herb.Abstr., Hort.Abstr., INIS Atomind., Ind.Med. (1959-), Ind.Vet., Maize Abstr., Ornam.Hort., Pig News & Info., Plant Breed.Abstr., Plant Gen.Res.Abstr., Plant Grow.Reg.Abstr., Potato Abstr., Protozool.Abstr., Ref.Zh., Rev.Appl.Entomol., Rev.Arom.& Med.Plants, Rev.Med.& Vet.Mycol., Rev.Plant Path., Sci.Cit.Ind. (coverage dropped), Seed Abstr., Soils & Fert., Triticale Abstr., Zoo.Rec.
—CASDDS, CISTI, East View, GNLM, KNAW, Linda Hall. **CCC.**
Published by: (Rossiiskaya Akademiya Nauk/Russian Academy of Sciences), M A I K Nauka - Interperiodica, S.-Peterburgskoe Otdelenie, Mendeleevskaya liniya 1, St Petersburg 199034, Russian Federation. Ed. N N Nikol'skii. Pub. S V Valchuk. Adv. contact N Ya. Shubina. page USD 100. Circ: 600. **US dist. addr.:** East View Publications, 3020 Harbor Ln N, Minneapolis, MN 55447. TEL 612-550-0961.

TSITOLOGIYA I GENETIKA; mezhdunarodnyi nauchnyi zhurnal. see *BIOLOGY—Genetics*

ZHONGGUO XIUFU CHONGJIAN WAIKE ZAZHI/CHINESE JOURNAL OF REPARATIVE AND RECONSTRUCTIVE SURGERY. see *MEDICAL SCIENCES—Surgery*

BIOLOGY—Entomology

see also AGRICULTURE—Crop Production And Soil
ENGINEERING—Chemical Engineering

ABSTRACTS OF ENTOMOLOGY. see *BIOLOGY—Abstracting, Bibliographies, Statistics*

THE ANNALS OF MEDICAL ENTOMOLOGY. see *MEDICAL SCIENCES*

BIOCONTROL SCIENCE AND TECHNOLOGY. see *AGRICULTURE—Crop Production And Soil*

595.7 DEU ISSN 0179-5295
CODEN: BIZEE6
BIOLOGISCHE ZEITSCHRIFT. Text in German. 1986. irreg. price varies. adv. bk.rev.
Indexed: Arts & Hum.Cit.Ind. (coverage dropped), Zoo.Rec. (until 19??).
Published by: Research and Consulting Institute, Lister Weg 40, Hamburg 22117, Germany. Ed. R Sergel.

595.7 NLD
CATALOGUE OF PALAEARCTIC DIPTERA. Text in Dutch. 1984. irreg., latest vol.7, 1991. price varies. illus. *Refereed.* **Document type:** *Monographic series, Catalog, Academic/Scholarly.* **Description:** Catalogs the main taxonomic nomenclatorial and distribution data of some 25,000 fly species from the arctic regions.
Published by: Elsevier Science BV, PO Box 211, Amsterdam 1000 AE, Netherlands. TEL 31-20-485-3757, 31-20-485-3911, FAX 31-20-485-3432, 31-20-485-3598, nlinfo-f@elsevier.nl; usinfo-f@elsevier.com; forinfo-kyf04035@niftyserve.or.jp, http://www.elsevier.nl/. Eds. A Soos, L Papp. **Subscr. in Australasia and the Far East to:** Elsevier Science (Singapore) Pte Ltd, No.1 Temasek Ave, 17-01 Millenia Tower, Singapore 039192, Singapore. TEL 65-434-3727, FAX 65-337-2230, asiainfo@elsevier.com.sg; **Subscr. in Japan to:** Elsevier Science Inc - Japan Regional Office, 9-15 Higashi-Azabu 1-chome, Minato-ku, Tokyo 106-0044, Japan. TEL 81-3-5561-5033, FAX 81-3-5561-5047, info@elsevier.co.jp; **Subscr. in the Americas to:** Elsevier Science, PO Box 945, New York, NY 10159-0945. TEL 212-633-3730, 888-437-4636, FAX 212-633-3680, usinfo-f@elsevier.com, http://www.elsevier.com

595.7 DEU ISSN 0344-9084
QL461
DEUTSCHE GESELLSCHAFT FUER ALLGEMEINE UND ANGEWANDTE ENTOMOLOGIE. MITTEILUNGEN. Text in English, German. 1978. irreg. (approx. biennial). price varies. back issues avail. **Document type:** *Bulletin, Academic/Scholarly.*
Indexed: Agroforest.Abstr., Bio-Contr.News & Info., Fababean Abstr., Forest Prod.Abstr., Forest.Abstr., Helminthol.Abstr., Maize Abstr., Postharvest, Potato Abstr., Protozool.Abstr., Ref.Zh., Rev.Appl.Entomol., Rev.Plant Path., Weed Abstr., Zoo.Rec.
—BLDSC (5839.380000).
Published by: Deutsche Gesellschaft fuer Allgemeine und Angewandte Entomologie, Schicklerstr 5, Eberswalde 16225, Germany. TEL 49-3334-589818, FAX 49-3334-212379, blank@dei-eberswalde.de, http://www.dgaae.de.

595.7 USA ISSN 0273-7353
E S A NEWSLETTER. Text in English. 1978. m. USD 18 domestic to individuals; USD 24 foreign to individuals; USD 35 domestic to institutions; USD 41 foreign to institutions (effective 2001). adv. back issues avail. **Document type:** *Newsletter, Academic/Scholarly.* **Description:** Contains feature articles, meeting announcements, listing of employment opportunities, notices of grants and awards, member profiles, and branch and section news.
Published by: Entomological Society of America, 9301 Annapolis Rd, Lanham, MD 20706. TEL 301-731-4535, FAX 301-731-4538, esa@entsoc.org, http://www.entsoc.org. Circ: 9,000 (paid).

595.7 USA ISSN 0013-8746
QL461 CODEN: AESAAI
ENTOMOLOGICAL SOCIETY OF AMERICA. ANNALS; devoted to the interest of classical entomology. Text in English. 1908. bi-m. USD 84 domestic to individuals; USD 104 foreign to individuals; USD 162 domestic to institutions; USD 182 foreign to institutions (effective 2000). adv. bk.rev. abstr, bibl, charts, illus. index. reprints avail. *Refereed.* **Document type:** *Journal, Academic/Scholarly.* **Description:** Devoted to the basic aspects of the biology of insects.
Related titles: Microform ed.: (from MIM,PQC,PMC); ♦ Online - full content ed.: Entomological Society of America. Annals Online; Online - full text ed.: (from Institute for Scientific Information).
Indexed: ASCA, Abstr.Hyg., AgBiotech, Agri.Eng.Abstr., Agricola, Anim.Behav.Abstr., Appl.Ecol.Abstr., Aqua.Sci.& Fish.Abstr., Bibl.Agri., Bio-Contr.News & Info., Biodet.Abstr., Biol.& Agr.Ind. (Mar.1983-), Biol.Abstr., Chem.Abstr., Chem.Indus.Notes, Chem.Titles, Chemorec.Abstr., Cott.& Trop.Fibr.Abstr., Curr.Adv.Cell & Devel.Biol., Curr.Adv.Ecol.Sci., Curr.Cont., Curr.Ind.Stat., Derwent Biotech.Abstr., Ecol.Abstr., Entomol.Abstr., Environ.Per.Bibl. (1972-), Environ.Sci.Poll.Mgmt., Excerp.Med., Field Crop Abstr., Forest.Abstr., Genet.Abstr., Geol.Abstr., Helminthol.Abstr., Hort.Abstr., Hum.Gen.Abstr., INIS Atomind., Ind.Sci.Rev., Ind.Vet., Maize Abstr., Plant Breed.Abstr., Postharvest, Potato Abstr., Poult.Abstr., Protozool.Abstr., Rev.Appl.Entomol., Rev.Med.& Vet.Mycol., Rev.Plant Path., Sci.Cit.Ind., Seed Abstr., Soils & Fert., Soyabean Abstr., Sport Fish.Abstr., Triticale Abstr., Trop.Dis.Bull., Vet.Bull., Weed Abstr., Wild.Rev., Zoo.Rec.
—BLDSC (1025.000000), CASDDS, CISTI, GNLM, IDS, Infotrieve, ingenta, Linda Hall. **CCC.**
Published by: Entomological Society of America, 9301 Annapolis Rd, Lanham, MD 20706. TEL 301-731-4535, FAX 301-731-4538, esa@entsoc.org, http://www.entsoc.org/pubs. Eds. Carl W Schaefer, Leo Lachance. Circ: 2,800. **Subscr. to:** PO Box 177, Hyattsville, MD 20781-0177.

595.7 USA
ENTOMOLOGICAL SOCIETY OF AMERICA. ANNALS ONLINE. Text in English. bi-m. USD 124 to individuals; USD 242 to institutions (effective 2000). *Refereed.* **Document type:** *Academic/Scholarly.*
Media: Online - full content (from BioOne). **Related titles:** Microform ed.: (from MIM,PQC,PMC); Online - full text ed.: (from Institute for Scientific Information); ♦ Print ed.: Entomological Society of America. Annals. ISSN 0013-8746.
Published by: Entomological Society of America, 9301 Annapolis Rd, Lanham, MD 20706. TEL 301-731-4535, FAX 301-731-4538, esa@entsoc.org, http://www.entsoc.org/pubs.

ENTOMOLOGY ABSTRACTS. see *BIOLOGY—Abstracting, Bibliographies, Statistics*

595.7 USA ISSN 0046-225X
SB599 CODEN: EVETBX
ENVIRONMENTAL ENTOMOLOGY. Text in English. 1972. bi-m. USD 90 domestic to individuals; USD 110 foreign to individuals; USD 194 domestic to institutions; USD 214 foreign to institutions; USD 25 domestic to members; USD 45 foreign to members (effective 2000). adv. abstr, bibl, charts, illus, stat. index. reprint service avail. from PQC. *Refereed.* **Document type:** *Journal, Academic/Scholarly.* **Description:** Reports of research on the interaction of insects with the biological, chemical, and physical aspects of their environment.
Related titles: Microform ed.: (from MIM,PQC); Online - full text ed.: (from BioOne, Institute for Scientific Information); ♦ Print ed.: Environmental Entomology Online.
Indexed: ASCA, AgBiotech, Agri.& Environ.Biotech.Abstr., Agri.Eng.Abstr., Agricola, Agroforest.Abstr., Anim.Behav.Abstr., Apic.Abstr., Appl.Ecol.Abstr., Aqua.Sci.& Fish.Abstr., Bibl.Agri., Bio-Contr.News & Info., Biol.& Agr.Ind. (Apr.1983-), Biol.Abstr., Chem.Abstr., Chem.Indus.Notes, Chem.Titles, Chemorec.Abstr., Cott.& Trop.Fibr.Abstr., Crop Physiol.Abstr., Curr.Adv.Ecol.Sci., Curr.Adv.Plant Sci., Curr.Cont., Curr.Ind.Stat., Ecol.Abstr., Energy Info.Abstr., Entomol.Abstr., Environ.Abstr., Environ.Per.Bibl. (1972-), Environ.Sci.Poll.Mgmt., Excerp.Med., Fababean Abstr., Field Crop Abstr., Forest Prod.Abstr., Forest.Abstr., Genet.Abstr., Helminthol.Abstr., Herb.Abstr., Hort.Abstr., Hum.Gen.Abstr., INIS Atomind., Ind.Sci.Rev., Ind.Vet., Int.Abstr.Biol.Sci., Irr.& Drain.Abstr., Maize Abstr., Microbiol.Abstr., Nutr.Abstr., Plant Breed.Abstr., Plant Sci., Pollut.Abstr., Postharvest, Potato Abstr., Poult.Abstr., Protozool.Abstr., Rev.Appl.Entomol., Rev.Med.& Vet.Mycol., Rev.Plant Path., Rice Abstr., Sci.Cit.Ind., Seed Abstr., Soils & Fert., Sorghum & Millets Abstr., Soyabean Abstr., Sport Fish.Abstr., Triticale Abstr., Vet.Bull., Weed Abstr., Wild.Rev., Zoo.Rec.
—BLDSC (3791.464000), CASDDS, CISTI, EMDOCS, IDS, ingenta, Linda Hall. **CCC.**
Published by: Entomological Society of America, 9301 Annapolis Rd, Lanham, MD 20706. TEL 301-731-4535, FAX 301-731-4538, esa@entsoc.org, http://www.entsoc.org. Circ: 3,100.

595.7 USA
ENVIRONMENTAL ENTOMOLOGY ONLINE. Text in English. bi-m. USD 130 to individuals; USD 274 to institutions (effective 2000). *Refereed.* **Document type:** *Academic/Scholarly.*

Related titles: ♦ Print ed.: Environmental Entomology. ISSN 0046-225X.
Published by: Entomological Society of America, 9301 Annapolis Rd, Lanham, MD 20706. TEL 301-731-4535, FAX 301-731-4538, esa@entsoc.org, http://www.entsoc.org/pubs.

595.7 CZE ISSN 1210-5759
QL461 CODEN: EJENE2
EUROPEAN JOURNAL OF ENTOMOLOGY. Text and summaries in English. 1904. q. USD 65 in Europe to individuals; USD 85 elsewhere to individuals; USD 160 in Europe to institutions; USD 180 elsewhere to institutions (effective 2001). adv. bk.rev. bibl, charts, illus. 128 p./no. *Refereed.* **Document type:** *Journal, Academic/Scholarly.* **Description:** Includes articles on all aspects of entomology (taxonomy, morphology, physiology, ecology, zoogeography, applied entomology), Myriapoda, Chelicerata and terrestrial Crustacea.
Formerly (until vol.90, 1993): Acta Entomologica Bohemoslovaca (0001-5601)
Related titles: Online - full text ed.: (from Institute for Scientific Information).
Indexed: ASCA, Anim.Behav.Abstr., Apic.Abstr., Appl.Ecol.Abstr., Aqua.Sci.& Fish.Abstr., Bio-Contr.News & Info., Biol.Abstr., Biotech.& Bioeng.Abstr. (coverage dropped), Chem.Abstr., Chem.Indus.Notes, Chem.Titles, Chemorec.Abstr., Curr.Adv.Ecol.Sci., Curr.Adv.Gen.& Molec.Biol., Curr.Cont., Ecol.Abstr., Entomol.Abstr., Environ.Sci.Poll.Mgmt., Forest.Abstr., Genet.Abstr. (coverage dropped), Geol.Abstr., Helminthol.Abstr., Hort.Abstr., Hum.Gen.Abstr., IBR, Microbiol.Abstr., Plant Gen.Res.Abstr., Postharvest, Ref.Zh., Rev.Appl.Entomol., Rev.Med.& Vet.Mycol., Sci.Cit.Ind., Triticale Abstr., Weed Abstr., Zoo.Rec.
—BLDSC (3829.728850), CASDDS, CISTI, IDS, ingenta, Linda Hall.
Published by: Ceska Akademie Ved, Entomologicky Ustav/Czech Academy of Sciences, Institute of Entomology, Branisovska 31, Ceske Budejovice 37005, Czech Republic. TEL 420-38-7775213, FAX 420-38-5300354, eje@entu.cas.cz, http://www.entu.cas.cz/eje. Eds. Ivo Hodek, Petr Svacha TEL 420-38-7775258. R&P Petr Svacha adv.: page USD 100; 17 x 24.7. Circ: 400.

595.70948 NLD ISSN 0106-8377
CODEN: FESCDE
FAUNA ENTOMOLOGICA SCANDINAVICA. Text in English. 1973. irreg., latest vol.35, 1998. price varies. illus. back issues avail. *Refereed.* **Document type:** *Monographic series, Academic/Scholarly.* **Description:** Scholarly studies aiding in the identification and study of specific insect classes indigenous to Fennoscandia and Denmark.
Indexed: Aqua.Sci.& Fish.Abstr., Biol.Abstr., Genet.Abstr. (coverage dropped), Hum.Gen.Abstr., Zoo.Rec.
—BLDSC (3897.945000).
Published by: (Societas Entomologica Scandinavica), Brill Academic Publishers, PO Box 9000, Leiden 2300 PA, Netherlands. TEL 31-71-535-3500, FAX 31-71-531-7532, cs@brill.nl. Ed. N P Kristensen. R&P Elizabeth Venekamp.

595.7 MEX ISSN 0430-8603
QL477 CODEN: FEMXAA
FOLIA ENTOMOLOGICA MEXICANA. Text and summaries in English, Spanish. 1961. 3/yr. MXP 250 domestic; USD 35 foreign (effective 2001). adv. bk.rev. abstr, bibl, charts, illus. index, cum.index: 1961-1971. *Refereed.* **Document type:** *Journal, Academic/Scholarly.* **Description:** Presents papers on physiology, morphology, systematics, ecology, and all experimental and applied branches of entomology, arachnology and acarology.
Related titles: Microfilm ed.: (from OMN).
Indexed: Apic.Abstr., Aqua.Sci.& Fish.Abstr., Bio-Contr.News & Info., Biol.Abstr., Entomol.Abstr., Genet.Abstr., Hort.Abstr., Hum.Gen.Abstr., Maize Abstr., Poult.Abstr., Ref.Zh., Rev.Appl.Entomol., Rev.Med.& Vet.Mycol., Soils & Fert., Zoo.Rec.
—Linda Hall.
Published by: Sociedad Mexicana de Entomologia, A.C., Consejo Editorial Folia Entomologica Mexicana, Apdo. Postal 63, Xalapa, VERACRUZ 91000, Mexico. TEL 52-28-421800, FAX 52-28-187809, folia@ecologia.edu.mx, http://www.ecologia.edu.mx/folentmex. Ed., R&P Sergio Ibanez-Bernal. Adv. contact Arturo Bonet Ceballos. Circ: 800.

HESSISCHE FAUNISTISCHE BRIEFE. see *BIOLOGY—Zoology*

595.7 FRA ISSN 0245-0151
INSECTES. Text in French. 1979. q. FRF 185; FRF 50 newsstand/cover (effective 1998). **Description:** Covers different aspects of entomology from biology, environmental protection to agricultural techniques.
Indexed: Zoo.Rec.
Published by: Office pour l'Information Eco-Entomologique, BP 9, Guyancourt Cedex 78041, France. TEL 33-1-30441343. Ed. Remi Coutin. Pub. Robert Guilbot.

595.7 USA
INSECTIMES✱ . Text in English. q.
Published by: Nor-Am Chemical Company, PO Box 12014, Research Triangle Park, NC 27709-2014. TEL 302-477-3014, FAX 302-477-3013. Circ: 19,000.

595.7 BEL ISSN 0374-6232
CODEN: BIETBB
INSTITUT ROYAL DES SCIENCES NATURELLES DE BELGIQUE. BULLETIN. SERIE ENTOMOLOGIE. Text in English. 1930. a., latest vol.70, 2000. BEF 1,500, USD 30 domestic; BEF 1,750 foreign (effective 2000). bibl, charts, illus. cum.index. back issues avail. **Document type:** *Academic/Scholarly.*
Indexed: Biol.Abstr., GeoRef, Ref.Zh., Rev.Appl.Entomol., Sport Fish.Abstr., Wild.Rev., Zoo.Rec.
—Linda Hall.
Published by: Koninklijk Belgisch Instituut voor Natuurwetenschappen/Institut Royal des Sciences Naturelles de Belgique, Vautierstraat 29, Brussels 1000, Belgium. TEL 32-2-6274211, FAX 32-2-6274113, rib@naturalsciences.be, http://www.naturalsciences.be. Ed. L Baert. Circ: 1,500.

632.7 GBR ISSN 0020-8256
SB950 CODEN: IPCLBZ
INTERNATIONAL PEST CONTROL; crop protection, public health, wood preservation. Text in English. 1959. bi-m. GBP 79, USD 142 (effective 2000). adv. bk.rev. charts, illus, tr.lit. index. **Document type:** *Academic/Scholarly.* **Description:** Deals with all aspects of pest eradication and prevention.
Indexed: Abstr.Hyg., Agri.& Environ.Biotech.Abstr. (coverage dropped), Agri.Eng.Abstr., Agroforest.Abstr., Bio-Contr.News & Info., Biol.& Agr.Ind. (Jan.1983-Jan.1989), Biol.Abstr., CBNB (1985-), Chem.Abstr., Chem.Indus.Notes, Chem.Titles, Derwent Biotech.Abstr., Environ.Per.Bibl. (1972-), Excerp.Med., Field Crop Abstr., Forest Prod.Abstr., Forest.Abstr., Herb.Abstr., Hort.Abstr., Ind.Vet., Maize Abstr., PROMT, Postharvest, Poult.Abstr., Rev.Appl.Entomol., Rev.Arom.& Med.Plants, Rev.Med.& Vet.Mycol., Rev.Plant Path., Seed Abstr., Small Anim.Abstr., Soils & Fert., Soyabean Abstr., Sport Fish.Abstr., Triticale Abstr., Trop.Dis.Bull., Vet.Bull., Weed Abstr., Wild.Rev., Zoo.Rec.
—BLDSC (4544.910000), CASDDS, ingenta, Linda Hall.
Published by: Research Information Ltd., 222 Maylands Ave, Hemel Hempstead Rd, Hemel Hempstead, Herts HP3 8LA, United Kingdom. TEL 44-20-8328-2471, FAX 44-1442-259395, info@resinf.co.uk, http://www.users.globalnet.co.uk/~resinf. Ed. David Macdonald. Pub. Kumar Patel. Adv. contact Ras Patel. B&W page GBP 576. Circ: 4,800.

595.7 USA ISSN 0022-0493
SB599 CODEN: JEENAI
JOURNAL OF ECONOMIC ENTOMOLOGY. Text in English. 1908. bi-m. USD 95 domestic to individuals; USD 115 foreign to individuals; USD 194 domestic to institutions; USD 214 foreign to institutions; USD 25 domestic to members; USD 45 foreign to members (effective 2000). adv. bk.rev. bibl, charts, illus. index. back issues avail.; reprints avail. *Refereed.* **Document type:** *Journal, Academic/Scholarly.* **Description:** Reports on the economic significance of insects.
Related titles: Microform ed.: (from PQC,PMC); ♦ Online - full content ed.: Journal of Economic Entomology Online; Online - full text ed.: (from BioOne, Institute for Scientific Information).
Indexed: ASCA, Abstr.Hyg., AgBiotech, Agri.& Environ.Biotech.Abstr., Agri.Eng.Abstr., Agricola, Agroforest.Abstr., Anim.Behav.Abstr., Apic.Abstr., Appl.Ecol.Abstr., Aqua.Sci.& Fish.Abstr., Bibl.Agri., Bio-Contr.News & Info., Biol.& Agr.Ind. (Feb.1983-), Biol.Abstr., Biol.Dig., Chem.Abstr., Chem.Indus.Notes, Chem.Titles, Chemorec.Abstr., Cott.& Trop.Fibr.Abstr., Crop Physiol.Abstr., Curr.Adv.Gen.& Molec.Biol., Curr.Adv.Plant Sci., Curr.Cont., Curr.Ind.Stat., Dairy Sci.Abstr., Derwent Biotech.Abstr., Entomol.Abstr., Environ.Per.Bibl. (1972-), Environ.Sci.Poll.Mgmt., Excerp.Med., Field Crop Abstr., Food Sci.& Tech.Abstr., Forest Prod.Abstr., Forest.Abstr., Genet.Abstr., Helminthol.Abstr., Herb.Abstr., Hort.Abstr., Hum.Gen.Abstr., INIS Atomind., Ind.Med. (1908-), Ind.Sci.Rev., Ind.Vet., Int.Abstr.Biol.Sci., Irr.& Drain.Abstr., Maize Abstr., Microbiol.Abstr., Nutr.Abstr., Ornam.Hort., Plant Breed.Abstr., Plant Gen.Res.Abstr., Plant Grow.Reg.Abstr., Plant Sci., Postharvest, Potato Abstr., Poult.Abstr., Protozool.Abstr., Psychol.Abstr., Rev.Appl.Entomol., Rev.Arom.& Med.Plants, Rev.Med.& Vet.Mycol., Rev.Plant Path., Rice Abstr., Risk Abstr., Rural Recreat.Tour.Abstr., SSCI (coverage dropped), Sci.Cit.Ind., Seed Abstr., Small Anim.Abstr., Soils & Fert., Sorghum & Millets Abstr., Soyabean Abstr., Sport Fish.Abstr., Sugar Ind.Abstr., THA, Triticale Abstr., Trop.Dis.Bull., Trop.Oil Seeds Abstr., VITIS, Vet.Bull., Weed Abstr., Wild.Rev., World Ag.Econ.& Rur.Soc.Abstr., Zoo.Rec.
—BLDSC (4973.000000), CASDDS, CISTI, EMDOCS, GNLM, IDS, ingenta, Linda Hall. **CCC.**
Published by: Entomological Society of America, 9301 Annapolis Rd, Lanham, MD 20706. TEL 301-731-4535, FAX 301-731-4538, esa@entsoc.org, http://www.entsoc.org/pubs. Circ: 4,300.

595.7 616.968 USA ISSN 0022-2585
RA639.5 CODEN: JMENA6
JOURNAL OF MEDICAL ENTOMOLOGY. Text in English. 1964. bi-m. USD 84 domestic to individuals; USD 104 foreign to individuals; USD 1,620 domestic to institutions; USD 182 foreign to institutions; USD 25 domestic to members; USD 45 foreign to members (effective 2000). adv. bk.rev. bibl, charts, illus, maps. index. back issues avail.; reprint service avail. from PQC. *Refereed.* **Document type:** *Journal, Academic/Scholarly.* **Description:** Covers all phases of medical entomology.
Related titles: Microform ed.: (from PQC); ♦ Online - full content ed.: Journal of Medical Entomology Online; Online - full text ed.: (from BioOne, Institute for Scientific Information).
Indexed: ASCA, Abstr.Hyg., AgBiotech, Agri.& Environ.Biotech.Abstr. (coverage dropped), Agricola, Agroforest.Abstr., Anim.Behav.Abstr., Appl.Ecol.Abstr. (coverage dropped), Aqua.Sci.& Fish.Abstr., Bibl.Agri., Bio-Contr.News & Info., Biol.Abstr., Biol.Dig., Chem.Abstr., Chem.Titles, Chemorec.Abstr., Curr.Adv.Ecol.Sci., Curr.Cont., Dent.Ind., Derwent Biotech.Abstr., Entomol.Abstr., Environ.Per.Bibl. (1993-1994), Environ.Sci.Poll.Mgmt., Excerp.Med., Focus on: Vet.Sci.& Med., Genet.Abstr., Helminthol.Abstr., Hum.Gen.Abstr., INIS Atomind., Ind.Med. (1964-), Ind.Sci.Rev., Ind.Vet., Maize Abstr., Poult.Abstr., Protozool.Abstr., Ref.Zh., Rev.Appl.Entomol., Rev.Arom.& Med.Plants, Rev.Med.& Vet.Mycol., Rice Abstr., Sci.Cit.Ind., Small Anim.Abstr., So.Pac.Per.Ind., Sport Fish.Abstr., Trop.Dis.Bull., Vet.Bull., Weed Abstr., Wild.Rev., Zoo.Rec.
—BLDSC (5017.060000), CASDDS, CISTI, GNLM, IDS, ingenta, Linda Hall. **CCC.**
Published by: Entomological Society of America, 9301 Annapolis Rd, Lanham, MD 20706. TEL 301-731-4538, FAX 301-731-4538, esa@entsoc.org, http://www.entsoc.org/pubs. Eds. C Dayton Steelman, William K Reisen. Circ: 1,600. **Subscr. to:** Allen Press Inc., PO Box 1897, Lawrence, KS 66044-8897.

595.7 616.968 USA
JOURNAL OF MEDICAL ENTOMOLOGY ONLINE. Text in English. bi-m. USD 124 to individuals; USD 242 to institutions (effective 2000). *Refereed.* **Document type:** *Academic/Scholarly.*
Media: Online - full content. **Related titles:** ♦ Print ed.: Journal of Medical Entomology. ISSN 0022-2585.
Published by: Entomological Society of America, 9301 Annapolis Rd, Lanham, MD 20706. TEL 301-731-4535, FAX 301-731-4538, esa@entsoc.org, http://www.entsoc.org/pubs.

595.7 USA ISSN 0022-8567
QL461 CODEN: JKESA7
KANSAS ENTOMOLOGICAL SOCIETY. JOURNAL. Text in English. 1928. q. USD 85 to institutions; USD 88 in Canada & Mexico to institutions; USD 100 elsewhere to institutions (effective 1999). bk.rev. abstr, bibl, charts, illus. index. back issues avail.; reprint service avail. from PQC. *Refereed.* **Document type:** *Academic/Scholarly.* **Description:** Covers research on all aspects of the science of entomology.
Related titles: Microform ed.: (from PQC); Online - full text ed.: (from Institute for Scientific Information).
Indexed: ASCA, Agricola, Appl.Ecol.Abstr. (coverage dropped), Aqua.Sci.& Fish.Abstr., Bio-Contr.News & Info., Biol.Abstr., Chem.Abstr., Chemorec.Abstr., Curr.Adv.Ecol.Sci., Curr.Cont., Ecol.Abstr., Entomol.Abstr. (coverage dropped), Forest Prod.Abstr., Forest.Abstr., Helminthol.Abstr., Herb.Abstr., Hort.Abstr., Maize Abstr., Plant Breed.Abstr., Postharvest, Protozool.Abstr., Rev.Appl.Entomol., Rev.Med.& Vet.Mycol., Sci.Cit.Ind., Seed Abstr., Soils & Fert., Sorghum & Millets Abstr., Soyabean Abstr., Sport Fish.Abstr., Triticale Abstr., Weed Abstr., Wild.Rev., Zoo.Rec.
—BLDSC (4810.400000), CISTI, ingenta, Linda Hall.
Published by: Kansas Entomological Society, PO Box 1897, Lawrence, KS 66044-8897. TEL 785-843-1235, FAX 785-843-1274, orders@allenpress.com, http://www.allenpress.com. Ed. Leonard Ferrington. Circ: 800. **Subscr. to:** Allen Press Inc., PO Box 1897, Lawrence, KS 66044-8897. **Co-sponsor:** Central States Entomological Society.

595.7 CHN ISSN 0454-6296
QL461 CODEN: KCHPA2
KUNCHONG XUEBAO/ACTA ENTOMOLOGICA SINICA. Text in Chinese; Summaries in English. 1950. q. USD 96 (effective 2000). adv. index. *Refereed.* **Document type:** *Academic/Scholarly.* **Description:** Contains theses dealing with insect faunistics, systematics, morphology, physiology, ecology, insecticide toxicology, and pathology, especially concerning injurious and beneficial insects in agriculture, forestry, animal husbandry, and medicine.
Indexed: ASCA, Apic.Abstr., Aqua.Sci.& Fish.Abstr., Bio-Contr.News & Info., Biol.Abstr., Chem.Abstr., Chem.Indus.Notes, Chem.Titles, Cott.& Trop.Fibr.Abstr., Curr.Adv.Ecol.Sci., Ecol.Abstr., Entomol.Abstr. (coverage dropped), Fababean Abstr., Forest.Abstr., GeoRef, Geol.Abstr., Helminthol.Abstr., Hort.Abstr., Ind.Vet., Maize Abstr., Plant Breed.Abstr., Ref.Zh., Rev.Appl.Entomol., Rev.Med.& Vet.Mycol., Rev.Plant Path., Rice Abstr., Sci.Cit.Ind. (coverage dropped), Trop.Oil Seeds Abstr., Weed Abstr., Zoo.Rec.
—BLDSC (0615.500000), CASDDS, CISTI, Linda Hall.
Published by: (Chinese Academy of Sciences/Zhongguo Kexueyuan), Kexue Chubanshe/Science Press, 16 Donghuang Cheng Genbei Jie, Beijing 100717, China. Ed. Qin Junde. Circ: 11,000.

MEDICAL & VETERINARY ENTOMOLOGY. see *MEDICAL SCIENCES*

▼ **MEDICAL & VETERINARY ENTOMOLOGY ONLINE.** see *MEDICAL SCIENCES*

OSAKA-SHIRITSU SHIZENSHI HAKUBUTSUKAN SHUZO SHIRYO MOKUROKU/OSAKA MUSEUM OF NATURAL HISTORY. SPECIAL PUBLICATIONS. see *BIOLOGY*

PARASITICA. see *BIOLOGY*

REVIEW OF MEDICAL AND VETERINARY ENTOMOLOGY. see *MEDICAL SCIENCES—Abstracting, Bibliographies, Statistics*

595.7 JPN ISSN 0915-2652
SF542.75.J3 CODEN: SKNHEK
SANSHI KONCHU NOGYO GIJUTSU KENKYUSHO HOKOKU/NATIONAL INSTITUTE OF SERICULTURAL AND ENTOMOLOGICAL SCIENCE. BULLETIN. Text in Japanese. 1990. irreg. (1-2/yr).
Indexed: Ref.Zh., Zoo.Rec.
—BLDSC (2640.532000).
Published by: National Institute of Sericultural and Entomological Science, 1-2 Owashi, Tsukuba-shi, Ibaraki-ken 305-0851, Japan.

595.7 ITA ISSN 0037-8747
SOCIETA ENTOMOLOGICA ITALIANA. MEMORIE. Text in Italian. 1922. a. ITL 50,000 domestic; ITL 75,000 foreign.
Indexed: Aqua.Sci.& Fish.Abstr., Entomol.Abstr., Genet.Abstr. (coverage dropped), Hum.Gen.Abstr., Rev.Appl.Entomol., Zoo.Rec.
—CISTI, Linda Hall.
Published by: Societa Entomologica Italiana, Via Brigata Liguria, 9, Genoa, GE 16121, Italy.

595.7 FRA
STATION BIOLOGIQUE DE BESSE EN CHANDESSE. ANNALES. Text in English, French, German. 1966. a. FRF 100, USD 15. back issues avail.
Indexed: Aqua.Sci.& Fish.Abstr., Aquacult.Abstr., Biol.Abstr., Curr.Adv.Ecol.Sci., Environ.Sci.Poll.Mgmt.
Published by: Universite Clermont II, Station Biologique Besse, BP 45, Aubiere 63170, France.

595.7 DNK ISSN 1398-8700
WORLD CATALOGUE OF INSECTS. Text in English. 1998. irreg., latest vol.2, 1999. price varies. bibl. *Refereed.* **Document type:** *Catalog, Academic/Scholarly.* **Description:** Features Worldscale, authoritative catalogues of monophyletic insect taxa containing standard nomenclatural information on all names pertaining to the taxon treated, including type locality and distribution to the extent this is relevant.
Indexed: Zoo.Rec.
Published by: Apollo Books Aps, Kirkeby Sand 19, Stenstrup 5771, Denmark. TEL 45-62-26-37-37, FAX 45-62-26-37-80, apollobooks@vip.cybercity.dk, http://www.apollobooks.com. Ed. M Hansen.

BIOLOGY—Genetics

576.5 YUG ISSN 0534-0012
QH431.A1 CODEN: GNTKDF
ACTA BIOLOGICA IUGOSLAVICA. SERIJA F: GENETIKA*. Key Title: Genetika. Text in Serbo-Croatian. 1969. 3/yr. price varies. **Document type:** *Academic/Scholarly.*
Indexed: Chem.Abstr., Curr.Adv.Ecol.Sci., Curr.Cont. (coverage dropped).
—CASDDS, CISTI, Linda Hall.
Published by: Unija Bioloskih Naucnih Drustava Jugoslavije/Yugoslav Union of Biological Sciences, Kneza Milosa 101-111, Belgrade 11000, Yugoslavia. TEL 381-11-615315, pedja@bf.bio.bg.ac.yu. Ed. Dr. Vitko Soric. **Co-sponsor:** Drustvo Geneticara Jugoslavije.

576.5 URY ISSN 0797-6852
ACTA GENETICA ET TERATOLOGICA. Text in Spanish; Summaries in English. 1991. a. USD 20. illus. index. back issues avail. **Document type:** *Academic/Scholarly.*
Published by: Fernando Mane-Garzon, Ed. & Pub., Casilla de Correo 157, Montevideo, Uruguay. Circ: 500.

599.9 ITA ISSN 0001-5660
CODEN: AGMGAK
ACTA GENETICAE MEDICAE ET GEMELLOLOGIAE: TWIN RESEARCH. Text in Italian. 1952. q. USD 300 (effective 1998 & 1999). adv. bk.rev. abstr, bibl, charts, illus. index. reprint service avail. from ISI.
Formerly (until 1979): Acta Geneticae Medicae et Gemellologiae (1120-9623)
Related titles: Microfilm ed.
Indexed: A.I.C.P., ASCA, Abstr.Anthropol., Biol.Abstr., Curr.Adv.Ecol.Sci., Curr.Cont. (coverage dropped), Dairy Sci.Abstr., Dent.Ind., Excerp.Med., Helminthol.Abstr., INIS Atomind., Ind.Med. (1952-), Ind.Sci.Rev., PsycInfo, Psychol.Abstr. (1976-), SSCI (coverage dropped), Sci.Cit.Ind. (coverage dropped), e-psyche.
—BLDSC (0618.000000), CISTI, EMDOCS, GNLM, ingenta, KNAW.
Published by: Associazione Istituto di Genetica Medica e Gemellologia Gregorio Mendel, Piazza Galeno, 5, Rome, RM 00161, Italy. TEL 39-6-8554658, FAX 39-6-44291069, mendel@mclink.it, http://www.mendel.it. Ed. Luigi Gedda.

576.5 CZE ISSN 0085-0748
CODEN: FMDLAJ
ACTA MUSEI MORAVIAE. SUPPLEMENTUM: FOLIA MENDELIANA. Text in English, French, German; Summaries in English. 1966. a. USD 18 (effective 2000). **Document type:** *Academic/Scholarly.*
Related titles: ♦ Supplement to: Moravske Zemske Muzeum. Casopis. Vedy Biologicke. ISSN 1211-8788.
Indexed: A.I.C.P., Biol.Abstr.
—KNAW, Linda Hall.
Published by: Moravske Zemske Muzeum, Zelny trh 6, Brno 65937, Czech Republic. TEL 42-5-42321205, FAX 42-5-42212792, mzm@mzm.anet.cz, mzm.@mzm.anet.cz. Ed. Anna Matalova.

576.5 USA ISSN 0065-2660
QH431.A1 CODEN: ADGEAV
ADVANCES IN GENETICS. Text in English. 1947. irreg., latest vol.37, 1997. reprint service avail. from ISI. *Refereed.* **Document type:** *Monographic series.*
Incorporates (1991-1995): Molecular Genetic Medicine (1057-2805)
Related titles: Online - full text ed.: (from Institute for Scientific Information); ♦ Supplement: Advances in Genetics. Supplement. ISSN 0065-2679.
Indexed: ASCA, Abstr.Hyg., Anim.Breed.Abstr., Aqua.Sci.& Fish.Abstr., Biol.& Agr.Ind. (Jan.1984-), Biol.Abstr., Biotech.& Bioeng.Abstr., Biotech.Cit.Ind., Chem.Abstr., Chem.Indus.Notes, Chem.Titles, Cott.& Trop.Fibr.Abstr., Curr.Adv.Ecol.Sci., Derwent Biotech.Abstr., Genet.Abstr., Hum.Gen.Abstr., INIS Atomind., Ind.Med. (1947-), Ind.Sci.Rev., Nuc.Acids Abstr., Plant Breed.Abstr., Poult.Abstr., Rev.Appl.Entomol., Sci.Cit.Ind., Sport Fish.Abstr., Telegen, Trop.Dis.Bull.
—BLDSC (0708.000000), CASDDS, CISTI, GNLM, ingenta, Linda Hall. **CCC.**
Published by: Academic Press, Inc., Journal Division (Subsidiary of: Harcourt Brace & Company), 525 B St, Ste 1900, San Diego, CA 92101-4495. TEL 619-231-0926, FAX 619-699-6715. Ed. M Demerec. **Subscr. to:** Order Dept., 6277 Sea Harbor Dr, 4th Fl, Orlando, FL 32887. TEL 800-321-5068.

576.5 USA ISSN 0065-2679
ADVANCES IN GENETICS. SUPPLEMENT. Text in English. 1966. irreg. price varies. **Document type:** *Monographic series.*
Related titles: ♦ Supplement to: Advances in Genetics. ISSN 0065-2660.
—CISTI, Linda Hall.
Published by: Academic Press, Inc., Journal Division (Subsidiary of: Harcourt Brace & Company), 525 B St, Ste 1900, San Diego, CA 92101-4495. TEL 619-230-1840, FAX 619-699-6800. **Subscr. to:** Order Dept., 6277 Sea Harbor Dr, 4th Fl, Orlando, FL 32887. TEL 800-321-5068.

572.86 USA ISSN 1067-5701
QH447 CODEN: AGBIE9
ADVANCES IN GENOME BIOLOGY. Text in English. 1992. irreg. USD 128.50 per vol.. **Document type:** *Academic/Scholarly.*
Indexed: Chem.Abstr., Chem.Indus.Notes, Chem.Titles.
—CASDDS, CISTI, GNLM, Infotrieve. **CCC.**
Published by: J A I Press Inc., 100 Prospect St, Box 811, Stamford, CT 06904-0811. TEL 203-323-9606, FAX 203-357-8446. Ed. Ram Verma.

599.9 USA ISSN 0065-275X
QH431.A1 CODEN: ADHGA8
ADVANCES IN HUMAN GENETICS. Text in English. 1970. irreg., latest vol.23, 1998. price varies. *Refereed.* **Document type:** *Monographic series.*
Related titles: Online - full text ed.: (from Institute for Scientific Information).
Indexed: ASCA, Biol.& Agr.Ind. (Jan.1989-Jan.1994), Biol.Abstr., Biotech.Cit.Ind., Chem.Abstr., Chem.Indus.Notes, Curr.Adv.Ecol.Sci., Excerp.Med., INIS Atomind., Ind.Med. (1970-), Ind.Sci.Rev., Int.Abstr.Biol.Sci., Sci.Cit.Ind.
—CASDDS, CISTI, EMDOCS, GNLM, IDS, ingenta, KNAW, Linda Hall. **CCC.**
Published by: Kluwer Academic - Plenum Publishers (Subsidiary of: Wolters Kluwer N.V.), 233 Spring St, New York, NY 10013-1578. TEL 212-620-8000, 800-221-9369, FAX 212-463-0742, info@plenum.com, http://www.plenum.com. Eds. K Hirschhorn, R J Desnick.

576.5 NGA ISSN 0795-6762
AFRICAN JOURNAL OF GENETICS. Text in English. q. USD 15. **Document type:** *Academic/Scholarly.*
Related titles: French ed.: Journal Africain de Genetique.
Published by: Global Press, Ugbowo, PO Box 10123, Benin City, Nigeria. TEL 234-52-200250, TELEX 41365. Ed. O S A Aromose.

599.9 USA ISSN 0002-9297
QH431.A1 CODEN: AJHGAG
AMERICAN JOURNAL OF HUMAN GENETICS; a record of research, review and bibliographic material relating to heredity in man. Text in English. 1948. m., latest vol.68, 2001, Jan. USD 695 in United States to institutions All subscribers; USD 783.65 in Canada to institutions All subscribers; USD 735 elsewhere to institutions All subscribers; USD 61.90 newsstand/cover All subscribers (effective Sep. 2002). adv. bk.rev. charts, illus, stat. index. reprints avail. *Refereed.* **Document type:** *Academic/Scholarly.* **Description:** Examines research into and the application of genetic principles in medicine, psychology, anthropology, and social services, as well as in related areas of molecular and cell biology.
Related titles: Microform ed.: (from MIM,PQC); Online - full text ed.: (from EBSCO Publishing, Gale Group, Institute for Scientific Information).

B

Indexed: A.I.C.P., ASCA, Abstr.Anthropol., Abstr.Hyg., Anim.Breed.Abstr., Bibl.Asian Stud. (1971), Bibl.Dev.Med.& Child Neur., Biol.& Agr.Ind. (Jan.1990-), Biol.Abstr., Biostat., Biotech.& Bioeng.Abstr., Biotech.Cit.Ind., Chem.Abstr., Chem.Indus.Notes, Chem.Titles, Chic.Per.Ind., Curr.Adv.Cancer Res., Curr.Adv.Ecol.Sci., Curr.Adv.Gen.& Molec.Biol., Curr.Cont., Curr.Ind.Stat., DSH Abstr., Dairy Sci.Abstr., Excerp.Med., Focus on: Mol.Med., Gen.Sci.Ind. (Jul.1997-), Genet.Abstr., Helminthol.Abstr., Hum.Gen.Abstr., INIS Atomind., Ind.Med. (1949-), Ind.Sci.Rev., Inpharma, Int.Abstr.Biol.Sci., Med.& Surg.Dermat., Neurosci.Abstr., Neurosci.Cit.Ind., Nuc.Acids Abstr., Pharm.&Out.News, Reac., Sci.Cit.Ind., So.Pac.Per.Ind., Sociol.Abstr., Sport Fish.Abstr., THA, Telegen.
—BLDSC (0825.000000), ADONIS, CASDDS, CISTI, EMDOCS, GNLM, IDS, ingenta, KNAW, Linda Hall. **CCC.**

Published by: (American Society of Human Genetics), University of Chicago Press, Journals Division, PO Box 37005, Chicago, IL 60637. TEL 773-702-7600, FAX 312-702-0694, subscriptions@journals.uchicago.edu, subscriptions@press.uchicago.edu, http://www.journals.uchicago.edu/AJHG/home.html. Ed. Stephen T. Warren. adv.: page USD 385; trim 10.88 x 8.25. Circ: 3,000 (paid).

576.5 USA ISSN 0148-7299
RB155 CODEN: AJMGDA

AMERICAN JOURNAL OF MEDICAL GENETICS. Text in English. 1977. 36/yr. USD 7,850 in United States; USD 8,250 in Canada & Mexico; USD 8,590 elsewhere; USD 8,243 combined subscription in United States for print and online eds.; USD 8,643 combined subscription in Canada & Mexico for print and online eds.; USD 8,983 combined subscription elsewhere for print and online eds. (effective 2002). adv. bk.rev. charts, illus. index. back issues avail.; reprint service avail. from ISI. *Refereed.* **Document type:** *Academic/Scholarly.* **Description:** Covers all the biological and medical aspects of genetic disorders.

Related titles: Microform ed.: (from PQC); Online - full text ed.: ISSN 1096-8628. USD 7,850 in United States; USD 7,850 in Canada & Mexico; USD 7,850 elsewhere (effective 2002) (from EBSCO Publishing, Wiley InterScience, Institute for Scientific Information); ♦ Supplement: American Journal of Medical Genetics. Supplement. ISSN 1040-3787.

Indexed: ASCA, Bibl.Dev.Med.& Child Neur., Biol.Abstr., Biotech.& Bioeng.Abstr. (coverage dropped), Biotech.Cit.Ind., Cal.Tiss.Abstr., Curr.Adv.Ecol.Sci., Curr.Adv.Gen.& Molec.Biol., Curr.Cont., Dent.Ind., Environ.Sci.Poll.Mgmt., Excerp.Med., Fam.Ind., Genet.Abstr. (coverage dropped), Helminthol.Abstr., Hum.Gen.Abstr., INIS Atomind., Ind.Med. (1977-), Ind.Sci.Rev., Inpharma, Kidney, Med.& Surg.Dermat., Neurosci.Abstr. (coverage dropped), Neurosci.Cit.Ind., Nuc.Acids Abstr., Nutr.Abstr., Pharm.&Out.News, Reac., Ref.Zh., Risk Abstr., SSCI (coverage dropped), Sci.Cit.Ind., THA.
—BLDSC (0827.900000), CISTI, EMDOCS, GNLM, IDS, ingenta, KNAW. **CCC.**

Published by: John Wiley & Sons, Inc., Journals (Subsidiary of: Wiley InterScience), 605 Third Ave, New York, NY 10158. TEL 212-850-6645, FAX 212-850-6021, subinfo@jwiley.com, uscs-wis@wiley.com, http://www.wiley.co.uk, http://www.wiley.com. Ed. John M Opitz. adv.: B&W page GBP 640, color page GBP 1,515; trim 210 x 279. Circ: 150. **Subscr. outside the Americas to:** John Wiley & Sons Ltd., Baffins Ln, Chichester, Sussex PO19 IUD, United Kingdom. TEL 44-1243-779777, FAX 44-1243-843232, cs-journals@wiley.co.uk, http://www.wiley.co.uk.

599.9 USA ISSN 1040-3787
CODEN: AJMSED

AMERICAN JOURNAL OF MEDICAL GENETICS. SUPPLEMENT. Text in English. 1986. irreg. **Document type:** *Monographic series.*

Related titles: ♦ Supplement to: American Journal of Medical Genetics. ISSN 0148-7299.

Indexed: INIS Atomind., Ind.Med. (until 1999, dropped).
—CISTI.

Published by: John Wiley & Sons, Inc., Journals (Subsidiary of: Wiley InterScience), 605 Third Ave, New York, NY 10158. TEL 212-850-6000, FAX 212-850-6088, SUBINFO@JWILEY.COM. **Subscr. outside the Americas to:** John Wiley & Sons Ltd., Baffins Ln, Chichester, Sussex PO19 IUD, United Kingdom. FAX 44-1243-776128.

599.9 NZL ISSN 1175-2203

▼ **AMERICAN JOURNAL OF PHARMACOGENOMICS.** Text in English. 2001. q. USD 95 to individuals Print or Online ed.; USD 114 to individuals Print & Online eds.; USD 695 to institutions Print or Online ed.; USD 834 to institutions Print & Online eds. (effective 2001). abstr. **Document type:** *Academic/Scholarly.* **Description:** Includes articles on cutting edge developments and clinical implications of genomic research and technology.

Related titles: Online - full text ed.: (from Ovid Technologies, Inc.).

Published by: Adis International Limited, Mairangi Bay, Private Bag 65901, Auckland 1010, New Zealand. TEL 64-9-477-0700, FAX 64-9-477-0766, pharmacogenomics@adis.co.nz, http://www.adis.com. Ed. Anne Bardsley-Elliot.

575.1 GBR ISSN 0268-9146
WMLC 93/3020 CODEN: ANGEE3

ANIMAL GENETICS. Text in English. 1970. bi-m., latest vol.33, 2002. GBP 318 in Europe; USD 504 in North America; GBP 350 elsewhere (effective 2002). adv. bk.rev. illus. index. back issues avail. *Refereed.* **Document type:** *Journal, Academic/Scholarly.*

Formerly (until 1986): Animal Blood Groups and Biochemical Genetics (0003-3480)

Related titles: Microform ed.: (from PQC); Online - full text ed.: ISSN 1365-2052. GBP 287 in Europe; USD 454 in North America; GBP 287 elsewhere (effective 2002) (from Ovid Technologies, Inc., EBSCO Publishing, O C L C Online Computer Library Center, Inc., RoweCom Information Quest, ingenta, Munksgaard & Blackwell Science's Synergy, Swets Blackwell, Institute for Scientific Information).

Indexed: ASCA, AgBiotech, Agricola, Anim.Breed.Abstr., Aqua.Sci.& Fish.Abstr., Biol.Abstr., Biotech.& Bioeng.Abstr., Biotech.Cit.Ind., Chem.Abstr., Chem.Indus.Notes, Chem.Titles, Curr.Adv.Ecol.Sci., Curr.Cont., Dairy Sci.Abstr., Excerp.Med., Focus on: Vet.Sci.& Med., Genet.Abstr., Hum.Gen.Abstr., Ind.Med. (1986-), Ind.Sci.Rev., Ind.Vet., Inpharma, Int.Abstr.Biol.Sci., Nuc.Acids Abstr., Pig News & Info., Plant Breed.Abstr., Poult.Abstr., Protozool.Abstr., Reac., Sci.Cit.Ind., Sport Fish.Abstr., Vet.Bull., Wild.Rev., Zoo.Rec.
—BLDSC (0903.572000), CASDDS, CISTI, EMDOCS, GNLM, IDS, Infotrieve, ingenta, Linda Hall. **CCC.**

Published by: (International Society for Animal Genetics), Blackwell Science Ltd., PO Box 88, Oxford OX2 0NE, United Kingdom. TEL 44-1865-206180, 44-1865-206002, FAX 44-1865-206219, jnl.orders@blacksci.co.uk, http://www.blackwell-science.com/~cgilib/jnlpage.asp?Journal=agen&File=agen, http://www.blackwellpublishing.com. Ed. Dr. A Archibald. Pub. Amanda McLean Inglis. R&P Sophie Savage. Adv. contact Jenny Applin. Circ: 515.

576.5 FRA ISSN 0003-3995
CODEN: AGTQAH

ANNALES DE GENETIQUE. Text and summaries in English, French. 1957. q. EUR 287 in Europe to institutions; JPY 38,000 in Japan to institutions; USD 321 in United States to institutions (effective 2002). bk.rev. charts, illus. *Refereed.* **Document type:** *Academic/Scholarly.*

Related titles: Online - full text ed.: (from ingenta, ScienceDirect, Institute for Scientific Information).

Indexed: ASCA, Abstr.Anthropol., Anim.Breed.Abstr., Bibl.Dev.Med.& Child Neur., Biol.Abstr., Biotech.Cit.Ind., Chem.Abstr., Curr.Adv.Cancer Res., Curr.Adv.Ecol.Sci., Curr.Adv.Gen.& Molec.Biol., Curr.Cont., Dairy Sci.Abstr., Dent.Ind., Excerp.Med., GeoRef, Helminthol.Abstr., INIS Atomind., Ind.Med. (1958-), Ind.Sci.Rev., Inpharma, Int.Abstr.Biol.Sci., Reac., Ref.Zh., SSCI (coverage dropped), Sci.Cit.Ind., Sport Fish.Abstr., Wild.Rev., Zoo.Rec.
—BLDSC (0975.300000), CASDDS, CISTI, EMDOCS, GNLM, IDS, ingenta. **CCC.**

Published by: (Semaine des Hopitaux), Elsevier Paris, Editions Scientifiques et Medicales (Subsidiary of: Reed Elsevier plc. group), 23 rue Linois, Paris 75015, France. http://www.elsevier.com/locate/angen. Eds. C Stoll, R Berger. Circ: 1,000.

599.9 GBR ISSN 0003-4800
HQ750.A1 CODEN: ANHGAA

ANNALS OF HUMAN GENETICS. Text in English. 1925. bi-m. GBP 314 to institutions (effective 2002). adv. bk.rev. charts, illus. index. back issues avail.; reprint service avail. from SWZ. *Refereed.* **Document type:** *Academic/Scholarly.* **Description:** Concerned with the application of scientific techniques to the study of human inheritance, such as gene mapping, cytogenetics, clinical genetics or mathematical models.

Formerly: Annals of Eugenics

Related titles: Microform ed.: (from PQC); Online - full text ed.: (from EBSCO Publishing, O C L C Online Computer Library Center, Inc., RoweCom Information Quest, Swets Blackwell, Institute for Scientific Information).

Indexed: A.I.C.P., ASCA, Abstr.Anthropol., Abstr.Hyg., AgBiotech, Anim.Breed.Abstr., Anthropol.Lit., Bibl.Dev.Med.& Child Neur., Biol.Abstr., Biotech.Cit.Ind., Chem.Abstr., Curr.Adv.Ecol.Sci., Curr.Cont., Curr.Ind.Stat., Dairy Sci.Abstr., Excerp.Med., Helminthol.Abstr., INIS Atomind., Ind.Med. (1954-), Ind.Sci.Rev., Inpharma, Int.Abstr.Biol.Sci., Math.R., Nutr.Abstr., Plant Breed.Abstr., Psychol.Abstr., Reac., Ref.Zh., Rev.Appl.Entomol., SSCI (coverage dropped), Sci.Cit.Ind., Stat.Theor.Meth.Abstr., THA, Trop.Dis.Bull.
—BLDSC (1041.000000), CASDDS, CISTI, EMDOCS, GNLM, IDS, ingenta, Linda Hall. **CCC.**

Published by: Cambridge University Press, Edinburgh Bldg, Shaftesbury Rd, Cambridge CB2 2RU, United Kingdom. FAX 44-1223-315052, information@cup.cam.ac.uk, information@cambridge.org, http://www.cup.org/journals/CUPJNLS.html. Eds. C A B Smith, D A Hopkinson, Sue Povey. R&P Linda Nicol. Adv. contact Rebecca Symons.

576.5 USA ISSN 0066-4197
QH431.A1 CODEN: ARVGB7

ANNUAL REVIEW OF GENETICS. Text in English. 1967. a. USD 60 domestic to individuals; USD 65 foreign to individuals; USD 120 domestic to institutions; USD 130 foreign to institutions (effective 1999). adv. bibl, charts. index, cum.index. back issues avail.; reprints avail. *Refereed.* **Document type:** *Academic/Scholarly.* **Description:** Reviews synthesize and filter primary research in order to identify the principal contributions in the field of genetics.

Related titles: Microfilm ed.: (from PQC); Online - full text ed.: (from Gale Group, HighWire Pr., Northern Light Technology, Inc., EBSCO Publishing, H. W. Wilson, Institute for Scientific Information).

Indexed: ASCA, Abstr.Anthropol., Abstr.Hyg., AgBiotech, Agri.& Environ.Biotech.Abstr. (coverage dropped), Anim.Behav.Abstr., Anim.Breed.Abstr., Appl.Ecol.Abstr., Aqua.Sci.& Fish.Abstr., Bibl.Agri., Biol.& Agr.Ind. (Jan.1983-), Biol.Abstr., Biol.Dig., Biotech.Cit.Ind., Chem.Abstr., Chem.Indus.Notes, Chem.Titles, Curr.Adv.Biochem., Curr.Adv.Cell & Devel.Biol., Curr.Adv.Ecol.Sci., Curr.Adv.Gen.& Molec.Biol., Curr.Cont., Derwent Biotech.Abstr., Diar.Dis.Res., Entomol.Abstr., Environ.Sci.Poll.Mgmt., Excerp.Med., Forest Prod.Abstr., Forest.Abstr., Gen.Sci.Ind. (Jun.1992-), Genet.Abstr., Helminthol.Abstr., Hum.Gen.Abstr., INIS Atomind., Ind.Med. (1967-), Ind.Sci.Rev., Inpharma, Int.Abstr.Biol.Sci., Media Rev.Dig., Microbiol.Abstr., Neurosci.Abstr., Nuc.Acids Abstr., Plant Breed.Abstr., Plant Gen.Res.Abstr., Protozool.Abstr., Reac., Rev.Appl.Entomol., Rev.Med.& Vet.Mycol., Rev.Plant Path., Sci.Cit.Ind., THA, Trop.Dis.Bull., Zoo.Rec.
—BLDSC (1522.565000), ADONIS, CASDDS, CISTI, EMDOCS, GNLM, IDS, ingenta, KNAW, Linda Hall. **CCC.**

Published by: Annual Reviews Inc., 4139 El Camino Way, Box 10139, Palo Alto, CA 94303-0139. TEL 650-493-4400, 800-523-8635, FAX 650-424-0910, service@annurev.org; orders@allenpress.com, http://www.annualreviews.org. Ed. Samuel Gubins. R&P, Adv. contact Swati Aneja TEL 650-843-6634. **Subscr. to:** Allen Press Inc., PO Box 1897, Lawrence, KS 66044-8897.

576.5 USA ISSN 1087-2906
QP623.5.A58 CODEN: ANADF5

ANTISENSE AND NUCLEIC ACID DRUG DEVELOPMENT. Text in English. 1991. bi-m. USD 178 domestic to individuals; USD 294 foreign to individuals; USD 214 domestic to individuals print and online eds. combined; USD 329 foreign to individuals print and online eds. combined; USD 298 domestic to institutions; USD 400 foreign to institutions; USD 358 domestic to institutions print and online eds. combined; USD 460 foreign to institutions print and online eds. combined (effective 2002). adv. back issues avail.; reprints avail. *Refereed.* **Document type:** *Journal, Academic/Scholarly.* **Description:** Deals with man-made substances and their effects on gene expression at the RNA and DNA levels both in vitro and in vivo.

Formerly (until 1997): Antisense Research and Development (1050-5261)

Related titles: Online - full content ed.: USD 178 to individuals; USD 298 to institutions (effective 2002); Online - full text ed.: (from CatchWord Ltd., Institute for Scientific Information, RoweCom Information Quest).

Indexed: ASCA, AgBiotech, Biotech.Cit.Ind., Chem.Abstr., Chem.Indus.Notes, Chem.Titles, Curr.Cont., Derwent Biotech.Abstr., Excerp.Med. (1993-), Genet.Abstr. (coverage dropped), Ind.Med. (1996-), Ind.Sci.Rev., Ind.Vet., Inpharma, Med.& Pharm.Biotech.Abstr., Nuc.Acids Abstr., Pharm.&Out.News, Reac., Sci.Cit.Ind., Vet.Bull.
—BLDSC (1551.690000), CASDDS, CISTI, EMDOCS, GNLM, IDS, ingenta, KNAW. **CCC.**
Published by: Mary Ann Liebert, Inc. Publishers, 2 Madison Ave, Larchmont, NY 10538. TEL 914—834-3100, FAX 914-834-1388, info@liebertpub.com, www.liebertpub.com/ard, http://www.liebertpub.com. Eds. Arthur M Krieg, C A Stein.

572.8 USA ISSN 1056-5191
RB155.6
APPLIED CYTOGENETICS. Text in English. 1975. bi-m. USD 105. adv. bk.rev. back issues avail. **Document type:** *Trade.* **Description:** Covers clinical cytogenetics and molecular cytogenetics for laboratory and medical personnel.
Formerly (until 1990): Karyogram (0732-8745)
—KNAW.
Published by: Association of Cytogenetic Technologists, c/o A C T Association Manager, Box 15945-288, Lenexa, KS 66285. TEL 913-541-9077, FAX 931-541-0156. Ed. Barbara J Kaplan. Adv. contact Leslee Urhahn. Circ: 1,700.

576.5 USA ISSN 0271-7107
CODEN: AGNEEN
APPLIED GENETICS NEWS. Text in English. 1980. m. USD 415 (effective 1999). **Document type:** *Proceedings.* **Description:** Covers the biotechnology industry from technical and economic perspectives.
Related titles: Online - full text ed.: (from Data-Star, The Dialog Corporation, Gale Group, NewsNet, Northern Light Technology, Inc., LexisNexis, Factiva).
Indexed: BPIA, Curr.Biotech.Abstr., P.N.I.
—CISTI, Infotrieve. **CCC.**
Published by: Business Communications Co., Inc. (Norwalk), 25 Van Zant St, Ste 13, Norwalk, CT 06855-1781. TEL 203-853-4266, FAX 203-853-0348. Ed. Philip Rotheim.

APPLIED MICROBIOLOGY AND BIOTECHNOLOGY. see *BIOLOGY—Biotechnology*

ARCHIVES OF MICROBIOLOGY. see *BIOLOGY—Microbiology*

576.5 ITA ISSN 0066-9830
CODEN: AAGNA3
ASSOCIAZIONE GENETICA ITALIANA. ATTI. Text and summaries in English, Italian. 1955. a. ITL 20,000, USD 7.
Indexed: Anim.Breed.Abstr., Biol.Abstr., Curr.Adv.Ecol.Sci., Curr.Cont. (coverage dropped), INIS Atomind.
—CISTI, Linda Hall.
Published by: Associazione Genetica Italiana, c/o Istituto di Biologia Animale, Via Leonardo Loredan, 10, Padua, PD 35131, Italy. Ed. G A Danieli. Circ: 300.

AUSTRALIAN AND NEW ZEALAND DIRECTORY OF GENETICS SUPPORT GROUPS, SERVICES AND INFORMATION. see *BIOLOGY—Abstracting, Bibliographies, Statistics*

576.5 NLD ISSN 0167-4781
B B A - GENE STRUCTURE AND EXPRESSION. Text in Dutch. 1962. 18/yr. EUR 2,277 in Europe to institutions; JPY 302,400 in Japan to institutions; USD 2,548 elsewhere to institutions (effective 2002). back issues avail. *Refereed.* **Document type:** *Academic/Scholarly.* **Description:** Examines DNA and RNA structures. Includes sequence data, nucleic acid and protein interaction, DNA modifying enzymes and replication. Explores transcription mechanisms and factors as well as control of gene expression.
Related titles: Microform ed.: (from PQC); Online - full text ed.: (from EBSCO Publishing, ingenta, Swets Blackwell, ScienceDirect, Institute for Scientific Information).
Indexed: ASCA, AgBiotech, Anim.Breed.Abstr., BBCI, Biodet.Abstr., Biol.Abstr., Biotech.Cit.Ind., Chem.Abstr., Crop Physiol.Abstr., Curr.Cont., Dairy Sci.Abstr., Derwent Biotech.Abstr., Excerp.Med., Helminthol.Abstr., INIS Atomind., Ind.Chem. (coverage dropped), Ind.Med. (coverage dropped), Inpharma, Int.Abstr.Biol.Sci., Nutr.Abstr., Plant Breed.Abstr., Protozool.Abstr., Reac., Ref.Zh., Rev.Appl.Entomol., Rev.Med.& Vet.Mycol., Rev.Plant Path., Rice Abstr., Sci.Cit.Ind., Seed Abstr., Soils & Fert., Triticale Abstr.
—ADONIS, CISTI, EMDOCS, IDS. **CCC.**
Published by: Elsevier Science BV, PO Box 211, Amsterdam 1000 AE, Netherlands. TEL 31-20-485-2911, FAX 31-20-485-2457, nlinfo-f@elsevier.nl, http://www.elsevier.com/locate/bbaexp. Eds. J D Gralla, P C van der Vliet. **Subscr. in Australasia and the Far East to:** Elsevier Science (Singapore) Pte Ltd, No.1 Temasek Ave, 17-01 Millenia Tower, Singapore 039192, Singapore. TEL 65-434-3727, FAX 65-337-2230; **Subscr. in Japan to:** Elsevier Science Inc - Japan Regional Office, 9-15 Higashi-Azabu 1-chome, Minato-ku, Tokyo 106-0044, Japan. TEL 81-3-5561-5033; **Subscr. in the Americas to:** Elsevier Science, PO Box 945, New York, NY 10159-0945. TEL 212-633-3730, FAX 212-633-3680.

599.9 NLD ISSN 0925-4439
CODEN: BBADEX
B B A - MOLECULAR BASIS OF DISEASE. Text in Dutch. 9/yr. EUR 1,042 in Europe to institutions; JPY 138,300 in Japan to institutions; USD 1,165 elsewhere to institutions (effective 2002). *Refereed.* **Document type:** *Academic/Scholarly.* **Description:** Focuses on a fundamental biochemical and genetic approach to understanding dysfunction in human disease states and their models.
Related titles: Microfilm ed.: (from PQC); Online - full text ed.: (from EBSCO Publishing, ingenta, Swets Blackwell, ScienceDirect, Institute for Scientific Information).
Indexed: ASCA, BBCI, Curr.Cont., Derwent Biotech.Abstr., Excerp.Med., Focus on: Mol.Med., Helminthol.Abstr., Ind.Vet., Inpharma, Int.Abstr.Biol.Sci., Nutr.Abstr., Protozool.Abstr., Reac., Ref.Zh., Rev.Med.& Vet.Mycol., Sci.Cit.Ind., Vet.Bull.
—ADONIS, CISTI, EMDOCS, IDS. **CCC.**
Published by: Elsevier Science BV, PO Box 211, Amsterdam 1000 AE, Netherlands. TEL 31-20-485-2911, FAX 31-20-485-2457, nlinfo-f@elsevier.nl, http://www.elsevier.com/locate/bbadis, http://www.elsevier.nl. Eds. J R Riordan, P E Fraser. **Subscr. in Australasia and the Far East to:** Elsevier Science (Singapore) Pte Ltd, No.1 Temasek Ave, 17-01 Millenia Tower, Singapore 039192, Singapore. TEL 65-434-3727, FAX 65-337-2230; **Subscr. in Japan to:** Elsevier Science Inc - Japan Regional Office, 9-15 Higashi-Azabu 1-chome, Minato-ku, Tokyo 106-0044, Japan. TEL 81-3-5561-5033; **Subscr. in the Americas to:** Elsevier Science, PO Box 945, New York, NY 10159-0945. TEL 212-633-3730, FAX 212-633-3680.

591.35 FRA ISSN 0153-6281
B T I A; la revue francaise de la genetique et de la reproduction. (Bulletin Technique de l'Insemination Artificielle) Text in French. 1976. q. FRF 211 domestic to individuals; FRF 288 foreign to individuals (effective 1999). adv. bk.rev. **Document type:** *Bulletin.* **Description:** For specialists in the reproduction and insemination of cattle, including veterinarians and owners of livestock.
Published by: (Association pour l'Information en Insemination Artificielle), Societe de Diffusion de la Presse Agricole, BP 47, Lempdes 63370, France. TEL 33-4-73421717, FAX 33-4-73913560, TELEX 397-467. Ed. Maurice Lacroix. Adv. contact Jeanne Fischer.

BABRAHAM INSTITUTE. CORPORATE PLAN. see *BIOLOGY—Physiology*

BABRAHAM INSTITUTE. REPORT. see *BIOLOGY—Physiology*

576.5 BGR ISSN 1311-0160
BALKAN JOURNAL OF MEDICAL GENETICS. Text in English. 1998. q. USD 120 foreign (effective 2002). **Document type:** *Journal, Academic/Scholarly.*
Published by: Meditsinski Universitet - Sofia, Tsentur za Informatsiia po Meditsina/Medical University - Sofia, Medical Information Center, 1 Sv Georgi Sofiiski ul, Sofia 1431, Bulgaria. TEL 359-2-9522342, FAX 359-2-9522393, mutafov@medun.acad.bg, http://www.medun.acad.bg. **Dist. by:** Sofia Books, Ul Silivria 16, Sofia 1404, Bulgaria. TEL 359-2-9586257, sofiabooks@hotmail.com, http://www.sofiabooks.hit.bg.

576.5 610 USA ISSN 0001-8244
CODEN: BHGNAT
BEHAVIOR GENETICS; an international journal devoted to research in the inheritance of behavior in animals and man. Text in English. 1970. bi-m. EUR 746, USD 747 to institutions for print or online ed.; EUR 143, USD 144 to individuals for print or online ed.; EUR 895.20, USD 896.40 to institutions for print & online eds. combined (effective 2002). adv. bk.rev. bibl, charts, illus, stat. index. back issues avail. *Refereed.* **Document type:** *Academic/Scholarly.* **Description:** Explores the genetic analysis of complex traits.
Related titles: Microfilm ed.: (from PQC); Online - full text ed.: (from Ovid Technologies, Inc., EBSCO Publishing, O C L C Online Computer Library Center, Inc., Swets Blackwell, Kluwer Online, Institute for Scientific Information, RoweCom Information Quest).
Indexed: ASCA, Abstr.Anthropol., Addic.Abstr., AgBiotech, Anim.Behav.Abstr., Anim.Breed.Abstr., Apic.Abstr., Biol.Abstr., Chemorec.Abstr., Child Devel.Abstr., Curr.Adv.Ecol.Sci., Curr.Cont., Curr.Ind.Stat., Dairy Sci.Abstr., Entomol.Abstr., Excerp.Med., Fam.Ind., Genet.Abstr., Hum.Gen.Abstr., INIS Atomind., Ind.Med. (1970-), Ind.Sci.Rev., Inpharma, Int.Abstr.Biol.Sci., Neurosci.Cit.Ind., Nuc.Acids Abstr., Nutr.Abstr., PsycInfo, Psychol.Abstr. (1970-), Reac., Ref.Zh., Rev.Appl.Entomol., Rev.Med.& Vet.Mycol., Russ.Acad.Sci.Bibl., SSCI, Sci.Cit.Ind., Sport Fish.Abstr., Wild.Rev., Zoo.Rec., e-psyche.
—BLDSC (1876.691000), CISTI, EMDOCS, GNLM, IDS, ingenta, KNAW. **CCC.**
Published by: (Behavior Genetics Association), Kluwer Academic - Plenum Publishers (Subsidiary of: Wolters Kluwer N.V.), 233 Spring St, New York, NY 10013-1578. TEL 212-620-8000, 800-221-9369, FAX 212-463-0742, http://www.wkap.nl/journalhome.htm/0001-8244. Ed. Dr. Norman Henderson. R&P Rose Luongo TEL 781-871-6311.

BILTEN ZA TRANSFUZIOLOGIJU. see *MEDICAL SCIENCES—Hematology*

576.5 USA ISSN 0006-2928
QH431 CODEN: BIGEBA
BIOCHEMICAL GENETICS. Text in English. 1967. m. USD 875, EUR 873.50 to institutions for print or online ed.; USD 1,050, EUR 1,048.80 to institutions for print & online eds. combined (effective 2002). adv. back issues avail. *Refereed.* **Document type:** *Academic/Scholarly.* **Description:** Publishes original research results in biochemical genetics.
Related titles: Microfilm ed.: (from PQC); Online - full text ed.: (from CatchWord Ltd., EBSCO Publishing, O C L C Online Computer Library Center, Inc., RoweCom Information Quest, Swets Blackwell, Kluwer Online, Institute for Scientific Information).
Indexed: ASCA, Abstr.Anthropol., AgBiotech, Agri.& Environ.Biotech.Abstr. (coverage dropped), Agricola, Anim.Breed.Abstr., Aqua.Sci.& Fish.Abstr., BBCI, Bibl.Agri., Biol.& Agr.Ind. (Feb.1983-), Biol.Abstr., Biotech.& Bioeng.Abstr., Biotech.Cit.Ind., Chem.Abstr., Chem.Indus.Notes, Chem.Titles, Curr.Adv.Ecol.Sci., Curr.Cont., Dairy Sci.Abstr., Dent.Ind., Derwent Biotech.Abstr., Entomol.Abstr., Excerp.Med., Forest.Abstr., Genet.Abstr., Helminthol.Abstr., Hort.Abstr., Hum.Gen.Abstr., INIS Atomind., Ind.Med. (1967-), Ind.Sci.Rev., Inpharma, Int.Abstr.Biol.Sci., Maize Abstr., Nuc.Acids Abstr., Ornam.Hort., Pig News & Info., Plant Breed.Abstr., Plant Gen.Res.Abstr., Plant Grow.Reg.Abstr., Poult.Abstr., Psychol.Abstr., Reac., Ref.Zh., Rev.Appl.Entomol., Rev.Med.& Vet.Mycol., Rev.Plant Path., Sci.Cit.Ind., Seed Abstr., Sorghum & Millets Abstr., Soyabean Abstr., Sport Fish.Abstr., Triticale Abstr., Wild.Rev., Zoo.Rec.
—BLDSC (2066.980000), CASDDS, CatchWord, CISTI, EMDOCS, GNLM, IDS, ingenta, Linda Hall. **CCC.**
Published by: Kluwer Academic - Plenum Publishers (Subsidiary of: Wolters Kluwer N.V.), 233 Spring St, New York, NY 10013-1578. TEL 212-620-8000, 800-221-9369, FAX 212-463-0742, http://www.wkap.nl/journalhome.htm/0006-2928. Ed. Hugh S Forrest. R&P Rose Luongo TEL 781-871-6311.

BIOMOLECULAR ENGINEERING. see *BIOLOGY—Biotechnology*

576.5 ARG ISSN 0067-9720
QH442
BOLETIN GENETICO. Text and summaries in English, Spanish. 1965. irreg., latest vol.15, 1989. USD 15; or exchange.
Indexed: Biol.Abstr.
Published by: Instituto Nacional de Tecnologia Agropecuaria, Centro de Investigaciones en Ciencias Agronomicas, Departamento de Genetica, Casilla de Correos 25, Castelar, Buenos Aires 1712, Argentina.

576.5 PRT ISSN 0870-7235
CODEN: BRGED7
BROTERIA GENETICA. Text in English, French, German, Italian, Portuguese, Spanish. 1902. q. USD 19. bk.rev. bibl, charts, illus. index, cum.index: 1902-1917; 1918-1959. **Document type:** *Academic/Scholarly.*
Supersedes (in 1980): Broteria: Ciencias Naturais (0007-2427)
Related titles: Microfiche ed.: (from IDC).
Indexed: Biol.Abstr., Chem.Abstr., M.L.A., Pig News & Info., Sport Fish.Abstr., Wild.Rev., Zoo.Rec.
—BLDSC (2351.020000), CISTI, Linda Hall.

B

Published by: (Sociedade Portuguesa de Genetica), Edicoes Broteria, Rua Maestro Antonio Taborda 14, Lisbon Codex 1293, Portugal. TEL 351-1-3961660. Ed. Luis J Archer. Circ: 1,000.

C A S BIOTECH UPDATES. GENETIC ENGINEERING. see *BIOLOGY—Abstracting, Bibliographies, Statistics*

CANCER GENE THERAPY. see *MEDICAL SCIENCES—Oncology*

CANCER GENETICS & CYTOGENETICS. see *MEDICAL SCIENCES—Oncology*

576.5 DEU ISSN 0009-5915
QH301 CODEN: CHROAU
CHROMOSOMA; biology of the nucleus. Text in English. 1939. 8/yr. EUR 1,210 domestic; EUR 1,197.90 in Germany; EUR 177 newsstand/cover foreign (effective 2002). adv. bibl, charts, illus. index. back issues avail.; reprint service avail. from ISI. *Refereed.* **Document type:** *Journal, Academic/Scholarly.* **Description:** Publishes original papers and current review articles relating the molecular structure and function of chromosomes to that of the nucleus.
Related titles: Microform ed.: (from PQC); Online - full text ed.: ISSN 1432-0886 (from EBSCO Publishing, RoweCom Information Quest, Swets Blackwell, Springer LINK, Institute for Scientific Information).
Indexed: ASCA, Abstr.Anthropol., AgBiotech, Agricola, Anim.Breed.Abstr., Aqua.Sci.& Fish.Abstr., Bibl.Agri., Bio-Contr.News & Info., Biol.Abstr., Biotech.& Bioeng.Abstr., Biotech.Cit.Ind., Chem.Abstr., Chem.Indus.Notes, Chem.Titles, Curr.Adv.Cell & Devel.Biol., Curr.Adv.Ecol.Sci., Curr.Adv.Gen.& Molec.Biol., Curr.Cont., Dent.Ind., Excerp.Med., Genet.Abstr., Helminthol.Abstr., Hum.Gen.Abstr., INIS Atomind., Ind.Med. (1939-), Ind.Sci.Rev., Inpharma, Int.Abstr.Biol.Sci., Maize Abstr., Microbiol.Abstr., Nuc.Acids Abstr., Ornam.Hort., Plant Breed.Abstr., Reac., Ref.Zh., Rev.Appl.Entomol., Sci.Cit.Ind., Sport Fish.Abstr., Triticale Abstr., Wild.Rev., Zoo.Rec.
—BLDSC (3184.000000), CASDDS, CISTI, EMDOCS, GNLM, IDS, ingenta, Linda Hall. **CCC.**
Published by: Springer-Verlag (Subsidiary of: BertelsmannSpringer), Tiergartenstr 17, Heidelberg 69121, Germany. TEL 49-6221-345-0, FAX 49-6221-345229, subscriptions@springer.de, http://link.springer.de/link/service/journals/00412/index.htm, http://www.springer.de. **Subscr. in N. America to:** Springer-Verlag New York Inc., PO Box 2485, Secaucus, NJ 07096-2485. TEL 212-460-1500, FAX 212-473-6272.

CLINICAL CYTOGENETICS. see *BIOLOGY—Abstracting, Bibliographies, Statistics*

576.5 DNK ISSN 0009-9163
RB155 CODEN: CLGNAY
CLINICAL GENETICS; an international journal of genetics and molecular medicine. Text in English. 1970. m. USD 540 in the Americas to institutions print & online eds. combined; GBP 375 elsewhere to institutions print & online eds. combined (effective 2002). adv. bibl, charts, illus. reprint service avail. from SWZ,ISI. *Refereed.* **Document type:** *Academic/Scholarly.*
Related titles: Online - full text ed.: ISSN 1399-0004. GBP 338 (2002) (from Ovid Technologies, Inc., EBSCO Publishing, O C L C Online Computer Library Center, Inc., RoweCom Information Quest, ingenta, Munksgaard & Blackwell Science's Synergy, Swets Blackwell, Institute for Scientific Information).
Indexed: ASCA, Abstr.Anthropol., Bibl.Dev.Med.& Child Neur., Biol.Abstr., Biotech.& Bioeng.Abstr., Biotech.Cit.Ind., Chem.Abstr., Curr.Adv.Ecol.Sci., Curr.Adv.Gen.& Molec.Biol., Curr.Cont., Curr.Tit.Dent., Dairy Sci.Abstr., Dent.Ind., Dok.Arbeitsmed., Excerp.Med., Genet.Abstr., Hum.Gen.Abstr., INIS Atomind., Ind.Med. (1970-), Ind.Sci.Rev., Inpharma, Int.Abstr.Biol.Sci., Med.& Surg.Dermat., Neurosci.Cit.Ind., Nuc.Acids Abstr., Nutr.Abstr., Pharm.&Out.News, Reac., Risk Abstr., SSCI (coverage dropped), Sci.Cit.Ind.
—BLDSC (3286.287000), CASDDS, CISTI, EMDOCS, GNLM, IDS, ingenta, KNAW. **CCC.**
Published by: Blackwell Munksgaard, Noerre Soegade 35, PO Box 2148, Copenhagen K 1016, Denmark. TEL 45-77-33-33-33, FAX 45-77-33-33-77, customerservice@munksgaard.dk, http://journals.munksgaard.dk/clinicalgenetics, http://www.munksgaard.dk. Ed. Michael R Hayden. Adv. contact Eric Rozario TEL 45-77-33-33-01. Circ: 1,100.

660.65 USA ISSN 1536-2302
CODEN: CLONFB
▼ **CLONING AND STEM CELLS.** Text in English. 1999. q. USD 197 domestic to individuals; USD 258 foreign to individuals; USD 236 domestic to individuals print and online eds. combined; USD 297 foreign to individuals print and online eds. combined; USD 343 domestic to institutions; USD 426 foreign to institutions; USD 412 domestic to institutions print and online eds. combined; USD 494 foreign to institutions print and online eds. combined (effective 2002). adv. back issues avail.; reprints avail. *Refereed.* **Document type:** *Journal, Academic/Scholarly.* **Description:** Covers all aspects of cloning research and applications.
Formerly (until Aug. 2001): Cloning (1520-4553)
Related titles: Online - full text ed.: USD 197 worldwide to individuals; USD 343 worldwide to institutions (effective 2002) (from EBSCO Publishing, O C L C Online Computer Library Center, Inc., RoweCom Information Quest, Swets Blackwell).
Indexed: Agri.& Environ.Biotech.Abstr., Aqua.Sci.& Fish.Abstr., Biotech.& Bioeng.Abstr., Environ.Sci.Poll.Mgmt., Genet.Abstr., Med.& Pharm.Biotech.Abstr.
—BLDSC (3286.692200), CatchWord. **CCC.**
Published by: Mary Ann Liebert, Inc. Publishers, 2 Madison Ave, Larchmont, NY 10538. TEL 914—834-3100, FAX 914-834-1388, info@liebertpub.com, www.liebertpub.com/clo, http://www.liebertpub.com. Ed. Ian Wilmut.

599.9 CHE ISSN 1422-2795
CODEN: COGEFX
COMMUNITY GENETICS. Text in English. 1998. q. CHF 621 in Europe to institutions; CHF 632.60 overseas to institutions; EUR 444.20 in Europe to institutions; USD 483 overseas to institutions (effective 2002). adv. back issues avail. **Document type:** *Journal, Academic/Scholarly.* **Description:** International forum for research in the expanding field of community genetics, an area of medical care responding to the explosion of developments in human genetics which impact both the individual and society.
Related titles: Online - full text ed.: ISSN 1422-2833. CHF 58 to institutions with print edition (effective 2001); EUR 42, USD 45 to institutions with print edition (effective 2002) (from EBSCO Publishing, O C L C Online Computer Library Center, Inc., RoweCom Information Quest, Swets Blackwell).
—BLDSC (3363.627500), GNLM, KNAW.
Published by: S. Karger AG, Allschwilerstr 10, PO Box, Basel 4009, Switzerland. TEL 41-61-306-1111, FAX 41-61-306-1234, karger@karger.ch, http://www.online.karger.com/journals/cmg, http://www.karger.com. Ed. L P Ten Kate. adv.: page USD 1,185.

576.8 333.95 NLD ISSN 1566-0621
▼ **CONSERVATION GENETICS.** Text in English. 2000. q. USD 60, EUR 63.50 to individuals for print or online ed.; USD 218, EUR 217 to institutions for print or online ed.; EUR 260.40 combined subscription to institutions print & online eds. (effective 2002). *Refereed.* **Document type:** *Journal, Academic/Scholarly.*
Related titles: Online - full text ed.: (from O C L C Online Computer Library Center, Inc., Swets Blackwell, Kluwer Online, RoweCom Information Quest).
Indexed: Appl.Ecol.Abstr., Biotech.& Bioeng.Abstr., Entomol.Abstr., Genet.Abstr.
—BLDSC (3418.058000).
Published by: Kluwer Academic Publishers Group (Subsidiary of: Wolters Kluwer N.V.), Spuiboulevard 50, PO Box 17, Dordrecht 3300 AA, Netherlands. TEL 31-78-639-2392, FAX 31-78-654-2254, services@wkap.nl, http://kapis1.wkap.nl/journalhome.htm/1568-0621, http://www.wkap.nl. Ed. A R Hoelzel. Pub. Ad Plaizier TEL 31-78-639-2234. **Subscr. in the Americas to:** Kluwer Academic - Plenum Publishers, 233 Spring St, New York, NY 10013-1578. TEL 212-620-8468, FAX 212-807-1047; **Subscr. to:** Journals Department, PO Box 322, Dordrecht 3300 AH, Netherlands. TEL 31-78-639-2392, FAX 31-78-654-6474.

576.5 NLD ISSN 0929-712X
CONTEMPORARY ISSUES IN GENETICS AND EVOLUTION. Text in English. 1993. irreg., latest vol.4, 1995. price varies. *Refereed.* **Document type:** *Monographic series.*
—BLDSC (3425.184215), KNAW.
Published by: Kluwer Academic Publishers Group (Subsidiary of: Wolters Kluwer N.V.), Spuiboulevard 50, PO Box 17, Dordrecht 3300 AA, Netherlands. FAX 31-78-639-2254, services@wkap.nl, http://www.wkap.nl. **Dist. by:** Journals Department, PO Box 322, Dordrecht 3300 AH, Netherlands. FAX 31-78-654-6474.

576.5 USA ISSN 1045-4403
QH450 CODEN: CRGEEJ
CRITICAL REVIEWS IN EUKARYOTIC GENE EXPRESSION. Text in English. 1990. q. USD 94 to individuals; USD 411 to institutions (effective 2000). adv. *Refereed.* **Document type:** *Academic/Scholarly.* **Description:** Assimilates and presents timely concepts and experimental approaches that contribute to the advances in understanding gene regulation, organization and structure.
Related titles: Online - full text ed.: (from Institute for Scientific Information).
Indexed: ASCA, Agricola, Biotech.& Bioeng.Abstr., Biotech.Cit.Ind., Chem.Abstr., Chem.Indus.Notes, Chem.Titles, Genet.Abstr., Hum.Gen.Abstr., Ind.Med. (1990-), Int.Abstr.Biol.Sci., Microbiol.Abstr., Nuc.Acids Abstr.
—BLDSC (3487.475300), CASDDS, CISTI, EMDOCS, GNLM, IDS, Infotrieve, ingenta, KNAW, Linda Hall. **CCC.**
Published by: Begell House Inc., 79 Madison Ave, Ste 1205, New York, NY 10016-7892. TEL 212-725-1999, FAX 212-213-8368, begellhouse@worldnet.att.net, orders@begellhouse.com. Pub. William Begell. R&P, Adv. contact Jung K Ra.

CURRENT ADVANCES IN GENETICS AND MOLECULAR BIOLOGY. see *BIOLOGY—Abstracting, Bibliographies, Statistics*

CURRENT DIRECTIONS IN AUTOIMMUNITY. see *MEDICAL SCIENCES—Allergology And Immunology*

576.5 DEU ISSN 0172-8083
QH426 CODEN: CUGED5
CURRENT GENETICS; eukaryotes with emphasis on yeasts, fungi, protists, cell organelles. Text in English. 1980. m. EUR 1,481 domestic; EUR 1,470.70 in Germany; EUR 145 newsstand/cover foreign (effective 2002). adv. reprint service avail. from ISI. *Refereed.* **Document type:** *Journal, Academic/Scholarly.* **Description:** Covers the genetics of eukaryotes, with an emphasis on yeasts, other fungi, protists, and cell organelles.
Related titles: Microform ed.: (from PQC); Online - full text ed.: ISSN 1432-0983 (from EBSCO Publishing, RoweCom Information Quest, Swets Blackwell, Springer LINK, Institute for Scientific Information).
Indexed: ASCA, AgBiotech, Agri.& Environ.Biotech.Abstr. (coverage dropped), Agricola, Anim.Breed.Abstr., Aqua.Sci.& Fish.Abstr., Bibl.Agri., Bio-Contr.News & Info., Biotech.Cit.Ind., Chem.Abstr., Chem.Indus.Notes, Chem.Titles, Crop Physiol.Abstr., Curr.Adv.Ecol.Sci., Curr.Biotech.Abstr., Curr.Cont., Dairy Sci.Abstr., Derwent Biotech.Abstr., Entomol.Abstr., Environ.Sci.Poll.Mgmt., Excerp.Med., Fababean Abstr., Food Sci.& Tech.Abstr., Forest.Abstr., Genet.Abstr., Hum.Gen.Abstr., INIS Atomind., Ind.Med. (1979-), Ind.Sci.Rev., Inpharma, Int.Abstr.Biol.Sci., Maize Abstr., Microbiol.Abstr., Nuc.Acids Abstr., Nutr.Abstr., Plant Breed.Abstr., Plant Gen.Res.Abstr., Potato Abstr., Protozool.Abstr., Reac., Rev.Appl.Entomol., Rev.Med.& Vet.Mycol., Rev.Plant Path., Rice Abstr., Sci.Cit.Ind., Soils & Fert., Sorghum & Millets Abstr., Soyabean Abstr., Triticale Abstr., Weed Abstr., Zoo.Rec.
—BLDSC (3496.960000), CASDDS, CISTI, EMDOCS, GNLM, IDS, ingenta, Linda Hall. **CCC.**
Published by: Springer-Verlag (Subsidiary of: BertelsmannSpringer), Tiergartenstr 17, Heidelberg 69121, Germany. TEL 49-6221-345-0, FAX 49-6221-345229, subscriptions@springer.de, http://link.springer.de/link/service/journals/00294/index.htm, http://www.springer.de. Ed. L A Grivell. **Subscr. in N. America to:** Springer-Verlag New York Inc., PO Box 2485, Secaucus, NJ 07096-2485. TEL 212-460-1500, FAX 212-473-6272.

576.5 USA ISSN 1389-2029
▼ **CURRENT GENOMICS.** Text in English. 2000 (Jun.). q. USD 110, USD 600 to institutions (effective 2000). adv. *Refereed.* **Document type:** *Academic/Scholarly.* **Description:** Features reviews in genomics, functional genomics and related areas.
Related titles: Online - full text ed.: (from Swets Blackwell).
Indexed: Entomol.Abstr., Genet.Abstr., Med.& Pharm.Biotech.Abstr.
Published by: Bentham Science Publishers, 102 N.E. 2nd St, Mail Box 135, Boca Raton, FL 33432. FAX 561-393-7229, m.bentham@inter.nl.net. Adv. contact Tom Lucas.

CURRENT ISSUES IN MOLECULAR BIOLOGY. see *BIOLOGY—Biochemistry*

576.5 GBR ISSN 0959-437X
QH426 CODEN: COGDET
CURRENT OPINION IN GENETICS & DEVELOPMENT. Text in English. 1991. bi-m. EUR 170 in Europe to individuals; JPY 20,600 in Japan to individuals; USD 184 elsewhere to individuals; EUR 213 in Europe to qualified personnel; JPY 25,700 in Japan to qualified personnel; USD 230 elsewhere to qualified personnel; EUR 908 in Europe to institutions; JPY 125,900 in Japan to institutions; USD 1,015 elsewhere to institutions (effective 2002). adv. bibl, illus. back issues avail. *Refereed.* **Document type:** *Academic/Scholarly.* **Description:** Directed toward researchers, educators and students of genetics and development. Presents review articles, followed by annotated bibliographies of references consulted. Includes a "Paper Alert" section, giving brief summaries of relevant papers recently published in other journals.
Related titles: CD-ROM ed.; Online - full text ed.: USD 227 in North America to individuals; USD 247 in North America to individuals with print ed; GBP 137 elsewhere to individuals; GBP 150 elsewhere to individuals with print ed; USD 822 in North America to institutional members includes print ed; GBP 500 elsewhere to institutional members includes print ed (effective 1999 & 2000) (from EBSCO Publishing, ingenta, Swets Blackwell, ScienceDirect, Institute for Scientific Information).
Indexed: ASCA, AgBiotech, Anim.Breed.Abstr., Aqua.Sci.& Fish.Abstr., Biotech.Cit.Ind., Chem.Abstr., Chem.Indus.Notes, Chem.Titles, Curr.Cont., Excerp.Med. (1993-), Genet.Abstr., Helminthol.Abstr., Hum.Gen.Abstr., Ind.Med. (1991-), Ind.Sci.Rev., Inpharma, Int.Abstr.Biol.Sci., Neurosci.Abstr., Nuc.Acids Abstr., Oncog.G.F.Abstr. (coverage dropped), Pharm.&Out.News, Reac., Sci.Cit.Ind., Zoo.Rec.
—BLDSC (3500.775100), ADONIS, CASDDS, CISTI, EMDOCS, GNLM, IDS, ingenta. **CCC.**
Published by: Elsevier Science Ltd., Elsevier Trends Journals, 84 Theobald's Rd, London WC1X 8RR, United Kingdom. TEL 44-20-7611-4400, FAX 44-20-7611-4468, cbiol@cursci.co.uk, info@current-opinion.com, http://www.elsevier.com/locate/gde, http://www.current-opinion.com. Circ: 20,000. **Subscr. to:** PO Box 331, Haywards Heath, West Sussex RH16 3FG, United Kingdom. TEL 44-1444-475650, FAX 44-1444-445423.

599.9 USA
CURRENT PROTOCOLS IN HUMAN GENETICS. Text in English. 2 base vols. plus q. updates. USD 575 (effective 2001); USD 610 combined subscription for base vol. & update; USD 330 updates for base vol. & update (effective 2002). **Document type:** *Academic/Scholarly.*
Related titles: CD-ROM ed.: USD 565 (effective 2001); USD 595 combined subscription for base vol. & update; USD 325 renewals for base vol. & update (effective 2002).
Published by: John Wiley & Sons, Inc., Journals (Subsidiary of: Wiley InterScience), 605 Third Ave, New York, NY 10158. TEL 212-850-6645, FAX 212-850-6021, subinfo@jwiley.com, uscs-wis@wiley.com, http://www.wiley.com. **Subscr. to:** John Wiley & Sons Ltd., Baffins Ln, Chichester, Sussex PO19 IUD, United Kingdom. TEL 44-1243-779777, FAX 44-1243-843232, cs-journals@wiley.co.uk.

576.5 CHE ISSN 1424-8581
QH431 CODEN: CGCGBR
CYTOGENETIC AND GENOME RESEARCH. Text in English, French, German. 1962. 16/yr. (in 4 vols.). CHF 3,248 in Europe to institutions; CHF 3,294 overseas to institutions; EUR 2,320.80 in Europe to institutions; USD 2,520 overseas to institutions (effective 2002). adv. charts, illus. index. reprint service avail. from PSC. *Refereed.* **Document type:** *Journal, Academic/Scholarly.*
Former titles: Cytogenetics and Cell Genetics (0301-0171); Cytogenetics (0011-4537)
Related titles: Microform ed.; Online - full text ed.: ISSN 1424-859X. CHF 232, EUR 168, USD 180 to institutions with print edition (effective 2002) (from EBSCO Publishing, O C L C Online Computer Library Center, Inc., RoweCom Information Quest, ProQuest Information & Learning, Swets Blackwell, Institute for Scientific Information).
Indexed: ASCA, Abstr.Anthropol., Abstr.Hyg., AgBiotech, Anim.Breed.Abstr., Aqua.Sci.& Fish.Abstr., BBCI, Biol.Abstr., Biotech.& Bioeng.Abstr., Biotech.Cit.Ind., Chem.Abstr., Chem.Indus.Notes, Chem.Titles, Curr.Adv.Ecol.Sci., Curr.Cont., Dairy Sci.Abstr., Excerp.Med., Genet.Abstr., Helminthol.Abstr., Hum.Gen.Abstr., INIS Atomind., Ind.Med. (1973-), Ind.Sci.Rev., Ind.Vet., Inpharma, Int.Abstr.Biol.Sci., Microbiol.Abstr., Neurosci.Cit.Ind., Nuc.Acids Abstr., Pharm.&Out.News, Pig News & Info., Plant Breed.Abstr., Poult.Abstr., Reac., Sci.Cit.Ind., Sport Fish.Abstr., Trop.Dis.Bull., Vet.Bull., Zoo.Rec.
—BLDSC (3506.770000), CASDDS, CISTI, EMDOCS, GNLM, IDS, Infotrieve, KNAW, Linda Hall. **CCC.**
Published by: S. Karger AG, Allschwilerstr 10, PO Box, Basel 4009, Switzerland. TEL 41-61-306-1111, FAX 41-61-306-1234, karger@karger.ch, http://www.online.karger.com/journals/ccg, http://www.karger.com. Eds. H P Klinger, M Schmid. adv.: page USD 1,195. Circ: 1,800.

572.8 GBR ISSN 1043-4666
QR185.8.C95 CODEN: CYTIE9
CYTOKINE. Text in English. 1989. m. GBP 655 to institutions (effective 2001). adv. reprint service avail. from SWZ. *Refereed.* **Document type:** *Academic/Scholarly.* **Description:** Publishes original work on all cytokines including interleukins, cytotoxins, hematopoietic factors, transforming growth factors, interferons, and other known or new cytokines.
Related titles: Online - full text ed.: (from EBSCO Publishing, O C L C Online Computer Library Center, Inc., RoweCom Information Quest, ingenta, Swets Blackwell, IDEAL Online Library, Institute for Scientific Information).
Indexed: ASCA, BBCI, Biol.Abstr., Chem.Abstr., Chem.Indus.Notes, Chem.Titles, Curr.Cont., Excerp.Med. (1993-), INIS Atomind., Ind.Med. (1989-), Ind.Sci.Rev., Inpharma, Pharm.&Out.News, Reac., Rev.Appl.Entomol., Sci.Cit.Ind.
—BLDSC (3506.778000), ADONIS, CASDDS, CISTI, EMDOCS, GNLM, IDS, Infotrieve, ingenta, KNAW. **CCC.**
Published by: (International Cytokine Society), Academic Press (Subsidiary of: Harcourt Publishers Ltd.), 24 Oval Rd, London NW1 7DX, United Kingdom. TEL 44-20-7267-4466, FAX 44-20-7482-2293, apsubs@acad.com, http://www.academicpress.com/cytokine; http://www.europe.idealibrary.com/. Eds. Gordon W Duff, Scott K Durum. R&P Catherine John. Adv. contact Nik Screen. **Subscr. to:** Harcourt Publishers Ltd., Foots Cray High St, Sidcup, Kent DA14 5HP, United Kingdom. TEL 44-20-8300-3322, FAX 44-20-8309-0807.

576.5 USA ISSN 0095-4527
QH426 CODEN: CYGEDX
CYTOLOGY AND GENETICS. Text in English. 1974. bi-m. USD 1,645 in US & Canada; USD 1,840 elsewhere (effective 2002). bibl, charts, illus. index. *Refereed.* **Document type:** *Journal, Academic/Scholarly.* **Description:** Covers genetic structure of populations, genotoxic effects in plants, animals and humans, heredity, breeding, and genetic diagnostics.
Related titles: ♦ Translation of: Tsitologiya i Genetika. ISSN 0564-3783.
Indexed: Biol.Abstr., Excerp.Med., Sport Fish.Abstr., Wild.Rev., Zoo.Rec.
—BLDSC (0411.088000), CISTI, GNLM, Infotrieve, ingenta. **CCC.**
Published by: (Natsional'na Akademiya Nauk Ukrainy UKR), Allerton Press, Inc., 18 W 27th St, New York, NY 10001. TEL 646-424-9686, FAX 646-424-9695, journals@allertonpress.com, http://www.allertonpress.com/. Ed. Yuri Y. Gleba.

581.3 CZE ISSN 1212-1975
CODEN: SUSLDO
CZECH JOURNAL OF GENETICS AND PLANT BREEDING. Text and summaries in Czech, Slovak, English. 1965. q. USD 62 in Europe; USD 64 elsewhere (effective 2000). bk.rev. back issues avail. **Description:** Publishes original scientific studies concerning genetics, plant selection, seed growing, biology of plants, and phytopathology.
Former titles (until 1998): Genetika a Slechteni (0862-8629); (until 1989): U V T I Z Sbornik - Genetika a Slechteni (0036-5378)
Indexed: AgBiotech, Bibl.Agri., Biol.Abstr., Chem.Abstr., Crop Physiol.Abstr., Field Crop Abstr., Helminthol.Abstr., Herb.Abstr., Hort.Abstr., INIS Atomind., Maize Abstr., Plant Breed.Abstr., Plant Gen.Res.Abstr., Plant Grow.Reg.Abstr., Potato Abstr., Ref.Zh., Rev.Appl.Entomol., Rev.Plant Path., Seed Abstr., Soyabean Abstr., Triticale Abstr., VITIS, Weed Abstr.
—BLDSC (3507.371470), CASDDS, CISTI.
Published by: Ustav Zemedelskych a Potravinarskych Informaci/Institute of Agricultural and Food Information, Slezska 7, Prague, 2 120 56, Czech Republic. TEL 420-2-24253489, FAX 420-2-24253938, editor@uzpi.cz. Ed. Marie Cerna. Circ: 300. **Co-sponsor:** Ceska Akademie Zemedelskych Ved.

D N A PROBES. see *BIOLOGY—Abstracting, Bibliographies, Statistics*

DEVELOPMENTAL AND COMPARATIVE IMMUNOLOGY; ontogeny - phylogeny - aging. see *MEDICAL SCIENCES—Allergology And Immunology*

576.5 USA ISSN 0070-7333
QL537.M6
DROSOPHILA INFORMATION SERVICE. Text in English. 1934. a. USD 15 domestic; USD 18 foreign (effective 2000). **Document type:** *Academic/Scholarly.* **Description:** Publishes research articles, descriptions of new mutations, stock lists, directory information, as well as general interest topics for Drosophila researchers.
Indexed: Curr.Adv.Ecol.Sci., Zoo.Rec.
Address: Department of Zoology, 730 Van Vleet Oval, University of Oklahoma, Norman, OK 73019. TEL 405-325-4821, FAX 405-325-7560, jthompson@ou.edu. Ed. James N Thompson Jr. Circ: 1,200.

B

576.5 GBR ISSN 1469-221X
▼ **E M B O REPORTS.** (European Molecular Biology Organization) Text in English. 2000 (Jul). m. GBP 72, USD 119 to individuals; GBP 345, USD 560 to institutions (effective 2002). adv. bk.rev. back issues avail. *Refereed.* **Document type:** *Journal, Academic/Scholarly.* **Description:** Intended for rapid publications of short, high quality papers in all areas of molecular biology.
Related titles: Online - full text ed.: E M B O Reports Online. ISSN 1469-3178. 2000. GBP 310, USD 504 to institutions Online only (effective 2002) (from HighWire Pr., Swets Blackwell, Institute for Scientific Information, RoweCom Information Quest).
Indexed: BBCI, Biotech.Cit.Ind., Curr.Cont.
—BLDSC (3733.086000).
Published by: (European Molecular Biology Organization), Oxford University Press, Academic Division, Great Clarendon St, Oxford OX2 6DP, United Kingdom. TEL 44-1865-267907, FAX 44-1865-267835, jnl.info@oup.co.uk, http://www.embo-reports.oupjournals.org, http://www.oup.co.uk/journals. Ed. Frank Gannon. Pub. David Prosser. R&P Fionna Willis. adv.: page GBP 260, page USD 470. Circ: 1,000. **Subscr. addr. in the US:** Oxford University Press, Journals, 2001 Evans Rd, Cary, NC 27513. TEL 800-852-7323, FAX 919-677-1714, jnlorders@oup-usa.org; **Subscr. to:** Journals Marketing, Great Clarendon St, Oxford OX2 6DP, United Kingdom.

576.5 EGY ISSN 0046-161X
QH426 CODEN: EJGCA9
EGYPTIAN JOURNAL OF GENETICS AND CYTOLOGY. Text in Arabic. 1972. s-a. USD 50 to individuals; USD 150 to institutions (effective 2001). adv. abstr. reprint service avail. from PQC. **Document type:** *Proceedings, Academic/Scholarly.*
Indexed: Anim.Breed.Abstr., Biol.Abstr., Cott.& Trop.Fibr.Abstr., Curr.Adv.Ecol.Sci., Curr.Cont. (coverage dropped), Dairy Sci.Abstr., Excerp.Med. (until 19??), Fababean Abstr., Genet.Abstr. (coverage dropped), Maize Abstr., Seed Abstr., Soyabean Abstr., Triticale Abstr., Weed Abstr., Zoo.Rec.
—CISTI.
Published by: Egyptian Society of Genetics and Cytology, University of Cairo, Faculty of Agriculture, Department of Genetics, Giza, Egypt. Eds. A R Selim, Dr. S. H. Hassanien. R&P Dr. S. H. Hassanien. Adv. contact Dr. Fatthy M. Abdel-Tawab. Circ: 500.

576.5 AUT ISSN 1020-5209
EMERGING TECHNOLOGY SERIES: GENETIC ENGINEERING AND BIOTECHNOLOGY. Text in German. 1982. q. USD 40; free in developing nations.
Formerly (until 1996): Genetic Engineering and Biotechnology: Monitor (1012-537X)
—CISTI.
Published by: United Nations Industrial Development Organization, Statistical and Networking, Postfach 300, Vienna, W 1400, Austria. TEL 43-1-26026-3736, FAX 43-1-2606-6843, drhind@unido.org, http://www.unido.org. Ed. V Campbell. Circ: 1,800.

ENDOCYTOBIOSIS AND CELL RESEARCH. see *BIOLOGY—Cytology And Histology*

ENTREZ DOCUMENT RETRIEVAL SYSTEM. see *BIOLOGY—Abstracting, Bibliographies, Statistics*

576.549 USA ISSN 0893-6692
QH465.C5 CODEN: EMMUEG
ENVIRONMENTAL AND MOLECULAR MUTAGENESIS. Text in English. 1979. 9/yr. USD 575 in United States; USD 665 in Canada & Mexico; USD 741 elsewhere; USD 604 combined subscription in United States for print and online eds.; USD 694 combined subscription in Canada & Mexico for print and online eds.; USD 770 combined subscription elsewhere for print and online eds. (effective 2002). adv. bk.rev. bibl, illus. *Refereed.* **Document type:** *Academic/Scholarly.* **Description:** Provides an international forum for research on basic mechanisms of mutation, the detection of mutagens, and the implications of environmental mutagens for human health.
Formerly: Environmental Mutagenesis (0192-2521)
Related titles: Online - full text ed.: ISSN 1098-2280. USD 575 in United States; USD 575 in Canada & Mexico; USD 575 elsewhere (effective 2002) (from EBSCO Publishing, Wiley InterScience, Institute for Scientific Information); ♦ Supplement: Environmental and Molecular Mutagenesis. Supplement. ISSN 0898-3003.
Indexed: ASCA, Anim.Breed.Abstr., Aqua.Sci.& Fish.Abstr., Biol.Abstr., Biotech.& Bioeng.Abstr., CSNB, Chem.Abstr., Chem.Indus.Notes, Chem.Titles, Curr.Adv.Cancer Res., Curr.Adv.Ecol.Sci., Curr.Adv.Gen.& Molec.Biol., Curr.Cont., Dok.Arbeitsmed., Environ.Sci.Poll.Mgmt., Excerp.Med., Food Sci.& Tech.Abstr., Genet.Abstr., Helminthol.Abstr., Hum.Gen.Abstr., INIS Atomind., Ind.Med. (1987-), Ind.Sci.Rev., Inpharma, Int.Abstr.Biol.Sci., Lab.Haz.Bull., NRN, Nuc.Acids Abstr., Nutr.Abstr., Pharm.&Out.News, Pollut.Abstr., Reac., Ref.Zh., Rev.Appl.Entomol., Rev.Med.& Vet.Mycol., Sci.Cit.Ind., Sel.Water Res.Abstr., Sport Fish.Abstr., Tox.Abstr., Weed Abstr., Wild.Rev.
—BLDSC (3791.383100), CASDDS, CISTI, EMDOCS, GNLM, IDS, ingenta, Linda Hall. **CCC.**
Published by: (Environmental Mutagen Society), John Wiley & Sons, Inc., Journals (Subsidiary of: Wiley InterScience), 605 Third Ave, New York, NY 10158. TEL 212-850-6645, FAX 212-850-6021, subinfo@wiley.com, uscs-wis@wiley.com, http://www.wiley.com. Ed. Errol Zeiger. adv.: B&W page GBP 640, color page GBP 1,515; trim 174 x 254. Circ: 1,500. **Subscr. outside the Americas to:** John Wiley & Sons Ltd., Baffins Ln, Chichester, Sussex PO19 IUD, United Kingdom. TEL 44-1243-779777, FAX 44-1243-843232, cs-journals@wiley.co.uk, http://www.wiley.co.uk.

576.549 USA ISSN 0898-3003
ENVIRONMENTAL AND MOLECULAR MUTAGENESIS. SUPPLEMENT. Text in English. 1987. irreg. back issues avail. **Document type:** *Academic/Scholarly.*
Related titles: ♦ Supplement to: Environmental and Molecular Mutagenesis. ISSN 0893-6692.
Indexed: Biol.Abstr., Excerp.Med., Ind.Med. (coverage dropped).
—BLDSC (3791.383110), CISTI.
Published by: (Environmental Mutagen Society), John Wiley & Sons, Inc., Journals (Subsidiary of: Wiley InterScience), 605 Third Ave, New York, NY 10158. **Subscr. outside the Americas to:** John Wiley & Sons Ltd., Baffins Ln, Chichester, Sussex PO19 IUD, United Kingdom. FAX 44-1243-776128.

613.94 USA
EUGENICS SPECIAL INTEREST GROUP BULLETIN. Text in English. 1970. irreg. USD 6. **Document type:** *Bulletin.*
Published by: Eugenics Special Interest Group, PO Box 138, East Schodack, NY 12163. TEL 518-732-2390, willardh2@juno.com. Ed. Willard Hoyt.

572.8 FRA ISSN 1148-5493
CODEN: ECYNEJ
EUROPEAN CYTOKINE NETWORK. Text in English. 1990. 4/yr. FRF 1,300 domestic to individuals; EUR 210 in Europe to individuals; USD 245 elsewhere to individuals; FRF 2,100 domestic to institutions; EUR 332 in Europe to institutions; USD 382 elsewhere to institutions; FRF 525 newsstand/cover (effective 2001). *Refereed.* **Document type:** *Academic/Scholarly.* **Description:** Serves as a link between immunological, biological, molecular, hematological and oncological researchers and clinicians.
Related titles: Online - full text ed.: FRF 1,300 in Europe to individuals; USD 220 elsewhere to individuals; FRF 2,100 in Europe to institutions; USD 350 elsewhere to institutions (effective 2001) (from Institute for Scientific Information).
Indexed: ASCA, BBCI, Chem.Abstr., Chem.Indus.Notes, Chem.Titles, Curr.Cont., Excerp.Med. (1993-), Ind.Med. (1990-), Ind.Sci.Rev., Inpharma, Int.Abstr.Biol.Sci., Pharm.&Out.News, Protozool.Abstr., Reac., Rev.Appl.Entomol., Sci.Cit.Ind., Trop.Dis.Bull.
—BLDSC (3829.688820), ADONIS, CASDDS, EMDOCS, GNLM, IDS, KNAW.
Published by: John Libbey Eurotext, 127 av. de la Republique, Montrouge 92120, France. TEL 1-46-73-06-60, FAX 1-40-84-09-99, marketing@jle.com, http://www.john-libbey-eurotext.fr/. Eds. Didier Fradelizi, Jacques Bertoglio. **Subscr. to:** A T E I, 3 av. Pierre Kerautret, Romainville 92230, France. TEL 33-1-48408686, FAX 33-1-48400731, atei@club-internet.fr.

599.9 GBR ISSN 1018-4813
CODEN: EJHGEU
EUROPEAN JOURNAL OF HUMAN GENETICS. Text in English. 1993. 8/yr. GBP 320 in Europe to individuals for print or online ed.; USD 480 rest of world to individuals for print or online ed.; GBP 352 combined subscription in Europe to individuals print & online; USD 528 combined subscription rest of world to individuals print & online; GBP 715 in Europe to institutions for print or online ed.; USD 1,073 rest of world to institutions for print or online ed.; GBP 743 combined subscription in Europe to institutions print & online; USD 1,115 combined subscription rest of world to institutions print & online (effective 2002). adv. charts, illus, stat. back issues avail. *Refereed.* **Document type:** *Journal, Academic/Scholarly.* **Description:** Contains information on the development of research, education and medical application in the field of human genetics.
Related titles: Microform ed.: (from PQC); Online - full text ed.: (from EBSCO Publishing, O C L C Online Computer Library Center, Inc., RoweCom Information Quest, ingenta, Swets Blackwell, Institute for Scientific Information).
Indexed: ASCA, Biotech.Cit.Ind., Chem.Abstr., Chem.Indus.Notes, Chem.Titles, Curr.Cont., Excerp.Med. (1994-), Ind.Med. (1992-), Inpharma, Pharm.&Out.News, Reac., Sci.Cit.Ind.
—BLDSC (3829.730020), CASDDS, CISTI, EMDOCS, GNLM, IDS, Infotrieve, KNAW. **CCC.**
Published by: (European Society of Human Genetics), Nature Publishing Group Specialist Journals (Subsidiary of: Holtzbrink Publishers), Houndmills, Basingstoke, Hants RG21 6XS, United Kingdom. TEL 44-1256-329242, FAX 44-1256-328339, subscriptions@nature.com, http://www.nature.com/ejhg. Ed. G.-J. Van Ommen. Pub. Katy Christomanou. R&P Trace Noel. Adv. contact Robert Sloan TEL 44-20-8882-7199.

576.5 GBR ISSN 0960-7420
QR184 CODEN: EJOIE3
EUROPEAN JOURNAL OF IMMUNOGENETICS. Text in English. 1974. bi-m., latest vol.29, 2002. GBP 500 in Europe; USD 790 in North America; GBP 548 elsewhere (effective 2002). adv. bk.rev. abstr, bibl, illus. index. back issues avail.; reprint service avail. from ISI. *Refereed.* **Document type:** *Academic/Scholarly.* **Description:** Publishes original contributions on the genetic control of components of the immune system and their interactions in both humans and experimental animals.
Formerly: Journal of Immunogenetics (0305-1811)
Related titles: Microform ed.: (from PQC); Online - full text ed.: ISSN 1365-2370. GBP 450 in Europe; USD 711 in North America; GBP 450 elsewhere (effective 2002) (from Ovid Technologies, Inc., EBSCO Publishing, O C L C Online Computer Library Center, Inc., RoweCom Information Quest, ingenta, Munksgaard & Blackwell Science's Synergy, Swets Blackwell, Institute for Scientific Information); Supplement: European Journal of Immunogenetics. Supplement. ISSN 1367-3661. 1997.
Indexed: AIDS & Cancer Res., Abstr.Hyg., Anim.Breed.Abstr., Biol.Abstr., Biotech.& Bioeng.Abstr., Biotech.Cit.Ind., Chem.Abstr., Chem.Indus.Notes, Chem.Titles, Curr.Adv.Ecol.Sci., Curr.Biotech.Abstr., Curr.Cont., Dairy Sci.Abstr., Excerp.Med., Genet.Abstr., Helminthol.Abstr., Hum.Gen.Abstr., INIS Atomind., Immun.Abstr., Ind.Med. (1991-), Ind.Sci.Rev., Ind.Vet., Inpharma, Int.Abstr.Biol.Sci., Nuc.Acids Abstr., Pharm.&Out.News, Reac., Sci.Cit.Ind., Trop.Dis.Bull., Vet.Bull.
—BLDSC (3829.730050), ADONIS, CASDDS, CISTI, EMDOCS, GNLM, IDS, ingenta, KNAW. **CCC.**
Published by: Blackwell Science Ltd., PO Box 88, Oxford OX2 0NE, United Kingdom. TEL 44-1865-206180, 44-1865-206002, FAX 44-1865-206219, jnl.orders@blacksci.co.uk, http://www.blackwell-science.com/~cgilib/jnlpage.asp?Journal=ejimm&File=ejimm, http://www.blackwellpublishing.com. Ed. E D Albert. Pub. Allen Stevens. R&P Sophie Savage. Adv. contact Jenny Applin. Circ: 435.

576.8 USA ISSN 0014-3820
QH301 CODEN: EVOLAO
EVOLUTION; international journal of organic evolution. Text in English. 1947. m. USD 65 domestic to individuals; USD 70 foreign to individuals; USD 190 domestic to institutions; USD 200 foreign to institutions; USD 60 in developing nations to institutions (effective 2001). adv. bk.rev. bibl, charts, illus, stat. index. back issues avail.; reprints avail. *Refereed.* **Document type:** *Academic/Scholarly.* **Description:** Reports observations and perspectives in evolutionary biology.
Related titles: Microform ed.: (from PQC); Online - full text ed.: (from Gale Group, BioOne, Northern Light Technology, Inc., H. W. Wilson, JSTOR (Web-based Journal Archive), Institute for Scientific Information).
Indexed: ASCA, Abstr.Anthropol., AgBiotech, Agricola, Agroforest.Abstr., Anim.Behav.Abstr., Anim.Breed.Abstr., Apic.Abstr., Appl.Ecol.Abstr., Aqua.Sci.& Fish.Abstr., Aquacult.Abstr., Bibl.Agri., Bio-Contr.News & Info., Biol.& Agr.Ind. (Jan.1983-), Biol.Abstr., Br.Tech.Ind., Chem.Abstr., Chem.Indus.Notes, Chem.Titles, Curr.Adv.Ecol.Sci., Curr.Adv.Plant Sci., Curr.Cont., Curr.Ind.Stat., Deep Sea Res.& Oceanogr.Abstr., Ecol.Abstr., Entomol.Abstr., Environ.Sci.Poll.Mgmt., Excerp.Med., Field Crop Abstr., Food Sci.& Tech.Abstr., Forest Prod.Abstr., Forest.Abstr., Gen.Sci.Ind. (Nov.1982-), Genet.Abstr., GeoRef, Geol.Abstr., Helminthol.Abstr., Herb.Abstr., Hum.Gen.Abstr., INIS Atomind., Ind.Med., Ind.Sci.Rev., Ind.Vet., Inpharma, Int.Abstr.Biol.Sci., Int.Aerosp.Abstr., Key Word Ind.Wildl.Res., Maize Abstr., Microbiol.Abstr., Nuc.Acids Abstr., Nutr.Abstr., Ocean.Abstr., Ornam.Hort., Pharm.&Out.News, Plant Breed.Abstr., Plant Gen.Res.Abstr., Plant Sci., Poult.Abstr., Protozool.Abstr., Reac., Ref.Zh., Rev.Appl.Entomol., Rev.Med.& Vet.Mycol., Rev.Plant Path., SSCI (coverage dropped), Sci.Cit.Ind., Seed Abstr., Sh.& Vib.Dig., So.Pac.Per.Ind., Soyabean Abstr., Sport Fish.Abstr., Triticale Abstr., Vet.Bull., Weed Abstr., Wild.Rev., Zoo.Rec.
—BLDSC (3834.000000), CASDDS, CISTI, EMDOCS, ingenta, Linda Hall.
Published by: Society for the Study of Evolution, c/o Allen Press, Inc, Box 1897, Lawrence, KS 66044-8897. TEL 785-843-1235, 800-627-0629, FAX 785-843-1274, ssoe@allenpress.com, http://www.lsvl.la.asu.edu/evolution. Ed. Donald M Waller. Circ: 4,500.

576.8 USA ISSN 0071-3260
QH366.A1 CODEN: EVBIAI
EVOLUTIONARY BIOLOGY. Text in English. 1967. irreg., latest vol.32. price varies. *Refereed.* **Document type:** *Monographic series.*
Related titles: Online - full text ed.: (from Institute for Scientific Information).
Indexed: ASCA, Abstr.Anthropol., Biol.Abstr., Biol.Dig., Chem.Abstr., Chem.Indus.Notes, Chem.Titles, Curr.Adv.Ecol.Sci., Deep Sea Res.& Oceanogr.Abstr., GeoRef, Ind.Sci.Rev., SSCI (coverage dropped), Sci.Cit.Ind., Sport Fish.Abstr., Wild.Rev., Zoo.Rec.
—BLDSC (3834.400000), CASDDS, CISTI, IDS, Infotrieve, ingenta, KNAW, Linda Hall. **CCC.**
Published by: Kluwer Academic - Plenum Publishers (Subsidiary of: Wolters Kluwer N.V.), 233 Spring St, New York, NY 10013-1578. TEL 212-620-8000, 800-221-9369, FAX 212-463-0742, info@plenum.com, http://www.plenum.com. Eds. Bruce Wallace, Max Hecht.

EXCERPTA MEDICA. SECTION 22: HUMAN GENETICS. see *BIOLOGY—Abstracting, Bibliographies, Statistics*

▼ **F E M S YEAST RESEARCH.** see *BIOLOGY—Microbiology*

▼ **FAMILIAL CANCER.** see *MEDICAL SCIENCES—Oncology*

GATHERED VIEW; national newsletter of the Prader-Willi syndrome Assn. (USA). see *MEDICAL SCIENCES*

GENBANK. see *BIOLOGY—Biochemistry*

GENE; an international journal focusing on gene cloning and gene structure and function. see *BIOLOGY—Biotechnology*

576.5 572.8 USA ISSN 1052-2166
QH450 CODEN: GEEXEJ

GENE EXPRESSION; international journal of molecular and cellular science. Text in English. 1991. bi-m. USD 625 domestic; USD 655 foreign (effective 2001). adv. back issues avail. *Refereed.* **Document type:** *Academic/Scholarly.* **Description:** Publishes papers on all aspects of gene including its structure, function and regulation in prokaryotes, eukaryotes and viruses. Topics on DNA replication, DNA repair, gene transcription, transcriptional control, RNA processing, posttranscriptional control, oncogenes, molecular mechanisms of action of hormones, molecular mechanisms of cellular differentiation, growth and development, protein syntheses, and posttranslational control.
Related titles: Online - full text ed.: (from Institute for Scientific Information).
Indexed: Agricola, Aqua.Sci.& Fish.Abstr., Biotech.Cit.Ind., Entomol.Abstr., Environ.Sci.Poll.Mgmt., Genet.Abstr., Ind.Med. (1991-), Int.Abstr.Biol.Sci., Microbiol.Abstr., Nuc.Acids Abstr.
—BLDSC (4096.402395), CASDDS, CISTI, GNLM, IDS, Infotrieve, KNAW. **CCC.**
Published by: Cognizant Communication Corporation, 3 Hartsdale Rd, Elmsford, NY 10523-3701. TEL 914-592-7720, FAX 914-592-8981, cogcomm@aol.com, http://www.cognizantcommunication.com. Ed. Samson Jacob. Pub., R&P Robert N Miranda. Adv. contact Lori Miranda.

576.5 NLD ISSN 1567-133X

▼ **GENE EXPRESSION PATTERNS.** Text in English. 2001. q. EUR 327 in Europe to institutions; JPY 43,500 in Japan to institutions; USD 367 elsewhere to institutions (effective 2002).
—ADONIS.
Published by: Elsevier Science BV, Sara Burgerhartstraat 25, Amsterdam 1055 KV, Netherlands. TEL 31-20-485-2911, FAX 31-20-485-2457, nlinfo-f@elsevier.nl, http://www.elsevier.com/locate/bresg, http://www.elsevier.nl. Ed. M Frenkel.

576.5 USA

THE GENE LETTER. Text in English. 1996. bi-m. **Document type:** *Newsletter.* **Description:** Covers the scientific, ethical, legal and social aspects of genetics.
Media: Online - full text.
Published by: (Shriver Center, Inc.), Shriver Center, 200 Trapelo Rd, Waltham, MA 02452. TEL 781-642-0292, FAX 781-642-0292, dwertz@shriver.org; webmaster@shriver.org, http://www.geneletter.org. Eds. Dorothy C Wertz, Philip R Reilly. R&P Dorothy C Wertz. Circ: 25,500.

576.5 660 NLD ISSN 1388-9532

▼ **GENE THERAPY AND REGULATION**; an international interdisciplinary journal. Text in English. 1999. q. EUR 212, USD 245 includes online ed. (effective 2002). back issues avail. *Refereed.* **Document type:** *Journal, Academic/Scholarly.* **Description:** Explores all aspects of research on gene therapy and ancillary basic cell- and molecular biology approaches, including molecular cloning, sequencing, and gene regulation.
Related titles: Online - full content ed.: 2000 (from EBSCO Publishing, Swets Blackwell); Online - full text ed.: (from CatchWord Ltd.).
Published by: V S P (Subsidiary of: Brill Academic Publishers), PO Box 346, Zeist 3700 AH, Netherlands. TEL 31-30-692-5790, FAX 31-30-693-2081, vsppub@compuserve.com, http://www.vsppub.com/journals/jn-GenTheReg.html. Ed. Roger Bertolotti TEL 33-4-93817381.

GENE THERAPY (SHEFFIELD). see *BIOLOGY—Abstracting, Bibliographies, Statistics*

576.5 USA ISSN 0890-9369
QH426 CODEN: GEDEEP

GENES & DEVELOPMENT. Text in English. 1987. s-m. USD 140 domestic to individuals; USD 216 in Canada & Mexico to individuals; USD 248 elsewhere to individuals; USD 850 domestic to institutions; USD 926 in Canada & Mexico to institutions; USD 958 elsewhere to institutions (effective 2001). adv. illus. Index. back issues avail.; reprints avail. *Refereed.* **Document type:** *Journal, Academic/Scholarly.* **Description:** Publishes research papers of general interest and biological significance in molecular biology, molecular genetics, and related areas.
Related titles: Online - full text ed.: 1997 (from HighWire Pr., EBSCO Publishing, Gale Group, Institute for Scientific Information).
Indexed: ASCA, Abstr.Anthropol., AgBiotech, Anim.Breed.Abstr., Aqua.Sci.& Fish.Abstr., Biol.& Agr.Ind. (Jan.1996-), Biol.Dig., Biotech.Cit.Ind., Chem.Abstr., Chem.Indus.Notes, Chem.Titles, Crop Physiol.Abstr., Curr.Adv.Cell & Devel.Biol., Curr.Adv.Gen.& Molec.Biol., Curr.Cont., Dairy Sci.Abstr., Entomol.Abstr., Environ.Sci.Poll.Mgmt., Field Crop Abstr., Gen.Sci.Ind. (Jul.1997-), Genet.Abstr., Helminthol.Abstr., Hum.Gen.Abstr., INIS Atomind., Ind.Med. (1987-), Ind.Sci.Rev., Ind.Vet., Inpharma, Int.Abstr.Biol.Sci., Maize Abstr., Microbiol.Abstr., Neurosci.Abstr., Nuc.Acids Abstr., Nutr.Abstr., Oncog.G.F.Abstr. (coverage dropped), Ornam.Hort., Plant Breed.Abstr., Plant Grow.Reg.Abstr., Poult.Abstr., Protozool.Abstr., Reac., Ref.Zh., Rev.Appl.Entomol., Rev.Plant Path., Rice Abstr., SSCI (coverage dropped), Sci.Cit.Ind., Seed Abstr., Telegen, Weed Abstr., Wild.Rev.
—BLDSC (4111.759700), CASDDS, CISTI, EMDOCS, GNLM, IDS, ingenta, Linda Hall. **CCC.**
Published by: (Genetics Society), Cold Spring Harbor Laboratory Press, Publications Department, 10 Skyline Dr, Plainview, NY 11803. TEL 516-349-1930, FAX 516-349-1946, cshpress@cshl.org, http://www.genesdev.org, http://www.cshl.org. Eds. D Solter, T Grodzicker.

576.5 JPN ISSN 1341-7568
QH426 CODEN: GGSYF5

GENES & GENETIC SYSTEMS. Text in English. 1921. bi-m. USD 130. adv. bk.rev. back issues avail. *Refereed.* **Document type:** *Academic/Scholarly.* **Description:** Covers a wide range in the field of genetics: general genetics, molecular genetics, cytogenetics, population genetics and evolution, and genome research.
Formerly (until vol.70, no.6, 1996): Japanese Journal of Genetics - Idengaku Zasshi (0021-504X)
Related titles: Online - full text ed.: (from Institute for Scientific Information).
Indexed: AgBiotech, Agrindex, Anim.Breed.Abstr., Aqua.Sci.& Fish.Abstr., Aquacult.Abstr., Biol.Abstr., Biotech.Cit.Ind., Chem.Abstr., Chem.Indus.Notes, Chem.Titles, Curr.Cont., Entomol.Abstr., Environ.Sci.Poll.Mgmt., Excerp.Med., Fababean Abstr., Field Crop Abstr., Forest.Abstr., Genet.Abstr., Helminthol.Abstr., Hort.Abstr., Hum.Gen.Abstr., INIS Atomind., Ind.Med. (1996-), Ind.Sci.Rev., Ind.Vet., Inpharma, JTA, Jap.Per.Ind., Nuc.Acids Abstr., Ornam.Hort., Plant Breed.Abstr., Plant Gen.Res.Abstr., Reac., Rev.Appl.Entomol., Rev.Plant Path., Rice Abstr., Sci.Cit.Ind., Seed Abstr., Soyabean Abstr., Sport Fish.Abstr., Triticale Abstr., Weed Abstr., Wild.Rev., Zoo.Rec.
—CASDDS, CISTI, EMDOCS, GNLM, IDS, Infotrieve, ingenta, Linda Hall. **CCC.**
Published by: Genetics Society of Japan/Nihon Iden Gakkai, c/o National Institute of Genetics, 1111 Yata, Mishima-shi, Shizuoka-ken 411-0801, Japan. TEL 81-6-6879-8317, FAX 81-6-6879-8320, shinagaw@biken.osaka-u.ac.jp. Ed., R&P Hideo Shinagawa. Circ: 2,000. **Dist. by:** Business Center for Academic Societies Japan, 5-16-9 Honkomagome, Bunkyo-ku, Tokyo 113-0021, Japan. TEL 81-3-5814-5811.

576.5 GBR ISSN 1466-4879

▼ **GENES AND IMMUNITY**; genetics, genomics and function. Text in English. 1999. bi-m. GBP 68 to individuals; GBP 290 in Europe to institutions; GBP 310 rest of world to institutions; GBP 75 to individuals Print & Online eds.; GBP 319 in Europe to institutions Print & Online eds.; GBP 341 rest of world to institutions Print & Online eds. (effective 2001). **Document type:** *Academic/Scholarly.*
Related titles: Online - full text ed.: GBP 68 to individuals; GBP 290 to institutions (effective 2001) (from ingenta, Swets Blackwell, Institute for Scientific Information, RoweCom Information Quest).
Indexed: Biotech.& Bioeng.Abstr., Biotech.Cit.Ind., Immun.Abstr., Ind.Med.
—BLDSC (4111.762200).
Published by: Nature Publishing Group Specialist Journals (Subsidiary of: Holtzbrink Publishers), Houndmills, Basingstoke, Hants RG21 6XS, United Kingdom. TEL 44-1256-329242, FAX 44-1256-328339, subscriptions@nature.com, http://www.nature.com/gene.

576.5 DNK ISSN 1601-1848

▼ **GENES, BRAIN AND BEHAVIOR.** Text in English. 2001. q. USD 209 in the Americas to institutions print & online eds. combined; GBP 131 elsewhere to institutions print & online eds. combined (2002). adv. **Document type:** *Academic/Scholarly.* **Description:** Covers the analysis of the behavioral and neural phenotypes with the unifying theme being the genetic approach as a tool to increase our understanding of these phenotypes.
Related titles: Online - full content ed.: ISSN 1601-183X. forthcoming 2002.
Published by: (International Behavioural and Neural Genetics Society GBR), Munksgaard (Subsidiary of: Blackwell Science Ltd.), 35 Norre Sogade, PO Box 2148, Copenhagen K 1016, Denmark. TEL 45-7733-3333, FAX 45-7733-3377, headoffice@munksgaard.dk, http://www.munksgaard.dk/. Ed. Wim E Crusio. Adv. contact Eric Rozario TEL 45-7733-3301. B&W page DKK 4,000, B&W page USD 580, color page DKK 14,500, color page USD 1,890; trim 210 x 280.

572.8 USA ISSN 1045-2257
RC268.4 CODEN: GCCAES

GENES, CHROMOSOMES & CANCER. Text in English. 1989. m. USD 1,295 in United States; USD 1,415 in Canada & Mexico; USD 1,517 elsewhere; USD 1,360 combined subscription in United States for print and online eds.; USD 1,480 combined subscription in Canada & Mexico for print and online eds.; USD 1,582 combined subscription elsewhere for print and online eds. (effective 2002). adv. back issues avail. *Refereed.* **Document type:** *Academic/Scholarly.* **Description:** Covers all aspects of genomic abnormalities related to neoplasia. Particular emphasis is placed on work combining molecular and cytogenetic analysis of the acquired genetic alterations of cancer cells.
Related titles: Microform ed.: (from PQC); Online - full text ed.: ISSN 1098-2264. USD 1,295 in United States; USD 1,295 in Canada & Mexico; USD 1,295 elsewhere (effective 2002) (from EBSCO Publishing, Wiley InterScience, Institute for Scientific Information).
Indexed: ASCA, Biotech.& Bioeng.Abstr., Biotech.Cit.Ind., Chem.Abstr., Chem.Indus.Notes, Chem.Titles, Curr.Cont., Genet.Abstr., Hum.Gen.Abstr., Ind.Med. (1989-), Ind.Sci.Rev., Inpharma, Int.Abstr.Biol.Sci., Nuc.Acids Abstr., Oncog.G.F.Abstr., Pharm.&Out.News, Reac., Ref.Zh., Sci.Cit.Ind.
—BLDSC (4111.763000), CASDDS, CISTI, EMDOCS, GNLM, IDS, ingenta, KNAW.
Published by: John Wiley & Sons, Inc., Journals (Subsidiary of: Wiley InterScience), 605 Third Ave, New York, NY 10158. TEL 212-850-6645, FAX 212-850-6021, subinfo@wiley.com, http://www.wiley.com. Eds. Felix Mitelman, Janet D Rowley. adv.: B&W page GBP 640, color page GBP 1,515; trim 210 x 279. Circ: 800. **Subscr. outside the Americas to:** John Wiley & Sons Ltd., Baffins Ln, Chichester, Sussex PO19 IUD, United Kingdom. TEL 44-1243-779777, FAX 44-1243-843232, cs-journals@wiley.co.uk, http://www.wiley.co.uk.

576.5 GBR ISSN 1356-9597
QH441.5 CODEN: GECEFL

GENES TO CELLS. Text in English. 1996. m., latest vol.7, 2002. GBP 95 in Europe to individuals; USD 152 in North America to individuals; GBP 105 elsewhere to individuals; GBP 683 in Europe to institutions; USD 1,083 in North America to institutions; GBP 752 elsewhere to institutions (effective 2002). adv. *Refereed.* **Document type:** *Academic/Scholarly.* **Description:** Provides an international forum for papers relating to physiological, biophysical, and evolutionary ecology.
Related titles: Online - full text ed.: ISSN 1365-2443. GBP 86 in Europe to individuals; USD 137 in North America to individuals; GBP 86 elsewhere to individuals; GBP 615 in Europe to institutions; USD 975 in North America to institutions; GBP 615 elsewhere to institutions (effective 2002) (from EBSCO Publishing, O C L C Online Computer Library Center, Inc., RoweCom Information Quest, ingenta, Munksgaard & Blackwell Science's Synergy, Swets Blackwell, Institute for Scientific Information).
Indexed: AgBiotech, Aqua.Sci.& Fish.Abstr., Biotech.& Bioeng.Abstr., Biotech.Cit.Ind., Chem.Abstr., Chem.Indus.Notes, Chem.Titles, Crop Physiol.Abstr., Curr.Cont., Genet.Abstr., Hum.Gen.Abstr., Ind.Med. (1996-), Microbiol.Abstr., Neurosci.Abstr. (coverage dropped), Nuc.Acids Abstr., Oncog.G.F.Abstr. (coverage dropped), Plant Breed.Abstr., Sci.Cit.Ind.
—BLDSC (4111.762500), CASDDS, CISTI, GNLM, IDS, Infotrieve, KNAW. **CCC.**
Published by: (Molecular Biology Society of Japan), Blackwell Science Ltd., PO Box 88, Oxford OX2 0NE, United Kingdom. TEL 44-1865-206180, 44-1865-206002, FAX 44-1865-206219, jnl.orders@blacksci.co.uk, http://www.blackwell-science.com/~cgilib/jnlpage.asp?Journal=gtc&File=gtc, http://www.blackwellpublishing.com. Ed. Dr. Jun Ichi Tomizawa. Pub. Sue Hewitt. R&P Sophie Savage. Adv. contact Martine Cariou Keen. Circ: 695.

B

B

599.9 GBR ISSN 1466-920X
▼ **GENESCREEN**; an international journal of medical genomics. Text in English. 2000. q., latest vol.2, 2002. GBP 60 in Europe to individuals; USD 102 in North America to individuals; GBP 66 elsewhere to individuals; GBP 255 in Europe to institutions; USD 432 in North America to institutions; GBP 280 elsewhere to institutions (effective 2002). **Description:** Contains original scientific contributions in the field of Medical Genomics with an emphasis on the exploitation of genomic information to improve health and the quality of life. Developments in genomics within the wider scope of medicine are encouraged, with a willingness to present methodological breakthroughs which may or may not be related to specific diseases.
Related titles: Online - full text ed.: ISSN 1466-9218. GBP 54 in Europe to individuals; USD 92 in North America to individuals; GBP 54 elsewhere to individuals; GBP 230 in Europe to institutions; USD 389 in North America to institutions; GBP 230 elsewhere to institutions (effective 2002) (from EBSCO Publishing, ingenta, Munksgaard & Blackwell Science's Synergy, Swets Blackwell).
—BLDSC (4111.764000).
Published by: Blackwell Science Ltd., PO Box 88, Oxford OX2 0NE, United Kingdom. TEL 44-1865-206180, 44-1865-206002, FAX 44-1865-206219, jnl.orders@blacksci.co.uk, http://www.blackwell-science.com/~cgilib/jnlpage.asp?Journal=gsc&File=gsc, http://www.blackwellpublishing.com. Eds. G Duff, I Peake. Pub. Allen Stevens. R&P Sophie Savage. Adv. contact Jenny Applin. Circ: 500.

576.5 USA ISSN 1526-954X
QH453 CODEN: DGNTDW
GENESIS: THE JOURNAL OF GENETICS AND DEVELOPMENT. Text in English. 1979. 8/yr. USD 1,499 in United States; USD 1,619 in Canada & Mexico; USD 1,721 elsewhere; USD 1,574 in United States for print and online eds.; USD 1,694 in Canada & Mexico for print and online eds.; USD 1,796 elsewhere for print and online eds. (effective 2002). adv. bk.rev. bibl, illus. back issues avail. *Refereed.* **Document type:** *Academic/Scholarly.* **Description:** Covers molecular and developmental genetics and provides a forum for research on all organisms, including prokaryotes, plants, insects, worms, and mammals.
Formerly (until 2000): Developmental Genetics (0192-253X)
Related titles: Microform ed.: (from PQC); Online - full text ed.: ISSN 1526-968X. USD 1,499 in United States; USD 1,499 in Canada & Mexico; USD 1,499 elsewhere (effective 2002) (from EBSCO Publishing, Wiley InterScience, Institute for Scientific Information).
Indexed: ASCA, AgBiotech, Agricola, Anim.Breed.Abstr., Aqua.Sci.& Fish.Abstr., Bibl.Agri., Biol.Abstr., Biotech.Cit.Ind., Chem.Abstr., Chem.Indus.Notes, Chem.Titles, Crop Physiol.Abstr., Curr.Adv.Biochem., Curr.Adv.Cell & Devel.Biol., Curr.Adv.Ecol.Sci., Curr.Adv.Gen.& Molec.Biol., Curr.Cont., Dairy Sci.Abstr., Excerp.Med., Field Crop Abstr., Forest.Abstr., Genet.Abstr., Helminthol.Abstr., Hum.Gen.Abstr., INIS Atomind., Ind.Med. (2000-), Ind.Sci.Rev., Inpharma, Int.Abstr.Biol.Sci., Maize Abstr., Microbiol.Abstr., Nuc.Acids Abstr., Nutr.Abstr., Pig News & Info., Plant Breed.Abstr., Plant Grow.Reg.Abstr., Poult.Abstr., Reac., Ref.Zh., Rev.Appl.Entomol., Rice Abstr., Sci.Cit.Ind., Seed Abstr., Weed Abstr., Zoo.Rec.
—BLDSC (4111.807500), CASDDS, CISTI, EMDOCS, GNLM, IDS, ingenta. **CCC.**
Published by: John Wiley & Sons, Inc., Journals (Subsidiary of: Wiley InterScience), 605 Third Ave, New York, NY 10158. TEL 212-850-6645, FAX 212-850-6021, subinfo@wiley.com, uscs-wis@wiley.com, http://www.wiley.com. Ed. Gerald M Kidder. adv.: B&W page GBP 640, color page GBP 1,515; trim 210 x 279. Circ: 550. **Subscr. outside the Americas to:** John Wiley & Sons Ltd., Baffins Ln, Chichester, Sussex PO19 IUD, United Kingdom. TEL 44-1243-779777, FAX 44-1243-843232, cs-journals@wiley.co.uk, http://www.wiley.co.uk.

GENETHICS NEWS. see *BIOLOGY—Biotechnology*

576.5 CHE ISSN 1015-8146
RB155.7 CODEN: GECOEG
GENETIC COUNSELING. Summaries in English, French, German. 1952. 4/yr. CHF 225, EUR 146.10 to individuals; CHF 295, EUR 191.55 to institutions (effective 2002). adv. bk.rev. abstr, charts, illus, stat. index, cum.index. Supplement avail.; reprint service avail. from IRC. *Refereed.* **Document type:** *Journal, Academic/Scholarly.*
Formerly (until 1990): Journal de Genetique Humaine (0021-7743)
Related titles: Online - full text ed.: (from Institute for Scientific Information).
Indexed: ASCA, Anthropol.Lit. (coverage dropped), Bibl.Dev.Med.& Child Neur., Biol.Abstr., Biotech.Cit.Ind., Chem.Abstr., Curr.Cont., Dent.Ind., Excerp.Med., Ind.Med. (1990-), Ind.Sci.Rev., Int.Nurs.Ind., SSCI (coverage dropped), Sci.Cit.Ind. (coverage dropped).
—BLDSC (4111.845000), CISTI, EMDOCS, GNLM, IDS, Infotrieve, ingenta, KNAW, Linda Hall. **CCC.**
Published by: Editions Medecine et Hygiene, Case Postale 456, Geneva, 4 1211, Switzerland. TEL 41-22-7029311, FAX 41-22-7029355, abonnements@medhyg.ch, http://www.medhyg.ch. Circ: 800.

576.5 JPN
GENETIC ENGINEERING. Text in English. 1985. irreg.
Published by: Associazione Biologica Italo-Giapponese/ Nichii Seibutsugaku Kyokai, Nagoya Daigaku Rigakubu Rinkai Jikkenjo, Furo-cho, Chikusa-ku, Nagoya-shi, Aichi-ken 464-0814, Japan.

GENETIC ENGINEERING; principles and methods. see *BIOLOGY—Biotechnology*

576.5 USA ISSN 0270-6377
TP248.6 CODEN: GENNDX
GENETIC ENGINEERING NEWS; the information source of the biotechnology industry. Text in English. 1981. 21/yr., latest vol.21, 2001. USD 479 domestic; USD 587 foreign (effective 2002). adv. bk.rev. pat, stat, tr.lit. *Refereed.* **Document type:** *Newspaper, Trade.* **Description:** Covers the biotechnology-bioprocess industry. Examines significant issues, regulatory and scale-up guidelines, R&D, financial news including public offerings, mergers, and venture capital, corporate profiles, reports, and news.
Related titles: Online - full text ed.: (from Gale Group, Factiva, Institute for Scientific Information).
Indexed: ASCA, AgBiotech, Agricola, Anim.Breed.Abstr., Bibl.Agri., Biotech.Cit.Ind., Bus.& Indus. (May 1994-), Chem.Abstr., Chem.Indus.Notes, Chem.Titles, Ind.Vet., SSCI (coverage dropped), Telegen.
—CASDDS, CISTI, GNLM, IDS.
Published by: Mary Ann Liebert, Inc. Publishers, 2 Madison Ave, Larchmont, NY 10538. TEL 914—834-3100, FAX 914-834-1388, info@liebertpub.com, www.genengnews.com, http://www.genegnews.com.

576.5 USA ISSN 0741-0395
GENETIC EPIDEMIOLOGY. Text in English. bi-m. USD 1,785 in United States; USD 1,865 in Canada & Mexico; USD 1,933 elsewhere; USD 1,875 combined subscription in United States for print and online eds.; USD 1,955 combined subscription in Canada & Mexico for print and online eds.; USD 2,023 combined subscription elsewhere for print and online eds. (effective 2002). adv. bk.rev. back issues avail. *Refereed.* **Document type:** *Academic/Scholarly.* **Description:** Provides a forum for research concerned with the etiology, distribution, and control of disease in groups of relatives and with the inherited predisposition to, or causes of, diseases in populations.
Related titles: Microform ed.: (from PQC); Online - full text ed.: ISSN 1098-2272. USD 1,785 in United States; USD 1,785 in Canada & Mexico; USD 1,785 elsewhere (effective 2002) (from EBSCO Publishing, Wiley InterScience, Institute for Scientific Information).
Indexed: ASCA, Anim.Breed.Abstr., Biol.Abstr., Biotech.Cit.Ind., Chem.Abstr., Curr.Adv.Ecol.Sci., Curr.Adv.Gen.& Molec.Biol., Curr.Cont., Environ.Sci.Poll.Mgmt., Excerp.Med., Genet.Abstr., Hum.Gen.Abstr., Ind.Med. (1984-), Ind.Sci.Rev., Inpharma, Nuc.Acids Abstr., Pharm.&Out.News, Reac., Ref.Zh., Risk Abstr., SSCI (coverage dropped), Sci.Cit.Ind., THA.
—BLDSC (4111.848000), CISTI, EMDOCS, GNLM, IDS, ingenta, KNAW. **CCC.**
Published by: John Wiley & Sons, Inc., Journals (Subsidiary of: Wiley InterScience), 605 Third Ave, New York, NY 10158. TEL 212-850-6645, FAX 212-850-6021, subinfo@wiley.com, uscs-wis@wiley.com, http://www.wiley.com. Eds. A Chakravarti, J M Mulvihill. adv.: B&W page GBP 640, color page GBP 1,515; trim 174 x 254. Circ: 850. **Subscr. outside the Americas to:** John Wiley & Sons Ltd., Baffins Ln, Chichester, Sussex PO19 IUD, United Kingdom. TEL 44-1243-779777, FAX 44-1243-843232, cs-journals@wiley.co.uk, http://www.wiley.co.uk.

GENETIC EPISTEMOLOGIST. see *PSYCHOLOGY*

576.5 USA
GENETIC RESOURCE. Text in English. 1983. s-a. USD 15. bk.rev. **Document type:** *Newsletter.* **Description:** Covers clinical genetics and related public health policy issues for lay and professional readers.
Published by: New England Regional Genetics Group, PO Box 670, Mount Desert, ME 04660-0670. TEL 207-839-5324, FAX 207-839-8637. Ed. Robin J R Blatt. R&P Joseph Robinson TEL 207-288-2704. Circ: 7,000.

576.5 NLD ISSN 0925-9864
SB123.3 CODEN: GRCEE9
GENETIC RESOURCES AND CROP EVOLUTION; an international journal. Short title: G R A C E. Text in English. 1953. bi-m. EUR 628, USD 628 to institutions for print & online ed.; EUR 753, USD 753.60 to institutions for print or online eds. combined (effective 2001). back issues avail. *Refereed.* **Document type:** *Journal, Academic/Scholarly.* **Description:** Publishes original articles on taxonomical, morphological, cytological, ethnobotanical and biochemical research of genetic resources, including contributions on broader issues in gene-bank management, such as collection, storage, maintenance and documentation.
Formerly (until 1992): Kulturpflanze (0075-7209)
Related titles: Microform ed.: (from PQC); Online - full text ed.: (from EBSCO Publishing, O C L C Online Computer Library Center, Inc., RoweCom Information Quest, Swets Blackwell, Kluwer Online, Institute for Scientific Information).
Indexed: ASCA, AgBiotech, Agri.& Environ.Biotech.Abstr., Agricola, Agroforest.Abstr., Apic.Abstr., Biol.Abstr., Chem.Abstr., Compumath, Curr.Adv.Plant Sci., Curr.Cont., Ecol.Abstr., Environ.Sci.Poll.Mgmt., Field Crop Abstr., Forest.Abstr., Genet.Abstr., Helminthol.Abstr., Herb.Abstr., Hort.Abstr., Hum.Gen.Abstr., IDA, Int.Abstr.Biol.Sci., Maize Abstr., Microbiol.Abstr., Nuc.Acids Abstr., Ornam.Hort., Plant Breed.Abstr., Plant Gen.Res.Abstr., Plant Sci., Potato Abstr., Rev.Appl.Entomol., Rev.Arom.& Med.Plants, Rev.Plant Path., Rice Abstr., Seed Abstr., Soils & Fert., Soyabean Abstr., Triticale Abstr., VITIS, Weed Abstr.
—BLDSC (4111.907000), CASDDS, CISTI, EMDOCS, IDS, Infotrieve, ingenta. **CCC.**
Published by: Kluwer Academic Publishers Group (Subsidiary of: Wolters Kluwer N.V.), Spuiboulevard 50, PO Box 17, Dordrecht 3300 AA, Netherlands. TEL 31-78-639-2392, FAX 31-78-654-2254, services@wkap.nl, http://www.wkap.nl/journalhome.htm/0925-9864. Eds. K Pistrick, Karl Hammer. **Subscr. in the Americas to:** Kluwer Academic - Plenum Publishers, 233 Spring St, New York, NY 10013-1578. TEL 212-620-8468, FAX 212-807-1047**; Subscr. to:** Journals Department, PO Box 322, Dordrecht 3300 AH, Netherlands. TEL 31-78-639-2392, FAX 31-78-654-6474.

576.5 USA ISSN 0272-9032
CODEN: GTNEEA
GENETIC TECHNOLOGY NEWS. Text in English. 1981. w. (51/yr). USD 885 in North America to institutions; USD 985 elsewhere to institutions (effective 2001). abstr, bibl, charts, pat, stat, tr.lit. back issues avail. **Document type:** *Newsletter.* **Description:** Explores genetic engineering and its uses in the chemical, pharmaceutical, food processing and energy industries, as well as in agriculture, animal breeding and medicine.
Related titles: Online - full text ed.; Supplement: Patent Update; Strategic Partners Report; Market Forecast.
Indexed: Chem.Abstr., Chem.Indus.Notes, Chem.Titles, Curr.Biotech.Abstr.
—BLDSC (4111.923000), CASDDS, CISTI, Infotrieve. **CCC.**
Published by: Technical Insights (Subsidiary of: John Wiley & Sons, Inc., Journals), 605 3rd Ave, New York, NY 10158-0012. TEL 212-850-8600, FAX 212-850-8800, insights@wiley.com, http://www.wiley.com/technical_insights. Ed. Peter Savage. Pub. Paul Majchrzyk.

576.5 USA ISSN 1090-6576
CODEN: GETEF4
GENETIC TESTING. Text in English. 1997. q. USD 148 domestic to individuals; USD 228 foreign to individuals; USD 178 domestic to individuals print and online eds. combined; USD 258 foreign to individuals print and online eds. combined; USD 349 domestic to institutions print and online eds. combined; USD 449 foreign to institutions print and online eds. combined (effective 2002). back issues avail.; reprints avail. *Refereed.* **Document type:** *Journal, Academic/Scholarly.* **Description:** Focuses on all aspects of genetic testing, including prenatal diagnosis, risk assessment, methodologies, ethical and legal uses.
Related titles: Online - full text ed.: USD 178 to individuals; USD 349 to institutions (effective 2002) (from CatchWord Ltd., EBSCO Publishing, O C L C Online Computer Library Center, Inc., RoweCom Information Quest, Swets Blackwell, Institute for Scientific Information).
Indexed: Curr.Cont., Excerp.Med., Focus on: Mol.Med., Ind.Med. (1997-), Int.Nurs.Ind.
—BLDSC (4111.926000), CASDDS, CatchWord, IDS, Infotrieve. **CCC.**

Published by: Mary Ann Liebert, Inc. Publishers, 2 Madison Ave, Larchmont, NY 10538. TEL 914—834-3100, FAX 914-834-1388, info@liebertpub.com, www.liebertpub.com/gte, http://www.liebertpub.com. Ed. Dr. Fred Gilbert.

576.5 NLD ISSN 0016-6707
QH301 CODEN: GENEA3
GENETICA; the international journal on genetics. Text in English. 1919. 9/yr. EUR 1,520, USD 1,522 to institutions for print or online ed.; EUR 1,824, USD 1,826.40 to institutions for print & online eds. combined (effective 2002). adv. illus. back issues avail.; reprint service avail. from SWZ. *Refereed.* **Document type:** *Journal, Academic/Scholarly.*
Related titles: Microform ed.: (from PQC); Online - full text ed.: (from EBSCO Publishing, O C L C Online Computer Library Center, Inc., RoweCom Information Quest, Swets Blackwell, Kluwer Online, Institute for Scientific Information).
Indexed: ASCA, AgBiotech, Anim.Breed.Abstr., Aqua.Sci.& Fish.Abstr., Bio-Contr.News & Info., Biol.Abstr., Biotech.Cit.Ind., Chem.Abstr., Chem.Indus.Notes, Chem.Titles, Curr.Adv.Ecol.Sci., Curr.Cont., Entomol.Abstr., Excerp.Med., Field Crop Abstr., Food Sci.& Tech.Abstr., Forest.Abstr., Genet.Abstr., Helminthol.Abstr., Herb.Abstr., Hum.Gen.Abstr., INIS Atomind., Ind.Med. (1919-), Ind.Sci.Rev., Inpharma, Int.Abstr.Biol.Sci., Maize Abstr., Nuc.Acids Abstr., Plant Breed.Abstr., Plant Gen.Res.Abstr., Reac., Ref.Zh., Rev.Appl.Entomol., Rev.Med.& Vet.Mycol., SSCI (coverage dropped), Sci.Cit.Ind., Seed Abstr., Small Anim.Abstr., Sport Fish.Abstr., Triticale Abstr., Weed Abstr., Wild.Rev., Zoo.Rec.
—BLDSC (4112.000000), CASDDS, CISTI, EMDOCS, GNLM, IDS, Infotrieve, ingenta, Linda Hall. **CCC.**
Published by: Kluwer Academic Publishers Group (Subsidiary of: Wolters Kluwer N.V.), Spuiboulevard 50, PO Box 17, Dordrecht 3300 AA, Netherlands. TEL 31-78-639-2392, FAX 31-78-654-2254, services@wkap.nl, http://www.wkap.nl/journalhome.htm/0016-6707. Eds. Pierre Capy, Ronny C Woodruff. **Subscr. in the Americas to:** Kluwer Academic - Plenum Publishers, 233 Spring St, New York, NY 10013-1578. TEL 212-620-8468, FAX 212-807-1047; **Subscr. to:** Journals Department, PO Box 322, Dordrecht 3300 AH, Netherlands. TEL 31-78-639-2392, FAX 31-78-654-6474.

576.5 GBR ISSN 0016-6723
QH431.A1 CODEN: GENRA8
GENETICAL RESEARCH. Text in English. 1960. bi-m. GBP 440 to institutions (effective 2002). adv. bk.rev. charts, illus. index. back issues avail.; reprint service avail. from SWZ,PQC. *Refereed.* **Document type:** *Academic/Scholarly.* **Description:** Covers current research in all branches of genetics: for geneticists, molecular and developmental biologists, and plant and animal breeders.
Related titles: Microform ed.: (from PQC); Online - full text ed.: (from EBSCO Publishing, O C L C Online Computer Library Center, Inc., RoweCom Information Quest, Swets Blackwell, Institute for Scientific Information).
Indexed: ASCA, Abstr.Anthropol., Abstr.Hyg., AgBiotech, Agri.& Environ.Biotech.Abstr. (coverage dropped), Agricola, Anim.Breed.Abstr., Aqua.Sci.& Fish.Abstr., Bibl.Agri., Biol.& Agr.Ind. (Feb.1983-Apr.1989), Biol.Abstr., Biostat., Biotech.Cit.Ind., Chem.Abstr., Chem.Indus.Notes, Chem.Titles, Curr.Adv.Biochem., Curr.Adv.Ecol.Sci., Curr.Adv.Gen.& Molec.Biol., Curr.Biotech.Abstr., Curr.Cont., Curr.Ind.Stat., Dairy Sci.Abstr., Dent.Ind., Derwent Biotech.Abstr., Entomol.Abstr. (coverage dropped), Environ.Sci.Poll.Mgmt., Excerp.Med., Forest.Abstr., Genet.Abstr., Helminthol.Abstr., Hum.Gen.Abstr., INIS Atomind., Ind.Med. (1960-), Ind.Sci.Rev., Ind.Vet., Inpharma, Int.Abstr.Biol.Sci., Maize Abstr., Math.R., Microbiol.Abstr., Nuc.Acids Abstr., Nutr.Abstr., Pig News & Info., Plant Breed.Abstr., Plant Gen.Res.Abstr., Postharvest, Protozool.Abstr., Reac., Ref.Zh., Rev.Appl.Entomol., Rev.Med.& Vet.Mycol., Rev.Plant Path., Sci.Cit.Ind., Soils & Fert., Sport Fish.Abstr., Telegen, Triticale Abstr., Trop.Dis.Bull., Vet.Bull., Weed Abstr., Wild.Rev., Zoo.Rec.
—BLDSC (4114.250000), CASDDS, CISTI, GNLM, IDS, ingenta, Linda Hall. **CCC.**
Published by: Cambridge University Press, Edinburgh Bldg, Shaftesbury Rd, Cambridge CB2 2RU, United Kingdom. FAX 44-1223-315052, information@cup.cam.ac.uk, information@cambridge.org, http://www.cup.cam.ac.uk, http://www.uk.cambridge.org/journals/pmu. Eds. D. J. Finnegan, Trudy F.C. Mackay, W.G. Hill. R&P Linda Nicol. Adv. contact Rebecca Symons.

576.5 USA ISSN 0016-6731
QH431 CODEN: GENTAE
GENETICS; a periodical record of investigations bearing on heredity and variation. Text in English. 1916. m. USD 600 domestic to institutions; USD 620 foreign to institutions (effective 2001). adv. abstr, bibl, charts, illus. index. back issues avail.; reprint service avail. from PQC. *Refereed.* **Description:** Aims to facilitate communication among scientists and professors who are involved in research and education relative to the study of special organisms.
Related titles: Microform ed.: (from MIM,PQC,PMC); Online - full text ed.: (from HighWire Pr., EBSCO Publishing, RoweCom Information Quest, Gale Group, Factiva, Institute for Scientific Information).
Indexed: ASCA, Abstr.Anthropol., Abstr.Hyg., AgBiotech, Agri.& Environ.Biotech.Abstr. (coverage dropped), Agricola, Agroforest.Abstr., Anim.Behav.Abstr., Anim.Breed.Abstr., Apic.Abstr., Aqua.Sci.& Fish.Abstr., Aquacult.Abstr., Bio-Contr.News & Info., Biol.& Agr.Ind. (Jan.1983-), Biol.Abstr., Biol.Dig., Biotech.& Bioeng.Abstr., Biotech.Cit.Ind., Chem.Abstr., Chem.Indus.Notes, Chem.Titles, Chemorec.Abstr., Compumath, Cott.& Trop.Fibr.Abstr., Curr.Adv.Biochem., Curr.Adv.Cell & Devel.Biol., Curr.Adv.Ecol.Sci., Curr.Adv.Gen.& Molec.Biol., Curr.Cont., Curr.Ref.Fish Res., Dairy Sci.Abstr., Derwent Biotech.Abstr., Entomol.Abstr., Environ.Sci.Poll.Mgmt., Excerp.Med., Fababean Abstr., Food Sci.& Tech.Abstr., Forest.Abstr., Gen.Sci.Ind. (Apr.1984-), Genet.Abstr., Helminthol.Abstr., Hum.Gen.Abstr., INIS Atomind., Ind.Med. (1916-), Ind.Sci.Rev., Int.Abstr.Biol.Sci., Maize Abstr., Microbiol.Abstr., Neurosci.Abstr. (coverage dropped), Nuc.Acids Abstr., Ocean.Abstr., Ornam.Hort., Pig News & Info., Plant Breed.Abstr., Plant Gen.Res.Abstr., Plant Grow.Reg.Abstr., Postharvest, Potato Abstr., Poult.Abstr., Protozool.Abstr., Ref.Zh., Rev.Appl.Entomol., Rev.Arom.& Med.Plants, Rev.Med.& Vet.Mycol., Rev.Plant Path., Rice Abstr., Sci.Cit.Ind., Seed Abstr., Soils & Fert., Sorghum & Millets Abstr., Soyabean Abstr., Sport Fish.Abstr., Triticale Abstr., Trop.Dis.Bull., VITIS, Weed Abstr., Wild.Rev., Zoo.Rec.
—BLDSC (4115.000000), CASDDS, CISTI, GNLM, IDS, Infotrieve, ingenta, Linda Hall. **CCC.**
Published by: Genetics Society of America, 9650 Rockville Pike, Bethesda, MD 20814. TEL 301-530 7029, FAX 301-571 5728, genetics-gsa@andrew.cmu.edu; staff@dues.faseb.org, http://www.genetics.org. Ed. Elizabeth W Jones. Circ: 5,000. **Subscr. to:** FASEB, Subscriptions, Rm L2310, 9650 Rockville Pike, Bethesda, MD 20814. TEL 301-530-7026.

GENETICS ABSTRACTS. see *BIOLOGY—Abstracting, Bibliographies, Statistics*

576.5 BRA ISSN 1415-4757
QH426 CODEN: GMBIFG
GENETICS AND MOLECULAR BIOLOGY. Text in English; Summaries in English, Portuguese. 1978. q. BRL 60 domestic to individuals; USD 50 foreign to individuals; BRL 70 domestic to institutions; USD 90 foreign to institutions (effective 1999). adv. bk.rev. abstr. index. back issues avail. *Refereed.* **Document type:** *Academic/Scholarly.* **Description:** Publishes the results of original research in evolution, genetics, molecular biology and their application to the improvement of plants, animals and human well-being.
Formerly (until 1998): Brazilian Journal of Genetics (0100-8455)
Related titles: Online - full text ed.: (from SciELO, Institute for Scientific Information).
Indexed: AgBiotech, Agroforest.Abstr., Anim.Breed.Abstr., Bio-Contr.News & Info., Biol.Abstr., Biotech.Cit.Ind., Chem.Abstr., Chem.Indus.Notes, Chem.Titles, Crop Physiol.Abstr., Curr.Adv.Ecol.Sci., Curr.Cont., Dairy Sci.Abstr., Derwent Biotech.Abstr., Excerp.Med., Field Crop Abstr., Forest.Abstr., Genet.Abstr. (coverage dropped), Herb.Abstr., Hort.Abstr., INIS Atomind., Ind.Vet., Inpharma, Int.Abstr.Biol.Sci., Maize Abstr., Nutr.Abstr., Pharm.&Out.News, Pig News & Info., Plant Breed.Abstr., Plant Gen.Res.Abstr., Plant Grow.Reg.Abstr., Poult.Abstr., Reac., Ref.Zh., Rev.Appl.Entomol., Rev.Med.& Vet.Mycol., Rev.Plant Path., Rice Abstr., Sci.Cit.Ind. (coverage dropped), Seed Abstr., Sorghum & Millets Abstr., Soyabean Abstr., Sport Fish.Abstr., Triticale Abstr., Trop.Dis.Bull., Vet.Bull., Weed Abstr., Zoo.Rec.
—BLDSC (4115.091500), CASDDS, CISTI, EMDOCS, GNLM, IDS, KNAW, Linda Hall.
Published by: Sociedade Brasileira de Genetica, Rua Capitao Adelmio Norberto da Silva 736, At B Vista, Ribeirao Preto, SP 14025-670, Brazil. TEL 55-16-6218540, FAX 55-16-6201253, rbg@genbov.fmrp.usp.br, http://www.scielo.br/. Ed. Francisco A. Moura Duarte. R&P Francisco A Moura Duarte. Circ: 2,000.

576.5 USA ISSN 1098-3600
GENETICS IN MEDICINE. Text in English. 1998. bi-m. USD 254 domestic to individuals; USD 290 elsewhere to individuals; USD 498 domestic to institutions; USD 534 foreign to institutions; USD 84 newsstand/cover (effective 2002). adv. *Refereed.* **Document type:** *Journal.* **Description:** Offers an unprecedented forum for the presentation of innovative, practice-focused papers in contemporary genetics medicine, including such areas as clinical genetics, biochemical genetics, cytogenetics, molecular genetics, public health genetics, genetic epidemiology, common disease genetics, genetic counseling, and genetic education.
Related titles: Online - full text ed.: USD 647.40 domestic academic site license; USD 683.40 foreign academic site license; USD 722.10 domestic corporate site license; USD 758.10 foreign corporate site license (2002) (from Ovid Technologies, Inc., Institute for Scientific Information).
Indexed: Biotech.Cit.Ind., Curr.Cont.
—BLDSC (4115.151000).
Published by: (American College of Medical Genetics), Lippincott Williams & Wilkins (Baltimore) (Subsidiary of: Wolters Kluwer N.V.), 351 W Camden St, Baltimore, MD 21201-2436. TEL 410-528-4000, http://www.wwilkins.com/GIM/. Ed. Richard A King TEL 612-626-4224. **Subscr. to:** Lippincott Williams & Wilkins, Order Dept, 16522 Hunters Green Pkwy, Hagerstown, MD 21740. TEL 301-714-2334, 800-638-3030, FAX 301-824-7390.

599.9 GBR ISSN 1471-3624
GENETICS LAW MONITOR. Text in English. bi-m. GBP 187 to individuals; GBP 140 academic rate (effective 2001). **Description:** Presents papers about the legal, ethical and social implications of human genetics.
—BLDSC (4115.145000).
Published by: Monitor Press Ltd. (Subsidiary of: Informa Group PLC), Suffolk House, Church Field Rd, Sudbury, Suffolk CO10 2YA, United Kingdom. TEL 44-1787-378607, FAX 44-1787-880201, http://www.geneticslawmonitor.com/, http://www.monitorpress.co.uk. Ed. Iain Goldrein. R&P Zoe Turner.

576.5 ZAF ISSN 0259-0301
GENETICS NEWSLETTER/GENETIKA NUUSBRIEF. Text in Afrikaans, English. 1968. q. membership. bk.rev.
Media: Duplicated (not offset).
Published by: South African Genetic Society, c/o Department of Genetics, University of Stellenbosch, Stellenbosch, South Africa. Ed. Dr. A E Retief. Circ: (controlled).

591.35 636.081 FRA ISSN 0999-193X
SF105 CODEN: GSEVE9
GENETICS, SELECTION, EVOLUTION. Text in English; Summaries in English, French. 1969. bi-m. EUR 267 domestic; FRF 2,045, EUR 312 in the European Union; FRF 2,146, EUR 327 elsewhere (2001). bk.rev. charts, illus. index. reprint service avail. from ISI. *Refereed.* **Document type:** *Academic/Scholarly.* **Description:** International journal open to original research papers in the field of animal genetics and evolution. Areas of interest include all aspects related to cytogenetics: cellular, biotechnical, factorial, mathematical, quantitative and population genetics.
Former titles (until 1989): Genetique, Selection, Evolution (0754-0264); (until 1983): Annales de Genetique et de Selection Animale (0003-4002)
Related titles: Online - full text ed.: Genetics, Selection, Evolution Online. ISSN 1297-9686 (from EBSCO Publishing, ingenta, Swets Blackwell, RoweCom Information Quest, Institute for Scientific Information,PQC).
Indexed: ASCA, AgBiotech, Anim.Breed.Abstr., Aqua.Sci.& Fish.Abstr., Biol.Abstr., Chem.Abstr., Chem.Indus.Notes, Chem.Titles, Curr.Adv.Ecol.Sci., Curr.Cont., Dairy Sci.Abstr., Ecol.Abstr., Entomol.Abstr., Environ.Sci.Poll.Mgmt., Food Sci.& Tech.Abstr., Forest.Abstr., Genet.Abstr., Hum.Gen.Abstr., Ind.Vet., Int.Abstr.Biol.Sci., Microbiol.Abstr., Nuc.Acids Abstr., Nutr.Abstr., Pig News & Info., Plant Breed.Abstr., Plant Gen.Res.Abstr., Poult.Abstr., Protozool.Abstr., Rev.Appl.Entomol., Rev.Plant Path., Rice Abstr., Sci.Cit.Ind., Sport Fish.Abstr., Triticale Abstr., Vet.Bull., Wild.Rev., Zoo.Rec.
—BLDSC (4115.158000), CASDDS, CISTI, EMDOCS, IDS, Infotrieve, ingenta, Linda Hall. **CCC.**
Published by: (France. Institut National de la Recherche Agronomique), E D P Sciences, 7 av. du Hoggar, B.P. 112, P.A. de Courtaboeuf, Les Ulis Cedex A 91944, France. TEL 33-1-69187575, FAX 33-1-69288491, subscribers@edpsciences.org, http://www.edpsciences.org. Eds. B Bibe, J R David. Circ: 2,000.

B

B

576.5 GBR
GENETICS SOCIETY. NEWSLETTER. Text in English. 2/yr. GBP 25 to membership (effective 2000 & 2001). Website rev. illus. back issues avail. **Document type:** *Newsletter, Academic/Scholarly.* **Description:** Updates members of the Genetical Society of Great Britain to important and noteworthy news and events.
Formerly: Genetical Society. Newsletter
Published by: Genetics Society, Roslin Biocentre, Roslin Institute, Roslin EH25 9PS, United Kingdom. john.armour@nottingham.ac.uk, mail@genetics.org.uk, http://www.genetics.org.uk/newsletter/welcome.htm. Ed. John Armour. Adv. contact Jayne Richards TEL 44-131-5274472.

576.5 CAN ISSN 0316-4357
QH426
GENETICS SOCIETY OF CANADA BULLETIN. Text in English. 1959. q. CND 25; CND 30 foreign (effective 1999). adv. bk.rev. **Document type:** *Bulletin.*
—CISTI, Linda Hall.
Published by: Genetics Society of Canada, 141 Laurier Av W, Ste 1112, Ottawa, ON K1P 5J3, Canada. TEL 613-232-9459, FAX 613-594-5190. Ed., Pub., R&P, Adv. contact Michael Bentley TEL 403-220-6794. Circ: 450.

GENETICS SOCIETY OF JAPAN. ABSTRACTS OF THE ANNUAL MEETING/NIHON IDEN GAKKAI TAIKAI PUROGURAMU YOKOSHU. see *BIOLOGY—Abstracting, Bibliographies, Statistics*

576.5 RUS ISSN 0016-6758
CODEN: GNKAA5
GENETIKA. Text in Russian. 1965. m. RUR 345 per month (effective 2001). bk.rev. index. **Document type:** *Academic/Scholarly.* **Description:** Investigates genetic processes at the molecular, cellular, organismic, and population levels, with articles on the impact of modern genetics and environmental concerns.
Related titles: Online - full text ed.; ♦ English Translation: Russian Journal of Genetics. ISSN 1022-7954.
Indexed: Abstr.Hyg., AgBiotech, Agri.& Environ.Biotech.Abstr. (coverage dropped), Anim.Breed.Abstr., Bibl.Dev.Med.& Child Neur., Bio-Contr.News & Info., Biol.Abstr., Chem.Abstr., Chem.Indus.Notes, Chem.Titles, Cott.& Trop.Fibr.Abstr., Crop Physiol.Abstr., Curr.Adv.Ecol.Sci., Curr.Cont. (coverage dropped), Dairy Sci.Abstr., Dent.Ind., Derwent Biotech.Abstr., Excerp.Med., Field Crop Abstr., Forest.Abstr., Helminthol.Abstr., Hort.Abstr., INIS Atomind., Ind.Med. (1965-), Ind.Sci.Rev., Ind.Vet., Inpharma, Maize Abstr., Pig News & Info., Plant Breed.Abstr., Plant Gen.Res.Abstr., Plant Grow.Reg.Abstr., Potato Abstr., Poult.Abstr., Reac., Ref.Zh., Rev.Appl.Entomol., Rev.Arom.& Med.Plants, Rev.Med.& Vet.Mycol., Rev.Plant Path., Risk Abstr., SSCI (coverage dropped), Sci.Cit.Ind. (coverage dropped), Seed Abstr., Soils & Fert., Sport Fish.Abstr., Triticale Abstr., Vet.Bull., Weed Abstr., Wild.Rev., Zoo.Rec.
—BLDSC (0047.080000), CASDDS, CISTI, East View, GNLM, IDS, KNAW, Linda Hall. **CCC.**
Published by: (Rossiiskaya Akademiya Nauk/Russian Academy of Sciences), M A I K Nauka - Interperiodica, Mezhdunarodnyi Otdel, Profsoyuznaya ul 90, Moscow 117864, Russian Federation. TEL 7-095-3661600, FAX 7-095-336-0666, compmg@maik.ru, http://www.maik.rssi.ru/journals/geneng.htm. Ed. G P Georgiev. **US dist. addr.:** Kluwer Academic Publishers, PO Box 17, Dordrecht 3300 AH, Netherlands. TEL 31-78-392392, http://www.wkap.nl.

581.3 BGR ISSN 0016-6766
CODEN: GESKAC
GENETIKA I SELEKTSIIA/GENETICS AND PLANT BREEDING. Text in Bulgarian; Summaries in English, Russian. 1968. bi-m. BGL 1.40 per issue. bk.rev. bibl, charts, illus. back issues avail.; reprint service avail. from IRC.
Indexed: Anim.Breed.Abstr., Aqua.Sci.& Fish.Abstr., BSL Biol., Biol.Abstr., Chem.Abstr., Curr.Adv.Ecol.Sci., Dairy Sci.Abstr., Genet.Abstr., Hort.Abstr., Hum.Gen.Abstr., INIS Atomind., Ind.Vet., Maize Abstr., Pig News & Info., Plant Grow.Reg.Abstr., Poult.Abstr., Seed Abstr., Weed Abstr.
—CASDDS, CISTI, Linda Hall.
Published by: (Akademiia na Selskostopanskite Nauki), Publishing House of the Bulgarian Academy of Sciences, Akad G Bonchev 6, Sofia 1113, Bulgaria. Ed. Khristo Daskalov. Circ: 1,010. **Dist. by:** Hemus, 6 Rouski blvd, Sofia 1000, Bulgaria.

576.5 USA ISSN 0740-9737
CODEN: GEWAE6
GENEWATCH. Text in English. 1982. bi-m. USD 35 domestic to individuals; USD 30 in Canada & Mexico to libraries; USD 17 elsewhere to students; USD 50 domestic to non-profit organizations; USD 100 in Canada & Mexico to corporations (effective 1999). bk.rev., video rev. charts, bibl, illus, maps. 20 p./no. 3 cols./p. back issues avail. *Refereed.* **Document type:** *Newsletter, Journal, Academic/Scholarly.* **Description:** Contains articles, commentary, international news, and legislative updates on social issues pertaining to genetic engineering and biotechnology.
Indexed: Alt.Press Ind., Telegen.
—IDS.
Published by: Council for Responsible Genetics (CRG), 5 Upland Rd, Ste 3, Cambridge, MA 02140-2717. TEL 617-868-0870, FAX 617-491-5344, suzanne@gene-watch.org, crg@essential.org, www.gene-watch.org, http://www.essential.org/crg. Ed. Martin Teitel. R&P Kimberly Wilson. Circ: 2,000 (paid).

576.8 CAN ISSN 0831-2796
QH431.A1 CODEN: GENOE3
GENOME. Text mainly in English; Text occasionally in French. 1957. bi-m. CND 142 domestic to individuals; USD 142 foreign to individuals; CND 377 domestic to institutions; USD 377 foreign to institutions (effective 1999). adv. charts, illus, stat. index. back issues avail. *Refereed.* **Document type:** *Academic/Scholarly.* **Description:** Publishes papers in applied and basic genetics and cytology.
Formerly: Canadian Journal of Genetics and Cytology - Journal Canadien de Genetique et de Cytologie (0008-4093)
Related titles: Microfiche ed.: (from MML); Microfilm ed.: (from PMC); Microform ed.: (from MML); Online - full text ed.: ISSN 1480-3321 (from EBSCO Publishing, O C L C Online Computer Library Center, Inc., RoweCom Information Quest, ProQuest Information & Learning, CISTI, LexisNexis, Swets Blackwell, Institute for Scientific Information).
Indexed: ASCA, Abstr.Anthropol., AgBiotech, Anim.Breed.Abstr., Aqua.Sci.& Fish.Abstr., Bio-Contr.News & Info., Biol.& Agr.Ind. (Jan.1996-), Biol.Abstr., Biotech.Cit.Ind., CBCA Ref., Chem.Abstr., Chem.Indus.Notes, Chem.Titles, Cott.& Trop.Fibr.Abstr., Curr.Adv.Cell & Devel.Biol., Curr.Adv.Ecol.Sci., Curr.Adv.Gen.& Molec.Biol., Curr.Adv.Plant Sci., Curr.Biotech.Abstr., Curr.Cont., Derwent Biotech.Abstr., Entomol.Abstr., Excerp.Med., Forest.Abstr., Genet.Abstr., Helminthol.Abstr., Hort.Abstr., Hum.Gen.Abstr., INIS Atomind., Ind.Med. (1987-), Ind.Sci.Rev., Ind.Vet., Inpharma, Int.Abstr.Biol.Sci., Maize Abstr., Nuc.Acids Abstr., Ocean.Abstr. (coverage dropped), Ornam.Hort., Plant Breed.Abstr., Plant Gen.Res.Abstr., Plant Grow.Reg.Abstr., Plant Sci., Pollut.Abstr., Potato Abstr., Reac., Rev.Appl.Entomol., Rev.Plant Path., Rice Abstr., Sci.Cit.Ind., Seed Abstr., Sorghum & Millets Abstr., Soyabean Abstr., Sport Fish.Abstr., Triticale Abstr., VITIS, Vet.Bull., Weed Abstr., Wild.Rev., Zoo.Rec.
—BLDSC (4116.312000), ADONIS, CASDDS, CISTI, EMDOCS, GNLM, IDS, ingenta, KNAW, Linda Hall. **CCC.**
Published by: (Genetics Society of Canada), N R C Research Press, Building M 55, Ottawa, ON K1A 0R6, Canada. TEL 613-993-9084, FAX 613-952-7656, http://www.nrc.ca/cisti/journals/. Ed. Dr. Peter Moens. Adv. contact Judy Heyman. B&W page CND 675; trim 11 x 8.5. Circ: 1,138.

572.86 USA ISSN 1088-9051
QP606.D46 CODEN: GEREFS
GENOME RESEARCH. Text in English. 1991. m. USD 117 domestic to individuals; USD 156 in Canada & Mexico to individuals; USD 173 elsewhere to individuals; USD 780 domestic to institutions; USD 819 in US & Canada to institutions; USD 836 elsewhere to institutions (effective 2001). adv. illus. back issues avail. *Refereed.* **Document type:** *Journal, Academic/Scholarly.* **Description:** Focuses on genome studies in all species, including genetic and physical mapping, DNA sequencing, gene discovery, informatics, statistical and mathematical methods and genome structure as well as technological innovations and applications.
Formerly (until Aug 1995): P C R Methods and Applications (Polymerase Chain Reaction) (1054-9803)
Related titles: Online - full text ed.: 1997 (from HighWire Pr., EBSCO Publishing, Institute for Scientific Information).
Indexed: ASCA, AgBiotech, Anim.Breed.Abstr., Biotech.Cit.Ind., Chem.Abstr., Chem.Indus.Notes, Chem.Titles, Curr.Cont., Excerp.Med. (1993-), Food Sci.& Tech.Abstr., Genet.Abstr., Helminthol.Abstr., Hum.Gen.Abstr., Ind.Med. (1995-), Ind.Vet., Inpharma, Int.Abstr.Biol.Sci., Maize Abstr., Nuc.Acids Abstr., Nutr.Abstr., Oncog.G.F.Abstr. (coverage dropped), Pharm.&Out.News, Pig News & Info., Plant Breed.Abstr., Poult.Abstr., Protozool.Abstr., Reac., Rev.Appl.Entomol., Rev.Med.& Vet.Mycol., Rev.Plant Path., Rice Abstr., Sci.Cit.Ind., Soils & Fert., Triticale Abstr., Vet.Bull.
—BLDSC (4116.313800), CASDDS, CISTI, EMDOCS, GNLM, IDS, Infotrieve, ingenta, KNAW, Linda Hall. **CCC.**
Published by: Cold Spring Harbor Laboratory Press, Publications Department, 10 Skyline Dr, Plainview, NY 11803. TEL 516-349-1930, 800-843-4388, FAX 516-349-1946, cshpress@cshl.org, http://www.genome.org, http://www.cshl.org. Ed. L Goodman. Adv. contact Marcie Ebenstein.

599.9 USA ISSN 0888-7543
QH445.2 CODEN: GNMCEP
GENOMICS; international journal for analysis of the human and other genomes. Text in English. 1987. s-m. USD 1,999 in US & Canada to institutions; USD 2,300 elsewhere to institutions (effective 2001). back issues avail. *Refereed.* **Document type:** *Academic/Scholarly.* **Description:** Emphasizes the integration of basic and applied research in human and comparative gene mapping, molecular cloning, large-scale restriction mapping, and DNA sequencing and computational analysis.
Related titles: Online - full text ed.: (from EBSCO Publishing, O C L C Online Computer Library Center, Inc., RoweCom Information Quest, ingenta, Swets Blackwell, IDEAL Online Library, Institute for Scientific Information).
Indexed: ASCA, Abstr.Anthropol., AgBiotech, Agricola, Anim.Breed.Abstr., BBCI, Bibl.Agri., Biotech.& Bioeng.Abstr., Biotech.Cit.Ind., Chem.Abstr., Chem.Indus.Notes, Chem.Titles, Curr.Adv.Cell & Devel.Biol., Curr.Adv.Gen.& Molec.Biol., Curr.Cont., Curr.Ind.Stat., Derwent Biotech.Abstr., Genet.Abstr., Helminthol.Abstr., Hum.Gen.Abstr., INIS Atomind., Ind.Med. (1987-), Ind.Sci.Rev., Ind.Vet., Inpharma, Int.Abstr.Biol.Sci., Neurosci.Abstr. (coverage dropped), Neurosci.Cit.Ind., Nuc.Acids Abstr., Nutr.Abstr., Pharm.&Out.News, Plant Breed.Abstr., Poult.Abstr., Protozool.Abstr., Reac., SSCI (coverage dropped), Sci.Cit.Ind., Telegen, Vet.Bull.
—BLDSC (4116.314000), ADONIS, CASDDS, CISTI, EMDOCS, GNLM, IDS, ingenta, Linda Hall. **CCC.**
Published by: Academic Press, Inc., Journal Division (Subsidiary of: Harcourt Brace & Company), 525 B St, Ste 1900, San Diego, CA 92101-4495. TEL 619-230-1840, FAX 619-699-6800, apsubs@acad.com, http://www.academicpress.com/genomics.

572.86 USA
GENOMICS SOURCE BOOK. Text in English. 1997. a. USD 349; USD 379 foreign (effective 1999). **Document type:** *Trade.*
Published by: American Health Consultants (Subsidiary of: Medical Economics Co., Inc.), 3525 Piedmont Rd, N E, 6 Piedmont Center, Ste 400, Atlanta, GA 30305. TEL 404-262-5476, custserv@ahcpub.com, http://www.ahcpub.com.

576.5 KOR ISSN 0254-5934
QH426 CODEN: KJGEDG
HAN'GUG YUJEON HAGHOEJI/KOREAN JOURNAL OF GENETICS. Text in Korean. 1979. q. KRW 70,000 domestic; USD 100 foreign. adv. bk.rev. *Refereed.* **Document type:** *Proceedings, Academic/Scholarly.* **Description:** Publishes original reports on any field of genetics.
Related titles: Online - full text ed.: (from Institute for Scientific Information).
Indexed: ASCA, Biol.Abstr., Biotech.Cit.Ind., Chem.Abstr., Chem.Indus.Notes, Chem.Titles, Curr.Adv.Gen.& Molec.Biol., Genet.Abstr. (coverage dropped), Sport Fish.Abstr., Zoo.Rec.
—BLDSC (5113.551000), CASDDS, CISTI.
Published by: Han'gug Yujeon Haghoe/Genetics Society of Korea, Seoul National University, Dept. of Biology, College of Natural Science, Sinlimdong Sab 56-1, Kwanakguseoul 151-742, Korea, S.. TEL 82-53-950-6353, FAX 82-53-943-2762, yselee@kyungpook.ac.kr, http://www.bric.postech.ac.kr/gsk/. Circ: 500.

599.9 USA ISSN 1063-0627
CODEN: HAIRE4
HARVARD AIDS INSTITUTE SERIES ON GENE REGULATION OF HUMAN RETROVIRUSES. Text in English. 1991. irreg. price varies. reprint service avail. from PQC. *Refereed.* **Document type:** *Proceedings.*
Indexed: Chem.Abstr., Chem.Indus.Notes, Chem.Titles.
—CASDDS, CISTI.
Published by: (Harvard AIDS Institute), Lippincott Williams & Wilkins (Philadelphia) (Subsidiary of: Wolters Kluwer N.V.), 530 Walnut St, Philadelphia, PA 19106-3621. TEL 301-223-2300, 800-638-3030, FAX 301-223-2400.

576.5 SWE ISSN 0018-0661
QH431.A1 CODEN: HEREAY
HEREDITAS; a periodical devoted to the publication of original research in all aspects of genetics and cytology. Text in English. 1920. bi-m. USD 216 in the Americas to institutions print & online eds. combined; GBP 150 elsewhere to institutions print & online eds. combined (effective 2002). adv. abstr, bibl, illus. index, cum.index: vols.1-40. back issues avail. *Refereed.* **Document type:** *Academic/Scholarly.*
Formerly: Hereditas-Genetiskt Arkiv
Related titles: Microfilm ed.: (from PQC); Online - full text ed.: (from Institute for Scientific Information).
Indexed: Abstr.Anthropol., AgBiotech, Agroforest.Abstr., Anim.Behav.Abstr., Anim.Breed.Abstr., Appl.Ecol.Abstr., Aqua.Sci.& Fish.Abstr., Bio-Contr.News & Info., Biol.Abstr., Biotech.Cit.Ind., Chem.Abstr., Chem.Indus.Notes, Chem.Titles, Crop Physiol.Abstr., Curr.Adv.Ecol.Sci., Curr.Cont., Dent.Ind., Entomol.Abstr., Excerp.Med., Fababean Abstr., Field Crop Abstr., Forest.Abstr., Genet.Abstr., Helminthol.Abstr., Herb.Abstr., Hum.Gen.Abstr., INIS Atomind., Ind.Med. (1920-), Ind.Sci.Rev., Ind.Vet., Inpharma, Int.Abstr.Biol.Sci., Maize Abstr., Nuc.Acids Abstr., Pig News & Info., Plant Breed.Abstr., Plant Gen.Res.Abstr., Plant Grow.Reg.Abstr., Poult.Abstr., Protozool.Abstr., Reac., Ref.Zh., Rev.Appl.Entomol., Rev.Med.& Vet.Mycol., Rev.Plant Path., Rice Abstr., Sci.Cit.Ind., Seed Abstr., Soils & Fert., Sport Fish.Abstr., Telegen, Triticale Abstr., Trop.Dis.Bull., Vet.Bull., Weed Abstr., Wild.Rev., Zoo.Rec.
—BLDSC (4299.000000), CASDDS, CISTI, GNLM, ingenta, Linda Hall.
Published by: (Scandinavian Association of Geneticists), Mendelian Society of Lund, Department of Genetics, Lund 22362, Sweden. TEL 46-46-222784, FAX 46-46-147874, Lars.Davring@gen.lu.se. Ed. Ulf Gyllensten. Adv. contact Lars Davring. Circ: 1,000. **Subscr. to:** Hereditas-Distribution, Fack 1601, Lund 22101, Sweden.

576.5 GBR ISSN 0018-067X
QH431 CODEN: HDTYAT
HEREDITY; an international journal of genetics. Text in English. 1947. m. GBP 348 in Europe; USD 590 in North America; GBP 383 elsewhere; GBP 382.80 in Europe print & online eds.; USD 649 in North America print & online eds.; GBP 421.30 elsewhere print & online eds. (effective 2001). adv. bk.rev. bibl, charts, illus. index. back issues avail.; reprints avail. *Refereed.* **Document type:** *Journal, Academic/Scholarly.* **Description:** Publishes articles in all areas of genetics, focusing on the genetics of eukaryotes.
Related titles: Microform ed.: (from PQC); Online - full text ed.: ISSN 1365-2540. USD 531 in North America; GBP 314 elsewhere (effective 2001) (from Ovid Technologies, Inc., EBSCO Publishing, O C L C Online Computer Library Center, Inc., RoweCom Information Quest, ingenta, Gale Group, Munksgaard & Blackwell Science's Synergy, Swets Blackwell, Institute for Scientific Information).
Indexed: ASCA, Abstr.Anthropol., Abstr.Hyg., AgBiotech, Agricola, Agroforest.Abstr., Anim.Breed.Abstr., Apic.Abstr., Appl.Ecol.Abstr., Aqua.Sci.& Fish.Abstr., Bio-Contr.News & Info., Biol.& Agr.Ind. (Feb.1983-), Biol.Abstr., Biotech.Cit.Ind., Chem.Abstr., Chem.Indus.Notes, Chem.Titles, Curr.Adv.Cell & Devel.Biol., Curr.Adv.Ecol.Sci., Curr.Adv.Gen.& Molec.Biol., Curr.Cont., Curr.Ind.Stat., Curr.Ref.Fish Res., Ecol.Abstr., Entomol.Abstr., Environ.Sci.Poll.Mgmt., Excerp.Med., Field Crop Abstr., Food Sci.& Tech.Abstr., Forest.Abstr., Gen.Sci.Ind. (Jul.1997-), Genet.Abstr., Helminthol.Abstr., Herb.Abstr., Hort.Abstr., Hum.Gen.Abstr., INIS Atomind., Ind.Med. (1947-), Ind.Sci.Rev., Ind.Vet., Inpharma, Int.Abstr.Biol.Sci., Maize Abstr., Nuc.Acids Abstr., Ornam.Hort., Pig News & Info., Plant Breed.Abstr., Plant Gen.Res.Abstr., Postharvest, Potato Abstr., Poult.Abstr., Reac., Ref.Zh., Rev.Appl.Entomol., Rev.Med.& Vet.Mycol., Rev.Plant Path., Rice Abstr., Sci.Cit.Ind., Seed Abstr., Soils & Fert., Soyabean Abstr., Sport Fish.Abstr., THA, Triticale Abstr., Trop.Dis.Bull., Vet.Bull., Weed Abstr., Wild.Rev., Zoo.Rec.
—BLDSC (4300.000000), CASDDS, CISTI, EMDOCS, GNLM, IDS, Infotrieve, ingenta, Linda Hall. **CCC.**
Published by: Blackwell Science Ltd., Osney Mead, Oxford OX2 0EL, United Kingdom. TEL 44-1865-206206, FAX 44-1865-721205, journals.cs@blacksci.co.uk, http://www.blackwell-science.com/products/journals/hered.htm. Ed. J F Y Brookfield. Pub. Amanda McLean Inglis. R&P Sophie Savage. Adv. contact Jenny Applin. Circ: 1,075.

576.549 JPN ISSN 0918-5976
CODEN: MMGCEK
HONYU DOBUTSU SHIKEN BUNKAKAI KAIHO/MAMMALIAN MUTAGENICITY STUDY GROUP COMMUNICATIONS. Text in English, Japanese. 1988. a. JPY 2,000. adv. bk.rev. *Refereed.* **Document type:** *Academic/Scholarly.* **Description:** Contains papers reporting results (including negative data) of original research concerning mutagenesis, chromosome breakage, and related subjects in mammalian cells and mammals.
Indexed: Chem.Abstr., Chem.Indus.Notes, Chem.Titles.
—CASDDS.
Published by: Nihon Kankyo Hen'igen Gakkai, Honyu Dobutsu Shiken Bunkakai/Environmental Mutagen Society of Japan, Mammalian Mutagenicity Study Group, Shokuhin Yakuhin Anzen Senta Hadano Kenkyujo, 729-5 Ochiai, Hadano-shi, Kanagawa-ken 257-0025, Japan. Ed. Makoto Hayashi.

599.935 USA ISSN 1063-2158
HUMAN EVOLUTION, BEHAVIOR, AND INTELLIGENCE. Text in English. 1992. irreg. price varies. **Document type:** *Monographic series.*
Indexed: e-psyche.
Published by: Praeger Publishers (Subsidiary of: Greenwood Publishing Group Inc.), 88 Post Rd W, Box 5007, Westport, CT 06881-5007. TEL 203-226-3571, FAX 203-222-1502.

599.9 USA ISSN 1043-0342
RB155.8 CODEN: HGTHE3
HUMAN GENE THERAPY. Text in English. 1990. 18/yr., latest vol.12, 2001. USD 549 domestic to individuals; USD 799 foreign to individuals; USD 659 domestic to individuals print and online eds. combined; USD 909 foreign to individuals print and online eds. combined; USD 1,480 domestic to institutions; USD 1,667 foreign to institutions; USD 1,776 domestic to institutions print and online eds. combined; USD 1,963 foreign to institutions print and online eds. combined (effective 2002). back issues avail.; reprints avail. *Refereed.* **Document type:** *Journal, Academic/Scholarly.* **Description:** Publishes papers on the transfer of genes in mammals, including humans. Covers improvements in vector development, delivery systems and animal models, as well as ethical, legal, and regulatory issues.
Related titles: Online - full text ed.: USD 549 to individuals; USD 1,480 to institutions (effective 2002) (from CatchWord Ltd., EBSCO Publishing, O C L C Online Computer Library Center, Inc., RoweCom Information Quest, Swets Blackwell, Institute for Scientific Information).
Indexed: ASCA, AgBiotech, Anim.Breed.Abstr., Biotech.Cit.Ind., Chem.Abstr., Chem.Indus.Notes, Chem.Titles, Curr.Cont., Derwent Biotech.Abstr., Environ.Sci.Poll.Mgmt., Excerp.Med. (1993-), Focus on: Mol.Med., Genet.Abstr., Hum.Gen.Abstr., Ind.Med. (1990-), Ind.Sci.Rev., Ind.Vet., Inpharma, Int.Abstr.Biol.Sci., Med.& Pharm.Biotech.Abstr., Neurosci.Abstr., Nuc.Acids Abstr., Pharm.&Out.News, Protozool.Abstr., Reac., Saf.Sci.Abstr., Sci.Cit.Ind.
—BLDSC (4336.092000), ADONIS, CASDDS, CatchWord, CISTI, EMDOCS, GNLM, IDS, ingenta, KNAW. **CCC.**
Published by: Mary Ann Liebert, Inc. Publishers, 2 Madison Ave, Larchmont, NY 10538. TEL 914—834-3100, FAX 914-834-1388, info@liebertpub.com, www.liebertpub.com/hum, http://www.liebertpub.com/blr. Ed. Dr. W French Anderson.

599.9 DEU ISSN 0340-6717
CODEN: HUGEDQ
HUMAN GENETICS. Text in English. 1964. m. EUR 3,021 domestic; EUR 3,010.70 in Germany; EUR 299 newsstand/cover foreign (effective 2002). adv. charts, illus. back issues avail.; reprint service avail. from ISI. *Refereed.* **Document type:** *Journal, Academic/Scholarly.* **Description:** Covers human genetics, cytogenetics, biochemical genetics, population genetics, immunogenetics, pharmacogenetics, genetic diagnosis and counseling.
Continues: Humangenetik (0018-7348)
Related titles: Microform ed.: (from PQC); Online - full text ed.: ISSN 1432-1203 (from EBSCO Publishing, RoweCom Information Quest, Swets Blackwell, Springer LINK, Institute for Scientific Information).
Indexed: ASCA, Anim.Breed.Abstr., Bibl.Asian Stud. (1970-1971), Bibl.Dev.Med.& Child Neur., Biol.Abstr., Biotech.& Bioeng.Abstr., Biotech.Cit.Ind., Chem.Abstr., Chem.Indus.Notes, Chem.Titles, Curr.Adv.Cancer Res., Curr.Adv.Ecol.Sci., Curr.Cont., Excerp.Med., Focus on: Mol.Med., Genet.Abstr., Hum.Gen.Abstr., INIS Atomind., Ind.Med. (1976-), Ind.Sci.Rev., Inpharma, Int.Abstr.Biol.Sci., Med.& Surg.Dermat., Pharm.&Out.News, Reac., Rev.Appl.Entomol., SSCI (coverage dropped), Sci.Cit.Ind.
—BLDSC (4336.095000), CASDDS, CISTI, EMDOCS, GNLM, IDS, ingenta, KNAW, Linda Hall. **CCC.**
Published by: Springer-Verlag (Subsidiary of: BertelsmannSpringer), Tiergartenstr 17, Heidelberg 69121, Germany. TEL 49-6221-345-0, FAX 49-6221-345229, subscriptions@springer.de, http://link.springer.de/link/service/journals/00439/index.htm, http://www.springer.de. **Subscr. in N. America to:** Springer-Verlag New York Inc., PO Box 2485, Secaucus, NJ 07096-2485. TEL 212-460-1500, FAX 212-473-6272.

599.9 USA ISSN 0172-7699
HUMAN GENETICS. SUPPLEMENT. Text in English. 1978. irreg. price varies. reprint service avail. from ISI. **Document type:** *Academic/Scholarly.*
Related titles: Microform ed.: (from PQC).
Indexed: Ind.Med. (coverage dropped).
—CISTI.
Published by: Springer-Verlag, Journals (Subsidiary of: BertelsmannSpringer), 175 Fifth Ave, New York, NY 10010. TEL 212-460-1500, FAX 212-473-6272.

599.935 USA ISSN 1050-6101
QH447
HUMAN GENOME NEWS. Text in English. 1989. bi-m. free per issue. bk.rev., Website rev. charts, illus. 16 p./no. back issues avail. *Refereed.* **Document type:** *Newsletter, Government, Academic/Scholarly.* **Description:** Facilitates communication among life sciences researchers and informs persons interested in genetic research. Provides resource and technology updates to stimulate genomic applications.
Related titles: Online - full text ed.: (from Institute for Scientific Information).
Indexed: ASCA, Biotech.Cit.Ind., SSCI (coverage dropped).
—BLDSC (4336.097600), IDS.
Published by: Human Genome Management Information System, Oak Ridge National Laboratory, 1060 Commerce Park, Oak Ridge, TN 37830. TEL 865-576-6669, FAX 865-574-9888, mansfieldbk@ornl.gov, http://www.ornl.gov/hgmis. Ed. Betty K Mansfield. R&P Anne Anderson. Circ: 14,300 (controlled). **Subscr. to:** Oak Ridge National Laboratory, 1060 Commerce Park, Oak Ridge, TN 37830. **Co-sponsor:** U.S. Department of Energy.

611.01816 USA
HUMAN GENOME PROGRAM REPORT. Text in English. 1990. biennial. free per issue. **Document type:** *Government.*
Related titles: Online - full text ed.
Published by: U.S. Department of Energy, Human Genome Program, Office of Health and Environmental Research, ER 72 GTN, Washington, DC 20585. TEL 301-903-6488, FAX 301-903-5051, adamsonae@ornl.gov, http://www.ornl.gov/hgmis. Eds. Anne E Adamson, Daniel W Drell. R&P Betty Mansfield TEL 423-576-6669. Circ: 12,300; 12,300 (controlled). **Orders to:** National Technical Information Service, Government Research Center. FAX 703-321-8547. **Co-sponsor:** Oak Ridge National Laboratory. Human Genome Management Information System.

599.935 CHE ISSN 0001-5652
RB155 CODEN: HUHEAS
HUMAN HEREDITY; international journal of human and medical genetics. Text in English. 1950. 8/yr. CHF 1,286, EUR 918.40 in Europe to institutions; CHF 1,309.20, USD 1,000 elsewhere to institutions (effective 2002). adv. bibl, charts, illus, stat. index. back issues avail. *Refereed.* **Document type:** *Journal, Academic/Scholarly.* **Description:** Devoted to methodological and applied research on the genetics of human populations, linkage analysis, and the genetic mechanisms of disease.
Formerly: Acta Genetica et Statistica Medica
Related titles: Microform ed.; Online - full text ed.: ISSN 1423-0062. CHF 116, EUR 84, USD 90 to institutions with print edition (effective 2002) (from EBSCO Publishing, O C L C Online Computer Library Center, Inc., RoweCom Information Quest, Swets Blackwell, Institute for Scientific Information).

B

Indexed: A.I.C.P. (1969-), ASCA, Abstr.Anthropol., Abstr.Hyg., Anim.Breed.Abstr., Anthropol.Lit., Bibl.Dev.Med.& Child Neur., Biol.Abstr., Biotech.Cit.Ind., Chem.Abstr., Chem.Indus.Notes, Chem.Titles, Curr.Adv.Ecol.Sci., Curr.Cont., Curr.Ind.Stat., Dok.Arbeitsmed., Excerp.Med., Ind.Med. (1969-), Ind.Sci.Rev., Inpharma, Nutr.Abstr., Pharm.&Out.News, Reac., Rural Recreat.Tour.Abstr., Sci.Cit.Ind., THA, World Ag.Econ.& Rur.Soc.Abstr.
—BLDSC (4336.150000), CASDDS, CISTI, GNLM, IDS, ingenta, KNAW, Linda Hall. **CCC.**
Published by: S. Karger AG, Allschwilerstr 10, PO Box, Basel 4009, Switzerland. TEL 41-61-306-1111, FAX 41-61-306-1234, karger@karger.ch, http://www.online.karger.com/journals/hhe, http://www.karger.com. Ed. J Ott. adv.: page USD 1,195. Circ: 1,000.

B

599.9 GBR ISSN 0964-6906
RB155.5 CODEN: HMGEE5
HUMAN MOLECULAR GENETICS. Text in English. 1992. 26/yr. GBP 225, USD 336 to individuals; GBP 835, USD 1,450 to institutions (effective 2002). adv. back issues avail.; reprint service avail. from SWZ. *Refereed.* **Document type:** *Journal, Academic/Scholarly.* **Description:** Concentrates on full-length research papers covering a wide range of topics in all aspects of human molecular genetics.
Related titles: Online - full text ed.: ISSN 1460-2083. 1999. GBP 751, USD 1,305 to institutions Online only (effective 2002) (from HighWire Pr., EBSCO Publishing, O C L C Online Computer Library Center, Inc., RoweCom Information Quest, ingenta, Swets Blackwell, Institute for Scientific Information).
Indexed: ASCA, Biotech.& Bioeng.Abstr., Biotech.Cit.Ind., Chem.Abstr., Chem.Indus.Notes, Chem.Titles, Curr.Cont., Derwent Biotech.Abstr., Excerp.Med. (1993-), Focus on: Mol.Med., Genet.Abstr., Hum.Gen.Abstr., Ind.Med. (1992-), Ind.Sci.Rev., Inpharma, Int.Abstr.Biol.Sci., Neurosci.Abstr., Neurosci.Cit.Ind., Pharm.&Out.News, Reac., Sci.Cit.Ind.
—BLDSC (4336.198000), CASDDS, CISTI, EMDOCS, GNLM, IDS, ingenta, Linda Hall. **CCC.**
Published by: Oxford University Press, Academic Division, Great Clarendon St, Oxford OX2 6DP, United Kingdom. TEL 44-1865-267907, FAX 44-1865-267835, jnl.info@oup.co.uk, http://www.hmg.oupjournals.org, http://www.oup.co.uk/journals. Eds. H F Willard, K E Davies. Pubs. David Prosser, Martin Richardson. R&P Fionna Willis. adv.: page GBP 445, page USD 800. Circ: 2,000. **Subscr. in US to:** Oxford University Press, Journals, 2001 Evans Rd, Cary, NC 27513. TEL 800-852-7323, FAX 919-677-1714, jnlorders@oup-usa.org; **Subscr. to:** Journals Marketing, Great Clarendon St, Oxford OX2 6DP, United Kingdom.

576.549 USA ISSN 1059-7794
RB155.5 CODEN: HUMUE3
HUMAN MUTATION. Text in English. 1992. 12/yr. (in 2 vols., 6 nos./vol.). USD 835 in United States; USD 955 in Canada & Mexico; USD 1,057 elsewhere; USD 877 combined subscription in United States for print and online eds.; USD 997 combined subscription in Canada & Mexico for print and online eds.; USD 1,099 combined subscription elsewhere for print and online eds. (effective 2002). adv. bk.rev. back issues avail. *Refereed.* **Document type:** *Academic/Scholarly.* **Description:** Publishes original research articles, mutation updates, briefs on new mutations and reviews on broad aspects of mutation research as related to understanding the human genome and medical aspects of genetic disorders. For molecular, human and medical geneticists in academic, industrial and clinical research settings.
Related titles: Microform ed.: (from PQC); Online - full text ed.: ISSN 1098-1004. 1996. USD 835 in United States; USD 835 in Canada & Mexico; USD 835 elsewhere (effective 2002) (from EBSCO Publishing, Wiley InterScience, Institute for Scientific Information).
Indexed: ASCA, Biotech.& Bioeng.Abstr. (coverage dropped), Biotech.Cit.Ind., Chem.Abstr., Chem.Indus.Notes, Chem.Titles, Curr.Cont., Excerp.Med. (1993-), Focus on: Mol.Med., Genet.Abstr (coverage dropped), Hum.Gen.Abstr., Ind.Med. (1992-), Inpharma, Int.Abstr.Biol.Sci., Pharm.&Out.News, Reac., Ref.Zh., Sci.Cit.Ind.
—BLDSC (4336.217000), CASDDS, CISTI, EMDOCS, GNLM, IDS, Infotrieve, KNAW. **CCC.**
Published by: John Wiley & Sons, Inc., Journals (Subsidiary of: Wiley InterScience), 605 Third Ave, New York, NY 10158. TEL 212-850-6645, FAX 212-850-6021, subinfo@wiley.com, uscs-wis@wiley.com, http://www.wiley.com. Eds. Haig H Kazazian Jr., R G H Cotton. adv.: B&W page GBP 640, color page GBP 1,515; trim 210 x 279. Circ: 750. **Subscr. outside the Americas to:** John Wiley & Sons Ltd., Baffins Ln, Chichester, Sussex PO19 IUD, United Kingdom. TEL 44-1243-779777, FAX 44-1243-843232, cs-journals@wiley.co.uk, http://www.wiley.co.uk.

I E E E TRANSACTIONS ON EVOLUTIONARY COMPUTATION. see *BIOLOGY—Computer Applications*

ICHTHYOSIS FOCUS. see *MEDICAL SCIENCES—Dermatology And Venereology*

599.935 JPN ISSN 0387-0022
CODEN: IDENBZ
IDEN/HEREDITY. Text in Japanese. 1947. m. JPY 900 per issue. Supplement avail.
Indexed: Chem.Abstr., Chem.Indus.Notes, Chem.Titles, GeoRef, INIS Atomind.
—BLDSC (4300.020000), CASDDS, CISTI.
Published by: (Idengaku Fukyukai/Association for Propagation of the Knowledge of Genetics), Shokabo Publisher Co. Ltd., 8-1 Yonban-cho, Chiyoda-ku, Tokyo 102-0081, Japan.

576.5 DEU ISSN 0093-7711
QR184 CODEN: IMNGBK
IMMUNOGENETICS. Text in English. 1974. m. EUR 1,421.10 domestic; EUR 1,410.70 in Germany; EUR 139 newsstand/cover foreign (effective 2001). reprint service avail. from ISI. *Refereed.* **Document type:** *Journal, Academic/Scholarly.* **Description:** Covers the areas of immunogenetics of cell interaction and tissue differentiation and development, phylogeny of alloantigens, and genetic control of immune response and disease susceptibility.
Related titles: Microform ed.: (from PQC); Online - full text ed.: ISSN 1432-1211 (from EBSCO Publishing, RoweCom Information Quest, Swets Blackwell, Springer LINK, Institute for Scientific Information).
Indexed: AIDS & Cancer Res., ASCA, AgBiotech, Agri.& Environ.Biotech.Abstr. (coverage dropped), Anim.Breed.Abstr., Biol.Abstr., Biotech.Cit.Ind., Chem.Abstr., Chem.Indus.Notes, Chem.Titles, Curr.Adv.Ecol.Sci., Curr.Adv.Gen.& Molec.Biol., Curr.Cont., Dent.Ind., Derwent Biotech.Abstr., Excerp.Med., Genet.Abstr., Helminthol.Abstr., Hum.Gen.Abstr., INIS Atomind., Immun.Abstr., Ind.Med. (1974-), Ind.Sci.Rev., Ind.Vet., Inpharma, Int.Abstr.Biol.Sci., Nuc.Acids Abstr., Pig News & Info., Poult.Abstr., Protozool.Abstr., Reac., Rev.Appl.Entomol., Rev.Med.& Vet.Mycol., Sci.Cit.Ind., Small Anim.Abstr., Sport Fish.Abstr., Vet.Bull., Wild.Rev., Zoo.Rec.
—BLDSC (4369.665000), ADONIS, CASDDS, CISTI, GNLM, IDS, ingenta, KNAW. **CCC.**
Published by: Springer-Verlag (Subsidiary of: BertelsmannSpringer), Tiergartenstr 17, Heidelberg 69121, Germany. TEL 49-6221-345-0, FAX 49-6221-345229, subscriptions@springer.de, http://link.springer.de/link/service/journals/00251/index.htm, http://www.springer.de. Ed. R E Bontrop. **Subscr. in N. America to:** Springer-Verlag New York Inc., PO Box 2485, Secaucus, NJ 07096-2485. TEL 212-460-1500, FAX 212-473-6272.

IN VITRO CELLULAR & DEVELOPMENTAL BIOLOGY - PLANT. see *BIOLOGY—Botany*

INDIAN JOURNAL OF GENETICS AND PLANT BREEDING. see *BIOLOGY—Botany*

599.9 IND ISSN 0971-6866
INDIAN JOURNAL OF HUMAN GENETICS. Text in English. s-a. **Document type:** *Journal, Academic/Scholarly.*
—BLDSC (4415.230000).
Published by: The Indian Society of Human Genetics, Department of Genetics, Osmania University, Hyderabad 500 007, India. TEL 91-040-7018951 ext. 335, FAX 91-040-7172614. Ed. T Padma.

599.9 IND ISSN 0378-8156
GN49 CODEN: IJPGDB
INDIAN JOURNAL OF PHYSICAL ANTHROPOLOGY AND HUMAN GENETICS. Text in English. 1975-1994; N.S. 1997. s-a. INR 200, USD 30 (effective 2000). adv. bk.rev. bibl, charts. cum.index every 10 yrs. *Refereed.* **Document type:** *Academic/Scholarly.* **Description:** Serves as a medium for scholarly studies devoted to biological aspects of human populations including genetics, evolution, ecology, dermography, growth, physiology, biochemistry, pharmacology, disease patterns and behaviour of individuals comprising them.
Indexed: A.I.C.P. (1975-), Anthropol.Lit., Bibl.Asian Stud. (1975-1991), Biol.Abstr., Curr.Adv.Ecol.Sci.
—GNLM, Linda Hall.
Published by: Ethnographic & Folk Culture Society, L-II-31 Sector B, Aliganj Housing Scheme, P O Box 209, Lucknow, Uttar Pradesh 226 024, India. TEL 91-522-372362. Ed. B R K Shukla. R&P Nadeem Hasnain. Adv. contact Kamal Kishore. page INR 1,000; 195 x 145. Circ: 350.

▼ **INFECTION, GENETICS AND EVOLUTION.** see *MEDICAL SCIENCES*

576.5 NLD ISSN 1567-7257
INFECTION, GENETICS AND EVOLUTION ONLINE. Text in English. q. USD 297 to institutions (effective 2001).
Media: Online - full text. **Related titles:** ♦ Print ed.: Infection, Genetics and Evolution. ISSN 1567-1348.
Published by: Elsevier Science BV, Sara Burgerhartstraat 25, Amsterdam 1055 KV, Netherlands. TEL 31-20-485-2911, FAX 31-20-485-2457, nlinfo-f@elsevier.nl, http://www.elsevier.com/locate/meegon, http://www.elsevier.nl.

576.5 CUB ISSN 0138-6832
INFORMACION EXPRESS. SERIE: GENETICA Y REPRODUCCION. Text in Spanish. 1977. 3/yr. USD 6; in N. America; S. America $9; Europe $10; others $14; or exchange basis.
Indexed: Agrindex.
—CISTI.
Published by: Centro de Informacion y Documentacion Agropecuario, Gaveta Postal 4149, Havana 4, Cuba. **Dist. by:** Ediciones Cubanas, Obispo No. 527, Apdo. 605, Havana, Cuba.

576.5 USA
INSIDE THE JACKSON LABORATORY. Text in English. 1952. q. free per issue. charts, illus.
Former titles: Jax (0021-5570); Jackson Laboratory News
Published by: Jackson Laboratory, 600 Main St, Bar Harbor, ME 04609. TEL 207-288-6051. Ed. Luther Young. Circ: 14,000.

INSTITUT PASTEUR. ANNALES. ACTUALITES. see *BIOLOGY—Microbiology*

INSTITUTE OF PRIMATE RESEARCH. ANNUAL REPORT. see *BIOLOGY—Zoology*

599.90285 JPN
INTERNATIONAL JOURNAL OF EVOLUTIONARY OPTIMIZATION. Text in Japanese. irreg. **Description:** Aims to collect and disseminate the progressive body of knowledge on evolutionary optimization and other areas of machine learning, via a single organized medium. Includes genetic algorithms, genetic programming, evolutionary programming and evolution strategies.
Related titles: Online - full text ed.
Published by: Kanazawa University, Department of Human and Mechanical Systems Engineering, Bionic Design Laboratory, Kanazawa 920, Japan. TEL 81-762-34-4758, FAX 81-762-34-4668, sourav@kenroku.ipc.kanazawa-u.ac.jp, http://genetic.hm.t.kanazawa-u.ac.jp/evopt/. Ed. Sourav Kundu.

576.5 SGP ISSN 0218-1932
QH447 CODEN: IJGREY
INTERNATIONAL JOURNAL OF GENOME RESEARCH. Text in English. 1992. bi-m. USD 240 to institutions; USD 120 to individuals. **Document type:** *Academic/Scholarly.* **Description:** Publishes research on human genomes, as well as other organisms and simple genomes such as those of Drosophila melanogaster and bacteria.
Indexed: Food Sci.& Tech.Abstr., Genet.Abstr. (coverage dropped), Hum.Gen.Abstr., SSCI (coverage dropped).
—CASDDS, GNLM, IDS. **CCC.**
Published by: World Scientific Publishing Co Pte Ltd, Farrer Rd, PO Box 128, Singapore 912805, Singapore. TEL 65-3825663, FAX 65-3825919.

576.5 RUS ISSN 0301-391X
ITOGI NAUKI I TEKHNIKI. GENETIKA CHELOVEKA. Text in Russian. irreg., latest vol.6, 1982. price varies.
Published by: Vserossiiskii Institut Nauchnoi i Tekhnicheskoi Informatsii (VINITI), Usievicha ul 20-a, Moscow 125315, Russian Federation. TEL 7-095-1526441, FAX 7-095-943-0060. **Dist. by:** Mezhdunarodnaya Kniga, B Yakimanka 39, Moscow 117049, Russian Federation. TEL 7-095-2384967, FAX 7-095-2384634; **US dist. addr.:** East View Publications, 3020 Harbor Ln N, Minneapolis, MN 55447. TEL 612-550-0961.

576.5 RUS ISSN 0202-7097
CODEN: INTGDP
ITOGI NAUKI I TEKHNIKI. OBSHCHAYA GENETIKA. Text in Russian. irreg. **Document type:** *Academic/Scholarly.*
—CASDDS, Linda Hall.
Published by: Vserossiiskii Institut Nauchnoi i Tekhnicheskoi Informatsii (VINITI), Usievicha ul 20-a, Moscow 125315, Russian Federation. TEL 7-095-1526441, FAX 7-095-943-0060. **US dist. addr.:** East View Publications, 3020 Harbor Ln N, Minneapolis, MN 55447. TEL 612-550-0961.

599.9 USA ISSN 0447-3353
CODEN: JALEBX
JAMES ARTHUR LECTURE ON THE EVOLUTION OF THE HUMAN BRAIN. Text in English. 1956. irreg., latest vol.68, 1998. price varies. **Document type:** *Monographic series.*
Indexed: Biol.Abstr., e-psyche.
—BLDSC (4645.500000), CISTI.
Published by: American Museum of Natural History, Central Park West at 79th St, New York, NY 10024-5192. TEL 212-769-5000, FAX 212-769-5233, scipubs.@amnh.org, scipubs@amnh.org, http://www.amnh.org. Ed. Brenda Jones. Circ: 1,000.

JOURNAL OF APPLIED GENETICS; an international journal of genetics and breeding. see *BIOLOGY—Botany*

JOURNAL OF BASIC MICROBIOLOGY; an international journal on biochemistry, physiology, genetics, morphology and ecology of microorganisms. see *BIOLOGY—Microbiology*

JOURNAL OF BIOSOCIAL SCIENCE. see *SOCIOLOGY*

576.5 DNK ISSN 0270-4145
QL991 CODEN: JCGBDF
JOURNAL OF CRANIOFACIAL GENETICS AND DEVELOPMENTAL BIOLOGY. Text in English. 1981. q. DKK 2,300; DKK 2,530 print & online eds. combined (effective 2001). adv. bibl, charts, illus. index. reprints avail. *Refereed.* **Document type:** *Academic/Scholarly.*
Related titles: ♦ Online - full text ed.: Journal of Craniofacial Genetics and Developmental Biology Online.
Indexed: ASCA, Abstr.Anthropol., Aqua.Sci.& Fish.Abstr., Biol.Abstr., Biotech.& Bioeng.Abstr., Cal.Tiss.Abstr., Chem.Abstr., Chem.Indus.Notes, Curr.Cont., Curr.Tit.Dent., Dent.Ind., Excerp.Med., Genet.Abstr., Hum.Gen.Abstr., INIS Atomind., Ind.Med. (1981-), Ind.Sci.Rev., Inpharma, Nuc.Acids Abstr., Reac., Sci.Cit.Ind.
—ADONIS, CASDDS, CISTI, EMDOCS, GNLM, IDS, ingenta, KNAW. **CCC.**
Published by: (Society of Craniofacial Genetics), Blackwell Munksgaard, Noerre Soegade 35, PO Box 2148, Copenhagen K 1016, Denmark. TEL 45-77-33-33-33, FAX 45-77-33-33-77, customerservice@munksgaard.dk, http://journals.munksgaard.dk/craniofacialgenetics, http://www.munksgaard.dk. Eds. Harold C Slavkin, Michael Melnick. Circ: 400.

576.5 DNK
JOURNAL OF CRANIOFACIAL GENETICS AND DEVELOPMENTAL BIOLOGY ONLINE. Text in English. q. DKK 2,070 (effective 2001). **Document type:** *Academic/Scholarly.*
Media: Online - full text (from EBSCO Publishing, ingenta, Swets Blackwell). **Related titles:** ♦ Print ed.: Journal of Craniofacial Genetics and Developmental Biology. ISSN 0270-4145.
Published by: Blackwell Munksgaard, Noerre Soegade 35, PO Box 2148, Copenhagen K 1016, Denmark. TEL 45-77-33-33-33, FAX 45-77-33-33-77, fsub@mail.munksgaard.dk, http://www.ingenta.com/journals/browse/mksg/cgd, http://www.munksgaard.dk.

576.5 IND ISSN 0253-7605
CODEN: JCGEDO
THE JOURNAL OF CYTOLOGY AND GENETICS. Text in English. 1966. s-a. USD 45; INR 200 domestic to individuals; INR 500 domestic to institutions; INR 2,000 domestic life-member (effective 2001). bk.rev. 100 p./no. 1 cols./p. back issues avail.; reprints avail. *Refereed.* **Document type:** *Journal, Academic/Scholarly.*
Indexed: Chem.Abstr., Curr.Cont. (coverage dropped), Helminthol.Abstr., Plant Breed.Abstr., Zoo.Rec.
—CASDDS, CISTI, ingenta, Linda Hall.
Published by: Society of Cytologists and Geneticists, 261 7th Main Vijayanagar II Stage, Bangalore 560040, India. TEL 91-81-3387421, bhmn@hotmail.com. Ed., Pub., R&P, Adv. contact B H M Nijalingappa. Circ: 350 (controlled). **Dist. by:** H P C Publishers Distributors Pvt. Ltd., 1st Fl., Flats 1 & 2, Darya Ganj, 4805-24 Bharat Ram Rd., New Delhi 110 002, India. TEL 91-11-3254401, FAX 91-11-6192511.

▼ **JOURNAL OF ENDOCRINE GENETICS.** see *MEDICAL SCIENCES—Endocrinology*

576.8 GBR ISSN 1010-061X
QH359 CODEN: JEBIEQ
JOURNAL OF EVOLUTIONARY BIOLOGY. Text in English. 1988. bi-m., latest vol.15, 2002. GBP 630 in Europe; USD 998 in North America; GBP 693 elsewhere (effective 2002). adv. index. back issues avail. *Refereed.* **Document type:** *Academic/Scholarly.* **Description:** Covers both micro- and macro-evolution of all types of organisms, integrating perspective across molecular and microbial evolution, behavior, genetics, ecology, life histories, development, paeolntology, systematics and morphology.
Related titles: Online - full text ed.: ISSN 1420-9101. GBP 567 in Europe; USD 899 in North America; GBP 567 elsewhere (effective 2002) (from EBSCO Publishing, O C L C Online Computer Library Center, Inc., RoweCom Information Quest, ingenta, Munksgaard & Blackwell Science's Synergy, Swets Blackwell, Springer LINK, Institute for Scientific Information).
Indexed: ASCA, AgBiotech, Anim.Behav.Abstr., Anim.Breed.Abstr., Appl.Ecol.Abstr., Aqua.Sci.& Fish.Abstr., Bio-Contr.News & Info., Biol.Abstr., Chem.Abstr., Chem.Indus.Notes, Chem.Titles, Curr.Adv.Biochem., Curr.Adv.Cell & Devel.Biol., Curr.Adv.Gen.& Molec.Biol., Curr.Cont., Ecol.Abstr., Entomol.Abstr., Environ.Sci.Poll.Mgmt., Genet.Abstr., Hum.Gen.Abstr., Ind.Sci.Rev., Int.Abstr.Biol.Sci., Microbiol.Abstr., Nuc.Acids Abstr., Plant Breed.Abstr., Plant Gen.Res.Abstr., Postharvest, Poult.Abstr., Protozool.Abstr., Rev.Appl.Entomol., Rev.Arom.& Med.Plants, Rev.Med.& Vet.Mycol., Rev.Plant Path., Sci.Cit.Ind., Seed Abstr., Sport Fish.Abstr., Weed Abstr., Zoo.Rec.
—BLDSC (4979.642100), CASDDS, CISTI, EMDOCS, IDS, ingenta. **CCC.**
Published by: (European Society for Evolutionary Biology), Blackwell Science Ltd., PO Box 88, Oxford OX2 0NE, United Kingdom. TEL 44-1865-206180, 44-1865-206002, FAX 44-1865-206219, jnl.orders@blacksci.co.uk, http://www.blackwell-science.com/~cgilib/jnlpage.asp?Journal=jeb&File=jeb, http://www.blackwellpublishing.com. Ed. P H van Tienderen. Pub. Amanda McLean Inglis. R&P Tracey Davies. Adv. contact Jenny Applin. Circ: 630.

THE JOURNAL OF GENDER-SPECIFIC MEDICINE. see *MEDICAL SCIENCES*

576.5 USA ISSN 1099-498X
CODEN: JGMEFG
▼ **JOURNAL OF GENE MEDICINE.** Text in English. 1999. bi-m. USD 445 in United States; USD 445 in Canada & Mexico; USD 445 elsewhere; USD 468 combined subscription in United States for print and online eds.; USD 468 combined subscription in Canada & Mexico for print and online eds.; USD 468 combined subscription elsewhere for print and online eds. (effective 2002). bk.rev. *Refereed.* **Document type:** *Academic/Scholarly.* **Description:** Presents articles on all aspects of gene therapy, including design and production of vectors, research into mechanisms and underlying gene transfer, precilinical studies and clinical trials.
Related titles: Online - full text ed.: ISSN 1521-2254. USD 445 in United States; USD 445 in Canada & Mexico; USD 445 elsewhere (effective 2002) (from EBSCO Publishing, Wiley InterScience, Institute for Scientific Information).
Indexed: Biotech.& Bioeng.Abstr., Biotech.Cit.Ind., Curr.Cont., Genet.Abstr., Ind.Med. (1999-), Med.& Pharm.Biotech.Abstr., Nuc.Acids Abstr.
—BLDSC (4987.668000).
Published by: (European Society of Gene Therapy), John Wiley & Sons, Inc., Journals (Subsidiary of: Wiley InterScience), 605 Third Ave, New York, NY 10158. TEL 212-850-6645, FAX 212-850-6021, subinfo@wiley.com, uscs-wis@wiley.com, http://www.wiley.com. Eds. Kay E Davies, Olivier Danos, Richard Mulligan. **Subscr. in the Americas to:** John Wiley & Sons Ltd., Baffins Ln, Chichester, Sussex PO19 IUD, United Kingdom. TEL 44-1243-779777, FAX 44-1243-843232, cs-journals@wiley.co.uk, http://www.wiley.co.uk.

576.5 USA ISSN 0022-1325
L11 CODEN: JGPYAI
THE JOURNAL OF GENETIC PSYCHOLOGY; developmental and clinical psychology. Text in English. 1891. q., latest vol.163, 2002. USD 136 domestic; USD 149 foreign; USD 34 (effective 2001 - 2002). adv. bibl, charts. index. back issues avail.; reprint service avail. from SWZ,PSC,SCH. *Refereed.* **Document type:** *Academic/Scholarly.* **Description:** Devoted to research and theory in developmental, clinical and educational psychology.
Related titles: CD-ROM ed.: (from ProQuest Information & Learning); Microfilm ed.: (from PMC); Online - full text ed.: (from ProQuest Information & Learning, Gale Group, Northern Light Technology, Inc., H. W. Wilson, Factiva, Institute for Scientific Information).
Indexed: ASCA, Adol.Ment.Hlth.Abstr., AgeLine, Bibl.Dev.Med.& Child Neur., Biol.Abstr., C.I.J.E. (coverage dropped), Child Devel.Abstr., Crim.Just.Abstr., Curr.Adv.Ecol.Sci., Curr.Cont., DSH Abstr., ERA, Except.Child Educ.Abstr., Excerp.Med., Fam.Ind., IBR, IBZ, INIS Atomind., Ind.Med. (1954-), Ind.Philos., Indian Psychol.Abstr., Int.Nurs.Ind., Lang.& Lang.Behav.Abstr., Mid.East: Abstr.& Ind., Mult.Ed.Abstr., P C I, PsycInfo, Psychol.Abstr. (1932-), Psycscan D.P., Ref.Zh., Russ.Acad.Sci.Bibl., SOPODA, SSCI, Soc.Sci.Ind. (Jun.1982-), Soc.Work Res.& Abstr., Sociol.Abstr., Sociol.Educ.Abstr., Sp.Ed.Needs Abstr., Stud.Wom.Abstr., e-psyche.
—BLDSC (4989.900000), CISTI, GNLM, IDS, ingenta. **CCC.**
Published by: (Helen Dwight Reid Educational Foundation), Heldref Publications, 1319 Eighteenth St, N W, Washington, DC 20036-1802. TEL 202-296-6267, 800-365-9753, FAX 202-293-6130, gnt@heldref.org, http://www.heldref.org. Ed. Elizabeth Bruce. Circ: 1,000. **Subscr. to:** Allen Press Inc., PO Box 1897, Lawrence, KS 66044-8897.

591.35 ITA ISSN 0394-9257
SB123 CODEN: JGBREX
JOURNAL OF GENETICS & BREEDING; a journal devoted to agricultural genetics. Text in English. 1946. q. ITL 200,000 (effective 2000). adv. bk.rev. charts, illus. index. *Refereed.* **Document type:** *Academic/Scholarly.* **Description:** Focuses on biochemical and molecular genetics, genetic fundamentals of breeding, breeding methodology and genetic aspects of "in vitro" culture.
Formerly: Genetica Agraria (0016-6685)
Indexed: AgBiotech, Anim.Breed.Abstr., Biol.Abstr., Chem.Abstr., Chem.Indus.Notes, Chem.Titles, Cott.& Trop.Fibr.Abstr., Crop Physiol.Abstr., Curr.Adv.Gen.& Molec.Biol., Curr.Adv.Plant Sci., Fababean Abstr., Field Crop Abstr., Food Sci.& Tech.Abstr., Forest.Abstr., Helminthol.Abstr., Herb.Abstr., Hort.Abstr., INIS Atomind., Int.Abstr.Biol.Sci., Irr.& Drain.Abstr., Maize Abstr., Ornam.Hort., Plant Breed.Abstr., Plant Gen.Res.Abstr., Plant Grow.Reg.Abstr., Plant Sci., Postharvest, Potato Abstr., Rev.Appl.Entomol., Rev.Arom.& Med.Plants, Rev.Plant Path., Rice Abstr., Seed Abstr., Sorghum & Millets Abstr., Soyabean Abstr., Triticale Abstr.
—BLDSC (4990.200000), CASDDS, CISTI, EMDOCS.
Published by: Istituto Sperimentale per la Cerealicoltura, Via Cassia, 176, Rome, RM 00191, Italy. TEL 39-6-3295705-6-7, FAX 39-6-36308761, isc.pian@iol.it, http://hosting.iol.it/isc. Eds. A Bianchi, A J Pryor. Circ: 300 (controlled).

599.9 GBR ISSN 0047-2484
GN281 CODEN: JHEVAT
JOURNAL OF HUMAN EVOLUTION. Text in English. 1972. m. GBP 637 to institutions (effective 2001). adv. bk.rev. charts, illus. index. reprint service avail. from SWZ. *Refereed.* **Document type:** *Academic/Scholarly.* **Description:** Concentrates on papers covering all aspects of human evolution.
Related titles: Online - full text ed.: (from EBSCO Publishing, O C L C Online Computer Library Center, Inc., RoweCom Information Quest, ingenta, Swets Blackwell, IDEAL Online Library, Institute for Scientific Information).

Indexed: A.I.C.P. (1972-), ASCA, Abstr.Anthropol., Anthropol.Lit., Appl.Ecol.Abstr. (coverage dropped), Arts & Hum.Cit.Ind. (coverage dropped), Biol.Abstr., Biostat., Br.Archaeol.Abstr., Cal.Tiss.Abstr., Curr.Adv.Ecol.Sci., Curr.Cont., Ecol.Abstr., Environ.Sci.Poll.Mgmt., Excerp.Med., Geo.Abstr.H.G., Geo.Abstr.P.G., GeoRef, Geol.Abstr., Ind.Med. (1972-), Ind.Sci.Rev., Intl.Bibl.Soc.Sci., Mid.East: Abstr.& Ind., NAA, SSCI, Sci.Cit.Ind., Wild.Rev., Zoo.Rec.
—BLDSC (5003.415000), GNLM, IDS, ingenta, Linda Hall. **CCC.**
Published by: Academic Press (Subsidiary of: Harcourt Publishers Ltd.), 24 Oval Rd, London NW1 7DX, United Kingdom. TEL 44-20-7267-4466, FAX 44-20-7482-2293, apsubs@acad.com, http://www.academicpress.com/jhevol. R&P Catherine John. Adv. contact Nik Screen. **Subscr. to:** Harcourt Publishers Ltd., Foots Cray High St, Sidcup, Kent DA14 5HP, United Kingdom. TEL 44-20-8300-3322, FAX 44-20-8309-0807.

599.9 JPN ISSN 1434-5161
QH431 CODEN: JHGEFR
JOURNAL OF HUMAN GENETICS. Text in English. 1956. m. (in 1 vol., 12 nos./vol.). EUR 353.70 domestic; EUR 350.20 in Germany; EUR 30 foreign for Print & Online Eds. (effective 2002). adv. bk.rev. *Refereed.* **Document type:** *Academic/Scholarly.* **Description:** Covers all aspects of human genetics, including gene cloning and mapping, linkage analysis, mutational analysis, evolution, cancer genetics, and gene therapy, as well as genetic and functional analysis of animal models of disease or behavior.
Former titles (until Oct. 1997): Japanese Journal of Human Genetics (0916-8478); (until 1992): Jinrui Idengaku Zasshi (0021-5074)
Related titles: Online - full text ed.: ISSN 1435-232X (from EBSCO Publishing, RoweCom Information Quest, Swets Blackwell, Springer LINK, Institute for Scientific Information).
Indexed: ASCA, Abstr.Anthropol., Biol.Abstr., Biotech.& Bioeng.Abstr., Biotech.Cit.Ind., Chem.Abstr., Chem.Indus.Notes, Chem.Titles, Curr.Adv.Cancer Res., Curr.Cont., Excerp.Med., Genet.Abstr., Helminthol.Abstr., Hum.Gen.Abstr., INIS Atomind., INSPEC (coverage dropped), Ind.Med. (1998-), Ind.Sci.Rev., Inpharma, Int.Abstr.Biol.Sci., Jap.Per.Ind., Pharm.&Out.News, Reac., Sci.Cit.Ind., THA.
—BLDSC (5003.415500), CASDDS, CISTI, GNLM, IDS, ingenta, KNAW, Linda Hall.
Published by: (Japan Society of Human Genetics), Springer-Verlag Tokyo, Eastern Book Service, Inc. (Subsidiary of: BertelsmannSpringer), 3-13 Hongo 3-chome, Bunkyo-ku, Tokyo 113-0033, Japan. TEL 81-3-38120331, FAX 81-3-3812-0719, yusuke@ims.u-tokyo.ac.jp; access@link.springer.de, http://link.springer-ny.com/link/service/journals/10038/index.htm, http://link.springer.de. Ed. Yusuke Nakamura. Circ: 1,200. **Subscr. in N. America to:** Springer-Verlag New York Inc., PO Box 2485, Secaucus, NJ 07096-2485. TEL 800-777-4643, 212-460-1526, FAX 201-348-4505, orders@springer-ny.com; **Subscr. outside of N. America & Japan to:** Springer-Verlag, c/o Gabriele Kubitza, Haberstrasse 7, Heidelberg 69126, Germany. TEL 49-6221-345242, FAX 49-30-82787448, 49-6221-345229, subscriptions@springer.de, http://link.springer-ny.com; **Subscr. to:** Eastern Book Service, Inc., 3-13 Hongo 3-chome, Bunkyo-ku, Tokyo 113-8480, Japan. TEL 81-3-3818-0861, FAX 81-3-3818-0864, orders@svt-ebs.co.jp.

599.9 GBR ISSN 0022-2593
QH431 CODEN: JMDGAE
JOURNAL OF MEDICAL GENETICS. Text in English. 1964. m. GBP 137, USD 221 combined subscription to individuals includes print & online eds.; GBP 293, USD 478 to institutions for print only (effective 2002). adv. bk.rev. charts, illus. index. reprint service avail. from PQC. *Refereed.* **Document type:** *Journal, Academic/Scholarly.* **Description:** Devoted to all areas of medical genetics, including clinical applications of molecular genetics, dysmorphology (the delineation and genetic basis of new syndromes), ethical and social aspects of medical genetics, and the development of medical genetic services.
Related titles: CD-ROM ed.: (from Ovid Technologies, Inc.); Microform ed.: (from PQC); Online - full text ed.: J M G Online. ISSN 1468-6244. USD 99, GBP 65 to individuals (effective 2002); Institutions please contact publisher for online rates. (from Ovid Technologies, Inc., HighWire Pr., Northern Light Technology, Inc., EBSCO Publishing, O C L C Online Computer Library Center, Inc., RoweCom Information Quest, ProQuest Information & Learning, ingenta, Swets Blackwell, Institute for Scientific Information).
Indexed: ASCA, Abstr.Anthropol., Abstr.Hyg., Anim.Breed.Abstr., Arts & Hum.Cit.Ind. (coverage dropped), Bibl.Dev.Med.& Child Neur., Biol.Abstr., Biotech.& Bioeng.Abstr., Biotech.Cit.Ind., Chem.Abstr., Chem.Indus.Notes, Chem.Titles, Curr.Adv.Cell & Devel.Biol., Curr.Adv.Ecol.Sci., Curr.Adv.Gen.& Molec.Biol., Curr.Cont., Dent.Ind., Excerp.Med., Genet.Abstr., Helminthol.Abstr., Hum.Gen.Abstr., INIS Atomind., Ind.Med. (1964-), Ind.Sci.Rev., Ind.Vet., Inpharma, Int.Abstr.Biol.Sci., Med.& Surg.Dermat., Neurosci.Abstr. (coverage dropped), Neurosci.Cit.Ind., Nutr.Abstr., Pharm.&Out.News, Reac., Risk Abstr., SSCI (coverage dropped), Sci.Cit.Ind., So.Pac.Per.Ind., Trop.Dis.Bull., Vet.Bull.
—BLDSC (5017.070000), ADONIS, CASDDS, CISTI, GNLM, IDS, ingenta, KNAW. **CCC.**
Published by: B M J Publishing Group, B M A House, Tavistock Sq, London WC1H 9JR, United Kingdom. TEL 44-20-7387-4499, FAX 44-20-7383-6400, info.norththames@bma.org.uk, http://www.jmedgenet.com, http://www.bma.org.uk. Ed. Eamonn R Maher. Pub. Alex Williamson. R&P Carol Torselli TEL 44-20-7383-6674. Adv. contact Euan Currer TEL 44-20-7383-6181.

576.8 USA ISSN 0022-2844
QH366.A1 CODEN: JMEVAU
JOURNAL OF MOLECULAR EVOLUTION. Text mainly in English. 1971. m. (in 2 vols., 6 nos./vol.). USD 1,522.70 domestic for Print & Online Eds.; USD 1,469.30 in Germany for Print & Online Eds.; USD 141.50 newsstand/cover foreign (effective 2002). adv. reprint service avail. from ISI. *Refereed.* **Document type:** *Academic/Scholarly.* **Description:** Covers molecular evolution and molecular biology. Includes a new focus on the evolutionary aspects of molecular population genetics.
Related titles: Microform ed.: (from PQC); Online - full text ed.: ISSN 1432-1432 (from EBSCO Publishing, RoweCom Information Quest, Swets Blackwell, Springer LINK, Institute for Scientific Information).
Indexed: ASCA, AgBiotech, Agricola, Anim.Breed.Abstr., Aqua.Sci.& Fish.Abstr., BBCI, Bibl.Agri., Bio-Contr.News & Info., Biol.& Agr.Ind. (Mar.1983-Jul.1989), Biotech.Cit.Ind., Chem.Abstr., Chem.Cit.Ind., Chem.Titles, Curr.Adv.Ecol.Sci., Curr.Cont., Curr.Ind.Stat., Dairy Sci.Abstr., Eng.Ind., Excerp.Med., Food Sci.& Tech.Abstr., Genet.Abstr., GeoRef, Helminthol.Abstr., Hum.Gen.Abstr., INIS Atomind., Ind.Med. (1971-), Ind.Sci.Rev., Inpharma, Int.Abstr.Biol.Sci., Int.Aerosp.Abstr., Maize Abstr., Nuc.Acids Abstr., Plant Breed.Abstr., Poult.Abstr., Protozool.Abstr., Reac., Ref.Zh., Rev.Appl.Entomol., Sci.Cit.Ind., Seed Abstr., Soyabean Abstr., Sport Fish.Abstr., Weed Abstr., Wild.Rev., Zoo.Rec.
—BLDSC (5020.710000), ADONIS, CASDDS, CISTI, Ei, GNLM, IDS, Linda Hall. **CCC.**
Published by: (International Society of Molecular Evolution), Springer-Verlag, Journals (Subsidiary of: BertelsmannSpringer), 175 Fifth Ave, New York, NY 10010. TEL 212-460-1500, FAX 212-473-6272, orders@springer-ny.com, http://www.springer-ny.com. Ed. Emile Zuckerkandl. R&P Ian Gross. Adv. contact Brian Skepton. **N. American subscr. to:** Journal Fulfillment Services, PO Box 2485, Secaucus, NJ 07096-2485. TEL 800-777-4643, FAX 201-348-4505.

▼ **JOURNAL OF MOLECULAR MICROBIOLOGY AND BIOTECHNOLOGY.** see *BIOLOGY—Microbiology*

599.9 CHE ISSN 1422-6251
QH431 CODEN: MOHGAD
KEY ISSUES IN HUMAN GENETICS. Text in English. 1966. irreg., latest vol.14. CHF 180 in Europe; DEM 215 in Germany; USD 160 in United States (2001). reprint service avail. from ISI. *Refereed.* **Document type:** *Monographic series, Academic/Scholarly.* **Description:** Publishes sophisticated genetic studies transformed into clear interpretations of their medical importance.
Formerly: Monographs in Human Genetics (0077-0876)
Related titles: Online - full text ed.: (from Institute for Scientific Information).
Indexed: Biol.Abstr., Chem.Abstr., Chem.Indus.Notes, Chem.Titles, Curr.Cont. (coverage dropped), Ind.Med. (coverage dropped).
—CASDDS, CISTI, GNLM, KNAW. **CCC.**
Published by: S. Karger AG, Allschwilerstr 10, PO Box, Basel 4009, Switzerland. TEL 41-61-306-1111, FAX 41-61-306-1234, karger@karger.ch, http://www.karger.com/bookseries/KIHUG.

576.5 JPN ISSN 0080-8539
CODEN: SEZIA3
KIHARA SEIBUTSUGAKU KENKYUJO. SEIKEN JIHO/KIHARA INSTITUTE FOR BIOLOGICAL RESEARCH. REPORT. Text in Japanese. 1941. a. JPY 1,000, USD 8 to members. **Document type:** *Bulletin.*
Indexed: Agrindex, Biol.Abstr., INIS Atomind., Jap.Per.Ind., VITIS.
—CISTI.
Published by: Yokohama City University, Kihara Institute for Biological Research/Yokohama Shiritsu Daigaku Kihara Seibutsugaku Kenkyujo, 22-2 Seto Kanazawa-ku, Minami-ku, Yokohama, Kanagawa-ken 232-0000, Japan.

576.5 JPN
KIKAN KEISEI KENKYUKAI KAISHI/JAPANESE SOCIETY FOR BASIC AND APPLIED ORGAN RESEARCH. BULLETIN. Text in Japanese. a.
Published by: Kikan Keisei Kenkyukai, Nagoya Daigaku Igakubu, Koku Gekagaku Kyoshitsu, 65 Tsurumai-cho, Showa-ku, Nagoya-shi, Aichi-ken 466-0065, Japan.

KIKAN KEISEI KENKYUKAI KOEN YOSHISHU/JAPANESE SOCIETY FOR BASIC AND APPLIED ORGAN RESEARCH. ABSTRACTS OF THE MEETING. see *BIOLOGY—Abstracting, Bibliographies, Statistics*

576.5 JPN
KIKAN KEISEI NYUSU/JAPANESE SOCIETY FOR BASIC AND APPLIED ORGAN RESEARCH. NEWS. Text in Japanese. 1989. irreg.
Indexed: Russ.Acad.Sci.Bibl.
Published by: Kikan Keisei Kenkyukai, Nagoya Daigaku Igakubu, Koku Gekagaku Kyoshitsu, 65 Tsurumai-cho, Showa-ku, Nagoya-shi, Aichi-ken 466-0065, Japan.

599.935 USA ISSN 0938-8990
QL738.5 CODEN: MAMGEC
MAMMALIAN GENOME. Text in English. 1991. m. USD 936 domestic; USD 923.30 in Germany; USD 86.90 combined subscription per issue foreign (effective 2002). adv. back issues avail.; reprint service avail. from ISI. *Refereed.* **Document type:** *Academic/Scholarly.* **Description:** Presents articles on experimental, theoretical, and technical aspects of genome organization, the evolution of mice, humans, and other mammalian species.
Incorporates (1949-1997): Mouse Genome (0959-0587)
Related titles: Microform ed.: (from PQC); Online - full text ed.: ISSN 1432-1777 (from EBSCO Publishing, RoweCom Information Quest, Swets Blackwell, Springer LINK, Institute for Scientific Information).
Indexed: ASCA, AgBiotech, Anim.Breed.Abstr., Aqua.Sci.& Fish.Abstr., Biotech.& Bioeng.Abstr., Biotech.Cit.Ind., Chem.Abstr., Chem.Titles, Curr.Cont., Dairy Sci.Abstr., Focus on: Vet.Sci.& Med., Genet.Abstr., Helminthol.Abstr., Hum.Gen.Abstr., Ind.Med. (1991-), Ind.Vet., Inpharma, Int.Abstr.Biol.Sci., Neurosci.Abstr., Nuc.Acids Abstr., Nutr.Abstr., Pig News & Info., Plant Breed.Abstr., Pollut.Abstr., Poult.Abstr., Protozool.Abstr., Reac., Sci.Cit.Ind., Vet.Bull., Wild.Rev.
—BLDSC (5357.450000), ADONIS, CASDDS, CISTI, GNLM, IDS, ingenta, KNAW. **CCC.**
Published by: (International Mammalian Genome Society), Springer-Verlag, Journals (Subsidiary of: BertelsmannSpringer), 175 Fifth Ave, New York, NY 10010. TEL 212-460-1500, FAX 212-473-6272, orders@springer-ny.com, http://www.springer-ny.com. R&P Ian Gross. Adv. contact Brian Skepton. **N. American subscr. to:** Journal Fulfillment Services, PO Box 2485, Secaucus, NJ 07096-2485. TEL 800-777-4643, FAX 201-348-4505.

MANKIND QUARTERLY; an international quarterly journal dealing with both physical and cultural anthropology including related subjects such as psychology, demography, genetics, linguistics and mythology. see *ANTHROPOLOGY*

576.5 DEU ISSN 0936-5931
CODEN: MGENEZ
MEDIZINISCHE GENETIK. Text in German. 1989. 4/yr. DEM 220, EUR 120 (effective 2001). adv. bk.rev. bibl. *Refereed.* **Document type:** *Journal, Academic/Scholarly.* **Description:** Contains case reports on genetic counseling, ethics, diagnoses, patenting, and other questions.
Indexed: Excerp.Med. (1994-).
—BLDSC (5535.076700), EMDOCS, GNLM.
Published by: Berufsverband Medizinische Genetik e.V., Goethestr 29, Munich 80336, Germany. TEL 49-89-55027855, FAX 49-89-55027856, verlag@medgenetik.de, http://www.medgenetik.de. Ed., R&P Christine Scholz. Pub. Jan Murken. Adv. contact Wolfgang Kroner. color page DEM 3,680; trim 210 x 297. Circ: 1,850. **Co-sponsor:** Gesellschaft fuer Humangenetik e.V.

576.5 IND ISSN 0970-9649
MENDEL; multidisciplinary international journal of science. Text in English. 1984. q. INR 200, USD 100 to individuals; INR 500, USD 200 to institutions (effective 2001). adv. bk.rev. 100 p./no. back issues avail.; reprints avail. *Refereed.* **Document type:** *Yearbook, Academic/Scholarly, Abstract/Index.* **Description:** Publishes papers and general articles of common interest in all fields of science and medicine.
Published by: Mendelian Society of India, 194-B S K Puri, Patna, Bihar 800 001, India. TEL 91-612-233741. Ed. R N Trivedi. Circ: 750 (controlled).

576.5 ARG ISSN 0325-223X
MENDELIANA. Text in Spanish; Summaries in English. 1976. s-a. ARS 15 domestic; USD 20 foreign (effective 1999). bk.rev. back issues avail. *Refereed.* **Document type:** *Academic/Scholarly.* **Description:** Covers all areas of genetics.
Indexed: Biol.Abstr., Excerp.Med., Genet.Abstr. (coverage dropped).
—KNAW.
Published by: Sociedad Argentina de Genetica, CC 25, Castelar, Buenos Aires 1712, Argentina. FAX 54-111-1917. Ed. Sol L Rabasa. Circ: 650.

576.5 USA ISSN 1067-2389
CODEN: MEMGE6
METHODS IN MOLECULAR GENETICS. Text in English. 1993. irreg., latest vol.8, 1996. **Document type:** *Monographic series.*
Indexed: Chem.Abstr., Chem.Titles.
—BLDSC (5748.202200), CASDDS, CISTI, Infotrieve. **CCC.**
Published by: Academic Press, Inc., Journal Division (Subsidiary of: Harcourt Brace & Company), 525 B St, Ste 1900, San Diego, CA 92101-4495. TEL 619-230-1840, FAX 619-699-6800, http://www.apnet.com.

576.5 DEU ISSN 1617-4615
QH431 CODEN: MGGEAE
MOLECULAR GENETICS AND GENOMICS; an international journal. Short title: M G G. Text in English. 1908. m. EUR 3,043.90 domestic; EUR 3,024.70 in Germany; EUR 299.80 newsstand/cover foreign (effective 2002). adv. charts, illus. Index. back issues avail.; reprint service avail. from ISI. *Refereed.* **Document type:** *Journal, Academic/Scholarly.* **Description:** For biotechnicians, microbiologists, virologists, and biochemists. Covers the genetics of prokaryotes, including plastids, mitochondria, plasmids, "jumping genes," and transposable elements. Provides background research on the molecular genetics of eukaryotes, and its practical applications in genetic engineering.
Former titles (until 2001): Molecular and General Genetics (0026-8925); Zeitschrift fuer Vererbungslehre
Related titles: Microform ed.: (from PQC); Online - full text ed.: ISSN 1617-4623 (from EBSCO Publishing, RoweCom Information Quest, Swets Blackwell, Springer LINK, Institute for Scientific Information).
Indexed: ASCA, AgBiotech, Agri.& Environ.Biotech.Abstr. (coverage dropped), Agricola, Anim.Breed.Abstr., Aqua.Sci.& Fish.Abstr., BBCI, Bibl.Agri., Bio-Contr.News & Info., Biol.& Agr.Ind. (Jul.2001-), Biol.Abstr., Biotech.& Bioeng.Abstr., Biotech.Cit.Ind., CEABA, Chem.Abstr., Chem.Indus.Notes, Chem.Titles, Cott.& Trop.Fibr.Abstr., Crop Physiol.Abstr., Curr.Adv.Biochem., Curr.Adv.Ecol.Sci., Curr.Adv.Gen.& Molec.Biol., Curr.Biotech.Abstr., Curr.Cont., Dairy Sci.Abstr., Derwent Biotech.Abstr., Entomol.Abstr. (coverage dropped), Environ.Sci.Poll.Mgmt., Excerp.Med., Field Crop Abstr., Food Sci.& Tech.Abstr., Forest.Abstr., Genet.Abstr., Helminthol.Abstr., Hort.Abstr., Hum.Gen.Abstr., INIS Atomind., Ind.Med. (1967-), Ind.Sci.Rev., Ind.Vet., Int.Abstr.Biol.Sci., Maize Abstr., Microbiol.Abstr., Nuc.Acids Abstr., Nutr.Abstr., Ornam.Hort., Plant Breed.Abstr., Plant Gen.Res.Abstr., Plant Grow.Reg.Abstr., Postharvest, Potato Abstr., Poult.Abstr., Rev.Appl.Entomol., Rev.Arom.& Med.Plants, Rev.Med.& Vet.Mycol., Rev.Plant Path., Rice Abstr., Sci.Cit.Ind., Seed Abstr., Soils & Fert., Soyabean Abstr., Sugar Ind.Abstr., Triticale Abstr., VITIS, Weed Abstr., Wild.Rev., Zoo.Rec.
—BLDSC (5900.764000), ADONIS, CASDDS, CISTI, GNLM, IDS, ingenta, Linda Hall. **CCC.**
Published by: Springer-Verlag (Subsidiary of: BertelsmannSpringer), Tiergartenstr 17, Heidelberg 69121, Germany. TEL 49-6221-345-0, FAX 49-6221-345229, subscriptions@springer.de, http://link.springer.de/link/service/journals/00438/index.htm, http://www.springer.de. Eds. C P Hollenberg, W Arber. **Subscr. in N. America to:** Springer-Verlag New York Inc., PO Box 2485, Secaucus, NJ 07096-2485. TEL 212-460-1500, FAX 212-473-6272.

MOLECULAR GENETICS, MICROBIOLOGY AND VIROLOGY. see *BIOLOGY—Microbiology*

MOLECULAR NEUROBIOLOGY; a review journal. see *BIOLOGY—Biochemistry*

576.5 USA ISSN 1055-7903
QH367.5 CODEN: MPEVEK
MOLECULAR PHYLOGENETICS AND EVOLUTION. Text in English. 1992. m. USD 435 in US & Canada to institutions; USD 499 elsewhere to institutions (effective 2001). adv. back issues avail. *Refereed.* **Document type:** *Academic/Scholarly.* **Description:** Provides a forum for molecular studies that advance our understanding of phylogeny and evolution. Encourages collaboration of molecular biologists and computer scientists, with systematic and evolutionary biologists.
Related titles: Online - full text ed.: (from EBSCO Publishing, O C L C Online Computer Library Center, Inc., RoweCom Information Quest, ingenta, Swets Blackwell, IDEAL Online Library, Institute for Scientific Information).
Indexed: ASCA, AgBiotech, Anim.Breed.Abstr., BBCI, Bio-Contr.News & Info., Chem.Abstr., Chem.Indus.Notes, Chem.Titles, Curr.Cont., Forest.Abstr., Ind.Med. (1992-), Ind.Vet., Plant Breed.Abstr., Plant Gen.Res.Abstr., Rev.Appl.Entomol., Rev.Med.& Vet.Mycol., Rev.Plant Path., Sci.Cit.Ind., Sport Fish.Abstr., Zoo.Rec.
—BLDSC (5900.819800), ADONIS, CASDDS, CISTI, GNLM, IDS, Infotrieve, ingenta. **CCC.**
Published by: Academic Press, Inc., Journal Division (Subsidiary of: Harcourt Brace & Company), 525 B St, Ste 1900, San Diego, CA 92101-4495. TEL 619-230-1840, FAX 619-699-6800, apsubs@acad.com, http://www.academicpress.com/mpe. Ed. Morris Goodman.

MOLEKULYARNAYA GENETIKA, MIKROBIOLOGIYA I VIRUSOLOGIYA/MOLECULAR GENETICS, MICROBIOLOGY AND VIRUSOLOGY. see *BIOLOGY—Microbiology*

576.5 USA ISSN 0341-5376
MONOGRAPHS ON THEORETICAL AND APPLIED GENETICS. Text in English. 1975. irreg., latest vol.21, 1994. price varies. reprint service avail. from ISI. **Document type:** *Monographic series.*
Indexed: Biol.Abstr.
—CISTI, Infotrieve. **CCC.**
Published by: Springer-Verlag, Journals (Subsidiary of: BertelsmannSpringer), 175 Fifth Ave, New York, NY 10010. TEL 212-460-1500, FAX 212-473-6272.

576.549 GBR ISSN 0267-8357
QH465.A1 CODEN: MUTAEX
MUTAGENESIS. Text in English. 1986. bi-m. GBP 360, USD 600 (effective 2002). adv. bk.rev. illus. index. 128 p./no. back issues avail.; reprint service avail. from SWZ. *Refereed.* **Document type:** *Journal, Academic/Scholarly.* **Description:** International, multi-disciplinary journal for genetic toxicology research. Includes genetic mutation studies, mutagenicity testing guidelines, test program results, letters, and reviews.
Related titles: Online - full text ed.: ISSN 1464-3804. GBP 324, USD 540 to institutions Online only (effective 2002) (from HighWire Pr., EBSCO Publishing, O C L C Online Computer Library Center, Inc., RoweCom Information Quest, ingenta, Swets Blackwell, Institute for Scientific Information).
Indexed: ASCA, AgBiotech, Anim.Breed.Abstr., Aqua.Sci.& Fish.Abstr., Biol.Abstr., Biotech.& Bioeng.Abstr., Chem.Abstr., Chem.Indus.Notes, Chem.Titles, Curr.Adv.Ecol.Sci., Curr.Cont., Dairy Sci.Abstr., Environ.Sci.Poll.Mgmt., Excerp.Med., Genet.Abstr., Helminthol.Abstr., Hum.Gen.Abstr., INIS Atomind., Ind.Med. (1986-), Ind.Sci.Rev., Ind.Vet., Inpharma, Int.Abstr.Biol.Sci., Nuc.Acids Abstr., Nutr.Abstr., Oncog.G.F.Abstr. (coverage dropped), Plant Breed.Abstr., Plant Grow.Reg.Abstr., Protozool.Abstr., Reac., Rev.Appl.Entomol., Rev.Arom.& Med.Plants, Rev.Med.& Vet.Mycol., Sci.Cit.Ind., Tox.Abstr., Triticale Abstr., Vet.Bull., W.R.C.Inf., Weed Abstr.
—BLDSC (5991.895500), CASDDS, CISTI, EMDOCS, GNLM, IDS, ingenta, KNAW, Linda Hall. **CCC.**
Published by: (U.K. Environmental Mutagen Society), Oxford University Press, Academic Division, Great Clarendon St, Oxford OX2 6DP, United Kingdom. TEL 44-1865-267907, FAX 44-1865-267835, jnl.info@oup.co.uk, http://www.mutage.oupjournals.org/, http://www.oup.co.uk/journals. Eds. J M Parry, Dr. J L Schwartz, M Hayashi. Pub. David Prosser. R&P Fionna Willis. adv.: B&W page GBP 220, B&W page USD 420; trim 178 x 255. Circ: 600. **Subscr. in U.S. to:** Oxford University Press, Journals, 2001 Evans Rd, Cary, NC 27513. TEL 800-852-7323, FAX 919-677-1714, jnlorders@oup-usa.org.

576.549 NLD ISSN 0921-8262
MUTATION RESEARCH; international journal on mutagenesis, chromosome breakage and related subjects. Text in English, French, German. 1964. w. (59/yr.). NLG 15,340, EUR 6,960.99 in Europe; USD 7,787 elsewhere (effective 1999). adv. charts, illus. *Refereed.* **Document type:** *Academic/Scholarly.*
Incorporates: Environmental Mutagen Society Newsletter (0013-9319)
Related titles: Microform ed.: (from PQC); Online - full text ed.; ♦ Special ed.: Mutation Research - D N A Repair. ISSN 0921-8777; ♦ Mutation Research Letters. ISSN 0165-7992; ♦ Mutation Research - Reviews in Genetic Toxicology. ISSN 0165-1110; ♦ Mutation Research - Fundamental and Molecular Mechanisms of Mutagenesis. ISSN 0027-5107; ♦ Mutation Research - Reviews in Mutation Research. ISSN 1383-5742.
Indexed: Abstr.Anthropol., Anim.Breed.Abstr., Biol.Abstr., Biotech.& Bioeng.Abstr. (coverage dropped), C.I.S. Abstr., Chem.Abstr., Chem.Cit.Ind., Chem.Indus.Notes, Chem.Titles, Crop Physiol.Abstr., Curr.Adv.Cell & Devel.Biol., Curr.Adv.Ecol.Sci., Curr.Adv.Gen.& Molec.Biol., Curr.Cont. (coverage dropped), Dairy Sci.Abstr., Dent.Ind., Dok.Arbeitsmed., Excerp.Med., Fababean Abstr., Field Crop Abstr., Food Sci.& Tech.Abstr., Genet.Abstr. (coverage dropped), Helminthol.Abstr., INIS Atomind., Ind.Med. (coverage dropped), Ind.Sci.Rev., Ind.Vet., Int.Nurs.Ind., Lab.Haz.Bull., Maize Abstr., Microbiol.Abstr., Nuc.Acids Abstr., Plant Breed.Abstr., Plant Grow.Reg.Abstr., Poult.Abstr., Protozool.Abstr., Rev.Appl.Entomol., Rev.Med.& Vet.Mycol., Rev.Plant Path., Risk Abstr., SSCI (coverage dropped), Sci.Cit.Ind. (coverage dropped), Seed Abstr., Sel.Water Res.Abstr., Soils & Fert., Sport Fish.Abstr., Triticale Abstr., Trop.Dis.Bull., W.R.C.Inf., Weed Abstr., Wild.Rev., Zoo.Rec.
—CISTI, IDS, Linda Hall. **CCC.**
Published by: Elsevier Science BV, PO Box 211, Amsterdam 1000 AE, Netherlands. TEL 31-20-485-3757, TELEX 18582 ESPA NL, nlinfo-f@elsevier.nl, http://www.elsevier.nl/. **Subscr. in Australasia and the Far East to:** Elsevier Science (Singapore) Pte Ltd, No.1 Temasek Ave, 17-01 Millenia Tower, Singapore 039192, Singapore. TEL 65-434-3727, FAX 65-337-2230, asiainfo@elsevier.com.sg; **Subscr. in Japan to:** Elsevier Science Inc - Japan Regional Office, 9-15 Higashi-Azabu 1-chome, Minato-ku, Tokyo 106-0044, Japan. TEL 81-3-5561-5033, FAX 81-3-5561-5047, info@elsevier.co.jp; **Subscr. in the Americas to:** Elsevier Science, PO Box 945, New York, NY 10159-0945. TEL 212-633-3730, FAX 212-633-3680, usinfo-f@elsevier.com.

576.549 NLD ISSN 0027-5107
QH431 CODEN: MUREAV
MUTATION RESEARCH - FUNDAMENTAL AND MOLECULAR MECHANISMS OF MUTAGENESIS. Text in English, French, German. 1964. 16/yr. (in 8 vols.). NLG 17,601, EUR 7,989.99 in Europe to institutions Full Set; JPY 1,105,700 in Japan to institutions Full Set; USD 8,934 elsewhere to institutions Full Set (effective 2001). adv. charts, illus. index. back issues avail. *Refereed.* **Document type:** *Academic/Scholarly.* **Description:** Publishes complete research papers in the are of mutation research which focus on fundamental mechanism, underlying phenotypic and genotypic expression of genetic damage.
Related titles: Microform ed.: (from PQC); Online - full text ed.: (from ingenta, ScienceDirect, Swets Blackwell, Institute for Scientific Information); ♦ Special ed. of: Mutation Research. ISSN 0921-8262.

B

Indexed: ASCA, AgBiotech, Anim.Breed.Abstr., Aqua.Sci.& Fish.Abstr., BBCI, Biol.Abstr., Biotech.& Bioeng.Abstr., Biotech.Cit.Ind., Chem.Abstr., Curr.Cont., Dairy Sci.Abstr., Environ.Sci.Poll.Mgmt., Excerp.Med., Food Sci.& Tech.Abstr., Genet.Abstr., Hum.Gen.Abstr., INIS Atomind., Ind.Med. (1964-), Ind.Sci.Rev., Ind.Vet., Inpharma, Int.Abstr.Biol.Sci., Microbiol.Abstr., Nuc.Acids Abstr., Nutr.Abstr., Oncog.G.F.Abstr. (coverage dropped), Pollut.Abstr., Reac., Ref.Zh., Rev.Appl.Entomol., Rev.Med.& Vet.Mycol., Rev.Plant Path., Sci.Cit.Ind., Weed Abstr.

—BLDSC (5991.900000), ADONIS, CASDDS, CISTI, IDS, ingenta, Linda Hall. **CCC.**

Published by: Elsevier Science BV, PO Box 211, Amsterdam 1000 AE, Netherlands. TEL 31-20-485-3757, TELEX 18582 ESPA NL, nlinfo-f@elsevier.nl; usinfo-f@elsevier.com; forinfo-kyf04035@niftyserve.or.jp, http://www.elsevier.com/locate/mrmolmech, http://www.elsevier.nl. **Subscr. in Australasia and the Far East to:** Elsevier Science (Singapore) Pte Ltd, No.1 Temasek Ave, 17-01 Millenia Tower, Singapore 039192, Singapore. TEL 65-434-3727, FAX 65-337-2230; **Subscr. in Japan to:** Elsevier Science Inc - Japan Regional Office, 9-15 Higashi-Azabu 1-chome, Minato-ku, Tokyo 106-0044, Japan. TEL 81-3-5561-5033, FAX 81-3-5561-5047; **Subscr. in the Americas to:** Elsevier Science, PO Box 945, New York, NY 10159-0945. TEL 212-633-3730, FAX 212-633-3680.

576.549 NLD ISSN 1383-5718
CODEN: MRGTE

MUTATION RESEARCH - GENETIC TOXICOLOGY AND ENVIRONMENTAL MUTAGENESIS. Text in Dutch. 1988. 18/yr. EUR 3,369 in Europe to institutions; JPY 447,300 in Japan to institutions; USD 3,768 elsewhere to institutions (effective 2002). back issues avail. *Refereed.* **Document type:** *Academic/Scholarly.* **Description:** Covers all aspects of genetic toxicology and biomonitoring of environmental and occupational exposure to mutagens.

Former titles (until 1997): Mutation Research - Genetic Toxicology; (until 1994): Mutation Research - Genetic Toxicology Testing (0165-1218); Incorporates (in 1996): Mutation Research - Environmental Mutagenesis and Related Subjects; Which had former titles (until 1994): Mutation Research - Section on Environmental Mutagenesis and Related Subjects including Methodology; Mutation Research - Section on Environmental Mutagenesis and Related Subjects (0165-1161)

Related titles: Microform ed.: (from PQC); Online - full text ed.: (from EBSCO Publishing, ingenta, ScienceDirect, Swets Blackwell, Institute for Scientific Information).

Indexed: ASCA, Abstr.Hyg., Anim.Breed.Abstr., Aqua.Sci.& Fish.Abstr., BBCI, Biotech.& Bioeng.Abstr., Curr.Cont., Dairy Sci.Abstr., Environ.Sci.Poll.Mgmt., Excerp.Med., Food Sci.& Tech.Abstr., Forest Prod.Abstr., Genet.Abstr., Hum.Gen.Abstr., INIS Atomind., Ind.Med. (coverage dropped), Ind.Sci.Rev., Ind.Vet., Inpharma, Int.Abstr.Biol.Sci., Microbiol.Abstr., Nuc.Acids Abstr., Nutr.Abstr., Oncog.G.F.Abstr. (coverage dropped), Plant Breed.Abstr., Reac., Ref.Zh., Rev.Appl.Entomol., Rev.Arom.& Med.Plants, Rev.Med.& Vet.Mycol., Rev.Plant Path., Sci.Cit.Ind., Tox.Abstr., Triticale Abstr., Trop.Dis.Bull., Vet.Bull., Weed Abstr.

—ADONIS, CISTI, IDS. **CCC.**

Published by: Elsevier Science BV, PO Box 211, Amsterdam 1000 AE, Netherlands. TEL 31-20-485-2911, FAX 31-20-485-2457, http://www.elsevier.com/locate/mrgentox. Ed. F H Sobels. **Subscr. in Australasia and the Far East to:** Elsevier Science (Singapore) Pte Ltd, No.1 Temasek Ave, 17-01 Millenia Tower, Singapore 039192, Singapore. TEL 65-434-3727, FAX 65-337-2230; **Subscr. in Japan to:** Elsevier Science Inc - Japan Regional Office, 9-15 Higashi-Azabu 1-chome, Minato-ku, Tokyo 106-0044, Japan. TEL 81-3-5561-5033; **Subscr. in the Americas to:** Elsevier Science, PO Box 945, New York, NY 10159-0945. TEL 212-633-3730, FAX 212-633-3680, usinfo-f@elsevier.com.

576.549 NLD ISSN 0165-7992
CODEN: MRLED

MUTATION RESEARCH LETTERS. Text in Dutch. 1988. a. (in 3 vols., 4 nos./vol.). NLG 1,326, USD 698 (effective 1995). back issues avail. *Refereed.* **Document type:** *Academic/Scholarly.* **Description:** Specializes in the rapid publication of short communications on progressive work in the field of mutation research.

Related titles: Microform ed.: (from PQC); Online - full text ed.: (from ingenta); ♦ Special ed. of: Mutation Research. ISSN 0921-8262.

Indexed: ASCA, Aqua.Sci.& Fish.Abstr., Biotech.& Bioeng.Abstr. (coverage dropped), Curr.Cont. (coverage dropped), Environ.Sci.Poll.Mgmt., Excerp.Med., Food Sci.& Tech.Abstr., Genet.Abstr., Hum.Gen.Abstr., INIS Atomind., Ind.Med. (coverage dropped), Microbiol.Abstr., Nuc.Acids Abstr., Oncog.G.F.Abstr. (coverage dropped).

—CISTI, IDS, Infotrieve. **CCC.**

Published by: Elsevier Science BV, PO Box 211, Amsterdam 1000 AE, Netherlands. TEL 31-20-485-3757, TELEX 18582 ESPA NL, nlinfo-f@elsevier.nl; usinfo-f@elsevier.com; forinfo-kyf04035@niftyserve.or.jp, http://www.elsevier.nl/. **Subscr. in Australasia and the Far East to:** Elsevier Science (Singapore) Pte Ltd, No.1 Temasek Ave, 17-01 Millenia Tower, Singapore 039192, Singapore. TEL 65-434-3727, FAX 65-337-2230; **Subscr. in Japan to:** Elsevier Science Inc - Japan Regional Office, 9-15 Higashi-Azabu 1-chome, Minato-ku, Tokyo 106-0044, Japan. TEL 81-3-5561-5033, FAX 81-3-5561-5047, info@elsevier.co.jp; **Subscr. in the Americas to:** Elsevier Science, PO Box 945, New York, NY 10159-0945. TEL 212-633-3730, FAX 212-633-3680, http://www.elsevier.com.

576.549 NLD ISSN 0165-1110

MUTATION RESEARCH - REVIEWS IN GENETIC TOXICOLOGY. Text in Dutch. 1988. bi-m. NLG 938, USD 572 (effective 1996). back issues avail. *Refereed.* **Document type:** *Academic/Scholarly.* **Description:** Provides a medium for the dissemination of advanced reviews in the field of genetic toxicology.

Related titles: Microform ed.: (from PQC); ♦ Special ed. of: Mutation Research. ISSN 0921-8262.

Indexed: ASCA, Biol.Abstr., Biotech.& Bioeng.Abstr. (coverage dropped), Chem.Abstr., Curr.Cont. (coverage dropped), Excerp.Med., Hum.Gen.Abstr. (coverage dropped), INIS Atomind., Ind.Med. (coverage dropped), Ind.Sci.Rev., Soyabean Abstr., Tox.Abstr. (coverage dropped).

—CISTI, GNLM, IDS. **CCC.**

Published by: Elsevier Science BV, PO Box 211, Amsterdam 1000 AE, Netherlands. TEL 31-20-485-3757, TELEX 18582 ESPA NL, nlinfo-f@elsevier.nl; usinfo-f@elsevier.com; forinfo-kyf04035@niftyserve.or.jp, http://www.elsevier.nl/. **Subscr. in Australasia and the Far East to:** Elsevier Science (Singapore) Pte Ltd, No.1 Temasek Ave, 17-01 Millenia Tower, Singapore 039192, Singapore. TEL 65-434-3727, FAX 65-337-2230; **Subscr. in Japan to:** Elsevier Science Inc - Japan Regional Office, 9-15 Higashi-Azabu 1-chome, Minato-ku, Tokyo 106-0044, Japan. TEL 81-3-5561-5033, FAX 81-3-5561-5047, info@elsevier.co.jp; **Subscr. in the Americas to:** Elsevier Science, PO Box 945, New York, NY 10159-0945. TEL 212-633-3730, FAX 212-633-3680, http://www.elsevier.com.

576.549 NLD ISSN 1383-5742

MUTATION RESEARCH - REVIEWS IN MUTATION RESEARCH. Text in English. bi-m. EUR 726 in Europe to institutions; JPY 96,400 in Japan to institutions; USD 812 elsewhere to institutions (effective 2002). back issues avail. *Refereed.* **Document type:** *Academic/Scholarly.* **Description:** Encompasses the entire spectrum of the science of mutation research and its applications.

Related titles: Online - full text ed.: (from EBSCO Publishing, ingenta, ScienceDirect, Swets Blackwell, Institute for Scientific Information); ♦ Special ed. of: Mutation Research. ISSN 0921-8262.

Indexed: Aqua.Sci.& Fish.Abstr., BBCI, Curr.Cont., Dairy Sci.Abstr., Entomol.Abstr. (coverage dropped), Environ.Sci.Poll.Mgmt., Forest Prod.Abstr., Genet.Abstr., Hum.Gen.Abstr., Inpharma, Int.Abstr.Biol.Sci., Microbiol.Abstr., Nutr.Abstr., Plant Breed.Abstr., Reac., Ref.Zh., Rev.Med.& Vet.Mycol., Sci.Cit.Ind., Trop.Dis.Bull.

—ADONIS, IDS. **CCC.**

Published by: Elsevier Science BV, PO Box 211, Amsterdam 1000 AE, Netherlands. TEL 31-20-485-3757, TELEX 18582 ESPA NL, nlinfo-f@elsevier.nl, http://www.elsevier.com/locate/mrrev, http://www.elsevier.nl. **Subscr. in Australasia and the Far East to:** Elsevier Science (Singapore) Pte Ltd, No.1 Temasek Ave, 17-01 Millenia Tower, Singapore 039192, Singapore. TEL 65-434-3727, FAX 65-337-2230; **Subscr. in Japan to:** Elsevier Science Inc - Japan Regional Office, 9-15 Higashi-Azabu 1-chome, Minato-ku, Tokyo 106-0044, Japan. TEL 81-3-5561-5033, FAX 81-3-5561-5047; **Subscr. in the Americas to:** Elsevier Science, PO Box 945, New York, NY 10159-0945. TEL 212-633-3730, FAX 212-633-3680.

576.5 USA ISSN 1060-8788

N C B I NEWS. Text in English. 1991. 4/yr. free per issue. **Document type:** *Newsletter, Government.* **Description:** Informs the biomedical community about N.C.B.I. research activities and the availability of molecular biology database and software services.

Related titles: Online - full text ed.

Published by: U.S. National Center for Biotechnology Information, National Library of Medicine, Bldg 38A, Rm 8N 803, 8600 Rockville Pike, Bethesda, MD 20894. TEL 301-496-2475, FAX 301-480-9241, info@ncbi.nlm.nih.gov, http://www.ncbi.nlm.nih.gov/Web/Newsltr/. Circ: 25,000.

576.5 JPN ISSN 0077-4995
QH431.A1

NATIONAL INSTITUTE OF GENETICS. ANNUAL REPORT (ENGLISH EDITION). Text in English. 1949. a. free per issue.

Related titles: ♦ Japanese ed.: Kokuritsu Idengaku Kenkyujo Nenpo.

Indexed: Anim.Breed.Abstr., Aqua.Sci.& Fish.Abstr., Aquacult.Abstr., Biotech.& Bioeng.Abstr., Environ.Sci.Poll.Mgmt., Genet.Abstr., Hum.Gen.Abstr., INIS Atomind., Rev.Appl.Entomol.

—CISTI, Linda Hall.

Published by: Ministry of Education, National Institute of Genetics/Monbusho Kokuritsu Idengaku Kenkyujo, 1111 Yata, Mishima-shi, Shizuoka-ken 411-0801, Japan. Circ: 600.

576.5 USA ISSN 1061-4036
QH431 CODEN: NGENEC

NATURE GENETICS. Text in English. 1992. m. USD 199 domestic to individuals; GBP 185 foreign to individuals; USD 710 domestic to institutions; GBP 520 foreign to institutions (effective 2001). adv. illus. Index. back issues avail.; reprints avail. *Refereed.* **Document type:** *Academic/Scholarly.* **Description:** Comprehensive coverage of new developments and issues in all branches of genetics, with particular emphasis on the human genome project and genetic aspects of disease.

Related titles: Online - full text ed.: (from EBSCO Publishing, ingenta, Institute for Scientific Information); ♦ Supplement to: Nature. ISSN 0028-0836.

Indexed: ASCA, AgBiotech, Anim.Breed.Abstr., Aqua.Sci.& Fish.Abstr., Arts & Hum.Cit.Ind. (coverage dropped), Bibl.Agri., Biol.& Agr.Ind. (Jan.1996-), Biol.Dig., Biotech.Cit.Ind., Cal.Tiss.Abstr., Chem.Abstr., Chem.Indus.Notes, Chem.Titles, Chemorec.Abstr., Curr.Cont., Dairy Sci.Abstr., Derwent Biotech.Abstr., Diab.Cont., Entomol.Abstr., Environ.Sci.Poll.Mgmt., Excerp.Med. (1993-), Genet.Abstr., Helminthol.Abstr., Hum.Gen.Abstr., Immun.Abstr. (coverage dropped), Ind.Med. (1992-), Ind.Sci.Rev., Inpharma, Int.Abstr.Biol.Sci., Jrnl.Watch Derm., Mass Spectr.Bull., Neurosci.Abstr., Nuc.Acids Abstr., Nutr.Abstr., Oncog.G.F.Abstr. (coverage dropped), Pharm.&Out.News, Plant Breed.Abstr., Protozool.Abstr., Reac., Ref.Zh., SSCI (coverage dropped), Sci.Cit.Ind., Tox.Abstr. (coverage dropped), Wild.Rev.

—BLDSC (6046.625000), CASDDS, CISTI, EMDOCS, GNLM, IDS, ingenta. **CCC.**

Published by: Macmillan Magazines Ltd. (Subsidiary of: Macmillan Publishers Ltd.), 1234 National Press Bldg, Washington, DC 20045. TEL 202-626-2513, subscriptions@natureny.com, http://www.genetics.nature.com. Ed. Bette Phimister. Pub. Adrian Ivinson. Adv. contact Marion Delancy. Circ: 3,000. **Subscr. in UK and Europe to:** Macmillan Magazines Ltd, Brunel Rd, Basingstoke, Hants RG21 6XT, United Kingdom. TEL 44-1256-29242, FAX 44-1256-812358; **Subscr. to:** Allen Press Inc., PO Box 1897, Lawrence, KS 66044-8897. TEL 800-524-0384, FAX 615-377-0525.

599.9 DEU ISSN 1364-6745
CODEN: NEROFX

NEUROGENETICS. Text in German. 1997. q. EUR 414.40 domestic; EUR 410.60 in Germany; EUR 120 newsstand/cover foreign (effective 2002). *Refereed.* **Document type:** *Journal, Academic/Scholarly.* **Description:** Publishes findings that contribute to a better understanding of the genetic basis of normal and abnormal function of the nervous system.

Related titles: Online - full text ed.: ISSN 1364-6753 (from EBSCO Publishing, RoweCom Information Quest, Swets Blackwell, Springer LINK, Institute for Scientific Information).

Indexed: Biotech.Cit.Ind., Focus on: Mol.Med., Ind.Med. (1997-), Neurosci.Cit.Ind., e-psyche.

—BLDSC (6081.371550), CASDDS, IDS.

Published by: Springer-Verlag (Subsidiary of: BertelsmannSpringer), Tiergartenstr 17, Heidelberg 69121, Germany. TEL 49-6221-345-0, FAX 49-6221-345229, subscriptions@springer.de, http://link.springer.de/link/service/journals/10048/index.htm, http://www.springer.de. Eds. M B Graeber, U Mueller. **Subscr. in US to:** Springer-Verlag New York Inc., PO Box 2485, Secaucus, NJ 07096-2485.

599.9 GBR ISSN 1463-6778
TP248.13 CODEN: GEBIER
NEW GENETICS AND SOCIETY. Text in English. 1981. 3/yr. GBP 66, USD 123 to individuals; GBP 300, USD 518 to institutions (effective 2002). adv. bk.rev. *Refereed.* **Document type:** *Academic/Scholarly.*
Description: Provides an international platform for discussion of key issues raised by the exploitation of the new genetics. Publishes social science research alongside theoretical and methodological contributions.
Former titles: Genetic Engineer and Biotechnologist (0959-020X); (until 1990): International Industrial Biotechnology (0269-7815); (until 1986): Industrial Biotechnology (0268-3024); (until 1985): Industrial Biotechnology Wales (0266-9854)
Related titles: Online - full content ed.: ISSN 1469-9915 (from EBSCO Publishing, O C L C Online Computer Library Center, Inc., ProQuest Information & Learning, Swets Blackwell); Online - full text ed.: (from CatchWord Ltd., Institute for Scientific Information, RoweCom Information Quest); Supplement: European Bio Patent Watch.
Indexed: ASCA, AgBiotech, Agri.& Environ.Biotech.Abstr., Agri.Eng.Abstr., Anim.Breed.Abstr., Aqua.Sci.& Fish.Abstr., Biotech.& Bioeng.Abstr., Biotech.Cit.Ind., CEABA, Curr.Adv.Biochem., Curr.Biotech.Abstr., Derwent Biotech.Abstr., Eng.Ind., Environ.Sci.Poll.Mgmt., Food Sci.& Tech.Abstr., Genet.Abstr., Hum.Gen.Abstr., Med.& Pharm.Biotech.Abstr., Microbiol.Abstr., Ref.Zh., Risk Abstr., SSCI (coverage dropped), Saf.Sci.Abstr., Soils & Fert., Telegen, World Ag.Econ.& Rur.Soc.Abstr.
—BLDSC (6084.211700), ADONIS, CASDDS, CatchWord, CISTI, Ei, GNLM, IDS, Infotrieve. **CCC.**
Published by: (G B Biotechnology Ltd.), Carfax Publishing Limited (Subsidiary of: Taylor & Francis Group), PO Box 25, Abingdon, Oxon OX14 3UE, United Kingdom. TEL 44-1235-401000, FAX 44-1235-401550, enquiries@carfax.co.uk, enquiry@tandf.co.uk, http://www.carfax.co.uk. Eds. Harry Rothman, Peter Glasner.

NIHON JINRUI IDEN GAKKAI TAIKAI SHOROKUSHU/ JAPAN SOCIETY OF HUMAN GENETICS. ABSTRACTS OF THE ANNUAL MEETING. see *BIOLOGY—Abstracting, Bibliographies, Statistics*

576.5 GBR
NORWICH RESEARCH PARK NEWSLETTER. Text in English. 1987. s-a. USD 10. back issues avail. **Document type:** *Newsletter.*
Formerly: Biological Research in Norwich
Published by: University of East Anglia, School of Biological Sciences, Norwich, Norfolk NR4 7TJ, United Kingdom. TEL 0603-592197, FAX 0603-259492. Ed. Richard James. Circ: 600.

NUCLEUS; international journal of cytology and allied topics. see *BIOLOGY—Cytology And Histology*

572.86 611.01816 USA
QH442 CODEN: MCGEFP
O M I C S: A JOURNAL OF INTEGRATIVE BIOLOGY. Text in English. 1994. q. USD 139 domestic to individuals; USD 217 foreign to individuals; USD 167 domestic to individuals print and online eds. combined; USD 245 foreign to individuals print and online eds. combined; USD 394 domestic to institutions; USD 508 foreign to institutions; USD 473 domestic to institutions print and online eds. combined; USD 587 foreign to institutions print and online eds. combined (effective 2002). back issues avail.; reprints avail. *Refereed.* **Document type:** *Journal, Academic/Scholarly.*
Description: Offers a unique repository for genome and DNA sequencing; mapping, informatics, biological interpretations, human disease, ethical, legal, and social issues, new technology, and computational approaches.
Former titles (until 2001): Microbial & Comparative Genomics (1090-6592); (until 1996): Genome Science and Technology (1070-2830)
Related titles: Online - full text ed.: USD 394 to institutions; USD 139 to individuals (effective 2002) (from Swets Blackwell, RoweCom Information Quest).
Indexed: Agricola, Aqua.Sci.& Fish.Abstr., Chem.Abstr., Chem.Indus.Notes, Chem.Titles, Environ.Sci.Poll.Mgmt., Genet.Abstr., Hum.Gen.Abstr., Ind.Med. (1996-), Microbiol.Abstr., Nuc.Acids Abstr.
—BLDSC (5756.910500), CASDDS, CISTI, Infotrieve. **CCC.**
Published by: Mary Ann Liebert, Inc. Publishers, 2 Madison Ave, Larchmont, NY 10538. TEL 914—834-3100, FAX 914-834-1388, info@liebertpub.com, www.liebertpub.com/mcg, http://www.liebertpub.com. Ed. Dr. Glen A Evans.

ONCOGENE. see *MEDICAL SCIENCES—Oncology*

572.8 GBR
OXFORD MONOGRAPHS ON MOLECULAR GENETICS. Text in English. 1966. irreg., latest vol.34, 1997. price varies. *Refereed.* **Document type:** *Monographic series.*
Formerly (until 1997): Oxford Monographs on Medical Genetics (1352-240X)
—BLDSC (6321.007500).
Published by: Oxford University Press, Great Clarendon St, Oxford OX2 6DP, United Kingdom. TEL 44-1865-56767, FAX 44-1865-56646, TELEX 837330 OXPRES G, jnlorders@oup.co.uk, http://www.oup.co.uk. **Orders in N. America to:** Oxford University Press, Journals. TEL 919-677-0977, FAX 919-677-1714, http://www.oup.co.uk.

576.8 GBR ISSN 0265-072X
QH359 CODEN: OSEBE3
OXFORD SURVEYS IN EVOLUTIONARY BIOLOGY. Text in English. 1984. a. price varies. bk.rev. **Document type:** *Academic/Scholarly.*
Indexed: Anim.Breed.Abstr., Curr.Adv.Gen.& Molec.Biol., GeoRef, Sport Fish.Abstr., Wild.Rev., Zoo.Rec.
—CISTI, Infotrieve, ingenta. **CCC.**
Published by: Oxford University Press, Oxford Journals, Walton St, Oxford OX2 6DP, United Kingdom. FAX 44-1865-267773, jnlorders@oup.co.uk, jnl.orders@oup.co.uk, http://www.oup.co.uk. **Subscr. in N. America to:** Oxford University Press, Journals. TEL 919-677-0977, FAX 919-677-1714, http://www.oup.co.uk.

576.5 GBR ISSN 0265-0738
QH426 CODEN: OSEGEI
OXFORD SURVEYS ON EUKARYOTIC GENES. Text in English. 1984. a. price varies. **Document type:** *Academic/Scholarly.* **Description:** Forum for authoritative reviews of particular genes or gene families whose structure or function is better understood as a result of recent research.
Indexed: Anim.Breed.Abstr., Ind.Med. (coverage dropped), Pig News & Info., Sport Fish.Abstr.
—CASDDS, CISTI, GNLM, Linda Hall.
Published by: Oxford University Press, Oxford Journals, Walton St, Oxford OX2 6DP, United Kingdom. FAX 44-1865-267773, jnl.orders@oup.co.uk, http://www.oup.co.uk. Ed. Norman Maclean. **Subscr. in N. America to:** Oxford University Press, Journals. TEL 919-677-0977, FAX 919-677-0977, http://www.oup.co.uk.

576.5 IND
PERSPECTIVES IN CYTOLOGY & GENETICS; proceedings of the all India Congress of cytology and genetics. Text in English. 1971. triennial. INR 325; USD 100 foreign. *Refereed.* **Document type:** *Academic/Scholarly.* **Description:** Contains proceedings of the all India Congress of cytology and genetics.
Indexed: Zoo.Rec.
—BLDSC (6428.140000).
Published by: (Calcutta University, Department of Botany), All India Congress of Cytology & Genetics, c/o G.K. Manna, B10 - 250 Kalyani, Kalyani, West Bengal 41235, India. TEL 91-33-5829113. Ed. G K Manna. Circ: 300 (paid).

576.5 USA ISSN 0960-314X
CODEN: PHMCEE
PHARMACOGENETICS. Text in English. 1991. 9/yr., latest vol.11. USD 244 domestic to individuals print & online eds. combined; USD 244 foreign to individuals print & online eds. combined; USD 855 per issue domestic to institutions; USD 855 per issue foreign to institutions; USD 87 newsstand/cover (effective 2002). adv. index. back issues avail.; reprints avail. *Refereed.* **Document type:** *Academic/Scholarly.* **Description:** Devoted to the rapid publication of research papers, brief review articles, and short communications on genetic variation in response to drugs and other chemicals.
Related titles: Online - full text ed.: USD 1,111.50 domestic academic site license; USD 1,111.50 foreign academic site license; USD 1,239.75 domestic corporate site license; USD 1,239.75 foreign corporate site license (2002) (from Ovid Technologies, Inc., EBSCO Publishing, Institute for Scientific Information).
Indexed: ASCA, BBCI, Biotech.Cit.Ind., Chem.Abstr., Chem.Titles, Curr.Cont., Derwent Biotech.Abstr., Excerp.Med. (1993-), Ind.Med. (1991-), Inpharma, Int.Abstr.Biol.Sci., Pharm.&Out.News, Reac., SSCI (coverage dropped), Sci.Cit.Ind.
—BLDSC (6446.249000), ADONIS, CASDDS, CISTI, EMDOCS, GNLM, IDS, KNAW.
Published by: Lippincott Williams & Wilkins (Philadelphia) (Subsidiary of: Wolters Kluwer N.V.), 530 Walnut St, Philadelphia, PA 19106-3621. TEL 215-521-8300, FAX 215-521-8902, www.jpharmacogenetics.com, http://www.lww.com. Circ: 180. **Subscr. to:** PO Box 1600, Hagerstown, MD 21740-1600. TEL 800-777-2295, FAX 301-824-7390.

576.5 USA ISSN 0733-9003
CODEN: PTCYDB
PROGRESS AND TOPICS IN CYTOGENETICS. Text in English. 1981. irreg., latest vol.8, 1989. price varies. *Refereed.*
Indexed: Biol.Abstr., Chem.Abstr., Chem.Indus.Notes, Chem.Titles.
—CASDDS, CISTI, KNAW.
Published by: John Wiley & Sons, Inc., Journals (Subsidiary of: Wiley InterScience), 605 Third Ave, New York, NY 10158. TEL 212-475-7700.

576.5 USA ISSN 0955-8829
CODEN: PSGEEX
PSYCHIATRIC GENETICS. Text in English. 1990. q., latest vol.11. USD 221 domestic to individuals; USD 221 foreign to individuals; USD 527 per issue domestic to institutions; USD 527 per issue foreign to institutions; USD 120 newsstand/cover (effective 2002). adv. bk.rev. index. *Refereed.* **Document type:** *Academic/Scholarly.*
Description: Forum for novel approaches using new technologies to better understand the normal and abnormal brain.
Related titles: CD-ROM ed.; Online - full text ed.: USD 685.10 domestic academic site license; USD 685.10 foreign academic site license; USD 764.15 domestic corporate site license; USD 764.15 foreign corporate site license (2002) (from EBSCO Publishing, Institute for Scientific Information).
Indexed: ASCA, Biotech.Cit.Ind., Excerp.Med. (1993-), Ind.Med. (1990-), Inpharma, Int.Abstr.Biol.Sci., Neurosci.Cit.Ind., Pharm.&Out.News, PsycInfo, Psychol.Abstr. (1990-), Reac., SSCI (coverage dropped), e-psyche.
—BLDSC (6946.214050), ADONIS, CISTI, EMDOCS, GNLM, IDS, KNAW.
Published by: Lippincott Williams & Wilkins (Philadelphia) (Subsidiary of: Wolters Kluwer N.V.), 530 Walnut St, Philadelphia, PA 19106-3621. TEL 215-521-8300, FAX 215-521-8902, http://www.psychgenetics.com, http://www.lww.com. Ed. Dr. John I Nurnberger Jr. Adv. contact Gemma Heiser. Circ: 800. **Subscr. to:** PO Box 1600, Hagerstown, MD 21740-1600. TEL 800-777-2295, FAX 301-824-7390.

R N A. (Ribonucleic Acid) see *BIOLOGY—Biochemistry*

REFERATIVNYI ZHURNAL. GENETIKA CHELOVEKA. see *BIOLOGY—Abstracting, Bibliographies, Statistics*

REFERATIVNYI ZHURNAL. GENETIKA I SELEKTSIYA MIKROORGANIZMOV. see *BIOLOGY—Abstracting, Bibliographies, Statistics*

REFERATIVNYI ZHURNAL. GENETIKA I SELEKTSIYA SEL'SKOKHOZYAISTVENNYKH ZHIVOTNYKH. see *BIOLOGY—Abstracting, Bibliographies, Statistics*

REFERATIVNYI ZHURNAL. GENETIKA I SELEKTSIYA VOZDELYVAEMYKH RASTENII. see *BIOLOGY—Abstracting, Bibliographies, Statistics*

REFERATIVNYI ZHURNAL. GENETIKA: TSITOLOGIYA. see *BIOLOGY—Abstracting, Bibliographies, Statistics*

REFERATIVNYI ZHURNAL. OBSHCHAYA GENETIKA. see *BIOLOGY—Abstracting, Bibliographies, Statistics*

576.5 DNK ISSN 1398-1714
▼ **REVIEWS IN IMMUNOGENETICS.** Text in English. ceased; resumed 1999. q. DKK 790 to individuals; DKK 869 to individuals print & online eds. combined; DKK 2,100 to institutions; DKK 2,310 to institutions print & online eds. combined (effective 2001). adv. *Refereed.* **Document type:** *Journal, Academic/Scholarly.*
Description: Provides up-to-date information relevant to all aspects of immunogenetics. Topics range from basic science to laboratory testing and clinical applications.
—BLDSC (7790.769950).
Published by: Blackwell Munksgaard, Noerre Soegade 35, PO Box 2148, Copenhagen K 1016, Denmark. FAX 45-77-33-33-77, fsub@munksgaard.dk, http://journals.munksgaard.dk/reviewsimmunogenetics, http://www.munksgaard.dk. Ed. J. Hansen.

REVISTA DE DERECHO Y GENOMA HUMANO/LAW AND THE HUMAN GENOME REVIEW. see *LAW*

B

576.5 RUS ISSN 1022-7954
QH431 CODEN: RJGEEQ
RUSSIAN JOURNAL OF GENETICS. Text in English. 1965. m. EUR 2,666 to institutions for print or online ed.; EUR 3,199.20 to institutions print & online eds.combined (effective 2002). back issues avail. *Refereed.* **Document type:** *Academic/Scholarly.* **Description:** Investigates genetic processes at the molecular, cellular, organismic, and population levels, with articles on the impact of modern genetics and environmental concerns.
Formerly (until 1994): Soviet Genetics (0038-5409)
Related titles: Microfilm ed.: (from PQC); Online - full text ed.: ISSN 1608-3369 (from Swets Blackwell, Kluwer Online, Institute for Scientific Information, RoweCom Information Quest); ♦ Translation of: Genetika. ISSN 0016-6758.
Indexed: Biol.Abstr., Biotech.Cit.Ind., Chem.Abstr., Chem.Indus.Notes, Chem.Titles, Curr.Adv.Ecol.Sci., Curr.Cont., Excerp.Med., INIS Atomind., Ind.Med. (coverage dropped), Int.Abstr.Biol.Sci., Sci.Cit.Ind., Sport Fish.Abstr., Wild.Rev.
—BLDSC (0420.760960), CASDDS, CISTI, GNLM, Infotrieve, ingenta. **CCC.**
Published by: (Rossiiskaya Akademiya Nauk/Russian Academy of Sciences), M A I K Nauka - Interperiodica, Mezhdunarodnyi Otdel, Profsoyuznaya ul 90, Moscow 117864, Russian Federation. TEL 7-095-336-1600, FAX 7-095-336-0666, compmg@maik.ru, compmg@maik.rssi.ru; info@plenum.com, http://www.maik.rssi.ru/journals/geneng.htm; http://www.plenum.com. Ed. G P Georgiev. **Dist. by:** Kluwer Academic Publishers, PO Box 17, Dordrecht 3300 AH, Netherlands. TEL 31-78-392392, http://www.wkap.nl.

SILVAE GENETICA; Zeitschrift fuer Forstgenetik und Forstpflanzenzuechtung. see *BIOLOGY—Botany*

613.94 USA ISSN 0037-766X
HQ750.A1 CODEN: SOBIAL
SOCIAL BIOLOGY. Text in English. 1954. 2/yr. USD 105 (effective 2001). bk.rev. abstr, charts, illus. index. back issues avail.; reprint service avail. from PQC. *Refereed.* **Document type:** *Academic/Scholarly.* **Description:** Furthers knowledge of the biological and cultural forces affecting human populations and their evolution.
Formerly: Eugenics Quarterly (0097-2762)
Related titles: Microform ed.: (from PQC); Online - full text ed.: (from Gale Group, Factiva, Institute for Scientific Information).
Indexed: ASCA, ASSIA, Abstr.Anthropol., Abstr.Hyg., AgeLine, Anthropol.Lit., Arts & Hum.Cit.Ind. (coverage dropped), Biol.& Agr.Ind. (coverage dropped), Biol.Abstr., Biol.Dig., Chem.Abstr., Curr.Adv.Ecol.Sci., Curr.Cont., Curr.Lit.Fam.Plan., Dairy Sci.Abstr., Diar.Dis.Res., Environ.Sci.Poll.Mgmt., Excerp.Med., Fam.Ind., IBR, INIS Atomind., Ind.Med. (1969-), Indian Psychol.Abstr., Intl.Bibl.Soc.Sci., Lang.& Lang.Behav.Abstr., Nutr.Abstr., P.A.I.S. (coverage dropped), Pollut.Abstr., Popul.Ind., PsycInfo, Psychol.Abstr. (1969-), Risk Abstr., SOPODA, SSCI, Saf.Sci.Abstr., Soc.Sci.Ind. (Apr.1982-Dec.1993), Soc.Serv.Abstr., Sociol.Abstr., Trop.Dis.Bull., World Ag.Econ.& Rur.Soc.Abstr., e-psyche.
—BLDSC (8318.055000), CISTI, GNLM, IDS, ingenta.
Published by: Society for the Study of Social Biology, 1129 E 8th St, Box 2349, Port Angeles, WA 98362. TEL 360-457-6530, FAX 360-457-6530, osb-rb@olympus.net, http://www.allenpress.com. Ed. Richard H Osborne. Circ: 1,650. **Subscr. to:** Allen Press Inc., PO Box 1897, Lawrence, KS 66044-8897.

SOCIETY FOR IN VITRO BIOLOGY. MONOGRAPH SERIES. see *BIOLOGY—Biotechnology*

576.5 USA ISSN 0740-7750
QH426 CODEN: SCMGDN
SOMATIC CELL AND MOLECULAR GENETICS. Text in English. 1975. bi-m. EUR 849 to institutions for print or online ed.; USD 1,020, USD 1,018.80 to institutions print & online eds. combined (effective 2002). adv. *Refereed.* **Document type:** *Academic/Scholarly.* **Description:** Publishes original research conducted in the fields of cellular and molecular genetics of higher eukaryotic systems.
Formerly (until 1984): Somatic Cell Genetics (0098-0366)
Related titles: Microfilm ed.: (from PQC); Online - full text ed.: (from O C L C Online Computer Library Center, Inc., Swets Blackwell, Kluwer Online, Institute for Scientific Information).
Indexed: ASCA, AgBiotech, Agri.& Environ.Biotech.Abstr. (coverage dropped), Anim.Breed.Abstr., Aqua.Sci.& Fish.Abstr., Biol.Abstr., Biotech.& Bioeng.Abstr., Biotech.Cit.Ind., Chem.Abstr., Chem.Indus.Notes, Chem.Titles, Curr.Adv.Biochem., Curr.Adv.Cell & Devel.Biol., Curr.Adv.Ecol.Sci., Curr.Adv.Gen.& Molec.Biol., Curr.Cont., Derwent Biotech.Abstr., Excerp.Med., Genet.Abstr., Hum.Gen.Abstr., INIS Atomind., Ind.Med. (1984-), Ind.Sci.Rev., Inpharma, Int.Abstr.Biol.Sci., Microbiol.Abstr., Nuc.Acids Abstr., Oncog.G.F.Abstr. (coverage dropped), Reac., Sci.Cit.Ind., Telegen.
—BLDSC (8327.808800), CASDDS, CISTI, EMDOCS, GNLM, IDS, ingenta, Linda Hall. **CCC.**
Published by: Kluwer Academic - Plenum Publishers (Subsidiary of: Wolters Kluwer N.V.), 233 Spring St, New York, NY 10013-1578. TEL 212-620-8000, 800-221-9369, FAX 212-463-0742, services@wkap.nl, http://www.wkap.nl/journalhome.htm/0740-7750. Ed. Richard L Davidson. R&P Rose Luongo TEL 781-871-6311.

576.5 USA ISSN 0081-4148
QH431.A1 CODEN: SGSYBV
STADLER GENETICS SYMPOSIUM. PROCEEDINGS. Text in English. 1971. irreg., latest vol.21, 2000. price varies. *Refereed.* **Document type:** *Proceedings.*
Indexed: Anim.Breed.Abstr., Biol.Abstr., Chem.Abstr., Rice Abstr.
—CASDDS, CISTI, Infotrieve, KNAW, Linda Hall. **CCC.**
Published by: Kluwer Academic - Plenum Publishers (Subsidiary of: Wolters Kluwer N.V.), 233 Spring St, New York, NY 10013-1578. TEL 212-620-8000, 800-221-9369, FAX 212-463-0742, info@plenum.com, http://www.plenum.com.

▼ **THALAMUS AND RELATED SYSTEMS.** see *BIOLOGY*

576.5 DEU ISSN 0040-5752
SB123 CODEN: THAGA6
THEORETICAL AND APPLIED GENETICS; international journal of breeding research. Short title: T A G. Text in English. 1929. 16/yr. DEM 7,062 domestic; DEM 7,102 foreign (effective 2001). back issues avail.; reprint service avail. from ISI. *Refereed.* **Document type:** *Journal, Academic/Scholarly.* **Description:** Reflects the continuing progress of plant and animal breeding genetics, including fundamental and applied aspects.
Supersedes: Zuechter
Related titles: Microform ed.: (from PQC); Online - full text ed.: ISSN 1432-2242 (from EBSCO Publishing, RoweCom Information Quest, Swets Blackwell, Springer LINK, Institute for Scientific Information).
Indexed: ASCA, Abstr.Bull.Inst.Pap.Chem., AgBiotech, Agri.& Environ.Biotech.Abstr., Agricola, Agroforest.Abstr., Anim.Breed.Abstr., Apic.Abstr., Aqua.Sci.& Fish.Abstr., Bibl.Agri., Biol.Abstr., Biotech.Cit.Ind., CEABA, Chem.Abstr., Chem.Indus.Notes, Chem.Titles, Cott.& Trop.Fibr.Abstr., Crop Physiol.Abstr., Curr.Adv.Ecol.Sci., Curr.Adv.Gen.& Molec.Biol., Curr.Adv.Plant Sci., Curr.Biotech.Abstr., Curr.Cont., Curr.Ind.Stat., Dairy Sci.Abstr., Derwent Biotech.Abstr., Eng.Ind., Entomol.Abstr., Environ.Sci.Poll.Mgmt., Excerp.Med., Fababean Abstr., Field Crop Abstr., Food Sci.& Tech.Abstr., Forest Prod.Abstr., Forest.Abstr., Genet.Abstr., Helminthol.Abstr., Herb.Abstr., Hort.Abstr., Hum.Gen.Abstr., INIS Atomind., Ind.Sci.Rev., Inpharma, Int.Abstr.Biol.Sci., Irr.& Drain.Abstr., Maize Abstr., Nuc.Acids Abstr., Nutr.Abstr., Ornam.Hort., Plant Breed.Abstr., Plant Gen.Res.Abstr., Plant Grow.Reg.Abstr., Plant Sci., Postharvest, Potato Abstr., Poult.Abstr., Reac., Rev.Appl.Entomol., Rev.Arom.& Med.Plants, Rev.Plant Path., Rice Abstr., Sci.Cit.Ind., Seed Abstr., Soils & Fert., Sorghum & Millets Abstr., Soyabean Abstr., Sport Fish.Abstr., Triticale Abstr., Trop.Oil Seeds Abstr., VITIS, Weed Abstr., Wild.Rev., World Ag.Econ.& Rur.Soc.Abstr., Zoo.Rec.
—BLDSC (8814.552000), CASDDS, CISTI, EMDOCS, GNLM, IDS, ingenta, Linda Hall. **CCC.**
Published by: Springer-Verlag (Subsidiary of: BertelsmannSpringer), Tiergartenstr 17, Heidelberg 69121, Germany. TEL 49-6221-345-0, FAX 49-6221-345229, subscriptions@springer.de, http://link.springer.de/link/service/journals/00122/index.htm, http://www.springer.de. Eds. C Moellers, H C Becker. **Subscr. in N. America to:** Springer-Verlag New York Inc., PO Box 2485, Secaucus, NJ 07096-2485. TEL 212-460-1500, FAX 212-473-6272.

576.549 USA ISSN 0888-7519
CODEN: TCMUE9
TOPICS IN CHEMICAL MUTAGENESIS. Text in English. 1984. irreg., latest vol.2. price varies. back issues avail. *Refereed.* **Document type:** *Monographic series.*
Indexed: Chem.Abstr.
—CASDDS, CISTI.
Published by: Kluwer Academic - Plenum Publishers (Subsidiary of: Wolters Kluwer N.V.), 233 Spring St, New York, NY 10013-1578. TEL 212-620-8000, 800-221-9369, FAX 212-463-0742, info@plenum.com, http://www.plenum.com. Ed. Frederick J de Serres.

576.6 NLD ISSN 0962-8819
QH442.6 CODEN: TRSEES
TRANSGENIC RESEARCH. Text in Dutch. 1991. bi-m. EUR 830 to institutions for print or online ed.; EUR 996 to institutions print & online eds.combined (effective 2002). adv. bk.rev. reprints avail. *Refereed.* **Document type:** *Academic/Scholarly.* **Description:** Provides the rapid publication of research in transgenic higher organisms, including their production and properties resulting from the transgenic state, use as experimental tools, exploitation and application, and environmental impact.
Related titles: Online - full text ed.: (from EBSCO Publishing, O C L C Online Computer Library Center, Inc., RoweCom Information Quest, Swets Blackwell, Kluwer Online, Institute for Scientific Information).
Indexed: ASCA, AgBiotech, Agri.& Environ.Biotech.Abstr., Agricola, Anim.Breed.Abstr., BBCI, Bibl.Agri., Biotech.Cit.Ind., Chem.Abstr., Chem.Indus.Notes, Crop Physiol.Abstr., Curr.Adv.Plant Sci., Curr.Cont., Dairy Sci.Abstr., Derwent Biotech.Abstr., Environ.Sci.Poll.Mgmt., Forest.Abstr., Genet.Abstr., Hum.Gen.Abstr., Ind.Med. (1991-), Ind.Sci.Rev., Ind.Vet., Inpharma, Int.Abstr.Biol.Sci., Maize Abstr., Med.& Pharm.Biotech.Abstr., Nuc.Acids Abstr., Nutr.Abstr., Plant Breed.Abstr., Plant Grow.Reg.Abstr., Plant Sci., Potato Abstr., Poult.Abstr., Reac., Rev.Appl.Entomol., Rev.Plant Path., Rice Abstr., Sci.Cit.Ind., Seed Abstr., Triticale Abstr., VITIS, Weed Abstr.
—BLDSC (9020.713000), ADONIS, CASDDS, CISTI, EMDOCS, GNLM, IDS, Infotrieve. **CCC.**
Published by: Kluwer Academic Publishers Group (Subsidiary of: Wolters Kluwer N.V.), Spuiboulevard 50, PO Box 17, Dordrecht 3300 AA, Netherlands. FAX 31-78-639-2254, TELEX 290164 CHAPMA G, services@wkap.nl, http://www.wkap.nl. Eds. C A Pinkert, R Forster. Adv. contact Gemma Heiser. **Dist. by:** Journals Department, PO Box 322, Dordrecht 3300 AH, Netherlands. TEL 781-871-6600, FAX 31-78-654-6474.

576.5 GBR ISSN 0168-9525
QH426 CODEN: TRGEE2
TRENDS IN GENETICS; DNA, differentiation and development. Text in English. 1985. m. GBP 92, EUR 115 in Europe to individuals; JPY 14,000 in Japan to individuals; USD 126 elsewhere to individuals; EUR 908 in Europe to institutions; JPY 125,900 in Japan to institutions; USD 1,015 elsewhere to institutions (effective 2002); GBP 47 in Europe to students (effective 2001); JPY 10,100 in Japan to students; USD 78 elsewhere to students; USD 1,308 to institutions Print & online eds. combined; EUR 144 in Europe to qualified personnel; JPY 17,500 in Japan to qualified personnel; USD 157 elsewhere to qualified personnel (effective 2002). adv. bk.rev. index. back issues avail.; reprint service avail. from SWZ. *Refereed.* **Document type:** *Academic/Scholarly.* **Description:** Covers all aspects of genetics - molecular genetics, differentiation, development, clinical genetics, recombinant DNA.
Related titles: Online - full text ed.: (from ingenta, Swets Blackwell, Institute for Scientific Information, ScienceDirect).
Indexed: ASCA, AgBiotech, Anim.Breed.Abstr., Aqua.Sci.& Fish.Abstr., Bibl.Agri., Biol.Abstr., Biotech.Cit.Ind., Chem.Abstr., Crop Physiol.Abstr., Curr.Adv.Biochem., Curr.Adv.Cell & Devel.Biol., Curr.Adv.Gen.& Molec.Biol., Curr.Cont., Derwent Biotech.Abstr., Entomol.Abstr., Excerp.Med., Food Sci.& Tech.Abstr., Genet.Abstr., Helminthol.Abstr., Hum.Gen.Abstr., Ind.Med. (1985-), Ind.Sci.Rev., Inpharma, Int.Abstr.Biol.Sci., Maize Abstr., Neurosci.Abstr., Nuc.Acids Abstr., Oncog.G.F.Abstr. (coverage dropped), Pharm.&Out.News, Plant Breed.Abstr., Plant Grow.Reg.Abstr., Potato Abstr., Poult.Abstr., Protozool.Abstr., Reac., Ref.Zh., Rev.Appl.Entomol., Rev.Med.& Vet.Mycol., Rev.Plant Path., Sci.Cit.Ind., Weed Abstr., Wild.Rev., Zoo.Rec.
—BLDSC (9049.598000), ADONIS, CASDDS, CISTI, GNLM, IDS. **CCC.**

Published by: Elsevier Science Ltd., Elsevier Trends Journals, 68 Hills Rd, Cambridge CB2 1LA, United Kingdom. TEL 44-1223-315961, FAX 44-1223-464460, TIG@elsevier.co.uk, http://www.elsevier.com/locate/issn/01689525. Eds. J Alfred, M Thorne. Pub. Peter Desmond. Adv. contact Thelma Reid. **Subscr. in Australasia and the Far East to:** Elsevier Science (Singapore) Pte Ltd, No.1 Temasek Ave, 17-01 Millenia Tower, Singapore 039192, Singapore. TEL 65-434-3727, FAX 65-337-2230; **Subscr. in the Americas to:** Elsevier Science, PO Box 945, New York, NY 10159-0945. TEL 212-633-3730, FAX 212-633-3680; **Subscr. to:** Elsevier Current Trends Subscriptions, PO Box 331, Haywards Heath, W Sussex RH16 3FG, United Kingdom. TEL 44-1444-475650, FAX 44-1444-445423.

TRENDS IN MICROBIOLOGY. see *BIOLOGY—Microbiology*

TRISOMY 21; an international, multidisciplinary journal of Downs Syndrome. see *MEDICAL SCIENCES—Psychiatry And Neurology*

576.5 UKR ISSN 0564-3783
CODEN: TGANAK

TSITOLOGIYA I GENETIKA; mezhdunarodnyi nauchnyi zhurnal. Text in Ukrainian. 1965. bi-m. USD 209 (effective 2001).
Related titles: ♦ English Translation: Cytology and Genetics. ISSN 0095-4527.
Indexed: AgBiotech, Anim.Breed.Abstr., Aqua.Sci.& Fish.Abstr., Aquacult.Abstr., Bio-Contr.News & Info., Biol.Abstr., Chem.Abstr., Chem.Indus.Notes, Chem.Titles, Cott.& Trop.Fibr.Abstr., Crop Physiol.Abstr., Curr.Adv.Ecol.Sci., Dent.Ind., Environ.Sci.Poll.Mgmt., Excerp.Med., Field Crop Abstr., Forest.Abstr., Herb.Abstr., Hort.Abstr., INIS Atomind., Ind.Med (1967-), Int.Aerosp.Abstr., Maize Abstr., Pig News & Info., Plant Breed.Abstr., Plant Gen.Res.Abstr., Plant Grow.Reg.Abstr., Potato Abstr., Poult.Abstr., Rev.Arom.& Med.Plants, Rev.Med.& Vet.Mycol., Rev.Plant Path., Seed Abstr., Sorghum & Millets Abstr., Soyabean Abstr., Triticale Abstr., Weed Abstr., Zoo.Rec.
—BLDSC (0397.030000), CASDDS, CISTI, East View, EMDOCS, GNLM, Infotrieve, Linda Hall. **CCC.**
Published by: Natsional'na Akademiya Nauk Ukrainy, Institut Klitynnoi Biologii ta Genetychnoi Inzhenerii, Vul Akad Zabolotnogo 148, Kiev 252143, Ukraine. TEL 380-44-2667109, cytogen@iicb.kiev.ua, glazko@biotech.kiev.ua. Ed. Yu. Yu. Gleba. **Co-sponsor:** Ukrainska Akademiya Agrarnykh Nauk, Institut Agroecologii i Biotechnologii.

599.9 AUS ISSN 1369-0523
CODEN: TWREFP

TWIN RESEARCH. Text in English. 1998. q. AUD 384 in Australia & New Zealand to institutions; AUD 480 elsewhere to institutions (effective 2001); Includes online access.. adv. back issues avail. **Document type:** *Academic/Scholarly.*
Related titles: Online - full text ed.: (from EBSCO Publishing, O C L C Online Computer Library Center, Inc., RoweCom Information Quest, ingenta, CatchWord Ltd., Swets Blackwell).
Indexed: Ind.Med. (1998-).
—BLDSC (9076.957150). **CCC.**
Published by: (International Society for Twin Studies), Australian Academic Press Pty. Ltd., 32 Jeays St, Bowen Hills, QLD 4006, Australia. TEL 61-7-32571176, FAX 61-7-32525908, australianacademicpress@compuserve.com, http://www.australianacademicpress.com.au/Publications/TR/TR.html. Ed. Nick Martin TEL 61-7-3362-0278.

576.5 SVK

UNIVERZITA KOMENSKEHO. PEDAGOGICKA FAKULTA V TRNAVE. PRIRODNE VEDY: BIOLOGIA-GENETIKA. Text in Slovak. irreg. (approx. a.). price varies.
Published by: Univerzita Komenskeho, Pedagogicka Fakulta v Trnave, c/o Study and Information Center, Safarikova nam 6, Bratislava 81806, Slovakia.

VIRUS GENES. see *BIOLOGY—Microbiology*

599.935 CHN ISSN 0253-9772
QH426 CODEN: ICHUDW

YICHUAN/HEREDITAS. Text in Chinese. 1972. bi-m. USD 78 (effective 2000). adv. bk.rev. **Document type:** *Academic/Scholarly.* **Description:** Contains research reports, breeding work based on genetic theories, information on study results in stages, exchange of teaching instructions, and stories and news tidbits on personalities.
Indexed: AgBiotech, Anim.Breed.Abstr., Chem.Abstr., Chem.Indus.Notes, Chem.Titles, Helminthol.Abstr., Maize Abstr., Plant Breed.Abstr., Rev.Appl.Entomol., Rev.Plant Path., Rice Abstr., Seed Abstr., Soyabean Abstr., Triticale Abstr., Zoo.Rec.
—CASDDS, Linda Hall.
Published by: Kexue Chubanshe/Science Press, 16 Donghuang Cheng Genbei Jie, Beijing 100717, China. Circ: 31,000.

576.5 CHN ISSN 0379-4172
QH431 CODEN: ICHPCG

YICHUAN XUEBAO/ACTA GENETICA SINICA. Text in Chinese; Summaries in English. 1974. m. CNY 14 per issue domestic; USD 112 (effective 2000). adv. back issues avail. *Refereed.* **Document type:** *Academic/Scholarly.* **Description:** Covers genetics research in mainland China, including molecular genetics, genetic engineering, medical genetics, and genetics of plants, animals and microorganisms.
Indexed: Anim.Breed.Abstr., Biol.Abstr., Chem.Abstr., Chem.Indus.Notes, Cott.& Trop.Fibr.Abstr., Curr.Adv.Biochem., Curr.Adv.Gen.& Molec.Biol., Excerp.Med., Fababean Abstr., Field Crop Abstr., GeoRef, Helminthol.Abstr., Ind.Med. (1974-), Maize Abstr., Ornam.Hort., Pig News & Info., Plant Breed.Abstr., Plant Grow.Reg.Abstr., Poult.Abstr., Rice Abstr., Seed Abstr., Sorghum & Millets Abstr., Soyabean Abstr., Sport Fish.Abstr., Triticale Abstr., Zoo.Rec.
—CASDDS, CISTI, GNLM, Linda Hall.
Published by: (Yichuan Yanjiusuo), Kexue Chubanshe/Science Press, 16 Donghuang Cheng Genbei Jie, Beijing 100717, China. Ed. Li Huang Zhu. Circ: 16,000. **Co-sponsor:** Zhongguo Yichuan Xuehui.

ZHONGGUO YOUSHENG YOUYU/JOURNAL OF IMPROVING BIRTH OUTCOME AND CHILD DEVELOPMENT OF CHINA. see *BIRTH CONTROL*

616.042 CHN ISSN 1003-9406

ZHONGHUA YIXUE YICHUANXUE ZAZHI/CHINESE JOURNAL OF MEDICAL GENETICS. Text in Chinese. 1984. bi-m. USD 37.80; USD 6.30 newsstand/cover (effective 2001). **Document type:** *Academic/Scholarly.*
Formerly (until 1991): Yichuan yu Jibing / Heredity and Disease (1002-0756)
Indexed: Eng.Ind., Ind.Med.
—BLDSC (3180.425800).
Published by: Huaxi Yike Daxue/West China University of Medical Sciences, 17 Renmin Nanlu 3 Duan, Chengdu, Sichuan 610041, China. TEL 581130. Ed. Liu Zudong. **Dist. by:** China International Book Trading Corp, 35, Chegongzhuang Xilu, Haidian District, Beijing 100044, China. TEL 86-1-68413849, FAX 86-1-68412048, cibtc@mail.cibtc.com.cn, http://www.cibtc.com.cn.

576.5 GBR ISSN 0967-1994
QH491 CODEN: ZYGOEB

ZYGOTE; the biology of gametes and early embryos. Text in English. 1993. q. USD 248 to institutions (effective 2002). adv. bk.rev. back issues avail. *Refereed.* **Document type:** *Academic/Scholarly.* **Description:** Provides a multidisciplinary forum for reports on all aspects of early developmental biology. Concentrates on the programming of developmental information during gametogenesis, through its modification at fertilization to the integration of the maternal and embryonic genomes.
Related titles: Online - full text ed.: (from EBSCO Publishing, O C L C Online Computer Library Center, Inc., RoweCom Information Quest, Swets Blackwell, Institute for Scientific Information).
Indexed: ASCA, AgBiotech, Agricola, Anim.Breed.Abstr., Curr.Cont. (coverage dropped), Hort.Abstr., Ind.Med. (1993-), Inpharma, Ornam.Hort., Pig News & Info., Reac., Zoo.Rec.
—BLDSC (9538.885000), CASDDS, CISTI, GNLM, IDS, Infotrieve, ingenta, KNAW. **CCC.**
Published by: Cambridge University Press, Edinburgh Bldg, Shaftesbury Rd, Cambridge CB2 2RU, United Kingdom. FAX 44-1223-315052, information@cup.cam.ac.uk, information@cambridge.org, http://www.cup.cam.ac.uk, http://www.uk.cambridge.org/journals/pmu. Ed. Brian Dale. R&P Linda Nicol. Adv. contact Rebecca Symons.

BIOLOGY—Microbiology

579 USA ISSN 0044-7897
CODEN: ASMNBO

A S M NEWS (WASHINGTON). Text in English. 1935. m. USD 50 domestic to non-members; USD 50 in Canada to non-members; USD 50 in Europe to non-members; USD 54 in Latin America to non-members; USD 55 elsewhere to non-members (effective 2001); members free. adv. bk.rev. stat. index. back issues avail.; reprint service avail. from PQC. *Refereed.* **Document type:** *Trade.* **Description:** Provides information on a broad range of scientific and policy issues to microbiologists; letters; opinion pieces; meetings calendar; reports of legislative activity; and classified employment listings.
Related titles: Microform ed.: (from PQC); Online - full text ed.: (from Institute for Scientific Information).
Indexed: Biodet.Abstr., Biol.Abstr., Biotech.Cit.Ind., CAD CAM Abstr., Environ.Abstr., Environ.Sci.Poll.Mgmt., Ind.Med. (coverage dropped), Ind.Vet., Microbiol.Abstr., Poult.Abstr., Rev.Med.& Vet.Mycol., SSCI (coverage dropped), Telegen, Virol.Abstr. (coverage dropped).
—BLDSC (1745.171000), CISTI, IDS. **CCC.**
Published by: American Society for Microbiology, 1325 Massachusetts Ave, N W, Washington, DC 20005-4171. TEL 202-737-3600, 800-633-4931, Asmnews@asmusa.org, subscriptions@asmusa.org, http://www.asmusa.org. Ed. Michael I Goldberg. Circ: 42,000. **Subscr. to:** PO Box 11127, Birmingham, AL 35201-1127.

579.2 USA
QR383

A T C C ANIMAL VIRUSES AND ANTISERA, CHLAMYDIAE, AND RICKETTSIAE. Text in English. 1975. irreg., latest vol.7, 1996. USD 36 in North America; USD 48 elsewhere. **Document type:** *Catalog.*
Formerly: A T C C Catalogue of Animal Viruses and Antisera, Chlamydiae, and Rickettsiae (1057-6495); Which supersedes in part (in 1990): American Type Culture Collection. Catalogue of Animal and Plant Viruses, Chlamydiae, Rickettsiae and Virus Antisera (0898-4182); Which supersedes in part (in 1986): American Type Culture Collection. Catalogue of Strains 2: Animal Cell Lines, Animal Viruses, Bacterial Viruses, Mycoviruses, Plant Viruses, Rickettsiae, Chlamydiae (0363-2989)
—CISTI, Infotrieve. **CCC.**
Published by: American Type Culture Collection, 10801 University Blvd, Manassas, VA 20110. TEL 800-638-6597, FAX 301-816-4361, sales@atcc.org. Eds. C Buck, G Paulino.

579.3 USA

A T C C BACTERIA & BACTERIOPHAGES. Text in English. 1985. irreg., latest vol.19, 1996. USD 45 in North America; USD 55 elsewhere. **Document type:** *Catalog.*
Formerly: A T C C Catalogue of Bacteria and Bacteriophages (1050-8120); Which supersedes in part: American Type Culture Collection. Catalogue of Strains 1
Published by: American Type Culture Collection, 10801 University Blvd, Manassas, VA 20110. TEL 800-638-6597, FAX 301-816-4361, sales@atcc.org.

579.2 USA

A T C C CATALOGUE OF PLANT VIRUSES AND ANTISERA. Text in English. 1975. irreg., latest vol.7, 1993. USD 5. **Document type:** *Catalog.*
Supersedes in part (in 1990): American Type Culture Collection. Catalogue of Animal and Plant Viruses, Chlamydiae, Rickettsiae and Virus Antisera (0898-4182); Which supersedes in part (in 1986): American Type Culture Collection. Catalogue of Strains 2: Animal Cell Lines, Animal Viruses, Bacterial Viruses, Mycoviruses, Plant Viruses. Rickettsiae, Chlamydiae (0363-2989)
—CISTI, Infotrieve. **CCC.**
Published by: American Type Culture Collection, 10801 University Blvd, Manassas, VA 20110. TEL 800-638-6597, FAX 301-816-4361, Sales@ATCC.org.

579.2 USA

A T C C CATALOGUE OF PROTISTS. ALGAE - PROTOZOA. Text in English. 1985. irreg., latest vol.18, 1993. USD 5. **Document type:** *Catalog.*
Published by: American Type Culture Collection, 10801 University Blvd, Manassas, VA 20110. TEL 800-638-6597, FAX 301-816-4361, Sales@ATCC.org. Ed. T A Nerad.

B

579.2 USA

A T C C CONNECTION. Text in English. 1981. q. free per issue. **Document type:** *Newsletter.* **Description:** Characterization, preservation, and use of biological cultures.
Former titles: A T C C Quarterly Newsletter (0894-9026); (until 1985): American Type Culture Collection. Quarterly Newsletter (0743-4758)
Indexed: Telegen.
—CCC.
Published by: American Type Culture Collection, 10801 University Blvd, Manassas, VA 20110. TEL 800-638-6597, FAX 301-816-4361, news@atcc.org. Ed. E M Brown. Circ: 18,500.

A T C C FILAMENTOUS FUNGI. see *BIOLOGY—Botany*

A T C C YEASTS. see *BIOLOGY—Botany*

B

579 YUG ISSN 0581-1538
QR1 CODEN: MIKJAT

ACTA BIOLOGICA IUGOSLAVICA. SERIJA B: MIKROBIOLOGIJA✱. Text in Serbo-Croatian. 1964. s-a. price varies. back issues avail. **Document type:** *Academic/Scholarly.*
Indexed: Abstr.Hyg., Agri.& Environ.Biotech.Abstr. (coverage dropped), Aqua.Sci.& Fish.Abstr., Biol.Abstr., Chem.Abstr., Dairy Sci.Abstr., Environ.Sci.Poll.Mgmt., Excerp.Med., Hort.Abstr., Ind.Med. (coverage dropped), Ind.Vet., Microbiol.Abstr., Nutr.Abstr., Rev.Appl.Entomol., Soils & Fert., Trop.Dis.Bull., Vet.Bull.
—BLDSC (5761.630000), CASDDS, CISTI, Linda Hall.
Published by: Unija Bioloskih Naucnih Drustava Jugoslavije/Yugoslav Union of Biological Sciences, Kneza Milosa 101-111, Belgrade 11000, Yugoslavia. TEL 381-11-615315, pedja@bf.bio.bf.ac.yu. Ed. Dr. Vitko Soric.

579 HUN ISSN 1217-8950
QR1 CODEN: AMIHEF

ACTA MICROBIOLOGICA ET IMMUNOLOGICA HUNGARICA. Text in English. 1954. q. USD 198 (effective 2002). adv. bk.rev. bibl, charts, illus, abstr. index. 120 p./no. back issues avail. **Document type:** *Journal, Academic/Scholarly.* **Description:** Publishes research on medical and veterinary bacteriology, bacterial genetics, virology, mycology, parasitology. Includes immunology and epidemiology, agricultural and industrial microbiology.
Former titles (until 1994): Acta Microbiologica Hungarica (0231-4622); (until 1982): Academiae Scientiarum Hungaricae. Acta Microbiologica (0001-6187)
Related titles: Online - full text ed.
Indexed: ASCA, Abstr.Hyg., Aqua.Sci.& Fish.Abstr., Aquacult.Abstr., Bio-Contr.News & Info., Biol.Abstr., CEABA, Chem.Abstr., Chem.Indus.Notes, Chem.Titles, Crop Physiol.Abstr., Curr.Adv.Ecol.Sci., Curr.Biotech.Abstr., Curr.Cont. (coverage dropped), Dairy Sci.Abstr., Dent.Ind., Derwent Biotech.Abstr., Environ.Sci.Poll.Mgmt., Excerp.Med., Field Crop Abstr., Helminthol.Abstr., Hort.Abstr., INIS Atomind., Ind.Med. (1994-), Ind.Sci.Rev., Ind.Vet., NPU, Pig News & Info., Plant Grow.Reg.Abstr., Postharvest, Rev.Appl.Entomol., Rev.Med.& Vet.Mycol., Rev.Plant Path., Sci.Cit.Ind. (coverage dropped), Soils & Fert., Soyabean Abstr., Triticale Abstr., Trop.Dis.Bull., Vet.Bull., Weed Abstr.
—BLDSC (0637.978000), CASDDS, CISTI, GNLM, Infotrieve, ingenta, KNAW, Linda Hall. **CCC.**
Published by: (Magyar Tudomanyos Akademia, Semmelweis University, Institute of Medical Microbiology), Akademiai Kiado Rt., PO Box 245, Budapest 1519, Hungary. TEL 36-1-4648233, FAX 36-1-4648297, journals@akkrt.hu, http://www.akkrt.hu. Ed. Istvan Nasz.

579 POL ISSN 0137-1320
CODEN: AMPOAX

ACTA MICROBIOLOGICA POLONICA. Text and summaries in English. 1952. q., latest vol.50, 2001. PLZ 50 domestic; USD 140 foreign (effective 2002). bk.rev. charts, illus. index. 100 p./no. 1 cols./p. reprints avail. **Document type:** *Journal, Academic/Scholarly.*
Formed by the 1976 merger of: Acta Microbiologica Polonica. Series A: Microbiologica Generalis (0567-7815); Acta Microbiologica Polonica. Series B: Microbiologica Applicata (0567-7823); Which both superseded (in 1969): Acta Microbiologica Polonica (0001-6195)
Related titles: Online - full text ed.
Indexed: ASCA, Abstr.Hyg., AgBiotech, Agri.& Environ.Biotech.Abstr. (coverage dropped), AgroAgen, AgroLibrex, Aqua.Sci.& Fish.Abstr., Bio-Contr.News & Info., Biodet.Abstr., Biol.Abstr., CEABA, Chem.Abstr., Chem.Indus.Notes, Chem.Titles, Curr.Adv.Ecol.Sci., Curr.Biotech.Abstr., Curr.Cont. (coverage dropped), Dairy Sci.Abstr., Derwent Biotech.Abstr., Environ.Sci.Poll.Mgmt., Excerp.Med., Field Crop Abstr., Food Sci.& Tech.Abstr., Helminthol.Abstr., Herb.Abstr., Hort.Abstr., INIS Atomind., Ind.Med. (1976-), Ind.Sci.Rev., Ind.Vet., Maize Abstr., Microbiol.Abstr., Pig News & Info., Plant Breed.Abstr., Pollut.Abstr., Poult.Abstr., Rev.Appl.Entomol., Rev.Med.& Vet.Mycol., Rev.Plant Path., Rural Recreat.Tour.Abstr., Sci.Cit.Ind. (coverage dropped), Seed Abstr., Sel.Water Res.Abstr., Soils & Fert., Sugar Ind.Abstr., Triticale Abstr., Vet.Bull., Weed Abstr., World Ag.Econ.& Rur.Soc.Abstr.
—BLDSC (0638.000000), CASDDS, CISTI, GNLM, IDS, ingenta, KNAW, Linda Hall.
Published by: Polskie Towarzystwo Mikrobiologow/Polish Society of Microbiologists, Ul Chocimska 24, Warsaw 00791, Poland. TEL 48-22-5421400, FAX 48-22-5541302, pzh@medstat.waw.pl, http://www.microbiology.pl/amp. Ed., Adv. contact Krystyna I Wolska. Circ: 750. **Dist. by:** Ars Polona, Krakowskie Przedmiescie 7, Warsaw, Poland. TEL 48-22-8261201.

579.65 POL ISSN 1230-2821
QL757 CODEN: ACTPEO

ACTA PARASITOLOGICA. Text and summaries in English. 1953. q. USD 150 (effective 2000). adv. bk.rev. bibl, illus. index. *Refereed.* **Document type:** *Academic/Scholarly.* **Description:** Presents original papers and research reports on theoretical and practical questions on parasitologic research.
Formerly (until vol.37, 1992): Acta Parasitologica Polonica (0065-1478)
Related titles: Online - full text ed.: (from Institute for Scientific Information).
Indexed: Abstr.Hyg., AgBiotech, AgroAgen, AgroLibrex, Anim.Breed.Abstr., Bio-Contr.News & Info., Biol.Abstr., Chem.Abstr., Chem.Indus.Notes, Chem.Titles, Curr.Adv.Ecol.Sci., Curr.Cont., Excerp.Med., Helminthol.Abstr., INIS Atomind., Ind.Vet., Int.Abstr.Biol.Sci., Key Word Ind.Wildl.Res., Pig News & Info., Poult.Abstr., Protozool.Abstr., Rev.Appl.Entomol., Rev.Med.& Vet.Mycol., Sport Fish.Abstr., Trop.Dis.Bull., Vet.Bull., Zoo.Rec.
—BLDSC (0643.300000), CASDDS, CISTI, GNLM, IDS, ingenta, KNAW.
Published by: Polska Akademia Nauk, Instytut Parazytologii im. Witolda Stefanskiego/Polish Academy of Sciences, Witold Stefanski Institute of Parasitology, Ul Twarda 51-55, Warsaw 00818, Poland. TEL 48-22-6206226, FAX 48-22-6206227, actapar@twarda.pan.pl, http://www.ipar.pan.pl/acta. Ed., R&P Katarzyna Niewiadomska. Adv. contact Anna Pucilowska. Circ: 350. **Dist. by:** Ars Polona, Krakowskie Przedmiescie 7, Warsaw, Poland.

579.4 POL ISSN 0065-1583
CODEN: ACPZAU

ACTA PROTOZOOLOGICA. Text in English. 1963. q. USD 200 (effective 2002). illus. reprint service avail. from ISI. *Refereed.* **Document type:** *Journal, Academic/Scholarly.*
Related titles: Online - full text ed.: (from Institute for Scientific Information).
Indexed: ASCA, Abstr.Hyg., AgroAgen, AgroLibrex, Aqua.Sci.& Fish.Abstr., Bio-Contr.News & Info., Biol.Abstr., Chem.Abstr., Chem.Indus.Notes, Chem.Titles, Curr.Adv.Ecol.Sci., Curr.Cont., Deep Sea Res.& Oceanogr.Abstr., Entomol.Abstr., Environ.Sci.Poll.Mgmt., Excerp.Med., GeoRef, Helminthol.Abstr., INIS Atomind., Ind.Sci.Rev., Ind.Vet., Int.Abstr.Biol.Sci., Microbiol.Abstr., Postharvest, Protozool.Abstr., Ref.Zh., Rev.Appl.Entomol., Rev.Med.& Vet.Mycol., Sci.Cit.Ind., Soils & Fert., Trop.Dis.Bull., Vet.Bull., Zoo.Rec.
—BLDSC (0661.370000), CASDDS, CISTI, EMDOCS, IDS, ingenta, Linda Hall.
Published by: Polska Akademia Nauk, Instytut Biologii Doswiadczalnej im. M. Nenckiego/Polish Academy of Sciences, M. Nencki Institute of Experimental Biology, Ul Pasteura 3, Warsaw 02093, Poland. TEL 48-22-659-8571, FAX 48-22-8225342, jurek@nencki.gov.pl, http://www.nencki.gov.pl/public.htm. Ed., R&P Jerzy Sikora. Circ: 460. **Dist. by:** Ars Polona, Krakowskie Przedmiescie 7, Warsaw, Poland.

579.2 SVK ISSN 0001-723X
CODEN: AVIRA2

ACTA VIROLOGICA; international journal. Text and summaries in English. 1957. bi-m. USD 198 (effective 2001 - 2002). bk.rev. charts, illus. index. *Refereed.* **Document type:** *Academic/Scholarly.* **Description:** Devoted to original experimental papers in all fields of general virology and molecular biology of viruses, as well as of human and veterinary virology and rickettsiology.
Related titles: Online - full text ed.: (from Institute for Scientific Information).
Indexed: AIDS & Cancer Res., ASCA, Abstr.Hyg., AgBiotech, Agri.& Environ.Biotech.Abstr. (coverage dropped), Aqua.Sci.& Fish.Abstr., Bio-Contr.News & Info., Biol.Abstr., Chem.Abstr., Chem.Indus.Notes, Chem.Titles, Crop Physiol.Abstr., Curr.Adv.Ecol.Sci., Curr.Cont., Dairy Sci.Abstr., Dent.Ind., Derwent Biotech.Abstr., Excerp.Med., INIS Atomind., Ind.Med. (1957-), Ind.Sci.Rev., Ind.Vet., Inpharma, Int.Abstr.Biol.Sci., Microbiol.Abstr., Pharm.&Out.News, Pig News & Info., Potato Abstr., Poult.Abstr., Protozool.Abstr., Reac., Rev.Appl.Entomol., Rev.Med.& Vet.Mycol., Rev.Plant Path., Rice Abstr., Sci.Cit.Ind., Seed Abstr., Sport Fish.Abstr., Telegen, Trop.Dis.Bull., Vet.Bull., Virol.Abstr., Weed Abstr., Wild.Rev., Zoo.Rec.
—BLDSC (0671.500000), CASDDS, CISTI, EMDOCS, GNLM, IDS, ingenta, KNAW. **CCC.**
Published by: (Slovak Academy of Sciences, Institute of Virology), Slovak Academic Press Ltd., Nam Slobody 6, PO Box 57, Bratislava 81005, Slovakia. viruacta@savba.savba.sk, http://www.europe.idealibrary.com/. Ed. J Zemla. Circ: 1,200.

579.37 ITA
QR82.A35 CODEN: ACTID2

ACTINOMYCETES (ONLINE EDITION). Text in Italian. 1965. 3/yr. USD 20 to individuals; USD 60 to institutions (effective 1997). adv. bk.rev. illus. back issues avail. **Document type:** *Newspaper.*
Former titles (until 1999): Actinomycetes (Print Edition) (0732-0574); Biology of the Actinomycetes and Related Organisms; Nocardial Biology
Media: Online - full content.
Indexed: Bio-Contr.News & Info., Biol.Abstr., Chem.Abstr., Rev.Med.& Vet.Mycol., Rev.Plant Path.
—CASDDS, CISTI.
Published by: Centro per l'Ecologia Teorica e Applicata, Via Vittorio Veneto, 19, Gorizia, GO 34170, Italy. TEL 39-481-536466, FAX 39-432-536470, bio@biostrat.demon.co.uk, http://bioline.bdt.org.br/ac. Ed. Romano Locci. Adv. contact Fulvio Bisani. Circ: 250. **Subscr. to:** Prof. R. Locci, c/o Chair of Mycology, University of Udine, Aera Rizzi, Via Delle Scienze, 208, Udine, UD 33100, Italy. **Co-sponsor:** Dipartimento Biologia Applicata alla Difesa delle Pianti.

579 USA ISSN 0065-2164
QR1 CODEN: ADAMAP

ADVANCES IN APPLIED MICROBIOLOGY. Text in English. 1959. irreg., latest vol.46, 1997. index. reprint service avail. from ISI. *Refereed.*
Related titles: Online - full text ed.: (from Institute for Scientific Information).
Indexed: ASCA, Aqua.Sci.& Fish.Abstr., Biol.& Agr.Ind. (Jan.1983-), Biol.Abstr., Biotech.Cit.Ind., CEABA, Chem.Abstr., Chem.Indus.Notes, Chem.Titles, Curr.Adv.Ecol.Sci., Curr.Biotech.Abstr., Dairy Sci.Abstr., Deep Sea Res.& Oceanogr.Abstr., Derwent Biotech.Abstr., Eng.Ind., Environ.Sci.Poll.Mgmt., Excerp.Med., Food Sci.& Tech.Abstr., Ind.Med. (1959-), Ind.Sci.Rev., Ind.Vet., Int.Abstr.Biol.Sci., Plant Breed.Abstr., Pollut.Abstr., Rev.Appl.Entomol., Sci.Cit.Ind., Telegen, Vet.Bull., Weed Abstr., World Ag.Econ.& Rur.Soc.Abstr.
—BLDSC (0699.100000), CASDDS, CISTI, Ei, EMDOCS, GNLM, ingenta, Linda Hall. **CCC.**
Published by: Academic Press, Inc., Journal Division (Subsidiary of: Harcourt Brace & Company), 525 B St, Ste 1900, San Diego, CA 92101-4495. TEL 619-231-0926, FAX 619-699-6715. Ed. Wayne W Umbreit. **Subscr. to:** Order Dept., 6277 Sea Harbor Dr, 4th Fl, Orlando, FL 32887. TEL 800-321-5068.

579.17 USA ISSN 0147-4863
QR100 CODEN: AMIED5

ADVANCES IN MICROBIAL ECOLOGY. Text in English. 1977. irreg., latest vol.16. price varies. *Refereed.* **Document type:** *Monographic series.*
Related titles: Online - full text ed.: (from Institute for Scientific Information).
Indexed: ASCA, Agricola, Appl.Ecol.Abstr., Aqua.Sci.& Fish.Abstr., Chem.Abstr., Chem.Indus.Notes, Chem.Titles, Curr.Adv.Ecol.Sci., Deep Sea Res.& Oceanogr.Abstr., Environ.Sci.Poll.Mgmt., Genet.Abstr., GeoRef, Hum.Gen.Abstr., Ind.Sci.Rev., Microbiol.Abstr., Nutr.Abstr., Rev.Plant Path., Sci.Cit.Ind., Soils & Fert., Vet.Bull.

—BLDSC (0709.415000), CASDDS, CISTI, ingenta, KNAW, Linda Hall. **CCC.**
Published by: Kluwer Academic - Plenum Publishers (Subsidiary of: Wolters Kluwer N.V.), 233 Spring St, New York, NY 10013-1578. TEL 212-620-8000, 800-221-9369, FAX 212-463-0742, info@plenum.com, http://www.plenum.com. Eds. K C Marshall, M Alaxander.

579 USA ISSN 0065-2911
QR84 CODEN: AMIPB2
ADVANCES IN MICROBIAL PHYSIOLOGY. Text in English. 1967. irreg., latest vol.39, 1997. reprint service avail. from ISI. *Refereed.* **Document type:** *Monographic series.*
Related titles: Online - full text ed.: (from Institute for Scientific Information).
Indexed: ASCA, Abstr.Hyg., Aqua.Sci.& Fish.Abstr., BBCI, Biol.& Agr.Ind. (Jan.1996-), Biol.Abstr., Chem.Abstr., Chem.Indus.Notes, Chem.Titles, Curr.Adv.Ecol.Sci., Deep Sea Res.& Oceanogr.Abstr., Environ.Sci.Poll.Mgmt., Excerp.Med., Ind.Med. (1967-), Ind.Sci.Rev., Int.Abstr.Biol.Sci., Microbiol.Abstr., Rev.Med.& Vet.Mycol., Sci.Cit.Ind., Trop.Dis.Bull.
—BLDSC (0709.420000), CASDDS, CISTI, GNLM, ingenta, KNAW, Linda Hall. **CCC.**
Published by: Academic Press, Inc., Journal Division (Subsidiary of: Harcourt Brace & Company), 525 B St, Ste 1900, San Diego, CA 92101-4495. TEL 619-231-0926, FAX 619-699-6715. Eds. A H Rose, J F Wilkinson. **Subscr. to:** Order Dept., 6277 Sea Harbor Dr, 4th Fl, Orlando, FL 32887. TEL 800-321-5068.

579.2 USA ISSN 0065-3527
QR360 CODEN: AVREA8
ADVANCES IN VIRUS RESEARCH. Text in English. 1953. irreg., latest vol.50, 1998. index. reprint service avail. from ISI. *Refereed.*
Related titles: Online - full text ed.: (from Institute for Scientific Information).
Indexed: AIDS & Cancer Res., ASCA, Abstr.Hyg., Biol.Abstr., Biotech.& Bioeng.Abstr., Chem.Abstr., Chem.Indus.Notes, Chem.Titles, Curr.Adv.Ecol.Sci., Environ.Sci.Poll.Mgmt., Excerp.Med., Forest.Abstr., Hort.Abstr., Ind.Med. (1953-), Ind.Sci.Rev., Ind.Vet., Microbiol.Abstr., Neurosci.Abstr., Pollut.Abstr., Rev.Appl.Entomol., Rev.Plant Path., Sci.Cit.Ind., Trop.Dis.Bull., Vet.Bull., Virol.Abstr.
—BLDSC (0712.000000), CASDDS, CISTI, GNLM, ingenta, Linda Hall. **CCC.**
Published by: Academic Press, Inc., Journal Division (Subsidiary of: Harcourt Brace & Company), 525 B St, Ste 1900, San Diego, CA 92101-4495. TEL 619-231-0926, FAX 619-699-6715. **Subscr. to:** Order Dept., 6277 Sea Harbor Dr, 4th Fl, Orlando, FL 32887. TEL 800-321-5068.

579 ITA ISSN 1121-9750
CODEN: AAMJEP
ALPE ADRIA MICROBIOLOGY JOURNAL. Abbreviated title: A A M J. Text in Italian. 1992. q. DEM 60 to individuals; DEM 150 to institutions (effective 1999). adv. abstr. *Refereed.* **Document type:** *Academic/Scholarly.* **Description:** Publishes review articles, original papers, correspondence, and congress proceedings in the field of pathogenesis of infections, diagnostic microbiology, epidemiology of infectious diseases, and mechanisms of action of antimicrobial agents.
Indexed: Chem.Abstr., Chem.Indus.Notes, Chem.Titles, Environ.Sci.Poll.Mgmt., Excerp.Med. (1994-), Helminthol.Abstr., Ind.Vet., Int.Abstr.Biol.Sci., Microbiol.Abstr., Rev.Appl.Entomol., Rev.Med.& Vet.Mycol., Zoo.Rec.
—BLDSC (0801.953000), CASDDS, EMDOCS, GNLM.
Published by: (Associazione Microbiologici Clinici Italiani), Biomedia s.r.l., Via Carlo Farini, 70, Milan, MI 20159, Italy. TEL 39-2-69001316, FAX 39-2-69001311, giuseppe.botta@drmm.uniud.it, http://www.mf.uni.lj.si/~gubina/aamj.html. Ed. Bela Lanyi. Circ: 2,500.

AMERICAN SOCIETY FOR MICROBIOLOGY. ABSTRACTS OF THE GENERAL MEETING. see *BIOLOGY—Abstracting, Bibliographies, Statistics*

579.3149 GBR ISSN 1075-9964
QH518.5 CODEN: ANAEF8
ANAEROBE. Text in English. 1995. bi-m. GBP 225 to institutions (effective 2001). reprint service avail. from SWZ. *Refereed.* **Document type:** *Academic/Scholarly.* **Description:** Focuses on studies pertaining to obligate and facultative anaerobes. Seeks to foster communication among a variety of disciplines.
Related titles: Online - full text ed.: (from EBSCO Publishing, O C L C Online Computer Library Center, Inc., RoweCom Information Quest, ingenta, Swets Blackwell, IDEAL Online Library, Institute for Scientific Information).
Indexed: ASCA, AgBiotech, Chem.Abstr., Chem.Indus.Notes, Chem.Titles, Curr.Cont., Excerp.Med. (1996-), Inpharma, Int.Abstr.Biol.Sci., Nutr.Abstr., Pharm.&Out.News, Protozool.Abstr., Reac., Ref.Zh., Sci.Cit.Ind.
—BLDSC (0859.882000), ADONIS, CASDDS, CISTI, EMDOCS, GNLM, IDS, Infotrieve. **CCC.**
Published by: Academic Press (Subsidiary of: Harcourt Publishers Ltd.), 24 Oval Rd, London NW1 7DX, United Kingdom. TEL 44-20-7482-2893, FAX 44-20-7267-0362, apsubs@acad.com, http://www.academicpress.com/anaerobe. Ed. Larry Barton. **Subscr. to:** Harcourt Publishers Ltd., Foots Cray High St, Sidcup, Kent DA14 5HP, United Kingdom. TEL 44-20-8300-3322, FAX 44-20-8309-0807.

579 JPN
ANNUAL REVIEW MEN'EKI/ANNUAL REVIEW. IMMUNITY. Text in Japanese. 1988. a. JPY 8,925 (effective 1998). adv. **Document type:** *Academic/Scholarly.*
Published by: Chugai Igakusha, 62 Yarai-cho, Shinjuku-ku, Tokyo 162-0805, Japan. R&P M Takahashi. Adv. contact M. Takahashi.

579 USA ISSN 0066-4227
QR1 CODEN: ARMIAZ
ANNUAL REVIEW OF MICROBIOLOGY. Text in English. 1947. a. USD 60 domestic to individuals; USD 65 foreign to individuals; USD 120 domestic to institutions; USD 130 foreign to institutions (effective 1999). adv. bibl, charts. index, cum.index. back issues avail.; reprints avail. *Refereed.* **Document type:** *Academic/Scholarly.* **Description:** Reviews filter and synthesize primary research to identify the principal contributions in microbiology.
Related titles: Microfilm ed.: (from PQC); Online - full text ed.: (from Gale Group, HighWire Pr., Northern Light Technology, Inc., EBSCO Publishing, H. W. Wilson, Factiva, Institute for Scientific Information).
Indexed: AESIS, ASCA, Abstr.Bull.Inst.Pap.Chem., Abstr.Hyg., Agri.& Environ.Biotech.Abstr. (coverage dropped), Amer.Bibl.Slavic & E.Eur.Stud., Aqua.Sci.& Fish.Abstr., Biodet.Abstr., Biol.& Agr.Ind. (Jan.1989-), Biol.Abstr., Biol.Dig., CEABA, Chem.Abstr., Chem.Indus.Notes, Chem.Titles, Curr.Adv.Ecol.Sci., Curr.Biotech.Abstr., Curr.Cont., Dairy Sci.Abstr., Deep Sea Res.& Oceanogr.Abstr., Derwent Biotech.Abstr., Diar.Dis.Res., Environ.Sci.Poll.Mgmt., Excerp.Med., Food Sci.& Tech.Abstr., Forest Prod.Abstr., Forest.Abstr., Gen.Sci.Ind. (Jun.1992-), Helminthol.Abstr., INIS Atomind., Ind.Med. (1947-), Ind.Sci.Rev., Ind.Vet., Inpharma, Int.Abstr.Biol.Sci., Media Rev.Dig., Microbiol.Abstr., Nutr.Abstr., Plant Breed.Abstr., Protozool.Abstr., Reac., Rev.Appl.Entomol., Rev.Med.& Vet.Mycol., Rev.Plant Path., Rice Abstr., Sci.Cit.Ind., Soils & Fert., Sugar Ind.Abstr., THA, Trop.Dis.Bull., VITIS, Vet.Bull., Virol.Abstr. (coverage dropped), Zoo.Rec.
—BLDSC (1523.000000), ADONIS, CASDDS, CINDOC, CISTI, EMDOCS, GNLM, IDS, ingenta, KNAW, Linda Hall. **CCC.**
Published by: Annual Reviews Inc., 4139 El Camino Way, Box 10139, Palo Alto, CA 94303-0139. TEL 650-493-4400, 800-523-8635, FAX 650-424-0910, service@annurev.org; orders@allenpress.com, http://www.annualreviews.org. Ed. Samuel Gubins. R&P, Adv. contact Swati Aneja TEL 650-843-6634. **Subscr.to:** Allen Press Inc., PO Box 1897, Lawrence, KS 66044-8897.

579 USA ISSN 0066-4804
RM265 CODEN: AACHAX
ANTIMICROBIAL AGENTS AND CHEMOTHERAPY. Text in English. 1972. m. USD 325 domestic to non-members; USD 348 in Canada to non-members; USD 380 in Europe to non-members; USD 384 in Latin America to non-members; USD 387 elsewhere to non-members; USD 55 domestic to members; USD 82 domestic to members Print & online eds.; USD 83 in Canada to members; USD 110 in Canada to members Print & online eds.; USD 98 in Europe to members; USD 125 in Europe to members Print & online eds.; USD 101 in Latin America to members; USD 128 in Latin America to members Print & online eds.; USD 113 elsewhere to members; USD 140 elsewhere to members Print & online eds. (effective 2001). adv. index. back issues avail.; reprint service avail. from PQC. *Refereed.* **Document type:** *Academic/Scholarly.* **Description:** Forum for new work relating to antimicrobial, antiviral, antiparasitic, and anticancer agents and chemotherapy.
Related titles: CD-ROM ed.; Microform ed.: (from PQC); Online - full text ed.: ISSN 1098-6596. USD 260 to non-members; USD 41 to members (effective 2001) (from HighWire Pr., EBSCO Publishing, Institute for Scientific Information).
Indexed: AIDS Abstr., ASCA, Abstr.Hyg., Abstr.Inter.Med., AgBiotech, Agri.& Environ.Biotech.Abstr. (coverage dropped), Biol.Abstr., Chem.Abstr., Chem.Cit.Ind., Chem.Indus.Notes, Chem.Titles, Curr.Adv.Cancer Res., Curr.Adv.Ecol.Sci., Curr.Adv.Gen.& Molec.Biol., Curr.Cont., Dairy Sci.Abstr., Dent.Ind., Derwent Biotech.Abstr., Diar.Dis.Res., Environ.Sci.Poll.Mgmt., Excerp.Med., Genet.Abstr. (coverage dropped), Helminthol.Abstr., Hum.Gen.Abstr., INIS Atomind., I.P.A., Ind.Med. (1972-), Ind.Sci.Rev., Ind.Vet., Inpharma, Jrnl.Watch Inf.Dis., Kidney, Med.& Pharm.Biotech.Abstr., Med.& Surg.Dermat., Microbiol.Abstr., Neurosci.Cit.Ind., Nuc.Acids Abstr., Nutr.Abstr., Pharm.&Out.News, Pig News & Info., Poult.Abstr., Protozool.Abstr., Reac., Rev.Appl.Entomol., Rev.Arom.& Med.Plants, Rev.Med.& Vet.Mycol., Rev.Plant Path., Sci.Cit.Ind., Small Anim.Abstr., Telegen, Trop.Dis.Bull., Vet.Bull., Virol.Abstr.
—BLDSC (1549.151000), CASDDS, CISTI, EMDOCS, GNLM, IDS, ingenta, KNAW, Linda Hall. **CCC.**
Published by: American Society for Microbiology, 1752 N St N W, Washington, DC 20036-2904. TEL 202-737-3600, 800-633-4931, FAX 202-942-9319, subscriptions@amsusa.org, http://journals.asm.org/, http://www.asmusa.org. Ed. George M Eliopoulos. Circ: 6,400 (paid).

579.2 NLD ISSN 0166-3542
CODEN: ARSRDR
ANTIVIRAL RESEARCH; a multidisciplinary journal of antiviral agents, natural host defence mechanisms, interferons and antiviral vaccines. Text in English. 1981. m. EUR 1,590 in Europe to institutions; JPY 211,200 in Japan to institutions; USD 1,779 elsewhere to institutions (effective 2002). adv. bk.rev. illus, abstr. index. back issues avail.; reprint service avail. from SWZ. *Refereed.* **Document type:** *Academic/Scholarly.* **Description:** Publishes full-length original articles, short definitive papers and review articles, pertaining to the effective control of virus infections in animals and hunans, as well as in plants or lower organisms.
Formerly: Journal of Antiviral Research
Related titles: Microform ed.: (from PQC); Online - full text ed.: (from ingenta, Swets Blackwell, ScienceDirect, Institute for Scientific Information).
Indexed: AIDS & Cancer Res., AIDS Abstr., ASCA, Abstr.Hyg., Biol.Abstr., Chem.Abstr., Chem.Indus.Notes, Chem.Titles, Curr.Adv.Ecol.Sci., Curr.Adv.Gen.& Molec.Biol., Curr.Cont., Dairy Sci.Abstr., Derwent Biotech.Abstr., Environ.Sci.Poll.Mgmt., Excerp.Med., Forest Prod.Abstr., Ind.Med. (1981-), Ind.Sci.Rev., Ind.Vet., Inpharma, Int.Abstr.Biol.Sci., Med.& Pharm.Biotech.Abstr., Microbiol.Abstr., Nutr.Abstr., Pharm.&Out.News, Pig News & Info., Potato Abstr., Poult.Abstr., Reac., Ref.Zh., Rev.Appl.Entomol., Rev.Arom.& Med.Plants, Rev.Med.& Vet.Mycol., Rev.Plant Path., Sci.Cit.Ind., Small Anim.Abstr., Vet.Bull., Virol.Abstr.
—BLDSC (1552.830000), ADONIS, CASDDS, CISTI, EMDOCS, GNLM, IDS, ingenta, Linda Hall. **CCC.**
Published by: (International Society for Antiviral Research), Elsevier Science BV, PO Box 211, Amsterdam 1000 AE, Netherlands. TEL 31-20-485-2911, FAX 31-20-485-2457, nlinfo-f@elsevier.nl, http://www.elsevier.com/locate/antiviral. Eds. E de Clerq, R J Whitley. **Subscr. in Australasia and the Far East to:** Elsevier Science (Singapore) Pte Ltd, No.1 Temasek Ave, 17-01 Millenia Tower, Singapore 039192, Singapore. TEL 65-434-3727, FAX 65-337-2230; **Subscr. in Japan to:** Elsevier Science Inc - Japan Regional Office, 9-15 Higashi-Azabu 1-chome, Minato-ku, Tokyo 106-0044, Japan. TEL 81-3-5561-5033; **Subscr. in the Americas to:** Elsevier Science, PO Box 945, New York, NY 10159-0945. TEL 212-633-3730, FAX 212-633-3680.

ANTIVIRAL THERAPY. see *MEDICAL SCIENCES—Communicable Diseases*

ANTIVIRAL WEEKLY. see *MEDICAL SCIENCES—Allergology And Immunology*

ANTONIE VAN LEEUWENHOEK; international journal of general and molecular microbiology. see *BIOLOGY—Biotechnology*

579 USA ISSN 0099-2240
QR1 CODEN: AEMIDF
APPLIED AND ENVIRONMENTAL MICROBIOLOGY. Text in English. 1953. m. USD 421 domestic to non-members; USD 448 in Canada to non-members; USD 484 in Europe to non-members; USD 489 in Latin America to non-members; USD 503 elsewhere to non-members; USD 64 domestic to members; USD 95 domestic to members Print & online eds.; USD 98 in Canada to members; USD 129 in Canada to members Print & online eds.; USD 123 in Europe to members; USD 154 in Europe to members Print & online eds.; USD 136 in Latin America to members; USD 167 in Latin America to members Print & online eds.; USD 151 elsewhere to members; USD 182 elsewhere to members Print & online eds. (effective 2001). adv. bibl, charts, illus. index. back issues avail.; reprint service avail. from PQC. *Refereed.* **Document type:** *Academic/Scholarly.* **Description:** Addresses all aspects of applied and environmental microbiology, including biotechnology, food microbiology, industrial microbiology, and microbial ecology.
Formerly (until 1976): Applied Microbiology (0003-6919)
Related titles: Microform ed.: (from PQC); Online - full text ed.: ISSN 1098-5336. USD 337 to non-members (effective 2001) (from HighWire Pr., EBSCO Publishing, Gale Group, Factiva, Institute for Scientific Information).
Indexed: AESIS, ASCA, Abstr.Bull.Inst.Pap.Chem., Abstr.Hyg., AgBiotech, Agri.& Environ.Biotech.Abstr., Agri.Eng.Abstr., Agricola, Agroforest.Abstr., Appl.Ecol.Abstr., Aqua.Sci.& Fish.Abstr., Bibl.Agri., Bio-Contr.News & Info., Biodet.Abstr., Biol.& Agr.Ind. (Nov.1982-), Biol.Abstr., Biotech.Cit.Ind., CEABA, C.I.S. Abstr., Chem.Abstr., Chem.Cit.Ind., Chem.Indus.Notes, Chem.Titles, Comput.Dtbs., Crop Physiol.Abstr., Curr.Adv.Biochem., Curr.Adv.Ecol.Sci., Curr.Adv.Gen.& Molec.Biol., Curr.Biotech.Abstr., Curr.Cont., Curr.Pack.Abstr., Dairy Sci.Abstr., Dent.Ind., Derwent Biotech.Abstr., Diar.Dis.Res., E & P Hlth. (1993-), Ecol.Abstr., Energy Info.Abstr., Eng.Ind., Entomol.Abstr., Environ.Abstr., Environ.Per.Bibl. (1975-), Environ.Sci.Poll.Mgmt., Excerp.Med., Field Crop Abstr., Fluidex, Food Sci.& Tech.Abstr., Forest Prod.Abstr., Forest.Abstr., Gas Process.& Ppl. (1993-), Gen.Sci.Ind. (Mar.1984-Jun.1992), Genet.Abstr., Geo.Abstr.P.G., GeoRef, Geol.Abstr., Helminthol.Abstr., Herb.Abstr., Hort.Abstr., Hum.Gen.Abstr., IBR, INIS Atomind., I.P.A., Ind.Med. (1976-), Ind.Sci.Rev., Ind.Vet., Int.Abstr.Biol.Sci., Irr.& Drain.Abstr., Maize Abstr., Mass Spectr.Bull., Mat.Sci.Cit.Ind. (coverage dropped), Microbiol.Abstr., Nonwov.Abstr., Nuc.Acids Abstr., Nutr.Abstr., Ocean.Abstr., Off.Tech. (1993-), Paper & Bd.Abstr., Petrol.Abstr. (1977-, dropped), Pig News & Info., Plant Breed.Abstr., Plant Gen.Res.Abstr., Plant Grow.Reg.Abstr., Pollut.Abstr., Postharvest, Potato Abstr., Poult.Abstr., Protozool.Abstr., Ref.Zh., Repindex, Rev.Appl.Entomol., Rev.Arom.& Med.Plants, Rev.Med.& Vet.Mycol., Rev.Plant Path., Rice Abstr., Risk Abstr., Saf.Sci.Abstr., Sci.Cit.Ind., Seed Abstr., Sel.Water Res.Abstr., Soils & Fert., Soyabean Abstr., Sport Fish.Abstr., Sugar Ind.Abstr., Telegen, Triticale Abstr., Trop.Dis.Bull., VITIS, Vet.Bull., Virol.Abstr. (coverage dropped), W.R.C.Inf., WasteInfo, Weed Abstr., Wild.Rev., World Text.Abstr., Zoo.Rec.
—BLDSC (1571.440000), CASDDS, CINDOC, CISTI, Ei, EMDOCS, GNLM, IDS, ingenta, Linda Hall. **CCC.**
Published by: American Society for Microbiology, 1752 N St N W, Washington, DC 20036-2904. TEL 202-737-3600, 800-633-4931, subscriptions@amsusa.org, journals.asm.org, http://aem.asm.org/, http://www.asmusa.org. Ed. Judy D Wall. Circ: 7,100 (paid).

APPLIED BIOCHEMISTRY AND MICROBIOLOGY. see *BIOLOGY—Biochemistry*

APPLIED MICROBIOLOGY AND BIOTECHNOLOGY. see *BIOLOGY—Biotechnology*

579.2 USA ISSN 1041-245X
CODEN: AVREEC
APPLIED VIROLOGY RESEARCH. Text in English. 1988. irreg., latest vol.3, 1994. price varies. back issues avail. *Refereed.* **Document type:** *Monographic series.*
—BLDSC (1580.113200), CISTI, KNAW.
Published by: Kluwer Academic - Plenum Publishers (Subsidiary of: Wolters Kluwer N.V.), 233 Spring St, New York, NY 10013-1578. TEL 212-620-8000, 800-221-9369, FAX 212-463-0742, info@plenum.com, http://www.plenum.com. Ed. E Kurstak.

579 DEU ISSN 0948-3055
QR106 CODEN: MMFWE7
AQUATIC MICROBIAL ECOLOGY. Text in English. 1985. 6/yr. (in 2 vols., 3 nos./vol.). EUR 356 domestic; EUR 365 foreign (effective 2002). bk.rev. back issues avail. *Refereed.* **Document type:** *Journal, Academic/Scholarly.* **Description:** Presents original papers, short notes and reviews on basic and applied research devoted to aquatic microbial ecology.
Formerly (until 1995): Marine Microbial Food Webs (0297-8148)
Related titles: ♦ Online - full text ed.: Aquatic Microbial Ecology Online. ISSN 1616-1564.
Indexed: ASCA, Appl.Ecol.Abstr., Aqua.Sci.& Fish.Abstr., Aquacult.Abstr., Curr.Cont., Ecol.Abstr., Environ.Sci.Poll.Mgmt., Genet.Abstr., Geo.Abstr.P.G., Hum.Gen.Abstr., Ind.Sci.Rev., Microbiol.Abstr., Ocean.Abstr., Sci.Cit.Ind., Soils & Fert., Zoo.Rec.
—BLDSC (1582.395000), CASDDS, CISTI, Infotrieve. **CCC.**
Published by: Inter-Research, Nordbuente 23, Oldendorf 21385, Germany. TEL 49-4132-7127, FAX 49-4132-8883, marita@int-res.com, http://www.int-res.com.

579 DEU ISSN 1616-1564
AQUATIC MICROBIAL ECOLOGY ONLINE. Text in English. 9/yr. EUR 317 (effective 2002). *Refereed.* **Document type:** *Academic/Scholarly.*
Media: Online - full text (from Institute for Scientific Information). **Related titles:** ♦ Print ed.: Aquatic Microbial Ecology. ISSN 0948-3055.
Published by: Inter-Research, Nordbuente 23, Oldendorf 21385, Germany. TEL 49-4132-7127, FAX 49-4132-8883, webmaster@int-res.com, marita@int-res.com, http://www.int-res.com/journals/ame/index.html.

579 DEU ISSN 0302-8933
QR1 CODEN: AMICCW
ARCHIVES OF MICROBIOLOGY. Text in English. 1939. m. EUR 2,329.10 domestic; EUR 2,318.70 in Germany; EUR 229.80 foreign (effective 2002). adv. bibl, charts, illus. index. back issues avail.; reprint service avail. from ISI. *Refereed.* **Document type:** *Journal, Academic/Scholarly.* **Description:** Publishes papers on all areas of basic research in microbiology using biochemical, genetic, microbiological, molecular biological, physiological or physical methods, or combinations thereof.
Formerly: Archiv fuer Mikrobiologie (0003-9276)
Related titles: Microform ed.: (from PQC); Online - full text ed.: ISSN 1432-072X (from EBSCO Publishing, RoweCom Information Quest, Swets Blackwell, Springer LINK, Institute for Scientific Information).
Indexed: ASCA, AgBiotech, Agri.& Environ.Biotech.Abstr. (coverage dropped), Agricola, Agroforest.Abstr., Aqua.Sci.& Fish.Abstr., Bibl.Agri., Biodet.Abstr., Biol.Abstr., Biotech.Cit.Ind., CEABA, Chem.Abstr., Chem.Indus.Notes, Chem.Titles, Curr.Adv.Ecol.Sci., Curr.Biotech.Abstr., Curr.Cont., Dairy Sci.Abstr., Deep Sea Res.& Oceanogr.Abstr., Dent.Ind., Derwent Biotech.Abstr., Environ.Sci.Poll.Mgmt., Excerp.Med., Field Crop Abstr., Food Sci.& Tech.Abstr., Forest Prod.Abstr., Forest.Abstr., GeoRef, Helminthol.Abstr., INIS Atomind., Ind.Med. (1974-), Ind.Sci.Rev., Ind.Vet., Inpharma, Int.Abstr.Biol.Sci., Irr.& Drain.Abstr., Med.& Surg.Dermat., Microbiol.Abstr., Nutr.Abstr., Pharm.&Out.News, Plant Breed.Abstr., Pollut.Abstr., Protozool.Abstr., Reac., Rev.Med.& Vet.Mycol., Rev.Plant Path., Sci.Cit.Ind., Sel.Water Res.Abstr., Soils & Fert., Soyabean Abstr., Sport Fish.Abstr., Triticale Abstr., Vet.Bull., W.R.C.Inf., Weed Abstr.
—BLDSC (1637.940000), ADONIS, CASDDS, CISTI, EMDOCS, GNLM, IDS, Infotrieve, ingenta, Linda Hall. **CCC.**
Published by: Springer-Verlag (Subsidiary of: BertelsmannSpringer), Tiergartenstr 17, Heidelberg 69121, Germany. TEL 49-6221-345-0, FAX 49-6221-345229, subscriptions@springer.de, http://link.springer.de/link/service/journals/00203/index.htm, http://www.springer.de. **Subscr. in N. America to:** Springer-Verlag New York Inc., PO Box 2485, Secaucus, NJ 07096-2485. TEL 212-460-1500, FAX 212-473-6272.

579.2 AUT ISSN 0304-8608
QR360 CODEN: ARVIDF
ARCHIVES OF VIROLOGY. Text in English. 1939. m. EUR 2,162.80; EUR 2,143.50 in Germany; EUR 210 newsstand/cover (effective 2002). adv. charts, illus. index. reprint service avail. from ISI. *Refereed.* **Document type:** *Journal, Academic/Scholarly.* **Description:** Publishes original contributions from all branches of research on viruses, virus-like agents, and virus infections of humans, animals, plants, insects, and bacteria.
Formerly: Archiv fuer die Gesamte Virusforschung (0003-9012)
Related titles: Microform ed.: (from PQC); Online - full text ed.: ISSN 1432-8798 (from EBSCO Publishing, RoweCom Information Quest, Swets Blackwell, Springer LINK, Institute for Scientific Information); ♦ Supplement: Archives of Virology. Supplementum. ISSN 0939-1983.
Indexed: AIDS & Cancer Res., AIDS Abstr., ASCA, Abstr.Hyg., AgBiotech, Agri.& Environ.Biotech.Abstr. (coverage dropped), Agricola, Agroforest.Abstr., Aqua.Sci.& Fish.Abstr., Bibl.Agri., Bio-Contr.News & Info., Biol.Abstr., Biotech.& Bioeng.Abstr., Chem.Abstr., Chem.Indus.Notes, Chem.Titles, Curr.Adv.Ecol.Sci., Curr.Cont., Dairy Sci.Abstr., Dent.Ind., Derwent Biotech.Abstr., Excerp.Med., Food Sci.& Tech.Abstr., Genet.Abstr., Hum.Gen.Abstr., INIS Atomind., Ind.Med. (1975-), Ind.Sci.Rev., Ind.Vet., Inpharma, Int.Abstr.Biol.Sci., Maize Abstr., Med.& Surg.Dermat., Neurosci.Cit.Ind., Nuc.Acids Abstr., Pharm.&Out.News, Pig News & Info., Plant Breed.Abstr., Potato Abstr., Poult.Abstr., Protozool.Abstr., Reac., Rev.Appl.Entomol., Rev.Arom.& Med.Plants, Rev.Med.& Vet.Mycol., Rev.Plant Path., Rice Abstr., Sci.Cit.Ind., Small Anim.Abstr., Soyabean Abstr., Sport Fish.Abstr., Triticale Abstr., Trop.Dis.Bull., Vet.Bull., Virol.Abstr., Wild.Rev., Zoo.Rec.
—BLDSC (1643.600000), ADONIS, CASDDS, CISTI, EMDOCS, GNLM, IDS, Infotrieve, ingenta. **CCC.**
Published by: Springer-Verlag Wien (Subsidiary of: BertelsmannSpringer), Sachsenplatz 4-6, PO Box 89, Vienna, W 1201, Austria. TEL 43-1-3302415-0, FAX 43-1-330242665, journals@springer.at, http://www.springer.at/archivirol. Ed. M.H. Van Regenmortel. R&P Angela Foessl TEL 43-1-3302415517. Adv. contact Michael Katzenberger TEL 43-1-3302415220. B&W page XEU 1,000; 170 x 230. **Subscr. in N. America to:** Springer-Verlag, Journals, 175 Fifth Ave, New York, NY 10010. TEL 212-460-1500, FAX 212-473-6272, orders@springer-ny.com, http://www.springer-ny.com.

579.2 AUT ISSN 0939-1983
CODEN: AVISE9
ARCHIVES OF VIROLOGY. SUPPLEMENTUM. Text in English. 1991. irreg. adv. abstr. reprints avail. *Refereed.* **Document type:** *Monographic series, Academic/Scholarly.* **Description:** Publishes original papers from all branches of research on viruses, virus-like agents, and virus infections of humans, animals, plants, insects and bacteria.
Related titles: ♦ Supplement to: Archives of Virology. ISSN 0304-8608.
Indexed: Agricola, Ind.Med. (1991-), Poult.Abstr.
—BLDSC (1643.610000), ADONIS, CASDDS, CISTI. **CCC.**
Published by: Springer-Verlag Wien (Subsidiary of: BertelsmannSpringer), Sachsenplatz 4-6, PO Box 89, Vienna, W 1201, Austria. TEL 43-1-3302415-0, FAX 43-1-330242665, books@springer.at, http://www.springer.at/archivirol. Eds. C H Calisher, G Siegl. R&P Angela Foessl TEL 43-1-3302415517. Adv. contact Michael Katzenberger TEL 43-1-3302415220. B&W page XEU 1,000; 170 x 230. **Subscr. in N. America to:** Springer-Verlag, Journals, 175 Fifth Ave, New York, NY 10010. TEL 212-460-1500, FAX 212-473-6272, orders@springer-ny.com, books@springer.at, http://www.springer-ny.com.

B B A - MOLECULAR CELL RESEARCH. see *BIOLOGY—Cytology And Histology*

579.3 ROM ISSN 1220-3696
CODEN: BVPED
BACTERIOLOGIA, VIRUSOLOGIA, PARAZITOLOGIA, EPIDEMIOLOGIA. Text in Romanian; Summaries in English, French. 1956. 4/yr., latest vol.46, 2001. ROL 600,000 domestic; USD 80 foreign; USD 20 per issue (effective 2001). adv. bk.rev. abstr, bibl, charts, illus. Index. back issues avail. *Refereed.* **Document type:** *Journal, Internal, Bibliography.*
Former titles (until 1990): Revista de Igiena, Bacteriologie, Virusologie, Parazitologie, Epidemiologie, Pneumoftiziologie: Bacteriologia, Virusologia, Parazitologia, Epidemiologia (0376-4494); (until 1974): Bacteriologie, Virusologie, Parazitologie, Epidemiologie (0301-7338); (until 1973): Microbiologie, Parazitologie, Epidemiologie (0026-2609); (until 1957): Revista de Microbiologie, Parazitologie, Epidemiologie (1220-0956)
Indexed: Biol.Abstr., Chem.Abstr., Excerp.Med. (until 1990), Ind.Med. (1990-), Ind.Vet., Nutr.Abstr., Pig News & Info., Poult.Abstr., Protozool.Abstr., Trop.Dis.Bull., Vet.Bull.
—BLDSC (1854.950000), CASDDS, CISTI, GNLM.
Published by: Romanian Medical Association, Str. Ionel Perlea Nr.10, Bucharest 70754, Romania. TEL 401-3141062, FAX 401-4115672. Pub., R&P Marian Negut. Circ: 200 (paid and controlled). **Subscr. to:** ILEXIM, Str. 13 Decembrie 3, PO Box 136-137, Bucharest 70116, Romania.

579.3 USA
BERGEY'S MANUAL OF DETERMINATIVE BACTERIOLOGY. Text in English. a. USD 65 (effective 1999). *Refereed.* **Document type:** *Academic/Scholarly.*
Published by: Williams & Wilkins, Book Division (Subsidiary of: Waverly International), 351 W Camden St, Baltimore, MD 21201-2436. TEL 410-528-4000, FAX 410-528-4312, http://www.wwilkins.com.

BIOFORUM. see *BIOLOGY*

579.3 JPN ISSN 0385-5201
RM409 CODEN: BOBODP
BOKIN BOBAI/JOURNAL OF ANTIBACTERIAL AND ANTIFUNGAL AGENTS. Text in Japanese; Summaries in English. 1973. m. JPY 10,000 (effective 2000). adv. **Document type:** *Academic/Scholarly, Abstract/Index.*
Indexed: Chem.Abstr., Chem.Indus.Notes, Chem.Titles, Excerp.Med., Food Sci.& Tech.Abstr., INIS Atomind.
—CASDDS, EMDOCS, GNLM. **CCC.**
Published by: Nihon Bokin Bobai Gakkai/Society for Antibacterial and Antifungal Agents, Japan, 9th Fl, Shin-Kousan Bldg, 13-38, Nishimotocho 1-chome, Nishi-ku, Osaka-shi 550-0005, Japan. Ed. Tetsuaki Tsuchido. Pub. K. Arai. R&P K Arai TEL 81-6-6538-2166. Adv. contact Iwao Yamamoto.

579.65 CHL ISSN 0365-9402
CODEN: BCPRAH
BOLETIN CHILENO DE PARASITOLOGIA. Text in Spanish; Abstracts in English. 1946. s-a. USD 20 domestic; USD 25 foreign (effective 1999). adv. bk.rev. charts, illus. index. *Refereed.* **Document type:** *Bulletin, Academic/Scholarly.* **Description:** Includes subjects dealing with biology, epidemiology, clinics, laboratory and prevention of parasitoses.
Related titles: Online - full text ed.
Indexed: Abstr.Hyg., Biol.Abstr., Chem.Abstr., Excerp.Med., Helminthol.Abstr., INIS Atomind., Ind.Med. (1954-), Ind.Vet., Pig News & Info., Poult.Abstr., Protozool.Abstr., Rev.Appl.Entomol., Rev.Med.& Vet.Mycol., Rural Devel.Abstr., Small Anim.Abstr., Sport Fish.Abstr., Trop.Dis.Bull., Vet.Bull., Wild.Rev., Zoo.Rec.
—CISTI, EMDOCS, GNLM, Linda Hall.
Published by: Universidad de Chile, Departamento de Parasitologia, Casilla 9183, Santiago, Chile. TEL 56-2-6786252 ext. 6252, FAX 56-2-7356579. Ed. Hugo Schenone. Circ: 1,000.

579 ITA ISSN 0394-9877
CODEN: BMILE4
BOLLETTINO DI MICROBIOLOGIA ED INDAGINI DI LABORATORIO. Text in Italian. 1981. q. ITL 90,000 domestic; ITL 120,000 foreign (effective 2000). adv. bk.rev. index. *Refereed.*
Published by: Sirse S.r.l., Via Confu 51, Brescia, BS 25124, Italy. TEL 39-03-0221522, info@sirse.com. Ed. Dr. A Turano. Circ: 2,000.

579 BRA ISSN 1517-8382
QR6 CODEN: RMBGBP
BRAZILIAN JOURNAL OF MICROBIOLOGY. Text in English. 1970. q. membership; BRL 35 newsstand/cover. adv. bk.rev. index. back issues avail.; reprint service avail. from ISI. *Refereed.* **Document type:** *Academic/Scholarly.* **Description:** Publishes original research papers, research notes, and reviews, covering all aspects of microbiology.
Formerly (until 2000): Revista de Microbiologia (0001-3714)
Related titles: Online - full text ed.: (from SciELO, Institute for Scientific Information).
Indexed: ASCA, Abstr.Hyg., Aqua.Sci.& Fish.Abstr., Bio-Contr.News & Info., Biol.Abstr., Chem.Abstr., Chem.Titles, Curr.Adv.Ecol.Sci., Curr.Cont., Dairy Sci.Abstr., Environ.Sci.Poll.Mgmt., Excerp.Med., Field Crop Abstr., Food Sci.& Tech.Abstr., Forest.Abstr., Helminthol.Abstr., Hort.Abstr., INIS Atomind., Ind.Med. (coverage dropped), Ind.Vet., Int.Abstr.Biol.Sci., Irr.& Drain.Abstr., Maize Abstr., Microbiol.Abstr., Nutr.Abstr., Pig News & Info., Postharvest, Ref.Zh., Rev.Appl.Entomol., Rev.Med.& Vet.Mycol., Rev.Plant Path., Soils & Fert., Sugar Ind.Abstr., Trop.Dis.Bull., Vet.Bull.
—BLDSC (7866.425000), CASDDS, CISTI, GNLM, IDS, KNAW.
Published by: Sociedade Brasileira de Microbiologia/Brazilian Society for Microbiology, c/o Bernadette Franco, Ed., Depto. de Microbiologia, Instituto de Ciencias Biomedicas USP, Av. Prof. Lineu Prestes, 1374, Sao Paulo, SP 05508-900, Brazil. TEL 55-11-8139647, FAX 55-11-8139647, revmicro@icb.usp.br. Eds. Benedito Correa, Bernadette D G M Franco. Pub., Adv. contact Bernadette Franco. Circ: 1,500.

C A S BIOTECH UPDATES. PHARMACEUTICAL APPLICATIONS. see *BIOLOGY—Abstracting, Bibliographies, Statistics*

C A SELECTS. ANTIFUNGAL & ANTIMYCOTIC AGENTS. see *BIOLOGY—Abstracting, Bibliographies, Statistics*

C A SELECTS. MONOCLONAL ANTIBODIES. see *BIOLOGY—Abstracting, Bibliographies, Statistics*

C A SELECTS. VIRUCIDES & VIRUSTATS. see *BIOLOGY—Abstracting, Bibliographies, Statistics*

579 CAN ISSN 0008-4166
QR1 CODEN: CJMIAZ
CANADIAN JOURNAL OF MICROBIOLOGY/JOURNAL CANADIEN DE MICROBIOLOGIE. Text mainly in English; Text occasionally in French. 1954. m. CND 151 domestic to individuals; USD 151 foreign to individuals; CND 422 domestic to institutions; USD 422 foreign to institutions (effective 1999). adv. bibl, illus. index. back issues avail.; reprint service avail. from PQC. *Refereed.* **Document type:** *Academic/Scholarly.*
Related titles: Microfiche ed.: (from MML); Microform ed.: (from PQC,PMC,MML); Online - full text ed.: ISSN 1480-3275 (from EBSCO Publishing, O C L C Online Computer Library Center, Inc., RoweCom Information Quest, ProQuest Information & Learning, CISTI, LexisNexis, Swets Blackwell, Institute for Scientific Information).
Indexed: ASCA, Abstr.Bull.Inst.Pap.Chem., Abstr.Hyg., AgBiotech, Agri.& Environ.Biotech.Abstr. (coverage dropped), Agricola, Agroforest.Abstr., Aqua.Sci.& Fish.Abstr., Aquacult.Abstr., Bibl.Agri., Bio-Contr.News & Info., Biodet.Abstr., Biol.& Agr.Ind. (Jan.1983-), Biol.Abstr., CBCA Ref., CEABA, Chem.Abstr., Chem.Indus.Notes, Chem.Titles, Crop Physiol.Abstr., Curr.Adv.Biochem., Curr.Adv.Ecol.Sci., Curr.Biotech.Abstr., Curr.Cont., Dairy Sci.Abstr., Deep Sea Res.& Oceanogr.Abstr., Dent.Ind., Derwent Biotech.Abstr., Diar.Dis.Res., Ecol.Abstr., Eng.Ind., Environ.Abstr., Environ.Sci.Poll.Mgmt., Excerp.Med., Field Crop Abstr., Food Sci.& Tech.Abstr., Forest Prod.Abstr., Forest.Abstr., Geol.Abstr., Helminthol.Abstr., Herb.Abstr., Hort.Abstr., IDA, INIS Atomind., Ind.Med. (1954-), Ind.Sci.Rev., Ind.Vet., Inpharma, Int.Abstr.Biol.Sci., Int.Aerosp.Abstr., Irr.& Drain.Abstr., Maize Abstr., Microbiol.Abstr., NPU, Nutr.Abstr., Ocean.Abstr. (coverage dropped), Ornam.Hort., Pharm.&Out.News, Pig News & Info., Plant Breed.Abstr., Plant Grow.Reg.Abstr., Pollut.Abstr., Postharvest, Poult.Abstr., Protozool.Abstr., Reac., Rev.Appl.Entomol., Rev.Med.& Vet.Mycol., Rev.Plant Path., Rice Abstr., Sci.Cit.Ind., Seed Abstr., Sel.Water Res.Abstr., Small Anim.Abstr., Soils & Fert., Soyabean Abstr., Sport Fish.Abstr., Sugar Ind.Abstr., Telegen, Triticale Abstr., Trop.Dis.Bull., Trop.Oil Seeds Abstr., Vet.Bull., W.R.C.Inf., Weed Abstr., World Text.Abstr.
—BLDSC (3033.000000), ADONIS, CASDDS, CISTI, EMDOCS, GNLM, IDS, ingenta, Linda Hall. **CCC.**
Published by: N R C Research Press, Building M 55, Ottawa, ON K1A 0R6, Canada. TEL 613-993-9084, FAX 613-952-7656, research.journals@nrc.ca;, http://www.nrc.ca/cisti/journals/. Eds. H G Deneer, Dr. Jim J Germida. Adv. contact Judy Heyman. B&W page CND 675; trim 11 x 8.5. Circ: 1,341.

579 CZE ISSN 0009-0646
CESKOSLOVENSKA SPOLECNOST MIKROBIOLOGICKA. BULLETIN. Text in Czech. 1960. q. membership. bk.rev. bibl, charts, stat. **Document type:** *Bulletin.*
Published by: Ceskoslovenska Spolecnost Mikrobiologicka, Videnska 1083, Prague 14220, Czech Republic. TEL 42-2-4752494, FAX 42-2-4713221. Ed. C John. adv.: page CZK 10,000. Circ: 1,150.

579 JPN ISSN 0914-8221
QR245
CHIBA DAIGAKU SHINKAKU BISEIBUTSU KENKYU SENTA HOKOKU/CHIBA UNIVERSITY. RESEARCH CENTER FOR PATHOGENIC FUNGI AND MICROBIAL TOXICOSES. ANNUAL REPORT. Text in Japanese. 1987. a.
—BLDSC (1407.630000).
Published by: Chiba Daigaku, Shinkaku Biseibutsu Kenkyu Senta/Chiba University. Research Center for Pathogenic Fungi and Microbial Toxicoses, 8-1 Inohana 1-chome, Chuo-ku, Chiba-shi 260-0856, Japan.

CLINICAL AND DIAGNOSTIC LABORATORY IMMUNOLOGY. see *MEDICAL SCIENCES—Allergology And Immunology*

CLINICAL MICROBIOLOGY AND INFECTION. see *MEDICAL SCIENCES*

579 USA ISSN 0196-4399
CODEN: CMNEEJ
CLINICAL MICROBIOLOGY NEWSLETTER. Text in English. 1983. 24/yr. EUR 47 in Europe to individuals; JPY 6,300 in Japan to individuals; USD 53 elsewhere to individuals; EUR 306 in Europe to institutions; JPY 40,600 in Japan to institutions; USD 342 elsewhere to institutions (effective 2002). back issues avail. **Document type:** *Newsletter.* **Description:** For clinical microbiologists, clinical pathologists, laboratory technologists and technicians.
Related titles: Microform ed.: (from PQC); Online - full text ed.: (from ingenta, Swets Blackwell, ScienceDirect).
Indexed: Abstr.Hyg., Diar.Dis.Res., Environ.Sci.Poll.Mgmt., Excerp.Med., Ind.Vet., Microbiol.Abstr., Pollut.Abstr., Protozool.Abstr., Rev.Appl.Entomol., Rev.Med.& Vet.Mycol., Risk Abstr., Saf.Sci.Abstr., Trop.Dis.Bull.
—BLDSC (3286.305600), GNLM, Infotrieve, ingenta, KNAW. **CCC.**
Published by: Elsevier Science, 655 Ave of the Americas, New York, NY 10010. TEL 212-989-5800, FAX 212-633-3990, usinfo-f@elsevier.com, http://www.elsevier.com/locate/clinmicnews. Ed. Mary Jane Ferraro. **Subscr. in Australasia and the Far East to:** Elsevier Science (Singapore) Pte Ltd, No.1 Temasek Ave, 17-01 Millenia Tower, Singapore 039192, Singapore. TEL 65-434-3727, FAX 65-337-2230; **Subscr. in Japan to:** Elsevier Science Inc - Japan Regional Office, 9-15 Higashi-Azabu 1-chome, Minato-ku, Tokyo 106-0044, Japan. TEL 81-3-5561-5033, FAX 81-3-5561-5047; **Subscr. outside the Americas to:** Elsevier Science BV, PO Box 211, Amsterdam 1000 AE, Netherlands. TEL 31-20-485-3757, FAX 31-20-485-3432, nlinfo-f@elsevier.nl, http://www.elsevier.nl.

579 USA ISSN 0893-8512
QR67 CODEN: CMIREX
CLINICAL MICROBIOLOGY REVIEWS. Text in English. 1988. q. USD 295 domestic to non-members; USD 299 in Canada to non-members; USD 314 in Europe to non-members; USD 315 in Latin America to non-members; USD 316 elsewhere to non-members (effective 2001). adv. illus. index. back issues avail.; reprint service avail. from PQC. *Refereed.* **Document type:** *Academic/Scholarly.* **Description:** Addresses reviews on all aspects of clinical and medical microbiology, including immunology.
Related titles: CD-ROM ed.; Microform ed.: (from PQC); Online - full text ed.: ISSN 1098-6618 (from HighWire Pr., EBSCO Publishing, Institute for Scientific Information).
Indexed: ASCA, Abstr.Hyg., AgBiotech, Biodet.Abstr., Biol.Abstr., Chem.Abstr., Chem.Indus.Notes, Chem.Titles, Curr.Cont., Diar.Dis.Res., Environ.Sci.Poll.Mgmt., Excerp.Med., Food Sci.& Tech.Abstr., Genet.Abstr., Helminthol.Abstr., Ind.Med. (1988-), Ind.Vet., Inpharma, Int.Abstr.Biol.Sci., Microbiol.Abstr., Pharm.&Out.News, Pollut.Abstr., Poult.Abstr., Protozool.Abstr., Reac., Rev.Appl.Entomol., Rev.Med.& Vet.Mycol., Risk Abstr., Saf.Sci.Abstr., Sci.Cit.Ind., Trop.Dis.Bull., Virol.Abstr. (coverage dropped).
—BLDSC (3286.305650), CASDDS, CISTI, EMDOCS, GNLM, IDS, ingenta, KNAW. **CCC.**
Published by: American Society for Microbiology, 1325 Massachusetts Ave, N W, Washington, DC 20005-4171. TEL 202-737-3600, 800-633-4931, subscriptions@asmusa.org, http://cmr.asm.org/, http://www.asmusa.org. Ed. Betty A Forbes. Circ: 9,200.

579 GBR
COMMUNICABLE DISEASE AND PUBLIC HEALTH. Text in English. 1998. q. GBP 88 domestic; GBP 110 foreign (effective 2000). bk.rev. *Refereed.* **Document type:** *Academic/Scholarly.* **Description:** Aims to meet the needs of a wide range of readers who share concern in the management, prevention, and control of communicable diseases.
Formed by the merger of (1983-1998): P H L S Microbiology Digest (0265-3400); (1967-1998): Communicable Disease Report Review (1350-9349); Which superseded in part (in 1991): Communicable Disease Report. Weekly Edition (0144-3186)
Indexed: Abstr.Hyg., Dairy Sci.Abstr., Food Sci.& Tech.Abstr., Ind.Med. (1998-), Ind.Vet., Int.Nurs.Ind., Nutr.Abstr., Protozool.Abstr., Rural Recreat.Tour.Abstr., Small Anim.Abstr., Trop.Dis.Bull., Vet.Bull.
—BLDSC (3341.341900), GNLM.
Published by: Public Health Laboratory Service, 61 Colindale Ave, London NW9 5HT, United Kingdom. TEL 44-20-8200-6868, FAX 44-20-8200-7868, shandysi@phls.co.uk, http://www.phls.co.uk/cdsc. Ed. Dr. Stuart Handysides. Circ: 1,500.

B

579 GBR ISSN 0147-9571
CODEN: CIMIDV

COMPARATIVE IMMUNOLOGY, MICROBIOLOGY AND INFECTIOUS DISEASES; the international journal for medical and veterinary researchers and practitioners. Text in English. 1978. q. NLG 1,271, EUR 663 in Europe to institutions; JPY 88,000 in Japan to institutions; USD 742 elsewhere to institutions (effective 2002). adv. index. *Refereed.* **Document type:** *Academic/Scholarly.* **Description:** Provides a forum for physicians and veterinarians specializing in immunology, immunopathology, microbiology and infectious diseases in both humans and animals.
Related titles: Microfilm ed.: (from PQC); Online - full text ed.: (from ingenta, ScienceDirect, Institute for Scientific Information).
Indexed: AIDS & Cancer Res., ASCA, Abstr.Hyg., AgBiotech, Aqua.Sci.& Fish.Abstr., Biol.Abstr., Curr.Adv.Ecol.Sci., Curr.Cont., Dairy Sci.Abstr., Derwent Biotech.Abstr., Environ.Sci.Poll.Mgmt., Excerp.Med., Focus on: Vet.Sci.& Med., Helminthol.Abstr., Immun.Abstr., Ind.Med. (1978-), Ind.Sci.Rev., Ind.Vet., Int.Abstr.Biol.Sci., Microbiol.Abstr., Nutr.Abstr., Pig News & Info., Poult.Abstr., Protozool.Abstr., Ref.Zh., Rev.Appl.Entomol., Rev.Arom.& Med.Plants, Rev.Med.& Vet.Mycol., Sci.Cit.Ind., Trop.Dis.Bull., Vet.Bull., Wild.Rev., Zoo.Rec.
—BLDSC (3363.782600), CISTI, GNLM, IDS, Infotrieve, ingenta, KNAW. **CCC.**
Published by: Pergamon (Subsidiary of: Elsevier Science), The Boulevard, Langford Ln, East Park, Kidlington, Oxford OXB 1GB, United Kingdom. FAX 44-1865-843010, http://www.elsevier.com/locate/cimid. Ed. Charles Pilet. Circ: 1,000. **Subscr. in Australasia and the Far East to:** Elsevier Science (Singapore) Pte Ltd, No.1 Temasek Ave, 17-01 Millenia Tower, Singapore 039192, Singapore. TEL 65-434-3727, FAX 65-337-2230; **Subscr. in the Americas to:** Elsevier Science, PO Box 945, New York, NY 10159-0945. TEL 212-633-3730, FAX 212-633-3680; **Subscr. to:** Elsevier Science BV, PO Box 211, Amsterdam 1000 AE, Netherlands. TEL 31-20-485-3757, nlinfo-f@elsevier.nl, http://www.elsevier.nl.

579 CHE ISSN 1420-9519
QR1 CODEN: CMICFN

CONTRIBUTIONS TO MICROBIOLOGY. Text in English. 1973. irreg., latest vol.9. CHF 200 in Europe; DEM 240 in Germany; USD 200 in United States (2001). reprint service avail. from ISI. *Refereed.* **Document type:** *Monographic series, Academic/Scholarly.*
Formerly (until 1998): Contributions to Microbiology and Immunology (0301-3081); Which supersedes: Bibliotheca Microbiologia (0067-8058)
Indexed: Biol.Abstr., Chem.Abstr., Chem.Indus.Notes, Chem.Titles, Curr.Cont. (coverage dropped), Ind.Med. (1998-), Ind.Vet., Protozool.Abstr., Vet.Bull.
—BLDSC (3458.830000), CASDDS, CISTI, GNLM, Linda Hall. **CCC.**
Published by: S. Karger AG, Allschwilerstr 10, PO Box, Basel 4009, Switzerland. TEL 41-61-306-1111, FAX 41-61-306-1234, karger@karger.ch, http://www.karger.com/bookseries/COMII. Ed. Axel Schmidt.

579 USA ISSN 1040-841X
QR1 CODEN: CRVMAC

CRITICAL REVIEWS IN MICROBIOLOGY. Text in English. 1971. q. USD 375 (effective 1998). bibl, charts, illus. back issues avail. *Refereed.* **Document type:** *Academic/Scholarly.* **Description:** Reviews the many diverse fields of microbiology: viruses, rickettsiae, mycoplasmas, bacteria, fungi, algae, and protozoa.
Formerly: C R C Critical Reviews in Microbiology (0045-6454)
Related titles: Online - full text ed.: (from O C L C Online Computer Library Center, Inc., Swets Blackwell, ScienceDirect, Institute for Scientific Information).
Indexed: ASCA, Agricola, Aqua.Sci.& Fish.Abstr., Biol.Abstr., Chem.Abstr., Chem.Indus.Notes, Chem.Titles, Curr.Adv.Ecol.Sci., Curr.Biotech.Abstr., Curr.Cont., Deep Sea Res.& Oceanogr.Abstr., Derwent Biotech.Abstr., Entomol.Abstr., Environ.Sci.Poll.Mgmt., Food Sci.& Tech.Abstr., Helminthol.Abstr., Ind.Med. (1980-), Ind.Sci.Rev., Inpharma, Int.Abstr.Biol.Sci., Microbiol.Abstr., NRN, Nutr.Abstr., Pharm.&Out.News, Protozool.Abstr., Reac., Rev.Appl.Entomol., Rev.Med.& Vet.Mycol., Sci.Cit.Ind., Soils & Fert., Telegen, Weed Abstr., Zoo.Rec.
—BLDSC (3487.478000), CASDDS, CISTI, EMDOCS, GNLM, IDS, ingenta, Linda Hall. **CCC.**
Published by: C R C Press, LLC, 2000 Corporate Blvd, N W, Boca Raton, FL 33431. TEL 561-994-0555, 800-272-7737, FAX 561-998-9784. Ed. Ronald M Atlas. Circ: 620.

CURRENT ADVANCES IN APPLIED MICROBIOLOGY & BIOTECHNOLOGY. see *BIOLOGY—Abstracting, Bibliographies, Statistics*

579 616.01 GBR ISSN 1466-531X

▼ **CURRENT ISSUES IN INTESTINAL MICROBIOLOGY.** Text in English. 2000. s-a. GBP 75, USD 150 to individuals; GBP 130, USD 260 to institutions (effective 2002). *Refereed.* **Document type:** *Academic/Scholarly.* **Description:** Publishes high-quality review papers in all areas of intestinal microbiology pertaining to human and other animal systems including, microbial ecology, pathogenic organisms, probiotics and prebiotics.
Related titles: Online - full text ed.: Current Issues in Intestinal Microbiology Online. ISSN 1466-5328. 2000. GBP 40, USD 80 to individuals; GBP 80, USD 160 to institutions (effective 2002).
Indexed: Biotech.& Bioeng.Abstr., Environ.Sci.Poll.Mgmt., Virol.Abstr.
—BLDSC (3499.072600).
Published by: Horizon Scientific Press, 32 Hewitts Ln, PO Box 1, Wymondham, Norfolk NR18 0EA, United Kingdom. TEL 44-1953-601106, FAX 44-1953-603068, mail@horizonpress.com, orders@horizonpress.com, http://www.ciim.net, http://www.horizonpress.com/. Ed. Gerald W Tannock.

CURRENT ISSUES IN MOLECULAR BIOLOGY. see *BIOLOGY—Biochemistry*

579 USA ISSN 0343-8651
QR1 CODEN: CUMIDD

CURRENT MICROBIOLOGY; an international journal. Text in English. 1978. m. (in 2 vols., 6 nos./vol.). USD 702 domestic for print & online eds.; USD 750.30 in Germany for print & online eds.; USD 69.60 newsstand/cover foreign (effective 2002). adv. illus. reprint service avail. from ISI. *Refereed.* **Document type:** *Academic/Scholarly.* **Description:** Keeps readers up-to-date in all areas of microbiology, both medical and nonmedical.
Related titles: Microform ed.: (from PQC); Online - full text ed.: ISSN 1432-0991 (from EBSCO Publishing, RoweCom Information Quest, Swets Blackwell, Springer LINK, Institute for Scientific Information).
Indexed: ASCA, Abstr.Hyg., AgBiotech, Agri.& Environ.Biotech.Abstr. (coverage dropped), Agricola, Aqua.Sci.& Fish.Abstr., Aquacult.Abstr., Bio-Contr.News & Info., CEABA, Chem.Abstr., Chem.Indus.Notes, Chem.Titles, Curr.Adv.Biochem., Curr.Adv.Ecol.Sci., Curr.Adv.Gen.& Molec.Biol., Curr.Biotech.Abstr., Curr.Cont., Dairy Sci.Abstr., Deep Sea Res.& Oceanogr.Abstr., Derwent Biotech.Abstr., Diar.Dis.Res., Environ.Sci.Poll.Mgmt., Excerp.Med., Food Sci.& Tech.Abstr., Forest Prod.Abstr., Forest.Abstr., Genet.Abstr., Helminthol.Abstr., Hort.Abstr., Hum.Gen.Abstr., Ind.Med. (1978-), Ind.Sci.Rev., Ind.Vet., Inpharma, Maize Abstr., Microbiol.Abstr., Nuc.Acids Abstr., Nutr.Abstr., Pharm.&Out.News, Pig News & Info., Plant Breed.Abstr., Plant Grow.Reg.Abstr., Postharvest, Poult.Abstr., Protozool.Abstr., Reac., Rev.Appl.Entomol., Rev.Med.& Vet.Mycol., Rev.Plant Path., Sci.Cit.Ind., Small Anim.Abstr., Soils & Fert., Sport Fish.Abstr., Sugar Ind.Abstr., Trop.Dis.Bull., Vet.Bull., Weed Abstr.
—BLDSC (3500.420000), CASDDS, CISTI, EMDOCS, GNLM, IDS, Infotrieve, ingenta, Linda Hall. **CCC.**
Published by: Springer-Verlag, Journals (Subsidiary of: BertelsmannSpringer), 175 Fifth Ave, New York, NY 10010. TEL 212-460-1500, FAX 212-473-6272, orders@springer-ny.com, http://www.springer-ny.com. Ed. A Balows. R&P Ian Gross. Adv. contact Brian Skepton. Circ: 1,000. **N. American subscr. to:** Journal Fulfillment Services, PO Box 2485, Secaucus, NJ 07096-2485. TEL 800-777-2491, FAX 201-348-4505.

CURRENT PROTOCOLS IN IMMUNOLOGY. see *MEDICAL SCIENCES—Allergology And Immunology*

579 USA ISSN 0070-217X
QR1 CODEN: CTMIA3

CURRENT TOPICS IN MICROBIOLOGY AND IMMUNOLOGY. Text in English. irreg., latest vol.208, 1996. price varies. reprint service avail. from ISI. *Refereed.* **Document type:** *Monographic series.* **Description:** Publishes research and studies in microbiology and immunology.
Formerly: Ergebnisse der Mikrobiologie und Immunitaetsforschung
Related titles: Online - full text ed.: (from Institute for Scientific Information).
Indexed: AIDS & Cancer Res., AIDS Abstr., ASCA, Abstr.Hyg., Biol.Abstr., Chem.Abstr., Chem.Indus.Notes, Chem.Titles, Curr.Adv.Ecol.Sci., Environ.Sci.Poll.Mgmt., Excerp.Med., Genet.Abstr., Hum.Gen.Abstr., Immun.Abstr., Ind.Med. (1967-), Ind.Sci.Rev., Ind.Vet., Int.Abstr.Biol.Sci., Microbiol.Abstr., Nuc.Acids Abstr., Protozool.Abstr., Sci.Cit.Ind., Trop.Dis.Bull., Vet.Bull., Virol.Abstr. (coverage dropped).
—BLDSC (3504.890000), CASDDS, CISTI, EMDOCS, GNLM, IDS, ingenta, KNAW, Linda Hall. **CCC.**
Published by: Springer-Verlag, Journals (Subsidiary of: BertelsmannSpringer), 175 Fifth Ave, New York, NY 10010. TEL 212-460-1500, FAX 212-473-6272, orders@springer-ny.com, http://www.springer-ny.com.

CURRENTS IN HEMATOIMMUNOLOGY. see *MEDICAL SCIENCES—Allergology And Immunology*

DEVELOPMENTAL AND COMPARATIVE IMMUNOLOGY; ontogeny - phylogeny - aging. see *MEDICAL SCIENCES—Allergology And Immunology*

579.2 NLD ISSN 0167-8256
CODEN: DMVIDD

DEVELOPMENTS IN MOLECULAR VIROLOGY. Text in English. 1981. irreg. price varies. *Refereed.* **Document type:** *Monographic series.*
Indexed: Chem.Abstr., Chem.Indus.Notes, Chem.Titles.
—CASDDS, CISTI, KNAW.
Published by: Kluwer Academic Publishers Group (Subsidiary of: Wolters Kluwer N.V.), Spuiboulevard 50, PO Box 17, Dordrecht 3300 AA, Netherlands. FAX 31-78-639-2254, services@wkap.nl, http://www.wkap.nl. **Dist. by:** Journals Department, PO Box 322, Dordrecht 3300 AH, Netherlands. FAX 31-78-654-6474.

579 USA ISSN 0732-8893
RB37.A1 CODEN: DMIDDZ

DIAGNOSTIC MICROBIOLOGY AND INFECTIOUS DISEASE. Text in English. 1983. m. EUR 388 in Europe to individuals; JPY 51,300 in Japan to individuals; USD 434 elsewhere to individuals; EUR 1,024 in Europe to institutions; JPY 135,900 in Japan to institutions; USD 1,146 elsewhere to institutions (effective 2002). adv. bk.rev. abstr. index. back issues avail. *Refereed.* **Document type:** *Academic/Scholarly.* **Description:** Provides information on latest developments in clinical microbiology and the diagnosis and treatment of infectious diseases.
Related titles: Microform ed.: (from PQC); Online - full text ed.: (from ingenta, Swets Blackwell, ScienceDirect, Institute for Scientific Information).
Indexed: Biol.Abstr., Chem.Abstr., Chem.Indus.Notes, Chem.Titles, Curr.Adv.Ecol.Sci., Curr.Cont., Diar.Dis.Res., Excerp.Med., INIS Atomind., INSPEC (coverage dropped), Ind.Med. (1983-), Ind.Sci.Rev., Inpharma, Int.Abstr.Biol.Sci., Int.Nurs.Ind., Jrnl.Watch Inf.Dis., Med.& Surg.Dermat., Pharm.&Out.News, Protozool.Abstr., Reac., Sci.Cit.Ind.
—BLDSC (3579.662000), ADONIS, CASDDS, CISTI, EMDOCS, GNLM, IDS, ingenta, KNAW. **CCC.**
Published by: Elsevier Science, PO Box 945, New York, NY 10159-0945. TEL 212-989-5800, FAX 212-633-3990, usinfo-f@elsevier.com, http://www.elsevier.com/locate/diagmicrobio. Ed. Dr. Ronald N Jones. **Subscr. in Australasia and the Far East to:** Elsevier Science (Singapore) Pte Ltd, No.1 Temasek Ave, 17-01 Millenia Tower, Singapore 039192, Singapore. TEL 65-434-3727, FAX 65-337-2230; **Subscr. in Japan to:** Elsevier Science Inc - Japan Regional Office, 9-15 Higashi-Azabu 1-chome, Minato-ku, Tokyo 106-0044, Japan. TEL 81-3-5561-5033; **Subscr. outside the Americas to:** Elsevier Science BV, PO Box 211, Amsterdam 1000 AE, Netherlands. TEL 31-20-485-3757, http://www.elsevier.nl.

DRUG RESISTANCE UPDATE. see *MEDICAL SCIENCES*

579 USA

ECONOMIC MICROBIOLOGY. Text in English. 1977. irreg., latest vol.8, 1983. reprint service avail. from ISI. *Refereed.*
Indexed: Chem.Abstr., Food Sci.& Tech.Abstr.
Published by: Academic Press, Inc., Journal Division (Subsidiary of: Harcourt Brace & Company), 525 B St, Ste 1900, San Diego, CA 92101-4495. TEL 619-231-0926, FAX 619-699-6715. Ed. A H Rose. **Subscr. to:** Order Dept., 6277 Sea Harbor Dr, 4th Fl, Orlando, FL 32887. TEL 800-321-5068.

579 EGY ISSN 0301-8172
QR1 CODEN: EJMBA2
EGYPTIAN JOURNAL OF MICROBIOLOGY/MAGALLAH AL-MISRIYAH LIL-MIKRUBIYULUGIYA. Text in English; Summaries in Arabic, English. 1966. q. USD 147 (effective 2000). charts, illus. reprint service avail. from IRC. **Document type:** *Academic/Scholarly.*
Formerly: Journal of Microbiology of the United Arab Republic (0022-2704)
Indexed: Bio-Contr.News & Info., Biol.Abstr., Chem.Abstr., Chem.Indus.Notes, Chem.Titles, Curr.Adv.Ecol.Sci., Curr.Biotech.Abstr., Dairy Sci.Abstr., Diar.Dis.Res., Field Crop Abstr., Food Sci.& Tech.Abstr., Forest.Abstr., Herb.Abstr., Ind.Vet., Maize Abstr., Nutr.Abstr., Postharvest, Potato Abstr., Protozool.Abstr., Rev.Appl.Entomol., Rev.Med.& Vet.Mycol., Rev.Plant Path., Seed Abstr., Soils & Fert., Soyabean Abstr., Sugar Ind.Abstr., Triticale Abstr.
—BLDSC (3664.405000), CASDDS, CISTI, ingenta, Linda Hall.
Published by: (Society of Applied Microbiology, Research Department), National Information and Documentation Centre (NIDOC), Tahrir St., Dokki, Awqaf P.O., Cairo, Egypt. TEL 20-2-3371696. Ed. M S Foda. Circ: 1,000.

ENFERMEDADES INFECCIOSAS Y MICROBIOLOGIA. see *MEDICAL SCIENCES—Communicable Diseases*

579 GBR ISSN 1462-2912
QR100 CODEN: ENMIFM
▼ **ENVIRONMENTAL MICROBIOLOGY.** Text in English. 1999. bi-m., latest vol.4, 2002. GBP 110 in Europe to individuals; USD 175 in North America to individuals; GBP 121 elsewhere to individuals; GBP 507 in Europe to institutions; USD 804 in North America to institutions; GBP 558 elsewhere to institutions (effective 2002). adv. *Refereed.* **Document type:** *Academic/Scholarly.* **Description:** Devoted to the study of microbial processes in the environment, microbial communities and microbial interactions.
Related titles: Online - full text ed.: ISSN 1462-2920. GBP 99 in Europe to individuals; USD 158 in North America to individuals; GBP 99 elsewhere to individuals; GBP 457 in Europe to institutions; USD 724 in North America to institutions; GBP 457 elsewhere to institutions (effective 2002) (from EBSCO Publishing, O C L C Online Computer Library Center, Inc., RoweCom Information Quest, ingenta, Munksgaard & Blackwell Science's Synergy, Swets Blackwell, Institute for Scientific Information).
Indexed: AgBiotech, Bio-Contr.News & Info., Biotech.Cit.Ind., Curr.Cont., Dairy Sci.Abstr., Field Crop Abstr., Forest.Abstr., Hort.Abstr., Ind.Med., Irr.& Drain.Abstr., Maize Abstr., Nutr.Abstr., Potato Abstr., Protozool.Abstr., Rev.Appl.Entomol., Rev.Plant Path., Rice Abstr., Soils & Fert., Soyabean Abstr., Weed Abstr., Zoo.Rec.
—BLDSC (3791.522600), CASDDS, Infotrieve. **CCC.**
Published by: (Society for Applied Microbiology), Blackwell Science Ltd., PO Box 88, Oxford OX2 0NE, United Kingdom. TEL 44-1865-206180, 44-1865-206002, FAX 44-1865-206219, jnl.orders@blacksci.co.uk, http://www.blackwell-science.com/~cgilib/jnlpage.asp?Journal=emi&File=emi, http://www.blackwellpublishing.com. Eds. D Stahl, K Timmis. Pub. Amanda McLean Inglis. R&P Sophie Savage. Adv. contact Jenny Applin. Circ: 900.

ENZYME AND MICROBIAL TECHNOLOGY; biotechnology research and reviews. see *BIOLOGY—Biotechnology*

579 CZE ISSN 1210-7913
QR1 CODEN: EMIME6
EPIDEMIOLOGIE, MIKROBIOLOGIE, IMUNOLOGIE. Text in Czech, Slovak; Summaries in Czech, English. 1952. q. EUR 84, USD 112 (effective 2001). adv. bk.rev. abstr, bibl, charts, illus, stat. index. *Refereed.*
Formerly (until 1994): Ceskoslovenska Epidemiologie, Mikrobiologie, Imunologie (0009-0522)
Indexed: Abstr.Hyg., Biol.Abstr., C.I.S. Abstr., Chem.Abstr., Curr.Adv.Ecol.Sci., Dairy Sci.Abstr., Dok.Arbeitsmed., Excerp.Med., INIS Atomind., Ind.Med. (coverage dropped), Ind.Vet., Nutr.Abstr., Poult.Abstr., Protozool.Abstr., Rev.Appl.Entomol., Rev.Med.& Vet.Mycol., Trop.Dis.Bull., Vet.Bull.
—BLDSC (3793.573000), CASDDS, CISTI, GNLM. **CCC.**
Published by: (Ceska Lekarska Spolecnost J.E. Purkyne/Czech Medical Association), Nakladatelske Stredisko C L S J.E. Purkyne, Sokolska 31, Prague 12026, Czech Republic. TEL 42-2-24911420, FAX 42-2-24911420, nts@iol.cz, http://www.clsjep.cz, http://www.medical.cz. Ed. Dr. B Tichacek. adv.: B&W page CZK 25,100, color page CZK 35,200; 250 x 170. Circ: 750. **Dist. by:** Abont s.r.o., Chlumova 17, Prague, 3 130 00, Czech Republic; **Dist. in Western Countries by:** Kubon & Sagner, Hesstr 39-41, Munich 80798, Germany.

579.65 GBR ISSN 0950-2688
RA421 CODEN: EPINEU
EPIDEMIOLOGY AND INFECTION. Text in English. 1901. bi-m. USD 472 to institutions (effective 2002). adv. bk.rev. charts, illus. index. back issues avail.; reprint service avail. from PQC. *Refereed.* **Document type:** *Academic/Scholarly.* **Description:** Contains original findings in the fields of microbiology and infectious disease. Emphasis is on epidemiology, prevention and control.
Formerly (until 1987): Journal of Hygiene (0022-1724)
Related titles: Microform ed.: (from PQC,PMC); Online - full text ed.: (from EBSCO Publishing, O C L C Online Computer Library Center, Inc., RoweCom Information Quest, Swets Blackwell, Institute for Scientific Information).
Indexed: AIDS Abstr., ASCA, Abstr.Health Care Manage.Stud., Abstr.Hyg., Addic.Abstr., AgBiotech, Aqua.Sci.& Fish.Abstr., Aquacult.Abstr., Art.Hosp.& Tour., Biodet.Abstr., Biol.Abstr., Biostat., Br.Tech.Ind., Brit.Nur.Ind., Chem.Abstr., Chem.Indus.Notes, Chem.Titles, Curr.Adv.Ecol.Sci., Curr.Adv.Gen.& Molec.Biol., Curr.Cont., Curr.Ind.Stat., Dairy Sci.Abstr., Diar.Dis.Res., Environ.Sci.Poll.Mgmt., Excerp.Med., Food Sci.& Tech.Abstr., Helminthol.Abstr., INIS Atomind., Ind.Med. (1987-), Ind.Sci.Rev., Ind.Vet., Inpharma, Int.Abstr.Biol.Sci., Int.Nurs.Ind., Lab.Haz.Bull., Microbiol.Abstr., NRN, Nutr.Abstr., Pharm.&Out.News, Pig News & Info., Pollut.Abstr., Poult.Abstr., Protozool.Abstr., Reac., Ref.Zh., Rev.Appl.Entomol., Rev.Med.& Vet.Mycol., Rev.Plant Path., Rice Abstr., Risk Abstr., Saf.Sci.Abstr., Sci.Cit.Ind., Sel.Water Res.Abstr., Small Anim.Abstr., Sport Fish.Abstr., THA, Trop.Dis.Bull., Vet.Bull., Virol.Abstr. (coverage dropped), W.R.C.Inf., Wild.Rev., Zoo.Rec.
—BLDSC (3793.600000), CASDDS, CISTI, EMDOCS, GNLM, IDS, Infotrieve, KNAW, Linda Hall. **CCC.**
Published by: Cambridge University Press, Edinburgh Bldg, Shaftesbury Rd, Cambridge CB2 2RU, United Kingdom. FAX 44-1223-315052, information@cup.cam.ac.uk; journals_subscriptions@cup.org, http://www.cup.cam.ac.uk, http://www.uk.cambridge.org/journals/pmu. Ed. B Drasar. R&P Linda Nicol. Adv. contact Rebecca Symons.

579 DEU ISSN 0934-9723
CODEN: EJCDEU
EUROPEAN JOURNAL OF CLINICAL MICROBIOLOGY & INFECTIOUS DISEASES; an international journal on pathogenesis, diagnosis, epidemiology, therapy, and prevention of infectious diseases. Text in German. 1982. m. EUR 411.10 domestic; EUR 780.70 in Germany; EUR 38 newsstand/cover foreign (effective 2002). adv. *Refereed.* **Document type:** *Journal, Academic/Scholarly.* **Description:** Presents information and opinions in the fields of clinical microbiology and infectious diseases.
Formerly: European Journal of Clinical Microbiology
Related titles: Online - full text ed.: ISSN 1435-4373 (from EBSCO Publishing, RoweCom Information Quest, Swets Blackwell, Springer LINK, Institute for Scientific Information).
Indexed: ASCA, Abstr.Hyg., Abstr.Inter.Med., Biol.Abstr., Chem.Abstr., Chem.Indus.Notes, Chem.Titles, Curr.Adv.Ecol.Sci., Curr.Cont., Dairy Sci.Abstr., Dent.Ind., Diar.Dis.Res., Environ.Sci.Poll.Mgmt., Excerp.Med., Forest Prod.Abstr., Forest.Abstr., Ind.Med. (1988-), Ind.Sci.Rev., Ind.Vet., Inpharma, Int.Abstr.Biol.Sci., Int.Nurs.Ind., Jrnl.Watch Inf.Dis., Med.& Surg.Dermat., Microbiol.Abstr., NRN, Nutr.Abstr., Pharm.&Out.News, Protozool.Abstr., Reac., Rev.Appl.Entomol., Rev.Med.& Vet.Mycol., Sci.Cit.Ind., Trop.Dis.Bull.
—BLDSC (3829.727700), ADONIS, CASDDS, CISTI, EMDOCS, GNLM, IDS, Infotrieve, ingenta, KNAW. **CCC.**
Published by: Springer-Verlag (Subsidiary of: BertelsmannSpringer), Tiergartenstr 17, Heidelberg 69121, Germany. TEL 49-6221-345-0, FAX 49-6221-345229, subscriptions@springer.de, http://link.springer.de/link/service/journals/10096/index.htm, http://www.springer.de. Ed. I Braveny. Circ: 3,000.

EUROPEAN JOURNAL OF PROTISTOLOGY. see *PALEONTOLOGY*

EXCERPTA MEDICA. ABSTRACT JOURNALS. see *BIOLOGY—Abstracting, Bibliographies, Statistics*

EXCERPTA MEDICA. SECTION 4: MICROBIOLOGY: BACTERIOLOGY, MYCOLOGY, PARASITOLOGY AND VIROLOGY. see *BIOLOGY—Abstracting, Bibliographies, Statistics*

579.2 USA
EXPERIMENTAL VIROLOGY. Text in English. 1978. irreg., latest vol.4, 1983. reprint service avail. from ISI. *Refereed.*
Published by: Academic Press, Inc., Journal Division (Subsidiary of: Harcourt Brace & Company), 525 B St, Ste 1900, San Diego, CA 92101-4495. TEL 619-231-0926, FAX 619-699-6715. Eds. F Brown, T W Tinsley. **Subscr. to:** Order Dept., 6277 Sea Harbor Dr, 4th Fl, Orlando, FL 32887. TEL 800-321-5068.

616.01 NLD ISSN 0928-8244
QR46 CODEN: FIMIEV
F E M S IMMUNOLOGY AND MEDICAL MICROBIOLOGY. Text in English. 12/m. NLG 2,043, EUR 927.07 in Europe to institutions; JPY 130,500 in Japan to institutions; USD 1,037 elsewhere to institutions; NLG 10,973, EUR 4,979.33 in Europe to institutions Full Set FEMS Microbiology; JPY 698,000 in Japan to institutions Full Set FEMS Microbiology; USD 5,570 elsewhere to institutions Full Set FEMS Microbiology (effective 2001). back issues avail. *Refereed.* **Document type:** *Academic/Scholarly.* **Description:** Focuses on works describing the mechanisms of immunity and how these can be exploited in the diagnosis and treatment of disease.
Formerly (until 1993): F E M S Microbiology Immunology (0920-8534)
Related titles: Microform ed.: (from PQC); Online - full text ed.: (from ingenta, Swets Blackwell, ScienceDirect, Institute for Scientific Information).
Indexed: AIDS & Cancer Res., ASCA, Abstr.Hyg., AgBiotech, Agricola, Bibl.Agri., Chem.Indus.Notes, Chem.Titles, Curr.Cont., Dairy Sci.Abstr., Environ.Sci.Poll.Mgmt., Excerp.Med. (1988-), Immun.Abstr., Ind.Med. (1993-), Ind.Sci.Rev., Ind.Vet., Inpharma, Int.Abstr.Biol.Sci., Microbiol.Abstr., Nutr.Abstr., Pharm.&Out.News, Pig News & Info., Poult.Abstr., Protozool.Abstr., Reac., Rev.Appl.Entomol., Rev.Med.& Vet.Mycol., Sci.Cit.Ind., Telegen, Trop.Dis.Bull., Vet.Bull.
—BLDSC (3905.291000), ADONIS, CASDDS, CISTI, EMDOCS, GNLM, IDS, ingenta, KNAW, Linda Hall. **CCC.**
Published by: (Federation of European Microbiological Societies GBR), Elsevier Science BV, PO Box 211, Amsterdam 1000 AE, Netherlands. TEL 31-20-485-2911, FAX 31-20-485-2457, nlinfo-f@elsevier.nl, http://www.elsevier.com/locate/femsim. Ed. Loek van Alphen. **Subscr. in Australasia and the Far East to:** Elsevier Science (Singapore) Pte Ltd, No.1 Temasek Ave, 17-01 Millenia Tower, Singapore 039192, Singapore. TEL 65-434-3727, FAX 65-337-2230; **Subscr. in Japan to:** Elsevier Science Inc - Japan Regional Office, 9-15 Higashi-Azabu 1-chome, Minato-ku, Tokyo 106-0044, Japan. TEL 81-3-5561-5033; **Subscr. in the Americas to:** Elsevier Science, PO Box 945, New York, NY 10159-0945. TEL 212-633-3730, FAX 212-633-3680.

579.072 NLD ISSN 0921-8254
F E M S MICROBIOLOGY. Text in English. 1977. 57/yr. (in 22 vols.). USD 5,570 (effective 2001). cum.index. back issues avail. *Refereed.* **Document type:** *Academic/Scholarly.* **Description:** Publishes reports on microbiological research.
Related titles: Microform ed.: (from PQC).
Indexed: Apic.Abstr., Biol.Abstr., Chem.Abstr., Curr.Cont. (coverage dropped), Excerp.Med.
Published by: (Federation of European Microbiological Societies GBR), Elsevier Science BV, PO Box 211, Amsterdam 1000 AE, Netherlands. TEL 31-20-485-3911, FAX 31-20-485-2457, nlinfo-f@elsevier.nl; usinfo-f@elsevier.com; forinfo-kyf04035@niftyserve.or.jp, http://www.elsevier.nl/. **Subscr. in Australasia and the Far East to:** Elsevier Science (Singapore) Pte Ltd, No.1 Temasek Ave, 17-01 Millenia Tower, Singapore 039192, Singapore. TEL 65-434-3727, FAX 65-337-2230; **Subscr. in U.S. and Canada to:** Elsevier Science, PO Box 945, New York, NY 10159-0945. TEL 212-633-3730, FAX 212-633-3680.

579.17 NLD ISSN 0168-6496
CODEN: FMECEZ
F E M S MICROBIOLOGY ECOLOGY. Text in English. m. EUR 988 in Europe to institutions; JPY 131,200 in Japan to institutions; USD 1,105 elsewhere to institutions (effective 2002). back issues avail. *Refereed.* **Document type:** *Academic/Scholarly.* **Description:** Details fundamental aspects of the ecology of micro-organisms in a variety of environments and situations.
Related titles: Microform ed.: (from PQC); Online - full text ed.: (from EBSCO Publishing, ingenta, Swets Blackwell, ScienceDirect, Institute for Scientific Information).

B

Indexed: ASCA, Abstr.Hyg., AgBiotech, Agricola, Appl.Ecol.Abstr., Aqua.Sci.& Fish.Abstr., Bibl.Agri., Bio-Contr.News & Info., Biodet.Abstr., Chem.Abstr., Chem.Indus.Notes, Chem.Titles, Crop Physiol.Abstr., Curr.Cont., Dairy Sci.Abstr., Ecol.Abstr., Environ.Abstr., Environ.Sci.Poll.Mgmt., Excerp.Med., Field Crop Abstr., Forest Prod.Abstr., Forest.Abstr., Geo.Abstr.P.G., Geol.Abstr., Ind.Sci.Rev., Ind.Vet., Inpharma, Int.Abstr.Biol.Sci., Irr.& Drain.Abstr., Microbiol.Abstr., Nutr.Abstr., Ocean.Abstr., Plant Breed.Abstr., Pollut.Abstr., Potato Abstr., Protozool.Abstr., Reac., Rev.Appl.Entomol., Rev.Med.& Vet.Mycol., Rev.Plant Path., Rice Abstr., Russ.Acad.Sci.Bibl., Sci.Cit.Ind., Seed Abstr., Sel.Water Res.Abstr., Soils & Fert., Soyabean Abstr., Telegen, Triticale Abstr., Weed Abstr., Zoo.Rec.
—BLDSC (3905.296000), ADONIS, CASDDS, CISTI, GNLM, IDS, ingenta, Linda Hall. **CCC.**
Published by: (Federation of European Microbiological Societies GBR), Elsevier Science BV, PO Box 211, Amsterdam 1000 AE, Netherlands. TEL 31-20-485-3911, FAX 31-20-485-2457, nlinfo-f@elsevier.nl; usinfo-f@elsevier.com; forinfo-kyf04035@niftyserve.or.jp, http://www.elsevier.com/locate/femsecol, http://www.elsevier.nl. Eds. P Bavoli, T Chakraborty. **Subscr. in Australasia and the Far East to:** Elsevier Science (Singapore) Pte Ltd, No.1 Temasek Ave, 17-01 Millenia Tower, Singapore 039192, Singapore. TEL 65-434-3727, FAX 65-337-2230**; Subscr. in Japan to:** Elsevier Science Inc - Japan Regional Office, 9-15 Higashi-Azabu 1-chome, Minato-ku, Tokyo 106-0044, Japan. TEL 81-3-5561-5033**; Subscr. in the Americas to:** Elsevier Science, PO Box 945, New York, NY 10159-0945. TEL 212-633-3730, FAX 212-633-3680.

579 NLD ISSN 0378-1097
QR1 CODEN: FMLED7
F E M S MICROBIOLOGY LETTERS. Text in English. 1977. 24/yr. EUR 3,428 in Europe to institutions; JPY 454,800 in Japan to institutions; USD 3,833 elsewhere to institutions (effective 2002). adv. back issues avail.; reprint service avail. from SWZ,ISI. *Refereed.* **Document type:** *Academic/Scholarly.* **Description:** Covers all aspects of microbiology and microbial chemistry.
Related titles: Microform ed.: (from PQC); Online - full text ed.: (from ingenta, Swets Blackwell, ScienceDirect, Institute for Scientific Information).
Indexed: ASCA, AgBiotech, Agri.& Environ.Biotech.Abstr., Agricola (coverage dropped), Aqua.Sci.& Fish.Abstr., BBCI, Bibl.Agri., Bio-Contr.News & Info., Biodet.Abstr., Biol.Abstr., Biotech.Cit.Ind., CEABA, Chem.Abstr., Chem.Indus.Notes, Chem.Titles, Curr.Adv.Biochem., Curr.Adv.Ecol.Sci., Curr.Adv.Gen.& Molec.Biol., Curr.Biotech.Abstr., Curr.Cont., Dairy Sci.Abstr., Deep Sea Res.& Oceanogr.Abstr., Derwent Biotech.Abstr., Environ.Abstr., Environ.Sci.Poll.Mgmt., Excerp.Med., Field Crop Abstr., Food Sci.& Tech.Abstr., Forest Prod.Abstr., Forest.Abstr., Genet.Abstr., GeoRef, Helminthol.Abstr., Hort.Abstr., Hum.Gen.Abstr., INIS Atomind., Ind.Med. (1977-), Ind.Sci.Rev., Ind.Vet., Inpharma, Int.Abstr.Biol.Sci., Mass Spectr.Bull., Microbiol.Abstr., Nuc.Acids Abstr., Nutr.Abstr., Pig News & Info., Plant Breed.Abstr., Plant Gen.Res.Abstr., Poult.Abstr., Protozool.Abstr., Reac., Rev.Appl.Entomol., Rev.Arom.& Med.Plants, Rev.Med.& Vet.Mycol., Rev.Plant Path., Rice Abstr., Sci.Cit.Ind., Soils & Fert., Sport Fish.Abstr., Sugar Ind.Abstr., Telegen, Trop.Dis.Bull., Vet.Bull., Virol.Abstr. (coverage dropped), Weed Abstr., Wild.Rev., Zoo.Rec.
—BLDSC (3905.300000), ADONIS, CASDDS, CISTI, EMDOCS, GNLM, IDS, ingenta, Linda Hall. **CCC.**
Published by: (Federation of European Microbiological Societies GBR), Elsevier Science BV, PO Box 211, Amsterdam 1000 AE, Netherlands. TEL 31-20-485-3911, FAX 31-20-485-3598, http://www.elsevier.com/locate/femslett, http://www.elsevier.nl. Ed. F G Priest. **Subscr. in Australasia and the Far East to:** Elsevier Science (Singapore) Pte Ltd, No.1 Temasek Ave, 17-01 Millenia Tower, Singapore 039192, Singapore. TEL 65-434-3727, FAX 65-337-2230**; Subscr. in Japan to:** Elsevier Science Inc - Japan Regional Office, 9-15 Higashi-Azabu 1-chome, Minato-ku, Tokyo 106-0044, Japan. TEL 81-3-5561-5033**; Subscr. in the Americas to:** Elsevier Science, PO Box 945, New York, NY 10159-0945. TEL 212-633-3730, FAX 212-633-3680.

579 NLD ISSN 0168-6445
QR1 CODEN: FMREE4
F E M S MICROBIOLOGY REVIEWS. Text in English. 1977. 5/yr. EUR 382 in Europe to institutions (effective 2001); JPY 50,800 in Japan to institutions; USD 427 elsewhere to institutions (effective 2002). back issues avail. *Refereed.* **Document type:** *Academic/Scholarly.* **Description:** Covers the entire field of microbiology with an emphasis on topicality and readability.
Related titles: Microform ed.: (from PQC); Online - full text ed.: (from EBSCO Publishing, ingenta, Swets Blackwell, ScienceDirect, Institute for Scientific Information).
Indexed: AESIS, ASCA, Agri.& Environ.Biotech.Abstr., Agricola, Aqua.Sci.& Fish.Abstr., BBCI, Biodet.Abstr., Biol.Abstr., Biotech.Cit.Ind., CEABA, Chem.Abstr., Chem.Cit.Ind., Curr.Cont., Derwent Biotech.Abstr., Environ.Abstr., Environ.Sci.Poll.Mgmt., Excerp.Med., Food Sci.& Tech.Abstr., Ind.Med. (1985-), Ind.Sci.Rev., Inpharma, Int.Abstr.Biol.Sci., Mat.Sci.Cit.Ind. (coverage dropped), Microbiol.Abstr., Protozool.Abstr., Reac., Ref.Zh., Sci.Cit.Ind., Zoo.Rec.
—BLDSC (3905.305000), ADONIS, CASDDS, CISTI, GNLM, IDS, ingenta, Linda Hall. **CCC.**
Published by: (Federation of European Microbiological Societies GBR), Elsevier Science BV, PO Box 211, Amsterdam 1000 AE, Netherlands. TEL 31-20-485-2911, FAX 31-20-485-2457, nlinfo-f@elsevier.nl; usinfo-f@elsevier.com; forinfo-kyf04035@niftyserve.or.jp, http://www.elsevier.com/locate/femsrev. Ed. N Brown. **Subscr. in Australasia and the Far East to:** Elsevier Science (Singapore) Pte Ltd, No.1 Temasek Ave, 17-01 Millenia Tower, Singapore 039192, Singapore. TEL 65-434-3727, FAX 65-337-2230**; Subscr. in Japan to:** Elsevier Science Inc - Japan Regional Office, 9-15 Higashi-Azabu 1-chome, Minato-ku, Tokyo 106-0044, Japan. TEL 81-3-5561-5033**; Subscr. in the Americas to:** Elsevier Science, PO Box 945, New York, NY 10159-0945. TEL 212-633-3730, FAX 212-633-3680.

579 571 576.5 NLD ISSN 1567-1356
▼ **F E M S YEAST RESEARCH.** Text in English. 2001. q. EUR 222 in Europe to institutions; JPY 29,400 in Japan to institutions; USD 248 elsewhere to institutions (effective 2002). back issues avail. **Document type:** *Journal, Academic/Scholarly.* **Description:** Publishes original research papers and mini-reviews that cover both yeast and yeast-like organisms.
Related titles: Online - full text ed.: Federation of European Microbiological Societies Yeast Research Online. ISSN 1567-1364. NLG 286, EUR 129.78 in Europe to institutions; JPY 18,000 in Japan to institutions; USD 146 elsewhere to institutions (effective 2001).
—BLDSC (3905.325000), ADONIS.
Published by: (Federation of European Microbiological Societies GBR), Elsevier Science BV, PO Box 211, Amsterdam 1000 AE, Netherlands. TEL 31-20-485-2911, FAX 31-20-485-2457, http://www.elsevier.com/locate/femsyr, http://www.elsevier.nl. Ed. Lex Scheffers.

FOLIA PARASITOLOGICA. see *MEDICAL SCIENCES—Communicable Diseases*

579 GBR ISSN 0740-0020
QR115 CODEN: FOMIE5
FOOD MICROBIOLOGY. Text in English. 1984. bi-m. GBP 384 to institutions (effective 2001). adv. bk.rev. reprint service avail. from SWZ. *Refereed.* **Document type:** *Academic/Scholarly.* **Description:** Publishes primary research papers, short research communications, reviews, reports of meetings, and news items dealing with all aspects of the microbiology of foods.
Related titles: Online - full text ed.: (from EBSCO Publishing, O C L C Online Computer Library Center, Inc., RoweCom Information Quest, ingenta, Swets Blackwell, IDEAL Online Library, Institute for Scientific Information).
Indexed: ASCA, Agricola, Aqua.Sci.& Fish.Abstr., Bibl.Agri., Biodet.Abstr., Biotech.Cit.Ind., Chem.Abstr., Chem.Indus.Notes, Chem.Titles, Curr.Adv.Ecol.Sci., Curr.Cont., Dairy Sci.Abstr., Environ.Sci.Poll.Mgmt., Excerp.Med., Food Sci.& Tech.Abstr., Forest Prod.Abstr., Forest.Abstr., Ind.Vet., Int.Abstr.Biol.Sci., Microbiol.Abstr., Nutr.Abstr., Pig News & Info., Pollut.Abstr., Postharvest, Poult.Abstr., Ref.Zh., Rev.Med.& Vet.Mycol., Rev.Plant Path., Risk Abstr., Saf.Sci.Abstr., Sci.Cit.Ind., Sugar Ind.Abstr., Vet.Bull.
—BLDSC (3981.300000), ADONIS, CASDDS, CISTI, EMDOCS, GNLM, IDS, Infotrieve, ingenta, Linda Hall. **CCC.**
Published by: Academic Press (Subsidiary of: Harcourt Publishers Ltd.), 24 Oval Rd, London NW1 7DX, United Kingdom. TEL 44-20-7267-4466, FAX 44-20-7482-2293, apsubs@acad.com, http://www.academicpress.com/foodmicro; http://www.europe.idealibrary.com/. Ed. C A Batt. R&P Catherine John. Adv. contact Nik Screen. **Subscr. to:** Harcourt Publishers Ltd., Foots Cray High St, Sidcup, Kent DA14 5HP, United Kingdom. TEL 44-20-8300-3322, FAX 44-20-8309-0807.

579.2 DEU
FRONTIERS OF VIROLOGY. Text in English. irreg., latest vol.2. **Document type:** *Academic/Scholarly.*
Published by: Springer-Verlag (Subsidiary of: BertelsmannSpringer), Haber Str 7, Heidelberg 69126, Germany. FAX 49-30-82787448, subscriptions@springer.de, http://www.springer.de, http://link.springer-ny.com. Eds. Gholamreza Darai, Yechiel Becker.

579 USA ISSN 0149-0451
QR103 CODEN: GEJODG
GEOMICROBIOLOGY JOURNAL; an international journal of geomicrobiology and microbial biogeochemistry. Text in English. 1978. bi-m. GBP 113, USD 186 to individuals; GBP 365, USD 602 to institutions (effective 2002). adv. bk.rev. abstr. index. *Refereed.* **Document type:** *Academic/Scholarly.* **Description:** Explores the geologic impact of microbial transformations of materials that make up the Earth's crust, oceans, sea lakes, bottom sediments, soils, mineral deposits, and rocks.
Related titles: Online - full text ed.: ISSN 1521-0529 (from CatchWord Ltd., EBSCO Publishing, O C L C Online Computer Library Center, Inc., RoweCom Information Quest, Swets Blackwell, Institute for Scientific Information).
Indexed: AESIS, ASCA, Aqua.Sci.& Fish.Abstr., Biol.Abstr., Chem.Abstr., Chem.Indus.Notes, Chem.Titles, Curr.Adv.Ecol.Sci., Curr.Biotech.Abstr., Curr.Cont., Deep Sea Res.& Oceanogr.Abstr., E & P Hlth. (1993-), Ecol.Abstr., Environ.Sci.Poll.Mgmt., Forest.Abstr., Gas Process.& Ppl. (1993-), Geo.Abstr.P.G., GeoRef, Geol.Abstr., Geomech.Abstr., Hort.Abstr., INIS Atomind., Ind.Sci.Rev., Microbiol.Abstr., Off.Tech. (1993-), Ornam.Hort., Petrol.Abstr. (1989-, dropped), Pollut.Abstr., Rev.Plant Path., SSCI (coverage dropped), Sci.Cit.Ind., Sel.Water Res.Abstr., Soils & Fert., W.R.C.Inf.
—BLDSC (4147.590000), CASDDS, CatchWord, CISTI, EMDOCS, IDS, ingenta, Linda Hall. **CCC.**
Published by: Taylor & Francis Ltd. (Subsidiary of: Taylor & Francis Group), 325 Chestnut St, Suite 800, Philadelphia, PA 19016. TEL 215-625-8900, FAX 215-625-2940, info@taylorandfrancis.com, http://www.taylorandfrancis.com/. Ed. William C Ghiorse. **Subscr. addr. in Europe:** Taylor & Francis Group, Journals Customer Service, Rankine Rd, Basingstoke, Hants RG24 8PR, United Kingdom. TEL 44-1256-813000, FAX 44-1256-479438, enquiry@tanf.co.uk, http://www.tandf.co.uk/journals.

579 ITA ISSN 0390-5462
CODEN: GBVID3
GIORNALE DI BATTERIOLOGIA, VIROLOGIA ED IMMUNOLOGIA. Text in Italian. 1926. s-a. abstr.
Supersedes: Giornale di Batteriologia, Virologia ed Immunologia ed Annali dell'Ospedale Maria Vittoria di Torino. Parte 1. Microbiologia (0301-1453); Which superseded in part: Giornale di Batteriologia, Virologia ed Immunologia ed Annali dell'Ospedale Maria Vittoria di Torino (0017-0267)
Indexed: Biol.Abstr., Chem.Abstr., Chem.Indus.Notes, Chem.Titles, Ind.Med. (coverage dropped), Ind.Vet., Rev.Med.& Vet.Mycol., Trop.Dis.Bull., Vet.Bull.
—CASDDS, CISTI, GNLM.
Published by: Ospedale Maria Vittoria, Via Luigi Cibrario, 72, Turin, TO 10144, Italy. TEL 74 92 345.

579 ITA ISSN 0017-0380
GIORNALE DI MICROBIOLOGIA. Text in English, French, German, Italian, Spanish. 1955. q. index.
Indexed: Biol.Abstr., Chem.Abstr., Excerp.Med., INIS Atomind.
—CISTI, GNLM, Linda Hall.
Published by: Istituto Microbiologia, Via Luigi Mangiagalli, 31, Milan, MI 20133, Italy. Ed. Romolo Deotto. Circ: 650.

GLYCOCONJUGATE JOURNAL. see *BIOLOGY—Biochemistry*

579.3 CHN ISSN 1001-1072
GUOWAI YIXUE (JISHENGBING FENCE)/FOREIGN MEDICAL SCIENCES (PARASITOSIS). Text in Chinese. 1979. bi-m. USD 10.20; USD 1.70 newsstand/cover (effective 2001). **Document type:** *Academic/Scholarly.*
Published by: Zhongguo Yufang Yixue Kexueyuan, Jishengchongbing Yanjiusuo/Chinese Academy of Preventive Medicine, Institute of Parasitic Diseases, 207 Ruijin 2 Lu, Shanghai 200025, China. TEL 86-21-6437-7008. Ed. Xiao Shuhua. **Dist. by:** China International Book Trading Corp, 35, Chegongzhuang Xilu, Haidian District, Beijing 100044, China. TEL 86-1-68413849, FAX 86-1-68412048, cibtc@mail.cibtc.com.cn, http://www.cibtc.com.cn.

579 616.3 616.99 USA ISSN 1083-4389
HELICOBACTER. Text in English. 1996. q., latest vol.7, 2002. GBP 99 per issue in Europe to individuals; USD 143 per issue in North America to individuals; GBP 99 per issue elsewhere to individuals; GBP 354 per issue in Europe to institutions; USD 562 per issue elsewhere to institutions; GBP 390 per issue in North America to institutions (effective 2002). adv. reprints avail. *Refereed.* **Document type:** *Academic/Scholarly.* **Description:** Investigates the critical role Helicobacter plays in peptic ulcers, gastric adenocarcinoma, and primary gastric lymphoma.
Related titles: Online - full text ed.: ISSN 1523-5378. GBP 90 in Europe to individuals; USD 129 in North America to individuals; GBP 90 elsewhere to individuals; GBP 319 in Europe to institutions; USD 506 in North America to institutions; GBP 319 elsewhere to institutions (effective 2002) (from EBSCO Publishing, O C L C Online Computer Library Center, Inc., RoweCom Information Quest, ingenta, Munksgaard & Blackwell Science's Synergy, Swets Blackwell, Institute for Scientific Information).
Indexed: Curr.Cont., Ind.Med. (1996-), Int.Nurs.Ind., Sci.Cit.Ind.
—BLDSC (4285.102500), CISTI, GNLM, IDS, Infotrieve. **CCC.**
Published by: Blackwell Science Ltd., PO Box 88, Oxford OX2 0NE, United Kingdom. TEL 44-1865-206180, 44-1865-206002, FAX 44-1865-206219, jnl.orders@blacksci.co.uk, http://www.blackwell-science.com/~cgilib/jnlpage.asp?Journal=xheli&File=xheli, http://www.blackwellpublishing.com. Ed. D Graham. Pub. Allen Stevens. R&P Sophie Savage. Adv. contact Jenny Applin. Circ: 1,000.

IMMUNOHISTOCHEMISTRY. see *BIOLOGY—Abstracting, Bibliographies, Statistics*

579 IND ISSN 0046-8991
QR1 CODEN: IJMBAC
INDIAN JOURNAL OF MICROBIOLOGY. Text in English. 1961. q. USD 100 (effective 2001). adv. bk.rev. **Document type:** *Academic/Scholarly.*
Related titles: Online - full text ed.: (from Institute for Scientific Information).
Indexed: Agri.& Environ.Biotech.Abstr. (coverage dropped), Agroforest.Abstr., Aqua.Sci.& Fish.Abstr., Aquacult.Abstr., Bio-Contr.News & Info., Biol.Abstr., Chem.Abstr., Crop Physiol.Abstr., Dairy Sci.Abstr., Derwent Biotech.Abstr., Diar.Dis.Res., Environ.Sci.Poll.Mgmt., Excerp.Med., Field Crop Abstr., Food Sci.& Tech.Abstr., Forest.Abstr., Hort.Abstr., INIS Atomind., Ind.Med. (coverage dropped), Ind.Vet., Nutr.Abstr., Plant Breed.Abstr., Plant Grow.Reg.Abstr., Poult.Abstr., Protozool.Abstr., Rev.Appl.Entomol., Rev.Med.& Vet.Mycol., Rev.Plant Path., Rice Abstr., Soils & Fert., Soyabean Abstr., Sugar Ind.Abstr., Triticale Abstr., Trop.Dis.Bull., Vet.Bull., Weed Abstr.
—BLDSC (4417.300000), CASDDS, CISTI, GNLM, ingenta, Linda Hall.
Published by: (Association of Microbiologists of India), Scientific Publishers, 5-A New Pali Rd., P O Box 91, Jodhpur, Rajasthan 342 001, India. TEL 91-291-433323, FAX 91-291-512580, scienti@sancharnet.in, http://www.scientificpub.com. Ed. Dr. K S Gopalkrishnan. Circ: 2,000. **Dist. by:** H P C Publishers Distributors Pvt. Ltd., 1st Fl., Flats 1 & 2, Darya Ganj, 4805-24 Bharat Ram Rd., New Delhi 110 002, India. TEL 91-11-3254401, FAX 91-11-619-3511, hpcpd@hpc.cc, http://www.bizdelhi.com/publisher/hpc, http://www.hpc.cc.

579 IND ISSN 0377-4929
CODEN: IJPMDT
INDIAN JOURNAL OF PATHOLOGY & MICROBIOLOGY. Text in English. 1949. q. INR 2,000; INR 4,000 foreign (effective 1999). adv. bk.rev. abstr, bibl, charts, illus. index. back issues avail.; reprint service avail. from IRC. *Refereed.* **Document type:** *Academic/Scholarly.*
Formerly: Indian Journal of Pathology and Bacteriology (0019-5448)
Related titles: CD-ROM ed.; Diskette ed.
Indexed: Biol.Abstr., Chem.Abstr., Curr.Adv.Ecol.Sci., Dent.Ind., Diar.Dis.Res., Excerp.Med., ExtraMED, Food Sci.& Tech.Abstr., INIS Atomind., Ind.Med. (1975-), Ind.Vet., Nutr.Abstr., Rev.Med.& Vet.Mycol., Rev.Plant Path., Vet.Bull.
—BLDSC (4417.950000), CISTI, EMDOCS, GNLM, ingenta, KNAW.
Published by: Indian Association of Pathologists and Microbiologists, Department of Microbiology, Indira Gandhi Institute of Medical Sciences, Patna, Bihar 800 014, India. TEL 91-0612-287631, 91-212-331139. Ed. S K Shahi. R&P, Adv. contact S.K. Shahi. page INR 7,000. Circ: 4,500. **Subscr. to:** Dr. A.M. Phatak, Treasurer, I A P M, Dept. of Pathology, T.N. Medical College and BYL Nair Hospital, Dr. A.L. Nair Rd., Mumbai, Maharashtra 400 008, India.

INFECTOLOGIA Y MICROBIOLOGIA CLINICA. see *MEDICAL SCIENCES—Communicable Diseases*

579.3 FRA ISSN 0924-4204
QR1 CODEN: AIPAEZ
INSTITUT PASTEUR. ANNALES. ACTUALITES. Text in French. 1990. q. EUR 97 in Europe to institutions; USD 122 elsewhere to institutions (effective 2002). bk.rev. back issues avail. *Refereed.* **Document type:** *Academic/Scholarly.* **Description:** Presents the scientific activities of the institute, which is involved in many fields from medical bacteriology to sophisticated genetics through embryogenesis and neurobiology.
Related titles: Microform ed.: (from PQC); Online - full text ed.: (from ingenta, Swets Blackwell, ScienceDirect).
Indexed: Excerp.Med. (1993-), Int.Abstr.Biol.Sci.
—BLDSC (0926.500000), CISTI, EMDOCS, GNLM, Infotrieve. **CCC.**
Published by: (Institut Pasteur), Elsevier Paris, Editions Scientifiques et Medicales (Subsidiary of: Reed Elsevier plc. group), 23 rue Linois, Paris 75015, France. TEL 33-1-45589110, FAX 33-1-45589419, academic@elsevier-fr.com, http://www.elsevier.com/locate/aipact. Ed. Georges N Cohen.

579.2 DZA ISSN 0020-2460
INSTITUT PASTEUR D'ALGERIE. ARCHIVES. Text in English, French. 1921. a. DZD 30, USD 6. bibl, charts, illus, stat. index.
Related titles: Microfilm ed.
Indexed: Bio-Contr.News & Info., Biol.Abstr., Dairy Sci.Abstr., Excerp.Med., Helminthol.Abstr., Ind.Med. (1923-), Ind.Vet., Protozool.Abstr., Rev.Appl.Entomol., Trop.Dis.Bull., Vet.Bull., Zoo.Rec.
—CISTI, GNLM, Linda Hall.
Published by: Institut Pasteur d'Algerie, Rue du Docteur Laveran, Algiers, Algeria. TEL 67-25-02, TELEX 65337. Circ: 1,000.

579.2 SEN ISSN 0377-3418
QR64.S382
INSTITUT PASTEUR DE DAKAR. RAPPORT SUR LE FONCTIONNEMENT TECHNIQUE. Text in French. 1938. a. free. **Document type:** *Yearbook, Corporate, Academic/Scholarly.* **Description:** Reports on medical research activities in virology, immunology and vaccinology, epidemiology and entomology, bacteriology.
Indexed: Biol.Abstr.
Published by: Institut Pasteur Dakar, 36 av Pasteur, PO Box 220, Dakar, Senegal. TEL 221-839-9201, FAX 221-839-9210, mathiot@pasteur.sn. Ed., Pub., R&P, Adv. contact Christian Mathiot. Circ: 600.

579.65 GRC ISSN 0004-6620
CODEN: AINPAW
INSTITUT PASTEUR HELLENIQUE. ARCHIVES. Text in French; Summaries in English, Greek. 1923. a. free per issue. adv.
Indexed: Abstr.Hyg., Biol.Abstr., Ind.Vet., Trop.Dis.Bull., Vet.Bull.
—CASDDS, GNLM.
Published by: Institut Pasteur Hellenique, 127 Reine Sophie Ave, Athens 618, Greece. Ed. Charles Serie. Circ: 1,500.

579 JPN ISSN 0073-8751
QR1
INSTITUTE FOR FERMENTATION, OSAKA. RESEARCH COMMUNICATIONS/HAKKO KENKYUJO HOKOKU. Text and summaries in English. 1963. biennial, latest vol.18, 1997. JPY 1,300 per issue. cum.index. back issues avail. **Document type:** *Bulletin.* **Description:** Provides information on the institute's taxonomical research studies of microorganisms, basic studies on animal cells, and on the culture collection of the institute.
Formerly (until no.4, 1969): Institute for Fermentation, Osaka. Annual Report
Indexed: Biol.Abstr., Curr.Biotech.Abstr., Ref.Zh., Rev.Appl.Entomol., Rev.Med.& Vet.Mycol., Rev.Plant Path.
—BLDSC, CISTI.
Published by: Institute for Fermentation Osaka/Hakko Kenkyujo, 17-85 Juso-Hon-Machi 2-chome, Yodogawa-ku, Osaka-shi 532-0024, Japan. FAX 81-6-6300-6814, yo@mb.infoweb.ne.jp, http://www.soc.nacsis.ac.jp/yo/index.html. Ed. Masao Takeuchi. Circ: 1,300.

579 BRA ISSN 0073-9855
R25 CODEN: RIALA6
INSTITUTO ADOLFO LUTZ. REVISTA. Text in English, Portuguese; Summaries in English, Portuguese. 1941. s-a. exchange basis. bibl, charts, illus. index. *Refereed.* **Document type:** *Government.* **Description:** Original papers in experimental and laboratory medicine or public health laboratory with emphasis on microbiology, epidemiology, chemistry and food chemistry.
Indexed: Abstr.Hyg., Agrindex, Anal.Abstr., Aqua.Sci.& Fish.Abstr., Biol.Abstr., Chem.Abstr., Chem.Titles, Dairy Sci.Abstr., Environ.Sci.Poll.Mgmt., Excerp.Med., Food Sci.& Tech.Abstr., Helminthol.Abstr., Ind.Med. (coverage dropped), Ind.Vet., Maize Abstr., Microbiol.Abstr., Nutr.Abstr., Postharvest, Poult.Abstr., Protozool.Abstr., Ref.Zh., Rev.Appl.Entomol., Rev.Med.& Vet.Mycol., Soyabean Abstr., Sugar Ind.Abstr., Tox.Abstr. (coverage dropped), Triticale Abstr., Trop.Dis.Bull., Vet.Bull., Virol.Abstr. (coverage dropped), Zoo.Rec.
—BLDSC (7816.000000), CASDDS.
Published by: Instituto Adolfo Lutz, Diretoria Geral, Ave. Dr Arnaldo, 355, Centro, Caixa Postal 7027, Sao Paulo, SP 01064-970, Brazil. TEL 55-11-8510111, FAX 55-11-8533505. Ed. Luiz Carlos Meneguetti. Circ: 1,200.

B

579 USA ISSN 0276-1076
QR187.5 CODEN: INRFDC
INTERFERON. Text in English. 1979. irreg., latest vol.9, 1987. reprint service avail. from ISI.
Indexed: Curr.Adv.Ecol.Sci.
—CASDDS, CISTI, GNLM.
Published by: Academic Press, Inc., Journal Division (Subsidiary of: Harcourt Brace & Company), 525 B St, Ste 1900, San Diego, CA 92101-4495. TEL 619-231-0926, FAX 619-699-6715. Ed. I Gresser. **Subscr. to:** Order Dept., 6277 Sea Harbor Dr, 4th Fl, Orlando, FL 32887. TEL 800-321-5068.

INTERNATIONAL ANTIVIRAL NEWS. see *MEDICAL SCIENCES—Communicable Diseases*

INTERNATIONAL JOURNAL FOR PARASITOLOGY. see *MEDICAL SCIENCES—Communicable Diseases*

579 NLD ISSN 0924-8579
CODEN: IAAGEA
INTERNATIONAL JOURNAL OF ANTIMICROBIAL AGENTS. Text in English. 1991. 12/yr. EUR 1,042 in Europe to institutions; JPY 138,400 in Japan to institutions; USD 1,165 elsewhere to institutions (effective 2002). adv. back issues avail. *Refereed.* **Document type:** *Academic/Scholarly.* **Description:** Provides information on the physical, chemical, pharmacological, in vitro and clinical properties of individual antimicrobial agents, and immunotherapy.
Related titles: Microform ed.: (from PQC); Online - full text ed.: (from ingenta, Swets Blackwell, ScienceDirect, Institute for Scientific Information).
Indexed: ASCA, Abstr.Hyg., Agri.& Environ.Biotech.Abstr., Agroforest.Abstr., Chem.Abstr., Chem.Indus.Notes, Chem.Titles, Curr.Cont., Derwent Biotech.Abstr., Environ.Sci.Poll.Mgmt., Excerp.Med., Ind.Med. (1991-), Ind.Sci.Rev., Ind.Vet., Inpharma, Int.Abstr.Biol.Sci., Int.Nurs.Ind., Med.& Pharm.Biotech.Abstr., Microbiol.Abstr., Nutr.Abstr., Pharm.&Out.News, Pig News & Info., Poult.Abstr., Protozool.Abstr., Reac., Rev.Appl.Entomol., Rev.Arom.& Med.Plants, Rev.Med.& Vet.Mycol., Saf.Sci.Abstr., Sci.Cit.Ind., Trop.Dis.Bull., Vet.Bull., Virol.Abstr. (coverage dropped).
—BLDSC (4542.084000), CASDDS, CISTI, EMDOCS, GNLM, IDS, Infotrieve, KNAW. **CCC.**
Published by: (International Society of Chemotherapy BRD), Elsevier Science BV, PO Box 211, Amsterdam 1000 AE, Netherlands. TEL 31-20-485-3911, FAX 31-20-485-3598, nlinfo-f@elsevier.nl, http://www.elsevier.com/locate/ijantimicag. Ed. David Williams. **Subscr. in Australasia and the Far East to:** Elsevier Science (Singapore) Pte Ltd, No.1 Temasek Ave, 17-01 Millenia Tower, Singapore 039192, Singapore. TEL 65-434-3727, FAX 65-337-2230; **Subscr. in Japan to:** Elsevier Science Inc - Japan Regional Office, 9-15 Higashi-Azabu 1-chome, Minato-ku, Tokyo 106-0044, Japan. TEL 81-3-5561-5033; **Subscr. in the Americas to:** Elsevier Science, PO Box 945, New York, NY 10159-0945. TEL 212-633-3730, FAX 212-633-3680.

579 NLD ISSN 0168-1605
CODEN: IJFMDD
INTERNATIONAL JOURNAL OF FOOD MICROBIOLOGY. Text and summaries in English. 1984. 24/yr. EUR 136 in Europe to qualified personnel; JPY 17,600 in Japan to qualified personnel; USD 151 elsewhere to qualified personnel; EUR 2,374 in Europe to institutions; JPY 315,200 in Japan to institutions; USD 2,655 elsewhere to institutions (effective 2002). adv. bk.rev. abstr, bibl, charts, illus. back issues avail. *Refereed.* **Document type:** *Academic/Scholarly.* **Description:** Covers all aspects of microbiological safety, quality and acceptability of foods.
Related titles: Microform ed.: (from PQC); Online - full text ed.: (from ingenta, Swets Blackwell, ScienceDirect, Institute for Scientific Information).
Indexed: ASCA, Abstr.Hyg., Agri.& Environ.Biotech.Abstr., Agricola, Apic.Abstr., Aqua.Sci.& Fish.Abstr., Bibl.Agri., Bio-Contr.News & Info., Biotech.Cit.Ind., Curr.Adv.Ecol.Sci., Curr.Cont., Dairy Sci.Abstr., Eng.Ind., Environ.Sci.Poll.Mgmt., Excerp.Med., Food Sci.& Tech.Abstr., Hort.Abstr., Ind.Med. (1984-), Ind.Sci.Rev., Ind.Vet., Int.Abstr.Biol.Sci., Int.Nurs.Ind., Irr.& Drain.Abstr., Maize Abstr., Microbiol.Abstr., Nutr.Abstr., Ocean.Abstr., Pig News & Info., Pollut.Abstr., Postharvest, Poult.Abstr., Protozool.Abstr., Rev.Med.& Vet.Mycol., Rev.Plant Path., Risk Abstr., SSCI (coverage dropped), Saf.Sci.Abstr., Sci.Cit.Ind., Seed Abstr., Soils & Fert., Soyabean Abstr., Sugar Ind.Abstr., Triticale Abstr., Vet.Bull., World Ag.Econ.& Rur.Soc.Abstr.
—BLDSC (4542.253000), CASDDS, CISTI, Ei, GNLM, IDS, Infotrieve, ingenta, Linda Hall. **CCC.**
Published by: (International Union of Microbiological Societies), Elsevier Science BV, PO Box 211, Amsterdam 1000 AE, Netherlands. TEL 31-20-485-3911, FAX 31-20-485-3598, nlinfo-f@elsevier.nl, http://www.elsevier.com/locate/ijfoodmicro. Ed. M Jakobsen. Circ: 700. **Subscr. in Australasia and the Far East to:** Elsevier Science (Singapore) Pte Ltd, No.1 Temasek Ave, 17-01 Millenia Tower, Singapore 039192, Singapore. TEL 65-434-3727, FAX 65-337-2230; **Subscr. in Japan to:** Elsevier Science Inc - Japan Regional Office, 9-15 Higashi-Azabu 1-chome, Minato-ku, Tokyo 106-0044, Japan. TEL 81-3-5561-5033; **Subscr. in the Americas to:** Elsevier Science, PO Box 945, New York, NY 10159-0945. TEL 212-633-3730, FAX 212-633-3680. **Co-sponsor:** International Committee on Food Microbiology and Hygiene.

INTERNATIONAL JOURNAL OF MEDICAL MICROBIOLOGY. see *MEDICAL SCIENCES—Communicable Diseases*

579.3 GBR ISSN 1466-5026
QR1 CODEN: IJSBA8
INTERNATIONAL JOURNAL OF SYSTEMATIC AND EVOLUTIONARY MICROBIOLOGY. Text in English. 1951. q. USD 395 in North America; GBP 240 rest of world (effective 2000). adv. bk.rev. bibl, charts, illus. index. back issues avail.; reprint service avail. from PQC. *Refereed.* **Document type:** *Academic/Scholarly.* **Description:** Publishes papers concerned with the systematics of bacteria, yeasts, and yeastlike organisms, including taxonomy, nomenclature, identification, characterization, and culture preservation.
Former titles (until 1999): International Journal of Systematic Bacteriology (0020-7713); (until 1966): International Bulletin of Bacteriological Nomenclature and Toxonomy
Related titles: CD-ROM ed.; Microform ed.: (from PQC); Online - full text ed.: ISSN 1466-5034 (from HighWire Pr., EBSCO Publishing, Institute for Scientific Information).
Indexed: ASCA, Abstr.Bull.Inst.Pap.Chem., Abstr.Hyg., AgBiotech, Agricola, Aqua.Sci.& Fish.Abstr., Bio-Contr.News & Info., Biol.Abstr., Chem.Abstr., Chem.Indus.Notes, Chem.Titles, Curr.Cont., Dairy Sci.Abstr., Deep Sea Res.& Oceanogr.Abstr., Environ.Sci.Poll.Mgmt., Excerp.Med., Food Sci.& Tech.Abstr., Forest.Abstr., Genet.Abstr., Helminthol.Abstr., Ind.Med. (2000-), Ind.Sci.Rev., Ind.Vet., Inpharma, Int.Abstr.Biol.Sci., Maize Abstr., Microbiol.Abstr., Nutr.Abstr., Pig News & Info., Potato Abstr., Poult.Abstr., Protozool.Abstr., Reac., Rev.Appl.Entomol., Rev.Med.& Vet.Mycol., Rev.Plant Path., Sci.Cit.Ind., Small Anim.Abstr., Soils & Fert., Soyabean Abstr., Sport Fish.Abstr., Sugar Ind.Abstr., Trop.Dis.Bull., Vet.Bull., W.R.C.Inf., Weed Abstr., Zoo.Rec.
—BLDSC (4542.688000), CASDDS, CISTI, GNLM, IDS, ingenta, Linda Hall. **CCC.**
Published by: (International Union of Microbiological Societies NLD, International Committee on Systematic Bacteriology), Society for General Microbiology, Marlborough House, Basingstoke Rd, Spencers Wood, Reading, Berks RG7 1AG, United Kingdom. TEL 44-118-9881815, FAX 44-118-988-1834, ijsb@socgenmicrobiol.org.uk, http://www.socgenmicrobiol.org.uk/ijsbmain.htm; http://ijs.sgmjournals.org. Ed. Erko Stackebrandt. R&P Kendra Waite. Adv. contact Aidan Parte. B&W page USD 656, color page USD 1,312. Circ: 1,100.

579 ESP ISSN 1139-6709
INTERNATIONAL MICROBIOLOGY. Text in English. 1998. q. EUR 254.40 domestic; EUR 252 in Germany; EUR 73.50 newsstand/cover foreign (effective 2002). **Document type:** *Academic/Scholarly.* **Description:** Publishes original research papers, short communications, critical reviews and opinion letters dealing with all fields of microbiology and addressed to the international scientific community.
Indexed: Abstr.Hyg., AgBiotech, Field Crop Abstr., Ind.Med., Ind.Vet., Plant Breed.Abstr., Protozool.Abstr., Rev.Appl.Entomol., Rev.Med.& Vet.Mycol., Rev.Plant Path., Soils & Fert., Soyabean Abstr., Weed Abstr.
—BLDSC (4544.178500), CINDOC.
Published by: (Spanish Society for Microbiology), Springer-Verlag Iberica S.A. (Subsidiary of: BertelsmannSpringer), Provenca, 388 1a planta, Barcelona 08025, Spain. TEL 34-93-457-0227, FAX 34-93-457-1502. Ed. Ricard Guerrero. Circ: 2,100.

579 USA ISSN 0733-6373
CODEN: POCHES
INTERSCIENCE CONFERENCE ON ANTIMICROBIAL AGENTS AND CHEMOTHERAPY. PROGRAM AND ABSTRACTS. Abbreviated title: I C A A C Program and Abstracts. Text in English. 1961. a. USD 25. back issues avail. *Refereed.* **Document type:** *Proceedings.*
Related titles: Online - full text ed.: (from Institute for Scientific Information).
—BLDSC (0564.529000), IDS, Linda Hall.
Published by: American Society for Microbiology, 1325 Massachusetts Ave, N W, Washington, DC 20005-4171. TEL 202-737-3600.

579.2 CHE ISSN 0300-5526
QR355 CODEN: IVRYAK
INTERVIROLOGY; international journal of basic and medical virology. Text in English. 1973. bi-m. CHF 1,089, EUR 777.80 in Europe to institutions; CHF 1,106.40, USD 846 elsewhere to institutions (effective 2002). adv. bk.rev. bibl, charts, illus. back issues avail. *Refereed.* **Document type:** *Journal, Academic/Scholarly.* **Description:** Covers progress in both basic and clinical virus research, and aims to provide a forum of exchange among the various disciplines with virology.
Related titles: Microform ed.; Online - full text ed.: ISSN 1423-0100. CHF 58 to institutions with print edition; EUR 42, USD 45 to institutions wirh print edition (effective 2002) (from Northern Light Technology, Inc., EBSCO Publishing, O C L C Online Computer Library Center, Inc., RoweCom Information Quest, ProQuest Information & Learning, Swets Blackwell, Institute for Scientific Information).
Indexed: AIDS & Cancer Res., AIDS Abstr., Abstr.Hyg., AgBiotech, Biol.Abstr., Chem.Abstr., Chem.Indus.Notes, Chem.Titles, Curr.Cont., Dairy Sci.Abstr., Excerp.Med., Forest.Abstr., Ind.Med. (1973-), Ind.Vet., Inpharma, Int.Sci.Rev., Pharm.&Out.News, Pig News & Info., Poult.Abstr., Reac., Rev.Appl.Entomol., Rev.Med.& Vet.Mycol., Rev.Plant Path., Sci.Cit.Ind., Trop.Dis.Bull., Vet.Bull., Virol.Abstr.
—BLDSC (4557.472000), CASDDS, CISTI, EMDOCS, GNLM, IDS, Infotrieve, ingenta, KNAW, Linda Hall. **CCC.**
Published by: S. Karger AG, Allschwilerstr 10, PO Box, Basel 4009, Switzerland. TEL 41-61-306-1111, FAX 41-61-306-1234, karger@karger.ch, http://www.online.karger.com/journals/int, http://www.karger.com. Ed. R W Braun. adv.: page USD 1,185. Circ: 1,200.

579 RUS ISSN 0130-6758
ITOGI NAUKI I TEKHNIKI. MIKROBIOLOGIYA. Text in Russian. irreg. **Document type:** *Academic/Scholarly.*
—Linda Hall.
Published by: Vserossiiskii Institut Nauchnoi i Tekhnicheskoi Informatsii (VINITI), Usievicha ul 20-a, Moscow 125315, Russian Federation. TEL 7-095-1526441, FAX 7-095-943-0060. **US dist. addr.:** East View Publications, 3020 Harbor Ln N, Minneapolis, MN 55447. TEL 612-550-0961.

579 RUS ISSN 0321-2181
ITOGI NAUKI I TEKHNIKI. VIRUSOLOGIYA. Text in Russian. irreg. **Document type:** *Academic/Scholarly.*
—Linda Hall.
Published by: Vserossiiskii Institut Nauchnoi i Tekhnicheskoi Informatsii (VINITI), Usievicha ul 20-a, Moscow 125315, Russian Federation. TEL 7-095-1526441, FAX 7-095-943-0060. **US dist. addr.:** East View Publications, 3020 Harbor Ln N, Minneapolis, MN 55447. TEL 612-550-0961.

616.015 JPN ISSN 0916-4804
CODEN: NIGZE4
JAPANESE JOURNAL OF MEDICAL MYCOLOGY/NIHON ISHINKIN GAKKAI ZASSHI. Text in English. 1960. q. JPY 10,300. adv. bk.rev. index. back issues avail. **Document type:** *Academic/Scholarly.*
Formerly (until 1990): Shinkin to Shinkinsho (0583-0516)
Indexed: Ind.Med. (1990-), Ind.Vet., Rev.Med.& Vet.Mycol., Small Anim.Abstr., Soils & Fert., Vet.Bull.
—CASDDS, CISTI, EMDOCS, GNLM.
Published by: (Japanese Society for Medical Mycology), Business Center for Academic Societies Japan/Nihon Gakkai Jimu Senta, 5-16-9 Honkomagome, Bunkyo-ku, Tokyo 113-0021, Japan. TEL 81-3-5814-5811, FAX 81-3-5814-5822, TELEX 2722268 BCJSP J. Circ: 1,000.

616.01 USA ISSN 1054-2744
QR46
JAWETZ, MELNICK & ADELBERG'S MEDICAL MICROBIOLOGY✶. Text in English. 1954. biennial, latest vol.20, 1995. USD 37.95 (effective 1998). *Refereed.* **Document type:** *Academic/Scholarly.* **Description:** Descriptions of basic microbiology and virology; covers developments in the fields of biochemistry, genetics, pharmacology and immunology.
Former titles (until 1991): Medical Microbiology; (until 1989): Review of Medical Microbiology (0486-6118)
—CISTI, Infotrieve. **CCC.**
Published by: Appleton & Lange, Journal Division (Subsidiary of: Simon & Schuster Company), 11 W 19th St, New York, CT 10011-4209. TEL 203-406-4500, FAX 203-406-4600.

579.3 GBR ISSN 1364-5072
QR1 CODEN: JAMIFK
JOURNAL OF APPLIED MICROBIOLOGY. Text in English. 1938. m., latest vol.92, 2002. GBP 978 in Europe; USD 1,550 in North America; GBP 1,076 elsewhere (effective 2002). adv. bk.rev. abstr, bibl. index. back issues avail. *Refereed.* **Document type:** *Academic/Scholarly.* **Description:** Publishes papers on all aspects of applied microbiology, including environmental, food, agricultural, medical, pharmaceutical, veterinary, taxonomy, soil, water and biodeterioration.
Former titles (until 1997): Journal of Applied Bacteriology (0021-8847); Society for Applied Bacteriology. Proceedings
Related titles: Microform ed.: (from PQC); Online - full text ed.: ISSN 1365-2672. GBP 881 in Europe; USD 1,395 in North America; GBP 881 elsewhere (effective 2002) (from Ovid Technologies, Inc., EBSCO Publishing, O C L C Online Computer Library Center, Inc., RoweCom Information Quest, ingenta, Munksgaard & Blackwell Science's Synergy, Swets Blackwell, Institute for Scientific Information); ♦ Supplement: Letters in Applied Microbiology. ISSN 0266-8254.
Indexed: ASCA, Abstr.Hyg., AgBiotech, Agri.& Environ.Biotech.Abstr., Agricola, Aqua.Sci.& Fish.Abstr., Aquacult.Abstr., Bio-Contr.News & Info., Biol.& Agr.Ind. (Jan.1997-), Biol.Abstr., Biotech.Cit.Ind., CEABA, Chem.Abstr., Curr.Biotech.Abstr., Curr.Cont., Curr.Leather Lit., Dairy Sci.Abstr., Deep Sea Res.& Oceanogr.Abstr., Dent.Ind., Derwent Biotech.Abstr., Ecol.Abstr., Eng.Ind., Environ.Sci.Poll.Mgmt., Excerp.Med., Field Crop Abstr., Food Sci.& Tech.Abstr., Forest Prod.Abstr., Forest.Abstr., Genet.Abstr., Geo.Abstr.P.G., GeoRef, Helminthol.Abstr., Herb.Abstr., Hort.Abstr., Hum.Gen.Abstr., IDA, INIS Atomind., Ind.Med. (1997-), Ind.Sci.Rev., Ind.Vet., Inpharma, Int.Abstr.Biol.Sci., Irr.& Drain.Abstr., Maize Abstr., Mass Spectr.Bull., Microbiol.Abstr., Nutr.Abstr., Ocean.Abstr. (coverage dropped), Ornam.Hort., Packag.Sci.Tech., Pharm.&Out.News, Pig News & Info., Plant Grow.Reg.Abstr., Pollut.Abstr., Postharvest, Potato Abstr., Poult.Abstr., Protozool.Abstr., Reac., Rev.Appl.Entomol., Rev.Arom.& Med.Plants, Rev.Med.& Vet.Mycol., Rev.Plant Path., Risk Abstr., Saf.Sci.Abstr., Sci.Cit.Ind., Seed Abstr., Sel.Water Res.Abstr., Soils & Fert., Soyabean Abstr., Sport Fish.Abstr., Sugar Ind.Abstr., Telegen, Triticale Abstr., Trop.Dis.Bull., Vet.Bull., W.R.C.Inf., Weed Abstr., Zoo.Rec.
—BLDSC (4943.070000), ADONIS, CASDDS, CISTI, Ei, EMDOCS, GNLM, IDS, Infotrieve, ingenta, Linda Hall. **CCC.**

Published by: (Society for Applied Bacteriology), Blackwell Science Ltd., PO Box 88, Oxford OX2 0NE, United Kingdom. TEL 44-1865-206180, 44-1865-206002, FAX 44-1865-206219, jnl.orders@blacksci.co.uk, http://www.blackwell-science.com/~cgilib/jnlpage.asp?Journal=jam&File=jam, http://www.blackwellpublishing.com. Ed. Duncan E S Stewart Tull. Pub. Amanda McLean Inglis. R&P Sophie Savage. Adv. contact Jenny Applin. Circ: 2,770.

579.3 USA ISSN 0021-9193
QR1 CODEN: JOBAAY

JOURNAL OF BACTERIOLOGY. Text in English. 1916. fortn. USD 688 domestic to non-members; USD 731 in Canada to non-members; USD 772 in Europe to non-members; USD 781 in Latin America to non-members; USD 803 elsewhere to non-members (effective 2001). adv. abstr, bibl, illus. index. back issues avail.; reprint service avail. from PQC. *Refereed.* **Document type:** *Academic/Scholarly.* **Description:** Devoted to the advancement of fundamental knowledge concerning bacteria and other microorganisms, including fungi and other unicellular, eucaryotic organisms.

Related titles: CD-ROM ed.: USD 500 in North America; USD 524 elsewhere (effective 1999); Microform ed.: (from PQC); Online - full text ed.: ISSN 1098-5530 (from HighWire Pr., EBSCO Publishing, Gale Group, Factiva, Institute for Scientific Information).

Indexed: ASCA, Abstr.Bull.Inst.Pap.Chem., Abstr.Hyg., AgBiotech, Agri.& Environ.Biotech.Abstr., Agricola, Aqua.Sci.& Fish.Abstr., BBCI, Bibl.Agri., Bio-Contr.News & Info., Biol.& Agr.Ind. (Jan.1983-), Biol.Abstr., Biol.Dig., Biotech.& Bioeng.Abstr., Biotech.Cit.Ind., Chem.Abstr., Chem.Cit.Ind., Chem.Indus.Notes, Chem.Titles, Curr.Adv.Biochem., Curr.Adv.Gen.& Molec.Biol., Curr.Biotech.Abstr., Curr.Cont., Dairy Sci.Abstr., Deep Sea Res.& Oceanogr.Abstr., Dent.Ind., Derwent Biotech.Abstr., Diar.Dis.Res., Environ.Sci.Poll.Mgmt., Field Crop Abstr., Food Sci.& Tech.Abstr., Gen.Sci.Ind. (Jun.1984-), Genet.Abstr., Helminthol.Abstr., Herb.Abstr., Hort.Abstr., Hum.Gen.Abstr., INIS Atomind., Immun.Abstr. (coverage dropped), Ind.Med. (1916-), Ind.Sci.Rev., Ind.Vet., Inpharma, Int.Abstr.Biol.Sci., Int.Aerosp.Abstr., Maize Abstr., Med.& Surg.Dermat., Microbiol.Abstr., Nuc.Acids Abstr., Nutr.Abstr., Ocean.Abstr. (coverage dropped), Pharm.&Out.News, Pig News & Info., Plant Breed.Abstr., Plant Grow.Reg.Abstr., Poult.Abstr., Protozool.Abstr., Reac., Ref.Zh., Rev.Appl.Entomol., Rev.Med.& Vet.Mycol., Rev.Plant Path., Rice Abstr., Sci.Cit.Ind., Seed Abstr., Soils & Fert., Soyabean Abstr., Sport Fish.Abstr., Sugar Ind.Abstr., Telegen, Triticale Abstr., Trop.Dis.Bull., Vet.Bull., Virol.Abstr. (coverage dropped), W.R.C.Inf., Weed Abstr.

—BLDSC (4951.000000), CASDDS, CISTI, GNLM, IDS, ingenta, Linda Hall. **CCC.**

Published by: American Society for Microbiology, 1752 N St N W, Washington, DC 20036-2904. TEL 202-737-3600, 800-633-4931, subscriptions@asmusa.org, http://jb.asm.org/, http://www.asmusa.org. Ed. Graham C Walker. Circ: 5,400 (paid).

579 DEU ISSN 0233-111X
QR1 CODEN: JBMIEQ

JOURNAL OF BASIC MICROBIOLOGY; an international journal on biochemistry, physiology, genetics, morphology and ecology of microorganisms. Text in English. 1960. 6/yr. EUR 558 in Europe; CHF 958 in Switzerland & Liechtenstein; USD 728 elsewhere; EUR 586 combined subscription in Europe for print and online eds.; CHF 1,006 combined subscription in Switzerland & Liechtenstein, for print and online eds.; USD 765 combined subscription elsewhere for print and online eds. (effective 2002). adv. bk.rev. abstr, charts, illus. index. *Refereed.* **Document type:** *Journal, Academic/Scholarly.* **Description:** Publishes results of fundamental research on procariotic and eucariotic microorganisms.

Formerly: Zeitschrift fuer Allgemeine Mikrobiologie (0044-2208)

Related titles: Online - full text ed.: ISSN 1521-4028. EUR 558 in Europe; CHF 958 in Switzerland & Liechtenstein; USD 728 elsewhere (effective 2002) (from EBSCO Publishing, Wiley InterScience, Institute for Scientific Information).

Indexed: ASCA, Abstr.Hyg., Bio-Contr.News & Info., Biol.Abstr., Chem.Abstr., Chem.Indus.Notes, Chem.Titles, Curr.Adv.Biochem., Curr.Biotech.Abstr., Curr.Cont., Dairy Sci.Abstr., Deep Sea Res.& Oceanogr.Abstr., Derwent Biotech.Abstr., Excerp.Med., Food Sci.& Tech.Abstr., Forest.Abstr., Helminthol.Abstr., Herb.Abstr., INIS Atomind., Ind.Med. (1985-), Ind.Vet., Inpharma, Int.Abstr.Biol.Sci., Plant Grow.Reg.Abstr., Postharvest, Protozool.Abstr., Reac., Rev.Appl.Entomol., Rev.Med.& Vet.Mycol., Rev.Plant Path., Rice Abstr., SSCI (coverage dropped), Sci.Cit.Ind., Soils & Fert., Soyabean Abstr., Sugar Ind.Abstr., Triticale Abstr., Trop.Dis.Bull., Vet.Bull., W.R.C.Inf.

—BLDSC (4951.125000), CASDDS, CISTI, EMDOCS, GNLM, IDS, ingenta, Linda Hall. **CCC.**

Published by: Wiley - V C H, Postfach 101161, Weinheim 69451, Germany. FAX 49-6201-606-117, adsales@wiley-vch.de, subservice@wiley-vch.de, http://www.interscience.wiley.com. Ed. H Malke. R&P Claudia Rutz. Adv. contact Aenne Anders TEL 49-6201-606552. **Subscr. in the Americas to:** John Wiley & Sons, Inc., Journals. TEL 44-1243-779777, 212-850-6645, FAX 212-850-6021; **Subscr. outside Germany, Austria & Switzerland to:** John Wiley & Sons Ltd., Baffins Ln, Chichester, Sussex PO19 IUD, United Kingdom. TEL 44-1243-779777, FAX 44-1243-843232.

JOURNAL OF CLINICAL MICROBIOLOGY. see *MEDICAL SCIENCES*

579.5 USA ISSN 1369-1082
QR115 CODEN: JFMYFZ

JOURNAL OF FOOD MYCOLOGY. Text in English. 1998. q. USD 309 domestic; USD 330 foreign (effective 2000). adv. *Refereed.* **Document type:** *Academic/Scholarly.* **Description:** Publishes reviews and original papers on all aspects of food mycology including food-born fungi, mycotoxin formation, and biochemical properties of fungi.

Related titles: Online - full text ed.

—CASDDS. **CCC.**

Published by: (International Commission of Food Mycology), Aspen Publishers, Inc., 200 Orchard Ridge Dr, Ste 200, Gaithersburg, MD 20878. TEL 301-417-7500, 800-638-8437, FAX 301-695-7931, customer.service@aspenpubl.com, http://www.aspenpub.com. Ed. J I Pitt. Adv. contact Gemma Heiser. **Dist. by:** Aspen Publishers Inc., Distribution Center, 7201 McKinney Circle, Frederick, MD 21701. TEL 301-698-7100, FAX 301-417-7550.

579 JPN ISSN 0022-1260
QR1 CODEN: JGAMA9

THE JOURNAL OF GENERAL AND APPLIED MICROBIOLOGY. Text in English. 1955. bi-m. JPY 8,000; USD 85 foreign. charts, illus. reprint service avail. from PQC. *Refereed.* **Document type:** *Academic/Scholarly.* **Description:** Devoted to the publication of original papers pertaining to general and applied microbiology.

Related titles: Microform ed.: (from PQC); Online - full text ed.: (from Institute for Scientific Information).

Indexed: AESIS, ASCA, Agri.& Environ.Biotech.Abstr., Aqua.Sci.& Fish.Abstr., Bio-Contr.News & Info., Biol.Abstr., Biotech.Cit.Ind., CEABA, Chem.Abstr., Chem.Indus.Notes, Chem.Titles, Curr.Adv.Ecol.Sci., Curr.Biotech.Abstr., Curr.Cont., Dairy Sci.Abstr., Derwent Biotech.Abstr., Eng.Ind., Environ.Sci.Poll.Mgmt., Excerp.Med., Field Crop Abstr., Food Sci.& Tech.Abstr., Forest.Abstr., Helminthol.Abstr., Herb.Abstr., Hort.Abstr., INIS Atomind., Ind.Sci.Rev., Ind.Vet., Inpharma, Int.Abstr.Biol.Sci., JTA, Microbiol.Abstr., Nutr.Abstr., Pharm.&Out.News, Plant Breed.Abstr., Pollut.Abstr., Reac., Ref.Zh., Rev.Med.& Vet.Mycol., Rev.Plant Path., Sci.Cit.Ind., Sel.Water Res.Abstr., Soils & Fert., Sport Fish.Abstr., Sugar Ind.Abstr., Vet.Bull., W.R.C.Inf.

—BLDSC (4987.700000), CASDDS, CISTI, Ei, GNLM, IDS, ingenta, Linda Hall. **CCC.**

Published by: Microbiology Research Foundation/Oyo Biseibutsugaku Kenkyu Shoreikai, Japan Academic Societies Center Bldg, 4-16 Yayoi 2-chome, Bunkyo-ku, Tokyo 113-0032, Japan. TEL 81-3-3817-5821, FAX 81-3-3817-5820. Ed. Junta Sugiyama. Circ: 680. **Dist. by:** Maruzen Co., Ltd., International Division, Export Dept, P.O. Box 5050, Tokyo International 100-3191, Japan. TEL 81-3-3273-3234, FAX 81-3-3271-6076.

579.2 GBR ISSN 0022-1317
QR360 CODEN: JGVIAY

JOURNAL OF GENERAL VIROLOGY. Text in English. 1967. m., latest vol.82, 2001. USD 1,100 in North America; EUR 655 elsewhere (effective 2002). adv. bibl, charts, illus. index. 3000 p./no. 2 cols./p. back issues avail.; reprints avail. *Refereed.* **Document type:** *Journal, Academic/Scholarly.* **Description:** Topical research on all aspects of viruses & prions.

Related titles: Online - full text ed.: (from HighWire Pr., EBSCO Publishing, Institute for Scientific Information).

Indexed: AIDS & Cancer Res., AIDS Abstr., ASCA, Abstr.Hyg., AgBiotech, Agri.& Environ.Biotech.Abstr. (coverage dropped), Agricola, Anim.Breed.Abstr., Aqua.Sci.& Fish.Abstr., Bibl.Agri., Bio-Contr.News & Info., Biol.Abstr., Biotech.& Bioeng.Abstr., Biotech.Cit.Ind., CEABA, Chem.Abstr., Chem.Indus.Notes, Chem.Titles, Curr.Adv.Cancer Res., Curr.Adv.Ecol.Sci., Curr.Adv.Gen.& Molec.Biol., Curr.Biotech.Abstr., Curr.Cont., Dairy Sci.Abstr., Dent.Ind., Derwent Biotech.Abstr., Diar.Dis.Res., Environ.Sci.Poll.Mgmt., Excerp.Med., Food Sci.& Tech.Abstr., Genet.Abstr., Helminthol.Abstr., Hort.Abstr., Hum.Gen.Abstr., INIS Atomind., Immun.Abstr., Ind.Med. (1967-), Ind.Sci.Rev., Ind.Vet., Inpharma, Int.Abstr.Biol.Sci., Neurosci.Cit.Ind., Nuc.Acids Abstr., Nutr.Abstr., Pharm.&Out.News, Pig News & Info., Plant Breed.Abstr., Potato Abstr., Poult.Abstr., Reac., Rev.Appl.Entomol., Rev.Med.& Vet.Mycol., Rev.Plant Path., Rice Abstr., Sci.Cit.Ind., Small Anim.Abstr., Soils & Fert., Sport Fish.Abstr., Triticale Abstr., Trop.Dis.Bull., Trop.Oil Seeds Abstr., Vet.Bull., Virol.Abstr., W.R.C.Inf., Wild.Rev., Zoo.Rec.

—BLDSC (4989.300000), CASDDS, CISTI, GNLM, IDS, ingenta, Linda Hall. **CCC.**

Published by: Society for General Microbiology, Marlborough House, Basingstoke Rd, Spencers Wood, Reading, Berks RG7 1AG, United Kingdom. TEL 44-118-988-1813, 44-188-988-1833, FAX 44-118-988-1834, 44-188-988-1834, jgv@sgm.ac.uk, http://vir.sgmjournals.org, http://vir.sgmjournalshorg. Ed. S Siddell. R&P Marianne Asbury TEL 44-188-988-1825. Adv. contact John Brimelow TEL 44-188-988-1808. Circ: 1,550.

JOURNAL OF HUMAN VIROLOGY. see *MEDICAL SCIENCES—Communicable Diseases*

JOURNAL OF INDUSTRIAL MICROBIOLOGY AND BIOTECHNOLOGY. see *BIOLOGY—Biotechnology*

579 NLD ISSN 0167-7012
QR65 CODEN: JMIMDQ

JOURNAL OF MICROBIOLOGICAL METHODS. Text in English. 1983. m. EUR 1,555 in Europe to institutions; JPY 206,400 in Japan to institutions; USD 1,739 elsewhere to institutions (effective 2002). abstr. back issues avail. *Refereed.* **Document type:** *Academic/Scholarly.* **Description:** Publishes original papers and short reviews covering methods on all aspects of microbiology, excluding virology.

Related titles: Microform ed.: (from PQC); Online - full text ed.: (from ingenta, ScienceDirect, Swets Blackwell, Institute for Scientific Information).

Indexed: ASCA, Abstr.Bull.Inst.Pap.Chem., Abstr.Hyg., AgBiotech, Agri.& Environ.Biotech.Abstr., Agroforest.Abstr., Aqua.Sci.& Fish.Abstr., Biodet.Abstr., Biol.Abstr., Biotech.Cit.Ind., CEABA, Chem.Abstr., Chem.Indus.Notes, Chem.Titles, Curr.Adv.Biochem., Curr.Adv.Ecol.Sci., Curr.Biotech.Abstr., Curr.Cont., Dairy Sci.Abstr., Derwent Biotech.Abstr., Environ.Sci.Poll.Mgmt., Excerp.Med., Food Sci.& Tech.Abstr., INIS Atomind., Ind.Med. (1983-), Ind.Sci.Rev., Ind.Vet., Inpharma, Int.Abstr.Biol.Sci., Mass Spectr.Bull., Microbiol.Abstr., Nutr.Abstr., Pig News & Info., Pollut.Abstr., Poult.Abstr., Protozool.Abstr., Reac., Rev.Appl.Entomol., Rev.Arom.& Med.Plants, Rev.Med.& Vet.Mycol., Rev.Plant Path., Sci.Cit.Ind., Sel.Water Res.Abstr., Soils & Fert., Vet.Bull., W.R.C.Inf.

—BLDSC (5019.260000), ADONIS, CASDDS, CISTI, GNLM, IDS, Infotrieve, ingenta, Linda Hall. **CCC.**

Published by: Elsevier Science BV, PO Box 211, Amsterdam 1000 AE, Netherlands. TEL 31-20-485-3911, FAX 31-20-485-3598, nlinfo-f@elsevier.nl, http://www.elsevier.com/locate/jmicmeth. Eds. D White, A Fox. **Subscr. in Australasia and the Far East to:** Elsevier Science (Singapore) Pte Ltd, No.1 Temasek Ave, 17-01 Millenia Tower, Singapore 039192, Singapore. TEL 65-434-3727, FAX 65-337-2230; **Subscr. in Japan to:** Elsevier Science Inc - Japan Regional Office, 9-15 Higashi-Azabu 1-chome, Minato-ku, Tokyo 106-0044, Japan. TEL 81-3-5561-5033; **Subscr. in the Americas to:** Elsevier Science, PO Box 945, New York, NY 10159-0945. TEL 212-633-3730, FAX 212-633-3680.

JOURNAL OF MICROBIOLOGY AND BIOTECHNOLOGY. see *BIOLOGY—Biotechnology*

579 TWN
QR1 CODEN: CKWCD9

JOURNAL OF MICROBIOLOGY, IMMUNOLOGY AND INFECTION/WEIMIAN YU GANRAN ZAZHI. Text in English. 1968. q., latest vol.33. USD 90 (effective 2001). adv. abstr. index. 100 p./no. *Refereed.* **Document type:** *Academic/Scholarly.*

B

Former titles: Chinese Journal of Microbiology and Immunology (0253-2662); (until 1980): Chinese Journal of Microbiology (0009-4587)
Related titles: CD-ROM ed.
Indexed: Abstr.Hyg., Aqua.Sci.& Fish.Abstr., Aquacult.Abstr., Biodet.Abstr., Biol.Abstr., Cal.Tiss.Abstr., Chem.Abstr., Environ.Sci.Poll.Mgmt., Excerp.Med., ExtraMED, Food Sci.& Tech.Abstr., Helminthol.Abstr., Ind.Med. (coverage dropped), Ind.Vet., Nutr.Abstr., Protozool.Abstr., Rev.Appl.Entomol., Rev.Med.& Vet.Mycol., Trop.Dis.Bull., Vet.Bull., Virol.Abstr.
—BLDSC (5019.320000), CASDDS, CISTI, GNLM.
Published by: Chinese Society of Microbiology, National Taiwan University, College of Medicine, 1, Jenai Rd, Sec1, Taipei, Taiwan. TEL 886-2-28757532, 886-2-23562220, FAX 886-2-28730052, 886-2-23915180. Ed. Yu Tien Liu. Pub. Czau Sium Yang. Circ: 4,000. **Co-sponsor:** Chinese Society of Immunology, Infectious Diseases Society of Republic of China.

549 GBR ISSN 1464-1801
▼ **JOURNAL OF MOLECULAR MICROBIOLOGY AND BIOTECHNOLOGY.** Text in English. 1999. q. GBP 130, USD 260 to individuals; GBP 360, USD 720 to institutions (effective 2002). back issues avail. *Refereed.* **Document type:** *Academic/Scholarly.* **Description:** Publishes high-quality primary research papers, along with reviews and written symposia, in the fields of molecular microbiology and biotechnology.
Related titles: Online - full text ed.: ISSN 1475-3774. GBP 80, USD 160 to individuals; GBP 250, USD 500 to institutions (effective 2002) (from Institute for Scientific Information).
Indexed: AIDS & Cancer Res., AgBiotech, Agri.& Environ.Biotech.Abstr., Aqua.Sci.& Fish.Abstr., Biotech.& Bioeng.Abstr., Biotech.Cit.Ind., Crop Physiol.Abstr., Dairy Sci.Abstr., Environ.Sci.Poll.Mgmt., Genet.Abstr., Ind.Med., Maize Abstr., Med.& Pharm.Biotech.Abstr., Microbiol.Abstr., Nuc.Acids Abstr., Plant Breed.Abstr., Soils & Fert., Sugar Ind.Abstr., Tox.Abstr., Virol.Abstr., Zoo.Rec.
—BLDSC (5020.716250).
Published by: Horizon Scientific Press, 32 Hewitts Ln, PO Box 1, Wymondham, Norfolk NR18 0EA, United Kingdom. TEL 44-1953-601106, FAX 44-1953-603068, mail@horizonpress.com, orders@horizonpress.com, http://www.jmmb.net, http://www.horizonpress.com/. Ed. Milton H Saier.

JOURNAL OF PARASITOLOGY. see *MEDICAL SCIENCES—Communicable Diseases*

JOURNAL OF VETERINARY PARASITOLOGY. see *VETERINARY SCIENCE*

579.2 NLD ISSN 0166-0934
CODEN: JVMEDH
JOURNAL OF VIROLOGICAL METHODS. Text in English. 1980. 16/yr. EUR 2,822 in Europe to institutions; JPY 374,400 in Japan to institutions; USD 3,157 elsewhere to institutions (effective 2002). adv. back issues avail.; reprint service avail. from ISI. *Refereed.* **Document type:** *Academic/Scholarly.* **Description:** Publishes original papers covering techniques on all aspects of virology.
Related titles: Microform ed.: (from PQC,PMC); Online - full text ed.: (from ingenta, ScienceDirect, Swets Blackwell, Institute for Scientific Information).
Indexed: AIDS & Cancer Res., AIDS Abstr., ASCA, Abstr.Hyg., AgBiotech, Agri.Eng.Abstr., Aqua.Sci.& Fish.Abstr., Bio-Contr.News & Info., Biol.Abstr., Biotech.& Bioeng.Abstr., Biotech.Cit.Ind., Chem.Abstr., Chem.Indus.Notes, Chem.Titles, Curr.Adv.Ecol.Sci., Curr.Adv.Gen.& Molec.Biol., Curr.Cont., Dairy Sci.Abstr., Environ.Sci.Poll.Mgmt., Excerp.Med., INIS Atomind., Ind.Med. (1980-), Ind.Sci.Rev., Ind.Vet., Inpharma, Int.Abstr.Biol.Sci., Med.& Pharm.Biotech.Abstr., Microbiol.Abstr., Pharm.&Out.News, Pig News & Info., Potato Abstr., Poult.Abstr., Reac., Rev.Appl.Entomol., Rev.Med.& Vet.Mycol., Rev.Plant Path., Rice Abstr., Sci.Cit.Ind., Small Anim.Abstr., Sport Fish.Abstr., Triticale Abstr., Trop.Dis.Bull., Vet.Bull., Virol.Abstr.
—BLDSC (5072.486000), ADONIS, CASDDS, CISTI, EMDOCS, GNLM, IDS, ingenta. **CCC.**
Published by: Elsevier Science BV, PO Box 211, Amsterdam 1000 AE, Netherlands. TEL 31-20-485-3911, FAX 31-20-485-3598, nlinfo-f@elsevier.nl; usinfo-f@elsevier.com; forinfo-kyf04035@niftyserve.or.jp, http://www.elsevier.com/locate/jviromet. Eds. A J Zuckerman, S Giles. **Subscr. in Australasia and the Far East to:** Elsevier Science (Singapore) Pte Ltd, No.1 Temasek Ave, 17-01 Millenia Tower, Singapore 039192, Singapore. TEL 65-434-3727, FAX 65-337-2230; **Subscr. in Japan to:** Elsevier Science Inc - Japan Regional Office, 9-15 Higashi-Azabu 1-chome, Minato-ku, Tokyo 106-0044, Japan. TEL 81-3-5561-5033; **Subscr. in the Americas to:** Elsevier Science, PO Box 945, New York, NY 10159-0945. TEL 212-633-3730, FAX 212-633-3680.

579.2 USA ISSN 0022-538X
QR360 CODEN: JOVIAM
JOURNAL OF VIROLOGY. Text in English. 1967. fortn. USD 772 domestic to non-members; USD 830 in Canada to non-members; USD 901 in Europe to non-members; USD 911 in Latin America to non-members; USD 944 elsewhere to non-members (effective 2001). adv. charts, illus. s-a. index. back issues avail.; reprint service avail. from PQC. *Refereed.* **Document type:** *Academic/Scholarly.* **Description:** Covers viruses obtained in studies using cross-disciplinary approaches of biochemistry, biophysics, cell biology, genetics, immunology, molecular biology, morphology, physiology, pathogenesis, and immunity.
Related titles: CD-ROM ed.: USD 500 in North America; USD 524 elsewhere; Microform ed.: (from PQC); Online - full text ed.: ISSN 1098-5514 (from HighWire Pr., EBSCO Publishing, Institute for Scientific Information).
Indexed: AIDS & Cancer Res., AIDS Abstr., ASCA, AgBiotech, Agri.& Environ.Biotech.Abstr. (coverage dropped), Agricola, Aqua.Sci.& Fish.Abstr., BBCI, Bibl.Agri., Bio-Contr.News & Info., Biol.& Agr.Ind. (Jan.1996-), Biol.Abstr., Biotech.& Bioeng.Abstr., Chem.Abstr., Chem.Titles, Curr.Adv.Biochem., Curr.Adv.Cancer Res., Curr.Adv.Ecol.Sci., Curr.Adv.Gen.& Molec.Biol., Curr.Biotech.Abstr., Curr.Cont., Dairy Sci.Abstr., Dent.Ind., Derwent Biotech.Abstr., Diar.Dis.Res., Environ.Sci.Poll.Mgmt., Excerp.Med., Food Sci.& Tech.Abstr., Genet.Abstr., Helminthol.Abstr., Hort.Abstr., Hum.Gen.Abstr., INIS Atomind., Immun.Abstr., Ind.Med. (1967-), Ind.Sci.Rev., Ind.Vet., Inpharma, Int.Abstr.Biol.Sci., Jrnl.Watch Inf.Dis., Med.& Pharm.Biotech.Abstr., Neurosci.Abstr., Neurosci.Cit.Ind., Nuc.Acids Abstr., Oncog.G.F.Abstr., Pharm.&Out.News, Pig News & Info., Plant Breed.Abstr., Potato Abstr., Poult.Abstr., Protozool.Abstr., Reac., Ref.Zh., Rev.Appl.Entomol., Rev.Med.& Vet.Mycol., Rev.Plant Path., Rice Abstr., Saf.Sci.Abstr., Sci.Cit.Ind., Small Anim.Abstr., Sport Fish.Abstr., Telegen, Trop.Dis.Bull., Vet.Bull., Virol.Abstr., Wild.Rev.
—BLDSC (5072.490000), CASDDS, CISTI, GNLM, IDS, ingenta, Linda Hall. **CCC.**
Published by: American Society for Microbiology, 1752 N St N W, Washington, DC 20036-2904. TEL 202-737-3600, 800-633-4931, FAX 202-942-9319, subscriptions@asmusa.org, http://asmusa.edo.com/jvi/, http://www.asmusa.org. Ed. Thomas E Shenk. Circ: 4,300 (paid).

KISEICHU BUNRUI KEITAI DANWAKAI KAIHO/JAPANESE SOCIETY FOR SYSTEMATIC PARASITOLOGY. CIRCULAR. see *MEDICAL SCIENCES—Communicable Diseases*

579.2 JPN ISSN 0075-7357
QR360 CODEN: ARIVAK
KYOTO UNIVERSITY. INSTITUTE FOR VIRUS RESEARCH. ANNUAL REPORT✶ /KYOTO DAIGAKU UIRUSU KENKYUJO NENKAN KIYO. Text in English. 1958. a.
Indexed: Biol.Abstr., Chem.Abstr., INIS Atomind.
—BLDSC (1306.800000), CASDDS.
Published by: (Kyoto University, Institute for Virus Research), Kyoto University Press, Yoshidahon-Machi, Sakyo-ku, Kyoto-shi 606-8317, Japan. Ed. Seiich Matsumoto. Circ: (controlled).

579.3 GBR
LACTIC ACID BACTERIA. Text in English. 1992. irreg. price varies. bibl. *Refereed.* **Document type:** *Monographic series.* **Description:** Scholarly monographs pertaining to the bacteriology and microbiology of lactic acid bacteria in dairy products and related substances, incorporating relevant aspects of toxicological studies.
Published by: Pergamon (Subsidiary of: Elsevier Science), The Boulevard, Langford Ln, East Park, Kidlington, Oxford OXB 1GB, United Kingdom. FAX 44-1865-843010, nlinfo-f@elsevier.nl; usinfo-f@elsevier.com; forinfo-kyf04035@niftyserve.or.jp, http://www.elsevier.nl/. **Subscr. in Australasia and the Far East to:** Elsevier Science (Singapore) Pte Ltd, No.1 Temasek Ave, 17-01 Millenia Tower, Singapore 039192, Singapore. TEL 65-434-3727, FAX 65-337-2230; **Subscr. in the Americas to:** Elsevier Science, PO Box 945, New York, NY 10159-0945. TEL 212-633-3730, FAX 212-633-3680; **Subscr. to:** Elsevier Science BV, PO Box 211, Amsterdam 1000 AE, Netherlands. TEL 31-20-485-3757, nlinfo-f@elsevier.nl, http://www.elsevier.nl.

579 FRA ISSN 0023-7302
CODEN: LAITAG
LE LAIT. Text in French; Text and summaries in English, French. 1921. bi-m. FRF 1,971 in the European Union; FRF 2,045 elsewhere (effective 2001); FRF 1,687 domestic; EUR 316 in the European Union; EUR 327 elsewhere (effective 2001). adv. *Refereed.* **Document type:** *Academic/Scholarly.* **Description:** Includes scientific articles on the microbiology, biochemistry and physiochemistry of milk and its derivatives, or on transformation procedures.
Related titles: Microform ed.: (from PMC); Online - full text ed.: ISSN 1297-9694 (from EBSCO Publishing, ingenta, Swets Blackwell, Institute for Scientific Information, RoweCom Information Quest).
Indexed: ASCA, Biol.Abstr., Chem.Abstr., Chem.Indus.Notes, Chem.Titles, Curr.Cont., Dairy Sci.Abstr., Excerp.Med., Food Sci.& Tech.Abstr., INIS Atomind., Ind.Vet., Nutr.Abstr., Sci.Cit.Ind.
—BLDSC (5143.800000), CASDDS, CINDOC, CISTI, IDS, Infotrieve, Linda Hall. **CCC.**
Published by: (France. Institut National de la Recherche Agronomique), E D P Sciences, 7 av. du Hoggar, B.P. 112, P.A. de Courtaboeuf, Les Ulis Cedex A 91944, France. TEL 33-1-69187575, FAX 33-1-69288491, subscribers@edpsciences.org, http://www.edpsciences.org. Ed. J L Maubois. Circ: 2,500.

579 GBR ISSN 0266-8254
QR1 CODEN: LAMIE7
LETTERS IN APPLIED MICROBIOLOGY. Text in English. 1985. m. GBP 828 in Europe; USD 1,448 in United States; GBP 911 rest of world (effective 2000); includes Journal of Applied Microbiology & Annual Symposium. adv. *Refereed.* **Document type:** *Academic/Scholarly.* **Description:** Reflects developments in biotechnology in such fields as applied microbial genetics, immunodiagnosis, cell culture and fermentation science.
Related titles: Online - full text ed.: ISSN 1472-765X (from Ovid Technologies, Inc., EBSCO Publishing, O C L C Online Computer Library Center, Inc., RoweCom Information Quest, ingenta, Swets Blackwell, Institute for Scientific Information); ♦ Supplement to: Journal of Applied Microbiology. ISSN 1364-5072.
Indexed: ASCA, Abstr.Hyg., AgBiotech, Agri.& Environ.Biotech.Abstr., Agri.Eng.Abstr., Agricola, Agroforest.Abstr., Aqua.Sci.& Fish.Abstr., Aquacult.Abstr., Bibl.Agri., Bio-Contr.News & Info., Biotech.Cit.Ind., CEABA, Chem.Abstr., Chem.Indus.Notes, Chem.Titles, Curr.Cont., Dairy Sci.Abstr., Derwent Biotech.Abstr., Ecol.Abstr., Environ.Sci.Poll.Mgmt., Fluidex, Food Sci.& Tech.Abstr., Forest.Abstr., Helminthol.Abstr., INIS Atomind., Ind.Med. (1985-), Ind.Vet., Inpharma, Int.Abstr.Biol.Sci., Maize Abstr., Microbiol.Abstr., Nutr.Abstr., Pig News & Info., Pollut.Abstr., Postharvest, Potato Abstr., Poult.Abstr., Protozool.Abstr., Reac., Rev.Appl.Entomol., Rev.Arom.& Med.Plants, Rev.Med.& Vet.Mycol., Rev.Plant Path., Risk Abstr., Saf.Sci.Abstr., Sci.Cit.Ind., Sel.Water Res.Abstr., Soils & Fert., Soyabean Abstr., Sport Fish.Abstr., Sugar Ind.Abstr., Triticale Abstr., Trop.Dis.Bull., Vet.Bull., W.R.C.Inf., World Text.Abstr.
—BLDSC (5185.126700), ADONIS, CASDDS, CISTI, EMDOCS, GNLM, IDS, ingenta, Linda Hall. **CCC.**
Published by: (Society for Applied Bacteriology), Blackwell Science Ltd., Osney Mead, Oxford OX2 0EL, United Kingdom. TEL 44-1865-206206, FAX 44-1865-721205, journals.cs@blacksci.co.uk, http://www.blackwell-science.com. Eds. C R Harwood, D M Gibson. Pub. Amanda McLean Inglis. R&P Sophie Savage. Adv. contact Jenny Applin.

LA LETTRE DE L'INFECTIOLOGUE; de la microbiologie a la clinique. see *MEDICAL SCIENCES—Communicable Diseases*

MEDICAL MICROBIOLOGIST. see *MEDICAL SCIENCES*

579 POL ISSN 0025-8601
R91 CODEN: MDMIAZ
MEDYCYNA DOSWIADCZALNA I MIKROBIOLOGIA. Text in Multiple languages. 1949. q. PLZ 40 domestic; USD 120 foreign (effective 2002). **Document type:** *Academic/Scholarly.*
Indexed: Abstr.Hyg., AgroLibrex, Biol.Abstr., Chem.Abstr., Chem.Titles, Dent.Ind., Excerp.Med., INIS Atomind., I.P.A., Ind.Med. (1949-), Ind.Vet., Mass Spectr.Bull., Rev.Appl.Entomol., Rev.Med.& Vet.Mycol., Rev.Plant Path., Vet.Bull.
—BLDSC (5536.000000), CASDDS, CISTI, GNLM.
Published by: Panstwowy Zaklad Higieny/National Institute of Hygiene, Ul Chocimska 24, Warsaw 00791, Poland. TEL 48-22-8497781, FAX 48-22-8497484, pzh@medstat.waw.pl. Ed. Stanislaw Kaluzewski. R&P Jolanta Szych. **Dist. by:** Ars Polona, Krakowskie Przedmiescie 7, Warsaw, Poland. TEL 48-22-8261201, FAX 48-22-8268673. **Co-sponsor:** Polskie Towarzystwo Mikrobiologow/Polish Society of Microbiologists.

579 USA ISSN 0580-9517
QR65 CODEN: MMICEU
METHODS IN MICROBIOLOGY. Text in English. 1969. irreg., latest vol.25, 1998. *Refereed.* **Document type:** *Monographic series.*
Related titles: Online - full text ed.: (from Institute for Scientific Information).
Indexed: Chem.Abstr., Chem.Indus.Notes, Chem.Titles, Sci.Cit.Ind.
—BLDSC (5748.201000), CASDDS, CISTI, GNLM, ingenta. **CCC.**
Published by: Academic Press, Inc., Journal Division (Subsidiary of: Harcourt Brace & Company), 525 B St, Ste 1900, San Diego, CA 92101-4495. TEL 619-230-1840, FAX 619-699-6800, http://www.apnet.com.

579.3 FRA ISSN 1286-4579
CODEN: RESVEY
▼ **MICROBES AND INFECTION**; a journal on infectious agents and host defenses. Text in English. 1999. 15/yr. EUR 790 in Europe to institutions; JPY 104,700 in Japan to institutions; USD 883 elsewhere to institutions (effective 2002). adv. bk.rev. index. back issues avail.; reprint service avail. from ISI. *Refereed.* **Document type:** *Bulletin, Academic/Scholarly.* **Description:** Presents reviews on all aspects of microbiology, immunology and infectious diseases, and aims at providing researchers and teaching staff in these fields.
Formed by the merger of (1903-1999): Institut Pasteur. Bulletin (0020-2452); (1989-1999): Research in Virology (0923-2516); Which was formerly (until 1988): Institut Pasteur. Annales. Virologie (0769-2617); (1980-1985): Annales de Virologie (0242-5017); (1989-1999): Research in Immunology (0923-2494); Which was formerly (until 1988): Institut Pasteur. Annales. Immunologie (0769-2625); (until 1985): Annales d'Immunologie (0300-4910); Which superseded in part (1887-1972): Institut Pasteur. Annales (0020-2444)
Related titles: Microform ed.: (from PQC,PMC); Online - full text ed.: (from ingenta, Swets Blackwell, ScienceDirect, Institute for Scientific Information).
Indexed: AIDS & Cancer Res., ASCA, Abstr.Hyg., AgBiotech, Agri.& Environ.Biotech.Abstr., Aqua.Sci.& Fish.Abstr., Biol.Abstr., Chem.Abstr., Chem.Indus.Notes, Chem.Titles, Curr.Adv.Ecol.Sci., Curr.Cont., Dairy Sci.Abstr., Derwent Biotech.Abstr., Environ.Sci.Poll.Mgmt., Excerp.Med., Helminthol.Abstr., INIS Atomind., Immun.Abstr., Ind.Med. (1999-), Ind.Sci.Rev., Ind.Vet., Inpharma, Int.Abstr.Biol.Sci., Microbiol.Abstr., Pig News & Info., Plant Breed.Abstr., Pollut.Abstr., Protozool.Abstr., Reac., Rev.Appl.Entomol., Rev.Med.& Vet.Mycol., Rev.Plant Path., Risk Abstr., Saf.Sci.Abstr., Sci.Cit.Ind., Soils & Fert., Tox.Abstr., Trop.Dis.Bull., Vet.Bull., Virol.Abstr.
—BLDSC (5756.909000), ADONIS, CASDDS, CISTI, EMDOCS, GNLM, IDS, Infotrieve, Linda Hall. **CCC.**
Published by: (Institut Pasteur), Elsevier Paris, Editions Scientifiques et Medicales (Subsidiary of: Reed Elsevier plc. group), 23 rue Linois, Paris 75015, France. TEL 33-1-45589110, FAX 33-1-45589419, a.dore@elsevier.fr; academic@elsevier-fr.com; mccoull@bond.rz-berlin, http://www.elsevier.com/locate/micinf, http://www.elsevier.fr; http://www.pasteur.fr. Eds. A Sher, Stefan H E Kaufmann. Circ: 1,300.

579 GBR ISSN 0966-6796
MICROBIAL CLEAN-UP. Text in English. 1992. 10/yr. GBP 250, USD 295. back issues avail. **Description:** Covers developments in the use of microbes to eliminate pollutants, effluents, and waste.
Address: 2-3 Cornwall Terr, Regent's Park, London NW1 4QP, United Kingdom. TEL 0171-935-2382, FAX 0171-486-7083.

MICROBIAL DRUG RESISTANCE; mechanism, epidemiology, and disease. see *MEDICAL SCIENCES*

579 USA ISSN 0095-3628
QR100 CODEN: MCBEBU
MICROBIAL ECOLOGY; an international journal. Text in English. 8/yr. (in 2 vols., 4 nos./vol.). USD 779.80 domestic for Print & Online Eds.; USD 744.20 in Germany for Print & Online Eds.; USD 106.20 newsstand/cover foreign (effective 2002). adv. reprint service avail. from SWZ,ISI. *Refereed.* **Document type:** *Academic/Scholarly.* **Description:** Publishes original articles in all areas of ecology involving microorganisms.
Related titles: Microform ed.: (from PQC); Online - full text ed.: ISSN 1432-184X (from EBSCO Publishing, RoweCom Information Quest, Swets Blackwell, Springer LINK, Institute for Scientific Information).
Indexed: ASCA, Agricola, Appl.Ecol.Abstr., Aqua.Sci.& Fish.Abstr., Aquacult.Abstr., Bio-Contr.News & Info., Biol.& Agr.Ind. (Jan.1996-), Biol.Abstr., Chem.Abstr., Chem.Indus.Notes, Chem.Titles, Curr.Adv.Ecol.Sci., Curr.Cont., Dairy Sci.Abstr., Deep Sea Res.& Oceanogr.Abstr., Ecol.Abstr., Entomol.Abstr. (coverage dropped), Environ.Sci.Poll.Mgmt., Excerp.Med., Field Crop Abstr., Forest Prod.Abstr., Forest.Abstr., Genet.Abstr., Geo.Abstr.H.G., Geo.Abstr.P.G., GeoRef, Helminthol.Abstr., Hum.Gen.Abstr., IBR, INIS Atomind., Ind.Sci.Rev., Ind.Vet., Int.Abstr.Biol.Sci., Irr.& Drain.Abstr., Maize Abstr., Microbiol.Abstr., Nutr.Abstr., Ocean.Abstr., Pollut.Abstr., Rev.Appl.Entomol., Rev.Plant Path., Rice Abstr., Sci.Cit.Ind., Seed Abstr., Sel.Water Res.Abstr., Soils & Fert., Soyabean Abstr., Sport Fish.Abstr., Triticale Abstr., Vet.Bull., W.R.C.Inf., Weed Abstr.
—BLDSC (5756.920000), CASDDS, CISTI, EMDOCS, IDS, ingenta, Linda Hall. **CCC.**
Published by: Springer-Verlag, Journals (Subsidiary of: BertelsmannSpringer), 175 Fifth Ave, New York, NY 10010. TEL 212-460-1500, FAX 212-473-6272, orders@springer-ny.com, http://link.springer.de/link/service/journals/00248/index.htm. Ed. James K Fredrickson. R&P Ian Gross. Adv. contact Brian Skepton. **N. American subscr. to:** Journal Fulfillment Services, PO Box 2485, Secaucus, NJ 07096-2485. TEL 800-777-4643, FAX 201-348-4505.

MICROBIAL ECOLOGY IN HEALTH & DISEASE. see *MEDICAL SCIENCES—Communicable Diseases*

MICROBIOLOGIA MEDICA. see *MEDICAL SCIENCES*

579.072 DEU ISSN 0944-5013
QR51 CODEN: MCRSEJ
MICROBIOLOGICAL RESEARCH. Text in English. 1895. 4/yr. EUR 128, GBP 94 to individuals; EUR 315, GBP 225 to institutions (effective 2002). adv. bk.rev. bibl, charts, illus. index. reprint service avail. from ISI. *Refereed.* **Document type:** *Journal, Academic/Scholarly.* **Description:** Publishes original research papers and short communications on prokaryotic and eukaryotic micro-organisms.
Former titles (until 1993): Zentralblatt fuer Mikrobiologie (0232-4393); Zentralblatt fuer Bakteriologie, Parasitenkunde, Infektionskrankheiten und Hygiene: Zweite Abteilung - Naturwissenschaft
Related titles: Online - full text ed.: (from Institute for Scientific Information).
Indexed: ASCA, Aqua.Sci.& Fish.Abstr., Bio-Contr.News & Info., CEABA, Chem.Abstr., Chem.Titles, Curr.Adv.Biochem., Curr.Adv.Gen.& Molec.Biol., Curr.Cont., Dairy Sci.Abstr., Derwent Biotech.Abstr., Ecol.Abstr., Environ.Sci.Poll.Mgmt., Field Crop Abstr., Fluidex, Food Sci.& Tech.Abstr., Forest.Abstr., Geo.Abstr.P.G., Helminthol.Abstr., Hort.Abstr., INIS Atomind., Ind.Med. (1994-), Ind.Vet., Int.Abstr.Biol.Sci., Microbiol.Abstr., Nutr.Abstr., Plant Grow.Reg.Abstr., Postharvest, Potato Abstr., Rev.Appl.Entomol., Rev.Arom.& Med.Plants, Rev.Med.& Vet.Mycol., Rev.Plant Path., Rice Abstr., Seed Abstr., Soils & Fert., Soyabean Abstr., Sugar Ind.Abstr., Triticale Abstr., Trop.Oil Seeds Abstr., Vet.Bull., Weed Abstr.
—BLDSC (5757.590000), CASDDS, CISTI, EMDOCS, GNLM, IDS, Infotrieve, ingenta, Linda Hall. **CCC.**
Published by: Urban & Fischer Verlag, Loebdergraben 14A, Jena 07743, Germany. TEL 49-3641-626444, FAX 49-3641-626500, info@urbanfischer.de, http://www.urbanfischer.de. Eds. Dr. Gabriele Diekert, J Woestemeyer. R&P Martin Huber TEL 49-3641-626430. Adv. contact Sabine Schroeter. page DEM 750; trim 280 x 210. Circ: 350.

579 USA ISSN 0889-3381
THE MICROBIOLOGICAL UPDATE. Text in English. 1982. m., latest vol.19. USD 220 domestic; USD 240 foreign (effective 2001). bk.rev. back issues avail. *Refereed.* **Document type:** *Newsletter.* **Description:** Keeps readers abreast of the latest literature and discussions of microbiological control, along with issues relevant to the pharmaceutical, cosmetics, and medical-device industries.
—BLDSC (5757.630000).
Published by: Microbiological Applications, Inc., 132 San Remo Dr, Islamorada, FL 33036. TEL 305-664-8513, FAX 305-664-8597. Ed. Murray S Cooper. R&P, Adv. contact Claire Sandberg.

579 GBR ISSN 1350-0872
QR1 CODEN: MROBEO
MICROBIOLOGY. Text in English. 1947. m. GBP 580, USD 995 (effective 2000). adv. bibl, charts, illus. index. back issues avail.; reprints avail. *Refereed.* **Document type:** *Academic/Scholarly.* **Description:** Original work on microorganisms in the laboratory and in the field; emphasis on fundamental studies.
Formerly (until 1993): Journal of General Microbiology (0022-1287)
Related titles: Microfilm ed.: (from PMC); Online - full text ed.: (from HighWire Pr., EBSCO Publishing, Gale Group, Kluwer Online, Institute for Scientific Information).
Indexed: ASCA, Abstr.Hyg., AgBiotech, Agri.& Environ.Biotech.Abstr., Agricola, Agroforest.Abstr., Aqua.Sci.& Fish.Abstr., BBCI, Bio-Contr.News & Info., Biol.& Agr.Ind. (Jan.1994-), Biol.Abstr., Biol.Dig., Biotech.Cit.Ind., CEABA, Chem.Abstr., Chem.Cit.Ind., Chem.Titles, Curr.Adv.Biochem., Curr.Adv.Ecol.Sci., Curr.Adv.Gen.& Molec.Biol., Curr.Biotech.Abstr., Curr.Cont., Dairy Sci.Abstr., Deep Sea Res.& Oceanogr.Abstr., Dent.Ind., Derwent Biotech.Abstr., Environ.Sci.Poll.Mgmt., Excerp.Med., Field Crop Abstr., Food Sci.& Tech.Abstr., Forest Prod.Abstr., Gen.Sci.Ind. (Jan.1994-), GeoRef, Helminthol.Abstr., Herb.Abstr., Hort.Abstr., INIS Atomind., Ind.Med. (1994-), Ind.Sci.Rev., Ind.Vet., Inpharma, Maize Abstr., Mass Spectr.Bull., Med.& Surg.Dermat., Microbiol.Abstr., Nutr.Abstr., Pig News & Info., Plant Breed.Abstr., Plant Gen.Res.Abstr., Potato Abstr., Poult.Abstr., Protozool.Abstr., Reac., Ref.Zh., Rev.Appl.Entomol., Rev.Med.& Vet.Mycol., Rev.Plant Path., Rice Abstr., Sci.Cit.Ind., Seed Abstr., Small Anim.Abstr., Soils & Fert., Soyabean Abstr., Sport Fish.Abstr., Sugar Ind.Abstr., Triticale Abstr., Trop.Dis.Bull., Vet.Bull., W.R.C.Inf., Weed Abstr.
—BLDSC (5757.750500), CASDDS, CISTI, EMDOCS, GNLM, IDS, ingenta, Linda Hall. **CCC.**
Published by: Society for General Microbiology, Marlborough House, Basingstoke Rd, Spencers Wood, Reading, Berks RG7 1AG, United Kingdom. TEL 44-118-988-1804, FAX 44-118-988-1834, mic-fb@highwire.stanford.edu, http://www.socgenmicrobiol.org.uk/mic_main.html; http://mic.sgmjournals.org. Ed. J R Saunders. Adv. contact C Sinclair. Circ: 2,440.

579 RUS ISSN 0026-2617
QR1 CODEN: MIBLAO
MICROBIOLOGY. Text in Russian. 1932. bi-m. EUR 2,737 to institutions for print or online ed.; EUR 3,284.40 to institutions print & online eds.combined (effective 2002). charts, illus. index. back issues avail. *Refereed.* **Document type:** *Academic/Scholarly.* **Description:** Investigates a wide range of problems in the areas of fundamental and applied microbiology.
Related titles: Microfilm ed.: (from PQC); Online - full text ed.: (from Swets Blackwell, Kluwer Online, Institute for Scientific Information, RoweCom Information Quest); ♦ Translation of: Mikrobiologiya. ISSN 0026-3656.
Indexed: ASCA, Biol.Abstr., Biotech.Cit.Ind., Chem.Titles, Curr.Adv.Ecol.Sci., Curr.Biotech.Abstr., Curr.Cont., Dairy Sci.Abstr., Deep Sea Res.& Oceanogr.Abstr., Food Sci.& Tech.Abstr., Forest.Abstr., INIS Atomind., Ind.Med. (coverage dropped), Ind.Sci.Rev., Int.Abstr.Biol.Sci., Rev.Plant Path., Sci.Cit.Ind., Soils & Fert., Weed Abstr.
—BLDSC (0416.200000), CASDDS, CISTI, GNLM, IDS, ingenta, Linda Hall. **CCC.**
Published by: (Rossiiskaya Akademiya Nauk/Russian Academy of Sciences), M A I K Nauka - Interperiodica, Mezhdunarodnyi Otdel, Profsoyuznaya ul 90, Moscow 117864, Russian Federation. TEL 7-095-336-1600, FAX 7-095-336-0666, compmg@maik.ru, http://www.maik.rssi.ru/journals/micbio.htm. Ed. M V Ivanov. **Dist. by:** Kluwer Academic Publishers, PO Box 17, Dordrecht 3300 AH, Netherlands. TEL 31-78-639-2392, FAX 31-78-654-6474, http://www.wkap.nl.

▼ **MICROBIOLOGY**; Royal Australasian College of Dental Surgeons. Lecture notes in microbiology. see *MEDICAL SCIENCES—Dentistry*

MICROBIOLOGY ABSTRACTS: SECTION A. INDUSTRIAL & APPLIED MICROBIOLOGY. see *BIOLOGY—Abstracting, Bibliographies, Statistics*

MICROBIOLOGY ABSTRACTS: SECTION B. BACTERIOLOGY. see *BIOLOGY—Abstracting, Bibliographies, Statistics*

B

MICROBIOLOGY ABSTRACTS: SECTION C. ALGOLOGY, MYCOLOGY AND PROTOZOOLOGY. see *BIOLOGY—Abstracting, Bibliographies, Statistics*

579 JPN ISSN 0385-5600
QR1 CODEN: MIIMDV
MICROBIOLOGY AND IMMUNOLOGY. Text in English. 1957. m. USD 255. adv. charts, illus. *Refereed.* **Document type:** *Academic/Scholarly.*
Formerly (until vol. 21, 1977): Japanese Journal of Microbiology (0021-5139)
Related titles: Microform ed.: (from PMC); Online - full text ed.: (from Institute for Scientific Information).
Indexed: AIDS & Cancer Res., ASCA, Abstr.Hyg., AgBiotech, Agri.& Environ.Biotech.Abstr. (coverage dropped), Biol.Abstr., Chem.Abstr., Chem.Indus.Notes, Chem.Titles, Curr.Adv.Cancer Res., Curr.Adv.Ecol.Sci., Curr.Adv.Gen.& Molec.Biol., Curr.Biotech.Abstr., Curr.Cont., Dairy Sci.Abstr., Dent.Ind., Derwent Biotech.Abstr., Diar.Dis.Res., Environ.Sci.Poll.Mgmt., Excerp.Med., Helminthol.Abstr., INIS Atomind., Immun.Abstr., Ind.Med. (1977-), Ind.Sci.Rev., Ind.Vet., Inpharma, Int.Abstr.Biol.Sci., Microbiol.Abstr., Nutr.Abstr., Pharm.&Out.News, Pig News & Info., Poult.Abstr., Protozool.Abstr., Reac., Ref.Zh., Rev.Appl.Entomol., Rev.Arom.& Med.Plants, Rev.Med.& Vet.Mycol., Rev.Plant Path., Sci.Cit.Ind., Soils & Fert., Sport Fish.Abstr., Telegen, Trop.Dis.Bull., Vet.Bull., Virol.Abstr. (coverage dropped), W.R.C.Inf.
—BLDSC (5757.791000), CASDDS, CISTI, EMDOCS, GNLM, IDS, Linda Hall. **CCC.**
Published by: (Japanese Society for Bacteriology/Nihon Saikin Gakkai), Center for Academic Publications Japan, 2-4-16 Yayoi, Bunkyo-ku, Tokyo 113-0032, Japan. TEL 81-3-3817-5821, FAX 81-3-3817-5820, capj@crisscross.com. Circ: 1,500. **Dist. by:** Business Center for Academic Societies Japan, 5-16-9 Honkomagome, Bunkyo-ku, Tokyo 113-0021, Japan. TEL 81-3-5814-5811, FAX 81-3-5814-5822. **Co-sponsors:** Japanese Society for Immunology; Society of Japanese Virologists/Nihon Uirusu Gakkai.

579 USA ISSN 1092-2172
QR1 CODEN: MMBRF7
MICROBIOLOGY AND MOLECULAR BIOLOGY REVIEWS. Text in English. 1937. q. USD 48 domestic to members; USD 320 domestic to non-members; USD 326 in Canada to non-members; USD 343 in Europe to non-members; USD 344 in Latin America to non-members; USD 345 elsewhere to non-members (effective 2001). adv. bibl. index. back issues avail.; reprint service avail. from PQC. *Refereed.* **Document type:** *Academic/Scholarly.* **Description:** Presents broad-based reviews on the expanding disciplines of microbiolgy, immunology, and molecular and cellular biology.
Former titles (until 1997): Microbiological Reviews (0146-0749); (until 1978): Bacteriological Reviews (0005-3678)
Related titles: CD-ROM ed.: USD 300 in North America; USD 324 elsewhere (effective 1999); Microform ed.: (from PQC); Online - full text ed.: ISSN 1098-5557 (from HighWire Pr., EBSCO Publishing, Gale Group, Factiva, Institute for Scientific Information).
Indexed: ASCA, Abstr.Bull.Inst.Pap.Chem., Abstr.Hyg., Agri.& Environ.Biotech.Abstr. (coverage dropped), Aqua.Sci.& Fish.Abstr., Aquacult.Abstr., Bio-Contr.News & Info., Biol.& Agr.Ind. (Mar.1997-), Biol.Abstr., Biol.Dig., CEABA, Chem.Abstr., Chem.Indus.Notes, Chem.Titles, Crop Physiol.Abstr., Curr.Adv.Ecol.Sci., Curr.Biotech.Abstr., Curr.Cont., Dairy Sci.Abstr., Deep Sea Res.& Oceanogr.Abstr., Derwent Biotech.Abstr., Diar.Dis.Res., Environ.Sci.Poll.Mgmt., Excerp.Med., Field Crop Abstr., Food Sci.& Tech.Abstr., Gen.Sci.Ind. (Mar.1997-), Genet.Abstr., Helminthol.Abstr., Hort.Abstr., Hum.Gen.Abstr., INIS Atomind., Ind.Med. (1997-), Ind.Sci.Rev., Ind.Vet., Inpharma, Int.Abstr.Biol.Sci., Microbiol.Abstr., Nuc.Acids Abstr., Nutr.Abstr., Potato Abstr., Protozool.Abstr., Reac., Rev.Appl.Entomol., Rev.Med.& Vet.Mycol., Rev.Plant Path., Sci.Cit.Ind., Soils & Fert., Telegen, Trop.Dis.Bull., Vet.Bull., Virol.Abstr. (coverage dropped), W.R.C.Inf., Zoo.Rec.
—BLDSC (5757.791300), CASDDS, CISTI, GNLM, IDS, Infotrieve, ingenta, Linda Hall. **CCC.**
Published by: American Society for Microbiology, 1752 N St N W, Washington, DC 20036-2904. TEL 202-737-3600, 800-633-4931, subscriptions@asmusa.org, http://mmbr.asm.org/, http://www.asmusa.org. Ed. Catherine L Squires. Circ: 8,200 (paid).

579 USA ISSN 0092-6027
CODEN: MSERDS
MICROBIOLOGY SERIES. Text in English. irreg., latest vol.18, 1987. price varies. adv. *Refereed.* **Document type:** *Monographic series.*
Indexed: Diar.Dis.Res., GeoRef.
—CASDDS, CISTI.
Published by: Marcel Dekker, Inc., Attn: Eridania Perrez, 270 Madison Ave, New York, NY 10016-0602. TEL 212-889-9595, 800-228-1160, FAX 212-658-4540, marketing@dekker.com, http://www.dekker.com. Ed. Allan I Laskin. R&P Julia Mulligan. Adv. contact Eridania Perez.

579 GBR ISSN 1464-0570
QR1
MICROBIOLOGY TODAY. Text in English. 1974. q. GBP 50, USD 85 (effective 2002). adv. bk.rev. 64 p./no. back issues avail. **Document type:** *Magazine, Academic/Scholarly.* **Description:** Publishes articles on microbiology; also includes information on society activities.
Former titles (until 1999): Society for General Microbiology. Quarterly (0142-7547); Society for General Microbiology Proceedings (0306-2708)
Related titles: Online - full text ed.: (from EBSCO Publishing).
Indexed: Abstr.Hyg., Aqua.Sci.& Fish.Abstr., Curr.Adv.Ecol.Sci., Dairy Sci.Abstr., Environ.Sci.Poll.Mgmt., Ind.Vet., Microbiol.Abstr., Nutr.Abstr., Plant Breed.Abstr., Pollut.Abstr., Potato Abstr., Res.High.Educ.Abstr., Rev.Med.& Vet.Mycol., Rev.Plant Path., Vet.Bull.
—BLDSC (5757.798550), CISTI, Infotrieve, ingenta, Linda Hall. **CCC.**
Published by: Society for General Microbiology, Marlborough House, Basingstoke Rd, Spencers Wood, Reading, Berks RG7 1AG, United Kingdom. TEL 44-118-988-1802, FAX 44-118-988-5656, mtoday@sgm.ac.uk, http://www.sgm.ac.uk. Ed. M. Jones. R&P Janice Meekings. Adv. contact Julie Lander. Circ: 5,500 (paid).

579 GBR ISSN 0026-2633
QR46 CODEN: MCBIA7
MICROBIOS; a prestige international biomedical research journal of chemical and general microbiology. Text in English. 1969. m. GBP 350; includes supplements. adv. bk.rev. abstr. bibl. charts, illus. index. Supplement avail. *Refereed.* **Description:** Devoted to fundamental studies of viruses, bacteria, micro-fungi, microscopic algae, and protozoa.
Related titles: Online - full text ed.: (from Institute for Scientific Information).
Indexed: ASCA, Abstr.Hyg., AgBiotech, Agri.& Environ.Biotech.Abstr. (coverage dropped), Aqua.Sci.& Fish.Abstr., Biol.Abstr., Biol.Dig., Chem.Abstr., Chem.Titles, Curr.Adv.Biochem., Curr.Adv.Ecol.Sci., Curr.Adv.Gen.& Molec.Biol., Curr.Biotech.Abstr., Curr.Cont., Dairy Sci.Abstr., Deep Sea Res.& Oceanogr.Abstr., Derwent Biotech.Abstr., Environ.Sci.Poll.Mgmt., Excerp.Med., Field Crop Abstr., Forest Prod.Abstr., Helminthol.Abstr., Hort.Abstr., INIS Atomind., Ind.Med. (1969-), Ind.Sci.Rev., Ind.Vet., Inpharma, Maize Abstr., Microbiol.Abstr., Nutr.Abstr., Ornam.Hort., Pharm.&Out.News, Plant Breed.Abstr., Plant Grow.Reg.Abstr., Poult.Abstr., Protozool.Abstr., Reac., Ref.Zh., Rev.Appl.Entomol., Rev.Arom.& Med.Plants, Rev.Med.& Vet.Mycol., Rev.Plant Path., Rice Abstr., Sci.Cit.Ind., Soils & Fert., Soyabean Abstr., Sugar Ind.Abstr., Triticale Abstr., Trop.Dis.Bull., Vet.Bull., Weed Abstr., Zoo.Rec.
—BLDSC (5757.800000), CASDDS, CISTI, GNLM, ingenta. **CCC.**
Published by: Faculty Press, 88 Regent St, Cambridge CB2 1DP, United Kingdom. FAX 44-1553-840695.

MICROCIRCULATION. see *MEDICAL SCIENCES*

616.01 579 DNK
MIKROBIOLOGI-NYT. Text in Danish. 1983. q. USD 10. adv. bk.rev. **Document type:** *Newsletter.*
Formerly: Hurtigmetode-nyt (0109-0763)
Published by: Mikrobiologisk Gruppe-Levnedsmiddelselskabet, Ingenioerhuset, Vester Farimagsgade 29, Copenhagen V 1780, Denmark. TEL 45-53-15-65-65, FAX 45-33-15-37-37. Ed. Poul Sigsgaard. R&P Kalvebad Brygge.

579 616.9 UKR ISSN 0201-8462
QR1 CODEN: MZHUDX
MIKROBIOLOGICHNYI ZHURNAL; nauchnyi zhurnal. Text and summaries in English, Russian, Ukrainian. 1934. bi-m. USD 45 domestic; USD 102 foreign (effective 2001). bk.rev. bibl. abstr. illus. index. 75 p./no. reprints avail. **Document type:** *Journal, Academic/Scholarly.*
Related titles: Diskette ed.; Online - full content ed.
Indexed: Abstr.Hyg., Agri.& Environ.Biotech.Abstr. (coverage dropped), Aqua.Sci.& Fish.Abstr., Aquacult.Abstr., Bio-Contr.News & Info., Biol.Abstr., Chem.Abstr., Crop Physiol.Abstr., Dairy Sci.Abstr., Derwent Biotech.Abstr., Djerelo, Environ.Sci.Poll.Mgmt., Excerp.Med., Field Crop Abstr., GeoRef, Herb.Abstr., Ind.Med. (coverage dropped), Ind.Vet., Maize Abstr., Microbiol.Abstr., Nutr.Abstr., Pig News & Info., Potato Abstr., Protozool.Abstr., Rev.Appl.Entomol., Rev.Med.& Vet.Mycol., Rev.Plant Path., Seed Abstr., Soils & Fert., Triticale Abstr., Vet.Bull.
—CASDDS, CISTI, East View, GNLM, KNAW, Linda Hall. **CCC.**
Published by: Natsional'na Akademiya Nauk Ukrainy, Institut Mikrobiologii i Virusologii im. D.K. Zabolotnogo/National Ukrainian Academy of Sciences Zabolotny, Institut of Microbiology and Virology, Vul Akad Zabolotnogo 154, Kyiv 03143, Ukraine. TEL 380-44-2663487, FAX 380-44-2662379, smirnov@imv.kiev.ua. Ed. V V Smirnov.

579 TUR ISSN 0374-9096
CODEN: MIBUBI
MIKROBIYOLOJI BULTENI/BULLETIN OF MICROBIOLOGY. Text in Turkish; Summaries in English. 1965. q. USD 100 foreign (effective 2001). adv. abstr. *Refereed.* **Document type:** *Academic/Scholarly.* **Description:** Covers microbiology, medical microbiology, infectious diseases and chemotherapy. Includes case reports and discussions of practical medical microbiology.
Indexed: Apic.Abstr., Chem.Abstr., Chem.Titles, Excerp.Med., Ind.Med. (until 1994, dropped).
—BLDSC (5761.665000), CASDDS, CISTI, EMDOCS, GNLM.
Published by: Ankara Microbiology Society, Hacettepe University Faculty of Medicine, Dept. of Clinical Microbiology, Ankara 06100, Turkey. TEL 90-312-3051560, FAX 90-312-3115250, hutfm-e@servis2.net.tr. Ed. Dr. Ayfer Gunalp. Pub. Durdal Us. R&P, Adv. contact Burcin Sener. Circ: 350 (paid).

579 DEU ISSN 0026-3680
QH201 CODEN: MKKSA2
MIKROKOSMOS; Zeitschrift fuer angewandte Mikroskopie, Mikrobiologie, Mikrochemie und mikroskopische Technik. Text in German. 1907. 6/yr. EUR 63 (effective 2002). adv. bk.rev. bibl. charts, illus. index. *Refereed.* **Document type:** *Journal, Academic/Scholarly.* **Description:** Covers applied microscopy, microbiology, microchemistry, and microscopal technology.
Indexed: Biol.Abstr., Chem.Abstr., Excerp.Med., GeoRef, Zoo.Rec.
—CASDDS, CISTI, Infotrieve, Linda Hall. **CCC.**
Published by: Urban & Fischer Verlag, Loebdergraben 14A, Jena 07743, Germany. TEL 49-3641-626444, FAX 49-3641-626421, info@urbanfischer.de, http://www.urbanfischer.de. Ed. K Hausmann. Adv. contact Sabine Schroeter. Circ: 1,600.

579 571.6 NLD ISSN 1567-7249
▼ **MITOCHONDRION.** Text in English. 2001. bi-m. EUR 300 in Europe to institutions; JPY 39,800 in Japan to institutions; USD 336 elsewhere to institutions (effective 2002). *Refereed.*
Published by: (Mitochondria Research Society USA), Elsevier Science BV, Sara Burgerhartstraat 25, Amsterdam 1055 KV, Netherlands. TEL 31-20-485-2911, FAX 31-20-485-2457, nlinfo-f@elsevier.nl, http://www.elsevier.com/locate/mito, http://www.elsevier.nl. Eds. B Chance, K K Singh.

579 JPN ISSN 0026-8054
MODERN MEDIA/MODAN MEDIA. Text in Japanese. 1955. m. bk.rev. charts, illus.
Indexed: Chem.Abstr., Chem.Titles, Ref.Zh.
—BLDSC (5889.700000).
Published by: Eiken Chemical Co. Ltd./Eiken Kagaku K. K., 5-26-20 O-Ji, Kita-ku, Tokyo 114-0002, Japan. TEL 81-3-3913-6231, FAX 81-3-3914-7027. Ed. Hiromitsu Enomoto. Circ: (controlled).

MOLECULAR AND BIOCHEMICAL PARASITOLOGY. see *BIOLOGY—Biochemistry*

MOLECULAR CARCINOGENESIS. see *MEDICAL SCIENCES—Oncology*

579 USA ISSN 0891-4168
QH506
MOLECULAR GENETICS, MICROBIOLOGY AND VIROLOGY. Text in English. 1986. bi-m. USD 1,140 in US & Canada; USD 1,335 elsewhere (effective 2002). abstr, charts, illus. *Refereed.* **Document type:** *Journal, Academic/Scholarly.* **Description:** Covers microbiology, virology, genetic engineering, immunology, DNA, and the methodology of molecular genetics.
Related titles: ♦ Translation of: Molekulyarnaya Genetika, Mikrobiologiya i Virusologiya. ISSN 0208-0613.
—BLDSC (0416.235500), CISTI, GNLM. **CCC.**
Published by: (Biotechnologicheskya Akademiya RUS), Allerton Press, Inc., 18 W 27th St, New York, NY 10001. TEL 646-424-9686, FAX 646-424-9695, journals@allertonpress.com, http://www.allertonpress.com/. Ed. E D Sverdlov.

579 GBR ISSN 0950-382X
QR74 CODEN: MOMIEE
MOLECULAR MICROBIOLOGY. Text in English. 23/yr., latest vol.43, 2002. GBP 192 in Europe to individuals; USD 306 in North America to individuals; GBP 212 elsewhere to individuals; GBP 1,738 in Europe to institutions; USD 2,754 in North America to institutions; GBP 1,912 elsewhere to institutions (effective 2002). adv. bibl, illus. index. back issues avail. *Refereed.* **Document type:** *Academic/Scholarly.* **Description:** Publishes original research and review articles reporting new developments in the genetics, molecular biology and biochemistry of prokaryotic and eukaryotic microorganisms, and covers the most important advances in bacterial pathogenicity.
Incorporates: Microbiological Sciences (0265-1351)
Related titles: Microform ed.: USD 2,456 in North America to institutions; USD 284 in North America to individuals; GBP 1,449 elsewhere to institutions; GBP 167 elsewhere to individuals (effective 2001) (from EBSCO Publishing, O C L C Online Computer Library Center, Inc.); Online - full text ed.: Molecular Microbiology Online. ISSN 1365-2958. 1998. GBP 173 in Europe to individuals; USD 276 in North America to individuals; GBP 173 elsewhere to individuals; GBP 1,565 in Europe to institutions; USD 2,479 in North America to institutions; GBP 1,565 elsewhere to institutions (effective 2002) (from ingenta, Munksgaard & Blackwell Science's Synergy, Swets Blackwell, Institute for Scientific Information, RoweCom Information Quest, Ovid Technologies, Inc.,PQC).
Indexed: ASCA, AgBiotech, Agricola, Aqua.Sci.& Fish.Abstr., BBCI, Bibl.Agri., Biotech.Cit.Ind., Chem.Abstr., Chem.Indus.Notes, Chem.Titles, Crop Physiol.Abstr., Curr.Adv.Biochem., Curr.Adv.Gen.& Molec.Biol., Curr.Cont., Dairy Sci.Abstr., Derwent Biotech.Abstr., Environ.Sci.Poll.Mgmt., Field Crop Abstr., Food Sci.& Tech.Abstr., Genet.Abstr., Hort.Abstr., Hum.Gen.Abstr., Ind.Med. (1987-), Ind.Sci.Rev., Ind.Vet., Inpharma, Int.Abstr.Biol.Sci., Maize Abstr., Microbiol.Abstr., Nuc.Acids Abstr., Nutr.Abstr., Pharm.&Out.News, Plant Breed.Abstr., Plant Grow.Reg.Abstr., Poult.Abstr., Protozool.Abstr., Reac., Ref.Zh., Rev.Appl.Entomol., Rev.Med.& Vet.Mycol., Rev.Plant Path., Sci.Cit.Ind., Soils & Fert., Soyabean Abstr., Sugar Ind.Abstr., Telegen, Vet.Bull., Weed Abstr.
—BLDSC (5900.817960), ADONIS, CASDDS, CISTI, EMDOCS, GNLM, IDS, ingenta, Linda Hall. **CCC.**
Published by: Blackwell Science Ltd., PO Box 88, Oxford OX2 0NE, United Kingdom. TEL 44-1865-206180, 44-1865-206002, FAX 44-1865-206219, jnl.orders@blacksci.co.uk, http://www.blackwell-science.com/~cgilib/jnlpage.asp?Journal=mole&File=mole, http://www.blackwellpublishing.com. Ed. C Higgins. Pub. Amanda McLean Inglis. R&P Sophie Savage. Adv. contact Jenny Applin. Circ: 1,600.

MOLECULAR PLANT - MICROBE INTERACTIONS. see *BIOLOGY—Biochemistry*

MOLECULAR REPRODUCTION AND DEVELOPMENT. see *BIOLOGY—Biochemistry*

579 RUS ISSN 0208-0613
QR74 CODEN: MGMVDU
MOLEKULYARNAYA GENETIKA, MIKROBIOLOGIYA I VIRUSOLOGIYA/MOLECULAR GENETICS, MICROBIOLOGY AND VIRUSOLOGY. Text in Russian; Summaries in English. 1983. q. USD 132 foreign (effective 2000). adv. Website rev. abstr. reprints avail. **Document type:** *Journal, Academic/Scholarly.* **Description:** Deals with fundamental and applied problems of molecular genetics, molecular microbiology and molecular virology.
Related titles: ♦ English Translation: Molecular Genetics, Microbiology and Virology. ISSN 0891-4168.
Indexed: Biol.Abstr., Chem.Abstr., Chem.Titles, Curr.Cont. (coverage dropped), INIS Atomind., Ind.Med. (1983-), Ref.Zh.
—CASDDS, CISTI, East View, GNLM, Linda Hall.
Published by: Izdatel'stvo Meditsina, Petroverigskii per 6-8, Moscow 101000, Russian Federation. TEL 7-095-9248785, 7-095-928-86-48, FAX 7-095-9211355, 7-095-9286003, meditsina@iname.com, http://www.medit.ru. Ed. Ye D Sverdlov. Pub. A M Stochik. R&P I Izmailova. Adv. contact O A Fadeeva TEL 7-095-923-51-40. Circ: 500. **Dist. by:** Mezhdunarodnaya Kniga, B Yakimanka 39, Moscow 117049, Russian Federation. TEL 7-095-2384967, FAX 7-095-2384634; **US dist. addr.:** East View Publications, 3020 Harbor Ln N, Minneapolis, MN 55447. TEL 612-550-0961.

579.65 POL ISSN 0540-6722
MONOGRAFIE PARAZYTOLOGICZNE. Text in Polish. 1959. irreg., latest vol.14, 1988. price varies. bibl, illus. back issues avail. **Document type:** *Monographic series.*
Indexed: Biol.Abstr., Zoo.Rec.
Published by: Polskie Towarzystwo Parazytologiczne/Polish Parasitological Society, Ul Grochowska 272, Warsaw 03849, Poland. niewiadk@twarda.pan.pl. Ed. Katarzyna Niewiadomska. Circ: 400. **Dist. by:** Ars Polona, Krakowskie Przedmiescie 7, Warsaw, Poland.

579.2 CHE ISSN 0077-0965
CODEN: MONVAK
MONOGRAPHS IN VIROLOGY. Text in English. 1967. irreg., latest vol.23. CHF 180 in Europe; DEM 220 in Germany; USD 160 in United States (effective 2001). reprint service avail. from ISI. *Refereed.* **Document type:** *Monographic series, Academic/Scholarly.* **Description:** Reference tools for virologists and non-virologists alike.
Related titles: Online - full text ed.: (from Institute for Scientific Information).
Indexed: Biol.Abstr., Chem.Abstr., Curr.Cont. (coverage dropped), Ind.Med. (coverage dropped).
—BLDSC (5917.780000), CISTI, GNLM, Infotrieve, ingenta, KNAW. **CCC.**
Published by: S. Karger AG, Allschwilerstr 10, PO Box, Basel 4009, Switzerland. TEL 41-61-306-1111, FAX 41-61-306-1234, karger@karger.ch, http://www.karger.com/bookseries/MOVIR. Ed. H W Doerr.

MYCOBACTERIA. see *BIOLOGY—Abstracting, Bibliographies, Statistics*

MYCOPATHOLOGIA. see *BIOLOGY—Botany*

NEDERLANDS TIJDSCHRIFT VOOR MEDISCHE MICROBIOLOGIE. see *MEDICAL SCIENCES*

579 ITA ISSN 1121-7138
CODEN: MIBLDR
THE NEW MICROBIOLOGICA; quarterly journal of microbiological sciences. Text and summaries in English. 1978. q. ITL 190,000. adv. bk.rev. *Refereed.* **Document type:** *Academic/Scholarly.*
Formerly (until 1992): Microbiologica (0391-5352)
Related titles: Online - full text ed.: (from Institute for Scientific Information).
Indexed: Aqua.Sci.& Fish.Abstr., Bio-Contr.News & Info., Biol.Abstr., Curr.Adv.Ecol.Sci., Curr.Cont., Environ.Sci.Poll.Mgmt., Excerp.Med., Food Sci.& Tech.Abstr., Ind.Med. (1993-), Ind.Vet., Inpharma, Microbiol.Abstr., Nutr.Abstr., Pharm.&Out.News, Pig News & Info., Protozool.Abstr., Reac., Rev.Appl.Entomol., Rev.Med.& Vet.Mycol., Rev.Plant Path., Sci.Cit.Ind. (coverage dropped), Sugar Ind.Abstr., Telegen, Trop.Dis.Bull., Vet.Bull.
—BLDSC (5757.400000), CASDDS, CISTI, GNLM, IDS, ingenta, KNAW.
Published by: (University of Bologna, Institute of Microbiology), Luigi Penzie e Figlio Publishers, Via D da Catalogna, 1-3, Pavia, PV 27100, Italy. TEL 0382-35000, TELEX 0382-304435. Ed. Michele La Placa. Circ: 500.

NIHON BOKIN BOBAI GAKKAI. NENJI TAIKAI YOSHISHU/SOCIETY FOR ANTIBACTERIAL AND ANTIFUNGAL AGENTS, JAPAN. ABSTRACTS OF THE MEETING. see *BIOLOGY—Abstracting, Bibliographies, Statistics*

579 JPN ISSN 0914-5818
CODEN: ACTIF4
NIHON HOSENKIN GAKKAISHI/ACTINOMYCETOLOGICA. Text in English, Japanese; Summaries in English. 1962. s-a. JPY 7,000 (effective 1999). **Document type:** *Academic/Scholarly.*
Indexed: Chem.Abstr., Chem.Indus.Notes, Chem.Titles.
—BLDSC (0675.405500), CASDDS.
Published by: Nihon Hosenkin Gakkai/Society for Actinomycetes, Japan, Biseibutsu Kagaku Kenkyujo, 14-23 Kami-Osaki 3-chome, Shinagawa-ku, Tokyo 141-0021, Japan. Ed. Sueharu Horinouchi. R&P Nihon Hosenkin Gakkai.

579.2 JPN
NIHON UIRUSU GAKKAI HOKKAIDO SHIBU KAIHO/SOCIETY OF JAPANESE VIROLOGISTS. HOKKAIDO BRANCH. NEWS. Text in Japanese. a.
Published by: Nihon Uirusu Gakkai, Hokkaido Shibu/Society of Japanese Virologists, Hokkaido Branch, Hokkaido Daigaku Juigakubu Jui Koshu Eiseigaku Koza, Nishi 9-chome, Kita 18-jo, Kita-ku, Sapporo-shi, Hokkaido 060, Japan.

579.2 JPN
NIHON UIRUSU GAKKAI KAIHO/SOCIETY OF JAPANESE VIROLOGISTS. BULLETIN. Text in Japanese. s-a.
Published by: Nihon Uirusu Gakkai, Nihon Gakkai Jimu Senta, 16-9 Honkomagome 5-chome, Bunkyo-ku, Tokyo 113-0021, Japan.

B

579.2 JPN
NIHON UIRUSU GAKKAI SOKAI ENZETSU SHOROKU/SOCIETY OF JAPANESE VIROLOGISTS. PROCEEDINGS OF THE ANNUAL MEETING. Text in Japanese. 1953. a. **Document type:** *Proceedings.*
Published by: Nihon Uirusu Gakkai, Nihon Gakkai Jimu Senta, 16-9 Honkomagome 5-chome, Bunkyo-ku, Tokyo 113-0021, Japan.

O M I C S: A JOURNAL OF INTEGRATIVE BIOLOGY. see *BIOLOGY—Genetics*

579 GBR ISSN 1362-6809
OPINION: SPECIALIST REVIEWS OF KEY PAPERS IN MICROBIOLOGY. Abbreviated title: Opinion: Micro. Text in English. 1996. 3/yr. **Document type:** *Academic/Scholarly.*
Published by: Hayward Medical Communications Ltd., Covent Garden, Seven Dials Warehouse, 44 Earlham St, London WC2H 9LA, United Kingdom. TEL 44-20-7240-4493, FAX 44-20-7240-4479, admin@hayward.co.uk, http://www.hayward.co.uk. Ed. Tom Rogers. Circ: 1,800. **Subscr. to:** Rosemary House, Lanwades Park, Kentford, Near, Newmarket, Suffolk CB8 7PW, United Kingdom. TEL 44-1638-751515, FAX 44-1638-751517.

579 DNK ISSN 0902-0055
CODEN: OMIMEE
ORAL MICROBIOLOGY AND IMMUNOLOGY. Text in English. 1987. bi-m. USD 360 in the Americas to institutions print & online eds. combined; GBP 250 elsewhere to institutions print & online eds. combined (effective 2002). illus. *Refereed.* **Document type:** *Academic/Scholarly.*
Related titles: Online - full text ed.: DKK 1,242 to individuals; DKK 2,412 to institutions (effective 2001) (from Ovid Technologies, Inc., EBSCO Publishing, O C L C Online Computer Library Center, Inc., RoweCom Information Quest, ingenta, Munksgaard & Blackwell Science's Synergy, Swets Blackwell, Institute for Scientific Information).
Indexed: AIDS & Cancer Res., ASCA, Biol.Abstr., Chem.Abstr., Chem.Indus.Notes, Chem.Titles, Curr.Cont., Curr.Tit.Dent., Environ.Sci.Poll.Mgmt., Immun.Abstr., Ind.Sci.Rev., Inpharma, Int.Abstr.Biol.Sci., Microbiol.Abstr., Reac., Rev.Med.& Vet.Mycol., Sci.Cit.Ind.
—BLDSC (6277.590000), CASDDS, CISTI, EMDOCS, GNLM, IDS, ingenta, KNAW. **CCC.**
Published by: Blackwell Munksgaard, Noerre Soegade 35, PO Box 2148, Copenhagen K 1016, Denmark. TEL 45-77-33-33-33, FAX 45-77-33-33-77, customerservice@munksgaard.dk, http://journals.munksgaard.dk/omi, http://www.munksgaard.dk. Ed. Joergen Slots. Circ: 625.

579 ITA ISSN 0390-5454
OSPEDALE MARIA VITTORIA DI TORINO. ANNALI. Text in Italian. s-a.
Supersedes: Giornale di Batteriologia, Virologia ed Immunologia ed Annali dell'Ospedale Maria Vittoria di Torino. Parte 2. Sezione Clinica (0301-1445); Which superseded in part: Giornale di Batteriologia, Virologia ed Immunologia ed Annali dell'Ospedale Maria Vittoria di Torino (0017-0267)
Indexed: Biol.Abstr., Dent.Ind., Trop.Dis.Bull.
—CISTI, GNLM.
Published by: Ospedale Maria Vittoria, Via Luigi Cibrario, 72, Turin, TO 10144, Italy. TEL 74 92 345.

579 GBR ISSN 0141-9692
P H L S DIRECTORY. Text in English. 1980. irreg. GBP 5.95 (effective 2000). **Document type:** *Directory.*
Published by: Public Health Laboratory Service, 61 Colindale Ave, London NW9 5HT, United Kingdom. TEL 44-20-8200-4400, FAX 44-20-8200-7875. Circ: 10,000.

664.001579 GBR ISSN 0968-1280
P H L S FOOD AND ENVIRONMENT BULLETIN. Text in English. 1991. m., latest vol.10, 2001. GBP 58 in United Kingdom; GBP 74 in Europe; GBP 94 elsewhere (effective 2002). **Document type:** *Bibliography.* **Description:** Covers food, water, environmental microbiology related to prevention of infection.
Formerly (until 1992): P H L S Food and Environmental Microbiology Bulletin
Related titles: E-mail ed.
Published by: Public Health Laboratory Service, 61 Colindale Ave, London NW9 5HT, United Kingdom. TEL 44-20-8200-4400, FAX 44-20-8200-7875. Ed. Margaret Clennett.

P H L S LIBRARY BULLETIN. see *BIOLOGY—Abstracting, Bibliographies, Statistics*

579.65 FRA ISSN 1252-607X
QL757 CODEN: PASIED
PARASITE. Text and summaries in English, French. 1923. q. EUR 185 in Europe to individuals; EUR 250 elsewhere to individuals; EUR 145 in Europe to students; EUR 220 in Europe to institutions; EUR 300.88 elsewhere to institutions; EUR 55 newsstand/cover (effective 2002). bk.rev. illus. index. reprint service avail. from ISI. *Refereed.* **Document type:** *Academic/Scholarly.* **Description:** Contains original work in parasitology research: protozoology, helminthology, entomology, therapeutics, immunology, molecular biology, genetics, epidemiology.
Formerly (until 1994): Annales de Parasitologie Humaine et Comparee (0003-4150)
Related titles: Microform ed.: (from PQC); Online - full text ed.: (from Institute for Scientific Information).
Indexed: ABI Inform. (Mar.1992-, dropped), ASCA, Abstr.Hyg., Aqua.Sci.& Fish.Abstr., Biol.Abstr., Chem.Abstr., Chem.Indus.Notes, Chem.Titles, Curr.Adv.Ecol.Sci., Curr.Cont., Dairy Sci.Abstr., Entomol.Abstr., Environ.Sci.Poll.Mgmt., Excerp.Med., Helminthol.Abstr., Ind.Med. (1994-), Ind.Sci.Rev., Ind.Vet., Microbiol.Abstr., Pig News & Info., Pollut.Abstr., Protozool.Abstr., Rev.Appl.Entomol., Rev.Arom.& Med.Plants, Rev.Med.& Vet.Mycol., Rev.Plant Path., Risk Abstr., Saf.Sci.Abstr., Sci.Cit.Ind., Trop.Dis.Bull., Vet.Bull., Zoo.Rec.
—BLDSC (6404.939000), CISTI, GNLM, IDS, Infotrieve, ingenta, Linda Hall. **CCC.**
Published by: (Societe Francaise de Parasitologie), Princeps Editions, 64 av. du General de Gaulle, Issy-les-Moulineaux 92130, France. TEL 33-01-46382414, FAX 33-01-40957215. Ed. Dr. J M Dumas. Circ: 700.

579.65 CHL ISSN 0716-0720
RC119
PARASITOLOGIA AL DIA. Text in Spanish; Summaries in English. 1977. q. USD 55 (effective 1996 & 1997). adv. bk.rev. charts, illus. *Refereed.* **Document type:** *Academic/Scholarly.*
Related titles: Online - full text ed.: (from SciELO).
Indexed: Abstr.Hyg., Bio-Contr.News & Info., Dairy Sci.Abstr., Helminthol.Abstr., Ind.Med. (coverage dropped), Ind.Vet., Poult.Abstr., Protozool.Abstr., Rev.Appl.Entomol., Rev.Med.& Vet.Mycol., Trop.Dis.Bull., Vet.Bull.
Published by: Sociedad Chilena de Parasitologia, Casilla 50470, Santiago 1, Chile. FAX 56-2-5416840, TELEX JUMAR. Ed. Hector Alcaino A. Circ: 3,000. **Co-sponsor:** Federacion Latinoamericano de Parasitologos.

579.65 DEU ISSN 0932-0113
QL757 CODEN: PARREZ
PARASITOLOGY RESEARCH. Text in English, French, German; Summaries in English. 1928. 12/yr. EUR 2,095.90 domestic; EUR 2,076.70 in Germany; EUR 205 newsstand/cover foreign (effective 2002). adv. charts, illus. back issues avail.; reprint service avail. from ISI. *Refereed.* **Document type:** *Journal, Academic/Scholarly.* **Description:** Presents information on the latest developments in parasitology research, with special emphasis on practical aspects such as immunodiagnosis, chemotherapy, and epidemiology. Includes review articles that provide an overview of current advances.
Formerly: Zeitschrift fuer Parasitenkunde (0044-3255)
Related titles: Microform ed.: (from PQC); Online - full text ed.: ISSN 1432-1955 (from EBSCO Publishing, RoweCom Information Quest, Swets Blackwell, Springer LINK, Institute for Scientific Information).
Indexed: ASCA, Abstr.Hyg., AgBiotech, Agri.& Environ.Biotech.Abstr. (coverage dropped), Agroforest.Abstr., Aqua.Sci.& Fish.Abstr., Aquacult.Abstr., Bio-Contr.News & Info., Biol.Abstr., Chem.Abstr., Curr.Adv.Ecol.Sci., Curr.Cont., Dairy Sci.Abstr., Derwent Biotech.Abstr., Environ.Sci.Poll.Mgmt., Excerp.Med., Focus on: Vet.Sci.& Med., Helminthol.Abstr., INIS Atomind., Ind.Med. (1987-), Ind.Sci.Rev., Ind.Vet., Inpharma, Nutr.Abstr., Pig News & Info., Poult.Abstr., Protozool.Abstr., Rev.Appl.Entomol., Rev.Arom.& Med.Plants, Rev.Med.& Vet.Mycol., Rev.Plant Path., SSCI (coverage dropped), Sci.Cit.Ind., Sport Fish.Abstr., Trop.Dis.Bull., Vet.Bull., Weed Abstr., Wild.Rev., Zoo.Rec.
—BLDSC (6406.120000), ADONIS, CASDDS, CISTI, GNLM, IDS, Infotrieve, ingenta, Linda Hall. **CCC.**
Published by: (Deutschen Gesellschaft fuer Parasitologie), Springer-Verlag (Subsidiary of: BertelsmannSpringer), Tiergartenstr 17, Heidelberg 69121, Germany. TEL 49-6221-345-0, FAX 49-6221-345229, subscriptions@springer.de, http://link.springer.de/link/service/journals/00436/index.htm, http://www.springer.de. Eds. B Chobotar, H Mehlhorn. **Subscr. in N. America to:** Springer-Verlag New York Inc., PO Box 2485, Secaucus, NJ 07096-2485. TEL 212-460-1500, FAX 212-473-6272.

PARASITOLOGY (SHEFFIELD). see *BIOLOGY—Abstracting, Bibliographies, Statistics*

PARAZITOLOGIYA/PARASITOLOGY. see *MEDICAL SCIENCES—Communicable Diseases*

PATHOBIOLOGY; journal of immunopathology, molecular and cellular biology. see *MEDICAL SCIENCES—Allergology And Immunology*

PENDIK VETERINER MIKROBIYOLOJI DERGISI. see *VETERINARY SCIENCE*

579 POL ISSN 0079-4252
QR1 CODEN: PMKMAV
POSTEPY MIKROBIOLOGII. Text in Polish; Summaries in English, Polish. 1962. q. PLZ 44 domestic; USD 70 foreign (effective 2001). adv. **Document type:** *Monographic series.*
Indexed: Abstr.Hyg., AgroLibrex, CEABA, Chem.Abstr., Chem.Indus.Notes, Chem.Titles, Curr.Adv.Ecol.Sci., Dairy Sci.Abstr., Excerp.Med., INIS Atomind., Ind.Vet., Rev.Appl.Entomol., Rev.Med.& Vet.Mycol., Rev.Plant Path., Soils & Fert.
—CASDDS, CISTI.
Published by: Polskie Towarzystwo Mikrobiologow/Polish Society of Microbiologists, Ul Chocimska 24, Warsaw 00791, Poland. TEL 48-22-5421400, FAX 48-22-5541302, pzh@medstat.waw.pl. Ed. Jerzy Hrebenda. Circ: 1,150. **Dist. by:** Ars Polona, Krakowskie Przedmiescie 7, Warsaw, Poland. TEL 48-22-8261201, FAX 48-22-8268673.

PRIKLADNAYA BIOKHIMIYA I MIKROBIOLOGIYA. see *BIOLOGY—Biochemistry*

579.65 616.96 PAK ISSN 1018-2500
PROCEEDINGS OF PARASITOLOGY. Text in English. 1985. s-a. USD 120 foreign to individuals; USD 160 foreign to institutions; PKR 1,000 domestic to individuals; PKR 2,000 domestic to institutions (effective 2001). adv. bk.rev. abstr, bibl, illus, maps. 80 p./no. back issues avail. *Refereed.* **Document type:** *Journal, Academic/Scholarly.* **Description:** Studies the prevalence and histopathology of diseases in Pakistan. Publishes information about paristic diseases in other countries.
Indexed: Helminthol.Abstr., Ind.Vet., Protozool.Abstr., Rev.Appl.Entomol., Zoo.Rec.
—BLDSC (6848.730600).
Published by: Baqai Medical University, Department of Parisitology, Karachi 74600, Pakistan. TEL 92-21-6637951, FAX 92-21-4547045, baqaiuniv@hotmail.com, baqaiuni@hotmail.com. Ed., Pub. Dr. Fatima Mujib Bilqees. adv.: B&W page USD 200, color page USD 400. Circ: 1,200. **Dist. by:** Al-Haseeb, A-314, Block D, N. Nazimabad, Karachi 74700, Pakistan. TEL 92-21-4937503.

579 NLD ISSN 0079-6352
QR53 CODEN: PIMRAS
PROGRESS IN INDUSTRIAL MICROBIOLOGY. Text in Dutch. 1959. irreg., latest vol.34, 1995. price varies. *Refereed.* **Document type:** *Monographic series, Academic/Scholarly.* **Description:** Examines in depth several culture media used in food science laboratories.
Indexed: AESIS, Biol.Abstr., CEABA, Chem.Abstr., Chem.Indus.Notes, Chem.Titles, Curr.Biotech.Abstr., Derwent Biotech.Abstr., Food Sci.& Tech.Abstr.
—BLDSC (6868.500000), CASDDS, CISTI, GNLM, Infotrieve, ingenta, Linda Hall. **CCC.**
Published by: Elsevier Science BV, PO Box 211, Amsterdam 1000 AE, Netherlands. TEL 31-20-485-3757, 31-20-485-3911, FAX 31-20-485-3432, 31-20-485-3598, nlinfo-f@elsevier.nl; usinfo-f@elsevier.com; forinfo-kyf04035@niftyserve.or.jp, http://www.elsevier.nl/. Ed. M E Bushell. **Subscr. in Australasia and the Far East to:** Elsevier Science (Singapore) Pte Ltd, No.1 Temasek Ave, 17-01 Millenia Tower, Singapore 039192, Singapore. TEL 65-434-3727, FAX 65-337-2230, asiainfo@elsevier.com.sg; **Subscr. in Japan to:** Elsevier Science Inc - Japan Regional Office, 9-15 Higashi-Azabu 1-chome, Minato-ku, Tokyo 106-0044, Japan. TEL 81-3-5561-5033, FAX 81-3-5561-5047, info@elsevier.co.jp; **Subscr. in the Americas to:** Elsevier Science, PO Box 945, New York, NY 10159-0945. TEL 212-633-3730, 888-437-4636, FAX 212-633-3680, usinfo-f@elsevier.com, http://www.elsevier.com

PROGRESS IN MEDICAL VIROLOGY. see *MEDICAL SCIENCES—Communicable Diseases*

REFERATIVNYI ZHURNAL. MIKROBIOLOGIYA SANITARNAYA I MEDITSINSKAYA. see *BIOLOGY—Abstracting, Bibliographies, Statistics*

REFERATIVNYI ZHURNAL. VIRUSOLOGIYA. see *BIOLOGY—Abstracting, Bibliographies, Statistics*

REFERATIVNYI ZHURNAL. VIRUSOLOGIYA. MIKROBIOLOGIYA. see *BIOLOGY—Abstracting, Bibliographies, Statistics*

RESEARCH COMMUNICATIONS IN BIOCHEMISTRY AND CELL & MOLECULAR BIOLOGY. see *BIOLOGY—Biochemistry*

579.072 FRA ISSN 0923-2508
QR1 CODEN: ANMBCM
RESEARCH IN MICROBIOLOGY. Text in English; Abstracts in English, French. 1887. 10/yr. EUR 573 in Europe to institutions; JPY 82,300 in Japan to institutions; USD 660 in the Americas to institutions (effective 2002). adv. bk.rev. abstr, illus. index. back issues avail.; reprint service avail. from ISI. *Refereed.* **Document type:** *Academic/Scholarly.* **Description:** Publishes original reports, brief notes and position papers on general and molecular microbiology, physiology and microbial genetics, environmental and applied microbiology, industrial microbiology, mycology and medical microbiology.
Former titles (until 1989): Institut Pasteur. Annales. Microbiologie (0769-2609); (until 1985): Annales de Microbiologie (0300-5410); Which superseded in part (in 1972): Institut Pasteur. Annales (0020-2444)
Related titles: Microform ed.: (from RPI,PMC); Online - full text ed.: (from ingenta, Institute for Scientific Information, ScienceDirect).
Indexed: ASCA, Abstr.Hyg., Agri.& Environ.Biotech.Abstr. (coverage dropped), Aqua.Sci.& Fish.Abstr., Biol.Abstr., Chem.Abstr., Chem.Indus.Notes, Chem.Titles, Curr.Adv.Biochem., Curr.Adv.Ecol.Sci., Curr.Adv.Gen.& Molec.Biol., Curr.Cont., Dairy Sci.Abstr., Derwent Biotech.Abstr., Environ.Sci.Poll.Mgmt., Excerp.Med., Food Sci.& Tech.Abstr., Genet.Abstr. (coverage dropped), INIS Atomind., Ind.Med. (1989-), Ind.Sci.Rev., Ind.Vet., Inpharma, Microbiol.Abstr., Pharm.&Out.News, Pig News & Info., Poult.Abstr., Reac., Rev.Appl.Entomol., Rev.Med.& Vet.Mycol., Sci.Cit.Ind., Soils & Fert., Trop.Dis.Bull., Vet.Bull., Weed Abstr.
—BLDSC (7742.720000), ADONIS, CASDDS, CISTI, EMDOCS, GNLM, IDS, Infotrieve, ingenta, Linda Hall. **CCC.**
Published by: (Institut Pasteur), Elsevier Paris, Editions Scientifiques et Medicales (Subsidiary of: Reed Elsevier plc. group), 23 rue Linois, Paris 75015, France. TEL 33-1-45589110, FAX 33-1-45589419, a.dore@elsevier.fr; mhofnung@pasteur.fr; academic@elsevier-fr.com, http://www.elsevier.nl/locate/issn/09232508. Ed. M Hofnung. Circ: 2,100.

REVIEWS IN MEDICAL MICROBIOLOGY. see *MEDICAL SCIENCES*

B

579.2 GBR ISSN 1052-9276
CODEN: RMVIEW
REVIEWS IN MEDICAL VIROLOGY. Text in English. 1991. q. USD 690 in United States; USD 690 in Canada & Mexico; USD 690 elsewhere; USD 725 combined subscription in United States for print and online eds.; USD 725 combined subscription in Canada & Mexico for print and online eds.; USD 725 combined subscription elsewhere for print and online eds. (effective 2002). adv. back issues avail.; reprint service avail. from SWZ. *Refereed.* **Document type:** *Academic/Scholarly.* **Description:** Reviews current research and new information on all viruses of medical importance.
Related titles: Microform ed.: (from PQC); Online - full text ed.: ISSN 1099-1654. 1996. USD 690 in United States; USD 690 in Canada & Mexico; USD 690 elsewhere (effective 2002) (from EBSCO Publishing, ingenta, Wiley InterScience, Institute for Scientific Information).
Indexed: AIDS & Cancer Res., ASCA, Abstr.Hyg., Chem.Abstr., Chem.Indus.Notes, Chem.Titles, Curr.Cont., Environ.Sci.Poll.Mgmt., Excerp.Med. (1994-), Genet.Abstr. (coverage dropped), Ind.Med. (1991-), Ind.Sci.Rev., Inpharma, Int.Abstr.Biol.Sci., Microbiol.Abstr., Nuc.Acids Abstr., Pharm.&Out.News, Poult.Abstr., Reac., Rev.Med.& Vet.Mycol., Saf.Sci.Abstr., Sci.Cit.Ind., Trop.Dis.Bull., Virol.Abstr.
—BLDSC (7792.500000), CASDDS, GNLM, IDS, Infotrieve, KNAW. **CCC.**
Published by: Wiley Europe Ltd., Baffins Ln, Chichester, W Sussex PO19 1UD, United Kingdom. TEL 44-1243-779777, FAX 44-1243-843232, customer@wiley.co.uk, http://www.wiley.co.uk. Ed. Paul Griffiths. Pub. Richard Baggaley. R&P Diane Southern TEL 44-1243-770347. adv.: B&W page GBP 650, color page GBP 1,550; trim 210 x 297. Circ: 400. **Subscr. in the Americas to:** John Wiley & Sons, Inc., Journals, 605 Third Ave, New York, NY 10158. TEL 212-850-6645, FAX 212-850-6021, uscs-wis@wiley.com; **Subscr. to:** John Wiley & Sons Ltd., Baffins Ln, Chichester, Sussex PO19 IUD, United Kingdom. cs-journals@wiley.co.uk.

579 ARG ISSN 0325-7541
QR1 CODEN: RAMID4
REVISTA ARGENTINA DE MICROBIOLOGIA. Text in English, Spanish. 1968. q. USD 45 domestic; USD 55 foreign (effective 1999). adv. *Refereed.* **Document type:** *Academic/Scholarly.*
Indexed: Abstr.Hyg., AgBiotech, Bio-Contr.News & Info., Biol.Abstr., Chem.Abstr., Chem.Indus.Notes, Chem.Titles, Dairy Sci.Abstr., Excerp.Med., Field Crop Abstr., Food Sci.& Tech.Abstr., INIS Atomind., Ind.Med. (1979-), Ind.Vet., Maize Abstr., Nutr.Abstr., Pig News & Info., Postharvest, Protozool.Abstr., Rev.Appl.Entomol., Rev.Med.& Vet.Mycol., Rev.Plant Path., Soils & Fert., Soyabean Abstr., Trop.Dis.Bull., Vet.Bull., Weed Abstr.
—BLDSC (7841.400000), CASDDS, CISTI, GNLM.
Published by: Asociacion Argentina de Microbiologia, P.B. B, Bulnes, 44, Capital Federal, Buenos Aires 1176, Argentina. TEL 54-114-9584888, FAX 54-114-9824888, aam@drwebsa.com.ar, http://www.drwebsa.com.ar/aam/. Ed. Dr. Elsa Damonte. Circ: 1,500.

REVISTA IBEROAMERICANA DE MICOLOGIA. see *MEDICAL SCIENCES*

579 MEX ISSN 0187-4640
QR1 CODEN: RLMIAA
REVISTA LATINOAMERICANA DE MICROBIOLOGIA. Text in Spanish. 1958. q. USD 40. bk.rev. **Document type:** *Academic/Scholarly.* **Description:** Original papers in medical bacteriology, virology, immunology, genetics and molecular biology, parasitology, and industrial and agricultural microbiology.
Former titles (until 1970): Revista Latinoamericana de Microbiologia y Parasitologia (0370-5986); (until 1966): Revista Latinoamericana de Microbiologia (0034-9771)
Indexed: Abstr.Hyg., Aqua.Sci.& Fish.Abstr., Bio-Contr.News & Info., Biol.Abstr., Cal.Tiss.Abstr., Chem.Abstr., Chem.Titles, Chemorec.Abstr., Dairy Sci.Abstr., Deep Sea Res.& Oceanogr.Abstr., Environ.Sci.Poll.Mgmt., Excerp.Med., Field Crop Abstr., Food Sci.& Tech.Abstr., GeoRef, Helminthol.Abstr., Ind.Med. (1958-), Ind.Vet., Int.Abstr.Biol.Sci., Maize Abstr., Microbiol.Abstr., Neurosci.Abstr. (coverage dropped), Pollut.Abstr., Protozool.Abstr., Ref.Zh., Rev.Appl.Entomol., Rev.Med.& Vet.Mycol., Rev.Plant Path., Soils & Fert., Sugar Ind.Abstr., Trop.Dis.Bull., Vet.Bull., Zoo.Rec.
—BLDSC (7863.500000), CASDDS, CISTI, GNLM, KNAW, Linda Hall.
Published by: (Asociacion Mexicana de Microbiologia), Asociacion Latinoamericana de Microbiologia, Apdo. Postal 4-862, Mexico City, DF 06400, Mexico. TEL 525-3414795, FAX 525-3963503. Ed. Dr. Jorge Ortigoza Ferado. Circ: 2,500.

REVISTA MEXICANA DE MICOLOGIA. see *BIOLOGY—Botany*

579 PRY ISSN 0556-6908
QR22.P37
REVISTA PARAGUAYA DE MICROBIOLOGIA. Text in Spanish; Summaries in English. 1966. a. USD 10. illus.
Indexed: Excerp.Med., Ind.Vet., Rev.Appl.Entomol., Trop.Dis.Bull., Vet.Bull.
Published by: Universidad Nacional de Asuncion, Facultad de Ciencias Medicas, Catedra de Bacteriologia y Parasitologia, Casilla de Correos 1102, Asuncion, Paraguay. Ed. Dr. Arquimedes Canese.

REVUE ROUMAINE DE VIROLOGIE/RUMANIAN JOURNAL OF VIROLOGY. see *MEDICAL SCIENCES—Communicable Diseases*

579.65 ITA ISSN 0035-6387
QL757 CODEN: RPSTAX
RIVISTA DI PARASSITOLOGIA. Text in English, French, German, Italian, Spanish. 1937. 3/yr. USD 60. adv. bk.rev. charts, illus. index.
Indexed: Abstr.Hyg., Aqua.Sci.& Fish.Abstr., Biol.Abstr., Chem.Abstr., Environ.Sci.Poll.Mgmt., Excerp.Med., Helminthol.Abstr., Ind.Vet., Microbiol.Abstr., Pollut.Abstr., Rev.Appl.Entomol., Rev.Med.& Vet.Mycol., Trop.Dis.Bull., Vet.Bull., Zoo.Rec.
—BLDSC (7992.200000), CASDDS, CISTI, GNLM, ingenta.
Published by: Istituto di Parassitologia, Universita di Messina, Via Cesare Battisti, 48, Messina, ME 98168, Italy. TEL 090-673136. Circ: 600.

579 ROM ISSN 1220-8485
CODEN: RAMIE5
ROMANIAN ARCHIVES OF MICROBIOLOGY AND IMMUNOLOGY. Text in English; Summaries in English, French. 1928. q. USD 150 (effective 1993). bk.rev. charts, illus, abstr. index. 96 p./no. back issues avail.; reprints avail. **Document type:** *Journal, Academic/Scholarly.*
Formerly (until 1991): Archives Roumaines de Pathologie Experimentale et de Microbiologie (0004-0037)
Indexed: Abstr.Hyg., Aqua.Sci.& Fish.Abstr., Biol.Abstr., Chem.Abstr., Excerp.Med., INIS Atomind., Ind.Med. (1991-), Ind.Vet., Protozool.Abstr., Ref.Zh., Rev.Appl.Entomol., Trop.Dis.Bull., Vet.Bull.
—BLDSC, CASDDS, CISTI, GNLM.
Published by: Institutul Cantacuzino, Spl. Independentei 103, PO Box 1-525, Bucharest 70100, Romania. TEL 40-01-4113800, FAX 40-01-4115672, office@cantacuzino.ro, http://www.cantacuzino.ro. Circ: 1,000.

SCHWEIZERISCHE ZEITSCHRIFT FUER PILZKUNDE/BOLLETTINO SVIZZERO DI MICOLOGIA/BULLETIN SUISSE DE MYCOLOGIE. see *BIOLOGY—Botany*

579 JPN ISSN 0919-3758
TP500 CODEN: SEKAEA
SEIBUTSU KOGAKU KAISHI. Text in Japanese; Summaries in English. 1977. m. JPY 12,000 (effective 1999). adv. abstr. *Refereed.* **Document type:** *Academic/Scholarly.*
Formerly (until 1993): Hakkokogaku (0385-6151)
Related titles: Online - full text ed.: (from Institute for Scientific Information).
Indexed: ASCA, AgBiotech, Biol.Abstr., Biotech.Cit.Ind., Chem.Abstr., Chem.Indus.Notes, Chem.Titles, Curr.Cont., Derwent Biotech.Abstr., Excerp.Med., Food Sci.& Tech.Abstr., INIS Atomind., Int.Abstr.Biol.Sci., Plant Breed.Abstr.
—BLDSC (8219.044000), CASDDS, CISTI, IDS, Infotrieve, Linda Hall. **CCC.**
Published by: The Society for Fermentation and Bioengineering Japa/Seibutsu Kogakkai, Business office c/o Faculty of Engineering Osaka University, 2-1 Yamada-Oka, Suita-shi, Osaka-fu 565-0871, Japan. TEL 81-6-6876-2731, FAX 81-6-6879-2034, sfbj@ijnet.or.jp, http://wwwsoc.nacsis.ac.jp/sfbj. Ed. Sakayu Shimizu. Pub. Tohru Kobayashi. Adv. contact Takekuma Kuroki.

579 FRA ISSN 0081-1068
SOCIETE FRANCAISE DE MICROBIOLOGIE. ANNUAIRE. Text in French. 1961. triennial. membership.
Published by: (Societe Francaise de Microbiologie), Institut Pasteur, 28 rue du Docteur Roux, Paris 75015, France.

579.3 USA
SOCIETY FOR APPLIED BACTERIOLOGY. TECHNICAL SERIES. Text in English. irreg., latest vol.21, 1985. reprint service avail. from ISI. *Refereed.*
Indexed: Biol.Abstr., Chem.Abstr., Chem.Indus.Notes, Chem.Titles, Food Sci.& Tech.Abstr.
Published by: Academic Press, Inc., Journal Division (Subsidiary of: Harcourt Brace & Company), 525 B St, Ste 1900, San Diego, CA 92101-4495. TEL 619-231-0926, FAX 619-699-6715. **Subscr. to:** Order Dept., 6277 Sea Harbor Dr, 4th Fl, Orlando, FL 32887. TEL 800-321-5068.

579.3 GBR ISSN 1467-4734
SOCIETY FOR APPLIED MICROBIOLOGY. SYMPOSIUM SERIES. Text in English. 1971. irreg., latest vol.12, 1984. reprint service avail. from ISI. *Refereed.*
Formerly (until 1998): Society for Applied Bacteriology. Symposium Series (0300-9610)
Indexed: Biol.Abstr., Chem.Abstr., Chem.Indus.Notes, Chem.Titles, Curr.Adv.Ecol.Sci., Food Sci.& Tech.Abstr., Ind.Med. (1998-), Ind.Vet., Rev.Appl.Entomol., Rev.Plant Path., Soils & Fert., Vet.Bull.
Published by: (Society for Applied Microbiology), Blackwell Science Ltd., Osney Mead, Oxford OX2 0EL, United Kingdom. TEL 44-1865-206206, FAX 44-1865-721205, http://blackwell-science.com.

579 GBR ISSN 0081-1394
QR1 CODEN: SSGMAI
SOCIETY FOR GENERAL MICROBIOLOGY. SYMPOSIUM. Text in English. 1961. irreg. price varies. index. **Document type:** *Proceedings.*
Indexed: Biol.Abstr., Chem.Abstr., Chem.Indus.Notes, Chem.Titles, Curr.Biotech.Abstr., Rev.Plant Path.
—BLDSC (8585.010000), CASDDS, KNAW. **CCC.**
Published by: (Society for General Microbiology USA), Cambridge University Press, Edinburgh Bldg, Shaftesbury Rd, Cambridge CB2 2RU, United Kingdom. FAX 44-1223-315052, information@cup.cam.ac.uk, information@cambridge.org, http://www.cup.cam.ac.uk, http://www.uk.cambridge.org/journals/pmu. R&P Linda Nicol.

▼ **SURGICAL INFECTIONS.** see *MEDICAL SCIENCES—Surgery*

579 DEU ISSN 0723-2020
QR1 CODEN: SAMIDF
SYSTEMATIC AND APPLIED MICROBIOLOGY. Text in English. 1980. irreg. (4 nos./vol.). EUR 304, GBP 210 to individuals; EUR 524, GBP 426 to institutions (effective 2002). *Refereed.* **Document type:** *Journal, Academic/Scholarly.* **Description:** Covers aspects of the systematics of microorganisms and agricultural, food, industrial and ecological microbiology.
Formerly: Zentralblatt fuer Bakteriologie, Mikrobiologie und Hygiene (0172-5564)
Related titles: Online - full text ed.: (from Institute for Scientific Information).
Indexed: AESIS, ASCA, Abstr.Hyg., AgBiotech, Agri.& Environ.Biotech.Abstr., Agricola, Aqua.Sci.& Fish.Abstr., Bio-Contr.News & Info., Biol.Abstr., Biotech.Cit.Ind., Chem.Abstr., Chem.Indus.Notes, Chem.Titles, Curr.Adv.Ecol.Sci., Curr.Cont., Dairy Sci.Abstr., Deep Sea Res.& Oceanogr.Abstr., Derwent Biotech.Abstr., Environ.Sci.Poll.Mgmt., Excerp.Med., Food Sci.& Tech.Abstr., Forest.Abstr., GeoRef, Helminthol.Abstr., Ind.Med. (1983-), Ind.Sci.Rev., Ind.Vet., Inpharma, Int.Abstr.Biol.Sci., Microbiol.Abstr., Nutr.Abstr., Plant Breed.Abstr., Postharvest, Potato Abstr., Reac., Ref.Zh., Rev.Appl.Entomol., Rev.Med.& Vet.Mycol., Rev.Plant Path., Rice Abstr., Sci.Cit.Ind., Soils & Fert., Soyabean Abstr., Vet.Bull., Weed Abstr.
—BLDSC (8589.176000), CASDDS, CISTI, EMDOCS, GNLM, IDS, Infotrieve, ingenta, Linda Hall. **CCC.**
Published by: Urban & Fischer Verlag, Loebdergraben 14A, Jena 07743, Germany. TEL 49-3641-626444, FAX 49-3641-626421, info@urbanfischer.de, http://www.urbanfischer.de. Eds. K H Schleifer, M Teuber.

579 KOR ISSN 0253-3162
QR1 CODEN: TMHCDX
TAEHAN MISAENGMUL HAKHOE CHI* /KOREAN SOCIETY FOR MICROBIOLOGY. JOURNAL. Text in Korean; Abstracts and contents page in English. 1957. bi-m. USD 70. adv. bibl, charts. **Document type:** *Academic/Scholarly.* **Description:** Devoted to the dissemination of new knowledge concerning the microbiological aspects of human and animal infections, particularly regarding their etiologic agents, diagnosis, pathogenesis, epidemiology, and antimicrobial agents and chemotherapy.
Indexed: Chem.Abstr., Chem.Indus.Notes, Chem.Titles, Excerp.Med. (until 1993), Ind.Vet., Protozool.Abstr., Rev.Appl.Entomol., Vet.Bull.
—BLDSC (4812.346200), CASDDS, GNLM. **CCC.**

B

Published by: Korean Society for Microbiology/Taehan Misaengmul Hakhoe, c/o Dept. of Microbiology Yonsei University College of Medicine, Seodaemun-gu, 134 Shinchon dong, Seoul 120749, Korea, S.. TEL 82-2-293-2111, FAX 82-2-293-1629. Ed. Pyung Woo Lee. Circ: 400.

579 GBR ISSN 0966-842X
QR1 CODEN: TRMIEA

TRENDS IN MICROBIOLOGY. Text in English. 1993. m. GBP 92, EUR 115 in Europe to individuals; JPY 14,000 in Japan to individuals; USD 126 elsewhere to individuals; EUR 908 in Europe to institutions; JPY 125,900 in Japan to institutions; USD 1,015 elsewhere to institutions; GBP 47 in Europe to students; JPY 10,100 in Japan to students; USD 78 elsewhere to students; USD 1,308 to institutions Print & online eds. combined; JPY 17,500 in Japan to qualified personnel; USD 157 elsewhere to qualified personnel (effective 2002). adv. bk.rev. abstr, bibl. index. back issues avail.; reprints avail. *Refereed.* **Document type:** *Academic/Scholarly.* **Description:** Provides a forum for the discussion of all aspects of infection, covering dynamics, cell biology, immunology, genetics and evolution of infectious organisms, including fungi, and bacteria and viruses, as well as their plant and animal hosts.
Related titles: Microform ed.: (from PQC); Online - full text ed.: (from ingenta, Swets Blackwell, Institute for Scientific Information, ScienceDirect).
Indexed: ASCA, Agri.& Environ.Biotech.Abstr., Appl.Ecol.Abstr. (coverage dropped), Aqua.Sci.& Fish.Abstr., BBCI, Derwent Biotech.Abstr., Environ.Sci.Poll.Mgmt., Excerp.Med. (1993-), Food Sci.& Tech.Abstr., Ind.Med. (1993-), Ind.Vet., Int.Abstr.Biol.Sci., Microbiol.Abstr., Nuc.Acids Abstr., Protozool.Abstr., Ref.Zh., Rev.Appl.Entomol., Rev.Med.& Vet.Mycol., Rev.Plant Path., Sci.Cit.Ind., Seed Abstr., Soils & Fert., Trop.Dis.Bull., Virol.Abstr. (coverage dropped).
—BLDSC (9049.664000), ADONIS, CISTI, EMDOCS, GNLM, IDS, Infotrieve, ingenta. **CCC.**
Published by: Elsevier Science Ltd., Elsevier Trends Journals, 68 Hills Rd, Cambridge CB2 1LA, United Kingdom. TEL 44-1223-315961, FAX 44-1223-464430, TIM@elsevier.co.uk, http://www.elsevier.com/locate/issn/0966842X. Eds. D P O'Connell, S Clarkson. Adv. contact Thelma Reid. **Subscr. in Australasia and the Far East to:** Elsevier Science (Singapore) Pte Ltd, No.1 Temasek Ave, 17-01 Millenia Tower, Singapore 039192, Singapore. TEL 65-434-3727, FAX 65-337-2230; **Subscr. in the Americas to:** Elsevier Science, PO Box 945, New York, NY 10159-0945. TEL 212-633-3730, FAX 212-633-3680; **Subscr. to:** Elsevier Current Trends Subscriptions, PO Box 331, Haywards Heath, W Sussex RH16 3FG, United Kingdom. TEL 44-1444-475650, FAX 44-1444-445423.

616.96 GBR ISSN 1471-4922
CODEN: PATOE2

TRENDS IN PARASITOLOGY. Text in English. 1985. m. GBP 92, EUR 115 in Europe to individuals; JPY 14,000 in Japan to individuals; USD 126 elsewhere to individuals; NLG 1,908, EUR 908 in Europe to institutions; JPY 125,900 in Japan to institutions; USD 1,015 elsewhere to institutions; GBP 47 in Europe to students; JPY 10,100 in Japan to students; USD 78 elsewhere to students; EUR 1,168.94 in Europe to institutions Print & online eds. combined; JPY 162,200 in Japan to institutions Print & online eds. combined; USD 1,308 elsewhere to institutions Print & online eds. combined; EUR 144 in Europe to qualified personnel; JPY 17,500 in Japan to qualified personnel; USD 157 elsewhere to qualified personnel (effective 2002). bk.rev. illus, abstr. index. back issues avail.; reprints avail. *Refereed.* **Document type:** *Journal, Academic/Scholarly.* **Description:** Provides an interdisciplinary forum for communications in all aspects of current field and laboratory research in parasitology from molecular biology to ecology.
Formerly: Parasitology Today (0169-4758)
Related titles: Online - full text ed.: (from ingenta, ScienceDirect, Swets Blackwell, Institute for Scientific Information).
Indexed: AIDS & Cancer Res., ASCA, Abstr.Hyg., AgBiotech, Anim.Breed.Abstr., Aqua.Sci.& Fish.Abstr., Bio-Contr.News & Info., Biol.Abstr., Chem.Abstr., Chem.Titles, Curr.Adv.Ecol.Sci., Curr.Cont., Dairy Sci.Abstr., Derwent Biotech.Abstr., Diar.Dis.Res., Entomol.Abstr., Environ.Sci.Poll.Mgmt., Excerp.Med., Genet.Abstr. (coverage dropped), Helminthol.Abstr., Immun.Abstr., Ind.Med. (2001-), Ind.Sci.Rev., Ind.Vet., Inpharma, Microbiol.Abstr., Pharm.&Out.News, Poult.Abstr., Protozool.Abstr., Reac., Rev.Appl.Entomol., Rev.Arom.& Med.Plants, Rev.Med.& Vet.Mycol., Rural Devel.Abstr., Sci.Cit.Ind., Sport Fish.Abstr., Trop.Dis.Bull., Vet.Bull., Wild.Rev., Zoo.Rec.
—BLDSC (9049.669500), ADONIS, CASDDS, CISTI, GNLM, IDS. **CCC.**
Published by: Elsevier Science Ltd., Elsevier Trends Journals, 68 Hills Rd, Cambridge CB2 1LA, United Kingdom. TEL 44-1223-315961, FAX 44-1223-464430, parasites@current-trends.com, PT@elsevier.co.uk, http://www.trends.com/pt/default.htm. Eds. Linsey Stapley, Sally Hirst. Circ: 4,600. **Subscr. in Australasia and the Far East to:** Elsevier Science (Singapore) Pte Ltd, No.1 Temasek Ave, 17-01 Millenia Tower, Singapore 039192, Singapore. TEL 65-434-3727, FAX 65-337-2230; **Subscr. in the Americas to:** Elsevier Science, PO Box 945, New York, NY 10159-0945. TEL 212-633-3730, FAX 212-633-3680; **Subscr. to:** Elsevier Current Trends Subscriptions, PO Box 331, Haywards Heath, W Sussex RH16 3FG, United Kingdom. TEL 44-1444-475650, FAX 44-1444-445423.

UNIVERSITY OF TOKYO. INSTITUTE OF APPLIED MICROBIOLOGY. REPORTS. see *BIOLOGY—Abstracting, Bibliographies, Statistics*

UNIVERSITY OF WAIKATO. ANTARCTIC RESEARCH UNIT. REPORT. see *EARTH SCIENCES—Geology*

579 NLD ISSN 0378-1135
CODEN: VMICDQ

VETERINARY MICROBIOLOGY; an international journal. Text in English. 1976. 24/yr. EUR 1,575 in Europe to institutions; JPY 209,300 in Japan to institutions; USD 1,757 elsewhere to institutions (effective 2002). adv. bk.rev. bibl, illus. index. *Refereed.* **Document type:** *Academic/Scholarly.* **Description:** Concerned with microbiological diseases of all animals that are useful to man. Publishes information on pathogenesis, host responses, immunology, epidemiology, disease prevention, treatment, control and comparative studies of diseases affecting man and animals, as well as laboratory studies of the causal agents of diseases of animals.
Related titles: Microform ed.: (from PQC); Online - full text ed.: (from ingenta, Swets Blackwell, Institute for Scientific Information, ScienceDirect).
Indexed: AESIS, ASCA, Abstr.Hyg., AgBiotech, Agri.& Environ.Biotech.Abstr., Agricola, Aqua.Sci.& Fish.Abstr., Aquacult.Abstr., Biol.Abstr., Chem.Abstr., Chem.Indus.Notes, Curr.Adv.Ecol.Sci., Curr.Cont., Dairy Sci.Abstr., Dent.Ind., Derwent Biotech.Abstr., Environ.Sci.Poll.Mgmt., Excerp.Med., Focus on: Vet.Sci.& Med., Food Sci.& Tech.Abstr., Helminthol.Abstr., INIS Atomind., Ind.Med. (1976-), Ind.Sci.Rev., Ind.Vet., Inpharma, Int.Abstr.Biol.Sci., Microbiol.Abstr., Pharm.&Out.News, Pig News & Info., Poult.Abstr., Protozool.Abstr., Reac., Rev.Appl.Entomol., Rev.Med.& Vet.Mycol., Sci.Cit.Ind., Small Anim.Abstr., Sport Fish.Abstr., Trop.Dis.Bull., Vet.Bull., Virol.Abstr. (coverage dropped), Wild.Rev., World Ag.Econ.& Rur.Soc.Abstr., Zoo.Rec.
—BLDSC (9229.120000), ADONIS, CASDDS, CISTI, EMDOCS, GNLM, IDS, Infotrieve, ingenta, Linda Hall. **CCC.**
Published by: Elsevier Science BV, PO Box 211, Amsterdam 1000 AE, Netherlands. TEL 31-20-485-3911, FAX 31-20-485-3598, nlinfo-f@elsevier.nl, http://www.elsevier.nl/inca/publications/store/5/0/3/3/2/0/. Eds. J F Prescott, Dr. J G Songer, M C Horzinek. **Subscr. in Australasia and the Far East to:** Elsevier Science (Singapore) Pte Ltd, No.1 Temasek Ave, 17-01 Millenia Tower, Singapore 039192, Singapore. TEL 65-434-3727, FAX 65-337-2230; **Subscr. in Japan to:** Elsevier Science Inc - Japan Regional Office, 9-15 Higashi-Azabu 1-chome, Minato-ku, Tokyo 106-0044, Japan. TEL 81-3-5561-5033; **Subscr. in the Americas to:** Elsevier Science, PO Box 945, New York, NY 10159-0945. TEL 212-633-3730, FAX 212-633-3680.

579.2 FRA ISSN 1267-8694

VIROLOGIE. Text in French. 1997. 6/yr. FRF 670 domestic to individuals; EUR 114 in Europe to individuals; FRF 790 elsewhere to individuals; FRF 1,120 domestic to institutions; EUR 183 in Europe to institutions; FRF 1,240 elsewhere to institutions; FRF 470 domestic to students; EUR 84 in Europe to students; FRF 590 elsewhere to students; FRF 190 newsstand/cover (effective 2001). **Description:** Publishes review articles of the latest research done in basic medical, animal and plant virology.
Related titles: CD-ROM ed.: FRF 590 domestic; FRF 620 foreign (effective 2001); Online - full text ed.: FRF 670 in Europe to individuals; FRF 690 elsewhere to individuals; FRF 1,120 to institutions; FRF 470 to students (effective 2001).
—BLDSC (9240.405000).
Published by: John Libbey Eurotext, 127 av. de la Republique, Montrouge 92120, France. TEL 33-01-46730660, FAX 33-01-40840999, marketing@jle.com, http://www.john-libbey-eurotext.fr/. **Subscr. to:** A T E I, 3 av. Pierre Kerautret, Romainville 92230, France. TEL 33-1-48408686, FAX 33-1-48400731, atei@club-internet.fr.

579.2 USA ISSN 0042-6822
QR360 CODEN: VIRLAX

VIROLOGY. Text in English. 1955. 26/yr. USD 3,900 in US & Canada to institutions; USD 4,200 rest of world to institutions (effective 2001). adv. bibl, charts, illus. index. back issues avail.; reprints avail. *Refereed.* **Document type:** *Academic/Scholarly.* **Description:** Publishes the results of basic research in all branches of virology, including the viruses of vertebrates and invertebrates, plants, bacteria, and yeast and fungi.
Related titles: CD-ROM ed.: ISSN 1089-862X; Online - full text ed.: (from EBSCO Publishing, O C L C Online Computer Library Center, Inc., RoweCom Information Quest, ingenta, Swets Blackwell, IDEAL Online Library, Institute for Scientific Information).
Indexed: AIDS & Cancer Res., AIDS Abstr., ASCA, Abstr.Hyg., AgBiotech, Agri.& Environ.Biotech.Abstr. (coverage dropped), Agricola, Anim.Breed.Abstr., Aqua.Sci.& Fish.Abstr., BBCI, Bibl.Agri., Bio-Contr.News & Info., Biol.& Agr.Ind. (Nov.1982-), Biol.Abstr., Biotech.& Bioeng.Abstr., Chem.Abstr., Chem.Indus.Notes, Chem.Titles, Curr.Adv.Cancer Res., Curr.Adv.Ecol.Sci., Curr.Adv.Gen.& Molec.Biol., Curr.Cont., Dairy Sci.Abstr., Dent.Ind., Derwent Biotech.Abstr., Environ.Sci.Poll.Mgmt., Excerp.Med., Food Sci.& Tech.Abstr., Genet.Abstr., Helminthol.Abstr., Hort.Abstr., Hum.Gen.Abstr., INIS Atomind., Immun.Abstr., Ind.Med. (1955-), Ind.Sci.Rev., Ind.Vet., Inpharma, Int.Abstr.Biol.Sci., Maize Abstr., Neurosci.Abstr., Neurosci.Cit.Ind., Nuc.Acids Abstr., Nutr.Abstr., Pharm.&Out.News, Pig News & Info., Plant Breed.Abstr., Potato Abstr., Poult.Abstr., Protozool.Abstr., Reac., Ref.Zh., Rev.Appl.Entomol., Rev.Med.& Vet.Mycol., Rev.Plant Path., Rice Abstr., Sci.Cit.Ind., Small Anim.Abstr., So.Pac.Per.Ind., Sport Fish.Abstr., Triticale Abstr., Trop.Dis.Bull., Vet.Bull., Virol.Abstr., W.R.C.Inf., Wild.Rev.
—BLDSC (9240.500000), ADONIS, CASDDS, CISTI, GNLM, IDS, ingenta, Linda Hall. **CCC.**
Published by: Academic Press, Inc., Journal Division (Subsidiary of: Harcourt Brace & Company), 525 B St, Ste 1900, San Diego, CA 92101-4495. TEL 619-230-1840, FAX 619-688-6800, apsubs@acad.com, http://www.apnet.com/www/journal/vy.htm; http://www.idealibrary.com/. Ed. Robert Lamb.

VIROLOGY AND AIDS ABSTRACTS. see *BIOLOGY—Abstracting, Bibliographies, Statistics*

579.2 USA ISSN 0083-6591
QR360 CODEN: VIRMB3

VIROLOGY MONOGRAPHS/VIRUSFORSCHUNG IN EINZELDARSTELLUNGEN. Text in English. 1968. irreg., latest vol.18, 1981. price varies. reprint service avail. from ISI. **Document type:** *Monographic series.*
Formerly: Handbuch der Virusforschung
Indexed: Biol.Abstr., Ind.Med. (coverage dropped).
—CISTI, GNLM.
Published by: Springer-Verlag, Journals (Subsidiary of: BertelsmannSpringer), 175 Fifth Ave, New York, NY 10010. TEL 212-460-1500, FAX 212-473-6272.

579.2 JPN ISSN 0042-6857
CODEN: UIRUAF

VIRUS/UIRUSU. Text in Japanese; Summaries in English. 1951. s-a. adv. bk.rev. abstr, charts, illus. index.
Indexed: Biol.Abstr., Chem.Abstr., Chem.Titles, Excerp.Med., Ind.Med. (1951-), Ind.Vet., Jap.Per.Ind., Ref.Zh., Rev.Plant Path., Vet.Bull.
—BLDSC (9240.850000), CASDDS, CISTI, GNLM.
Published by: Society of Japanese Virologists/Nihon Uirusu Gakkai, Nihon Gakkai Jimu Senta, 16-9 Honkomagome 5-chome, Bunkyo-ku, Tokyo 113-0021, Japan. Ed. Dr. Isao Yoshioka. Circ: 1,200. **Overseas Distributor:** Japan Publications Trading Co., Ltd., PO Box 5030, Tokyo International, Tokyo 100-31, Japan.

579.2 USA ISSN 0920-8569
CODEN: VIGEET

VIRUS GENES. Text in English. 1987. bi-m. USD 560, EUR 559 to institutions for print or online ed.; USD 672, EUR 670.80 to institutions print & online eds. combined (effective 2002). adv. bk.rev. back issues avail.; reprint service avail. from SWZ,PQC. *Refereed.* **Document type:** *Academic/Scholarly.* **Description:** Publishes the results of studies on the structure and function of virus genes (animal, insect, plant and bacterial).

Related titles: Microform ed.: (from PQC); Online - full text ed.: (from EBSCO Publishing, O C L C Online Computer Library Center, Inc., RoweCom Information Quest, Swets Blackwell, Kluwer Online, Institute for Scientific Information).

Indexed: AIDS & Cancer Res., ASCA, Abstr.Hyg., AgBiotech, Aqua.Sci.& Fish.Abstr., Bio-Contr.News & Info., Biol.Abstr., Biotech.& Bioeng.Abstr., Biotech.Cit.Ind., Chem.Abstr., Chem.Indus.Notes, Curr.Cont., Dairy Sci.Abstr., Excerp.Med., Genet.Abstr., Hum.Gen.Abstr., Ind.Med. (1987-), Ind.Sci.Rev., Ind.Vet., Inpharma, Int.Abstr.Biol.Sci., Nuc.Acids Abstr., Pharm.&Out.News, Pig News & Info., Plant Breed.Abstr., Potato Abstr., Poult.Abstr., Reac., Rev.Appl.Entomol., Rev.Med.& Vet.Mycol., Rev.Plant Path., Rice Abstr., Sci.Cit.Ind., Vet.Bull., Virol.Abstr., Weed Abstr.

—BLDSC (9240.850500), ADONIS, CASDDS, CISTI, EMDOCS, GNLM, IDS, ingenta. **CCC.**

Published by: Kluwer Academic Publishers Boston, 101 Philip Dr, Assinippi Park, Norwell, MA 02061. TEL 781-871-6600, FAX 781-871-9045, services@wkap.nl, http://www.wkap.nl/journalhome.htm/0920-8569. Ed. Yechiel Becker. R&P Rose Luongo TEL 781-871-6311. **Subscr. outside the Americas:** Kluwer Academic Publishers Group, Journals Department, PO Box 322, Dordrecht 3300 AH, Netherlands. TEL 31-78-639-2392, FAX 31-78-654-6474**; Subscr. to:** Kluwer Academic - Plenum Publishers, 233 Spring St, New York, NY 10013-1578. TEL 212-620-8468, FAX 212-807-1047.

579.2 NLD ISSN 0168-1702
CODEN: VIREDF

VIRUS RESEARCH; an international journal of molecular and cellular virology. Text in English. 1984. 16/yr. EUR 1,141 in Europe to institutions; JPY 151,500 in Japan to institutions; USD 1,276 elsewhere to institutions; USD 3,299 includes Journal of Clinical Virology (effective 2002). adv. bk.rev. bibl, charts, illus. index. back issues avail.; reprint service avail. from ISI. *Refereed.* **Document type:** *Academic/Scholarly.* **Description:** Publishes original papers on fundamental research concerning virus structure, replication, and pathogenesis.

Related titles: Microform ed.: (from PQC); Online - full text ed.: (from ingenta, Swets Blackwell, Institute for Scientific Information, ScienceDirect).

Indexed: AIDS & Cancer Res., AIDS Abstr., ASCA, Abstr.Hyg., AgBiotech, Aqua.Sci.& Fish.Abstr., Bio-Contr.News & Info., Biol.Abstr., Chem.Abstr., Chem.Indus.Notes, Chem.Titles, Curr.Adv.Ecol.Sci., Curr.Adv.Gen.& Molec.Biol., Curr.Cont., Dairy Sci.Abstr., Excerp.Med., Genet.Abstr. (coverage dropped), INIS Atomind., Ind.Med. (1984-), Ind.Sci.Rev., Ind.Vet., Inpharma, Int.Abstr.Biol.Sci., Mass Spectr.Bull., Nuc.Acids Abstr., Pharm.&Out.News, Pig News & Info., Plant Breed.Abstr., Poult.Abstr., Reac., Ref.Zh., Rev.Appl.Entomol., Rev.Med.& Vet.Mycol., Rev.Plant Path., Sci.Cit.Ind., Trop.Dis.Bull., Vet.Bull., Virol.Abstr., Wild.Rev.

—BLDSC (9240.852000), ADONIS, CASDDS, CISTI, GNLM, IDS, ingenta, Linda Hall. **CCC.**

Published by: Elsevier Science BV, PO Box 211, Amsterdam 1000 AE, Netherlands. TEL 31-20-485-3911, FAX 31-20-485-3598, nlinfo-f@elsevier.nl, http://www.elsevier.nl/locate/virusres. Eds. B W J Mahy, R W Compans, U Desselberger. Circ: 1,000. **Subscr. in Australasia and the Far East to:** Elsevier Science (Singapore) Pte Ltd, No.1 Temasek Ave, 17-01 Millenia Tower, Singapore 039192, Singapore. TEL 65-434-3727, FAX 65-337-2230**; Subscr. in Japan to:** Elsevier Science Inc - Japan Regional Office, 9-15 Higashi-Azabu 1-chome, Minato-ku, Tokyo 106-0044, Japan. TEL 81-3-5561-5033**; Subscr. in the Americas to:** Elsevier Science, PO Box 945, New York, NY 10159-0945. TEL 212-633-3730, FAX 212-633-3680.

579.2 RUS ISSN 0507-4088
CODEN: VVIRAT

VOPROSY VIRUSOLOGII/PROBLEMS OF VIROLOGY. Text in Russian; Summaries in English. 1956. bi-m. USD 224 foreign (effective 2000). adv. bk.rev. **Document type:** *Journal, Academic/Scholarly.* **Description:** Deals with advances achieved in virology in Russia and abroad. Publishes papers about viral diseases of man, animals and plants.

Indexed: AIDS & Cancer Res., ASCA, Abstr.Hyg., AgBiotech, Agri.& Environ.Biotech.Abstr. (coverage dropped), Aqua.Sci.& Fish.Abstr., Bio-Contr.News & Info., Biol.Abstr., Chem.Abstr., Chem.Indus.Notes, Chem.Titles, Curr.Adv.Ecol.Sci., Curr.Cont. (coverage dropped), Dairy Sci.Abstr., Dent.Ind., Derwent Biotech.Abstr., Excerp.Med., INIS Atomind., Ind.Med. (1956-), Ind.Vet., Inpharma, Nutr.Abstr., Pharm.&Out.News, Pig News & Info., Poult.Abstr., Reac., Ref.Zh., Rev.Appl.Entomol., Rev.Med.& Vet.Mycol., Sci.Cit.Ind. (coverage dropped), Small Anim.Abstr., Trop.Dis.Bull., Vet.Bull., Virol.Abstr., Zoo.Rec.

—BLDSC (0041.900000), CASDDS, CISTI, EMDOCS, GNLM, IDS, Infotrieve, KNAW. **CCC.**

Published by: Izdatel'stvo Meditsina, Petroverigskii per 6-8, Moscow 101000, Russian Federation. TEL 7-095-9246740, FAX 7-095-9232074, 7-095-9211355, meditsina@iname.com. Ed. D K Lvov. Pub. A M Stochik. R&P T Kurushina. Adv. contact O A Fadeeva TEL 7-095-923-51-40. Circ: 850. **Dist. by:** Mezhdunarodnaya Kniga, B Yakimanka 39, Moscow 117049, Russian Federation. TEL 7-095-2384967, FAX 7-095-2384634.

579 FIN ISSN 0358-6758

WALTER AND ANDREE DE NOTTBECK FOUNDATION SCIENTIFIC REPORTS. Text and summaries in English. 1976. irreg. free per issue. back issues avail. *Refereed.* **Document type:** *Academic/Scholarly.* **Description:** Deals with the algae, bacteria, zooplankton and other biota of marine areas, especially the Baltic Sea.

Published by: Walter and Andree de Nottbeck Foundation, c/o Department of Ecology and Systematics, University of Helsinki, Unionsgatan 44, PL 70, Helsinki 00014, Finland. TEL 358-9-191-86-01, FAX 358-0-191-86-56, carl-adam.haeggstrom@helsinki.fi. Ed. Carl Adam Haeggstrom. Circ: 500. **Dist. by:** Tvarminne Zoological Station, Hangoe 10900, Finland.

579 CHN ISSN 1002-056X

WEISHENGWU XUE ZAZHI/JOURNAL OF MICROBIOLOGY. Text in Chinese. 1979. q. USD 20.

—BLDSC (5019.285600).

Published by: Liaoning Weishengwu Yanjiusuo/Liaoning Institute of Microbiology, No22, Wenhua Lu 2 Duan, Chaoyang, Liaoning 122000, China. TEL 0421-2814613. Ed. Ding Jian.

579 CHN ISSN 0001-6209
QR1 CODEN: WSHPA8

WEISHENGWU XUEBAO/ACTA MICROBIOLOGICA SINICA. Text in Chinese; Summaries in English. 1953. bi-m. USD 116 (effective 2000). adv. charts, illus. *Refereed.* **Document type:** *Academic/Scholarly.* **Description:** Contains theses on the theory and application of microbiology in industrial, agricultural, medical, and veterinary sciences, as well as virology (including taxomorphology, physio-biochemistry, genetics, and serology.).

Indexed: AgBiotech, Aqua.Sci.& Fish.Abstr., Bio-Contr.News & Info., Biodet.Abstr., Biol.Abstr., Chem.Abstr., Chem.Indus.Notes, Curr.Adv.Biochem., Curr.Adv.Ecol.Sci., Curr.Adv.Gen.& Molec.Biol., Dairy Sci.Abstr., Environ.Sci.Poll.Mgmt., Helminthol.Abstr., Hort.Abstr., Ind.Med. (1953-), Ind.Vet., Microbiol.Abstr., Pig News & Info., Poult.Abstr., Rev.Appl.Entomol., Rev.Med.& Vet.Mycol., Rev.Plant Path., Rice Abstr., Soils & Fert., Soyabean Abstr., Vet.Bull.

—BLDSC (0638.500000), CASDDS, CISTI, GNLM, KNAW, Linda Hall.

Published by: (Chinese Academy of Sciences/Zhongguo Kexueyuan), Kexue Chubanshe/Science Press, 16 Donghuang Cheng Genbei Jie, Beijing 100717, China. Circ: 11,000.

579 CHN ISSN 0253-2654
QR1 CODEN: WSWPDI

WEISHENGWUXUE TONGBAO/MICROBIOLOGY. Text in Chinese. 1973. bi-m. USD 86 (effective 2000). adv. **Document type:** *Academic/Scholarly.* **Description:** Aims to expand the reader's knowledge of microbiology. Carries information on new results, techniques, and methods from the spheres of industry, agriculture, medicine, and veterinary medicine.

Indexed: Chem.Abstr., Chem.Indus.Notes, Chem.Titles, Cott.& Trop.Fibr.Abstr.

—BLDSC (5757.730000), CASDDS.

Published by: (Chinese Academy of Sciences/Zhongguo Kexueyuan), Kexue Chubanshe/Science Press, 16 Donghuang Cheng Genbei Jie, Beijing 100717, China. Circ: 16,000.

579 CHN ISSN 1000-0674
QE719 CODEN: WEXUE9

WEITI GUSHENGWU XUEBAO/ACTA MICROPALAEONTOLOGICA SINICA. Text in Chinese; Summaries in English. 1984. q. USD 130.80 (effective 2000). adv. bk.rev. *Refereed.* **Document type:** *Academic/Scholarly.* **Description:** Publishes the latest results of studies in morphology, taxonomy, systematics, evolution, stratigraphy, paleobiogeography, and paleoecology. Covers various groups of microfossils, and provides news about academic activities, both in China and abroad.

Indexed: GeoRef, Ref.Zh., Zoo.Rec.

Published by: (Zhongguo Kexueyuan/Chinese Academy of Sciences), Kexue Chubanshe/Science Press, 16 Donghuang Cheng Genbei Jie, Beijing 100717, China. Circ: 6,000.

WORLD JOURNAL OF MICROBIOLOGY AND BIOTECHNOLOGY. see *BIOLOGY—Biotechnology*

579 USA ISSN 1054-772X
QR46

YEAR BOOK OF CLINICAL MICROBIOLOGY. Text in English. 1991. a.

—GNLM.

Published by: C R C Press, LLC, 2000 Corporate Blvd, N W, Boca Raton, FL 33431. TEL 561-994-0555, 800-272-7737, FAX 561-998-9784.

YEAST; a forum for yeast researchers. see *BIOLOGY—Botany*

579.2 CHN ISSN 1003-5125
CODEN: BIZAES

ZHONGGUO BINGDUXUE/VIROLOGICA SINICA. Text in Chinese. 1986. q. USD 5.40 per issue domestic; USD 89 (effective 2000). adv. *Refereed.* **Document type:** *Academic/Scholarly.* **Description:** Aims to present mainland China's main achievements in virology to the specialized reader. Contains research papers, communications, and notes, as well as reviews and discussions.

Formerly: Bingduxue Zazhi (1000-3223)

Related titles: Online - full content ed.: (from WanFang Data Corp.).

Indexed: AIDS & Cancer Res., Chem.Abstr., Chem.Indus.Notes, Chem.Titles, Derwent Biotech.Abstr., Virol.Abstr.

—BLDSC (9240.350000), CASDDS.

Published by: (Zhongguo Kexueyuan, Wuhan Bingdu Yanjiusuo), Kexue Chubanshe/Science Press, 16 Donghuang Cheng Genbei Jie, Beijing 100717, China. Circ: 6,000.

579.3 CHN ISSN 1000-7423
CODEN: ZJYZET

ZHONGGUO JISHENGCHONGXUE YU JISHENGCHONGBING ZAZHI/CHINESE JOURNAL OF PARASITOLOGY AND PARASITIC DISEASES. Text in Chinese. bi-m. adv. **Document type:** *Academic/Scholarly.*

Indexed: AgBiotech, Bio-Contr.News & Info., Helminthol.Abstr., Ind.Med. (1987-), Ind.Vet., Pig News & Info., Poult.Abstr., Protozool.Abstr., Rev.Appl.Entomol., Rev.Med.& Vet.Mycol., Rural Devel.Abstr., Trop.Dis.Bull., Vet.Bull., Zoo.Rec.

—BLDSC (3180.465000), GNLM.

Published by: Zhongguo Yufang Yixue Kexueyuan, Jishengchongbing Yanjiusuo/Chinese Academy of Preventive Medicine, Institute of Parasitic Diseases, 207 Ruijin 2 Lu, Shanghai 200025, China. TEL 86-21-6437-7008. Ed., R&P Feng Zheng. Adv. contact Minyi Yao.

572.3 CHN ISSN 1002-2694

ZHONGGUO RENSHOU GONGHUANBING ZAZHI/CHINESE JOURNAL OF ZOONOSES. Text in Chinese; Summaries in English. 1985. bi-m. USD 48; USD 4.50 newsstand/cover (effective 2001). adv. bk.rev. *Refereed.* **Document type:** *Academic/Scholarly.* **Description:** Discusses and examines bacteria and diseases common both to human beings and animals.

Related titles: Online - full content ed.: (from WanFang Data Corp.).

Indexed: Abstr.Hyg., AgBiotech, Aqua.Sci.& Fish.Abstr., Aquacult.Abstr., Dairy Sci.Abstr., Environ.Sci.Poll.Mgmt., Ind.Vet., Nutr.Abstr., Pig News & Info., Poult.Abstr., Protozool.Abstr., Rev.Appl.Entomol., Rev.Med.& Vet.Mycol., Trop.Dis.Bull., Vet.Bull., Virol.Abstr., Zoo.Rec.

—BLDSC (3180.710000).

B

Published by: Fujian-sheng Weisheng Fangyi Zhan, Jintai Lu 76, Fuzhou, Fujian 350001, China. TEL 86-591-7552018, rsghb@pub2.fz.fj.cn, http://zrsz.chinajournal.net.cn, http://www.si.net.cn/publicat. Eds. Enshu Yu TEL 86-591-7563582, Longsan Xu. R&P Enshu Yu TEL 86-591-7563582. Adv. contact Huang Feng. **Dist. overseas by:** China International Book Trading Corp, 35, Chegongzhuang Xilu, Haidian District, Beijing 100044, China. TEL 86-1-68413849, FAX 86-1-68412048, cibtc@mail.cibtc.com.cn, http://www.cibtc.com.cn. **Co-sponsor:** Zhongguo Weishengwu Xuehui/Chinese Microbiology Society.

579 RUS ISSN 0372-9311
QR1 CODEN: ZMEIAV
ZHURNAL MIKROBIOLOGII, EPIDEMIOLOGII I IMMUNOBIOLOGII/JOURNAL OF MICROBIOLOGY, EPIDEMIOLOGY AND IMMUNOBIOLOGY. Text in Russian; Summaries in English. 1924. bi-m. RUR 300 domestic; USD 169 foreign (effective 2000). bk.rev. illus. **Description:** Presents original scientific studies and surveys on etiology, laboratory diagnosis and pathogenesis of infectious diseases, theoretical and applied immunology, epidemiology of infectious diseases and methods of their control.
Indexed: Abstr.Hyg., Biol.Abstr., Chem.Abstr., Chem.Indus.Notes, Chem.Titles, Curr.Adv.Ecol.Sci., Curr.Cont. (coverage dropped), Dairy Sci.Abstr., Dent.Ind., Environ.Sci.Poll.Mgmt., Helminthol.Abstr., Ind.Med. (1935-), Ind.Vet., Pig News & Info., Protozool.Abstr., Ref.Zh., Rev.Appl.Entomol., Rev.Med.& Vet.Mycol., Rev.Plant Path., Saf.Sci.Abstr., Sci.Cit.Ind. (coverage dropped), Trop.Dis.Bull., Vet.Bull., Zoo.Rec.
—BLDSC (0060.900000), CASDDS, CISTI, East View, EMDOCS, GNLM, IDS, Infotrieve, Linda Hall. **CCC.**
Published by: Rossiiskaya Akademiya Meditsinskikh Nauk, Institut Vakcin i Sivorotok im. I.I. Mechnikova/Russian Academy of Medical Sciences, Mechnikova Institute for Vaccines & Sera, ZHMEI, A-ya 42, Moscow 125284, Russian Federation. TEL 7-095-917-4900, FAX 7-095-017-5460, instmech@iitp.ru. Ed. B F Semenov. Circ: 1,200 (paid). **Subscr. to:** Mezhdunarodnaya Kniga, B Yakimanka 39, Moscow 117049, Russian Federation. **US dist. addr.:** East View Publications, 3020 Harbor Ln N, Minneapolis, MN 55447. TEL 612-550-0961.

BIOLOGY—Microscopy

570.282 GBR ISSN 1052-0295
QH613 CODEN: BIHIEU
BIOTECHNIC AND HISTOCHEMISTRY; a journal for microtechnic and histochemistry. Variant title: Biotech & Histochem. Text in English. 1926. bi-m. USD 120 in North America to individuals for Print & Online Eds.; USD 162, GBP 108 rest of world to individuals for Print & Online Eds.; USD 220 in North America to institutions for Print & Online Eds.; USD 255, GBP 170 rest of world to institutions for Print & Online Eds. (effective 2001). adv. bk.rev. bibl, charts, illus, stat. index. *Refereed.* **Document type:** *Journal, Academic/Scholarly.* **Description:** Covers new materials, apparatus, and methods involved in the preparation of biological specimens.
Formerly: Stain Technology (0038-9153)
Related titles: Microfilm ed.; Online - full content ed.: 2001. USD 198 in North America; USD 230, USD 153 rest of world (effective 2001); Online - full text ed.: (from CatchWord Ltd., Institute for Scientific Information).
Indexed: ASCA, Abstr.Bull.Inst.Pap.Chem., Abstr.Hyg., Agricola, Anim.Breed.Abstr., BBCI, Biol.Abstr., Chem.Abstr., Chem.Indus.Notes, Chem.Titles, Curr.Adv.Ecol.Sci., Curr.Cont., Dent.Ind., Excerp.Med., Field Crop Abstr., Forest.Abstr., GeoRef, Helminthol.Abstr., Hort.Abstr., INIS Atomind., Ind.Med. (1991-), Ind.Sci.Rev., Ind.Vet., Inpharma, Int.Abstr.Biol.Sci., Int.Aerosp.Abstr., Nutr.Abstr., Plant Breed.Abstr., Plant Grow.Reg.Abstr., Potato Abstr., Poult.Abstr., Protozool.Abstr., Reac., Rev.Appl.Entomol., Rev.Med.& Vet.Mycol., Rev.Plant Path., SSCI (coverage dropped), Sci.Cit.Ind., Seed Abstr., Soils & Fert., Trop.Dis.Bull., Vet.Bull.
—BLDSC (2089.777000), CASDDS, CISTI, EMDOCS, GNLM, IDS, ingenta, Linda Hall.
Published by: (Biological Stain Commission USA), BIOS Scientific Publishers Ltd., 9 Newtec Pl, Magdalen Rd, Oxford, Berks OX4 1RE, United Kingdom. TEL 44-1865-726286, FAX 44-1865-200386, cic@bios.co.uk, nigel.farrar@bios.co.uk, www.bios.co.uk/journals/bh/index.htm, http://www.bios.co.uk. Eds. G S Nettleton TEL 502-852-7546, William E Grizzle TEL 205-934-4214. Pub. Nigel Farrar. Adv. contact Amanda Whiting. B&W page USD 565. Circ: 1,362; 1,318 (paid). **Dist. by:** Turpin Distribution Services Ltd.

570.282 NLD ISSN 0923-0475
CODEN: EMBME5
ELECTRON MICROSCOPY IN BIOLOGY AND MEDICINE. Text in English. 1984. irreg., latest vol.9, 1991. price varies. *Refereed.* **Document type:** *Monographic series.*
—CISTI.
Published by: Kluwer Academic Publishers Group (Subsidiary of: Wolters Kluwer N.V.), Spuiboulevard 50, PO Box 17, Dordrecht 3300 AA, Netherlands. FAX 31-78-639-2254, services@wkap.nl, http://www.wkap.nl. **Dist. by:** Journals Department, PO Box 322, Dordrecht 3300 AH, Netherlands. FAX 31-78-654-6474.

502.82 DEU ISSN 0936-6911
ELEKTRONENMIKROSKOPIE. Text in German. 1989. irreg. (2-3/yr.). EUR 37.07 domestic; EUR 38.99 in Europe; EUR 45.98 elsewhere; EUR 18 newsstand/cover (effective 2002). **Document type:** *Journal, Academic/Scholarly.*
Published by: (Deutsche Gesellschaft fuer Elektronenmikroskopie e.V.), Wissenschaftliche Verlagsgesellschaft mbH, Postfach 101061, Stuttgart 70009, Germany. TEL 49-711-2582-0, FAX 49-711-2582-290, service@wissenschaftliche-verlagsgesellschaft.de, http://www.wissenschaftliche-verlagsgesellschaft.de.

502.82 ISR ISSN 0071-2647
EUROPEAN CONGRESS ON ELECTRON MICROSCOPY. Text in English. quadrennial, latest 1976, 6th, Jerusalem. **Document type:** *Proceedings.*
Published by: (Israel Society of Electron Microscopy), Tal International, Inquire: Prof. D. Danon, Weizmann Institute of Science, Rehovot, Israel.

570.282 MKD ISSN 0015-9298
CODEN: FRBAAB
FRAGMENTA BALCANICA MUSEI MACEDONICI SCIENTIARUM NATURALIUM✱ . Text in Macedonian. 1954. irreg. (5-9/yr.).
Indexed: Biol.Abstr., Curr.Adv.Ecol.Sci., Deep Sea Res.& Oceanogr.Abstr., GeoRef, Rev.Appl.Entomol., Zoo.Rec.
Published by: Prirodonaucen Muzej na Makedonija, Bulevar Ilinden 66, Skopje 91000, Macedonia.

570.282 GBR ISSN 0022-0744
QC373.E4 CODEN: JELJA7
JOURNAL OF ELECTRON MICROSCOPY. Text in English. 1953. bi-m. GBP 100, USD 160 to individuals; GBP 220, USD 350 to institutions (effective 2002). adv. bk.rev. abstr, charts, illus, stat. back issues avail. *Refereed.* **Document type:** *Journal, Academic/Scholarly.*
Related titles: Microform ed.: (from PQC); Online - full text ed.: (from Institute for Scientific Information).
Indexed: ASCA, Abstr.Bull.Inst.Pap.Chem., Alloys Ind., Aqua.Sci.& Fish.Abstr., Aquacult.Abstr., Biol.Abstr., Chem.Abstr., Chem.Cit.Ind., Chem.Indus.Notes, Chem.Titles, Crop Physiol.Abstr., Curr.Cont., Dairy Sci.Abstr., Deep Sea Res.& Oceanogr.Abstr., Dent.Ind., Eng.Ind., Eng.Mat.Abstr., Environ.Sci.Poll.Mgmt., Excerp.Med., Helminthol.Abstr., INIS Atomind., INSPEC (1968-), Ind.Med. (1953-), Ind.Sci.Rev., Ind.Vet., Inpharma, Int.Abstr.Biol.Sci., JTA, Mat.Sci.Cit.Ind. (coverage dropped), Met.Abstr., Met.Abstr.Ind., Nonfer.Met.Alert, PCC Alert, Pharm.&Out.News, Plant Breed.Abstr., Reac., Ref.Zh., Rev.Appl.Entomol., Sci.Cit.Ind., Steels Alert, Vet.Bull., W.R.C.Inf., World Alum.Abstr., Zoo.Rec.
—BLDSC (4974.880000), AskIEEE, CASDDS, CISTI, Ei, GNLM, IDS, ingenta, Linda Hall. **CCC.**
Published by: (Japanese Society of Electron Microscopy), Oxford University Press, Academic Division, Great Clarendon St, Oxford OX2 6DP, United Kingdom. TEL 44-1865-267907, FAX 44-1865-267835, jnl.info@oup.co.uk, http://www3.oup.co.uk/jmicro/, http://www.oup.co.uk/journals. Ed. M Tanaka. Pubs. David Prosser, Toyoshi Onji. Circ: 3,900. **Subscr. in US to:** Oxford University Press, Journals, 2001 Evans Rd, Cary, NC 27513. TEL 800-852-7323, FAX 919-677-1714, jnlorders@oup-usa.org; **Subscr. to:** Journals Marketing, Great Clarendon St, Oxford OX2 6DP, United Kingdom.

570.282 GBR ISSN 0022-2720
CODEN: JMICAR
JOURNAL OF MICROSCOPY. Text in English. 1878. m., latest vol.205, 2002. GBP 660 in Europe; USD 1,046 in North America; GBP 726 elsewhere (effective 2002). adv. bk.rev. abstr, bibl, charts, illus. index. back issues avail.; reprint service avail. from ISI. *Refereed.* **Document type:** *Academic/Scholarly.*
Formerly (until 1969): Royal Microscopical Society. Journal (0368-3974)
Related titles: Microform ed.: (from PQC); Online - full text ed.: ISSN 1365-2818. GBP 594 in Europe; USD 942 in North America; GBP 594 elsewhere (effective 2002) (from Ovid Technologies, Inc., EBSCO Publishing, O C L C Online Computer Library Center, Inc., RoweCom Information Quest, ingenta, Munksgaard & Blackwell Science's Synergy, Swets Blackwell, Institute for Scientific Information).
Indexed: ASCA, Abstr.Bull.Inst.Pap.Chem., AgBiotech, Alloys Ind., Aqua.Sci.& Fish.Abstr., Bio-Contr.News & Info., Biol.Abstr., C.I.S. Abstr., Chem.Abstr., Chem.Cit.Ind., Chem.Titles, Compumath, Crop Physiol.Abstr., Curr.Adv.Cancer Res., Curr.Adv.Ecol.Sci., Curr.Cont., Curr.Ind.Stat., Deep Sea Res.& Oceanogr.Abstr., Dent.Ind., Eng.Mat.Abstr., Environ.Sci.Poll.Mgmt., Excerp.Med., Field Crop Abstr., Forest.Abstr., GeoRef, Helminthol.Abstr., Herb.Abstr., Hort.Abstr., INIS Atomind., INSPEC (Feb.1972-), Ind.Med. (1969-), Ind.Sci.Rev., Ind.Vet., Inpharma, Int.Abstr.Biol.Sci., Int.Aerosp.Abstr., METADEX, Maize Abstr., Mat.Sci.Cit.Ind. (coverage dropped), Met.Abstr., Met.Abstr.Ind., Nonfer.Met.Alert, Ornam.Hort., PCC Alert, Photo.Abstr., Phys.Ber., Plant Breed.Abstr., Plant Grow.Reg.Abstr., Pollut.Abstr., Protozool.Abstr., Reac., Rev.Appl.Entomol., Rev.Med.& Vet.Mycol., Rev.Plant Path., Sci.Cit.Ind., Seed Abstr., Soils & Fert., Soyabean Abstr., Steels Alert, Triticale Abstr., Weed Abstr., World Alum.Abstr.
—BLDSC (5019.695000), ADONIS, AskIEEE, CASDDS, CISTI, GNLM, IDS, Infotrieve, ingenta, Linda Hall. **CCC.**
Published by: (Royal Microscopical Society), Blackwell Science Ltd., PO Box 88, Oxford OX2 0NE, United Kingdom. TEL 44-1865-206180, 44-1865-206002, FAX 44-1865-206219, jnl.orders@blacksci.co.uk, http://www.blackwell-science.com/~cgilib/jnlpage.asp?Journal=jms&File=jms, http://www.blackwellpublishing.com. Ed. P Echlin. Pub. Sue Hewitt. R&P Sophie Savage. Adv. contact Jenny Applin. Circ: 1,255.

502.82 USA ISSN 1059-910X
QH212.E4 CODEN: MRTEEO
JOURNAL OF MICROSCOPY RESEARCH AND TECHNIQUE. Text in English. 1984. 24/yr. USD 4,995 in United States; USD 5,235 in Canada & Mexico; USD 5,439 elsewhere; USD 5,245 combined subscription in United States for print and online eds.; USD 5,485 combined subscription in Canada & Mexico for print and online eds.; USD 5,689 combined subscription elsewhere for print and online eds. (effective 2002). adv. bk.rev. bibl, illus. back issues avail. *Refereed.* **Document type:** *Academic/Scholarly.* **Description:** Encompasses all aspects of advanced microscopy, focusing on equipment, methodology, and applications in the biological, materials, and medical sciences.
Formerly: Journal of Electron Microscopy Technique (0741-0581)
Related titles: Microform ed.: (from PQC); Online - full text ed.: ISSN 1097-0029. 1996. USD 4,995 in United States; USD 4,995 in Canada & Mexico; USD 4,995 elsewhere (effective 2002) (from EBSCO Publishing, Wiley InterScience, Institute for Scientific Information).
Indexed: Abstr.Bull.Inst.Pap.Chem., Agri.& Environ.Biotech.Abstr., Aqua.Sci.& Fish.Abstr., Biotech.& Bioeng.Abstr., Cal.Tiss.Abstr., Chem.Abstr., Chem.Indus.Notes, Chem.Titles, Curr.Adv.Cell & Devel.Biol., Curr.Cont., Environ.Sci.Poll.Mgmt., Excerp.Med., Genet.Abstr., GeoRef, Hum.Gen.Abstr., INIS Atomind., Ind.Med. (1992-), Ind.Vet., METADEX, Med.& Pharm.Biotech.Abstr., Protozool.Abstr., Ref.Zh., Rev.Appl.Entomol., Rev.Med.& Vet.Mycol., Sci.Cit.Ind.
—BLDSC (5760.600850), CASDDS, CISTI, EMDOCS, GNLM, IDS, ingenta, Linda Hall. **CCC.**
Published by: John Wiley & Sons, Inc., Journals (Subsidiary of: Wiley InterScience), 605 Third Ave, New York, NY 10158. TEL 212-850-6645, FAX 212-850-6021, subinfo@wiley.com, uscs-wis@wiley.com, http://www.wiley.com. Ed. John Johnson Jr. adv.: B&W page GBP 640, color page GBP 1,515; trim 210 x 279. Circ: 700. **Subscr. outside the Americas to:** John Wiley & Sons Ltd., Baffins Ln, Chichester, Sussex PO19 IUD, United Kingdom. TEL 44-1243-779777, FAX 44-1243-843232, cs-journals@wiley.co.uk.

570.282 JPN ISSN 0918-4287
RB43.5 CODEN: MELMEJ
MEDICAL ELECTRON MICROSCOPY. Text in English. 1993. q. (in 1 vol., 4 nos./vol.). EUR 196.40 domestic; EUR 192.80 in Germany; EUR 52.80 newsstand/cover foreign for Print & Online Eds. (effective 2002). **Document type:** *Academic/Scholarly.* **Description:** Investigates the electron microsopic examination of structures, molecules, organelles, cells, tissues, and organs.
Supersedes the English part of: Nihon Rinsho Denshi Kenbikyo Gakkaishi (0021-4981)

Related titles: Online - full text ed.: ISSN 1437-773X (from EBSCO Publishing, RoweCom Information Quest, Swets Blackwell, Springer LINK).
Indexed: Chem.Abstr., Chem.Indus.Notes, Chem.Titles.
—BLDSC (5527.192500), CASDDS, CISTI, EMDOCS, GNLM, Infotrieve. **CCC.**
Published by: (Clinical Electron Microscopy Society of Japan/Nippon Rinsho Denshi Kenbikyo Gakkai), Springer-Verlag Tokyo (Subsidiary of: BertelsmannSpringer), 3-13 Hongo 3-chome, Bunkyo-ku, Tokyo 113-0033, Japan. FAX 81-3-3812-0719, orders@svt-ebs.co.jp, http://link.springer-ny.com/link/service/journals/00795/index.htm, http://www.springer.ny.com. Ed. M Mori. **Subscr. in N. America to:** Springer-Verlag New York Inc., PO Box 2485, Secaucus, NJ 07096-2485. TEL 800-777-4643, 212-460-1526, FAX 201-348-4505, orders@springer-ny.com. **Dist. outside N. America & Japan by:** Springer-Verlag, Haber Str 7, Heidelberg 69126, Germany. TEL 49-30-82787-0, subscriptions@springer.de, http://link.springer.de, http://link.springer-ny.com.

MEDITSINSKI PREGLED. KLINICHNA LABORATORIIA. see *BIOLOGY—Biochemistry*

570.282 DEU ISSN 0076-6771
METHODENSAMMLUNG DER ELEKTRONENMIKROSKOPIE/METHODS OF ELECTRON MICROSCOPY. Text in German. 1970. irreg., latest vol.11, 1984. DEM 817 to non-members; DEM 653.60 to members (effective 2001). **Document type:** *Monographic series, Academic/Scholarly.*
Published by: (Deutsche Gesellschaft fuer Elektronenmikroskopie e.V.), Wissenschaftliche Verlagsgesellschaft mbH, Postfach 101061, Stuttgart 70009, Germany. TEL 49-711-2582-0, FAX 49-711-2582-290, service@wissenschaftliche-verlagsgesellschaft.de, http://www.wissenschaftliche-verlagsgesellschaft.de. Eds. G Schimmel, W Vogell.

502.282 GBR ISSN 0968-4328
QH201 CODEN: MCONEN
MICRON; the international research and review journal for microscopy. Text in English. 1969. 8/yr. EUR 1,053 in Europe to institutions; JPY 139,800 in Japan to institutions; USD 1,178 elsewhere to institutions (effective 2002). back issues avail. *Refereed.* **Document type:** *Academic/Scholarly.* **Description:** Publishes original research and reviews covering the design, application, practice or theory of microscopy and microanalysis; also covers optical and electron beam systems linked to computer image processing and other image analytical methods.
Incorporates (1987-1992): Electron Microscopy Reviews (0892-0354); Formerly (until 1993): Micron and Microscopica Acta (0739-6260); Supersedes: Micron (0047-7206)
Related titles: Microfilm ed.: (from PQC); Online - full text ed.: (from ingenta, ScienceDirect, Swets Blackwell, Institute for Scientific Information).
Indexed: ASCA, Abstr.Bull.Inst.Pap.Chem., Alloys Ind., Br.Ceram.Abstr., Chem.Abstr., Chem.Titles, Curr.Adv.Ecol.Sci., Curr.Cont., Deep Sea Res.& Oceanogr.Abstr., GeoRef, INIS Atomind., INSPEC (1971-1991, dropped), Ind.Med. (1993-), Ind.Sci.Rev., Inpharma, Int.Abstr.Biol.Sci., Met.Abstr., Met.Abstr.Ind., Nonfer.Met.Alert, PCC Alert, Reac., Ref.Zh., Rev.Appl.Entomol., Rev.Plant Path., Sci.Cit.Ind., Steels Alert, W.R.C.Inf., World Alum.Abstr., Zoo.Rec.
—BLDSC (5759.300000), CASDDS, CISTI, EMDOCS, GNLM, IDS, Infotrieve, ingenta, Linda Hall. **CCC.**
Published by: Pergamon (Subsidiary of: Elsevier Science), The Boulevard, Langford Ln, East Park, Kidlington, Oxford OXB 1GB, United Kingdom. FAX 44-1865-843010, nlinfo-f@elsevier.nl; usinfo-f@elsevier.com; forinfo-kyf04035@niftyserve.or.jp, http://www.elsevier.com/locate/micron. Eds. D J Cockayne, R W Horne. **Subscr. in Australasia and the Far East to:** Elsevier Science (Singapore) Pte Ltd, No.1 Temasek Ave, 17-01 Millenia Tower, Singapore 039192, Singapore. TEL 65-434-3727, FAX 65-337-2230; **Subscr. in the Americas to:** Elsevier Science, PO Box 945, New York, NY 10159-0945. TEL 212-633-3730, FAX 212-633-3680; **Subscr. to:** Elsevier Science BV, PO Box 211, Amsterdam 1000 AE, Netherlands. TEL 31-20-485-3757, nlinfo-f@elsevier.nl.

MICROSCOPE. see *CHEMISTRY—Analytical Chemistry*

570.282 USA ISSN 1041-0716
MICROSCOPE TECHNOLOGY & NEWS✱. Text in English. 1990. m. USD 197. **Document type:** *Newsletter.*
—**CCC.**
Published by: Cambrex Group, 112 Washington St, Ste 2, Marblehead, MA 01945-3554. TEL 617-742-8290, FAX 617-742-4942.

570.282 CAN ISSN 0383-1825
CODEN: BMSCDQ
MICROSCOPICAL SOCIETY OF CANADA. BULLETIN. Text in English. 1973. q. CND 40, USD 42. adv. bk.rev. bibl, charts, illus, tr.lit. back issues avail. *Refereed.* **Document type:** *Bulletin.* **Description:** Presents new developments in microscopy-instrumentation, applications, and biological and materials sciences.
—CISTI.
Published by: Microscopical Society of Canada/Societe de Microscopie du Canada, c/o F Leggett, 2918 13th Ave S, Lethbridge, AB T1K 0T2, Canada. TEL 403-327-4342, FAX 403-382-3156, leggett@em.agr.ca. R&P Pierre Charest. Adv. contact Dianne Moyles. page CND 399; trim 9 x 6. Circ: 500 (paid).

570.282 CAN ISSN 0381-1751
CODEN: PMSCDA
MICROSCOPICAL SOCIETY OF CANADA. PROCEEDINGS. Text in English. 1974. a. CND 25 domestic; USD 25 foreign. adv. **Document type:** *Proceedings.*
Indexed: Biol.Abstr., GeoRef.
—CASDDS, Linda Hall.
Published by: Microscopical Society of Canada/Societe de Microscopie du Canada, c/o F Leggett, 2918 13th Ave S, Lethbridge, AB T1K 0T2, Canada. TEL 403-327-4342, FAX 403-382-3156, leggett@em.agr.ca. Circ: 650.

502.82 ZAF
CODEN: VESADE
MICROSCOPY SOCIETY OF SOUTHERN AFRICA. PROCEEDINGS/MIKROSKOPIEVERENIGING VAN SUIDELIKE AFRIKA. VERRIGTINGS. Text in English; Text occasionally in Afrikaans. 1971. a. ZAR 220. back issues avail. *Refereed.* **Document type:** *Proceedings, Abstract/Index.* **Description:** Publishes abstracts accepted for presentation at the annual conference.
Former titles: Electron Microscopy Society of Southern Africa. Proceedings (0250-0418); Southern African Electron Microscopy Society. Conference Proceedings
Indexed: Biol.Abstr., Chem.Abstr., Chem.Indus.Notes, Chem.Titles, Curr.Adv.Ecol.Sci., Excerp.Med., INSPEC (coverage dropped), Sport Fish.Abstr., Zoo.Rec.
—BLDSC (6757.660000), CASDDS, KNAW.
Published by: Microscopy Society of Southern Africa, Unit for Electron Microscopy, Faculty of Biological & Agricultural Sciences, University of Pretoria, Pretoria 0002, South Africa. TEL 27-12-4202075, FAX 27-12-4203266, hall@scientia.up.ac.za, ahall@nsnper1.up.ac.za. Ed. R H M Cross. Circ: 200.

502.82 NLD ISSN 0165-201X
CODEN: PMEMD4
PRACTICAL METHODS IN ELECTRON MICROSCOPY. Text in Dutch. 1973. irreg., latest vol.14, 1992. price varies. back issues avail. *Refereed.* **Document type:** *Monographic series, Academic/Scholarly.* **Description:** Discusses new methods for using electron microscopes in life sciences research.
Indexed: Chem.Abstr., Chem.Indus.Notes, Chem.Titles, GeoRef.
—BLDSC (6595.080000), CASDDS.
Published by: Elsevier Science BV, PO Box 211, Amsterdam 1000 AE, Netherlands. TEL 31-20-485-3757, 31-20-485-3911, FAX 31-20-485-3432, 31-20-485-3598, nlinfo-f@elsevier.nl; usinfo-f@elsevier.com; forinfo-kyf04035@niftyserve.or.jp, http://www.elsevier.nl/. Ed. Audrey M Glauert. **Subscr. in Australasia and the Far East to:** Elsevier Science (Singapore) Pte Ltd, No.1 Temasek Ave, 17-01 Millenia Tower, Singapore 039192, Singapore. TEL 65-434-3727, FAX 65-337-2230, asiainfo@elsevier.com.sg; **Subscr. in Japan to:** Elsevier Science Inc - Japan Regional Office, 9-15 Higashi-Azabu 1-chome, Minato-ku, Tokyo 106-0044, Japan. TEL 81-3-5561-5033, FAX 81-3-5561-5047, info@elsevier.co.jp; **Subscr. in the Americas to:** Elsevier Science, PO Box 945, New York, NY 10159-0945. TEL 212-633-3730, 888-437-4636, FAX 212-633-3680, usinfo-f@elsevier.com, http://www.elsevier.com

570.282 616 GBR ISSN 0969-3823
QH201 CODEN: QJMIEN
QUEKETT JOURNAL OF MICROSCOPY. Text in English. 1868. s-a. GBP 35 in Europe to non-members; GBP 40, USD 72 elsewhere to non-members (effective 2000). adv. bk.rev. illus. *Refereed.* **Document type:** *Academic/Scholarly.* **Description:** Covers all aspects of light microscopy, it's history, practical application in all branches of science, the instrument, design and usage including photo and video microscopy.
Formerly (until 1993): Microscopy (0026-2838)
Related titles: CD-ROM ed.
Indexed: Bibl.Agri., Biol.Abstr., Chem.Abstr., Deep Sea Res.& Oceanogr.Abstr., Excerp.Med., GeoRef, Hort.Abstr., Ref.Zh., W.R.C.Inf., Zoo.Rec.
—CISTI, ingenta, Linda Hall.
Published by: Quekett Microscopical Club, 90 The Fairway, South Ruislip, Mddx HA4 0SQ, United Kingdom. TEL 44-1367-710223, FAX 44-1367-718963, qmc@thomashope.freeserve.co.uk. Ed. Dr. B Bracegirdle. Circ: 650.

570.282 GBR
ROYAL MICROSCOPICAL SOCIETY. ANNUAL IMMUNOCYTOCHEMISTRY MEETING. Text in English. a. **Document type:** *Proceedings.*
—BLDSC (1086.249000).
Published by: Royal Microscopical Society, 37-38 St Clements St, Oxford, Berks OX4 1AJ, United Kingdom. TEL 44-1865-248768, FAX 44-1865-791237.

570.282 GBR ISSN 0035-9017
QH201
ROYAL MICROSCOPICAL SOCIETY. PROCEEDINGS. Text in English. 1966. q., latest vol.37, 2002. GBP 190 in Europe; USD 301 in North America; GBP 209 elsewhere (effective 2002). adv. abstr, illus. index. back issues avail.; reprint service avail. from ISI. **Document type:** *Proceedings, Academic/Scholarly.* **Description:** Contain a lively mix of articles, news, views and reports of society business.
Related titles: Online - full text ed.
Indexed: Curr.Adv.Cell & Devel.Biol., Deep Sea Res.& Oceanogr.Abstr., Excerp.Med., Fuel & Energy Abstr., METADEX.
—BLDSC (6799.500000), CISTI, Infotrieve, Linda Hall. **CCC.**
Published by: Blackwell Science Ltd., Osney Mead, Oxford OX2 0EL, United Kingdom. TEL 44-1865-206206, FAX 44-1865-721205, journals.cs@blacksci.co.uk, http://www.blackwell-science.com. Ed. P J Evenett. Pub. Sue Hewitt. R&P Sophie Savage. Adv. contact Jenny Applin. Circ: 2,000.

570.282 GBR
ROYAL MICROSCOPICAL SOCIETY. U K ANNUAL SCANNED PROBE MICROSCOPY MEETING. Text in English. a. **Document type:** *Proceedings.*
Published by: Royal Microscopical Society, 37-38 St Clements St, Oxford, Berks OX4 1AJ, United Kingdom. TEL 44-1865-248768, FAX 44-1865-791237.

570.282 USA ISSN 0161-0457
QH212.S3 CODEN: SCNNDF
SCANNING; journal of scanning microscopies. Text in English. 1978. 6/yr., latest vol.23, 2001. USD 200 domestic to individuals; USD 210 foreign to individuals; USD 350 domestic to institutions; USD 395 foreign to institutions (effective 2001). adv. bk.rev. index. 80 p./no. back issues avail.; reprints avail. *Refereed.* **Document type:** *Journal, Academic/Scholarly.*
Related titles: Online - full text ed.: (from EBSCO Publishing, Institute for Scientific Information).
Indexed: ASCA, CEABA, Chem.Abstr., Chem.Indus.Notes, Chem.Titles, Curr.Adv.Ecol.Sci., Curr.Cont., Dairy Sci.Abstr., Eng.Ind., Field Crop Abstr., Food Sci.& Tech.Abstr., GeoRef, Hort.Abstr., INSPEC (1979-), Ind.Med. (1978-), Ind.Sci.Rev., Inpharma, Maize Abstr., Mass Spectr.Bull., Mat.Sci.Cit.Ind. (coverage dropped), Photo.Abstr., Plant Breed.Abstr., Postharvest, Protozool.Abstr., Reac., Ref.Zh., Rev.Appl.Entomol., Rev.Arom.& Med.Plants, Rev.Plant Path., Sci.Cit.Ind., Seed Abstr.
—BLDSC (8087.704000), AskIEEE, CASDDS, CISTI, Ei, GNLM, IDS, Infotrieve, ingenta, Linda Hall. **CCC.**
Published by: (Foundation for Advances in Medicine & Science, Inc.), F A M S, Inc., PO Box 832, Mahwah, NJ 07430-0832. TEL 201-818-1010, FAX 201-818-0086, scanning@fams.org, http://www.scanning-fams.org, http://www.scanning.org. Ed. David C Joy. Pub. Tony Bourgholtzer. R&P Phaedra McGuinness. Adv. contact Judi Cupit. Circ: 6,984.

502.82 USA ISSN 0891-7035
QH212.S3 CODEN: SCMIEU
SCANNING MICROSCOPY; an international journal of scanning electron microscopy, related techniques, and applications. Text in English. 1968. q. USD 164; USD 189 foreign. cum.index. back issues avail. *Refereed.* **Document type:** *Academic/Scholarly.* **Description:** Theory, instruments, advancements and physical and biological applications related to scanning microscopes and related techniques.
Supersedes (in 1986): Scanning Electron Microscopy (0586-5581); Which incorporated: Scanning Electron Microscope Symposium. Proceedings
Related titles: ♦ Supplement: Scanning Microscopy Supplement. ISSN 0892-953X.

Indexed: AESIS, ASCA, Abstr.Bull.Inst.Pap.Chem., Alloys Ind., Anal.Abstr., Bioeng.Abstr., Biol.Abstr., Chem.Abstr., Chem.Titles, Comput.& Info.Sys., Curr.Cont. (coverage dropped), Dairy Sci.Abstr., Deep Sea Res.& Oceanogr.Abstr., Dent.Ind., Electron.& Communic.Abstr.J., Eng.Mat.Abstr., Excerp.Med., Food Sci.& Tech.Abstr., GeoRef, INIS Atomind., INSPEC (1979-1986, Mar.1987-), ISMEC, Ind.Med. (1987-), Ind.Sci.Rev., Int.Abstr.Biol.Sci., Mass Spectr.Bull., Mat.Sci.Cit.Ind. (coverage dropped), Met.Abstr., Met.Abstr.Ind., Meteor.& Geoastrophys.Abstr., Nonfer.Met.Alert, PCC Alert, Rev.Plant Path., SSCI (coverage dropped), Sci.Cit.Ind. (coverage dropped), Solid St.Abstr., Sport Fish.Abstr., Steels Alert, World Alum.Abstr., Zoo.Rec.
—BLDSC (8087.705300), AskIEEE, CASDDS, CISTI, Ei, EMDOCS, GNLM, IDS, ingenta, Linda Hall. **CCC.**
Published by: Scanning Microscopy International, Inc., AMF O Hare, PO Box 66507, Chicago, IL 60666-0507. TEL 708-529-6677, FAX 708-980-6698. Ed. Om Johari. Circ: 1,500.

502.82 USA ISSN 0892-953X
CODEN: SMSUEU
SCANNING MICROSCOPY SUPPLEMENT; proceedings of the Pfefferkorn Conference. Text in English. 1987. a. price varies. back issues avail. **Document type:** *Proceedings.* **Description:** Covers fundamental problems of interest to electron microscopists and users of related techniques.
Supersedes (1982-1985): Pfefferkorn Conference. Proceedings
Related titles: ♦ Supplement to: Scanning Microscopy. ISSN 0891-7035.
Indexed: Chem.Abstr., Chem.Indus.Notes, Chem.Titles, Eng.Ind., INIS Atomind., INSPEC (1990-), Ind.Med. (1987-), Zoo.Rec.
—BLDSC (8087.705330), AskIEEE, CASDDS, CISTI, KNAW, Linda Hall. **CCC.**
Published by: Scanning Microscopy International, Inc., AMF O Hare, PO Box 66507, Chicago, IL 60666-0507. TEL 708-529-6677, FAX 708-980-6677. Ed. Om Johari. Circ: 1,000.

SCHWEIZERISCHE ZEITSCHRIFT FUER PILZKUNDE/BOLLETTINO SVIZZERO DI MICOLOGIA/BULLETIN SUISSE DE MYCOLOGIE. see *BIOLOGY—Botany*

570.282 NLD ISSN 0304-3991
QH212.E4 CODEN: ULTRD6
ULTRAMICROSCOPY; journal devoted to the technical and theoretical advancement of structural research. Text in Dutch. 1975. 16/yr. EUR 1,712 in Europe to institutions; JPY 227,200 in Japan to institutions; USD 1,915 elsewhere to institutions (effective 2002). back issues avail.; reprint service avail. from SWZ. *Refereed.* **Document type:** *Academic/Scholarly.* **Description:** Covers all fundamental and technical aspects pertaining to ultramicroscopic elucidation of structure, ranging from particle optics to radiation interaction.
Related titles: Microform ed.: (from PQC); Online - full text ed.: (from EBSCO Publishing, ingenta, Swets Blackwell, Institute for Scientific Information, ScienceDirect).
Indexed: ASCA, Alloys Ind., Bioeng.Abstr., Biol.Abstr., Biotech.& Bioeng.Abstr., Chem.Abstr., Chem.Cit.Ind., Compumath, Comput.& Info.Sys., Curr.Adv.Biochem., Curr.Adv.Cell & Devel.Biol., Curr.Adv.Ecol.Sci., Curr.Cont., Dairy Sci.Abstr., Electron.& Communic.Abstr.J., Eng.Ind., Eng.Mat.Abstr., Excerp.Med., GeoRef, Helminthol.Abstr., INIS Atomind., INSPEC (Jul.1975-), Ind.Med. (1975-), Ind.Sci.Rev., Inpharma, METADEX, Mat.Sci.Cit.Ind. (coverage dropped), Met.Abstr., Met.Abstr.Ind., Nonfer.Met.Alert, PCC Alert, Photo.Abstr., Phys.Ber., Reac., Sci.Cit.Ind., Steels Alert, World Alum.Abstr.
—BLDSC (9082.783000), AskIEEE, CASDDS, CISTI, Ei, EMDOCS, IDS, Infotrieve, ingenta, Linda Hall. **CCC.**
Published by: North-Holland (Subsidiary of: Elsevier Science BV), PO Box 211, Amsterdam 1000 AE, Netherlands. TEL 31-20-485-3911, FAX 31-20-485-3598, http://www.elsevier.com/locate/issn/03043991, http://www.elsevier.nl. Eds. E Zeitler, P Kruit, S M Lindsay. **Subscr. in Australasia and the Far East to:** Elsevier Science (Singapore) Pte Ltd, No.1 Temasek Ave, 17-01 Millenia Tower, Singapore 039192, Singapore. TEL 65-434-3727, FAX 65-337-2230; **Subscr. in Japan to:** Elsevier Science Inc - Japan Regional Office, 9-15 Higashi-Azabu 1-chome, Minato-ku, Tokyo 106-0044, Japan. TEL 81-3-5561-5033; **Subscr. in the Americas to:** Elsevier Science, PO Box 945, New York, NY 10159-0945. TEL 212-633-3730, FAX 212-633-3680, usinfo-f@elsevier.com.

BIOLOGY—Ornithology

see also AGRICULTURE—Poultry And Livestock; PETS

598.41 USA ISSN 0892-6387
AMERICAN PHEASANT AND WATERFOWL SOCIETY MAGAZINE. Text in English. 1975. 10/yr. USD 25 domestic; USD 35 foreign (effective 2000). adv. bk.rev. **Document type:** *Newsletter.*
Published by: American Pheasant and Waterfowl Society, W 2270 US Hwy 10, Granton, WI 54436. TEL 715-238-7291. Ed., R&P Lloyd Ure. Circ: 1,800 (paid).

AVIAN DISEASES. see *VETERINARY SCIENCE*

598 152 USA ISSN 0156-1383
QL698.3 CODEN: BBEHDU
BIRD BEHAVIOR; an international and interdisciplinary multimedia journal. Text in English. 1977. s-a. USD 40 domestic to individuals; USD 55 foreign to individuals; USD 120 domestic to institutions; USD 145 foreign to institutions; USD 30 domestic to students; USD 43 foreign to students (effective 2001). adv. bk.rev. illus, stat. index. back issues avail.; reprint service avail. from PQC. **Document type:** *Academic/Scholarly.* **Description:** Research on descriptive and quantitative analyses of behavior, behavior ecology, experimental psychology and behavioral physiology of birds.
Formerly: Babbler (0314-5921)
Related titles: Microform ed.
Indexed: Anim.Behav.Abstr., Appl.Ecol.Abstr. (coverage dropped), Aqua.Sci.& Fish.Abstr., Aus.Sci.Ind., Biol.Abstr., Curr.Adv.Ecol.Sci., Curr.Cont. (coverage dropped), Ecol.Abstr., Environ.Per.Bibl. (1991-), Ind.Sci.Rev., Psychol.Abstr., Sci.Cit.Ind. (coverage dropped), Sport Fish.Abstr., Vet.Bull., Wild.Rev., Zoo.Rec., e-psyche.
—Infotrieve, Linda Hall. **CCC.**
Published by: Cognizant Communication Corporation, 3 Hartsdale Rd, Elmsford, NY 10523-3701. TEL 914-592-7720, FAX 914-592-8981, cogcomm@aol.com, http://www.cognizantcommunication.com. Ed. Dr. David B Miller. Pub., R&P Robert N Miranda. Adv. contact Lori Miranda. Circ: 300.

598 USA ISSN 0895-495X
QL671
BIRDER'S WORLD; exploring birds in the field and backyard. Text in English. 1987. bi-m. USD 22.50 (effective 2001); USD 4.50 newsstand/cover (effective 1999). adv. **Document type:** *Consumer.*
Related titles: Online - full text ed.: (from Gale Group).
Indexed: Biol.Dig., Sport Fish.Abstr., Wild.Rev.
—ingenta, Linda Hall.
Published by: Kalmbach Publishing Co., PO Box 1612, Waukesha, WI 53187-1612. TEL 262-796-8776, 888-558-1544, FAX 262-796-0126, mail@birdersworld.com, http://www.birdersworld.com. Ed. Diane Jolie. Pub. Deborah Hufford. Adv. contact Dina Johnston. B&W page USD 2,312, color page USD 3,237. Circ: 71,745. **Dist. by:** Hearst Distribution Group Inc., 250 W 55th St, Ste 1115, New York, NY 10019. TEL 212-649-4447, FAX 212-262-1239; **Dist. in UK by:** Comag, Tavistock Works, Tavistock Rd, W Drayton, Middx UB7 7QX, United Kingdom. TEL 44-1895-433600, FAX 44-189-543-3606.

598 USA ISSN 1041-6676
BIRDSCOPE. Text in English. 1987. 4/yr. membership. **Document type:** *Newsletter.* **Description:** Explains research programs of the laboratory in lay terms.
Formerly: Cornell University. Cooperative Research Newsletter
Indexed: Wild.Rev., Zoo.Rec.
—Linda Hall.
Published by: Cornell University, Laboratory of Ornithology, 159 Sapsucker Woods Rd, Ithaca, NY 14850. TEL 607-254-2473, FAX 607-254-2415. Ed. Tim Gallagher. Circ: 40,000.

598 USA
NEW HAMPSHIRE BIRD RECORDS. Text in English. 1982. q. USD 15 to non-members; USD 10 to members (effective 2000). **Document type:** *Bulletin.* **Description:** Describes bird sightings in New Hampshire.
Published by: Audubon Society of New Hampshire, 3 Silk Farm Rd, Box 528 B, Concord, NH 03301. TEL 603-224-9909, FAX 603-226-0902, http://www.nhaudubon.org. Ed. Becky Suomala. Circ: 300.

598 IND ISSN 0031-3297
QL671 CODEN: PAVOA8
PAVO; the Indian journal of ornithology. Text in English. 1963. s-a. INR 95; USD 25 foreign. adv. bk.rev. charts, illus. index. **Document type:** *Academic/Scholarly.*
Indexed: Aqua.Sci.& Fish.Abstr., Biol.Abstr., Chem.Abstr., Curr.Adv.Ecol.Sci., IBR, Nutr.Abstr., Zoo.Rec.
—CASDDS.
Published by: Society of Animal Morphologists & Physiologists, c/o Maharaja Sayajirao University of Baroda, Dept. of Zoology, Faculty of Science, Baroda, Gujarat 390 002, India. Ed. Bonny Pilo. Circ: 200.

598 DEU ISSN 0722-2947
QL671
SEEVOEGEL. Text in English, German. 1980. q. DEM 48 to members (effective 1999). adv. bk.rev. **Document type:** *Academic/Scholarly.*
Indexed: Aqua.Sci.& Fish.Abstr., Aquacult.Abstr., Environ.Sci.Poll.Mgmt., Key Word Ind.Wildl.Res., Ref.Zh., Zoo.Rec.
Published by: Verein Jorsand zum Schutze der Seevoegel und der Natur e.V., c/o Uwe Schneider, Haus der Natur Wulfsdorf, Ahrensburg 22926, Germany. TEL 49-4102-32656, FAX 49-4102-31983. Ed. Nicolaus Peters. Adv. contact Uwe Schneider. Circ: 6,000.

598 DEU ISSN 0173-0266
VOGEL UND UMWELT; Zeitschrift fuer Vogelkunde und Naturschutz in Hessen. Text in German. 1980. 3/yr. DEM 25 (effective 2001). bk.rev. 240 p./no. 2 cols./p. back issues avail. **Document type:** *Journal, Government.*
Indexed: Key Word Ind.Wildl.Res.
Published by: Hessisches Ministerium fuer Umwelt, Landwirtschaft und Forsten, Hoelderlinstr 1-3, Wiesbaden 65187, Germany. TEL 49-611-817-0, FAX 49-611-8172181, info@vsw-ffm.hlf-net.de. Circ: 2,000.

BIOLOGY—Physiology

see also MEDICAL SCIENCES

13C IGAKU/SOCIETY FOR THE MEDICAL APPLICATION OF CARBON THIRTEEN. BULLETIN. see *MEDICAL SCIENCES*

612.044 USA ISSN 1097-9743
A S E P NEWSLETTER. Text in English. m. back issues avail. **Document type:** *Newsletter.* **Description:** Covers news, opinions, excercise physiology professionals, and events that shape exercise physiology.
Media: Online - full text.
Published by: American Society of Exercise Physiologists, College of St Scholastica, 1200 Kenwood Ave, Duluth, MN 55811. TEL 218-723-6297, FAX 218-723-6472, tboone2@css.edu, http://www.css.edu/users/tboone2/asep/toc.htm. Ed. Tommy Boone. Adv. contact Tomy Boone.

571 BGR ISSN 0323-9950
CODEN: APPBDI
ACTA PHYSIOLOGICA ET PHARMACOLOGICA BULGARICA. Text in English. 1974. q. USD 52 foreign (effective 2002). reprints avail. **Document type:** *Journal, Academic/Scholarly.* **Description:** Publishes original experimental studies, theoretical papers and reviews in the area of clinical physiology and pharmacology.
Supersedes: Bulgarska Akademiia na Naukite, Sofia, Institut po Fiziologiia. Izvestiia
Indexed: Abstr.Bulg.Sci.Med.Lit., BSL Biol., Biol.Abstr., Chem.Abstr., Chem.Indus.Notes, Chem.Titles, Curr.Adv.Ecol.Sci., Dairy Sci.Abstr., Excerp.Med., GeoRef, INIS Atomind., Ind.Med. (1974-), Ref.Zh.
—BLDSC (0650.900000), CASDDS, CISTI, EMDOCS, GNLM, ingenta, KNAW, Linda Hall.
Published by: (Bulgarska Akademiia na Naukite/Bulgarian Academy of Sciences), Publishing House of the Bulgarian Academy of Sciences, Akad G Bonchev 6, Sofia 1113, Bulgaria. Circ: 456. **Dist. by:** Hemus, 6 Rouski blvd, Sofia 1000, Bulgaria.

571 HUN ISSN 0231-424X
QP1 CODEN: APHHDU
ACTA PHYSIOLOGICA HUNGARICA. Text in English. 1950. q. USD 198 (effective 2002). adv. bk.rev. bibl, charts, illus, abstr. index. 120 p./no. back issues avail. **Document type:** *Journal, Academic/Scholarly.* **Description:** Publishes new research papers in experimental medical sciences, covering physiology, pathophysiology and pharmacology.
Formerly (until 1982): Academiae Scientiarum Hungaricae. Acta Physiologica (0001-6756)
Related titles: Online - full text ed.: (from PMC).

Indexed: ASCA, Agri.& Environ.Biotech.Abstr. (coverage dropped), Anim.Breed.Abstr., Biol.Abstr., Chem.Abstr., Chem.Indus.Notes, Chem.Titles, Curr.Adv.Ecol.Sci., Curr.Cont. (coverage dropped), Derwent Biotech.Abstr., Environ.Sci.Poll.Mgmt., Excerp.Med., INIS Atomind., Ind.Med. (1983-), Ind.Sci.Rev., Ind.Vet., Mass Spectr.Bull., Neurosci.Cit.Ind., Nutr.Abstr., Pollut.Abstr., Poult.Abstr., Risk Abstr., Saf.Sci.Abstr., Sci.Cit.Ind. (coverage dropped), Vet.Bull.
—BLDSC (0652.500000), CASDDS, CISTI, EMDOCS, GNLM, IDS, ingenta, KNAW, Linda Hall. **CCC.**
Published by: (Magyar Tudomanyos Akademia), Akademiai Kiado Rt., PO Box 245, Budapest 1519, Hungary. TEL 36-1-4648233, FAX 36-1-4648297, journals@akkrt.hu. Ed. Emil Monos.

571 ARG ISSN 0327-6309
CODEN: APTLEZ
ACTA PHYSIOLOGICA PHARMACOLOGICA ET THERAPEUTICA LATINOAMERICANA; fisiologia, farmacologia, bioquimica y ciencias afines. Text in English, French, Portuguese, Spanish; Abstracts in English, Spanish. 1950. q. USD 140. adv. charts, illus. index. **Document type:** *Academic/Scholarly.*
Former titles (until 1990): Acta Physiologica et Pharmacologica Latino Americana (0326-6656); (until 1984): Acta Physiologica Latinoamericana (0001-6764)
Related titles: Microfilm ed.
Indexed: Biol.Abstr., Chem.Abstr., Chem.Indus.Notes, Chem.Titles, Curr.Adv.Ecol.Sci., Curr.Cont. (coverage dropped), Dairy Sci.Abstr., Excerp.Med., Ind.Med. (1991-), Ind.Sci.Rev., Nutr.Abstr., Sci.Cit.Ind. (coverage dropped).
—BLDSC (0653.500000), CASDDS, CISTI, EMDOCS, GNLM, KNAW, Linda Hall.
Published by: Asociacion Latinoamericana de Ciencias Fisiologicas, Serrano, 669, Capital Federal, Buenos Aires 1414, Argentina. TEL 54-114-8557204, FAX 54-114-8562751. Ed., Adv. contact Dr. Enri S Borda. Circ: 1,000. **Co-sponsor:** Asociacion Latinoamericana de Farmacologia.

571 GBR ISSN 0001-6772
QP1 CODEN: APSCAX
ACTA PHYSIOLOGICA SCANDINAVICA. Text in English. 1940. m., latest vol.174, 2002. GBP 120 in Europe to individuals; USD 160 in North America to individuals; GBP 120 elsewhere to individuals; GBP 280.50 in Europe to institutions; USD 445 in North America to institutions; GBP 308.50 elsewhere to institutions (effective 2002). adv. abstr, bibl, charts, illus. back issues avail.; reprint service avail. from SWZ. *Refereed.* **Document type:** *Academic/Scholarly.* **Description:** Provides readers with original reports on physiology and biological pharmacology.
Formerly: Skandinavisches Archiv fur Physiologie
Related titles: Microform ed.: (from PQC); Online - full text ed.: ISSN 1365-201X. GBP 108 in Europe to individuals; USD 144 in North America to individuals; GBP 108 elsewhere to individuals; GBP 253 in Europe to institutions; USD 401 in North America to institutions; GBP 253 elsewhere to institutions (effective 2002) (from Ovid Technologies, Inc., EBSCO Publishing, O C L C Online Computer Library Center, Inc., RoweCom Information Quest, ingenta, Munksgaard & Blackwell Science's Synergy, Swets Blackwell, Institute for Scientific Information).
Indexed: AMED, ASCA, Agri.& Environ.Biotech.Abstr. (coverage dropped), Anim.Breed.Abstr., Aqua.Sci.& Fish.Abstr., Biol.Abstr., C.I.S. Abstr., Chem.Abstr., Chem.Indus.Notes, Chem.Titles, Curr.Adv.Ecol.Sci., Curr.Cont., Dairy Sci.Abstr., Dent.Ind., Derwent Biotech.Abstr., Excerp.Med., Helminthol.Abstr., INIS Atomind., Ind.Med. (1940-), Ind.Sci.Rev., Ind.Vet., Inpharma, Int.Abstr.Biol.Sci., Neurosci.Cit.Ind., Nutr.Abstr., Pharm.&Out.News, Pig News & Info., Poult.Abstr., Reac., Sci.Cit.Ind., Sport Fish.Abstr., Sugar Ind.Abstr., THA, Vet.Bull., Wild.Rev., Zoo.Rec.
—BLDSC (0654.800000), ADONIS, CASDDS, CISTI, EMDOCS, GNLM, IDS, ingenta, KNAW, Linda Hall. **CCC.**
Published by: (Scandinavian Physiological Society), Blackwell Science Ltd., PO Box 88, Oxford OX2 0NE, United Kingdom. TEL 44-1865-206180, 44-1865-206002, FAX 44-1865-206219, jnl.orders@blacksci.co.uk, http://www.blackwell-science.com/products/journals/aps.htm, http://www.blackwellpublishing.com. Ed. B Uvnas. Pub. Allen Stevens. R&P Sophie Savage. Adv. contact Jenny Applin. Circ: 1,300.

571 GBR ISSN 0302-2994
QP1 CODEN: APSSAD
ACTA PHYSIOLOGICA SCANDINAVICA. SUPPLEMENTUM. Text in English. 1940. irreg. adv. **Document type:** *Academic/Scholarly.*
Formerly: Skandinavisches Archiv fur Physiologie. Supplementum
Related titles: Online - full text ed.: (from Ovid Technologies, Inc.).
Indexed: Chem.Abstr., Chem.Indus.Notes, Chem.Titles, Environ.Sci.Poll.Mgmt., Excerp.Med., Ind.Med. (1940-), Int.Abstr.Biol.Sci., Nutr.Abstr., Pollut.Abstr., Risk Abstr., Saf.Sci.Abstr., Sport Fish.Abstr., Wild.Rev., Zoo.Rec.
—BLDSC (0655.000000), ADONIS, CASDDS, CISTI, EMDOCS, ingenta, KNAW, Linda Hall.
Published by: (Scandinavian Physiological Society), Blackwell Science Ltd., Osney Mead, Oxford OX2 0EL, United Kingdom. TEL 44-1865-206206, FAX 44-1865-721205, journals.cs@blacksci.co.uk, http://www.blackwell-science.com. Pub. Allen Stevens. R&P Sophie Savage. Adv. contact Jenny Applin.

571.1 636.08 DEU ISSN 0301-2743
CODEN: FTPTAG
ADVANCES IN ANIMAL PHYSIOLOGY AND ANIMAL NUTRITION/FORTSCHRITTE IN DER TIERPHYSIOLOGIE UND TIERERNAEHRUNG. Text and summaries in English, French, German. 1972. irreg., latest vol.23, 1996. price varies. bibl, illus. index. reprint service avail. from ISI. **Document type:** *Monographic series.*
Related titles: ♦ Supplement to: Journal of Animal Physiology and Animal Nutrition. ISSN 0931-2439.
Indexed: Agri.& Environ.Biotech.Abstr. (coverage dropped), Biol.Abstr., Chem.Abstr., Dairy Sci.Abstr., Food Sci.& Tech.Abstr., Ind.Med. (coverage dropped), Ind.Vet., Nutr.Abstr., Zoo.Rec.
—CASDDS, CISTI, GNLM.
Published by: Blackwell Wissenschafts Verlag GmbH, Kurfuerstendamm 57, Berlin 10707, Germany. TEL 49-30-32790627, FAX 49-30-32790610, aboverwalt@blackwis.de, abo@blackwis.de, http://www.blackwell.de. Ed. Wolfgang Boettuw.

ADVANCES IN ELECTROMAGNETIC FIELDS IN LIVING SYSTEMS. see *BIOLOGY—Biophysics*

573.6 NLD
ADVANCES IN ORGAN BIOLOGY. Text in English. irreg. **Description:** Summarizes new knowledge by researchers seeking to unravel the complex mechanisms of the maintenance and termination of pregnancy. Chapters are devoted to the best studied animal models of parturition.
—BLDSC (0709.559000).
Published by: Elsevier Science BV, Sara Burgerhartstraat 25, Amsterdam 1055 KV, Netherlands. TEL 31-20-485-2911, FAX 31-20-485-2457, nlinfo-f@elsevier.nl. Ed. E Edward Bittar.

612.007 USA ISSN 1043-4046
CODEN: APEDF5
ADVANCES IN PHYSIOLOGY EDUCATION. Text in English. 1989. a. USD 25 domestic to non-members; USD 30 in Canada & Mexico to non-members; USD 35 elsewhere to non-members; USD 35 domestic to institutions; USD 40 in Canada & Mexico to institutions; USD 45 elsewhere to institutions; USD 15 newsstand/cover (effective 2002); free to members (print & online eds.). adv. bibl, charts, illus. back issues avail. *Refereed.* **Document type:** *Academic/Scholarly.* **Description:** Concerned with issues of education in physiology at all educational levels, covering scholarly essays on the direction and scope of physiology training, as well as practical aids to teaching.
Related titles: Online - full text ed.: Advances in Physiology Education Online. ISSN 1522-1229. free (from HighWire Pr., EBSCO Publishing, Factiva, Institute for Scientific Information).
Indexed: ASCA, C.I.J.E., Ind.Med. (1989-), Ref.Zh.
—BLDSC (0710.045000), CISTI, IDS. **CCC.**
Published by: American Physiological Society, 9650 Rockville Pike, Bethesda, MD 20814-3991. TEL 301-530-7071, FAX 301-571-1814, info@aps.faseb.org, info@the-aps.org, http://www.ajpadvan.org, http://www.the-aps.org/. Ed. D U Silverthorn. adv.: B&W page USD 1,250, color page USD 2,345. Circ: 11,790 (controlled).

AGING. see *BIOLOGY—Abstracting, Bibliographies, Statistics*

571 DNK ISSN 0105-3639
CODEN: ABSYB2
ALFRED BENZON SYMPOSIUM. PROCEEDINGS. Text in Danish. 1969. irreg. price varies. **Document type:** *Proceedings.*
Indexed: Biol.Abstr., Chem.Abstr., Chem.Indus.Notes, Chem.Titles.
—CASDDS, KNAW. **CCC.**
Published by: Blackwell Munksgaard, Book Division, Noerre Soegade 35, PO Box 2148, Copenhagen K 1016, Denmark. FAX 45-77-33-33-77. Ed. Hanne Terp.

571.6 USA ISSN 0363-6143
QH631
AMERICAN JOURNAL OF PHYSIOLOGY: CELL PHYSIOLOGY. Text in English. 1977. m. USD 340 domestic to non-members; USD 380 in Canada & Mexico to non-members; USD 420 elsewhere to non-members; USD 510 domestic to institutions; USD 550 in Canada & Mexico to institutions; USD 590 elsewhere to institutions; USD 355 domestic to non-members for print & onlin eds.; USD 395 in Canada & Mexico to non-members for print & onlin eds.; USD 435 elsewhere to non-members for print & onlin eds. (effective 2001); USD 140 domestic to members for print & onlin eds.; USD 180 in Canada & Mexico to members for print & onlin eds.; USD 220 elsewhere to members for print & onlin eds.; USD 535 domestic to institutions for print & onlin eds.; USD 575 in Canada & Mexico to institutions for print & onlin eds.; USD 615 elsewhere to institutions for print & onlin eds.; USD 60 newsstand/cover (effective 2002). adv. back issues avail.; reprint service avail. from PQC. *Refereed.* **Document type:** *Academic/Scholarly.* **Description:** Provides original, innovative work about normal and abnormal cell functions. Stringently reviewed, thorough and thought-provoking papers are published on the structure and function of cell membranes, contractile systems, and cellular organelles. Audience: Cell biologists, Physiologists, Biochemists and Biophysicists.
Related titles: Microform ed.: (from PQC); Online - full text ed.: A J P: Cell Physiology Online. ISSN 1522-1563. USD 290 to non-members; USD 435 to institutions (effective 2002) (from HighWire Pr., EBSCO Publishing, Factiva, Institute for Scientific Information).
Indexed: ASCA, Abstr.Hyg., Agri.& Environ.Biotech.Abstr. (coverage dropped), BBCI, Biol.& Agr.Ind. (coverage dropped), Biol.Abstr., Chem.Abstr., Curr.Cont., Dent.Ind., Excerp.Med., Helminthol.Abstr., Ind.Med. (1977-), Ind.Sci.Rev., Ind.Vet., Inpharma, Int.Abstr.Biol.Sci., Key Word Ind.Wildl.Res., Nutr.Abstr., Pharm.&Out.News, Reac., Sci.Cit.Ind., Trop.Dis.Bull., Vet.Bull.
—CISTI, EMDOCS, IDS, Infotrieve. **CCC.**
Published by: American Physiological Society, 9650 Rockville Pike, Bethesda, MD 20814-3991. TEL 301-530-7071, FAX 301-571-1814, info@aps.faseb.org, info@the-aps.org, http://www.ajpcell.org, http://www.the-aps.org/. Ed. K E Barrett. adv.: B&W page USD 980, color page USD 2,075. Circ: 3,467 (paid).

571 USA ISSN 0002-9513
QP1 CODEN: AJPHAP
AMERICAN JOURNAL OF PHYSIOLOGY (CONSOLIDATED). (Consolidates papers published in all 7 American Journal of Physiology specialty journals.) Text in English. 1898. m. USD 1,815 domestic to non-members; USD 1,945 in Canada & Mexico to non-members; USD 2,190 elsewhere to non-members; USD 2,725 domestic to institutions; USD 2,855 in Canada & Mexico to institutions; USD 3,100 elsewhere to institutions; USD 1,900 domestic to non-members for print & online eds.; USD 2,030 in Canada & Mexico to non-members for print & online eds.; USD 2,275 elsewhere to non-members for print & online eds.; USD 705 domestic to members for print & online eds.; USD 835 in Canada & Mexico to members for print & online eds.; USD 1,080 elsewhere to members for print & online eds.; USD 2,855 domestic to institutions for print & online eds.; USD 2,985 in Canada & Mexico to institutions for print & online eds.; USD 3,230 elsewhere to institutions for print & online eds.; USD 240 newsstand/cover (effective 2002). adv. bibl, charts, illus. index, cum.index. back issues avail.; reprint service avail. from PQC,ISI. *Refereed.* **Document type:** *Academic/Scholarly.* **Description:** Includes seven sections: Cell physiology, Endocrinology and metabolism, Gastrointestinal and liver physiology, Heart and circulatory physiology, Lung celluar and molecular physiology, Regulatory, integrative and comparative physiology, Renal physiology.
Related titles: Microform ed.: (from PQC,PMC); Online - full text ed.: A J P Online. USD 2,315 to institutions (effective 2001); USD 1,560 to non-members; USD 2,340 to institutions (effective 2002) (from Gale Group).

B

B

Indexed: Abstr.Hyg., AgBiotech, Agri.& Environ.Biotech.Abstr. (coverage dropped), Agricola, Anim.Breed.Abstr., Aqua.Sci.& Fish.Abstr., Bibl.Agri., Biol.& Agr.Ind. (Nov.1982-), Biol.Abstr., Chem.Abstr., Chem.Indus.Notes, Chem.Titles, Chemorec.Abstr., Curr.Adv.Biochem., Curr.Adv.Cell & Devel.Biol., Curr.Adv.Ecol.Sci., Curr.Adv.Gen.& Molec.Biol., Curr.Cont. (coverage dropped), Curr.Ref.Fish Res., Dairy Sci.Abstr., Dent.Ind., Derwent Biotech.Abstr., Gen.Sci.Ind. (Jun.1992-), Helminthol.Abstr., INIS Atomind., Ind.Med. (coverage dropped), Ind.Sci.Rev., Ind.Vet., Int.Abstr.Biol.Sci., Key Word Ind.Wildl.Res., Kidney, Maize Abstr., Mass Spectr.Bull., Neurosci.Abstr. (coverage dropped), Neurosci.Cit.Ind., Nutr.Abstr., Pig News & Info., Poult.Abstr., Protozool.Abstr., Ref.Zh., Rev.Appl.Entomol., Rev.Arom.& Med.Plants, SSCI (coverage dropped), Sci.Cit.Ind. (coverage dropped), Small Anim.Abstr., Soyabean Abstr., Sport Fish.Abstr., Sugar Ind.Abstr., Trop.Dis.Bull., Vet.Bull., Weed Abstr., Wild.Rev., Zoo.Rec.

—BLDSC (0834.000000), CASDDS, CISTI, GNLM, IDS, ingenta, KNAW, Linda Hall. **CCC.**

Published by: American Physiological Society, 9650 Rockville Pike, Bethesda, MD 20814-3991. TEL 301-530-7180, FAX 301-571-8305, info@the-aps.org, http://ajpcon.physiology.org/, http://www.the-aps.org/. adv.: B&W page USD 775, color page USD 1,125. Circ: 2,500.

573.4 USA ISSN 0193-1849
QP187.A1

AMERICAN JOURNAL OF PHYSIOLOGY: ENDOCRINOLOGY AND METABOLISM. Text in English. 1977. m. USD 235 domestic to non-members; USD 275 in Canada & Mexico to non-members; USD 295 elsewhere to non-members; USD 355 domestic to institutions; USD 395 in Canada & Mexico to institutions; USD 415 elsewhere to institutions; USD 250 domestic to non-members for print & online eds.; USD 290 in Canada & Mexico to non-members for print & online eds.; USD 310 elsewhere to non-members for print & online eds.; USD 100 domestic to members for print & online eds.; USD 140 in Canada & Mexico to members for print & online eds.; USD 160 elsewhere to members for print & online eds.; USD 370 domestic to institutions for print & online eds.; USD 410 in Canada & Mexico to institutions for print & online eds.; USD 430 elsewhere to institutions for print & online eds.; USD 60 newsstand/cover none (effective 2002). back issues avail.; reprint service avail. from PQC. *Refereed.* **Document type:** *Academic/Scholarly.* **Description:** Examines organisms at all levels of endocrine and metabolic systems development, from the subcellular and molecular to the level of whole animal.

Supersedes in part (in 1980): American Journal of Physiology: Endocrinology, Metabolism and Gastrointestinal Physiology (0363-6100)

Related titles: Microform ed.: (from PQC); Online - full text ed.: A J P: Endocrinology and Metabolism Online. ISSN 1522-1555. USD 300 to institutions (effective 2001); USD 205 to non-members; USD 305 to institutions (effective 2002) (from HighWire Pr., EBSCO Publishing, Factiva, Institute for Scientific Information).

Indexed: ASCA, Abstr.Hyg., Agri.& Environ.Biotech.Abstr. (coverage dropped), Anim.Breed.Abstr., BBCI, Biol.& Agr.Ind. (coverage dropped), Biol.Abstr., Chem.Abstr., Curr.Cont., Dairy Sci.Abstr., Dent.Ind., Excerp.Med., Ind.Med. (1980-), Ind.Sci.Rev., Ind.Vet., Inpharma, Int.Abstr.Biol.Sci., Key Word Ind.Wildl.Res., Nutr.Abstr., Pharm.&Out.News, Reac., Sci.Cit.Ind., Trop.Dis.Bull., Vet.Bull.

—CISTI, EMDOCS, IDS, Infotrieve. **CCC.**

Published by: American Physiological Society, 9650 Rockville Pike, Bethesda, MD 20814-3991. TEL 301-530-7071, FAX 301-571-1814, info@aps.faseb.org, info@the-aps.org, http://www.ajpendo.org, http://www.the-aps.org/. Ed. M Mueckler. Circ: 3,553 (paid).

573.3 USA ISSN 0193-1857
QP145

AMERICAN JOURNAL OF PHYSIOLOGY: GASTROINTESTINAL AND LIVER PHYSIOLOGY. Text in English. 1977. m. USD 255 domestic to non-members; USD 295 in Canada & Mexico to non-members; USD 315 elsewhere to non-members; USD 380 domestic to institutions; USD 420 in Canada & Mexico to institutions; USD 440 elsewhere to institutions; USD 265 domestic to non-members for print & online eds.; USD 305 in Canada & Mexico to non-members for print & online eds.; USD 325 elsewhere to non-members for print & online eds.; USD 100 domestic to members for print & online eds.; USD 140 in Canada & Mexico to members for print & online eds.; USD 160 elsewhere to members for print & online eds.; USD 400 domestic to institutions for print & online eds.; USD 440 in Canada & Mexico to institutions for print & online eds.; USD 460 elsewhere to institutions for print & online eds.; USD 60 newsstand/cover (effective 2002). abstr. back issues avail. *Refereed.* **Document type:** *Academic/Scholarly.* **Description:** Presents original papers dealing with normal or abnormal function of the alimentary canal and its accessory organs including the salivary glands, pancreas, gallbladder, and liver.

Supersedes in part (in 1980): American Journal of Physiology: Endocrinology, Metabolism and Gastrointestinal Physiology (0363-6100)

Related titles: Online - full text ed.: A J P: Gastrointestinal and Liver Physiology Online. ISSN 1522-1547. USD 325 to institutions (effective 2001); USD 220 to non-members; USD 330 to institutions (effective 2002) (from HighWire Pr., EBSCO Publishing, Factiva, Institute for Scientific Information).

Indexed: ASCA, Abstr.Hyg., Agri.& Environ.Biotech.Abstr. (coverage dropped), BBCI, Biol.& Agr.Ind. (coverage dropped), Biol.Abstr., Chem.Abstr., Curr.Cont., Dairy Sci.Abstr., Dent.Ind., Excerp.Med., Helminthol.Abstr., Ind.Med. (1980-), Ind.Sci.Rev., Ind.Vet., Inpharma, Int.Abstr.Biol.Sci., Key Word Ind.Wildl.Res., Nutr.Abstr., Pharm.&Out.News, Reac., Sci.Cit.Ind., Trop.Dis.Bull., Vet.Bull.

—CISTI, EMDOCS, IDS, Infotrieve. **CCC.**

Published by: American Physiological Society, 9650 Rockville Pike, Bethesda, MD 20814-3991. TEL 301-530-7071, FAX 301-571-1814, info@aps.faseb.org, info@the-aps.org, http://www.ajpgi.org, http://www.the-aps.org/. Ed. M F Kagnoff. Circ: 3,588 (paid).

573.1 USA ISSN 0363-6135
QP101.2

AMERICAN JOURNAL OF PHYSIOLOGY: HEART AND CIRCULATORY PHYSIOLOGY. Text in English. 1977. m. USD 470 domestic to non-members; USD 520 in Canada & Mexico to non-members; USD 570 elsewhere to non-members; USD 705 domestic to institutions; USD 755 in Canada & Mexico to institutions; USD 805 elsewhere to institutions; USD 490 domestic to non-members for print & online eds.; USD 540 in Canada & Mexico to non-members for print & online eds.; USD 590 elsewhere to non-members for print & online eds.; USD 195 domestic to members for print & online eds.; USD 245 in Canada & Mexico to members for print & online eds.; USD 295 elsewhere to members for print & online eds.; USD 740 domestic to institutions for print & online eds.; USD 790 in Canada & Mexico to institutions for print & online eds.; USD 840 elsewhere to institutions for print & online eds.; USD 65 newsstand/cover (effective 2002). abstr. back issues avail.; reprint service avail. from PQC. *Refereed.* **Document type:** *Academic/Scholarly.* **Description:** Presents experimental and theoretical studies of cardiovascular function at all levels of organization ranging from the intact animal to the cellular, subcellular, and molecular levels.

Related titles: CD-ROM ed.; Microform ed.: (from PQC); Online - full text ed.: A J P: Heart and Circulatory Physiology Online. ISSN 1522-1539. USD 600 to institutions (effective 2001); USD 405 to non-members; USD 605 to institutions (effective 2002) (from HighWire Pr., EBSCO Publishing, Factiva, Institute for Scientific Information).

Indexed: ASCA, Abstr.Hyg., Agri.& Environ.Biotech.Abstr. (coverage dropped), BBCI, Biol.& Agr.Ind. (coverage dropped), Biol.Abstr., Chem.Abstr., Curr.Cont., Dent.Ind., Excerp.Med., Helminthol.Abstr., INIS Atomind., Ind.Med. (1977-), Ind.Sci.Rev., Ind.Vet., Inpharma, Int.Abstr.Biol.Sci., Key Word Ind.Wildl.Res., Nutr.Abstr., Pharm.&Out.News, Reac., Sci.Cit.Ind., Trop.Dis.Bull., Vet.Bull.

—CISTI, EMDOCS, IDS, Infotrieve. **CCC.**

Published by: American Physiological Society, 9650 Rockville Pike, Bethesda, MD 20814-3991. TEL 301-530-7164, FAX 301-571-8305, info@aps.faseb.org, info@the-aps.org, http://www.ajpheart.org, http://www.the-aps.org/. Ed. D R Harder. Circ: 950.

571 USA ISSN 1040-0605
QP121.A1 CODEN: APLPE7

AMERICAN JOURNAL OF PHYSIOLOGY: LUNG CELLULAR AND MOLECULAR PHYSIOLOGY. Text in English. 1989. m. USD 230 domestic to non-members; USD 270 in Canada & Mexico to non-members; USD 310 elsewhere to non-members; USD 345 domestic to institutions; USD 385 in Canada & Mexico to institutions; USD 425 elsewhere to institutions; USD 240 domestic to non-members print & online eds.; USD 280 in Canada & Mexico to non-members print & online eds.; USD 320 elsewhere to non-members print & online eds.; USD 95 domestic to members print & online eds.; USD 135 in Canada & Mexico to members print & online eds.; USD 175 elsewhere to members print & online eds.; USD 360 domestic to institutions print & online eds.; USD 400 in Canada & Mexico to institutions print & online eds.; USD 440 elsewhere to institutions print & online eds.; USD 60 newsstand/cover (effective 2002). abstr. back issues avail. *Refereed.* **Document type:** *Academic/Scholarly.* **Description:** Presents original investigative and theoretical papers dealing with molecular, cellular, and morphological aspects of normal and abnormal function and response of respiratory cell components of the respiratory system.

Related titles: Online - full text ed.: A J P: Lung Cellular and Molecular Physiology Online. ISSN 1522-1504. USD 295 to institutions (effective 2001); USD 195 to non-members; USD 295 to institutions (effective 2002) (from HighWire Pr., EBSCO Publishing, Factiva, Institute for Scientific Information).

Indexed: ASCA, BBCI, Curr.Cont., Ind.Med. (1989-), Ind.Sci.Rev., Inpharma, Int.Abstr.Biol.Sci., Pharm.&Out.News, Reac., Sci.Cit.Ind.

—CISTI, EMDOCS, GNLM, IDS, Infotrieve. **CCC.**

Published by: American Physiological Society, 9650 Rockville Pike, Bethesda, MD 20814-3991. TEL 301-530-7164, FAX 301-571-8305, info@aps.faseb.org, info@the-aps.org, http://www.ajplung.org, http://www.the-aps.org/. Ed. A B Malik. Circ: 1,150.

571 USA ISSN 0363-6119
QP33

AMERICAN JOURNAL OF PHYSIOLOGY: REGULATORY, INTEGRATIVE AND COMPARATIVE PHYSIOLOGY. Text in English. 1977. m. USD 325 domestic to non-members; USD 365 in Canada & Mexico to non-members; USD 405 elsewhere to non-members; USD 490 domestic to institutions; USD 530 in Canada & Mexico to institutions; USD 570 elsewhere to institutions; USD 340 domestic to non-members print & online eds.; USD 380 in Canada & Mexico to non-members print & online eds.; USD 420 elsewhere to non-members print & online eds.; USD 125 domestic to members print & online eds.; USD 165 in Canada & Mexico to members print & online eds.; USD 205 elsewhere to members print & online eds.; USD 510 domestic to institutions print & online eds.; USD 550 in Canada & Mexico to institutions print & online eds.; USD 590 elsewhere to institutions print & online eds.; USD 60 newsstand/cover (effective 2002). abstr. back issues avail.; reprint service avail. from PQC. *Refereed.* **Document type:** *Academic/Scholarly.* **Description:** Presents original articles that emphasize relationships between organ systems and control of physiological processes in the whole organism, and articles on comparative physiology.

Related titles: Microform ed.: (from PQC); Online - full text ed.: A J P: Regulatory, Integrative and Comparative Physiology Online. ISSN 1522-1490. USD 415 to institutions (effective 2001); USD 280 to non-members; USD 420 to institutions (effective 2002) (from HighWire Pr., EBSCO Publishing, Factiva, Institute for Scientific Information).
Indexed: ASCA, Abstr.Hyg., Agri.& Environ.Biotech.Abstr. (coverage dropped), BBCI, Biol.& Agr.Ind. (coverage dropped), Biol.Abstr., Chem.Abstr., Curr.Cont., Dent.Ind., Excerp.Med., Helminthol.Abstr., Ind.Med. (1977-), Ind.Sci.Rev., Ind.Vet., Inpharma, Int.Abstr.Biol.Sci., Key Word Ind.Wildl.Res., Nutr.Abstr., Pharm.&Out.News, Reac., Sci.Cit.Ind., Trop.Dis.Bull., Vet.Bull.
—CISTI, EMDOCS, IDS, Infotrieve. **CCC.**
Published by: American Physiological Society, 9650 Rockville Pike, Bethesda, MD 20814-3991. TEL 301-530-7164, FAX 301-571-3813, info@aps.faseb.org, info@the-aps.org, http://www.ajpregu.org, http://www.the-aps.org/. Ed. P B Persson. Circ: 500.

573.49 USA
QP249
AMERICAN JOURNAL OF PHYSIOLOGY: RENAL PHYSIOLOGY. Text in English. 1977. m. USD 235 domestic to non-members; USD 275 in Canada & Mexico to non-members; USD 295 elsewhere to non-members; USD 355 domestic to institutions; USD 395 in Canada & Mexico to institutions; USD 415 elsewhere to institutions; USD 250 domestic to non-members for print & online eds.; USD 290 in Canada & Mexico to non-members for print & online eds.; USD 310 elsewhere to non-members for print & online eds.; USD 110 domestic to members for print & online eds.; USD 150 in Canada & Mexico to members for print & online eds.; USD 170 elsewhere to members for print & online eds.; USD 370 domestic to institutions for print & online eds.; USD 410 in Canada & Mexico to institutions for print & online eds.; USD 430 elsewhere to institutions for print & online eds.; USD 60 newsstand/cover (effective 2002). abstr. back issues avail.; reprint service avail. from PQC. *Refereed.* **Document type:** *Academic/Scholarly.* **Description:** Covers subject matter relating to the kidney, urinary tract, and epithelial cell layers. Also covers body fluid volume control and composition.
Formerly (until Jan. 1997): American Journal of Physiology: Renal, Fluid and Electrolyte Physiology (0363-6127)
Related titles: Microform ed.: (from PQC); Online - full text ed.: A J P: Renal Physiology Online. ISSN 1522-1466. USD 300 to institutions (effective 2001); USD 205 to non-members; USD 305 to institutions (effective 2002) (from HighWire Pr., EBSCO Publishing, Institute for Scientific Information).
Indexed: ASCA, Abstr.Hyg., Agri.& Environ.Biotech.Abstr. (coverage dropped), BBCI, Biol.& Agr.Ind. (coverage dropped), Biol.Abstr., Chem.Abstr., Curr.Cont., Dent.Ind., Excerp.Med., Helminthol.Abstr., INIS Atomind., Ind.Med. (1997-), Ind.Sci.Rev., Ind.Vet., Inpharma, Int.Abstr.Biol.Sci., Key Word Ind.Wildl.Res., Nutr.Abstr., Pharm.&Out.News, Reac., Sci.Cit.Ind., Trop.Dis.Bull., Vet.Bull.
—CISTI, EMDOCS, IDS, Infotrieve. **CCC.**
Published by: American Physiological Society, 9650 Rockville Pike, Bethesda, MD 20814-3991. TEL 301-530-7164, FAX 301-571-3813, info@aps.faseb.org, info@the-aps.org, http://www.ajprenal.org, http://www.the-aps.org/. Ed. J M Sands. Circ: 3,830 (paid).

612 ZAF
ANATOMIESE VERENIGING VAN SUIDER-AFRIKA. KONGRESVERRIGTINGE/ANATOMICAL SOCIETY OF SOUTHERN AFRICA. PROCEEDINGS OF ANNUAL CONGRESS. Text in Afrikaans, English. 197?. a., latest 1994, 24th, Pretoria. price varies. **Document type:** *Proceedings.*
Published by: Anatomiese Vereniging van Suider-Afrika/Anatomical Society of Southern Africa, c/o Dr HB Groenwald, Dept. Anatomie Fakulteit Veerartsenykunde, Privaatsak X04, Onderstepoort, Pretoria 0110, South Africa.

571 DEU ISSN 0340-2061
QL951 CODEN: ANEMDG
ANATOMY AND EMBRYOLOGY. Text in English. 1892. m. EUR 2,875.90 foreign; EUR 2,856.70 in Germany; EUR 283 newsstand/cover foreign (effective 2002). adv. bibl, charts, illus. back issues avail.; reprint service avail. from ISI. *Refereed.* **Document type:** *Journal, Academic/Scholarly.* **Description:** Publishes original and review articles on the morphology and developmental biology of vertebrates, with an emphasis on mammals.
Former titles: Journal of Anatomy and Embryology; Zeitschrift fuer Anatomie und Entwicklungsgeschichte (0044-2232)
Related titles: Microform ed.: (from PQC); Online - full text ed.: ISSN 1432-0568 (from EBSCO Publishing, RoweCom Information Quest, Swets Blackwell, Springer LINK, Institute for Scientific Information).
Indexed: ASCA, Anim.Breed.Abstr., Biol.Abstr., Chem.Abstr., Curr.Adv.Cell & Devel.Biol., Curr.Adv.Ecol.Sci., Curr.Cont., Dairy Sci.Abstr., Dent.Ind., Excerp.Med., INIS Atomind., Ind.Med. (1974-), Ind.Sci.Rev., Ind.Vet., Inpharma, Int.Abstr.Biol.Sci., Neurosci.Cit.Ind., Pig News & Info., Poult.Abstr., Reac., Sci.Cit.Ind., Vet.Bull., Zoo.Rec.
—BLDSC (0900.030000), ADONIS, CASDDS, CISTI, EMDOCS, GNLM, IDS, Infotrieve, ingenta, Linda Hall. **CCC.**
Published by: Springer-Verlag (Subsidiary of: BertelsmannSpringer), Tiergartenstr 17, Heidelberg 69121, Germany. TEL 49-6221-345-0, FAX 49-6221-345229, subscriptions@springer.de, http://link.springer.de/link/service/journals/00429/index.htm, http://www.springer.de. **Subscr. in N. America to:** Springer-Verlag New York Inc., PO Box 2485, Secaucus, NJ 07096-2485. TEL 212-460-1500, FAX 212-473-6272.

571.8 USA ISSN 0090-5348
HQ768
ANNUAL EDITIONS: HUMAN DEVELOPMENT. Text in English. 1972. a. USD 12.25. illus. *Refereed.* **Document type:** *Academic/Scholarly.*
Published by: Dushkin - McGraw-Hill, Sluice Dock, Guilford, CT 06437-9989. TEL 203-453-4351, FAX 203-453-6000. Ed. Karen Fieberg. Pub. Ian Nielsen. R&P Cheryl Greenleaf.

571 USA ISSN 0066-4278
QP1 CODEN: ARPHAD
ANNUAL REVIEW OF PHYSIOLOGY. Text in English. 1939. a. USD 62 domestic to individuals; USD 67 foreign to individuals; USD 124 domestic to institutions; USD 134 foreign to institutions (effective 1999). adv. bibl, charts. index, cum.index. back issues avail.; reprints avail. *Refereed.* **Document type:** *Academic/Scholarly.* **Description:** Synthesizes and filters primary research to identify the principal contributions in the field of physiology.
Related titles: Microfilm ed.: (from PQC); Online - full text ed.: (from HighWire Pr., EBSCO Publishing, H. W. Wilson, Gale Group, Institute for Scientific Information).
Indexed: ASCA, Abstr.Hyg., Anim.Breed.Abstr., Aqua.Sci.& Fish.Abstr., Biol.& Agr.Ind. (Jan.1983-), Biol.Abstr., Biotech.& Bioeng.Abstr., Cal.Tiss.Abstr., Chem.Abstr., Chem.Indus.Notes, Chem.Titles, Chemorec.Abstr., Curr.Adv.Ecol.Sci., Curr.Cont., Dairy Sci.Abstr., Deep Sea Res.& Oceanogr.Abstr., Dent.Ind., Diar.Dis.Res., Entomol.Abstr., Excerp.Med., Focus on: Sports Sci.& Med., Gen.Sci.Ind. (Jul.1997-), Helminthol.Abstr., INIS Atomind., Ind.Med. (1939-), Ind.Sci.Rev., Ind.Vet., Inpharma, Int.Abstr.Biol.Sci., Media Rev.Dig., Neurosci.Abstr., Nutr.Abstr., PsycInfo, Psychol.Abstr. (1939-), Reac., SSCI (coverage dropped), Sci.Cit.Ind., THA, Zoo.Rec., e-psyche.
—BLDSC (1527.000000), ADONIS, CASDDS, CISTI, EMDOCS, GNLM, IDS, ingenta, KNAW, Linda Hall. **CCC.**
Published by: Annual Reviews Inc., 4139 El Camino Way, Box 10139, Palo Alto, CA 94303-0139. TEL 650-493-4400, 800-523-8635, FAX 650-424-0910, service@annurev.org; orders@allenpress.com, http://www.biomedical.annualreviews.org. Ed. Samuel Gubins. R&P, Adv. contact Swati Aneja TEL 650-843-6634. **Subscr.to:** Allen Press Inc., PO Box 1897, Lawrence, KS 66044-8897.

612 NLD ISSN 0920-5268
CODEN: AAPAED
APPLIED CARDIOPULMONARY PATHOPHYSIOLOGY; the interface between laboratory and clinical practice. Abbreviated title: A C P. Text in English. 1988. q. NLG 385 domestic to institutions; USD 197.50 in United States to institutions. *Refereed.* **Document type:** *Academic/Scholarly.*
Related titles: Microform ed.: (from PQC); Online - full text ed.: (from EBSCO Publishing).
Indexed: ASCA, Curr.Cont. (coverage dropped), Eng.Ind., Excerp.Med. (1992-), Ind.Sci.Rev., Inpharma, Pharm.&Out.News, Reac., Sci.Cit.Ind. (coverage dropped).
—BLDSC (1571.921330), CASDDS, CISTI, Ei, EMDOCS, GNLM, IDS, Infotrieve. **CCC.**
Published by: Kluwer Academic Publishers Group (Subsidiary of: Wolters Kluwer N.V.), Spuiboulevard 50, PO Box 17, Dordrecht 3300 AA, Netherlands. FAX 31-78-639-2254, services@wkap.nl, http://www.wkap.nl. Ed. Omar Prakash. **Dist. by:** Journals Department, PO Box 322, Dordrecht 3300 AH, Netherlands. TEL 781-871-6600, FAX 31-78-654-6474.

599.9 JPN ISSN 1341-3473
APPLIED HUMAN SCIENCE; journal of physiological anthropology. Text in English. 1982. m. JPY 3,500. **Description:** Contains original articles, reviews, reports, technical reports and brief communications.
Formerly: Annals of Physiological Anthropology (0287-8429)
Indexed: Biol.Abstr., Ergon.Abstr., Excerp.Med., Ind.Med. (coverage dropped).
—GNLM, KNAW.
Published by: Japan Society of Physiological Anthropology/Seiri Jinrui Gakkai, c/o Business Center for Academic Societies Japan, 5-16-9 Honkomagome, Bunkyo-ku, Tokyo 113-0021, Japan. TEL 81-3-5814-5801, FAX 81-3-5814-5820, iwanaga@dergo2.tech.chiba-u.ac.jp. Eds. L Harada, N Nagai.

ARCHIVES ITALIENNES DE BIOLOGIE; journal of neuroscience. see *MEDICAL SCIENCES—Psychiatry And Neurology*

571 NLD ISSN 1381-3455
QP1 CODEN: APBIF5
ARCHIVES OF PHYSIOLOGY AND BIOCHEMISTRY. Text in English, French. 1904. 5/yr., latest vol.109, 2001. NLG 933 to institutions includes supplement & online ed.; USD 491 to institutions includes supplement & online ed (effective 2001). adv. charts, illus. index, cum.index. Supplement avail.; back issues avail. *Refereed.* **Document type:** *Journal, Academic/Scholarly.* **Description:** Publishes original research papers relating to the various parts of the physiological and biochemical sciences.
Former titles (until vol.104): Archives Internationales de Physiologie, de Biochimie et de Biophysique (0778-3124); Archives Internationales de Physiologie et de Biochimie (0003-9799)
Related titles: Microfilm ed.: (from PMC); Online - full text ed.: (from EBSCO Publishing, O C L C Online Computer Library Center, Inc., RoweCom Information Quest, Swets Blackwell, Institute for Scientific Information).
Indexed: Anim.Breed.Abstr., Aqua.Sci.& Fish.Abstr., Aquacult.Abstr., BBCI, Biol.Abstr., Chem.Abstr., Chem.Indus.Notes, Curr.Adv.Ecol.Sci., Curr.Cont. (coverage dropped), Dairy Sci.Abstr., Environ.Sci.Poll.Mgmt., Excerp.Med., Helminthol.Abstr., Hort.Abstr., INIS Atomind., Ind.Med. (1995-), Ind.Sci.Rev., Ind.Vet., Inpharma, Int.Abstr.Biol.Sci., Nutr.Abstr., Pharm.&Out.News, Pig News & Info., Reac., Sci.Cit.Ind. (coverage dropped), Vet.Bull., Zoo.Rec.
—BLDSC (1639.570000), ADONIS, CASDDS, CISTI, EMDOCS, GNLM, IDS, Infotrieve, ingenta, KNAW, Linda Hall. **CCC.**
Published by: Swets & Zeitlinger BV, PO Box 825, Lisse 2160 SZ, Netherlands. TEL 31-252-435111, FAX 31-252-415888, orders@swets.nl, http://www.swets.nl/sps/journals/apb.html. Eds. E Marani, J A Maassen. R&P J van der Valk. **Dist. in N. America by:** Swets & Zeitlinger, PO Box 582, Downingtown, PA 19335-998. TEL 800-477-9387, FAX 610-524-5366.

571 ITA ISSN 0004-0096
QP1 CODEN: ARFIAY
ARCHIVIO DI FISIOLOGIA. Text in Italian. 1904. q. ITL 10,000. bk.rev.
Related titles: Microfiche ed.: (from BHP).
Indexed: Biol.Abstr., Chem.Abstr., Excerp.Med., Ind.Med. (coverage dropped), Nutr.Abstr.
—CISTI, GNLM.
Published by: Societa Italiana di Fisiologia, Viale Margagni 65, Florence, FI, Italy.

571 AUS
CODEN: PAPPCH
AUSTRALIAN PHYSIOLOGICAL AND PHARMACOLOGICAL SOCIETY. PROCEEDINGS (ONLINE EDITION). Text in English. 1970. 2/yr. adv. bk.rev. **Document type:** *Proceedings.*
Former titles: Australian Physiological and Pharmacological Society. Proceedings (Print Edition) (0067-2084); Australian Physiological Society. Proceedings
Media: Online - full content.
Indexed: Biol.Abstr., Chem.Abstr., INIS Atomind.
—BLDSC (6655.500000), CASDDS, CISTI, GNLM, ingenta, KNAW.
Published by: Australian Physiological and Pharmacological Society (APPS), c/o Dr Ian McCance, APPS Office of Publications, PO Box 2371, Mt. Waverley, VIC 3149, Australia. FAX 61-6-2492687, http://www.med.monash.edu.au/physiology/APPS/Proceedings/proceedings.html, http://www.apps.org.au. Ed. I McCance. Adv. contact C E Hill. page AUD 330. Circ: 550.

B

573.8 CHE ISSN 1047-5125
CODEN: ANSYEL
AUTONOMIC NERVOUS SYSTEM. Text in English. irreg., latest vol.12. price varies. *Refereed.* **Document type:** *Monographic series.*
Indexed: e-psyche.
—BLDSC (1835.053000). **CCC.**
Published by: Gordon and Breach - Harwood Academic (Subsidiary of: Taylor & Francis Group), PO Box 531, Lausanne 1000, Switzerland. Ed. Geoffrey Burnstock. **Subscr. addr. in US:** International Publishers Direct, PO Box 32160, Newark, NJ 07102. FAX 215-750-6343.

571.1 GBR ISSN 1359-1533
BABRAHAM INSTITUTE. CORPORATE PLAN. Text in English. 1995. irreg. price varies. stat, charts, illus. back issues avail. **Document type:** *Corporate.* **Description:** Presents a five-year plan for the institute that includes discussion of the mission statement, research strategy, education and training programs, and institute structure and finance.
Published by: Babraham Institute, Babraham Institute, Babraham Hall, Babraham, Cambridge CB2 4AT, United Kingdom. TEL 44-1223-496000, FAX 44-1223-496020, babraham.contact@bbsrc.ac.uk, http://www.babraham.ac.uk. Eds. Caroline Edmonds, Mary Read, Richard Dyer. Pub. Caroline Edmonds. Circ: 1,500 (controlled).

571.1 GBR ISSN 1354-8425
BABRAHAM INSTITUTE. REPORT. Text in English. 1960. a. price varies. illus. **Document type:** *Corporate.*
Former titles (until 1994): Institute of Animal Physiology and Genetics Research. Report (0959-5783); Institute of Animal Physiology. Report (0065-4507)
Related titles: Online - full text ed.
Indexed: Anim.Breed.Abstr.
—BLDSC (1854.610700).
Published by: Babraham Institute, Babraham Institute, Babraham Hall, Babraham, Cambridge CB2 4AT, United Kingdom. TEL 44-1223-496000, FAX 44-1223-496020, babraham.contact@bbsrc.ac.uk, http://www.babraham.ac.uk. Eds. Don Powell, Mary Read. Pub. Caroline Edmonds. Circ: 1,500.

571 NLD ISSN 1567-8466
▼ **BIOCOMPLEXITY**; from molecular interaction to the living cell. Text in English. 2001. q. EUR 181.50, USD 182 to institutions for print or online ed.; EUR 218.40, USD 218.40 combined subscription to institutions for print & online eds. (effective 2002). **Document type:** *Journal, Academic/Scholarly.*
Related titles: Online - full content ed.; Online - full text ed.: (from RoweCom Information Quest).
Published by: Kluwer Academic Publishers Group (Subsidiary of: Wolters Kluwer N.V.), Spuiboulevard 50, PO Box 17, Dordrecht 3300 AA, Netherlands. TEL 31-78-639-2392, FAX 31-78-654-2254, services@wkap.nl, http://www.wkap.nl/journalhome.htm/1567-8466. Ed. Hans V Westerhoff. **Subscr. in N America to:** Kluwer Academic - Plenum Publishers, 233 Spring St, New York, NY 10013-1578. TEL 212-620-8468, 800-221-9369, FAX 212-807-1047; **Subscr. to:** Journals Department, PO Box 322, Dordrecht 3300 AH, Netherlands. TEL 31-78-639-2392, FAX 31-78-654-6474.

573.6 USA ISSN 0523-6754
CODEN: BIRSB5
BIOLOGY OF REPRODUCTION. SUPPLEMENT. Text in English. 1969. a. USD 18. back issues avail. **Document type:** *Academic/Scholarly.*
Related titles: ♦ Supplement to: Biology of Reproduction. ISSN 0006-3363.
Indexed: Biol.Abstr.
—**CCC.**
Published by: Society for the Study of Reproduction, 1603 Monroe St, Madison, WI 53711-2021. TEL 608-256-2777, FAX 608-256-4610, http://www.ssr.org/bor.

BIOLOGY OF SPORT; a quarterly journal of sport and exercise sciences. see *MEDICAL SCIENCES—Sports Medicine*

THE BREAST JOURNAL. see *MEDICAL SCIENCES—Obstetrics And Gynecology*

THE BREAST JOURNAL ONLINE. see *MEDICAL SCIENCES—Obstetrics And Gynecology*

BUREIN SAIENSU/BRAIN SCIENCE. see *MEDICAL SCIENCES—Psychiatry And Neurology*

BUREIN SAIENSU SAIZENSEN/FRONTIERS OF BRAIN SCIENCE. see *MEDICAL SCIENCES—Psychiatry And Neurology*

612 JPN ISSN 0917-6225
BYOTAI SEIRI TO SHINDAN CHIRYO/SANWA KAGAKU CO. MEDICAL REPORT. Text in Japanese. 1980. s-a.
Published by: Sanwa Kagaku Kenkyujo/Sanwa Kagaku Co., Ltd., 35 Higashi-Sotobori-cho, Higashi-ku, Nagoya-shi, Aichi-ken 461-0017, Japan.

571 JPN ISSN 0387-9666
BYOTAI SEIRI (TOKYO)/JOURNAL OF PATHOLOGICAL PHYSIOLOGY. Text in Japanese. 1964. irreg.
—**CCC.**
Published by: Tokyo Hokenkai, Byotai Seiri Kenkyujo/Tokyo Hokenkai Foundation, Pathological Physiology Laboratory, 47-11 Kumano-cho, Itabashi-ku, Tokyo 173-0025, Japan.

571 GBR ISSN 0951-077X
CODEN: CESSDT
CAMBRIDGE TEXTS IN THE PHYSIOLOGICAL SCIENCES. Text in English. 1979. irreg. price varies. **Document type:** *Monographic series.*
Indexed: Biol.Abstr.
Published by: Cambridge University Press, Edinburgh Bldg, Shaftesbury Rd, Cambridge CB2 2RU, United Kingdom. FAX 44-1223-315052, information@cup.cam.ac.uk, information@cambridge.org, http://www.cup.cam.ac.uk, http://www.uk.cambridge.org/journals/pmu. R&P Linda Nicol.

571 CAN ISSN 0008-4212
CODEN: CJPPA3
CANADIAN JOURNAL OF PHYSIOLOGY AND PHARMACOLOGY/JOURNAL CANADIEN DE PHYSIOLOGIE ET PHARMACOLOGIE. Text mainly in English; Text occasionally in French. 1929. m. CND 167 domestic to individuals; USD 167 foreign to individuals; CND 498 domestic to institutions; USD 498 foreign to institutions (effective 1999). adv. bibl, illus. index. back issues avail.; reprint service avail. from PQC. *Refereed.* **Document type:** *Academic/Scholarly.*
Formerly (until 1964): Canadian Journal of Biochemistry and Physiology (0576-5544); Which supersedes in part (in 1954): Canadian Journal of Medical Sciences (0316-4403); Which was formerly (until 1951): Canadian Journal of Research. Section E: Medical Sciences (0366-743X)
Related titles: Microfiche ed.: (from MML); Microform ed.: (from PQC,PMC,MML); Online - full text ed.: ISSN 1205-7541 (from EBSCO Publishing, O C L C Online Computer Library Center, Inc., RoweCom Information Quest, ProQuest Information & Learning, CISTI, Swets Blackwell, Institute for Scientific Information).
Indexed: ASCA, AgBiotech, Agri.& Environ.Biotech.Abstr. (coverage dropped), Anal.Abstr., Anim.Breed.Abstr., Apic.Abstr., Biodet.Abstr., Biol.Abstr., CBCA Ref., Chem.Abstr., Chem.Indus.Notes, Chem.Titles, Curr.Adv.Cell & Devel.Biol., Curr.Adv.Ecol.Sci., Curr.Cont., Dairy Sci.Abstr., Dent.Ind., Derwent Biotech.Abstr., Dok.Arbeitsmed., Environ.Sci.Poll.Mgmt., Excerp.Med., Helminthol.Abstr., Hort.Abstr., INIS Atomind., Ind.Med. (1964-), Ind.Sci.Rev., Ind.Vet., Inpharma, Int.Abstr.Biol.Sci., Med.& Surg.Dermat., Neurosci.Cit.Ind., Nutr.Abstr., Pharm.&Out.News, Pig News & Info., Pollut.Abstr., Poult.Abstr., Reac., Rev.Arom.& Med.Plants, Rev.Med.& Vet.Mycol., Risk Abstr., Saf.Sci.Abstr., Sci.Cit.Ind., Sugar Ind.Abstr., THA, Vet.Bull., Wild.Rev.
—BLDSC (3034.300000), ADONIS, CASDDS, CINDOC, CISTI, EMDOCS, GNLM, IDS, Infotrieve, ingenta, Linda Hall. **CCC.**
Published by: N R C Research Press, Building M 55, Ottawa, ON K1A 0R6, Canada. TEL 613-993-9084, FAX 013-952-7656, research.journals@nrc.ca, http://www.nrc.ca/cisti/journals/. Eds. Kanji Nakatsu, S Jacobs Kaufman. Adv. contact Judy Heyman. B&W page CND 675; trim 11 x 8.5. Circ: 854.

CARBOHYDRATE LETTERS. see *BIOLOGY—Biochemistry*

571.1 CZE ISSN 1210-6313
QP1 CODEN: CEFYAD
CESKOSLOVENSKA FYZIOLOGIE/CZECHOSLOVAK PHYSIOLOGY. Text in Czech. 1952. q. EUR 84, USD 112 (effective 2001). adv. bk.rev. charts, illus. index, cum.index every 11 yrs. *Refereed.* **Description:** Review articles on topics of current interest in human and animal physiology, pathological physiology, biochemistry, pharmacology and perspectives in biology and medicine; reports of new methods.
Formerly (until 1993): Ceskoslovenska Fyziologie (0009-0557)
Indexed: Biol.Abstr., C.I.S. Abstr., Chem.Abstr., Chem.Indus.Notes, Chem.Titles, INIS Atomind., Ind.Med. (1952-), Nutr.Abstr.
—BLDSC (3122.050000), CASDDS, CISTI, GNLM, Linda Hall.
Published by: (Ceska Lekarska Spolecnost J.E. Purkyne/Czech Medical Association), Nakladatelske Stredisko C L S J.E. Purkyne, Sokolska 31, Prague 12026, Czech Republic. TEL 42-2-24911420, FAX 42-2-24911420, nts@iol.cz, http://www.clsjep.cz, http://www.medical.cz. Ed. Jan Mares. adv.: B&W page CZK 17,700, color page CZK 26,600; 246 x 167. Circ: 1,200. **Dist. by:** Abont s.r.o., Chlumova 17, Prague, 3 130 00, Czech Republic; **Dist. in Western Countries by:** Kubon & Sagner, Hesstr 39-41, Munich 80798, Germany.

571 GBR ISSN 0379-864X
QP455 CODEN: CHSED8
CHEMICAL SENSES. Text in English. 1974. 9/yr. GBP 165, USD 275 to individuals; GBP 395, USD 650 to institutions (effective (No. 2002). adv. bk.rev. illus. index. 96 p./no. back issues avail.; reprint service avail. from SWZ. *Refereed.* **Document type:** *Journal, Academic/Scholarly.* **Description:** International forum for chemoreception research at morphological, biochemical, physiological and psychophysical levels. Covers development and specific application of new methods.
Formerly: Chemical Senses and Flavour (0302-2471)
Related titles: Online - full text ed.: ISSN 1464-3553. GBP 355, USD 585 to institutions Online only (effective 2002) (from HighWire Pr., EBSCO Publishing, O C L C Online Computer Library Center, Inc., RoweCom Information Quest, ingenta, Swets Blackwell, Institute for Scientific Information).
Indexed: ASCA, Anim.Behav.Abstr., Anim.Breed.Abstr., Aqua.Sci.& Fish.Abstr., Chem.Abstr., Chem.Indus.Notes, Chem.Titles, Chemorec.Abstr., Curr.Adv.Ecol.Sci., Curr.Cont., Curr.Ref.Fish Res., Entomol.Abstr., Excerp.Med., Food Sci.& Tech.Abstr., Ind.Med. (1980-), Ind.Sci.Rev., Ind.Vet., Inpharma, Maize Abstr., Neurosci.Abstr., Neurosci.Cit.Ind., Nutr.Abstr., Potato Abstr., PsycInfo, Psychol.Abstr. (1974-), Reac., Rev.Appl.Entomol., Rev.Med.& Vet.Mycol., SSCI (coverage dropped), Sci.Cit.Ind., Sport Fish.Abstr., Sugar Ind.Abstr., Vet.Bull., Zoo.Rec., e-psyche.
—BLDSC (3151.510000), CASDDS, CISTI, EMDOCS, GNLM, IDS, Infotrieve, ingenta, Linda Hall. **CCC.**
Published by: (European Chemoreception Organization), Oxford University Press, Academic Division, Great Clarendon St, Oxford OX2 6DP, United Kingdom. TEL 44-1865-267907, FAX 44-1865-267835, jnl.info@oup.co.uk, http://chemse.oupjournals.org/, http://www.oup.co.uk/journals. Eds. Barry Ache, R A Steinbrecht, Dr. R. Hudson. Pub. David Prosser. R&P Fionna Willis. adv.: B&W page USD 415, B&W page GBP 230; trim 178 x 255. Circ: 1,000. **U.S. subscr. to:** Oxford University Press, Journals, 2001 Evans Rd, Cary, NC 27513. TEL 800-852-7323, FAX 919-677-1714, jnlorders@oup-usa.org; **Subscr. to:** Journals Marketing, Great Clarendon St, Oxford OX2 6DP, United Kingdom. **Co-sponsor:** Association for Chemoreception Sciences.

571 CHN ISSN 0258-6428
CHINESE JOURNAL OF PHYSIOLOGICAL SCIENCES. Text in English. 1985. q. USD 145 domestic to individuals; USD 165 foreign to individuals; USD 245 domestic to institutions; USD 265 foreign to institutions (effective 1999). adv. 96 p./no. *Refereed.* **Document type:** *Academic/Scholarly.*
Related titles: ♦ Chinese ed.: Shengli Xuebao. ISSN 0371-0874.
—CISTI, EMDOCS, GNLM, KNAW.
Published by: (Shanghai Institute of Physiology), Kexue Chubanshe/Science Press, 16 Donghuang Cheng Genbei Jie, Beijing 100717, China. Circ: 6,000. **Overseas dist. by:** Science Press New York Ltd.

571 TWN ISSN 0304-4920
QP1 CODEN: CJPHDG
CHINESE JOURNAL OF PHYSIOLOGY/CHUNG-KUO SHENG LI HSUEH TSA CHIH. Text in English. 1927. q. TWD 1,600, USD 80. adv. abstr, bibl, charts, illus. **Document type:** *Academic/Scholarly.* **Description:** Contains original papers concerned with all fields of physiology, pharmacology, anatomy, and biochemistry.
Related titles: Online - full text ed.: (from Institute for Scientific Information).
Indexed: Chem.Abstr., Chem.Indus.Notes, Chem.Titles, Excerp.Med., Ind.Med. (1927-).
—BLDSC (3180.550000), CASDDS, EMDOCS, GNLM, IDS, KNAW.
Published by: Chinese Physiological Society/Chung-kuo Sheng Li Hsueh Hui, Department of Physiology, National Yan-Ming Medical College, Shih-pai, Taipei 11221, Taiwan. FAX 02-826-4049. Ed. Paulus S Wang. Circ: 1,000.

612.8 JPN ISSN 0300-0338
CHOKAKU GENGO SHOGAI/COMMUNICATION DISORDER RESEARCH. Text in Japanese; Summaries in English. 1972. q. JPY 4,000.
Indexed: e-psyche.
Published by: Chokaku Gengo Shogai Kenkyukai/Research Association of Communication Disorder, Tokyo Gakugei Daigaku Tokushu Kyoiku Shisetsu, 1-1 Nukui-Kita-Machi 4-chome, Koganei-shi, Tokyo-to 184-0015, Japan.

571 ITA ISSN 0392-3436
CINESIOLOGIA. Variant title: Quaderni di Cinesiologia. Text in Italian. 1971. q. ITL 8,000.
Published by: Edizioni Quattroventi, Via Dini, 16, Casella Postale 156, Urbino, PS 61029, Italy. TEL 39-722-2588, FAX 39-722-320998. Ed. Osvaldo Cappellini.

571 AUS ISSN 0305-1870
RM1 CODEN: CEXPB9
CLINICAL AND EXPERIMENTAL PHARMACOLOGY & PHYSIOLOGY. Text in English. 1974. m. AUD 1,099 domestic to institutions; AUD 999 in New Zealand to institutions; USD 1,010 elsewhere to institutions; AUD 1,209 domestic to institutions paper & online eds. combined; AUD 1,099 in New Zealand to institutions paper & online eds. combined; USD 1,111 elsewhere to institutions paper & online eds. combined (effective 2001). adv. back issues avail.; reprint service avail. from PQC. *Refereed.* **Document type:** *Academic/Scholarly.* **Description:** Compiles original contributions relating to the broad fields of pharmacology and physiology.
Incorporates: Australian Society for Medical Research. Proceedings (0067-2130); Which superseded (1961-1965): Medical Research (0311-9556)
Related titles: Online - full text ed.: ISSN 1440-1681. AUD 990 domestic to institutions; AUD 900 in New Zealand to institutions; USD 909 elsewhere to institutions (effective 2001) (from Ovid Technologies, Inc., EBSCO Publishing, O C L C Online Computer Library Center, Inc., RoweCom Information Quest, ingenta, Munksgaard & Blackwell Science's Synergy, Swets Blackwell, Institute for Scientific Information); ♦ Supplement: Clinical and Experimental Pharmacology & Physiology. Supplement. ISSN 0143-9294.
Indexed: ASCA, AgBiotech, Agri.& Environ.Biotech.Abstr. (coverage dropped), Anim.Breed.Abstr., Cal.Tiss.Abstr., Chem.Abstr., Chem.Indus.Notes, Chem.Titles, Curr.Adv.Ecol.Sci., Curr.Cont., Dent.Ind., Derwent Biotech.Abstr., Excerp.Med., INIS Atomind., Ind.Med. (1974-), Ind.Sci.Rev., Ind.Vet., Inpharma, Int.Abstr.Biol.Sci., Neurosci.Cit.Ind., Nutr.Abstr., Pharm.&Out.News, Pig News & Info., Reac., Rev.Arom.& Med.Plants, Sci.Cit.Ind., THA, Vet.Bull., Weed Abstr.
—BLDSC (3286.252000), ADONIS, CASDDS, CISTI, EMDOCS, GNLM, IDS, ingenta, KNAW, Linda Hall. **CCC.**
Published by: (Australasian Society of Clinical and Experimental Pharmacologists), Blackwell Science Asia Pty Ltd, PO Box 378, Carlton South, VIC 3053, Australia. TEL 61-3-9347-0300, FAX 61-3-9347-5001, info@blacksci-asia.com.au; cepp@med.monash.edu.au, http://www.blacksci.co.uk. Ed. Warwick P Anderson. Adv. contact Kathryn O'Brien. B&W page AUD 1,012, color page AUD 2,057; trim 210 x 275. Circ: 650.

571 AUS ISSN 0143-9294
CLINICAL AND EXPERIMENTAL PHARMACOLOGY & PHYSIOLOGY. SUPPLEMENT. Text in English. 1974. irreg.
Related titles: ♦ Supplement to: Clinical and Experimental Pharmacology & Physiology. ISSN 0305-1870.
Indexed: Ind.Med. (1974-).
—BLDSC (3286.252500).
Published by: Blackwell Science Asia Pty Ltd, PO Box 378, Carlton South, VIC 3053, Australia. TEL 61-3-9347-0300, FAX 61-3-9347-5001.

CLINICAL DYSMORPHOLOGY. see *BIOLOGY*

571 USA ISSN 1520-8702
CLINICAL EXERCISE PHYSIOLOGY. Text in English. q. USD 48 domestic to individuals; USD 144 domestic to institutions; USD 30 domestic to students (effective 2001). **Description:** Dedicated to practical exercise physiology related research in clinical settings.
Indexed: AMED.
—BLDSC (3286.285500).
Published by: Human Kinetics Publishers, Inc., PO Box 5076, Champaign, IL 61825-5076. TEL 800-747-4457, FAX 217-351-1549, http://www.humankinetics.com. Ed. Steven J Keteyian TEL 313-972-1920. Adv. contact David Kotarba TEL 800-747-4457 x 2389.

CLINICAL PHYSIOLOGY AND FUNCTIONAL IMAGING. see *MEDICAL SCIENCES*

571 USA
CLINICAL PHYSIOLOGY SERIES. Text in English. 1977. irreg. price varies. **Document type:** *Academic/Scholarly.* **Description:** Series is designed as a bridge between basic science and clinical medicine.
Published by: American Physiological Society, 9650 Rockville Pike, Bethesda, MD 20814-3991. TEL 301-530-7164, FAX 301-571-8305, info@aps/faseb.org, info@the-aps.org, http://www.faseb.org/aps.

571.1 AUS
COMMONWEALTH SCIENTIFIC AND INDUSTRIAL RESEARCH ORGANISATION. DIVISION OF LIVESTOCK INDUSTRIES. DIVISIONAL INFORMATION SHEETS. Text in English. 1969. irreg. free per issue. **Document type:** *Government.*
Former titles (until 2000): Commonwealth Scientific and Industrial Research Organisation. Division of Animal Production. Divisional Information Sheets; (until 1993): C.S.I.R.O. Division of Animal Production. Technical Report; (until 1975): C.S.I.R.O. Division of Animal Physiology. Technical Report (0084-9014)
Published by: C S I R O, Division of Livestock Industries, Public Affairs & Communication, Delivery Centre, Locked Bag 1, Blacktown, NSW 2148, Australia. TEL 61-2-98402700, FAX 61-2-98402940, catherine.young@li.csiro.au, http://www.li.csiro.au. R&P Pat Wilson TEL 61-2-98402741.

575.1 AUS
COMMONWEALTH SCIENTIFIC AND INDUSTRIAL RESEARCH ORGANIZATION. DIVISION OF ANIMAL PRODUCTION. DIVISIONAL INFORMATION. Text in English. irreg. **Document type:** *Corporate.*
Former titles (until 1993): C.S.I.R.O. Division of Animal Production. Research Report (0155-7742); (until 1976): C.S.I.R.O. Division of Animal Physiology. Report (0069-7281)
Indexed: Biol.Abstr.
—CISTI.
Published by: C S I R O, Division of Livestock Industries, Public Affairs & Communication, Delivery Centre, Locked Bag 1, Blacktown, NSW 2148, Australia. TEL 61-2-98402700, FAX 61-2-98402940, p.wilson@prospect.anprod.csiro.au, catherine.young@li.csiro.au, http://www.anprod.csiro.au, http://www.li.csiro.au. Ed., R&P Pat Wilson TEL 61-2-98402741.

571 USA ISSN 1095-6433
QP33 CODEN: CBPAB5
COMPARATIVE BIOCHEMISTRY AND PHYSIOLOGY. PART A: MOLECULAR & INTEGRATIVE PHYSIOLOGY. Text and summaries in English, French, German. 1961. m. EUR 4,208 in Europe to institutions; JPY 558,900 in Japan to institutions; USD 4,707 elsewhere to institutions (effective 2002). adv. bk.rev. bibl, charts, illus. back issues avail. *Refereed.* **Document type:** *Journal, Academic/Scholarly.* **Description:** Original research on the biochemistry and physiology of animals.
Former titles (until 1997): Comparative Biochemistry and Physiology. Part A: Physiology (1096-4940); (until 1994): Comparative Biochemistry and Physiology. Part A: Comparative Physiology (0300-9629)
Related titles: Microfiche ed.: (from MIM); Microfilm ed.: (from PQC); Online - full text ed.: (from ingenta, Swets Blackwell, ScienceDirect, Institute for Scientific Information).
Indexed: ASCA, AgBiotech, Agricola, Anim.Behav.Abstr., Anim.Breed.Abstr., Apic.Abstr., Aqua.Sci.& Fish.Abstr., BBCI, Bibl.Agri., Bio-Contr.News & Info., Biol.Abstr., Cal.Tiss.Abstr., Chem.Abstr., Chemorec.Abstr., Crop Physiol.Abstr., Curr.Adv.Cancer Res., Curr.Adv.Ecol.Sci., Curr.Cont., Curr.Ref.Fish Res., Dairy Sci.Abstr., Deep Sea Res.& Oceanogr.Abstr., Dent.Ind., Entomol.Abstr., Environ.Sci.Poll.Mgmt., Excerp.Med., Field Crop Abstr., Food Sci.& Tech.Abstr., Helminthol.Abstr., Herb.Abstr., Hort.Abstr., INIS Atomind., Ind.Med. (1998-), Ind.Sci.Rev., Ind.Vet., Inpharma, Int.Abstr.Biol.Sci., Key Word Ind.Wildl.Res., Maize Abstr., Neurosci.Abstr. (coverage dropped), Neurosci.Cit.Ind., Nutr.Abstr., Ocean.Abstr., Pharm.&Out.News, Pig News & Info., Plant Breed.Abstr., Pollut.Abstr., Poult.Abstr., Protozool.Abstr., Reac., Rev.Appl.Entomol., Rev.Med.& Vet.Mycol., Sci.Cit.Ind., Seed Abstr., Sel.Water Res.Abstr., Small Anim.Abstr., Soils & Fert., Soyabean Abstr., Sport Fish.Abstr., Vet.Bull., Weed Abstr., Wild.Rev., Zoo.Rec.
—BLDSC (3363.751000), ADONIS, CISTI, EMDOCS, GNLM, ingenta, Linda Hall. **CCC.**
Published by: Elsevier Science, Box 945, New York, NY 10159-0945. TEL 212-989-5800, FAX 212-633-3990, usinfo-f@elsevier.com, http://www.elsevier.com/locate/cbpa. Eds. Peter W Hochachka, Thomas P Mommsen. adv.: B&W page USD 550, color page USD 1,350. Circ: 2,000. **Subscr. in Australasia and the Far East to:** Elsevier Science (Singapore) Pte Ltd, No.1 Temasek Ave, 17-01 Millenia Tower, Singapore 039192, Singapore. TEL 65-434-3727, FAX 65-337-2230; **Subscr. in Japan to:** Elsevier Science Inc - Japan Regional Office, 9-15 Higashi-Azabu 1-chome, Minato-ku, Tokyo 106-0044, Japan. TEL 81-3-5561-5033; **Subscr. outside the Americas to:** Elsevier Science BV, PO Box 211, Amsterdam 1000 AE, Netherlands. TEL 31-20-485-3757, FAX 31-20-485-3432.

COMPARATIVE BIOCHEMISTRY AND PHYSIOLOGY. PART B: BIOCHEMISTRY & MOLECULAR BIOLOGY. see *BIOLOGY—Biochemistry*

B

571.3 IND ISSN 0379-0436
QH540 CODEN: CPECDM
COMPARATIVE PHYSIOLOGY AND ECOLOGY. Text in English. 1976. q. USD 28.
Indexed: Appl.Ecol.Abstr. (coverage dropped), Aqua.Sci.& Fish.Abstr., Aquacult.Abstr., Bio-Contr.News & Info., Biol.Abstr., Chem.Abstr., Curr.Adv.Ecol.Sci., Curr.Cont. (coverage dropped), Curr.Ref.Fish Res., Entomol.Abstr., Environ.Sci.Poll.Mgmt., Excerp.Med., Field Crop Abstr., Genet.Abstr., Helminthol.Abstr., Hort.Abstr., Hum.Gen.Abstr., INIS Atomind., Ind.Sci.Rev., Ind.Vet., Ocean.Abstr., Poult.Abstr., Rice Abstr., Sci.Cit.Ind. (coverage dropped), Soils & Fert., Vet.Bull., Weed Abstr.
—CASDDS, CISTI, Infotrieve, Linda Hall. **CCC.**
Published by: Impex India, M-S Premier Publication, 863 Sadarpura, Behind Syndicate Bank, Jodhpur, Rajasthan 342 003, India.

571 GBR ISSN 0143-2044
CODEN: CRLED9
CRYOLETTERS. Text in English. 1979. bi-m. GBP 48, USD 80 to individuals; GBP 96, USD 160 to institutions (effective 2002). adv. bk.rev. index. Supplement avail. *Refereed.* **Document type:** *Newsletter, Proceedings, Academic/Scholarly.* **Description:** Contains original research reports, authoritative reviews, technical developments and commissioned book reviews of studies involving low temperature techniques in the investigation of physical chemical, biological and ecological problems, or the effects produced by low temperatures in a wide variety of scientific and technical processes.
Related titles: Online - full text ed.: (from Institute for Scientific Information).
Indexed: ASCA, AgBiotech, Agricola, Anim.Breed.Abstr., Bibl.Agri., Biol.Abstr., Chem.Abstr., Chem.Indus.Notes, Chem.Titles, Crop Physiol.Abstr., Curr.Adv.Biochem., Curr.Adv.Cell & Devel.Biol., Curr.Adv.Ecol.Sci., Curr.Adv.Plant Sci., Curr.Cont., Field Crop Abstr., Forest.Abstr., Hort.Abstr., Ind.Sci.Rev., Inpharma, Int.Abstr.Biol.Sci., Maize Abstr., Plant Breed.Abstr., Plant Gen.Res.Abstr., Plant Grow.Reg.Abstr., Plant Sci., Potato Abstr., Reac., Ref.Zh., Rev.Appl.Entomol., Rev.Med.& Vet.Mycol., Rice Abstr., Sci.Cit.Ind., Seed Abstr., Sport Fish.Abstr., Sugar Ind.Abstr., Zoo.Rec.
—BLDSC (3490.133000), CASDDS, CISTI, EMDOCS, IDS, ingenta. **CCC.**
Address: Royal Veterinary College, Dept. of Veterinary Basic Sciences, Royal College St, London NW1 0TU, United Kingdom. FAX 44-20-7388-1027, cryoletters@rvc.ac.uk, http://www.rvc.ac.uk/cryoletters/home.htm. Ed., Pub., R&P, Adv. contact P F Watson. Circ: 250 (paid).

CURRENT MEDICAL LITERATURE. G H AND GROWTH FACTORS. see *MEDICAL SCIENCES*

CURRENT OPINION IN NEUROBIOLOGY. see *MEDICAL SCIENCES—Psychiatry And Neurology*

CURRENT TOPICS IN NEUROBIOLOGY. see *MEDICAL SCIENCES—Psychiatry And Neurology*

612.821 USA ISSN 1053-0797
BF1074 CODEN: DRMGEW
DREAMING. Text in English. 1991. q. USD 322 to institutions for print or online ed.; EUR 321 to institutions for print or online eds.; USD 366.40, EUR 365.20 to institutions for print & online eds.combined (effective 2002). adv. *Refereed.* **Document type:** *Journal, Academic/Scholarly.* **Description:** Provides a forum for biological and physiological studies involving sleep and dream research, psychological studies, psychoanalytic investigations, and papers on the link between dreams and art, literature, and other human activities.
Related titles: Online - full text ed.: (from EBSCO Publishing, O C L C Online Computer Library Center, Inc., RoweCom Information Quest, Swets Blackwell, Kluwer Online, Institute for Scientific Information).
Indexed: ASCA, Arts & Hum.Cit.Ind. (coverage dropped), Curr.Cont., Fam.Ind., PsycInfo, Psychol.Abstr. (1991-), SSCI, e-psyche.
—BLDSC (3623.341400), GNLM, IDS, ingenta. **CCC.**
Published by: (Association for the Study of Dreams), Kluwer Academic - Plenum Publishers (Subsidiary of: Wolters Kluwer N.V.), 233 Spring St, New York, NY 10013-1578. TEL 212-620-8000, 800-221-9369, FAX 212-463-0742, services@wkap.nl, info@plenum.com, http://www.wkap.nl/journalhome.htm/1053-0797. Ed. Deirdre L Barrett. **Subscr. outside the Americas to:** Kluwer Academic Publishers Group, Journals Department, PO Box 322, Dordrecht 3300 AH, Netherlands. TEL 31-78-639-2392, FAX 31-78-654-6474.

571 EGY ISSN 0301-8660
QH301
EGYPTIAN JOURNAL OF PHYSIOLOGICAL SCIENCE. Text in English; Summaries in Arabic, English. 1974. 3/yr. USD 112 (effective 2000). abstr, charts, illus. back issues avail.; reprint service avail. from IRC. **Document type:** *Academic/Scholarly.*
Formerly: Egyptian Journal of Physiology
Indexed: Biol.Abstr., Chem.Abstr., Chem.Indus.Notes, Chem.Titles, Crop Physiol.Abstr., Dairy Sci.Abstr., Field Crop Abstr., Hort.Abstr., Ind.Vet., Maize Abstr., Nutr.Abstr., Ornam.Hort., Plant Breed.Abstr., Plant Grow.Reg.Abstr., Rev.Appl.Entomol., Rev.Med.& Vet.Mycol., Rev.Plant Path., Seed Abstr., Soils & Fert., Soyabean Abstr., Triticale Abstr., Vet.Bull., Weed Abstr.
—BLDSC (3664.417000), CASDDS, CISTI, GNLM, Linda Hall.
Published by: (Egyptian Physiological Society, Research Department), National Information and Documentation Centre (NIDOC), Tahrir St., Dokki, Awqaf P.O., Cairo, Egypt. TEL 20-2-3371696. Ed. M M El Fouly. Circ: 1,000.

ELECTROMYOGRAPHY AND CLINICAL NEUROPHYSIOLOGY. see *MEDICAL SCIENCES—Psychiatry And Neurology*

ENDOCRINE. see *MEDICAL SCIENCES—Endocrinology*

ENDOTHELIUM. see *BIOLOGY—Abstracting, Bibliographies, Statistics*

EUROPEAN JOURNAL OF ANATOMY. see *MEDICAL SCIENCES*

571 DEU ISSN 1439-6319
QP1 CODEN: EJAPCK
EUROPEAN JOURNAL OF APPLIED PHYSIOLOGY. Text in English. m. EUR 2,611.10 domestic; EUR 2,600.70 in Germany; EUR 258 newsstand/cover foreign (effective 2002). reprint service avail. from ISI. *Refereed.* **Document type:** *Journal, Academic/Scholarly.* **Description:** Contains articles with an emphasis on environmental and work physiology.
Former titles (until vol.81, no.3): European Journal of Applied Physiology and Occupational Physiology (0301-5548); Internationale Zeitschrift fuer Angewandte Physiologie Einschliesslich Arbeitsphysiologie (0020-9376)
Related titles: Microform ed.: (from PQC); Online - full text ed.: ISSN 1439-6327 (from EBSCO Publishing, RoweCom Information Quest, Swets Blackwell, Springer LINK, Institute for Scientific Information).
Indexed: AMED, ASCA, Biol.Abstr., C.I.S. Abstr., Chem.Abstr., Chem.Indus.Notes, Chem.Titles, Curr.Adv.Biochem., Curr.Adv.Ecol.Sci., Curr.Cont., Environ.Sci.Poll.Mgmt., Ergon.Abstr., Excerp.Med., Focus on: Sports Sci.& Med., HRIS, INIS Atomind., Ind.Med. (coverage dropped), Ind.Sci.Rev., Inpharma, Neurosci.Cit.Ind., Nutr.Abstr., Pharm.&Out.News, Phys.Ed.Ind., Pollut.Abstr., Reac., Risk Abstr., SSCI (coverage dropped), Saf.Sci.Abstr., Sci.Cit.Ind., Sportsearch (1975-), Sugar Ind.Abstr., THA, Trop.Dis.Bull.
—BLDSC (3829.722450), CASDDS, CISTI, EMDOCS, GNLM, IDS, ingenta. **CCC.**
Published by: Springer-Verlag (Subsidiary of: BertelsmannSpringer), Tiergartenstr 17, Heidelberg 69121, Germany. TEL 49-6221-345-0, FAX 49-6221-345229, subscriptions@springer.de, http://link.springer.de/link/service/journals/00421/index.htm, http://www.springer.de. Ed. P E de Prampero. **Subscr. in N. America to:** Springer-Verlag New York Inc., PO Box 2485, Secaucus, NJ 07096-2485. TEL 212-460-1500, FAX 212-473-6272.

EUROPEAN JOURNAL OF MORPHOLOGY; incorporating european archives & biology. see *BIOLOGY*

EXCERPTA MEDICA. SECTION 1: ANATOMY, ANTHROPOLOGY, EMBRYOLOGY & HISTOLOGY. see *BIOLOGY—Abstracting, Bibliographies, Statistics*

EXCERPTA MEDICA. SECTION 2: PHYSIOLOGY. see *MEDICAL SCIENCES—Abstracting, Bibliographies, Statistics*

EXCERPTA MEDICA. SECTION 21: DEVELOPMENTAL BIOLOGY AND TERATOLOGY. see *BIOLOGY—Abstracting, Bibliographies, Statistics*

571.1 GBR ISSN 0958-0670
QP1 CODEN: EXPHEZ
EXPERIMENTAL PHYSIOLOGY. Text in English. 1908. bi-m. USD 471 to institutions (effective 2002). adv. bk.rev. Supplement avail.; back issues avail. *Refereed.* **Document type:** *Academic/Scholarly.* **Description:** Contains research papers on all aspects of experimental physiology from molecular to animal studies.
Former titles: Quarterly Journal of Experimental Physiology; Quarterly Journal of Experimental Physiology and Cognate Medical Sciences (0144-8757)
Related titles: Microform ed.: (from PQC,PMC); Online - full text ed.: ISSN 1469-445X (from EBSCO Publishing, O C L C Online Computer Library Center, Inc., RoweCom Information Quest, Swets Blackwell, Institute for Scientific Information).
Indexed: ASCA, Anim.Breed.Abstr., Biol.Abstr., Chem.Abstr., Chem.Indus.Notes, Chem.Titles, Curr.Adv.Biochem., Curr.Adv.Ecol.Sci., Curr.Cont., Dairy Sci.Abstr., Excerp.Med., Ind.Med. (1990-), Ind.Sci.Rev., Ind.Vet., Inpharma, Int.Abstr.Biol.Sci., Neurosci.Cit.Ind., Nutr.Abstr., Pharm.&Out.News, Pig News & Info., Poult.Abstr., Reac., Ref.Zh., Rev.Arom.& Med.Plants, Rice Abstr., Sci.Cit.Ind., Small Anim.Abstr., THA, Vet.Bull.
—BLDSC (3840.040000), CASDDS, CISTI, EMDOCS, GNLM, IDS, ingenta, KNAW, Linda Hall.
Published by: (Physiological Society), Cambridge University Press, Edinburgh Bldg, Shaftesbury Rd, Cambridge CB2 2RU, United Kingdom. FAX 44-1223-315052, information@cup.cam.ac.uk, information@cambridge.org, http://www.cup.cam.ac.uk/, http://www.uk.cambridge.org/journals/pmu. Eds. J Gillespie, J.H. Coote. R&P Linda Nicol. Adv. contact Rebecca Symons. Circ: 750.

▼ **F E M S YEAST RESEARCH.** see *BIOLOGY—Microbiology*

571 UKR ISSN 0533-1153
CODEN: FAVUAI
FIZIOLOGICHESKI AKTIVNYE VESHCHESTVA; respublikanskii mezhvedomstvennyi sbornik nauchnykh trudov. Text in Russian. 1966. a.
Indexed: Chem.Abstr., Chem.Indus.Notes, Chem.Titles.
—CASDDS, Infotrieve, Linda Hall. **CCC.**
Published by: Natsional'na Akademiya Nauk Ukrainy, Institut Organicheskoi Khimii, Vul Tereshchenkivska 3, Kiev 252601, Ukraine. TEL 044-224-4068, FAX 044-224-7060, iochkiev@sovam.com. **Dist. by:** Mezhdunarodnaya Kniga, B Yakimanka 39, Moscow 117049, Russian Federation.

571 RUS
QP1 CODEN: FZLZAM
FIZIOLOGICHESKII ZHURNAL IM. SECHENOVA/ SECHENOV PHYSIOLOGICAL JOURNAL. Text in Russian; Summaries in English. 1917. m. USD 310. bk.rev. bibl, charts, illus. index.
Formerly: Fiziologicheskii Zhurnal S.S.S.R. im. Sechenova (0015-329X)
Indexed: Anim.Breed.Abstr., Biol.Abstr., Chem.Abstr., Curr.Adv.Ecol.Sci., Dent.Ind., Excerp.Med., Helminthol.Abstr., Ind.Med. (coverage dropped), Int.Aerosp.Abstr., Nutr.Abstr., Poult.Abstr., PsycInfo, Psychol.Abstr. (1932-), Ref.Zh., Russ.Acad.Sci.Bibl., SSCI (coverage dropped), Sci.Cit.Ind. (coverage dropped), Vet.Bull., e-psyche.
—CASDDS, CISTI, East View, GNLM, Infotrieve, Linda Hall. **CCC.**
Published by: (Rossiiskaya Akademiya Nauk/Russian Academy of Sciences), M A I K Nauka - Interperiodica, S.-Peterburgskoe Otdelenie, Mendeleevskaya liniya 1, St Petersburg 199034, Russian Federation. TEL 812-218-37-12. Ed. Y V Natochin. Circ: 2,000. **Dist. by:** Mezhdunarodnaya Kniga, B Yakimanka 39, Moscow 117049, Russian Federation. TEL 7-095-2384967, FAX 7-095-2384634; **US dist. addr.:** East View Publications, 3020 Harbor Ln N, Minneapolis, MN 55447. TEL 612-550-0961.

571 UKR ISSN 0201-8489
QP1 CODEN: FIZHDO
FIZIOLOGICHESKII ZHURNAL (KIEV)/FIZIOLOGICHNYI ZHURNAL; nauchno-teoreticheskii zhurnal. Text in Russian, Ukrainian; Summaries in English. 1955. bi-m. USD 42. bk.rev. illus. index.
Formerly (until 1978): Fiziologichnyi Zhurnal (0015-3311)
Indexed: Biol.Abstr., Chem.Abstr., Djerelo, Excerp.Med., INIS Atomind., Ind.Med. (coverage dropped), Ind.Sci.Rev., Neurosci.Cit.Ind., Poult.Abstr., Ref.Zh., Vet.Bull.
—CASDDS, CISTI, East View, GNLM, Infotrieve, KNAW, Linda Hall. **CCC.**
Published by: Natsional'na Akademiya Nauk Ukrainy, Institut Fiziologii im. Bogomol'tsya, Vul Bogomol'tsya 4, Kiev 252601, Ukraine. TEL 380-44-2930745. Ed. Ph N Serkov. **Dist. by:** Mezhdunarodnaya Kniga, B Yakimanka 39, Moscow 117049, Russian Federation. TEL 7-095-2384967, FAX 7-095-2384634; **US dist. addr.:** East View Publications, 3020 Harbor Ln N, Minneapolis, MN 55447. TEL 612-550-0961.

571 RUS ISSN 0131-1646
QP34.5 CODEN: FICHDB
FIZIOLOGIYA CHELOVEKA. Text in Russian. 1975. bi-m. USD 236. illus. **Description:** Publishes studies on the physiology of work, speech, and sport, emphasizing their relationship to the physiology of the brain and the neurophysiology of psychological activity.
Related titles: Online - full text ed.; ♦ English Translation: Human Physiology. ISSN 0362-1197.
Indexed: Biol.Abstr., Chem.Abstr., Chem.Indus.Notes, Chem.Titles, INIS Atomind., Ind.Med. (1975-), Int.Aerosp.Abstr., Ref.Zh.
—CASDDS, CISTI, East View, GNLM, KNAW, Linda Hall.
Published by: (Rossiiskaya Akademiya Nauk/Russian Academy of Sciences), M A I K Nauka - Interperiodica, Mezhdunarodnyi Otdel, Profsoyuznaya ul 90, Moscow 117864, Russian Federation. TEL 7-095-336-1600, FAX 7-095-336-0666, compmg@maik.ru, http://www.maik.rssi.ru/journals/humphys.htm. Ed. Vsevolod I Medvedev. **Dist. by:** Mezhdunarodnaya Kniga, B Yakimanka 39, Moscow 117049, Russian Federation; **US dist. addr.:** Kluwer Academic Publishers, PO Box 17, Dordrecht 3300 AH, Netherlands. TEL 31-78-392392, FAX 31-78-546474, http://www.wkap.nl.

571 UKR ISSN 0256-1425
QK710 CODEN: FBKRAT
FIZIOLOGIYA I BIOKHIMIYA KUL'TURNYKH RASTENII/PHYSIOLOGY AND BIOCHEMISTRY OF CULTIVATED PLANTS; nauchno-teoreticheskii zhurnal. Text in Russian; Summaries in English, Russian, Ukrainian. 1969. bi-m. UAK 31.80 domestic; USD 97.04 foreign (effective 2001). abstr. 92 p./no. **Description:** Covers fundamental aspects of theoretical and experimental plant physiology and biochemistry, physiological genetics and genetic engineering. Publishes the results of original research, reviews, short communications, and methodological articles concerning the aforementioned subjects as well as cell and molecular biology, biotechnology and ecology. Also includes information on conferences, congresses and symposia.
Media: Large Type (10 pt.).
Indexed: Biol.Abstr., Chem.Abstr., Chem.Indus.Notes, Chem.Titles, Cott.& Trop.Fibr.Abstr., Crop Physiol.Abstr., Curr.Adv.Ecol.Sci., Djerelo, Field Crop Abstr., Herb.Abstr., Hort.Abstr., INIS Atomind., Ind.Sci.Rev., Maize Abstr., Plant Breed.Abstr., Plant Grow.Reg.Abstr., Potato Abstr., Rev.Arom.& Med.Plants, Rev.Plant Path., Rice Abstr., Sci.Cit.Ind. (coverage dropped), Seed Abstr., Soils & Fert., Soyabean Abstr., Triticale Abstr., Weed Abstr.
—BLDSC (0390.250000), CISTI, Linda Hall.
Published by: (Institut Fiziologii Roslin ta Genetiki, Natsional'na Akademiya Nauk Ukrainy), Izdatel'stvo Logos, Vul Vasyl'kivs'ka 31-17, Kiev, Ukraine. TEL 380-44-2630114, FAX 380-44-2635150, plant@ifrg.freenet.kiev.ua. Ed. V V Morgun. **Dist. by:** Mezhdunarodnaya Kniga, B Yakimanka 39, Moscow 117049, Russian Federation; **Dist. in U.S. by:** Victor Kamkin Inc., 4956 Boiling Brook Pkwy, Rockville, MD 20852.

GENE; an international journal focusing on gene cloning and gene structure and function. see *BIOLOGY—Biotechnology*

571 SVK ISSN 0231-5882
QP1 CODEN: GPBIE2
GENERAL PHYSIOLOGY AND BIOPHYSICS. Text in English. 1982. q. USD 215 (effective 2000). bk.rev. back issues avail. *Refereed.* **Document type:** *Academic/Scholarly.* **Description:** Publishes original scientific studies within the sphere of general physiology, biophysics and biochemistry at the cellular and molecular levels, along with papers relating the progress and development of the respective research techniques and methods.
Related titles: E-mail ed.; Fax ed.; Online - full text ed.: (from Institute for Scientific Information).
Indexed: ASCA, BBCI, Chem.Abstr., Chem.Indus.Notes, Chem.Titles, Curr.Adv.Ecol.Sci., Curr.Cont., Dairy Sci.Abstr., Ind.Med. (1982-), Ind.Sci.Rev., Inpharma, Pharm.&Out.News, Reac., Ref.Zh., Sci.Cit.Ind., Soils & Fert., Zoo.Rec.
—BLDSC (4106.725000), CASDDS, CISTI, EMDOCS, GNLM, IDS, ingenta, KNAW.
Published by: Slovak Academy of Sciences, Institute of Molecular Physiology and Genetics, Vlarska 5, Bratislava 83334, Slovakia. TEL 421-7-54772111, FAX 421-7-54773666, umfguhrk@savba.savba.sk, http://www.savba.sk/logos/journals/gpb/gpb.html. Ed. Branislav Uhrik. **Dist. by:** Raud D. Print, Gwerkovej 6, Bratislava 85104, Slovakia; Karger Libri AG, Petersgraben 31, Basel 4011, Switzerland.

571 JPN
GIFU DAIGAKU IGAKUBU HANSHA KENKYU SHISETSU GYOSEKISHU/GIFU UNIVERSITY. SCHOOL OF MEDICINE. INSTITUTE OF EQUILIBRIUM RESEARCH. BULLETIN. Text in English, Japanese. 1974. every 3 yrs.
Published by: Gifu Daigaku, Igakubu/Gifu University, School of Medicine, Hansha Kenkyu Shisetsu Hansha Seirigaku Bumon, 40 Tsukasa-Machi, Gifu-shi 500-8705, Japan. TEL 81-58-265-1241 ext 2300, FAX 81-58-267-2954.

571 CHE ISSN 0897-7194
QP552.G76 CODEN: GRFAEC
GROWTH FACTORS. Text in English. 1989. 4/yr. GBP 107, USD 129, EUR 142 to individuals; GBP 483, USD 632, EUR 643 to institutions; GBP 791, USD 1,036, EUR 1,055 to corporations (effective 2002). *Refereed.* **Document type:** *Journal, Academic/Scholarly.*
Related titles: CD-ROM ed.; Microform ed.; Online - full text ed.: (from RoweCom Information Quest, Institute for Scientific Information).
Indexed: AIDS & Cancer Res., ASCA, BBCI, Curr.Cont., Food Sci.& Tech.Abstr., Ind.Med. (1988-), Ind.Sci.Rev., Inpharma, Int.Abstr.Biol.Sci., Oncog.G.F.Abstr., Reac., Sci.Cit.Ind.
—BLDSC (4223.032950), CISTI, EMDOCS, GNLM, ingenta, KNAW. **CCC.**
Published by: Gordon and Breach - Harwood Academic (Subsidiary of: Taylor & Francis Group), PO Box 531, Lausanne 1000, Switzerland. TEL 41-21-6411280, FAX 41-21-6411281, info@gbhap.com, http://www.gbhap.com/Growth_Factors/. Ed. A W Burgess. **Subscr. addr. in US:** International Publishers Direct, PO Box 32160, Newark, NJ 07102. FAX 215-750-6343.

H F S P WORKSHOP. see *MEDICAL SCIENCES*

571 USA ISSN 0072-9876
HANDBOOK OF PHYSIOLOGY. Text in English. 1959. irreg. price varies. *Refereed.* **Document type:** *Monographic series.* **Description:** Provides a comprehensive but critical presentation of the state of knowledge in the various fields of functional biology.
Indexed: Biol.Abstr.
Published by: American Physiological Society, 9650 Rockville Pike, Bethesda, MD 20814-3991. TEL 301-530-7164, FAX 301-571-8305, info@aps.faseb.org, info@the-aps.org, http://www.faseb.org/aps.

571 JPN ISSN 0385-5716
HEIKO SHINKEI KAGAKU/EQUILIBRIUM RESEARCH. Text in Japanese; Summaries in English. 1957. bi-m. JPY 10,000. back issues avail. *Refereed.* **Document type:** *Academic/Scholarly.* **Description:** Contains review and original articles on vestibular neuroscience and medicine.
Indexed: Excerp.Med.
—BLDSC (3794.509700), EMDOCS, GNLM.
Published by: Nihon Heiko Shinkeika Gakkai/Japan Society for Equilibrium Research, 39 Kawabata-Higashi Marutamachi-dori, Sakyo-ku, Kyoto-shi 606-8395, Japan. TEL 81-75-751-0068, FAX 81-75-751-0068, js-er@mbox.kyoto-inet.or.jp. Ed. Yu Yoshimoto. Circ: 2,000.

571 JPN ISSN 0916-0337
HEIKO SHINKEI KAGAKU. SUPPLEMENT/EQUILIBRIUM RESEARCH. SUPPLEMENT. Text in Japanese; Summaries in English. 1987. irreg.
—BLDSC (3794.509710).
Published by: Nihon Heiko Shinkeika Gakkai/Japan Society for Equilibrium Research, 30 Kawabata-higashi Marutamachi-dori, Sakyo-ku, Kyoto-shi 606-8395, Japan. TEL 81-75-751-0068, FAX 81-75-751-0068, js-er@mbox.kyoto-inet.or.jp.

HUMAN BRAIN MAPPING. see *MEDICAL SCIENCES—Psychiatry And Neurology*

HUMAN DEVELOPMENT. see *MEDICAL SCIENCES*

HUMAN PHYSIOLOGY. see *MEDICAL SCIENCES*

HUMAN REPRODUCTION UPDATE. see *BIOLOGY—Abstracting, Bibliographies, Statistics*

616.178059 USA ISSN 1077-3975
IN VITRO REPORT. Text in English. 1950. bi-m. USD 40; USD 55 foreign (effective 1998). adv. *Refereed.* **Document type:** *Monographic series, Proceedings, Academic/Scholarly.* **Description:** Contains news and notes about branches, sections, committees, and members of the society, placement service, notice of events of interest, and short articles.
Formerly (until 1994): T C A Report (0163-772X)
Published by: Society for In Vitro Biology, 9315 Largo Dr. W., Ste. 255, Largo, MD 20774. TEL 301-324-5054, FAX 301-324-5057, sivb@sivb.org, http://www.sivb.org. Ed. Sandra Schneider. Adv. contact Denise McCall. Circ: 2,100. **Subscr. to:** PO Box 73230, Baltimore, MD 21273.

571 IND ISSN 0019-5499
QP1 CODEN: IJPPAZ
INDIAN JOURNAL OF PHYSIOLOGY AND PHARMACOLOGY. Text in English. 1957. q. INR 2,000, USD 100 (effective 2000). adv. bk.rev. bibl, charts, illus. index. back issues avail. *Refereed.* **Document type:** *Academic/Scholarly.*
Related titles: CD-ROM ed.
Indexed: Appl.Mech.Rev., Biol.Abstr., Chem.Abstr., Chem.Indus.Notes, Chem.Titles, Curr.Adv.Ecol.Sci., Excerp.Med., ExtraMED, INIS Atomind., Ind.Med. (1957-), Rev.Med.& Vet.Mycol., Vet.Bull.
—BLDSC (4420.130000), CASDDS, CISTI, GNLM, ingenta, KNAW, Linda Hall.
Published by: Association of Physiologists and Pharmacologists of India, Department of Physiology, All India Institute of Medical Sciences, Ansari Nagar, New Delhi 110 029, India. TEL 91-11-6594812, FAX 91-11-6862663, TELEX 31-73042 AIMS IN, rambij@medinst.ernet.in. Ed., Pub., R&P, Adv. contact D Ghosh TEL 91-11-6963826. Circ: 20,000. **Dist. by:** H P C Publishers Distributors Pvt. Ltd., 1st Fl., Flats 1 & 2, Darya Ganj, 4805-24 Bharat Ram Rd., New Delhi 110 002, India. TEL 91-11-325-4402, FAX 91-11-686-3511.

612 611 GBR
▼ **INSIDE THE HUMAN BODY.** Text in English. 1999. w. GBP 1.70 newsstand/cover (effective 2000). **Document type:** *Academic/Scholarly, Consumer.* **Description:** Provides a comprehensive and up-to-date collection of everything one ever wanted to know about the human body - how it works, what can go wrong, and how it is treated.
Published by: Bright Star Publishing plc, 179 Dalling Rd, London W6 0ES, United Kingdom. subs@midsubs.com, http://www.brightstar.co.uk. **Dist. by:** Comag, Tavistock Works, Tavistock Rd, W Drayton, Middx UB7 7QX, United Kingdom. TEL 44-1895-444055, FAX 44-1895-433602.

INTEGRATIVE PHYSIOLOGICAL AND BEHAVIORAL SCIENCE. see *MEDICAL SCIENCES—Psychiatry And Neurology*

INVERTEBRATE NEUROBIOLOGY. see *BIOLOGY—Abstracting, Bibliographies, Statistics*

571 RUS ISSN 0134-2673
QP1 CODEN: INTFCL
ITOGI NAUKI I TEKHNIKI. FIZIOLOGIYA CHELOVEKA I ZHIVOTNYKH. Text in Russian. irreg., latest vol.38, 1989.
—Linda Hall.
Published by: Vserossiiskii Institut Nauchnoi i Tekhnicheskoi Informatsii (VINITI), Usievicha ul 20-a, Moscow 125315, Russian Federation. TEL 7-095-1526441, FAX 7-095-943-0060. **Dist. by:** Mezhdunarodnaya Kniga, B Yakimanka 39, Moscow 117049, Russian Federation. TEL 7-095-2384967, FAX 7-095-2384634; **US dist. addr.:** East View Publications, 3020 Harbor Ln N, Minneapolis, MN 55447. TEL 612-550-0961.

571 RUS ISSN 0202-7186
CODEN: ITFRDU
ITOGI NAUKI I TEKHNIKI. FIZIOLOGIYA RASTENII. Text in Russian. irreg.
—CASDDS, Linda Hall.
Published by: Vserossiiskii Institut Nauchnoi i Tekhnicheskoi Informatsii (VINITI), Usievicha ul 20-a, Moscow 125315, Russian Federation. TEL 7-095-1526441, FAX 7-095-943-0060. **US dist. addr.:** East View Publications, 3020 Harbor Ln N, Minneapolis, MN 55447. TEL 612-550-0961.

571 JPN ISSN 0021-521X
QP1 CODEN: JJPHAM
JAPANESE JOURNAL OF PHYSIOLOGY. Text in English. 1951. bi-m. USD 160. *Refereed.* **Document type:** *Academic/Scholarly.*
Related titles: Online - full text ed.: (from Institute for Scientific Information).
Indexed: ASCA, Aqua.Sci.& Fish.Abstr., Biol.Abstr., Chem.Abstr., Chem.Indus.Notes, Chem.Titles, Curr.Cont., Dairy Sci.Abstr., Dent.Ind., Excerp.Med., INIS Atomind., Ind.Med. (1950-), Ind.Sci.Rev., Inpharma, Int.Abstr.Biol.Sci., Neurosci.Cit.Ind., Nutr.Abstr., Pharm.&Out.News, Reac., SSCI (coverage dropped), Sci.Cit.Ind., THA, Zoo.Rec.
—BLDSC (4658.000000), CASDDS, CISTI, GNLM, IDS, ingenta, KNAW, Linda Hall. **CCC.**
Published by: (Physiological Society of Japan), Center for Academic Publications Japan, 2-4-16 Yayoi, Bunkyo-ku, Tokyo 113-0032, Japan. TEL 03-3817-5821, FAX 03-3817-5830, capj@crisscross.com. Ed. Hiroyuki Suga. Circ: 1,600. **Dist. by:** Business Center for Academic Societies Japan, 5-16-9 Honkomagome, Bunkyo-ku, Tokyo 113-0021, Japan. TEL 03-5814-5811, FAX 03-5814-5822.

JOURNAL OF ANIMAL MORPHOLOGY AND PHYSIOLOGY. see *BIOLOGY*

571.1 DEU ISSN 0931-2439
SF95 CODEN: ZTTFAA
JOURNAL OF ANIMAL PHYSIOLOGY AND ANIMAL NUTRITION/ZEITSCHRIFT FUER TIERPHYSIOLOGIE UND TIERERNAEHRUNG. Text in English; Summaries in English, German. 1938. bi-m. DEM 1,507.95 in Europe; DEM 1,537.28 elsewhere; DEM 1,658.75 in Europe print & online eds. combined; DEM 1,691.01 elsewhere print & online eds. combined (effective 2001). adv. bk.rev. abstr, bibl, charts, illus. index. back issues avail. *Refereed.* **Document type:** *Journal, Academic/Scholarly.* **Description:** Publishes research in the fields of animal physiology, physiology and biochemistry of nutrition, animal feeding, feed technology, and food preservation.
Formerly (until 1986): Zeitschrift fuer Tierphysiologie, Tierernaehrung und Futtermittelkunde (0044-3565)
Related titles: ♦ Online - full text ed.: Journal of Animal Physiology and Animal Nutrition Online. ISSN 1439-0396; ♦ Supplement: Advances in Animal Physiology and Animal Nutrition. ISSN 0301-2743.
Indexed: ASCA, Agri.& Environ.Biotech.Abstr. (coverage dropped), Anim.Breed.Abstr., Aqua.Sci.& Fish.Abstr., Aquacult.Abstr., Biol.Abstr., Chem.Abstr., Chem.Indus.Notes, Chem.Titles, Curr.Cont., Dairy Sci.Abstr., Derwent Biotech.Abstr., Environ.Sci.Poll.Mgmt., Excerp.Med., Fababean Abstr., Field Crop Abstr., Focus on: Vet.Sci.& Med., Food Sci.& Tech.Abstr., Genet.Abstr., Helminthol.Abstr., Herb.Abstr., Hum.Gen.Abstr., INIS Atomind., Ind.Sci.Rev., Ind.Vet., Key Word Ind.Wildl.Res., Maize Abstr., Nutr.Abstr., Pig News & Info., Pollut.Abstr., Potato Abstr., Poult.Abstr., Psychol.Abstr., Ref.Zh., Rev.Appl.Entomol., Sci.Cit.Ind., Seed Abstr., Soyabean Abstr., Sport Fish.Abstr., Sugar Ind.Abstr., Triticale Abstr., Vet.Bull., Weed Abstr., Wild.Rev., Zoo.Rec.
—BLDSC (4936.600000), CASDDS, CISTI, GNLM, IDS, Infotrieve, ingenta. **CCC.**

B

Published by: Blackwell Wissenschafts Verlag GmbH, Kurfuerstendamm 57, Berlin 10707, Germany. TEL 49-30-32790665, FAX 49-30-32790610, abo@blackwis.de, http://www.blackwell.de. Ed. M Kirchgessner. adv.: B&W page DEM 560; trim 122 x 190. Circ: 400.

571.1 DEU ISSN 1439-0396
JOURNAL OF ANIMAL PHYSIOLOGY AND ANIMAL NUTRITION ONLINE. Text in English, German. 10/yr. DEM 1,358 (effective 2001). **Document type:** *Academic/Scholarly.*
Media: Online - full text (from EBSCO Publishing, O C L C Online Computer Library Center, Inc., ingenta, Munksgaard & Blackwell Science's Synergy, Swets Blackwell, Institute for Scientific Information). **Related titles:** ♦ Print ed.: Journal of Animal Physiology and Animal Nutrition. ISSN 0931-2439.
Published by: Blackwell Wissenschafts Verlag GmbH, Kurfuerstendamm 57, Berlin 10707, Germany. TEL 49-30-32790665, FAX 49-30-32790610, abo@blackwis.de, http://www.blackwell.de.

B

573.6 USA
JOURNAL OF ANIMAL SCIENCE. SUPPLEMENT. BIENNIAL SYMPOSIUM ON ANIMAL REPRODUCTION. Text in English. irreg., latest vol.76, no.3, 1997. USD 20 (effective 1999). *Refereed.* **Document type:** *Monographic series.*
Formerly: Journal of Animal Science. Supplement (0075-4129)
Indexed: Ind.Med. (coverage dropped).
Published by: American Society of Animal Science, 1111 N Dunlap Ave, Savoy, IL 61874. TEL 217-356-3192, FAX 217-398-4119, asas@assochq.org, http://www.asas.org.

571.43 612 USA ISSN 1065-8483
RC1235
JOURNAL OF APPLIED BIOMECHANICS. Abbreviated title: J A B. Text in English. 1985. q. USD 45 to individuals; USD 135 to institutions; USD 30 to students (effective 2001). adv. bk.rev. bibl, charts, stat, illus. index. back issues avail.; reprint service avail. from PSC. *Refereed.* **Document type:** *Academic/Scholarly.* **Description:** Designed to stimulate and communicate research and theory on the forces affecting human movement in sport exercise and rehabilitation.
Formerly (until 1992): International Journal of Sport Biomechanics (0740-2082)
Related titles: Online - full text ed.: (from Institute for Scientific Information).
Indexed: AMED, A.S.& T.Ind. (Jan.2001-), ASCA, CINAHL, Curr.Cont., Eng.Ind., Ergon.Abstr., Excerp.Med. (1995-), Focus on: Sports Sci.& Med., IBZ, Inpharma, Phys.Ed.Ind., Reac., SSCI (coverage dropped), Sportsearch (1985-).
—BLDSC (4940.653000), GNLM, IDS, Infotrieve, ingenta. **CCC.**
Published by: (International Society of Biomechanics), Human Kinetics Publishers, Inc., PO Box 5076, Champaign, IL 61825-5076. TEL 217-351-5076, FAX 217-351-2674. Ed. Mark Grabiner. Pub. Rainer Martens. R&P Cheri Banks TEL 217-351-5076 ext 2275. Adv. contact Patty Rodriguiz. Circ: 1,088 (paid).
Co-sponsor: International Society for the Biomechanics of Sport.

571 USA ISSN 8750-7587
QP1 CODEN: JAPHEV
JOURNAL OF APPLIED PHYSIOLOGY. Text in English. 1948. m. USD 575 domestic to non-members; USD 625 in Canada & Mexico to non-members; USD 675 elsewhere to non-members; USD 865 domestic to institutions; USD 915 in Canada & Mexico to institutions; USD 965 elsewhere to institutions; USD 605 domestic to non-members for print & online eds.; USD 655 in Canada & Mexico to non-members for print & online eds.; USD 705 elsewhere to non-members for print & online eds.; USD 255 domestic to members for print & online eds.; USD 305 in Canada & Mexico to members for print & online eds.; USD 355 elsewhere to members for print & online eds.; USD 905 domestic to institutions for print & online eds.; USD 955 in Canada & Mexico to institutions for print & online eds.; USD 1,005 elsewhere to institutions for print & online eds.; USD 80 newsstand/cover (effective 2002). adv. bibl, charts, illus. index, cum.index: vols.1-39 (1948-1975). back issues avail.; reprint service avail. from PQC. *Refereed.* **Document type:** *Academic/Scholarly.* **Description:** Presents original papers that deal with normal or abnormal function in four areas: respiratory physiology, environmental physiology, exercise physiology, and temperature regulation.
Former titles: Journal of Applied Physiology: Respiratory, Environmental and Exercise Physiology (0161-7567); (until 1977): Journal of Applied Physiology (0021-8987)
Related titles: Microform ed.: (from PQC); Online - full text ed.: Journal of Applied Physiology Online. ISSN 1522-1601. USD 750 to institutions (effective 2001); USD 495 to non-members; USD 740 to institutions (effective 2002) (from HighWire Pr., Institute for Scientific Information, RoweCom Information Quest).
Indexed: AMED, ASCA, Abstr.Anthropol., AgeLine, Agri.& Environ.Biotech.Abstr. (coverage dropped), Anim.Breed.Abstr., Aqua.Sci.& Fish.Abstr., Aquacult.Abstr., Biol.& Agr.Ind. (Nov.1982-), Biol.Abstr., C.I.S. Abstr., Chem.Abstr., Chem.Indus.Notes, Chem.Titles, Chemorec.Abstr., Curr.Cont., Dairy Sci.Abstr., Dent.Ind., Derwent Biotech.Abstr., Environ.Sci.Poll.Mgmt., Ergon.Abstr., Excerp.Med., Focus on: Sports Sci.& Med., Helminthol.Abstr., INIS Atomind., INSPEC (pre-1969-Aug.1989, dropped), Ind.Med. (1985-), Ind.Vet., Inpharma, Int.Abstr.Biol.Sci., Int.Aerosp.Abstr., Neurosci.Abstr. (coverage dropped), Neurosci.Cit.Ind., Nutr.Abstr., Pharm.&Out.News, Phys.Ed.Ind., Pollut.Abstr., Reac., Rev.Appl.Entomol., Risk Abstr., SSCI (coverage dropped), Saf.Sci.Abstr., Sci.Cit.Ind., Sport Fish.Abstr., Sportsearch (1974-), Sugar Ind.Abstr., Trop.Dis.Bull., Vet.Bull., Wild.Rev., Zoo.Rec.
—BLDSC (4946.000000), CASDDS, CISTI, EMDOCS, GNLM, IDS, Infotrieve, ingenta, KNAW, Linda Hall. **CCC.**
Published by: American Physiological Society, 9650 Rockville Pike, Bethesda, MD 20814-3991. TEL 301-530-7071, FAX 301-571-1814, info@aps.faseb.org, info@the-aps.org, http://www.the-aps.org/publications/specialcalls/pub_sc2.html. Ed. Gary C Sieck. adv.: page USD 1,090. Circ: 3,286 (paid and free).

573.8 DEU ISSN 0340-7594
QP1 CODEN: JCPADN
JOURNAL OF COMPARATIVE PHYSIOLOGY. A: SENSORY, NEURAL, AND BEHAVIORAL PHYSIOLOGY. Text in English. 1924. m. EUR 3,145.90 domestic; EUR 3,126.70 in Germany; EUR 310 newsstand/cover foreign (effective 2002). adv. charts, illus. cum.index. reprint service avail. from ISI. *Refereed.* **Document type:** *Journal, Academic/Scholarly.* **Description:** Concerned with invertebrates, vertebrates, and non-human mammals, particularly with the sense organs, neural processes, as well as with the experimental analysis of behavior.
Supersedes in part (in 1984): Zeitschrift fuer Vergleichende Physiologie (0044-362X)
Related titles: Microform ed.: (from PQC,PMC); Online - full text ed.: ISSN 1432-1351 (from EBSCO Publishing, RoweCom Information Quest, Swets Blackwell, Springer LINK, Institute for Scientific Information).
Indexed: ASCA, Agricola, Anim.Behav.Abstr., Anim.Breed.Abstr., Apic.Abstr., Aqua.Sci.& Fish.Abstr., Bibl.Agri., Bio-Contr.News & Info., Biol.Abstr., Biotech.& Bioeng.Abstr., Chem.Abstr., Chem.Indus.Notes, Chem.Titles, Chemorec.Abstr., Curr.Adv.Biochem., Curr.Adv.Cell & Devel.Biol., Curr.Cont., Curr.Ref.Fish Res., Dairy Sci.Abstr., Deep Sea Res.& Oceanogr.Abstr., Dent.Ind., Entomol.Abstr., Excerp.Med., Forest.Abstr., Helminthol.Abstr., INIS Atomind., Ind.Med. (1984-), Ind.Sci.Rev., Ind.Vet., Inpharma, Int.Abstr.Biol.Sci., Neurosci.Abstr., Neurosci.Cit.Ind., Nutr.Abstr., Poult.Abstr., Reac., Rev.Appl.Entomol., Rev.Med.& Vet.Mycol., SSCI (coverage dropped), Sci.Cit.Ind., Sport Fish.Abstr., Vet.Bull., Wild.Rev., Zoo.Rec., e-psyche.
—BLDSC (4963.210000), CASDDS, CISTI, EMDOCS, GNLM, IDS, ingenta, Linda Hall. **CCC.**
Published by: Springer-Verlag (Subsidiary of: BertelsmannSpringer), Tiergartenstr 17, Heidelberg 69121, Germany. TEL 49-6221-345-0, FAX 49-6221-345229, subscriptions@springer.de, http://link.springer.de/link/service/journals/00359/index.htm, http://www.springer.de. Ed. F G Barth. **Subscr. in N. America to:** Springer-Verlag New York Inc., PO Box 2485, Secaucus, NJ 07096-2485. TEL 212-460-1500, FAX 212-473-6272.

571 DEU ISSN 0174-1578
QP33 CODEN: JPBPDL
JOURNAL OF COMPARATIVE PHYSIOLOGY. B: BIOCHEMICAL, SYSTEMIC, AND ENVIRONMENTAL PHYSIOLOGY. Text in English. 1924. 8/yr. EUR 1,518.80 domestic; EUR 1,513.80 in Germany; EUR 225 newsstand/cover foreign (effective 2002). adv. charts, illus. cum.index. reprint service avail. from ISI. *Refereed.* **Document type:** *Journal, Academic/Scholarly.* **Description:** Provides information from the molecular level up to the organismic levels of animals, including comparative aspects of metabolism and enzymology, physiology of body fluids, and muscular physiology.
Formerly: Journal of Comparative Physiology. B. Systematic and Environmental Physiology (0340-7616); Supersedes in part (in 1984): Zeitschrift fuer Vergleichende Physiologie (0044-362X)
Related titles: Microform ed.: (from PQC,PMC); Online - full text ed.: ISSN 1432-136X (from EBSCO Publishing, RoweCom Information Quest, Swets Blackwell, Springer LINK, Institute for Scientific Information).
Indexed: ASCA, Agricola, Anim.Behav.Abstr., Anim.Breed.Abstr., Apic.Abstr., Aqua.Sci.& Fish.Abstr., Biol.Abstr., Chem.Abstr., Chem.Indus.Notes, Chem.Titles, Curr.Cont., Dairy Sci.Abstr., Deep Sea Res.& Oceanogr.Abstr., Excerp.Med., Forest.Abstr., Helminthol.Abstr., INIS Atomind., Ind.Med. (1984-), Ind.Sci.Rev., Ind.Vet., Inpharma, Int.Abstr.Biol.Sci., Neurosci.Abstr., Nutr.Abstr., Poult.Abstr., Reac., Rev.Appl.Entomol., Sci.Cit.Ind., Soils & Fert., Sport Fish.Abstr., Wild.Rev., Zoo.Rec.
—BLDSC (4963.211000), CASDDS, CISTI, GNLM, IDS, ingenta, Linda Hall. **CCC.**
Published by: Springer-Verlag (Subsidiary of: BertelsmannSpringer), Tiergartenstr 17, Heidelberg 69121, Germany. TEL 49-6221-345-0, FAX 49-6221-345229, subscriptions@springer.de, http://link.springer.de/link/service/journals/00360/index.htm, http://www.springer.de. Eds. I D Hume, L C Wang. **Subscr. in N. America to:** Springer-Verlag New York Inc., PO Box 2485, Secaucus, NJ 07096-2485. TEL 212-460-1500, FAX 212-473-6272.

573.8 GBR ISSN 0307-5095
JOURNAL OF ELECTROPHYSIOLOGICAL TECHNOLOGY. Text in English. 1949. q. GBP 10; GBP 20 foreign. adv. bk.rev. abstr, bibl, charts, illus. index. *Refereed.* **Document type:** *Academic/Scholarly, Abstract/Index.* **Description:** Publishes original articles and reviews on all technical and clinical aspects of human neurophysiology, particularly EEG, EPs and EMG.
Formerly: Electrophysiological Technologists' Association. Proceedings and Journal (0013-4597)
Indexed: Excerp.Med., Ind.Med. (coverage dropped), e-psyche.
—BLDSC (4976.150000), CISTI, GNLM, ingenta.
Published by: Electrophysiological Technologists' Association, c/o E.E.G. Department, St Bartholomew's Hospital, W Smithfield, London EC1A 7BE, United Kingdom. TEL 44-171-601-8859, FAX 44-171-601-7875. Eds. C R Green, R Pottinger. R&P Christopher Green. Adv. contact L O'Neill. Circ: 700.

JOURNAL OF EVOLUTIONARY BIOCHEMISTRY AND PHYSIOLOGY. see *BIOLOGY—Biochemistry*

612.044 USA ISSN 1097-9751
QP301
JOURNAL OF EXERCISE PHYSIOLOGY. Abbreviated title: J E P. Text in English. 1998. q. bk.rev. back issues avail. *Refereed.* **Document type:** *Academic/Scholarly.* **Description:** Includes scientific research by exercise physiologists in such areas as body composition, environmental exercise physiology, exercise and health, fitness and training, research design and statistics, and much more.
Related titles: Online - full text ed.
Published by: American Society of Exercise Physiologists, College of St Scholastica, 1200 Kenwood Ave, Duluth, MN 55811. TEL 218-723-6297, FAX 218-723-6472, tboone2@css.edu, http://www.css.edu/users/tboone2/asep/fldr/fldr.htm. Ed. Tommy Boone.

571 USA ISSN 0022-1295
QP1 CODEN: JGPLAD
JOURNAL OF GENERAL PHYSIOLOGY. Text in English. 1918. m. (in 2 vols., 6 nos./vol.). USD 535 in US & Canada to institutions print ed.; USD 630 elsewhere to institutions print ed.; USD 430 to institutions online ed.; USD 965 in US & Canada to institutions print and online ed.; USD 1,060 elsewhere to institutions print and online ed. (effective 2001). adv. bibl, illus, charts. index. 90 p./no. reprint service avail. from PQC,ISI. *Refereed.* **Document type:** *Journal, Academic/Scholarly.* **Description:** Articles that elucidate basic biological, chemical, or physical mechanisms of broad physiological significance.
Related titles: Microform ed.: (from PQC); Online - full text ed.: (from HighWire Pr., EBSCO Publishing, RoweCom Information Quest, Gale Group, Factiva, Institute for Scientific Information).
Indexed: ASCA, Abstr.Hyg., Aqua.Sci.& Fish.Abstr., Aquacult.Abstr., Biol.& Agr.Ind. (May 1983-), Biol.Abstr., Chem.Abstr., Chem.Indus.Notes, Chem.Titles, Curr.Adv.Ecol.Sci., Curr.Cont., Excerp.Med., Gen.Sci.Ind. (Jun.1984-), INIS Atomind., INSPEC (coverage dropped), Ind.Med. (1918-), Ind.Sci.Rev., Ind.Vet., Inpharma, Int.Abstr.Biol.Sci., Neurosci.Cit.Ind., Nutr.Abstr., Pharm.&Out.News, Reac., Ref.Zh., Rev.Appl.Entomol., Rev.Med.& Vet.Mycol., Sci.Cit.Ind., Sport Fish.Abstr., Trop.Dis.Bull., Vet.Bull., Wild.Rev., Zoo.Rec.
—BLDSC (4989.000000), CASDDS, CISTI, GNLM, IDS, ingenta, Linda Hall. **CCC.**

Published by: (Society of General Physiologists), Rockefeller University Press, 1114 First Ave, New York, NY 10021. TEL 212-327-8522, FAX 212-327-8513, JGP@rockefeller.edu, rupress@rockefeller.edu, http://www.jgp.org; http://www.rockefeller.edu/rupress. Ed. Dr. Olaf S Andersen. adv.: B&W page USD 545, color page USD 1,945; 7.75 x 10.25. Circ: 1,186.

573.679 USA ISSN 1083-3021
CODEN: JMBNFU

JOURNAL OF MAMMARY GLAND BIOLOGY AND NEOPLASIA. Text in English. 1996. q. USD 338, EUR 337 to institutions for print or online ed.; USD 405.60, EUR 404.40 to institutions for print & online eds.combined (effective 2002). *Refereed.* **Document type:** *Journal, Academic/Scholarly.* **Description:** Publishes concise state-of-the-art research papers and reviews on all aspects of the biology and pathology of the mammary gland.

Related titles: Online - full text ed.: (from CatchWord Ltd., EBSCO Publishing, O C L C Online Computer Library Center, Inc., RoweCom Information Quest, Swets Blackwell, Kluwer Online, Institute for Scientific Information).

Indexed: Anim.Breed.Abstr., Curr.Cont., Dairy Sci.Abstr., Ind.Med. (1996-), Sci.Cit.Ind.

—BLDSC (5011.020000), CatchWord, CISTI, GNLM, IDS, Infotrieve, ingenta. **CCC.**

Published by: Kluwer Academic - Plenum Publishers (Subsidiary of: Wolters Kluwer N.V.), 233 Spring St, New York, NY 10013-1578. TEL 212-620-8000, 800-221-9369, FAX 212-463-0742, info@plenum.com, http://www.wkap.nl/journalhome.htm/1083-3021. Eds. Gary C Chamness, Kermit L Carraway. R&P Rose Luongo TEL 781-871-6311. **Subscr. outside the Americas to:** Kluwer Academic Publishers Group, Journals Department, PO Box 322, Dordrecht 3300 AH, Netherlands. TEL 31-78-639-2392, FAX 31-78-654-6474.

573.8 USA ISSN 0022-3034
QP351 CODEN: JNEUBZ

JOURNAL OF NEUROBIOLOGY; an international journal. Text in English. 1969. 16/yr. USD 3,250 in United States; USD 3,410 in Canada & Mexico; USD 3,546 elsewhere; USD 3,413 combined subscription in United States for print and online eds.; USD 3,573 combined subscription in Canada & Mexico for print and online eds.; USD 3,709 combined subscription elsewhere for print and online eds. (effective 2002). adv. bk.rev. back issues avail.; reprint service avail. from PQC. *Refereed.* **Document type:** *Academic/Scholarly.* **Description:** Covers neuroscience from molecular, genetic and cellular approaches. Vertebrate and invertebrate nervous systems are examined at the levels of the individual cell, the ensemble, and overall behavior.

Related titles: Microform ed.: (from PQC); Online - full text ed.: ISSN 1097-4695. USD 3,250 in United States; USD 3,250 in Canada & Mexico; USD 3,250 elsewhere (effective 2002) (from EBSCO Publishing, Wiley InterScience, Institute for Scientific Information).

Indexed: ASCA, Apic.Abstr., Aqua.Sci.& Fish.Abstr., Biol.Abstr., Cal.Tiss.Abstr. (coverage dropped), Chem.Abstr., Chem.Titles, Chemorec.Abstr., Curr.Adv.Ecol.Sci., Curr.Cont., Dent.Ind., Entomol.Abstr. (coverage dropped), Excerp.Med., Helminthol.Abstr., INIS Atomind., Ind.Med. (1969-), Ind.Sci.Rev., Inpharma, Int.Abstr.Biol.Sci., Neurosci.Abstr., Neurosci.Cit.Ind., Reac., Rev.Appl.Entomol., Sci.Cit.Ind., Sport Fish.Abstr., THA, Tox.Abstr. (coverage dropped), Wild.Rev., Zoo.Rec., e-psyche.

—BLDSC (5021.450000), CASDDS, CISTI, GNLM, IDS, ingenta, Linda Hall. **CCC.**

Published by: John Wiley & Sons, Inc., Journals (Subsidiary of: Wiley InterScience), 605 Third Ave, New York, NY 10158. TEL 212-850-6645, FAX 212-850-6021, subinfo@wiley.com, uscs-wis@wiley.com, http://www.wiley.com. Eds. Darcy B Kelley, Eduardo Macagno. adv.: B&W page GBP 640, color page GBP 1,515; trim 210 x 279. Circ: 750. **Subscr. outside the Americas to:** John Wiley & Sons Ltd., Baffins Ln, Chichester, Sussex PO19 IUD, United Kingdom. TEL 44-1243-779777, FAX 44-1243-843232, cs-journals@wiley.co.uk.

573.8 USA ISSN 0022-3077
QP351 CODEN: JONEA4

JOURNAL OF NEUROPHYSIOLOGY. Text in English. 1938. m. USD 655 domestic to non-members; USD 715 in Canada & Mexico to non-members; USD 775 elsewhere to non-members (effective 2001); USD 985 domestic to institutions; USD 1,045 in Canada & Mexico to institutions; USD 1,105 elsewhere to institutions; USD 685 domestic to non-members for print & online eds.; USD 745 in Canada & Mexico to non-members for print & online eds.; USD 805 elsewhere to non-members for print & online eds.; USD 255 domestic to members for print & online eds.; USD 315 in Canada & Mexico to members for print & online eds.; USD 375 elsewhere to members for print & online eds.; USD 1,030 domestic to institutions for print & online eds.; USD 1,090 in Canada & Mexico to institutions for print & online eds.; USD 1,150 elsewhere to institutions for print & online eds.; USD 90 newsstand/cover (effective 2002). adv. abstr, charts, illus. index. back issues avail.; reprint service avail. from PQC. *Refereed.* **Document type:** *Academic/Scholarly.* **Description:** Presents original articles on the function of the nervous system. Articles report on investigations that use the techniques of electro-physiology, experimental neuroanatomy, electron microscopy and tissue culture.

Related titles: Microfilm ed.: (from PQC,PMC); Online - full text ed.: Journal of Neurophysiology Online. ISSN 1522-1598. USD 855 to institutions (effective 2001); USD 565 to non-members; USD 845 to institutions (effective 2002) (from HighWire Pr., EBSCO Publishing, RoweCom Information Quest, Institute for Scientific Information).

Indexed: ASCA, Agri.& Environ.Biotech.Abstr. (coverage dropped), Aqua.Sci.& Fish.Abstr., Biol.Abstr., Cal.Tiss.Abstr. (coverage dropped), Chem.Abstr., Chem.Titles, Chemorec.Abstr., Compumath, Curr.Adv.Cell & Devel.Biol., Curr.Adv.Ecol.Sci., Curr.Cont., Dent.Ind., Derwent Biotech.Abstr., Excerp.Med., INIS Atomind., Ind.Med. (1938-), Ind.Sci.Rev., Inpharma, Int.Abstr.Biol.Sci., Neurosci.Abstr., Neurosci.Cit.Ind., Nutr.Abstr., PsycInfo, Psychol.Abstr. (1938-), Reac., SSCI (coverage dropped), Sci.Cit.Ind., Sport Fish.Abstr., Tox.Abstr. (coverage dropped), Zoo.Rec., e-psyche.

—BLDSC (5022.000000), CASDDS, CISTI, GNLM, IDS, ingenta, KNAW, Linda Hall. **CCC.**

Published by: American Physiological Society, 9650 Rockville Pike, Bethesda, MD 20814-3991. TEL 301-530-7164, FAX 301-571-3813, info@aps.faseb.org, info@the-aps.org, http://www.jn.org, http://www.the-aps.org/. Ed. P L Strick. adv.: B&W page USD 525, color page USD 878. Circ: 2,002.

571 GBR ISSN 0022-3751
QP1 CODEN: JPHYA7

JOURNAL OF PHYSIOLOGY. Text in English. 1878. s-m. (plus proceedings 5/yr.). USD 2,560 to institutions (effective 2002). adv. bibl, charts, illus. index, cum.index. back issues avail.; reprints avail. *Refereed.* **Document type:** *Academic/Scholarly.* **Description:** Covers physiological research in vertebrates: respiration, circulation, excretion, reproduction, digestion and homeostasis. Emphasis is on neurophysiology and muscle contraction.

Related titles: Microform ed.: (from PQC,PMC); Online - full text ed.: (from EBSCO Publishing, O C L C Online Computer Library Center, Inc., RoweCom Information Quest, HighWire Pr., Institute for Scientific Information).

Indexed: ASCA, Agri.& Environ.Biotech.Abstr. (coverage dropped), Anim.Breed.Abstr., Apic.Abstr., Aqua.Sci.& Fish.Abstr., Aquacult.Abstr., Biol.& Agr.Ind. (Nov.1982-), Biol.Abstr., Cal.Tiss.Abstr., Chem.Abstr., Chem.Indus.Notes, Chem.Titles, Chemorec.Abstr., Curr.Adv.Biochem., Curr.Adv.Ecol.Sci., Curr.Cont., Curr.Ref.Fish Res., Dairy Sci.Abstr., Deep Sea Res.& Oceanogr.Abstr., Dent.Ind., Derwent Biotech.Abstr., Environ.Sci.Poll.Mgmt., Ergon.Abstr., Excerp.Med., Helminthol.Abstr., INIS Atomind., INSPEC (1968-1969, dropped), Ind.Med. (1878-), Ind.Sci.Rev., Ind.Vet., Inpharma, Int.Abstr.Biol.Sci., Mass Spectr.Bull., Neurosci.Abstr. (coverage dropped), Neurosci.Cit.Ind., Nutr.Abstr., Pharm.&Out.News, Pig News & Info., Poult.Abstr., Protozool.Abstr., Reac., Ref.Zh., Rev.Appl.Entomol., Rev.Med.& Vet.Mycol., SSCI (coverage dropped), Sci.Cit.Ind., Small Anim.Abstr., Sport Fish.Abstr., Vet.Bull., Wild.Rev., Zoo.Rec., e-psyche.

—BLDSC (5039.000000), CASDDS, CISTI, GNLM, IDS, ingenta, Linda Hall.

Published by: (Physiological Society, London), Cambridge University Press, Edinburgh Bldg, Shaftesbury Rd, Cambridge CB2 2RU, United Kingdom. FAX 44-1223-315052, information@cup.cam.ac.uk, information@cambridge.org, http://www.cup.cam.ac.uk/, http://www.uk.cambridge.org/journals/pmu. Eds. Barry Hirst, D A Eisner. R&P Linda Nicol. Adv. contact Rebecca Symons. Circ: 3,100.

JOURNAL OF PHYSIOLOGY AND BIOCHEMISTRY. see *MEDICAL SCIENCES*

571 POL ISSN 0867-5910
QP1 CODEN: JPHPEI

JOURNAL OF PHYSIOLOGY AND PHARMACOLOGY. Text in English. 1950. q. PLZ 100; USD 115 foreign (effective 1999). bk.rev. illus. *Refereed.* **Document type:** *Academic/Scholarly.*

Formerly (until 1991): Acta Physiologica Polonica (0044-6033)

Related titles: Online - full text ed.: (from Institute for Scientific Information).

Indexed: ASCA, AgroAgen, AgroLibrex, Apic.Abstr., Biol.Abstr., Chem.Abstr., Chem.Indus.Notes, Chem.Titles, Curr.Cont., Excerp.Med., INIS Atomind., INSPEC (Jan.1973-Aug.1983, dropped), Ind.Med. (1991-), Inpharma, Nutr.Abstr., Pharm.&Out.News, Reac., Vet.Bull.

—BLDSC (5039.500000), CASDDS, CISTI, EMDOCS, GNLM, ingenta, KNAW, Linda Hall.

Published by: Polskie Towarzystwo Fizjologiczne/Polish Physiological Society, Ul Grzegorzecka 16, Krakow 31531, Poland. TEL 48-12-4211006, FAX 48-12-4211578. Ed. Jan Bugajski. Circ: 600.

JOURNAL OF PHYSIOLOGY (PARIS); an integrative neuroscience journal. see *MEDICAL SCIENCES—Psychiatry And Neurology*

JOURNAL OF SEROTONIN RESEARCH. see *MEDICAL SCIENCES—Psychiatry And Neurology*

573.8 NLD ISSN 0957-4271
QP471 CODEN: JVEREH

JOURNAL OF VESTIBULAR RESEARCH: EQUILIBRIUM AND ORIENTATION; an international journal of experimental and clinical vestibular science. Text in English. 1991. bi-m. EUR 530, USD 481 to institutions (effective 2002). adv. bk.rev. back issues avail. *Refereed.* **Document type:** *Journal, Academic/Scholarly.* **Description:** Includes experimental and observational studies and theoretical papers based on the current knowledge of vestibular science.

Related titles: Online - full text ed.: (from ingenta, Swets Blackwell, Institute for Scientific Information, RoweCom Information Quest).

Indexed: ASCA, Excerp.Med. (1994-), Focus on: Sports Sci.& Med., INSPEC (1990-), Ind.Med. (1991-), Int.Abstr.Biol.Sci., Neurosci.Abstr., Neurosci.Cit.Ind., PsycInfo, Psychol.Abstr. (1990-), SSCI (coverage dropped), e-psyche.

—BLDSC (5072.340000), ADONIS, AskIEEE, CISTI, EMDOCS, GNLM, IDS, Infotrieve, KNAW. **CCC.**

Published by: I O S Press, Nieuwe Hemweg 6B, Amsterdam 1013 BG, Netherlands. TEL 31-20-688-3355, FAX 31-20-620-3419, market@iospress.nl, http://www.iospress.nl. Eds. Desmond J Ireland TEL 204-257-2444, Ralph M Jell. R&P C Koolbergen TEL 31-20-638-2189. Adv. contact M Janmaat. **Subscr. in Australasia and the Far East to:** Kinokuniya Company Ltd, Shinjuku 3-chome, Shinjuku-ku, Tokyo 160-0022, Japan. FAX 81-3-3439-1094, journal@kinokuniya.co.jp, http://www.kinokuniya.co.jp**; Subscr.in the Americas to:** I O S Press, Inc, 5795-G Burke Centre Pkwy, Burke, VA 22015. TEL 703-323-5554, FAX 703-323-3668, iosbooks@iospress.com.

573.7 NLD ISSN 0968-0160
RD561 CODEN: KNEEF2

THE KNEE. Text in English. 1994. q. EUR 103 in Europe to individuals; JPY 13,600 in Japan to individuals; USD 115 elsewhere to individuals; EUR 297 in Europe to institutions; JPY 39,400 in Japan to institutions; USD 332 elsewhere to institutions (effective 2002). adv. back issues avail. *Refereed.* **Document type:** *Academic/Scholarly.* **Description:** Publishes studies on the clinical treatment and fundamental biomechanical characteristics of the knee.

Related titles: Microfilm ed.: (from PQC); Online - full text ed.: (from ingenta, ScienceDirect, Swets Blackwell, Institute for Scientific Information).

Indexed: Focus on: Sports Sci.& Med.

—BLDSC (5099.863500), CISTI, GNLM, IDS, Infotrieve. **CCC.**

Published by: Elsevier Science BV, PO Box 211, Amsterdam 1000 AE, Netherlands. http://www.elsevier.com/locate/knee. Eds. John H Newman, Richard S Laskin. **Subscr. in Australasia and the Far East to:** Elsevier Science (Singapore) Pte Ltd, No.1 Temasek Ave, 17-01 Millenia Tower, Singapore 039192, Singapore. TEL 65-434-3727, FAX 65-337-2230; **Subscr. in Japan to:** Elsevier Science Inc - Japan Regional Office, 9-15 Higashi-Azabu 1-chome, Minato-ku, Tokyo 106-0044, Japan. TEL 81-3-5561-5033; **Subscr. in the Americas to:** Elsevier Science, PO Box 945, New York, NY 10159-0945. TEL 212-633-3730, FAX 212-633-3680, usinfo-f@elsevier.com.

571 USA
LIPPINCOTT-RAVEN PRESS SERIES IN PHYSIOLOGY. Text in English. irreg. reprint service avail. from PQC. *Refereed.* **Document type:** *Monographic series.*
Former titles: Raven Press Series in Physiology; Raven Press Series in Experimental Physiology
Published by: Lippincott - Raven Publishers (Subsidiary of: Wolters Kluwer N.V.), 530 Walnut St, Philadelphia, PA 19106. TEL 215-521-8300, FAX 215-521-8902, http:/www.lrpub.com. R&P Alice McElhinney. **Subscr. to:** Box 1600, Hagerstown, MD 21741-1600. TEL 800-777-2295, FAX 301-824-7390.

LOOSE CONNECTIONS. see *SOCIAL SERVICES AND WELFARE*

573.25 USA ISSN 0362-3181
CODEN: LBHDD7
LUNG BIOLOGY IN HEALTH AND DISEASE. Text in English. 1976. irreg., latest vol.133, 1999. price varies. adv. *Refereed.* **Document type:** *Monographic series.*
Indexed: Biol.Abstr., Chem.Abstr., Chem.Indus.Notes, Chem.Titles, Mass Spectr.Bull.
—BLDSC (5307.240000), CASDDS, CISTI. **CCC.**
Published by: Marcel Dekker, Inc., Attn: Eridania Perrez, 270 Madison Ave, New York, NY 10016-0602. TEL 212-696-9000, 800-228-1160, FAX 212-685-4540, marketing@dekker.com, http://www.dekker.com. Pub. Russell Dekker. R&P Jullia Mulligan. Adv. contact Eridania Perez.

MAMMARY GLAND. see *BIOLOGY—Abstracting, Bibliographies, Statistics*

573.1 NLD ISSN 0168-1745
MICROCIRCULATION REVIEWS. Text in English. 1982. irreg. price varies. *Refereed.* **Document type:** *Monographic series.*
—CISTI.
Published by: Kluwer Academic Publishers Group (Subsidiary of: Wolters Kluwer N.V.), Spuiboulevard 50, PO Box 17, Dordrecht 3300 AA, Netherlands. FAX 31-78-639-2254, services@wkap.nl, http://www.wkap.nl. **Dist. by:** Journals Department, PO Box 322, Dordrecht 3300 AH, Netherlands. FAX 31-78-654-6474.

573.8 UKR ISSN 0028-2561
QP361 CODEN: NEFZB2
NEIROFIZIOLOGIYA/NEUROPHYSIOLOGY; nauchno-teoreticheskii zhurnal. Text in Russian; Summaries in English. 1969. bi-m. USD 95. bk.rev. illus.
Related titles: ♦ English Translation: Neurophysiology. ISSN 0090-2977.
Indexed: Biol.Abstr., Chem.Abstr., Chem.Indus.Notes, Chem.Titles, Dent.Ind., Djerelo, Excerp.Med., Ind.Med. (until 1992, dropped), Neurosci.Cit.Ind., e-psyche.
—CASDDS, CISTI, GNLM, KNAW, Linda Hall.
Published by: Natsional'na Akademiya Nauk Ukrainy, Institut Fiziologii im. Bogomol'tsya, Vul Bogomol'tsya 4, Kiev 252601, Ukraine. TEL 38-44-2930745. Ed. P G Kostyuk. Circ: 900. **US dist. addr.:** East View Publications, 3020 Harbor Ln N, Minneapolis, MN 55447. TEL 612-550-0961.

571.878 USA ISSN 0197-4580
QP376 CODEN: NEAGDO
NEUROBIOLOGY OF AGING; experimental and clinical research. Text in English. 1980. bi-m. EUR 189 in Europe to qualified personnel; JPY 25,100 in Japan to qualified personnel; USD 211 elsewhere to qualified personnel; EUR 1,221 in Europe to institutions; JPY 162,100 in Japan to institutions; USD 1,366 elsewhere to institutions (effective 2002). abstr. illus. index. back issues avail.; reprint service avail. from PQC,ISI. *Refereed.* **Document type:** *Academic/Scholarly.*
Description: Fosters better understanding and treatment of functional changes associated with aging.
Related titles: Microfilm ed.: (from PQC); Online - full text ed.: (from ingenta, ScienceDirect, Swets Blackwell, Institute for Scientific Information).
Indexed: ASCA, Biol.Abstr., Chem.Abstr., Chem.Indus.Notes, Chem.Titles, Chemorec.Abstr., Curr.Adv.Ecol.Sci., Curr.Cont., Excerp.Med., INIS Atomind., Ind.Med. (1980-), Ind.Sci.Rev., Inpharma, Int.Abstr.Biol.Sci., Neurosci.Abstr., Neurosci.Cit.Ind., Nutr.Abstr., Pharm.&Out.News, PsycInfo, Psychol.Abstr. (1980-), Reac., Rev.Appl.Entomol., SSCI (coverage dropped), Sci.Cit.Ind., THA, e-psyche.
—BLDSC (6081.311000), ADONIS, CASDDS, CISTI, GNLM, IDS, ingenta, KNAW. **CCC.**
Published by: Elsevier Science, 655 Ave of the Americas, New York, NY 10010. TEL 212-989-5800, FAX 212-633-3990, http://www.elsevier.com/locate/neuaging. Ed. Paul D Coleman. **Subscr. in Australasia and the Far East to:** Elsevier Science (Singapore) Pte Ltd, No.1 Temasek Ave, 17-01 Millenia Tower, Singapore 039192, Singapore. TEL 65-434-3727, FAX 65-337-2230; **Subscr. in Japan to:** Elsevier Science Inc - Japan Regional Office, 9-15 Higashi-Azabu 1-chome, Minato-ku, Tokyo 106-0044, Japan. TEL 81-3-5561-5033; **Subscr. outside the Americas to:** Elsevier Science BV, PO Box 211, Amsterdam 1000 AE, Netherlands. TEL 31-20-485-3757, nlinfo-f@elsevier.nl.

NEUROBIOLOGY OF DISEASE. see *MEDICAL SCIENCES—Psychiatry And Neurology*

573.8 USA
NEUROMETHODS. Text in English. 1985. irreg. price varies. **Document type:** *Monographic series, Academic/Scholarly.* **Description:** Presents detailed methods and techniques for neuroscientists.
Formerly: Neuromethods. Series 1: Neurochemistry (1048-6089)
Indexed: Chem.Abstr., Chem.Indus.Notes, Chem.Titles, Neurosci.Abstr., e-psyche.
—BLDSC (6081.503500).
Published by: Humana Press Inc., 999 Riverview Dr, Ste 208, Totowa, NJ 07512. TEL 973-256-1699, FAX 973-256-8341, humana@humanapr.com, http://humanapress.com.

NEUROPHYSIOLOGY. see *BIOLOGY—Abstracting, Bibliographies, Statistics*

NEUROPSYCHOBIOLOGY; international journal of experimental and clinical research in biological psychiatry, pharmacopsychiatry, biological psychology, pharmacopsychology and pharmacoelectroencephalography. see *MEDICAL SCIENCES—Psychiatry And Neurology*

571 USA ISSN 0886-1714
QP1 CODEN: NEPSEY
NEWS IN PHYSIOLOGICAL SCIENCES; an international journal of physiology. Abbreviated title: N I P S. Text in English. 1986. bi-m. USD 110 domestic to non-members; USD 115 in Canada & Mexico to non-members; USD 120 elsewhere to non-members; USD 165 domestic to institutions; USD 170 in Canada & Mexico to institutions; USD 175 elsewhere to institutions; USD 115, USD 120, USD 125 to non-members for print & online eds.; USD 170, USD 175, USD 180 to institutions for print & online eds.; USD 30 newsstand/cover (effective 2002); free to members (print & online eds.). adv. charts, illus. index. back issues avail.; reprint service avail. from PQC. *Refereed.* **Document type:** *Academic/Scholarly.*
Description: Designed to keep physiologists informed about current developments in their field.
Related titles: Microfiche ed.; Microform ed.: (from PQC); Online - full text ed.: News in Physiological Sciences Online. ISSN 1522-161X. USD 145 to institutions (effective 2001); USD 95 to non-members; USD 140 to institutions (effective 2002) (from HighWire Pr., EBSCO Publishing, RoweCom Information Quest, Institute for Scientific Information).
Indexed: ASCA, Biol.Dig., Chem.Abstr., Chem.Indus.Notes, Chem.Titles, Curr.Cont., Inpharma, Neurosci.Cit.Ind., Reac., SSCI (coverage dropped), Sci.Cit.Ind.
—BLDSC (6105.385000), CASDDS, CISTI, GNLM, IDS, Infotrieve, ingenta, KNAW, Linda Hall. **CCC.**
Published by: American Physiological Society, 9650 Rockville Pike, Bethesda, MD 20814-3991. TEL 301-530-7071, FAX 301-571-1814, info@the-aps.org, http://nips.physiology.org/, http://www.the-aps.org/. Ed. S G Schultz. adv.: B&W page USD 1,250, color page USD 2,345. Circ: 9,909. **Subscr. to:** Subscription Department. **Co-publisher:** International Union of Physiological Sciences.

NEWSLETTER: FRONTIER RESEARCH PROGRAM. see *MEDICAL SCIENCES—Psychiatry And Neurology*

612.4 JPN ISSN 0916-1104
NIHON DAEKISEN GAKKAISHI/JAPAN SALIVARY GLAND SOCIETY. JOURNAL. Text in English, Japanese. 1959. a.
—BLDSC (4805.870000).
Published by: Nihon Daekisen Gakkai, 1604 Shimo-Sakunobe, Takatsu-ku, Kawasaki-shi, Kanagawa-ken 213-0033, Japan.

NIHON SEIRI JINRUI GAKKAI TAIKAI SHOROKUSHU/JAPAN SOCIETY OF PHYSIOLOGICAL ANTHROPOLOGY. ABSTRACTS OF THE MEETING. see *BIOLOGY—Abstracting, Bibliographies, Statistics*

571 JPN ISSN 0031-9341
CODEN: NISEAV
NIHON SEIRIGAKU ZASSHI/PHYSIOLOGICAL SOCIETY OF JAPAN. JOURNAL. Text in Japanese; Summaries in English. 1937. m. JPY 1,000 per issue. adv. bk.rev. stat. cum.index.
Related titles: Microform ed.
Indexed: ASCA, Biol.Abstr., Chem.Abstr., Curr.Adv.Ecol.Sci., Dent.Ind., Excerp.Med., INIS Atomind., Ind.Med. (1936-).
—CASDDS, CISTI, GNLM.
Published by: Nihon Seiri Gakkai, 30-10 Hongo 3-chome, Bunkyo-ku, Tokyo 113-0033, Japan. TEL 81-3-3815-1624, FAX 81-3-5684-2539. Ed. Akimichi Kaneko. Circ: 3,500 (paid).

571 JPN ISSN 0911-2057
NIHON SHIKKAN MODERU DOBUTSU KENKYUKAI KIROKU/JAPANESE ASSOCIATION OF ANIMAL MODELS FOR HUMAN DISEASES. PROCEEDINGS. Text in Japanese; Summaries in English. 1985. a. **Document type:** *Proceedings.*
Published by: Nihon Shikkan Moderu Dobutsu Kenkyukai, Wakayama Kenritsu Ika Daigaku, Dai 2 Seirigaku Kyoshitsu, 9, 9 Bancho, Wakayama-shi, Wakayama-ken 640, Japan.

571 JPN ISSN 0446-6578
CODEN: NTAZAD
NIHON TAISHITSUGAKU ZASSHI/JAPANESE JOURNAL OF CONSTITUTIONAL MEDICINE. Text in Japanese; Summaries in English. 1932. a. adv. **Document type:** *Academic/Scholarly.*
Indexed: INIS Atomind.
—CASDDS.
Published by: Nihon Taishitsu Gakkai/Japanese Society of Constitutional Medicine, c/o Kumamoto Daigaku Igakubu, Fuzoku Iden Igaku Kenkyu Shisetsu, 24-1 kuhon-Ji 4-chome, Kumamoto-shi 862-0976, Japan. Ed. Hiromichi Okuda. Adv. contact Norio Fujiki.

NO NO IGAKU SEIBUTSUGAKU KONWAKAI SHOROKU/ABSTRACTS OF CONFERENCE ON MEDICINE AND BIOLOGY OF THE BRAIN. see *BIOLOGY—Abstracting, Bibliographies, Statistics*

THE NOETIC JOURNAL; an international forum on the cosmology of consciousness. see *PHYSICS*

571 JPN ISSN 0387-494X
OSAKA SHIKA DAIGAKU SEIRIGAKU KYOSHITSU RONBUNSHU/OSAKA DENTAL UNIVERSITY. DEPARTMENT OF PHYSIOLOGY. COLLECTION OF PAPERS. Text in English, Japanese. irreg.
Published by: Osaka Shika Daigaku, Seirigaku Kyoshitsu, 1-47, Kyobashi, Higashi-ku, Osaka-shi 540, Japan.

573.6 GBR ISSN 0260-0854
QP251 CODEN: ORRBDQ
OXFORD REVIEWS OF REPRODUCTIVE BIOLOGY. Text in English. 1979. a. USD 120. illus. *Refereed.* **Document type:** *Academic/Scholarly.*
Related titles: Microform ed.: (from PQC); Online - full text ed.: (from Institute for Scientific Information).
Indexed: ASCA, Chem.Abstr., Curr.Adv.Biochem., Curr.Adv.Cell & Devel.Biol., Curr.Adv.Gen.& Molec.Biol., Ind.Sci.Rev., Ind.Vet., Poult.Abstr., Sci.Cit.Ind., Vet.Bull.
—CASDDS, CISTI, GNLM, ingenta, Linda Hall. **CCC.**
Published by: Oxford University Press, Oxford Journals, Walton St, Oxford OX2 6DP, United Kingdom. TEL 44-1865-56767, FAX 44-1865-56646, jnlorders@oup.co.uk, jnl.orders@oup.co.uk, http://www.oup.co.uk. Ed. C A Finn. **Subscr. in N. America to:** Oxford University Press, Journals. TEL 919-677-0977, FAX 919-677-1714, http://www.oup.co.uk.

PAKISTAN JOURNAL OF PATHOLOGY. see *MEDICAL SCIENCES*

PANCREATIC AND SALIVARY SECRETION. see *BIOLOGY—Abstracting, Bibliographies, Statistics*

612 NLD ISSN 0928-4680
CODEN: PTHOE7

PATHOPHYSIOLOGY. Text in English. 1994. q. EUR 357 in Europe to institutions; JPY 47,400 in Japan to institutions; USD 400 elsewhere to institutions (effective 2002). back issues avail.; reprints avail. *Refereed.* **Document type:** *Academic/Scholarly.* **Description:** Publishes original interdisciplinary papers on the etiology, development and elimination of pathological processes.

Incorporates (1995-1999): Physiological Medicine

Related titles: Microform ed.: (from PQC); Online - full text ed.: (from ingenta, ScienceDirect, Swets Blackwell).

Indexed: Chem.Abstr., Chem.Titles, Excerp.Med. (1995-).

—BLDSC (6412.834000), CASDDS, CISTI, EMDOCS, GNLM, Infotrieve, KNAW. **CCC.**

Published by: (International Society for Pathophysiology), Elsevier Science BV, PO Box 211, Amsterdam 1000 AE, Netherlands. TEL 31-20-485-3911, FAX 31-20-485-3598, nlinfo-f@elsevier.nl, http://www.elsevier.nl/locate/pathophys. Eds. D N Granger, T Yoshikawa. **Subscr. in Australasia and the Far East to:** Elsevier Science (Singapore) Pte Ltd, No.1 Temasek Ave, 17-01 Millenia Tower, Singapore 039192, Singapore. TEL 65-434-3727, FAX 65-337-2230**; Subscr. in Japan to:** Elsevier Science Inc - Japan Regional Office, 9-15 Higashi-Azabu 1-chome, Minato-ku, Tokyo 106-0044, Japan. TEL 81-3-5561-5033**; Subscr. in the Americas to:** Elsevier Science, PO Box 945, New York, NY 10159-0945. TEL 212-633-3730, FAX 212-633-3680.

PERSPECTIVES ON DEVELOPMENTAL NEUROBIOLOGY. see *MEDICAL SCIENCES—Psychiatry And Neurology*

PFLUEGERS ARCHIV/EUROPEAN JOURNAL OF PHYSIOLOGY; european journal of physiology. see *MEDICAL SCIENCES*

573.8 CZE ISSN 0862-8408
QP1 CODEN: PHRSEJ

PHYSIOLOGICAL RESEARCH. Text in English. 1952. bi-m. CZK 600 domestic; GBP 158 foreign (effective 2001). charts, illus. index. *Refereed.* **Document type:** *Academic/Scholarly.* **Description:** Publishes articles dealing with normal and pathological physiology, biochemistry, biophysics, pharmacology, toxicology, cell biology, experimental medicine, endocrinology and cardiovascular diseases. Preference is given to papers concerning ontogenetic aspects of the above topics.

Formerly (until 1991): Physiologia Bohemoslovaca (0369-9463)

Related titles: Online - full text ed.: (from Institute for Scientific Information).

Indexed: ASCA, Biol.Abstr., C.I.S. Abstr., Chem.Abstr., Chem.Indus.Notes, Chem.Titles, Curr.Adv.Ecol.Sci., Curr.Cont., Dairy Sci.Abstr., Dent.Ind., Excerp.Med., Helminthol.Abstr., INIS Atomind., Ind.Med. (1991-), Ind.Sci.Rev., Ind.Vet., Inpharma, Int.Abstr.Biol.Sci., Neurosci.Cit.Ind., Nutr.Abstr., Pharm.&Out.News, Pig News & Info., Psychol.Abstr., Reac., Ref.Zh., Sci.Cit.Ind., Vet.Bull., e-psyche.

—BLDSC (6484.950000), CASDDS, CISTI, EMDOCS, GNLM, IDS, Infotrieve. **CCC.**

Published by: Ceska Akademie Ved, Fyziologicky Ustav/Czech Academy of Sciences, Institute of Physiology, Physiological Research, Albertov 5, Prague, 2 128 00, Czech Republic. TEL 420-2-29420590, FAX 420-2-29420590, kunes@sun1.biomed.cas.cz, physres@biomed.cas.cz, http://www.lf2.cuni.cz/physiolres/physiolres.htm. Ed. Dr. J Kunes. Circ: 250. **Dist. by:** Harcourt Publishers Ltd.

571 USA ISSN 0031-9333
QP1 CODEN: PHREA7

PHYSIOLOGICAL REVIEWS. Text in English. 1921. q. USD 215 domestic to non-members; USD 235 in Canada & Mexico to non-members; USD 255 elsewhere to non-members; USD 325 domestic to institutions; USD 345 in Canada & Mexico to institutions; USD 365 elsewhere to institutions; USD 230 domestic to non-members for print & online eds.; USD 250 in Canada & Mexico to non-members for print & online eds.; USD 270 elsewhere to non-members for print & online eds.; USD 100 domestic to members for print & online eds.; USD 120 in Canada & Mexico to members for print & online eds.; USD 140 elsewhere to members for print & online eds.; USD 340 domestic to institutions for print & online eds.; USD 360 in Canada & Mexico to institutions for print & online eds.; USD 380 elsewhere to institutions for print & online eds.; USD 90 newsstand/cover (effective 2002). adv. bibl, charts, illus. cum.index: 1936-1951, 1952-1966, 1967-1981. back issues avail.; reprint service avail. from PQC. *Refereed.* **Document type:** *Academic/Scholarly.* **Description:** Contains invited critical reviews of physiological topics, as well as reviews in biochemistry, nutrition, general physiology, biophysics, and neuroscience.

Related titles: Microfilm ed.: (from PQC,PMC); Online - full text ed.: Physiological Reviews Online. ISSN 1522-1210. USD 285 to institutions (effective 2001); USD 185 to non-members; USD 280 to institutions (effective 2002) (from Gale Group, HighWire Pr., Northern Light Technology, Inc., EBSCO Publishing, RoweCom Information Quest, Factiva, Institute for Scientific Information); Supplement: Physiology of Cystic Fibrosis. USD 60 to non-members; USD 30 to members (effective 2001); USD 60 to institutions (effective 2002).

Indexed: ASCA, Agri.& Environ.Biotech.Abstr. (coverage dropped), Anim.Breed.Abstr., Aqua.Sci.& Fish.Abstr., Biol.& Agr.Ind. (Apr.1983-), Biol.Abstr., Chem.Abstr., Chem.Titles, Curr.Adv.Ecol.Sci., Curr.Cont., Dairy Sci.Abstr., Dent.Ind., Derwent Biotech.Abstr., Excerp.Med., Focus on: Sports Sci.& Med., Gen.Sci.Ind. (Apr.1984-), INIS Atomind., Ind.Med. (1921-), Ind.Sci.Rev., Inpharma, Int.Abstr.Biol.Sci., Neurosci.Abstr., Nutr.Abstr., Reac., Ref.Zh., SSCI (coverage dropped), Sci.Cit.Ind., Sport Fish.Abstr., Trop.Dis.Bull., Weed Abstr., Wild.Rev., Zoo.Rec.

—BLDSC (6485.000000), CASDDS, CISTI, GNLM, IDS, ingenta, Linda Hall. **CCC.**

Published by: American Physiological Society, 9650 Rockville Pike, Bethesda, MD 20814-3991. TEL 301-530-7164, FAX 301-571-8305, info@aps.faseb.org/aps, info@the-aps.org, http://physrev.physiology.org, http://www.the-aps.org/. Ed. S L Hamilton. Circ: 3,352.

571 USA ISSN 0031-9376
QP1 CODEN: PYSOAP

THE PHYSIOLOGIST. Text in English. 1958. bi-m. USD 50 domestic to non-members; USD 55 in Canada & Mexico to non-members; USD 60 elsewhere to non-members; USD 75 domestic to institutions; USD 80 in Canada & Mexico to institutions; USD 85 elsewhere to institutions; USD 15 newsstand/cover (effective 2002); free to members (print & online eds.). adv. charts, illus. back issues avail.; reprint service avail. from PQC. *Refereed.* **Document type:** *Academic/Scholarly.* **Description:** Contains articles on the society's affairs and announcements, as well as articles of importance to physiologists that are not suitable for other society publications.

Related titles: Microform ed.: (from PQC); Online - full text ed.

Indexed: Biol.Abstr., C.I.J.E. (coverage dropped), Chem.Abstr., Dent.Ind., Excerp.Med., INIS Atomind., Ind.Med. (1957-), Int.Aerosp.Abstr., Sport Fish.Abstr.

—BLDSC (6487.200000), CISTI, GNLM, ingenta, Linda Hall. **CCC.**

Published by: American Physiological Society, 9650 Rockville Pike, Bethesda, MD 20814-3991. TEL 301-530-7164, FAX 301-571-8305, info@aps.faseb.org, info@the-aps.org, http://www.faseb.org/aps/tphys.htm, http://www.the-aps.org/. Ed. M Frank. adv.: B&W page USD 950, color page USD 1,300. Circ: 9,764.

▼ **PHYSIOLOGY**; Royal Australasian College of Dental Surgeons. Lecture notes in physiology. see *MEDICAL SCIENCES—Dentistry*

573.8 USA ISSN 0031-9384
QP351 CODEN: PHBHA4

PHYSIOLOGY AND BEHAVIOR; an international journal. Text in English. 1966. 15/yr. EUR 313 in Europe to qualified personnel; JPY 41,700 in Japan to qualified personnel; USD 351 elsewhere to qualified personnel; EUR 3,107 in Europe to institutions; JPY 412,500 in Japan to institutions; USD 3,475 elsewhere to institutions (effective 2002). adv. bk.rev. charts, illus, stat. index. back issues avail.; reprint service avail. from PQC. *Refereed.* **Document type:** *Journal, Academic/Scholarly.* **Description:** Publishes original research contributions in the areas of neural control of eating, drinking, body composition and body fluids; hormonal control of behavior; sleep activity; rhythms; taste and olfaction; and learning and memory.

Related titles: Microfiche ed.: (from MIM); Microfilm ed.: (from PQC); Online - full text ed.: (from ingenta, Swets Blackwell, Institute for Scientific Information, ScienceDirect).

Indexed: ASCA, Agri.Eng.Abstr., Anim.Behav.Abstr., Anim.Breed.Abstr., Apic.Abstr., Aqua.Sci.& Fish.Abstr., Biol.Abstr., Biotech.& Bioeng.Abstr., Chem.Abstr., Chem.Titles, Chemorec.Abstr., Curr.Adv.Ecol.Sci., Curr.Cont., Curr.Ind.Stat., Dairy Sci.Abstr., Dent.Ind., Excerp.Med., Food Sci.& Tech.Abstr., IBR, INIS Atomind., Ind.Med. (1966-), Ind.Sci.Rev., Ind.Vet., Indian Psychol.Abstr., Inpharma, Int.Abstr.Biol.Sci., Lang.& Lang.Behav.Abstr., Maize Abstr., Neurosci.Abstr. (coverage dropped), Neurosci.Cit.Ind., Nutr.Abstr., Pharm.&Out.News, Pig News & Info., Potato Abstr., Poult.Abstr., Protozool.Abstr., PsycInfo, Psychol.Abstr. (1966-), Reac., Rev.Appl.Entomol., Rev.Arom.& Med.Plants, Rev.Med.& Vet.Mycol., Russ.Acad.Sci.Bibl., SSCI, Sci.Cit.Ind., Soils & Fert., Soyabean Abstr., Sport Fish.Abstr., Sugar Ind.Abstr., THA, Vet.Bull., Wild.Rev., Zoo.Rec., e-psyche.

—BLDSC (6488.100000), ADONIS, CASDDS, CISTI, GNLM, IDS, ingenta. **CCC.**

Published by: Elsevier Science, Box 945, New York, NY 10159-0945. TEL 212-989-5800, FAX 212-633-3990, usinfo-f@elsevier.com, http://www.elsevier.nl/locate/physbeh, http://www.elsevier.com. Eds. Jaap M Koolhass, Matthew J Wayner, Stephen C Woods. adv.: B&W page USD 550, color page USD 1,350. Circ: 1,800. **Subscr. in Australasia and the Far East to:** Elsevier Science (Singapore) Pte Ltd, No.1 Temasek Ave, 17-01 Millenia Tower, Singapore 039192, Singapore. TEL 65-434-3727, FAX 65-337-2230**; Subscr. in Japan to:** Elsevier Science Inc - Japan Regional Office, 9-15 Higashi-Azabu 1-chome, Minato-ku, Tokyo 106-0044, Japan. TEL 81-3-5561-5033**; Subscr. outside the Americas to:** Elsevier Science BV, PO Box 211, Amsterdam 1000 AE, Netherlands. TEL 31-20-485-3757.

571 JPN ISSN 0370-9612
QH188 CODEN: PEJAE6

PHYSIOLOGY AND ECOLOGY JAPAN. Text in English. 1947. s-a. USD 30 to individuals; USD 60 to institutions. bk.rev. back issues avail. **Description:** Covers all fields of physiology and ecology.

Indexed: Biol.Abstr., Curr.Adv.Ecol.Sci., Ecol.Abstr., Sel.Water Res.Abstr.

—CISTI.

Published by: Physiology and Ecology Japan Editorial Office/Seiri Seitai Kankokai, Kyoto Daigaku Rigakubu Dobutsugaku Kyoshitsu, Kitashirakawa, Sakyo-ku, Kyoto-shi 606, Japan. FAX 075-751-6149, TELEX J-5422302-SCIKYU. Ed. Hiroya Kawanabe. Circ: 700.

PHYSIOLOGY CANADA. see *MEDICAL SCIENCES*

571 ZAF ISSN 1022-1220

PHYSIOLOGY SOCIETY OF SOUTHERN AFRICA. PROCEEDINGS. Text in English. 1993. a. **Document type:** *Proceedings.*

Published by: Physiology Society of Southern Africa, c/o University of Pretoria, Faculty of Medicine, Dept. of Physiology, Pretoria 0002, South Africa.

PLATELETS (SHEFFIELD). see *BIOLOGY—Abstracting, Bibliographies, Statistics*

B

571 USA ISSN 1099-5862
PROFESSIONALIZATION OF EXERCISE PHYSIOLOGY; an international electronic journal for exercise physiologists. Text in English. 1998. m. bk.rev. back issues avail. *Refereed.* **Document type:** *Journal, Academic/Scholarly.* **Description:** Focuses on articles that provide a rationale for the professionalization of exercise physiology and to increase awareness of exercise physiology as a developing profession.
Media: Online - full text.
Published by: College of St. Scholastica, Department of Exercise Physiology, 1200 Kenwood Ave., Duluth, MN 55811. TEL 218-723-6297, tboone2@css.edu, http://www.css.edu/users/tboone2/asep/fldr/pro1a.htm. Ed. Tommy Boone.

573.8 GBR ISSN 0301-0082
QP356 CODEN: PGNBA5
PROGRESS IN NEUROBIOLOGY; an international review journal. Text in English. 1973. 18/yr. EUR 2,301 in Europe to institutions; JPY 305,700 in Japan to institutions; USD 2,574 elsewhere to institutions (effective 2002). back issues avail. *Refereed.* **Document type:** *Academic/Scholarly.* **Description:** Reviews advances in the field of neurobiology with coverage of all relevant disciplines.
Related titles: Microfilm ed.: (from PQC); Online - full text ed.: (from ingenta, Swets Blackwell, Institute for Scientific Information, ScienceDirect).
Indexed: ASCA, Anim.Behav.Abstr., Biol.Abstr., Cal.Tiss.Abstr., Chem.Abstr., Chem.Indus.Notes, Chem.Titles, Chemorec.Abstr., Curr.Adv.Cell & Devel.Biol., Curr.Adv.Ecol.Sci., Curr.Cont., Excerp.Med., Ind.Med. (1973-), Ind.Sci.Rev., Inpharma, Int.Abstr.Biol.Sci., Neurosci.Abstr., Neurosci.Cit.Ind., Nutr.Abstr., Pharm.&Out.News, Psychol.Abstr. (1994-), Reac., Sci.Cit.Ind., Sport Fish.Abstr., THA, Wild.Rev., Zoo.Rec., e-psyche.
—BLDSC (6870.300000), ADONIS, CASDDS, CISTI, EMDOCS, GNLM, IDS, ingenta, Linda Hall. **CCC.**
Published by: Pergamon (Subsidiary of: Elsevier Science), The Boulevard, Langford Ln, East Park, Kidlington, Oxford OXB 1GB, United Kingdom. FAX 44-1865-843010, info-f@elsevier.nl; usinfo-f@elsevier.com; forinfo-kyf04035@niftyserve.or.jp, http://www.elsevier.com/locate/pneurobio, http://www.elsevier.nl/. Ed. M J Zigmond. **Subscr. in Australasia and the Far East to:** Elsevier Science (Singapore) Pte Ltd, No.1 Temasek Ave, 17-01 Millenia Tower, Singapore 039192, Singapore. TEL 65-434-3727, FAX 65-337-2230; **Subscr. in the Americas to:** Elsevier Science, PO Box 945, New York, NY 10159-0945. TEL 212-633-3730, FAX 212-633-3680; **Subscr. to:** Elsevier Science BV, PO Box 211, Amsterdam 1000 AE, Netherlands. TEL 31-20-485-3757, FAX 31-20-485-3432.

PSYCHOPHYSIOLOGY; an international journal. see *MEDICAL SCIENCES—Psychiatry And Neurology*

571 GBR ISSN 0265-1742
RECENT ADVANCES IN PHYSIOLOGY. Text in English. 1925. irreg., latest vol.10. **Document type:** *Monographic series, Academic/Scholarly.*
Published by: Churchill Livingstone (Subsidiary of: Harcourt Publishers Ltd.), Robert Stevenson House, 1-3 Baxter's Pl, Leith Walk, Edinburgh, Midlothian EH1 3AF, United Kingdom. TEL 44-131-556-2424, FAX 44-131-459-1177, http://www.churchillmed.com. **US subscr. to:** Churchill Livingstone, 650 Ave of the Americas, New York, NY 10011. TEL 212-206-5000.

REDOX REPORT. see *PHARMACY AND PHARMACOLOGY*

REFERATIVNYI ZHURNAL. FIZIOLOGIYA I MORFOLOGIYA CHELOVEKA I ZHIVOTNYKH. see *BIOLOGY—Abstracting, Bibliographies, Statistics*

RENAL PHYSIOLOGY. see *BIOLOGY—Abstracting, Bibliographies, Statistics*

RENIN, ANGIOTENSIN & KININS. see *BIOLOGY—Abstracting, Bibliographies, Statistics*

REPRODUCTION. ABSTRACT SERIES. see *BIOLOGY—Abstracting, Bibliographies, Statistics*

573.6 GBR
CODEN: JRFSAR
REPRODUCTION. SUPPLEMENT. Text in English. 1966. irreg., latest vol.57. price varies. adv. back issues avail. *Refereed.* **Document type:** *Monographic series, Academic/Scholarly.*
Formerly (until 2001): Journal of Reproduction and Fertility. Supplement (0449-3087)
Related titles: ◆ Supplement to: Journal of Reproduction and Fertility. ISSN 0022-4251.
Indexed: AgBiotech, Agricola, Anim.Breed.Abstr., Biol.Abstr., Chem.Abstr., Chem.Indus.Notes, Chem.Titles, Dairy Sci.Abstr., Ind.Med. (1966-), Nutr.Abstr., Sport Fish.Abstr., Wild.Rev., Zoo.Rec.
—BLDSC (5049.601000), CASDDS, CISTI, ingenta, KNAW, Linda Hall. **CCC.**
Published by: Journals of Reproduction & Fertility Ltd, 22 Newmarket Rd, Cambridge CB5 8DT, United Kingdom. TEL 44-1223-351809, FAX 44-1223-359754, jrf@journals-of-reproduction.org.uk, http://www.journals-of-reproduction.org.uk. Adv. contact Mrs. C H Clarke. **Dist. by:** Portland Press Ltd.

573.6 USA ISSN 0890-6238
CODEN: REPTED
REPRODUCTIVE TOXICOLOGY. Text in English. 1988. bi-m. EUR 168 in Europe to qualified personnel; JPY 22,300 in Japan to qualified personnel; USD 188 elsewhere to qualified personnel; EUR 902 in Europe to institutions; JPY 119,700 in Japan to institutions; USD 1,009 elsewhere to institutions (effective 2002). back issues avail. *Refereed.* **Document type:** *Academic/Scholarly.* **Description:** Publishes original research on the influence of chemical and physical agents on reproduction, focusing on the application of in vitro, animal and clinical research to the practice of clinical medicine.
Related titles: Microfilm ed.: (from PQC); Online - full text ed.: (from ingenta, Swets Blackwell, Institute for Scientific Information, ScienceDirect).
Indexed: ASCA, Aqua.Sci.& Fish.Abstr., Chem.Abstr., Chem.Indus.Notes, Chem.Titles, Curr.Cont., Environ.Sci.Poll.Mgmt., Fam.Ind., Ind.Med. (1987-), Ind.Sci.Rev., Inpharma, Int.Abstr.Biol.Sci., Lab.Haz.Bull., NRN, Nutr.Abstr., Pharm.&Out.News, Pollut.Abstr., Reac., Rev.Appl.Entomol., Rev.Arom.& Med.Plants, Rev.Med.& Vet.Mycol., Risk Abstr., SSCI (coverage dropped), Saf.Sci.Abstr., Sci.Cit.Ind., Tox.Abstr., Weed Abstr.
—BLDSC (7713.706500), CASDDS, CISTI, GNLM, IDS, Infotrieve, ingenta, KNAW. **CCC.**
Published by: (Reproductive Toxicology Center), Elsevier Science, PO Box 945, New York, NY 10159-0945. TEL 212-989-5800, FAX 212-633-3990, usinfo-f@elsevier.com, http://www.elsevier.nl/locate/reprotox. Ed. Dr. Anthony R Scialli. **Subscr. in Australasia and the Far East to:** Elsevier Science (Singapore) Pte Ltd, No.1 Temasek Ave, 17-01 Millenia Tower, Singapore 039192, Singapore. TEL 65-434-3727, FAX 65-337-2230; **Subscr. in Japan to:** Elsevier Science Inc - Japan Regional Office, 9-15 Higashi-Azabu 1-chome, Minato-ku, Tokyo 106-0044, Japan. TEL 81-3-5561-5033; **Subscr. outside the Americas to:** Elsevier Science BV, PO Box 211, Amsterdam 1000 AE, Netherlands. TEL 31-20-485-3757.

573.2 NLD ISSN 0034-5687
QP121.A1 CODEN: RSPYAK
RESPIRATION PHYSIOLOGY. Text in Dutch. 1966. 15/yr. EUR 99 in Europe to qualified personnel; JPY 13,000 in Japan to qualified personnel; USD 110 elsewhere to qualified personnel; EUR 1,619 in Europe to institutions; JPY 215,000 in Japan to institutions; USD 1,811 elsewhere to institutions (effective 2002). illus. reprints avail. *Refereed.* **Document type:** *Academic/Scholarly.* **Description:** For researchers in respiratory, pulmonary and circulatory physiology.
Related titles: Microform ed.: (from PQC); Online - full text ed.: (from ingenta, Swets Blackwell, Institute for Scientific Information, ScienceDirect).
Indexed: ASCA, Biol.Abstr., C.I.S. Abstr., Chem.Abstr., Chem.Indus.Notes, Chem.Titles, Curr.Adv.Biochem., Curr.Adv.Ecol.Sci., Curr.Cont., Dent.Ind., Excerp.Med., Ind.Med. (1966-), Ind.Sci.Rev., Ind.Vet., Inpharma, Int.Abstr.Biol.Sci., Neurosci.Cit.Ind., Pig News & Info., Poult.Abstr., Reac., Risk Abstr., Sci.Cit.Ind., Sport Fish.Abstr., THA, Vet.Bull., Wild.Rev., Zoo.Rec.
—BLDSC (7777.650000), CASDDS, CISTI, GNLM, IDS, ingenta, KNAW. **CCC.**
Published by: Elsevier Science BV, PO Box 211, Amsterdam 1000 AE, Netherlands. TEL 31-20-485-3757, FAX 31-20-485-3432, TELEX 18582 ESPA NL, http://www.elsevier.nl/locate/resphysiol. Ed. P Scheid. **Subscr. in Australasia and the Far East to:** Elsevier Science (Singapore) Pte Ltd, No.1 Temasek Ave, 17-01 Millenia Tower, Singapore 039192, Singapore. TEL 65-434-3727, FAX 65-337-2230; **Subscr. in Japan to:** Elsevier Science Inc - Japan Regional Office, 9-15 Higashi-Azabu 1-chome, Minato-ku, Tokyo 106-0044, Japan. TEL 81-3-5561-5033, FAX 81-3-5561-5047; **Subscr. in the Americas to:** Elsevier Science, PO Box 945, New York, NY 10159-0945. TEL 212-633-3730, FAX 212-633-3680, usinfo-f@elsevier.com, http://www.elsevier.com.

612 USA ISSN 0892-1253
REVIEW OF MEDICAL PHYSIOLOGY. Text in English. 1963. biennial. **Document type:** *Monographic series, Academic/Scholarly.*
—BLDSC (7792.400000), CISTI.
Published by: Appleton & Lange, Journal Division (Subsidiary of: Simon & Schuster Company), 11 W 19th St, New York, CT 10011-4209. TEL 203-406-4500, FAX 203-406-4600.

571 USA ISSN 0303-4240
QP1 CODEN: RPBEA5
REVIEWS OF PHYSIOLOGY, BIOCHEMISTRY AND PHARMACOLOGY. Text in English. irreg. price varies. reprint service avail. from ISI. *Refereed.* **Document type:** *Monographic series.*
Formerly: Ergebnisse der Physiologie, Biologischen Chemie und Experimentellen Pharmakologie (0080-2042)
Related titles: Online - full text ed.: (from Institute for Scientific Information).
Indexed: ASCA, BBCI, Biol.Abstr., Chem.Abstr., Chem.Indus.Notes, Chem.Titles, Curr.Adv.Ecol.Sci., Ind.Med. (1974-), Ind.Sci.Rev., Sci.Cit.Ind.
—BLDSC (7794.020000), CASDDS, CISTI, GNLM, IDS, ingenta, KNAW, Linda Hall. **CCC.**
Published by: Springer-Verlag, Journals (Subsidiary of: BertelsmannSpringer), 175 Fifth Ave, New York, NY 10010. TEL 212-460-1500, FAX 212-473-6272.

REVISTA BRASILEIRA DE MASTOLOGIA. see *MEDICAL SCIENCES—Oncology*

571 ROM ISSN 1220-840X
CODEN: RMEPDZ
REVUE ROUMAINE DE PHYSIOLOGIE/ROMANIAN JOURNAL OF PHYSIOLOGY. Text in English, French, German, Russian, Spanish. q. bk.rev. charts, illus. index. **Document type:** *Academic/Scholarly.*
Formerly (until 1990): Physiologie (1011-6206); Which supersedes in part (in 1975): Revue Roumaine de Morphologie et de Physiologie (0377-4953); Which was formed by the 1974 merger of: Revue Roumaine de Physiologie (0035-399X); Revue Roumaine de Morphologie et d'Embryologie (0377-4945); Which was formed by the 1973 merger of: Morfologia Normala si Patologia (0027-1063); Revue Roumaine d'Embryologie et de Cytologie. Serie de Cytologie (0556-8056); Revue Roumaine d'Embryologie (0300-063X); Which was formerly (1964-1972): Revue Roumaine d'Embryologie et de Cytologie. Serie d'Embryologie (0035-4007)
Indexed: Biol.Abstr., Chem.Abstr., Chem.Indus.Notes, Chem.Titles, Curr.Adv.Ecol.Sci., Excerp.Med. (until 1993), Ind.Med. (coverage dropped).
—BLDSC, CASDDS, CISTI, GNLM, KNAW, Linda Hall.
Published by: (Academia de Stiinte Medicale), Editura Academiei Romane, Calea 13 Septembrie 13, Bucharest 76117, Romania. Ed. P Groza. Circ: 600. **Dist. by:** Rodipet S.A.. TEL 401-618-5103, FAX 401-222-6407.

RINSHO KOKYU SEIRI/JOURNAL OF CLINICAL RESPIRATORY PHYSIOLOGY. see *MEDICAL SCIENCES—Respiratory Diseases*

571 JPN ISSN 0285-3299
CODEN: SGKHEB
SEIRIGAKU GIJUTSU KENKYUKAI HOKOKU/REPORT OF PHYSIOLOGICAL TECHNOLOGY. Text in Japanese. 1979. a.
Indexed: Chem.Abstr., Chem.Indus.Notes, Chem.Titles.
—CASDDS.
Published by: Okazaki Kokuritsu Kyodo Kenkyu Kiko, Seirigaku Kenkyujo/Okazaki National Research Institutes, National Institute for Physiological Sciences, 38 Saigo-Naka-Myodaiji, Okazaki-shi, Aichi-ken 444-0000, Japan.

571 JPN ISSN 0913-0322
CODEN: SGHOEH
SEIRIGAKU KENKYUJO GIJUTSUKA HOKOKU/NATIONAL INSTITUTE FOR PHYSIOLOGICAL SCIENCES. TECHNICAL DIVISION. ANNUAL REPORT. Text in Japanese. 1986. a.
Indexed: Chem.Abstr.
—CASDDS.
Published by: Okazaki Kokuritsu Kyodo Kenkyu Kiko, Seirigaku Kenkyujo/Okazaki National Research Institutes, National Institute for Physiological Sciences, 38 Saigo-Naka-Myodaiji, Okazaki-shi, Aichi-ken 444-0000, Japan.

571 JPN
SEIRIGAKU KENKYUJO NENPO/NATIONAL INSTITUTE FOR PHYSIOLOGICAL SCIENCES. ANNUAL REPORT. Text in English, Japanese. 1980. a.

Published by: Okazaki Kokuritsu Kyodo Kenkyu Kiko, Seirigaku Kenkyujo/Okazaki National Research Institutes, National Institute for Physiological Sciences, 38 Saigo-Naka-Myodaiji, Okazaki-shi, Aichi-ken 444-0000, Japan.

571 JPN
SEIRIKEN SAKYURA/OKAZAKI NATIONAL RESEARCH INSTITUTES. NATIONAL INSTITUTE FOR PHYSIOLOGICAL SCIENCES. CIRCULAR. Text in Japanese. 1978. a.
Published by: Okazaki Kokuritsu Kyodo Kenkyu Kiko, Seirigaku Kenkyujo/Okazaki National Research Institutes, National Institute for Physiological Sciences, 38 Saigo-Naka-Myodaiji, Okazaki-shi, Aichi-ken 444-0000, Japan.

571.978 GBR ISSN 1044-579X
CODEN: SECBE7
SEMINARS IN CANCER BIOLOGY. Text in English. 1989. bi-m. GBP 235 to institutions (effective 2001). adv. reprint service avail. from SWZ. *Refereed.* **Document type:** *Academic/Scholarly.*
Related titles: Online - full text ed.: (from EBSCO Publishing, O C L C Online Computer Library Center, Inc., RoweCom Information Quest, ingenta, Swets Blackwell, IDEAL Online Library, Institute for Scientific Information).
Indexed: AIDS & Cancer Res., ASCA, Biotech.& Bioeng.Abstr., Chem.Abstr., Chem.Titles, Curr.Cont., Genet.Abstr., Hum.Gen.Abstr., Ind.Med. (1990-), Ind.Sci.Rev., Inpharma, Nuc.Acids Abstr., Oncog.G.F.Abstr., Pharm.&Out.News, Reac., Sci.Cit.Ind.
—BLDSC (8239.448340), ADONIS, CASDDS, CISTI, GNLM, IDS, Infotrieve, ingenta, KNAW. **CCC.**
Published by: Academic Press (Subsidiary of: Harcourt Publishers Ltd.), 24 Oval Rd, London NW1 7DX, United Kingdom. TEL 44-20-7267-4466, FAX 44-20-7482-2293, apsubs@acad.com, http://www.academicpress.com/semcancer; http://www.europe.idealibrary.com/. R&P Catherine John. Adv. contact Nik Screen. **Subscr. to:** Harcourt Publishers Ltd., Foots Cray High St, Sidcup, Kent DA14 5HP, United Kingdom. TEL 44-20-8300-3322, FAX 44-20-8309-0807.

SENSORY NEURON; the international interdisciplinary journal reporting basic and clinical research on sensory receptors and primary afferent neurons. see *MEDICAL SCIENCES—Psychiatry And Neurology*

571 CHN ISSN 0559-7765
QP1 CODEN: SLKHA8
SHENGLI KEXUE JINZHAN/PROGRESS IN PHYSIOLOGICAL SCIENCES. Text in Chinese; Abstracts in English. 1957. q. USD 20 (effective 1999). adv. bk.rev. *Refereed.* **Document type:** *Academic/Scholarly.* **Description:** Covers physiology, biochemistry, molecular biology, pharmacology, biophysics, pathophysiology and nutrition.
Indexed: Chem.Abstr., Chem.Indus.Notes, Chem.Titles, ExtraMED, Ind.Med. (1957-).
—BLDSC (6873.490000), CASDDS, GNLM, Linda Hall.
Published by: Neuroscience Research Institute, Beijing Medical University, 38 Xueyuan Rd, Beijing 100083, China. TEL 86-1-6209-1150, FAX 86-1-6202-9252, hanjs@iname.com. Ed. Han Jisheng. Adv. contact Lazhi Feng. Circ: 3,000 (paid).

571 CHN ISSN 0371-0874
QP1 CODEN: SLHPAH
SHENGLI XUEBAO/ACTA PHYSIOLOGICA SINICA. Text in Chinese; Summaries in English. 1927. bi-m. USD 80 (effective 2000). adv. *Refereed.* **Document type:** *Academic/Scholarly.* **Description:** Contains mostly original research papers on physiology. Also includes short communications and reviews.
Related titles: ♦ English ed.: Chinese Journal of Physiological Sciences. ISSN 0258-6428.
Indexed: Biol.Abstr., Chem.Abstr., Chem.Titles, Excerp.Med., Ind.Med. (1953-), Psychol.Abstr. (1965-), Ref.Zh.
—BLDSC (0655.500000), CASDDS, CISTI, EMDOCS, GNLM, Linda Hall.
Published by: (Shanghai Institute of Physiology), Kexue Chubanshe/Science Press, 16 Donghuang Cheng Genbei Jie, Beijing 100717, China. Circ: 7,000.

SIGNAL'NAYA INFORMATSIYA. FIZIOLOGIYA I MORFOLOGIYA CHELOVEKA I ZHIVOTNYKH: KROV' I LIMFA. see *BIOLOGY—Abstracting, Bibliographies, Statistics*

616.178059 USA
QH585
SOCIETY FOR IN VITRO BIOLOGY. PROCEEDINGS. Text in English. irreg. price varies. *Refereed.* **Document type:** *Proceedings.* **Description:** Publishes the proceedings of various meetings and specific topics of interest to tissue culture researchers.
Formerly: Tissue Culture Association. Proceedings of the Annual Meeting (0272-6564)
Published by: Society for In Vitro Biology, 9315 Largo Dr. W., Ste. 255, Largo, MD 20774. TEL 301-324-5054, FAX 301-324-5057, sivb@sivb.org, http://www.sivb.org.

612 301 GBR ISSN 0954-7800
CODEN: SHUBAC
SOCIETY FOR THE STUDY OF HUMAN BIOLOGY. SYMPOSIUM SERIES. Text in English. 1960. irreg. price varies. *Refereed.* **Document type:** *Proceedings.*
Formerly (until 1986): Society for the Study of Human Biology. Symposia (0081-153X)
Indexed: Biol.Abstr., Curr.Adv.Ecol.Sci., GeoRef.
—CASDDS. **CCC.**
Published by: (Society for the Study of Human Biology), Cambridge University Press, Edinburgh Bldg, Shaftesbury Rd, Cambridge CB2 2RU, United Kingdom. FAX 44-1223-315052, information@cup.cam.ac.uk, information@cambridge.org, http://www.cup.cam.ac.uk, http://www.uk.cambridge.org/journals/pmu. R&P Linda Nicol. Circ: 200.

573.8 GBR ISSN 0899-0220
QP450 CODEN: SMOREZ
SOMATOSENSORY AND MOTOR RESEARCH. Text in English. 1983. q. GBP 117, USD 175 to individuals; GBP 292, USD 482 to institutions (effective 2002). adv. charts, illus. index. back issues avail.; reprint service avail. from PQC. *Refereed.* **Document type:** *Academic/Scholarly.* **Description:** Original research on somatic sensation and its neural mechanisms. Experimental and descriptive studies.
Formerly: Somatosensory Research (0736-7244)
Related titles: Online - full text ed.: ISSN 1369-1651 (from CatchWord Ltd., EBSCO Publishing, O C L C Online Computer Library Center, Inc., RoweCom Information Quest, Institute for Scientific Information).
Indexed: ASCA, Anim.Behav.Abstr., Aqua.Sci.& Fish.Abstr., Biol.Abstr., Chem.Abstr., Curr.Adv.Cell & Devel.Biol., Curr.Adv.Ecol.Sci., Curr.Cont., Excerp.Med., Ind.Med. (1988-), Ind.Sci.Rev., Inpharma, Int.Abstr.Biol.Sci., Neurosci.Abstr., Neurosci.Cit.Ind., PsycInfo, Psychol.Abstr. (1983-), Reac., Ref.Zh., SSCI (coverage dropped), Sci.Cit.Ind., e-psyche.
—BLDSC (8327.809150), ADONIS, CASDDS, CatchWord, CISTI, EMDOCS, GNLM, IDS, Infotrieve, ingenta, KNAW. **CCC.**
Published by: Carfax Publishing Limited (Subsidiary of: Taylor & Francis Group), c/o Sue Dommett, PO Box 25, Abingdon, Oxford OX14 3UE, United Kingdom. TEL 44-1235-401000, FAX 44-1235-401550, enquiries@carfax.co.uk, enquiries@carfax.co.uk/, http://www.carfax.co.uk. Ed. Thomas Woolsey. Circ: 500.

571 CHE ISSN 0888-4803
QH301 CODEN: SRFREP
SOVIET SCIENTIFIC REVIEWS SERIES. SECTION F: PHYSIOLOGY AND GENERAL BIOLOGY REVIEWS. Text in English. irreg., latest vol.12. EUR 164; price varies. *Refereed.* **Document type:** *Monographic series, Academic/Scholarly.*
Related titles: Microform ed.
—CISTI. **CCC.**
Published by: Gordon and Breach - Harwood Academic (Subsidiary of: Taylor & Francis Group), PO Box 531, Lausanne 1000, Switzerland. Ed. T M Turpaev. **Subscr. addr. in US:** PTT, PO Box 566, Williston, VT 05495-0080. TEL 800-326-8917, FAX 802-864-7626.

STUDIES IN FERTILITY AND STERILITY. see *MEDICAL SCIENCES*

612 NLD ISSN 0926-9738
STUDIES IN HUMAN BIOLOGY. Text in English. 1990. irreg. price varies. **Document type:** *Monographic series.*
—KNAW.
Published by: Kluwer Academic Publishers Group (Subsidiary of: Wolters Kluwer N.V.), Spuiboulevard 50, PO Box 17, Dordrecht 3300 AA, Netherlands. FAX 31-78-639-2254, services@wkap.nl, http://www.wkap.nl. **Dist. by:** Journals Department, PO Box 322, Dordrecht 3300 AH, Netherlands. FAX 31-78-654-6474.

571 GBR ISSN 0969-8116
STUDIES IN PHYSIOLOGY. Text in English. 1993. irreg., latest vol.4, 2000. GBP 22, USD 37.40 (effective 2002). *Refereed.* **Document type:** *Monographic series, Academic/Scholarly.*
—CISTI.
Published by: Portland Press Ltd., 59 Portland Pl, London W1N 3AJ, United Kingdom. TEL 44-20-7580-5530, FAX 44-20-7323-1136, sales@portland-service.com, http://www.portlandpress.com/bst/default.htm. R&P Adam Marshall. **Subscr. to:** Commerce Way, Colchester, Essex CO2 8HP, United Kingdom. TEL 44-1206-796351, FAX 44-1206-796351.

TOKYO SHIKA DAIGAKU SEIRIGAKU KYOSHITSU GYOSEKISHU/TOKYO DENTAL COLLEGE. DEPARTMENT OF PHYSIOLOGY. BIBLIOGRAPHY. see *BIOLOGY—Abstracting, Bibliographies, Statistics*

571 ITA ISSN 0392-8470
UNIVERSITA DI FERRARA. ANNALI. SEZIONE 1: ANATOMIA UMANA. Text in Italian. 1951. a.
Published by: (Universita di Ferrara), Casa Editrice Leo S. Olschki, Viuzzo Del Pozzetto, Florence, FI 50126, Italy. TEL 39-55-6530684, FAX 39-55-6530214.

571 ITA ISSN 0373-5915
UNIVERSITA DI FERRARA. ANNALI. SEZIONE 13: ANATOMIA E FISIOLOGIA COMPARATA. Text in Italian. 1956. irreg.
Published by: (Universita di Ferrara), Casa Editrice Leo S. Olschki, Viuzzo Del Pozzetto, Florence, FI 50126, Italy. TEL 39-55-6530684, FAX 39-55-6530214.

571 CHN ISSN 1000-6834
CODEN: ZYSZE2
ZHONGGUO YINGYONG SHENGLIXUE ZAZHI/CHINESE JOURNAL OF APPLIED PHYSIOLOGY. Text in Chinese; Abstracts and contents page in English. 1985. q. CNY 40 domestic; USD 28.53 foreign (effective 2001). adv. *Refereed.* **Document type:** *Academic/Scholarly.* **Description:** Covers environmental physiology, pathophysiology, clinical physiology, cellular physiology, molecular physiology, ergonomics, work and exercise physiology, medical engineering and veterinary physiology.
Indexed: Ind.Med. (1985-).
—BLDSC (3180.294400), CASDDS.
Published by: (Zhongguo Shengli Xuehui/Chinese Association for Physiological Sciences), Zhongguo Yingyong Shenglixue Zazhi Bianjibu, One Da Li Dao, Tianjin 300050, China. TEL 86-22-84655184, FAX 86-22-3314818. Ed. Lu Yongda. Adv. contact Dengyun Xu TEL 86-22-28256563. page USD 500. Circ: 4,000 (paid). **Dist. outside China by:** China International Book Trading Corp, 35 Chegongzhuang Xilu, Haidian District, Beijing 100044, China.

ZHURNAL EVOLYUTSIONNOI BIOKHIMII I FIZIOLOGII. see *BIOLOGY—Biochemistry*

573.8 RUS ISSN 0044-4677
CODEN: ZVNDAM
ZHURNAL VYSSHEI NERVNOI DEYATEL'NOSTI. Text in Russian; Summaries in English. 1951. bi-m. USD 247.50. bk.rev. index. *Refereed.*
Related titles: Online - full text ed.: (from Institute for Scientific Information).
Indexed: ASCA, Biol.Abstr., C.C.M.J., Chem.Abstr., Chem.Indus.Notes, Chem.Titles, Curr.Adv.Ecol.Sci., Curr.Cont. (coverage dropped), Dent.Ind., Excerp.Med., INIS Atomind., Ind.Med. (1951-), Inpharma, Neurosci.Cit.Ind., Psychol.Abstr. (1951-), Reac., Ref.Zh., Russ.Acad.Sci.Bibl., SSCI (coverage dropped), Sci.Cit.Ind. (coverage dropped), Zoo.Rec., e-psyche.
—CASDDS, CISTI, East View, GNLM, IDS, Infotrieve, KNAW, Linda Hall. **CCC.**
Published by: (Otdelenie Fiziologii im. I.P. Pavlova, Rossiiskaya Akademiya Nauk/Russian Academy of Sciences), M A I K Nauka - Interperiodica, Mezhdunarodnyi Otdel, Profsoyuznaya ul 90, Moscow 117864, Russian Federation. TEL 7-095-3360266, FAX 7-095-420-2220. Ed. P V Simonov. **Dist. in U.S. by:** Victor Kamkin Inc., 4956 Boiling Brook Pkwy, Rockville, MD 20852.

BIOLOGY—Zoology

see also PETS; VETERINARY SCIENCE

594 USA ISSN 1041-5300
A M U NEWS. Text in English. 1960. s-a. USD 25 to members. bk.rev. back issues avail. **Document type:** *Newsletter.* **Description:** Focuses on the study of mollusks.

B

Published by: American Malacological Union, Inc., c/o Dr Raymond W Neck, Houston Museum of Natural Science, One Hermann Circle Dr, Houston, TX 77030. TEL 713-639-4678, FAX 713-523-4125. Circ: 800. **Subscr. to:** c/o David Hargreave, Department of Science Studies, Western Michigan University, Kalamazoo, MI 49008. TEL 616-387-2723.

A T C C ANIMAL VIRUSES AND ANTISERA, CHLAMYDIAE, AND RICKETTSIAE. see *BIOLOGY—Microbiology*

590 POL ISSN 0001-530X
QL1 CODEN: ABCZAQ
ACTA BIOLOGICA CRACOVIENSIA. ZOOLOGIA. Text in English. 1958. a. price varies. charts, illus. index. **Document type:** *Academic/Scholarly.* **Description:** Original research papers. Forum for zoologists involved in investigating function and structure of animals from cell level.
Indexed: ASCA, AgroAgen, AgroLibrex, Anim.Breed.Abstr., Biol.Abstr., Chem.Abstr., Curr.Adv.Ecol.Sci., Curr.Cont. (coverage dropped), Helminthol.Abstr., IBR, INIS Atomind., Ind.Vet., Key Word Ind.Wildl.Res., Sci.Cit.Ind. (coverage dropped), Vet.Bull., Zoo.Rec.
—BLDSC (0602.420000), CASDDS, CISTI, ingenta, KNAW, Linda Hall.
Published by: (Polska Akademia Nauk/Polish Academy of Sciences, Oddzial w Krakowie, Komisja Biologiczna), Ossolineum Publishing House of the Polish Academy of Sciences, Pl Solny 14 a, Wroclaw 50062, Poland. TEL 48-71-343-6961, FAX 48-71-448-103, TELEX 0712771 OSS PL. Ed. Cz Jura. Circ: 780.

571.9 DEU ISSN 0873-9749
ACTA ETHOLOGICA. Text in English. 1998. 2/yr. EUR 106.10 domestic; EUR 104.20 in Germany; EUR 59.40 newsstand/cover foreign (effective 2002). back issues avail. *Refereed.* **Document type:** *Journal, Academic/Scholarly.* **Description:** Publishes original contributions, reviews, short notes and commentaries in the entire field of the behavioral biology of both humans and other animals.
Related titles: Microform ed.; ♦ Online - full text ed.: Acta Ethologica Online. ISSN 1437-9546.
Indexed: Zoo.Rec.
—BLDSC (0615.547700).
Published by: (Instituto Superior de Psicologia Aplicada PRT), Springer-Verlag (Subsidiary of: BertelsmannSpringer), Tiergartenstr 17, Heidelberg 69121, Germany. TEL 49-6221-345-0, FAX 49-6221-345229, subscriptions@springer.de, http://link.springer.de/link/service/journals/10211/index.htm, http://www.springer.de. Ed. Rui Oliveira. **Subscr. to:** Springer-Verlag New York Inc., PO Box 2485, Secaucus, NJ 07096-2485. TEL 212-460-1500, FAX 212-473-6272.

590 GBR ISSN 1463-6395
ACTA ZOOLOGICA ONLINE. Text in English. q. GBP 45 in Europe to individuals (effective 2002); USD 72 in North America to individuals; GBP 45 elsewhere to individuals; GBP 297 in Europe to institutions; USD 470 in North America to institutions; GBP 297 elsewhere to institutions (effective 2001). **Document type:** *Academic/Scholarly.*
Media: Online - full text (from EBSCO Publishing, Munksgaard & Blackwell Science's Synergy, O C L C Online Computer Library Center, Inc., RoweCom Information Quest, ingenta, Swets Blackwell, Institute for Scientific Information). **Related titles:** Microform ed.: (from PQC); ♦ Print ed.: Acta Zoologica. ISSN 0001-7272.
Published by: Blackwell Science Ltd., Osney Mead, Oxford OX2 0EL, United Kingdom. TEL 44-1685-206206, FAX 44-1685-721205, website@blacksci.com, http://www.blackwell-science.com.

ADVANCES IN ANIMAL PHYSIOLOGY AND ANIMAL NUTRITION/FORTSCHRITTE IN DER TIERPHYSIOLOGIE UND TIERERNAEHRUNG. see *BIOLOGY—Physiology*

599.657 CAN ISSN 0835-5851
ALCES; a journal devoted to the biology and management of moose. Text in English. 1963. q. CND 38, USD 30 (effective 2000). charts, illus. back issues avail. *Refereed.* **Document type:** *Academic/Scholarly.* **Description:** Original research relating in the broadest sense to the biology and management of moose.
Formerly (until 1981): North American Moose Conference. Proceedings (0836-8716)
Related titles: Microfiche ed.
Indexed: Anim.Breed.Abstr., Dairy Sci.Abstr., Environ.Abstr., Forest Prod.Abstr., Forest.Abstr., Helminthol.Abstr., Herb.Abstr., Ind.Vet., Key Word Ind.Wildl.Res., Nutr.Abstr., Rev.Appl.Entomol., Sport Fish.Abstr., Vet.Bull., Wild.Rev., Zoo.Rec.
—BLDSC (0786.716000), CISTI, Infotrieve, ingenta. **CCC.**
Address: Lakehead University Bookstore, 855 Oliver Rd, Thunder Bay, ON P7B 5E1, Canada. TEL 807-343-8528, FAX 807-346-7796, mlankest@lakeheadu.ca. Eds. A Rodgers, W Ballard. R&P M Lankester. Circ: 300.

599.8 USA ISSN 0275-2565
QL737.P9 CODEN: AJPTDU
AMERICAN JOURNAL OF PRIMATOLOGY. Text in English. 1981. m. USD 2,095 in United States; USD 2,225 in Canada & Mexico; USD 2,335 elsewhere; USD 2,200 combined subscription in United States for print and online eds.; USD 2,330 combined subscription in Canada & Mexico for print and online eds.; USD 2,440 combined subscription elsewhere for print and online eds. (effective 2002). adv. bk.rev. bibl, charts, illus. index. back issues avail. *Refereed.* **Document type:** *Academic/Scholarly.* **Description:** Examines topics relevant to the study of primates, including all aspects of their anatomy, behavior, development, ecology, evolution, genetics, nutrition, physiology, reproduction, systematics, conservation, husbandry, and use in biomedical research.
Related titles: Microform ed.: (from PQC); Online - full text ed.: ISSN 1098-2345. USD 2,095 in United States; USD 2,095 in Canada & Mexico; USD 2,095 elsewhere (effective 2002) (from EBSCO Publishing, Wiley InterScience, Institute for Scientific Information).
Indexed: ASCA, Abstr.Anthropol., Anim.Behav.Abstr., Anthropol.Lit., Appl.Ecol.Abstr., Biol.Abstr., Biotech.& Bioeng.Abstr., Chem.Abstr., Chem.Indus.Notes, Chem.Titles, Curr.Adv.Biochem., Curr.Adv.Ecol.Sci., Curr.Cont., Ecol.Abstr., Environ.Sci.Poll.Mgmt., Excerp.Med., Focus on: Vet.Sci.& Med., Forest.Abstr., Genet.Abstr., GeoRef, Hum.Gen.Abstr., Ind.Med. (1981-), Ind.Sci.Rev., Ind.Vet., Inpharma, Int.Abstr.Biol.Sci., Intl.Bibl.Soc.Sci., Nutr.Abstr., PsycInfo, Psychol.Abstr. (1981-), Reac., Rev.Appl.Entomol., Rev.Med.& Vet.Mycol., SSCI (coverage dropped), Sci.Cit.Ind., Sport Fish.Abstr., Sugar Ind.Abstr., Vet.Bull., Wild.Rev., Zoo.Rec., e-psyche.
—BLDSC (0834.400000), CASDDS, EMDOCS, IDS, ingenta, Linda Hall. **CCC.**
Published by: John Wiley & Sons, Inc., Journals (Subsidiary of: Wiley InterScience), 605 Third Ave, New York, NY 10158. TEL 212-850-6645, FAX 212-850-6021, subinfo@jwiley.com, uscs-wis@wiley.com, http://wiley.co.uk, http://www.wiley.com. Ed. M J Raleigh. adv.: B&W page GBP 640, color page GBP 1,515; trim 174 x 254. Circ: 650. **Subscr. outside the Americas to:** John Wiley & Sons Ltd., Baffins Ln, Chichester, Sussex PO19 IUD, United Kingdom. TEL 44-1243-779777, FAX 44-1243-843232, cs-journals@wiley.co.uk, http://www.wiley.co.uk.

590.74 USA ISSN 0003-0082
QL1 CODEN: AMUNAL
AMERICAN MUSEUM NOVITATES. Short title: Notivates. Text in English. 1921. irreg., latest no.3332, 2001, Apr. price varies. bibl, illus, maps. back issues avail. *Refereed.* **Document type:** *Monographic series, Academic/Scholarly.* **Description:** Contains brief professional research papers in paleontology and zoology, primarily systematics and evolutionary biology.
Related titles: Online - full text ed.: (from BioOne).
Indexed: AESIS, Apic.Abstr., Aqua.Sci.& Fish.Abstr., Aquacult.Abstr., Biol.Abstr., Deep Sea Res.& Oceanogr.Abstr., Environ.Sci.Poll.Mgmt., GeoRef, Helminthol.Abstr., Key Word Ind.Wildl.Res., Ref.Zh., Rev.Appl.Entomol., Zoo.Rec.
—CISTI, Linda Hall.
Published by: American Museum of Natural History Library, Scientific Publications Distribution, Central Park W at 79th St, New York, NY 10024-5192. TEL 212-769-5545, FAX 212-769-5009, scipubs@amnh.org, http://nimidi.amnh.org. Ed. Brenda Jones. Circ: 1,000.

ANIMAL BEHAVIOR ABSTRACTS. see *BIOLOGY—Abstracting, Bibliographies, Statistics*

591.5 GBR ISSN 0003-3472
QL750 CODEN: ANBEA8
ANIMAL BEHAVIOUR. Text in English. 1952. m. GBP 520 to institutions (effective 2001). adv. bk.rev. illus. index. reprint service avail. from SWZ. *Refereed.* **Document type:** *Academic/Scholarly.* **Description:** Contains critical reviews, original papers, and research articles about all aspects of animal behavior for biologists and veterinarians.
Related titles: Microform ed.: (from PQC,PMC); Online - full text ed.: (from EBSCO Publishing, O C L C Online Computer Library Center, Inc., RoweCom Information Quest, ingenta, Gale Group, Swets Blackwell, IDEAL Online Library, Factiva, Institute for Scientific Information).
Indexed: ASCA, Acad.Ind., AgBiotech, Agri.& Environ.Biotech.Abstr. (coverage dropped), Agricola, Anim.Behav.Abstr., Anim.Breed.Abstr., Apic.Abstr., Appl.Ecol.Abstr., Aqua.Sci.& Fish.Abstr., Bibl.Agri., Bio-Contr.News & Info., Biol.& Agr.Ind. (May 1983-), Biol.Abstr., Chem.Abstr., Chemorec.Abstr., Child Devel.Abstr., Curr.Adv.Ecol.Sci., Curr.Cont., Curr.Ref.Fish Res., Dairy Sci.Abstr., Deep Sea Res.& Oceanogr.Abstr., Ecol.Abstr., Entomol.Abstr., Environ.Sci.Poll.Mgmt., Excerp.Med., Food Sci.& Tech.Abstr., Forest.Abstr., Gen.Sci.Ind. (May 1984-), Helminthol.Abstr., Ind.Med. (coverage dropped), Ind.Sci.Rev., Ind.Vet., Inpharma, Int.Abstr.Biol.Sci., Key Word Ind.Wildl.Res., MLA Intl.Bibl., Nutr.Abstr., Ocean.Abstr., Pig News & Info., Pollut.Abstr., Poult.Abstr., PsycInfo, Psychol.Abstr. (1953-), Reac., Rev.Appl.Entomol., Rev.Med.& Vet.Mycol., Risk Abstr., SSCI (coverage dropped), Sci.Cit.Ind., Seed Abstr., Small Anim.Abstr., Sport Fish.Abstr., Vet.Bull., Wild.Rev., World Ag.Econ.& Rur.Soc.Abstr., Zoo.Rec., e-psyche.
—BLDSC (0902.950000), ADONIS, CASDDS, CISTI, EMDOCS, GNLM, IDS, ingenta, Linda Hall. **CCC.**
Published by: (Association for the Study of Animal Behaviour), Academic Press (Subsidiary of: Harcourt Publishers Ltd.), 24 Oval Rd, London NW1 7DX, United Kingdom. TEL 44-20-7267-4466, FAX 44-20-7482-2293, apsubs@acad.com, http://www.hbuk.co.uk/ap/anbehav; http://www.europe.idealibrary.com/. Eds. B G Galef Jr., C J Barnard. R&P Catherine John. Adv. contact Nik Screen. **Subscr. to:** Harcourt Publishers Ltd., Foots Cray High St, Sidcup, Kent DA14 5HP, United Kingdom. TEL 44-20-8300-3322, FAX 44-20-8309-0807.
Co-sponsor: Animal Behaviour Society.

ANIMAL GENETICS. see *BIOLOGY—Genetics*

ANIMAL NATURAL HISTORY SERIES. see *SCIENCES: COMPREHENSIVE WORKS*

590.724 USA ISSN 0892-7936
QL85
ANTHROZOOS; a multidisciplinary journal on the interactions of people and animals. Text in English. 1987. q. USD 40 domestic to individuals; USD 50 foreign to individuals; USD 55 domestic to institutions; USD 65 foreign to institutions (effective 1999). adv. bk.rev. abstr, illus. index. back issues avail.; reprints avail. *Refereed.* **Document type:** *Academic/Scholarly.* **Description:** Explore impact of animals on human health and culture.
Related titles: Online - full text ed.: (from Institute for Scientific Information).
Indexed: ASCA, AgeLine, Agricola, Anim.Behav.Abstr. (coverage dropped), Arts & Hum.Cit.Ind. (coverage dropped), Bibl.Agri., Curr.Cont., Environ.Abstr., Environ.Per.Bibl. (1989-), Focus on: Vet.Sci.& Med., Ind.Vet., InterActions Bibl. (1989-), Key Word Ind.Wildl.Res., Lang.& Lang.Behav.Abstr., PsycInfo, Psychol.Abstr. (1987-), Rural Devel.Abstr., SOPODA, SSCI, Sci.Cit.Ind. (coverage dropped), Small Anim.Abstr., Sociol.Abstr., Sport Fish.Abstr., Vet.Bull., Wild.Rev., e-psyche.
—BLDSC (1546.670000), CIS, IDS, Infotrieve, ingenta. **CCC.**
Published by: Delta Society, 289 Perimeter Rd E, Renton, WA 98055-1329. TEL 425-226-7357, FAX 425-235-1076, http://www.petsforum.com/deltasociety/dsc900.htm, http://www.dumedia.com/delta.html. Ed. A L Podberscek. Circ: 1,200.

591.5 NLD ISSN 0168-1591
CODEN: AABSEV
APPLIED ANIMAL BEHAVIOUR SCIENCE; an international scientific journal reporting on the application of ethology to animals used by man. Text in English. 1975. 20/yr. EUR 1,478 in Europe to institutions; JPY 196,500 in Japan to institutions; USD 1,653 elsewhere to institutions (effective 2002). adv. bk.rev. bibl, illus, abstr. index. back issues avail.; reprint service avail. from SWZ. *Refereed.* **Document type:** *Academic/Scholarly.* **Description:** Deals with the behaviour of domesticated and utilized animals.
Formerly (until 1985): Applied Animal Ethology (0304-3762)
Related titles: Microform ed.: (from PQC); Online - full text ed.: (from ingenta, Swets Blackwell, ScienceDirect, Institute for Scientific Information).

Indexed: ASCA, AgBiotech, Agri.Eng.Abstr., Agricola, Agroforest.Abstr., Anim.Behav.Abstr., Anim.Breed.Abstr., Aqua.Sci.& Fish.Abstr., Bibl.Agri., Biol.Abstr., Curr.Adv.Ecol.Sci., Curr.Cont., Dairy Sci.Abstr., Ecol.Abstr., Field Crop Abstr., Focus on: Vet.Sci.& Med., Geo.Abstr.H.G., Geo.Abstr.P.G., Herb.Abstr., Ind.Sci.Rev., Ind.Vet., Int.Abstr.Biol.Sci., InterActions Bibl. (1989-), Key Word Ind.Wildl.Res., Maize Abstr., Nutr.Abstr., Pig News & Info., Poult.Abstr., PsycInfo, Psychol.Abstr., Psycscan B.A.& T., Rev.Med.& Vet.Mycol., SSCI (coverage dropped), Sci.Cit.Ind., Small Anim.Abstr., Sport Fish.Abstr., Triticale Abstr., Vet.Bull., Wild.Rev., Zoo.Rec., e-psyche.
—BLDSC (1571.446000), CISTI, EMDOCS, IDS, Infotrieve, ingenta. **CCC.**
Published by: Elsevier Science BV, PO Box 211, Amsterdam 1000 AE, Netherlands. TEL 31-20-485-3911, FAX 31-20-485-3598, nlinfo-f@elsevier.nl, http://www.elsevier.com/locate/applanim. Eds. H Gonyou, P Jensen. **Subscr. in Australasia and the Far East to:** Elsevier Science (Singapore) Pte Ltd, No.1 Temasek Ave, 17-01 Millenia Tower, Singapore 039192, Singapore. TEL 65-434-3727, FAX 65-337-2230; **Subscr. in Japan to:** Elsevier Science Inc - Japan Regional Office, 9-15 Higashi-Azabu 1-chome, Minato-ku, Tokyo 106-0044, Japan. TEL 81-3-5561-5033; **Subscr. in the Americas to:** Elsevier Science, PO Box 945, New York, NY 10159-0945. TEL 212-633-3730, FAX 212-633-3680.

595.4 FRA ISSN 0763-1901
ARACHNOLOGIA - BULLETIN D'INFORMATION ET DE LIAISON DU C I D A. Key Title: Arachnologia. Text in French. 1984. a. FRF 40, USD 7. **Document type:** *Bulletin.*
Formerly: Centre International de Documentation Arachnologique. Bulletin d'Information et de Liaison.
Published by: Centre International de Documentation Arachnologique, 61 rue de Buffon, Paris 75005, France. FAX 40-79-38-63, arachne@mnhn.fr.

596 GBR ISSN 0003-9969
RK1 CODEN: AOBIAR
ARCHIVES OF ORAL BIOLOGY; a multidisciplinary journal in oral research. Text in English, French, German. 1959. m. EUR 116 in Europe to individuals; JPY 15,400 in Japan to individuals; USD 130 elsewhere to individuals; EUR 19,557 in Europe to institutions; JPY 259,900 in Japan to institutions; USD 2,189 elsewhere to institutions (effective 2002). adv. bk.rev. charts, illus. index. back issues avail. *Refereed.* **Document type:** *Academic/Scholarly.* **Description:** Publishes research results on every aspect of the oral and dental tissues and bone from the entire range of vertebrates.
Related titles: Microfilm ed.: (from PQC); Online - full text ed.: (from ingenta, Swets Blackwell, ScienceDirect, Institute for Scientific Information).
Indexed: ASCA, Abstr.Anthropol., AgBiotech, Anim.Breed.Abstr., Biol.Abstr., Chem.Abstr., Chem.Indus.Notes, Chem.Titles, Curr.Adv.Biochem., Curr.Adv.Cell & Devel.Biol., Curr.Adv.Ecol.Sci., Curr.Cont., Curr.Tit.Dent., Dairy Sci.Abstr., Dent.Ind., Excerp.Med., GeoRef, INIS Atomind., Ind.Med. (1959-), Ind.Sci.Rev., Ind.Vet., Inpharma, Int.Abstr.Biol.Sci., Mass Spectr.Bull., Med.& Surg.Dermat., NRN, Neurosci.Cit.Ind., Nutr.Abstr., Pharm.&Out.News, Reac., Rev.Appl.Entomol., Rev.Arom.& Med.Plants, Rev.Med.& Vet.Mycol., Rev.Plant Path., SSCI (coverage dropped), Sci.Cit.Ind., Small Anim.Abstr., Sugar Ind.Abstr., Triticale Abstr., Trop.Dis.Bull., Vet.Bull.
—BLDSC (1638.475000), CASDDS, CISTI, EMDOCS, GNLM, IDS, ingenta, KNAW, Linda Hall. **CCC.**
Published by: Pergamon (Subsidiary of: Elsevier Science), The Boulevard, Langford Ln, East Park, Kidlington, Oxford OXB 1GB, United Kingdom. FAX 44-1865-843010, http://www.elsevier.com/locate/archoralbio. Ed. D B Ferguson. Circ: 1,250. **Subscr. in Australasia and the Far East to:** Elsevier Science (Singapore) Pte Ltd, No.1 Temasek Ave, 17-01 Millenia Tower, Singapore 039192, Singapore. TEL 65-434-3727; **Subscr. in the Americas to:** Elsevier Science, PO Box 945, New York, NY 10159-0945. TEL 212-633-3730, FAX 212-633-3680; **Subscr. to:** Elsevier Science BV, PO Box 211, Amsterdam 1000 AE, Netherlands. TEL 31-20-485-3757, nlinfo-f@elsevier.nl, http://www.elsevier.nl.

590 JPN ISSN 0389-1836
CODEN: ADJHDO
AZABU DAIGAKU JUIGAKUBU KENKYU HOKOKU/AZABU UNIVERSITY. VETERINARY MEDICINE. BULLETIN. Text in English, Japanese; Summaries in English. 1954-1986; resumed 1988. s-a. per issue exchange basis. **Document type:** *Bulletin, Academic/Scholarly.*
Formerly: Azabu Veterinary College. Bulletin
Indexed: Biol.Abstr., Dairy Sci.Abstr., Ind.Vet., Rev.Med.& Vet.Mycol., Rev.Plant Path., Small Anim.Abstr., Vet.Bull.
—CASDDS.
Published by: Azabu University, School of Veterinary Medicine/Azabu Daigaku Juigakubu, 1-17-71 Fuchinobe, Sagamihara-shi, Kanagawa-ken 229-0006, Japan. TEL 81-427-54-7111, FAX 81-427-54-7661. Ed. Kiyoshi Tabuchi. Circ: 800.

591.5 NLD ISSN 0005-7959
BF671 CODEN: BEHAA8
BEHAVIOUR; an international journal of behaviourial biology. Text in English, German. 1947. 12/yr. EUR 514, USD 596 to individuals includes online ed. (effective 2002). bibl, charts, illus. cum.index: vols.1-132. back issues avail.; reprint service avail. from SCH,PSC. *Refereed.* **Document type:** *Journal, Academic/Scholarly.* **Description:** Covers the scientific study of animal behavior.
Related titles: Microform ed.: (from PMC,SWZ); Online - full content ed.: 1999 (from EBSCO Publishing, O C L C Online Computer Library Center, Inc., Swets Blackwell); Online - full text ed.: (from CatchWord Ltd., Institute for Scientific Information).
Indexed: ASCA, Abstr.Anthropol., Anim.Behav.Abstr., Anim.Breed.Abstr., Appl.Ecol.Abstr., Aqua.Sci.& Fish.Abstr., Bio-Contr.News & Info., Biol.Abstr., Chem.Abstr., Curr.Adv.Ecol.Sci., Curr.Cont., Dairy Sci.Abstr., Deep Sea Res.& Oceanogr.Abstr., Ecol.Abstr., Entomol.Abstr., Environ.Sci.Poll.Mgmt., Food Sci.& Tech.Abstr., Ind.Sci.Rev., Ind.Vet., Key Word Ind.Wildl.Res., M.L.A., MLA Intl.Bibl., Nutr.Abstr., Ocean.Abstr. (coverage dropped), Poult.Abstr., PsycInfo, Psychol.Abstr. (1950-), Rev.Appl.Entomol., Rev.Med.& Vet.Mycol., Russ.Acad.Sci.Bibl., SSCI (coverage dropped), Sci.Cit.Ind., Sport Fish.Abstr., Vet.Bull., Wild.Rev., Zoo.Rec., e-psyche.
—BLDSC (1876.650000), CatchWord, CISTI, IDS, ingenta, Linda Hall. **CCC.**
Published by: Brill Academic Publishers, PO Box 9000, Leiden 2300 PA, Netherlands. TEL 31-71-535-3500, FAX 31-71-531-7532, cs@brill.nl, http://www.vsppub.com/journals/jn-Beh.html, http://www.brill.nl. Eds. J G van Rhijn, M Daly. R&P Elizabeth Venekamp.

BIOLOGICAL SOCIETY OF WASHINGTON. PROCEEDINGS. see *BIOLOGY*

BRAZILIAN JOURNAL OF VETERINARY RESEARCH AND ANIMAL SCIENCE. see *VETERINARY SCIENCE*

590 IND ISSN 0970-0765
QL1 CODEN: BPAAS:A
BULLETIN OF PURE & APPLIED SCIENCES. SECTION A: ZOOLOGY. Text in English. 1982. s-a. (in 20 vols.). INR 300, USD 50 (effective 2001). adv. bk.rev. 100 p./no. back issues avail.; reprints avail. *Refereed.* **Document type:** *Journal, Academic/Scholarly.* **Description:** Research papers related to Zoological Science.
Media: Large Type (11 pt.).
Indexed: Zoo.Rec.
—CISTI, Infotrieve, Linda Hall. **CCC.**
Published by: A.K. Sharma, Ed. & Pub., 19-A, D D A Flats, Mansarover Park, Shahdara, New Delhi 110 032, India. TEL 91-11-2117408, bulletin@mantraonline.com, bulletin@satyam.net.in. R&P, Adv. contact A K Sharma. B&W page INR 1,000, B&W page USD 50, color page INR 2,000, color page USD 100. Circ: 600.

C A SELECTS. ANIMAL LONGEVITY AND AGING. see *BIOLOGY—Abstracting, Bibliographies, Statistics*

CENTRE INTERNATIONAL DE DOCUMENTATION ARACHNOLOGIQUE. LISTE DES TRAVAUX ARACHNOLOGIQUES. see *BIOLOGY—Abstracting, Bibliographies, Statistics*

590.724 USA ISSN 1532-0820
SF77 CODEN: LBASAE
COMPARATIVE MEDICINE (MEMPHIS). Text in English. 1950. bi-m. USD 150 domestic; USD 165 in Canada & Mexico; USD 190 elsewhere (effective 2001). adv. charts, illus. index. back issues avail. *Refereed.* **Document type:** *Academic/Scholarly.* **Description:** Covers comparative medicine and laboratory animal science with articles about animal models, animal behavior, animal biotechnology and related topics.
Former titles (until 2000): Laboratory Animal Science (0023-6764); (until 1971): Laboratory Animal Care (0094-5331); (until 1963): Animal Care Panel. Proceedings (0097-076X)
Related titles: Microform ed.: (from PMC); Online - full text ed.: (from Institute for Scientific Information).
Indexed: ASCA, AgBiotech, Agri.& Environ.Biotech.Abstr. (coverage dropped), Agricola, Anim.Breed.Abstr., Biol.Abstr., Chem.Abstr., Chem.Indus.Notes, Chem.Titles, Curr.Adv.Ecol.Sci., Curr.Cont., Dairy Sci.Abstr., Dent.Ind., Derwent Biotech.Abstr., Diar.Dis.Res., Excerp.Med., Focus on: Vet.Sci.& Med., Helminthol.Abstr., INIS Atomind., Ind.Med. (coverage dropped), Ind.Sci.Rev., Ind.Vet., Inpharma, Int.Abstr.Biol.Sci., Nutr.Abstr., Pig News & Info., Poult.Abstr., Protozool.Abstr., Reac., Rev.Appl.Entomol., Rev.Med.& Vet.Mycol., Rev.Plant Path., Sci.Cit.Ind., Small Anim.Abstr., Soyabean Abstr., Sport Fish.Abstr., Vet.Bull., Wild.Rev., Zoo.Rec.
—BLDSC (3363.790200), CASDDS, CISTI, GNLM, IDS, ingenta, KNAW.
Published by: American Association for Laboratory Animal Science, 9190 Crestwyn Hills Drive, Memphis, TN 38125. TEL 901-754-8620, FAX 901-753-0046, info@aalas.org, http://www.aalas.org. Ed. Robert O Jacoby. R&P, Adv. contact Chris Lyons. Circ: 3,000.

594.1477 ITA ISSN 0394-0152
QL401
LA CONCHIGLIA/SHELL; international shell magazine. Text in Italian, English. 1969. q. ITL 58.81, EUR 55 (effective 2002). adv. bk.rev., video rev. bibl. illus. index. 64 p./no. Supplement avail.; back issues avail.; reprints avail. *Refereed.* **Document type:** *Magazine, Yearbook.* **Description:** Presents papers on taxonomy, ethology, and environmental issues related to malacology. Lists events, shows and symposia.
Related titles: CD-ROM ed.; English ed.
Indexed: Zoo.Rec.
Published by: Evolver S.r.l., Via Cesare Federici, 1, Rome, RM 00147, Italy. TEL 39-06-5132536, FAX 39-06-5132796, conchiglia@evolver.it, http://www.evolver.it. Ed., Adv. contact Maria Antonietta Fontana. R&P Paolo Angioy. B&W page USD 500; trim 600 x 870. Circ: 1,500. **Subscr. to:** Via Focilide, 31, Rome, RM 00125, Italy.

CYPRIS; international ostracoda newsletter. see *PALEONTOLOGY*

597.92 USA ISSN 0191-3875
QL666.C584
DESERT TORTOISE COUNCIL. PROCEEDINGS OF SYMPOSIUM. Text in English. 1976. a. USD 15 to non-members; USD 10 to members. **Document type:** *Proceedings.*
Indexed: Zoo.Rec.
Published by: Desert Tortoise Council, PO Box 3141, Wrightwood, CA 92397. Ed. Breck Bartholonew. R&P Ed Larue. Circ: 600.

590 JPN ISSN 0916-8419
QL750 CODEN: DSKEEN
DOBUTSU SHINRIGAKU KENKYU/JAPANESE JOURNAL OF ANIMAL PSYCHOLOGY. Text in English, Japanese; Summaries in English. 1947. s-a. JPY 1,700 per issue (effective 1999). adv. index. back issues avail. **Document type:** *Academic/Scholarly.*
Formerly (until 1990): Dobutsu Shinrigaku Nenpo - Annual of Animal Psychology (0003-5130)
Indexed: Biol.Abstr., Jap.Per.Ind., PsycInfo, Psychol.Abstr. (1956-), Zoo.Rec., e-psyche.
Published by: Nihon Dobutsu Shinri Gakkai/Japanese Society for Animal Psychology, c/o University of Tsukuba, Institute of Psychology, 1-1-1 Tenno-Dai, Tsukuba-shi, Ibaraki-ken 305-0006, Japan. TEL 81-298-53-4720, FAX 81-298-53-4720, makinoju@human.tsukuba.ac.jp. Ed. Hiroshige Okaichi. Adv. contact Junshiro Makino. Circ: 500 (controlled). **Subscr. to:** Japan Publications Trading Co. Ltd., Tokyo International, PO Box 5030, Tokyo 100-31, Japan.

590 CHN ISSN 1000-0739
QL351 CODEN: DFXUEB
DONGWU FENLEI XUEBAO/ACTA ZOOTAXONOMICA SINICA. Text in Chinese; Summaries in English. 1964. q. CNY 16 domestic; USD 96 foreign (effective 2000). adv. *Refereed.* **Description:** Contains theses on zootaxonomy, its theory and practice, scientific notes and academic discussions.
Related titles: Online - full content ed.: (from WanFang Data Corp.).
Indexed: Apic.Abstr., Bio-Contr.News & Info., Forest.Abstr., Helminthol.Abstr., Poult.Abstr., Protozool.Abstr., Ref.Zh., Rev.Appl.Entomol., Rev.Arom.& Med.Plants, Rev.Med.& Vet.Mycol., Soils & Fert., Zoo.Rec.
—CISTI, Linda Hall.
Published by: (Zhongguo Kexueyuan, Chengdu Shengwu Yanjiusuo), Kexue Chubanshe/Science Press, 16 Donghuang Cheng Gen Beijie, Beijing 100707, China. Ed. Jian-Ming Zhao. Circ: 6,000.

B

590 CHN ISSN 0001-7302
QL1 CODEN: TWHPA3
DONGWU XUEBAO/ACTA ZOOLOGICA SINICA. Text in Chinese; Summaries in English. 1935. q. CNY 18 domestic; USD 89 foreign (effective 2000). adv. charts, illus, maps. *Refereed.* **Document type:** *Academic/Scholarly.* **Description:** Contains original theses on zoology, including taxonomy, faunistics, morphology, ecology, and experimental zoology. Also includes information about research progress and discussions among various schools of research and academic viewpoints.
Related titles: Online - full content ed.: (from WanFang Data Corp.).
Indexed: Aqua.Sci.& Fish.Abstr., Aquacult.Abstr., Bio-Contr.News & Info., Biol.Abstr., Chem.Abstr., Chem.Indus.Notes, Chem.Titles, Curr.Adv.Ecol.Sci., Curr.Cont. (coverage dropped), Ecol.Abstr., Environ.Sci.Poll.Mgmt., GeoRef, Geol.Abstr., Helminthol.Abstr., Ind.Sci.Rev., Ind.Vet., Key Word Ind.Wildl.Res., Ocean.Abstr. (coverage dropped), Pig News & Info., Poult.Abstr., Protozool.Abstr., Ref.Zh., Sci.Cit.Ind. (coverage dropped), Sport Fish.Abstr., Vet.Bull., Wild.Rev., Zoo.Rec.
—CASDDS, CISTI, KNAW, Linda Hall.
Published by: (Zhongguo Kexueyuan, Dongwu Yanjiusuo), Kexue Chubanshe/Science Press, 16 Donghuang Cheng Genbei Jie, Beijing 100717, China. Ed. Zu Wang Wang. Circ: 11,000.

590 JPN ISSN 0912-1129
DOSEI KYOKAI KAIHO/JAPANESE ASSOCIATION OF VETERINARY BIOLOGISTS. BULLETIN. Text in Japanese. 1968. q.
Published by: Dobutsuyo Seibutsugakuteki Seizai Kyokai, 11 Kanda-Mikura-cho, Chiyoda-ku, Tokyo 101-0038, Japan.

599.665 USA ISSN 0149-0672
SF277
EQUUS. Text in English. 1977. m. USD 19.95 domestic; USD 31.95 foreign (effective 2001). adv. bk.rev. illus. index. reprint service avail. from PQC. **Document type:** *Trade.* **Description:** Provides the latest information from the world's top veterinarians, equine researchers, riders and trainers on understanding and influencing equine behavior, recognizing the warning signs of illness and disease, and solving riding and training problems.
Related titles: Microform ed.: (from PQC).
Indexed: Farm & Garden Ind., Sports Per.Ind., Sportsearch (1978-), Zoo.Rec.
—CISTI, ingenta.
Published by: Primedia Enthusiast Group (Subsidiary of: Primedia Consumer Media & Magazine Group), 656 Quince Orchard Rd, Gaithersburg, MD 20878. adv.: B&W page USD 4,155, color page USD 6,640. Circ: 150,328 (paid).

591.5 DEU ISSN 0179-1613
QL750 CODEN: ETHOEM
ETHOLOGY. Text in English. 1937. m. DEM 1,949.97 in Europe; DEM 2,002.77 elsewhere; DEM 2,144.97 in Europe print & online eds. combined; DEM 2,203.05 elsewhere print & online eds. combined (effective 2001). adv. bk.rev. illus, stat. index. back issues avail. *Refereed.* **Document type:** *Journal, Academic/Scholarly.* **Description:** Contains contributions from all branches of behavior research on all species of animals, both in the field and in the laboratory.
Formerly: Zeitschrift fuer Tierpsychologie (0044-3573)
Related titles: ♦ Online - full text ed.: Ethology Online. ISSN 1439-0310; ♦ Supplement: Advances in Ethology. ISSN 0931-4202.
Indexed: ASCA, Agricola, Anim.Behav.Abstr., Anim.Breed.Abstr., Apic.Abstr., Appl.Ecol.Abstr. (coverage dropped), Aqua.Sci.& Fish.Abstr., Aquacult.Abstr., Bio-Contr.News & Info., Biol.Abstr., Curr.Adv.Ecol.Sci., Curr.Cont., Dairy Sci.Abstr., Deep Sea Res.& Oceanogr.Abstr., Ecol.Abstr., Entomol.Abstr., Environ.Sci.Poll.Mgmt., Helminthol.Abstr., Ind.Med. (coverage dropped), Ind.Vet., Indian Psychol.Abstr., Inpharma, Int.Abstr.Biol.Sci., M.L.A., MLA Intl.Bibl., Nutr.Abstr., Pig News & Info., Poult.Abstr., PsycInfo, Psychol.Abstr. (1937-), Reac., Ref.Zh., Rev.Appl.Entomol., Rev.Med.& Vet.Mycol., SSCI (coverage dropped), Sci.Cit.Ind., So.Pac.Per.Ind., Sport Fish.Abstr., Vet.Bull., Wild.Rev., Zoo.Rec., e-psyche.
—BLDSC (3815.240000), CISTI, EMDOCS, IDS, ingenta. **CCC.**
Published by: Blackwell Wissenschafts Verlag GmbH, Kurfuerstendamm 57, Berlin 10707, Germany. TEL 49-30-32790665, FAX 49-30-32790610, abo@blackwis.de, http://www.blackwell.de. Ed. Michael Taborsky. adv.: B&W page DEM 560; trim 122 x 190. Circ: 650.

591.5 DEU ISSN 1439-0310
ETHOLOGY ONLINE. Text in English. m. DEM 1,755 (effective 2001). **Document type:** *Academic/Scholarly.*
Media: Online - full text (from EBSCO Publishing, O C L C Online Computer Library Center, Inc., RoweCom Information Quest, ingenta, Munksgaard & Blackwell Science's Synergy, Swets Blackwell, Institute for Scientific Information). **Related titles:** ♦ Print ed.: Ethology. ISSN 0179-1613.
Published by: Blackwell Wissenschafts Verlag GmbH, Kurfuerstendamm 57, Berlin 10707, Germany. TEL 49-30-32790665, FAX 49-30-32790610, abo@blackwis.de, http://www.blackwell.de.

591.5 ESP ISSN 1130-3204
QL750 CODEN: ETOLEE
ETOLOGIA. Text in English, Spanish. 1989. a. ESP 5,500 domestic to individuals; ESP 7,000 foreign to individuals; ESP 12,500 domestic to institutions; ESP 13,000 foreign to institutions (effective 2000). adv. bibl, charts, illus. *Refereed.* **Document type:** *Bulletin, Academic/Scholarly.* **Description:** Covers the field of animal behavior research, both theoretical and applied.
Indexed: Anim.Behav.Abstr., Aqua.Sci.& Fish.Abstr., Entomol.Abstr., Ind.SST, Rev.Appl.Entomol., Seed Abstr., Wild.Rev., Zoo.Rec., e-psyche.
—BLDSC (3816.344089), CINDOC.
Published by: Sociedad Espanola de Etologia, c/o Museu de Zoologia, Apartado 593, Barcelona 08080, Spain. TEL 34-3-3196912, FAX 34-3-3104999, jcsenar@intercom.es, http://www.uvigo.es/webs/c04/webc04/etologia/SEE.html. Eds. J C Senar, L Arias de Reyna. R&P, Adv. contact Maria Luisa Arroyo. Circ: 4,000.

595.42 NLD ISSN 0168-8162
QL458 CODEN: EAACEM
EXPERIMENTAL & APPLIED ACAROLOGY. Text in Dutch. 1985. m. EUR 1,232, USD 1,234 to institutions for print or online ed.; EUR 1,478.40, USD 1,480.80 to institutions for print & online eds. combined (effective 2002). adv. bk.rev. illus. index. back issues avail.; reprint service avail. from ISI. *Refereed.* **Document type:** *Journal, Academic/Scholarly.* **Description:** Brings together basic and applied research on various acarine groups, so that acarologists may more easily keep abreast of developments in related fields.
Related titles: Online - full text ed.: (from EBSCO Publishing, O C L C Online Computer Library Center, Inc., RoweCom Information Quest, Swets Blackwell, Kluwer Online, Institute for Scientific Information).
Indexed: ASCA, AgBiotech, Agricola, Apic.Abstr., Bio-Contr.News & Info., Biol.Abstr., Chem.Abstr., Chem.Indus.Notes, Chem.Titles, Chemorec.Abstr., Curr.Cont., Derwent Biotech.Abstr., Ecol.Abstr., Entomol.Abstr., Environ.Per.Bibl. (1991-1994), Excerp.Med., Fababean Abstr., Field Crop Abstr., Food Sci.& Tech.Abstr., Genet.Abstr., Hort.Abstr., Hum.Gen.Abstr., IDA, Ind.Med. (1985-), Ind.Vet., Int.Abstr.Biol.Sci., Postharvest, Potato Abstr., Poult.Abstr., Protozool.Abstr., Rev.Appl.Entomol., Rev.Med.& Vet.Mycol., Rev.Plant Path., Sci.Cit.Ind., Soils & Fert., Sport Fish.Abstr., Vet.Bull., Wild.Rev., Zoo.Rec.
—BLDSC (3838.620000), CASDDS, CISTI, EMDOCS, GNLM, IDS, Infotrieve, ingenta, Linda Hall. **CCC.**
Published by: Kluwer Academic Publishers Group (Subsidiary of: Wolters Kluwer N.V.), Spuiboulevard 50, PO Box 17, Dordrecht 3300 AA, Netherlands. TEL 31-78-639-2392, FAX 31-78-654-2254, services@wkap.nl, http://www.wkap.nl/journalhome.htm/0168-8162. Eds. F Jongejan, J Bruin, L P S van der Geest. Adv. contact Gemma Heiser. Circ: 1,000. **Subscr. in the Americas to:** Kluwer Academic - Plenum Publishers, 233 Spring St, New York, NY 10013-1578. TEL 212-620-8468, FAX 212-807-1047; **Subscr. to:** Journals Department, PO Box 322, Dordrecht 3300 AH, Netherlands. TEL 31-78-639-2392, FAX 31-78-654-6474.

591.993 NZL ISSN 0111-5383
QL340
FAUNA OF NEW ZEALAND. (no.1 Terebrantia, no.2 Osoriinae, no.3 Anthribdae, no.4 Eriophyoidea Except Eriophyinae, no.5 Eriophyinae, no.6 Hydraenidae, no.7 Cryptostigmata, no.8 Calliphoridae, no.9 Protura, no.10 Tubulifera, no.11 pseudococcidae, no.12 Pompilidae, no.13 Encyrtidae, no.14 Lepidoptera, no.15 Ambositrinae, no.16 Nepticulidae, no.17 Mymaridae, no.18 Chalcidoidea, no.19 Mantodea, no.20 Bibionidae, no.21 Margarodidae, no.22 Notonemouridae, no.23 Sciapodinae, Medeterinae, no.24 Therevidae, no.25 Cercopidae, no.26 Tenebrionidae, no.27 Antarctoperlinae, no.28 Larvae of Curculionoidea, no.29 Crytohynchinae, no.30 Hepialidae, no.31 Talitridae, no.32 Sphecidae, no.33 Moranilini, no.34 Anthicidae, no.35 Cydnidae, Acanthosomatidae, and Pentatomidae, no.36 Leptophlebiidae, no.37 Coleoptera, no.38 Naturalised Terrestrial Stylommatophora, no.39 Molytini, no.40 Cixiidae, no.41 Coccidae) Text in English. 1982. irreg., latest no.41. USD 850 for set of no.1-41 (effective 2000); price varies each no.. bibl, illus. back issues avail. *Refereed.* **Document type:** *Monographic series.* **Description:** Describes systematic taxonomy of New Zealand invertebrates.
Indexed: Aqua.Sci.& Fish.Abstr., Bio-Contr.News & Info., Biol.Abstr., Curr.Adv.Ecol.Sci., Entomol.Abstr., Rev.Appl.Entomol., Zoo.Rec.
—BLDSC (3899.254000), Linda Hall.
Published by: Manaaki Whenua Press, PO Box 40, Lincoln 8152, New Zealand. TEL 64-3-325-6700, FAX 64-3-325-2127, mwpress@landcare.cri.nz, http://www.landcare.cri.nz/mwpress/. Ed. Trevor Crosby. Pub., R&P Greg Comfort TEL 64-3-3256700. Circ: 400.

590 DEU ISSN 0430-1285
QH540 CODEN: FOEMA7
FAUNISTISCH-OEKOLOGISCHE MITTEILUNGEN. Text in German. 1952. irreg. DEM 8. **Document type:** *Academic/Scholarly.*
Formerly (until 1966): Faunistische Mitteilungen aus Norddeutschland (0933-6559)
Indexed: Aqua.Sci.& Fish.Abstr., Aquacult.Abstr., Environ.Sci.Poll.Mgmt., GeoRef, IBR, IBZ, Zoo.Rec.
Published by: (Faunistisch-Oekologische Arbeitsgemeinschaft), Wachholtz Verlag GmbH, Rungestr 4, Neumuenster 24537, Germany. TEL 49-4321-906276, FAX 49-4321-906275.

592.57 USA ISSN 0360-7550
CODEN: FPNCAT
FLORIDA. DEPARTMENT OF AGRICULTURE AND CONSUMER SERVICES. NEMATOLOGY CIRCULAR. Text in English. 1962. bi-m. free per issue. **Document type:** *Government.*
Indexed: Bio-Contr.News & Info., Biol.Abstr., Helminthol.Abstr., Ornam.Hort., Rev.Appl.Entomol., Rev.Plant Path., Weed Abstr., Zoo.Rec.
Published by: Department of Agriculture and Consumer Services, Division of Plant Industry, 1911 S W 34th St, Box 147100, Gainesville, FL 32614-7100. TEL 904-372-3505, FAX 904-955-2301. R&P Maeve McConnell.

FOLIA PARASITOLOGICA. see *MEDICAL SCIENCES—Communicable Diseases*

591.9489 DNK ISSN 0416-704X
GALATHEA REPORT; scientific results of the Danish deep-sea expedition round the world 1950-52. Text in English. 1956. irreg., latest vol.18, 2000. price varies. **Document type:** *Bulletin, Academic/Scholarly.*
Indexed: GeoRef, Zoo.Rec.
Published by: Apollo Books Aps, Kirkeby Sand 19, Stenstrup 5771, Denmark. TEL 45-62-26-37-37, FAX 45-62-26-37-80, apollobooks@vip.cybercity.dk. Ed. Torben Wolff.

590 BRA ISSN 0103-6076
QL242 CODEN: GOZOEV
GOELDIANA ZOOLOGIA. Text in Portuguese. 1990. irreg., latest vol.19, 1993. BRL 1.50 domestic; USD 2 foreign (effective 2000).
Indexed: Zoo.Rec.
Published by: Conselho Nacional de Desenvolvimento Cientifico e Tecnologico, Museu Paraense Emilio Goeldi, Comercio, Caixa Postal 399, Belem, PA 66017-970, Brazil. TEL 091-274-2195, FAX 091-274-1811, mgdoc@musu-goeldi.br.

599.884 USA
GORILLA. Text in English. 1976. s-a. USD 25; USD 30 foreign (effective 2000). bk.rev. back issues avail. **Document type:** *Newsletter, Consumer.* **Description:** Reports of the results and progress of ongoing study of gorilla behavior and interspecies communication, with other topics relating to the preservation and captive maintenance of gorillas.
Indexed: Wild.Rev., e-psyche.
Published by: Gorilla Foundation, PO Box 620530, Woodside, CA 94062. TEL 650-216-6450, FAX 650-365-7906, hanabiko@earthlink.net, koko@koko.org, http://www.gorilla.org, http://www.koko.org. Ed. Dr. Francine Patterson. R&P Kevin Connelly. Circ: 30,000.

GRAELLSIA; revista de zoologia. see *BIOLOGY*

GRASDUINEN. see *BIOLOGY—Botany*

592.3 SVK ISSN 0440-6605
QL392 CODEN: HMTGA4
HELMINTHOLOGIA. Text in English. 1959. 4/yr. USD 156 (effective 2001 - 2002). adv. bk.rev. illus. index. 60 p./no. *Refereed.* **Document type:** *Academic/Scholarly.* **Description:** For physicians, students of medicine, and other scientific and specialized workers engaged in parasitology.
Related titles: Online - full text ed.: (from Institute for Scientific Information).
Indexed: ASCA, Abstr.Bulg.Sci.Med.Lit., Abstr.Hyg., AgBiotech, Bio-Contr.News & Info., Biol.Abstr., Chem.Abstr., Chem.Indus.Notes, Chem.Titles, Curr.Cont., Excerp.Med. (until 19??), Helminthol.Abstr., Ind.Vet., Nutr.Abstr., Pig News & Info., Poult.Abstr., Protozool.Abstr., Rev.Appl.Entomol., Rev.Med.& Vet.Mycol., Sport Fish.Abstr., Trop.Dis.Bull., Vet.Bull., Wild.Rev., Zoo.Rec.
—BLDSC (4285.900000), CASDDS, CISTI, IDS, ingenta.
Published by: (Slovak Academy of Sciences, Parasitological Institute), Slovak Academic Press Ltd., Nam Slobody 6, PO Box 57, Bratislava 81005, Slovakia. helminth@linuxl.saske.sk, http://www.elis.sk. Ed., Adv. contact Pavol Dubinsky TEL 421-55-6334455. R&P Milan Rybos TEL 421-55-633141113. Circ: 700. **Subscr. to:** Slovak Academic Press Ltd. **Dist. also by:** Mezhdunarodnaya Kniga, B Yakimanka 39, Moscow 117049, Russian Federation. TEL 7-095-2384967, FAX 7-095-2384634.; **Dist. by:** Slovart.

HELMINTHOLOGICAL ABSTRACTS. see *BIOLOGY—Abstracting, Bibliographies, Statistics*

590 DEU ISSN 0721-6874
HESSISCHE FAUNISTISCHE BRIEFE. Text in German. 1981. q. DEM 30 (effective 2000). adv. bk.rev. **Document type:** *Academic/Scholarly.*
Indexed: Ref.Zh., Zoo.Rec.
Published by: Naturwissenschaftlicher Verein Darmstadt e.V., Bessungerstr 125-C, Darmstadt 64295, Germany. TEL 49-6151-133288. Ed. Michael Hoellwarth. Circ: 500.

590 JPN ISSN 0285-3760
HOKURIKU JOURNAL OF ZOOTECHNICAL SCIENCE. Text in Japanese. 1951. s-a. JPY 600. back issues avail.
Published by: Japan Zootechnical Society, Hokuriku Branch, c/o Department of Animal Husbandry, Faculty of Agriculture, Niigata University, Niigata 950-21, Japan. TEL 025-262-6662, FAX 025-263-1659. Ed. K Yamamoto. Circ: 800.

599 JPN ISSN 0916-7625
HONYU DOBUTSU RANSHI GAKKAISHI/JOURNAL OF MAMMALIAN OVA RESEARCH. Text in English, Japanese. 1984. s-a. membership.
Published by: Honyu Dobutsu Ranshi Gakkai/Japanese Society of Mammalian Ova Research, Nihon Daigaku Nojuigakubu Jui Serigaku Kyoshitsu, 1866 Kameino, Fujisawa-shi, Kanagawa-ken 252-0813, Japan.

HONYU DOBUTSU SHIKEN BUNKAKAI KAIHO/MAMMALIAN MUTAGENICITY STUDY GROUP COMMUNICATIONS. see *BIOLOGY—Genetics*

▼ **I E H ASSESSMENT ON THE ECOLOGICAL SIGNIFICANCE OF ENDOCRINE DISRUPTION.** see *ENVIRONMENTAL STUDIES—Pollution*

590.724 USA ISSN 1084-2020
QL55
I L A R JOURNAL. Text in English. 1957. q. USD 50 to individuals; USD 500 to institutions; USD 20 to students (effective 2000). bk.rev. bibl, illus. back issues avail. *Refereed.* **Document type:** *Academic/Scholarly.* **Description:** Articles on animal models, along with issues of interest to animal care and use committees. Information on alternatives, adjuncts and refinements to the use of animals, with letters to the editor, announcements of new books and meetings.
Former titles: I L A R News (0018-9960); Information on Laboratory Animals for Research
Indexed: Agricola, Bibl.Agri., Ind.Vet., Ref.Zh., Sport Fish.Abstr., Vet.Bull., Wild.Rev.
—BLDSC (4364.040000), CISTI, Infotrieve, ingenta. **CCC.**
Published by: Institute for Laboratory Animal Research, 2101 Constitution Ave, N W, Washington, DC 20418. TEL 202-334-2590, FAX 202-334-1687, ilarj@nas.edu, http://www.national-academies.org/ILAR. Ed. Gerald Rebhart. R&P Susan Vaupel. Circ: 3,500.

590 USA
I W R C PROCEEDINGS. Text in English. 1991. a. price varies. back issues avail. **Document type:** *Proceedings.* **Description:** Publishes papers presented at the annual IWRC conference.
Published by: International Wildlife Rehabilitation Council, 4437 Central Pl., Ste. B4, Suisun, CA 94585-1663. TEL 707-864-1761, FAX 707-864-3106, iwrc@inreach.com, http://www.iwrc-online.org.

590 USA
I W R C SKILLS SEMINARS. Text in English. irreg., latest vol.10. price varies. illus. back issues avail. **Document type:** *Monographic series, Academic/Scholarly, Trade.* **Description:** Covers various aspects on rehabilitating wild birds and animals.
Published by: International Wildlife Rehabilitation Council, 4437 Central Pl., Ste. B4, Suisun, CA 94585-1663. TEL 707-864-1761, FAX 707-864-3106, iwrc@inreach.com, http://www.iwrc-online.org.

597 DEU ISSN 0936-9902
CODEN: IEFRES
ICHTHYOLOGICAL EXPLORATION OF FRESHWATERS; international journal for field-orientated ichthyology. Text in German. 1990. q. DEM 150 to individuals; DEM 280 to institutions. index. back issues avail. **Document type:** *Academic/Scholarly.*
Indexed: Aqua.Sci.& Fish.Abstr., Aquacult.Abstr., Environ.Per.Bibl. (1991-1993), Environ.Sci.Poll.Mgmt., Sport Fish.Abstr., Zoo.Rec.
—BLDSC (4361.950950).
Published by: Verlag Dr. Friedrich Pfeil, Postfach 650086, Munich 81214, Germany. TEL 49-89-742827-0, FAX 49-89-7242772. Ed. Maurice Kottelat. Circ: 500.

IN VITRO CELLULAR & DEVELOPMENTAL BIOLOGY - ANIMAL. see *MEDICAL SCIENCES*

599.935 KEN
INSTITUTE OF PRIMATE RESEARCH. ANNUAL REPORT. Text in English. 1981. a.
Published by: Institute of Primate Research, Karen, PO Box 24481, Nairobi, Kenya. FAX 254-2-882546, TELEX 254-2-22892.

590 USA
INTERNATIONAL WILDLIFE REHABILITATION COUNCIL. INDIVIDUAL PAPERS. Text in English. irreg. price varies. back issues avail. **Document type:** *Monographic series, Academic/Scholarly.* **Description:** Discusses the rehabilitation of specific birds and mammals.
Published by: International Wildlife Rehabilitation Council, 4437 Central Pl., Ste. B4, Suisun, CA 94585-1663. TEL 707-864-1761, FAX 707-864-3106, iwrc@inreach.com, http://www.iwrc-online.org.

592 USA ISSN 1077-8306
QH201 CODEN: TAMSAJ
INVERTEBRATE BIOLOGY. Text in English. 1880. q. USD 85 in US & Canada to institutions; USD 110 elsewhere to institutions (effective 2001). adv. bk.rev. bibl, illus. index, cum.index: vols.1-80 (1880-1961). back issues avail. *Refereed.* **Document type:** *Academic/Scholarly.* **Description:** It publishes papers on all aspects of the biology of invertebrates-protozoans and metazoans, aquatic and terrestrial, free-living and symbiotic.
Formerly: American Microscopical Society. Transactions (0003-0023)
Related titles: Microfilm ed.: (from PMC); Online - full text ed.: (from Institute for Scientific Information).
Indexed: ASCA, Abstr.Bull.Inst.Pap.Chem., Anim.Behav.Abstr., Aqua.Sci.& Fish.Abstr., Biol.& Agr.Ind. (Apr.1983-Oct.1994), Biol.Abstr., Chem.Abstr., Curr.Adv.Ecol.Sci., Curr.Cont., Dairy Sci.Abstr., Deep Sea Res.& Oceanogr.Abstr., Entomol.Abstr., Forest.Abstr., Genet.Abstr. (coverage dropped), GeoRef, Helminthol.Abstr., Hum.Gen.Abstr., INIS Atomind., Ind.Med. (coverage dropped), Ind.Sci.Rev., Ind.Vet., Inpharma, Neurosci.Abstr. (coverage dropped), Ocean.Abstr. (coverage dropped), Pollut.Abstr., Protozool.Abstr., Reac., Rev.Appl.Entomol., Rev.Med.& Vet.Mycol., Sci.Cit.Ind., Soils & Fert., Sport Fish.Abstr., Vet.Bull., Wild.Rev., Zoo.Rec.
—BLDSC (4557.703195), CASDDS, CISTI, GNLM, IDS, Infotrieve, ingenta, KNAW, Linda Hall. **CCC.**
Published by: American Microscopical Society, Dept of Biology, Winthrop University, Rock Hill, SC 29733. ams@allen press.com, http://www.invertebratebiology.org. Ed. Dr. Vicki Pearse. R&P Julian Smith. Circ: 1,200. **Subscr. to:** Allen Press Inc., PO Box 1897, Lawrence, KS 66044-8897. **Co-sponsor:** American Society of Zoologists, Division of Invertebrate Zoology.

B

592 DEU ISSN 1354-2516
CODEN: INNEFP
INVERTEBRATE NEUROSCIENCE. Text in English. 1995. q. EUR 334.40 domestic; EUR 330.60 in Germany; EUR 96 newsstand/cover foreign (effective 2002). adv. *Refereed.* **Document type:** *Journal, Academic/Scholarly.* **Description:** Publishes articles on invertebrate neuroscience, including studies of molecular biology, development, neurogenetics, neurotoxicology and neuronal networks.
Related titles: ♦ Online - full text ed.: Invertebrate Neuroscience Online. ISSN 1439-1104.
Indexed: Aqua.Sci.& Fish.Abstr., Chem.Abstr., Chem.Indus.Notes, Chem.Titles, Chemorec.Abstr., Curr.Cont. (coverage dropped), Entomol.Abstr. (coverage dropped), Helminthol.Abstr., Ind.Med. (1995-), Inpharma, Neurosci.Abstr., Ocean.Abstr., Reac., Rev.Appl.Entomol., Zoo.Rec.
—BLDSC (4557.703530), CASDDS, CISTI, IDS, Linda Hall.
Published by: Springer-Verlag (Subsidiary of: BertelsmannSpringer), Tiergartenstr 17, Heidelberg 69121, Germany. TEL 49-6221-345-0, FAX 49-6221-345229, subscriptions@springer.de, http://link.springer.de/link/service/journals/10158/index.htm, http://www.springer.de. Ed. L M Hall. **Subscr. to:** Springer-Verlag New York Inc., PO Box 2485, Secaucus, NJ 07096-2485. TEL 212-460-1500, FAX 212-473-6272.

592 DEU ISSN 1439-1104
INVERTEBRATE NEUROSCIENCE ONLINE. Text in English. q. **Document type:** *Journal, Academic/Scholarly.*
Media: Online - full text (from EBSCO Publishing, RoweCom Information Quest, Swets Blackwell, Springer LINK). **Related titles:** ♦ Print ed.: Invertebrate Neuroscience. ISSN 1354-2516.
Published by: Springer-Verlag (Subsidiary of: BertelsmannSpringer), Haber Str 7, Heidelberg 69126, Germany. TEL 49-30-82787-0, FAX 49-30-82787301, service@springer.de, http://www.springer.de.

590 AUS
INVERTEBRATE SYSTOMATICS (ONLINE EDITION). Text in English. bi-m. AUD 660, USD 570 (effective 2002). back issues avail. **Document type:** *Journal, Academic/Scholarly.*
Formerly (until 2001): Invertebrate Taxonomy (Online Edition) (1445-4572)
Media: Online - full text (from EBSCO Publishing, Swets Blackwell, Institute for Scientific Information). **Related titles:** Microfiche ed.: (from PQC); ♦ Print ed.: Invertebrate Systomatics (Print Edition). ISSN 1445-5226.
Published by: C S I R O Publishing, 150 Oxford St, Collingwood, VIC 3066, Australia. TEL 61-3-96627629, FAX 61-3-9662-7611, publishing@csiro.au, http://www.publish.csiro.au/journal/is. Ed. Camilla Myers.

571.3 AUS ISSN 1445-5226
QL362.5 CODEN: ITAXEO
INVERTEBRATE SYSTOMATICS (PRINT EDITION); Australian journal of scientific research. Text in English. 1971. bi-m. AUD 730 combined subscription domestic for print & online eds.; AUD 640 combined subscription foreign for print & online eds. (effective 2002). adv. index. back issues avail. *Refereed.* **Document type:** *Journal, Academic/Scholarly.* **Description:** Covers taxonomy and systematics of invertebrates of the southern hemisphere and Indo-Pacific Region.
Former titles (until 2001): Invertebrate Taxonomy (Print Edition) (0818-0164); (until 1987): Australian Journal of Zoology, Supplementary Series (0310-9089)

Related titles: Microfiche ed.: (from PQC); ♦ Online - full text ed.: Invertebrate Systematics (Online Edition).

Indexed: Agroforest.Abstr., Aqua.Sci.& Fish.Abstr., Bio-Contr.News & Info., Biol.Abstr., Curr.Cont., Ecol.Abstr., Entomol.Abstr., Forest Prod.Abstr., Forest.Abstr., GeoRef, Geol.Abstr., Helminthol.Abstr., Int.Abstr.Biol.Sci., Rev.Appl.Entomol., Rev.Med.& Vet.Mycol., Sci.Cit.Ind., Zoo.Rec.

—BLDSC (4557.703700), CISTI, IDS, Infotrieve, ingenta, Linda Hall. **CCC.**

Published by: (C S I R O Australia), C S I R O Publishing, 150 Oxford St, Collingwood, VIC 3066, Australia. TEL 61-3-96627629, FAX 61-3-9662-7611, camilla.myers@publish.csiro.au, publishing@csiro.au, http://www.publish.csiro.au/journals/is. Ed. Camilla Myers. Circ: 500. **Co-sponsor:** Australian Academy of Science.

B

590 JPN ISSN 0424-7086
QL461 CODEN: ESDBAK

JAPANESE JOURNAL OF SANITARY ZOOLOGY/EISEI DOBUTSU. Text in English, Japanese. 1950. q. JPY 10,300. back issues avail. **Document type:** *Academic/Scholarly.*

Indexed: Abstr.Hyg., Aqua.Sci.& Fish.Abstr., Bio-Contr.News & Info., Biol.Abstr., Chem.Abstr., Derwent Biotech.Abstr., Entomol.Abstr. (coverage dropped), Helminthol.Abstr., Ind.Vet., Protozool.Abstr., Ref.Zh., Rev.Appl.Entomol., So.Pac.Per.Ind., Trop.Dis.Bull., Vet.Bull.

—BLDSC (5527.330000), CASDDS, CISTI, Infotrieve, ingenta. **CCC.**

Published by: (Japan Society of Sanitary Zoology), Business Center for Academic Societies Japan/Nihon Gakkai Jimu Senta, 5-16-9 Honkomagome, Bunkyo-ku, Tokyo 113-0021, Japan. TEL 81-3-5814-5811, FAX 81-3-5814-5822, TELEX 2722268 BCJSP J. Circ: 1,000.

599.74 JPN

JAPANESE PELAGIC INVESTIGATION ON FUR SEALS. Text in Japanese. 1958. a. free per issue to qualified personnel.

Published by: National Research Institute of Far Seas Fisheries, 5-7-1 Ori-Do, shimizu-shi, Shizuoka-ken 424-0902, Japan. TEL 0543-340-715, FAX 0543-359-642. Circ: 100.

JOURNAL OF ANIMAL ECOLOGY. see *BIOLOGY*

JOURNAL OF ANIMAL PHYSIOLOGY AND ANIMAL NUTRITION/ZEITSCHRIFT FUER TIERPHYSIOLOGIE UND TIERERNAEHRUNG. see *BIOLOGY—Physiology*

JOURNAL OF ANIMAL PHYSIOLOGY AND ANIMAL NUTRITION ONLINE. see *BIOLOGY—Physiology*

595.3 USA ISSN 0278-0372
QL435.A1 CODEN: JCBIDB

JOURNAL OF CRUSTACEAN BIOLOGY. Text in English. 1981. q. USD 105 in North America; USD 125 elsewhere (effective 2001). bk.rev. back issues avail. *Refereed.* **Document type:** *Academic/Scholarly.* **Description:** Provides international exchange of information among persons interested in any aspect of crustacean studies.

Related titles: Online - full text ed.: (from Institute for Scientific Information).

Indexed: ASCA, Anim.Behav.Abstr. (coverage dropped), Appl.Ecol.Abstr. (coverage dropped), Aqua.Sci.& Fish.Abstr., Aquacult.Abstr., Biol.Abstr., Chem.Abstr., Curr.Cont., Deep Sea Res.& Oceanogr.Abstr., Ecol.Abstr., Entomol.Abstr., Environ.Sci.Poll.Mgmt., Genet.Abstr., GeoRef, Ind.Sci.Rev., Int.Abstr.Biol.Sci., Mar.Sci.Cont.Tab., Ocean.Abstr., Protozool.Abstr., Ref.Zh., Rev.Med.& Vet.Mycol., Sci.Cit.Ind., Sport Fish.Abstr., Zoo.Rec.

—BLDSC (4965.680000), CASDDS, EMDOCS, IDS, ingenta, Linda Hall.

Published by: Crustacean Society, 810 E 10th St, Box 1897, Lawrence, KS 66044. TEL 913-843-1221, FAX 913-843-1274. Ed. Arthur G Humes. Circ: 1,100.

590.724 USA ISSN 0022-104X
QL1 CODEN: JEZOAO

JOURNAL OF EXPERIMENTAL ZOOLOGY. Text in English. 1904. 18/yr. USD 5,270 in United States; USD 5,450 in Canada & Mexico; USD 5,603 elsewhere; USD 5,534 combined subscription in United States for print and online eds.; USD 5,714 combined subscription in Canada & Mexico for print and online eds.; USD 5,867 combined subscription elsewhere for print and online eds. (effective 2002). adv. abstr, bibl, charts, illus. index. back issues avail.; reprint service avail. from SWZ. *Refereed.* **Document type:** *Academic/Scholarly.* **Description:** Reports research results; includes investigations of all levels of biological organization, from the molecular to the organismal.

Related titles: Microform ed.: (from PMC,PQC,SWZ); Online - full text ed.: ISSN 1097-010X. 1998. USD 5,270 in United States; USD 5,270 in Canada & Mexico; USD 5,270 elsewhere (effective 2002) (from EBSCO Publishing, Wiley InterScience, Institute for Scientific Information); ♦ Supplement: Journal of Experimental Zoology. Supplement. ISSN 1059-8324.

Indexed: ASCA, AgBiotech, Anim.Breed.Abstr., Aqua.Sci.& Fish.Abstr., Bio-Contr.News & Info., Biol.& Agr.Ind. (Mar.1983-), Biol.Abstr., Cal.Tiss.Abstr., Chem.Abstr., Chem.Indus.Notes, Chem.Titles, Curr.Adv.Biochem., Curr.Adv.Cell & Devel.Biol., Curr.Adv.Gen.& Molec.Biol., Curr.Cont., Curr.Ref.Fish Res., Dairy Sci.Abstr., Deep Sea Res.& Oceanogr.Abstr., Entomol.Abstr., Excerp.Med. (until 1992), Helminthol.Abstr., INIS Atomind., Ind.Med. (1904-), Ind.Sci.Rev., Ind.Vet., Inpharma, Int.Abstr.Biol.Sci., Key Word Ind.Wildl.Res., Maize Abstr., Neurosci.Abstr., Neurosci.Cit.Ind., Nutr.Abstr., Pig News & Info., Plant Breed.Abstr., Plant Gen.Res.Abstr., Poult.Abstr., Protozool.Abstr., Reac., Ref.Zh., Rev.Appl.Entomol., Rev.Med.& Vet.Mycol., Sci.Cit.Ind., Soils & Fert., Sport Fish.Abstr., Triticale Abstr., Vet.Bull., Wild.Rev., Zoo.Rec.

—BLDSC (4983.000000), CASDDS, CISTI, EMDOCS, GNLM, IDS, ingenta, Linda Hall. **CCC.**

Published by: John Wiley & Sons, Inc., Journals (Subsidiary of: Wiley InterScience), 605 Third Ave, New York, NY 10158. TEL 212-850-6645, FAX 212-850-6021, subinfo@wiley.com, uscs-wis@wiley.com, http://www.wiley.com. Ed. Francis Ruddle. adv.: B&W page GBP 640, color page GBP 1,515; trim 210 x 279. Circ: 1,200. **Subscr. outside the Americas to:** John Wiley & Sons Ltd., Baffins Ln, Chichester, Sussex PO19 IUD, United Kingdom. TEL 44-1243-779777, FAX 44-1243-843232, cs-journals@wiley.co.uk, http://www.wiley.co.uk.

590.724 USA ISSN 1059-8324
CODEN: JEZSE6

JOURNAL OF EXPERIMENTAL ZOOLOGY. SUPPLEMENT. Text in English. 1987. irreg. (approx a.). back issues avail. *Refereed.* **Document type:** *Academic/Scholarly.*

Related titles: ♦ Supplement to: Journal of Experimental Zoology. ISSN 0022-104X.

Indexed: Ind.Med. (coverage dropped), Sport Fish.Abstr., Wild.Rev., Zoo.Rec.

—CISTI.

Published by: John Wiley & Sons, Inc., Journals (Subsidiary of: Wiley InterScience), 605 Third Ave, New York, NY 10158. **Subscr. outside the Americas to:** John Wiley & Sons Ltd., Baffins Ln, Chichester, Sussex PO19 IUD, United Kingdom. FAX 44-1243-776128.

597.8 587.9 USA

JOURNAL OF HERPETOLOGICAL MEDICINE AND SURGERY. Text in English. 1992. q. USD 110 in North America to institutions; USD 125 elsewhere to institutions (effective 2001). adv. back issues avail. *Refereed.* **Document type:** *Bulletin, Academic/Scholarly.* **Description:** Aims to improve reptilian and amphibian husbandary and veterinary care through education, exchange of ideas and research.

Formerly (until 2000): Association of Reptilian and Amphibian Veterinarians. Bulletin (1076-3139)

Indexed: Derwent Biotech.Abstr., Wild.Rev., Zoo.Rec.

—BLDSC (4998.070000).

Published by: (Association of Reptilian and Amphibian Veterinarians), Allen Press Inc., PO BOx 1897, Lawrence, KS 66044. TEL 785-843-1235, FAX 785-843-1274, arav@allenpress.com, http://www.allenpress.com. Ed. Thomas H Boyer.

599 USA ISSN 1064-7554
QL708.5 CODEN: JMEVEY

JOURNAL OF MAMMALIAN EVOLUTION. Text in English. 1993. q. USD 283, EUR 283 to institutions for print or online ed.; EUR 339.60, USD 339.60 to institutions for print & online eds. combined (effective 2002). bk.rev. *Refereed.* **Document type:** *Journal, Academic/Scholarly.* **Description:** Investigates all aspects of the comparative and evolutionary biology of mammals, with contributions from specialists in the fields of paleontology, molecular biology, comparative anatomy, developmental biology and cytogenics.

Related titles: Microfilm ed.: (from PQC); Online - full text ed.: (from EBSCO Publishing, O C L C Online Computer Library Center, Inc., Swets Blackwell, Kluwer Online, RoweCom Information Quest).

Indexed: Aqua.Sci.& Fish.Abstr., Ecol.Abstr., Genet.Abstr., Hum.Gen.Abstr., Ref.Zh., Wild.Rev., Zoo.Rec.

—BLDSC (5010.880000), CISTI, Infotrieve, ingenta. **CCC.**

Published by: (Society for the Study of Mammalian Evolution), Kluwer Academic - Plenum Publishers (Subsidiary of: Wolters Kluwer N.V.), 233 Spring St, New York, NY 10013-1578. TEL 212-620-8000, 800-221-9369, FAX 212-463-0742, info@plenum.com, http://www.wkap.nl/journalhome.htm/1064-7554. Eds. Jean Louis Hartenberger, W Patrick Luckett. R&P Rose Luongo TEL 781-871-6311. **Subscr. outside the Americas to:** Kluwer Academic Publishers Group, Journals Department, PO Box 322, Dordrecht 3300 AH, Netherlands. TEL 31-78-639-2392, FAX 31-78-654-6474.

599 USA ISSN 0022-2372
QL700 CODEN: JOMAAL

JOURNAL OF MAMMALOGY. Text in English. 1919. q. USD 170 (effective 2001). adv. bk.rev. bibl, charts, illus. index. back issues avail.; reprint service avail. from PQC. *Refereed.* **Document type:** *Academic/Scholarly.* **Description:** It publishes original research on both terrestrial and marine mammals. All aspects of the biology of mammals, including paleontology, are covered in the worldwide scope of this journal.

Related titles: Microform ed.: (from PQC,PMC); Online - full text ed.: (from Northern Light Technology, Inc., ProQuest Information & Learning, Gale Group, BioOne, Factiva, Institute for Scientific Information).

Indexed: ABSEARCH Mammal. (1950-), ASCA, Abstr.Anthropol., Agricola, Anim.Behav.Abstr., Anim.Breed.Abstr., Appl.Ecol.Abstr., Aqua.Sci.& Fish.Abstr., Bibl.Agri., Bio-Contr.News & Info., Biol.& Agr.Ind. (Feb.1983-), Biol.Abstr., Biotech.& Bioeng.Abstr., Chemorec.Abstr., Curr.Adv.Ecol.Sci., Curr.Cont., Dairy Sci.Abstr., Deep Sea Res.& Oceanogr.Abstr., Ecol.Abstr., Environ.Sci.Poll.Mgmt., Forest Prod.Abstr., Forest.Abstr., Gen.Sci.Ind. (Aug.1984-), Genet.Abstr., Geo.Abstr.H.G., GeoRef, Geol.Abstr., Hum.Gen.Abstr., INIS Atomind., Ind.Med. (coverage dropped), Ind.Sci.Rev., Ind.Vet., Int.Abstr.Biol.Sci., Key Word Ind.Wildl.Res., Nutr.Abstr., Ocean.Abstr., Pollut.Abstr., Ref.Zh., Rev.Appl.Entomol., SSCI (coverage dropped), Sci.Cit.Ind., Seed Abstr., Sel.Water Res.Abstr., So.Pac.Per.Ind., Sport Fish.Abstr., Vet.Bull., Weed Abstr., Wild Life Rev., Wild.Rev., Zoo.Rec.

—BLDSC (5011.000000), CISTI, EMDOCS, GNLM, ingenta, Linda Hall.

Published by: American Society of Mammalogists, c/o Dr H Duane Smith, Sec -Treas, Monte L Bean Life Science Museum, Brigham Young University, Provo, UT 84602-0200. TEL 801-378-2492, asm@allenpress.com, orders@allenpress.com, http://www.mammalogy.org. Ed. David M Leslie. R&P H Duane Smith. Adv. contact Cheryl A Schmidt. **Subscr. to:** Allen Press Inc., PO Box 1897, Lawrence, KS 66044-8897.

594 USA ISSN 1053-6388
CODEN: JMAMEL

JOURNAL OF MEDICAL AND APPLIED MALACOLOGY. Text in English, Spanish. 1989. a. USD 50 to non-members. abstr, bibl, charts, illus, stat. back issues avail. **Description:** Contains original research on mollusks that are of medical, veterinary, agricultural and economic importance.

—CISTI.

Published by: International Society for Medical and Applied Malacology, PO Box 2715, Ann Arbor, MI 48106. TEL 313-764-0470. Ed. John B Burch. Circ: 200.

579.9 615.49 BRA ISSN 0104-7930
CODEN: JVTOFG

JOURNAL OF VENOMOUS ANIMALS AND TOXINS. Text in English. 1995. s-a. BRL 35 domestic; USD 30 foreign (effective 2001). adv. bk.rev. abstr, bibl, charts, illus, maps. index. back issues avail. *Refereed.* **Document type:** *Academic/Scholarly.* **Description:** Devoted to research on different aspects of toxins, venomous animals, their products and derivatives.

Media: Diskette (from SciELO). **Related titles:** Online - full text ed.: (from SciELO).
Indexed: Aqua.Sci.& Fish.Abstr., Chem.Abstr., Chem.Indus.Notes, Chem.Titles, Entomol.Abstr. (coverage dropped), Environ.Sci.Poll.Mgmt., Excerp.Med. (1996-), INIS Atomind., Ind.Vet., Int.Abstr.Biol.Sci., Neurosci.Abstr. (coverage dropped), Pollut.Abstr., Rev.Appl.Entomol., Rev.Med.& Vet.Mycol., Rev.Plant Path., Saf.Sci.Abstr., Tox.Abstr., Triticale Abstr., Wild.Rev., Zoo.Rec.
—BLDSC (5072.285000), CASDDS, EMDOCS.
Published by: Universidade Estadual Paulista, Centro de Estudos de Venenos e Animais Peconhentos/Center for the Study of Venoms and Venomous Animals, Rubiao Junior, S/N Botucatu, Sao Paulo, SP 18618-000, Brazil. TEL 55-14-68213963, FAX 55-14-68026054, cevap@cevap.org.br, http://www.scielo.br/jvat, http://www.cevap.org.br. Ed., R&P, Adv. contact Benedito Barraviera. page USD 60. Circ: 1,300.
Co-sponsor: Microsoft Informatica Ltda.

590 USA ISSN 1071-2232
SF996.45
JOURNAL OF WILDLIFE REHABILITATION. Text in English. 1977. q. USD 40 domestic to individual members; USD 46 in Canada & Mexico to individual members; USD 50 elsewhere to individual members; USD 52 domestic to institutions; USD 60 in Canada & Mexico to institutions; USD 62 elsewhere to institutions; USD 30 domestic to libraries; USD 38 in Canada & Mexico to libraries; USD 40 elsewhere to libraries; USD 30 domestic to students; USD 38 in Canada & Mexico to students; USD 40 elsewhere to students (effective 2000). bk.rev. illus. index. back issues avail.; reprints avail. *Refereed.* **Document type:** *Trade.* **Description:** Dedicated to the dissemination of information related to the field of wildlife rehabilitation.
Formerly (until 1993): Wildlife Journal (0893-6560)
Related titles: Online - full text ed.: (from Institute for Scientific Information).
Indexed: ASCA, Focus on: Vet.Sci.& Med., Sport Fish.Abstr., Wild.Rev., Zoo.Rec.
—BLDSC (5072.630500), IDS, ingenta.
Published by: International Wildlife Rehabilitation Council, 4437 Central Pl., Ste. B4, Suisun, CA 94585-1663. TEL 707-864-1761, FAX 707-864-3106, iwrc@inreach.com, http://www.iwrc-online.org. Ed. Jan Ambrosini. R&P Mary Reynolds. Circ: 2,000.

590.7 DEU ISSN 1439-0469
JOURNAL OF ZOOLOGICAL SYSTEMATICS AND EVOLUTIONARY RESEARCH ONLINE. Text in English, French, German. 4/yr. USD 856 (effective 2001). **Document type:** *Academic/Scholarly.*
Media: Online - full text (from EBSCO Publishing, O C L C Online Computer Library Center, Inc., ingenta, Munksgaard & Blackwell Science's Synergy, Swets Blackwell, Institute for Scientific Information). **Related titles:** ♦ Print ed.: Journal of Zoological Systematics and Evolutionary Research. ISSN 0947-5745.
Published by: Blackwell Wissenschafts Verlag GmbH, Kurfuerstendamm 57, Berlin 10707, Germany. TEL 49-30-32790679, FAX 49-30-32790610, abo@blackwis.de, http://www.blackwell.de.

590.724 GBR ISSN 0023-6772
SF405.5 CODEN: LBANAX
LABORATORY ANIMALS. Text in English. 1966. q. GBP 118 in Europe to institutions; USD 200 in United States to institutions; GBP 123 elsewhere to institutions (effective 2002). adv. bk.rev. charts, illus. index. *Refereed.* **Document type:** *Journal, Academic/Scholarly.* **Description:** Provides an international forum for the publication of research carried out by scientists primarily concerned with the care, welfare and science of laboratory animals.
Related titles: Online - full text ed.: (from CatchWord Ltd., Swets Blackwell, Institute for Scientific Information, RoweCom Information Quest).
Indexed: ASCA, AgBiotech, Agricola, Anim.Breed.Abstr., Bibl.Agri., Biol.Abstr., Chem.Abstr., Chem.Indus.Notes, Chem.Titles, Curr.Adv.Cell & Devel.Biol., Curr.Adv.Ecol.Sci., Curr.Cont., Dairy Sci.Abstr., Excerp.Med., Focus on: Vet.Sci.& Med., Helminthol.Abstr., Ind.Med. (1967-), Ind.Sci.Rev., Ind.Vet., Inpharma, Int.Abstr.Biol.Sci., Nutr.Abstr., Pig News & Info., Poult.Abstr., Protozool.Abstr., Reac., Ref.Zh., Rev.Arom.& Med.Plants, Rev.Med.& Vet.Mycol., Rev.Plant Path., Sci.Cit.Ind., Soyabean Abstr., Sport Fish.Abstr., Vet.Bull., Wild.Rev., Zoo.Rec.
—BLDSC (5138.600000), ADONIS, CASDDS, CISTI, GNLM, IDS, ingenta, Linda Hall. **CCC.**
Published by: (Laboratory Animal Science Association), Royal Society of Medicine Press Ltd, 1 Wimpole St, London W1M 8AE, United Kingdom. TEL 44-20-7290-2921, FAX 44-20-7290-2929, rsmjournals@rsm.ac.uk, http://www.roysocmed.ac.uk/pub/la.htm. R&P Caroline McLaughlin. Circ: 1,700.

LIBRARY NEWS FOR ZOOS AND AQUARIUMS. see *LIBRARY AND INFORMATION SCIENCES*

599.6362 USA ISSN 0887-9923
LLAMAS MAGAZINE; information for camelid lovers everywhere. Text in English. 1979. 5/yr. USD 20 domestic; USD 25 in Canada; USD 30 elsewhere (effective 1999). adv. bk.rev. illus. cum.index: 1982-1997. back issues avail.; reprints avail. **Document type:** *Trade.*
Formerly: 3 L Llama Magazine (0739-1064)
—ingenta.
Published by: Clay Press, Inc., PO Box 250, Jackson, CA 95642-2322. TEL 209-295-7800, FAX 209-295-7878, claypres@volcano.net, http://www.llamapaedia.com/resources/resources.html. Ed., R&P Cheryl Dal Porto. Pub. Cleave Dal Porto. Adv. contact Tina Dal Porto. Circ: 5,000 (paid).

597.9 639.9 GBR ISSN 0839-7708
MARINE TURTLE NEWSLETTER. Text in English. 1976. q. free (effective 2001). bk.rev. back issues avail. *Refereed.* **Document type:** *Newsletter, Academic/Scholarly.* **Description:** Provides a forum for exchange of information about all aspects of marine turtle biology and conservation. Alerts interested people to particular threats to marine turtles, as they arise.
Related titles: Online - full content ed.; Spanish ed.: Noticiero de Tortugas Marinas. ISSN 1463-9335. 1976.
Indexed: Ocean.Abstr., Zoo.Rec.
Published by: Marine Turtle Research Group, School of Biological Sciences, University of Wales Swansea, Singleton Park, Swansea SA2 8PP, United Kingdom. TEL 44-1792-205678 ext 4411, FAX 44-1792-295447, MTN@swan.ac.uk, http://www.seaturtle.org/mtn. Eds. Annette Broderick, Brendan Godley. Circ: 2,500.

590 DEU ISSN 0934-6643
MERTENSIELLA. Text in English, German. 1988. irreg., latest vol.11, 1999. price varies. illus. **Document type:** *Monographic series, Academic/Scholarly.*
Related titles: ♦ Supplement to: Salamandra. ISSN 0036-3375.
Indexed: Zoo.Rec.
—BLDSC (5682.281963).
Published by: Deutsche Gesellschaft fuer Herpetologie und Terrarienkunde e.V., Postfach 1421, Rheinbach 53351, Germany. TEL 49-2225-703333, FAX 49-2225-703338, gs@dght.de, http://www.dght.de. Circ: 2,000.

▼ **MOLECULAR BIOLOGY TODAY.** see *BIOLOGY—Botany*

599.8 USA ISSN 0740-9729
CODEN: MONPD5
MONOGRAPHS IN PRIMATOLOGY. Text in English. 1983. irreg., latest vol.13, 1990. price varies. *Refereed.* **Document type:** *Monographic series.*
Indexed: Biol.Abstr.
—CISTI.
Published by: John Wiley & Sons, Inc., Journals (Subsidiary of: Wiley InterScience), 605 Third Ave, New York, NY 10158.

590.74 PRT ISSN 0870-3876
DP702.M11 CODEN: BMMFA2
MUSEU MUNICIPAL DO FUNCHAL. BOLETIM. Text in Portuguese. 1945. a. per issue exchange basis. illus, maps, stat. back issues avail. **Document type:** *Bulletin.*
Related titles: Diskette ed.
Indexed: Aqua.Sci.& Fish.Abstr., Aquacult.Abstr., Biol.Abstr., Curr.Adv.Ecol.Sci., Deep Sea Res.& Oceanogr.Abstr., Environ.Sci.Poll.Mgmt., Sport Fish.Abstr., Wild.Rev., Zoo.Rec.
—BLDSC (2139.000000).
Published by: Camara Municipal do Funchal, Museo Municipal do Funchal Historia Natural, RUA DA MOURARIA, 31, Funchal, Madeira 9004-546, Portugal. TEL 351-91-229761, FAX 351-91-225180. Ed. Antonio Domingos Abreu. Circ: 750.

590.7 BRA
MUSEU PARAENSE EMILIO GOELDI. BOLETIM. NOVA SERIE ZOOLOGIA. Text mainly in Portuguese; Text occasionally in English, French. 1957; N.S. 1984. s-a. BRL 12 per issue domestic; USD 15 per issue foreign (effective 2000). abstr, bibl, illus. **Description:** Original papers in zoological research.
Formerly (until 1983, no.124): Museu Paraense Emilio Goeldi. Boletim. Nova Serie: Zoologia (0077-2232)
Indexed: Biol.Abstr., Curr.Adv.Ecol.Sci., GeoRef, Rev.Med.& Vet.Mycol., Rural Devel.Abstr., Wild.Rev., World Ag.Econ.& Rur.Soc.Abstr., Zoo.Rec.
—BLDSC (2143.500000).
Published by: Conselho Nacional de Desenvolvimento Cientifico e Tecnologico, Museu Paraense Emilio Goeldi, Comercio, Caixa Postal 399, Belem, PA 66017-970, Brazil. TEL 091-274-2195, FAX 091-274-1811, mgdoc@musu-goeldi.br. Circ: 1,000.

590 DEU ISSN 0173-7481
CODEN: AVNHAV
NATURWISSENSCHAFTLICHER VEREIN IN HAMBURG. ABHANDLUNGEN* . Text in German. 1937. irreg. price varies. bk.rev. bibl, illus. index. reprint service avail. from ISI. **Document type:** *Monographic series, Academic/Scholarly.*
Supersedes in part: Naturwissenschaftlicher Verein in Hamburg. Abhandlungen und Verhandlungen (0301-2697)
Indexed: Biol.Abstr., Chem.Abstr., GeoRef, Zoo.Rec.
—CISTI, Linda Hall.
Published by: Naturwissenschaftlicher Verein Hamburg, Martin-Luther-King-Platz 3, Hamburg 20146, Germany. TEL 49-40-41233927.

NEMATOLOGICAL ABSTRACTS. see *BIOLOGY—Abstracting, Bibliographies, Statistics*

NIHON JIKKEN DOBUTSU GAKKAI SOKAI KOEN YOSHISHU/JAPANESE ASSOCIATION FOR LABORATORY ANIMAL SCIENCE. ABSTRACTS OF GENERAL MEETING. see *BIOLOGY—Abstracting, Bibliographies, Statistics*

590.724 JPN ISSN 0913-2139
NIHON JIKKEN DOBUTSU GIJUTSUSHA KYOKAI HOKKAIDO SHIBU KAISHI/JAPANESE ASSOCIATION FOR EXPERIMENTAL ANIMAL TECHNOLOGISTS. HOKKAIDO BRANCH. JOURNAL. Text in Japanese. 1977. a.
Published by: Nihon Jikken Dobutsu Gijutsusha Kyokai, Hokkaido Shibu/Japanese Association for Experimental Animal Technologists, Hokkaido Branch, Hokkaido Daigaku Igakubu Fuzoku Dobutsu Jikken Shisetsu, Nishi 7-chome, Kita 15-jo, Kita-ku, Sapporo-shi, Hokkaido 060, Japan.

591.5 USA ISSN 0738-4394
QL750
PERSPECTIVES IN ETHOLOGY. Text in English. 1973. irreg., latest vol.12, 1998. price varies. back issues avail. *Refereed.* **Document type:** *Monographic series.*
Indexed: Zoo.Rec.
—KNAW. **CCC.**
Published by: Kluwer Academic - Plenum Publishers (Subsidiary of: Wolters Kluwer N.V.), 233 Spring St, New York, NY 10013-1578. TEL 212-620-8000, 800-221-9369, FAX 212-463-0742, info@plenum.com, http://www.plenum.com. Eds. P H Klopfer, P P G Bateson.

PRIMATE EYE. see *ANTHROPOLOGY*

599.8 JPN ISSN 0032-8332
QL737.P9 CODEN: PRMTBU
PRIMATES; journal of primatology. Text in English. 1957. q. JPY 15,000 foreign to individuals; JPY 22,000 to institutions (effective 2001). bk.rev. abstr, charts, illus, stat. *Refereed.* **Document type:** *Academic/Scholarly.*
Related titles: Online - full text ed.: (from Institute for Scientific Information).
Indexed: Abstr.Anthropol., Anim.Behav.Abstr., Anthropol.Lit., Appl.Ecol.Abstr., Curr.Cont., Environ.Sci.Poll.Mgmt., Focus on: Vet.Sci.& Med., Genet.Abstr., GeoRef, Helminthol.Abstr., Hum.Gen.Abstr., Ind.Sci.Rev., Ind.Vet., Intl.Bibl.Soc.Sci., PsycInfo, Psychol.Abstr. (1966-), SSCI (coverage dropped), Sci.Cit.Ind., Sport Fish.Abstr., Vet.Bull., Wild.Rev., Zoo.Rec.
—BLDSC (6612.925000), CASDDS, CISTI, IDS, ingenta, Linda Hall.
Published by: Japan Monkey Centre/Nihon Monki Senta, 26 Kanrin, Inuyama-shi, Aichi-ken 484-0081, Japan. TEL 81-568-61-2327, FAX 81-568-62-6823, ldz05366@nifty.ne.jp, http://www.meitetsu.co.jp/japan-monkeycentre/. Ed. Yukimaru Sugiyama. R&P Mitsuo Iwamoto. Circ: 600.

591 JPN
PROBLEMS IN MODERN ZOOLOGY. Text in Japanese. irreg.?. **Document type:** *Monographic series.*
Published by: Zoological Society of Japan/Nihon Dobutsu Gakkai, Toshin Bldg 2F, 2-27-2 Hongo, Bunkyo-ku, Tokyo 113-0033, Japan. TEL 81-3-5814-5811, FAX 81-3-3814-5352. Ed. Seiichiro Kawashima.

PROTOZOOLOGICAL ABSTRACTS. see *BIOLOGY—Abstracting, Bibliographies, Statistics*

B

590 POL ISSN 0033-247X
QL1 CODEN: PZOOAC
PRZEGLAD ZOOLOGICZNY. Text in Polish; Abstracts and contents page in English. 1957. q. PLZ 16 (effective 2000). adv. bk.rev. bibl, illus. index. **Document type:** *Academic/Scholarly.*
Indexed: AgroLibrex, Aqua.Sci.& Fish.Abstr., Aquacult.Abstr., Biol.Abstr., Chem.Abstr., Deep Sea Res.& Oceanogr.Abstr., Environ.Sci.Poll.Mgmt., GeoRef, Ind.Vet., Ref.Zh., Vet.Bull., Zoo.Rec.
—CASDDS, CISTI, Linda Hall.
Published by: Polskie Towarzystwo Zoologiczne, Ul Sienkiewicza 21, Wroclaw 50335, Poland. TEL 48-71-225041, FAX 48-71-222817. Ed., Adv. contact Romuald J Pomorski. R&P Jerzy Turzanski. Circ: 1,420. **Dist. by:** ORPAN, Palac Kultury i Nauki, Warsaw 00901, Poland.

590 RUS
REFERATIVNYI ZHURNAL. ZOOPARAZITOLOGIYA. Text in Russian. 1960. m. **Document type:** *Academic/Scholarly.*
Published by: Vserossiiskii Institut Nauchnoi i Tekhnicheskoi Informatsii (VINITI), Usievicha ul 20-a, Moscow 125315, Russian Federation. TEL 7-095-1526441, FAX 7-095-943-0060. **US dist. addr.:** East View Publications, 3020 Harbor Ln N, Minneapolis, MN 55447. TEL 612-550-0961.

REVISTA VETERINARIA Y ZOOTECNICA DE CALDAS. see *VETERINARY SCIENCE*

595.4 FRA ISSN 0398-4346
REVUE ARACHNOLOGIQUE. Text in English, French; Summaries in French. 1977. irreg., latest vol.12, 1998. FRF 180, EUR 27.44. back issues avail. *Refereed.*
Indexed: Biol.Abstr., Ref.Zh., Zoo.Rec.
Address: rue du Ruisseau, Solignac-sur-Loire 43370, France. Ed. J.C. Ledoux. Pub. J C Ledoux.

590 RUS
ROSSIISKII NEMATOLOGICHESKII ZHURNAL. Text in Russian. s-a. USD 75 in United States. **Document type:** *Academic/Scholarly.*
Published by: Institut Parazitologii, Leninskii pr-t 38, Moscow 117334, Russian Federation. TEL 7-095-2367162. **US dist. addr.:** East View Publications, 3020 Harbor Ln N, Minneapolis, MN 55447. TEL 612-550-0961.

SEA GRANT ABSTRACTS; publications from the nation's Sea Grant programs. see *BIOLOGY—Abstracting, Bibliographies, Statistics*

SHE ZHI/JOURNAL OF SNAKE. see *MEDICAL SCIENCES*

599 CHN ISSN 1000-1050
SHOULEI XUEBAO/ACTA THERIOLOGICA SINICA. Text in Chinese; Summaries in English. 1981. q. USD 70 (effective 2000). adv. bk.rev. *Refereed.* **Document type:** *Academic/Scholarly.* **Description:** Contains original theses on basic theories and applications of mammalian zoology. Includes taxonomy, morphology, ecology, physiology, biochemistry, paleontology and evolution, raising, domestication, natural protection, hunting, and prevention of cruelty.
Indexed: Ecol.Abstr., Geol.Abstr., Ref.Zh., Zoo.Rec.
Published by: (Xibei Gaoyuan Shengwu Yanjiusuo), Kexue Chubanshe/Science Press, 16 Donghuang Cheng Genbei Jie, Beijing 100717, China. Ed. Wang Zuwang. Circ: 5,500.

590 JPN
SHUKAN ASAHI HYAKKA/WEEKLY ASAHI ENCYCLOPEDIA. Text in Japanese. 1975. w.
Published by: Asahi Shimbun Publishing Co., 3-2 Tsuki-Ji 5-chome, Chuo-ku, Tokyo 104-0045, Japan. Ed. Tsuyosi Nogami. **Order to:** Oversea Courier Service Co. Ltd., 9 Shibaura 2-chome, Minato-ku, Tokyo 108-0023, Japan.

599.5 USA
SKYHOPPER. Text in English. 1980. q. USD 35 to members (effective 2000). **Document type:** *Newsletter.* **Description:** Current information on whale and dolphin research, education, and conservation.
Formerly: Whale News (1061-5970)
Published by: American Cetacean Society, PO Box 1391, San Pedro, CA 90733-1391. TEL 310-548-6279, FAX 310-548-6950, acs@pobox.com. Ed. Shirley Brim. R&P Kathleen Owston. Circ: 1,000.

590 FRA ISSN 0750-6848
CODEN: BSLBBS
SOCIETE LINNEENNE DE BORDEAUX. BULLETIN. Text in French; Summaries in English. 1971. q. FRF 250, USD 17 (effective 1999). bk.rev. back issues avail. **Document type:** *Bulletin.*
Indexed: Aqua.Sci.& Fish.Abstr., Aquacult.Abstr., Biol.Abstr., Environ.Sci.Poll.Mgmt., GeoRef, Zoo.Rec.
—Linda Hall.
Published by: Societe Linneenne de Bordeaux, 1 Place Bardineau, Bordeaux 33000, France. TEL 33-5-56379782. Ed. Michel Laguerre. Circ: 600.

SOCIETE LINNEENNE DE PROVENCE. BULLETIN. see *BIOLOGY—Botany*

590 FRA ISSN 0750-747X
SOCIETE ZOOLOGIQUE DE FRANCE. MEMOIRES. Text in French; Text occasionally in English; Summaries in English, French. 1888. irreg. price varies. index. back issues avail. *Refereed.* **Document type:** *Academic/Scholarly.*
Indexed: GeoRef, Sport Fish.Abstr.
Published by: Societe Zoologique de France, 195 rue Saint Jacques, Paris 75005, France. TEL 33-1-40793110. Ed. Jean-Loup d'Hondt.

590 ROM ISSN 1220-5273
QH301 CODEN: SCBADI
STUDII SI CERCETARI DE BIOLOGIE. SERIA BIOLOGIE ANIMALA. Text in Romanian. 1948. s-a. **Document type:** *Academic/Scholarly.*
Formerly (until 1989): Studii si Cercetari de Biologie. Seria Zoologia (1220-1634); Supersedes in part (in 1975): Studii si Cercetari de Biologie (1015-2237); Which was formed by the merger of (1958-1973): Studii si Cercetari de Biologie. Seria Botanica (0370-8934); Which was formerly (until 1963): Studii si Cercetari de Biologie. Seria Biologie Vegetala (0365-5997); (1958-1973): Studii si Cercetari de Biologie. Seria Zoologie (0370-8950)
Indexed: Biol.Abstr., Chem.Abstr., Chem.Indus.Notes, Chem.Titles, Ind.Vet., Sport Fish.Abstr., Vet.Bull., Wild.Rev., Zoo.Rec.
—CASDDS, CISTI, Linda Hall.
Published by: (Academia Romana), Editura Academiei Romane, Calea 13 Septembrie 13, Bucharest 76117, Romania. Ed. Mihai Bacescu. **Dist. by:** Rodipet S.A.. TEL 401-618-5103, FAX 401-226407.

591.9561 TUR ISSN 1300-0179
CODEN: DTZDEY
TURKISH JOURNAL OF ZOOLOGY/TURK ZOOLOJI DERGISI. Text in English, Turkish. 1976. 4/yr. USD 100 (effective 1999). *Refereed.* **Document type:** *Journal, Academic/Scholarly.*
Formerly (until 1994): Doga Turkish Journal of Zoology - Doga Turk Zooloji Dergisi (1011-0895)
Related titles: Online - full text ed.
Indexed: Anim.Breed.Abstr., Bio-Contr.News & Info., Ecol.Abstr., Food Sci.& Tech.Abstr., Forest.Abstr., Geo.Abstr.P.G., Geol.Abstr., Ind.Vet., Irr.& Drain.Abstr., Nutr.Abstr., Potato Abstr., Poult.Abstr., Protozool.Abstr., Rev.Appl.Entomol., Rev.Arom.& Med.Plants, Rev.Med.& Vet.Mycol., Soils & Fert., Vet.Bull., Weed Abstr., Zoo.Rec.
—BLDSC (9072.498000), CASDDS, CISTI, Linda Hall.
Published by: Scientific and Technical Research Council of Turkey - TUBITAK/Turkiye Bilimsel ve Teknik Arastirma Kurumu, Ataturk Bulvari No. 221, Kavaklidere, Ankara 06100, Turkey. TEL 90-312-468-5300, FAX 90-312-426-8073, bdym@tubitak.gov.tr, http://www.tubitak.gov.tr/journals/zoology/. Ed. Aykut Kence.

590 ESP ISSN 0213-3997
QL1 CODEN: ABBAEI
UNIVERSIDAD DE MURCIA. ANALES DE BIOLOGIA. SECCION BIOLOGIA ANIMAL. Text mainly in English, Spanish. 1984. a., latest vol.22, 1999, for the year 1997. ESP 2,000 (effective 2001). bk.rev. back issues avail. **Document type:** *Academic/Scholarly.*
Indexed: Bio-Contr.News & Info., Ind.SST.
—CISTI.
Published by: Universidad de Murcia, Servicio de Publicaciones, C Actor Isidoro Maiquez 9, Murcia 30007, Spain. TEL 34-68-363207, FAX 34-68-835418, vgm@um.es, http://www.um.es/spumweb. Ed. Diego Jose Rivera Nunez TEL 34-968-364958. Circ: 606.

591.972 MEX ISSN 0368-8720
UNIVERSIDAD NACIONAL AUTONOMA DE MEXICO. INSTITUTO DE BIOLOGIA. ANALES: SERIE ZOOLOGIA. Text in English, French, Spanish; Summaries in English, French, Spanish. 1967. s-a. MXP 100, USD 30 per issue (effective 2000). adv. abstr, charts, illus, stat. back issues avail. **Document type:** *Monographic series.* **Description:** Publishes articles in the area of Zoology.
Supersedes in part: Universidad Nacional Autonoma de Mexico. Instituto de Biologia. Anales (0076-7174)
Indexed: Aqua.Sci.& Fish.Abstr., Aquacult.Abstr., Ecol.Abstr., Entomol.Abstr. (coverage dropped), Environ.Sci.Poll.Mgmt., Helminthol.Abstr., Ind.Vet., Maize Abstr., Pollut.Abstr., Postharvest, Protozool.Abstr., Rev.Appl.Entomol., Rice Abstr., Zoo.Rec.
—Linda Hall.
Published by: Universidad Nacional Autonoma de Mexico, Instituto de Biologia, Ciudad Universitaria, Apdo Postal 70-233, Mexico City, DF 04510, Mexico. TEL 52-5-622-5690, FAX 52-5-622-5687, javierd@mail.ibiologia.unam.mx, http://www.ibiologia.unam.mx. Ed. Alfonso N Garcia Aldrete. Adv. contact Javier Dominguez Galicia. Circ: 1,500.

590 IND ISSN 0256-971X
QL1
UTTAR PRADESH JOURNAL OF ZOOLOGY. Text and summaries in English. 1981. 3/yr. INR 100, USD 20 to individuals; INR 200, USD 30 to institutions. adv. bk.rev. back issues avail. *Refereed.* **Document type:** *Academic/Scholarly.*
Indexed: Agroforest.Abstr., Anim.Breed.Abstr., Bio-Contr.News & Info., Biol.Abstr., Field Crop Abstr., Forest.Abstr., Helminthol.Abstr., Ind.Vet., Nutr.Abstr., Plant Breed.Abstr., Postharvest, Potato Abstr., Protozool.Abstr., Rev.Appl.Entomol., Rice Abstr., Seed Abstr., Triticale Abstr., Weed Abstr., Zoo.Rec.
—BLDSC (9135.619000).
Published by: Uttar Pradesh Zoological Society, c/o PG Dept. of Zoology, Muzaffarnagar 251 001, India. TEL 91-131-409053, FAX 91-131-402510. Circ: 225.

VETERINARSKI ARHIV. see *VETERINARY SCIENCE*

590 USA ISSN 0736-6094
Z6674
WILDLIFE DISEASE REVIEW. Text in English. 1983. m. USD 225; USD 255 foreign. index.
Address: P.O. Box 1522, Ft. Collins, CO 80522. TEL 303-484-6267, FAX 303-482-6184, TELEX 820567. Ed. B Zimmerman. Circ: 150.

WILDLIFE REHABILITATION. see *CONSERVATION*

590 NLD
WORLD ANIMAL SCIENCE. (Consists of: Series A, Basic Information; Series B, Disciplinary Approach; Series C, Production System Approach) Text in English. 1981. irreg., latest vol.10, 1996. price varies. back issues avail. *Refereed.* **Document type:** *Monographic series, Academic/Scholarly.* **Description:** Provides zoologists with a complete, coherent, up-to-date picture of the entire field of animal production science.
—BLDSC.
Published by: Elsevier Science BV, PO Box 211, Amsterdam 1000 AE, Netherlands. TEL 31-20-485-2911, FAX 31-20-485-2457, nlinfo-f@elsevier.nl; usinfo-f@elsevier.com; forinfo-kyf04035@niftyserve.or.jp, http://www.elsevier.nl/. Eds. A Neimann-Sorensen, D E Tribe. **Subscr. in Australasia and the Far East to:** Elsevier Science (Singapore) Pte Ltd, No.1 Temasek Ave, 17-01 Millenia Tower, Singapore 039192, Singapore. TEL 65-434-3727; **Subscr. in Japan to:** Elsevier Science Inc - Japan Regional Office, 9-15 Higashi-Azabu 1-chome, Minato-ku, Tokyo 106-0044, Japan. TEL 81-3-5561-5033, FAX 81-3-5561-5047, info@elsevier.co.jp; **Subscr. in the Americas to:** Elsevier Science, PO Box 945, New York, NY 10159-0945. TEL 212-633-3730, FAX 212-633-3680, http://www.elsevier.com.

599.32 FRA ISSN 1257-5011
WORLD RABBIT SCIENCE. Text in French. 1992. q. FRF 533 domestic; FRF 552, EUR 84.15 in Europe; FRF 672 elsewhere (effective 2001). adv. bibl, illus.
Formed by the merger of (1980-1992): Journal of Applied Rabbit Research (0738-9760); (1983-1992): Cuni - Sciences (0984-7847)
Indexed: AgBiotech, Anim.Breed.Abstr., Dairy Sci.Abstr., Food Sci.& Tech.Abstr., Ind.Vet., Nutr.Abstr., Poult.Abstr., Protozool.Abstr., Rev.Med.& Vet.Mycol., Soyabean Abstr., Triticale Abstr., Trop.Oil Seeds Abstr., Vet.Bull., World Ag.Econ.& Rur.Soc.Abstr.
—BLDSC (9358.560000), CISTI.

Published by: Association Francaise de Cuniculture, BP 50, Lempdes 63370, France. TEL 33-4-73920152, FAX 33-4-73928680, asfrcuni@easynet.fr, http://www.rabbit-science.com. Ed. F Lebas. Circ: 1,500.

590.73 DEU
ZOO - NACHRICHTEN; Allwetterzoo - Nachrichten. Text in German. 1980. 2/yr. DEM 20 (effective 2000). adv. bk.rev. back issues avail. **Document type:** *Magazine, Consumer.* **Description:** Reports and news about animals and events at the Allwetterzoo.
Published by: Westfaelischer Zoologischer Garten Muenster GmbH, Sentruper Str 315, Muenster 48161, Germany. TEL 49-251-89040, FAX 49-251-890490. Ed. Ilona Zuehlke. Circ: 5,000.

590 ESP ISSN 1130-4251
QL293
ZOOLOGICA BAETICA. Text in Spanish. 1989. a. price varies. **Document type:** *Academic/Scholarly.*
Indexed: Aqua.Sci.& Fish.Abstr., Entomol.Abstr., Ind.SST, Rev.Appl.Entomol., Zoo.Rec.
—CINDOC.
Published by: (Departamento de Biologia Animal, Ecologia y Genetica, Universidad de Granada), Editorial Universidad de Granada, Antiguo Colegio Maximo, Campus de Cartuja, Granada 18071, Spain. TEL 34-58-243930, FAX 34-58-243931. Ed. Felipe Pascual Torres.

ZOOLOGICAL RECORD. see *BIOLOGY—Abstracting, Bibliographies, Statistics*

590 TWN ISSN 1021-5506
QL307.2 CODEN: ZOSTEG
ZOOLOGICAL STUDIES. Summaries in Chinese. 1962. q. USD 60 to individuals; free per issue to institutions (effective 2001). 150 p./no. reprint service avail. from ISI. *Refereed.* **Document type:** *Journal, Academic/Scholarly.* **Description:** Publishes original research papers covering major issues in Zoology.
Formerly (until 1994): Academia Sinica. Institute of Zoology. Bulletin (0001-3943)
Related titles: Online - full text ed.: (from Institute for Scientific Information).
Indexed: AgBiotech, Anim.Breed.Abstr., Aqua.Sci.& Fish.Abstr., Aquacult.Abstr., Biol.Abstr., Chem.Abstr., Chem.Indus.Notes, Chem.Titles, Curr.Adv.Ecol.Sci., Curr.Cont., Entomol.Abstr., Environ.Sci.Poll.Mgmt., Genet.Abstr., Helminthol.Abstr., Hum.Gen.Abstr., Ind.Vet., Math.R., Ocean.Abstr., Protozool.Abstr., Rev.Appl.Entomol., Rev.Med.& Vet.Mycol., Sci.Cit.Ind., Soils & Fert., Sport Fish.Abstr., Vet.Bull., Wild.Rev., Zoo.Rec.
—BLDSC (9520.250000), CASDDS, CISTI, IDS, ingenta, Linda Hall.
Published by: Academia Sinica, Institute of Zoology/Chung Yang Yen Chiu Yuan, Tung Wu Hsueh Yen Chiu So, Nankang, Taipei 11529, Taiwan. TEL 886-2-27899529, 886-2-27899550, FAX 886-2-27899529, 886-2-27858059, zoolstud@gate.sinica.edu.tw, http://www.sinica.edu.tw/zool. Circ: 700 (controlled).

590 DEU ISSN 0944-2006
QL1 CODEN: ZOLGEA
ZOOLOGY; analysis of complex systems. Text in English. 1886. 4/yr. EUR 102, GBP 74 to individuals; EUR 349, GBP 280 to institutions (effective 2002). adv. bk.rev. bibl, charts, illus. index. reprint service avail. from ISI. *Refereed.* **Document type:** *Journal, Academic/Scholarly.* **Description:** Takes a system-oriented approach to the study of animals while placing particular emphasis on the comparative aspects of animal biology.
Supersedes (in 1993): Zoologische Jahrbuecher. Abteilung fuer Allgemeine Zoologie und Physiologie der Tiere (0044-5185); Zoologische Jahrbuecher. Abteilung fuer Anatomie und Ontogenie der Tiere (0044-5177)
Related titles: Online - full text ed.: (from Institute for Scientific Information).
Indexed: ASCA, Anim.Breed.Abstr., Apic.Abstr., Biol.Abstr., Chem.Abstr., Chem.Indus.Notes, Chem.Titles, Curr.Cont., Deep Sea Res.& Oceanogr.Abstr., Ecol.Abstr., GeoRef, Ind.Sci.Rev., Neurosci.Cit.Ind., Rev.Appl.Entomol., SSCI (coverage dropped), Sci.Cit.Ind., Soils & Fert., Sport Fish.Abstr., VITIS, Zoo.Rec.
—BLDSC (9529.330000), CASDDS, CISTI, IDS, Infotrieve, Linda Hall. **CCC.**
Published by: Urban & Fischer Verlag, Loebdergraben 14A, Jena 07743, Germany. TEL 49-3641-626444, FAX 49-3641-626500, info@urbanfischer.de, http://www.urbanfischer.de. Ed. J Matthias Starck. R&P Martin Huber TEL 49-3641-626430. Adv. contact Sabine Schroeter. page DEM 750; trim 280 x 210. Circ: 330.

ZOOMORPHOLOGY; an international journal of comparative and functional morphology. see *BIOLOGY*

BIOPHYSICS

see BIOLOGY—Biophysics

CELLULAR & MOLECULAR BIOLOGY LETTERS; an international journal. see *BIOLOGY*

BIOTECHNOLOGY

see BIOLOGY—Biotechnology

BABRAHAM INSTITUTE. CORPORATE PLAN. see *BIOLOGY—Physiology*

BIRTH CONTROL

see also POPULATION STUDIES

613.9 340.5 GBR
A L R A NEWSLETTER. Text in English. q. GBP 15 to members (effective 2000). adv. bk.rev. **Document type:** *Newsletter.* **Description:** Presents a pro-choice forum for the association.
Former titles (until 1995): Breaking Chains (0309-7978); (until 1977): A L R A Newsletter
Published by: Abortion Law Reform Association, 2-12 Pentonville Rd, London N1 9FP, United Kingdom. TEL 020-7278-5539, FAX 020-7278-5236, alra@mailbox.co.uk, http://www.alramailbox.co.uk. Ed. Jane Roe. Circ: 2,000.

613.942 USA
A V S C NEWS*. Text in English. 1963. q. membership. illus, stat. **Document type:** *Newsletter.* **Description:** Reports news and information related to family planning and reproductive health worldwide.
Formerly: A V S News (0001-2904)
Indexed: Curr.Lit.Fam.Plan.
Published by: (Association for Voluntary Surgical Contraception), A V S C International, 440 9th Ave Frnt 2, New York, NY 10001-1620. TEL 212-561-8000, FAX 212-779-9439, info@avsc.org, http://www.avsc.org. Ed. Karen Landovitz. R&P Pamela Beyer Harper TEL 212-561-8043. Circ: 8,000.

ABORTION REVIEW. see *WOMEN'S HEALTH*

613.94 USA ISSN 1012-8689
CODEN: ACDSEL
ADVANCES IN CONTRACEPTIVE DELIVERY SYSTEMS. Text in English. 1980. q. USD 180 to individuals; USD 190 foreign to individuals; USD 200 to institutions; USD 210 foreign to institutions. adv. bk.rev. charts, illus. index. *Refereed.* **Document type:** *Academic/Scholarly.*
Formerly (until 1984): Contraceptive Delivery Systems (0143-6112)
Related titles: Microform ed.
Indexed: Biol.Abstr., Chem.Abstr., Chem.Indus.Notes, Chem.Titles, Curr.Cont. (coverage dropped), Excerp.Med., Ind.Sci.Rev., Sci.Cit.Ind. (coverage dropped).
—CASDDS, CISTI, EMDOCS, GNLM, ingenta.
Published by: (World Federation of Contraception - Health), Reproductive Health Center, 78 Surfsong Rd., Kiawah Island, SC 29455. TEL 803-768-5556, FAX 803-769-6494. Ed. E Hafez. Circ: 500.

338.96 KEN ISSN 0250-698X
AFRICA LINK. Text in English, French. 1971. s-a. free per issue. bk.rev. **Document type:** *Newsletter.* **Description:** Covers the activities of the family planning associations in Sub-Saharan Africa. Addresses sexual and reproductive health issues.
Media: Duplicated (not offset). **Related titles:** ♦ French ed.: Africa Link. Edition Francaise. ISSN 1012-5019.
Indexed: CWI.
—BLDSC (0732.160800).
Published by: Africa Regional Office, Planned Parenthood Federation, Madison Insurance House, Upper Hill, PO Box 30234, Nairobi, Kenya. TEL 254-2-720280, FAX 254-2-726596, ippfaro@ken.healthnet.org, info@ippfaro.org. Ed. Justice Pobi. R&P Kodjo Efu. Circ: 3,000 (controlled).

338.96 KEN ISSN 1012-5019
AFRICA LINK. EDITION FRANCAISE. Text in French. 1988. s-a.
Media: Duplicated (not offset). **Related titles:** ♦ English ed.: Africa Link. ISSN 0250-698X.
Published by: Africa Regional Office, Planned Parenthood Federation, Madison Insurance House, Upper Hill, PO Box 30234, Nairobi, Kenya.

ASIAN AND PACIFIC WOMEN'S RESOURCE AND ACTION SERIES. see *WOMEN'S INTERESTS*

301.426 PAN
BOLETIN CONCIENCIA. Text in Spanish. 1967. s-a. free per issue. adv. illus. **Document type:** *Bulletin.*
Formerly: Conciencia
Published by: Asociacion Panamena para el Planeamiento de la Familia, Apdo. Postal 4637, Panama City 5, Panama. TEL 507-2607005, FAX 507-2362979, aplafa@sinfo.net. Ed., Adv. contact Monica Fabrega. Pub. Alfonso Lavergne. Circ: 5,000.

B

613.9 ATG
CARIBBEAN FAMILY PLANNING AFFILIATION. ANNUAL REPORT. Text in English. 1981. a. free per issue to qualified personnel. **Description:** Report on the year's activities in family life education and family planning.
Published by: (International Planned Parenthood Federation, Western Hemisphere Region), Caribbean Family Planning Affiliation Limited, Airport and Factory Rds., PO Box 419, St John's, Antigua. FAX 809-462-1187. Circ: 2,000.

613.9 312 USA
CELEBRATE LIFE (STAFFORD). Text in English. 1978. bi-m. USD 12.95 (effective 1998). adv. bk.rev. index. **Document type:** *Consumer.* **Description:** Covers abortion, euthanasia, life and family issues from a pro-life perspective.
Formerly (until 1994): All About Issues (0733-1231)
Published by: American Life League, Inc., 1179 Courthouse Rd, Box 1350, Stafford, VA 22555. TEL 504-659-4171, FAX 504-659-2586, clmag@all.org. Eds. Cathy Kenyon, Rich Gelina. Pub. Judie Brown. Circ: 130,000.

301.426 IND
CENTRE CALLING. Text in English. 1966. m. free per issue. bk.rev.
Published by: Department of Family Welfare, Kotla Rd., P O Box 5410, New Delhi 110 002, India. Ed. Uma Shankar Mishra. Circ: 40,000. **Subscr. to:** Editor, P O Box 5410, New Delhi 110 002, India.

CHOICES; sexual and reproductive health and rights in Europe. see *POPULATION STUDIES*

613.943 USA ISSN 0010-7824
RG136.A1 CODEN: CCPTAY
CONTRACEPTION. Text in English. 1970. 12/yr. EUR 214 in Europe to individuals; JPY 29,600 in Japan to individuals; USD 238 elsewhere to individuals (effective 2002); NLG 1,231 in Europe to institutions (effective 2001); EUR 594 in Europe to institutions; JPY 80,600 in Japan to institutions; USD 664 elsewhere to institutions (effective 2002). adv. bibl, charts, illus, abstr. s-a. index. back issues avail.; reprint service avail. from PQC. *Refereed.* **Document type:** *Journal, Academic/Scholarly.* **Description:** Research reports in clinical and experimental contraception.
Related titles: Microfilm ed.: (from PQC); Online - full text ed.: (from ingenta, Swets Blackwell, ScienceDirect, Institute for Scientific Information).
Indexed: ASCA, Agri.& Environ.Biotech.Abstr. (coverage dropped), Agroforest.Abstr., Anim.Breed.Abstr., Bibl.Repro., Biol.Abstr., Chem.Abstr., Chem.Indus.Notes, Chem.Titles, Cott.& Trop.Fibr.Abstr., Curr.Adv.Cancer Res., Curr.Adv.Ecol.Sci., Curr.Cont., Curr.Lit.Fam.Plan., Dairy Sci.Abstr., Derwent Biotech.Abstr., Environ.Sci.Poll.Mgmt., Excerp.Med., Fam.Ind., Field Crop Abstr., Hort.Abstr., INIS Atomind., I.P.A., Ind.Med. (1970-), Ind.Sci.Rev., Inpharma, Int.Abstr.Biol.Sci., Int.Nurs.Ind., Intl.Polym.Sci.& Tech., Jrnl.Watch Wom.Hlth., Nutr.Abstr., Pharm.&Out.News, Pollut.Abstr., Popul.Ind., Protozool.Abstr., RAPRA (1981-), Reac., Rev.Arom.& Med.Plants, Rev.Med.& Vet.Mycol., Risk Abstr., Rural Devel.Abstr., SSCI (coverage dropped), Saf.Sci.Abstr., Sci.Cit.Ind., Seed Abstr., Trop.Dis.Bull.
—BLDSC (3425.750000), ADONIS, CASDDS, CINDOC, CISTI, EMDOCS, GNLM, IDS, ingenta, KNAW. **CCC.**

Published by: Elsevier Science, Box 945, New York, NY 10159-0945. FAX 212-633-3990, usinfo-f@elsevier.com, http://www.elsevier.com/locate/contraception. Eds. A Lawson, F Nakamura. **Subscr. in Australasia and the Far East to:** Elsevier Science (Singapore) Pte Ltd, No.1 Temasek Ave, 17-01 Millenia Tower, Singapore 039192, Singapore. TEL 65-434-3727, FAX 65-337-2230; **Subscr. in Japan to:** Elsevier Science Inc - Japan Regional Office, 9-15 Higashi-Azabu 1-chome, Minato-ku, Tokyo 106-0044, Japan. TEL 81-3-5561-5033; **Subscr. outside the Americas to:** Elsevier Science BV, PO Box 211, Amsterdam 1000 AE, Netherlands. TEL 31-20-485-3757.

B

301.426 613.9 GBR
CONTRACEPTIVE EDUCATION BULLETIN. Text in English. 1976. q. GBP 15; GBP 18 foreign (effective 2001). adv. bk.rev., Website rev. bibl. 6 p./no. 3 cols./p. **Document type:** *Bulletin.* **Description:** Contains news, information, and commentary about contraception, reproductive health and sexual health issues.
Supersedes (in 1996): Family Planning Today (0309-1112); Which supersedes: Family Planning (0014-7338)
Indexed: Biol.Abstr., Curr.Lit.Fam.Plan., Russ.Acad.Sci.Bibl.
Published by: Family Planning Association, 2-12, Pentonville Rd, London N1 9FP, United Kingdom. TEL 44-20-7837-5432, FAX 44-20-7837-3042, joannac@fpa.org.uk, http://www.fpa.org.uk. Ed., R&P Joanna Clarke-Jones TEL 44-20-7923-5721. Circ: 5,000.

613.9 USA ISSN 0091-9721
RG136.A1
CONTRACEPTIVE TECHNOLOGY. Text in English. biennial.
—BLDSC (3425.770000).
Published by: Irvington Publishers, Inc., 522 E 82nd St, Ste 1, New York, NY 10028.

613.9 USA ISSN 0274-726X
CONTRACEPTIVE TECHNOLOGY UPDATE. Text in English. 1980. m. USD 377 domestic; USD 407 foreign; USD 63 newsstand/cover (effective 2001). bk.rev. back issues avail.; reprints avail. *Refereed.* **Document type:** *Newsletter.* **Description:** Addresses the needs of family planning professionals and is oriented toward clinical information.
Incorporates (1993-1999): Women's Health Center Management (1082-863X); Incorporates (1989-1991): Reproductive Technology Update (1050-8740)
Related titles: Microfilm ed.: (from PQC); Online - full text ed.: (from Northern Light Technology, Inc., Gale Group).
Indexed: CINAHL, Curr.Lit.Fam.Plan.
—BLDSC (3425.773000).
Published by: American Health Consultants (Subsidiary of: Medical Economics Co., Inc.), 3525 Piedmont Rd, N E, 6 Piedmont Center, Ste 400, Atlanta, GA 30305. TEL 404-262-5476, 404-262-7436, 800-688-2421, FAX 404-262-7837, 800-284-3291, custserv@ahcpub.com, http://www.ahcpub.com. Circ: 1,710.

DZIECKO. see *WOMEN'S HEALTH*

301.4 EGY
E P F P R. (Egyptian Population and Family Planning Review) Text in Arabic, English. 1968. 2/yr. EGP 5, USD 30 (effective 1999). bk.rev. bibl, stat. **Document type:** *Academic/Scholarly.*
Indexed: Popul.Ind.
Published by: Cairo University, Institute of Statistical Studies and Research, Tharwat St., Orman, Cairo, Egypt. FAX 20-2-3482533. Ed. Ibrahim Farag Eissa. Circ: 400.

613.9 USA ISSN 1092-2687
EDUCATOR'S UPDATE. Text in English. 1996. bi-m. USD 24. bk.rev., video rev. bibl, illus. reprints avail.
Published by: Planned Parenthood Federation of America, Inc., Education Department, 810 Seventh Ave, New York, NY 10019. library@ppfa.org, http://www.plannedparenthood.org/library/PPFA-LIBRARY/EdUpIndex.htm. Ed. Gloria A Roberts. Circ: 150.

301.426 COL
ESTUDIOS DE PLANIFICACION FAMILIAR. Text in Spanish. 1975 (vol.9). 2/yr.
Published by: Asociacion Colombiana para al Estudio Cientifico de la Poblacion, Canal Ramirez-Antares, Carrera 18, 33-95, Bogota, CUND, Colombia. Ed. Dr. Guillermo Lopez Escobar.

613.943 GBR ISSN 1362-5187
CODEN: ECRCFK
EUROPEAN JOURNAL OF CONTRACEPTION AND REPRODUCTIVE HEALTH CARE. Text in English. 1996. q. GBP 75, USD 130 to individuals; GBP 130, USD 210 to institutions (effective 2000). adv. *Refereed.* **Document type:** *Academic/Scholarly.*
Related titles: Online - full text ed.: ISSN 1473-0782 (from CatchWord Ltd.).
Indexed: Ind.Med. (1996-), Int.Nurs.Ind.
—BLDSC (3829.728227), ADONIS, CASDDS, GNLM, Infotrieve. **CCC.**
Published by: (European Society of Contraception), Parthenon Publishing Group (Subsidiary of: C R C Press (New York)), Casterton Hall, Casterton, Carnforth, Lancs LA6 2LA, United Kingdom. TEL 44-1524-272084, FAX 44-1524-271587, mail@parthpub.com, http://www.parthpub.com/contra/home.html.

613.9 BGD
F P A B HIGHLIGHTS. Text in English. 1978. q. 4 p./no. back issues avail. **Document type:** *Newsletter.*
Published by: Family Planning Association of Bangladesh, 2 Naya Paltan, Dhaka 2, Bangladesh. TEL 88-2-316134, 88-2-8311423, 88-2-8319343, FAX 88-2-8313008, TELEX 632379 IFIC BJ, fpab1@citechoo.net. Eds. Ahmad Neaz, M Emamul Haque. Pub. Ahmad Neaz. Circ: 1,000.

301.426 TWN
F P A C MONTHLY REPORT✶. Text in Chinese, English. 1961. m. free per issue.
Published by: Family Planning Association of China, No1, Ln 160, Fuhsing S. Rd Sec 2, Taipei 106, Taiwan.

301.4 PAK
F P A P ANNUAL REPORT. Text in English. 1964. a. **Document type:** *Corporate.*
Former titles: F P A P Biennial Report (0071-3759)
Published by: Family Planning Association of Pakistan, 3-A Temple Rd., Lahore, Pakistan. Circ: 1,000 (controlled).

613.9 PHL
THE F P O P BULLETIN. Text in English. 1969. q. free per issue. **Document type:** *Bulletin.*
Published by: Family Planning Organization of the Philippines, 50 Dona Magdalina Hemady Ave, New Manila, Quezon City, Philippines. TEL 721-71-01, FAX 721-40-67. Ed. Javier Gil C Montemayor. Circ: 2,000.

613.9 FJI
FAMILY PLANNING ASSOCIATION OF FIJI. NEWS. Text in English. 1976 (no.37). bi-m. charts, illus.
Published by: Family Planning Association of Fiji, PO Box 619, Suva, Fiji.

301.42 IND ISSN 0377-7774
FAMILY PLANNING ASSOCIATION OF INDIA. REPORT. Text in English. 1950. a. free per issue. illus.
Published by: Family Planning Association of India, Bajaj Bhavan, Nariman Point, Mumbai, Maharashtra 400 021, India. TEL 91-22-202-9080, FAX 91-22-202-9038, fpai@giasbm01.vsnl.net.in. Ed., R&P Jyoti Moodbidri. Circ: 2,000.

301.42 KEN
FAMILY PLANNING ASSOCIATION OF KENYA. ANNUAL REPORT. Key Title: Annual Report - Family Planning Association of Kenya. Text in English. 1971. a. free per issue. illus. **Document type:** *Corporate.*
Published by: Family Planning Association of Kenya, Harabee P, Haile Selassie Ave., PO Box 30581, Nairobi, Kenya. Ed. Inzoberi John. Circ: 2,000.

362.8 NPL ISSN 0303-4755
HQ766.5.N37
FAMILY PLANNING ASSOCIATION OF NEPAL. ANNUAL REPORT. Text in English. 1960. a. free per issue. stat. **Description:** Provides information on the programs and activities of the FPAN throughout the year.
Published by: Family Planning Association of Nepal, P O Box 486, Katmandu, Nepal. TEL 977-1-524440, FAX 977-1-524211, TELEX 2307 FPAN NP. Circ: 75.

362.8 NPL
FAMILY PLANNING ASSOCIATION OF NEPAL. NEWSLETTER. Text in English. 1973. bi-m. free per issue. **Document type:** *Newsletter.* **Description:** Provides news and information of the association.
Published by: Family Planning Association of Nepal, P O Box 486, Katmandu, Nepal. TEL 977-1-524440, FAX 977-1-524211.

FAMILY PLANNING PERSPECTIVES. see *MEDICAL SCIENCES—Obstetrics And Gynecology*

362.8 USA ISSN 0095-3121
HQ766.5.U5
FAMILY PLANNING PROGRAMS IN OKLAHOMA; annual statistical report. Text in English. 1971. a. illus. **Document type:** *Government.*
Published by: Department of Health, Maternal and Child Health Service, 1000 N E 10th St, Oklahoma City, OK 73117-1299. TEL 405-271-4476. Circ: 450.

613.94 GMB ISSN 0796-0174
THE GAMBIA FAMILY PLANNING ASSOCIATION NEWSLETTER. Text in English. 1972. q. free per issue. adv. **Document type:** *Newsletter.* **Description:** Reports on workshops, training programs, resource development and association activities.
Former titles: Family Planning Association of the Gambia; (until 1987): What's On
Published by: Gambia Family Planning Association, PO Box 325, Banjul, Gambia. TEL 220-370325, FAX 220-392463, gfpa@commit.gm. Ed., Pub. Yankubba Dibba. Circ: 150.

613.9 GRD
GRENADA PLANNED PARENTHOOD ASSOCIATION. ANNUAL REPORT. Text in English. a. **Document type:** *Corporate.*
Published by: Grenada Planned Parenthood Association, Scott St., St. George's, Grenada. FAX 809-440-8057. Circ: 300.

613.9 CHN ISSN 1001-3490
GUOWAI YIXUE (JIHUA SHENGYU FENCE)/FOREIGN MEDICAL SCIENCES (BIRTH CONTROL). Text in Chinese. q.
Published by: Tianjin Yixue Keji Qingbao Yanjiusuo/Tianjin Medical Science and Technology Information Institute, 131 Chengdu Dao, Heping-qu, Tianjin 300050, China. TEL 302570. Ed. Yu Aifeng.

613.9 362.1 USA ISSN 1096-7699
HQ766.5.U5
THE GUTTMACHER REPORT ON PUBLIC POLICY. Text in English. 1998. bi-m. USD 36 domestic to individuals; USD 45 domestic to institutions (effective 2001). **Document type:** *Bulletin.* **Description:** Review of reproductive health and public policy.
Related titles: Online - full text ed.: (from LexisNexis).
Indexed: P.A.I.S.
Published by: Alan Guttmacher Institute, 120 Wall St, 21st Fl, New York, NY 10005. TEL 212-248-1111, FAX 212-248-1951, http://www.agi-usa.org. Ed. Cory Richards. Circ: 3,000 (paid).

GYNECOLOGIE OBSTETRIQUE ET FERTILITE. see *MEDICAL SCIENCES—Obstetrics And Gynecology*

HANDLING PREGNANCY AND BIRTH CASES. see *LAW—Family And Matrimonial Law*

301.426 IND ISSN 0253-6803
RA529
HEALTH AND POPULATION: PERSPECTIVES AND ISSUES. Text in English. 1972. q. USD 60 (effective 2000). adv. bk.rev. **Document type:** *Academic/Scholarly.* **Description:** Focuses on family planning.
Formed by the merger of: N I H A E Bulletin (0378-6196); Journal of Population Research (0377-0478); Which was formerly: National Institute of Family Planning. Newsletter
Related titles: CD-ROM ed.
Indexed: Abstr.Hyg., Bibl.Asian Stud. (1978-1995), Diar.Dis.Res., Environ.Sci.Poll.Mgmt., Excerp.Med., ExtraMED, Pollut.Abstr., Popul.Ind., Risk Abstr., Saf.Sci.Abstr., Trop.Dis.Bull.
Published by: National Institute of Health and Family Welfare, New Mehrauli Rd., Munirka, New Delhi 110 067, India. Ed. Somnath Roy. Circ: 1,000. **Dist. by:** H P C Publishers Distributors Pvt. Ltd., 1st Fl., Flats 1 & 2, Darya Ganj, 4805-24 Bharat Ram Rd., New Delhi 110 002, India. TEL 91-11-325-4401, FAX 91-11-686-3511.

613.9 USA ISSN 0194-8032
HQ767
HEARTBEAT (ORLANDO). Text in English. 1978. q. USD 25; includes Pulse. adv. bk.rev. charts, illus.
Published by: Institute for Women and Children, 4680 Lake Underhill Rd, Orlando, FL 32807. TEL 407-277-1942, FAX 407-381-0907. Circ: 4,000.

613.9 IDN
I P P A NEWSLETTER. Text in English. 1977. q. IDR 8,000, USD 5. stat. **Document type:** *Newsletter.* **Description:** Discusses methods used to curtail population growth.
Indexed: Curr.Lit.Fam.Plan.
Published by: Indonesian Planned Parenthood Association, Jalan Hang Jebat 111-F3, Kebayaran Baru, PO Box 18, Jakarta 12120, Indonesia. TEL 62-21-715905, FAX 62-21-7394088. Ed. Kustiniyati Muchtar. Circ: 2,000.

363.96 612.6 GBR
I P P F ANNUAL REPORT. Text in English, French, Spanish; Summaries in Japanese, German. 1974. a. free per issue. illus. **Document type:** *Corporate.*
Former titles: I P P F in Action; International Planned Parenthood Federation. Annual Report (0307-6857)
Related titles: Online - full content ed.
Published by: International Planned Parenthood Federation, Regent's College, Inner Circle, Regents Park, London NW1 4NS, United Kingdom. info@ippf.org, http://www.ippf.org.

325 613.9 GBR ISSN 0019-0357 CODEN: IPPMAY
I P P F MEDICAL BULLETIN. Text in English, French, Spanish. 1966. bi-m. free per issue to qualified personnel. **Document type:** *Bulletin, Academic/Scholarly.* **Description:** Provides up-to-date information on clinical aspects and developments in the field of family planning practice.
Related titles: Online - full content ed.; French ed.: Bulletin Medicale de l'I P P F. ISSN 0306-7815. 1966; Spanish ed.: Boletin Medico de I P P F. ISSN 0306-7823. 1966.
Indexed: Abstr.Hyg., Excerp.Med., Inpharma, Pharm.&Out.News, Reac., Trop.Dis.Bull.
—BLDSC (4567.450000), GNLM.
Published by: International Planned Parenthood Federation, Regent's College, Inner Circle, Regents Park, London NW1 4NS, United Kingdom. TELEX 919573 IPEPEE G, info@ippf.org, http://www.ippf.org. Circ: 30,000 (controlled).

I U S S P NEWSLETTER/U I E S P BULLETIN DE LIAISON. see *POPULATION STUDIES*

I U S S P PAPERS/U I E S P DOCUMENTS DE L'UNION. see *POPULATION STUDIES*

613.94 ECU
INFORME ANUAL DE LAS ACTIVIDADES DE LAS UNIDADES OPERATIVAS DE SALUD EN EL PROGRAMA DE PLANIFICACION FAMILIAR DEL MINISTERIO DE SALUD. Text in Spanish. a.
Published by: Ministerio de Salud Publica, Departamento Nacional de Poblacion, Quito, Pichincha, Ecuador.

301.426 IND
INSTITUTE OF ECONOMIC RESEARCH. PUBLICATIONS ON FAMILY PLANNING. Text in English. irreg. price varies.
Published by: Institute of Economic Research, Director, Vidyagiri, Dharwar, Karnataka 580 004, India. FAX 836-41001.

INTERNATIONAL FAMILY PLANNING PERSPECTIVES. see *MEDICAL SCIENCES—Obstetrics And Gynecology*

INTERNATIONAL POPULATION CONFERENCE. PROCEEDINGS. see *POPULATION STUDIES*

363.96 USA
J A M A CONTRACEPTION NEWSLINE. (Journal of the American Medical Association) Text in English. 1998. w. back issues avail. *Refereed.*
Media: Online - full text.
Published by: American Medical Association, J A M A Information Centers, 515 N State St, Chicago, IL 60610. TEL 312-464-5000, 800-262-2350, FAX 312-464-4181, contraception@ama-assn.org, http://www.ama-assn.org/special/contra/contra.htm.

301.426 JPN ISSN 0911-0755
J O I C F P NEWS. Text in English. 1974. m. free per issue. bk.rev. **Document type:** *Newsletter, Academic/Scholarly.* **Description:** Reports on reproductive health and family planning activities in Japan and the world, with a focus on the Integrated Project, promoted worldwide by JOICFP.
—BLDSC (4672.195750).
Published by: Japanese Organization for International Cooperation in Family Planning Inc., Hoken Kaikan Shinkan Bldg, 1-10 Ichi-Gayata-Machi, Shinjuku-ku, Tokyo 162-0843, Japan. TEL 81-3-3268-5875, FAX 81-3-3235-7090, joicfp@i.bekkoame.ne.jp, info@joicfp.or.jp, http://www.bekkoame.ne.jp/i/joicfp. Ed. Yasuo Kon. Circ: 5,000.

JOHNS HOPKINS UNIVERSITY. POPULATION INFORMATION PROGRAM. POPULATION REPORTS. ENGLISH EDITION. see *POPULATION STUDIES*

JOHNS HOPKINS UNIVERSITY. POPULATION INFORMATION PROGRAM. POPULATION REPORTS. FRENCH EDITION. see *POPULATION STUDIES*

JOHNS HOPKINS UNIVERSITY. POPULATION INFORMATION PROGRAM. POPULATION REPORTS. PORTUGUESE EDITION. see *POPULATION STUDIES*

JOHNS HOPKINS UNIVERSITY. POPULATION INFORMATION PROGRAM. POPULATION REPORTS. SPANISH EDITION. see *POPULATION STUDIES*

613.9 GBR ISSN 1471-1893 CODEN: BJFPDD
JOURNAL OF FAMILY PLANNING AND REPRODUCTIVE HEALTH CARE. Text in English. 1975. q. GBP 45 domestic to individuals; GBP 50 foreign to individuals; GBP 90 domestic to institutions; GBP 110 foreign to institutions (effective 2002). adv. bk.rev. illus. *Refereed.* **Document type:** *Journal, Academic/Scholarly.* **Description:** Presents original papers and review articles by leading authorities on all aspects of reproductive health care.
Formerly: British Journal of Family Planning (0144-8625)
Related titles: Online - full text ed.: (from CatchWord Ltd.).
Indexed: ASCA, ASSIA, Biol.Abstr., Brit.Nur.Ind., CINAHL, Curr.Cont., Curr.Lit.Fam.Plan., Excerp.Med., Fam.Ind., Ind.Med. (197?-), Int.Nurs.Ind., SSCI.
—BLDSC (4983.722500), GNLM, IDS, Infotrieve, KNAW. **CCC.**
Published by: Faculty of Family Planning and Reproductive Health Care, 11 Cornwall Ter, London NWI 4QP, United Kingdom. journal@ffprhc.org.uk, http://www.ffprhc.org.uk/. Circ: 11,000.

613.9 IND ISSN 0022-1074
HQ750.A2
JOURNAL OF FAMILY WELFARE. Text in English. 1954. s-a. INR 100; USD 35 foreign. bk.rev. abstr. charts. reprint service avail. from ISI. **Document type:** *Academic/Scholarly, Abstract/Index.*
Related titles: CD-ROM ed.
Indexed: ASCA, AgeLine, Bibl.Asian Stud. (1971-1995), Curr.Cont. (coverage dropped), Curr.Lit.Fam.Plan., ERA, ExtraMED, Fam.Ind., IMFL, Mult.Ed.Abstr., Popul.Ind., SSCI (coverage dropped), Stud.Wom.Abstr.
—BLDSC (4983.750000), IDS, ingenta.
Published by: Family Planning Association of India, Bajaj Bhavan, Nariman Point, Mumbai, Maharashtra 400 021, India. TEL 91-22-202-9080, FAX 91-22-202-9038, fpai@giasbm01.vsnl.net.in, http://www.fpaindia.com/. Eds. Smt Avabai B Wadia, Jyoti Moodbidri. R&P Jyoti Moodbidri. Circ: 1,500.

301.42 KOR ISSN 0259-9112
JOURNAL OF POPULATION AND HEALTH STUDIES. Text in English, Korean. 1974. s-a. free per issue. stat. **Description:** Covers planned parenthood issues.
Former titles: Journal of Population and Health; Family Planning Quarterly; Journal of Family Planning Studies
Indexed: Bibl.Asian Stud. (1989), IDA, Popul.Ind., Rural Recreat.Tour.Abstr., World Ag.Econ.& Rur.Soc.Abstr.
Published by: Korea Institute for Population and Health, SAN 42-14 Bulgwang-Dong, Eunpyung-Ku, Seoul 122, Korea, S.. Ed. Joung Joo Lee. Circ: (controlled).

JOURNAL OF PRENATAL & PERINATAL PSYCHOLOGY & HEALTH. see *MEDICAL SCIENCES—Obstetrics And Gynecology*

613.9 IDN ISSN 0216-0269
KABAR. Text in Indonesian. 1980. q. IDR 9,600, USD 6.
Indexed: So.Pac.Per.Ind.
Published by: Indonesian Planned Parenthood Association, Jalan Hang Jebat 111-F3, Kebayaran Baru, PO Box 18, Jakarta 12120, Indonesia. TEL 62-21-715905, FAX 62-21-7394088. Circ: 5,000.

613.9 GBR
KEY NOTE MARKET REPORT: CONTRACEPTIVES. Variant title: Contraceptives. Text in English. 1993. irreg. GBP 265 (effective 1999). **Document type:** *Trade.*
Formerly: Key Note Report: Contraceptives (1352-6561)
Related titles: CD-ROM ed.; Online - full text ed.
Published by: Key Note Ltd., Field House, 72 Oldfield Rd, Hampton, Mddx TW12 2HQ, United Kingdom. TEL 44-20-8481-8750, FAX 44-20-8783-0049, http://www.keynote.co.uk.

179 306.874 USA ISSN 0882-116X
L F L REPORTS. Text in English. 1981. irreg. donation. bk.rev. back issues avail. **Document type:** *Newsletter.* **Description:** Focuses on the issue of abortion from a non-religious, libertarian pro-life perspective, and the philosophical foundation of parental obligation.
Published by: Libertarians for Life, 13424 Hathaway Dr., Wheaton, MD 20906. TEL 301-460-4141, DORIS.GORDON@IAD.BLKCAT.COM, http://www.cris.com/~bwjass/lfl. Ed. John Walker. Circ: 1,000.

MALAYSIAN JOURNAL OF REPRODUCTIVE HEALTH. see *MEDICAL SCIENCES—Obstetrics And Gynecology*

618 IDN ISSN 0216-4027
MANTAP: MAJALAH ILMAIH P K M I/INDONESIAN ASSOCIATION FOR SECURE CONTRACEPTION. JOURNAL. Text mainly in Indonesian; Text occasionally in English. 1981. q. USD 200. reprint service avail. from IRC. **Document type:** *Academic/Scholarly.*
Published by: Perkumpulan Kontrasepsi Mantap Indonesia (PKMI)/Indonesian Association for Secure Contraception, Jalan Kramat Sentiong 49 A, Jakarta 10450, Indonesia. TEL 62-21-3155122, FAX 62-21-3155125. Ed. Azrul Azwar. Circ: 1,000.

B

304.6 BOL
MONOGRAFIAS DE POBLACION Y DESARROLLO. Text in Spanish. 1974. irreg., latest vol.23, 1985. price varies. **Document type:** *Monographic series, Academic/Scholarly.*
Published by: Centro de Investigaciones Sociales, Casilla 6931 - C.C., La Paz, Bolivia. TEL 591-2-352931. Ed. Antonio Cisneros.

301.42 IND ISSN 0077-4944
N I F P GENERAL SERIES. Text in English. 1965. irreg., latest vol.22, 1977.
Published by: National Institute of Health and Family Welfare, New Mehrauli Rd., Munirka, New Delhi 110 067, India. Ed. S Pramanik. Circ: 3,000.

301.42 IND ISSN 0077-4952
N I F P MANUAL SERIES. Text in English. 1966. irreg. free or on exchange basis.
Published by: National Institute of Health and Family Welfare, New Mehrauli Rd., Munirka, New Delhi 110 067, India. Ed. S Pramanik. Circ: 3,000.

301.42 IND ISSN 0077-4960
N I F P MONOGRAPH SERIES. Text in English. 1966. irreg., latest vol.19, 1973. free per issue.
Published by: National Institute of Health and Family Welfare, New Mehrauli Rd., Munirka, New Delhi 110 067, India. Ed. S Pramanik. Circ: 3,000.

301.42 IND ISSN 0077-4979
N I F P REPORT SERIES. Text in English. 1966. irreg., latest vol.12, 1973. on exchange basis.
Published by: National Institute of Health and Family Welfare, New Mehrauli Rd., Munirka, New Delhi 110 067, India. Ed. S Pramanik. Circ: 3,000.

301.42 IND ISSN 0077-4987
N I F P TECHNICAL PAPER SERIES. Text in English. 1966. irreg., latest vol.17, 1973. on exchange basis.
Published by: National Institute of Health and Family Welfare, New Mehrauli Rd., Munirka, New Delhi 110 067, India. Ed. S Pramanik. Circ: 3,000.

613.9 618 616.95 USA ISSN 0270-3637
NETWORK (DURHAM). Text in English. 1979. q. free per issue to qualified personnel. back issues avail. **Document type:** *Newsletter, Academic/Scholarly.* **Description:** Covers contraceptive methods, concern for maternal and child mortality; AIDS; sexually transmitted diseases.
Related titles: Online - full text ed.: (from LexisNexis); French ed.; Spanish ed.
Indexed: CWI, P.A.I.S.
—CISTI.
Published by: Family Health International, Research Triangle Park Branch, PO Box 13950, Durham, NC 27709. FAX 919-544-7040, http://www.fhi.org. Ed. Nash Herndon. Circ: 65,000 (controlled).

NEW PARENT. see *MEDICAL SCIENCES—Obstetrics And Gynecology*

613.9 DNK ISSN 1396-8165
NYHEDSBREV - FORENINGEN SEX OG SAMFUND. Key Title: Nyhedsbrev - Foreningen Sex & Samfund. Text in Danish. 1982. q. DKK 125 to membership; DKK 500 to institutions; DKK 75 to students (effective 2001). bk.rev. **Document type:** *Newsletter, Abstract/Index, Consumer, Government.* **Description:** Information and articles about sexual and reproductive health and rights.
Former titles (until 1996): Nyhedsbrev - Foreningen for Familieplanlaegning. Sex og Samfund (1396-8157); (until 1994): Familieplanlaegning (0108-8793)
Published by: Foreningen Sex og Samfund, c/o Bjarne B Christensen, Skindergade 28 A, A., Copenhagen K 1159, Denmark. TEL 45-33-93-10-10, FAX 45-33-93-10-09, danish-fpa@sexogsamfund.dk, http://www.sexogsamfund.dk. Circ: 6,000.

ON THE ISSUES; the progressive woman's quarterly. see *WOMEN'S INTERESTS*

301.426 IND
ORISSA FAMILY PLANNING BULLETIN. Text in English. 1971. m. free per issue. charts.
Published by: State Family Welfare Bureau, Directorate of Family Welfare, Bhubaneswar, Orissa, India. Ed. Dr. N N Parida. Circ: 1,200.

OUTLOOK (SEATTLE); reproductive health. see *PUBLIC HEALTH AND SAFETY*

613.9 AUS ISSN 1323-675X
OVULATION METHOD RESEARCH AND REFERENCE CENTRE OF AUSTRALIA. BULLETIN. Text in English. 1974. q. AUD 25 (effective 2001). bk.rev. cum.index every 2 yrs. back issues avail. *Refereed.* **Document type:** *Bulletin.* **Description:** Covers philosophy and theology of marriage, scientific research into reproductive biology pertaining to natural family planning, and the teaching of natural family planning.
Formerly (until vol.22, no.1, 1995): Natural Family Planning Council of Victoria. Bulletin (0312-7567)
Published by: Ovulation Method Research and Reference Centre of Australia, Billings Family Life Centre, Melbourne, 27 Alexandra Parade, Fitzroy North, VIC 3068, Australia. TEL 61-3-94811722, FAX 61-3-94824208, 61-3-94824208. Ed. John J Billings. R&P J J Billings TEL 61-3-94811722. Circ: 3,000.

613.9 USA
OVULATION METHOD TEACHERS ASSOCIATION (PUBLICATION). Text in English. 1975. q. USD 10. adv. bk.rev. back issues avail. **Description:** Covers ovulation method of natural family planning and related health issues.
Published by: Ovulation Method Teachers Association, PO Box 10 1780, Anchorage, AK 99510-1780. TEL 907-343-4623, FAX 907-344-8606. Circ: 500.

PASSAGES (WASHINGTON, D.C.). see *CHILDREN AND YOUTH—About*

PERSPECTIVAS INTERNACIONALES EN PLANIFICACION FAMILIAR. see *MEDICAL SCIENCES—Obstetrics And Gynecology*

PERSPECTIVES INTERNATIONALES SUR LE PLANNING FAMILIAL. see *MEDICAL SCIENCES—Obstetrics And Gynecology*

613.94 IND
PLANNED PARENTHOOD. Text in English. 1953. m. free per issue. **Document type:** *Bulletin.*
Related titles: Microfilm ed.: (from PQC).
Published by: Family Planning Association of India, Bajaj Bhavan, Nariman Point, Mumbai, Maharashtra 400 021, India. TEL 91-22-202-9080, FAX 91-22-202-9038, fpai@giasbm01.vsnl.net.in, http://www.fpaindia.com/. Ed., R&P Jaishree Kochavara. Circ: 5,000.

613.94 USA
PLANNED PARENTHOOD TODAY; news from the most trusted advocate for reproductive choice. Text in English. q. illus. **Description:** Reports on topics of reproductive freedom and other issues affecting the health of women.
Published by: Planned Parenthood Federation of America, Inc., 810 Seventh Ave, New York, NY 10019. TEL 212-541-7800, members_services@ppfa.org, http://www.ppfa.org. Ed. Danielle T Leigh. **Subscr. to:** PPFA, PO Box 4447, New York, NY 10164-0359. TEL 212-261-4677.

PRO FAMILIA MAGAZIN; die Zeitschrift fuer Sexualpaedagogik, Sexualberatung und Familienplanung. see *PSYCHOLOGY*

363.46 USA
PRO-LIFE ACTION NEWS. Text in English. 1981. q. USD 10 donation (effective 2000). adv. bk.rev. **Document type:** *Newspaper.* **Description:** Includes material relating to pro-life activism such as protests and sidewalk counseling.
Published by: Pro-Life Action League, 6160 N Cicero Ave, Ste 600, Chicago, IL 60646. TEL 773-777-2900, FAX 773-777-3061, scheidl@ibm.net, http://www.prolifeaction.org. Ed., Adv. contact Ann Scheidler. Circ: 7,500.

613.9 USA
PULSE (ORLANDO). Text in English. q. USD 29 includes Heartbeat.
Published by: Institute for Women and Children, 4680 Lake Underhill Rd, Orlando, FL 32807. TEL 407-277-1942, FAX 407-381-0907.

RE PRODUCTIONS. see *PHYSICAL FITNESS AND HYGIENE*

RENKOUXUE YU JIHUA SHENGYU/DEMOGRAPHY AND FAMILY PLANNING. see *POPULATION STUDIES*

REPORTER ON HUMAN REPRODUCTION & THE LAW; cases, statutes and materials on law and life sciences. see *LAW*

612.6 CHN ISSN 1001-7844
REPRODUCTION AND CONTRACEPTION. Text in English. 1989. q. USD 80 (effective 2001). back issues avail. **Document type:** *Journal, Academic/Scholarly.*
Related titles: Online - full content ed.; ♦ Chinese ed.: Shengzhi yu Biyun. ISSN 0253-357X.
Published by: Shengzhi yu Biyun Bianjibu, 2140 Xietu Lu, Shanghai 200032, China. TEL 86-21-4049215, FAX 85-21-4046128, randc@sippr.stc.sh.cn, http://www.repacon.com/. R&P Lixi Wang. Circ: 500 (paid); 100 (controlled).

REPRODUKTIONSMEDIZIN. see *MEDICAL SCIENCES—Obstetrics And Gynecology*

RESUMENES SOBRE POBLACION DOMINICANA. see *POPULATION STUDIES*

613.9 CHN ISSN 0253-357X CODEN: SCYYDZ
SHENGZHI YU BIYUN. Text in Chinese. 1980. bi-m. CNY 21 domestic; USD 60 foreign (effective 2001). 200 p./no. **Document type:** *Academic/Scholarly.* **Description:** Covers birth control related issues in China.
Related titles: Online - full content ed.; ♦ English ed.: Reproduction and Contraception. ISSN 1001-7844.
Indexed: Chem.Abstr., Chem.Indus.Notes, Chem.Titles. —BLDSC (7713.598300), CASDDS, GNLM.
Published by: (Shanghai Jihua Shengyu Kexue Yanjiusuo/Shanghai Institute of Planned Parenthood Research), Shengzhi yu Biyun Bianjibu, 2140 Xietu Lu, Shanghai 200032, China. TEL 86-21-4049215, FAX 85-21-4046128, randc@sippr.stc.sh.cn, http://www.repacon.com/. Ed. Ersheng Gao. R&P Lixi Wang. Adv. contact Liang Qi TEL 86-21-64184195. Circ: 4,000. **Dist. overseas by:** China International Book Trading Corp, 35 Chegongzhuang Xilu, Haidian District, Beijing 100044, China.

SINGAPORE JOURNAL OF OBSTETRICS & GYNAECOLOGY. see *MEDICAL SCIENCES—Obstetrics And Gynecology*

618 614 USA
U.S. CENTERS FOR DISEASE CONTROL. ABORTION SURVEILLANCE. ANNUAL SUMMARY. Text in English. a. free per issue. **Document type:** *Academic/Scholarly.*
Formerly: Abortion Surveillance
Indexed: Curr.Lit.Fam.Plan.
Published by: U.S. Centers for Disease Control, 1600 Clifton Rd, Atlanta, GA 30333. TEL 404-639-3311.

362.8 USA ISSN 0094-4424
HQ763
U.S. CENTERS FOR DISEASE CONTROL. FAMILY PLANNING SERVICES: ANNUAL SUMMARY. Key Title: Family Planning Services; Annual Survey. Text in English. a. stat. **Document type:** *Government.*
Published by: U.S. Centers for Disease Control, Atlanta, GA 30333. TEL 404-639-3311.

WOMEN'S GLOBAL NETWORK FOR REPRODUCTIVE RIGHTS. NEWSLETTER. see *WOMEN'S HEALTH*

613.9 USA
WORLD FEDERATION OF HEALTH AGENCIES FOR THE ADVANCEMENT OF VOLUNTARY SURGICAL CONTRACEPTION. COMMUNIQUE✶. Text in Arabic, English, French, Spanish. 2/yr. free per issue. illus.
Published by: World Federation of Health Agencies for the Advancement of Voluntary Surgical Contraception, 440 9th Ave, FRNT 2, New York, NY 10001-1620. TEL 212-351-2525, FAX 212-599-0959, TELEX 425604 AVS UI. Ed. Lynn Bakamjian. Circ: 5,500.

363.96 CHN ISSN 1004-8189
ZHONGGUO JIHUA ZHENGYUXUE ZAZHI/CHINESE JOURNAL OF FAMILY PLANNING. Text in Chinese. 1992. m. USD 20.40; USD 1.70 newsstand/cover (effective 2001). **Document type:** *Academic/Scholarly.*
Published by: China International Book Trading Corp/Zhongguo Guoji Tushu Maoyi Zonggongsi cibtc@mail.cibtc.com.cn, http://www.cibtc.com.cn. **Dist. by:** 35, Chegongzhuang Xilu, Haidian District, Beijing 100044, China.

613.9 CHN
ZHONGGUO YOUSHENG YOUYU/JOURNAL OF IMPROVING BIRTH OUTCOME AND CHILD DEVELOPMENT OF CHINA. Text in Chinese. q. USD 11.60; USD 2.90 newsstand/cover (effective 2001). **Document type:** *Academic/Scholarly.*
Published by: China International Book Trading Corp/Zhongguo Guoji Tushu Maoyi Zonggongsi cibtc@mail.cibtc.com.cn, http://www.cibtc.com.cn. **Dist. by:** 35, Chegongzhuang Xilu, Haidian District, Beijing 100044, China.

BIRTH CONTROL—Abstracting, Bibliographies, Statistics

613.9 GBR ISSN 0140-5314
HQ767.5.G7
GREAT BRITAIN. GOVERNMENT STATISTICAL SERVICE. ABORTION STATISTICS. Text in English. 1974. irreg. **Document type:** *Government.* —BLDSC (6237.634000).
Published by: (Puerto Rico. Department of Health USA, Great Britain. Statistics Division), Government Statistical Service, SD2, Rm 804, Hannibal House, Elephant and Castle, London SE1 6TE, United Kingdom. TEL 0171-972-2193. **Orders to:** Department of Health and Social Security (Leaflets), PO Box 21, Stanmore, Mddx HA7 1AY, United Kingdom.

301 USA ISSN 0095-3105
HQ767.5.U5
NEBRASKA STATISTICAL REPORT OF ABORTIONS. Text in English. a. free per issue. **Document type:** *Government.*
Published by: Data Management, PO Box 95007, Lincoln, NE 68509. TEL 402-471-2871, mark.miller@hhss.state.ne.us, http://www.hhs.state.ne.us. Ed. Mark Miller.

301.426 016 IND ISSN 0028-4327
NEW BOOKS ON FAMILY PLANNING. Text in English. 1968. bi-m. per issue exchange basis. bibl.
Media: Duplicated (not offset).
Published by: National Institute of Health and Family Welfare, New Mehrauli Rd., Munirka, New Delhi 110 067, India. Circ: 1,250 (controlled).

613.9 SEN
SENEGAL. MINISTERE DE L'ECONOMIE, DES FINANCES ET DU PLAN. ENQUETE SUR LA PLANIFICATION FAMILIALE. Text in French. 1990. irreg. XOF 5,000; XOF 7,000 foreign (effective 1998). **Document type:** *Government.*
Published by: Ministere de l'Economie des Finances et du Plan, Direction de la Prevision et de la Statistique, BP 116, Dakar, Senegal. TEL 221-21-03-01. Pub. Ibrahima Sarr.

613.94 618.88 DNK ISSN 0106-7729
STATISTIK OM PRAEVENTION OG ABORTER. (Included in the series: Vitalstatistik) Text in Danish; Summaries in English. 1978. biennial. DKK 60.
Formerly: Statistik om Legale Aborter
Published by: Sundhedsstyrelsen, Amaliegade 13, PO Box 2020, Copenhagen K 1012, Denmark. **Subscr. to:** Statens Informationt, PO Box 1003, Copenhagen K 1009, Denmark.

618 USA ISSN 0300-6972
U.S. CENTERS FOR DISEASE CONTROL. ABORTION SURVEILLANCE REPORT. Text in English. 1969. q. free per issue. stat. **Document type:** *Government.*

Published by: U.S. Centers for Disease Control, 1600 Clifton Rd, Atlanta, GA 30333. TEL 404-639-3311. Circ: (controlled).

BOTANY

see BIOLOGY—Botany

BUILDING AND CONSTRUCTION

see also ARCHITECTURE; ENGINEERING—Civil Engineering; HEATING, PLUMBING AND REFRIGERATION; HOUSING AND URBAN PLANNING

ARBOUW JOURNAAL. see *OCCUPATIONAL HEALTH AND SAFETY*

690 628 LCA ISSN 1010-5700
B T - L M & S. (Building Technology - Land Management & Safety) Text in English. 1985. q. USD 10. adv. **Document type:** *Academic/Scholarly, Consumer.* **—CCC.**
Published by: A L K I M Communication Production Company, Box MA 020, Marchand Post Office, Castries, St. Lucia. Ed., Adv. contact Albert Deterville. Circ: 5,000.

▼ **CONSTRUCTION & ENGINEERING MAGAZINE**; OSHA news, legal issues, workers' comp, safety issues, products, services. see *OCCUPATIONAL HEALTH AND SAFETY*

EVALUATING YOUR FIRM'S INJURY & ILLNESS RECORD. CONSTRUCTION INDUSTRIES. see *OCCUPATIONAL HEALTH AND SAFETY*

FIBROUS MATERIALS IN THE ENVIRONMENT. see *ENVIRONMENTAL STUDIES—Toxicology And Environmental Safety*

G I - GESUNDHEITS INGENIEUR; Haustechnik - Bauphysik - Umwelttechnik. see *PUBLIC HEALTH AND SAFETY*

I E Q STRATEGIES; a guide to the practical control of indoor air problems. (Indoor Environmental Quality) see *ENVIRONMENTAL STUDIES—Pollution*

JIANZHU ANQUAN/CONSTRUCTION SAFETY. see *OCCUPATIONAL HEALTH AND SAFETY*

KENSETSU KOJI SAIGAI BOSHI TEIANSHU/ PROPOSALS FOR INDUSTRIAL SAFETY OF CONSTRUCTION. see *OCCUPATIONAL HEALTH AND SAFETY*

393 SWE
M E - TIDNINGEN. Text in Swedish. 1957. m. (10/yr.). SEK 240. adv. bk.rev. abstr, charts, illus, stat, tr.lit. **Document type:** *Trade.*
Former titles: Maskinentreprenoeren (0284-7140); (until 1986): S E R - Tidningen (0037-2080)
Published by: Maskinentreprenoernas Foerlags AB/Swedish Earth Moving Machine Owners Association, Fack 1609, Stockholm 11186, Sweden. TEL 46-8-762-70-65, FAX 46-8-611-85-41. Ed. Dag Af Ekenstam. Pub. Nils Jakobsson. Adv. contact Christer Holmquist. B&W page SEK 11,250, color page SEK 18,250; trim 270 x 185. Circ: 6,900.

690 690 DEU ISSN 0172-2514
WUERTTEMBERGISCHE BAU-BERUFSGENOSSENSCHAFT. MITTEILUNGEN. Text in German. 1960. 4/yr. adv. bk.rev. charts, illus. **Document type:** *Trade.* **Description:** Covers safety and health protection in the building industry. Features accident prevention, safety rules, reports of events, lists of courses in safety, forthcoming events and exhibitions.
Formerly: Bau (0005-6413)
Indexed: C.I.S. Abstr.
Published by: Wuerttembergische Bau-Berufsgenossenschaft, Friedrich-Gerstlacher-Str 15, Boeblingen 71032, Germany. TEL 49-7031-625-0, FAX 49-7031-625-100. Ed. Horst Haun. Circ: 24,000.

BUSINESS AND ECONOMICS

see also ADVERTISING AND PUBLIC RELATIONS; BUSINESS AND ECONOMICS—Accounting; BUSINESS AND ECONOMICS—Banking And Finance; BUSINESS AND ECONOMICS—Domestic Commerce; BUSINESS AND ECONOMICS—Economic Situation And Conditions; BUSINESS AND ECONOMICS—Economic Systems And Theories, Economic History; BUSINESS AND ECONOMICS—International Commerce; BUSINESS AND ECONOMICS—International Development And Assistance; BUSINESS AND ECONOMICS—Investments; BUSINESS AND ECONOMICS—Labor And Industrial Relations; BUSINESS AND ECONOMICS—Management; BUSINESS AND ECONOMICS—Marketing And Purchasing; BUSINESS AND ECONOMICS—Office Equipment And Services; BUSINESS AND ECONOMICS—Personnel Management; BUSINESS AND ECONOMICS—Production Of Goods And Services; BUSINESS AND ECONOMICS—Public Finance, Taxation; BUSINESS AND ECONOMICS—Small Business; BUSINESS AND ECONOMICS—Trade And Industrial Directories; CONSUMER EDUCATION AND PROTECTION; INSURANCE; LABOR UNIONS; OCCUPATIONS AND CAREERS; REAL ESTATE; see also specific industries

368.382 USA ISSN 1054-5913
RA413.5.U5
A A P P O JOURNAL. Text in English. 1991. bi-m. USD 50; USD 80 foreign. adv. back issues avail. *Refereed.* **Description:** Highlights research and trends within managed health care.
Indexed: I.P.A.
Published by: (American Association of Preferred Provider Organizations), Health Care Communications, 1 Bridge Plaza, Ft. Lee, NJ 07024. TEL 201-947-5545, FAX 201-947-8406. Ed. Douglas L Elden. Circ: 23,000.

A W H P ACTION. see *PHYSICAL FITNESS AND HYGIENE*

AIDS WEEKLY PLUS. see *MEDICAL SCIENCES—Communicable Diseases*

ARZNEIMITTEL ZEITUNG. see *PHARMACY AND PHARMACOLOGY*

BIOPHOENIX DATABASE ON CD-ROM. see *MEDICAL SCIENCES*

BIOTECH MARKET NEWS & LEGAL STRATEGIES. see *BIOLOGY—Biotechnology*

DENTAL ECONOMICS; revista de la gestion de la clinica dental. see *MEDICAL SCIENCES—Dentistry*

362.10258 USA ISSN 1526-6052
▼ **E-HEALTHCARE MARKET REPORTER.** Text in English. 1999. 24/yr. USD 577 via email only (effective 2000). Index. back issues avail. **Description:** An executive briefing delivered via email on the latest developments in the proliferation of electronic commerce among healthcare and managed care organizations.
Published by: Managed Care Information Center, 1913 Atlantic Ave, Ste F4, Manasquan, NJ 08736. TEL 888-843-6242, FAX 888-329-6242, info@themcic.com, mcic@themcic.com, http://www.themcic.com. Pub. Robert K Jenkins.

EUROPEAN PHARMACEUTICAL REVIEW; the quarterly review of pharmaceutical business and technology. see *PHARMACY AND PHARMACOLOGY*

GEZONDHEIDSZORG, BELEID EN ORGANIZATIE. see *HEALTH FACILITIES AND ADMINISTRATION*

HEALTH CARE BUSINESS DIGEST. see *MEDICAL SCIENCES*

HOMECARE. see *MEDICAL SCIENCES—Nurses And Nursing*

▼ **INTERNATIONAL JOURNAL OF HEALTH CARE FINANCE AND ECONOMICS.** see *PUBLIC HEALTH AND SAFETY*

JOURNAL OF BUSINESS & PSYCHOLOGY. see *PSYCHOLOGY*

330 USA
▼ **L O H A S JOURNAL.** Variant title: Natural Business LOHAS Journal. Text in English. 2000. bi-m. USD 30 (effective 2000). adv. **Document type:** *Journal, Trade.* **Description:** Tracks business and consumer trends involving products produced with a concern for health and the environment.
Published by: Natural Business Communications LLC, PO Box 7370, Boulder, CO 80306-7370. TEL 303-442-8983, FAX 303-440-7741, info@lohasjournal.com, http://www.lohasjournal.com. Adv. contact Rod Rubino. B&W page USD 3,000, color page USD 5,000; trim 8.375 x 10.875.

LOSINKA. see *PUBLIC ADMINISTRATION—Municipal Government*

330 610 USA
M X; business strategies for medical technology executives. Text in English. bi-m. free to qualified personnel; USD 50 newsstand/cover (effective 2001). adv. **Document type:** *Trade.* **Description:** Provides business news and information relevant to medical device executives.
Formerly (until 1999): Medical Device Executive Portfolio
Published by: Canon Communications LLC, 11444 W Olympic Blvd, Ste 900, Los Angeles, CA 90064-1549. TEL 310-445-4200, FAX 310-445-4299, feedback@devicelink.com, http://www.devicelink.com/mx. Ed. Steve Halasey. Pub. William F Cobert. Adv. contact Carolyn Dale. B&W page USD 4,065, color page USD 5,265. Circ: 15,000 (controlled).

MANAGED CARE MEDICINE. see *MEDICAL SCIENCES*

338.473621 USA
MEDICAL ECONOMICS MAGAZINE; the business magazine of the medical profession. Text in English. irreg. USD 99.95 (effective 1999). adv. back issues avail. **Document type:** *Trade.*
Related titles: Online - full text ed.
Published by: Medical Economics Co., Inc., 5 Paragon Dr, Montvale, NJ 07645-1742. TEL 201-358-7500, 800-223-0581, FAX 201-358-7252, http://www.pdr.net/memag/index.htm. Ed. Jeff Forster. Pub. Frank Lederer. Adv. contact Kevin Bolum.

MIND MATTERS REVIEW. see *PSYCHOLOGY*

NUTRITION BUSINESS JOURNAL. see *NUTRITION AND DIETETICS*

PHARMACEUTICAL BUSINESS NEWS; the executive newsletter for the pharmaceutical industry. see *PHARMACY AND PHARMACOLOGY*

PHARMACEUTICAL COMPANY PROFILES. see *PHARMACY AND PHARMACOLOGY*

PHARMACOECONOMICS. see *PHARMACY AND PHARMACOLOGY*

SAMSOM ARTSENPRAKTIJK. see *MEDICAL SCIENCES*

330 GBR ISSN 1356-9627
SELF-ASSESSMENT* ; the magazine of continuous quality improvement. Text in English. q. GBP 120; GBP 140 foreign. adv. bk.rev. illus. **Document type:** *Trade.* **Description:** Examines how the use of self-assessment leads to continuous improvement, superior competitive performance, and achievement of world-class status.
Published by: I F S International Ltd., Wolseley Business Park, Kempston, Beds MK42 7PW, United Kingdom. TEL 44-1234-853605, FAX 44-1234-854499. Ed. Dan M Boland. Pub. Roy L Chase. R&P, Adv. contact David Watts.

330 660 USA
SPECTRUM (WALTHAM). Text in English. a. USD 500 (effective 2000). **Description:** Provides clients with expert opinion and analysis of business and technology issues affecting current global and regional markets as well as the companies participating in these markets. It publishes more than 80 reports per year. The reports are arranged by topic into five portfolios. It offers concise, insightful and informative analysis of current and prospective opportunities and challenges vital to corporate growth.
Published by: Decision Resources, Inc., Bay Colony Corporate Center, 1100 Winter St, Waltham, MA 02154-1238. TEL 781-487-3737, FAX 781-487-3735, carbone@deresources.com, carbone@dresources.com, http://www.dresources.com.

B

BUSINESS AND ECONOMICS—Abstracting, Bibliographies, Statistics

330.1 BWA
BOTSWANA. CENTRAL STATISTICS OFFICE. DEMOGRAPHIC AND HEALTH SURVEY. Text in English. a., latest 1996. charts. back issues avail. **Document type:** *Government.* **Description:** Provides demographic profiles of family planning, pregnancy, infant and childhood mortality, and child care.
Related titles: E-mail ed.; Fax ed.
Published by: Central Statistics Office, c/o Government Statistician, Private Bag 0024, Gaborone, Botswana. TEL 267-31-352200, FAX 267-31-352201, csobots@gov.bw. Ed. G M Charumbira. Pub. J G Segwe. **Orders to:** Government Printer, Private Bag 0081, Gaborone, Botswana. TEL 267-353202, FAX 267-312001, http://www.gov.bw.

DIRECTORY OF EUROPEAN MEDICAL ORGANISATIONS. see *MEDICAL SCIENCES—Abstracting, Bibliographies, Statistics*

338.91 610 551 DEU ISSN 0722-0111
Z7164.U5
ENTWICKLUNGSLAENDER-STUDIEN; Bibliographie entwicklungslaenderbezogener Forschungsarbeiten. Text in German. 1966. a. index. back issues avail. **Document type:** *Bibliography.*
Indexed: GeoRef, Rural Devel.Abstr., World Ag.Econ.& Rur.Soc.Abstr.
—BLDSC (3791.040000).
Published by: Deutsche Stiftung fuer Internationale Entwicklung, Zentrale Dokumentation/German Foundation for International Development, Hans-Boeckler-Str 5, Bonn 53225, Germany. TEL 49-228-4001-0, FAX 49-228-4001-111. Ed. Herbert H Henselek.

FRITZ-HUESER-INSTITUT FUER DEUTSCHE UND AUSLAENDISCHE ARBEITERLITERATUR. INFORMATIONEN. see *LITERATURE—Abstracting, Bibliographies, Statistics*

L M S ALERT. PHARMACOECONOMICS. (Literature Monitoring and Evaluation Service) see *PHARMACY AND PHARMACOLOGY—Abstracting, Bibliographies, Statistics*

657.75 331.252 GBR ISSN 0309-0078
NATIONAL ASSOCIATION OF PENSION FUNDS. ANNUAL SURVEY. Text in English. 1975. a. GBP 125 to non-members; GBP 75 to members (effective 2000). **Document type:** *Bulletin.* **Description:** Provides a source of statistics on occupational pension plans in the UK including contributions, benefits, investments and other topical issues.
Published by: National Association of Pension Funds, NIOC House, 4 Victoria St, London SW1H 0NE, United Kingdom. TEL 020 7808 1300, FAX 020 7222 7585, http://www.napf.co.uk. Ed. Mike Brown.

657.75 331.252 GBR ISSN 0144-2589
NATIONAL ASSOCIATION OF PENSION FUNDS. YEAR BOOK. Text in English. 1979. a. GBP 65 to non-members; GBP 35 to members (effective 2000). **Document type:** *Directory.* **Description:** Provides information on the NAPF and its members including a breakdown of the largest UK funds.
Related titles: Online - full text ed.: (may not contain a full list of members).
Published by: National Association of Pension Funds, NIOC House, 4 Victoria St, London SW1H 0NE, United Kingdom. TEL 44-171-730-0585, FAX 44-171-730-2595, http://www.napf.co.uk. Ed. Sheila Longley. Circ: 4,000.

NETHERLANDS. CENTRAAL BUREAU VOOR DE STATISTIEK. LEEFSITUATIE VAN DE NEDERLANDSE BEVOLKING, DEEL 1: GEZONDHEID EN KWALITEIT VAN DE ARBEID. see *PUBLIC HEALTH AND SAFETY—Abstracting, Bibliographies, Statistics*

PHARMACOECONOMICS AND OUTCOMES NEWS; rapid alerts to world pharmacoeconomic news, views and practical application. see *PHARMACY AND PHARMACOLOGY—Abstracting, Bibliographies, Statistics*

338.4 316.8 ZAF
SOUTH AFRICA. STATISTICS SOUTH AFRICA. CENSUS OF PROFESSIONAL AND BUSINESS SERVICES - ACCOUNTING, AUDITING AND BOOK-KEEPING SERVICES. Text in English. irreg., latest 1987. ZAR 10 (effective 2000). **Document type:** *Government.*
Former titles: South Africa. Statistics South Africa. Census of Business Services - Accounting, Auditing and Book-keeping Services; (until Aug. 1998): South Africa. Central Statistical Service. Census of Business Services - Accounting, Auditing and Book-keeping Services
Published by: Statistics South Africa/Statistieke Suid-Afrika, Private Bag X44, Pretoria 0001, South Africa. TEL 27-12-310-8911, FAX 27-12-310-8500, info@statssa.pwv.gov.za, http://www.statssa.gov.za.

004.021 ZAF
SOUTH AFRICA. STATISTICS SOUTH AFRICA. CENSUS OF PROFESSIONAL AND BUSINESS SERVICES - DATA PROCESSING SERVICES. Text in English. irreg., latest 1993. ZAR 10 (effective 2000). **Document type:** *Government.*
Former titles: South Africa. Statistics South Africa. Census of Business Services - Data Processing Services; (until Aug. 1998): South Africa. Central Statistical Service. Census of Business Services - Data Processing Services
Published by: Statistics South Africa/Statistieke Suid-Afrika, Private Bag X44, Pretoria 0001, South Africa. TEL 27-12-310-8911, FAX 27-12-310-8500, info@statssa.pwv.gov.za, http://www.statssa.gov.za.

BUSINESS AND ECONOMICS—Accounting

657 150 USA ISSN 1050-4753
HF5601
BEHAVIORAL RESEARCH IN ACCOUNTING. Text in English. 1989. a. USD 20 (effective 1999). back issues avail.; reprint service avail. from PSC,SCH. **Description:** Publishes original research related to accounting and how it affects and is affected by individuals and organizations.
Related titles: Microform ed.: (from PQC); Online - full text ed.: (from ProQuest Information & Learning).
Indexed: Account.Ind., J.of Econ.Lit., e-psyche.
—BLDSC (1877.780000).
Published by: American Accounting Association, 5717 Bessie Dr, Sarasota, FL 34233. TEL 941-921-7747, FAX 941-923-4093, http://www.hsb.baylor.edu/html/davisc/abo/bria/briahome.htm. Ed. Don W Finn. R&P Mary Cole.

THE HOSPITAL ACCOUNTS RECEIVABLE ANALYSIS. see *HEALTH FACILITIES AND ADMINISTRATION*

657 USA
MEDICAL CLIENT NEWSLETTER. Text in English. q. **Description:** Information on members' services to clients.
Published by: C P A Associates International, Inc., Meadows Office Complex, 201 Rte 17 N, Rutherford, NJ 07070-2574. TEL 212-804-8686.

PATIENT ACCOUNTS. see *HEALTH FACILITIES AND ADMINISTRATION*

658 USA ISSN 1060-0418
THE RECEIVABLES REPORT; the monthly newsletter for America's health care financial manager. Text in English. 1986. m. USD 345 to individuals; USD 35 newsstand/cover (effective 2002). **Document type:** *Newsletter, Trade.* **Description:** Includes actual profit-improvement examples from facilities nationwide, secrets for successfully challenging denials, tips for using automation to increase cash flow, and strategies that are currently being used to prepare for health care reform.
—CCC.
Published by: Aspen Publishers, Inc., 200 Orchard Ridge Dr, Ste 200, Gaithersburg, MD 20878. TEL 301-417-7500, 800-638-8437, FAX 301-695-7931, customer.service@aspenpul.com, http://www.aspenpub.com. Ed. Joann Petaschnick. **Dist. by:** Aspen Publishers Inc., Distribution Center, 7201 McKinney Circle, Frederick, MD 21701. TEL 301-698-7100, FAX 301-417-7550.

BUSINESS AND ECONOMICS—Banking And Finance

see also BUSINESS AND ECONOMICS—Economic Situation And Conditions; BUSINESS AND ECONOMICS—Investments; INSURANCE

AUDIT COMMISSION. HEALTH INFORMATION BULLETIN. see *PUBLIC ADMINISTRATION—Municipal Government*

AUDIT COMMISSION. LOCAL GOVERNMENT INFORMATION BULLETIN. see *PUBLIC ADMINISTRATION—Municipal Government*

332.1 GBR
AUDIT COMMISSION. LOCAL GOVERNMENT REPORTS. Text in English. irreg. (approx. 35-50/yr.). GBP 600 (effective 1999). **Document type:** *Monographic series, Government.*
Published by: Audit Commission for Local Authorities and the National Health Service in England and Wales, 1 Vincent Sq, London SW1P 2PN, United Kingdom. TEL 44-207- 8281212, http://www.audit-commission.gov.uk. **Orders to:** Bookpoint. FAX 44-1235-404454.

332.1 GBR
AUDIT COMMISSION. REPORTS. Text in English. irreg. price varies. adv. **Document type:** *Monographic series, Government.*
Supersedes (in 1999): Audit Commission. Occasional Papers (0959-2571)
Published by: Audit Commission for Local Authorities and the National Health Service in England and Wales, 1 Vincent Sq, London SW1P 2PN, United Kingdom. TEL 44-20-7828-1212, http://www.audit-commission.gov.uk. Adv. contact B Dewar. **Orders to:** Bookpoint, 39 Milton Park, Milton, Abingdon, Oxon OX14 4TD, United Kingdom. TEL 44-123-5400400, FAX 44-123-5400454.

330 USA ISSN 1530-7271
▼ **DENTIST'S MONEY DIGEST.** Text in English. 2000. bi-m. free domestic; USD 80 in Canada; USD 132 elsewhere (effective 2001). adv. *Refereed.* **Document type:** *Journal, Consumer.*
Published by: Medical World Communications, 241 Forsgate Dr, Jamesburg, NJ 08831. TEL 732-656-1143, FAX 732-656-1148, http://www.dentallearning.com. Ed., R&P Randy Robbin. Pub. Dan Perkins. Adv. contact Margaret Pagel TEL 847-205-5660. B&W page USD 9,930, color page USD 11,630; trim 10.1875 x 13.3875. Circ: 127,000.

ECUADOR. INSTITUTO NACIONAL DE ESTADISTICA Y CENSOS. CUENTAS NACIONALES DE LA SALUD. see *BUSINESS AND ECONOMICS—Public Finance, Taxation*

305.26 USA
ELDERCARE FORUM. Text in English. 1994. q. USD 14. **Document type:** *Trade.* **Description:** Educates and informs caregivers about issues related to aging and taking care of an aging parent. Focuses on personal financial management, health and medical issues, housing, government programs, and resources for caregivers.
Related titles: Online - full text ed.
Published by: ElderCare Financial Management, Inc., 170 Elaine Dr, Roswell, GA 30075. TEL 770-518-2767, hwlj87a@prodigy.com, http://www.mindspung.com/~eldercare/elderweb.htm. Ed., R&P Laura Beller. Circ: 15,000 (paid).

▼ **JOURNAL OF PSYCHOLOGY AND FINANCIAL MARKETS.** see *PSYCHOLOGY*

332 610 USA ISSN 8750-9407
PHYSICIANS FINANCIAL NEWS. Text in English. 1983. 16/yr. USD 105 domestic; USD 145 foreign; USD 10 newsstand/cover (effective 2001). adv. **Document type:** *Newspaper, Trade.* **Description:** Helps primary care physicians manage their money and run their practices more efficiently.
Incorporates: Computer News for Physicians
Related titles: ♦ Supplement: Physicians Lifestyle Magazine. ISSN 1049-6610.
Published by: Rogers Media, One Harmon Meadow Blvd, Secaucus, NJ 07094. TEL 201-864-2400, FAX 201-864-3626, editorial@pfnpublishing.com, http://pfnpublishing.com. Ed. Noreen Perrotta. Pub. Jeannette Brandofino. Adv. contact Irene Stewart. B&W page USD 9,170, color page USD 10,920; bleed 11.125 x 15.375. Circ: 140,000 (controlled).

PRIME TIMES MAGAZINE (MADISON). see *CONSUMER EDUCATION AND PROTECTION*

REIMBURSEMENT ADVISOR. see *HEALTH FACILITIES AND ADMINISTRATION*

SURGICAL NEWS (ONLINE). see *EDUCATION—Higher Education*

TAX, ESTATE & FINANCIAL PLANNING FOR THE ELDERLY. see *GERONTOLOGY AND GERIATRICS*

B

BUSINESS AND ECONOMICS—Domestic Commerce

PHARMACEUTICAL: LATIN AMERICAN INDUSTRIAL REPORT. see *PHARMACY AND PHARMACOLOGY*

BUSINESS AND ECONOMICS—Economic Situation And Conditions

ADVANCES IN BEHAVIORAL ECONOMICS. see *PSYCHOLOGY*

BOTSWANA. CENTRAL STATISTICS OFFICE. DEMOGRAPHIC AND HEALTH SURVEY. see *BUSINESS AND ECONOMICS—Abstracting, Bibliographies, Statistics*

330.9 658 USA ISSN 0739-8034
RA410.53
HEALTH CARE COSTS. Text in English. 1981. q.
Published by: D R I - McGraw-Hill, 24 Hartwell Ave, Lexington, MA 02173. TEL 617-863-5100, FAX 617-860-6332. Ed. Sheila Smith.

HEALTH CARE STRATEGIST. see *MEDICAL SCIENCES*

JOURNAL OF RESEARCH IN PHARMACEUTICAL ECONOMICS. see *PHARMACY AND PHARMACOLOGY*

L M S ALERT. PHARMACOECONOMICS. (Literature Monitoring and Evaluation Service) see *PHARMACY AND PHARMACOLOGY—Abstracting, Bibliographies, Statistics*

MEDICAL BUSINESS REVIEW; medical business analysis for the doctor-executive. see *BUSINESS AND ECONOMICS—Management*

NETHERLANDS. CENTRAAL BUREAU VOOR DE STATISTIEK. LEEFSITUATIE VAN DE NEDERLANDSE BEVOLKING, DEEL 1: GEZONDHEID EN KWALITEIT VAN DE ARBEID. see *PUBLIC HEALTH AND SAFETY—Abstracting, Bibliographies, Statistics*

O T C BULLETIN; the business newsletter for Europe's consumer healthcare industry. (Over the Counter) see *PHARMACY AND PHARMACOLOGY*

PHARMACEUTICAL COMPANIES ANALYSIS. see *PHARMACY AND PHARMACOLOGY*

PHARMACEUTICAL STRATEGIC ALLIANCES; the drug and biotech alliances reference guide. see *PHARMACY AND PHARMACOLOGY*

330.9 615.19 FRA
PREVISIONS GLISSANTES DETAILLEES EN PERSPECTIVES SECTORIELLES (VOL.22): PARACHIMIE. Text in French. 1959. a. (in 42 vols.). FRF 7,000 per vol.; FRF 50,000 per set. charts, stat.
Formerly: Previsions Glissantes Detaillees en Perspectives Sectorielles (Vol.19): Parachimie et Pharmacie; Supersedes in part: Economie Francaise en Perspectives Sectorielles (Vols.1-5); Which supersedes in part: Prevision a Un An de l'Economie Francaise
Published by: B I P E Conseil, L'Atrium - 6 Place Abel Gance, Boulogne-Billancourt Cedex 92652, France. TEL 33-1-46944522, FAX 33-1-46944599, 100332.644@compuserve.com.

330.9 610 FRA
PREVISIONS GLISSANTES DETAILLEES EN PERSPECTIVES SECTORIELLES (VOL.38): PHARMACIE - SANTE. Text in French. 1959. a. (in 42 vols.). FRF 7,000 per vol.; FRF 50,000 per set. charts, stat.
Formerly: Previsions Glissantes Detaillees en Perspectives Sectorielles (Vol.35): Sante; Supersedes in part: Economie Francaise en Perspectives Sectorielles (Vols.1-5); Which supersedes in part: Prevision a Un An de l'Economie Francaise
Published by: B I P E Conseil, L'Atrium - 6 Place Abel Gance, Boulogne-Billancourt Cedex 92652, France. TEL 33-1-46944522, FAX 33-1-46944599, 100332.644@compuserve.com.

330.9 USA ISSN 1075-7848
REIMBURSEMENT UPDATE. Text in English. 1984. q. USD 105. **Document type:** *Newsletter.*
Address: 355 Oak Trail Dr., Louisville, TX 75067. TEL 817-491-3593. Ed. Frederic R Curtiss.

START-UP; Windhover's review of emerging medical ventures. see *MEDICAL SCIENCES*

STRATEGIC COMMENTARY. see *MEDICAL SCIENCES*

WEEKLY PHARMACY REPORTS: THE GREEN SHEET. see *PHARMACY AND PHARMACOLOGY*

WINDHOVER'S IN VIVO; the business and medicine report. see *MEDICAL SCIENCES*

BUSINESS AND ECONOMICS—Economic Systems And Theories, Economic History

153.83 330 USA ISSN 0895-5646
HB615 CODEN: JRUNEN
JOURNAL OF RISK AND UNCERTAINTY. Text in English. 1988. bi-m. USD 555, EUR 554 to institutions for print or online ed.; USD 666, EUR 664.80 to institutions for print & online eds.combined (effective 2002). adv. reprint service avail. from SWZ,PQC. *Refereed.* **Document type:** *Journal, Academic/Scholarly.* **Description:** Publishes original theoretical and empirical contributions dealing with the analysis of risk-bearing behavior and decision making under uncertainty.
Related titles: Microform ed.: (from PQC); Online - full text ed.: (from EBSCO Publishing, O C L C Online Computer Library Center, Inc., RoweCom Information Quest, Swets Blackwell, Kluwer Online, Institute for Scientific Information).
Indexed: ASCA, Curr.Cont., Environ.Sci.Poll.Mgmt., Intl.Bibl.Soc.Sci., J.of Econ.Lit., Lang.& Lang.Behav.Abstr., Oper.Res.Manage.Sci., Qual.Contr.Appl.Stat., Risk Abstr., SOPODA, SSCI, Saf.Sci.Abstr., Sociol.Abstr., Stat.Theor.Meth.Abstr. (1996-), Zent.Math., e-psyche.
—BLDSC (5052.101000), IDS, ingenta. **CCC.**
Published by: Kluwer Academic Publishers Boston, 101 Philip Dr, Assinippi Park, Norwell, MA 02061. TEL 781-871-6600, FAX 781-871-9045, services@wkap.nl, http://www.wkap.nl/journalhome.htm/0895-5646. Ed. W Kip Viscusi. R&P Rose Luongo TEL 781-871-6311. **Subscr. outside the Americas to:** Kluwer Academic Publishers Group, Journals Department, PO Box 322, Dordrecht 3300 AH, Netherlands. TEL 31-78-639-2392, FAX 31-78-654-6474; **Subscr. to:** Kluwer Academic - Plenum Publishers, 233 Spring St, New York, NY 10013-1578. TEL 212-620-8468, FAX 212-807-1047.

330.1 USA
STUDIES IN HEALTH AND HUMAN VALUES. Text in English. 1989. irreg. price varies. **Document type:** *Monographic series.*
Published by: Praeger Publishers (Subsidiary of: Greenwood Publishing Group Inc.), 88 Post Rd W, Box 5007, Westport, CT 06881-5007. TEL 203-226-3571, FAX 203-222-1502.

BUSINESS AND ECONOMICS—International Commerce

B B I N: MEDICAL DEVICE WEEK. (Biomedical Business International Newsletter) see *MEDICAL SCIENCES*

THE B B I NEWSLETTER. see *MEDICAL SCIENCES*

PROVEN TRADE CONTACTS. see *MEDICAL SCIENCES*

BUSINESS AND ECONOMICS—International Development And Assistance

338.91 USA
C H R I A NEWS. Text in English. 1983. q. USD 35 to membership. bk.rev. *Refereed.* **Document type:** *Newsletter.*
Formerly: C H R I C A News
Published by: Committee for Health Rights in the Americas, 474 Valencia St, Ste 120, San Francisco, CA 94103-3415. TEL 415-431-7760, FAX 415-431-7768. Ed., R&P Shannon Coughlin.

ENTWICKLUNGSLAENDER-STUDIEN; Bibliographie entwicklungslaenderbezogener Forschungsarbeiten. see *BUSINESS AND ECONOMICS—Abstracting, Bibliographies, Statistics*

338.91 IRL
IRISH AID ANNUAL REPORT; food - human rights - health - water - education. Text in English. a. illus, stat. **Document type:** *Government, Corporate.* **Description:** Reports on the efforts of Irish Aid (with and without the cooperation of international organizations) to administer development and emergency relief. Discusses water and sanitation, food security, health, education, and human rights in the recipient countries.
Related titles: Online - full text ed.
Published by: Department of Foreign Affairs, Development Co-operation Division, Irish Aid, 76-78 Harcourt St., Dublin 2, Ireland. TEL 353-1-478-0822, http://www.irlgov.ie/iveagh/foreignaffairs/irishaid/.

M A P NEWS. see *SOCIAL SERVICES AND WELFARE*

615.1 GBR ISSN 1469-3828
▼ **MULTINATIONAL PHARMACEUTICAL COMPANIES.** Text in English. 1999. a. GBP 345, USD 550 (effective 2001). **Description:** Research and marketing directory of worldwide professionals in the pharmaceutical field.
Related titles: CD-ROM ed.: GBP 580, USD 930 (effective 2001).
Published by: Business Monitor International Ltd., Commercial Intelligence Service, 179 Queen Victoria St, London EC4V 4DU, United Kingdom. TEL 44-20-7248-0468, FAX 44-20-7248-0467, http://www.businessmonitor.com.

T R A C NEWSLETTER. (Transvaal Rural Action Committee) see *POLITICAL SCIENCE—Civil Rights*

WORLDWATCH READER. see *ENVIRONMENTAL STUDIES*

BUSINESS AND ECONOMICS—Investments

BIONICS. see *MEDICAL SCIENCES—Experimental Medicine, Laboratory Technique*

332.6322 USA ISSN 1092-8995
BIOTECH NAVIGATOR. Text in English. 1997. m. USD 199 in US & Canada; USD 235 elsewhere (effective 2000). back issues avail. **Document type:** *Newsletter.* **Description:** Gives detailed rationale explaining the logic behind each biotechnology stock evaluation, whether positive or negative.
Media: Online - full text.
Address: PO Box 7274, Beaverton, OR 97007-7274. TEL 503-649-1355, FAX 503-649-4490, info@biotechnav.com, nwong@biotechnav.com, http://www.biotechnav.com. Ed. Nadine Wong.

GENERIC LINE. see *PHARMACY AND PHARMACOLOGY*

332.6 USA ISSN 1065-996X
MEDICAL TECHNOLOGY STOCK LETTER. Text in English. 1983. bi-w. USD 320 domestic; USD 350 foreign (effective 2000). back issues avail. **Document type:** *Newsletter.* **Description:** Investment advisory providing specific buy and sell recommendations on medical and biotechnology stocks.
Published by: Piedmont Venture Group, PO Box 40460, Berkeley, CA 94704. TEL 510-843-1857, FAX 510-843-0901, mtsl@bioinvest.com, http://www.bioinvest.com. Ed. Jim McCamant.

332 USA
N A R I STETHOSCOPE. Text in English. 1961. s-a. membership. adv. charts, illus. **Document type:** *Newsletter.*
Published by: National Association of Residents and Interns, 350 Fairway Dr, Ste 200, Deerfield Beach, FL 33441-1834. TEL 954-571-1877, http://www.nari-assn.com. Ed. B Lydia Young. Adv. contact Joe Santoli. Circ: 15,000.

332.6 615.1 USA ISSN 1076-9382
PHARMACEUTICAL VENTURES. Text in English. 1991. 48/yr. USD 415 (effective 1999). back issues avail. **Document type:** *Newsletter.* **Description:** For sophisticated investors. Covers the financial markets of the pharmaceutical manufacturers and researchers.
Indexed: ABC, Inpharma, Reac.
Published by: Scitec Services, 5324 Sinclair Rd, Columbus, OH 43229. TEL 614-433-0648, FAX 614-433-0432. Ed., Pub. Frank McKim.

THE PHYSICIAN'S PERSONAL ADVISORY. see *HEALTH FACILITIES AND ADMINISTRATION*

B

332.62 USA ISSN 1092-9711
VENTURE CAPITAL AND HEALTH CARE. Text in English. 1997. m. USD 595 domestic; USD 655 foreign (effective 2000). adv. charts, stat. back issues avail. **Document type:** *Newsletter.* **Description:** Explores the business of private equity investment in the trillion dollar health care market. For venture capitalists, private investors, investment banks, health care companies and entrepreneurs.
Published by: Asset Alternatives, Inc., 170 Linden St, 2nd Fl, Wellesley, MA 02482. TEL 781-304-1400, FAX 781-304-1440, info@assetnews.com, http://www.assetnews.com. Ed., Pub. Steven P Galante. R&P, Adv. contact Doreen C Purvis. B&W page USD 1,000, color page USD 1,200; trim 11 x 8.5. Circ: 612 (paid).

332.6 610 GBR ISSN 1357-4388
YOUR PRIVATE HEALTH OPTION. Text in English. 1994. q. GBP 2.50 newsstand/cover. adv. **Document type:** *Consumer.* **Description:** Provides consumers with the information they need to select the private health care plan that best meets their needs.
Formerly (until 1995): Which Private Health Option (1354-9936)
Published by: Matching Hat Ltd., 143 Charing Cross Rd, Penthouse Ste., London WC1H OEE, United Kingdom. TEL 44-171-478-4600, FAX 44-171-478-4619. Ed. Andrew Stuart. Pub. Bharat Sagar. Adv. contact James Toward. Circ: 50,000 (paid).

BUSINESS AND ECONOMICS—Labor And Industrial Relations

see also LABOR UNIONS

AMERICANS WITH DISABILITIES ACT: EMPLOYEE RIGHTS AND EMPLOYER OBLIGATIONS. see *HANDICAPPED*

331 DEU ISSN 0341-0900
ANGEWANDTE ARBEITSWISSENSCHAFT. Text in German. 1975. q. DEM 28.20 (effective 2001). index. **Document type:** *Journal, Academic/Scholarly.*
Indexed: IBZ.
—**CCC.**
Published by: (Institut fuer Angewandte Arbeitswissenschaft e.V.), Wirtschaftsverlag Bachem GmbH, Ursulaplatz 1, Cologne 50668, Germany. TEL 49-221-1619155, FAX 49-221-1619231, bachem-verlagsgruppe@netcologne.de, http://www.bachem-verlagsgruppe.de. Ed. Joachim Schauer. Circ: 4,000.

AUSTRALIAN JOURNAL OF MANAGEMENT AND ORGANISATIONAL BEHAVIOUR. see *PSYCHOLOGY*

C I R NEWS. see *MEDICAL SCIENCES*

331 SVN ISSN 1408-3760
DELO + VARNOST; revija za varstvo pri delu. Text in Slovenian. 1956. bi-m., latest vol.46. SIT 19,800 domestic; DEM 180 (effective 1999). adv. bk.rev. 52 p./no. back issues avail. **Document type:** *Journal.*
Indexed: C.I.S. Abstr.
Published by: Zavod za Varstvo Pri Delu, Bohoriceva 22-a, Ljubljana 61000, Slovenia. TEL 386-1-4320253, FAX 386-1-2312562, inof@zvd.si, info@zvd.si, http://www.zvd.si. Ed. Tatjana Srol. Circ: 1,000.

331 FRA ISSN 0767-2187
DICTIONNAIRE PERMANENT: SECURITE ET CONDITIONS DE TRAVAIL. Text in French. 2 base vols. plus m. updates. FRF 1,730 (effective 1998). **Description:** Focuses on working conditions, on-site safety and hygiene.
Related titles: CD-ROM ed.
Published by: Editions Legislatives, 80 av. de la Marne, Montrouge Cedex 92546, France. TEL 33-1-40926868, FAX 33-1-46560015, el@editions-legislatives.fr, http://www.editions-legislatives.fr. Pub. Michel Vaillant.

DRUG DETECTION REPORT; the newsletter on drug testing in the workplace. see *BUSINESS AND ECONOMICS—Personnel Management*

E I R E C KENKYU HOKOKUSHU. see *MEDICAL SCIENCES—Physical Medicine And Rehabilitation*

EVALUATING YOUR FIRM'S INJURY & ILLNESS RECORD. CONSTRUCTION INDUSTRIES. see *OCCUPATIONAL HEALTH AND SAFETY*

EVALUATING YOUR FIRM'S INJURY & ILLNESS RECORD. SERVICE INDUSTRIES. see *OCCUPATIONAL HEALTH AND SAFETY*

EVALUATING YOUR FIRM'S INJURY & ILLNESS RECORD. TRANSPORTATION & PUBLIC UTILITIES INDUSTRIES. see *OCCUPATIONAL HEALTH AND SAFETY*

EVALUATING YOUR FIRM'S INJURY & ILLNESS RECORD. WHOLESALE & RETAIL TRADE INDUSTRIES. see *OCCUPATIONAL HEALTH AND SAFETY*

H R PRACTITIONERS GUIDE. see *BUSINESS AND ECONOMICS—Personnel Management*

HADSHOT KUPPOT HOLIM. see *INSURANCE*

HEALTH CARE LABOR MANUAL. see *HEALTH FACILITIES AND ADMINISTRATION*

344.01 USA ISSN 0890-9245
KF3580.H4
HEALTH EMPLOYMENT LAW UPDATE. Text in English. 1985. 12/yr. USD 125 (effective 2001). index. 8 p./no. back issues avail. **Document type:** *Newsletter.* **Description:** Presents advice covering current legislation and legal decisions, issues and trends, policy concerns and authoritative legal analysis for human resource executives.
Published by: Rutkowski & Associates Inc., PO Box 15250, Evansville, IN 47716-0250. TEL 812-476-4520. R&P Barbara Lang Rutkowski.

HOSPITAL EMPLOYEE HEALTH. see *HEALTH FACILITIES AND ADMINISTRATION*

INTERNATIONAL JOURNAL OF ORGANISATIONAL BEHAVIOUR. see *PSYCHOLOGY*

INTERNATIONAL SOCIETY FOR OCCUPATIONAL ERGONOMICS AND SAFETY. NEWSLETTER. see *OCCUPATIONAL HEALTH AND SAFETY*

MAINE. DEPARTMENT OF LABOR. BUREAU OF LABOR STANDARDS. SUBSTANCE ABUSE TESTING REPORT. see *DRUG ABUSE AND ALCOHOLISM*

MEDICAL PRACTICES COMMITTEE. RECRUITMENT SURVEY (YEAR). see *MEDICAL SCIENCES*

331.1 MEX
MEXICO. CENTRO DE INFORMACION TECNICA Y DOCUMENTACION. INDICE DE ARTICULOS SOBRE SEGURIDAD E HIGIENE INDUSTRIAL. Text in Spanish. 1979. 3/yr. MXP 140, USD 13.
Published by: Servicio Nacional de Adiestramiento Rapido de la Mano de Obra en la Industria, Centro de Informacion Tecnica y Documentacion, Calzada Atzcapotzalco-la Villa 209, Apdo. 16-099, Mexico City, DF, Mexico. Ed. Javier Pedraza Garcia. Circ: 2,000.

NETHERLANDS. CENTRAAL BUREAU VOOR DE STATISTIEK. LEEFSITUATIE VAN DE NEDERLANDSE BEVOLKING, DEEL 1: GEZONDHEID EN KWALITEIT VAN DE ARBEID. see *PUBLIC HEALTH AND SAFETY—Abstracting, Bibliographies, Statistics*

NEUE B S. (Betriebs Sicherheit) see *OCCUPATIONAL HEALTH AND SAFETY*

OCCUPATIONAL ERGONOMICS. see *OCCUPATIONAL HEALTH AND SAFETY*

OFFICIAL DISABILITY GUIDELINES. see *OCCUPATIONAL HEALTH AND SAFETY*

PSICOLOGIA E LAVORO. see *PSYCHOLOGY*

PUBLIC SERVICE ASSOCIATION JOURNAL. see *PUBLIC ADMINISTRATION*

RAGGED EDGE. see *HANDICAPPED—Visually Impaired*

331 363.7 360 DNK ISSN 1399-1442
▼ **TIDSSKRIFT FOR ARBEJDSLIV.** Text in Danish; Summaries in English. 1999. q. DKK 400 to individuals; DKK 600 to institutions; DKK 130 per issue (effective 2001). abstr, bibl. 128 p./no. 2 cols./p. back issues avail. *Refereed.* **Document type:** *Journal, Abstract/Index.* **Description:** Multidisciplinary studies of the labor market, working life and working environment.
Formerly (until 1999): Nyt om Arbejdsliv (0909-1203)
Related titles: Online - full text ed.
Published by: (Roskilde Universitet, Center for Studier i Arbejdsliv), Tidsskrift for Arbejdsliv, Fibigerstraede 13, Aalborg OE 9220, Denmark. http://www.nyt-om-arbejdsliv.dk. Eds. Joergen Burchardt, Herman Knudsen. Circ: 800. **Co-publisher:** Odense University Press.

LE TRAVAIL HUMAIN. see *PSYCHOLOGY*

344.01 USA ISSN 1054-7819
WORKERS' COMP ADVISOR∗ ; helping doctors, lawyers, and employers cope with the workers' comp system. Text in English. 1987. m. USD 197. adv. bk.rev. back issues avail. **Document type:** *Newsletter.* **Description:** Covers the workers compensation industry.
—**CCC.**
Published by: Genesis Publishing, 550 Torrey Point Rd, Del Mar, CA 92014-3630. TEL 619-453-0858. Ed. Donna Buys Hawkins.

WORKERS' COMP MANAGED CARE. see *INSURANCE*

331 CAN ISSN 0834-292X
WORKLIFE REPORT. Text in English. 1981. bi-m. CND 35; CND 39 foreign. bk.rev. reprint service avail. from PQC. **Description:** Aims to promote awareness of research, issues and trends in labor relations, personnel, and other work-related areas.
Related titles: Online - full text ed.: (from ProQuest Information & Learning, Northern Light Technology, Inc., Gale Group, Factiva).
Indexed: ABI Inform. (1982-), CBCA Bus. (1996-), CBCA Ref., P.A.I.S.
—BLDSC (9351.222000). **CCC.**
Published by: I R Research Services, P O Box 1092, Kingston, ON K7L 4Y5, Canada. TEL 613-542-5596. Ed. L A Kelly. Circ: 1,500.

BUSINESS AND ECONOMICS—Management

ADULT DAY SERVICES LETTER. see *GERONTOLOGY AND GERIATRICS*

AMBULATORY OUTREACH. see *MEDICAL SCIENCES*

APOTHEKEN-PRAXIS; Forum fuer Marketing und Management. see *PHARMACY AND PHARMACOLOGY*

AUSTRALIAN DENTAL PRACTICE MAGAZINE. see *MEDICAL SCIENCES—Dentistry*

BRITISH JOURNAL OF CLINICAL GOVERNANCE. see *MEDICAL SCIENCES*

658 USA ISSN 0164-9914
CHAIN DRUG REVIEW; the reporter for the chain drug store industry. Text in English. 1978. fortn. (except m. in May, Dec. & Jul.). USD 136; USD 8.36 newsstand/cover (effective 2000). adv. **Document type:** *Magazine, Trade.*
Related titles: Online - full text ed.: (from Northern Light Technology, Inc., Gale Group, Factiva).
Indexed: Bus.& Indus. (May 1994-).
—BLDSC (3128.734150).
Published by: Racher Press, Inc., 220 Fifth Ave, 18th Fl, New York, NY 10001. TEL 212-213-6000, FAX 212-213-6106. Ed. David Pinto. adv.: B&W page USD 10,189, color page USD 13,070. Circ: 44,826.

CHANGING MEDICAL MARKETS; the international monthly newsletter for executives in the healthcare and biotechnology industries. see *MEDICAL SCIENCES*

CLINICAL LEADERSHIP & MANAGEMENT REVIEW. see *MEDICAL SCIENCES—Experimental Medicine, Laboratory Technique*

THE CLINICIAN IN MANAGEMENT. see *MEDICAL SCIENCES*

CRONER'S HEALTH & SAFETY MANAGER. see *OCCUPATIONAL HEALTH AND SAFETY*

DENTAL PRACTICE MANAGEMENT. see *MEDICAL SCIENCES—Dentistry*

DISEASE MANAGEMENT NEWS. see *MEDICAL SCIENCES*

▼ **DRUG COST MANAGEMENT REPORT.** see *PHARMACY AND PHARMACOLOGY*

ESSENTIALS OF MANAGED HEALTH CARE. see *INSURANCE*

F & W - FUEHREN UND WIRTSCHAFTEN IM KRANKENHAUS. see *HEALTH FACILITIES AND ADMINISTRATION*

FINANCIAL MANAGEMENT STRATEGIES FOR MEDICAL OFFICES. see *HEALTH FACILITIES AND ADMINISTRATION*

FITNESS MANAGEMENT. see *PHYSICAL FITNESS AND HYGIENE*

GEDRAG & ORGANISATIE. see *HEALTH FACILITIES AND ADMINISTRATION*

GREAT BRITAIN. HEALTH & SAFETY EXECUTIVE. TECHNOLOGY AND HEALTH SCIENCES DIVISION. SPECIALIST INSPECTOR REPORTS. see *PUBLIC HEALTH AND SAFETY*

GROUP PRACTICE SOLUTIONS. see *HEALTH FACILITIES AND ADMINISTRATION*

THE GUIDE TO HOSPITAL PERFORMANCE. see *HEALTH FACILITIES AND ADMINISTRATION*

HEALTH CARE MANAGEMENT HANDBOOK (YEAR). see *MEDICAL SCIENCES*

HEALTH CARE MANAGEMENT REVIEW. see *HEALTH FACILITIES AND ADMINISTRATION*

HEALTH CARE MANAGEMENT SCIENCE. see *HEALTH FACILITIES AND ADMINISTRATION*

658 USA ISSN 1060-0434
THE HEALTH CARE REGISTRATION; the newsletter for health care registration professionals. Text in English. 1991. m. USD 320 to individuals; USD 32 newsstand/cover (effective 2002). **Document type:** *Newsletter, Trade.* **Description:** Offers simple, straightforward information, with tips on how to run the department more efficiently. Focuses on patient relations, with regular information on up-front collections, problems in admitting areas, employee management issues, and productivity.
—**CCC.**
Published by: Aspen Publishers, Inc., 200 Orchard Ridge Dr, Ste 200, Gaithersburg, MD 20878. TEL 301-417-7500, 800-638-8437, FAX 301-695-7931, customer.service@aspenpubl.com, http://www.aspenpub.com. Ed. Laura J Merisalo. **Dist. by:** Aspen Publishers Inc., Distribution Center, 7201 McKinney Circle, Frederick, MD 21701. TEL 301-698-7100, FAX 301-417-7550.

HEALTHCARE LEADERSHIP REVIEW. see *HEALTH FACILITIES AND ADMINISTRATION*

HEALTHCARE RISK CONTROL SYSTEM; an information and consultation system. see *HEALTH FACILITIES AND ADMINISTRATION*

HOSPITAL MANAGEMENT INTERNATIONAL. see *HEALTH FACILITIES AND ADMINISTRATION*

HOSPITAL MATERIALS MANAGEMENT; the newsletter for materials management and group purchasing. see *HEALTH FACILITIES AND ADMINISTRATION*

658 FRA
IMPACT MEDECIN; les dossiers de F M C du praticien. Text in French. 45/yr. FRF 600. **Document type:** *Newspaper.*
Address: 1 rue Paul Cezanne, Paris Cedex 8 75375, France. Ed. Jean de Charon. Circ: 90,000.

658.8 USA
INNOVATIVE LEADER (ONLINE); monthly tool to increase creativity and productivity. Text in English. 1992. m. free. adv. bk.rev. illus. back issues avail. **Document type:** *Newsletter, Trade.* **Description:** Provides a resource for managers to stimulate creativity and productivity.
Former titles (until Mar. 2001): Innovative Leader (Print) (1092-2156); (until Mar. 1997): R and D Innovator (1061-1894)
Media: Online - full content.
Published by: Winston J Brill Associates, 4134 Cherokee Dr, Madison, WI 53711. TEL 608-231-6766, FAX 608-231-6794, wbrill@winstonbrill.com, http://www.WinstonBrill.com, http://www.winstonbrill.com. Ed., Pub., R&P, Adv. contact Winston J Brill.

INSTITUTE OF PHARMACY MANAGEMENT INTERNATIONAL. INSTITUTE NEWS. see *PHARMACY AND PHARMACOLOGY*

INTAND NEWSLETTER; the newsletter of the international network for transactional analysis, neuro-linguistic programming. see *PSYCHOLOGY*

INTERNATIONAL HOSPITAL & AGED CARE JOURNAL. see *HEALTH FACILITIES AND ADMINISTRATION*

650.13 USA ISSN 1044-4068
HD42 CODEN: IOCMEY
INTERNATIONAL JOURNAL OF CONFLICT MANAGEMENT. Text in English. 1990. q. USD 69 domestic to individuals; USD 84 foreign to individuals; USD 189 domestic to institutions; USD 204 foreign to institutions (effective 2000). adv. bk.rev. *Refereed.* **Document type:** *Academic/Scholarly.* **Description:** Publishes original empirical and conceptual articles, case studies, simulations, and teaching notes on various aspects of conflict management.
Related titles: Online - full text ed.: (from Northern Light Technology, Inc., ProQuest Information & Learning, Factiva, Institute for Scientific Information).
Indexed: ABI Inform. (Jan.1996-), ASCA, Curr.Cont., Environ.Sci.Poll.Mgmt., Fam.Ind., Lang.& Lang.Behav.Abstr., Per.Islam. (1990-), Pollut.Abstr., PsycInfo, Risk Abstr., SOPODA, SSCI, Soc.Serv.Abstr., Sociol.Abstr., e-psyche.
—BLDSC (4542.175700), IDS, ingenta. **CCC.**
Published by: Center for Advanced Studies in Management, 1574 Mallory Ct, Bowling Green, KY 42103-1300. TEL 502-782-2601, FAX 502-782-2601, mgt2000@aol.com, http://members.aol.com/mgt2000/ijcm.htm/. Ed. M Afzalur Rahim. R&P, Adv. contact Masuda Rahim. Circ: 999 (paid).

658 158 GBR ISSN 0268-3946
JOURNAL OF MANAGERIAL PSYCHOLOGY. Text in English. 1986. 8/yr. USD 6,969 in North America; EUR 7,389 in Europe; AUD 8,569 in Australasia; GBP 4,349 in the UK & rest of the world (effective 2002). abstr. back issues avail.; reprint service avail. from SWZ. **Document type:** *Journal, Academic/Scholarly.* **Description:** Offers practical guidance for personnel and training managers. Provides personnel managers with an essential digest of the latest legislation, research and publications affecting their profession.
Related titles: Online - full text ed.: (from Gale Group, EBSCO Publishing, O C L C Online Computer Library Center, Inc., RoweCom Information Quest, ingenta, Swets Blackwell).
Indexed: ABI Inform. (1986-1995), Br.Educ.Ind., ERA, Emerald, Emrld.Intell., Environ.Sci.Poll.Mgmt., Ergon.Abstr., Human Resour.Abstr., Mgmt.& Market.Abstr., Pollut.Abstr., Risk Abstr., SOMA, Saf.Sci.Abstr., Tech.Educ.Abstr., Tr.& Dev.Alert, e-psyche.
—BLDSC (5011.530000). **CCC.**
Published by: Emerald, 60-62 Toller Ln, Bradford, W Yorks BD8 9BY, United Kingdom. TEL 44-1274-777700, FAX 44-1274-785200, info@emeraldinsight.com, http://www.emeraldinsight.com/jmp.htm, http://www.emeraldinsight.com/journals/. Ed. Yochanan Altman.

JOURNAL OF NURSING MANAGEMENT. see *MEDICAL SCIENCES—Nurses And Nursing*

JOURNAL OF PHARMACEUTICAL MARKETING AND MANAGEMENT. see *PHARMACY AND PHARMACOLOGY*

JOURNAL OF PUBLIC HEALTH MANAGEMENT AND PRACTICE. see *PUBLIC HEALTH AND SAFETY*

JOURNAL OF RISK AND UNCERTAINTY. see *BUSINESS AND ECONOMICS—Economic Systems And Theories, Economic History*

KWALITEIT IN BEELD. see *HEALTH FACILITIES AND ADMINISTRATION*

658 USA ISSN 1048-9843
HD57.7 CODEN: LEQUEN
THE LEADERSHIP QUARTERLY; an international journal of political, social and behavioral science. Text in English. 1990. q. EUR 106 in Europe to individuals; JPY 14,000 in Japan to individuals; USD 118 elsewhere to individuals; EUR 295 in Europe to institutions; JPY 39,200 in Japan to institutions; USD 330 elsewhere to institutions (effective 2002). bk.rev. back issues avail. *Refereed.* **Document type:** *Academic/Scholarly.* **Description:** Publishes timely leadership research and applications.
Related titles: Microform ed.: (from PQC); Online - full text ed.: (from ingenta, ScienceDirect, Institute for Scientific Information).
Indexed: ABI Inform. (Win.1997-), ASCA, Curr.Cont., Emerald, Lang.& Lang.Behav.Abstr., PsycInfo, Psychol.Abstr. (1990-), SOPODA, SSCI, Soc.Serv.Abstr., Sociol.Abstr., e-psyche.
—BLDSC (5162.866600), Infotrieve. **CCC.**
Published by: Elsevier Science, PO Box 945, New York, NY 10159-0945. TEL 212-989-5800, FAX 212-633-3990, usinfo-f@elsevier.com, http://www.elsevier.com/locate/leader. Eds. Bernard M Bass, J G Hunt. **Subscr. in Australasia and the Far East to:** Elsevier Science (Singapore) Pte Ltd, No.1 Temasek Ave, 17-01 Millenia Tower, Singapore 039192, Singapore. TEL 65-434-3727, FAX 65-337-2230; **Subscr. in Japan to:** Elsevier Science Inc - Japan Regional Office, 9-15 Higashi-Azabu 1-chome, Minato-ku, Tokyo 106-0044, Japan. TEL 81-3-5561-5033, FAX 81-3-5561-5047; **Subscr. outside the Americas to:** Elsevier Science BV, PO Box 211, Amsterdam 1000 AE, Netherlands. TEL 31-20-485-3757, FAX 31-20-485-3432, nlinfo-f@elsevier.nl.

MANAGED DENTAL CARE. see *MEDICAL SCIENCES—Dentistry*

MANAGEMENT UND KRANKENHAUS; Informationsdienst fuer alle Fuehrungskraefte im Krankenhaus. see *HEALTH FACILITIES AND ADMINISTRATION*

MARKET PROFILES FOR MEDICARE RISK CONTRACTING. see *HEALTH FACILITIES AND ADMINISTRATION*

MASSACHUSETTS PSYCHOLOGIST. see *PSYCHOLOGY*

MEDICAL BUSINESS GULF COAST EDITION. see *MEDICAL SCIENCES*

658 330.9 610 USA
MEDICAL BUSINESS REVIEW* ; medical business analysis for the doctor-executive. Text in English. 1981. m. USD 144. bk.rev. back issues avail.
Published by: Cast, Hursh & Associates, 4401 Taylor Rd, Fort Wayne, IN 46804-1913. TEL 219-436-3036. Ed. William Cast. Circ: 2,000.

658 USA ISSN 1052-4894
MEDICAL OFFICE MANAGER; the newsletter for physician office administrators. Text in English. 1987. m. USD 217 (effective 2001). bk.rev. index. back issues avail. **Document type:** *Newsletter.* **Description:** Covers issues and regulations affecting the management of medical practices.
Published by: Ardmore Publishing Company, PO Box 52843, Atlanta, GA 30355. TEL 404-367-1991, FAX 404-367-1995. Ed., Pub., R&P Susan Crawford. Circ: 4,200 (paid and controlled).

MEDICAL OFFICE STAFF MANAGEMENT STRATEGIES. see *HEALTH FACILITIES AND ADMINISTRATION*

658 615 USA
N A C D S ANNUAL REPORT. Text in English. 19??. a. membership. back issues avail. **Document type:** *Directory, Corporate, Trade.* **Description:** Offers information about the association.
Related titles: CD-ROM ed.; Online - full text ed.
Published by: National Association of Chain Drug Stores, 413 N Lee St, Box 1417 D49, Alexandria, VA 22313-1417. TEL 703-549-3001, FAX 703-836-4869, jcovert@nacds.org, http://www.nacds.org. Ed. John Covert.

658 615 USA ISSN 1079-8641
N A C D S SOURCEBOOK. Text in English. 19??. a. USD 25 to members (effective 1999). **Document type:** *Directory, Bibliography, Trade.* **Description:** Contains listings of boards of pharmacy and publications serving the chain drug store industry.
Related titles: CD-ROM ed.; Online - full text ed.
Published by: National Association of Chain Drug Stores, 413 N Lee St, Box 1417 D49, Alexandria, VA 22313-1417. TEL 703-549-3001, FAX 703-836-4869, jcovert@nacds.org, http://www.nacds.org. Ed. John Covert.

658 615 USA ISSN 1079-1116
NATIONAL ASSOCIATION OF CHAIN DRUG STORES. EXECUTIVE NEWSLETTER. Variant title: N A C D S Executive Newsletter. Text in English. bi-w. USD 100 (effective 1999). **Document type:** *Newsletter.* **Description:** Contains government and pharmacy activities on issues of concern to top level chain drug store executives. Includes member news, as well as activities of the Association.
Published by: National Association of Chain Drug Stores, 413 N Lee St, Box 1417 D49, Alexandria, VA 22313-1417. TEL 703-549-3001, FAX 703-836-4869, jcovert@nacds.org, http://www.nacds.org. Ed. John Covert. Circ: 3,000.

O B G MANAGEMENT. (Obstetrics and Gynecology) see *MEDICAL SCIENCES—Obstetrics And Gynecology*

ORGANIZATION & ENVIRONMENT. see *OCCUPATIONAL HEALTH AND SAFETY*

658 USA ISSN 0749-5978
BF636.A1 CODEN: OBDPFO
ORGANIZATIONAL BEHAVIOR AND HUMAN DECISION PROCESSES; a journal of fundamental research and theory in applied psychology. Text in English. 1966. bi-m. USD 1,175 in US & Canada to institutions; USD 1,275 elsewhere to institutions (effective 2001). adv. bibl, charts, stat, illus. Index. back issues avail.; reprints avail. *Refereed.* **Document type:** *Academic/Scholarly.* **Description:** Features articles that describe original empirical research and theoretical developments in all areas of human decision processes and organizational psychology.
Formerly (until 1985): Organizational Behavior and Human Performance (0030-5073)
Related titles: Online - full text ed.: (from EBSCO Publishing, O C L C Online Computer Library Center, Inc., RoweCom Information Quest, ingenta, Gale Group, Swets Blackwell, IDEAL Online Library, Factiva, Institute for Scientific Information).
Indexed: ABI Inform. (Sep.1971-), ASCA, ASSIA, AgeLine, B.P.I. (Apr.1982-Dec.1984), BPIA, Bus.Ind., CINAHL, Commun.Abstr., Cont.Pg.Manage., Curr.Cont., Curr.Ind.Stat., Fam.Ind., IBZ, Ind.Philos., Int.Lab.Doc., Intl.Bibl.Soc.Sci., L.R.I., Lang.& Lang.Behav.Abstr., Mid.East: Abstr.& Ind., PsycInfo, Psychol.Abstr. (1966-), Psycscan A.P., Rel.Ind.One, Rel.Ind.Two, Risk Abstr., Russ.Acad.Sci.Bibl., SCIMP, SOPODA, SSCI, Sociol.Abstr., Tr.& Indus.Ind., e-psyche.
—BLDSC (6290.749000), IDS. **CCC.**
Published by: Academic Press, Inc., Journal Division (Subsidiary of: Harcourt Brace & Company), 525 B St, Ste 1900, San Diego, CA 92101-4495. TEL 619-230-1840, FAX 619-699-6800, apsubs@acad.com, http://www.academicpress.com/obhdp. Ed. Daniel R Ilgen.

658 USA
OTO'S SCOPE✱. Text in English. 1983. 3/yr. membership. **Document type:** *Newsletter.*
Published by: Association of Otolaryngology Administrators, P O Box 503269, Saint Louis, MO 63150-0001. TEL 319-356-2371. Ed. Richard M Harding. Circ: 600.

▼ **PHARMAVOICE.** see *PHARMACY AND PHARMACOLOGY*

330 USA
PHYSICIAN COMPENSATION REPORT. Text in English. m. USD 379 (effective 2001). **Description:** Includes data, benchmarks, and the specifics of hundresds of actual physician pay plans, plus news and strategies that can help medical groups enhance revenues.
Published by: Atlantic Information Services, Inc., 1100 17th St, N W, Ste 300, Washington, DC 20036. Pub. Richard Biehl. **Co-publisher:** Medical Group Management Association.

THE PHYSICIAN'S ADVISORY. see *HEALTH FACILITIES AND ADMINISTRATION*

PHYSICIAN'S MANAGEMENT MANUALS. see *MEDICAL SCIENCES*

PHYSICIAN'S PRACTICE DIGEST. see *MEDICAL SCIENCES*

Q I - T Q M. (Quality Improvement - Total Quality Management) see *HEALTH FACILITIES AND ADMINISTRATION*

628 614 DNK ISSN 0906-270X
RENT I DANMARK. Text in Danish. 1974. 8/yr. DKK 236. adv. bk.rev.
Formerly: Renhold Vedligehold (0900-856X)
Published by: Forlaget Thorsgaard ApS, Holmensvej 5, PO Box 5, Frederikssund 3600, Denmark. TEL 42-31-21-05, FAX 47-38-36-33, post@thorsgaard.dk. Ed. Kim Thorsgaard. Pub. Forlaget Thorsgaard. Adv. contact Erik Hvalsoe. B&W page DKK 13,450, color page DKK 16,450; trim 297 x 210. Circ: 6,350 (controlled).

SAFETY MANAGEMENT. see *OCCUPATIONAL HEALTH AND SAFETY*

658 GBR ISSN 0963-2638
SELECTION AND DEVELOPMENT REVIEW. Text in English. 1984. bi-m. GBP 37, USD 50 (effective 2000). adv. bk.rev. back issues avail. *Refereed.* **Document type:** *Academic/Scholarly.* **Description:** Focuses on selection and development issues for professional people whose job it is to assess other people.
Formerly: Guidance and Assessment Review (0265-1610)
Indexed: e-psyche.
—BLDSC (8235.144870).
Published by: The British Psychological Society, St Andrews House, 48 Princess Rd E, Leicester LE1 7DR, United Kingdom. FAX 44-116-254-8824, mail@bps.org.uk, http://www.bps.org.uk. Eds. John Boddy, Tuvia Melamed. R&P, Adv. contact Lorraine Brookes TEL 44-116-254-9568.

BUSINESS AND ECONOMICS—Marketing And Purchasing

see also ADVERTISING AND PUBLIC RELATIONS

ANALGESICS: THE INTERNATIONAL MARKET. see *PHARMACY AND PHARMACOLOGY*

AUSTRALIAN DENTAL PRACTICE MAGAZINE. see *MEDICAL SCIENCES—Dentistry*

658 USA ISSN 1064-4180
BIOMEDICAL MARKET NEWSLETTER. Text in English. 1991. m. USD 695; USD 790 foreign; USD 995 by email. charts, illus, stat, tr.lit. *Refereed.* **Document type:** *Newsletter.* **Description:** Covers business, financial, regulations and marketing on medical equipment, devices, clinical tests, supplies and instruments worldwide.
Related titles: Online - full text ed.: (from Dow Jones Interactive, Gale Group, Northern Light Technology, Inc.).
Indexed: Bus.& Indus. (Jan.1996-).
Published by: Biomedical Market Newsletter, Inc., 3237 Idaho Pl, Costa Mesa, CA 92626-2207. TEL 714-434-9500, 800-875-8181, FAX 714-434-9755. Pub., R&P David G Anast.

BUSINESS RATIO. PHARMACEUTICAL MANUFACTURERS & DEVELOPERS. see *PHARMACY AND PHARMACOLOGY*

BUSINESS RATIO REPORT: THE MEDICAL EQUIPMENT INDUSTRY; an industry sector analysis. see *MEDICAL SCIENCES*

BUSINESS RATIO. RETAIL AND WHOLESALE CHEMISTS. see *PHARMACY AND PHARMACOLOGY*

BUSINESS RATIO. THE OPTICAL INDUSTRY. see *PHYSICS—Optics*

362 USA ISSN 1529-1863
▼ **C O R HEALTHCARE MARKET STRATEGIST.** Text in English; Summaries in English. 2000. m. USD 266 domestic; USD 278 foreign; USD 35 newsstand/cover (effective 2001). bk.rev., Website rev. abstr, bibl, charts, illus, stat. Index. back issues avail.; reprints avail. **Document type:** *Newsletter, Trade.* **Description:** Covers strategic marketing issues in healthcare organizations.
Formed by the merger of: Healthcare Market Strategist; Healthcare Marketing Abstracts (0891-5016)
Related titles: Online - full content ed.; Online - full text ed.
Published by: C O R Health, LLC, PO Box 50507, Santa Barbara, CA 93150. TEL 805-564-2177, FAX 805-564-2146, info@corhealth.com, http://www.corhealth.com. Ed. Bridget Meaney. Pub. Dean H. Anderson.

COMMUNITY PHARMACY. see *PHARMACY AND PHARMACOLOGY*

368.382 USA ISSN 1073-6816
COMPETITIVE HEALTHCARE MARKET REPORTER. Text in English. 1993. 24/yr. USD 457 (effective 2000). adv. index. back issues avail. **Document type:** *Newsletter.* **Description:** Helps keep readers abreast of this fiercely competitive market. Get the facts and details you'll need on strategic issues, market facts, mergers and acquisitions, economics, network alliances and plan affiliations.
—CCC.
Published by: Managed Care Information Center, 1913 Atlantic Ave, Ste F4, Manasquan, NJ 08736. TEL 888-843-6242, FAX 888-329-6242, mcic@themcic.com, http://www.themcic.com. Ed. Joseph Schmidt. Pub. Robert K Jenkins. R&P Catherine Casavillo. Adv. contact Suzanne Baker.

COUGH AND COLD REMEDIES: THE INTERNATIONAL MARKET. see *PHARMACY AND PHARMACOLOGY*

D & A. see *MEDICAL SCIENCES—Orthopedics And Traumatology*

DIGESTIVE REMEDIES: THE INTERNATIONAL MARKET. see *PHARMACY AND PHARMACOLOGY*

EVALUATING YOUR FIRM'S INJURY & ILLNESS RECORD. WHOLESALE & RETAIL TRADE INDUSTRIES. see *OCCUPATIONAL HEALTH AND SAFETY*

EXCERPTA MEDICA. SECTION 36: HEALTH POLICY, ECONOMICS AND MANAGEMENT. see *HEALTH FACILITIES AND ADMINISTRATION—Abstracting, Bibliographies, Statistics*

EYEWEAR: THE INTERNATIONAL MARKET. see *MEDICAL SCIENCES—Orthopedics And Traumatology*

658 615 USA
FAMILY ALMANAC. Text in English. 1915. a. free at participating pharmacies. illus. **Document type:** *Consumer.*
Former titles: N A R D Almanac and Health Guide; N A R D Almanac
Published by: Creative Publishing, 1608 South Dakota Ave, Sioux Falls, SD 57105. TEL 605-336-9434, 800-423-7158, FAX 605-338-3501, kal1303567@aol.com. Ed. Ken Alvine. Circ: 125,000 (controlled).

HEALTHCARE MARKETER'S EXECUTIVE BRIEFING. see *MEDICAL SCIENCES*

HOMECARE MONDAY. see *MEDICAL SCIENCES—Nurses And Nursing*

INNOVATIVE LEADER (ONLINE); monthly tool to increase creativity and productivity. see *BUSINESS AND ECONOMICS—Management*

▼ **INTERNATIONAL JOURNAL OF MEDICAL MARKETING;** facilitating excellence in device, diagnostic and pharmaceutical marketing. see *PHARMACY AND PHARMACOLOGY*

658 USA ISSN 0899-8620
JOURNAL OF CONSUMER SATISFACTION, DISSATISFACTION AND COMPLAINING BEHAVIOR. Variant title: C S - D & C B. Text in English. 1988. a. USD 15 domestic; USD 18 foreign (effective 2000 & 2001). 2 cols./p. back issues avail. *Refereed.* **Document type:** *Journal, Academic/Scholarly.*
Indexed: Ind.S.A.Per., e-psyche.
—BLDSC (4965.216000), ingenta.
Published by: Consumer Satisfaction, Dissatisfaction and Complaining Behavior, Inc., Marriott School of Management, 632 TNRB, Brigham Young University, Provo, UT 84602. FAX 801-226-7650, hkhunt@byu.edu, http://www.csdcb.org. Ed. H Keith Hunt.

658.8 150 NLD ISSN 0167-4870
HB74.P8
THE JOURNAL OF ECONOMIC PSYCHOLOGY. Text in English. 1981. bi-m. EUR 145 in Europe to individuals; JPY 19,200 in Japan to individuals; USD 163 elsewhere to individuals; EUR 402 in Europe to institutions; JPY 53,300 in Japan to institutions; USD 450 elsewhere to institutions (effective 2002). adv. index. back issues avail.; reprint service avail. from SWZ. *Refereed.* **Document type:** *Academic/Scholarly.* **Description:** Presents research on behavioral, especially socio-psychological, aspects of economic phenomena and processes.
Related titles: Microform ed.: (from PQC); Online - full text ed.: (from ingenta, Gale Group, ScienceDirect, Swets Blackwell, Factiva, Institute for Scientific Information).

Indexed: ABI Inform. (Dec.1984-), ASCA, BPIA, C.R.E.J., Curr.Cont., Emerald, Fam.Ind., Food Sci.& Tech.Abstr., HRIS, Indian Psychol.Abstr., Intl.Bibl.Soc.Sci., J.of Econ.Lit., Manage.Cont., PSI, Polit.Sci.Abstr., PsycInfo, Psychol.Abstr. (1981-), Russ.Acad.Sci.Bibl., SSCI, Tr.& Indus.Ind., e-psyche.
—BLDSC (4973.054100), IDS, ingenta. **CCC.**
Published by: (Society "European Research in Economic Psychology"), North-Holland (Subsidiary of: Elsevier Science BV), PO Box 211, Amsterdam 1000 AE, Netherlands. TEL 31-20-485-3911, FAX 31-20-485-3598, http://www.elsevier.nl/locate/joep. Eds. P Earl, S E G Lea. **Subscr. in Australasia and the Far East to:** Elsevier Science (Singapore) Pte Ltd, No.1 Temasek Ave, 17-01 Millenia Tower, Singapore 039192, Singapore. TEL 65-434-3727, FAX 65-337-2230; **Subscr. in Japan to:** Elsevier Science Inc - Japan Regional Office, 9-15 Higashi-Azabu 1-chome, Minato-ku, Tokyo 106-0044, Japan. TEL 81-3-5561-5033; **Subscr. in the Americas to:** Elsevier Science, PO Box 945, New York, NY 10159-0945. TEL 212-633-3730, FAX 212-633-3680, usinfo-f@elsevier.com.

658.8 USA
RA965.5
JOURNAL OF HOSPITAL MARKETING & PUBLIC RELATIONS. Text in English. 1987. s-a. USD 75 to individuals; USD 101 in Canada to individuals; USD 109 elsewhere to individuals; USD 150 to institutions; USD 203 in Canada to institutions; USD 218 elsewhere to institutions; USD 325 to libraries; USD 439 in Canada to libraries; USD 471 elsewhere to libraries (effective Aug. 2001). adv. bk.rev. back issues avail.; reprint service avail. from HAW. *Refereed.* **Document type:** *Journal, Academic/Scholarly.* **Description:** Presents new and effective ways of marketing hospital services. Shares current marketing applications and methodologies by professional hospital marketing consultants and educators.
Formerly (until 2001): Journal of Hospital Marketing (0883-7570)
Related titles: Microfiche ed.: (from PQC); Microform ed.
Indexed: CINAHL, Curr.Cont. (coverage dropped), Excerp.Med., Hosp.Lit.Ind., Med.Care Rev.
—EMDOCS, GNLM, Haworth.
Published by: Haworth Press, Inc., 10 Alice St, Binghamton, NY 13904-1580. TEL 607-722-5857, 800-429-6784, FAX 607-722-6362, 800-895-0582, getinfo@haworthpressinc.com, http://www.haworthpress.com/journals/journallist.asp. Ed. Tony Carter. Pub. William Cohen. R&P Ruthann Heath TEL 607-723-5857 ext 316. Adv. contact Jackie Blakeslee TEL 607-722-5857 ext 346. B&W page USD 315, color page USD 550; trim 6 x 8.5. Circ: 380.

658.8 610 615 NGA ISSN 0331-0124
JOURNAL OF MEDICAL AND PHARMACEUTICAL MARKETING. Text in English. 1972. bi-m. USD 115.20. adv. illus.
Related titles: Online - full text ed.
Indexed: I.P.A.
Published by: Fred Atoki Publishing Co. Ltd., Plot 25 Kekere-Ekun St., Orile-Iganmu, PO Box 7313, Lagos, Nigeria. Circ: 16,000.

JOURNAL OF PHARMACEUTICAL MARKETING AND MANAGEMENT. see *PHARMACY AND PHARMACOLOGY*

KEY NOTE MARKET REVIEW: U K PHARMACEUTICAL INDUSTRY. see *PHARMACY AND PHARMACOLOGY*

L M S; new developments in laboratory equipment. (Laboratory Marketing Spectrum) see *MEDICAL SCIENCES—Experimental Medicine, Laboratory Technique*

M P R EXCHANGE. see *HEALTH FACILITIES AND ADMINISTRATION*

THE MARKET FOR O T C HEALTHCARE IN ASIA. (Over the Counter) see *PHARMACY AND PHARMACOLOGY*

THE MARKET FOR O T C HEALTHCARE IN CHINA AND HONG KONG. (Over the Counter) see *PHARMACY AND PHARMACOLOGY*

THE MARKET FOR O T C HEALTHCARE IN EASTERN EUROPE. (Over the Counter) see *PHARMACY AND PHARMACOLOGY*

THE MARKET FOR O T C HEALTHCARE IN LATIN AMERICA. (Over the Counter) see *PHARMACY AND PHARMACOLOGY*

▼ **THE MARKET FOR O T C HEALTHCARE IN WESTERN EUROPE.** (Over the Counter) see *PHARMACY AND PHARMACOLOGY*

658.8 613.7 USA ISSN 1094-1304
RA410.A1
MARKETING HEALTH SERVICES. Text in English. 1981. q. USD 70 domestic to individuals; USD 90 foreign to individuals; USD 90 domestic to institutions; USD 110 foreign to institutions; USD 45 to members (effective 2000). adv. bk.rev. abstr, bibl, charts, illus, stat. index. back issues avail.; reprint service avail. from PQC. **Document type:** *Academic/Scholarly.* **Description:** Geared to meet the needs of health care marketers with articles from professionals on provocative and relevant topics.
Formerly (until 1996): Journal of Health Care Marketing (0737-3252)
Related titles: Microfiche ed.: (from MIM,PQC); Online - full text ed.: (from LexisNexis, H. W. Wilson, Northern Light Technology, Inc., ProQuest Information & Learning, Gale Group, Factiva, Institute for Scientific Information).
Indexed: ABI Inform. (Fall 1983-), B.P.I. (Mar.1997-), Curr.Cont., Excerp.Med., Int.Nurs.Ind., P.A.I.S.
—BLDSC (5381.645800), EMDOCS, GNLM, IDS, Infotrieve, ingenta, KNAW. **CCC.**
Published by: American Marketing Association, 311 S Wacker Dr, Ste 5800, Chicago, IL 60606. TEL 312-542-9000, 800-262-1150, FAX 312-542-9001, info@ama.org, http://www.ama.org. Ed. Chris Brennan. R&P Rochelle Amos TEL 312-542-9022. Adv. contact Richard Ballschmiede. Circ: 4,000.

MARKETING RESULTS; vakblad voor verkopers van drogisterijartikelen. see *PHARMACY AND PHARMACOLOGY*

658.8 615.19 USA ISSN 1067-733X
MED AD NEWS. Text in English. 1982. m. USD 150 in United States; USD 270 elsewhere (effective 1999). adv. charts, illus, stat. back issues avail. *Refereed.* **Document type:** *Trade.*
Formerly: Medical Advertising News (0745-0907)
Related titles: Online - full text ed.: (from Northern Light Technology, Inc., Gale Group, Factiva).
Indexed: Bus.& Indus. (Jan.1995-).
—BLDSC (5424.621800). **CCC.**
Published by: Engel Publishing Partners, 820 Bear Tavern Rd, W, Trenton, NJ 08628. TEL 609-530-0044, FAX 609-530-1274, www@engelpub.com. Ed. Styli Engel. Pub., Adv. contact Lisa Banket. R&P Miriam Rodriguez. Circ: 3,000 (paid); 10,000 (controlled).

MEDICAL MARKETING & MEDIA. see *PHARMACY AND PHARMACOLOGY*

659.1 USA ISSN 1054-3066
MEDICAL NEWS REPORT. Text in English. 1991. m. USD 150. **Document type:** *Newsletter.* **Description:** Aimed at health care public relations professionals; reports on crisis communications, medical topics making news, media relations, and public relations management.
Published by: Standish Publishing Co., PO Box 335, Ardmore, PA 19003. TEL 610-519-9220, FAX 610-519-9221. Ed. Kim Standish. Circ: 500 (paid).

MEDICAL PRODUCTS SALES. see *MEDICAL SCIENCES*

MEDICATED SKINCARE: THE INTERNATIONAL MARKET. see *PHARMACY AND PHARMACOLOGY*

MEDISTAT. see *INSTRUMENTS*

N A P W NEWS/N V F G NUUS. see *PHARMACY AND PHARMACOLOGY*

613.2 USA ISSN 0164-338X
CODEN: NFMEEI
NATURAL FOODS MERCHANDISER; new ideas, trends, products for the natural and organic foods industry. Text in English. 1979. 12/yr. USD 95 domestic; USD 110 in Canada; USD 125 elsewhere; USD 15 newsstand/cover (effective 2000). adv. bk.rev. charts, illus, mkt, pat, stat, tr.lit. back issues avail. *Refereed.* **Document type:** *Magazine, Trade.* **Description:** Provides information to companies involved in the development, marketing, sales and distribution of natural and organic products and dietary supplements.
Related titles: Online - full text ed.
Indexed: Bus.& Indus. (Jun.1996-).
Published by: New Hope Natural Media (Subsidiary of: Penton Media, Inc.), 1401 Pearl St, Boulder, CO 80302. TEL 303-939-8440, http://www.healthwell.com. adv.: B&W page USD 5,150, color page USD 8,060; trim 10.75 x 14.75. Circ: 500 (paid); 15,000 (controlled).

NATURAL PRODUCTS INDUSTRY INSIDER. see *NUTRITION AND DIETETICS*

NEW PRODUCT REVIEW. see *NUTRITION AND DIETETICS*

O T C BUSINESS NEWS. see *PHARMACY AND PHARMACOLOGY*

O T C HEALTHCARE: A WORLD SURVEY. (Over The Counter) see *PHARMACY AND PHARMACOLOGY*

PHARMA BUSINESS; the international magazine of pharmaceutical business and marketing. see *PHARMACY AND PHARMACOLOGY*

658 659.1 DEU ISSN 0721-5665
PHARMA-MARKETING JOURNAL. Text in German. 1976. bi-m. DEM 135 (effective 2001). adv. bk.rev. 36 p./no. **Document type:** *Journal, Trade.*
—GNLM.
Published by: I F A M Institut, Kaiser-Wilhelm-Ring 43, Duesseldorf 40545, Germany. TEL 49-211-55986-0, FAX 49-211-575043, info@ifam-online.de. Ed. Malte W Wilkes. Adv. contact Uwe Rothstein. Circ: 1,100.

PHARMACEUTICAL MARKETERS DIRECTORY. see *PHARMACY AND PHARMACOLOGY*

PHARMACIES AND DRUGSTORES: A WORLD SURVEY. see *PHARMACY AND PHARMACOLOGY*

PHARMACY RETAILER. see *PHARMACY AND PHARMACOLOGY*

PRACTICE BUILDERS. see *ADVERTISING AND PUBLIC RELATIONS*

PRODUCT ALERT. see *FOOD AND FOOD INDUSTRIES*

659.1 615 USA ISSN 1078-6937
HF5415.15
PRODUCT MANAGEMENT TODAY. Text in English. 1990. m. USD 45. adv. **Document type:** *Trade.* **Description:** Covers marketing, product management, managed care marketing and career development issues affecting the product management team, service healthcare manufacturers and service sector companies.
—CCC.
Published by: Product Management Today, Inc., 28 Jones Ave, Flourtown, PA 19031. TEL 215-233-9384, FAX 215-233-9320. Ed. Peter Ciszewski. Pub. Thomas Lyons Drake. Circ: 9,600 (controlled).

PSYCHOLOGY & MARKETING. see *PSYCHOLOGY*

RECRUITMENT, RETENTION & RESTRUCTURING REPORT; strategies for recruiters, managers, R&R committees, & human resource directors. see *MEDICAL SCIENCES—Nurses And Nursing*

RETAIL NEWS. see *PHARMACY AND PHARMACOLOGY*

658 USA ISSN 0749-5153
STRATEGIC HEALTH CARE MARKETING. Text in English. 1984. m. USD 269 (effective 2001). bk.rev. index. back issues avail. **Document type:** *Newsletter.* **Description:** Covers strategies and techniques in a wide range of service settings - from hospitals to physicians' offices.
—CCC.
Published by: Health Care Communications, 11 Heritage Lane, Box 594, Rye, NY 10580. TEL 914-967-6741, FAX 914-967-3054, healthcomm@aol.com, http://www.strategichealthcare.com. Ed., Pub. Michele von Dambrowski.

THETA MARKET RESEARCH REPORTS. see *MEDICAL SCIENCES*

VETERINARY INDUSTRY NEWSLETTER; reporting on the business of veterinary products and animal health biotech. see *VETERINARY SCIENCE*

VISION MONDAY. see *MEDICAL SCIENCES—Ophthalmology And Optometry*

VITAMINS & DIETARY SUPPLEMENTS: THE INTERNATIONAL MARKET. see *PHARMACY AND PHARMACOLOGY*

WORLD HEALTHCARE MARKETING DIRECTORY. see *MEDICAL SCIENCES*

THE WORLD MARKET FOR EYEWEAR. see *MEDICAL SCIENCES—Orthopedics And Traumatology*

▼ **THE WORLD MARKET FOR O T C HEALTHCARE.** (Over the Counter) see *PHARMACY AND PHARMACOLOGY*

THE WORLD MARKET FOR ORAL HYGIENE. see *BEAUTY CULTURE*

THE WORLD MARKET FOR SKIN CARE AND SUN CARE. see *BEAUTY CULTURE*

BUSINESS AND ECONOMICS—Office Equipment And Services

651.3 331.8 DNK ISSN 0903-7497
LAEGESEKRETAER NYT. Text in Danish. 1968. 11/yr. adv.
Published by: Dansk Laegesekretaerforening - H K, H C Andersens Boulevard 50, Copenhagen V 1780, Denmark. TEL 45-33-30-43-43, FAX 45-33-30-44-49, www.dl-hk.dk. Ed. Niels Stoktoft Overgaard. adv.: color page DKK 6,600; 175 x 245. Circ: 9,600.

651.3 SWE ISSN 0345-746X
LAEKARSEKRETERAREN. Text in Swedish. 1964. 10/yr. SEK 300 (effective 2000). **Document type:** *Trade.*
Published by: Sveriges Laekarsekreterarfoerbund (LSF), Sandsjoen 48, Lockryd, Svenljunga 51291, Sweden. TEL 46-33-280566, FAX 46-33-280505, http://www.lakarsekreterarforbundet.a.se. Ed. Ewalena Sternfeldt.

BUSINESS AND ECONOMICS—Personnel Management

ABHIGYAN; the journal of foundation for organization research and education. see *SOCIAL SCIENCES: COMPREHENSIVE WORKS*

APPLIED H.R.M. RESEARCH. (Human Resources Management) see *PSYCHOLOGY*

658.3 USA
BENEFITS GUIDE. Text in English. base vol. plus bi-m. updates (and m. newsletter). USD 340 (effective 1998). **Document type:** *Trade.* **Description:** Provides current information that deals with managed care (for AIDS and other catastrophic diseases), flexible benefits, cafeteria plans, family leave, COBRA, health care, continuation coverage and retiree health benefits. Includes federal and state laws.
Formerly: Managing Employee Benefits (1057-3364)
Published by: Warren, Gorham and Lamont, 395 Hudson St, New York, NY 10014. TEL 212-367-6300, FAX 212-367-6718, http://www.InsideHR.com. Ed. Martin Censor. **Subscr. to:** The Park Square Bldg., 31 St James Ave, Boston, MA 02116-4112. TEL 800-950-1207.

658.3 GBR
BLUEPRINT (NOTTINGHAM). Text in English. 1970. 10/yr. free to current employees. back issues avail. **Description:** Informs employees of Boots The Chemests in the UK and overseas.
Formerly (until 1995): Boots Company News
Published by: Boots The Chemests, 1 Thane Rd W., Nottingham NG2 3AA, United Kingdom. TEL 44-115-959-2365, FAX 44-115-959-5684. Ed., R&P David Shelton. Circ: 32,000 (controlled).

364 USA ISSN 1055-6281
DRUG DETECTION REPORT; the newsletter on drug testing in the workplace. Text in English. 1991. bi-w. USD 310; USD 326 out of North America (effective 2000). **Document type:** *Newsletter.* **Description:** Provides information to help protect companies and employees with coverage of key issues surrounding drug and alcohol testing in the workplace.
Related titles: E-mail ed.; Online - full text ed.: (from Gale Group, Northern Light Technology, Inc., Factiva).
Published by: Business Publishers, Inc., 8737 Colesville Rd, 11th Fl, Silver Spring, MD 20910-3928. TEL 301-587-6300, 800-274-6737, FAX 301-589-8493, bpinews@bpinews.com, http://www.bpinews.com. Ed. Beth McConnell. Pub. Leonard A Eiserer.

658.3 157.6 USA ISSN 0749-0003
HF5549.5.A4
EMPLOYEE ASSISTANCE QUARTERLY. Text in English. 1985. q. USD 75 to individuals; USD 101 in Canada to individuals; USD 109 elsewhere to individuals; USD 150 to institutions; USD 203 in Canada to institutions; USD 218 elsewhere to institutions; USD 450 to libraries; USD 608 in Canada to libraries; USD 653 elsewhere to libraries (effective Aug. 2001). adv. bk.rev. illus. back issues avail.; reprint service avail. from HAW. *Refereed.* **Document type:** *Journal, Academic/Scholarly.* **Description:** Covers development of scholarly and research literature regarding work-based alcoholism programs and the employee assistance movement.
Formerly (until 1985): Labor Management Alcoholism Journal
Related titles: Microfiche ed.: (from PQC); Microform ed.
Indexed: Excerp.Med., Human Resour.Abstr., IBZ, IMFL, Lang.& Lang.Behav.Abstr., P.A.I.S., Peace Res.Abstr., PsycInfo, Psychol.Abstr. (1985-), Ref.Zh., SOPODA, Sage Urb.Stud.Abstr., Soc.Serv.Abstr., Soc.Work Res.& Abstr., Sociol.Abstr., Viol.& Abuse Abstr., e-psyche. —BLDSC (3737.032400), EMDOCS, Haworth, ingenta.
Published by: Haworth Press, Inc., 10 Alice St, Binghamton, NY 13904-1580. TEL 607-722-5857, 800-429-6784, FAX 607-722-6362, 800-895-0582, getinfo@haworthpressinc.com, http://www.haworthpress.com/journals/journallist.asp. Ed. Keith McClellan. Pub. William Cohen. R&P Ruthann Heath TEL 607-723-5857 ext 316. Adv. contact Jackie Blakeslee TEL 607-722-5857 ext 346. B&W page USD 315, color page USD 550; trim 6 x 8.5. Circ: 1,080.

658.3 158 USA ISSN 1097-6221
EMPLOYEE ASSISTANCE REPORT; supporting EAP and HR professionals. Text in English. m. USD 189 (effective 2000). **Document type:** *Newsletter.* **Description:** Offers employee-assistance and human-resources professionals tips on how to best serve company employees. Covers relevant issues and developments in the field.
Indexed: e-psyche.
Published by: Impact Publications, Inc., E3430 Mountain View Lane, Box 322, Waupaca, WI 54981. TEL 715-258-2448, FAX 715-258-9048, impact@gglbbs.com, http://www.gglbbs.com/impact. Ed. Karen Kolpien. Pub., R&P Scott Kolpien.

658.3 362.128 USA ISSN 0889-5422
KF3457.3.A15
EMPLOYEE TESTING & THE LAW; reporting legal, technical, and business developments in employee testing. Text in English. 1986. m. USD 295. bk.rev. index. back issues avail. **Description:** Covers legal and business issues involved in polygraphs, paper and pencil, drug and AIDS testing.
Related titles: Microform ed.: (from PQC).
Indexed: CJPI, e-psyche.
Published by: Vanguard Information Publications, PO Box 667, Chapel Hill, NC 27514. TEL 919-967-2420, FAX 919-967-6294. Ed. Ted Shults. Circ: 2,000.

THE EXECUTIVE REPORT ON MANAGED CARE. see *INSURANCE*

EXECUTIVE REPORT ON PHYSICIAN ORGANIZATIONS. see *INSURANCE*

F & W - FUEHREN UND WIRTSCHAFTEN IM KRANKENHAUS. see *HEALTH FACILITIES AND ADMINISTRATION*

658.3 USA
H R PRACTITIONERS GUIDE. Text in English. m.
Media: CD-ROM.
Published by: The Bureau of National Affairs, Inc., 1231 25th St, N W, Washington, DC 20037. TEL 800-372-1033, http://www.bna.com. **Subscr. to:** 9435 Key West Ave, Rockville, MD 20850.

HOME HEALTH EXECUTIVE COMPENSATION REPORT. see *HEALTH FACILITIES AND ADMINISTRATION*

HOSPITAL AND HEALTH CARE REPORT. see *HEALTH FACILITIES AND ADMINISTRATION*

HUMAN RESOURCES MANAGEMENT - O S H A COMPLIANCE. see *OCCUPATIONAL HEALTH AND SAFETY*

INTAND NEWSLETTER; the newsletter of the international network for transactional analysis, neuro-linguistic programming. see *PSYCHOLOGY*

658.3 USA ISSN 0749-2685
HD69.C6
INTERNATIONAL REGISTRY OF ORGANIZATION DEVELOPMENT PROFESSIONALS AND ORGANIZATION DEVELOPMENT HANDBOOK. Text in English. 1973. a. USD 25 (effective 2000). **Document type:** *Directory.* **Description:** Lists over 400 pages of member's credentials, criteria for becoming a registered O.D. professional, descriptions of all O.D. and O.B. academic programs, O.D. networks and the O.D. international code of ethics, a statement on the knowledge and skill necessary to be competent in the field, and a variety of additional information.
Published by: Organization Development Institute, 11234 Walnut Ridge Rd, Chesterland, OH 44026. TEL 440-729-7419, donwcole@aol.com, http://members.aol.com/odinst. Ed. Donald W Cole. Circ: 500.

658.3 USA ISSN 1057-5073
HG9395
JOURNAL OF HEALTH CARE BENEFITS. Text in English. 1991. bi-m. USD 131.98; USD 207.75 foreign. **Document type:** *Trade.* **Description:** Provides strategies for designing health care plans effectively and economically.
—Infotrieve. **CCC.**
Published by: Warren, Gorham and Lamont, 395 Hudson St, New York, NY 10014. TEL 212-367-6300, FAX 212-367-6718. Eds. Jeffrey D Mamorsky, Joseph W Duva. **Subscr. to:** The Park Square Bldg., 31 St James Ave, Boston, MA 02116-4112. TEL 800-950-1207.

JOURNAL OF MULTICULTURAL COUNSELING AND DEVELOPMENT. see *PSYCHOLOGY*

JOURNAL OF ORGANIZATIONAL BEHAVIOR MANAGEMENT. see *PSYCHOLOGY*

658.3 150 DEU
ORGANISATIONSBERATUNG, SUPERVISION, COACHING. Text in German. 1994. q. EUR 50 domestic; EUR 53.50 foreign; EUR 38.75 domestic to students; EUR 42.25 foreign to students; EUR 12.50 newsstand/cover (effective 2002). **Document type:** *Journal, Academic/Scholarly.*
Formerly: Organisationsberatung, Supervision, Clinical Management (0946-9834)
Indexed: IBZ, e-psyche.
Published by: Verlag Leske und Budrich GmbH, Postfach 300551, Leverkusen 51334, Germany. TEL 49-2171-4907-0, FAX 49-2171-4907-11, leske-budrich@t-online.de, http://www.leske-budrich.de.

PERSONNEL PSYCHOLOGY. see *PSYCHOLOGY*

658.3 DEU
R K W KONTAKT. Text in German. 1955. bi-m. free to members. bk.rev. **Document type:** *Newsletter, Trade.*
Published by: Rationalisierungs- und Innovationszentrum der Deutschen Wirtschaft e.V., Landesgruppe Bayern, Gustav-Heinemann-Ring 212, Munich 81739, Germany. TEL 49-89-670040-0, FAX 49-89-67004040, info@rkw-bayern.de, http://www.rkw-bayern.de. Ed. Rudolf Donnert. Circ: 2,500.

WORK AND STRESS. see *PSYCHOLOGY*

658.3 346 USA
WORKER'S COMPENSATION GUIDE. Text in English. base vol. plus s-a. updates. USD 180. **Document type:** *Trade.* **Description:** Serves as a resource of ideas and techniques for reducing worker's compensation costs. Includes federal regulations and state compensation laws.
Published by: Warren, Gorham and Lamont, 395 Hudson St, New York, NY 10014. TEL 212-367-6300, FAX 212-367-6718, http://www.InsideHR.com. Ed. Steve Levinson. **Subscr. to:** The Park Square Bldg., 31 St James Ave, Boston, MA 02116-4112. TEL 800-950-1207.

WORKLIFE REPORT. see *BUSINESS AND ECONOMICS—Labor And Industrial Relations*

WORKSITE WELLNESS WORKS. see *PUBLIC HEALTH AND SAFETY*

BUSINESS AND ECONOMICS—Production Of Goods And Services

BAYER ALKALIZER. see *BIOLOGY*

CLEANER PRODUCTION. see *OCCUPATIONAL HEALTH AND SAFETY*

338.473621 GBR ISSN 1356-9007
ECONOMICS, MEDICINES, & HEALTH. Text in English. 1994. irreg. (1-2/yr.). GBP 37.50; GBP 9.50 newsstand/cover. adv. charts, illus. back issues avail. **Document type:** *Academic/Scholarly.* **Description:** Analyses, reviews, and explains the economics and politics of health care. For pharmaceutical executives, pharmacists, general practitioners, and National Health Service medical directors, advisors, and executives.
Published by: Catalyst Healthcare Communications, The Folly, Pinner Hill Rd, Pinner, Mddx HA5 3YQ, United Kingdom. TEL 44-1233-266-2623, FAX 44-181-429-0112, catalyst@dial.pipex.com. Ed. Mark Greener. Pub., Adv. contact Dr. Julian Guest. page USD 1,425; 210 x 297. Circ: 3,000.

F D C CONTROL NEWSLETTER. (Food, Drug, and Cosmetics) see *FOOD AND FOOD INDUSTRIES*

F T BIOTECHNOLOGY & PHARMACEUTICAL COMPANIES DATABASE CD-ROM (YEARS). (Financial Times) see *BIOLOGY—Biotechnology*

FOOD AND DRUG LETTER. see *PHARMACY AND PHARMACOLOGY*

THE I E A JOURNAL OF ERGONOMICS. see *ENGINEERING*

LIFE SCIENCE TODAY. see *PHARMACY AND PHARMACOLOGY*

THE MARKET FOR O T C HEALTHCARE IN ASIA. (Over the Counter) see *PHARMACY AND PHARMACOLOGY*

THE MARKET FOR O T C HEALTHCARE IN CHINA AND HONG KONG. (Over the Counter) see *PHARMACY AND PHARMACOLOGY*

THE MARKET FOR O T C HEALTHCARE IN EASTERN EUROPE. (Over the Counter) see *PHARMACY AND PHARMACOLOGY*

THE MARKET FOR O T C HEALTHCARE IN LATIN AMERICA. (Over the Counter) see *PHARMACY AND PHARMACOLOGY*

▼ **THE MARKET FOR O T C HEALTHCARE IN WESTERN EUROPE.** (Over the Counter) see *PHARMACY AND PHARMACOLOGY*

O T C HEALTHCARE: A WORLD SURVEY. (Over The Counter) see *PHARMACY AND PHARMACOLOGY*

PHARMACEUTICALS (YEAR): INTERNATIONAL YEARBOOK. see *PHARMACY AND PHARMACOLOGY*

PRODUCT SAFETY LETTER. see *PUBLIC HEALTH AND SAFETY*

REHABILITATION INDUSTRIES CORPORATION. ANNUAL REPORT. see *MEDICAL SCIENCES—Physical Medicine And Rehabilitation*

▼ **THEORETICAL ISSUES IN ERGONOMICS SCIENCE.** see *ENGINEERING*

WASHINGTON DRUG LETTER (WASHINGTON, 1979). see *PHARMACY AND PHARMACOLOGY*

▼ **THE WORLD MARKET FOR O T C HEALTHCARE.** (Over the Counter) see *PHARMACY AND PHARMACOLOGY*

BUSINESS AND ECONOMICS—Public Finance, Taxation

CHARTERED INSTITUTE OF PUBLIC FINANCE AND ACCOUNTANCY. CEMETERIES STATISTICS. ACTUALS. see *PUBLIC HEALTH AND SAFETY—Abstracting, Bibliographies, Statistics*

CHARTERED INSTITUTE OF PUBLIC FINANCE AND ACCOUNTANCY. CREMATORIA STATISTICS. ACTUALS. see *PUBLIC HEALTH AND SAFETY—Abstracting, Bibliographies, Statistics*

CHARTERED INSTITUTE OF PUBLIC FINANCE AND ACCOUNTANCY. ENVIRONMENTAL HEALTH STATISTICS. ACTUALS. see *PUBLIC HEALTH AND SAFETY—Abstracting, Bibliographies, Statistics*

336 ECU
ECUADOR. INSTITUTO NACIONAL DE ESTADISTICA Y CENSOS. CUENTAS NACIONALES DE LA SALUD. Text in Spanish. irreg. **Document type:** *Government.*
Related titles: Diskette ed.
Published by: Instituto Nacional de Estadistica y Censos, Juan Larrea N15-36 y Jose Riofrio, Quito, Ecuador. TEL 593-2-529858, FAX 593-2-509836, inec1@ecnet.ec, http://www.inec.gov.ec.

336.2 USA
▼ **GUIDE TO AUDITING HEALTH CARE BILLING PRACTICES.** Text in English. 1999. base vol. updates 12/yr. USD 321 (effective 2001). **Description:** Includes step-by-step guidance on recognizing problems, auditing components of the billing process, auditing IS billing systems, special billing problems and more.
Published by: Atlantic Information Services, Inc., 1100 17th St, N W, Ste 300, Washington, DC 20036. Ed. Frances Fernald. Pub. Richard Biehl.

HEALTH CARE FINANCING REVIEW. see *MEDICAL SCIENCES*

HEALTH CARE FINANCING REVIEW. SUPPLEMENT. see *PUBLIC HEALTH AND SAFETY*

MEDICAL AND DISABILITY APPEAL TRIBUNALS: THE LEGISLATION. see *SOCIAL SERVICES AND WELFARE*

330 NZL
NEW ZEALAND. STATISTICS NEW ZEALAND. PUBLIC HEALTH FINANCIAL STATISTICS. Text in English. q. stat. **Document type:** *Government.* **Description:** Describes the financial performance and financial position of Hospital and Health Service providers.
Published by: Statistics New Zealand/Te Tari Tatau, PO Box 2922, Wellington, New Zealand. TEL 64-4-495-4600, FAX 64-4-473-2626, info@stats.govt.nz, http://www.stats.govt.nz.

STEUER-BRIEF FUER AERZTE UND ZAHNAERZTE. see *MEDICAL SCIENCES*

BUSINESS AND ECONOMICS—Small Business

RISK MANAGEMENT FOR EXECUTIVE WOMEN. see *INSURANCE*

338 636.089 USA ISSN 0042-4862
VETERINARY ECONOMICS; business solutions for practicing veterinarians. Text in English. 1960. m. USD 42 domestic; USD 59 in Canada & Mexico; USD 83 elsewhere; USD 10 newsstand/cover (effective 2001). adv. bk.rev. charts, illus, stat, tr.lit. index. reprints avail. *Refereed.* **Document type:** *Trade.* **Description:** Covers all aspects of veterinary practice management and finance.
Related titles: Microform ed.: (from PQC); Online - full text ed.: (from Northern Light Technology, Inc., ProQuest Information & Learning, Institute for Scientific Information).
Indexed: ASCA, Account.Ind. (1974-), Focus on: Vet.Sci.& Med., Helminthol.Abstr., Ind.Vet., SRI, Vet.Bull.
—BLDSC (9227.070000), CISTI, IDS, Infotrieve, ingenta. **CCC.**
Published by: Veterinary Medicine Publishing Group (Subsidiary of: Medical Economics Co., Inc.), 15333 W. 95th, Lenexa, KS 66219. TEL 913-492-4300, 800-255-6864, FAX 913-492-4157, ve@vetmedpub.com., http://www.vetmedpub.com/ve/index.html. Ed. Marnette Denell Falley. Pub., R&P Rebecca Turner Chapman. Circ: 50,000.

BUSINESS AND ECONOMICS—Trade And Industrial Directories

A B H I DIRECTORY. see *MEDICAL SCIENCES*

A V M A DIRECTORY. see *VETERINARY SCIENCE*

670.29 FRA
ANNUAIRE FOURNI-LABO PHARMACIE (YEAR); cosmetique et alimentaire. Text in French. a. FRF 460 (effective 1999). index. **Description:** For researchers, technicians, laboratory managers and pharmacy industry executives.
Published by: Moreux, 190 bd. Haussmann, Paris 75008, France. TEL 33-1-44959950, FAX 33-1-49539016, moreux@club-internet.fr.

ANNUARIO DEI FORNITORI DELLA SANITA IN ITALIA. see *HEALTH FACILITIES AND ADMINISTRATION*

681.4029 ITA
ANNUARIO OTTICO ITALIANO. Text in Italian. 1970. a. ITL 150,000 per issue (effective 2001). adv. **Document type:** *Directory.* **Description:** Provides addresses of suppliers and retail sellers of optics, frame, and optical instrument industries in Italy.
Related titles: CD-ROM ed.
Published by: Edizioni Ariminum, Via Negroli, 51, Milan, MI 20133, Italy. TEL 39-02-730091, FAX 39-02-717346, welcome@vedere.it, http://www.vedere.it. adv.: color page XEU 1,300.

ANTIBACTERIAL PRODUCTS AND MARKETS. see *PHARMACY AND PHARMACOLOGY*

610.29 AUS ISSN 1323-0824
AUSTRALIAN HEALTH AND MEDICAL INDUSTRY GUIDE. Text in English. 1992. a. AUD 85 (effective 2000). **Document type:** *Directory.* **Description:** Outlines exporters of Australian health and medical equipment and services. Indicates areas of expertise, contact details, where they export to, etc.
Formerly: Australian Health and Medical Exports
Published by: (Austrade), A P N Business Information Group (Subsidiary of: A P N News & Media Ltd), 46-48 Porter St Prahran, Melburne, VIC 3181, Australia. TEL 61-3-9245-7777, FAX 61-3-9245-7840, info@kompass.com.au, http://www.kompass.com. Circ: 8,000.

▼ **BIOCOMMERCE DATA'S BUSINESS PROFILE SERIES. VOLUME 1: THE U S BIOTECHNOLOGY DIRECTORY.** see *BIOLOGY—Biotechnology*

▼ **BIOCOMMERCE DATA'S BUSINESS PROFILE SERIES. VOLUME 2. THE EUROPEAN BIOTECHNOLOGY DIRECTORY.** see *BIOLOGY—Biotechnology*

▼ **BIOCOMMERCE DATA'S BUSINESS PROFILE SERIES. VOLUME 3: THE INTERNATIONAL BIOTECHNOLOGY DIRECTORY.** see *BIOLOGY—Biotechnology*

BIOCOMMERCE DATA'S BUSINESS PROFILE SERIES. VOLUME 4: THE U K BIOTECHNOLOGY DIRECTORY. see *BIOLOGY—Biotechnology*

BUYERS GUIDE FOR THE HEALTH CARE MARKET; a directory of products and service for health care institutions. see *HEALTH FACILITIES AND ADMINISTRATION*

CHEMIST & DRUGGIST DIRECTORY. see *PHARMACY AND PHARMACOLOGY*

613.029 COL ISSN 0121-800X
DIRECTORIO DE PROVEEDORES DE LA SALUD. Text in Spanish. 1992. a. free per issue. adv. **Description:** Lists suppliers for clinics and hospitals.
Published by: Publicar S.A., Ave. 68, 75-A-50 of. 314,, Apartado Aereo 8010, Santa Fe de Bogota, CUND, Colombia. TEL 57-1-225-5555, FAX 57-1-3115645, colombiaexport@publicor.com, http://www.colombiaexport.com. R&P, Adv. contact Jaime Concha. page USD 2,400. Circ: 20,000.

659.1029 GBR
DIRECTORY OF ADVERTISING AGENCIES. Text in English. s-a. GBP 75 newsstand/cover (effective 2000). adv. **Document type:** *Directory, Trade.*
Published by: Pharmaceutical Marketing Limited, Vincent House, Vincent Ln, Dorking, Surrey RH4 3JD, United Kingdom. TEL 44-1306-740777, FAX 44-1306-741069, info@pharmark.co.uk. Ed. Andy Rice. Pub. Mark Savage. R&P Keith Shilson. Adv. contact Zoe Almeida.

660.6029 AUS ISSN 1327-1482
DIRECTORY OF AUSTRALIAN BIOTECHNOLOGY COMPANIES. Text in English. 1989. biennial. AUD 25. adv. back issues avail. **Document type:** *Directory, Trade.* **Description:** Provides full-page company profiles of 38 biotech companies and listings of companies serving the industry.
Formerly: Australian and New Zealand Biotechnology Directory (1032-8068)
Media: Online - full text.
Published by: Australian Biotechnology Association Ltd., PO Box 4, Gardenvale, VIC 3185, Australia. TEL 61-3-95968879, FAX 61-3-95968874, aba@netspace.net.au, http://biotech.isr.gov.au. Eds. Barbara Arnold, Martin Playne. Adv. contact Gary Dolder. Circ: 3,000.

613.029 USA ISSN 1049-9253
DIRECTORY OF HEALTH CARE PROFESSIONALS. Text in English. 1990. a. **Document type:** *Directory.*
Published by: American Hospital Association, One North Franklin, Chicago, IL 60606-3421. TEL 312-422-3395, FAX 312-422-4583.

613.029 USA ISSN 1064-8496
RA971.33
DIRECTORY OF HEALTHCARE GROUP PURCHASING ORGANIZATIONS. Text in English. 1983. a. USD 325 (effective 2000). adv. **Document type:** *Directory.* **Description:** Provides information on over 500 group purchasing organizations.
Related titles: Online - full text ed.: (from The Dialog Corporation).
Published by: Medical Economics Co., Inc., 5 Paragon Dr, Montvale, NJ 07645-1742. TEL 201-358-7657, 800-745-2601, FAX 201-722-2662, mdr@medec.com. Ed. Bill Shaughnessy.

615.1029 USA ISSN 1054-3082
HD9666.3
DIRECTORY OF HIGH VOLUME INDEPENDENT DRUG STORES (YEAR). Text in English. 1992. a. USD 290 (effective 1999). **Document type:** *Directory.* **Description:** Profiles approximately 8,800 one-unit drug retailers and the names and titles of over 16,500 key executives within those companies (including owner, president, head pharmacist and general buyer). Company listings provide sales volume, product lines carried, square footage, indicates computerized Rx, year founded and more.
Related titles: Diskette ed.; Magnetic Tape ed.
Published by: C S G Information Services (Subsidiary of: Lebhar-Friedman, Inc.), 3922 Coconut Palm Dr, Tampa, FL 33619. TEL 813-664-6800, FAX 813-664-6882. Ed. Debbie Scruggs.

362.11029 USA ISSN 0885-9671
RA977
DIRECTORY OF HOSPITAL PERSONNEL. Text in English. 1986. a. USD 275 (effective 2001). **Document type:** *Directory, Trade.*
Related titles: Online - full text ed.: (from The Dialog Corporation).
Published by: Grey House Publishing, 185 Millerton Rd, PO Box 860, Millerton, NY 12546. TEL 518-789-8700, 800-562-2139, FAX 518-789-0556, books@greyhouse.com, http://www.greyhouse.com. Ed. Laura Mars. Pub. Leslie E Mackenzie.

362.11029 GBR ISSN 1472-1945
DIRECTORY OF HOSPITALS AND TRUSTS (YEAR). Text in English. 1987. a. GBP 90; USD 144 in United States. adv. **Document type:** *Directory.* **Description:** Provides an up-to-date reference guide to the key practitioners and professionals in the UK health service.
Former titles (until 2000): Directory of Hospitals and N H S Trusts (Year) (1365-9391); (until 1993): Directory of Hospitals (Year) (0963-6099)
—BLDSC (3593.944200).
Published by: Informa Publishing, 69-77 Paul St, London EC2A 4IQ, United Kingdom. TEL 44-171-553-1000, FAX 44-171-553-1593, liz@pearson-pro.com, http://www.fthealthcare.com.

DIRECTORY OF SURGICAL SPECIALISTS. see *MEDICAL SCIENCES—Surgery*

DIRECTORY OF WORKERS' COMPENSATION MANAGED CARE ORGANIZATIONS. see *LAW—Corporate Law*

THE EUROPEAN HOSPITALS DATABASE ON CD-ROM. see *HEALTH FACILITIES AND ADMINISTRATION*

EXECUTIVE MANAGED CARE DIRECTORY. see *HEALTH FACILITIES AND ADMINISTRATION*

F T BIOTECHNOLOGY & PHARMACEUTICAL COMPANIES DATABASE CD-ROM (YEARS). (Financial Times) see *BIOLOGY—Biotechnology*

615.19029 GBR
FINANCIAL SURVEY. THE PHARMACEUTICAL INDUSTRY. Text in English. a. GBP 249 (effective 2001). charts, stat. **Document type:** *Directory, Trade.* **Description:** Contains financial information and contact data for companies in the industry.
Former titles (until 199?): Financial Survey. Pharmaceutical Manufacturers & Distributors; (until 1991): Financial Survey Company Directory. Pharmaceutical Manufacturers and Distributors (0952-4819)
Related titles: Diskette ed.: GBP 424 (effective 2001).
Published by: The Prospect Shop Ltd., Field House, 72 Oldfield Rd, Hampton, Middx TW12 2HQ, United Kingdom. TEL 44-20-8461-8730, 44-20-8481-8720, FAX 44-20-8783-1940, info@theprospectshop.co.uk.

THE FITZHUGH DIRECTORY OF INDEPENDENT HEALTHCARE AND LONG TERM CARE. FINANCIAL INFORMATION. see *MEDICAL SCIENCES*

GENERAL MEDICAL COUNCIL. MEDICAL REGISTER. see *MEDICAL SCIENCES*

H I D A MANUFACTURERS DIRECTORY. see *MEDICAL SCIENCES*

362.1 USA ISSN 0887-4484
H M O - P P O DIRECTORY. (Health Maintenance Organization - Preferred Provider Organization) Text in English. 1986. a. USD 250; USD 499 print & CD-ROM eds.; USD 495 print & online eds. (effective 2001 & 2002). **Document type:** *Directory, Trade.* **Description:** Provides comprehensive information on over 1,600 health maintenance and preferred provider organizations arranged alphabetically.
Related titles: CD-ROM ed.; Online - full text ed.
Published by: Grey House Publishing, 185 Millerton Rd, PO Box 860, Millerton, NY 12546. TEL 518-789-8700, 800-562-2139, FAX 518-789-0556, books@greyhouse.com, http://www.greyhouse.com. Ed. Laura Mars. Pub. Leslie E Mackenzie.

HANDBUCH FUER DAS GESUNDHEITSWESEN IN SCHLESWIG-HOLSTEIN. see *MEDICAL SCIENCES*

613.029 GBR
HEALTH & SAFETY MARKETGUIDE. Text in English; Summaries in French, German, Italian, Spanish. 1981. a. GBP 45 (effective 2001). adv. back issues avail. **Document type:** *Directory.*
Former titles (until Dec. 2000): European Health & Safety Marketguide (0962-385X); (until 1990): Health and Safety Marketguide (0261-8036)
Published by: Aydee Marketing Ltd., Nithsdale House, 159 Cambridge St, Aylesbury, Bucks HP20 1BQ, United Kingdom. TEL 44-1296-434381, FAX 44-1296-436936, info@aydee.com, http://www.aydee.com. Ed., Pub. Richard Salmon. Adv. contact Muriel Scutt. page GBP 1,195; trim 184 x 260. Circ: 6,000 (paid).

HEALTH DATA DIRECTORY. see *MEDICAL SCIENCES—Computer Applications*

HEALTHCARE FOODSERVICE WHO'S WHO. see *FOOD AND FOOD INDUSTRIES*

362.1 USA
HEALTHCARE GROUP PURCHASING ORGANIZATIONS. Text in English. a. USD 325; USD 650 print & online eds. (effective 2002). **Document type:** *Directory, Trade.* **Description:** Provides comprehensive information on over 550 group healthcare purchasing organizations.
Related titles: Online - full text ed.
Published by: Grey House Publishing, 185 Millerton Rd, PO Box 860, Millerton, NY 12546. TEL 518-789-8700, 800-562-2139, FAX 518-789-0556, books@greyhouse.com, http://www.greyhouse.com. Ed. Laura Mars. Pub. Leslie E Mackenzie.

I N A S P HEALTH DIRECTORY (YEAR). see *MEDICAL SCIENCES*

382.029 USA
INTERNATIONAL DIRECTORY OF DRUGS AND PHARMACEUTICALS IMPORTERS. Text in English. 1978. a., latest 2002. USD 260 for Print or CD-ROM ed.; USD 310 combined subscription for both Print and CD-ROM ed. (effective 2001). **Document type:** *Directory, Trade.* **Description:** Provides information for manufacturers, exporters and trading firms; includes complete name and address; name of contact person; email address; year established; number of employees; telephone and fax numbers, bank reference, as well as a listing of drugs and pharmaceuticals currently being imported. In addition, the directory features a comprehensive classified section where importers are listed by product.
Related titles: CD-ROM ed.
Published by: Interdata, 1741 Kekamek, Poulsbo, WA 98370. TEL 360-779-1511, 800-818-0140, FAX 360-697-4696, interdat@export-leads.com, http://www.importersnet.com/. **Dist. by:** Current Pacific Ltd., PO Box 36-536, Northcote, Auckland, New Zealand. TEL 64-9-480-1388, FAX 64-9-480-1387, info@cplnz.com, http://www.cplnz.com.

382.029 USA
INTERNATIONAL DIRECTORY OF MEDICAL, HOSPITAL AND SURGICAL EQUIPMENT IMPORTERS. Text in English. a., latest 2001. USD 295 for Print or CD-ROM ed.; USD 345 combined subscription for both Print & CD-ROM eds. (effective 2001). **Document type:** *Directory, Trade.* **Description:** Provides information for manufacturers, exporters and trading firms; includes complete name and address; name of contact person; email address; year established; number of employees; telephone and fax numbers, bank reference, as well as a listing of medical, hospital and surgical equipment currently being imported. In addition, the directory features a comprehensive classified section where importers are listed by product.
Related titles: CD-ROM ed.
Published by: Interdata, 1741 Kekamek, Poulsbo, WA 98370. TEL 360-779-1511, 800-818-0140, FAX 360-697-4696, interdat@export-leads.com, http://www.importersnet.com/. **Dist. by:** Current Pacific Ltd., PO Box 36-536, Northcote, Auckland, New Zealand. TEL 64-9-480-1388, FAX 64-9-480-1387, info@cplnz.com, http://www.cplnz.com.

382.029 USA
INTERNATIONAL DIRECTORY OF OPTICAL GOODS AND INSTRUMENTS IMPORTERS. Text in English. 1978. a., latest 2001. USD 220 for Print or CD-ROM ed.; USD 270 combined subscription for both Print & CD-ROM eds. (effective 2001). **Document type:** *Directory, Trade.* **Description:** Provides information for manufacturers, exporters and trading firms; includes complete name and address; name of contact person; email address; year established; number of employees; telephone and fax numbers, bank reference, as well as a listing of optical goods and instruments currently being imported. In addition, the directory features a comprehensive classified section where importers are listed by product.
Related titles: CD-ROM ed.
Published by: Interdata, 1741 Kekamek, Poulsbo, WA 98370. TEL 360-779-1511, 800-818-0140, FAX 360-697-4696, interdat@export-leads.com, http://www.importersnet.com/. **Dist. by:** Current Pacific Ltd., PO Box 36-536, Northcote, Auckland, New Zealand. TEL 64-9-480-1388, FAX 64-9-480-1387, info@cplnz.com, http://www.cplnz.com.

382.029 USA
INTERNATIONAL DIRECTORY OF SAFETY, SECURITY AND FIRE FIGHTING EQUIPMENT IMPORTERS. Text in English. 1978. a., latest 2001. USD 220 for Print or CD-ROM ed.; USD 270 combined subscription for Print & CD-ROM eds. (effective 2001). **Document type:** *Directory, Trade.* **Description:** Provides information for manufacturers, exporters and trading firms; includes complete name and address; name of contact person; email address; year established; number of employees; telephone and fax numbers, bank reference, as well as a listing of safety, security and fire fighting equipment currently being imported. In addition, the directory features a comprehensive classified section where importers are listed by product.
Related titles: CD-ROM ed.
Published by: Interdata, 1741 Kekamek, Poulsbo, WA 98370. TEL 360-779-1511, 800-818-0140, FAX 360-697-4696, interdat@export-leads.com, http://www.importersnet.com/. **Dist. by:** Current Pacific Ltd., PO Box 36-536, Northcote, Auckland, New Zealand. TEL 64-9-480-1388, FAX 64-9-480-1387, info@cplnz.com, http://www.cplnz.com.

INTERNATIONAL MED-TECH DIRECTORY; the international financial guide to over 800 publicly traded healthcare companies. see *MEDICAL SCIENCES*

338.0029 JPN ISSN 1341-6162
IRYO KIKI GYOSHA NENKAN/JAPANESE MEDICAL INDUSTRY DIRECTORY. Text in English, Japanese. 1995. biennial, latest no.6, 2000. USD 50 newsstand/cover (effective 2001). 128 p./no. **Document type:** *Trade.* **Description:** Lists approximately 1,300 medical industry companies operating in Japan: makers, importers, exporters, distributors, associations, etc.
Published by: Genyosha Publications Inc., 4-7 Shibuya 2-chome, Shibuya-ku, Tokyo 150-0002, Japan. TEL 81-3-3407-7521, FAX 81-3-3407-7902, info@genyosha.co.jp, http://www.genyosha.com. Ed., Pub. K Eda. Circ: 7,000.

JAPAN PHARMACEUTICAL REPORT. see *PHARMACY AND PHARMACOLOGY*

670.29 CAN
LABORATORY YELLOW PAGES. Text in English. 1990. a. CND 40. adv. **Document type:** *Directory.*

Published by: Jesmar Communications Inc., 30 E Beaver Creek Rd, Ste 220, Richmond, ON L4B 1J2, Canada. TEL 416-886-5040, FAX 416-886-6615. Ed. Kathleen Hurd. Circ: 32,140.

658.0029 GBR
MAJOR PHARMACEUTICAL COMPANIES OF THE WORLD (YEAR). Text in English. a. GBP 490 (effective 2001). **Document type:** *Directory.* **Description:** Provides essential business profiles for 2,500 of the largest pharmaceutical companies worldwide in the pharmaceutical industry. Over 12,500 named senior executives.
Published by: Graham & Whiteside, Tuition House, 5-6 Francis Grove, London SW19 4DT, United Kingdom. TEL 44-20-8947-1011, FAX 44-20-8947-1163, sales@graham-whiteside.com, http://www.graham-whiteside.com. **Dist. by:** Current Pacific Ltd., PO Box 36-536, Northcote, Auckland, New Zealand. TEL 64-9-480-1388, FAX 64-9-480-1387, info@cplnz.com, http://www.cplnz.com.

MANAGED HEALTH CARE DIRECTORY. see *HEALTH FACILITIES AND ADMINISTRATION*

613.029 TWN
MEDICAL & HEALTH EQUIPMENT BUYERS' GUIDE. Text in English. 1995. s-a. USD 30 per vol. (effective 2001). **Document type:** *Catalog, Trade.* **Description:** Product catalogs and supplier directories for all kinds of medical and health-related equipment and supplies.
Formerly: Taiwan Medical & Health Equipment Buyers' Guide (1025-7799)
Related titles: CD-ROM ed.: USD 20 (effective 2000).
Published by: Trade Winds Inc., No 7 Ln 75, Yung Kang St, Taipei 106, Taiwan. TEL 886-2-2393-2718, FAX 886-2-2395-2901, tradwind@ms2.hinet.net, http://www.medequipb2b.com, http://www.medical-equip-guide.com. Ed. Daniel Foong. Pub. Herbert Chen. R&P Donald Shapiro. Adv. contact Melody Lin TEL 886-2-2351-3180. **Subscr. in US to:** Trade Winds Inc., PO Box 820519, Dallas, TX 75382. TEL 877-861-1188, FAX 972-699-1189, twinds8888@aol.com.

362.1029 USA ISSN 0146-8022
HD9994.U5
MEDICAL AND HEALTHCARE MARKETPLACE GUIDE*. Text in English. 1973. a. USD 670 domestic; USD 745 foreign. adv. **Document type:** *Directory.* **Description:** Profiles approximately 5,500 "high visibility" manufacturers, service organizations, dealers and distributors in the medical and healthcare marketplace. Analyzes over 100 market segments.
Formerly (until 1975): Medical and Healthcare Stock Market Guide (0097-4870)
Related titles: CD-ROM ed.; Online - full text ed.: (from LexisNexis).
Indexed: Bus.& Indus. (1995-).
Published by: Dorland Healthcare Information, 1500 Walnut St Ste 1000, Philadelphia, PA 19102. Circ: 1,000.

MEDICAL PRODUCTS OF JAPAN; medical equipment directory. see *MEDICAL SCIENCES*

N D A PIPELINE. (New Drug Approval) see *PHARMACY AND PHARMACOLOGY*

615.534029 USA
NATIONAL DIRECTORY OF CHIROPRACTIC. Text in English. 1989. a., latest 12th ed. USD 45. adv. **Document type:** *Directory.* **Description:** Provides information on the chiropractic profession: lists providers of chiropractic supplies and services; chiropractic colleges; information on chiropractors; state by state information on licensing, examination, societies and organizations.
Related titles: Diskette ed.
Published by: National Directory of Chiropractic Foundation, PO Box 10056, Olathe, KS 66051. TEL 800-888-7914, FAX 913-780-0658, directory@sprintmail.com, http://www.chirodirectory.com, http://www.nationaldirectoryofchiro.com. Ed., R&P Larry Glavas. Pub. Ross S Trivas. Adv. contact Scott Fletcher. page USD 1,995. Circ: 6,800 (paid); 31,200 (controlled).

(YEAR) NATIONAL DIRECTORY OF FIRE CHIEFS & E M S ADMINISTRATORS. see *FIRE PREVENTION*

380 615 NZL
NEW ZEALAND GAZETTE TRADE LISTS. REGISTER OF PHARMACIES. Text in English. irreg. **Document type:** *Government, Trade.*
Published by: GP Legislation Services, P.O. Box 12418, Thorndon, Wellington, New Zealand. TEL 64-4-496-5655, FAX 64-4-496-5698, http://www.gplegislation.co.nz.

OCCUPATIONAL HEALTH & SAFETY NEWS. see *OCCUPATIONAL HEALTH AND SAFETY*

613.029 GBR
ORGANISATIONS CONCERNED WITH HEALTH AND SAFETY INFORMATION. Text in English. a. **Document type:** *Directory.* **Description:** Contains details of organizations concerned with health and safety and related areas.
Formerly (until 1998): Directory of Organisations Concerned with Health and Safety Information
Published by: Health and Safety Executive, Rose Ct, 2 Southwark Bridge, London SE1 9HS, United Kingdom. TEL 44-1541-545500, FAX 44-114-289-2333, http://www.open.gov.uk/hse/org/org98.htm. Ed. Anne Darvill.

615.1029 JPN
PHARMACEUTICAL MANUFACTURERS OF JAPAN. Text in Japanese. 1981. biennial. JPY 15,000. **Description:** Addresses and research figures of Japanese pharmaceutical companies.
Published by: Yakugyo Jiho Co. Ltd., 2-36 Kanda-Jinbo-cho, Chiyoda-ku, Tokyo 101-0051, Japan.

PHARMACEUTICALS (YEAR): INTERNATIONAL YEARBOOK. see *PHARMACY AND PHARMACOLOGY*

380.1029 USA
PHYSICIANS & SURGEONS DIRECTORY. Text in English. a. USD 695 (effective 2001). back issues avail.
Related titles: CD-ROM ed.; Diskette ed.; E-mail ed.; Fax ed.; Magnetic Tape ed.; Online - full text ed.
Published by: American Business Directories (Subsidiary of: American Business Information, Inc.), 5711 S 86th Circle, Box 27347, Omaha, NE 68127. TEL 888-260-7943, FAX 402-331-5481, karen.peters@infousa.com, http://www.directoriesusa.com.

613.029 USA
PLUNKETT'S HEALTH CARE INDUSTRY ALMANAC. Text in English. 1985. a. USD 199.99 (effective 2001); includes CD-ROM. **Document type:** *Directory, Trade.* **Description:** Complete reference guide to the American health care industry and its leading corporations.
Related titles: CD-ROM ed.
Published by: Plunkett Research, Ltd, PO Drawer 541737, Houston, TX 77254-1737. TEL 713-932-0000, FAX 713-932-7080, info@plunkettresearch.com, http://www.plunkettresearch.com. Ed., Pub. Jack W Plunkett.

658.564029 GBR
TECHNOMARK REGISTER. CONTRACT PACKAGERS & MANUFACTURERS - EUROPE. Text in English. a. GBP 320, USD 576. adv. **Document type:** *Directory.* **Description:** Listing organizations which undertake, as a primary objective, medical, scientific or technical work on a commercial basis involving packaging and manufacturing in the European pharmaceutical and healthcare industries.
Related titles: CD-ROM ed.: GBP 475.
Published by: Technomark Consulting Services Ltd., King House, 5-11 Westbourne Grove, London W2 4UA, United Kingdom. TEL 44-171-229-9239, FAX 44-171-792-2587, info@technomark.com, http://www.technomark.co.uk. Ed. R G Hughes. R&P Marianne Searle. Adv. contact Allan Tappenden.

690.029 GBR
TECHNOMARK REGISTER. CONTRACT RESEARCH ORGANISATIONS - NORTH AMERICA. Text in English. a. GBP 400, USD 720. adv. **Document type:** *Directory.* **Description:** Listing organizations which undertake, as a primary objective, medical, scientific or technical work on a commercial basis in the North American pharmaceutical or healthcare industries.
Published by: Technomark Consulting Services Ltd., King House, 5-11 Westbourne Grove, London W2 4UA, United Kingdom. TEL 44-171-229-9239, info@technomark, http://www.technomark.co.uk. Ed. R G Hughes. R&P Marianne Searle. Adv. contact Allan Tappenden.

615.9029 GBR
TECHNOMARK REGISTER. EUROPEAN CONTRACT RESEARCH ORGANISATIONS. CLINICAL RESEARCH. Text in English. 1988. a. GBP 400 (effective 1999); USD 720. adv. **Document type:** *Directory.* **Description:** Listing organizations which undertake, as a primary objective, medical, scientific or technical work on a commercial basis.
Related titles: CD-ROM ed.: GBP 600, USD 1,080.
Published by: Technomark Consulting Services Ltd., King House, 5-11 Westbourne Grove, London W2 4UA, United Kingdom. TEL 44-171-229-9239, FAX 44-171-792-2587, info@technomark.com, http://www.technomark.co.uk. Ed. R G Hughes. R&P Marianne Searle. Adv. contact Allan Tappenden. Circ: 400.

571.95029 GBR
TECHNOMARK REGISTER. EUROPEAN CONTRACT RESEARCH ORGANISATIONS. TOXICOLOGY & ANALYSIS. Text in English. a. GBP 320, USD 576. adv. **Document type:** *Directory.* **Description:** Listing organizations which undertake, as a primary objective, medical,scientific or technical work on a commercial basis in the pharmaceutical or healthcare industries.
Related titles: CD-ROM ed.: GBP 475.
Published by: Technomark Consulting Services Ltd., King House, 5-11 Westbourne Grove, London W2 4UA, United Kingdom. TEL 44-171-229-9239, FAX 44-171-792-2587, info@technomark.com, http://www.technomark.co.uk. Ed. R G Hughes. R&P Marianne Searle. Adv. contact Allen Tappenden.

WORLD HEALTHCARE MARKETING DIRECTORY. see *MEDICAL SCIENCES*

WORLD PHARMACEUTICAL DIRECTORY. see *PHARMACY AND PHARMACOLOGY*

C

CARDIOVASCULAR DISEASES

see MEDICAL SCIENCES—Cardiovascular Diseases

CERAMICS, GLASS AND POTTERY

see also ART; ARTS AND HANDICRAFTS

CHEMICAL ENGINEERING

see ENGINEERING—Chemical Engineering

CHEMISTRY

see also CHEMISTRY—Analytical Chemistry; CHEMISTRY—Computer Applications; CHEMISTRY—Crystallography; CHEMISTRY—Inorganic Chemistry; CHEMISTRY—Organic Chemistry; CHEMISTRY—Physical Chemistry

ACADEMIE SERBE DES SCIENCES ET DES ARTS. CLASSE DES SCIENCES MATHEMATIQUES ET NATURELLES. BULLETIN SCIENCES NATURELLES. see *SCIENCES: COMPREHENSIVE WORKS*

ACTA PHARMACEUTICA TURCICA. see *PHARMACY AND PHARMACOLOGY*

ADVANCES IN MEDICINAL CHEMISTRY. see *MEDICAL SCIENCES*

542 USA ISSN 0172-4967
ANLEITUNG FUER DIE CHEMISCHE LABORATORIUMSPRAXIS - CHEMICAL LABORATORY PRACTICE. Text in English. 1970. irreg., latest vol.24, 1989. price varies. reprint service avail. from ISI. **Document type:** *Monographic series.*
Formerly: Anleitung fuer die Chemische Laboratoriumspraxis (0066-1910)
Published by: Springer-Verlag, Journals (Subsidiary of: BertelsmannSpringer), 175 Fifth Ave, New York, NY 10010. TEL 212-460-1500, FAX 212-473-6272. Ed. H Mayer Kaupp.

ARCHEIA TES PHARMAKEUTIKES (ATHENS). see *PHARMACY AND PHARMACOLOGY*

ASSOCIATION OF MARINE LABORATORIES OF THE CARIBBEAN. PROCEEDINGS. see *EARTH SCIENCES—Oceanography*

540 ITA
B C F INTERNATIONAL. (Bollettino Chimico Farmaceutico) Text in English. bi-m. USD 120 foreign (effective 2000).
Published by: Societa Editoriale Farmaceutica s.r.l., Via Ausonio, 12, Milan, MI 20123, Italy. TEL 39-2-89404545, FAX 39-2-89401168.

BAYER REPORT. see *PHARMACY AND PHARMACOLOGY*

BRAGANTIA. see *AGRICULTURE*

C A SELECTS. OMEGA-3 FATTY ACIDS & FISH OIL. see *CHEMISTRY—Abstracting, Bibliographies, Statistics*

C A SELECTS. PHOSPHOLIPIDS (CHEMICAL ASPECTS). see *CHEMISTRY—Abstracting, Bibliographies, Statistics*

C Y R I C ANNUAL REPORT. (Cyclotron Radioisotope Center) see *MEDICAL SCIENCES—Radiology And Nuclear Medicine*

CHEMECOLOGY; covering health, safety and the environment. see *ENVIRONMENTAL STUDIES*

540 615 JPN ISSN 0009-2363
RS1.N56 CODEN: CPBTAL
CHEMICAL & PHARMACEUTICAL BULLETIN. Text in English. 1953. m. USD 125 to members. adv. charts, tr.mk. index. 150 p./no. *Refereed.* **Document type:** *Bulletin, Academic/Scholarly.*
Formerly: Pharmaceutical Bulletin
Related titles: Microfilm ed.: (from PMC); Online - full text ed.: (from Institute for Scientific Information).
Indexed: ASCA, Agri.& Environ.Biotech.Abstr. (coverage dropped), Anal.Abstr., Aqua.Sci.& Fish.Abstr., Bio-Contr.News & Info., Biol.Abstr., Chem.Abstr., Chem.Cit.Ind., Chem.Indus.Notes, Chem.Infd., Chem.Titles, Crop Physiol.Abstr., Curr.Adv.Cancer Res., Curr.Adv.Ecol.Sci., Curr.Chem.React., Curr.Cont., Dairy Sci.Abstr., Dent.Ind., Derwent Biotech.Abstr., Environ.Sci.Poll.Mgmt., Excerp.Med., Field Crop Abstr., Forest Prod.Abstr., Forest.Abstr., Helminthol.Abstr., Herb.Abstr., Hort.Abstr., INIS Atomind., I.P.A., Ind.Chem., Ind.Med. (1958-), Ind.Sci.Rev., Ind.Vet., Inpharma, MOS, Mass Spectr.Bull., Mat.Sci.Cit.Ind. (coverage dropped), Microbiol.Abstr., NPU, Nuc.Acids Abstr., Nutr.Abstr., Ornam.Hort., Pharm.&Out.News, Plant Grow.Reg.Abstr., Pollut.Abstr., Protozool.Abstr., RCI, Reac., Ref.Zh., Rev.Appl.Entomol., Rev.Arom.& Med.Plants, Rev.Med.& Vet.Mycol., Rev.Plant Path., Risk Abstr., Saf.Sci.Abstr., Sci.Cit.Ind., Seed Abstr., Soils & Fert., Sugar Ind.Abstr., Vet.Bull., Weed Abstr.
—BLDSC (3138.800000), CASDDS, CINDOC, CISTI, GNLM, IDS, ingenta, KNAW, Linda Hall. **CCC.**
Published by: Pharmaceutical Society of Japan/Nihon Yakugakkai, 2-12-15, Shibuya, Shibuya-ku, Tokyo 150-0002, Japan. TEL 81-3-3406-3321, FAX 81-3-3498-1835, ronb@pharm.or.jp, http://cpb.pharm.or.jp. Ed. Kenji Koga. Circ: 3,650.

540 660 NLD ISSN 0927-0841
CHEMICAL SAFETY SHEETS. Text in English. 1991. a. price varies. stat. **Description:** Specifies health hazards and precautionary measures associated with more than 950 chemicals.
Published by: (Nederlandse Institut voor Arbeitsomstandigheden), Kluwer Academic Publishers Group (Subsidiary of: Wolters Kluwer N.V.), Spuiboulevard 50, PO Box 17, Dordrecht 3300 AA, Netherlands. FAX 31-78-639-2254, services@wkap.nl, http://www.wkap.nl. Circ: 5,000. **Dist. by:** Journals Department, PO Box 322, Dordrecht 3300 AH, Netherlands. FAX 31-78-654-6474. **Co-sponsor:** Vereniging van de Nederlandse Chemische Industrie/Association of the Dutch Chemical Industry.

540 530 616.075 JPN
CHEMICAL SOCIETY OF JAPAN. SYMPOSIUM ON PHYSICAL AND CHEMICAL ASPECTS OF ULTRASOUND. PROCEEDINGS/ONPA NO BUSSEI TO KAGAKU TORONKAI KOEN RONBUNSHU. Text in Japanese. a. **Document type:** *Proceedings.*
Published by: Chemical Society of Japan/Nippon Kagakukai, 1-5, Kanda-Surugadai 1-Chome, Chiyoda-ku, Tokyo 101-0062, Japan.

540 660 615 CHE ISSN 0009-2983
CODEN: CHRUAE
CHEMISCHE RUNDSCHAU; Zeitung fuer Chemie, Lebensmitteltechnologie, Pharmazie und Biotechnologie. Text in German. 1947. fortn. CHF 128; CHF 159 foreign (effective 1999). adv. bk.rev. illus, mkt. **Document type:** *Newspaper.*
Related titles: Online - full text ed.: (from Gale Group, Factiva).
Indexed: CBNB (1985-), CEABA, C.I.S. Abstr., Chem.Abstr., Chem.Indus.Notes, Chem.Titles, Key to Econ.Sci., PROMT.
—CASDDS.
Published by: Vogt-Schild AG, Zuchwilerstr 21, Solothurn, 1 4501, Switzerland. TEL 41-32-6247111, FAX 41-32-6247444, a.widmer@vsonline.ch, http://www.chemische-rundschau.ch. Ed. Alfred Widmer. Adv. contact Hansruedi Spiri. B&W page CHF 6,230.4, color page CHF 7,330.4; trim 290 x 440. Circ: 18,500 (controlled).

530 GBR ISSN 1074-5521
QP501 CODEN: CBOLE2
CHEMISTRY & BIOLOGY. Text in English. 1994. m. EUR 226 in Europe to qualified personnel; JPY 30,000 in Japan to qualified personnel; USD 253 elsewhere to qualified personnel; EUR 1,043 in Europe to institutions; JPY 138,500 in Japan to institutions; USD 1,169 elsewhere to institutions (effective 2002). adv. bk.rev. illus. back issues avail. *Refereed.* **Document type:** *Academic/Scholarly.* **Description:** Directed toward researchers, educators and students of signaling, molecular recognition and structure-based design. Features original research and reviews.
Related titles: Online - full text ed.: (from EBSCO Publishing, ingenta, Swets Blackwell, ScienceDirect, Institute for Scientific Information).
Indexed: AIDS & Cancer Res., ASCA, Agri.& Environ.Biotech.Abstr., Aqua.Sci.& Fish.Abstr., BBCI, Biol.Dig., Chem.Abstr., Chem.Indus.Notes, Chem.Titles, Curr.Cont., Environ.Sci.Poll.Mgmt., Genet.Abstr., Hum.Gen.Abstr., Immun.Abstr., Ind.Med. (1994-), Ind.Sci.Rev., Inpharma, Med.& Pharm.Biotech.Abstr., Microbiol.Abstr., Nuc.Acids Abstr., Nutr.Abstr., Oncog.G.F.Abstr., Protozool.Abstr., Reac., Rev.Appl.Entomol., Rev.Med.& Vet.Mycol., Sci.Cit.Ind.
—BLDSC (3168.890000), ADONIS, CASDDS, CISTI, EMDOCS, GNLM, IDS, Infotrieve, ingenta. **CCC.**
Published by: Elsevier Science BV, Sara Burgerhartstraat 25, Amsterdam 1055 KV, Netherlands. http://www.elsevier.com/locate/chembiol. Eds. K C Nicolaou, Stuart L Schreiber. adv.: B&W page USD 750, color page USD 1,950; trim 11 x 8.5. Circ: 4,700. **Dist. by:** Turpin Distribution Services Ltd., Blackhorse Rd, Letchworth, Herts SG6 1HN, United Kingdom. FAX 44-1462-480947.

540 577 CHE ISSN 0275-7540
QH545.A1 CODEN: CHECDY
CHEMISTRY AND ECOLOGY. Text in English. 1982. 4/yr. GBP 270, USD 325, EUR 359 to individuals; GBP 766, USD 990, EUR 1,020 to institutions; GBP 1,239, USD 1,621, EUR 1,654 to corporations (effective 2002). *Refereed.* **Document type:** *Journal, Academic/Scholarly.*
Related titles: CD-ROM ed.; Microform ed.; Online - full text ed.: (from EBSCO Publishing, RoweCom Information Quest).
Indexed: Aqua.Sci.& Fish.Abstr., Aquacult.Abstr., Chem.Abstr., Ecol.Abstr., Environ.Abstr., Environ.Sci.Poll.Mgmt., Food Sci.& Tech.Abstr., Geo.Abstr.H.G., Geo.Abstr.P.G., GeoRef, Geol.Abstr., IDA, Pollut.Abstr., Sel.Water Res.Abstr., Sport Fish.Abstr., Wild.Rev., Zoo.Rec.
—BLDSC (3169.500000), CISTI, Infotrieve. **CCC.**
Published by: Gordon and Breach - Harwood Academic (Subsidiary of: Taylor & Francis Group), PO Box 531, Lausanne 1000, Switzerland. TEL 41-21-6411280, FAX 41-21-6411281, info@gbhap.com, http://www.gbhap.com. Ed. Gwyneth Howells. **Subscr. addr. in US:** International Publishers Direct, PO Box 32160, Newark, NJ 07102. FAX 215-750-6343.

632.9 571.2 USA ISSN 0937-2148
CODEN: CPLPET
CHEMISTRY OF PLANT PROTECTION SERIES. Text in English. 1986. irreg., latest vol.12, 1995. price varies. reprint service avail. from ISI. **Document type:** *Monographic series.*
Indexed: Chem.Abstr., Chem.Indus.Notes, Chem.Titles, GeoRef.
—CASDDS, CISTI. **CCC.**
Published by: Springer-Verlag, Journals (Subsidiary of: BertelsmannSpringer), 175 Fifth Ave, New York, NY 10010. TEL 212-460-1500, FAX 212-473-6272.

CHEMOSPHERE; chemistry, biology and toxicology as related to environmental problems. see *ENVIRONMENTAL STUDIES—Toxicology And Environmental Safety*

540 ITA ISSN 0392-839X
CODEN: CHOGDS
CHIMICA OGGI/CHEMISTRY TODAY. Text in English. 1982. 10/yr. ITL 150,000 domestic to individuals; USD 190 foreign to individuals; ITL 185,000 domestic to institutions; USD 255 foreign to institutions. adv. bk.rev. Index. back issues avail. *Refereed.* **Document type:** *Journal, Trade.*
Related titles: Online - full text ed.: (from Factiva, Institute for Scientific Information).
Indexed: ASCA, Agri.Eng.Abstr., CBNB (1987-), CEABA, Chem.Abstr., Chem.Cit.Ind., Chem.Indus.Notes, Chem.Titles, Curr.Biotech.Abstr., Eng.Ind., I.P.A., Rev.Appl.Entomol., Rev.Plant Path., Soils & Fert., Weed Abstr.
—BLDSC (3175.100000), CASDDS, CISTI, Ei, IDS.
Published by: Teknoscienze s.r.l., Via Aurelio Saffi, 23, Milan, MI 20123, Italy. TEL 39-02-4818118, FAX 39-02-4818070, mickycar@tin.it, http://www.teknoscienze.com. Ed. Carla Scesa. R&P, Adv. contact Michaela Carmagnola. B&W page USD 2,050; trim 210 x 297. Circ: 8,000.

540 FRA
CODEN: ICHEDI
CHIMIE HEBDO; chimie, parachimie, pharmacie. Text in French; Summaries in English, German. w. (42/yr.). FRF 3,680; FRF 4,150 foreign (effective 1999). **Description:** Devoted to the chemicals, specialty chemical and pharmaceutical industries in France and throughout the world.
Formerly (until Apr. 1998): Informations Chimie Hebdo (0339-6045)
Related titles: Online - full text ed.: (from Factiva); ♦ Supplement to: Informations - Chimie. ISSN 0020-045X.
Indexed: CBNB (1985-), Chem.Abstr., Chem.Indus.Notes, Chem.Titles.
—BLDSC (3179.230000), CASDDS.
Published by: Societe d'Expansion Technique et Economique S.A., 4 rue de Seze, Paris 75009, France. TEL 33-1-44945060, FAX 33-1-44945075, http://www.infochimie.presse.fr. Ed. Dmitri Savostianoff.

CLINICA CHIMICA ACTA; international journal of clinical chemistry and medical biochemistry. see *MEDICAL SCIENCES*

CLINICAL CHEMISTRY AND ENZYMOLOGY COMMUNICATIONS. see *BIOLOGY—Biochemistry*

540 USA ISSN 1386-2073
CODEN: CCHSFU
COMBINATORIAL CHEMISTRY & HIGH THROUGHPUT SCREENING. Text in English. 1998. bi-m. USD 225 to individuals; USD 800 to institutions; effective 2000. adv. *Refereed.* **Document type:** *Academic/Scholarly.* **Description:** Publishes original research articles describing various topics in combinatorial chemistry and/or high throughput screening. Ancillary subjects, such as robotics and informatics, are also covered.
Related titles: Online - full text ed.: (from ingenta, Swets Blackwell, Institute for Scientific Information).
Indexed: Aqua.Sci.& Fish.Abstr., Biotech.& Bioeng.Abstr., Chem.Abstr., Chem.Cit.Ind., Curr.Cont., Ind.Med. (1998-), Mass Spectr.Bull., Med.& Pharm.Biotech.Abstr., RCI.
—BLDSC (3324.739000), CASDDS, IDS, Infotrieve. **CCC.**
Published by: Bentham Science Publishers, 102 N.E. 2nd St, Mail Box 135, Boca Raton, FL 33432. FAX 561-393-7229, m.bentham@inter.nl.net, http://www.bscipubl.demon.co.uk/cchts. Ed. Richard B Breemen. Adv. contact Tom Lucas.

COMMENTATIONES PHYSICO-MATHEMATICAE ET CHEMICO-MEDICAE. see *PHYSICS*

CRYOLETTERS. see *BIOLOGY—Physiology*

CURRENT TOPICS IN ENVIRONMENTAL AND TOXICOLOGICAL CHEMISTRY. see *ENVIRONMENTAL STUDIES—Toxicology And Environmental Safety*

FARBE AKTUELL PLUS. see *PHARMACY AND PHARMACOLOGY*

FARMACI. see *PHARMACY AND PHARMACOLOGY*

FOOD AND CHEMICAL TOXICOLOGY. see *ENVIRONMENTAL STUDIES—Toxicology And Environmental Safety*

HANDBOOK OF CHEMICAL NEUROANATOMY. see *MEDICAL SCIENCES—Psychiatry And Neurology*

C

540 USA ISSN 0897-8026
TP669 CODEN: IFRMEC
I N F O R M: INTERNATIONAL NEWS ON FATS, OILS & RELATED MATERIALS. Text in English. 1990. m. USD 120 domestic; USD 135 foreign (effective 2002). adv. bk.rev. charts, illus. back issues avail.; reprints avail. **Document type:** *Magazine, Trade.* **Description:** News and information of interest to professionals interested in the science and technology of fats and oils, surfactants, detergents, proteins, oleochemicals, and related substances.
Related titles: Online - full text ed.: (from Gale Group, Factiva).
Indexed: Abstr.Bull.Inst.Pap.Chem., AgBiotech, Agri.Eng.Abstr., Chem.Abstr., Chem.Indus.Notes, Chem.Titles, Dairy Sci.Abstr., Eng.Ind., Food Sci.& Tech.Abstr., Forest Prod.Abstr., Hort.Abstr., Maize Abstr., Nutr.Abstr., P.A.I.S., Plant Breed.Abstr., Plant Gen.Res.Abstr., Postharvest, Ref.Zh., Rev.Arom.& Med.Plants, Seed Abstr., Soyabean Abstr., Text.Tech.Dig. (1990-1994), Triticale Abstr., VITIS, World Ag.Econ.& Rur.Soc.Abstr.
—BLDSC (4478.882000), CASDDS, CISTI, Ei, GNLM, Infotrieve, ingenta, Linda Hall. **CCC.**
Published by: (American Oil Chemists' Society), A O C S Press, 2211 W Bradley Ave, Champaign, IL 61821. TEL 217-359-2344, FAX 217-351-8091, publications@aocs.org, http://www.aocs.org, http://www.aocs.org/press. Ed. J Rattray. R&P Connie Winslow. Adv. contact Trish Sipes. B&W page USD 1,500, color page USD 2,730; 8.25 x 11.

I U P A C SERIES ON ANALYTICAL AND PHYSICAL CHEMISTRY OF ENVIRONMENTAL SYSTEMS. see *ENVIRONMENTAL STUDIES—Toxicology And Environmental Safety*

THE IMMUNOASSAY KIT DIRECTORY. SERIES A: CLINICAL CHEMISTRY. see *MEDICAL SCIENCES—Allergology And Immunology*

THE IMMUNOASSAY KIT DIRECTORY. SERIES B: INFECTIOUS DISEASES. see *MEDICAL SCIENCES—Allergology And Immunology*

540 DEU
INFORMATION SOURCES IN CHEMISTRY. Text in English. irreg., latest vol.5, 2000. USD 100 in North America (effective 2001). bibl. **Document type:** *Directory, Bibliography.* **Description:** Evaluates specific materials - professional journals, government publications, gray literature for the pure and industrial chemist. Covers inorganic chemistry to pharmaceuticals.
Published by: K.G. Saur Verlag (Subsidiary of: Gale Group), Ortlerstr 8, Munich 81373, Germany. TEL 49-89-76902-0, FAX 49-89-76902150, info@saur.de, http://www.saur.de. Eds. J F Rowland, R T Bottle.

540 IND ISSN 0020-3254
TP1 CODEN: JOICA7
INSTITUTION OF CHEMISTS (INDIA). JOURNAL. Text in English. 1929. bi-m. USD 25. adv. bk.rev. charts, illus. index. back issues avail. *Refereed.* **Document type:** *Proceedings, Academic/Scholarly.*
Supersedes in part: Institution of Chemists (India). Journal and Proceedings
Indexed: Chem.Abstr., Chem.Indus.Notes, Chem.Titles, Dairy Sci.Abstr., Eng.Ind., Food Sci.& Tech.Abstr.
—BLDSC (4791.300000), CASDDS, CISTI, Ei, ingenta, Linda Hall.
Published by: Institution of Chemists (India), 11-4 Dr. Biresh Guha Rd., Kolkata, West Bengal 700 017, India. TEL 91-33-240-3832. Ed. Debi Chakravarti. R&P Arun K Chakravarti. Adv. contact Hony Secretary. B&W page USD 30; trim 234 x 180. Circ: 1,500.

540 IND ISSN 0369-8599
INSTITUTION OF CHEMISTS (INDIA). PROCEEDINGS. Text in English. q. **Document type:** *Proceedings, Academic/Scholarly.*
Supersedes in part: Institution of Chemists (India). Journal and Proceedings
Indexed: Chem.Abstr.
Published by: Institution of Chemists (India), 11-4 Dr. Biresh Guha Rd., Kolkata, West Bengal 700 017, India. TEL 91-33-240-3832. Ed. Debi Chakravarti. R&P Arun R Chakravarti. Circ: 2,000.

INTERNATIONAL JOURNAL OF OCCUPATIONAL SAFETY AND ERGONOMICS. see *OCCUPATIONAL HEALTH AND SAFETY*

541.3 615.8 HUN ISSN 0865-0497
TK9400 CODEN: IZDIE2
IZOTOPTECHNIKA, DIAGNOSZTIKA/ISOTOPE TECHNICS, DIAGNOSTICS. Short title: I T D. Text in Hungarian; Summaries in English. 1958. 4/yr. USD 30. adv. bk.rev. **Document type:** *Academic/Scholarly.* **Description:** Covers the application of stable and radio-isotopes in medicine, industry, agriculture and basic research.
Former titles (until 1989): Izotoptechnika (0004-7201); Atomtechnikai Tajekoztato
Indexed: Biol.Abstr., Chem.Abstr., Chem.Indus.Notes, Chem.Titles, INIS Atomind., INSPEC (1979-1984, 1992-1994, dropped).
—AskIEEE, CASDDS, CISTI.
Published by: Izotop Intezet Kft., PO Box 77, Budapest 1525, Hungary. TEL 361-169-9499, FAX 361-169-5087, TELEX 225360. Ed. Istvan Mucha. adv.: page USD 100. Circ: 350 (controlled).

JAPANESE WEEKLY ON PHARMACY AND CHEMISTRY/YAKUGYO SHINBUN. see *PHARMACY AND PHARMACOLOGY*

540 USA ISSN 1058-5834
QD502 CODEN: JCBKEI
JOURNAL OF CHEMICAL AND BIOCHEMICAL KINETICS. Text in English. 1991. q. USD 300 (effective 1999). **Document type:** *Academic/Scholarly.* **Description:** Presents original research on the development and use of kinetic methods, in the study of mechanisms and kinetics of chemical and biochemical processes.
Indexed: Chem.Abstr., Chem.Indus.Notes, Chem.Titles.
—CASDDS, CISTI, ingenta, Linda Hall.
Published by: Nova Science Publishers, Inc., 227 Main St, Ste 100, Huntington, NY 11743-6907. TEL 631-424-6682, FAX 631-425-5933, novascience@earthlink.net, http://www.nexusworld.com/nova. Ed. Gennady E Zaikov.

544.92 NLD ISSN 1387-2273
QD271 CODEN: JCBADL
JOURNAL OF CHROMATOGRAPHY. B, BIOMEDICAL SCIENCES AND APPLICATIONS. Text in English, French, German; Summaries in English. 1977. 32/yr. EUR 4,058 in Europe to institutions; JPY 539,200 in Japan to institutions; USD 4,539 elsewhere to institutions (effective 2002). adv. bk.rev. charts, illus. index. back issues avail.; reprint service avail. from PQC. *Refereed.* **Document type:** *Academic/Scholarly.* **Description:** Addresses developments in and applications of separation Science related to drugs and other pharmacologically active compounds, and to research in biomedical sciences.
Formerly (until 1997): Journal of Chromatography - Biomedical Applications (0378-4347)
Related titles: Microform ed.: (from PQC); Online - full text ed.: (from ingenta, ScienceDirect, Swets Blackwell, Institute for Scientific Information); ♦ Supplement to: The Journal of Chromatography A. ISSN 0021-9673.
Indexed: ASCA, Agri.& Environ.Biotech.Abstr. (coverage dropped), Anal.Abstr., BBCI, Biol.Abstr., C.I.S. Abstr., Chem.Abstr., Chem.Cit.Ind., Chem.Titles, Chromat.Abstr., Curr.Adv.Biochem., Curr.Cont., Curr.Leather Lit., Dairy Sci.Abstr., Derwent Biotech.Abstr., Eng.Ind., Environ.Per.Bibl., Excerp.Med., Food Sci.& Tech.Abstr., Helminthol.Abstr., I.P.A., Ind.Med. (1997-), Ind.Sci.Rev., Ind.Vet., Inpharma, Int.Abstr.Biol.Sci., Mass Spectr.Bull., Neurosci.Cit.Ind., Nutr.Abstr., Pig News & Info., Protozool.Abstr., RCI, Reac., Ref.Zh., Rev.Plant Path., Sci.Cit.Ind., THA, Vet.Bull., Weed Abstr.
—BLDSC (4958.350300), ADONIS, CASDDS, CINDOC, CISTI, EMDOCS, GNLM, IDS, ingenta, Linda Hall. **CCC.**
Published by: Elsevier Science BV, PO Box 211, Amsterdam 1000 AE, Netherlands. nlinfo-f@elsevier.nl, http://www.elsevier.nl/locate/jchromb. Eds. D K Lloyd, W Lindner. adv.: B&W page USD 1,020, color page USD 2,205; trim 192 x 262. Circ: 1,500. **Subscr. in Australasia and the Far East to:** Elsevier Science (Singapore) Pte Ltd, No.1 Temasek Ave, 17-01 Millenia Tower, Singapore 039192, Singapore; **Subscr. in Japan to:** Elsevier Science Inc - Japan Regional Office, 9-15 Higashi-Azabu 1-chome, Minato-ku, Tokyo 106-0044, Japan. TEL 81-3-5561-5033; **Subscr. in the Americas to:** Elsevier Science, PO Box 945, New York, NY 10159-0945. TEL 212-633-3730, FAX 212-633-3680.

JOURNAL OF LUMINESCENCE; an interdisciplinary journal of research on excited state processes in condensed matter. see *PHYSICS—Optics*

KHIMIKO-FARMATSEVTICHESKII ZHURNAL. see *PHARMACY AND PHARMACOLOGY*

LEBENSMITTEL- UND BIOTECHNOLOGIE; die oesterreichische Fachzeitschrift fuer Lebensmittelindustrie und -forschung. see *FOOD AND FOOD INDUSTRIES*

LEBENSMITTELCHEMIE; Zeitschrift des Lebensmittelchemischen Gesellschaft. see *FOOD AND FOOD INDUSTRIES*

540 CHE ISSN 0278-6281
QP501 CODEN: LCHRDM
LIFE CHEMISTRY REPORTS. Text in English. irreg. EUR 696, USD 766 to institutions; EUR 1,070, USD 1,177 to corporations (effective 2000). *Refereed.* **Document type:** *Monographic series.*
Related titles: CD-ROM ed.: ISSN 1026-8030; Online - full text ed.: ISSN 1029-2489 (from EBSCO Publishing, RoweCom Information Quest); ♦ Supplement: Life Chemistry Reports. Supplement Series. ISSN 0892-0419.
Indexed: Chem.Abstr.
—BLDSC (5208.921250), CISTI, GNLM, Infotrieve, ingenta. **CCC.**
Published by: Gordon and Breach - Harwood Academic (Subsidiary of: Taylor & Francis Group), PO Box 531, Lausanne 1000, Switzerland. Eds. A M Michelson, J V Bannister. **Subscr. addr. in US:** International Publishers Direct, PO Box 32160, Newark, NJ 07102. FAX 215-750-6343.

540 CHE ISSN 0892-0419
LIFE CHEMISTRY REPORTS. SUPPLEMENT SERIES. Text in French, English. 1983. irreg.
Related titles: ♦ Supplement to: Life Chemistry Reports. ISSN 0278-6281.
—BLDSC (5208.921260).
Published by: Gordon and Breach - Harwood Academic (Subsidiary of: Taylor & Francis Group), PO Box 531, Lausanne 1000, Switzerland. TEL 41-21-6411280, FAX 41-21-6411281.

C

MEDICINAL CHEMISTRY RESEARCH; an international journal for rapid communications on design and mechanisms of action of biologically active agents. see *MEDICAL SCIENCES*

540 USA ISSN 1389-5575
▼ **MINI - REVIEWS IN MEDICINAL CHEMISTRY.** Text in English. 2000 (Jun.). bi-m. USD 139, USD 900 to institutions (effective 2000). adv. *Refereed.* **Document type:** *Academic/Scholarly.* **Description:** Features mini-reviews on medicinal chemistry and related areas.
Published by: Bentham Science Publishers, 102 N.E. 2nd St, Mail Box 135, Boca Raton, FL 33432. FAX 561-393-7229, m.bentham@inter.nl.net. Adv. contact Tom Lucas.

MOLECULAR AND CELLULAR PROBES; the location, diagnosis, and monitoring of disease by nucleic acid techniques. see *MEDICAL SCIENCES—Experimental Medicine, Laboratory Technique*

N C F. see *PHARMACY AND PHARMACOLOGY*

NAPRALERT ON CD-ROM. see *PHARMACY AND PHARMACOLOGY*

NATURE BIOTECHNOLOGY. see *BIOLOGY—Biotechnology*

570 610 USA ISSN 0195-7198
CODEN: PSSBDF
NAUKOVE TOVARYSTVO IMENI SHEVCHENKA. PROCEEDINGS OF THE SECTION OF CHEMISTRY, BIOLOGY AND MEDICINE. Text in English, Ukrainian. 1973 (vol.7). irreg. price varies. **Document type:** *Proceedings.*
Supersedes in part: Naukove Tovarystvo Imeni Shevchenka. Proceedings of the Section of Mathematics, Natural Sciences and Medicine (0470-5017)
Published by: Shevchenko Scientific Society, 63 Fourth Ave, New York, NY 10003. TEL 212-254-5130.

540 NLD ISSN 1380-3689
CODEN: NTKCFX
NEDERLANDS TIJDSCHRIFT VOOR KLINISCHE CHEMIE. Text in Dutch. 1976. bi-m. NLG 160; NLG 175 foreign (effective 1999). adv. bk.rev. index. back issues avail. **Document type:** *Academic/Scholarly.*
Formerly: Nederlandse Vereniging voor Klinische Chemie. Tijdschrift (0168-8472)
Indexed: Chem.Abstr., Chem.Indus.Notes, Chem.Titles, Excerp.Med., Int.Abstr.Biol.Sci.
—BLDSC (6071.950000), CASDDS, CISTI, GNLM, KNAW.

Published by: Nederlandse Vereniging voor Klinische Chemie, Vredenburg 134, 2nd Fl., Utrecht 3511 BG, Netherlands. TEL 31-30-232-8623, FAX 31-30-231-1178. Circ: 800.

NEUROCHEMISTRY INTERNATIONAL; the international journal for the rapid publication of critical reviews, original and rapid research communications in neurochemistry. see *MEDICAL SCIENCES—Psychiatry And Neurology*

NEW TRENDS IN SYNTHETIC MEDICINAL CHEMISTRY. see *MEDICAL SCIENCES*

NIPPON KAYAKU. ANNUAL REPORT. see *PHARMACY AND PHARMACOLOGY*

NUCLEUS. see *ENERGY—Nuclear Energy*

ORIGINS OF LIFE AND EVOLUTION OF THE BIOSPHERE. see *BIOLOGY*

PHARMACEUTICAL CHEMISTRY JOURNAL. see *PHARMACY AND PHARMACOLOGY*

PHARMACOCHEMISTRY LIBRARY. see *PHARMACY AND PHARMACOLOGY*

540 570 USA ISSN 0363-499X
QH515 CODEN: PPHRDL
PHOTOCHEMICAL & PHOTOBIOLOGICAL REVIEWS. Text in English. 1976. irreg., latest vol.7, 1983. back issues avail. *Refereed.* **Document type:** *Monographic series.*
—CASDDS, CISTI, GNLM, Linda Hall. **CCC.**
Published by: Kluwer Academic - Plenum Publishers (Subsidiary of: Wolters Kluwer N.V.), 233 Spring St, New York, NY 10013-1578. TEL 212-620-8000, 800-221-9369, FAX 212-463-0742, info@plenum.com, http://www.plenum.com. Ed. K C Smith.

541.35 USA ISSN 0031-8655
QD601.A1 CODEN: PHCBAP
PHOTOCHEMISTRY AND PHOTOBIOLOGY. Text in English. 1962. 12/yr. (in 2 vols.). USD 590 to institutions Print & online eds. (effective 2001). adv. bk.rev. bibl, charts, illus. back issues avail. *Refereed.* **Document type:** *Academic/Scholarly.* **Description:** Publishes original reports and reviews on current topics in photobiology and in photobiologically relevant photochemistry.
Related titles: CD-ROM ed.; Microfilm ed.: (from PQC); Online - full text ed.: (from ProQuest Information & Learning, BioOne, Institute for Scientific Information).
Indexed: AMED, ASCA, Agri.Eng.Abstr., Agricola, Aqua.Sci.& Fish.Abstr., BBCI, Bibl.Agri., Biol.Abstr., Biwk.Pap.Rad.Chem.& Photochem., Chem.Abstr., Chem.Cit.Ind., Chem.Titles, Crop Physiol.Abstr., Curr.Adv.Biochem., Curr.Adv.Cancer Res., Curr.Adv.Ecol.Sci., Curr.Adv.Gen.& Molec.Biol., Curr.Adv.Plant Sci., Curr.Cont., Dairy Sci.Abstr., Deep Sea Res.& Oceanogr.Abstr., Eng.Ind., Environ.Sci.Poll.Mgmt., Excerp.Med., Field Crop Abstr., Forest.Abstr., Genet.Abstr., Helminthol.Abstr., Herb.Abstr., Hort.Abstr., Hum.Gen.Abstr., INIS Atomind., Ind.Med. (1962-), Ind.Sci.Rev., Ind.Vet., Inpharma, Int.Abstr.Biol.Sci., Int.Aerosp.Abstr., Jrnl.Watch Derm., Mass Spectr.Bull., Med.& Surg.Dermat., Microbiol.Abstr., Neurosci.Cit.Ind., Nuc.Acids Abstr., Nutr.Abstr., Ornam.Hort., Pharm.&Out.News, Plant Breed.Abstr., Plant Grow.Reg.Abstr., Plant Sci., Protozool.Abstr., Reac., Ref.Zh., Rev.Appl.Entomol., Rev.Arom.& Med.Plants, Rev.Plant Path., Rice Abstr., Sci.Cit.Ind., Triticale Abstr., Vet.Bull., Weed Abstr.
—BLDSC (6465.985000), CASDDS, CISTI, Ei, EMDOCS, GNLM, IDS, ingenta, Linda Hall. **CCC.**
Published by: American Society for Photobiology, BioTech Park, Ste 9, 1021 15th St, Augusta, GA 30901. TEL 706-722-7511, FAX 706-722-7515, maps@csranet.com; orders@allenpress.com, phot@allenpress.com, http://www.photobiology.org; http://www.pol-us.net; http://www.allenpress.com. Ed. J C Scaiano. Adv. contact Sarah A Stephens. Circ: 2,100. **Subscr. to:** Allen Press Inc., PO Box 1897, Lawrence, KS 66044-8897.

PODSTAWY I METODY OCENY SRODOWISKA PRACY/PRINCIPLES AND METHODS OF ASSESSING THE WORKING ENVIRONMENT. see *PUBLIC HEALTH AND SAFETY*

540 610 NLD ISSN 0079-6468
RM30 CODEN: PMDCAY
PROGRESS IN MEDICINAL CHEMISTRY. Text in English. 1961. irreg., latest vol.36, 1999. price varies. back issues avail. *Refereed.* **Document type:** *Monographic series, Academic/Scholarly.* **Description:** Explores research and developments in the subspecialty of medicinal chemistry.
Indexed: Agri.& Environ.Biotech.Abstr. (coverage dropped), Biol.Abstr., Chem.Abstr., Chem.Indus.Notes, Chem.Titles, Derwent Biotech.Abstr., Ind.Med. (1961-), Ind.Sci.Rev.
—BLDSC (6868.970000), CASDDS, CISTI, GNLM, ingenta, KNAW, Linda Hall. **CCC.**
Published by: Elsevier Science BV, PO Box 211, Amsterdam 1000 AE, Netherlands. TEL 31-20-485-3757, 31-20-485-3911, FAX 31-20-485-3432, 31-20-485-3598, nlinfo-f@elsevier.nl; usinfo-f@elsevier.com; forinfo-kyf04035@niftyserve.or.jp, http://www.elsevier.nl/. Eds. A W Oxford, F D King. **Subscr. in Australasia and the Far East to:** Elsevier Science (Singapore) Pte Ltd, No.1 Temasek Ave, 17-01 Millenia Tower, Singapore 039192, Singapore. TEL 65-434-3727, FAX 65-337-2230, asiainfo@elsevier.com.sg; **Subscr. in Japan to:** Elsevier Science Inc - Japan Regional Office, 9-15 Higashi-Azabu 1-chome, Minato-ku, Tokyo 106-0044, Japan. TEL 81-3-5561-5033, FAX 81-3-5561-5047, info@elsevier.co.jp; **Subscr. in the Americas to:** Elsevier Science, PO Box 945, New York, NY 10159-0945. TEL 212-633-3730, 888-437-4636, FAX 212-633-3680, usinfo-f@elsevier.com, http://www.elsevier.com

R T E C S. (Registry of Toxic Effects of Chemical Substances) see *ENVIRONMENTAL STUDIES—Toxicology And Environmental Safety*

541.3884 JPN ISSN 0033-8303
R895.A1 CODEN: RAISAB
RADIOISOTOPES. Text in English, Japanese; Summaries in English. 1952. m. JPY 15,000 (effective 2000). adv. abstr, bibl, charts, illus. index. **Document type:** *Academic/Scholarly.*
Indexed: Art & Archaeol.Tech.Abstr., Biol.Abstr., Chem.Abstr., Chem.Indus.Notes, Chem.Titles, Dairy Sci.Abstr., Dent.Ind., Excerp.Med., Food Sci.& Tech.Abstr., INIS Atomind., INSPEC (Dec.1979-), Ind.Med. (coverage dropped), JTA, Mass Spectr.Bull., Ref.Zh.
—BLDSC (7237.300000), AskIEEE, CASDDS, CISTI, GNLM, Linda Hall.
Published by: Japan Radioisotope Association/Nihon Aisotope Kyokai, 28-45 Honkomagome 2-chome, Bunkyo-ku, Tokyo 113-0021, Japan. TEL 81-3-3946-7110, FAX 81-3-3946-2640. Ed. Tatsuyi Hamada. Circ: 5,000.

RESEARCH. see *PHARMACY AND PHARMACOLOGY*

RESEARCH. SPANISH EDITION. see *PHARMACY AND PHARMACOLOGY*

REVISTA COLOMBIANA DE CIENCIAS QUIMICO FARMACEUTICAS. see *PHARMACY AND PHARMACOLOGY*

570 USA ISSN 0081-9603
CODEN: SFSSA5
SURFACTANT SCIENCE SERIES. Text in English. 1966. irreg., latest vol.83, 1999. price varies. adv. *Refereed.* **Document type:** *Monographic series.*
Indexed: Biol.Abstr., Chem.Abstr., Chem.Indus.Notes, Chem.Titles.
—BLDSC (8548.100000), CASDDS, CISTI. **CCC.**
Published by: Marcel Dekker, Inc., Attn: Eridania Perrez, 270 Madison Ave, New York, NY 10016-0602. TEL 212-696-9000, 800-228-1160, FAX 212-685-4540, marketing@dekker.com, http://www.dekker.com. Eds. F M Fowkes, M J Schick. R&P Julia Mulligan. Adv. contact Eridania Perez.

TAKEDA RESEARCH LABORATORIES. JOURNAL. see *BIOLOGY*

540 USA ISSN 0082-2531
QD61 CODEN: TQCMAT
TECHNIQUES OF CHEMISTRY. Text in English. 1971. irreg., latest vol.22, 1992. price varies. *Refereed.* **Document type:** *Monographic series.*
Incorporates: Technique of Inorganic Chemistry; Technique of Organic Chemistry (0082-240X)
Indexed: Chem.Abstr., Chem.Indus.Notes, Chem.Titles.
—BLDSC (8743.870000), CASDDS, CISTI, Infotrieve. **CCC.**
Published by: John Wiley & Sons, Inc., Journals (Subsidiary of: Wiley InterScience), 605 Third Ave, New York, NY 10158. TEL 212-850-6000, FAX 212-850-6088. Ed. A Weissberger.

▼ **THALAMUS AND RELATED SYSTEMS.** see *BIOLOGY*

TOXICOLOGICAL AND ENVIRONMENTAL CHEMISTRY. see *ENVIRONMENTAL STUDIES—Toxicology And Environmental Safety*

WEST AFRICAN JOURNAL OF BIOLOGICAL AND APPLIED CHEMISTRY. see *BIOLOGY—Biochemistry*

CHEMISTRY—Abstracting, Bibliographies, Statistics

540 610 USA ISSN 0895-6499
CODEN: CBUCE5
C A S BIOTECH UPDATES. ANTIBODY CONJUGATES. Text in English. s-w. USD 270 (effective 2001). **Document type:** *Abstract/Index.* **Description:** Covers preparation and uses of antibody conjugates, including disease diagnosis and therapy; immunochemical techniques and antibody immobilization studies.
Published by: Chemical Abstracts Service (Subsidiary of: American Chemical Society), 2540 Olentangy River Rd, Box 3012, Columbus, OH 43210-0012. TEL 614-447-3600, 800-753-4227, FAX 614-447-3751.

C A S BIOTECH UPDATES. ENVIRONMENTAL BIOTECHNOLOGY. see *ENVIRONMENTAL STUDIES—Abstracting, Bibliographies, Statistics*

540 011 USA ISSN 1040-7103
CODEN: CUPSEP
C A S BIOTECH UPDATES. PRODUCT PURIFICATION & SEPARATION. Text in English. s-w. USD 270 (effective 2001). **Document type:** *Abstract/Index.* **Description:** Covers methods and apparatus for the purification and separation of products of such processes as chemical and enzymic syntheses, fermentation, and genetic engineering; including purification and natural sources.
Published by: Chemical Abstracts Service (Subsidiary of: American Chemical Society), 2540 Olentangy River Rd, Box 3012, Columbus, OH 43210-0012. TEL 614-447-3600, 800-753-4227, FAX 614-447-3751.

540 016 USA
C A SELECTS. Text in English. 1976. s-w. USD 275 domestic to non-members; USD 83 domestic to members; USD 319 foreign to non-members; USD 127 foreign to members (effective 2001). **Document type:** *Abstract/Index.*
Related titles: Online - full text ed.
Published by: Chemical Abstracts Service (Subsidiary of: American Chemical Society), 2540 Olentangy River Rd, Box 3012, Columbus, OH 43210-0012. TEL 614-447-3600, 800-333-9511, FAX 614-447-3751, http://www.cas.org/. Ed. David W Weisgerber.

540 USA ISSN 1045-8522
CODEN: CSDAEX
C A SELECTS. ANTIBACTERIAL AGENTS. Text in English. s-w. USD 275 (effective 2001). **Document type:** *Abstract/Index.* **Description:** Covers design, synthesis, therapeutic use, mode of action, and structure-activity relationships of antibacterial agents.
Formerly (until 1989): C A Selects. Bactericides, Disinfectants and Antiseptics (0890-1848)
Published by: Chemical Abstracts Service (Subsidiary of: American Chemical Society), 2540 Olentangy River Rd, Box 3012, Columbus, OH 43210-0012. TEL 614-447-3600, 800-753-4227, FAX 614-447-3751.

541.37 USA ISSN 0146-4442
CODEN: CSERDK
C A SELECTS. ELECTROCHEMICAL REACTIONS. Text in English. s-w. USD 275 (effective 2001). **Document type:** *Abstract/Index.* **Description:** Covers electrolysis, electrooxidation, electroreduction, polarography; electrochemical reactions in biochemistry, organic, macromolecular, applied, and inorganic chemistry.
Published by: Chemical Abstracts Service (Subsidiary of: American Chemical Society), 2540 Olentangy River Rd, Box 3012, Columbus, OH 43210-0012. TEL 614-447-3600, 800-753-4227, FAX 614-447-3751.

540 USA ISSN 0895-5808 CODEN: CSEAE4
C A SELECTS. ENZYME ASSAYS. Text in English. 1988. s-w. USD 275 (effective 2001). **Document type:** *Abstract/Index.* **Description:** Covers quantitative and qualitative methods (e.g., spectrophotometric, radiometric, immunochemical, histochemical, cytochemical) for the determination of enzymes and for the use of enzymes in laboratory or clinical analysis.
Published by: Chemical Abstracts Service (Subsidiary of: American Chemical Society), 2540 Olentangy River Rd, Box 3012, Columbus, OH 43210-0012. TEL 614-447-3600, 800-753-4227, FAX 614-447-3751.

664 615.9 USA ISSN 0162-7813 CODEN: CSFTDV
C A SELECTS. FOOD TOXICITY. Text in English. s-w. USD 275 (effective 2001). **Document type:** *Abstract/Index.* **Description:** Covers mutagenicity, teratogenicity, carcinogenicity, toxic side effects, and health hazards of foods and additives; contamination of foods by agrochemicals, nitroso compounds, heavy metals, aromatic hydrocarbons, and other toxicants.
Published by: Chemical Abstracts Service (Subsidiary of: American Chemical Society), 2540 Olentangy River Rd, Box 3012, Columbus, OH 43210-0012. TEL 614-447-3600, 800-753-4227, FAX 614-447-3751.

546 USA ISSN 0195-5012 CODEN: CIOMDJ
C A SELECTS. INORGANIC & ORGANOMETALLIC REACTION SYSTEMS. Text in English. s-w. USD 275 (effective 2001). **Document type:** *Abstract/Index.* **Description:** Covers mechanistic and kinetic aspects of reactions of inorganic, organometallic and organometalloidal compounds.
Published by: Chemical Abstracts Service (Subsidiary of: American Chemical Society), 2540 Olentangy River Rd, Box 3012, Columbus, OH 43210-0012. TEL 614-447-3600, 800-753-4227, FAX 614-447-3751.

016.6165 USA ISSN 1047-8086 CODEN: CSLEEH
C A SELECTS. LEUKOTRIENES. Text in English. 1985. s-w. USD 275 (effective 2001). **Document type:** *Abstract/Index.* **Description:** Covers the synthesis, chemistry, biochemistry, physiology and pathology, and pharmacology, including pharmaceutical formulation of leukotrienes and slow-reacting substances of anaphylaxis.
Formerly (until 1989): BIOSIS CAS Selects: Leukotrienes and Slow-Reacting Substances
Published by: Chemical Abstracts Service (Subsidiary of: American Chemical Society), 2540 Olentangy River Rd, Box 3012, Columbus, OH 43210-0012. TEL 614-447-3600, 800-753-4227, FAX 614-447-3751.

540 USA ISSN 1040-7197 CODEN: CAMSE6
C A SELECTS. MEMBRANE SEPARATION. Text in English. 1989. s-w. USD 275 (effective 2001). **Document type:** *Abstract/Index.* **Description:** Covers theory and technology of dialysis, electrodialysis, electroosmosis, gas separation by membrane permeation and pervaporation.
Published by: Chemical Abstracts Service (Subsidiary of: American Chemical Society), 2540 Olentangy River Rd, Box 3012, Columbus, OH 43210-0012. TEL 614-447-3600, 800-753-4227, FAX 614-447-3751.

669 USA ISSN 0160-9114 CODEN: CSMCDF
C A SELECTS. METALLO ENZYMES & METALLO COENZYMES. Text in English. s-w. USD 275 (effective 2001). **Document type:** *Abstract/Index.* **Description:** Covers preparation, analysis, and biochemical effects of enzymes and coenzymes that contain metals (cobalt, copper, iron, zinc, and molybdenum); metalloproteins, metal-containing vitamins; mechanisms by which metals are bound to enzymes.
Published by: Chemical Abstracts Service (Subsidiary of: American Chemical Society), 2540 Olentangy River Rd, Box 3012, Columbus, OH 43210-0012. TEL 614-447-3600, 800-753-4227, FAX 614-447-3751.

016.547042 USA ISSN 1052-1976 CODEN: CSOOES
C A SELECTS. OLEOCHEMICALS CONTAINING NITROGEN. Text in English. 1990. s-w. USD 275 (effective 2001). **Document type:** *Abstract/Index.* **Description:** Covers analysis, preparation, properties, reactions, and uses of amides, amines, betaines, imidazoles, imidazolines, nitriles, and quaternary ammonium compounds derived from fats and oils.
Published by: Chemical Abstracts Service (Subsidiary of: American Chemical Society), 2540 Olentangy River Rd, Box 3012, Columbus, OH 43210-0012. TEL 614-447-3600, 800-753-4227, FAX 614-447-3751.

016.54 USA ISSN 1052-1984 CODEN: CSONEP
C A SELECTS. OMEGA-3 FATTY ACIDS & FISH OIL. Text in English. 1990. s-w. USD 275 (effective 2001). **Document type:** *Abstract/Index.* **Description:** Covers all aspects of the chemistry of omega-3 fatty acids, freshwater and marine fish oils, and oils from other marine animals.
Published by: Chemical Abstracts Service (Subsidiary of: American Chemical Society), 2540 Olentangy River Rd, Box 3012, Columbus, OH 43210-0012. TEL 614-447-3600, 800-753-4227, FAX 614-447-3751.

547.3 USA ISSN 0275-7117 CODEN: COACDT
C A SELECTS. ORGANIC ANALYTICAL CHEMISTRY. Text in English. s-w. USD 275 (effective 2001). **Document type:** *Abstract/Index.* **Description:** Covers methods, reagents, apparatus; detection and determination of elements, radicals, and compounds in organic materials; and analysis of organometallic compounds.
Published by: Chemical Abstracts Service (Subsidiary of: American Chemical Society), 2540 Olentangy River Rd, Box 3012, Columbus, OH 43210-0012. TEL 614-447-3600, 800-753-4227, FAX 614-447-3751.

540 USA ISSN 0885-0186 CODEN: CSOMEM
C A SELECTS. ORGANIC OPTICAL MATERIALS. Text in English. s-w. USD 275 (effective 2001). **Document type:** *Abstract/Index.* **Description:** Covers optical materials based on organic compounds.
Published by: Chemical Abstracts Service (Subsidiary of: American Chemical Society), 2540 Olentangy River Rd, Box 3012, Columbus, OH 43210-0012. TEL 614-447-3600, 800-753-4227, FAX 614-447-3751.

540 USA ISSN 0195-508X CODEN: CORSDQ
C A SELECTS. ORGANIC STEREOCHEMISTRY. Text in English. s-w. USD 275 (effective 2001). **Document type:** *Abstract/Index.* **Description:** Covers conformational and configurational analysis; steric factors in organic reactions and properties of organic compounds; asymmetric synthesis, preparation of specific stereoisomers, and stereoselectivity of organic reactions.
Published by: Chemical Abstracts Service (Subsidiary of: American Chemical Society), 2540 Olentangy River Rd, Box 3012, Columbus, OH 43210-0012. TEL 614-447-3600, 800-753-4227, FAX 614-447-3751.

016.54 USA ISSN 1051-3930 CODEN: CAPSEL
C A SELECTS. PHOSPHOLIPIDS (CHEMICAL ASPECTS). Text in English. 1990. s-w. USD 275 (effective 2001). **Document type:** *Abstract/Index.* **Description:** Covers analysis, properties, preparation, reactions, and uses in food, feed, pharmaceuticals, cosmetics, and membrane models of phospholipids.
Published by: Chemical Abstracts Service (Subsidiary of: American Chemical Society), 2540 Olentangy River Rd, Box 3012, Columbus, OH 43210-0012. TEL 614-447-3600, 800-753-4227, FAX 614-447-3751.

016.572 USA ISSN 0148-2335 CODEN: CSPHDB
C A SELECTS. PHOTOBIOCHEMISTRY. Text in English. s-w. USD 275 (effective 2001). **Document type:** *Abstract/Index.* **Description:** Covers photochemistry of biological materials, their constituents, and molecular structure.
Published by: Chemical Abstracts Service (Subsidiary of: American Chemical Society), 2540 Olentangy River Rd, Box 3012, Columbus, OH 43210-0012. TEL 614-447-3600, 800-753-4227, FAX 614-447-3751.

547 USA ISSN 1084-2314 CODEN: CPCCFE
C A SELECTS PLUS. CARBOHYDRATES (CHEMICAL ASPECTS). Text in English. s-w. USD 275 (effective 2001). **Document type:** *Abstract/Index.* **Description:** Characterization, reactions, structure analysis, and nonindustrial synthesis of carbohydrates and their derivatives and polymers.
Formerly: C A Selects. Carbohydrates (Chemical Aspects) (0740-0756)
Published by: Chemical Abstracts Service (Subsidiary of: American Chemical Society), 2540 Olentangy River Rd, Box 3012, Columbus, OH 43210-0012. TEL 614-447-3600, 800-753-4227, FAX 614-447-3751.

540 USA ISSN 1084-2330 CODEN: CPCTFV
C A SELECTS PLUS. CONTROLLED RELEASE TECHNOLOGY. Text in English. s-w. USD 275 (effective 2001). **Document type:** *Abstract/Index.* **Description:** Covers the science and technology of controlled release of biologically active materials (drugs, agrochemicals).
Formerly: C A Selects. Controlled Release Technology (0740-0748)
Published by: Chemical Abstracts Service (Subsidiary of: American Chemical Society), 2540 Olentangy River Rd, Box 3012, Columbus, OH 43210-0012. TEL 614-447-3600, 800-753-4227, FAX 614-447-3751.

614.19 USA ISSN 1084-2365 CODEN: CSFCFG
C A SELECTS PLUS. FORENSIC CHEMISTRY. Text in English. s-w. USD 275 (effective 2001). **Document type:** *Abstract/Index.* **Description:** Covers the chemistry of investigative science.
Formerly: C A Selects. Forensic Chemistry (0362-9880)
Published by: Chemical Abstracts Service (Subsidiary of: American Chemical Society), 2540 Olentangy River Rd, Box 3012, Columbus, OH 43210-0012. TEL 614-447-3600, 800-753-4227, FAX 614-447-3751.

540 USA ISSN 0195-5136 CODEN: CLPODH
C A SELECTS. PORPHYRINS. Text in English. s-w. USD 275 (effective 2001). **Document type:** *Abstract/Index.* **Description:** Covers chemical and biochemical aspects of porphyrins.
Published by: Chemical Abstracts Service (Subsidiary of: American Chemical Society), 2540 Olentangy River Rd, Box 3012, Columbus, OH 43210-0012. TEL 614-447-3600, 800-753-4227, FAX 614-447-3751.

540 USA ISSN 0148-2343 CODEN: CSEPDE
C A SELECTS. PROSTAGLANDINS. Text in English. s-w. USD 275 (effective 2001). **Document type:** *Abstract/Index.* **Description:** Covers the chemistry of prostaglandins, prostacyclins, thromboxanes, leukotrienes; enzymes of prostaglandin metabolism.
Published by: Chemical Abstracts Service (Subsidiary of: American Chemical Society), 2540 Olentangy River Rd, Box 3012, Columbus, OH 43210-0012. TEL 614-447-3600, 800-753-4227, FAX 614-447-3751.

540 USA ISSN 0146-4523 CODEN: CSRCD6
C A SELECTS. RADIATION CHEMISTRY. Text in English. s-w. USD 275 (effective 2001). **Document type:** *Abstract/Index.* **Description:** Covers radiation chemistry and biochemistry; radiation chemistry in aqueous and non-aqueous systems; energy transfer and ionic reactions.
Published by: Chemical Abstracts Service (Subsidiary of: American Chemical Society), 2540 Olentangy River Rd, Box 3012, Columbus, OH 43210-0012. TEL 614-477-3600, 800-753-4227, FAX 614-447-3751.

540 USA ISSN 0749-7342 CODEN: CSRCE7
C A SELECTS. RADIATION CURING. Text in English. s-w. USD 275 (effective 2001). **Document type:** *Abstract/Index.* **Description:** Covers treatment of polymers with electron beams, gamma rays, and other forms of ionizing radiation.
Published by: Chemical Abstracts Service (Subsidiary of: American Chemical Society), 2540 Olentangy River Rd, Box 3012, Columbus, OH 43210-0012. TEL 614-447-3600, 800-753-4227, FAX 614-447-3751.

615 USA ISSN 0160-9181 CODEN: CSASD3
C A SELECTS. STEROIDS (CHEMICAL ASPECTS). Text in English. s-w. USD 275 (effective 2001). **Document type:** *Abstract/Index.* **Description:** Covers isolation and synthesis of steroids, their chemical reactions and transformations.
Published by: Chemical Abstracts Service (Subsidiary of: American Chemical Society), 2540 Olentangy River Rd, Box 3012, Columbus, OH 43210-0012. TEL 614-447-3600, 800-753-4227, FAX 614-447-3751.

540 USA ISSN 0895-5816
CODEN: CSSREN

C A SELECTS. STRUCTURE - ACTIVITY RELATIONSHIPS. Text in English. 1988. s-w. USD 275 (effective 2001). **Document type:** *Abstract/Index.* **Description:** Covers structure-activity relationships of therapeutic agents and compounds that have potential therapeutic uses.
Published by: Chemical Abstracts Service (Subsidiary of: American Chemical Society), 2540 Olentangy River Rd, Box 3012, Columbus, OH 43210-0012. TEL 614-447-3600, 800-753-4227, FAX 614-447-3751.

536 USA ISSN 0162-7864
CODEN: CSTHDV

C A SELECTS. THERMOCHEMISTRY. Text in English. s-w. USD 275 (effective 2001). **Document type:** *Abstract/Index.* **Description:** Covers chemical thermodynamics: heat capacities and thermodynamic functions such as enthalpies, free energies, and entropies for physicochemical and biochemical processes.
Published by: Chemical Abstracts Service (Subsidiary of: American Chemical Society), 2540 Olentangy River Rd, Box 3012, Columbus, OH 43210-0012. TEL 614-447-3600, 800-753-4227, FAX 614-447-3751.

CHEMICAL HAZARDS IN INDUSTRY. see *OCCUPATIONAL HEALTH AND SAFETY—Abstracting, Bibliographies, Statistics*

CHEMICAL SAFETY NEWSBASE. see *OCCUPATIONAL HEALTH AND SAFETY—Abstracting, Bibliographies, Statistics*

540 GBR ISSN 0885-1980

CURRENT ADVANCES IN CLINICAL CHEMISTRY. Text in English. 1974. m. EUR 120 in Europe to qualified personnel; JPY 16,275 in Japan to qualified personnel; USD 135 elsewhere to qualified personnel; EUR 1,070 in Europe to institutions; JPY 141,843 in Japan to institutions; USD 1,197 elsewhere to institutions (effective 2002). adv. bk.rev. **Document type:** *Abstract/Index.* **Description:** Provides a current awareness service for clinical chemists, research workers, teachers and students in the field of clinical chemistry. Lists titles of papers published throughout the world classified into 29 main areas and provides a comprehensive listing of review articles.
Formerly: Current Clinical Chemistry (0305-0165)
Related titles: Diskette ed.; Microform ed.: (from PQC); Online - full text ed.
—BLDSC (3494.062500), GNLM, Infotrieve. **CCC.**
Published by: (Association of Clinical Biochemists), Elsevier Science BV, PO Box 211, Amsterdam 1000 AE, Netherlands. TEL 31-20-485-2911, FAX 31-20-485-2457, nlinfo-f@elsevier.nl, http://www.elsevier.com/locate/caclinchem, http://www.elsevier.nl. Circ: 2,400. **Subscr. in Australasia and the Far East to:** Elsevier Science (Singapore) Pte Ltd, No.1 Temasek Ave, 17-01 Millenia Tower, Singapore 039192, Singapore. TEL 65-434-3727, FAX 65-337-2230; **Subscr. in Japan to:** Elsevier Science Inc - Japan Regional Office, 9-15 Higashi-Azabu 1-chome, Minato-ku, Tokyo 106-0044, Japan. TEL 81-3-5561-5033; **Subscr. in the Americas to:** Elsevier Science, PO Box 945, New York, NY 10159-0945. TEL 212-633-3730, FAX 212-633-3680.

HIGH PERFORMANCE LIQUID CHROMATOGRAPHY. see *PHARMACY AND PHARMACOLOGY—Abstracting, Bibliographies, Statistics*

IMMUNOASSAY. see *MEDICAL SCIENCES—Abstracting, Bibliographies, Statistics*

CHEMISTRY—Analytical Chemistry

ANALYSES OF HAZARDOUS SUBSTANCES IN BIOLOGICAL MATERIALS. see *ENVIRONMENTAL STUDIES—Toxicology And Environmental Safety*

ANNALES DE BIOCHIMIE CLINIQUE DU QUEBEC. see *MEDICAL SCIENCES—Experimental Medicine, Laboratory Technique*

BIOMEDICAL CHROMATOGRAPHY. see *MEDICAL SCIENCES—Experimental Medicine, Laboratory Technique*

547.3 USA ISSN 1075-4261
QP519.9.S6 CODEN: BIOSFS

BIOSPECTROSCOPY; an international interdisciplinary journal. Text in English. 1995. 7/yr. USD 225; USD 347.50 foreign (effective 1999). adv. back issues avail.; reprints avail. *Refereed.* **Document type:** *Academic/Scholarly.* **Description:** Provides a forum for molecular spectroscopists and researchers. Emphasizes the benefits of applying molecular spectroscopy to biomolecular problems.
Related titles: Microform ed.: (from PQC); Online - full text ed.: ISSN 1520-6343. 1997 (from EBSCO Publishing, Wiley InterScience).
Indexed: ASCA, Aqua.Sci.& Fish.Abstr., BBCI (coverage dropped), Chem.Abstr., Chem.Cit.Ind., Chem.Indus.Notes, Chem.Titles, Curr.Cont. (coverage dropped), Ind.Med. (1995-), Inpharma, Reac., Rev.Med.& Vet.Mycol.
—CASDDS, CISTI, GNLM, IDS, Infotrieve, ingenta. **CCC.**
Published by: John Wiley & Sons, Inc., Journals (Subsidiary of: Wiley InterScience), 605 Third Ave, New York, NY 10158. subinfo@jwiley.com, http://www.interscience.wiley.com/japges/1075-4261/, http://www.wiley.co.uk. Ed. Laurence A Nafie. Adv. contact Roberta Frederick. B&W page GBP 640, color page GBP 1,515; trim 216 x 279. Circ: 850. **Overseas subscr. to:** John Wiley & Sons Ltd., Baffins Ln, Chichester, Sussex PO19 IUD, United Kingdom. FAX 44-1243-776128, http://www.wiley.co.uk.

COSMETIC SCIENCE MONOGRAPHS. see *BEAUTY CULTURE—Perfumes And Cosmetics*

CURRENT OPINION IN DRUG DISCOVERY & DEVELOPMENT. see *PHARMACY AND PHARMACOLOGY*

542 DEU ISSN 0070-315X
CODEN: DMDGAG

DECHEMA MONOGRAPHIEN. Text in German. irreg., latest vol.121, 1990. price varies. index. reprint service avail. from ISI. **Document type:** *Monographic series, Academic/Scholarly.*
Indexed: CEABA, Chem.Abstr., Chem.Indus.Notes, Chem.Titles, Dairy Sci.Abstr., Food Sci.& Tech.Abstr., GeoRef, Mass Spectr.Bull.
—BLDSC (3535.995000), CASDDS, CISTI, Infotrieve, Linda Hall. **CCC.**
Published by: (Deutsche Gesellschaft fuer Chemisches Apparatewesen e.V. - DECHEMA), Wiley - V C H, Postfach 101161, Weinheim 69451, Germany. TEL 49-6201-606-0, FAX 49-6201-606-328, subservice@wiley-vch.de, http://www.wiley-vch.de. **Subscr. in N. America to:** John Wiley & Sons, Inc., Journals, 605 Third Ave, New York, NY 10158. TEL 44-1243-779777, 212-850-6645, FAX 212-850-6021; **Subscr. outside Germany, Austria & Switzerland to:** John Wiley & Sons Ltd., Baffins Ln, Chichester, Sussex PO19 IUD, United Kingdom. TEL 44-1243-779777, FAX 44-1243-843232.

543 JPN ISSN 0385-1516
CODEN: DONED9

DOJIN NYUSU/DOJIN NEWS. Text in Japanese; Summaries in English. 1976. 6/yr. free per issue. **Document type:** *Newsletter.* **Description:** Covers topics in chemistry and their applications in pharmacology.
Indexed: Biol.Abstr., Chem.Abstr., Chem.Indus.Notes, Chem.Titles.
—CASDDS.
Published by: Dojindo Laboratories, Kumamoto Techno Research Park, 2025-5 Tabaru, Kamimashiki-gun, Mashiki-machi, Kumamoto-ken 861-2202, Japan. TEL 81-96-286-1515, FAX 81-96-286-1525, info@dojindo.co.jp; order@dojindo.co.jp, http://www.dojindo.co.jp.

615.19 JPN ISSN 0919-9322

DONJINDO NEWSLETTER. Text in English. 1992. 3/yr. free per issue. adv. **Document type:** *Newsletter.* **Description:** Covers topics in chemistry and their application in pharmacology.
Published by: Dojindo Laboratories, Kumamoto Techno Research Park, 2025-5 Tabaru, Kamimashiki-gun, Mashiki-machi, Kumamoto-ken 861-2202, Japan. TEL 096-286-1515, FAX 096-286-1525, info@dojindo.co.jp; order@dojindo.co.jp, http://www.dojindo.co.jp. Ed. Meiko Sato. R&P Mikihiko Saito. Adv. contact Ken'yu Kina.

EXPERIMENTAL AND MOLECULAR PATHOLOGY. see *MEDICAL SCIENCES*

FOLIA MICROBIOLOGICA. see *BIOLOGY—Biochemistry*

543 USA ISSN 1073-9149
QD53 CODEN: ISCTEF

INSTRUMENTATION SCIENCE & TECHNOLOGY. Text in English. 1973. 5/yr. USD 145 to individuals print and online eds.; USD 875 to institutions print only (effective 2002). adv. bk.rev. bibl, charts, illus. *Refereed.* **Document type:** *Academic/Scholarly.* **Description:** Dedicated to publishing papers dealing with instrument design innovations and applications in the areas of chemistry, biotechnology, and environemntal science.
Former titles (until 1994): Analytical Instrumentation (0743-5797); (until 1984): Chemical, Biomedical and Environmental Instrumentation (0190-4094); Chemical Instrumentation (0009-2592)
Related titles: Microform ed.: (from RPI); Online - full text ed.: (from EBSCO Publishing, O C L C Online Computer Library Center, Inc., RoweCom Information Quest, Swets Blackwell, Institute for Scientific Information).
Indexed: ASCA, Abstr.Bull.Inst.Pap.Chem., Anal.Abstr., Bioeng.Abstr., Biol.Abstr., Biotech.& Bioeng.Abstr., Chem.Abstr., Chem.Cit.Ind., Chem.Indus.Notes, Chem.Titles, Curr.Cont., Curr.Tit.Electrochem., Eng.Ind., Excerp.Med., GeoRef, INIS Atomind., INSPEC (1971-1977, 1979-), Int.Sci.Rev., Mass Spectr.Bull., Sci.Cit.Ind.
—BLDSC (4529.043800), AskIEEE, CASDDS, CISTI, Ei, IDS, Infotrieve, ingenta, Linda Hall. **CCC.**
Published by: Marcel Dekker Inc., 270 Madison Ave, New York, NY 10016. TEL 212-696-9000, 800-228-1160, FAX 212-685-4540, http://www.dekker.com/servlet/product/productid/CI. Ed. Jack Cazes. R&P Julia Mulligan. Adv. contact Diane Saulon. B&W page USD 800. Circ: 325. **Subscr. to:** Marcel Dekker Journals.

543 USA
RB46.5 CODEN: JOUIDK

JOURNAL OF IMMUNOASSAY AND IMMUNOCHEMISTRY. Text in English. 1980. 4/yr. USD 115 to individuals print & online eds.; USD 795 to institutions print only (effective 2002). *Refereed.* **Document type:** *Academic/Scholarly.* **Description:** Presents coverage of this rapidly expanding field, providing practical, hands-on information with an emphasis on applications.
Formerly (until 2001): Journal of Immunoassay (0197-1522)
Related titles: Microform ed.: (from RPI); Online - full content ed.; Online - full text ed.: (from Institute for Scientific Information, RoweCom Information Quest).
Indexed: AIDS & Cancer Res., ASCA, Abstr.Hyg., Anal.Abstr., Aqua.Sci.& Fish.Abstr., BBCI, Biol.Abstr., Biotech.& Bioeng.Abstr., Biotech.Cit.Ind., Chem.Abstr., Chem.Indus.Notes, Chem.Titles, Curr.Adv.Ecol.Sci., Curr.Cont., Excerp.Med., INIS Atomind., Immun.Abstr., Ind.Med. (1980-), Ind.Sci.Rev., Ind.Vet., Inpharma, Int.Abstr.Biol.Sci., Med.& Pharm.Biotech.Abstr., Microbiol.Abstr., Protozool.Abstr., Reac., Ref.Zh., Sci.Cit.Ind., Telegen, Vet.Bull., Virol.Abstr.
—BLDSC (5004.560000), CASDDS, CISTI, GNLM, IDS, ingenta, KNAW. **CCC.**
Published by: Marcel Dekker Inc., 270 Madison Ave, New York, NY 10016. TEL 212-696-9000, 800-228-1160, FAX 212-685-4540, journals@dekker.com, http://www.dekker.com/servlet/product/productid/IAS. Ed. Jack Cazes. R&P Julia Mulligan. Adv. contact Diane Saulon. Circ: 350.

544.92 HUN ISSN 0933-4173
QD79.C8 CODEN: JPCTE5

JOURNAL OF PLANAR CHROMATOGRAPHY - MODERN TLC (JPC). Text in English. 1987. bi-m., latest vol.14, 2001. USD 296; USD 51 newsstand/cover (effective 2001). adv. bk.rev. index. 80 p./no. back issues avail. *Refereed.* **Document type:** *Journal, Academic/Scholarly.* **Description:** Publishes papers on analytical and preparative planar chromatography in the pharmaceutical and chemical industries.
Related titles: Online - full text ed.: (from Institute for Scientific Information).
Indexed: ASCA, Anal.Abstr., Chem.Abstr., Chem.Cit.Ind., Chem.Indus.Notes, Chem.Titles, Chromat.Abstr., Curr.Cont., Eng.Ind., Excerp.Med. (1995-), Mass Spectr.Bull., Nutr.Abstr., Sci.Cit.Ind., Sugar Ind.Abstr., Weed Abstr.
—BLDSC (5073.675000), CASDDS, CISTI, Ei, GNLM, IDS, Infotrieve, ingenta, Linda Hall. **CCC.**
Published by: Research Institute for Medicinal Plants, Lupaszigeti utca 4, PO Box 11, Budakalasz 2011, Hungary. TEL 36-26-340203, FAX 36-26-340426, rimp@mail.matav.hu. Ed., R&P, Adv. contact Szabolcs Nyiredy. page DEM 3,000; 178 x 240. Circ: 1,450 (paid); 220 (controlled).

LUMINESCENCE; journal of biological and chemical luminescence. see *CHEMISTRY—Physical Chemistry*

544 615 ISR ISSN 0793-0291
RS431.M45 CODEN: MBADEI
METAL-BASED DRUGS. Text in English. 1994. 6/yr., latest vol.8. USD 360 to institutions (effective 2002). **Document type:** *Academic/Scholarly.*
Indexed: Chem.Abstr., Chem.Titles.
—BLDSC (5683.686000), CASDDS, EMDOCS, GNLM, KNAW.
Published by: Freund Publishing House, Ltd., P O Box 35010, Tel Aviv 61350, Israel. TEL 972-3-562-8538, FAX 972-3-562-8540, h_freund@netvision.net.il, http://www.angelfire.com/il/freund. Ed. M Gielen.

502.82 USA ISSN 0026-282X
QH201 CODEN: MICRAD
MICROSCOPE. Text in English. 1937. q. USD 75 (effective 2001). adv. bk.rev. bibl, charts, illus, pat, stat, tr.lit. index, cum.index. back issues avail. *Refereed.* **Description:** Dedicated to the advancement of all forms of microscopy for the biologist, mineralogist, metallographer or chemist.
Indexed: Abstr.Bull.Inst.Pap.Chem., Alloys Ind., Art & Archaeol.Tech.Abstr., Chem.Abstr., Curr.Cont. (coverage dropped), Deep Sea Res.& Oceanogr.Abstr., Eng.Mat.Abstr., Excerp.Med., GeoRef, INIS Atomind., INSPEC (Jul.1968-), METADEX, Met.Abstr., Met.Abstr.Ind., Nonfer.Met.Alert, PCC Alert, Ref.Zh., Sci.Cit.Ind. (coverage dropped), Steels Alert, World Alum.Abstr.
—BLDSC (5760.000000), AskIEEE, CASDDS, CISTI, ingenta, Linda Hall. **CCC.**
Published by: McCrone Research Institute, 2820 S Michigan Ave, Chicago, IL 60616-3292. TEL 312-842-7100, FAX 312-842-1078, dstoney@mcri.org, http://www.mcri.org. Ed. David Stoney. Adv. contact Nancy Daerr. Circ: 1,200.

N M R IN BIOMEDICINE. (Nuclear Magnetic Resonance) see *MEDICAL SCIENCES—Radiology And Nuclear Medicine*

544.6 NLD ISSN 0079-6565
QC762 CODEN: PNMRAT
PROGRESS IN NUCLEAR MAGNETIC RESONANCE SPECTROSCOPY. Text in English. 1966. 8/yr. EUR 890 in Europe to institutions; JPY 118,200 in Japan to institutions; USD 996 elsewhere to institutions (effective 2002). index. *Refereed.* **Document type:** *Academic/Scholarly.* **Description:** Publishes review articles covering applications of NMR in chemistry, biochemistry and biological science, as well as fundamental theory and instrumental developments.
Related titles: Microfilm ed.: (from PQC); Online - full text ed.: (from ingenta, Swets Blackwell, Institute for Scientific Information, ScienceDirect).
Indexed: ASCA, Bioeng.Abstr., Biotech.& Bioeng.Abstr., Chem.Abstr., Chem.Cit.Ind., Chem.Indus.Notes, Chem.Titles, Curr.Cont., Eng.Ind., INIS Atomind., INSPEC (1975-), Ind.Sci.Rev., Met.Abstr., Sci.Cit.Ind., World Alum.Abstr.
—BLDSC (6870.750000), ADONIS, AskIEEE, CASDDS, CISTI, Ei, GNLM, IDS, Linda Hall. **CCC.**
Published by: Elsevier Science BV, PO Box 211, Amsterdam 1000 AE, Netherlands. TEL 31-20-485-2911, FAX 31-20-485-2457, http://www.elsevier.com/locate/pnmrs. Eds. J Feeney, J W Emsley, L H Sutcliffe. **Subscr. in Australasia and the Far East to:** Elsevier Science (Singapore) Pte Ltd, No.1 Temasek Ave, 17-01 Millenia Tower, Singapore 039192, Singapore. TEL 65-434-3727, FAX 65-337-2230; **Subscr. in Japan to:** Elsevier Science Inc - Japan Regional Office, 9-15 Higashi-Azabu 1-chome, Minato-ku, Tokyo 106-0044, Japan. TEL 81-3-5561-5033; **Subscr. in the Americas to:** Elsevier Science, PO Box 945, New York, NY 10159-0945. TEL 212-633-3730, FAX 212-633-3680, usinfo-f@elsevier.com, http://www.elsevier.com.

547.593 GBR ISSN 0933-4807
CODEN: PTRDEO
PTERIDINES. Text in English. 1989. 4/yr. adv. bk.rev. index. *Refereed.* **Document type:** *Academic/Scholarly.* **Description:** Multi-disciplinary study of pteridines and related materials.
Related titles: Online - full text ed.: (from Institute for Scientific Information).
Indexed: ASCA, BBCI, Chem.Abstr., Chem.Cit.Ind., Chem.Indus.Notes, Chem.Titles, Excerp.Med. (1994-), Int.Abstr.Biol.Sci.
—BLDSC (6946.579300), CASDDS, CISTI, EMDOCS, GNLM, IDS, Infotrieve, Linda Hall. **CCC.**
Published by: International Society of Pteridinology, Portsmouth, Hants PO3 6AD, United Kingdom. TEL 44-1705-822331.

543 616.075 GBR ISSN 0926-2040
QC762 CODEN: SSNRE4
SOLID STATE NUCLEAR MAGNETIC RESONANCE; an international journal. Abbreviated title: S S N M R. Text in English. 1992. irreg. (in 2 vols.). USD 802 (effective 2001). back issues avail. *Refereed.* **Document type:** *Academic/Scholarly.* **Description:** Covers experimental and theoretical aspects of solid state NMR, including advances in instrumentation, techniques and methodology, simulation and applications.
Related titles: Microform ed.: 1992 (from PQC); Online - full text ed.: (from RoweCom Information Quest, ingenta, Swets Blackwell, IDEAL Online Library, Institute for Scientific Information, ScienceDirect).
Indexed: ASCA, Alloys Ind., Bioeng.Abstr., Biotech.& Bioeng.Abstr., Chem.Abstr., Chem.Cit.Ind., Chem.Indus.Notes, Chem.Titles, Curr.Cont., Eng.Ind., Eng.Mat.Abstr., INSPEC (Feb.1992-), Ind.Med. (1992-), Ind.Sci.Rev., METADEX, Met.Abstr., Met.Abstr.Ind., Nonfer.Met.Alert, PCC Alert, Sci.Cit.Ind., Steels Alert, World Alum.Abstr.
—BLDSC (8327.391000), AskIEEE, CASDDS, CISTI, Ei, GNLM, IDS, Infotrieve. **CCC.**
Published by: Academic Press (Subsidiary of: Harcourt Publishers Ltd.), 32 Jamestown Rd, London NW1 7BY, United Kingdom. apssubs@acad.com, http://www.academicpress.com/snmr, http://www.academicpress.com/jcp.

643 NLD ISSN 0168-6461
STUDIES IN ANALYTICAL CHEMISTRY. Text in English. 1981. irreg., latest vol.8, 1989. price varies. *Refereed.* **Document type:** *Monographic series, Academic/Scholarly.* **Description:** Reviews topics in analytical chemistry.
Indexed: INSPEC (coverage dropped).
Published by: Elsevier Science BV, PO Box 211, Amsterdam 1000 AE, Netherlands. TEL 31-20-485-3757, 31-20-485-3911, FAX 31-20-485-3432, 31-20-485-3598, nlinfo-f@elsevier.nl, http://www.elsevier.nl. **Subscr. in Australasia and the Far East to:** Elsevier Science (Singapore) Pte Ltd, No.1 Temasek Ave, 17-01 Millenia Tower, Singapore 039192, Singapore. TEL 65-434-3727, FAX 65-337-2230, asiainfo@elsevier.com.sg; **Subscr. in Japan to:** Elsevier Science Inc - Japan Regional Office, 9-15 Higashi-Azabu 1-chome, Minato-ku, Tokyo 106-0044, Japan. TEL 81-3-5561-5033, FAX 81-3-5561-5047, info@elsevier.co.jp; **Subscr. in the Americas to:** Elsevier Science, PO Box 945, New York, NY 10159-0945. TEL 212-633-3730, 888-437-4636, FAX 212-633-3680, usinfo-f@elsevier.com, http://www.elsevier.com

UNIVERSIDAD CENTRAL DE VENEZUELA. FACULTAD DE FARMACIA. REVISTA. see *PHARMACY AND PHARMACOLOGY*

CHEMISTRY—Computer Applications

541.220285 USA ISSN 1093-3263
QD461 CODEN: JMGRDV
JOURNAL OF MOLECULAR GRAPHICS AND MODELLING. Text in English. 1983. bi-m. EUR 265 in Europe to qualified personnel; JPY 35,200 in Japan to qualified personnel; USD 296 elsewhere to qualified personnel; EUR 823 in Europe to institutions; JPY 109,200 in Japan to institutions; USD 920 elsewhere to institutions (effective 2002). adv. bk.rev. abstr, illus. index. back issues avail. *Refereed.* **Document type:** *Academic/Scholarly.* **Description:** Practical and theoretical research on the use of computer graphics for the investigation of molecular structure, function and interaction.
Formerly: Journal of Molecular Graphics (0263-7855)
Related titles: Microform ed.: (from PQC); Online - full text ed.: (from ingenta, ScienceDirect, Swets Blackwell, Institute for Scientific Information).
Indexed: Aqua.Sci.& Fish.Abstr., BBCI, Bioeng.Abstr., Biotech.Cit.Ind., Chem.Abstr., Chem.Cit.Ind., Chem.Indus.Notes, Chem.Titles, Comput.& Info.Sys., Comput.Cont., Curr.Cont. (coverage dropped), Eng.Ind., Excerp.Med. (1992-), INSPEC, Ind.Med. (1997-), Ind.Sci.Rev., Int.Abstr.Biol.Sci., RCI, Sci.Cit.Ind., Solid St.Abstr.
—BLDSC (5020.713100), ADONIS, CASDDS, CISTI, Ei, EMDOCS, GNLM, IDS, Infotrieve, ingenta, Linda Hall. **CCC.**
Published by: (Molecular Graphics and Modelling Society), Elsevier Science, PO Box 945, New York, NY 10159-0945. TEL 212-989-5800, FAX 212-633-3990, usinfo-f@elsevier.com, http://www.elsevier.com/locate/jmgm. Eds. Vivian Cody, W G Richards. **Subscr. in Australasia and the Far East to:** Elsevier Science (Singapore) Pte Ltd, No.1 Temasek Ave, 17-01 Millenia Tower, Singapore 039192, Singapore. TEL 65-434-3727, FAX 65-337-2230; **Subscr. in Japan to:** Elsevier Science Inc - Japan Regional Office, 9-15 Higashi-Azabu 1-chome, Minato-ku, Tokyo 106-0044, Japan. TEL 81-3-5561-5033; **Subscr. outside the Americas to:** Elsevier Science BV, PO Box 211, Amsterdam 1000 AE, Netherlands. TEL 31-20-485-3757.

CHEMISTRY—Crystallography

ACTA BIOPHYSICS SINICA. see *BIOLOGY—Biophysics*

MICROSCOPE. see *CHEMISTRY—Analytical Chemistry*

CHEMISTRY—Inorganic Chemistry

JOURNAL OF INORGANIC BIOCHEMISTRY; an interdisciplinary journal. see *BIOLOGY—Biochemistry*

CHEMISTRY—Organic Chemistry

547 615.7 USA ISSN 0099-9598
QD421.A1 CODEN: ALKAAR
THE ALKALOIDS; chemistry and biology. Text in English. 1950. irreg., latest vol.51, 1998. reprint service avail. from ISI. *Refereed.* **Document type:** *Monographic series.*
Indexed: Chem.Abstr., Chem.Indus.Notes, Chem.Titles, Mass Spectr.Bull.
—BLDSC (0788.529000), CASDDS, CISTI, GNLM. **CCC.**
Published by: Academic Press, Inc., Journal Division (Subsidiary of: Harcourt Brace & Company), 525 B St, Ste 1900, San Diego, CA 92101-4495. TEL 619-231-0926, FAX 619-699-6715. **Subscr. to:** Order Dept., 6277 Sea Harbor Dr, 4th Fl, Orlando, FL 32887. TEL 800-321-5068.

BIOCHEMICAL PHARMACOLOGY. see *PHARMACY AND PHARMACOLOGY*

547 610 GBR ISSN 0968-0896
QP550 CODEN: BMECEP
BIOORGANIC & MEDICINAL CHEMISTRY. Text in English. 1993. m. EUR 1,453 in Europe to institutions; JPY 193,000 in Japan to institutions; USD 1,625 elsewhere to institutions; EUR 178 in Europe to qualified personnel; JPY 23,700 in Japan to qualified personnel; USD 200 elsewhere to qualified personnel (effective 2002). back issues avail. *Refereed.* **Document type:** *Academic/Scholarly.* **Description:** Publishes full original research papers and critical reviews on biomolecular chemistry, medicinal chemistry and related disciplines.
Related titles: Microfilm ed.: (from PQC); Online - full text ed.: ISSN 1464-3391 (from EBSCO Publishing, ingenta, Swets Blackwell, ScienceDirect, Institute for Scientific Information).
Indexed: BBCI, Chem.Abstr., Chem.Cit.Ind., Chem.Indus.Notes, Chem.Titles, Curr.Cont., Derwent Biotech.Abstr., Excerp.Med. (1995-), INIS Atomind., Ind.Med. (1993-), Int.Abstr.Biol.Sci., Mass Spectr.Bull., Ref.Zh., Sci.Cit.Ind.
—BLDSC (2089.325000), CASDDS, CINDOC, CISTI, EMDOCS, GNLM, IDS, Infotrieve, Linda Hall. **CCC.**
Published by: Pergamon (Subsidiary of: Elsevier Science), The Boulevard, Langford Ln, East Park, Kidlington, Oxford OXB 1GB, United Kingdom. FAX 44-1865-843010, nlinfo-f@elsevier/nl; usinfo-f@elsevier.com; forinfo-kyf04035@niftyserve.or.jp, http://www.elsevier.com/locate/tetonline, http://www.elsevier.nl/. Ed. Chi Huey Wong. **Subscr. in Australasia and the Far East to:** Elsevier Science (Singapore) Pte Ltd, No.1 Temasek Ave, 17-01 Millenia Tower, Singapore 039192, Singapore. TEL 65-434-3727, FAX 65-337-2230; **Subscr. in the Americas to:** Elsevier Science, PO Box 945, New York, NY 10159-0945. TEL 212-633-3730, FAX 212-633-3680, usinfo-f@elsevier.com, http://www.elsevier.com; **Subscr. to:** Elsevier Science BV, PO Box 211, Amsterdam 1000 AE, Netherlands. TEL 31-20-485-3757, FAX 31-20-485-3432, nlinfo-f@elsevier.nl, http://www.elsevier.nl.

C

547 610 GBR ISSN 0960-894X
QP501 CODEN: BMCLE8
BIOORGANIC & MEDICINAL CHEMISTRY LETTERS; for rapid dissemination of preliminary communications on all aspects of bioorganic chemistry, medicinal chemistry and related disciplines. Text in English. 1991. s-m. EUR 257 in Europe to qualified personnel; JPY 34,200 in Japan to qualified personnel; USD 288 elsewhere to qualified personnel; EUR 1,956 in Europe to institutions; JPY 259,800 in Japan to institutions; USD 2,188 elsewhere to institutions (effective 2002). back issues avail. *Refereed.* **Document type:** *Academic/Scholarly.* **Description:** Publishes preliminary communications and theoretical research results in bioorganic and medicinal chemistry.
Related titles: Microfilm ed.: (from PQC); Online - full text ed.: ISSN 1464-3405 (from EBSCO Publishing, ingenta, Swets Blackwell, ScienceDirect, Institute for Scientific Information).
Indexed: ASCA, BBCI, Chem.Abstr., Chem.Cit.Ind., Chem.Indus.Notes, Chem.Titles, Curr.Cont., Derwent Biotech.Abstr., Excerp.Med. (1992-), Ind.Med. (1991-), Ind.Sci.Rev., Ind.Vet., Inpharma, Int.Abstr.Biol.Sci., MOS, Mass Spectr.Bull., NPU, Neurosci.Cit.Ind., Pharm.&Out.News, Protozool.Abstr., Reac., Ref.Zh., Rev.Appl.Entomol., Rev.Arom.& Med.Plants, Rev.Med.& Vet.Mycol., Rev.Plant Path., Rice Abstr., Sci.Cit.Ind., Soils & Fert., Vet.Bull., Weed Abstr.
—BLDSC (2089.330000), ADONIS, CASDDS, CINDOC, CISTI, EMDOCS, GNLM, IDS, ingenta, Linda Hall. **CCC.**
Published by: Pergamon (Subsidiary of: Elsevier Science), The Boulevard, Langford Ln, East Park, Kidlington, Oxford OXB 1GB, United Kingdom. FAX 44-1865-843010, nlinfo-f@elsevier/nl; usinfo-f@elsevier.com; forinfo-kyf04035@niftyserve.or.jp, http://www.elsevier.com/locate/tetonline, http://www.elsevier.nl/. Ed. D L Boger. **Subscr. in Australasia and the Far East to:** Elsevier Science (Singapore) Pte Ltd, No.1 Temasek Ave, 17-01 Millenia Tower, Singapore 039192, Singapore. TEL 65-434-3727, FAX 65-337-2230; **Subscr. in the Americas to:** Elsevier Science, PO Box 945, New York, NY 10159-0945. TEL 212-633-3730, FAX 212-633-3680, usinfo-f@elsevier.com, http://www.elsevier.com; **Subscr. to:** Elsevier Science BV, PO Box 211, Amsterdam 1000 AE, Netherlands. TEL 31-20-485-3757, FAX 31-20-485-3432, nlinfo-f@elsevier.nl, http://www.elsevier.nl.

547 RUS ISSN 0132-3423
QD415.A1 CODEN: BIKHD7
BIOORGANICHESKAYA KHIMIYA. Text in Russian; Summaries in English. 1975. bi-m. RUR 345 for 2 mos. (effective 2001). illus. *Refereed.* **Document type:** *Academic/Scholarly.* **Description:** Publishes reviews and the results of original experimental and theoretical investigations on the structure, structure-activity relationships, and synthesis of biopolymers such as proteins, nucleic acids, polysaccharides, mixed biopolymers and their more highly organized complexes and low molecular mass bioregulators such as peptides, lipids, and antibiotics.
Related titles: Online - full text ed.; ♦ Russian Translation: Russian Journal of Bioorganic Chemistry. ISSN 1068-1620.
Indexed: ASCA, AgBiotech, Agri.& Environ.Biotech.Abstr. (coverage dropped), BBCI, Biol.Abstr., Chem.Abstr., Chem.Cit.Ind., Chem.Indus.Notes, Chem.Titles, Curr.Adv.Ecol.Sci., Curr.Cont. (coverage dropped), Dairy Sci.Abstr., Derwent Biotech.Abstr., Excerp.Med., INIS Atomind., Ind.Med. (1975-), Ind.Sci.Rev., Ind.Vet., Inpharma, MOS, Mass Spectr.Bull., NPU, Nutr.Abstr., Plant Breed.Abstr., Plant Grow.Reg.Abstr., RCI, Reac., Ref.Zh., Rev.Appl.Entomol., Rev.Med.& Vet.Mycol., Rev.Plant Path., Sci.Cit.Ind., Sugar Ind.Abstr., Zoo.Rec.
—CASDDS, CISTI, East View, GNLM, IDS, Infotrieve, KNAW, Linda Hall. **CCC.**
Published by: (Rossiiskaya Akademiya Nauk/Russian Academy of Sciences), M A I K Nauka - Interperiodica, Mezhdunarodnyi Otdel, Profsoyuznaya ul 90, Moscow 117864, Russian Federation. FAX 7-095-336-0666, rjbc@ibch.siobc.ras.ru, http://www.maik.rssi.ru/journals/biochem.htm, http://rjbc.siobc.ras.ru. Ed. Vadim T Ivanov. **Dist. by:** Mezhdunarodnaya Kniga, B Yakimanka 39, Moscow 117049, Russian Federation.

C A SELECTS. OLEOCHEMICALS CONTAINING NITROGEN. see *CHEMISTRY—Abstracting, Bibliographies, Statistics*

547 NLD ISSN 0969-0239
TS933.C4 CODEN: CELLE8
CELLULOSE. Text in Dutch. 1994. q. USD 493 in the Americas to institutions for print or online ed.; EUR 492 elsewhere to institutions for print or online ed.; USD 591.60 in the Americas to institutions for print & online eds. combined; EUR 590.40 elsewhere to institutions for print & online eds. combined (effective 2002). adv. reprints avail. *Refereed.* **Document type:** *Journal, Academic/Scholarly.* **Description:** Contains research and review papers relating to scientific progress in the field of cellulose, especially the chemistry, biochemistry, physics, and materials science of cellulose and its derivatives.
Related titles: Online - full text ed.: (from EBSCO Publishing, O C L C Online Computer Library Center, Inc., RoweCom Information Quest, Swets Blackwell, Kluwer Online, Institute for Scientific Information).
Indexed: ASCA, Chem.Cit.Ind., Derwent Biotech.Abstr., Eng.Ind., Fluidex, Mat.Sci.Cit.Ind., Nonwov.Abstr., Paper & Bd.Abstr., World Text.Abstr.
—BLDSC (3098.059800), CASDDS, IDS. **CCC.**
Published by: (Cellulose Division USA, American Chemical Society USA), Kluwer Academic Publishers Group (Subsidiary of: Wolters Kluwer N.V.), Spuiboulevard 50, PO Box 17, Dordrecht 3300 AA, Netherlands. TEL 31-78-639-2392, FAX 31-78-654-2254, services@wkap.nl, http://www.wkap.nl/journalhome.htm/0969-0239. Ed. Wolfgang Glasser. Adv. contact Gemma Heiser. **Subscr. in the Americas to:** Kluwer Academic - Plenum Publishers, 233 Spring St, New York, NY 10013-1578. TEL 212-620-8468, FAX 212-807-1047; **Subscr. to:** Journals Department, PO Box 322, Dordrecht 3300 AH, Netherlands. TEL 31-78-639-2392, FAX 31-78-654-6474. **Co-sponsor:** Japanese Cellulose Research Society.

577 547 CHE ISSN 0937-7409
QH541.15.C44 CODEN: CHMOE9
CHEMOECOLOGY; evolutionary, mechanistic and environmental approaches to chemically-mediated interactions. Text in English. 1990-199?; N.S. 1998. q. CHF 448, USD 156 to individuals; CHF 456, USD 327 to institutions; CHF 134, USD 96.70 newsstand/cover to institutions (effective 2002). back issues avail. *Refereed.* **Document type:** *Journal, Academic/Scholarly.* **Description:** Publishes papers dealing with the manifold interactions between organisms (between animals or animal and plant) caused by chemical substances and their interactions.
Related titles: Online - full text ed.: ISSN 1423-0445. N.S. (from EBSCO Publishing, Swets Blackwell, Springer LINK, Institute for Scientific Information).
Indexed: BBCI, Bio-Contr.News & Info., Chem.Abstr., Chem.Indus.Notes, Chem.Titles, Crop Physiol.Abstr., Curr.Cont., Field Crop Abstr., Forest Prod.Abstr., Forest.Abstr., Rev.Appl.Entomol., Rev.Med.& Vet.Mycol., Seed Abstr., Triticale Abstr., Weed Abstr., Zoo.Rec.
—BLDSC (3172.258000), CASDDS, CISTI, Infotrieve, ingenta. **CCC.**
Published by: Birkhaeuser Verlag AG (Subsidiary of: BertelsmannSpringer), Klosterberg, Postfach 133, Basel 4010, Switzerland. TEL 41-61-2050730, FAX 41-61-2050792, subscriptions@birkhauser.ch, http://link.springer.de/link/service/journals/00049/index.htm, http://www.birkhauser.ch/journals. Eds. D Daloze, J Pasteels. Circ: 400. **Dist. in N.America by:** Springer-Verlag, 333 Meadowlands Parkway, Secaucus, NJ 07094. TEL 800-777-4643, FAX 201-348-4505.

547 USA ISSN 1022-0178
RS201.C64 CODEN: PCRMEY
CONTROLLED RELEASE SOCIETY. INTERNATIONAL SYMPOSIUM ON CONTROLLED RELEASE OF BIOACTIVE MATERIALS. PROCEEDINGS. Text in English. 1973. a. USD 85 to members (effective 1999). back issues avail. **Document type:** *Proceedings.*
Related titles: CD-ROM ed.
Indexed: Chem.Abstr., Chem.Indus.Notes, Excerp.Med. (1993-).
—BLDSC (6846.782860), CASDDS, KNAW.
Published by: Controlled Release Society, Inc., 1020 Milwaukee Ave, Ste 335, Deerfield, IL 60015-3500. TEL 847-808-7071. Circ: 3,000.

EUROPEAN JOURNAL OF MEDICINAL CHEMISTRY. see *BIOLOGY—Biochemistry*

FITOTERAPIA; journal for the study of medicinal plants - rivista di studi ed applicazioni delle piante medicinali. see *BIOLOGY—Botany*

547 668.4 GBR ISSN 1468-5736
▼ **FOCUS ON POLYVINYL CHLORIDE.** Text in English. 2000. m. EUR 654 in Europe to institutions; JPY 86,900 in Japan to institutions; USD 732 elsewhere to institutions (effective 2002). **Document type:** *Newsletter, Trade.* **Description:** Monitors all commercial and technical developments in the PVC sector, from supply to production, including new end-uses and applications of rigid and plasticised PVC.
Indexed: CBNB (2000-).
Published by: Elsevier Advanced Technology (Subsidiary of: Elsevier Science), The Boulevard, Langford Ln, Kidlington, Oxon OX5 2BG, United Kingdom. TEL 44-1865-843750, FAX 44-1865-843971, eatsales@elsevier.co.uk, http://www.elsevier.com/locate/fopc, http://www.elsevier.nl/.

FOLIA MICROBIOLOGICA. see *BIOLOGY—Biochemistry*

547 USA ISSN 0163-9102
QP751 CODEN: HLREDI
HANDBOOK OF LIPID RESEARCH. Text in English. 1978. irreg., latest vol.8, 1996. price varies. back issues avail. *Refereed.* **Document type:** *Monographic series.*
—BLDSC (4250.850000), CASDDS, CISTI, Infotrieve, KNAW. **CCC.**
Published by: Kluwer Academic - Plenum Publishers (Subsidiary of: Wolters Kluwer N.V.), 233 Spring St, New York, NY 10013-1578. TEL 212-620-8000, 800-221-9369, FAX 212-463-0742, info@plenum.com, http://www.plenum.com. Ed. Fred Snyder.

547 615.9 362.1 GBR
I E H SPECIAL REPORT ON ORGANOPHOSPHORUS ESTERS; an evaluation of chronic neurotoxic effects. Text in English. 1998. irreg. GBP 12.50 (effective 2000). **Document type:** *Monographic series, Academic/Scholarly.* **Description:** Evaluates the chronic neurotoxic effects resulting from exposure to organophosphorus pesticide, a group of chemicals, including some agents used for sheep dipping.
Published by: Institute for Environment and Health, University of Leicester, 94 Regent Rd, Leicester, Leics LE1 7DD, United Kingdom. TEL 44-116-223-1600, FAX 44-116-223-1601, msto1@le.ac.uk, http://www.le.ac.uk/ieh/. R&P Ruth Gardener.

547 GBR ISSN 0952-3499
QP517.M67 CODEN: JMORE4
JOURNAL OF MOLECULAR RECOGNITION. Text in English. 1988. 7/yr. USD 995 in United States; USD 995 in Canada & Mexico; USD 995 elsewhere; USD 1,045 combined subscription in United States for print and online eds.; USD 1,045 combined subscription in Canada & Mexico for print and online eds.; USD 1,045 combined subscription elsewhere for print and online eds. (effective 2002). adv. bk.rev. back issues avail.; reprint service avail. from SWZ. *Refereed.* **Document type:** *Academic/Scholarly.* **Description:** Covers the research on the basic principles, characterization, and application of specific molecular interactions in chemistry, biology, biotechnology and medicine.
Related titles: Microform ed.: (from PQC); Online - full text ed.: ISSN 1099-1352. USD 995 in United States; USD 995 in Canada & Mexico; USD 995 elsewhere (effective 2002) (from EBSCO Publishing, Wiley InterScience, Institute for Scientific Information).
Indexed: ASCA, BBCI, Chem.Abstr., Chem.Titles, Curr.Cont., Eng.Ind., Ind.Med. (1988-), Int.Abstr.Biol.Sci., Ref.Zh.
—BLDSC (5020.725000), CASDDS, CISTI, Ei, EMDOCS, GNLM, IDS, ingenta. **CCC.**
Published by: Wiley Europe Ltd., Baffins Ln, Chichester, W Sussex PO19 1UD, United Kingdom. TEL 44-1243-779777, FAX 44-1243-775878, customer@wiley.co.uk, http://www.wiley.co.uk. adv.: B&W page GBP 650, color page GBP 1,550; trim 210 x 279. **Subscr. in the Americas to:** John Wiley & Sons, Inc., Journals, 605 Third Ave, New York, NY 10158. TEL 212-850-6021, 212-850-6645, subinfo@jwiley.com.

547 GBR ISSN 1075-2617
CODEN: JPSIEI
JOURNAL OF PEPTIDE SCIENCE. Text in English. 1994. 8/yr. USD 795 in United States; USD 795 in Canada & Mexico; USD 795 elsewhere; USD 835 combined subscription in United States for print and online eds.; USD 835 combined subscription in Canada & Mexico for print and online eds.; USD 835 combined subscription elsewhere for print and online eds. (effective 2002). adv. back issues avail. *Refereed.* **Document type:** *Academic/Scholarly.*
Related titles: Microform ed.: (from PQC); Online - full text ed.: ISSN 1099-1387. USD 795 in United States; USD 795 in Canada & Mexico; USD 795 elsewhere (effective 2002) (from EBSCO Publishing, Wiley InterScience, Institute for Scientific Information).

C

Indexed: BBCI, Chem.Abstr., Chem.Indus.Notes, Chem.Titles, Curr.Cont., INIS Atomind., INSPEC (Apr.1999-), Ind.Med. (1995-), Mass Spectr.Bull., Sci.Cit.Ind.
—BLDSC (5030.530000), CASDDS, CISTI, IDS, Infotrieve. **CCC.**
Published by: (European Peptide Society), Wiley Europe Ltd., Baffins Ln, Chichester, W Sussex PO19 1UD, United Kingdom. TEL 44-1243-779777, FAX 44-1243-775878, customer@wiley.co.uk, http://www.wiley.co.uk. adv.: B&W page GBP 650, color page GBP 1,550; trim 210 x 279. **Subscr. in the Americas to:** John Wiley & Sons, Inc., Journals, 605 Third Ave, New York, NY 10158. TEL 212-850-6021, 212-850-6645, subinfo@jwiley.com.

547 GBR
NATURAL PRODUCTS NEWS. Text in English. 1994. 12/yr. GBP 59; GBP 69 in Europe; GBP 79 elsewhere (effective 2001). adv. bk.rev. 80 p./no. back issues avail. **Document type:** *Magazine, Trade.* **Description:** Aims to inform and entertain health food retailers, suppliers and others in the natural healthcare movement by communicating news, opinions and ideas from all sectors of the industry.
Published by: Full Moon Communications, 58 High St, Steyning BN44 3RD, United Kingdom. TEL 44-1903-817300, FAX 44-1903-817310, info@naturalproducts.co.uk, http://www.naturalproducts.co.uk. Ed. Jim Manson. Pub. Robin Bines. Adv. contact Philip Daniell TEL 44-1903-817301. color page GBP 2,150; trim 245 x 342. Circ: 800 (paid); 2,100 (controlled).

571.95 DEU
ORGANOHALOGEN COMPOUNDS. Text in English. irreg., latest vol.30. DEM 200. **Document type:** *Academic/Scholarly.*
Indexed: Chem.Abstr., Chem.Titles, Mass Spectr.Bull., Zoo.Rec.
—BLDSC (6291.076000).
Published by: (Verein zur Foerderung der Umweltforschung, -Erziehung und Oeffentlichkeitsarbeit e.V.), Eco-Informa Press, Jean-Paul-Str 30, Bayreuth 95444, Germany. TEL 49-921-552156, FAX 49-921-54626. Ed. Dr. O Hutzinger.

668.9 610 POL ISSN 0370-0747
CODEN: PMYMAX
POLIMERY W MEDYCYNIE. Text in Polish. 1965. 4/yr. USD 58 foreign (effective 2000). adv. bk.rev. *Refereed.* **Document type:** *Academic/Scholarly.*
Formerly (until 1971): Tworzywa Sztuczne w Medycynie (0372-3356)
Indexed: Chem.Abstr., Chem.Titles, Ind.Med. (1970-).
—BLDSC (6547.742600), CASDDS, CISTI, GNLM.
Published by: Akademia Medyczna we Wroclawiu, Zaklad Chirurgii Eksperymentalnej i Badania Biomaterialow, Ul Poniatowskiego 2, Wroclaw 50326, Poland. TEL 48-71-3226310, FAX 48-71-215729. Ed., Adv. contact Roman Rutowski. R&P Urszula Tomczyk. Circ: 800 (paid); 200 (controlled).

547 GBR ISSN 1472-7781
QD241 CODEN: JCPRB4
ROYAL CHEMICAL SOCIETY. JOURNAL. PERKIN TRANSACTIONS 1. Key Title: Journal of the Chemical Society. Perkin Transactions 1. Text in English. 1972. s-m. GBP 1,138, USD 1,898 to individuals (effective 2002); includes free online access. adv. charts, illus, abstr. index. back issues avail.; reprints avail. *Refereed.* **Document type:** *Academic/Scholarly.* **Description:** Contains papers on all aspects of organic and bio-organic chemistry.
Former titles (until 2001): Perkin 1 (1470-4358); Incorporates in part (in Jan. 2000): Acta Chemica Scandinavica (0904-213X); Which was formed by the 1989 merger of: Acta Chemica Scandinavica. Series A: Physical and Inorganic Chemistry (0904-6437); Acta Chemica Scandinavica. Series B: Organic Chemistry and Biochemistry (0904-6445); Which superseded in part (1947-1973): Acta Chemica Scandinavica (0001-5393); Former titles (until 1999): Royal Society of Chemistry. Journal: Perkin Transactions 1 (0300-922X); Incorporates: Contemporary Organic Synthesis (1350-4894); (until 1971): Chemical Society, London. Journal. Section C: Organic Chemistry (0022-4952)
Related titles: Online - full text ed.: ISSN 1364-5463. GBP 1,105, USD 1,898 (effective 2001) (from CatchWord Ltd., Royal Society of Chemistry, EBSCO Publishing, O C L C Online Computer Library Center, Inc., RoweCom Information Quest, Swets Blackwell, Institute for Scientific Information).
Indexed: ASCA, Abstr.Bull.Inst.Pap.Chem., Agri.& Environ.Biotech.Abstr. (coverage dropped), Aqua.Sci.& Fish.Abstr., Aquacult.Abstr., Art & Archaeol.Tech.Abstr., Biol.Abstr., Cadscan, Chem.Abstr., Chem.Cit.Ind., Chem.Indus.Notes, Chem.Titles, Curr.Adv.Biochem., Curr.Adv.Ecol.Sci., Curr.Chem.React., Curr.Cont., Derwent Biotech.Abstr., Environ.Sci.Poll.Mgmt., Food Sci.& Tech.Abstr., GeoRef, Hort.Abstr., INIS Atomind., Ind.Chem., Ind.Med. (coverage dropped), Inpharma, Lead Abstr., MOS, Mass Spectr.Bull., NPU, RCI, Reac., Ref.Zh., Rev.Plant Path., Sci.Cit.Ind., Soils & Fert., Sugar Ind.Abstr., Zincscan.
—BLDSC (6426.487500), ADONIS, CASDDS, CatchWord, CINDOC, CISTI, Ei, IDS, ingenta, Linda Hall. **CCC.**
Published by: Royal Society of Chemistry, Thomas Graham House, Science Park, Milton Rd, Cambridge CB4 4WF, United Kingdom. TEL 44-1223-432360, FAX 44-1223-423429, perkin@rsc.org, sales@rsc.org, advertising@rsc.org, http://www.rsc.org/perkin1. Ed. S R Buxton. R&P Sharon Bellard. Circ: 2,000. **Subscr. to:** Turpin Distribution Services Ltd., Blackhorse Rd, Letchworth, Herts SG6 1HN, United Kingdom. TEL 44-1462-672555, FAX 44-1462-480947.

547 RUS ISSN 1068-1620
QD415.A1 CODEN: RJBCET
RUSSIAN JOURNAL OF BIOORGANIC CHEMISTRY. Text in Russian. 1975. m. EUR 1,745 to institutions for print or online ed.; EUR 2,094 to institutions print & online eds.combined (effective 2002). back issues avail. *Refereed.* **Document type:** *Academic/Scholarly.* **Description:** Disseminates the results of original experimental and theoretical investigations on the structure, structure-activity relationships, and synthesis of biopolymers and low-molecular-mass bioregulators.
Formerly (until 1993): Soviet Journal of Bioorganic Chemistry (0360-4497)
Related titles: Microfilm ed.: (from PQC); Online - full text ed.: ISSN 1608-330X (from Swets Blackwell, Kluwer Online, Institute for Scientific Information, RoweCom Information Quest); ♦ Translation of: Bioorganicheskaya Khimiya. ISSN 0132-3423.
Indexed: Biol.Abstr., Chem.Titles, Curr.Cont., INIS Atomind., Ind.Vet., Mass Spectr.Bull., RCI (coverage dropped), Rev.Med.& Vet.Mycol.
—BLDSC (0420.760700), CISTI, Infotrieve, ingenta. **CCC.**
Published by: (Rossiiskaya Akademiya Nauk/Russian Academy of Sciences), M A I K Nauka - Interperiodica, Mezhdunarodnyi Otdel, Profsoyuznaya ul 90, Moscow 117864, Russian Federation. rjbc@ibch.ru, http://www.maik.rssi.ru/journals/biochem.htm, http://rjbc.siobc.ras.ru. Ed. Vadim T Ivanov. **Dist. by:** Kluwer Academic Publishers, PO Box 17, Dordrecht 3300 AH, Netherlands. TEL 31-78-392392, http://www.wkap.nl.

UNIVERSIDAD CENTRAL DE VENEZUELA. FACULTAD DE FARMACIA. REVISTA. see *PHARMACY AND PHARMACOLOGY*

CHEMISTRY—Physical Chemistry

572 574.192 USA ISSN 1057-8943
QH345 CODEN: ABCHEA
ADVANCES IN BIOPHYSICAL CHEMISTRY. Text in English. 1990. irreg., latest vol.6, 1997. USD 112.50. **Document type:** *Monographic series.*
Indexed: Chem.Abstr., Chem.Cit.Ind., Chem.Indus.Notes, Chem.Titles.
—BLDSC (0700.258000), CASDDS, CISTI, Infotrieve. **CCC.**
Published by: J A I Press Inc., 100 Prospect St, Box 811, Stamford, CT 06904-0811. TEL 203-323-9606, FAX 203-357-8446, jai@jaipress.com. Ed. C Allen Bush.

541 NLD ISSN 0001-8686
QD506 CODEN: ACISB9
ADVANCES IN COLLOID AND INTERFACE SCIENCE. Text in English, French, German. 1965. 15/yr. EUR 1,653 in Europe to institutions; JPY 219,800 in Japan to institutions; USD 1,849 elsewhere to institutions (effective 2002). adv. bk.rev. charts. back issues avail.; reprints avail. *Refereed.* **Document type:** *Journal, Academic/Scholarly.* **Description:** Covers all traditional and other subjects in the realm of colloid and surface science.
Related titles: Microform ed.: (from PQC); Online - full text ed.: (from ingenta, Swets Blackwell, ScienceDirect, Institute for Scientific Information).
Indexed: AESIS, ASCA, Abstr.Bull.Inst.Pap.Chem., Acoust.Abstr., Alloys Ind. (1986-1992), Bioeng.Abstr., Chem.Abstr., Chem.Cit.Ind., Chem.Indus.Notes, Chem.Titles, Comput.& Info.Sys., Curr.Cont., Dairy Sci.Abstr., Electron.& Communic.Abstr.J., Eng.Ind., INIS Atomind., INSPEC (Feb.1974-Nov.1983, dropped), ISMEC, Ind.Med. (1967-), Ind.Sci.Rev., Mat.Sci.Cit.Ind., Met.Abstr. (1986-1992), Met.Abstr.Ind. (1986-1992), Nonfer.Met.Alert (1986-1992), PCC Alert (1986-1992), Photo.Abstr., Phys.Ber., Ref.Zh., Sci.Cit.Ind., Steels Alert (1986-1992), World Surf.Coat.
—BLDSC (0703.950000), CASDDS, CISTI, Ei, GNLM, IDS, ingenta, Linda Hall. **CCC.**
Published by: Elsevier Science BV, PO Box 211, Amsterdam 1000 AE, Netherlands. TEL 31-20-485-3757, FAX 31-20-485-3432, TELEX 18582 ESPA NL, nlinfo-f@elsevier.nl, http://www.elsevier.com/locate/cis, http://www.elsevier.nl. Eds. J Berg, T Tadros. **Subscr. in Australasia and the Far East to:** Elsevier Science (Singapore) Pte Ltd, No.1 Temasek Ave, 17-01 Millenia Tower, Singapore 039192, Singapore. TEL 65-434-3727, FAX 65-337-2230, asiainfo@elsevier.com.sg; **Subscr. in Japan to:** Elsevier Science Inc - Japan Regional Office, 9-15 Higashi-Azabu 1-chome, Minato-ku, Tokyo 106-0044, Japan. TEL 81-3-5561-5033, FAX 81-3-5561-5047, info@elsevier.co.jp; **Subscr. in the Americas to:** Elsevier Science, PO Box 945, New York, NY 10159-0945. TEL 212-633-3730, 888-437-4636, FAX 212-633-3680, usinfo-f@elsevier.com, http://www.elsevier.com. **Dist. by:** Elsevier Science (Brazil).

331.88 541.3 NOR ISSN 0801-6828
BIOINGENIOEREN; the medical laboratory technologist. Text in Norwegian. 1965. m. NOK 480; NOK 540 in Europe; NOK 600 elsewhere (effective 2001). adv. bk.rev. illus, stat, tr.lit. index. **Document type:** *Magazine, Academic/Scholarly.*
Formerly (until 1987): Fysiokjemikeren (0333-0796)
Indexed: INIS Atomind.
—CCC.
Published by: Bioingeniorfaglig Institutt/Norwegian Institute of Biomedical Science, PO Box 9100 Groenland, Oslo 0133, Norway. TEL 47-22-05-35-00, FAX 47-22-17-06-04. Ed. Patricia Melsom. Adv. contact Anita Madsuns TEL 47-62-94-69-05. B&W page NOK 8,100, color page NOK 12,700; trim 185 x 260. Circ: 5,000.

662 541 CHE ISSN 0010-2202
QD516 CODEN: CBSTB9
COMBUSTION SCIENCE AND TECHNOLOGY. Text in English. 1969. 12/yr. (in 12 vols., 6 nos./vol.). GBP 1,535, USD 2,206, EUR 2,514 to individuals; GBP 3,591, USD 5,179, EUR 5,166 to institutions; GBP 5,379, USD 7,985, EUR 8,011 to corporations (effective 2002). adv. charts, illus. index. *Refereed.* **Document type:** *Journal, Academic/Scholarly.*
Incorporates (in 1975): Pyrodynamics
Related titles: CD-ROM ed.; Microform ed.; Online - full text ed.: (from EBSCO Publishing, RoweCom Information Quest, Institute for Scientific Information).
Indexed: AESIS, A.S.& T.Ind. (Jan.1983-Sep.1993), ASCA, Appl.Mech.Rev., Aqua.Sci.& Fish.Abstr., Chem.Abstr., Chem.Cit.Ind., Chem.Eng.Abstr., Curr.Cont., Electron.& Communic.Abstr.J., Eng.Ind., Environ.Per.Bibl., Environ.Sci.Poll.Mgmt., Excerp.Med., Fuel & Energy Abstr., Gas Abstr., INIS Atomind., INSPEC (coverage dropped), ISMEC, Ind.Sci.Rev., Int.Aerosp.Abstr., Mat.Sci.Cit.Ind. (coverage dropped), Pollut.Abstr., Sci.Cit.Ind., Solid St.Abstr.
—CISTI, ingenta. **CCC.**
Published by: Gordon and Breach - Harwood Academic (Subsidiary of: Taylor & Francis Group), PO Box 531, Lausanne 1000, Switzerland. TEL 41-21-6411280, FAX 41-21-6411281, info@gbhap.com, http://www.gbhap.com. Ed. R A Yetter. **Subscr. addr. in US:** International Publishers Direct, PO Box 32160, Newark, NJ 07102. FAX 215-750-6343.

CONCEPTS IN MAGNETIC RESONANCE; an educational quarterly. see *MEDICAL SCIENCES—Radiology And Nuclear Medicine*

541.3 NLD ISSN 0075-3696
CODEN: JSQCA7
JERUSALEM SYMPOSIA ON QUANTUM CHEMISTRY AND BIOCHEMISTRY. Text in English. 1969. irreg., latest vol.27, 1995. price varies. *Refereed.* **Document type:** *Proceedings.*
Indexed: Biol.Abstr., Chem.Abstr., Chem.Indus.Notes, Chem.Titles, Eng.Ind.
—CASDDS, CISTI, Infotrieve. **CCC.**

C

Published by: (Section on Sciences ISR, Israel Academy of Sciences and Humanities ISR), Kluwer Academic Publishers Group (Subsidiary of: Wolters Kluwer N.V.), Spuiboulevard 50, PO Box 17, Dordrecht 3300 AA, Netherlands. FAX 31-78-639-2254, services@wkap.nl, http://www.wkap.nl. Ed. B Pullman. **Dist. by:** Journals Department, PO Box 322, Dordrecht 3300 AH, Netherlands. FAX 31-78-654-6474.

JOURNAL OF PLANAR CHROMATOGRAPHY - MODERN TLC (JPC). see *CHEMISTRY—Analytical Chemistry*

541.3 GBR ISSN 1522-7235
QH641 CODEN: LUMIFC
LUMINESCENCE; journal of biological and chemical luminescence. Text in English. 1987. bi-m. USD 1,115 in United States; USD 1,115 in Canada & Mexico; USD 1,115 elsewhere; USD 1,171 combined subscription in United States for print and online eds.; USD 1,171 combined subscription in Canada & Mexico for print and online eds.; USD 1,171 combined subscription elsewhere for print and online eds. (effective 2002). adv. back issues avail.; reprint service avail. from SWZ. *Refereed.* **Document type:** *Academic/Scholarly.* **Description:** Provides a forum for the publication of original scientific papers, short communications, technical notes and reviews on fundamental and applied aspects of all forms of luminescence.
Formerly (until 1999): Journal of Bioluminescence and Chemiluminescence (0884-3996)
Related titles: Microform ed.: (from PQC); Online - full text ed.: ISSN 1522-7243. USD 1,115 in United States; USD 1,115 in Canada & Mexico; USD 1,115 elsewhere (effective 2002) (from EBSCO Publishing, Wiley InterScience, Institute for Scientific Information).
Indexed: ASCA, Anal.Abstr., Aqua.Sci.& Fish.Abstr., BBCI, CEABA, Cal.Tiss.Abstr., Chem.Abstr., Chem.Indus.Notes, Chem.Titles, Curr.Biotech.Abstr., Curr.Cont., Eng.Ind., Environ.Sci.Poll.Mgmt., INSPEC (Apr.1988-), Ind.Med. (1999-), Inpharma, Pollut.Abstr., Reac., Ref.Zh., Sci.Cit.Ind., Telegen.
—BLDSC (5304.782850), AskIEEE, CASDDS, CISTI, Ei, GNLM, IDS, ingenta, Linda Hall. **CCC.**
Published by: Wiley Europe Ltd., Baffins Ln, Chichester, W Sussex PO19 1UD, United Kingdom. TEL 44-1243-779777, FAX 44-1243-775878, customer@wiley.co.uk, http://www.wiley.co.uk. adv.: B&W page GBP 650, color page GBP 1,550; trim 210 x 279. **Subscr. in N. America to:** John Wiley & Sons, Inc., Journals, 605 Third Ave, New York, NY 10158. TEL 212-850-6021, 212-850-6645, subinfo@jwiley.com.

541.3 615.842 RUS ISSN 0033-8311
CODEN: RADKAU
RADIOKHIMIYA. Text in Russian. 1959. bi-m. index. **Document type:** *Academic/Scholarly.* **Description:** Examines the theoretical and applied aspects of radiochemistry.
Related titles: ♦ English Translation: Radiochemistry. ISSN 1066-3622.
Indexed: Chem.Abstr., Chem.Indus.Notes, Chem.Titles, Curr.Cont. (coverage dropped), Eng.Ind., Fuel & Energy Abstr., INIS Atomind., METADEX, Ocean.Abstr. (coverage dropped), Ref.Zh.
—BLDSC (0139.500000), CASDDS, CISTI, East View, Linda Hall.
Published by: (Rossiiskaya Akademiya Nauk/Russian Academy of Sciences), M A I K Nauka - Interperiodica, S.-Peterburgskoe Otdelenie, Mendeleevskaya liniya 1, St Petersburg 199034, Russian Federation. TEL 7-812-3507249, compmg@maik.ru, http://www.maik.rssi.ru/journals/radchem.htm. Ed. Boris F Myasoedov. **US dist. addr.:** Kluwer Academic Publishers, PO Box 17, Dordrecht 3300 AH, Netherlands. TEL 31-78-639-2392, FAX 31-78-654-6474, http://www.wkap.nl.

CHILDREN AND YOUTH—About

see also EDUCATION; MEDICAL SCIENCES—Pediatrics

155.4 AUS
A E C A RESEARCH IN PRACTICE. Text in English. 1978. q. AUD 41.55; AUD 44 foreign (effective 2000). bibl, charts, illus. back issues avail. *Refereed.* **Document type:** *Monographic series.* **Description:** Contains practical information to workers in all early childhood settings.
Former titles: A E C A Resource Book Series (1320-2170); Australian Early Childhood Resource Booklets (0156-0999)
Indexed: Aus.Educ.Ind., e-psyche.
Published by: Australian Early Childhood Association Inc., Knox St, PO Box 105, Watson, ACT 2602, Australia. TEL 61-2-6241-6900, FAX 61-2-6241-5547, national@aeca.org.au. R&P Louise Tigchelaar. Circ: 2,500.

ACTA MEDICA AUXOLOGICA. see *MEDICAL SCIENCES—Endocrinology*

155.4 USA ISSN 0737-5166
ACTA PAEDOLOGICA✱ ; an international journal of child development. Text in English. 1984. q. adv. bk.rev. abstr, charts, illus. index.
Indexed: Psychol.Abstr., e-psyche.
Published by: Eterna International, Inc., PO Box 5731, Hauppauge, NY 11788-0154. Ed. Howard M Bahr.

ADOLESCENCE. see *MEDICAL SCIENCES—Psychiatry And Neurology*

370.15 USA ISSN 0001-8449
HQ793 CODEN: ADOLAO
ADOLESCENCE (SAN DIEGO); an international quarterly devoted to the physiological, psychological, psychiatric, sociological, and educational aspects of the second decade of human life. Text in English. 1966. q. USD 86 to individuals; USD 121 to institutions (effective 2000). adv. bk.rev. bibl, charts, illus, stat. index, cum.index. 256 p./no. back issues avail.; reprint service avail. from PQC,SCH,PSC,ISI. *Refereed.* **Document type:** *Journal, Academic/Scholarly.* **Description:** Articles cover a variety of viewpoints on topics relating to adolescence.
Related titles: CD-ROM ed.; Microform ed.: (from PQC); Online - full text ed.: (from ProQuest Information & Learning, Gale Group, H. W. Wilson, Factiva, Institute for Scientific Information).
Indexed: ASCA, ASSIA, Abstr.Anthropol., Abstr.Crim.& Pen., Adol.Ment.Hlth.Abstr., AgeLine, Amer.Bibl.Slavic & E.Eur.Stud., Bibl.Agri., Biol.Abstr., C.I.J.E., CINAHL, Child.Lit.Abstr., Crim.Just.Abstr., Curr.Cont., Curr.Lit.Fam.Plan., ERA, Educ.Admin.Abstr., Educ.Ind. (Jan.1983-), Environ.Sci.Poll.Mgmt., Except.Child Educ.Abstr., Excerp.Med., High.Educ.Abstr., IBR, IBZ, IMFL, INIS Atomind., Ind.Med. (1966-), Ind.Philos., Lang.& Lang.Behav.Abstr., Mid.East: Abstr.& Ind., Mult.Ed.Abstr., P C I, Pollut.Abstr., PsycInfo, Psychol.Abstr. (1966-), Psycscan D.P., Rel.Ind.One, Rel.Ind.Two, Risk Abstr., SOPODA, SSCI, Saf.Sci.Abstr., Sage Fam.Stud.Abstr., Sage Race Rel.Abstr., Soc.Sci.Ind. (Mar.1987-), Soc.Serv.Abstr., Soc.Work Res.& Abstr., Sociol.Abstr., Sociol.Educ.Abstr., Sp.Ed.Needs Abstr., Stud.Wom.Abstr., THA, Tech.Educ.Abstr., Viol.& Abuse Abstr., e-psyche.
—BLDSC (0696.581000), GNLM, IDS, ingenta. **CCC.**
Published by: Libra Publishers, Inc., 3089C Clairemont Dr,, PMB 383, San Diego, CA 92117. TEL 858-571-1414. Ed., Adv. contact William Kroll. R&P Jon Kroll. page USD 300. Circ: 3,000.

ADOLESCENT PSYCHIATRY; annals of the American Society for Adolescent Psychiatry. see *MEDICAL SCIENCES—Psychiatry And Neurology*

▼ ADULTSPAN. see *PSYCHOLOGY*

ADVANCES IN LEARNING AND BEHAVIORAL DISABILITIES. see *EDUCATION—Special Education And Rehabilitation*

ADVANCES IN MOTOR DEVELOPMENT RESEARCH. see *PHYSICAL FITNESS AND HYGIENE*

AERZTLICHER RATGEBER FUER JUNGE ELTERN. see *MEDICAL SCIENCES—Pediatrics*

AIDS BOOK REVIEW JOURNAL. see *MEDICAL SCIENCES—Communicable Diseases*

362.7 157.61 DEU ISSN 0720-3551
AKTION JUGENDSCHUTZ. INFORMATIONEN. Short title: A J S Informationen. Text in German. 1965. bi-m. DEM 6, USD 5. adv. bk.rev. bibl, charts, illus, stat. back issues avail. **Document type:** *Government.*
Published by: Aktion Jugendschutz Landesarbeitsstelle Baden-Wuerttemberg, Stafflenbergstr 44, Stuttgart 70184, Germany. TEL 49-711-237370, FAX 49-711-2373730. Ed. Birgit Ebbert. Circ: 20,000.

AMBULATORY CHILD HEALTH. see *MEDICAL SCIENCES—Pediatrics*

AMBULATORY CHILD HEALTH ONLINE. see *MEDICAL SCIENCES—Pediatrics*

AMERICAN ACADEMY OF CHILD AND ADOLESCENT PSYCHIATRY. JOURNAL. see *MEDICAL SCIENCES—Psychiatry And Neurology*

AMERICAN JOURNAL OF ORTHOPSYCHIATRY. see *PSYCHOLOGY*

ANNUAL EDITIONS: CHILD GROWTH & DEVELOPMENT. see *MEDICAL SCIENCES—Pediatrics*

THE ARC INSIGHT. see *SOCIAL SERVICES AND WELFARE*

155.4 616.8 USA ISSN 1077-0305
ASSOCIATION FOR CHILD PSYCHOANALYSIS. NEWSLETTER. Text in English. 1980. q. free. bk.rev. abstr, bibl. back issues avail. **Document type:** *Newsletter, Academic/Scholarly.* **Description:** Publishes abstracts of scientific meetings and reports on the activities of the members of the association.
Indexed: e-psyche.
Published by: Association for Child Psychoanalysis, Inc., PO Box 253, Ramsey, NJ 07446. TEL 201-825-3138, FAX 201-825-3138, childanalysis@compuserve.com. Eds. Barbara Streeter, Denia Barrett. Circ: 700.

649 618.9 USA
▼ BABY (KENNESAW). Text in English. 2001. bi-m. USD 19.99; USD 5.99 newsstand/cover (effective 2002). adv. **Document type:** *Consumer.*
Published by: Highbury House Communications, Inc., 1925 Vaughn Rd Ste 235, Kennesaw, GA 30411. TEL 770-422-3225. Ed. Jeanine Cox. Pub. Michael Meyers.

BABY MAGAZINE INFANT CARE GUIDE. see *MEDICAL SCIENCES—Pediatrics*

649 618.92 DEU ISSN 0724-1119
BABY POST. Text in German. bi-m. DEM 4.95 newsstand/cover (effective 2000). adv. **Document type:** *Magazine, Consumer.*
Published by: Marken-Verlag GmbH, Hugo-Junkers-Str 20, Cologne 50739, Germany. TEL 49-221-957427-0, FAX 49-221-95742777, marken-info@markenverlag.de, http://www.markenverlag.de. adv.: B&W page DEM 13,400, color page DEM 24,120. Circ: 90,000 (paid and controlled).

649 618.92 DEU
BABY - UNSER GLUECK. Text in German. 1984. 2/yr. DEM 6.50 newsstand/cover (effective 2000). adv. **Document type:** *Magazine, Consumer.* **Description:** Contains articles and information for parents and those wishing to become parents.
Published by: Marken-Verlag GmbH, Hugo-Junkers-Str 20, Cologne 50739, Germany. TEL 49-221-957427-0, FAX 49-221-95742777, marken-info@markenverlag.de, http://www.markenverlag.de. adv.: page DEM 15,800. Circ: 100,000 (paid and controlled).

BABYCARE BOOK. see *MEDICAL SCIENCES—Pediatrics*

BABYFIRST. see *MEDICAL SCIENCES—Pediatrics*

649.1 USA ISSN 1520-7730
BEFORE BIRTH AND BEYOND; community newsletter. Text in English. s-m. free per issue. adv. **Document type:** *Newsletter.* **Description:** Presents articles on pregnancy, infant and child health, reader tips, freebies and information of interest to parents and persons who work in the areas of pregnancy, childbirth, breastfeeding, parenting and pediatrics.
Related titles: Online - full text ed.
Published by: Doerr Consulting, StorkNet, 3702 S Virginia St, No G 12 235, Reno, NV 89502. storknet@storknet.org, http://www.storknet.org/newsletter/index.html. Ed. Maribeth Doerr. Circ: 1,500.

155.4 367 DEU ISSN 0067-5105
BEITRAEGE ZUR KINDERPSYCHOTHERAPIE. Text in German. 1965. irreg., latest vol.32, 1998. price varies. index. **Document type:** *Monographic series, Academic/Scholarly.*
—GNLM.
Published by: Ernst Reinhardt Verlag, Kemnatenstr 46, Munich 80639, Germany. TEL 49-89-1780160, FAX 49-89-17801630. Eds. Gerd Biermann, Manfred Endres.

BOERNE- OG UNGDOMSTANDPLEJEN I DANMARK. see *MEDICAL SCIENCES—Dentistry*

BRAILLE CHESS MAGAZINE. see *SPORTS AND GAMES*

C

362.7 USA ISSN 1058-1073
HQ767.8
BROWN UNIVERSITY CHILD AND ADOLESCENT BEHAVIOR LETTER; monthly reports on the problems of children and adolescents growing up. Text in English. 1984. m. USD 167 domestic to individuals; USD 197 domestic to institutions; USD 207 in Canada to institutions; USD 227 elsewhere to institutions (effective 2001). bk.rev. abstr, bibl, stat. 8 p./no. back issues avail.; reprints avail. **Document type:** *Newsletter.* **Description:** Offers practical interventions, professional commentary and hands on techniques for working with troubled children and adolescents.
Incorporates (in 1992): Children and Teens Today (0882-942X); Which was formerly (until 1985): Children and Teens in Crisis (0732-7420); Formerly (until 1991): Brown University Child Behavior and Development Letter (0898-2562)
Related titles: Online - full text ed.: (from Gale Group).
Indexed: e-psyche.
—CCC.
Published by: Manisses Communications Group, Inc., PO Box 9758, Providence, RI 02906-9758. TEL 401-831-6020, 800-333-7771, FAX 401-861-6370, manissesCS@manisses.com, http://www.manisses.com. Ed. Dr. Gregory K Fritz. Pub. Betty R Lang.

BROWN UNIVERSITY CHILD & ADOLESCENT PSYCHOPHARMACOLOGY; updates on research, use of psychotropic medications and specific interventions with children & adolescents. see *MEDICAL SCIENCES—Pediatrics*

C C B D NEWSLETTER. see *EDUCATION—Special Education And Rehabilitation*

362.76 USA
C H I L D NEWSLETTER. Text in English. 1984. q. USD 25 domestic to members; USD 35 foreign to members (effective 2001). bk.rev. *Refereed.* **Document type:** *Newsletter.* **Description:** Seeks to end the child abuse and neglect associated with the practices of certain religious groups.
Published by: (Children's Healthcare Is a Legal Duty), C H I L D, Inc., PO Box 2604, Sioux City, IA 51106. TEL 712-948-3500, FAX 712-948-3704, childinc@netins.net, http://www.childrenshealthcare.org. Ed., R&P Rita Swan. Circ: 440 (controlled).

CAHIERS ALFRED BINET; education, psychologie et sciences de l'enfance. see *PSYCHOLOGY*

CANADIAN INTRAMURAL RECREATION ASSOCIATION. BULLETIN; the voice of intramurals in Canada. see *PHYSICAL FITNESS AND HYGIENE*

CANDLELIGHTERS CHILDHOOD CANCER FOUNDATION YOUTH NEWSLETTER. see *MEDICAL SCIENCES—Oncology*

CARNEGIE-MELLON SYMPOSIA ON COGNITION SERIES. see *PSYCHOLOGY*

155.4 USA ISSN 0894-7988
CHILD; the essential guide for parents. Text in English. 1986. 10/yr. USD 12.97 domestic; USD 28.94 in Canada; USD 44 elsewhere; USD 2.95 newsstand/cover domestic; GBP 2.20 newsstand/cover in United Kingdom; CND 3.50 newsstand/cover in Canada (effective 2000). adv. bk.rev. illus. reprints avail. **Document type:** *Magazine, Consumer.* **Description:** Offers information on child rearing and includes articles on child development, behavior, health, nutrition, fitness, and education. Covers new products and services for children and their parents, as well as travel, fashion, food and beauty topics.
Formerly (until 1986): For Today's Children
Published by: Gruner + Jahr U.S.A. Publishing (Subsidiary of: Gruner und Jahr AG & Co.), 375 Lexington Ave, New York, NY 10017-5514. TEL 212-499-2000, 800-727-3682, FAX 212-499-2160, childmail@childmagazine.com, backtalk@childmagazine.com, http://www.childmagazine.com. Ed. Miriam Aronz. Pub. Sharon Summer. Adv. contact Steven Sigler. B&W page USD 51,315, color page USD 61,525; trim 10.5 x 7.88. Circ: 923,175 (paid). **Subscr. to:** PO Box 3176, Harlan, IA 51593-0367. **Dist. in UK by:** Comag, Tavistock Works, Tavistock Rd, W Drayton, Middx UB7 7QX, United Kingdom. TEL 44-1895-444055, FAX 44-1895-433602.

362.76 GBR ISSN 0145-2134
HV713 CODEN: CABND3
CHILD ABUSE & NEGLECT. Text in English. 1977. m. EUR 167 in Europe to qualified personnel; JPY 22,100 in Japan to qualified personnel; USD 186 elsewhere to qualified personnel; EUR 1,171 in Europe to institutions; JPY 155,500 in Japan to institutions; USD 1,310 elsewhere to institutions (effective 2002). adv. bk.rev. illus. index. back issues avail.; reprints avail. *Refereed.* **Document type:** *Academic/Scholarly.* **Description:** Provides an international multidisciplinary forum on all aspects of child abuse and neglect, including sexual abuse, with emphasis on prevention and treatment.
Formerly: International Journal on Child Abuse and Neglect
Related titles: Microfilm ed.: (from PQC); Online - full text ed.: (from ingenta, Gale Group, Swets Blackwell, ScienceDirect, Factiva, Institute for Scientific Information).
Indexed: ASCA, ASSIA, Abstr.Crim.& Pen., Adol.Ment.Hlth.Abstr., Bibl.Dev.Med.& Child Neur., Br.Educ.Ind., C.I.J.E., Child Devel.Abstr., Crim.Just.Abstr., Curr.Cont., Educ.Ind. (Jun.1992-), Environ.Sci.Poll.Mgmt., Except.Child Educ.Abstr., Excerp.Med., Fam.Ind., IBZ, Ind.Med. (1977-), Ind.Per.Art.Relat.Law, Ind.Philos., Ind.U.S.Gov.Per., Indian Psychol.Abstr., Int.Nurs.Ind., Intl.Bibl.Soc.Sci., Lang.& Lang.Behav.Abstr., P C I, Pollut.Abstr., PsycInfo, Psychol.Abstr. (1980-), Risk Abstr., SOPODA, SSCI, Saf.Sci.Abstr., Soc.Sci.Ind. (Jan.1994-), Soc.Serv.Abstr., Soc.Work Res.& Abstr., Sociol.Abstr., Viol.& Abuse Abstr., e-psyche.
—BLDSC (3172.912500), EMDOCS, GNLM, IDS, ingenta, KNAW. **CCC.**
Published by: (International Society for Prevention of Child Abuse and Neglect), Pergamon (Subsidiary of: Elsevier Science), The Boulevard, Langford Ln, East Park, Kidlington, Oxford OXB 1GB, United Kingdom. FAX 44-1865-843010, nlinfo-f@elsevier/nl; usinfo-f@elsevier.com; forinfo-kyf04035@niftyserve.or.jp, http://www.elsevier.com/locate/chiabuneg, http://www.elsevier.nl/homepage/. Ed. Richard D Krugman. Circ: 1,500. **Subscr. in Australasia and the Far East to:** Elsevier Science (Singapore) Pte Ltd, No.1 Temasek Ave, 17-01 Millenia Tower, Singapore 039192, Singapore. TEL 65-434-3727, FAX 65-337-2230; **Subscr. in the Americas to:** Elsevier Science, PO Box 945, New York, NY 10159-0945. TEL 212-633-3730, FAX 212-633-3680, usinfo-f@elsevier.com; **Subscr. to:** Elsevier Science BV, PO Box 211, Amsterdam 1000 AE, Netherlands. TEL 31-20-485-3757, FAX 31-20-485-3432, nlinfo-f@elsevier.nl, http://www.elsevier.nl.

CHILD ABUSE PREVENTION; national child protection clearing house newsletter. see *SOCIAL SERVICES AND WELFARE*

CHILD & ADOLESCENT HEALTH CARE. see *MEDICAL SCIENCES—Pediatrics*

CHILD AND ADOLESCENT SOCIAL WORK JOURNAL. see *SOCIOLOGY*

155.4 USA ISSN 1053-1890
HV701 CODEN: CYCFEH
CHILD AND YOUTH CARE FORUM; an independent journal of day and residential child and youth care practice. Text in English. 1971. bi-m. USD 496 in the Americas to institutions for print or online ed.; EUR 495 elsewhere to institutions for print or online ed.; USD 595.20 in the Americas to institutions for print & online eds. combined; EUR 594 elsewhere to institutions for print & online eds. combined (effective 2002). adv. bk.rev. bibl, illus. index. back issues avail.; reprint service avail. from PQC,PSC,SCH,ISI. *Refereed.* **Document type:** *Journal, Academic/Scholarly.* **Description:** Covers the training of personnel and psychological testing.
Former titles (until 1990): Child and Youth Care Quarterly (0893-0848); (until 1987): Child Care Quarterly (0045-6632)
Related titles: Microform ed.: (from PQC); Online - full text ed.: (from EBSCO Publishing, O C L C Online Computer Library Center, Inc., Swets Blackwell, Kluwer Online, RoweCom Information Quest).
Indexed: ASCA, ASSIA, Abstr.Crim.& Pen., Adol.Ment.Hlth.Abstr., Bibl.Agri., C.I.J.E. (coverage dropped), Child Devel.Abstr., Community Ment.Health Rev., Curr.Cont. (coverage dropped), ERA, Educ.Ind. (Dec.1982-Dec.1986), Except.Child Educ.Abstr., IMFL, Mid.East: Abstr.& Ind., Mult.Ed.Abstr., PsycInfo, Psychol.Abstr. (1965-), Psycscan D.P., SOMA, SSCI (coverage dropped), Sage Fam.Stud.Abstr., Sage Urb.Stud.Abstr., Soc.Work Res.& Abstr., Sociol.Educ.Abstr., Sp.Ed.Needs Abstr., Viol.& Abuse Abstr., e-psyche.
—BLDSC (3172.915800), GNLM, IDS, Infotrieve, ingenta. **CCC.**
Published by: Kluwer Academic - Plenum Publishers (Subsidiary of: Wolters Kluwer N.V.), 233 Spring St, New York, NY 10013-1578. TEL 212-620-8000, 800-221-9369, FAX 212-463-0742, services@wkap.nl, info@plenum.com, http://www.wkap.nl/journalhome.htm/1053-1890. Eds. Doug Magnuson, Jerome Beker, Sibylle Artz. **Subscr. outside the Americas to:** Kluwer Academic Publishers Group, Journals Department, PO Box 322, Dordrecht 3300 AH, Netherlands. TEL 31-78-639-2392, FAX 31-78-654-6474.

155.4 USA ISSN 1055-0518
CHILD ASSESSMENT NEWS. Text in English. 1991. 6/yr. USD 75 domestic to individuals; USD 85 foreign to individuals; USD 105 domestic to institutions; USD 115 foreign to institutions (effective 2000). **Document type:** *Newsletter.*
Indexed: e-psyche.
Published by: Guilford Publications, Inc., 72 Spring St, 4th Fl, New York, NY 10012. TEL 212-431-9800, 800-365-7006, FAX 212-966-6708, info@guilford.com. Pub. Robert Matloff. R&P Kathy Kuehl.

649 155.4 USA ISSN 0009-3920
HQ750.A1 CODEN: CHDEAW
CHILD DEVELOPMENT. Text in English. 1930. bi-m. GBP 232 to institutions in UK & Europe; USD 328 to institutions in the Americas & Caribbean; GBP 232 elsewhere to institutions (effective 2002). adv. bk.rev. illus. index. back issues avail.; reprint service avail. from PSC,SCH. *Refereed.* **Document type:** *Journal, Academic/Scholarly.* **Description:** Publishes original articles on all aspects of child development, from the prenatal period through adolescence.
Related titles: Microform ed.: (from PQC); Online - full text ed.: (from Gale Group, Institute for Scientific Information, RoweCom Information Quest).
Indexed: AMED, ASCA, ASSIA, Abstr.Anthropol., Abstr.Crim.& Pen., Acad.Ind., Adol.Ment.Hlth.Abstr., AgeLine, Behav.Med.Abstr., Bibl.Agri., Bibl.Asian Stud. (1971), Bibl.Dev.Med.& Child Neur., Biol.Abstr., Bk.Rev.Ind. (1977-1980), C.I.J.E., Chic.Per.Ind., Child Devel.Abstr., Child.Bk.Rev.Ind. (1977-1980), Commun.Abstr., Cont.Pg.Educ., Crim.Just.Abstr., Curr.Adv.Ecol.Sci., Curr.Cont., Curr.Ind.Stat., DSH Abstr., Dent.Ind., ERA, Educ.Ind. (coverage dropped), Environ.Sci.Poll.Mgmt., Fam.Ind., Hlth.Ind., IBR, IBZ, IMFL, Ind.Med. (1930-), Ind.Philos., Intl.Bibl.Soc.Sci., Lang.& Lang.Behav.Abstr., Ling.Abstr., M.L.A., MLA Intl.Bibl., Mid.East: Abstr.& Ind., Mult.Ed.Abstr., Neurosci.Cit.Ind., Nutr.Abstr., P C I, Peace Res.Abstr., Pollut.Abstr., PsycInfo, Psychol.Abstr. (1930-), Psycscan D.P., Risk Abstr., Rural Recreat.Tour.Abstr., Russ.Acad.Sci.Bibl., SOMA, SOPODA, SSCI, Saf.Sci.Abstr., Sage Fam.Stud.Abstr., Sage Race Rel.Abstr., Soc.Sci.Ind. (Feb.1982-), Soc.Serv.Abstr., Sociol.Abstr., Sociol.Educ.Abstr., Sp.Ed.Needs Abstr., Stud.Wom.Abstr., Viol.& Abuse Abstr., Yrbk.Assoc.Educ.& Rehab.Blind, e-psyche.
—BLDSC (3172.940000), CISTI, GNLM, IDS, ingenta, KNAW. **CCC.**
Published by: (Society for Research in Child Development), Blackwell Publishers, 350 Main St, Malden, MA 02148. TEL 781-388-8200, FAX 718-388-8232, subscript@blackwellpub.com, http://www.srcd.org/cd, http://www.blackwellpublishers.co.uk/journals/diph. Ed. Marc H Bornstein. R&P Gretchen Voter TEL 781-388-0423. Adv. contact Anne Marie Sheehy TEL 781-388-0427. Circ: 8,600.

331.31 363.1 346.01 USA ISSN 1060-6661
HD6228
CHILD LABOR MONITOR. Text in English. 1991. q. USD 15 (effective 1998). back issues avail. **Document type:** *Newsletter.* **Description:** Focuses on state, national, and international efforts to end child labor exploitation, and to ensure the health, education and well being of working minors.
Published by: National Consumers League, Inc., 1701 K St, N W, Ste 1200, Washington, DC 20006. TEL 202-835-3323, FAX 202-835-0747, info@nclnet.org, http://www.nclnet.org. Ed. Darlene Adkins.

362.7 USA ISSN 1077-5595
RC569.5.C55 CODEN: CMALFA
CHILD MALTREATMENT. Text in English. 1996. q. USD 75 to individuals; USD 295 to institutions; USD 25 newsstand/cover to individuals; USD 75 newsstand/cover to institutions (effective 2002). adv. illus. Index. back issues avail.; reprints avail. *Refereed.* **Document type:** *Academic/Scholarly.* **Description:** Reports the latest scientific information and technical innovations relating to child abuse.
Related titles: Online - full text ed.: (from EBSCO Publishing, O C L C Online Computer Library Center, Inc., RoweCom Information Quest, ProQuest Information & Learning, ingenta, Swets Blackwell).

C

Indexed: ASSIA, CINAHL, Child Devel.Abstr., Crim.Just.Abstr., ERA, Environ.Sci.Poll.Mgmt., IBZ, Ind.Med., Lang.& Lang.Behav.Abstr., Pollut.Abstr., PsycInfo, Risk Abstr., SOPODA, Saf.Sci.Abstr., Sage Fam.Stud.Abstr., Soc.Serv.Abstr., Sociol.Abstr., Viol.& Abuse Abstr., e-psyche.

—BLDSC (3172.944770), ingenta. **CCC.**

Published by: (American Professional Society on the Abuse of Children), Sage Publications, Inc., 2455 Teller Rd, Thousand Oaks, CA 91320. TEL 818-597-4867, FAX 818-597-4879, info@sagepub.com, http://www.sagepub.com. Ed. Mark Chaffin. Pub. Sara Miller McCune. R&P Tanya Udin. Adv. contact DeAnna Vega Hammersley. page USD 275. Circ: 4,000 (paid). **Overseas subscr. to:** Sage Publications Ltd., 6 Bonhill St, London EC2A 4PU, United Kingdom; Sage Publications India Pvt. Ltd., 4215, New Delhi 110 048, India.

CHILD STUDY JOURNAL. see *EDUCATION*

305.23 GBR ISSN 0907-5682
HQ767.8 CODEN: CHILFF

CHILDHOOD; a global journal of child research. Text in English. 1993. q. GBP 41 to individuals; GBP 210 to institutions; GBP 11 newsstand/cover to individuals; GBP 54 newsstand/cover to institutions (effective 2002). adv. bk.rev. charts, illus. reprints avail. *Refereed.* **Document type:** *Academic/Scholarly.* **Description:** Interdisciplinary forum for research relating to children in contemporary global society that spans divisions between geographical regions, disciplines, social and cultural contexts, and applied and basic research.

Related titles: Online - full text ed.: (from EBSCO Publishing, O C L C Online Computer Library Center, Inc., RoweCom Information Quest, ingenta, Swets Blackwell, Institute for Scientific Information).

Indexed: ASSIA, Brit.Nur.Ind., C.I.J.E., Curr.Cont., Indian Psychol.Abstr., Lang.& Lang.Behav.Abstr., PsycInfo, Psychol.Abstr., SOPODA, SSCI, Sage Fam.Stud.Abstr., Soc.Serv.Abstr., Sociol.Abstr., Viol.& Abuse Abstr., e-psyche.

—BLDSC (3172.951500), IDS, Infotrieve. **CCC.**

Published by: (Norwegian Centre for Child Research), Sage Publications Ltd., 6 Bonhill St, London EC2A 4PU, United Kingdom. TEL 44-20-7374-0645, FAX 44-20-7374-8741, market@sagepub.co.uk, http://www.sagepub.co.uk. Eds. Chris Jenks, Irene Rizzini, Jens Qvortrup. Adv. contact Jenny Kirby. page GBP 195; trim 192 x 114. Circ: 700.

649 GBR ISSN 0951-0605
HQ767.8

CHILDREN & SOCIETY. Text in English. 1987. 5/yr. USD 270 in United Kingdom; USD 270 in Canada & Mexico; USD 270 elsewhere; USD 284 combined subscription in United States for print and online eds.; USD 284 combined subscription in Canada & Mexico for print and online eds.; USD 284 combined subscription elsewhere for print and online eds. (effective 2002). adv. bk.rev. index. back issues avail. **Document type:** *Academic/Scholarly.* **Description:** Covers all aspects of child health, education, care and development.

Related titles: Online - full text ed.: ISSN 1099-0860. USD 270 in United States; USD 270 in Canada & Mexico; USD 270 elsewhere (effective 2002) (from EBSCO Publishing, ingenta, Wiley InterScience).

Indexed: ASSIA, Abstr.Crim.& Pen., Br.Educ.Ind., C.I.J.E., Cont.Pg.Educ., Crim.Just.Abstr., ERA, IBR, Intl.Bibl.Soc.Sci., Lang.& Lang.Behav.Abstr., Mult.Ed.Abstr., PsycInfo, Psychol.Abstr. (1987-), SOPODA, Soc.Serv.Abstr., Soc.Work Res.& Abstr., Sociol.Abstr., Sociol.Educ.Abstr., Sp.Ed.Needs Abstr., e-psyche.

—BLDSC (3172.961300). **CCC.**

Published by: (National Children's Bureau Enterprises Ltd.), Wiley Europe Ltd., Baffins Ln, Chichester, W Sussex PO19 1UD, United Kingdom. TEL 44-1243-779777, FAX 44-1243-775878, customer@wiley.co.uk, http://www.interscience.wiley.com/jpages/0951-0605/, http://www.wiley.co.uk. adv.: B&W page GBP 650, color page GBP 1,550; trim 200 x 260. Circ: 700. **Subscr. to:** John Wiley & Sons, Inc., Journals, 605 Third Ave, New York, NY 10158. TEL 212-850-6021, 212-850-6645, subinfo@jwiley.com.

362.7 GBR ISSN 0190-7409
HV701

CHILDREN AND YOUTH SERVICES REVIEW; an international multidisciplinary review of the welfare of young people. Text in English. 1979. 12/yr. EUR 142 in Europe to qualified personnel; JPY 18,800 in Japan to qualified personnel; USD 158 elsewhere to qualified personnel; EUR 834 in Europe to institutions; JPY 110,700 in Japan to institutions; USD 932 elsewhere to institutions (effective 2002). bk.rev. illus. Index. back issues avail.; reprints avail. *Refereed.* **Document type:** *Academic/Scholarly.* **Description:** Provides a forum for the critical analysis and assessment of social service programs designed to serve young people throughout the world, including in-depth coverage of child welfare, foster care, adoptions, child abuse and neglect, income support, mental health services, and social policy.

Related titles: Microfilm ed.: (from PQC); Online - full text ed.: (from ingenta, Gale Group, Swets Blackwell, ScienceDirect, Institute for Scientific Information).

Indexed: ASCA, ASSIA, Abstr.Crim.& Pen., Abstr.Soc.Geront., Adol.Ment.Hlth.Abstr., C.I.J.E. (coverage dropped), Chic.Per.Ind., Child Devel.Abstr., Crim.Just.Abstr., Curr.Cont., Except.Child Educ.Abstr., Excerp.Med., Fam.Ind., Lang.& Lang.Behav.Abstr., PSI, PsycInfo, Psychol.Abstr. (1979-), Risk Abstr., SOPODA, SSCI, Sage Fam.Stud.Abstr., Sage Pub.Admin.Abstr., Soc.Sci.Ind. (Jul.1999-), Soc.Serv.Abstr., Soc.Work Res.& Abstr., Sociol.Abstr., Sp.Ed.Needs Abstr., Viol.& Abuse Abstr., e-psyche.

—BLDSC (3172.962000), IDS, ingenta. **CCC.**

Published by: Pergamon (Subsidiary of: Elsevier Science), The Boulevard, Langford Ln, East Park, Kidlington, Oxford OXB 1GB, United Kingdom. FAX 44-1865-843010, nlinfo-f@elsevier/nl; usinfo-f@elsevier.com; forinfo-kyf04035@niftyserve.or.jp, http://www.elsevier.com/locate/childyouth, http://www.elsevier.nl/. Ed. Dr. Duncan Lindsey. Circ: 1,200. **Subscr. in Australasia and the Far East to:** Elsevier Science (Singapore) Pte Ltd, No.1 Temasek Ave, 17-01 Millenia Tower, Singapore 039192, Singapore. TEL 65-434-3727, FAX 65-337-2230; **Subscr. in the Americas to:** Elsevier Science, PO Box 945, New York, NY 10159-0945. TEL 212-633-3730, FAX 212-633-3680, usinfo-f@elsevier.com, http://www.elsevier.com; **Subscr. to:** Elsevier Science BV, PO Box 211, Amsterdam 1000 AE, Netherlands. TEL 31-20-485-3757, FAX 31-20-485-3432, nlinfo-f@elsevier.nl, http://www.elsevier.nl.

CHILDREN'S ENVIRONMENTS; theory, research, policy and applications. see *PSYCHOLOGY*

649 362.1 USA

CHILDREN'S HEALTH & SAFETY. Text in English. bi-m. **Document type:** *Directory, Consumer.* **Description:** Sourcebook for parents of young children provides key health information.

Address: 103 Glen St, Glen Cove, NY 11542. TEL 516-656-0911, FAX 516-656-0904.

CHILDREN'S MENTAL HEALTH SERVICES. see *PSYCHOLOGY*

155.4 USA

CHILD'S PLAY. Text in English. 1984. q. USD 55 to membership (effective 2000). adv. bk.rev. back issues avail. **Document type:** *Newsletter.* **Description:** Covers toy libraries, toys, play and programs advantageous to the healthy development of children. Also provides a network among professionals who work with children in play settings.

Published by: U S A Toy Library Association, 1213 Wilmette Ave, Ste 201, Wilmette, IL 60091-2566. TEL 847-864-3330, FAX 847-864-3332, usatla@aol.com, http://www.sjccdc.cc.ca.us/toylibrary/, http://usatla.deltacollege.org. Ed., R&P, Adv. contact Judith Iacuzzi. Pub. Judith Q Iacuzzi. Circ: 700.

616.8 362 GBR ISSN 1359-1045
RJ499.A1 CODEN: CCPPFR

CLINICAL CHILD PSYCHOLOGY & PSYCHIATRY. Text in English. 1996. q. GBP 51 to individuals; GBP 250 to institutions; GBP 14 newsstand/cover to individuals; GBP 64 newsstand/cover to institutions (effective 2002). adv. bk.rev. *Refereed.* **Description:** Publishes papers that focus on clinical and therapeutic aspects of child and adolescent psychology and psychiatry.

Related titles: Online - full text ed.: (from EBSCO Publishing, O C L C Online Computer Library Center, Inc., RoweCom Information Quest, ingenta, Swets Blackwell).

Indexed: ASSIA, Abstr.Soc.Geront., Excerp.Med., Indian Psychol.Abstr., PsycInfo, Sage Fam.Stud.Abstr., Viol.& Abuse Abstr., e-psyche.

—BLDSC (3286.268400), GNLM.

Published by: Sage Publications Ltd., 6 Bonhill St, London EC2A 4PU, United Kingdom. TEL 44-20-7374-0645, FAX 44-20-7374-8741, market@sagepub.co.uk, http://www.sagepub.co.uk. Ed. Bryan Lask. Adv. contact Jenny Kirby. page GBP 250; trim 200 x 125. Circ: 1,150.

COMMUNICATION DISORDERS QUARTERLY. see *EDUCATION—Special Education And Rehabilitation*

▼ **COMMUNITY CARE REVIEW NEWSLETTER.** see *SOCIAL SERVICES AND WELFARE*

THE COMPLEAT MOTHER; the magazine of pregnancy, birth and breastfeeding. see *MEDICAL SCIENCES—Obstetrics And Gynecology*

CONCERN NEWS. see *SOCIAL SERVICES AND WELFARE*

CONTRIBUTIONS TO RESIDENTIAL TREATMENT. see *PSYCHOLOGY*

DOWN & UP. see *HANDICAPPED*

DZIECKO. see *WOMEN'S HEALTH*

362.7 CHE ISSN 0300-4430
HQ767.8 CODEN: ECDCAD

EARLY CHILD DEVELOPMENT AND CARE. Text in English. 1971. 6/yr. (in 6 vols., 1 no./vol.). GBP 383, USD 459, EUR 504 to individuals; GBP 1,125, USD 1,427, EUR 1,499 to institutions; GBP 2,457, USD 3,119, EUR 3,282 to corporations (effective 2002). adv. bk.rev. abstr, charts, illus. index. reprint service avail. from SCH,PSC. *Refereed.* **Document type:** *Journal, Academic/Scholarly.*

Related titles: Microform ed.

Indexed: ASSIA, Biol.Abstr., Br.Educ.Ind., C.I.J.E., Child Devel.Abstr., Cont.Pg.Educ., Educ.Ind. (Jan.1983-Jun.1997), Excerp.Med., IBZ, Ind.Philos., Indian Psychol.Abstr., Mult.Ed.Abstr., PsycInfo, Psychol.Abstr. (1973-), e-psyche.

—CISTI, ingenta. **CCC.**

Published by: Gordon and Breach - Harwood Academic (Subsidiary of: Taylor & Francis Group), PO Box 531, Lausanne 1000, Switzerland. TEL 41-21-6411280, FAX 41-21-6411281, info@gbhap.com, http://www.gbhap.com. Ed. Roy Evans. **Subscr. addr. in US:** International Publishers Direct, PO Box 32160, Newark, NJ 07102. FAX 215-750-6343.

EARLY CHILDHOOD EDUCATION JOURNAL. see *EDUCATION*

▼ **EARLY CHILDHOOD RESEARCH & PRACTICE.** see *EDUCATION*

EARLY INTERVENTION. see *EDUCATION—Special Education And Rehabilitation*

155.4 618.92 FRA ISSN 0013-7545
HQ768

ENFANCE; psychologie, pedagogie, neuro-psychiatrie, sociologie. Text in French. 1948. q. EUR 57 domestic to individuals; EUR 69 foreign to individuals (effective 2002). adv. bk.rev. index. **Description:** Publishes the works of well-known developmental psychologists.

Indexed: IBR, Lang.& Lang.Behav.Abstr., PsycInfo, Psychol.Abstr. (1948-), SOPODA, Sociol.Abstr., e-psyche.

—BLDSC (3747.869000).

Published by: (Laboratoire de Psycho-Biologie de l'Enfant), Presses Universitaires de France, Departement des Revues, 6 av. Reille, Paris 75685 Cedex 14, France. TEL 33-1-60873030, FAX 33-1-60792045, revues@puf.com. Ed. M Abdallah Pretreille. Pub. Helene Gratiot Alphandery. Circ: 2,000.

155.5 FRA ISSN 1286-5559

ENFANCE & PSY. Text in French. 1997. q. EUR 44 domestic to individuals; EUR 55 domestic to institutions; EUR 60 foreign (effective 2001).

Published by: Editions Eres, 11 rue des Alouettes, Ramonville Saint-Agne 31520, France. TEL 33-05-61751576, FAX 33-05-61735289, eres@editions-eres.com. Eds. Didier Lauru, Patrice Huerre, Jean-Louis Le Run.

ETABLISSEMENTS MEDICAUX POUR ENFANTS. see *HEALTH FACILITIES AND ADMINISTRATION*

EXCEPTIONAL CHILDREN. see *EDUCATION—Special Education And Rehabilitation*

EXCEPTIONAL PARENT; the magazine for families and professionals. see *EDUCATION—Special Education And Rehabilitation*

FAMILIE & CO. see *MEDICAL SCIENCES—Pediatrics*

649 AUT
FAMILIENMAGAZIN. Text in German, French, English, Chinese. 1957. 10/yr. ATS 1,200; ATS 1,664 foreign. adv. bk.rev. illus. **Document type:** *Consumer.*
Formerly: Elternblatt (0013-6441)
Indexed: e-psyche.
Published by: Oesterreichische Kinderfrennde, Rauhensteingasse 5-5, Vienna, W 1010, Austria. TEL 43-1-5121298, FAX 43-1-74095183, isr.zv@bohmann.co.at, http://www.isr.co.at. Ed., R&P Gerda Stockhammer TEL 43-1-74095456. Circ: 65,000.

FAMILY WAYS; education resources for pregnancy to parenthood. see *MEDICAL SCIENCES—Obstetrics And Gynecology*

348 USA
FIRST YEAR OF LIFE; a guide to your baby's growth and development month by month. Text in English. 1977. 3/yr. Dist. with The American Baby Basket for New Parents through participating hospitals only. adv. **Document type:** *Magazine, Consumer.* **Description:** Details physical, emotional and social growth of the baby during monthly stages.
Related titles: ♦ Issued with: American Baby. ISSN 0044-7544.
Indexed: CINAHL.
Published by: Primedia Consumer Media & Magazine Group, 249 W 17th St, New York, NY 10011-5300. TEL 212-462-3500, FAX 212-367-8333, http://www.primedia.com/. Ed. Judith Nolte. Pub. Bob Davidowitz. Adv. contact Jeff Christian. B&W page USD 124,500, color page USD 158,700; trim 10.5 x 7.88. Circ: 3,000,000 (controlled).

FOCAL POINT; a national bulletin on family support and children's mental health. see *HANDICAPPED*

FOCUS ON EXCEPTIONAL CHILDREN. see *EDUCATION—Special Education And Rehabilitation*

FOEDSEL & FOERAELDRASKAP. see *MEDICAL SCIENCES—Obstetrics And Gynecology*

649 DEU ISSN 0721-9121
FRUEHFOERDERUNG INTERDISZIPLINAER; Zeitschrift fuer Praxis und Theorie der fruehen Hilfe fuer behinderte und entwicklungsauffaellige Kinder. Text in German. 1982. q. DEM 69; DEM 55.20 to students (effective 2000). adv. bk.rev. index. back issues avail. **Document type:** *Academic/Scholarly.*
Indexed: Psychol.Abstr., e-psyche.
—GNLM. **CCC.**
Published by: Ernst Reinhardt Verlag, Kemnatenstr 46, Munich 80639, Germany. TEL 49-89-1780160, FAX 49-89-17801630. Adv. contact Sofie Bittlinger. Circ: 1,800.

362.7 USA ISSN 1054-8289
HV741 CODEN: FCHIEW
THE FUTURE OF CHILDREN. Text in English. 1991. 2/yr. free per issue. illus. reprints avail. *Refereed.* **Document type:** *Academic/Scholarly.* **Description:** Covers child health, education, and welfare public policy issues.
Related titles: Online - full text ed.: (from Northern Light Technology, Inc., ProQuest Information & Learning, Institute for Scientific Information).
Indexed: ASCA, C.I.J.E., CINAHL, Child Devel.Abstr., Crim.Just.Abstr., Curr.Cont., Fam.Ind., IMFL, Ind.Med. (1991-), Int.Nurs.Ind., Lang.& Lang.Behav.Abstr., PsycInfo, SOPODA, SSCI, Sage Race Rel.Abstr., Soc.Serv.Abstr., Soc.Work Res.& Abstr., Sociol.Abstr., e-psyche.
—BLDSC (4060.523000), GNLM, IDS, ingenta.
Published by: David and Lucile Packard Foundation, Center for the Future of Children, 300 Second St, Ste 102, Los Altos, CA 94022. TEL 415-948-3696, FAX 415-948-6498, http://www.futureofchildren.org. Ed. Richard E Behrman. R&P Dona M Leyva. Circ: 50,000.

GIFTED UNLIMITED. see *EDUCATION—Special Education And Rehabilitation*

155.5 JPN ISSN 0915-4965
GIFU SHISHUNKI KENKYU/GIFU SOCIETY OF ADOLESCENTOLOGY. JOURNAL. Text in Japanese. 1985. a. adv. **Document type:** *Bulletin.*
Indexed: e-psyche.
Published by: (Gifu Shishunki Kenkyukai), Gifuken Seishin Hoken Senta/Gifu Prefectural Mental Health Center, 8-1 Shimonara 2-chome, Gifu-shi 500-8385, Japan. Ed. Akihiko Shibata. Adv. contact Hiroyuki Koide.

GUILFORD SCHOOL PRACTITIONER SERIES. see *PSYCHOLOGY*

649 618 GBR
HAVING A BABY. Text in English. 1994. bi-m. GBP 2.60 newsstand/cover (effective 2000). adv. **Document type:** *Magazine, Consumer.*
Published by: National Magazine Company Ltd., Broadwick St, London W1V 2BP, United Kingdom. TEL 44-20-7439-5000, FAX 44-20-7439-5350.

HAWAII. DEPARTMENT OF HEALTH. MENTAL HEALTH SERVICES FOR CHILDREN AND YOUTH; children's MH services branch. see *SOCIAL SERVICES AND WELFARE*

649 USA ISSN 1076-1764
HEALTHY KIDS. Text in English. 1989. bi-m. USD 15.94 domestic; USD 25.94 foreign; USD 5 per issue; free per issue at pediatrician's office (effective 2000). adv. illus. **Document type:** *Magazine, Consumer.* **Description:** Provides for parents of children from birth to age ten, with information about children's physical and emotional well-being.
Formed by the merger of (1990-1994): Healthy Kids: 4-10 Years. (1062-4236); Which was formerly: American Baby's Healthy Kids: 4-10 Years; (1989-1994): Healthy Kids: Birth - 3 (1063-0945); Which was formerly: American Baby's Healthy Kids: Birth - 3; (until 1990): American Baby's Healthy Kids
Published by: (American Academy of Pediatrics), Primedia Consumer Media & Magazine Group, 249 W 17th St, New York, NY 10011-5300. TEL 212-745-0500, 800-678-1208, FAX 212-367-8332, http://www.healthykids.com/. Ed. Laura Broadwell. adv.: B&W page USD 62,300, color page USD 97,900; trim 10.5 x 7.88. Circ: 1,554,632.

158 362.7 GBR ISSN 1462-8260
HEALTHY MINDS. Text in English. 1998. s-a. free per issue. **Document type:** *Bulletin.* **Description:** Highlights the contributions of voluntary sector initiatives to the mental health and well-being of young people.
Indexed: e-psyche.
Published by: National Children's Bureau Enterprises Ltd., 8 Wakley St, London EC1V 7QE, United Kingdom. TEL 44-20-7843-6000, FAX 44-20-7278-9512, http://www.ncb.org.uk. Circ: 1,000.

HUMAN STRESS: CURRENT SELECTED RESEARCH. see *PSYCHOLOGY*

305.23 618.2 NLD
IN VERWACHTING. Text in Dutch. a. adv. charts, illus. **Document type:** *Magazine, Consumer.* **Description:** Offers expectant mothers important advice on caring for their unborn infants to provide the best chances for having a healthy baby.
Published by: V N U Tijdschriften B.V., Postbus 1900, Hoofddorp 2130 JH, Netherlands. TEL 31-23-556-6770, FAX 31-23-556-6771, ServiceTeam@tijdschriften.vnu.com, http://www.vnu.nl/vnu/organisatie.

305.232 USA ISSN 1525-0008
▼ **INFANCY.** Text in English. 2000. q. USD 55 in US & Canada to individuals; USD 85 elsewhere to individuals; USD 245 in US & Canada to institutions; USD 275 elsewhere to institutions (effective 2002). adv. **Document type:** *Journal, Academic/Scholarly.* **Description:** Provides original research on normal and aberrant infant development in the first two years, including both human and animal research.
Related titles: Online - full text ed.: (from CatchWord Ltd., RoweCom Information Quest).
—BLDSC (4478.256000), CatchWord.
Published by: (International Society on Infant Studies), Lawrence Erlbaum Associates, Inc., 10 Industrial Ave, Mahwah, NJ 07430-2262. TEL 201-760-3735, 800-926-6579, FAX 201-236-0072, journals@erlbaum.com, http://www.erlbaum.com/Journals/journals/IN/in.htm. Ed. Leslie B Cohen. adv.: page USD 375; trim 5 x 8.

INFANT AND CHILD DEVELOPMENT. see *PSYCHOLOGY*

INFANTS AND YOUNG CHILDREN; an interdisciplinary journal of special care practices. see *MEDICAL SCIENCES—Pediatrics*

155.4 ITA ISSN 0390-2420
INFANZIA. Text in Italian. 1973. m. ITL 63,000; ITL 74,000 foreign. adv. bk.rev.
Indexed: e-psyche.
Published by: Nuova Italia Editrice S.p.A, Via Ernesto Codignola, Scandicci, FI 50018, Italy. nib.reviews@lanuovaitalia.it, http://www.lanuovaitalia.it/. Ed. Pietro Bertolini.

▼ **INFORMASIAN.** see *HANDICAPPED—Visually Impaired*

362.7 155.4 GBR ISSN 0267-3843
INTERNATIONAL JOURNAL OF ADOLESCENCE AND YOUTH. Text in English. 1987. 4/yr. GBP 79, USD 159 (effective 2001). *Refereed.* **Document type:** *Journal, Academic/Scholarly.* **Description:** Covers psychological growth and development, health and medical care, social policy, education, employment, unemployment, leisure, sex education, family relationships, and homelessness.
Indexed: ASSIA, Br.Educ.Ind., Cont.Pg.Educ., ERA, Fam.Ind., IBZ, Ind.Philos., Lang.& Lang.Behav.Abstr., Mult.Ed.Abstr., PsycInfo, Psychol.Abstr. (1987-), SOPODA, Soc.Serv.Abstr., Sociol.Abstr., Sociol.Educ.Abstr., Sp.Ed.Needs Abstr., e-psyche.
—BLDSC (4541.562000).
Published by: A B Academic Publishers, PO Box 42, Bicester, Oxon OX26 6NW, United Kingdom. jrnls@abapubl.demon.co.uk. Ed. Roy Evans.

INTERNATIONAL JOURNAL OF CHILDREN'S SPIRITUALITY. see *PSYCHOLOGY*

362.76 345.025 616.858 USA ISSN 1043-8823
HV8079.C48 CODEN: ICCAEG
ISSUES IN CHILD ABUSE ACCUSATIONS. Text in English. 1989. biennial. USD 50; USD 70 foreign (effective 1998). bk.rev. back issues avail. *Refereed.* **Document type:** *Academic/Scholarly.* **Description:** Provides a multidisciplinary forum on all aspects of child abuse, with special emphasis on research and commentary that questions the methods and conventional wisdom of the child abuse establishment.
Indexed: Lang.& Lang.Behav.Abstr., SOPODA, Sociol.Abstr.
—GNLM, ingenta.
Published by: Institute for Psychological Therapies, 13200 Cannon City Blvd, Northfield, MN 55057. TEL 507-645-8881, FAX 507-645-8883, under006@gold.tc.umn.edu. Ed. Hollida Wakefield. Circ: 200 (paid).

ISSUES IN CHILD ABUSE PREVENTION. see *SOCIAL SERVICES AND WELFARE*

J D C - BROOKDALE INSTITUTE OF GERONTOLOGY AND HUMAN DEVELOPMENT. ANNUAL REPORT. see *GERONTOLOGY AND GERIATRICS*

J D C - BROOKDALE INSTITUTE OF GERONTOLOGY AND HUMAN DEVELOPMENT. RESEARCH SERIES. see *GERONTOLOGY AND GERIATRICS*

JA ZUM BABY; medizinischer Ratgeber fuer werdende und junge Eltern. see *MEDICAL SCIENCES—Pediatrics*

155.5 GBR ISSN 0140-1971
RJ499.A1
JOURNAL OF ADOLESCENCE. Text in English. 1978. bi-m. GBP 250 to institutions (effective 2001). adv. bk.rev. index. reprint service avail. from SWZ. *Refereed.* **Document type:** *Academic/Scholarly.* **Description:** International, broadly based, cross-disciplinary journal that addresses itself to issues of professional and academic importance.
Related titles: Online - full text ed.: (from EBSCO Publishing, O C L C Online Computer Library Center, Inc., RoweCom Information Quest, ingenta, Gale Group, Swets Blackwell, IDEAL Online Library, Factiva, Institute for Scientific Information).
Indexed: ASCA, ASSIA, Abstr.Crim.& Pen., Addic.Abstr., Bibl.Agri., Br.Educ.Ind., Brit.Nur.Ind., C.I.J.E., Crim.Just.Abstr., Curr.Cont., ERA, Environ.Sci.Poll.Mgmt., Excerp.Med., Fam.Ind., Hist.Abstr. (1986-, dropped), Hosp.Abstr., Ind.Med. (1978-), Indian Psychol.Abstr., Lang.& Lang.Behav.Abstr., P C I, Pollut.Abstr., PsycInfo, Psychol.Abstr. (1980-), Risk Abstr., SOMA, SOPODA, SSCI, Saf.Sci.Abstr., Sage Race Rel.Abstr., Soc.Sci.Ind. (Sep.1982-), Soc.Serv.Abstr., Sociol.Abstr., Sociol.Educ.Abstr., Stud.Wom.Abstr., Tech.Educ.Abstr., e-psyche.
—BLDSC (4918.942000), GNLM, IDS, ingenta, KNAW. **CCC.**

C

Published by: Academic Press (Subsidiary of: Harcourt Publishers Ltd.), 24 Oval Rd, London NW1 7DX, United Kingdom. TEL 44-20-7482-2293, 44-20-7267-4466, apsubs@acad.com, http://www.academicpress.com/adolescence; http://www.europe.idealibrary.com/. Ed. John Coleman. R&P Catherine John. Adv. contact Nik Screen. **Subscr. to:** Harcourt Publishers Ltd., Foots Cray High St, Sidcup, Kent DA14 5HP, United Kingdom. TEL 44-20-8300-3322, FAX 44-20-8309-0807.

JOURNAL OF ADOLESCENT HEALTH. see *MEDICAL SCIENCES*

JOURNAL OF ADOLESCENT RESEARCH. see *PSYCHOLOGY*

JOURNAL OF CHILD AND ADOLESCENT PSYCHIATRIC NURSING. see *MEDICAL SCIENCES—Nurses And Nursing*

JOURNAL OF CHILD & ADOLESCENT SUBSTANCE ABUSE. see *DRUG ABUSE AND ALCOHOLISM*

JOURNAL OF CHILD AND FAMILY STUDIES. see *PSYCHOLOGY*

155.4 GBR ISSN 0305-0009
P118

JOURNAL OF CHILD LANGUAGE. Text in English. 1974. 3/yr. GBP 77 to individuals; USD 240 to institutions (effective 2002). adv. bk.rev. back issues avail.; reprint service avail. from SWZ,PQC. *Refereed.* **Document type:** *Academic/Scholarly.* **Description:** Covers all aspects of the scientific study of language behavior in children and the underlying principles, including normal and pathological development of both monolingual and bilingual children.
Related titles: Microform ed.: (from PQC); Online - full text ed.: (from EBSCO Publishing, O C L C Online Computer Library Center, Inc., RoweCom Information Quest, Swets Blackwell, Institute for Scientific Information).
Indexed: AMED, ASCA, ASSIA, Abstr.Anthropol., Arts & Hum.Cit.Ind. (coverage dropped), Bibl.Dev.Med.& Child Neur., Bibl.Ling., Br.Educ.Ind., C.I.J.E., CINAHL, Child Devel.Abstr., Child.Lit.Abstr., Commun.Abstr., Cont.Pg.Educ., Curr.Cont., Educ.Ind. (Oct.1983-), Fam.Ind., IBZ, Ind.Med. (1974-), Int.Nurs.Ind., Lang.& Lang.Behav.Abstr. (1974-), Lang.Teach.& Ling.Abstr., Ling.Abstr., M.L.A., MLA Intl.Bibl., Mid.East: Abstr.& Ind., Mult.Ed.Abstr., P C I, PsycInfo, Psychol.Abstr. (1974-), Psycscan D.P., Russ.Acad.Sci.Bibl., SOPODA, SSCI, Sage Fam.Stud.Abstr., Sociol.Abstr., Stud.Wom.Abstr., Yrbk.Assoc.Educ.& Rehab.Blind, e-psyche.
—BLDSC (4957.600000), IDS, ingenta. **CCC.**
Published by: Cambridge University Press, Edinburgh Bldg, Shaftesbury Rd, Cambridge CB2 2RU, United Kingdom. FAX 44-1223-315052, information@cup.cam.ac.uk, information@cambridge.org, http://www.cup.cam.ac.uk, http://www.uk.cambridge.org/journals/pmu. Ed. Elena Lieven. R&P Linda Nicol. Adv. contact Rebecca Symons. Circ: 1,850.

JOURNAL OF CHILD SEXUAL ABUSE; research, treatment & program innovations for victims, survivors & offenders. see *SOCIAL SERVICES AND WELFARE*

JOURNAL OF CLINICAL CHILD AND ADOLESCENT PSYCHOLOGY. see *PSYCHOLOGY*

305.235 USA ISSN 0272-4316
HQ796

JOURNAL OF EARLY ADOLESCENCE. Text in English. 1981. q. USD 65 to individuals; USD 260 to institutions; USD 25 newsstand/cover to individuals; USD 70 newsstand/cover to institutions (effective 2002). adv. bk.rev., film rev. back issues avail.; reprint service avail. from PQC. *Refereed.* **Document type:** *Academic/Scholarly.* **Description:** Takes an interdisciplinary approach through research studies, reviews, and theoretical papers to the need for focus on the characteristics of persons 10-14 years old.
Related titles: Microform ed.; Online - full text ed.: (from EBSCO Publishing, O C L C Online Computer Library Center, Inc., RoweCom Information Quest, ProQuest Information & Learning, ingenta, Swets Blackwell, Institute for Scientific Information).
Indexed: ASCA, Adol.Ment.Hlth.Abstr., C.I.J.E. (coverage dropped), Child Devel.Abstr., Crim.Just.Abstr., Curr.Cont., Curr.Lit.Fam.Plan., Educ.Ind. (coverage dropped), Fam.Ind., IMFL, Lang.& Lang.Behav.Abstr., Mult.Ed.Abstr., Peace Res.Abstr., PsycInfo, Psychol.Abstr. (1981-), SOPODA, SSCI, Sage Fam.Stud.Abstr., Soc.Sci.Ind. (coverage dropped), Soc.Serv.Abstr., Soc.Work Res.& Abstr., Sociol.Abstr., Viol.& Abuse Abstr., e-psyche.
—BLDSC (4970.701000), IDS, ingenta. **CCC.**
Published by: Sage Publications, Inc., 2455 Teller Rd, Thousand Oaks, CA 91320. TEL 805-499-0721, FAX 805-499-0871, libraries@sagepub.com., libaries@sagepub.com, http://www.sagepub.com. Ed. E Ellen Thornburg. R&P Tanya Udin. Adv. contact DeAnna Vega Hammersley. Circ: 1,200. **Overseas subscr. to:** Sage Publications Ltd., 6 Bonhill St, London EC2A 4PU, United Kingdom; Sage Publications India Pvt. Ltd., 4215, New Delhi 110 048, India.

JOURNAL OF EARLY INTERVENTION. see *EDUCATION—Special Education And Rehabilitation*

JOURNAL OF EXPERIMENTAL CHILD PSYCHOLOGY. see *PSYCHOLOGY*

JOURNAL OF HIV - AIDS PREVENTION & EDUCATION FOR ADOLESCENTS & CHILDREN. see *MEDICAL SCIENCES—Communicable Diseases*

JOURNAL OF PRACTICAL APPROACHES TO DEVELOPMENTAL HANDICAP. see *EDUCATION—Special Education And Rehabilitation*

155.4 USA ISSN 1532-7795
HQ796 CODEN: JRADET

JOURNAL OF RESEARCH ON ADOLESCENCE. Text in English. 1991. q. adv. *Refereed.* **Document type:** *Journal, Academic/Scholarly.* **Description:** Publishes original researches pertinent to the development patterns inherent throughout adolescence.
Media: Online - full content. **Related titles:** Online - full text ed.: (from CatchWord Ltd., Institute for Scientific Information, RoweCom Information Quest).
Indexed: ASCA, ASSIA, Addic.Abstr., C.I.J.E., Curr.Cont., Environ.Sci.Poll.Mgmt., Fam.Ind., Lang.& Lang.Behav.Abstr., Mult.Ed.Abstr., PsycInfo, Psychol.Abstr. (1991-), Risk Abstr., SOPODA, SSCI, Saf.Sci.Abstr., Soc.Serv.Abstr., Sociol.Abstr., Sp.Ed.Needs Abstr., THA, e-psyche.
—BLDSC (5051.920000), CatchWord, Infotrieve, ingenta. **CCC.**
Published by: (Society for Research on Adolescence), Lawrence Erlbaum Associates, Inc., 10 Industrial Ave, Mahwah, NJ 07430-2262. TEL 201-760-3735, 800-926-6579, FAX 201-236-0072, journals@erlbaum.com, http://www.catchword.com/erlbaum/10508392/contp1-1.htm, http://www.erlbaum.com. Ed. Diane Scott Jones. adv.: page USD 400; trim 5 x 8.

JOURNAL OF SOCIAL WORK PRACTICE. see *SOCIAL SERVICES AND WELFARE*

155.4 USA ISSN 0047-2891
HQ796 CODEN: JYADA

JOURNAL OF YOUTH AND ADOLESCENCE; a multidisciplinary research publication. Text in English. 1972. bi-m. USD 660, EUR 659 to institutions for print or online ed.; USD 792 to institutions for print & online eds.combined; EUR 790.80 to institutions print & online eds.combined (effective 2002). adv. bibl, charts, illus. back issues avail.; reprints avail. *Refereed.* **Document type:** *Journal, Academic/Scholarly.* **Description:** Enables psychiatrists, psychologists, sociologists, social workers, counsellors, and educators to share ideas relevant to the subject of youth and adolescence.
Related titles: Microfilm ed.: (from PQC); Online - full text ed.: (from ProQuest Information & Learning, Gale Group, EBSCO Publishing, O C L C Online Computer Library Center, Inc., Swets Blackwell, Kluwer Online, Factiva, Institute for Scientific Information, RoweCom Information Quest).
Indexed: ASCA, ASSIA, Abstr.Crim.& Pen., Addic.Abstr., Adol.Ment.Hlth.Abstr., AgeLine, Bibl.Agri., CERDIC, C.I.J.E., Chic.Per.Ind., Child Devel.Abstr., Commun.Abstr., Crim.Just.Abstr., Curr.Cont., Curr.Lit.Fam.Plan., ERA, Educ.Admin.Abstr., Educ.Ind. (Feb.1983-Apr.1992), Excerp.Med., Fam.Ind., High.Educ.Abstr., IBZ, IMFL, Ind.Philos., Lang.& Lang.Behav.Abstr., Mid.East: Abstr.& Ind., Mult.Ed.Abstr., P C I, PsycInfo, Psychol.Abstr. (1972-), Psycscan D.P., Ref.Zh., SOMA, SOPODA, SSCI, Sage Fam.Stud.Abstr., Sage Race Rel.Abstr., Sage Urb.Stud.Abstr., Soc.Sci.Ind. (Feb.1987-), Soc.Serv.Abstr., Sociol.Abstr., Sociol.Educ.Abstr., Sp.Ed.Needs Abstr., Stud.Wom.Abstr., THA, Viol.& Abuse Abstr., e-psyche.
—BLDSC (5072.720000), GNLM, IDS, ingenta. **CCC.**
Published by: Kluwer Academic - Plenum Publishers (Subsidiary of: Wolters Kluwer N.V.), 233 Spring St, New York, NY 10013-1578. TEL 800-221-9369, info@plenum.com, http://www.wkap.nl/journalhome.htm/0047-2891. Ed. Daniel Offer. R&P Rose Luongo TEL 781-871-6311. **Subscr. outside the Americas to:** Kluwer Academic Publishers Group, Journals Department, PO Box 322, Dordrecht 3300 AH, Netherlands. TEL 31-78-639-2392, FAX 31-78-654-6474.

305.235 GBR ISSN 1367-6261

JOURNAL OF YOUTH STUDIES. Text in English. 1998. 4/yr. GBP 41, USD 66 to individuals; GBP 155, USD 255 to institutions (effective 2002). **Document type:** *Academic/Scholarly.* **Description:** Aims to serve as a multidisciplinary journal devoted to a theoretical and empirical understanding of young people's experiences and life contexts.
Related titles: Online - full text ed.: ISSN 1469-9680 (from CatchWord Ltd., EBSCO Publishing, O C L C Online Computer Library Center, Inc., RoweCom Information Quest, Swets Blackwell).
Indexed: Cont.Pg.Educ., Crim.Just.Abstr., Sage Race Rel.Abstr., Soc.Serv.Abstr., Sociol.Abstr., Stud.Wom.Abstr., e-psyche.
—BLDSC (5072.725000), CatchWord. **CCC.**
Published by: Carfax Publishing Limited (Subsidiary of: Taylor & Francis Group), PO Box 25, Abingdon, Oxon OX14 3UE, United Kingdom. TEL 44-1235-401000, FAX 44-1235-401550, enquiries@carfax.co.uk, enquiry@tandf.co.uk, http://www.carfax.co.uk. Ed. Andy Furlong.

JUNGE FAMILIE; das Baby-Journal. see *MEDICAL SCIENCES—Pediatrics*

362.7 AUS

KIDSAFE. Text in English. 1979. q. AUD 20 (effective 1998). adv. *Refereed.* **Document type:** *Consumer.* **Description:** Information on prevention of Children's injuries.
Former titles (until Autumn 1994): Safeguard (1038-3409); Safe Guard (0818-0474); (until 1986): Child Accident Prevention Foundation of Australia. Quarterly Journal (0725-9573); (until 1981): Child Accident Prevention Foundation of Australia. Journal (0728-8778)
Published by: Child Accident Prevention Foundation of Australia, Suite 4, Level 1, 280 Church St, Richmond, VIC 3121, Australia. TEL 61-3-94271008, FAX 61-3-94213831. Ed. Carol Taylor. Adv. contact Janine O'Longhlan. Circ: 3,000.

371.392 DEU ISSN 0945-5582

DAS KIND. Text in German. 1987. s-a. DEM 24. bk.rev. back issues avail. **Document type:** *Newsletter.*
Published by: Deutsche Montessori Gesellschaft e.V., Postfach 5461, Wuerzburg 97004, Germany. TEL 0931-8885560. Ed. Waltraud Harth Peter. Circ: 500.

KIND EN ADOLESCENT. see *MEDICAL SCIENCES—Pediatrics*

618 688.72 649 362.7 DEU

KINDER; fuer Eltern, Erzieher und Kinder. Text in German. 1971. 10/yr. EUR 13 domestic; EUR 17 foreign (effective 2002). adv. 55 p./no. 4 cols./p. back issues avail. **Document type:** *Magazine, Consumer.*
Published by: Junior-Verlag GmbH und Co. KG, Fehlandtstr 41, Hamburg 20354, Germany. TEL 49-40-344434, FAX 49-40-352540, info@junior-verlag.de, http://www.junior-verlag.de. Ed. Dagmar von Schweinitz. Pub., R&P Manfred Zedler. Adv. contact Birgit Koenig. B&W page XEU 9,000, color page XEU 16,200; trim 185 x 250. Circ: 280,000 (paid and controlled).

▼ **KINDER, KINDER**; sicher - gesund. see *PUBLIC HEALTH AND SAFETY*

KINDERANALYSE. see *PSYCHOLOGY*

618.92 362.7 NLD ISSN 0926-0838

KINDEROPVANG. Text in Dutch. 1969. m. (11/yr.). NLG 155 foreign. **Document type:** *Trade.* **Description:** Addresses all professionals involved in the care and teaching of children. Reviews toys and books for children and offers practical advice in all areas.
Formerly (until 1990): Kleine Wereld (0166-7106)
Published by: Elsevier Gezondheidszorg B.V., Tijdstroom (Subsidiary of: Reed Elsevier plc Group), Planetenbaan 1, Maarssen 3600 AK, Netherlands. TEL 31-346-577577, FAX 31-346-554287, http://www.tijdstroom.nl. **Subscr. to:** Elsevier Den Haag, Postbus 16500, The Hague 2500 BM, Netherlands. TEL 31-70-381-9900, FAX 31-70-333-8399.

LEARNING DISABILITIES RESEARCH AND PRACTICE. see *EDUCATION—Special Education And Rehabilitation*

649 618 GBR
THE LOCAL BABY DIRECTORY: BRISTOL & BATH. Text in English. a., latest 2001-2002. GBP 4.99 newsstand/cover (effective 2001). adv. Website rev. 150 p./no. **Document type:** *Directory, Consumer.* **Description:** Contains a definitive directory of resources throughout Bristol & Bath for parents and carers. Includes everything from acupuncture to zoos, from adventure playgrounds to yoga.
Published by: Baby Directory Ltd., 10 Grove Park Terrace, London W4 3QG, United Kingdom. TEL 44-20-8742-8724, FAX 44-20-8580-7085, editor@babydirectory.com, http://www.babydirectory.com. Ed. Gail Boulton.

649 618.2 GBR
▼ **THE LOCAL BABY DIRECTORY: HERTS & MIDDLESEX**; an a-z of everything for pregnant women, babies and children. Text in English. 1999. a. GBP 4.99 newsstand/cover (effective 2001). adv. Website rev. 150 p./no. *Refereed.* **Document type:** *Directory, Consumer.* **Description:** Provides a definitive directory of resources throughout Herts and Middlesex for parents and carers. Contains everything from acupuncture to zoos, from adventure playgrounds to yoga.
Published by: Baby Directory Ltd., 10 Grove Park Terrace, London W4 3QG, United Kingdom. TEL 44-20-8742-8724, FAX 44-20-8580-7085, editor@babydirectory.com, http://www.babydirectory.com. Ed., Adv. contact Brigid Phillips TEL 44-20-8429-1849. Pub., R&P Dr. Karen Liebreich. B&W page GBP 350, color page GBP 600;. Circ: 3,000 (paid).

649 618 GBR
THE LOCAL BABY DIRECTORY: OXFORDSHIRE, BERKS & BUCKS; an a-z of everything for pregnant women, babies and children. Text in English. a., latest 2001-2002. GBP 4.99 per issue (effective 2001). adv. Website rev. 150 p./no. **Document type:** *Consumer.* **Description:** Contains a definitive directory of resources throughout Oxfordshire, Berks & Bucks for parents and carers. Includes everything from acupuncture to zoos, from adventure playgrounds to yoga.
Published by: Baby Directory Ltd., 10 Grove Park Terrace, London W4 3QG, United Kingdom. TEL 44-20-8742-8724, FAX 44-20-8580-7085, editor@babydirectory.com, http://www.babydirectory.com. Ed. Francesca Lee.

649 618 GBR
THE LOCAL BABY DIRECTORY: SOUTH WALES; an a-z of everything for pregnant women, babies and children. Text in English. a., latest 2001-2002. GBP 4.99 newsstand/cover (effective 2001). adv. Website rev. 150 p./no. **Document type:** *Directory, Consumer.* **Description:** Contains a definitive directory of resources throughout South Wales for parents and carers. Includes everything from acupuncture to zoos, from adventure playgrounds to yoga.
Published by: Baby Directory Ltd., 10 Grove Park Terrace, London W4 3QG, United Kingdom. TEL 44-20-8742-8724, FAX 44-20-8580-7085, editor@babydirectory.com, http://www.babydirectory.com. Ed. Gail Boulton.

649 618 GBR
THE LOCAL BABY DIRECTORY: SURREY; an a-z everything for pregnant women, babies and children. Text in English. a., latest 2001-2002. GBP 4.99 newsstand/cover (effective 2001). adv. Website rev. 150 p./no. **Document type:** *Directory, Consumer.* **Description:** Contains a definitive directory of resources throughout Surrey for parents and carers. Includes everything from acupuncture to zoos, from adventure playgrounds to yoga.
Published by: Baby Directory Ltd., 10 Grove Park Terrace, London W4 3QG, United Kingdom. TEL 44-20-8742-8724, FAX 44-20-8580-7085, editor@babydirectory.com, http://www.babydirectory.com. Ed. Angela Thompson.

649 618 GBR
THE LOCAL BABY DIRECTORY: SUSSEX & HAMPSHIRE; an a-z of everything for pregnant women, babies and children. Text in English. a., latest 2001-2002. GBP 4.99 newsstand/cover (effective 2001). Website rev. 150 p./no. **Document type:** *Directory, Consumer.* **Description:** Contains a definitive directory of resources throughout Sussex & Hampshire for parents and carers. Includes everything from acupuncture to zoos, from adventure playgrounds to yoga.
Published by: Baby Directory Ltd., 10 Grove Park Terrace, London W4 3QG, United Kingdom. TEL 44-20-8742-8724, FAX 44-20-8580-7085, editor@babydirectory.com, http://www.babydirectory.com.

649 618.2 GBR ISSN 1369-9539
THE LONDON BABY DIRECTORY; an a-z of everything for pregnant women, babies and children. Text in English. 1997. a. GBP 6.99 newsstand/cover (effective 2001). adv. Website rev. index. **Document type:** *Directory, Consumer.* **Description:** Contains a definitive directory of resources throughout London for parents and carers. Includes everything from acupuncture to zoos, from adventure playgrounds to yoga.
Published by: Baby Directory Ltd., 10 Grove Park Terrace, London W4 3QG, United Kingdom. TEL 44-20-8742-8724, FAX 44-20-8580-7085, editor@babydirectory.com, http://www.babydirectory.com. Ed., Pub., R&P, Adv. contact Dr. Karen Liebreich. B&W page GBP 610, color page GBP 999;. Circ: 7,500 (paid).

M R D D EXPRESS. (Mental Retardation and Developmental Disabilities) see *EDUCATION—Special Education And Rehabilitation*

362.7 155.4 NLD ISSN 1382-4406
MANAGEMENT KINDEROPVANG. Text in Dutch. 1995. 10/yr. **Document type:** *Trade.* **Description:** Discusses all issues in managing daycare centers and nursery schools for directors as well as teacher, caregivers, assistants, and support personnel.
Published by: Elsevier Gezondheidszorg B.V., Tijdstroom (Subsidiary of: Reed Elsevier plc Group), Planetenbaan 1, Maarssen 3600 AK, Netherlands. TEL 31-346-577577, FAX 31-346-554287, http://www.tijdstroom.nl. **Subscr. to:** Elsevier Den Haag, Postbus 16500, The Hague 2500 BM, Netherlands. TEL 31-70-381-9900, FAX 31-70-333-8399.

MERRILL - PALMER QUARTERLY. see *PSYCHOLOGY*

362.7 618.92 FRA ISSN 1258-780X
METIERS DE LA PETITE ENFANCE. Text in French. 1994. 10/yr. EUR 60 in Europe to institutions; USD 67 elsewhere to institutions; EUR 60 in Europe to individuals (effective 2002). **Description:** Includes articles and research, professional news coverage, medical issues and practical mementos.
Published by: Elsevier Paris, Editions Scientifiques et Medicales (Subsidiary of: Reed Elsevier plc. group), 23 rue Linois, Paris 75015, France. http://www.elsevier.com/locate/mpenf. Circ: 10,000.

MOTDRAG; Accent. see *DRUG ABUSE AND ALCOHOLISM*

MOTHER & BABY. see *MEDICAL SCIENCES—Obstetrics And Gynecology*

MOTHER AND CHILD. see *WOMEN'S INTERESTS*

MOTHERING; the magazine of natural family living. see *WOMEN'S HEALTH*

NATIONAL DEAF CHILDREN'S SOCIETY. ANNUAL REPORT. see *HANDICAPPED—Hearing Impaired*

649 GBR
NATURAL PARENT. Text in English. 1998. bi-m. GBP 2.50 newsstand/cover (effective 2000). adv. **Document type:** *Magazine, Consumer.* **Description:** Contains information and advice on raising and nurturing a family using alternative and holistic methods.
Indexed: Gend.Watch.
Published by: Mothers Know Best Ltd., 77 Grosvenor Ave, London N5 2NN, United Kingdom. TEL 44-171-354-4592, FAX 44-171-354-8907.

NEUROPSYCHOLOGY, DEVELOPMENT, AND COGNITION. SECTION C: CHILD NEUROPSYCHOLOGY; a journal on normal and abnormal development in childhood and adolescence. see *PSYCHOLOGY*

618 649 CAN ISSN 1193-9397
NEW MOTHER. Text in English. 1979. s-a. free per issue. adv. **Description:** Provides articles on parenting the newborn, feeding, development and daily care issues.
Formerly (until 1992): Chatelaine's New Mother (0708-5303)
Related titles: French ed.: Mere Nouvelle. ISSN 1193-9389.
Indexed: CBCA Ref.
Published by: (Today's Parent Group), Professional Publishing Associates, 269 Richmond St W, Toronto, ON M5V 1X1, Canada. TEL 416-596-8680, FAX 416-596-1991. Ed. Holly Bennett. Circ: 160,000 (controlled).

OMVAARDAREN. see *SOCIAL SERVICES AND WELFARE*

790.019 370.15 USA ISSN 1055-1336
LC3991
OUR GIFTED CHILDREN. Text in English. 1991. m. USD 30; USD 40 foreign. adv. bk.rev. bibl, charts, illus, tr.lit. back issues avail. **Document type:** *Trade.* **Description:** Directed to those concerned with gifted children and covers psychology, schooling, work force, and leadership.
Indexed: e-psyche.
Published by: Royal Fireworks Press, PO Box 399, Unionville, NY 10988. TEL 914-726-4444, FAX 914-726-3824, rfpress@frontier.net. Ed. Michael Clay Thompson. Pub. T M Kemnitz. R&P Myrna Kaye.

OUR WAY. see *RELIGIONS AND THEOLOGY—Judaic*

PAEDIATRIC AND PERINATAL DRUG THERAPY. see *PHARMACY AND PHARMACOLOGY*

649 USA ISSN 0737-5158
PAEDONOSON✱ ; an international journal of chronic illness and disability in childhood. Text in English. 1984. q. adv. bk.rev. abstr, charts, illus. index.
Published by: Eterna International, Inc., PO Box 5731, Hauppauge, NY 11788-0154. Ed. Stephen B Parrish.

649 618.2 BRA ISSN 0030-9567
PAIS E FILHOS; revista mensal da familia moderna. Text in Portuguese. 1968. m. USD 42. adv. bk.rev., film rev. charts, illus. **Document type:** *Consumer.* **Description:** Contains information about pregnancy and children from birth to 12 years.
Published by: Bloch Editores S.A., Rua do Russell 766-804, Rio De Janeiro, RJ 22210-000, Brazil. TEL 021-5554000, FAX 021-2059998. Ed. Silvia Leal. Circ: 120,000.

C

649.155 USA
PARENTING FOR HIGH POTENTIAL. Text in English. 1996. q. USD 50 domestic; USD 60 foreign (effective 2001). adv. **Document type:** *Consumer, Academic/Scholarly.* **Description:** For parents and teachers who want to help develop the gifts and talents that will enable all children to reach their full potential.
Indexed: e-psyche.
Published by: National Association for Gifted Children, 1707 L St, N W, Ste 550, Washington, DC 20036-4201. TEL 202-785-4268, FAX 202-785-4268, nagc@nagc.org. Ed. Donald Treflinger. Adv. contact Cora Powers. page USD 1,500; 7.1875 x 10.

PARENTING'S HEALTHY PREGNANCY. see *MEDICAL SCIENCES—Obstetrics And Gynecology*

PARENTS PREGNANCY. see *MEDICAL SCIENCES—Obstetrics And Gynecology*

362.7 613.9 USA ISSN 1071-3158
PASSAGES (WASHINGTON, D.C.). Text in English, French, Spanish. 1978-2000; N.S. 2000 (Sep.). 3/yr. USD 24 (effective 1999). bk.rev., film rev. charts, illus, stat. back issues avail. **Document type:** *Newsletter.* **Description:** Includes summaries of projects on adolescent reproductive health.
Published by: Advocates for Youth, 1025 Vermont Ave, N W, Ste 200, Washington, DC 20005. TEL 202-347-5700, FAX 202-347-2263, TELEX 425900 SWIFT UI ATT CFP. Ed. Cate Lane.

PEDIATRICS FOR PARENTS; the monthly newsletter for caring adults. see *MEDICAL SCIENCES—Pediatrics*

PRAXIS SPIEL UND GRUPPE. see *EDUCATION*

PREGNANCY & BIRTH. see *MEDICAL SCIENCES—Obstetrics And Gynecology*

THE PREGNANCY BOOK. see *MEDICAL SCIENCES—Obstetrics And Gynecology*

028.5 CHN
QINGSHAONIAN YU JIANKANG/YOUTH AND HEALTH. Text in Chinese. m. USD 28.80; USD 2.40 newsstand/cover (effective 2001). **Document type:** *Academic/Scholarly.*

Published by: China International Book Trading Corp/Zhongguo Guoji Tushu Maoyi Zonggongsi cibtc@mail.cibtc.com.cn, http://www.cibtc.com.cn. **Dist. by:** 35, Chegongzhuang Xilu, Haidian District, Beijing 100044, China.

RECLAIMING CHILDREN AND YOUTH; the journal of emotional and behavioral problems. see *PSYCHOLOGY*

647 610 JPN ISSN 0386-8435
HQ767.8
RESEARCH AND CLINICAL CENTER FOR CHILD DEVELOPMENT. ANNUAL REPORT. Text and summaries in English. 1978. a. free per issue. cum.index. back issues avail. *Refereed.* **Document type:** *Academic/Scholarly.*
Indexed: Psychol.Abstr.
—BLDSC (1289.661000).
Published by: Hokkaido University, Research and Clinical Center for Child Development, Nishi 7-chome, Kita 11-jo, Kita-ku, Sapporo-shi 060-0081, Japan. TEL 81-11-706-2607, FAX 81-11-706-4946, schen@edu.hokudai.ac.jp. Ed. Shing Jen Chen. Pub. Takashi Morotomi. R&P Shing-Jen Chen. Circ: 500 (controlled).

RESIDENTIAL TREATMENT NEWS. see *PSYCHOLOGY*

649 618.92 DEU
RUND UMS BABY. Text in German. m. adv. **Document type:** *Consumer.* **Description:** Provides information and content on all aspects of pregnancy, birth and baby care for parents.
Media: Online - full text.
Published by: Ulrich Schneider Multimedia, Franziskanerstr 16, Olpe-Biggesee 57462, Germany. redaktion@rund-ums-baby.de, http://www.rund-ums-baby.de.

155.4 305.23 370.15 USA
S R C D NEWSLETTER. Text in English. 1958. quadrennial. free. **Document type:** *Newsletter, Academic/Scholarly.* **Description:** Reports on news and events of interest to members of the Society for Research in Child Development, including publications, meetings and symposia, memoirs, and reports on Federal legislation.
Media: Online - full content.
Published by: Society for Research in Child Development, 505 E Huron, Ste 301, Ann Arbor, MI 48104-1522. TEL 734-998-6578, FAX 734-998-6569, pamreid@umich.edu, srcd@umich.edu, http://www.srcd.org/news/default.shtml. Ed. Pam Trotman Reid.

364.4 053.6 NLD ISSN 0928-2041
SAMENWERKINGSVERBAND JEUGDHULPVERLENING UTRECHT. NIEUWSBRIEF. Key Title: Nieuwsbrief Jeugdhulpverlening. Short title: Nieuwsbrief S J U. Text in Dutch. 1991. m. NLG 60 (effective 1999). bk.rev. back issues avail. **Document type:** *Bulletin, Newsletter.* **Description:** Covers institutes for youth psychology and youth mental help.
Related titles: E-mail ed.; Fax ed.
Published by: Samenwerkingsverband Jeugdhulpverlening Utrecht, FC Dondersstraat 1, Utrecht 9572 JA, Netherlands. TEL 31-30-272-3794, FAX 31-30-272-3688, ssjumj@worldonline.nl. Pub. H Jumelet.

362.7 157.63 USA ISSN 0894-5152
SCHOOL INTERVENTION REPORT. Abbreviated title: S I R. Text in English. 1987. q. USD 22 domestic to non-members; USD 30 foreign to non-members. bk.rev. cum.index 1987-1990. back issues avail. **Document type:** *Newsletter.* **Description:** Covers students at risk from drugs, alcohol, dropping out, physical violence, and adolescent pregnancy.
Published by: Safe Schools Coalition, Inc., 5351 Gulf Dr, Holmes Beach, FL 35217-1338. TEL 941-778-9140, 800-537-4903, FAX 941-778-6818. Ed. Alan W McEvoy. Pub., R&P Edsel L Erickson. Circ: 3,000. **Subscr. to:** Box 1338, Dept S49, Holmes Beach, FL 34218-1338.

▼ **SEX EDUCATION.** see *EDUCATION*

613.0432 USA
SHAKEN BABY ALLIANCE; dedicated to prevention, support and justice. Text in English, French, German, Italian, Spanish. 1998. q. **Description:** Includes articles on shaken baby syndrome and child abuse.
Address: PO Box 150734, Ft. Worth, TX 76108. TEL 817-444-9357, jackson4@gte.net, http://www.shakenbaby.com.

362.41 USA
SIBLING INFORMATION NETWORK NEWSLETTER. Text in English. 1981. q. USD 8.50 to individuals; USD 15 to institutions. bk.rev. back issues avail. **Document type:** *Newsletter.*
Published by: A.J. Pappanikou Center, 249 Glenbrook Rd., Storrs, CT 06269-2064. TEL 860-486-4985, http://www.uconnced.org/pubs.htm. Ed., R&P Lisa Glidden. Circ: 1,500.

155.4 USA ISSN 0037-976X
LB1103 CODEN: MSCDA7
SOCIETY FOR RESEARCH IN CHILD DEVELOPMENT. MONOGRAPHS. Text in English. 1935. 3/yr. USD 222 in North America included with subscr to: Child Development; USD 244 out of North America included with subscr to: Child Development (effective 2000). adv. back issues avail.; reprint service avail. from PSC,SCH. *Refereed.* **Document type:** *Monographic series, Academic/Scholarly.* **Description:** Presents in-depth research studies and findings in child development and related disciplines.
Related titles: Microform ed.: (from PQC); Online - full text ed.: (from EBSCO Publishing, Institute for Scientific Information, RoweCom Information Quest).
Indexed: ASCA, Adol.Ment.Hlth.Abstr., Bibl.Dev.Med.& Child Neur., Biol.Abstr., C.I.J.E., Child Devel.Abstr., Crim.Just.Abstr., Curr.Cont. (coverage dropped), Educ.Ind. (Jan.1983-), IBR, IBZ, IMFL, Ind.Med. (1935-), Ind.Philos., Lang.& Lang.Behav.Abstr., Mid.East: Abstr.& Ind., PsycInfo, Psychol.Abstr., Psycscan D.P., SOPODA, SSCI, Sci.Cit.Ind. (coverage dropped), Sociol.Abstr., e-psyche.
—BLDSC (5914.820000), CISTI, GNLM, IDS, ingenta. **CCC.**
Published by: (Society for Research in Child Development), Blackwell Publishers, 350 Main St, Malden, MA 02148. TEL 781-388-8200, 800-835-6770, FAX 781-388-8232, subscript@blackwellpub.com, http://www.blackwellpub.com, http://www.blackwellpublishers.co.uk/journals/diph. Ed. Rachel K Clifton. R&P Gretchen Voter TEL 781-388-0423. Adv. contact Anne Marie Sheehy TEL 781-388-0427.

STUDENT ASSISTANCE JOURNAL. see *DRUG ABUSE AND ALCOHOLISM*

TANDLAEGERNES NYE TIDSSKRIFT. see *MEDICAL SCIENCES—Dentistry*

THEIR WORLD. see *EDUCATION—Special Education And Rehabilitation*

649 USA ISSN 0895-0784
TWIN SERVICES REPORTER. Text in English. 1983. biennial. adv. bk.rev. index. back issues avail. **Document type:** *Newsletter.* **Description:** Provides information about multiple births.
Formerly: Twinline Reporter
Address: PO Box 10066, Berkeley, CA 94709. TEL 510-524-0863, FAX 510-524-0863, twinservices@juno.com, http://www.twinservices.org. Ed. Patricia Malmstrom. Circ: 850.

YOU'ER ZHILI SHIJIE/INFANTS' INTELLIGENCE WORLD. see *PSYCHOLOGY*

YOUNG EXCEPTIONAL CHILDREN. see *EDUCATION—Special Education And Rehabilitation*

YOUNGMINDS MAGAZINE. see *MEDICAL SCIENCES—Psychiatry And Neurology*

649.1 CAN ISSN 1188-2360
YOUR BABY. Text in French. 1991. 3/yr. adv. **Document type:** *Consumer.* **Description:** Published for parents of babies and toddlers from birth to 24 months.
Related titles: French ed.: Mon Enfant. ISSN 1188-2379; ♦ Special ed. of: Today's Parent. ISSN 0823-9258.
Published by: (Today's Parent Group), Professional Publishing Associates, 269 Richmond St W, Toronto, ON M5V 1X1, Canada. TEL 416-596-8680, FAX 416-596-1991. Ed. Holly Bennett. Pub. Kathy Bergen. Adv. contact Lauren McFarlane. Circ: 190,000 (controlled).

CHILDREN AND YOUTH—Abstracting, Bibliographies, Statistics

BREASTFEEDING ABSTRACTS. see *MEDICAL SCIENCES—Abstracting, Bibliographies, Statistics*

CHILDREN AND YOUTH—For

028.5 616.861 USA ISSN 1054-1411
ALATEEN TALK. Text in English. 1964. q. USD 2.50 (effective 2001). illus. **Document type:** *Newsletter.* **Description:** Alateen members, young people whose lives have been affected by someone else's drinking, share their experiences. Targets young people and professionals working with adolescents.
Published by: (Al-Anon Family Group Headquarters, Inc.), A F G, Inc., 1600 Corporate Landing Pkwy, Virginia Beach, VA 23454-5617. TEL 757-563-1600, FAX 757-563-1655, wso@al-anon.org, http://www.al-anon.alateen.org. Ed., R&P Evalynn Bolles. Circ: 5,500 (paid and controlled).

AUTUMN SCHOOL OF STUDIES ON ALCOHOL & DRUGS. PROCEEDINGS OF SEMINARS. see *DRUG ABUSE AND ALCOHOLISM*

BLAST OFF. see *HANDICAPPED—Visually Impaired*

BOYS' LIFE (BRAILLE EDITION). see *HANDICAPPED—Visually Impaired*

BURBUJAS. see *HANDICAPPED—Visually Impaired*

028.5 362.4 DEU
CHRIS; Kinderzeitschrift der Christoffel-Blindenmission. Text in German. 1997. q. free. **Document type:** *Bulletin, Consumer.* **Description:** Concerns medical and rehabilitation projects in developing nations.
Published by: Christoffel-Blindenmission e.V., Nibelungenstr 124, Bensheim 64625, Germany. TEL 49-6251-131-0, FAX 49-6251-131-122, 101666.2434@compuserve.com, communications@cbm-i.org, http://www.cbmi.de. Circ: 90,000.

DO DO. see *BIOLOGY*

EXPECTATIONS. see *HANDICAPPED—Visually Impaired*

FUTURE REFLECTIONS. see *HANDICAPPED—Visually Impaired*

GOOD-NEWS-LETTER (WASHINGTON, 1990). see *NUTRITION AND DIETETICS*

HEALTHLINES SAY; support for the asthmatic youth. see *MEDICAL SCIENCES—Allergology And Immunology*

HYOGO KENRITSU KODOMO BYOIN NENPO/HYOGO PREFECTURAL KOBE CHILDREN'S HOSPITAL. ANNUAL REPORT. see *HEALTH FACILITIES AND ADMINISTRATION*

028.5 DEU
JUGENDROTKREUZ. Text in German. 1986. m. DEM 33.60. **Document type:** *Bulletin.* **Description:** Health information from the Red Cross, geared toward young children.
Formerly: Bernie
Published by: (Deutsches Rotes Kreuz/German Red Cross, Referat Jugendrotkreuz), D R K Werbung GmbH, Friedrich-Ebert-Allee 71, Bonn 53113, Germany. TEL 49-228-541278, FAX 49-228-541450. Ed. Hildegard Witteler.

KID'S HEALTH. see *MEDICAL SCIENCES—Pediatrics*

028.5 613.7 DEU
MEDIZINI. Text in German. m. adv. **Document type:** *Consumer.*
Published by: Wort und Bild Verlag Konradshoehe GmbH, Konradshoehe, Baierbrunn 82065, Germany. TEL 49-89-74433-0, FAX 49-89-74433150, http://www.wortundbild.de. Adv. contact Wolfgang Smeilus.

NATIONAL PEDICULOSIS ASSOCIATION. PROGRESS. see *PUBLIC HEALTH AND SAFETY*

NUTRIDATE. see *NUTRITION AND DIETETICS*

OESTERREICHISCHES JUGENDROTKREUZ. ARBEITSBLAETTER. see *SOCIAL SERVICES AND WELFARE*

SCHOLASTIC CHOICES; personal development & living skills. see *EDUCATION—Teaching Methods And Curriculum*

051 614 USA ISSN 1062-0095
STRAIGHT TALK (PLEASANTVILLE); a magazine for teens. Text in English. 1991. irreg. USD 19.95 4 issues; USD 8.95 newsstand/cover (effective 2001). illus. **Document type:** *Magazine.* **Description:** Deals with health and behavior yopics of concern to adolescents.
Formerly (until 1992): Rodale's Straight Talk
Related titles: Supplement: Discussion Leader's Magazine. 1991; Talking Straight With Your Teenager. 1998.
Published by: The Learning Partnership, Inc., PO Box 199, Pleasantville, NY 10570. TEL 914-769-0055, FAX 914-769-5676, stteenmag@aol.com. Ed. Rita V Fisher. Pub., R&P John H Fisher. Circ: 1,000,000 (paid).

028.5 340 360 AUS
STREETWIZE COMMUNICATIONS; youth rights comics. Text in English. 1984. irreg. free to membership. **Document type:** *Consumer.* **Description:** Provides health, legal and survival information, passed on to young disadvantaged people in an entertaining format.
Formerly: Streetwize Comics (0815-0486)
Published by: Streetwize Comics Ltd., Ste 7, 24 S Chalmer St, Redfern, NSW 2016, Australia. TEL 61-2-9319-0220, FAX 61-2-9319-5553, stwize@streetwize.com.au, http://www.streetwize.com. Ed. Liz Stelton. Circ: 10,000.

TEAM OF ADVOCATES FOR SPECIAL KIDS NEWSLETTER. see *HANDICAPPED*

VITA DELL'INFANZIA. see *EDUCATION*

VRIEND. see *HANDICAPPED—Hearing Impaired*

028.5 570 RUS ISSN 0205-5767
YUNYI NATURALIST. Text in Russian. 1928. m. RUR 192 for 6 mos. (effective 2000). adv. bk.rev. illus. index. **Document type:** *Magazine, Consumer.* **Description:** For children in 4th - 10th grades who are interested in biology.
—East View.
Published by: Izdatel'stvo Molodaya Gvardiya, Novodmitrovskaya ul 5-a, Moscow 125015, Russian Federation. TEL 7-095-285-3948, FAX 7-095-285-3948, unnat@dateline.ru. Ed. Ludmila Samsonova. Circ: 16,500. **Dist. by:** Mezhdunarodnaya Kniga, B Yakimanka 39, Moscow 117049, Russian Federation. TEL 7-095-2384967, FAX 7-095-2384634; **US dist. addr.:** East View Publications, 3020 Harbor Ln N, Minneapolis, MN 55447. TEL 612-550-0961.

CHIROPRACTIC, HOMEOPATHY, OSTEOPATHY

see MEDICAL SCIENCES—Chiropractic, Homeopathy, Osteopathy

CIVIL DEFENSE

see also MILITARY

363.347 NLD ISSN 0920-3168
UA929.N2
ALERT* ; maandblad voor rampenbestrijding en crisisbeheersing. Text in Dutch. 1984. m. NLG 159 domestic (effective 2001). adv. bk.rev. abstr, illus, tr.lit. **Document type:** *Trade.* **Description:** Covers all aspects of disaster planning and relief, crisis management and related public safety topics.
Incorporates (1954-1984): Paladijn (0031-0166); (1957-1984): Netherlands. Ministerie van Binnelandse Zaken. Inspectie voor het Brandweerwezen. Maandelijkse Mededelingen (0020-2045); (in 1984): Noodzaak (0165-1471); Which was formerly (1952-1973): Civiele Verdediging (0009-7802)
Indexed: C.I.S. Abstr., Excerp.Med., INIS Atomind.
—KNAW.
Published by: Uitgeverijten Brink Meppel BV/Elsevier Business Information, The Hague (Subsidiary of: Reed Elsevier plc), Postbus 16500, The Hague 2500 BK, Netherlands. TEL 31-70-4415000, FAX 31-70-4415900. Circ: 2,334.

363.347 AUS ISSN 1324-1540
THE AUSTRALIAN JOURNAL OF EMERGENCY MANAGEMENT. Text in English. 1986. q. free. 64 p./no. back issues avail. *Refereed.* **Document type:** *Academic/Scholarly.*
Formerly (until 1995): Macedon Digest (0817-4024)
Published by: Heuristic Enterprises, 32 Ferrier St, Mt Macedon, VIC 3441, Australia. TEL 61-3-5421-5214, FAX 61-3-5421-5272, fleming@netcon.net.au, http://www.ema.gov.au/. Ed., Pub. Rob Fleming.

363.347 USA ISSN 0164-1875
D R C BOOK & MONOGRAPH SERIES. (Disaster Research Center) Text in English. 1968. irreg., latest vol.28, 1994. price varies. **Document type:** *Monographic series.*
Formerly: Ohio State University. Disaster Research Center. D R C - T R (0078-4109)
Indexed: Lang.& Lang.Behav.Abstr., SOPODA, Sociol.Abstr.
Published by: University of Delaware, Disaster Research Center, Newark, DE 19716. TEL 302-831-6618, FAX 302-831-2091, TELEX 70 99 85, castelli@udel.edu, http://www.udel.edu/DRC/homepage.htm.

363.347 USA
DISASTER PLANNING SOURCEBOOK. Text in English. 1997. a. USD 269; USD 229 foreign (effective 1999). **Document type:** *Trade.*
Published by: American Health Consultants (Subsidiary of: Medical Economics Co., Inc.), 3525 Piedmont Rd, N E, 6 Piedmont Center, Ste 400, Atlanta, GA 30305. TEL 404-262-5476, custserv@ahcpub.com, http://www.ahcpub.com.

DOCTORS FOR DISASTER PREPAREDNESS NEWSLETTER. see *MEDICAL SCIENCES*

363.347 USA
HAZARD TECHNOLOGY. Text in English. 1980. q. free per issue. adv. **Document type:** *Newspaper.* **Description:** Covers the use of technology in the field of emergency and environmental management.
Formerly: Hazard Monthly (0742-6410); Incorporates: Corporate Emergency Management
Related titles: Online - full text ed.
Published by: Emergency Information System, International, 1401 Rockville Pike, Ste 500, Rockville, MD 20852. TEL 301-738-6900, 800-999-5009, FAX 301-738-1026, info@eisint.com, http://www.eisintl.com. Ed. K C Chartrand. Pub. James W Morentz. Circ: 55,000.

363.348 344.05348 SWE ISSN 1400-3120
STUDIES ON EMERGENCIES AND DISASTER RELIEF. Text in English. 1992. irreg., latest vol.7, 1998. SEK 60 per issue (effective 2000). **Document type:** *Monographic series, Academic/Scholarly.*
Formerly (until 1994): Sida Studies on Emergencies and Disaster Relief (1103-4858)
—BLDSC (8490.480200).
Published by: Nordiska Afrikainstitutet/Nordic Africa Institute, PO Box 1703, Uppsala 75147, Sweden. TEL 46-18-562200, FAX 46-18-562290, orders@nai.uu.se, http://www.nai.uu.se. **Co-sponsors:** Sida; University of Oxford, Refugee Studies Programme.

363.347 USA
UNIVERSITY OF DELAWARE. DISASTER RESEARCH CENTER. MISCELLANEOUS REPORTS. Text in English. 1978 (no.20). irreg., latest vol.48, 1994. **Document type:** *Monographic series.*
Formerly: Ohio State University, Columbus. Disaster Research Center. Miscellaneous Reports
Published by: University of Delaware, Disaster Research Center, Newark, DE 19716. TEL 302-831-6618, FAX 302-831-2091, susan.castelli@news.udel.edu, http://www.udel.edu/DRC/drc/htm.

363.347 USA
UNIVERSITY OF DELAWARE. DISASTER RESEARCH CENTER. REPORT SERIES. Text in English. 1968. irreg., latest vol.19, 1989. *Refereed.* **Document type:** *Monographic series.*
Formerly: Ohio State University. Disaster Research Center. Report Series (0078-4133)
Published by: University of Delaware, Disaster Research Center, Newark, DE 19716. TEL 302-831-6618, FAX 302-831-2091, susan.castelli@mvs.udel.edu, http://www.udel.edu/DRC/drc/htm.

CIVIL ENGINEERING

see ENGINEERING—Civil Engineering

CIVIL LAW

see LAW—Civil Law

CIVIL RIGHTS

see POLITICAL SCIENCE—Civil Rights

CLASSICAL STUDIES

see also ARCHAEOLOGY; HISTORY; LINGUISTICS; LITERATURE; MUSEUMS AND ART GALLERIES

CLEANING AND DYEING

see also TEXTILE INDUSTRIES AND FABRICS

CLOTHING TRADE

see also CLOTHING TRADE—Fashions; TEXTILE INDUSTRIES AND FABRICS

687.19 USA
SUNGLASS ASSOCIATION OF AMERICA. NEWSLETTER. Text in English. m. membership only. **Document type:** *Newsletter.* **Description:** Association and industry news with updates on new members and address corrections.
Published by: Sunglass Association of America, 49 East Ave, Norwalk, CT 06851. TEL 203-845-9015, FAX 203-847-1304, http://www.sunglassassociation.com. Ed. Swea Nightingale.

CLOTHING TRADE—Fashions

COTTET MAGAZINE. see *MEDICAL SCIENCES—Ophthalmology And Optometry*

CLUBS

see also COLLEGE AND ALUMNI

BOYS' LIFE (BRAILLE EDITION). see *HANDICAPPED—Visually Impaired*

367 615 USA ISSN 0746-3979
COMMUNICATOR (ATHENS). Text in English. 1889. q. USD 10 (effective 1999). adv. back issues avail. **Document type:** *Trade.*
Published by: Phi Delta Chi Pharmacy Fraternity, PO Box 1883, Athens, GA 30603-1883. TEL 706-613-0300, FAX 706-613-0200, phidexnatl@aol.com, http://www.umich.edu/~jbonasso/pdcnew/home.htm. Ed. Thomas Ellington. R&P, Adv. contact Anthony D Chaffee. Circ: 4,500.

DOMINANT NEWSLETTER. see *PSYCHOLOGY*

367 610.73 USA
REFLECTIONS ON NURSING LEADERSHIP. Text in English. 1975. q. USD 20 domestic; USD 30 foreign (effective 2001). adv. back issues avail. **Document type:** *Newsletter.* **Description:** Highlights the meetings, conferences, seminars, and national and international events of the organization.
Formerly (until 2000): Reflections (Indianapolis) (0885-8144)
Indexed: Int.Nurs.Ind.
Published by: Sigma Theta Tau International Honor Society of Nursing, 550 W North St, Indianapolis, IN 46202. TEL 317-634-8171, FAX 317-634-8188. Ed. Jeff Burnham. Adv. contact Rachael McLaughlin.

367 153 USA
SINISTRALIAN. Text in English. 1977. q. USD 5.75. bk.rev. back issues avail. **Description:** Provides information on the recent developments in left-handedness studies for Mensans.
Indexed: e-psyche.
Published by: Sinistral SIG, 200 Emmett Ave, Derby, CT 06418. TEL 203-735-1759. Ed. Sharlene McEvoy. Circ: 100.

COLLEGE AND ALUMNI

see also CLUBS; EDUCATION—Higher Education; LITERARY AND POLITICAL REVIEWS; LITERATURE

378 USA
ALLIANCE (CHARLESTON). Text in English. 1985. a. USD 15 to members (effective 1997). **Document type:** *Newsletter.* **Description:** News, information, and announcements for the alumni of the Medical University of South Carolina, College of Health-Related Professions.

C

Published by: Medical University of South Carolina, College of Health Related Professions, Alumni Association, 171 Ashley Ave, Charleston, SC 29425. Ed. Wanda Hancock. Circ: 3,200.

ALUMNUS (NEW YORK). see *MEDICAL SCIENCES—Orthopedics And Traumatology*

C C H S NEWS. see *MEDICAL SCIENCES—Respiratory Diseases*

CHRISTIAN MEDICAL COLLEGE VELLORE ALUMNI JOURNAL. see *MEDICAL SCIENCES*

CORNELL MEDICINE. see *MEDICAL SCIENCES*

DARTMOUTH MEDICINE. see *MEDICAL SCIENCES*

DENTAL IMAGES. see *MEDICAL SCIENCES—Dentistry*

371.85 610 USA
GOZZLE NIPPER. Text in English. 1915. a. **Document type:** *Bulletin.* **Description:** Includes information on the medical professional fraternity.
Published by: (Iota Tau Sigma Fraternity), Journal Publishing Corp., PO Box 792, Kirksville, MO 63501-0792. TEL 816-665-9808, FAX 816-665-0331. Ed. James J Woodruff. Circ: 15,000 (controlled).

378 610 USA ISSN 0191-7757
R747
HARVARD MEDICAL ALUMNI BULLETIN. Text in English. 1891. q. free per issue. adv. bk.rev. illus. index. **Document type:** *Academic/Scholarly.*
—BLDSC (4268.230000).
Published by: Harvard Medical School Alumni Association, 25 Shattuck St, Boston, MA 02115. FAX 617-432-0013, bulletin@warren.med.harvard.edu. Ed. William Ira Bennett. Adv. contact Sarah Jane Nelson. Circ: 15,000.

C

378 615.1 ITA
ISTITUTO DI RICERCHE FARMACOLOGICHE MARIO NEGRI. ALUMNI NEWS. Text in Italian. 1998. m. free per issue. **Document type:** *Bulletin.* **Description:** Presents news about the institute and its activities.
Media: Online - full text.
Published by: Istituto di Ricerche Farmacologiche Mario Negri, Via Eritrea, 62, Milan, MI 20157, Italy. TEL 39-2-390141, FAX 39-2-3546277, http://www.irfmn.mnegri.it/perp/aa/.

LOS ANGELES COLLEGE OF CHIROPRACTIC. NEWS & ALUMNI REPORT. see *MEDICAL SCIENCES—Chiropractic, Homeopathy, Osteopathy*

378.198 610 USA
LOYOLA MEDICINE. Text in English. 1986. s-a. free per issue. back issues avail. **Document type:** *Academic/Scholarly.*
Formerly: Stritch M.D. (1054-7649)
Published by: Loyola University, Stritch School of Medicine, 2160 S First Ave, Maywood, IL 60153. TEL 708-216-6700, FAX 708-216-8199, http://www.lumc.edu. Circ: 5,500 (controlled). **Co-sponsor:** Loyola University Medical Center.

378 610 DEU
M H H - INFO. Text in German. 1972. m. bk.rev. **Document type:** *Newsletter.*
Published by: Medizinische Hochschule Hannover, Carl-Neuberg-Str 1, Hannover 30625, Germany. TEL 49-511-532-6771, FAX 49-511-532-3852, TELEX 0922044-MEDHO-D. Circ: 2,600.

MASSACHUSETTS COLLEGE OF PHARMACY. BULLETIN. see *PHARMACY AND PHARMACOLOGY*

610 USA
MEDICINE ON THE MIDWAY. Variant title: University of Chicago. Pritzker School of Medicine. Alumni Association. Magazine. Text in English. 1944. 3/yr. free per issue. illus. *Refereed.* **Document type:** *Bulletin.* **Description:** Covers news of graduates and their achievements, and updates alumni and alumnae of events of interest at the University of Chicago Hospital.
Formerly: University of Chicago. Pritzker School of Medicine. Alumni Association. Bulletin (0009-3734)
Published by: University of Chicago Hospitals, Office of Public Affairs, 5841 S Maryland Ave, Mail Code 6063, Chicago, IL 60637. TEL 773-702-7322, FAX 773-702-3171. Ed., R&P Carmen Marti. Circ: 14,000 (controlled).

NEGRI NEWS. see *PHARMACY AND PHARMACOLOGY*

NURSING PROGRESS. see *MEDICAL SCIENCES—Nurses And Nursing*

371.85 USA ISSN 0022-3581
R745
PHI RHO SIGMA. JOURNAL. Key Title: Journal of Phi Rho Sigma. Text in English. 1900. q. membership only. bk.rev. bibl. illus.
Published by: Phi Rho Sigma Medical Society, PO Box 90264, Indianapolis, IN 46290-0264. TEL 317-255-4379, FAX 317-253-5067. Ed. Dr. James Jackson. Circ: 16,000 (controlled).

TULANE MEDICINE. see *MEDICAL SCIENCES*

UNIVERSITY COLLEGE LONDON. EASTMAN ACADEMY. NEWSLETTER. see *MEDICAL SCIENCES—Dentistry*

378 617.6 USA ISSN 1088-9108
UNIVERSITY OF ILLINOIS AT CHICAGO. COLLEGE OF DENTISTRY. ALUMNI REPORT. Text in English. 1985. s-a. USD 6 (effective 2000). bk.rev. **Document type:** *Bulletin.*
Published by: University of Illinois at Chicago, College of Dentistry, 801 S Paulina St, Chicago, IL 60612-7211. TEL 312-413-2927, FAX 312-413-2927, billbike@uic.edu. Ed., R&P William Bike TEL 312-996-8495. Pub. Irwin Robinson. Circ: 5,500 (controlled).

378.18 CAN ISSN 0830-5315
VOX ME D A L. Text in English. 1958. s-a. free per issue to members. adv. bk.rev. back issues avail. **Document type:** *Newsletter, Academic/Scholarly.* **Description:** Contains programs and services of the Dalhousie Medical Alumni Association and activities of faculty, students and staff.
Formerly (until 1988): Me D A L (0318-0735)
Related titles: Online - full text ed.
Published by: Dalhousie University, Dalhousie Medical Alumni Association, Dalhousie University, First Floor, Tupper Bldg, Halifax, NS B3H 4H7, Canada. TEL 902-494-8800, FAX 902-494-2033, dilly.macfarlane@dal.ca, http://www.medicine.dal.ca/dmaa. Ed. Dr. D C S Brown. R&P D.E. MacFarlane. Adv. contact D E MacFarlane. color page CND 7,000; trim 11 x 8.5. Circ: 6,700 (controlled).

COMMUNICABLE DISEASES

see MEDICAL SCIENCES—Communicable Diseases

COMMUNICATIONS

see also COMMUNICATIONS—Postal Affairs; COMMUNICATIONS—Radio; COMMUNICATIONS—Telephone And Telegraph; COMMUNICATIONS—Television And Cable; COMMUNICATIONS—Video; JOURNALISM

362.1 USA ISSN 1040-7316
9-1-1 MAGAZINE. Text in English. 1988. bi-m. USD 24 domestic; USD 38 in Canada & Mexico; USD 46 elsewhere (effective 2000). adv. bk.rev. back issues avail. *Refereed.* **Document type:** *Trade.* **Description:** Provides technical information for senior personnel in emergency safety communications and response. Includes news of technical conferences, product evaluations and field reports.
Published by: Official Publications, Inc., PO Box 11788, Santa Ana, CA 92711-1788. TEL 714-544-7776, 800-231-8911, FAX 714-838-9233, publisher@9-1-1magazine.com, http://www.9-1-1magazine.com. Ed. Randall Larson. Pub. James E Voelkl. R&P Jackie Voelkl. Adv. contact Pam Martin. B&W page USD 1,960. Circ: 13,000.

BACON'S MEDICAL & HEALTH MEDIA DIRECTORY. see *MEDICAL SCIENCES*

JOURNAL OF HEALTH COMMUNICATION. see *MEDICAL SCIENCES*

PUBLIC SAFETY COMMUNICATIONS. see *PUBLIC HEALTH AND SAFETY*

TELEMEDICINE & TELEHEALTH NETWORK. see *MEDICAL SCIENCES*

TELEMEDICINE BUSINESS NEWSLETTER. see *MEDICAL SCIENCES*

TELEMEDICINE TODAY. see *MEDICAL SCIENCES*

COMMUNICATIONS—Abstracting, Bibliographies, Statistics

SAFETY ABSTRACTS. see *PUBLIC HEALTH AND SAFETY—Abstracting, Bibliographies, Statistics*

COMMUNICATIONS—Postal Affairs

383.4 GBR ISSN 0269-1396
PRATIQUE; newsletter of the disinfected mail study circle. Text in English. 1974. 3/yr., latest vol.26 (Normally one volume per year). GBP 12 in British Isles to membership; GBP 15 in Europe to membership; GBP 20, USD 32 elsewhere to membership (effective 2001). adv. bk.rev. charts, maps. 36 p./no. back issues avail. **Document type:** *Journal, Academic/Scholarly.* **Description:** Focuses on accounts of the treatment of mail, worldwide. Also includes related topics such as maritime and other certificates of health, ships' documents, public health proclamations restricting or restoring the freedom to trade with ports or regions suspected of harbouring infections diseases, and vaccination ephemera.
Published by: Disinfected Mail Study Circle, 25 Sinclair Grove, London NW11 9JH, United Kingdom. TEL 44-20-8455-9190. Ed., R&P, Adv. contact V. Denis Vandervelde TEL 20 8455 9190. Pub. V Denis Vandervelde. B&W page GBP 75. Circ: 140 (paid); 20 (controlled).

COMMUNICATIONS—Radio

BRAILLE RADIO TIMES. see *HANDICAPPED—Visually Impaired*

621.3673 616.07572 AUS
SPECTRUM (COLLINGWOOD). Text in English. 1994. 10/yr. AUD 100 (effective 2000). adv. back issues avail. **Document type:** *Newsletter, Academic/Scholarly.*
Published by: Australian Institute of Radiography, c/o E.M. Hughes Sec., PO Box 1169, Collingwood, VIC 3066, Australia. TEL 61-3-94193336, FAX 61-3-94160783, air@a-i-r.com/au. R&P E M Hughes. adv.: page AUD 550; trim 210 x 297.

COMMUNICATIONS—Telephone And Telegraph

T D I NATIONAL DIRECTORY OF T T Y NUMBERS (YEAR). see *HANDICAPPED—Hearing Impaired*

COMMUNICATIONS—Television And Cable

354.55 USA
CAPTION✶. Text in English. 1980. a. free per issue.
Published by: National Captioning Institute, Inc., 1900 Gallows Rd, Ste 3000, Vienna, VA 22182-3865. FAX 703-998-2450. Ed. Morgan Bramlet. Circ: 100,000 (controlled).

COMMUNICATIONS—Video

ADAM GAY VIDEO DIRECTORY. see *HOMOSEXUALITY*

COMPUTER APPLICATIONS

see COMPUTERS

COMPUTERS

see also COMPUTERS—Artificial Intelligence; COMPUTERS—Automation; COMPUTERS—Computer Security; COMPUTERS—Data Communications And Data Transmission Systems; COMPUTERS—Electronic Data Processing; COMPUTERS—Information Science And Information Theory; COMPUTERS—Internet; COMPUTERS—Microcomputers; COMPUTERS—Personal Computers; COMPUTERS—Robotics; COMPUTERS—Software

ASSISTIVE TECHNOLOGY RESEARCH SERIES. see *HANDICAPPED—Computer Applications*

▼ **E-HEALTHCARE MARKET REPORTER.** see *BUSINESS AND ECONOMICS*

004 USA ISSN 0737-0024
QA76.9.S88 CODEN: HCINE6
HUMAN - COMPUTER INTERACTION (MAHWAH); a journal of theoretical, empirical, and methodological issues of user psychology and of system design. Text in English. 1985. q. USD 55 in US & Canada to individuals; USD 85 elsewhere to individuals; USD 395 in US & Canada to institutions; USD 425 elsewhere to institutions (effective 2002). adv. bk.rev. *Refereed.* **Document type:** *Journal, Academic/Scholarly.* **Description:** Publishes theoretical, empirical and methodological articles on user psychology and computer system design as it affects the user. Reports on helping to define the issues.
Related titles: Online - full text ed.: ISSN 1532-7051. USD 49.50 to individuals; USD 355.50 to institutions (effective 2002) (from CatchWord Ltd., EBSCO Publishing, O C L C Online Computer Library Center, Inc., RoweCom Information Quest, Swets Blackwell, Institute for Scientific Information).
Indexed: ASCA, Abstr.Hum.Comp.Inter., C.I.J.E., Compumath, Comput.& Info.Sys., Comput.Lit.Ind., Curr.Cont., Electron.& Communic.Abstr.J., Environ.Sci.Poll.Mgmt., IBZ, INSPEC (1987-), LISA, Pollut.Abstr., PsycInfo, Psychol.Abstr. (1985-), Risk Abstr., Saf.Sci.Abstr., Sci.Cit.Ind., e-psyche.
—BLDSC (4336.043450), AskIEEE, CASDDS, CatchWord, CISTI, Ei, ingenta, Linda Hall. **CCC.**
Published by: Lawrence Erlbaum Associates, Inc., 10 Industrial Ave, Mahwah, NJ 07430-2262. TEL 201-760-3735, 800-926-6579, FAX 201-236-0072, journals@erlbaum.com, http://www.erlbaum.com/Journals/journals/HCI/hci.htm. Ed. Thomas P Moran. adv.: page USD 500; trim 5 x 8. Circ: 1,200.

004 570 610 USA
I E E E - E M B S CONFERENCE ON INFORMATION TECHNOLOGY APPLICATIONS IN BIOMEDICINE. PROCEEDINGS. Text in English. a. USD 102 (effective 2001). **Document type:** *Proceedings.*
Published by: Institute of Electrical and Electronics Engineers, Inc., 3 Park Ave, 17th Fl, New York, NY 10017. TEL 800-678-4333, customer.service@ieee.org, http://www.ieee.org.

INFORMATICS AND MEDICAL COMPUTING NEWS. see *MEDICAL SCIENCES*

004 614 USA ISSN 0020-5419
INTERFACE (BETHESDA)* . Text in English. 1968. 9/yr. free per issue. bk.rev. index.
Published by: U.S. National Institutes of Health, Division of Computer Research and Technology, Computer Center, Bldg 12A, Rm 4039, Bethesda, MD 20892. TEL 301-496-5381. Ed. Joseph D Naughton. Circ: 3,000.

▼ **INTERNATIONAL JOURNAL OF COGNITION & TECHNOLOGY**; co-existence, convergence and co-evolution. see *PSYCHOLOGY*

▼ **NUOVE TECNOLOGIE IN MEDICINA, INFORMATICA, TELEMATICA APPLICAZIONI.** see *MEDICAL SCIENCES—Experimental Medicine, Laboratory Technique*

24 X 7. see *HEALTH FACILITIES AND ADMINISTRATION*

COMPUTERS—Artificial Intelligence

006.3 USA ISSN 1059-7123
QL750 CODEN: ADBEEA
ADAPTIVE BEHAVIOR; animals, animats, software agents, robots, adaptive systems. Text in English. 1992-1998 (vol.6, no.3-4); resumed 2001. q. GBP 175 UK, Europe, Middle East & Africa; USD 250 elsewhere (effective 2002). back issues avail. *Refereed.* **Document type:** *Academic/Scholarly.* **Description:** International journal providing a forum for experimental and theoretical research on adaptive behavior in animals and autonomous artificial systems, with emphasis on mechanism, organizational principles, and architectures that can be expressed in computational, physical, or mathematical models.
Related titles: Microfilm ed.: suspended (from PQC); Online - full text ed.: (from Institute for Scientific Information).
Indexed: Anim.Behav.Abstr. (coverage dropped), Aqua.Sci.& Fish.Abstr., Compumath, Comput.Abstr., Curr.Cont., Ecol.Abstr., Entomol.Abstr., Ergon.Abstr., INSPEC (Sum.1992-), Int.Aerosp.Abstr., Neurosci.Abstr. (coverage dropped), PsycInfo, Psychol.Abstr. (1992-), SSCI, Wild.Rev., Zoo.Rec., e-psyche.
—BLDSC (0678.309000), AskIEEE, CISTI, IDS, Infotrieve, ingenta, Linda Hall. **CCC.**
Published by: (International Society for Adaptive Behavior), Sage Publications Ltd., 6 Bonhill St, London EC2A 4PU, United Kingdom. TEL 44-20-7374-0645, FAX 44-20-7374-8741, info@sagepub.co.uk, http://www.sagepub.co.uk/. Ed. John Hallam. **Affiliates:** Sage Publications, Inc.; Sage Publications India Pvt. Ltd.

006.361 NLD ISSN 0933-3657
R859.7.A78 CODEN: AIMEEW
ARTIFICIAL INTELLIGENCE IN MEDICINE. Text in Dutch. 1989. 9/yr. EUR 544 in Europe to institutions; JPY 72,300 in Japan to institutions; USD 608 elsewhere to institutions (effective 2002). adv. bk.rev. back issues avail. *Refereed.* **Document type:** *Academic/Scholarly.* **Description:** Publishes original articles from a wide variety of interdisciplinary perspectives concerning the theory and practice of medical artificial intelligence.
Related titles: Microform ed.: (from PQC); Online - full text ed.: (from EBSCO Publishing, ingenta, Swets Blackwell, ScienceDirect, Institute for Scientific Information).
Indexed: ASCA, Bioeng.Abstr., Compumath, Comput.& Info.Sys., Comput.Abstr., Comput.Lit.Ind., Curr.Cont., Electron.& Communic.Abstr.J., Eng.Ind., Environ.Sci.Poll.Mgmt., Excerp.Med. (1992-), INSPEC (1989-), Ind.Med. (1989-), Ind.Sci.Rev., Inpharma, Int.Nurs.Ind., LISA, Pharm.&Out.News, Pollut.Abstr., Reac., Risk Abstr., SSCI (coverage dropped), Saf.Sci.Abstr., Sci.Cit.Ind.
—BLDSC (1735.036800), AskIEEE, CISTI, Ei, EMDOCS, GNLM, IDS, Infotrieve. **CCC.**
Published by: Elsevier Science BV, PO Box 211, Amsterdam 1000 AE, Netherlands. TEL 31-20-485-2911, FAX 31-20-485-2457, nlinfo-f@elsevier.nl, http://www.elsevier.com/locate/artmed. Ed. K S Sadegh Zadeh. Circ: 1,500. **Subscr. in Australasia and the Far East to:** Elsevier Science (Singapore) Pte Ltd, No.1 Temasek Ave, 17-01 Millenia Tower, Singapore 039192, Singapore. TEL 65-434-3727, FAX 65-337-2230; **Subscr. in Japan to:** Elsevier Science Inc - Japan Regional Office, 9-15 Higashi-Azabu 1-chome, Minato-ku, Tokyo 106-0044, Japan. TEL 81-3-5561-5033, FAX 81-3-5561-5047; **Subscr. in the Americas to:** Elsevier Science, PO Box 945, New York, NY 10159-0945. TEL 212-633-3730, FAX 212-633-3680, usinfo-f@elsevier.com.

006.3 591.5 USA ISSN 1064-5462
QH324.2 CODEN: ARLIEY
ARTIFICIAL LIFE. Text in English. 1993. q. USD 54 in US & Canada to individuals; USD 74 elsewhere to institutions; USD 188 in US & Canada to individuals; USD 208 elsewhere to institutions (effective 2001). **Document type:** *Academic/Scholarly.* **Description:** Acts as a primary forum for international scientific and engineering research in the new discipline of synthetic biological work. Covers topics from the origin of life, through self-reproduction, to evolution, growth and development all the way to the dynamics of whole ecosystems. Presents articles and reviews on synthetic approaches to the spectrum of biological phenomena.
Related titles: Microfiche ed.: (from PQC); Online - full content ed.: ISSN 1530-9185. USD 49 in US & Canada to individuals; USD 169 in US & Canada to institutions; USD 69 elsewhere to individuals; USD 189 elsewhere to institutions (effective 2001) (from EBSCO Publishing, O C L C Online Computer Library Center, Inc., Swets Blackwell); Online - full text ed.: (from CatchWord Ltd., Institute for Scientific Information, RoweCom Information Quest).
Indexed: Compumath, Comput.Abstr., Curr.Cont., INSPEC (Win.1999-), Ind.Med. (1994-), Sci.Cit.Ind., Zoo.Rec.
—BLDSC (1735.045000), CatchWord, CISTI.
Published by: (Santa Fe Institute), M I T Press, 5 Cambridge Center, Cambridge, MA 02142-1407. TEL 617-253-2866, FAX 617-577-1545, editor@alife.santafe.edu, journals-orders@mit.edu, http://mitpress.mit.edu/ALIFE, http://mitpress.mit.edu/alife. R&P Paul Dzus. Circ: 1,000 (paid).

006.35 USA ISSN 0161-4126
COMMUNICATION OUTLOOK; focusing on communication aids and techniques. Text in English. 1978. 4/yr. USD 18; USD 24 foreign. adv. bk.rev. back issues avail. **Description:** Covers technological developments for persons who experience communication handicaps due to neurological, sensory or neuromuscular conditions.
Related titles: Microform ed.: (from PQC).
Indexed: INSPEC (Win.1984-), Rehabil.Lit., Yrbk.Assoc.Educ.& Rehab.Blind, e-psyche.
—BLDSC (3361.600000), AskIEEE.
Published by: Artificial Language Laboratory, 405 Computer Center, Michigan State University, E, Lansing, MI 48824-1042. TEL 517-353-0870, FAX 517-353-4766, co@all.cps.msu.edu. Ed., R&P John Eulenber. Adv. contact Carolyn Watt. Circ: 1,000.

006.32 SGP ISSN 0129-0657
QA76.87 CODEN: IJSZEG
INTERNATIONAL JOURNAL OF NEURAL SYSTEMS. Text in English. 1989. 6/yr. SGD 230, USD 148 to individuals; USD 690 to institutions; SGD 413, USD 244 in developing nations to institutions (effective 2001); SGD 288 to individuals in Asia Pacific & Australasia except Hong Kong and China; USD 160 elsewhere to individuals; SGD 793 to institutions in Asia Pacific & Australasia except Hong Kong and China; USD 441 elsewhere to institutions; SGD 475 in developing nations to institutions in Asia Pacific & Australasia except Hong Kong and China; USD 264 in developing nations to institutions (effective 2002). back issues avail. **Document type:** *Academic/Scholarly.* **Description:** Contains original contributions on all aspects of information processing in natural and artificial neural systems.
Related titles: Online - full text ed.: (from EBSCO Publishing, Swets Blackwell, ScienceDirect).
Indexed: ASCA, Aqua.Sci.& Fish.Abstr., Comput.Abstr., INSPEC (1989-), Ind.Med. (1989-), Neurosci.Abstr. (coverage dropped), Neurosci.Cit.Ind., SSCI (coverage dropped).
—BLDSC (4542.373700), AskIEEE, CISTI, IDS, Infotrieve, ingenta. **CCC.**
Published by: World Scientific Publishing Co Pte Ltd, Farrer Rd, PO Box 128, Singapore 912805, Singapore. wspc@wspc.com.sg, http://www.worldscientific.com. Eds. Benny Lautrup, S Brunak. Circ: 300.

▼ **JOURNAL OF COGNITIVE SYSTEMS RESEARCH.** see *PSYCHOLOGY*

JOURNAL OF COMPUTATIONAL NEUROSCIENCE. see *MEDICAL SCIENCES—Psychiatry And Neurology*

006.361 NLD ISSN 0928-9119
MEDICAL ARTIFICIAL INTELLIGENCE. Text in English. 1992. irreg., latest vol.2, 1995. price varies. *Refereed.* **Document type:** *Monographic series, Academic/Scholarly.*
—BLDSC (5526.245000).
Published by: Elsevier Science BV, PO Box 211, Amsterdam 1000 AE, Netherlands. TEL 31-20-485-3757, 31-20-485-3911, FAX 31-20-485-3432, 31-20-485-3598, nlinfo-f@elsevier.nl; usinfo-f@elsevier.com; forinfo-kyf04035@niftyserve.or.jp, http://www.elsevier.nl/. Ed. K S Zadeh. **Subscr. in Australasia and the Far East to:** Elsevier Science (Singapore) Pte Ltd, No.1 Temasek Ave, 17-01 Millenia Tower, Singapore 039192, Singapore. TEL 65-434-3727, FAX 65-337-2230, asiainfo@elsevier.com.sg; **Subscr. in Japan to:** Elsevier Science Inc - Japan Regional Office, 9-15 Higashi-Azabu 1-chome, Minato-ku, Tokyo 106-0044, Japan. TEL 81-3-5561-5033, FAX 81-3-5561-5047, info@elsevier.co.jp; **Subscr. in the Americas to:** Elsevier Science, PO Box 945, New York, NY 10159-0945. TEL 212-633-3730, 888-437-4636, FAX 212-633-3680, usinfo-f@elsevier.com, http://www.elsevier.com

006.32 616.8 USA ISSN 0899-7667
QA76.5 CODEN: NEUCEB
NEURAL COMPUTATION. Text in English. 1989. m. USD 88 in United States to individuals for print or online ed.; USD 94.16 in Canada to individuals for print or online ed.; USD 136 elsewhere to individuals for print or online ed.; USD 506 in United States to institutions for print or online ed.; USD 541.42 in Canada to institutions for print or online ed.; USD 554 elsewhere to institutions for print or online ed.; USD 60 in United States to students for print or online ed.; USD 64.20 in Canada to students for print or online ed.; USD 108 elsewhere to students for print or online ed. (effective 2002). back issues avail.; reprint service avail. from PQC. *Refereed.* **Document type:** *Academic/Scholarly.* **Description:** Provides interdisciplinary forum for the dissemination of research results and for reviews of research in neural computation.
Related titles: Microform ed.: (from PQC); Online - full text ed.: ISSN 1530-888X (from CatchWord Ltd., HighWire Pr., Swets Blackwell, Institute for Scientific Information, RoweCom Information Quest).
Indexed: A.I.Abstr., ASCA, Acoust.Abstr., Compumath, Comput.Abstr., Comput.Lit.Ind., Curr.Cont., Eng.Ind., INSPEC (Spr.1989-), Ind.Med. (1989-), Ind.Sci.Rev., Inpharma, Neurosci.Abstr., Neurosci.Cit.Ind., PsycInfo, Psychol.Abstr. (1989-), Reac., Ref.Zh., Sci.Cit.Ind., Zent.Math., e-psyche.
—BLDSC (6081.280200), AskIEEE, CatchWord, CISTI, Ei, GNLM, IDS, ingenta. **CCC.**
Published by: (Salk Institute), M I T Press, 5 Cambridge Center, Cambridge, MA 02142-1407. TEL 617-253-2866, FAX 617-258-5028, journals-info@mit.edu, http://mitpress.mit.edu/NECO. Ed. Terrence Sejnowski. R&P Paul Dzus. Circ: 1,800.

C

006.3 CZE ISSN 1210-0552
QA76.87 CODEN: NNWOFJ
NEURAL NETWORK WORLD; international journal on non-standard artificial intelligence. Text in English. 1991. bi-m. USD 250, USD 480 (effective 2001). back issues avail. *Refereed.* **Document type:** *Journal, Academic/Scholarly.* **Description:** Covers the latest developments in the field of information technology, focusing on neurocomputing based on applications of artificial neural networks. Also covers related fields such as brain and neurophysiological research, artificial intelligence and massive parallel information processing.
Indexed: Bioeng.Abstr., Biotech.& Bioeng.Abstr., Eng.Ind., INSPEC (1996-), e-psyche.
—BLDSC (6081.280620), AskIEEE, CISTI, Ei.
Published by: Ceska Akademie Ved, Ustav Informatiky/Czech Academy of Sciences, Institute of Information and Computing Technology, Pod Vodarenskou Vezi 2, Prague, 1 182 071, Czech Republic. TEL 420-2-66052080, 420-2-24221721-Ext 418, FAX 420-2-8585789, nnw@cs.cas.cz, mirko@fd.cvut.cz, http://www.cs.cas.cz/nnw;. Ed. Mirko Novak. **Co-publisher:** V S P. **Co-sponsor:** Ceske Uceni Technicke v Praze.

006.32 GBR ISSN 0893-6080
QA76.5 CODEN: NNETEB
NEURAL NETWORKS. Text in English. 1988. 10/yr. EUR 221 in Europe to qualified personnel; JPY 29,400 in Japan to qualified personnel; USD 247 elsewhere to qualified personnel; EUR 1,150 in Europe to institutions; JPY 152,700 in Japan to institutions; USD 1,287 elsewhere to institutions (effective 2002). adv. bk.rev. illus. back issues avail.; reprints avail. *Refereed.* **Document type:** *Academic/Scholarly.* **Description:** Covers the modelling of brain and behavioral processes, and the application of these processes to computer and related technologies.
Related titles: Microfilm ed.: (from PQC); Online - full text ed.: (from EBSCO Publishing, ingenta, ScienceDirect, Swets Blackwell, Institute for Scientific Information).
Indexed: A.I.Abstr., A.S.& T.Ind. (Jan.1991-), ASCA, Abstr.Hum.Comp.Inter., Acoust.Abstr., Bioeng.Abstr., Biostat., Compumath, Comput.& Info.Sys., Comput.Abstr., Comput.Lit.Ind., Curr.Cont., Curr.Ind.Stat., Eng.Ind., Excerp.Med. (1995-), INSPEC (1988-), ISMEC, Ind.Med., Ind.Sci.Rev., Int.Abstr.Biol.Sci., Neurosci.Abstr. (coverage dropped), Neurosci.Cit.Ind., Oper.Res.Manage.Sci., PsycInfo, Psychol.Abstr. (1989-), Qual.Contr.Appl.Stat., Russ.Acad.Sci.Bibl., SSCI (coverage dropped), Sci.Cit.Ind., Telegen, Zent.Math., e-psyche.
—BLDSC (6081.280800), AskIEEE, CISTI, Ei, GNLM, IDS, ingenta, Linda Hall. **CCC.**
Published by: (International Neural Networks Society), Pergamon (Subsidiary of: Elsevier Science), The Boulevard, Langford Ln, East Park, Kidlington, Oxford OXB 1GB, United Kingdom. FAX 44-1865-843010, http://www.elsevier.com/locate/neunet, http://www.elsevier.com/locate/elecacc. Eds. Mitsuo Kawato, Stephen Grossberg, John Taylor TEL 44-171-873-2214, Mitsuo Kawato, Dr. Stephen Grossberg TEL 617-353-7857. adv.: B&W page USD 600, color page USD 1,400. Circ: 3,000. **Subscr. in Australasia and the Far East to:** Elsevier Science (Singapore) Pte Ltd, No.1 Temasek Ave, 17-01 Millenia Tower, Singapore 039192, Singapore. TEL 65-434-3727, FAX 65-337-2230; **Subscr. in the Americas to:** Elsevier Science, PO Box 945, New York, NY 10159-0945. TEL 212-633-3730, FAX 212-633-3680, usinfo-f@elsevier.com; **Subscr. to:** Elsevier Science BV, PO Box 211, Amsterdam 1000 AE, Netherlands. TEL 31-20-485-3757. **Co-sponsors:** European Neural Networks Society; Japanese Neural Networks Society.

006.32 USA ISSN 1370-4621
QA76.87 CODEN: NPLEFG
NEURAL PROCESSING LETTERS. Text in English. 1994. bi-m. USD 485, EUR 485 to institutions for print or online ed.; USD 582, EUR 582 to institutions for print & online eds.combined (effective 2002). reprint service avail. from SWZ. *Refereed.* **Document type:** *Journal, Academic/Scholarly.* **Description:** Promotes fast exchange of information in the community of neural network researchers and users, and publishes research results and innovative ideas in all fields of artificial neural networks.
Related titles: Online - full text ed.: (from EBSCO Publishing, O C L C Online Computer Library Center, Inc., RoweCom Information Quest, Swets Blackwell, Kluwer Online, Institute for Scientific Information).
Indexed: ASCA, Compumath, Comput.Abstr., Comput.Lit.Ind., Eng.Ind., Environ.Eng.Abstr., Environ.Sci.Poll.Mgmt., INSPEC (Sep.1994-Nov.1995, Apr.1996-), Inform.Sci.Abstr., Neurosci.Cit.Ind., e-psyche.
—BLDSC (6081.281020), AskIEEE, IDS. **CCC.**
Published by: Kluwer Academic Publishers Boston, 101 Philip Dr, Assinippi Park, Norwell, MA 02061. TEL 781-871-6600, FAX 781-871-9045, services@wkap.nl, http://www.wkap.nl/journalhome.htm/1370-4621. Eds. Francois Blayo, Michael Verleysen, Mohamad Hassoum. R&P Rose Luongo TEL 781-871-6311. **Subscr. outside the Americas to:** Kluwer Academic Publishers Group, Journals Department, PO Box 322, Dordrecht 3300 AH, Netherlands. TEL 31-78-639-2392, FAX 31-78-654-6474; **Subscr. to:** Kluwer Academic - Plenum Publishers, 233 Spring St, New York, NY 10013-1578. TEL 212-620-8468, FAX 212-807-1047.

SEMIOTIC AND COGNITIVE STUDIES. see *PHILOSOPHY*

TRENDS IN COGNITIVE SCIENCES. see *PSYCHOLOGY*

COMPUTERS—Automation

629.89 NLD ISSN 1387-5825
PROCESS CONTROL; vakblad voor procesbesturing en analysetechniek. Text in Dutch. 1996. 10/yr. NLG 120 (effective 1999). adv. illus, tr.lit. back issues avail. **Document type:** *Journal, Trade.* **Description:** Covers laboratory technology and process automation.
Formerly (until 1997): L T i P A (1385-1837); Which was formed by the 1996 merger of: I en P A (0928-1177); L T en I (0928-1185)
Published by: Array Publications BV, Postbus 615, Alphen aan den Rijn 2400 AP, Netherlands. TEL 31-172-424177, FAX 31-172-424381, pc@array.nl, http://array.nl/lp, http://www.array.nl. Ed. N Heijna. Adv. contact Jos Raaphorst. B&W page NLG 2,850, color page NLG 4,550; trim 297 x 210. Circ: 4,500 (controlled).

COMPUTERS—Computer Assisted Instruction

see also *EDUCATION—Computer Applications*

COMPUTERS—Computer Industry, Vocational Guidance

see also *EDUCATION; OCCUPATIONS AND CAREERS*

COMPUTERS—Computer Networks

see also *COMPUTERS—Internet*

COMPUTERS—Computer Programming

see also *COMPUTERS—Software*

COMPUTERS—Computer Sales

see also *BUSINESS AND ECONOMICS—Marketing And Purchasing*

COMPUTERS—Computer Security

HEALTHCARE DATA SECURITY MANUAL. see *HEALTH FACILITIES AND ADMINISTRATION*

COMPUTERS—Cybernetics

see also *COMPUTERS—Artificial Intelligence*

COMPUTERS—Data Communications And Data Transmission Systems

362 004.6 USA
ADVANCE FOR HEALTH INFORMATION EXECUTIVES. Text in English. m. Free to qualified subscribers. adv. **Document type:** *Magazine, Trade.* **Description:** Publishes solutions and strategies for health information systems, such as computer-based patient records systems.
Related titles: Online - full content ed.
Published by: Merion Publications, Inc., 2900 Horizon Dr, PO Box 61556, King Of Prussia, PA 19406. TEL 800-355-5627, FAX 610-278-1421, 610-278-1425, firving@merion.com, http://www.advanceforhie.com, http://www.advanceweb.com.

COMPUTERS—Electronic Data Processing

PHARMACY ELECTRONIC COMMUNICATIONS STANDARD. see *PHARMACY AND PHARMACOLOGY*

SOUTH AFRICA. STATISTICS SOUTH AFRICA. CENSUS OF PROFESSIONAL AND BUSINESS SERVICES - DATA PROCESSING SERVICES. see *BUSINESS AND ECONOMICS—Abstracting, Bibliographies, Statistics*

COMPUTERS—Information Science And Information Theory

see also *COMPUTERS*

H I C. (Health Informatics Conference) see *MEDICAL SCIENCES—Computer Applications*

003 NLD ISSN 0923-8433
HUMAN FACTORS IN INFORMATION TECHNOLOGY. Text in English. 1989. irreg., latest vol.13, 1999. price varies. back issues avail. *Refereed.* **Document type:** *Monographic series, Academic/Scholarly.* **Description:** Surveys a wide range of topics dealing with all aspects of human factors in the application of information technology.
Indexed: Zent.Math., e-psyche.
—BLDSC (4336.081300).
Published by: Elsevier Science BV, PO Box 211, Amsterdam 1000 AE, Netherlands. TEL 31-20-485-3757, 31-20-485-3911, FAX 31-20-485-3432, 31-20-485-3598, nlinfo-f@elsevier.nl; usinfo-f@elsevier.com; forinfo-kyf04035@niftyserve.or.jp, http://www.elsevier.nl/. Eds. Hans Jorg Bullinger, Peter G Polson. **Subscr. in Australasia and the Far East to:** Elsevier Science (Singapore) Pte Ltd, No.1 Temasek Ave, 17-01 Millenia Tower, Singapore 039192, Singapore. TEL 65-434-3727, FAX 65-337-2230, asiainfo@elsevier.com.sg; **Subscr. in Japan to:** Elsevier Science Inc - Japan Regional Office, 9-15 Higashi-Azabu 1-chome, Minato-ku, Tokyo 106-0044, Japan. TEL 81-3-5561-5033, FAX 81-3-5561-5047, info@elsevier.co.jp; **Subscr. in the Americas to:** Elsevier Science, PO Box 945, New York, NY 10159-0945. TEL 212-633-3730, 888-437-4636, FAX 212-633-3680, usinfo-f@elsevier.com, http://www.elsevier.com

INFORMATICS IN HEATHCARE AUSTRALIA. see *MEDICAL SCIENCES—Computer Applications*

IRYO JOHO SHISUTEMU KENKYU KAIHATSU HOKOKUSHO/REPORT OF RESEARCH AND DEVELOPMENT OF MEDICAL INFORMATION SYSTEM. see *MEDICAL SCIENCES*

▼ **THE NEW REVIEW OF HEALTH INFORMATICS.** see *PHYSICAL FITNESS AND HYGIENE*

STUDIES IN VISUAL INFORMATION PROCESSING. see *MEDICAL SCIENCES—Psychiatry And Neurology*

COMPUTERS—Internet

C O R E-HEALTH TREND WATCH. see *MEDICAL SCIENCES*

C O R HEALTHCARE STRATEGIST TREND WATCH. see *HEALTH FACILITIES AND ADMINISTRATION*

616.8584 USA ISSN 1094-9313
CODEN: CYBEFA
CYBERPSYCHOLOGY & BEHAVIOR; the impact of the Internet, multi-media & virtual reality on behavior & society. Text in English. 1998. bi-m. USD 119 domestic to individuals; USD 179 foreign to individuals; USD 143 domestic to individuals print and online eds. combined; USD 203 foreign to individuals print and online eds. combined; USD 218 domestic to institutions; USD 283 foreign to institutions; USD 262 domestic to institutions print and online eds. combined; USD 326 foreign to institutions print and online eds. combined (effective 2002). adv. back issues avail.; reprints avail. *Refereed.* **Document type:** *Journal, Academic/Scholarly.* **Description:** Explores the impact of the Internet, multimedia, and virtual reality on behavior and society.
Related titles: Online - full text ed.: USD 119 to individuals; USD 218 to institutions (effective 2002) (from CatchWord Ltd., EBSCO Publishing, O C L C Online Computer Library Center, Inc., RoweCom Information Quest, Swets Blackwell, Institute for Scientific Information).
Indexed: Curr.Cont., Ergon.Abstr., Excerp.Med., SSCI.
—BLDSC (3506.400270), CatchWord. **CCC.**

C

Published by: Mary Ann Liebert, Inc. Publishers, 2 Madison Ave, Larchmont, NY 10538. TEL 914—834-3100, FAX 914-834-1388, info@liebertpub.com, www.liebertpub.com/cpb, http://www.liebertpub.com. Ed. Dr. Mark Wiederhold.

▼ **FAMILY MEDICINE NET GUIDE**; your guide to the internet. see *MEDICAL SCIENCES*

▼ **FAMILY MEDICINE NET GUIDE ENEWSLETTER.** see *MEDICAL SCIENCES*

▼ **FAMILY MEDICINE NET GUIDE ONLINE.** see *MEDICAL SCIENCES*

025.04362 USA ISSN 1089-4187
RA773.6 CODEN: HCINF7
HEALTH CARE ON THE INTERNET; a journal for medical professionals, consumers & librarians. Text in English. 1997. q. USD 50 to individuals; USD 68 in Canada to individuals; USD 73 elsewhere to individuals; USD 125 to institutions; USD 169 in Canada to institutions; USD 181 elsewhere to institutions (effective Aug. 2001). adv. back issues avail.; reprint service avail. from HAW. **Document type:** *Journal, Academic/Scholarly.* **Description:** Discusses topics relating to internet-accessible materials on health care.
Related titles: Microform ed.: (from PQC); Online - full text ed.: free with print ed. (effective 2001).
Indexed: ASSIA, AgeLine, CINAHL, Comput.Lit.Ind., Environ.Sci.Poll.Mgmt., INSPEC (1997-), Inform.Sci.Abstr., LISA, Microcomp.Ind. (Mar.1998-), Pollut.Abstr., Ref.Zh., Risk Abstr., Saf.Sci.Abstr. —BLDSC (4274.942510), AskIEEE, Haworth.
Published by: Haworth Press, Inc., 10 Alice St, Binghamton, NY 13904-1580. TEL 607-722-5857, 800-429-6784, FAX 607-722-6362, 800-895-0582, getinfo@haworthpressinc.com, http://www.haworthpress.com/journals/journallist.asp. Ed. M Sandra Wood. Pub. William Cohen. R&P Ruthann Heath TEL 607-723-5857 ext 316. Adv. contact Jackie Blakeslee TEL 607-722-5857 ext 346. B&W page USD 315, color page USD 550; trim 4.375 x 7.125. Circ: 600.

HEALTH INFORMATION ON THE INTERNET. see *MEDICAL SCIENCES*

025.4 600 USA
▼ **IHEALTHCARE WEEKLY.** Text in English. 2000. d. adv. **Document type:** *Trade.* **Description:** Covers news and events affecting traditional and Internet healthcare services and providers.
Media: Online - full text.
Published by: Rising Tide Studios, 307 W 36th St, 10th Fl, New York, NY 10018-6403. TEL 646-473-2222, FAX 646-473-2223, subscribe@ihealthcareweekly.com, http://www.ihealthcareweekly.com. Ed. Jason McCabe Calacanis. Pub. Karol Martesko-Fenster. Adv. contact Keith Long.

INFONET GAZETTE. see *MEDICAL SCIENCES*

INTERNET - MEDICINA. see *MEDICAL SCIENCES—Computer Applications*

004.678 USA ISSN 1086-5691
INTERNET MEDICINE. Text in English. 1996. m., latest vol.6. USD 114 domestic to individuals; USD 114 foreign to individuals; USD 175 per issue domestic to institutions; USD 175 per issue foreign to institutions; USD 15 newsstand/cover (effective 2002). **Document type:** *Newsletter.*
Related titles: Online - full text ed.: USD 227.50 domestic for academic site license; USD 227.50 foreign for academic site license; USD 253.75 domestic for corporate site license; USD 253.75 foreign for corporate site license (effective 2002).
Indexed: CINAHL, Inform.Sci.Abstr., Microcomp.Ind. (Jul.1999-).
Published by: Lippincott Williams & Wilkins (Philadelphia) (Subsidiary of: Wolters Kluwer N.V.), 530 Walnut St, Philadelphia, PA 19106-3621. TEL 215-521-8300, FAX 215-521-8902, http://www.lww.com. Eds. Barbara Ward, Dr. Luis G Pareras. **Subscr. to:** PO Box 1600, Hagerstown, MD 21740-1600.

▼ **JOURNAL OF TECHNOLOGY IN COUNSELING.** see *PSYCHOLOGY*

▼ **MD NET GUIDE**; physician's internet directory. see *MEDICAL SCIENCES*

▼ **MD NET GUIDE ENEWSLETTER.** see *MEDICAL SCIENCES*

▼ **MD NET GUIDE ONLINE**; physician's internet directory. see *MEDICAL SCIENCES*

▼ **ONCOLOGY NET GUIDE**; internet guide to cancer sites. see *MEDICAL SCIENCES—Oncology*

▼ **ONCOLOGY NET GUIDE ENEWSLETTER.** see *MEDICAL SCIENCES—Oncology*

▼ **ONCOLOGY NET GUIDE ONLINE**; internet guide to cancer sites. see *MEDICAL SCIENCES—Oncology*

COMPUTERS—Microcomputers

see also COMPUTERS—Personal Computers

ACCESS (RESEARCH TRIANGLE PARK). see *COMPUTERS—Personal Computers*

COMPUTERTALK; for contemporary pharmacy management. see *PHARMACY AND PHARMACOLOGY—Computer Applications*

COMPUTERTALK PHARMACY SYSTEMS BUYERS GUIDE. see *PHARMACY AND PHARMACOLOGY—Computer Applications*

CYBERLOG; library of applied medical software. see *MEDICAL SCIENCES—Computer Applications*

DENTAL COMPUTER NEWSLETTER. see *MEDICAL SCIENCES—Computer Applications*

004.14 SGP ISSN 0219-581X
▼ **INTERNATIONAL JOURNAL OF NANOSCIENCE.** Text in English. forthcoming 2002. bi-m. SGD 202, USD 112 to individuals; SGD 504, USD 280 combined subscription to institutions for print & online eds.; SGD 302, USD 168 combined subscription in developing nations to institutions for print & online eds. (effective 2001 - 2002). *Refereed.* **Document type:** *Journal, Academic/Scholarly.* **Description:** Covers all aspects of nanometer scale science and technology, including subjects from basic science of nanoscale physics and chemistry to nanostructured materials and applications in nanodevices, quantum engineering and quantum computing.
Published by: World Scientific Publishing Co Pte Ltd, Farrer Rd, PO Box 128, Singapore 912805, Singapore. TEL 65-382-5663, FAX 65-382-5919, wspcsl@singnet.com.sg, http://www.worldscinet.com/journals/ijn/ijn.shtml, http://www.wspc.com. **Subscr. in the US to:** 1060 Main St, River Edge, NJ 07661. TEL 888-977-2665, sales@wspc.com.

620.5 USA ISSN 1533-4880
▼ **JOURNAL OF NANOSCIENCE AND NANOTECHNOLOGY.** Text and summaries in English. 2001. q. USD 149 to individuals; USD 575 to institutions (effective 2001). abstr. back issues avail. *Refereed.* **Document type:** *Journal, Academic/Scholarly, Corporate, Government.* **Description:** Covers research activities in all areas of nanoscience and nanotechnology, containing original full research articles, rapid communications of important new scientific and technological findings, reviews with author's photo and short biography, and current research news encompassing the fundamental and applied research in all disciplines of science, engineering and medicine.
Related titles: Online - full text ed.: (from CatchWord Ltd.).
Indexed: INSPEC.
—CCC.
Published by: American Scientific Publishers, 25650 N Lewis Way, Stevenson Ranch, CA 91381-1439. TEL 661-254-0807, FAX 661-254-1207, jnn@aspbs.com, order@aspbs.com, http://aspbs.com/jnn/, http://www.aspbs.com. Ed., R&P H S Nalwa.

MICRO MEDICAL NEWSLETTER. see *MEDICAL SCIENCES—Computer Applications*

COMPUTERS—Personal Computers

see also COMPUTERS—Microcomputers

004.16 USA
A P H TECHNOLOGY UPDATE; technology for people who are visually impaired. Text in English. 1985. s-a. free. **Document type:** *Newsletter.* **Description:** Contains articles about computer products designed for visually impaired users.
Former titles: Access Abilities; Micro Materials Update (1081-518X)
Related titles: Audio cassette/tape ed.; Braille ed.; CD-ROM ed.
Published by: American Printing House for the Blind, Inc., 1839 Frankfort Ave, Louisville, KY 40206. TEL 502-895-2405, FAX 502-899-2274, info@aph.org, http://www.aph.org/techup. Ed. Larry Skutchan. Circ: 8,800.

004.16 USA ISSN 0733-8074
QA76.5 CODEN: ACCSEG
ACCESS (RESEARCH TRIANGLE PARK)*. Text in English. 1982. 6/yr. USD 21. adv. bk.rev. **Description:** Features technical articles on applications to engineering and science. Regular columns include statistics column, numerical analysis, scientific use of Amiga and Macintosh.
Indexed: INSPEC (May 1985-Feb.1990, dropped), Oper.Res.Manage.Sci., Qual.Contr.Appl.Stat. —ingenta.
Published by: L E D S Publishing Co. Inc., 1014 Evergreen Dr, Durham, NC 27712-2214. TEL 919-477-3690. Ed. Leslie E Sparks. Circ: 4,000.

CYBERLOG; library of applied medical software. see *MEDICAL SCIENCES—Computer Applications*

MICRO MEDICAL NEWSLETTER. see *MEDICAL SCIENCES—Computer Applications*

COMPUTERS—Robotics

see also COMPUTERS—Artificial Intelligence

▼ **INTERNATIONAL JOURNAL OF NANOSCIENCE.** see *COMPUTERS—Microcomputers*

▼ **JOURNAL OF MICROMECHATRONICS.** see *ENGINEERING—Electrical Engineering*

▼ **JOURNAL OF NANOSCIENCE AND NANOTECHNOLOGY.** see *COMPUTERS—Microcomputers*

COMPUTERS—Software

BIOTECH SOFTWARE AND INTERNET REPORT; the computer software journal for scientists. see *BIOLOGY—Biotechnology*

CYBERLOG; library of applied medical software. see *MEDICAL SCIENCES—Computer Applications*

MEDICAL SOFTWARE REVIEWS; the leading resource for objective evaluations of medical software. see *MEDICAL SCIENCES—Computer Applications*

T E S S. (The Educational Software Selector) see *EDUCATION—Computer Applications*

CONSERVATION

see also ENERGY; ENVIRONMENTAL STUDIES; FISH AND FISHERIES; FORESTS AND FORESTRY; WATER RESOURCES

577 AUS ISSN 1320-145X
C A L M SCIENCE. (Conservation and Land Management) Variant title: CALMScience. Text in English. 1994. irreg. (approx. 2/yr.). AUD 30 per issue. Supplement avail.; back issues avail. *Refereed.* **Description:** For those interested in nature conservation, sustainable utilization and land management.
Formed by the merger of (1985-1994): Western Australia. Department of Conservation and Land Management. Technical Report (0816-6757); Which was formerly: Western Australia. Department of Conservation and Land Management. Occasional Paper (0816-9675); (1986-1994): Western Australia. Department of Conservation and Land Management. Research Bulletin (1032-8106); Which was formerly (until 1986): Western Australia. Department of Conservation and Land Management. Bulletin (0816-9675); Western Australia. Forest Department. Bulletin (0085-8129)
Indexed: Aus.Sci.Ind., Biol.Abstr., Ecol.Abstr., Forest Prod.Abstr., Forest.Abstr., Rev.Plant Path., Rural Recreat.Tour.Abstr., Seed Abstr., Sport Fish.Abstr., Wild.Rev., Zoo.Rec. —BLDSC (3015.446000), CISTI.
Published by: Department of Conservation and Land Management, Locked Bag 29, Bentley Delivery Centre, W.A. 6893, Australia. TEL 61-89334-0333, FAX 61-89334-0498, http://www.calm.wa.gov.au. Ed. K Keannelly. Circ: 500.

C

CARIBBEAN RESEARCH INSTITUTE. REPORT. see *HISTORY—History Of North And South America*

COMPARATIVE PHYSIOLOGY AND ECOLOGY. see *BIOLOGY—Physiology*

577 USA ISSN 0888-8892
QH75.A1 CODEN: CBIOEF
CONSERVATION BIOLOGY. Text in English; Abstracts in Spanish. 1986. bi-m. USD 205 domestic to individuals; USD 215 in Canada & Mexico to individuals; USD 240 elsewhere to individuals; USD 395 domestic to institutions; USD 405 in Canada & Mexico to institutions; USD 430 elsewhere to institutions; USD 225 to individuals print & online eds. combined; USD 434.50 to institutions print & online eds. combined (effective 2001). adv. illus. index. back issues avail.; reprints avail. *Refereed.* **Document type:** *Academic/Scholarly.*
Related titles: Online - full text ed.: ISSN 1523-1739. USD 185 to individuals; USD 356 to institutions (effective 2001) (from Ovid Technologies, Inc., EBSCO Publishing, O C L C Online Computer Library Center, Inc., RoweCom Information Quest, JSTOR (Web-based Journal Archive), ingenta, Gale Group, Munksgaard & Blackwell Science's Synergy, Swets Blackwell, Institute for Scientific Information).
Indexed: ABSEARCH Conserv.Biol. (1987-), ASCA, Agricola, Agroforest.Abstr., Anim.Behav.Abstr., Anim.Breed.Abstr., Appl.Ecol.Abstr., Aqua.Sci.& Fish.Abstr., Bibl.Agri., Bio-Contr.News & Info., Biol.& Agr.Ind. (Jan.1996-), Curr.Adv.Plant Sci., Curr.Cont., Ecol.Abstr., Entomol.Abstr., Environ.Abstr., Environ.Ind., Environ.Per.Bibl. (1989-), Environ.Sci.Poll.Mgmt., Forest Prod.Abstr., Forest.Abstr., Gen.Sci.Ind. (Jul.1997-), Genet.Abstr., Geo.Abstr.H.G., Geo.Abstr.P.G., GeoRef, Geol.Abstr., Helminthol.Abstr., Herb.Abstr., Hum.Gen.Abstr., IDA, Ind.Sci.Rev., Ind.Vet., Int.Abstr.Biol.Sci., Irr.& Drain.Abstr., Key Word Ind.Wildl.Res., Ocean.Abstr., Pig News & Info., Plant Breed.Abstr., Plant Gen.Res.Abstr., Plant Sci., Rev.Appl.Entomol., Rev.Med.& Vet.Mycol., Rice Abstr., Rural Devel.Abstr., Rural Recreat.Tour.Abstr., SSCI (coverage dropped), Sci.Cit.Ind., Seed Abstr., Sel.Water Res.Abstr., Soils & Fert., Sport Fish.Abstr., Weed Abstr., Wild.Rev., Wildlife & Conserv.Biol.Abstr. (1986-), World Ag.Econ.& Rur.Soc.Abstr., Zoo.Rec.
—BLDSC (3417.999000), CISTI, EMDOCS, IDS, ingenta. **CCC.**
Published by: (Society for Conservation Biology), Blackwell Science Inc., Commerce Pl, 350 Main St, Malden, MA 02148-5018. TEL 781-388-8250, FAX 781-388-8255, journals@blacksci.com, http://www.blackwell-science.com. Ed. Reed Noss. R&P Tracey Davies. Adv. contact Jenny Applin. Circ: 5,000.

▼ **CONSERVATION GENETICS.** see *BIOLOGY—Genetics*

COUNTRY ROAD CHRONICLES. see *NATIVE AMERICAN STUDIES*

ECOLOGIA. see *BIOLOGY*

ECOLOGICAL PSYCHOLOGY. see *PSYCHOLOGY*

THE ECOLOGISTS. see *BIOLOGY*

ENVIRONMENT ABSTRACTS. see *CONSERVATION—Abstracting, Bibliographies, Statistics*

ENVIRONMENTAL OPPORTUNITIES. see *ENVIRONMENTAL STUDIES*

333.72 USA
ILLINOIS. NATURAL HISTORY SURVEY. REPORTS. Text in English. 1962. 6/yr. free per issue. **Document type:** *Newsletter, Trade.* **Description:** Reports current research undertaken at the Illinois Natural History Survey, for a non-specialist audience.
Indexed: Biol.Dig., Ref.Zh., Sport Fish.Abstr., Wild.Rev.
Published by: Department of Natural Resources, Natural History Survey, Natural Resources Bldg, 607 E Peabody Dr, Champaign, IL 61820. TEL 217-244-2115, FAX 217-333-4949. Ed. Charles Warwick. Circ: 2,200.

JOURNAL OF RANGE MANAGEMENT; covering the study, management, and use of rangeland ecosystems and range resources. see *BIOLOGY*

JOURNAL OF WILDLIFE DISEASES. see *VETERINARY SCIENCE*

MARINE CONSERVATION. see *BIOLOGY*

MARINE TURTLE NEWSLETTER. see *BIOLOGY—Zoology*

N B I A NEWSLETTER. see *AGRICULTURE*

N E C N P NEWSLETTER. see *ENERGY*

NOTICIAS DE GALAPAGOS. see *SCIENCES: COMPREHENSIVE WORKS*

333.72 DEU ISSN 0032-6542
AM1 CODEN: PPTRAA
DER PRAEPARATOR. Text in English, German. 1955. q. DEM 40; DEM 48 foreign (effective 1996). adv. bk.rev. charts, illus. index every 2 yrs. **Document type:** *Bulletin.*
Indexed: Art & Archaeol.Tech.Abstr., BHA, Chem.Abstr., GeoRef, Russ.Acad.Sci.Bibl., Zoo.Rec.
—GNLM.
Published by: Verband Deutscher Praeparatoren e.V., Middeweg 36, Bottrop 46240, Germany. TEL 49-2041-96651, FAX 49-2041-29716. Ed. Siegfried Eckardt. Circ: 2,000.

PRIMATE EYE. see *ANTHROPOLOGY*

SHOKUCHU SHOKUBUTSU KENKYUKAI KAISHI/INSECTIVOROUS PLANT SOCIETY. JOURNAL. see *BIOLOGY—Botany*

SKYHOPPER. see *BIOLOGY—Zoology*

TORONTO FIELD NATURALIST. see *BIOLOGY*

333.72 AUS
TURNING THE TIDE. Text in English. 1978. s-a. AUD 35 (effective 2000). bk.rev. **Document type:** *Bulletin, Consumer.* **Description:** Contains commentary on Australian marine and coastal conservation issues, particularly the management of marine protected areas, including the Great Barrier Reef and Australian tidal wetlands.
Former titles: Australian Marine Conservation Society. Bulletin; Australian Littoral Society. Bulletin (0157-308X)
Published by: Australian Marine Conservation Society Inc., PO Box 3139, Yeronga, QLD 4104, Australia. FAX 61-7-38925814, ames@ozemail.com.au, http://www.ozemail.com.au/~amcs. Ed. Kris Plowman. R&P Anne Clarke TEL 61-7-38485235. Adv. contact Carol Deane. Circ: 2,000.

VOGEL UND UMWELT; Zeitschrift fuer Vogelkunde und Naturschutz in Hessen. see *BIOLOGY—Ornithology*

333.9 USA ISSN 0273-4419
QL737.C4
WHALEWATCHER. Text in English. 1967. q. USD 35 to members (effective 2000). adv. bk.rev. charts, illus. index. **Document type:** *Academic/Scholarly.*
Indexed: GeoRef, Zoo.Rec.
—BLDSC (9309.554500).
Published by: American Cetacean Society, PO Box 1391, San Pedro, CA 90733-1391. TEL 310-548-6279, FAX 310-548-6950, acs@pobox.com. Ed. Shirley Brim. R&P Kathleen Owston. Circ: 1,000.

333.95416 USA
WILDLIFE REHABILITATION. Text in English. 1996 (vol.14). a. USD 25 to members; USD 30 to non-members. **Document type:** *Proceedings.*
Indexed: Zoo.Rec.
—BLDSC.
Published by: National Wildlife Rehabilitators Association, 14 N. 7th Ave., St. Cloud, MN 56303. TEL 320-259-4086, nwra@cloudnet.com, http://www.nwrawildlife.org.

WILDLIFE REHABILITATION TODAY. see *VETERINARY SCIENCE*

CONSERVATION—Abstracting, Bibliographies, Statistics

016.33372 USA ISSN 0093-3287
GF1
ENVIRONMENT ABSTRACTS. Text in English. 1975. m. price varies. illus. Index. reprints avail. **Document type:** *Abstract/Index.* **Description:** Addresses the impact of humankind and technology on the environment with attention to air, water, and noise pollution; solid and toxic wastes; radiological contamination; toxicological effects; control technologies; resource management; population; endangered species; and geophysical and climatic change. Information is abstracted and indexed from scientific, technical, and business journals; conference and symposium proceedings; and academic and government reports.
Incorporates (1985-1991): Acid Rain Abstracts (0882-1402); Formerly: Environment Information Access (0013-9181)
Related titles: CD-ROM ed.; Online - full text ed.: (from Data-Star, The Dialog Corporation, F I Z Technik, Questel Orbit Inc.).
—BLDSC (3791.095010), Infotrieve, Linda Hall. **CCC.**
Published by: Congressional Information Service, Inc. (Subsidiary of: LexisNexis), 4520 East West Hwy, Bethesda, MD 20814. TEL 301-654-1550, 800-638-8380, FAX 301-654-4033, cisinfo@lexis-nexis.com., http://www.cispubs.com. Ed. Larry Sheridan.

CONSUMER EDUCATION AND PROTECTION

ASHES TO DUST. see *PUBLIC HEALTH AND SAFETY*

AUSTRALIAN RECALLS AND CANCELLATIONS. see *PUBLIC HEALTH AND SAFETY*

CHOICE HEALTH READER. see *PHYSICAL FITNESS AND HYGIENE*

363.19 640.73 USA
CONSUMER PRODUCT SAFETY REVIEW. Text in English. 1976. q. USD 16 domestic; USD 20 foreign (effective 2001). **Document type:** *Government, Consumer.* **Description:** Informs consumers, public health and medical professionals, and industry about injuries and deaths associated with consumer products.
Former titles (until 1996): N E I S S Data Highlights; N E I S S News (0364-6475)
Related titles: Online - full text ed.
Indexed: Amer.Stat.Ind. (1996-).
Published by: U.S. Consumer Product Safety Commission, Washington, DC 220207. TEL 202-512-1800, http://www.cpsc.gov/cpscpub/pubs/cpsr.html. Ed. Nancy Sachs TEL 301-504-0554. Circ: 1,300 (paid). **Subscr. to:** U.S. Government Printing Office, Superintendent of Documents, PO Box 371954, Pittsburgh, PA 15250-7954. TEL 202-512-1800, FAX 202-512-2250, orders@gpo.gov, http://www.access.gpo.gov.

CONSUMER REPORTS ON HEALTH. see *PHYSICAL FITNESS AND HYGIENE*

640.73 362.11 USA ISSN 1070-2644
CONSUMERS' GUIDE TO HOSPITALS. Text in English. 1988. irreg. (approx. biennial). USD 12 (effective 1999). adv. charts, illus, stat. back issues avail. **Document type:** *Consumer.* **Description:** Gives death rates at 5500 US hospitals as well as information on how to choose a hospital, how to get the best care wherever you go, and how to keep costs down.
Published by: Center for the Study of Services, 733 15th St, N W, Ste 820, Washington, DC 20005-2112. TEL 202-347-9612, 800-475-7283, http://www.checkbook.org. Pub. Robert Krughoff. R&P Kevin Brassler. Adv. contact Tara Eberly.

353.84 USA ISSN 0362-1332
HD9000.9.U5 CODEN: FDACBH
F D A CONSUMER. (Food and Drug Administration) Text in English. 1967. bi-m. USD 13.50 (effective 2001). illus. cum.index: vols. 1-22. back issues avail.; reprint service avail. from PQC. **Document type:** *Government, Consumer.* **Description:** Contains information for consumers about Food and Drug Administration regulatory and scientific decisions, and about the safe use of products regulated by FDA.
Formerly: F D A Papers (0014-5750)
Related titles: Microform ed.: (from PQC); Online - full text ed.: (from The Dialog Corporation, Gale Group, ProQuest Information & Learning, H. W. Wilson, Factiva, Institute for Scientific Information).
Indexed: Acad.Ind., AgBiotech, AgeLine, Agricola, BPIA, Bibl.Agri., Biol.Dig., CHNI, Consum.Ind. (1989-), Curr.Lit.Fam.Plan., Curr.Pack.Abstr., Excerp.Med., Food Sci.& Tech.Abstr., Gen.Sci.Ind. (Jun.1992-), Hlth.Ind., INIS Atomind., I.P.A., Ind.U.S.Gov.Per., Ind.Vet., Inpharma, L.R.I., MEDOC, Mag.Ind., NRN, Nutr.Abstr., P.A.I.S., PMR, Pharm.&Out.News, R.G. (Feb.1983-), R.G.Abstr. (Feb.1983-), Reac., Rev.Appl.Entomol., Sugar Ind.Abstr., Telegen.
—BLDSC (3901.292000), CISTI, GNLM, IDS, ingenta, Linda Hall.
Published by: U.S. Food and Drug Administration, Office of Public Affairs, 5600 Fishers Ln, Rockville, MD 20857. TEL 301-443-3220. Ed., R&P Dori Stehlin. Circ: 28,000 (paid). **Subscr. to:** U.S. Government Printing Office, Superintendent of Documents, PO Box 371954, Pittsburgh, PA 15250-7954. TEL 202-512-1800, FAX 202-512-2250, orders@gpo.gov, http://www.access.gpo.gov.

640.73 USA
F D A WEEK. (Food and Drug Administration) Text in English. w. USD 645 in US & Canada; USD 695 elsewhere (effective 2001). **Document type:** *Newsletter.*
Related titles: E-mail ed.
Published by: Inside Washington Publishers, PO Box 7167, Ben Franklin Sta, Washington, DC 20044-7167. TEL 703-416-8500, FAX 703-416-8543, service@iwpnews.com.

FAMILY ECONOMICS AND NUTRITION REVIEW. see *HOME ECONOMICS*

571.959 USA
FOOD & WATER JOURNAL. Text in English. 1992. q. USD 25 domestic; USD 40 in Canada; USD 45 elsewhere (effective 2001). bk.rev. charts, illus. back issues avail. **Document type:** *Magazine, Consumer.* **Description:** Aims to stimulate the necessary efforts to build local, safe, and sustainable alternatives in food production as well as provide the language, philosophy and strategic imperatives for lasting fundamental change.
Formerly: Safe Food News
Indexed: Alt.Press Ind.
Published by: Food and Water, Inc., 389 VT Rte. 215, Walden, VT 05873. TEL 802-563-3300, FAX 802-563-3310, info@foodandwater.org, http://www.foodandwater.org/journal.asp. Ed. Michael Colby. Circ: 15,000.

▼ **FOOD SAFETY SOURCEBOOK.** see *FOOD AND FOOD INDUSTRIES*

HEALTH LETTER (WASHINGTON). see *MEDICAL SCIENCES*

640.73 614 NLD ISSN 1566-0974
HC79.C63
INJURY PREVENTION AND SAFETY PROMOTION. Text in English. 1994. q. NLG 223, USD 124 to individuals; NLG 628, USD 330 to institutions includes online ed. (effective 2000). adv. bk.rev. back issues avail.; reprint service avail. from SWZ. *Refereed.* **Document type:** *Academic/Scholarly.* **Description:** Publishes original papers, review articles, short communications and news items relating to research in the etiology of accidents in everyday life, policy development and implementation of prevention strategies.
Former titles (until 2000): International Journal for Consumer and Product Safety (1387-3059); (until 1998): International Journal for Consumer Safety (0929-8347); Which superseded: E C O S A Newsletter
Related titles: Online - full text ed.: (from EBSCO Publishing, O C L C Online Computer Library Center, Inc., RoweCom Information Quest, Swets Blackwell).
Indexed: Environ.Sci.Poll.Mgmt., Ergon.Abstr., Pollut.Abstr., Risk Abstr., Saf.Sci.Abstr.
—BLDSC (4514.410000). **CCC.**
Published by: (European Consumer Safety Association), Aeolus Press (Subsidiary of: Swets & Zeitlinger BV), PO Box 825, Lisse 2160 SZ, Netherlands. FAX 31-344-572562, orders@swets.nl, http://www.swets.nl/sps/AEolus/ijcps.html. Ed. Wim Rogmans. Pub. J K W van Leeuwen. R&P C E van Leeuwen-Meyren. Adv. contact Patrick Kleian. **Subscr. to:** Swets & Zeitlinger BV, PO Box 825, Lisse 2160 SZ, Netherlands. TEL 31-252-435111, FAX 31-252-415888, orders@swets.nl. **Dist. in N. America by:** Swets & Zeitlinger, PO Box 582, Downingtown, PA 19335-998. TEL 610-524-9387.

MASS CYCLIST. see *SPORTS AND GAMES—Bicycles And Motorcycles*

614 640.73 360 USA ISSN 0736-4873
PEOPLE'S MEDICAL SOCIETY NEWSLETTER. Text in English. 1983. bi-m. USD 24 to membership (effective 2001). bk.rev. charts, stat, illus. index. back issues avail.; reprints avail. **Document type:** *Newsletter.* **Description:** Provides medical consumers with previously unavailable medical information so that they can make informed decisions about their own health care.
Related titles: CD-ROM ed.; Online - full text ed.: (from Gale Group, Northern Light Technology, Inc., ProQuest Information & Learning, Factiva).
Indexed: CHNI, CINAHL, Hlth.Ind.
Published by: People's Medical Society, 462 Walnut St, Allentown, PA 18102-5488. TEL 610-770-1670, FAX 610-770-0607, info@peoplesmed.org, http://www.peoplesmed.org. Ed., R&P Karla Morales. Circ: 65,000.

640.73 332 USA ISSN 0195-5934
PRIME TIMES MAGAZINE (MADISON)* . Text in English. 1978. bi-m. USD 25 to non-members. adv. **Document type:** *Consumer.* **Description:** Covers consumer education, health, travel, lifestyle, and money management for credit union members 50 and over.
Published by: (MEMBERS Prime Club, Inc.), Grote Publishing, 802 W Broadway Ste 306, Madison, WI 53713-1890. TEL 608-257-4640, FAX 608-257-4670. Ed. Mary Carel Verden. Pub. Mary-Carel Verden. R&P, Adv. contact Frances Healy. Circ: 80,000 (controlled).

PRODUCT ALERT. see *FOOD AND FOOD INDUSTRIES*

▼ **REAL HEALTHCARE.** see *HEALTH FACILITIES AND ADMINISTRATION*

SCHOLASTIC CHOICES; personal development & living skills. see *EDUCATION—Teaching Methods And Curriculum*

SHEDDING LIGHT ON LEGISLATION. see *PUBLIC HEALTH AND SAFETY*

TEST SANTE. see *PUBLIC HEALTH AND SAFETY*

TOPICS IN SAFETY, RISK, RELIABILITY AND QUALITY. see *OCCUPATIONAL HEALTH AND SAFETY*

VEGETARIAN JOURNAL. see *NUTRITION AND DIETETICS*

640.73 USA
R726.C66
VOICES (WASHINGTON). Text in English. 1975. q. USD 35. bk.rev. illus. **Document type:** *Newsletter.*
Former titles (until 2000): Choices (Washington) (1079-2953); (until 1994): Choice in Dying News; Concern for Dying - Society for the Right to Die Newsletter; (until 1985): Concern for Dying Newsletter (0192-1096); (until 1978): Euthanasia News (0164-1581)
Related titles: Online - full text ed.
Indexed: R.G. (1992-, dropped), R.G.Abstr. (Aug.1992-).
Published by: Partnership for Caring, 1035 30th St, N W, Washington, DC 20007-3823. TEL 202-338-9790, 800-989-WILL, FAX 202-338-0242, pfc@partnershipforcaring.org, http://www.partnershipforcaring.org. Ed., R&P Karen Kaplan. Circ: 80,000.

CONSUMER EDUCATION AND PROTECTION—Abstracting, Bibliographies, Statistics

016.64073 USA ISSN 1053-1424
CONSUMERS REFERENCE DISC. Text in English. 199?. q. USD 695 (effective 2000). **Document type:** *Abstract/Index, Bibliography.* **Description:** Provides access to abstracted articles from Consumers Index and Consumer Health & Nutrition Index from 1985 to the present.
Media: CD-ROM (from National Information Services Corp. (NISC)). **Related titles:** Magnetic Tape ed.; Online - full text ed.; ♦ Print ed.: Consumers Index. ISSN 0094-0534.
Published by: National Information Services Corporation (NISC), Wyman Towers, 3100 St Paul St, Baltimore, MD 28218. TEL 410-243-0797, FAX 410-243-0982, sales@nisc.com, http://www.nisc.com. Pub. Fred Durr.

CORPORATE LAW

see LAW—Corporate Law

CRIMINAL LAW

see LAW—Criminal Law

CRIMINOLOGY AND LAW ENFORCEMENT

see also CRIMINOLOGY AND LAW ENFORCEMENT—Security; EDUCATION—Special Education And Rehabilitation; MEDICAL SCIENCES—Forensic Sciences

364 340.6 614.19 JPN ISSN 0302-0029
CODEN: HAZAAY
ACTA CRIMINOLOGIAE ET MEDICINAE LEGALIS JAPONICA/HANZAIGAKU ZASSHI. Text in English, Japanese. 1928. bi-m. USD 55 (effective 1992). adv. bk.rev. **Document type:** *Academic/Scholarly.*
Indexed: Abstr.Crim.& Pen., Biol.Abstr., Chem.Abstr., Chem.Indus.Notes, Chem.Titles, Excerp.Med. (1996-), Jap.Per.Ind.
—CASDDS, EMDOCS, GNLM.
Published by: Japanese Association of Criminology/Nihon Hanzai Gakkai, c/o Department of Criminal Psychiatry, Medical and Dental University, 2-3-10 Kanda-Surugadai, Chiyoda-ku, Tokyo 101-0062, Japan. FAX 03-3291-5799. Ed. A Yamagami. Circ: 800.

365 616.8 USA
AMERICAN ASSOCIATION OF MENTAL HEALTH PROFESSIONALS IN CORRECTIONS. MONOGRAPH SERIES. Text in English. 1940. q. USD 60. **Document type:** *Monographic series, Academic/Scholarly.* **Description:** For professionals working in correctional settings.
Indexed: e-psyche.
Published by: (American Association of Mental Health Professionals in Corrections), Martin Psychiatric Research Foundation, PO Box 3365, Fairfield, CA 94533. TEL 707-864-0910, FAX 707-964-0910. Ed. Dr. Clyde Verne Martin. Circ: 4,000.

364.128 USA
AMERICAN POLYGRAPH ASSOCIATION NEWSLETTER. Text in English. 1966. bi-m. USD 80 domestic; USD 100 foreign (effective 2000). adv. bk.rev. back issues avail.; reprint service avail. from PQC. **Document type:** *Newsletter.* **Description:** Covers current cases, legal changes, news of technical interest, worldwide activities, and training.
Related titles: Microform ed.: (from PQC).
Indexed: e-psyche.
Published by: (American Polygraph Association), Seridan Press, PO Box 8037, Chattanooga, TN 37414-0037. TEL 423-892-3992, 800-272-8037. Ed. Donald Krapohl. R&P, Adv. contact Robbie Bennett. Circ: 3,500.

ARCHIVOS DE CRIMINOLOGIA, NEURO-PSIQUIATRIA Y DISCIPLINAS CONEXAS. see *MEDICAL SCIENCES—Psychiatry And Neurology*

ARCHIWUM MEDYCYNY SADOWEJ I KRIMINOLOGII. see *MEDICAL SCIENCES—Forensic Sciences*

364.4 NLD ISSN 0005-4259
BALANS; personeelsblad van de Directie Delinquentenzord en Jeugdinrichtingen. Text in Dutch. 1970. m. NLG 5. adv. bk.rev. charts, illus.
Published by: Ministerie van Justitie, Redactie Balans, Terminal Noord Kamer 452, Postbus 20301, The Hague 2500 EH, Netherlands. TEL 31-70-3702613. Circ: 5,400.

BOLLETTINO PER LE FARMACODIPENDENZE E L'ALCOOLISMO. see *DRUG ABUSE AND ALCOHOLISM*

364 GBR ISSN 0007-0955
HV6001 CODEN: BJCDAR
THE BRITISH JOURNAL OF CRIMINOLOGY; delinquency and deviant social behaviour. Text in English. 1950. q. GBP 45, USD 79 to individuals; GBP 133, USD 220 to institutions (effective 2002). adv. bk.rev. abstr, bibl, illus. index. 212 p./no. back issues avail.; reprint service avail. from SWZ,WSH,PSC,SCH. *Refereed.* **Document type:** *Journal, Academic/Scholarly.* **Description:** Focuses on British and international criminology, including social deviance.
Supersedes (in 1960): British Journal of Delinquency
Related titles: Microform ed.; Online - full text ed.: ISSN 1464-3529. GBP 119, USD 198 to institutions Online only (effective 2002) (from Gale Group, Northern Light Technology, Inc., EBSCO Publishing, O C L C Online Computer Library Center, Inc., RoweCom Information Quest, ingenta, Swets Blackwell, Factiva, Institute for Scientific Information).
Indexed: ASCA, ASSIA, Abstr.Crim.& Pen., Addic.Abstr., Adol.Ment.Hlth.Abstr., AgeLine, Br.Educ.Ind., Br.Hum.Ind., CJPI, Crim.Just.Abstr., Curr.Adv.Ecol.Sci., Curr.Cont., ERA, Environ.Sci.Poll.Mgmt., Euro.LJI, IBR, IMFL, Intl.Bibl.Soc.Sci., LJI, L.R.I. (Jan.1980-), Lang.& Lang.Behav.Abstr., Leg.Per. (coverage dropped), Mid.East: Abstr.& Ind., Mult.Ed.Abstr., P C I, P.A.I.S. (coverage dropped), PsycInfo, Psychol.Abstr. (1960-), Risk Abstr., Russ.Acad.Sci.Bibl., SOPODA, SSCI, Saf.Sci.Abstr., Soc.Sci.Ind. (Oct.1982-), Soc.Serv.Abstr., Sociol.Abstr., Stud.Wom.Abstr., e-psyche.
—BLDSC (2307.300000), IDS, ingenta. **CCC.**

C

Published by: (Institute for the Study and Treatment of Delinquency), Oxford University Press, Academic Division, Great Clarendon St, Oxford OX2 6DP, United Kingdom. TEL 44-1865-267907, FAX 44-1865-267835, jnl.info@oup.co.uk, http://www3.oup.co.uk/crimin/, http://www.oup.co.uk/journals. Eds. G Pearson, Richard Sparks. Pub. Martin Green. R&P Fionna Willis. Adv. contact Helen Pearson TEL 44-1235-201904. page GBP 275; trim 150 x 210. Circ: 1,700. **U.S. subscr. to:** Oxford University Press, Journals. TEL 800-852-7323, FAX 919-677-1714, jnlorders@oup-usa.org; **Subscr. to:** Journals Marketing, Great Clarendon St, Oxford OX2 6DP, United Kingdom.

364 302 TTO ISSN 1025-5591
CARIBBEAN JOURNAL OF CRIMINOLOGY & SOCIAL PSYCHOLOGY. Text in English. 1996. s-a. (Jan., July). TTD 130 domestic to individuals; USD 25 foreign to individuals; TTD 170 domestic to institutions; USD 30 foreign to institutions; TTD 70 newsstand/cover domestic to individuals; USD 15 newsstand/cover foreign to individuals; TTD 90 newsstand/cover domestic to institutions; USD 20 newsstand/cover foreign to institutions (effective 2000). adv. bk.rev. *Refereed.* **Document type:** *Academic/Scholarly.* **Description:** Encourages cross-cultural, multidisciplinary research in this area of criminology. Makes policy recommendations both within the Caribbean and worldwide.
Indexed: Crim.Just.Abstr., P.A.I.S., PsycInfo, Soc.Serv.Abstr., Sociol.Abstr., e-psyche.
—BLDSC (3053.029500).
Published by: University of the West Indies, Centre for Criminology & Criminal Justice, St. Augustine Campus, St. Augustine, Trinidad & Tobago. TEL 868-662-2002 ext 3352, FAX 868-645-1020, crimrd@trinidad.net, http://web.carib-link.net/soc-sci/centres/journal.htm. Ed. Ramesh Deosaran. Circ: 121 (paid). **Dist. by:** Gaunt Inc., Gaunt Bldg, 3011 Gulf Dr, Holmes Beach, FL 34217-2199. TEL 800-942-8683, 941-778-5211, 941-778-5252, info@guant.com, http://www.guant.com.

C

COMPOSITE ART MANUAL. see *MEDICAL SCIENCES—Forensic Sciences*

CONTROLLED SUBSTANCES REGULATION. see *DRUG ABUSE AND ALCOHOLISM*

CORHEALTH. see *MEDICAL SCIENCES*

CRIMINAL BEHAVIOUR AND MENTAL HEALTH. see *MEDICAL SCIENCES—Psychiatry And Neurology*

364 150 USA ISSN 0093-8548
HV9261 CODEN: CJBHAB
CRIMINAL JUSTICE & BEHAVIOR. Text in English. 1973. bi-m. USD 70 to individuals; USD 380 to institutions; USD 20 newsstand/cover to individuals; USD 70 newsstand/cover to institutions (effective 2002). adv. bk.rev. illus. index. back issues avail.; reprint service avail. from PSC,PQC,WSH,SCH. *Refereed.* **Document type:** *Academic/Scholarly.* **Description:** Covers criminal justice relating to mental health, personality assessment, and changes. Advances the knowledge and expertise of professionals and academics involved in forensic psychology, with a concentration in correctional psychology.
Supersedes: Correctional Psychologist (0589-8218)
Related titles: Microfiche ed.: (from WSH); Microfilm ed.: (from PQC,WSH,PMC); Online - full text ed.: (from EBSCO Publishing, O C L C Online Computer Library Center, Inc., RoweCom Information Quest, ProQuest Information & Learning, Gale Group, ingenta, Swets Blackwell, Institute for Scientific Information).
Indexed: ASCA, ASSIA, Abstr.Bk.Rev.Curr.Leg.Per., Abstr.Crim.& Pen., AgeLine, C.I.J.E. (coverage dropped), CJPI, C.L.I., Crim.Just.Abstr., Curr.Cont., Environ.Sci.Poll.Mgmt., Excerp.Med., Fam.Ind., Human Resour.Abstr., Ind.Per.Art.Relat.Law, L.R.I. (Mar.1980-), Leg.Cont., Mid.East: Abstr.& Ind., Mult.Ed.Abstr., P.A.I.S. (coverage dropped), Peace Res.Abstr., PsycInfo, Psychol.Abstr. (1974-), Psychol.R.G., Risk Abstr., Russ.Acad.Sci.Bibl., SSCI, Saf.Sci.Abstr., Sage Fam.Stud.Abstr., Sage Pub.Admin.Abstr., Sage Urb.Stud.Abstr., Soc.Sci.Ind. (Nov.1982-), Soc.Serv.Abstr., Sociol.Abstr., Sp.Ed.Needs Abstr., Viol.& Abuse Abstr., e-psyche.
—BLDSC (3487.348000), IDS, ingenta. **CCC.**

Published by: (American Association of Correctional Psychologists), Sage Publications, Inc., 2455 Teller Rd, Thousand Oaks, CA 91320. TEL 818-597-4867, FAX 818-597-4879, info@sagepub.com, http://www.sagepub.co.uk/. Ed. Dr. Curt R Bartol. Pub. Sara Miller McCune. R&P Tanya Udin. Adv. contact DeAnna Vega Hammersley. page USD 275. Circ: 1,950 (paid). **Overseas subscr. to:** Sage Publications Ltd., 6 Bonhill St, London EC2A 4PU, United Kingdom; Sage Publications India Pvt. Ltd., 4215, New Delhi 110 048, India. **Affiliate:** American Correctional Association.

DEVIANT BEHAVIOR. see *SOCIOLOGY*

364 301 150 USA
▼ **DOMESTIC VIOLENCE AND CHILD ABUSE SOURCEBOOK.** Text in English. 1999 (May). irreg., latest 2001. USD 78 per issue (effective 2001). charts, bibl. master index master index. **Description:** Contains basic information about spousal/partner, child, and elder physical, emotional, and sexual abuse, teen dating violence, and stalking. Includes information about hotlines, safe houses, safety plans, and other resources for support and assistance, community initiative, and reports on current directions in research and treatment, along with a glossary, sources for further reading, and governmental and non-governmental organizations contact information.
Published by: Omnigraphics, Inc., 615 Griswold St, Detroit, MI 48226. TEL 313-961-1340, 800-234-1340, FAX 313-961-1383, 800-875-1340, info@omnigraphics.com, http://www.omnigraphics.com. Ed. Helene Henderson.

DRUG DETECTION REPORT; the newsletter on drug testing in the workplace. see *BUSINESS AND ECONOMICS—Personnel Management*

DRUG ENFORCEMENT ADMINISTRATION REGISTRATION FILE - ACTIVE. see *MEDICAL SCIENCES*

EMPLOYEE TESTING & THE LAW; reporting legal, technical, and business developments in employee testing. see *BUSINESS AND ECONOMICS—Personnel Management*

364 USA ISSN 1057-9397
F D A ENFORCEMENT REPORT. (Food and Drug Administration) Text in English. w. USD 97; USD 121.25 foreign (effective 1998). **Document type:** *Government.* **Description:** Lists actions taken in connection with agency regulatory activities.
Related titles: Online - full text ed.: (from Gale Group).
Indexed: Consum.Ind. (1989-).
Published by: U.S. Food and Drug Administration, Office of Public Affairs, 5600 Fishers Ln, Rockville, MD 20857. TEL 301-443-3285. **Subscr. to:** U.S. Government Printing Office, Superintendent of Documents.

363.24 614.19 GBR ISSN 0951-1288
FINGERPRINT WORLD. Text in English. 1975. q. GBP 17 in the European Union to individuals; USD 40 elsewhere to individuals; GBP 20 in the European Union to institutions; USD 60 elsewhere to institutions. adv. bk.rev. **Document type:** *Academic/Scholarly.*
Published by: Fingerprint Society, Merseyside Police, Fingerprint Bureau, Canning Pl., Liverpool, Merseyside L1 8JX, United Kingdom. Ed., R&P Graham Hughes. Adv. contact Steve Mewett. Circ: 1,200. **Subscr. to:** Vivienne Galloway, The Fingerprint Society, 5 Slate Close, Glenfield, Leics LE3 8QQ, United Kingdom.

364.1 USA ISSN 1088-7679
HV6515
HOMICIDE STUDIES; an interdisciplinary & international journal. Text in English. 1997. q. USD 70 to individuals; USD 320 to institutions; USD 25 newsstand/cover to individuals; USD 85 newsstand/cover to institutions (effective 2002). illus. reprints avail. *Refereed.* **Document type:** *Academic/Scholarly.* **Description:** Devoted to the dissemination of information concerning research, public policy and applied knowledge relating to the study of homicide.
Related titles: Online - full text ed.: (from EBSCO Publishing, O C L C Online Computer Library Center, Inc., RoweCom Information Quest, ingenta, Swets Blackwell).
Indexed: Abstr.Soc.Geront., Crim.Just.Abstr., Environ.Sci.Poll.Mgmt., IBZ, Peace Res.Abstr., Pollut.Abstr., Risk Abstr., Saf.Sci.Abstr., Sage Fam.Stud.Abstr., Sage Pub.Admin.Abstr., Sage Urb.Stud.Abstr., Soc.Serv.Abstr., Sociol.Abstr., Viol.& Abuse Abstr.
—BLDSC (4326.177900). **CCC.**

Published by: Sage Publications, Inc., 2455 Teller Rd, Thousand Oaks, CA 91320. TEL 805-499-0721, FAX 805-499-0871, order@sagepub.com, info@sagepub.com, http://www.sagepub.com. Ed. M Dwayne Smith. R&P Tanya Udin. Adv. contact DeAnna Vega Hammersley. **Overseas subscr. to:** Sage Publications Ltd., 6 Bonhill St, London EC2A 4PU, United Kingdom; Sage Publications India Pvt. Ltd., 4215, New Delhi 110 048, India.

INSTITUTO NACIONAL DE MEDICINA LEGAL DE COLOMBIA. REVISTA. see *MEDICAL SCIENCES—Forensic Sciences*

INTERNATIONAL DIRECTORY OF SAFETY, SECURITY AND FIRE FIGHTING EQUIPMENT IMPORTERS. see *BUSINESS AND ECONOMICS—Trade And Industrial Directories*

364.4 USA ISSN 0148-4648
HV5800
INTERNATIONAL DRUG REPORT. Text in English. 1960. q. USD 35 domestic; USD 50 foreign (effective 2001). bk.rev., film rev. charts, stat. index. **Document type:** *Newsletter.*
Supersedes: International Narcotic Conference. Report: Proceedings of Annual Conference (0074-7114); Former titles: International Narcotic Report (0020-806X); International Drug Reporter
Published by: International Narcotic Enforcement Officers Association, 112 State St, Ste 1200, Albany, NY 12207. TEL 518-463-6232. Ed., R&P Celeste Morga. Circ: 10,000.

616.8 364.3 USA ISSN 0306-624X
HV9261 CODEN: IOTCAH
INTERNATIONAL JOURNAL OF OFFENDER THERAPY AND COMPARATIVE CRIMINOLOGY. Text in English. 1957. bi-m. USD 55 to individuals; USD 340 to institutions; USD 20 newsstand/cover to individuals; USD 65 newsstand/cover to institutions (effective 2002). adv. bk.rev. bibl, stat, illus. index, cum.index: 1957-1975. back issues avail.; reprint service avail. from WSH,PSC,SCH. *Refereed.* **Description:** International forum for research, discussion, and treatment of variables associated with crime and delinquency, with an emphasis on the theoretical and clinical treatment of the offender.
Former titles (until 1972): International Journal of Offender Therapy (0020-7497); (until 1966): Journal of Offender Therapy; (until 1961): Association for Psychiatric Treatment of Offenders. Journal
Related titles: Microfilm ed.: (from PQC); Online - full text ed.: (from EBSCO Publishing, O C L C Online Computer Library Center, Inc., RoweCom Information Quest, ProQuest Information & Learning, Gale Group, ingenta, Swets Blackwell, Institute for Scientific Information).
Indexed: ASCA, ASSIA, Abstr.Bk.Rev.Curr.Leg.Per., Abstr.Crim.& Pen., AgeLine, Amer.Bibl.Slavic & E.Eur.Stud., CJPI, C.L.I., Crim.Just.Abstr., Curr.Cont., Environ.Sci.Poll.Mgmt., IBZ, IMFL, Ind.Per.Art.Relat.Law, Ind.Philos., Intl.Bibl.Soc.Sci., L.R.I. (Apr.1980-), Lang.& Lang.Behav.Abstr., Leg.Per. (coverage dropped), Mid.East: Abstr.& Ind., Pollut.Abstr., PsycInfo, Psychol.Abstr. (1967-), Ref.Zh., Risk Abstr., SOPODA, SSCI, Saf.Sci.Abstr., Sage Fam.Stud.Abstr., Sage Urb.Stud.Abstr., Soc.Sci.Ind. (Jan.1994-), Soc.Serv.Abstr., Sociol.Abstr., Viol.& Abuse Abstr., e-psyche.
—BLDSC (4542.424000), GNLM, IDS, Infotrieve, ingenta. **CCC.**
Published by: Sage Publications, Inc., 2455 Teller Rd, Thousand Oaks, CA 91320. TEL 818-597-4867, FAX 818-597-4879, info@sagepub.com, http://www.sagepub.co.uk/. Ed. George Palermo. Pub. Sara Miller McCune. R&P Tanya Udin. Adv. contact DeAnna Vega Hammersley. page USD 225. Circ: 1,000. **Overseas subscr. to:** Sage Publications Ltd., 6 Bonhill St, London EC2A 4PU, United Kingdom; Sage Publications India Pvt. Ltd., 4215, New Delhi 110 048, India.

364.4 USA
INTERNATIONAL NARCOTIC ENFORCEMENT OFFICERS ASSOCIATION DIRECTORY. Text in English. a. membership only. **Document type:** *Directory.*
Published by: International Narcotic Enforcement Officers Association, 112 State St, Ste 1200, Albany, NY 12207. TEL 518-463-6232. Ed. Celeste Morga. Circ: 10,000.

364 USA
INTERNATIONAL SYMPOSIUM ON FINGERPRINT DETECTION AND IDENTIFICATION. PROCEEDINGS. Text in English. irreg. 435 p./no. **Document type:** *Proceedings, Academic/Scholarly.*

Published by: International Association for Identification, c/o Joseph Polski, 2535 Pilot Knob Rd, Ste 117, Mendota Heights, MN 55120-1120. TEL 651-681-8566, FAX 651-681-8443, iaisecty@theiai.org, http://www.theiai.org/. Eds. Eliot Springer, Joseph Almog.

ISSUES IN CHILD ABUSE ACCUSATIONS. see *CHILDREN AND YOUTH—About*

JOURNAL OF ADDICTIONS & OFFENDER COUNSELING. see *PSYCHOLOGY*

JOURNAL OF CLINICAL FORENSIC MEDICINE. see *MEDICAL SCIENCES—Forensic Sciences*

JOURNAL OF CORRECTIONAL HEALTH CARE. see *MEDICAL SCIENCES*

306.85 USA ISSN 0885-7482
HQ809 CODEN: JFVIEV

JOURNAL OF FAMILY VIOLENCE. Text in English. 1986. q. USD 418, EUR 417 to institutions for print or online ed.; USD 501.60, EUR 500.40 to institutions for print & online eds. combined. (effective 2002). adv. bk.rev. illus. Index. back issues avail.; reprints avail. *Refereed.* **Document type:** *Journal, Academic/Scholarly.* **Description:** Examines clinical and investigative efforts concerning all forms of family violence; includes case studies and reviews.
Related titles: Microfilm ed.: (from PQC); Online - full text ed.: (from EBSCO Publishing, O C L C Online Computer Library Center, Inc., RoweCom Information Quest, Gale Group, Swets Blackwell, Kluwer Online, Factiva, Institute for Scientific Information).
Indexed: ASCA, ASSIA, Abstr.Soc.Geront., AgeLine, Crim.Just.Abstr., Curr.Cont., Environ.Sci.Poll.Mgmt., Fam.Ind., IBZ, IMFL, Ind.Per.Art.Relat.Law, Ind.Philos., Intl.Bibl.Soc.Sci., Lang.& Lang.Behav.Abstr., Peace Res.Abstr., Pollut.Abstr., PsycInfo, Psychol.Abstr. (1986-), Rel.Ind.One, Rel.Ind.Two, Risk Abstr., Russ.Acad.Sci.Bibl., SOPODA, SSCI, Saf.Sci.Abstr., Sage Fam.Stud.Abstr., Sage Urb.Stud.Abstr., Soc.Sci.Ind. (Jan.1994-), Soc.Serv.Abstr., Sociol.Abstr., Viol.& Abuse Abstr., e-psyche.
—BLDSC (4983.746000), IDS, Infotrieve, ingenta. **CCC.**
Published by: Kluwer Academic - Plenum Publishers (Subsidiary of: Wolters Kluwer N.V.), 233 Spring St, New York, NY 10013-1578. TEL 212-620-8000, 800-221-9369, FAX 212-463-0742, info@plenum.com, http://www.wkap.nl/journalhome.htm/0885-7482. Eds. Michel Hersen, Vincent B Van Hasselt. R&P Rose Luongo TEL 781-871-6311. **Subscr. outside the Americas to:** Kluwer Academic Publishers Group, Journals Department, PO Box 322, Dordrecht 3300 AH, Netherlands. TEL 31-78-639-2392, FAX 31-78-654-6474.

364 USA ISSN 0886-2605
WMLC 93/799

JOURNAL OF INTERPERSONAL VIOLENCE; concerned with the study and treatment of victims and perpetrators of physical and sexual violence. Text in English. 1986. m. USD 145 to individuals; USD 550 to institutions; USD 20 newsstand/cover to individuals; USD 60 newsstand/cover to institutions (effective 2002). adv. illus. Index. back issues avail.; reprints avail. *Refereed.* **Document type:** *Academic/Scholarly.* **Description:** Provides a forum for the discussion of the concerns and activities of professionals and researchers working in domestic violence, child sexual abuse, rape and sexual assault, physical child abuse, and other violent crimes.
Related titles: Online - full text ed.: (from EBSCO Publishing, O C L C Online Computer Library Center, Inc., RoweCom Information Quest, ProQuest Information & Learning, Gale Group, ingenta, Swets Blackwell, Institute for Scientific Information).
Indexed: ASCA, ASSIA, Abstr.Crim.& Pen., Abstr.Soc.Geront., Addic.Abstr., AgeLine, C.I.J.E., CJPI, Crim.Just.Abstr., Curr.Cont., Environ.Sci.Poll.Mgmt., Fam.Ind., IBZ, IMFL, Int.Nurs.Ind., Lang.& Lang.Behav.Abstr., Mult.Ed.Abstr., PsycInfo, Psychol.Abstr. (1986-), Risk Abstr., Russ.Acad.Sci.Bibl., SOPODA, SSCI, Saf.Sci.Abstr., Sage Fam.Stud.Abstr., Sage Race Rel.Abstr., Soc.Sci.Ind. (Jan.1994-), Soc.Serv.Abstr., Soc.Work Res.& Abstr., Sociol.Abstr., Sp.Ed.Needs Abstr., Stud.Wom.Abstr., Viol.& Abuse Abstr., e-psyche.
—BLDSC (5007.693500), IDS, Infotrieve, ingenta. **CCC.**
Published by: Sage Publications, Inc., 2455 Teller Rd, Thousand Oaks, CA 91320. TEL 818-597-4867, FAX 818-597-4879, info@sagepub.com, http://www.sagepub.com. Ed. Jon R Conte. Pub. Sara Miller McCune. R&P Tanya Udin. Adv. contact DeAnna Vega Hammersley. page USD 275. Circ: 3,250 (paid). **Overseas subscr. to:** Sage Publications Ltd., 6 Bonhill St, London EC2A 4PU, United Kingdom. TEL 44-20-7374-0645, FAX 44-20-7374-8741; Sage Publications India Pvt. Ltd., 4215, New Delhi 110 048, India. TEL 91-11-641-9884, FAX 91-11-647-2426.

364 362.8 USA ISSN 1050-9674
HV9261 CODEN: JOFHEB

JOURNAL OF OFFENDER REHABILITATION; a multidisciplinary journal of innovation in research, services, and programs in corrections and criminal justice. Text in English. 1976. q. USD 75 to individuals; USD 101 in Canada to individuals; USD 109 elsewhere to individuals; USD 150 to institutions; USD 203 in Canada to institutions; USD 218 elsewhere to institutions; USD 300 to libraries; USD 405 in Canada to libraries; USD 435 elsewhere to libraries (effective Aug. 2001). adv. bk.rev. illus. index. back issues avail.; reprint service avail. from HAW. *Refereed.* **Document type:** *Journal, Academic/Scholarly.* **Description:** Publishes research and concepts on the rehabilitation of criminal offenders, both in custodial and community settings.
Former titles (until 1990): Journal of Offender Counseling, Services and Rehabilitation (0195-6116); (until 1980): Offender Rehabilitation (0364-3093)
Related titles: Microfiche ed.: (from PQC); Microform ed.; Online - full text ed.: (from Gale Group).
Indexed: Abstr.Crim.& Pen., Adol.Ment.Hlth.Abstr., Alt.Press Ind., Behav.Abstr., CERDIC, C.I.J.E., CJPI, Chic.Per.Ind., Chicago Psychoanal.Lit.Ind., Crim.Just.Abstr., Curr.Cont. (coverage dropped), Environ.Sci.Poll.Mgmt., Human Resour.Abstr., IBZ, IMFL, Lang.& Lang.Behav.Abstr., Past.Care & Couns.Abstr., Peace Res.Abstr., Pollut.Abstr., Psychol.Abstr. (1976-), Ref.Zh., Risk Abstr., SOPODA, Saf.Sci.Abstr., Sage Fam.Stud.Abstr., Sage Pub.Admin.Abstr., Sage Urb.Stud.Abstr., Soc.Sci.Ind. (Jul.1999-), Soc.Serv.Abstr., Soc.Work Res.& Abstr., Sociol.Abstr., Stud.Wom.Abstr., Viol.& Abuse Abstr., e-psyche.
—BLDSC (5026.218000), Haworth, ingenta.
Published by: Haworth Press, Inc., 10 Alice St, Binghamton, NY 13904-1580. TEL 607-722-5857, 800-429-6784, FAX 607-722-6362, 800-895-0582, getinfo@haworthpressinc.com, http://www.haworthpress.com/journals/journallist.asp. Ed. Nathaniel J Pallone. Pub. William Cohen. R&P Ruthann Heath TEL 607-723-5857 ext 316. Adv. contact Jackie Blakeslee TEL 607-722-5857 ext 346. B&W page USD 315, color page USD 550; trim 6 x 8.5. Circ: 450.

364 USA ISSN 0882-0783
HV6001

JOURNAL OF POLICE AND CRIMINAL PSYCHOLOGY. Text in English. 1985. s-a. USD 50 to individuals; USD 75 to institutions (effective 2000). *Refereed.* **Document type:** *Academic/Scholarly.*
Related titles: Microfilm ed.: (from PQC).
Indexed: CJPI, Crim.Just.Abstr., Curr.Lit.Traf.& Trans., e-psyche.
—ingenta.
Published by: Society of Police and Criminal Psychology, c/o Dr Wayman Mullins, Southwest Texas State University, Hines Academic Center, Rm 120, San Marcos, TX 78666. TEL 512-245-2174, FAX 512-245-8063. R&P Wayman C Mullins. Circ: 200.

JOURNAL OF SEXUAL AGGRESSION. see *PSYCHOLOGY*

LEGAL AND CRIMINOLOGICAL PSYCHOLOGY. see *PSYCHOLOGY*

NARC OFFICER. see *LAW*

363.23 USA

NATIONAL LAW ENFORCEMENT AND CORRECTIONS TECHNOLOGY NEWS SUMMARY. Text in English. 1998. w. back issues avail. **Document type:** *Government.* **Description:** Provides a service to law enforcement, corrections, and forensic science practitioners.
Media: Online - full text.
Published by: National Law Enforcement and Corrections Technology Center, PO Box 1160, Rockville, MD 20849-1160. TEL 800-148-2742, dengler@nlectc.org, http://www.nlectc.org/inthenews/NewsSummary/weeklynews.html. Ed. Donna Engler.

080 362.127 USA ISSN 0197-7024
HV8078.A1

POLYGRAPH. Text in English. 1972. q. USD 80 domestic; USD 100 foreign (effective 2001 - 2002). adv. bk.rev. charts. index. reprint service avail. from PQC. **Document type:** *Academic/Scholarly.* **Description:** Discusses forensic psychophysiology, polygraph operations, research, history, psychology, physiology, instrumentation, law notes, abstracts, and training.
Supersedes: American Polygraph Association. Journal (0003-0562)
Related titles: Microfilm ed.: (from PQC).
Indexed: Abstr.Crim.& Pen., Art & Archaeol.Tech.Abstr., CJPI, Crim.Just.Abstr., Paper & Bd.Abstr., e-psyche.
Published by: (American Polygraph Association), Sheridan Press, PO Box 8037, Chattanooga, TN 37414-0037. TEL 423-892-3992, 800-272-8037. Ed. Donald Krapohl. R&P, Adv. contact Robbie Bennett. Circ: 3,500.

PSYCHOLOGY, CRIME AND LAW. see *PSYCHOLOGY*

PUBLIC SAFETY AND JUSTICE POLICIES - STATE CAPITALS. see *LAW*

363.24 614.19 GBR ISSN 0951-645X

RIDGE DETAIL IN NATURE. Text in English. 1979. a. USD 5. **Document type:** *Trade.*
Published by: Fingerprint Society, Merseyside Police, Fingerprint Bureau, Canning Pl., Liverpool, Merseyside L1 8JX, United Kingdom. Ed. John Berry. Circ: 100. **Subscr. to:** The Fingerprint Society, Vivienne Galloway, 5 Slate Close, Glenfield, Leicester LE3 8QQ, United Kingdom.

SEXUAL ABUSE; a journal of research and treatment. see *PSYCHOLOGY*

364 158.7 USA

STRESS MANAGEMENT FOR LAW ENFORCEMENT; behind the shield: combating trauma. Text in English. 199?. irreg., latest 1999. USD 19.95 (effective 2000). **Document type:** *Trade.* **Description:** Handbook covering stress and trauma associated with the law enforcement and criminal justice professional. Includes related topics dealing with this growing problem.
Published by: Gould Publications, Inc., 1333 N US Hwy 17 92, Longwood, FL 32750-3724. TEL 800-717-7917, FAX 407-695-2906, info@gouldlaw.com, http://www.gouldlaw.com. Ed. Peter Pranzo.

364 USA ISSN 0361-5170
HV6250

VICTIMOLOGY; an international journal. Text in English. 1976. irreg., latest 1996 (vols.11-13). USD 115 (effective 1996). adv. bk.rev. back issues avail. **Document type:** *Academic/Scholarly.*
Indexed: Abstr.Crim.& Pen., Adol.Ment.Hlth.Abstr., CJPI, C.L.I., Chicago Psychoanal.Lit.Ind., Crim.Just.Abstr., Hlth.Ind., IBR, L.R.I. (Mar.1980-Jan.1985), Leg.Cont., Mid.East: Abstr.& Ind., P C I, P.A.I.S., Past.Care & Couns.Abstr., Psychol.Abstr., Russ.Acad.Sci.Bibl., Soc.Sci.Ind. (1983-, dropped), Sociol.Abstr., Stud.Wom.Abstr., Viol.& Abuse Abstr., e-psyche.
—Infotrieve. **CCC.**
Published by: (National Institute of Victimology), Victimology, Inc., 2333 N Vernon St, Arlington, VA 22207. TEL 703-528-3387. Ed. Emilio C Viano. Circ: 2,000.

VIOLENCE AND VICTIMS. see *SOCIOLOGY*

WOUND BALLISTICS REVIEW. see *MEDICAL SCIENCES—Forensic Sciences*

WUJING YIXUE/MEDICAL JOURNAL OF THE CHINESE PEOPLE'S ARMED POLICE FORCES. see *MEDICAL SCIENCES*

CRIMINOLOGY AND LAW ENFORCEMENT—Abstracting, Bibliographies, Statistics

364 614.19 USA

CRIMINALIST'S SOURCE BOOK. Text in English. a. USD 25.
Published by: International Reference Organization in Forensic Medicine & Sciences, PO Box 8282, Wichita, KS 67208. TEL 316-685-7612.

CRIMINOLOGY AND LAW ENFORCEMENT—Security

see also COMPUTERS—Computer Security

C

GUIDE TO HEALTH DATA SECURITY. see *MEDICAL SCIENCES—Computer Applications*

HEALTHCARE DATA SECURITY MANUAL. see *HEALTH FACILITIES AND ADMINISTRATION*

364.4 USA ISSN 0745-1148
HOSPITAL SECURITY AND SAFETY MANAGEMENT. Text in English. 1980. m. USD 249 domestic; USD 274 foreign (effective 2001). tr.lit. back issues avail.; reprints avail. **Document type:** *Newsletter.* **Description:** Newsletter on hospital security and safety management for security directors at hospitals and medical centers.
Indexed: Int.Nurs.Ind.
Published by: Rusting Publications, PO Box 190, Port Washington, NY 11050. TEL 516-883-1440, FAX 516-883-1683, rustingpubs@aol.com, www.rustingpubs.com. Eds. Robert R Rusting, Susan Krivin. Circ: 1,200.

364.4 613 IRL
IRISH SECURITY NEWS. Text in English. 3/yr.
Published by: Security Media, Baldoyle, PO Box 1822, Dublin 13, Ireland. TEL 391115, FAX 735934. Ed. Fionnuala Tattersall. Circ: 3,000.

JOURNAL OF HEALTHCARE PROTECTION MANAGEMENT. see *HEALTH FACILITIES AND ADMINISTRATION*

SAFETY REMINDER. see *OCCUPATIONAL HEALTH AND SAFETY*

363.22 DEU ISSN 0937-2555
SCHUTZ AKTUELL; magazin fuer sicherheit. Text in German. 1986. q. DEM 30. adv. bk.rev. back issues avail. **Document type:** *Consumer.*
Formerly: Katastrophenschutz Aktuell (0930-1240)
Published by: Thome Verlag GmbH, Goethestr 21, Munich 80336, Germany. TEL 089-591964, FAX 089-553079. Ed. Angela Christiane Grond. Adv. contact Doris Tegethoff. Circ: 6,500.

364.4 GBR
SECURITY SPECIFIER. Text in English. 1984. 6/yr. GBP 24 (effective 2000). **Document type:** *Trade.*
Published by: Specifiers Journals Ltd, 32 Portland St, Cheltenham, Glos GL52 2PB, United Kingdom. TEL 44-1242-583222, FAX 44-1242-222331. Ed. D G Constantine. Adv. contact Christopher Musk. Circ: 14,803.

D

CROP PRODUCTION AND SOIL

see AGRICULTURE—Crop Production And Soil

CRYSTALLOGRAPHY

see CHEMISTRY—Crystallography

CYTOLOGY AND HISTOLOGY

see BIOLOGY—Cytology And Histology

DAIRYING AND DAIRY PRODUCTS

see AGRICULTURE—Dairying And Dairy Products

DANCE

see also MUSIC; THEATER

A D T A NEWSLETTER. see *MEDICAL SCIENCES—Physical Medicine And Rehabilitation*

793.33 USA
ABILITY BALLROOM DANCE JOURNAL✶. Text in English. q. USD 25. **Description:** Covers news, interviews, sports medicine and health products.
Published by: World Dance and Dance Sport Council, 301 W 55th St, Ste 4, New York, NY 10019-4532. Ed. Richard Diaz.

AEROBIC BEAT. see *PHYSICAL FITNESS AND HYGIENE*

AMERICAN DANCE THERAPY ASSOCIATION. (NO.) ANNUAL CONFERENCE PROCEEDINGS. see *MEDICAL SCIENCES—Physical Medicine And Rehabilitation*

792.8 USA ISSN 0146-3721
RC489.D3
AMERICAN JOURNAL OF DANCE THERAPY. Text in English. 1968. s-a. USD 256, EUR 256 to institutions for print or online ed.; USD 50, EUR 50 to individuals for print or online ed.; USD 307.20, EUR 307.20 to institutions for print and online eds. combined (effective 2002). adv. bk.rev. abstr, bibl, illus. Index. back issues avail.; reprint service avail. from PSC,SCH. *Refereed.* **Document type:** *Journal, Academic/Scholarly.* **Description:** Covers clinical use of dance therapy, theoretical considerations which provide a framework for dance therapy intervention, and research in dance therapy.
Supersedes (in 1977): American Dance Therapy Association. Monograph
Related titles: Online - full text ed.: NLG 517, EUR 234.50 to institutions; NLG 620.40, EUR 281.40 to institutions for online & print edition (effective 2001) (from EBSCO Publishing, O C L C Online Computer Library Center, Inc., Swets Blackwell, Kluwer Online, RoweCom Information Quest).
Indexed: ASCA, AgeLine, Arts & Hum.Cit.Ind. (coverage dropped), Curr.Cont. (coverage dropped), Excerp.Med., Fam.Ind., IIPA, Ind.Dance Per., PsycInfo, Psychol.Abstr. (1977-), SSCI (coverage dropped), e-psyche.
—BLDSC (0824.220000), GNLM, IDS, Infotrieve, ingenta. **CCC.**
Published by: (American Dance Therapy Association), Kluwer Academic - Human Sciences Press (Subsidiary of: Wolters Kluwer N.V.), 233 Spring St, New York, NY 10013-1578. TEL 212-620-8000, FAX 212-807-1047, info@plenum.com, http://www.wkap.nl/journalhome.htm/0146-3721, http://www.kluweronline.nl.

CONTRIBUTIONS TO THE STUDY OF MUSIC AND DANCE. see *MUSIC*

DANCE MEDICINE - HEALTH NEWSLETTER. see *MEDICAL SCIENCES—Physical Medicine And Rehabilitation*

I D E A FITNESS MANAGER. see *PHYSICAL FITNESS AND HYGIENE*

MEDICAL PROBLEMS OF PERFORMING ARTISTS. see *MEDICAL SCIENCES*

DATA COMMUNICATIONS AND DATA TRANSMISSION SYSTEMS

see COMPUTERS—Data Communications And Data Transmission Systems

DENTISTRY

see MEDICAL SCIENCES—Dentistry

▼ **DENTIST'S MONEY DIGEST.** see *BUSINESS AND ECONOMICS—Banking And Finance*

DERMATOLOGY AND VENEREOLOGY

see MEDICAL SCIENCES—Dermatology And Venereology

DOMESTIC COMMERCE

see BUSINESS AND ECONOMICS—Domestic Commerce

DRUG ABUSE AND ALCOHOLISM

see also PHARMACY AND PHARMACOLOGY

616.86 USA
A D A M H A NEWS. (Alcohol, Drug Abuse, and Mental Health Administration) Text in English. 1976. bi-m. USD 6.
Indexed: Ind.U.S.Gov.Per., MEDOC, Med.Care Rev., e-psyche.
Published by: U.S. Department of Health and Human Services, Alcohol, Drug Abuse, and Mental Health Administration, Parklawn Bldg, Rm 13C 05, 5600 Fishers Ln, Rockville, MD 20857. TEL 301-443-0746, FAX 301-443-9050. Eds. Bernardine A Moore, Deborah Goodman. Circ: 12,000.

616.86 USA
A S A M NEWS. Text in English. 1985. bi-m. USD 50 to non-members. adv. bk.rev. *Refereed.* **Document type:** *Newsletter.* **Description:** Covers health care reform; current information related to alcohol, tobacco, and other addicting drugs; association news.
Formerly: American Medical Society on Alcoholism and Other Drug Dependencies. Newsletter (0889-9215)
Related titles: Online - full text ed.
Published by: American Society of Addiction Medicine, 4601 N Park Ave, Ste U101, Chevy Chase, MD 20815-4519. TEL 703-538-2285, FAX 703-536-6186, bbwilford@aol.com, http://www.asam.org. Ed., R&P Bonnie B Wilford. Adv. contact Dennis Matos. Circ: 3,200.

616.86 CHE ISSN 1420-2999
ABHAENGIGKEITEN. Text in German. 1995. 3/yr. CHF 45 domestic to individuals; DEM 59 in Germany to individuals; CHF 50 elsewhere to individuals; CHF 63 domestic to institutions; DEM 83 in Germany to institutions; CHF 68 elsewhere to institutions; CHF 20 newsstand/cover domestic; DEM 30 newsstand/cover in Germany; CHF 25 newsstand/cover elsewhere (effective 2001). adv. bk.rev. abstr, bibl. *Refereed.* **Document type:** *Bulletin, Consumer.* **Description:** Provides experts and other interested people with results of the latest research and information on the prevention and treatment of alcoholism and other addictions.
Formed by the merger of (1977-1995): Drogalkohol (0250-6815); (1932-1995): Suchtprobleme und Sozialarbeit (1420-3065); Which was formerly (until 1980): Fuersorger (0016-3139)
Indexed: Ref.Zh.
—GNLM.
Published by: Schweizerische Fachstelle fuer Alkohol- und Andere Drogenprobleme, Postfach 870, Lausanne 1010, Switzerland. TEL 41-21-3212976, FAX 41-21-3212940, hfahrenkrug@sfa-ispa.ch, http://www-sfa-ispa.ch. Ed. Hermann Fahrenkrug. Adv. contact Madelene Gentil. Circ: 1,100.

616.86 157.63 SWE ISSN 0345-0406
ACCENT. Text in Swedish. 1879. 12/yr. SEK 175 (effective 2001). adv. bk.rev. **Document type:** *Magazine, Consumer.*
Formerly (until 1974): Accent, Unga Tankar
Published by: I O G T - N T O, U N F, S L N, Stora Essingen, Gammelgaerdsvaegen 38-42, Stockholm 10536, Sweden. TEL 46-8-6726000, FAX 46-8-6726001, accent@iogt.se, info@iogt.se, http://www.iogt.se. Ed. Eva Aahlstroem. adv.: color page SEK 10,500; trim 210 x 275. Circ: 44,500 (controlled).

616.86 GBR ISSN 0965-2140
HV5800 CODEN: ADICE5
ADDICTION. Text in English. 1884. m., latest vol.97, 2002. GBP 220 in Europe to individuals for paper ed.; USD 349 in North America to individuals for paper ed.; GBP 242 rest of world to individuals for paper ed.; GBP 702 in Europe to institutions for paper ed.; USD 1,114 in North America to institutions for paper ed.; GBP 773 elsewhere to institutions for paper ed. (effective 2002). adv. bk.rev. charts, illus, stat. index. back issues avail. *Refereed.* **Document type:** *Journal, Academic/Scholarly.*
Former titles (until 1993): British Journal of Addiction (0952-0481); (until 1980): British Journal of Addiction to Alcohol and Other Drugs (0007-0890); (until 1947): British Journal of Inebriety (0366-0796)
Related titles: Microfiche ed.; Online - full text ed.: ISSN 1360-0443. GBP 198 in Europe to individuals; USD 315 in North America to individuals; GBP 198 elsewhere to individuals; GBP 632 in Europe to institutions; USD 1,003 in North America to institutions; GBP 632 elsewhere to institutions (effective 2002) (from CatchWord Ltd., Northern Light Technology, Inc., EBSCO Publishing, O C L C Online Computer Library Center, Inc., RoweCom Information Quest, ProQuest Information & Learning, Swets Blackwell, Institute for Scientific Information).
Indexed: ASCA, ASSIA, Abstr.Crim.& Pen., Abstr.Hyg., Addic.Abstr., Adol.Ment.Hlth.Abstr., AgeLine, Arts & Hum.Cit.Ind. (coverage dropped), Biol.Abstr., Brit.Nur.Ind., Chem.Abstr., Crim.Just.Abstr., Curr.Adv.Ecol.Sci., Curr.Cont., ERA, Environ.Sci.Poll.Mgmt., Excerp.Med., Fam.Ind., IMFL, I.P.A., Ind.Med. (1993-), Ind.Sci.Rev., Indian Psychol.Abstr., Inpharma, Intl.Bibl.Soc.Sci., Lang.& Lang.Behav.Abstr., Mid.East: Abstr.& Ind., Mult.Ed.Abstr., NRN, Nutr.Abstr., Pharm.&Out.News, Pollut.Abstr., PsycInfo, Psychol.Abstr. (1971-), Reac., Ref.Zh., Risk Abstr., Rural Recreat.Tour.Abstr., SOPODA, SSCI, Saf.Sci.Abstr., Sci.Cit.Ind., Soc.Serv.Abstr., Sociol.Abstr., Sp.Ed.Needs Abstr., Stud.Wom.Abstr., THA, Trop.Dis.Bull., e-psyche.

—BLDSC (0678.548000), ADONIS, CatchWord, EMDOCS, GNLM, IDS, ingenta, KNAW. **CCC.**

Published by: (Society for the Study of Addiction), Blackwell Science Ltd., PO Box 88, Oxford OX2 0NE, United Kingdom. TEL 44-1865-206180, 44-1865-206002, FAX 44-1865-206219, jnl.orders@blacksci.co.uk, http://www.blackwell-science.com/~cgilib/jnlpage.asp?Journal=add&File=add, http://www.blackwellpublishing.com.

616.86 GBR ISSN 0968-7610

ADDICTION ABSTRACTS. Text in English. 1994. q. USD 252, GBP 153 to individuals; USD 524, GBP 318 to institutions (effective 2002). adv. index. **Document type:** *Abstract/Index.*

Related titles: Microfiche ed.; Online - full content ed.: ISSN 1469-2856 (from Swets Blackwell); Online - full text ed.: ISSN 1469-2856 (from ProQuest Information & Learning).

—CCC.

Published by: Carfax Publishing Limited (Subsidiary of: Taylor & Francis Group), PO Box 25, Abingdon, Oxon OX14 3UE, United Kingdom. TEL 44-1235-401000, FAX 44-1235-401550, enquiries@carfax.co.uk, enquiry@tandf.co.uk, http://www.carfax.co.uk. Ed. Mike Gossop.

616.86 GBR ISSN 1355-6215
RC563 CODEN: ADBIFN

ADDICTION BIOLOGY. Text in English. 1996. q. USD 256, GBP 157 to individuals; USD 566, GBP 343 to institutions (effective 2002). *Refereed.* **Document type:** *Academic/Scholarly.*

Related titles: Online - full text ed.: ISSN 1369-1600 (from CatchWord Ltd., Northern Light Technology, Inc., EBSCO Publishing, O C L C Online Computer Library Center, Inc., RoweCom Information Quest, ProQuest Information & Learning, Swets Blackwell, Institute for Scientific Information).

Indexed: Cal.Tiss.Abstr., Curr.Cont., Environ.Sci.Poll.Mgmt., Focus on: Psychophar., Inpharma, Neurosci.Abstr., Neurosci.Cit.Ind., Pharm.&Out.News, Pollut.Abstr., Reac., Ref.Zh., Risk Abstr., Rural Recreat.Tour.Abstr., Saf.Sci.Abstr., Tox.Abstr.

—BLDSC (0678.557000), ADONIS, CASDDS, CatchWord, GNLM, IDS, Infotrieve, KNAW. **CCC.**

Published by: Carfax Publishing Limited (Subsidiary of: Taylor & Francis Group), PO Box 25, Abingdon, Oxon OX14 3UE, United Kingdom. TEL 44-1235-401000, FAX 44-1235-401550, enquiries@carfax.co.uk, enquiry@tandf.co.uk, http://www.carfax.co.uk.

616.86 CHE ISSN 1058-6989
CODEN: AREREQ

ADDICTION RESEARCH AND THEORY. Text in English. 1993. 6/yr. GBP 96, USD 117 to individuals; GBP 228, USD 300 to corporations (effective 2002). *Refereed.* **Document type:** *Journal, Academic/Scholarly.* **Description:** Cross-disciplinary journal examining the effects of context on the use and misuse of substances, and on the nature of intoxications of all kinds.

Related titles: Microform ed.

Indexed: Addic.Abstr., AgeLine, Crim.Just.Abstr., Curr.Cont., Fam.Ind., Lang.& Lang.Behav.Abstr., PsycInfo, SOPODA, SSCI, Soc.Serv.Abstr., Sociol.Abstr., e-psyche.

—BLDSC (0678.590000), GNLM, Infotrieve. **CCC.**

Published by: Gordon and Breach - Harwood Academic (Subsidiary of: Taylor & Francis Group), PO Box 531, Lausanne 1000, Switzerland. TEL 41-21-6411280, FAX 41-21-6411281, info@gbhap.com, http://www.gbhap.com. Eds. E Drucker, J B Davies. **Subscr. addr. in US:** International Publishers Direct, PO Box 32160, Newark, NJ 07102. FAX 215-750-6343.

616.86 USA

ADDICTION TREATMENT FORUM. Text in English. 1994. q. **Document type:** *Newsletter.* **Description:** For addiction treatment community - both professionals and patients. Focuses on opiate addiction and the benefits of methadone treatment.

Media: Online - full text.

Address: 1759 E Golf Rd, Ste 320, Schaumburg, IL 60173. http://www.atforum.com/.

616.86 GBR ISSN 0306-4603
RC565

ADDICTIVE BEHAVIORS; an international journal. Text in English. 1976. bi-m. EUR 147 in Europe to individuals; JPY 19,500 in Japan to individuals; USD 165 elsewhere to individuals; EUR 916 in Europe to institutions; JPY 121,600 in Japan to institutions; USD 1,025 elsewhere to institutions (effective 2002); NLG 2,157, EUR 978.80 in Europe to institutions Includes Eating Behaviors; JPY 135,000 in Japan to institutions Includes Eating Behaviors; USD 1,104 elsewhere to institutions Includes Eating Behaviors (effective 2001). adv. bk.rev. charts, illus. index. reprint service avail. from PSC,SCH. *Refereed.* **Document type:** *Academic/Scholarly.* **Description:** Publishes original research and theoretical papers in the area of substance abuse, with particular emphasis on alcohol and drug abuse, smoking and problems associated with eating.

Incorporates (1990-1994): Annual Review of Addictions Research and Treatment (0955-663X)

Related titles: Microform ed.: (from PQC); Online - full text ed.: (from ingenta, Gale Group, Swets Blackwell, ScienceDirect, Factiva, Institute for Scientific Information).

Indexed: ASCA, Abstr.Anthropol., Abstr.Crim.& Pen., Addic.Abstr., Adol.Ment.Hlth.Abstr., AgeLine, Behav.Med.Abstr., Bibl.Ind., Biol.Abstr., Chic.Per.Ind., Curr.Adv.Ecol.Sci., Curr.Cont., Dairy Sci.Abstr., Environ.Sci.Poll.Mgmt., Excerp.Med., Fam.Ind., HRIS, High.Educ.Abstr., Ind.Med. (1975-), Int.Nurs.Ind., Mid.East: Abstr.& Ind., Nutr.Abstr., PsycInfo, Psychol.Abstr. (1976-), Risk Abstr., Rural Recreat.Tour.Abstr., SSCI, Saf.Sci.Abstr., Soc.Sci.Ind. (Jan.1994-), e-psyche.

—BLDSC (0678.750000), CISTI, EMDOCS, GNLM, IDS, Infotrieve, ingenta, KNAW. **CCC.**

Published by: Pergamon (Subsidiary of: Elsevier Science), The Boulevard, Langford Ln, East Park, Kidlington, Oxford OXB 1GB, United Kingdom. FAX 44-1865-843010, nlinfo-f@elsevier/nl; usinfo-f@elsevier.com; forinfo-kyf04035@niftyserve.or.jp, http://www.elsevier.com/locate/addictbeh. Ed. Peter M Miller. Circ: 1,200. **Subscr. in Australasia and the Far East to:** Elsevier Science (Singapore) Pte Ltd, No.1 Temasek Ave, 17-01 Millenia Tower, Singapore 039192, Singapore. TEL 65-434-3727, FAX 65-337-2230; **Subscr. in the Americas to:** Elsevier Science, PO Box 945, New York, NY 10159-0945. TEL 212-633-3730, FAX 212-633-3680, usinfo-f@elsevier.com; **Subscr. to:** Elsevier Science BV, PO Box 211, Amsterdam 1000 AE, Netherlands. TEL 31-20-485-3757, FAX 31-20-485-3432, nlinfo-f@elsevier.nl.

362.29 USA ISSN 1531-5754

ADDICTIVE DISORDERS & THEIR TREATMENT. Text in English. q. USD 76 in North America to individuals; USD 80 elsewhere to individuals; USD 157 in North America to institutions; USD 161 elsewhere to institutions; USD 39 newsstand/cover (effective 2002). bk.rev. *Refereed.* **Document type:** *Journal, Academic/Scholarly.* **Description:** Devoted to practical clinical research and treatment issues related to the misuse of alcohol and licit and illicit drugs and the study and treatment of addictive disorders and their behaviors.

Related titles: Online - full text ed.: USD 195 academic site license; USD 217.50 corporate site license (effective 2002).

Published by: Lippincott Williams & Wilkins (Philadelphia) (Subsidiary of: Wolters Kluwer N.V.), 530 Walnut St, Philadelphia, PA 19106-3621. TEL 215-521-8300, FAX 215-521-8902, custserv@lww.com, http://www.addictiondisorders.com, http://www.lww.com/. Ed. Dr. Pedro Ruiz. **Subscr. to:** PO Box 1600, Hagerstown, MD 21740-1600. TEL 800-638-3030, FAX 310-223-2400.

616.8 ESP ISSN 0214-4840

ADICCIONES. Text in Spanish. 1989. q. ESP 6,000, EUR 36 domestic to individuals; USD 55, EUR 55 foreign to individuals; ESP 14,000, EUR 84 domestic to institutions; USD 123, EUR 123 foreign to institutions (effective 2002). adv. bk.rev. *Refereed.* **Document type:** *Academic/Scholarly.* **Description:** Journal on drug issues for Spanish-speaking audience.

Indexed: Addic.Abstr., Excerp.Med. (1994-).

—BLDSC (0681.401000), CINDOC, EMDOCS.

Published by: Socidrogalcohol, La Rambla, 15, 2a 3a, Palma De Mallorca, Baleares 07003, Spain. TEL 34-97-1727434, FAX 34-97-1213306, adicciones@socidrogalcohol.org. Ed., R&P, Adv. contact Amador Calafat. Circ: 2,000.

AKTION JUGENDSCHUTZ. INFORMATIONEN. see *CHILDREN AND YOUTH—About*

616.86 SWE

AKTUELLT. Text in Swedish. 1922. 4/yr. SEK 95 (effective 2001). adv. bk.rev. illus. **Document type:** *Newspaper.* **Description:** Presents articles on social work from a Christian perspective.

Former titles (until 1996): Drogfritt Liv (1101-7015); (until vol.5, 1989): Folkets Vael (0015-5861)

Published by: Hela Manniskan, Sundbyberg 17299, Sweden. TEL 46-8-453-68-50, FAX 46-8-453-68-60. Ed. Carl Johan Friman. Pub. Karin Israelsson. Circ: 7,000.

616.861 USA ISSN 1054-1446

AL-ANON SPEAKS OUT; a community resource for professionals. Text in English, Spanish, French. 1978. s-a. free. **Document type:** *Newsletter.* **Description:** Informs members of the helping professions about the help available to the families and friends of alcoholics through Al-Anon - Alateen program.

Published by: (Al-Anon Family Group Headquarters, Inc.), A F G, Inc., 1600 Corporate Landing Pkwy, Virginia Beach, VA 23454-5617. TEL 757-563-1600, FAX 757-563-1655, http://www.al-anon.alateen.org. Ed., R&P Claire Ricewasser. Circ: 9,000.

353.9 USA
HV5297.A4

ALASKA. DEPARTMENT OF HEALTH AND SOCIAL SERVICES. DIVISION OF ALCOHOLISM AND DRUG ABUSE. REPORT. Text in English. a. free per issue. illus.

Formerly: Alaska. Department of Health and Social Services. Office of Alcoholism. Report (0095-3318)

Published by: Department of Health and Social Services, Division of Alcoholism and Drug Abuse, PO Box 110607, Juneau, AK 99811-0607. TEL 907-465-2071, FAX 907-465-2185.

ALATEEN TALK. see *CHILDREN AND YOUTH—For*

616.861 GBR ISSN 0735-0414
HV5441 CODEN: ALALDD

ALCOHOL & ALCOHOLISM. Text in English. 1963. bi-m. GBP 370, USD 605 to individuals; GBP 370, USD 605 to institutions (effective 2002). bk.rev. charts, stat. index. 112 p./no. Supplement avail.; back issues avail.; reprint service avail. from PQC. *Refereed.* **Document type:** *Journal, Academic/Scholarly.* **Description:** Publishes research from all clinical disciplines of medicine, the basic medical sciences, psychology, sociology, and epidemiology.

Former titles (until 1983): British Journal on Alcohol and Alcoholism (0309-1635); (until 1976): Journal of Alcoholism: Bulletin of Alcoholism (0021-8685)

Related titles: Microfilm ed.: (from PQC); Online - full text ed.: ISSN 1464-3502. 199?. GBP 330, USD 540 to institutions (effective 2002) (from HighWire Pr., EBSCO Publishing, O C L C Online Computer Library Center, Inc., RoweCom Information Quest, ingenta, Swets Blackwell, Institute for Scientific Information).

Indexed: ASCA, ASSIA, Abstr.Crim.& Pen., Abstr.Hyg., Addic.Abstr., Anim.Behav.Abstr., Biol.Abstr., Chem.Abstr., Chem.Indus.Notes, Chem.Titles, Curr.Adv.Ecol.Sci., Curr.Cont., Environ.Sci.Poll.Mgmt., Excerp.Med., Focus on: Psychophar., Ind.Med. (1983-), Ind.Sci.Rev., Inpharma, Int.Abstr.Biol.Sci., Lang.& Lang.Behav.Abstr., NRN, Neurosci.Abstr. (coverage dropped), Neurosci.Cit.Ind., Nutr.Abstr., Pharm.&Out.News, PsycInfo, Psychol.Abstr. (1983-), Reac., Risk Abstr., SOPODA, SSCI (coverage dropped), Saf.Sci.Abstr., Sci.Cit.Ind., Soc.Serv.Abstr., Sociol.Abstr., THA, Tox.Abstr., Trop.Dis.Bull., e-psyche.

—BLDSC (0786.754800), CASDDS, CISTI, EMDOCS, GNLM, IDS, ingenta, KNAW. **CCC.**

Published by: (Medical Council on Alcoholism), Oxford University Press, Academic Division, Great Clarendon St, Oxford OX2 6DP, United Kingdom. TEL 44-1865-267907, FAX 44-1865-267835, jnl.info@oup.co.uk, http://alcalc.oupjournals.org/, http://www.oup.co.uk/journals. Eds. Abdulla Badawy, Gian Luigi Gessa, Margaret Brown. Pub. Mandy Sketch. R&P Fionna Willis. Circ: 850. **U.S. subscr. to:** Oxford University Press, Journals, 2001 Evans Rd, Cary, NC 27513. TEL 800-852-7323, FAX 919-677-1714, jnlorders@oup-usa.org; **Subscr. to:** Journals Marketing, Great Clarendon St, Oxford OX2 6DP, United Kingdom. **Co-sponsor:** European Society for Biomedical Research on Alcoholism.

ALCOHOL ISSUES INSIGHTS. see *BEVERAGES*

D

616.861 USA ISSN 0741-8329
QP801 CODEN: ALCOEX
ALCOHOL (NEW YORK); an international biomedical journal. Text in English. 1984. 9/yr. EUR 195 in Europe to individuals; JPY 25,800 in Japan to individuals; USD 218 elsewhere to individuals; EUR 1,213 in Europe to institutions; JPY 161,100 in Japan to institutions; USD 1,356 elsewhere to institutions (effective 2002). adv. illus, abstr. index. back issues avail.; reprints avail. *Refereed.* **Document type:** *Academic/Scholarly.* **Description:** Publishes original research articles and reviews on biomedical aspects of alcohol abuse and alcoholism.
Incorporates: Alcohol and Drug Research; Former titles (until 1986): Substance and Alcohol Actions - Misuse (0191-8877); Substance and Alcohol Misuse
Related titles: Microform ed.: (from PQC); Online - full text ed.: (from ingenta, Swets Blackwell, ScienceDirect, Institute for Scientific Information).
Indexed: Anim.Behav.Abstr. (coverage dropped), Biol.Abstr., Chem.Abstr., Chem.Indus.Notes, Chem.Titles, Curr.Adv.Ecol.Sci., Curr.Cont., Environ.Sci.Poll.Mgmt., Excerp.Med., Focus on: Psychophar., INIS Atomind., Ind.Med. (1984-), Ind.Sci.Rev., Indian Psychol.Abstr., Int.Abstr.Biol.Sci., NRN, Neurosci.Abstr. (coverage dropped), Neurosci.Cit.Ind., Nutr.Abstr., PsycInfo, Psychol.Abstr. (1984-), Risk Abstr., Saf.Sci.Abstr., Sci.Cit.Ind., Tox.Abstr., e-psyche.
—BLDSC (0786.754600), CASDDS, CISTI, EMDOCS, GNLM, IDS, ingenta, KNAW. **CCC.**
Published by: Elsevier Science, 655 Ave of the Americas, New York, NY 10010. TEL 212-989-5800, FAX 212-633-3990, nlinfo-f@elsevier.nl; usinfo-f@elsevier.com; forinfo-kyf04035@niftyserve.or.jp, http://www.elsevier.com/locate/alcohol. Eds. R Jerrells, S Borg. Circ: 1,500. **Subscr. in Australasia and the Far East to:** Elsevier Science (Singapore) Pte Ltd, No.1 Temasek Ave, 17-01 Millenia Tower, Singapore 039192, Singapore. TEL 65-434-3727, FAX 65-337-2230; **Subscr. in Japan to:** Elsevier Science Inc - Japan Regional Office, 9-15 Higashi-Azabu 1-chome, Minato-ku, Tokyo 106-0044, Japan. TEL 81-3-5561-5033, FAX 81-3-5561-5047; **Subscr. outside the Americas to:** Elsevier Science BV, PO Box 211, Amsterdam 1000 AE, Netherlands. TEL 31-20-485-3757, FAX 31-20-485-3432, nlinfo-f@elsevier.nl.

616.861 157.61 USA
HV5285 CODEN: AHRWDZ
ALCOHOL RESEARCH & HEALTH. Text in English. 1975. q. USD 22 domestic (effective 2001). bibl, charts, illus, abstr. Index. back issues avail.; reprints avail. *Refereed.* **Document type:** *Government, Academic/Scholarly.* **Description:** Presents current research findings and contains articles on the effects, prevention and treatment of alcohol abuse and alcoholism.
Formerly (until 1999): Alcohol Health & Research World (0090-838X)
Related titles: Online - full text ed.: (from Gale Group, H. W. Wilson, Factiva, Institute for Scientific Information).
Indexed: ASCA, Adol.Ment.Hlth.Abstr., AgeLine, Amer.Stat.Ind. (1973-), CINAHL, Chem.Abstr., Curr.Cont., Fam.Ind., HRIS, Hlth.Ind., Ind.Med. (1999-), Ind.U.S.Gov.Per., Indian Psychol.Abstr., MEDOC, Mid.East: Abstr.& Ind., NRN, P.A.I.S., PsycInfo, Psychol.Abstr. (1985-), SSCI, Soc.Sci.Ind. (Jan.1999-), Soc.Work Res.& Abstr., e-psyche.
—BLDSC (0786.781400), CASDDS, GNLM, IDS, ingenta.
Published by: U.S. National Institute on Alcohol Abuse and Alcoholism, 6000 Executive Blvd, Bethesda, MD 20892-7003. TEL 301-443-3860, FAX 301-480-1726, http://www.niaaa.nih.gov. Ed. Dianne M Welsh. R&P Barbara Vann TEL 202-842-7600. Circ: 3,700 (paid). **Subscr. to:** U.S. Government Printing Office, Superintendent of Documents, PO Box 371954, Pittsburgh, PA 15250-7954. TEL 202-512-1800, FAX 202-512-2250, orders@gpo.gov, http://www.access.gpo.gov; **Subscr. to:** National Technical Information Service, Government Research Center. FAX 703-321-8547.

616.86 HRV ISSN 0002-502X
CODEN: ALCMAN
ALCOHOLISM; journal on alcoholism and related addictions. Text in English; Summaries in Croatian, English. 1965. s-a., latest vol.37, 2001. USD 30 (effective 2002). adv. bk.rev. charts, illus, stat. index. 96 p./no. reprint service avail. from PQC. *Refereed.* **Document type:** *Academic/Scholarly.* **Description:** Publishes original scientific papers, short communications, professional papers concerning man's use and misuse of ethyl alcohol and other substance dependency.
Related titles: CD-ROM ed.; E-mail ed.; Fax ed.; Microfilm ed.: (from Northern Light Technology, Inc.); Online - full text ed.: USD 30 (effective 2002); ♦ Supplement: Alcoholism. Supplement. ISSN 1330-6170.
Indexed: ASCA, Addic.Abstr., Biol.Abstr., CHNI, Excerp.Med., Fam.Ind., NRN, P.A.I.S., Trop.Dis.Bull., e-psyche.
—ADONIS, GNLM, KNAW.
Published by: Centar za Proucavanje i Suzbijanje Alkoholizma i Drugih Ovisnosti/Centre for Study and Control of Alcoholism and Other Addictions, Vinogradska 29, Zagreb 10000, Croatia. FAX 385-1-3768287, vlatko.thaller@zg.tel.hr, http://www.mzt.hr. Ed., R&P, Adv. contact Vlatko Thaller. Circ: 1,000. **Co-sponsor:** International Council on Alcoholism and Addictions.

616.863 USA ISSN 1042-1394
ALCOHOLISM & DRUG ABUSE WEEKLY; news for policy and program decision-makers. Text in English. 1986. 48/yr., latest vol.13, 2001 (48/yr.). USD 499 domestic to individuals; USD 619 domestic to institutions; USD 639 in Canada to institutions; USD 649 elsewhere to institutions (effective 2001). 8 p./no. back issues avail.; reprints avail. **Document type:** *Newsletter.* **Description:** Includes news and anlysis of federal and state public policy development funding, cutting-edge programs and legislation in the addiction field.
Incorporates (in 1991): Addictions Program Management; Formerly (until 1988): Drug Abuse Report (0889-7050)
Related titles: Online - full text ed.: (from Data-Star, The Dialog Corporation, Gale Group, Northern Light Technology, Inc., Factiva).
—Infotrieve. **CCC.**
Published by: Manisses Communications Group, Inc., PO Box 9758, Providence, RI 02906-9758. TEL 401-831-6020, 800-333-7771, FAX 401-861-6370, manissesCS@manisses.com, http://www.manisses.com. Ed. Gary A Enos. Pub. Betty R Lang.

616.861 USA ISSN 0145-6008
RC565 CODEN: ACRSDM
ALCOHOLISM: CLINICAL AND EXPERIMENTAL RESEARCH. Text in English. 1977. m. USD 312 domestic to individuals; USD 376 foreign to individuals; USD 600 domestic to institutions; USD 680 foreign to institutions; USD 81 newsstand/cover (effective 2002). adv. back issues avail. *Refereed.* **Document type:** *Academic/Scholarly.* **Description:** Presents original clinical and research studies on alcoholism, alcohol-induced syndromes and resultant organ damage.
Related titles: Microfilm ed.: (from WWS); Online - full text ed.: USD 780 domestic academic site license; USD 860 foreign academic site license; USD 870 domestic corporate site license; USD 950 foreign corporate site license (2002) (from Ovid Technologies, Inc., Institute for Scientific Information).
Indexed: Abstr.Hyg., Addic.Abstr., Adol.Ment.Hlth.Abstr., Behav.Med.Abstr., CINAHL, Chem.Indus.Notes, Chem.Titles, Chic.Per.Ind., Curr.Adv.Ecol.Sci., Curr.Cont., Excerp.Med., Focus on: Psychophar., INIS Atomind., Ind.Med. (1977-), Ind.Sci.Rev., Inpharma, Int.Abstr.Biol.Sci., Int.Nurs.Ind., Jrnl.Watch Psych., Neurosci.Cit.Ind., Nutr.Abstr., Pharm.&Out.News, Pig News & Info., PsycInfo, Psychol.Abstr. (1981-), Reac., Risk Abstr., SSCI (coverage dropped), Sci.Cit.Ind., THA, e-psyche.
—BLDSC (0786.789300), CASDDS, CISTI, EMDOCS, GNLM, IDS, ingenta, KNAW.
Published by: (Research Society on Alcoholism), Williams & Wilkins (Subsidiary of: Waverly International), 351 W Camden St, Baltimore, MD 21201-2436. TEL 410-528-4068, 800-222-3790, FAX 410-528-4452, djones@wwilkins.com, http://www.wwilkins.com, http://www.Lww.com. Ed. Dr. Marcus A Rothschild. Adv. contact David Jones. B&W page USD 450; trim 10.88 x 8.13. Circ: 1,426; 1,368 (paid). **Co-sponsor:** International Society for Biomedical Research on Alcoholism.

616.86 HRV ISSN 1330-6170
ALCOHOLISM. SUPPLEMENT. Text in English; Summaries in Croatian, English. 1967. irreg. USD 30 (effective 2002). bk.rev. charts, illus, stat. index. 96 p./no. *Refereed.* **Document type:** *Proceedings, Academic/Scholarly.*
Related titles: ♦ Supplement to: Alcoholism. ISSN 0002-502X.
Published by: Centar za Proucavanje i Suzbijanje Alkoholizma i Drugih Ovisnosti/Centre for Study and Control of Alcoholism and Other Addictions, Vinogradska 29, Zagreb 10000, Croatia. FAX 385-1-3768287, vlatko.thaller@zg.tel.hr, http://www.mzt.hr. Ed. Vlatko Thaller.

616.861 USA ISSN 0734-7324
ALCOHOLISM TREATMENT QUARTERLY; the practitioner's quarterly for individual, group, and family therapy. Text in English. 1984. q. USD 75 to individuals; USD 101 in Canada to individuals; USD 109 elsewhere to individuals; USD 200 to institutions; USD 270 in Canada to institutions; USD 290 elsewhere to institutions; USD 450 to libraries; USD 608 in Canada to libraries; USD 653 elsewhere to libraries (effective Aug. 2001). adv. bk.rev. abstr, bibl. back issues avail.; reprint service avail. from HAW. *Refereed.* **Document type:** *Journal, Trade.* **Description:** Geared toward the needs of clinicians who work with alcoholic clients and their families.
Formerly: Alcoholism Counseling and Treatment
Related titles: Microfiche ed.: (from PQC); Microform ed.
Indexed: A.D.& D., Abstr.Anthropol., Abstr.Crim.& Pen., Crim.Just.Abstr., Environ.Sci.Poll.Mgmt., Excerp.Med., IMFL, Ind.Per.Art.Relat.Law, Lang.& Lang.Behav.Abstr., Past.Care & Couns.Abstr., PsycInfo, Psychol.Abstr. (1984-), Ref.Zh., Rehabil.Lit., Risk Abstr., SOPODA, Saf.Sci.Abstr., Sage Fam.Stud.Abstr., Soc.Serv.Abstr., Soc.Work Res.& Abstr., Sociol.Abstr., Stud.Wom.Abstr., THA.
—BLDSC (0786.797000), EMDOCS, GNLM, Haworth, ingenta, KNAW.
Published by: Haworth Press, Inc., 10 Alice St, Binghamton, NY 13904-1580. TEL 607-722-5857, 800-429-6784, FAX 607-722-6362, 800-895-0582, getinfo@haworthpressinc.com, http://www.haworthpress.com/journals/journallist.asp. Ed. Thomas McGovern. Pub. William Cohen. R&P Ruthann Heath TEL 607-723-5857 ext 316. Adv. contact Jackie Blakeslee TEL 607-722-5857 ext 346. B&W page USD 315, color page USD 550; trim 6 x 8.5. Circ: 725.

616.861 362.29 344 ITA ISSN 0394-9826
ALCOLOGIA; European journal of alcohol studies. Text in English. 1989. 3/yr. ITL 90,000; ITL 35,000 newsstand/cover (effective 2001). adv. **Document type:** *Academic/Scholarly.* **Description:** Published under the auspices of Societa Italiana di Alcologia, it means to promote the exchange of opinions and information on alcohol and drug related pathologies and problems, behavior and lifestyles.
Indexed: Addic.Abstr., Excerp.Med. (1996-).
—BLDSC (0786.797300), EMDOCS.
Published by: Eurohealth Editors srl, Via Castiglione 28, Bologna 40124, Italy. TEL 39-051-263703, FAX 39-051-238564, mcccongress.tin.it. adv.: color page ITL 9,000,000. Circ: 1,100.

616.8 FRA ISSN 0002-5054
ALCOOL OU SANTE. Text in French. 1951. q. FRF 100 domestic to individuals; FRF 125 foreign to individuals; FRF 80 domestic to libraries; FRF 100 foreign to libraries (effective 2001). adv. bk.rev. abstr, bibl, charts, illus. index. **Document type:** *Consumer.* **Description:** Covers the different aspects of alcoholism such as prevention, trafficking, public health, foreign countries, general news.
Indexed: Ref.Zh.
Published by: Association Nationale de Prevention de l'Alcoolisme, 20 rue St. Fiacre, Paris 75002, France. TEL 33-1-42335104, FAX 33-1-45081702, contact@anpa.asso.fr, http://www.anpa.asso.fr. Ed. Patrick Elineau. R&P Elisabeth Francois. Circ: 7,000.

616.86 FRA ISSN 1620-4522
ALCOOLOGIE ET ADDICTOLOGIE. Text in French; Summaries in English, French. 1978. q. EUR 69 in Europe to individuals; EUR 89 elsewhere to individuals; EUR 50 in Europe to students; EUR 96 in Europe to institutions; EUR 115 elsewhere to institutions; EUR 24 newsstand/cover (effective 2002). **Description:** Transdisciplinary approach of alcoholism and other addictions.
Former titles (until 2000): Alcoologie (1142-1983); (until 1989): Societe Francaise d'Alcoologie. Bulletin (0245-6664)
Indexed: Addic.Abstr.
—BLDSC (0786.802000).
Published by: (Societe Française d'Alcoologie), Princeps Editions, 64 av. du General de Gaulle, Issy-les-Moulineaux 92130, France. TEL 33-01-46382414, FAX 33-01-40957215. Ed. J D Favre.

617.8 USA
ALERT (EWING); news on alcoholism and drug addiction services for persons who are hard of hearing. Text in English. 1989. s-a. free per issue. adv. back issues avail. **Document type:** *Newsletter.* **Description:** Disseminates local and national news on alcohol and drug use among persons who are deaf or hard of hearing. Contains information on service providers.

D

Published by: Sings of Sobriety, Inc., 865 Lower Ferry Rd., Ste. B-12, Ewing, NJ 08628. TEL 609-882-7177, 800-332-7677, FAX 609-882-6808, sosnj@juno.com, http://www.members.aol.com/sosnj. Ed. Steven Shevlin. R&P Lisetle Ortiz. Adv. contact Heather Bird. Circ: 2,000.

616.86 SWE ISSN 0345-0732
ALKOHOL OCH NARKOTIKA/ALCOHOL AND OTHER DRUGS. Text in Swedish; Summaries in English. 1906. 6/yr. SEK 250; SEK 48 newsstand/cover (effective 2001). adv. bk.rev. bibl, illus, stat. index, cum.index. **Document type:** *Magazine, Consumer.* **Description:** Monitors drug trends in Sweden.
Incorporates (in 1989): Forskningsnytt; Formerly (until 1973): Alkoholfraagen (0002-5518); Which was formed by the 1956 merger of: Tidskrift foer Systembolagen; Tirfing
—GNLM.
Published by: Centralfoerbundet foer Alkohol- och Narkotikaupplysning, Olof Palmes gata 17, Fack 704 12, Stockholm 10133, Sweden. TEL 46-8-412-46-00, FAX 46-8-10-46-41, staffan.hasselgren@can.se, http://www.can.se. Ed. Staffan Hasselgren. Circ: 6,000.

616.863 USA ISSN 0095-2990
HV5800 CODEN: AJDABD
AMERICAN JOURNAL OF DRUG AND ALCOHOL ABUSE. Text in English. 1975. q. USD 95 to individuals print & online eds.; USD 860 to institutions print ed. only (effective 2002). adv. bibl, charts, illus. *Refereed.* **Document type:** *Academic/Scholarly.* **Description:** Dedicated to the presentation of essential aspects of drug and alcohol abuse.
Related titles: Microform ed.: (from RPI); Online - full text ed.: (from Gale Group, EBSCO Publishing, O C L C Online Computer Library Center, Inc., RoweCom Information Quest, Swets Blackwell, Factiva, Institute for Scientific Information).
Indexed: ASCA, Addic.Abstr., Adol.Ment.Hlth.Abstr., AgeLine, Amer.Bibl.Slavic & E.Eur.Stud., Behav.Med.Abstr., Biol.Abstr., Crim.Just.Abstr., Curr.Adv.Ecol.Sci., Curr.Cont., Curr.Lit.Fam.Plan., Environ.Sci.Poll.Mgmt., Excerp.Med., Fam.Ind., Gen.Sci.Ind. (Jun.1992-), HRIS, I.P.A., Ind.Med. (1974-), Int.Nurs.Ind., Lang.& Lang.Behav.Abstr., Mid.East: Abstr.& Ind., NRN, Pollut.Abstr., PsycInfo, Psychol.Abstr. (1976-), Ref.Zh., Risk Abstr., Russ.Acad.Sci.Bibl., SOPODA, SSCI, Saf.Sci.Abstr., Soc.Sci.Ind. (Jan.1994-), Soc.Serv.Abstr., Soc.Work Res.& Abstr., Sociol.Abstr., THA, Tox.Abstr., e-psyche.
—BLDSC (0824.320000), CASDDS, CISTI, EMDOCS, GNLM, IDS, ingenta, KNAW. **CCC.**
Published by: Marcel Dekker Inc., 270 Madison Ave, New York, NY 10016. TEL 212-696-9000, 800-228-1160, FAX 212-685-4540, http://www.dekker.com/servlet/rpoduct/productid/ADA. Ed. Edward Kaufman. R&P Julia Mulligan. Adv. contact Diane Saulon. B&W page USD 800. Circ: 825.

616.8 USA ISSN 1055-0496
RC563 CODEN: AJADEA
AMERICAN JOURNAL ON ADDICTIONS. Text in English. 1992. q. GBP 82, USD 136 to individuals; GBP 171, USD 282 to institutions (effective 2002). adv. bk.rev. abstr, bibl, charts, illus, stat. index. *Refereed.* **Document type:** *Consumer, Academic/Scholarly.* **Description:** Presents original research related to the assessment and treatment of addictive disorders.
Related titles: Microform ed.: (from PQC); Online - full text ed.: ISSN 1521-0391 (from CatchWord Ltd., EBSCO Publishing, O C L C Online Computer Library Center, Inc., RoweCom Information Quest, ProQuest Information & Learning, Swets Blackwell, Institute for Scientific Information).
Indexed: ASCA, Addic.Abstr., Crim.Just.Abstr., Curr.Cont., Excerp.Med. (1994-), Ind.Med. (1992-), Jrnl.Watch Psych., PsycInfo, Psychol.Abstr. (1992-), SSCI, e-psyche.
—BLDSC (0820.947000), CatchWord, EMDOCS, GNLM, IDS, Infotrieve, ingenta, KNAW. **CCC.**
Published by: (American Academy of Psychiatrists in Alcoholism and Addictions), Taylor & Francis Ltd. (Subsidiary of: Taylor & Francis Group), 325 Chestnut St, Suite 800, Philadelphia, PA 19016. TEL 215-625-8900, FAX 215-625-2940, info@taylorandfrancis.com, http://www.taylorandfrancis.com/. Ed. Sheldon Miller. Circ: 1,300. **Subsr. addr. in Europe:** Taylor & Francis Group, Journals Customer Service, Rankine Rd, Basingstoke, Hants RG24 8PR, United Kingdom. TEL 44-1256-813000, FAX 44-1256-479438, enquiry@tanf.co.uk, http://www.tandf.co.uk/journals.

362.29 616.863 SWE ISSN 0280-512X
ANHOERIG* . Text in Swedish. 1981. bi-m.
Published by: Riksfoerbundet Foeraeldrafoereningen mod Narkotika, Pipersgatan 27, Stockholm 11228, Sweden.

616.861 USA
ANNUAL EDITIONS: DRUGS, SOCIETY & BEHAVIOR. Text in English. 1986. a. USD 12.25. illus. **Document type:** *Academic/Scholarly.*
Published by: Dushkin - McGraw-Hill, Sluice Dock, Guilford, CT 06437-9989. TEL 203-453-4351, FAX 203-453-6000. Ed. High Wilson. Pub. Ian Nielsen. R&P Cheryl Greenleaf.

362.29 616.863 SWE ISSN 0281-577X
ANONYMA ALKOHOLISTER. BULLETIN. Text in Swedish. 1965-1980; resumed 1982. bi-m. SEK 120 (effective 1994). **Document type:** *Bulletin.*
Published by: Anonyma Alkoholister, Fack 16387, Stockholm 10327, Sweden. TEL 47-8-642-26-09, FAX 47-8-714-82-24. Circ: 1,500.

616.861 JPN ISSN 0910-495X
ARUKORU IRYO KENKYU/JAPANESE STUDIES ON ALCOHOLISM TREATMENT. Text in Japanese. 1984. q. JPY 1,880.
Published by: (Shiheki Mondai Rinsho Kenkyujo), Seiwa Shoten Co. Ltd., 2-5 Kami-Takai-Do 1-chome, Suginami-ku, Tokyo 168-0074, Japan.

616.861 JPN ISSN 0389-4118
RC565 CODEN: AKYIDF
ARUKORU KENKYU TO YAKUBUTSU IZON/JAPANESE JOURNAL OF ALCOHOL STUDIES AND DRUG DEPENDENCE. Text in English, Japanese. 1966. q. adv. bk.rev. abstr, bibl, charts, illus. index. **Document type:** *Academic/Scholarly.*
Formerly (until 1981): Arukoru Kenkyu - Japanese Journal of Studies on Alcohol (0021-5244)
Indexed: Addic.Abstr., Biol.Abstr., Chem.Abstr., Excerp.Med., Ind.Med. (coverage dropped), Int.Nurs.Ind.
—CASDDS, EMDOCS, GNLM.
Published by: Nihon Arukoru Igakkai/Japanese Medical Society of Alcohol Studies, c/o Kyoto Furitsu Ika Daigaku Hoigaku Kyoshitsu, 465 Kajiicho, Hirokoji Agaru, Kawaramachi Dori, Kamigyo-ku, Kyoto-shi 602, Japan. Circ: 1,000.

ASHES TO DUST. see *PUBLIC HEALTH AND SAFETY*

616.861 AUS ISSN 0726-4607
AUSTRA-LINK. Text in English. 1981. m. AUD 12 domestic; AUD 25 foreign (effective 2001). 12 p./no. *Refereed.* **Document type:** *Magazine, Consumer.* **Description:** Recovering from effects of living with someone else's alcoholism, using the Al-Anon 12-step program.
Published by: Al-Anon Family Groups (Australia) Pty. Ltd., GPO Box 1002 H, Melbourne, VIC 3001, Australia. TEL 61-3-9654-8838, FAX 61-3-9654-8865, agso@alphalink.com.au, http://www.atanon.alateen.org/australia. Ed., R&P Mary Richards. Circ: 1,350.

AUSTRALIAN COUNCIL ON SMOKING AND HEALTH NEWSLETTER. see *PHYSICAL FITNESS AND HYGIENE*

178 AUS
AUTUMN SCHOOL OF STUDIES ON ALCOHOL & DRUGS. PROCEEDINGS OF SEMINARS. Text in English. 1966. a. AUD 18. back issues avail. **Document type:** *Proceedings.*
Published by: St. Vincent Hospital, Department of Drug and Alcohol Studies, Victoria Parade, Fitzroy, VIC 3065, Australia. TEL 61-3-288-2627, FAX 61-3-288-2642, TELEX SVHOSM AA 32229. Circ: 250.

B I M S. (Blaukreuz Information - Meinungen - Szene) see *RELIGIONS AND THEOLOGY—Protestant*

BEHAVIORAL HEALTH BUSINESS NEWS. see *INSURANCE*

616.86 USA ISSN 1075-6701
HV5285
BEHAVIORAL HEALTH MANAGEMENT. Text in English. 1980. bi-m. USD 78 domestic; USD 100 in Canada & Mexico; USD 110 elsewhere (effective 2000). adv. bk.rev. **Description:** Addresses the problems of providing cost-effective mental health and substance abuse treatment in an environment of managed care.
Former titles (until 1994): Addiction and Recovery (1052-4614); (until 1989): Alcoholism and Addiction and Recovery Life (1053-3923); (until 1988): Alcoholism and Addiction (0899-8043); (until 1987): Alcoholism and Addiction Magazine (0884-1403); (until 1985): Alcoholism (0275-9519)
Related titles: Online - full text ed.: (from Gale Group, ProQuest Information & Learning, Northern Light Technology, Inc., Factiva).
Indexed: Hlth.Ind., Soc.Sci.Ind. (Jan.1994-Nov.1998).
—Infotrieve, ingenta. **CCC.**
Published by: Medquest Communications, LLC, 629 Euclid Ave, Ste 1200, Cleveland, OH 44114-3003. TEL 216-522-9700, FAX 216-522-9707. Ed. Monica Oss. Pub. Mark Goodman III. Circ: 23,000.

362.29 616.863 SWE ISSN 0345-1577
BLAA BANDET; Blaabandsroerelsens tidning. Text in Swedish. 1883. 9/yr. SEK 75 (effective 1999). **Document type:** *Newsletter.*
Address: Fack 1233, Orebro 70112, Sweden. TEL 46-19-130575, FAX 46-19-121136. Ed. Per Olof Svensson.

362.29 616.863 SWE ISSN 0345-1585
BLAA KORSET; informationsblad. Text in Swedish. 1969. q. SEK 30 (effective 1990).
Address: Soergaarden, Koeping 73192, Sweden.

616.86 344 DEU ISSN 0006-5250
CODEN: BLALAL
BLUTALKOHOL; wissenschaftliche Zeitschrift fuer die medizinische und juristische Praxis. Text in English, German. 1961. bi-m. EUR 49.40 domestic; EUR 52.15 in Europe; EUR 53.65 elsewhere; EUR 8.70 newsstand/cover (effective 2002). adv. bk.rev. bibl, charts. s-a. index, cum.index: 1961-62. back issues avail. **Document type:** *Journal, Academic/Scholarly.*
Indexed: Abstr.Crim.& Pen., Biol.Abstr., Chem.Abstr., Chem.Indus.Notes, Chem.Titles, Excerp.Med., Mass Spectr.Bull.
—CASDDS, GNLM, Infotrieve, KNAW. **CCC.**
Published by: (Bund gegen Alkohol im Strassenverkehr e.V.), Steintor Verlag GmbH, Graphengiesserstr 30, Luebeck 23566, Germany. TEL 49-451-8798849, FAX 49-451-8798837, info@steintor-verlag.de. R&P R Jacobson. Circ: 3,200.

178 364 ITA ISSN 0392-3126
BOLLETTINO PER LE FARMACODIPENDENZE E L'ALCOOLISMO. Text in Italian. 1991. q. free per issue. bk.rev. **Document type:** *Bulletin, Government.*
—BLDSC (2236.530000).
Published by: (Settore Tossicodipendenze e Patologie, Italy. Ministero della Sanita), United Nations Interregional Crime and Justice Research Institute/Institut Interregional de Recherche des Nations Unies sur la Criminalite et la Justice, Via Giulia, 52, Rome, RM 00186, Italy. TEL 39-6-6877437, FAX 39-6-6892638, unicri@unicri.it. Ed. Dr. Carlo Vetere. Circ: 7,000.

616.863 USA ISSN 1040-6328
RC563
BROWN UNIVERSITY DIGEST OF ADDICTION THEORY & APPLICATION. Variant title: D A T A. Text in English. m., latest vol.20, 2001. USD 149 domestic to individuals; USD 227 domestic to institutions; USD 237 in Canada to institutions; USD 267 elsewhere to institutions (effective 2001). 8 p./no. back issues avail.; reprints avail. **Document type:** *Newsletter.* **Description:** News-style synopsis of critical research developments in the treatment and prevention of addiction.
Incorporates (in 1991): Addictions Alert (0887-8145)
Related titles: Online - full text ed.: (from Gale Group).
Indexed: Ref.Zh.
—Infotrieve. **CCC.**
Published by: Manisses Communications Group, Inc., PO Box 9758, Providence, RI 02906-9758. TEL 401-831-6020, 800-333-7771, FAX 401-861-6370, manissesCS@manisses.com, http://www.manisses.com. Ed. Dr. Timothy Mueller. Pub. Betty R Lang. R&P Barbara Deekle.

615.1 USA ISSN 0007-523X
HV5800 CODEN: BNUNA5
BULLETIN ON NARCOTICS. Text in English. 1949. q. USD 10 per issue. bibl, charts, illus. index. reprint service avail. from PQC. **Description:** Provides current information on all aspects of national and international drug control.
Formerly: Bulletin of Narcotic Drugs
Related titles: Microform ed.: (from PQC,PMC); Online - full text ed.; Arabic ed.: Nashrat al-Mukhaddirat. ISSN 0256-9000. 1985; Chinese ed.: Mazuipin Gongbao. ISSN 0251-8694; French ed.: Bulletin des Stupefiant. ISSN 0251-3706; Russian ed.: Byulleten' po Narkoticheskim Sredstvam. ISSN 0251-7094; Spanish ed.: Boletin de Estupefacientes. ISSN 0251-7086. 1952.

D

Indexed: ASSIA, Abstr.Crim.& Pen., Abstr.Hyg., Addic.Abstr., Adol.Ment.Hlth.Abstr., Agri.& Environ.Biotech.Abstr. (coverage dropped), Biol.Abstr., Chem.Abstr., Chem.Indus.Notes, Chem.Titles, Crim.Just.Abstr., Curr.Cont. (coverage dropped), Derwent Biotech.Abstr., Excerp.Med., HRIS, IIS, I.P.A., Ind.Med. (1949-), Ind.Sci.Rev., P.A.I.S., Psychol.Abstr., Russ.Acad.Sci.Bibl., SSCI (coverage dropped), Soc.Sci.Ind. (coverage dropped), Trop.Dis.Bull.
—BLDSC (2881.430000), CASDDS, GNLM, ingenta, Linda Hall. **CCC.**
Published by: United Nations Publications, Sales and Marketing Section, Room DC2 0853, New York, NY 10017. TEL 212-963-8302, 800-253-9646, FAX 212-963-3489, publications@un.org, http://www.un.org/publications. **Dist. by:** Distribution and Sales Section, Palais des Nations, Geneva CH-1211, Switzerland.

616.86 USA
C S A P PREVENTION MONOGRAPH. Text in English. irreg., latest vol.14, 1993. **Document type:** *Monographic series, Government.*
Published by: National Clearinghouse for Alcohol and Drug Information, Center for Substance Abuse Prevention, PO Box 2345, Rockville, MD 20847-2345. TEL 800-729-6686, FAX 301-468-6433, info@prevline.health.org, http://www.health.org.

616.86 157.63 CAN
CENTRE FOR ADDICTION AND MENTAL HEALTH. ANNUAL REPORT. Text in English. 1951. a. free per issue (2000). **Document type:** *Government.*
Former titles: Addiction Research Foundation of Ontario. Annual Report; Alcoholism and Drug Addiction Research Foundation. Annual Report (0065-6119)
—CISTI.
Published by: Centre for Addiction and Mental Health, 33 Russell St, Toronto, ON M5S 2S1, Canada. TEL 416-595-6059, FAX 416-593-4694, mkt@arf.org, http://www.arf.org. Circ: 2,000 (controlled).

616.86 USA
COMMUNITY OF RECOVERY. Text in English. 1998. q. free per issue to qualified personnel. **Document type:** *Newsletter, Trade.* **Description:** Provides mostly current information regarding the treatment of the disease of chemical dependency.
Published by: Sundown M. Ranch, 2280 State Rte 821, Yakima, WA 98284-0735. TEL 360-757-1606, 800-326-7444. Ed. Len Baltzer. R&P Len Balterzer. **Subscr. to:** Sundown M Ranch, PO Box 735, Sedro Wooley, WA 98284-9913.

616.861 CAN ISSN 0045-799X
CONCERNS. Text in English. 1902. q. CND 25 to members. bk.rev. illus. **Document type:** *Newsletter.* **Description:** Informs members of issues and programs involving the organization, its Board and staff.
Formerly: Advocate (Scarborough)
Indexed: Abstr.Bk.Rev.Curr.Leg.Per.
—Infotrieve. **CCC.**
Published by: Concerns Canada, 4500 Sheppard Ave., E., Ste. 112H, Agincourt, ON M1S 3R6, Canada. TEL 416-293-3400, FAX 416-293-1142. Ed. Karl N Burden. Circ: 16,000.

362.2 USA ISSN 0091-4509
HV5800
CONTEMPORARY DRUG PROBLEMS. Text in English. 1971. q. USD 30 to individuals; USD 36 domestic to institutions; USD 48 foreign to institutions (effective 2001). adv. bk.rev. back issues avail.; reprint service avail. from PQC,WSH,PSC,SCH. **Document type:** *Academic/Scholarly.* **Description:** Discusses contemporay drug problems.
Related titles: Microfilm ed.: (from PQC); Online - full text ed.: (from ProQuest Information & Learning, Gale Group, Factiva).
Indexed: Abstr.Crim.& Pen., Addic.Abstr., Adol.Ment.Hlth.Abstr., Amer.Bibl.Slavic & E.Eur.Stud., C.L.I., Crim.Just.Abstr., Curr.Cont. (coverage dropped), Excerp.Med., Hlth.Ind., I.P.A., Ind.Per.Art.Relat.Law, L.R.I. (Jan.1980-), Lang.& Lang.Behav.Abstr., Leg.Per. (coverage dropped), Mid.East: Abstr.& Ind., P C I, P.A.I.S., Psychol.Abstr., SOPODA, SSCI (coverage dropped), Sage Pub.Admin.Abstr., Soc.Sci.Ind. (Feb.1983-), Sociol.Abstr.
—BLDSC (3425.179000), GNLM, ingenta.
Published by: Federal Legal Publications, Inc., 157 Chambers St, New York, NY 10007. TEL 212-619-4949. Ed. Robin Room. Pub. Martin Greenberg. Circ: 1,800.

616.863 USA
CONTROLLED SUBSTANCES REGULATION. Text in English. 1972. q. USD 287. **Description:** Comprehensive guide to current Drug Enforcement Administration requirements for manufacturing, storing, securing, shipping and distributing controlled substances.
Formerly: Controlled Substances Handbook
Published by: Government Information Services (Subsidiary of: Thompson Publishing Group), 1725 K St, N W, 7th Fl, Washington, DC 20006. TEL 800-876-0226, FAX 202-759-9657. Ed. Ken Baumgartner.

COUNSELOR; the magazine for addiction professionals. see *PSYCHOLOGY*

616.863 ITA ISSN 1121-0311
DELFINO. Text in Italian. 1976. bi-m. ITL 30,000; ITL 55,000 foreign (effective 1994). adv. bk.rev., film rev. index. **Description:** Focuses its attention on the drug addict, includes interviews, looks at personal experiences of the drug addict, family and friends. Also looks at other addictions such as alcoholism, smoking and other forms of drugs.
Published by: Centro Italiano di Solidarieta, Via Attilio Ambrosini, 129, Rome, RM 00147, Italy. TEL 39-6-541951, FAX 6-5407306, ceis@inroma.roma.it. Ed. Enzo Caffarelli. Adv. contact Simona Cordeschi. **Subscr. to:** Piazza Benedetto Cairoli, 118, Rome, RM 00186, Italy.

616.86 800 USA ISSN 1044-4149
DIONYSOS; journal of literature and addiction. Text in English. 1989-1994; resumed 1995. 2/yr. USD 8 to individuals; USD 12 to institutions (effective 1999). bk.rev., play rev., tel.rev. back issues avail. *Refereed.* **Document type:** *Academic/Scholarly.* **Description:** Contains news notes and articles dealing with the cultural and aesthetic side of intoxication. Covers both the creative and destructive role of drinking and drug use in the lives and works of writers and artists.
Former titles: Addiction; Intoxication
Indexed: MLA Intl.Bibl.
Published by: Seattle University, Addiction Studies Program, 900 Broadway, Seattle, WA 98122-4490. TEL 206-296-5351, FAX 206-296-2141, jimharb@seattleu.edu. Ed., R&P James Harbaugh. Circ: 150 (paid).

616.8 AUS
DIRECTORY OF AL-ANON AND ALATEEN MEETINGS IN AUSTRALIA. Text in English. 1991. s-a. AUD 1 domestic; AUD 2 foreign (effective 2001). back issues avail. **Document type:** *Directory.*
Published by: Al-Anon Family Groups (Australia) Pty. Ltd., GPO Box 1002 H, Melbourne, VIC 3001, Australia. TEL 61-3-9654-8838, FAX 61-3-9654-8865, http://www.al-anon.alateen.org/australia. Ed. Beryl Stone. Circ: 50.

616.86 USA ISSN 1067-814X
DRUG, ALCOHOL, AND OTHER ADDICTIONS. Text in English. 1989. irreg. **Document type:** *Directory.*
Related titles: Magnetic Tape ed.
Published by: Oryx Press, 4041 N Central Ave, 700, Phoenix, AZ 85012-3397. TEL 602-265-2651, FAX 602-265-6250, info@oryxpress.com, http://www.oryxpress.com/. Eds. Jennifer Ashley, Anne Thompson. Pub. Phyllis Steckler.

616.86 USA ISSN 1053-3818
CODEN: DAAREM
DRUG AND ALCOHOL ABUSE REVIEWS. Text in English. 1991. irreg., latest vol.8. price varies. illus, stat. back issues avail. *Refereed.* **Document type:** *Monographic series, Academic/Scholarly.* **Description:** Examines the effects of drugs and alcohol on various systems in the human body, along with issues in the treatment and prevention of drug and alcohol abuse and misuse.
—Infotrieve. **CCC.**
Published by: Humana Press Inc., 999 Riverview Dr, Ste 208, Totowa, NJ 07512. TEL 973-256-1699, FAX 973-256-8341, humana@humanapr.com, humana@humnaapr.com, http://humanapress.com. Ed. Ronald R Watson. R&P Richard Hruska.

616.86 157.6 IRL ISSN 0376-8716
RC566.A1 CODEN: DADEDV
DRUG AND ALCOHOL DEPENDENCE; an international journal on biomedical and psychosocial approaches. Text in English. 1975. m. EUR 1,052 in Europe to institutions; JPY 168,800 in Japan to institutions; USD 1,423 elsewhere to institutions (effective 2002). bk.rev. abstr. back issues avail. *Refereed.* **Document type:** *Academic/Scholarly.* **Description:** For workers in the fields of biomedical, as well as clinical, epidemiological, psychosocial, socio-cultural, educational and medico-legal research.
Related titles: Microform ed.: (from PQC); Online - full text ed.: (from ingenta, Swets Blackwell, ScienceDirect, Institute for Scientific Information).
Indexed: ASCA, ASSIA, Abstr.Crim.& Pen., Addic.Abstr., Adol.Ment.Hlth.Abstr., Biol.Abstr., Chem.Abstr., Chem.Indus.Notes, Chem.Titles, Chic.Per.Ind., Community Ment.Health Rev., Crim.Just.Abstr., Curr.Adv.Ecol.Sci., Curr.Cont., Dairy Sci.Abstr., Environ.Sci.Poll.Mgmt., Excerp.Med., Focus on: Psychophar., HRIS, I.P.A., Ind.Med. (1975-), Ind.Sci.Rev., Inpharma, Int.Abstr.Biol.Sci., Int.Nurs.Ind., Lang.& Lang.Behav.Abstr., Mid.East: Abstr.& Ind., Neurosci.Abstr. (coverage dropped), Neurosci.Cit.Ind., Pharm.&Out.News, Pollut.Abstr., PsycInfo, Psychol.Abstr. (1975-), Reac., Risk Abstr., SOPODA, SSCI (coverage dropped), Saf.Sci.Abstr., Sci.Cit.Ind., Soc.Serv.Abstr., Sociol.Abstr., THA, Trop.Dis.Bull., e-psyche.
—BLDSC (3627.890000), ADONIS, CASDDS, CISTI, EMDOCS, GNLM, IDS, ingenta, KNAW. **CCC.**
Published by: (International Council on Alcohol and Addictions), Elsevier Science Ireland Ltd, Elsevier House, Brookvale Plaza, E. Park, Shannon, Co. Clare, Ireland. TEL 353-61-471944, FAX 353-61-472144, http://www.elsevier.com/locate/drugalcdep. Eds. I Stolerman, R Balster. **Subscr. in Australasia and the Far East to:** Elsevier Science (Singapore) Pte Ltd, No.1 Temasek Ave, 17-01 Millenia Tower, Singapore 039192, Singapore. TEL 65-434-3727, FAX 65-337-2230; **Subscr. in the Americas to:** Elsevier Science, PO Box 945, New York, NY 10159-0945. TEL 212-989-5800, FAX 212-633-3680, usinfo-f@elsevier.com; **Subscr. to:** Elsevier Science BV, PO Box 211, Amsterdam 1000 AE, Netherlands. TEL 31-20-485-3757. **Co-sponsor:** College on Problems of Drug Dependence.

616.86 GBR
DRUG AND ALCOHOL FINDINGS. Text in English. q. GBP 60 (effective 2000).
—BLDSC (3627.891000).
Published by: The Findings Partnership, c/o DrugScope, 32-36 Loman St, London SE1 0EE, United Kingdom. FAX 44-20-8888-6277, findings@mashton.cix.co.uk. Ed. Mike Ashton.

178 GBR ISSN 0959-5236
DRUG AND ALCOHOL REVIEW. Text in English. 1982. q. GBP 131, USD 211 to individuals; GBP 452, USD 745 to institutions (effective 2002). bk.rev. index. back issues avail. *Refereed.* **Document type:** *Academic/Scholarly.* **Description:** Reviews the clinical, biomedical, psychological and sociological aspects of alcohol, tobacco, and drug use.
Former titles (until Jan. 1990): Australian Drug and Alcohol Review; Australian Alcohol - Drug Review (0726-4550)
Related titles: Online - full text ed.: ISSN 1465-3362 (from CatchWord Ltd., EBSCO Publishing, O C L C Online Computer Library Center, Inc., RoweCom Information Quest, ProQuest Information & Learning, Swets Blackwell, Institute for Scientific Information).
Indexed: ASCA, ASSIA, Addic.Abstr., Crim.Just.Abstr., Curr.Cont., ERA, Environ.Sci.Poll.Mgmt., Mult.Ed.Abstr., Pollut.Abstr., PsycInfo, Psychol.Abstr. (1994-), Risk Abstr., SSCI, Saf.Sci.Abstr., Sage Fam.Stud.Abstr., Stud.Wom.Abstr., Tox.Abstr., Viol.& Abuse Abstr., e-psyche.
—BLDSC (3627.895000), CatchWord, IDS, Infotrieve, ingenta, KNAW. **CCC.**
Published by: (Australian Medical and Professional Society on Alcohol and Drug Related Problems AUS), Carfax Publishing Limited (Subsidiary of: Taylor & Francis Group), PO Box 25, Abingdon, Oxon OX14 3UE, United Kingdom. TEL 44-1235-401000, FAX 44-1235-401550, enquiries@carfax.co.uk, enquiry@tandf.co.uk, http://www.carfax.co.uk. Ed. John B Saunders.

DRUG DETECTION REPORT; the newsletter on drug testing in the workplace. see *BUSINESS AND ECONOMICS—Personnel Management*

D

362.29 371.7 GBR ISSN 1461-8842
DRUG EDUCATION MATTERS. Text in English. 1998. 3/yr. GBP 15 to individuals; GBP 25 to institutions (effective 2000). bk.rev. **Document type:** *Newsletter.* **Description:** Covers the recent developments in drug education and contains features on drug education in practice.
Published by: National Children's Bureau Enterprises Ltd., 8 Wakley St, London EC1V 7QE, United Kingdom. TEL 44-20-7843-6038, FAX 44-20-7278-9512, def@ncb.org.uk, http://www.ucb.org.uk, http://www.ncb.org.uk. Circ: 2,000.

DRUG INDUCED DISORDERS. see *PHARMACY AND PHARMACOLOGY*

616.863 157.63 GBR ISSN 0305-4349
DRUGLINK. Text in English. 1976. bi-m. GBP 51; GBP 64 foreign (effective 1999). adv. bk.rev. bibl. back issues avail. **Document type:** *Newsletter.* **Description:** Examines the abuse and misuse of drugs.
Indexed: ASSIA.
Published by: Institute for the Study of Drug Dependence, Waterbridge House, Institute For The Study Of Drug Dependence (I S D, 32-36 Loman St, London SE1 0EE, United Kingdom. TEL 44-207-928-1211, FAX 44-207-928-1771, services@isdd.co.uk, http://www.isdd.co.uk. Ed. Neil Bell. R&P Harry Shapiro. Adv. contact Jan Hodgman. page GBP 220; 181 x 264. Circ: 2,300.

616.863 USA ISSN 0744-2823
HV5825
DRUGS & DRUG ABUSE EDUCATION. NEWSLETTER*. Text in English. 1969. m. USD 79. bk.rev. charts. **Description:** Covers treatment, prevention education, congressional and agency developments, and state and local programs.
Incorporates: Alcoholism and Alcohol Education (0044-7226); Formerly: Washington Drug Review (0146-728X)
Published by: Editorial Resources, Inc., PO Box 20754, Scattle, WA 98102-1754. TEL 206-322-8387. Ed. David L Howell.

345.027 340 USA
DRUGS AND THE LAW; detection, recognition & investigation. Text in English. 1992. irreg. USD 44.95 (effective 2000). **Document type:** *Government.* **Description:** A publication for anyone involved with the problem of drug abuse. Covers topics such as current patterns in drug abuse. Drugs, crime and violence, addiction and behavior, drug law enforcement, drug treatment, rehabilitation, prevention, education and more.
Published by: Gould Publications, Inc., 1333 N US Hwy 17 92, Longwood, FL 32750-3724. TEL 407-695-9500, 800-717-7917, FAX 407-695-2906, info@gouldlaw.com, http://www.gouldlaw.com.

616.86 GBR ISSN 0968-7637
CODEN: DEPPEH
DRUGS: EDUCATION, PREVENTION & POLICY. Text in English. 1994. 4/yr. GBP 93, USD 153 to individuals; GBP 360, USD 594 to institutions (effective 2002). adv. bk.rev. index. *Refereed.* **Document type:** *Academic/Scholarly.* **Description:** Publishes multidisciplinary papers on the prevention of substance abuse and related problems. Provides a forum for those concerned with education and prevention policy and its application in the community, and promotes dialogue with those affected by such applications and community practice.
Related titles: Microfiche ed.; Online - full text ed.: ISSN 1465-3370 (from CatchWord Ltd., EBSCO Publishing, O C L C Online Computer Library Center, Inc., RoweCom Information Quest, ProQuest Information & Learning, Swets Blackwell, Institute for Scientific Information).
Indexed: ASCA, ASSIA, Addic.Abstr., Br.Educ.Ind., Crim.Just.Abstr., Curr.Cont., ERA, Environ.Sci.Poll.Mgmt., Lang.& Lang.Behav.Abstr., Mult.Ed.Abstr., Pollut.Abstr., PsycInfo, Risk Abstr., SOPODA, SSCI, Saf.Sci.Abstr., Sage Race Rel.Abstr., Soc.Serv.Abstr., Sociol.Abstr., e-psyche.
—BLDSC (3629.818000), CatchWord, IDS, Infotrieve. **CCC.**
Published by: Carfax Publishing Limited (Subsidiary of: Taylor & Francis Group), PO Box 25, Abingdon, Oxon OX14 3UE, United Kingdom. TEL 44-1235-401000, FAX 44-1235-401550, enquiries@carfax.co.uk, enquiry@tandf.co.uk, http://www.carfax.co.uk. Ed. Stuart Ware.

362.29 AUS ISSN 1036-9864
DRUGS IN SOCIETY. Text in English. 1986. q. back issues avail.
Formerly (1986-1991): Channel A D F Q (1030-8342)
Related titles: Online - full text ed.
Published by: Alcohol and Drug Foundation, PO Box 332, Spring Hill, QLD 4004, Australia. TEL 61-7-38323798, FAX 61-7-38322527, dinie@ats.com.au, http://www.adfq.org. Ed. Craig Ashdown.

616.86 USA ISSN 0273-8910
HF5549.5.E42 CODEN: EAPDEW
E A P DIGEST. (Employee Assistance Programs) Text in English. 1980. bi-m. USD 36 domestic; USD 45 in Canada; USD 55 elsewhere. adv. bk.rev. **Document type:** *Trade.*
Indexed: Soc.Work Res.& Abstr., e-psyche.
—ingenta.
Published by: Performance Resource Press, Inc., 1270 Rankin Dr, Ste F, Troy, MI 48083-2843. TEL 810-588-7733, FAX 810-588-6633. Ed. Brent Chartier. Circ: 10,000.

EMPLOYEE ASSISTANCE QUARTERLY. see *BUSINESS AND ECONOMICS—Personnel Management*

362.29 616.86 CHE ISSN 1022-6877
CODEN: EADREE
EUROPEAN ADDICTION RESEARCH. Text in English. 1995. q. CHF 501 in Europe to institutions; CHF 512.60 overseas to institutions; EUR 358.20 in Europe to institutions; USD 391 overseas to institutions (effective 2002). adv. back issues avail. *Refereed.* **Document type:** *Journal, Academic/Scholarly.* **Description:** International forum for the exchange of interdisciplinary information and expert opinions on all aspects of addiction research. Coverage ranges from clinical and research advances in the fields of psychiatry, biology, pharmacology and epidemiology to the social, and legal implications of political decisions.
Related titles: Online - full text ed.: ISSN 1421-9891. CHF 58, EUR 42, USD 45 to institutions with print edition (effective 2002) (from EBSCO Publishing, O C L C Online Computer Library Center, Inc., RoweCom Information Quest, Swets Blackwell, Institute for Scientific Information).
Indexed: Addic.Abstr., Crim.Just.Abstr., Curr.Cont., Excerp.Med. (1996-), Ind.Med. (1995-), SSCI.
—BLDSC (3829.482945), EMDOCS, GNLM, IDS, Infotrieve, KNAW. **CCC.**
Published by: S. Karger AG, Allschwilerstr 10, PO Box, Basel 4009, Switzerland. TEL 41-61-306-1111, FAX 41-61-306-1234, karger@karger.ch, http://www.online.karger.com/journals/ear, http://www.karger.com. Eds. A Uchtenhagen, M Krausz. adv.: page USD 1,195.

616.863 DEU
FAMILIEN-KALENDER. Text in German. 1902. a. DEM 6.80 (effective 2000). bk.rev. back issues avail. **Document type:** *Bulletin.*
Published by: Blaukreuz Verlag, Freiligrathstr 27, Wuppertal 42289, Germany. Ed. Claudius Schillinger. Circ: 16,000.

345.0277 340 345 614.19 USA ISSN 1048-8731
FORENSIC DRUG ABUSE ADVISOR; a monthly digest of information on the forensic aspects of drug abuse. Text in English. 1989. m. USD 197 (effective 2000). bk.rev. stat. back issues avail. *Refereed.* **Document type:** *Newsletter.* **Description:** An information source for medical, legal, and substance abuse professionals and libraries. Emphasizes latest scientific discoveries in drug abuse, work place testing, federal regulations, and the law.
Published by: Forensic Drug Abuse Advisor, Inc., PO Box 5139, Berkeley, CA 94705-5139. TEL 510-849-0923, FAX 510-849-0958, fdaa@batnet.com. Ed. Steven B Karch. Pub. Donna Leonti. Circ: 800 (paid).

616.86 USA ISSN 0194-8121
THE FORUM (VIRGINIA BEACH). Text in English. 1952. m. USD 10 domestic; USD 11 foreign (effective 2001). index. back issues avail. **Description:** Family members and friends of alcoholics relate personal experiences regarding Twelve Step program of recovery.
Related titles: Braille ed.; Large type ed. 22 pt.
Published by: (Al-Anon Family Group Headquarters, Inc.), A F G, Inc., 1600 Corporate Landing Pkwy, Virginia Beach, VA 23454-5617. TEL 757-563-1600, FAX 757-563-1655, http://www.al-anon.alateen.org. Ed. Patrick Quiggle. R&P Caryn Johnson. Circ: 40,000.

178 CAN
FORWARD. Text in English. 1894. m. CND 2, USD 2.25. adv. illus.
Published by: (Grand Division Sons of Temperance of Nova Scotia), David Allbon & Co. Ltd., P O Box 1090, Windsor, NS B0N 2T0, Canada. TEL 902-798-2456. Ed. Annie L Bird. Circ: 600.

FREIE FAHRT/ROUTE LIBRE. see *PUBLIC HEALTH AND SAFETY*

616.861 DEU ISSN 0342-4685
FUEREINANDER. Text in German. 1971. s-m. DEM 22.80 (effective 2000). reprint service avail. from SCH,PSC. **Document type:** *Bulletin.*
Incorporated (1906-1999): Rettung (0048-7430)
—CCC.
Published by: (Blaues Kreuz in Deutschland e.V.), Blaukreuz Verlag, Freiligrathstr 27, Wuppertal 42289, Germany. Ed. Claudius Schillinger. Circ: 14,000.

616.86 362.1 NLD ISSN 0166-2880
DE GEHEEL-ONTHOUDER. Text in Dutch. 1901. bi-m. NLG 15.50; NLG 22.50 foreign (effective 1999). adv. bk.rev. illus, stat. back issues avail. *Refereed.* **Document type:** *Journal, Academic/Scholarly, Consumer.* **Description:** Reports new facts on the medical, criminological, and sociological aspects of drug and alcohol abuse to increase public awareness of this problem.
Related titles: Fax ed.
Published by: Algemeen Nederlandse Geheel-Onthouders Bond (ANGOB), Stationsweg 11, Maarssen 3603 ED, Netherlands. TEL 31-346-562563, FAX 31-346-562563, dkorf@worldmail.nl. Ed., R&P D. Korf. Adv. contact W Matla. B&W page NLG 1,650; trim 270 x 184. Circ: 1,020 (paid). **Dist. by:** Drukkerij Banda, PO Box 14, Kollum 9290, Netherlands. TEL 31-511-451341, FAX 31-511-451312.

616.86 USA
GUILFORD SUBSTANCE ABUSE SERIES. Text in English. irreg. (approx. 2/yr.). **Document type:** *Monographic series.* **Description:** Provides therapies and theories that can be used to treat and understand people with alcohol and drug problems and their families.
Published by: Guilford Publications, Inc., 72 Spring St, New York, NY 10012. TEL 212-431-9800, 800-365-7006, FAX 212-966-6708, info@guilford.com. Ed. Seymour Weingarten. Pub. Robert Matloff. R&P David Mitchell. Adv. contact Christine Luberto.

616.86 USA
HAZELDEN VOICE; news and opinion for recovering people and professionals. Text in English. 1990. 2/yr. free per issue. bk.rev. **Document type:** *Newsletter.* **Description:** Covers a broad range of issues for professionals in the chemical health field and for those in recovery from chemical dependency and other related addictive behaviors.
Formerly (until 1996): Hazelden News and Professional Update
Published by: Hazelden Foundation, PO Box 11, Center City, MN 55012-0011. TEL 651-213-4455, FAX 651-213-4344. Ed., R&P Marty Duda. Circ: 95,000 (free).

178 GBR
THE HERALD (BRISTOL). Text in English. 1836. 2/yr. free per issue. **Document type:** *Bulletin.* **Description:** Facts, views, comments from Christian viewpoint, on the alcohol-drug scene.
Formerly: Western Temperance Herald (0049-7517)
Published by: Western Alcohol and Drugs Education Society, Upper, 6 Gloucester St, Eastville, Bristol BS5 6QE, United Kingdom. TEL 0272-512187. Ed. Raymond Foster. Circ: 3,500.

HIGHLIFE; tijdschrift voor levensgenieters. see *LITERARY AND POLITICAL REVIEWS*

362.2 HKG
HONG KONG NARCOTICS REPORT. Text in Chinese. 1965. a. free per issue to qualified personnel. illus.
Former titles: Action Committee Against Narcotics. Annual Report; Narcotics Progress Report
Published by: Action Committee Against Narcotics, c/o Narcotics Division Government Secretariat, Queensway Governnment Offices, High Block, 66 Queensway, Hong Kong, Hong Kong. FAX 852-2521-7761. Circ: 10,000.

178 CHE
I C A A PUBLICATIONS. Text in English. 1982. irreg. price varies. **Document type:** *Monographic series, Academic/Scholarly.* **Description:** Discusses innovations in treatment, education and control of substance abuse.
Published by: International Council on Alcohol and Addictions, Case Postale 189, Lausanne 1001, Switzerland. TEL 41-21-3209865, FAX 41-21-3209817, infoconf@icaa.ch, http://www.icaa.ch. Ed., R&P Christian Pellet.

D

613.8 USA ISSN 1016-0477
I C A D T S REPORTER. Text in English. 1990. q. free.
Document type: *Newsletter, Academic/Scholarly.*
Description: Aims to reduce mortality and morbidity brought about by misuse of alcohol and drugs by operators of vehicles in all modes of transportation.
Published by: International Committee on Alcohol, Drugs and Traffic Safety, 3798 Mosswood Dr, Lafayette, CA 94549. TEL 925-962-1810, FAX 925-962-1810, http://raru.adelaide.edu.au/icadts. Eds. Barry Sweedler, Kathryn Stewart.

613.81 CHE
INTERNATIONAL CONGRESS ON ALCOHOLISM AND DRUG DEPENDENCE. PROCEEDINGS. Text in Multiple languages. triennial. CHF 175. **Document type:** *Proceedings, Academic/Scholarly.*
Former titles: International Congress on Alcoholism and Addictions. Proceedings; International Congress on Alcohol and Alcoholism. Proceedings
Published by: International Council on Alcohol and Addictions, Case Postale 189, Lausanne 1001, Switzerland. TEL 41-21-3209865, FAX 41-21-3209817, infoconf@icaa.ch, http://www.icaa.ch. Ed., R&P Dr. Joerg Spieldenner.

INTERNATIONAL DRUG REPORT. see *CRIMINOLOGY AND LAW ENFORCEMENT*

613.81 CHE
HV5801 CODEN: PIIDD3
INTERNATIONAL INSTITUTE ON THE PREVENTION AND TREATMENT OF DEPENDENCIES. SELECTED PAPERS. Text in English. 1970. irreg. **Document type:** *Monographic series, Academic/Scholarly.*
Former titles (until 1996): International Institutes on the Prevention and Treatment of Addictions. Selected Papers (0254-2536); International Institute on the Prevention and Treatment of Drug Dependence. Selected Papers
Indexed: Chem.Abstr.
—CASDDS.
Published by: International Council on Alcohol and Addictions, Case Postale 189, Lausanne 1001, Switzerland. TEL 41-21-3209865, FAX 41-21-3209817, infoconf@icaa.ch, http://www.icaa.ch. Ed., R&P Dr. Joerg Spieldenner. Circ: 1,000.

616.86 NLD ISSN 0955-3959
HV5800 CODEN: IJDPED
INTERNATIONAL JOURNAL OF DRUG POLICY. Text in English. 1989. bi-m. EUR 151 in Europe to individuals; JPY 20,000 in Japan to individuals; USD 168 elsewhere to individuals; EUR 362 in Europe to institutions; JPY 48,000 in Japan to institutions; USD 405 elsewhere to institutions (effective 2002). adv. bk.rev. *Refereed.*
Document type: *Academic/Scholarly.* **Description:** Presents current research, reliable information and in-depth policy analyses of the global drugs debate.
Related titles: Online - full text ed.: (from ingenta, Swets Blackwell, ScienceDirect).
Indexed: ASSIA, Abstr.Crim.& Pen., Abstr.Hyg., Addic.Abstr., CINAHL, Crim.Just.Abstr., I.P.A., Soc.Serv.Abstr., Sociol.Abstr., Trop.Dis.Bull.
—BLDSC (4542.188500), ADONIS, KNAW.
Published by: Elsevier Science BV, Regional Sales Office, PO Box 211, Amsterdam 1000 AE, Netherlands. TEL 31-20-485-2911, nlinfo-f@elsevier.nl, http://www.elsevier.com/locate/drugpo. Eds. G Stimson, T Rhodes. Adv. contact Maggy Park. page GBP 225. Circ: 400. **Subscr. in Australasia and the Far East to:** Elsevier Science (Singapore) Pte Ltd, No.1 Temasek Ave, 17-01 Millenia Tower, Singapore 039192, Singapore. TEL 65-434-3727, FAX 65-337-2230; **Subscr. in Japan to:** Elsevier Science Inc - Japan Regional Office, 9-15 Higashi-Azabu 1-chome, Minato-ku, Tokyo 106-0044, Japan. TEL 81-3-5561-5033; **Subscr. in the Americas to:** Elsevier Science, PO Box 945, New York, NY 10159-0945. TEL 212-633-3730, FAX 212-633-3680.

INTERNATIONAL NARCOTIC ENFORCEMENT OFFICERS ASSOCIATION DIRECTORY. see *CRIMINOLOGY AND LAW ENFORCEMENT*

INTERNATIONAL NARCOTICS CONTROL BOARD. REPORT FOR (YEAR). see *PHARMACY AND PHARMACOLOGY*

616.86 CHE
INTERNATIONALES SYMPOSIUM GEGEN DROGEN IN DER SCHWEIZ. Text in German. 1991. irreg.
Document type: *Proceedings.*
Indexed: e-psyche.
Published by: Verein zur Foerderung der Psychologischen Menschenkenntnis, Susenbergstr 53, Zuerich 8044, Switzerland.

362.2 USA
IOWA SUBSTANCE ABUSE REPORT (YEAR). Text in English. 1973. a. free per issue. **Document type:** *Government.*
Former titles: Iowa Comprehensive State Plan for Substance Abuse (Year); Iowa Comprehensive State Plan for Substance Abuse Prevention: Annual Performance Report; (until 1980): Iowa Comprehensive State Plan for Drug Abuse Prevention: Annual Performance Report (0363-4507)
Published by: Department of Public Health, Division of Substance Abuse, Lucas State Office Bldg, 321 E 12th St, Des Moines, IA 50319. TEL 515-281-3641, FAX 515-281-4535. Circ: 1,000.

616.8 DEU ISSN 0940-4910
JAHRBUCH SUCHT. Text in German. 1958. a. DEM 27 (effective 2001). adv. **Document type:** *Yearbook, Academic/Scholarly.*
Former titles: Jahrbuch zur Frage der Suchtgefahren (0170-7337); Jahrbuch zur Alkohol- und Tabakfrage (0075-2827)
Indexed: IBZ.
—GNLM.
Published by: (Deutsche Hauptstelle gegen die Suchtgefahren), Neuland Verlagsgesellschaft mbH, Markt 24-26, Geesthacht 21502, Germany. TEL 49-4152-81342, FAX 49-4152-81343, vertrieb@neuland.com, http://www.neuland.com. Circ: 7,000.

616.86 CAN ISSN 1481-3122
THE JOURNAL OF ADDICTION AND MENTAL HEALTH. Text in English, French. 1998. bi-m. CND 24.95 domestic; CND 36.95 foreign (effective 2000). adv. bk.rev. abstr. index. back issues avail. **Document type:** *Newsletter, Trade, Government.* **Description:** Covers the latest developments in the mental health and addications fields for professionals and consumers.
Formed by the merger of (1972-1998): Addiction and Mental Health Services Corporation. Journal (0044-6203); (1994-1998): Fondation de la Recherche sur la Toxicomanie. Journal (1201-2572)
Media: Microfiche. **Related titles:** CD-ROM ed.; Online - full text ed.: (from LexisNexis); French ed.: Le Journal de Toxicomanie et de Sante Mentale. ISSN 1481-3254.
Indexed: CBCA Ref., Can.B.P.I., Can.Per.Ind.
—CCC.
Published by: Centre for Addiction and Mental Health, 33 Russell St, Toronto, ON M5S 2S1, Canada. TEL 416-595-6714, 800-661-1111, FAX 416-595-6892, adubey@arf.org, http://www.camh.net/journal. Ed., R&P Anita Dubey. Adv. contact Doreen Grbic. B&W page CND 1,300. Circ: 8,000; 1,000 (paid); 1,500 (controlled).

JOURNAL OF ADDICTIONS NURSING. see *MEDICAL SCIENCES—Nurses And Nursing*

616.86 USA ISSN 1055-0887
HV5800 CODEN: JADDER
JOURNAL OF ADDICTIVE DISEASES; the official journal of the American Society of Addictive Medicine. Text in English. 1981. q. USD 85 to individuals; USD 115 in Canada to individuals; USD 123 elsewhere to individuals; USD 150 to institutions; USD 203 in Canada to institutions; USD 218 elsewhere to institutions; USD 500 to libraries; USD 675 in Canada to libraries; USD 725 elsewhere to libraries (effective Aug. 2001). adv. bk.rev. bibl. back issues avail.; reprint service avail. from HAW. *Refereed.* **Document type:** *Journal, Academic/Scholarly.* **Description:** Covers current topics in alcoholism and substance abuse field and devotes an entire issue to each topic.
Formerly (until 1991): Advances in Alcohol and Substance Abuse (0270-3106); Supersedes (1977-1981): Drug Abuse and Alcoholism Review (0149-5968)
Related titles: Microfiche ed.: (from PQC); Microform ed.; Online - full text ed.: (from Institute for Scientific Information).
Indexed: ASCA, Abstr.Anthropol., Abstr.Crim.& Pen., Addic.Abstr., Adol.Ment.Hlth.Abstr., Biol.Abstr., CJPI, Chem.Abstr., Child Devel.Abstr., Crim.Just.Abstr., Curr.Adv.Ecol.Sci., Curr.Cont., Environ.Sci.Poll.Mgmt., Excerp.Med., Fam.Ind., IMFL, INIS Atomind., I.P.A., Ind.Med. (1991-), Int.Nurs.Ind., Lang.& Lang.Behav.Abstr., Past.Care & Couns.Abstr., Pollut.Abstr., PsycInfo, Psychol.Abstr. (1981-), Risk Abstr., SOPODA, SSCI, Saf.Sci.Abstr., Sage Race Rel.Abstr., Soc.Serv.Abstr., Soc.Work Res.& Abstr., Sociol.Abstr., Stud.Wom.Abstr., THA, Tox.Abstr., e-psyche.
—BLDSC (4918.934050), CASDDS, EMDOCS, GNLM, Haworth, IDS, ingenta, KNAW.
Published by: (American Society of Addiction Medicine), Haworth Press, Inc., 10 Alice St, Binghamton, NY 13904-1580. TEL 607-722-5857, 800-429-6784, FAX 607-722-6362, 800-895-0582, getinfo@haworthpressinc.com, http://www.haworthpress.com/journals/journallist.asp. Ed. Dr. Barry Stimmel. Pub. William Cohen. R&P Ruthann Heath TEL 607-723-5857 ext 316. Adv. contact Jackie Blakeslee TEL 607-722-5857 ext 346. B&W page USD 375, color page USD 650; trim 6 x 8.5. Circ: 4,000.

616.86 USA ISSN 0090-1482
HV5128.U5 CODEN: JADEDT
JOURNAL OF ALCOHOL AND DRUG EDUCATION. Short title: J.A.D.E. Text in English. 1955. 3/yr. USD 45 domestic; USD 55 foreign (effective 2001). back issues avail.; reprint service avail. from PQC. *Refereed.*
Document type: *Academic/Scholarly.* **Description:** Serves as a forum for various educational philosophies and differing points of view in regard to alcohol and drugs. Reports teacher experience and experiments and provides a reference for actual teaching materials, factual guide for prevention, techniques and procedures.
Formerly: Journal of Alcohol Education (0021-8677)
Related titles: Microform ed.: (from PQC); Online - full text ed.: (from H. W. Wilson, ProQuest Information & Learning, Institute for Scientific Information).
Indexed: ASCA, Addic.Abstr., Adol.Ment.Hlth.Abstr., AgeLine, C.I.J.E., CINAHL, Cont.Pg.Educ., Crim.Just.Abstr., Curr.Cont., ERA, Educ.Ind. (Jan.1983-), Environ.Sci.Poll.Mgmt., Fam.Ind., HRIS, High.Educ.Abstr., Mult.Ed.Abstr., Pollut.Abstr., PsycInfo, Psychol.Abstr. (1972-), Risk Abstr., Russ.Acad.Sci.Bibl., SSCI, Saf.Sci.Abstr., Sp.Ed.Needs Abstr., Tech.Educ.Abstr., e-psyche.
—BLDSC (4926.720000), GNLM, IDS, ingenta.
Published by: American Alcohol and Drug Information Foundation (Lansing), 1120 East Oakland, P O Box 10212, Lansing, MI 48901-0212. TEL 517-484-2636, FAX 517-484-0444, dcorbin@coe.unomaha.edu, http://www.unomaha.edu/~healthed/JADE.html. Eds. David E Corbin, Manoj Sharma, Allen B Rice II. R&P Kenton L Owens.

JOURNAL OF BEHAVIORAL HEALTH SERVICES AND RESEARCH. see *PUBLIC HEALTH AND SAFETY*

616.863 USA ISSN 0885-4734
RC563
JOURNAL OF CHEMICAL DEPENDENCY TREATMENT; the official journal of the national association of addiction treatment providers. Text in English. 1987. s-a. USD 75 to individuals; USD 101 in Canada to individuals; USD 109 elsewhere to individuals; USD 150 to institutions; USD 203 in Canada to institutions; USD 218 elsewhere to institutions; USD 225 to libraries; USD 304 in Canada to libraries; USD 326 elsewhere to libraries (effective Aug. 2001). adv. back issues avail.; reprint service avail. from HAW. *Refereed.* **Document type:** *Journal, Academic/Scholarly.* **Description:** Provides direct clinical services. Each issue examines a specific chemical dependency problem. Stresses clinical techniques and methods while integrating theory and research.
Related titles: Microfiche ed.: (from PQC); Microform ed.
Indexed: Crim.Just.Abstr., Environ.Sci.Poll.Mgmt., IMFL, Pollut.Abstr., Psychol.Abstr., Risk Abstr., Saf.Sci.Abstr., Soc.Work Res.& Abstr., THA.
—BLDSC (4955.900000), GNLM, Haworth.
Published by: Haworth Press, Inc., 10 Alice St, Binghamton, NY 13904-1580. TEL 607-722-5857, 800-429-6784, FAX 607-722-6362, 800-895-0582, getinfo@haworthpressinc.com, http://www.haworthpress.com/journals/journallist.asp. Eds. David Powell, Gerald Shulman. Pub. William Cohen. R&P Ruthann Heath TEL 607-723-5857 ext 316. Adv. contact Jackie Blakeslee TEL 607-722-5857 ext 346. B&W page USD 315, color page USD 550; trim 6 x 8.5. Circ: 825.

616.863 USA ISSN 1067-828X
RJ506.D78 CODEN: JCAAFI
JOURNAL OF CHILD & ADOLESCENT SUBSTANCE ABUSE. Text in English. 1989. q. USD 60 to individuals; USD 81 in Canada to individuals; USD 87 elsewhere to individuals; USD 95 to institutions; USD 128 in Canada to institutions; USD 138 elsewhere to institutions; USD 225 to libraries; USD 304 in Canada to libraries; USD 326 elsewhere to libraries (effective Aug. 2001). adv. bk.rev. back issues avail.; reprint service avail. from HAW. *Refereed.* **Document type:** *Journal, Academic/Scholarly.* **Description:** Provides realistic and usable strategies in a clear and concise manner for the chemically dependent adolescent and his or her family.
Formerly (until 1994): Journal of Adolescent Chemical Dependency (0896-7768)

Related titles: Microfiche ed.: (from PQC); Microform ed.; Online - full text ed.: (from Institute for Scientific Information).
Indexed: ASCA, Biol.Dig., C.I.J.E., CINAHL, Chem.Abstr., Child Devel.Abstr., Crim.Just.Abstr., Curr.Cont., ERA, Environ.Sci.Poll.Mgmt., Except.Child Educ.Abstr., Fam.Ind., IMFL, Ind.Med. (coverage dropped), Lang.& Lang.Behav.Abstr., PsycInfo, Psychol.Abstr. (1991-), SOPODA, SSCI, Sage Fam.Stud.Abstr., Soc.Serv.Abstr., Soc.Work Res.& Abstr., Sociol.Abstr., Sp.Ed.Needs Abstr., THA, Viol.& Abuse Abstr., e-psyche.
—BLDSC (4957.425300), GNLM, Haworth, IDS, KNAW.
Published by: Haworth Press, Inc., 10 Alice St, Binghamton, NY 13904-1580. TEL 607-722-5857, 800-429-6784, FAX 607-722-6362, 800-895-0582, getinfo@haworthpressinc.com, http://www.haworthpress.com/journals/journallist.asp. Eds. Brad Donohue, Vincent B Van Hasselt. Pub. William Cohen. R&P Ruthann Heath TEL 607-723-5857 ext 316. Adv. contact Jackie Blakeslee TEL 607-722-5857 ext 346. B&W page USD 315, color page USD 550; trim 6 x 8.5.

362.293 USA ISSN 0047-2379
HV5808 CODEN: JDGEBT
JOURNAL OF DRUG EDUCATION. Text in English. 1970. q. USD 56 to individuals; USD 218 to institutions (effective 2001). adv. bk.rev. abstr, charts, illus. back issues avail.; reprint service avail. from SCH,PSC. *Refereed.* **Document type:** *Journal, Academic/Scholarly.* **Description:** Contains current, authoritative and practical articles on the latest developments in preventive practices, and issues and trends in drug education and addiction management.
Related titles: Online - full text ed.: (from Institute for Scientific Information).
Indexed: ASCA, ASSIA, Abstr.Anthropol., Adol.Ment.Hlth.Abstr., AgeLine, Biol.Abstr., C.I.J.E., Chic.Per.Ind., Cont.Pg.Educ., Crim.Just.Abstr., Curr.Cont., ERA, Educ.Ind. (Jan.1983-), Educ.Tech.Abstr., Environ.Sci.Poll.Mgmt., Excerp.Med., Fam.Ind., I.P.A., Ind.Med. (1971-), Lang.& Lang.Behav.Abstr., Mid.East: Abstr.& Ind., Mult.Ed.Abstr., Pollut.Abstr., PsycInfo, Psychol.Abstr. (1971-), Ref.Zh., Risk Abstr., SOPODA, SSCI, Saf.Sci.Abstr., Soc.Serv.Abstr., Sociol.Abstr., Sp.Ed.Needs Abstr., Stud.Wom.Abstr., Tech.Educ.Abstr., e-psyche.
—BLDSC (4970.550000), CISTI, EMDOCS, GNLM, IDS, Infotrieve, ingenta, KNAW. **CCC.**
Published by: Baywood Publishing Co., Inc., 26 Austin Ave, Box 337, Amityville, NY 11701. TEL 631-691-1270, 800-638-7819, FAX 631-691-1770, info@baywood.com, baywood@baywood.com, http://baywood.com/search/PreviewJournal.asp?qsRecord=13. R&P Julie Krempa. Adv. contact Joi Tamber-Brooks.

616.86 USA ISSN 0022-0426
HV5800 CODEN: JDGIA6
JOURNAL OF DRUG ISSUES. Text in English. 1971. q. USD 80 to individuals; USD 90 foreign to individuals; USD 105 to institutions; USD 115 foreign to institutions (effective 1999 - 2000). adv. bk.rev. bibl, charts. index, cum.index. reprint service avail. from WSH,PQC,PSC,SCH. *Refereed.* **Document type:** *Academic/Scholarly.* **Description:** Critical commentary on a wide range of drug policy issues.
Related titles: Microfilm ed.: (from PQC); Online - full text ed.: (from Northern Light Technology, Inc., H. W. Wilson, ProQuest Information & Learning, Gale Group, Factiva, Institute for Scientific Information).
Indexed: ASCA, ASSIA, Abstr.Crim.& Pen., Addic.Abstr., Adol.Ment.Hlth.Abstr., AgeLine, Behav.Abstr., Biol.Abstr., C.L.I., Crim.Just.Abstr., Curr.Cont., Environ.Sci.Poll.Mgmt., Excerp.Med., IBZ, IMFL, I.P.A., Ind.Per.Art.Relat.Law, Lang.& Lang.Behav.Abstr., Leg.Per. (coverage dropped), Mid.East: Abstr.& Ind., P C I, Pollut.Abstr., PsycInfo, Psychol.Abstr. (1972-), Ref.Zh., Rel.Ind.One, Rel.Ind.Two, Risk Abstr., SOPODA, SSCI, Saf.Sci.Abstr., Soc.Sci.Ind. (Jan.1987-), Soc.Serv.Abstr., Soc.Work Res.& Abstr., Sociol.Abstr., THA, e-psyche.
—BLDSC (4970.570000), GNLM, IDS, ingenta, KNAW. **CCC.**
Published by: Florida State University, School of Criminology & Criminal Justice, PO Box 66696, Tallahassee, FL 32313-6696. TEL 850-664-7368, FAX 850-644-9614. Ed. Bruce Bullington. R&P Claire Knox TEL 850-644-6157. Circ: 1,000.

616.863 USA ISSN 1533-2640
HV5800 CODEN: DRSOEI
JOURNAL OF ETHNICITY IN SUBSTANCE ABUSE. Text in English. 1986. q. USD 50 to individuals; USD 68 in Canada to individuals; USD 73 elsewhere to individuals; USD 125 to institutions; USD 169 in Canada to institutions; USD 181 elsewhere to institutions; USD 275 to libraries; USD 371 in Canada to libraries; USD 399 elsewhere to libraries (effective Aug. 2001). adv. bk.rev. reprint service avail. from HAW. *Refereed.* **Document type:** *Academic/Scholarly.* **Description:** Provides current information pertaining to the field of substance abuse. Directed toward researchers, professionals, and practitioners in substance abuse related fields and to students seeking to enter the field.
Formerly (until 2001): Drugs & Society (8756-8233)
Related titles: Microfiche ed.: (from PQC); Microform ed.; Online - full text ed.: (from Gale Group).
Indexed: ASSIA, Abstr.Anthropol., CJPI, Child Devel.Abstr., Crim.Just.Abstr., Environ.Sci.Poll.Mgmt., Excerp.Med., IBZ, IMFL, I.P.A., Int.Polit.Sci.Abstr., Lang.& Lang.Behav.Abstr., P.A.I.S., Pollut.Abstr., PsycInfo, Psychol.Abstr. (1986-), Ref.Zh., SOPODA, Soc.Sci.Ind. (Jan.2002-), Soc.Serv.Abstr., Soc.Work Res.& Abstr., Sociol.Abstr., Tox.Abstr., e-psyche.
—BLDSC (3629.652000), EMDOCS, GNLM, Haworth, ingenta.
Published by: Haworth Press, Inc., 10 Alice St, Binghamton, NY 13904-1580. TEL 607-722-5857, 800-429-6784, FAX 607-722-6362, 800-895-0582, getinfo@haworthpressinc.com, http://www.haworthpress.com/journals/journallist.asp. Ed. Peter Myers. Pub. William Cohen. R&P Ruthann Heath TEL 607-723-5857 ext 316. Adv. contact Jackie Blakeslee TEL 607-722-5857 ext 346. B&W page USD 315, color page USD 550; trim 6 x 8.5. Circ: 350.

616.863 USA ISSN 1091-1332
RC568.M4
JOURNAL OF MAINTENANCE IN THE ADDICTIONS; innovations in research, theory, & practice. Text in English. 1996. q. USD 45 to individuals; USD 61 in Canada to individuals; USD 65 elsewhere to individuals; USD 50 to institutions; USD 68 in Canada to institutions; USD 73 elsewhere to institutions; USD 95 to libraries; USD 128 in Canada to libraries; USD 138 elsewhere to libraries (effective Aug. 2001). adv. reprint service avail. from HAW. *Refereed.* **Document type:** *Journal, Academic/Scholarly.* **Description:** Provides cutting-edge articles that assist in the understanding of clinical management at the most practical level.
Related titles: Microfiche ed.: (from PQC); Microform ed.; Online - full text ed.
—BLDSC (5010.797500), Haworth.
Published by: Haworth Press, Inc., 10 Alice St, Binghamton, NY 13904-1580. TEL 607-722-5857, 800-429-6784, FAX 607-722-6362, 800-895-0582, getinfo@haworthpressinc.com, http://www.haworthpress.com/journals/journallist.asp. Eds. Ira Marion, Dr. J Thomas Payte, Joan Zweben, Peter DeMaria. Pub. William Cohen. R&P Ruthann Heath TEL 607-723-5857 ext 316. Adv. contact Jackie Blakeslee TEL 607-722-5857 ext 346. B&W page USD 315, color page USD 550; trim 6 x 8.5.

JOURNAL OF MINISTRY IN ADDICTION & RECOVERY. see *RELIGIONS AND THEOLOGY*

301 616.8 615 USA ISSN 0279-1072
BF207 CODEN: JPDRD3
JOURNAL OF PSYCHOACTIVE DRUGS; a multidisciplinary forum. Text in English. 1967. q. USD 90 to individuals; USD 160 to institutions (effective 2001). adv. bk.rev. charts, illus, stat. reprint service avail. from PQC,SCH,PSC,ISI. *Refereed.* **Document type:** *Journal, Academic/Scholarly.* **Description:** Focuses on human use and abuse of alcohol and other drugs, as well as related issues, such as treatment modalities, AIDS, and dual diagnosis.
Formerly (until vol.13, 1981): Journal of Psychedelic Drugs (0022-393X)
Related titles: Microform ed.: (from PQC); Online - full text ed.: (from Northern Light Technology, Inc., ProQuest Information & Learning, Institute for Scientific Information).
Indexed: ASCA, Addic.Abstr., Adol.Ment.Hlth.Abstr., AgeLine, Biol.Abstr., Chem.Abstr., Chic.Per.Ind., Crim.Just.Abstr., Curr.Cont., Excerp.Med., Fam.Ind., HRIS, IMFL, Ind.Med. (1981-), Int.Nurs.Ind., PsycInfo, Psychol.Abstr. (1971-), Ref.Zh., SSCI, Sage Fam.Stud.Abstr., Sage Race Rel.Abstr., Soc.Sci.Ind. (coverage dropped), THA, Viol.& Abuse Abstr., e-psyche.
—BLDSC (5043.263000), CASDDS, CISTI, EMDOCS, GNLM, IDS, Infotrieve, ingenta, KNAW. **CCC.**

Published by: Haight-Ashbury Publications, 612 Clayton St, San Francisco, CA 94117. TEL 415-565-1904, FAX 415-864-6162, hapjpd@hafreeclinics.org, http://www.hafci.org/hafci/index.,html. Eds. Richard B Seymour, Terry Chambers. Circ: 800.

JOURNAL OF PUBLIC HEALTH POLICY. see *PUBLIC HEALTH AND SAFETY*

362.29 USA ISSN 1065-2019
JOURNAL OF RATIONAL RECOVERY. Text in English. 1988. bi-m. USD 32 domestic; USD 50 foreign; USD 11 base vol(s). per issue (effective 2001). **Document type:** *Journal, Academic/Scholarly.*
Published by: Rational Recovery Systems, Inc., Box 800, Lotus, CA 95651 . TEL 530-621-4374, 530-621-2667, http://www.rational.org/.

JOURNAL OF SOCIAL WORK PRACTICE. see *SOCIAL SERVICES AND WELFARE*

▼ **JOURNAL OF SOCIAL WORK PRACTICE IN THE ADDICTIONS.** see *SOCIAL SERVICES AND WELFARE*

616.861 016 USA ISSN 0096-882X
RC565 CODEN: JSALDP
JOURNAL OF STUDIES ON ALCOHOL. Text in English. 1940. bi-m. USD 140 domestic to individuals; USD 155 foreign to individuals; USD 175 domestic to institutions; USD 190 foreign to institutions (effective 2000). adv. bk.rev. abstr, bibl, charts, illus. index. back issues avail.; reprint service avail. from PSC,SCH. *Refereed.* **Document type:** *Academic/Scholarly.* **Description:** Contributes to knowledge about alcohol, its use, misuse and its biomedical, behavioral and sociocultural effects.
Formerly (until 1974): Quarterly Journal of Studies on Alcohol (0033-5649)
Related titles: Microform ed.: (from PQC); Online - full text ed.: (from Northern Light Technology, Inc., H. W. Wilson, Gale Group, Factiva, Institute for Scientific Information).
Indexed: ASCA, ASSIA, Abstr.Crim.& Pen., Addic.Abstr., Adol.Ment.Hlth.Abstr., AgeLine, Aqua.Sci.& Fish.Abstr., Behav.Med.Abstr., Bibl.Asian Stud. (1970), Biol.Abstr., C.I.S. Abstr., Chem.Abstr., Crim.Just.Abstr., Curr.Adv.Ecol.Sci., Curr.Cont., Dent.Ind., Dok.Arbeitsmed., Environ.Sci.Poll.Mgmt., Excerp.Med., Fam.Ind., HRIS, High.Educ.Abstr., Hist.Abstr. (coverage dropped), Ind.Med. (1975-), Ind.Sci.Rev., Int.Abstr.Biol.Sci., Int.Nurs.Ind., Jrnl.Watch Psych., Lang.& Lang.Behav.Abstr., Mid.East: Abstr.& Ind., Neurosci.Cit.Ind., Nutr.Abstr., P C I, P.A.I.S., Pollut.Abstr., PsycInfo, Psychol.Abstr. (1940-), Psychopharmacol.Abstr., Ref.Zh., Risk Abstr., Russ.Acad.Sci.Bibl., SSCI, Saf.Sci.Abstr., Sage Race Rel.Abstr., Sci.Cit.Ind., Soc.Sci.Ind. (May 1982-), Soc.Serv.Abstr., Soc.Work Res.& Abstr., Sociol.Abstr., THA, Tox.Abstr., VITIS, e-psyche.
—BLDSC (5066.895000), CASDDS, GNLM, IDS, ingenta, KNAW, Linda Hall. **CCC.**
Published by: (Rutgers Center of Alcohol Studies), Alcohol Research Documentation, Inc., c/o Charles Rouse, Bus Admin, Rutgers Center of Alcohol Studies, 607 Allison Rd, Piscataway, NJ 08854-8001. TEL 732-445-2190, FAX 732-445-3500. Ed. Marc A Schuckit. R&P Pat Castellano TEL 908-445-3510. Adv. contact Charles Rouse. Circ: 2,000 (paid).

616.86 GBR ISSN 0899-3289
RC563 CODEN: JSABEU
JOURNAL OF SUBSTANCE ABUSE. Text in English. 1988. q. NLG 215, EUR 97.56 in Europe to individuals; JPY 13,500 in Japan to individuals; USD 109 elsewhere to individuals; NLG 508, EUR 230.52 in Europe to institutions; JPY 31,900 in Japan to institutions; USD 258 elsewhere to institutions (effective 2001). index. back issues avail. *Refereed.* **Document type:** *Academic/Scholarly.* **Description:** Publishes articles pertaining to alcohol abuse, drug abuse, smoking, and eating disorders.
Related titles: Online - full text ed.: (from ingenta, ScienceDirect, Swets Blackwell, Institute for Scientific Information).
Indexed: Addic.Abstr., AgeLine, Curr.Cont., Environ.Sci.Poll.Mgmt., Excerp.Med. (1995-), Focus on: Psychophar., IMFL, Ind.Med. (1988-), Lang.& Lang.Behav.Abstr., Mult.Ed.Abstr., Pollut.Abstr., PsycInfo, Psychol.Abstr. (1989-), SOPODA, SSCI, Saf.Sci.Abstr., Soc.Work Res.& Abstr., Sociol.Abstr., Stud.Wom.Abstr., THA, Tox.Abstr., e-psyche.
—BLDSC (5066.931000), GNLM, Infotrieve, ingenta, KNAW. **CCC.**
Published by: Elsevier Science, The Boulevard, Langford Ln, Kidlington, Oxon OX5 1GB, United Kingdom. TEL 44-1865-843000, FAX 44-1865-843010, usinfo-f@elsevier.com, http://www.elsevier.com/locate/jsubab. Ed. Ted D Nirenberg. Circ: 350.

D

363 USA ISSN 0740-5472
RC563 CODEN: JSATEG
JOURNAL OF SUBSTANCE ABUSE TREATMENT. Text in English. 1984. 8/yr. EUR 162 in Europe to individuals; JPY 21,400 in Japan to individuals; USD 181 elsewhere to individuals; EUR 500 in Europe to institutions; JPY 66,400 in Japan to institutions; USD 559 elsewhere to institutions (effective 2002). adv. bk.rev. index. back issues avail. *Refereed.* **Document type:** *Academic/Scholarly.* **Description:** Features original contributions and articles on the clinical treatment of substance abuse and alcoholism.
Related titles: Microfilm ed.: (from PQC); Online - full text ed.: (from ingenta, Gale Group, ScienceDirect, Swets Blackwell, Factiva, Institute for Scientific Information).
Indexed: ASCA, Abstr.Anthropol., Addic.Abstr., Crim.Just.Abstr., Curr.Adv.Ecol.Sci., Curr.Cont., Environ.Sci.Poll.Mgmt., Fam.Ind., Ind.Med. (1984-), Int.Nurs.Ind., Lang.& Lang.Behav.Abstr., Pollut.Abstr., PsycInfo, Psychol.Abstr. (1984-), Risk Abstr., SOPODA, SSCI, Saf.Sci.Abstr., Soc.Serv.Abstr., Sociol.Abstr., THA, e-psyche.
—BLDSC (5066.932000), EMDOCS, GNLM, IDS, ingenta, KNAW. **CCC.**
Published by: (North Shore University Hospital), Elsevier Science, PO Box 945, New York, NY 10159-0945. TEL 212-989-5800, FAX 212-633-3990, nlinfo-f@elsevier.nl; usinfo-f@elsevier.com; forinfo-kyf04035@niftyserve.or.jp, http://www.elsevier.com/locate/jsat. Eds. John Imhof, Robert Hirsch. **Subscr. in Australasia and the Far East to:** Elsevier Science (Singapore) Pte Ltd, No.1 Temasek Ave, 17-01 Millenia Tower, Singapore 039192, Singapore. TEL 65-434-3727, FAX 65-337-2230; **Subscr. in Japan to:** Elsevier Science Inc - Japan Regional Office, 9-15 Higashi-Azabu 1-chome, Minato-ku, Tokyo 106-0044, Japan. TEL 81-3-5561-5033, FAX 81-3-5561-5047; **Subscr. outside the Americas to:** Elsevier Science BV, PO Box 211, Amsterdam 1000 AE, Netherlands. TEL 31-20-485-3757, FAX 31-20-485-3432, nlinfo-f@elsevier.nl.

616.8 610.73 GBR ISSN 1465-9891
CODEN: JSMIFA
JOURNAL OF SUBSTANCE USE; for nursing, health and social care. Text in English. 1996. q. GBP 49, USD 80 to individuals; GBP 172, USD 284 to institutions (effective 2002). adv. back issues avail. *Refereed.* **Document type:** *Academic/Scholarly.*
Formerly (until 1999): Journal of Substance Misuse (1357-5007)
Related titles: Online - full content ed.; Online - full text ed.: (from CatchWord Ltd.).
Indexed: ASSIA, Brit.Nur.Ind., CINAHL, Environ.Sci.Poll.Mgmt., Pollut.Abstr., Risk Abstr., Saf.Sci.Abstr., Tox.Abstr.
—BLDSC (5066.932700), EMDOCS, GNLM.
Published by: Radcliffe Medical Press Ltd., 18 Marcham Rd, Abingdon, Oxon OX14 1AA, United Kingdom. TEL 44-1235-528820, FAX 44-1235-528830, contact-us@radcliffemed.com, http://www.radcliffe-oxford.com/. Ed. Richard Pates.

JOURNAL OF TOXICOLOGY. CLINICAL TOXICOLOGY. see *PHARMACY AND PHARMACOLOGY*

616.861 DEU ISSN 0935-6223
KRANKENTRANSPORT UND RETTUNGSWESEN. Text in German. 1978. irreg. DEM 286 (effective 2000). **Document type:** *Monographic series, Trade.*
Published by: Erich Schmidt Verlag GmbH & Co. (Berlin), Genthiner Str 30G, Berlin 10785, Germany. TEL 49-30-250085-0, FAX 49-30-25008511, esv@esvmedien.de, http://www.erich-schmidt-verlag.de.

616.863 331 USA
MAINE. DEPARTMENT OF LABOR. BUREAU OF LABOR STANDARDS. SUBSTANCE ABUSE TESTING REPORT. Text in English. 1990. a. free. **Document type:** *Government.* **Description:** Contains results of the annual substance abuse testing survey.
Published by: Department of Labor, Bureau of Labor Standards, 45 State House Station, Augusta, ME 04333-0045. TEL 207-624-6440, FAX 207-624-6449, webmaster_bls@state.me.us. Ed., R&P Ruth A Ladd. Circ: 251.

616.8 340 USA ISSN 1010-9595
HD9665.3
MANUFACTURE OF NARCOTIC DRUGS AND PSYCHOTROPIC SUBSTANCES UNDER INTERNATIONAL CONTROL. Text in English, French, Spanish. 1948. a.
Formed by the 1987 merger of: Manufacture of Narcotic Drugs and Psychotropic Substances (0251-6713); Fabrication de Stupefiants et de Substances Psychotropes (0251-673X); Fabricacion de Estupefacientes y Sustancias Sicotropicas (0251-6721)
Published by: (United Nations Commission on Narcotic Drugs), United Nations Publications, Sales and Marketing Section, Room DC2 0853, New York, NY 10017. TEL 212-963-8302, 800-253-9646, FAX 212-963-3489, publications@un.org, http://www.un.org/publications.

MEDITSINSKI PREGLED. NEVROLOGIIA I PSICHIATRIIA. see *MEDICAL SCIENCES—Psychiatry And Neurology*

616.861 USA ISSN 0891-8651
MONDAY MORNING REPORT. Text in English. 1977. s-m. USD 60 domestic; USD 70 foreign (effective 2000 - 2001). **Document type:** *Newsletter.* **Description:** Covers significant issues, events, and opinions in the alcohol problems field.
Published by: Alcohol Research Information Service, 1106 E Oakland Ave, Lansing, MI 48906. TEL 517-485-9900, FAX 517-485-1928. Ed. Robert Hammond. Circ: 1,000.

362.2 USA
MONTANA COMPREHENSIVE CHEMICAL DEPENDENCY PLAN. Text in English. 1972. a. free per issue. **Document type:** *Government.*
Formerly: Montana State Plan for Alcohol Abuse and Alcoholism Prevention, Treatment and Rehabilitation (0090-3809)
Published by: Department of Corrections and Human Services, 1539 11th Ave, Helena, MT 59620. TEL 406-449-3930. Circ: 100.

306 362.29 616.89 SWE ISSN 0280-3348
MOTDRAG; Accent. Text in Swedish. 1980. bi-m. SEK 70 (effective 1990).
Incorporates (in 1988): Accent Ung; Former titles (until 1982): Motdrag foer Drogfrihet; (until 1981): Klartext om Droger (0349-408X)
Published by: U N F - Ungdomens Nykterhetsfoerbund, Fack 1747, Stockholm 11187, Sweden. TEL 46-8-789-49-50, FAX 46-8-20-43-54. Ed. Helena Karlsson.

362 USA ISSN 1046-5421
THE N A WAY MAGAZINE. (Narcotics Anonymous) Text in English. 1982. m. USD 15 domestic; USD 20 in Canada. illus. back issues avail. **Description:** Covers drug addiction, the N A recovery fellowship and more.
Formerly (until 1988): N.A. Way (0896-9116)
Published by: Narcotics Anonymous, World Service Office, PO Box 9999, Van Nuys, CA 91409. TEL 818-773-9999, FAX 818-700-0700. Ed. Cynthia Tooredman. Circ: 10,000.

N C A A DRUG TESTING PROGRAM. see *SPORTS AND GAMES*

616.863 USA ISSN 0048-0673
N C I CATALYST∗ ; interfaith action on alcohol and other drug problems. Text in English. 1967. s-a. USD 15. bk.rev. bibl. illus. **Document type:** *Newsletter.*
Published by: North Conway Institute, Inc., 168 Mount Vernon St, West, Newton, MA 02165-2517. TEL 617-742-0424. Ed. Priscilla Martin. Circ: 2,500.

616.861 USA ISSN 0147-0515
N I A A A - R U C A S ALCOHOLISM TREATMENT SERIES. (National Institute on Alcohol Abuse and Alcoholism - Rutgers University Center of Alcohol Studies) Text in English. 1978. irreg. price varies. index. **Document type:** *Monographic series, Academic/Scholarly.*
Formerly: N.I.A.A.A. - R.U.C.A.S. Alcoholism Treatment Monographs
Indexed: Psychol.Abstr.
Published by: Rutgers Center of Alcohol Studies, Publications Division, c/o Charles Rouse, Bus Admin, 607 Allison Rd, Piscataway, NJ 08854-8001. TEL 732-445-2190. Ed. Marc Schuckit.

616.863 616.863 USA ISSN 1046-9516
CODEN: MIDAD
N I D A RESEARCH MONOGRAPH. Text in English. 1975. irreg., latest vol.121, 1992. free per issue. bibl. charts. back issues avail.
Formerly (until 1976): U.S. National Institute on Drug Abuse. Research Monograph Series (0361-8595)
Related titles: Microfiche ed.
Indexed: Chem.Abstr., Chem.Indus.Notes, Chem.Titles, Curr.Cont. (coverage dropped), Excerp.Med., INIS Atomind., Ind.Med. (1976-), Psychol.Abstr., Psychopharmacol.Abstr.
—BLDSC (6110.170000), CASDDS, CISTI, EMDOCS, GNLM, KNAW.
Published by: U.S. National Institute on Drug Abuse, 5600 Fishers Ln, Rm 111, Rockville, MD 20857. TEL 301-443-6245. Circ: 3,000.

NARC OFFICER. see *LAW*

362.29 616.863 SWE ISSN 0281-3629
NARCONON-NYTT. Text in Swedish. 1977-1978; resumed 1982. q. SEK 100 (effective 1990). **Document type:** *Newspaper.*
Published by: Riksorganisationen Narconon i Sverige (RONS), Fack 3081, Varby 14303, Sweden. Ed. Haakan Larsson.

616.86 USA ISSN 0094-3991
HV5800
NARCOTICS AND DRUG ABUSE A TO Z. Text in English. 1971. base vol. plus q. updates. USD 100 (effective 1999). bibl. **Document type:** *Directory.* **Description:** Lists narcotics and drugs and treatment centers arranged by state.
Published by: Croner Publications, Inc., 10951 Sorrento Valley Rd, Ste 1 D, San Diego, CA 92121-1613. TEL 619-546-1894, 800-441-4033, FAX 619-546-1955, paul@croner.com, http://www.sdic.net/croner.

616.861 616.863 USA
NATIONAL DIRECTORY OF DRUG ABUSE AND ALCOHOLISM TREATMENT AND PREVENTION PROGRAMS. Text in English. 1979. a. free per issue. **Document type:** *Directory, Government.*
Published by: U.S. Substance Abuse and Mental Health Services Administration, Office of Applied Studies, 5600 Fishers Ln, Rm 16 105, Rockville, MD 20857. TEL 301-443-7934, FAX 301-443-9847. Circ: 12,500.

178 DEU
NEUES VON SYNANON; der nuechterne Weg. Text in German. q. free. back issues avail. **Document type:** *Bulletin.* **Description:** News and information from Synanon, a self-help group of former drug addicts and alcoholics.
Published by: Stiftung Synanon, Bernburger Str 10, Berlin 10963, Germany. TEL 49-30-55000-0, FAX 49-30-55000220. Ed., R&P, Adv. contact Michael Frommhold. Circ: 50,000.

▼ **NICOTINE & TOBACCO RESEARCH.** see *TOBACCO*

362.29 616.8632 FIN ISSN 1455-0725
HV5516 CODEN: NANTFY
NORDISK ALKOHOL- & NARKOTIKATIDSKRIFT/NORDIC STUDIES ON ALCOHOL AND DRUGS. Text in Swedish, Danish, Norwegian; Summaries in English. 1984. 6/yr. FIM 150 (effective 2000). adv. bk.rev. stat. back issues avail. **Document type:** *Academic/Scholarly.* **Description:** Presents articles in the social science of drug and alcohol abuse in Nordic society.
Former titles (until 1997): Nordisk Alkoholtidskrift (0789-6069); (until 1991): Alkoholpolitik (0782-9671)
Indexed: Addic.Abstr., Lang.& Lang.Behav.Abstr., SOPODA, Soc.Serv.Abstr., Sociol.Abstr.
—BLDSC (6117.945300).
Published by: Stakes Forsknings-och Utvecklingscentralen foer Social- och Haelsovaarden, PL 220, Helsinki 00531, Finland. TEL 358-9-3967-2198, FAX 358-9-3967-2191, nat@stakes.fi. Ed., Pub., R&P Kerstin Stenius TEL 358-9-3967-2197. Circ: 1,700.

362.29 616.86 344 SWE ISSN 1102-9021
OBEROENDE. Text in Swedish. 1969. q. SEK 145 (effective 1998).
Former titles (until 1992): Slaa Tillbaka (0349-2958); (until 1980): RFHL Kontakt (0345-9993)
Published by: R F H L - Riksfoerbundet foer Hjaelp aat Laekemedelsmissbrukare, Fack 23076, Stockholm 10435, Sweden. TEL 46-8-34-15-65. Ed. Birgitta Bergmark. Adv. contact Arne Borgren.

616.863 USA
P R I D E QUARTERLY NEWSLETTER. Text in English. q. bk.rev. **Description:** Covers activities of PRIDE and information concerning drug education and prevention.
Published by: (National Parents' Resource Institute for Drug Education, Inc.), Standard Press, 1210 Menlo Dr, Atlanta, GA 30318. TEL 404-351-6780. Ed. Doug Hall. **Subscr. to:** PRIDE, The Hurt Bldg, Ste 210, 50 Hurt Plaza, Atlanta, GA 30303.

178 IRL
PIONEER. Text in English. 1948. m. IEP 12.50 in Ireland; IEP 13 in United Kingdom; IEP 21.50 elsewhere (effective 2001). adv. bk.rev. charts, illus. **Document type:** *Newsletter.*

D

Former titles: New Pioneer (0332-1827); (until vol.33, Sep. 1980): Pioneer (0031-997X)
Published by: Pioneer Total Abstinence Association, 27 Upper Sherrard St., Dublin 1, Ireland. TEL 353-1-8749464, FAX 353-1-8748485, pioneer@s-j.ie, http://www.pioneertotal.ie, http://www.pioneertotal.com. Ed. Maureen Manning. adv.: B&W page IEP 600, color page IEP 780; trim 210 x 297. Circ: 16,000.

616.86 USA ISSN 1040-9882
HV5285
PREVENTION PIPELINE; an alcohol and drug awareness service. Variant title: C S A P Prevention Pipeline. Text in English. 1982. bi-m. USD 28; USD 32 foreign (effective 1999). **Document type:** *Government.* **Description:** Intended to stimulate an exchange of information and experiences among specialists in the field of drug and alcohol abuse prevention, focusing on the announcement of programmatic resources and selected scientific and technical literature, upcoming conferences, and news from the field.
Formerly (until 1987): Alcohol Awareness Service
Indexed: HRIS.
Published by: National Clearinghouse for Alcohol and Drug Information, Center for Substance Abuse Prevention, PO Box 2345, Rockville, MD 20847-2345. TEL 800-729-6686, FAX 301-468-6433, info@prevline.health.org, http://www.health.org. Ed. Barbara Ryan. R&P Craig Steinberg TEL 301-468-2600. Circ: 3,200 (paid).

362.292 POL ISSN 0032-9495
PROBLEMY ALKOHOLIZMU. Text in Polish; Summaries in English. 1975. m. PLZ 60,000. bk.rev. abstr. back issues avail.
Supersedes in part (in 1976): Problemy Alkoholizmu, Zdrowie i Trzezwosc (0137-3889); Which was formed by the merger of (1957-1975): Zdrowie i Trzezwosc (0867-3632); (1966-1975): Problemy Alkoholizmu (0239-4308); Which was formerly (1953-1965): Walka z Alkoholizmem (0509-5948)
Indexed: Russ.Acad.Sci.Bibl.
Published by: Spoleczny Komitet Przeciwalkoholowy, Ul Lwowska 5, Warsaw 00660, Poland. TEL 48-22-256626. Ed. Jan Brodzki. Circ: 6,000.

616.86 NLD ISSN 0921-8742
PROGRESS IN ALCOHOL RESEARCH. Text in English. 1985. irreg., latest vol.2, 1990. price varies. back issues avail. **Document type:** *Monographic series, Academic/Scholarly.* **Description:** Reports on the effects of alcoholism on ultrastructural and neurochemical levels.
—KNAW.
Published by: V S P (Subsidiary of: Brill Academic Publishers), PO Box 346, Zeist 3700 AH, Netherlands. TEL 31-30-692-5790, FAX 31-30-693-2081, vsppub@compuserve.com, http://www.vsppub.com/books/bs14.html. Ed. H Ollat. **Dist. in US & Canada by:** Books International, PO Box 605, Herndon, VA 20172. TEL 703-661-1500, FAX 703-661-1501.

616.86 CAN ISSN 0229-2947
PROJECTION (TORONTO)✶ ; an audio-visual review service. Text in English. 1971. bi-m. CND 18; CND 23 foreign. film rev.
Published by: (Addiction Research Foundation of Ontario, Subscription - Marketing Department), Canadian Centre on Substance Abuse/Centre Canadien de Lutte Contre l'Alcoholisme et les Toxicomanies, 75 Albert St., Ste 300, Ottawa, ON K1P 5E7, Canada. Ed. Debbie Monkman. Circ: 750.

616.86 USA ISSN 0893-164X
RC563 CODEN: PABEEI
PSYCHOLOGY OF ADDICTIVE BEHAVIORS. Text in English. 1987. q. USD 62 domestic to non-members; USD 77 foreign to non-members; USD 55 domestic to members; USD 65 foreign to members; USD 90 domestic to institutions; USD 122 foreign to institutions (effective 2001). adv. bk.rev. back issues avail. *Refereed.* **Document type:** *Academic/Scholarly.* **Description:** Covers alcoholism, drug abuse, eating disorders, smoking and nicotine addiction, and other compulsive behaviors such as gambling.
Former titles (until 1987): Society of Psychologists in Addictive Behaviors. Bulletin; Society of Psychologists in Substance Abuse. Bulletin
Related titles: Online - full text ed.: (from Institute for Scientific Information).
Indexed: ASCA, ASSIA, Addic.Abstr., Crim.Just.Abstr., Curr.Cont., Excerp.Med. (1995-), Fam.Ind., Ind.Med. (1987-), PsycInfo, Psychol.Abstr. (1981-), SSCI, Soc.Work Res.& Abstr., e-psyche.
—BLDSC (6946.535315), IDS, Infotrieve, ingenta. **CCC.**
Published by: American Psychological Association, 750 First St., N.E., Washington, DC 20002-4242. TEL 202-336-5600, 800-374-3721, FAX 202-336-5568, subscriptions@apa.org, http://www.apa.org/journals/adb.html. Ed. Thomas Brandon. Circ: 1,700.

PSYCHOTHERAPY NETWORKER. see *PSYCHOLOGY*

PUBLIC HEALTH REVIEWS; an international quarterly. see *PUBLIC HEALTH AND SAFETY*

616.863 USA ISSN 0738-422X
HV5001 CODEN: RDALE9
RECENT DEVELOPMENTS IN ALCOHOLISM. Text in English. irreg., latest vol.15. price varies. *Refereed.* **Document type:** *Monographic series.*
Indexed: Chem.Abstr., Chem.Indus.Notes, Chem.Titles, Dent.Ind., Ind.Med. (1983-), Psychol.Abstr.
—BLDSC (7304.104500), CASDDS, GNLM, KNAW. **CCC.**
Published by: (American Medical Society on Alcoholism), Kluwer Academic - Plenum Publishers (Subsidiary of: Wolters Kluwer N.V.), 233 Spring St, New York, NY 10013-1578. TEL 212-620-8000, 800-221-9369, FAX 212-463-0742, info@plenum.com, http://www.plenum.com. Ed. Dr. Marc Galanter. **Co-sponsor:** Research Society on Alcoholism.

616.86 USA ISSN 1061-7191
RECOVERY TODAY; the newsmagazine for today's recovering community. Text in English. 1990. m. USD 15. **Description:** Focuses on recovery from alcoholism, drug addiction and eating disorders. Promotes personal growth.
Indexed: e-psyche.
Address: 1313 S Military Tr, Ste 314, Deerfield Beach, FL 33442. TEL 407-488-6362. Ed. Kathleen Low. Circ: 30,000.

616.861 USA
REPORT ON ALCOHOL, DRUGS, AND DISABILITY. Text in English. 1992. q. free per issue. bk.rev. **Document type:** *Newsletter.* **Description:** Includes a calendar of events and activities, legislative updates, successful program descriptions, editorial opinion, leadership profiles, and networking opportunities.
Related titles: Audio cassette/tape ed.
Published by: National Association on Alcohol, Drugs, and Disability, 2165 Bunker Hill Dr, San Mateo, CA 94402-3801. TEL 650-578-8047. Ed. John De Miranda. Circ: 1,500.

RESEARCH COMMUNICATIONS IN ALCOHOL & SUBSTANCES OF ABUSE. see *PHARMACY AND PHARMACOLOGY*

616.861 AUS
REVIVER. Text in English. 1954. m. AUD 24. *Refereed.* **Document type:** *Directory, Consumer.*
Published by: Alcoholics Anonymous Central Service Office, 127 Edwin St, Croydon, NSW 2132, Australia. TEL 61-2-97991199, FAX 61-2-9716754. Circ: 2,500 (paid).

616.86 NOR ISSN 0809-2834
RUS & AVHENGIGHET. Text in Norwegian. 1980. 6/yr. NOK 285 to individuals; NOK 560, USD 105 to institutions; NOK 180 to students; NOK 100, USD 20 per issue (effective 2001). adv. bk.rev. **Document type:** *Academic/Scholarly.* **Description:** Presents information and debate on drug problems in Norway and internationally.
Formerly (until 1998): Stoffmisbruk (0333-144X)
—CCC.
Published by: Scandinavian University Press (Subsidiary of: Taylor & Francis Ltd.), Postboks 2959, Toeyen, Oslo 0608, Norway. FAX 47-22-57-53-53, www.universitetsforlaget.no/tidsskrifter. Ed. Martin Blindheim. Circ: 5,000.

616.8 USA
RUTGERS CENTER OF ALCOHOL STUDIES. MONOGRAPH. Text in English. 1958. irreg., latest vol.14, 1981. price varies. index. **Document type:** *Monographic series, Academic/Scholarly.*
Formerly: Rutgers University. Center of Alcohol Studies. Monograph (0080-4983)
Indexed: Biol.Abstr.
Published by: Rutgers Center of Alcohol Studies, Publications Division, c/o Charles Rouse, Bus Admin, 607 Allison Rd, Piscataway, NJ 08854-8001. TEL 732-445-2190. Ed. Marc Schuckit.

S A L I S DIRECTORY. see *LIBRARY AND INFORMATION SCIENCES*

616.861 USA
S A M H S A NEWS. Text in English. bi-m. USD 9.50; USD 11.90 foreign (effective 1995). back issues avail. **Document type:** *Newsletter, Government.* **Description:** Publishes articles on agency-related issues, such as AIDS, alcoholism, drug abuse, and general mental health. Publicizes agency events.
Published by: U.S. Substance Abuse and Mental Health Services Administration, Office of Applied Studies, 5600 Fishers Ln, Rm 16 105, Rockville, MD 20857. TEL 301-443-7934, FAX 301-443-9847. **Subscr. to:** U.S. Government Printing Office, Superintendent of Documents.

SCHOOL INTERVENTION REPORT. see *CHILDREN AND YOUTH—About*

SMOKE; cigars, pipes and life's other burning desires. see *GENERAL INTEREST PERIODICALS—United States*

SMOKING AND HEALTH NEWSLETTER. see *PHYSICAL FITNESS AND HYGIENE*

616.86 USA ISSN 1059-6259
SOBER TIMES✶ ; the recovery magazine. Text in English. 1987. bi-m. USD 16.50; USD 39 foreign. adv. bk.rev. **Document type:** *Consumer.* **Description:** Focuses on ways to maintain happy, healthy lives, free of substance abuse and compulsive behavior.
Address: PO Box 13013, Mill Creek, WA 98082-1013. Ed. Cliff Creager. Pub. Jerauld D Miller. Adv. contact Joe Wooley. Circ: 80,000 (controlled).

362.292 USA ISSN 1071-4111
SOBERING THOUGHTS. Text in English. 1976. m. USD 14.95 domestic; CND 21.95 in Canada; USD 26.95 elsewhere (effective 2001). bk.rev. index. 16 p./no. back issues avail. **Document type:** *Newsletter.* **Description:** For women who are recovering alcoholics. Contains personal reminiscences, inspirational articles, and news of self-help groups worldwide.
Formerly: Women for Sobriety. Newsletter
Published by: Women for Sobriety, Inc., PO Box 618, Quakertown, PA 18951. TEL 215-536-8026, FAX 215-538-9026, newlife@nni.com, http://www.womenforsobriety.org. Ed., R&P Rebecca M Fenner. Circ: 2,000 (paid).

616.86 CAN ISSN 0845-924X
HD9390.C23
SOCIETE DES ALCOOLS DU QUEBEC. RAPPORT ANNUEL. Text in English. 1971. a. free per issue. **Document type:** *Government, Corporate.*
Former titles (until 1985): Societe des Alcools du Quebec. Rapport d'Activite (0715-8254); (until 1982): Societe des Alcools du Quebec. Rapport Annuel (0715-884X); Which has English editions (1972-1974): Quebec Liquor Corporation. Annual Report (0715-8858); (1962-1971): Quebec. Liquor Board. Annual Report (0481-2875)
Published by: Societe des Alcools du Quebec, 905 DeLorimier, Montreal, PQ H2K 3V9, Canada. TEL 514-873-3844, info@saq.qc.ca, http://www.saq.com. Ed. Lyne Bellavance. R&P Nicole Creamer.

STRAIGHT TALK (PLEASANTVILLE); a magazine for teens. see *CHILDREN AND YOUTH—For*

616.863 USA ISSN 0735-6544
RM301.15
STREET PHARMACOLOGIST. Text in English. 1978. 4/yr. USD 25. bk.rev., film rev. bibl, charts, illus, stat. index, cum.index: 1978-1983. back issues avail. **Description:** Discusses substance abuse trends and other drug-related issues.
Published by: Up Front, Inc., 5701 Biscayne Blvd, Ste 602, Miami, FL 33137. TEL 305-757-2566, FAX 305-758-4676. Ed. James N Hall. Circ: 1,500.

STREETWIZE COMMUNICATIONS; youth rights comics. see *CHILDREN AND YOUTH—For*

616.86 USA ISSN 1042-6388
STUDENT ASSISTANCE JOURNAL. Text in English. 1988. 5/yr. USD 34 domestic; USD 43 in Canada; USD 52 elsewhere. film rev. tr.lit. back issues avail. **Document type:** *Trade.* **Description:** Looks at the various personal problems of students and how they affect their behavior at school. Emphasis is on drug abuse and alcoholism.
Indexed: Soc.Work Res.& Abstr., e-psyche.
Published by: Performance Resource Press, Inc., 1270 Rankin Dr, Ste F, Troy, MI 48083-2843. TEL 810-588-7733, FAX 810-588-6633. Ed. Gerri Andrews. Circ: 10,000.

D

616.863 USA ISSN 0889-7077
SUBSTANCE ABUSE. Text in English. 1984. q. EUR 368 to institutions for print or online ed.; EUR 441.60 to institutions print & online eds.combined (effective 2002). bk.rev. back issues avail. *Refereed.* **Document type:** *Academic/Scholarly.* **Description:** Publishes international, interdisciplinary forum for the publication of original empirical research papers and reviews in the field of addiction and substance abuse. Topics covered include clinical and preclinical research, education, health-service delivery, and policy.
Related titles: Online - full text ed.: (from EBSCO Publishing, O C L C Online Computer Library Center, Inc., RoweCom Information Quest, Swets Blackwell, Kluwer Online).
Indexed: Addic.Abstr., CINAHL, PsycInfo, e-psyche.
—BLDSC (8503.481000), Infotrieve, ingenta. **CCC.**
Published by: (Association for Medical Education and Research in Substance Abuse), Kluwer Academic - Plenum Publishers (Subsidiary of: Wolters Kluwer N.V.), 233 Spring St, New York, NY 10013-1578. TEL 212-620-8000, 800-221-9369, FAX 212-463-0742, services@wkap.nl, http://www.wkap.nl/journalhome.htm/0889-7077. Ed. Dr. Marc Galanter. R&P Rose Luongo TEL 781-871-6311. Circ: 600.

616.863 USA ISSN 1040-4163
SUBSTANCE ABUSE REPORT✱ ; twice-monthly newsletter covering all aspects of drug abuse: its prevention, detection and treatment. Text in English. 1970. s-m. USD 275. bk.rev. **Document type:** *Trade.* **Description:** Analyzes developments in the field of substance abuse treatment. Contains news and information on treatment programs, medical research and laboratory breakthroughs written for a professional audience.
Former titles: Addiction and Substance Abuse Report (0160-967X); Addiction and Drug Abuse Report (0001-8074)
Related titles: Online - full text ed.: (from Gale Group).
Indexed: CJPI.
Published by: Business Research Publications, Inc, 210 E 39th St, New York, NY 10016-2754. TEL 212-673-4700, FAX 212-475-1790. Ed. Alison Knopf.

616.86 157.6 USA ISSN 1082-6084
RC566.A1 CODEN: SUMIFL
SUBSTANCE USE AND MISUSE. Text in English. 1966. 14/yr. USD 255 to individuals print & online eds.; USD 2,275 to institutions print only (effective 2002). adv. charts. *Refereed.* **Document type:** *Academic/Scholarly.* **Description:** Disseminates facts, theories, points of view, and highlighting of critical unresolved issues in related areas of substance use, misuse and dependency, eating disorders, and gambling.
Formerly (until vol.31, 1996): International Journal of the Addictions (0020-773X)
Related titles: Microform ed.; Online - full content ed.; Online - full text ed.: (from Institute for Scientific Information, RoweCom Information Quest).
Indexed: ASCA, ASSIA, Abstr.Crim.& Pen., Addic.Abstr., Adol.Ment.Hlth.Abstr., AgeLine, Biol.Abstr., Chem.Abstr., Chic.Per.Ind., Crim.Just.Abstr., Curr.Cont., Environ.Sci.Poll.Mgmt., Excerp.Med., Fam.Ind., IBZ, I.P.A., Ind.Med. (1996-), Ind.Sci.Rev., Indian Psychol.Abstr., Inpharma, Int.Nurs.Ind., Lang.& Lang.Behav.Abstr., Mid.East: Abstr.& Ind., NRN, Pharm.&Out.News, Pollut.Abstr., PsycInfo, Psychol.Abstr. (1971-), Reac., Ref.Zh., Risk Abstr., SOPODA, SSCI, Saf.Sci.Abstr., Sci.Cit.Ind., Soc.Serv.Abstr., Soc.Work Res.& Abstr., Sociol.Abstr., Tox.Abstr., e-psyche.
—BLDSC (8503.493000), CISTI, EMDOCS, GNLM, IDS, Infotrieve, ingenta, KNAW. **CCC.**
Published by: Marcel Dekker Inc., 270 Madison Ave, New York, NY 10016. TEL 212-696-9000, 800-228-1160, FAX 212-685-4540, journals@dekker.com, http://www.dekker.com/servlet/product/productid/JA. Ed. Stanley Einstein. R&P Julia Mulligan. Adv. contact Diane Saulon. page USD 800. Circ: 650 (paid and free).

616.861 DEU ISSN 0939-5911
SUCHT. Text in German. 1955. bi-m. DEM 168 domestic; DEM 234 foreign (effective 2001). adv. bk.rev. index. 72 p./no. *Refereed.* **Document type:** *Journal, Academic/Scholarly.*
Formerly (until 1991): Suchtgefahren (0491-421X)
Indexed: Addic.Abstr., Excerp.Med., IBZ.
—BLDSC (8505.640000), EMDOCS, GNLM, KNAW. **CCC.**
Published by: (Deutsche Hauptstelle gegen die Suchtgefahren), Neuland Verlagsgesellschaft mbH, Markt 24-26, Geesthacht 21502, Germany. TEL 49-4152-81342, FAX 49-4152-81343, vertrieb@neuland.com, http://www.neuland.com. Ed. Rolf Huellinghorst. R&P, Adv. contact Jens Burmester. Circ: 3,000.

178 DEU ISSN 0930-8350
SUCHTREPORT. Text in German. 6/yr. DEM 54 domestic; DEM 60 in Europe; DEM 64 elsewhere (effective 2000). **Document type:** *Bulletin.*
—GNLM.
Published by: Stiftung Synanon, Bernburger Str 10, Berlin 10963, Germany. TEL 49-30-55000255, FAX 49-30-55000282. Ed., R&P, Adv. contact Michael Frommhold.

178 DEU ISSN 1439-9903
▼ **SUCHTTHERAPIE.** Text in German. 2000. q. EUR 98.80 domestic to institutions; EUR 102.80 in Europe to institutions; EUR 105.80 elsewhere to institutions; EUR 29 newsstand/cover (effective 2002). **Document type:** *Journal, Academic/Scholarly.*
Related titles: Online - full text ed.
Published by: Georg Thieme Verlag, Ruedigerstr 14, Stuttgart 70469, Germany. TEL 49-711-8931-0, FAX 49-711-8931298, kunden.service@thieme.de, http://www.thieme.de.

TABAC ET SANTE; tabagisme. see *PHYSICAL FITNESS AND HYGIENE*

616.863 USA
TAKING SIDES: CLASHING VIEWS ON CONTROVERSIAL ISSUES IN DRUGS AND SOCIETY. Text in English. 1993. irreg., latest vol.3, 1997. USD 13. illus. **Document type:** *Academic/Scholarly.*
Published by: Dushkin - McGraw-Hill, Sluice Dock, Guilford, CT 06437-9989. TEL 203-453-4351. Ed. Raymond Goldberg. Pub. David Dean. R&P Cheryl Greenleaf.

616.86 NLD ISSN 0378-2778
RC566.A1
TIJDSCHRIFT VOOR ALCOHOL, DRUGS EN ANDERE PSYCHOTROPE STOFFEN. Text in Dutch; Summaries in Dutch, English. 1975. 4/yr. NLG 100; NLG 85 to students. adv. bk.rev. back issues avail. **Document type:** *Academic/Scholarly.*
Indexed: Abstr.Crim.& Pen., Addic.Abstr., PsycInfo, Psychol.Abstr. (1984-), e-psyche.
—BLDSC (8837.860000), EMDOCS, GNLM, Infotrieve, KNAW. **CCC.**
Published by: Stichting T A D P, PO Box 725, Utrecht 3500 AS, Netherlands. Circ: 1,500.

615.9 ARG ISSN 0325-3961
TOXICOMANIAS. Text in Spanish. 1974. 3/yr.
Address: Paraguay, 2155, Capital Federal, Buenos Aires 1121, Argentina.

616.863 USA
TWELVE STEP RAG. Variant title: The Rag. Text in English. 1972. bi-m., latest vol.35, 2001. USD 4.50 domestic; USD 10.50 foreign (effective 2000). back issues avail. **Document type:** *Newsletter.* **Description:** Provides an information source for families and friends affected by someone else's use of drugs, alcohol or related behavioral problems.
Published by: Families Anonymous, Inc., PO Box 3475, Culver City, CA 90231-3475. TEL 310-815-8010, 800-736-9805, FAX 310-815-9682, famanon@familiesanonymous.org, http://www.familiesanonymous.org. Circ: 2,500.

616.863 610 USA ISSN 0098-311X
RA1242.T6
U.S. SURGEON GENERAL. REPORT. (Includes sub-series: Health Benefits of Smoking Cessation; Health Consequences of Involuntary Smoking; Health Consequences of Smoking; Health Consequences of Smoking for Women; Preventing Tobacco Use Among Young People; Reducing the Health Consequences of Smoking; Smoking and Health in the Americas) Text in English. 1964. a. free per issue. bibl, charts, illus, stat. index, cum.index: 1964-1982. **Document type:** *Consumer, Government.* **Description:** Addresses the prevention and cessation of tobacco use and the protection of nonsmokers.
—CISTI.
Published by: U.S. Centers for Disease Control, National Center for Chronic Disease Prevention and Health Promotion, Office on Smoking and Health, 4770 Buford Hwy, NE, MS K 50, Atlanta, GA 30341-3724. TEL 404-488-5705, 800-CDC-1311, FAX 404-488-5939. Circ: (controlled). **Orders to:** U.S. Government Printing Office, Superintendent of Documents.

616.86 362.29 SWE ISSN 0346-427X
VI LAENKAR. Text in Swedish. 1957. 9/yr. SEK 100 (effective 1998). 56 p./no. 3 cols./p.
Published by: Laenkarnas Riksfoerbund, Blommensbergsvaegen 178, Haegersten 12652, Sweden. TEL 46-8-18-96-880, FAX 46-8-18-29-89. Ed. Sven Erik Johansson. Pub. Ingemar Rosen. adv.: B&W page SEK 6,000; trim 248 x 171. Circ: 2,300.

362.295 GBR ISSN 1358-6912
WEED WORLD. Text in English. bi-m. GBP 18 domestic; GBP 22 in Europe; USD 32.35 in United States; CND 43.15 in Canada (effective 2001). back issues avail. **Document type:** *Magazine, Consumer.* **Description:** Covers cannabis smokin, growing, legal news, political change, travel info, competitions, new products, medical breakthroughs and more.
Address: PO Box 1332, Coventry CV8 3YA, United Kingdom. editor@weedworld.co.uk, http://www.weedworld.co.uk/. **Subscr. to:** DirectMag, PO Box 2165, Williamsville, NY 14231. TEL 877-474-3321, FAX 905-619-2903.

178 USA ISSN 0043-4965
WHITE RIBBON BULLETIN. Text in English. 1883. q. USD 7 (effective 1998). bk.rev. *Refereed.* **Document type:** *Newsletter.*
Published by: (World's Woman's Christian Temperance Union), M & D Printing Co., R I Box 43, Lowpoint, IL 61545. TEL 309-443-5275, FAX 309-364-3355. Ed. Mrs. Melvin Christ. Circ: 4,250.

616.8 USA ISSN 0043-5937
WINNER. Text in English. 1957. m. (during school term). USD 17.97 (effective 1999). charts, illus. **Description:** Drug education for grades four to six.
Published by: Health Connection, 55 W Oak Ridge Dr, Hagerstown, MD 21740. TEL 800-548-8700, FAX 1-888-294-8405. Ed. Lincoln Steed. Circ: 35,000.

616.863 362.29 USA
HV4997
WORKPLACE SUBSTANCE ABUSE ADVISOR. Text in English. 1986. bi-w. USD 377 (effective 1998). index. back issues avail. **Document type:** *Newsletter.* **Description:** Reviews federal, state, local laws and regulations involving alcohol and drug use, testing policies, EAP's, court decisions, and drug enforcement budgets.
Formerly (until 1996): National Report on Substance Abuse (0891-5709)
Related titles: Online - full text ed.: (from Human Resources Information Network, LexisNexis).
—**CCC.**
Published by: L R P Publications, 747 Dresher Rd, Box 980, Horsham, PA 19044. TEL 215-784-0941, 800-341-7874, FAX 215-784-9639, custserve@lrp.com, http://www.lrp.com. Ed. Valerie Jones.

178 360 USA
WORLD'S WOMAN'S CHRISTIAN TEMPERANCE UNION. TRIENNIAL REPORT. Text in English. 1891. triennial. USD 5. bk.rev. index. **Document type:** *Proceedings.*
Formerly: World's Woman's Christian Temperance Union. Convention Report (0084-2540)
Published by: World's Woman's Christian Temperance Union, HCR 3, Box 155, Wannaska, MN 56761. Ed. Pearl Loe. Circ: 600.

616.86 POL ISSN 0513-8809
ZDROWIE I TRZEZWOSC✱ . Text in Polish. 1976. m. PLZ 180,000. back issues avail.
Supersedes in part (in 1976): Problemy Alkoholizmu, Zdrowie i Trzezwosc (0137-3889); Which was formed by the merger of (1957-1975): Zdrowie i Trzezwosc (0867-3632); (1966-1975): Problemy Alkoholizmu (0239-4308); Which was formerly (1953-1965): Walka z Alkoholizmem (0509-5948)
Published by: Polska Liga "Trzezwosc", Ul Kopernika 36-40, Warsaw 00924, Poland. TEL 48-22-6358620. Ed. Henryk Babendich. Circ: 70,000.

616.863 CHN ISSN 1007-9718
ZHONGGUO YAOWU YILAIXING ZAZHI/CHINESE JOURNAL OF DRUG DEPENDENCE. Text in Chinese. 1992. q. CNY 40 domestic; USD 20.80 foreign; CNY 10 newsstand/cover domestic; USD 5.20 newsstand/cover foreign (effective 2001). back issues avail. **Document type:** *Journal, Academic/Scholarly.* **Description:** Publishes scientific research on drug dependence, the social issue of addiction, prevention and treatment of drug abuse.
Related titles: Online - full content ed.: (from WanFang Data Corp.).
—BLDSC (3180.317120).

Published by: Zhongguo Yaowu Yilaixing Yanjiusuo/National Institute on Drug Dependence, Peking Xueyuan Lu 38 Hao, 280 Xinxiang, Beijing 100083, China. TEL 86-10-62032625, FAX 68-10-62032624, niddbmu@public3.bta.net.cn, lyh509@21cn.com, http://www.periodicals.com.cn/gyjs.asp?ID=297699, http://www.nidd.ac.cn/. **Dist. by:** China International Book Trading Corp, 35 Chegongzhuang Xilu, Haidian District, Beijing 100044, China. cibtc@mail.cibtc.com.cn, http://www.cibtc.com.cn.

DRUG ABUSE AND ALCOHOLISM—Abstracting, Bibliographies, Statistics

616.861 157.61 016 USA ISSN 0161-1267
BOTTOM LINE (LANSING); on alcohol in society. Text in English. 1974. q. USD 40 domestic; USD 50 foreign (effective 2000 - 2001). bk.rev. **Document type:** *Academic/Scholarly.* **Description:** Deals with research, issues, events and opinions relating to public policy in the field of alcohol problems, with special emphasis on prevention.
Formed by the 1977 merger of: Alcohol Abstracts; Report on Alcohol (0002-7774); Viewpoint
Published by: Alcohol Research Information Service, 1106 E Oakland Ave, Lansing, MI 48906. TEL 517-485-9900, FAX 517-485-1928. Ed., R&P Robert Hammond. Circ: 5,000.

DRUG FILE UPDATE; a current awareness index to publications on drugs and doping in sport. see *SPORTS AND GAMES—Abstracting, Bibliographies, Statistics*

016.61383 NLD ISSN 0925-5958
CODEN: DRDPA
EXCERPTA MEDICA. SECTION 40: DRUG DEPENDENCE, ALCOHOL ABUSE AND ALCOHOLISM. Text in English. 1973. bi-m. EUR 1,052 in Europe to institutions; JPY 139,482 in Japan to institutions; USD 1,177 elsewhere to institutions (effective 2002). adv. index, cum.index. **Document type:** *Abstract/Index, Academic/Scholarly, Trade.* **Description:** Provides a comprehensive current-awareness service for trade and scholarly articles covering all aspects of the abuse of drugs, alcohol and organic solvents and includes material relating to the experimental pharmacology of addiction.
Formerly: Excerpta Medica. Section 40: Drug Dependence (0304-4041)
Related titles: CD-ROM ed.: (from SilverPlatter Information, Inc.); Online - full text ed.: (from DIMDI, Data-Star, The Dialog Corporation, JICST).
—GNLM, Infotrieve, Linda Hall. **CCC.**
Published by: Excerpta Medica Medical Communications BV (Subsidiary of: Reed Elsevier plc), Rooseveltweg 15, Almere-Stad 1314 SJ, Netherlands. TEL 31-36-538-5600, FAX 31-36-538-5650, http://www.elsevier.com/locate/drug, http://www.excerptamedica.com. **Subscr. in Australasia and the Far East to:** Elsevier Science (Singapore) Pte Ltd, No.1 Temasek Ave, 17-01 Millenia Tower, Singapore 039192, Singapore. TEL 65-434-3727, FAX 65-337-2230; **Subscr. in Japan to:** Elsevier Science Inc - Japan Regional Office, 9-15 Higashi-Azabu 1-chome, Minato-ku, Tokyo 106-0044, Japan. TEL 81-3-5561-5033, FAX 81-3-5561-5047; **Subscr. in the Americas to:** Elsevier Science, PO Box 945, New York, NY 10159-0945. TEL 212-633-3730, 888-437-4636, FAX 212-633-3680, usinfo-f@elsevier.com, http://www.elsevier.com. **Dist. by:** Elsevier Science (Brazil).; Elsevier Science BV, PO Box 211, Amsterdam 1000 AE, Netherlands. TEL 31-20-485-3757, FAX 31-20-485-3432.

616.861 016 USA ISSN 0074-204X
INTERNATIONAL BIBLIOGRAPHY OF STUDIES ON ALCOHOL. Text in English. 1966. irreg. price varies. bibl. index. **Document type:** *Monographic series, Bibliography.*
Published by: Rutgers Center of Alcohol Studies, Publications Division, c/o Charles Rouse, Bus Admin, 607 Allison Rd, Piscataway, NJ 08854-8001. TEL 732-445-2190. Ed. Marc Schuckit.

INTERNATIONAL NARCOTICS CONTROL BOARD. PSYCHOTROPIC SUBSTANCES; assessments of medical and scientific requirements for substances in schedules II, III and IV. Requirements of import authorization for substances in schedules III and IV. see *PHARMACY AND PHARMACOLOGY—Abstracting, Bibliographies, Statistics*

016.15761 RUS
REFERATIVNYI ZHURNAL. ALKOGOL'NAYA BOLEZN. Text in Russian. 1997. m. USD 175 in United States. **Document type:** *Academic/Scholarly.*
Published by: Vserossiiskii Institut Nauchnoi i Tekhnicheskoi Informatsii (VINITI), Usievicha ul 20-a, Moscow 125315, Russian Federation. TEL 7-095-1526441, FAX 7-095-943-0060. **US dist. addr.:** East View Publications, 3020 Harbor Ln N, Minneapolis, MN 55447. TEL 612-550-0961.

016.616863 RUS
REFERATIVNYI ZHURNAL. NARKOLOGICHESKAYA TOKSIKOLOGIYA. Text in Russian. m. USD 435 in United States. **Document type:** *Abstract/Index.*
Published by: Vserossiiskii Institut Nauchnoi i Tekhnicheskoi Informatsii (VINITI), Usievicha ul 20-a, Moscow 125315, Russian Federation. TEL 7-095-1526441, FAX 7-095-943-0060. **US dist. addr.:** East View Publications, 3020 Harbor Ln N, Minneapolis, MN 55447. TEL 612-550-0961.

EARTH SCIENCES

see also EARTH SCIENCES—Geology; EARTH SCIENCES—Hydrology; EARTH SCIENCES—Oceanography

ANTARCTIC SCIENCE. see *BIOLOGY*

ARCTIC, ANTARCTIC AND ALPINE RESEARCH. see *SCIENCES: COMPREHENSIVE WORKS*

550 CHE ISSN 0374-6402
BULLETIN DE LA MURITHIENNE. Text in French, German; Summaries in English, German. 1861. a. CHF 20 (effective 2001). bk.rev. abstr, bibl, charts, illus, maps. back issues avail. *Refereed.* **Document type:** *Bulletin, Academic/Scholarly.*
Indexed: Biol.Abstr., Zoo.Rec.
Published by: Societe Valaisanne des Sciences Naturelles, Case Postale 2251, Sion 1950, Switzerland. TEL 41-27-6064732, lamurithienne@admin.ch, http://www.murithienne.unibe.ch. Ed. Jean Claude Praz. Circ: 850.

500 USA
CHIHUAHUAN DESERT DISCOVERY. Text in English. 1975. s-a. membership. **Document type:** *Newsletter.* **Description:** Presents articles on the natural sciences in the Chihuahan Desert region of the United States and Mexico.
Published by: Chihuahuan Desert Research Institute, PO Box 905, Ft. Davis, TX 79734. TEL 915-364-2499, manager@cdri.org. Circ: 1,000.

550 570 USA
CHIHUAHUAN DESERT NEWSBRIEFS. Text in English. 1983. s-a. free per issue. **Document type:** *Newsletter.*
Published by: Chihuahuan Desert Research Institute, PO Box 905, Ft. Davis, TX 79734. TEL 915-364-2499, manager@cdri.org. R&P Dennis J Miller. Circ: 5,000.

CONTRIBUTIONS IN MARINE SCIENCE. see *BIOLOGY*

DECHENIANA-BEIHEFTE (BONN). see *BIOLOGY*

DORTMUNDER BEITRAEGE ZUR LANDESKUNDE. see *BIOLOGY*

ECOLOGIA EN BOLIVIA. see *BIOLOGY*

ELECTRICITE DE FRANCE. DIRECTION DES ETUDES ET RECHERCHES. COLLECTION DE NOTES INTERNES. BIOLOGIE, SCIENCES DE LA TERRE ET ENVIRONNEMENT. see *BIOLOGY*

FLORIDA MUSEUM OF NATURAL HISTORY. BULLETIN. see *BIOLOGY*

FOUNDATION FOR SCIENTIFIC RESEARCH IN THE CARIBBEAN REGION. PUBLICATION. see *BIOLOGY*

GEOBIOS; an international journal of life sciences on earth. see *BIOLOGY*

GEOBIOS NEW REPORTS; biannual journal of life sciences. see *BIOLOGY*

KEVO SUBARCTIC RESEARCH INSTITUTE. REPORTS. see *BIOLOGY*

KONGELIGE DANSKE VIDENSKABERNES SELSKAB. BIOLOGISKE SKRIFTER. see *BIOLOGY*

NATUR UND MENSCH: JAHRESMITTEILUNGEN DER NATURHISTORISCHEN GESELLSCHAFT NUERNBERG. see *BIOLOGY*

NATURWISSENSCHAFTLICHE ZEITSCHRIFT FUER NIEDERBAYERN. see *BIOLOGY*

NATURWISSENSCHAFTLICHER VEREIN ZU BREMEN. ABHANDLUNGEN. see *BIOLOGY*

011.4309982 DNK
QH84.1
POLARFRONTEN. Text in Danish. 1997. q. free per issue. bk.rev. illus. cum.index. back issues avail. **Document type:** *Academic/Scholarly.* **Description:** Polar research.
Formerly (until 1997): Forskning i Groenland-Tusaat (0105-7502)
Published by: Danish Polar Center, Strandgade 100 H, Copenhagen K 1401, Denmark. TEL 45-32-88-01-00, FAX 45-32-88-01-01, polarfronten@dpc.dk, http://www.dpc.dk. Eds. Poul-Erik Philbert, Henning Thing. Circ: 5,000.

550 570 DEU ISSN 0341-9665
CODEN: MIPOD4
POLLICHIA. MITTEILUNGEN. Summaries in English, French, German. 1888. a. DEM 50 (effective 2000). back issues avail. **Document type:** *Academic/Scholarly.*
Indexed: Biol.Abstr., GeoRef, IBR, Zoo.Rec.
—CISTI, Infotrieve, Linda Hall. **CCC.**
Published by: Pollichia Verein fuer Naturforschung und Landespflege, Hermann Schaefer Str 17, Bad Duerkheim 67098, Germany. stapf@mail.uni-mainz.de. Ed. Karl Stapf. Circ: 3,000.

SOCIETE DES NATURALISTES LUXEMBOURGEOIS. BULLETIN. see *BIOLOGY*

UNIVERSITY OF WISCONSIN-MILWAUKEE. FIELD STATION BULLETIN. see *BIOLOGY*

WASEDA DAIGAKU KYOIKUGAKUBU GAKUJUTSU KENKYU. SEIBUTSUGAKU, CHIGAKU HEN/WASEDA UNIVERSITY. SCHOOL OF EDUCATION. SCIENTIFIC RESEARCHES: BIOLOGY, GEOLOGY. see *BIOLOGY*

EARTH SCIENCES—Abstracting, Bibliographies, Statistics

A S F A MARINE BIOTECHNOLOGY ABSTRACTS. (Aquatic Sciences & Fisheries Abstracts) see *BIOLOGY—Abstracting, Bibliographies, Statistics*

BIBLIOGRAPHY ON COLD REGIONS SCIENCE & TECHNOLOGY. see *ENGINEERING—Abstracting, Bibliographies, Statistics*

551.46 USA
UNDERWATER AND HYPERBARIC MEDICINE: ABSTRACTS FROM THE LITERATURE. Text in English. bi-m. USD 100; USD 50 diskette (effective 2000). **Document type:** *Academic/Scholarly, Abstract/Index.*
Former titles: Underwater Medicine: Abstracts from the Literature (0886-3474); Underwater Physiology Abstracts
Related titles: Diskette ed.
Published by: Undersea and Hyperbaric Medical Society, Inc., 10531 Metropolitan Ave, Kensington, MD 20895. TEL 301-942-2980, FAX 301-942-7804, uhms@uhms.org, http://www.uhms.org. Ed. Leon J Greenbaum Jr. Circ: 250.

EARTH SCIENCES—Geology

see also MINES AND MINING INDUSTRY

ALTENBURGER NATURWISSENSCHAFTLICHE FORSCHUNGEN. see *BIOLOGY*

ASSOCIATION OF MARINE LABORATORIES OF THE CARIBBEAN. PROCEEDINGS. see *EARTH SCIENCES—Oceanography*

BADISCHER LANDESVEREIN FUER NATURKUNDE UND NATURSCHUTZ, FREIBURG. MITTEILUNGEN. NEUE FOLGE. see *BIOLOGY*

BEITRAEGE ZUR NATURKUNDE IN OSTHESSEN. see *BIOLOGY*

BIOLOGY AND ENVIRONMENT; proceedings of the Royal Irish Academy. see *BIOLOGY*

E

BRAGANTIA. see *AGRICULTURE*

CANADIAN MINING JOURNAL. see *MINES AND MINING INDUSTRY*

551.22 CHN
DIZHEN KANAN ANQUAN. Text in Chinese. 1994 (Feb.). q. CNY 4 domestic (effective 2000). **Document type:** *Academic/Scholarly.*
Related titles: Online - full content ed.: (from WanFang Data Corp.).
Published by: Zhongguo Dizhi Daxue/China University of Geosciences, Yujiashan, Wuhan, Hubei 430074, China. TEL 86-27-87482270. Ed. Xiu-quan Wei.

ENTWICKLUNGSLAENDER-STUDIEN; Bibliographie entwicklungslaenderbezogener Forschungsarbeiten. see *BUSINESS AND ECONOMICS—Abstracting, Bibliographies, Statistics*

HOKKAIDO KYOIKU DAIGAKU KIYO. DAI-2-BU, B. SEIBUTSUGAKU, CHIGAKU, NOGAKU-HEN/ HOKKAIDO UNIVERSITY OF EDUCATION. JOURNAL. SECTION 2 B. BIOLOGY, GEOLOGY, AND AGRICULTURE. see *BIOLOGY*

INTERNATIONAL PEAT JOURNAL. see *BIOLOGY—Botany*

MOSKOVSKOE OBSHCHESTVO ISPYTATELEI PRIRODA. BIOLOGICHESKII OTDEL. BYULLETEN/MOSCOW SOCIETY OF NATURALISTS. BIOLOGICAL SERIES. BULLETIN. see *BIOLOGY*

NATUR UND MENSCH: JAHRESMITTEILUNGEN DER NATURHISTORISCHEN GESELLSCHAFT NUERNBERG. see *BIOLOGY*

NATURAL HAZARDS REVIEW. see *ENVIRONMENTAL STUDIES*

REAL SOCIEDAD ESPANOLA DE HISTORIA NATURAL. BOLETIN. ACTAS. see *BIOLOGY*

REVUE DES SCIENCES NATURELLES D'AUVERGNE. see *BIOLOGY*

SENCKENBERGISCHE NATURFORSCHENDE GESELLSCHAFT. ABHANDLUNGEN. see *BIOLOGY*

SOCIETE LINNEENNE DE BORDEAUX. BULLETIN. see *BIOLOGY—Zoology*

551 570 USA ISSN 0275-0120
CODEN: TBGBDG
TOPICS IN GEOBIOLOGY. Text in English. 1980. irreg., latest vol.16, 2000. price varies. *Refereed.* **Document type:** *Monographic series.*
Indexed: GeoRef, Zoo.Rec.
—BLDSC (8867.441000), CASDDS, CISTI, Infotrieve. **CCC.**
Published by: Kluwer Academic - Plenum Publishers (Subsidiary of: Wolters Kluwer N.V.), 233 Spring St, New York, NY 10013-1578. TEL 212-620-8000, 800-221-9369, FAX 212-463-0742, info@plenum.com, http://www.plenum.com. Eds. D S Jones, Neil Landman.

TURUN YLIOPISTO. JULKAISUJA. SARJA A. II. BIOLOGICA - GEOGRAPHICA - GEOLOGICA/ ANNALES UNIVERSITATIS TURKUENSIS. see *BIOLOGY*

559.8 597 551.9 NZL ISSN 0110-2192
QE350 CODEN: RUWADY
UNIVERSITY OF WAIKATO. ANTARCTIC RESEARCH UNIT. REPORT. Text in English. 1972. a. free per issue. **Document type:** *Academic/Scholarly.*
Indexed: Chem.Abstr., GeoRef.
Published by: University of Waikato, Antarctic Research Unit, Private Bag 3105, Hamilton, New Zealand. Circ: 350.

EARTH SCIENCES—Hydrology

ALGOLOGICAL STUDIES; Archiv fuer Hydrobiologie, Supplementbaende. see *BIOLOGY*

ARCHIV FUER HYDROBIOLOGIE. see *BIOLOGY*

ARCHIV FUER HYDROBIOLOGIE. SUPPLEMENT-BAND: ARBEITEN AUS DEM LIMNOLOGISCHEN INSTITUT DER UNIVERSITAET KONSTANZ. see *BIOLOGY*

ARCHIV FUER HYDROBIOLOGIE. SUPPLEMENT-BAND: LARGE RIVERS. see *BIOLOGY*

ARCHIV FUER HYDROBIOLOGIE. SUPPLEMENT-BAND: UNTERSUCHUNGEN DES ELBE-AESTUARS. see *BIOLOGY*

ARCHIV FUER HYDROBIOLOGIE. SUPPLEMENT VOLUMES, MONOGRAPHIC STUDIES. see *BIOLOGY*

551.48 DEU ISSN 0067-8643
QH96.A1 CODEN: BNGWAU
DIE BINNENGEWAESSER; Einzeldarstellungen aus der Limnologie und ihren Grenzgebieten. Text in English, German. 1926. irreg. price varies. **Document type:** *Monographic series, Academic/Scholarly.*
Indexed: Biol.Abstr., Deep Sea Res.& Oceanogr.Abstr. —CISTI.
Published by: E. Schweizerbart'sche Verlagsbuchhandlung, Johannesstr 3A, Stuttgart 70176, Germany. TEL 49-711-625001, FAX 49-711-625005, mail@schweizerbart.de, schweizerbart@schweizerbart.de, http://www.schweizerbart.de. Ed. W Lampert.

DEVELOPMENTS IN HYDROBIOLOGY. see *BIOLOGY*

GIDROBIOLOGICHESKII ZHURNAL; nauchnyi zhurnal. see *BIOLOGY*

HYDROBIOLOGIA; the international journal on limnology and marine sciences. see *BIOLOGY*

HYDROBIOLOGICAL JOURNAL. see *BIOLOGY*

REPORTS OF INVESTIGATIONS ABOUT LAKE BIWA. see *PUBLIC HEALTH AND SAFETY*

SHUISHENG SHENGWU XUEBAO/ACTA HYDROBIOLOGICA SINICA. see *BIOLOGY*

U N A M. INSTITUTO DE CIENCIAS DEL MAR Y LIMNOLOGIA. ANALES. see *EARTH SCIENCES—Oceanography*

EARTH SCIENCES—Oceanography

A S F A MARINE BIOTECHNOLOGY ABSTRACTS. (Aquatic Sciences & Fisheries Abstracts) see *BIOLOGY—Abstracting, Bibliographies, Statistics*

ADVANCES IN MARINE BIOLOGY. see *BIOLOGY*

578.77 PRI
ASSOCIATION OF MARINE LABORATORIES OF THE CARIBBEAN. PROCEEDINGS. Text in English. 1957. irreg., latest vol.22, 1989. USD 5.
Formerly: Association of Island Marine Laboratories of the Caribbean. Proceedings (0066-9571)
Indexed: Aqua.Sci.& Fish.Abstr., Aquacult.Abstr., Environ.Sci.Poll.Mgmt.
Published by: Association of Marine Laboratories of the Caribbean, University of Puerto Rico, Dept of Marine Sciences, Mayaguez, PR 00708. FAX 787-265-2880, TELEX UPR MAY 3452024. Ed. Lucy Bunkley Williams. Circ: 500.

BIOLOGIYA MORYA/MARINE BIOLOGY. see *BIOLOGY*

578.77 FRA ISSN 0007-8603
C M A S BULLETIN D'INFORMATION/C M A S NEWSLETTER. (Confederation Mondiale des Activites) Text in French. 1959. 4/yr. FRF 80. bk.rev. illus. **Document type:** *Newsletter.*
Published by: World Underwater Federation, Viale Tiziano, 74, Rome, RM 00196, Italy. Circ: 2,000.

FISHES OF THE WESTERN NORTH ATLANTIC. MEMOIRS. see *BIOLOGY*

578.77 FRA ISSN 0020-7918
I M S NEWSLETTER. (International Marine Science) Text in English. 1963. q. (online ed. biennial). free per issue to qualified personnel. **Document type:** *Newsletter.*
Formerly (until 1970): International Marine Science (1013-2813)
Related titles: Online - full text ed.; Arabic ed.; Chinese ed.; Russian ed.; Spanish ed.: Boletin Internacional de Ciencias del Mar. ISSN 0379-5276; French ed.: Bulletin International des Sciences de la Mer. ISSN 0251-4451.
Indexed: Curr.Adv.Ecol.Sci., Meteor.& Geoastrophys.Abstr., Russ.Acad.Sci.Bibl., Sport Fish.Abstr.
—CISTI, Linda Hall.
Published by: (Environment and Development in Coastal Regions and in Small Islands), UNESCO S C - C S I, 1 rue Miollis, Paris Cedex 15 75732, France. TEL 33-1-45683934, FAX 33-1-45685808, g.archibald@unesco.org, http://www/unesco.org/ioc/IMSNewsletteron-line. Ed. Gail Archibald. Circ: 5,000 (controlled).

JOURNAL OF PLANKTON RESEARCH. see *BIOLOGY*

MARINE BIOLOGICAL ASSOCIATION OF INDIA. JOURNAL. see *BIOLOGY*

MARINE ENVIRONMENTAL RESEARCH. see *ENVIRONMENTAL STUDIES—Pollution*

MEMOIRS OF THE HOURGLASS CRUISES. see *BIOLOGY*

578.77 ITA ISSN 0390-492X
QH152 CODEN: MBMOA5
MEMORIE DI BIOLOGIA MARINA E DI OCEANOGRAFIA. Text and summaries in English, French, German, Italian. 1930-1940; N.S. 1971. bi-m. ITL 10,000. adv. bk.rev. back issues avail.
Indexed: Aqua.Sci.& Fish.Abstr., Biol.Abstr., Chem.Abstr., Deep Sea Res.& Oceanogr.Abstr., Environ.Sci.Poll.Mgmt., Ocean.Abstr. (coverage dropped), Sport Fish.Abstr.
—Linda Hall.
Published by: Universita degli Studi di Messina, Istituto di Zoologia, Stazione di Biologia Marina, Messina, ME, Italy. Ed. Carmelo Cavallaro. Circ: 350.

578.77 GBR ISSN 0078-3218
GC1 CODEN: OCMBAT
OCEANOGRAPHY AND MARINE BIOLOGY: AN ANNUAL REVIEW*. Text in English. 1963. a. price varies.
Related titles: Online - full text ed.: (from Institute for Scientific Information).
Indexed: ASCA, Aqua.Sci.& Fish.Abstr., Aquacult.Abstr., Biol.Abstr., Chem.Abstr., Curr.Adv.Ecol.Sci., Deep Sea Res.& Oceanogr.Abstr., Environ.Sci.Poll.Mgmt., GeoRef, Helminthol.Abstr., Meteor.& Geoastrophys.Abstr., Ocean.Abstr., Pollut.Abstr., Sci.Cit.Ind., Sport Fish.Abstr., Zoo.Rec.
—BLDSC (6233.996000), CASDDS, CISTI, ingenta, Linda Hall.
Published by: Aberdeen University Press, University of Aberdeen, Old Aberdeen, Aberdeen AB9 1FX, United Kingdom. Ed. Margaret Barnes.

551.46 570 DZA ISSN 0031-4137
PELAGOS. Text in French; Summaries in English. 1963. s-a. DZD 60. illus. **Document type:** *Academic/Scholarly.*
Indexed: Biol.Abstr., Ocean.Abstr. (coverage dropped), Pollut.Abstr.
—Linda Hall.
Published by: Institut des Sciences de la Mer et de l'Ameagement du Littoral, Sidi Fredj, B P 54, Algiers 42321, Algeria. **Dist. in U.S. by:** African Imprint Library Services, 236 Main St, Falmouth, MA 02540. TEL 508-540-5378.

551.46 GBR
QH91.A1
SCOTTISH ASSOCIATION FOR MARINE SCIENCE. DUNSTAFFNAGE MARINE LABORATORY. ANNUAL REPORT. Text in English. 1896. a. **Document type:** *Corporate.*
Former titles: Dunstaffnage Marine Laboratory and Scottish Marine Biological Association. Annual Reports; Scottish Marine Biological Association. Annual Report (0375-2062)
Related titles: Microfiche ed.
Indexed: Aqua.Sci.& Fish.Abstr., Aquacult.Abstr., Biol.Abstr., Ocean.Abstr. (coverage dropped).
Published by: Scottish Association for Marine Science, Dunstaffnage Marine Laboratory, PO Box 3, Oban, Argyll PA34 4AD, United Kingdom. TEL 44-1631-562244, FAX 44-1631-565518, ew@wpo.nerc.ac.uk, http://www.nerc-oban.ac.uk/dml/index.html. Circ: 1,000.

578.77 DEU ISSN 0080-889X
QE39 CODEN: SEMADJ
SENCKENBERGIANA MARITIMA. Text and summaries in German, English. 1969. 6/yr. DEM 98 (effective 2001). back issues avail.; reprints avail. *Refereed.* **Document type:** *Journal, Academic/Scholarly.* **Description:** Contains papers on marine geology, biology, paleontology, and ecology of the marine environment.

E

Indexed: Aqua.Sci.& Fish.Abstr., Aquacult.Abstr., Biol.Abstr., Curr.Adv.Ecol.Sci., Deep Sea Res.& Oceanogr.Abstr., Ecol.Abstr., Environ.Sci.Poll.Mgmt., Geo.Abstr.P.G., GeoRef, IBR, IBZ, Ocean.Abstr. (coverage dropped), Pollut.Abstr., Ref.Zh., Sport Fish.Abstr., Zoo.Rec.
—BLDSC (8241.040000), CISTI, Linda Hall. **CCC.**
Published by: (Deutsche Forschungsgemeinschaft, Senckenbergische Naturforschende Gesellschaft), E. Schweizerbart'sche Verlagsbuchhandlung, Johannesstr 3A, Stuttgart 70176, Germany. TEL 49-711-625001, FAX 49-711-625005, schweizerbart@schweizerbart.de, http://www.schweizerbart.de. Ed. G Hertweck. R&P Peter Koenigshof TEL 49-69-7542257. Circ: 650.

551.46 578.77 SEN ISSN 0850-1602
SENEGAL. CENTRE DE RECHERCHE OCEANOGRAPHIQUE. DOCUMENT SCIENTIFIQUE. Text in French. 1966. irreg., latest vol.146, 1997. XOF 75,000, USD 130 (effective 1998). adv. bibl. back issues avail. **Document type:** *Monographic series, Proceedings.*
Related titles: Microfiche ed.
Published by: Centre de Recherche Oceanographique de Dakar-Thiaroye, BP 2241, Dakar, Senegal. TEL 221-8340536, FAX 221-8342792, adiallo@crodt.isra.sn. R&P, Adv. contact Anis Diallo.

SHUISHENG SHENGWU XUEBAO/ACTA HYDROBIOLOGICA SINICA. see *BIOLOGY*

THALASSAS; revista de ciencias del mar. see *BIOLOGY*

551.48 MEX ISSN 0185-3287
U N A M. INSTITUTO DE CIENCIAS DEL MAR Y LIMNOLOGIA. ANALES. Text in Spanish. 1967. a. MXP 25, USD 3 newsstand/cover (effective 2000). back issues avail.
Supersedes (in 1980): U N A M. Centro de Ciencias del Mar y Limnologia. Anales (0186-3428); Which was formerly (until 1970): U N A M. Instituto de Biologia. Anales. Serie Ciencias del Mar y Limnologia
Related titles: Online - full text ed.
Indexed: Aqua.Sci.& Fish.Abstr., Aquacult.Abstr., Environ.Sci.Poll.Mgmt.
—CISTI, Linda Hall.
Published by: Universidad Nacional Autonoma de Mexico, Biblioteca del Instituto de Ciencias del Mar y Limnologia, Unidad de Bibliotecas, Circuito Exterior, Ciudad Universitaria, Mexico, DF 04510, Mexico. TEL 52-5-6225804, FAX 52-5-6225804. Ed. Agustin A Castanares.

UNIVERSIDADE FEDERAL DE PERNAMBUCO. DEPARTAMENTO DE OCEANOGRAFIA. CENTRO DE TECNOLOGIA. TRABALHOS OCEANOGRAFICOS. see *BIOLOGY*

ECONOMIC SITUATION AND CONDITIONS

see BUSINESS AND ECONOMICS—Economic Situation And Conditions

ECONOMIC SYSTEMS AND THEORIES, ECONOMIC HISTORY

see BUSINESS AND ECONOMICS—Economic Systems And Theories, Economic History

ECONOMICS

see BUSINESS AND ECONOMICS

EDUCATION

see also CHILDREN AND YOUTH—About; EDUCATION—Adult Education; EDUCATION—Computer Applications; EDUCATION—Guides To Schools And Colleges; EDUCATION—Higher Education; EDUCATION—International Education Programs; EDUCATION—School Organization And Administration; EDUCATION—Special Education And Rehabilitation; EDUCATION—Teaching Methods And Curriculum

613.7 AUS ISSN 1321-0394
GV201
A C H P E R HEALTHY LIFESTYLES JOURNAL. Text in English. 1954. q. AUD 44 domestic; AUD 60 foreign (effective 2001). adv. bk.rev., film rev. charts, illus, stat. back issues avail.; reprint service avail. from PQC. **Document type:** *Consumer.* **Description:** For specialists in physical education, health, dance, community fitness, and recreation, doctors, physiotherapists, university lecturers, schools and colleges.
Former titles (until 1994): A C H P E R National Journal (0813-2283); (until 1983): A J H P E R. Australian Journal for Health, Physical Education and Recreation (0813-2275); (until 1977): Australian Journal for Health, Physical Education and Recreation (0312-827X); (until 1975): Australian Journal of Physical Education (0312-8261); Which was formerly (until 1960): Physical Education Journal (0004-9492)
Related titles: Microform ed.: (from PQC).
Indexed: Aus.Educ.Ind., Cont.Pg.Educ., ERA, Nutr.Abstr., Rural Recreat.Tour.Abstr., SOMA, Sociol.Educ.Abstr., Sportsearch (1983-), Tech.Educ.Abstr., World Ag.Econ.& Rur.Soc.Abstr.
—BLDSC (0576.545000), Infotrieve, ingenta. **CCC.**
Published by: Australian Council for Health Physical Education and Recreation Inc., PO Box 304, Hindmarsh, SA 5007, Australia. TEL 61-8-8340-3388, FAX 61-8-8340-3399, membership@achper.org.au, http://www.achper.org.au/. Adv. contact Lyndall Bryden. Circ: 3,500.

370.72 USA
A V K O NEWSLETTER. Text in English. 1974. q. USD 25 to members (effective 2000). bk.rev. back issues avail. **Document type:** *Newsletter.* **Description:** Contains news and information to assist members of the foundation.
Published by: A V K O Educational Research Foundation, Inc., 3084 W Willard Rd, Ste C, Clio, MI 48420-7801. TEL 810-686-9283, FAX 810-686-1101. Ed. R J Rayl.

ADOLESCENCE (SAN DIEGO); an international quarterly devoted to the physiological, psychological, psychiatric, sociological, and educational aspects of the second decade of human life. see *CHILDREN AND YOUTH—About*

370.15 USA
ADVANCES IN COGNITION AND EDUCATIONAL PRACTICE. Text in English. 1992. a. USD 78.50. **Document type:** *Academic/Scholarly.*
Indexed: e-psyche.
—BLDSC.
Published by: J A I Press Inc., 100 Prospect St, Box 811, Stamford, CT 06904-0811. TEL 203-323-9606, FAX 203-357-8446, jai@jaipress.com. Ed. Jerry Carlson.

ADVANCES IN PHYSIOLOGY EDUCATION. see *BIOLOGY—Physiology*

AFFINITY. see *RELIGIONS AND THEOLOGY—Other Denominations And Sects*

371.15 150 JPN
AIIKU TSUSHIN/LETTERS OF HUMAN GROWTH. Text in Japanese. 1975. q. JPY 4,000 (effective 2001). bk.rev. 8 p./no. **Document type:** *Newsletter, Academic/Scholarly.* **Description:** Contains Dr. Kokubu Yasutaka's editorial on humanistic psychology and Dr. Hori Shinichiro's presentation of his thoughts and practice at Kinokuni Kodomonomura Gakuen (Japanese Summer Hill School), Wakayama-ken, Japan. Also included are member reports of their application of humanistic philosophy in living and working areas.
Indexed: e-psyche.
Published by: Shin Aiiku Shinri Kenkyukai/Japanese Study Group of Humanistic Education, c/o Mr Masahiro Makino, 3-41-39 kugayama, Suginami-ku, Tokyo 168-0082, Japan. makino@kgc.keio.ac.jp. Ed. Yasutaka Kokubu. R&P Mr. Masahiro Makino.

AMERICAN ASSOCIATION FOR MEDICAL TRANSCRIPTION. JOURNAL. see *MEDICAL SCIENCES*

370.15 POL ISSN 0867-2040
ANNALES UNIVERSITATIS MARIAE CURIE-SKLODOWSKA. SECTIO J. PAEDAGOGIA - PSYCHOLOGIA. Text and summaries in English, Polish. 1988. a. price varies. **Document type:** *Academic/Scholarly.*
Indexed: Lang.& Lang.Behav.Abstr., SOPODA, Sociol.Abstr., e-psyche.
Published by: Uniwersytet Marii Curie-Sklodowskiej, Wydawnictwo, Pl M Curie Sklodowskiej 5, Lublin 20031, Poland. TEL 48-81-375304, FAX 48-81-336699. Ed. Stanislaw Popek. Circ: 500.

370.15 USA ISSN 0731-1141
LB1051
ANNUAL EDITIONS: EDUCATIONAL PSYCHOLOGY. Text in English. 1981. a. USD 12.25. illus. *Refereed.* **Document type:** *Academic/Scholarly.*
Indexed: e-psyche.
Published by: Dushkin - McGraw-Hill, Sluice Dock, Guilford, CT 06437-9989. TEL 203-453-4351, FAX 203-453-6000. Pub. Ian Nielsen. R&P Cheryl Greenleaf.

ANNUAL REPORT ON ALLIED DENTAL HEALTH EDUCATION. see *MEDICAL SCIENCES—Dentistry*

ANNUAL REPORT ON DENTAL EDUCATION. see *MEDICAL SCIENCES—Dentistry*

370.15 IND ISSN 0971-2909
ASIAN JOURNAL OF PSYCHOLOGY AND EDUCATION. Text in English. 1976. 6/yr. USD 39.50. adv. bk.rev. reprint service avail. from ISI.
Indexed: IBR, Psychol.Abstr., e-psyche.
—BLDSC (1742.570000).
Published by: Agra Psychological Research Cell, Tiwari Kothi, Belanganj, Agra, Uttar Pradesh 282 004, India. Eds. B V Patel, N S Chauhan.

AUSTRALIAN TEACHER OF THE DEAF. see *HANDICAPPED—Hearing Impaired*

BEHAVIOROLOGY. see *PSYCHOLOGY*

BIOTECHNOLOGY EDUCATION. see *BIOLOGY—Biotechnology*

BRITISH JOURNAL OF EDUCATIONAL PSYCHOLOGY. see *PSYCHOLOGY*

CANADIAN JOURNAL OF BEHAVIOURAL SCIENCE/REVUE CANADIENNE DES SCIENCES DU COMPORTEMENT. see *PSYCHOLOGY*

CANADIAN JOURNAL OF COUNSELLING/REVUE CANADIENNE DE COUNSELING. see *PSYCHOLOGY*

370.15 CAN ISSN 0829-5735
CANADIAN JOURNAL OF SCHOOL PSYCHOLOGY. Text in English. 1985. 2/yr. CND 42 to individuals; CND 80 to institutions. adv. bk.rev. back issues avail. **Document type:** *Academic/Scholarly.* **Description:** For psychologists, counsellors, teachers and administrators involved in any type of work in schools or other educational institutions.
Related titles: Microfiche ed.: (from MML); Microform ed.: (from MML).
Indexed: Can.Educ.Ind., PsycInfo, Psychol.Abstr. (1993-), e-psyche.
—BLDSC (3035.518000). **CCC.**
Published by: Canadian Association of School Psychologists, Faculty of Education Clinic, University of Alberta, Edmonton, AB T6G 2G5, Canada. TEL 403-492-5718, FAX 403-492-1318. Ed., R&P, Adv. contact Jeffrey Derevensky TEL 514-398-4249. Circ: 500.

155.4 USA ISSN 0009-4005
LB1101 CODEN: CSJOD2
CHILD STUDY JOURNAL. Text in English. 1970. q. USD 17 domestic to individuals (effective 1999); USD 34 domestic to institutions; USD 39 foreign (effective 2000). bk.rev. illus. index. back issues avail.; reprint service avail. from PQC,PSC,SCH. *Refereed.* **Document type:** *Academic/Scholarly.* **Description:** Serves as a venue to discuss theory and research on child and adolescent development.
Formerly: Child Study Center Bulletin
Related titles: Microfilm ed.: (from PQC); Online - full text ed.: (from H. W. Wilson, Gale Group).
Indexed: AgeLine, C.I.J.E., Child Devel.Abstr., Cont.Pg.Educ., Curr.Cont. (coverage dropped), ERA, Educ.Ind. (Jan.1983-), Except.Child Educ.Abstr., Fam.Ind., IBZ, IMFL, Ind.Philos., Lang.& Lang.Behav.Abstr., Mult.Ed.Abstr., P C I, PsycInfo, Psychol.Abstr. (1970-), Psycscan D.P., Ref.Zh., SOPODA, SSCI (coverage dropped), Soc.Serv.Abstr., Sociol.Abstr., Sp.Ed.Needs Abstr., e-psyche.
—BLDSC (3172.949000), ingenta.
Published by: State University of New York at Buffalo, Behavioral and Humanistic Studies, Bacon Hall 306, 1300 Elmwood Ave, Buffalo, NY 14222-1095. TEL 716-878-5302, FAX 716-878-5833. Ed. Donald E Carter. R&P Glenda Leyonmark. Circ: 500.

E

370.15 POL ISSN 0137-706X
CHOWANNA. Text in Polish; Summaries in English. 1929; N.S. 1993. s-a. PLZ 14 (effective 2000). *Refereed.* **Document type:** *Academic/Scholarly.* **Description:** Covers theoretical and applied aspects of pedagogy and psychology.
Indexed: e-psyche.
Published by: Wydawnictwa Szkolne i Pedagogiczne, Ul Bankowa 12 B, Katowice 40007, Poland. TEL 48-32-596915, FAX 48-32-599-605, wydawus@us.edu.pl, http://www.us.edu.pl/uniwersytet/jednostki/ogolne. R&P Barbara Woznica. Circ: 275.

COGNITION AND INSTRUCTION. see *PSYCHOLOGY*

COGNITION AND LANGUAGE; a series in psycholinguistics. see *LINGUISTICS*

370.15 FRA ISSN 0246-4950
COLLECTION ORIENTATIONS* . Text in French. irreg. price varies.
Indexed: e-psyche.
Published by: Editions Scientifiques et Psychologiques, c/o Office de Justification de la Diffusion Controle (O J D), 40 Bd. Malesherbes, Paris 75008, France. TEL 46-45-38-12, FAX 40-95-73-32. Ed. G Pihouee.

370.15 USA ISSN 0361-476X
LB1051
CONTEMPORARY EDUCATIONAL PSYCHOLOGY. Text in English. 1976. q. USD 430 in US & Canada to institutions; USD 450 elsewhere to institutions (effective 2001). illus. index. back issues avail. *Refereed.* **Document type:** *Academic/Scholarly.* **Description:** Journal of empirical research and theory that demonstrates the application of psychological methods and research to problems in education. Covers the process of education through the life span, and presents a clear relationship of topic to data and theory.
Related titles: Online - full text ed.: (from EBSCO Publishing, O C L C Online Computer Library Center, Inc., RoweCom Information Quest, ingenta, Swets Blackwell, IDEAL Online Library, Institute for Scientific Information).
Indexed: ASCA, Arts & Hum.Cit.Ind. (coverage dropped), C.I.J.E. (coverage dropped), Chic.Per.Ind., Child Devel.Abstr., Cont.Pg.Educ., Curr.Cont., ERA, Educ.Ind. (Jul.1983-), Educ.Tech.Abstr., IBR, Mult.Ed.Abstr., PsycInfo, Psychol.Abstr. (1976-), Res.High.Educ.Abstr., SOMA, SSCI, Sp.Ed.Needs Abstr., Tech.Educ.Abstr., e-psyche.
—BLDSC (3425.181000), IDS, ingenta. **CCC.**
Published by: Academic Press, Inc., Journal Division (Subsidiary of: Harcourt Brace & Company), 525 B St, Ste 1900, San Diego, CA 92101-4495. TEL 619-230-1840, FAX 619-699-6800, apsubs@acad.com, http://www.academicpress.com/cep. Ed. James M Royer.

371.4 USA ISSN 0011-0035
CODEN: CESUDZ
COUNSELOR EDUCATION AND SUPERVISION. Text in English. 1961. q. USD 50 domestic to institutions; USD 70 foreign to institutions (effective 2001). adv. bk.rev. illus, abstr, bibl. index. 80 p./no. back issues avail.; reprint service avail. from PQC,SCH,PSC. *Refereed.* **Document type:** *Journal, Academic/Scholarly.* **Description:** Covers theory, practice and research on pre-service and in-service preparation and supervision.
Related titles: Microform ed.: (from PQC); Online - full text ed.: (from H. W. Wilson, ProQuest Information & Learning).
Indexed: A.D.& D., AgeLine, C.I.J.E., Cont.Pg.Educ., Curr.Cont. (coverage dropped), ERA, Educ.Ind. (Jun.1983-), Educ.Tech.Abstr., Fam.Ind., Mult.Ed.Abstr., PsycInfo, Psychol.Abstr. (1966-), SSCI (coverage dropped), Sp.Ed.Needs Abstr., e-psyche.
—BLDSC (3481.350000), ingenta. **CCC.**
Published by: (Association for Counselor Education and Supervision), American Counseling Association, 5999 Stevenson Ave, Alexandria, VA 22304-3300. TEL 703-823-9800, FAX 703-823-0252, http://www.counseling.org, http://www.ncda.org. Ed. Marlowe H Smaby. R&P Cynthia Peay TEL 703-823-9800 x 249. Adv. contact Kathy Maguire TEL 703-823-9800 ext 207. Circ: 3,500.

370.15 USA ISSN 0093-5263
CREATIVITY IN ACTION. Text in English. 1972. bi-m. USD 50 domestic; USD 55 in Canada & Mexico; USD 60 elsewhere (effective 2000). bk.rev. illus. back issues avail. **Document type:** *Newsletter.* **Description:** Helps readers learn more about and practice more of many important ideas and techniques that enhance creative thinking and action.
Related titles: Online - full text ed.
Indexed: e-psyche.
Published by: Creative Education Foundation, Inc., 1050 Union Rd, Buffalo, NY 14224. TEL 716-675-3181, FAX 716-675-3209, cefhq@cef-cpsi.org, http://www.cef-cpsi.org. R&P Grace Guzzutta. Circ: 500.

370.15 POL ISSN 0239-3271
H8
CZLOWIEK I SPOLECZENSTWO. Text in Polish; Text occasionally in English. 1984. a., latest vol.14, 1996. bk.rev. back issues avail. **Document type:** *Monographic series, Academic/Scholarly.* **Description:** Covers psychology, sociology and education.
Indexed: e-psyche.
Published by: (Adam Mickiewicz University, Institute of Sociology), Adam Mickiewicz University Press, Nowowiejskiego 55, Poznan 61734, Poland. TEL 48-61-527380, FAX 48-61-527701. Pub. Maria Jankowska. R&P Malgorzata Bis. Circ: 300.

370.15 USA
DREAM SWITCHBOARD. Text in English. 1988. 4/yr. USD 10 (effective 1999). adv. bk.rev., film rev., play rev. *Refereed.* **Document type:** *Newsletter.* **Description:** Provides elementary and secondary school classroom assistance to help students understand dreams.
Indexed: e-psyche.
Published by: (Community Dreamsharing Network), Dream Switchboard, PO Box 8032, Hicksville, NY 11802-8032. TEL 516-735-1969, FAX 516-731-2395, comdreamnt@aol.com. Ed. Harold R Ellis. Circ: 500 (paid).

372.21 USA ISSN 1082-3301
LB1139.25 CODEN: ECEJFA
EARLY CHILDHOOD EDUCATION JOURNAL. Text in English. 1973. q. USD 322, EUR 321 to institutions for print or online ed.; USD 386.40, EUR 365.20 to institutions for print & online eds.combined (effective 2002). adv. bk.rev. illus. back issues avail.; reprint service avail. from PQC,SCH,PSC,ISI. *Refereed.* **Document type:** *Journal, Academic/Scholarly.* **Description:** Provides a practical and lively forum for early childhood teachers, program administrators, day care workers, and other professionals concerned with the education of young children.
Formerly (until 1995): Day Care and Early Education (0092-4199)
Related titles: Microform ed.: (from PQC); Online - full text ed.: (from EBSCO Publishing, O C L C Online Computer Library Center, Inc., Swets Blackwell, Kluwer Online, RoweCom Information Quest).
Indexed: Behav.Abstr., Bk.Rev.Ind., C.I.J.E., Cont.Pg.Educ., ERA, Educ.Admin.Abstr., Educ.Ind. (Oct.1995-), Except.Child Educ.Abstr., Excerp.Med., Fam.Ind., Lang.& Lang.Behav.Abstr., Media Rev.Dig., Mult.Ed.Abstr., SOPODA, Soc.Work Res.& Abstr., Sociol.Abstr., Sp.Ed.Needs Abstr.
—BLDSC (3642.957300), Infotrieve, ingenta. **CCC.**
Published by: (Early Childhood Education Journal), Kluwer Academic - Plenum Publishers (Subsidiary of: Wolters Kluwer N.V.), 233 Spring St, New York, NY 10013-1578. TEL 212-620-8000, 800-221-9369, FAX 212-463-0742, services@wkap.nl, info@plenum.com, http://www.wkap.nl. Ed. Dr. Mary Jalongo. Circ: 10,000 (paid). **Subscr. outside the Americas to:** Kluwer Academic Publishers Group, Journals Department, PO Box 322, Dordrecht 3300 AH, Netherlands. TEL 31-78-639-2392, FAX 31-78-654-6474.

155.4 USA ISSN 1524-5039
▼ **EARLY CHILDHOOD RESEARCH & PRACTICE.** Text in English. 1999. s-a. free per issue. *Refereed.* **Document type:** *Journal, Academic/Scholarly.* **Description:** Features articles related to the development and care of children from birth to approximately age 8.
Media: Online - full text.
Published by: E R I C Clearinghouse on Elementary and Early Childhood Education, 51 Gerty Dr, University of Illinois at Urbana, Champaign, IL 61820-7469. l-preece@uiuc.edu, http://ecrp.uiuc.edu/. Ed. Lilian G Katz.

EARLY CHILDHOOD UPDATE. see *PSYCHOLOGY*

370.15 USA ISSN 1040-9289
LB1101 CODEN: EEDEF4
EARLY EDUCATION AND DEVELOPMENT. Text in English. 1989. q. USD 145; USD 155 foreign (effective 1999). adv. bk.rev. **Document type:** *Academic/Scholarly.* **Description:** Presents empirical research in early childhood education and child development, with emphasis on practical implications for practitioners.
Indexed: C.I.J.E., Child Devel.Abstr., Educ.Ind. (Jul.1997-), Lang.& Lang.Behav.Abstr., PsycInfo, Psychol.Abstr. (1993-), SOPODA, Sociol.Abstr., e-psyche.
—BLDSC (3642.964800), ingenta.
Published by: Wide Range Inc., PO Box 3410, Wilmington, DE 19804-0250. TEL 302-652-4990, 800-221-9728, FAX 302-652-1644, eed@widerange.com. Ed. Richard R Abidin. Pub., R&P, Adv. contact Jean McWatters. Circ: 350.

EDUCACION MEDICA; aprender y ensenar en las profesiones sanitarias. see *MEDICAL SCIENCES*

EDUCATION AND AGEING. see *GERONTOLOGY AND GERIATRICS*

370 150 IND ISSN 0046-1385
EDUCATION AND PSYCHOLOGY REVIEW. Text in English. 1961. q. INR 10, USD 3. bk.rev. stat.
Indexed: Bibl.Asian Stud. (1971, 1975-1979), Cont.Pg.Educ., Psychol.Abstr., e-psyche.
Published by: Maharaja Sayajirao University of Baroda, Faculty of Education and Psychology, Baroda, Gujarat 390 002, India. Ed. D M Desai. Circ: 400.

370.15 SWE ISSN 0070-9263
LB1051 CODEN: EPINDT
EDUCATIONAL AND PSYCHOLOGICAL INTERACTIONS. Text in English. 1964. irreg. back issues avail. **Document type:** *Journal, Academic/Scholarly.*
Indexed: Child Devel.Abstr., Cont.Pg.Educ., Educ.Tech.Abstr., Mult.Ed.Abstr., Psychol.Abstr., Sociol.Abstr., Sp.Ed.Needs Abstr., e-psyche.
—BLDSC (3661.365000).
Published by: Malmoe University, Department of Education, Fack 23501, Malmo 20045, Sweden. FAX 46-40-325-210.

EDUCATIONAL AND PSYCHOLOGICAL MEASUREMENT; devoted to the development and application of measures of individual differences. see *PSYCHOLOGY*

EDUCATIONAL PSYCHOLOGIST. see *PSYCHOLOGY*

370.15 GBR ISSN 0144-3410
LB1051 CODEN: EDPSFV
EDUCATIONAL PSYCHOLOGY; an international journal of experimental educational psychology. Text in English. 1981. 5/yr. GBP 123, USD 198 to individuals; GBP 496, USD 962 to institutions (effective 2002). adv. bk.rev. stat. index. reprint service avail. from PSC,SCH. *Refereed.* **Document type:** *Academic/Scholarly.*
Related titles: Microfiche ed.; Online - full text ed.: ISSN 1469-5820 (from CatchWord Ltd., Northern Light Technology, Inc., EBSCO Publishing, O C L C Online Computer Library Center, Inc., RoweCom Information Quest, ProQuest Information & Learning, Swets Blackwell).
Indexed: Bibl.Asian Stud. (1971, 1998), Br.Educ.Ind., C.I.J.E., Child Devel.Abstr., Child.Lit.Abstr., Cont.Pg.Educ., ERA, Educ.Tech.Abstr., Ind.Philos., Lang.& Lang.Behav.Abstr., Mult.Ed.Abstr., PsycInfo, Psychol.Abstr. (1981-), Res.High.Educ.Abstr., SOMA, SOPODA, Sociol.Abstr., Sociol.Educ.Abstr., Sp.Ed.Needs Abstr., Stud.Wom.Abstr., Tech.Educ.Abstr.
—BLDSC (3661.535000), CatchWord, ingenta. **CCC.**
Published by: Carfax Publishing Limited (Subsidiary of: Taylor & Francis Group), PO Box 25, Abingdon, Oxon OX14 3UE, United Kingdom. TEL 44-1235-401000, FAX 44-1235-401550, enquiries@carfax.co.uk, enquiry@tandf.co.uk, http://www.carfax.co.uk. Eds. Kevin Wheldall, Richard Riding. Circ: 1,000.

370.15 USA ISSN 0266-7363
EDUCATIONAL PSYCHOLOGY IN PRACTICE. Text in English. 4/yr. GBP 48, USD 81 to individuals; GBP 143, USD 235 to institutions (effective 2002). adv. bk.rev. bibl, illus. index. back issues avail.; reprint service avail. from PQC. *Refereed.* **Document type:** *Academic/Scholarly.* **Description:** Features new ideas and the latest developments, plus informational articles about the practical aspects of educational psychology.
Formerly: A E P Journal (0309-3573)
Related titles: Microfilm ed.; Online - full text ed.: ISSN 1469-5839 (from CatchWord Ltd., EBSCO Publishing, O C L C Online Computer Library Center, Inc., Swets Blackwell, RoweCom Information Quest).
Indexed: Br.Educ.Ind., Cont.Pg.Educ., ERA, Educ.Admin.Abstr., Mult.Ed.Abstr., PsycInfo, Psychol.Abstr. (1974-), Sp.Ed.Needs Abstr., Tech.Educ.Abstr., Viol.& Abuse Abstr., e-psyche.
—BLDSC (3661.540000), CatchWord, Infotrieve, ingenta. **CCC.**
Published by: (Association of Educational Psychologists GBR), Carfax Publishing Co. (Subsidiary of: Taylor & Francis Group), 325 Chestnut St, Ste 800, Philadelphia, PA 19106. TEL 800-354-1420, http://www.tandf.co.uk/journals/carfax/02667363.html. Ed. Jeremy Monsen. Circ: 2,800.

370.15 USA ISSN 1040-726X
LB1051 CODEN: EPSREO
EDUCATIONAL PSYCHOLOGY REVIEW. Text in English. 1989. q. USD 358, EUR 357 to institutions for print or online ed.; USD 429.60, EUR 428.40 to institutions for print & online eds.combined (effective 2002). adv. illus. back issues avail.; reprints avail. *Refereed.* **Document type:** *Journal, Academic/Scholarly.* **Description:** Publishes review articles in general education psychology: learning, cognition, measurement, school-related counseling, and development.
Related titles: Microfilm ed.: (from PQC); Online - full text ed.: (from EBSCO Publishing, O C L C Online Computer Library Center, Inc., Swets Blackwell, Kluwer Online, Institute for Scientific Information, RoweCom Information Quest).
Indexed: ASCA, Cont.Pg.Educ., Crim.Just.Abstr., Curr.Cont., ERA, Educ.Ind. (Jun.1992-), Educ.Tech.Abstr., Lang.& Lang.Behav.Abstr., Mult.Ed.Abstr., PsycInfo, Psychol.Abstr. (1989-), SOMA, SOPODA, SSCI, Sociol.Abstr., Sociol.Educ.Abstr., Sp.Ed.Needs Abstr., Tech.Educ.Abstr., e-psyche.
—BLDSC (3661.545000), IDS, Infotrieve, ingenta. **CCC.**
Published by: Kluwer Academic - Plenum Publishers (Subsidiary of: Wolters Kluwer N.V.), 233 Spring St, New York, NY 10013-1578. TEL 212-620-8000, FAX 212-463-0742, services@wkap.nl, info@plenum.com, http://www.wkap.nl/journalhome.htm/1040-726X. Ed. Kenneth A Kierwa. R&P Rose Luongo TEL 781-871-6311. **Subscr. outside the Americas to:** Kluwer Academic Publishers Group, Journals Department, PO Box 322, Dordrecht 3300 AH, Netherlands. TEL 31-78-639-2392, FAX 31-78-654-6474.

372 155.4 USA ISSN 0013-5984
L11 CODEN: ELSJA2
THE ELEMENTARY SCHOOL JOURNAL. Abbreviated title: E S J. Text in English. 1900. 5/yr., latest vol.99, 1998, Sep. USD 37 in United States to individuals; USD 45.59 in Canada to individuals; USD 43 elsewhere to individuals; USD 110 in United States to institutions; USD 123.70 in Canada to institutions; USD 116 elsewhere to institutions; USD 24 in United States to students; USD 31.68 in Canada to students; USD 30 elsewhere to students; USD 11.40 newsstand/cover to individuals; USD 26 newsstand/cover to institutions (effective 2002). adv. bk.rev. abstr, illus. index. back issues avail.; reprint service avail. from PQC,SCH,PSC,ISI. *Refereed.* **Document type:** *Academic/Scholarly.* **Description:** Covers student and teacher behavior and interactions in elementary school settings, discusses curricula.
Related titles: Microform ed.: (from PQC,PMC); Online - full text ed.: (from ProQuest Information & Learning, Gale Group, Factiva, Institute for Scientific Information).
Indexed: ASCA, Acad.Ind., C.I.J.E., Chic.Per.Ind., Cont.Pg.Educ., Curr.Cont., DSH Abstr., ERA, Educ.Admin.Abstr., Educ.Ind. (Mar.1983-), Educ.Tech.Abstr., Except.Child Educ.Abstr., Fam.Ind., Lang.& Lang.Behav.Abstr., Mult.Ed.Abstr., P C I, PsycInfo, Psychol.Abstr. (1965-), SOMA, SOPODA, SSCI, Sage Race Rel.Abstr., Sociol.Abstr., Sociol.Educ.Abstr., Sp.Ed.Needs Abstr., Tech.Educ.Abstr., e-psyche.
—BLDSC (3727.200000), IDS, Infotrieve, ingenta. **CCC.**
Published by: University of Chicago Press, Journals Division, PO Box 37005, Chicago, IL 60637. TEL 773-753-3347, FAX 773-753-0811, subscriptions@journals.uchicago.edu, orders@press.uchicago.edu, http:// www.journals.uchicago.edu/ESJ/. Ed. Thomas L Good. adv.: B&W page USD 385; trim 10 x 6.75. Circ: 3,637 (paid).

ESPRIT LIBRE. see *PSYCHOLOGY*

370.15 DEU ISSN 0256-2928
CODEN: EJPDER
EUROPEAN JOURNAL OF PSYCHOLOGY OF EDUCATION. Text in English. 1986. q. DEM 309 domestic; DEM 310 foreign (effective 2001). adv. bk.rev. bibl, charts. *Refereed.* **Document type:** *Journal, Academic/Scholarly.* **Description:** Publishes empirical research results, theoretical and methodological articles and critical literature reviews with a focus on the psychological perspective in education.
Related titles: Online - full text ed.: (from Institute for Scientific Information).
Indexed: ASCA, C.I.J.E., Child Devel.Abstr., Cont.Pg.Educ., Curr.Cont., ERA, Educ.Admin.Abstr., Educ.Tech.Abstr., Lang.& Lang.Behav.Abstr., Mult.Ed.Abstr., PsycInfo, Psychol.Abstr. (1986-), SOMA, SOPODA, SSCI, Sociol.Abstr., Sociol.Educ.Abstr., Sp.Ed.Needs Abstr., Tech.Educ.Abstr., e-psyche.
—BLDSC (3829.738000), IDS.
Published by: (Instituto Superior de Psicologia Aplicada PRT, Universite de Provence FRA), Springer-Verlag (Subsidiary of: BertelsmannSpringer), Tiergartenstr 17, Heidelberg 69121, Germany. TEL 49-6221-345-0, FAX 49-6221-345229, subscriptions@springer.de, http://www.springer.de. Ed. M Gilly. **Co-sponsor:** University of Neuchatel.

EXCEPTIONAL CHILDREN. see *EDUCATION—Special Education And Rehabilitation*

FAMILIENMAGAZIN. see *CHILDREN AND YOUTH—About*

FAMILY MEDICINE. see *MEDICAL SCIENCES*

370.15 HRV ISSN 0352-6798
B1 CODEN: RFFPEQ
FILOZOFSKI FAKULTET - ZADAR. RAZDIO FILOZOFIJE, PSIHOLOGIJE, SOCIOLOGIJE I PEDAGOGIJE. RADOVI. Text in Croatian, English; Summaries in English. 1985. a. USD 20 foreign (effective 2000). index, cum.index no.1-2. back issues avail. *Refereed.* **Document type:** *Academic/Scholarly.* **Description:** Interdisciplinary journal covers philosophy, psychology, sociology, and education.
Indexed: Lang.& Lang.Behav.Abstr., Ling.Abstr., Russ.Acad.Sci.Bibl., SOPODA, Soc.Serv.Abstr., Sociol.Abstr., e-psyche.
Published by: Sveuciliste u Splitu, Filozofski Fakultet Zadar, Obala P Kresimira IV 2, Zadar 23000, Croatia. TEL 385-23-316-311, FAX 385-23-316882, radovi-razdio_fpsp@ffzd.hr. Ed. Erma Ivos Niksic. Circ: 500. **Co-sponsor:** Ministarstva Znanosti i Tehnologije Republike Hrvatske.

370.15 USA ISSN 1059-6011
HM134 CODEN: GOSTDA
GROUP & ORGANIZATION MANAGEMENT; an international journal. Text in English. 1976. q. USD 75 to individuals; USD 335 to institutions; USD 25 newsstand/cover to individuals; USD 90 newsstand/cover to institutions (effective 2002). adv. bk.rev. illus. index. back issues avail.; reprint service avail. from PQC,PSC,SCH. *Refereed.* **Document type:** *Academic/Scholarly.* **Description:** Aims to bridge the gap between research and practice for psychologists, group facilitators, educators, and consultants involved in the broad field of human relations training.
Formerly (until Mar. 1992): Group and Organization Studies (0364-1082)
Related titles: Microform ed.: (from PQC); Online - full text ed.: (from Gale Group, EBSCO Publishing, O C L C Online Computer Library Center, Inc., RoweCom Information Quest, ProQuest Information & Learning, ingenta, Swets Blackwell, Institute for Scientific Information).
Indexed: ABI Inform. (Mar.1981-), ASCA, BPIA, Bus.Ind., C.I.J.E. (coverage dropped), CINAHL, Commun.Abstr., Curr.Cont., Emerald, Environ.Sci.Poll.Mgmt., Ergon.Abstr., Human Resour.Abstr., IMFL, Lang.& Lang.Behav.Abstr., Manage.Cont., Pers.Lit., Polit.Sci.Abstr., PsycInfo, Psychol.Abstr. (1976-), Psycscan A.P., Risk Abstr., SSCI, Saf.Sci.Abstr., Sage Fam.Stud.Abstr., Sage Pub.Admin.Abstr., Sociol.Abstr., Stud.Wom.Abstr., Tech.Educ.Abstr., Viol.& Abuse Abstr., e-psyche.
—BLDSC (4220.173900), CISTI, IDS, ingenta. **CCC.**
Published by: (Eastern Academy of Management), Sage Publications, Inc., 2455 Teller Rd, Thousand Oaks, CA 91320. TEL 805-499-9774, 800-818-7243, FAX 805-499-0871, info@sagepub.com, http:// www.sagepub.com. Ed. Christopher J Earley. R&P Tanya Udin. Adv. contact DeAnna Vega Hammersley. Circ: 1,300. **Overseas subscr. to:** Sage Publications Ltd., 6 Bonhill St, London EC2A 4PU, United Kingdom; Sage Publications India Pvt. Ltd., 4215, New Delhi 110 048, India.

613.7 370 JPN ISSN 0018-3350
HEALTH AND PHYSICAL EDUCATION/HOKEN TAIIKU KYOSHITSU. Text in Japanese. 1967. q. JPY 300 per issue. adv. bk.rev. charts. **Document type:** *Academic/Scholarly.*
Published by: Taishukan Publishing Co. Ltd., 3-24 Kanda-Nishiki-cho, Chiyoda-ku, Tokyo 101-8466, Japan. FAX 81-3-3295-4108, physic-edu@taishukan.co.jp, hanbai@fa.mbn.or.jp, http://www.taishukan.co.jp. Eds. Kazuyuki Suzuki, Shoichi Tamaki. Pub. Shigeo Suzuki. Circ: 5,000 (controlled).

370.15 IND
I S P T JOURNAL OF RESEARCH IN EDUCATIONAL & PSYCHOLOGICAL TESTING & MEASUREMENT. Text in English. 1977. s-a. INR 200, USD 250. adv. bk.rev. back issues avail. **Document type:** *Academic/Scholarly.* **Description:** Devoted to the fields of educational, psychological measurement, evaluation, testing and other allied subjects.
Formerly: I S P T Journal of Research in Educational and Psychological Measurement (0251-0146)
Indexed: Indian Psychol.Abstr., e-psyche.
Published by: Institute for Studies in Psychological Testing, 101 Doon, Jakhan, Rajpur Rd., Dehra Dun, Uttar Pradesh 248 001, India. TEL 91-135-684551. Ed. S P Kulshrestha. Circ: 500.

IGAKU KYOIKU/MEDICAL EDUCATION. see *MEDICAL SCIENCES*

INDIAN JOURNAL OF PSYCHOMETRY AND EDUCATION. see *PSYCHOLOGY*

370.15 ESP ISSN 0210-3702
LB1051
INFANCIA Y APRENDIZAJE/JOURNAL FOR THE STUDY OF EDUCATION AND DEVELOPMENT. Text in English, Spanish. 1978. q. ESP 2,800 per issue foreign. adv. *Refereed.* **Document type:** *Academic/Scholarly.* **Description:** Concerned with the psychology of development-education processes. Publishes original articles on empirical research and literary reviews and theoretical essays.
Related titles: Online - full text ed.: (from CatchWord Ltd.).
Indexed: Child Devel.Abstr., PsycInfo, Psychol.Abstr. (1982-), e-psyche.
—CINDOC. **CCC.**
Published by: Fundacion Infancia y Aprendizaje, Cr Canillas, 138, 2o 16C, Madrid 28043, Spain. TEL 34-91-388-3874, FAX 34-91-300-3527. Ed. Cesar Coll. Circ: 3,000.

370.15 ROM
INSTITUTUL DE SUBINGINERI ORADEA. LUCRARI STIINTIFICE: SERIA PEDAGOGIE, PSIHOLOGIE, METODICA. Text in Romanian; Text occasionally in English, French; Summaries in English, French, German, Romanian. 1967. irreg. **Document type:** *Academic/Scholarly.*
Formerly: Institutul Pedagogic Oradea. Lucrari Stiintifice: Seria Pedagogie, Psihologie, Metodica; Which superseded in part (in 1973): Institutul Pedagogica Oradea. Lucrari Stiintifice: Seria Istorie, Stiinte Sociale, Pedagogie; Which superseded in part (in 1971): Institutul Pedagogica Oradea. Lucrari Stiintifice: Seria A si Seria B; Which was formerly (until 1969): Institutul Pedagogic Oradea. Lucrari Stiintifice
Indexed: e-psyche.
Published by: Institutul de Subingineri Oradea, Calea Armatei Rosii 5, Oradea 3700, Romania.

370.15 RUS
INTEGRAL'NOE ISSLEDOVANIE INDIVIDUAL'NOSTI. Text in Russian. 1977. irreg.
Indexed: e-psyche.
Published by: Permskii Gosudarstvennyi Pedagogicheskii Institut, Perm, Russian Federation. TEL 32-85-90. Ed. Bronislaw Aleksandrovich Vyatkin. Circ: 700.

INTERNATIONAL JOURNAL OF CHILDREN'S SPIRITUALITY. see *PSYCHOLOGY*

INTERNATIONAL JOURNAL OF HEALTH PROMOTION AND EDUCATION. see *PHYSICAL FITNESS AND HYGIENE*

370.117 150 USA ISSN 1530-5058
▼ **INTERNATIONAL JOURNAL OF TESTING.** Text in English. 2001. q. USD 50 in US & Canada to individuals; USD 80 elsewhere to individuals; USD 150 in US & Canada to institutions; USD 180 elsewhere to institutions (effective 2002). adv. *Refereed.* **Document type:** *Journal, Academic/Scholarly.* **Description:** Dedicated to the advancement of theory, research, and practice in testing and assessment in psychology, education, counseling, human resource management, and related disciplines.
Related titles: Online - full text ed.: USD 45 per issue to individuals; USD 135 per issue to institutions (2002) (from CatchWord Ltd.).
Published by: (International Test Commission), Lawrence Erlbaum Associates, Inc., 10 Industrial Ave, Mahwah, NJ 07430-2262. TEL 201-760-3735, 800-926-6579, FAX 201-236-0072, journals@erlbaum.com, http://www.erlbaum.com/Journals/journals/IJT/ijt.htm. Ed. Norbert Tanzer. adv.: page USD 300; trim 5 x 8.

E

JAPANESE JOURNAL OF EDUCATIONAL PSYCHOLOGY. see *PSYCHOLOGY*

JOHANN WILHELM KLEIN; literarische Zeitschrift fuer Blinde. see *HANDICAPPED—Visually Impaired*

370.113 USA ISSN 0195-7597
JOURNAL FOR VOCATIONAL SPECIAL NEEDS EDUCATION. Text in English. 1978. 3/yr. USD 24; USD 30 foreign. adv. bk.rev. charts, stat, illus. back issues avail.; reprints avail. *Refereed.* **Document type:** *Academic/Scholarly.*
Related titles: Microform ed.: 1978 (from PQC).
Indexed: C.I.J.E., Cont.Pg.Educ., ERA, Educ.Tech.Abstr., Mult.Ed.Abstr., Sp.Ed.Needs Abstr., Tech.Educ.Abstr.
—BLDSC (5072.512500), ingenta.
Address: c/o John Gugerty, Center for Education and Work, Univ of Wisconsin, 1025 W Johnson St, 964, Madison, WI 53706-1796. rojewski@uga.cc.uga.edu, http://www.cew.wisc.edu/jvsne/. Ed. John Gugerty. Circ: 2,000 (paid).

JOURNAL OF APPLIED DEVELOPMENTAL PSYCHOLOGY; an international lifespan journal. see *PSYCHOLOGY*

370.153 USA ISSN 1053-0819
LB1060.2 CODEN: JBEDE5
JOURNAL OF BEHAVIORAL EDUCATION. Text in English. 1991. q. USD 295, EUR 294.50 to institutions for print or online ed.; USD 354, EUR 354 to institutions for print & online eds. combined (effective 2002). adv. *Refereed.* **Document type:** *Journal, Academic/Scholarly.* **Description:** Serves as a forum for research on the application of behavioral principles and technology to education.
Related titles: Online - full text ed.: (from O C L C Online Computer Library Center, Inc., Swets Blackwell, Kluwer Online, RoweCom Information Quest).
Indexed: Cont.Pg.Educ., ERA, Educ.Ind. (Jul.1997-), Intl.Bibl.Soc.Sci., Mult.Ed.Abstr., PsycInfo, Psychol.Abstr. (1991-), Psycscan B.A.& T., SOMA, Sp.Ed.Needs Abstr., e-psyche.
—BLDSC (4951.260000), Infotrieve, ingenta. **CCC.**
Published by: Kluwer Academic - Plenum Publishers (Subsidiary of: Wolters Kluwer N.V.), 233 Spring St, New York, NY 10013-1578. TEL 212-620-8000, 800-221-9369, FAX 212-463-0742, info@plenum.com, http://www.wkap.nl/journalhome.htm/1053-0819. Ed. Mark Wolery. **Subscr. outside the Americas to:** Kluwer Academic Publishers Group, Journals Department, PO Box 322, Dordrecht 3300 AH, Netherlands. TEL 31-78-639-2392, FAX 31-78-654-6474.

JOURNAL OF BIOLOGICAL EDUCATION. see *BIOLOGY*

JOURNAL OF BLACK STUDIES. see *SOCIAL SCIENCES: COMPREHENSIVE WORKS*

370.152 GBR ISSN 1360-6352
JOURNAL OF COGNITIVE EDUCATION. Text in English. 1990. 3/yr. GBP 30 domestic to individuals; GBP 32 in Europe to individuals; GBP 34 elsewhere to individuals; GBP 60 domestic to institutions; GBP 64 in Europe to institutions; GBP 68 elsewhere to institutions (effective 2000). **Document type:** *Academic/Scholarly.* **Description:** Disseminates theory, research and methodology, policies, and practices relating to cognitive education, taken in the broadest sense.
Formerly: International Journal of Cognitive Education and Mediated Learning (0957-4964)
Related titles: Online - full text ed.
Indexed: Cont.Pg.Educ., Except.Child Educ.Abstr., PsycInfo, Soc.Work Res.& Abstr., e-psyche.
Published by: Questions Publishing Company Ltd., 27 Frederick St, Hockley, Birmingham, Warks B1 3HH, United Kingdom. TEL 44-121-212-0919, FAX 44-121-212-0959, http://www.education-quest.com. Ed. Adrian Ashman. Circ: 350.

150 370 USA ISSN 0022-0175
BF408
THE JOURNAL OF CREATIVE BEHAVIOR. Text in English. 1967. q., latest vol.36, 2002. USD 75 to individuals; USD 85 elsewhere to individuals; USD 95 to institutions; USD 110 elsewhere to institutions (effective 2002). adv. bk.rev. bibl, charts, illus, stat. index. reprint service avail. from PQC,PSC,SCH. *Refereed.* **Document type:** *Academic/Scholarly.*
Related titles: Microform ed.: (from PQC); Online - full text ed.: (from Institute for Scientific Information).
Indexed: ASCA, ASSIA, Adol.Ment.Hlth.Abstr., Amer.Bibl.Slavic & E.Eur.Stud., C.I.J.E., Commun.Abstr., Cont.Pg.Educ., Curr.Cont., ERA, Educ.Ind. (Jan.1983-), Educ.Tech.Abstr., Except.Child Educ.Abstr., Lang.& Lang.Behav.Abstr., Mult.Ed.Abstr., P C I, Pers.Lit., PsycInfo, Psychol.Abstr., Ref.Zh., Russ.Acad.Sci.Bibl., SOPODA, SSCI, Soc.Sci.Ind. (coverage dropped), Soc.Work Res.& Abstr., Sociol.Abstr., e-psyche.
—BLDSC (4965.500000), IDS, ingenta, Linda Hall.
Published by: Creative Education Foundation, Inc., 1050 Union Rd, Buffalo, NY 14224. TEL 716-675-3181, FAX 716-675-3209, cefhq@cef-cpsi.org, http://www.cef-cpsi.org/pubs.html. Ed. Thomas B Ward. R&P Grace Guzzutta. Circ: 2,000.

JOURNAL OF DRUG EDUCATION. see *DRUG ABUSE AND ALCOHOLISM*

370 150 IND ISSN 0022-0590
L61
JOURNAL OF EDUCATION AND PSYCHOLOGY. Text in English. 1943. q. INR 60, USD 30 (effective 1995-96). adv. bk.rev. index. *Refereed.* **Document type:** *Academic/Scholarly.*
Indexed: Bibl.Asian Stud. (1975-1977), Curr.Cont. (coverage dropped), e-psyche.
Published by: Sardar Patel University, Department of Education, Vallabh Vidyanagar 388 120, India. TEL 91-2792-30379. Ed. Jayendra K Dave. Circ: 300 (paid).

370.15 USA ISSN 1047-4412
LB2799 CODEN: JEPCFB
JOURNAL OF EDUCATIONAL AND PSYCHOLOGICAL CONSULTATION. Text in English. 1990. q. USD 45 in US & Canada to individuals; USD 75 elsewhere to individuals; USD 380 in US & Canada to institutions; USD 410 elsewhere to institutions (effective 2002). adv. bk.rev. *Refereed.* **Document type:** *Journal, Academic/Scholarly.* **Description:** Serves as a forum for the exchange of ideas, theories, and research among the fields of school psychology, special education, and reading.
Related titles: Online - full text ed.: ISSN 1532-768X. USD 40.50 to individuals (effective 2001 - 2002); USD 342 to institutions (effective 2002) (from CatchWord Ltd., EBSCO Publishing, O C L C Online Computer Library Center, Inc., RoweCom Information Quest, Swets Blackwell, Institute for Scientific Information).
Indexed: ASCA, C.I.J.E. (coverage dropped), Cont.Pg.Educ., Curr.Cont., ERA, Except.Child Educ.Abstr., IMFL, Lang.& Lang.Behav.Abstr., Mult.Ed.Abstr., PsycInfo, Psychol.Abstr. (1990-), SOMA, SOPODA, SSCI, Sociol.Abstr., Sociol.Educ.Abstr., Sp.Ed.Needs Abstr., e-psyche.
—BLDSC (4973.154050), CatchWord, Infotrieve, ingenta. **CCC.**
Published by: (Association for Educational and Psychological Consultants), Lawrence Erlbaum Associates, Inc., 10 Industrial Ave, Mahwah, NJ 07430-2262. TEL 201-236-9500, 800-926-6579, FAX 201-236-0072, journals@erlbaum.com, http://www.erlbaum.com/Journals/journals/JEPC/jepc.htm. Ed. Joseph Zins. adv.: page USD 375; trim 5 x 8.

370.15 USA ISSN 0022-0663
LB1051.A2
JOURNAL OF EDUCATIONAL PSYCHOLOGY. Text in English. 1910. q. USD 118 domestic to non-members; USD 133 foreign to non-members; USD 59 domestic to members; USD 69 foreign to members; USD 255 domestic to institutions; USD 287 foreign to institutions (effective 2001). adv. bibl, charts, illus. index. reprint service avail. from PQC,PSC,SCH. *Refereed.* **Document type:** *Academic/Scholarly.* **Description:** Deals with learning and cognition, psychological development, relationships, and adjustment of the individual, especially as related to the problems of instruction. Articles pertain to all levels of education and to all age groups.
Related titles: Microform ed.: (from PQC,PMC); Online - full text ed.: (from Gale Group, Factiva, Institute for Scientific Information).
Indexed: ASCA, Acad.Ind., Adol.Ment.Hlth.Abstr., AgeLine, Arts & Hum.Cit.Ind. (coverage dropped), Bibl.Dev.Med.& Child Neur., Biol.Abstr., C.I.J.E. (coverage dropped), Commun.Abstr., Cont.Pg.Educ., Curr.Cont., Curr.Ind.Stat., ERA, Educ.Admin.Abstr., Educ.Ind. (Oct.1982-), Educ.Tech.Abstr., Except.Child Educ.Abstr., Fam.Ind., High.Educ.Abstr., High.Educ.Curr.Aware.Bull., IBR, IBZ, Ind.Med. (coverage dropped), Ind.Philos., Lang.Teach.& Ling.Abstr., Mid.East: Abstr.& Ind., Mult.Ed.Abstr., P C I, PsycInfo, Psychol.Abstr. (1926-), Psycscan D.P., Res.High.Educ.Abstr., Russ.Acad.Sci.Bibl., SOMA, SSCI, Sage Fam.Stud.Abstr., Soc.Serv.Abstr., Sociol.Abstr., Sp.Ed.Needs Abstr., Stud.Wom.Abstr., Tech.Educ.Abstr., e-psyche.
—BLDSC (4973.200000), IDS, ingenta. **CCC.**
Published by: American Psychological Association, 750 First St., N.E., Washington, DC 20002-4242. TEL 202-336-5600, 800-374-2721, FAX 202-336-5568, subscriptions@apa.org, http://www.apa.org/journals/edu.html. Ed. Michael Pressley. Circ: 4,600.

JOURNAL OF HUMANISTIC COUNSELING, EDUCATION AND DEVELOPMENT. see *PSYCHOLOGY*

370.15 USA ISSN 0094-1956
LB1051
JOURNAL OF INSTRUCTIONAL PSYCHOLOGY. Text in English. 1974. q. USD 27 to individuals; USD 37 foreign to individuals; USD 33 to institutions; USD 43 foreign to institutions (effective 2000). bk.rev. back issues avail.; reprint service avail. from PQC. **Document type:** *Academic/Scholarly.*
Related titles: Microform ed.: (from PQC); Online - full text ed.: (from H. W. Wilson).
Indexed: C.I.J.E. (coverage dropped), Chic.Per.Ind., Cont.Pg.Educ., ERA, Educ.Ind. (Jun.1983-), Educ.Tech.Abstr., High.Educ.Abstr., Lang.& Lang.Behav.Abstr., Mult.Ed.Abstr., PsycInfo, Psychol.Abstr. (1974-), Ref.Zh., SOMA, SOPODA, Sociol.Abstr., Sociol.Educ.Abstr., Sp.Ed.Needs Abstr., Tech.Educ.Abstr., e-psyche.
—BLDSC (5007.513000), ingenta.
Published by: Project Innovation, Inc., PO Box 8826, Spring Hill Sta, Mobile, AL 36608. TEL 334-343-1878. Ed. George E Uhlig. Circ: 400 (paid).

370.15 USA ISSN 1060-6041
LB1025.3
JOURNAL OF INVITATIONAL THEORY AND PRACTICE. Text in English. 1992. s-a. USD 35 (effective 2000). bk.rev. back issues avail. *Refereed.* **Document type:** *Trade.* **Description:** Invitational theory and practice in schools and other organizations. Theory founded on self-concept and perceptual psychology.
Indexed: C.I.J.E., e-psyche.
—BLDSC (5008.055000).
Published by: International Alliance for Invitational Education, School of Education, University of North Carolina at Greensboro, Box 26171, Greensboro, NC 27402-6171. TEL 336-334-3431, FAX 336-334-3433, http://www.uncg.edu/ced/iaie01.htm. Ed., R&P Phil Riner. Circ: 3,000.

JOURNAL OF MOTOR BEHAVIOR. see *PSYCHOLOGY*

JOURNAL OF NUTRITION EDUCATION. see *NUTRITION AND DIETETICS*

370.15 155.4 530.8 USA ISSN 1090-655X
R853.O87
JOURNAL OF OUTCOME MEASUREMENT; dedicated to health, education, and social science. (JOM) Text in English. 1997. q., latest vol.5, ends 2002. USD 35 domestic to individuals; USD 59 foreign to individuals; USD 100 domestic to institutions; USD 124 foreign to institutions ((No. 2001). adv. bk.rev. abstr, charts. 1 cols./p. back issues avail. *Refereed.* **Document type:** *Journal, Academic/Scholarly.* **Description:** Publishes scholarly research from all disciplines relative to outcome measurement, the measurement of the results of any intervention designed to alter the physical or mental state of an individual.
Related titles: Duplicated (not offset) ed.
Indexed: C.I.J.E., Ind.Med. (1997-), e-psyche.
—BLDSC (5027.728500).
Published by: Rehabilitation Foundation, Inc., PO Box 675, Wheaton, IL 60189. TEL 630-462-4102, FAX 630-462-4547, JOMEA@rfi.org, http://www.rfi.org. Ed., R&P Dr. Richard Harvey. Adv. contacts Gail Goford, Jo Ruff TEL 630-221-1200. page USD 400, 1/2 page USD 275, 1/4 page USD 240. Circ: 200 (paid).

370.15 USA ISSN 0734-2829
LB1131 CODEN: JPSAES
JOURNAL OF PSYCHOEDUCATIONAL ASSESSMENT. Text in English. 1982. q., latest vol.19, 2001 (March, June, September, and December). USD 160 domestic; USD 174 foreign (effective 2001). adv. bk.rev. bibl, charts, illus. index. back issues avail. *Refereed.* **Document type:** *Monographic series, Academic/Scholarly.*
Related titles: Online - full text ed.: (from Institute for Scientific Information).
Indexed: ASCA, Chic.Per.Ind., Curr.Cont., Fam.Ind., IBR, Lang.& Lang.Behav.Abstr., PsycInfo, Psychol.Abstr. (1983-), Ref.Zh., SOPODA, SSCI, Sociol.Abstr., e-psyche.
—BLDSC (5043.275000), ingenta. **CCC.**

E

Published by: Psychoeducational Corporation, 505 22nd St, Knoxville, TN 37916. TEL 423-546-9651, FAX 423-546-0148, http://www.people.memphis.edu/~brackenba/home.html. Ed. Peter Chapman. R&P R Steve McCallum. Circ: 700.

JOURNAL OF SCHOOL HEALTH. see *PUBLIC HEALTH AND SAFETY*

JOURNAL OF SCHOOL NURSING. see *MEDICAL SCIENCES—Nurses And Nursing*

370.15 USA ISSN 1050-8406
L11 CODEN: JLSBE3
JOURNAL OF THE LEARNING SCIENCES; a journal of ideas and their applications. Text in English. 1991. q. USD 50 in US & Canada to individuals; USD 80 elsewhere to individuals; USD 390 in US & Canada to institutions; USD 420 elsewhere to institutions (effective 2002). adv. *Refereed.* **Document type:** *Journal, Academic/Scholarly.* **Description:** Provides a multidisciplinary forum for the presentation and discussion of research on teaching and learning.
Related titles: Online - full text ed.: ISSN 1532-7809. USD 45 to individuals; USD 351 to institutional members (effective 2002) (from CatchWord Ltd., EBSCO Publishing, O C L C Online Computer Library Center, Inc., RoweCom Information Quest, Swets Blackwell, Institute for Scientific Information).
Indexed: ASCA, C.I.J.E., Cont.Pg.Educ., Curr.Cont., ERA, Educ.Tech.Abstr., Fam.Ind., Lang.& Lang.Behav.Abstr., Mult.Ed.Abstr., PsycInfo, Psychol.Abstr. (1991-), SOMA, SOPODA, SSCI, Sociol.Abstr., Tech.Educ.Abstr., e-psyche.
—BLDSC (5010.231000), CatchWord, ingenta. **CCC.**
Published by: Lawrence Erlbaum Associates, Inc., 10 Industrial Ave, Mahwah, NJ 07430-2262. TEL 201-760-3735, 800-926-6579, FAX 201-236-0072, journals@erlbaum.com, http://www.erlbaum.com/Journals/journals/JLS/jls.htm. Ed. Janet L Kolodner. adv.: page USD 350; trim 5 x 8.

JOURNAL OF YOUTH STUDIES. see *CHILDREN AND YOUTH—About*

370.15 FIN ISSN 0075-4625
CODEN: JYSEAV
JYVASKYLA STUDIES IN EDUCATION, PSYCHOLOGY AND SOCIAL RESEARCH. Text in English, Finnish; Summaries in English. 1962. irreg. price varies. **Document type:** *Monographic series.*
Indexed: Cont.Pg.Educ., Psychol.Abstr., Russ.Acad.Sci.Bibl., e-psyche.
—BLDSC (5078.500000).
Published by: Jyvaskylan Yliopisto/University of Jyvaskyla, Publications Center, PL 35, Jyvaeskylae 40100, Finland. TEL 941-601-211, FAX 603-371, TELEX 28219JYK SF. Eds. Paula Lyytinen, Paula Maatta. Circ: 450.

KINDEROPVANG. see *CHILDREN AND YOUTH—About*

KOGNITION OG PAEDAGOGIK. see *PSYCHOLOGY*

370.15 JPN ISSN 0452-9650
KYOIKU SHINRIGAKU NENPO/ANNUAL REPORT OF EDUCATIONAL PSYCHOLOGY IN JAPAN. Text in Japanese. 1961. a. JPY 4,000 (effective 2000). adv. **Document type:** *Academic/Scholarly.*
Indexed: e-psyche.
—BLDSC (1511.030000).
Published by: Japanese Association of Educational Psychology/Nihon Kyoiku Shinri Gakkai, 5-26-5-701 Hongo, Bunkyo-ku, Tokyo 113-0033, Japan. Ed. Akio Kikuchi. Adv. contact Seijun Takano.

370.15 GBR ISSN 1041-6080
LB1051 CODEN: LIDIEI
LEARNING AND INDIVIDUAL DIFFERENCES; a multidisciplinary journal in education. Text in English. 1989. q. EUR 114 in Europe to individuals; JPY 15,100 in Japan to individuals; USD 127 elsewhere to individuals; EUR 273 in Europe to institutions; JPY 36,300 in Japan to institutions; USD 306 elsewhere to institutions (effective 2002). back issues avail. *Refereed.* **Document type:** *Academic/Scholarly.* **Description:** Devoted to publishing articles that make a substantial contribution to an understanding of individual differences within an educational context.
Related titles: Microform ed.: (from PQC); Online - full text ed.: (from ingenta, ScienceDirect, Swets Blackwell, Institute for Scientific Information).
Indexed: ASCA, AgeLine, Child Devel.Abstr., Cont.Pg.Educ., Curr.Cont., Educ.Ind. (Jul.1997-), Lang.& Lang.Behav.Abstr., PsycInfo, Psychol.Abstr. (1989-), SOPODA, SSCI, Sociol.Abstr., e-psyche.
—BLDSC (5179.325880), IDS, ingenta. **CCC.**
Published by: Elsevier Science, The Boulevard, Langford Ln, Kidlington, Oxon OX5 1GB, United Kingdom. TEL 44-1865-843000, FAX 44-1865-843010, usinfo-f@elsevier.com, http://www.elsevier.com/locate/lindif. Eds. H Lee Swanson, J B Cooney.

370.1523 GBR ISSN 0959-4752
LA620 CODEN: LEAIE9
LEARNING AND INSTRUCTION. Text in English. 1991. bi-m. EUR 440 in Europe to institutions; JPY 58,400 in Japan to institutions; USD 492 elsewhere to institutions (effective 2002). index. back issues avail. *Refereed.* **Document type:** *Academic/Scholarly.* **Description:** Presents papers and review articles on the processes of learning, development, instruction, and teaching representing a variety of theoretical perspectives, and different methodological approaches.
Related titles: Microfilm ed.: (from PQC); Online - full text ed.: (from ingenta, ScienceDirect, Swets Blackwell, Institute for Scientific Information).
Indexed: Br.Educ.Ind., C.I.J.E., Cont.Pg.Educ., Curr.Cont., Educ.Tech.Abstr., Mult.Ed.Abstr., PsycInfo, Psychol.Abstr. (1991-), Res.High.Educ.Abstr., SOMA, SSCI, Sp.Ed.Needs Abstr., Tech.Educ.Abstr., e-psyche.
—BLDSC (5179.325890), IDS, Infotrieve, ingenta. **CCC.**
Published by: (European Association for Research on Learning and Instruction), Pergamon (Subsidiary of: Elsevier Science), The Boulevard, Langford Ln, East Park, Kidlington, Oxford OXB 1GB, United Kingdom. FAX 44-1865-843010, nlinfo-f@elsevier.nl; usinfo-f@elsevier.com; forinfo-kyf04035@niftyserve.or.jp, http://www.elsevier.com/locate/learninstruc. Eds. Erik Decorte, K Littleton. **Subscr. in Australasia and the Far East to:** Elsevier Science (Singapore) Pte Ltd, No.1 Temasek Ave, 17-01 Millenia Tower, Singapore 039192, Singapore. TEL 65-434-3727, FAX 65-337-2230; **Subscr. in the Americas to:** Elsevier Science, PO Box 945, New York, NY 10159-0945. TEL 212-633-3730, FAX 212-633-3680, usinfo-f@elsevier.com; **Subscr. to:** Elsevier Science BV, PO Box 211, Amsterdam 1000 AE, Netherlands. TEL 31-20-485-3757, nlinfo-f@elsevier.nl.

150 370 USA ISSN 0023-9690
BF1 CODEN: LNMVAV
LEARNING AND MOTIVATION. Text in English. 1970. q. USD 425 in US & Canada to institutions; USD 550 elsewhere to institutions (effective 2001). adv. charts, illus. back issues avail. *Refereed.* **Document type:** *Academic/Scholarly.* **Description:** Features original experimental research studies devoted to the analysis of basic phenomena and mechanisms of learning, memory, and motivation.
Related titles: Online - full text ed.: (from EBSCO Publishing, O C L C Online Computer Library Center, Inc., RoweCom Information Quest, ingenta, Gale Group, Swets Blackwell, IDEAL Online Library, Factiva, Institute for Scientific Information).
Indexed: ASCA, Adol.Ment.Hlth.Abstr., Anim.Behav.Abstr., Aqua.Sci.& Fish.Abstr., Biol.Abstr., Biotech.& Bioeng.Abstr., Chemorec.Abstr., Commun.Abstr., Cont.Pg.Educ., Curr.Cont., IBZ, Ind.Philos., Lang.& Lang.Behav.Abstr., Mid.East: Abstr.& Ind., Neurosci.Abstr. (coverage dropped), Neurosci.Cit.Ind., P C I, PsycInfo, Psychol.Abstr. (1970-), Psycscan B.A.& T., Russ.Acad.Sci.Bibl., SOPODA, SSCI, Soc.Sci.Ind. (Aug.1982-), Sociol.Abstr., Stud.Wom.Abstr., Tech.Educ.Abstr., e-psyche.
—ADONIS, IDS, ingenta. **CCC.**
Published by: Academic Press, Inc., Journal Division (Subsidiary of: Harcourt Brace & Company), 525 B St, Ste 1900, San Diego, CA 92101-4495. TEL 619-230-1840, FAX 619-699-6800, apsubs@acad.com, http://www.academicpress.com/l&m. Ed. Steven F Maier.

MABAT SHELANU/OUR REVIEW. see *HANDICAPPED—Hearing Impaired*

MANAGEMENT KINDEROPVANG. see *CHILDREN AND YOUTH—About*

370 DEU ISSN 0173-3842
MATERIALIEN AUS DER BILDUNGSFORSCHUNG. Text in German, English; Summaries in English. 1972. irreg., latest vol.71, 2001. price varies. **Document type:** *Monographic series, Academic/Scholarly.* **Description:** Monographic series of reports on works-in-progress at the institute.
Published by: Max-Planck-Institut fuer Bildungsforschung, Lentzeallee 94, Berlin 14195, Germany. TEL 49-30-82406-0.

▼ **MATHEMATICAL THINKING AND LEARNING**; an international journal. see *MATHEMATICS*

MATHEMATICS EDUCATION LIBRARY. see *LIBRARY AND INFORMATION SCIENCES*

371.4 USA ISSN 0748-1756
LB1027.5
MEASUREMENT AND EVALUATION IN COUNSELING AND DEVELOPMENT. Text in English. 1968. q. USD 55 (effective 2001). adv. bk.rev. abstr, charts, stat, bibl. index. 64 p./no. back issues avail.; reprint service avail. from PQC. *Refereed.* **Document type:** *Journal, Academic/Scholarly.* **Description:** Focuses on the latest research and applications for counselors, administrators, educators, researchers and students.
Formerly (until 1984): Measurement and Evaluation in Guidance (0025-6307)
Related titles: Microform ed.: (from PQC); Online - full text ed.: (from ProQuest Information & Learning, Institute for Scientific Information, H. W. Wilson).
Indexed: ASCA, AgeLine, C.I.J.E., Curr.Cont., Educ.Ind. (Apr.1983-Apr.1984), Fam.Ind., High.Educ.Abstr., IMFL, PsycInfo, Psychol.Abstr. (1968-), SSCI, Soc.Work Res.& Abstr., Sp.Ed.Needs Abstr., e-psyche.
—BLDSC (5413.560800), IDS, ingenta. **CCC.**
Published by: (Association for Measurement and Evaluation in Counseling and Development), American Counseling Association, 5999 Stevenson Ave, Alexandria, VA 22304-3300. TEL 703-823-9800, FAX 703-823-0252, http://www.counseling.org. Ed. Patricia B Elmore. R&P Cynthia Peay TEL 703-823-9800 x 249. Adv. contact Kathy Maguire TEL 703-823-9800 ext 207. Circ: 2,000.

MEDICAL EDUCATION ONLINE. see *MEDICAL SCIENCES*

MEDICAL TEACHER. see *MEDICAL SCIENCES*

▼ **MEDUCATOR.** see *MEDICAL SCIENCES*

MEGAMOT; behavioural sciences journal. see *SOCIOLOGY*

MERRILL - PALMER QUARTERLY. see *PSYCHOLOGY*

MIMESIS (BAURU); revista da area de ciencias humanas. see *SOCIAL SCIENCES: COMPREHENSIVE WORKS*

370.1 USA ISSN 0027-6987
N R T A BULLETIN. Text in English. 1970 (vol.11). m. membership. adv. illus. **Document type:** *Trade.* **Description:** Focuses on subjects of interest to retired teachers, such as educational trends, pension plans, developments from Congress and state legislatures.
Indexed: AgeLine.
Published by: (National Retired Teachers Association), A A R P, Research, 601 E St, N W, Washington, DC 20049. TEL 202-434-2277, FAX 202-434-6408, http://www.aarp.org. Ed. Elliot Carlson. adv.: B&W page USD 299,180, color page USD 331,500. Circ: 28,000,000.

372.86 USA
NEBRASKA JOURNAL. Text in English. s-a. USD 10. adv. back issues avail.
Indexed: Phys.Ed.Ind.
Published by: Nebraska Association for Health, Physical Education, Recreation & Dance, Dept of Health, Kinesiology and Leisure Studies, Lambert Gym, Purdue University, West Lafayette, IN 47907-1362. TEL 402-554-2670. Ed. Tom Sharpe. Circ: 350.

371.912 DEU
DIE NEUE SONDERSCHULE. Text in German. 1956. bi-m. EUR 39; EUR 25.50 to students; EUR 7 newsstand/cover (effective 2002). adv. bk.rev. abstr, charts, illus. index. reprint service avail. from SCH,PSC. **Document type:** *Journal, Academic/Scholarly.*
Formerly: Sonderschule (0323-4592)
Indexed: IBR, IBZ, Lang.& Lang.Behav.Abstr.
Published by: Hermann Luchterhand Verlag GmbH, Heddesdorfer Str 31, Neuwied 56564, Germany. TEL 49-2631-801-0, FAX 49-2631-801204, info@luchterhand.de, http://www.luchterhand.de. Ed. Hannelore Ruppe. Adv. contact Gabriele Pannwitz. Circ: 9,500.

NEW YORK STATE ASSOCIATION OF SCHOOL NURSES COMMUNICATOR. see *MEDICAL SCIENCES—Nurses And Nursing*

▼ **NORTH AMERICAN JOURNAL OF PSYCHOLOGY.** see *PSYCHOLOGY*

▼ **NURSE EDUCATION IN PRACTICE.** see *MEDICAL SCIENCES—Nurses And Nursing*

▼ **NURSING AND HEALTH SCIENCE EDUCATION.** see *MEDICAL SCIENCES—Nurses And Nursing*

370.1523 USA ISSN 1092-5619
PALO ALTO REVIEW; journal of ideas. Text in English. 1992. s-a. USD 10; USD 5 newsstand/cover (effective 1999). bk.rev., film rev., software rev., tel.rev., video rev. illus. back issues avail. *Refereed.* **Document type:** *Academic/Scholarly.* **Description:** Contains articles, poems, and stories about people, places, and events dealing with living and learning.
Indexed: e-psyche.
Published by: Palo Alto College, 1400 W Villaret Blvd, San Antonio, TX 78224-2499. TEL 210-921-5017, FAX 210-921-5008. Eds. Bob Richmond, Ellen Shull. Circ: 600.

370.15 IND ISSN 0971-1562
PERSPECTIVES IN PSYCHOLOGICAL RESEARCHES. Text in English, Hindi. 1978. s-a. free per issue. adv. bk.rev. stat. **Document type:** *Academic/Scholarly.*
Indexed: Indian Psychol.Abstr., e-psyche.
—BLDSC (6428.161200).
Address: 53 Dalsingar, Azamgarh 276 001, India. TEL 91-546-222006. Ed. Dr. Ramji Srivastava. Circ: 1,000.

370.15 DEU ISSN 0934-5256
PRAXIS SPIEL UND GRUPPE. Text in German. q. DEM 47; DEM 42.80 to students (effective 2001). adv. back issues avail. **Document type:** *Magazine, Academic/Scholarly.*
Formerly (until 1988): Schwalbacher Blaetter
Indexed: e-psyche.
Published by: Matthias Gruenewald Verlag GmbH, Max-Hufschmidt-Str 4A, Mainz 55130, Germany. TEL 49-6131-9286-0, FAX 49-6131-928626, mail@gruenewaldverlag.de, http://www.engagementbuch.de. Ed. Hiltraud Laubach. Adv. contact Antje Weber TEL 49-6131-928613. B&W page DEM 1,050; trim 135 x 200. Circ: 1,200.

371.4 USA ISSN 1096-2409
LB1027.5
PROFESSIONAL SCHOOL COUNSELING. Text in English. 1997. 5/yr. USD 75 domestic to institutions; USD 100 foreign to institutions (effective 2000). adv. bk.rev. illus. Index. reprint service avail. from PQC,PSC,SCH. *Refereed.* **Document type:** *Academic/Scholarly, Trade.* **Description:** Keeps the reader up-to-date with ideas and techniques on how to deal with current issues in elementary, middle, and secondary school counseling.
Formed by the merger of (1965-1997): Elementary School Guidance and Counseling (0013-5976); (1954-1997): School Counselor (0036-6536); Which superseded (1953-1954): Elementary Counselor (0013-5941)
Related titles: Microform ed.: 1997 (from PQC); Online - full text ed.: (from Northern Light Technology, Inc., H. W. Wilson, ProQuest Information & Learning).
Indexed: AgeLine, C.I.J.E., Chic.Per.Ind., Cont.Pg.Educ., ERA, Educ.Ind. (May 1983-Aug.1997), Fam.Ind., Mult.Ed.Abstr., PsycInfo, Psychol.Abstr. (1968-), Sage Fam.Stud.Abstr., Soc.Work Res.& Abstr., Sociol.Educ.Abstr., Sp.Ed.Needs Abstr., Tech.Educ.Abstr., e-psyche.
—BLDSC (6864.220100), ingenta. **CCC.**
Published by: (American School Counselor Association), American Counseling Association, c/o Randall Parker, Special Education D5300, The University of Texas, Austin, TX 78712. asca@erols.com, http://www.schoolcounselor.org/profjourn.html. Ed. Stanley Baker. **Subscr. to:** 750 First St N E, Washington, DC 20002.

370.15 ITA ISSN 0392-680X
PSICOLOGIA E SCUOLA; giornale italiano di psicologia dell'educazione e pedagogia sperimentale. Text in Italian. 1980. 5/yr. ITL 44,000 domestic; ITL 57,000 foreign (effective 2001). charts, illus, stat. back issues avail. **Description:** Covers a variety of topics in educational psychology: research and theory in the field, implications of psychology for education, teacher training, and practical tools for teachers.
Indexed: Ind.Philos., e-psyche.
Published by: Giunti Gruppo Editoriale S.p.A., Via Bolognese, 165, Florence, FI 50139, Italy. TEL 39-55-5062236, FAX 39-55-5062397, periodici@giunti.it, http://www.giunti.it. Ed. Massimo Casini.

370.15 USA ISSN 1091-4781
PSYCH DISCOURSE. Text in English. 1970. m. USD 95 to individuals; USD 110 to institutions (effective 2000); free to members of ABPsi. adv. back issues avail. **Document type:** *Newsletter, Trade.* **Description:** Covers news of member and chapter activities. Includes original articles, letters and essays.
Formerly: Association of Black Psychologists Newsletter
Indexed: e-psyche.
Published by: Association of Black Psychologists, PO Box 55999, Washington, DC 20040-5999. TEL 202-722-0808, 202-722-0808. Ed., R&P Dr. Halford H Fairchild. Adv. contact Rosa Wright. page USD 650; trim 9 x 7. Circ: 1,500.

PSYCHOLOGIA A PATOPSYCHOLOGIA DIETATA. see *PSYCHOLOGY*

370.15 FRA ISSN 1148-9502
PSYCHOLOGIE & EDUCATION. Text in French. 1962. q. FRF 350 (effective 2000). bk.rev. back issues avail. **Document type:** *Academic/Scholarly.*
Former titles (until 1990): Psychologie Scolaire (0291-8382); (until 1969): Association Francaise des Psychologues Scolaires. Bulletin (0999-2243)
Indexed: e-psyche.
Published by: Association Francaise des Psychologues Scolaires, c/o Alain Brabant, 3 rue des 4 Assiettes, Smarves 86240, France. TEL 33-5-49559927, FAX 33-5-49559927, afps@infonie.fr, http://webhome.infonie.fr/afps/. Ed. Michel Monville. R&P Alma Braban. Circ: 2,000.

PSYCHOLOGY & EDUCATION; an interdisciplinary journal. see *PSYCHOLOGY*

PSYCHOLOGY IN THE SCHOOLS. see *PSYCHOLOGY*

370.15 GBR ISSN 1463-9807
THE PSYCHOLOGY OF EDUCATION REVIEW. Text in English. 1979. s-a. GBP 8 to non-members (effective 2000). bk.rev. reprint service avail. from ISI. *Refereed.* **Description:** Publishes material in educational psychology likely to be of general interest to members. Includes the "open dialogue" section in which there is a simultaneous exchange of views on an issue of substantial interest. This consists of an initial paper, peer review, and an author's reply.
Formerly (until 1998): British Psychological Society. Education Section. Review (0262-4087)
Indexed: Br.Educ.Ind., Cont.Pg.Educ., SOMA, e-psyche.
—BLDSC (6946.535584).
Published by: The British Psychological Society, St Andrews House, 48 Princess Rd E, Leicester LE1 7DR, United Kingdom. TEL 44-116-254-9568, FAX 44-116-247-0787, mail@bps.org.uk. Eds. Pam Maras, Susan Hallam. R&P, Adv. contact Z Terry TEL 44-116-252-9562. Circ: 850.

PSYKOLOGISK PAEDAGOGISK RAADGIVNING/ JOURNAL OF SCHOOL PSYCHOLOGY; tidsskrift for paedagogisk psykologi og raadgivning. see *PSYCHOLOGY*

370.15 ITA
QUALE SCUOLA?; periodico di educazione per una scuola diversa. Text in Italian. 1982. q. ITL 30,000; ITL 60,000 foreign (effective 1995). **Description:** Covers primary and elementary education and the psychological development of children.
Indexed: e-psyche.
Address: Traversa T. de Amicis 41 2-A, Naples, NA 80145, Italy. TEL 39-81-5466406. Ed. Salvatore Alosco.

READING AND WRITING; an interdisciplinary journal. see *LINGUISTICS*

370.15 USA ISSN 0270-2711
BF456.R2 CODEN: RRPSDW
READING PSYCHOLOGY; an international quarterly. Text in English. 1979. q. GBP 76, USD 123 to individuals; GBP 153, USD 253 to institutions (effective 2002). adv. bk.rev. bibl, charts, stat. index. back issues avail.; reprint service avail. from PSC,SCH,PQC. *Refereed.* **Document type:** *Academic/Scholarly.* **Description:** Publishes original manuscripts in the field of literacy, reading, and related psychology disciplines.
Related titles: Online - full text ed.: ISSN 1521-0685 (from CatchWord Ltd., EBSCO Publishing, O C L C Online Computer Library Center, Inc., RoweCom Information Quest, Swets Blackwell).
Indexed: AgeLine, C.I.J.E., Child Devel.Abstr., Cont.Pg.Educ., ERA, Educ.Tech.Abstr., Lang.& Lang.Behav.Abstr., M.L.A., MLA Intl.Bibl., Mult.Ed.Abstr., PsycInfo, Psychol.Abstr. (1979-), SOPODA, Sociol.Abstr., Sp.Ed.Needs Abstr., Stud.Wom.Abstr., Tech.Educ.Abstr., e-psyche.
—BLDSC (7301.260000), CatchWord, ingenta. **CCC.**
Published by: (University of North Texas, College of Education, Pupil Appraisal Center), Taylor & Francis Ltd. (Subsidiary of: Taylor & Francis Group), 325 Chestnut St, Suite 800, Philadelphia, PA 19016. TEL 215-625-8900, FAX 215-625-2940, info@taylorandfrancis.com, http://www.taylorandfrancis.com/. Ed. William H Rupley. Circ: 275. **Subscr. addr. in Europe:** Taylor & Francis Group, Journals Customer Service, Rankine Rd, Basingstoke, Hants RG24 8PR, United Kingdom. TEL 44-1256-813000, FAX 44-1256-479438, enquiry@tanf.co.uk, http://www.tandf.co.uk/journals.

371 USA ISSN 1046-3364
RESEARCH AND TEACHING IN DEVELOPMENTAL EDUCATION. Short title: R T D E. Text in English. 1984. s-a. USD 35 to members; USD 30 to institutions. adv. bk.rev. *Refereed.* **Document type:** *Academic/Scholarly.* **Description:** Interdisciplinary journal which focuses on theoretically based articles on pedagogy, evaluation, program design and delivery in the areas of mathematics, writing and reading.
Indexed: C.I.J.E., Cont.Pg.Educ., ERA, Educ.Tech.Abstr., Sp.Ed.Needs Abstr., Tech.Educ.Abstr.
—BLDSC (7716.075000), ingenta.
Published by: New York College Learning Skills Association, Finger Lakes Community College, 4355 Lake Shore Dr, Canandaigua, NY 14424. TEL 716-394-3500, FAX 716-394-5005. Ed., R&P, Adv. contact Patricia A Malinowski. Circ: 800.

REVIEW (WASHINGTON); rehabilitation and education for blindness and visual impairment. see *HANDICAPPED—Visually Impaired*

370.15 ARG
REVISTA ARGENTINA DE PSICOPEDAGOGIA. Text in Portuguese, Spanish; Abstracts in English. 1981. q. USD 30 (effective 2000). adv. bk.rev. abstr, bibl. **Document type:** *Academic/Scholarly.*
Supersedes (1975-1981): Revista de Psicopedagogia
Published by: Fundacion Suzuki, Charlone, 1689, San Miguel, Buenos Aires 1663, Argentina. TEL 54-11-664-0771, FAX 54-11-667-1476. Ed. Elizabeth J Calvo de Suzuki. Circ: 500.

REVISTA DE PSICOLOGIA EDUCATIVA; revista de los psicologos de la educacion. see *PSYCHOLOGY*

370.15 CAN ISSN 0080-2492
REVUE CANADIENNE DE PSYCHO-EDUCATION. Text in French; Summaries in English, French. 1964. biennial. CND 25 to individuals; CND 35 to institutions. bk.rev. bibl.
Indexed: PsycInfo, Psychol.Abstr. (1982-), Pt.de Rep., e-psyche.
—BLDSC (7896.219000). **CCC.**
Published by: Universite de Montreal, Ecole de Psycho-Education, Succ Centre Ville, C P 6128, Montreal, PQ H3C 3J7, Canada. FAX 514-343-6951, rcpe@videotrom.ca. Ed. Serge Larivee. Circ: 600.

370.15 COD
REVUE ZAIROISE DE PSYCHOLOGIE ET DE PEDAGOGIE. Text in French; Abstracts occasionally in English. 1972. 2/yr. USD 8 per issue.
Indexed: e-psyche.
Published by: Universite de Kisangani, Faculte de Psychologie et des Sciences de l'Education, BP 1386, Kisangani, Congo, Dem. Republic. Ed. Bamwisho Mihia.

ROLLSTUHLSPORT. see *SPORTS AND GAMES*

S R C D NEWSLETTER. see *CHILDREN AND YOUTH—About*

SCHOOL NURSE NEWS; current issues affecting school nurses. see *MEDICAL SCIENCES—Nurses And Nursing*

SCHOOL PSYCHOLOGY QUARTERLY. see *PSYCHOLOGY*

370.15 USA
THE SERIES ON SOCIAL EMOTIONAL LEARNING. Text and summaries in English. irreg. price varies. illus. **Document type:** *Monographic series, Academic/Scholarly.* **Description:** Examines the psychological aspects of issues in teaching and learning.

E

Published by: Teachers College Press, Teachers College, Columbia University, 525 W 120th St, Box 303, New York, NY 10027-6694. http://tc-press.tc.columbia.edu. **Dist. by:** Eurospan University Press Group, Order Dept, 3 Henrietta St, London WC2E 8LU, United Kingdom. TEL 44-20-7240-0856, FAX 44-20-7379-0609, http://www.eurospan.co.uk; Pademelon Press, Pty Ltd, 7-10 Anella Ave, PO Box 229, Castle Hill, NSW 2154, Australia. TEL 61-2-9634-2558, FAX 61-2-9680-4634; Transdex International, Pte Ltd, Block 1, Farrer Rd 307-05, Singapore 268817, Singapore. TEL 65-468-6242, FAX 65-462-5457.

613.9071 GBR ISSN 1468-1811
▼ **SEX EDUCATION.** Text in English. 2001. 3/yr. GBP 35, USD 57 to individuals; GBP 105, USD 172 to institutions (effective 2002). **Document type:** *Academic/Scholarly.* **Description:** Covers the research into sex education in educational institutions, families, media influence, peer influence and other areas.
Related titles: Online - full text ed.: (from CatchWord Ltd., RoweCom Information Quest).
Indexed: Br.Educ.Ind.
Published by: Carfax Publishing Limited (Subsidiary of: Taylor & Francis Group), PO Box 25, Abingdon, Oxon OX14 3UE, United Kingdom. FAX 44-1325-401550, http://www.tandf.co.uk/journals/frameloader.html?http://www.tandf.co.uk/journals/carfax/14681811.html, http://www.carfax.co.uk. Ed. Michael Reiss.

370 610 RUS
SHKOLA ZDOROV'YA. Text in Russian. q. USD 85 in United States.
Indexed: Ref.Zh.
Published by: Izdatel'stvo Dyagnostika Adaptatsiya Razvitie, Ul Arkhitektora Vlasova 19, Moscow 117335, Russian Federation. TEL 7-095-1283987, FAX 7-095-1284865. Ed. V N Kasatkin. **US dist. addr.:** East View Publications, 3020 Harbor Ln N, Minneapolis, MN 55447. TEL 612-550-0961.

370.15 IND
SIKSHA. Text in Bengali. m.
Indexed: e-psyche.
Published by: Aijtkumar Basu, 1 A College Rd., Kolkata, West Bengal 700 009, India.

370.15 NLD ISSN 1381-2890
LC189.8 CODEN: SPEDFX
SOCIAL PSYCHOLOGY OF EDUCATION; an international journal. Text in English. 1996. q. EUR 346 to institutions for print or online ed.; EUR 415.20 to institutions print & online eds.combined (effective 2002). *Refereed.* **Document type:** *Academic/Scholarly.* **Description:** Fills the gap between the disciplines of psychology and sociology, covering a wide variety of content concerns, theoretical interests and research methods.
Related titles: Online - full text ed.: (from EBSCO Publishing, O C L C Online Computer Library Center, Inc., RoweCom Information Quest, Swets Blackwell, Kluwer Online).
Indexed: Aus.Educ.Ind., Cont.Pg.Educ., PsycInfo, Soc.Serv.Abstr., Sociol.Abstr., e-psyche.
—BLDSC (8318.146100). **CCC.**
Published by: Kluwer Academic Publishers Group (Subsidiary of: Wolters Kluwer N.V.), Spuiboulevard 50, PO Box 17, Dordrecht 3300 AA, Netherlands. FAX 31-78-639-2254, services@wkap.nl, http://www.wkap.nl. Ed. Bruce J Biddle. **Dist. by:** Journals Department, PO Box 322, Dordrecht 3300 AH, Netherlands. TEL 781-871-6600, FAX 31-78-654-6474.

SOCIETY FOR RESEARCH IN CHILD DEVELOPMENT. MONOGRAPHS. see *CHILDREN AND YOUTH—About*

370.15 ITA ISSN 0393-6163
STUDI DI PSICOLOGIA DELL'EDUCAZIONE. Text in Italian. 1982. q. ITL 55,000 domestic; ITL 80,000 foreign (effective 2000). bibl, charts, illus, stat. **Document type:** *Academic/Scholarly.*
Indexed: Ind.Philos., Psychol.Abstr., e-psyche.
Published by: (Pontificia Universita della Santa Croce), Casa Editrice Armando s.r.l., Viale Trastevere, 236, Rome, RM 00153, Italy. TEL 39-6-5817245, FAX 39-6-5818564, armando@palomar.it, http://www.armando.it. Ed. Roberto Truzoli.

370.15 SWE ISSN 0346-5926
STUDIA PSYCHOLOGICA ET PAEDAGOGICA; series altera. Text in English, Swedish; Summaries in English. 1947. irreg. price varies. back issues avail. **Document type:** *Journal, Academic/Scholarly.*
Indexed: e-psyche.
Published by: Malmoe University, Department of Education, Fack 23501, Malmo 20045, Sweden. FAX 46-40-325-210. **Co-sponsor:** Malmoe Institute of Education.

370.15 ROM ISSN 1221-8111
STUDIA UNIVERSITATIS "BABES-BOLYAI". PSYCHOLOGIA - PAEDAGOGIA. Text in English, Romanian; Summaries in English, French, German. 1990. s-a. per issue exchange basis. **Document type:** *Academic/Scholarly.*
Indexed: Russ.Acad.Sci.Bibl., e-psyche.
Published by: Universitatea "Babes-Bolyai", Biblioteca Centrala Universitara, Str. Gh. Bilascu 24, Cluj-Napoca 3400, Romania. TEL 40-64-194315, FAX 40-64-191906, puc@hera.ubbcluj.ro. Ed. A Marga.

370 DEU ISSN 0076-5627
STUDIEN UND BERICHTE. Text mainly in German; Summaries in English. 1965. irreg., latest vol.68, 2000. price varies. **Document type:** *Monographic series, Academic/Scholarly.*
Published by: Max-Planck-Institut fuer Bildungsforschung, Lentzeallee 94, Berlin 14195, Germany. TEL 49-30-82406-0.

370.15 SWE ISSN 0348-291X
STUDIES IN EDUCATION AND PSYCHOLOGY. Text in English. 1977. irreg. price varies. **Document type:** *Academic/Scholarly.*
Indexed: e-psyche.
Published by: (Stockholm University, Institute of Education), H L S Foerlag, Fack 34103, Stockholm 10026, Sweden.

THE SURVEY KIT. see *MEDICAL SCIENCES*

370.15 HRV ISSN 0353-4448
SVEUCILISTE U ZAGREBU. FILOZOFSKI FAKULTET. INSTITUT ZA PEDAGOGIJSKA ISTRAZIVANJA. ZBORNIK RADOVA∗. Text in Croatian; Summaries in English, Russian. 1981. a. USD 5.
Formerly: Odgoj i Samoupravljanje (0351-4889)
Indexed: Ref.Zh., e-psyche.
Published by: Sveuciliste u Zagrebu, Filozofski Fakultet, Institut za Pedagogijska Istrazivanja, Savska 77, Zagreb 10000, Croatia. Circ: 1,000.

370.15 AUT
TIROLER SCHULE. Text in German. 1890. q. ATS 100; USD 10 foreign. bk.rev., tel.rev., video rev. bibl, illus, abstr. back issues avail. *Refereed.* **Document type:** *Monographic series, Newsletter, Newspaper, Academic/Scholarly, Bibliography.*
Indexed: e-psyche.
Published by: Katholischer Tiroler Lehrerverein, Riedgasse 9, Innsbruck, T 6020, Austria. TEL 43-512-2230521. Pub. Paul Larpl. Circ: 3,000. **Subscr. to:** Paul Lampl, Aflingerstrasse 7a-4, Voels, T 6176, Austria. TEL 43-512-302427.

TODAY'S SCHOOL PSYCHOLOGIST. see *PSYCHOLOGY*

▼ **UNDERSTANDING STATISTICS**; statistical issues in psychology, education, and the social sciences. see *STATISTICS*

370.15 POL ISSN 0083-4254
UNIWERSYTET IM. ADAMA MICKIEWICZA. PSYCHOLOGIA-PEDAGOGIKA. Text in Polish. 1961. irreg., latest vol.110, 1996. price varies. bk.rev. **Document type:** *Monographic series, Academic/Scholarly.* **Description:** Contains current research results of one author in the field of psychology, including monographs and Ph.D. works.
Formerly: Uniwersytet im. Adama Mickiewicza w Poznaniu. Wydzial Historyczny. Prace. Seria Psychologia-Pedagogika (0860-1380)
Indexed: Psychol.Abstr., e-psyche.
Published by: Adam Mickiewicz University Press, Nowowiejskiego 55, Poznan 61734, Poland. TEL 48-61-527380, FAX 48-61-527701. Pub. Maria Jankowska. R&P Malgorzata Bis.

370 ITA ISSN 0042-7241
VITA DELL'INFANZIA. Text in Italian. 1952. m. ITL 50,000 domestic; ITL 70,000 foreign (effective 2000). adv. bk.rev. bibl, illus. index, cum.index.
Indexed: Ind.Philos., e-psyche.
Published by: Opera Nazionale Montessori, Via Di San Gallicano, 7, Rome, RM 00153, Italy. TEL 39-6-5883320, info@montessori.it, http://www.montessori.it. Ed. Elena Dompe. adv.: B&W page ITL 180,000. Circ: 8,000.

370.15 SVK ISSN 0139-6919
VYCHOVAVATEL. Text in Slovak. 1955. 10/yr.
Indexed: Russ.Acad.Sci.Bibl., e-psyche.
Published by: (Slovakia. Ministry of Education of the Slovak Socialist Republic), Vydavatel'stvo Edocatio, Sasinkova 5, Bratislava 81560, Slovakia. TEL 21-42-49. Ed. Jan Farkas. Circ: 12,500. **Subscr. to:** Slovart, Gottwaldovo nam 48, Bratislava 805 32, Czechoslovakia.

WASHINGTON COUNSELETTER. see *OCCUPATIONS AND CAREERS*

370.15 IND
WEST BENGAL. BUREAU OF EDUCATIONAL AND PSYCHOLOGICAL RESEARCH. Text in English. 1971. s-a. free per issue.
Indexed: e-psyche.
Published by: Bureau of Educational and Psychological Research, 25-3 Ballygunge Circular Rd., Kolkata, Maharashtra 700 019, India. Ed. Maya Mukherjee.

YISHI JINXIU ZAZHI/JOURNAL OF POSTGRADUATES OF MEDICINE. see *MEDICAL SCIENCES*

ZEITSCHRIFT FUER ENTWICKLUNGSPSYCHOLOGIE UND PAEDAGOGISCHE PSYCHOLOGIE. see *PSYCHOLOGY*

ZHONGYI JIAOYU/EDUCATION OF TRADITIONAL CHINESE MEDICINE. see *ALTERNATIVE MEDICINE*

EDUCATION—Abstracting, Bibliographies, Statistics

016.3719 GBR
BRITISH INSTITUTE OF LEARNING DISABILITIES. CURRENT AWARENESS SERVICE. Variant title: C A S. Text in English. 1979. m. GBP 44 to individuals; GBP 55 to institutions (effective 2001). adv. back issues avail. **Document type:** *Bibliography.* **Description:** Bibliography of current books, articles, educational events, and audiovisual materials covering all aspects of learning disabilities.
Formerly: British Institute of Mental Handicap. Current Awareness Service (0143-0289)
Published by: British Institute of Learning Disabilities, Wolverhampton Rd, Kidderminster, Worcs DY10 3PP, United Kingdom. TEL 44-1562-850251, FAX 44-1562-851970, bild@bild.demon.co.uk. Ed. Linda Averill. Circ: 1,000.

016.3719 USA ISSN 0160-4309
Z5814.C52
EXCEPTIONAL CHILD EDUCATION RESOURCES. Text in English. 1969. q. USD 89 to non-members; USD 69 to members; USD 26 newsstand/cover (effective 2001). adv. illus. reprints avail. **Document type:** *Abstract/Index.* **Description:** Computerized database containing more than 85,000 abstracts in the field of special education. Every citation gives author, title, source, publication date, availability date, subject terms, and a descriptive summary of the document or journal article.
Formerly (until May 1977): Exceptional Child Education Abstracts (0014-4010)
Related titles: CD-ROM ed.: (from SilverPlatter Information, Inc.).
Published by: Council for Exceptional Children, 1110 N. Glebe Rd., Arlington, VA 22201-5704. TEL 703-620-3660, http://www.cec.sped.org/. Ed. Kathleen McLane. R&P Melinda MacDonald. Adv. contact Victor Erickson. Circ: 1,000 (paid).

016.370117 GBR ISSN 0260-9770
LC1099
MULTICULTURAL EDUCATION ABSTRACTS. Text in English. 1982. q. GBP 161, USD 292 to individuals; GBP 410, USD 720 to institutions (effective 2002). adv. bk.rev. cum.index. back issues avail. **Document type:** *Abstract/Index.*
Related titles: Microfiche ed.; Online - full content ed.: ISSN 1467-5854 (from Northern Light Technology, Inc., ProQuest Information & Learning).
—**CCC.**
Published by: Carfax Publishing Limited (Subsidiary of: Taylor & Francis Group), PO Box 25, Abingdon, Oxon OX14 3UE, United Kingdom. TEL 44-1235-401000, FAX 44-1235-401550, enquiries@carfax.co.uk, enquiry@tandf.co.uk, http://www.carfax.co.uk. Ed. Derek Cherrington.

E

016.6137 USA ISSN 0191-9202
GV201
PHYSICAL EDUCATION INDEX. Text in English. 1978. q. USD 240 (effective 2002). index. back issues avail.; reprints avail. **Document type:** *Abstract/Index.* **Description:** Subject index to health, physical education, recreation, dance, sports, and sports medicine literature in over 180 journals.
Published by: Cambridge Scientific Abstracts, 7200 Wisconsin Ave., Suite 601, Bethesda, MD 20814. TEL 301-961-6798, FAX 301-961-6799, journals@csa.com, http://www.csa.com/journals.

016.3719 GBR ISSN 0954-0822
SPECIAL EDUCATIONAL NEEDS ABSTRACTS. Text in English. 1989. q. GBP 153, USD 271 to individuals; GBP 442, USD 730 to institutions (effective 2002). adv. bk.rev. **Document type:** *Abstract/Index.*
Related titles: Microfiche ed.; Online - full content ed.: ISSN 1467-5889 (from Northern Light Technology, Inc., ProQuest Information & Learning).
—CCC.
Published by: Carfax Publishing Limited (Subsidiary of: Taylor & Francis Group), PO Box 25, Abingdon, Oxon OX14 3UE, United Kingdom. TEL 44-1235-401000, FAX 44-1235-401550, enquiries@carfax.co.uk, enquiry@tandf.co.uk, http://www.carfax.co.uk. Ed. Derek Cherrington.

016.6137 GBR ISSN 0142-1794
SPORTS DOCUMENTATION MONTHLY BULLETIN. Text in English, Multiple languages; Summaries in English. 1971. m. GBP 58 in United Kingdom to individuals; GBP 79 in United Kingdom to institutions; GBP 79 elsewhere (effective 2002). index, cum.index. back issues avail. **Document type:** *Bulletin, Abstract/Index.* **Description:** Lists recent periodical articles and conference papers on the scientific and medical aspects of sport, physical education, and recreation, with indexes of authors and subject matter.
Formerly (until 1974): Sports Information Monthly Bulletin
Indexed: Ergon.Abstr.
—BLDSC (8419.834000).
Published by: Centre for Sports Science and History, Main Library, University of Birmingham, Edgbaston, Birmingham B15 2TT, United Kingdom. TEL 44-121-414-5843, FAX 44-121-471-4691, CENSSAH@bham.ac.uk. Circ: 330.

EDUCATION—Adult Education

APPROVED PROVIDERS OF CONTINUING PHARMACEUTICAL EDUCATION. see *PHARMACY AND PHARMACOLOGY*

C M E; South Africa's continuing medical education journal. (Continuing Medical Education) see *MEDICAL SCIENCES*

CANADIAN JOURNAL OF CONTINUING MEDICAL EDUCATION. see *MEDICAL SCIENCES*

374.8 USA ISSN 0736-1920
HF5381.A1
CAREER PLANNING AND ADULT DEVELOPMENT JOURNAL. Text in English. 1982. q. USD 59 to membership includes Career Planning and Adult Development Network (effective 2001). adv. bk.rev., film rev. illus. back issues avail.; reprints avail. *Refereed.* **Description:** Articles on group and individual career counseling techniques, assessment, and job search skills for career counselors.
Indexed: C.I.J.E., Tr.& Dev.Alert.
—BLDSC (3051.762000), ingenta.
Published by: Career Planning and Adult Development Network, 4965 Sierra Rd, San Jose, CA 95132. TEL 408-441-9100, FAX 408-441-9101, info@careertrainer.com. Ed. Steven E Beasley. Circ: 1,000.

374.8 USA ISSN 0898-1353
CAREER PLANNING AND ADULT DEVELOPMENT NETWORK NEWSLETTER; a newsletter for career counselors, educators, and human resource specialists. Text in English. 1979. bi-m. USD 49 domestic to non-members includes Career Planning & Adult Development Journal; USD 64 foreign to non-members includes Career Planning & Adult Development Journal (effective 2001). bk.rev., film rev. back issues avail. **Document type:** *Newsletter.* **Description:** Listing of workshops, conferences, films, books and counseling techniques for career counselors.
Formerly: Career Planning and Adult Development Newsletter (0898-1345)
Indexed: C.I.J.E. (coverage dropped).
Published by: Career Planning and Adult Development Network, 4965 Sierra Rd, San Jose, CA 95132. TEL 408-441-9100, FAX 408-441-9101, info@careertrainor.com, http://www.careernetwork.org/career_newsletter.html. Ed. Richard L Knowdell. Circ: 1,500 (paid and controlled).

CONTINUING MEDICAL EDUCATION DIRECTORY. see *MEDICAL SCIENCES*

374.22 USA
EDUCATION SPECIAL INTEREST SECTION QUARTERLY. Text in English. 1991. q. USD 20 (effective 1999). **Document type:** *Newsletter.*
Formerly: Education Special Interest Section Newsletter (1059-0595)
Published by: American Occupational Therapy Association, Inc., 4720 Montgomery Lane, Bethesda, MD 20814-3425. TEL 301-652-2682, FAX 301-652-7711.

EDUCATIONAL GERONTOLOGY; an international journal. see *GERONTOLOGY AND GERIATRICS*

HEALTH EDUCATION & BEHAVIOR. see *PUBLIC HEALTH AND SAFETY*

374 JPN ISSN 0912-1420
HOKEN KANRI SENTA DAYORI. Text in Japanese. 1975. 3/yr. **Document type:** *Bulletin.* **Description:** Contains news of the center.
Published by: Nara Joshi Daigaku, Hoken Kanri Senta/Nara Women's University, Health Administration Center, Kita-Uoyahigashi-Machi, Nara-shi 630-8285, Japan. Ed. Kimihiro Yamamoto. Circ: 3,000.

INTAND NEWSLETTER; the newsletter of the international network for transactional analysis, neuro-linguistic programming. see *PSYCHOLOGY*

JOURNAL OF CONTINUING EDUCATION IN THE HEALTH PROFESSIONS. see *MEDICAL SCIENCES*

NARA JOSHI DAIGAKU HOKEN KANRI SENTA NENPO/NARA WOMEN'S UNIVERSITY. HEALTH ADMINISTRATION CENTER. ARCHIVES OF HEALTH CARE. see *PUBLIC HEALTH AND SAFETY*

NETWORK NEWS (SHERMAN). see *POLITICAL SCIENCE—Civil Rights*

EDUCATION—Computer Applications

CLOSING THE GAP. see *EDUCATION—Special Education And Rehabilitation*

370.285 USA
LB1028.7
T E S S. (The Educational Software Selector) Text in English. 1984. a. USD 82.50 for base vol (1996); USD 32.50 for update. index. back issues avail. **Document type:** *Directory, Trade.* **Description:** Contains descriptions of software for all grade levels, preschool through postgraduate.
Former titles: Latest and Best of T E S S; Educational Software Selector (8755-5107)
Media: CD-ROM.
Published by: Educational Products Information Exchange (EPIE) Institute, 103 3 W Montauk Hwy, 3, Hampton, NY 11946-4006. TEL 516-728-9100, FAX 516-728-9228.

EDUCATION—Guides To Schools And Colleges

ADMISSION REQUIREMENTS OF U S AND CANADIAN DENTAL SCHOOLS. see *MEDICAL SCIENCES—Dentistry*

610.711 USA
R840
AMERICAN MEDICAL ASSOCIATION. GRADUATE MEDICAL EDUCATION DIRECTORY (YEARS). Variant title: Graduate Medical Education Directory (Years). Text in English. 1914. a. USD 70 (effective 2000). reprint service avail. from PQC. **Document type:** *Directory, Trade.*
Former titles (until 1993): American Medical Association. Directory of Graduate Medical Education Programs Accredited by the Accreditation Council for Graduate Medical Education (0892-0109); American Medical Association. Directory of Residency Training Accredited by the Accreditation Council for Graduate Medical Education (0164-1670); American Medical Association. Directory of Residency Training Programs (0097-899X); American Medical Association. Directory of Accredited Residencies; American Medical Association. Directory of Approved Residencies; (until 1975): American Medical Association. Directory of Approved Internships and Residencies (0419-2141)
Related titles: CD-ROM ed.
—BLDSC (4206.836800), GNLM, Infotrieve. **CCC.**
Published by: American Medical Association, 515 N State St, P O Box 10946, Chicago, IL 60610-0946. TEL 312-464-5000, 800-262-8335, FAX 312-464-5600.

DIRECTORY OF HIGHER EDUCATION NURSING COURSES. see *MEDICAL SCIENCES—Nurses And Nursing*

DIRECTORY OF OSTEOPATHIC POSTDOCTORAL EDUCATION. see *MEDICAL SCIENCES—Chiropractic, Homeopathy, Osteopathy*

GRADUATE STUDY IN PSYCHOLOGY. see *PSYCHOLOGY*

HEALTH PROFESSIONS CAREER AND EDUCATION DIRECTORY. see *MEDICAL SCIENCES*

INSIDER'S GUIDE TO GRADUATE PROGRAMS IN CLINICAL AND COUNSELING PSYCHOLOGY (YEARS). see *PSYCHOLOGY*

371.025 371.9 GBR ISSN 1472-0744
ISBI.COM. (Independent or Fee-paying Schools in the British Isles) Text in English. 1996. s-a. GBP 18 worldwide (effective 2001). **Document type:** *Directory, Academic/Scholarly.* **Description:** Directory of all the independent and fee-paying schools and residential special needs schools in the British Isles, special language schools, summer schools and educational suppliers, organizations and consultants.
Former titles (until 2000): I S B I, the Education Database (1463-3574); (until 1998): I S B I, the Database (1366-4654)
Media: CD-ROM.
Published by: (Independent Schools of the British Isles), Which School Ltd., Tilshead House, High St, Tilshead, Salisbury, Wilts SP3 4RX, United Kingdom. TEL 44-1980-620575, FAX 44-1980-621090, cdrom@isbi.com, http://www.isbi.com. Ed. Richard Essberger. Adv. contact Mrs. Pamela Wickham TEL 44-1926-641231.

NATIONAL DIRECTORY OF EDUCATIONAL PROGRAMS IN GERONTOLOGY AND GERIATRICS. see *GERONTOLOGY AND GERIATRICS*

OPPORTUNITIES FOR MINORITY STUDENTS IN THE U.S. DENTAL SCHOOLS. see *EDUCATION—Higher Education*

570.71025 USA ISSN 1088-9434
L901
PETERSON'S GRADUATE AND PROFESSIONAL PROGRAMS: THE BIOLOGICAL SCIENCES (YEAR) (BOOK 3). Text in English. 1966. a. USD 44.95. **Document type:** *Directory.* **Description:** Covers nearly 4,000 programs in such areas as oncology, conservation, biology, pharmacology, and zoology in the United States and Canada.
Former titles: Peterson's Guide to Graduate Programs in the Biological and Agricultural Sciences (Year) (Book 3) (0894-9360); (until 1989): Peterson's Annual Guides - Graduate Study. Book 3. Graduate Programs in the Biological, Agricultural, and Health Sciences (0887-8412); (until 1984): Peterson's Annual Guides to Graduate Study. Book 3. Biological, Agricultural, and Health Sciences. (0278-5358); (1976-1977): Peterson's Annual Guides to Graduate Study. Book 3: Biological and Health Sciences (0887-8404)
Related titles: CD-ROM ed.: (from SilverPlatter Information, Inc.); Online - full text ed.: (from The Dialog Corporation).
Published by: Peterson's Magazine Group, 202 Carnegie Center, PO Box 2123, Princeton, NJ 08543-2123. TEL 609-243-9111, FAX 609-243-9150, http://www.petersons.com. Ed. Barbara Lawrence.

PETERSON'S GUIDE TO NURSING PROGRAMS. see *MEDICAL SCIENCES—Nurses And Nursing*

E

378.0025 GBR
WHICH DEGREE. SCIENCES, MEDICINE, MATHEMATICS. Text in English. 196?. a. GBP 20.95 per issue (effective 2002). **Document type:** *Directory.* **Description:** Guides students and career counselors to degree programs in the natural sciences, along with medicine and mathematics, with concise course descriptions.
Published by: (Careers Research and Advisory Centre), Hobsons PLC, Challenger House, 42 Adler St, London E1 1EE, United Kingdom. TEL 44-1223-460366, FAX 44-1223-301506. **Dist. by:** Biblios Publishers' Distribution Services Ltd., Star Rd, Partridge Green, W Sussex RH13 8LD, United Kingdom. TEL 44-1403-710851, FAX 44-1403-711143.

EDUCATION—Higher Education

378.3 AUS
DIRECTORY OF FUNDING SOURCES. Text in English. a. AUD 40 to non-members; AUD 35 to members. back issues avail. **Document type:** *Directory.* **Description:** Lists funding agencies throughout Australia.
Formerly (until 1989): Directory of Funding Sources for Nursing Projects, Grants and Scholarships (1030-3618)
Media: Diskette.
Published by: Royal College of Nursing Australia, 1 Napier Close, Deakin, ACT 2600, Australia. TEL 61-2-6282-5633, FAX 61-2-6282-3565. Adv. contact Joanne Ramadge.

571.9 USA ISSN 0070-6086
RB123
DIRECTORY OF PATHOLOGY TRAINING PROGRAMS (YEAR). Text in English. 1968. a. USD 25 (effective 2000). **Document type:** *Directory.* **Description:** Describes residency programs and postgraduate subspecialty fellowships in anatomic and clinical pathology in the US and Canada, and post-sophomore fellowships.
—GNLM.
Published by: Intersociety Committee on Pathology Information, 9650 Rockville Pike, Bethesda, MD 20814. TEL 301-571-1880, FAX 301-571-1879, icpi@pathol.faseb.org, http://www.pathologytraining.org. Ed. Eileen Lavine. R&P Frances Pitlick. Circ: 2,500.

378.198287 GBR
DISABLED GRADUATES CASEBOOK. Text in English. 1994. a. GBP 9.99 per issue (effective 2002). **Document type:** *Directory.* **Description:** Recent graduates discuss their careers.
Formerly: Careers for Disabled Graduates
Published by: (Careers Research and Advisory Centre), Hobsons PLC, Challenger House, 42 Adler St, London E1 1EE, United Kingdom. TEL 44-1223-354551, FAX 44-1223-323154. **Dist. by:** Biblios Publishers' Distribution Services Ltd., Star Rd, Partridge Green, W Sussex RH13 8LD, United Kingdom. TEL 44-1403-710851, FAX 44-1403-711143.

378.3 AUS
GUIDE TO SUCCESSFUL GRANT APPLICATIONS. Text in English. a. AUD 12 to non-members; AUD 10 to members. **Document type:** *Trade.* **Description:** Provides practical advice on how to develop high-quality grant applications.
Published by: Royal College of Nursing Australia, 1 Napier Close, Deakin, ACT 2600, Australia. TEL 61-2-6282-5633, FAX 61-2-6282-3565. Ed. Helen Hamilton. R&P Lisa Howdin. Adv. contact Joanne Ramadge.

617.6071 USA ISSN 0022-0337
RK71
JOURNAL OF DENTAL EDUCATION. Text in English. 1936. m. USD 75 domestic; USD 100 in Canada; USD 125 elsewhere (effective 2000). adv. bk.rev. charts, illus, stat. index. reprints avail. **Document type:** *Academic/Scholarly.* **Description:** Contains articles on dental educational research, teaching methods and materials, curriculum, and administration of educational programs.
Related titles: Microform ed.
Indexed: AgeLine, Biol.Abstr., C.I.J.E., Cont.Pg.Educ., Curr.Tit.Dent., Dent.Abstr., Dent.Ind., ERA, High.Educ.Abstr., INIS Atomind., Ind.Med. (1936-), Res.High.Educ.Abstr., Tech.Educ.Abstr.
—BLDSC (4968.450000), CISTI, GNLM, ingenta, KNAW.
Published by: American Association of Dental Schools, 1625 Massachusetts Ave, N W, Washington, DC 20036-2212. TEL 202-667-9433. Ed. Dr. James D Bader. R&P Sue Sandmeyer. Circ: 4,300.

617.6071 USA
OPPORTUNITIES FOR MINORITY STUDENTS IN THE U.S. DENTAL SCHOOLS. Text in English. 1995. biennial. USD 10 (effective 2000). **Document type:** *Directory.* **Description:** Provides information on programs available to minority students at U.S. dental schools, admission requirements, admission and graduation statistics.
Published by: American Association of Dental Schools, 1625 Massachusetts Ave, N W, Washington, DC 20036-2212. TEL 202-667-9433, FAX 202-667-0642, aads@aads.jhu.edu, http://www.adds.jhu.edu. Ed. Sue Sandmeyer. Circ: 3,000.

E

617 AUS
SURGICAL NEWS (ONLINE). Text in English. 1980. 3/yr. bk.rev. charts, illus. back issues avail. **Document type:** *Bulletin.* **Description:** Publishes financial and related issues concerning the Royal College.
Formerly (until 2000): R A C S Bulletin (Print Edition) (0728-1048)
Media: Online - full content.
Published by: Royal Australasian College of Surgeons, Spring St, Melbourne, VIC 3000, Australia. TEL 61-3-9249-1200, FAX 61-3-9249-1219, surgical.news@surgeons.org, http://www.medeserv.com.au/racs/open/surgical_news/surg_news.cfm, http://www.surgeons.org/. Ed. Fiona Gillies. Circ: 6,300.

TEACHING AND LEARNING IN MEDICINE; an international journal. see *MEDICAL SCIENCES*

UNIVERSITIES SAFETY ASSOCIATION. DIGEST. see *PUBLIC HEALTH AND SAFETY*

UNIVERSITY OF TECHNOLOGY, SYDNEY. FACULTY OF NURSING, MIDWIFERY AND HEALTH HANDBOOK. see *MEDICAL SCIENCES—Nurses And Nursing*

WHICH DEGREE. SCIENCES, MEDICINE, MATHEMATICS. see *EDUCATION—Guides To Schools And Colleges*

WORLD MEDICAL JOURNAL. see *MEDICAL SCIENCES*

EDUCATION—International Education Programs

MULTICULTURAL EDUCATION ABSTRACTS. see *EDUCATION—Abstracting, Bibliographies, Statistics*

370.116 USA
OVER THE RAINBOW. Text in English. 1982. s-a. membership. adv. bk.rev. back issues avail. **Document type:** *Newsletter.* **Description:** Provides information on the latest opportunities concerning travel and international exchange programs, and provides information on scholarships,and new publications. Provides details on MIUSA's community service programs and international exchanges.
Related titles: Audio cassette/tape ed.
Published by: Mobility International U S A, PO Box 10767, Eugene, OR 97440-2767. TEL 541-343-1284, FAX 541-343-6812, info@miusa.org, http://www.miusa.org. Ed. Susan Sygall. Adv. contact Pamela Houston TEL 541-343-1284. Circ: 300.

SUBTLE ENERGIES AND ENERGY MEDICINE; an interdisciplinary journal of energetic and informational interactions. see *PHYSICS*

EDUCATION—School Organization And Administration

371.6 USA
AMERICAN SCHOOL AND HOSPITAL MAINTENANCE. Text in English. 1978. q. adv. **Document type:** *Magazine, Trade.* **Description:** Focuses on the renovation, maintenance, energy, and security of the physical plant and grounds.
Published by: A S & H M, 100-6 Coolidge Hill Rd, Watertown, MA 02472-5031. TEL 617-923-8158, FAX 617-926-7174, http://www.facilitymanagement.com/ashmmag.htm. adv.: B&W page USD 2,750; trim 8.125 x 10.875. Circ: 34,305.

371.223 USA ISSN 0883-5330
R850.A1
DIRECTORY OF BIOMEDICAL AND HEALTH CARE GRANTS. Text in English. 1985. a. USD 84.50 domestic; USD 101.40 foreign (effective 2000). **Document type:** *Directory.* **Description:** Lists more than 3,000 federal, state and private grants and funding programs in health and related fields, including sponsoring organizations, application procedures, addresses, and restrictions.
Related titles: Online - full text ed.: (from The Dialog Corporation).
Published by: Oryx Press, PO Box 33889, Phoenix, AZ 85067-3889. TEL 602-265-2651, 800-279-6799, FAX 602-265-6250, info@oryxpress.com, http://www.oryxpress.com/. Eds. Millie Hannnum, Anne Thompson. Pub. Phyllis Steckler. R&P Lori Cavanaugh TEL 602-265-2651 ext 662.

DIRECTORY OF GRANTS FOR ORGANIZATIONS SERVING PEOPLE WITH DISABILITIES; a guide to sources of funding in the United States for programs & services for persons with disabilities. see *EDUCATION—Special Education And Rehabilitation*

371.71 GBR ISSN 0265-1602
EDUCATION AND HEALTH. Text in English. 1983. q. GBP 16 (effective 2001). adv. bk.rev. charts. *Refereed.* **Document type:** *Journal.* **Description:** For teachers and health-care professionals.
Indexed: Art.Hosp.& Tour., Br.Educ.Ind., Brit.Nur.Ind., Cont.Pg.Educ.
—BLDSC (3661.187000).
Published by: Schools Health Education Unit, Renslade House, Bonhay Rd, Exeter, Devon EX4 3AY, United Kingdom. TEL 44-1392-667272, FAX 44-1392-667269, sheu@sheu.org.uk, www.sheu.org.uk. Ed., R&P David McGeorge. Adv. contact Michelle Dickinson. Circ: 5,250 (controlled).

363.119371 GBR ISSN 0262-5229
GREAT BRITAIN. DEPARTMENT OF EDUCATION AND SCIENCE. SAFETY IN EDUCATION✶. Text in English. 1981. irreg. free per issue. bk.rev. bibl, charts, illus, stat. back issues avail. **Document type:** *Government.* **Description:** Accounts of local governments' good practice in educational building and management.
—**CCC.**
Published by: Department of Education and Science, Sanctuary Bldg, Great Switer St, London SW1P 3BT, United Kingdom. Ed. Bernard McDonnell. Circ: 100,000.

371.716 USA
TX945
JOURNAL OF CHILD NUTRITION & MANAGEMENT. Text in English. 1977. s-a. USD 30; USD 32 foreign (effective 1999). bk.rev. index. back issues avail. *Refereed.* **Description:** Covers research concerning school food service and child nutrition.
Formerly (until 1997): School Food Service Research Review (0149-6808)
Indexed: Agricola, Hospit.Ind., Lod.Restr.& Tour.Ind.
—BLDSC (4957.630000), CISTI, ingenta.
Published by: American School Food Service Association, 700 S Washington St Ste 300, Alexandria, VA 22314-4287. TEL 703-739-3900, FAX 703-739-3915, asfsa@asfsa.org, http://www.asfsa.org. Ed. Jeannie Sneed. Circ: 250.

371.2 371.9 362.1 USA
MAINTAINING SAFE SCHOOLS - SCHOOL VIOLENCE ALERT. Text in English. m. USD 135 (effective 1999). back issues avail. **Document type:** *Newsletter.* **Description:** Provides strategies for mediation and crisis management that have worked in schools, security measures being taken by schools to curb violence. Highlights special rules that apply to disciplining students with disabilities.
Published by: L R P Publications, 747 Dresher Rd, Box 980, Horsham, PA 19044. TEL 800-341-7874, FAX 215-784-9639, custserve@lrp.com, http://www.lrp.com. Pub. Kenneth F Kahn.

REVISTA BRASILEIRA DE SAUDE ESCOLAR/ BRAZILIAN JOURNAL OF SCHOOL HEALTH. see *PUBLIC HEALTH AND SAFETY*

371.6 CAN ISSN 0834-0455
S I E C C A N NEWSLETTER. Text in English. 1965. irreg. (2-3/yr.). CND 45 in Canada to individuals; CND 50 in United States to individuals; CND 70 elsewhere to individuals; CND 65 in Canada to institutions; CND 70 in United States to institutions; CND 90 elsewhere to institutions; CND 30 in Canada to students; CND 35 in United States to students; CND 55 elsewhere to students (effective 2001). adv. bk.rev., film rev. *Refereed.* **Document type:** *Newsletter.* **Description:** Features practical teaching and counselling ideas, articles, media reports and reviews.
Formerly: S I E C C A N Newsletter Toronto (0381-873X)
Indexed: CINAHL.
Published by: Sex Information and Education Council of Canada, 850 Coxwell Ave, York, ON M4C 5R1, Canada. TEL 416-446-5304, FAX 416-778-0785, sieccan@web.net, http://www.sieccan.org. Ed. F Michael Barrett. R&P, Adv. contact Alex McKay. Circ: 1,000.

371.716 USA ISSN 1075-3885
LB3475.A1 CODEN: SFNUEO
SCHOOL FOODSERVICE AND NUTRITION. Text in English. 1946. 11/yr. USD 75 to non-members; USD 125 foreign to non-members (effective 2001). adv. bk.rev. tr.lit. index. **Description:** Covers legislative and management issues concerning school food service and child nutrition.
Former titles (until Jun. 1994): School Food Service Journal (0160-6271); School Lunch Journal (0036-6641)
Indexed: Agricola.
—CISTI, ingenta.
Published by: American School Food Service Association, 700 S. Washington St., Ste. 300, Alexandria, VA 22314-4287. TEL 703-739-3900, FAX 703-739-3915, asfsa@asfsa.org, http://www.asfsa.org. Ed. Patricia L Fitzgerald. Pub. Barbara S Borschow. R&P Patrick White. Adv. contact Maria Robertson. Circ: 60,000 (paid).

SCHOOL LAW BRIEFINGS. see *EDUCATION—Special Education And Rehabilitation*

EDUCATION—Special Education And Rehabilitation

see also CRIMINOLOGY AND LAW ENFORCEMENT; HANDICAPPED; SOCIAL SERVICES AND WELFARE

371.928 USA
A C R M D ON THE RECORD. (Association for Children with Retarded Mental Development) Text in English. 1960. s-a. free.
Published by: Association for C R M D, Inc., 345 Hudson St, 3rd Fl, New York, NY 10014. TEL 212-627-8318. Ed. Philip Vassallo. Circ: 3,500.

A H R C CHRONICLE. see *MEDICAL SCIENCES—Psychiatry And Neurology*

371.9 USA ISSN 0736-5829
GV445
ADAPTED PHYSICAL ACTIVITY QUARTERLY. Short title: A P A Q. Text in English. 1984. q. USD 45 to individuals; USD 135 to institutions; USD 30 to students (effective 2001). adv. bk.rev. abstr, bibl, charts, stat, illus. index. back issues avail.; reprint service avail. from PSC. *Refereed.* **Document type:** *Academic/Scholarly.* **Description:** Communicates scholarly inquiries related to physical activity for at-risk infants, pre-schoolers, and students who receive special educations.
Related titles: Online - full text ed.: (from Institute for Scientific Information).
Indexed: AMED, CINAHL, ERA, Except.Child Educ.Abstr., Excerp.Med., Focus on: Sports Sci.& Med., IBZ, Phys.Ed.Ind., PsycInfo, Psychol.Abstr. (1984-), SSCI (coverage dropped), Sp.Ed.Needs Abstr., Sportsearch (1984-), e-psyche.
—BLDSC (0678.308000), EMDOCS, GNLM, IDS, Infotrieve, ingenta. **CCC.**
Published by: (International Federation for Adapted Physical Activity), Human Kinetics Publishers, Inc., PO Box 5076, Champaign, IL 61825-5076. TEL 217-351-5076, FAX 217-351-2674, http://www.humankinetics.com. Ed. Claudine Sherrill. Pub. Rainer Martens. R&P Cheri Banks TEL 217-351-5076 ext 2275. Adv. contact Patty Rodriguiz. Circ: 977 (paid and free).

371.94 USA ISSN 0735-004X
RJ506.L4
ADVANCES IN LEARNING AND BEHAVIORAL DISABILITIES. Text in English. 1982. a. USD 78.50 to institutions. *Refereed.*
Indexed: IBZ, Lang.& Lang.Behav.Abstr., Psychol.Abstr., SOPODA, Sociol.Abstr., e-psyche.
—BLDSC (0709.258000), GNLM. **CCC.**
Published by: J A I Press Inc., 100 Prospect St, Box 811, Stamford, CT 06904-0811. FAX 203-357-8446. Ed. Kenneth D Gadow.

371.928 USA ISSN 0742-6313
ADVANCES IN MENTAL RETARDATION AND DEVELOPMENTAL DISABILITIES. Text in English. 1983. irreg. **Document type:** *Monographic series.*
Indexed: e-psyche.
Published by: Taylor & Francis Ltd. (Subsidiary of: Taylor & Francis Group), 325 Chestnut St, Suite 800, Philadelphia, PA 19016. TEL 215-625-8900, FAX 215-625-2940, info@taylorandfrancis.com, http://www.taylorandfrancis.com/. **Subscr. to:** Taylor & Francis Group, Journals Customer Service, Rankine Rd, Basingstoke, Hants RG24 8PR, United Kingdom. TEL 44-1256-813000, FAX 44-1256-479438, enquiry@tanf.co.uk, http://www.tandf.co.uk/journals.

371.94 USA
ADVOCATE (BETHESDA). Text in English. 1968. bi-m. USD 25 domestic to individual members; USD 40 foreign to individual members; USD 200 to institutions (effective 2000). adv. bk.rev. *Refereed.* **Document type:** *Newsletter.* **Description:** Provides the latest news on autism. Features include personal stories. Includes information on medical research and legislative issues.
Formerly (1979): N S A C Newsletter (0047-9101)
Media: Duplicated (not offset).
Indexed: e-psyche.
Published by: Autism Society of America, 7910 Woodmont Ave, Ste 300, Bethesda, MD 20814-3015. TEL 301-657-0881, 800-328-8476, FAX 301-657-0869, http://www.autism-society.org. Circ: 24,000 (paid).

ALL INDIA INSTITUTE OF SPEECH AND HEARING. JOURNAL. see *HANDICAPPED—Hearing Impaired*

AMERICAN ANNALS OF THE DEAF. see *HANDICAPPED—Hearing Impaired*

AMERICAN JOURNAL OF ART THERAPY; art in psychotherapy, education, and rehabilitation. see *MEDICAL SCIENCES—Physical Medicine And Rehabilitation*

AMERICAN PRINTING HOUSE FOR THE BLIND. DEPARTMENT OF EDUCATIONAL AND TECHNICAL RESEARCH. REPORT OF RESEARCH AND DEVELOPMENT ACTIVITIES. see *HANDICAPPED—Visually Impaired*

371.91 USA ISSN 0362-4048
HD7255.A2
AMERICAN REHABILITATION. Text in English. 1975. q. USD 15 (effective 2001). bk.rev. illus. Index. back issues avail.; reprints avail. **Document type:** *Academic/Scholarly, Government.* **Description:** Comments on all aspects of life affecting persons with handicaps, bringing program, treatment, news, and legislative affairs to interested professional and consumer groups.
Related titles: Microform ed.: (from PQC); Online - full text ed.: (from ProQuest Information & Learning, Gale Group, Northern Light Technology, Inc.).
Indexed: AMED, AgeLine, CINAHL, Except.Child Educ.Abstr., Hlth.Ind., Ind.U.S.Gov.Per., L.R.I., MEDOC, Med.Care Rev., Rehabil.Lit.
—BLDSC (0853.541000), GNLM.
Published by: (U.S. Rehabilitation Services Administration), U.S. Department of Education, Mary E Switzer Bldg, Rm 3030, 330 C St, S W, Washington, DC 20202. TEL 202-205-8266, frank_romano@ed.gov, http://www.ed.gov/pubs/AmericanRehab. Ed. Frank Romano. Circ: 8,000. **Subscr. to:** U.S. Government Printing Office, Superintendent of Documents, PO Box 371954, Pittsburgh, PA 15250-7954. TEL 202-512-1800, FAX 202-512-2250, orders@gpo.gov, http://www.access.gpo.gov.

AMERICAN SOCIETY FOR ADOLESCENT PSYCHIATRY. NEWSLETTER. see *MEDICAL SCIENCES—Psychiatry And Neurology*

371.913 USA ISSN 0736-9387
RJ496.A5 CODEN: ORSBBT
ANNALS OF DYSLEXIA; an interdisciplinary journal of specific language disability. Text in English. 1951. a. USD 55 to members. reprint service avail. from PQC. *Refereed.* **Document type:** *Academic/Scholarly.*
Formerly (until 1981): Orton Society. Bulletin (0474-7534)
Related titles: Microform ed.: (from PQC); Online - full text ed.: (from H. W. Wilson, ProQuest Information & Learning, Institute for Scientific Information).
Indexed: ASCA, C.I.J.E., Child Devel.Abstr., Curr.Cont., DSH Abstr., Educ.Ind. (Jan.1983-), Except.Child Educ.Abstr., Lang.& Lang.Behav.Abstr., PsycInfo, Psychol.Abstr. (1963-), SOPODA, SSCI, Sociol.Abstr., e-psyche.
—BLDSC (1040.357500), IDS, ingenta.
Published by: International Dyslexia Association, 8600 LaSalle Rd, Ste 382, Chester Bldg, Baltimore, MD 21286-2044. TEL 410-296-0232. Ed., R&P Cindy Cressi. Circ: 10,000.

371.9 USA
ARKANSAS. DIVISION OF REHABILITATION SERVICES. ANNUAL REPORT. Text in English. 1940. a. free. illus, stat.
Published by: Division of Rehabilitation Services, PO Box 3781, Little Rock, AR 72203. TEL 501-628-8168. Circ: 1,000.

371.9 USA ISSN 1040-0435
RM698 CODEN: ASTEF2
ASSISTIVE TECHNOLOGY. Text in English. 1989. s-a. USD 65 in US & Canada to individuals; USD 80 elsewhere to individuals; USD 75 in US & Canada to institutions; USD 90 elsewhere to institutions (effective 2001). adv. back issues avail. *Refereed.* **Description:** Seeks to foster communications among researchers, developers, clinicians, educators, consumers and others working in all aspects of the assistive technology arena.
Related titles: Online - full text ed.: (from Institute for Scientific Information).
Indexed: AgeLine, CINAHL, Curr.Cont., Excerp.Med. (1996-), INSPEC (1993-), SSCI.
—AskIEEE, Ei, EMDOCS, GNLM, IDS, ingenta.
Published by: R E S N A, 1700 N Moore St, Ste 1540, Arlington, VA 22209-1903. TEL 703-524-6686, orders@allenpress.com, info@resna.org, http://www.allenpress.com, http://www.resna.org. Ed. Lawrence Trachtman. Circ: 1,900. **Subscr. to:** Allen Press Inc., PO Box 1897, Lawrence, KS 66044-8897.

371.91 AUS ISSN 1324-8928
AUSTRALIAN JOURNAL OF LEARNING DISABILITIES. Text in English. 1969. q. AUD 73; AUD 75 to New Zealand & SE Asia; AUD 81 elsewhere (effective 2001). adv. bk.rev., software rev. index. back issues avail.; reprints avail. *Refereed.* **Document type:** *Journal, Magazine, Academic/Scholarly.* **Description:** Covers all aspects of special education. Looks at learning disabilities and the intelligent underachiever.
Former titles (until June 1996): Australian Journal of Remedial Education (0311-1954); Remedial Education (0048-7236)
Indexed: Aus.Educ.Ind., Aus.P.A.I.S. (Coverage Dropped), Cont.Pg.Educ., ERA, Except.Child Educ.Abstr., Lang.& Lang.Behav.Abstr., SOPODA, Sociol.Abstr., Sp.Ed.Needs Abstr., Tech.Educ.Abstr.
—ingenta.
Published by: Learning Difficulties Australia (LDA), 4 Canterbury Rd, Toorak, VIC 3142, Australia. TEL 61-3-9826-0371, FAX 61-3-9826-2696, davidson@area.org.au, http://www.netspace.net.au/~area. Ed., R&P, Adv. contact Christopher Davidson. page AUD 320. Circ: 1,000.

BACK TO WORK. see *OCCUPATIONAL HEALTH AND SAFETY*

371.9 DEU ISSN 0170-902X
DAS BAND. Text in German. 1970. bi-m. DEM 22 (effective 1999). adv. bk.rev., play rev. abstr, illus, tr.lit. **Document type:** *Newsletter.*
Indexed: Ref.Zh.
Published by: Bundesverband fuer Koerper- und Mehrfachbehinderte e.V., Brehmstr 5-7, Duesseldorf 40239, Germany. TEL 49-211-64004-0, FAX 49-211-6400420, bv-km@t-online.de, http://www.paritaet.org/bvkm. Ed. Stephanie Wilken Dapper. Circ: 20,000.

371.94 USA ISSN 0198-7429
RJ506.B44
BEHAVIORAL DISORDERS. Text in English. 1976. q. USD 20 to individuals; USD 50 to institutions (effective 1999). adv. bk.rev. reprint service avail. from PQC,PSC,SCH. *Refereed.* **Document type:** *Academic/Scholarly.* **Description:** Directed to educators, parents, mental health personnel and others concerned with the education and well-being of children and youth with behavioral and emotional disorders.
Related titles: Microform ed.: (from PQC); Online - full text ed.: (from ProQuest Information & Learning, Institute for Scientific Information).
Indexed: ASCA, C.I.J.E., Crim.Just.Abstr., Curr.Cont., Educ.Ind. (Nov.1983-), Except.Child Educ.Abstr., Fam.Ind., Mult.Ed.Abstr., PsycInfo, Psychol.Abstr. (1976-), SSCI, Sp.Ed.Needs Abstr., e-psyche.
—BLDSC (1877.370000), ingenta.
Published by: (Council for Children with Behavioral Disorders), Council for Exceptional Children, 1920 Association Drive, Reston, VA 22091. TEL 703-620-3660, FAX 703-264-9494, http://www.cec.sped.org/bk/17.htm, http://www.unr.edu/educ/ceds/indexceds.html. Eds. Gary Sasso, Jo Hendrickson. R&P Robert Gable. Circ: 9,000.

371.9 DEU ISSN 0171-9718
BEHINDERTENHILFE DURCH ERZIEHUNG, UNTERRICHT UND THERAPIE. Text in German. 1977. irreg., latest vol.18, 1993. price varies. **Document type:** *Monographic series.*
Published by: Ernst Reinhardt Verlag, Kemnatenstr 46, Munich 80639, Germany. TEL 49-89-1780160, FAX 49-89-17801630. Ed. Otto Speck.

371.9 USA
BETHPHAGE MESSENGER. Text in English. 3/yr.
Published by: Bethphage, Lind Center, South 118th St. Suite A, Omaha, NE 681372221. TEL 800-279-1234, 402-896-3884, FAX 402-894-4784, http://www.bethphage.org/organization/newsletter.html. Ed. Carrie L Reed. Circ: 100,000.

BRITISH ASSOCIATION OF TEACHERS OF THE DEAF. ASSOCIATION MAGAZINE. see *HANDICAPPED—Hearing Impaired*

BRITISH INSTITUTE OF LEARNING DISABILITIES. CURRENT AWARENESS SERVICE. see *EDUCATION—Abstracting, Bibliographies, Statistics*

371.92 GBR ISSN 0969-7950
RC569.7 CODEN: BJDDE2
BRITISH JOURNAL OF DEVELOPMENTAL DISABILITIES. Abbreviated title: B J D D. Text in English. 1952. s-a. GBP 18; USD 49 in United States; CND 69 in Canada; AUD 73 in Australia; GBP 22 elsewhere (effective 2000). adv. bk.rev. charts, illus. cum.index every 2 yrs. *Refereed.* **Document type:** *Journal, Academic/Scholarly, Trade.* **Description:** Provides an international forum for a multidisciplinary approach to the problems posed by mental handicaps and learning disabilities.
Former titles (until 1992): British Journal of Mental Subnormality (0374-633X); Journal of Mental Subnormality (0022-2666)
Related titles: Online - full text ed.: (from Institute for Scientific Information).
Indexed: ASCA, ASSIA, Adol.Ment.Hlth.Abstr., AgeLine, Bibl.Dev.Med.& Child Neur., Biol.Abstr., Br.Educ.Ind., Brit.Nur.Ind., Curr.Cont., Excerp.Med., Lang.& Lang.Behav.Abstr., Mid.East: Abstr.& Ind., PsycInfo, Psychol.Abstr. (1971-), SOPODA, SSCI, Sociol.Abstr., Sp.Ed.Needs Abstr., e-psyche.
—BLDSC (2307.450000), GNLM, IDS, ingenta, KNAW.
Published by: (British Society for Developmental Disabilities), S E F A (Publications) Ltd., The Globe, 4 Great William St, Stratford-upon-Avon, Warks CV37 6RY, United Kingdom. editor@bjdd.org, walter.guenzburg@vu-wien.ac.at, http://www.bjdd.org. Ed. A L Guenzburg. Pub. W H Guenzburg. R&P W.H. Guenzburg. Adv. contact B Salmons. Circ: 1,500 (paid).

371.9 GBR ISSN 0952-3383
LC3986.G7 CODEN: BJSPEB
BRITISH JOURNAL OF SPECIAL EDUCATION; a journal of the National Association for Special Educational Needs. Text in English. 1974. q. GBP 98 to institutions in UK & Europe; USD 215 to institutions in the Americas & Caribbean; GBP 134 elsewhere to institutions (effective 2002). adv. bk.rev. cum.index: 1974-1983. back issues avail.; reprint service avail. from SCH,PSC. **Document type:** *Academic/Scholarly.*
Formerly (until 1985): Special Education - Forward Trends (0305-7526); Which was formed by the 1974 merger of: Special Education (0038-6707); Forward Trends (0015-8658)
Related titles: Microfiche ed.; Microfilm ed.; Online - full text ed.: ISSN 1467-8578 (from EBSCO Publishing, O C L C Online Computer Library Center, Inc., RoweCom Information Quest, ingenta, Swets Blackwell).
Indexed: ASSIA, Br.Educ.Ind., C.I.J.E., Child Devel.Abstr., Child.Lit.Abstr., Cont.Pg.Educ., Curr.Adv.Ecol.Sci., ERA, Educ.Tech.Abstr., Except.Child Educ.Abstr., High.Educ.Curr.Aware.Bull., Lang.& Lang.Behav.Abstr., Lang.Teach.& Ling.Abstr., Russ.Acad.Sci.Bibl., SOMA, SOPODA, Sociol.Abstr., Sociol.Educ.Abstr., Sp.Ed.Needs Abstr., e-psyche.
—BLDSC (2324.850000), GNLM, ingenta. **CCC.**
Published by: (National Association for Special Education Needs), Blackwell Publishers Ltd., 108 Cowley Rd, Oxford OX4 1JF, United Kingdom. TEL 44-1865-791100, FAX 44-1865-791347, nasen@bbnc.org.uk; jnlinfo@blackwellpublishers.co.uk, http://www.blackwellpublishers.co.uk/journals/bjse/. Ed. Christina Tilstone.

BRITISH JOURNAL OF VISUAL IMPAIRMENT. see *HANDICAPPED—Visually Impaired*

371.91 DEU ISSN 0172-0996
DAS BRUDERHAUS. Text in German. 1949. s-a. free per issue.
Published by: Gustav Werner Stiftung, Ringelbachstr 211, Reutlingen 72762, Germany. FAX 07121-278300. Ed. I Steudle. Circ: 20,000.

371.9 DEU
BUNDESARBEITSGEMEINSCHAFT HILFE FUER BEHINDERTE. BERICHTE. JAHRESSPIEGEL. Text in German. a. free per issue. **Document type:** *Academic/Scholarly.*

E

Formerly: Bundesarbeitsgemeinschaft Hilfe fuer Behinderte. Jahrespiegel
Published by: Bundesarbeitsgemeinschaft Hilfe fuer Behinderte e.V., Kirchfeldstr 149, Duesseldorf 40215, Germany. Ed. Elfriede Loebel.

C A E D H H JOURNAL/ASSOCIATION CANADIENNE DES ENSEIGNANTS(ES) DES SOURDS(ES) ET DES MALENTENDANTS(ES). REVUE. see *HANDICAPPED—Hearing Impaired*

371.9 USA
C C B D NEWSLETTER. Text in English. 1987. 4/yr. membership only. **Document type:** *Newsletter.* **Description:** Gives information on the council and its activities; includes news, legislation and other developments in the field.
Published by: (Council for Children with Behavioral Disorders), Council for Exceptional Children, 1920 Association Drive, Reston, VA 22091. TEL 703-620-3660, FAX 703-264-9494. Ed. Brenda Scheuermann. R&P Robert Gable. Circ: 8,400.

C P D NEWS. (Center for Persons with Disabilities) see *HANDICAPPED*

371.9 BRN ISSN 0827-3391
CANADIAN JOURNAL OF SPECIAL EDUCATION. Text in English. 1984. s-a. BND 25. **Document type:** *Academic/Scholarly.*
Related titles: Microfiche ed.: (from MML); Microform ed.: (from MML).
Indexed: C.I.J.E. (coverage dropped), Can.Educ.Ind., Except.Child Educ.Abstr.
—ingenta. **CCC.**
Published by: Center for Human Development and Research, c/o Dr. Marg Csapo, Special Education Unit, Ministry of Education, Bandar Seri Begawan, Brunei Darussalam. TEL 673-446-553.

THE CAPSTONE (TOWSON); news from the Council, and its accreditation and evaluation systems and ProLerna. see *HANDICAPPED*

371.95 USA ISSN 0885-7288
LC3981
CAREER DEVELOPMENT FOR EXCEPTIONAL INDIVIDUALS. Text in English. 1978. s-a. USD 20; USD 24 foreign (effective 1999). bk.rev. illus. reprints avail. **Document type:** *Academic/Scholarly.* **Description:** Contains articles on the latest research activities, model programs, and issues in career development and transition planning for exceptional individuals.
Related titles: Microform ed.: (from PQC).
Indexed: C.I.J.E., Except.Child Educ.Abstr.
—ingenta.
Published by: Council for Exceptional Children, 1920 Association Drive, Reston, VA 22091. TEL 703-620-3660, FAX 703-264-9494, http://www.ed.uiuc.edu/sped/dcdt/cdei.html. Eds. Michael Benz, Michael Bullis. Circ: 2,700.

CHICOREL INDEX SERIES. see *BIBLIOGRAPHIES*

371.9 GBR ISSN 0265-6590
LC4704.5
CHILD LANGUAGE TEACHING AND THERAPY. Text in English. 1985. 3/yr., latest vol.16. GBP 48 in Europe to individuals; USD 89 in North America to individuals; GBP 54 rest of world to individuals; GBP 102 rest of world to institutions; USD 202 in North America to institutions; GBP 118 rest of world to institutions; GBP 39 in Europe to members Applies to members of NAPLIC and TESOL (North America) AAAL and BAAL; USD 74 in North America to members Applies to members of NAPLIC and TESOL (North America) AAAL and BAAL; GBP 41 rest of world to members Applies to members of NAPLIC and TESOL (North America) AAAL and BAAL; GBP 59 in developing nations; GBP 39 newsstand/cover in Europe; USD 69 newsstand/cover in North America; GBP 41 newsstand/cover rest of world (effective 2002). adv. bk.rev. back issues avail.; reprints avail. *Refereed.* **Document type:** *Journal, Academic/Scholarly.* **Description:** Helps persons involved with children handicapped by an inadequate command of the spoken or written language.
Related titles: Online - full text ed.: (from EBSCO Publishing, O C L C Online Computer Library Center, Inc., RoweCom Information Quest, ingenta, Swets Blackwell).
Indexed: ASSIA, Br.Educ.Ind., CINAHL, Chic.Per.Ind., Child Devel.Abstr., Cont.Pg.Educ., ERA, Educ.Tech.Abstr., IBZ, Lang.& Lang.Behav.Abstr. (1985-), Lang.Teach.& Ling.Abstr., MLA Intl.Bibl., P C I, Psyclnfo, Psychol.Abstr. (1992-), Ref.Zh., SOPODA, Sociol.Abstr., Sp.Ed.Needs Abstr., Tech.Educ.Abstr., e-psyche.
—BLDSC (3172.944690), ingenta. **CCC.**
Published by: Arnold Publishers (Subsidiary of: Hodder Headline plc.), 338 Euston Rd, London NW1 3BH, United Kingdom. TEL 44-20-7873-6337, FAX 44-20-7873-6325, arnoldjournals@hodder.co.uk, http://www.arnoldpublishers.com/journals/journtitles.htm, http://www.palliativemedjournal.com. Eds. Carol Miller, Jannet Wright. Adv. contact Mary Attree. **Subscr. to:** Turpin Distribution Services Ltd., Blackhorse Rd, Letchworth, Herts SG6 1HN, United Kingdom. TEL 44-1462-488900, FAX 44-1462-483011, custservturpin@turpinltd.com.

CHILD PSYCHIATRY AND HUMAN DEVELOPMENT. see *MEDICAL SCIENCES—Psychiatry And Neurology*

371.9 JPN ISSN 0916-2682
CHIRYO KYOIKU KENKYU KIYO/GIFU UNIVERSITY. DEPARTMENT OF REMEDIAL EDUCATION. REPORT. Text in Japanese. 1979. a.
Published by: Gifu Daigaku, Kyoikugakubu/Gifu University, Faculty of Education, Chiryo Kyoikugaku Kenkyushitsu, 1-1 Yanagi-To, Gifu 501-1112, Japan.

CLINICAL CHILD AND FAMILY PSYCHOLOGY REVIEW. see *PSYCHOLOGY*

371.9142 USA ISSN 0890-409X
RJ496.C67
CLINICAL CONNECTION; idea source for the speech and language specialist working with the young communicator. Text in English. 1986. q. USD 39 domestic; USD 43 in Canada; USD 49 elsewhere. bk.rev. back issues avail. **Document type:** *Academic/Scholarly.* **Description:** Forum for speech and language pathologists to share practical clinical ideas.
Published by: A A D of Northern Virginia, 708 Pendleton St, Alexandria, VA 22314-1819. TEL 703-549-5126, FAX 703-548-5563. Ed. Georgina Ruley Parks. Circ: 6,000.

CLINICAL LINGUISTICS & PHONETICS. see *MEDICAL SCIENCES—Psychiatry And Neurology*

371.9025 USA ISSN 0886-1935
HV1569.5
CLOSING THE GAP. Text in English. 1982. bi-m. USD 32 domestic; USD 47 in Canada; USD 63 elsewhere (effective 2000). adv. bk.rev. **Document type:** *Journal, Academic/Scholarly.* **Description:** Aimed at people working with persons with disabilities and those interested in the use of micro-computers in special education and rehabilitation. Each issue contains information emphasizing the practical applications of micro-computers as personal tools and educational aids for the handicapped.
Related titles: Online - full text ed.: (from Northern Light Technology, Inc.).
Indexed: CWI, SoftBase (Dec.1991-Aug.1992).
Address: PO Box 68, Henderson, MN 56044. TEL 507-248-3294, FAX 507-248-3810, info@closingthegap.com, http://www.closingthegap.com. Ed. Budd Hagen. Adv. contact Maryann Harty. Circ: 10,000.

371.9142 USA ISSN 1525-7401
RJ496.C67
COMMUNICATION DISORDERS QUARTERLY. Text in English. 1977. 4/yr., latest vol.22, Sum. USD 43 in North America to individuals; USD 71 elsewhere to individuals; USD 109 in North America to institutions; USD 138 elsewhere to institutions (effective 2002). adv. bk.rev. 64 p./no. back issues avail. *Refereed.* **Document type:** *Journal, Academic/Scholarly.* **Description:** Discusses many aspects of communication disorders: speech, hearing, language, and learning disabilities.
Former titles: Journal of Children's Communication Development (1093-5703); (until 1995): Journal of Childhood Communication Disorders (0735-3170)
Related titles: Online - full text ed.: (from ProQuest Information & Learning, CatchWord Ltd.).
Indexed: C.I.J.E. (coverage dropped), Except.Child Educ.Abstr., Lang.& Lang.Behav.Abstr. (1988-), Psychol.Abstr. (1991-), SOPODA, Sociol.Abstr., e-psyche.
—BLDSC (3359.821000), ingenta.
Published by: (Council for Exceptional Children), Pro-Ed Inc., 8700 Shoal Creek Blvd, Austin, TX 78757-6897. TEL 512-451-3246, FAX 512-302-9129, proed1@aol.com, http://www.proedinc.com. R&P Barbara Rivera TEL 512-451-3246 ext 653. Circ: 2,200.

371.94 GBR ISSN 0045-7663
COMMUNICATION (LONDON, 1967); the magazine of the National Autistic Society. Text in English. 1967. 3/yr. GBP 11 domestic to members; GBP 16 foreign to members (effective 2001). adv. bk.rev. 32 p./no. **Document type:** *Magazine.*
Indexed: Curr.Cont. (coverage dropped), Lang.& Lang.Behav.Abstr., SSCI (coverage dropped).
—BLDSC (3354.818000).
Published by: National Autistic Society, 393 City Rd, London EC1V 1NG, United Kingdom. TEL 44-20-7833-2299, FAX 44-20-7833-9666, communication@nas.org.uk, http://www.nas.org.uk. Ed., R&P Anne Cooper. Circ: 10,000 (paid).

371.912 USA
COURAGE NEWS. Text in English. q. free per issue. back issues avail.
Published by: Courage Center, 3915 Golden Valley Rd., Golden Valley, MN 55422. TEL 612-520-0520, FAX 612-520-0577.

371.91 USA ISSN 1059-8243
CUED SPEECH JOURNAL. Short title: C S Journal. Text in English. 1985. a. USD 5 to non-members (effective 2000). adv. abstr, bibl, charts, stat. 80 p./no. back issues avail. *Refereed.* **Document type:** *Journal, Academic/Scholarly.* **Description:** Discusses professional use of and research on Cued Speech, a system of communication for people with hearing, speech and language needs.
Formerly: Cued Speech Annual (1041-6226)
Published by: National Cued Speech Association, 23970 Hermitage Rd., Shaker Heights, OH 44122. TEL 216-292-6213, 800-459-3529, cuedspdisc@aol.com, http://www.cuedspeech.org. Ed., R&P, Adv. contact Pam Beck. Circ: 500.

371.9 USA
D L D TIMES. Text in English. 1984. 3/yr. membership only. **Document type:** *Newsletter.* **Description:** Provides information and news in the field of learning disabilities, and the activities of the division.
Published by: Council for Exceptional Children, Division for Learning Disabilities, 1920 Association Drive, Reston, VA 22091. TEL 703-620-3660, FAX 703-264-9494. Ed. Dr. Kate Garnett. Circ: 12,500.

371.9 USA
D P H D NEWSLETTER. (Council for Exceptional Children) Text in English. 1980. q. membership only. adv. **Document type:** *Newsletter.* **Description:** Provides information on the division and its activities. Includes news about education for children with physical or health disabilities.
Published by: Council for Exceptional Children, Division for Physical & Health Disabilities, 1920 Association Dr, Reston, VA 20191-1589. TEL 703-620-3660, FAX 703-264-9494, http://www.cec.org, http://www.cec.sped.org. Ed. Sherwood Best. Circ: 1,500.

371.9 DNK ISSN 0908-1755
DANISH CENTRE FOR TECHNICAL AIDS FOR REHABILITATION AND EDUCATION. NEWSLETTER. Text in Danish. 1989. 2/yr. free per issue. bk.rev. **Document type:** *Newsletter.*
Formerly (until 1992): Datch Information (0905-0221)
Published by: Danish Centre for Technical Aids for Rehabilitation and Special Education, Gregersensvej, Taastrup 2630, Denmark. TEL 45-43-99-33-22, FAX 45-43-52-70-72. Ed. Joergen Bisgaard.

DEAF - BLIND PERSPECTIVES. see *HANDICAPPED—Visually Impaired*

DEAFNESS AND EDUCATION INTERNATIONAL. see *HANDICAPPED—Hearing Impaired*

371.9 DEU ISSN 0939-4702
DEUTSCHE BEHINDERTENZEITSCHRIFT. Abbreviated title: D B Z. Text in German. 1964. bi-m. DEM 29. bk.rev. **Document type:** *Bulletin.*
Former titles: Behindertenzeitschrift (0175-5854); Behinderte Kind (0005-7991)
Indexed: e-psyche.
—GNLM, Infotrieve. **CCC.**
Published by: Reha-Verlag GmbH, Roonstr 30, Bonn 53175, Germany. TEL 49-228-352328, FAX 49-228-359569. Ed. Leo Sparty. adv.: B&W page DEM 1,500; trim 297 x 210. Circ: 10,000.

DEVELOPMENTAL DISABILITIES BULLETIN. see *MEDICAL SCIENCES—Psychiatry And Neurology*

DEVELOPMENTAL DISABILITIES SPECIAL INTEREST SECTION QUARTERLY. see *PSYCHOLOGY*

371.95 GBR
DEVON COUNTY COUNCIL. SPECIAL EDUCATIONAL NEEDS SERIES. Text in English. 1993 (no.2). irreg. **Document type:** *Monographic series, Government.*
Indexed: e-psyche.
Published by: Devon County Council, Education, County Hall, Devon County Council, Topsham Rd, Exeter, Devon EX2 4QQ, United Kingdom.

371.95 USA ISSN 0737-2477
LB3050
DIAGNOSTIQUE. Text in English. 1976. q. USD 28; USD 32 foreign (effective 1999). adv. bk.rev. illus. back issues avail.; reprints avail. **Document type:** *Academic/Scholarly.* **Description:** Directed to psychologists, diagnosticians, and special educators who use methods of educational measurement in evaluating exceptional individuals.
Related titles: Microform ed.: (from PQC).
Indexed: C.I.J.E., Cont.Pg.Educ., Except.Child Educ.Abstr., e-psyche.
—BLDSC (3579.671900).
Published by: (Council for Educational Diagnostic Services), Council for Exceptional Children, 1920 Association Drive, Reston, VA 22091. TEL 703-620-3660, FAX 703-264-9494, http://www.unr.edu/educ/ceds/indexceds.html. Ed., R&P Ronald Taylor. Circ: 1,800.

371.95 USA ISSN 0070-5012
LC4007
DIRECTORY FOR EXCEPTIONAL CHILDREN; a listing of educational and training facilities. Text in English. 1954. irreg., latest vol.14, 2001. USD 75 (effective 2001). adv. illus, stat. index. 1056 p./no. **Document type:** *Directory, Consumer, Trade.* **Description:** Includes 3,000 schools, facilities and organizations across the US serving children and young adults with developmental, emotional, physical and medical disabilities.
Indexed: e-psyche.
Published by: Porter Sargent Publishers, Inc., 11 Beacon St, Ste 1400, Boston, MA 02108. TEL 617-523-1670, FAX 617-523-1021, info@portersargent.com, http://www.portersargent.com. Ed. Daniel P. McKeever. Adv. contact John Yonce. page USD 540; 4.25 x 7. Circ: 3,000.

371.22 USA ISSN 1077-3282
HV1553
DIRECTORY OF GRANTS FOR ORGANIZATIONS SERVING PEOPLE WITH DISABILITIES; a guide to sources of funding in the United States for programs & services for persons with disabilities. Text in English. 1978. biennial, latest vol.10, 1996. USD 59.50 (effective 1998). bk.rev. **Document type:** *Directory.* **Description:** Lists funding sources for programs and services for organizations serving people who are disabled. Provides extensive profiles on foundations and includes essays on grantsmanship to help guide the reader through the intricate process of securing a grant.
Formerly (until 1993): Handicapped Funding Directory (0733-4753)
Published by: Research Grant Guides, PO Box 1214, Loxahatchee, FL 33470. TEL 561-795-6129, FAX 561-795-7794. Ed. Richard M Eckstein.

DIVISION ON VISUAL IMPAIRMENTS QUARTERLY. see *HANDICAPPED—Visually Impaired*

DOWN & UP. see *HANDICAPPED*

371.9144 GBR ISSN 1076-9242
RC394.W6D952 CODEN: DYSLEO
DYSLEXIA. Text in English. 1995. q. USD 265 in United States; USD 265 in Canada & Mexico; USD 265 elsewhere; USD 279 combined subscription in United States for print and online eds.; USD 279 combined subscription in Canada & Mexico for print and online eds.; USD 279 combined subscription elsewhere for print and online eds. (effective 2002). adv. back issues avail. *Refereed.* **Document type:** *Academic/Scholarly.* **Description:** Provides reviews and reports of research, assessment and intervention practice.
Related titles: Microform ed.: (from PQC); Online - full text ed.: ISSN 1099-0909. USD 265 in United States; USD 265 in Canada & Mexico; USD 265 elsewhere (effective 2002) (from EBSCO Publishing, ingenta, Wiley InterScience).
Indexed: ASSIA, Br.Educ.Ind., ERA, Ind.Med. (1995-), e-psyche.
—BLDSC (3637.234000), Infotrieve. **CCC.**
Published by: (British Dyslexia Association), Wiley Europe Ltd., Baffins Ln, Chichester, W Sussex PO19 1UD, United Kingdom. TEL 44-1243-779777, FAX 44-1243-775878, customer@wiley.co.uk, http://www.wiley.co.uk. adv.: B&W page GBP 650, color page GBP 1,550; trim 165 x 248. **Subscr. in the Americas to:** John Wiley & Sons, Inc., Journals, 605 Third Ave, New York, NY 10158. TEL 212-850-6021, 212-850-6645, subinfo@jwiley.com.

371.9144 GBR
DYSLEXIA HANDBOOK. Text in English. a.
—BLDSC (3637.237000).
Published by: British Dyslexia Association, 98 London Rd, Reading RG1 5AU, United Kingdom. TEL 44-118-966-2677, FAX 44-118-966-8271, info@dyslexiahelp-bda.demon.co.uk, http://www.bda-dyslexia.org.uk. Ed. Ian Smythe.

371.9 USA ISSN 1058-8396
EARLY INTERVENTION. Text in English. 1986. q. free per issue. bk.rev. back issues avail. **Document type:** *Newsletter.*
Published by: (Illinois Early Childhood Intervention Clearinghouse), Illinois Public Health Association, 223 S Third St, Springfield, IL 62701. TEL 217-522-5687. Ed. Chet Brandt. Circ: 4,900 (controlled). **Subscr. to:** 830 S Spring St, Springfield, IL 62701.

371.9 CAN ISSN 1482-8383
EASTER SEALS - MARCH OF DIMES NATIONAL COUNCIL. ANNUAL REPORT. Text in English, French. 1963. a. free per issue. **Document type:** *Corporate.* **Description:** Information on rehabilitation, fund raising services and the network of organizations improving the quality of life for the disabled.
Formerly: Canadian Rehabilitation Council for the Disabled. Annual Report (0068-9580)
Published by: Easter Seals - March of Dimes National Council, 90 Eglington Ave E, Ste 511, Toronto, ON M4P 2Y3, Canada. TEL 416-932-8382, FAX 416-932-9844, national.council@esmodnc.org, http://www.esmodnc.org. Circ: 2,000.

371.95 USA
EDUCATION AND PSYCHOLOGY OF THE GIFTED SERIES. Text in English. irreg. price varies. charts, illus. back issues avail. **Document type:** *Monographic series, Academic/Scholarly, Trade.*
Published by: Teachers College Press, Teachers College, Columbia University, 525 W 120th St, Box 303, New York, NY 10027-6694. http://www.teacherscollegepress.com. Pub. Carole Saltz. R&P Amy Detjen. **Dist. by:** Eurospan University Press Group, Order Dept, 3 Henrietta St, London WC2E 8LU, United Kingdom. TEL 44-20-7240-0856, FAX 44-20-7379-0609, http://www.eurospan.co.uk; Pademelon Press, Pty Ltd, 7-10 Anella Ave, PO Box 229, Castle Hill, NSW 2154, Australia. TEL 61-2-9634-2558, FAX 61-2-9680-4634; Transdex International, Pte Ltd, Block 1, Farrer Rd 307-05, Singapore 268817, Singapore. TEL 65-468-6242, FAX 65-462-5457.

371.928 USA ISSN 1079-3917
HV894
EDUCATION AND TRAINING IN MENTAL RETARDATION AND DEVELOPMENTAL DISABILITIES. Text in English. 1966. q. USD 30 domestic to individuals; USD 75 domestic to institutions; USD 79.50 foreign to institutions; USD 20 newsstand/cover (effective 2001). adv. bk.rev. illus. index. reprint service avail. from PQC,SCH,PSC. **Document type:** *Academic/Scholarly.* **Description:** Publishes research into the theory and methodology of teaching students with severe developmental disabilties.
Former titles (until 1993): Education and Training in Mental Retardation (1042-9859); (until Dec. 1986): Education and Training of the Mentally Retarded (0013-1237)
Related titles: Microform ed.: (from PQC); Online - full text ed.: (from H. W. Wilson, Institute for Scientific Information).
Indexed: ASCA, Adol.Ment.Hlth.Abstr., AgeLine, Behav.Med.Abstr., C.I.J.E., Cont.Pg.Educ., Curr.Cont., Educ.Admin.Abstr., Educ.Ind. (Apr.1983-Dec.1986), Except.Child Educ.Abstr., Excerp.Med., Fam.Ind., Lang.& Lang.Behav.Abstr., Mid.East: Abstr.& Ind., PsycInfo, Psychol.Abstr. (1971-), Rehabil.Lit., SOPODA, SSCI, Soc.Serv.Abstr., Soc.Work Res.& Abstr., Sociol.Abstr., Sp.Ed.Needs Abstr., e-psyche.
—BLDSC (3661.201000), GNLM, IDS, ingenta.
Published by: Council for Exceptional Children, Division on Mental Retardation and Developmental Disabilities, 1110 N Glebe Rd., Ste 300, Arlington, VA 22201-5704. TEL 703-620-3660, FAX 703-264-9494, http://www.mrddcec.org/publications.htm, http://www.cec.sped.org/. Ed. H Stanley Zucker. Circ: 8,000 (controlled).

371.9 USA
THE EDUCATIONAL THERAPIST. Text in English. 3/yr. USD 25 to non-members; USD 50 to institutions (effective 2000). *Refereed.* **Description:** Covers learning disabilities issues. For readers on the graduate level in the various disciplines that work with a learning disabled population.
Published by: Association of Educational Therapists, 1804 West Burbank Blvd, Burbank, CA 91506. TEL 818-843-1183, FAX 818-843-7423, aetla@aol.com. Ed. Li Moon.

371.9 GBR ISSN 0964-8690
EDUCATIONAL THERAPY & THERAPEUTIC TEACHING. Text in English. 1985. s-a. GBP 6 to non-members (effective 2000). bk.rev. index. back issues avail. **Document type:** *Academic/Scholarly.* **Description:** Explores the theory of educational therapy, a mode of treatment for persons with learning disabilities. Disseminates knowledge in the field among professionals and students in education, educational psychology, and related disciplines.
Formerly (until 1992): Journal of Educational Therapy (0952-4339)
Indexed: Br.Educ.Ind., Cont.Pg.Educ.
—BLDSC (3662.570000).
Published by: Forum for the Advancement of Educational Therapy and Therapeutic Teaching, Caspare House, 1 Noel Rd, London NI 8HQ, United Kingdom. TEL 020 7704 1977. Eds. Lee Marsden, Sue Davies.

EDUCAZIONE DEI SORDI. see *HANDICAPPED—Hearing Impaired*

371.94 GBR ISSN 1363-2752
EMOTIONAL AND BEHAVIOURAL DIFFICULTIES. Text in English. 1959. q. GBP 40 to individuals; GBP 11 newsstand/cover to individuals; GBP 132 to institutions; GBP 34 newsstand/cover to institutions (effective 2002). adv. bk.rev. *Refereed.* **Document type:** *Academic/Scholarly.* **Description:** Covers interests of disturbed children and promotes communication between professional workers involved with them. Regional and national events; monographs on specific topics.
Former titles (until 1996): Therapeutic Care and Education (0968-1728); Maladjustment and Therapeutic Education (0264-4614); New Growth (0261-0477); Therapeutic Education (0305-7860); Association of Workers for Maladjusted Children. Journal
Related titles: Online - full text ed.: (from O C L C Online Computer Library Center, Inc., ingenta, RoweCom Information Quest).
Indexed: ASSIA, Br.Educ.Ind., Cont.Pg.Educ., ERA, PsycInfo, Psychol.Abstr. (1984-), Sp.Ed.Needs Abstr., Tech.Educ.Abstr., e-psyche.
—BLDSC (3733.567500), GNLM.
Published by: (Association of Workers for Children with Emotional and Behavioral Difficulties), Sage Publications Ltd., 6 Bonhill St, London EC2A 4PU, United Kingdom. TEL 44-20-7374-0645, FAX 44-20-7374-8741, market@sagepub.co.uk, http://www.sagepub.co.uk. Ed., R&P, Adv. contact Paul Cooper TEL 44-1223-369631. Circ: 2,000. **Subscr. to:** Allan Rimmer, Administrative Officer, AWCEBD, Sutton, Charlton Ct, E, Maidstone, Kent ME17 3DQ, United Kingdom. TEL 44-1622-843104, FAX 44-1622-844220; **Subscr. to:** Sage Publications India Pvt. Ltd., P O Box 4215, New Delhi 110 048, India; Sage Publications, Inc., 2455 Teller Rd, Thousand Oaks, CA 91320.

371.928 USA
ENCOR RESPONDENCE. Text in English. q. free. **Document type:** *Newsletter.*
Published by: Eastern Nebraska Community Office of Retardation, 900 S 74th Plz, Ste 200, Omaha, NE 68114. Ed. Billie Dawson. Circ: 800 (free).

371.92 CAN ISSN 0829-8815
ENTOURAGE; the magazine promoting community living. Text in English, French. 1958. q. CND 19.26. adv. bk.rev. *Refereed.* **Document type:** *Consumer.* **Description:** Explores the issues affecting people with disabilities, their families and the advocates working for them. Keeps readers up-to-date on developments in the disability movement across Canada and around the world.

Incorporates (in Jun. 1988): Information Exchange Bulletin; Former titles (until 1986): Revue Canadienne de la Deficience Mentale - Canadian Journal on Mental Retardation; Deficience Mentale - Mental Retardation (0011-7668)
Indexed: C.I.J.E. (coverage dropped), Can.Educ.Ind., Can.Per.Ind. (Jan.1988-), Except.Child Educ.Abstr., GeoRef, Psychol.Abstr., Sp.Ed.Needs Abstr.
Published by: Roeher Institute at York University, c/ o Becker Associates, P O Box 507, Station Q, Toronto, ON M4T 2M5, Canada. TEL 416-661-9611, FAX 416-661-5701. Ed. Marguerite Martindale. Circ: 4,000.

371.9 DEU ISSN 0942-8623
ERGOTHERAPIE UND REHABILITATION. Text in German. 1962. 7/yr. DEM 80. adv. bk.rev. abstr, charts, illus. index. back issues avail. **Document type:** *Trade.*
Formerly (until 1993): Beschaeftigungstherapie und Rehabilitation (0340-529X)
Indexed: IBZ.
—GNLM.
Published by: (Deutscher Verband der Ergotherapeuten e.V.), Schulz - Kirchner Verlag GmbH, Mollweg 2, Idstein 65510, Germany. TEL 49-6126-9320-0, FAX 49-6126-9320-50. Ed. Christa Berting Hueneke. Adv. contact Doris Zimmermann. page DEM 2,030; trim 260 x 180. Circ: 13,350.

EXCEPTIONAL CHILD EDUCATION RESOURCES. see *EDUCATION—Abstracting, Bibliographies, Statistics*

371.9 155.4 USA ISSN 0014-4029
CODEN: EXCCAJ
EXCEPTIONAL CHILDREN. Text in English. 1934. q. USD 58; USD 66 foreign (effective 1999). adv. bibl, illus. index. reprint service avail. from PQC,PSC,SCH. *Refereed.* **Document type:** *Academic/Scholarly.* **Description:** Publishes current articles on critical and controversial issues in special education, as well as credible articles on research and developments in the field.
Related titles: Microfilm ed.: (from PQC); Online - full text ed.: (from Gale Group, ProQuest Information & Learning, Northern Light Technology, Inc., H. W. Wilson, Factiva, Institute for Scientific Information).
Indexed: ASCA, ASSIA, Acad.Ind., Adol.Ment.Hlth.Abstr., Bibl.Dev.Med.& Child Neur., C.I.J.E., Cont.Pg.Educ., Crim.Just.Abstr., Curr.Cont., ERA, Educ.Admin.Abstr., Educ.Ind. (Apr.1983-), Educ.Tech.Abstr., Except.Child Educ.Abstr., Excerp.Med., Fam.Ind., IBR, IBZ, IMFL, Ind.Med. (coverage dropped), L.R.I., Lang.& Lang.Behav.Abstr., Media Rev.Dig. (Jan.1989-Dec.1991), Mult.Ed.Abstr., PsycInfo, Psychol.Abstr. (1935-), Psycscan D.P., Rehabil.Lit., SOMA, SOPODA, SSCI, Soc.Work Res.& Abstr., Sociol.Abstr., Sociol.Educ.Abstr., Sp.Ed.Needs Abstr., Tech.Educ.Abstr., e-psyche.
—BLDSC (3835.300000), GNLM, IDS, ingenta.
Published by: Council for Exceptional Children, 1920 Association Drive, Reston, VA 22091. TEL 703-620-3660, FAX 703-264-9494, cecpubs@cec.sped.org, http://www.cec.sped.org/ec-jour.htm. Eds. Bob Algozzine, Martha Thurlow. R&P Melinda MacDonald. Adv. contact Victor Erickson. Circ: 58,000.

371.91 362.4 USA ISSN 0046-9157
EXCEPTIONAL PARENT; the magazine for families and professionals. Text in English. 1971. m. USD 36 domestic; USD 47 in Canada (effective 2001). adv. bk.rev. illus. Index. back issues avail.; reprint service avail. from PQC,PSC,SCH. **Document type:** *Consumer.* **Description:** Source of help and guidance for the parents of children and young adults with disabilities and special health needs and the professionals who serve them.
Related titles: Microfilm ed.: (from PQC); Online - full text ed.: (from Gale Group, ProQuest Information & Learning, Northern Light Technology, Inc., H. W. Wilson, Factiva).
Indexed: C.I.J.E. (coverage dropped), CINAHL, Educ.Ind. (Apr.1983-), Except.Child Educ.Abstr., Fam.Ind., Hlth.Ind., IMFL, Ind.Med. (coverage dropped), Ment.Retard.Abstr., Psychol.Abstr., Rehabil.Lit., Sp.Ed.Needs Abstr., Yrbk.Assoc.Educ.& Rehab.Blind.
—BLDSC (3835.500000), ingenta. **CCC.**
Published by: Psy-Ed. Corp., 555 Kinderkamack Road, Oradell, NJ 07649-1517. TEL 201-634-6550, epmag12@aol.com, http://families.com. Ed. Rick Rader. Pub. Joseph M Valenzano. R&P Bridget M Lyne. Circ: 65,000 (paid); 33,000 (controlled).

371.95 CAN ISSN 1183-322X
EXCEPTIONALITY EDUCATION CANADA. Text in English. 1991. 3/yr. CND 30 domestic to individuals; USD 30 foreign to individuals; CND 50 domestic to institutions; USD 50 foreign to institutions; CND 20 domestic to students; USD 20 foreign to students. *Refereed.* **Document type:** *Academic/Scholarly.* **Description:** Provides a forum for scholarly exchange among Canadian professionals in education and related disciplines who are involved with students across the spectrum of exceptionality.
Related titles: Microform ed.: (from MML).
Indexed: Can.Educ.Ind., Except.Child Educ.Abstr.
—BLDSC (3835.570000). **CCC.**
Published by: University of Prince Edward Island, c/o Vianne Timmons, Dean of Education, 550 University Ave, Charlottetown, PE C1A 4P3, Canada. Ed., R&P Vianne Timmons TEL 902-566-0330. Circ: 250.

371.91 USA ISSN 0015-4288
HV1796
FLORIDA SCHOOL HERALD. Text in English. 1891. 6/yr. USD 6 (effective 2000). abstr, illus. **Document type:** *Newsletter.* **Description:** Highlights education of the deaf and blind.
Published by: Florida School for the Deaf and the Blind, 207 North San Marco Ave., St. Augustine, FL 32084-2799. TEL 904-827-2219, FAX 904-827-2218, http://www.fsdb.k12.fl.us. Ed. Kathy Gillespie. Circ: 1,550 (controlled).

FOCAL POINT; a national bulletin on family support and children's mental health. see *HANDICAPPED*

FOCUS ON AUTISM AND OTHER DEVELOPMENTAL DISABILITIES. see *MEDICAL SCIENCES—Psychiatry And Neurology*

371.95 USA ISSN 0015-511X
FOCUS ON EXCEPTIONAL CHILDREN. Text in English. 1969. 9/yr. (Sep.-May). USD 36 (effective 2001). adv. bk.rev. illus. index. 16 p./no. back issues avail.; reprint service avail. from PQC. **Document type:** *Academic/Scholarly.*
Related titles: CD-ROM ed.; Microform ed.: (from PQC); Online - full text ed.: (from Northern Light Technology, Inc., H. W. Wilson, ProQuest Information & Learning, Institute for Scientific Information).
Indexed: ASCA, C.I.J.E., Cont.Pg.Educ., Curr.Cont., Educ.Ind. (May 1983-), Except.Child Educ.Abstr., Rehabil.Lit., SSCI.
—BLDSC (3964.215000), IDS, ingenta.
Published by: Love Publishing Co., PO Box 22353, Denver, CO 80222. TEL 303-221-7333, FAX 303-221-7444. Ed. Stanley F Love. Circ: 3,000.

FUTURE REFLECTIONS. see *HANDICAPPED—Visually Impaired*

371.9 DEU ISSN 0932-934X
G W G - ZEITSCHRIFT. Text in German. 1971. q. DEM 40. adv. bk.rev. back issues avail.
Formerly: G W G-Info
—GNLM.
Published by: Gesellschaft fuer Wissenschaftliche Gespraechspsychotherapie e.V., Richard-Wagner-Str 12, Cologne 51145, Germany. TEL 0221-252917. Ed. Michael Behr. Circ: 8,000.

GATHERED VIEW; national newsletter of the Prader-Willi syndrome Assn. (USA). see *MEDICAL SCIENCES*

371.928 DEU ISSN 0173-9573
GEISTIGE BEHINDERUNG; Fachzeitschrift der Lebenshilfe fuer geistig Behinderte. Text in German. 1962. q. DEM 44 (effective 2001). adv. bk.rev. illus. index. **Document type:** *Journal, Academic/Scholarly.* **Description:** Directed to specialists working with the mentally retarded. Focus is on development, education, social adaptation, special problems. Also lists available positions.
Formerly (until 1980): Lebenshilfe (0023-995X)
Indexed: IBR, IBZ, e-psyche.
—GNLM.
Published by: Bundesvereinigung Lebenshilfe fuer Menschen mit Geistiger Behinderung e.V., Postfach 701163, Marburg 35020, Germany. TEL 49-6421-491-0, FAX 49-6421-491167. Ed. Theo Fruehauf. Adv. contact Ursula Dahlstroem. Circ: 8,500.

371.95 USA ISSN 0016-9862
LC3991 CODEN: GICQAC
GIFTED CHILD QUARTERLY. Text in English. 1957. q. USD 50 domestic to membership; USD 60 foreign to membership (effective 1999). adv. bk.rev. illus. back issues avail.; reprint service avail. from SCH,PSC. *Refereed.* **Document type:** *Academic/Scholarly.* **Description:** For educational researchers, administrators, teachers and parents of gifted children. Publishes research and theoretical papers on the nature and needs of high-ability children.
Related titles: Microfilm ed.: (from PQC); Online - full text ed.: (from Gale Group, Factiva, Institute for Scientific Information).
Indexed: ASCA, ASSIA, Acad.Ind., Arts & Hum.Cit.Ind. (coverage dropped), C.I.J.E., Child Devel.Abstr., Cont.Pg.Educ., Curr.Cont., Educ.Ind. (Apr.1983-), Except.Child Educ.Abstr., Fam.Ind., IMFL, L.R.I., PsycInfo, Psychol.Abstr. (1958-), SSCI, e-psyche.
—BLDSC (4175.300000), ingenta.
Published by: National Association for Gifted Children, 1707 L St, N W, Ste 550, Washington, DC 20036-4201. TEL 202-785-4268, FAX 202-785-4268, nagc@nagc.org, http://www.nagc.org/publications/giftedchild/index.html. Ed. Tracy L Cross. R&P Peter Rosenstein. Adv. contact Cora Powers. B&W page USD 700; trim 11 x 8.5. Circ: 6,500 (paid).

371.95 USA ISSN 0740-560X
GIFTED UNLIMITED. Text in English. m. USD 25 includes membership. **Document type:** *Newsletter.*
Published by: Northwest Gifted Child Association, PO Box 1226, Bellevue, WA 98009. TEL 206-649-8546, 800-864-2073. Ed. Howard Modell. Circ: 375.

GONG; mesicnik sluchove postizenych. see *HANDICAPPED—Hearing Impaired*

371.91 USA ISSN 1090-3364
THE GRAM. Text in English. 1968. q. USD 15 domestic; USD 30 foreign (effective 2000). adv. bk.rev., film rev., software rev. charts. *Refereed.* **Document type:** *Newsletter.*
Formerly: C A N H C - Gram (California Association for Neurologically Handicapped Children)
Published by: Learning Disabilities Association of California (L D A - C A), 655 Lewelling Blvd, Ste 355, San Leandro, CA 94579. TEL 916-725-7881, FAX 916-725-8786, Theamclean@aol.com, http://www.LDACA.org. Ed., Pub., R&P, Adv. contact Betty G Schiemenz. B&W page USD 500; trim 7.5 x 9.25. Circ: 3,600. **Dist. by:** Thea McLean, 6060 Sunrise Vista Dr., Ste.1550, Citrus Heights, CA 95610. TEL 510-352-9469, FAX 510-352-8283.

371.91 NOR
HANDICAP IDRETT. Text in Norwegian. bi-m. adv.
Published by: (Norges Handicapidrettsforbund), Per Sletholt og Co., Postboks 57, Tveita, Oslo, 6, Norway.

HEIDELBERGER BEITRAEGE ZUR GEHOERLOSENBILDUNG UND SCHWERHOERIGENBILDUNG. see *HANDICAPPED—Hearing Impaired*

HEILPAEDAGOGISCHE FORSCHUNG; Zeitschrift fuer Paedagogik und Psychologie Behinderter. see *MEDICAL SCIENCES—Psychiatry And Neurology*

371.95 GBR ISSN 1359-8139
LC3991
HIGH ABILITY STUDIES. Text in English. 1990. 2/yr. GBP 43, USD 66 to individuals; GBP 146, USD 241 to institutions (effective 2002). **Document type:** *Academic/Scholarly.* **Description:** Offers a medium of scientific, scholarly and practical communication among researchers and practitioners in the field of giftedness.
Formerly (until vol.7): European Journal for High Ability (0937-4450)
Related titles: Online - full text ed.: ISSN 1469-834X (from CatchWord Ltd., Northern Light Technology, Inc., EBSCO Publishing, ProQuest Information & Learning, Swets Blackwell, Institute for Scientific Information, RoweCom Information Quest).
Indexed: Br.Educ.Ind., Cont.Pg.Educ., Curr.Cont., ERA, Except.Child Educ.Abstr., PsycInfo, Res.High.Educ.Abstr., SSCI, Stud.Wom.Abstr., e-psyche.
—BLDSC (4307.283450), CatchWord. **CCC.**
Published by: (European Council for High Ability), Carfax Publishing Limited (Subsidiary of: Taylor & Francis Group), Carfax Publishing Co, PO Box 24, Abingdon, Oxon OX14 3UE, United Kingdom. TEL 44-1235-401000, FAX 44-1235-401550, enquiries@carfax.co.uk, enquiries@carfax.co.uk/, http://www.carfax.co.uk. Ed. A Cropley.

E

371.91 DNK ISSN 1395-1912
HIT. Text in Danish. 1988. 5/yr. (includes 1 book). DKK 375 (effective 2001). adv. bk.rev. **Document type:** *Academic/Scholarly.*
Former titles (until 1995): Via Datch (0903-9821); (until 1988): Mikronyt i Specialundervisningen (0900-6230)
Published by: Danish Centre for Rehabilitation and Special Education, Graham Bells Vej 1 A, Aarhus N 8200, Denmark. TEL 45-86-78-37-00, FAX 45-86-78-37-30, tb.mikkelsen@hmi.dk. Eds. Marianne Henriksen, Trine Bjerre Mikkelsen. Adv. contact Trine G Bak. Circ: 1,700.

HOERGESCHAEDIGTE KINDER. see *HANDICAPPED—Hearing Impaired*

HOME CARE FAMILY NEWSLETTER. see *SOCIAL SERVICES AND WELFARE*

HYDROCEPHALUS NEWS & NOTES. see *MEDICAL SCIENCES—Psychiatry And Neurology*

371.93 AUS ISSN 0810-6398
HYPER ACTIVITIES. Text in English. 1976. 8/yr. AUD 15 (effective 1999). adv. bk.rev. index. back issues avail. **Document type:** *Newsletter.* **Description:** Discusses diet behavior management, medication, hyperactivity, attention deficit disorder.
Indexed: e-psyche.
Published by: Hyperactivity Attention Deficit Association (N.S.W.), 15-29 Bertram St, Chatswood, NSW 2067, Australia. hyperadd@bigpond.com. Ed., Pub., R&P, Adv. contact Roslyn Mitchell. page AUD 200. Circ: 500.

I F H O H JOURNAL. see *HANDICAPPED—Hearing Impaired*

371.9 FRA
INTERNATIONAL ASSOCIATION OF WORKERS FOR TROUBLED CHILDREN AND YOUTH. CONGRESS REPORTS. Text in English, French. 1955. quadrennial. USD 30. **Document type:** *Proceedings, Bulletin.*
Formerly: International Association of Workers for Maladjusted Children. Congress Report (0074-1787)
Published by: International Association of Workers for Troubled Children and Youth, E.E.S., 22 rue Halevy, Lille 59000, France.

371.91 362.4 GBR ISSN 1034-912X
LC4661 CODEN: IJDEFF
INTERNATIONAL JOURNAL OF DISABILITY, DEVELOPMENT AND EDUCATION. Text in English. 1954. q. GBP 74, USD 122 to individuals; GBP 199, USD 326 to institutions (effective 2002). adv. bk.rev. bibl, charts, illus. Index. reprint service avail. from PSC. *Refereed.* **Document type:** *Academic/Scholarly.* **Description:** Reflects a variety of topics, disciplines, research methods and cultural perspectives. Various orientations are represented including special education, psychology, and social work.
Former titles (until 1990): Exceptional Child (0156-6555); Slow Learning Child (0037-704X)
Related titles: Microfilm ed.: (from NRP); Online - full text ed.: ISSN 1465-346X (from CatchWord Ltd., EBSCO Publishing, H. W. Wilson, O C L C Online Computer Library Center, Inc., RoweCom Information Quest, Swets Blackwell).
Indexed: AMED, ASSIA, Aus.Educ.Ind., C.I.J.E., Cont.Pg.Educ., Curr.Cont. (coverage dropped), ERA, Educ.Ind. (Jun.1992-), Educ.Tech.Abstr., Except.Child Educ.Abstr., Ind.Philos., Lang.& Lang.Behav.Abstr., Mid.East: Abstr.& Ind., Mult.Ed.Abstr., PsycInfo, Psychol.Abstr. (1964-), Res.High.Educ.Abstr., SOMA, SOPODA, SSCI (coverage dropped), Sociol.Abstr., Sociol.Educ.Abstr., Sp.Ed.Needs Abstr., e-psyche.
—BLDSC (4542.185450), CatchWord, ingenta. **CCC.**
Published by: (Fred and Eleanor Schonell Educational Research Centre), Carfax Publishing Limited (Subsidiary of: Taylor & Francis Group), PO Box 25, Abingdon, Oxon OX14 3UE, United Kingdom. TEL 44-1235-401000, FAX 44-1235-401550, enquiries@carfax.co.uk, enquiry@tandf.co.uk, http://www.carfax.co.uk/ijd-ad.htm. Adv. contact Robert Brown. Circ: 1,400.

INTERNATIONAL JOURNAL OF LANGUAGE AND COMMUNICATION DISORDERS. see *MEDICAL SCIENCES—Otorhinolaryngology*

INTERNATIONAL JOURNAL OF REHABILITATION RESEARCH. see *MEDICAL SCIENCES—Physical Medicine And Rehabilitation*

371.9 BRN ISSN 0827-3383
INTERNATIONAL JOURNAL OF SPECIAL EDUCATION. Text in English. 1985. s-a. USD 30 to individuals; USD 45 to institutions (effective 1999). adv. **Document type:** *Academic/Scholarly.* **Description:** Descriptive research articles on special education worldwide.
Related titles: Microfiche ed.: (from MML); Microform ed.: (from MML).
Indexed: Can.Educ.Ind., Cont.Pg.Educ., ERA, Except.Child Educ.Abstr., Sp.Ed.Needs Abstr.
—BLDSC (4542.665000). **CCC.**
Published by: International Association of Special Education, c/o Dr. Marg Csapo, Special Education Unit, Ministry of Education, Bandar Seri Begawan, Brunei Darussalam. TEL 673-446-553, csapobru@ppl.brunet.bn. Ed. Marg Csapo. adv.: B&W page USD 100. Circ: 500.

INTERNATIONAL REVIEW OF RESEARCH IN MENTAL RETARDATION. see *MEDICAL SCIENCES—Psychiatry And Neurology*

371.9 USA ISSN 1053-4512
LC4001 CODEN: ISCLEP
INTERVENTION IN SCHOOL AND CLINIC. Text in English. 1965. 5/yr. USD 39 in North America to individuals; USD 71 elsewhere to individuals; USD 109 in North America to institutions; USD 150 elsewhere to institutions (effective 2002). bk.rev. bibl, charts, illus. Index. back issues avail.; reprint service avail. from SCH,PSC. *Refereed.* **Document type:** *Journal, Academic/Scholarly.* **Description:** Interdisciplinary journal directed to an international audience of teachers, parents, educational therapists and specialists in all fields, who deal with the day-to-day aspects of special and remedial education.
Formerly: Academic Therapy (0001-396X)
Related titles: Microfilm ed.: (from PQC); Online - full text ed.: (from H. W. Wilson, ProQuest Information & Learning, Institute for Scientific Information, CatchWord Ltd.).
Indexed: ASCA, ASSIA, Arts & Hum.Cit.Ind. (coverage dropped), C.I.J.E., Cont.Pg.Educ., Curr.Cont., DSH Abstr., ERA, Educ.Ind. (Sep.1990-), Except.Child Educ.Abstr., Fam.Ind., IBZ, Lang.& Lang.Behav.Abstr., Psychol.Abstr., Rehabil.Lit., SOPODA, SSCI, Sociol.Abstr., Sp.Ed.Needs Abstr., e-psyche.
—BLDSC (4557.471850), GNLM, IDS, Infotrieve, ingenta. **CCC.**
Published by: Pro-Ed Inc., 8700 Shoal Creek Blvd, Austin, TX 78757-6897. TEL 512-451-3246, FAX 512-302-9129, proed1@aol.com, http://www.proedinc.com. Ed. Brenda Smith Myles. Pub. Donald D Hammill. Adv. contact Allison Turrell. Circ: 2,800.

ISBI.COM. (Independent or Fee-paying Schools in the British Isles) see *EDUCATION—Guides To Schools And Colleges*

ITALIAN JOURNAL OF INTELLECTIVE IMPAIRMENT/RIVISTA ITALIANA DEL DISTURBO INTELLETTIVO. see *MEDICAL SCIENCES—Psychiatry And Neurology*

JAHRBUCH FUER BLINDENFREUNDE. see *HANDICAPPED—Visually Impaired*

JOURNAL OF ABNORMAL CHILD PSYCHOLOGY. see *PSYCHOLOGY*

JOURNAL OF ATTENTION DISORDERS. see *MEDICAL SCIENCES—Psychiatry And Neurology*

371.94 USA ISSN 0162-3257
RJ499.A1 CODEN: JADDDQ
JOURNAL OF AUTISM AND DEVELOPMENTAL DISORDERS. Text in English. 1971. bi-m. USD 649, EUR 648 to institutions for print or online ed.; USD 89, EUR 89 to individuals for pirnt or online ed.; USD 778.80, EUR 777.60 to institutions for print & online eds. combined (effective 2002). adv. bk.rev. abstr, charts, illus, stat. index. back issues avail.; reprint service avail. from PSC,SCH. *Refereed.* **Document type:** *Journal, Academic/Scholarly.* **Description:** Includes research covering the psychopathologies in childhood, including autism and childhood schizophrenia. Publishes experimental studies on the biochemical, neurological, and genetic aspects of a particular disorder; the implications for normal development; and the interaction between disordered behavior of individuals and social or group factors.
Formerly (until 1979): Journal of Autism and Childhood Schizophrenia (0021-9185)
Related titles: Microfilm ed.: (from PQC); Online - full text ed.: (from Ovid Technologies, Inc., EBSCO Publishing, O C L C Online Computer Library Center, Inc., RoweCom Information Quest, Swets Blackwell, Kluwer Online, Institute for Scientific Information).
Indexed: AMED, ASCA, ASSIA, Bibl.Dev.Med.& Child Neur., Biol.Abstr., C.I.J.E., CINAHL, Chem.Abstr., Child Devel.Abstr., Curr.Cont., Educ.Ind. (Jun.1983-), Except.Child Educ.Abstr., Excerp.Med., Fam.Ind., IMFL, INIS Atomind., Ind.Med. (1979-), Mid.East: Abstr.& Ind., Neurosci.Cit.Ind., PsycInfo, Psychol.Abstr. (1971-), Psycscan D.P., Ref.Zh., Risk Abstr., SSCI, Soc.Work Res.& Abstr., e-psyche.
—BLDSC (4949.552000), CISTI, GNLM, IDS, Infotrieve, ingenta, KNAW. **CCC.**
Published by: (Autism Society of America), Kluwer Academic - Plenum Publishers (Subsidiary of: Wolters Kluwer N.V.), 233 Spring St, New York, NY 10013-1578. TEL 212-620-8000, 800-221-9369, FAX 212-463-0742, info@plenum.com, http://www.wkap.nl/journalhome.htm/0162-3257. Ed. Gary B Mesibov. R&P Rose Luongo TEL 781-871-6311. **Subscr. outside the Americas to:** Kluwer Academic Publishers Group, Journals Department, PO Box 322, Dordrecht 3300 AH, Netherlands. TEL 31-78-639-2392, FAX 31-78-654-6474.

JOURNAL OF CHILD AND ADOLESCENT PSYCHIATRIC NURSING. see *MEDICAL SCIENCES—Nurses And Nursing*

JOURNAL OF COMMUNICATION DISORDERS. see *PSYCHOLOGY*

JOURNAL OF DEVELOPMENTAL AND PHYSICAL DISABILITIES. see *HANDICAPPED*

371.95 USA ISSN 1053-8151
LC4019.2
JOURNAL OF EARLY INTERVENTION. Text in English. 1979. q. USD 50 domestic to individuals; USD 74 foreign to individuals; USD 70 domestic to institutions; USD 74 foreign to institutions (effective 2001). adv. bk.rev. illus. Index. back issues avail.; reprints avail. *Refereed.* **Document type:** *Journal, Academic/Scholarly, Trade.* **Description:** Features current research, exemplary practices, family involvement, personnel preparation, collaborative efforts, legislation, and technology for professionals.
Formerly (until 1989): Council of Exceptional Children. Division for Early Childhood. Journal (0885-3460)
Related titles: Online - full text ed.: (from Institute for Scientific Information).
Indexed: ASCA, C.I.J.E., Cont.Pg.Educ., Curr.Cont., ERA, Except.Child Educ.Abstr., Fam.Ind., Mult.Ed.Abstr., PsycInfo, Psychol.Abstr. (1989-), SSCI, Sp.Ed.Needs Abstr., e-psyche.
—BLDSC (4970.705000), IDS, ingenta.
Published by: Council for Exceptional Children, Division for Early Childhood, 1380 Lawrence St Ste 650, Denver, CO 80204. TEL 303-556-3328, FAX 303-556-3310, http://www.fpg.unc.edu/~jei/. Ed. R A McWilliam. Adv. contact Robin McWilliam. B&W page USD 300. Circ: 7,000. **Subscr. to:** Allen Press Inc., PO Box 1897, Lawrence, KS 66044-8897.

JOURNAL OF EMOTIONAL AND BEHAVIORAL DISORDERS. see *MEDICAL SCIENCES—Psychiatry And Neurology*

371.9 GBR ISSN 1469-0047
JOURNAL OF LEARNING DISABILITIES. Text in English. 1997. q. GBP 37 to individuals; GBP 210 to institutions; GBP 10 newsstand/cover to individuals; GBP 54 newsstand/cover to institutions (effective 2002). bk.rev. *Refereed.* **Document type:** *Academic/Scholarly.* **Description:** Provides a medium for the exchange of best practice, knowledge, and research between the academic and professional disciplines of education, social and health care, who are committed to the advancement of services for people with learning disabilities.
Formerly (until 2000): Journal of Learning Disabilities for Nursing, Health and Social Care (1362-0177)
Related titles: Online - full text ed.: (from ingenta, Swets Blackwell, RoweCom Information Quest).
Indexed: Br.Educ.Ind., Brit.Nur.Ind., Fam.Ind., MLA Intl.Bibl. (coverage dropped).
—BLDSC (5010.230050).
Published by: Sage Publications Ltd., 6 Bonhill St, London EC2A 4PU, United Kingdom. TEL 44-20-7330-1266, FAX 44-20-7374-8741, market@sagepub.co.uk, http://www.sagepub.co.uk. Ed. Bob Gates.

E

371.91 USA ISSN 0022-2194
LB1134 CODEN: JLDIAD
JOURNAL OF LEARNING DISABILITIES. Text in English. 1967. bi-m., latest vol.34. USD 54 in North America to individuals; USD 88 elsewhere to individuals; USD 138 in North America to institutions; USD 161 elsewhere to institutions (effective 2002). adv. bibl, charts, illus. index. back issues avail.; reprint service avail. from PSC,SCH. *Refereed.* **Document type:** *Journal, Academic/Scholarly.* **Description:** Contains articles on practice, research, and theory related to learning disabilities.
Related titles: Microform ed.: (from NRP,PQC); Online - full text ed.: (from H. W. Wilson, ProQuest Information & Learning, Gale Group, Institute for Scientific Information, CatchWord Ltd.).
Indexed: AMED, ASCA, ASSIA, Adol.Ment.Hlth.Abstr., Bibl.Dev.Med.& Child Neur., Biol.Abstr., Bk.Rev.Ind. (1975-1990), C.I.J.E., CINAHL, Child Devel.Abstr., Cont.Pg.Educ., Curr.Cont., Educ.Admin.Abstr., Educ.Ind. (Apr.1983-), Educ.Tech.Abstr., Except.Child Educ.Abstr., Excerp.Med., High.Educ.Abstr., High.Educ.Curr.Aware.Bull., IBR, IBZ, IMFL, Ind.Med. (1968-), Ind.Philos., Int.Nurs.Ind., Lang.& Lang.Behav.Abstr., MLA Intl.Bibl., Mid.East: Abstr.& Ind., Mult.Ed.Abstr., Neurosci.Cit.Ind., P.A.I.S., PsycInfo, Psychol.Abstr. (1968-), Psycscan D.P., Rehabil.Lit., SOMA, SOPODA, SSCI, Sociol.Abstr., Sp.Ed.Needs Abstr., Tech.Educ.Abstr., Yrbk.Assoc.Educ.& Rehab.Blind.
—BLDSC (5010.230000), GNLM, IDS, ingenta. **CCC.**
Published by: Pro-Ed Inc., 8700 Shoal Creek Blvd, Austin, TX 78757-6897. TEL 512-451-3246, FAX 512-302-9129, proed1@aol.com, http://www.proedinc.com. Ed. Wayne P. Hresko. Pub. Donald D Hammill. adv.: B&W page USD 800, color page USD 1,000. Circ: 7,000.

JOURNAL OF OUTCOME MEASUREMENT; dedicated to health, education, and social science. (JOM) see *EDUCATION*

371.91 CAN ISSN 0707-7807
JOURNAL OF PRACTICAL APPROACHES TO DEVELOPMENTAL HANDICAP. Text in English. 1977. s-a. CND 11 to individuals; CND 14 to institutions. adv. bk.rev. abstr, illus, stat. back issues avail. *Refereed.* **Document type:** *Academic/Scholarly.* **Description:** Concerned with disability, practice and applied research in the field of rehabilitation.
Related titles: Microfiche ed.: (from MML); Microform ed.: (from MML).
Indexed: ASSIA, Sp.Ed.Needs Abstr.
—Infotrieve. **CCC.**
Published by: University of Calgary, Rehabilitation Studies, c/o Rehabilitation Studies, Education Tower 4th Fl, University of Calgary, 2500 University Dr, N W, Calgary, AB T2N 1N4, Canada. TEL 403-220-7429, FAX 403-284-5569, aneufeld@acs.ucalgary.ca. Ed. Aldred Neufeldt. Circ: 450. **Co-sponsor:** Vocational and Rehabilitation Research Institute.

371.9 USA ISSN 0022-4669
LC4001 CODEN: JSPEB9
THE JOURNAL OF SPECIAL EDUCATION. Text in English. 1966. q., latest vol.35. USD 43 in North America to individuals; USD 71 elsewhere to individuals; USD 109 in North America to institutions; USD 138 elsewhere to institutions (effective 2002). adv. abstr, bibl, charts, illus, stat. index. back issues avail.; reprint service avail. from SCH,PSC. *Refereed.* **Document type:** *Journal, Academic/Scholarly.* **Description:** Contains research articles in all subspecialities of special education for individuals with disabilities from mild to severe.
Related titles: Microform ed.: (from NRP,PQC); Online - full text ed.: (from H. W. Wilson, ProQuest Information & Learning, Gale Group, Institute for Scientific Information, CatchWord Ltd.).
Indexed: ASCA, ASSIA, C.I.J.E., Child Devel.Abstr., Cont.Pg.Educ., Curr.Cont., Curr.Ind.Stat., Curr.Lit.Fam.Plan., ERA, Educ.Admin.Abstr., Educ.Ind. (Mar.1983-), Educ.Tech.Abstr., Except.Child Educ.Abstr., Excerp.Med., Fam.Ind., High.Educ.Curr.Aware.Bull., IBZ, Lang.& Lang.Behav.Abstr., Ment.Retard.Abstr., Mult.Ed.Abstr., P.A.I.S., PsycInfo, Psychol.Abstr. (1966-), Rehabil.Lit., SOPODA, SSCI, Soc.Serv.Abstr., Sociol.Abstr., Sociol.Educ.Abstr., Tech.Educ.Abstr., Yrbk.Assoc.Educ.& Rehab.Blind, e-psyche.
—BLDSC (5066.120000), IDS, ingenta. **CCC.**
Published by: Pro-Ed Inc., 8700 Shoal Creek Blvd, Austin, TX 78757-6897. TEL 512-451-3246, FAX 512-302-9129, proed1@aol.com, http://www.proedinc.com. Ed. Douglas Fuchs. Pub. Donald D Hammill. Adv. contact Allison Turrell. B&W page USD 400. Circ: 4,000 (paid and free).

JOURNAL ON DEVELOPMENTAL DISABILITIES/ JOURNAL SUR LES HANDICAPS DU DEVELOPPEMENT. see *MEDICAL SCIENCES—Psychiatry And Neurology*

371.9 USA ISSN 0739-909X
L D A NEWSBRIEFS; items of interest on learning disabilities. Text in English. 1978 (no.118). bi-m. USD 15; USD 35 foreign (effective 1999). adv. bk.rev. **Document type:** *Newsletter.* **Description:** Provides information on learning disabilities to the community of educators and others who are interested.
Formerly: A C L D Newsbriefs (Association for Children and Adults with Learning Disabilities)
Published by: Learning Disabilities Association of America, 4156 Library Rd, Pittsburgh, PA 15234. TEL 412-341-1515, FAX 412-344-0224, ldnatl@usaor.net, http://www.danatl.org. Ed., R&P Lynne Cannon. Adv. contact Andrea Turkheimer. Circ: 50,000.

371.91 USA
THE L D READER. (Learning Disabilities) Text in English. 1995. irreg., latest vol.61. free (effective 2000). back issues avail. **Document type:** *Newsletter.* **Description:** Offers persons with learning disabilities and their families support in dealing with their condition. Seeks to foster public awareness and understanding of learning disabilities by disseminating practical information and dispelling common myths.
Media: Online - full text.
Indexed: e-psyche.
Published by: L D Reader, 202 Lake Rd, New, Preston, CT 06777. TEL 860-868-3214, ldr@ldresources.com; richard@ldresources.com, http://www.ldresources.com. Ed. Richard Wanderman.

371.928 USA ISSN 0163-2205
L I N K S. (Living in New Kinds of Situations) Text in English. 1970. m. adv. bk.rev. **Document type:** *Newspaper, Trade.* **Description:** A publication for private providers serving people with disabilities.
Indexed: Cont.Pg.Educ.
Published by: (American Network for Community Options Resources), A N C O R, 1101 King St. Suite 380, Alexandria, VA 22314. TEL 703-535-7850, FAX 703-535-7860, http://www.ancor.org/links.html. adv.: page USD 600. Circ: 7,000.

LANGUAGE, SPEECH AND HEARING SERVICES IN SCHOOLS. see *MEDICAL SCIENCES—Otorhinolaryngology*

371.9 USA ISSN 1046-6819
LEARNING DISABILITIES (PITTSBURGH); a multidisciplinary journal. Text in English. 1989. s-a. USD 25 (effective 1999). *Refereed.* **Description:** Covers all forms of learning disabilities from a multidisciplinary perspective.
Indexed: C.I.J.E.
—BLDSC (5179.326380).
Published by: Learning Disabilities Association of America, 4156 Library Rd, Pittsburgh, PA 15234. TEL 412-341-1515, FAX 412-344-0224. Ed. Dr. Janet Learner. Circ: 800 (paid).

371.9 USA ISSN 0938-8982
LC4704 CODEN: LDRPE6
LEARNING DISABILITIES RESEARCH AND PRACTICE. Text in English. 1991. q. USD 120 single user; USD 395 multi user; USD 96 to members (effective 2002). adv. **Document type:** *Journal, Academic/Scholarly.* **Description:** Covers current research of interest to teachers, teacher educators and researchers.
Formed by the merger of (1985-1991): Learning Disabilities Research (0892-502X); (1985-1991): Learning Disabilities Focus (0892-5011)
Media: Online - full content. **Related titles:** Online - full text ed.: (from RoweCom Information Quest, CatchWord Ltd.).
Indexed: C.I.J.E., Cont.Pg.Educ., Except.Child Educ.Abstr., PsycInfo, Psychol.Abstr. (1991-), Sp.Ed.Needs Abstr., Tech.Educ.Abstr., e-psyche.
—CCC.
Published by: (Division for Learning Disabilities, Council for Exceptional Children), Lawrence Erlbaum Associates, Inc., 10 Industrial Ave, Mahwah, NJ 07430-2262. TEL 201-760-3735, 800-926-6579, FAX 201-236-0072, journals@erlbaum.com, http://alidoro.catchword.com/vl=2250773/cl=14/nw=1/rpsv/cw/erlbaum/09388982/contp1.htm, http://www.erlbaum.com. Eds. Deborah L Speece, Sharon Vaughn. adv.: page USD 550; trim 7 x 10. Circ: 14,000.

371.9 GBR ISSN 1465-8712
▼ **LEARNING DISABILITY PRACTICE.** Text in English. 1999. bi-m. GBP 60 in Europe to institutions; GBP 76 elsewhere to institutions (effective 2002). adv. **Document type:** *Academic/Scholarly.* **Description:** Provides material that is accessible, topical and jargon-free for the specialist nurse and care giver.
Indexed: Brit.Nur.Ind., e-psyche.
—BLDSC (5179.326485).
Published by: (Royal College of Nursing), R C N Publishing Co. (Subsidiary of: B M J Publishing Group), R C N Direct, Copse Walk, Cardiff Gate Business Park, Cardiff CF23 8XG, United Kingdom. TEL 44-29-2054-6450, FAX 44-29-2054-6401, directjournalsteam@rcn.org.uk, http://www.rcn.org.uk/. Ed. John Turnbull. Adv. contact Phil Whomes. Circ: 900 (controlled).

371.9 DEU
LEBENSHILFE AKTUELL. Text in German. 1975. bi-m. adv. back issues avail. **Document type:** *Journal, Academic/Scholarly.* **Description:** Provides information about mental handicaps.
Published by: Bundesvereinigung Lebenshilfe fuer Menschen mit Geistiger Behinderung e.V., Postfach 701163, Marburg 35020, Germany. TEL 49-6421-491-0, FAX 49-6421-491167. Eds. Dr. Bernhard Conrads, Juergen Reuter. Adv. contact Ursula Dahlstroem. Circ: 125,000.

LIGHT (WHEATON). see *HANDICAPPED—Visually Impaired*

LOGOPEDIE EN FONIATRIE; vaktijdschrift voor logopedie (stem-, spraak-, taal- en gehoorstoornissen). see *HANDICAPPED—Hearing Impaired*

LOGOPEDNYTT. see *MEDICAL SCIENCES—Psychiatry And Neurology*

371.928 USA
M R D D EXPRESS. (Mental Retardation and Developmental Disabilities) Text in English. 1984. s-a. membership only. **Document type:** *Newsletter.* **Description:** Presents information on the division and its activities. Includes news in the field of mental retardation.
Former titles: C E C - M R Newsletter; C E C - M Report
Published by: Council for Exceptional Children, Division on Mental Retardation and Developmental Disabilities, 1110 N Glebe Rd., Ste 300, Arlington, VA 22201-5704. TEL 703-620-3660, FAX 703-264-9494, http://www.cec.sped.org/. Ed. Phil Parette. Circ: 7,000 (controlled).

MAINTAINING SAFE SCHOOLS - SCHOOL VIOLENCE ALERT. see *EDUCATION—School Organization And Administration*

MARBURGER BUECHERLISTEN. see *HANDICAPPED—Visually Impaired*

371.95 USA ISSN 0025-9551
BF412
MENSA RESEARCH JOURNAL. Text in English. 3/yr. USD 21 (effective 2001). adv. bk.rev. back issues avail. **Document type:** *Journal, Academic/Scholarly.* **Description:** Covers research on intelligence; aimed particularly at the gifted.
Published by: Mensa Education and Research Foundation, 1229 Corporate Dr W, Arlington, TX 76006-6103. TEL 817-607-0060, FAX 817-649-5232. Ed. Phyllis Miller. R&P Annette Kovac TEL 817-607-0060. Circ: 1,000.

371.928 USA ISSN 0047-6765
RC569.7 CODEN: MRTDAH
MENTAL RETARDATION. Text in English. 1963. bi-m. USD 115; USD 121 in Canada; USD 130 elsewhere (effective 1999). adv. bk.rev. illus. index. back issues avail.; reprint service avail. from PSC,SCH. *Refereed.* **Document type:** *Academic/Scholarly.* **Description:** Seeks effective ways to help people with mental retardation and their families.
Related titles: Microfilm ed.; Online - full text ed.: (from H. W. Wilson, Institute for Scientific Information).
Indexed: ASCA, Adol.Ment.Hlth.Abstr., AgeLine, Bibl.Dev.Med.& Child Neur., Biol.Abstr., C.I.J.E., Child Devel.Abstr., Curr.Cont., Curr.Lit.Fam.Plan., Dent.Ind., Educ.Ind. (Jun.1983-), Excerp.Med., Hosp.Lit.Ind., INIS Atomind., Ind.Med. (1963-), Int.Nurs.Ind., Lang.& Lang.Behav.Abstr., Mult.Ed.Abstr., PsycInfo, Psychol.Abstr. (1953-), Rehabil.Lit., SOPODA, SSCI, Soc.Serv.Abstr., Sociol.Abstr., Sp.Ed.Needs Abstr., e-psyche.
—BLDSC (5678.655000), CISTI, GNLM, IDS, ingenta, KNAW. **CCC.**

E

Published by: American Association on Mental Retardation, 444 N Capitol St, Washington, DC 20001-1512. TEL 202-387-1968, 800-424-3688, FAX 202-387-2193, orders@allenpress.com, http://www.allenpress.com. Ed. Steven Taylor. Pub. M Doreen Croser. R&P Stephen Stidinger. Circ: 11,500. **Subscr. to:** Allen Press Inc., PO Box 1897, Lawrence, KS 66044-8897.

MILL NECK FOUNDATION NEWSLETTER. see *HANDICAPPED—Hearing Impaired*

MINNESOTA SPEECH - LANGUAGE - HEARING ASSOCIATION. NEWSLETTER. see *MEDICAL SCIENCES—Otorhinolaryngology*

MISSOURI RECORD. see *HANDICAPPED—Hearing Impaired*

371.9 USA

N A P S E C MEMBERSHIP DIRECTORY. Text in English. 1980. biennial. USD 32. **Document type:** *Directory.* **Description:** Lists and describes over 200 member schools that have populations of students with disabilities, including day, residential, summer, clinical programs, and hospital affiliated programs.

Published by: National Association of Private Schools for Exceptional Children, 1522 K St, N W, Ste 1032, Washington, DC 20005. TEL 202-408-3338, FAX 202-408-3340. Ed. Sherry L Kolbe. Circ: 500.

371.91 GBR

NATIONAL ASSOCIATION FOR SPECIAL EDUCATIONAL NEEDS. PUBLICATIONS. Text in English. 1983. irreg. **Document type:** *Monographic series.*

Formerly: National Council for Special Education. Occasional Publications

Published by: National Association for Special Educational Needs, NASEN House, 4-5 Amber Business Village, Amber Village, Amington, Tamworth, Warks B77 4RP, United Kingdom. TEL 44-1827-311500, FAX 44-1827-313005, welcome@nasen.org.uk.

371.9 USA ISSN 1043-2167
LC3981

NATIONAL FORUM OF SPECIAL EDUCATION JOURNAL - ELECTRONIC. Abbreviated title: N F S E Journal. Text in English. 1989. irreg., latest vol.14, 2001. USD 36 domestic to individuals; USD 72 domestic to institutions; USD 144 foreign to institutions (effective 2001). adv. index. back issues avail. *Refereed.* **Document type:** *Journal, Academic/Scholarly.*

Media: Online - full text.

Indexed: Except.Child Educ.Abstr.

—CCC.

Published by: (National Forum Society of Educators), National Forum Journals, 4000 Locke Ln, Ste 9, Lake Charles, LA 70605-2244. TEL 337-477-0008, FAX 337-562-2848, http://www.nationalforum.com. Ed., Pub., R&P, Adv. contact William Kritsonis TEL 337-477-0008. Circ: 7,500.

371.91 CAN ISSN 0709-1370

NATIONAL (OTTAWA, 1970). Text in English. 1970. q. USD 20 (effective 1998). adv. bk.rev. **Document type:** *Newsletter.* **Description:** Covers the Association's national activities: projects, federal government liaison; reports on provincial, territorial associations' initiatives; includes articles and resources about learning disabilities.

Former titles: Post (0380-7967); Perceptual Post (0380-7975)

Related titles: French ed.

Indexed: Can.Educ.Ind.

Published by: Learning Disabilities Association of Canada, Kildare House, 323 Chapel St, Ottawa, ON K1N 7Z2, Canada. TEL 613-238-5721, FAX 613-235-5391, LDACTAAC@fox.nstn.ca, http://educ.queensu.ca/~lda. Ed. P Mantha. Circ: 8,000.

NEW LITERATURE ON VISUAL IMPAIRMENT. see *HANDICAPPED—Abstracting, Bibliographies, Statistics*

NEW MEXICO PROGRESS. see *HANDICAPPED—Hearing Impaired*

NORDISK TIDSKRIFT FOER DOEVUNDERVISNINGEN. see *HANDICAPPED—Hearing Impaired*

371.9 NOR ISSN 0048-0509
LC3950 CODEN: NTSPFA

NORDISK TIDSSKRIFT FOR SPESIALPEDAGOGIKK. Text in Danish, Norwegian, Swedish; Summaries in English. 1923. q. NOK 290 to individuals; NOK 480, USD 85 to institutions; NOK 225 to students; NOK 130, USD 22 per issue (effective 2001). adv. bk.rev. illus. index. **Document type:** *Academic/Scholarly.* **Description:** Provides information on current research and development within special education.

Indexed: Lang.& Lang.Behav.Abstr., SOPODA, Sociol.Abstr., e-psyche.

Published by: Scandinavian University Press (Subsidiary of: Taylor & Francis Ltd.), Postboks 2959, Toeyen, Oslo 0608, Norway. FAX 47-22-57-53-53, www.universitetsforlaget.no/tidsskrifter. Ed. Christine Moe Hovind. Circ: 2,000.

NORTH DAKOTA STATE PLAN FOR REHABILITATION FACILITIES AND WORKSHOPS; annual modification. see *MEDICAL SCIENCES—Physical Medicine And Rehabilitation*

371.9142 CAN ISSN 1207-5639

THE O S L A CONNECTION. Text in English. 1960. 3/yr. membership. adv. *Refereed.* **Document type:** *Newsletter.*

Former titles (until 1995): O S L A Newsletter (0836-4362); (until 1987): O.S.H.A. Ontario Speech and Hearing Association (0705-8713); (until 1976): Ontario Speech and Hearing Association. Journal (0705-8888)

Published by: Ontario Association of Speech - Language Pathologists and Audiologists, 410 Jarvis St, Toronto, ON M4Y 2G6, Canada. TEL 416-920-3676, FAX 416-920-6214, http://www.osla.on.ca. Ed. Liz Brady. R&P, Adv. contact Lucy Robinson. Circ: 1,500 (controlled).

371.912 USA
HV2510 CODEN: PEDEFN

ODYSSEY: NEW DIRECTIONS IN DEAF EDUCATION. Text in English. 1982. q. free. adv. bk.rev., film rev. illus. index. back issues avail.; reprints avail. *Refereed.* **Document type:** *Academic/Scholarly.* **Description:** Directed to professionals and families involved with educating deaf and hard-of-hearing students. Provides a forum for exchange of creative approaches to classroom teaching; gives views about current issues in deafness and education.

Former titles (until 2000): Perspectives in Education and Deafness (1051-6204); (until 1989): Perspectives for Teachers of the Hearing Impaired (0735-6315)

Indexed: C.I.J.E., Comput.Lit.Ind., Except.Child Educ.Abstr., Fam.Ind., Lang.& Lang.Behav.Abstr., SOPODA, Soc.Sci.Ind. (coverage dropped), Sociol.Abstr.

—ingenta.

Published by: Gallaudet University, Laurent Clerc National Deaf Education Center, 800 Florida Ave, N E, Washington, DC 20002-3695. TEL 202-651-5340, 800-526-9105, FAX 202-651-5708, http://clerccenter.gallaudet.edu/Odyssey/index.html. Ed. Cathryn Carroll. Adv. contact Susan Flanigan. Circ: 4,000.

OKEE. see *MEDICAL SCIENCES—Psychiatry And Neurology*

371.91 USA ISSN 1041-6234

ON CUE. Text in English. 1984. q. membership. adv. bk.rev. illus. 12 p./no. **Document type:** *Newsletter, Consumer.* **Description:** Information for professionals and families regarding the use of Cued Speech, a system of communication for people with hearing, speech and language needs.

Published by: National Cued Speech Association, 23970 Hermitage Rd., Shaker Heights, OH 44122. TEL 216-292-6213, 800-459-3529, cuedspdisc@aol.com, http://www.cuedspeech.org. Ed., R&P, Adv. contact Pam Beck. Circ: 350.

ONE IN SEVEN. see *HANDICAPPED—Hearing Impaired*

OREGON OUTLOOK. see *HANDICAPPED—Hearing Impaired*

371.91 USA ISSN 8756-5811

PALAESTRA; forum of sport, physical education and recreation for those with disabilities. Text in English. 1984. q. USD 19 domestic to individuals; USD 25 in Canada to individuals; USD 32 elsewhere to individuals; USD 25 domestic to institutions; USD 31 in Canada to institutions; USD 38 elsewhere to institutions (effective 2001). adv. bk.rev. illus. Index. back issues avail.; reprints avail. *Refereed.* **Document type:** *Consumer.* **Description:** Provides technical, "how-to" articles and practical research on recreation and physical education activities for individuals with a disability. Covers national and international sports events and looks at equipment and facility modification.

Related titles: Microform ed.: (from PQC); Online - full text ed.: (from Gale Group, Northern Light Technology, Inc., ProQuest Information & Learning, Factiva).

Indexed: Hlth.Ind., Phys.Ed.Ind., Sports Per.Ind., Sportsearch (1984-).

—BLDSC (6345.214200), ingenta.

Published by: Challenge Publications, Ltd., Circulation Department, PO Box 508, Macomb, IL 61455-0508. TEL 309-833-1902, FAX 309-833-1902, challpub@macomb.com, http://www.palaestra.com. Ed. David P Beaver. adv.: B&W page USD 1,270, color page USD 2,045. Circ: 5,500. **Co-sponsors:** Committee on Sports for the Disabled of the United States Olympic Committee; Adapted Physical Activity Council of the American Alliance for Health, Physical Education, Recreation and Dance.

371.928 USA ISSN 0031-4609

PENNSYLVANIA MESSAGE. Text in English. 1965. q. USD 20. adv. bk.rev. abstr. 16 p./no. back issues avail.

Indexed: e-psyche.

Published by: The Arc of Pennsylvania, 2001 N Front St, Ste 221, Harrisburg, PA 17102-2104. TEL 717-234-2621, FAX 717-234-7615, komyers@usa.net, http://www.thearcpa.org. Ed. Kristi O'Connell Myers. Circ: 8,500 (controlled).

371.92 USA ISSN 0731-566X

PEOPLE WITH SPECIAL NEEDS - DOWN SYNDROME REPORT✶ **.** Text in English. 1985. 6/yr. USD 5 (effective 2000). bk.rev., film rev. bibl, charts, stat. **Document type:** *Newsletter.*

Published by: The Arc, Upper Valley, PO Box 12420, Grand Forks, ND 58308-2420. Robjohns@sendit.sendit.nodak.edu. Circ: 6,000.

PERSPECTIVES (BALTIMORE). see *MEDICAL SCIENCES—Psychiatry And Neurology*

371.91 USA

PHYSICAL DISABILITIES - EDUCATION & RELATED SERVICES. Text in English. 1978. s-a. membership only. adv. bk.rev. **Document type:** *Directory, Trade.* **Description:** Provides educational and support services information for individuals with physical or health disabilities.

Formerly: D P H Journal

Indexed: C.I.J.E., Except.Child Educ.Abstr.

Published by: Council for Exceptional Children, Division for Physical & Health Disabilities, 1920 Association Dr, Reston, VA 20191-1589. TEL 703-620-3660, FAX 703-264-9494, http://www.cec.sped.org. Ed. Barbara Kulik. Circ: 1,500.

PINE CONE. see *MEDICAL SCIENCES—Psychiatry And Neurology*

▼ **PLENUM SERIES ON HUMAN EXCEPTIONALITY.** see *PSYCHOLOGY*

371.91 JPN

PRACTICAL EDUCATION FOR THE HANDICAPPED/ JISSEN SHOGAIJI KYOIKU. Text in Japanese. 1973. m. JPY 4,800.

Formerly: Education for the Handicapped

Published by: Gakken Co. Ltd., 40-5 Kami-Ikedai 4-chome, Ota-ku, Tokyo 145-0064, Japan. Ed. Yukio Nakayama.

371.91 USA ISSN 1045-988X
HV888

PREVENTING SCHOOL FAILURE; for special class teachers and parents of the handicapped. Text in English. 1976. q., latest vol.46, 2001. USD 45 domestic to individuals; USD 58 foreign to individuals; USD 93 domestic to institutions; USD 106 foreign to institutions; USD 23.25 newsstand/cover (effective 2001 - 2002). adv. bk.rev. charts, illus. index. back issues avail.; reprint service avail. from PQC. *Refereed.* **Document type:** *Academic/Scholarly.*

Formerly: Pointer (Washington) (0554-4246)

E

Related titles: CD-ROM ed.: (from ProQuest Information & Learning); Microform ed.; Online - full text ed.: (from H. W. Wilson, ProQuest Information & Learning, Gale Group).
Indexed: Behav.Abstr., C.I.J.E., Cont.Pg.Educ., ERA, Educ.Ind. (Sep.1989-), Except.Child Educ.Abstr., Fam.Ind., Psychol.Abstr., Rehabil.Lit., Sp.Ed.Needs Abstr.
—BLDSC (6612.727400), ingenta. **CCC.**
Published by: (Helen Dwight Reid Educational Foundation), Heldref Publications, 1319 Eighteenth St, N W, Washington, DC 20036-1802. TEL 202-296-6267, FAX 202-296-5149, http://www.heldref.org/. Ed. Mary O'Donnell. Adv. contact Grant Williams. Circ: 700.

PURE FACTS. see *MEDICAL SCIENCES—Psychiatry And Neurology*

QUALITY OF CARE. see *MEDICAL SCIENCES—Psychiatry And Neurology*

371.91 USA
R E S N A NEWS. (Rehabilitation Engineering and Assistive Technology Society of North America) Text in English. 1982. bi-m. USD 25. adv. bk.rev. back issues avail. **Document type:** *Newsletter, Academic/Scholarly.* **Description:** Aims for the dissemination and utilization of knowledge of rehabilitative and assistive technology.
Formerly (until 1990): Rehabilitation Technology Review (0882-2476)
Published by: R E S N A, 1700 N Moore St, Ste 1540, Arlington, VA 22209-1903. TEL 703-524-6686, FAX 703-524-6630, info@resna.org, http://www.resna.org. Ed. Marian Hall. Circ: 2,000.

RAAKPUNT. see *MEDICAL SCIENCES—Psychiatry And Neurology*

371.9144 GBR ISSN 1366-2031
REACH NEWSLETTER. Text in English. 1985. 3/yr. GBP 25 to individuals; GBP 35 to institutions (effective 2001). bk.rev., software rev. **Document type:** *Newsletter.* **Description:** Contains articles for people who work with children who have reading disabilities.
Former titles (until 1996): National Library for the Handicapped Child. Newsletter (0952-9705); Blyton Handi Read Centre Newsletter
Published by: Reach Advice Centre (Subsidiary of: REACH: National Advice Centre for Children with Reading Difficulties), California Country Park, Nine Mile Ride, Finchampstead, Wokingham, Berks RG40 4HT, United Kingdom. TEL 44-118-973-7575, FAX 44-118-973-7105, reach@reach-reading.demon.co.uk, http://www.reach-reading.demon.co.uk. Ed., R&P Beverley Mathias. Circ: 1,500.

371.9 USA ISSN 1080-0220
HV1
REFLECTIONS: NARRATIVES OF PROFESSIONAL HELPING. Text in English. 1995. q. USD 30 domestic to individuals; USD 45 foreign to individuals; USD 45 domestic to libraries; USD 60 foreign to libraries (effective 2000). adv. film rev. index. back issues avail. *Refereed.* **Document type:** *Academic/Scholarly.* **Description:** Publishes personal narratives by and for persons in the helping and academic professions - anyone engaged in bringing about social change.
Indexed: Soc.Serv.Abstr., Soc.Work Res.& Abstr., Sociol.Abstr., e-psyche.
Published by: University Press, California State University, Long Beach, c/o Dept of Social Work, Long Beach, CA 90840-0902. TEL 562-985-4626, FAX 562-985-5514, reflect@csulb.edu, http://www.csulb.edu/depts/socialwk/refections/call.htm. Ed., R&P Mary Ann Jimenez. Adv. contact Paul Abels.

371.9 USA ISSN 0889-7018
HD7255.5
REHABILITATION EDUCATION. Text in English. 1987. q. USD 25 domestic to individuals; USD 40 foreign to individuals; USD 90 domestic to institutions; USD 105 foreign to institutions; USD 10 domestic to students; USD 25 foreign to students. adv. *Refereed.* **Document type:** *Academic/Scholarly.* **Description:** Features original contributions dealing with all aspects of rehabilitation education, including curriculum development, information about instruction materials, education media, and issues related to licensing, certification and accreditation.
Indexed: AMED, CINAHL, Cont.Pg.Educ., Mult.Ed.Abstr., PsycInfo, Psychol.Abstr. (1993-), Sociol.Educ.Abstr., Tech.Educ.Abstr., e-psyche.
—BLDSC (7350.236200), GNLM, ingenta. **CCC.**
Published by: (National Council on Rehabilitation Education), Elliott & Fitzpatrick, Inc., 1135 Cedar Shoals Dr, Athens, GA 30605. TEL 706-548-8161, 800-843-4977, FAX 706-546-8417. Ed. Dr. Douglas C Strohmer. Adv. contact Tim Field. page USD 250; 7.63 x 5.38. Circ: 675.

REHABILITATION GAZETTE; international journal of independent living by and for persons with a disability. see *HANDICAPPED*

REHABILITATION INDUSTRIES CORPORATION. ANNUAL REPORT. see *MEDICAL SCIENCES—Physical Medicine And Rehabilitation*

371.9 USA ISSN 0741-9325
LC3950
REMEDIAL AND SPECIAL EDUCATION. Text in English. 1984. bi-m., latest vol.22. USD 43 in North America to individuals; USD 77 elsewhere to individuals; USD 127 in North America to institutions; USD 150 elsewhere to institutions (effective 2002). adv. bk.rev. illus. Index. 64 p./no. back issues avail.; reprint service avail. from SCH,PSC. *Refereed.* **Document type:** *Journal, Academic/Scholarly.* **Description:** Features articles on all topics in the field, bridging the gap between theory and practice. Two special issues each year provide in-depth coverage of a single topic.
Formed by the merger of (1981-1984): Topics in Learning and Learning Disabilities (0271-1494); (1980-1984): Exceptional Education Quarterly (0196-6960); (1978-1983): Journal for Special Educators (0197-5323); Which was formed by the 1978 merger of: Special Children (0160-3248); Journal for Special Educators of the Mentally Retarded (0012-2807); Which was formerly: Digest of the Mentally Retarded; Incorporates: Retarded Adult
Related titles: Microfilm ed.: (from PQC); Online - full text ed.: (from H. W. Wilson, ProQuest Information & Learning, Institute for Scientific Information, CatchWord Ltd.).
Indexed: ASCA, ASSIA, C.I.J.E., Cont.Pg.Educ., Crim.Just.Abstr., Curr.Cont., Curr.Lit.Fam.Plan., ERA, Educ.Ind. (Jan.1984-), Educ.Tech.Abstr., Except.Child Educ.Abstr., Fam.Ind., IBZ, Lang.& Lang.Behav.Abstr., Mult.Ed.Abstr., PsycInfo, Psychol.Abstr. (1984-), SOMA, SOPODA, SSCI, Sociol.Abstr., Sp.Ed.Needs Abstr., Tech.Educ.Abstr., e-psyche.
—BLDSC (7356.760000), IDS, Infotrieve, ingenta. **CCC.**
Published by: Pro-Ed Inc., 8700 Shoal Creek Blvd, Austin, TX 78757-6897. TEL 512-451-3246, FAX 512-302-9129, proed1@aol.com, http://www.proedinc.com. Ed. Edward Polloway. Pub. Donald D Hammill. R&P Barbara Rivera TEL 512-451-3246 ext 653. adv.: B&W page USD 400. Circ: 2,200 (paid and free).

REPORT ON DISABILITY PROGRAMS. see *SOCIAL SERVICES AND WELFARE*

RESEARCH IN DEVELOPMENTAL DISABILITIES; a multidisciplinary journal. see *MEDICAL SCIENCES—Psychiatry And Neurology*

RIABILITAZIONE E APPRENDIMENTO. see *MEDICAL SCIENCES—Physical Medicine And Rehabilitation*

371.9142 GBR
ROYAL COLLEGE OF SPEECH AND LANGUAGE THERAPISTS. BULLETIN. Text in English. 1945. m. GBP 40; GBP 45 overseas; GBP 70 with European Journal of Disorders of Communication; GBP 85 overseas with European Journal of Disorders of Communication (effective 1999). adv. bk.rev. Supplement avail. **Document type:** *Bulletin, Academic/Scholarly.* **Description:** Contains research papers, practice reports, correspondence and Royal College news of interest to students and professionals in speech-language pathology and audiology.
Former titles: College of Speech and Language Therapists. Bulletin (0953-6086); College of Speech Therapists. Bulletin
—BLDSC (2700.250000).
Published by: Royal College of Speech and Language Therapists, 7 Bath Pl, London EC2 3DR, United Kingdom. TEL 44-20-7613-3855, FAX 44-20-7613-3854. Ed. Jenny Sheridan. R&P Jenny Shendan TEL 44-20-7613-6404. Adv. contact Vivien Robinson. Circ: 8,000 (controlled).

371.9 USA ISSN 8756-8705
RURAL SPECIAL EDUCATION QUARTERLY. Text in English. 1984. q. USD 50; USD 56 foreign (effective Sep. 1995). illus. Index. back issues avail.; reprints avail. **Document type:** *Academic/Scholarly.* **Description:** Covers pre-service training, administration and curriculum for pre-service educators and direct service providers.
Indexed: Agricola, Bibl.Agri., C.I.J.E.
—BLDSC (8052.631000), ingenta.
Published by: American Council on Rural Special Education, Kansas State University, 2323 Anderson Ave., Ste. 226, Manhattan, KS 66502-2912. TEL 785-532-2737, FAX 785-532-7732, http://www.ksu.edu/acres/pub.html. Ed. Barbara Ludlow TEL 304-293-3450 ext. 1127. Circ: 650.

371.9 USA
RURALINK. Text in English. 6/yr. membership. **Document type:** *Newsletter.* **Description:** Covers resources and information on rural special education.
Published by: American Council on Rural Special Education, Kansas State University, 2323 Anderson Ave., Ste. 226, Manhattan, KS 66502-2912. TEL 785-532-2737, FAX 785-532-7732, acres@ksu.edu. Ed. Barbara Ludlow TEL 304-293-3450 ext. 1127. Circ: 600.

371.9 GBR ISSN 1367-2460
S L D EXPERIENCE. Text in English. 1992. 3/yr. GBP 21.50 domestic to individuals; GBP 50 foreign to institutions (effective 2001). adv. bk.rev. *Refereed.* **Document type:** *Academic/Scholarly.*
Indexed: e-psyche.
—BLDSC (8309.428970).
Published by: BILD Publications, Wolverhampton Rd, Kidderminster, Worcs DY10 3PP, United Kingdom. TEL 44-1562-850251, FAX 44-1562-851970, bild@bild.demon.co.uk, http://www.bild.org.uk. Ed. Beryl Smith. Circ: 1,500 (paid).

371.9 AUS ISSN 1328-682X
S P E L D BULLETIN. Text in English. 1970. 2/yr. AUD 35 to members (effective 2000). adv. bk.rev. **Document type:** *Bulletin.*
Formerly: D.A.W.A. Bulletin
Indexed: Aus.Educ.Ind.
Published by: Specific Learning Difficulties Association of Victoria Inc., 494 Brunswick St, Fitzroy North, VIC 3068, Australia. TEL 61-3-94894344, FAX 61-3-94862437, spelolvic@telstra.easymail.com.au, http://www.vicnet.net.au/~speld. Ed., R&P, Adv. contact Christopher Davidson TEL 61-3-9826-0371. Circ: 700.

371.9 AUS
S P E L D NEWS. Text in English. 1969. q. AUD 25 to membership; AUD 35 foreign to membership (effective 1999). bk.rev. back issues avail. **Document type:** *Newsletter.* **Description:** Contains articles relating to recent research into specific learning difficulties and related subjects.
Published by: Specific Learning Difficulties Association of New South Wales, 33-41 Linfield Ave, Lindfield, NSW 2070, Australia. TEL 61-2-9416-9100, FAX 61-2-9416-9277, http://www.edfac.usyd.edu.au/projects/speld. Ed., R&P Valentine Badham. Circ: 1,500.

SAGGI; neuropsicologia infantile psicopedagogia riabilitazione. see *MEDICAL SCIENCES—Psychiatry And Neurology*

371.9 371.2 USA ISSN 1094-3749
SCHOOL LAW BRIEFINGS. Text in English. m. USD 130 (effective 1999). back issues avail. **Document type:** *Newsletter.* **Description:** Summaries of general education, special education and early childhood court cases, as well as administrative hearings. Each issue includes a brief overview of all the court cases and administrative hearings.
Formerly: School Law Bulletin
—CCC.
Published by: L R P Publications, 747 Dresher Rd, Box 980, Horsham, PA 19044. TEL 800-341-7874, FAX 215-784-9639, custserve@lrp.com, http://www.lrp.com. Pub. Kenneth F Kahn.

SEMINARS IN SPEECH AND LANGUAGE. see *MEDICAL SCIENCES—Otorhinolaryngology*

SERCE I TROSKA. see *HANDICAPPED*

371.91 JPN ISSN 0037-3990
SHITAI FUJIYU KYOIKU/JAPANESE JOURNAL OF EDUCATION OF THE HANDICAPPED. Text in Japanese. 1970. 5/yr. JPY 3,600. **Description:** Includes rehabilitation techniques.
Published by: Japanese Society for Disabled Children/Nihon Shitai Fujiyuji Kyokai, 1-7 Komone 1-chome, Itabashi-ku, Tokyo 173-0037, Japan. Circ: 4,500.

SIGHTS AND SOUNDS. see *HANDICAPPED—Hearing Impaired*

THE SILENT ADVOCATE. see *HANDICAPPED—Hearing Impaired*

SMITH - KETTLEWELL TECHNICAL FILE; a biannual technical journal for the blind and visually impaired. see *HANDICAPPED—Visually Impaired*

371.9 DEU ISSN 0342-7366
SONDERPAEDAGOGIK; Vierteljahresschrift ueber aktuelle Probleme der Behinderten in Schule und Gesellschaft. Text in German. 1964. q. DEM 48; DEM 38.40 to students (effective 1999). adv. bk.rev. **Document type:** *Academic/Scholarly.*
Indexed: IBR, IBZ.
—CCC.
Published by: Wissenschaftsverlag Volker Spiess GmbH, Gneisenaustr 33, Berlin 10961, Germany. TEL 49-30-6917073, FAX 49-30-6914067. Ed. Heinz Neukaeter.

371.9 USA
SOWER. Text in English. 1981. q. free per issue. back issues avail. **Document type:** *Newsletter.*
Formerly: Broadcaster
Published by: Beatrice State Development Center, Department of Public Institutions, 3000 Lincoln Blvd, Beatrice, NE 68310. TEL 402-223-2302. Ed. Jerry Crisp. Circ: 6,000.

371.9 GBR ISSN 0966-4831
SPECIAL. Text in English. 1992. 3/yr. **Document type:** *Academic/Scholarly.*
Published by: National Association for Special Educational Needs, NASEN House, 4-5 Amber Business Village, Amber Village, Amington, Tamworth, Warks B77 4RP, United Kingdom. TEL 44-1827-311500, FAX 44-1827-313005, welcome@nasen.org.uk.

371.9 371.3 USA ISSN 1094-3773
SPECIAL EDUCATION LAW MONTHLY. Text in English. m. USD 120 (effective 1999). back issues avail. **Document type:** *Newsletter.* **Description:** Covers court decisions and administrative rulings affecting the education of students with disabilities. Brief overviews and case summaries are included.
—CCC.
Published by: L R P Publications, 747 Dresher Rd, Box 980, Horsham, PA 19044. TEL 800-341-7874, FAX 215-784-9639, custserve@lrp.com, http://www.lrp.com. Pub. Kenneth F Kahn.

371.9 USA
SPECIAL EDUCATION REPORT; the independent bi-weekly news service on legislation, programs and funding for special education. Text in English. 1975. bi-w. USD 350 to individuals; USD 16 newsstand/cover (effective 2002). s-a. index. **Document type:** *Newsletter.* **Description:** Covers federal and state legislation and LRE policy issues. Looks at innovations and research in the field.
Formerly (until 1992): Education of the Handicapped (0194-2255)
Indexed: Rehabil.Lit.
—ingenta.
Published by: Aspen Publishers, Inc., 200 Orchard Ridge Dr, Ste 200, Gaithersburg, MD 20878. TEL 301-417-7500, FAX 301-695-7931, customer.service@aspenpubl.com, http://www.aspenpub.com. Ed. William J Cahir. Pub. Marjorie Weiner. **Dist. by:** Aspen Publishers Inc., Distribution Center, 7201 McKinney Circle, Frederick, MD 21701. TEL 301-698-7100, FAX 301-417-7550.

SPECIAL EDUCATIONAL NEEDS ABSTRACTS. see *EDUCATION—Abstracting, Bibliographies, Statistics*

371.9 USA ISSN 0739-9820
SPECIAL SERVICES IN THE SCHOOLS. Text in English. 1984. q. USD 60 to individuals; USD 81 in Canada to individuals; USD 87 elsewhere to individuals; USD 150 to institutions; USD 203 in Canada to institutions; USD 218 elsewhere to institutions; USD 250 to libraries; USD 338 in Canada to libraries; USD 363 elsewhere to libraries (effective Aug. 2001). adv. bk.rev. back issues avail.; reprint service avail. from HAW. *Refereed.* **Document type:** *Journal, Academic/Scholarly.* **Description:** Disseminates state-of-the-art material to education professionals of children with special needs in public schools and related educational settings.
Related titles: Microfiche ed.: (from PQC); Microform ed.
Indexed: C.I.J.E., Child Devel.Abstr., Cont.Pg.Educ., ERA, Educ.Tech.Abstr., Except.Child Educ.Abstr., Mult.Ed.Abstr., Psychol.Abstr. (1984-), Soc.Work Res.& Abstr., Sociol.Educ.Abstr., Sp.Ed.Needs Abstr., e-psyche.
—BLDSC (8404.023000), Haworth.
Published by: Haworth Press, Inc., 10 Alice St, Binghamton, NY 13904-1580. TEL 607-722-5857, 800-429-6784, FAX 607-722-6362, 800-895-0582, getinfo@haworthpressinc.com, http://www.haworthpress.com/journals/journallist.asp. Ed. Charles A Maher. Pub. William Cohen. R&P Ruthann Heath TEL 607-723-5857 ext 316. Adv. contact Jackie Blakeslee TEL 607-722-5857 ext 346. B&W page USD 315, color page USD 550; trim 6 x 8.5. Circ: 275.

371.9142 GBR ISSN 1368-2105
SPEECH & LANGUAGE THERAPY IN PRACTICE. Text in English. 1985. q. GBP 24 domestic to individuals; GBP 28 in Europe to individuals; GBP 32 elsewhere to individuals; GBP 40 domestic to institutions; GBP 44 in Europe to institutions. adv. bk.rev. **Document type:** *Academic/Scholarly.* **Description:** Contains practical information for speech and language therapists and associated professionals.
Former titles (until 1997): Human Communication (0968-1108); (until 1991): Speech Therapy in Practice (0269-0527)
—BLDSC (8411.195820).
Published by: Avril Nicoll Ed. & Pub., Lynwood Cottage, High St, Drumlithie, Stonehaven AB39 3YZ, United Kingdom. avrilnicoll@sol.co.uk, http://www.sol.co.uk/s/speechnag. R&P Avril Nicoll. adv.: B&W page GBP 450, color page GBP 600. Circ: 1,300 (paid).

371.9 DEU ISSN 0342-0477
SPRACHE - STIMME - GEHOER; Zeitschrift fuer Kommunikationsstoerungen. Text in German; Summaries in English, German. 1977. q. EUR 64.80 domestic to institutions; EUR 68.80 in Europe to institutions; EUR 71.80 elsewhere to institutions; EUR 37 to students; EUR 18 newsstand/cover (effective 2002). adv. bk.rev. index. back issues avail.; reprint service avail. from PQC. *Refereed.* **Document type:** *Journal, Academic/Scholarly.*
Related titles: Online - full text ed.: ISSN 1439-1260.
Indexed: Curr.Cont. (coverage dropped), Excerp.Med.
—EMDOCS, GNLM, Infotrieve. **CCC.**
Published by: Georg Thieme Verlag, Ruedigerstr 14, Stuttgart 70469, Germany. TEL 49-711-8931-0, FAX 49-711-8931298, kunden.service@thieme.de, http://www.thieme.de/ssg. Ed. M Ptok. R&P Peter Eich. adv.: page DEM 2,000; 175 x 250. Circ: 2,500.

371.9 DEU ISSN 0584-9470
DIE SPRACHHEILARBEIT. Text in German. 1956. q. DEM 68 (effective 1999). **Document type:** *Academic/Scholarly.*
Indexed: IBR, IBZ.
—GNLM.
Published by: Verlag Modernes Lernen - Dortmund, Hohe Str 39, Dortmund 44139, Germany. TEL 49-231-128048, FAX 49-231-128009. Circ: 7,200.

371.95 DEU
STUDIENSTIFTUNG. JAHRESBERICHT. Text in German. 1970. a. free per issue. illus, stat. **Document type:** *Corporate.* **Description:** Report of the society which enables specially gifted students to further their education and receive scholarships. Includes report on activities and statistics.
Published by: Studienstiftung des Deutschen Volkes, Mirbachstr 7, Bonn 53173, Germany. Ed. Klaus H Kohrs. Circ: 35,000.

STUDIES IN SPEECH PATHOLOGY AND CLINICAL LINGUISTICS. see *MEDICAL SCIENCES—Psychiatry And Neurology*

371.9 GBR ISSN 0268-2141
LB1029.R4
SUPPORT FOR LEARNING. Text in English. 1967. q. GBP 98 to institutions in UK & Europe; USD 215 to institutions in the Americas & Caribbean; GBP 134 elsewhere to institutions (effective 2002). **Document type:** *Academic/Scholarly.*
Formerly (until 1986): Remedial Education (0034-4214)
Related titles: Microform ed.: (from SWZ); Online - full text ed.: (from EBSCO Publishing, O C L C Online Computer Library Center, Inc., RoweCom Information Quest, ingenta, Swets Blackwell).
Indexed: Br.Educ.Ind., Child.Lit.Abstr., Cont.Pg.Educ., ERA, Educ.Tech.Abstr., Except.Child Educ.Abstr., High.Educ.Curr.Aware.Bull., Lang.Teach.& Ling.Abstr., PsycInfo, Psychol.Abstr. (1986-), Sp.Ed.Needs Abstr., Tech.Educ.Abstr., e-psyche.
—BLDSC (8547.638300), ingenta. **CCC.**
Published by: (National Association for Special Educational Needs), Blackwell Publishers Ltd., 108 Cowley Rd, Oxford OX4 1JF, United Kingdom. TEL 44-1865-791100, FAX 44-1865-791347, nasen@bbcnc.org.uk; jnlinfo@blackwellpublishers.co.uk, http://www.blackwellpublishers.co.uk. Ed. Caroline Roaf. Circ: 5,500.

SWIAT CISZY; czasopismo polskich inwalidow sluchu. see *HANDICAPPED—Hearing Impaired*

T C H I UPDATE. see *HANDICAPPED—Hearing Impaired*

371.95 AUS ISSN 0815-8150
TALENTED. Text in English. 1983. 4/yr. AUD 40, USD 28 (effective 1999). bk.rev. back issues avail. *Refereed.* **Document type:** *Newsletter.* **Description:** For teachers and parents on the education of the gifted and talented.
Indexed: Aus.Educ.Ind.
Published by: University of New England, School of Curriculum Studies, Armidale, NSW 2351, Australia. TEL 61-67-733832, FAX 61-67-735078, sbailey@metz.une.edu.au. Ed. Linley Lloyd. R&P Stan Bailey. Circ: 500 (paid).

371.9 USA ISSN 0888-4064
LC3969.45
TEACHER EDUCATION AND SPECIAL EDUCATION. Text in English. 1977. q. USD 18 domestic to individuals; USD 23 foreign to individuals; USD 35 domestic to institutions; USD 40 foreign to institutions. adv. bk.rev. back issues avail.; reprint service avail. from PSC,SCH. **Document type:** *Academic/Scholarly, Trade.* **Description:** Contains reports of original research, evaluations of personnel preparation programs or components thereof, and theoretically based discussions of personnel preparation practices.
Related titles: Microform ed.: (from PQC); Online - full text ed.: (from H. W. Wilson).
Indexed: C.I.J.E., Cont.Pg.Educ., ERA, Educ.Ind. (Oct.1983-), Educ.Tech.Abstr., Except.Child Educ.Abstr., SOMA, Sp.Ed.Needs Abstr., Tech.Educ.Abstr.
—BLDSC (8613.440000), ingenta.
Published by: Council for Exceptional Children, Division of Teacher Education, 1920 Association Drive, Reston, VA 22091. TEL 703-620-3660, FAX 703-264-9494. Eds. Anne Bauer, Lawrence Johnson. Adv. contact Victor Erickson. Circ: 3,300. **Subscr. to:** Boyd Printing, 49 Sheridan Ave, Albany, NY 12210.

371.92 GBR ISSN 0040-0572
TEACHING & TRAINING. Text in English. 1962. q. GBP 1.65. adv. bk.rev., film rev. illus.
Indexed: High.Educ.Curr.Aware.Bull.
Published by: National Association of Teachers of the Mentally Handicapped, c/o Edward R.D. Myer, 77 Highfield, Bromham, Chippenham, Wilts SN15 2HT, United Kingdom. Circ: 1,600.

TEAM OF ADVOCATES FOR SPECIAL KIDS NEWSLETTER. see *HANDICAPPED*

371.9 USA
THEIR WORLD. Text in English. 1970. a. USD 6. adv. bk.rev. abstr.
Published by: National Center for Children with Learning Disabilities, 381 Park Ave S, 1420, New York, NY 10016-8806. TEL 212-545-7510. Ed. Sheldon H Horowitz. Circ: 70,000.

371.9142 USA ISSN 0271-8294
RC423.A1
TOPICS IN LANGUAGE DISORDERS. Text in English. 1981. q. USD 135 to individuals; USD 41 newsstand/cover (effective 2002). adv. bk.rev. illus. reprint service avail. from PSC,SCH. *Refereed.* **Document type:** *Journal, Trade.* **Description:** Provides information that bridges the gap between theory, research and everyday practice.
Related titles: Online - full text ed.: (from ProQuest Information & Learning, Institute for Scientific Information).
Indexed: AMED, ASCA, AgeLine, C.I.J.E., CINAHL, Curr.Cont., Educ.Ind. (Nov.1983-), Except.Child Educ.Abstr., Lang.& Lang.Behav.Abstr., PsycInfo, Psychol.Abstr. (1981-), SOPODA, SSCI, Sociol.Abstr., e-psyche.
—BLDSC (8867.458500), GNLM, IDS, ingenta. **CCC.**
Published by: Aspen Publishers, Inc., 200 Orchard Ridge Dr, Ste 200, Gaithersburg, MD 20878. TEL 301-417-7500, 800-638-8437, FAX 301-417-7550, customer.service@aspenpubl.com, http://www.aspenpublishers.com. Ed. Katherine G Butler. Pub. Jack Bruggeman. Circ: 4,550 (paid). **Dist. by:** Aspen Publishers Inc., Distribution Center, 7201 McKinney Circle, Frederick, MD 21701. TEL 301-698-7100.

E

TOWERS. see *HANDICAPPED—Visually Impaired*

371.9 CAN ISSN 0381-9612
THE TRUST. Text in English. 1967. q. free with membership. bk.rev. bibl. back issues avail. **Document type:** *Newsletter.* **Description:** Provides information with intellectual disabilities in the areas of education, housing, recreation and employment for parents and caregivers.
Published by: Regina and District Association for Community Living Inc., 2216 Smith St, Regina, SK S4P 2P4, Canada. TEL 306-790-5680, FAX 306-586-7899, racl@sk.sympatico.ca. Ed., R&P Elyse Fisher. Circ: 500.

371.9 USA ISSN 0070-6736
LC4019
U S C ANNUAL DISTINGUISHED LECTURE SERIES MONOGRAPHS IN SPECIAL EDUCATION AND REHABILITATION. Text in English. 1962. a. price varies. **Document type:** *Monographic series.*
Indexed: C.I.J.E. (coverage dropped), Except.Child Educ.Abstr., Rehabil.Lit.
Published by: (University of Southern California, School of Education), University of Southern California Press, c/o Bookstore, University Park, Los Angeles, CA 90007. TEL 213-743-5371. Ed. James F Magary. Circ: 3,000.

371.9 CHE ISSN 0017-9655
VIERTELJAHRESSCHRIFT FUER HEILPAEDAGOGIK UND IHRE NACHBARGEBIETE. Text in German; Summaries in English, French, German. 1932. q. CHF 52 domestic; EUR 33 Germany & Austria; CHF 56 elsewhere; CHF 28 domestic to students; EUR 18 to students Germany & Austria; CHF 35 elsewhere to students (effective 2002). adv. bk.rev. **Document type:** *Journal, Academic/Scholarly.*
Formerly: Heilpaedagogische Werkblaetter
Indexed: IBZ, PsycInfo, Psychol.Abstr. (1952-), e-psyche.
Published by: Heilpaedagogisches Institut der Universitaet Freiburg, Petrus Kanisius Gasse 21, Fribourg 1700, Switzerland. TEL 41-26-3007700, FAX 41-26-3009749, christina.amrein@unifr.ch, http://pedcurmac13.unifr.ch/. Ed., Adv. contact Christina Amrein. Pub. Urs Haeberlin. Circ: 2,000.

371.92 FRA ISSN 1152-6653
VIVRE ENSEMBLE. Text in French. 1962. bi-m. FRF 170; FRF 200 foreign (effective 1999). adv. bk.rev., film rev. bibl, stat. **Document type:** *Newspaper.*
Formerly (until 1990): Epanouir (0182-4651)
Published by: Union Nationale des Associations de Parents et Amis de Personnes Handicapees Mentales, 15 rue Coysevox, Paris Cedex 18 75876, France. TEL 33-1-44855050, FAX 33-1-44855060, public@unapei.org, http://www.unapei.org. Ed., Pub., R&P Patrick Gohet. Adv. contact Christophe Magnant. Circ: 75,250 (controlled).

371.9 USA
VOCATIONAL REHABILITATION REVIEW✶. Text in English. 1982. w. membership.
Published by: National Association of Rehabilitation Facilities, 206 S 6th St, Springfield, IL 62701-1530. Ed. Charles W Harles. Circ: 545. **Subscr. to:** PO Box 17675, Washington, DC 20041.

THE VOLTA REVIEW. see *HANDICAPPED—Hearing Impaired*

VOLTA VOICES. see *HANDICAPPED—Hearing Impaired*

371.9 USA
WASHINGTON (STATE). DIVISION OF VOCATIONAL REHABILITATION. STATE FACILITIES DEVELOPMENT PLAN. Text in English. 1969. every 3 yrs. free.
Former titles: Washington (State). Vocational Rehabilitation Services Division. State Facilities Development Plan; Washington (State). Vocational Rehabilitation Services Division. State Facilities Plan (0092-5543)
Published by: Department of Social and Health Services, Division of Vocational Rehabilitation, OB 2, Olympia, WA 98504. TEL 206-753-0767, FAX 206-586-6505. Circ: 1,000.

371.912 USA ISSN 0199-8293
WORLD AROUND YOU. Text in English. 1978. 5/yr. USD 10 domestic; USD 15 foreign (effective 2000). adv. back issues avail. **Document type:** *Journal, Academic/Scholarly.* **Description:** News magazine for hearing impaired teens.
Related titles: ♦ Special ed.: World Around You. Teacher's Edition. ISSN 1059-9894.
Published by: Gallaudet University, National Deaf Educ Network & Clearinghouse, 800 Florida Ave, N E, KDES PAS 6, Washington, DC 20002-3695. TEL 202-651-5340, FAX 202-651-5708, cmcarrol@gallux.gallaudet.edu, http://clerccenter.gallaudet.edu/WorldAroundYou/. Ed. Cathryn Carroll. Adv. contact Susan Flanigan. Circ: 6,500.

371.95 USA
WORLD COUNCIL FOR GIFTED AND TALENTED CHILDREN. YEARBOOK. Text in English. 1981. biennial. USD 15. back issues avail. **Document type:** *Proceedings.* **Description:** Describes the proceedings of the world conferences held by the council.
Published by: World Council for Gifted and Talented Children, PO Box 10034, Beaumont, TX 77710. TEL 409-880-8046, FAX 409-880-8685.

371.9 USA ISSN 1096-2506
LC4019.3
YOUNG EXCEPTIONAL CHILDREN. Text in English. 1997. q. USD 20 to individuals; USD 35 to institutions. bk.rev. *Refereed.* **Document type:** *Academic/Scholarly.* **Description:** Provides practical ideas for teachers, early-care and education personnel, administrators, therapists, family members, and others who work with or on behalf of children from birth through age 8 who have disabilities or developmental delays, are gifted and talented, or are at risk for future developmental problems.
Incorporates: D E C Communicator
Published by: Council for Exceptional Children, Division for Early Childhood, 1380 Lawrence St Ste 650, Denver, CO 80204. TEL 303-556-3328, FAX 303-556-3310, ostrosky@uiuc.edu, http://www.dec-sped.org. Ed. Michaelene Ostrosky. Circ: 6,600.

EDUCATION—Teaching Methods And Curriculum

see also specific subjects

610.71 USA ISSN 0092-0371
R745
A A M C CURRICULUM DIRECTORY. Text in English. 1972. a. USD 35 (effective 1999). reprint service avail. from PQC. **Document type:** *Directory.* **Description:** Describes the academic programs of medical schools in the Unites States, Canada, and Puerto Rico. Includes information on curriculum characteristics and current trends and innovations of interest to applicants, other students, faculties, and deans.
Published by: Association of American Medical Colleges, 2450 N St N W, Washington, DC 20037-1126. TEL 202-828-0416, FAX 202-828-1123. R&P Cynthia Bennett.

613.7 USA ISSN 0890-4073
RA440.A1
ADVANCES IN HEALTH EDUCATION: CURRENT RESEARCH. Text in English. 1988. a. USD 37.50. bk.rev. index. back issues avail. *Refereed.* **Description:** Contains original research on current issues, both biological and behavioral, in the field of health education.
Indexed: e-psyche.
Published by: A M S Press, Inc., 56 E 13th St, New York, NY 10003. TEL 212-777-4700, FAX 212-995-5413. Ed. James H Humphrey.

370.15 USA
BEHAVIORAL EDUCATOR. Text in English. 1980. q. USD 5 to individuals; USD 3 to students. adv. bk.rev. back issues avail.
Indexed: e-psyche.
Published by: Special Interest Group in Education, c/o Deborah A Shanley, Ed, 330 E 71st St, New York, NY 10021. TEL 212-734-8401. Circ: 110. **Subscr. to:** Theodore A. Hoch, 509 Allen Hall, West Virginia University, Box 6122, Morgantown, WV 26506-6122. **Co-sponsor:** Association for Behavior Analysis in Education.

613.7 GBR
BRITISH JOURNAL OF PHYSICAL EDUCATION. RESEARCH SUPPLEMENT. Text in English. q. membership. *Refereed.* **Document type:** *Academic/Scholarly.* **Description:** Publishes original research on all aspects of physical and health education, outdoor activities, and sports and dance.
Published by: Physical Education Association of the United Kingdom, Ling House, Building 25., London Rd, Reading, Berks RG1 5AQ, United Kingdom. TEL 44-1189-316240, FAX 44-1189-316242, pea.uk@cableol.co.uk, http://www.teleschool.org.uk/pea. Ed. Neil Armstrong.

BUROS - NEBRASKA SERIES ON MEASUREMENT AND TESTING. see *PSYCHOLOGY*

CANADIAN INTRAMURAL RECREATION ASSOCIATION. BULLETIN; the voice of intramurals in Canada. see *PHYSICAL FITNESS AND HYGIENE*

CAROLINA TIPS. see *BIOLOGY*

CHILD LANGUAGE TEACHING AND THERAPY. see *EDUCATION—Special Education And Rehabilitation*

371.33 USA ISSN 0199-820X
CURRENT HEALTH 1; the beginning guide to health education. Text in English. 1974. 8/yr. (m., Sep.-May). USD 33.95 (effective 2002). charts, illus. reprint service avail. from PQC. **Description:** Provides students in grades 4-7 with today's essential health information in a stimulating magazine format. Includes a separate teacher's guide.
Related titles: Microform ed.: (from PQC); Online - full text ed.: (from Northern Light Technology, Inc., H. W. Wilson, ProQuest Information & Learning).
Indexed: Ind.Child.Mag., Jun.High Mag.Abstr., Mag.Ind., PMR, R.G. (coverage dropped), R.G.Yng.Pple. (Sep.1999-).
—ingenta.
Published by: Weekly Reader Corporation, 200 First Stamford Pl, Box 120023, Stamford, CT 06912-0023. TEL 800-446-3355, FAX 609-786-3360, customerservice@weeklyreader.com, http://www.weeklyreader.com/features/wrch.html. Ed. Andrew Casino TEL 203-705-3569. Pub. Peter Bergen. R&P Aimee Knoller TEL 203-705-3569. Circ: 165,783 (paid).

371.33 USA ISSN 0163-156X
CURRENT HEALTH 2; the continuing guide to health education. Text in English. 8/yr. (m., Sep.-May). USD 33.95 (effective 2002). **Description:** Provides middle- and high-school students with today's essential health information in a stimulating magazine format that students relate to. Includes a separate teacher's guide.
Related titles: CD-ROM ed.: (from ProQuest Information & Learning); Microfiche ed.: (from NBI); Online - full text ed.: (from Gale Group, ProQuest Information & Learning, Northern Light Technology, Inc., H. W. Wilson, Factiva); ♦ Supplement: Human Sexuality Supplement. ISSN 0196-061X.
Indexed: Acad.Ind., Hlth.Ind., Jun.High Mag.Abstr., R.G. (Sep.1982-), R.G.Abstr. (Sep.1982-), R.G.Yng.Pple. (Sep.1998-).
—ingenta.
Published by: Weekly Reader Corporation, 200 First Stamford Pl, Box 120023, Stamford, CT 06912-0023. TEL 800-446-3355, FAX 609-786-3360, http://www.weeklyreader.com, http://www.weeklyreader.com/features/wrch.html. Ed. Andrew Casino TEL 203-705-3569. Pub. Peter Berger. R&P Aimee Knoller TEL 203-705-3569. Circ: 229,274 (paid).

DIAGNOSTIQUE. see *EDUCATION—Special Education And Rehabilitation*

DRUG EDUCATION MATTERS. see *DRUG ABUSE AND ALCOHOLISM*

371.334 USA ISSN 1068-7378
EFFECTIVE SCHOOL PRACTICES. Text in English. 1981. q. USD 25 (effective 2000). adv. bk.rev. **Document type:** *Academic/Scholarly.* **Description:** Publishes research, training methods, and experiences of teachers in research-based effective technology practices.
Formerly (until 1992): A D I News
Indexed: Cont.Pg.Educ.
Published by: Association for Direct Instruction, PO Box 10252, Eugene, OR 97440. TEL 541-485-1293, FAX 541-683-7543, erica@adihome.org, http://www.adihome.org. Ed. Bonnie Grossen. R&P Erica Eden. Adv. contact Bryan Wickman. Circ: 3,000.

EQUINE VETERINARY EDUCATION. see *VETERINARY SCIENCE*

371.33 USA ISSN 0196-061X
HUMAN SEXUALITY SUPPLEMENT. Text in English. 8/yr. (m., Sep.-May). USD 3.30 (effective 2000).
Description: Contains current information on the sexual aspects of health and well-being. Includes a separate teacher's guide.
Related titles: ♦ Supplement to: Current Health 2. ISSN 0163-156X.
Published by: Weekly Reader Corporation, 200 First Stamford Pl, Box 120023, Stamford, CT 06912-0023. TEL 800-446-3355, FAX 609-786-3360, http://www.weeklyreader.com. Ed. Andrew Casino TEL 203-705-3569. Pub. Peter Bergen. R&P Aimee Knoller TEL 203-705-3569.

371.393 USA
INTERNATIONAL CONFERENCE ON PIAGETIAN THEORY AND THE HELPING PROFESSIONS. PROCEEDINGS. Text in English. 1978 (8th). a. price varies. **Document type:** *Proceedings.*
Published by: (Children's Hospital of Los Angeles, University Affiliated Program), University of Southern California, Department of Sociology and Social Research, University Park, KAP 352, Los Angeles, CA 90089-2539. TEL 213-740-3533, FAX 213-740-3535. Ed. Barry Glassner.

JOURNAL OF AUDIO VISUAL MEDIA IN MEDICINE. see *MEDICAL SCIENCES*

JOURNAL OF EARLY INTERVENTION. see *EDUCATION—Special Education And Rehabilitation*

JOURNAL OF PHARMACY TEACHING. see *PHARMACY AND PHARMACOLOGY*

JOURNAL OF STRUCTURAL LEARNING AND INTELLIGENT SYSTEMS. see *PSYCHOLOGY*

613.7 USA ISSN 0273-5024
GV363
JOURNAL OF TEACHING IN PHYSICAL EDUCATION. Text in English. 1981. q. USD 45 to individuals; USD 135 to institutions; USD 30 to students (effective 2001). adv. bk.rev. bibl, charts, stat, illus. index. back issues avail.; reprint service avail. from PSC,SCH. *Refereed.* **Document type:** *Academic/Scholarly.* **Description:** Designed to stimulate and communicate research and practical applications in the field of physical education. Offers new teaching methods and ideas to help students, teachers, teacher educators, and administrators at all levels.
Related titles: Online - full text ed.: (from Institute for Scientific Information).
Indexed: ASCA, C.I.J.E., Cont.Pg.Educ., Curr.Cont., ERA, Educ.Ind. (Jul.1997-), Educ.Tech.Abstr., Focus on: Sports Sci.& Med., IBZ, Phys.Ed.Ind., PsycInfo, Psychol.Abstr. (1989-), Rural Recreat.Tour.Abstr., SOMA, SSCI, Sociol.Educ.Abstr., Sp.Ed.Needs Abstr., Sportsearch (1982-), Tech.Educ.Abstr., e-psyche.
—BLDSC (5068.285700), IDS, ingenta. **CCC.**
Published by: Human Kinetics Publishers, Inc., PO Box 5076, Champaign, IL 61825-5076. TEL 217-351-5076, FAX 217-351-2674, http://www.humankinetics.com. Eds. Deborah Tannehill, Hans van der Mars. Pub. Rainer Martens. R&P Cheri Banks TEL 217-351-5076 ext 2275. Adv. contact David Kotarba TEL 800-747-4457 x 2389. Circ: 1,183 (paid).

JOURNAL OF THEORY CONSTRUCTION AND TESTING. see *MEDICAL SCIENCES—Nurses And Nursing*

DAS KIND. see *CHILDREN AND YOUTH—About*

MENTAL MEASUREMENTS YEARBOOK. see *PSYCHOLOGY*

371.39 153.9 USA
▼ **MULTIPLE INTELLIGENCES NEWSLETTER.** Text in English. 1999. irreg. (approx s-m.). free per issue. back issues avail. **Document type:** *Newsletter.* **Description:** Explores on ways to apply the theory of multiple intelligences, pioneered by Dr. Howard Gardner, in teaching and assessing students.
Media: Online - full text. **Related titles:** E-mail ed.
Published by: Multiple Intelligences Research and Consulting, 1316 S Lincoln St, Kent, OH 44240. TEL 330-673-8024, mi_news_subscribe@topica.com, http://www.topica.com/t/16. Ed. Clifford Morris. Pub. C Branton Shearer. Circ: 2,600.

371.3 POL ISSN 0077-653X
LB1043.2.P6
NEODIDAGMATA. Text in Polish; Text occasionally in English, French, German; Summaries in English, French, Russian. 1970. irreg., latest vol.23, 1997. price varies. **Document type:** *Monographic series, Academic/Scholarly.* **Description:** Contains papers of the university's specialists in the field of psychology, pedagogics and sociology.
Indexed: Psychol.Abstr., e-psyche.
Published by: (Uniwersytet im. Adama Mickiewicza), Adam Mickiewicz University Press, Nowowiejskiego 55, Poznan 61734, Poland. TEL 48-61-527380, FAX 48-61-527701. Ed. Waclaw Strykowski. Pub. Maria Jankowska. R&P Malgorzata Bis. Circ: 400.

NURSE EDUCATOR. see *MEDICAL SCIENCES—Nurses And Nursing*

NUTRIDATE. see *NUTRITION AND DIETETICS*

PEER COUNSELLOR JOURNAL. see *SOCIAL SERVICES AND WELFARE*

▼ **PHARMACY EDUCATION.** see *PHARMACY AND PHARMACOLOGY*

PHYSICAL EDUCATION INDEX. see *EDUCATION—Abstracting, Bibliographies, Statistics*

613.7 NZL ISSN 1172-5958
PHYSICAL EDUCATION NEW ZEALAND. JOURNAL. Text in English. 1953. 4/yr. NZD 45 domestic; USD 30 foreign (effective 2000). adv. bk.rev. cum.index: 1953-1967. reprint service avail. from PQC. *Refereed.* **Document type:** *Academic/Scholarly.*
Formerly: New Zealand Journal of Health, Physical Education and Recreation (0028-8314)
Related titles: Microform ed.: (from PQC); Online - full text ed.: (from ProQuest Information & Learning).
Indexed: Cont.Pg.Educ., Ind.N.Z.Per., Phys.Ed.Ind., Rural Recreat.Tour.Abstr., Sportsearch (1973-).
—BLDSC (5036.206500), GNLM, Infotrieve, ingenta. **CCC.**
Published by: Physical Education New Zealand Inc., Johnsonville, PO Box 13396, Wellington, New Zealand. TEL 64-4-477-6300, FAX 64-4-478-5237, admin@penz.org.nz. Ed. Mike Boyes. R&P Chris Tait. Circ: 800.

POSTGRADUATE INSTITUTE OF MEDICAL EDUCATION AND RESEARCH, CHANDIGARH. BULLETIN. see *MEDICAL SCIENCES*

613.7 USA ISSN 0033-6297
GV201
QUEST (CHAMPAIGN). Text in English. 1963. q. USD 45 to individuals; USD 135 to institutions; USD 30 to students (effective 2001). adv. bk.rev. bibl, charts, illus, stat. back issues avail.; reprint service avail. from PSC,SCH. *Refereed.* **Document type:** *Academic/Scholarly.* **Description:** Examines issues facing today's physical education faculty and students. Synthesizes research in the sports sciences and other subdisciplines of human movement.
Related titles: Microform ed.: (from PQC); Online - full text ed.: (from Institute for Scientific Information).
Indexed: CERDIC, C.I.J.E., Cont.Pg.Educ., Curr.Cont., ERA, Educ.Ind. (Jan.1983-), Educ.Tech.Abstr., Focus on: Sports Sci.& Med., IBZ, Mult.Ed.Abstr., Phys.Ed.Ind., Rural Recreat.Tour.Abstr., SSCI, Sociol.Educ.Abstr., Sportsearch (1975-), Tech.Educ.Abstr.
—BLDSC (7216.146400), IDS, ingenta. **CCC.**
Published by: (National Association for Physical Education in Higher Education), Human Kinetics Publishers, Inc., PO Box 5076, Champaign, IL 61825-5076. TEL 217-351-5076, 800-747-4457, FAX 217-351-2674, http://www.humankinetics.com. Ed. John M Dunn. Pub. Rainer Martens. R&P Cheri Banks TEL 217-351-5076 ext 2275. Adv. contact Patty Rodriguiz. Circ: 1,330 (paid and free). **Co-sponsor:** American Academy of Physical Education.

RESEARCH QUARTERLY FOR EXERCISE AND SPORT. see *PHYSICAL FITNESS AND HYGIENE*

613.7 BRA ISSN 0102-8464
REVISTA DE EDUCACAO FISICA. Text in Portuguese. 1932. s-a. free per issue. **Document type:** *Academic/Scholarly.* **Description:** Covers physical training, sports, physical fitness, health and education.
Related titles: Diskette ed.
Published by: Centro de Capacitacao Fisica do Exercito, Av. Joao Luis s-n - URLA, Rio De Janeiro, RJ 22291-090, Brazil. TEL 55-21-543-3323, FAX 55-21-543-3323. Ed. Maj Josue Morisson de Maraes. Circ: 5,000.

S I E C U S REPORT. see *SOCIOLOGY*

028.5 USA ISSN 0883-475X
TX1
SCHOLASTIC CHOICES; personal development & living skills. Text in English. 1956. 8/yr. (m., during school year). USD 10.75; USD 21.75 for Teacher's ed. (effective 2001). adv. illus. index. reprint service avail. from PQC. **Document type:** *Magazine, Consumer.* **Description:** Allows for high- and middle-school students, grades 7-12, to make informed decisions on health, fitness, drugs, sex, family life, careers, and consumer products.
Incorporates (in 1999): Health Choices; Supersedes (in 1985): Co-Ed (0009-9724); Incorporates (in 1991): Forecast for the Home Economist (0890-9849); Which superseded (in 1986): Forecast for Home Economics (0015-7090); (1963-1966): Practical Forecast for Home Economics (0742-8693)
Related titles: Microform ed.: (from PQC); Online - full text ed.: (from The Dialog Corporation, H. W. Wilson, ProQuest Information & Learning).
Indexed: Educ.Ind. (Sep.1986-Apr.1991), Ind.Child.Mag., Mag.Ind., Media Rev.Dig. (Jan.1989-Dec.1991), R.G.Yng.Pple. (Sep.1999-).
—CISTI, ingenta.
Published by: Scholastic Inc., 555 Broadway, 2nd Fl, New York, NY 10012-3999. TEL 212-343-6100, 800-724-6528, choicesmag@scholastic.com, http://www.scholastic.com, http://www.coachadguide.com. Ed. Denise Rinaldo. Circ: 185,562. **Subscr. to:** Scholastic Magazines, 2931 E McCarthy St, Box 3710, Jefferson City, MO 65102. TEL 800-325-6149.

370.15 GBR ISSN 0143-0343
LB1051
SCHOOL PSYCHOLOGY INTERNATIONAL. Text in English. 1979. q. GBP 46 to individuals; GBP 345 to institutions; GBP 13 newsstand/cover to individuals; GBP 87 newsstand/cover to institutions (effective 2002). adv. bk.rev. illus. back issues avail. *Refereed.* **Document type:** *Academic/Scholarly.* **Description:** Highlights the concerns of those who provide quality mental health, educational, therapeutic and support services to schools and communities throughout the world.
Related titles: Online - full text ed.: (from EBSCO Publishing, O C L C Online Computer Library Center, Inc., RoweCom Information Quest, ingenta, Swets Blackwell, Institute for Scientific Information).
Indexed: ASCA, ASSIA, Br.Educ.Ind., C.I.J.E. (coverage dropped), Chic.Per.Ind., Child Devel.Abstr., Cont.Pg.Educ., Curr.Cont., ERA, Educ.Admin.Abstr., Fam.Ind., IBR, IBZ, Ind.Philos., Lang.& Lang.Behav.Abstr., Mult.Ed.Abstr., PsycInfo, Psychol.Abstr. (1979-), SOMA, SOPODA, SSCI, Sage Fam.Stud.Abstr., Sociol.Abstr., Sociol.Educ.Abstr., Sp.Ed.Needs Abstr., Tech.Educ.Abstr., Viol.& Abuse Abstr., e-psyche.
—BLDSC (8092.926300), IDS, Infotrieve, ingenta. **CCC.**
Published by: Sage Publications Ltd., 6 Bonhill St, London EC2A 4PU, United Kingdom. TEL 44-20-7374-0645, FAX 44-20-7374-8741, market@sagepub.co.uk, http://www.sagepub.co.uk/. Eds. C S McLoughlin, R L Burden. Adv. contact Jenny Kirby. page GBP 195; trim 185 x 115. Circ: 700.

SCHOOL SCIENCE REVIEW. see *SCIENCES: COMPREHENSIVE WORKS*

613.7 CHN ISSN 1006-2076
SHANDONG TIYU XUEYUAN XUEBAO/SHANDONG PHYSICAL EDUCATION INSTITUTE. JOURNAL. Text in Chinook; Abstracts and contents page in English. 1985. q. *Refereed.* **Document type:** *Journal, Academic/Scholarly.*
—BLDSC (4874.730050).
Published by: Shandong Tiyu Xueyuan/Shandong Physical Education Institute, 2 Wenhua Xi Rd, Jinan, Shandong 250063, China. Ed. Zhaobiao Fan.

SPECIAL EDUCATION LAW MONTHLY. see *EDUCATION—Special Education And Rehabilitation*

SPORTS DOCUMENTATION MONTHLY BULLETIN. see *EDUCATION—Abstracting, Bibliographies, Statistics*

E

617.1 USA ISSN 0892-4562
GV223
STRATEGIES (RESTON); a journal for physical and sport educators. Text in English. 1987. bi-m. USD 40 to individuals; USD 80 in US & Canada to libraries; USD 14 newsstand/cover (effective 2001). adv. charts, illus. index, cum.index: 1987-1997. back issues avail.; reprints avail. *Refereed.* **Document type:** *Academic/Scholarly.* **Description:** Geared toward physical and sports educators, including teachers, coaches, administrators, and athletic directors. Emphasis is placed on applying research to daily practice and on the collaboration between practitioners in the field and university-based educators.
Indexed: C.I.J.E., Educ.Ind. (Jul.1992-).
—BLDSC (8474.034210), ingenta.
Published by: (National Association for Girls and Women in Sport), American Alliance for Health, Physical Education, Recreation, and Dance, 1900 Association Dr, Reston, VA 20191-1599. TEL 703-476-3451, 800-213-7193, FAX 703-476-9527, info@aahperd.org, http://www.aahperd.org/aahperd/publications-strategies.html. Eds. Dora Schield, Judith C Young. Adv. contact Nancy Jones. page USD 700; trim 10 x 7.25. Circ: 7,500 (paid). **Co-sponsor:** National Association for Sport and Physical Education.

STUDENT UND PRAKTIKANT; Forum fuer die Pharmazeutische Ausbildung. see *PHARMACY AND PHARMACOLOGY*

TEACHER EDUCATION AND SPECIAL EDUCATION. see *EDUCATION—Special Education And Rehabilitation*

TEACHING OF PSYCHOLOGY. see *PSYCHOLOGY*

TESTS IN PRINT. see *PSYCHOLOGY*

TODAY'S SCHOOL PSYCHOLOGIST. see *PSYCHOLOGY*

TRAINING IN COUNSELLING & PSYCHOTHERAPY. see *PSYCHOLOGY*

UNTERRICHT BIOLOGIE; Beitraege zu seiner Gestaltung. see *BIOLOGY*

VERPLEEGKUNDE; Nederlandse-Vlaams tijdschrift voor verpleegkundigen. see *MEDICAL SCIENCES—Nurses And Nursing*

WYZSZA SZKOLA PEDAGOGICZNA IM. KOMISJI EDUKACJI NARODOWEJ W KRAKOWIE. ROCZNIK NAUKOWO-DYDAKTYCZNY. PRACE PSYCHOLOGICZNE. see *PSYCHOLOGY*

WYZSZA SZKOLA PEDAGOGICZNA IM. KOMISJI EDUKACJI NARODOWEJ W KRAKOWIE. ROCZNIK NAUKOWO-DYDAKTYCZNY. PRACE Z DYDAKTYKI BIOLOGII. see *BIOLOGY*

YOUNG EXCEPTIONAL CHILDREN. see *EDUCATION—Special Education And Rehabilitation*

ELECTRICAL ENERGY

see ENERGY—Electrical Energy

ELECTRICAL ENGINEERING

see ENGINEERING—Electrical Engineering

ELECTRICITY

see PHYSICS—Electricity

ELECTRONIC DATA PROCESSING

see COMPUTERS—Electronic Data Processing

ELECTRONICS

ELECTROMEDICA (DEUTSCHE AUSGABE). see *MEDICAL SCIENCES*

610 621.381 USA ISSN 1087-9447
MEDICAL ELECTRONICS MANUFACTURING. Text in English. 1992. s-a. free to qualified personnel; USD 40 newsstand/cover (effective 2001). adv. **Document type:** *Trade.* **Description:** Provides information and resources for the design and devlopment of medical electronics products.
Published by: Canon Communications LLC, 11444 W Olympic Blvd, Ste 900, Los Angeles, CA 90064-1549. TEL 310-445-4200, FAX 310-445-4299, feedback@devicelink.com, http://www.devicelink.com/mem. Ed. Sherrie Steward. Pub. William F Cobert. Adv. contact Kevin O'Grady TEL 310-445-3700. B&W page USD 3,740, color page USD 5,280. Circ: 20,000 (controlled).

ENCYCLOPEDIAS AND GENERAL ALMANACS

613.7 610 USA ISSN 0890-4480
RA431
WORLD BOOK HEALTH AND MEDICAL ANNUAL✱. Text in English. 1987. a. price varies. adv. cum.index. **Document type:** *Consumer.* **Description:** Provides new health facts and medical discoveries of the previous year. Aims to give insight into health topics from family health to medical and safety alerts. Includes a directory of health resources.
Published by: World Book, Inc., 233 N Michigan Ave, Ste 2000, Chicago, IL 60601-5805. TEL 800-967-5325, FAX 312-258-3950, http://www.worldbook.com. Ed. Robert J Janus. Pub. Michael N Ross. R&P Janet T Peterson TEL 312-258-3874. Adv. contact Mark Willy. **Subscr. to:** World Book Direct Marketing, Annuals Supplement Service, Box 11207, Des Moines, IA 50340-1207.

ENDOCRINOLOGY

see MEDICAL SCIENCES—Endocrinology

ENERGY

see also ENERGY—Electrical Energy; ENERGY—Nuclear Energy

ANNUAL REPORT ON PIPELINE SAFETY. see *ENVIRONMENTAL STUDIES—Toxicology And Environmental Safety*

ENVIRONMENTAL BIOLOGY. see *ENVIRONMENTAL STUDIES*

333.79 DNK ISSN 0106-2557
FORSKNINGSCENTER RISOE. AARSBERETNING. Text in Danish. 1957. a. free per issue.
Former titles: Forsoegsanlaeg Risoe. Aarsberetning; Formerly (until 1977): Beretning om Atomenergikommissionens Virksomhed (0415-326X)
Indexed: Food Sci.& Tech.Abstr., Potato Abstr.
Published by: Forskningscenter Risoe, Materials Department, Roskilde, Denmark.

531.64 333.7 539.7 614.8 USA ISSN 0738-9477
N E C N P NEWSLETTER. Text in English. 1971. q. USD 25 to membership Individual; USD 40 to membership Family (effective 2000). bk.rev., film rev. abstr, bibl, charts, illus, stat. back issues avail. **Description:** Explores and educates the public on safe, clean alternatives to nuclear power.
Formerly: On the Watch
Published by: New England Coalition on Nuclear Pollution, Inc., PO Box 545, Brattleboro, VT 05302. TEL 802-257-0336, necnp@necnp.org, http://www.necnp.org/. Eds. Cornelia W Iselin, Diana P Sidebotham. Circ: 1,000.

NUCLEAR LEMONS; an assessment of America's worst commercial nuclear reactors. see *ENERGY—Nuclear Energy*

NUCLEAR PLANT JOURNAL. see *ENERGY—Nuclear Energy*

333.79 USA ISSN 0888-5729
NUCLEUS (CAMBRIDGE). Text in English. 1976. q. USD 25 (effective 2001). back issues avail. **Document type:** *Newsletter, Magazine.* **Description:** Examines energy and transportation policy, arms control, nuclear power safety, and global environmental problems such as global warming.
Related titles: Online - full text ed.
Published by: Union of Concerned Scientists, Two Brattle Sq, Box 9105, Cambridge, MA 02238-9105. TEL 617-547-5552, FAX 617-864-9405, ucs@ucsusa.org, http://www.ucsusa.org/publications/pubs-home.html. Eds. Anita S Speiss, Stuart Kiang. R&P Anita S Speiss. Circ: 60,000.

PULSE OF THE PLANET. see *ENVIRONMENTAL STUDIES*

U.S. NUCLEAR REGULATORY COMMISSION. REPORT TO CONGRESS ON ABNORMAL OCCURRENCES. see *ENERGY—Nuclear Energy*

ENERGY—Electrical Energy

343.73 347.3 621.3 USA ISSN 1069-6695
KF1256.A53
ELECTROMAGNETIC FIELD LITIGATION REPORTER. Text in English. 1986. m. USD 775 (effective 1999). adv. index. back issues avail. **Document type:** *Newsletter.* **Description:** Covers the legal actions involving electromagnetic radiation from power lines.
Related titles: Online - full text ed.: (from LexisNexis).
Published by: Andrews Publications, 175 Strafford Ave, Bldg 4, Ste 140, Wayne, PA 19087. TEL 610-225-0510, 800-345-1101, FAX 610-225-0501, http://www.andrewspub.com. Ed. Ronald V Baker. Pub., R&P Robert Maroldo. Adv. contact Sofia Pables.

ENERGY—Nuclear Energy

621.48 USA ISSN 0736-492X
QC770
ARIZONA RADIATION REGULATORY AGENCY. ANNUAL REPORT. Text in English. 1965. a. **Document type:** *Government.* **Description:** Annual summary of agency program activities.
Published by: Radiation Regulatory Agency, 4814 S 40th St, Phoenix, AZ 85040. TEL 602-255-4845. Ed. Athrur Nunez.

621.48 614.85 DEU ISSN 0937-4426
B F S - BERICHTE. (Bundesamt fuer Strahlenschutz) Text in German. 1990. irreg., latest vol.13, 1997. **Document type:** *Monographic series, Government.*
Indexed: GeoRef.
Published by: (Bundesamt fuer Strahlenschutz), Wirtschaftsverlag N W GmbH, Buergermeister-Smidt-Str 74-76, Bremerhaven 27568, Germany. TEL 49-471-94544-0, FAX 49-471-9454488, vertrieb@nw-verlag.de, http://www.nw-verlag.de.

621.48 614.85 DEU ISSN 0949-2216
B F S - E T. (Bundesamt fuer Strahlenschutz - Entsorgung und Transport) Text in German. irreg., latest vol.27, 1998. DEM 22.50 per issue. **Document type:** *Monographic series, Government.*
Former titles (until 1995): E T - Berichte (0937-4434); (until 1990): P T B - Berichte (0721-0892)
Indexed: GeoRef.
Published by: (Bundesamt fuer Strahlenschutz), Wirtschaftsverlag N W GmbH, Buergermeister-Smidt-Str 74-76, Bremerhaven 27568, Germany. TEL 49-471-94544-0, FAX 49-471-9454488, vertrieb@nw-verlag.de, http://www.nw-verlag.de.

621.48 614.85 DEU
B F S - I A R. (Bundesamt fuer Strahlenschutz - Atmosphaerische Radioaktivitaet) Text in German. 1990. irreg., latest vol.3, 1998. **Document type:** *Monographic series, Government.*
Indexed: GeoRef.
Published by: (Bundesamt fuer Strahlenschutz), Wirtschaftsverlag N W GmbH, Buergermeister-Smidt-Str 74-76, Bremerhaven 27568, Germany. TEL 49-471-94544-0, FAX 49-471-9454488, vertrieb@nw-verlag.de, http://www.nw-verlag.de.

621.48 614.85 DEU ISSN 0949-2224
CODEN: BIBEFN
B F S - I S H BERICHTE. Text in German. 1983. irreg., latest vol.184, 1999. **Document type:** *Monographic series, Government.*
Former titles (until 1994): I S H Berichte (0937-4558); (until 1989): I S H Heft (0175-4254); Which was formed by the merger of (197?-1983): S T H Berichte (0172-0198); (1981-1983): I S H Berichte (0721-4634)
Indexed: Chem.Abstr., Chem.Indus.Notes, Chem.Titles, GeoRef, Ref.Zh.
—BLDSC (1947.486270), CASDDS, CISTI, GNLM.
Published by: (Bundesamt fuer Strahlenschutz), Wirtschaftsverlag N W GmbH, Buergermeister-Smidt-Str 74-76, Bremerhaven 27568, Germany. TEL 49-471-94544-0, FAX 49-471-9454488, vertrieb@nw-verlag.de, http://www.nw-verlag.de. **Co-sponsor:** Institut fuer Strahlenhygiene.

621.48 614.85 DEU ISSN 0949-3204
B F S - K T. (Bundesamt fuer Strahlenschutz - Kerntechnische Sicherheit) Text in German. 1992. irreg., latest vol.22, 1999. **Document type:** *Monographic series, Government.*
Formerly (until 1995): K T - Berichte (0937-4442)
Indexed: GeoRef.

Published by: (Bundesamt fuer Strahlenschutz), Wirtschaftsverlag N W GmbH, Buergermeister-Smidt-Str 74-76, Bremerhaven 27568, Germany. TEL 49-471-94544-0, FAX 49-471-9454488, vertrieb@nw-verlag.de, http://www.nw-verlag.de.

621.48 614.85 DEU ISSN 0949-3212
B F S - S T. (Bundesamt fuer Strahlenschutz - Strahlenschutz) Text in German. 1964. irreg., latest vol.16, 1999. **Document type:** *Monographic series, Government.*
Former titles (until 1995): S T - Berichte (0939-3285); (until 1992): Staatliches Amt fuer Atomsicherheit und Strahlenschutz der DDR. Report (0138-2551); (until 1974): Staatliche Zentrale fuer Strahlenschutz. Report (0138-2500)
Indexed: GeoRef, Ref.Zh.
Published by: (Bundesamt fuer Strahlenschutz), Wirtschaftsverlag N W GmbH, Buergermeister-Smidt-Str 74-76, Bremerhaven 27568, Germany. TEL 49-471-94544-0, FAX 49-471-9454488, vertrieb@nw-verlag.de, http://www.nw-verlag.de.

621.48 614.85 DEU ISSN 0937-4469
B F S - SCHRIFTEN. (Bundesamt fuer Strahlenschutz) Text in German. 1990. irreg., latest vol.18, 1998. **Document type:** *Monographic series, Government.*
Indexed: GeoRef.
Published by: (Bundesamt fuer Strahlenschutz), Wirtschaftsverlag N W GmbH, Buergermeister-Smidt-Str 74-76, Bremerhaven 27568, Germany. TEL 49-471-94544-0, FAX 49-471-9454488, vertrieb@nw-verlag.de, http://www.nw-verlag.de.

BEZPIECZENSTWO JADROWE I OCHRONA RADIOLOGICZNA. see *PUBLIC HEALTH AND SAFETY*

C Y R I C ANNUAL REPORT. (Cyclotron Radioisotope Center) see *MEDICAL SCIENCES—Radiology And Nuclear Medicine*

612.01455 NLD ISSN 0926-9770
EURO COURSES. HEALTH PHYSICS AND RADIATION PROTECTION. Text in English. 1991. irreg., latest vol.2, 1993. price varies. *Refereed.* **Document type:** *Proceedings.*
Published by: (Commission of the European Communities BEL), Kluwer Academic Publishers Group (Subsidiary of: Wolters Kluwer N.V.), Spuiboulevard 50, PO Box 17, Dordrecht 3300 AA, Netherlands. FAX 31-78-639-2254, services@wkap.nl, http://www.wkap.nl. **Dist. by:** Journals Department, PO Box 322, Dordrecht 3300 AH, Netherlands. FAX 31-78-654-6474.

I A E A SAFETY STANDARDS SERIES. see *PUBLIC HEALTH AND SAFETY*

JOURNAL OF NUCLEAR AGRICULTURE AND BIOLOGY. see *AGRICULTURE—Crop Production And Soil*

539.7 GBR ISSN 0952-4746
CODEN: JRPREA
JOURNAL OF RADIOLOGICAL PROTECTION. Text in English. 1981. q. USD 417 to institutions; USD 313 microfiche (effective 2000). adv. bk.rev. **Document type:** *Academic/Scholarly.* **Description:** Covers dosimetry, instrument development, specialized measuring techniques, biological effects, environmental impact assessment.
Formerly: Society for Radiological Protection. Journal (0260-2814)
Related titles: Microform ed.: (from AIP); Online - full text ed.: (from EBSCO Publishing, RoweCom Information Quest).
Indexed: Aqua.Sci.& Fish.Abstr., Bioeng.Abstr., Biol.Abstr., Chem.Abstr., Chem.Indus.Notes, Chem.Titles, Eng.Ind., Environ.Sci.Poll.Mgmt., Excerp.Med., INIS Atomind., INSPEC (Spr.1981-Win.1987, Mar.1988-), Ind.Med. (1988-), Pollut.Abstr., Risk Abstr., Saf.Sci.Abstr., Sel.Water Res.Abstr., Tox.Abstr.
—BLDSC (5043.950000), AskIEEE, CASDDS, CISTI, Ei, EMDOCS, GNLM, Infotrieve, ingenta, KNAW, Linda Hall. **CCC.**
Published by: (Institute of Physics), I O P Publishing Ltd., Dirac House, Temple Back, Bristol BS1 6BE, United Kingdom. TEL 44-117-929-7481, FAX 44-117-929-4318, custserv@ioppublishing.co.uk, http://www.iop.org/journals/jr, http:/www.iop.org. Ed. R Wakeford. Adv. contact Chris Manning. Circ: 226. **Subscr. addr. in US:** American Institute of Physics, Subscriber Service, Ste 1N01, 2 Huntingdon Quadrangle, Melville, NY 11747-4502. TEL 516-576-2200. **Co-sponsor:** Society for Radiological Protection.

N E C N P NEWSLETTER. see *ENERGY*

333.792 614.8 USA
NUCLEAR LEMONS; an assessment of America's worst commercial nuclear reactors. Text in English. 1979. irreg., latest vol.4, 1993. USD 40; USD 60 with Data supplement. back issues avail. **Description:** Reviews accidents, management lapses, fines, emergency plant shutdowns and other mishaps at US commercial nuclear power plants.
Formerly: Nuclear Power Safety Report
Published by: Public Citizen's Critical Mass Energy Project, 215 Pennsylvania Ave, S E, Washington, DC 20003. TEL 202-546-4996, FAX 202-547-7392. **Subscr. to:** Public Citizen, Inc., 1600 20th St, N W, Washington, DC 20009. TEL 202-588-1000, FAX 202-588-7798.

539.7 614.8 USA ISSN 0892-2055
TK1078
NUCLEAR PLANT JOURNAL. Text in English. 1983. bi-m. USD 120; USD 150 foreign (effective 1999). adv. bk.rev. charts, illus, stat, tr.lit. back issues avail. *Refereed.* **Document type:** *Trade.* **Description:** Includes technical papers, articles and departments aimed at developing better methods, systems, products, and services in the nuclear power industry.
Formerly (until 1987): Nuclear Plant Safety (0742-4868)
Related titles: Online - full text ed.: (from Institute for Scientific Information).
Indexed: ASCA, Eng.Ind., Environ.Sci.Poll.Mgmt., ISMEC, Pollut.Abstr., Risk Abstr., Saf.Sci.Abstr., Solid St.Abstr.
—BLDSC (6182.430000), CISTI, Ei, IDS, Infotrieve, ingenta, Linda Hall. **CCC.**
Published by: (International Nuclear Power Industry), E Q E S, Inc., 799 Roosevelt Rd, Bldg 6, Ste 208, Glen Ellyn, IL 60137-5925. TEL 630-858-6161 ext. 14, FAX 630-858-8787. Ed., Pub., R&P Newal K Agnihotri. Adv. contact Eileen Frederickson. Circ: 20,000.

333.792 PHL ISSN 0115-2300
NUCLEUS* . Text in English. 1960. a. PHP 20, USD 20. **Document type:** *Academic/Scholarly.*
Indexed: INIS Atomind.
—Linda Hall.
Published by: Radioisotope Society of the Philippines, c/o Philippine Nuclear Research Institute, Commonwealth Ave, Diliman, Quezon City, Philippines. Ed. Aida D Davila Eugenio. Circ: 500.

621.48 USA ISSN 0748-4151
TK9152
U.S. NUCLEAR REGULATORY COMMISSION. REPORT TO CONGRESS ON ABNORMAL OCCURRENCES. Key Title: Report to Congress on Abnormal Occurrences. Text in English. 1975. a. USD 6.50; USD 8.15 foreign (effective 1995). back issues avail. **Document type:** *Government.* **Description:** Reports unscheduled events N.R.C. has deemed important for public health and safety.
Published by: U.S. Nuclear Regulatory Commission, 1 White Flint North Bldg, 11555 Rockville Pike, Rockville, MD 20852-2738.

VITAL SIGNS (CAMBRIDGE). see *PUBLIC HEALTH AND SAFETY*

ZHONGHUA FANGSHE YIXUE YU FANGHU ZAZHI/CHINESE JOURNAL OF RADIOLOGICAL MEDICINE AND PROTECTION. see *MEDICAL SCIENCES—Radiology And Nuclear Medicine*

ENGINEERING

see also ENGINEERING—Chemical Engineering; ENGINEERING—Civil Engineering; ENGINEERING—Computer Applications; ENGINEERING—Electrical Engineering; ENGINEERING—Engineering Mechanics And Materials; ENGINEERING—Hydraulic Engineering; ENGINEERING—Industrial Engineering; ENGINEERING—Mechanical Engineering

ADVANCES IN OCCUPATIONAL ERGONOMICS AND SAFETY. see *OCCUPATIONAL HEALTH AND SAFETY*

AMERICAN INTERNATIONAL JOURNAL OF ARTS, SCIENCES, ENGINEERING AND MEDICINE. see *ART*

ANNUAL CONFERENCE ON ACTIVATED SLUDGE PROCESS CONTROL. PROCEEDINGS. see *PUBLIC HEALTH AND SAFETY*

620.8 GBR ISSN 0003-6870
TA166 CODEN: AERGBW
APPLIED ERGONOMICS; human factors in technology and society. Text in English. 1969. bi-m. EUR 183 in Europe to qualified personnel; JPY 24,300 in Japan to qualified personnel; USD 205 elsewhere to qualified personnel; EUR 735 in Europe to institutions; JPY 97,600 in Japan to institutions; USD 822 elsewhere to institutions (effective 2002). adv. bk.rev. abstr, illus. index. back issues avail.; reprint service avail. from PSC,SCH. *Refereed.* **Document type:** *Academic/Scholarly.* **Description:** Covers applications of ergonomics in the office, in industry consumer products, information technology and military design.
Related titles: Microform ed.: (from PQC); Online - full text ed.: (from ingenta, Gale Group, Swets Blackwell, ScienceDirect, Factiva, Institute for Scientific Information).
Indexed: ASCA, Abstr.Hum.Comp.Inter., Acoust.Abstr., AgeLine, Agri.Eng.Abstr., BMT, Br.Tech.Ind., C.I.S. Abstr., Curr.Cont., Cyb.Abstr., Dok.Arbeitsmed., Eng.Ind., Environ.Sci.Poll.Mgmt., Ergon.Abstr., Excerp.Med., Fam.Ind., HRIS, IBR, INIS Atomind., INSPEC (Jun.1971-Dec.1983, dropped), ISMEC, Ind.Med. (1969-), Int.Nurs.Ind., Noise Pollut.Publ.Abstr., PsycInfo, Psychol.Abstr. (1971-), Psycscan A.P., SSCI, Saf.Sci.Abstr., Sci.Cit.Ind., Trop.Dis.Bull.
—BLDSC (1572.500000), CISTI, Ei, EMDOCS, IDS, ingenta, Linda Hall. **CCC.**
Published by: Pergamon (Subsidiary of: Elsevier Science), The Boulevard, Langford Ln, East Park, Kidlington, Oxford OXB 1GB, United Kingdom. FAX 44-1865-843010, nlinfo-f@elsevier/nl; usinfo-f@elsevier.com; forinfo-kyf04035@niftyserve.or.jp, http://www.elsevier.com/locate/apergo. Eds. J R Wilson, K C Parsons. **Subscr. in Australasia and the Far East to:** Elsevier Science (Singapore) Pte Ltd, No.1 Temasek Ave, 17-01 Millenia Tower, Singapore 039192, Singapore. TEL 65-434-3727, FAX 65-337-2230; **Subscr. in the Americas to:** Elsevier Science, PO Box 945, New York, NY 10159-0945. TEL 212-633-3730, FAX 212-633-3680, usinfo-f@elsevier.com; **Subscr. to:** Elsevier Science BV, PO Box 211, Amsterdam 1000 AE, Netherlands. TEL 31-20-485-3757, FAX 31-20-485-3432, nlinfo-f@elsevier.nl.

B M E S BULLETIN. see *MEDICAL SCIENCES*

BIO-MEDICAL MATERIALS AND ENGINEERING; an international journal. see *BIOLOGY—Bioengineering*

C S P DIRECTORY AND INTERNATIONAL REGISTRY OF CERTIFIED SAFETY PROFESSIONALS. see *OCCUPATIONAL HEALTH AND SAFETY*

620.86 GBR ISSN 1365-5531
CLEANROOM TECHNOLOGY. Text in English. 1996. 8/yr. GBP 65 in Europe; USD 95 in United States; GBP 4.50 newsstand/cover (effective 2002). adv. **Document type:** *Magazine, Trade.* **Description:** Provides up-to-date news, events, buyers' guides, new facility developments and more in-depth features on technical subjects.
Indexed: Eng.Ind., INSPEC (Spr.1996-).
Published by: Polygon Media Ltd. (Subsidiary of: United Business Media), Tubs Hill House, London Rd, Seven Oaks, Kent TN13 1BY, United Kingdom. TEL 44-1732-470000, FAX 44-1732-470049, http://www.cleanroom-technology.co.uk. Ed. Versha Miyanger. Adv. contact Sandra Sterling. B&W page GBP 1,890, color page GBP 2,540; trim 105 x 150. Circ: 9,000 (controlled).

▼ **CONSTRUCTION & ENGINEERING MAGAZINE**; OSHA news, legal issues, workers' comp, safety issues, products, services. see *OCCUPATIONAL HEALTH AND SAFETY*

620.8 GBR ISSN 0267-4718
TA166
CONTEMPORARY ERGONOMICS. Text in English. 1984. a. GBP 712 (effective 1999). adv. **Document type:** *Monographic series.* **Description:** Information for those who have an interest in people's interaction with their working and leisure environment, including designers, manufacturing and production engineers, health and safety specialists, psychologists, and applied physiologists.
Indexed: e-psyche.
—BLDSC (3425.181600), Infotrieve. **CCC.**
Published by: Taylor & Francis Group, Taylor & Francis Ltd., 11 New Fetter Ln, London EC4P 4EE, United Kingdom. TEL 44-20-7583-9855, FAX 44-20-7842-2298, info@tandf.co.uk, http://www.tandf.co.uk. Ed. M A Hanson. **Subscr. in N. America to:** Taylor & Francis Ltd., 325 Chestnut St, Suite 800, Philadelphia, PA 19016. TEL 800-354-1420, FAX 215-625-8914, info@taylorandfrancis.com, http://www.taylorandfrancis.com/.

620.8 158.7 ITA ISSN 1123-7651
ERGONOMIA; prodotti, lavoro, ricerca. Text in Italian. 1992. q. ITL 40,000 domestic to individuals; ITL 70,000 foreign to individuals; ITL 100,000 to institutions. **Document type:** *Monographic series.* **Description:** Information on products, work, and research in ergonomics.
Indexed: Ergon.Abstr., IBZ, e-psyche.
Published by: (Societa Italiana de Ergonomia), Moretti e Vitalli Editori, Via Betty Ambiveri 15, Bergamo, BG 24126, Italy. TEL 39-35-321588, FAX 39-35-321647. Ed. Enrico Moretti.

620.8 GBR ISSN 0014-0139
TA166 CODEN: ERGOAX
ERGONOMICS; an international journal of research and practice in human factors and ergonomics. Text in English. 1957. 15/yr. GBP 1,370, USD 2,260 to institutions (effective 2002). adv. bk.rev. abstr, bibl, illus. index. cum.index: 1968-1979. back issues avail.; reprint service avail. from PSC,SCH. *Refereed.* **Document type:** *Academic/Scholarly.* **Description:** Concerned with the diverse interactions of humans with their working environment and equipment. Explores the psychological, physiological and engineering-design aspects of human factors as they relate to work performance and efficiency.
Related titles: Microform ed.: (from NRP); Online - full text ed.: ISSN 1366-5847. 1997 (from CatchWord Ltd., EBSCO Publishing, O C L C Online Computer Library Center, Inc., RoweCom Information Quest, Gale Group, Swets Blackwell, Factiva, Institute for Scientific Information).
Indexed: AMED, A.S.& T.Ind. (Jan.1991-), Abstr.Anthropol., Abstr.Hum.Comp.Inter., Acoust.Abstr., AgeLine, Appl.Mech.Rev., BMT, Bibl.Asian Stud. (1970), Bioeng.Abstr., Biol.Abstr., Br.Rail.Bd., Br.Tech.Ind., CINAHL, C.I.S. Abstr., Chem.Abstr., Compumath, Comput.& Info.Sys., Comput.Lit.Ind., Curr.Cont., Cyb.Abstr., Dent.Ind., Electron.& Communic.Abstr.J., Emerald, Eng.Ind., Environ.Sci.Poll.Mgmt., Ergon.Abstr., Excerp.Med., HRIS, IBZ, INIS Atomind., ISMEC, Ind.Med. (1957-), Ind.Philos., Ind.Sci.Rev., Int.Aerosp.Abstr., Lab.Haz.Bull., Mgmt.& Market.Abstr., Neurosci.Cit.Ind., Noise Pollut.Publ.Abstr., Nutr.Abstr., P.A.I.S., Psyclnfo, Psychol.Abstr. (1957-), Psycscan A.P., Risk Abstr., SSCI, Saf.Sci.Abstr., Sci.Cit.Ind., Trop.Dis.Bull., e-psyche.
—BLDSC (3808.500000), CatchWord, CISTI, Ei, GNLM, IDS, ingenta, Linda Hall. **CCC.**
Published by: (Ergonomics Society), Taylor & Francis Group, Taylor & Francis Ltd., 11 New Fetter Ln, London EC4P 4EE, United Kingdom. TEL 44-20-7583-9855, FAX 44-20-7842-2298, info@tandf.co.uk, http://www.tandf.co.uk. Ed. Rob Stammers. **Subscr. in N. America to:** Taylor & Francis Ltd., 325 Chestnut St, Suite 800, Philadelphia, PA 19016. TEL 800-354-1420, FAX 215-625-8914, info@taylorandfrancis.com, http://www.taylorandfrancis.com/.

620 616.89 USA ISSN 1064-8046
TA166 CODEN: ERDEFR
ERGONOMICS IN DESIGN; the magazine of human factors applications. Text in English. 1993. q., latest vol.9, 2001, Fall. USD 41 to non-members (effective 2001). adv. bk.rev., software rev. Index. 32 p./no. back issues avail. *Refereed.* **Document type:** *Magazine, Academic/Scholarly.* **Description:** Designed to serve the needs of scientists, researchers, and practitioners concerned with the usability of products, systems and environments. Provides up-to-date demonstrations of the importance of ergonomics principles in design and implementation.
Related titles: Microform ed.: (from PQC).
Indexed: Eng.Ind., Environ.Sci.Poll.Mgmt., Ergon.Abstr., INSPEC (Jan.1996-), Pollut.Abstr., Risk Abstr., Saf.Sci.Abstr., e-psyche.
—BLDSC (3808.560000), AskIEEE, ingenta. **CCC.**
Published by: Human Factors and Ergonomics Society, PO Box 1369, Santa Monica, CA 90406-1369. TEL 310-394-1811, FAX 310-394-2410, info@hfes.org, nfes@compuserve.com, http://hfes.org. Eds. John B Shafer, John F. Kelley. Adv. contact Lois Smith. Circ: 5,300.

620.8 GBR ISSN 0268-5639
THE ERGONOMIST. Text in English. 1965. m. membership. bk.rev. **Document type:** *Newsletter.* **Description:** Covers society events and alerts readers to forthcoming conferences and events.
Indexed: Ergon.Abstr., Lab.Haz.Bull., e-psyche.
Published by: Ergonomics Society, Devonshire House, Devonshire Sq, Loughborough, Leics LE11 3DW, United Kingdom. TEL 44-1865-311776. Ed. Dr. A Kaye C Simmons. adv.: page GBP 670; trim 190 x 240. Circ: 1,300.

ESCUELA TECNICA SUPERIOR DE INGENIEROS DE MONTES. BIBLIOTECA. BOLETIN BIBLIOGRAFICO Y DOCUMENTAL. INFORMACION FORESTAL. SERIE A: MONOGRAFIAS. see *FORESTS AND FORESTRY—Abstracting, Bibliographies, Statistics*

ESCUELA TECNICA SUPERIOR DE INGENIEROS DE MONTES. BIBLIOTECA. BOLETIN BIBLIOGRAFICO Y DOCUMENTAL. INFORMACION FORESTAL. SERIE B: PUBLICACIONES PERIODICAS. see *FORESTS AND FORESTRY—Abstracting, Bibliographies, Statistics*

FRONTIERS OF MEDICAL AND BIOLOGICAL ENGINEERING. see *BIOLOGY—Bioengineering*

HAZARDOUS WASTE CONSULTANT. see *ENVIRONMENTAL STUDIES—Waste Management*

HAZARDOUS WASTE REGULATORY ANALYSIS SERVICE. see *ENVIRONMENTAL STUDIES—Waste Management*

158.7 620.8 USA ISSN 0018-7208
T58.A2 CODEN: HUFAA6
HUMAN FACTORS. Text in English. 1958. q. USD 176 domestic (effective 2002). illus. index; cum.index every 5 years. 176 p./no. back issues avail.; reprint service avail. from PQC,PSC,SCH. *Refereed.* **Document type:** *Journal, Academic/Scholarly.* **Description:** Presents papers of scientific merit that contribute to the understanding and advancement of the systematic consideration of people in relation to machines and environments.
Related titles: Microform ed.: (from PQC); Online - full text ed.: (from Northern Light Technology, Inc., H. W. Wilson, ProQuest Information & Learning, Gale Group, Factiva, Institute for Scientific Information).
Indexed: A.S.& T.Ind. (Aug.1983-), ASCA, Abstr.Anthropol., Abstr.Hum.Comp.Inter., AgeLine, Agri.Eng.Abstr., Aqua.Sci.& Fish.Abstr., BMT, Bioeng.Abstr., Biol.Abstr., C.I.S. Abstr., Commun.Abstr., Comput.& Info.Sys., Curr.Cont., Dok.Arbeitsmed., Electron.& Communic.Abstr.J., Eng.Ind., Environ.Sci.Poll.Mgmt., Ergon.Abstr., HRIS, Human Resour.Abstr., IBZ, INIS Atomind., INSPEC (Dec.1968-), ISMEC, Ind.Med. (1958-), Ind.Philos., Ind.Sci.Rev., Inform.Sci.Abstr., Lanc.Ind., Mgmt.& Market.Abstr., Pollut.Abstr., Psyclnfo, Psychol.Abstr. (1958-), Psycscan A.P., Ref.Zh., Risk Abstr., Russ.Acad.Sci.Bibl., SSCI, Saf.Sci.Abstr., Sage Urb.Stud.Abstr., Sci.Cit.Ind., e-psyche.
—BLDSC (4336.075000), AskIEEE, CISTI, Ei, GNLM, IDS, ingenta, Linda Hall. **CCC.**
Published by: Human Factors and Ergonomics Society, PO Box 1369, Santa Monica, CA 90406-1369. TEL 310-394-1811, FAX 310-394-2410, lois@hfes.org, http://www.hfes.org. Eds. Eduardo Salas, W C Howell. Circ: 6,200.

620.8 301.1 USA ISSN 1071-1813
TA166 CODEN: PHFSDQ
HUMAN FACTORS AND ERGONOMICS SOCIETY ANNUAL MEETING. PROCEEDINGS. Text in English. 1972. a., latest vol.45, 2001, Fall. USD 95 to non-members (effective 2000). 1500 p./no. reprint service avail. from PQC. *Refereed.* **Document type:** *Proceedings, Academic/Scholarly.*
Former titles: Human Factors Society Annual Meeting (0163-5182); Human Factors Society. Proceedings of the Annual Meeting (0363-9797)
Related titles: CD-ROM ed.; Microform ed.: (from PQC); Online - full text ed.: (from ProQuest Information & Learning).
Indexed: Bioeng.Abstr., Comput.& Info.Sys., ISMEC, Int.Aerosp.Abstr., e-psyche.
—BLDSC (6844.113600), Ei, GNLM, Infotrieve. **CCC.**
Published by: Human Factors and Ergonomics Society, PO Box 1369, Santa Monica, CA 90406-1369. TEL 310-394-1811, FAX 310-394-2410, info@hfes.org, hfes@compuserve.com, http://hfes.org. Circ: 1,700 (paid).

620.8 158.7 USA ISSN 1527-3660
Q300
HUMAN FACTORS AND ERGONOMICS SOCIETY BULLETIN. Text in English. 1958. m., latest vol.44, 2001, Dec. USD 42 to non-members (effective 2000). adv. 8 p./no. back issues avail. **Document type:** *Newsletter, Trade, Academic/Scholarly.* **Description:** Serves as a forum for readers to keep abreast of current technology and events in the world of human factors - ergonomics, as well as world events of interest to members.
Formerly (until 1993): Human Factors Society Bulletin (0438-1629)
Indexed: Abstr.Hum.Comp.Inter., AgeLine, Ergon.Abstr., Psychol.Abstr., e-psyche.
—BLDSC (2555.353900), Infotrieve. **CCC.**
Published by: Human Factors and Ergonomics Society, PO Box 1369, Santa Monica, CA 90406-1369. TEL 310-394-1811, FAX 310-394-2410, info@hfes.org, hfes@compuserve.com, http://hfes.org. Adv. contact Lois Smith. Circ: 5,000.

620 SGP
THE I E A JOURNAL OF ERGONOMICS. Text in English. 1998. q. free. back issues avail. *Refereed.* **Document type:** *Academic/Scholarly.* **Description:** Offers a Web based platform for the rapid dissemination of research in the fields of ergonomics: cognition, including HCI, biomechanics, organizational design, and job design.
Media: Online - full content.
Published by: International Ergonomics Association, c/o Martin G Helander, School of Mechanical and Production Engineering, Nanyang Technological University, Singapore 639798, Singapore. TEL 65-790-6398, FAX 65-791-1859, mahel@ntu.edu.sg, http://ergonomics-iea.org/iea/journal/journal, http://ergonomics-iea.org/iea/main.html. Eds. Martin G Helander, Waldemar Karwowski.

INSTITUTE OF ENVIRONMENTAL SCIENCES AND TECHNOLOGY. ANNUAL TECHNICAL MEETING. PROCEEDINGS. see *ENVIRONMENTAL STUDIES*

INSTITUTE OF ENVIRONMENTAL SCIENCES. TUTORIAL SERIES. see *ENVIRONMENTAL STUDIES*

320.8 GBR
INTERNATIONAL CONFERENCE ON ENGINEERING PSYCHOLOGY AND COGNITIVE ERGONOMICS. Text in English. a.
—BLDSC (3766.565000).
Published by: Ashgate Publishing Ltd (Subsidiary of: Gower Publishing Co. Ltd.), Gower House, Croft Rd, Aldershot, Hants GU11 3HR, United Kingdom. TEL 44-1252-331551, FAX 44-1252-317446, info@ashgate.com, http://www.ashgate.com.

INTERNATIONAL SOCIETY FOR OCCUPATIONAL ERGONOMICS AND SAFETY. NEWSLETTER. see *OCCUPATIONAL HEALTH AND SAFETY*

▼ **JOURNAL OF NANOSCIENCE AND NANOTECHNOLOGY.** see *COMPUTERS—Microcomputers*

JOURNAL OF PRODUCTS AND TOXICS LIABILITY. see *LAW*

JOURNAL OF REHABILITATION RESEARCH AND DEVELOPMENT. see *MEDICAL SCIENCES—Orthopedics And Traumatology*

628 USA ISSN 0748-2116
QC789.2.U62
LOGOS (ARGONNE). Text in English. 3/yr. free per issue. bk.rev. bibl, illus. reprint service avail. from SCH. **Document type:** *Academic/Scholarly.* **Description:** Reports on selected research programs conducted at Argonne National Laboratory, focusing on engineering research, biomedical and environmental science and technology.
Indexed: Energy Info.Abstr., Environ.Abstr.
—ingenta.
Published by: Argonne National Laboratory, Office of Public Affairs, 9700 S. Cass Ave., Bldg. 200, Argonne, IL 60439. TEL 630-252-5575, FAX 630-252-5274. Ed. Evelyn Brown.

620 610 GBR
MEDICAL AND BIOMEDICAL ENGINEERING REPORTS. Text in English. irreg. price varies. back issues avail. **Document type:** *Academic/Scholarly.*
Published by: Royal Academy of Engineering, 29 Great Peter St, Westminster, London SW1P 3LW, United Kingdom. TEL 44-20-7222-2688, FAX 44-20-7233-0054, http://www.raeng.org.uk.

620 USA
▼ **MEDICAL DESIGN NEWS.** Text in English. 2001. bi-m. Free to qualified personnel. adv. **Document type:** *Magazine, Trade.* **Description:** Targets design engineers, engineering managers, and related technical personnel who design, develop, and manufacture components and manufacturing equipment for the medical and biomedical industry.
Published by: Penton Media, Inc. (Subsidiary of: Pittway Company), 1300 E 9th St, Cleveland, OH 44114-1503. FAX 212-931-9799, http://www.medicaldesignnews.com, http://www.penton.com. adv.: B&W page USD 3,995, color page USD 5,245; trim 7.25 x 10.5. Circ: 35,000 (paid and controlled).

E

620 USA ISSN 0361-7904
T55.A1
NATIONAL DIRECTORY OF SAFETY CONSULTANTS. Text in English. 1974. biennial. updated quarterly. **Document type:** *Directory.* **Description:** Covers credentials and expertise areas of hundreds of safety and health consultants, cross-referenced by geography, education, professional designation and expertise.
Media: Online - full text.
Published by: American Society of Safety Engineers, 1800 E Oakton St, Des Plaines, IL 60018-2187. TEL 847-768-3433, FAX 847-296-9221, http://www.asse.org. Eds. David deVries, Rennie Heath. Circ: 1,000.

NORTHEAST BIOENGINEERING CONFERENCE. PROCEEDINGS. see *BIOLOGY—Bioengineering*

OCCUPATIONAL ERGONOMICS. see *OCCUPATIONAL HEALTH AND SAFETY*

620 621 USA ISSN 0273-8139
PHARMACEUTICAL ENGINEERING. Text in English. 1980. bi-m. USD 60; USD 78 foreign (effective 1999). adv. bk.rev. tr.lit. back issues avail. *Refereed.* **Document type:** *Trade.* **Description:** For professionals in the pharmaceutical, biotechnology, medical device and diagnostic manufacturing industries.
Indexed: I.P.A.
—BLDSC (6443.670000), EMDOCS, GNLM, ingenta, Linda Hall.
Published by: International Society for Pharmaceutical Engineering, Inc., 3816 W Linebaugh Ave, Ste 412, Tampa, FL 33624-4702. TEL 813-960-2105, FAX 813-264-2816, ispehq@ispe.org, http://www.ispe.org. Ed., R&P, Adv. contact Gloria Esoda. Circ: 17,000.

RESOURCE DIRECTORY OF SCIENTISTS AND ENGINEERS WITH DISABILITIES. see *BIOGRAPHY*

SANGYO ANZEN KENKYUJO GIJUTSU SHISHIN/NATIONAL INSTITUTE OF INDUSTRIAL SAFETY. TECHNICAL RECOMMENDATION. see *OCCUPATIONAL HEALTH AND SAFETY*

620 GBR ISSN 1463-922X
▼ **THEORETICAL ISSUES IN ERGONOMICS SCIENCE.** Abbreviated title: T I E S. Text in English. 2000. q. GBP 95, USD 150 to individuals; USD 326, GBP 197 to institutions (effective 2002). bk.rev. bibl, charts. *Refereed.* **Document type:** *Journal, Academic/Scholarly.* **Description:** Offers a theoretical basis for the science of ergonomics, publishing experiments and applied research.
Related titles: Online - full text ed.: ISSN 1464-536X (from EBSCO Publishing, O C L C Online Computer Library Center, Inc., Swets Blackwell, CatchWord Ltd., RoweCom Information Quest).
Indexed: Ergon.Abstr.
—BLDSC (8814.559400), CatchWord.
Published by: (International Ergonomics Association USA), Taylor & Francis Group, Taylor & Francis Ltd., 11 New Fetter Ln, London EC4P 4EE, United Kingdom. TEL 44-20-7583-9855, FAX 44-20-7842-2298, info@tandf.co.uk, http://www.tandf.co.uk/journals. Ed. Waldemar Karwowski. **Subscr. addr. in the US:** Taylor & Francis Ltd., 325 Chestnut St, Suite 800, Philadelphia, PA 19016. TEL 800-354-1420, FAX 215-625-8914, info@taylorandfrancis.com, http://www.taylorandfrancis.com/.

ENGINEERING—Abstracting, Bibliographies, Statistics

624 551.4 551 USA ISSN 0149-3825
GB2401
BIBLIOGRAPHY ON COLD REGIONS SCIENCE & TECHNOLOGY. Text in English. 1951. a. USD 30.50 (effective 1999). bibl. index, cum.index. back issues avail. **Document type:** *Government, Bibliography.*
Related titles: CD-ROM ed.: (from National Information Services Corp. (NISC)); Microfiche ed.; Online - full text ed.
Published by: U.S. Army, Cold Regions Research and Engineering Laboratory, 72 Lyme Rd, Hanover, NH 03755-1290. TEL 603-646-4221, FAX 603-646-4712, http://www.lcweb.loc.gov/rr/scitech/coldregions/welcome.html. Ed. Sharon Tahirkheli.

016.66 USA ISSN 0749-7318
CODEN: CASHE3
C A SELECTS. NOVEL PESTICIDES & HERBICIDES. Text in English. s-w. USD 275 (effective 2001). **Document type:** *Abstract/Index.* **Description:** Covers newly prepared or published compounds that have activity, are being tested, or are to be tested as pesticides.
Published by: Chemical Abstracts Service (Subsidiary of: American Chemical Society), 2540 Olentangy River Rd, Box 3012, Columbus, OH 43210-0012. TEL 614-447-3600, 800-753-4227, FAX 614-447-3751.

DIRECTORY OF PUBLISHED PROCEEDINGS. SERIES S E M T - SCIENCE, ENGINEERING, MEDICINE AND TECHNOLOGY. see *SCIENCES: COMPREHENSIVE WORKS—Abstracting, Bibliographies, Statistics*

620 016 GBR ISSN 0046-2446
TA166
ERGONOMICS ABSTRACTS. Text in English. 1968. 2/yr. GBP 1,194, USD 1,969 to institutions (effective 2002). adv. bk.rev. illus. Index. reprint service avail. from SCH,PSC. *Refereed.* **Document type:** *Abstract/Index.* **Description:** Provides an abstracting service for all areas of ergonomics and human factors. Invaluable source of information for everyone who needs up-to-date information in human-computer interaction, psychology, physiology, biomechanics and work design.
Related titles: CD-ROM ed.: ISSN 1357-5422. 199?; Microform ed.; Online - full content ed.: ISSN 1464-5084. 199? (from JSTOR (Web-based Journal Archive), O C L C Online Computer Library Center, Inc., Swets Blackwell); Online - full text ed.: (from RoweCom Information Quest).
Indexed: Comput.Lit.Ind.
Published by: (Ergonomics Information Analysis Centre), Taylor & Francis Group, Taylor & Francis Ltd., 11 New Fetter Ln, London EC4P 4EE, United Kingdom. TEL 44-20-7583-9855, FAX 44-20-7842-2298, info@tandf.co.uk, http://www.tandf.co.uk. Ed. Christine Stapleton. **Subscr. in N. America to:** Taylor & Francis Ltd., 325 Chestnut St, Suite 800, Philadelphia, PA 19016. TEL 800-354-1420, FAX 215-625-8914, info@taylorandfrancis.com, http://www.taylorandfrancis.com/.

SAFETY ABSTRACTS. see *PUBLIC HEALTH AND SAFETY—Abstracting, Bibliographies, Statistics*

ENGINEERING—Chemical Engineering

see also PLASTICS

660.2 542 USA ISSN 0569-5473
A I CH E EQUIPMENT TESTING PROCEDURES SERIES. Text in English. 1952. irreg., latest 1992. price varies. back issues avail. *Refereed.* **Document type:** *Trade.* **Description:** Prepared for the engineer involved in installing equipment and testing practices evaluation.
Related titles: Microform ed.: (from ISI).
Indexed: Eng.Ind.
—CCC.
Published by: American Institute of Chemical Engineers, Equipment Testing Procedures Committee, 3 Park Ave, New York, NY 10016-5901. TEL 800-242-4363, FAX 212-591-8888, http://www.aiche.org.

C A SELECTS. NOVEL PESTICIDES & HERBICIDES. see *ENGINEERING—Abstracting, Bibliographies, Statistics*

660.2 DEU ISSN 1436-2597
C I T PLUS. (Chemie Ingenieur Technik) Text in German. 1998. 12/yr. DEM 268 domestic to institutions; EUR 137 in Europe to institutions; CHF 238 to institutions Switzerland & Liechtenstein; USD 158 elsewhere to institutions (effective 2001). 68 p./no. **Document type:** *Journal, Academic/Scholarly.* **Description:** Covers all aspects of chemical engineering and allied academic fields.
Related titles: Online - full text ed.: (from Wiley InterScience).
Indexed: API Abstr.
—BLDSC (3267.699000).
Published by: Wiley - V C H, Postfach 101161, Weinheim 69451, Germany. TEL 49-6201-606-0, FAX 49-6201-606-328, subservice@wiley-vch.de, http://www.wiley-vch.de/vch/home/citplus. Ed. W Siess. R&P Claudia Rutz. Adv. contact Roland Thome.

660.2 665.5 IND
CHEMICALS, DRUGS, PHARMACEUTICALS, PETROLEUM, PETROCHEMICALS, FERTILIZERS. Text in English. 1967. w. INR 715, USD 85 (effective 1999). bk.rev. **Document type:** *Newsletter.* **Description:** Includes topics such as chemicals and pharmaceuticals and its use in India.
Formed by the merger of: Chemical Process Engineering. Drugs - Pharmaceuticals (0047-0910); Dyestuff Industry and Chemicals (0047-0929); Petroleum - Petrochemicals - Fertilisers - Agricultural Chemistry (0047-1046); Scientific Instruments, Laboratory Equipment and Chemicals (0047-1070)
Media: Duplicated (not offset).
Published by: International Press Cutting Service, PO Box 121, Allahabad, Uttar Pradesh 211 001, India. TEL 91-532-622392. Ed. Nandi Khanna. Circ: 1,200.

660.2 DEU ISSN 0009-286X
TP1 CODEN: CITEAH
CHEMIE-INGENIEUR-TECHNIK; Verfahrenstechnik, Technische Chemie, Apparatewaren, Biotechnologie. Abbreviated title: C I T. Text in German. 1928. m. EUR 1,248 in Europe; CHF 2,368 in Switzerland & Liechtenstein; USD 1,668 elsewhere; EUR 1,311 combined subscription in Europe for print and online eds.; CHF 2,487 combined subscription in Switzerland & Liechtenstein, for print and online eds.; USD 1,752 combined subscription elsewhere for print and online eds. (effective 2002). adv. bk.rev. charts, illus, mkt, tr.lit. index. 130 p./no. 2 cols./p. reprint service avail. from ISI. *Refereed.* **Document type:** *Journal, Academic/Scholarly.* **Description:** Contains research and application orientated articles describing the latest findings in industry, development, construction and production.
Related titles: Microfiche ed.; Microfilm ed.: (from VCI); Online - full text ed.: ISSN 1522-2640. EUR 1,248 in Europe; CHF 2,368 in Switzerland & Liechtenstein; USD 1,668 elsewhere (effective 2002) (from Wiley InterScience, Institute for Scientific Information).
Indexed: API Abstr., API Catal., API Hlth.& Environ., API Oil., API Pet.Ref., API Pet.Subst., ASCA, Agri.& Environ.Biotech.Abstr. (coverage dropped), Alloys Ind., Appl.Mech.Rev., CEABA, Chem.Abstr., Chem.Cit.Ind., Chem.Indus.Notes, Chem.Infd., Chem.Titles, Curr.Cont., Derwent Biotech.Abstr., Dok.Arbeitsmed., Eng.Ind., Eng.Mat.Abstr., Excerp.Med., Fluidex, Forest Prod.Abstr., Foul.Prev.Res.Dig., INIS Atomind., INSPEC (Jul.1971-Nov.1990, dropped), Ind.Sci.Rev., Intl.Polym.Sci.& Tech., Lab.Haz.Bull., Mat.Sci.Cit.Ind. (coverage dropped), Met.Abstr., Met.Abstr.Ind., Nonfer.Met.Alert, PCC Alert, PROMT, Petrol.Abstr. (coverage dropped), RAPRA (1962-1998), Ref.Zh., Risk Abstr., SSCI (coverage dropped), Sci.Cit.Ind., Sel.Water Res.Abstr., Steels Alert, Sugar Ind.Abstr., W.R.C.Inf., World Alum.Abstr.
—BLDSC (3157.000000), AskIEEE, CASDDS, CISTI, Ei, IDS, Infotrieve, ingenta, Linda Hall. **CCC.**
Published by: (Gesellschaft Deutscher Chemiker), Wiley - V C H, Postfach 101161, Weinheim 69451, Germany. TEL 49-6201-606-147, FAX 49-6201-606-117, subservice@wiley-vch.de, http://www.wiley-vch.de/home/cit. Ed. B Boeck. R&P Claudia Rutz. Adv. contact Roland Thome. page XEU 3,200; trim 180 x 260. Circ: 5,850. **Subscr. in the Americas to:** John Wiley & Sons, Inc., Journals. TEL 44-1243-779777, 212-850-6645, FAX 212-850-6021; **Subscr. outside Germany, Austria & Switzerland to:** John Wiley & Sons Ltd., Baffins Ln, Chichester, Sussex PO19 IUD, United Kingdom. TEL 44-1243-779777, FAX 44-1243-843232. **Co-sponsors:** Deutsche Gesellschaft fuer Chemisches Apparatewesen, Chemische Technik und Biotechnologie; Gesellschaft Verfahrenstechnik und Chemieingenieurwesen.

CRYOGAS INTERNATIONAL; the source of timely and relevant information for the industrial gas and cryogenics industries. see *ENGINEERING—Mechanical Engineering*

660.2 574.28 IRL
EUROPEAN SYMPOSIUM ON BIOCHEMICAL ENGINEERING SCIENCE. PROCEEDINGS. Text in English. 1996. irreg. **Document type:** *Proceedings.*
Published by: Dublin City University, Faculty of Science and Paramedical Studies, Dublin 9, Ireland. **Co-sponsor:** European Federation of Biotechnology.

GLOBAL PESTICIDE CAMPAIGNER. see *ENVIRONMENTAL STUDIES—Toxicology And Environmental Safety*

660 614.85 GBR ISSN 0260-9576
LOSS PREVENTION BULLETIN. Text in English. 1974. bi-m. GBP 260 in United Kingdom to institutions; EUR 497.28 to institutions in Euro Zone; USD 494.32 elsewhere to institutions (effective 2001). bk.rev. cum.index. back issues avail. *Refereed.* **Document type:** *Bulletin.* **Description:** Includes articles and case studies on all aspects of safety for the process industries. Contains legal updates and news on conferences and events worldwide.
Related titles: Online - full content ed.: (from EBSCO Publishing, O C L C Online Computer Library Center, Inc., Swets Blackwell); Online - full text ed.: (from CatchWord Ltd., RoweCom Information Quest).
Indexed: CEABA, CSNB, Lab.Haz.Bull.
—BLDSC (5294.742000), CISTI, Linda Hall.

E

Published by: Institution of Chemical Engineers, George E Davis Bldg, 165-189 Railway Terr, Rugby, Warks CV21 3HQ, United Kingdom. TEL 44-1788-578214, FAX 44-1788-560833, http://www.icheme.org/learning/. R&P Tracey Donaldson. Adv. contact Jo Cheshire. Circ: 1,000 (paid).

660 JPN ISSN 0385-1559
CODEN: NNGADV

NIPPON NOYAKU GAKKAISHI. Text in Japanese. 1976. 4/yr. JPY 6,000, USD 40 (effective 1993). adv. bk.rev. index. back issues avail. *Refereed.* **Document type:** *Academic/Scholarly.* **Description:** Contains articles on research results on pesticide science in general, agrochemistry and chemistry of biologically active natural products.

Related titles: Online - full text ed.: (from Institute for Scientific Information); ♦ English ed.: Journal of Pesticide Science (International Edition). ISSN 0916-9962.

Indexed: Aqua.Sci.& Fish.Abstr., Chem.Abstr., Chem.Indus.Notes, Chem.Titles, Crop Physiol.Abstr., Curr.Cont., Curr.Ref.Fish Res., Derwent Biotech.Abstr., Entomol.Abstr. (coverage dropped), Environ.Sci.Poll.Mgmt., Field Crop Abstr., Food Sci.& Tech.Abstr., Hort.Abstr., Maize Abstr., Plant Grow.Reg.Abstr., Pollut.Abstr., RCI, Rev.Appl.Entomol., Rice Abstr., Sci.Cit.Ind., Seed Abstr., Sel.Water Res.Abstr., Soils & Fert., Tox.Abstr., Weed Abstr.

—BLDSC (5030.981000), CASDDS, CISTI, IDS, Infotrieve, Linda Hall. **CCC.**

Published by: Pesticide Science Society of Japan/Nippon Noyaku Gakkai, 1-43-11 Komagome, Toshima-ku, Tokyo 170-8484, Japan. Ed. Ko Wakabayshi. Circ: 2,000.

540 USA ISSN 0272-6351
TP156.P3 CODEN: PTCHDS

PARTICULATE SCIENCE AND TECHNOLOGY; an international journal. (Includes: Fine Particle Society. Proceedings) Text in English. 1983. q. GBP 104, USD 172 to individuals; GBP 263, USD 434 to institutions (effective 2002). adv. bk.rev. bibl, charts, illus. index. back issues avail.; reprint service avail. from PQC. *Refereed.* **Document type:** *Academic/Scholarly.* **Description:** Disseminates theoretical and applied aspects of particle sizing, separation, health hazards.

Related titles: Online - full text ed.: (from Institute for Scientific Information).

Indexed: ASCA, Alloys Ind., Appl.Mech.Rev., Aqua.Sci.& Fish.Abstr., Chem.Abstr., Chem.Eng.Abstr., Chem.Indus.Notes, Chem.Titles, Curr.Cont., Eng.Ind., Eng.Mat.Abstr., Environ.Sci.Poll.Mgmt., METADEX, Met.Abstr., Met.Abstr.Ind., Nonfer.Met.Alert, PCC Alert, Pollut.Abstr., Saf.Sci.Abstr., Steels Alert, T.C.E.A., World Alum.Abstr.

—BLDSC (6407.557000), CASDDS, CISTI, Ei, IDS, ingenta, Linda Hall. **CCC.**

Published by: (Fine Particle Society), Taylor & Francis Ltd. (Subsidiary of: Taylor & Francis Group), 325 Chestnut St, Suite 800, Philadelphia, PA 19016. TEL 215-625-8900, FAX 215-625-2940, info@taylorandfrancis.com, http://www.taylorandfrancis.com/. Eds. Malay K Mazumder, Virendra M Puri. Circ: 600. **Subscr. addr. in Europe:** Taylor & Francis Group, Journals Customer Service, Rankine Rd, Basingstoke, Hants RG24 8PR, United Kingdom. TEL 44-1256-813000, FAX 44-1256-479438, enquiry@tanf.co.uk, http://www.tandf.co.uk/journals.

PESTICIDE ANALYTICAL MANUAL. see *PUBLIC HEALTH AND SAFETY*

660 615.19 DEU

PROCHEM. Text in German. a. adv. **Document type:** *Directory.*

Published by: G I T Verlag GmbH, Roesslerstr 90, Darmstadt 64293, Germany. TEL 49-6151-8090-0, FAX 49-6151-8090183, gitverlaggmbh@gitverlag.com, http://www.gitverlag.com. Adv. contact Michael Klinge.

PROFESSIONAL PEST CONTROLLER. see *PUBLIC HEALTH AND SAFETY*

615.9 GBR ISSN 0887-6142
QP801.P38 CODEN: PPBTDV

PROGRESS IN PESTICIDE BIOCHEMISTRY AND TOXICOLOGY. Text in English. 1981. irreg. price varies. illus. **Document type:** *Monographic series, Academic/Scholarly.* **Description:** Addresses what happens to pesticides in the environment after they are applied.

Formerly: Progress in Pesticide Biochemistry (0730-1898)

Indexed: Chem.Abstr., Chem.Indus.Notes, Chem.Titles, Sport Fish.Abstr., Wild.Rev., Zoo.Rec.

—CASDDS, CISTI.

Published by: Wiley Europe Ltd., Baffins Ln, Chichester, W Sussex PO19 1UD, United Kingdom. TEL 44-1243-779777, FAX 44-1243-843232, cs-journals@wiley.co.uk, http://www.wiley.co.uk. Eds. D H Hutson, T R Roberts.

SPECTRUM (WALTHAM). see *BUSINESS AND ECONOMICS*

368.11 DEU ISSN 0042-1804

V F D B: ZEITSCHRIFT FUER FORSCHUNG UND TECHNIK IM BRANDSCHUTZ. Text in German; Summaries in English, French. q. EUR 78, CHF 152.60; EUR 20.90, CHF 50 newsstand/cover (effective 2002). adv. charts, illus. index. **Document type:** *Journal, Trade.*

Formerly: V F D B Zeitschrift

Indexed: C.I.S. Abstr., Chem.Abstr., INIS Atomind.

—CISTI, Infotrieve. **CCC.**

Published by: (Vereinigung zur Foerderung des Deutschen Brandschutzes e.V.), W. Kohlhammer GmbH, Hessbruehlstr 69, Stuttgart 70565, Germany. TEL 49-711-7863-1, FAX 49-711-7863263, info@kohlhammer-katalog.de, http://www.kohlhammer.de. Circ: 1,000.

ENGINEERING—Civil Engineering

see also BUILDING AND CONSTRUCTION; TRANSPORTATION—Roads And Traffic

CURRENT TOPICS IN TRANSPORT. see *TRANSPORTATION—Roads And Traffic*

DIZHEN KANAN ANQUAN. see *EARTH SCIENCES—Geology*

624 614 USA ISSN 8755-3457

DRINKING WATER & BACKFLOW PREVENTION. Text in English. 1984. m. USD 36 domestic; USD 48 in Canada & Mexico; USD 50 elsewhere (effective 1999). adv. bk.rev. back issues avail. **Document type:** *Trade.* **Description:** Dedicated to water system safety everywhere.

Formerly: Backflow Prevention

Indexed: W.R.C.Inf.

Published by: Asay & Associates, PO Box 33209, Northglenn, CO 80233. TEL 303-451-0978, FAX 303-452-9776. Ed. Kristi M James. Circ: 3,200 (paid).

T R L NEWS. (Transport Research Laboratory) see *TRANSPORTATION—Roads And Traffic*

ENGINEERING—Computer Applications

THE I E A JOURNAL OF ERGONOMICS. see *ENGINEERING*

▼ **THEORETICAL ISSUES IN ERGONOMICS SCIENCE.** see *ENGINEERING*

ENGINEERING—Electrical Engineering

E M F HEALTH & SAFETY DIGEST. (Electric and Magnetic Field) see *OCCUPATIONAL HEALTH AND SAFETY*

HEALTH & SAFETY NEWSLINE; for the engineering industry (UK). see *PUBLIC HEALTH AND SAFETY*

621.3 629.892 NLD ISSN 1389-2258

▼ **JOURNAL OF MICROMECHATRONICS.** Text in English. 1999. q. EUR 185, USD 214 includes online ed. (effective 2002). back issues avail. *Refereed.* **Document type:** *Journal, Academic/Scholarly.* **Description:** Examines the theory and applications of microtechnology, with emphasis on the integration and mechatronic aspects of diverse micromechatronic systems.

Related titles: Online - full content ed.: 2000 (from EBSCO Publishing, Swets Blackwell); Online - full text ed.: (from CatchWord Ltd.).

Published by: V S P (Subsidiary of: Brill Academic Publishers), PO Box 346, Zeist 3700 AH, Netherlands. TEL 31-30-692-5790, FAX 31-30-693-2081, vsppub@compuserve.com, http://www.vsppub.com/journals/jn-JouMic.html. Eds. Paolo Dario, Ronald Fearing, Toshio Fukuda.

NEUROELECTRIC NEWS. see *MEDICAL SCIENCES—Psychiatry And Neurology*

SANGYO ANZEN KENKYUJO GIJUTSU SHISHIN/NATIONAL INSTITUTE OF INDUSTRIAL SAFETY. TECHNICAL RECOMMENDATION. see *OCCUPATIONAL HEALTH AND SAFETY*

SELENIUM - TELLURIUM DEVELOPMENT ASSOCIATION. BULLETIN. see *METALLURGY*

ENGINEERING—Engineering Mechanics And Materials

620 610 USA

ANNUAL BOOK OF A S T M STANDARDS. VOLUME 13.01. MEDICAL DEVICES; EMERGENCY MEDICAL SERVICES. Text in English. 1986. a. USD 202 in North America; USD 222 elsewhere (effective 2001). reprint service avail. from PQC. **Document type:** *Trade.*

Formerly: Annual Book of A S T M Standards. Volume 13.01. Medical Devices

Related titles: CD-ROM ed.; Microfiche ed.

Published by: American Society for Testing and Materials, 100 Barr Harbor Dr, West Conshohocken, PA 19428-2959. TEL 610-832-9500, FAX 610-832-9555, service@astm.org, http://www.astm.org.

BIOMATERIALS. see *MEDICAL SCIENCES*

CLINICAL ENGINEERING SECTION NEWSLETTER. see *INSTRUMENTS*

620.1 610 USA ISSN 0957-4530
R857.M3 CODEN: JSMMEL

JOURNAL OF MATERIALS SCIENCE: MATERIALS IN MEDICINE. Text in English. m. USD 915, EUR 912 to institutions for print or online ed.; USD 1,098, EUR 1,094.40 to institutions for print & online eds.combined (effective 2002). adv. illus. back issues avail.; reprint service avail. from PQC,ISI. *Refereed.* **Document type:** *Journal, Academic/Scholarly.* **Description:** Publishes papers on the science and technology of biomaterials and their applications as medical or dental implants, prostheses and devices, and biological materials.

Related titles: Online - full text ed.: (from EBSCO Publishing, O C L C Online Computer Library Center, Inc., RoweCom Information Quest, Swets Blackwell, Kluwer Online, Institute for Scientific Information).

Indexed: A.S.& T.Ind. (Jan.2000-), ASCA, Alloys Ind., Bioeng.Abstr., Biotech.& Bioeng.Abstr., Br.Ceram.Abstr., Br.Tech.Ind., Chem.Abstr., Chem.Cit.Ind., Chem.Titles, Curr.Cont., Eng.Ind., Eng.Mat.Abstr., Excerp.Med. (1993-), INIS Atomind., INSPEC (Jun.1990-), ISMEC, Int.Aerosp.Abstr., Intl.Polym.Sci.& Tech., METADEX, Mat.Sci.Cit.Ind., Met.Abstr., Met.Abstr.Ind., Nonfer.Met.Alert, PCC Alert, RAPRA (1990-), Ref.Zh., Steels Alert, World Alum.Abstr.

—BLDSC (5012.258000), ADONIS, AskIEEE, CASDDS, CISTI, Ei, EMDOCS, GNLM, IDS, Infotrieve, Linda Hall. **CCC.**

Published by: (European Society for Biomaterials GBR), Kluwer Academic Publishers Boston, 101 Philip Dr, Assinippi Park, Norwell, MA 02061. TEL 781-871-6600, FAX 781-871-9045, services@wkap.nl, http://www.wkap.nl/journalhome.htm/0957-4530. Ed. William Bonfield. R&P Rose Luongo TEL 781-871-6311. Adv. contact Gemma Heiser TEL 781-871-6600. **Subscr. outside the Americas to:** Kluwer Academic Publishers Group, Journals Department, PO Box 322, Dordrecht 3300 AH, Netherlands. TEL 31-78-639-2392, FAX 31-78-654-6474; **Subscr. to:** Kluwer Academic - Plenum Publishers, 233 Spring St, New York, NY 10013-1578. TEL 212-620-8468, FAX 212-807-1047.

ENGINEERING—Hydraulic Engineering

AMERICAN SOCIETY OF SANITARY ENGINEERING. YEAR BOOK. see *HEATING, PLUMBING AND REFRIGERATION*

SAFETY NEWS. see *WATER RESOURCES*

E

ENGINEERING—Industrial Engineering

620.82 363.11 USA ISSN 1090-8471
TS155.6 CODEN: HFEMF5
HUMAN FACTORS AND ERGONOMICS IN MANUFACTURING. Text in English. 1991. q. USD 599 in United States; USD 639 in Canada & Mexico; USD 673 elsewhere; USD 629 combined subscription in United States for print and online eds.; USD 669 combined subscription in Canada & Mexico for print and online eds.; USD 703 combined subscription elsewhere for print and online eds. (effective 2002). adv. back issues avail. *Refereed.* **Document type:** *Academic/Scholarly.* **Description:** Provides a forum for the dissemination of scientific work on the human aspects of advanced manufacturing technologies; focuses on the design, management, and operation of advanced manufacturing systems.
Formerly (until 1997): International Journal of Human Factors in Manufacturing (1045-2699)
Related titles: Microform ed.: (from PQC); Online - full text ed.: ISSN 1520-6564. 1996. USD 599 in United States; USD 599 in Canada & Mexico; USD 599 elsewhere (effective 2002) (from EBSCO Publishing, Wiley InterScience, Institute for Scientific Information).
Indexed: ASCA, Bioeng.Abstr., Curr.Cont., Eng.Ind., Environ.Sci.Poll.Mgmt., Ergon.Abstr., INSPEC (Jan.1991-), Pollut.Abstr., Risk Abstr., SSCI, Saf.Sci.Abstr., e-psyche.
—BLDSC (4336.077500), AskIEEE, Ei, IDS, Infotrieve, ingenta. **CCC.**
Published by: John Wiley & Sons, Inc., Journals (Subsidiary of: Wiley InterScience), 605 Third Ave, New York, NY 10158. TEL 212-850-6645, FAX 212-850-6021, subinfo@wiley.com, uscs-wis@wiley.com, http://www.wiley.com. Eds. Gavriel Salvendy, Waldemar Karwowski. adv.: B&W page GBP 640, color page GBP 1,515; trim 178 x 254. Circ: 475. **Subscr. outside the Americas to:** John Wiley & Sons Ltd., Baffins Ln, Chichester, Sussex PO19 IUD, United Kingdom. TEL 44-1243-779777, FAX 44-1243-843232, cs-journals@wiley.co.uk, http://www.wiley.co.uk.

INDUSTRIAL SAFETY SERIES. see *OCCUPATIONAL HEALTH AND SAFETY*

N P R A NATIONAL SAFETY CONFERENCE. PROCEEDINGS. see *PETROLEUM AND GAS*

ENGINEERING—Mechanical Engineering

ADAPTIVE BEHAVIOR; animals, animats, software agents, robots, adaptive systems. see *COMPUTERS—Artificial Intelligence*

AMERICAN SOCIETY FOR HOSPITAL ENGINEERING TECHNICAL DOCUMENT SERIES. see *HEALTH FACILITIES AND ADMINISTRATION*

621 USA ISSN 1052-0139
HD9660.G37
CRYOGAS INTERNATIONAL; the source of timely and relevant information for the industrial gas and cryogenics industries. Text in English. 1963. m. (11/yr.). USD 150 domestic; USD 200 foreign (effective 2000). adv. bk.rev. abstr, pat. index. **Document type:** *Trade.* **Description:** Reports developments in technology, market development, and new products for the industrial gases and cryogenic equipment industries, including non-cryogenic gas production processes and specialty and medical gases.
Formerly (until Nov. 1990): Cryogenic Information Report (0011-2259)
—CISTI, Infotrieve, ingenta. **CCC.**
Published by: J.R. Campbell & Associates, Inc., 5 Militia Dr, Lexington, MA 02173. TEL 781-862-0624, FAX 781-863-9411, cryogas@cryogas.com, http://www.cryogas.com. Ed. Bob Keeley. Pub. John R Campbell. Adv. contact John Miaskowski. B&W page USD 974, color page USD 1,524; trim 8.5 x 11. Circ: 544 (paid and controlled).

HEALTH & SAFETY NEWSLINE; for the engineering industry (UK). see *PUBLIC HEALTH AND SAFETY*

INSTITUTION OF MECHANICAL ENGINEERS. PROCEEDINGS. PART H: JOURNAL OF ENGINEERING IN MEDICINE. see *BIOLOGY—Bioengineering*

362.1 614 CHE
JOURNAL OF CRASH PREVENTION AND INJURY CONTROL. Text in English. q. GBP 65, USD 79, EUR 95 to individuals; GBP 280, USD 340, USD 345 to institutions; GBP 411, USD 508, EUR 519 to corporations (effective 2002).
Published by: Gordon and Breach - Harwood Academic (Subsidiary of: Taylor & Francis Group), PO Box 531, Lausanne 1000, Switzerland. TEL 41-21-6411280, FAX 41-21-6411281, info@gbhap.com, http://www.gbhap.com/Crash_Prevention_Injury_Control/. Ed. Walter Pilkey. **Dist. by:** International Publishers Direct.

621 USA ISSN 1065-3090
TA357 CODEN: JFVPEI
JOURNAL OF FLOW VISUALIZATION AND IMAGE PROCESSING. Text in English. 1993. q. USD 45 to individuals; USD 315 to institutions (effective 2000). adv. index. *Refereed.* **Document type:** *Academic/Scholarly.* **Description:** Publishes original papers to disseminate and exchange the knowledge and information obtained through research on the principles and applications of flow visualization techniques including flow image processing.
Indexed: Appl.Mech.Rev., Eng.Ind.
—BLDSC (4984.440000), CISTI, ingenta. **CCC.**
Published by: Begell House Inc., 79 Madison Ave, Ste 1205, New York, NY 10016-7892. TEL 212-725-1999, FAX 212-213-8368, begellhouse@worldnet.att.net, orders@begellhouse.com. Eds. R Reznicek, Wen Jei Yang. Pub. William Begell. R&P, Adv. contact Jung K Ra.

▼ **JOURNAL OF MICROMECHATRONICS.** see *ENGINEERING—Electrical Engineering*

531.1134 USA ISSN 0022-4901
TX341 CODEN: JTXSBU
JOURNAL OF TEXTURE STUDIES; an international journal of rheology, psychorheology, physical and sensory testing of foods and pharmaceuticals. Text in English. 1969. bi-m., latest vol.32, 2001. USD 148. adv. bk.rev. illus, abstr, bibl, stat. index. back issues avail.; reprints avail. *Refereed.* **Document type:** *Journal, Academic/Scholarly.* **Description:** Covers textural subjects for those interested in texture as part of commodity work and for rheologists attempting to relate fundamental measurements to textural attributes.
Related titles: Online - full text ed.: (from Institute for Scientific Information).
Indexed: ASCA, Agri.Eng.Abstr., Agricola, Biol.Abstr., Chem.Abstr., Curr.Adv.Ecol.Sci., Curr.Cont., Dairy Sci.Abstr., Eng.Ind., Food Sci.& Tech.Abstr., Hort.Abstr., Ind.Sci.Rev., Postharvest, Sci.Cit.Ind.
—BLDSC (5069.055000), CASDDS, CISTI, Ei, IDS, ingenta, Linda Hall.
Published by: Food & Nutrition Press, Inc., 6527 Main St, PO Box 374, Trumbull, CT 06611. TEL 203-261-8587, FAX 203-261-9724, foodpress@worldnet.att.net, http://www.foodscipress.com. Eds. M C Bourne, T Van Uliet, V.N.M. Rao. Adv. contact John J O'Neil.

PARTICULATE SCIENCE AND TECHNOLOGY; an international journal. see *ENGINEERING—Chemical Engineering*

620.86 363.1 345.0242 USA ISSN 1041-9489
SAFETY BRIEF. Text in English. 1981. q. free per issue. back issues avail. **Document type:** *Academic/Scholarly.*
Published by: Triodyne Inc., 5950 W Touhy Ave, Niles, IL 60714-4610. TEL 847-677-4730, FAX 847-647-2047, infoserv@triodyne.com, http://www.triodyne.com. Ed. Paula L Barnett.

SHOBO KENKYUJO HOKOKU/FIRE RESEARCH INSTITUTE OF JAPAN. REPORT. see *FIRE PREVENTION*

TRIODYNE SAFETY BULLETIN. see *OCCUPATIONAL HEALTH AND SAFETY*

ENTOMOLOGY

see BIOLOGY—Entomology

ENVIRONMENTAL STUDIES

see also BIOLOGY; CONSERVATION; ENVIRONMENTAL STUDIES—Pollution; ENVIRONMENTAL STUDIES—Toxicology And Environmental Safety; ENVIRONMENTAL STUDIES—Waste Management; PUBLIC HEALTH AND SAFETY; WATER RESOURCES

577 ITA ISSN 1122-178X
A A M TERRA NUOVA; rivista ecoalternativa. (Agricoltura Alimentazione Medicina) Text in Italian. 1977. m. ITL 50,000 (effective 1998). back issues avail. **Document type:** *Consumer.* **Description:** Covers alternative medicine, natural food, ecology, environment, and psychology.
Published by: Associazione A A M Terra Nuova, Via Don L Sturzo, 19, Borgo San Lorenzo, FI 50032, Italy. TEL 39-055-8456116. Ed. John Masnovo.

A S H E S. see *HEALTH FACILITIES AND ADMINISTRATION*

A S H E S ANNUAL CONFERENCE. PROCEEDINGS MANUAL. see *HEALTH FACILITIES AND ADMINISTRATION*

ACTA BIOLOGICA IUGOSLAVICA. SERIJA D: EKOLOGIJA. see *BIOLOGY*

363.7 ITA ISSN 0393-0521
AMBIENTE RISORSE SALUTE; scienza, tecnica e cultura per uno sviluppo di qualita. Text in Italian; Summaries in English. 1982. m. ITL 100,000. adv. bk.rev. charts, stat. back issues avail. **Document type:** *Newsletter.* **Description:** Environmental pollution, utilization of resources and development of new and clean technologies are considered with special reference to community medicine and law.
Indexed: CEABA, INIS Atomind.
Published by: Centro Studi "l'Uomo e l'Ambiente", Via Delle Palme, 13, Padua, PD 35137, Italy. TEL 049-8759622, FAX 049-8761945, ars@csinternational.com, http://www.csinternational.com/ars. Ed. Franco Spelzini. R&P Domenico Ceravolo. Adv. contact Fernando Fujani. B&W page ITL 2,800,000, color page ITL 3,300,000; 297 x 210. Circ: 6,000.

333.72 BGR
ANTROPO-EKOLOGIIA. Text in Bulgarian; Summaries in Bulgarian, English. 1978. q., latest vol.24, 2001. BGL 14 domestic; USD 30 foreign (effective 2001 - 2002). adv. abstr. index. 63 p./no. back issues avail. *Refereed.* **Document type:** *Academic/Scholarly, Abstract/Index, Bibliography.* **Description:** Provides original articles and abstracts of foreign publications on environmental studies, occupational medicine, adolescent hygiene.
Formerly: Chovekat i Negovata Zhiznena Sreda (0204-9708)
Indexed: Abstr.Bulg.Sci.Med.Lit.
Published by: Meditsinski Universitet - Sofia, Tsentur za Informatsiia po Meditsina/Medical University - Sofia, Medical Information Center, 1 Sv Georgi Sofiiski ul, Sofia 1431, Bulgaria. TEL 359-2-9522342, FAX 359-2-9522393, mutafov@sun.medunacad.bg, mutafov@sun.medun.acad.bg, http://www.medun.acad.bg. Ed. Dr. A Monov. R&P, Adv. contact Dr. Christo Mutafov. B&W page USD 50, color page USD 150; 12 x 18. Circ: 200.

AQUILO. SERIE BOTANICA. see *BIOLOGY—Botany*

363.7 USA ISSN 0003-9896
RC963 CODEN: AEHLAU
ARCHIVES OF ENVIRONMENTAL HEALTH. Text in English. 1950. bi-m., latest vol.57, 2002. USD 170 domestic; USD 190 foreign (effective 2001 - 2002). adv. bk.rev. charts, illus. index. back issues avail.; reprints avail. *Refereed.* **Document type:** *Academic/Scholarly.* **Description:** Consolidates the latest research from such varying fields as epidemiology, toxicology, biostatistics, and biochemistry.
Related titles: CD-ROM ed.: (from ProQuest Information & Learning); Microform ed.; Online - full text ed.: (from Gale Group, Ovid Technologies, Inc., Northern Light Technology, Inc., H. W. Wilson, ProQuest Information & Learning, Factiva, Institute for Scientific Information).

E

Indexed: AESIS, AIM, API Abstr., API Catal., API Hlth.& Environ., API Oil., API Pet.Ref., API Pet.Subst., API Transport., A.S.& T.Ind. (coverage dropped), ASCA, Abstr.Hyg., Acid Pre.Dig., Acoust.Abstr., AgeLine, Agri.& Environ.Biotech.Abstr. (coverage dropped), Biodet.Abstr., Biol.& Agr.Ind. (Jul.1989-), Biol.Abstr., Br.Ceram.Abstr., C.I.S. Abstr., CSNB, Cadscan, Chem.Abstr., Chem.Indus.Notes, Chem.Titles, Curr.Adv.Cancer Res., Curr.Adv.Ecol.Sci., Curr.Cont., Dairy Sci.Abstr., Dent.Ind., Derwent Biotech.Abstr., Diar.Dis.Res., Energy Info.Abstr., Energy Rev., Environ.Abstr., Environ.Ind., Environ.Per.Bibl. (1972-), Environ.Sci.Poll.Mgmt., Excerp.Med., Forest Prod.Abstr., Fuel & Energy Abstr., G.Soc.Sci.& Rel.Per.Lit., Gas Abstr., GeoRef, Helminthol.Abstr., Hosp.Lit.Ind., INIS Atomind., Ind.Hyg.Dig., Ind.Med. (1960-), Ind.Sci.Rev., Ind.Vet., Inpharma, Int.Abstr.Biol.Sci., Intl.Polym.Sci.& Tech., Lab.Haz.Bull., Lead Abstr., METADEX, Med.& Surg.Dermat., Microbiol.Abstr., NRN, Nutr.Abstr., Pharm.&Out.News, Pollut.Abstr., RAPRA (1964-1999), Reac., Repindex, Rev.Appl.Entomol., Rev.Med.& Vet.Mycol., Rev.Plant Path., Risk Abstr., Rural Devel.Abstr., SSCI (coverage dropped), Saf.Sci.Abstr., Sci.Cit.Ind., Sel.Water Res.Abstr., Small Anim.Abstr., So.Pac.Per.Ind., THA, Tox.Abstr., Trop.Dis.Bull., Vet.Bull., W.R.C.Inf., Weed Abstr., Zincscan.
—BLDSC (1634.250000), CASDDS, CISTI, EMDOCS, GNLM, IDS, ingenta. **CCC.**
Published by: (Helen Dwight Reid Educational Foundation), Heldref Publications, 1319 Eighteenth St, N W, Washington, DC 20036-1802. TEL 202-296-6267, 800-365-9753, FAX 202-293-6130, aeh@heldref.org; orders@allenpress.com, http://www.heldref.org; http://www.allenpress.com. Ed. Patricia McCready. Adv. contact Grant Williams. Circ: 2,000. **Subscr. to:** Allen Press Inc., PO Box 1897, Lawrence, KS 66044-8897.

363.7 PHL ISSN 0116-2993
CODEN: ASENEL
ASIAN ENVIRONMENT; journal of environmental science and technology for balanced development. Text and summaries in English. 1978. q. USD 30. adv. bk.rev. index. back issues avail. **Document type:** *Academic/Scholarly.*
Indexed: Bibl.Asian Stud. (1984-1992), Chem.Abstr., Chem.Indus.Notes, Chem.Titles, Ecol.Abstr., Eng.Ind., Environ.Per.Bibl. (1990-1994), Environ.Sci.Poll.Mgmt., Excerp.Med., Geo.Abstr.H.G., Geo.Abstr.P.G., GeoRef, Geol.Abstr., HR Rep., IDA, Pollut.Abstr., W.R.C.Inf.
—CASDDS, CISTI, Ei, EMDOCS.
Published by: Asian Environment Journals, P.O. Box 90, Makati, Philippines. TELEX 63199-ETPI-MO-PH-OUANTECH. Ed. E A R Ouano. Circ: 2,000. **Co-sponsors:** Pollution Control Association of Philippines; Philippine Society of Sanitary Engineers; Indonesian Society of Sanitary Engineers.

ATMOSPHERIC ENVIRONMENT. see *ENVIRONMENTAL STUDIES—Pollution*

AWARENESS MAGAZINE. see *ALTERNATIVE MEDICINE*

344.046 USA ISSN 1065-8084
B N A'S FEDERAL ENVIRONMENT & SAFETY REGULATORY MONITORING REPORT. Text in English. 1993. bi-w. USD 548 (effective 2001). back issues avail. **Description:** Summarizes all regulatory activities from EPA and OSHA, as well as DOT hazardous materials transportation issues.
Related titles: Online - full text ed.: (from Bureau of National Affairs, Inc., (BNA), The).
—CCC.
Published by: The Bureau of National Affairs, Inc., 1231 25th St, N W, Washington, DC 20037. TEL 202-452-4200, 800-372-1033, 800-452-7773, FAX 202-822-8092, customercare@bna.com, bnaplus@bna.com, http://www.bna.com/. Ed. Susan Korn. Pub. Gregory McCaffery.

344.046 USA ISSN 1065-8076
KF3775.Z95
B N A'S STATE ENVIRONMENT & SAFETY REGULATORY MONITORING REPORT. Text in English. 1993. bi-w. USD 1,121 (effective 2001). back issues avail. **Description:** Covers regulatory developments for all 50 states and the District of Columbia.
Related titles: Online - full text ed.: (from Bureau of National Affairs, Inc., (BNA), The).
—CCC.
Published by: The Bureau of National Affairs, Inc., 1231 25th St, N W, Washington, DC 20037. TEL 202-452-4200, 800-372-1033, 800-452-7773, FAX 202-822-8092, customercare@bna.com, bnaplus@bna.com, http://www.bna.com/. Ed. Susan Korn. Pub. Gregory McCaffery.

BATIMENT - ENTRETIEN. see *OCCUPATIONAL HEALTH AND SAFETY*

577 DEU ISSN 0340-5443
QL750 CODEN: BESOD6
BEHAVIORAL ECOLOGY AND SOCIOBIOLOGY. Text in English. 1976. m. EUR 1,978.20 domestic; EUR 1,970.70 in Germany; EUR 195 newsstand/cover foreign (effective 2002). reprint service avail. from ISI. *Refereed.* **Document type:** *Journal, Academic/Scholarly.* **Description:** Deals with quantitative, empirical and theoretical studies in the field of analysis of animal behavior at the levels of the individual, population and community.
Related titles: Microform ed.: (from PQC); Online - full text ed.: ISSN 1432-0762 (from EBSCO Publishing, RoweCom Information Quest, Swets Blackwell, Springer LINK, Institute for Scientific Information).
Indexed: ASCA, Abstr.Anthropol., Agricola, Anim.Behav.Abstr., Anim.Breed.Abstr., Apic.Abstr., Appl.Ecol.Abstr., Aqua.Sci.& Fish.Abstr., Bibl.Agri., Bio-Contr.News & Info., Biol.Abstr., Biotech.& Bioeng.Abstr., Curr.Adv.Ecol.Sci., Curr.Cont., Deep Sea Res.& Oceanogr.Abstr., Ecol.Abstr., Entomol.Abstr., Environ.Per.Bibl. (1985-), Environ.Sci.Poll.Mgmt., Forest.Abstr., Genet.Abstr., Helminthol.Abstr., Hum.Gen.Abstr., Ind.Sci.Rev., Int.Abstr.Biol.Sci., Key Word Ind.Wildl.Res., Nutr.Abstr., Ocean.Abstr., Postharvest, Poult.Abstr., Protozool.Abstr., PsycInfo, Psychol.Abstr. (1982-), Rev.Appl.Entomol., Rev.Med.& Vet.Mycol., Russ.Acad.Sci.Bibl., SSCI (coverage dropped), Sci.Cit.Ind., Soils & Fert., Sport Fish.Abstr., Weed Abstr., Wild.Rev., Zoo.Rec., e-psyche.
—BLDSC (1877.400000), CISTI, EMDOCS, IDS, ingenta, Linda Hall. **CCC.**
Published by: Springer-Verlag (Subsidiary of: BertelsmannSpringer), Tiergartenstr 17, Heidelberg 69121, Germany. TEL 49-6221-345-0, FAX 49-6221-345229, subscriptions@springer.de, http://link.springer.de/link/service/journals/00265/index.htm, http://www.springer.de. Ed. T Czeschlik. **Subscr. in N. America to:** Springer-Verlag New York Inc., PO Box 2485, Secaucus, NJ 07096-2485. TEL 212-460-1500, FAX 212-473-6272.

BEZPIECZENSTWO JADROWE I OCHRONA RADIOLOGICZNA. see *PUBLIC HEALTH AND SAFETY*

BIOMEDICAL RESEARCH. see *MEDICAL SCIENCES*

BIONYT/BIO-NEWS; populaer forskning. see *BIOLOGY*

BIOTECHNOLOGY AND BIOTECHNOLOGICAL EQUIPMENT; international scientific-theoretical and applied publication. see *BIOLOGY—Biotechnology*

577 JPN ISSN 0289-0011
BIOTRONICS; environment control and environmental biology. Text in English. 1972. a. free per issue to qualified personnel. charts. **Document type:** *Academic/Scholarly.* **Description:** Contains original contributions, information on environment control and environmental biology for biological researchers, and news.
Indexed: Agri.Eng.Abstr., Biol.Abstr., Crop Physiol.Abstr., Curr.Adv.Ecol.Sci., Curr.Adv.Plant Sci., Ecol.Abstr., Field Crop Abstr., Forest.Abstr., Hort.Abstr., Maize Abstr., Ornam.Hort., Ref.Zh., Rev.Arom.& Med.Plants, Soyabean Abstr., Triticale Abstr., Weed Abstr.
—CISTI, ingenta.
Published by: (Slovakia. Ministry of Education KEN), Kyushu University, Biotron Institute, Kyushu University 12, Fukuoka-shi 812-8581, Japan. TEL 81-92-642-3060, FAX 81-92-642-3069. Ed. Nobuyuki Yamasaki. Circ: 1,000.

C A L M SCIENCE. (Conservation and Land Management) see *CONSERVATION*

363.7 BEL
C O N C A W E REVIEW. Text in English. 1992. 2/yr. free per issue. **Description:** Contains news about CONCAWE, descriptions of its technical reports and introductory articles on topics in the fields of environment, health, and safety such as sulfur dioxide emissions controls, oil pipeline integrity and prevention of major accidents.
Indexed: API Abstr.
Published by: C O N C A W E, Boulevard du Souverain 165, Brussels B-1160, Belgium. TEL 32-2-5669160, FAX 32-2-5669181, http://www.concawe.be. Ed., R&P Jean-Francois Larive. Circ: 4,000.

363.7 GBR ISSN 1369-376X
CERAM ENVIRONMENT BULLETIN. Text in English. 1991. q. **Document type:** *Bulletin.* **Description:** Includes environmental and health issues.
Formerly (until 1997): CERAM Research. Environmental Information Service. Bulletin (0965-2477)
Related titles: Online - full text ed.
Published by: Ceram Research, Queens Rd, Penkhull, Stoke-on-Trent, Staffs ST4 7LQ, United Kingdom. TEL 44-1762-764444, FAX 44-1762-412331, info@ceram.co.uk, http://www.ceram.co.uk. Ed. Joanne Dawson. Circ: 400.

628 USA ISSN 0738-7776
CODEN: CHMCE7
CHEMECOLOGY; covering health, safety and the environment. Text in English. 1967. m. free per issue. illus. back issues avail. **Document type:** *Academic/Scholarly.* **Description:** Articles on issues and concerns in contemporary environmental health and safety affecting the American public.
Formerly (until 1972): Currents (0011-4006)
Indexed: Biol.Dig., C.I.J.E., Energy Ind., Energy Info.Abstr., Environ.Abstr., Environ.Per.Bibl. (1990-1995), Ind.Hyg.Dig., Telegen.
Published by: Chemical Manufacturers Association, 1300 Wilson Blvd, Arlington, VA 22209. TEL 703-741-5000, FAX 703-741-6095. Circ: 75,000.

CHEMISTRY AND ECOLOGY. see *CHEMISTRY*

CHILDREN'S ENVIRONMENTS; theory, research, policy and applications. see *PSYCHOLOGY*

▼ **CLINICS IN OCCUPATIONAL AND ENVIRONMENTAL MEDICINE.** see *MEDICAL SCIENCES*

577 USA
CONSCIOUS CHOICE; the journal of ecology and natural living. Text in English. 1988. bi-m. USD 18 (effective 1999). **Document type:** *Consumer.* **Description:** Reports on environmental issues and natural alternatives in health care, food, and nutrition.
Related titles: Online - full text ed.
Address: 920 N Franklin, Ste 202, Chicago, IL 60610-3121. TEL 312-440-4373, cc@consciouschoice.com, http://www.consciouschoice.com. Ed. Sheri Reda. Pub. Jim Slama. R&P James Faber.

CONTRIBUTIONS IN MARINE SCIENCE. see *BIOLOGY*

363.7 GBR
CRONER'S ENVIRONMENTAL MANAGEMENT. Text in English. 1991. base vol. plus q. updates. GBP 360; GBP 279 updates. **Document type:** *Trade.* **Description:** Covers the implications to organizations of U.K. and E.C. environmental protection legislation and how effective environmental management can be achieved.
Incorporates (in Aug. 1998): Environmental Case Law
Related titles: Diskette ed.
Indexed: WasteInfo.
—BLDSC (3487.817700).
Published by: Croner Publications Ltd. (Subsidiary of: Wolters Kluwer N.V.), Croner House, 173 Kingston Rd, New Malden, Surrey KT3 3SS, United Kingdom. TEL 44-208-547-3333, FAX 44-20-8547-2637, info@croner.co.uk, info@croner.cch.co.uk, http://www.croner.co.uk. Ed. K Hunter. Pub. Dr. Brian Kellard.

CURRENT TOPICS IN ENVIRONMENTAL AND TOXICOLOGICAL CHEMISTRY. see *ENVIRONMENTAL STUDIES—Toxicology And Environmental Safety*

DIZHEN KANAN ANQUAN. see *EARTH SCIENCES—Geology*

363.72 USA ISSN 1078-0475
CODEN: EHPSEO
E H P SUPPLEMENTS. (Environmental Health Perspectives) Text in English. 1972. m. USD 75; USD 93.75 foreign (effective 1999). adv. bibl, charts, illus. reprint service avail. from PQC. *Refereed.* **Document type:** *Proceedings, Government, Academic/Scholarly.* **Description:** Includes original, peer-reviewed monographs on conference and workshop proceedings, perspective statements on selected problem areas, toxicologic information summaries, overviews of areas on environmental health, and reviews on specific environmental problems and agents.
Supersedes in part (in 1993): E H P (0091-6765)
Related titles: Microform ed.: (from PQC,PMC); Online - full text ed.: (from Institute for Scientific Information, H. W. Wilson).

Indexed: Abstr.Hyg., Acid Pre.Dig., Biol.Abstr., Biol.Dig., C.I.S. Abstr., Cadscan, Chem.Abstr., Chem.Indus.Notes, Chem.Titles, Curr.Adv.Ecol.Sci., Curr.Cont. (coverage dropped), Deep Sea Res.& Oceanogr.Abstr., Dent.Ind., Environ.Abstr., Environ.Ind., Environ.Per.Bibl. (1993-), Excerp.Med., Food Sci.& Tech.Abstr., INIS Atomind., Ind.Hyg.Dig., Ind.Med. (coverage dropped), Ind.Sci.Rev., Ind.U.S.Gov.Per., Lead Abstr., NRN, Pollut.Abstr., Poult.Abstr., Rev.Med.& Vet.Mycol., Risk Abstr., Saf.Sci.Abstr., Sel.Water Res.Abstr., Tox.Abstr. (coverage dropped), Vet.Bull., W.R.C.Inf., Zincscan.

—BLDSC (3791.499300), CASDDS, CINDOC, CIS, CISTI, GNLM, IDS, ingenta, Linda Hall.

Published by: U.S. Department of Health and Human Services, National Institute of Environmental Health Sciences, Environmental Health Information Service, PO Box 12233, Research Triangle Park, NC 27709. TEL 919-541-3406, FAX 919-541-0273, surak@niehs.nih.gov, http://ehis.niehs.nih.gov/. Ed. Gary E.R. Hook. Pub. Gary E R Hook. R&P Linda Roberts. Adv. contact Nancy Surak. Circ: 2,900. **Subscr. to:** O C R Subscription Services Inc., PO Box 12510, Research Triangle Park, NC 22708. TEL 800-315-3010, FAX 919-541-0763.

E M F HEALTH & SAFETY DIGEST. (Electric and Magnetic Field) see *OCCUPATIONAL HEALTH AND SAFETY*

577 DNK ISSN 0906-7590
QH84.1 CODEN: ECOGEG

ECOGRAPHY; pattern and diversity in ecology. Text in English. 1978. bi-m. USD 192 in the Americas to institutions print & online eds. combined; GBP 133 elsewhere to institutions print & online eds. combined (effective 2002). adv. bk.rev. charts, illus. index. reprint service avail. from ISI. *Refereed.* **Document type:** *Academic/Scholarly.*

Formerly (until 1992): Holarctic Ecology (0105-9327)

Related titles: Online - full text ed.: DKK 173 (effective 2002) (from EBSCO Publishing, ingenta, Swets Blackwell, Institute for Scientific Information).

Indexed: ASCA, Anim.Behav.Abstr. (coverage dropped), Anim.Breed.Abstr., Appl.Ecol.Abstr., Aqua.Sci.& Fish.Abstr., Bio-Contr.News & Info., Biol.Abstr., Chem.Abstr., Curr.Adv.Ecol.Sci., Curr.Adv.Plant Sci., Curr.Cont., Curr.Ref.Fish Res., Deep Sea Res.& Oceanogr.Abstr., Ecol.Abstr., Entomol.Abstr., Environ.Per.Bibl. (1991-), Environ.Sci.Poll.Mgmt., Forest Prod.Abstr., Forest.Abstr., GeoRef, Helminthol.Abstr., Herb.Abstr., INIS Atomind., Ind.Sci.Rev., Int.Abstr.Biol.Sci., Key Word Ind.Wildl.Res., Nutr.Abstr., Plant Sci., Rev.Appl.Entomol., Rev.Med.& Vet.Mycol., Rev.Plant Path., Sci.Cit.Ind., Seed Abstr., Sel.Water Res.Abstr., Soils & Fert., Sport Fish.Abstr., Triticale Abstr., Weed Abstr., Wild.Rev., Zoo.Rec.

—BLDSC (3648.627000), CASDDS, CISTI, EMDOCS, IDS, Infotrieve, ingenta, Linda Hall. **CCC.**

Published by: (Nordic Society Oikos), Blackwell Munksgaard, Noerre Soegade 35, PO Box 2148, Copenhagen K 1016, Denmark. TEL 45-77-33-33-33, FAX 45-77-33-33-77, TELEX 19431-MUNKS-DK, customerservice@munksgaard.dk, http://www.blackwellmunksgaard.com/ecography. Eds. Martin Zobel, Tartu Esoma. Circ: 625. **Co-sponsor:** Nordic Publishing Board in Science.

577 USA ISSN 1051-0761
QH540 CODEN: ECAPE7

ECOLOGICAL APPLICATIONS. Text in English. 1991. 6/yr. USD 190 in North America; USD 229 elsewhere (effective 2001). adv. bibl, charts, illus. index. back issues avail. *Refereed.* **Document type:** *Academic/Scholarly.* **Description:** Publishes articles on the ecological basis for decision making and policy in the areas of global change, biogeochemistry, conservation biology, ecotoxicology, pollution ecology, fisheries and wildlife ecology, forestry, agroecosystems, range management, soils, hydrology and groundwater, landscape ecology, and epidemiology.

Related titles: Microfilm ed.: (from PQC); Online - full text ed.: (from JSTOR (Web-based Journal Archive), Gale Group, Institute for Scientific Information).

Indexed: ABSEARCH Ecol.& Plant Sci. (1945-), ASCA, Agricola, Agroforest.Abstr., Anim.Behav.Abstr., Appl.Ecol.Abstr., Aqua.Sci.& Fish.Abstr., Bibl.Agri., Bio-Contr.News & Info., Crop Physiol.Abstr., Curr.Adv.Plant Sci., Curr.Cont., Curr.Ind.Stat., Ecol.Abstr., Ecol.Zoo.& Plant Sci.Abstr. (1991-), Entomol.Abstr., Environ.Per.Bibl. (1990-), Environ.Sci.Poll.Mgmt., Field Crop Abstr., Food Sci.& Tech.Abstr., Forest.Abstr., Genet.Abstr., Geo.Abstr.P.G., GeoRef, Geol.Abstr., Helminthol.Abstr., Herb.Abstr., Hort.Abstr., Hum.Gen.Abstr., IDA, INIS Atomind., Ind.Sci.Rev., Int.Abstr.Biol.Sci., Irr.& Drain.Abstr., Meteor.& Geoastrophys.Abstr., Ornam.Hort., Plant Grow.Reg.Abstr., Plant Sci., Pollut.Abstr., Rev.Appl.Entomol., Rev.Med.& Vet.Mycol., Rev.Plant Path., SSCI (coverage dropped), Sci.Cit.Ind., Seed Abstr., Sel.Water Res.Abstr., Soils & Fert., Sport Fish.Abstr., Weed Abstr., Wild.Rev., World Ag.Econ.& Rur.Soc.Abstr., Zoo.Rec.

—BLDSC (3648.855000), CISTI, ingenta, Linda Hall.

Published by: Ecological Society of America, 1707 H St. N.W. Suite 400, Washington, DC 20006. TEL 202-833-8773, FAX 202-833-8775, esahq@esa.org; orders@allenpress.com, http://www.sdsc.edu/~ESA/; http://www.allenpress.com. Ed. Louis F Pitelka. R&P Katherine McCarter. Adv. contact Liz Endres. Circ: 4,200. **Subscr. to:** Allen Press Inc., PO Box 1897, Lawrence, KS 66044-8897.

577 USA ISSN 0012-9615
QH540 CODEN: ECMOAQ

ECOLOGICAL MONOGRAPHS. Text in English. 1931. q. USD 110 in North America; USD 136 elsewhere (effective 2001). adv. bibl, charts, illus. index, irreg. cum.index. back issues avail. *Refereed.* **Document type:** *Monographic series, Academic/Scholarly.* **Description:** Publishes major research papers dealing with all aspects of ecology, as well as discussions and essays that develop ecological theory.

Related titles: Microfiche ed.: (from IDC); Microform ed.: (from PQC,PMC); Online - full text ed.: (from ProQuest Information & Learning, Gale Group, JSTOR (Web-based Journal Archive), Institute for Scientific Information).

Indexed: ABSEARCH Ecol.& Plant Sci. (1945-), ASCA, Agricola, Anim.Behav.Abstr., Appl.Ecol.Abstr., Aqua.Sci.& Fish.Abstr., Bibl.Agri., Biol.& Agr.Ind. (Jun.1983-), Biol.Abstr., Chem.Abstr., Curr.Adv.Ecol.Sci., Curr.Cont., Curr.Ind.Stat., Curr.Ref.Fish Res., Deep Sea Res.& Oceanogr.Abstr., Ecol.Abstr., Ecol.Zoo.& Plant Sci.Abstr. (1945-), Energy Ind., Energy Info.Abstr., Energy Rev., Entomol.Abstr., Environ.Per.Bibl. (1989-), Environ.Sci.Poll.Mgmt., Excerp.Med., Field Crop Abstr., Forest Prod.Abstr., Forest.Abstr., Gen.Sci.Ind. (Jun.1984-), Geo.Abstr.H.G., Geo.Abstr.P.G., GeoRef, Geol.Abstr., Helminthol.Abstr., Herb.Abstr., IBR, INIS Atomind., Ind.Sci.Rev., Int.Abstr.Biol.Sci., Key Word Ind.Wildl.Res., Meteor.& Geoastrophys.Abstr., Nutr.Abstr., Ocean.Abstr., P C I, Plant Breed.Abstr., Pollut.Abstr., Rev.Appl.Entomol., Sci.Cit.Ind., Seed Abstr., Sel.Water Res.Abstr., Soils & Fert., Sport Fish.Abstr., Weed Abstr., Wild.Rev., Zoo.Rec.

—BLDSC (3649.000000), CASDDS, CISTI, IDS, ingenta, Linda Hall.

Published by: Ecological Society of America, 1707 H St. N.W. Suite 400, Washington, DC 20006. TEL 202-833-8773, FAX 202-833-8775, esahq@esa.org. Ed. Robert K Peet. Adv. contact Liz Endres. Circ: 3,400. **Subscr. to:** Allen Press Inc., PO Box 1897, Lawrence, KS 66044-8897.

577 USA ISSN 0012-9623
QH540 CODEN: BECLAG

ECOLOGICAL SOCIETY OF AMERICA. BULLETIN. Text in English. 1917. q. USD 35 (effective 1999). adv. bk.rev. abstr. **Document type:** *Bulletin.* **Description:** Publishes brief articles about the science of ecology, including news, meeting arrangements, reviews of meetings and software, and awards of the Ecological Society of America.

Indexed: Biol.Abstr., Deep Sea Res.& Oceanogr.Abstr., Field Crop Abstr., GeoRef, Herb.Abstr., Hort.Abstr., INIS Atomind., Sport Fish.Abstr., Wild.Rev., Zoo.Rec.

—BLDSC (2498.200000), CISTI, ingenta, Linda Hall.

Published by: Ecological Society of America, 1707 H St. N.W. Suite 400, Washington, DC 20006. TEL 202-833-8773, FAX 202-833-8775, esahq@esa.org, http://www.sdsc.edu/~esa/. Ed. Allen Solomon. R&P Katherine McCarter. Adv. contact J David Baldwin. Circ: 7,300.

577 USA ISSN 0012-9658
QH540 CODEN: ECOLAR

ECOLOGY. Text in English. 1920. m. USD 470 in North America; USD 548 elsewhere (effective 2001). adv. bk.rev. bibl, charts, illus. index, cum.index. back issues avail.; reprints avail. *Refereed.* **Document type:** *Academic/Scholarly.* **Description:** Deals with all aspects of ecology, as well as discussions and essays that develop ecological theory.

Related titles: Microfiche ed.: (from IDC); Microfilm ed.: (from PMC); Microform ed.: (from PQC); Online - full text ed.: (from ProQuest Information & Learning, Gale Group, JSTOR (Web-based Journal Archive), Factiva, Institute for Scientific Information).

Indexed: ABSEARCH Ecol.& Plant Sci. (1945-), ASCA, Abstr.Anthropol., Acid Pre.Dig., Agricola, Anim.Behav.Abstr., Anim.Breed.Abstr., Apic.Abstr., Appl.Ecol.Abstr., Aqua.Sci.& Fish.Abstr., Bio-Contr.News & Info., Biol.& Agr.Ind. (Feb.1983-), Biol.Abstr., Bk.Rev.Ind. (1991-), Chem.Abstr., Child.Bk.Rev.Ind. (1991-), Compumath, Crop Physiol.Abstr., Curr.Cont., Curr.Ind.Stat., Curr.Ref.Fish Res., Deep Sea Res.& Oceanogr.Abstr., Ecol.Abstr., Ecol.Zoo.& Plant Sci.Abstr. (1945-), Energy Ind., Energy Info.Abstr., Energy Rev., Entomol.Abstr., Environ.Per.Bibl. (1973-), Environ.Sci.Poll.Mgmt., Excerp.Med., Field Crop Abstr., Food Sci.& Tech.Abstr., Forest Prod.Abstr., Forest.Abstr., Gen.Sci.Ind. (May 1984-), Genet.Abstr., Geo.Abstr.P.G., GeoRef, Helminthol.Abstr., Herb.Abstr., Hort.Abstr., Hum.Gen.Abstr., IBR, INIS Atomind., Ind.Sci.Rev., Ind.Vet., Int.Abstr.Biol.Sci., Irr.& Drain.Abstr., Key Word Ind.Wildl.Res., Meteor.& Geoastrophys.Abstr., Microbiol.Abstr., Mid.East: Abstr.& Ind., Nutr.Abstr., Ocean.Abstr., Ornam.Hort., P C I, Plant Breed.Abstr., Plant Gen.Res.Abstr., Pollut.Abstr., Poult.Abstr., Ref.Zh., Rel.Ind.One, Rel.Ind.Two, Rev.Appl.Entomol., Rev.Arom.& Med.Plants, Rev.Med.& Vet.Mycol., Rev.Plant Path., Rice Abstr., Risk Abstr., SSCI (coverage dropped), Sci.Cit.Ind., Seed Abstr., Sel.Water Res.Abstr., Soils & Fert., Sport Fish.Abstr., W.R.C.Inf., Weed Abstr., Wild.Rev., Zoo.Rec.

—BLDSC (3650.000000), CASDDS, CISTI, ingenta, Linda Hall.

Published by: Ecological Society of America, 1707 H St. N.W. Suite 400, Washington, DC 20006. TEL 202-833-8773, FAX 202-833-8775, esahq@esa.org, http://www.sdsc.edu/projects/ESA/public.htmlipubsE.M.html; http://www.allenpress.com. Ed. Robert K Peet. Circ: 6,400. **Subscr. to:** Allen Press Inc., PO Box 1897, Lawrence, KS 66044-8897.

577 USA ISSN 0098-6615
QH104

ECOLOGY U S A. Text in English. 1972. bi-w. USD 135 (effective 2000). illus. **Document type:** *Newsletter.* **Description:** Provides comprehensive coverage of the ecosystem as a whole with its complex interrelationships.

Indexed: Bio-Contr.News & Info., Field Crop Abstr., Forest.Abstr., Herb.Abstr., Maize Abstr., Seed Abstr., Soils & Fert., Triticale Abstr., Weed Abstr.

—CCC.

Published by: Business Publishers, Inc., 8737 Colesville Rd, 11th Fl, Silver Spring, MD 20910-3928. TEL 301-587-6300, 800-274-6737, FAX 301-589-8493, bpinews@bpinews.com, http://www.bpinews.com. Ed. Elaine Eiserer. Pub. Leonard A Eiserer.

ELECTRICITE DE FRANCE. DIRECTION DES ETUDES ET RECHERCHES. COLLECTION DE NOTES INTERNES. BIOLOGIE, SCIENCES DE LA TERRE ET ENVIRONNEMENT. see *BIOLOGY*

333.714 NLD ISSN 0929-0788

ENVIRONMENT & ASSESSMENT. Text in English. 1990. irreg., latest vol.5, 1993. price varies. *Refereed.* **Document type:** *Monographic series.*

Indexed: GeoRef.

—BLDSC (3791.096900).

Published by: Kluwer Academic Publishers Group (Subsidiary of: Wolters Kluwer N.V.), Spuiboulevard 50, PO Box 17, Dordrecht 3300 AA, Netherlands. FAX 31-78-639-2254, services@wkap.nl, http://www.wkap.nl. **Dist. by:** Journals Department, PO Box 322, Dordrecht 3300 AH, Netherlands. FAX 31-78-654-6474.

363.7 GBR ISSN 0964-9131

ENVIRONMENT AND SAFETY BRIEFING. Text in English. 1991. w. GBP 675. bk.rev. **Document type:** *Bulletin.* **Description:** Provides concise summaries of newly published U.K. and E.C. legislation, reports, and authoritative information concerning the environment and health and safety.

Related titles: Diskette ed.; Online - full text ed.

Published by: Barbour Index, New Lodge, Drift Rd, Winkfield, Windsor, Berks SL4 4RQ, United Kingdom. TEL 44-1344-884121, FAX 44-1344-884845. Ed. D Denton.

363.7 GBR ISSN 0160-4120
TD169 CODEN: ENVIDV
ENVIRONMENT INTERNATIONAL; a journal of environmental science, risk & health. Text in English. 1978. 8/yr. EUR 1,025 in Europe to institutions; JPY 136,100 in Japan to institutions; USD 1,146 elsewhere to institutions (effective 2002). adv. bk.rev. charts, stat. index. back issues avail.; reprints avail. *Refereed.* **Document type:** *Academic/Scholarly.* **Description:** Provides a forum for original environmental literature. Includes data, causes of pollution, methods for protection and various topics of environmental protection.
Formerly (until 1978): International Journal of the Environment
Related titles: Microfilm ed.: (from PQC); Online - full text ed.: (from ingenta, Swets Blackwell, ScienceDirect, Institute for Scientific Information).
Indexed: AESIS, ASCA, Abstr.Hyg., Acid Pre.Dig., Anim.Breed.Abstr., Appl.Ecol.Abstr. (coverage dropped), Aqua.Sci.& Fish.Abstr., Biodet.Abstr., Bioeng.Abstr., Biol.Abstr., Chem.Abstr., Chem.Indus.Notes, Chem.Titles, Curr.Adv.Ecol.Sci., Curr.Cont., Deep Sea Res.& Oceanogr.Abstr., Ecol.Abstr., Energy Info.Abstr., Energy Res.Abstr., Energy Rev., Eng.Ind., Environ.Abstr., Environ.Ind., Environ.Per.Bibl. (1980-), Environ.Sci.Poll.Mgmt., Excerp.Med., Field Crop Abstr., Forest.Abstr., Geo.Abstr.H.G., Geo.Abstr.P.G., GeoRef, Geol.Abstr., Herb.Abstr., IDA, I.M.M.Abstr., INIS Atomind., Ind.Med., Ind.Vet., Irr.& Drain.Abstr., Mass Spectr.Bull., Meteor.& Geoastrophys.Abstr., Microbiol.Abstr., Nutr.Abstr., Pig News & Info., Pollut.Abstr., Ref.Zh., Rev.Appl.Entomol., Rev.Plant Path., Risk Abstr., SSCI (coverage dropped), Saf.Sci.Abstr., Sci.Cit.Ind. (coverage dropped), Sel.Water Res.Abstr., Soils & Fert., Sport Fish.Abstr., Tox.Abstr., Triticale Abstr., Vet.Bull., W.R.C.Inf., WasteInfo, Weed Abstr., Wild.Rev., World Ag.Econ.& Rur.Soc.Abstr., Zoo.Rec.
—BLDSC (3791.330000), CASDDS, CISTI, Ei, GNLM, IDS, Infotrieve, ingenta, Linda Hall. **CCC.**
Published by: Pergamon (Subsidiary of: Elsevier Science), The Boulevard, Langford Ln, East Park, Kidlington, Oxford OXB 1GB, United Kingdom. TEL 44-1865-843565, FAX 44-1865-843976, http://www.elsevier.com/locate/envint. Ed. Ruth E Alcock. Circ: 2,000. **Subscr. in Australasia and the Far East to:** Elsevier Science (Singapore) Pte Ltd, No.1 Temasek Ave, 17-01 Millenia Tower, Singapore 039192, Singapore. TEL 65-434-3727, FAX 65-337-2230; **Subscr. in the Americas to:** Elsevier Science, PO Box 945, New York, NY 10159-0945. TEL 212-633-3730, 888-437-4636, FAX 212-633-3680, usinfo-f@elsevier.com; **Subscr. to:** Elsevier Science Inc - Japan Regional Office, 9-15 Higashi-Azabu 1-chome, Minato-ku, Tokyo 106-0044, Japan. TEL 81-3-5561-5033, FAX 81-3-5561-5047. **Subscr. to:** Elsevier Science BV, PO Box 211, Amsterdam 1000 AE, Netherlands. TEL 31-20-485-3757, FAX 31-20-485-3432.; **Dist. by:** Elsevier Science (Brazil).

577 USA ISSN 0094-7237
CODEN: EVBLBS
ENVIRONMENTAL BIOLOGY. Text in English. 1972. irreg. USD 3 per issue. back issues avail. **Document type:** *Monographic series, Academic/Scholarly.*
Indexed: Biol.Abstr.
Published by: Cornell University, Department of Entomology, 6126 Comstock Hall, Ithaca, NY 14853. TEL 607-255-2212, FAX 607-255-0939, dp18@cornell.edu. Ed. David Pimentel.

ENVIRONMENTAL HEALTH. see *PUBLIC HEALTH AND SAFETY*

628 USA
▼ **ENVIRONMENTAL HEALTH & SAFETY INTERNET GAZETTE.** Text in English. 1999. m. free per issue. adv. **Document type:** *Newsletter.* **Description:** Covers environmental health and safety topics.
Media: Online - full text.
Published by: E H S Marketplace, 4505 Infirmary Rd, PO Box 250, Dayton, OH 45449. TEL 937-859-6287, FAX 937-859-9132, news@ehsn.com, http://www.ehsmarketplace.com. Ed. Tammy Devilbiss. Adv. contact Gary Bramble.

616.98 CHE ISSN 0250-863X
RA1190 CODEN: EHCRDN
ENVIRONMENTAL HEALTH CRITERIA. Text in English. 1976. irreg. (approximately 6 volumes). CHF 242 (effective 2001). back issues avail. **Document type:** *Monographic series.* **Description:** Examines the risks to human health and the environment of selected chemicals and environmental pollutants.
Related titles: French ed.: Criteres d'Hygiene de l'Environnement. ISSN 0250-846X; Russian ed.: Kriterii Sanitarno-Gigienicheskogo Sostoyaniya Okruzhayushchei Sredy. ISSN 0250-8648; Spanish ed.: Criterios de Salud Ambiental. ISSN 0250-8478.
Indexed: Abstr.Hyg., Dairy Sci.Abstr., Diar.Dis.Res., Eng.Ind., Environ.Abstr., Excerp.Med., Food Sci.& Tech.Abstr., GeoRef, Ind.Vet., Rev.Appl.Entomol., Rev.Med.& Vet.Mycol., Rev.Plant Path., Vet.Bull.
—BLDSC (3791.491000), CISTI, Ei, EMDOCS, GNLM, KNAW, Linda Hall.
Published by: World Health Organization, Marketing and Dissemination, Geneva, 27 1211, Switzerland. TEL 41-22-791-2476, FAX 41-22-791-4857, publications@who.ch, http://www.who.int. Circ: 5,000.

363.7 USA
ENVIRONMENTAL HEALTH MONTHLY. Text in English. 1988. m. USD 35 (effective 1999). back issues avail. **Document type:** *Academic/Scholarly.*
Published by: Center for Health, Environment, and Justice, Marcoin Building, 150 South Washington St, Ste 300, Box 6806, Falls Church, VA 22046-6806. TEL 703-237-2249, FAX 703-237-8389, cchw@essential.org, http://www.essential.org/cchw; www.sustain.org/hcwh. Ed. Stephen U Lester. Circ: 700.

363.72 USA
ENVIRONMENTAL HEALTH NEWS. Text in English. 1951. 3/yr. free per issue. bk.rev. bibl, illus. back issues avail. *Refereed.* **Document type:** *Newsletter.* **Description:** Informs researchers, teachers, and workers about current news and issues in environmental health.
Supersedes (in 1987): Environmental Health and Safety News; Formerly: Occupational Health Newsletter (0029-7925)
Related titles: Online - full content ed.
Indexed: CSNB, Lab.Haz.Bull., WasteInfo.
—BLDSC (3791.498100).
Published by: University of Washington, Department of Environmental Health, PO Box 354695, Seattle, WA 98105-6099. TEL 206-685-6737, FAX 206-685-3872, kjhall@u.washington.edu, http://depts.washington.edu/envhlth/info/publications.html. Ed. Kathy Hall. Circ: 4,000.

363.7 USA
RA565.A1 CODEN: EVHPAZ
ENVIRONMENTAL HEALTH PERSPECTIVES. Text in English. 1993. m. USD 249 to individuals; USD 1,369 Corporate Institutions; USD 849 Educational & Government Institutions; USD 45 to students (effective 2001). adv. illus. Supplement avail.; reprints avail. *Refereed.* **Document type:** *Government, Academic/Scholarly.* **Description:** Includes original peer-reviewed scientific articles concerning all aspects of environmental health and science, up-to-date news items and articles on important and controversial environmental issues.
Supersedes in part (in 1993): E H P (0091-6765)
Related titles: Online - full text ed.: USD 65 (effective 2001) (from Institute for Scientific Information, H. W. Wilson); ♦ Supplement: Environmental Health Perspectives Supplement.
Indexed: ASCA, Abstr.Hyg., Agri.Eng.Abstr., Anim.Breed.Abstr., Aqua.Sci.& Fish.Abstr., Aquacult.Abstr., Bio-Contr.News & Info., CSNB, Chem.Abstr., Chem.Cit.Ind., Chem.Indus.Notes, Chem.Titles, Compumath, Curr.Cont. (coverage dropped), Curr.Ind.Stat., Dairy Sci.Abstr., Environ.Abstr., Environ.Per.Bibl. (1974-), Environ.Sci.Poll.Mgmt., Excerp.Med., Food Sci.& Tech.Abstr., Forest Prod.Abstr., Forest.Abstr., Gen.Sci.Ind. (Jul.1997-, dropped), Ind.Med. (coverage dropped), Ind.Sci.Rev., Ind.Vet., Inpharma, Int.Abstr.Biol.Sci., Int.Nurs.Ind., Irr.& Drain.Abstr., Lab.Haz.Bull., Microbiol.Abstr., NRN, Nutr.Abstr., Pig News & Info., Pollut.Abstr., Reac., Ref.Zh., Rev.Appl.Entomol., Rev.Med.& Vet.Mycol., Rev.Plant Path., Risk Abstr., Rural Devel.Abstr., SSCI (coverage dropped), Saf.Sci.Abstr., Sci.Cit.Ind. (coverage dropped), Sel.Water Res.Abstr., Soils & Fert., THA, Tox.Abstr. (coverage dropped), Trop.Dis.Bull., W.R.C.Inf., WasteInfo, Weed Abstr., Wild.Rev., World Ag.Econ.& Rur.Soc.Abstr., Zoo.Rec.
—BLDSC (3791.499000), CASDDS, CINDOC, CIS, CISTI, GNLM, IDS, ingenta, Linda Hall.
Published by: U.S. Department of Health and Human Services, National Institute of Environmental Health Sciences, PO Box 12233, Research Triangle Park, NC 27709. TEL 919-541-3406, FAX 919-541-0273, ehis@niehs.nih.gov, http://ehis.niehs.nih.gov/. Ed. Gary E R Hook. R&P Linda Roberts. Adv. contact Nancy Surak. Circ: 6,500. **Subscr. to:** O C R Subscription Services Inc., PO Box 12510, Research Triangle Park, NC 22708. TEL 800-315-3010, FAX 919-541-0763; **Subscr. to:** U.S. Government Printing Office, Superintendent of Documents, PO Box 371954, Pittsburgh, PA 15250-7954.

363.7 USA
ENVIRONMENTAL HEALTH PERSPECTIVES SUPPLEMENT. Text in English. bi-m. USD 85; USD 20 newsstand/cover domestic; USD 25 newsstand/cover foreign (effective 2001). **Document type:** *Academic/Scholarly.* **Description:** Presents conference, workshop, and symposium proceedings as well as in-depth perspective reviews.
Related titles: ♦ Supplement to: Environmental Health Perspectives.
Indexed: Environ.Per.Bibl.
Published by: U.S. Department of Health and Human Services, National Institute of Environmental Health Sciences, PO Box 12233, Research Triangle Park, NC 27709. **Subscr. to:** U.S. Government Printing Office, Superintendent of Documents, PO Box 371954, Pittsburgh, PA 15250-7954. TEL 202-512-1800, FAX 202-512-2250, orders@gpo.gov, http://www.access.gpo.gov.

ENVIRONMENTAL HEALTH REPORT (YEAR). see *PUBLIC HEALTH AND SAFETY*

ENVIRONMENTAL HEALTH REVIEW. see *PUBLIC HEALTH AND SAFETY*

616.98 GBR ISSN 0956-6163
RA565.A1 CODEN: EMHEEB
ENVIRONMENTAL MANAGEMENT & HEALTH. Text in English. 1990. 5/yr. USD 6,379 in North America (effective 2001); EUR 6,779 in Europe; AUD 7,749 in Australasia; GBP 3,989 in the UK & rest of the World (effective 2002). reprint service avail. from SWZ. **Document type:** *Academic/Scholarly.* **Description:** Examines environmental factors and their impact on human health.
Related titles: Online - full text ed.: (from EBSCO Publishing, O C L C Online Computer Library Center, Inc., RoweCom Information Quest, ingenta, Swets Blackwell).
Indexed: ABI Inform. (1992-1995), Agri.Eng.Abstr., Aqua.Sci.& Fish.Abstr., Emerald, Emrld.Intell., Environ.Per.Bibl. (1990-), Environ.Sci.Poll.Mgmt., INIS Atomind., Pollut.Abstr., Potato Abstr., Protozool.Abstr., Rev.Appl.Entomol., Rev.Med.& Vet.Mycol., Risk Abstr., Rural Recreat.Tour.Abstr., Saf.Sci.Abstr., Sel.Water Res.Abstr., Soils & Fert., Trop.Dis.Bull., Weed Abstr., World Ag.Econ.& Rur.Soc.Abstr.
—BLDSC (3791.519200), Infotrieve. **CCC.**
Published by: Emerald, 60-62 Toller Ln, Bradford, W Yorks BD8 9BY, United Kingdom. TEL 44-1274-777700, FAX 44-1274-785200, info@emeraldinsight.com, http://www.emeraldinsight.com/emh.htm, http://www.mcb.co.uk/. Ed. Walter Leal Filho TEL 49-40-766180-56.

363.7063 USA
ENVIRONMENTAL MANAGEMENT NEWS. Text in English. 1969. 4/yr. USD 150 to members. index. **Document type:** *Newsletter.* **Description:** Includes articles on facilities planning and design, internal building systems, maintenance and operations, and building services.
Former titles: Environmental Management (Englewood) (1051-2837); Professional Sanitation Management (0033-0191)
Indexed: Energy Info.Abstr., Environ.Abstr., Ocean.Abstr. (coverage dropped), Pollut.Abstr., Russ.Acad.Sci.Bibl., Sport Fish.Abstr., Wild.Rev.
—Linda Hall.
Published by: Environmental Management Association, 1721 Pheasant Lane, Jeffersonville, PA 19403-3333. TEL 610-539-8588, FAX 610-539-8588. Ed. Barry M Dressler.

ENVIRONMENTAL MEDICINE. see *MEDICAL SCIENCES*

333.72 USA ISSN 0736-9603
ENVIRONMENTAL OPPORTUNITIES. Text in English. 1982. m. USD 49 (effective 1999). adv. back issues avail. **Document type:** *Newsletter.*
Address: 103 Roxbury St, 5, Keene, NH 03431. TEL 603-357-5940, FAX 603-357-5940. Ed. Sanford Berry. Circ: 1,500.

363.7 USA ISSN 0509-769X
RA569 CODEN: ERSSD6
ENVIRONMENTAL RADIATION SURVEILLANCE IN WASHINGTON STATE. ANNUAL REPORT. Text in English. 1961. a. illus. *Refereed.* **Document type:** *Government.*
Published by: Department of Health, Division of Radiation Protection, Box 47827, Olympia, WA 98504-7827. TEL 206-586-3306, FAX 206-753-1496. Ed. John L Erickson. Circ: 500.

E

363.70072 USA ISSN 0013-9351
RA565 CODEN: ENVRAL
ENVIRONMENTAL RESEARCH; a journal of environmental medicine and the environmental sciences. Text in English. 1967. 8/yr. USD 1,535 in US & Canada to institutions; USD 1,760 elsewhere to institutions (effective 2001). adv. bk.rev. illus. index. back issues avail.; reprints avail. *Refereed.* **Document type:** *Academic/Scholarly.* **Description:** Publishes original reports describing studies of the toxic effects of environmental agents in humans and animals.
Related titles: Online - full text ed.: (from EBSCO Publishing, O C L C Online Computer Library Center, Inc., RoweCom Information Quest, ingenta, Swets Blackwell, IDEAL Online Library, Institute for Scientific Information).
Indexed: AESIS, API Abstr., API Catal., API Hlth.& Environ., API Oil., API Pet.Ref., API Pet.Subst., API Transport., A.S.& T.Ind. (Oct.1983-), ASCA, Anim.Breed.Abstr., Appl.Ecol.Abstr. (coverage dropped), Aqua.Sci.& Fish.Abstr., Biol.& Agr.Ind. (Jan.1996-), Biol.Abstr., C.I.S. Abstr., Cadscan, Chem.Abstr., Curr.Adv.Ecol.Sci., Curr.Cont., Dairy Sci.Abstr., Ecol.Abstr., Entomol.Abstr. (coverage dropped), Environ.Abstr., Environ.Ind., Environ.Per.Bibl., Environ.Sci.Poll.Mgmt., Excerp.Med., Field Crop Abstr., GeoRef, Helminthol.Abstr., INIS Atomind., Ind.Med. (1967-), Ind.Sci.Rev., Ind.Vet., Inpharma, Int.Abstr.Biol.Sci., Lead Abstr., Meteor.& Geoastrophys.Abstr., NRN, Noise Pollut.Publ.Abstr., Nutr.Abstr., Ocean.Abstr., Pharm.&Out.News, Pollut.Abstr., Poult.Abstr., Reac., Ref.Zh., Rev.Appl.Entomol., Risk Abstr., SSCI (coverage dropped), Saf.Sci.Abstr., Sci.Cit.Ind., Sel.Water Res.Abstr., Soc.Sci.Ind. (coverage dropped), Soils & Fert., Sport Fish.Abstr., Tox.Abstr., Trop.Dis.Bull., Vet.Bull., W.R.C.Inf., Wild.Rev., Zincscan, Zoo.Rec.
—BLDSC (3791.590000), ADONIS, CASDDS, CISTI, GNLM, IDS, ingenta, Linda Hall. **CCC.**
Published by: Academic Press, Inc., Journal Division (Subsidiary of: Harcourt Brace & Company), 525 B St, Ste 1900, San Diego, CA 92101-4495. TEL 619-230-1840, FAX 619-699-6800, apsubs@acad.com, http://www.academicpress.com/er. Ed. Ellen K Silbergeld.

ESTONIAN ACADEMY OF SCIENCES. PROCEEDINGS. BIOLOGY - ECOLOGY/EESTI TEADUSTE AKADEEMIA. TOIMETISED. BIOLOOGIA. OKOLOOGIA. see *BIOLOGY*

ESTUARIES; a journal of research on any aspect of natural science and management applied to estuaries. see *BIOLOGY*

EVERYONE'S BACKYARD. see *ENVIRONMENTAL STUDIES—Waste Management*

F E M S MICROBIOLOGY ECOLOGY. see *BIOLOGY—Microbiology*

G I - GESUNDHEITS INGENIEUR; Haustechnik - Bauphysik - Umwelttechnik. see *PUBLIC HEALTH AND SAFETY*

363.7 NLD ISSN 0925-9406
GELUID. Text in Dutch. q. **Description:** Follows latest developments in noise control.
Formerly (until 1991): Geluid en Omgeving (0165-2982)
Published by: (Nederlands Stichting Geluidshinder), Samsom H.D. Tjeenk Willink B.V. (Subsidiary of: Wolters Kluwer N.V.), Postbus 316, Alphen aan den Rijn 2400 AH, Netherlands. TEL 31-1720-66822, FAX 31-1720-66639.

THE GIST. see *FOOD AND FOOD INDUSTRIES*

HARVARD MEDICAL SCHOOL. CENTER FOR HEALTH AND THE GLOBAL ENVIRONMENT. NEWSLETTER. see *PUBLIC HEALTH AND SAFETY*

HAZARD TECHNOLOGY. see *CIVIL DEFENSE*

613.1 AUS
HEALTH AND ENVIRONMENT REVIEW. Text in English. fortn. **Document type:** *Abstract/Index.* **Description:** Provides reports excerpted from scientific literature on environmental and occupational health and safety, nutrition, lifestyle, fitness and health, and a host of related issues.
Media: Online - full text.
Published by: Ecol Data, Australia. magi@imagic.com.au, http://www.imagic.com.au/~magi/ecol/ecol.html.

HEALTHY OPTIONS. see *PHYSICAL FITNESS AND HYGIENE*

616.98 CHN ISSN 1001-5914
HUANJING YU JIANKANG ZAZHI/JOURNAL OF ENVIRONMENT AND HEALTH. Text in Chinese. 1984. bi-m. USD 22.20; USD 3.70 newsstand/cover (effective 2001). adv. **Document type:** *Academic/Scholarly.*
Published by: Tianjin Shi Weisheng Fangbing Zhongxin/Tianjin Municipal Center of Health and Disease Prevention, 76 Tianshanshe Dajie, Hedong-qu, Tianjin 300011, China. TEL 86-22-2441-4403, FAX 86-22-2432-9940. Ed., Pub., R&P, Adv. contact Dong Shanheng. Circ: 4,000. **Dist. by:** China International Book Trading Corp, 35, Chegongzhuang Xilu, Haidian District, Beijing 100044, China. TEL 86-1-68413849, FAX 86-1-68412048, cibtc@mail.cibtc.com.cn, http://www.cibtc.com.cn.

363.72 GBR ISSN 0951-1504
CODEN: IESAD7
I E & S NEWS. Text in English. 1978. q. GBP 80, USD 132 (effective 2000). back issues avail. **Document type:** *Newsletter.* **Description:** Intended for environmental and safety officers.
Formerly (until 1982): International Environment and Safety (0141-4836)
Indexed: C.I.S. Abstr., Chem.Abstr., INIS Atomind., Int.Packag.Abstr., Lab.Haz.Bull.
—CASDDS, CISTI.
Published by: International Labmate Ltd., 12 Alban Park, Hatfield Rd, St Albans, Herts AL4 0JJ, United Kingdom. TEL 44-1727-855574, FAX 44-1727-841694. Ed. Michael H Pattison. Circ: 10,500.

616.98 GBR
I E H ASSESSMENT. Text in English. irreg., latest vol.5, 1998. price varies. **Document type:** *Monographic series, Academic/Scholarly.* **Description:** Examines and evaluates important issues in environmental health.
Published by: Institute for Environment and Health, University of Leicester, 94 Regent Rd, Leicester, Leics LE1 7DD, United Kingdom. TEL 44-116-223-1600, FAX 44-116-223-1601, msto1@le.ac.uk, http://www.le.ac.uk/ieh/. R&P Miriam Turner-Oswick.

363.7 GBR
I E H REPORT. Text in English. 1993. irreg., latest vol.10, 1998. price varies. **Document type:** *Monographic series, Academic/Scholarly.*
Published by: Institute for Environment and Health, University of Leicester, 94 Regent Rd, Leicester, Leics LE1 7DD, United Kingdom. TEL 44-116-223-1600, FAX 44-116-223-1601, msto1@le.ac.uk, http://www.le.ac.uk/ieh/. R&P Ruth Gardener.

616.98 GBR
I E H SPECIAL REPORT. Text in English. irreg., latest vol.5, 1998. price varies. **Document type:** *Monographic series, Academic/Scholarly.*
Published by: Institute for Environment and Health, University of Leicester, 94 Regent Rd, Leicester, Leics LE1 7DD, United Kingdom. TEL 44-116-223-1600, FAX 44-116-223-1601, msto1@le.ac.uk, http://www.le.ac.uk/ieh/. R&P Ruth Gardener.

IAN RAMSEY CENTRE. PUBLICATIONS. see *PHILOSOPHY*

INDIAN JOURNAL OF ENVIRONMENTAL HEALTH. see *PUBLIC HEALTH AND SAFETY*

363.7 USA ISSN 1526-8403
▼ **INDOOR ENVIRONMENT CONNECTIONS**; the newspaper for the iaq marketplace. (indoor air quality) Text in English. 1999. m. USD 48 domestic; USD 68 foreign (effective 2000). adv. **Document type:** *Newspaper, Trade.* **Description:** Provides a forum where individuals, companies, and organizations representing various disciplines can unite to share expertise to solve indoor environmental problems.
Published by: Indoor Environment Communications, 10400 Connecticut Ave, Ste 510, Kensington, MD 20895. TEL 301-962-5070, FAX 301-962-5125, iecnews@aol.com, http://www.ieconnections.com. Ed. Joshua Hull. Pubs. Glenn Fellman, Susan Valenti. Adv. contact Diane Chester. B&W page USD 1,890; 10 x 12.5.

363.7 ITA ISSN 1122-0481
INFORMAZIONE INNOVATIVA; agenzia quindicinale di documentazione internazionale servizio di informazione innovativa scientifica tecnologica legislativa per la produzione, l'ambiente, la sanita. Short title: Inf-Inn. Text in Italian; Summaries in English. 1985. fortn. ITL 600,000. adv. bk.rev. back issues avail. **Document type:** *Bulletin.* **Description:** Covers clean technologies, energy sources, technology of new materials, waste treatments, waste water treatment, agroindustrial biotechnology.
Published by: Centro Studi "l'Uomo e l'Ambiente", Via Delle Palme, 13, Padua, PD 35137, Italy. TEL 39-49-8759622, FAX 39-49-8761945. Ed. Franco Spelzini. R&P Domenico Ceravolo. Adv. contact Giuseppina Vittadello. Circ: 1,000.

INGENIERIA SANITARIA. see *PUBLIC HEALTH AND SAFETY*

577 USA
CODEN: IESPAF
INSTITUTE OF ENVIRONMENTAL SCIENCES AND TECHNOLOGY. ANNUAL TECHNICAL MEETING. PROCEEDINGS. Text in English. 1960. a. USD 175 to non-members; USD 145 to members (effective 2000). adv. reprint service avail. from PQC. **Document type:** *Proceedings, Trade.*
Formerly (until 1998): Institute of Environmental Sciences. Annual Technical Meeting. Proceedings (0073-9227)
Related titles: Microfilm ed.: (from PQC).
Indexed: Bioeng.Abstr., Biol.Abstr., Chem.Abstr., Chem.Indus.Notes, Chem.Titles, Comput.& Info.Sys., Electron.& Communic.Abstr.J., Eng.Ind., GeoRef, ISMEC, Mass Spectr.Bull., Sh.& Vib.Dig., Solid St.Abstr.
—BLDSC (1535.805000), CASDDS, Ei. **CCC.**
Published by: Institute of Environmental Sciences and Technology, 940 E. Northwest Hwy., Mt. Prospect, IL 60056-3422. TEL 847-255-1561, FAX 847-255-1699, InstEnvSci@aol.com, iest@iest.org, http://instenvsci.org, http://www.iest.org. Ed. Roberta Burrows. R&P Julie Kendrick. Adv. contact Donna Sullivan.

363.7 USA ISSN 0073-9251
INSTITUTE OF ENVIRONMENTAL SCIENCES. TUTORIAL SERIES. Text in English. irreg. price varies. **Description:** Represents material used for classes in environmental science and is intended specifically for course attendants.
Published by: Institute of Environmental Sciences and Technology, 940 E. Northwest Hwy., Mt. Prospect, IL 60056-3422. TEL 847-255-1561, FAX 847-255-1561.

628 IND ISSN 0251-110X
TD1 CODEN: JEEEDS
INSTITUTION OF ENGINEERS (INDIA). ENVIRONMENTAL ENGINEERING DIVISION. JOURNAL. Text in English. 1920. s-a. INR 80, USD 25 (effective 2000). adv. charts, illus. index. *Refereed.* **Document type:** *Academic/Scholarly.*
Formerly: Institution of Engineers (India). Public Health Engineering Division. Journal (0020-3416)
Indexed: Chem.Abstr., Chem.Indus.Notes, Chem.Titles, Eng.Ind., Environ.Eng.Abstr., Environ.Sci.Poll.Mgmt., GeoRef, INIS Atomind., Ocean.Abstr. (coverage dropped), Pollut.Abstr.
—BLDSC (4794.021000), CASDDS, CISTI, Ei, Linda Hall.
Published by: Institution of Engineers (India), Environmental Engineering Division, 8 Gokhale Rd., Kolkata, West Bengal 700 020, India. TEL 91-33-2238334, FAX 91-33-2238345. Ed., Pub. B C Thakurta. Adv. contact S S Basu. Circ: 8,000.

616.98 GBR ISSN 0960-3123
RA565.A1 CODEN: IJEREO
INTERNATIONAL JOURNAL OF ENVIRONMENTAL HEALTH RESEARCH. Text in English. 1991. q. GBP 131, USD 216 to individuals; GBP 329, USD 543 to institutions (effective 2002). back issues avail. *Refereed.* **Document type:** *Academic/Scholarly.* **Description:** Examines the interaction between the environment and human health, as it relates to the natural environment, the built environment, and communicable diseases.
Related titles: Online - full text ed.: ISSN 1369-1619 (from CatchWord Ltd., EBSCO Publishing, O C L C Online Computer Library Center, Inc., RoweCom Information Quest, Swets Blackwell, Institute for Scientific Information).
Indexed: ASCA, Abstr.Hyg., Aqua.Sci.& Fish.Abstr., Brit.Nur.Ind., Chem.Abstr., Chem.Indus.Notes, Chem.Titles, Curr.Cont., Dairy Sci.Abstr., Ecol.Abstr., Environ.Per.Bibl. (1993-), Environ.Sci.Poll.Mgmt., Excerp.Med. (1993-), Fluidex, Food Sci.& Tech.Abstr., Geo.Abstr.H.G., Geo.Abstr.P.G., Helminthol.Abstr., Ind.Med., Ind.Vet., Int.Abstr.Biol.Sci., Irr.& Drain.Abstr., Microbiol.Abstr., Nutr.Abstr., Pig News & Info., Pollut.Abstr., Protozool.Abstr., Rev.Appl.Entomol., Rev.Med.& Vet.Mycol., Rev.Plant Path., Risk Abstr., SSCI (coverage dropped), Saf.Sci.Abstr., Sel.Water Res.Abstr., Soils & Fert., Sport Fish.Abstr., Tox.Abstr., Trop.Dis.Bull., Vet.Bull., Weed Abstr., Wild.Rev., Zoo.Rec.
—BLDSC (4542.242000), ADONIS, CASDDS, CatchWord, CISTI, EMDOCS, GNLM, IDS, Infotrieve, ingenta. **CCC.**

E

Published by: Carfax Publishing Limited (Subsidiary of: Taylor & Francis Group), PO Box 25, Abingdon, Oxon OX14 3UE, United Kingdom. TEL 44-1235-401000, FAX 44-1235-401550, enquiries@carfax.co.uk, enquiry@tandf.co.uk, http://www.carfax.co.uk.

INTERNATIONAL JOURNAL OF MEDICINE, BIOLOGY AND THE ENVIRONMENT. see *MEDICAL SCIENCES—Oncology*

577 JPN ISSN 0021-5007
QH540 CODEN: NSGSAF

JAPANESE JOURNAL OF ECOLOGY/NIPPON SEITAI GAKKAISHI. Text in Japanese; Summaries in English. 1954. 3/yr. JPY 9,000. bk.rev. charts, illus. index. **Document type:** *Academic/Scholarly.*

Indexed: Abstr.Hyg., Agrindex, Anim.Behav.Abstr. (coverage dropped), Appl.Ecol.Abstr., Aqua.Sci.& Fish.Abstr., Bio-Contr.News & Info., Biol.Abstr., Chem.Abstr., Crop Physiol.Abstr., Deep Sea Res.& Oceanogr.Abstr., Ecol.Abstr., Entomol.Abstr. (coverage dropped), Environ.Sci.Poll.Mgmt., Field Crop Abstr., Forest Prod.Abstr., Forest.Abstr., Genet.Abstr., Geo.Abstr.P.G., GeoRef, Herb.Abstr., Hum.Gen.Abstr., Jap.Per.Ind., Pollut.Abstr., Ref.Zh., Rev.Appl.Entomol., Rev.Med.& Vet.Mycol., Rev.Plant Path., Rice Abstr., Rural Recreat.Tour.Abstr., Seed Abstr., Sel.Water Res.Abstr., Soils & Fert., Sport Fish.Abstr., W.R.C.Inf., Weed Abstr., Wild.Rev., Zoo.Rec.

—CASDDS, CISTI, Infotrieve, ingenta, Linda Hall. **CCC.**

Published by: Ecological Society of Japan/Nihon Seitai Gakkai, c/o Dept of Biology, Tokyo Metropolitan University, 1-1 Minami-osawa, Hachioji 192-0397, Japan. Ed. Yasunori Watanabe. Circ: 3,300.

577 IND ISSN 0254-8704
CODEN: JEBIDP

JOURNAL OF ENVIRONMENTAL BIOLOGY; an international research journal of environmental sciences & toxicology. Text in English. 1980. q., latest vol.23, 2002. USD 140 foreign to individuals (effective 2002). adv. bk.rev. back issues avail. *Refereed.* **Document type:** *Academic/Scholarly.* **Description:** Serves as the exclusive research journal in India concerned with environmental pollution and toxicology.

Related titles: Online - full text ed.: (from Institute for Scientific Information).

Indexed: ASCA, Anim.Behav.Abstr. (coverage dropped), Anim.Breed.Abstr., Appl.Ecol.Abstr. (coverage dropped), Aqua.Sci.& Fish.Abstr., Aquacult.Abstr., Biol.Abstr., Cadscan, Chem.Abstr., Chem.Indus.Notes, Chem.Titles, Crop Physiol.Abstr., Curr.Adv.Ecol.Sci., Curr.Cont., Curr.Ref.Fish Res., Ecol.Abstr., Energy Info.Abstr., Entomol.Abstr., Environ.Abstr., Environ.Sci.Poll.Mgmt., Excerp.Med., Field Crop Abstr., Forest.Abstr., Hort.Abstr., Ind.Med., Ind.Vet., Indian Sci.Abstr., Int.Abstr.Biol.Sci., Irr.& Drain.Abstr., Lead Abstr., Plant Breed.Abstr., Pollut.Abstr., Poult.Abstr., Rev.Appl.Entomol., Rev.Med.& Vet.Mycol., Rev.Plant Path., Rice Abstr., Saf.Sci.Abstr., Seed Abstr., Sel.Water Res.Abstr., Soils & Fert., Sugar Ind.Abstr., Tox.Abstr. (coverage dropped), Triticale Abstr., Vet.Bull., Weed Abstr., World Text.Abstr., Zincscan, Zoo.Rec.

—BLDSC (4979.359000), CASDDS, CIS, CISTI, EMDOCS, IDS.

Address: 1/206 Vikas Nagar, Lucknow, Uttar Pradesh 226 022, India. TEL 0522-769181, 0522-769181, http://www.geocities.com/j_biol. Ed., R&P R C Dalela TEL 91-522-768752. Pub., Adv. contact Kiran Dalela. B&W page USD 600, color page USD 1,000; trim 21 x 27. Circ: 50,000.

363.72 USA ISSN 0022-0892
RA565.A1 CODEN: JEVHAH

JOURNAL OF ENVIRONMENTAL HEALTH. Text in English. 1938. 10/yr. USD 75 in US & Canada to membership; USD 115 elsewhere to membership; USD 90 in US & Canada to institutions; USD 165 in India to institutions; USD 135 elsewhere to institutions (effective 2001). adv. bk.rev. charts, illus. index. back issues avail.; reprints avail. *Refereed.* **Document type:** *Academic/Scholarly.* **Description:** Covers all phases of environmental health, protection and sanitation.

Related titles: Microfilm ed.: (from PQC); Online - full text ed.: (from ProQuest Information & Learning, Gale Group, Northern Light Technology, Inc., H. W. Wilson, Factiva, Institute for Scientific Information).

Indexed: A.S.& T.Ind. (Sep.1983-), ASCA, Aqua.Sci.& Fish.Abstr., Bibl.Agri., Biol.Abstr., C.I.J.E. (coverage dropped), CINAHL, C.I.S. Abstr., Cadscan, Chem.Abstr., Chem.Indus.Notes, Chem.Titles, Curr.Cont., Dairy Sci.Abstr., Energy Info.Abstr., Energy Rev., Environ.Abstr., Environ.Per.Bibl. (1972-), Environ.Sci.Poll.Mgmt., Excerp.Med., Fluidex, Food Sci.& Tech.Abstr., Gen.Sci.Ind. (Jul.1984-), Geo.Abstr.H.G., Geo.Abstr.P.G., GeoRef, Helminthol.Abstr., Hosp.Lit.Ind., INIS Atomind., Ind.Med., Ind.Sci.Rev., Lead Abstr., Microbiol.Abstr., Noise Pollut.Publ.Abstr., Nutr.Abstr., Ocean.Abstr. (coverage dropped), Pollut.Abstr., Protozool.Abstr., Repindex, Rev.Appl.Entomol., Rev.Med.& Vet.Mycol., Risk Abstr., SSCI (coverage dropped), Saf.Sci.Abstr., Sci.Cit.Ind. (coverage dropped), Sel.Water Res.Abstr., Soils & Fert., Tox.Abstr., W.R.C.Inf., Wild.Rev., Zincscan.

—BLDSC (4979.380000), CASDDS, CIS, CISTI, GNLM, IDS, ingenta, Linda Hall. **CCC.**

Published by: National Environmental Health Association, 720 S Colorado Blvd, S Tower, Ste 970, Denver, CO 80246. TEL 303-756-9090, FAX 303-691-9490, staff@neha.org, http://www.neha.org. Ed. Nelson Fabian. R&P Julie Collins. Adv. contact Veronika Clark. Circ: 6,000 (paid).

628 GBR ISSN 0265-931X
CODEN: JERAEE

JOURNAL OF ENVIRONMENTAL RADIOACTIVITY. Text in English. 1984. 18/yr. EUR 162 in Europe to qualified personnel; JPY 21,600 in Japan to qualified personnel; USD 182 elsewhere to qualified personnel; EUR 1,337 in Europe to institutions; JPY 177,234 in Japan to institutions; USD 1,496 elsewhere to institutions (effective 2002). adv. back issues avail. *Refereed.* **Document type:** *Academic/Scholarly.* **Description:** International forum for original research on any aspect of radioactivity in natural systems.

Related titles: Online - full text ed.: (from ingenta, ScienceDirect, Swets Blackwell, Institute for Scientific Information).

Indexed: ASCA, Abstr.Hyg., Aqua.Sci.& Fish.Abstr., Bioeng.Abstr., Biol.Abstr., Chem.Abstr., Chem.Cit.Ind., Chem.Indus.Notes, Chem.Titles, Crop Physiol.Abstr., Curr.Cont., Dairy Sci.Abstr., Deep Sea Res.& Oceanogr.Abstr., Ecol.Abstr., Energy Rev., Eng.Ind., Environ.Abstr., Environ.Per.Bibl. (1994-), Environ.Sci.Poll.Mgmt., Excerp.Med., Field Crop Abstr., Food Sci.& Tech.Abstr., Forest Prod.Abstr., Forest.Abstr., Geo.Abstr.H.G., Geo.Abstr.P.G., GeoRef, Geol.Abstr., Geomech.Abstr., Herb.Abstr., Hort.Abstr., INIS Atomind., INSPEC (1986-), ISMEC, Ind.Med. (1984-), Ind.Vet., Int.Abstr.Biol.Sci., Irr.& Drain.Abstr., Nutr.Abstr., Pollut.Abstr., Potato Abstr., Poult.Abstr., Ref.Zh., Rice Abstr., Risk Abstr., Saf.Sci.Abstr., Sel.Water Res.Abstr., Soils & Fert., Sport Fish.Abstr., Tox.Abstr. (coverage dropped), Triticale Abstr., Trop.Dis.Bull., Weed Abstr., Wild.Rev., World Ag.Econ.& Rur.Soc.Abstr., Zoo.Rec.

—BLDSC (4979.392000), AskIEEE, CASDDS, CISTI, Ei, EMDOCS, IDS, ingenta, Linda Hall. **CCC.**

Published by: (University of Glasgow, Department of Chemistry), Pergamon (Subsidiary of: Elsevier Science), The Boulevard, Langford Ln, East Park, Kidlington, Oxford OXB 1GB, United Kingdom. FAX 44-1865-843010, usinfo-f@elsevier.com, http://www.elsevier.com/locate/jenvrad. Eds. M S Baxter, T G Hinton. **Subscr. in Australasia and the Far East to:** Elsevier Science (Singapore) Pte Ltd, No.1 Temasek Ave, 17-01 Millenia Tower, Singapore 039192, Singapore. TEL 65-434-3727, FAX 65-337-2230; **Subscr. in the Americas to:** Elsevier Science, PO Box 945, New York, NY 10159-0945. TEL 212-633-3730, FAX 212-633-3680; **Subscr. to:** Elsevier Science BV, PO Box 211, Amsterdam 1000 AE, Netherlands. TEL 31-20-485-3757.

JOURNAL OF ENVIRONMENTAL SCIENCE AND HEALTH. PART A: TOXIC HAZARDOUS SUBSTANCES AND ENVIRONMENTAL ENGINEERING. see *ENVIRONMENTAL STUDIES—Toxicology And Environmental Safety*

363.72 USA ISSN 0360-1234
QH545.A1 CODEN: JPFCD2

JOURNAL OF ENVIRONMENTAL SCIENCE AND HEALTH. PART B: PESTICIDES, FOOD CONTAMINANTS, AND AGRICULTURAL WASTES. Text in English. 1966. bi-m. USD 145 to individuals print & online eds.; USD 1,125 to institutions print only (effective 2002). adv. *Refereed.* **Document type:** *Academic/Scholarly.* **Description:** Provides an outlet for original research reports on analytical techniques or improvements on existing methods applicable to residues of pestidices, food contaminants and other contaminants and their metabolites in the ecosphere.

Supersedes in part: Environmental Letters (0013-9300)

Related titles: Microform ed.: (from RPI); Online - full content ed.; Online - full text ed.: (from Institute for Scientific Information, RoweCom Information Quest).

Indexed: ASCA, Agri.& Environ.Biotech.Abstr. (coverage dropped), Agri.Eng.Abstr., Agricola, Agroforest.Abstr., Anal.Abstr., Aqua.Sci.& Fish.Abstr., Bibl.Agri., Bio-Contr.News & Info., Bioeng.Abstr., Biol.Abstr., Cadscan, Chem.Abstr., Chem.Indus.Notes, Chem.Titles, Cott.& Trop.Fibr.Abstr., Crop Physiol.Abstr., Curr.Cont., Dairy Sci.Abstr., Derwent Biotech.Abstr., Dok.Arbeitsmed., Ecol.Abstr., Eng.Ind., Entomol.Abstr., Environ.Abstr., Environ.Per.Bibl. (1977-), Environ.Sci.Poll.Mgmt., Excerp.Med., Field Crop Abstr., Fluidex, Food Sci.& Tech.Abstr., Forest Prod.Abstr., Forest.Abstr., Geo.Abstr.H.G., Geo.Abstr.P.G., GeoRef, Helminthol.Abstr., Hort.Abstr., IDA, INIS Atomind., ISMEC, Ind.Med. (1976-), Ind.Sci.Rev., Ind.Vet., Int.Abstr.Biol.Sci., Irr.& Drain.Abstr., Lead Abstr., Maize Abstr., Microbiol.Abstr., Nutr.Abstr., Ocean.Abstr. (coverage dropped), Pig News & Info., Pollut.Abstr., Postharvest, Poult.Abstr., Ref.Zh., Rev.Appl.Entomol., Rev.Arom.& Med.Plants, Rev.Med.& Vet.Mycol., Rev.Plant Path., Rice Abstr., Risk Abstr., Saf.Sci.Abstr., Sci.Cit.Ind., Seed Abstr., Sel.Water Res.Abstr., Soils & Fert., Soyabean Abstr., Sport Fish.Abstr., Sugar Ind.Abstr., Tox.Abstr., Triticale Abstr., Vet.Bull., W.R.C.Inf., WasteInfo, Weed Abstr., Wild.Rev., Zincscan, Zoo.Rec.

—BLDSC (4979.394000), CASDDS, CIS, CISTI, Ei, EMDOCS, GNLM, IDS, Infotrieve, ingenta, Linda Hall. **CCC.**

Published by: Marcel Dekker Inc., 270 Madison Ave, New York, NY 10016. TEL 212-696-9000, 800-228-1160, FAX 212-685-4540, journals@dekker.com, http://www.dekker.com/servlet/product/productid/PFC. Ed. Shahamat U Khan. R&P Julia Mulligan. Adv. contact Anne Mullins. B&W page USD 800. Circ: 325.

JOURNAL OF ENVIRONMENTAL SCIENCE AND HEALTH. PART C: ENVIRONMENTAL CARCINOGENESIS & ECOTOXICOLOGY REVIEWS. see *ENVIRONMENTAL STUDIES—Toxicology And Environmental Safety*

616.98 GBR ISSN 1053-4245
RA565.A1 CODEN: JEAEE9

JOURNAL OF EXPOSURE ANALYSIS AND ENVIRONMENTAL EPIDEMIOLOGY. Text in English. 1991. 6/yr. GBP 303 in Europe to institutions for print or online ed.; USD 445 elsewhere to institutions for print or online ed.; GBP 334 combined subscription in Europe to institutions print & online; USD 501 combined subscription elsewhere to institutions print & online (effective 2002). adv. bk.rev. illus, charts, stat. index. back issues avail.; reprints avail. *Refereed.* **Document type:** *Journal, Academic/Scholarly.* **Description:** Covers new and emerging areas of human exposure assessment: measurement; monitoring methods; modeling; dose-effect relationships; multimedia exposure assessment; biomakers; and environmental and epidemiological studies involving molecular biomarkers.

Related titles: Online - full text ed.: (from EBSCO Publishing, O C L C Online Computer Library Center, Inc., RoweCom Information Quest, ingenta, Swets Blackwell, Institute for Scientific Information).

Indexed: ASCA, Chem.Abstr., Chem.Indus.Notes, Chem.Titles, Curr.Cont., Excerp.Med. (1993-), INIS Atomind., Ind.Med. (1991-), Int.Abstr.Biol.Sci., Lab.Haz.Bull., Nutr.Abstr., Rev.Appl.Entomol., Rev.Med.& Vet.Mycol., SSCI (coverage dropped), Soils & Fert., Weed Abstr.

—BLDSC (4983.085000), CASDDS, CISTI, EMDOCS, GNLM, IDS, Infotrieve. **CCC.**

Published by: (International Society of Exposure Analysis), Nature Publishing Group Specialist Journals (Subsidiary of: Holtzbrink Publishers), Houndmills, Basingstoke, Hants RG21 6XS, United Kingdom. TEL 44-1256-329242, FAX 44-1256-328339, subscriptions@nature.com, http://www.nature.com/jea. Ed. Edo Pellizzari. Pub. Julia Schulhof. adv.: page USD 400. Circ: 700. **Affiliate:** Nature Publishing Group Specialist Journals.

JOURNAL OF OCCUPATIONAL AND ENVIRONMENTAL MEDICINE. see *MEDICAL SCIENCES*

JOURNAL OF RADIOLOGICAL PROTECTION. see *ENERGY—Nuclear Energy*

▼ **JOURNAL OF THE I C R U.** see *PHYSICS—Nuclear Physics*

E

614.7 570 KOR ISSN 1226-8399
JOURNAL OF TOXICOLOGY AND PUBLIC HEALTH. Text in Korean. bi-m. KRW 20,000, USD 100. **Document type:** *Academic/Scholarly.* **Description:** For toxicologists, molecular biologists, geneticists, biochemists, pharmacologists, clinical researchers and epidemiologists with a global view on public well-being through toxicological research.
Formerly (until 1997): Korean Journal of Toxicology (0258-2368)
—BLDSC (5069.735500).
Published by: Korean Society of Toxicology, BBRC-KIST, Sungbuk-gu, 39-1 Hawolgok dong, Seoul 136791, Korea, S.. TEL 82-2-958-5055, FAX 82-2-958-5059. **Subscr. to:** Department of Biological Sciences, KAIST, 373-1 Kusung dong, Yusung Gu Taejo 305701, Korea, S.

KEVO SUBARCTIC RESEARCH INSTITUTE. REPORTS. see *BIOLOGY*

LABORATORY SAFETY & ENVIRONMENTAL MANAGEMENT. see *PUBLIC HEALTH AND SAFETY*

LIETUVOS MOKSLU AKADEMIJA. EKOLOGIJA. see *BIOLOGY*

LOGOS (ARGONNE). see *ENGINEERING*

MANAGEMENT O H S & E. see *OCCUPATIONAL HEALTH AND SAFETY*

MEDDELELSER OM GROENLAND, BIOSCIENCE. see *BIOLOGY*

616.98 SWE ISSN 1100-9535
MILJOEMEDICIN/ENVIRONMENTAL MEDICINE. Text in Swedish. 1987. 4/yr. free per issue. **Document type:** *Newsletter.*
Published by: Institutet foer Miljoemedicin (IMM)/Institute of Environmental Medicine, Fack 210, Stockholm 17177, Sweden. TEL 46-8-728-64-00, FAX 46-8-33-69-81.

MIND MATTERS REVIEW. see *PSYCHOLOGY*

363.7 NLD ISSN 1381-2386
MITIGATION AND ADAPTATION STRATEGIES FOR GLOBAL CHANGE; an international journal devoted to scientific, engineering, socio-economic and policy responses to environmental change. Text in English. 1995. q. EUR 263 to institutions for print or online ed.; EUR 315.60 to institutions print & online eds.combined (effective 2002). *Refereed.* **Document type:** *Academic/Scholarly.* **Description:** Covers technical and policy options for coping with issues such as global climate change, stratospheric ozone depletion, acid deposition, as well as other emerging environmental problems.
Related titles: Online - full text ed.: (from EBSCO Publishing, O C L C Online Computer Library Center, Inc., RoweCom Information Quest, Swets Blackwell, Kluwer Online).
Indexed: Aqua.Sci.& Fish.Abstr., Environ.Per.Bibl. (1996-), Environ.Sci.Poll.Mgmt., Forest.Abstr., Geo.Abstr.P.G., INIS Atomind., Meteor.& Geoastrophys.Abstr., Pollut.Abstr., Soils & Fert.
—BLDSC (5829.740000), Infotrieve. **CCC.**
Published by: Kluwer Academic Publishers Group (Subsidiary of: Wolters Kluwer N.V.), Spuiboulevard 50, PO Box 17, Dordrecht 3300 AA, Netherlands. FAX 31-78-639-2254, services@wkap.nl, http://www.wkap.nl. Ed. Robert K Dixon. **Dist. by:** Journals Department, PO Box 322, Dordrecht 3300 AH, Netherlands. TEL 781-871-6600, FAX 31-78-654-6474.

N B I A NEWSLETTER. see *AGRICULTURE*

577 DEU
NATUR UND KOSMOS. Text in German. 1981. m. DEM 98.40 domestic; DEM 103.80 foreign; DEM 9.50 newsstand/cover (effective 2001 & 2002). adv. bk.rev. 130 p./no. **Document type:** *Magazine, Consumer.* **Description:** Focuses mainly on ecological and environmental subjects. Frequently publishes stories on biology, zoology, and ecology of animals and plants, on medical and psychological topics, consumer information, and articles dealing with chemical and nuclear industries and their dangers.
Formerly: Natur (0723-5038)
Related titles: Online - full text ed.
Indexed: INIS Atomind., Key Word Ind.Wildl.Res.
—Linda Hall.
Published by: Natur Media GmbH, Belfortstr 8, Munich 81667, Germany. TEL 49-89-458727-0, FAX 49-89-45872724, redaktion@natur.de, http://www.natur.de. Ed. Gerd Pfitzenmaier. adv.: B&W page DEM 10,790, color page DEM 17,960; trim 176 x 250. Circ: 104,417 (controlled).

363.7 GBR ISSN 0072-7008 CODEN: NERRB4
NATURAL ENVIRONMENT RESEARCH COUNCIL. REPORT. Text in English. 1967. a. GBP 12.
Indexed: Aqua.Sci.& Fish.Abstr., Aquacult.Abstr., Br.Archaeol.Abstr., Environ.Sci.Poll.Mgmt., Field Crop Abstr., GeoRef, Herb.Abstr.
—Linda Hall.
Published by: Natural Environment Research Council, Polaris House, North Star Ave, Swindon, Wilts SN2 1EU, United Kingdom. TEL 44-1793-411500, FAX 44-1793-411501, TELEX 444293 ENVRE G, nerccomm@wpo.nerc.ac.uk. Ed. B H Knowles.

628 551 362.1 USA ISSN 1527-6988
NATURAL HAZARDS REVIEW. Text in English. q. USD 43 domestic to members for print and online eds.; USD 53 foreign to members for print and online eds.; USD 65 domestic to individuals for print and online eds.; USD 80 foreign to individuals for print and online eds.; USD 193 domestic to institutions for print and online eds.; USD 203 foreign to institutions for print and online eds. (effective 2001). bk.rev. back issues avail. *Refereed.* **Document type:** *Magazine, Academic/Scholarly.* **Description:** Provides innovative and practical solutions to the problems and challenges faced by the hazards community - government, academic, private sector and non-governmental organizations.
Related titles: CD-ROM ed.: USD 43 to members for CD-ROM and online eds.; USD 65 to individuals for CD-ROM and online eds.; USD 193 to institutions for CD-ROM and online eds. (effective 2001); Online - full text ed.: USD 37 to members; USD 55 to individuals; USD 164 to institutions (effective 2001) (from EBSCO Publishing).
Indexed: EEA, Environ.Sci.Poll.Mgmt.
—BLDSC (6037.890000), Linda Hall.
Published by: American Society of Civil Engineers, 1801 Alexander Graham Bell Dr., Reston, VA 20191-4400. TEL 703-295-6300, 800-548-2723, FAX 703-295-6222, marketing@asce.org, http://www.pubs.asce.org/journals/nh.html. Eds. Dennis S Mileti, James E Beavers.

363.7 USA ISSN 1051-8096
NEW OHIO JOURNAL* . Text in English. 1990. bi-m. USD 20. **Description:** Covers personal and environmental health.
Published by: David Smigelski, Ed. & Pub., 4518 N E 28th Ave, Portland, OR 97211-7110.

NEW SOLUTIONS; a journal of environmental and occupational health policy. see *OCCUPATIONAL HEALTH AND SAFETY*

NUCLEUS (CAMBRIDGE). see *ENERGY*

628 USA
O S H A REQUIRED SAFETY TRAINING FOR SUPERVISORS. (Occupational Safety and Health Administration) Text in English. 1982. m. USD 99 (effective 1998). adv. index. back issues avail. **Document type:** *Newsletter.* **Description:** Reports on right-to-know regulations and OSHA details.
Former titles: SafetyWorks for Supervisors (1083-4516); (until 1995): O S H A Training Bulletin for Supervisors (0896-9957); (until 1988): Hazardous Materials Training Bulletin for Supervisors (0887-9125); Hazardous Waste Training Bulletin for Supervisors (0744-4168)
—CCC.
Published by: Business & Legal Reports, Inc., 39 Academy St, Madison, CT 06443-1513. TEL 203-318-0000, 800-727-5257, FAX 203-245-2559. Ed. John F Brady. Pub. Robert L Brady. R&P Kathy Long. Adv. contact Paul Conderino. Circ: 1,500.

OCCUPATIONAL HAZARDS; magazine of health & environment. see *OCCUPATIONAL HEALTH AND SAFETY*

OCCUPATIONAL SAFETY & ENVIRONMENTAL NEWS. see *OCCUPATIONAL HEALTH AND SAFETY*

PHYSIOLOGY AND ECOLOGY JAPAN. see *BIOLOGY—Physiology*

628 POL ISSN 0084-2869
POLITECHNIKA WROCLAWSKA. INSTYTUT INZYNIERII OCHRONY SRODOWISKA. PRACE NAUKOWE. MONOGRAFIE. Text in Polish; Summaries in English, French, German, Russian. 1969. irreg., latest vol.38, 1998. price varies. adv. **Document type:** *Monographic series.*
Indexed: INIS Atomind., INSPEC (1994-).
—AskIEEE, Ei, Linda Hall.
Published by: (Instytut Inzynierii Ochrony Srodowiska, Politechnika Wroclawska), Oficyna Wydawnicza Politechniki Wroclawskiej, Wybrzeze Wyspianskiego 27, Wroclaw 50370, Poland. TEL 48-71-3282940, FAX 48-71-3282940, oficwyd@pwr.wroc.pl. R&P Halina Dudek. **Dist. by:** Ars Polona, Krakowskie Przedmiescie 7, Warsaw, Poland.

363.7 USA ISSN 1041-6773
PULSE OF THE PLANET. Text in English. 1989. 4/yr. USD 20 (effective 2000). bk.rev. **Document type:** *Monographic series, Academic/Scholarly.* **Description:** Constitutes an environmental research journal focusing on alternative energy research applications of Wilhelm Reich's work, with translations of related papers from Germany and other countries.
Published by: Orgone Biophysical Research Laboratory, PO Box 1148, Ashland, OR 97520. TEL 541-552-0118, FAX 541-552-0118, demeo@mind.net, http://www.orgonelab.org/xdpulse.htm. Ed., R&P James DeMeo.

616.98 USA ISSN 1078-103X
RACHEL'S ENVIRONMENT & HEALTH WEEKLY. Text in English. 1986. w. USD 25 to individuals; USD 45 to libraries; USD 400 to corporations (effective 2000). **Document type:** *Newsletter.* **Description:** Covers international and US hazardous waste issues, including air pollution, landfills, incineration and public health, radiation and nuclear wastes, environmental justice, pollution prevention, regulatory actions, and citizen law-reform campaigns.
Formerly: Rachel's Hazardous Waste News (1065-4623)
Related titles: Diskette ed.; Online - full text ed.
Indexed: Alt.Press Ind.
Published by: Environmental Research Foundation, PO Box 5036, Annapolis, MD 21403-7036. TEL 410-263-1584, FAX 410-263-8944, erf@rachel.org, http://www.rachel.org. Ed. Peter Montague. R&P Carrie Jantz.

RADIATION PROTECTION DOSIMETRY. see *PHYSICS—Nuclear Physics*

RAUM UND ZEIT; die neue Dimension der Wissenschaft. see *MEDICAL SCIENCES*

REPINDEX. see *ENVIRONMENTAL STUDIES—Abstracting, Bibliographies, Statistics*

REVIEWS OF ENVIRONMENTAL CONTAMINATION AND TOXICOLOGY. see *ENVIRONMENTAL STUDIES—Toxicology And Environmental Safety*

616.98 ISR ISSN 0048-7554
RA565.A1 CODEN: REVHA3
REVIEWS ON ENVIRONMENTAL HEALTH. Text in English. 1972. q., latest vol.17. USD 290 (effective 2002). adv. bk.rev. index. back issues avail. **Document type:** *Academic/Scholarly.*
Indexed: Abstr.Hyg., Chem.Abstr., Chem.Indus.Notes, Chem.Titles, Curr.Adv.Ecol.Sci., Curr.Cont. (coverage dropped), Dok.Arbeitsmed., Energy Rev., Environ.Per.Bibl., Excerp.Med., I.P.A., Ind.Med. (1972-).
—BLDSC (7790.525000), CASDDS, CISTI, GNLM, ingenta, Linda Hall.
Published by: Freund Publishing House, Ltd., P O Box 35010, Tel Aviv 61350, Israel. TEL 972-3-562-8540, FAX 972-3-562-8538, h_freund@netvision.net.il, http://www.angelfire.com/il/freund. Ed. V Buchner.

363.7 615.9 ROM ISSN 1224-3183
REVISTA DE ECOLOGIE INDUSTRIALA; Labor and Environmental Protection Magazine. Text in Romanian; Abstracts in English, Romanian. 1993. q. USD 30 (effective 2001). **Document type:** *Trade.*
Indexed: METADEX.
Published by: Oficiul de Informare si Documentare pentru Industria Constructoare de Masini, Sos. Oltenitei 103, Sector 4, OP8, Bucharest 75651, Romania. TEL 40-01-3324301, FAX 40-01-3320775, oid@mec.ictcm.ro. Eds. Doru Marculescu, Elena Baican. Pub. Speranta Stomff.

RIVISTA DI IDROBIOLOGIA. see *BIOLOGY*

E

SAFETY AND HEALTH; the international safety, health and environmental magazine. see *OCCUPATIONAL HEALTH AND SAFETY*

SAFETY MANAGEMENT; the bigger picture in occupational safety, health and environmental risk management. see *OCCUPATIONAL HEALTH AND SAFETY*

SAFETY RESOURCES; middle management to CEO issues. see *OCCUPATIONAL HEALTH AND SAFETY*

SATYA; magazine of vegetarianism, environmentalism, and animal advocacy. see *NUTRITION AND DIETETICS*

333.72 NLD ISSN 0048-9697
RA565 CODEN: STENDL
THE SCIENCE OF THE TOTAL ENVIRONMENT; an international journal for scientific research into the environment and its relationship with man. Text in Dutch. 1972. 54/yr. EUR 4,166 in Europe to institutions; JPY 552,600 in Japan to institutions; USD 4,661 elsewhere to institutions (effective 2002). adv. bk.rev. charts, illus. index. reprint service avail. from SWZ. *Refereed.* **Document type:** *Academic/Scholarly.* **Description:** Publishes research into man-made changes in the environment, especially disturbances of the natural levels and distribution of chemical elements and compounds and the impact of this on the living world. Particular emphasis is given to applications of environmental chemistry to nutrition, pollution control, environmental medicine, planning and policy.
Related titles: Microform ed.: (from PQC); Online - full text ed.: (from ingenta, Swets Blackwell, Institute for Scientific Information, ScienceDirect).
Indexed: ASCA, Acid Pre.Dig., Agri.& Environ.Biotech.Abstr. (coverage dropped), Agri.Eng.Abstr., Anal.Abstr., Anim.Breed.Abstr., Aqua.Sci.& Fish.Abstr., Arts & Hum.Cit.Ind. (coverage dropped), Biol.Abstr., C.I.S. Abstr., Chem.Abstr., Chem.Cit.Ind., Chem.Titles, Crop Physiol.Abstr., Curr.Adv.Biochem., Curr.Adv.Ecol.Sci., Curr.Cont., Dairy Sci.Abstr., Deep Sea Res.& Oceanogr.Abstr., Derwent Biotech.Abstr., Dok.Arbeitsmed., Ecol.Abstr., Energy Ind., Energy Info.Abstr., Energy Rev., Eng.Ind., Entomol.Abstr., Environ.Abstr., Environ.Ind., Environ.Per.Bibl. (1972-), Environ.Sci.Poll.Mgmt., Excerp.Med., Field Crop Abstr., Fluidex, Food Sci.& Tech.Abstr., Forest.Abstr., Geo.Abstr.H.G., Geo.Abstr.P.G., GeoRef, Geol.Abstr., Geomech.Abstr., Hort.Abstr., IDA, INIS Atomind., Ind.Med. (1972-), Ind.Sci.Rev., Ind.Vet., Int.Abstr.Biol.Sci., Irr.& Drain.Abstr., Key Word Ind.Wildl.Res., METADEX, Maize Abstr., Mass Spectr.Bull., Meteor.& Geoastrophys.Abstr., Microbiol.Abstr., Mid.East: Abstr.& Ind., Nutr.Abstr., Ocean.Abstr., Ornam.Hort., Pollut.Abstr., Potato Abstr., Rev.Appl.Entomol., Rev.Plant Path., Rice Abstr., Risk Abstr., SSCI (coverage dropped), Saf.Sci.Abstr., Sci.Cit.Ind., Sel.Water Res.Abstr., Soils & Fert., Sport Fish.Abstr., Tox.Abstr., Triticale Abstr., Vet.Bull., W.R.C.Inf., Wastelnfo, Weed Abstr., Wild.Rev., Zoo.Rec.
—BLDSC (8165.030000), CASDDS, CISTI, Ei, EMDOCS, GNLM, IDS, ingenta, Linda Hall. **CCC.**
Published by: Elsevier Science BV, PO Box 211, Amsterdam 1000 AE, Netherlands. TEL 31-20-485-3757, FAX 31-20-485-3432, TELEX 18582 ESPA NL, nlinfo-f@elsevier.nl; usinfo-f@elsevier.com; forinfo-kyf04035@niftyserve.or.jp, http://www.elsevier.nl/locate/issn/00489697. Ed. E Hamilton. **Subscr. in Australasia and the Far East to:** Elsevier Science (Singapore) Pte Ltd, No.1 Temasek Ave, 17-01 Millenia Tower, Singapore 039192, Singapore. TEL 65-434-3727, FAX 65-337-2230, asiainfo@elsevier.com.sg; **Subscr. in Japan to:** Elsevier Science Inc - Japan Regional Office, 9-15 Higashi-Azabu 1-chome, Minato-ku, Tokyo 106-0044, Japan. TEL 81-3-5561-5033, FAX 81-3-5561-5047, info@elsevier.co.jp; **Subscr. in the Americas to:** Elsevier Science, PO Box 945, New York, NY 10159-0945. TEL 212-633-3730, FAX 212-633-3680, usinfo-f@elsevier.com, http://www.elsevier.com.

SEEVOEGEL. see *BIOLOGY—Ornithology*

363.7 JPN ISSN 0037-1025
CODEN: STKADC
SEIKATSU TO KANKYO* /LIFE AND ENVIRONMENT. Text in Japanese. 1956. m. adv. charts, illus. index.
Indexed: Chem.Abstr., Chem.Indus.Notes, Chem.Titles.
—CASDDS.
Published by: Nihon Kankyo Eisei Senta/Japan Environmental Sanitation Center, 10-6 Yotsuya-Kami-cho, Kawasaki-ku, Kawasaki-shi, Kanagawa-ken 210-0828, Japan. Ed. Kazumi Kuroda. Circ: 10,000.

SOCIETY & ANIMALS; social scientific studies of the human experience of other animals. see *ANIMAL WELFARE*

STRAALEVERNRAPPORT/N R P A REPORT. see *PUBLIC HEALTH AND SAFETY*

363.7 USA ISSN 1083-7639
GE170 CODEN: SYREFS
SYNTHESIS - REGENERATION: A MAGAZINE OF GREEN SOCIAL THOUGHT. Text in English. 1992. 3/yr., latest vol.25. USD 12 domestic to individuals; USD 15 in Canada to individuals; USD 20 elsewhere to individuals; USD 25 domestic to institutions; USD 28 in Canada to institutions; USD 33 elsewhere to institutions (effective 2001). bk.rev. illus. 48 p./no. 2 cols./p. back issues avail. **Document type:** *Magazine, Academic/Scholarly.* **Description:** Covers the environment, social and labor. Features discussions of electoral strategies and proposals for legal and constitutional changes.
Former titles (until 1993): Regeneration: A Magazine of Left Green Social Thought; (until 1991): Workers' Democracy; Green Synthesis; Synthesis
Related titles: CD-ROM ed.; Microfiche ed.: (from CIS); Online - full text ed.
Indexed: Alt.Press Ind., Environ.Abstr., Lang.& Lang.Behav.Abstr., P.A.I.S., SOPODA, Sociol.Abstr.
Published by: W D Press, PO Box 24115, St. Louis, MO 63130. TEL 314-727-5393, gpusa@igc.apc.org, http://www.greens.org/. Ed., R&P Don Fitz TEL 314-727-8554. Circ: 3,000 (paid).

T R A C NEWSLETTER. (Transvaal Rural Action Committee) see *POLITICAL SCIENCE—Civil Rights*

TASMANIAN NATURALIST. see *BIOLOGY*

TECHNICAL LITERATURE ABSTRACTS: HEALTH & ENVIRONMENT. see *ENVIRONMENTAL STUDIES—Abstracting, Bibliographies, Statistics*

363.7 DEU ISSN 0942-5675
CODEN: TERAFN
TERRATECH; Zeitschrift fuer Altlasten und Bodenschutz. Text in German. 1992. 6/yr. EUR 78 domestic; EUR 84 foreign (effective 2002). adv. **Document type:** *Magazine, Trade.*
Indexed: CEABA, GeoRef.
—BLDSC (8794.814000), CASDDS. **CCC.**
Published by: Vereinigte Fachverlage GmbH, Lise-Meitner-Str 2, Mainz 55129, Germany. TEL 49-6131-992-0, FAX 49-6131-992-100, info@vfmz.de, http://www.industrie-service.de. Ed. Hans Joachim Schmitz. Adv. contact Michael Kiefer. B&W page DEM 3,200, color page DEM 4,700; trim 185 x 265. Circ: 2,500 (controlled).

THIRD WORLD SCIENCE & ENVIRONMENT PERSPECTIVES. see *ENVIRONMENTAL STUDIES—Toxicology And Environmental Safety*

TRENDS IN ECOLOGY AND EVOLUTION. see *BIOLOGY*

TUBERKULEZ I EKOLOGIYA. see *MEDICAL SCIENCES—Respiratory Diseases*

UMWELTSCHUTZ. see *PUBLIC HEALTH AND SAFETY*

UNIVERSIDAD DE MURCIA. ANALES DE BIOLOGIA. SECCION BIOLOGIA AMBIENTAL. see *BIOLOGY*

363.7 USA ISSN 0899-1405
WARY CANARY; a news network for allergics, "sensitive birds," & environmental health advocates. Text in English. 1986. q. USD 20 domestic (effective 1999); USD 24 in Canada; USD 27 elsewhere. adv. **Document type:** *Consumer.* **Description:** Covers preventive self-care and recovery from environmentally and chemically induced illness, toxic-response syndrome and allergies, including geographic relocation for health, sources and resources of nontoxic materials, dietary strategies and nontraditional medical alternatives.
Indexed: Environ.Abstr.
Published by: Wary Canary Press, PO Box 2204, Ft. Collins, CO 80522. TEL 303-224-0083. Ed., R&P Suzanne Randegger TEL 970-493-8089. Adv. contact Ed Randegger. Circ: 750.

WOHNUNG & GESUNDHEIT; Fachzeitschrift fuer oekologisches Bauen & Leben. see *ARCHITECTURE*

WORKERS LIFE (PRETORIA). see *OCCUPATIONAL HEALTH AND SAFETY*

324.2187 USA
WORLDWATCH READER. Text in English. irreg., latest 1998. USD 14.95 per issue (effective 2000). **Document type:** *Consumer.* **Description:** Covers the most important problems facing humanity: energy production, transportation, and environmentally friendly heating systems; how to reverse the declining health of the oceans, forests, and freshwater resourcess; and what to do about the the new social instabilities that result from environmental distress.
Published by: Worldwatch Institute, 1776 Massachusetts Ave, N W, Washington, DC 20036. wwpub@worldwatch.org, http://www.worldwatch.org. Eds. Ed Ayres, Lester R Brown.

YAMAGUCHIKEN EISEI KOGAI KENKYU SENTA GYOSEKI HOKOKU. see *PUBLIC HEALTH AND SAFETY*

ZHIWU SHENGTAI XUEBAO/ACTA PHYTOECOLOGICA SINICA. see *BIOLOGY—Botany*

ENVIRONMENTAL STUDIES—Abstracting, Bibliographies, Statistics

016.6159 IND ISSN 0970-440X
ABSTRACTS OF CURRENT LITERATURE IN TOXICOLOGY. Text in English. 1988. q. INR 250, USD 25 to individuals; INR 400, USD 40 to institutions (effective 2000). bk.rev. **Document type:** *Abstract/Index.* **Description:** Includes selected original scientific research work published in 250 journals received in ITRC library.
Published by: Industrial Toxicology Research Centre, Mahatma Gandhi Marg, P O Box 80, Lucknow, Uttar Pradesh 226 001, India. TEL 91-522-220107, FAX 91-522-228227, TELEX 0535-2456 ITRC IN, sna@itrc.ernet.in, intox@itrc.sirnetd.ernet.in. Ed. Saad-uz Zaman.

016.66 USA ISSN 0884-7452
CODEN: CBEBEO
C A S BIOTECH UPDATES. ENVIRONMENTAL BIOTECHNOLOGY. Text in English. s-w. USD 270 (effective 2001). **Document type:** *Abstract/Index.* **Description:** Covers treatment and disposal of industrial, municipal, domestic, and laboratory wastes and sewage; biochemical implications in water treatment, air pollution, and industrial hygiene.
Published by: Chemical Abstracts Service (Subsidiary of: American Chemical Society), 2540 Olentangy River Rd, Box 3012, Columbus, OH 43210-0012. TEL 614-447-3600, 800-753-4227, FAX 614-447-3751.

016.3637392 USA ISSN 1047-8213
CODEN: CSIPEZ
C A SELECTS. INDOOR AIR POLLUTION. Text in English. 1988. s-w. USD 275 (effective 2001). **Document type:** *Abstract/Index.* **Description:** Covers the air pollution of indoor environments. Includes pollution from chemical contaminants, particulates, and biological agents.
Formerly (until 1989): BIOSIS CAS Selects: Indoor Air Pollution
Published by: Chemical Abstracts Service (Subsidiary of: American Chemical Society), 2540 Olentangy River Rd, Box 3012, Columbus, OH 43210-0012. TEL 614-447-3600, 800-753-4227, FAX 614-447-3751.

016.6159 GBR ISSN 0965-0512
Z6665.A1
CURRENT ADVANCES IN TOXICOLOGY. Text in English. 1984. m. EUR 120 in Europe to qualified personnel; JPY 16,275 in Japan to qualified personnel; USD 135 elsewhere to qualified personnel; EUR 1,243 in Europe to institutions; JPY 164,730 in Japan to institutions; USD 1,390 elsewhere to institutions (effective 2002). adv. **Document type:** *Abstract/Index.* **Description:** Provides a current awareness service in the sphere of toxicology. Gives listings of titles of toxicological papers published throughout the world, classified into 127 main subject areas, and provides a comprehensive listing of review articles.
Formerly (until 1992): Current Advances in Pharmacology and Toxicology (0741-1685)
Related titles: Diskette ed.; Microfilm ed.: (from PQC); Online - full text ed.
—BLDSC (3494.068200), Infotrieve. **CCC.**

E

Published by: Elsevier Science BV, PO Box 211, Amsterdam 1000 AE, Netherlands. TEL 31-20-485-2911, FAX 31-20-485-2457, http://www.elsevier.com/locate/catox. adv.: B&W page USD 550, color page USD 1,350. Circ: 1,100. **Subscr. in Australasia and the Far East to:** Elsevier Science (Singapore) Pte Ltd, No.1 Temasek Ave, 17-01 Millenia Tower, Singapore 039192, Singapore. TEL 65-434-3727, FAX 65-337-2230; **Subscr. in Japanto:** Elsevier Science Inc - Japan Regional Office, 9-15 Higashi-Azabu 1-chome, Minato-ku, Tokyo 106-0044, Japan. TEL 81-3-5561-5033; **Subscr. in the Americas to:** Elsevier Science, PO Box 945, New York, NY 10159-0945. TEL 212-633-3730, FAX 212-633-3680, usinfo-f@elsevier.com.

E & P HEALTH, SAFETY AND ENVIRONMENT. (Exploration and Production) see *PETROLEUM AND GAS—Abstracting, Bibliographies, Statistics*

016.6159 DEU ISSN 1431-679X
ENVIRONMENTAL AND SAFETY TECHNOLOGY. Text in English. m. GBP 184; USD 310 in United States. **Document type:** *Abstract/Index.* **Description:** Provides coverage of environmental and safety aspects of interest to chemical and process engineers.
Formerly (until 1996): Environmental Protection and Process Safety (0948-9916); Safety, Environmental Protection and Analysis (0938-5215)
Published by: DECHEMA e.V., Postfach 150104, Frankfurt Am Main D-60061, Germany. TEL 49-69-7564-349, FAX 49-69-7564-201, forsyth@dechema.de, http://www.dechema.de. **Dist. by:** Turpin Distribution Services Ltd., Blackhorse Rd, Letchworth, Herts SG6 1HN, United Kingdom. FAX 44-1462-480947.

016.6137 NLD ISSN 0300-5194
CODEN: EHPCA6
EXCERPTA MEDICA. SECTION 46: ENVIRONMENTAL HEALTH AND POLLUTION CONTROL. Text in English. 1971. 16/yr. EUR 2,442 in Europe to institutions; JPY 323,752 in Japan to institutions; USD 2,732 elsewhere to institutions (effective 2002). adv. index, cum.index. **Document type:** *Abstract/Index, Academic/Scholarly.* **Description:** Provides a comprehensive current-awareness service covering the medical aspects of air, soil and water pollution, noise hindrance and radioactivity as related to the general environment.
Formerly (until 1971): Excerpta Medica. Section 46: Environmental Health (0046-2268)
Related titles: CD-ROM ed.: (from SilverPlatter Information, Inc.); Online - full text ed.: (from DIMDI, Data-Star, The Dialog Corporation, JICST).
—GNLM, Infotrieve, Linda Hall. **CCC.**
Published by: Excerpta Medica Medical Communications BV (Subsidiary of: Reed Elsevier plc), Rooseveltweg 15, Almere-Stad 1314 SJ, Netherlands. http://www.elsevier.com/locate/envheapolcon. **Subscr. in Australasia and the Far East to:** Elsevier Science (Singapore) Pte Ltd, No.1 Temasek Ave, 17-01 Millenia Tower, Singapore 039192, Singapore. TEL 65-434-3727, FAX 65-337-2230; **Subscr. in Japan to:** Elsevier Science Inc - Japan Regional Office, 9-15 Higashi-Azabu 1-chome, Minato-ku, Tokyo 106-0044, Japan. TEL 81-3-5561-5033, FAX 81-3-5561-5047; **Subscr. in the Americas to:** Elsevier Science, PO Box 945, New York, NY 10159-0945. TEL 212-633-3730, 888-437-4636, FAX 212-633-3680, usinfo-f@elsevier.com. **Dist. by:** Elsevier Science (Brazil).; Elsevier Science BV, PO Box 211, Amsterdam 1000 AE, Netherlands. TEL 31-20-485-3757, FAX 31-20-485-3432.

016.6159 NLD ISSN 0167-8353
CODEN: TXICDD
EXCERPTA MEDICA. SECTION 52: TOXICOLOGY. Text in English. 1983. 20/yr. NLG 3,950, EUR 1,792.43 in Europe to institutions; JPY 243,000 in Japan to institutions; USD 2,006 elsewhere to institutions (effective 2001). adv. index, cum.index. **Document type:** *Abstract/Index, Academic/Scholarly.* **Description:** Provides a comprehensive current-awareness service of clinical and professional articles covering the toxic mechanisms and effects of both medicinal and non-medicinal substances.
Related titles: CD-ROM ed.: (from SilverPlatter Information, Inc.); Online - full text ed.: (from DIMDI, Data-Star, The Dialog Corporation, JICST).
—GNLM, Linda Hall. **CCC.**
Published by: Excerpta Medica Medical Communications BV (Subsidiary of: Reed Elsevier plc), Rooseveltweg 15, Almere-Stad 1314 SJ, Netherlands. TEL 31-36-538-5600, FAX 31-36-538-5650, http://www.elsevier.nl/inca/publications/store/5/0/6/0/1/4/, http://www.excerptamedica.com. **Subscr. in Australasia and the Far East to:** Elsevier Science (Singapore) Pte Ltd, No.1 Temasek Ave, 17-01 Millenia Tower, Singapore 039192, Singapore. TEL 65-434-3727, FAX 65-337-2230; **Subscr. in Japan to:** Elsevier Science Inc - Japan Regional Office, 9-15 Higashi-Azabu 1-chome, Minato-ku, Tokyo 106-0044, Japan. TEL 81-3-5561-5033, FAX 81-3-5561-5047; **Subscr. in the Americas to:** Elsevier Science, PO Box 945, New York, NY 10159-0945. TEL 212-633-3730, 888-437-4636, FAX 212-633-3680, usinfo-f@elsevier.com, http://www.elsevier.com. **Dist. by:** Elsevier Science (Brazil).; Elsevier Science BV, PO Box 211, Amsterdam 1000 AE, Netherlands. TEL 31-20-485-3757, FAX 31-20-485-3432.

016.571959 USA ISSN 0093-3295
RA1270.P4
PESTICIDES ABSTRACTS. Text in English. m. USD 21. index. reprint service avail. from PQC.
Continues: Health Aspects of Pesticides: Abstract Bulletin
Related titles: Microform ed.: (from PQC,MIM).
Indexed: Rev.Appl.Entomol., Weed Abstr.
—CISTI, GNLM, Linda Hall.
Published by: U.S. Environmental Protection Agency, Office of Pesticides and Toxic Substances, Washington, DC 20460. TEL 919-655-4000. **Subscr. to:** Supt. of Documents, Govt Printing Office, Washington, DC 20402.

016.3637 PER ISSN 0252-7987
REPINDEX. Text in English, Spanish; Abstracts in Spanish. 1982. 3/yr. USD 120 (effective 1999). bibl. **Document type:** *Abstract/Index.* **Description:** Reproduces some full-text documents and indexes others in the fields of sanitation engineering and environmental sciences.
Related titles: Online - full text ed.: ISSN 1564-0884.
Published by: Organizacion Panamericana de la Salud, Centro Panamericano de Ingenieria Sanitaria y Ciencias del Ambiente, Los Pinos 259, Urb. Camacho, Casilla Postal 4337, Lima 100, Peru. TEL 511-4371077, FAX 511-4378289, cepis@cepis.ops-oms.org, http://www.cepis.ops-oms.org.

016.6284 USA ISSN 0824-3336
HD61
RISK ABSTRACTS. Text in English. 1984. q. USD 445 for print & online combined (effective 2001). bk.rev. abstr, bibl, illus. index. back issues avail.; reprints avail. **Document type:** *Abstract/Index.* **Description:** Covers risk from industrial, technological, environmental, medical and other sources, with emphasis on risk assessment and management.
Related titles: Online - full text ed.: USD 355 (effective 2002) (from CSA).
Indexed: Russ.Acad.Sci.Bibl.
Published by: (Institute for Risk Research CAN, University of Waterloo CAN), Cambridge Scientific Abstracts, 7200 Wisconsin Ave., Suite 601, Bethesda, MD 20814. TEL 301-961-6798, FAX 301-961-6799, journals@csa.com, http://www.csa.com/journals. Ed. Craig Emerson. Pub. Ted Caris.

016.6131 USA ISSN 1087-1411
CODEN: THENFI
TECHNICAL LITERATURE ABSTRACTS: HEALTH & ENVIRONMENT. Text in English. w. USD 350. **Document type:** *Abstract/Index.* **Description:** Reports on air, water, and land pollution and the sources, effects and control of, measurement methods, pollution control catalysts; solid and liquid waste recovery, treatment and disposal, and related topics.
Former titles: Literature Abstracts: Health and Environment (1065-0490); (until 1991): A P I Abstracts - Health and Environment
Related titles: Online - full text ed.: A P I EnCompass: Environment (from The Dialog Corporation, Questel Orbit Inc., S T N International).
Published by: Elsevier Engineering Information, Inc., A P I EnCompass, 1 Castle Point Ter, Hoboken, NJ 07030-5906. TEL 212-366-4040, FAX 212-366-4298, info@apiencompass.org, http://www.apiencompass.org.

016.6159 USA ISSN 0140-5365
RA1190
TOXICOLOGY ABSTRACTS. Text in English. 1978. m. USD 1,285 for print & online combined (effective 2002). adv. bk.rev. abstr. index. back issues avail. **Document type:** *Abstract/Index.* **Description:** Covers all aspects of toxicology including substance abuse, radiation, and toxicity testing.
Related titles: Online - full text ed.: USD 965 (effective 2002) (from The Dialog Corporation, S T N International, CSA).
Published by: Cambridge Scientific Abstracts, 7200 Wisconsin Ave., Suite 601, Bethesda, MD 20814. TEL 301-961-6798, FAX 301-961-6799, journals@csa.com, http://www.csa.com/journals. Ed. Roberta Gardner. Pub. Ted Caris.

ENVIRONMENTAL STUDIES—Pollution

ADVANCES IN NOISE RESEARCH. see *MEDICAL SCIENCES—Otorhinolaryngology*

363.7384 USA ISSN 1068-2643
ASBESTOS & LEAD ABATEMENT REPORT; inspection - analysis - removal - maintenance - alternatives. Text in English. 1987. m. USD 357; USD 365 out of North America (effective 2000). **Document type:** *Newsletter.* **Description:** Covers areas of control techniques, worksite health and safety, new federal standards, medical research efforts, state and local regulations, waste disposal, insurance, documentation, financing, contract management, analysis technology, and certification rules.
Incorporates (1988-1997): Indoor Pollution News (0896-8594); Former titles (until 1993): Asbestos Abatement Report (0893-858X); (until 1991): Asbestos Control Report (0893-4533)
Related titles: Online - full text ed.: (from Gale Group, Northern Light Technology, Inc., Factiva).
—**CCC.**
Published by: Business Publishers, Inc., 8737 Colesville Rd, 11th Fl, Silver Spring, MD 20910-3928. TEL 301-587-6300, 800-274-6737, FAX 301-589-8493, bpinews@bpinews.com, http://www.bpinews.com. Ed. Bill Pritchard. Pub. Leonard A Eiserer.

628.53 GBR ISSN 1352-2310
TD881 CODEN: AENVEQ
ATMOSPHERIC ENVIRONMENT. Text in English, French, German. 1967. 36/yr. EUR 346 in Europe to qualified personnel; JPY 45,900 in Japan to qualified personnel; USD 387 elsewhere to qualified personnel; EUR 4,191 in Europe to institutions; JPY 556,600 in Japan to institutions; USD 4,688 elsewhere to institutions (effective 2002). adv. bk.rev. charts, illus. index. Supplement avail.; back issues avail. *Refereed.* **Document type:** *Academic/Scholarly.* **Description:** Covers all subjects related to the atmosphere and human interactions with it.
Formed by the 1993 merger of: Atmospheric Environment. Part A, General Topics (0960-1686); Atmospheric Environment. Part B, Urban Atmosphere (0957-1272); Each of which superseded in part (in 1990): Atmospheric Environment (0004-6981)
Related titles: CD-ROM ed.; Microfiche ed.: (from MIM); Microfilm ed.: (from PQC); Online - full text ed.: (from ingenta, Swets Blackwell, ScienceDirect, Institute for Scientific Information).
Indexed: AESIS, API Abstr., API Catal., API Hlth.& Environ., API Oil., API Pet.Ref., API Pet.Subst., API Transport., A.S.& T.Ind. (Jan.1990-Dec.1993), ASCA, Abstr.Hyg., Acid Pre.Dig., Agri.Eng.Abstr., Anal.Abstr., Appl.Mech.Rev., Aqua.Sci.& Fish.Abstr., Bioeng.Abstr., Biol.& Agr.Ind. (coverage dropped), Biol.Abstr., CAD CAM Abstr., CEABA, C.I.S. Abstr., Cadscan, Chem.Abstr., Chem.Cit.Ind., Chem.Eng.Abstr., Chem.Indus.Notes, Chem.Titles, Crop Physiol.Abstr., Curr.Cont., Curr.Ind.Stat., Deep Sea Res.& Oceanogr.Abstr., Ecol.Abstr., Electron.& Communic.Abstr.J., Energy Info.Abstr., Energy Rev., Eng.Ind., Environ.Abstr., Environ.Ind., Environ.Per.Bibl. (1972-), Environ.Sci.Poll.Mgmt., Excerp.Med., Field Crop Abstr., Fluidex, Forest Prod.Abstr., Forest.Abstr., Fuel & Energy Abstr., Geo.Abstr.H.G., Geo.Abstr.P.G., Geol.Abstr., Geomech.Abstr., Herb.Abstr., Hort.Abstr., IDA, INIS Atomind., INSPEC (Jan.1972-1992, dropped), ISMEC, Ind.Med. (coverage dropped), Ind.Sci.Rev., Int.Abstr.Biol.Sci., Intl.Civil Eng.Abstr., Lead Abstr., Mass Spectr.Bull., Meteor.& Geoastrophys.Abstr., Ocean.Abstr., Ornam.Hort., Pig News & Info., Pollut.Abstr., Repindex, Rev.Appl.Entomol., Rev.Med.& Vet.Mycol., Rev.Plant Path., Risk Abstr., SSCI (coverage dropped), Saf.Sci.Abstr., Sci.Cit.Ind., Sel.Water Res.Abstr., Soft.Abstr.Eng., Soils & Fert., Solid St.Abstr., T.C.E.A., Triticale Abstr., W.R.C.Inf., WasteInfo, Weed Abstr., Zincscan.
—BLDSC (1767.120000), CASDDS, CINDOC, CISTI, Ei, EMDOCS, GNLM, IDS, Infotrieve, ingenta, Linda Hall. **CCC.**

E

Published by: Pergamon (Subsidiary of: Elsevier Science), The Boulevard, Langford Ln, East Park, Kidlington, Oxford OXB 1GB, United Kingdom. FAX 44-1865-843010, nlinfo-f@elsevier/nl; usinfo-f@elsevier.com; forinfo-kyf04035@niftyserve.or.jp, http://www.elsevier.com/locate/atmosenv, http://www.elsevier.nl:80/inca/publications/store/2/4/6/. Eds. M Benarie, P Brimblecombe. Circ: 2,600. **Subscr. in Australasia and the Far East to:** Elsevier Science (Singapore) Pte Ltd, No.1 Temasek Ave, 17-01 Millenia Tower, Singapore 039192, Singapore. TEL 65-434-3727, FAX 65-337-2230**; Subscr. in the Americas to:** Elsevier Science, PO Box 945, New York, NY 10159-0945. TEL 212-633-3730, FAX 212-633-3680, usinfo-f@elsevier.com**; Subscr. to:** Elsevier Science BV, PO Box 211, Amsterdam 1000 AE, Netherlands. TEL 31-20-485-3757, nlinfo-f@elsevier.nl.

C A SELECTS. INDOOR AIR POLLUTION. see *ENVIRONMENTAL STUDIES—Abstracting, Bibliographies, Statistics*

CHEMECOLOGY; covering health, safety and the environment. see *ENVIRONMENTAL STUDIES*

E H & S PRODUCTS. (Environmental, Health & Safety) see *OCCUPATIONAL HEALTH AND SAFETY*

EXCERPTA MEDICA. SECTION 46: ENVIRONMENTAL HEALTH AND POLLUTION CONTROL. see *ENVIRONMENTAL STUDIES—Abstracting, Bibliographies, Statistics*

HAZARDOUS SUBSTANCES & PUBLIC HEALTH. see *PUBLIC HEALTH AND SAFETY*

363.7392 GBR
HEALTH EFFECTS OF OZONE AND NITROGEN OXIDES IN AN INTEGRATED ASSESSMENT OF AIR POLLUTION. Text in English. 1997. irreg. **Document type:** *Monographic series, Academic/Scholarly.* **Description:** Summarizes the proceedings of a workshop on the health effects of ozone and nitrogen oxide, particularly in relation to long-range transboundary are pollution.
Published by: Institute for Environment and Health, University of Leicester, 94 Regent Rd, Leicester, Leics LE1 7DD, United Kingdom. TEL 44-116-223-1600, FAX 44-116-223-1601, msto1@le.ac.uk, http://www.le.ac.uk/ieh/. R&P Ruth Gardener.

628.53 363.1791 614.4 GBR
I E H ASSESSMENT INDOOR AIR QUALITY IN THE HOME: CARBON MONOXIDE. Text in English. 1998. irreg. GBP 25 (effective 2000). **Document type:** *Monographic series, Academic/Scholarly.* **Description:** Evaluates the risks to health and well-being of exposure to carbon monoxide in homes. It reviews carbon monoxide levels in the home and the health effects caused by carbon monoxide, including a discussion of susceptible groups.
Published by: Institute for Environment and Health, University of Leicester, 94 Regent Rd, Leicester, Leics LE1 7DD, United Kingdom. TEL 44-116-223-1600, FAX 44-116-223-1601, msto1@le.ac.uk, http://www.le.ac.uk/ieh/. R&P Ruth Gardener.

571.95 GBR
▼ **I E H ASSESSMENT ON THE ECOLOGICAL SIGNIFICANCE OF ENDOCRINE DISRUPTION.** Text in English. 1999. irreg. GBP 20 (effective 2000). **Document type:** *Monographic series, Academic/Scholarly.* **Description:** Evaluates the evidence from around the world that environmental chemicals may be causing endocrine disruption in wildlife.
Published by: Institute for Environment and Health, University of Leicester, 94 Regent Rd, Leicester, Leics LE1 7DD, United Kingdom. TEL 44-116-223-1600, FAX 44-116-223-1601, msto1@le.ac.uk, http://www.le.ac.uk/ieh/. R&P Ruth Gardener.

304.28 GBR
I E H REPORT ON HEALTH EFFECTS OF WASTE COMBUSTION PRODUCTS. Text in English. 1997. irreg. GBP 15 (effective 2000). **Document type:** *Monographic series, Academic/Scholarly.* **Description:** Reviews the health effects of ten pollutants produced during the combustion of chemical, clinical, municipal and sewage waste. The substances are cadmium, mercury, arsenic, chromium, nickel, dioxins, polycyclic aromatic hydrocarbons, polychlorinated biphenyls, particulate matter and sulphur dioxide. The report discusses the likelihood of adverse health effects in populations living near waste incinerators, based on toxicological evaluations and epidemiological studies and makes recommendations for further research required to improve risk assessment.
Published by: Institute for Environment and Health, University of Leicester, 94 Regent Rd, Leicester, Leics LE1 7DD, United Kingdom. TEL 44-116-223-1600, FAX 44-116-223-1601, msto1@le.ac.uk, http://www.le.ac.uk/ieh/. R&P Ruth Gardener.

304.28 GBR
I E H REPORT ON THE USE OF BIOMARKERS IN ENVIRONMENTAL EXPOSURE ASSESSMENT. Text in English. 1996. irreg. GBP 20 per issue (effective 2000). **Document type:** *Monographic series, Academic/Scholarly.* **Description:** Summarizes the outcome of an expert workshop held by IEH at the end of 1995 examining the use of biomarkers to measure human exposure to chemical pollutants in the environment. It includes six short papers on key topics related to the use of biomarkers.
Published by: Institute for Environment and Health, University of Leicester, 94 Regent Rd, Leicester, Leics LE1 7DD, United Kingdom. TEL 44-116-223-1600, 44-116-223-1600, msto1@le.ac.uk, http://www.le.ac.uk/ieh/. R&P Ruth Gardener.

628.53 690 USA
I E Q STRATEGIES; a guide to the practical control of indoor air problems. (Indoor Environmental Quality) Text in English. 1988. m. USD 297 domestic; USD 357 foreign (effective 2000). charts, illus. back issues avail. **Document type:** *Newsletter.* **Description:** Covers current research, case studies, trends, and news in the field of indoor air quality (IAQ). Includes resource reviews, information exchange, industry events, and feature articles.
Formerly (until 1998): Indoor Air Quality Update (1040-5313)
Related titles: Online - full text ed.
—CISTI.
Published by: Cutter Information Corp., 37 Broadway, Ste 1, Arlington, MA 02474. TEL 781-641-5718, FAX 781-648-1950, http://www.cutter.com. Ed. John Lempesis.

363.7382 GBR
I M O - U N E P GUIDELINES ON OIL SPILL DISPERSENT APPLICATION; including environmental considerations. Text in English. 1982. irreg., latest vol.2, 1995.
Published by: International Maritime Organization/ Organisation Maritime Internationale, 4 Albert Embankment, London SE1 7SR, United Kingdom. **Co-sponsor:** United Nations Environment Programme.

JOURNAL OF ECOTOXICOLOGY & ENVIRONMENTAL MONITORING; an international journal for scientific research on toxicology and pollution. see *ENVIRONMENTAL STUDIES—Toxicology And Environmental Safety*

363.7384 USA ISSN 0893-357X
SB950.2.A1
JOURNAL OF PESTICIDE REFORM. Text in English. 1979. q. USD 15 domestic to individuals; USD 25 foreign to individuals; USD 25 to institutions (effective 1999). bk.rev., video rev. charts, illus. back issues avail.; reprints avail. **Document type:** *Newsletter, Academic/Scholarly.* **Description:** Comprehensive publication covering citizen reform actions, legal issues, research results, progressive pesticide legislation, alternatives to pesticide use, and documented cases of successful sustainable pest management.
Formerly (until 1985): N C A P News
Indexed: Agri.Eng.Abstr., Agricola, Bibl.Agri., Bio-Contr.News & Info., Environ.Per.Bibl. (1989-), Forest Prod.Abstr., Forest.Abstr., Helminthol.Abstr., Hort.Abstr., Ornam.Hort., Rev.Appl.Entomol., Rev.Med.& Vet.Mycol., Rev.Plant Path., Soils & Fert., Weed Abstr.
—BLDSC (5030.975000), CISTI, ingenta.
Published by: Northwest Coalition for Alternatives to Pesticides, PO Box 1393, Eugene, OR 97440-1393. TEL 541-344-5044, FAX 541-344-6923, info@pesticide.org, http://www.pesticide.org, http://www.efn.org/~ncap. Ed. Caroline Cox. R&P Pollyanna Lind. Circ: 2,000 (paid).

628.168 GBR ISSN 0141-1136
QH545.W3 CODEN: MERSDW
MARINE ENVIRONMENTAL RESEARCH. Text in English. 1978. 10/yr. EUR 1,139 in Europe to institutions; JPY 151,200 in Japan to institutions; USD 1,274 elsewhere to institutions (effective 2002). adv. bk.rev. illus. index. back issues avail.; reprints avail. *Refereed.* **Document type:** *Academic/Scholarly.* **Description:** Provides research papers on chemical, physical and biological interactions in the oceans and coastal waters. Serves as a forum for new information on biology, chemistry and toxicology.
Incorporates (in 1991): Oil and Chemical Pollution (0269-8579); Which was formerly (until 1982): Journal of Oil and Petrochemical Pollution (0143-7127)
Related titles: Microform ed.: (from PQC); Online - full text ed.: (from ingenta, ScienceDirect, Swets Blackwell, Institute for Scientific Information).
Indexed: API Abstr., API Catal., API Hlth.& Environ., API Oil., API Pet.Ref., API Pet.Subst., API Transport., ASCA, Anim.Breed.Abstr., Appl.Ecol.Abstr. (coverage dropped), Aqua.Sci.& Fish.Abstr., Aquacult.Abstr., Biol.Abstr., Cadscan, Chem.Abstr., Chem.Titles, Curr.Adv.Ecol.Sci., Curr.Cont., Curr.Ref.Fish Res., Deep Sea Res.& Oceanogr.Abstr., E & P Hlth. (1993-), Ecol.Abstr., Energy Ind., Energy Info.Abstr., Energy Rev., Eng.Ind., Environ.Abstr., Environ.Per.Bibl. (1985-), Environ.Sci.Poll.Mgmt., Excerp.Med., Food Sci.& Tech.Abstr., Forest Prod.Abstr., Gas Process.& Ppl. (1993-), Geo.Abstr.H.G., GeoRef, Geol.Abstr., Herb.Abstr., INIS Atomind., Ind.Med. (1978-), Ind.Sci.Rev., Ind.Vet., Irr.& Drain.Abstr., Lead Abstr., Mar.Sci.Cont.Tab., Mass Spectr.Bull., Microbiol.Abstr., Nutr.Abstr., Ocean.Abstr., Off.Tech. (1993-), Petrol.Abstr. (1981-), Pollut.Abstr., Rev.Appl.Entomol., Risk Abstr., Sci.Cit.Ind., Sel.Water Res.Abstr., Soils & Fert., Sport Fish.Abstr., Tox.Abstr., Vet.Bull., W.R.C.Inf., Weed Abstr., Zincscan, Zoo.Rec.
—BLDSC (5375.270000), CASDDS, CISTI, Ei, IDS, Infotrieve, ingenta, Linda Hall, PADDS. **CCC.**
Published by: Pergamon (Subsidiary of: Elsevier Science), The Boulevard, Langford Ln, East Park, Kidlington, Oxford OXB 1GB, United Kingdom. FAX 44-1865-843010, nlinfo-f@elsevier.nl; usinfo-f@elsevier.com; forinfo-kyf04035@niftyserve.or.jp, nlinfo-f@elsevier/nl; usinfo-f@elsevier.com; forinfo-kyf04035@niftyserve.or.jp, http://www.elsevier.nl/locate/marenvrev. Eds. G Roesijadi, R B Spies. **Subscr. in Australasia and the Far East to:** Elsevier Science (Singapore) Pte Ltd, No.1 Temasek Ave, 17-01 Millenia Tower, Singapore 039192, Singapore. TEL 65-434-3727, FAX 65-337-2230**; Subscr. in the Americas to:** Elsevier Science, PO Box 945, New York, NY 10159-0945. TEL 212-633-3730, FAX 212-633-3680, usinfo-f@elsevier.com**; Subscr. to:** Elsevier Science BV, PO Box 211, Amsterdam 1000 AE, Netherlands. TEL 31-20-485-3757, FAX 31-20-485-3432, nlinfo-f@elsevier.nl.

NOISE & HEALTH; an inter-disciplinary journal. see *MEDICAL SCIENCES—Otorhinolaryngology*

NONSMOKERS' VOICE. see *TOBACCO*

PESTICIDES ABSTRACTS. see *ENVIRONMENTAL STUDIES—Abstracting, Bibliographies, Statistics*

THE SCIENCE OF THE TOTAL ENVIRONMENT; an international journal for scientific research into the environment and its relationship with man. see *ENVIRONMENTAL STUDIES*

ENVIRONMENTAL STUDIES—Toxicology And Environmental Safety

571.95 AUS
A S E NEWSLETTER. Text in English. 1995. q.?. AUD 60 (effective 2001). 30 p./no. **Document type:** *Newsletter.* **Description:** Reports on issues of interest to ASE membership.
Published by: Australian Society for Ecotoxicology, Centre for Ecotoxicology, c/o University of Technology Sydney, Westbourne St, Gore Hill, NSW 2065, Australia. TEL 61-2-6250-7559, FAX 61-2-6250-7554, grippon@ea.gov.au, http://www.bio.uts.edu.au/ase. Ed. Greg Rippon. Adv. contact Russ Hyne TEL 61-2-9514-4138.

E

ABSTRACTS OF CURRENT LITERATURE IN TOXICOLOGY. see *ENVIRONMENTAL STUDIES—Abstracting, Bibliographies, Statistics*

615.9 ITA ISSN 0393-635X
CODEN: ATTHEH
ACTA TOXICOLOGICA ET THERAPEUTICA; international journal of toxicology, pharmacology and therapy. Text in English; Summaries in Italian. 1980. q. ITL 80,000; ITL 160,000 foreign (effective 1998). index.
Indexed: Chem.Abstr., Chem.Indus.Notes, Chem.Titles, Excerp.Med.
—BLDSC (0665.600000), CASDDS, EMDOCS, GNLM, KNAW.
Published by: Casa Editrice Maccari, Via Palermo, 44, Parma, PR 43100, Italy. TEL 39-521-771268. Ed. M Esposito. Circ: 1,200.

615.9 USA ISSN 0899-7195
RA1247.C65
ADVANCES IN COMBUSTION TOXICOLOGY. Text in English. 1988. irreg. price varies. **Document type:** *Monographic series, Academic/Scholarly.* **Description:** Scientific reports on toxicology from fires.
—CISTI.
Published by: C R C Press, LLC, 2000 Corporate Blvd, N W, Boca Raton, FL 33431. TEL 800-272-7737, FAX 800-374-3401, orders@crcpress.com, http://www.crcpress.com. Ed. Gordon E Hartzell.

ADVERSE DRUG REACTIONS AND TOXICOLOGICAL REVIEWS. see *PHARMACY AND PHARMACOLOGY*

571.95 351 USA
AGENT ORANGE REVIEW; for veterans who served in Vietnam. Text in English. 1982. irreg. (approx. 1-2/yr.). free per issue. **Document type:** *Newsletter, Government.* **Description:** Provides information on Agent Orange exposure, examination, compensation, and other related matters including legislation for Vietnam veterans, families, and others concerned about the effects of herbicides used in Vietnam.
Related titles: Online - full content ed.
Published by: U.S. Department of Veterans Affairs, Environmental Agents Service - 131, V A Headquarters, 810 Vermont Ave, N W, Washington, DC 20420. TEL 202-273-8580, 202-273-8580. Ed. Donald J Rosenblum. Circ: (controlled).

AGRICULTURAL AND BIOLOGICAL RESEARCH. see *AGRICULTURE*

ALTLASTEN - SPEKTRUM; Erfassung - Bewertung - Sanierung. see *ENVIRONMENTAL STUDIES—Waste Management*

571.95 DEU ISSN 0179-7247
RA1229.4 CODEN: AHSMEB
ANALYSES OF HAZARDOUS SUBSTANCES IN BIOLOGICAL MATERIALS. Text in English. 1985. irreg. **Document type:** *Monographic series, Academic/Scholarly.*
Indexed: Chem.Abstr., Chem.Indus.Notes, Chem.Titles.
—BLDSC (0890.967000), CASDDS, CISTI, Infotrieve. **CCC.**
Published by: Wiley - V C H, Postfach 101161, Weinheim 69451, Germany. TEL 49-6201-606-0, FAX 49-6201-606-328, subservice@wiley-vch.de, http://www.wiley-vch.de. **Subscr. in N. America to:** John Wiley & Sons, Inc., Journals, 605 Third Ave, New York, NY 10158. TEL 44-1243-779777, 212-850-6645, FAX 212-850-6021; **Subscr. outside Germany, Austria & Switzerland to:** John Wiley & Sons Ltd., Baffins Ln, Chichester, Sussex PO19 IUD, United Kingdom. TEL 44-1243-779777, FAX 44-1243-843232.

363.7 USA
ANDERSON'S OHIO E P A ON CD-ROM. Text in English. irreg. **Document type:** *Trade.* **Description:** provides easy access to Ohio Revised Code statutes and Ohio Administrative Code Compiles regulations relating to the Ohio EPA and to the Ohio Fire Marshal?s oversight of underground storage tanks, as well as the Low Level Radioactive Waste Development Authority regulations. Includes annotations of federal, state, Environmental Review Appeals Commission decisions, Ohio Attorney General opinions, and cross-references to related statutory and regulatory provisions.
Media: CD-ROM.
Published by: (Ohio Environmental Protection Agency), Anderson Publishing Co, 2035 Reading Rd, Cincinnati, OH 45202. TEL 513-421-4142, 800-582-7295, FAX 513-562-8116, mail@andersonpublishing.com, http://www.andersonpublishing.com/pubcats/legalsoft/2.shtml.

615.9 FRA ISSN 0242-6110
TX501 CODEN: AFETDF
ANNALES DES FALSIFICATIONS DE L'EXPERTISE CHIMIQUE ET TOXICOLOGIQUE. Text in French. 1907. q. FRF 647; FRF 810 foreign (effective 1998). adv. **Document type:** *Academic/Scholarly.*
Supersedes (in 1979): Annales des Falsifications et de l'Expertise Chimique (0003-4274); Annales des Falsifications et des Fraudes
Indexed: Biol.Abstr., Chem.Abstr., Chem.Indus.Notes, Chem.Titles, Dairy Sci.Abstr., Food Sci.& Tech.Abstr., GeoRef, INIS Atomind., Nutr.Abstr., Packag.Sci.Tech., Sugar Ind.Abstr.
—BLDSC (0972.980000), CASDDS, CISTI, Linda Hall.
Published by: Librairie Lavoisier, 11 rue Lavoisier, Paris Cedex 8 75384, France. group@lavoisier.fr, http://www.lavoisier.fr. Circ: 2,000. **Subscr. to:** Lavoisier Abonnements, 14 rue de Provigny, Cachan Cedex 94236, France. TEL 33-1-47406700, FAX 33-1-47406703.

363.7 USA ISSN 0277-3287
TN880.5
ANNUAL REPORT ON PIPELINE SAFETY. Text in English. a. **Document type:** *Government.*
Published by: U.S. Department of Transportation, Research & Special Programs Administration, 400 Seventh St, S W, Rm 8410, Washington, DC 20590. TEL 202-366-4000.

ANNUAL REVIEW OF PHARMACOLOGY AND TOXICOLOGY. see *PHARMACY AND PHARMACOLOGY*

615.9 NLD ISSN 0166-445X
QH545.W3 CODEN: AQTODG
AQUATIC TOXICOLOGY. Text in English. 1981. 20/yr. EUR 1,516 in Europe to institutions; JPY 201,500 in Japan to institutions; USD 1,696 elsewhere to institutions (effective 2002). adv. charts, illus, stat, abstr. index. back issues avail.; reprint service avail. from SWZ. *Refereed.* **Document type:** *Academic/Scholarly.* **Description:** Provides information for environmental toxicologists, ecotoxicologists, marine biologists, biochemical toxicologists, environmental monitoring researchers, and conservationists.
Related titles: Online - full text ed.: (from ingenta, Swets Blackwell, ScienceDirect, Institute for Scientific Information).
Indexed: ASCA, Agricola, Anim.Breed.Abstr., Aqua.Sci.& Fish.Abstr., Biol.Abstr., Chem.Abstr., Curr.Adv.Ecol.Sci., Curr.Cont., Derwent Biotech.Abstr., Ecol.Abstr., Energy Ind., Energy Info.Abstr., Environ.Sci.Poll.Mgmt., Excerp.Med., Food Sci.& Tech.Abstr., INIS Atomind., Ind.Med., Int.Abstr.Biol.Sci., METADEX, Mar.Sci.Cont.Tab., Nutr.Abstr., Ocean.Abstr., Pollut.Abstr., Ref.Zh., Rev.Appl.Entomol., Sci.Cit.Ind., Sel.Water Res.Abstr., Sport Fish.Abstr., Tox.Abstr., W.R.C.Inf., Wild.Rev., Zoo.Rec.
—BLDSC (1582.480000), CASDDS, CISTI, EMDOCS, GNLM, IDS, Infotrieve, ingenta, Linda Hall. **CCC.**
Published by: Elsevier Science BV, PO Box 211, Amsterdam 1000 AE, Netherlands. TEL 31-20-485-2911, FAX 31-20-485-2457, nlinfo-f@elsevier.nl, http://www.elsevier.com/locate/aquatox, http://www.elsevier.nl. Ed. D E Hinton. **Subscr. in Australasia and the Far East to:** Elsevier Science (Singapore) Pte Ltd, No.1 Temasek Ave, 17-01 Millenia Tower, Singapore 039192, Singapore. TEL 65-434-3727, FAX 65-337-2230; **Subscr. in Japan to:** Elsevier Science Inc - Japan Regional Office, 9-15 Higashi-Azabu 1-chome, Minato-ku, Tokyo 106-0044, Japan. TEL 81-3-5561-5033, FAX 81-3-5561-5047; **Subscr. in the Americas to:** Elsevier Science, PO Box 945, New York, NY 10159-0945. TEL 212-633-3730, FAX 212-633-3680, usinfo-f@elsevier.com, http://www.elsevier.com.

615.902 USA ISSN 0090-4341
QH545.P4 CODEN: AECTCV
ARCHIVES OF ENVIRONMENTAL CONTAMINATION AND TOXICOLOGY. Text in English. 1972. 8/yr. (in 2 vols., 4 nos./vol.). USD 933.80 for Print & Online Eds.; USD 898.20 in Germany for Print & Online Eds.; USD 129 newsstand/cover (effective 2002). adv. charts. reprint service avail. from ISI. *Refereed.* **Document type:** *Academic/Scholarly.* **Description:** Contains detailed reports of important advances and discoveries in the fields of air, water, and soil contamination and pollution.
Related titles: Microform ed.: (from PQC); Online - full text ed.: ISSN 1432-0703 (from EBSCO Publishing, RoweCom Information Quest, Swets Blackwell, Springer LINK, Institute for Scientific Information).
Indexed: AESIS, ASCA, Abstr.Hyg., Acid Pre.Dig., Agri.& Environ.Biotech.Abstr. (coverage dropped), Agri.Eng.Abstr., Agricola, Anal.Abstr., Appl.Ecol.Abstr., Aqua.Sci.& Fish.Abstr., Bio-Contr.News & Info., Biodet.Abstr., Biol.& Agr.Ind. (Jan.1996-), Cadscan, Chem.Abstr., Chem.Cit.Ind., Chem.Indus.Notes, Chem.Titles, Crop Physiol.Abstr., Curr.Adv.Ecol.Sci., Curr.Cont., Dairy Sci.Abstr., Deep Sea Res.& Oceanogr.Abstr., Derwent Biotech.Abstr., Dok.Arbeitsmed., Ecol.Abstr., Eng.Ind., Entomol.Abstr. (coverage dropped), Environ.Abstr., Environ.Ind., Environ.Per.Bibl. (1991-), Environ.Sci.Poll.Mgmt., Excerp.Med., Field Crop Abstr., Food Sci.& Tech.Abstr., Forest Prod.Abstr., Forest.Abstr., Geo.Abstr.P.G., GeoRef, Geol.Abstr., Herb.Abstr., Hort.Abstr., Ind.Med. (1973-), Ind.Sci.Rev., Ind.Vet., Inpharma, Int.Abstr.Biol.Sci., Irr.& Drain.Abstr., Key Word Ind.Wildl.Res., Lab.Haz.Bull., Lead Abstr., Maize Abstr., Mass Spectr.Bull., Microbiol.Abstr., NRN, Nutr.Abstr., Ocean.Abstr., Pollut.Abstr., Poult.Abstr., Reac., Rev.Appl.Entomol., Rev.Med.& Vet.Mycol., Rev.Plant Path., Risk Abstr., Saf.Sci.Abstr., Sci.Cit.Ind., Seed Abstr., Sel.Water Res.Abstr., Soils & Fert., Soyabean Abstr., Sport Fish.Abstr., Tox.Abstr., Triticale Abstr., Vet.Bull., W.R.C.Inf., Weed Abstr., Wild.Rev., Zincscan, Zoo.Rec.
—BLDSC (1634.240000), CASDDS, CIS, CISTI, Ei, EMDOCS, GNLM, IDS, ingenta, Linda Hall. **CCC.**
Published by: Springer-Verlag, Journals (Subsidiary of: BertelsmannSpringer), 175 Fifth Ave, New York, NY 10010. TEL 212-460-1500, FAX 212-473-6272, orders@springer-ny.com; helpdesk@link.springer.de, http://www.springer-ny.com. Ed. H M Bolt. R&P Ian Gross. Adv. contact Brian Skepton. **N. American subscr. to:** Journal Fulfillment Services, PO Box 2485, Secaucus, NJ 07096-2485. TEL 800-777-4643, FAX 201-348-4505.

571.95 DEU ISSN 0340-5761
CODEN: ARTODN
ARCHIVES OF TOXICOLOGY. Text in English. 1930. m. EUR 1,621.10 domestic; EUR 1,610.70 in Germany; EUR 159 newsstand/cover foreign (effective 2002). adv. bibl, charts, illus. back issues avail.; reprint service avail. from ISI. *Refereed.* **Document type:** *Journal, Academic/Scholarly.* **Description:** Provides up-to-date information on the latest advances in toxicology, including toxic activities at the molecular level in humans and experimental animals.
Former titles: Archiv fuer Toxikologie (0003-9446); Fuehner-Wieland's Sammlung von Vergiftungsfaellen
Related titles: Microform ed.: (from PQC); Online - full text ed.: ISSN 1432-0738 (from EBSCO Publishing, RoweCom Information Quest, Swets Blackwell, Springer LINK, Institute for Scientific Information).
Indexed: ASCA, Agri.& Environ.Biotech.Abstr. (coverage dropped), Aqua.Sci.& Fish.Abstr., Biol.Abstr., C.I.S. Abstr., Chem.Abstr., Chem.Indus.Notes, Chem.Titles, Curr.Adv.Ecol.Sci., Curr.Cont., Dairy Sci.Abstr., Dent.Ind., Derwent Biotech.Abstr., Dok.Arbeitsmed., Environ.Abstr., Environ.Sci.Poll.Mgmt., Excerp.Med., Forest Prod.Abstr., Helminthol.Abstr., INIS Atomind., Ind.Med. (1974-), Ind.Sci.Rev., Ind.Vet., Inpharma, Int.Abstr.Biol.Sci., Lab.Haz.Bull., Mass Spectr.Bull., NRN, Neurosci.Abstr. (coverage dropped), Neurosci.Cit.Ind., Nutr.Abstr., Pharm.&Out.News, Pollut.Abstr., Protozool.Abstr., Reac., Rev.Appl.Entomol., Rev.Med.& Vet.Mycol., Rev.Plant Path., Risk Abstr., Saf.Sci.Abstr., Sci.Cit.Ind., Sport Fish.Abstr., Tox.Abstr., Vet.Bull., Weed Abstr., Wild.Rev., Zoo.Rec.
—BLDSC (1643.510000), ADONIS, CASDDS, CISTI, EMDOCS, GNLM, IDS, Infotrieve, ingenta. **CCC.**
Published by: (Deutsche Gesellschaft fuer experimentelle und klinische Pharmakologie und Toxikologie), Springer-Verlag (Subsidiary of: BertelsmannSpringer), Tiergartenstr 17, Heidelberg 69121, Germany. TEL 49-6221-345-0, FAX 49-6221-345229, subscriptions@springer.de; helpdesk@link.springer.de, http://link.springer.de/link/service/journals/00204/index.htm, http://www.springer.de. Eds. H M Bolt, P H Bach. **Subscr. in N. America to:** Springer-Verlag New York Inc., PO Box 2485, Secaucus, NJ 07096-2485. TEL 212-460-1500, FAX 212-473-6272. **Co-sponsor:** Deutsche Gesellschaft fuer Rechtsmedizin.

ARCHIVES OF TOXICOLOGY. SUPPLEMENT. see *PHARMACY AND PHARMACOLOGY*

E

615.9 HRV ISSN 0004-1254
RA1211 CODEN: AHRTAN
ARHIV ZA HIGIJENU RADA I TOKSIKOLOGIJU/ ARCHIVES OF INDUSTRIAL HYGIENE AND TOXICOLOGY. Text in Croatian, English. 1950. q. HRK 250 domestic to individuals; HRK 75 domestic to institutions; USD 70 in Europe; USD 85 elsewhere. adv. bk.rev. abstr, bibl, charts, illus, stat. index. Supplement avail.; back issues avail. *Refereed.* **Document type:** *Academic/Scholarly.* **Description:** Covers occupational health, related epidemiological and laboratory research, toxicology, genotoxicology, environmental health, radiation protection, ergonomics, air pollution (indoor and outdoor), chemical agents in war, occupational and accidental exposure, monitoring, and more related topics.
Indexed: Biodet.Abstr., Biol.Abstr., C.I.S. Abstr., Chem.Abstr., Chem.Indus.Notes, Chem.Titles, Curr.Adv.Ecol.Sci., Dok.Arbeitsmed., Environ.Sci.Poll.Mgmt., Ergon.Abstr., Excerp.Med., INIS Atomind., Ind.Hyg.Dig., Ind.Med. (1956-), Int.Abstr.Biol.Sci., Pollut.Abstr., Risk Abstr., Saf.Sci.Abstr., Tox.Abstr.
—BLDSC (1666.200000), CASDDS, CISTI, EMDOCS, GNLM, KNAW.
Published by: Institut za Medicinska Istrazivanja i Medicinu Rada/Institute for Medical Research and Occupational Health, Ksaverska cesta 2, pp 291, Zagreb 10001, Croatia. TEL 385-1-4673188, FAX 385-1-4673303, arhiv@imi.hr, http://mimi.imi.hr/arhiv/oarhivu.html, http://mimi.imi.hr/arhiv/oarhivu.html; http://www.mimi.imi.hr/archiv/arhonline.html. Ed. Radovana Plestina. R&P, Adv. contact Dado Cakalo. Circ: 800 (paid); 200 (controlled). **Co-sponsor:** Ministry of Science and Technology.

AUSTRALASIAN COLLEGE OF NUTRITIONAL AND ENVIRONMENTAL MEDICINE. JOURNAL. see *MEDICAL SCIENCES*

571.95 AUS ISSN 1323-3475
AUSTRALASIAN JOURNAL OF ECOTOXICOLOGY. Text in English. 1995. s-a. AUD 100 (effective 2001). bk.rev. illus, abstr, charts. 75 p./no. back issues avail. *Refereed.* **Document type:** *Academic/Scholarly.* **Description:** Publishes research and reviews in toxicology and environmental safety.
Indexed: Appl.Ecol.Abstr. (coverage dropped), Aquacult.Abstr., Sel.Water Res.Abstr.
—BLDSC (1794.930000).
Published by: Australian Society for Ecotoxicology, Centre for Ecotoxicology, c/o University of Technology Sydney, Westbourne St, Gore Hill, NSW 2065, Australia. TEL 61-2-9514-4151, FAX 61-2-6250-7554, http://www.bio.uts.edu.au/ase. Ed., R&P John C Chapman. Adv. contact Ms. Narelle Richardson TEL 61-2-9514-4071.

615.9 AUS ISSN 1035-0764
AUSTRALIAN TOXIC NETWORK NEWS. Text in English. 1986. q. AUD 25. *Refereed.* **Document type:** *Newsletter.* **Description:** Covers toxicity of chemicals, health issues, pollution and waste.
Published by: Toxic Chemical Committee, Total Environment Centre, 1-88 Cumberland St, Sydney, NSW 2000, Australia. TEL 61-2-92478476, FAX 61-2-92471178. Ed., R&P Barbara Macdonald. Circ: 250.

363 USA ISSN 1092-4736
B E L L E NEWSLETTER. (Biological Effects of Low Level Exposures) Text in English. 1992. irreg. (3-4/yr.). free per issue. **Document type:** *Consumer.*
—BLDSC (1890.349250).
Published by: Northeast Regional Environmental Public Health Center, University of Massachusetts, School of Public Health, Amherst, MA 01003. TEL 413-545-3164, FAX 413-545-4692, edwardc@schoolph.umass.edu, http://www.belleonline.com. Circ: 9,000.

615.9 CHE ISSN 0892-7014
QH91.8.M3 CODEN: BFOUEC
BIOFOULING; the journal of bioadhesion and biofilm research. Text in English. 1988. 4/yr. GBP 160, USD 193, EUR 212 to individuals; GBP 675, USD 900, EUR 900 to institutions; GBP 1,137, USD 1,474, EUR 1,517 to corporations (effective 2002). back issues avail. *Refereed.* **Document type:** *Journal, Academic/Scholarly.* **Description:** Provides a forum for publishing pure and applied work on microbial, plant or animal fouling and its control, as well as studies of all kinds on bioadhesion.
Related titles: CD-ROM ed.; Microform ed.; Online - full text ed.: (from EBSCO Publishing, RoweCom Information Quest, Institute for Scientific Information).
Indexed: ASCA, Aqua.Sci.& Fish.Abstr., Biodet.Abstr., Biotech.Cit.Ind., Curr.Cont. (coverage dropped), Ecol.Abstr., Environ.Per.Bibl. (1992-), Environ.Sci.Poll.Mgmt., Fluidex, Food Sci.& Tech.Abstr., Inpharma, Int.Abstr.Biol.Sci., METADEX, Microbiol.Abstr., Ocean.Abstr., Pollut.Abstr., Reac., Sel.Water Res.Abstr., World Surf.Coat., Zoo.Rec.
—BLDSC (2072.146500), CISTI, EMDOCS, Infotrieve. **CCC.**
Published by: Gordon and Breach - Harwood Academic (Subsidiary of: Taylor & Francis Group), PO Box 531, Lausanne 1000, Switzerland. TEL 41-21-6411280, FAX 41-21-6411281, info@gbhap.com, http://www.gbhap.com. Ed. Len Evans. **Subscr. addr. in US:** International Publishers Direct, PO Box 32160, Newark, NJ 07102. FAX 215-750-6343.

615.9 USA ISSN 0007-4861
RA565.A1 CODEN: BECTA6
BULLETIN OF ENVIRONMENTAL CONTAMINATION AND TOXICOLOGY. Text in English. 1966. m. (in 2 vols., 6 nos./vol.). USD 760 domestic for Print & Online Eds.; USD 747.30 in Germany for Print & Online Eds.; USD 69.30 newsstand/cover domestic (effective 2002). adv. back issues avail.; reprint service avail. from ISI. *Refereed.* **Document type:** *Academic/Scholarly.* **Description:** Disseminates advances and discoveries in the areas of soil, air, and food contamination and pollution.
Related titles: Microform ed.: (from PQC); Online - full text ed.: ISSN 1432-0800 (from EBSCO Publishing, RoweCom Information Quest, Swets Blackwell, Springer LINK, Institute for Scientific Information).
Indexed: AESIS, ASCA, Abstr.Bull.Inst.Pap.Chem., Acid Pre.Dig., Agri.& Environ.Biotech.Abstr. (coverage dropped), Agri.Eng.Abstr., Agricola, Agroforest.Abstr., Anal.Abstr., Anim.Breed.Abstr., Appl.Ecol.Abstr. (coverage dropped), Aqua.Sci.& Fish.Abstr., Aquacult.Abstr., Bibl.Agri., Bio-Contr.News & Info., Biodet.Abstr., Biol.& Agr.Ind. (Jan.1983-), Biol.Abstr., CSNB, Cadscan, Chem.Abstr., Chem.Indus.Notes, Chem.Titles, Crop Physiol.Abstr., Curr.Adv.Ecol.Sci., Curr.Cont., Curr.Ref.Fish Res., Dairy Sci.Abstr., Deep Sea Res.& Oceanogr.Abstr., Derwent Biotech.Abstr., Dok.Arbeitsmed., E & P Hlth. (1993-), Ecol.Abstr., Energy Rev., Eng.Ind., Environ.Abstr., Environ.Ind., Environ.Per.Bibl., Environ.Sci.Poll.Mgmt., Excerp.Med., Field Crop Abstr., Food Sci.& Tech.Abstr., Forest Prod.Abstr., Forest.Abstr., Gas Process.& Ppl. (1993-), Geo.Abstr.H.G., Geo.Abstr.P.G., GeoRef, Geol.Abstr., Helminthol.Abstr., Herb.Abstr., Hort.Abstr., IDA, INIS Atomind., Ind.Med. (1966-), Ind.Sci.Rev., Ind.Vet., Int.Abstr.Biol.Sci., Irr.& Drain.Abstr., Key Word Ind.Wildl.Res., Lab.Haz.Bull., Lead Abstr., Maize Abstr., Mass Spectr.Bull., Microbiol.Abstr., NRN, Nutr.Abstr., Ocean.Abstr., Off.Tech. (1993-), Ornam.Hort., Petrol.Abstr. (1981-, dropped), Pig News & Info., Pollut.Abstr., Postharvest, Poult.Abstr., Ref.Zh., Rev.Appl.Entomol., Rev.Arom.& Med.Plants, Rev.Med.& Vet.Mycol., Rev.Plant Path., Rice Abstr., Risk Abstr., SSCI (coverage dropped), Saf.Sci.Abstr., Sci.Cit.Ind., Seed Abstr., Sel.J.Water, Sel.Water Res.Abstr., Soils & Fert., Soyabean Abstr., Sport Fish.Abstr., Sugar Ind.Abstr., Tox.Abstr., Triticale Abstr., Trop.Dis.Bull., Vet.Bull., W.R.C.Inf., Weed Abstr., Wild.Rev., Zincscan, Zoo.Rec.
—BLDSC (2853.300000), CASDDS, CIS, CISTI, Ei, EMDOCS, GNLM, IDS, ingenta, Linda Hall, PADDS. **CCC.**
Published by: Springer-Verlag, Journals (Subsidiary of: BertelsmannSpringer), 175 Fifth Ave, New York, NY 10010. TEL 212-460-1500, FAX 212-473-6272, link@springer-ny.com, http://link.springer.de/link/service/journals/00128/index.htm. Ed. H N Nigg. R&P Ian Gross. Adv. contact Brian Skepton. **N. American subscr. to:** Journal Fulfillment Services, PO Box 2485, Secaucus, NJ 07096-2485. TEL 800-777-4643, FAX 201-348-4505.

615.902 USA ISSN 8755-4259
C I I T ACTIVITIES. Key Title: Activities - Chemical Industry Institute of Toxicology. Text in English. 1981. m. free per issue to qualified personnel. *Refereed.* **Document type:** *Newsletter.*
Indexed: CSNB.
—BLDSC (3198.237600).
Published by: Chemical Industry Institute of Toxicology, 6 Davis Dr, Box 12137, Durham, NC 27709. TEL 919-558-1200, FAX 919-558-1300, nellis@ciit.org, http://www.ciit.org. Ed. Dr. Barbara Kuyper. Circ: 8,000 (controlled).

363.7 USA
C R C P D NEWSBRIEF. Text in English. bi-m. USD 35 (effective 1999). adv. back issues avail. **Document type:** *Newsletter.* **Description:** Contains technical information on radiation control, CRCPD activities, and job announcements.
Related titles: E-mail ed.
Published by: Conference of Radiation Control Program Directors, 205 Capitol Ave, Frankfort, KY 40601-2832. TEL 502-227-4543, FAX 502-227-7862, chopkins@crcpd.org, Cariganlin@aol.com, http://www.crcpd.org. Ed., R&P Curt Hopkins TEL 502-227-4543. Circ: 800.

571.95 NLD ISSN 0742-2091
QH573 CODEN: CBTOE2
CELL BIOLOGY AND TOXICOLOGY; an international journal devoted to research at the cellular level. Text in Dutch. 1984. bi-m. USD 390 in the Americas to institutions for print or online ed.; EUR 390 elsewhere to institutions for print or online ed.; USD 468 in the Americas to institutions for print & online eds. combined; EUR 468 elsewhere to institutions for print & online eds. combined (effective 2002). adv. index. *Refereed.* **Document type:** *Journal, Academic/Scholarly.* **Description:** Provides a rapid publication outlet for papers of high scientific standards in the areas of cell biology, genetic, molecular and cellular toxicology.
Related titles: Online - full text ed.: (from EBSCO Publishing, O C L C Online Computer Library Center, Inc., RoweCom Information Quest, Swets Blackwell, Kluwer Online, Institute for Scientific Information).
Indexed: ASCA, Aqua.Sci.& Fish.Abstr., Biol.Abstr., Chem.Abstr., Chem.Indus.Notes, Chem.Titles, Curr.Cont., Environ.Sci.Poll.Mgmt., Excerp.Med., INIS Atomind., Ind.Med. (1984-), Ind.Sci.Rev., Ind.Vet., Inpharma, Int.Abstr.Biol.Sci., Pharm.&Out.News, Pollut.Abstr., Reac., Rev.Med.& Vet.Mycol., Sci.Cit.Ind., Tox.Abstr., Weed Abstr.
—BLDSC (3097.706000), CASDDS, CISTI, EMDOCS, GNLM, IDS, ingenta, KNAW. **CCC.**
Published by: Kluwer Academic Publishers Group (Subsidiary of: Wolters Kluwer N.V.), Spuiboulevard 50, PO Box 17, Dordrecht 3300 AA, Netherlands. TEL 31-78-639-2392, FAX 31-78-654-2254, services@wkap.nl, http://www.wkap.nl/journalhome.htm/0742-2091. Ed. Andre Guillouzo. Circ: 1,000. **Subscr. in the Americas to:** Kluwer Academic - Plenum Publishers, 233 Spring St, New York, NY 10013-1578. TEL 212-620-8468, FAX 212-807-1047; **Subscr. to:** Journals Department, PO Box 322, Dordrecht 3300 AH, Netherlands. TEL 31-78-639-2392, FAX 31-78-654-6474.

615.9 GBR
CHAPMAN & HALL ECOTOXICOLOGY SERIES. Text in English. 1994. irreg., latest vol.2, 1994. price varies. back issues avail. **Document type:** *Monographic series.*
Indexed: GeoRef, Zoo.Rec.
Published by: Chapman & Hall Ltd. (Subsidiary of: International Thomson Publishing Group), Journals Department, Chapman & Hall, 2-6 Boundary Row, London SE1 8HN, United Kingdom. TEL 44-20-7865-0066, FAX 44-20-7522-9623. Eds. Brenda Sanders, Michael H Depledge. **Subscr. to:** International Thompson Publishing Services Ltd.

615.9 USA ISSN 1074-9098
CODEN: CHLSEG
CHEMICAL HEALTH AND SAFETY. Text in English. 1994. bi-m. EUR 301 in Europe to institutions; JPY 39,900 in Japan to institutions; USD 337 elsewhere to institutions (effective 2002). adv. bk.rev. charts, illus, stat. index. back issues avail. *Refereed.* **Document type:** *Academic/Scholarly.* **Description:** Covers topics in the safe handling and manufacture of chemicals.
Related titles: Microfiche ed.; Microfilm ed.; Online - full text ed.: (from EBSCO Publishing, ingenta, Swets Blackwell, ScienceDirect).
Indexed: CSNB, Chem.Abstr., Chem.Indus.Notes, Chem.Titles, Lab.Haz.Bull.
—BLDSC (3146.588500), CASDDS, Infotrieve. **CCC.**
Published by: (Division of Chemical Health and Safety, American Chemical Society), Elsevier Science, 655 Ave of the Americas, New York, NY 10010. TEL 212-989-5800, FAX 212-633-3990, usinfo-f@elsevier.com, http://www.elsevier.com/locate/chs. Ed. H J Elston. Pub. Anthony Durniak. Circ: 2,600 (paid).

615.9 USA ISSN 0893-228X
RA1190 CODEN: CRTOEC
CHEMICAL RESEARCH IN TOXICOLOGY. Text in English. 1988. m. USD 756 in North America to institutions; USD 807 elsewhere to institutions; USD 907 in North America to institutions Print & online eds.; USD 958 elsewhere to institutions Print & online eds. (effective 2002); for additional pricing options for print and web editions contact inside sales specialist, Ms. Chako Dickinson, at 202-872-4063. back issues avail. *Refereed.* **Document type:** *Journal, Academic/Scholarly.* **Description:** Publishes full papers, rapid communications, and invited reviews on structural, mechanistic, and technological advances in research concerned with the toxicological effects of chemical agents.
Related titles: Microform ed.: (from PQC); Online - full text ed.: ISSN 1520-5010. USD 794 to institutions (effective 2002) (from EBSCO Publishing, Institute for Scientific Information).
Indexed: ASCA, Aqua.Sci.& Fish.Abstr., BBCI, Chem.Abstr., Chem.Cit.Ind., Chem.Indus.Notes, Chem.Titles, Curr.Adv.Gen.& Molec.Biol., Curr.Cont., Environ.Abstr., Environ.Sci.Poll.Mgmt., Excerp.Med., INIS Atomind., Ind.Med. (1988-), Ind.Sci.Rev., Inpharma, Int.Abstr.Biol.Sci., Mass Spectr.Bull., Nutr.Abstr., Ocean.Abstr., Pharm.&Out.News, Pollut.Abstr., Reac., Ref.Zh., Rev.Appl.Entomol., Rev.Med.& Vet.Mycol., Sci.Cit.Ind., Sel.Water Res.Abstr., Telegen.
—BLDSC (3150.465000), CASDDS, CISTI, EMDOCS, GNLM, IDS, ingenta, Linda Hall. **CCC.**
Published by: American Chemical Society, 1155 16th St, N W, Washington, DC 20036. TEL 202-332-5544, 800-333-9511, FAX 202-332-4559, service@acs.org, http://pubs.acs.org/crt. Ed. Lawrence J Marnett. Circ: 950. **Subscr. to:** American Chemical Society, Member and Subscriber Services, PO Box 3337, Columbus, OH 43210. TEL 614-447-3674, FAX 614-447-3671.

615.9 IRL ISSN 0009-2797
QP501 CODEN: CBINA8
CHEMICO-BIOLOGICAL INTERACTIONS; a journal of molecular and biochemical toxicology. Text in English. 1969. 18/yr. EUR 2,364 in Europe to institutions; JPY 313,800 in Japan to institutions; USD 2,644 elsewhere to institutions (effective 2002). bibl, charts, illus. back issues avail. *Refereed.* **Document type:** *Academic/Scholarly.* **Description:** Contains articles devoted to the mechanism by which exogenous chemicals produce changes in biological systems.
Related titles: Microform ed.: (from PQC); Online - full text ed.: (from ingenta, Swets Blackwell, ScienceDirect, Institute for Scientific Information).
Indexed: ASCA, Aqua.Sci.& Fish.Abstr., BBCI, Chem.Abstr., Chem.Cit.Ind., Chem.Indus.Notes, Chem.Titles, Crop Physiol.Abstr., Curr.Adv.Biochem., Curr.Adv.Cancer Res., Curr.Adv.Ecol.Sci., Curr.Cont., Deep Sea Res.& Oceanogr.Abstr., Derwent Biotech.Abstr., Environ.Sci.Poll.Mgmt., Excerp.Med., Field Crop Abstr., Helminthol.Abstr., Hort.Abstr., INIS Atomind., Ind.Med. (1969-), Ind.Sci.Rev., Ind.Vet., Inpharma, Int.Abstr.Biol.Sci., Lab.Haz.Bull., Neurosci.Cit.Ind., Pharm.&Out.News, Pig News & Info., Potato Abstr., Reac., Rev.Appl.Entomol., Rev.Med.& Vet.Mycol., Rev.Plant Path., Sci.Cit.Ind., Sport Fish.Abstr., Vet.Bull., Weed Abstr.
—BLDSC (3155.500000), ADONIS, CASDDS, CISTI, EMDOCS, GNLM, IDS, ingenta, Linda Hall. **CCC.**
Published by: Elsevier Science Ireland Ltd, Elsevier House, Brookvale Plaza, E. Park, Shannon, Co. Clare, Ireland. TEL 353-61-709600, FAX 353-61-709100, http://www.elsevier.com/locate/chembioint, http://www.elsevier.nl. Eds. Ian Cotgreave, James A Bond. R&P Annette Moloney. **Subscr. in Australasia and the Far East to:** Elsevier Science (Singapore) Pte Ltd, No.1 Temasek Ave, 17-01 Millenia Tower, Singapore 039192, Singapore. TEL 65-434-3727, FAX 65-337-2230, asiainfo@elsevier.com.sg; **Subscr. in the Americas to:** Elsevier Science, PO Box 945, New York, NY 10159-0945. TEL 212-633-3730, FAX 212-633-3680, usinfo-f@elsevier.com; **Subscr. to:** Elsevier Science Inc - Japan Regional Office, 9-15 Higashi-Azabu 1-chome, Minato-ku, Tokyo 106-0044, Japan. TEL 81-3-5561-5033, FAX 81-3-5561-5047, info@elsevier.co.jp. **Subscr. to:** Elsevier Science BV, PO Box 211, Amsterdam 1000 AE, Netherlands. TEL 31-20-485-3757, FAX 31-20-485-3432, nlinfo-f@elsevier.nl.

615.9 GBR ISSN 0045-6535
QH540 CODEN: CMSHAF
CHEMOSPHERE; chemistry, biology and toxicology as related to environmental problems. Text in English, French, German. 1972. 32/yr. EUR 365 in Europe to qualified personnel; JPY 48,400 in Japan to qualified personnel; USD 408 elsewhere to qualified personnel; EUR 3,292 in Europe to institutions; JPY 437,200 in Japan to institutions; USD 3,684 elsewhere to institutions (effective 2002). adv. *Refereed.* **Document type:** *Academic/Scholarly.* **Description:** Publishes original research in environmental protection from the fields of chemistry, biology, physics, toxicology and interrelated disciplines.
Incorporates (2000-2002): Chemosphere - Global Change Science (1465-9972)
Related titles: Microfilm ed.: (from PQC); Online - full text ed.: (from ingenta, Swets Blackwell, ScienceDirect, Institute for Scientific Information).
Indexed: ASCA, Abstr.Bull.Inst.Pap.Chem., Abstr.Hyg., Acid Pre.Dig., Agri.& Environ.Biotech.Abstr. (coverage dropped), Agri.Eng.Abstr., Agricola, Agroforest.Abstr., Anal.Abstr., Anim.Breed.Abstr., Appl.Ecol.Abstr. (coverage dropped), Aqua.Sci.& Fish.Abstr., Aquacult.Abstr., Bibl.Agri., Bio-Contr.News & Info., Biodet.Abstr., Biol.Abstr., C.I.S. Abstr., Cadscan, Chem.Abstr., Chem.Cit.Ind., Chem.Indus.Notes, Chem.Titles, Chromat.Abstr., Crop Physiol.Abstr., Curr.Adv.Ecol.Sci., Curr.Cont., Curr.Ref.Fish Res., Dairy Sci.Abstr., Deep Sea Res.& Oceanogr.Abstr., Derwent Biotech.Abstr., Ecol.Abstr., Energy Ind., Energy Rev., Eng.Ind., Environ.Abstr., Environ.Per.Bibl. (1975-), Environ.Sci.Poll.Mgmt., Excerp.Med., Field Crop Abstr., Fluidex, Food Sci.& Tech.Abstr., Forest Prod.Abstr., Forest.Abstr., Geo.Abstr.H.G., Geo.Abstr.P.G., GeoRef, Geol.Abstr., Geomech.Abstr., Helminthol.Abstr., Herb.Abstr., Hort.Abstr., IDA, INIS Atomind., Ind.Med. (1972-), Ind.Sci.Rev., Ind.Vet., Int.Abstr.Biol.Sci., Irr.& Drain.Abstr., LISA, Lab.Haz.Bull., Lead Abstr., Maize Abstr., Mass Spectr.Bull., Mat.Sci.Cit.Ind. (coverage dropped), Meteor.& Geoastrophys.Abstr., Nonwov.Abstr., Nutr.Abstr., Ocean.Abstr., Ornam.Hort., Paper & Bd.Abstr., Pig News & Info., Pollut.Abstr., Potato Abstr., Poult.Abstr., Protozool.Abstr., Ref.Zh., Rev.Appl.Entomol., Rev.Arom.& Med.Plants, Rev.Med.& Vet.Mycol., Rev.Plant Path., Rice Abstr., Risk Abstr., Rural Devel.Abstr., SSCI (coverage dropped), Saf.Sci.Abstr., Sci.Cit.Ind., Seed Abstr., Sel.Water Res.Abstr., Soils & Fert., Sport Fish.Abstr., Tox.Abstr., Triticale Abstr., Vet.Bull., W.R.C.Inf., WasteInfo, Weed Abstr., Wild.Rev., World Text.Abstr., Zincscan, Zoo.Rec.
—BLDSC (3172.280000), CASDDS, CISTI, Ei, EMDOCS, GNLM, IDS, ingenta, Linda Hall. **CCC.**
Published by: Pergamon (Subsidiary of: Elsevier Science), The Boulevard, Langford Ln, East Park, Kidlington, Oxford OXB 1GB, United Kingdom. FAX 44-1865-843010, nlinfo-f@elsevier/nl; usinfo-f@elsevier.com; forinfo-kyf04035@niftyserve.or.jp, http://www.elsevier.com/locate/chemosphere, http://www.elsevier.nl/. Ed. Otto Hutzinger. Circ: 1,000. **Subscr. in Australasia and the Far East to:** Elsevier Science (Singapore) Pte Ltd, No.1 Temasek Ave, 17-01 Millenia Tower, Singapore 039192, Singapore. TEL 65-434-3727, FAX 65-337-2230; **Subscr. in the Americas to:** Elsevier Science, PO Box 945, New York, NY 10159-0945. TEL 212-633-3730, FAX 212-633-3680, usinfo-f@elsevier.com, http://www.elsevier.com; **Subscr. to:** Elsevier Science BV, PO Box 211, Amsterdam 1000 AE, Netherlands. TEL 31-20-485-3757, FAX 31-20-485-3432, nlinfo-f@elsevier.nl, http://www.elsevier.nl.

615.9 CHE ISSN 0886-5140
CODEN: COTXEI
COMMENTS ON TOXICOLOGY. Text in English. 1986. bi-m. GBP 167, USD 203, USD 223 to individuals; GBP 656, USD 840, EUR 845 to institutions; GBP 991, USD 1,288, EUR 1,292 to corporations (effective 2002). **Document type:** *Academic/Scholarly.*
Related titles: Microform ed.
Indexed: Aqua.Sci.& Fish.Abstr., Environ.Sci.Poll.Mgmt., Excerp.Med. (1996-), Int.Abstr.Biol.Sci., Pollut.Abstr., Rev.Med.& Vet.Mycol., Risk Abstr., Saf.Sci.Abstr., Soils & Fert., Tox.Abstr.
—BLDSC (3336.042500), CISTI, EMDOCS, GNLM, Infotrieve. **CCC.**
Published by: Gordon and Breach - Harwood Academic (Subsidiary of: Taylor & Francis Group), PO Box 531, Lausanne 1000, Switzerland. Ed. A Wallace Hayes. **Subscr. addr. in US:** International Publishers Direct, PO Box 32160, Newark, NJ 07102. FAX 215-750-6343.

COMPARATIVE BIOCHEMISTRY AND PHYSIOLOGY. TOXICOLOGY & PHARMACOLOGY. see *BIOLOGY—Biochemistry*

COMPARATIVE HAEMATOLOGY INTERNATIONAL. see *MEDICAL SCIENCES—Hematology*

COSMETIC SCIENCE MONOGRAPHS. see *BEAUTY CULTURE—Perfumes And Cosmetics*

615.9 USA ISSN 1040-8444
RA1190 CODEN: CRTXB2
CRITICAL REVIEWS IN TOXICOLOGY. Text in English. 1971. bi-m. USD 495 (effective 1998). bibl, charts, illus. back issues avail. *Refereed.* **Document type:** *Academic/Scholarly.* **Description:** Aimed at making available critical assessments of subjects that are part of the advancing frontiers of toxicology and related basic scientific disciplines.
Formerly: C R C Critical Reviews in Toxicology (0045-6446)
Related titles: Online - full text ed.: (from Northern Light Technology, Inc., O C L C Online Computer Library Center, Inc., ProQuest Information & Learning, Swets Blackwell, ScienceDirect, Institute for Scientific Information); (from EBSCO Publishing).
Indexed: ASCA, Aqua.Sci.& Fish.Abstr., Biol.Abstr., CSNB, Chem.Abstr., Chem.Cit.Ind., Chem.Titles, Curr.Adv.Ecol.Sci., Curr.Cont., Dok.Arbeitsmed., Entomol.Abstr., Environ.Abstr., Environ.Per.Bibl. (1992-), Environ.Sci.Poll.Mgmt., Excerp.Med., Food Sci.& Tech.Abstr., INIS Atomind., Ind.Med. (1980-), Ind.Sci.Rev., Ind.Vet., Inpharma, Int.Abstr.Biol.Sci., Lab.Haz.Bull., NRN, Neurosci.Abstr., Nutr.Abstr., Pharm.&Out.News, Pollut.Abstr., Reac., Rev.Appl.Entomol., Risk Abstr., Saf.Sci.Abstr., Sci.Cit.Ind., Sport Fish.Abstr., THA, Trop.Dis.Bull., Wild.Rev.
—BLDSC (3487.484000), ADONIS, CASDDS, CIS, CISTI, EMDOCS, GNLM, IDS, ingenta, Linda Hall. **CCC.**
Published by: C R C Press, LLC, 2000 Corporate Blvd, N W, Boca Raton, FL 33431. TEL 561-994-0555, 800-272-7737, FAX 561-998-9784. Ed. Dr. Roger O McClellan. Circ: 640.

CURRENT ADVANCES IN TOXICOLOGY. see *ENVIRONMENTAL STUDIES—Abstracting, Bibliographies, Statistics*

615.9 USA
CURRENT ISSUES IN TOXICOLOGY. Text in English. 1984. irreg. price varies. reprint service avail. from ISI. **Document type:** *Monographic series.*
Published by: (International Life Science Institute), Springer-Verlag, Journals (Subsidiary of: BertelsmannSpringer), 175 Fifth Ave, New York, NY 10010. TEL 212-460-1500, FAX 212-473-6272.

615.9 CHE ISSN 0275-2581
CURRENT TOPICS IN ENVIRONMENTAL AND TOXICOLOGICAL CHEMISTRY. Text in English. 1976. irreg., latest vol.16. price varies. *Refereed.* **Document type:** *Monographic series.*
Indexed: GeoRef.
—BLDSC (3504.882000), CISTI.
Published by: Gordon and Breach - Harwood Academic (Subsidiary of: Taylor & Francis Group), PO Box 531, Lausanne 1000, Switzerland. Eds. O Hutzinger, Roland W Frei. **Subscr. addr. in US:** International Publishers Direct, PO Box 32160, Newark, NJ 07102. FAX 215-750-6343.

CURRENT TOPICS IN TRANSPORT. see *TRANSPORTATION—Roads And Traffic*

344.046334 USA
DEFENDING PESTICIDES IN LITIGATION. Text in English. a. USD 208 per issue (effective 2000). **Document type:** *Trade.* **Description:** Providess technical data concerning pesticides and regulations.
Published by: West Group (Subsidiary of: Thomson Corporation, The), 620 Opperman Dr., Eagan, MN 55123. TEL 800-344-5008, FAX 800-340-9378, http://www.westgroup.com.

615.9 GBR
DIALOG ONDISC ENVIRONMENTAL CHEMISTRY, HEALTH AND SAFETY. Text in English. 1993. base vol. plus q. updates. USD 1,695 (effective 2002). **Document type:** *Abstract/Index.* **Description:** Provides comprehensive business, scientific and technical information on environmental chemistry, health and safety.
Former titles: K R OnDisc Environmental Chemistry, Health and Safety; Dialog OnDisc Environmental Chemistry, Health and Safety
Media: CD-ROM (from The Dialog Corporation).

E

Published by: Royal Society of Chemistry, Thomas Graham House, Science Park, Milton Rd, Cambridge CB4 4WF, United Kingdom. TEL 44-1223-432360, FAX 44-1223-423429, sales@rsc.org, http://www.rsc.org/csnb. **Subscr. to:** The Dialog Corp. Plc., OnDisc Europe, 2 Des Roches Sq, Witan Way, Witney, Oxon OX8 6BE, United Kingdom. TEL 44-1993-899300, FAX 44-1993-899333.

615.902 GBR
THE DICTIONARY OF SUBSTANCES AND THEIR EFFECTS. Text in English. 1996. irreg. (2nd ed., 1999). GBP 1,295 per vol. (effective 2002); (includes free access to a fully searchable web database). back issues avail. **Document type:** *Academic/Scholarly.* **Description:** Toxicological and environmental information on chemicals.
Related titles: CD-ROM ed.: (from SilverPlatter Information, Inc.); Online - full text ed.: (from The Dialog Corporation).
Published by: Royal Society of Chemistry, Thomas Graham House, Science Park, Milton Rd, Cambridge CB4 4WF, United Kingdom. TEL 44-1223-432360, FAX 44-1223-423429, sales@rsc.org, http://www.rsc.org/dose. Eds. M L Richardson, S Gangolli.

628 USA
DIRECTORY OF PERSONNEL RESPONSIBLE FOR RADIOLOGICAL HEALTH PROGRAMS. Text in English. a. USD 30 (effective 1999). **Document type:** *Directory.* **Description:** Lists professional personnel in state and local government agencies who administer radiation control activities, as well as personnel in selected federal agencies in certain U.S. territories, Canada, and Mexico who have responsibility for certain radiation protection activities.
Published by: Conference of Radiation Control Program Directors, 205 Capitol Ave, Frankfort, KY 40601-2832. TEL 502-227-4543, FAX 502-227-7862, ssmith@crcpd.org, http://www.crcpd.org.

DRUG AND CHEMICAL TOXICOLOGY; an international journal for rapid communication. see *PHARMACY AND PHARMACOLOGY*

DRUG AND CHEMICAL TOXICOLOGY SERIES. see *PHARMACY AND PHARMACOLOGY*

571.97 BEL ISSN 1013-9516
E C E T O C DOCUMENT. Text in English. irreg., latest vol.42, 2001. EUR 125 per vol. to non-members. back issues avail. *Refereed.* **Document type:** *Monographic series, Academic/Scholarly.* **Description:** Addresses emerging issues in ecotoxicology in humans and the environment.
—BLDSC (3647.345000).
Published by: European Centre for Ecotoxicology and Toxicology of Chemicals, Ave E Van Nieuwenhuyse 4, Bte 6, Brussels 1160, Belgium. TEL 32-2-675-3600, FAX 32-2-675-3625, info@ecetoc.org, http://www.ecetoc.org/pages/Publications.cmm.

571.95 BEL ISSN 0773-6347
E C E T O C MONOGRAPH. Text in English. 1979. irreg., latest vol.29, 2000. EUR 125 per vol. to non-members. back issues avail. *Refereed.* **Document type:** *Monographic series, Academic/Scholarly.* **Description:** Evaluates important issues relating to the application of sound scientific methods in evaluating risks of chemicals and compounds to human health and the general environment.
—BLDSC (5914.595500).
Published by: European Centre for Ecotoxicology and Toxicology of Chemicals, Ave E Van Nieuwenhuyse 4, Bte 6, Brussels 1160, Belgium. TEL 32-2-675-3600, FAX 32-2-675-3625, info@ecetoc.org, http://www.ecetoc.org/pages/Publications.cfm.

571.95 BEL ISSN 1373-7244
E C E T O C SPECIAL REPORT (NEW SERIES). Text in English. N.S. 1994. irreg., latest vol.16, 1999. EUR 125 per vol. to non-members. charts, stat. back issues avail. *Refereed.* **Document type:** *Monographic series, Academic/Scholarly.* **Description:** Compiles data regarding specific regulatory issues or demands.
Published by: European Centre for Ecotoxicology and Toxicology of Chemicals, Ave E Van Nieuwenhuyse 4, Bte 6, Brussels 1160, Belgium. TEL 32-2-675-3600, FAX 32-2-675-3625, info@ecetoc.org, http://www.ecetoc.org/pages/Publications.cfm.

571.95 BEL ISSN 0773-8072
E C E T O C TECHNICAL REPORT. Text in English. 1981. irreg., latest vol.79, 2001. EUR 125 per vol.. back issues avail. *Refereed.* **Document type:** *Monographic series, Academic/Scholarly.* **Description:** Addresses specific applications of ecotoxicology in evaluating hazards and risks of chemicals to humans and the environment.
—BLDSC (8715.261000).
Published by: European Centre for Ecotoxicology and Toxicology of Chemicals, Ave E Van Nieuwenhuyse 4, Bte 6, Brussels 1160, Belgium. TEL 32-2-675-3600, FAX 32-2-675-3625, info@ecetoc.org, http://www.ecetoc.org/pages/Publications.htm.

577.27 USA ISSN 0963-9292
RA565.A1 CODEN: ECOTEL
ECOTOXICOLOGY. Text in English. 1992. bi-m. EUR 594, USD 594 to institutions for print or online ed.; EUR 712.80, USD 712.80 to institutions for print & online eds.combined (effective 2002). adv. reprints avail. *Refereed.* **Document type:** *Journal, Academic/Scholarly.* **Description:** Covers the fundamental research on the effects of toxic chemicals on populations, communities and terrestrial, fresh water and marine ecosystems.
Related titles: Online - full text ed.: (from EBSCO Publishing, O C L C Online Computer Library Center, Inc., RoweCom Information Quest, Swets Blackwell, Kluwer Online, Institute for Scientific Information).
Indexed: ASCA, Appl.Ecol.Abstr., Aqua.Sci.& Fish.Abstr., Chem.Abstr., Chem.Indus.Notes, Chem.Titles, Curr.Cont., Ecol.Abstr., Environ.Abstr., Environ.Per.Bibl., Environ.Sci.Poll.Mgmt., Excerp.Med. (1994-), Forest.Abstr., Geo.Abstr.P.G., Geol.Abstr., Hort.Abstr., Ind.Med., Ind.Sci.Rev., Int.Abstr.Biol.Sci., Maize Abstr., Ornam.Hort., Pollut.Abstr., Rev.Appl.Entomol., Sci.Cit.Ind., Sel.Water Res.Abstr., Soils & Fert., Sport Fish.Abstr., Tox.Abstr., Weed Abstr., Wild.Rev., Zoo.Rec.
—BLDSC (3659.553500), ADONIS, CASDDS, CISTI, EMDOCS, IDS, Infotrieve, ingenta. **CCC.**
Published by: Kluwer Academic Publishers Boston, 101 Philip Dr, Assinippi Park, Norwell, MA 02061. TEL 781-871-6600, FAX 781-871-9045, services@wkap.nl, http://www.wkap.nl/journalhome.htm/0963-9292. Eds. David B Peakall, Lee R Shugart. Adv. contact Gemma Heiser. **Subscr. outside the Americas to:** Kluwer Academic - Plenum Publishers, 233 Spring St, New York, NY 10013-1578. TEL 212-620-8468, FAX 212-807-1047; **Subscr. to:** Kluwer Academic Publishers Group, Journals Department, PO Box 322, Dordrecht 3300 AH, Netherlands. TEL 31-78-639-2392, FAX 31-78-654-6474.

615.9 USA ISSN 0147-6513
QH545.A1 CODEN: EESADV
ECOTOXICOLOGY AND ENVIRONMENTAL SAFETY. Variant title: Environmental Research. Section B. Text in English. 1977. 9/yr. USD 750 in US & Canada to institutions; USD 865 elsewhere to institutions (effective 2001). adv. index. back issues avail. *Refereed.* **Document type:** *Academic/Scholarly.* **Description:** Examines the biologic and toxic effects of natural or synthetic chemical pollutants on animal, plant, or microbial ecosystems, and their routes into the affected organisms.
Related titles: Online - full text ed.: Ecotoxicology and Environmental Safety - Online. ISSN 1090-2414 (from EBSCO Publishing, O C L C Online Computer Library Center, Inc., RoweCom Information Quest, ingenta, Swets Blackwell, IDEAL Online Library, Institute for Scientific Information).
Indexed: ASCA, Abstr.Hyg., Agricola, Agroforest.Abstr., Aqua.Sci.& Fish.Abstr., Bibl.Agri., Biodet.Abstr., Cadscan, Chem.Abstr., Chem.Indus.Notes, Chem.Titles, Crop Physiol.Abstr., Curr.Cont., Curr.Ref.Fish Res., Dairy Sci.Abstr., Ecol.Abstr., Eng.Ind., Entomol.Abstr., Environ.Abstr., Environ.Ind., Environ.Sci.Poll.Mgmt., Excerp.Med., Field Crop Abstr., Food Sci.& Tech.Abstr., Forest Prod.Abstr., Forest.Abstr., Geo.Abstr.H.G., Geo.Abstr.P.G., Geol.Abstr., Helminthol.Abstr., Hort.Abstr., INIS Atomind., Ind.Med. (1977-), Ind.Sci.Rev., Ind.Vet., Inpharma, Int.Abstr.Biol.Sci., Irr.& Drain.Abstr., Lead Abstr., Maize Abstr., Microbiol.Abstr., Nutr.Abstr., Ocean.Abstr., Plant Breed.Abstr., Pollut.Abstr., Postharvest, Poult.Abstr., Protozool.Abstr., Reac., Ref.Zh., Rev.Appl.Entomol., Rev.Arom.& Med.Plants, Rev.Med.& Vet.Mycol., Rev.Plant Path., Rice Abstr., Risk Abstr., Saf.Sci.Abstr., Sci.Cit.Ind., Seed Abstr., Sel.Water Res.Abstr., Soils & Fert., Soyabean Abstr., Sport Fish.Abstr., Tox.Abstr., Triticale Abstr., Vet.Bull., W.R.C.Inf., Weed Abstr., Wild.Rev., Zincscan, Zoo.Rec.
—BLDSC (3659.555000), ADONIS, CASDDS, CISTI, Ei, GNLM, IDS, ingenta, Linda Hall. **CCC.**
Published by: (International Society of Ecotoxicology and Environmental Safety), Academic Press, Inc., Journal Division (Subsidiary of: Harcourt Brace & Company), 525 B St, Ste 1900, San Diego, CA 92101-4495. TEL 619-250-1840, FAX 619-699-6800, apsubs@acad.com, http://www.academicpress.com/ees. Eds. Frederick Coulston, Friedhelm Korte. **Co-sponsor:** International Academy of Enfironmental Safety.

EKSPERIMENTAL'NAYA I KLINICHESKAYA FARMAKOLOGIYA. see *PHARMACY AND PHARMACOLOGY*

ELECTRICAL SENSITIVITY NEWS. see *PUBLIC HEALTH AND SAFETY*

EMERGENCY RESPONSE GUIDANCE FOR AIRCRAFT INCIDENTS INVOLVING DANGEROUS GOODS. see *TRANSPORTATION—Air Transport*

613.62 615.902 FRA ISSN 1155-1925
ENCYCLOPEDIE MEDICO-CHIRURGICALE. TRAITE DE TOXICOLOGIE - PATHOLOGIE PROFESSIONELLE. Cover title: Traite de Toxicologie - Pathologie Professionelle. Variant title: Encyclopedie Medico-Chirurgicale, Instantanes Medicaux. Toxicologie - Pathologie Professionelle. Text in French. 1937. 3 base vols. plus q. updates. bibl, charts, illus. *Refereed.* **Document type:** *Academic/Scholarly.* **Description:** Provides a comprehensive, up-to-date reference for diagnosing and treating ailments involving poisoning occurring in the work place.
Former titles (until 1991): Encyclopedie Medico-Chirurgicale. Intoxications, Pathologie du Travail, Maladies par Agents Physiques (1154-290X); (until 1990): Encyclopedie Medico-Chirurgicale. Pathologie du Travail, Intoxications, Maladies par Agents Physiques (0246-0653); (until 1962): Encyclopedie Medico-Chirurgicale. Medecine du Travail, Intoxications, Maladies par Agents Physiques (0246-0734); (until 1952): Encyclopedie Medico-Chirurgicale. Intoxications et Maladies par Agents Physiques (0246-0726)
Published by: Elsevier Paris, Editions Scientifiques et Medicales (Subsidiary of: Reed Elsevier plc. group), 23 rue Linois, Paris 75015, France. TEL 31-1-45589110, FAX 33-1-45589425, redaction-emc@elsevier.fr, redacion-emc@elsevier.fr, http://www.elsevier.fr, http://www.elsevier.com.

363.7 USA
ENVIRONMENT, HEALTH & SAFETY MANAGEMENT. Text in English. 1990. bi-w. USD 427; USD 467 foreign (effective 1999). tr.lit. back issues avail. **Document type:** *Newsletter, Trade.* **Description:** Provides timely advice on regulations, management trends, international standards, and case studies for senior environmental, health and safety managers in multinational companies.
Related titles: E-mail ed.
Published by: (Environmental Group, Inc.), J. Gary Taylor, Ed. & Pub., 50 Sution Pl, S 14 C, New York, NY 10022. TEL 212-308-4666, FAX 212-308-1160, thmder@pipeline.com. **Subscr. to:** Performance Marketing, 3120 Cottonwood Dr., Laughlin, NY 89029. TEL 702-299-0011, FAX 702-299-0224.

ENVIRONMENT INFORMATION BULLETIN. see *PUBLIC HEALTH AND SAFETY*

ENVIRONMENTAL AND MOLECULAR MUTAGENESIS. see *BIOLOGY—Genetics*

ENVIRONMENTAL AND MOLECULAR MUTAGENESIS. SUPPLEMENT. see *BIOLOGY—Genetics*

ENVIRONMENTAL AND SAFETY TECHNOLOGY. see *ENVIRONMENTAL STUDIES—Abstracting, Bibliographies, Statistics*

344.046 USA
ENVIRONMENTAL AND TOXIC TORT TRIALS. Text in English. 1991. base vol. plus irreg. updates. USD 85.
Indexed: Ref.Zh.
Published by: Lexis Law Publishing (Subsidiary of: Reed Elsevier plc), PO Box 7587, Charlottesville, VA 22906-7587. TEL 804-972-7600, 800-562-1197, FAX 804-972-7666, llp.customer.support@lexis-nexis.com, http://www.lexislawpublishing.com. Ed. Allan Kanner.

▼ **ENVIRONMENTAL HEALTH & SAFETY INTERNET GAZETTE.** see *ENVIRONMENTAL STUDIES*

615.9 USA ISSN 1529-9201

ENVIRONMENTAL PROTECTION NEWS. Text in English. 1985. s-m. USD 399 (effective 2001). **Document type:** *Newsletter.* **Description:** Provides news and regulatory developments in the environmental field.

Former titles: Environmental Protection Week (1524-0630); (until 1999): Environmental Protection News (1057-171X); (until 1990): Environmental Protection Week (1050-7124); (until 198?): Environmental Management News (0893-3413)

Indexed: AESIS.

—Infotrieve. **CCC.**

Published by: Stevens Publishing Corporation, 5151 Beltline Rd, 10th fl, Dallas, TX 75240. TEL 972-687-6753, FAX 972-687-6770, anelson@stevenspublishing.com. Ed. Angela Garcia Nelson.

615.9 USA ISSN 1520-4081
QH90.57.B5 CODEN: ETOXFH

ENVIRONMENTAL TOXICOLOGY; an international journal. Text in English. 1986. bi-m. USD 650 in United States; USD 710 in Canada & Mexico; USD 761 elsewhere; USD 683 combined subscription in United States for print and online eds.; USD 743 combined subscription in Canada & Mexico for print and online eds.; USD 794 combined subscription elsewhere for print and online eds. (effective 2002). adv. back issues avail. *Refereed.* **Document type:** *Academic/Scholarly.* **Description:** Presents original research papers on all aspects of environmental toxicology and water quality research, monitoring, standards and policies.

Former titles (until 1999): Environmental Toxicology and Water Quality (1053-4725); (until 1991): Toxicity Assessment (0884-8181)

Related titles: Microform ed.: (from PQC); Online - full text ed.: ISSN 1522-7278. USD 650 in United States; USD 650 in Canada & Mexico; USD 650 elsewhere (effective 2002) (from EBSCO Publishing, Wiley InterScience, Institute for Scientific Information).

Indexed: ASCA, Agricola, Aqua.Sci.& Fish.Abstr., Chem.Abstr., Chem.Indus.Notes, Chem.Titles, Curr.Cont., Ecol.Abstr., Eng.Ind., Environ.Per.Bibl. (1991-), Environ.Sci.Poll.Mgmt., Excerp.Med., Food Sci.& Tech.Abstr., Geo.Abstr.P.G., GeoRef, Ind.Med., Int.Abstr.Biol.Sci., Mass Spectr.Bull., Microbiol.Abstr., Pollut.Abstr., Repindex, Rev.Appl.Entomol., Sci.Cit.Ind., Sel.Water Res.Abstr., Sport Fish.Abstr., Tox.Abstr., W.R.C.Inf., Weed Abstr., Zoo.Rec.

—BLDSC (3791.784000), CASDDS, CISTI, Ei, EMDOCS, GNLM, IDS, Infotrieve, ingenta, Linda Hall. **CCC.**

Published by: John Wiley & Sons, Inc., Journals (Subsidiary of: Wiley InterScience), 605 Third Ave, New York, NY 10158. TEL 212-850-6645, FAX 212-850-6021, subinfo@wiley.com, uscs-wis@wiley.com, http://www.wiley.com. Eds. Bernard J Dutka, Dickson Liu. adv.: B&W page GBP 640, color page GBP 1,515; trim 153 x 229. Circ: 500. **Outside the Americas subscr. to:** John Wiley & Sons Ltd., Baffins Ln, Chichester, Sussex PO19 IUD, United Kingdom. TEL 44-1243-779777, FAX 44-1243-843232, cs-journals@wiley.co.uk, http://www.wiley.co.uk.

615.902 USA ISSN 0730-7268
QH545.A1 CODEN: ETOCDK

ENVIRONMENTAL TOXICOLOGY AND CHEMISTRY. Text in English. 1982. 12/yr. USD 725 domestic; USD 745 in Canada & Mexico; USD 765 elsewhere; USD 835 domestic Print & online eds.; USD 855 in Canada & Mexico Print & online eds.; USD 875 elsewhere Print & online eds. (effective 2001). adv. index. back issues avail. *Refereed.* **Document type:** *Academic/Scholarly.* **Description:** Covers environmental chemistry, environmental toxicology and hazard assessment.

Related titles: Microfilm ed.: (from PQC); Online - full text ed.: USD 725 (effective 2001) (from Institute for Scientific Information).

Indexed: ASCA, Abstr.Bull.Inst.Pap.Chem., AgBiotech, Agri.& Environ.Biotech.Abstr. (coverage dropped), Agri.Eng.Abstr., Agricola, Anal.Abstr., Anim.Breed.Abstr., Appl.Ecol.Abstr., Aqua.Sci.& Fish.Abstr., Aquacult.Abstr., Bibl.Agri., Bio-Contr.News & Info., Biodet.Abstr., Bioeng.Abstr., Biol.Abstr., Biotech.& Bioeng.Abstr., Chem.Abstr., Chem.Cit.Ind., Chem.Indus.Notes, Chem.Titles, Crop Physiol.Abstr., Curr.Adv.Ecol.Sci., Curr.Cont., Dairy Sci.Abstr., Derwent Biotech.Abstr., Ecol.Abstr., Energy Ind., Energy Info.Abstr., Eng.Ind., Entomol.Abstr., Environ.Abstr., Environ.Per.Bibl. (1990-), Environ.Sci.Poll.Mgmt., Excerp.Med., Field Crop Abstr., Food Sci.& Tech.Abstr., Forest Prod.Abstr., Forest.Abstr., Genet.Abstr., Geo.Abstr.P.G., GeoRef, Geol.Abstr., Helminthol.Abstr., Herb.Abstr., Hort.Abstr., Hum.Gen.Abstr., INIS Atomind., Ind.Med., Ind.Sci.Rev., Ind.Vet., Int.Abstr.Biol.Sci., Irr.& Drain.Abstr., Key Word Ind.Wildl.Res., METADEX, Microbiol.Abstr., Nonwov.Abstr., Nutr.Abstr., Paper & Bd.Abstr., Pollut.Abstr., Poult.Abstr., Ref.Zh., Rev.Appl.Entomol., Rev.Med.& Vet.Mycol., Rev.Plant Path., Rice Abstr., Risk Abstr., Rural Recreat.Tour.Abstr., Sci.Cit.Ind., Seed Abstr., Sel.Water Res.Abstr., Soils & Fert., Solid St.Abstr., Soyabean Abstr., Sport Fish.Abstr., Tox.Abstr., Triticale Abstr., Vet.Bull., W.R.C.Inf., Weed Abstr., Wild.Rev., World Ag.Econ.& Rur.Soc.Abstr., Zoo.Rec.

—BLDSC (3791.785000), CASDDS, CISTI, Ei, EMDOCS, GNLM, IDS, ingenta, Linda Hall. **CCC.**

Published by: Society of Environmental Toxicology and Chemistry, 1010 N 12th St, Pensacola, FL 32501-3370. TEL 850-469-1500, FAX 850-469-9778, setac@setac.org, http://www.setac.org, http://www.ruf.rice.edu:80/~etcj/. Ed. Calvin Herbert Ward. R&P, Adv. contact Cheri Mertins. **Subscr. to:** Allen Press Inc., PO Box 1897, Lawrence, KS 66044-8897.

615.9 NLD ISSN 1382-6689
RA1226 CODEN: ETOPFR

ENVIRONMENTAL TOXICOLOGY AND PHARMACOLOGY. Text in English. 1992; N.S. 1996. 6/yr. EUR 821 in Europe to institutions; JPY 136,100 in Japan to institutions; USD 1,146 elsewhere to institutions (effective 2002). abstr. back issues avail. *Refereed.* **Document type:** *Academic/Scholarly.* **Description:** Publishes research in mechanistic studies concerning the toxic effects in man and vertebrate animals of drugs and environmental contaminants.

Formerly (until 1996): European Journal of Pharmacology. Environmental Toxicology and Pharmacology Section (0926-6917)

Related titles: Microform ed.: N.S. (from PQC); Online - full text ed.: N.S. (from ingenta, Swets Blackwell, ScienceDirect, Institute for Scientific Information).

Indexed: ASCA, Aqua.Sci.& Fish.Abstr., BBCI, Biol.Abstr., Cal.Tiss.Abstr., Chem.Abstr., Chem.Indus.Notes, Chem.Titles, Curr.Cont., Derwent Biotech.Abstr., Environ.Per.Bibl., Environ.Sci.Poll.Mgmt., Excerp.Med. (1993-), Ind.Med. (coverage dropped), Ind.Sci.Rev., Inpharma, Int.Abstr.Biol.Sci., Neurosci.Abstr. (coverage dropped), Neurosci.Cit.Ind., Nutr.Abstr., Pharm.&Out.News, Pollut.Abstr., Reac., Rev.Appl.Entomol., Rev.Med.& Vet.Mycol., Risk Abstr., Saf.Sci.Abstr., Sci.Cit.Ind., Sel.Water Res.Abstr., Soyabean Abstr., THA, Tox.Abstr., Triticale Abstr., Weed Abstr.

—BLDSC (3791.785500), ADONIS, CASDDS, CISTI, EMDOCS, GNLM, IDS, Infotrieve, ingenta. **CCC.**

Published by: Elsevier Science BV, PO Box 211, Amsterdam 1000 AE, Netherlands. TEL 31-20-485-2911, FAX 31-20-485-2457, nlinfo-f@elsevier.nl, http://www.elsevier.com/locate/etap. Eds. J H Koeman, N P E Vermeulen. **Subscr. in Australasia and the Far East to:** Elsevier Science (Singapore) Pte Ltd, No.1 Temasek Ave, 17-01 Millenia Tower, Singapore 039192, Singapore. TEL 65-434-3727, FAX 65-337-2230; **Subscr. in Japan to:** Elsevier Science Inc - Japan Regional Office, 9-15 Higashi-Azabu 1-chome, Minato-ku, Tokyo 106-0044, Japan. TEL 81-3-5561-5033; **Subscr. in the Americas to:** Elsevier Science, PO Box 945, New York, NY 10159-0945. TEL 212-633-3730, FAX 212-633-3680.

615.902 NLD

ETHEL BROWNING'S TOXICITY AND METABOLISM OF INDUSTRIAL SOLVENTS. Text in English. 1987. irreg., latest vol.3, 1992. price varies. back issues avail. *Refereed.* **Document type:** *Monographic series, Academic/Scholarly.* **Description:** Reviews the environmental toxicity and metabolism of industrial solvents.

Published by: Elsevier Science BV, PO Box 211, Amsterdam 1000 AE, Netherlands. TEL 31-20-485-3757, 31-20-485-3911, FAX 31-20-485-3432, 31-20-485-3598, nlinfo-f@elsevier.nl; usinfo-f@elsevier.com; forinfo-kyf04035@niftyserve.or.jp, http://www.elsevier.nl/. **Subscr. in Australasia and the Far East to:** Elsevier Science (Singapore) Pte Ltd, No.1 Temasek Ave, 17-01 Millenia Tower, Singapore 039192, Singapore. TEL 65-434-3727, FAX 65-337-2230, asiainfo@elsevier.com.sg; **Subscr. in Japan to:** Elsevier Science Inc - Japan Regional Office, 9-15 Higashi-Azabu 1-chome, Minato-ku, Tokyo 106-0044, Japan. TEL 81-3-5561-5033, FAX 81-3-5561-5047, info@elsevier.co.jp; **Subscr. in the Americas to:** Elsevier Science, PO Box 2129, Marion, OH 43305-2129

EXCERPTA MEDICA. SECTION 30: CLINICAL AND EXPERIMENTAL PHARMACOLOGY. see *PHARMACY AND PHARMACOLOGY—Abstracting, Bibliographies, Statistics*

EXCERPTA MEDICA. SECTION 46: ENVIRONMENTAL HEALTH AND POLLUTION CONTROL. see *ENVIRONMENTAL STUDIES—Abstracting, Bibliographies, Statistics*

EXPERIMENTAL AND TOXICOLOGIC PATHOLOGY. see *MEDICAL SCIENCES*

571.95 363.7 GBR

FIBROUS MATERIALS IN THE ENVIRONMENT. Text in English. 1997. irreg. GBP 30 (effective 2000). **Document type:** *Monographic series, Academic/Scholarly.* **Description:** Reviews the likely public health impact of fibrous materials found in the built environment. Compiled with the assistance of the Building Research Establishment, sources and uses of both asbestos and man-made mineral fibers are described in detail, and an assessment of the evidence for health effects caused by these fibers are presented. Estimates are made of human exposure in buildings, including exposures arising on human health are evaluated. Finally, a number of strategies for managing fibrous materials are recommended.

Published by: Institute for Environment and Health, University of Leicester, 94 Regent Rd, Leicester, Leics LE1 7DD, United Kingdom. TEL 44-116-223-1600, FAX 44-116-223-1601, msto1@le.ac.uk, http://www.le.ac.uk/ieh/. R&P Ruth Gardener.

571.959 USA

FOCUS ON PESTICIDES. Text in English. irreg. **Document type:** *Bulletin.* **Description:** Summarizes topics regarding pesticide health risks, exposure and policy.

Related titles: Online - full text ed.

Published by: Environmental Advocates, 353 Hamilton St, Albany, NY 12210. TEL 518-462-5526, FAX 518-427-0381, webmistress@envadvocates.org, http://www.envadvocates.org.

615.9 USA ISSN 0899-7845
RM388

FOCUS ON PULMONARY PHARMACOLOGY AND TOXICOLOGY. Text in English. 1989. a.

—CISTI.

Published by: C R C Press, LLC, 2000 Corporate Blvd, N W, Boca Raton, FL 33431. TEL 561-994-0555, 800-272-7737, FAX 561-994-9784.

615.9 GBR ISSN 0278-6915
RA1190 CODEN: FCTOD7

FOOD AND CHEMICAL TOXICOLOGY. Text in English, French, German. 1963. m. EUR 247 in Europe to qualified personnel; JPY 32,800 in Japan to qualified personnel; USD 276 elsewhere to qualified personnel; EUR 1,931 in Europe to institutions; JPY 256,400 in Japan to institutions; USD 2,160 elsewhere to institutions (effective 2002). adv. bk.rev. charts, illus, abstr. index. back issues avail.; reprints avail. *Refereed.* **Document type:** *Academic/Scholarly.* **Description:** Reports of research on the metabolism and toxicology of foods and food additives, as well as studies of carcinogens, mutagens, and drug-nutrient interactions.

Formerly (until 1982): Food and Cosmetics Toxicology (0015-6264)

Related titles: Microfilm ed.: (from PQC); Online - full text ed.: (from ingenta, Swets Blackwell, ScienceDirect, Institute for Scientific Information).

E

Indexed: ASCA, Abstr.Hyg., AgBiotech, Agri.& Environ.Biotech.Abstr. (coverage dropped), Agricola, Anal.Abstr., Anim.Breed.Abstr., Aqua.Sci.& Fish.Abstr., Bibl.Agri., Biol.Abstr., CSNB, Chem.Abstr., Chem.Indus.Notes, Chem.Titles, Curr.Adv.Ecol.Sci., Curr.Cont., Curr.Pack.Abstr., Dairy Sci.Abstr., Dent.Ind., Derwent Biotech.Abstr., Dok.Arbeitsmed., Environ.Per.Bibl., Environ.Sci.Poll.Mgmt., Excerp.Med., Fababean Abstr., Field Crop Abstr., Food Sci.& Tech.Abstr., Hort.Abstr., INIS Atomind., Ind.Med. (1982-), Ind.Sci.Rev., Ind.Vet., Inpharma, Int.Abstr.Biol.Sci., Lab.Haz.Bull., Maize Abstr., Mass Spectr.Bull., Microbiol.Abstr., NRN, Nutr.Abstr., Packag.Sci.Tech., Pig News & Info., Pollut.Abstr., Postharvest, Potato Abstr., Poult.Abstr., Reac., Rev.Appl.Entomol., Rev.Arom.& Med.Plants, Rev.Med.& Vet.Mycol., Rev.Plant Path., Risk Abstr., SSCI (coverage dropped), Saf.Sci.Abstr., Sci.Cit.Ind., Sel.Water Res.Abstr., Soyabean Abstr., Sugar Ind.Abstr., Tox.Abstr., Triticale Abstr., Vet.Bull., W.R.C.Inf., Weed Abstr., World Surf.Coat.
—BLDSC (3977.026900), ADONIS, CASDDS, CISTI, EMDOCS, GNLM, IDS, ingenta, Linda Hall. **CCC.**
Published by: (British Industrial Biological Research Association), Pergamon (Subsidiary of: Elsevier Science), The Boulevard, Langford Ln, East Park, Kidlington, Oxford OXB 1GB, United Kingdom. FAX 44-1865-843010, http://www.elsevier.com/locate/foodchemtox. Eds. F Borzelleca, H Verhagen. Circ: 1,900. **Subscr. in Australasia and the Far East to:** Elsevier Science (Singapore) Pte Ltd, No.1 Temasek Ave, 17-01 Millenia Tower, Singapore 039192, Singapore. TEL 65-434-3727, FAX 65-337-2230; **Subscr. in the Americas to:** Elsevier Science, PO Box 945, New York, NY 10159-0945. TEL 212-633-3730, FAX 212-633-3680, usinfo-f@elsevier.com; **Subscr. to:** Elsevier Science BV, PO Box 211, Amsterdam 1000 AE, Netherlands. TEL 31-20-485-3757.

FOOD & WATER JOURNAL. see *CONSUMER EDUCATION AND PROTECTION*

FORSKNINGSCENTER RISOE. AARSBERETNING. see *ENERGY*

571.959 USA ISSN 1055-548X
SB950.9
GLOBAL PESTICIDE CAMPAIGNER✱ . Text in English. 1990. q. USD 25 to individuals; USD 50 to libraries; USD 100 to corporations. bk.rev. illus. reprints avail. **Document type:** *Bulletin.* **Description:** Provides information for the international pesticide reform movement. Brings together expert information and strategic ideas for environmental, public health, social justice and sustainable development advocacy.
Indexed: Alt.Press Ind., Ref.Zh.
Published by: Pesticide Action Network, North America Regional Center, 49 Powell St, 500, San Francisco, CA 94102-2811. TEL 415-541-9140, FAX 415-541-9253, panna@panna.org, http://www.panna.org/panna. Ed., R&P Ellen Hickey. Circ: 1,800.

571.95 351 USA
GULF WAR REVIEW; information for veterans who served in Desert Shield - Desert Storm. Text in English. 1992. irreg., latest vol.9, no.2, 2001 (approx. 4/yr.). free per issue. back issues avail. **Document type:** *Newsletter, Government.* **Description:** Addresses the concerns of U.S. veterans of the Persian Gulf War, along with those of their families and others interested in the possible long-term health implications of exposure to various potential environmental hazards during their tour of duty. Describes the actions the Department of Veterans Affairs and other agencies are taking in response to these concerns.
Formerly: Persian Gulf Review
Published by: U.S. Department of Veterans Affairs, Environmental Agents Service - 131, V A Headquarters, 810 Vermont Ave, N W, Washington, DC 20420. TEL 202-273-8580. Ed. Donald J Rosenblum.

344.0462 363.725 BEL
HANDHAVINGSZAKBOEKJE. Text in Dutch. biennial. BEF 1,295 (effective 2002). **Document type:** *Trade, Government.* **Description:** Comprehensive treatment of the legal code pertaining to waste management, with additional useful information.
Formerly: Afvalvademecum
Published by: Kluwer Belgie (Subsidiary of: Wolters Kluwer N.V.), Santvoortbeeklaan 21-25, Antwerp 2100, Belgium. info@kluwer.be, http://www.kluwer.be. Eds. Frans Geysels, Jan Vanheule, Rudy Meeuws.

363.7 388.324 USA
HAZARDOUS MATERIALS REGULATION GUIDE. Text in English. 1977. s-a. USD 199 (effective 2001). **Document type:** *Trade.* **Description:** Reference guide covering hazardous materials regulations.
Formerly: Hazardous Regulation Guide
Published by: J.J. Keller & Associates, Inc., 3003 W Breezewood Lane, Box 368, Neenah, WI 54957-0368. TEL 800-327-6868, FAX 800-727-7516, sales@jjkeller.com, http://www.jjkeller.com. Ed. Webb Shaw. Pub. John J Keller.

HAZARDOUS SUBSTANCES & PUBLIC HEALTH. see *PUBLIC HEALTH AND SAFETY*

HAZARDOUS WASTE REGULATORY ANALYSIS SERVICE. see *ENVIRONMENTAL STUDIES—Waste Management*

363.7 GBR ISSN 1353-1638
HEALTH, SAFETY AND ENVIRONMENT BULLETIN. Text in English. 1976. m. GBP 235; GBP 250 foreign. reprint service avail. from PQC. **Document type:** *Trade.* **Description:** Covers topics in occupational and environmental health and safety.
Incorporates in part (in 1995): Health and Safety Bulletin (1358-2208); Which was formerly (until 1994): Health and Safety Information Bulletin (0142-9086)
Related titles: ♦ Supplement: Environment Information Bulletin. ISSN 0964-5322.
Indexed: Br.Ceram.Abstr., CSNB, Cadscan, Euro.LJI, INIS Atomind., LJI, L.R.I. (Jan.1995-), Lab.Haz.Bull., Lead Abstr., Mgmt.& Market.Abstr., World Surf.Coat., Zincscan.
—BLDSC (4274.844100).
Published by: Eclipse Group Ltd., Industrial Relations Services, 18 Highbury Park, London N5 2AB, United Kingdom. TEL 44-20-7354-5858, FAX 44-207-226-8618.

615.9 GBR ISSN 0960-3271
RA1190 CODEN: HETOEA
HUMAN & EXPERIMENTAL TOXICOLOGY; an international journal. Text in English. 1981. m. GBP 319 in Europe to individuals; USD 458 in North America to individuals; GBP 322 rest of world to individuals; GBP 551 in Europe to institutions; USD 791 in North America to institutions; GBP 557 rest of world to institutions; GBP 255 in Europe to members of BTS, SOT; USD 366 in North America to members of BTS, SOT; GBP 258 rest of world to members of BTS, SOT; GBP 278 in developing nations; GBP 60 newsstand/cover in Europe; USD 87 newsstand/cover in North America; GBP 64 newsstand/cover rest of world (effective 2002). adv. index. back issues avail.; reprints avail. *Refereed.* **Document type:** *Journal, Academic/Scholarly.* **Description:** Covers all aspects of experimental and clinical studies of functional, biochemical and structural disorder, their causes and antidotes and other therapies using animal and human tissue, in vitro systems and medical and veterinary patients.
Formerly: Human Toxicology (0144-5952)
Related titles: Microform ed.: (from PQC); Online - full text ed.: GBP 385 (effective 1999) (from EBSCO Publishing, O C L C Online Computer Library Center, Inc., RoweCom Information Quest, ingenta, Swets Blackwell, Institute for Scientific Information).
Indexed: ASCA, Abstr.Hyg., Chem.Abstr., Chem.Indus.Notes, Chem.Titles, Crop Physiol.Abstr., Curr.Adv.Ecol.Sci., Curr.Adv.Gen.& Molec.Biol., Curr.Cont., Dairy Sci.Abstr., Dent.Ind., Dok.Arbeitsmed., Energy Ind., Energy Info.Abstr., Environ.Sci.Poll.Mgmt., Excerp.Med., Field Crop Abstr., INIS Atomind., Ind.Med. (1990-), Ind.Sci.Rev., Ind.Vet., Inpharma, Int.Abstr.Biol.Sci., Lab.Haz.Bull., Microbiol.Abstr., NRN, Neurosci.Abstr., Nutr.Abstr., Pharm.&Out.News, Pollut.Abstr., Reac., Ref.Zh., Rev.Appl.Entomol., Rev.Arom.& Med.Plants, Rev.Med.& Vet.Mycol., Risk Abstr., Saf.Sci.Abstr., Sci.Cit.Ind., Small Anim.Abstr., Tox.Abstr., Trop.Dis.Bull., Vet.Bull., Weed Abstr.
—BLDSC (4335.973000), CASDDS, CISTI, GNLM, IDS, ingenta, KNAW. **CCC.**
Published by: (British Toxicology Society), Arnold Publishers (Subsidiary of: Hodder Headline plc.), 338 Euston Rd, London NW1 3BH, United Kingdom. TEL 44-20-7873-6337, FAX 44-20-7873-6325, arnoldjournals@hodder.co.uk, http://www.arnoldpublishers.com/journals/Journpages/09603271.htm, http://www.arnoldpublishers.com/journals/journtitles.htm. Eds. A Wallace Hayes, Robert Kroes.

I E H ASSESSMENT INDOOR AIR QUALITY IN THE HOME: CARBON MONOXIDE. see *ENVIRONMENTAL STUDIES—Pollution*

571.95 614.85 614.4 GBR
▼ **I E H REPORT ON APPROACHES TO PREDICTING TOXICITY FROM OCCUPATIONAL EXPOSURE TO DUSTS.** Text in English. 1999. irreg. GBP 25 (effective 2000). **Document type:** *Monographic series, Academic/Scholarly.* **Description:** Addresses the scientific and medical uncertainties that are emerging in current risk assessments of the so-called "low toxicity" dusts encountered in the working environment. Individual articles are written by acknowledged international experts, who contributed to an overview of the current situation and the recommendations for future research.
Published by: Institute for Environment and Health, University of Leicester, 94 Regent Rd, Leicester, Leics LE1 7DD, United Kingdom. TEL 44-116-223-1600, FAX 44-116-223-1601, msto1@le.ac.uk, http://www.le.ac.uk/ieh/. Eds. Len Levy, Linda Shuker. R&P Ruth Gardener.

571.95 GBR
▼ **I E H REPORT ON BENZENE IN THE ENVIRONMENT.** Text in English. 1999. irreg. GBP 15 (effective 2000). **Document type:** *Monographic series, Academic/Scholarly.* **Description:** The aim of this report was to look at available data on contemporary sources and population exposure to benzene in the UK, together with information on the known human health effects (in particular leukemia), and assess any likely risks. The report summarizes and presents all the relevant data and provides an overall evaluation of the risks to public health of benzene in the environment.
Published by: Institute for Environment and Health, University of Leicester, 94 Regent Rd, Leicester, Leics LE1 7DD, United Kingdom. TEL 44-116-223-1600, FAX 44-116-223-1601, msto1@le.ac.uk, http://www.le.ac.uk/ieh/.

571.95 363.1791 GBR
I E H REPORT ON FACTORS AFFECTING THE ABSORPTION OF TOXIC METALS FROM THE DIET. Text in English. 1998. irreg. GBP 14 (effective 2000). **Document type:** *Monographic series, Academic/Scholarly.* **Description:** Aimed at individuals or groups involved in risk assessment of metals, especially from the diet. In particular, systematic reviews of the evidence for the effects of a number of factors on uptake of four metals, lead, cadmium, mercury and arsenic, from the gastrointestinal tract including: dose and speciation, other nutrients and constituents of the diet; pregnancy and lactation; extremities of age. medication; and gastrointestinal microflora are presented.
Published by: Institute for Environment and Health, University of Leicester, 94 Regent Rd, Leicester, Leics LE1 7DD, United Kingdom. TEL 44-116-223-1600, FAX 44-116-223-1601, msto1@le.ac.uk, http://www.le.ac.uk/ieh/. R&P Ruth Gardener.

616.8 571.95 GBR
I E H REPORT ON PERINATEL DEVELOPMENTAL NEUROTOXCITY. Text in English. 1997. irreg. GBP 25 (effective 2000). **Document type:** *Monographic series, Academic/Scholarly.* **Description:** An IEH workshop was recently held under the MRC's Neurosciences Approach to Human Health initiative. This report is based on the workshop and provides information on the state of understanding of developmental neurotoxicology, key research questions and research needs.
Published by: Institute for Environment and Health, University of Leicester, 94 Regent Rd, Leicester, Leics LE1 7DD, United Kingdom. TEL 44-116-223-1600, FAX 44-116-223-1601, msto1@le.ac.uk, http://www.le.ac.uk/ieh/. R&P Ruth Gardener.

363.1791 616.15 614.4 GBR
▼ **I E H REPORT ON U K BLOOD LEAD SURVEYS.** Text in English. 1999. irreg. GBP 25 (effective 2000). **Document type:** *Monographic series, Academic/Scholarly.* **Description:** Presents findings from part of the Health Survey for England 1995 that investigated blood lead levels, and the possible association of blood lead level and blood pressure. Recommendations are made for further research in a number of areas, particularly that of exposure measurements.
Published by: Institute for Environment and Health, University of Leicester, 94 Regent Rd, Leicester, Leics LE1 7DD, United Kingdom. TEL 44-116-223-1600, FAX 44-116-223-1601, msto1@le.ac.uk, http://www.le.ac.uk/ieh/. R&P Ruth Gardener.

I E H SPECIAL REPORT ON ORGANOPHOSPHORUS ESTERS; an evaluation of chronic neurotoxic effects. see *CHEMISTRY—Organic Chemistry*

E

I M O - U N E P GUIDELINES ON OIL SPILL DISPERSENT APPLICATION; including environmental considerations. see *ENVIRONMENTAL STUDIES—Pollution*

615.902 GBR
I U P A C SERIES ON ANALYTICAL AND PHYSICAL CHEMISTRY OF ENVIRONMENTAL SYSTEMS. Text in English. irreg., latest vol.5, 1998. **Document type:** *Monographic series, Academic/Scholarly.*
Indexed: GeoRef, Mass Spectr.Bull.
—BLDSC (4588.961000).
Published by: (International Union of Pure and Applied Chemistry USA), John Wiley & Sons Ltd., Baffins Ln, Chichester, Sussex PO19 IUD, United Kingdom. cs-books@wiley.co.uk, http://www.wiley.co.uk. Eds. Herman van Leeuwen, Jacques Buffle. **Subscr. in the Americas to:** John Wiley & Sons, Inc., Journals, 605 Third Ave, New York, NY 10158. TEL 44-1243-779777, 212-850-6645, FAX 212-850-6021, http://www.wiley.co.uk; **Subscr. to:** TEL 44-1243-779777, 212-850-6645, FAX 44-1243-843232, http://www.wiley.co.uk.

615.9 IND ISSN 0971-8613
INDUSTRIAL TOXICOLOGY RESEARCH CENTRE. ANNUAL REPORT. Text in English. 1966. a.
Formerly: Industrial Toxicology Research Centre. Scientific Report (0970-4469)
—BLDSC (1302.487220).
Published by: Industrial Toxicology Research Centre, Mahatma Gandhi Marg, P O Box 80, Lucknow, Uttar Pradesh 226 001, India. TEL 91-522-220107, FAX 91-522-228227, intox@itrc.sirnetd.ernet.in. Pub. P K Seth.

615.9 USA ISSN 0895-8378
CODEN: INHTE5
INHALATION TOXICOLOGY. Text in English. 1989. m. GBP 219, USD 362 to individuals; GBP 552, USD 910 to institutions (effective 2002). reprint service avail. from PQC. *Refereed.* **Document type:** *Academic/Scholarly.* **Description:** Presents the latest advances in all aspects of pulmonary toxicology.
Related titles: Microform ed.: (from PQC); Online - full text ed.: ISSN 1091-7691 (from CatchWord Ltd., EBSCO Publishing, O C L C Online Computer Library Center, Inc., RoweCom Information Quest, Swets Blackwell, Institute for Scientific Information).
Indexed: ASCA, CSNB, Chem.Abstr., Chem.Indus.Notes, Chem.Titles, Curr.Cont., Environ.Abstr., Environ.Sci.Poll.Mgmt., Ind.Med. (1989-), Ind.Sci.Rev., Inpharma, Int.Abstr.Biol.Sci., Lab.Haz.Bull., Pollut.Abstr., Reac., Risk Abstr., Saf.Sci.Abstr., Sci.Cit.Ind.
—BLDSC (4513.340800), CASDDS, CatchWord, CIS, EMDOCS, GNLM, IDS, Infotrieve, KNAW. **CCC.**
Published by: Taylor & Francis Ltd. (Subsidiary of: Taylor & Francis Group), 325 Chestnut St, Suite 800, Philadelphia, PA 19016. TEL 215-625-8900, FAX 215-625-2940, info@taylorandfrancis.com, http://www.taylorandfrancis.com/. Ed. Donald E Gardner. **Subscr. addr. in Europe:** Taylor & Francis Group, Journals Customer Service, Rankine Rd, Basingstoke, Hants RG24 8PR, United Kingdom. TEL 44-1256-813000, FAX 44-1256-479438, enquiry@tanf.co.uk, http://www.tandf.co.uk/journals.

INTERNATIONAL JOURNAL OF CLINICAL PHARMACOLOGY AND THERAPEUTICS. see *PHARMACY AND PHARMACOLOGY*

615.9 GBR ISSN 1091-5818
RA1190 CODEN: IJTOFN
INTERNATIONAL JOURNAL OF TOXICOLOGY. Text in English. 1982. bi-m. GBP 208, USD 343 to individuals; GBP 294, USD 485 to institutions (effective 2002). adv. *Refereed.* **Document type:** *Academic/Scholarly.* **Description:** Includes safety evaluation and risk assessment, carcinogenesis, mechanisms of toxicity, quality assurance, and general, developmental, reproductive, clinical, genetic, forensic, immuno-, and veterinary toxicology.
Formerly (until 1997): American College of Toxicology. Journal (0730-0913); Incorporates: Acute Toxicity Data (1044-2049)
Related titles: Online - full text ed.: ISSN 1092-874X (from CatchWord Ltd., EBSCO Publishing, O C L C Online Computer Library Center, Inc., RoweCom Information Quest, Swets Blackwell, Institute for Scientific Information).
Indexed: ASCA, Aqua.Sci.& Fish.Abstr., CSNB, Chem.Abstr., Chem.Indus.Notes, Chem.Titles, Curr.Adv.Ecol.Sci., Curr.Cont. (coverage dropped), Energy Info.Abstr., Environ.Abstr., Environ.Sci.Poll.Mgmt., Excerp.Med., Ind.Med., Ind.Sci.Rev., Int.Abstr.Biol.Sci., Lab.Haz.Bull., NRN, Pollut.Abstr., Risk Abstr., Saf.Sci.Abstr., Sci.Cit.Ind. (coverage dropped), Tox.Abstr.
—BLDSC (4542.695830), CASDDS, CatchWord, CISTI, EMDOCS, GNLM, IDS, Infotrieve, KNAW. **CCC.**
Published by: (American College of Toxicology), Taylor & Francis Group, Taylor & Francis Ltd., 11 New Fetter Ln, London EC4P 4EE, United Kingdom. TEL 44-20-7583-9855, FAX 44-20-7842-2298, info@tandf.co.uk, http://www.tandf.co.uk. Ed. Harihara M Mehendale. **Subscr. in N. America to:** Taylor & Francis Ltd., 325 Chestnut St, Suite 800, Philadelphia, PA 19016. TEL 800-354-1420, FAX 215-625-8914, info@taylorandfrancis.com, http://www.taylorandfrancis.com/.

ISSUES IN NUTRITION AND TOXICOLOGY SERIES. see *NUTRITION AND DIETETICS*

571.95 BEL
J A C C REPORT. (Joint Assessment of Commodity Chemicals) Text in English. 1983. irreg., latest vol.40, 2001. EUR 125 per vol. to non-members. back issues avail. *Refereed.* **Document type:** *Monographic series, Academic/Scholarly.*
Published by: European Centre for Ecotoxicology and Toxicology of Chemicals, Ave E Van Nieuwenhuyse 4, Bte 6, Brussels 1160, Belgium. TEL 32-2-675-3600, FAX 32-2-675-3625, info@ecetoc.org, http://www.ecetoc.org/pages/Publications.cfm.

577.27 JPN ISSN 0918-1091
J E T O C INFORMATION SHEET. Text in English. 1991. q. **Document type:** *Newsletter.*
Published by: Japan Chemical Industry Ecology - Toxicology Information Center/Nihon Kagaku Busshitsu Anzen Joho Senta, 19-4 Nishi-Shinbashi 1-chome, Minato-ku, Tokyo 105-0003, Japan. TEL 81-3-3593-1190, FAX 81-3-3593-1166, http://www.jetoc.or.jp. Ed. Takao Sawada.

JAPANESE JOURNAL OF FORENSIC TOXICOLOGY/HO CHUDOKU. see *MEDICAL SCIENCES—Forensic Sciences*

615.9 JPN ISSN 0914-3777
JAPANESE JOURNAL OF TOXICOLOGY/CHUDOKU KENKYU. Text in English, Japanese. 1988. 4/yr. JPY 1,500 per issue.
Indexed: Ind.Med., Inpharma, Pharm.&Out.News, Reac.
—BLDSC (4658.904000), GNLM.
Published by: (Japanese Association of Clinical Toxicology/Yakuji Kenkyukai), Yakugyo Jiho Co. Ltd., 2-36 Kanda-Jinbo-cho, Chiyoda-ku, Tokyo 101-0051, Japan.

615.9 USA ISSN 0146-4760
RA1221 CODEN: JATOD3
JOURNAL OF ANALYTICAL TOXICOLOGY. Text in English. 1977. 8/yr. USD 375 domestic; USD 395 foreign (effective 2001). adv. bk.rev. charts, illus. index. back issues avail.; reprints avail. *Refereed.* **Document type:** *Journal, Academic/Scholarly.* **Description:** Publishes all new product and literature descriptions that are applicable to the field, and contains articles submitted by research and technical staff chemists.
Related titles: Microfiche ed.; Microfilm ed.: (from MML); Online - full text ed.: (from ingenta, Institute for Scientific Information).
Indexed: ASCA, Anal.Abstr., Aqua.Sci.& Fish.Abstr., Biol.Abstr., CSNB, Chem.Abstr., Chem.Cit.Ind., Chem.Indus.Notes, Chem.Titles, Chromat.Abstr., Curr.Cont., Dairy Sci.Abstr., Dent.Ind., Environ.Sci.Poll.Mgmt., Excerp.Med., Food Sci.& Tech.Abstr., HRIS, INIS Atomind., Ind.Med. (1977-), Ind.Sci.Rev., Ind.Vet., Inpharma, Int.Abstr.Biol.Sci., Mass Spectr.Bull., Microbiol.Abstr., Nutr.Abstr., Pharm.&Out.News, Pollut.Abstr., Reac., Ref.Zh., Rev.Appl.Entomol., Rev.Med.& Vet.Mycol., Risk Abstr., Saf.Sci.Abstr., Sci.Cit.Ind., Sel.Water Res.Abstr., Small Anim.Abstr., Tox.Abstr., Vet.Bull., Weed Abstr.
—BLDSC (4928.700000), CASDDS, CISTI, GNLM, IDS, ingenta, Linda Hall. **CCC.**
Published by: Preston Publications, Inc., 6600 W Touhy Ave, Box 48312, Niles, IL 60714. http://www.jatox.com/, http://www.prestonpub.com/. Ed. Dr. Bruce Goldberger. Pub., Adv. contact S Tinsley Preston TEL 847-647-2900 ext 333. R&Ps Janice Gordon TEL 847-647-2900 ext 321, Kevin Bailey TEL 847-647-2900 ext 302. B&W page USD 530, color page USD 1,330. Circ: 1,100 (paid).

615.9 GBR ISSN 0260-437X
RA1190 CODEN: JJATDK
JOURNAL OF APPLIED TOXICOLOGY. Text in English. 1981. bi-m. USD 1,425 in United States; USD 1,425 in Canada & Mexico; USD 1,425 elsewhere; USD 1,497 combined subscription in United States for print and online eds.; USD 1,497 combined subscription in Canada & Mexico for print and online eds.; USD 1,497 combined subscription elsewhere for print and online eds. (effective 2002). adv. bk.rev. index. back issues avail.; reprint service avail. from SWZ. *Refereed.* **Document type:** *Academic/Scholarly.* **Description:** Encompasses, but is not limited to, the study of the toxic effects of chemicals and materials in the field of teratology, reproduction, mutagenesis, carcinogenesis, health, the environment, pathology, pharmacokinetics and biochemical mechanisms.
Related titles: Microform ed.: (from PQC); Online - full text ed.: ISSN 1099-1263. 1997. USD 1,425 in United States; USD 1,425 in Canada & Mexico; USD 1,425 elsewhere (effective 2002) (from EBSCO Publishing, Wiley InterScience, Institute for Scientific Information).
Indexed: AESIS, ASCA, Aqua.Sci.& Fish.Abstr., CSNB, Chem.Abstr., Chem.Indus.Notes, Chem.Titles, Curr.Adv.Cancer Res., Curr.Adv.Gen.& Molec.Biol., Curr.Cont., Dok.Arbeitsmed., Energy Info.Abstr., Environ.Abstr., Environ.Per.Bibl. (1990-), Environ.Sci.Poll.Mgmt., Excerp.Med., Ind.Hyg.Dig., Ind.Med. (1981-), Ind.Sci.Rev., Inpharma, Int.Abstr.Biol.Sci., Lab.Haz.Bull., NRN, Neurosci.Abstr., Petrol.Abstr. (coverage dropped), Pharm.&Out.News, Pollut.Abstr., Reac., Rev.Appl.Entomol., Risk Abstr., Saf.Sci.Abstr., Sci.Cit.Ind., Sport Fish.Abstr., Tox.Abstr., Wild.Rev., World Surf.Coat.
—BLDSC (4947.130000), CASDDS, CISTI, EMDOCS, GNLM, IDS, ingenta, Linda Hall. **CCC.**
Published by: Wiley Europe Ltd., Baffins Ln, Chichester, W Sussex PO19 1UD, United Kingdom. TEL 44-1243-779777, FAX 44-1243-775878, customer@wiley.co.uk, http://www.interscience.wiley.com/jpages/0260-437X/, http://www.wiley.co.uk. Ed. Harry Salem TEL 410-436-3034. adv.: B&W page GBP 750, color page GBP 1,650; trim 210 x 297. Circ: 500. **Subscr. in the Americas to:** John Wiley & Sons, Inc., Journals, 605 Third Ave, New York, NY 10158. TEL 212-850-6021, 212-850-6645, subinfo@jwiley.com.

577.27 IND ISSN 0971-0965
CODEN: JEEMEJ
JOURNAL OF ECOTOXICOLOGY & ENVIRONMENTAL MONITORING; an international journal for scientific research on toxicology and pollution. Text in English. 1991. q., latest vol.11, 2001. INR 600 domestic to institutions; USD 250 foreign to institutions (effective 2001). adv. bk.rev. charts, illus, abstr, bibl. indexed in many leading abstracting. 80 p./no. 10 cols./p. back issues avail. *Refereed.* **Document type:** *Journal, Academic/Scholarly.* **Description:** Reports laboratory and field researches pertaining to toxicology and environmental pollution.
Indexed: Agroforest.Abstr., Aqua.Sci.& Fish.Abstr., Bio-Contr.News & Info., Crop Physiol.Abstr., Dairy Sci.Abstr., Entomol.Abstr., Environ.Sci.Poll.Mgmt., Field Crop Abstr., Forest.Abstr., Helminthol.Abstr., Hort.Abstr., Ind.Vet., Maize Abstr., Microbiol.Abstr., Nutr.Abstr., Plant Breed.Abstr., Pollut.Abstr., Postharvest, Rev.Appl.Entomol., Rev.Med.& Vet.Mycol., Rev.Plant Path., Rice Abstr., Risk Abstr., Saf.Sci.Abstr., Seed Abstr., Sel.Water Res.Abstr., Soils & Fert., Soyabean Abstr., Sugar Ind.Abstr., Tox.Abstr., Triticale Abstr., Weed Abstr., Zoo.Rec.
—BLDSC (4973.095800), CASDDS, ingenta, Linda Hall.
Published by: Palani Paramount Publications, 57, Anna Nagar, Palani, Tamil Nadu 624 602, India. TEL 91-04545-42332, FAX 91-04545-45919, spalani1@md4.vsnl.net.in. Ed., R&P S Palanichamy. Adv. contact P Sarojini. page USD 125. Circ: 400. **Dist. by:** H P C Publishers Distributors Pvt. Ltd., 1st Fl., Flats 1 & 2, Darya Ganj, 4805-24 Bharat Ram Rd., New Delhi 110 002, India. TEL 91-11-325-4401, FAX 91-11-619- 511.

JOURNAL OF ENVIRONMENTAL MEDICINE. see *MEDICAL SCIENCES*

615.9 USA ISSN 0731-8898
RA1190 CODEN: JEPOEC
JOURNAL OF ENVIRONMENTAL PATHOLOGY, TOXICOLOGY AND ONCOLOGY. Text in English. 1981. q. USD 94 to individuals; USD 397 to institutions (effective 2000). adv. bk.rev. index. back issues avail. *Refereed.* **Document type:** *Academic/Scholarly.* **Description:** Provides an international forum for works that relate to toxicology, pathology and oncology.
Formerly: Journal of Environmental Pathology and Toxicology (0146-4779)
Related titles: Microfiche ed.

E

Indexed: Aqua.Sci.& Fish.Abstr., Chem.Abstr., Chem.Indus.Notes, Chem.Titles, Curr.Adv.Cancer Res., Curr.Cont. (coverage dropped), Dok.Arbeitsmed., Environ.Per.Bibl. (1993-), Environ.Sci.Poll.Mgmt., Excerp.Med., GeoRef, INIS Atomind., Ind.Med. (1984-), Ind.Sci.Rev., Ind.Vet., Int.Abstr.Biol.Sci., Microbiol.Abstr., Ocean.Abstr. (coverage dropped), Pollut.Abstr., Rev.Plant Path., Risk Abstr., Saf.Sci.Abstr., Sel.Water Res.Abstr., Soils & Fert., Sport Fish.Abstr., Vet.Bull., Wild.Rev., Zoo.Rec.
—BLDSC (4979.384400), CASDDS, CISTI, EMDOCS, GNLM, ingenta, KNAW. **CCC.**
Published by: (International Society for Environmental Toxicology and Cancer), Begell House Inc., 79 Madison Ave, Ste 1205, New York, NY 10016-7892. TEL 212-725-1999, FAX 212-213-8368, begellhouse@worldnet.att.net, orders@begellhouse.com. Ed. Edgar M Moran. Circ: 1,000.

363.72 USA ISSN 1093-4529
TD1 CODEN: JESHE6
JOURNAL OF ENVIRONMENTAL SCIENCE AND HEALTH. PART A: TOXIC HAZARDOUS SUBSTANCES AND ENVIRONMENTAL ENGINEERING. Text in English. 1966. 10/yr. USD 225 to individuals print & online eds.; USD 1,650 to institutions print only (effective 2002). *Refereed.* **Document type:** *Academic/Scholarly.* **Description:** Offers answers to serious contemporary environmental issues.
Former titles: Journal of Environmental Science and Health. Part A: Environmental Science and Engineering and Toxicology (1077-1204); Journal of Environmental Science and Health. Part A: Environmental Science and Engineering (0360-1226); Supersedes in part: Environmental Letters (0013-9300)
Related titles: Microform ed.: (from RPI); Online - full content ed.; Online - full text ed.: (from Institute for Scientific Information, RoweCom Information Quest).
Indexed: ASCA, Agri.Eng.Abstr., Anal.Abstr., Anim.Breed.Abstr., Aqua.Sci.& Fish.Abstr., Aquacult.Abstr., Bibl.Agri., Bioeng.Abstr., Biol.Abstr., Cadscan, Chem.Abstr., Chem.Cit.Ind., Chem.Indus.Notes, Chem.Titles, Crop Physiol.Abstr., Curr.Cont., Dairy Sci.Abstr., Energy Info.Abstr., Energy Rev., Eng.Ind., Environ.Abstr., Environ.Ind., Environ.Per.Bibl. (1977-), Environ.Sci.Poll.Mgmt., Excerp.Med., Field Crop Abstr., Forest Prod.Abstr., Forest.Abstr., GeoRef, Herb.Abstr., Hort.Abstr., INIS Atomind., Ind.Med., Ind.Sci.Rev., Ind.Vet., Int.Abstr.Biol.Sci., Irr.& Drain.Abstr., Lab.Haz.Bull., Lead Abstr., Maize Abstr., Microbiol.Abstr., NRN, Nutr.Abstr., Ocean.Abstr. (coverage dropped), Ornam.Hort., Plant Breed.Abstr., Plant Grow.Reg.Abstr., Pollut.Abstr., Poult.Abstr., Protozool.Abstr., Ref.Zh., Rev.Appl.Entomol., Rev.Plant Path., Rice Abstr., Risk Abstr., SSCI (coverage dropped), Saf.Sci.Abstr., Sci.Cit.Ind., Seed Abstr., Sel.Water Res.Abstr., Soils & Fert., Sport Fish.Abstr., Sugar Ind.Abstr., Tox.Abstr., Triticale Abstr., Trop.Dis.Bull., Vet.Bull., W.R.C.Inf., Weed Abstr., Wild.Rev., Zincscan, Zoo.Rec.
—BLDSC (4979.393300), CASDDS, CIS, CISTI, EMDOCS, GNLM, Infotrieve, ingenta, Linda Hall. **CCC.**
Published by: Marcel Dekker Inc., 270 Madison Ave, New York, NY 10016. TEL 212-696-9000, 800-228-1160, FAX 212-685-4540, http://www.dekker.com/servlet/product/productid/ESE. Ed. Shahamat U Khan. R&P Julia Mulligan. Adv. contact Diane Saulon. Circ: 300.

616.98 USA ISSN 1059-0501
RC268.5 CODEN: JSHREB
JOURNAL OF ENVIRONMENTAL SCIENCE AND HEALTH. PART C: ENVIRONMENTAL CARCINOGENESIS & ECOTOXICOLOGY REVIEWS. Key Title: Environmental Carcinogenesis & Ecotoxicology Reviews. Text in English. 1983. s-a. USD 60 to individuals print & online eds.; USD 550 to institutions print only (effective 2002). adv. *Refereed.* **Document type:** *Academic/Scholarly.* **Description:** Covers various areas of environmental carcinogenesis.
Former titles (until 1991): Environmental Carcinogenesis Reviews (0882-8164); (until 1984): Journal of Environmental Science and Health. Part C: Environmental Carcinogenesis Reviews (0736-3001); Journal of Environmental Science and Health. Part C: Environmental Health Sciences (0360-1242); Supersedes in part: Environmental Letters (0013-9300)
Related titles: Microform ed.: (from RPI); Online - full content ed.; Online - full text ed.: (from Institute for Scientific Information, RoweCom Information Quest).
Indexed: ASCA, Abstr.Hyg., Aqua.Sci.& Fish.Abstr., Cadscan, Chem.Abstr., Chem.Indus.Notes, Chem.Titles, Curr.Cont., Eng.Ind., Environ.Abstr., Environ.Per.Bibl. (1983-), Environ.Sci.Poll.Mgmt., Excerp.Med., Geo.Abstr.H.G., INIS Atomind., Ind.Sci.Rev., Inpharma, Int.Abstr.Biol.Sci., Lead Abstr., NRN, Pollut.Abstr., Reac., Ref.Zh., Sci.Cit.Ind., Sel.Water Res.Abstr., Tox.Abstr., Zincscan.
—BLDSC (4979.394300), CASDDS, CIS, CISTI, EMDOCS, GNLM, IDS, Infotrieve, ingenta, Linda Hall. **CCC.**
Published by: Marcel Dekker Inc., 270 Madison Ave, New York, NY 10016. TEL 212-696-9000, 800-228-1160, FAX 212-685-4540, http://www.dekker.com/servlet/product/productid/GNC. Ed. Yin Tak Woo. R&P Julia Mulligan. Adv. contact Diane Saulon. Circ: 250.

615.902 JPN ISSN 1344-9702
CODEN: JJTHEC
JOURNAL OF HEALTH SCIENCE/EISEI KAGAKU. Text in English. 1955. bi-m. USD 56 to members (effective 2001). adv. charts, stat. index. 100 p./no. back issues avail. *Refereed.* **Document type:** *Academic/Scholarly.* **Description:** Covers all aspects of health science.
Formerly (until 1998): Journal of Hygienic Chemistry / Eisei Kagaku (0013-273X); Which had variant title: Japanese Journal of Toxicology and Environmental Health / Koshu Eisei Nempo
Related titles: Online - full text ed.: (from Institute for Scientific Information).
Indexed: ASCA, Anal.Abstr., Aqua.Sci.& Fish.Abstr., Biol.Abstr., C.I.S. Abstr., Chem.Abstr., Chem.Indus.Notes, Chem.Titles, Curr.Adv.Ecol.Sci., Curr.Cont. (coverage dropped), Dairy Sci.Abstr., Environ.Sci.Poll.Mgmt., Excerp.Med., Food Sci.& Tech.Abstr., INIS Atomind., Ind.Med. (coverage dropped), Int.Abstr.Biol.Sci., Mass Spectr.Bull., Microbiol.Abstr., Nutr.Abstr., Pollut.Abstr., Rev.Appl.Entomol., Rev.Plant Path., Risk Abstr., Saf.Sci.Abstr., Seed Abstr., Sel.Water Res.Abstr., Soils & Fert., Sugar Ind.Abstr., Tox.Abstr., W.R.C.Inf., Weed Abstr.
—BLDSC (4996.870250), CASDDS, CISTI, GNLM, IDS, Infotrieve, KNAW. **CCC.**
Published by: Pharmaceutical Society of Japan/Nihon Yakugakkai, 2-12-15, Shibuya, Shibuya-ku, Tokyo 150-0002, Japan. TEL 81-3-3406-3321, FAX 81-3-3498-1835, ronb@pharm.or.jp, naganuma@mail.pharm.tohoku.ac.jp, http://jhs.pharm.or.jp. Ed. Manabu Kunimoto. Circ: 1,250 (controlled).

JOURNAL OF NATURAL TOXINS. see *PHARMACY AND PHARMACOLOGY*

615.9 USA ISSN 1056-8719
QP901 CODEN: JPTMEZ
JOURNAL OF PHARMACOLOGICAL AND TOXICOLOGICAL METHODS. Text in English. 1978. 6/yr. EUR 972 in Europe to institutions; JPY 129,000 in Japan to institutions; USD 1,086 elsewhere to institutions (effective 2002). abstr. back issues avail. *Refereed.* **Document type:** *Academic/Scholarly.* **Description:** Publishes original articles on current methods of investigation used in pharmacology and toxicology.
Formerly (until 1992): Journal of Pharmacological Methods (0160-5402)
Related titles: Microform ed.: (from PQC); Online - full text ed.: (from ingenta, ScienceDirect, Swets Blackwell, Institute for Scientific Information).
Indexed: ASCA, Agri.& Environ.Biotech.Abstr. (coverage dropped), Aqua.Sci.& Fish.Abstr., Biol.Abstr., Chem.Abstr., Chem.Indus.Notes, Chem.Titles, Compumath, Curr.Adv.Ecol.Sci., Curr.Cont., Dent.Ind., Derwent Biotech.Abstr., Environ.Sci.Poll.Mgmt., Excerp.Med., INIS Atomind., I.P.A., Ind.Med. (1992-), Ind.Sci.Rev., Inpharma, Int.Abstr.Biol.Sci., Neurosci.Abstr. (coverage dropped), Neurosci.Cit.Ind., Pollut.Abstr., Reac., Risk Abstr., Saf.Sci.Abstr., Sci.Cit.Ind., THA, Tox.Abstr.
—BLDSC (5032.650000), ADONIS, CASDDS, CISTI, EMDOCS, GNLM, IDS, Infotrieve, ingenta, KNAW, Linda Hall. **CCC.**
Published by: Elsevier Science, 655 Ave of the Americas, New York, NY 10010. TEL 212-989-5800, FAX 212-633-3990, usinfo-f@elsevier.com, http://www.elsevier.com/locate/jpharmtox. Eds. J H McNeill, P S Spencer. **Subscr. in Australasia and the Far East to:** Elsevier Science (Singapore) Pte Ltd, No.1 Temasek Ave, 17-01 Millenia Tower, Singapore 039192, Singapore. TEL 65-434-3727, FAX 65-337-2230; **Subscr. in Japan to:** Elsevier Science Inc - Japan Regional Office, 9-15 Higashi-Azabu 1-chome, Minato-ku, Tokyo 106-0044, Japan. TEL 81-3-5561-5033; **Subscr. outside the Americas to:** Elsevier Science BV, PO Box 211, Amsterdam 1000 AE, Netherlands. TEL 31-20-485-3757.

615.9 JPN ISSN 0914-9198
CODEN: JTPAE7
JOURNAL OF TOXICOLOGIC PATHOLOGY. Text in Japanese. s-a. **Document type:** *Academic/Scholarly.* **Description:** Publishes original papers, notes, and review articles from the members of the society.
Indexed: Chem.Abstr., Chem.Indus.Notes, Chem.Titles.
—BLDSC (5069.732000), CASDDS.
Published by: Japanese Society of Toxicologic Pathology, c/o Eisei Ishikawa, Ed., 3-25-8 Nishi-Shinbashi, Minato-ku, Tokyo 105-0000, Japan.

615.9 JPN ISSN 0388-1350
CODEN: JTSCDR
JOURNAL OF TOXICOLOGICAL SCIENCES. Text in English, Japanese. 1976. q. JPY 7,000. Supplement avail.
Indexed: Biol.Abstr., Chem.Abstr., Chem.Indus.Notes, Chem.Titles, Excerp.Med., INIS Atomind., Ind.Med. (1976-), Int.Abstr.Biol.Sci.
—BLDSC (5069.733000), CASDDS, CISTI, EMDOCS, GNLM, ingenta, KNAW. **CCC.**
Published by: Japanese Society of Toxicological Sciences/Nihon Doku Kagakkai, Gakkai CTR Bldg 4th Fl, 2-4-16 Yayoi, Bunkyo-ku, Tokyo 113-0032, Japan. TEL 03-3812-3093, FAX 03-3812-3552.

615.9 USA ISSN 1528-7394
RA1190 CODEN: JTEHD6
JOURNAL OF TOXICOLOGY AND ENVIRONMENTAL HEALTH. PART A. Text in English. 1975. s-m. GBP 688, USD 1,135 to individuals; GBP 1,602, USD 2,643 to institutions (effective 2002). adv. abstr, bibl, charts, illus. index. back issues avail.; reprint service avail. from PQC. *Refereed.* **Document type:** *Academic/Scholarly.* **Description:** Contains original research in environmental toxicology.
Supersedes in part (in 1998): Journal of Toxicology and Environmental Health (0098-4108)
Related titles: Microform ed.: (from PQC); Online - full text ed.: ISSN 1087-2620 (from CatchWord Ltd., EBSCO Publishing, Swets Blackwell, Institute for Scientific Information, RoweCom Information Quest).
Indexed: ASCA, Abstr.Hyg., AgBiotech, Agri.& Environ.Biotech.Abstr. (coverage dropped), Anim.Breed.Abstr., Aqua.Sci.& Fish.Abstr., Biol.Abstr., Biol.Dig., C.I.S. Abstr., CSNB, Cadscan, Chem.Abstr., Chem.Indus.Notes, Chem.Titles, Curr.Adv.Cell & Devel.Biol., Curr.Adv.Ecol.Sci., Curr.Cont., Dairy Sci.Abstr., Deep Sea Res.& Oceanogr.Abstr., Dent.Ind., Environ.Abstr., Environ.Ind., Environ.Per.Bibl. (1977-), Environ.Sci.Poll.Mgmt., Excerp.Med., Food Sci.& Tech.Abstr., Helminthol.Abstr., INIS Atomind., Ind.Hyg.Dig., Ind.Med. (1998-), Ind.Sci.Rev., Ind.Vet., Inpharma, Lab.Haz.Bull., Lead Abstr., Maize Abstr., NRN, Neurosci.Abstr., Neurosci.Cit.Ind., Nutr.Abstr., Ocean.Abstr., Pollut.Abstr., Poult.Abstr., Reac., Rev.Appl.Entomol., Rev.Med.& Vet.Mycol., Rev.Plant Path., Risk Abstr., Rural Recreat.Tour.Abstr., Saf.Sci.Abstr., Sci.Cit.Ind., Sel.Water Res.Abstr., Soyabean Abstr., Sport Fish.Abstr., Telegen, Trop.Dis.Bull., Trop.Oil Seeds Abstr., Vet.Bull., Weed Abstr., Wild.Rev., Zincscan, Zoo.Rec.
—BLDSC (5069.735100), ADONIS, CASDDS, CatchWord, CIS, CISTI, GNLM, IDS, ingenta. **CCC.**
Published by: Taylor & Francis Ltd. (Subsidiary of: Taylor & Francis Group), 325 Chestnut St, Suite 800, Philadelphia, PA 19016. TEL 215-625-8900, FAX 215-625-2940, info@taylorandfrancis.com, http://www.taylorandfrancis.com/. Ed. Sam Kacew. Circ: 1,000. **Subscr. addr. in Europe:** Taylor & Francis Group, Journals Customer Service, Rankine Rd, Basingstoke, Hants RG24 8PR, United Kingdom. TEL 44-1256-813000, FAX 44-1256-479438, enquiry@tanf.co.uk, http://www.tandf.co.uk/journals.

615.9 USA ISSN 1093-7404
RA1190 CODEN: JTEHD6
JOURNAL OF TOXICOLOGY AND ENVIRONMENTAL HEALTH. PART B: CRITICAL REVIEWS. Text in English. 1975. q. GBP 79, USD 130 to individuals; GBP 241, USD 397 to institutions (effective 2002). *Refereed.* **Document type:** *Academic/Scholarly.*
Supersedes in part (in 1998): Journal of Toxicology and Environmental Health (0098-4108)
Related titles: Online - full text ed.: ISSN 1521-6950 (from CatchWord Ltd., EBSCO Publishing, O C L C Online Computer Library Center, Inc., RoweCom Information Quest, Swets Blackwell, Institute for Scientific Information).
Indexed: Anim.Breed.Abstr., Aqua.Sci.& Fish.Abstr., CSNB, Chem.Indus.Notes, Curr.Cont., Environ.Sci.Poll.Mgmt., Ind.Med. (1998-), Neurosci.Abstr., Ocean.Abstr., Pollut.Abstr., Rev.Med.& Vet.Mycol., Saf.Sci.Abstr., Sci.Cit.Ind., Sel.Water Res.Abstr., Tox.Abstr.
—BLDSC (5069.735200), ADONIS, CASDDS, CatchWord, CIS, CISTI, GNLM, IDS, Infotrieve, ingenta. **CCC.**

E

Published by: Taylor & Francis Ltd. (Subsidiary of: Taylor & Francis Group), 325 Chestnut St, Suite 800, Philadelphia, PA 19016. TEL 215-625-8900, FAX 215-625-2940, info@taylorandfrancis.com, http://www.taylorandfrancis.com/. Ed. Sam Kacew. **Subscr. addr. in Europe:** Taylor & Francis Group, Journals Customer Service, Rankine Rd, Basingstoke, Hants RG24 8PR, United Kingdom. TEL 44-1256-813000, FAX 44-1256-479438, enquiry@tanf.co.uk, http://www.tandf.co.uk/journals.

JOURNAL OF TOXICOLOGY. CUTANEOUS AND OCULAR TOXICOLOGY. see *PHARMACY AND PHARMACOLOGY*

JOURNAL OF TOXICOLOGY. TOXIN REVIEWS. see *PHARMACY AND PHARMACOLOGY*

615.9 JPN ISSN 0914-4579
KIKANSHI J E T O C. Text in Japanese. 1980. m.
Published by: Japan Chemical Industry Ecology - Toxicology Information Center/Nihon Kagaku Busshitsu Anzen Joho Senta, 19-4 Nishi-Shinbashi 1-chome, Minato-ku, Tokyo 105-0003, Japan. TEL 81-3-3593-1190, FAX 81-3-3593-1166, http://www.jetoc.or.jp. Ed. Takao Sawada.

LACTIC ACID BACTERIA. see *BIOLOGY—Microbiology*

LAMY ENVIRONNEMENT L'EAU. see *LAW*

344.046 USA
LAW OF TOXIC TORTS. Text in English. base vol. plus irreg. updates. USD 686 (effective 2000). **Document type:** *Trade.* **Description:** Covers liability, litigation and major issues of toxic tort.
Published by: West Group (Subsidiary of: Thomson Corporation, The), 620 Opperman Dr., Eagan, MN 55123. TEL 800-344-5008, FAX 800-340-9378, http://www.westgroup.com.

LEAD ACTION NEWS. see *PUBLIC HEALTH AND SAFETY*

615.9 JPN
CODEN: MAIKD3
MAIKOTOKISHIN✶ /MYCOTOXINS. Text in English, Japanese; Summaries in English. 1975. s-a. JPY 4,000. adv. **Document type:** *Proceedings.*
Formerly (until no.37, 1993): Japanese Association of Mycotoxicology. Proceedings (0285-1466)
Indexed: Chem.Abstr., Chem.Titles, Food Sci.& Tech.Abstr., Postharvest, Rev.Appl.Entomol., Rev.Med.& Vet.Mycol., Rev.Plant Path.
—BLDSC (5995.762200), CASDDS.
Published by: Japanese Association of Mycotoxicology, Inohana 1-8-1, Chuo-ku, Chiba 260-8672, Japan. Ed. S Akao.

363.7 DEU ISSN 0936-4544
MESSUNG VON GEFAHRSTOFFEN. Text in German. 1989. irreg. DEM 268 (effective 2000). **Document type:** *Bulletin, Trade.*
Published by: Erich Schmidt Verlag GmbH & Co. (Berlin), Genthiner Str 30G, Berlin 10785, Germany. TEL 49-30-250085-0, FAX 49-30-25008511, esv@esvmedien.de, http://www.erich-schmidt-verlag.de.

615.9 USA ISSN 1063-3677
CODEN: MTTOEY
METHODS IN TOXICOLOGY. Text in English. 1993. irreg. **Document type:** *Monographic series.*
Indexed: Chem.Abstr., Chem.Indus.Notes, Chem.Titles.
—BLDSC (5748.208300), CASDDS, KNAW. **CCC.**
Published by: Academic Press, Inc., Journal Division (Subsidiary of: Harcourt Brace & Company), 525 B St, Ste 1900, San Diego, CA 92101-4495. TEL 619-230-1840, FAX 619-699-6800, http:// www.apnet.com.

MUTATION RESEARCH - GENETIC TOXICOLOGY AND ENVIRONMENTAL MUTAGENESIS. see *BIOLOGY—Genetics*

MUTATION RESEARCH - REVIEWS IN GENETIC TOXICOLOGY. see *BIOLOGY—Genetics*

615.95295 DEU ISSN 0178-7888
CODEN: MYREET
MYCOTOXIN RESEARCH. Text in English. 1985. s-a. DEM 73.50. adv. bk.rev.
Indexed: Chem.Abstr., Chem.Indus.Notes, Chem.Titles, Food Sci.& Tech.Abstr., Ind.Vet., Maize Abstr., Nutr.Abstr., Postharvest, Poult.Abstr., Rev.Appl.Entomol., Rev.Med.& Vet.Mycol., Rev.Plant Path., Rice Abstr., Triticale Abstr.
—BLDSC (5995.762000), CASDDS, CISTI, GNLM, ingenta. **CCC.**
Address: Postfach 3628, Mainz 55026, Germany. TEL 06131-320071, FAX 06131-381314. Ed. Dr. Rainer Schmidt. Circ: 1,000.

N I O S H MANUAL OF ANALYTICAL METHODS. see *OCCUPATIONAL HEALTH AND SAFETY*

N I O S H POCKET GUIDE TO CHEMICAL HAZARDS. see *OCCUPATIONAL HEALTH AND SAFETY*

571.95 USA ISSN 1056-9014
QP631 CODEN: NATOEE
NATURAL TOXINS. Text in English. 1992. bi-m. USD 495 (effective 2000). adv. bk.rev. back issues avail. *Refereed.* **Document type:** *Academic/Scholarly.* **Description:** Provides a forum for original research on the occurrence, isolation, identification, and characterization of natural products with toxic activities.
Related titles: Microform ed.: (from PQC); Online - full text ed.: ISSN 1522-7189. 1997 (from EBSCO Publishing, Wiley InterScience, Institute for Scientific Information).
Indexed: AgBiotech, Agricola, Aqua.Sci.& Fish.Abstr., BBCI, Biotech.& Bioeng.Abstr., Chem.Abstr., Chem.Indus.Notes, Chem.Titles, Dairy Sci.Abstr., Environ.Abstr., Environ.Per.Bibl. (1994-), Environ.Sci.Poll.Mgmt., Excerp.Med. (1993-), Field Crop Abstr., Food Sci.& Tech.Abstr., Forest.Abstr., Helminthol.Abstr., Herb.Abstr., Ind.Med. (1994-, dropped), Ind.Vet., Int.Abstr.Biol.Sci., Maize Abstr., Mass Spectr.Bull., Pig News & Info., Plant Grow.Reg.Abstr., Pollut.Abstr., Postharvest, Poult.Abstr., Rev.Appl.Entomol., Rev.Arom.& Med.Plants, Rev.Med.& Vet.Mycol., Rev.Plant Path., Rice Abstr., Saf.Sci.Abstr., Sel.Water Res.Abstr., Soils & Fert., Soyabean Abstr., Tox.Abstr., Triticale Abstr., Trop.Dis.Bull., Vet.Bull., Weed Abstr., Zoo.Rec.
—BLDSC (6041.515000), CASDDS, EMDOCS, GNLM, Infotrieve, KNAW. **CCC.**
Published by: John Wiley & Sons, Inc., Journals (Subsidiary of: Wiley InterScience), 605 Third Ave, New York, NY 10158. TEL 212-692-6645, subinfo@wiley.com, http://www.wiley.com. Eds. J David Miller, John A Simon. adv.: B&W page GBP 640, color page GBP 1,515; trim 210 x 279. Circ: 400. **Subscr. outside the Americas to:** John Wiley & Sons Ltd., Baffins Ln, Chichester, Sussex PO19 IUD, United Kingdom. TEL 44-1243-779777, FAX 44-1243-843232, cs-journals@wiley.co.uk.

NAUNYN-SCHMIEDEBERG'S ARCHIVES OF PHARMACOLOGY. see *PHARMACY AND PHARMACOLOGY*

NEUROTOXICOLOGY AND TERATOLOGY. see *MEDICAL SCIENCES—Psychiatry And Neurology*

NEUROTOXICOLOGY (LITTLE ROCK); an international journal. see *MEDICAL SCIENCES—Psychiatry And Neurology*

NEW SOLUTIONS; a journal of environmental and occupational health policy. see *OCCUPATIONAL HEALTH AND SAFETY*

571.95 FRA ISSN 1607-310X
O E C D GUIDELINES FOR THE TESTING OF CHEMICALS. (Organization for Economic Cooperation and Development) Text in English. a. USD 106, EUR 121, FRF 793.70, DEM 236.65, GBP 72, JPY 11,500 (effective 2001). **Description:** Provides information on the internationally agreed testing methods used by government, industry and independent laboratories to identify and characterize potential hazards of new and existing chemical substances, chemical preparations and chemical mixtures.
Media: Online - full content (from Swets Blackwell). **Related titles:** Print ed.: ISSN 1607-3096.
Published by: Organization for Economic Cooperation and Development, 2 rue Andre Pascal, Paris Cedex 16 75775, France. TEL 33-1-45248167, FAX 33-1-45241950, sales@oecd.org, http://www.oecd.org.

ORGANOHALOGEN COMPOUNDS. see *CHEMISTRY—Organic Chemistry*

571.959 USA
PESTICIDE LITIGATION MANUAL. Text in English. a. USD 193 (effective 1998). **Document type:** *Trade.* **Description:** Contains detailed analysis of pesticide litigation issues, including theories of liability, methods of apportioning liability, issues frequently briefed in pesticide cases, and analysis of damage theories.
Published by: West Group (Subsidiary of: Thomson Corporation, The), 620 Opperman Dr., Eagan, MN 55123. TEL 651-687-8000, 800-328-4880, FAX 651-687-7302, http://www.westgroup.com. Eds. George W Ware, John M Johnson.

PESTICIDES ABSTRACTS. see *ENVIRONMENTAL STUDIES—Abstracting, Bibliographies, Statistics*

571.959 632.9 GBR ISSN 1466-5670
PESTICIDES MONITOR; a monthly listing of UK approvals and other announcements on pesticides. Text and summaries in English. 1989. m. GBP 85; GBP 7.95 per issue (effective 1999). bk.rev. charts, illus. 3 cols./p. back issues avail. **Document type:** *Newsletter, Bulletin, Government.* **Description:** Reports on UK government approvals and other actions regarding agricultural pesticides and their use and safety.
Supersedes (in 1999): Pesticides Register (0955-7458)
Indexed: CBNB (1992-), Rural Devel.Abstr.
—BLDSC (6428.768000).
Published by: H.M.S.O., Publications Centre, PO Box 276, London SW8 5DT, United Kingdom. **Co-sponsors:** Ministry of Agriculture, Fisheries and Food, Pesticides Safety Directorate; Health and Safety Executive, Pesticides Registration Section.

▼ **PESTICIDES, PEOPLE AND NATURE.** see *AGRICULTURE—Crop Production And Soil*

PHARMACOLOGY AND THERAPEUTICS. see *PHARMACY AND PHARMACOLOGY*

PHARMACOLOGY & TOXICOLOGY. see *PHARMACY AND PHARMACOLOGY*

PHARMACOLOGY & TOXICOLOGY ONLINE. see *PHARMACY AND PHARMACOLOGY*

PHARMACOLOGY & TOXICOLOGY. SUPPLEMENTUM. see *PHARMACY AND PHARMACOLOGY*

PHARMACOLOGY, BIOCHEMISTRY AND BEHAVIOR. see *PHARMACY AND PHARMACOLOGY*

PROGRESS IN PESTICIDE BIOCHEMISTRY AND TOXICOLOGY. see *ENGINEERING—Chemical Engineering*

615.9 USA
RA1215
R T E C S. (Registry of Toxic Effects of Chemical Substances) Text in English. q. abstr, bibl. index. **Description:** Provides information on known toxic and biological effects of chemical substances for use by employers, employees, physicians, industrial hygienists, toxicologists, researchers, and others concerned with the safe handling of chemicals. Includes CODEN files.
Media: Online - full text (from NISC, Canadian Centre for Occupational Health & Safety). **Related titles:** CD-ROM ed.: (from SilverPlatter Information, Inc.); Magnetic Tape ed.
Indexed: MEDOC.
Published by: U.S. National Institute for Occupational Safety and Health, Attn: Publications, 4676 Columbia Pkwy, Cincinnati, OH 45226. TEL 800-356-4674, pubstaft@cdc.gov. Circ: 10,000.

571.959 FRA
RECOMMENDATIONS ON THE SAFE USE OF PESTICIDES IN SHIPS. Text in English. a. GBP 5; GBP 6 foreign. **Description:** Discusses the safe use of pesticides aboard ships.
Related titles: French ed.; Spanish ed.
Published by: International Maritime Organization/ Organisation Maritime Internationale, 4 Albert Embankment, London SE1 7SR, United Kingdom. TEL 071-735-7611, FAX 071-587-3210.

615.9 USA ISSN 0273-2300
RA1190 CODEN: RTOPDW
REGULATORY TOXICOLOGY AND PHARMACOLOGY. Text in English. 1981. bi-m. USD 545 in US & Canada to institutions; USD 615 elsewhere to institutions (effective 2001). adv. index. back issues avail. *Refereed.* **Document type:** *Academic/Scholarly.* **Description:** Reports the concepts and problems involved with the generation, evaluation, and interpretation of experimental animal and human data in the large perspective of the societal considerations of protecting human health and the environment.
Related titles: Online - full text ed.: (from EBSCO Publishing, O C L C Online Computer Library Center, Inc., RoweCom Information Quest, ingenta, Swets Blackwell, IDEAL Online Library, Institute for Scientific Information).

E

Indexed: ASCA, Aqua.Sci.& Fish.Abstr., Bibl.Agri., Chem.Abstr., Chem.Indus.Notes, Chem.Titles, Curr.Adv.Cancer Res., Curr.Adv.Ecol.Sci., Curr.Cont., Dok.Arbeitsmed., Energy Ind., Energy Info.Abstr., Environ.Sci.Poll.Mgmt., Excerp.Med., Helminthol.Abstr., INIS Atomind., Ind.Med. (1981-), Ind.Sci.Rev., Ind.Vet., Inpharma, Int.Abstr.Biol.Sci., Lab.Haz.Bull., NRN, Nutr.Abstr., Pharm.&Out.News, Pollut.Abstr., Postharvest, Reac., Rev.Appl.Entomol., Rev.Med.& Vet.Mycol., Rev.Plant Path., Risk Abstr., Saf.Sci.Abstr., Sci.Cit.Ind., Sel.Water Res.Abstr., Sugar Ind.Abstr., Tox.Abstr., W.R.C.Inf., Weed Abstr.
—BLDSC (7350.040000), ADONIS, CASDDS, CISTI, EMDOCS, GNLM, IDS, ingenta, KNAW, Linda Hall. **CCC.**
Published by: Academic Press, Inc., Journal Division (Subsidiary of: Harcourt Brace & Company), 525 B St, Ste 1900, San Diego, CA 92101-4495. TEL 619-230-1840, FAX 619-699-6800, apsubs@acad.com, http://www.academicpress.com/rtp. Eds. Albert C Kolbye Jr., Frederick Coulston.

RET - INFO. see *PUBLIC HEALTH AND SAFETY*

615.9 NLD ISSN 1382-6980
RA1190 CODEN: RPETEZ
REVIEWS IN TOXICOLOGY. Text in English. 1996. s-a. EUR 172, USD 161 to institutions (effective 2000). *Refereed.* **Document type:** *Journal, Academic/Scholarly.* **Description:** Publishes timely reviews of all aspects of toxicology, including fundamental toxicology, environmental and pesticide toxicology, risk assessment and methodological issues.
Formed by the merger of (1979-1996): Reviews in Biochemical Toxicology (0163-7673); (1984-1996): Reviews in Environmental Toxicology (0168-7255); (1991-1996): Reviews in Pesticide Toxicology (1062-3965)
Related titles: Online - full text ed.: (from RoweCom Information Quest).
Indexed: Agricola, Aqua.Sci.& Fish.Abstr., Chem.Abstr., Chem.Indus.Notes, Chem.Titles, Ecol.Abstr., Environ.Sci.Poll.Mgmt., Excerp.Med., Ind.Med. (coverage dropped), Ind.Sci.Rev., Int.Abstr.Biol.Sci., Microbiol.Abstr., Neurosci.Abstr. (coverage dropped), Pollut.Abstr., Tox.Abstr. (coverage dropped).
—BLDSC (7797.310000), ADONIS, CASDDS, CISTI, GNLM, Infotrieve, Linda Hall. **CCC.**
Published by: I O S Press, Nieuwe Hemweg 6B, Amsterdam 1013 BG, Netherlands. TEL 31-20-688-3355, FAX 31-20-620-3419, market@iospress.nl, http://www.iospress.nl. Ed. Ernest Hodgson TEL 919-515-5295. **Subscr. to:** I O S Press, Inc, 5795-G Burke Centre Pkwy, Burke, VA 22015. TEL 703-323-5554, FAX 703-323-3668, iosbooks@iospress.com; Kinokuniya Company Ltd, Shinjuku 3-chome, Shinjuku-ku, Tokyo 160-0022, Japan. FAX 81-3-3439-1094, journal@kinokuniya.co.jp, http://www.kinokuniya.co.jp; Globe Publication Pvt. Ltd., C-62 Inderpuri, New Delhi 100 012, India. TEL 91-11-579-3211, 91-11-579-3212, FAX 91-11-579-8876, custserve@globepub.com, http://www.globepub.com. **Co-publisher:** Toxicology Communications, Inc.

615.9 USA ISSN 0179-5953
TX501 CODEN: RCTOE4
REVIEWS OF ENVIRONMENTAL CONTAMINATION AND TOXICOLOGY. Text in English; Text occasionally in German, French. 1962. irreg., latest vol.145, 1995. price varies. reprint service avail. from ISI. **Document type:** *Monographic series.*
Supersedes (in 1987): Residue Reviews (0080-181X)
Related titles: Online - full text ed.: (from Institute for Scientific Information).
Indexed: ASCA, Agri.& Environ.Biotech.Abstr. (coverage dropped), Agricola, Biol.& Agr.Ind. (1987-), Biol.Abstr., Chem.Abstr., Chem.Cit.Ind., Chem.Indus.Notes, Chem.Titles, Dairy Sci.Abstr., Derwent Biotech.Abstr., Excerp.Med., Food Sci.& Tech.Abstr., GeoRef, Helminthol.Abstr., Hort.Abstr., INIS Atomind., Ind.Med. (1987-), Ind.Sci.Rev., Ind.Vet., Nutr.Abstr., Pollut.Abstr., Postharvest, Rev.Appl.Entomol., Rev.Plant Path., Rice Abstr., Sci.Cit.Ind., Soils & Fert., Sport Fish.Abstr., Vet.Bull., Weed Abstr., Wild.Rev., Zoo.Rec.
—BLDSC (7790.522000), CASDDS, CISTI, GNLM, IDS, ingenta, KNAW, Linda Hall. **CCC.**
Published by: Springer-Verlag, Journals (Subsidiary of: BertelsmannSpringer), 175 Fifth Ave, New York, NY 10010. TEL 212-460-1500, FAX 212-473-6272.

REVISTA DE ECOLOGIE INDUSTRIALA; Labor and Environmental Protection Magazine. see *ENVIRONMENTAL STUDIES*

REVISTA DE TOXICOLOGIA. see *PHARMACY AND PHARMACOLOGY*

RISK ABSTRACTS. see *ENVIRONMENTAL STUDIES—Abstracting, Bibliographies, Statistics*

RUSSIAN JOURNAL OF EXPERIMENTAL AND CLINICAL PHARMACOLOGY. see *PHARMACY AND PHARMACOLOGY*

S H E ALERT. (Safety, Health and the Environment) see *PAINTS AND PROTECTIVE COATINGS*

THE SCIENCE OF THE TOTAL ENVIRONMENT; an international journal for scientific research into the environment and its relationship with man. see *ENVIRONMENTAL STUDIES*

SENSITIVITY MATTERS. see *MEDICAL SCIENCES—Allergology And Immunology*

SEPSIS. see *MEDICAL SCIENCES—Communicable Diseases*

623.8 387.2 FRA
SHIP SAFETY AND POLLUTION PREVENTION - SHIP MANAGEMENT AND PORT STATE CONTROL. Text in English. irreg. GBP 5; GBP 6.50 foreign.
Related titles: French ed.; Spanish ed.
Published by: International Maritime Organization/ Organisation Maritime Internationale, 4 Albert Embankment, London SE1 7SR, United Kingdom. TEL 071-735-7611, FAX 071-587-3210.

577.27 GBR
SOLAS - INTERNATIONAL CONVENTION FOR THE SAFETY OF LIFE AT SEA. AMENDMENTS. Text in English. irreg. price varies. illus. **Description:** Discusses I.M.O. amendments to the 1974 legislation.
Related titles: Arabic ed.; Chinese ed.; French ed.; Russian ed.; Spanish ed.
Published by: International Maritime Organization/ Organisation Maritime Internationale, 4 Albert Embankment, London SE1 7SR, United Kingdom. TEL 44-20-7735-7611, FAX 44.20-7587-3210, TELEX 23588 IMOLDN G.

SPILL REPORTING PROCEDURES GUIDE. see *ENVIRONMENTAL STUDIES—Waste Management*

615.9 DEU
STRAHLENTELEX MIT ELEKTROSMOG-REPORT; unabhaengiger Informationsdienst zu Radioaktivitaet, Strahlung und Gesundheit. Text in German. 1987. m. DEM 109.53, EUR 56 (effective 2001). bk.rev. index. 12 p./no. back issues avail.; reprints avail. **Document type:** *Newsletter, Trade.* **Description:** Presents independent and critical information on radioactive pollution of the environment and electromagnetic fields.
Formerly: Strahlentelex (0931-4288)
Address: Rauxeler Weg 6, Berlin 13507, Germany. TEL 49-30-4352840, FAX 49-30-4352840, strahlentelex@t-online.de, http://www.strahlentelex.de. Ed., Pub. Thomas Dersee. Circ: 1,000 (controlled).

T R L NEWS. (Transport Research Laboratory) see *TRANSPORTATION—Roads And Traffic*

TECHNICAL INSTRUCTIONS FOR THE SAFE TRANSPORT OF DANGEROUS GOODS BY AIR. see *TRANSPORTATION—Air Transport*

TERATOLOGY; the international journal of abnormal development. see *BIOLOGY*

363.7 IND ISSN 0970-860X
Q180.D44
THIRD WORLD SCIENCE & ENVIRONMENT PERSPECTIVES. Text in English. 1989. q. INR 80 domestic to individuals; USD 20 foreign to individuals; INR 120 domestic to institutions; USD 25 foreign to institutions. **Document type:** *Academic/Scholarly.* **Description:** Features research articles in various aspects of science and environment policies in the Third World countries.
Published by: Centre for Science Technology and Environmental Policy Studies, C-5, Jangpura Extension, New Delhi 110 014, India. Ed. Ashok Raj.

571.95 RUS ISSN 0869-7922
TOKSIKOLOGICHESKII VESTNIK. Text in Russian. 1993. bi-m. RUR 60; USD 195 foreign. adv. bk.rev.
Indexed: Ref.Zh.
—BLDSC (0180.889000), East View.
Published by: Rossiiskii Registr Potentsyal'no Opasnykh Khimicheskikh i Biologicheskikh Veshchestv, Vadkovskii per 18-20, Moscow 101479, Russian Federation. TEL 7-095-9733021, FAX 7-095-9732657. Ed. B A Kurlyandskii. R&P K K Sidorov. Adv. contact L A Pomogayeva. Circ: 1,000. **US dist. addr.:** East View Publications, 3020 Harbor Ln N, Minneapolis, MN 55447. TEL 612-550-0961.

615.9 GBR
TOXIC EXPOSURE ADVISORY NEWSLETTER. Text in English. 1997. m. GBP 242, USD 400 to institutions; GBP 152, USD 250 to individuals. adv. **Document type:** *Newsletter.* **Description:** Provides health, legal, and environmental professionals with clear, concise, and timely information on recent toxicological developments.
Published by: Taylor & Francis Group, Taylor & Francis Ltd., Journals Customer Service, Rankine Rd, Basingstoke, Hants RG24 8PR, United Kingdom. **Subscr. in N. America to:** Taylor & Francis Ltd., 325 Chestnut St, Suite 800, Philadelphia, PA 19016. TEL 800-354-1420, FAX 215-625-8914, info@taylorandfrancis.com, http://www.taylorandfrancis.com/.

615.9 USA ISSN 0883-0576
KF3958
TOXIC SUBSTANCES CONTROL ACT - TEST SUBMISSION DATABASE. Short title: T S C A - T S C A T S. Text in English. 1981. irreg. USD 1,440 domestic; USD 2,880 in Canada & Mexico (effective 1999). **Document type:** *Government.*
Media: Microfiche.
Published by: (U.S. Environmental Protection Agency), U.S. National Technical Information Service, 5285 Port Royal Rd, Springfield, VA 22161. TEL 703-605-6060, FAX 703-605-6880, orders@ntis.fedworld.gov, http://www.ntis.gov.

346.038 USA
TOXIC TORT AND HAZARDOUS SUBSTANCE LITIGATION. Text in English. 1995. base vol. plus a. updates. USD 105. **Description:** Explains the most significant litigation issues in environmental exposure cases. Examines both common law and statutory developments.
Published by: Lexis Law Publishing (Subsidiary of: Reed Elsevier plc), PO Box 7587, Charlottesville, VA 22906-7587. TEL 804-972-7666, 800-562-1197, FAX 804-972-7666, llp.customer.support@lexis-nexis.com, http://www.lexislawpublishing.com. Eds. Charles D Case, L Neal Ellis Jr.

615.9 USA ISSN 0192-6233
RB1 CODEN: TOPADD
TOXICOLOGIC PATHOLOGY. Text in English. 1973. bi-m. GBP 127, USD 210 to individuals; GBP 157, USD 259 to institutions (effective 2002). adv. bk.rev. charts, illus. back issues avail. *Refereed.* **Document type:** *Academic/Scholarly.* **Description:** It is the leading publication in the recognition and definition of xenobiotic induced changed in animal, including human, tissue and body fluids as well as the application of these learnings in risk assessment.
Formerly (until vol.6, no.2, 1978): Society of Pharmacological and Environmental Pathologists. Bulletin (0094-1824)
Related titles: Online - full text ed.: (from CatchWord Ltd., Institute for Scientific Information).
Indexed: ASCA, Biol.Abstr., Chem.Abstr., Curr.Cont., Excerp.Med., INIS Atomind., Ind.Med. (1978-), Inpharma, Int.Abstr.Biol.Sci., Mass Spectr.Bull., Pharm.&Out.News, Reac., Rev.Med.& Vet.Mycol., Wild.Rev.
—BLDSC (8873.015000), CASDDS, CISTI, GNLM, IDS, Infotrieve, ingenta, KNAW. **CCC.**
Published by: (Society of Toxicologic Pathologists), Taylor & Francis Ltd. (Subsidiary of: Taylor & Francis Group), 325 Chestnut St, Suite 800, Philadelphia, PA 19016. TEL 215-625-8900, http://www.toxpath.org. Ed. Gordon C Hard. R&P Melissa Cleveland. Adv. contact Jill Franklin. page USD 480. Circ: 845 (controlled).

615.902 CHE ISSN 0277-2248
RA1190 CODEN: TECSDY
TOXICOLOGICAL AND ENVIRONMENTAL CHEMISTRY. Text in English. 12/yr. (in 6 vols., 4 nos./vol.). GBP 4,050, USD 4,950, EUR 5,400 to institutions; GBP 9,034, USD 10,296, EUR 11,232 to corporations (effective 2002). adv. *Refereed.* **Document type:** *Academic/Scholarly.*
Formerly: Toxicological and Environmental Chemistry Reviews (0092-9867)
Related titles: CD-ROM ed.; Microform ed.; Online - full text ed.: (from EBSCO Publishing, RoweCom Information Quest).

Indexed: ASCA, Aqua.Sci.& Fish.Abstr., Bioeng.Abstr., Biol.Abstr., Chem.Abstr., Chem.Cit.Ind., Comput.& Info.Sys., Curr.Adv.Ecol.Sci., Ecol.Abstr., Energy Ind., Energy Info.Abstr., Eng.Ind., Environ.Abstr., Environ.Per.Bibl. (1991-), Environ.Sci.Poll.Mgmt., Excerp.Med., Fluidex, Food Sci.& Tech.Abstr., Geo.Abstr.P.G., GeoRef, Geol.Abstr., INIS Atomind., Int.Abstr.Biol.Sci., METADEX, Microbiol.Abstr., Pollut.Abstr., Saf.Sci.Abstr., Sci.Cit.Ind. (coverage dropped), Sel.Water Res.Abstr., Tox.Abstr., W.R.C.Inf.
—CISTI, EMDOCS, GNLM, Infotrieve, ingenta, Linda Hall. **CCC.**
Published by: Gordon and Breach - Harwood Academic (Subsidiary of: Taylor & Francis Group), PO Box 531, Lausanne 1000, Switzerland. http://www.gbhap.com/ Toxicological_Env ironmental_Chemistry/. Ed. Hartmut Frank. **Subscr. addr. in US:** International Publishers Direct, PO Box 32160, Newark, NJ 07102. FAX 215-750-6343.

615.9 DEU
TOXICOLOGICAL EVALUATIONS. Text in English. irreg., latest vol.7, 1994. **Document type:** *Monographic series.*
—BLDSC.
Published by: (Berufsgenossenschaft der Chemischen Industrie), Springer-Verlag (Subsidiary of: BertelsmannSpringer), Haber Str 7, Heidelberg 69126, Germany. FAX 49-30-82787448, subscriptions@springer.de, http://www.springer.de, http://link.springer-ny.com.

615.9 USA ISSN 1096-6080
RA1190 CODEN: FAATDF
TOXICOLOGICAL SCIENCES. Text in English. 1980. m. GBP 730, USD 990, GBP 180, USD 240 to institutions (effective 2002). adv. abstr. index. back issues avail. *Refereed.* **Document type:** *Journal, Academic/Scholarly.* **Description:** Presents current articles and reports relating to those broad aspects of toxicology relevant to assessing the risk of exposure of toxic agents (chemicals, including drugs and natural products or forms of energy) to humans and other animals.
Formerly (until Dec. 1997): Fundamental and Applied Toxicology (0272-0590)
Related titles: Online - full text ed.: ISSN 1096-0929. GBP 657, USD 891 to institutions online only (effective 2002) (from HighWire Pr., EBSCO Publishing, ingenta, Swets Blackwell, IDEAL Online Library, Institute for Scientific Information, RoweCom Information Quest).
Indexed: ASCA, Aqua.Sci.& Fish.Abstr., Bibl.Agri., Bio-Contr.News & Info., CSNB, Chem.Abstr., Chem.Indus.Notes, Chem.Titles, Curr.Adv.Ecol.Sci., Curr.Adv.Gen.& Molec.Biol., Curr.Cont., Dairy Sci.Abstr., Derwent Biotech.Abstr., Dok.Arbeitsmed., Environ.Sci.Poll.Mgmt., Excerp.Med., INIS Atomind., Ind.Hyg.Dig., Ind.Med. (1998-), Ind.Sci.Rev., Ind.Vet., Inpharma, Int.Abstr.Biol.Sci., Lab.Haz.Bull., Mass Spectr.Bull., Microbiol.Abstr., NRN, Neurosci.Abstr., Neurosci.Cit.Ind., Nutr.Abstr., Pharm.&Out.News, Pig News & Info., Pollut.Abstr., Reac., Rev.Appl.Entomol., Rev.Med.& Vet.Mycol., Risk Abstr., Saf.Sci.Abstr., Sci.Cit.Ind., Sel.Water Res.Abstr., Small Anim.Abstr., Sport Fish.Abstr., Tox.Abstr., Vet.Bull., Weed Abstr., Wild.Rev.
—BLDSC (8873.031900), CASDDS, CISTI, EMDOCS, GNLM, IDS, ingenta, Linda Hall. **CCC.**
Published by: (Society of Toxicology), Oxford University Press, Academic Division, Great Clarendon St, Oxford OX2 6DP, United Kingdom. TEL 44-1865-267907, FAX 44-1865-267835, jnlorders@oup-usa.org, jnl.info@oup.co.uk, http://toxsci.oupjournals.org/, http://www.oup.co.uk/journals. Pub. J Fox. adv.: page GBP 475, page USD 850. **Subscr. outside the Americas to:** Journals Marketing, Great Clarendon St, Oxford OX2 6DP, United Kingdom.

615.9 IRL ISSN 0300-483X
RA1190 CODEN: TXCYAC
TOXICOLOGY; an international journal concerned with the effects of chemicals on living systems. Text in English. 1973. 33/yr. EUR 3,891 in Europe to institutions; JPY 517,000 in Japan to institutions; USD 4,352 elsewhere to institutions (effective 2002). adv. charts, illus. index. *Refereed.* **Document type:** *Academic/Scholarly.* **Description:** Publishes original scientific papers on the biological effects arising from the administration of chemical compounds, principally to animals, tissues or cells, but also to man.
Related titles: Microform ed.: (from PQC); Online - full text ed.: (from ingenta, Swets Blackwell, Institute for Scientific Information, ScienceDirect).
Indexed: ASCA, Agri.& Environ.Biotech.Abstr. (coverage dropped), Aqua.Sci.& Fish.Abstr., Biol.Abstr., Chem.Abstr., Chem.Indus.Notes, Chem.Titles, Curr.Adv.Cancer Res., Curr.Adv.Ecol.Sci., Curr.Cont., Dairy Sci.Abstr., Dent.Ind., Derwent Biotech.Abstr., Dok.Arbeitsmed., Energy Ind., Energy Info.Abstr., Environ.Abstr., Environ.Per.Bibl. (1991-1993), Environ.Sci.Poll.Mgmt., Excerp.Med., Food Sci.& Tech.Abstr., INIS Atomind., Ind.Med. (1973-), Ind.Sci.Rev., Ind.Vet., Inpharma, Int.Abstr.Biol.Sci., Lab.Haz.Bull., Neurosci.Abstr., Nutr.Abstr., Pharm.&Out.News, Pig News & Info., Pollut.Abstr., Poult.Abstr., Reac., Rev.Appl.Entomol., Rev.Med.& Vet.Mycol., Risk Abstr., Saf.Sci.Abstr., Sci.Cit.Ind., Small Anim.Abstr., Sport Fish.Abstr., THA, Trop.Dis.Bull., Vet.Bull., Weed Abstr., Wild.Rev., Zoo.Rec.
—BLDSC (8873.035000), ADONIS, CASDDS, CISTI, EMDOCS, GNLM, IDS, ingenta, Linda Hall. **CCC.**
Published by: Elsevier Science Ireland Ltd, Elsevier House, Brookvale Plaza, E. Park, Shannon, Co. Clare, Ireland. TEL 353-61-471944, FAX 353-61-472144, http://www.elsevier.com/locate/toxicol. Eds. H W J Marquardt, J Descotes, K Wallace. **Subscr. in Australasia and the Far East to:** Elsevier Science (Singapore) Pte Ltd, No.1 Temasek Ave, 17-01 Millenia Tower, Singapore 039192, Singapore. TEL 65-434-3727, FAX 65-337-2230; **Subscr. in the Americas to:** Elsevier Science, PO Box 945, New York, NY 10159-0945. TEL 212-633-3730, FAX 212-633-3680; **Subscr. to:** Elsevier Science BV, PO Box 211, Amsterdam 1000 AE, Netherlands. TEL 31-20-485-3757, FAX 31-20-485-3432.

TOXICOLOGY ABSTRACTS. see *ENVIRONMENTAL STUDIES—Abstracting, Bibliographies, Statistics*

615.9 USA ISSN 0041-008X
RA1190 CODEN: TXAPA9
TOXICOLOGY AND APPLIED PHARMACOLOGY; for those working in the fields of toxicology, pharmacology, biochemistry, nutrition, veterinary medicine. Text in English. 1959. 24/yr. USD 2,420 in US & Canada to institutions; USD 2,700 elsewhere to institutions (effective 2001). adv. bk.rev. bibl, charts. cum.index every 5 yrs. back issues avail. *Refereed.* **Document type:** *Academic/Scholarly.* **Description:** Covers scientific research pertaining to action on tissue structure or function resulting from administration of chemicals, drugs, or natural products to animals and humans.
Related titles: Online - full text ed.: (from EBSCO Publishing, O C L C Online Computer Library Center, Inc., RoweCom Information Quest, ingenta, Swets Blackwell, IDEAL Online Library, Institute for Scientific Information).
Indexed: ASCA, Abstr.Hyg., AgBiotech, Agri.& Environ.Biotech.Abstr. (coverage dropped), Agricola, BBCI, Biol.Abstr., C.I.S. Abstr., CSNB, Chem.Abstr., Chem.Titles, Curr.Adv.Ecol.Sci., Curr.Adv.Gen.& Molec.Biol., Curr.Cont., Dairy Sci.Abstr., Dent.Ind., Derwent Biotech.Abstr., Dok.Arbeitsmed., Environ.Abstr., Environ.Sci.Poll.Mgmt., Excerp.Med., Food Sci.& Tech.Abstr., Helminthol.Abstr., INIS Atomind., I.P.A., Ind.Hyg.Dig., Ind.Med. (1959-), Ind.Sci.Rev., Ind.Vet., Inpharma, Int.Abstr.Biol.Sci., Lab.Haz.Bull., NRN, Neurosci.Abstr., Neurosci.Cit.Ind., Nutr.Abstr., Ocean.Abstr. (coverage dropped), Pharm.&Out.News, Pollut.Abstr., Protozool.Abstr., Reac., Rev.Appl.Entomol., Rev.Arom.& Med.Plants, Rev.Med.& Vet.Mycol., Rev.Plant Path., Risk Abstr., Saf.Sci.Abstr., Sci.Cit.Ind., Sel.Water Res.Abstr., Sport Fish.Abstr., Sugar Ind.Abstr., THA, Vet.Bull., W.R.C.Inf., Weed Abstr., Wild.Rev., Zoo.Rec.
—BLDSC (8873.040000), ADONIS, CASDDS, CINDOC, CISTI, GNLM, IDS, ingenta, KNAW, Linda Hall. **CCC.**
Published by: Academic Press, Inc., Journal Division (Subsidiary of: Harcourt Brace & Company), 525 B St, Ste 1900, San Diego, CA 92101-4495. TEL 619-230-1840, FAX 619-699-6800, apsubs@acad.com, http://www.academicpress.com/tap. Ed. Edward Beresnick.

571.95 GBR ISSN 1364-8543
RA1190 CODEN: TENRFK
TOXICOLOGY AND ECOTOXICOLOGY NEWS - REVIEWS. Text in English. 1994. bi-m. GBP 179, USD 296 to institutions. adv. **Document type:** *Academic/Scholarly.*
Formerly (until 1997): Toxicology and Ecotoxicology News (1350-4592)
Indexed: Chem.Abstr., Chem.Indus.Notes, Food Sci.& Tech.Abstr.
—BLDSC (8873.040270), CASDDS, GNLM. **CCC.**
Published by: Taylor & Francis Group, Taylor & Francis Ltd., Journals Customer Service, Rankine Rd, Basingstoke, Hants RG24 8PR, United Kingdom. **Subscr. in N. America to:** Taylor & Francis Ltd., 325 Chestnut St, Suite 800, Philadelphia, PA 19016. TEL 800-354-1420, FAX 215-625-8914, info@taylorandfrancis.com, http:// www.taylorandfrancis.com/.

615.902 GBR ISSN 0748-2337
RA1199 CODEN: TIHEEC
TOXICOLOGY AND INDUSTRIAL HEALTH; an international journal. Text in English. 1985. 10/yr. GBP 164 in Europe to individuals; USD 228 in North America to individuals; GBP 169 rest of world to individuals; GBP 435 in Europe to institutions; USD 598 in North America to institutions; GBP 444 rest of world to institutions; GBP 131 in Europe to members bts, sot; USD 182 in North America to members bts, sot; GBP 135 rest of world to members bts, sot; GBP 222 in developing nations; GBP 60 newsstand/cover in Europe; USD 87 newsstand/cover in North America; GBP 64 newsstand/cover rest of world (effective 2002). adv. bk.rev. illus. index. back issues avail.; reprints avail. *Refereed.* **Document type:** *Journal, Academic/Scholarly.* **Description:** Publishes basic and applied research in the fields of toxicology, biochemical toxicology, genetic and cellular toxicology, including risk assessment associated with hazardous wastes and ground water contamination.
Related titles: Online - full text ed.: (from EBSCO Publishing, O C L C Online Computer Library Center, Inc., RoweCom Information Quest, ingenta, Swets Blackwell, Institute for Scientific Information).
Indexed: ASCA, CSNB, Chem.Abstr., Chem.Indus.Notes, Environ.Sci.Poll.Mgmt., INIS Atomind., Ind.Med. (1985-), Int.Abstr.Biol.Sci., Lab.Haz.Bull., METADEX, NRN, Pollut.Abstr., Risk Abstr., SSCI (coverage dropped), Saf.Sci.Abstr., Sci.Cit.Ind. (coverage dropped), Sel.Water Res.Abstr., Tox.Abstr.
—BLDSC (8873.040500), CASDDS, CISTI, EMDOCS, GNLM, IDS, ingenta, KNAW. **CCC.**
Published by: Arnold Publishers (Subsidiary of: Hodder Headline plc.), 338 Euston Rd, London NW1 3BH, United Kingdom. TEL 44-20-7873-6337, FAX 44-20-7873-6325, arnoldjournals@hodder.co.uk, http://www.arnoldpublishers.com/journals/Journpages/ 07482337.htm, http://www.arnoldpublishers.com/ journals/journtitles.htm. Ed. Dr. Ronald Hart. adv.: page USD 400. Circ: 500.

615.9 GBR ISSN 0887-2333
RA1199.4.I5 CODEN: TIVIEQ
TOXICOLOGY IN VITRO. Text in English. 1987. bi-m. EUR 86 in Europe to qualified personnel; JPY 11,500 in Japan to qualified personnel; USD 97 elsewhere to qualified personnel; EUR 764 in Europe to institutions; JPY 101,400 in Japan to institutions; USD 854 elsewhere to institutions (effective 2002). abstr. back issues avail. *Refereed.* **Document type:** *Academic/Scholarly.* **Description:** Research on the use of in vitro techniques for determining the toxic effects of chemicals and elucidating their mechanisms of action.
Related titles: Microfilm ed.: (from PQC); Online - full text ed.: (from ingenta, Swets Blackwell, Institute for Scientific Information, ScienceDirect).
Indexed: ASCA, Aqua.Sci.& Fish.Abstr., Chem.Abstr., Chem.Titles, Curr.Cont., Environ.Sci.Poll.Mgmt., Excerp.Med., Food Sci.& Tech.Abstr., Helminthol.Abstr., Ind.Med., Ind.Sci.Rev., Ind.Vet., Inpharma, Int.Abstr.Biol.Sci., Lab.Haz.Bull., Neurosci.Cit.Ind., Nutr.Abstr., Pollut.Abstr., Protozool.Abstr., Reac., Rev.Appl.Entomol., Rev.Med.& Vet.Mycol., Risk Abstr., Saf.Sci.Abstr., Sci.Cit.Ind., Weed Abstr.
—BLDSC (8873.043400), ADONIS, CASDDS, CISTI, EMDOCS, GNLM, IDS, Infotrieve. **CCC.**
Published by: (British Industrial Biological Research Association), Pergamon (Subsidiary of: Elsevier Science), The Boulevard, Langford Ln, East Park, Kidlington, Oxford OXB 1GB, United Kingdom. FAX 44-1865-843010, http://www.elsevier.com/locate/toxinvit. Eds. Bas J Blaauboer, Daniel Acosta, Stuart E Jaggers. **Subscr. in Australasia and the Far East to:** Elsevier Science (Singapore) Pte Ltd, No.1 Temasek Ave, 17-01 Millenia Tower, Singapore 039192, Singapore. TEL 65-434-3727, FAX 65-337-2230; **Subscr. in the Americas to:** Elsevier Science, PO Box 945, New York, NY 10159-0945. TEL 212-633-3730, FAX 212-633-3680, usinfo-f@elsevier.com; **Subscr. to:** Elsevier Science BV, PO Box 211, Amsterdam 1000 AE, Netherlands. TEL 31-20-485-3757.

E

615.9 IRL ISSN 0378-4274
CODEN: TOLED5
TOXICOLOGY LETTERS; an international journal for the rapid publication of short reports on biochemical mechanisms of mammalian toxicity. Text in English. 1977. 24/yr. EUR 2,930 in Europe to institutions; JPY 388,800 in Japan to institutions; USD 3,278 elsewhere to institutions (effective 2002). adv. abstr. back issues avail. *Refereed.* **Document type:** *Academic/Scholarly.* **Description:** Provides a forum for original and pertinent contributions in toxicology research.
Related titles: Microform ed.: (from PQC); Online - full text ed.: (from ingenta, Swets Blackwell, Institute for Scientific Information, ScienceDirect).
Indexed: ASCA, Agri.& Environ.Biotech.Abstr. (coverage dropped), Aqua.Sci.& Fish.Abstr., Biol.Abstr., CSNB, Chem.Abstr., Chem.Indus.Notes, Compumath, Curr.Adv.Biochem., Curr.Adv.Ecol.Sci., Curr.Cont., Curr.Ref.Fish Res., Dairy Sci.Abstr., Dent.Ind., Derwent Biotech.Abstr., Dok.Arbeitsmed., Energy Ind., Energy Info.Abstr., Environ.Sci.Poll.Mgmt., Excerp.Med., Food Sci.& Tech.Abstr., Forest Prod.Abstr., Helminthol.Abstr., INIS Atomind., I.P.A., Ind.Med. (1977-), Ind.Sci.Rev., Ind.Vet., Inpharma, Int.Abstr.Biol.Sci., Lab.Haz.Bull., Mass Spectr.Bull., NRN, Neurosci.Abstr. (coverage dropped), Neurosci.Cit.Ind., Nutr.Abstr., Pharm.&Out.News, Pollut.Abstr., Reac., Ref.Zh., Rev.Appl.Entomol., Rev.Arom.& Med.Plants, Rev.Med.& Vet.Mycol., Rev.Plant Path., Risk Abstr., SSCI (coverage dropped), Saf.Sci.Abstr., Sci.Cit.Ind., Sel.Water Res.Abstr., Sport Fish.Abstr., Vet.Bull., W.R.C.Inf., Weed Abstr., Wild.Rev., Zoo.Rec.
—BLDSC (8873.042000), ADONIS, CASDDS, CISTI, EMDOCS, GNLM, IDS, Infotrieve, ingenta, Linda Hall. **CCC.**
Published by: Elsevier Science Ireland Ltd, Elsevier House, Brookvale Plaza, E. Park, Shannon, Co. Clare, Ireland. TEL 353-61-471944, FAX 353-61-472144, http://www.elsevier.com/locate/toxlet. Eds. J P Kehrer, W Dekant. R&P Annette Moloney. **Subscr. in Australasia and the Far East to:** Elsevier Science (Singapore) Pte Ltd, No.1 Temasek Ave, 17-01 Millenia Tower, Singapore 039192, Singapore. TEL 65-434-3727, FAX 65-337-2230; **Subscr. in the Americas to:** Elsevier Science, PO Box 945, New York, NY 10159-0945. TEL 212-633-3730, FAX 212-633-3680; **Subscr. to:** Elsevier Science BV, PO Box 211, Amsterdam 1000 AE, Netherlands. TEL 31-20-485-3757.

615.9 USA ISSN 1051-7235
RA1221 CODEN: TOMEEB
TOXICOLOGY METHODS. Text in English. 1991. q., latest vol.11, 2001. GBP 93, USD 154 to individuals; GBP 327, USD 540 to institutions (effective 2002). charts, illus. reprint service avail. from PQC. *Refereed.* **Document type:** *Academic/Scholarly.* **Description:** Covers new methods and test designs in safety assessment, new in vivo and in vitro models, modifications to existing procedures, commentaries, and new technology and equipment.
Incorporates (in 2002): Toxic Substance Mechanisms (1076-9188); Which was formerly (1979-1995): Toxic Substances Journal (0199-3178)
Related titles: Microform ed.: (from PQC); Online - full text ed.: ISSN 1091-7667 (from CatchWord Ltd., EBSCO Publishing, O C L C Online Computer Library Center, Inc., RoweCom Information Quest, Swets Blackwell, Institute for Scientific Information).
Indexed: ASCA, Chem.Abstr., Chem.Titles, Compumath, Curr.Cont., Ind.Sci.Rev., Inpharma, Int.Abstr.Biol.Sci., Reac., Sci.Cit.Ind.
—BLDSC (8873.042100), CASDDS, CatchWord, GNLM, IDS, Infotrieve, ingenta, KNAW, Linda Hall. **CCC.**
Published by: Taylor & Francis Ltd. (Subsidiary of: Taylor & Francis Group), 325 Chestnut St, Suite 800, Philadelphia, PA 19016. TEL 215-625-8900, FAX 215-625-2940, info@taylorandfrancis.com, http://www.taylorandfrancis.com/. Ed. Steven I Baskin. Circ: 1,000. **Subscr. addr. in Europe:** Taylor & Francis Group, Journals Customer Service, Rankine Rd, Basingstoke, Hants RG24 8PR, United Kingdom. TEL 44-1256-813000, FAX 44-1256-479438, enquiry@tanf.co.uk, http://www.tandf.co.uk/journals.

TOXICON; an interdisciplinary journal on the toxins derived from animals, plants and microorganisms. see *PHARMACY AND PHARMACOLOGY*

615.9 NLD ISSN 0927-5215
CODEN: TMENEI
TRACE METALS IN THE ENVIRONMENT. Text in English. 1991. irreg., latest vol.3, 1993. price varies. back issues avail. *Refereed.* **Document type:** *Monographic series, Academic/Scholarly.*
Indexed: Chem.Abstr., Chem.Indus.Notes, Chem.Titles, GeoRef, Zoo.Rec.
—BLDSC (8876.879700), CASDDS. **CCC.**
Published by: Elsevier Science BV, PO Box 211, Amsterdam 1000 AE, Netherlands. TEL 31-20-485-3757, 31-20-485-3911, FAX 31-20-485-3432, 31-20-485-3598, nlinfo-f@elsevier.nl; usinfo-f@elsevier.com; forinfo-kyf04035@niftyserve.or.jp, http://www.elsevier.nl/. Ed. J O Nriagu. **Subscr. in Australasia and the Far East to:** Elsevier Science (Singapore) Pte Ltd, No.1 Temasek Ave, 17-01 Millenia Tower, Singapore 039192, Singapore. TEL 65-434-3727, FAX 65-337-2230, asiainfo@elsevier.com.sg; **Subscr. in Japan to:** Elsevier Science Inc - Japan Regional Office, 9-15 Higashi-Azabu 1-chome, Minato-ku, Tokyo 106-0044, Japan. TEL 81-3-5561-5033, FAX 81-3-5561-5047, info@elsevier.co.jp; **Subscr. in the Americas to:** Elsevier Science, PO Box 945, New York, NY 10159-0945. TEL 212-633-3730, 888-437-4636, FAX 212-633-3680, usinfo-f@elsevier.com, http://www.elsevier.com

TRENDS IN PHARMACOLOGICAL SCIENCES. see *PHARMACY AND PHARMACOLOGY*

U.S. NATIONAL TOXICOLOGY PROGRAM. REPORT ON CARCINOGENS. see *MEDICAL SCIENCES—Oncology*

615.9 USA ISSN 0145-6296
SF757.5 CODEN: VHTODE
VETERINARY AND HUMAN TOXICOLOGY. Text in English. 1958. bi-m., latest vol.43. USD 25 per issue domestic; USD 80 domestic; USD 90 in Canada; USD 100 elsewhere (effective 2002). adv. bk.rev. abstr, bibl, charts, illus. 68 p./no. 2 cols./p. back issues avail.; reprint service avail. from ISI. *Refereed.* **Document type:** *Journal, Academic/Scholarly.* **Description:** Contains contributions in the broad field of toxicology. Includes manuscripts of original research, scientific reviews, field observations in man or domestic and wild animals, papers presented at meetings, news items and announcements, and information of general educational value to toxicologists and related scientists.
Former titles (until 1976): Veterinary Toxicology (0091-5300); (until 1973): News from the American College of Veterinary Toxicologists
Related titles: Online - full text ed.: (from Institute for Scientific Information).
Indexed: ASCA, Abstr.Hyg., Agricola, Agroforest.Abstr., Aqua.Sci.& Fish.Abstr., Bibl.Agri., Biol.Abstr., Biol.Dig., Chem.Abstr., Chem.Indus.Notes, Chem.Titles, Curr.Adv.Ecol.Sci., Curr.Cont., Dairy Sci.Abstr., Dent.Ind., Derwent Biotech.Abstr., Energy Ind., Energy Info.Abstr., Environ.Sci.Poll.Mgmt., Excerp.Med., Focus on: Vet.Sci.& Med., Helminthol.Abstr., Herb.Abstr., Hort.Abstr., INIS Atomind., I.P.A., Ind.Med. (1977-), Ind.Sci.Rev., Ind.Vet., Inpharma, Int.Abstr.Biol.Sci., Maize Abstr., Med.Abstr., Nutr.Abstr., Ornam.Hort., Pollut.Abstr., Poult.Abstr., Protozool.Abstr., Reac., Rev.Appl.Entomol., Rev.Arom.& Med.Plants, Rev.Med.& Vet.Mycol., Rev.Plant Path., Risk Abstr., SSCI (coverage dropped), Saf.Sci.Abstr., Sci.Cit.Ind., Sport Fish.Abstr., Triticale Abstr., Trop.Dis.Bull., Vet.Bull., Weed Abstr., Wild.Rev., Zoo.Rec.
—BLDSC (9226.700000), CASDDS, CISTI, GNLM, IDS, ingenta, KNAW, Linda Hall. **CCC.**
Published by: (American Academy of Veterinary and Comparative Toxicology), Comparative Toxicology Laboratories, Publication Office, 1800 Denison Ave, Kansas State University, Manhattan, KS 66506-5606. TEL 785-532-4334, FAX 785-532-4481, TELEX 82 1034, oehme@vet.ksu.edu. Ed., Pub., R&P, Adv. contact Frederick W Oehme TEL 785-532-4334. Circ: 1,000 (paid).

YANBIAN - JIBIAN - TUBIAN/CARCINOGENSIS, TERATOGENSIS AND MUTAGENESIS. see *MEDICAL SCIENCES—Oncology*

615.9 CHN ISSN 1000-3002
CODEN: ZYYZEW
ZHONGGUO YAOLIXUE YU DULIXUE ZAZHI/CHINESE JOURNAL OF PHARMACOLOGY AND TOXICOLOGY. Text in Chinese, English. 1986. q. USD 31.20; CNY 10 newsstand/cover domestic; USD 5.20 newsstand/cover foreign (effective 2001). adv. *Refereed.* **Document type:** *Academic/Scholarly.* **Description:** To report the research achievements in the field of pharmacology and toxicology in China and other countries, including many branches such as pharmacology and toxicology of nervous, cardiovascular system, pharmacokinetics and toxicokinetics, etc. The readers are mainly pharmacologists, toxicologists, pharmacists, biochemists, from institutes and academies, universities.
Related titles: Microfiche ed.; Online - full content ed.: (from WanFang Data Corp.).
Indexed: Chem.Abstr., Chem.Indus.Notes, Chem.Titles, Excerp.Med., Int.Abstr.Biol.Sci.
—BLDSC (3180.474000), CASDDS, EMDOCS, GNLM.
Published by: Zhongguo Yaoli Xueyuan/Chinese Pharmacological Society, 27 Taiping Rd, Beijing 100850, China. TEL 86-10-823-2343, FAX 86-10-6821-1656, guol@nic.bmi.ac.cn. Ed. Rong Kangtai. Adv. contact Lu Zhengsu. B&W page USD 500, color page USD 980; trim 240 x 170. Circ: 4,000; 3,000 (paid). **Overseas subscr. to:** China International Book Trading Corp, 35, Chegongzhuang Xilu, Haidian District, Beijing 100044, China. TEL 86-1-68413849, FAX 86-1-68412048, cibtc@mail.cibtc.com.cn, http://www.cibtc.com.cn.

ENVIRONMENTAL STUDIES—Waste Management

604.7 DEU ISSN 0942-3818
CODEN: ALSPFF
ALTLASTEN - SPEKTRUM; Erfassung - Bewertung - Sanierung. Text in German. 1992. 6/yr. DEM 106.80; DEM 20 newsstand/cover (effective 2001). adv. **Document type:** *Newspaper, Trade.*
Indexed: CEABA, GeoRef, IBR, IBZ.
—CASDDS.
Published by: (Ingenieurtechnischer Verband Altlasten e.V.), Erich Schmidt Verlag GmbH & Co. (Berlin), Genthiner Str 30G, Berlin 10785, Germany. TEL 49-30-250085-0, FAX 49-30-25008521, redaktion@altlastenspektrum-itva.de, esv@esvmedien.de, http://www.erich-schmidt-verlag.de.

628.4 NLD ISSN 0923-9820
QR97.X46 CODEN: BIODEG
BIODEGRADATION. Text in English. 1990. bi-m. EUR 616, USD 617 to institutions for print or online ed.; EUR 331, USD 332 to individuals for pirnt or online ed.; EUR 739.20, USD 740.40 to institutions for print & online eds. combined (effective 2002). back issues avail.; reprint service avail. from SWZ. *Refereed.* **Document type:** *Journal, Academic/Scholarly.* **Description:** Presents papers on all aspects of science pertaining to the detoxification, recycling, amelioration or other treatment of waste materials and pollutants by naturally occurring or recombinant organisms.
Related titles: Microform ed.: (from PQC); Online - full text ed.: (from EBSCO Publishing, O C L C Online Computer Library Center, Inc., RoweCom Information Quest, Swets Blackwell, Kluwer Online, Institute for Scientific Information).
Indexed: ASCA, Agri.& Environ.Biotech.Abstr., Agricola, Aqua.Sci.& Fish.Abstr., Biol.Abstr., Biotech.Cit.Ind., Chem.Abstr., Chem.Indus.Notes, Chem.Titles, Curr.Cont., Deep Sea Res.& Oceanogr.Abstr., Derwent Biotech.Abstr., Ecol.Abstr., Eng.Ind., Environ.Abstr., Environ.Per.Bibl. (1993-), Environ.Sci.Poll.Mgmt., Field Crop Abstr., Fluidex, Geo.Abstr.P.G., Geol.Abstr., Ind.Med. (1990-), Int.Abstr.Biol.Sci., Irr.& Drain.Abstr., Microbiol.Abstr., Pollut.Abstr., Rev.Appl.Entomol., Rev.Plant Path., Sci.Cit.Ind., Sel.Water Res.Abstr., Soils & Fert., Sugar Ind.Abstr., W.R.C.Inf., Weed Abstr.
—BLDSC (2071.240000), CASDDS, CIS, CISTI, Ei, EMDOCS, GNLM, IDS, Infotrieve, ingenta, KNAW, Linda Hall. **CCC.**
Published by: Kluwer Academic Publishers Group (Subsidiary of: Wolters Kluwer N.V.), Spuiboulevard 50, PO Box 17, Dordrecht 3300 AA, Netherlands. TEL 31-78-639-2392, FAX 31-78-654-2254, services@wkap.nl, http://www.wkap.nl/journalhome.htm/0923-9820. Ed. Bruce E Rittmann. **Subscr. addr. in N America:** Kluwer Academic - Plenum Publishers, 233 Spring St, New York, NY 10013-1578. TEL 212-620-8468, 800-221-9369, FAX 212-807-1047; **Subscr. to:** Journals Department, PO Box 322, Dordrecht 3300 AH, Netherlands. TEL 31-78-639-2392, FAX 31-78-654-6474.

ENVIRONMENT, HEALTH & SAFETY MANAGEMENT. see *ENVIRONMENTAL STUDIES—Toxicology And Environmental Safety*

ENVIRONMENTAL COMPLIANCE & LITIGATION STRATEGY. see *LAW*

344.0462 USA ISSN 1056-3164
KF3775.A15
ENVIRONMENTAL REGULATORY ADVISOR. Text in English. 1991. m. USD 125 (effective 2001). **Description:** Provides information on congressional and regulatory activity to control, monitor and eliminate hazards created by pollutants, hazardous and toxic substances.
—ingenta.
Published by: J.J. Keller & Associates, Inc., 3003 W Breezewood Lane, Box 368, Neenah, WI 54957-0368. TEL 920-722-2848, 800-327-6868, FAX 920-727-7526, http://www.jjkeller.com.

E

604.7 USA ISSN 0749-3940
EVERYONE'S BACKYARD. Text in English. 1982. q. USD 35 (effective 1999). adv. bk.rev., film rev. charts, illus. back issues avail.; reprints avail. **Document type:** *Newsletter.*
Incorporates (1983-1990): Action Bulletin (0749-3959)
Indexed: Environ.Per.Bibl. (1989-).
Published by: Center for Health, Environment, and Justice, Marcoin Building, 150 South Washington St, Ste 300, Box 6806, Falls Church, VA 22046-6806. TEL 703-237-2249, FAX 703-237-8389, cchw@essential.org, http://www.essential.org/cchw; www.sustain.org/hcwh. Ed. Patty Lovera. R&P Barbara Sullivan. Adv. contact Joel Gysan. Circ: 6,000.

HAZARDOUS MATERIALS NEWSLETTER. see *PUBLIC HEALTH AND SAFETY*

363.7287 USA ISSN 0738-0232
TD811.5
HAZARDOUS WASTE CONSULTANT. Text in English. 1983. 8/yr. USD 798 to individuals; USD 120 newsstand/cover (effective 2002). bk.rev. back issues avail. *Refereed.* **Document type:** *Journal, Academic/Scholarly.* **Description:** Covers hazardous waste management topics by experts. Includes in-depth articles on technology, regulations and legal issues.
Related titles: Microform ed.: (from PQC); Online - full text ed.: (from ingenta, Swets Blackwell, Institute for Scientific Information).
Indexed: ASCA, Aqua.Sci.& Fish.Abstr., Curr.Cont., Eng.Ind., Environ.Abstr., Environ.Sci.Poll.Mgmt., Geo.Abstr.H.G., Geo.Abstr.P.G., Geol.Abstr., INIS Atomind., Pollut.Abstr., Sel.Water Res.Abstr., WasteInfo.
—BLDSC (4274.451440), Ei, EMDOCS, IDS, Linda Hall. **CCC.**
Published by: Aspen Publishers, Inc., 200 Orchard Ridge Dr, Ste 200, Gaithersburg, MD 20878. TEL 301-417-7500, FAX 301-695-7931. **Dist. by:** TEL 301-698-7100.

363.7287 USA ISSN 1087-0873
HAZARDOUS WASTE REGULATORY ANALYSIS SERVICE. Text in English. 1983. m. NLG 1,566, USD 795, EUR 710.62 (effective 2000). **Document type:** *Trade.* **Description:** Reviews and analyzes each proposed and final Resource Conservation and Recovery Act; Comprehensive Environmental Response, Compensation and Liability Act; and Superfund Admendments and Reauthorization Act regulation during the year.
Related titles: Online - full text ed.
Published by: Aspen Publishers, Inc., 200 Orchard Ridge Dr, Ste 200, Gaithersburg, MD 20878. TEL 301-417-7500, FAX 301-695-7931. **Dist. by:** TEL 301-698-7100.

I E H REPORT ON HEALTH EFFECTS OF WASTE COMBUSTION PRODUCTS. see *ENVIRONMENTAL STUDIES—Pollution*

363.17 USA
INFECTIOUS WASTES NEWS. Text in English. fortn.
Published by: Environmental Industry Associations, 4301 Connecticut Ave, N W, Ste 300, Washington, DC 20008. TEL 202-244-4700, FAX 202-966-4868. Ed. Michael Malloy.

LEAD ACTION NEWS. see *PUBLIC HEALTH AND SAFETY*

344.04622 USA
MEDICAL WASTE HANDBOOK. Text in English. a. USD 208 (effective 2000). **Document type:** *Trade.* **Description:** Provides comprehensive coverage of the medical waste laws from the federal and state regulations to agency structures.
Published by: West Group (Subsidiary of: Thomson Corporation, The), 620 Opperman Dr., Eagan, MN 55123. TEL 800-344-5008, FAX 800-340-9378, http://www.westgroup.com. Eds. David S Freeman, Gregory H Siskind, Sharon O Jacobs.

363.728 ITA ISSN 0394-5391
R S RIFIUTI SOLIDI. Text in Italian; Summaries in English, Italian. 1987. 6/yr. ITL 135,000 domestic; ITL 270,000 foreign (effective 2000). adv. 70 p./no. **Document type:** *Journal, Trade.* **Description:** Covers solid waste management.
Indexed: INIS Atomind.
—BLDSC (8036.703600).
Published by: (Centro di Ingegneria per la Protezione dell'Ambiente), C I P A s.a.s, Via Palladio, 26, Milan, MI 20135, Italy. TEL 39-02-58301528, FAX 39-02-58301550, cipami@tin.it. Ed. Raffaello Cossu. adv.: B&W page ITL 1,650,000, color page ITL 2,100,000; trim 210 x 297. Circ: 1,100.

RACHEL'S ENVIRONMENT & HEALTH WEEKLY. see *ENVIRONMENTAL STUDIES*

RADIATION PROTECTION NEWS AND NOTES. see *PUBLIC HEALTH AND SAFETY*

363.7287 USA ISSN 1056-5264
KF3945.Z9
SPILL REPORTING PROCEDURES GUIDE. Text in English. 1989. a. USD 215 (effective 2000). **Document type:** *Trade.* **Description:** For individuals responsible for reporting releases of hazardous substances.
—CCC.
Published by: B N A Books (Subsidiary of: The Bureau of National Affairs, Inc.), 1231 25th St, NW, Washington, DC 20037. TEL 202-452-4343, FAX 202-452-4997, books@bna.com, http://www.bna.com/bnabooks/publications/details/d_srp.htm. Ed. Jeffrey J Kimmel. Pub. Richard H Cornfield. **Subscr. to:** PO Box 7814, Edison, NJ 08818-7814. TEL 800-960-1220, FAX 732-346-1624.

TOXIC TORTS; litigation of hazardous substance cases. see *PUBLIC HEALTH AND SAFETY*

WATER SEWAGE AND EFFLUENT. see *WATER RESOURCES*

ETHNIC INTERESTS

A B N F JOURNAL. see *MEDICAL SCIENCES—Nurses And Nursing*

362.1 305.8 USA
A P A I T✱; HIV - AIDS from another angle. Text in English. 1994. q. free per issue. **Document type:** *Newsletter.*
Published by: Asian Pacific AIDS Intervention Team, 605 W Olympic Blvd, Ste 610, Los Angeles, CA 90015-1426. Ed. Noel Alumit.

AIDSIDA INFO. see *HOMOSEXUALITY*

AMERICAN INDIAN AND ALASKA NATIVE MENTAL HEALTH RESEARCH. see *NATIVE AMERICAN STUDIES*

COMPLEMENTARY CARE JOURNAL. see *SOCIOLOGY*

CONGREGATION NEWS. see *HANDICAPPED—Hearing Impaired*

ELDER VOICES. see *GERONTOLOGY AND GERIATRICS*

ETHNICITY & DISEASE. see *MEDICAL SCIENCES*

ETHNICITY AND HEALTH. see *PUBLIC HEALTH AND SAFETY*

HEALTHQUEST; total wellness for body, mind and spirit. see *NUTRITION AND DIETETICS*

HEART & SOUL. see *PHYSICAL FITNESS AND HYGIENE*

HELLENIC MEDICAL JOURNAL. see *MEDICAL SCIENCES*

HISPANIC JOURNAL OF BEHAVIORAL SCIENCES. see *PSYCHOLOGY*

JEWISH GUILD FOR THE BLIND. NEWSLETTER. see *HANDICAPPED—Visually Impaired*

JEWISH VEGETARIAN. see *NUTRITION AND DIETETICS*

JOURNAL OF BLACK PSYCHOLOGY. see *PSYCHOLOGY*

JOURNAL OF BLACK STUDIES. see *SOCIAL SCIENCES: COMPREHENSIVE WORKS*

▼ **JOURNAL OF IMMIGRANT HEALTH.** see *MEDICAL SCIENCES*

JOURNAL OF MULTICULTURAL COUNSELING AND DEVELOPMENT. see *PSYCHOLOGY*

JOURNAL OF MULTICULTURAL NURSING AND HEALTH. see *MEDICAL SCIENCES—Nurses And Nursing*

LIKUTIM; a journal of visual impairment and blindness. see *HANDICAPPED—Visually Impaired*

MEDICINA Y CULTURA. see *MEDICAL SCIENCES*

MEDICO INTERAMERICANO. see *MEDICAL SCIENCES*

MINORITY NURSE NEWSLETTER. see *MEDICAL SCIENCES—Nurses And Nursing*

N D A JOURNAL. see *MEDICAL SCIENCES—Dentistry*

NATIONAL CONGRESS OF JEWISH DEAF. QUARTERLY. see *HANDICAPPED—Hearing Impaired*

OESTERSJOEJUDISKT FORUM. see *POLITICAL SCIENCE—Civil Rights*

OPPORTUNITIES FOR MINORITY STUDENTS IN THE U.S. DENTAL SCHOOLS. see *EDUCATION—Higher Education*

OUT IN BLACK. see *HOMOSEXUALITY*

LA SALUD HISPANA; previniendo enfermedades. see *PHYSICAL FITNESS AND HYGIENE*

SHAMAN'S DRUM; a journal of experiential Shamanism. see *ANTHROPOLOGY*

SIDA; todo lo que usted debe saber. see *MEDICAL SCIENCES—Communicable Diseases*

SIDA AHORA. see *MEDICAL SCIENCES—Communicable Diseases*

306.766 USA
HA-YONAH/DOVE. Text in English. 1982. m. adv. illus. back issues avail. **Description:** Community interest for gay, lesbian and bisexual Jews.
Published by: Congregation Ahavat Shalom, PO Box 14392, San Francisco, CA 94114-0392. TEL 415-621-1020. Ed. David May. Circ: 350.

EXPERIMENTAL MEDICINE, LABORATORY TECHNIQUE

see MEDICAL SCIENCES—Experimental Medicine, Laboratory Technique

FAMILY AND MATRIMONIAL LAW

see LAW—Family And Matrimonial Law

FASHIONS

see CLOTHING TRADE—Fashions

FEED, FLOUR AND GRAIN

see AGRICULTURE—Feed, Flour And Grain

FIRE PREVENTION

628.92 DEU ISSN 0724-7443
112 - MAGAZIN DER FEUERWEHR. Text in German. 1975. m. DEM 87; DEM 115 foreign (effective 2000). adv. illus. **Document type:** *Magazine, Trade.*
Published by: E F B Verlagsgesellschaft mbH, Beethovenstr 27, Erlensee 63526, Germany. TEL 49-6183-3012, FAX 49-6183-3033. Ed. Helmut Raab. R&P Susanna Haus. Adv. contact Doris Wallow. B&W page DEM 3,870, color page DEM 5,670; trim 185 x 265. Circ: 30,000.

614.84 CAN ISSN 0838-679X
ATLANTIC FIREFIGHTER; the voice of the fire service in atlantic canada. Text in English. 1984. m. CND 11.95 (effective 1999). adv. bk.rev. 16 p./no. 6 cols./p. back issues avail. **Document type:** *Newspaper.* **Description:** Fire related stories-interest news related. Atlantic Canada. Information and interest to fire service. Fire marshall, fire department, EMS.
Published by: Hilden Publishing Ltd., P O Box 919, Amherst, NS B4H 4E1, Canada. TEL 902-667-3009, FAX 902-667-2868, atl.firefighter@ns.sympatico.ca. Ed. Terrance M Brown. Pub. Terrance Brown. R&P, Adv. contact Jennifer Brown TEL 902-667-3009. B&W page CND 1,199, color page CND 1,390. Circ: 7,000.

F

614.84 900 DEU ISSN 0006-9094
BRANDSCHUTZ; Deutsche Feuerwehr-Zeitung. Text in German. 1946. m. EUR 82.20, CHF 160.75; EUR 10.90, CHF 21.30 newsstand/cover (effective 2002). bk.rev. index. back issues avail. **Document type:** *Newspaper, Trade.*
Indexed: INIS Atomind., Ref.Zh.
—CISTI, Infotrieve. **CCC.**
Published by: W. Kohlhammer GmbH, Hessbruehlstr 69, Stuttgart 70565, Germany. TEL 49-711-7863-1, FAX 49-711-7863393, info@kohlhammer-katalog.de, http://www.kohlhammer.de. Circ: 14,500.

628.92 USA ISSN 1048-5074
CALIFORNIA FIRE SERVICE. Text in English. 1927. m. USD 50 (effective 1998). adv. bk.rev. charts, illus, stat, tr.lit. index, cum.index. back issues avail. **Document type:** *Trade.* **Description:** Firefighter news in the areas of fire suppression, prevention, emergency medical services, hazardous materials and disaster response.
Formerly (until 1990): California Fireman (0739-0114)
Published by: California State Firefighters' Association, 2701 K St, 201, Sacramento, CA 95816-5113. TEL 913-446-9880, FAX 916-446-9889. Ed. Gary C Giacomo. Adv. contact Colt Stewart. Circ: 30,000.

614.84 USA ISSN 0015-2552
TH9111
FIRE CHIEF; administration, training, operations. Text in English. 1956. m. USD 54; USD 114 foreign. adv. bk.rev. charts, illus. reprint service avail. from PQC. **Document type:** *Journal, Trade.* **Description:** Emphasizes helping fire administrators to solve their administrative and management problems and to meet today's challenges in five major areas of fire department responsibility: fire prevention, fire suppression, public education, emergency medical response and personal safety.
Incorporates: Volunteer Firefighter; Volunteer Fire Chief
Related titles: Microform ed.: (from PQC); Online - full text ed.: (from ProQuest Information & Learning, Gale Group).
—ingenta. **CCC.**
Published by: Primedia Business Magazines & Media, Inc. (Atlanta), 6151 Powers Ferry Rd, N W, Atlanta, GA 30339-2941. TEL 770-955-2500, FAX 770-955-0400, inquiries@primediabusiness.com, http://industryclick.com/magazine.asp?magazineid=157&siteid=26, http://www.primediabusiness.com/. Ed. Janet Wilmoth. Pub. Ray Anderson. Circ: 50,000. **Subscr. to:** Primedia Business Magazines & Media, Inc., PO Box 12914, Overland Park, KS 66282-2914. TEL 800-441-0294, FAX 913-967-1903.

628.92 USA ISSN 0889-5740
FIRE CONTROL DIGEST. Text in English. 1975. m. USD 195 domestic; USD 199 in Canada; USD 207 elsewhere (effective 2000). back issues avail. **Document type:** *Newsletter.* **Description:** Contains information about Federal and State programs, budgets, and emergency medical service for fire prevention professionals.
Published by: Washington Capital News Reports, Inc., 1745 Jefferson David Hwy, Ste 308, Arlington, VA 22202-3402. TEL 703-416-1950, FAX 703-416-1030. Ed. Susan O'Connell. Pub. Brian T Seehan. Circ: 300 (paid).

614.84 USA
FIRE FOCUS. Text in English. 1984. s-m. USD 30 (effective 2000); includes New Jersey State Fire Code. **Document type:** *Newsletter, Government.* **Description:** Trade news for fire service and related organizations.
Formerly: New Jersey Bureau of Fire Safety. Newsletter
Published by: Division of Fire Safety, Attn: Helen Kerr, Publication's Unit, P O Box 809, Trenton, NJ 08625-0809. TEL 609-633-6120, 609-633-6130, FAX 609-633-6744. Ed. Mike Matcho. Circ: 11,000.

614.84 USA ISSN 0015-2625
TH9111
FIRE NEWS. Text in English. 1916. 6/yr. membership. illus. **Document type:** *Newsletter.*
Indexed: C.I.S. Abstr.
—CISTI, Linda Hall.
Published by: National Fire Protection Association, 1 Batterymarch Park, Quincy, MA 02269. TEL 617-770-3500, http://www.wpi.edu/~fpe/nfpa.html, http://www.nfpa.org. Pub. Kathleen M Robinson. R&P Dennis Berry. Circ: 67,000 (controlled).

HEALTH & SAFETY NEWSLINE; for the engineering industry (UK). see *PUBLIC HEALTH AND SAFETY*

614.84 USA
ICHIEFS ON SCENE. Text in English. 1934. s-m. free to members; USD 3.50 newsstand/cover to non-members (effective 2001). adv. bk.rev., film rev. abstr, bibl, charts, illus, pat, stat, tr.lit. cum.index: 1970-1975. 8 p./no. back issues avail. **Document type:** *Newsletter.* **Description:** Provides an overview of the types of things that will affect change in the fire service field and gives specifics about where to obtain useful references. Reaches fire and EMS leaders in 40 countries worldwide.
Former titles (until 2000): I A F C On Scene (0893-3936); (until 1987): Washington Scene (0747-8992); (until 1987): International Fire Chief (0734-435X); (until 1979): International Association of Fire Chiefs. Official Publication (0161-2158); (until 1978): International Fire Chief (0364-8958)
Related titles: Online - full text ed.
—CISTI.
Published by: International Association of Fire Chiefs, 4025 Fair Ridge Dr, Fairfax, VA 22033-2868. TEL 703-273-0911, FAX 703-273-9363, onscene@ichiefs.org.org, http://www.iafc.org/. Ed., R&P, Adv. contact Mary Marshall. Circ: 12,000 (paid).

MAPFRE SEGURIDAD. see *OCCUPATIONAL HEALTH AND SAFETY*

628.922029 USA
TH9503
(YEAR) NATIONAL DIRECTORY OF FIRE CHIEFS & E M S ADMINISTRATORS. Text in English. 1992. a. USD 99 (effective 2000). adv. **Document type:** *Directory.*
Former titles: (Year) National Directory of Fire Chiefs & Emergency Departments (1522-7863); National Directory of Fire Chiefs, Rescue and Emergency Departments (1066-5609)
Related titles: CD-ROM ed.; Diskette ed.
Published by: Span Publishing, 3273 Church St, Ste 201, PO Box 365, Stevens Point, WI 54481-0365. TEL 715-345-2772, FAX 715-345-7288, http://www.safetysource.com. Ed. Laura Gross. Pub. Steve Cywinski. Circ: 2,500.

614.84 USA
TH9503
NATIONAL FIRE PROTECTION ASSOCIATION. REPORT ON COMMITTEES. Text in English. 1917. s-a. reprint service avail. from PQC.
Formerly: N F P A Technical Committee. Report (0077-4553)
Indexed: Text.Tech.Dig. (1977-1978).
Published by: National Fire Protection Association, 1 Batterymarch Park, Quincy, MA 02269. TEL 617-984-7565, 800-344-3555, FAX 617-984-7010.

614.84 USA
NEW JERSEY STATE FIRE CODE. Text in English. 1985. irreg. (plus s-a. update). USD 20; USD 30 with Newsletter. **Document type:** *Government.*
Published by: Division of Fire Safety, Attn: Helen Kerr, Publication's Unit, P O Box 809, Trenton, NJ 08625-0809. TEL 609-633-6130, FAX 609-633-6744.

628.9 NOR
NORWAY. DIREKTORATET FOR BRANN OG EKSPLOSJONSVERN. AARSBERETNING. Text in Norwegian; Summaries in English. 1915. a. free per issue. illus, stat. **Document type:** *Yearbook, Corporate, Government.*
Former titles: Norway. Statens Sprengstoffinspeksjon. Aarsberetning; Norway. Sprengstoffinspeksjonen. Aarsberetning
Published by: Direktoratet for Brann og Eksplosjonsvern, Postboks 355, Sentrum, Tonsberg 3101, Norway. TEL 47-33-39-88-00, FAX 47-33-31-06-60. Circ: 5,000.

614.84 JPN
OKINAWA PREFECTURE. ANNUAL REPORT OF FIRE AND DISASTER PREVENTION. Text in Japanese. 1973. a. free per issue. **Document type:** *Government.*
Published by: Okinawa-ken, 2-2 Izumizaki 1-chome, Naha-shi, Okinawa-ken 900-0000, Japan. TEL 81-98-866-2143, FAX 81-98-866-3204, http://www.okinawa.ttc.co.jp. Circ: 450.

352.3 628.92 BIH ISSN 0351-4714
POZAR EKSPLOZIJA PREVENTIVA; naucni, strucni i informativni casopis. Text in Serbo-Croatian. 1980. q. BAD 2,000. adv. bk.rev. abstr, bibl, charts, illus. index, cum.index. back issues avail.
Published by: Institut Zastite od Pozara i Eksplozije, Romanijska 10, Sarajevo 71000, Bosnia Herzegovina. TEL 071 538-480, FAX 071-468-108, TELEX 071-41667. Ed. Ratko Vujovic. Circ: 2,000.

344.053 352.3 USA
RHODE ISLAND FIRE LAW AND RULES ANNOTATED. Text in English. a., latest 1996. USD 38.50.
Published by: Lexis Law Publishing (Subsidiary of: Reed Elsevier plc), PO Box 7587, Charlottesville, VA 22906-7587. TEL 804-972-7566, 800-562-1197, FAX 800-643-1280, llp.customer.support@lexis-nexis.com, http://www.lexislawpublishing.com. Ed. George Harley.

353.979 JPN
SAIGAI NO JITTAI TO SHOBO NO GENKYO/ANNUAL REPORT OF FIRE AND DISASTER PREVENTION. Text and summaries in Japanese. 1967. a. free per issue.
Published by: General Affairs Department of Miyagi Prefecture, Fire and Disaster Prevention Section, 8-1 Honcho 3-chome, Aoba-ku, Sendai-shi, Miyagi-ken 980-0000, Japan. FAX 022-211-2399. Ed. Keisuke Kudo. Circ: 400.

628.92 621 JPN ISSN 0426-2700
CODEN: SHKHBF
SHOBO KENKYUJO HOKOKU/FIRE RESEARCH INSTITUTE OF JAPAN. REPORT. Text in Japanese; Summaries in English. 1950. s-a. free per issue. **Document type:** *Academic/Scholarly.*
Indexed: INIS Atomind.
—CASDDS, Linda Hall.
Published by: Fire Research Institute of Japan/Shobo Kenkyujo, 3-14-1 Nakahara, Mitaka-shi, Tokyo-to 181-0005, Japan. TEL 0422-44-8331, FAX 0422-42-7719. Circ: 881.

628.92 USA ISSN 0896-2685
SPRINKLER AGE. Text in English. 1981. m. USD 33.95 domestic; USD 150 foreign (effective 1999). adv. **Document type:** *Trade.* **Description:** Devoted to the professional development of the fire sprinkler industry.
Published by: American Fire Sprinkler Association, 12959 Jupiter Rd, Ste 142, Dallas, TX 75238. TEL 214-349-5965, FAX 214-343-8898, jknowles@firesprink.org, http://www.sprinklernet.com. Ed., R&P Janet Knowles. Pub. Janet R Knowles. Adv. contact Roger K Gragg. Circ: 3,900 (controlled).

614.84 USA
TURN OUT; the official magazine of the IFBA. Text in English. s-a. USD 15 to individuals (effective 2002). **Document type:** *Magazine.* **Description:** Promotes the well-being of fire departments and its members and related emergency support personnel.
Published by: International Fire Buff Association, PO Box 240144, Milwaukee, WI 53224-9007. turnout@ifba.org, http://www.ifba.org/turnout.

614.84 USA
VISITING FIREMAN. Text in English. a. USD 15 in US & Canada; USD 18 in Europe; USD 20 in Asia & the Pacific (effective 2002). **Document type:** *Directory, Trade.*
Address: N6271 Paradise Dr, Burlington, WI 53105.

614.84 USA ISSN 1071-1767
W F S QUARTERLY. Text in English. 1986. q. USD 40 domestic to individuals; USD 45 foreign to individuals; USD 50 domestic to institutions; USD 55 foreign to institutions (effective 2000). adv. bk.rev. index. back issues avail. **Document type:** *Newsletter.* **Description:** Discusses issues relevant to women involved in the fire service such as recruitment, physical agility testing, fitness training, firefighting techiques, reproductive safety, etc.
Published by: Women in the Fire Service, PO Box 5446, Madison, WI 53705. TEL 608-233-4768, FAX 608-233-4879, tfloren@wfsi.org, http://www.wfsi.org. Ed., Pub., Adv. contact Terese M Floren. R&P Terese Floren. Circ: 250 (paid).

614.84 USA ISSN 0042-9775
TH9111
W N Y F. (With New York Firefighters) Text in English. 1940. q. USD 18 domestic; USD 21 foreign (effective 2000). charts, illus. **Document type:** *Trade.* **Description:** Includes fire stories, technical articles, photos, and other job-related information for members of New York City Fire Department.
Published by: N Y C Fire Department, Public Information, 9 MetroTech Center, Brooklyn, NY 11201. TEL 718-999-1455, FAX 718-999-2789. Ed., R&P Janet Kimmerly. Circ: 14,000 (paid).

WHO'S WHO IN THE EMERGENCY & RESCUE SERVICES (YEAR). see *PUBLIC HEALTH AND SAFETY*

F

628.92 USA
WYOMING FIRE NEWS. Text in English. q. **Document type:** *Newsletter, Government.* **Description:** Provides information about fire prevention with advice, seminar schedules, public awareness tips, rulings, commentary, and a calendar of events.
Published by: Wyoming State Department of Fire Prevention, 122 W 25th St, Cheyenne, WY 82002. TEL 307-777-7288, FAX 307-777-7119. Ed. Elaine Codianne.

614.84 JPN ISSN 0910-4208
YOBO JIHO/ACCIDENT PREVENTION JOURNAL. Text in Japanese. 1950. q. free per issue. back issues avail. **Document type:** *Academic/Scholarly.*
Indexed: Ref.Zh.
Published by: Marine and Fire Insurance Association of Japan, 9 Kanda-Awaji-cho 2-chome, Chiyoda-ku, Tokyo 101-0063, Japan. FAX 03-3255-1236, LDB02422@niftyserve.or.jp. Ed. Nobuo Shioya. Circ: 14,600.

FIRE PREVENTION—Abstracting, Bibliographies, Statistics

614.84 GBR ISSN 0260-3098
FIRE STATISTICS UNITED KINGDOM. Text in English. 1946. a. price varies. **Document type:** *Government.*
Former titles (until 1977): United Kingdom Fire Statistics; United Kingdom Fire and Loss Statistics (0082-7959)
—CISTI, Infotrieve. **CCC.**
Published by: Home Office, 50 Queen Annes Gate, London SW1H 9AT, United Kingdom. TEL 081-760-2850. Circ: 900.

016.62892 RUS ISSN 0202-9901
REFERATIVNYI ZHURNAL. POZHARNAYA BEZOPASNOST'. Text in Russian. m. USD 285 in United States. **Document type:** *Abstract/Index.*
—East View.
Published by: Vserossiiskii Institut Nauchnoi i Tekhnicheskoi Informatsii (VINITI), Usievicha ul 20-a, Moscow 125315, Russian Federation. TEL 7-095-1526441, FAX 7-095-943-0060. Ed. B D Turkin. **US dist. addr.:** East View Publications, 3020 Harbor Ln N, Minneapolis, MN 55447. TEL 612-550-0961.

FISH AND FISHERIES

see also BIOLOGY—Zoology

578.77 UGA ISSN 0002-0036
SH1 CODEN: AJTHBC
AFRICAN JOURNAL OF TROPICAL HYDROBIOLOGY AND FISHERIES. Text in English, French. 1971-1976; resumed 1994. s-a. USD 50 to individuals; USD 75 to institutions; USD 25 to students (effective 2000). bk.rev. *Refereed.*
Indexed: Aqua.Sci.& Fish.Abstr., Aquacult.Abstr., Biol.Abstr., Environ.Sci.Poll.Mgmt., Sport Fish.Abstr.
—Linda Hall.
Published by: Lake Victoria Fisheries Organization, P O Box 1625, Jinja, Uganda. TEL 256-43-120205, FAX 256-43-130123, lvfo@source.co.ug, http://www.lvfo.org. Ed. M J Ntiba. Circ: 300 (paid and controlled).

639.34 DEU ISSN 1437-4854
AQUARISTIK - FACHMAGAZIN. Text in German. 1968. bi-m. EUR 29.50 (effective 2001). adv. bk.rev. 80 p./no. 3 cols./p. back issues avail. **Document type:** *Magazine, Trade.*
Former titles: T I (0942-5160); (until 1992): T I International (0176-3660)
Indexed: Zoo.Rec.
Published by: Tetra Verlag GmbH, Friedensweg 15, Bissendorf 49143, Germany. TEL 49-5402-8889, FAX 49-5402-8811, info@tetra-verlag.de, http://www.tetra-verlag.de. Ed. Hans Joachim Herrmann. Adv. contact Eckhard Grell. Circ: 10,000.

639 578.77 CAN ISSN 0706-6503
CODEN: CBFSDB
CANADIAN BULLETIN OF FISHERIES AND AQUATIC SCIENCES. Text in English. 1901. irreg., latest vol.227, 1994. price varies. **Document type:** *Monographic series, Government.*
Formerly: Canada. Fisheries Research Board. Bulletin (0068-7537)
Related titles: Microfiche ed.: (from MML); French ed.: ISSN 0706-6511.
Indexed: Aqua.Sci.& Fish.Abstr., Aquacult.Abstr., Arct.Bibl., Biol.Abstr., Chem.Abstr., Curr.Adv.Ecol.Sci., Deep Sea Res.& Oceanogr.Abstr., Environ.Sci.Poll.Mgmt., Food Sci.& Tech.Abstr., GeoRef, Helminthol.Abstr., Ocean.Abstr. (coverage dropped), Sel.Water Res.Abstr., Sport Fish.Abstr., Zoo.Rec.
—CASDDS, CISTI, Linda Hall. **CCC.**
Published by: National Research Council of Canada, Monograph Publishing Program, Building M 55, Ottawa, ON K1A 0R6, Canada. TEL 613-993-0151, http://www.nrc.ca/cisti/journals/. Ed. G J Neville. Circ: 1,000.

639.2 636.089 NCL ISSN 1025-4951
CIGUATERA. Text in English. 1991. irreg., latest vol.3, 1993. **Document type:** *Newsletter.*
Related titles: French ed.: ISSN 1025-7411.
Indexed: Aquacult.Abstr.
Published by: Secretariat of the Pacific Community, PO Box D5, Noumea Cedex 98848, New Caledonia. TEL 687-262000, FAX 687-263818, spc@spc.int, http://www.spc.int.

CONTRIBUTIONS IN MARINE SCIENCE. see *BIOLOGY*

639 578.77 DNK ISSN 1397-2464
SH267
DANMARKS FISKERIUNDERSOEGELSER. AARSBERETNING. Text in Danish. 1996. a. free per issue. **Document type:** *Government.*
Formed by the merger of (1966-1996): Danmark. Fiskeriministeriet. Forsoegslaboratorium. Aarsberetning (0070-3605); (1951-1996): Danmarks Fiskeri- og Havundersoegelser. Aarsberetning. (0416-9875); (1993-1996): Institut for Ferskvandsfiskeri og Fiskepleje. Aarsberetning (0908-1135)
Indexed: Aqua.Sci.& Fish.Abstr., Chem.Abstr., Food Sci.& Tech.Abstr.
Published by: Danmarks Fiskeriundersoegelser/Danish Institute for Fisheries Research, Jaegersborgvej 64-66, Lyngby 2800, Denmark. TEL 45-33-96-33-00, FAX 45-33-96-33-49, dir@dfu.min.dk, info@dfu.min.dk. Circ: 1,500.

639.8 BEL ISSN 0774-0689
EUROPEAN AQUACULTURE SOCIETY. SPECIAL PUBLICATIONS. Text in English. 1976. irreg. price varies. **Document type:** *Proceedings.* **Description:** Each issue focuses on a specific topic or area of research in aquaculture.
Indexed: Ocean.Abstr. (coverage dropped), Sport Fish.Abstr., Zoo.Rec.
—CISTI.
Published by: European Aquaculture Society (EAS), Slijkensesteenweg 4, Oostende 8400, Belgium. TEL 32-59-323859, FAX 32-59-321005, eas@unicall.be.

GIDROBIOLOGICHESKII ZHURNAL; nauchnyi zhurnal. see *BIOLOGY*

HYDROBIOLOGICAL JOURNAL. see *BIOLOGY*

639.3 636.089 USA ISSN 0899-7659
WMLC 93/306 CODEN: JAAHEO
JOURNAL OF AQUATIC ANIMAL HEALTH. Text in English. 1989. q. USD 175 in North America; USD 190 elsewhere; USD 190 in North America Print & online eds.; USD 205 elsewhere Print & online eds. (effective 2001). adv. charts, illus, stat. index. back issues avail. *Refereed.* **Document type:** *Academic/Scholarly.* **Description:** Carries research papers on the causes, effects, treatments and prevention of diseases, particularly of fish and shellfish.
Related titles: Online - full text ed.: USD 175 (effective 2001) (from EBSCO Publishing, Institute for Scientific Information).
Indexed: ABSEARCH Amer.Fish. (1989-), AgBiotech, Anim.Breed.Abstr., Aqua.Sci.& Fish.Abstr., Aquacult.Abstr., Curr.Cont., Derwent Biotech.Abstr., Environ.Abstr., Environ.Sci.Poll.Mgmt., Fish.Abstr. (1989-), Focus on: Vet.Sci.& Med., Helminthol.Abstr., Ind.Vet., Int.Abstr.Biol.Sci., Microbiol.Abstr., Nutr.Abstr., Ocean.Abstr., Pollut.Abstr., Protozool.Abstr., Rev.Appl.Entomol., Rev.Med.& Vet.Mycol., Sel.Water Res.Abstr., Sport Fish.Abstr., Vet.Bull., Wild.Rev., Zoo.Rec.
—BLDSC (4947.156800), CINDOC, CISTI, EMDOCS, IDS, Infotrieve, ingenta, Linda Hall. **CCC.**
Published by: American Fisheries Society, 5410 Grosvenor Ln, Ste 110, Bethesda, MD 20814-2199. TEL 301-897-8616, FAX 301-897-8096, main@fisheries.org, journals@fisheries.org, http://www.fisheries.org; http://afs.allenpress.com, http://www.afs.allenpress.com. Eds. Ronald P Hedrick, Stephen Kaatari. R&P Janet Harry. Adv. contact Hannelore Quigley. Circ: 1,500.

REVISTA DE BIOLOGIA MARINA Y OCEANOGRAFIA. see *BIOLOGY*

SINGAPORE JOURNAL OF PRIMARY INDUSTRIES. see *AGRICULTURE*

FOLKLORE

TAROT NETWORK NEWS. see *NEW AGE PUBLICATIONS*

FOOD AND FOOD INDUSTRIES

see also AGRICULTURE; FISH AND FISHERIES; FOOD AND FOOD INDUSTRIES—Bakers And Confectioners; FOOD AND FOOD INDUSTRIES—Grocery Trade; HOME ECONOMICS; HOTELS AND RESTAURANTS; NUTRITION AND DIETETICS

A Q I S BULLETIN. see *AGRICULTURE*

ADVANCES IN FOOD AND NUTRITION RESEARCH. see *NUTRITION AND DIETETICS*

664.0072 DEU ISSN 1431-7737
TX501 CODEN: CMTLBX
ADVANCES IN FOOD SCIENCES. Text in German. 3/yr. DEM 162.50 domestic; DEM 182.50 in Europe; DEM 202.50 elsewhere (effective 1999). **Document type:** *Academic/Scholarly.*
Formerly (until 1996): Chemie Mikrobiologie Technologie der Lebensmittel (0366-7154)
Indexed: Aqua.Sci.& Fish.Abstr., Biotech.& Bioeng.Abstr., Chem.Abstr., Chem.Indus.Notes, Chem.Titles, Chemorec.Abstr., Dairy Sci.Abstr., Environ.Sci.Poll.Mgmt., Excerp.Med., Food Sci.& Tech.Abstr., INIS Atomind., Mass Spectr.Bull., Microbiol.Abstr., Ref.Zh., VITIS.
—BLDSC (0707.020000), CASDDS, CINDOC, CISTI, Infotrieve, Linda Hall. **CCC.**
Published by: Technische Universitaet Muenchen, Institut fuer Lebensmitteltechnologie und Analytische Chemie, Weihenstephan 1, Freising 85350, Germany. TEL 49-8161-714296, FAX 49-8161-713668, leu@weihenstephan.de. Eds. G Leupold, H Parlar.

ALIMENTACION, NUTRICION Y SALUD. see *NUTRITION AND DIETETICS*

ALIMENTOS E NUTRICAO. see *NUTRITION AND DIETETICS*

ALLERGY HOTLINE. see *MEDICAL SCIENCES—Allergology And Immunology*

ANNUAL EDITIONS: NUTRITION. see *NUTRITION AND DIETETICS*

664 613.2 301 GBR
ANTHROPOLOGY OF FOOD AND NUTRITION. Text in English. irreg. price varies. bibl. Index.
—BLDSC (1546.502825).
Published by: Berghahn Books Ltd, 3 Newtec Pl, Magdalen Rd, Oxford OX4 1RE, United Kingdom. TEL 44-1865-250011, FAX 44-1865-250056, berghahnUK@aol.com, http://www.berghahnbooks.com. **Orders in the US & Rest of the World:** Berghahn Books Inc. **Orders in UK & Europe:** Estover Rd, Plymouth PL6 7PY, United Kingdom. TEL 44-1752-202301, FAX 44-1752-202333.

APPLIED AND ENVIRONMENTAL MICROBIOLOGY. see *BIOLOGY—Microbiology*

614 USA ISSN 0898-4131
HD9000.9.U5 CODEN: QBAODQ
ASSOCIATION OF FOOD AND DRUG OFFICIALS. JOURNAL. Text in English. 1937. q., latest vol.66, 2002. USD 80 in US & Canada; USD 90 elsewhere (effective 2002). adv. bibl. back issues avail.; reprint service avail. from ISI. *Refereed.* **Document type:** *Academic/Scholarly, Trade.* **Description:** Promotes and offers uniformity of laws affecting foods, drugs, cosmetics, devices, and product safety.
Former titles (until 1987): Association of Food and Drug Officials Quarterly Bulletin (0195-4865); (until 1975): Association of Food and Drug Officials of the United States. Quarterly Bulletin (0004-5721)
Related titles: Microfilm ed.: (from PMC).
Indexed: Curr.Adv.Ecol.Sci., Curr.Cont. (coverage dropped), Curr.Pack.Abstr., Dairy Sci.Abstr., Environ.Abstr., Food Sci.& Tech.Abstr., NRN.

F

—BLDSC (4704.160000), CASDDS, CISTI, GNLM, ingenta, Linda Hall.
Published by: Association of Food and Drug Officials, 2550 Kingston Rd Ste 311, York, PA 17402. TEL 717-757-2888, FAX 717-755-8089, afdo@afdo.org, http://www.afdo.org. Ed., R&P, Adv. contact Heinz Wilms. B&W page USD 500; trim 4.5 x 7.5. Circ: 900.

664 616.4 USA
▼ **BEST RECIPES DIABETIC COOKING.** Text in English. 2000. bi-m. USD 14.95; USD 3.50 newsstand/cover (effective 2001). adv. **Document type:** *Magazine, Consumer.*
Published by: Publications International Ltd., 7373 N Cicero Ave, Lincolnwood, IL 60646. TEL 847-329-5339. Ed. Susan Garard. Pub. Sara Armstrong Reddington.

664 BRA
TP368 CODEN: CITAC7
BRAZILIAN JOURNAL OF FOOD TECHNOLOGY. Text in English, Spanish, Portuguese. 1965. s-a. USD 30. bk.rev. *Refereed.* **Document type:** *Academic/Scholarly.*
Description: Publishes papers from around the world on a variety of topics in food science and technology, with an emphasis on applied knowledge.
Superseded (in 1998): Instituto de Tecnologia de Alimentos. Coletanea (0100-350X)
Indexed: Art.Hosp.& Tour., Biol.Abstr., Chem.Abstr., Chem.Indus.Notes, Chem.Titles, Dairy Sci.Abstr., Food Sci.& Tech.Abstr., Hort.Abstr., INIS Atomind., Nutr.Abstr.
—BLDSC (2277.407000), CASDDS, CISTI, Ei.
Published by: Instituto de Tecnologia de Alimentos, Centro, Caixa Postal 139, Campinas, SP 13012970, Brazil. TEL 19-2415222 ext. 130, FAX 19-2415034, bibital@ital.org.br, http://www.ital.org.br. Circ: 500.

664 GBR ISSN 0007-070X
TX501 CODEN: BFOJA9
BRITISH FOOD JOURNAL. Text in English. 1899. 11/yr. USD 7,989 in North America; EUR 8,499 in Europe; AUD 9,739 in Australasia; GBP 4,999 in United Kingdom & rest of the world (effective 2002). bk.rev. abstr, charts, illus, tr.lit. index. back issues avail.; reprint service avail. from SWZ. **Document type:** *Academic/Scholarly.* **Description:** Aims to foster a greater understanding of the methods and motives among all those involved in the food sector. Areas covered include food and sales law, consumer affairs, food marketing, production, nutrition and more.
Incorporates: Food Marketing (0267-4394); Formerly: British Food Journal and Hygienic Review
Related titles: Online - full text ed.: (from EBSCO Publishing, O C L C Online Computer Library Center, Inc., RoweCom Information Quest, ingenta, Swets Blackwell).
Indexed: ABI Inform. (1986-Dec.1987), AgBiotech, Agricola, Art.Hosp.& Tour., Biodet.Abstr., Chem.Abstr., Dairy Sci.Abstr., Emerald, Emrld.Intell., Environ.Sci.Poll.Mgmt., Food Sci.& Tech.Abstr., Ind.Vet., Microbiol.Abstr., Nutr.Abstr., Pig News & Info., Pollut.Abstr., Postharvest, Potato Abstr., Risk Abstr., Saf.Sci.Abstr., Sugar Ind.Abstr., Triticale Abstr., World Ag.Econ.& Rur.Soc.Abstr.
—BLDSC (2300.800000), CISTI, Infotrieve. **CCC.**
Published by: Emerald, 60-62 Toller Ln, Bradford, W Yorks BD8 9BY, United Kingdom. TEL 44-1274-777700, FAX 44-1274-785200, info@emeraldinsight.com, http://www.emeraldinsight.com/bfj.htm, http://www.mcb.co.uk/, http://www.emeraldinsight.com/journals/. Eds. David Jukes, Spencer Henson.

BUTTERWORTHS FOOD LAW. see *PUBLIC HEALTH AND SAFETY*

CALORIE CONTROL COMMENTARY. see *NUTRITION AND DIETETICS*

664 CAN
COMPENDIUM OF ANALYTICAL METHODS. Text in English. 4 base vols. plus s-a. updates. CND 200; CND 60 updates. **Document type:** *Government.*
Description: Covers the microbiological analysis of foods and water and the detection of extraneous materials in foods.
—BLDSC (3363.965200).
Published by: (Canada. Health and Welfare Canada, Canada. Health Protection Branch), Polyscience Publications Inc., Sta St Martin, P O Box 1606, Laval, PQ H7V 3P8, Canada. TEL 450-688-8484, 800-840-5870, FAX 450-688-1930, polyscience@aol.com, polysci@ietc.com. Ed. D Warburton. **Dist. in US by:** 100 Walnut St, Champlain, NY 12919.

CUADERNOS DE NUTRICION. see *NUTRITION AND DIETETICS*

664 614.85 USA
CURRENT ISSUES IN FOOD SAFETY. Text in English. base vol. plus q. updates. USD 545 (effective 2001). **Document type:** *Trade.*
Published by: John Wiley & Sons, Inc., Journals (Subsidiary of: Wiley InterScience), 605 Third Ave, New York, NY 10158. TEL 212-650-8000, FAX 212-850-6088, info@jwiley.com, http://www.wiley.com. **Subsr. outside the Americas:** John Wiley & Sons Ltd., Baffins Ln, Chichester, Sussex PO19 IUD, United Kingdom. TEL 44-1243-779777, FAX 44-1243-843232, cs-journals@wiley.co.uk.

D C A T DIGEST. see *PHARMACY AND PHARMACOLOGY*

363.192 USA ISSN 1043-3546
SF257 CODEN: DFESEC
DAIRY, FOOD AND ENVIRONMENTAL SANITATION; a publication for food safety professionals. Text in English. 1980. m., latest vol.21. USD 198 in United States; USD 208 in Canada & Mexico; USD 223 elsewhere (effective 2001). adv. bk.rev. abstr, charts, illus. index. 90 p./no. 3 cols./p. back issues avail.; reprint service avail. from PQC. *Refereed.* **Document type:** *Academic/Scholarly.* **Description:** Provides applied research information for food safety professionals in industry, regulatory or education.
Former titles: Dairy and Food Sanitation (0273-2866); Food and Fieldmen
Related titles: Microform ed.: (from PQC).
Indexed: Agricola, Bibl.Agri., Biodet.Abstr., Curr.Adv.Ecol.Sci., Dairy Sci.Abstr., Food Sci.& Tech.Abstr., Hort.Abstr., Ind.Vet., Nutr.Abstr., Pig News & Info., Postharvest, Potato Abstr., Poult.Abstr., Rev.Appl.Entomol., Rev.Plant Path., Sugar Ind.Abstr., Vet.Bull., World Ag.Econ.& Rur.Soc.Abstr.
—BLDSC (3514.712000), CISTI.
Published by: International Association for Food Protection, 6200 Aurora Ave, Ste 200W, Des Moines, IA 50322-2863. TEL 515-276-3344, FAX 515-276-8655, info@foodprotection.org, jcattanach@foodprotection.org, www.foodprotection.org, http://www.foodprotection.org. Ed., R&P Donna A Bahun. Adv. contact Dave Larson TEL 515-440-2810. Circ: 3,500.

DIETARY MANAGER MAGAZINE. see *NUTRITION AND DIETETICS*

613.2 FRA ISSN 0221-0347
CODEN: CAENDI
ECOLE NATIONALE SUPERIEURE DE BIOLOGIE APPLIQUEE A LA NUTRITION ET A L'ALIMENTATION. CAHIERS. Cover title: E N S B A N A Cahiers. Text in French. 1976. a. price varies. adv. bk.rev. bibl, charts, illus. **Document type:** *Monographic series.*
Former titles: Amis de l'E.N.S.B.A.N.A. (0221-0339); Amis de l'I.B.A.N.A. (Publication) (0003-1801)
Indexed: Chem.Abstr.
—CASDDS.
Published by: Ecole Nationale Superieure de Biologie Appliquee a la Nutrition et a l'Alimentation (ENSBANA), 11 rue Lavoisier, Paris Cedex 8 75384, France. TEL 42-65-39-95, FAX 42-65-02-46, TELEX LAVOISI 649404 F. Ed. Denis Lozinet. Circ: 3,000.

644.3 EGY ISSN 1110-0192
EGYPTIAN JOURNAL OF FOOD SCIENCE/AL-MAJALLAH AL-MISRIYYAH LI-ULUM AL-AGHDHIYA. Text in English; Summaries in Arabic, English. 1973. 2/yr. USD 77 (effective 2000). illus. reprint service avail. from IRC. **Document type:** *Academic/Scholarly.*
Related titles: CD-ROM ed.
Indexed: Apic.Abstr., Biol.Abstr., Chem.Abstr., Chem.Indus.Notes, Chem.Titles, Curr.Pack.Abstr., Dairy Sci.Abstr., ExtraMED, Food Sci.& Tech.Abstr., Hort.Abstr., Nutr.Abstr., Packag.Sci.Tech., Rev.Appl.Entomol., Rev.Arom.& Med.Plants, Rev.Plant Path., Sugar Ind.Abstr.
—BLDSC (3664.376000), Linda Hall.
Published by: (Society of Food Science and Technology, Research Department), National Information and Documentation Centre (NIDOC), Tahrir St., Dokki, Awqaf P.O., Cairo, Egypt. TEL 20-2-3371696. Ed. Azza A Ismail. Circ: 1,000.

ENVIRONMENTAL NUTRITION; the newsletter of food, nutrition and health. see *NUTRITION AND DIETETICS*

ERNAEHRUNG IM FOKUS; Zeitschrift fuer Fach-, Lehr- und Beratungskraefte im Bereich Ernaehrung. see *NUTRITION AND DIETETICS*

664 615 USA
F D A COMPLIANCE POLICY GUIDANCE. MANUAL. Text in English. base vol. plus unknown updates. USD 57 in North America; USD 114 elsewhere (effective 1999).
Description: Provides an organized system for issuing, filling and retrieving statements of FDA compliance policy, including those statements which contain regulatory action.
Formerly: F D A Compliance Policy Guide
Published by: (U.S.. U.S. Food and Drug Administration), U.S. National Technical Information Service, 5285 Port Royal Rd, Springfield, VA 22161. TEL 703-605-6060, 800-553-6847, FAX 703-605-6880, orders@ntis.fedworld.gov, http://www.ntis.gov.

F D A CONSUMER. (Food and Drug Administration) see *CONSUMER EDUCATION AND PROTECTION*

664 615 USA
F D A ENFORCEMENT MANUAL. (Food and Drug Administration) Text in English. 1993. m. **Document type:** *Trade.* **Description:** For professionals in the drug, medical device, food and cosmetic industries who are responsible for compliance with FDA's tough enforcement strategies. Provides current information on FDA enforcement practices, and gives practical step-by-step guidance on enforcement options.
Published by: Thompson Publishing Group, 1725 K St, N W, Ste 700, Washington, DC 20006. TEL 800-454-2959, FAX 800-999-5661.

664 615 USA
F D A INSPECTION OPERATIONS MANUAL. (Food and Drug Administration) Text in English. bi-m. USD 80 in North America; USD 160 elsewhere. **Document type:** *Government.* **Description:** Provides a system for the issuance of agencywide operating standards for inspectors and investigators. Includes necessary instructions and references, as well as excerpts of the authorities, responsibilities, objectives, policies and applicable guides.
Related titles: Supplement: F D A Inspection. Basic Manual.
Published by: U.S. Food and Drug Administration, Office of Public Affairs, 5600 Fishers Ln, Rockville, MD 20857. TEL 301-443-3220. **Subscr. to:** National Technical Information Service, Government Research Center. TEL 703-487-4630, FAX 703-321-8547.

F D A WEEK. (Food and Drug Administration) see *CONSUMER EDUCATION AND PROTECTION*

658.568 USA
F D C CONTROL NEWSLETTER. (Food, Drug, and Cosmetics) Text in English. 1974 (no.36). 3/yr. membership. bk.rev. charts.
Former titles: F D C Control; Food Quality Control (0532-0941)
Published by: American Society for Quality Control, Food, Drug and Cosmetic Division, 611 E Wisconsin Ave, Box 3005, Milwaukee, WI 53201-3005. TEL 414-272-8575. Ed. James B Kohnen. Circ: 3,000.

664 DNK ISSN 1398-0599
FOEDEVARENYT. Text in Danish. 1988. 6/yr. DKK 80 (effective 2001). **Document type:** *Newsletter, Government.* **Description:** Focuses on current activities of the National Food Agency of Denmark; features articles on toxicology, chemical contaminants in food, nutrition, and law dealing with food administration.
Formerly: L S T Nyt (0904-5198)
Published by: Ministeriet for Foedevarer Landbrug og Fiskeri, Foedevaredirektoratet/Ministry of Food, Agriculture and Fisheries. Veterinary and Food Administration, Morkhoej Bygade 19, Soborg 2860, Denmark. TEL 45-33-95-60-00, http://www.fdir.dk. Ed. K A Nielsen.

FOOD ADDITIVES AND CONTAMINANTS; analysis, surveillance, evaluation, control. see *PHARMACY AND PHARMACOLOGY*

▼ **FOOD ALLERGY AND INTOLERANCE JOURNAL**; a journal for the world food industry. see *MEDICAL SCIENCES—Allergology And Immunology*

FOOD AND CHEMICAL TOXICOLOGY. see *ENVIRONMENTAL STUDIES—Toxicology And Environmental Safety*

FOOD AND DRUG ADMINISTRATION. REGULATORY MANUAL. see *LAW*

FOOD & DRUG INSPECTION MONITOR. see *PHARMACY AND PHARMACOLOGY*

F

FOOD AND DRUG LAW JOURNAL. see *LAW*

FOOD & DRUG PACKAGING. see *PACKAGING*

FOOD & NUTRITION RESEARCH BRIEFS. see *NUTRITION AND DIETETICS*

FOOD & WATER JOURNAL. see *CONSUMER EDUCATION AND PROTECTION*

FOOD, DRINKS & DRUGS INDUSTRY BULLETIN. see *LAW*

FOOD, DRUG, COSMETIC, AND MEDICAL DEVICE LAW DIGEST. see *LAW*

FOOD FORUM. see *PUBLIC HEALTH AND SAFETY*

664 340 USA
FOOD LAW REPORTS. Text in English. 1938. w. USD 1,459 (effective 2001).
Formerly: Food Drug Cosmetic Law Reports (Food Edition) (0162-1130)
Related titles: CD-ROM ed.: USD 1,499 (effective 2000).
Published by: C C H Incorporated, 2700 Lake Cook Rd., Riverwoods, IL 60015. TEL 847-267-7000, 800-449-9525, FAX 773-866-3895, http://www.cch.com. Pub. Catherine Wolfe.

FOOD MICROBIOLOGY. see *BIOLOGY—Microbiology*

FOOD PROTECTION REPORT. see *PUBLIC HEALTH AND SAFETY*

FOOD SAFETY BRIEFING. see *OCCUPATIONAL HEALTH AND SAFETY*

FOOD SAFETY CONCERNS BULLETIN. see *PUBLIC HEALTH AND SAFETY*

664 362.1 USA
▼ **FOOD SAFETY SOURCEBOOK.** Text in English. 1999. irreg., latest 1999. USD 48 per issue (effective 2001). charts. Index. **Document type:** *Consumer.* **Description:** Basic consumer health information about the safe handling of meat, poultry, seafood, eggs, fruit juices, and other food items.
Published by: Omnigraphics, Inc., 615 Griswold St, Detroit, MI 48226. TEL 313-961-1340, 800-234-1340, FAX 313-961-1383, 800-875-1340, http://www.omnigraphics.com. Ed. Dawn Dawn D Matthews.

FOOD STRUCTURE. see *NUTRITION AND DIETETICS*

664 CAN ISSN 0715-6421
RA601
FOODBORNE AND WATERBORNE DISEASE IN CANADA. Text in English. a. CND 42. **Document type:** *Government.* **Description:** Summarizes information from federal, provisional and regional agencies on foodborne and waterborne disease occurring in Canada.
Formerly (until 1974): Food-Borne Diseases in Canada (0715-6413)
Related titles: French ed.: Intoxications Alimentaires et Maladies d'Origine Hydrique au Canada. ISSN 0715-6405.
—CISTI.
Published by: (Canada. Health and Welfare Canada, Canada. Health Protection Branch), Polyscience Publications Inc., Sta St Martin, P O Box 1606, Laval, PQ H7V 3P8, Canada. TEL 450-688-8484, 800-840-5870, FAX 450-688-1930, polyscience@aol.com, polysci@ietc.com. Ed. E Todd. Circ: 1,000. **Dist. in US by:** 100 Walnut St, Champlain, NY 12919.

▼ **FOODBORNE PATHOGENS AND DISEASE.** see *MEDICAL SCIENCES—Communicable Diseases*

664 613.2 USA ISSN 1072-429X
CODEN: FFFIE9
FRONTIERS IN FOODS AND FOOD INGREDIENTS. Text in English. 1993. irreg. price varies. bibl. **Document type:** *Monographic series.*
—BLDSC (4042.018000), CASDDS. **CCC.**
Published by: A T L Press, Inc., Science Publishers, PO Box 4563, T Sta, Shrewsbury, MA 01545.

664 NLD ISSN 0169-5959
THE GIST. Text in Dutch. q.
Published by: Royal Gist-brocades nv., Corporate Communications, PO Box 1, Delft 2600 MA, Netherlands.

664 NLD ISSN 0167-9112
GROOTKEUKEN; food magazine for care institutions. Text in Dutch. 1957. 11/yr. NLG 186.50 domestic; BEF 3,850 in Belgium; NLG 82.50 domestic to students; BEF 1,925 in Belgium to students (effective 2000). adv. illus. back issues avail. **Document type:** *Journal, Trade.* **Description:** Discusses food service in medical care institutions.
Related titles: E-mail ed.; Fax ed.
Published by: Keesing Noordervliet BV, De Molen 82, Houten 3995 AX, Netherlands. TEL 31-30-635-8585, FAX 31-30-635-8500, grootkeuken@keesing.nl, http://www.grootkeuken.nl, http://www.keesing.nl. Ed. C Blomsma. Pub. P T Both. Adv. contact P Scholten. B&W page NLG 2,665, color page NLG 4,615; trim 285 x 215. Circ: 2,029 (paid); 2,645 (controlled). **Subscr. to:** Abonneeservice, Antwoordnummer 10299, Amsterdam 1000 PA, Netherlands. TEL 31-20-564-1222, FAX 31-20-697-0305, service@keesing.nl.

H S R: HEALTH SUPPLEMENT RETAILER. see *NUTRITION AND DIETETICS*

HEALTH CARE FOOD & NUTRITION FOCUS. see *HEALTH FACILITIES AND ADMINISTRATION*

641.3 USA
HEALTH PRODUCTS BUSINESS; the business publication of the natural foods industry. Text in English. 1954. m. USD 60 (effective 2001). adv. bk.rev. illus. **Document type:** *Trade.* **Description:** Reaches health and natural foods retailers with news, information, purchasing guide, and surveys.
Formerly: Health Foods Business (0149-9602)
Related titles: Online - full text ed.: (from Gale Group, LexisNexis).
Indexed: Bus.& Indus. (May 1998-), Food Sci.& Tech.Abstr.
—BLDSC (4275.105060).
Published by: Cygnus Business Media Inc. (Melville), 445 Broad Hollow Rd, Ste 21, Melville, NY 11747-3601. Ed. Susanne Alberto. Pub. Bruce Leftakes. Circ: 16,000 (paid and controlled).

664 642.59 USA
HEALTHCARE FOODSERVICE MAGAZINE. Text in English. 1991. q. USD 25. adv. **Document type:** *Trade.* **Description:** For foodservice professionals in hospitals, nursing homes, hospices and treatment centers, contract caterers and restaurant and cafeteria operators in healthcare facilities in the US and Canada.
Related titles: Special ed.: Healthcare Foodservice Magazine. Annual Industry Directory.
Indexed: Int.Nurs.Ind.
Published by: International Publishing Company of America, 665 La Villa Dr, Miami, FL 33166. TEL 305-887-1700, FAX 305-885-1923. Pub., R&P Alexander C Morton. Adv. contact Barbara Coenson. Circ: 29,215.

363.7296 USA
HEALTHCARE FOODSERVICE WHO'S WHO. Text in English. 1979. triennial. USD 630. stat. index. **Document type:** *Directory.* **Description:** Provides food service data on hospitals with over 140 beds and nursing homes and long-term psychiatric and short-term mental health institutions in the US with more than 170 beds.
Related titles: Diskette ed.: USD 2,150.
Published by: Information Central Inc., PO Box 3900, Prescott, AZ 86302. TEL 520-778-1513, FAX 520-778-1513, awoodman@oldwest.net. Ed. Julie Woodman.

338.4764795 GBR ISSN 0968-5340
HYGIENE AND NUTRITION IN FOOD SERVICE AND CATERING; an international journal. Text in English. 1987. q. GBP 89, USD 179 (effective 1996). bk.rev. **Document type:** *Academic/Scholarly.* **Description:** Concerned with the nutritional and hygienic aspects of foodservice.
Formerly (until 1995): Catering and Health (0267-3851)
Indexed: Aqua.Sci.& Fish.Abstr., Art.Hosp.& Tour., Biotech.& Bioeng.Abstr., Environ.Sci.Poll.Mgmt., Food Sci.& Tech.Abstr., Microbiol.Abstr., Pollut.Abstr.
—BLDSC (4352.236500), GNLM.
Published by: A B Academic Publishers, PO Box 42, Bicester, Oxon OX26 6NW, United Kingdom. jrnls@abapubl.demon.co.uk. Eds. Michael Kipps, Dr. Robert H G Charles.

INGREDIENTS, HEALTH & NUTRITION. see *NUTRITION AND DIETETICS*

664 BRA ISSN 0074-0144
INSTITUTO DE TECNOLOGIA DE ALIMENTOS. INSTRUCOES PRATICAS. Text in Portuguese. 1968. irreg., latest vol.3, 1970. **Document type:** *Monographic series.*
Published by: Instituto de Tecnologia de Alimentos, Centro, Caixa Postal 139, Campinas, SP 13012970, Brazil. TEL 19-2415222 ext. 130, FAX 19-2415034, bibital@ital.org.br, http://www.ital.org.br.

664 BRA ISSN 0074-0152
INSTITUTO DE TECNOLOGIA DE ALIMENTOS. INSTRUCOES TECNICAS. Text in Portuguese. 1968. irreg. **Document type:** *Monographic series.*
Published by: Instituto de Tecnologia de Alimentos, Centro, Caixa Postal 139, Campinas, SP 13012970, Brazil. TEL 19-2415222 ext. 130, FAX 19-2415034, bibital@ital.org.br, http://www.ital.org.br.

INSTITUTO PANAMERICANO DE PROTECCION DE ALIMENTOS Y ZOONOSIS EN LAS AMERICAS. see *VETERINARY SCIENCE*

INSTITUTO PANAMERICANO DE PROTECCION DE ALIMENTOS Y ZOONOSIS. PUBLICACION TECNICA. see *VETERINARY SCIENCE*

664 GBR ISSN 0960-9784
INTERNATIONAL FOOD SAFETY NEWS. Text in English. 1992. 10/yr. GBP 245, USD 441 (effective 2000). adv. **Document type:** *Newsletter.* **Description:** Contains current and international news and analysis of information on food pathogens and all aspects of food safety for public health labs, hospitals, environmental health officers and food industry professionals.
Published by: Research Information Ltd., 222 Maylands Ave, Hemel Hempstead Rd, Hemel Hempstead, Herts HP3 8LA, United Kingdom. TEL 44-20-8328-2471, FAX 44-1442-259395, info@resinf.co.uk, http://www.foodsafetynews.com, http://www.users.globalnet.co.uk/~resinf. Eds. Paul Neaves, Tony Williams. Pub. Kumar Patel. Circ: 500.

INTERNATIONAL JOURNAL OF FOOD MICROBIOLOGY. see *BIOLOGY—Microbiology*

IRELAND. DEPARTMENT OF AGRICULTURE AND FOOD. PESTICIDE RESIDUES IN FOOD. see *PUBLIC HEALTH AND SAFETY*

JOINT F A O - W H O CODEX ALIMENTARIUS COMMISSION. REPORT OF THE SESSION. see *PUBLIC HEALTH AND SAFETY*

JOURNAL OF CHILD NUTRITION & MANAGEMENT. see *EDUCATION—School Organization And Administration*

JOURNAL OF FOOD MYCOLOGY. see *BIOLOGY—Microbiology*

363.192 USA ISSN 0362-028X
SF221 CODEN: JFPRDR
JOURNAL OF FOOD PROTECTION. Text in English. 1937. m. USD 293 in United States to individuals; USD 309 in Canada & Mexico; USD 338 elsewhere (effective 2001). adv. bk.rev. charts, illus. index. 125 p./no. 2 cols./p. back issues avail.; reprint service avail. from PQC. *Refereed.* **Document type:** *Academic/Scholarly.* **Description:** Publishes papers on topics in food science, related to food safety.
Formerly (until 1977): Journal of Milk and Food Technology (0022-2747)
Related titles: Microform ed.: (from PQC,PMC); Online - full text ed.: (from Institute for Scientific Information); Abridged ed.
Indexed: ASCA, Abstr.Hyg., AgBiotech, Agricola, Apic.Abstr., Aqua.Sci.& Fish.Abstr., Aquacult.Abstr., Bibl.Agri., Bio-Contr.News & Info., Biol.& Agr.Ind. (Jan.1983-), Biol.Abstr., Biotech.& Bioeng.Abstr., Chem.Abstr., Chem.Indus.Notes, Chem.Titles, Crop Physiol.Abstr., Curr.Adv.Ecol.Sci., Curr.Cont., Curr.Pack.Abstr., Dairy Sci.Abstr., Derwent Biotech.Abstr., Environ.Sci.Poll.Mgmt., Excerp.Med., Food Sci.& Tech.Abstr., Helminthol.Abstr., Hort.Abstr., INIS Atomind., Ind.Med. (1977-), Ind.Sci.Rev., Ind.Vet., Int.Abstr.Biol.Sci., Int.Packag.Abstr., Maize Abstr., Mass Spectr.Bull., Microbiol.Abstr., Nutr.Abstr., Packag.Sci.Tech., Pig News & Info., Pollut.Abstr., Postharvest, Potato Abstr., Poult.Abstr., Protozool.Abstr., Rev.Appl.Entomol., Rev.Arom.& Med.Plants, Rev.Med.& Vet.Mycol., Rev.Plant Path., Rice Abstr., Risk Abstr., Saf.Sci.Abstr., Sci.Cit.Ind., Seed Abstr., Soils & Fert., Sugar Ind.Abstr., Triticale Abstr., Vet.Bull., Weed Abstr., World Ag.Econ.& Rur.Soc.Abstr.
—BLDSC (4984.550000), CASDDS, CINDOC, CISTI, EMDOCS, IDS, ingenta, Linda Hall.

F

Published by: International Association for Food Protection, 6200 Aurora Ave, Ste 200W, Des Moines, IA 50322-2863. TEL 515-276-3344, FAX 515-276-8655, info.@foodprotection.org, http://www.foodprotection.org. Ed., R&P Bev Corron TEL 515-276-3344. Adv. contact Dave Larson TEL 515-440-2810. Circ: 3,500.

JOURNAL OF MEDICINAL FOOD. see *MEDICAL SCIENCES*

664 USA ISSN 1046-0756
TX556.M4 CODEN: JMFOEI
JOURNAL OF MUSCLE FOODS. Text in English. 1990. q., latest vol.12. USD 164 (effective 2001). bk.rev. *Refereed.* **Document type:** *Journal, Academic/Scholarly.* **Description:** Contains research and review manuscripts related to beef, lamb, veal, pork, seafood, poultry and muscle of other species that are consumed by humans.
Related titles: Online - full text ed.: (from Institute for Scientific Information).
Indexed: Curr.Cont., Food Sci.& Tech.Abstr., Nutr.Abstr., Pig News & Info., Poult.Abstr., Sci.Cit.Ind., Triticale Abstr.
—BLDSC (5021.110000), CISTI, IDS, ingenta, Linda Hall.
Published by: Food & Nutrition Press, Inc., 6527 Main St, PO Box 374, Trumbull, CT 06611. TEL 203-261-8587, FAX 203-261-9724, foodpress@worldnetatt.net, http://www.foodscipress.com. Eds. George J Flick, Norman G Marriott. Adv. contact John J O'Neil.

JOURNAL OF PALLIATIVE MEDICINE. see *MEDICAL SCIENCES*

JOURNAL OF SENSORY STUDIES. see *MEDICAL SCIENCES—Psychiatry And Neurology*

664 DEU ISSN 0174-6480
KUECHE IN KRANKENHAUS UND ALTENHEIM. Short title: K K A. Text in German. 1975. 8/yr. DEM 70; DEM 86 foreign (effective 2000). adv. bk.rev. **Document type:** *Newsletter, Trade.*
Published by: Gastro Manuscript Verlag GmbH, Waldstr 5, Huenstetten 65510, Germany. TEL 06438-2027, FAX 06438-4190. Ed. Werner Gros. Circ: 8,400.

664 AUT ISSN 0254-9298
CODEN: LEBIEE
LEBENSMITTEL- UND BIOTECHNOLOGIE; die oesterreichische Fachzeitschrift fuer Lebensmittelindustrie und -forschung. Text in German. 1984. 4/yr. ATS 40 domestic; EUR 51 foreign (effective 2001). adv. bk.rev. 32 p./no. 3 cols./p. back issues avail. **Document type:** *Journal, Trade.* **Description:** Examines the biotechnology methods, food industry, food analysis.
Indexed: CEABA, Chem.Abstr., Chem.Indus.Notes, Chem.Titles, Excerp.Med., Food Sci.& Tech.Abstr., INIS Atomind.
—BLDSC (5179.624500), CASDDS.
Published by: Fachverlag Wien, DOK 4, NW 21-22, Gross-Enzersdorf 2301, Austria. TEL 43-2249-4104, FAX 43-2249-7481, info@labor.at, http://www.labor.at. Ed. Dr. Sepp K. Fischer. adv.: page XEU 1,453; trim 185 x 258. Circ: 2,000.

664 614.19 DEU ISSN 0937-1478
TP372.5 CODEN: LEBEE2
LEBENSMITTELCHEMIE; Zeitschrift des Lebensmittelchemischen Gesellschaft. Text in German. 1946. bi-m. EUR 348 in Europe; CHF 578 in Switzerland & Liechtenstein; USD 438 elsewhere (effective 2002). adv. reprint service avail. from ISI. **Document type:** *Journal, Academic/Scholarly.* **Description:** Publishes articles describing new results in the analysis, investigation and technology of foods, , consumer goods and cosmetics.
Formerly (until 1990): Lebensmittel und Gerichtliche Chemie (0341-5309)
Related titles: Online - full text ed.: (from Wiley InterScience).
Indexed: Anal.Abstr., Biol.Abstr. (1991-), Chem.Abstr., Chem.Indus.Notes, Chem.Titles, Eng.Ind., Excerp.Med., Food Sci.& Tech.Abstr., Mass Spectr.Bull., Sugar Ind.Abstr., VITIS, Weed Abstr.
—BLDSC (5179.626000), CASDDS, CISTI, Ei, Infotrieve, Linda Hall. **CCC.**
Published by: (Lebensmittelchemie Gesellschaft - Fachgruppe in der Gesellschaft Deutscher Chemiker), Wiley - V C H, Postfach 101161, Weinheim 69451, Germany. FAX 49-6201-606-117, subservice@wiley-vch.de, http://www.wiley-vch.de. Ed. H Miethke. R&P Claudia Rutz. Adv. contact I Sinhoff. Circ: 3,420. **Subscr. in the Americas to:** John Wiley & Sons, Inc., Journals, 605 Third Ave, New York, NY 10158. TEL 212-850-6021, 212-850-6645; **Subscr. outside Germany, Austria & Switzerland to:** John Wiley & Sons Ltd., Baffins Ln, Chichester, Sussex PO19 IUD, United Kingdom. TEL 44-1243-779777, FAX 44-1243-843232.

MEAT AND POULTRY INSPECTION REGULATIONS; meat inspection, poultry inspection, rabbit inspection, voluntary inspection and certificate service of meat and poultry, humane slaughter of livestock. see *AGRICULTURE—Poultry And Livestock*

338.19 USA
N N F A TODAY. Text in English. 1986. 11/yr. USD 48. adv. bk.rev. **Document type:** *Newsletter.* **Description:** Provides practical information for natural product retailers and suppliers. Includes coverage of science, legislation, labeling and association developments.
Formerly (until Mar. 1993): N N F A Monitor; Which supersedes (1981?-1984): Food for Thought (Oceanside)
Published by: National Nutritional Foods Association, 3931 MacArthur Blvd, Ste 101, Newport Beach, CA 92660-3021. TEL 949-622-6272, FAX 949-622-6266, http://www.nnfa.org. Ed. Tracy A Taylor. Circ: 4,100 (controlled).

NATURAL FOOD TRADER. see *NUTRITION AND DIETETICS*

NUTRITION BULLETIN. see *NUTRITION AND DIETETICS*

THE NUTRITION FUNDING REPORT; a monthly guide to locating resources. see *NUTRITION AND DIETETICS*

NUTRITION LEGISLATION AND REGULATORY NEWS; a twice-monthly report of United States legislative, executive, and regulatory activities. see *NUTRITION AND DIETETICS*

613.2 ZMB ISSN 0078-284X
NUTRITION NEWS IN ZAMBIA. Text in English. 1969. q. free per issue. bk.rev. **Document type:** *Newsletter, Government.*
Media: Duplicated (not offset).
Published by: National Food and Nutrition Commission, PO Box 32669, Lusaka, Zambia. Circ: 5,000 (controlled).

NUTRITION SOCIETY OF INDIA. PROCEEDINGS. see *NUTRITION AND DIETETICS*

ORGANICA; a magazine of arts & activism. see *LITERATURE*

OUTPOST EXCHANGE; Milwaukee's food and wellness magazine. see *NUTRITION AND DIETETICS*

P H L S FOOD AND ENVIRONMENT BULLETIN. see *BIOLOGY—Microbiology*

PESTICIDE RESIDUES IN FOOD. see *PUBLIC HEALTH AND SAFETY*

PODRAVKA; znanstveno-strucni casopis. see *AGRICULTURE*

POSITIVE EATING. see *NUTRITION AND DIETETICS*

POTPOURRI FROM HERBAL ACRES. see *GARDENING AND HORTICULTURE*

664 CZE ISSN 0032-566X
POTRAVINAR. Text in Czech. 1946. m. CZK 9.60, USD 13.20.
Published by: N O S Pracovniku Potravinarskeho Prumyslu, Nam W Churchilla 2, Prague 11359, Czech Republic. Ed. Vladimir Marek. **Dist. by:** Artia, Ve Smeckach 30, Prague, 1 111 27, Czechoslovakia.

664 CZE
POTRAVINARSKE AKTUALITY. VYZIVA A LEGISLATIVA. Text in Czech. 1991. 5/yr. CZK 390 (effective 2000). **Document type:** *Consumer.*
Published by: Ustav Zemedelskych a Potravinarskych Informaci, Potravinarske Aktuality/Institute of Agricultural and Food Information, Slezska 7, Prague, 2 120 56, Czech Republic. TEL 420-2-24257939, FAX 420-2-22514003, insav@login.cz, insav@uzpi.cz, http://www.uzpi.cz. Eds. L Benesova, L Masakova.

PREVENTION OF FOOD ADULTERATION CASES. see *LAW*

663 USA ISSN 0740-3801
PRODUCT ALERT. Text in English. 1970. s-m. USD 700 (effective 2000). index. **Document type:** *Newsletter.* **Description:** Highlights reports on new consumer products, including foods, beverages, health and beauty aids, household and pet products.
Related titles: Online - full text ed.: (from CompuServe, Inc., Data-Star, The Dialog Corporation, Dow Jones Interactive, Gale Group, NewsNet, Factiva).
Indexed: Bus.& Indus. (Jan.1994-).
—Infotrieve. **CCC.**
Published by: Marketing Intelligence Service Ltd., 6473D Route 64, Naples, NY 14512-9726. TEL 716-374-6326, FAX 716-374-5217, mi@productscan.com, http://www.productscan.com. Eds. Daniel Smith, Thomas Vierhile. Pub., R&P Daniel Smith.

PURE FACTS. see *MEDICAL SCIENCES—Psychiatry And Neurology*

664 614 DEU ISSN 0178-2010
R F L. (Rundschau Fleischhygiene und Lebensmitteluebenwachung) Text in German. 1949. 12/yr. DEM 130.30; DEM 148.40 foreign (effective 2000). adv. bk.rev. bibl, illus. index. **Document type:** *Trade.*
Former titles (until 1986): R F L Rundschau fuer Fleischuntersuchung und Lebensmitteluebenwachung (0942-8143); (until 1985): Rundschau fuer Fleischuntersuchung und Lebensmitteluebenwachung (0341-0668); (until 1976): Rundschau fuer Fleischbeschauer, Trichinenschauer und Gluegelfleischkontrolleure (0340-1219); (until 1974): Rundschau fuer Fleischbeschauer und Trichinenschauer (0340-126X); Which incorporated (in 1991): Fleisch- und Lebensmittelhygiene (0933-2758); which was formerly (1978-1987): Fleischbeschau und Lebensmittelkontrolle (0170-8317)
Indexed: Ind.Vet., Vet.Bull.
—**CCC.**
Published by: Verlag M. und H. Schaper GmbH, Borsigstr 5, Alfeld 31061, Germany. TEL 49-5181-8009-0, FAX 49-5181-8009-33, info@schaper-verlag.de, http://www.schaper-verlag.de. Circ: 3,500.

REVISTA CUBANA DE ALIMENTACION Y NUTRICION. see *NUTRITION AND DIETETICS*

664 FRA
REVUE DE L'INDUSTRIE ALIMENTAIRE. Text in French. 1953. 10/yr. FRF 550. adv. **Document type:** *Corporate.*
Indexed: Food Sci.& Tech.Abstr.
Published by: Societe d'Edition et de Promotion Agro-Alimentaire Industrielle et Commerciales (SEPAIC), 8 Cite Paradis, Paris Cedex 10 75493, France. TEL 33-1-40227060, FAX 33-1-40227070. Ed. Jean Luc Jicquel. Adv. contact Muriel Case. Circ: 4,000.

SCHOOL FOODSERVICE AND NUTRITION. see *EDUCATION—School Organization And Administration*

664 MEX
SECTOR ALIMENTARIO EN MEXICO (YEAR). Text in Spanish. 1981. irreg., latest 1996. MXP 60 (effective 1999).
Published by: Instituto Nacional de Estadistica, Geografia e Informatica, Secretaria de Programacion y Presupuesto, Prol. Heroe de Nacozari 2301 Sur, Puerta 11, Acceso, Aguascalientes 20270, Mexico. TEL 52-4-918-1948, FAX 52-4-918-0739, http://www.inegi.gob.mx. Circ: 1,000.

SHIPIN KE-JI/FOOD SCIENCE. see *NUTRITION AND DIETETICS*

SODOBNO KMETIJSTVO. see *AGRICULTURE*

664 NCL ISSN 1018-0966
SOUTH PACIFIC FOODS LEAFLET. Text in English, French. 1980. irreg., latest 1994. **Document type:** *Monographic series.*
Related titles: French ed.: Aliments du Pacifique Sud. ISSN 1018-1296.

F

Published by: Secretariat of the Pacific Community, PO Box D5, Noumea Cedex 98848, New Caledonia. TEL 687-262000, FAX 687-263818, spc@spc.int, http://www.spc.int.

SPECIALTY COOKING; cookbook magazine. see *NUTRITION AND DIETETICS*

SPROUTLETTER. see *NUTRITION AND DIETETICS*

▼ **TRADITIONAL KITCHENS PRESENT**; Mary Dee's quick and tasty recipes. see *NUTRITION AND DIETETICS*

664 GBR ISSN 0968-0020
TRENDS IN FOOD SCIENCE AND TECHNOLOGY (REFERENCE EDITION). Text in English. 1990. a. GBP 345, USD 514; includes m. Trends in Food Science and Technology. back issues avail. *Refereed.* **Document type:** *Academic/Scholarly.* **Description:** Compendium of archival material from Trends in Food Science and Technology.
Related titles: ♦ Abridged ed. of: Trends in Food Science and Technology. ISSN 0924-2244.
Indexed: Curr.Cont. (coverage dropped), Nutr.Abstr.
—CISTI, Infotrieve. **CCC.**
Published by: Pergamon (Subsidiary of: Elsevier Science), The Boulevard, Langford Ln, East Park, Kidlington, Oxford OXB 1GB, United Kingdom. FAX 44-1865-843010, nlinfo-f@elsevier.nl; usinfo-f@elsevier.com; forinfo-kyf04035@niftyserve.or.jp, nlinfo-f@elsevier/nl; usinfo-f@elsevier.com; forinfo-kyf04035@niftyserve.or.jp, http://www.elsevier.nl/. Ed. Gillian Griffith. **Subscr. in Australasia and the Far East to:** Elsevier Science (Singapore) Pte Ltd, No.1 Temasek Ave, 17-01 Millenia Tower, Singapore 039192, Singapore. TEL 65-434-3727, FAX 65-337-2230; **Subscr. in the Americas to:** Elsevier Science, PO Box 945, New York, NY 10159-0945. TEL 212-633-3730, FAX 212-633-3680, usinfo-f@elsevier.com, http://www.elsevier.com; **Subscr. to:** Elsevier Science BV, PO Box 211, Amsterdam 1000 AE, Netherlands. TEL 31-20-485-3757, FAX 31-20-485-3432, nlinfo-f@elsevier.nl, http://www.elsevier.nl.

664 USA ISSN 0740-8609
U.S. DEPARTMENT OF AGRICULTURE. FOOD SAFETY AND INSPECTION SERVICE. MEAT AND POULTRY INSPECTION DIRECTORY. Text in English. s-a. USD 42 (effective 2001). **Document type:** *Directory, Government.*
Indexed: Consum.Ind. (1999-).
Published by: U.S. Department of Agriculture, Food Safety and Inspection Service, Rm 1140, South Bldg, 14th and Independence Ave, SW, Washington, DC 20250. TEL 202-720-2109, FAX 202-690-3023, fsis.foia@usda.gov, http://www.fsis.usda.gov/FOIA/popular.htm. **Subscr. to:** U.S. Government Printing Office, Superintendent of Documents, PO Box 371954, Pittsburgh, PA 15250-7954. TEL 202-512-1800, FAX 202-512-2250, orders@gpo.gov, http://www.access.gpo.gov.

UNIVERSIDAD CENTRAL DE VENEZUELA. FACULTAD DE FARMACIA. REVISTA. see *PHARMACY AND PHARMACOLOGY*

VEGETARIAN JOURNAL. see *NUTRITION AND DIETETICS*

VEGETARIAN JOURNAL'S FOODSERVICE UPDATE; healthy tips and recipes for institutions. see *NUTRITION AND DIETETICS*

VLEES IN VOEDING. see *NUTRITION AND DIETETICS*

664 NLD ISSN 1566-3310
▼ **VOEDINGSMIDDELENPRAKTIJK.** Variant title: Voedingsmiddelen Praktijk. Text in Dutch. 2000. q. NLG 40 domestic; BEF 750 in Belgium (effective 2000 & 2001); free with subscr to Voedingsmiddelentechnologie. adv. illus, mkt. back issues avail. **Document type:** *Journal, Newspaper-distributed.* **Description:** Informs readers on issues concerning food quality and safety.
Related titles: ♦ Supplement to: Voedingsmiddelentechnologie. ISSN 0042-7934.
Published by: Keesing Noordervliet BV, De Molen 82, Houten 3995 AX, Netherlands. TEL 31-30-635-8585, FAX 31-30-635-8500, http://www.vmt.nl, http://www.keesing.nl. **Subscr. to:** Abonneeservice, Antwoordnummer 10299, Amsterdam 1000 PA, Netherlands. TEL 31-20-564-1222, FAX 31-20-697-0305, service@keesing.nl.

664 POL
CODEN: AWAUEG
WARSAW AGRICULTURAL UNIVERSITY. S G G W. ANNALS. FOOD TECHNOLOGY AND NUTRITION. Text mainly in English; Text occasionally in French, German, Russian; Summaries in Polish. 1957. irreg. USD 10 per issue. **Document type:** *Academic/Scholarly.*
Former titles: Warsaw Agricultural University. S G G W - A R. Annals. Food Technology and Nutrition (0208-5755); (until 1980): Akademia Rolnicza, Warsaw. Zeszyty Naukowe. Technologia Rolno-Spozywcza; Szkola Glowna Gospodarstwa Wiejskiego w Warszawie. Zeszyty Naukowe. Technologia Rolno-Spozywcza (0137-7426)
Indexed: AgroLibrex, Chem.Abstr., Chem.Indus.Notes, Chem.Titles, Food Sci.& Tech.Abstr., Ref.Zh.
—CASDDS, CISTI, Linda Hall.
Published by: Szkola Glowna Gospodarstwa Wiejskiego (SGGW)/Warsaw Agricultural University, Ul Nowoursynowska 166, Warsaw 02766, Poland. Ed. W Roszkowski.

613.2 TWN ISSN 1021-9498
CODEN: YSFEEP
YAOWU SHIPIN FENXI/JOURNAL OF FOOD AND DRUG ANALYSIS. Text in Chinese, English. 1993. q. USD 60 (effective 2000). *Refereed.* **Document type:** *Academic/Scholarly.*
Related titles: Online - full text ed.: (from Institute for Scientific Information).
Indexed: ASCA, Anal.Abstr., Aqua.Sci.& Fish.Abstr., BBCI, Chem.Abstr., Chem.Cit.Ind., Chem.Indus.Notes, Dairy Sci.Abstr., Environ.Sci.Poll.Mgmt., Excerp.Med. (1994-), Field Crop Abstr., Food Sci.& Tech.Abstr., Hort.Abstr., Ind.Vet., Mass Spectr.Bull., Microbiol.Abstr., Nutr.Abstr., Pig News & Info., Pollut.Abstr., Postharvest, Poult.Abstr., Protozool.Abstr., Rev.Appl.Entomol., Rev.Arom.& Med.Plants, Rev.Med.& Vet.Mycol., Rice Abstr., Risk Abstr., Saf.Sci.Abstr., Soyabean Abstr., Sugar Ind.Abstr., Tox.Abstr., Trop.Dis.Bull., Vet.Bull., Weed Abstr.
—BLDSC (4984.537500), CASDDS, EMDOCS, IDS, KNAW.
Published by: National Laboratories of Foods and Drugs, 161-2 Kuen Yang St, Nankang, Taipei, Taiwan. TEL 886-2-7858283, http://www.nlfd.gov.tw/jfda/index_e.html. Ed. Tsi-Tee Suen. Pub. Chun-Heng Liao. Circ: 1,800.

613.2 ZMB ISSN 0084-4969
ZAMBIA. NATIONAL FOOD AND NUTRITION COMMISSION. ANNUAL REPORT. Text in English. 1968. a. free per issue. **Document type:** *Newsletter.*
Published by: National Food and Nutrition Commission, PO Box 32669, Lusaka, Zambia. Ed. Richard Mutemwa. Circ: 2,000.

FOOD AND FOOD INDUSTRIES—Abstracting, Bibliographies, Statistics

664 340 USA ISSN 1051-3914
CODEN: CAFAEJ
C A SELECTS. FOOD, DRUGS, & COSMETICS - LEGISLATIVE & REGULATORY ASPECTS. Text in English. 1990. s-w. USD 275 (effective 2001). **Document type:** *Abstract/Index.* **Description:** Covers government reports on food, drugs, and cosmetics, such as those found in the US Federal Register and those from governments of other countries. Includes information on standards of food, drugs, and cosmetics from non-government sources.
Published by: Chemical Abstracts Service (Subsidiary of: American Chemical Society), 2540 Olentangy River Rd, Box 3012, Columbus, OH 43210-0012. TEL 614-447-3600, 800-753-4227, FAX 614-447-3751.

C A SELECTS. FOOD TOXICITY. see *CHEMISTRY—Abstracting, Bibliographies, Statistics*

FOOD AND FOOD INDUSTRIES—Bakers And Confectioners

EESTI NAINE; a magazine for women. see *WOMEN'S INTERESTS*

FOOD AND FOOD INDUSTRIES—Grocery Trade

658.8 USA
CO-OP NEWS (HANOVER). Text in English. 1937. bi-m. USD 5 to non-members. bk.rev. illus. 16 p./no. 4 cols./p. back issues avail. **Document type:** *Newspaper, Consumer.* **Description:** Presents information on food issues, consumer affairs, co-operative membership, products, recipes, food history, and news of the Hanover Consumer Cooperative Society, along with its food stores and service centers.
Published by: Hanover Consumer Cooperative Society, Inc., 45 South Park St, Box 633, Hanover, NH 03755-0633. TEL 603-643-2667, FAX 603-643-1836, lisa@coopfoodstore.com, http://www.consumercoop.com. Ed. Rosemary Fifield. Circ: 11,500 (controlled).

FORENSIC SCIENCES

see MEDICAL SCIENCES—Forensic Sciences

FORESTS AND FORESTRY

see also CONSERVATION; FORESTS AND FORESTRY—Lumber And Wood

634.9 580 USA ISSN 0279-0106
ARBOR AGE. Text in English. 1981. m. USD 40; USD 65 foreign (effective 1999). adv. tr.lit. **Document type:** *Trade.* **Description:** Directed to the urban tree industry.
Related titles: Online - full text ed.: (from Gale Group).
Indexed: Agricola.
—BLDSC (1593.530000).
Published by: Adams Business Media, 2101 S Arlington Heights Rd, 150, Arlington, IL 60005. TEL 847-427-9512, FAX 847-882-6842, http://www.abm.net. Ed. Helen Stone. Pub. Colleen Long. Adv. contact Melissa Barrasso. Circ: 15,500.

BIOTECHNOLOGY AND BIOTECHNOLOGICAL EQUIPMENT; international scientific-theoretical and applied publication. see *BIOLOGY—Biotechnology*

BIOTECHNOLOGY IN AGRICULTURE AND FORESTRY. see *BIOLOGY—Biotechnology*

C A L M SCIENCE. (Conservation and Land Management) see *CONSERVATION*

FACULTAD NACIONAL DE AGRONOMIA MEDELLIN. REVISTA. see *AGRICULTURE*

582.16 634.9 635.977 SVK ISSN 0139-9144
QK474.8 CODEN: FODEDF
FOLIA DENDROLOGICA. Text in Slovak. irreg., latest vol.3, 1977. price varies. **Document type:** *Academic/Scholarly.*
Indexed: Biol.Abstr., Chem.Abstr., Forest Prod.Abstr., Forest.Abstr., Hort.Abstr., Irr.& Drain.Abstr., Soils & Fert.
—CASDDS, Linda Hall.
Published by: (Slovenska Akademia Vied/Slovak Academy of Sciences, Ustav Dendrobiologie), Veda Publishing House of the Slovak Academy of Sciences, Bradacova 7, Bratislava 85286, Slovakia. Ed. Frantisek Bencat. **Dist. by:** Slovart, Nam Slobody 6, Bratislava 81764, Slovakia. **Co-sponsor:** Arboretum Mlynany.

634.9 613.62 CAN ISSN 1198-1229
HEALTH & SAFETY RESOURCE. Text in English. 1955. bi-m. membership. **Document type:** *Government.* **Description:** Promotes health and safety in forest industries in Ontario.
Supersedes in part (in 1994): Tallyboard (0712-3094)
Related titles: ♦ French ed.: Ressource en Sante et en Securite. ISSN 1198-1237.
Indexed: Environ.Sci.Poll.Mgmt., Saf.Sci.Abstr.
Published by: Ontario Natural Resource Safety Association, 690 Mc Keown Ave, P O Box 2050, North Bay, ON P1B 9P1, Canada. TEL 705-472-4120, FAX 705-474-5800. Ed., R&P Susan Haldane. Circ: 10,000 (controlled).

363.11 CHN ISSN 1006-5091
LINYE LAODONG ANQUAN/FORESTRY LABOUR SAFETY. Text in Chinese. q. CNY 5 per issue domestic (effective 2000). back issues avail. **Document type:** *Academic/Scholarly.*
Related titles: Online - full content ed.: (from WanFang Data Corp.).

F

G

Published by: Linyebu Linye Chanyesi, Xuefu Lu 374 Hao, Ha'erbin 150086, China. TEL 86-451-6664063. Ed. Xiao-Guang Pan.

634.9 JPN ISSN 0387-9119
RINBOKU NO IKUSHU/FOREST TREE BREEDING. Text in Japanese; Summaries in English. 1957. q. JPY 4,000, USD 35. adv. bk.rev. **Document type:** *Bulletin.* **Description:** Contains research and information on forest tree breeding.
Indexed: Forest.Abstr., Plant Grow.Reg.Abstr., Ref.Zh.
Published by: Rinboku Ikushu Kyokai/Forest Tree Breeding Association, 7 Roku-Ban-cho, Chiyoda-ku, Tokyo 102-0085, Japan. TEL 81-3-3261-3433, FAX 81-3-3261-9406. Ed. Masashi Katsuta. Circ: 1,200.

TREE PHYSIOLOGY; an international botanical journal. see *BIOLOGY—Botany*

634.9 USA
TREEWORKER. Text in English. 1984. m. USD 15.95. **Document type:** *Newsletter.* **Description:** Deals with safety and educational issues pertinent to arboriculture: the care of trees.
Published by: National Arborist Association, PO Box 1094, Amherst, NH 03031-1094. TEL 603-673-3311, FAX 603-672-2613. Ed. Robert Rouse. Circ: 1,800.

UNIVERSITY OF DAR ES SALAAM. FACULTY OF AGRICULTURE, FORESTRY AND VETERINARY SCIENCE. ANNUAL RECORD OF RESEARCH. see *AGRICULTURE*

634.9 CHN ISSN 1001-7461
CODEN: XLIXE3
XIBEI LINXUEYUAN XUEBAO/NORTHWESTERN FORESTRY UNIVERSITY. JOURNAL. Text in Chinese. 1984. a. CNY 4 newsstand/cover domestic (effective 2000). **Document type:** *Academic/Scholarly.*
Related titles: Online - full content ed.: (from WanFang Data Corp.).
Indexed: Field Crop Abstr., Forest.Abstr., Hort.Abstr., Ornam.Hort., Postharvest, Rev.Plant Path., Rural Recreat.Tour.Abstr., Seed Abstr., Soils & Fert., Sugar Ind.Abstr.
—BLDSC (4834.407100).
Published by: Xibei Linxueyuan/Northwest Forestry College, Yangling, Shaanxi 712100, China. Ed. Xingyan Wang. **Dist. by:** China Education Books Import & Export Co., No15 Xueyuan Rd, Beijing, China.

FORESTS AND FORESTRY—Abstracting, Bibliographies, Statistics

634.9 574 ESP ISSN 0212-226X
ESCUELA TECNICA SUPERIOR DE INGENIEROS DE MONTES. BIBLIOTECA. BOLETIN BIBLIOGRAFICO Y DOCUMENTAL. INFORMACION FORESTAL. SERIE A: MONOGRAFIAS. Text in Spanish. 1969. q. ESP 1,600; ESP 2,000 foreign. bk.rev. **Document type:** *Monographic series, Bibliography.*
Supersedes in part: Escuela Tecnica Superior de Ingenieros de Montes. Biblioteca. Boletin Bibliografico y Documental (0210-1297)
Published by: (Universidad Politecnica de Madrid, Escuela Tecnica Superior de Ingenieros de Montes, Biblioteca), Fundacion Conde del Valle de Salazar, Ciudad Universitaria, S/N, Madrid 28040, Spain. TEL 91-336 70 85, FAX 91-453-95-57. Ed. Rosario Martin-Montalvo y San Gil.

634.9 570 ESP ISSN 0212-2278
ESCUELA TECNICA SUPERIOR DE INGENIEROS DE MONTES. BIBLIOTECA. BOLETIN BIBLIOGRAFICO Y DOCUMENTAL. INFORMACION FORESTAL. SERIE B: PUBLICACIONES PERIODICAS. Text in Spanish. 1969. q. ESP 1,600; ESP 2,000 foreign. **Document type:** *Bibliography.*
Supersedes in part: Escuela Tecnica Superior de Ingenieros de Montes. Biblioteca. Boletin Bibliografico y Documental
Published by: (Universidad Politecnica de Madrid, Escuela Tecnica Superior de Ingenieros de Montes, Biblioteca), Fundacion Conde del Valle de Salazar, Ciudad Universitaria, S/N, Madrid 28040, Spain. TEL 91-336 70 85, FAX 91-543-95-57. Ed. Rosario Martin-Montalvo y San Gil.

FORESTS AND FORESTRY—Lumber And Wood

WESTERN WOOD PRODUCTS ASSOCIATION. QUARTERLY INJURY & ILLNESS INCIDENCE REPORT. see *OCCUPATIONAL HEALTH AND SAFETY—Abstracting, Bibliographies, Statistics*

FUNERALS

393 DEU
BESTATTUNGSGEWERBE. Text in German. 1949. m. **Document type:** *Trade.*
Published by: Bundesverband des Deutschen Bestattungsgewerbes e.V., Schirmerstr 76, Duesseldorf 40211, Germany. TEL 49-211-1600810, FAX 49-211-1600850. Ed., R&P Juergen Bethke. Circ: 3,500.

FRONTIERES; les vivants et les morts. see *PSYCHOLOGY*

M E - TIDNINGEN. see *BUILDING AND CONSTRUCTION*

GARDENING AND HORTICULTURE

see also AGRICULTURE—Crop Production And/ Soil; BIOLOGY—Botany

ALOE, CACTUS & SUCCULENT SOCIETY OF ZIMBABWE. INGENS BULLETIN. see *BIOLOGY—Botany*

635 615.19 USA
AMERICAN HERB ASSOCIATION NEWSLETTER. Text in English. 1981. q. USD 20 domestic; USD 28 foreign (effective 2001). adv. bk.rev., film rev. abstr, bibl, charts, illus. back issues avail. **Document type:** *Newsletter.* **Description:** Covers current news, legal issues and events relating to medicinal plants. Written by professional herbalists.
Published by: American Herb Association, PO Box 1673, Nevada City, CA 95959-1673. TEL 530-265-9552, FAX 530-274-3140, http://www.jps.net/ahaherb. Ed. Kathi Keville. Adv. contact Marion Wyckoff. Circ: 12,000 (paid and controlled).

AQUARISTIK - FACHMAGAZIN. see *FISH AND FISHERIES*

635.9 USA ISSN 8756-7881
COMMON SENSE PEST CONTROL QUARTERLY. Text in English. 1984. q. USD 30 to individuals; USD 50 to institutions (effective 2000). adv. bk.rev. index. back issues avail. **Document type:** *Newsletter, Trade.* **Description:** Covers the least-toxic pest management in layperson's terms.
Indexed: Agricola, Bibl.Agri., Gard.Lit. (1992-1994).
—CISTI.
Published by: Bio Integral Resource Center, PO Box 7414, Berkeley, CA 94707. TEL 510-524-2567, FAX 510-524-1758. Ed. William Quarles. Circ: 1,200.

L'ERBORISTA. see *PHARMACY AND PHARMACOLOGY*

FOLIA DENDROLOGICA. see *FORESTS AND FORESTRY*

GARLIC TIMES; the newsletter of lovers of the stinking rose. see *NUTRITION AND DIETETICS*

635 GBR ISSN 0440-5757
HEATHER SOCIETY. YEARBOOK. Text in English. 1963. a. USD 28 to members (effective 2001). bk.rev. bibl, illus. cum.index: 1963-1972, 1972-1982, 1983-1993. back issues avail. **Document type:** *Yearbook.*
Indexed: Hort.Abstr., Ornam.Hort.
—CISTI.
Published by: Heather Society, Denbeigh, All Saints Rd, Creeting St Mary, Ipswich, Suffolk IP6 8PJ, United Kingdom. heathers@zetnet.co.uk, http://www.heathersociety.org.uk. Ed. Dr. E Charles Nelson. R&P, Adv. contact Arnold Stow TEL 44-1494-449397. Circ: 800.

635 USA ISSN 1048-3160
HERB, SPICE AND MEDICINAL PLANT DIGEST. Text in English. 1983. s-a. USD 10; USD 17 foreign (effective 1999). bk.rev. **Document type:** *Newsletter.* **Description:** Contains reports on the production, chemistry, and marketing of herbs, spices, and medicinal plants. For growers, merchants, and others with an interest in the culture and business related to aromatic and medicinal plant species.
Indexed: Gard.Lit. (1992-1994).
Published by: (Laboratories for Natural Products, Medicinal, and Aromatic Plants, University of Massachusetts), H S M P Press, Stockbridge Hall, Amherst, MA 01003. TEL 412-545-2347, FAX 413-545-3958, http://www-unix.oit.umass.edu/~herbdig/. Ed., R&P Lyle E Craker. Circ: 1,500.

635 580 USA ISSN 1049-6475
SB351.H5 CODEN: JHEPEF
JOURNAL OF HERBS, SPICES & MEDICINAL PLANTS. Text in English. 1991. q. USD 45 to individuals; USD 61 in Canada to individuals; USD 65 elsewhere to individuals; USD 65 to institutions; USD 88 in Canada to institutions; USD 94 elsewhere to institutions; USD 175 to libraries; USD 236 in Canada to libraries; USD 254 elsewhere to libraries (effective Aug. 2001). adv. bk.rev. illus. Index. back issues avail.; reprint service avail. from HAW. *Refereed.* **Document type:** *Journal, Academic/Scholarly.* **Description:** Features original articles and short reviews associated with the production and development of herbs, spices, and medicinal plants. Includes information related to such areas as physiology, breeding, productivity, commercial applications, and marketing.
Related titles: Microfiche ed.: (from PQC); Microform ed.
Indexed: AMED, AgBiotech, Agri.& Environ.Biotech.Abstr. (coverage dropped), Agricola, Aqua.Sci.& Fish.Abstr., Crop Physiol.Abstr., Environ.Sci.Poll.Mgmt., Food Sci.& Tech.Abstr., Forest Prod.Abstr., Forest.Abstr., Geo.Abstr.H.G., Helminthol.Abstr., Hort.Abstr., IDA, I.P.A., Ind.Vet., Irr.& Drain.Abstr., Nutr.Abstr., Per.Islam. (1992-), Plant Breed.Abstr., Plant Gen.Res.Abstr., Plant Grow.Reg.Abstr., Pollut.Abstr., Protozool.Abstr., Ref.Zh., Rev.Appl.Entomol., Rev.Arom.& Med.Plants, Rev.Plant Path., Rice Abstr., Risk Abstr., Saf.Sci.Abstr., Seed Abstr., Soils & Fert., Vet.Bull., Weed Abstr., World Ag.Econ.& Rur.Soc.Abstr.
—BLDSC (4997.800000), GNLM, Haworth.
Published by: Haworth Press, Inc., Food Products Press, 10 Alice St, Binghamton, NY 13904-1580. TEL 607-722-5857, 800-429-6784, FAX 607-722-6362, 800-895-0582, getinfo@haworthpressinc.com, http://www.haworthpress.com/journals/journallist.asp. Ed. Lyle E Craker. Pub. William Cohen. R&P Ruthann Heath TEL 607-723-5857 ext 316. Adv. contact Jackie Blakeslee TEL 607-722-5857 ext 346. B&W page USD 315, color page USD 550; trim 6 x 8.5.

635 615.82 USA ISSN 1088-3487
JOURNAL OF THERAPEUTIC HORTICULTURE. Text in English. 1986. a. USD 25 domestic to non-members; USD 30 in Canada to non-members; USD 35 elsewhere to non-members (effective 2000). bibl, charts, illus, stat. index. *Refereed.* **Document type:** *Academic/Scholarly.* **Description:** Devoted to using horticulture to enhance the lives of special populations through therapy and vocational rehabilitation.
Indexed: Gard.Lit. (1992-1994).
Published by: American Horticultural Therapy Association, 909 York St, Denver, CO 80206-3751. TEL 303-331-3862, FAX 303-331-0095, ahta@ahta.org, http://www.ahta.org. Ed. Jan Riggenbach. R&P Steven H Davis. Circ: 1,000.

635 DEU ISSN 0178-0166
KRAUT UND RUEBEN; biologisches Gaertnern und naturgemaesses Leben. Text in German. 1985. m. DEM 88 domestic; DEM 106 foreign; DEM 7.80 newsstand/cover (effective 2000). adv. bk.rev. **Document type:** *Magazine, Consumer.* **Description:** Focuses on organic gardening and holistic health.
—CCC.
Published by: B L V Verlagsgesellschaft mbH, Lothstr 29, Munich 80797, Germany. TEL 49-89-12705-0, FAX 49-89-12705354, redkraut-u-rueben@blv.de, blv.verlag@blv.de, http://www.blv.de/k&r. Ed. Wolfram Franke. Adv. contact Henning Stemmler. B&W page DEM 7,938, color page DEM 13,352; trim 186 x 210. Circ: 78,258 (paid).

635.73 USA ISSN 1048-8189
SB118.73
NURSERY BUSINESS RETAILER. Text in English. bi-m.
Supersedes in part (in 1990): Nursery Business (0029-6406)
—CISTI, ingenta.
Published by: Brantwood Publications, Inc., 2410 Northside Dr, Clearwater, FL 33761.

PEOPLE PLANT CONNECTION. see *PUBLIC HEALTH AND SAFETY*

635 664 USA ISSN 0197-4084
POTPOURRI FROM HERBAL ACRES. Text in English. 1979. q. USD 18. adv. bk.rev. charts. index. **Description:** Provides a forum to herbal experts for sharing their knowledge, crafts, culinary recipes, and the latest news about the world of herbs.
Published by: Pine Row Publications, PO Box 428, Washington, PA 18977. Ed. Phyllis V Shaudys. Circ: 2,000.

631.5 AUS ISSN 1320-3940
WARM EARTH; organic growing - healthy living. Text in English. 1993. q. AUD 26 domestic; AUD 32 in Asia & the Pacific; AUD 38 rest of world (effective 2000). adv. bk.rev. illus. back issues avail. *Refereed.* **Document type:** *Consumer.* **Description:** Provides information about organic gardening, care of the environment, obtaining good health.
Published by: Warm Earth Publishing, Kiah Cottage, Kenilworth, QLD 4754, Australia. TEL 61-74-460457, warmearth@powerup.com.au, http://www.powerup.com.au/~warmearth. Ed., Pub., R&P, Adv. contact Liz Sinnamon. B&W page AUD 200; trim 180 x 250. Circ: 10,000.

GASTROENTEROLOGY

see MEDICAL SCIENCES—Gastroenterology

GENEALOGY AND HERALDRY

GUIA DE FORNECEDORES HOSPITALARES. see *GERONTOLOGY AND GERIATRICS*

GENERAL INTEREST PERIODICALS—Germany

DER SONNTAGSBRIEF. see *GERONTOLOGY AND GERIATRICS*

GENERAL INTEREST PERIODICALS—Great Britain

LIGHT OF THE MOON. see *HANDICAPPED—Visually Impaired*

MOON MAGAZINE. see *HANDICAPPED—Visually Impaired*

PROGRESS. see *HANDICAPPED—Visually Impaired*

GENERAL INTEREST PERIODICALS—United States

051 USA ISSN 1049-6610
PHYSICIANS LIFESTYLE MAGAZINE✶ . Text in English. 1989. m. adv. bk.rev. back issues avail.
Related titles: ♦ Supplement to: Physicians Financial News. ISSN 8750-9407.
Published by: K & K Publishing, Inc., 1 Harmon Meadow Blvd, Ste 300, Secaucus, NJ 07094-3600. Ed. Emily Paulsen. Circ: (controlled).

051 USA ISSN 0048-9239
AP2 CODEN: SAEPAR
SATURDAY EVENING POST. Text in English. 1971. bi-m. USD 14.97 domestic; USD 19.97 foreign; USD 2.95 newsstand/cover (effective 2000). adv. illus. reprint service avail. from PQC. **Document type:** *Magazine, Consumer.* **Description:** Contains health-related articles, stories, and essays. Focuses on self-improvement, personal fitness, preventive medicine, and sports.
Related titles: Microfiche ed.: (from NBI); Microform ed.: (from PQC); Online - full text ed.: (from The Dialog Corporation, Gale Group, ProQuest Information & Learning, Northern Light Technology, Inc., H. W. Wilson, Factiva).
Indexed: Abr.R.G., Acad.Ind., Biog.Ind., Bk.Rev.Ind. (1974-), CCR, CINAHL, Child.Bk.Rev.Ind. (1974-), GeoRef, Hlth.Ind., Jun.High Mag.Abstr., Mag.Ind., PMR, R.G. (Jan.1983-), R.G.Abstr. (Jan.1983-), TOM.
—ingenta.
Published by: (Saturday Evening Post Society), Benjamin Franklin Literary and Medical Society, Inc., 1100 Waterway Blvd, PO Box 567, Indianapolis, IN 46206. TEL 317-636-8881, FAX 317-637-0126, drsutton@tcon.net, http://www.satevepost.org. Ed. Ted Kreiter. Pub. Dr. Cory Servaas. Adv. contact Don Sutton. B&W page USD 10,220, color page USD 13,440; trim 10 x 7. Circ: 400,000.

GENETICS

see BIOLOGY—Genetics

GEOGRAPHY

see also HISTORY; TRAVEL AND TOURISM

ANTARCTIC SCIENCE. see *BIOLOGY*

ARCTIC, ANTARCTIC AND ALPINE RESEARCH. see *SCIENCES: COMPREHENSIVE WORKS*

614.4 GBR ISSN 1353-8292
RA791 CODEN: HEPLFG
HEALTH & PLACE; an international journal. Variant title: Journal of Health and Place. Text mainly in English; Text occasionally in French, German; Abstracts in English. 1970; N.S. 1995. q. EUR 405 in Europe to institutions; JPY 53,700 in Japan to institutions; USD 453 elsewhere to institutions (effective 2002). adv. bk.rev. abstr, bibl, charts, illus, maps. back issues avail.; reprints avail. *Refereed.* **Document type:** *Academic/Scholarly.* **Description:** Reflects the convergences of the fields of medical geography, medical sociology, health policy, public health, and epidemiology.
Incorporates (in 1995): Geographia Medica (0300-807X); Which was formerly: Geographia Medica Hungarica (0435-3730)
Related titles: Online - full text ed.: N.S. (from ingenta, Swets Blackwell, ScienceDirect, Institute for Scientific Information).
Indexed: Biol.Abstr., CINAHL, Curr.Cont., Environ.Abstr., Excerp.Med., Geo.Abstr.H.G., IDA, Ind.Med. (coverage dropped), SSCI, Soc.Serv.Abstr., Sociol.Abstr., Stud.Wom.Abstr.
—BLDSC (4274.832700), CIS, EMDOCS, GNLM, Infotrieve. **CCC.**
Published by: Pergamon (Subsidiary of: Elsevier Science), The Boulevard, Langford Ln, East Park, Kidlington, Oxford OXB 1GB, United Kingdom. FAX 44-1865-843010, nlinfo-f@elsevier.nl; usinfo-f@elsevier.com; forinfo-kyf04035@niftyserve.or.jp, nlinfo-f@elsevier/nl; usinfo-f@elsevier.com; forinfo-kyf04035@niftyserve.or.jp, http://www.elsevier.com/locate/healthplace. Ed. Graham Moon. **Subscr. in:** Australasia Elsevier Science (Singapore) Pte Ltd, 1 Temasek Ave, 17-01 Millenia Tower, Singapore 039192, Singapore. TEL 65-337-2230, 65-434-3727; **Subscr. in the Americas to:** Elsevier Science, PO Box 945, New York, NY 10159-0945. TEL 212-633-3730, FAX 212-633-3680, usinfo-f@elsevier.com; **Subscr. to:** Elsevier Science BV, PO Box 211, Amsterdam 1000 AE, Netherlands. TEL 31-20-485-3757, FAX 31-20-485-3432, nlinfo-f@elsevier.nl.

KEVO SUBARCTIC RESEARCH INSTITUTE. REPORTS. see *BIOLOGY*

LUND STUDIES IN GEOGRAPHY. see *BIOLOGY*

POLAR BIOSCIENCE. see *BIOLOGY*

SIDAFRIQUE. see *MEDICAL SCIENCES—Communicable Diseases*

TURUN YLIOPISTO. JULKAISUJA. SARJA A. II. BIOLOGICA - GEOGRAPHICA - GEOLOGICA/ ANNALES UNIVERSITATIS TURKUENSIS. see *BIOLOGY*

ZEITSCHRIFT FUER ANGEWANDTE GEWASSEROEKOLOGIE. see *BIOLOGY*

GEOLOGY

see EARTH SCIENCES—Geology

AMERICAN MUSEUM NOVITATES. see *BIOLOGY—Zoology*

GERONTOLOGY AND GERIATRICS

306.38 ITA
50 & PIU. Text in Italian. 1979. m. ITL 35,000; ITL 3,500 newsstand/cover (effective 1999). **Document type:** *Newsletter, Consumer.*
Published by: Edizioni Cinquanta e Piu s.r.l., Via Del Melangolo, 26, Rome, RM 00186, Italy. TEL 39-6-68883245, FAX 39-6-6872597. Ed. Sergio Bille. adv.: color page ITL 50,000,000. Circ: 320,000.

305.26 USA ISSN 1044-1123
HQ1060
A A R P BULLETIN. Text in English. 1958. m. (11/yr.). USD 8 to members (effective 2000). adv. **Document type:** *Bulletin.* **Description:** Includes current news from the Executive Branch, Congress, courts, regulatory agencies and state legislatures. Reports on Washington activities and national trends that have a bearing on the lives of older people.
Formerly (until 1989): A A R P News Bulletin (0001-0200)
Indexed: CHNI.
Published by: A A R P, Research, 601 E St, N W, Washington, DC 20049. TEL 202-434-2277, FAX 202-434-6408, http://www.aarp.org. Ed. Elliot Carlson. adv.: B&W page USD 299,180, color page USD 331,500. Circ: 20,000,000.

306.38 USA ISSN 1092-342X
A A R P GLOBAL AGING REPORT. Text in English. 1996. bi-m. USD 40; USD 40 foreign (effective 1999). bk.rev. charts, maps, tr.lit. back issues avail. **Document type:** *Newsletter.* **Description:** Aims at professionals interested in aging issues around the world. Covers health, housing, returned planning, caregiving and other such issues.
Indexed: Ref.Zh.
Published by: (American Association of Retired Persons), A A R P, 601 E St, N W, Washington, DC 20049. TEL 202-434-2402, jprather@aarp.org, http://www.aarp.org. Ed. Johnie Prather. Circ: 1,000 (paid); 500 (controlled).

306.38 CAN ISSN 0826-497X
A C A NEWS; the provincial newsletter for seniors. Text in English. 1967. bi-m. USD 15 to individuals; USD 30 to institutions (effective 2002). adv. bk.rev. bibl, illus. back issues avail. **Document type:** *Newsletter.*
Former titles: Alberta Council on Aging News; Horizons (0018-4985)
Published by: Alberta Council on Aging, 1740 10130 103 St, Edmonton, AB T5J 3N9, Canada. TEL 403-423-7781, FAX 403-425-9246, acaging@compusmart.ab.ca. Ed. Chris Lawrence. Circ: 10,000.

305.26 USA ISSN 0890-278X
HQ1060
A G H E EXCHANGE✶ . Text in English. 1975. q. USD 25; USD 12 to students. adv. back issues avail. **Document type:** *Newsletter.* **Description:** Focuses on news of interest to gerontological educators. Sections include: Principles and Practices, Resource Briefs, Research and Training Notes, Policy Page, Research Reports, National News, Geriatric Education, Member Profiles and In and Around A G H E.
Formerly: A G H E Newsletter
Published by: Association for Gerontology in Higher Education, 1030 15th St N W, Ste 240, Washington, DC 20005. TEL 202-429-9277. Ed. Kathleen Segrist. R&P Cathy Tompkins. Adv. contact Derek Stepp. Circ: 3,500.

618.97 USA
A M D A REPORTS. Text in English. 1989. bi-m. membership. back issues avail.; reprints avail. **Document type:** *Newsletter.* **Description:** Covers issues for physicians who practice in long-term care facilities.
Published by: American Medical Directors Association, 10480 Little Patuxent Pkwy, Ste 760, Columbia, MD 21044. TEL 410-740-9743, FAX 410-740-4572, irenen@amda.com, http://www.amda.com. Ed. Joanne Kaldy. R&P Lorraine Tarnove. Circ: 6,200.

A S; maandblad voor de activiteitensector. (Activiteitensektor) see *SOCIAL SERVICES AND WELFARE*

618.97 ITA ISSN 0001-5741
ACTA GERONTOLOGICA. Text in Italian. 1950. q. ITL 80,000. adv. bk.rev.
Indexed: Biol.Abstr., Chem.Abstr., Excerp.Med., Ind.Med. (coverage dropped), Nutr.Abstr., Sci.Cit.Ind. (coverage dropped).
—CISTI, GNLM.
Published by: (Universita degli Studi di Pavia, Istituto Gerontologia e Geriatria), Tipografia del Libro, Via Cavallini, 15, Pavia, PV 27100, Italy. TEL 0382-21265, FAX 27419. Ed. Pietro de Nicola. Circ: 2,000.

155.67 USA ISSN 0192-4788
RC952.5 CODEN: AADADK
ACTIVITIES, ADAPTATION & AGING; the journal of activities management. Text in English. 1980. q. USD 60 to individuals; USD 81 in Canada to individuals; USD 87 elsewhere to individuals; USD 160 to institutions; USD 216 in Canada to institutions; USD 232 elsewhere to institutions; USD 420 to libraries; USD 567 in Canada to libraries; USD 609 elsewhere to libraries (effective Aug. 2001). adv. bk.rev. bibl, charts, illus. back issues avail.; reprint service avail. from HAW. *Refereed.* **Document type:** *Journal, Academic/Scholarly.* **Description:** Provides case studies, program evaluations, research and theory for activities directors and coordinators in nursing homes and community centers, as well as other professionals concerned with the enhancement of the lifestyles of the aged.

Related titles: Microfiche ed.: (from PQC); Microform ed.
Indexed: AMED, Abstr.Anthropol., Abstr.Soc.Geront., AgeLine, Behav.Abstr., Biol.Abstr., CINAHL, Chicago Psychoanal.Lit.Ind., ERA, Environ.Sci.Poll.Mgmt., Excerp.Med., IBZ, IMFL, Lang.& Lang.Behav.Abstr., Med.Care Rev., PSI, Past.Care & Couns.Abstr., Pollut.Abstr., PsycInfo, Psychol.Abstr. (1980-), Ref.Zh., Rehabil.Lit., Risk Abstr., Rural Recreat.Tour.Abstr., SOPODA, Saf.Sci.Abstr., Soc.Serv.Abstr., Soc.Work Res.& Abstr., Sociol.Abstr., Sp.Ed.Needs Abstr., Stud.Wom.Abstr., e-psyche.
—BLDSC (0676.470000), GNLM, Haworth, ingenta.
Published by: Haworth Press, Inc., 10 Alice St, Binghamton, NY 13904-1580. TEL 607-722-5857, 800-429-6784, FAX 607-722-6362, 800-895-0582, getinfo@haworthpressinc.com, http://www.haworthpress.com. Ed. Linnea Couture. Pub. William Cohen. R&P Ruthann Heath TEL 607-723-5857 ext 316. Adv. contact Jackie Blakeslee TEL 607-722-5857 ext 346. B&W page USD 315, color page USD 550; trim 6 x 8.5. Circ: 1,050.

306.38 362.6 USA ISSN 1524-2889
ACTIVITY DIRECTOR'S GUIDE; the complete guide of ideas, tips and techniques for the busy professional. Text in English. 1974. m. USD 28 (effective 2000). illus. back issues avail. **Document type:** *Journal, Trade.* **Description:** Provides practical, pre-tested programs, ideas and articles to keep the activities in nursing homes stimulating and worthwhile.
Published by: Eymann Publications, Inc, PO Box 3577, Reno, NV 89505-3577. TEL 775-358-1554, FAX 775-358-1476, eymann@care4elders.com, http://www.care4elders.com. Ed. Maureen Eng. Pub. Katie Eymann Pace.

610.7365 USA
ADULT DAY SERVICES LETTER. Text in English. 1985. 12/yr. USD 147 (effective 2001). adv. charts. index. 10 p./no. 2 cols./p. back issues avail. **Document type:** *Newsletter, Trade.* **Description:** Covers issues pertaining to the management and administration of adult day services, including financing strategies, staffing, program planning and marketing.
Formerly: Adult Day Care Letter (0885-4572)
Related titles: Online - full content ed.
—CCC.
Published by: Health Resources Publishing, 1913 Atlantic Ave, Ste F4, Manasquan, NJ 08736. TEL 732-292-1100, FAX 732-292-1111, hrp@healthrespubs.com, info@healthrespubs.com, http://www.healthrespubs.com. Ed. Beth-Ann Kerber. Pub. Robert K Jenkins. Adv. contact Judy Granholm.

ADVANCES (CHICAGO); progress in Alzheimer research and care. see *MEDICAL SCIENCES—Psychiatry And Neurology*

610.7365 USA
ADVANCES IN GERONTOLOGICAL NURSING. Text in English. 1996. irreg. USD 46.95; USD 50.80 foreign (effective 1999). **Document type:** *Academic/Scholarly.* **Description:** Discusses issues and concepts likely to be of major concern to geriatric nurses in the next century.
—BLDSC (0709.004000).
Published by: Springer Publishing Company, 536 Broadway, New York, NY 10012. TEL 212-431-4370, FAX 212-941-7842, springer@springerpub.com, http://www.springerpub.com. Eds. Elizabeth A Swanson, Toni Trip Reimer.

305.26 USA
ADVANCES IN LIFE COURSE RESEARCH. Text in English. 1985. a.
Formerly: Current Perspectives on Aging and Life Cycle (1040-2608)
—BLDSC (0709.278000).
Published by: Jai Press, Incorporated (Subsidiary of: Elsevier Science), 100 Prospect St., Stamford, CT 06904-0811. Ed. Timothy J Owens.

ADVANCES IN MOTOR DEVELOPMENT RESEARCH. see *PHYSICAL FITNESS AND HYGIENE*

305.26 DNK ISSN 0904-6216
AELDRE SAGEN. Text in Danish. 1967. 6/yr. adv.
Former titles (until 1988): Aktivt Otium (0902-5960); (until 1987): Otium (0108-5867)
Published by: Landsforeningen Aeldre Sagen, Vesterbrogade 97, Copenhagen V 1620, Denmark. TEL 45-31-23-44-11, FAX 45-31-23-46-23. Ed. Jesper Haller. Circ: 220,000.

618.97 GBR ISSN 0002-0729
RC952 CODEN: AANGAH
AGE AND AGEING. Text in English. 1972. bi-m. GBP 190, USD 315 to institutions; GBP 190, USD 315 to individuals (effective 2002). bk.rev. bibl, charts, illus. index. 108 p./no. back issues avail.; reprints avail. *Refereed.* **Document type:** *Journal, Academic/Scholarly.* **Description:** Covers biological gerontology and geriatrics, including research on ageing and the clinical, epidemiological and psychological aspects of medicine in old age.
Related titles: Online - full text ed.: ISSN 1468-2834. GBP 171, USD 280 to institutions (effective 2002) (from Gale Group, HighWire Pr., EBSCO Publishing, RoweCom Information Quest, ingenta, Swets Blackwell, Factiva, Institute for Scientific Information).
Indexed: AMED, ASCA, ASSIA, Abstr.Anthropol., Abstr.Health Care Manage.Stud., Abstr.Hyg., AgeLine, Bibl.Ind., Biol.Abstr., Brit.Nur.Ind., CINAHL, Chem.Abstr., Curr.Adv.Ecol.Sci., Curr.Cont., Dairy Sci.Abstr., Dent.Ind., Environ.Sci.Poll.Mgmt., Ergon.Abstr., Ind.Med. (1972-), Ind.Sci.Rev., Inpharma, Int.Nurs.Ind., NRN, Neurosci.Abstr. (coverage dropped), Neurosci.Cit.Ind., Nutr.Abstr., Pharm.&Out.News, Pollut.Abstr., Reac., Risk Abstr., SSCI (coverage dropped), Saf.Sci.Abstr., Sci.Cit.Ind., Soc.Sci.Ind. (Aug.1982-), Trop.Dis.Bull.
—BLDSC (0736.080000), CASDDS, CISTI, EMDOCS, GNLM, IDS, ingenta, KNAW. **CCC.**
Published by: (British Geriatrics Society), Oxford University Press, Academic Division, Great Clarendon St, Oxford OX2 6DP, United Kingdom. TEL 44-1865-267907, FAX 44-1865-267835, jnl.info@oup.co.uk, http://ageing.oupjournals.org/, http://www.oup.co.uk/journals. Ed. G P Mulley. Pub. Mandy Sketch. R&P Fionna Willis. Circ: 3,700. **U.S. subscr. to:** Oxford University Press, Journals, 2001 Evans Rd, Cary, NC 27513. TEL 800-852-7323, FAX 919-677-1714, jnlorders@oup-usa.org; **Subscr. to:** Journals Marketing, Great Clarendon St, Oxford OX2 6DP, United Kingdom. **Co-sponsor:** British Society for Research in Ageing.

362.6 GBR
AGE CONCERN INFORMATION BULLETIN. Text in English. 1974. m. GBP 23 in United Kingdom; GBP 32 in Europe; GBP 42 elsewhere (effective 2000). bk.rev. s-a index. **Document type:** *Bulletin.* **Description:** Covers news about legislation, policy and services affecting older persons. Reviews new books, reports and surveys.
Formerly: Age Concern Information Circular
Published by: Age Concern England, Astral House, 1268 London Rd, London SW16 4ER, United Kingdom. TEL 44-20-8765-7200, FAX 44-20-8765-7211, TELEX 24667 IMPEMP G, infodep@ace.org.uk. Ed. Cherry Ann Dowling. Circ: 2,000.

612.67 USA
AGE NEWS. Text in English. 1970. q. USD 50 to membership (effective 2000). Index. back issues avail. **Document type:** *Newsletter.* **Description:** Covers recent advances in aging research.
Published by: American Aging Association, 110 Chesley Dr, Media, PA 19063-1755. TEL 610-627-2626, FAX 610-565-9747, ameraging@aol.com, http://www.americanaging.org/. Eds. Dr. Gregory Fahy, Dr. Arthur K Balin. R&P Dr. Arthur K Balin.

362.6 GBR ISSN 0144-686X
HQ1060
AGEING AND SOCIETY. Text in English. 1981. bi-m. GBP 86 to individuals; USD 210 to institutions (effective 2002). adv. bk.rev. illus. Index. back issues avail.; reprints avail. *Refereed.* **Document type:** *Academic/Scholarly.* **Description:** Covers human ageing all over the world: theoretical and empirical research on such issues as life-styles in later life, work and retirement, mental illness, sexuality, demography, health care and the history of old age.
Related titles: Microform ed.: (from PQC); Online - full text ed.: (from EBSCO Publishing, O C L C Online Computer Library Center, Inc., RoweCom Information Quest, Gale Group, Swets Blackwell, Factiva, Institute for Scientific Information).
Indexed: AMED, ASCA, ASSIA, Abstr.Soc.Geront., AgeLine, Arts & Hum.Cit.Ind. (coverage dropped), Brit.Nur.Ind., Curr.Cont., Educ.Admin.Abstr., Geo.Abstr.H.G., Hist.Abstr. (1985-1989, dropped), IDA, Int.Polit.Sci.Abstr., Intl.Bibl.Soc.Sci., Lang.& Lang.Behav.Abstr., P C I, P.A.I.S., Ref.Zh., Rel.Ind.One, Rel.Ind.Two, SOPODA, SSCI, Soc.Sci.Ind. (Mar.1987-), Soc.Serv.Abstr., Sociol.Abstr., Stud.Wom.Abstr., Viol.& Abuse Abstr., World Bibl.Soc.Sec.
—BLDSC (0736.225770), CISTI, IDS, ingenta. **CCC.**
Published by: (British Society of Gerontology USA, Centre for Policy on Ageing), Cambridge University Press, Edinburgh Bldg, Shaftesbury Rd, Cambridge CB2 2RU, United Kingdom. FAX 44-1223-315052, information@cup.cam.ac.uk, information@cambridge.org, http://www.cup.cam.ac.uk, http://www.uk.cambridge.org/journals/pmu. Ed. Bill Rytheway. R&P Linda Nicol. Adv. contact Rebecca Symons. Circ: 1,050.

618.97 USA ISSN 0163-5158
HQ1060 CODEN: AGINFQ
AGEING INTERNATIONAL; information bulletin of the International Federation on Ageing. Variant title: Aging International. Text in English. 1973. q. USD 60 to individuals; USD 156 to institutions (effective 2001). adv. illus. Index. back issues avail.; reprints avail. **Document type:** *Academic/Scholarly.* **Description:** Dedicated to the well being of older persons worldwide. Focuses on social and economic issues, public policies, and use of resources.
Related titles: Online - full text ed.: (from CatchWord Ltd.).
Indexed: Abstr.Soc.Geront., AgeLine, C.I.J.E. (coverage dropped), Educ.Admin.Abstr., Environ.Sci.Poll.Mgmt., Fam.Ind., Lang.& Lang.Behav.Abstr., Pollut.Abstr., Risk Abstr., SOPODA, Saf.Sci.Abstr., Soc.Serv.Abstr., Sociol.Abstr., World Bibl.Soc.Sec.
—BLDSC (0736.225800), CISTI, GNLM, ingenta.
Published by: (International Federation on Ageing), Transaction Publishers, 35 Berrue Circle, Rutgers University, Piscataway, NJ 08854-8042. TEL 732-445-2280, FAX 732-445-3138, trans@transactionpub.com, http://www.who.ch/programmes/ina/ngo/ngo-83.htm. Ed. Blossom Wigdor. Pub. Mary Curtis. R&P Marlena Davidian TEL 732-445-2280 ext 100. Adv. contact Alicja Garbie. page USD 300; 4.5 x 7.75. Circ: 600. **Subscr. to:** Transaction Distribution Center, 390 Campus Dr, Somerset, NJ 08873. TEL 732-748-0300, FAX 732-748-1886.

612.67 IRL ISSN 1568-1637
▼ **AGEING RESEARCH REVIEWS.** Text in English. 2001. q. EUR 436 in Europe to institutions; JPY 57,900 in Japan to institutions; USD 487 elsewhere to institutions (effective 2002). **Document type:** *Journal, Academic/Scholarly.* **Description:** This is a source for critical reviews and viewpoints on emerging findings on mechanisms of aging and age-related disease.
Published by: Elsevier Science Ireland Ltd, Elsevier House, Brookvale Plaza, E. Park, Shannon, Co. Clare, Ireland. TEL 353-61-709600, FAX 353-61-709100, http://www.elsevier.nl.

305.26 USA ISSN 1088-5889
AGING AMERICA; an international newsletter featuring new developments in aging. Text in English. 1987. m. free for libraries and educational organizations. adv. bk.rev. index. back issues avail.; reprints avail. *Refereed.* **Document type:** *Newsletter, Academic/Scholarly, Consumer.* **Description:** A desk reference to new products, services and trends. Abstracts of new developments, including referenced sources for immediate follow-up for additional information.
Former titles (until 1996): Resources in Aging America (1086-9328); (until 1995): Resources in Aging (0892-0818)
Media: Online - full text.
—CCC.
Published by: Demko Publishing, 21946 Pine Trace, Boca Raton, FL 33428. TEL 561-482-6271, demko@demko.com, http://www.demko/newsleta.htm, http://www.demko.com. Ed., R&P Dr. David J Demko. Adv. contact Paul Harris. Circ: 60,000 (controlled and free).

616.89 GBR ISSN 1360-7863
CODEN: AMHTFD
AGING & MENTAL HEALTH. Text in English. 1997. q. GBP 76, USD 129 to individuals; GBP 267, USD 437 to institutions (effective 2002). back issues avail. *Refereed.* **Document type:** *Academic/Scholarly.* **Description:** Provides a forum for the rapidly expanding field that investigates the relationship between the aging process and mental health.
Related titles: Online - full text ed.: ISSN 1364-6915 (from CatchWord Ltd., EBSCO Publishing, O C L C Online Computer Library Center, Inc., RoweCom Information Quest, Swets Blackwell, Institute for Scientific Information).
Indexed: AgeLine, CINAHL, Curr.Cont., Environ.Sci.Poll.Mgmt., Lang.& Lang.Behav.Abstr., PsycInfo, Risk Abstr., SOPODA, SSCI, Saf.Sci.Abstr., Soc.Serv.Abstr., Sociol.Abstr., e-psyche.
—BLDSC (0736.354000), CatchWord, IDS, Infotrieve. **CCC.**

Published by: Carfax Publishing Limited (Subsidiary of: Taylor & Francis Group), PO Box 25, Abingdon, Oxon OX14 3UE, United Kingdom. TEL 44-1235-401000, FAX 44-1235-401550, enquiries@carfax.co.uk, enquiry@tandf.co.uk, http://www.carfax.co.uk/amh-ad.htm. Eds. Dan Blazer, Martin Orrell.

612.67 ITA ISSN 0394-9532
CODEN: AGNGET
AGING - CLINICAL AND EXPERIMENTAL RESEARCH. Text in English. 1989. bi-m. EUR 77.47 domestic; USD 100 foreign (effective 2002). *Refereed.* **Description:** Publishes original studies on gerontology, geriatrics and related fields.
Related titles: Online - full text ed.: EUR 38.73 (effective 2002) (from Institute for Scientific Information).
Indexed: ASCA, AgeLine, Curr.Cont., Ind.Med. (1989-), Inpharma, NRN, Nutr.Abstr., Reac., SSCI (coverage dropped).
—BLDSC (0736.295000), CASDDS, CISTI, EMDOCS, GNLM, IDS, KNAW.
Published by: Editrice Kurtis s.r.l., Via Luigi Zoja, 30, Milan, MI 20153, Italy. TEL 39-02-48202740, FAX 39-02-4820-1219, info@kurtis.it, http://www.kurtis.it. Ed. G Crepaldi.

THE AGING MALE. see *MEN'S HEALTH*

612.67 USA ISSN 0361-0179
AGING (NEW YORK). Text in English. 1975. irreg. price varies. reprint service avail. from PQC. *Refereed.* **Document type:** *Monographic series.*
Indexed: AgeLine, Biol.Abstr., Chem.Abstr., Curr.Cont. (coverage dropped), Mag.Ind., NRN, Sci.Cit.Ind. (coverage dropped).
Published by: Lippincott Williams & Wilkins (Philadelphia) (Subsidiary of: Wolters Kluwer N.V.), 530 Walnut St, Philadelphia, PA 19106-3621. TEL 301-223-2300, 800-638-3030, FAX 301-223-2400.

305.26 USA
AGING NEWS. Text in English. 1974. q. free per issue. bk.rev. charts, illus, stat. **Document type:** *Newsletter, Government.*
Formerly: New York (State). Office for the Aging. Newsletter; Supersedes: Cameo Newsletter (0008-2058)
Published by: Office for the Aging, 2 Empire State Plaza, Albany, NY 12223. FAX 518-474-0608. Ed. R Wendover. Circ: 35,000.

612.67 USA
AGING NEWS ALERT; the senior services & funding report. Text in English. 1982. s-m. USD 297 domestic (effective 2001); USD 307 in Canada; USD 337 elsewhere (2001). index. back issues avail. **Document type:** *Newsletter.* **Description:** For all professionals working with the elderly. Covers news and developments in the geriatric field.
Incorporates (1994-1996): Serving Elderly Clients; (1987-1992): Senior Care Professional (1051-6913); (1989-1992): Senior Law Report (1050-3250); Former titles: Aging Action Alert (1050-3188); Aging Alert
—CCC.
Published by: (Community Development Services, Inc.), C D Publications, 8204 Fenton St, Silver Spring, MD 20910-2889. TEL 301-588-6380, FAX 301-588-6385, ana@cdpublications.com, info@cdpublications.com, http://www.cdpublications.com. Ed. Brian Geller. Pub., R&P Mike Gerecht.

362.6 USA ISSN 0888-6830
HQ1060
AGING RESEARCH & TRAINING NEWS. Text in English. 1978. m. USD 277 (effective 2001). **Document type:** *Newsletter.* **Description:** Provides information on current grants and contracts for aging research and training.
Formerly (until 1987): Aging News (0197-4017)
Related titles: E-mail ed.
—CCC.
Published by: Business Publishers, Inc., 8737 Colesville Rd, 11th Fl, Silver Spring, MD 20910-3928. TEL 301-587-6300, 800-274-6737, FAX 301-589-8493, bpinews@bpinews.com, http://www.bpinews.com. Ed. Nancy Aldrich. Pub. Leonard A Eiserer.

612.67 JPN ISSN 0913-7602
AICHI IKA DAIGAKU KAREI IKAGAKU KENKYUJO KIYO/AICHI MEDICAL UNIVERSITY. INSTITUTE FOR MEDICAL SCIENCE OF AGING. BULLETIN. Text in English, Japanese. 1986. triennial. 100 p./no. **Document type:** *Bulletin, Academic/Scholarly.*
Published by: (Karei Ikagaku Kenkyujo/Institute for Medical Science of Aging), Aichi Ika Daigaku/Aichi Medical University, Karei Ikagaku Kenkyujo/Institute for Medical Science of Aging, Nagakute-cho, Aichi-gun, Aichi-ken 480-1195, Japan. TEL 81-52-264-4811, FAX 81-561-63-3531, yhashi@aichi-med-u.ac.jp. Ed. Dr. Yoshio Hashizume.

612.67 NOR ISSN 0801-9991
ALDRING OG ELDRE; gerontologisk magasin. Text in Norwegian, Danish, Swedish. 1984. q. NOK 265 to individuals; NOK 495, USD 94 to institutions; NOK 165 to students; NOK 135, USD 25 per issue (effective 2001). adv. bk.rev. **Document type:** *Academic/Scholarly.* **Description:** Focuses on professional gerontological issues for those who work or have an interest in the care of older people and their position in society.
Formerly (until 1988): Gerontologisk Magasin (0800-2509)
—CCC.
Published by: Scandinavian University Press (Subsidiary of: Taylor & Francis Ltd.), Postboks 2959, Toeyen, Oslo 0608, Norway. FAX 47-22-57-53-53, www.universitetsforlaget.no/tidsskrifter. Ed. Svein Olav Daatland. Circ: 2,500.

ALMSHOUSES GAZETTE. see *SOCIAL SERVICES AND WELFARE*

ALZHEIMER DISEASE AND ASSOCIATED DISORDERS. see *MEDICAL SCIENCES—Psychiatry And Neurology*

610.7365 362.6 USA ISSN 1070-5112
ALZHEIMER'S CARE GUIDE; published especially for those who care for people with Alzheimer's disease and related disorders. Text in English. 1993. m. USD 35 (effective 2000). illus. back issues avail. **Document type:** *Newsletter.* **Description:** Discusses caring for persons with Alzheimer's disease and related disorders. Covers effective care techniques dealing with difficult behaviors, research and breakthroughs, and activities.
Published by: Eymann Publications, Inc, PO Box 3577, Reno, NV 89505-3577. TEL 775-358-1554, FAX 775-358-1476, eymann@care4elders.com, http://www.care4elders.com. Ed. Maureen Eng. Pub. Katie Eymann Pace.

ALZHEIMER'S DISEASE SOURCEBOOK. see *MEDICAL SCIENCES—Psychiatry And Neurology*

610.7365 USA
ALZHEIMER'S HOME COMPANION. Text in English. 1998. m. USD 24.95 (effective 1999). **Document type:** *Newsletter.* **Description:** Provides care-givers with information, tips and insights into caring for someone with Alzheimer's disease.
Published by: Eymann Publications, Inc, PO Box 3577, Reno, NV 89505-3577. TEL 775-358-1554, FAX 775-358-1476, eymann@care4elders.com, http://www.care4elders.com. Ed. Maureen Eng. Pub. Katie Eymann Pace.

612.67 USA
CODEN: AGEEDB
AMERICAN AGING ASSOCIATION. JOURNAL. Text in English. 1978. q. USD 50 domestic; USD 90 foreign (effective 2000). bk.rev. index. *Refereed.* **Document type:** *Newsletter, Academic/Scholarly.* **Description:** Covers the effect of age on DNA, RNA, hormones, lysosomes, mitochondria, connective tissue, catecholamines, endoplasmic reticulum, and lipid metabolism.
Formerly (until Jan. 2000): Age (0161-9152)
Related titles: Online - full text ed.: (from Institute for Scientific Information).
Indexed: ASCA, AgeLine, Biol.Abstr., Chem.Abstr., Chem.Indus.Notes, Chem.Titles, Curr.Adv.Biochem., Curr.Cont., Environ.Sci.Poll.Mgmt., Excerp.Med., Helminthol.Abstr., Ind.Sci.Rev., NRN, Nutr.Abstr., Pollut.Abstr., Protozool.Abstr., Risk Abstr., SSCI (coverage dropped), Saf.Sci.Abstr., Sci.Cit.Ind.
—BLDSC (4683.748000), CASDDS, CISTI, EMDOCS, GNLM, IDS, ingenta, KNAW.
Published by: American Aging Association, 110 Chesley Dr, Media, PA 19063-1755. TEL 610-627-2626, FAX 610-565-9747. Ed., R&P, Adv. contact Dr. Arthur K Balin. Circ: 400.

618.97 USA ISSN 0002-8614
CODEN: JAGSAF
AMERICAN GERIATRICS SOCIETY. JOURNAL. Key Title: Journal of the American Geriatrics Society. Text in English. 1953. m. USD 182 domestic to individuals; USD 234 elsewhere to individuals; USD 330 domestic to institutions; USD 385 elsewhere to institutions; USD 200.20 to individuals print & online eds. combined; USD 363 to institutions print & online eds. combined (effective 2001). adv. bk.rev. abstr, charts, illus. index. reprint service avail. from PQC. *Refereed.* **Document type:** *Journal, Academic/Scholarly.* **Description:** Aims to provide latest clinical findings in geriatric medicine and gerontology.
Supersedes (in 1952): American Therapeutic Society. Transactions (0096-686X)
Related titles: Microfilm ed.: (from PQC,WWS); Online - full text ed.: ISSN 1532-5415. 2001. USD 164 to individuals; USD 297 to institutions (effective 2001) (from H. W. Wilson, Gale Group, Swets Blackwell, Factiva, Institute for Scientific Information, RoweCom Information Quest).
Indexed: AMED, ASCA, ASSIA, Abstr.Health Care Manage.Stud., Abstr.Soc.Geront., AgeLine, Agri.& Environ.Biotech.Abstr. (coverage dropped), Behav.Med.Abstr., Biol.Abstr., CINAHL, C.I.S. Abstr., Cal.Tiss.Abstr., Chem.Abstr., Chem.Indus.Notes, Chem.Titles, Curr.Adv.Ecol.Sci., Curr.Cont., Derwent Biotech.Abstr., Environ.Sci.Poll.Mgmt., Excerp.Med., Fam.Ind., Hosp.Lit.Ind., INIS Atomind., I.P.A., Ind.Med. (1953-), Ind.Sci.Rev., Inpharma, Int.Nurs.Ind., Jrnl.Watch, Jrnl.Watch Wom.Hlth., Lang.& Lang.Behav.Abstr., Med.& Surg.Dermat., NRN, Neurosci.Cit.Ind., Nutr.Abstr., Pharm.&Out.News, Pollut.Abstr., PsycInfo, Psychol.Abstr. (1953-), Reac., Risk Abstr., SOPODA, SSCI, Saf.Sci.Abstr., Sage Fam.Stud.Abstr., Sci.Cit.Ind., Soc.Sci.Ind. (Jan.1994-), Soc.Serv.Abstr., Soc.Work Res.& Abstr., Sociol.Abstr., THA, Viol.& Abuse Abstr., e-psyche.
—BLDSC (4686.300000), CASDDS, CISTI, GNLM, IDS, ingenta, KNAW.
Published by: (American Geriatrics Society), Blackwell Science Inc., Commerce Pl, 350 Main St, Malden, MA 02148-5018. TEL 781-388-8250, 888-661-5800, FAX 781-388-8255, journals@blacksci.com, http://www.blackwell-science.com. Ed. William Applegate. adv.: B&W page USD 1,300; trim 10.88 x 8.13. Circ: 9,018; 8,796 (paid).

618.97 USA
AMERICAN GERIATRICS SOCIETY NEWSLETTER. Text in English. 1972. q. membership. adv. **Document type:** *Newsletter.* **Description:** Covers news and activities of the society, and topical issues in geriatric medicine.
Published by: American Geriatrics Society, 350 5th Ave Ste 801, New York, NY 10118-0801. TEL 212-308-1414, FAX 212-832-8646, http://www.americangeriatrics.org. Ed., R&P Pamela W Ingham. Adv. contact Mike Guest. Circ: 10,000.

306.38 155 ISR
AMERICAN INSTITUTE OF GERONTOLOGY AND HUMAN DEVELOPMENT. BROOKDALE INSTITUTE OF GERONTOLOGY AND HUMAN DEVELOPMENT. RESEARCH REPORTS. Text in English, Hebrew. irreg. (7-8/yr.). **Document type:** *Academic/Scholarly.*
Former titles: American Institute of Gerontology and Human Development. Brookdale Institute of Gerontology and Human Development. Discussion Papers (0333-564X); Brookdale Institute of Gerontology. Discussion Papers
Published by: American Joint Distribution Committee, Brookdale Institute of Gerontology and Human Development, P O Box 13087, Jerusalem 91130, Israel. TEL 972-2-6557400, FAX 972-2-5635851.

618.97 USA ISSN 1082-5207
AMERICAN JOURNAL OF ALZHEIMER'S DISEASE. Text in English. 1986. bi-m. USD 136 domestic to individuals; USD 172 in Canada to individuals; USD 199 elsewhere to individuals; USD 193 domestic to institutions; USD 245 in Canada to institutions; USD 304 elsewhere to institutions (effective 2002). adv. bk.rev. abstr, bibl, charts, illus. 40 p./no. 2 cols./p. back issues avail. *Refereed.* **Document type:** *Academic/Scholarly.* **Description:** Publishes original articles and case studies on all aspects of Alzheimer's disease and care.
Former titles (until Mar. 1995): American Journal of Alzheimer's Care and Related Disorders and Research (0895-5336); (until 1987): American Journal of Alzheimer's Care and Related Disorders (0888-4897)
Indexed: Abstr.Soc.Geront., AgeLine, Biol.Dig., CINAHL, NRN, PsycInfo, Sage Fam.Stud.Abstr., Soc.Serv.Abstr., Sociol.Abstr., Viol.& Abuse Abstr., e-psyche.
—BLDSC (0820.995000), CISTI, GNLM, Infotrieve, KNAW. **CCC.**

G

Published by: Prime National Publishing Corp., 470 Boston Post Rd, Weston, MA 02493. TEL 781-899-2702, FAX 781-899-4900, alzheimers@pnpco.com, http://www.pnpco.com; http://www.alzheimersjournal.com. Ed. Dr. Daniel A Pollen. Pub., Adv. contact Richard A DeVito Sr. TEL 781-899-2702 ext. 107. R&P Dennis N Ricci. Circ: 3,000.

AMERICAN JOURNAL OF GERIATRIC CARDIOLOGY. see *MEDICAL SCIENCES—Cardiovascular Diseases*

618.97 USA ISSN 1064-7481
CODEN: AJGPE8
AMERICAN JOURNAL OF GERIATRIC PSYCHIATRY; official journal of the American Association for Geriatric Psychiatry. Text in English. 1993. q. USD 119 domestic to individuals Print & online eds.; USD 138 foreign to individuals Print & online eds.; USD 252 domestic to institutions Print & online eds.; USD 274 foreign to institutions Print & online eds. (effective 2001). adv. bk.rev. illus. Index. back issues avail.; reprints avail. *Refereed.* **Document type:** *Journal, Academic/Scholarly.* **Description:** Source of scientific and clinical information for the rapidly developing field of geriatric psychiatry.
Related titles: Microform ed.: (from PQC); Online - full text ed.: (from HighWire Pr., Northern Light Technology, Inc., EBSCO Publishing, RoweCom Information Quest, ProQuest Information & Learning, Institute for Scientific Information).
Indexed: ASCA, Abstr.Soc.Geront., AgeLine, Curr.Cont., Excerp.Med. (1994-), Ind.Med. (1993-), Int.Nurs.Ind., Jrnl.Watch Psych., PsycInfo, Psychol.Abstr. (1993-), SSCI, e-psyche.
—BLDSC (0824.657000), EMDOCS, GNLM, IDS, Infotrieve, KNAW. **CCC.**
Published by: American Psychiatric Press, Inc., Journals Division, 1400 K St, N W, Ste 1101, Washington, DC 20005. TEL 800-368-5777, FAX 202-682-6341, 202-789-2648, appi@psych.org, http://ajgp.psychiatryonline.org/, http://www.psychiatryonline.org, http://www.appi.org. Ed. Dr. Gene Cohen. R&P John McDuffie. Adv. contact Ryan Miller.

THE AMERICAN JOURNAL OF HOSPICE AND PALLIATIVE CARE. see *MEDICAL SCIENCES*

AMERICAN PARKINSON DISEASE ASSOCIATION. NEWSLETTER. see *SOCIAL SERVICES AND WELFARE*

618.97 FRA ISSN 0990-2295
ANNEE GERONTOLOGIQUE✱ . Text in French. 1987. a. price varies. adv. bk.rev. Supplement avail. **Document type:** *Monographic series, Academic/Scholarly.*
Related titles: ♦ English ed.: Facts and Research in Gerontology. ISSN 1163-0450; ♦ Supplement: Facts and Research in Gerontology Newsletter. ISSN 1167-4911.
—BLDSC (1049.085000).
Published by: SERDI, 45 chemin del Prat, Auzeville Tolosane 31320, France. FAX 33-5-61-751128. Eds. J L Albarede, P Vellas. Adv. contact Rachel Mayne.

305.26 USA ISSN 0272-3808
HQ1060
ANNUAL EDITIONS: AGING. Text in English. 1978. a. USD 12.25. illus. index. back issues avail. *Refereed.* **Document type:** *Academic/Scholarly.*
Formerly: Annual Editions. Focus: Aging (0162-3621)
Indexed: Bk.Rev.Ind.
Published by: Dushkin - McGraw-Hill, Sluice Dock, Guilford, CT 06437-9989. TEL 203-453-4351, FAX 203-453-6000. Ed. Harold Cox. Pub. Ian Nielsen. R&P Cheryl Greenleaf.

305.26 USA ISSN 0198-8794
RC952.A1
ANNUAL REVIEW OF GERONTOLOGY & GERIATRICS. Text in English. 1980. a., latest vol.18, 1998. USD 54; USD 61.80 foreign (effective 1999). back issues avail. **Document type:** *Academic/Scholarly.* **Description:** Explores the sociological and medical aspects of aging and treating the elderly. Focuses on intervention research.
—BLDSC (1522.565300), CISTI, GNLM, ingenta.
Published by: Springer Publishing Company, 536 Broadway, New York, NY 10012. TEL 212-431-4370, FAX 212-941-7842, springer@springerpub.com, http://www.springerpub.com. Eds. Cawton, Schulz. Circ: 800.

618.97 IRL ISSN 0167-4943
QP86 CODEN: AGGEDL
ARCHIVES OF GERONTOLOGY AND GERIATRICS; an international journal integrating experimental, clinical and social studies on ageing. Text in English. 1981. bi-m. EUR 1,237 in Europe to institutions; JPY 164,200 in Japan to institutions; USD 1,384 elsewhere to institutions (effective 2002). abstr. back issues avail. *Refereed.* **Document type:** *Academic/Scholarly.* **Description:** Provides a medium for the publication of papers from the fields of experimental gerontology and clinical and social geriatrics.
Related titles: Microform ed.: (from PQC); Online - full text ed.: (from ingenta, Swets Blackwell, ScienceDirect, Institute for Scientific Information); ♦ Supplement: Archives of Gerontology and Geriatrics. Supplement. ISSN 0924-7947.
Indexed: ASCA, Biol.Abstr., CINAHL, Chem.Abstr., Chem.Indus.Notes, Chem.Titles, Curr.Adv.Biochem., Curr.Adv.Cancer Res., Curr.Adv.Ecol.Sci., Curr.Cont., Environ.Sci.Poll.Mgmt., Excerp.Med., Fam.Ind., Ind.Med. (coverage dropped), Ind.Sci.Rev., Inpharma, Int.Abstr.Biol.Sci., NRN, Neurosci.Abstr. (coverage dropped), Neurosci.Cit.Ind., Pharm.&Out.News, Pollut.Abstr., PsycInfo, Psychol.Abstr. (1982-), Reac., Risk Abstr., SSCI (coverage dropped), Saf.Sci.Abstr., Sci.Cit.Ind., e-psyche.
—BLDSC (1634.401000), CASDDS, CISTI, EMDOCS, GNLM, IDS, Infotrieve, ingenta, KNAW. **CCC.**
Published by: Elsevier Science Ireland Ltd, Elsevier House, Brookvale Plaza, E. Park, Shannon, Co. Clare, Ireland. TEL 353-61-471944, FAX 353-61-472144, http://www.elsevier.com/locate/archger. Ed. I Zs.-Nagy. R&P Annette Moloney. **Subscr. in Australasia and the Far East to:** Elsevier Science (Singapore) Pte Ltd, No.1 Temasek Ave, 17-01 Millenia Tower, Singapore 039192, Singapore. TEL 65-434-3727, FAX 65-337-2230; **Subscr. in the Americas to:** Elsevier Science, PO Box 945, New York, NY 10159-0945. TEL 212-633-3730, FAX 212-633-3680; **Subscr. to:** Elsevier Science BV, PO Box 211, Amsterdam 1000 AE, Netherlands. TEL 31-20-485-3757, FAX 31-20-485-3432.

306.38 IRL ISSN 0924-7947
RC952.A1 CODEN: AGGSEU
ARCHIVES OF GERONTOLOGY AND GERIATRICS. SUPPLEMENT. Text in English. 1989. irreg. price varies. *Refereed.* **Document type:** *Academic/Scholarly.*
Related titles: ♦ Supplement to: Archives of Gerontology and Geriatrics. ISSN 0167-4943.
Indexed: Chem.Abstr., Chem.Indus.Notes, Chem.Titles.
—CASDDS, CISTI, Infotrieve, KNAW. **CCC.**
Published by: Elsevier Science Ireland Ltd, Elsevier House, Brookvale Plaza, E. Park, Shannon, Co. Clare, Ireland. TEL 353-61-471944, FAX 353-61-472144. R&P Annette Moloney. **Subscr. in Australasia and the Far East to:** Elsevier Science (Singapore) Pte Ltd, No.1 Temasek Ave, 17-01 Millenia Tower, Singapore 039192, Singapore. TEL 65-434-3727, FAX 65-337-2230; **Subscr. in the Americas to:** Elsevier Science, PO Box 945, New York, NY 10159-0945. TEL 212-633-3730, FAX 212-633-3680; **Subscr. to:** Elsevier Science BV, PO Box 211, Amsterdam 1000 AE, Netherlands. TEL 31-20-485-3757, FAX 31-20-485-3432.

618.97 BRA ISSN 1413-7615
CODEN: AGGEFN
ARQUIVOS DE GERIATRIA E GERONTOLOGIA. Text in Portuguese; Summaries in English, Portuguese. 1996. 3/yr. BRL 42, USD 72 (effective 2000). adv. bk.rev. bibl, charts. index, cum.index. back issues avail. **Document type:** *Academic/Scholarly.*
Indexed: Ref.Zh.
—KNAW.
Published by: (Sociedade Brasileira de Geriatria e Gerontologia), E C N - Editora Cientifica Nacional Ltda., Rua da Gloria, 366 Andar 3, Gloria, Rio De Janeiro, RJ 20241-180, Brazil. TEL 55-21-2213235, FAX 55-21-2213235, ecn@rj.sol.com.br. Ed. Vilma Camara. R&P, Adv. contact Maria Luiza Carvalho. Circ: 3,000.

ASSISTED LIVING BUSINESS REPORT. see *HEALTH FACILITIES AND ADMINISTRATION*

ASSISTED LIVING SUCCESS. see *HEALTH FACILITIES AND ADMINISTRATION*

612.67 JPN
ASU NO TOMO/FRIEND OF TOMORROW. Text in Japanese. 1973. bi-m. JPY 2,480. adv.
Published by: Fujin-no-Tomo Sha, 20-16, 2-chome, Nishi-Ikebukuro, Toshima-ku, Tokyo, Japan. FAX 03-3981-6747. Ed. Kouko Chiba. Pub. Susumu Miyake. Adv. contact Jun Nomura.

618.97 AUS
AUSTRALASIAN JOURNAL ON AGEING. Text in English. 1966. q. AUD 58 to individuals; AUD 65 to institutions (effective 1999). adv. bk.rev. *Refereed.* **Document type:** *Academic/Scholarly.* **Description:** Publishes original work that advances the understanding of gerontology and geriatrics.
Former titles (until 1998): Australian Journal on Ageing (0726-4240); (until 1980): Growing Older (0046-6492)
Indexed: ASCA, Abstr.Soc.Geront., AgeLine, Aus.P.A.I.S., Curr.Cont. (coverage dropped), PsycInfo, SSCI (coverage dropped), Soc.Serv.Abstr., Sociol.Abstr.
—BLDSC (1794.874000), GNLM, ingenta.
Published by: Council on the Ageing, Level 2, 3 Bowen Crescent, Melbourne, VIC 3004, Australia. TEL 61-3-98202655, cotaa@vicnet.net.au. Ed. Tony Jorm. R&P, Adv. contact Kathy Hogarty. Circ: 2,000.

B I F O C A L. (Bar Associations in Focus on Aging and the Law) see *LAW*

610.7365 USA ISSN 1094-6195
RA999.A35 CODEN: JLTAD4
BALANCE (ALEXANDRIA). Text in English. 1997. 8/yr. USD 80 to non-members; USD 90 foreign to non-members (effective 1999). adv. bk.rev., film rev. bibl, charts. index. back issues avail. **Document type:** *Trade.* **Description:** Publishes original research, practical information, trends and developments in long-term health care administration.
Former titles (until 1998): Continuum (1093-2704); Which was formed by the merger of (1972-1997): Journal of Long-Term Care Administration (0093-4445); (1967-1997): Long-Term Care Administrator (0146-275X)
Related titles: Microform ed.: (from PQC); Online - full text ed.: (from ProQuest Information & Learning).
Indexed: Abstr.Health Care Manage.Stud., Abstr.Soc.Geront., AgeLine, Biol.Abstr., CINAHL, Fam.Ind., Hosp.Lit.Ind., I.P.A., Int.Nurs.Ind., Med.Care Rev., Soc.Work Res.& Abstr.
—BLDSC (1860.440000), CISTI, GNLM, Infotrieve, ingenta. **CCC.**
Published by: American College of Health Care Administrators, 325 S Patrick St, Alexandria, VA 22314. TEL 703-739-7900, 888-882-2422, FAX 703-739-7901, info@achca.org, http://www.achca.org. Ed., R&P Jan Lamoglia TEL 703-739-7917. Adv. contact Pam Malloy. Circ: 6,900.

362.6 GBR ISSN 0964-0185
BASELINE. Text in English. ceased; resumed 1975. 3/yr. GBP 6. bk.rev. bibl. back issues avail.
Formerly (until 1990): Action Baseline (0959-4469)
Indexed: Artbibl.Mod., Brit.Nur.Ind., DAAI.
Published by: British Association for Service to the Elderly, 119 Hassell St, Newcastle-under-Lyme, Staffs ST5 1AX, United Kingdom. TEL 44-1782-661033, FAX 44-1782-712725. Ed. Dr. Frank Glendenning. Circ: 1,000.

306.38 CAN ISSN 0835-8702
LE BEL AGE. Text in French. 1979. 11/yr. CND 25.25 domestic (effective 2000). adv. bk.rev. back issues avail. **Document type:** *Consumer.*
Incorporates (in 1987): Temps de Vivre (0708-7632)
Indexed: Can.Per.Ind., Pt.de Rep. (1989-).
Published by: Senior Publications Inc., 5148 blvd Saint Laurent, Montreal, PQ H2T 1R8, Canada. TEL 514-273-9773, FAX 514-273-9268, belage@mail.transcontinental.ca. Ed., R&P Lucie Desaulniers. Pub. Francine Tremblay. Adv. contact Lucie Leduc. Circ: 136,028 (paid). **Subscr. to:** 1100 bd Rene Levesque O, 24e etage, Montreal, PQ H3B 4X9, Canada.

612.67 NLD ISSN 1389-5729
▼ **BIOGERONTOLOGY.** Text in English. 2000. bi-m. USD 296, EUR 295 to institutions for print or online ed.; USD 355.20, EUR 354 to institutions for print & online eds. combined (effective 2002). bk.rev. illus, abstr. *Refereed.* **Document type:** *Journal, Academic/Scholarly.* **Description:** Publishes original research reports, reviews, hypotheses, new methods and intervies, special issues on specific topics relating to aging, health and longevity.
Related titles: Online - full text ed.: (from EBSCO Publishing, O C L C Online Computer Library Center, Inc., Swets Blackwell, Kluwer Online, Institute for Scientific Information, RoweCom Information Quest).
Indexed: Curr.Cont.
—BLDSC (2072.174000).

Published by: Kluwer Academic Publishers Group (Subsidiary of: Wolters Kluwer N.V.), Postbus 17, Dordrecht 3300 AA, Netherlands. http://www.wkap.nl/journalhome.htm/1389-5729. Ed. Suresh I Rattan. **Subscr. addr. in N America:** Kluwer Academic - Plenum Publishers, 233 Spring St, New York, NY 10013-1578. TEL 212-620-8468, 800-221-9369, FAX 212-807-1047; **Subscr. to:** Journals Department, PO Box 322, Dordrecht 3300 AH, Netherlands. TEL 31-78-639-2392, FAX 31-78-654-6474.

BLAETTER AUS DEM HENRIETTENSTIFT. see *HEALTH FACILITIES AND ADMINISTRATION*

612.67 MLT ISSN 1016-5177
HQ1060
BOLD. Key Title: Bold Comment. Text in English. 1990. q. USD 50 to individuals; USD 60 to institutions. bk.rev. **Document type:** *Academic/Scholarly.*
Indexed: AgeLine.
—BLDSC (2122.615000).
Published by: International Institute on Ageing, 117 St. Paul St., Valletta VLT 07, Malta. TEL 356-243044, FAX 356-230248, TELEX 1990 AGEUN MW, inia@maltanet.net, http://www.inia.org.mt. Ed. Dr. Victor G Griffiths.

305.26 USA
BOSTON SENIORITY; serving Boston's elderly community. Text in English. 1977. m. free per issue. back issues avail. **Document type:** *Newsletter.* **Description:** Contains information on elderly issues and activities of the commission.
Published by: Mayor's Commission on Affairs of the Elderly, Boston City Hall, Rm 271, Boston, MA 02201. TEL 617-635-2712. Ed. Carrie W Dawe. Circ: 20,000.

618.97 USA
BROWN UNIVERSITY GERIATRIC PSYCHOPHARMACOLOGY UPDATE; updates on use of psychotropic medications in geriatrics and pertinent regulatory issues. Text in English. 1997. m., latest vol.5, 2001. USD 117 domestic to individuals; USD 217 domestic to institutions; USD 227 in Canada to institutions; USD 237 elsewhere to institutions (effective 2001). 8 p./no. back issues avail.; reprints avail. **Document type:** *Newsletter.* **Description:** Updates on research and use of psychotropic medications and specific interventions with aging.
Formerly: Brown University GeroPsych Report (1098-2450)
Related titles: E-mail ed.
Indexed: Ref.Zh.
Published by: Manisses Communications Group, Inc., PO Box 9758, Providence, RI 02906-9758. TEL 401-831-6020, 800-333-7771, FAX 401-861-6370, manissescs@manisses.com, manissesCS@manisses.com, http://www.manisses.com. Ed. Dr. Richard J Goldberg. Pub. Betty R Lang.

612.67 USA ISSN 0251-6802
HQ1060
BULLETIN ON AGEING. Text in English, French, Spanish. 1976. 3/yr. free per issue. bk.rev. back issues avail. **Document type:** *Bulletin.* **Description:** Provides information on ageing issues at the United Nations, along with government and nongovernment activities. Special annual thematic double issue.
Indexed: Abstr.Soc.Geront., AgeLine, World Bibl.Soc.Sec.
Published by: Department of Economic and Social Affairs, Division for Social Policy and Development, Programme on Ageing, DC2 1340, United Nations, New York, NY 10017. TEL 212-963-0500, FAX 212-963-3062. Circ: 3,000.

610.7365 USA ISSN 1093-6939
THE BULLETIN ON LONG-TERM CARE LAW. Text in English. 1997. 12/yr. USD 197 (effective 2001). adv. charts. index. 10 p./no. 2 cols./p. back issues avail. **Document type:** *Newsletter, Trade.* **Description:** Covers the legal and regulatory challenges to long-term care administrators. Follows changes to existing laws, proposed federal and state legislation, and legal cases that could affect long-term care facilities.
Related titles: Online - full content ed.
—CCC.
Published by: Health Resources Publishing, 1913 Atlantic Ave, Ste F4, Manasquan, NJ 08736. TEL 732-292-1100, FAX 732-292-1111, hrp@healthrespubs.com, info@healthrespubs.com, http://www.healthrespubs.com. Ed. Lew Gurman. Pub. Robert K Jenkins. Adv. contact Judy Granholm.

306.38 FRA ISSN 0184-6531
C L E I R P P A ANNEES - DOCUMENTS; annees a venir...annees d'avenir. Text in French. 1971. bi-m. FRF 520; FRF 580 foreign. adv. bk.rev., film rev. abstr, bibl, stat. index. back issues avail. **Document type:** *Academic/Scholarly.*
Formerly: Centre de Liaison, d'Etude, d'Information et de Recherche sur les Problemes des Personnes Agees. Annees Documents
Published by: Centre de Liaison d'Etude d'Information et de Recherche sur les Problemes des Personnes Agees, 15 rue Chateaubriand, Paris 75008, France. TEL 42-25-78-78, FAX 42-56-48-26. Ed. Naima Segret. Adv. contact Jean Michel Hote. Circ: 2,000.

306.38 FRA ISSN 1146-2965
C L E I R P P A INFOS; bulletin mensuel d'informations du CLEIRPPA. Text in French. 1983. m. FRF 520; FRF 580 foreign; includes CLEIRPPA Annees-Documents. adv. **Document type:** *Bibliography.*
Published by: Centre de Liaison d'Etude d'Information et de Recherche sur les Problemes des Personnes Agees, 15 rue Chateaubriand, Paris 75008, France. TEL 42-25-78-78, FAX 42-56-48-26. Ed. Naima Segret. Adv. contact Jean Michel Hote.

C M E JOURNAL - GERIATRIC MEDICINE. (Continuing Medical Education) see *MEDICAL SCIENCES*

612.67 CAN ISSN 0714-9808
HQ1060
CANADIAN JOURNAL ON AGING/REVUE CANADIENNE DU VIEILLISSEMENT. Text in English. 1982. q. CND 46 in Canada to individuals; USD 60 elsewhere to individuals; CND 65 in Canada to institutions; USD 75 elsewhere to institutions; CND 25 in Canada to students; USD 40 elsewhere to students (effective 2001). adv. bk.rev. charts, stat, illus. back issues avail.; reprints avail. *Refereed.* **Document type:** *Journal, Academic/Scholarly.* **Description:** Presents research findings, as well as conceptual, and theoretical papers from a variety of viewpoints including biology, and the health and social sciences.
Related titles: Online - full text ed.: (from Institute for Scientific Information).
Indexed: ASCA, Abstr.Soc.Geront., AgeLine, CBCA Ref., C.I.J.E., Can.B.P.I., Can.Per.Ind. (Mar.1988-), Can.Wom.Per.Ind., Curr.Cont., Excerp.Med., Fam.Ind., Lang.& Lang.Behav.Abstr., P.A.I.S., PsycInfo, Psychol.Abstr. (1982-), SOPODA, SSCI, Sage Fam.Stud.Abstr., Sage Race Rel.Abstr., Soc.Serv.Abstr., Soc.Work Res.& Abstr., Sociol.Abstr., e-psyche.
—BLDSC (3027.920000), CISTI, EMDOCS, GNLM, IDS, Infotrieve, ingenta, KNAW. **CCC.**
Published by: The Canadian Association on Gerontology/Association Canadienne de Gerontologie, 100-824 Meath St, Ottawa, ON K1Z 6E8, Canada. TEL 613-728-9347, FAX 613-728-8913, info@cagacg.ca, http://calj.icaap.org/calj/cja/, http://www.cagacg.ca/index.htm. Ed. Francois Beland. adv.: page CND 300. Circ: 1,600 (paid).

618.97 GBR
CARE; the journal of practice and development. Text in English. 1992. q. GBP 25; GBP 27.50 foreign. **Document type:** *Bulletin.*
Former titles: Journal of Practice and Staff Development; (until 1997): Elders (0964-6914); (until 1995): Journal of Training and Development (0959-7670)
Published by: Pepar Publications Ltd., The Gatehouse, Pepar Publications, 112 Park Hill Rd, Harborne, Staffs B17 9HD, United Kingdom. TEL 44-121-428-4474, FAX 44-121-428-4474, admin@pepar.demon.co.uk.

612.67 DEU ISSN 1435-9286
CARE KONKRET; Wochenzeitung fuer das Pflegemanagement. Text in German. m. EUR 90 (effective 2002). **Document type:** *Journal, Academic/Scholarly, Trade.*
Published by: Vincentz Verlag, Schiffgraben 43, Hannover 30175, Germany. TEL 49-511-9910000, FAX 49-511-9910099, info@vincentz.de, http://www.vincentz.de.

612.67 USA
CAREGIVER. Text in English. 1980. 3/yr. USD 10. bk.rev. **Document type:** *Newsletter.*
Indexed: CINAHL.
Published by: Duke Aging Center, Family Support Program, Duke Medical Center, Box 3600, Durham, NC 27710. TEL 919-660-7510, FAX 919-684-8569. Ed., R&P Lisa Gwyther. Circ: 8,000.

612.67 JPN ISSN 0910-3058
CHOJUGAKU KENKYU/RESEARCH OF LONGEVITY SCIENCE. Text in Japanese. 1984. s-a. JPY 1,500 per issue.
Published by: Kokusai Shizen Igakkai/International Natural Medicine Society, Seimei Kagaku Kyokai, 3-15 Hongo 1-chome, Bunkyo-ku, Tokyo 113-0033, Japan.

618.97 JPN
CHUJU KAGAKU SOGO KENKYU HOKOKU/ COMPREHENSIVE STUDIES ON SCIENCE OF AGING. Text in Japanese. 1991. a.
Published by: Choju Kagaku Shinko Zaidan/Japan Foundation for Aging and Health, 3-6 Toranomon 1-chome, Minato-ku, Tokyo 105-0001, Japan.

618.97 JPN ISSN 0918-533X
CHUOJU KAGAKU KOENKAI KIROKUSHU/LECTURES ON SCIENCE OF AGING. Text in Japanese. 1991. irreg.
Published by: Choju Kagaku Shinko Zaidan/Japan Foundation for Aging and Health, 3-6 Toranomon 1-chome, Minato-ku, Tokyo 105-0001, Japan.

618.97 USA ISSN 1095-1598
CLINICAL GERIATRICS. Text in English. 1993. 13/yr. *Refereed.* **Document type:** *Journal, Academic/Scholarly.* **Description:** Covers description, diagnoses and management of medical problems in the elderly, and offers continuing medical education credits.
Formerly: Clinical Geriatrics and Issues in Long-Term Care (1070-1389)
Indexed: CINAHL.
—BLDSC (3286.287500), GNLM.
Published by: MultiMedia Healthcare Inc., Office Center of Princeton Meadows, Bldg 300, Plainsboro, NJ 08536. TEL 609-275-3800, FAX 609-275-6076, info@mmhc.com, http://www.mmhc.com. Ed. Peter Ciszewki. Pub. Tioke Blazier. Circ: 85,000 (controlled).

155.67 USA ISSN 0731-7115
CLINICAL GERONTOLOGIST; the journal of aging and mental health. Text in English. 1977. q. USD 50 to individuals; USD 68 in Canada to individuals; USD 73 elsewhere to individuals; USD 125 to institutions; USD 169 in Canada to institutions; USD 181 elsewhere to institutions; USD 425 to libraries; USD 574 in Canada to libraries; USD 616 elsewhere to libraries (effective Aug. 2001). adv. bk.rev. abstr, bibl, illus. index. back issues avail.; reprint service avail. from HAW. *Refereed.* **Document type:** *Journal, Academic/Scholarly.* **Description:** Presents material relevant to the needs of mental health professionals and all practitioners who deal with the aged client.
Former titles: Journal of Aged Care (0270-3122); (until 1981): Aged Care and Services Review
Related titles: Microfiche ed.: (from PQC); Microform ed.
Indexed: ASSIA, Abstr.Anthropol., Abstr.Health Care Manage.Stud., Abstr.Soc.Geront., AgeLine, Behav.Abstr., Behav.Med.Abstr., Biol.Abstr., CINAHL, Chicago Psychoanal.Lit.Ind., Environ.Sci.Poll.Mgmt., Excerp.Med., Fam.Ind., Hosp.Abstr., Hosp.Lit.Ind., IMFL, Inpharma, Lang.& Lang.Behav.Abstr., Med.Care Rev., Past.Care & Couns.Abstr., Pharm.&Out.News, Pollut.Abstr., PsycInfo, Psychol.Abstr. (1982-), Reac., Ref.Zh., Rehabil.Lit., Risk Abstr., SOPODA, Saf.Sci.Abstr., Sage Fam.Stud.Abstr., Soc.Serv.Abstr., Soc.Work Res.& Abstr., Sociol.Abstr., Viol.& Abuse Abstr., e-psyche.
—BLDSC (3286.288000), EMDOCS, GNLM, Haworth, ingenta, KNAW.
Published by: Haworth Press, Inc., 10 Alice St, Binghamton, NY 13904-1580. TEL 607-722-5857, 800-429-6784, FAX 607-722-6362, 800-895-0582, getinfo@haworthpressinc.com, http://www.haworthpress.com/journals/journallist.asp. Ed. Terry L Brink. Pub. William Cohen. R&P Ruthann Heath TEL 607-723-5857 ext 316. Adv. contact Jackie Blakeslee TEL 607-722-5857 ext 346. B&W page USD 315, color page USD 550; trim 6 x 8.5. Circ: 750.

618.97 USA ISSN 0749-0690
RC952.A1
CLINICS IN GERIATRIC MEDICINE. Text in English. 1985. q. USD 134 domestic to individuals; USD 168 in Canada to individuals; USD 180 elsewhere to individuals; USD 192 domestic to institutions; USD 235 foreign to institutions; USD 59 per issue (effective 2001). back issues avail. *Refereed.* **Document type:** *Academic/Scholarly.* **Description:** Each issue discusses a single aspect of the psychiatric, psychological, physical, or medical treatment of elderly patients.
Related titles: Microfilm ed.; Online - full text ed.: (from Institute for Scientific Information).
Indexed: ASCA, Abstr.Soc.Geront., AgeLine, CINAHL, Curr.Cont., Excerp.Med., Fam.Ind., Ind.Med. (1985-), Inpharma, Int.Nurs.Ind., Nutr.Abstr., Reac., SSCI (coverage dropped).
—BLDSC (3286.562000), CISTI, EMDOCS, GNLM, IDS, ingenta, KNAW. **CCC.**

Published by: W.B. Saunders Co. (Subsidiary of: Harcourt Publishers Ltd.), 11830 Westline Industrial Dr, St Louis, MO 63146. TEL 800-325-4177, http://www.wbsaunders.com. Circ: 2,300. **Subscr. to:** Periodicals Fulfillment, W B Saunders Co, 6277 Sea Harbor Dr, 4th Fl, Orlando, FL 32891-4800.

CONDITION; Ratgebermagazin fuer Lauf- und Ausdauersport. see *SPORTS AND GAMES*

612.67 USA ISSN 0748-2760
RC952.A1
CONTEMPORARY GERIATRIC MEDICINE. Text in English. 1983. irreg., latest vol.3, 1988. price varies. back issues avail. *Refereed.* **Document type:** *Monographic series.*
Published by: Kluwer Academic - Plenum Publishers (Subsidiary of: Wolters Kluwer N.V.), 233 Spring St, New York, NY 10013-1578. TEL 212-620-8000, 800-221-9369, FAX 212-463-0742, info@plenum.com, http://www.plenum.com. Ed. Steven R Gambert.

618.97 USA ISSN 1069-0840
HQ1060
CONTEMPORARY GERONTOLOGY; a journal of reviews and critical discourse. Text in English. 1994. 4/yr., latest vol.7, 2001. USD 52 in United States to individuals; USD 88 for 2 yrs. in United States to individuals; USD 61 foreign to individuals; USD 104 for 2 yrs. foreign to individuals; USD 112 in United States to institutions; USD 190 for 2 yrs. in United States to institutions; USD 128 foreign to institutions; USD 218 for 2 yrs. foreign to institutions (effective 2001). adv. bk.rev. abstr. 36 p./no. back issues avail.; reprints avail. *Refereed.* **Document type:** *Journal, Academic/Scholarly.* **Description:** Contains 12 to 15 book reviews and occasional articles on critical discourse in gerontology intended to help gerontologists and allied professionals keep up with the growing literature on aging.
Indexed: AgeLine, Lang.& Lang.Behav.Abstr., SOPODA, Soc.Serv.Abstr., Sociol.Abstr.
—CCC.
Published by: (American Society on Aging), Springer Publishing Company, 536 Broadway, New York, NY 10012. TEL 212-431-4370, FAX 212-941-7842, springer@springerpub.com, http://www.springerpub.com. Ed. George L Maddox. Pub. Ursula Springer. R&P Dorothy Kouwenberg. Adv. contact Bob Friel. B&W page USD 300.

306.38 USA ISSN 0732-085X
CONTRIBUTIONS TO THE STUDY OF AGING. Text in English. 1982. irreg. price varies. index. **Document type:** *Monographic series.*
—BLDSC (3461.453300), CISTI.
Published by: Greenwood Press, Inc. (Subsidiary of: Greenwood Publishing Group Inc.), 88 Post Rd W, Box 5007, Westport, CT 06881. TEL 203-226-3571, FAX 203-226-1502.

303 CAN ISSN 0847-1797
D W D NEWSLETTER. Text in English. 1983. q. membership. bk.rev. charts, stat. **Document type:** *Newsletter.* **Description:** Discusses issues related to end of life decision making. Looks at ethical, legal, moral and social aspects of life-death concerns of Canadians.
Indexed: e-psyche.
Published by: Dying with Dignity, 55 Eglinton Ave E, Ste 705, Toronto, ON M4P 1G8, Canada. TEL 416-486-3998, FAX 416-489-9010, dwdca@web.net, http://www.web.net/dwd. Ed., R&P Kathy St. John. Circ: 5,000.

▼ **DEATH & DYING SOURCEBOOK.** see *PHILOSOPHY*

DEATH STUDIES; education - counseling - care - law - ethics. see *PSYCHOLOGY*

▼ **DEMENTIA.** see *MEDICAL SCIENCES—Psychiatry And Neurology*

DEMENTIA AND GERIATRIC COGNITIVE DISORDERS. see *MEDICAL SCIENCES—Psychiatry And Neurology*

305.26 ITA ISSN 1127-3909
DEMENZE. Text in Italian. 1998. q. ITL 70,000, USD 70; ITL 10,000 newsstand/cover (effective 2001). adv. **Document type:** *Magazine.* **Description:** Contains original articles and case reports on dementia and neuro-geriatric diseases with correlated matters addressed to Italian neurologists and geriatrics.
Published by: C I C Edizioni Internazionali s.r.l., Corso Trieste 42, Rome, RM 00198, Italy. TEL 39-06-8412673, FAX 39-06-8412688, info@gruppocic.it, 1160199510. adv.: B&W 1/8 page ITL 3,150,000, color page ITL 4,000,000; trim 210 x 290.

305.26 GBR
DIRECTORY FOR OLDER PEOPLE; a handbook of information & opportunities for the over-55s. Text in English. 1989. irreg., latest vol.2, 1992. USD 46.95 (effective 1999). **Document type:** *Directory.*
Published by: Prentice Hall - Harvester Wheatsheaf (Subsidiary of: Simon and Schuster International), Campus 400 Maylands Ave, Hemel Hempstead, Herts HP3 8LA, United Kingdom. TEL 44-1442-881900, FAX 44-1442-252544. Ed. Clare Grist. Pub. Rupert Knight. Circ: 1,400.

DIRECTORY OF AIDS FOR DISABLED AND ELDERLY PEOPLE. see *HANDICAPPED*

DIRECTORY OF FEDERAL AID FOR THE AGING. see *SOCIAL SERVICES AND WELFARE*

362.6 USA
HV1454.2.U6
DIRECTORY OF RETIREMENT FACILITIES. Text in English. 1985. a. USD 249 (effective 1999). **Document type:** *Directory.* **Description:** Lists more than 22,000 retirement facilities with contact names, addresses and telephone numbers, plus information about services and ownership.
Formerly: National Directory of Retirement Facilities (1053-6825)
Published by: H C I A Inc., 300 E Lombard St, Baltimore, MD 21202. TEL 800-568-3280, FAX 410-539-5220.

DRUGS & AGING. see *PHARMACY AND PHARMACOLOGY*

362.6 FRA ISSN 0243-0738
ECHO DE L'UNION. Text in French. 1978 (vol.32). m. FRF 60. adv. bk.rev. charts, illus, stat.
Former titles (until 1980): Echo; Echo des Vieux de France (0046-1083)
Published by: Union Nationale des Retraites et Personnes Agees (UNRPA), 50 rue Edouard Pailleron, Paris 75019, France. TEL 16-1-42-39-21-90.

305.2607 GBR ISSN 1352-8580
EDUCATION AND AGEING. Text in English. 1986. 3/yr. USD 55 to individuals; USD 260 to libraries (effective 2002). bk.rev. abstr, illus. back issues avail. *Refereed.* **Document type:** *Journal, Academic/Scholarly.* **Description:** Publishes scholarly articles which address the issues of learning in the later years, the teaching of gerontology, and the implications for education and educators of ageing society.
Formerly (until 1994): Journal of Educational Gerontology (0268-9987)
Related titles: Online - full text ed.
Indexed: AMED, AgeLine, Br.Educ.Ind., Cont.Pg.Educ., IBZ, Sociol.Abstr.
—BLDSC (3661.181600).
Published by: (Association for Education and Ageing), Triangle Journals Ltd., Attn: Roger Osborn-King, Publisher, PO Box 65, Wallingford, Oxfordshire OX10 0YG, United Kingdom. TEL 44-1491-838013, FAX 44-1491-834968, journals@triangle.co.uk, http://www.triangle.co.uk/eda. Eds. Jill Manthorpe, Pat Walker.

306.260715 USA ISSN 0360-1277
LC5201 CODEN: EDGEDA
EDUCATIONAL GERONTOLOGY; an international journal. Text in English. 1976. 10/yr. GBP 110, USD 182 to individuals; GBP 252, USD 416 to institutions (effective 2002). adv. bk.rev. abstr, bibl, charts. index. back issues avail.; reprint service avail. from PQC,SCH,PSC. *Refereed.* **Document type:** *Academic/Scholarly.* **Description:** Covers original advances in gerontology, adult education, and the social and behavioral sciences.
Related titles: Microform ed.: (from PQC); Online - full text ed.: ISSN 1521-0472 (from CatchWord Ltd., EBSCO Publishing, O C L C Online Computer Library Center, Inc., RoweCom Information Quest, Swets Blackwell, Institute for Scientific Information).
Indexed: A.D.& D., ASCA, Abstr.Soc.Geront., AgeLine, Biol.Abstr., C.I.J.E., CINAHL, Chic.Per.Ind., Cont.Pg.Educ., Curr.Cont., ERA, Educ.Admin.Abstr., Educ.Ind. (Jul.1983-), Educ.Tech.Abstr., Excerp.Med., Fam.Ind., Human Resour.Abstr., Intl.Bibl.Soc.Sci., Lang.& Lang.Behav.Abstr., Mult.Ed.Abstr., PsycInfo, Psychol.Abstr. (1976-), Res.High.Educ.Abstr., SOPODA, SSCI, Sage Fam.Stud.Abstr., Sage Pub.Admin.Abstr., Soc.Sci.Ind. (coverage dropped), Sociol.Abstr., Sociol.Educ.Abstr., Sp.Ed.Needs Abstr., Stud.Wom.Abstr., Tech.Educ.Abstr., Viol.& Abuse Abstr., e-psyche.
—BLDSC (3661.415000), CatchWord, GNLM, IDS, Infotrieve, ingenta, KNAW. **CCC.**
Published by: Taylor & Francis Ltd. (Subsidiary of: Taylor & Francis Group), 325 Chestnut St, Suite 800, Philadelphia, PA 19016. TEL 215-625-8900, FAX 215-625-2940, info@taylorandfrancis.com, http://www.taylorandfrancis.com/. Ed. D Barry Lumsden. Circ: 600. **Subscr. addr. in Europe:** Taylor & Francis Group, Journals Customer Service, Rankine Rd, Basingstoke, Hants RG24 8PR, United Kingdom. TEL 44-1256-813000, FAX 44-1256-479438, enquiry@tanf.co.uk, http://www.tandf.co.uk/journals.

EIJU SOGO BYOIN KIYO/EIJU GENERAL HOSPITAL. JOURNAL. see *MEDICAL SCIENCES—Experimental Medicine, Laboratory Technique*

306.38 USA
ELDER VOICES✱. Text in English. 1981. irreg.
Formerly: National Indian Council on Aging Quarterly
Indexed: AgeLine.
Published by: National Indian Council on Aging, Inc., 10501 Montgomery Blvd, N E, 210, Albuquerque, NM 87111-3846. TEL 505-888-3302.

ELDERCARE FORUM. see *BUSINESS AND ECONOMICS—Banking And Finance*

305.26 CAN ISSN 1480-7912
ELDERCARE QUARTERLY. Text in English. q. CND 13.62; USD 18 foreign. **Description:** Aimed primarily at the women and men facing the challenge of providing care to an elderly parent.
Address: 429 Danforth Ave, Ste 177, Toronto, ON M4K 1P1, Canada. TEL 416-463-8570, FAX 416-463-2282, robert.payne@canrem.com. Ed. Robert Payne.

612.67 GBR ISSN 1361-2700
ELDERLY CLIENT ADVISOR. Text in English. 1995. bi-m. GBP 195 domestic (effective Aug. 2001).
Related titles: Online - full content ed.
—BLDSC (3670.366300).
Published by: Ark Group Ltd, 4th Fl 200 Upper Richmond Rd, Zeeta House, London SW15 2SH, United Kingdom. TEL 44-20-8785-2700, FAX 44-20-8785-9373, info@ark.group.com, http://www.ecadviser.com. Ed. Nick Hussey.

612.67 USA ISSN 0891-9275
ELDERLY HEALTH SERVICES LETTER. Text in English. 1986. 12/yr. USD 197 (effective 2001). adv. charts. index. 10 p./no. 2 cols./p. back issues avail. **Document type:** *Newsletter, Trade.* **Description:** Covers issues pertaining to the management and administration of senior services programs, including financing strategies, staffing, and responding to the emergence of Medicare managed care and marketing.
Related titles: Online - full content ed.
—CCC.
Published by: Health Resources Publishing, 1913 Atlantic Ave, Ste F4, Manasquan, NJ 08736. TEL 732-292-1100, FAX 732-292-1111, hrp@healthrespubs.com, info@healthrespubs.com, http://www.healthrespubs.com. Ed. Jodi Kastel. Pub. Robert K Jenkins. Adv. contact Judy Granholm.

362.6 USA ISSN 1076-1616
K10 CODEN: JELAFJ
ETHICS, LAW, AND AGING REVIEW. Text in English. 1995. a., latest vol.7, 2001. USD 36 in United States to individuals; USD 66 for 2 yrs. in United States to individuals; USD 45 foreign to individuals; USD 77 for 2 yrs. foreign to individuals; USD 78 in United States to institutions; USD 133 for 2 yrs. in United States to institutions; USD 90 foreign to institutions; USD 153 for 2 yrs. foreign to institutions (effective 2001). adv. bk.rev., software rev., video rev., Website rev. illus. 250 p./no. reprints avail. *Refereed.* **Document type:** *Monographic series, Academic/Scholarly, Bibliography.* **Description:** Provides explanation and analysis of ethical and legal issues regarding aging and the aged for professionals who plan, administer, provide and finance health care and social services for older persons. Includes literature abstracts on selected current issues and a comprehensive bibliography..
Formerly: Journal of Ethics, Law, and Aging (1076-1616)
Indexed: AgeLine, CINAHL, Lang.& Lang.Behav.Abstr., P.A.I.S., SOPODA, Soc.Serv.Abstr., Soc.Work Res.& Abstr., Sociol.Abstr.
—BLDSC (3814.659270), Infotrieve, ingenta. **CCC.**
Published by: Springer Publishing Company, 536 Broadway, New York, NY 10012. TEL 212-431-4370, FAX 212-941-7842, springer@springerpub.com, http://www.springerpub.com. Ed. Marshall B Kapp. Pub. Ursula Springer. R&P Dorothy Kouwenberg. Adv. contact Bob Friel. B&W page USD 280; 5.5 x 8.5. Circ: 300 (paid).

362.6 GNQ ISSN 1023-6589
EUROLINK AGE BULLETIN. Text in English; Summaries in Dutch, Spanish, Italian. 1987. 3/yr. GBP 40 (effective 1999). bk.rev. *Refereed.* **Document type:** *Bulletin.*
Description: Promotes the interests of older people in the EU and ensures that issues on ageing are reflected in European wide policy and practice.
Related titles: French ed.: ISSN 1023-6570; German ed.: ISSN 1023-6562.
Published by: Eurolink Age, 1268 London Rd, London SW16 4ER, United Kingdom. TEL 44-181-765-7717, FAX 44-181-679-6727, eurolink@ace.org.uk, http://www.eurolinkage.org/euro/. Ed., R&P Liz Morall. Circ: 1,000.

618.97 DEU ISSN 1439-1147
CODEN: GEFOEV
EUROPEAN JOURNAL OF GERIATRICS. Text in English. 1991. bi-m. EUR 60 domestic; EUR 70 foreign (effective 2002). **Document type:** *Journal, Academic/Scholarly.*
Formerly (until 1999): Geriatrie Forschung (0940-6131)
Indexed: Excerp.Med. (1994-).
—EMDOCS, GNLM, KNAW.
Published by: Vincentz Verlag, Schiffgraben 43, Hannover 30175, Germany. TEL 49-511-9910000, FAX 49-511-9910099, info@vincentz.de, http://www.vincentz.de.

610.7365 DEU ISSN 0722-4737
EVANGELISCHE IMPULSE; Zeitschrift fuer die Arbeit mit alten Menschen. Text in German. 1979. 5/yr. DEM 31.90.
Published by: (Deutscher Evangelischer Verband duer Altenhilfe), Lithos Verlag GmbH, Hermannstr 5, Stuttgart 70178, Germany. TEL 0711-627023.

EXPERIENCE (CHICAGO). see *LAW*

EXPERIMENTAL AGING RESEARCH. see *PSYCHOLOGY*

612.67 USA ISSN 0531-5565
QP86 CODEN: EXGEAB
EXPERIMENTAL GERONTOLOGY. Text in English. 1965. 10/yr. NLG 316, EUR 143.39 in Europe to individuals; JPY 19,800 in Japan to individuals; USD 160 elsewhere to individuals; NLG 2,562, EUR 1,162.58 in Europe to institutions; JPY 160,900 in Japan to institutions; USD 1,300 elsewhere to institutions (effective 2001). adv. bk.rev. abstr. back issues avail. *Refereed.* **Document type:** *Academic/Scholarly.* **Description:** Publishes results of research in the processes of biological aging in plants, animals and humans from the molecular level to that of the entire organism.
Related titles: Microfilm ed.: (from PQC); Online - full text ed.: (from ingenta, Swets Blackwell, ScienceDirect, Institute for Scientific Information).
Indexed: ASCA, ASSIA, AgeLine, Biol.Abstr., Chem.Abstr., Chem.Indus.Notes, Chem.Titles, Curr.Adv.Biochem., Curr.Adv.Cell & Devel.Biol., Curr.Adv.Ecol.Sci., Curr.Cont., Excerp.Med., Forest.Abstr., Helminthol.Abstr., Hort.Abstr., INIS Atomind., Ind.Med. (1964-), Ind.Sci.Rev., Inpharma, Int.Abstr.Biol.Sci., Int.Nurs.Ind., NRN, Neurosci.Cit.Ind., Nutr.Abstr., Ornam.Hort., Pharm.&Out.News, Reac., Ref.Zh., Rev.Appl.Entomol., Rev.Arom.& Med.Plants, Rev.Plant Path., SSCI (coverage dropped), Sci.Cit.Ind.
—BLDSC (3839.340000), CASDDS, CISTI, EMDOCS, GNLM, IDS, ingenta, KNAW. **CCC.**
Published by: Elsevier Science, 655 Ave of the Americas, New York, NY 10010. TEL 212-989-5800, FAX 212-633-3990, http://www.elsevier.com/locate/expgero. Ed. Leonard Hayflick. Circ: 1,000. **Subscr. in Australasia and the Far East to:** Elsevier Science (Singapore) Pte Ltd, No.1 Temasek Ave, 17-01 Millenia Tower, Singapore 039192, Singapore. TEL 65-434-3727, FAX 65-337-2230; **Subscr. in Japan to:** Elsevier Science Inc - Japan Regional Office, 9-15 Higashi-Azabu 1-chome, Minato-ku, Tokyo 106-0044, Japan. TEL 81-3-5561-5033; **Subscr. outside the Americas to:** Elsevier Science BV, PO Box 211, Amsterdam 1000 AE, Netherlands. TEL 31-20-485-3757, nlinfo-f@elsevier.nl.

618.97 FRA ISSN 1163-0450
FACTS AND RESEARCH IN GERONTOLOGY. Text in English. 1992. a. price varies. **Document type:** *Monographic series, Academic/Scholarly.* **Description:** Provides a comprehensive collection of research on medical and psychological issues in the field of aging. Contributions are by European and American scholars.
Related titles: ♦ French ed.: Annee Gerontologique. ISSN 0990-2295.
—GNLM.
Published by: SERDI, 43 chemin del Prat, Auzeville-Tolosane 31320, France. FAX 33-5-61-751128, Springer@thorn.net, http://www.Liberty.com/Springer.html. Eds. Bruno Vellas, J L Albarede. **U.S. dist.:** Springer Publishing Company, 536 Broadway, New York, NY 10012.

612.67 FRA ISSN 1167-4911
FACTS AND RESEARCH IN GERONTOLOGY NEWSLETTER*. Text in English. 1992. m. adv. bk.rev. *Refereed.* **Document type:** *Newsletter.*
Related titles: French ed.: Lettre Mensuelle de l'Annee Gerontologique. ISSN 1146-0318. 1992; Spanish ed.: 1992; ♦ Supplement to: Annee Gerontologique. ISSN 0990-2295.
Indexed: Abstr.Anthropol.
—GNLM.
Published by: SERDI, 43 chemin del Prat, Auzeville-Tolosane 31320, France. FAX 33-5-61-751128. Ed. P Vellas. Adv. contact Rachel Mayne. Circ: 5,000.

305.42 USA
FIELD ADVOCATE. Text in English. m. USD 15. adv. **Document type:** *Bulletin.*
Published by: Older Women's League, 6660 11th St, N W, Ste 700, Washington, DC 20001-4512. TEL 202-783-6686. Ed. Lisa Lederer. Adv. contact Vicki O'Reilly. Circ: 20,000.

306.38 USA
FIFTY SOMETHING MAGAZINE. Text in English. 1990. bi-m. USD 10.95. adv. **Document type:** *Consumer.* **Description:** Provides information on travel, entertainment, finance, romance, health, nutrition, fitness and special events for the fifty-or-over reader. Includes feature stories on individuals, locally and nationally, and fiction.
Published by: Media Trends Publications, 1168 S Beachview Rd, Willoughby, OH 44094-7014. TEL 216-951-2468. Ed., R&P Linda L Lindeman. Adv. contact Kitty Kadas. Circ: 25,000.

FIT UND FUENFZIG. see *PHYSICAL FITNESS AND HYGIENE*

FOCUS: LIBRARY SERVICE TO OLDER ADULTS, PEOPLE WITH DISABILITIES. see *LIBRARY AND INFORMATION SCIENCES*

610.736 USA ISSN 0892-7103
FOCUS ON GERIATRIC CARE AND REHABILITATION. Text in English. 1987. 10/yr. USD 99; USD 12 newsstand/cover (effective 2001). **Document type:** *Newsletter.* **Description:** Covers common geriatric problems and offers hands-on tips and strategies that can be put to immediate use to improve the well-being of geriatric patients.
Related titles: Online - full text ed.: (from ProQuest Information & Learning).
Indexed: CINAHL.
—BLDSC (3964.215680). **CCC.**
Published by: Aspen Publishers, Inc., 200 Orchard Ridge Dr, Ste 200, Gaithersburg, MD 20878. TEL 301-417-7500, 800-638-8437, FAX 301-695-7931, customer.service@aspenpubl.com, http://www.aspenpub.com. Ed. Joan K Glickstein. **Dist. by:** Aspen Publishers Inc., Distribution Center, 7201 McKinney Circle, Frederick, MD 21701. TEL 301-698-7100, FAX 301-417-7550.

FORMULARY GERIATRICS. see *PHARMACY AND PHARMACOLOGY*

612.67 CAN ISSN 1188-181X
G R C NEWS. Text in English. 1990. q. free per issue. bk.rev. **Document type:** *Newsletter, Academic/Scholarly.* **Description:** Publishes news about the Centre and Canadian gerontological information.
Formerly: G R C Information Bulletin
Published by: Simon Fraser University, Gerontology Research Centre, 515 W Hastings St, Vancouver, BC V6B 5K3, Canada. TEL 604-291-5062, FAX 604-291-5066, gero@sfu.ca, http://harbour.sfu.ca/gero/grcnews/. Ed. Susannah Tredwell. Circ: 2,100.

306.38 USA ISSN 0738-7806
HQ1060 CODEN: GENREC
GENERATIONS (SAN FRANCISCO). Text in English. 1976. q. USD 38 (effective 2001). adv. bk.rev. illus. reprints avail. *Refereed.* **Description:** Each issue covers a specific topic in the field of aging with emphasis on practice, research and policy.
Related titles: Microform ed.: (from PQC); Online - full text ed.: (from H. W. Wilson, ProQuest Information & Learning, Gale Group, Institute for Scientific Information).
Indexed: Abstr.Anthropol., Abstr.Soc.Geront., AgeLine, Bk.Rev.Ind. (1984-), C.I.J.E., CINAHL, Child.Bk.Rev.Ind. (1984-), Curr.Cont., Human Resour.Abstr., Lang.& Lang.Behav.Abstr., P.A.I.S., Psychol.Abstr., Rel.Ind.One, Rel.Ind.Two, SOPODA, SSCI, Sage Fam.Stud.Abstr., Soc.Sci.Ind. (Jan.1994-), Soc.Serv.Abstr., Sociol.Abstr.
—BLDSC (4111.755300), IDS, ingenta.
Published by: American Society on Aging, 833 Market St, Ste 511, San Francisco, CA 94103-1824. TEL 415-974-9600, FAX 415-974-0300, info@asa.asaging.org, http://www.asaging.org. Ed. Mary Johnson. R&P Audrey Wong. Adv. contacts Julie Bennett, Susan Markey. page USD 1,225; trim 7.25 x 10. Circ: 10,000.

612.67 POL
GERENTOLOGIA POLSKA. Text in Polish. quadrennial. PLZ 28 (effective 2000).
Published by: (Polskie Towarzystwo Gerontologiczne), Medycyna Praktyczna, Ul Skawinska 8, Krakow 31066, Poland. TEL 48-12-4305520, FAX 48-12-4305536, listy@mp.pl, http://mp.pl/czasop.htm. Ed. Jozef Kocemba.

610.7365 AUS ISSN 1032-4410
GERIACTION*. Text in English. 1970. q. AUD 65. adv. bk.rev. back issues avail.
Indexed: CINAHL.
—BLDSC (4161.673000).
Published by: Geriaction Inc., 282 Victoria Ave, Chatswood, NSW 2067, Australia. FAX 02-411-6618. Ed. Raelene Allen. Circ: 1,500.

618.97 ITA ISSN 1122-5807
GERIATRIA. Text in Italian. 1989. bi-m. ITL 50,000 (effective 1996). bk.rev.
—BLDSC (4161.678000), EMDOCS, GNLM.
Published by: (Societa Italiana Geriatri Ospedalieri), Casa Editrice Scientifica Internazionale Periodici s.a.s., Via Cremona, 19, Rome, RM 00161, Italy. TEL 39-6-44290783, FAX 39-6-44241-598.

618.97 ITA ISSN 1121-8460
GERIATRIC AND MEDICAL INTELLIGENCE/MEDICINA E ANZIANI. Text in Italian; Abstracts in English. 1992. 2/yr. EUR 26 in Europe to individuals; USD 39 elsewhere to individuals; EUR 36 in Europe to institutions; USD 49 elsewhere to institutions (effective 2001). abstr. charts, illus, bibl, stat. 64 p./no. back issues avail.; reprints avail. *Refereed.* **Document type:** *Journal, Academic/Scholarly.*
—CISTI.
Published by: Wichtig Editore s.r.l., Via Friuli, 72, Milan, MI 20135, Italy. TEL 39-02-55195443, FAX 39-02-55195971, info@wichtig-publisher.com. Ed. Dr. Dario Cova. Pub. Dr. Diego Brancaccio. R&P Lucia Steele. Adv. contact Nella Bini. Circ: 2,050 (controlled); 2,000 (paid).

610.7365 362.6 USA ISSN 1524-2870
GERIATRIC CARE. Text in English. 1968. m. USD 87.50 (effective 2000); minimum sets of 25 subscr required. bk.rev. illus. **Document type:** *Newsletter.* **Description:** Includes articles and discussion questions written especially for those who work directly with the aged and emphasizes the psychosocial side of resident care.
Published by: Eymann Publications, Inc, PO Box 3577, Reno, NV 89505-3577. TEL 775-358-1554, FAX 775-358-1476, eymann@care4elders.com, http://www.care4elders.com. Ed. Maureen Eng. Pub. Katie Eymann Pace. Circ: 30,000.

618.97 USA ISSN 0891-2173
RA981.A2
GERIATRIC LENGTH OF STAY BY DIAGNOSIS AND OPERATION, UNITED STATES. Text in English. 1964. a. USD 295 (effective 1999). stat. back issues avail.
Related titles: Diskette ed.; Magnetic Tape ed.; Microfiche ed.
Indexed: SRI.
Published by: H C I A Inc., 300 E Lombard St, Baltimore, MD 21202. TEL 800-568-3280, FAX 410-539-5220.

618.97 GBR ISSN 0268-201X
GERIATRIC MEDICINE; midlife and beyond. Text in English. 1971. m. GBP 60 domestic; GBP 107 foreign (effective 2000). adv. bk.rev., video rev. charts, illus, stat. back issues avail. *Refereed.* **Document type:** *Academic/Scholarly, Bibliography, Trade.* **Description:** Covers new developments around the world in the study of disease conditions of midlife and beyond and the prevention and management of illness.

G

G

Incorporates (1989-1997): Care of the Elderly (0955-4262); Former titles (until 1985): Geriatrics for GP's (0267-8675); (until 1984): Geriatric Medicine (0143-3628); (until 1979): Modern Geriatrics (0026-7783)
Related titles: E-mail ed.; Fax ed.
Indexed: Brit.Nur.Ind.
—BLDSC (4161.690000), CISTI, GNLM, Infotrieve. **CCC.**
Published by: Medpress (Subsidiary of: Inside Communications Ltd.), 8th Fl, Tubs Hill House, London Rd, Sevenoaks, Kent TN13 1BL, United Kingdom. TEL 44-1732-464190, FAX 44-1732-740772, peter_sayer@mrn.co.uk, http://www.docnet.org.uk. Ed. Sue Lyon. Adv. contact Peter Sayer. Circ: 500 (paid); 20,000 (controlled).

610.7365 USA ISSN 0197-4572
RC954
GERIATRIC NURSING. Text in English. 1980. bi-m. USD 47 domestic to individuals; USD 74 foreign to individuals; USD 90 domestic to institutions; USD 117 foreign to institutions; USD 29 domestic to students; USD 53 foreign to students; USD 20 newsstand/cover (effective 2001). adv. bk.rev. charts, illus, tr.lit. index. reprint service avail. from PQC. *Refereed.*
Related titles: Microform ed.: (from PQC); Online - full text ed.: (from Ovid Technologies, Inc., EBSCO Publishing, IDEAL Online Library, Institute for Scientific Information, RoweCom Information Quest).
Indexed: AMED, ASCA, Abstr.Soc.Geront., AgeLine, Brit.Nur.Ind., CINAHL, Curr.Adv.Ecol.Sci., Curr.Cont., Hosp.Lit.Ind., I.P.A., Ind.Med. (coverage dropped), Int.Nurs.Ind., NRN, Nurs.Abstr., Psychol.Abstr., SSCI.
—BLDSC (4161.710000), GNLM, IDS, ingenta. **CCC.**
Published by: (National Gerontological Nursing Association), Mosby Year, Inc. (Subsidiary of: Harcourt General, Inc.), Mosby, MO 63146-3318. TEL 314-872-8370, 800-325-4177, FAX 314-432-1380, http://www.mosby.com/gerinurs, http://www.mosby.com/periodicals. Ed. Priscilla R Ebersole. Adv. contact Lynn Palazzolo. B&W page USD 1,480, color page USD 2,520; trim 10.88 x 8.13. Circ: 11,622.

610.7365 USA
▼ **GERIATRIC TIMES**; an interdisciplinary approach to healthy aging. Text in English. 2000. bi-m. adv. **Document type:** *Magazine, Consumer, Trade.* **Description:** Focuses on all aspects of geriatric healthcare and targets the full spectrum of healthcare providers in both independent and institutionalized settings.
Published by: C M E Inc., 2801 McGaw Ave, Irvine, CA 92614-5835. TEL 949-250-1008, 800-933-2632, FAX 949-250-0445, sales.manager@cmeinc.com, http://www.geriatrictimes.com. Ed. Dr. John L Schwartz.

618.97 USA ISSN 0016-867X
RC952.A1 CODEN: GERTAZ
GERIATRICS; medicine for midlife and beyond. Text in English. 1946. m., latest vol.56. USD 60 United States & Possessions; USD 85 in Canada & Mexico; USD 120 elsewhere; USD 6.50 newsstand/cover United States & Possessions (effective 2001). adv. bk.rev. abstr, bibl, charts, illus. Index. reprints avail. *Refereed.* **Document type:** *Trade.* **Description:** Examines the diagnosis and treatment of diseases and conditions associated with aging.
Related titles: Microform ed.; Online - full text ed.: (from Gale Group, ProQuest Information & Learning, Northern Light Technology, Inc., H. W. Wilson, Factiva, Institute for Scientific Information).
Indexed: AIM, AMED, ASCA, Abstr.Anthropol., Abstr.Soc.Geront., AgeLine, Agri.& Environ.Biotech.Abstr. (coverage dropped), Biol.Abstr., CINAHL, Chem.Abstr., Curr.Adv.Ecol.Sci., Curr.Cont., Dent.Ind., Derwent Biotech.Abstr., Environ.Sci.Poll.Mgmt., Excerp.Med., Gen.Sci.Ind. (Jun.1984-), Hosp.Lit.Ind., INIS Atomind., I.P.A., Ind.Med. (1946-), Ind.Sci.Rev., Inpharma, Int.Nurs.Ind., NRN, Nutr.Abstr., Pharm.&Out.News, Pollut.Abstr., Psychol.Abstr., Reac., Rev.Plant Path., Risk Abstr., SSCI (coverage dropped), Saf.Sci.Abstr., Sci.Cit.Ind.
—BLDSC (4161.800000), CASDDS, CISTI, GNLM, IDS, ingenta, KNAW. **CCC.**
Published by: Advanstar Communications Inc., 201 E Sandpointe Ave Ste 600, Santa Ana, CA 92707. TEL 440-891-2767, FAX 440-891-2683, geriatrics@advanstar.com, http://www.geri.com; http://www.modernmedicine.com/geri; http://www.advanstar.com. Ed. Alice V Luddington. Pub. Jennifer J Day. Circ: 55,571.

618.97 AUS ISSN 1444-1586
▼ **GERIATRICS & GERONTOLOGY INTERNATIONAL.** Text in English. 2001. q. (Launched with two issues published in the latter half of 2001 and will continue thereafter as a quarterly publication.). AUD 685 domestic; AUD 623 in New Zealand; JPY 45,650 in Japan; USD 380 elsewhere; AUD 754 domestic print & online eds.; AUD 686 in New Zealand print & online eds.; USD 418 elsewhere print & online eds. (effective 2001). adv. **Document type:** *Journal, Academic/Scholarly.*
Related titles: ♦ Online - full text ed.: Geriatrics & Gerontology International Online.
Published by: Blackwell Science Asia Pty Ltd, PO Box 378, Carlton South, VIC 3053, Australia. TEL 61-3-9347-0300, FAX 61-3-9347-5001, info@blacksci-asia.com.au, http://www.blacksci.co.uk/australi.

618.97 AUS
▼ **GERIATRICS & GERONTOLOGY INTERNATIONAL ONLINE.** Text in English. 2001. q. AUD 154 in Australia to individuals; AUD 140 in New Zealand to individuals; USD 81 elsewhere to individuals; AUD 341 in Australia to institutions; AUD 310 in New Zealand to institutions; JPY 22,140 in Japan to institutions; USD 171 elsewhere to institutions (effective 2002). **Document type:** *Academic/Scholarly.* **Description:** Covers the growing importance of the subject area in developed economies and its particular significance to a country like Japan with a large aging population.
Media: Online - full text (from Swets Blackwell). **Related titles:** ♦ Print ed.: Geriatrics & Gerontology International. ISSN 1444-1586.
Published by: Blackwell Science Asia Pty Ltd, PO Box 378, Carlton South, VIC 3053, Australia. TEL 61-3-9347-0300, FAX 61-3-9347-3016, info@blacksci-asia.com.au, http://www.blacksci.co.uk/australi.

618.97 CAN ISSN 1496-3892
GERIATRICS TODAY. Text in English. q. USD 34 to individuals; USD 64 to institutions (effective 2001). bk.rev. 45 p./no. back issues avail. *Refereed.* **Document type:** *Journal, Abstract/Index, Academic/Scholarly.* **Description:** Aims to provide current and optimal medical care to the vital, enlarging, aging population.
Formerly (until Jan. 2001): Mature Medicine Canada (1480-5537)
Related titles: Online - full text ed.: (from EBSCO Publishing).
—BLDSC (4161.870000).
Published by: (Canadian Geriatiac Society USA), F D Communications Inc., 5863 Leslie St., Box 1002, Toronto, ON M2H 1J8, Canada. TEL 416-224-5055, FAX 416-224-5455, medicine@sympatico.ca. Eds. Dr. Jean Triscott, Dr. William B Dalziel. Pub., Adv. contact Fran Deitel. R&P Dr. Mervyn Deitel TEL 416-750-9608. Circ: 18,000.

612.67 DEU ISSN 1439-1139
GERIATRIE JOURNAL; der aeltere Patient in Praxis und Klinik. Text in German. m. EUR 68 domestic; EUR 70 foreign (effective 2002). **Document type:** *Journal, Academic/Scholarly.*
Published by: Vincentz Verlag, Schiffgraben 43, Hannover 30175, Germany. TEL 49-511-9910000, FAX 49-511-9910099, info@vincentz.de, http://www.vincentz.de.

612.67 DEU ISSN 0936-7152
GERIATRIE PRAXIS. Text in German. 1989. m. DEM 69; DEM 42 to students. adv. **Document type:** *Academic/Scholarly.*
Incorporates (1993-1998): Home Care (0944-1360)
—CISTI, GNLM.
Published by: M M V Medien und Medizin Verlagsgesellschaft mbH Muenchen, St Alban Ring 248, PO Box 565, Basel 4020, Switzerland. TEL 41-61-3118700, FAX 41-61-3118732, jutta.brinkmann@bertelsmann.de, http://www.mmw.de. Ed. Brigitte Zoeller. Adv. contact Peter Esser. **Subscr. to:** MMV Subscription Service, Postfach 2125, Neu-Isenburg 63243, Germany. TEL 49-6102-506176, FAX 49-6102-506177.

612.67 ESP ISSN 0212-9744
CODEN: GERIE5
GERIATRIKA; revista iberoamericana de geriatria y gerontologia. Text in Spanish. 1984. bi-m. ESP 8,500 domestic; USD 85 in Europe; USD 105 elsewhere (effective 2001). adv. charts. *Refereed.* **Document type:** *Journal, Academic/Scholarly.* **Description:** Publishes original articles on geriatrics, gerontology, and clinical geriatrics.
Indexed: Excerp.Med.
—BLDSC (4161.911000), CINDOC, CISTI, EMDOCS, GNLM, KNAW.
Published by: (Sociedad Espanola de Geriatria y Gerontologia), Alpe Editores S.A., Pedro Rico, 27, Madrid 28029, Spain. TEL 34-91-733-8811, FAX 34-91-315-9652, alpeeditores@sistelcom.com. Ed. Dr. Jose Garay Lillo. Pub. Angeles Alvarez Sanchez. Adv. contact Ana Jurado. color page ESP 160,000; 280 x 210. Circ: 7,000 (controlled).

618.97 CAN ISSN 1205-9439
GERISOURCE LETTER; clinical tips and resources for geriatric long term care. Text in English. 1996. m. USD 36. bk.rev. illus. reprints avail.
Published by: Gerisource Consulting, 1928 Nelson St, Ste. 106, Vancouver, BC V6G 1N2, Canada. Ed. Christine Abney.

612.67 ESP ISSN 1134-928X
GEROKOMOS. Text in Spanish. 199?. q. ESP 7,010 to individuals; ESP 10,100 to institutions; ESP 5,600 to students (effective 2001). adv. back issues avail.; reprints avail. *Refereed.* **Document type:** *Academic/Scholarly.*
Related titles: Online - full text ed.
Published by: (Sociedad Espanola de Enfermeria Geriatrica y Gerontologica), Ediciones Doyma S.A., Traversa de Gracia, 17-21, Barcelona 08021, Spain. TEL 34-93-200-0711, gk@doyma.es, doyma@doyma.es, http://www.doyma.es/gk. Ed. Javier J Soldevilla Agreda. R&P Monica Barnes. Adv. contact Jose Antonio Hernandez. B&W page ESP 122,000, color page ESP 152,000; 280 x 210.

362.6 306.38 610.7365 NLD ISSN 1389-143X
▼ **GERON**; tijdschrift ouder worden en maatsarry. Text in Dutch. 1999. q. NLG 70 domestic; EUR 31.80 foreign (effective 2001). bk.rev. illus, stat. back issues avail. *Refereed.* **Document type:** *Journal, Academic/Scholarly.* **Description:** Offers news and advice for persons working with the elderly, whether through caring for them or research. Discusses issues about aging and working with this population.
Published by: Uitgeverij Coutinho, Slochterenlaan 7, Bussum 1405 AL, Netherlands. TEL 31-35-694-9991, FAX 31-35-694-7165, info@coutinho.nl, http://www.coutinho.nl. Ed., R&P Llse Karman. Pub. Dick Coutinho. Circ: 500.

306.38 DNK ISSN 0900-114X
GERONTOLOGI OG SAMFUND; nyt om aldring, alderdom og aeldrebefolkning. Text in Danish. 1985. q. DKK 256.25; DKK 308 foreign (effective 2000). bk.rev. illus. **Document type:** *Consumer.*
Published by: Dansk Gerontologisk Selskab, c/o Victor Hansen International Boghandel, M P Bruunsgade 45, Aarhus C 8000, Denmark. TEL 45-86-12-24-00, FAX 45-86-12-23-47. Ed. Christine Swane. Circ: 1,800.

618.97 BRA ISSN 0104-1258
GERONTOLOGIA. Text in Portuguese. 1992. q. adv. bk.rev. back issues avail. *Refereed.* **Document type:** *Academic/Scholarly.*
Related titles: Online - full text ed.
Published by: (Sociedade Brasileira de Geriatria e Gerontologia), Lemos Editorial & Graficos Ltda., Rua Rui Barbosa, 70, B Vista, Sao Paulo, SP 01326-010, Brazil. TEL 55-11-251-4300, FAX 55-11-251-4300, lemospl@netpoint.com.br, http://www.lemos.com.br. Ed. Dr. Wilson Jacob Filho. Adv. contact Paulo Lemos. Circ: 3,000 (controlled).

305.26 USA
GERONTOLOGICAL SOCIETY. MONOGRAPHS. Text in English. irreg. adv. reprint service avail. from PQC. **Document type:** *Academic/Scholarly.*
Published by: Gerontological Society of America, 1030 15th, N W, Ste 250, Washington, DC 20005-1503. TEL 202-842-1275, FAX 202-842-1150. Ed., Adv. contact Heather Worley. R&P Shirley Brown.

618.97 FRA ISSN 0016-9005
GERONTOLOGIE. Text in French. 1970. q. FRF 342.80; FRF 350 foreign (effective 1998). adv. bk.rev.
—GNLM.
Address: 14 passage du Guesclin, Paris 75015, France. TEL 33-1-47346463, FAX 33-1-47346463. Circ: 7,500.

618.97 FRA ISSN 0990-5669
GERONTOLOGIE PRATIQUE. Text in French. 1988. m. (10/yr.). EUR 39 domestic to individuals; EUR 53 foreign to individuals; EUR 27 domestic to libraries; EUR 42 foreign to libraries (effective 2002). **Document type:** *Newspaper.*

Published by: L E N Medical, 15 rue des Sablons, Paris 75116, France. TEL 33-1-47553131, FAX 33-1-47553132, lenmed@club-internet.fr, http://www.webmedguide.com. Ed. Dr. C Verny.

362.6 USA ISSN 0016-9013
HQ1060 CODEN: GRNTA3
THE GERONTOLOGIST. Text in English. 1961. bi-m. USD 93 to individuals; USD 103 foreign to individuals; USD 175 to institutions; USD 185 foreign to institutions (effective 2001). adv. bk.rev. bibl, charts, illus. index. reprint service avail. from PQC. *Refereed.* **Document type:** *Academic/Scholarly.* **Description:** Covers original research academics and gerontologists; using on two or three topics per issue. Includes program and abstracts for the annual meeting of the society.
Related titles: Microfilm ed.: (from PQC); Online - full text ed.: (from Northern Light Technology, Inc., ProQuest Information & Learning, Gale Group, HighWire Pr., Factiva, Institute for Scientific Information); Supplement: Annual Meeting Program.
Indexed: ASCA, ASSIA, Abstr.Health Care Manage.Stud., Abstr.Soc.Geront., Acad.Ind., AgeLine, Arts & Hum.Cit.Ind. (coverage dropped), Behav.Med.Abstr., Biol.Abstr., Brit.Nur.Ind., CERDIC, C.I.J.E., CINAHL, Chem.Abstr., Curr.Cont., Dok.Arbeitsmed., Ergon.Abstr., Excerp.Med., Fam.Ind., Gen.Sci.Ind. (Jul.1997-), Hlth.Ind., Hosp.Lit.Ind., I.P.A., Ind.Med. (1961-), Int.Nurs.Ind., Intl.Bibl.Soc.Sci., Mid.East: Abstr.& Ind., NRN, Neurosci.Cit.Ind., Past.Care & Couns.Abstr., PsycInfo, Psychol.Abstr. (1961-), Risk Abstr., SSCI, Sage Fam.Stud.Abstr., Sage Pub.Admin.Abstr., Sage Urb.Stud.Abstr., Soc.Sci.Ind. (Jun.1982-), Soc.Work Res.& Abstr., e-psyche.
—BLDSC (4162.300000), GNLM, IDS, ingenta, KNAW, Linda Hall. **CCC.**
Published by: Gerontological Society of America, 1030 15th St, N W, Ste 250, Washington, DC 20005-1503. TEL 202-842-1275, FAX 202-842-1150, jcampi@geron.org, hworley@geron.org; gerontologist@maxwell.syr.edu, http://gerontologist.gerontologyjournals.org/, http://www.geron.org. Ed. Laurence Branch. R&P Shirley Brown. adv.: B&W page USD 780, color page USD 1,650. Circ: 7,200 (paid). **Subscr. to:** PO Box 79151, Baltimore, MD 21279. **Co-sponsor:** Syracuse University, Maxwell School of Citizenship and Public Affairs, Center for Policy Research.

612.67 ISR ISSN 0334-2360
GERONTOLOGY. Text in Hebrew; Summaries in English. 1974. q. USD 80 (effective 1998). bk.rev. *Refereed.* **Document type:** *Academic/Scholarly.* **Description:** Publishes research covering biological, medical, social science and social work aspects of gerontology.
Related titles: Online - full text ed.: (from Northern Light Technology, Inc.).
Indexed: AgeLine, Curr.Cont. (coverage dropped), Ind.Heb.Per. (1977-), e-psyche.
Published by: Israel Gerontological Society, 8 Habonim St, Ramat Gan 52462, Israel. TEL 972-3-7513620, FAX 972-3-5756748. Ed. Dr. Hava Golander. Circ: 1,200.

612.67 CHE ISSN 0304-324X
CODEN: GERNDJ
GERONTOLOGY; international journal of experimental and clinical gerontology. Text in English. 1957. bi-m. CHF 870, EUR 621.80 in Europe to institutions; CHF 887.40, USD 677 elsewhere to institutions (effective 2002). adv. bk.rev. index. back issues avail. *Refereed.* **Document type:** *Journal, Academic/Scholarly.* **Description:** Includes experimental contributions from diverse medical, biological and behavioral disciplines, covering all aspects of aging in man and animals.
Formed by the 1976 merger of: Gerontologia (0016-898X); Gerontologia Clinica (0016-8998)
Related titles: Microfilm ed.; Online - full text ed.: ISSN 1423-0003. CHF 58 to institutions with print edition; EUR 42, USD 45 to institutions with print edityion (effective 2002) (from Northern Light Technology, Inc., EBSCO Publishing, O C L C Online Computer Library Center, Inc., RoweCom Information Quest, ProQuest Information & Learning, Swets Blackwell, Institute for Scientific Information).
Indexed: Biol.Abstr., Chem.Abstr., Chem.Indus.Notes, Chem.Titles, Curr.Adv.Ecol.Sci., Curr.Cont., Dent.Ind., Environ.Sci.Poll.Mgmt., Excerp.Med., Helminthol.Abstr., Ind.Med. (1976-), Ind.Sci.Rev., Inpharma, Int.Nurs.Ind., Med.& Surg.Dermat., Mid.East: Abstr.& Ind., NRN, Neurosci.Cit.Ind., Nutr.Abstr., Pharm.&Out.News, Pollut.Abstr., PsycInfo, Psychol.Abstr. (1990-), Reac., Risk Abstr., SSCI (coverage dropped), Saf.Sci.Abstr., Sci.Cit.Ind.
—BLDSC (4162.325000), CASDDS, CISTI, EMDOCS, GNLM, IDS, Infotrieve, ingenta, KNAW. **CCC.**
Published by: S. Karger AG, Allschwilerstr 10, PO Box, Basel 4009, Switzerland. TEL 41-61-306-1111, FAX 41-61-306-1234, karger@karger.ch, http://www.online.karger.com/journals/ger, http://www.karger.com. Ed. W Meier Ruge. adv.: page USD 1,185. Circ: 1,250.

362.6 USA ISSN 0270-1960
RC952.5
GERONTOLOGY & GERIATRICS EDUCATION. Text in English. 1980. q. USD 75 to individuals; USD 101 in Canada to individuals; USD 109 elsewhere to individuals; USD 200 to institutions; USD 270 in Canada to institutions; USD 290 elsewhere to institutions; USD 385 to libraries; USD 520 in Canada to libraries; USD 558 elsewhere to libraries (effective Aug. 2001). adv. bk.rev. charts, illus, stat. index. back issues avail.; reprint service avail. from HAW,SCH,PSC. *Refereed.* **Document type:** *Journal, Academic/Scholarly.* **Description:** Provides practical curriculum information for educators, trainers, and supervisors in the aging field.
Related titles: Microfiche ed.: (from PQC); Microform ed.
Indexed: Abstr.Anthropol., Abstr.Soc.Geront., AgeLine, CINAHL, Chicago Psychoanal.Lit.Ind., Cont.Pg.Educ., Dent.Ind., ERA, Educ.Admin.Abstr., Educ.Tech.Abstr., Excerp.Med., Fam.Ind., IBZ, IMFL, Ind.Med. (coverage dropped), Lang.& Lang.Behav.Abstr., Mult.Ed.Abstr., PSI, PsycInfo, Psychol.Abstr. (1984-), Ref.Zh., SOPODA, Sage Fam.Stud.Abstr., Soc.Serv.Abstr., Sociol.Abstr., Stud.Wom.Abstr., Tech.Educ.Abstr., Viol.& Abuse Abstr., e-psyche.
—BLDSC (4162.360000), GNLM, Haworth, ingenta.
Published by: Haworth Press, Inc., 10 Alice St, Binghamton, NY 13904-1580. TEL 607-722-5857, 800-429-6784, FAX 607-722-6362, 800-895-0582, getinfo@haworthpressinc.com, http://www.haworthpress.com/journals/journallist.asp. Ed. Pearl M. Mosher-Ashley. Pub. William Cohen. R&P Ruthann Heath TEL 607-723-5857 ext 316. Adv. contact Jackie Blakeslee TEL 607-722-5857 ext 346. B&W page USD 315, color page USD 550; trim 6 x 8.5. Circ: 500.

362.6 USA
GERONTOLOGY NEWS. Text in English. 1978. m. USD 50 domestic to non-members; USD 75 foreign to non-members (effective 2001). adv. reprint service avail. from PQC. **Document type:** *Newsletter.* **Description:** Reports on policy issues, fellowships and grants in the field of aging.
Incorporates (in 1990): Gerontology News. Grants - Fellowships - Jobs
Related titles: Online - full text ed.; ♦ Includes: Gerontology News. Conference Calendar.
Published by: Gerontological Society of America, 1030 15th St, N W, Ste 250, Washington, DC 20005-1503. TEL 202-842-1275, FAX 202-842-1150, sbrown@geron.org, http://www.geron.org/newsletter/news.html. R&P Shirley Brown. adv.: page USD 670. Circ: 5,200.

362.6 USA
GERONTOLOGY NEWS. CONFERENCE CALENDAR. Text in English. s-a. reprint service avail. from PQC. **Document type:** *Newsletter.*
Related titles: ♦ Issued with: Gerontology News.
Published by: Gerontological Society of America, 1030 15th St, N W, Ste 250, Washington, DC 20005-1503. TEL 202-842-1275, FAX 202-842-1150. Ed. Linda Krogh Harootyan. Circ: 6,500.

618.97 USA
GERONTOLOGY SPECIAL INTEREST SECTION QUARTERLY. Text in English. 1989. q. USD 20 (effective 1999). **Document type:** *Newsletter.*
Formerly (until 199?): Gerontology Special Interest Section Newsletter (0279-4101); Supersedes in part: American Occupational Therapy Association. Physical Disabilities Specialty Section. Newsletter (0194-6366)
Published by: American Occupational Therapy Association, Inc., 4720 Montgomery Lane, Bethesda, MD 20814-3425. TEL 301-652-2682, FAX 301-652-7711.

618.97 ITA ISSN 0017-0305
CODEN: GIGEAU
GIORNALE DI GERONTOLOGIA. Text in Italian; Summaries in English. 1952. m. ITL 220,000; ITL 300,000 foreign (effective 2001). adv. bk.rev. bibl, charts, illus. index. **Description:** Research papers on the science of aging and the care of the aging.
Indexed: Biol.Abstr., Chem.Abstr., Excerp.Med., Helminthol.Abstr., Ind.Med. (coverage dropped), Nutr.Abstr., Ref.Zh.
—BLDSC (4178.060000), CASDDS, CISTI, EMDOCS, GNLM, KNAW.
Published by: (Societa Italiana di Gerontologia e Geriatria), Pacini Editore, Via Alessandro Gherardesca, 1, Ospedaletto, PI 56121, Italy. TEL 39-050-313011, FAX 39-050-3130300, http://www.pacinieditore.it. Circ: 5,000.

306.38 DEU ISSN 0178-5109
GRAUER PANTHER. Text in German. 1983. m. DEM 30; DEM 3 newsstand/cover. adv. bk.rev. **Document type:** *Bulletin.*
Published by: (Senioren-Schutz-Bund "Graue Panther" e.V.), Klartext Verlag GmbH, Dickmannstr 2-4, Essen 45143, Germany. TEL 49-201-8620628, FAX 49-201-8620622. Circ: 10,000.

618.97 362.6 USA ISSN 1041-2352
GREAT IDEAS FOR LONG-TERM CARE. Text in English. m. USD 46 (effective 2000). illus. **Document type:** *Newsletter, Consumer.* **Description:** Provides ideas to save time and money, to serve residents better, and make operations in long-term care facilities run smoothly.
Formerly: Great Ideas Newsletter
Published by: Eymann Publications, Inc, PO Box 3577, Reno, NV 89505-3577. TEL 775-358-1554, FAX 775-358-1476, www.care4elders.com, eymann@care4elders.com, http://www.care4elders.com. Ed. Maureen Eng. Pub. Katie Eymann Pace. Circ: 1,000.

GROWTH, DEVELOPMENT & AGING. see *BIOLOGY*

610.7365 BRA ISSN 1414-1922
GUIA DE FORNECEDORES HOSPITALARES. Text in Portuguese. 1994. m. BRL 48, USD 48 (effective 1999). adv. back issues avail. **Document type:** *Consumer.* **Description:** Presents articles of interest to hospital workers. covers hospital instruments, medical sciences in general and products and equipment.
Related titles: Online - full text ed.
Published by: Editora Guia de Fornecedores Ltda., Av Doutor Adolfo Pinto, 109 Andar 4, B Funda, Sao Paulo, SP 01156-050, Brazil. TEL 55-11-3824-9655, FAX 55-11-826-9789, http://www.editoraguia.com.br. Ed. Eduardo David Airton. Adv. contact Camila Nunes. page USD 7,445; trim 14.1875 x 21.8333. Circ: 18,000.

618.97 CHN
GUOWAI YIXUE (LAONAN YIXUE FENCE)/FOREIGN MEDICAL SCIENCES (GERONTOLOGY). Text in Chinese. bi-m. USD 12; USD 2 newsstand/cover (effective 2001). **Document type:** *Academic/Scholarly.*
Published by: China International Book Trading Corp/Zhongguo Guoji Tushu Maoyi Zonggongsi cibtc@mail.cibtc.com.cn, http://www.cibtc.com.cn. **Dist. by:** 35, Chegongzhuang Xilu, Haidian District, Beijing 100044, China.

306.38 ISR
HA-GIL HE-HADASH. Text in Hebrew. 1980. q. free per issue. bk.rev. **Description:** Bulletin on the problems of retirement and aging in Israel and in the world.
Published by: Authority for Retirement and Aging, Sderot Weizmann 13, Jerusalem 91909, Israel. TEL 02-5386912, paz@nioi.gov.il. Eds. Zvi Lavie, Izit Regev. Circ: 9,000.

612.67 GBR ISSN 1365-4691
HEALTH & AGEING. Text in English. m. GBP 65 domestic; USD 120 foreign (effective 2000).
Published by: Medicom Publishing, Churston House, Portsmouth Rd, Esher, Surrey KT10 9AD, United Kingdom. TEL 44-1372-471671, FAX 44-1372-471672. Circ: 22,000 (controlled).

613.7 USA
HEALTHSMART MAGAZINE. Text in English. 1995. a. USD 4.95 (effective 1996 & 1997). adv. **Document type:** *Catalog.* **Description:** Discusses health and fitness issues for health-conscious persons over 50.
Published by: Healthsmart Publishing, 290 NE 5th Ave, Delray Beach, FL 33437. TEL 561-471-9003. Pub. Frank R Arena.

618.97 362.6 USA ISSN 1064-2080
HERE'S HELP. Text in English. m. USD 49 (effective 1999). illus. **Document type:** *Newsletter, Consumer.* **Description:** Contains inservice materials; three different one-hour activity programs every month that are mind-stimulating, easy to present, cost nothing to give and require absolutely no advanced preparation; and a lively selection of features and articles that can be used in newsletters or promotion pieces.
Formerly: Health Care Articles (1041-2174)

G

Published by: Eymann Publications, Inc, PO Box 3577, Reno, NV 89505-3577. TEL 775-358-1554, FAX 775-358-1476, eymann@care4elders.com, http://www.care4elders.com. Ed. Maureen Eng. Pub. Katie Eymann Pace. Circ: 1,000.

HOUSING THE ELDERLY REPORT. see *HOUSING AND URBAN PLANNING*

I H A FOCUS. see *HEALTH FACILITIES AND ADMINISTRATION*

INDEPENDENT HEALTHCARE ASSOCIATION. INITIAL DISCUSSION PAPER. see *HEALTH FACILITIES AND ADMINISTRATION*

618.97 IND ISSN 0971-4189
RC952
INDIAN JOURNAL OF GERONTOLOGY; a quarterly journal devoted to research on aging. Text in English. 1969. q. USD 50. adv. bibl. **Description:** Publishes research papers, popular and review articles and allied studies on aging.
Indexed: Indian Psychol.Abstr.
Published by: (Indian Gerontological Association), Rupa books Pvt. Ltd., S-12, Shopping Complex, Tilaknagar, Jaipur, Rajasthan 302 004, India. TEL 91-141-621531, FAX 91-141-621693, TELEX 0365-2631 KASA IN. Ed. K L Sharma.

362.6 DEU
INFORMATIONSDIENST ALTERSFRAGEN. Text in German. 1973. bi-m. DEM 48 (effective 1998). index. back issues avail. **Document type:** *Academic/Scholarly, Bibliography.*
Formerly (until 1997): Altenhilfe (0724-8849)
Published by: Deutsches Zentrum fuer Altersfragen e.V., Manfred-von-Richthofen-Str 2, Berlin 12101, Germany. TEL 49-30-786071, FAX 49-30-7854350. Ed. Roland Schmidt. Circ: 1,500.

305.26 USA
HQ1060
INNOVATIONS IN AGING. Text in English. 1972. q. membership. charts, illus, stat. **Document type:** *Consumer.*
Formerly (until 1997): Perspective on Aging (0096-2740)
Indexed: Abstr.Soc.Geront., AgeLine.
—ingenta.
Published by: National Council on the Aging, 409 Third St, S W, Washington, DC 20024. TEL 202-479-1200, http://www.ncoa.org. Pub. Michael Reinemer. Circ: 8,000.

305.26 USA
INSIDE A F A R. Text in English. m. **Document type:** *Newsletter, Consumer.* **Description:** Provides current news and information on aging research and related issues.
Published by: American Federation for Aging Research, 1414 Ave of the Americas, New York, NY 10019. TEL 212-752-2327, FAX 212-832-2298, amfedaging@aol.com, http://www.afar.org.

305.26 CHE ISSN 0074-1132
HQ1060 CODEN: ITGEAR
INTERDISCIPLINARY TOPICS IN GERONTOLOGY. Text in English. 1968. irreg., latest vol.30. CHF 200 in Europe; DEM 240 in Germany; USD 160 in United States price varies. reprint service avail. from ISI. *Refereed.* **Document type:** *Monographic series, Academic/Scholarly.*
Indexed: Biol.Abstr., Chem.Abstr., Curr.Adv.Ecol.Sci., Curr.Cont. (coverage dropped), Ind.Med. (coverage dropped).
—BLDSC (4533.360000), CASDDS, CISTI, GNLM, KNAW. **CCC.**
Published by: S. Karger AG, Allschwilerstr 10, PO Box, Basel 4009, Switzerland. TEL 41-61-306-1111, FAX 41-61-306-1234, karger@karger.ch, http://www.karger.com/bookseries/ITOGE. Eds. C Cassel, J Morrison.

INTERFACE (CHICAGO, 1984). see *MEDICAL SCIENCES—Dentistry*

INTERNATIONAL HOSPITAL & AGED CARE JOURNAL. see *HEALTH FACILITIES AND ADMINISTRATION*

305.26 USA ISSN 0091-4150
HQ1060 CODEN: IJADDT
INTERNATIONAL JOURNAL OF AGING & HUMAN DEVELOPMENT; a journal of psychosocial gerontology. Text in English. 1970. 8/yr. (in 2 vols.). USD 76 to individuals; USD 298 to institutions (effective 2001). adv. bk.rev. abstr, charts, illus, stat. Index. back issues avail.; reprints avail. *Refereed.* **Document type:** *Journal, Academic/Scholarly.* **Description:** Includes critical reviews, trendsetting reports, case histories, and essays covering the latest research and developments in intergenerational relations, institutionalization, work, and retirement.
Formerly (until 1973): Aging and Human Development (0002-0974)
Related titles: Online - full text ed.: (from Gale Group, Institute for Scientific Information).
Indexed: ASCA, ASSIA, Abstr.Anthropol., Abstr.Soc.Geront., AgeLine, Bibl.Asian Stud. (1981), Biol.Abstr., Bk.Rev.Ind. (1984-1986), C.I.J.E., Chic.Per.Ind., Commun.Abstr., Curr.Cont., Dent.Ind., Excerp.Med., Fam.Ind., Human Resour.Abstr., IMFL, Ind.Med. (1973-), Indian Psychol.Abstr., Int.Nurs.Ind., Lang.& Lang.Behav.Abstr., Mid.East: Abstr.& Ind., NRN, PSI, PsycInfo, Psychol.Abstr., Ref.Zh., SOPODA, SSCI, Sage Fam.Stud.Abstr., Soc.Sci.Ind. (Jan.1983-), Soc.Serv.Abstr., Soc.Work Res.& Abstr., Sociol.Abstr., e-psyche.
—BLDSC (4541.595000), CISTI, GNLM, IDS, Infotrieve, ingenta, KNAW. **CCC.**
Published by: Baywood Publishing Co., Inc., 26 Austin Ave, Box 337, Amityville, NY 11701. TEL 631-691-1270, 800-638-7819, FAX 631-691-1770, info@baywood.com, baywood@baywood.com, http://baywood.com/search/PreviewJournal.asp?qsRecord=5, http://baywood.com; http://literary.com/baywood/pages/AG/index.html. Eds. Bert Hayslip, Brian Devries. R&P Julie Krempa. Adv. contact Joi Tamber-Brooks.

612.67 USA
INTERNATIONAL JOURNAL OF ANTI-AGING MEDICINE. Variant title: I.J.A.A.M. Text in English. 1998. q. USD 89.95 (effective 1999). adv. *Refereed.* **Document type:** *Academic/Scholarly.* **Description:** Highlights emerging clinical technologies that promise significant improvement in longevity medicine, quality as well as quantity.
Published by: American Academy of Anti-Aging Medicine, 1341 West Fullerton, Ste 111, Chicago, IL 60614. TEL 800-558-1267, FAX 773-528-5390, a4m@worldhealth.net. Ed. Dr. Ronald Klatz. R&P, Adv. contact Rich Merner TEL 773-528-4333.

155.67 GBR ISSN 0885-6230
RC451.4.A5 CODEN: IJGPES
INTERNATIONAL JOURNAL OF GERIATRIC PSYCHIATRY. Text in English. 1986. m. USD 1,090 in United States; USD 1,090 in Canada & Mexico; USD 1,090 elsewhere; USD 1,145 combined subscription in United States for print and online eds.; USD 1,145 combined subscription in Canada & Mexico for print and online eds.; USD 1,145 combined subscription elsewhere for print and online eds. (effective 2002). adv. back issues avail.; reprint service avail. from SWZ. *Refereed.* **Document type:** *Academic/Scholarly.* **Description:** Communicates the results of original research in the causes, treatment and care of all forms of mental disorder that affect the elderly.
Related titles: Microform ed.: (from PQC); Online - full text ed.: ISSN 1099-1166. USD 1,090 in United States; USD 1,090 in Canada & Mexico; USD 1,090 elsewhere (effective 2002) (from EBSCO Publishing, Wiley InterScience, Institute for Scientific Information).
Indexed: ASCA, Abstr.Soc.Geront., AgeLine, Curr.Cont., Excerp.Med., Fam.Ind., Ind.Med. (1986-), Indian Psychol.Abstr., Int.Nurs.Ind., Neurosci.Cit.Ind., PsycInfo, Psychol.Abstr. (1987-), SSCI, Sage Fam.Stud.Abstr., e-psyche.
—BLDSC (4542.266600), EMDOCS, GNLM, IDS, Infotrieve, KNAW. **CCC.**
Published by: Wiley Europe Ltd., Baffins Ln, Chichester, W Sussex PO19 1UD, United Kingdom. TEL 44-1243-779777, FAX 44-1243-775878, customer@wiley.co.uk, http://www.wiley.co.uk. Ed. Alistair Burns. Pub. Deborah Reece. adv.: B&W page GBP 750, color page GBP 1,650; trim 200 x 260. Circ: 850. **Subscr. in the Americas to:** John Wiley & Sons, Inc., Journals, 605 Third Ave, New York, NY 10158. TEL 212-850-6645, FAX 212-850-6021, subinfo@jwiley.com.

INTERNATIONAL PSYCHOGERIATRICS; the official journal of the Interntional Psychogeriatric Association. see *MEDICAL SCIENCES—Psychiatry And Neurology*

618.97 USA
ISSUES ON AGING. Text in English. q. USD 75 domestic to non-members; USD 90 foreign to non-members (effective 2000). adv. **Document type:** *Academic/Scholarly.* **Description:** Provides information on the physical aspects of aging, including medical research, stuides, and events.
Indexed: CINAHL.
—BLDSC (4584.067000).
Published by: American Physical Therapy Association, Section on Geriatrics, 2920 East Ave S, Ste 200, La Crosse, WI 54601-7202. TEL 608-788-3982. Ed. Ron Scott. adv.: page USD 600.

618.97 ZAF ISSN 1017-2572
CODEN: JARDET
J A R D - JOURNAL OF AGE RELATED DISORDERS. Text in English. 1988. 6/yr. ZAR 73; ZAR 103 foreign (effective 1999). adv. abstr. back issues avail. *Refereed.* **Document type:** *Academic/Scholarly.* **Description:** Communicates results of high scientific quality in the causes, treatment and care of all forms of medical disorders in the elderly.
Formerly (until 1989): GeriatRx (1012-8182)
Indexed: Excerp.Med.
—BLDSC (4919.997650), EMDOCS, GNLM, KNAW.
Published by: (South African Geriatrics Society), Medical Media C C, PO Box 581, Kempton Park, Johannesburg 1620, South Africa. TEL 27-11-9756439, FAX 27-11-9702532. Ed., Pub. Greta Muller. R&P W D Middlemiss. Adv. contact W.D. Middlemiss. B&W page ZAR 3,800, color page ZAR 5,900; trim 210 x 297. Circ: 6,800. **Co-sponsor:** South African Gerontological Association.

305.26 362.17 649 ISR
J D C - BROOKDALE INSTITUTE OF GERONTOLOGY AND HUMAN DEVELOPMENT. ANNUAL REPORT. Text in English, Hebrew. a. USD 15 per issue (effective 2001). **Document type:** *Yearbook.* **Description:** Overview of research conducted in the past year and preview of program for coming year.
Formerly: Brookdale Institute. Annual Report
Published by: J D C - Brookdale Institute of Gerontology and Human Development in Israel, P O Box 13087, Jerusalem 91130, Israel. TEL 972-2-655-7400, FAX 972-2-563-5851.

306.38 ISR
J D C - BROOKDALE INSTITUTE OF GERONTOLOGY AND HUMAN DEVELOPMENT. RESEARCH SERIES. Text in English, Hebrew. irreg. USD 10 per issue (effective 2001). **Document type:** *Monographic series, Academic/Scholarly.*
Former titles: J D C - Brookdale Institute of Gerontology and Human Development. Special Series (0334-908X); Brookdale Institute of Gerontology. Special Series
Published by: J D C - Brookdale Institute of Gerontology and Human Development in Israel, P O Box 13087, Jerusalem 91130, Israel. TEL 972-2-56557400, FAX 972-2-563-5851.

618.97 JPN ISSN 0915-4620
JERONTOROJI/GERONTOLOGY. Text in Japanese. 4/yr. JPY 2,200 (effective 1998).
Published by: Medikaru Rebyusha/Medical Review Co., Ltd., 7-3 Hirano-Machi 1-chome, Chuo-ku, Osaka-shi 541-0046, Japan. TEL 81-6-223-1468, FAX 81-6-223-1245, medrev@osk2.3web.ne.jp.

362.6 USA ISSN 1042-1882
JOHNS HOPKINS MEDICAL LETTER HEALTH AFTER 50. Variant title: Health after 50. Text in English. 1989. m. illus. back issues avail.; reprints avail. *Refereed.* **Document type:** *Newsletter.*
Indexed: CHNI, CINAHL.
—BLDSC (4671.583000).
Published by: (Johns Hopkins Medical Institutions), Rebus Inc., 632 Broadway, 11th Fl, New York, NY 10012. TEL 212-505-2255, FAX 212-505-5462, health_after_50@enews.com. Ed. Patrice Benneward. Pub. Rodney Friedman. Circ: 475,000 (paid).

612.67 USA ISSN 0898-2643
RA564.8 CODEN: JAHEEG
JOURNAL OF AGING AND HEALTH; an interdisciplinary research forum. Text in English. 1989. q. USD 70 to individuals; USD 295 to institutions; USD 25 newsstand/cover to individuals; USD 80 newsstand/cover to institutions (effective 2002). adv. illus. Index. back issues avail.; reprints avail. *Refereed.* **Document type:** *Academic/Scholarly.* **Description:** Provides a forum for the presentation of research and scholarly exchange dealing with social and behavioral factors related to aging and health, with emphasis on health and the quality of life.

Related titles: Online - full text ed.: (from EBSCO Publishing, O C L C Online Computer Library Center, Inc., RoweCom Information Quest, ProQuest Information & Learning, ingenta, Swets Blackwell, Institute for Scientific Information).

Indexed: ASCA, Abstr.Soc.Geront., AgeLine, Behav.Med.Abstr., CINAHL, Curr.Cont., Environ.Sci.Poll.Mgmt., Fam.Ind., IMFL, Lang.& Lang.Behav.Abstr., Pollut.Abstr., PsycInfo, Psychol.Abstr. (1989-), SOPODA, SSCI, Saf.Sci.Abstr., Sage Race Rel.Abstr., Soc.Serv.Abstr., Sociol.Abstr., e-psyche.

—BLDSC (4919.997830), EMDOCS, GNLM, IDS, Infotrieve, ingenta, KNAW. **CCC.**

Published by: Sage Publications, Inc., 2455 Teller Rd, Thousand Oaks, CA 91320. TEL 805-499-0721, FAX 805-499-0871, info@sagepub.com, http://www.sagepub.com.uk/journals/usdetails/j0100.html. Ed. Kyriakos S Markides. R&P Tanya Udin. Adv. contact DeAnna Vega Hammersley. Circ: 1,250. **Overseas subscr. to:** Sage Publications Ltd., 6 Bonhill St, London EC2A 4PU, United Kingdom. TEL 44-20-7374-0645, FAX 44-20-7374-8741; Sage Publications India Pvt. Ltd., 4215, New Delhi 110 048, India. TEL 91-11-641-9884, FAX 91-11-647-2426.

612.67 USA ISSN 1087-3732
HQ1060 CODEN: JAIDFJ

JOURNAL OF AGING & IDENTITY. Text in English. 1996. q. EUR 217, USD 218 to institutions for print or online ed.; EUR 260.40, USD 261.60 to institutions for print & online eds. combined (effective 2002). *Refereed.* **Document type:** *Journal, Academic/Scholarly.* **Description:** Explores the phenomenon of aging, as represented in literature, popular culture, and the arts. Addresses compelling issues, such as attitudes toward aging, from a wide range of disciplines.

Related titles: Online - full text ed.: (from EBSCO Publishing, O C L C Online Computer Library Center, Inc., Swets Blackwell, Kluwer Online, RoweCom Information Quest).

Indexed: Lang.& Lang.Behav.Abstr., MLA Intl.Bibl., SOPODA, Soc.Serv.Abstr., Sociol.Abstr., e-psyche.

—BLDSC (4919.997840), Infotrieve, ingenta. **CCC.**

Published by: Kluwer Academic - Plenum Publishers (Subsidiary of: Wolters Kluwer N.V.), 233 Spring St, New York, NY 10013-1578. TEL 212-620-8000, 800-221-9369, FAX 212-463-0742, info@plenum.com, http://www.wkap.nl/journalhome.htm/1087-3732. Eds. Lagretta T Lenker, Larry Polivka. **Subscr. outside the Americas to:** Kluwer Academic Publishers Group, Journals Department, PO Box 322, Dordrecht 3300 AH, Netherlands. TEL 31-78-639-2392, FAX 31-78-654-6474.

JOURNAL OF AGING & PHARMACOTHERAPY. see *PHARMACY AND PHARMACOLOGY*

612.67 USA ISSN 1063-8652
QP86 CODEN: JAPAFB

JOURNAL OF AGING AND PHYSICAL ACTIVITY. Text in English. 1993. q. USD 45 to individuals; USD 135 to institutions; USD 30 to students (effective 2001). adv. abstr, bibl, charts, stat, illus. back issues avail.; reprints avail. *Refereed.* **Document type:** *Academic/Scholarly.* **Description:** Examines the relationship between physical activity and the aging process. Covers the development, implementation, and evaluation of physical activity programs for older adults.

Related titles: Online - full text ed.: (from Institute for Scientific Information).

Indexed: ASCA, Abstr.Anthropol., Abstr.Soc.Geront., AgeLine, CINAHL, Curr.Cont., Ergon.Abstr., Focus on: Sports Sci.& Med., IBZ, Lang.& Lang.Behav.Abstr., SOPODA, SSCI, Soc.Serv.Abstr., Sociol.Abstr.

—BLDSC (4919.997870), IDS, Infotrieve, ingenta. **CCC.**

Published by: Human Kinetics Publishers, Inc., PO Box 5076, Champaign, IL 61825-5076. TEL 217-351-5076, FAX 217-351-2674, http://www.humankinetics.com. Ed. Wojtek Chodzko Zajko. Pub. Rainer Martens. R&P Cheri Banks TEL 217-351-5076 ext 2275. Adv. contact Patty Rodriguiz. Circ: 745 (paid).

306.26 USA ISSN 0895-9420
HV1457 CODEN: JSPOE8

JOURNAL OF AGING & SOCIAL POLICY; a journal devoted to aging & social policy. Text in English. 1989. q. USD 60 domestic to individuals; USD 81 in Canada to individuals; USD 87 elsewhere to individuals; USD 120 domestic to institutions; USD 162 in Canada to institutions; USD 174 elsewhere to institutions; USD 275 domestic to libraries; USD 371 in Canada to libraries; USD 399 elsewhere to libraries (effective Aug. 2001). adv. bk.rev. illus. back issues avail.; reprint service avail. from HAW. *Refereed.* **Document type:** *Journal, Academic/Scholarly.* **Description:** Provides a forum for the analysis, argument, research, and advocacy of social policy as it affects the aging population.

Related titles: Microfiche ed.: (from PQC); Microform ed.; Online - full text ed.: (from Gale Group, Factiva).

Indexed: Abstr.Anthropol., Abstr.Soc.Geront., AgeLine, Biol.Dig., CINAHL, Environ.Sci.Poll.Mgmt., Fam.Ind., Geo.Abstr.H.G., Geo.Abstr.P.G., IBZ, IDA, IMFL, Lang.& Lang.Behav.Abstr., P.A.I.S., Pollut.Abstr., Ref.Zh., Risk Abstr., SOPODA, Saf.Sci.Abstr., Sage Fam.Stud.Abstr., Soc.Sci.Ind. (Jan.1994-), Soc.Serv.Abstr., Soc.Work Res.& Abstr., Sociol.Abstr.

—BLDSC (4919.997880), EMDOCS, GNLM, Haworth, ingenta.

Published by: Haworth Press, Inc., 10 Alice St, Binghamton, NY 13904-1580. TEL 607-722-5857, 800-429-6784, FAX 607-722-6362, 800-895-0582, getinfo@haworthpressinc.com, http://www.haworthpress.com/journals/journallist.asp. Eds. Francis G Caro, Robert Morris. Pub. William Cohen. R&P Ruthann Heath TEL 607-723-5857 ext 316. Adv. contact Jackie Blakeslee TEL 607-722-5857 ext 346. B&W page USD 315, color page USD 550; trim 6 x 8.5.

612.67 GBR ISSN 0890-4065
HQ1060

JOURNAL OF AGING STUDIES. Text in English. q. EUR 114 in Europe to individuals; JPY 15,100 in Japan to individuals; USD 127 elsewhere to individuals; EUR 273 in Europe to institutions; JPY 36,300 in Japan to institutions; USD 306 elsewhere to institutions (effective 2002). back issues avail. *Refereed.* **Document type:** *Academic/Scholarly.* **Description:** Covers the experience of aging from the perspectives of many disciplines offering new directions in theory and research and critiques of these approaches.

Related titles: Microform ed.: (from PQC); Online - full text ed.: (from H. W. Wilson, ingenta, Gale Group, Swets Blackwell, ScienceDirect, Institute for Scientific Information).

Indexed: ASCA, Abstr.Soc.Geront., AgeLine, Curr.Cont., Fam.Ind., IMFL, Indian Psychol.Abstr., Lang.& Lang.Behav.Abstr., P.A.I.S., PsycInfo, SOPODA, SSCI, Soc.Sci.Ind. (Jan.1994-), Soc.Serv.Abstr., Sociol.Abstr., e-psyche.

—BLDSC (4919.997900), ingenta. **CCC.**

Published by: Elsevier Science, The Boulevard, Langford Ln, Kidlington, Oxon OX5 1GB, United Kingdom. TEL 44-1865-843000, FAX 44-1865-843010, http://www.elsevier.com/locate/jaging. Eds. G Becker, R Adams.

618.97 USA ISSN 1094-5458
QP85 CODEN: JAMEF8

JOURNAL OF ANTI-AGING MEDICINE. Text in English. 1998. q. USD 149 domestic to individuals; USD 199 foreign to individuals; USD 179 domestic to individuals print and online eds. combined; USD 229 foreign to individuals print and online eds. combined; USD 221 domestic to institutions; USD 263 foreign to institutions; USD 265 domestic to institutions print and online eds. combined; USD 307 foreign to institutions print and online eds. combined (effective 2002). back issues avail.; reprints avail. *Refereed.* **Document type:** *Journal, Academic/Scholarly.* **Description:** Publishes papers from multiple fields, discussing gene and cell therapies. Covers new technologies for biomarker assay of the rate of human aging, enabling physicians to measure the effectiveness of one therapy against another for its ability to reverse or inhibit aging.

Related titles: Online - full content ed.: USD 149 to individuals; USD 221 to institutions (effective 2002) (from Swets Blackwell); Online - full text ed.: (from CatchWord Ltd., Institute for Scientific Information, RoweCom Information Quest).

Indexed: Curr.Cont., Excerp.Med., Focus on: Psychophar.

—BLDSC (4937.790000), CASDDS, CatchWord. **CCC.**

Published by: Mary Ann Liebert, Inc. Publishers, 2 Madison Ave, Larchmont, NY 10538. TEL 914—834-3100, FAX 914-834-1388, info@liebertpub.com, www.liebertpub.com/jaa, http://www.liebertpub.com. Ed. Dr. Michael Fossel.

618.97 USA ISSN 0733-4648
HQ1061

JOURNAL OF APPLIED GERONTOLOGY. Text in English. 1982. q. USD 73, GBP 61 to individuals; USD 350, GBP 252 to institutions; USD 25 newsstand/cover to individuals; USD 80 newsstand/cover to institutions (effective 2002). adv. bk.rev. illus. Index. back issues avail.; reprints avail. *Refereed.* **Document type:** *Academic/Scholarly.* **Description:** Covers all subdisciplines of aging with conclusions, findings, or suggestions immediately applicable to the problems encountered by older persons.

Related titles: Online - full text ed.: (from ProQuest Information & Learning, Gale Group, ingenta, Institute for Scientific Information).

Indexed: ASCA, Abstr.Soc.Geront., AgeLine, Chic.Per.Ind., Curr.Cont., Environ.Sci.Poll.Mgmt., Fam.Ind., Human Resour.Abstr., IMFL, Lang.& Lang.Behav.Abstr., NRN, Pollut.Abstr., PsycInfo, Psychol.Abstr. (1982-), Risk Abstr., SOPODA, SSCI, Saf.Sci.Abstr., Sage Fam.Stud.Abstr., Sage Race Rel.Abstr., Soc.Sci.Ind. (Jan.1994-), Soc.Serv.Abstr., Sociol.Abstr., Viol.& Abuse Abstr., e-psyche.

—BLDSC (4942.615000), EMDOCS, GNLM, IDS, ingenta, KNAW. **CCC.**

Published by: (Southern Gerontological Society), Sage Publications, Inc., 2455 Teller Rd, Thousand Oaks, CA 91320. TEL 805-499-0721, FAX 805-499-0871, libraries@sagepub.com., info@sagepub.com, http://www.sagepub.co.uk/journals/details/j0094.html, http://www.sagepub.com, http://www.sagepub.com/journals/usdetails/j0140.html. Ed. Larry C Mullins. R&P Tanya Udin. Adv. contact DeAnna Vega Hammersley. Circ: 1,600. **Overseas subscr. to:** Sage Publications Ltd., 6 Bonhill St, London EC2A 4PU, United Kingdom. TEL 44-20-7374-0645, FAX 44-20-7374-8741; Sage Publications India Pvt. Ltd., 4215, New Delhi 110 048, India. TEL 91-11-641-9884, FAX 91-11-647-2426.

618.97 USA ISSN 1079-9362
RC451.4.A5 CODEN: JCGEEP

JOURNAL OF CLINICAL GEROPSYCHOLOGY. Text in English. 1995. q. USD 286, EUR 285 to institutions for print or online ed.; USD 343.20, EUR 342 to institutions for print & online eds.combined (effective 2002). adv. *Refereed.* **Document type:** *Journal, Academic/Scholarly.* **Description:** Publishes original empirical, theoretical, review and clinical papers on the assessment, diagnosis, categorization, prevention and treatment of psychological problems in older adults.

Related titles: Microfilm ed.: (from PQC); Online - full text ed.: (from EBSCO Publishing, O C L C Online Computer Library Center, Inc., RoweCom Information Quest, Swets Blackwell, Kluwer Online).

Indexed: Fam.Ind., PsycInfo, e-psyche.

—BLDSC (4958.475000), GNLM, Infotrieve, ingenta. **CCC.**

Published by: Kluwer Academic - Plenum Publishers (Subsidiary of: Wolters Kluwer N.V.), 233 Spring St, New York, NY 10013-1578. TEL 212-620-8000, 800-221-9369, FAX 212-463-0742, info@plenum.com, http://www.wkap.nl/journalhome.htm/1079-9362. Eds. Michel Hersen, Vincent B Van Hasselt. R&P Rose Luongo TEL 781-871-6311. **Subscr. outside the Americas to:** Kluwer Academic Publishers Group, Journals Department, PO Box 322, Dordrecht 3300 AH, Netherlands. TEL 31-78-639-2392, FAX 31-78-654-6474.

612.67 NLD ISSN 0169-3816
HQ1060 CODEN: JCCGEB

JOURNAL OF CROSS-CULTURAL GERONTOLOGY. Text in English. 1986. q. EUR 299, USD 300 to institutions for print or online ed.; EUR 358.80, USD 360 to institutions for print & online eds.combined (effective 2002). adv. bk.rev. illus. index. back issues avail.; reprint service avail. from SWZ. *Refereed.* **Document type:** *Journal, Academic/Scholarly.* **Description:** Comprises a broad range of articles dealing with non-Western societies, written from the perspectives of history, anthropology, sociology, political science, psychology, population studies, health/biology, etc.

Related titles: Microform ed.: (from PQC); Online - full text ed.: (from EBSCO Publishing, O C L C Online Computer Library Center, Inc., RoweCom Information Quest, Swets Blackwell, Kluwer Online).

Indexed: Abstr.Soc.Geront., AgeLine, Anthropol.Lit., Biol.Abstr., Environ.Sci.Poll.Mgmt., Fam.Ind., IBR, IBZ, Ind.Med. (coverage dropped), Indian Psychol.Abstr., Intl.Bibl.Soc.Sci., Lang.& Lang.Behav.Abstr., PsycInfo, Psychol.Abstr. (1991-), Ref.Zh., Risk Abstr., SOPODA, Saf.Sci.Abstr., Sage Fam.Stud.Abstr., Soc.Serv.Abstr., Sociol.Abstr., e-psyche.

—BLDSC (4965.660000), GNLM, Infotrieve, ingenta. **CCC.**

Published by: Kluwer Academic Publishers Group (Subsidiary of: Wolters Kluwer N.V.), Spuiboulevard 50, PO Box 17, Dordrecht 3300 AA, Netherlands. TEL 31-78-639-2392, FAX 31-78-654-2254, services@wkap.nl, http://www.wkap.nl/journalhome.htm/0169-3816. Ed. J Neil Henderson. **Subscr. in the Americas to:** Kluwer Academic - Plenum Publishers, 233 Spring St, New York, NY 10013-1578. TEL 212-620-8468, FAX 212-807-1047; **Subscr. to.:** Journals Department, PO Box 322, Dordrecht 3300 AH, Netherlands. TEL 31-78-639-2392, FAX 31-78-654-6474.

THE JOURNAL OF DEMENTIA CARE; for all who work with people with dementia. see *MEDICAL SCIENCES—Psychiatry And Neurology*

362.6 USA ISSN 0894-6566
HV6626.3 CODEN: JEANE2

JOURNAL OF ELDER ABUSE & NEGLECT; an international journal. Text in English. 1988. q. USD 75 to individuals; USD 101 in Canada to individuals; USD 109 elsewhere to individuals; USD 175 to institutions; USD 236 in Canada to institutions; USD 254 elsewhere to institutions; USD 400 to libraries; USD 540 in Canada to libraries; USD 580 elsewhere to libraries (effective Aug. 2001). adv. bk.rev. illus. back issues avail.; reprint service avail. from HAW. *Refereed.* **Document type:** *Journal, Academic/Scholarly.* **Description:** Devoted to the study of causes, treatment, effects, and prevention of the mistreatment of older people. Provides a forum for the discussion of scientific investigation, program developments, policy initiatives, and personal commentary about elder abuse and neglect.
Related titles: Microfiche ed.: (from PQC); Microform ed.; Online - full text ed.: (from ProQuest Information & Learning, Gale Group, Factiva, Institute for Scientific Information).
Indexed: ASCA, Abstr.Crim.& Pen., Abstr.Soc.Geront., AgeLine, CINAHL, CJPI, Crim.Just.Abstr., Curr.Cont., Environ.Sci.Poll.Mgmt., Fam.Ind., IBZ, IMFL, Ind.Philos., Lang.& Lang.Behav.Abstr., Pollut.Abstr., Risk Abstr., SOPODA, SSCI, Saf.Sci.Abstr., Sage Fam.Stud.Abstr., Sage Urb.Stud.Abstr., Soc.Sci.Ind. (Jan.1994-Dec.1998), Soc.Serv.Abstr., Soc.Work Res.& Abstr., Sociol.Abstr., Viol.& Abuse Abstr.
—BLDSC (4973.293000), GNLM, Haworth, IDS, ingenta.
Published by: Haworth Press, Inc., 10 Alice St, Binghamton, NY 13904-1580. TEL 607-722-5857, 800-429-6784, FAX 607-722-6362, 800-895-0582, getinfo@haworthpressinc.com, http://www.haworthpress.com/journals/journallist.asp. Ed. Suzan McMurray Anderson. Pub. William Cohen. R&P Ruthann Heath TEL 607-723-5857 ext 316. Adv. contact Jackie Blakeslee TEL 607-722-5857 ext 346. B&W page USD 315, color page USD 550; trim 6 x 8.5.

JOURNAL OF GERIATRIC PSYCHIATRY; official journal of the Boston Society for Gerontological Psychiatry. see *MEDICAL SCIENCES—Psychiatry And Neurology*

618.97 CAN ISSN 0891-9887
CODEN: JGPNEN

JOURNAL OF GERIATRIC PSYCHIATRY AND NEUROLOGY; an interdisciplinary forum for clinicians and scientists. Text in English. 1988. q. USD 99 in US & Canada to individuals; USD 129 elsewhere to individuals; USD 155 in US & Canada to institutions; USD 179 elsewhere to institutions (effective 2001). adv. bk.rev. illus. back issues avail.; reprints avail. *Refereed.* **Document type:** *Journal, Academic/Scholarly.* **Description:** For physicians who treat aging patients as well as researchers in geriatric psychiatry and neurology.
Related titles: CD-ROM ed.; Online - full text ed.: (from ProQuest Information & Learning, Institute for Scientific Information).
Indexed: ASCA, Curr.Cont., Excerp.Med., Ind.Med. (1988-), Inpharma, Int.Nurs.Ind., Neurosci.Cit.Ind., Pharm.&Out.News, PsycInfo, Psychol.Abstr. (1988-), Reac., SSCI (coverage dropped), Sci.Cit.Ind., e-psyche.
—BLDSC (4995.081000), EMDOCS, GNLM, IDS, ingenta, KNAW. **CCC.**
Published by: (Alzheimer's Foundation), B.C. Decker Inc., 20 Hughson St S, LCD 1, P O Box 620, Hamilton, ON L8N 3K7, Canada. TEL 905-522-7017, 800-568-7281, FAX 905-522-7839, info@bcdecker.com, http://www.bcdecker.com. Ed. Alan Mellow. Pub. David LeGallais. R&P Paula Presutti. Adv. contact John Birkby. Circ: 450.

610.7365 USA ISSN 0098-9134
RC954

JOURNAL OF GERONTOLOGICAL NURSING; for nursing care of older adults. Text in English. 1974. m. USD 68 domestic to individuals (effective 2001); USD 75 in Canada to individuals; USD 108 elsewhere to individuals; USD 89 domestic to institutions (effective 2001); USD 85 in Canada to institutions; USD 129 elsewhere to institutions (effective 2001). adv. bk.rev. illus. index. reprint service avail. from PQC. *Refereed.* **Document type:** *Academic/Scholarly.* **Description:** Provides a forum for all aspects of gerontological nursing with original clinical articles and the latest research.
Related titles: Microform ed.: (from PQC); Online - full text ed.: (from Northern Light Technology, Inc., ProQuest Information & Learning).
Indexed: AMED, Abstr.Health Care Manage.Stud., Abstr.Soc.Geront., AgeLine, CINAHL, Fam.Ind., I.P.A., Int.Nurs.Ind., Nurs.Abstr., Psychol.Abstr., Sage Urb.Stud.Abstr., Viol.& Abuse Abstr.
—BLDSC (4995.094000), CISTI, GNLM, ingenta, KNAW. **CCC.**
Published by: Slack, Inc., 6900 Grove Rd, Thorofare, NJ 08086-9447. TEL 856-848-1000, 800-257-8290, FAX 856-853-5991, jgn@slackinc.com, http://www.slackinc.com/jgn.htm, http://www.slackinc.com/allied/jgn/jgnhome.htm. Ed. Dr. Kathleen C. Buckwalter. Pub. John C. Carter. adv.: B&W page USD 1,545, color page USD 2,830. Circ: 9,300 (paid).

306.38 USA ISSN 0163-4372
HV1451

JOURNAL OF GERONTOLOGICAL SOCIAL WORK. Text in English. 1978. q. (in 2 vols.). USD 50 to individuals; USD 68 in Canada to individuals; USD 73 elsewhere to individuals; USD 65 to institutions; USD 88 in Canada to institutions; USD 94 elsewhere to institutions; USD 350 to libraries; USD 473 in Canada to libraries; USD 508 elsewhere to libraries (effective Aug. 2001). adv. bk.rev. illus. back issues avail.; reprint service avail. from HAW. *Refereed.* **Document type:** *Journal, Academic/Scholarly.* **Description:** Covers social work practice, theory, administration, and consultation in the field of aging.
Related titles: Microfiche ed.: (from PQC); Microform ed.; Online - full text ed.: (from Gale Group, Factiva).
Indexed: ASCA, ASSIA, Abstr.Health Care Manage.Stud., Abstr.Soc.Geront., AgeLine, Behav.Abstr., Behav.Med.Abstr., CINAHL, Chic.Per.Ind., Commun.Abstr., Curr.Cont. (coverage dropped), Educ.Admin.Abstr., Excerp.Med., Fam.Ind., Human Resour.Abstr., IBZ, IMFL, Ind.Per.Art.Relat.Law, Lang.& Lang.Behav.Abstr., PsycInfo, Psychol.Abstr. (1978-), SOPODA, SSCI (coverage dropped), Soc.Sci.Ind. (Mar.1987-), Soc.Serv.Abstr., Soc.Work Res.& Abstr., Sociol.Abstr., Viol.& Abuse Abstr., Yrbk.Assoc.Educ.& Rehab.Blind, e-psyche.
—BLDSC (4995.094400), GNLM, Haworth, IDS, ingenta.
Published by: Haworth Press, Inc., 10 Alice St, Binghamton, NY 13904-1580. TEL 607-722-5857, 800-429-6784, FAX 607-722-6362, 800-895-0582, getinfo@haworthpressinc.com, http://www.haworthpress.com/journals/journallist.asp. Ed. Rose Dobrof. Pub. William Cohen. R&P Ruthann Heath TEL 607-723-5857 ext 316. Adv. contact Jackie Blakeslee TEL 607-722-5857 ext 346. B&W page USD 315, color page USD 550; trim 6 x 8.5. Circ: 1,540.

362.6 USA ISSN 0276-3893
HD7287.9

JOURNAL OF HOUSING FOR THE ELDERLY. Text in English. 1983. s-a. USD 60 to individuals; USD 81 in Canada to individuals; USD 87 elsewhere to individuals; USD 150 to institutions; USD 203 in Canada to institutions; USD 218 elsewhere to institutions; USD 325 to libraries; USD 439 in Canada to libraries; USD 471 elsewhere to libraries (effective Aug. 2001). adv. bk.rev. illus. reprint service avail. from HAW. *Refereed.* **Document type:** *Journal, Academic/Scholarly.* **Description:** Provides new research and synthesizes the cross-disciplinary efforts made in the area of residential environments for the elderly.
Related titles: Microfiche ed.: (from PQC); Microform ed.
Indexed: AMED, ASSIA, Abstr.Soc.Geront., AgeLine, Archit.Per.Ind., CINAHL, IBZ, IMFL, Lang.& Lang.Behav.Abstr., P.A.I.S., Peace Res.Abstr., Psychol.Abstr., SOPODA, Sage Fam.Stud.Abstr., Sage Urb.Stud.Abstr., Soc.Serv.Abstr., Sociol.Abstr., Urb.Aff.Abstr.
—BLDSC (5003.412000), Haworth, ingenta.

Published by: Haworth Press, Inc., 10 Alice St, Binghamton, NY 13904-1580. TEL 607-722-5857, 800-429-6784, FAX 607-722-6362, 800-895-0582, getinfo@haworthpressinc.com, http://www.haworthpress.com/journals/journallist.asp. Ed. Benyamin Schwarz. Pub. William Cohen. R&P Ruthann Heath TEL 607-723-5857 ext 316. Adv. contact Jackie Blakeslee TEL 607-722-5857 ext 346. B&W page USD 315, color page USD 550; trim 6 x 8.5. Circ: 360.

362.6 USA ISSN 1078-4470
CODEN: JMHAFL

JOURNAL OF MENTAL HEALTH AND AGING. Text in English. 1995. 4/yr. USD 52 in United States to individuals; USD 88 for 2 yrs. in United States to individuals; USD 61 foreign to individuals; USD 104 for 2 yrs. foreign to individuals; USD 112 in United States to institutions; USD 190 for 2 yrs. in United States to institutions; USD 128 foreign to institutions; USD 218 for 2 yrs. foreign to institutions (effective 2000). adv. bk.rev., software rev., video rev., Website rev. illus, abstr. 70 p./no. back issues avail.; reprints avail. *Refereed.* **Document type:** *Journal, Academic/Scholarly, Abstract/Index, Bibliography.* **Description:** Addresses issues in mental health for practitioners, educators, and researchers working with the elderly and their families.
Indexed: Abstr.Soc.Geront., AgeLine, CINAHL, Lang.& Lang.Behav.Abstr., P.A.I.S., PsycInfo, SOPODA, Soc.Serv.Abstr., Soc.Work Res.& Abstr., Sociol.Abstr., e-psyche.
—BLDSC (5017.686000), GNLM, Infotrieve, KNAW. **CCC.**
Published by: Springer Publishing Company, 536 Broadway, New York, NY 10012. TEL 212-431-4370, FAX 212-941-7842, springer@springerpub.com, http://www.springerpub.com. Ed. Donna Cohen. Pub. Ursula Springer. R&P Dorothy Kouwenberg. Adv. contact Bob Friel. B&W page USD 300; 5.5 x 8.5.

613.2 USA ISSN 0163-9366
TX361.A3 CODEN: JNELDA

JOURNAL OF NUTRITION FOR THE ELDERLY. Text in English. 1980. q. USD 60 to individuals; USD 81 in Canada to individuals; USD 87 elsewhere to individuals; USD 150 to institutions; USD 203 in Canada to institutions; USD 218 elsewhere to institutions; USD 435 to libraries; USD 587 in Canada to libraries; USD 631 elsewhere to libraries (effective Aug. 2001). adv. bk.rev. bibl, illus. reprint service avail. from HAW. *Refereed.* **Document type:** *Journal, Academic/Scholarly.* **Description:** Reports of dietary studies, systems and programs for providing nutritional care, and the cultural and behavioral aspects of nutrition for the elderly. Includes summaries of relevant articles in other journals.
Related titles: Microfiche ed.: (from PQC); Microform ed.
Indexed: Abstr.Anthropol., Abstr.Soc.Geront., AgeLine, Agricola, Bibl.Agri., Biol.Abstr., CINAHL, Chem.Abstr., Curr.Cont. (coverage dropped), Dairy Sci.Abstr., Environ.Sci.Poll.Mgmt., Excerp.Med., Food Sci.& Tech.Abstr., Hosp.Lit.Ind., IMFL, I.P.A., Int.Nurs.Ind., Med.Care Rev., NRN, Nutr.Abstr., Potato Abstr., PsycInfo, Psychol.Abstr. (1985-), Ref.Zh., Rehabil.Lit., Risk Abstr., Saf.Sci.Abstr., Soc.Work Res.& Abstr., e-psyche.
—BLDSC (5024.710000), GNLM, Haworth, ingenta, KNAW.
Published by: Haworth Press, Inc., Food Products Press, 10 Alice St, Binghamton, NY 13904-1580. TEL 607-722-5857, 800-429-6784, FAX 607-722-6362, 800-895-0582, getinfo@haworthpressinc.com, http://www.haworthpress.com/journals/journallist.asp. Ed. Annette B Natow. Pub. William Cohen. R&P Ruthann Heath TEL 607-723-5857 ext 316. Adv. contact Jackie Blakeslee TEL 607-722-5857 ext 346. B&W page USD 315, color page USD 550; trim 6 x 8.5. Circ: 725.

JOURNAL OF OCULAR PHARMACOLOGY AND THERAPEUTICS. see *MEDICAL SCIENCES—Ophthalmology And Optometry*

155.67 USA ISSN 1050-2289
BV4435 CODEN: JRGEES

JOURNAL OF RELIGIOUS GERONTOLOGY; the interdisciplinary journal of practice, theory & applied research. Text in English. 1985. q. USD 50 to individuals; USD 68 in Canada to individuals; USD 73 elsewhere to individuals; USD 200 to institutions; USD 270 in Canada to institutions; USD 290 elsewhere to institutions; USD 200 to libraries; USD 270 in Canada to libraries; USD 290 elsewhere to libraries (effective Aug. 2001). adv. bk.rev. illus. reprint service avail. from HAW. *Refereed.* **Document type:** *Journal, Academic/Scholarly.* **Description:** Provides articles that cut across denominational lines and academic disciplines to present a picture of the emerging field of religious gerentology.
Formerly (until vol.7, 1990): Journal of Religion and Aging (0738-6184)

Related titles: Microfiche ed.: (from PQC); Microform ed.
Indexed: ASSIA, Abstr.Soc.Geront., AgeLine, Chr.Per.Ind., G.Soc.Sci.& Rel.Per.Lit., Hist.Abstr. (1985-, dropped), IBZ, IMFL, Ind.Philos., Lang.& Lang.Behav.Abstr., Past.Care & Couns.Abstr., Per.Islam. (1991-), Psychol.Abstr., Rel.& Theol.Abstr. (1984-), Rel.Ind.One, Rel.Ind.Two, SOPODA, Sociol.Abstr.
—BLDSC (5049.354000), Haworth, ingenta.
Published by: Haworth Press, Inc., 10 Alice St, Binghamton, NY 13904-1580. TEL 607-722-5857, 800-429-6784, FAX 607-722-6362, 800-895-0582, getinfo@haworthpressinc.com, http://www.haworthpress.com/journals/journallist.asp. Ed. Rev. James Ellor. Pub. William Cohen. R&P Ruthann Heath TEL 607-723-5857 ext 316. Adv. contact Jackie Blakeslee TEL 607-722-5857 ext 346. B&W page USD 315, color page USD 550; trim 6 x 8.5. Circ: 875.

JOURNAL OF WOMEN AND AGING; the multidiciplinary quarterly of psychosocial practice, theory & research. see *WOMEN'S STUDIES*

612.67 USA ISSN 1079-5006
RC952.A1 CODEN: JGASFW
JOURNALS OF GERONTOLOGY. SERIES A: BIOLOGICAL SCIENCES & MEDICAL SCIENCES. Text in English. 1946. m. USD 222 domestic to individuals; USD 232 foreign to individuals; USD 485 domestic to institutions; USD 495 foreign to institutions (effective 2001). adv. bibl, charts, illus. Index. 112 p./no. 2 cols./p. reprint service avail. from PQC. *Refereed.* **Document type:** *Academic/Scholarly.* **Description:** Publishes original scientific and research papers on the biological and medical aspects of aging.
Supersedes in part (in 1995): Journal of Gerontology (0022-1422)
Related titles: Microfilm ed.: (from PQC); Online - full text ed.: (from ProQuest Information & Learning, Gale Group, HighWire Pr., Factiva, Institute for Scientific Information).
Indexed: AIM, ASCA, ASSIA, Abstr.Anthropol., Abstr.Health Care Manage.Stud., Abstr.Soc.Geront., AgeLine, Anim.Breed.Abstr., Arts & Hum.Cit.Ind. (coverage dropped), Biol.Abstr., Bk.Rev.Ind. (1984-), CERDIC, C.I.J.E. (coverage dropped), CINAHL, Chem.Abstr., Chem.Indus.Notes, Chem.Titles, Child.Bk.Rev.Ind. (1984-), Curr.Adv.Ecol.Sci., Curr.Cont., Dairy Sci.Abstr., Dent.Ind., Ergon.Abstr., Excerp.Med., Fam.Ind., Helminthol.Abstr., Hosp.Lit.Ind., Ind.Med. (1995-), Ind.Sci.Rev., Ind.Vet., Inpharma, Int.Nurs.Ind., Mid.East: Abstr.& Ind., Nutr.Abstr., P.A.I.S. (coverage dropped), Pharm.&Out.News, PsycInfo, Psychol.Abstr. (1946-), Reac., Rehabil.Lit., SSCI, Sage Fam.Stud.Abstr., Sage Urb.Stud.Abstr., Sci.Cit.Ind., Soc.Sci.Ind. (Jul.1982-, dropped), Soc.Work Res.& Abstr., Vet.Bull.
—BLDSC (4995.099000), CASDDS, CISTI, EMDOCS, GNLM, IDS, ingenta, KNAW. **CCC.**
Published by: Gerontological Society of America, 1030 15th St, N W, Ste 250, Washington, DC 20005-1503. TEL 202-842-1275, FAX 202-842-1150, http://biomed.gerontologyjournals.org/, http://www.geron.org. Eds. Dr. John A Faulkner, John Morley. R&P Shirley Brown. Adv. contact Heather Worley. B&W page USD 720, color page USD 1,455. Circ: 4,373 (paid and controlled).

155.67 USA ISSN 1079-5014
RC952.A1 CODEN: JGBSF3
JOURNALS OF GERONTOLOGY. SERIES B: PSYCHOLOGICAL SCIENCES & SOCIAL SCIENCES. Text in English. 1946. bi-m. USD 101 domestic to individuals; USD 111 foreign to individuals; USD 210 domestic to institutions; USD 220 foreign to institutions (effective 2001). adv. bibl, charts, illus. Index. 128 p./no. 2 cols./p. reprint service avail. from PQC. *Refereed.* **Document type:** *Academic/Scholarly.* **Description:** Publishes original scientific and research articles concerning psychological and social aspects of aging.
Supersedes in part (in 1995): Journal of Gerontology (0022-1422)
Related titles: Microfilm ed.: (from PQC); Online - full text ed.: (from Factiva, Institute for Scientific Information).
Indexed: AIM, ASCA, ASSIA, Abstr.Anthropol., Abstr.Health Care Manage.Stud., Abstr.Soc.Geront., AgeLine, Anim.Breed.Abstr., Arts & Hum.Cit.Ind. (coverage dropped), Biol.Abstr., Bk.Rev.Ind. (1984-), CERDIC, CINAHL, Chem.Abstr., Child.Bk.Rev.Ind. (1984-), Crim.Just.Abstr., Curr.Adv.Ecol.Sci., Curr.Cont., Dairy Sci.Abstr., Dent.Ind., Ergon.Abstr., Excerp.Med., Fam.Ind., Helminthol.Abstr., Hosp.Lit.Ind., Human Resour.Abstr., Ind.Med. (1995-), Ind.Sci.Rev., Indian Psychol.Abstr., Inpharma, Int.Nurs.Ind., Mid.East: Abstr.& Ind., Nutr.Abstr., P.A.I.S. (coverage dropped), Pharm.&Out.News, PsycInfo, Psychol.Abstr., Reac., Rehabil.Lit., SSCI, Sage Fam.Stud.Abstr., Sage Urb.Stud.Abstr., Sci.Cit.Ind., Soc.Sci.Ind. (Jan.1995-), Soc.Work Res.& Abstr., Viol.& Abuse Abstr., e-psyche.
—BLDSC (4995.099100), CASDDS, CISTI, EMDOCS, GNLM, IDS, Infotrieve, ingenta, KNAW. **CCC.**
Published by: Gerontological Society of America, 1030 15th St, N W, Ste 250, Washington, DC 20005-1503. TEL 202-842-1275, FAX 202-842-1150, http://www.geron.org. Eds. Fredric D Wolinsky, Margie Lachman. R&P Shirley Brown. Adv. contact Heather Worley. B&W page USD 695, color page USD 1,550. Circ: 6,459 (paid and controlled).

305.26 GBR ISSN 1365-9898
KEELE PAPERS IN GERIATRIC MEDICINE AND GERONTOLOGY. Text in English. 1997. irreg. **Document type:** *Academic/Scholarly.*
—BLDSC (5088.330670).
Published by: Keele University, Department of Geriatric Medicine, School of Postgraduate Medicine, Thornburrow Dr, Stoke-on-trent ST4 7QB, United Kingdom. Eds. Dr. Peter Crome, Salah Mahound.

610.7365 JPN ISSN 0912-8948
KISO ROKA GAKKAI SAKYURA/BIOMEDICAL GERONTOLOGY CIRCULAR. Text in Japanese. 1952. 3/yr.
Published by: Nihon Kiso Roka Gakkai/Japan Society for Biomedical Gerontology, Tokyoto Rojin Sogo Kenkyujo, 35-2 Sakae-cho, Itabashi-ku, Tokyo 173-0015, Japan.

612.67 RUS
KLINICHESKAYA GERONTOLOGIYA. Text in Russian. q. USD 85 in United States. **Document type:** *Journal, Academic/Scholarly, Trade.*
Indexed: Ref.Zh.
Published by: Mediko-Tekhnologicheskoe Predpriyatie N'iudyamed, Kolomenskii pr-t 4, Moscow 115446, Russian Federation. TEL 7-095-1187474, FAX 7-095-1187474. Ed. L I Dvoretskii. **US dist. addr.:** East View Publications, 3020 Harbor Ln N, Minneapolis, MN 55447. TEL 612-550-0961.

KYORIN IGAKKAI ZASSHI/KYORIN MEDICAL SOCIETY. JOURNAL. see *MEDICAL SCIENCES*

LAZARUS; Oesterreichs Zeitschrift fuer Kranken- und Altenpflege. see *MEDICAL SCIENCES—Nurses And Nursing*

LEARNING & MEMORY. see *MEDICAL SCIENCES—Psychiatry And Neurology*

305.26 USA
LIFELONG. Text in English. m. **Document type:** *Newsletter, Consumer.* **Description:** Provides a forum for information sharing between physicians and patients, serves as a credible source for synthesized physician-friendly analysis of current aging research, and helps improve the translation of this research into patient care applications.
Published by: American Federation for Aging Research, 1414 Ave of the Americas, New York, NY 10019. TEL 212-752-2327, FAX 212-832-2298, amfedaging@aol.com, http://www.afar.org.

362.6 610.7365 CAN ISSN 1183-1618
LONG TERM CARE. Text in English. 1991. q. CND 15, USD 21 (effective 2000). adv. back issues avail. **Document type:** *Academic/Scholarly.* **Description:** Features articles written by leading experts in the field of long-term care.
Published by: Ontario Nursing Home Association, 345 Renfrew Dr, Ste 202, Markham, ON L3R 9S9, Canada. TEL 905-470-8995, FAX 905-470-9595. Ed. Heather Lang Runtz. Adv. contact Michael Murton. page CND 1,250. Circ: 4,600.

610.7365 CAN ISSN 1180-2189
LONG TERM CARE MONITOR. Text in English. m. CND 107. **Document type:** *Trade.* **Description:** Provides practical information and news about ongoing issues in the long-term care sector, for administrators of facilities.
Published by: M P L Communications Inc., 133 Richmond St W, Ste 700, Toronto, ON M5H 3M8, Canada. TEL 416-869-1177, FAX 416-869-0456. Ed. John Hobel.

362.6 USA
LONG-TERM CARE NEWS* . Text in English. 1972. m. USD 10 to individuals; USD 125 to institutions. **Document type:** *Newsletter.*
Formerly (until 1992): Seniors in Sacramento
Published by: California Rural Legal Assistance Foundation, Public Interest Center on Long-Term Care, 2210 K St, 2nd Fl, Sacramento, CA 95816-4923. TEL 916-446-5085, FAX 916-446-3057. Ed. Thomas A Porter. Circ: 1,000.

305.26 ZAF ISSN 1021-4453
LONGEVITY. Text in English. 1993. m. adv. illus. **Document type:** *Consumer.*
Related titles: Microfiche ed.: (from NBI).
Published by: Longevity Magazine (Subsidiary of: General Media Publishing Group), PO Box 650663, Benmore, Johannesburg 2010, South Africa. TEL 27-11-884-7660, FAX 27-11-884-7660. Ed. Claudia Boffard. Adv. contact Ralph Boffard.

618.97 GBR ISSN 0964-5659
LONGEVITY REPORT. Text in English. bi-m. GBP 20 (effective 2000). **Document type:** *Newsletter.* **Description:** Covers the use of science and technology to extend healthy lifespan.
Published by: Reeves Telecommunications Laboratories, West Towan House, Porthtowan, Truro, Cornwall TR4 8AX, United Kingdom. john@longevb.demon.co.uk, longevityrpt@yahoo.com, http://ourworld.compuserve.com/homepages/johnder, http://geocities.yahoo.com/longevityrpt. Ed., Pub. John de Rivaz.

612.67 USA ISSN 0896-7032
LOOKING FORWARD. Text in English. q. USD 15; USD 30 foreign (effective 1999). illus. **Document type:** *Newsletter.* **Description:** Health care news and general health tips for retirees.
Published by: (Hope Heart Institute), International Health Awareness Center Inc., 350 E Michigan Ave, Ste 301, Kalamazoo, MI 49007-3851. TEL 616-343-0770, 800-334-4094, FAX 616-343-6260, hopeinfo@aol.com, http://www.hithoope.com. Ed. Carol P Garzona.

305.26 CAN ISSN 0831-3040
M S O S JOURNAL. Text in English. 1979. m. CND 20 (effective 2000). adv. bk.rev. **Document type:** *Newspaper.* **Description:** Official publication of the Manitoba Society of Seniors.
Published by: Manitoba Society of Seniors, 330 Portage Ave, Ste 1700, Winnipeg, MB R3C 0C4, Canada. FAX 204-943-1290, editor@msos.mb.ca. Ed. Matt Bellan. Adv. contact Bernie Bellan. Circ: 14,000.

306.38 USA ISSN 0742-0935
MATURE OUTLOOK; for vibrant people who enjoy life. Text in English. 1983. 8/yr. USD 19.95 to non-members; USD 3.25 newsstand/cover (effective 2000). adv. bk.rev. **Document type:** *Magazine, Consumer.* **Description:** Covers health and fitness, money, food and nutrition, travel and people.
Indexed: AgeLine.
Published by: Meredith Integrated Marketing, 1716 Locust St, Des Moines, IA 50309-3379. TEL 515-284-2007, FAX 515-284-2064. Ed. Peggy Person. Pub. Jim Carr. adv.: B&W page USD 31,080, color page USD 34,510; trim 10.5 x 8. Circ: 725,000. **Subscr. to:** PO Box 10448, Des Moines, IA 50306-0448.

MATURE YEARS. see *RELIGIONS AND THEOLOGY—Protestant*

MATURITAS; international journal for the study of the climacteric. see *MEDICAL SCIENCES—Obstetrics And Gynecology*

610.7365 USA ISSN 1048-3314
MCKNIGHT'S LONG-TERM CARE NEWS. Text in English. 1980. 16/yr. USD 47.95 in United States; USD 57.95 in Canada; USD 62.95 elsewhere; USD 5 newsstand/cover (effective 2001). adv. illus, stat. back issues avail. **Document type:** *Trade.* **Description:** Covers the entire continuum of long-term care including skilled nursing care, assisted living, special care units, retirement housing, adult day care, acute care and home health care at long-term care facilities nationwide.
Formerly (until Nov. 1989): Today's Nursing Home (1041-3189)
Related titles: Online - full text ed.: (from Gale Group).
—CCC.
Published by: McKnight Medical Communications (Subsidiary of: Medical Economics Publishing Co., Inc.), Two Northfield Plaza, Ste. 300, Northfield, IL 60093. TEL 847-441-3700, FAX 847-441-3701, ltcnews@medec.com, Hcn@medec.com, http://www.medec.com/ltcn/. Ed. John O'Connor. Pub. Suzanne M Powills. Adv. contact Deborah Tobiaski. Circ: 46,892 (paid and controlled).

612.67 IRL ISSN 0047-6374
QP86 CODEN: MAGDA3
MECHANISMS OF AGEING AND DEVELOPMENT. Text in English. 1972. 16/yr. EUR 2,652 in Europe to institutions; JPY 352,200 in Japan to institutions; USD 2,967 elsewhere to institutions (effective 2002). back issues avail.; reprints avail. *Refereed.* **Document type:** *Academic/Scholarly.* **Description:** Examines the fundamental mechanisms underlying the process of aging and development in biological systems, including man.
Related titles: Microform ed.: (from PQC); Online - full text ed.: (from ingenta, ScienceDirect, Swets Blackwell, Institute for Scientific Information).
Indexed: ASCA, AgeLine, Anim.Breed.Abstr., Biol.Abstr., Chem.Abstr., Chem.Titles, Curr.Adv.Biochem., Curr.Adv.Cell & Devel.Biol., Curr.Adv.Ecol.Sci., Curr.Cont., Dent.Ind., Excerp.Med., Helminthol.Abstr., Ind.Med. (1972-), Ind.Sci.Rev., Ind.Vet., Inpharma, Int.Abstr.Biol.Sci., Int.Aerosp.Abstr., Neurosci.Cit.Ind., Nutr.Abstr., Reac., Ref.Zh., SSCI (coverage dropped), Sci.Cit.Ind.
—BLDSC (5424.571000), ADONIS, CASDDS, CISTI, GNLM, IDS, ingenta, KNAW, Linda Hall. **CCC.**
Published by: Elsevier Science Ireland Ltd, Elsevier House, Brookvale Plaza, E. Park, Shannon, Co. Clare, Ireland. TEL 353-61-471944, FAX 353-61-472144, http://www.elsevier.nl/locate/mechagedev. Ed. B L Strehler. R&P Annette Moloney. **Subscr. in Australasia and the Far East to:** Elsevier Science (Singapore) Pte Ltd, No.1 Temasek Ave, 17-01 Millenia Tower, Singapore 039192, Singapore. TEL 65-434-3727, FAX 65-337-2230; **Subscr. in the Americas to:** Elsevier Science, PO Box 945, New York, NY 10159-0945. TEL 212-633-3730, FAX 212-633-3680, usinfo-f@elsevier.com; **Subscr. to:** Elsevier Science Inc - Japan Regional Office, 9-15 Higashi-Azabu 1-chome, Minato-ku, Tokyo 106-0044, Japan. TEL 81-3-5561-5033, FAX 81-3-5561-5047. **Subscr. to:** Elsevier Science BV, PO Box 211, Amsterdam 1000 AE, Netherlands. TEL 31-20-485-3757, FAX 31-20-485-3432.

618.97 614.58 ITA ISSN 0391-4844
CODEN: MGRCAT
MEDICINA GERIATRICA*. Text in Italian; Summaries in English, Italian. 1969. bi-m. ITL 50,000, USD 16 domestic; ITL 60,000 foreign. adv. bk.rev. bibl, illus, stat. index. back issues avail. **Document type:** *Academic/Scholarly.*
Indexed: Biol.Abstr.
—CISTI.
Published by: Societa Italiana Medici e Operatori Geriatrici, Casa Editrice Mattioli, Via Codura, 1 B, Fidenza, PR 43036, Italy. TEL 39-524-84547. Circ: 1,500.

346.013 USA
MENTAL CAPACITY: MEDICAL AND LEGAL ASPECTS OF THE AGING. Text in English. 1977. latest 1994, 2nd ed., base vol. plus a. updates. USD 115. **Description:** Covers the physiological and legal aspects of mental incompetence, including symptoms, causes and treatments of senility.
Indexed: e-psyche.
Published by: Shepard's (Subsidiary of: Reed Elsevier plc), 555 Middle Creek Pkwy, Colorado Springs, CO 80921. TEL 800-743-7393, customer_service@shepards.com, http://www.shepards.com.

612.67 USA
THE MERCK MANUAL OF GERIATRICS. Text in English. 1990. irreg., latest vol.3, 2000. **Document type:** *Monographic series, Trade.*
Published by: Merck Publishing Group, 126 E Lincoln Ave, PO Box 2000, Rahway, NJ 07065. TEL 732-594-4600, FAX 732-594-4600.

612.67 USA
MINNESOTA GERONTOLOGIST*. Text in English. 1977. 5/yr. USD 10. bk.rev. **Document type:** *Newsletter.* **Description:** Provides information on current issues in aging to its membership; it also provides information about MGS conferences and other activities of the society.
Published by: Minnesota Gerontological Society, 7550 France Ave, Ste 201, Minneapolis, MN 55435-4762. TEL 612-222-8233. Ed. Chris Osborn. Circ: 650.

612.67 USA ISSN 0275-360X
CODEN: MARDDR
MODERN AGING RESEARCH. Text in English. 1980. irreg., latest vol.9, 1990. price varies. *Refereed.*
Related titles: Online - full text ed.
Indexed: Biol.Abstr., Chem.Abstr., Chem.Indus.Notes, Chem.Titles.
—CASDDS.
Published by: John Wiley & Sons, Inc., Journals (Subsidiary of: Wiley InterScience), 605 Third Ave, New York, NY 10158. TEL 212-475-7700. Eds. Jay Roberts, Richard C Adelman.

618.97 ESP ISSN 0214-378X
MODERN GERIATRICS. Text in Spanish. 1988. 10/yr. USD 75 (effective 1996).
—GNLM.
Published by: Editorial Idepsa S.A., Principe de Vergara, 112 1o F, Madrid 28002, Spain. TEL 34-1-5637306, FAX 34-1-5632393.

305.26 USA ISSN 0026-8046
HQ1060
MODERN MATURITY. Text in English. 1958. bi-m. USD 10 membership only (effective 2000). adv. bk.rev. illus. back issues avail.; reprints avail. **Document type:** *Magazine, Consumer.* **Description:** Includes articles on finance, career options, travel, health, food, personalities, current affairs and fiction of interest to persons 50 and older.
Former titles (until 1960): We; Journal of Lifetime Living
Related titles: Microform ed.: (from PQC); Online - full text ed.: (from Gale Group, ProQuest Information & Learning, Factiva).
Indexed: AgeLine, CHNI, Consum.Ind. (1989-), Hlth.Ind., L.R.I., Mag.Ind., PMR, R.G. (1988-), R.G.Abstr. (1988-), Rehabil.Lit.
—ingenta.
Published by: A A R P, Research, 601 E St, N W, Washington, DC 20049. TEL 202-434-2277, FAX 202-434-6881, member@aarp.org, http://www.aarp.org/mmaturity/. Ed. J Hugh. Adv. contact Patricia Mondello. B&W page USD 240,510, color page USD 266,490. Circ: 20,000,000.

610.7365 USA ISSN 0889-4744
MONTHLY MINI-LESSONS IN CARE OF THE AGING; news, insights and updates on caring for elders. Text in English. 1986. m. USD 34 (effective 2000). illus. back issues avail. **Document type:** *Newsletter, Consumer.* **Description:** Covers care of the aging, with emphasis on inservice education for the staff in long-term care.
Published by: Eymann Publications, Inc, PO Box 3577, Reno, NV 89505-3577. TEL 775-358-1554, FAX 775-358-1476, eymann@care4elders.com, http://www.care4elders.com. Ed. Maureen Eng. Pub. Katie Eymann Pace.

305.42 USA
MOTHER'S DAY REPORT. Text in English. a. USD 8. adv. **Document type:** *Monographic series.*
Published by: Older Women's League, 666 11th St, N W, Ste 700, Washington, DC 20001-4512. TEL 202-783-6686. Ed. Lisa Lederer. Adv. contact Vicki O'Reilly. Circ: 20,000.

362.6 USA ISSN 1045-9073
N C O A NETWORKS. Text in English. 1989. bi-m. membership. adv. bk.rev. back issues avail. **Document type:** *Newspaper.* **Description:** Highlights activities of the various units of the council, reports legislative and regulatory activity and judicial decisions affecting older persons, and explores significant developments in the field of aging.
Formed by the 1989 merger of: Adult Day Care Quarterly; Community Care Quarterly; Older Worker News; Rural Aging Roundup; Senior Center Report; Senior Housing News; Update on Aging for the Voluntary Sector
Published by: National Council on the Aging, 409 Third St, S W, Washington, DC 20024. TEL 202-479-1200, FAX 202-479-0735. Ed., R&P, Adv. contact Elizabeth Joyce. Pub. Michael Reinemer. Circ: 8,000.

N R T A BULLETIN. see *EDUCATION*

305.26071 USA
HQ1060
NATIONAL DIRECTORY OF EDUCATIONAL PROGRAMS IN GERONTOLOGY AND GERIATRICS*. Text in English. 1976. triennial, latest vol.6, 1994. USD 85 (effective 1998). back issues avail. **Document type:** *Directory.* **Description:** Lists and describes some 1,000 gerontology programs and contact persons in accredited institutions of higher education in the US and Canada.
Formerly (until 1987): National Directory of Educational Programs in Gerontology (0148-4508)
Indexed: Abstr.Anthropol.
Published by: Association for Gerontology in Higher Education, 1001 Connecticut Ave, N W, Ste 410, Washington, DC 20036-5504. TEL 202-429-9277. Ed., R&P Derek Stepp. Circ: 1,000.

NATIONAL SENIOR CITIZENS LAW CENTER WASHINGTON WEEKLY. see *LAW*

NEUROPSYCHOLOGY, DEVELOPMENT AND COGNITION. SECTION B: AGING, NEUROPSYCHOLOGY AND COGNITION; a journal on normal and dysfunctional development. see *PSYCHOLOGY*

305.26 USA ISSN 1085-1003
HQ1060
NEW CHOICES; the magazine for your health, money & travel. Variant title: Living Even Better after 50. Text in English. 1960. 10/yr. USD 15; USD 2.95 newsstand/cover (effective 2001). adv. bk.rev. illus. index. reprint service avail. from PQC. **Document type:** *Magazine, Consumer.* **Description:** Contains practical and timely advice on travel, health, and personal finances for men and women from age 50 to retirement.
Former titles (until 1995): New Choices for Retirement Living (1061-2157); (until 1992): New Choices for the Best Years (1041-6277); (until 1989): 50 Plus (0163-2027); (1972-1978): Retirement Living (0090-4910); Harvest Years (0017-8209)
Related titles: Diskette ed.; Microform ed.: (from PQC); Online - full text ed.: (from H. W. Wilson, Gale Group, Factiva).
Indexed: AgeLine, CINAHL, Hlth.Ind., Mag.Ind., R.G. (Jan.1983-Nov.1988), R.G.Abstr. (Jan.1983-Dec.1991, Feb.1992-).
—ingenta. **CCC.**
Published by: Reader's Digest Association, Inc, Reader's Digest Rd, Pleasantville, NY 10570-7000. TEL 914-238-1000, FAX 914-244-5888, newchoices@readersdigest.com. Ed. Greg Daugherty. Pub. Peter Haeffner. adv.: B&W page USD 34,980, color page USD 47,650; trim 10 x 7. Circ: 619,352 (paid). **Subscr. to:** New Choices: Living Even Better After Fifty, Subscriptions, PO Box 5234, Harlan, IA 51593. TEL 800-678-2673.

306.38 CAN ISSN 0710-958X
NEWS FOR SENIORS. Text in English. 1984. m. CND 5, USD 15. back issues avail.
Published by: Society for the Retired & Semi-Retired, 15 Sir Winston Churchill Sq, 100th St & 102A Ave, Edmonton, AB T5J 2E5, Canada. TEL 403-489-4570. Ed. Irene Ramsell. Circ: 20,000.

362.6 NLD ISSN 1387-358X
NIEUWSBRIEF OF OUDERENZORG. Text in Dutch. 1998. 10/yr. included with Ouderenzorg. **Document type:** *Newsletter.* **Description:** Offers tips on the management and clinical aspects of caring for the elderly.
Related titles: ♦ Supplement to: Ouderenzorg. ISSN 1387-3571.
Published by: Elsevier Gezondheidszorg B.V., Tijdstroom (Subsidiary of: Reed Elsevier plc Group), Planetenbaan 1, Maarssen 3600 AK, Netherlands. TEL 31-346-577577, FAX 31-346-556287, http://www.tijdstroom.nl. Circ: 1,200. **Subscr. to:** Elsevier Den Haag, Postbus 16500, The Hague 2500 BM, Netherlands. TEL 31-70-381-9900, FAX 31-70-333-8399.

NIEUWSBRIEF W V G; informatie over voorzieningen voor gehandicapten en ouderen. (Wet Voorzieningen Gehandicapten) see *HANDICAPPED*

NIEUWSBRIEF ZORGVISIE. see *HEALTH FACILITIES AND ADMINISTRATION*

612.67 SWE ISSN 1403-2082
NORDISK GERIATRIK. Text in Swedish. 1998. q. adv. **Document type:** *Magazine, Trade.* **Description:** Covers all aspects of geriatric medicine that are clinically relevant to physicians and their practices.
Published by: Helix Communications AB, Baltzar von Platensgata 9, Stockholm 11242, Sweden. TEL 46-8-651-64-60, FAX 46-8-653-56-50, http://www.helixcom.se. Ed., Pub. Charles Garza. Adv. contact Ann Marie Sullivan. B&W page SEK 16,800, color page SEK 23,600.

054.1 FRA ISSN 0029-456X
NOTRE TEMPS; journal de la retraite heureuse. Text in French, Flemish. 1968. m. FRF 229 domestic; FRF 279 in Europe; FRF 20 newsstand/cover (effective 2000). adv. bk.rev. **Document type:** *Magazine, Consumer.* **Description:** General interest topics for people over 55.

Published by: Bayard Presse, 3 rue Bayard, Paris Cedex 8 75393, France. TEL 33-1-44356060, FAX 33-1-44356031, http://www.notretemps-mag.com, http://www.bayardpresse.fr. Ed. Jean-Paul Bury. Pub. Bernard Porte. adv.: B&W page FRF 156,000, color page FRF 173,500; trim 180 x 262. Circ: 1,000,000 (paid). **Subscr. to:** Bayard Presse International, BP 12, Paris Entreprise 99505, France. TEL 33-1-44216000, FAX 33-3-20274192.

610.7365 362.6 USA ISSN 1524-2900
NURSE AIDE - V I P; published especially for those very important people who care for the elderly. Text in English. 1989. m. USD 21 (effective 2000). back issues avail. **Document type:** *Newsletter, Trade.* **Description:** Provides practical advice, ideas, and suggestions for nurse aides working in long-term care, home health or any geriatric field.
Published by: Eymann Publications, Inc, PO Box 3577, Reno, NV 89505-3577. TEL 775-358-1554, FAX 775-358-1476, eymann@care4elders.com, http://www.care4elders.com. Ed. Maureen Eng. Pub. Katie Eymann Pace.

618.97 USA ISSN 1070-1370
NURSING HOME MEDICINE. Text in English. 12/yr. USD 95 domestic; USD 140 foreign; USD 60 to students. adv. bk.rev. back issues avail.; reprints avail. **Document type:** *Trade.* **Description:** Covers issues for long-term care.
Former titles: Journal of Medical Direction; (until 1990): Annual Medical Direction
Published by: MultiMedia Healthcare Inc., Office Center of Princeton Meadows, Bldg 300, Plainsboro, NJ 08536. TEL 609-275-3800, FAX 609-275-4779. Ed. Joanne Kaldy. Adv. contact Greg S Kloiber. Circ: 20,000.

NURSING HOMES; long term care management. see *MEDICAL SCIENCES—Nurses And Nursing*

610.7365 GBR ISSN 1472-0795
NURSING OLDER PEOPLE. Text in English. 1981. 10/yr. GBP 80 in Europe to institutions; GBP 96 elsewhere to institutions (effective 2002). adv. **Document type:** *Trade.*
Former titles (until 2000): Elderly Care (1369-1856); (until 1992): Nursing the Elderly (0956-8115); (until 1989): Geriatric Nursing and Home Care (0269-9079); British Journal of Geriatric Nursing (0262-5024)
Indexed: AMED, Brit.Nur.Ind., CINAHL, Int.Nurs.Ind.
—BLDSC (6187.107800), GNLM, Infotrieve. **CCC.**
Published by: (Royal College of Nursing), R C N Publishing Co. (Subsidiary of: B M J Publishing Group), R C N Direct, Copse Walk, Cardiff Gate Business Park, Cardiff CF23 8XG, United Kingdom. TEL 44-29-2054-6450, FAX 44-29-2054-6401, directjournalsteam@rcn.org.uk, http://www.rcn.org.uk/. Ed. Linda Thomas. Adv. contact Phil Whomes. Circ: 5,868.

305.4 USA
O W L OBSERVER. Text in English. q. USD 15. adv. **Document type:** *Newsletter, Consumer.*
Published by: Older Women's League, 666 11th St, N W, Ste 700, Washington, DC 20001-4512. TEL 202-783-6686, owlinfo@owl-national.org. Ed. Lisa Lederer. Adv. contact Vicki O'Reilly. Circ: 20,000.

353.537 USA
OHIO DEPARTMENT OF AGING. ANNUAL REPORT. Text in English. 1973. a. **Document type:** *Government.*
Formerly: Ohio. Commission on Aging. Annual Report (0363-9207)
Published by: Ohio Department of Aging, 50 W Broad St, 9th Fl, Columbus, OH 43215-5928. TEL 614-466-6191 TDD, 614-466-5500, FAX 614-466-5741. Ed. Suzanne Kashuba. Circ: 1,500.

362.6 GBR
OLD AGE: A REGISTER OF SOCIAL RESEARCH. Text in English. 1955. irreg., latest 1991, Nov. **Document type:** *Directory.* **Description:** Describes the projects of British universities, leading hospitals, research institutes and voluntary bodies on aging.
Published by: Centre for Policy on Ageing, Centre For Policy On Ageing, Flat 25, 19/23 Ironmonger Row, London EC1V 3QP, United Kingdom. TEL 44-20-7553-6500, FAX 44-20-7553-6501, ageinfo@cpa.org.uk, http://www.cpa.org.uk. Ed. Gillian Crosby.

306.38 USA ISSN 0738-9639
THE OLDER AMERICAN. Text in English. 1970. 3/yr. USD 15 to individual members (effective 1999); USD 50 to institutional members. adv. bk.rev. illus, stat. 48 p./no. 3 cols./p. back issues avail. **Document type:** *Newspaper, Consumer.* **Description:** Presents information relating to issues of advocacy, education, and training for intergenerational families and caregivers of the elderly.
Published by: (Massachusetts Association of Older Americans), Saltus Press, 108 Arlington St, Boston, MA 02116. TEL 617-426-0804, FAX 617-426-0070. Ed., R&P, Adv. contact Phyllis C Galante. B&W page USD 600; trim 11 x 8.5. Circ: 10,000.

OLDER AMERICANS REPORT. see *SOCIAL SERVICES AND WELFARE*

OPINION: SPECIALIST REVIEWS OF KEY PAPERS IN GENERAL & ELDERLY MEDICINE. see *MEDICAL SCIENCES*

362.6 USA
OPTIONS: NEWS FOR OLDER NEW YORKERS. Text in English. 1974. q. free per issue. bk.rev. **Document type:** *Newsletter, Government.* **Description:** Provides information on programs and services for senior citizens in New York City.
Published by: Department for the Aging, 2 Lafayette St, New York, NY 10007. TEL 212-442-1111, FAX 212-442-1096, http://www.ci.nyc.ny.us/aging. Ed. Helene S Wolff. Circ: 30,000.

OSTEOPOROSIS. see *MEDICAL SCIENCES—Abstracting, Bibliographies, Statistics*

362.6 NLD ISSN 1387-3571
OUDERENZORG. Text in Dutch. 1998. 10/yr. NLG 245; includes newsletter. adv. bk.rev. illus. index. **Document type:** *Trade.* **Description:** Covers the management and clincial aspects of caring for the elderly in the Netherlands and Belgium.
Formed by the 1998 merger of: Senior (0168-7492); Which was formerly (1955-1979): Bejaarden (0005-822X); Leeftijd (0165-3792); Which was formerly (1977-1979): Op Leeftijd (0030-333X)
Related titles: ♦ Supplement: Nieuwsbrief of Ouderenzorg. ISSN 1387-358X.
Published by: Elsevier Gezondheidszorg B.V., Tijdstroom (Subsidiary of: Reed Elsevier plc Group), Planetenbaan 1, Maarssen 3600 AK, Netherlands. TEL 31-346-577577, FAX 31-346-554287, http://www.tijdstroom.nl. Ed. A van der Marel. Pub. K Piebenga. Circ: 5,200. **Subscr. to:** Elsevier Den Haag, Postbus 16500, The Hague 2500 BM, Netherlands. TEL 31-70-381-9900, FAX 31-70-333-8399.

OVER 50 AND FIT; life before 50 is the warm-up. see *PHYSICAL FITNESS AND HYGIENE*

612.67 CAN ISSN 0831-7445
PERSPECTIVES (TORONTO). Text in English. 1977. q. CND 29.50 (effective 2000). adv. bk.rev. index. back issues avail. *Refereed.* **Document type:** *Academic/Scholarly.* **Description:** Covers clinical practice, education and research in gerontological nursing.
Indexed: CINAHL, Int.Nurs.Ind.
—BLDSC (6428.136800), GNLM.
Published by: Gerontological Nursing Association, P O BOX 368, STA K, Toronto, ON M4P 2G7, Canada. TEL 416-603-5800. Ed., R&P Petal Samuel. Adv. contact Heather Lang Runtz. Circ: 1,800.

▼ **PHYSICAL & MENTAL ISSUES IN AGING SOURCEBOOK.** see *MEDICAL SCIENCES*

618.97 USA ISSN 0270-3181
RC952.A1
PHYSICAL & OCCUPATIONAL THERAPY IN GERIATRICS; current trends in geriatric rehabilitation. Text in English. 1980. q. USD 60 to individuals; USD 81 in Canada to individuals; USD 87 elsewhere to individuals; USD 175 to institutions; USD 236 in Canada to institutions; USD 254 elsewhere to institutions; USD 400 to libraries; USD 540 in Canada to libraries; USD 580 elsewhere to libraries (effective Aug. 2001). adv. bk.rev. illus. back issues avail.; reprint service avail. from HAW. *Refereed.* **Document type:** *Journal, Academic/Scholarly.* **Description:** Provides a forum for allied health professionals to share information, clinical experience, research, and therapeutic practice in geriatrics.
Related titles: Microfiche ed.: (from PQC); Microform ed.
Indexed: AMED, Abstr.Soc.Geront., AgeLine, Biol.Abstr., CINAHL, Excerp.Med., IMFL, Int.Nurs.Ind., Med.Care Rev., P.A.I.S., Past.Care & Couns.Abstr., PsycInfo, Psychol.Abstr. (1982-), Rehabil.Lit., Soc.Work Res.& Abstr., Sociol.Abstr., e-psyche.
—BLDSC (6475.277000), EMDOCS, GNLM, Haworth, ingenta, KNAW.
Published by: Haworth Press, Inc., 10 Alice St, Binghamton, NY 13904-1580. TEL 607-722-5857, 800-429-6784, FAX 607-722-6362, 800-895-0582, getinfo@haworthpressinc.com, http://www.haworthpress.com/journals/journallist.asp. Ed. Ellen Dunleavey Taira. Pub. William Cohen. R&P Ruthann Heath TEL 607-723-5857 ext 316. Adv. contact Jackie Blakeslee TEL 607-722-5857 ext 346. B&W page USD 315, color page USD 550; trim 6 x 8.5. Circ: 850.

POST ACUTE CARE STRATEGY REPORT; the newsletter for integrating post acute services. see *MEDICAL SCIENCES—Nurses And Nursing*

618.97 FRA ISSN 0242-9772
PRACTICIENS ET TROISIEME AGE. Key Title: Practiciens et 3ieme Age. Text in French. 1977. 6/yr. EUR 72 domestic; EUR 80 foreign (effective 2002). adv. bibl, illus.
Formerly (until 1982): Medecine et Troisieme Age (0182-1377)
Indexed: Ref.Zh.
Published by: Societe Francaise d'Editions Medicales, 22-H rue du Chateau des Rentiers, Paris 75013, France. TEL 33-01-45835054, FAX 33-01-45831354, sfem96@mail.club-internet.fr. Ed. Colette Gallula.

610.7365 052 AUS ISSN 0729-5545
PRIME TIME. Text in English. bi-m. AUD 18; AUD 29 foreign (effective 2000). **Description:** Covers retirement planning, retirement living - health, finance, lifestyle as applied to 45 plus age group within Australia.
Published by: Diverse Publishing Co. Pty. Ltd., PO Box 370, North Melbourne, VIC 3051, Australia. TEL 61-3-93296040, FAX 61-3-93281116. Ed. Louise Chenana. Circ: 55,000.

612.67 UKR ISSN 0869-1703
PROBLEMY STARENIYA I DOLGOLETIYA/PROBLEMS OF AGING AND LONGEVITY. Text in Ukrainian. 1991. q. USD 85 (effective 1999). **Document type:** *Academic/Scholarly.* **Description:** Covers original research in the field of biology of aging, geriatrics, social gerontology and gerohygiene. Also publishes guidelines for practicioners, as well as lists of new books and other publications.
Published by: Akademiya Medychnykh Nauk Ukrainy, Institut Gerontologii, Vyshgorodskaya vul 67, Kiev 254114, Ukraine. TEL 380-44-430-4068, FAX 380-44-432-9956, direct@geront.freenet.kiev.ua. Ed. Vladislav V Bezrukov. **US dist. addr.:** East View Publications, 3020 Harbor Ln N, Minneapolis, MN 55447. TEL 612-550-0961.

155.67 USA ISSN 0882-7974
BF724.55.A35 CODEN: PAGIEL
PSYCHOLOGY AND AGING. Text in English. 1986. q. USD 107 domestic to non-members; USD 122 foreign to non-members; USD 53 domestic to members; USD 63 foreign to members; USD 238 domestic to institutions; USD 270 foreign to institutions (effective 2001). adv. charts, illus. index. back issues avail.; reprint service avail. from PSC,SCH. *Refereed.* **Document type:** *Academic/Scholarly.* **Description:** Publishes research on the psychological and behavioral aspects of aging.
Related titles: Microform ed.: (from PQC); Online - full text ed.: (from Gale Group, Factiva, Institute for Scientific Information).
Indexed: ASCA, ASSIA, Abstr.Soc.Geront., AgeLine, Behav.Med.Abstr., Curr.Cont., Excerp.Med. (1995-), Fam.Ind., IMFL, Ind.Med. (1986-), Int.Nurs.Ind., Neurosci.Cit.Ind., PsycInfo, Psychol.Abstr. (1986-), Russ.Acad.Sci.Bibl., SSCI, Soc.Sci.Ind. (Jan.1994-), Soc.Work Res.& Abstr., e-psyche.
—BLDSC (6946.535317), EMDOCS, GNLM, IDS, ingenta. **CCC.**
Published by: American Psychological Association, 750 First St., N.E., Washington, DC 20002-4242. TEL 202-336-5600, 800-374-2721, FAX 202-336-5568, subscriptions@apa.org, http://www.apa.org/journals/pag.html. Ed. Leah L Light. Circ: 2,800.

QUALITY CARE ADVOCATE. see *HEALTH FACILITIES AND ADMINISTRATION*

G

362.6 ITA ISSN 0486-0306
RASSEGNA GERIATRICA. Text in Italian; Summaries in English. 1964. q. ITL 45,000, USD 70 (effective 1999). **Description:** Contains original works, editorials, and scientific, medical, technical and sociological updates in the areas of gerontology and geriatrics.
Indexed: Excerp.Med.
—EMDOCS.
Published by: (Istituto Nazionale Riposo e Cura per Anziani), Casa Editrice Idelson, Via A. DeGasperi, 55, Naples, NA 80138, Italy. TEL 39-81-5524733, FAX 39-81-5518295, idelgno@tin.it, http://www.idelson-gnocchi.com. Ed. Luca Illuminati.

618.97 GBR ISSN 0144-0519
CODEN: RAGMDK
RECENT ADVANCES IN GERIATRIC MEDICINE. Text in English. 1978. irreg. **Document type:** *Monographic series, Academic/Scholarly.*
—CASDDS, CISTI, GNLM.
Published by: Churchill Livingstone (Subsidiary of: Harcourt Publishers Ltd.), Robert Stevenson House, 1-3 Baxter's Pl, Leith Walk, Edinburgh, Midlothian EH1 3AF, United Kingdom. TEL 44-131-556-2424, FAX 44-131-459-1177, http://www.churchillmed.com. **US subscr. to:** Churchill Livingstone, 650 Ave of the Americas, New York, NY 10011. TEL 212-206-5000.

RECENT ADVANCES IN PSYCHOGERIATRICS. see *MEDICAL SCIENCES—Psychiatry And Neurology*

612.67 BEL ISSN 0304-4408
CODEN: REJUDJ
REJUVENATION. Text in English. 1963. q. USD 100. adv. bk.rev. abstr, bibl, charts, illus, stat, tr.lit. index.
Former titles: International Association on the Artificial Prolongation of the Human Specific Lifespan. Official Journal (0301-5483); Acta Gerontologica et Geriatrica Belgica (0001-575X); Acta Gerontologica Belgica
Indexed: Abstr.Soc.Geront., Biol.Abstr., Chem.Abstr.
—CASDDS, CISTI, GNLM.
Published by: International Gerontological Think Tank, Center for Experimental Gerontology, c/o Dr H le Compte, Ed, Fabiolalaan 14, Knokke-Zoute 8300, Belgium. Circ: 1,000. **Co-sponsor:** Belgische Vereniging van Geriaters.

610.736 362.6 USA ISSN 1524-2897
REMEMBERING YESTERDAY; recalling those happy memories from the golden age of our past. Text in English. 1989. m. USD 17 (effective 2000). illus. back issues avail. **Document type:** *Newsletter, Consumer.* **Description:** Covers reminiscence groups in long term care or adult day care centers, and contains articles about the eras most residents like to remember.
Published by: Eymann Publications, Inc, PO Box 3577, Reno, NV 89505-3577. TEL 775-358-1554, FAX 775-358-1476, eymann@care4elders.com, http://www.care4elders.com. Ed. Maureen Eng. Pub. Katie Eymann Pace.

RESEARCH AND PRACTICE. see *MEDICAL SCIENCES—Psychiatry And Neurology*

612.67 USA ISSN 0164-0275
HQ1060
RESEARCH ON AGING; a quarterly of social gerontology and adult development. Text in English. 1979. bi-m. USD 80 to individuals; USD 380 to institutions; USD 20 newsstand/cover to individuals; USD 70 newsstand/cover to institutions (effective 2002). adv. bibl, charts, stat, abstr, illus. index. back issues avail.; reprints avail. *Refereed.* **Document type:** *Academic/Scholarly.* **Description:** Presents interdisciplinary research on current issues, methodological and research problems in the study of the elderly.
Related titles: Online - full text ed.: (from EBSCO Publishing, O C L C Online Computer Library Center, Inc., RoweCom Information Quest, ProQuest Information & Learning, Gale Group, ingenta, Swets Blackwell, Institute for Scientific Information).
Indexed: ASCA, Abstr.Anthropol., Abstr.Soc.Geront., AgeLine, Behav.Med.Abstr., Crim.Just.Abstr., Curr.Cont., Environ.Sci.Poll.Mgmt., Excerp.Med., Fam.Ind., Human Resour.Abstr., IMFL, Lang.& Lang.Behav.Abstr., NRN, Pollut.Abstr., PsycInfo, Psychol.Abstr. (1983-), Risk Abstr., SOPODA, SSCI, Sage Fam.Stud.Abstr., Soc.Sci.Ind. (Mar.1987-), Soc.Serv.Abstr., Soc.Work Res.& Abstr., Sociol.Abstr., World Bibl.Soc.Sec., e-psyche.
—BLDSC (7714.385000), GNLM, IDS, ingenta, KNAW. **CCC.**
Published by: Sage Publications, Inc., 2455 Teller Rd, Thousand Oaks, CA 91320. TEL 805-499-0721, FAX 805-499-0871, info@sagepub.com, http://www.sagepub.com. Ed. Angela O'Rand. R&P Tanya Udin. Adv. contact DeAnna Vega Hammersley. Circ: 1,400. **Overseas subscr. to:** Sage Publications Ltd., 6 Bonhill St, London EC2A 4PU, United Kingdom; Sage Publications India Pvt. Ltd., 4215, New Delhi 110 048, India.

306.38 USA
RETIREMENT LIFE (PORTLAND). Text in English. 1973. m. USD 10. adv. bk.rev. illus. **Document type:** *Newspaper.*
Formerly: Senior Citizen News
Address: 10211 S W Barbur, No 205A, Portland, OR 97219-5904. Ed. Dave Moody. Circ: 50,000.

306.38 GBR ISSN 0963-2417
RETIREMENT WORLD✱. Text in English. 1988. m. USD 15.10. **Description:** Features cooking and travel; financial, legal and medical advice.
Published by: Community Publishers Ltd., Brook House, Pennywell Rd, PO Box 215, Bristol, Avon BS99 7QX, United Kingdom. Ed. Tony Ferrand. Circ: 110,000.

612.67 GBR ISSN 0959-2598
RC952.A1 CODEN: RCGEEB
REVIEWS IN CLINICAL GERONTOLOGY. Text in English. 1991. q. GBP 110 to individuals; USD 342 to institutions (effective 2002). adv. **Document type:** *Academic/Scholarly.* **Description:** Dedicated to the advancement of knowledge and clinical practice in the health care of the elderly.
Related titles: Online - full text ed.: (from EBSCO Publishing, O C L C Online Computer Library Center, Inc., RoweCom Information Quest, Swets Blackwell).
Indexed: ASSIA, Abstr.Soc.Geront., CINAHL, Excerp.Med. (1993-), PsycInfo, Psychol.Abstr. (1991-), Sage Fam.Stud.Abstr., e-psyche.
—BLDSC (7788.979000), EMDOCS, GNLM, Infotrieve, KNAW. **CCC.**
Published by: Cambridge University Press, Edinburgh Bldg, Shaftesbury Rd, Cambridge CB2 2RU, United Kingdom. FAX 44-1223-315052, information@cup.cam.ac.uk, information@cambridge.org, http://www.cup.cam.ac.uk, http://www.uk.cambridge.org/journals/pmu. Eds. K. Woodhouse, Raymond Tallis. R&P Linda Nicol. Adv. contact Rebecca Symons.

612.67 ESP ISSN 1130-6882
REVISTA DE GERONTOLOGIA. Text in Spanish; Summaries in English. 1991. q. ESP 5,500, USD 100. adv. bk.rev. bibl, charts.
Published by: S G Editores, Casp, 79 5o, Barcelona 08013, Spain. TEL 343-232-82-51, FAX 343-232-40-20. Ed. Ricard Vinas.

612.67 ESP ISSN 0211-139X
CODEN: REGGDU
REVISTA ESPANOLA DE GERIATRIA Y GERONTOLOGIA. Text in Spanish. 1966. bi-m. ESP 14,900 to individuals; ESP 21,300 to institutions; ESP 11,920 to students (effective 2001). adv. bk.rev. abstr, bibl, charts, illus, stat. back issues avail.; reprints avail. *Refereed.* **Document type:** *Journal, Academic/Scholarly.*
Formerly (until 1976): Revista Espanola de Gerontologia (0034-9410)
Related titles: Online - full text ed.: 1996.
Indexed: Excerp.Med., Ind.Med.Esp., Ref.Zh.
—BLDSC (7854.002500), CINDOC.
Published by: (Sociedad Espanola de Geriatria y Gerontologia), Ediciones Doyma S.A., Traversa de Gracia, 17-21, Barcelona 08021, Spain. TEL 34-93-200-0711, regg@doyma.es, doyma@doyma.es, http://www.doyma.es/regg. Ed. J I Gonzalez Montalvo. R&P Monica Barnes. Adv. contact Jose Antonio Hernandez. B&W page ESP 122,000, color page ESP 152,000; 280 x 210. Circ: 3,000.

618.97 FRA ISSN 0397-7927
REVUE DE GERIATRIE. Text in French. 1954. m. (10/yr.). FRF 500 domestic to doctors; FRF 800 foreign to doctors (effective 2000). adv. bk.rev. charts, illus. index.
Former titles (until 1977): Revue de Gerontologie d'Expression Francaise (0375-975X); (until 1964): Revue Francaise de Gerontologie (0035-2896)
Indexed: Biol.Abstr., Curr.Cont. (coverage dropped), Excerp.Med., Ind.Med. (coverage dropped), Inpharma, Reac., Ref.Zh.
—BLDSC (7918.130000), CISTI, EMDOCS, GNLM, Infotrieve, KNAW. **CCC.**
Published by: Edimedica, 149 bd. Voltaire, Asniers 92600, France. TEL 33-47-935603, FAX 33-47-931728. Ed. F Vidal. Circ: 4,200.

RING DES WORTES; Seelsorgebrief fuer Hoergeschaedigte, Kranke und Senioren. see *RELIGIONS AND THEOLOGY—Roman Catholic*

618.97 ROM ISSN 0254-2307
CODEN: RJGGDV
ROMANIAN JOURNAL OF GERONTOLOGY AND GERIATRICS. Text in English, French. 1980. 4/yr. USD 58. adv. bk.rev. charts, stat. **Document type:** *Academic/Scholarly.*
Indexed: Abstr.Anthropol., Chem.Abstr., Curr.Adv.Ecol.Sci., Excerp.Med., Psychol.Abstr. (1993-).
—CASDDS, CISTI, EMDOCS, GNLM.
Published by: Institutul National de Gerontologie si Geriatrie, Str. Manastirea Caldarusani 9, Bucharest 79605, Romania. TEL 40-1-6665660. Ed. Alexandru Vrabiescu.

612.67 USA ISSN 1091-1146
RX REMEDY; prescriptions for a healthy life. Text in English. 1992. bi-m. USD 18 domestic; USD 36 foreign; USD 3 newsstand/cover (effective 1999). adv. back issues avail. *Refereed.* **Document type:** *Consumer.* **Description:** Provides health information for the over-50s.
Related titles: Online - full text ed.
Published by: MediZine, Inc., 298 Fifth Ave, 2nd Fl, New York, NY 10001. TEL 212-695-2223, FAX 212-695-2936, info@medizine.com, http://www.rxremedy.com/, http://www.medizine.com. adv.: color page USD 55,000; trim 10.5 x 8. Circ: 2,200,000 (controlled).

305.26 USA
▼ **SCIENTIFIC AMERICAN PRESENTS: THE QUEST TO BEAT AGING.** Text in English. 2000. q. USD 5.95 newsstand/cover (effective 2001). adv. **Document type:** *Consumer.*
Published by: Scientific American, Inc., 415 Madison Ave, New York, NY 10017-1111. http://www.sciam.com. Ed. John Rennie.

SEMINARS IN ARTHRITIS & RHEUMATISM. see *MEDICAL SCIENCES—Rheumatology*

SENIOR CITIZEN SENTINEL. see *SOCIAL SERVICES AND WELFARE*

305.26 USA
SENIOR CITIZENS POST. Text in English. 1971. q. membership. illus. **Document type:** *Newspaper.*
Published by: Coordinating Council for Senior Citizens, 807 S Duke St, Durham, NC 27701. TEL 919-688-8247, FAX 919-683-3406. Circ: 1,500 (controlled).

618.97 USA
SENIOR LIFE HEALTH MONITOR. Text in English. q. free. **Document type:** *Newsletter, Consumer.* **Description:** Covers senior citizen health issues such as healthy mind and body, nutrition, care and treatment.
Published by: Data Centrum Communications, Inc., 21 W 38th St, 4th fl, New York, NY 10018. Ed. Barbara Severs.

305.26 ZAF ISSN 0037-2234
SENIOR NEWS. Text in English. 1968; N.S. 1993. q. ZAR 10 (effective 1993). bk.rev. illus. **Document type:** *Newsletter.* **Description:** Articles concerning care of the elderly; news about international congresses.
Published by: (South African Council for the Aged), Public Eye, PO Box 1982, Parklands, Johannesburg 2121, South Africa. TEL 27-11-8809749. Ed. Pinky A C Vilakazi. Circ: 1,600.

362.6 USA
SENIOR NEWS. Text in English. 1988. m. USD 11 (effective 2000). adv. back issues avail. **Document type:** *Newspaper.* **Description:** Covers the many aspects of aging, including medical developments, estate planning, and consumer education.
Address: PO Box 23307, Waco, TX 76702. TEL 254-399-9811, news4srs@aol.com. Pub., Adv. contact Dan McNeil. Circ: 277,000 (controlled).

305.26 USA
SENIOR TIMES (COLUMBUS). Text in English. 1983. m. USD 12.95 (effective 2000). adv. 28 p./no. 6 cols./p. **Document type:** *Newspaper.* **Description:** Offers articles of general interest to senior citizens.
Published by: Senior Publishing Co., PO Box 30965, Columbus, OH 43230. TEL 614-337-2055, FAX 614-337-2059, SeniorTimes@iwaynet.net. Ed. Roberta Keck. Pub. Stephen Pinsky. Adv. contact Angela Miller. B&W page USD 2,100, color page USD 2,450; trim 15 x 11.38. Circ: 30,000.

362.6 USA
SENIOR WORLD OF ORANGE COUNTY; serving older adults in Orange County. Text in English. 1984. m. USD 10 (effective 1997). adv. **Document type:** *Newspaper.* **Description:** News, announcements, and information pertaining to the activities of older adults in this California county, with regular departments on dining, health, finance, travel, housing and lifestyle.
Published by: Kendell Communications Inc., 2000 Powell St Ste 1555, Emeryville, CA 94608-1861. TEL 714-898-2893. Ed. Laura Impastato. Adv. contact Resa Trent. Circ: 115,000.

362.6 USA
SENIOR WORLD OF SAN DIEGO; serving active older adults throughout San Diego County. Text in English. 1973. m. USD 10 (effective 1997). adv. **Document type:** *Newspaper.* **Description:** News, announcements, and information pertaining to the activities of older adults in this California county, with regular departments on dining, health, finance, travel, housing, lifestyle.
Related titles: Microfilm ed.: (from LIB).
Published by: Kendell Communications Inc., 2000 Powell St Ste 1555, Emeryville, CA 94608-1861. TEL 619-593-2900. Ed. Laura Impastato. Adv. contact Resa Trent. Circ: 92,000.

306.38 DEU
SENIOREN ECHO; Nachrichten fuer aeltere Bonner Buerger. Text in German. 1967. bi-m. bk.rev. **Document type:** *Newsletter.*
Published by: Stadtverwaltung Bonn, Stadthaus Amt 13, Berliner Platz, Bonn 53111, Germany. TEL 0228-773460, FAX 0228-772468. Ed. Werner D'hein. Circ: 16,000.

612.67 DEU ISSN 0934-9936
SENIOREN RATGEBER. Text in German. 1978. m. adv. **Document type:** *Consumer.*
Published by: Wort und Bild Verlag Konradshoehe GmbH, Konradshoehe, Baierbrunn 82065, Germany. TEL 49-89-74433-0, FAX 49-89-74433150, http://www.wortundbild.de. Adv. contact Wolfgang Smeilus.

306.38 USA ISSN 1087-9366
SILVER SENTINEL. Text in English. 1995. m. free per issue. bk.rev., music rev., play rev., tel.rev., video rev. charts, illus, stat. 16 p./no. 4 cols./p. **Document type:** *Newspaper.* **Description:** Covers health, finance, travel and senior issues for persons over 55.
Published by: Carousel Publishing Co., PO Box 896, Plaistow, NH 03865. FAX 603-382-2140, cardinal@bit-net, http://www.silversentinel.com. Ed. Joyce Driscoll. Pub., R&P Richard Driscoll. adv.: B&W page USD 790, color page USD 875; trim 15 x 10. Circ: 10,000.

618.97 USA ISSN 1096-0120
SKIN & AGING; the journal of geriatric dermatology. Text in English. 1993. m. USD 71.95; USD 111.95 foreign (effective 1999). adv. reprints avail. *Refereed.* **Document type:** *Trade.*
Formerly (until vol.5, no.8, 1997): Journal of Geriatric Dermatology (1072-8856)
Indexed: Med.& Surg.Dermat.
—BLDSC (8295.905000), CISTI.
Published by: H M P Communications, LLC, 950 W Valley Rd, Ste 2800, Wayne, PA 19087. TEL 610-688-8220, 800-237-7285, FAX 610-688-1060, jpersico@voicenet.com, http://www.medscape.com. Ed. Jack Persico. Pub. Thomas Gangemi. Adv. contact Sherry Shorten. B&W page USD 1,150, color page USD 1,900; trim 11 x 8.13. Circ: 6,902.

306.38 DEU ISSN 0174-0350
DER SONNTAGSBRIEF. Text in German. 1973. m. DEM 146.40. back issues avail.
Published by: Verlag Axel B. Trunkel, Landhausstr 82, Stuttgart 70190, Germany. TEL 0711-26863-0. Ed. Andrea Przyklenk. Circ: 30,000.

306.38 USA
SOUTHERN CALIFORNIA SENIOR LIFE. Text in English. 1983. m. USD 20 (effective 2001). adv. bk.rev. **Document type:** *Consumer.* **Description:** Covers health, travel, leisure, entertainment, financial affairs, legal matters, retirement living, housing, sports, employment, nutrition and political issues.
Published by: Senior Media, Inc., 6022 W Pico Blvd, 7, Los Angeles, CA 90035. TEL 323-933-9228, FAX 323-933-9261, seniorlife@aol.com. Ed. Herb Chase. Circ: 250,000.

612.67 USA ISSN 1070-6127
SOUTHWEST JOURNAL ON AGING. Text in English. 1984. s-a. USD 100 (effective 2000). adv. *Refereed.* **Document type:** *Academic/Scholarly.* **Description:** Each journal focuses on a special issue. Recent topics include: intergenerational issues, programs and policies, ethics and aging, and trends in adult day care.
Incorporates: Expressions; Formerly (until 1993): Southwestern (Denton) (1053-4911)
Indexed: AgeLine.
Published by: Southwest Society on Aging, Oklahoma State University, CHES Rm 139, Stillwater, OK 74078-6116. TEL 405-744-8280, FAX 405-744-6843, loriann@okstate.edu, http://www.swsaging.org. Ed. Ed Folts. R&P, Adv. contact Lance Robertson. Circ: 1,000.

612.67 USA ISSN 0272-5835
SPRINGER SERIES ON ADULTHOOD & AGING. Text in English. 1978. irreg., latest vol.25, 1990. price varies. **Document type:** *Monographic series.* **Description:** Explores issues in the medical and sociological aspects of aging.
Published by: Springer Publishing Company, 536 Broadway, New York, NY 10012. TEL 212-431-4370, FAX 212-941-7842, springer@springerpub.com, http://www.springerpub.com. Ed. Bernard D Starr. R&P Dorothy Kouwenberg.

362.6 USA
SPRINGER SERIES ON ETHICS, LAW, AND AGING. Text in English. 1994. irreg., latest vol.4, 1998. price varies. **Document type:** *Monographic series, Academic/Scholarly.*
Published by: Springer Publishing Company, 536 Broadway, New York, NY 10012. TEL 877-687-7476, FAX 212-941-7842, springer@springerpub.com, http://www.springerpub.com. R&P Dorothy Kouwenberg.

610.7365 USA
SPRINGER SERIES ON GERIATRIC NURSING. Text in English. 1991. irreg., latest vol.4, 1996. price varies. **Document type:** *Monographic series.* **Description:** Covers various aspects and issues of providing nursing for the elderly.
Published by: Springer Publishing Company, 536 Broadway, New York, NY 10012. TEL 212-431-4370, FAX 212-941-7842, springer@springerpub.com, http://www.springerpub.com. Ed. Mathy Mezey. R&P Dorothy Kouwenberg.

612.67 USA
SPRINGER SERIES ON LIFE STYLES & ISSUES ON AGING. Text in English. 1993. irreg., latest vol.5, 1997. price varies. **Document type:** *Monographic series.* **Description:** Explores various issues in the medical and sociological aspects of aging.
Published by: Springer Publishing Company, 536 Broadway, New York, NY 10012. TEL 212-431-4370, FAX 212-941-7842, springer@springerpub.com, http://www.springerpub.com. Ed. Bernard D Starr. R&P Dorothy Kouwenberg.

618.97 GBR
STUDIES IN EDUCATIONAL GERONTOLOGY. Text in English. irreg., latest vol.2, 1995. **Document type:** *Monographic series, Academic/Scholarly.*
—BLDSC.
Published by: Ashgate Publishing Ltd (Subsidiary of: Gower Publishing Co. Ltd.), Gower House, Croft Rd, Aldershot, Hants GU11 3HR, United Kingdom. TEL 44-1252-331551, FAX 44-1252-317446, info@ashgate.com, http://www.ashgate.com. Eds. Frank Glendenning, Ian Stuart Hamilton.

362.6 NLD ISSN 0167-0018
T V B. (Tijdschrift voor Verzorging en Beheer) Text in Dutch. 1971. bi-m. adv. illus. **Document type:** *Journal, Trade.*
Published by: APR Group, Postbus 2696, Amersfoort 3800 GE, Netherlands. TEL 31-33-456-7050, FAX 31-33-456-7433, info@aprgroup.nl, http://www.aprgroup.nl. Ed. Nettie van Doorn. Circ: 3,500 (controlled).

346.013 USA
TAX, ESTATE & FINANCIAL PLANNING FOR THE ELDERLY. Text in English. 1985. base vol. updates 2/yr. **Description:** Covers a broad spectrum of planning areas of special concern to the elderly and their families, including tax and financial planning for retirement; Medicare, Medicaid, nursing home and health care planning; estate planning and lifetime decision making.
Related titles: CD-ROM ed.
Published by: Matthew Bender & Co., Inc. (Subsidiary of: Lexis Law Publishing), 2 Park Ave, New York, NY 10016. TEL 212-448-2000, international@bender.com, http://www.bender.com.

THIS CARING BUSINESS. see *SOCIAL SERVICES AND WELFARE*

155.67 NLD ISSN 0167-9228
NDGEA CODEN: TGEGD
TIJDSCHRIFT VOOR GERONTOLOGIE EN GERIATRIE. Text in Dutch. 1970. bi-m. NLG 136 to individuals; NLG 100 to students (effective 1999). adv. bk.rev. *Refereed.* **Document type:** *Academic/Scholarly.*
Former titles (until 1982): Gerontologie (0168-8774); (until 1980): Nederlands Tijdschrift voor Gerontologie (0378-1186)
Indexed: Excerp.Med., Ind.Med. (1982-), Int.Nurs.Ind., PsycInfo, Psychol.Abstr., e-psyche.
—BLDSC (8841.530000), CISTI, GNLM, KNAW.
Published by: Nederlands Instituut voor Gerontologie, Postbus 222, Utrecht 3500 AE, Netherlands. TEL 31-30-276-9960, FAX 31-30-276-2880, tgg@nig.nl. Eds. Dr. H F A Diesfeldt, Dr. Th A M Vis. Adv. contact B Nitsche. Circ: 1,300.

618.97 USA ISSN 0882-7524
RC952.5
TOPICS IN GERIATRIC REHABILITATION. Text in English. 1985. q. USD 135 to individuals; USD 41 newsstand/cover (effective 2002). illus. reprints avail. *Refereed.* **Document type:** *Journal, Trade.* **Description:** Provides treatment-related information written by and for specialists in all aspects of geriatric care.
Related titles: Online - full text ed.: (from Ovid Technologies, Inc., ProQuest Information & Learning, Institute for Scientific Information).
Indexed: AMED, ASCA, Abstr.Soc.Geront., AgeLine, CINAHL, Curr.Cont., IMFL, SSCI, Viol.& Abuse Abstr.
—BLDSC (8867.441200), CISTI, EMDOCS, GNLM, IDS, Infotrieve, ingenta, KNAW. **CCC.**
Published by: Aspen Publishers, Inc., 200 Orchard Ridge Dr, Ste 200, Gaithersburg, MD 20878. TEL 301-417-7500, 800-638-8437, FAX 301-417-7550, customer.service@aspenpubl.com, http://www.aspenpublishers.com. Pub. Jack Bruggeman. Circ: 2,581 (paid). **Dist. by:** Aspen Publishers Inc., Distribution Center, 7201 McKinney Circle, Frederick, MD 21701. TEL 301-698-7100.

▼ **V O I C E**; victory over incontinence/continence education. see *PUBLIC HEALTH AND SAFETY*

306.38 CAN ISSN 0382-0068
VOICE OF UNITED SENIOR CITIZENS OF ONTARIO* . Text in English. 1969. m. (except July & Aug.). CND 10. adv. illus. **Document type:** *Newsletter.*
Formerly: United Senior Citizens of Ontario. Bulletin (0049-5441)
—CCC.
Published by: (United Senior Citizens of Ontario), Voice Association, 3033 Lakeshore Blvd West, Etobicoke, ON M8V 1K5, Canada. TEL 416-252-2021. Ed. Barb Skelton. Circ: 4,000.

306.38 FRA ISSN 0049-6707
VOIX DU RETRAITE* . Text in French. 1919. m. FRF 115. adv. index.
Published by: Societe de Presse d'Edition et de Diffusion d'Informations Sociales, 20 avenue Edouard Herriot, Le Plessis Robinson 92350, France. Ed. Philippe Agostini. Circ: 25,000.

610.7365 362.6 USA ISSN 1524-2919
VOLUNTEER AND VISTORS' GUIDE. Text in English. 1993. m. USD 29 (effective 2000). illus. back issues avail. **Document type:** *Newsletter, Consumer.* **Description:** Designed to help volunteers and visitors do all they can to help the elderly residents in long term care facilities. Provides insights, information and tips on the aging process, communication, understanding elders and more.
Published by: Eymann Publications, Inc, PO Box 3577, Reno, NV 89505-3577. TEL 775-358-1554, FAX 775-358-1476, eymann@care4elders.com, http://www.care4elders.com. Ed. Maureen Eng. Pub. Katie Eymann Pace.

305.26 USA ISSN 0083-8438
WEST VIRGINIA. COMMISSION ON AGING. ANNUAL PROGRESS REPORT. Text in English. 1961. a. free. **Document type:** *Government.*

Published by: West Virginia, Bureau of Senior Services, c/o James H Shock, Ed, 1900 Kanawha Blvd E, Holly Grove Bldg. 10, Charleston, WV 25305-0160. TEL 304-558-3317. Ed. James H Shock. Circ: 500 (controlled).

612.67 JPN
YOKUFUKAI CHOSA KENKYU KIYO/YOKUFUKAI GERIATRIC JOURNAL. Text in Japanese; Summaries in English. 1930. a. free per issue. **Document type:** *Academic/Scholarly.*
Formerly: Acta Gerontologica Japonica (0001-5768)
Indexed: Biol.Abstr., Chem.Abstr., Excerp.Med.
—BLDSC (9420.800000), GNLM.
Published by: Yokufukai Byoin/Yokufukai Geriatric Hospital, 1-12-1 Takaido-Nishi, Suginami-ku, Tokyo 168-0071, Japan.

612.67 DEU ISSN 0948-6704
RC952 CODEN: ZGERAG
ZEITSCHRIFT FUER GERONTOLOGIE UND GERIATRIE. Text in German; Summaries in English. 1968. bi-m. DEM 598, EUR 305.75, USD 400; USD 78.60 newsstand/cover (effective 2001). adv. bk.rev. illus, abstr. index. back issues avail.; reprint service avail. from ISI. *Refereed.* **Document type:** *Journal, Academic/Scholarly.*
Formerly: Zeitschrift fuer Gerontologie (0044-281X); Incorporates: Aktuelle Gerontologie (0300-5704)
Related titles: Microform ed.: (from PQC); Online - full text ed.: ISSN 1435-1269 (from EBSCO Publishing, RoweCom Information Quest, Swets Blackwell, Springer LINK, Institute for Scientific Information).
Indexed: ASCA, Biol.Abstr., Chem.Abstr., Curr.Cont., Dent.Ind., Excerp.Med., Ger.J.Psych., INIS Atomind., Ind.Med. (1995-), Inpharma, Int.Nurs.Ind., Neurosci.Cit.Ind., Nutr.Abstr., PsycInfo, Psychol.Abstr. (1968-), Reac., SSCI, Sci.Cit.Ind. (coverage dropped), e-psyche.
—BLDSC (9462.740050), CASDDS, CISTI, GNLM, IDS, Infotrieve, KNAW. **CCC.**
Published by: (Deutsche Gesellschaft fuer Gerontologie und Geriatrie), Dr. Dietrich Steinkopff Verlag (Subsidiary of: BertelsmannSpringer), Poststr 9, Darmstadt 64293, Germany. TEL 49-6151-82899-0, FAX 49-6151-82899-40, frey.steinkopff@springer.de, http://www.steinkopff.springer.de. Circ: 1,800. **Subscr. in N. America to:** Springer-Verlag, Journals; **Subscr. to:** Springer GmbH Auslieferungsgesellschaft, Haberstr 7, Heidelberg 69126, Germany. TEL 49-6221-345239, FAX 49-6221-345249, subscriptions@springer.de.

155.67 CHE ISSN 1011-6877
CODEN: ZGPSFB
ZEITSCHRIFT FUER GERONTOPSYCHOLOGIE UND PSYCHIATRIE. Text in English, German. 1988. q. CHF 118 domestic; CHF 148 foreign (effective 2001). adv. back issues avail. **Document type:** *Journal, Academic/Scholarly.*
Indexed: PsycInfo, Psychol.Abstr. (1992-), e-psyche.
—BLDSC (9462.740100), GNLM.
Published by: Hans Huber AG, Laengassstr 76, Bern, 9 3000, Switzerland. TEL 41-31-3004500, FAX 41-31-3004591, zeitschriften@hanshuber.com, http://www.hanshuber.com. Ed. W Oswald. Adv. contact Rene Waelchli. color page DEM 2,540; trim 170 x 250. Circ: 550.

616.716 CHN ISSN 1006-7108
ZHONGGUO GUZHI SHUSONG ZAZHI/CHINESE JOURNAL OF OSTEOPOROSIS. Text in Chinese. 1995 (Oct.). q. CNY 12.50 per issue domestic (effective 2000). back issues avail. **Document type:** *Academic/Scholarly.*
Related titles: Online - full content ed.: (from WanFang Data Corp.).
Published by: Zhongguo Guzhi Shusong Zazhishe, Zhaoyang-qu, Huixinli 38 Hao, Beijing 100029, China. TEL 86-1-64985881. Ed. Zhong Hou Liu. **Co-sponsor:** Zhongguo Laonian Xuehui, Guzhi Shusong Weiyuanhui.

306.38 CHN
ZHONGGUO LAONIAN BAO/CHINA ELDERLY JOURNAL. Text in Chinese. w. CNY 27.24. **Document type:** *Newspaper.*
Address: 34 Fuwai Dajie, Beijing 100832, China. TEL 86-10-831-8325. **Dist. overseas by:** China International Book Trading Corp, 35 Chegongzhuang Xilu, Haidian District, Beijing 100044, China.

618.97 CHN ISSN 0254-9026
ZHONGHUA LAONIAN YIXUE ZAZHI/CHINESE JOURNAL OF GERIATRICS. Text in Chinese; Abstracts in English. 1982. bi-m. CNY 45 domestic; USD 30.60 foreign; CNY 9.80 newsstand/cover domestic; USD 5.10 newsstand/cover foreign (effective 2001). 64 p./no. **Document type:** *Academic/Scholarly.*
Related titles: CD-ROM ed.; Online - full content ed.: (from WanFang Data Corp.).
Indexed: ExtraMED.
Published by: Zhonghua Yixuehui/Chinese Medical Association, Beijing Yiyuan (Beijing Hospital), 1 Dahua Lu, Beijing 100730, China. TEL 86-1-65132266 ext 3892. Ed. Wang Xinde. **Dist. overseas by:** China International Book Trading Corp, 35, Chegongzhuang Xilu, Haidian District, Beijing 100044, China. TEL 86-1-68413849, FAX 86-1-68412048, cibtc@mail.cibtc.com.cn, http://www.cibtc.com.cn.

ZORGVISIE. see *HEALTH FACILITIES AND ADMINISTRATION*

GERONTOLOGY AND GERIATRICS—Abstracting, Bibliographies, Statistics

016.30526 USA ISSN 1047-4862
Z7164.O4
ABSTRACTS IN SOCIAL GERONTOLOGY; current literature on aging. Text in English. 1957. q. USD 110 to individuals; USD 350 to institutions; USD 35 newsstand/cover to individuals; USD 90 newsstand/cover to institutions (effective 2002). illus. index. back issues avail.; reprints avail. **Document type:** *Abstract/Index, Bibliography, Government.* **Description:** Provides abstracts and bibliographies of major articles, books, reports, and other materials on all aspects of gerontology, including demography, economics, family relations, government policy, health, institutional care, physiology, psychiatric dysfunctions, psychology, societal attitudes, work and retirement.
Formerly (until 1990): Current Literature on Aging (0011-3662)
Related titles: Online - full text ed.: (from EBSCO Publishing, O C L C Online Computer Library Center, Inc., RoweCom Information Quest, ProQuest Information & Learning, ingenta, Swets Blackwell).
—CCC.
Published by: (National Council on the Aging), Sage Publications, Inc., 2455 Teller Rd, Thousand Oaks, CA 91320. TEL 805-499-9774, FAX 805-499-0871, info@sagepub.com, http://www.sagepub.com. R&P Tanya Udin. Adv. contact DeAnna Vega Hammersley. Circ: 8,300. **Overseas subscr. to:** Sage Publications Ltd., 6 Bonhill St, London EC2A 4PU, United Kingdom; Sage Publications India Pvt. Ltd., 4215, New Delhi 110 048, India.

016.30526 GBR ISSN 1358-1376
AGE.INFO CD-ROM. Text in English. 1996. 4/yr. GBP 600 (effective 2001 - 2002). **Document type:** *Bibliography.* **Description:** Contains 40,000 references to books, articles, central and local government reports, statistical sources, legislation, and research reports concerned with older age. Includes organisations database and database for calendar of events.
Media: CD-ROM.
Published by: Centre for Policy on Ageing, Centre For Policy On Ageing, Flat 25, 19/23 Ironmonger Row, London EC1V 3QP, United Kingdom. TEL 44-20-7553-6500, FAX 44-20-7553-6501, ageinfo@cpa.org.uk, http://www.cpa.org.uk. Ed. Gillian Crosby.

016.30526 USA
AGELINE. Text in English. 1978. bi-m. **Document type:** *Abstract/Index.* **Description:** Provides almost 60,000 abstracts of current literature on aging.
Media: Online - full text. **Related titles:** CD-ROM ed.: (from SilverPlatter Information, Inc.).
Published by: A A R P, Research, 601 E St, N W, Washington, DC 20049. TEL 202-434-6231, FAX 202-434-6408, ageline@aarp.org, http://research.aarp.org/ageline/about.html. Pub. Margaret N Eccles.

016.61897 USA ISSN 1045-0157
ASSOCIATION FOR GERONTOLOGY IN HIGHER EDUCATION. BRIEF BIBLIOGRAPHY✱. Variant title: Brief Bibliography Series: Selective Annotated Bibliographies for Gerontology Instruction. Text in English. 1985. irreg. USD 10 (effective 1998). back issues avail. *Refereed.* **Document type:** *Bibliography.* **Description:** Provides a series of brief annotated bibliographies on various subject areas related to gerontological instruction.
Published by: Association for Gerontology in Higher Education, 1030 15th St N W, Ste 240, Washington, DC 20005. TEL 202-429-9277. R&P Derek Stepp.

016.15567 BRA
BIBLIOGRAFIA DO IDOSO. Text in Portuguese. 1994. irreg. **Document type:** *Bibliography.* **Description:** Lists all material in the field of gerontology and geriatrics (e.g., books, magazines, articles, theses) available for students, researchers and others in the documentation center for the elderly at the Duarte Library.
Related titles: Diskette ed.
Address: Departamento de Bibl. Publicas, Rua Frei Caneca, 1402 Andar 7, Consolacao, Sao Paulo, SP 01307-002, Brazil. TEL 55-11-253-2331 ext. 264, FAX 55-11-289-4645, bp@prodam.pmsp.sp.gov.br. Circ: 1,500.

016.30526 USA ISSN 0743-7560
BIBLIOGRAPHIES AND INDEXES IN GERONTOLOGY. Text in English. 1985. irreg. price varies. **Document type:** *Monographic series, Bibliography.*
—BLDSC (1993.097370).
Published by: Greenwood Press, Inc. (Subsidiary of: Greenwood Publishing Group Inc.), 88 Post Rd W, Box 5007, Westport, CT 06881. TEL 203-226-3571, FAX 203-226-1502.

016.61897 GBR ISSN 1366-8544
CODEN: HCOPF9
CURRENT MEDICAL LITERATURE. HEALTH CARE OF OLDER PEOPLE. Text in English. 1988. q. USD 60 to individuals; USD 20 newsstand/cover to individuals; USD 140 to institutions; USD 40 newsstand/cover to institutions (effective 2002). back issues avail. **Document type:** *Abstract/Index.*
Formerly: Current Medical Literature. Geriatrics (0953-2501)
—CCC.
Published by: (Royal Society of Medicine), Current Medical Literature Ltd., 40-42 Osnaburgh St, London NW1 3ND, United Kingdom. TEL 44-20-7465-8377, FAX 44-20-7465-8380, enquiries@curmedlit.co.uk. **Dist. by:** Cassis Publishing Ltd., Realpage House, Abingdon Science Park, Barton Ln., Abingdon, Oxon OX13 3NB, United Kingdom. TEL 44-1235-537352, FAX 44-1235-537353.

016.61897 016.3626 NLD ISSN 0014-424X
CODEN: GERGB
EXCERPTA MEDICA. SECTION 20: GERONTOLOGY AND GERIATRICS. Text in English. 1958. 8/yr. EUR 1,084 in Europe to institutions; JPY 143,745 in Japan to institutions; USD 1,213 elsewhere to institutions (effective 2002). adv. index, cum.index. back issues avail. *Refereed.* **Document type:** *Abstract/Index, Academic/Scholarly.* **Description:** Provides a comprehensive current-awareness service of clinical and trade articles covering all clinical aspects of aging and experimental work on the aging process. Mental and emotional problems in the elderly and social and organizational aspects of health care for the aged are also included.
Related titles: CD-ROM ed.: (from SilverPlatter Information, Inc.); Online - full text ed.: (from DIMDI, Data-Star, The Dialog Corporation, JICST).
—GNLM, Infotrieve. **CCC.**
Published by: Excerpta Medica Medical Communications BV (Subsidiary of: Reed Elsevier plc), Rooseveltweg 15, Almere-Stad 1314 SJ, Netherlands. TEL 31-36-538-5600, FAX 31-36-538-5650, http://www.elsevier.com/locate/gerongeria, http://www.excerptamedica.com. **Subscr. in Australasia and the Far East to:** Elsevier Science (Singapore) Pte Ltd, No.1 Temasek Ave, 17-01 Millenia Tower, Singapore 039192, Singapore. TEL 65-434-3727, FAX 65-337-2230; **Subscr. in Japan to:** Elsevier Science Inc - Japan Regional Office, 9-15 Higashi-Azabu 1-chome, Minato-ku, Tokyo 106-0044, Japan. TEL 81-3-5561-5033, FAX 81-3-5561-5047; **Subscr. in the Americas to:** Elsevier Science, PO Box 945, New York, NY 10159-0945. TEL 212-633-3730, 888-437-4636, FAX 212-633-3680, usinfo-f@elsevier.com. **Dist. by:** Elsevier Science (Brazil).; Elsevier Science BV, PO Box 211, Amsterdam 1000 AE, Netherlands. TEL 31-20-485-3757.

016.3626 GBR ISSN 0140-2447
NEW LITERATURE ON OLD AGE. Text in English. 1977. 6/yr. GBP 27.50 domestic; GBP 33 foreign (effective 2000). adv. **Document type:** *Bibliography.* **Description:** Details on new books, government reports and periodical articles. Includes courses and conferences section.
—BLDSC (6084.465000).

Published by: Centre for Policy on Ageing, Centre For Policy On Ageing, Flat 25, 19/23 Ironmonger Row, London EC1V 3QP, United Kingdom. TEL 44-20-7553-6500, FAX 44-20-7553-6501, cpa@cpa.org.uk, gcrosby@cpa.org.uk, http://www.cpa.org.uk. Ed. Gillian Crosby. R&P, Adv. contact Angela Clark. **Subscr. to:** World Wide Subscription Service Ltd., Unit 4, Gibbs Reed Farm, Ticehurst, E Sussex TN5 7HE, United Kingdom.

016.61267 RUS
REFERATIVNYI ZHURNAL. GERONTOLOGIYA. GERIATRIYA. Text in Russian. 1997. bi-m. USD 99 in United States. **Document type:** *Abstract/Index.*
Published by: Vserossiiskii Institut Nauchnoi i Tekhnicheskoi Informatsii (VINITI), Usievicha ul 20-a, Moscow 125315, Russian Federation. TEL 7-095-1526441, FAX 7-095-943-0060. **US dist. addr.:** East View Publications, 3020 Harbor Ln N, Minneapolis, MN 55447. TEL 612-550-0961.

RESIDENTIAL CARE HOMES SCOTLAND. STATISTICAL INFORMATION NOTE. see *SOCIAL SERVICES AND WELFARE—Abstracting, Bibliographies, Statistics*

016.30526 GBR ISSN 0267-0348
SELECTED BIBLIOGRAPHIES ON AGEING. Text in English. 1984. irreg. **Document type:** *Bibliography.*
Published by: Centre for Policy on Ageing, Centre For Policy On Ageing, Flat 25, 19/23 Ironmonger Row, London EC1V 3QP, United Kingdom. TEL 44-20-7553-6500, FAX 44-20-7553-6501, ageinfo@cpa.org.uk, http://www.cpa.org.uk. Ed. Gillian Crosby.

016.61897 DEU ISSN 0721-1872
ZEITSCHRIFTENBIBLIOGRAPHIE GERONTOLOGIE. Text in German. 1977. a. DEM 48. back issues avail. **Document type:** *Bibliography.*
Published by: (Deutsches Zentrum fuer Altersfragen e.V.), Mabuse Verlag GmbH, Kasseler Str 1A, Frankfurt Am Main 60486, Germany. TEL 49-69-7074071, FAX 49-69-704152, mabuse@oeko-net.de, http://www.oeko-net.de/mabuse/. Circ: 1,500.

GIFTWARE AND TOYS

FAMILIE & CO. see *MEDICAL SCIENCES—Pediatrics*

JUNGE FAMILIE; das Baby-Journal. see *MEDICAL SCIENCES—Pediatrics*

KINDER; fuer Eltern, Erzieher und Kinder. see *CHILDREN AND YOUTH—About*

GROCERY TRADE

see FOOD AND FOOD INDUSTRIES—Grocery Trade

GUIDES TO SCHOOLS AND COLLEGES

see EDUCATION—Guides To Schools And Colleges

HANDICAPPED

see also EDUCATION—Special Education And Rehabilitation; HANDICAPPED—Computer Applications; HANDICAPPED—Hearing Impaired; HANDICAPPED—Physically Impaired; HANDICAPPED—Visually Impaired; SOCIAL SERVICES AND WELFARE

362.1 616.8 BEL ISSN 0777-4761
A B P CONTACT. Text in French. 1938. s-a. EUR 12.39 (effective (No. 2001). adv. bk.rev. illus. **Document type:** *Bulletin.* **Description:** Articles concerning activities of the association and information for disabled persons.
Former titles (until 1990): A B P Magazine (0777-4753); A B P - Association Belge des Paralyses. Bulletin (0001-0553)
Indexed: e-psyche.
Published by: Association Belge des Paralyses, Rue Ch De Meer 105-117, Brussels 1020, Belgium. TEL 32-2-421-6965, FAX 32-2-421-6960, daniel.peltzer@skynet.be, abp.asbl@skynet.be. Ed., Pub., R&P, Adv. contact Daniel Peltzer. Circ: 1,000.

362.4 USA
A H A NEWS. (American Hippotherapy Association) Text in English. 1992. 3/yr. membership. bk.rev. **Document type:** *Newsletter.* **Description:** Looks to promote research, education, and communication among physical and occupational therapists, and others utilizing the horse in a treatment approach based on principles of classic hippotherapy.
Indexed: InterActions Bibl. (1992-).
Published by: North American Riding for the Handicapped Association, Inc., American Hippotherapy Association, PO Box 33150, Denver, CO 80233. TEL 800-369-7433, FAX 303-252-4610, narha@narha.org, http://www.narha.org. Ed. Carol Huegel. R&P Pam Simons. Circ: 1,443.

362.4 CAN ISSN 0845-4469
ABILITIES; Canada's lifestyle magazine for people with disabilities. Text in English. 1986. q. CND 26 for 2 yrs. domestic to individuals; USD 26 for 2 yrs. in United States to individuals; USD 31 for 2 yrs. elsewhere to individuals; CND 34 for 2 yrs. domestic to institutions; USD 34 for 2 yrs. in United States to institutions; USD 39 for 2 yrs. elsewhere to institutions; CND 4 newsstand/cover (effective 2000). adv. **Document type:** *Consumer.* **Description:** Covers sports, travel, health, the arts, new technology, services, opportunities for people with disabilities.
Related titles: Audio cassette/tape ed.; Diskette ed.
Indexed: CBCA Ref., Can.Per.Ind. (Mar.1996-).
Published by: Canadian Abilities Foundation, 489 College St, Ste 501, Toronto, ON M6G 1A5, Canada. TEL 416-923-1885, FAX 416-923-9829, able@interlog.com, http://www.abilities.ca/. Ed., R&P Lisa Bendall. Adv. contact Raymond Cohen. Circ: 40,000.

617.087 CAN ISSN 1192-1188
ABILITY NETWORK MAGAZINE; Canada's cross-disability magazine. Text in English. 1991. q. CND 10, USD 18.50; CND 3.50 newsstand/cover (effective 1998). adv. bk.rev. illus. Index. back issues avail.; reprints avail. **Document type:** *Consumer.* **Description:** Written for, by, and about people with disabilities.
Related titles: Braille ed.; Diskette ed.; Online - full text ed.; Talking Book ed.
Published by: Ability Network Publishing Inc., 19 Mount Pleasant Ave, Dartmouth, NS B3A 3T3, Canada. TEL 902-461-9009, FAX 902-461-9484, anet@fox.nstn.ca, http://www.ability.ns.ca. Ed. Spencer Bevan John. Pub. Spencer Bevan-John. Adv. contact Anna Quon. B&W page CND 995; trim 10.5 x 8.5. Circ: 24,000. **Subscr. to:** 21 MicMac Blvd, P O Box 24045, Dartmouth, NS B3A 4T4, Canada.

362.40971 CAN ISSN 1206-0941
ACTIVE LIVING; the health, fitness and recreation magazine for people with a disability. Text in English. 1990. 6/yr. USD 19.97 domestic; USD 39.97 foreign; USD 5.50 newsstand/cover (effective 2000). adv. film rev., software rev. illus. back issues avail. *Refereed.* **Document type:** *Consumer.* **Description:** Contains information about health, fitness & recreation for people with a disability.
Formerly (until 1997): Disability Today (1186-9666)
Indexed: Diver.Y.World.
Published by: Disability Today Publishing Group, 132 Main St East, Ste 1, Grimsby, ON L3M 1P1, Canada. TEL 905-309-1639, FAX 905-309-1640, activeliv@aol.com. Ed. Theresa MacInnis. Pub. Jeffrey Tiessen. Circ: 75,000. **Dist. by:** International Press Publications Inc, 90 Nolan Ct, Ste 21, Markham, ON L3R 4L9, Canada. TEL 800-679-2514, FAX 905-946-9590.

362.4 ARE
AFAQ/HORIZONS. Text in Arabic. 1988. irreg. **Description:** Covers topics concerning the handicapped.
Published by: Center for the Supervision of the Handicapped, P O Box 216-809, Abu Dhabi, United Arab Emirates. TEL 668512. Ed. Amira Al Shibani. Circ: 1,000.

362.4 SWE ISSN 1103-8063
ALLT OM HJAELPMEDEL. Text in Swedish. 1946. 8/yr. SEK 350 (effective 2001). adv. bk.rev. charts, illus, stat. **Document type:** *Magazine, Consumer.* **Description:** Covers issues concerning technical aids for the handicapped in Sweden.
Formerly (until vol.6, 1992): Information om Rehabilitering (0020-0174)
Related titles: Audio cassette/tape ed.
Indexed: Excerp.Med.
Published by: Handikappinstitutet/Swedish Handicap Institute, Sorterargatan 23, Box 510, Vallingby 16215, Sweden. TEL 46-8-620-17-00, FAX 46-8-739-21-52, aoh@hi.se, http://www.hi.se/aoh/Index.asp. Ed. Elisabet Blomberg. Adv. contact Lars-Goeran Fransspn. B&W page SEK 10,900, color page SEK 14,200; trim 183 x 254. Circ: 3,300.

AMERICAN REHABILITATION. see *EDUCATION—Special Education And Rehabilitation*

331 USA
AMERICANS WITH DISABILITIES ACT: EMPLOYEE RIGHTS AND EMPLOYER OBLIGATIONS. Text in English. 1992. base vol. plus a. updates. **Description:** Practical, step-by-step guide to meeting all requirements of the ADA statute relating to the employer-employee relationship.
Related titles: CD-ROM ed.
Published by: Matthew Bender & Co., Inc. (Subsidiary of: Lexis Law Publishing), 2 Park Ave, New York, NY 10016. TEL 212-448-2000, international@bender.com, http://www.bender.com. Ed. Jonathan Mook.

362.4 340 USA
AMERICANS WITH DISABILITIES ACT: PUBLIC ACCOMMODATIONS AND COMMERCIAL FACILITIES. Text in English. 1996. base vol. plus a. updates. **Description:** Analyzes the requirements imposed upon by Title III of the ADA, with specific reference to facilities, goods, programs and services.
Related titles: CD-ROM ed.
Published by: Matthew Bender & Co., Inc. (Subsidiary of: Lexis Law Publishing), 2 Park Ave, New York, NY 10016. TEL 212-448-2000, international@bender.com, http://www.bender.com. Ed. Jonathan Mook.

500 AUS ISSN 1329-0517
ARTS ACCESS NEWS. Text in English. q. AUD 2,530 to individuals; AUD 55 to institutions (effective 2000). bk.rev. **Document type:** *Newsletter.* **Description:** Reports on events, activities, research and opportunities in the arts for people with disabilities and people disadvantaged by social conditions.
Formerly (until 1998): Access (Melbourne) (1038-2860)
Published by: Arts Access Society Inc., 24 Eastern Rd, South Melbourne, VIC 3205, Australia. TEL 61-3-9699-8299, FAX 61-3-9699-8868, artsacc@vicnet.net.au, info@artsaccess.com.au, http://vicnet.net.au/~artsacc, http://www.artsaccess.com.au. Ed., R&P Jane Haley. Circ: 1,500 (controlled).

DAS BAND. see *EDUCATION—Special Education And Rehabilitation*

617.03 USA
C P D NEWS. (Center for Persons with Disabilities) Text in English. 1992 (vol.15, no.2). q. free. **Document type:** *Newsletter, Academic/Scholarly.* **Description:** Designed for professionals and paraprofessionals.
Formerly: Exceptional News
Published by: Center for Persons with Disabilities, Outreach, Development & Dissemination Division, Utah State University, Logan, UT 84322-6845. TEL 435-797-1991, FAX 435-797-2044. Ed. Marlene Deer. Circ: 2,700.

362.4 USA
C S D NEWSLETTER. Text in English. 1978. q. membership. bk.rev.
Published by: Coalition on Sexuality and Disability, Inc., 122 E 23rd St, New York, NY 10010. TEL 212-242-3900. Ed. Pamela Boyle. Circ: 300.

362.4 USA
THE CAPSTONE (TOWSON); news from the Council, and its accreditation and evaluation systems and ProLerna. Text in English. 1980. q. free. **Document type:** *Newsletter.* **Description:** Provides highlights not only on the achievements made by the Council, but also individual stories depicting how personal outcomes have helped change the lives of people.
Formerly: Outlook on Quality and Leadership and Accreditation Council on Services for People with Disabilities: Update on Quality
Indexed: Diver.Y.World.
Published by: Council on Quality and Leadership in Supports for People with Disabilities, 100 West Rd., Ste. 406, Towson, MD 21204-2331. TEL 410-583-0060, FAX 410-583-0063, info@thecouncil.org, http://www.thecouncil.org. Ed. Shelly McLaughlin.

CARERS IN VICTORIA. see *SOCIAL SERVICES AND WELFARE*

H

D P H D NEWSLETTER. (Council for Exceptional Children) see *EDUCATION—Special Education And Rehabilitation*

362.4 UKR
DEFEKTOLOGIYA. Text in Ukrainian. q. USD 95 in United States.
Published by: Ministerstvo Prosveshcheniya Ukrainy, Pr Pobedy 10, Kiev, Ukraine. TEL 224-93-35. **US dist. addr.:** East View Publications, 3020 Harbor Ln N, Minneapolis, MN 55447. TEL 612-550-0961.

362.4 GBR ISSN 0309-4413
DIRECTORY FOR DISABLED PEOPLE. Text in English. 1977. irreg., latest vol.7, 1995. USD 46.95 (effective 1999). **Document type:** *Directory.* **Description:** Contains information and lists opportunities for disabled and handicapped people.
—BLDSC (3593.412000).
Published by: (Royal Association for Disability and Rehabilitation (RADAR)), Prentice Hall - Harvester Wheatsheaf (Subsidiary of: Simon and Schuster International), Campus 400 Maylands Ave, Hemel Hempstead, Herts HP3 8LA, United Kingdom. TEL 44-1442-881900, FAX 44-1442-252544, TELEX 82445. Ed. Clare Grist. Pub. Rupert Knight. Circ: 2,500.

362.4 GBR
DIRECTORY OF AIDS FOR DISABLED AND ELDERLY PEOPLE. Text in English. 1986. irreg. USD 45.95 (effective 1999). **Document type:** *Directory.* **Description:** A wide-ranging directory of equipment helpful to disabled people and others with difficulties in daily living.
Published by: Prentice Hall - Harvester Wheatsheaf (Subsidiary of: Simon and Schuster International), Campus 400 Maylands Ave, Hemel Hempstead, Herts HP3 8LA, United Kingdom. TEL 44-1442-881900, FAX 44-1442-252544. Ed. Clare Grist. Pub. Rupert Knight. Circ: 2,500.

362.4 CAN ISSN 1207-7267
DIRECTORY OF DISABILITY ORGANIZATIONS IN CANADA. Text in English. 1996. every 2 yrs. **Document type:** *Directory.*
Published by: Canadian Abilities Foundation, 489 College St, Ste 501, Toronto, ON M6G 1A5, Canada. TEL 416-923-1885, FAX 416-923-9829, able@interlog.com, http://www.abilities.ca/. Ed. Lisa Bendall.

DIRECTORY OF FEDERAL AID FOR THE HANDICAPPED. see *SOCIAL SERVICES AND WELFARE*

362.4 USA
DIRECTORY OF INFORMATION RESOURCES FOR THE HANDICAPPED. Text in English. irreg. **Document type:** *Directory.*
Published by: Ready Reference Press, PO Box 5169, Santa Monica, CA 90405.

617.087 615.8 GBR ISSN 0963-8288 CODEN: DREHET
DISABILITY AND REHABILITATION. Text in English. 1979. 18/yr. GBP 621, USD 1,024 to institutions (effective 2002). adv. bk.rev. *Refereed.* **Document type:** *Academic/Scholarly.* **Description:** Seeks to encourage a better understanding of all aspects of disability and to promote the rehabilitation process.
Former titles (until 1991): International Disability Studies (0259-9147); (until 1987): International Rehabilitation Medicine (0379-0797)
Related titles: Online - full text ed.: ISSN 1464-5165 (from CatchWord Ltd., EBSCO Publishing, O C L C Online Computer Library Center, Inc., RoweCom Information Quest, Swets Blackwell, Institute for Scientific Information).
Indexed: AMED, ASCA, AgeLine, CINAHL, Curr.Cont., ERA, Ergon.Abstr., Excerp.Med., Ind.Med. (1992-), Int.Nurs.Ind., PsycInfo, SSCI, Sp.Ed.Needs Abstr., e-psyche.
—BLDSC (3595.420300), CatchWord, CISTI, EMDOCS, GNLM, IDS, Infotrieve, ingenta, KNAW. **CCC.**
Published by: Taylor & Francis Group, Taylor & Francis Ltd., 11 New Fetter Ln, London EC4P 4EE, United Kingdom. TEL 44-20-7583-9855, FAX 44-20-7842-2298, info@tandf.co.uk, http://www.tandf.co.uk. Ed. Dave Muller. **Subscr. in N. America to:** Taylor & Francis Ltd., 325 Chestnut St, Suite 800, Philadelphia, PA 19016. TEL 800-354-1420, FAX 215-625-8914, info@taylorandfrancis.com, http://www.taylorandfrancis.com/.

368.3 344 USA ISSN 1055-9779
DISABILITY COMPLIANCE BULLETIN. Text in English. 1991. bi-w. USD 170 (effective 2000). bk.rev. back issues avail. **Document type:** *Newsletter.* **Description:** Reports & analysis of litigation brought under the Americans with Disabilities Act, Office for Civil Rights, Department of Transportation, Department of Health & Human Services & other relevant federal & state agencies.
Related titles: Online - full text ed.: (from LexisNexis).
—CCC.
Published by: L R P Publications, 747 Dresher Rd, Box 980, Horsham, PA 19044. TEL 215-784-0941, 800-341-7874, FAX 215-784-9014, custserve@lrp.com, http://www.lrp.com. Ed. Tom D'Agostino.

368.3 344 USA ISSN 1063-2506
DISABILITY LAW COMPLIANCE REPORT. Text in English. 1992. m. USD 168; USD 218 foreign. index. back issues avail. **Document type:** *Newsletter.* **Description:** Analyzes recent court interpretations of the Americans with Disabilities Act of 1990.
Related titles: Microfiche ed.: (from WSH).
Published by: Warren, Gorham and Lamont, 395 Hudson St, New York, NY 10014. TEL 212-367-6300, FAX 212-9367-6718. Ed. Gary S Marx. **Subscr. to:** The Park Square Bldg., 31 St James Ave, Boston, MA 02116-4112. TEL 800-950-1207.

617.087 362.4 618.2 GBR ISSN 0968-7653
DISABILITY, PREGNANCY & PARENTHOOD INTERNATIONAL; a forum for disabled parents and professionals to exchange information and experience. Text in English. 1993. q. GBP 15 in United Kingdom to individuals; GBP 17.50 to individuals rest of Europe; GBP 19.50 elsewhere to individuals; GBP 25 in United Kingdom to institutions; GBP 27.50 to institutions rest of Europe; GBP 29.50 elsewhere to institutions; GBP 10 in United Kingdom to disabled person; GBP 12.50 rest of Europe (to disabled person); GBP 14.50 elsewhere to disabled person (effective 2001). bk.rev., video rev., Website rev. back issues avail. *Refereed.* **Document type:** *Journal, Consumer, Trade.* **Description:** Promotes better awareness and support of disabled people in pregnancy and parenthood.
Related titles: Audio cassette/tape ed.: Free to registered blind.
—BLDSC (3595.421900).
Published by: D P P I, National Centre for Disabled Parents, Unit F9, 89/93 Fonthill Rd, London N4 3JH, United Kingdom. TEL 0800-018-4730 (helpline), 0800-018-9949 (text), 44-20-7263-3088, FAX 44-20-7263-6399, editor@dppi.org.uk, http://www.dppi.org.uk. Ed. Christine Winwood. Circ: 300 (paid); 115 (controlled).

362.4 020 USA ISSN 1070-7220
DISABILITY RESOURCES MONTHLY; the newsletter that monitors, reviews and reports on resources for independent living. Text in English. 1993. m. USD 30 domestic; USD 40 foreign (effective 2001). bk.rev. index. back issues avail. **Document type:** *Newsletter.* **Description:** Features short topical articles and news about books, pamphlets, periodicals, videotapes, online services, organizations and other resources for and about people with disabilities.
Related titles: Audio cassette/tape ed.
Published by: Disability Resources, 4 Glatter Ln, Centereach, NY 11720-1032. TEL 631-585-0290, FAX 631-585-0290, info@disabilityresources.org, http://www.disabilityresources.org. Ed. Julie Klauber.

362.4 GBR
DISABILITY UPDATE. Text in English. fortn. GBP 30; GBP 40 foreign. back issues avail. **Document type:** *Bulletin.* **Description:** Current awareness bulletin with media round-up.
Media: E-mail. **Related titles:** Audio cassette/tape ed.; Braille ed.; Diskette ed.
Published by: Greater London Association for the Disabled, London, 336 Brixton Rd, London SW9 7AA, United Kingdom. TEL 44-171-346-5813, FAX 44-171-346-5810, glad@btinternet.com. Ed. Steven Knopf. Circ: 300 (paid).

DISABLED GRADUATES CASEBOOK. see *EDUCATION—Higher Education*

362.4 616.858 NLD ISSN 1382-1903
DOWN & UP. Text in Dutch. 1988. q. EUR 25; EUR 30 foreign (effective 2001). adv. charts, illus. 64 p./no. back issues avail. **Document type:** *Newsletter, Consumer.* **Description:** Offers parents and caregivers of children with Down's syndrome advice and emotional support.
Indexed: e-psyche.
Published by: Stichting Down's Syndroom, Bovenboerseweg 41, Wanneperveen 7946 AL, Netherlands. TEL 31-522-281337, FAX 31-522-281799, info@downsyndroom.nl, http://www.downsyndroom.nl. Ed., Pub. Erik de Graaf. Adv. contact E de Graaf. B&W page NLG 1,000. Circ: 3,300 (paid).

EASTER SEALS - MARCH OF DIMES NATIONAL COUNCIL. ANNUAL REPORT. see *EDUCATION—Special Education And Rehabilitation*

EXCEPTIONAL PARENT; the magazine for families and professionals. see *EDUCATION—Special Education And Rehabilitation*

FLORIDA SCHOOL HERALD. see *EDUCATION—Special Education And Rehabilitation*

362.2 USA
FOCAL POINT; a national bulletin on family support and children's mental health. Text in English. s-a. free. back issues avail. *Refereed.* **Document type:** *Bulletin, Government.*
Media: Online - full text.
Published by: U.S. Department of Education, National Institute on Disability and Rehabilitation Research, Research and Training Center on Family Support and Children's Mental Health, RRI, Portland State University, PO Box 751, Portland, OR 97201-0751. TEL 503-725-4040, FAX 503-725-4175, schmitd@rri.pdx.edu, http://www.rtc.pdx.edu/fp/welcome.htm. Ed. Denise Schmidt. Circ: 25,000.

FOCUS: LIBRARY SERVICE TO OLDER ADULTS, PEOPLE WITH DISABILITIES. see *LIBRARY AND INFORMATION SCIENCES*

GUIA DE FORNECEDORES HOSPITALARES. see *GERONTOLOGY AND GERIATRICS*

362.4 617.087 NLD ISSN 1380-6661
HANDICAP & BELEID; tijdschrift voor beleidmakers en dienstverleners. Text in Dutch. 1954. 10/yr. free to qualified personnel. adv. bk.rev. illus. **Document type:** *Trade.* **Description:** Offers news, product information, analysis, opinion, and background information for policymakers, support personnel, and assistants in caring for persons with handicaps.
Supersedes (in 1994): Hefaistos (0928-6659); Which was formed by the merger of (1977-1992): Brandpunt (0166-3453); (1986-1992): Handicap Magazine (0920-4202); Which was formed by the merger of (1984-1986): Grip (0920-4261); And (1977-1986): R - Maandblad voor Revalidatie (0165-1382); Which was formerly (until 1976): Revalidatie (0304-503X); (1954-1971): Tijdscrift voor Revalidatie
Published by: Elsevier Gezondheidszorg B.V., Tijdstroom (Subsidiary of: Reed Elsevier plc Group), Planetenbaan 1, Maarssen 3600 AK, Netherlands. TEL 31-346-577577, FAX 31-346-554287, http://www.tijdstroom.nl. Ed. W Schepers. Pub. K Piebenga. Circ: 1,500. **Subscr. to:** Elsevier Den Haag, Postbus 16500, The Hague 2500 BM, Netherlands. TEL 31-70-381-9900, FAX 31-70-333-8399.

796.060489 DNK ISSN 0902-5618
HANDICAP IDRAET. Text in Danish. 1977. 8/yr. DKK 160. adv. **Document type:** *Bulletin.*
Formerly (until 1988): Handicap Information (0106-3197)
Published by: Dansk Handicap Idraets Forbund, Idraettens Hus, Brondby 2605, Denmark. Ed. Karin Moeller Olsen. Circ: 7,000.

HANDICAP IDRETT. see *EDUCATION—Special Education And Rehabilitation*

362.4 USA ISSN 0896-131X
HANDICAP NEWS. Text in English. 1984. m. USD 12.50; USD 35 foreign. adv. bk.rev.
Published by: Phyllis Burns, Ed. & Pub., 3060 E Bridge, Ste 342, Brighton, CO 80601-2724. Circ: 400.

362.4 BEL ISSN 0779-3367
HANDISCOOP. Text in Dutch. 1945. 10/yr. BEF 520 (effective 2000). adv. bk.rev. illus. **Document type:** *Newsletter.* **Description:** Covers issues relating to social services for the disabled and their integration into society.
Formerly (until 1993): K V G Blad (0779-3359)
Related titles: Audio cassette/tape ed.
Published by: Katholieke Vereniging Gehandicapten, Vormingsbeweging vzw, Arthur Goemaerelei 66, Antwerp 2018, Belgium. TEL 32-3-216-2990, FAX 32-3-248-1442. Ed., Adv. contact Lief Vanbael. Circ: 35,000.

I T - INVALIDITYOE. see *SOCIAL SERVICES AND WELFARE*

362.4 AUS ISSN 0815-2276
INDEPENDENT LIVING. Text in English. 1984. q. AUD 35; AUD 45 in New Zealand; AUD 52 elsewhere (effective 2000). adv. bk.rev. cum.index: 1994-1999. **Document type:** *Trade.* **Description:** Information on equipment, resources and environmental design for people with disabilities, caregivers, health professionals, builders and architects.
Published by: Independent Living Centre N.S.W. (Inc.), PO Box 3163, Putney, NSW 2112, Australia. TEL 61-2-9808-2233, FAX 61-2-9809-7132, ilcnsw@bigpond.com.au. Ed., R&P Jane Bringolf TEL 61-2-9807-3592. Adv. contact Elizabeth Kilian. Circ: 2,500.

362.4 ESP
INTEGRA; boletin de noticias. Text in Spanish. 1997. q. free per issue. back issues avail. **Document type:** *Newsletter.* **Description:** Undertakes specialized research and training offers and discusses efforts to offer technical support that promotes, increases, and facilitates living conditions for disadvantaged persons with physical, psychiatric, and sensory disabilities.
Related titles: Online - full text ed.
Published by: Universidad de Salamanca, Instituto Universitario de Integracion en la Comunidad (INICO)/University of Salamanca, Institute on Community Integration, Facultad de Psicologia, Avda Merced, 109-131, Salamanca 37005, Spain. TEL 34-923-294695, FAX 34-923-294685, davidapa@gugu.usal.es, http://www.usal.es/inico/newsletter/newsletter.html. Ed. David Aparicio Sanchez. Circ: 1,500.

362.4 658 USA ISSN 0732-8826
RD701.N8
INTERNATIONAL CENTER FOR THE DISABLED. ANNUAL REPORT. Text in English. 1972. a. **Document type:** *Corporate.*
Formerly (until 1980): I C D Rehabilitation and Research Center. Annual Report (0163-0806)
Published by: International Center for the Disabled, Public Relations, 340 E 24th St, New York, NY 10010.

INTERNATIONAL JOURNAL OF DISABILITY, DEVELOPMENT AND EDUCATION. see *EDUCATION—Special Education And Rehabilitation*

615.8 USA ISSN 1068-9591
RM930.A1 CODEN: IJRHEP
INTERNATIONAL JOURNAL OF REHABILITATION AND HEALTH. Text in English. 1994. q. USD 240, EUR 239.50 to institutions for print or online ed.; USD 288, EUR 288 to institutions for print & online eds. combimed (effective 2002). adv. *Refereed.* **Document type:** *Journal, Academic/Scholarly.* **Description:** Publishes articles and case studies addressing rehabilitation psychology and general rehabilitation issues, including diagnostic questions, physical, emotional, cognitive and sociological factors.
Formerly (until 1995): Journal of Rehabilitation & Health
Related titles: Microfilm ed.: (from PQC); Online - full text ed.: (from O C L C Online Computer Library Center, Inc., Swets Blackwell, Kluwer Online, RoweCom Information Quest).
Indexed: AMED, CINAHL, Excerp.Med. (1996-), e-psyche.
—BLDSC (4542.525900), EMDOCS, GNLM, Infotrieve, ingenta. **CCC.**
Published by: Kluwer Academic - Plenum Publishers (Subsidiary of: Wolters Kluwer N.V.), 233 Spring St, New York, NY 10013-1578. TEL 212-620-8000, 800-221-9369, FAX 212-463-0742, info@plenum.com, http://www.wkap.nl/journalhome.htm/1068-9591. Ed. Anthony J Goreczny. R&P Rose Luongo TEL 781-871-6311. **Subscr. outside the Americas to:** Kluwer Academic Publishers Group, Journals Department, PO Box 322, Dordrecht 3300 AH, Netherlands. TEL 31-78-639-2392, FAX 31-78-654-6474.

INTERNATIONAL JOURNAL OF REHABILITATION RESEARCH. see *MEDICAL SCIENCES—Physical Medicine And Rehabilitation*

362.3 USA ISSN 1056-263X
HV1551 CODEN: JDPDE6
JOURNAL OF DEVELOPMENTAL AND PHYSICAL DISABILITIES. Text in English. 1988. q. USD 355, NLG 781, EUR 354.50 to institutions for print or online ed.; USD 426, NLG 937.20, EUR 425.40 to institutions for print & online eds.combined (effective 2001). adv. bk.rev. bibl, charts, illus. index. back issues avail. *Refereed.* **Document type:** *Journal, Academic/Scholarly.* **Description:** Reports the latest developments, methodologies and technologies for professionals in all fields working with disabled persons, including comprehensive coverage of original research and clinical reports involving persons with multiple handicaps.
Formerly (until 1992): Journal of the Multihandicapped Person (0892-7561)
Related titles: Microfilm ed.: (from PQC); Online - full text ed.: (from EBSCO Publishing, O C L C Online Computer Library Center, Inc., RoweCom Information Quest, Swets Blackwell, Kluwer Online, Institute for Scientific Information).
Indexed: ASCA, Curr.Cont., Fam.Ind., IMFL, Indian Psychol.Abstr., PsycInfo, Psychol.Abstr. (1989-), SSCI, e-psyche.
—BLDSC (4969.290200), GNLM, IDS, Infotrieve, ingenta. **CCC.**
Published by: Kluwer Academic - Plenum Publishers (Subsidiary of: Wolters Kluwer N.V.), 233 Spring St, New York, NY 10013-1578. TEL 212-620-8000, 800-221-9369, FAX 212-463-0742, info@plenum.com, http://www.wkap.nl/journalhome.htm/1056-263X. Eds. Michel Hersen, Vincent B Van Hasselt. R&P Rose Luongo TEL 781-871-6311. **Subscr. outside the Americas to:** Kluwer Academic Publishers Group, Journals Department, PO Box 322, Dordrecht 3300 AH, Netherlands. TEL 31-78-639-2392, FAX 31-78-654-6474.

617.087 615.8 GBR ISSN 1470-8558
▼ **JOURNAL OF DISABILITY AND ORAL HEALTH.** Text in English. 2000. biennial.
Published by: British Society for Disability & Oral Health, The Dental School, Framlington Place, Newcastle-upon-Tyne NE2 4BW, United Kingdom. Ed. Dr. June Nunn.

362.4 340 USA ISSN 1044-2073
HV1551 CODEN: JDPSEH
JOURNAL OF DISABILITY POLICY STUDIES. Text in English. 1990. 4/yr., latest vol.12. USD 43 in North America to individuals; USD 71 elsewhere to individuals; USD 109 in North America to institutions; USD 138 elsewhere to institutions (effective 2002). adv. bk.rev. 64 p./no. back issues avail. *Refereed.* **Document type:** *Journal, Academic/Scholarly.* **Description:** Publishes research, discussion and review articles, and brief reports pertaining to both macro- and micro-policy issues affecting people with disabilities.
Related titles: Online - full text ed.: (from CatchWord Ltd.).
Indexed: Diver.Y.World, Except.Child Educ.Abstr., Lang.& Lang.Behav.Abstr., P.A.I.S., PsycInfo, Psychol.Abstr. (1993-), SOPODA, Soc.Serv.Abstr., Sociol.Abstr., e-psyche.
—Infotrieve, ingenta. **CCC.**
Published by: Pro-Ed Inc., 8700 Shoal Creek Blvd, Austin, TX 78757-6897. TEL 512-451-3246, FAX 512-451-8542, proed1@aol.com, http://www.proedinc.com. Ed. Kay Fletcher Schriner. R&P Barbara Rivera TEL 512-451-3246 ext 653. Adv. contact Melissa Tullos. Circ: 500.

JOURNAL OF LEARNING DISABILITIES. see *EDUCATION—Special Education And Rehabilitation*

JOURNAL OF REHABILITATION. see *MEDICAL SCIENCES—Physical Medicine And Rehabilitation*

JOURNAL OF RELIGION, DISABILITY & HEALTH; bridging clinical practice and spiritual supports. see *RELIGIONS AND THEOLOGY*

362.4 808 700 USA ISSN 0748-8742
PS153.P48
KALEIDOSCOPE (AKRON); exploring the experience of disability through literature and the fine arts. Text in English. 1979. s-a. USD 10 domestic to individuals; USD 15 in Canada to individuals; USD 18 elsewhere to individuals; USD 15 domestic to institutions; USD 20 in Canada to institutions; USD 23 elsewhere to institutions (effective 2001). bk.rev. back issues avail. **Document type:** *Consumer.* **Description:** Explores the experience of disability through literature and the fine arts. Expresses the experiences of disability from the perspective of individuals, families, healthcare professionals, and society as a whole.
Related titles: Audio cassette/tape ed.
Indexed: Amer.Hum.Ind. (1986-), Ind.Amer.Per.Verse.
—ingenta.
Published by: (United Disability Services), Kaleidoscope Press (Akron), 701 S Main St, Akron, OH 44311-1019. TEL 330-762-9755, FAX 330-762-0912, mshiplett@udsakron.org, pboerner@udsakron.org. Ed. Dr. Darshan Perusek. Pub. Gary M Knuth. R&P Gail Willmott. Circ: 1,000 (paid and controlled).

362.4 GBR
KEY NOTE MARKET REPORT: EQUIPMENT FOR THE DISABLED. Variant title: Equipment for the Disabled. Text in English. 1995. irreg., latest vol.2, 1999. GBP 265 (effective 1999). **Document type:** *Trade.*
Published by: Key Note Ltd., Field House, 72 Oldfield Rd, Hampton, Mddx TW12 2HQ, United Kingdom. TEL 44-20-8481-8750, FAX 44-20-8783-0049, http://www.keynote.co.uk. Ed. Donna Jones.

362.4 616.8 DEU
LEBENSWELTEN BEHINDERTER MENSCHEN. Text in German. 1997. irreg., latest vol.6, 1999. **Document type:** *Monographic series, Academic/Scholarly.*
Published by: Attempto Verlag, Dischingerweg 5, Tuebingen 72070, Germany. TEL 49-7071-9797-0, FAX 49-7071-75288, narr-francke@t-online.de, http://www.francke.de.

618.92 GBR ISSN 1360-323X
LINK (LONDON, 1966); the magazine for people with Spina Bifida and/or Hydrocephalus. Text in English. 1966. bi-m. GBP 4.80 domestic; GBP 7.50 foreign (effective 2001). adv. bk.rev. 24 p./no. back issues avail. **Document type:** *Magazine.*
Related titles: Audio cassette/tape ed.
Published by: Association for Spina Bifida and Hydrocephalus, 42 Park Rd, Peterborough, Cambs PE1 2UQ, United Kingdom. TEL 44-1733-555988, FAX 44-1733-555985, lizc@asbah.org, http://www.asbah.org/. Ed. Liz Cawthorne. Circ: 5,000.

362.4 GBR
LONDON DISABILITY NEWS. Text in English. 1989. m. GBP 6 to individuals; GBP 12 to institutions (effective 1999). adv. bk.rev., film rev., video rev. **Document type:** *Newspaper, Consumer, Trade.* **Description:** For disabled people and those who work with them. Includes news, letters, activities, and events.
Formerly (until 1989): G L A D Newsletter
Published by: Greater London Association for the Disabled, London, 336 Brixton Rd, London SW9 7AA, United Kingdom. TEL 44-171-346-5813, FAX 44-171-346-5810, glad@btinternet.com. adv.: page GBP 380. Circ: 5,000.

362.4 NLD ISSN 0925-0824
MAATGEVEND. Text in Dutch. 1989. 8/yr. NLG 30 (effective 1999). bk.rev. *Refereed.* **Document type:** *Newsletter.* **Description:** Deals with self-help groups, disabled organizations, and patient organizations.
Related titles: Diskette ed.
Published by: Stichting Symbiose, Unit P C G, Postbus 5086, Sittard 6130 PB, Netherlands. TEL 31-46-420-8000, FAX 31-46-420-8080, pvdh@symbiose.nl, http://www.symbiose.nl. Ed. Paul van der Hijden. Circ: 1,550.

362.4 USA
▼ **MAINSTREAM ONLINE**; news & advocacy in disability rights. Text in English. 2000. irreg. Free. **Document type:** *Magazine, Consumer.* **Description:** Contains news and issues related to disabilities and person with disabilities, covering such topics as law, medical and health issues.
Media: Online - full content.
Published by: Exploding Myths, Inc., 2973 Beech St, San Diego, CA 92102. editor@mainstream-mag.com, http://www.mainstream-mag.com/.

362.4 ARE
AL-MANAAL/HOPE. Text in Arabic. 1980. m. **Description:** Publishes research and articles on assistance to the handicapped in the U.A.E.
Published by: Human Services Office, PO Box 5696, Sharjah, United Arab Emirates. TEL 353072. Ed. Gamila M Al Qasimi. Circ: 2,000.

MEDICAL AND DISABILITY APPEAL TRIBUNALS: THE LEGISLATION. see *SOCIAL SERVICES AND WELFARE*

MENTAL RETARDATION AND DEVELOPMENTAL DISABILITIES (NEW YORK, 1995); research reviews. see *MEDICAL SCIENCES—Psychiatry And Neurology*

MISSOURI RECORD. see *HANDICAPPED—Hearing Impaired*

N A M I CALIFORNIA. JOURNAL. see *MEDICAL SCIENCES—Psychiatry And Neurology*

N A R H A NEWS. see *SPORTS AND GAMES—Horses And Horsemanship*

N A R H A STRIDES. see *SPORTS AND GAMES—Horses And Horsemanship*

371.9 020 USA
NATIONAL INFORMATION CENTER FOR CHILDREN AND YOUTH WITH DISABILITIES. TRANSITION SUMMARY. Text in English. 1985. a. price varies. back issues avail. **Document type:** *Newsletter.* **Description:** Discusses specific aspects of youth with disabilities making the transition from school to the adult world.
Formerly: National Information Center for Children and Youth with Handicaps. Transition Summary
Published by: National Information Center for Children and Youth with Disabilities (NICHCY), PO Box 1492, Washington, DC 20013. TEL 202-884-8200, 800-695-0285, FAX 202-884-8441, nichcy@aed.org, http://www.nichy.org. Ed. Lisa Kupper. Circ: 20,000.
Co-sponsor: U.S. Department of Education.

H

615.82 JPN ISSN 0285-1350
NATIONAL REHABILITATION CENTER FOR THE DISABLED. RESEARCH BULLETIN. Text in English, Japanese. 1980. a. free per issue. *Refereed.* **Document type:** *Bulletin, Academic/Scholarly.*
Published by: National Rehabilitation Center for the Disabled, 1 Namiki, 4 Chrome, Tokorozawa, Saitama 359-8555, Japan. TEL 81-429-95-3100, FAX 81-429-95-3102, head@rehab.go.up, http://www.rehab.go.jp. Ed. S Yamauchi. R&P Shigin Yamauchi. Circ: 500.

362.4 NLD
NEDERLANDS TIJDSCHRIFT VOOR DE ZORG AAN VERSTANDELIJK GEHANDICAPTEN. Text in Dutch. 1974. q. NLG 65 to individuals; NLG 100 to institutions. adv. bk.rev. back issues avail. *Refereed.* **Document type:** *Academic/Scholarly.*
Former titles (until 1995): Nederlands Tijdschrift voor Zwakzinnigenzorg (0923-2370); (until 1989): Ruit (0166-7270); Incorporates (in 1981): Tijdschrift voor Zwakzinnigheid, Autisme en Andere Ontwikkelingsstoornissen (0166-4085); Which was formerly (1963-1976): Tijdschrift voor Zwakzinnigheid en Zwakzinnigenzorg (0304-467X)
—KNAW.
Published by: Van Gorcum Publishers, PO Box 43, Assen 9400 AA, Netherlands. TEL 31-592-379555, FAX 31-592-379552, info@vangorcum.nl, assen@vgorchum.nl, http://www.vangorcum.nl, http://www.vgorcum.nl. Ed. Dr. M J M Schuurman. Adv. contact E Vankesteren.

362.43 617.087 USA ISSN 1086-4741
HV3011
NEW MOBILITY; total resource magazine for the disability community. Text in English. 1989. m. USD 27.95 domestic; USD 35.95 in Canada; USD 57.95 elsewhere (effective 2001). adv. bk.rev., Website rev. illus. back issues avail.; reprints avail. **Document type:** *Magazine, Consumer.* **Description:** Fosters a sense of community among the disabled, and reports medical and technical news of interest to families and health-care workers.
Former titles (until 1994): Spinal Network's New Mobility (1065-2124); (until 1992): Spinal Network EXTRA (1058-3483)
Related titles: Online - full text ed.
Published by: No Limits, Inc., PO Box 220, Horsham, PA 19044. TEL 215-675-9133, 888-850-0344 ext 108, FAX 215-675-9376, info@newmobility.com, http://www.newmobility.com. Ed. Jean Dobbs. Pub. Jeff Leonard. **Subscr. to:** PO Box 15518, North Hollywood, CA 91615-9773.

362.4 027.663 USA ISSN 0883-5845
NEWS ABOUT LIBRARY SERVICES FOR THE BLIND AND PHYSICALLY HANDICAPPED. Text in English. 1975. q. free per issue. bibl. 8 p./no. **Document type:** *Newsletter, Consumer.*
Media: Duplicated (not offset). **Related titles:** Audio cassette/tape ed.; Braille ed.; Large type ed.
Published by: State Library, Box 821, Columbia, SC 29202. TEL 803-734-4611, lbphbooks@leo.scsl.state.sc.us, http://www.state.sc.us/scs1/bpk. Ed. Naomi Bradey. Circ: 7,800 (controlled).

362.6 346.013 NLD ISSN 1380-6327
NIEUWSBRIEF W V G; informatie over voorzieningen voor gehandicapten en ouderen. (Wet Voorzieningen Gehandicapten) Text in Dutch. 1994. m. **Document type:** *Newsletter, Trade.* **Description:** Covers developments relating to the law governing handicapped persons in the Netherlands.
Published by: Elsevier Gezondheidszorg B.V., Tijdstroom (Subsidiary of: Reed Elsevier plc Group), Planetenbaan 1, Maarssen 3600 AK, Netherlands. TEL 31-346-577577, FAX 31-346-554287, http://www.tijdstroom.nl. Circ: 1,200. **Subscr. to:** Elsevier Den Haag, Postbus 16500, The Hague 2500 BM, Netherlands. TEL 31-70-381-9900, FAX 31-70-333-8399.

THE O S L A CONNECTION. see *EDUCATION—Special Education And Rehabilitation*

OSAKA SHIRITSU SHINSHIN SHOGAISHA RIHABIRITESHON SENTA KENKYU KIYO/OSAKA MUNICIPAL REHABILITATION CENTER FOR THE DISABLED. RESEARCH REPORTS. see *MEDICAL SCIENCES—Physical Medicine And Rehabilitation*

OVER THE RAINBOW. see *EDUCATION—International Education Programs*

PALAESTRA; forum of sport, physical education and recreation for those with disabilities. see *EDUCATION—Special Education And Rehabilitation*

PARAGRAPHIC. see *MEDICAL SCIENCES—Psychiatry And Neurology*

362.4 USA ISSN 1077-274X
PARENT NEWS. Text in English. 1992 (vol.15, no.3). q. free per issue. **Document type:** *Newsletter, Trade.* **Description:** Designed for parents and professionals.
Published by: Center for Persons with Disabilities, Outreach, Development & Dissemination Division, Utah State University, Logan, UT 84322-6845. TEL 435-797-1991, FAX 435-797-2044. Ed. Marlene Deer. Circ: 1,800.

362.4 USA
PEOPLE WITH DISABILITIES. Text in English. 1975. q. free per issue. reprint service avail. from PQC. **Document type:** *Government.*
Formerly (until 1992): Interface (Trenton) (0274-8940)
Related titles: Microform ed.: (from PQC).
Indexed: PROMT, RILM.
Published by: New Jersey Developmental Disabilities Council, CN 700, Roeblining Bldg, 7th Fl, 20 W State St, Trenton, NJ 08625. TEL 609-292-3745, FAX 609-292-7114. Ed. Ethan B Ellis. R&P Norman Reim. Circ: 10,000.

PHYSICAL DISABILITIES - EDUCATION & RELATED SERVICES. see *EDUCATION—Special Education And Rehabilitation*

362.3 USA
PHYSICAL DISABILITIES SPECIAL INTEREST SECTION QUARTERLY. Text in English. q. USD 20 (effective 1999). **Document type:** *Newsletter.*
Formerly (until 199?): Physical Disabilities Special Interest Section Newsletter (0279-411X); Which superseded in part: American Occupational Therapy Association. Physical Disabilities Specialty Section. Newsletter (0194-6366)
Published by: American Occupational Therapy Association, Inc., 4720 Montgomery Lane, Bethesda, MD 20814-3425. TEL 301-652-2682, FAX 301-652-7711.

PREVENTING SCHOOL FAILURE; for special class teachers and parents of the handicapped. see *EDUCATION—Special Education And Rehabilitation*

362.4 617.087 GBR ISSN 0954-237X
R A D A R BULLETIN. Text in English. m. (11/yr.). GBP 12 domestic; GBP 14.50 foreign. **Document type:** *Bulletin.*
Formerly: Royal Association for Disability and Rehabilitation
Published by: Royal Association for Disability and Rehabilitation, 12 City Forum., 250 City Rd, London EC1V 8AF, United Kingdom. TEL 44-171-250-3222, FAX 44-171-250-0212. Ed. Sue Pratt. Circ: 2,000.

362.43 USA
R E R REPORTS. Text in English. 1997. w. USD 295; USD 335 in Canada; USD 355 elsewhere. adv. **Document type:** *Trade.* **Description:** Provides the latest breaking rental equipment industry news, merger and acquisition activity, trends and analysis, plus much more.
Media: Fax.
Published by: Primedia Business Magazines & Media, Inc. (Subsidiary of: Primedia Inc.), 23815 Stuart Ranch Rd, Box 8987, Malibu, CA 90265-8987. TEL 310-317-4522, FAX 310-317-9644. Eds. Aaron Smith, Tom Nelson. Pub., Adv. contact Fred Jaegle. R&P Greg Vargas TEL 800-543-4116.

362.4 USA ISSN 1097-3052
RA790.65.I4
REACHING OUT. Text in English. 1977. bi-m. USD 25 (effective 1999). back issues avail. **Document type:** *Newsletter.* **Description:** Provides articles of general interest (medical and educational) to families and professionals caring for a child with CdLS; includes a medical column by doctors and letters from parents; source of current information on this syndrome.
Related titles: Fax ed.
Published by: Cornelia de Lange Syndrome Foundation, Inc., 302 W Main St, 100, Avon, CT 06001-3681. TEL 860-676-8166, 800-223-8355, FAX 860-676-8337, cdlsintl@iconn.net, www.cdlsoutreach.org. Ed. H Lawrence Jenkins. Circ: 5,000.

362.4 790 USA
RECREATION - ACCESS IN THE '90'S. Text in English. 1991. bi-m. USD 32 to non-members; USD 25 to members (effective 1999). **Description:** Presents information about disability awareness; product assessments; construction evaluations; issues pertaining to the accessibility of park and recreation facilities; programs for the handicapped.
Published by: National Recreation and Park Association, 22377 Belmont Ridge Rd, Ashburn, VA 20148-4501. Ed. Rikki S Epstein.

338.4768 USA
HD9995.P54
REHAB REPORT. Text in English. 1990. m. USD 36 domestic; USD 48 in Canada; USD 120 elsewhere (effective 1999). adv. bk.rev. tr.lit. reprints avail. **Document type:** *Trade.* **Description:** Provides the latest news concerning the rehabilitation industry, with information on new products, services, technology, market trends, and funding.
Formerly (until 1998): Team Rehab Report (1053-5926)
—CCC.
Published by: Primedia Business Magazines & Media, Inc. (Subsidiary of: Primedia Inc.), 23815 Stuart Ranch Rd, Box 8987, Malibu, CA 90265-8987. TEL 310-317-4522, FAX 310-317-9644, inquiries@primediabusiness.com, http://www.primediabusiness.com. Ed., R&P Van MacNeil. Pub., Adv. contact Sally Matteson. Circ: 12,000 (controlled).

REHABILITACION: PREVENCION Y INTEGRACION. see *MEDICAL SCIENCES—Physical Medicine And Rehabilitation*

362.4 616.8 USA ISSN 0034-3552
HD7255.A2 CODEN: RECBAQ
REHABILITATION COUNSELING BULLETIN. Text in English. 1957. q. USD 43 in North America to individuals; USD 71 elsewhere to individuals; USD 109 in North America to institutions; USD 138 elsewhere to institutions (effective 2002). bk.rev. charts, stat, illus. index. 64 p./no. back issues avail.; reprint service avail. from PQC. *Refereed.* **Document type:** *Journal, Academic/Scholarly, Trade.* **Description:** Discusses the psychological and social aspects of disability, psychiatric rehabilitation, developmental disabilities, career development and job placement of persons with special needs.
Related titles: Microform ed.: (from PQC); Online - full text ed.: (from H. W. Wilson, ProQuest Information & Learning, Institute for Scientific Information, CatchWord Ltd.).
Indexed: AMED, ASCA, AgeLine, C.I.J.E., Curr.Cont., Educ.Ind. (Jul.1992-), PsycInfo, Psychol.Abstr. (1963-), Rehabil.Lit., SSCI, Sage Pub.Admin.Abstr., Soc.Work Res.& Abstr., e-psyche.
—BLDSC (7350.230000), GNLM, IDS, ingenta, KNAW. **CCC.**
Published by: (American Rehabilitation Counseling Association), Pro-Ed Inc., 8700 Shoal Creek Blvd, Austin, TX 78757-6897. TEL 512-451-3246, FAX 512-302-9129, proed1@aol.com, http://www.counseling.org, http://www.proedinc.com. Ed. Douglas Strohmer. Pub. Donald D Hammill. R&P Barbara Rivera TEL 512-451-3246 ext 653. Circ: 4,100.

362.4 USA ISSN 0361-4166
HV1553 CODEN: RHGZA
REHABILITATION GAZETTE; international journal of independent living by and for persons with a disability. Text in English. 1958. s-a. USD 12 domestic to individuals; USD 16 foreign to individuals (effective 2001). abstr, illus. 8 p./no. 3 cols./p. back issues avail. **Document type:** *Newsletter, Consumer.* **Description:** News, features, and profiles pertaining to persons with disabilities, focusing on technologies for assuming independent living and pursuing careers and social opportunities.
Formerly: Toomey J Gazette (0495-8667)
Indexed: Except.Child Educ.Abstr., Excerp.Med.
Published by: Gazette International Networking Institute, 4207 Lindell Blvd., Ste. 110, St. Louis, MO 63108-2915. TEL 314-534-0475, FAX 314-534-5070, gini_intl@msn.com, http://www.post-polio.org/ivun.html. Ed. Joan Headley. Circ: 5,000.

REPORT ON ALCOHOL, DRUGS, AND DISABILITY. see *DRUG ABUSE AND ALCOHOLISM*

REPORT ON DISABILITY PROGRAMS. see *SOCIAL SERVICES AND WELFARE*

RESOURCE DIRECTORY OF SCIENTISTS AND ENGINEERS WITH DISABILITIES. see *BIOGRAPHY*

362.4 RUS
RUSSKII INVALID. Text in Russian. m. USD 129.95 in United States.
Related titles: Microfiche ed.: (from IDC).
Published by: Moskovskoe Gorodskoe Pravlenie, Vserossiiskogo Obshchestva Invalidov, Bersenevskaya nab 20-2, Moscow 103790, Russian Federation. TEL 7-095-2037734, FAX 7-095-9591024. Ed. N N Zhukov. **US dist. addr.:** East View Publications, 3020 Harbor Ln N, Minneapolis, MN 55447. TEL 612-550-0961.

617.03 POL ISSN 0867-7387
SERCE I TROSKA. Text in Polish. 1991. bi-m. PLZ 1 newsstand/cover. back issues avail. *Refereed.*
Published by: Polskie Towarzystwo Walki z Kalectwem, Ul Bohaterow Westerplatte 11, pok. 127, Zielona Gora 65034, Poland. TEL 48-68-3254231. Ed. Janusz Koniusz. adv.: page PLZ 300. Circ: 4,000. **Co-sponsors:** Polmozbyt; Panstwowy Fundusz Rehabilitacji Osob Niepelnosprawnych.

SEXUALITY AND DISABILITY; a journal devoted to the psychological and medical aspects of sexuality in rehabilitation and community settings. see *MEDICAL SCIENCES*

SPECIAL EDUCATION REPORT; the independent bi-weekly news service on legislation, programs and funding for special education. see *EDUCATION—Special Education And Rehabilitation*

362.3 BEL ISSN 0776-5827
DE STEM VAN DE OUDERS. Key Title: Amentia. De Stem van de Ouders. Text in Dutch. 1963. q. BEF 1,150. adv. bk.rev. bibl, illus. **Description:** Covers all aspects of mental retardation, both medical and social services.
Supersedes in part (in 1987): Amentia (0002-7022)
Indexed: e-psyche.
Published by: Nationale Vereniging voor Hulp aan Verstandelijk Gehandicapten v.z.w., Grensstraat 66, Brussels 1210, Belgium. TEL 32-2-219-8800, FAX 32-2-219-9061, anahm.nvhvg@skynet.be, http://users.skynet.be/anahm.nvhvg. Ed. E Buysse. Circ: 3,200.

371.92 USA
LC4631 CODEN: JPSHEF
T A S H JOURNAL. Text in English. 1975. q. USD 88 domestic to individuals; USD 98 in Canada to individuals; USD 113 elsewhere to individuals; USD 200 domestic to institutions; USD 210 in Canada to institutions; USD 225 elsewhere to institutions; USD 45 to students (effective 2000); membership. adv. bk.rev. illus. index. back issues avail.; reprint service avail. from PQC. *Refereed.* **Document type:** *Academic/Scholarly.* **Description:** Carries articles on topics such as inclusion, facilitated communication, supported living, supported employment, issues of early childhood, self-advocacy, positive behavioral practices, disability rights, and issues of concern to families.
Former titles: Association for Persons with Severe Handicaps. Journal (0749-1425); (until 1983): Association for the Severely Handicapped. Journal (JASH) (0274-9483); (until vol.5, no.1): A A E S P H Review (American Association for the Education of the Severely-Profoundly Handicapped) (0147-4375)
Related titles: Audio cassette/tape ed.; Microform ed.: (from PQC); Online - full text ed.: (from H. W. Wilson, Institute for Scientific Information).
Indexed: AMED, ASCA, AgeLine, C.I.J.E., Curr.Cont., Educ.Ind. (Sep.1983-Sep.1983), Except.Child Educ.Abstr., Fam.Ind., Lang.& Lang.Behav.Abstr., PsycInfo, SOPODA, SSCI, Sociol.Abstr., e-psyche. —BLDSC (4705.078000), IDS, ingenta.
Published by: T A S H, 29 W Susquehanna Ave, Ste 210, Baltimore, MD 21204-5201. TEL 410-828-8274, FAX 410-828-6706, http//www.tash.org, http://www.tash.org. Ed. Linda Bambara. Circ: 3,800.

362.4 USA
T A S H NEWSLETTER. Text in English. 10/yr. USD 88 domestic to individuals; USD 98 in Canada to individuals; USD 113 elsewhere to individuals; USD 200 domestic to institutions; USD 210 in Canada to institutions; USD 225 elsewhere to institutions; USD 45 to students (effective 2000); membership. reprint service avail. from PQC. **Document type:** *Newsletter.* **Description:** Carries articles on topics such as inclusion, facilitated communication, supported living, supported employment, issues of early childhood, self-advocacy, positive behavioral practices, disability rights, and issues of concern to families.
Formerly: Association for Persons with Severe Handicaps. Newsletter
Related titles: Audio cassette/tape ed.
—BLDSC.
Published by: T A S H, 29 W Susquehanna Ave, Ste 210, Baltimore, MD 21204-5201. TEL 410-828-8274, FAX 410-828-6706, info@tash.org, http://www.tash.org. Ed. Priscilla Newton. Circ: 4,800.

371.9 USA
TEAM OF ADVOCATES FOR SPECIAL KIDS NEWSLETTER. Text in English. 1984. bi-m. USD 25 to members (effective 2000). adv. bk.rev. **Document type:** *Newsletter.* **Description:** Provides information on educational, medical, and support services for parents of children with disabilities.
Published by: Team of Advocates for Special Kids (TASK), 100 W Cerritos Ave, Anaheim, CA 92805. TEL 714-533-8275, FAX 714-533-2533. Ed., Adv. contact Laura Grieef. R&P Eric Tellefsen. page USD 150. Circ: 630.

617.03 NLD ISSN 1055-4181
HV1551 CODEN: TEDIFB
TECHNOLOGY AND DISABILITY. Text in English. 1991. bi-m. (in 2 vols., 3 nos./vol.). EUR 279, USD 267 to institutions (effective 2002). illus. back issues avail. *Refereed.* **Document type:** *Journal, Academic/Scholarly.* **Description:** Deals with the application of rehabilitative and assistive technology for persons with disabilities.
Related titles: Microform ed.: (from PQC); Online - full text ed.: (from ingenta, Swets Blackwell, RoweCom Information Quest).
Indexed: AMED, ASCA, AgeLine, CINAHL, Ergon.Abstr., Except.Child Educ.Abstr., Excerp.Med., SSCI (coverage dropped).
—BLDSC (8758.612000), IDS. **CCC.**
Published by: I O S Press, Nieuwe Hemweg 6B, Amsterdam 1013 BG, Netherlands. TEL 31-20-688-3355, FAX 31-20-620-3419, market@iospress.nl, http://www.iospress.nl. Ed. Joseph P Lane TEL 716-829-3141. **Subscr. to:** I O S Press, Inc, 5795-G Burke Centre Pkwy, Burke, VA 22015. TEL 703-323-5554, FAX 703-323-3668, iosbooks@iospress.com; Kinokuniya Company Ltd, Shinjuku 3-chome, Shinjuku-ku, Tokyo 160-0022, Japan. FAX 81-3-3439-1094, journal@kinokuniya.co.jp, http://www.kinokuniya.co.jp; Globe Publication Pvt. Ltd., C-62 Inderpuri, New Delhi 100 012, India. TEL 91-11-579-3211, 91-11-579-3212, FAX 91-11-579-8876, custserve@globepub.com, http://www.globepub.com.

TOKYO METROPOLITAN REHABILITATION CENTER FOR THE PHYSICALLY AND MENTALLY HANDICAPPED. BULLETIN. see *MEDICAL SCIENCES—Physical Medicine And Rehabilitation*

617.8 JPN ISSN 0917-5601
UNDO SHOGAI/MOVEMENT DISORDER AND DISABILITY. Text in Japanese; Summaries in English, Japanese. 1991. s-a.
Published by: Undo Shogai Kenkyukai/Society of Movement Disorder and Disability, Jichi Ika Daigaku Iryo Senta Shinkei Naika, 1-847 Tenumacho, Omiya-shi, Saitama-ken 330-0000, Japan.

362.41 NLD ISSN 0929-4716
HET VAGGESCHIP. Text in Dutch. 1992. m. NLG 25 (effective 1999). adv. back issues avail. **Document type:** *Newsletter.* **Description:** For the deaf and blind, and professional and voluntary workers with deaf-blind people.
Media: Large Type (18 pt.). **Related titles:** Audio cassette/tape ed.; Braille ed.
Published by: Stichting het Vaggeschip, Hannie Schaftstraat 85, Hoofddorp 2135 KC, Netherlands. TEL 31-23-565-3378. Ed. J. Franken. R&P J Franken. Adv. contact D Hoogetoorn. B&W page NLG 100. Circ: 250.

362.3 BEL ISSN 0776-5835
LA VOIX DES PARENTS. Key Title: Amentia. La Voix des Parents. Text in French. 1963. q. BEF 900. adv. bk.rev. bibl, illus. **Document type:** *Bulletin.* **Description:** Covers all aspects of mental retardation.
Supersedes in part (in 1987): Amentia (0002-7022)
Published by: Association Francophone d'Aide aux Handicapes Mentaux a.s.b.l., Rue de la Limite 66, Brussels 1210, Belgium. TEL 32-2-2198800, FAX 32-2-2199061, anahm.nvhvg@skynet.be, http://users.skynet.be/anahm.nvhvg. Ed. Th Kempeneers Foulon. Circ: 3,200.

362.4 616.836 USA ISSN 0738-8012
WORD FROM WASHINGTON (WASHINGTON, D.C.). Text in English. 1969. bi-m. USD 25 disabled individuals; USD 55 to individuals. bk.rev. illus. **Document type:** *Newsletter.*
Indexed: Except.Child Educ.Abstr., Rehabil.Lit., e-psyche.
Published by: United Cerebral Palsy Associations, Inc., Governmental Activities Office, 1660 L St, N W, Ste 700, Washington, DC 20036-5602. TEL 202-776-0406, FAX 202-776-0414. Ed. Christopher Button. Circ: 8,000.

362.4 CHN ISSN 1003-1081
ZHONGGUO CANJIREN/DISABILITY IN CHINA. Text in Chinese. m. CNY 21.60. **Document type:** *Government.* **Description:** Introduces laws and policies concerning people with disabilities. Contains rehabilitation and special education information.
Published by: (Zhongguo Canjiren Lianhehui/China Disabled Persons' Federation), Disability in China Inc., A-8 Huixin Li Anwai, Chaoyang-qu, Beijing 100101, China. TEL 86-10-6496-8362. Ed. Li Zhiqi. **Dist. by:** Bureau pf Industrial and Commercial Administration, Chaoyang-qu, Beijing, China; **Dist. in US by:** China Books & Periodicals, Inc, 2929 24th St, San Francisco, CA 94110. TEL 415-282-2994.

HANDICAPPED—Abstracting, Bibliographies, Statistics

016.617 USA
ABSEARCH A S H A. (American Speech - Language - Hearing Association) Text in English. q. USD 89 to individuals; USD 150 to libraries; USD 250 universities; USD 350 region; USD 69 to students (effective 2001). **Document type:** *Abstract/Index.* **Description:** Contains 11,000+ records including citations and abstracts for all articles published from 1945 to present in the American Journal of Audiology; the American Journal of Speech - Language Pathology; the Journal of Speech, Language, and Hearing Research; Language, Speech, and Hearing Services in Schools.
Media: Online - full text. **Related titles:** CD-ROM ed.: USD 89 to students; USD 109 to individuals; USD 250 to libraries; USD 450 universities; USD 650 region (effective 2001).
Published by: ABSEARCH, Inc., 121 Sweet Ave, Moscow, ID 83843. TEL 208-885-3804, 800-867-1877, FAX 208-885-3803, custinfo@absearch.com, http://www.absearch.com.

016.36241 USA ISSN 0000-1120
Z5348
THE COMPLETE DIRECTORY OF LARGE PRINT BOOKS AND SERIALS. Text in English. 1970. a. USD 199 (effective 2001). **Document type:** *Directory, Bibliography.* **Description:** Provides finding and ordering information on large-print books, magazines and newspapers. Books are indexed by author, subject, and title.
Formerly (until 1988): Large Type Books in Print (0163-3198)
Media: Large Type (14 pt.). **Related titles:** CD-ROM ed.: (from Bowker Electronic Publishing); Magnetic Tape ed.; Microfiche ed.; Online - full text ed.
—CCC.
Published by: R.R. Bowker, 630 Central Ave., New Providence, NJ 07974. TEL 908-464-6800, FAX 908-655-3502, info@bowker.com, http://www.bowker.com.

011.63 USA ISSN 0889-6518
Z5346
MAGAZINES IN SPECIAL MEDIA. Text in English. biennial, latest 2000. free. **Document type:** *Directory, Government, Bibliography.* **Description:** Lists periodicals available throughout the country in special media to persons with visual and other physical handicaps.
Incorporates (1993-1995): Magazines (Washington) (0161-2689)
Media: Large Type (14 pt.). **Related titles:** Audio cassette/tape ed.; Braille ed.; Diskette ed.; Online - full text ed.
Published by: U.S. Library of Congress, National Library Service for the Blind and Physically Handicapped, Washington, DC 20542. TEL 202-707-5100, FAX 202-707-0712, nls@loc.gov, http://www.loc.gov/nls/reference/directories/index.html, http://lcweb.loc.gov/nls.

362 MWI
MALAWI. NATIONAL STATISTICAL OFFICE. SURVEY OF HANDICAPPED PERSONS. Text in English. 1983. irreg. MWK 40. **Document type:** *Government.*
Published by: National Statistical Office, Commissioner for Census and Statistics, PO Box 333, Zomba, Malawi. TEL 265-50-522377, FAX 265-50-523130.

011.36241 011.6177 GBR
NEW LITERATURE ON VISUAL IMPAIRMENT. Text in English. bi-m. GBP 20; GBP 30 foreign. **Document type:** *Directory, Bibliography.* **Description:** Keeps abreast of new books and periodicals covering all aspects of visual impairment, including persons who are deafblind and multiply disabled. Of use to all professionals involved with these populations, including social workers, special-education teachers, health care workers, and policy makers.
Related titles: Braille ed.
Published by: Royal National Institute for the Blind, 224 Great Portland St, London W1N 6AA, United Kingdom. FAX 44-1733-371555, cservices@rnib.org.uk, http://www.rnib.org.uk. **Subscr. to:** RNIB Customer Services, PO Box 173, Peterborough, Cambs PE2 6WS, United Kingdom. TEL 44-1733-370777, FAX 44-1733-317555.

027.6 016 362.4 USA
RECORDING FOR THE BLIND & DYSLEXIC. CATALOG OF BOOKS. Text in English. 1960. irreg. USD 69.95 (effective 1999). **Document type:** *Catalog.*
Formerly: Recording for the Blind. Catalog of Recorded Books (0484-1506)
Published by: Recording for the Blind & Dyslexic, Inc., 20 Roszel Rd, Princeton, NJ 08540. TEL 609-452-0606, FAX 609-987-8116. Circ: 15,000.

371.9 362.42 DEU
WER? WO? WAS? IN DER HOERGESCHAEDIGTENPAEDAGOGIK. Text in German. 1930. triennial. **Document type:** *Academic/Scholarly.*
Former titles: Statistische Nachrichten Bildungs- und Sozialeinrichtungen fuer Hoergeschaedigte in der Bundesrepublik Deutschland; Statistische Nachrichten ueber Bildungs- und Sozialeinrichtungen fuer Hoergeschaedigte im Deutschsprachigen Raum
Published by: (Bund Deutscher Hoergeschaedigtenpaedagogen), Median-Verlag von Killisch-Horn GmbH, Hauptstr 64, Heidelberg 69117, Germany. TEL 49-6221-90509-0, FAX 49-6221-9050920, median-verlag@t-online.de, http://www.median-verlag.de.

HANDICAPPED—Computer Applications

362.4 NLD ISSN 1383-813X
ASSISTIVE TECHNOLOGY RESEARCH SERIES. Text in English. 1995. irreg., latest vol.6, 1999. price varies. back issues avail. *Refereed.* **Document type:** *Monographic series, Proceedings, Academic/Scholarly.* **Description:** Reports on new applications and technologies for assisting persons with disabilities.
Indexed: Eng.Ind.
—BLDSC (1746.672062).
Published by: (Technology Initiative for Disabled and Elderly People BEL, Commission of the European Communities BEL), I O S Press, Van Diemenstraat 94, Amsterdam 1013 CN, Netherlands. TEL 31-20-638-2189, FAX 31-20-620-3419, market@iospress.nl, http://www.iospress.nl. **Subscr. to:** I O S Press, Inc, 5795-G Burke Centre Pkwy, Burke, VA 22015. TEL 703-323-5554, FAX 703-323-3668, iosbooks@iospress.com. **Dist. by:** Ohmsha Ltd, 3-1 Kanda-Nishiki-cho, Chiyoda-ku, Tokyo 101-0054, Japan. TEL 81-3-3233-0641, FAX 81-3-3233-2426, http://www.ohmsha.co.jp.

CLOSING THE GAP. see *EDUCATION—Special Education And Rehabilitation*

HANDICAPPED—Hearing Impaired

371.912 USA ISSN 0899-9228
HV2350 CODEN: JADAEI
A D A R A JOURNAL✱ ; journal of professionals networking for excellence in service delivery with individuals who are deaf or hard of hearing. Variant title: J A D A R A. Text in English. 1967. 3/yr. USD 60 domestic; USD 75 foreign. adv. bk.rev. back issues avail. **Document type:** *Newsletter, Academic/Scholarly.* **Description:** Deals with research findings (pragmatic application) program descriptions and articles on deafness and the disciplines of rehabilitation, social services, mental health, and other related areas.
Formerly: Journal of Rehabilitation of the Deaf (0730-1626)
Indexed: AMED, Curr.Cont. (coverage dropped), Except.Child Educ.Abstr., Lang.& Lang.Behav.Abstr., PsycInfo, Psychol.Abstr. (1972-), Rehabil.Lit., SOPODA, SSCI (coverage dropped), Sociol.Abstr.
—GNLM, ingenta.
Published by: (American Deafness & Rehabilitation Association), A D A R A, P O Box 727, Lusby, MD 20657-0727. TEL 650-372-0620. Ed. Gerard Walter. R&P, Adv. contact Elizabeth Charlson. Circ: 1,000.

617.8 USA
A D A R A NEWSLETTER✱. Text in English. 1970. q. USD 55 to membership; USD 70 foreign. adv. **Document type:** *Newsletter.* **Description:** For professionals networking for excellence in service delivery with individuals who are deaf or hard of hearing.
Published by: (American Deafness & Rehabilitation Association), A D A R A, P O Box 727, Lusby, MD 20657-0727. TEL 650-372-0620. Ed. Greg Mosher. R&P, Adv. contact Elizabeth Charlson. Circ: 1,100.

617.8 USA ISSN 0001-2475
RC423.A1
A S H A. Text in English. 1959. q. USD 70 domestic to individuals; USD 100 foreign to individuals; USD 110 domestic to institutions; USD 130 foreign to institutions. adv. bk.rev. illus. Index. back issues avail.; reprint service avail. from PQC. **Document type:** *Bulletin.* **Description:** Pertains to the professional and administrative activities of speech, language and hearing professions.
Related titles: Microfiche ed.: (from PQC); Online - full text ed.: (from ProQuest Information & Learning).
Indexed: AgeLine, Biol.Abstr., CINAHL, Child Devel.Abstr., Educ.Ind. (Sep.1983-Nov.1999), Except.Child Educ.Abstr., Ind.Med. (1959-), Noise Pollut.Publ.Abstr., Psychol.Abstr., Rehabil.Lit.
—CISTI, GNLM, ingenta. **CCC.**
Published by: American Speech - Language - Hearing Association, 10801 Rockville Pike, Rockville, MD 20852. TEL 301-897-5700, FAX 301-897-7358, sghoting@asha.org, http://www.asha.org/publications.html. Ed. Frederick T Spahr. Circ: 73,000.

617.89 USA ISSN 1085-9586
A S H A LEADER; building the future of the professions. Text in English. 1995. 22/yr., latest vol.6, 2001. USD 80 to non-members; USD 110 foreign to non-members; USD 125 to institutions; USD 150 foreign to institutions (effective 2002); includes Asha. adv. bk.rev., software rev., video rev. illus. **Document type:** *Newspaper, Corporate.* **Description:** Contains news related to audiology, speech-language pathology, and related professions.
Related titles: Online - full text ed.: (from Northern Light Technology, Inc., Gale Group).
Indexed: CINAHL.
—BLDSC (1742.027000). **CCC.**
Published by: American Speech - Language - Hearing Association, 10801 Rockville Pike, Rockville, MD 20852. TEL 301-897-5700, FAX 301-897-7358, sghoting@asha.org. Ed. Joanne Jessen. R&P Kirsten Gardner. Adv. contact Karmen Shum TEL 913-469-1110 ext 212. page USD 3,750; 10 x 12.5. Circ: 105,000.

362.41 AUS ISSN 0816-2220
ABILITIES. Text in English. 4/yr. free per issue. **Document type:** *Newsletter.*
Published by: Royal N S W Institute for Deaf and Blind Children, Deaf and Blind Children's Centre, 361-365 North Rocks Rd, N Rocks, NSW 2151, Australia. TEL 61-2-98711233. Circ: 49,000.

ACADEMY OF REHABILITATIVE AUDIOLOGY. JOURNAL. see *MEDICAL SCIENCES—Otorhinolaryngology*

362.42 ARG
AD VERBUM. Text in Spanish. 1969. q. free per issue. adv. bk.rev. bibl, illus, stat.
Published by: Confederacion Argentina de Sordomudos, Av. Pedro Medrano 1352, Buenos Aires, Argentina. Eds. Alvaro Daniel de Tomaso, Teodoro Manzanedo. Circ: 5,000 (controlled). **Co-sponsor:** Federacion Mondial de Sordos.

ADVANCES IN NOISE RESEARCH. see *MEDICAL SCIENCES—Otorhinolaryngology*

ALERT (EWING); news on alcoholism and drug addiction services for persons who are hard of hearing. see *DRUG ABUSE AND ALCOHOLISM*

371.912 IND ISSN 0377-0524
RC423.A1 CODEN: JAIHDT
ALL INDIA INSTITUTE OF SPEECH AND HEARING. JOURNAL. Text in English. 1970. a. INR 205, USD 30. **Document type:** *Academic/Scholarly.* **Description:** Pertains broadly to the studies of the normal processes and disorders of speech, language and hearing.
—GNLM.
Published by: All India Institute of Speech and Hearing, Manasagangotri, Mysore, Karnataka 570 006, India. TEL 91-821-514449, FAX 91-821-510515, nikam@aiish.ernet.in. Ed. S Nikam. Circ: 200.

371.912 USA ISSN 0002-726X
HV2510 CODEN: ANDFAL
AMERICAN ANNALS OF THE DEAF. Text in English. 1847. 5/yr. USD 50 domestic to individuals; USD 55 in Canada to individuals; USD 65 elsewhere to individuals; USD 60 domestic to institutions; USD 66 in Canada to institutions; USD 80 elsewhere to institutions (effective 2001). adv. bk.rev. bibl, charts, illus, stat. index. Supplement avail.; back issues avail.; reprint service avail. from PQC. *Refereed.* **Document type:** *Trade, Academic/Scholarly.* **Description:** For teachers, administrators, and researchers in the field of deaf education.
Formerly: American Annals of the Deaf and Dumb (0093-1284)
Related titles: Microfilm ed.: (from PQC); Online - full text ed.: (from Northern Light Technology, Inc., H. W. Wilson, ProQuest Information & Learning, Gale Group, Factiva, Institute for Scientific Information).
Indexed: ASCA, AgeLine, Bibl.Ind., Biol.Abstr., C.I.J.E., CINAHL, Child Devel.Abstr., Curr.Cont., ERA, Educ.Admin.Abstr., Educ.Ind. (Apr.1983-), Except.Child Educ.Abstr., Excerp.Med., Fam.Ind., Ind.Med. (1886-), Int.Nurs.Ind., Lang.& Lang.Behav.Abstr., Mult.Ed.Abstr., P.A.I.S., PsycInfo, Psychol.Abstr. (1928-), Rehabil.Lit., SOPODA, SSCI, Sociol.Abstr., Sp.Ed.Needs Abstr., e-psyche.
—BLDSC (0810.150000), GNLM, IDS, ingenta, KNAW. **CCC.**
Published by: Convention of American Instructors of the Deaf, FH, 409, 800 Florida Ave, N E, Washington, DC 20002. TEL 202-651-5530, FAX 202-651-5860, mary.carew@gallaudet.edu, http://sehs.gallaudet.edu/annals/. Ed. Dr. Donald Moores. adv.: B&W page USD 435. Circ: 4,000 (paid and controlled). **Co-sponsor:** Conference of Educational Administrators Serving the Deaf.

617.8 USA ISSN 1059-0889
RF286
AMERICAN JOURNAL OF AUDIOLOGY; a journal of clinical practice. Text in English. 1991. 3/yr. USD 45 domestic to individuals; USD 55 foreign to individuals; USD 125 domestic to institutions; USD 160 foreign to institutions (effective 2001). adv. charts, illus, bibl. 150 p./no. back issues avail.; reprints avail. **Document type:** *Journal, Academic/Scholarly.* **Description:** Addresses all aspects of clinical practice in audiology.
Related titles: Microform ed.: (from PQC); Online - full text ed.: (from ProQuest Information & Learning).
Indexed: ABSEARCH - ASHA (1945-), CINAHL, Educ.Ind., Ind.Med. (1991-).
—BLDSC (0821.800000), CISTI, GNLM, Infotrieve, ingenta. **CCC.**
Published by: American Speech - Language - Hearing Association, 10801 Rockville Pike, Rockville, MD 20852. TEL 301-897-5700, FAX 301-897-7358, sghoting@asha.org, http://professional.asha.org/publications/aja/htm. Ed. Gary Jacobson. R&P Kirsten Gardner. Adv. contact Karmen Shum TEL 913-469-1110 ext 212. Circ: 9,000.

362.42 USA ISSN 1058-0360
RC423.A1 CODEN: AJSPFZ
AMERICAN JOURNAL OF SPEECH - LANGUAGE PATHOLOGY; a journal of clinical practice. Text in English. 1991. 4/yr. USD 45 domestic to individuals (effective 2002); USD 55 foreign to individuals; USD 125 domestic to institutions; USD 160 foreign to institutions (2002). adv. charts, illus, bibl. back issues avail.; reprints avail. **Document type:** *Journal, Academic/Scholarly.* **Description:** Addresses all aspects of clinical practice in speech language pathology.
Related titles: Microform ed.: (from PQC); Online - full text ed.: (from ProQuest Information & Learning, Institute for Scientific Information).
Indexed: ABSEARCH - ASHA (1945-), CINAHL, Curr.Cont., Except.Child Educ.Abstr., Lang.& Lang.Behav.Abstr., SOPODA, SSCI, Sociol.Abstr.
—BLDSC (0838.350000), GNLM, IDS, Infotrieve, ingenta. **CCC.**
Published by: American Speech - Language - Hearing Association, 10801 Rockville Pike, Rockville, MD 20852. TEL 301-897-5700, FAX 301-897-7358, sghoting@asha.org. Ed. Richard K Peach. R&P Kirsten Gardner. Adv. contact Karmen Shum TEL 913-469-1110 ext 212. page USD 1,290; 7.1875 x 9.5. Circ: 33,000.

ASIA PACIFIC JOURNAL OF SPEECH, LANGUAGE AND HEARING. see *MEDICAL SCIENCES—Otorhinolaryngology*

362.42 CAN ISSN 1184-115X
ATLANTIC SILENT NEWS. Text in English. 1979. q. CND 5 domestic; CND 12 foreign. adv. illus. **Document type:** *Newsletter.*
Former titles: Coordination Council on Deafness of Nova Scotia. News; Access (Halifax) (0227-1435); Coordinating Council on Deafness of Nova Scotia. Newsletter (0227-1427)
Published by: Atlantic Ministry of the Deaf, 6225 Summit St, Halifax, NS B3L 1R6, Canada. TEL 902-443-3219. Eds. Frank O'Sullivan, Robert J Tupper. R&P, Adv. contact Robert J Tupper. Circ: 50. **Co-sponsors:** Society of Deaf and Hard of Hearing Nova Scotians; Co-Ordination Council on Deafness of Nova Scotia.

617.89 USA ISSN 0004-7473
AUDECIBEL. Text in English. 1952. bi-m. USD 35; USD 45 foreign (effective 1999). adv. bk.rev. charts, illus. index. reprint service avail. from PQC. **Document type:** *Trade.* **Description:** Provides technical and business information to help hearing instrument professionals serve hearing-impaired people.
Related titles: Microform ed.: (from PQC).
Indexed: Except.Child Educ.Abstr.
—ingenta.
Published by: International Hearing Society, 16880 Middlebelt Rd, 4, Livonia, MI 48154-3367. TEL 248-478-2610, FAX 734-522-0200, chlemsihs@aol.com. Ed. Glen Peacock. R&P, Adv. contact Cindy J Helms. Circ: 3,000.

362.42 FRA
AUDIO JOURNAL. Text in French. 1966. q. FRF 80; FRF 100 foreign. adv. illus.
Published by: Association pour l'Information des Troubles de l'Audition de la Parole et du Language, 18 rue Rene Baschet, Gagny 93220, France. TEL 43-81-40-57. Ed. Pierre Rosset. Circ: 15,000.

362.42 GBR ISSN 0004-8054
AURAL NEWS. Text in English. 1946. q. GBP 0.50. adv. bk.rev., film rev. charts, illus, stat.
Related titles: Microform ed.
Published by: Middlesex & Surrey League for the Hard of Hearing, 11 Josephs Rd, Guildford, Surrey GU1 DN1, United Kingdom. Ed. J W Penycate. Circ: 2,000.

617.89 SWE ISSN 0045-0030
AURIS; tidskrift for hoerselskadade. Text in Swedish. 1921. 8/yr. SEK 190 (effective 2001). adv. charts, illus, tr.lit. **Document type:** *Newspaper, Consumer.*
Former titles (until 1949): Meddelanden fraan Hoerselfraemjandet; (until vol.4, 1947): Meddelanden fraan Svenska Foereningen foer Doevas Vael
Related titles: Audio cassette/tape ed.
Published by: Hoerselskadades Riksfoerbund (HRF), Gaevlegatan 18A, Box 6605, Stockholm 11384, Sweden. TEL 46-8-4575500, FAX 46-8-313210, auris@kansli.hrf.se. Ed., Pub. Stefan Andersson. Adv. contact Elisabeth Skarboevik. B&W page SEK 10,700, color page SEK 14,500. Circ: 32,000.

617.89 AUS ISSN 0157-1532
AUSTRALIAN JOURNAL OF AUDIOLOGY. Text in English. 1979. s-a. AUD 30 to individuals; AUD 45 foreign to individuals; AUD 55 to institutions; AUD 80 foreign to institutions (effective 2000). back issues avail. **Document type:** *Academic/Scholarly.* **Description:** Publishes original, scientific articles on all aspects of audiology.
Indexed: Acoust.Abstr., Biol.Abstr., Excerp.Med., INSPEC (Nov.1982-May 1999, Nov.1999-), Noise Pollut.Publ.Abstr.
—AskIEEE, EMDOCS, GNLM, ingenta.
Published by: (Audiological Society of Australia), Australian Academic Press Pty. Ltd., 32 Jeays St, Bowen Hills, QLD 4006, Australia. TEL 61-7-32571176, FAX 61-7-32525908, australianacademicpress@compuserve.com, http://www.australianacademicpress.com.au.

371.912 AUS ISSN 0005-0334
AUSTRALIAN TEACHER OF THE DEAF✶. Text in English. 1956. a. AUD 15. adv. bk.rev. stat. cum.index.
Indexed: Aus.Educ.Ind., Cont.Pg.Educ., DSH Abstr., Sp.Ed.Needs Abstr.
Published by: Australian Association of Teachers of the Deaf, Cornwall St, Annerley, QLD 4103, Australia. Ed. Cathy Byrnes. Circ: 500.

362.42 ISR
BAT KOL. Text in Hebrew. 1986. s-a. adv. bk.rev. **Document type:** *Newsletter.*
Published by: Shema Parents' Association of Deaf & Hard of Hearing Children, Pelitei Hasefer 30, Tel Aviv 67894, Israel. TEL 972-3-5715656, FAX 972-3-5712017, http://www.batkol.virtual.co.il. Ed. Zevulun Gooreni.

371.912 GBR
BRITISH ASSOCIATION OF TEACHERS OF THE DEAF. ASSOCIATION MAGAZINE. Text in English. 1988. 5/yr. GBP 49.50 to members (effective 2001); includes Deafness and Education International (DEI); DEI is also available on subscription via Whurr Publishers. adv. bk.rev., software rev., Website rev. charts. index. **Document type:** *Magazine, Trade.* **Description:** Offers professional advice on practice and contains association news.
Supersedes in part: Teacher of the Deaf (0040-0459)
—ingenta.
Published by: British Association of Teachers of the Deaf, 41 The Orchard, Leven, E Yorkshire HU17 5QA, United Kingdom. magazine@batod.org.uk, batod@btinternet.com, www.batod.org.uk. Ed., R&P Ann Underwood TEL 44-1964-544243. Adv. contact Arnold Underwood. Circ: 1,800.

617.8 GBR ISSN 0300-5364
QP460 CODEN: BJAYAC
BRITISH JOURNAL OF AUDIOLOGY. Text in English. 1967. bi-m. USD 225 in North America to individuals; GBP 125 rest of world to individuals; USD 450 in North America to institutions; GBP 250 rest of world to institutions (effective 2001). adv. bk.rev. abstr. index. back issues avail.; reprint service avail. from SWZ,PQC. *Refereed.* **Document type:** *Journal, Academic/Scholarly.* **Description:** Examines the fundamental psychophysical and physiological aspects of hearing and hearing loss for the specialist and technologist; covers a broad spectrum of topics within the field of audiological studies.
Formerly: Sound (0038-1799)
Related titles: Microform ed.: (from PQC); Online - full content ed.: ISSN 1471-2849 (from ProQuest Information & Learning); Online - full text ed.: (from CatchWord Ltd., Institute for Scientific Information).
Indexed: ASCA, ASSIA, Acoust.Abstr., Biol.Abstr., CINAHL, Can.Mus.Per.Ind., Curr.Cont., Eng.Ind., Excerp.Med., INSPEC (Feb.2000-), Ind.Med. (1973-), Inpharma, Lang.& Lang.Behav.Abstr., NBA, Neurosci.Cit.Ind., Noise Pollut.Publ.Abstr., Pharm.&Out.News, Reac., SOPODA, Sci.Cit.Ind., Sociol.Abstr.
—BLDSC (2306.500000), ADONIS, CISTI, EMDOCS, GNLM, IDS, ingenta, KNAW, Linda Hall. **CCC.**
Published by: (British Society of Audiology), Whurr Publishers Ltd., 19b Compton Terr, London N1 2UN, United Kingdom. TEL 44-20-7359-5979, FAX 44-20-7226-5290, info@whurr.co.uk, http://www.whurr.co.uk. Ed. David Baguley. Adv. contact Lizzy Ewer. page GBP 410. **Subscr. in N. America to:** Whurr Publishers Ltd., PO Box 1897, Lawrence, KS 66044-8897. TEL 913-843-1221, FAX 913-843-1274, am&m@allenpress.com. **Subscr. to:** Turpin Distribution Services Ltd., Blackhorse Rd, Letchworth, Herts SG6 1HN, United Kingdom. TEL 44-1462-488900, FAX 44-1462-483011.

DAS BRUDERHAUS. see *EDUCATION—Special Education And Rehabilitation*

C A D CHAT. see *MEDICAL SCIENCES—Otorhinolaryngology*

371.912 CAN
HV2350
C A E D H H JOURNAL/ASSOCIATION CANADIENNE DES ENSEIGNANTS(ES) DES SOURDS(ES) ET DES MALENTENDANTS(ES). REVUE. Short title: Revue A C E S M. Text in English. 1974. 3/yr. CND 25 to individuals; CND 40 to institutions (effective 2000). adv. bk.rev. index. back issues avail. *Refereed.* **Document type:** *Academic/Scholarly.*
Former titles (until 1996): A C E H I Journal - Revue A C E D A (0382-7976); Canadian Teacher of the Deaf (0045-5431)
Related titles: Microfiche ed.: (from MML); Microform ed.: (from MML).
Indexed: C.I.J.E., Can.Educ.Ind., DSH Abstr., ERA, Except.Child Educ.Abstr., Sp.Ed.Needs Abstr.
—CCC.
Published by: (Canadian Association of Educators of the Deaf and Hard of Hearing), University of Alberta, Department of Educational Psychology, 6 102 Education North, Edmonton, AB T6G 2G5, Canada. TEL 403-492-4204, FAX 403-492-0390, rod.beattie@ualberta.ca; rod_beattie@psych.edu.ualberta.ca. Ed., R&P Rod G Beattie. Circ: 600.

H

362.42 USA ISSN 0885-7962
C O D A NEWSLETTER. Text in English. 1983. q. USD 20 (effective 2000 & 2001). adv. bk.rev. back issues avail. **Document type:** *Newsletter, Consumer.*
Published by: Children of Deaf Adults, PO Box 30715, Santa Barbara, CA 93130. TEL 805-682-0997, codanews@aol.com. Ed., Adv. contact Mark Whisenat. Circ: 500.

617.89 FRA ISSN 0980-3483
CAHIERS DE L'AUDITION. Text in French. 1961. q. FRF 360. adv. bk.rev. **Document type:** *Newspaper.*
Formerly: Audioprothesiste Francais
Published by: (Syndicat National Unifie des Audioprothesistes), Galatee s.a.r.l., 5 av. Joffre, Garches 92380, France. TEL 61-21-10-38, FAX 62-27-29-31. Ed. P Avan. Adv. contact F Degove.

371.912 CAN ISSN 0008-2805
CANADIAN (BELLEVILLE). Text in English. 1892. 4/yr. free per issue. illus.
Indexed: P C I.
Published by: Sir James Whitney School, 350 Dundas St W, Belleville, ON K8P 1B2, Canada. TEL 613-962-5361. Ed. G J Gervis. Circ: 644.

CAPTION. see *COMMUNICATIONS—Television And Cable*

CATALOG OF CAPTIONED FILMS FOR THE DEAF. see *MOTION PICTURES—Abstracting, Bibliographies, Statistics*

362.42 USA
CONGREGATION NEWS✶. Text in English. 1961. m. USD 10; USD 15 foreign. **Document type:** *Bulletin, Newsletter.* **Description:** Religion, Jewish education, recreation and workshops for the Jewish deaf.
Related titles: Microfilm ed.
Published by: Temple Beth Solomon of the Deaf, 5429 Lindley Ave, Tarzana, CA 91356-3703. TEL 818-899-2123, FAX 818-899-2202. Circ: 429.

362.4 USA
CONNECTICUT. COMMISSION ON THE DEAF AND HEARING-IMPAIRED. ANNUAL REPORT. (Included in Connecticut Administrative Reports) Text in English. 1974. a. free per issue. **Document type:** *Newsletter, Government.* **Description:** Provides advocacy, community education, counseling, interpreting, job development and placement, referral for deaf and hard of hearing persons.
Formerly: Connecticut. Commission to Study and Investigate the Problems of Deaf and Hearing-Impaired Persons. Annual Report (0094-727X)
Published by: Department of Human Resources, Commission on the Deaf and Hearing-Impaired, 1245 Farmington Ave, West Hartford, CT 06107-2668. TEL 860-561-0196, 800-708-6796, FAX 860-561-0162, cdhi@po.state.ct.us, http://www.state.ct.us/cdhi/index.htm, http://www.state.ct.us/cdhi/index/htm. Ed. Stacie J Mawson. Circ: 5,000.

362.42 IRL ISSN 1393-4805
CONTACT NEWS; voice of the Irish deaf. Text in English. 1979. 6/yr. IEP 7 domestic; USD 20 foreign (effective 2000). adv. bk.rev. back issues avail. **Document type:** *Newsletter, Consumer.* **Description:** Contains community events including sports, deaf issues, domestic and personal features, and social affairs.
Formerly (until 1996): Contact (0332-2491)
Address: 37 Offaly Rd., Cabra, Dublin 7, Ireland. TEL 353-1-8680202, FAX 353-1-8680202, tra7dun@eircom.net. Ed., R&P Stan Foran. Circ: 900.

COURAGE NEWS. see *EDUCATION—Special Education And Rehabilitation*

CUED SPEECH JOURNAL. see *EDUCATION—Special Education And Rehabilitation*

280.4 USA ISSN 0744-9100
DAILY DEVOTIONS FOR THE DEAF. Text in English. 1980. q. free. adv. illus. 96 p./no. 2 cols./p.
Description: Thematic devotion geared to hearing-impaired and deaf people.
Related titles: Large type ed. 14 pt.; Video ed.
Published by: Deaf Missions, 21199 Greenview Rd, Council Bluffs, IA 51503. TEL 712-322-5493, FAX 712-322-7792, deafmissions@deafmissions.com, http://www.deafmissions.com. Ed., R&P Duane King. Circ: 21,000.

DEAF - BLIND PERSPECTIVES. see *HANDICAPPED—Visually Impaired*

371.912 USA
DEAF CENTER NEWS✶. Text in English. 1989 (vol.9). m.
Description: Provides news and information for the deaf community and their hearing friends.
Published by: Lutheran Social Services, Deaf Center Services, 750 Kelly Dr, York, PA 17404-2433. TEL 717-848-6238.

362.42 ZAF
DEAF FEDERATION SOUTH AFRICA. SERVICE INFORMATION BOOKLET. Text in English. 1955. biennial. ZAR 7.50 (effective 1999). **Document type:** *Newsletter.*
Formerly: South African National Council for the Deaf. Service Information Booklet; Supersedes (in 1994): South African National Council for the Deaf. Annual Diary
Published by: South African National Council for the Deaf, Private Bag X4, Westhoven, Johannesburg 2142, South Africa. TEL 27-11-4821610, FAX 27-11-7265873. R&P K Kellerman. Circ: 4,000.

362.42 USA
DEAF SAN DIEGAN. Text in English. 1987-1990; resumed 1992. bi-m. USD 12. adv. bk.rev. **Document type:** *Newsletter.* **Description:** Focuses on community services for the deaf and hard-of-hearing in the San Diego area. Includes information on club activities.
Formerly (until 1990): Deaf Community Services Magazine of San Diego
Published by: Deaf Community Services of San Diego, Inc., 7851 Mission Center Ct, Ste 310, San Diego, CA 92108-1328. TEL 619-682-5001, FAX 619-692-5040. Adv. contact Mimi Francis. Circ: 3,000.

362.42 USA
DEAFDIGEST✶. Text in English. 1996. w. back issues avail. **Description:** For the deaf, hearing impaired, parents, friends and professionals that deal with the deaf.
Media: E-mail.
Published by: Silent News, Inc., 133 Gaither Dr., Ste. E, Mt. Laurel, NJ 08054-1710. barry@deafdigest.com, http://deafdigest.org, http://www.deafdigest.org. Ed. Barry M Strassler.

371.912 GBR ISSN 1464-3154
DEAFNESS AND EDUCATION INTERNATIONAL. Text in English. 1902. 3/yr. USD 115 in North America to individuals; GBP 60 rest of world to individuals; USD 144 in North America to institutions; GBP 80 rest of world to institutions (effective 2001). adv. charts. index. *Refereed.* **Document type:** *Academic/Scholarly.* **Description:** Provides a forum for peer-reviewed scholarly papers relevant to the education of deaf infants, children and young people, and reports original research on their linguistic, educational, social and cognitive development.
Former titles: Deafness and Education (1366-4379); (until 1997): British Association of Teachers of the Deaf. Journal (0266-4062); Which supersedes in part: Teacher of the Deaf (0040-0459)
Related titles: Online - full text ed.: (from Institute for Scientific Information).
Indexed: ASCA, Br.Educ.Ind., Cont.Pg.Educ., Curr.Cont., ERA, Educ.Tech.Abstr., High.Educ.Curr.Aware.Bull., Lang.& Lang.Behav.Abstr., SOPODA, SSCI, Sociol.Abstr., Sp.Ed.Needs Abstr., Tech.Educ.Abstr.
—BLDSC (3535.955970), ingenta.
Published by: (British Association of Teachers of the Deaf), Whurr Publishers Ltd., 19b Compton Terr, London N1 2UN, United Kingdom. TEL 44-20-7359-5979, FAX 44-20-7226-5290, info@whurr.co.uk, http://www.whurrjournals.co.uk/, http://www.whurr.co.uk. Ed. Clare Galloway. R&P Colin Whurr. Adv. contact Lizzy Ewer. B&W page GBP 300; trim 140 x 220. Circ: 2,100. **Subscr. in N. America to:** Whurr Publishers Ltd., PO Box 1897, Lawrence, KS 66044-8897. TEL 913-843-1221, FAX 913-843-1274, am&m@allenpress.com. **Subscr. to:** Turpin Distribution Services Ltd., Blackhorse Rd, Letchworth, Herts SG6 1HN, United Kingdom. TEL 44-1462-488900, FAX 44-1462-483011, custservturpin@turpinltd.com.

DEAFSPORTZINE. see *SPORTS AND GAMES*

371.912 DNK ISSN 0105-7723
DOEVES JUL. Text in Danish. 1957. a. DKK 30 (effective 2001). adv. bk.rev. **Document type:** *Yearbook.* **Description:** Christmas publication.
Published by: Danske Doeves Landsforbund, Rantzausgade 60, PO Box 704, Copenhagen N 2200, Denmark. TEL 45-35-24-09-10, FAX 45-35-24-09-20, lf@deaf.dk, http://www.deaf.dk. Ed. Thure Krarup. Adv. contact Gurli Andersen.

362.42 NOR ISSN 0332-6942
DOEVES TIDSSKRIFT. Text in Norwegian. 1920. bi-w. NOK 350 in Norway; NOK 380 elsewhere (effective 1999). adv. bk.rev. **Document type:** *Bulletin.* **Description:** Information about and for deaf people, their families and those working with the deaf; sign language, interpretation. News from the Norwegian Deaf Association and news from schools for the deaf.
Formerly (until 1968): Tegn og Tale (0332-7051)
—CCC.
Published by: Doeves Forlag AS, Postboks 3171, Bergen 5023, Norway. TEL 47-5-200747, FAX 47-5-200559, skaten@online.no; anda@online.no. Ed. Erling Jacobsen. Pub., R&P Rune Kvalheim. Adv. contact Leif Kallestad. B&W page NOK 5,000, color page NOK 9,000. Circ: 3,000.

DOTS AND TAPS; Canada's national magazine for the deaf-blind. see *HANDICAPPED—Visually Impaired*

371.912 ITA ISSN 1120-5393
EDUCAZIONE DEI SORDI. Text in Italian; Summaries in English, French, German, Spanish. 1872. q. ITL 30,000, USD 25, EUR 15.50. bk.rev.
Former titles (until 1952): Educazione del Sordomuti (1120-5628); (until 1938): Scuola dei Sordomuti (1120-561X); (until 1926): Educazione dei Sordomuti (0390-5993); (until 1884): Educazione del Sordomuti in Italia (1120-5601)
Address: Via Pendola, 35, Siena, SI 53100, Italy. FAX 39-05-7741923. Ed. Enrico Cimino. Circ: 500.

362.42 ITA ISSN 0013-2195
EFFETA; pubblicazione mensile dell'opera Gualandi. Text in Italian. 1905. m. ITL 40,000, USD 40. adv. bk.rev. illus.
Description: Covers psychology, history and pedagogy.
Related titles: CD-ROM ed.; Online - full text ed.
Indexed: Lang.& Lang.Behav.Abstr., SOPODA, Sociol.Abstr.
Published by: Istituto Gualandi per Sordomuti e Sordomute, Via Nosadella, 49, Bologna, BO 40123, Italy. TEL 39-51-330552, FAX 39-51-332878. Ed. Aldo Natali. Circ: 2,500.

362.42 USA ISSN 1526-8721
THE ENDEAVOR (GETTYSBURG). Text in English. 1967. q. USD 40 to members (effective 2001). adv. bk.rev. **Document type:** *Newsletter.* **Description:** Covers equipment for the deaf, activities of affiliates, and news pertinent to current concerns of the society and families with deaf children.
Incorporates: American Society for Deaf Children. President's Update
Published by: American Society for Deaf Children, P O Box 3355, Gettysburg, PA 17325. TEL 717-334-7922, 800-942-2732, FAX 717-334-8808, asdc1@aol.com, http://www.deafchildren.org/asdc2k/membership/endeavor.shtml, http://www.deafchildren.org/asdc2k/home/home.shtml. Ed. Margaret Finnegan. Pub., R&P Linda Zumbrun.

362.42 ESP
FARO DEL SILENCIO; la revista de todos los sordos Espanoles. Text in Spanish. 1977. bi-m. ESP 3,300, USD 42. adv. bk.rev. back issues avail. **Description:** Covers the association's activities and information related to deafness, including education, health and interpreting.
Published by: Confederacion Nacional de Sordos de Espana (C.N.S.E.), Alcala, 160, Madrid 28028, Spain. TEL 34-1-3565776, FAX 34-1-355-4336. Ed. Jesus Ayerra Blanco. Circ: 2,000.

617.8 ESP ISSN 1135-3511
FIAPAS. Text in Spanish. 1987. bi-m. ESP 2,500 domestic; ESP 5,000 foreign (effective 2001). adv. bk.rev. illus. **Document type:** *Newsletter, Corporate.* **Description:** Contains information for parents of deaf children, shares the experiences of professionals dealing with deafness, helps people who are deaf.
Published by: Federacion Espanola de Asociaciones de Padres y Amigos de los Sordos, Nunez de Balboa, 3, 1o Int., Madrid 28001, Spain. TEL 34-91-576-5149, FAX 34-91-576-5746, fiapas@jet.es, http://www.fiapas.es/. Ed. Carmen Danvila. Circ: 8,000 (paid).

FLORIDA SCHOOL HERALD. see *EDUCATION—Special Education And Rehabilitation*

362.42 USA ISSN 0739-9243
FRAT. Text in English. 1904. q. USD 8. adv. back issues avail. **Document type:** *Newspaper.* **Description:** Articles on life insurance and the deaf, with news from the divisions.
Published by: National Fraternal Society of the Deaf, 1118 S 6th St, Springfield, IL 62703. TEL 217-789-7429, FAX 217-789-7489. Ed., R&P, Adv. contact Al van Nevel. Circ: 7,500.

371.912 378 USA ISSN 0016-4089
HV2561
GALLAUDET TODAY. Text in English. 1970. q. USD 10; USD 12 foreign. bk.rev. illus. index. **Document type:** *Academic/Scholarly.* **Description:** Discusses issues concerning deafness.
Formerly: Gallaudet Bulletin
Indexed: Except.Child Educ.Abstr., Rehabil.Lit., Russ.Acad.Sci.Bibl.
Published by: Gallaudet University, Department of Publications and Production, 800 Florida Ave, N E, Washington, DC 20002-3695. TEL 202-651-5671, FAX 202-651-5670. Ed. Vickie Walter. Circ: 14,000.

371.912 CZE ISSN 0323-0732
GONG; mesicnik sluchove postizenych. Text in Czech. 1972. m. CZK 183. bk.rev. **Description:** Explores association activities, as well as deaf education and technical aids for the hard of hearing and deaf in the Czech Republic.
Published by: Asociace Organizaci Neslysicich, Nedoslychavych a Jejich Pratel (ASNEP)/Association of the Deaf, Hard of Hearing, and Friends, Habova 1571, Stodulky, Prague, 5 155 00, Czech Republic. TEL 42-2-6521412, FAX 42-2-6521411, gong@braillnet.cz. Circ: 3,300.

371.912 USA ISSN 1072-8791
GUILDER✶. Text in English. 1916. s-a. donation. adv. back issues avail. **Document type:** *Consumer.* **Description:** Presents information of interest to hard-of-hearing people; includes Guild activities.
Published by: Boston Guild for the Hard of Hearing, 1505 Commonwealth Ave, Ste 4, Brighton, MA 02135-3605. TEL 617-267-4730, FAX 617-267-9422. Ed., R&P Robert A Gilmore. Circ: 1,300.

617.89 IND ISSN 0971-0949
HEARING AID JOURNAL. Text in English. 1977. q. INR 300, USD 150 (effective 2002). adv. bk.rev. 28 p./no. 2 cols./p. **Document type:** *Journal, Academic/Scholarly.* **Description:** For audiologists, speech pathologists and hearing aid dealers.
Indexed: AgeLine, Psychol.Abstr.
—BLDSC (4275.271000).
Address: C4F/216, Janakpuri, New Delhi 110 058, India. TEL 91-11-5599839, FAX 91-11-5593216, kumars@vsnl.com. Ed. Satyendra Gupta. Pub., R&P Narendra Kumar. adv.: page USD 600; 6 x 8. Circ: 2,000.

362.42 GBR
HEARING CONCERN. Text in English. 1947. q. GBP 10 (effective 2001). bk.rev. back issues avail. **Document type:** *Trade, Consumer.* **Description:** Covers issues relating to hearing-impaired persons and professionals involved with them.
Formerly: Hark

Address: c/o Ed. Philip Barron, 7-11 Armstrong Rd, London W3 7JL, United Kingdom. TEL 44-181-743-1110, FAX 44-181-742-9043, hearing.concern@ukonline.co.uk, info@hearingconcern.com, http://web.ukonline.co.uk/hearing.concern, http://www.hearingconcern.com. Ed., R&P Philip Barron TEL 44-181-680-2229. Circ: 5,000 (controlled). **Dist. by:** Redesign, Jute Ln, Enfield, London EN3 7JL, United Kingdom. TEL 44-181-805-8585.

362.42 USA
HEARING HEALTH; the voice on hearing issues. Text in English. 1984. q. USD 24 domestic; USD 43 foreign; USD 4.95 newsstand/cover (effective 2001). adv. bk.rev., software rev. illus. 72 p./no. 3 cols./p. back issues avail. **Document type:** *Magazine, Consumer.* **Description:** Entertains and educates hearing impaired and deaf people nationwide on the issue of hearing loss.
Formerly (until 1992): Voice (0888-2517)
Related titles: Online - full text ed.
Indexed: Lang.& Lang.Behav.Abstr., SOPODA, Sociol.Abstr.
Published by: Voice International Publications, Inc., 2989 Main St, Box V, Ingleside, TX 78362-0500. TEL 361-776-7240, FAX 361-776-3278, ears2u@hearinghealthmag.com, http://www.hearinghealthmag.com. Ed., Pub. Paula Bonillas. R&P Dolores Stone TEL 361-776-7240. Adv. contact Lorraine Short TEL 361-529-6492. B&W page USD 4,000, color page USD 4,500; trim 10.88 x 8.75. Circ: 20,000.

617.89 USA ISSN 0745-7472
HEARING JOURNAL. Text in English. 1947. m. USD 89 domestic to individuals; USD 178 foreign to individuals; USD 106 domestic to institutions; USD 206 foreign to institutions (effective 2002). adv. bk.rev. charts, illus. index. **Document type:** *Journal, Trade.*
Former titles: Hearing Aid Journal (0091-2166); National Hearing Aid Journal (0027-9439)
Related titles: Online - full text ed.: (from Gale Group).
Indexed: CINAHL, Except.Child Educ.Abstr.
—BLDSC (4275.285500), GNLM, ingenta.
Published by: Lippincott Williams & Wilkins (Philadelphia) (Subsidiary of: Wolters Kluwer N.V.), 530 Walnut St, Philadelphia, PA 19106-3621. TEL 215-521-8300, FAX 215-521-8902, custserv@lww.com, http://www.lww.com/. Ed. David H. Kirkwood. Circ: 22,000 (controlled). **Dist. by:** PO Box 1600, Hagerstown, MD 21740-1600. TEL 800-638-3030, FAX 310-223-2400.

305.908162 USA ISSN 1090-6215
HEARING LOSS; the journal of self help for hard of hearing people. Text in English. 1980. bi-m. USD 25 to individuals; USD 40 in Canada & Mexico to individuals; USD 50 elsewhere to individuals (effective 2000). adv. bk.rev. back issues avail. **Description:** Contains information about hearing loss, assistance, technology, and coping techniques.
Former titles: S H H H Journal (1089-6716); Shhh (0883-1688)
Indexed: AgeLine, Except.Child Educ.Abstr.
Published by: Self Help for Hard of Hearing People, Inc., 7910 Woodmont Ave, Ste 1200, Bethesda, MD 20814. TEL 301-657-2248, FAX 301-913-9413, http://www.shhh.org. Ed., R&P Barbara Kelley. Circ: 30,000.

362.4 USA ISSN 0360-9278
HV2350
HEARING REHABILITATION QUARTERLY. Text in English. q. USD 35 (effective 1998). adv. bk.rev. **Document type:** *Academic/Scholarly, Consumer.*
Former titles (until 1975): Highlights (0360-9286); (until 1960): League for the Hard of Hearing. Quarterly Bulletin
Indexed: AgeLine, DSH Abstr., Except.Child Educ.Abstr., Psychol.Abstr., Rehabil.Lit.
—GNLM.
Published by: League for the Hard of Hearing, 71 W 23rd St, New York, NY 10010-4162. TEL 917-305-7700, FAX 917-305-7888, postmaster@lhh.org, http://www.lhh.org. Ed. Joseph F Brown. R&P Joseph Brown TEL 917-305-7810. Circ: 2,500.

371.92 DEU
HEIDELBERGER BEITRAEGE ZUR GEHOERLOSENBILDUNG UND SCHWERHOERIGENBILDUNG. Text in German. 1995. irreg., latest vol.3, 1998. DEM 42 per issue. **Document type:** *Monographic series, Academic/Scholarly.*
Published by: Median-Verlag von Killisch-Horn GmbH, Hauptstr 64, Heidelberg 69117, Germany. TEL 49-6221-90509-0, FAX 49-6221-9050920, median-verlag@t-online.de, http://www.median-verlag.de.

362.42 DNK ISSN 0018-4934
HOERELSEN. Text in Danish. 1913. 10/yr. DKK 120 (effective 1998). adv. bk.rev. charts, illus. index. **Document type:** *Newsletter, Consumer.*
Formerly: Tidsskrift for Tunghoere
Published by: Landsforeningen for Bedre Hoerelse/Danish Association for Better Hearing, Kloeverprisvej 10 B, Hvidovre 2650, Denmark. TEL 45-36-75-42-00, FAX 45-36-38-85-80. Ed. Henrik Boesen. Circ: 16,000.

371.912 DEU ISSN 0179-4728
HOEREN UND VERSTEHEN. Text in German. q. **Document type:** *Journal, Consumer.*
Published by: Median-Verlag von Killisch-Horn GmbH, Hauptstr 64, Heidelberg 69117, Germany. TEL 49-6221-90509-0, FAX 49-6221-9050920, median-verlag@t-online.de, http://www.median-verlag.de.

371.912 DEU ISSN 0018-3121
HOERGESCHAEDIGTE KINDER. Text in German. 1964. q. DEM 29.50 (effective 2000). adv. bk.rev. bibl, illus, stat. index. **Document type:** *Journal, Academic/Scholarly.*
Published by: (Deutsche Gesellschaft zur Foerderung der Gehoerlosen und Schwerhoerigen e.V.), Verlag Hoergeschaedigte Kinder GmbH, Bernadottestr 126, Hamburg 22605, Germany. TEL 49-40-8807031, FAX 49-40-8806793. Ed. Dr. Klaus B Guenther. Pub., R&P Ulf Mueller. Circ: 4,500.

371.912 DEU ISSN 0342-4898
HOERGESCHAEDIGTEN-PAEDAGOGIK. Text in German. 1946. 6/yr. EUR 57.80 domestic; EUR 67.10 foreign (effective 2002). adv. bk.rev. bibl, illus. index. **Document type:** *Journal, Academic/Scholarly.* **Description:** For educators of the deaf and hard-of-hearing.
Formerly: Neue Blaetter fuer Taubstummenbildung (0028-310X)
Related titles: ♦ Supplement: Hoergeschaedigten-Paedagogik. Beihefte.
Indexed: IBR, IBZ, Russ.Acad.Sci.Bibl.
—GNLM, Infotrieve. **CCC.**
Published by: (Berufsverband Deutscher Hoergeschaedigtenpaedagogen), Median-Verlag von Killisch-Horn GmbH, Hauptstr 64, Heidelberg 69117, Germany. TEL 49-6221-90509-0, FAX 49-6221-9050920, median-verlag@t-online.de, http://www.median-verlag.de. Ed. Manfred Breitinger. Circ: 1,500.

371.912 DEU
HOERGESCHAEDIGTEN-PAEDAGOGIK. BEIHEFTE. Text in German. irreg., latest vol.44, 2001. **Document type:** *Monographic series, Academic/Scholarly.*
Related titles: ♦ Supplement to: Hoergeschaedigten-Paedagogik. ISSN 0342-4898.
Published by: Median-Verlag von Killisch-Horn GmbH, Hauptstr 64, Heidelberg 69117, Germany. TEL 49-6221-90509-0, FAX 49-6221-9050920, median-verlag@t-online.de, http://www.median-verlag.de.

371.912 GBR ISSN 0255-0326
I F H O H JOURNAL. Text in English. 1980. 3/yr. USD 50 for 3 yrs. (effective 1999). adv. bk.rev. **Document type:** *Bulletin.* **Description:** News of the Federation and about the field of hearing loss.
Indexed: Russ.Acad.Sci.Bibl.
Published by: International Federation of the Hard of Hearing, PO Box 13, Abbots Langley, Herts WD5 0RQ, United Kingdom. TEL 44-1923-264584, FAX 44-1923-261635, c_shaw@compuserve.com. Ed., R&P, Adv. contact Christopher Shaw. Circ: 750.

371.912 USA ISSN 0745-1539
ILLINOIS ADVANCE. Text in English. 1870. 4/yr. free per issue. illus. **Document type:** *Newsletter.* **Description:** Serves as a learning project for students in the business education and printing classes, and as a means of communicating the school's affairs to family, friends, alumni, staff, and to sister schools in the U.S. and abroad.
Indexed: Rehabil.Lit.
Published by: Illinois School for the Deaf, 125 Webster Ave, Jacksonville, IL 62650. TEL 217-479-4257, FAX 217-479-4326. Ed. Ark Clodfelter. R&P Mark Clodfelter. Circ: 2,000.

362.42 BEL
INFO SOURDS JOURNAL. Text in French. 1984. 4/yr. BEF 300 domestic; BEF 500 foreign (effective 2000). adv. back issues avail. *Refereed.* **Document type:** *Bulletin.* **Description:** Presents news and facts of interest to the hard of hearing in Belgium. Includes calendar of events and puzzles.
Published by: Federation Francophone des Sourds de Belgique, Rue van Eyck 11 A-4, Brussels 1050, Belgium. TEL 32-2-6446844, FAX 32-2-6446844, infos@ffsb.be, http://www.ffsb.be. Ed. Martine Fraiture. Circ: 530; 332 (paid). **Dist. by:** Belgium.

INTERNATIONAL TINNITUS JOURNAL. see *MEDICAL SCIENCES—Otorhinolaryngology*

371.912 JPN
JAPANESE DEAF NEWS; newspaper of the deaf in Japan. Text in Japanese. 1948. m. JPY 3,800; JPY 250 newsstand/cover (effective 2001). adv. bk.rev. back issues avail. *Refereed.* **Document type:** *Newspaper.* **Description:** Contains news concerning the Japanese deaf community.
Formerly: Japan Hearing - Handicap News Paper
Published by: Japanese Federation of the Deaf, SK Bldg, 8th Fl, 130, Yamabuki-cho, Shinjuku-ku, Tokyo 162-0801, Japan. TEL 81-3-3268-8847, FAX 81-3-3267-3445, info@jfd.or.jp, http://www.jfd.or.jp. Ed., R&P, Adv. contact Eiichi Takada. Circ: 20,000 (paid). **Subscr. to:** c/o Seni-Kaiken, Muromachi-dori, Imadegawa Sagaru, Kamigyo-ku, Kyoto-shi 602, Japan. TEL 81-75-441-6079, FAX 81-75-441-6147.

H

371.912 USA ISSN 1081-4159
HV2350
THE JOURNAL OF DEAF STUDIES AND DEAF EDUCATION. Text in English. 1996. q. GBP 40, USD 60 to individuals; GBP 120, USD 175 to institutions; GBP 20, USD 30 to students (effective Mar. 2002). adv. back issues avail. *Refereed.* **Document type:** *Journal, Academic/Scholarly.* **Description:** Integrates and coordinates basic and applied research relating to individuals who are deaf, including cultural, developmental, linguistic, and educational topics.
Related titles: Online - full text ed.: ISSN 1465-7325. GBP 108, USD 157 to institutions Online only (effective Mar. 2002) (from HighWire Pr., EBSCO Publishing, O C L C Online Computer Library Center, Inc., RoweCom Information Quest, ingenta, Swets Blackwell).
—BLDSC (4967.818000). **CCC.**
Published by: Oxford University Press, Academic Division, Great Clarendon St, Oxford OX2 6DP, United Kingdom. TEL 44-1865-267907, FAX 44-1865-267835, jnlorders@oup-usa.org, jnl.info@oup.co.uk, http://deafed.oupjournals.org/, http://www.oup.co.uk/journals. Pub. J Fox. adv.: B&W page GBP 220, B&W page USD 420; trim 178 x 255. Circ: 900. **Subscr. outside the Americas to:** Journals Marketing, Great Clarendon St, Oxford OX2 6DP, United Kingdom.

371.912 USA ISSN 0882-7893
HV2402 CODEN: JOINEA
JOURNAL OF INTERPRETATION (ROCKVILLE). Text in English. 1981-1987; resumed. a. bk.rev. *Refereed.* **Document type:** *Academic/Scholarly.* **Description:** Presents articles and research related to the field of sign language interpreting.
Formerly (until 1985): Registry of Interpreters for the Deaf. Professional interpreting journal. (0277-6480)
Indexed: Lang.& Lang.Behav.Abstr., SOPODA, Sociol.Abstr.
Published by: (Registry of Interpreters for the Deaf, Inc.), R I D Publications, 8630 Fenton St, Ste 324, Silver Spring, MD 20910-3803. TEL 301-279-0555 V-TD, FAX 301-608-0508, views@rid.org, http://www.rid.org. Ed. Clay Nettles. Pub., R&P Stuart Nealy. Circ: 6,500.

362.42 USA ISSN 1092-4388
RC423 CODEN: JSPHAH
JOURNAL OF SPEECH, LANGUAGE, AND HEARING RESEARCH. Text in English. 1958. bi-m., latest vol.44, 2001. USD 105 to individuals; USD 135 foreign to individuals; USD 300 to institutions; USD 355 foreign to institutions (effective 2002). adv. bk.rev. bibl, charts, illus. Index. 218 p./no. back issues avail.; reprint service avail. from PQC,PSC,SCH. *Refereed.* **Document type:** *Journal, Academic/Scholarly.* **Description:** Includes papers pertaining to the process and disorder of hearing, language, and speech, and to the diagnosis and treatment of these disorders.
Formerly (until 1996): Journal of Speech and Hearing Research (0022-4685); Which incorporates (1948-1991): Journal of Speech and Hearing Disorders (0022-4677); Which was formerly (1936-1947): Journal of Speech Disorders (0885-9426)

Related titles: Microform ed.: (from PQC); Online - full text ed.: (from H. W. Wilson, ProQuest Information & Learning, Gale Group, Factiva, Institute for Scientific Information).
Indexed: ABSEARCH - ASHA (1945-), ASCA, ASSIA, AgeLine, Arts & Hum.Cit.Ind. (coverage dropped), Bibl.Dev.Med.& Child Neur., Biol.Abstr., C.I.J.E., CINAHL, Chem.Abstr., Curr.Cont., Dent.Ind., ERA, Educ.Ind. (Feb.1997-), Except.Child Educ.Abstr., Excerp.Med., Fam.Ind., INIS Atomind., INSPEC (Mar.1972-Dec.1996, Feb.1997-), Ind.Med. (1997-), Int.Nurs.Ind., Lang.& Lang.Behav.Abstr., Ling.Abstr., MLA Intl.Bibl., NBA, Noise Pollut.Publ.Abstr., PsycInfo, Psychol.Abstr., Rehabil.Lit., Russ.Acad.Sci.Bibl., SOPODA, SSCI, Soc.Sci.Ind. (Jul.1999-), Sociol.Abstr., Sp.Ed.Needs Abstr., e-psyche.
—BLDSC (5066.174000), AskIEEE, CISTI, GNLM, IDS, Infotrieve, ingenta, KNAW, Linda Hall. **CCC.**
Published by: American Speech - Language - Hearing Association, 10801 Rockville Pike, Rockville, MD 20852. TEL 301-897-5700, FAX 301-897-9358, sghoting@asha.org, http://professional.asha.org/publications/jslhr.htm. Eds. Charles Craig Formby, Claire Stathopoulos, Susan Ellis Weismer. R&P Kirsten Gardner. Adv. contact Karmen Shum TEL 913-469-1110 ext 212. Circ: 73,000.

H

371.912 USA
KA KULI O'HAWAI'I. Text in English. 1970. bi-m. USD 7.50 (effective 1998). back issues avail. **Document type:** *Newsletter.* **Description:** Community and educational news on the deaf.
Formerly: H A N D S (Hawaiian Aloha Needs Deaf Spirit)
Published by: Aloha State Association of Deaf, c/o Waikiki Community Center, 310 Paoakalani Ave, Rm 201 A, Honolulu, HI 96815-3738. TEL 808-926-8203, FAX 808-924-9664. Ed., R&P Steve Laracuente. Circ: 325.

362.42 FIN ISSN 0023-5741
KUULOVIESTI/HEARING NEWS. Text in Finnish; Summaries in English, Swedish. 1934. 8/yr. FIM 150 (effective 1997). adv. bk.rev. **Document type:** *Consumer.*
Published by: Kuulonhuoltoliitto/Finnish Federation of the Hard of Hearing, Iikantie 4, Helsinki 00400, Finland. FAX 5803770. Ed. Seppo Matinvesi. Adv. contact Taisto Vihavainen. B&W page FIM 6,000. Circ: 14,300.

617.89 USA
LISTENER. Text in English. 1956. q. free per issue. bk.rev., film rev. illus, stat. back issues avail. **Document type:** *Newsletter.* **Description:** Information and data for the hearing and speech impaired.
Published by: Hear Center, 301 E Del Mar Blvd, Pasadena, CA 91101. TEL 626-796-2016, FAX 626-796-2320. Ed., R&P Cheri Lee. Circ: 5,000.

616.885 NLD ISSN 0166-252X
LOGOPEDIE EN FONIATRIE; vaktijdschrift voor logopedie (stem-, spraak-, taal- en gehoorstoornissen). Text in Dutch. 1929. 11/yr. NLG 110; NLG 139.25 foreign. adv. bk.rev. **Document type:** *Academic/Scholarly.*
Published by: Nederlandse Vereniging voor Logopedie en Foniatrie, Postbus 3088, Gouda 2800 CD, Netherlands. TEL 31-182-524266, FAX 31-182-517655, logopedie@nvlf.nl. Pub. H Diemer. R&P L Elte. Adv. contact L Smith.

317.912 ISR
MABAT SHELANU. Text in English, Hebrew. q.
Published by: World Organization of Jewish Deaf, Helen Keller House, P O Box 9001, Tel Aviv 61090, Israel. TEL (03)303355.

362.42 ISR ISSN 0792-0814
MABAT SHELANU/OUR REVIEW. Text in Hebrew. 1969 (no.92). m. free per issue. adv. illus. **Document type:** *Newspaper.*
Former titles (until 1987): Demama Shelanu (0333-9319); Demama (0011-8176)
Published by: Association of the Deaf in Israel, Helen Keller Center, P O Box 9001, Tel Aviv 61090, Israel. TEL 972-3-7303355, FAX 972-3-7396419. Ed. Yoram Bar Yosef. Pub. Ahron Eini. Circ: 2,000.

371.912 USA
MILL NECK FOUNDATION NEWSLETTER. Text in English. 1951. q. free. **Document type:** *Newsletter.* **Description:** Covers education, employment and ministry for the deaf.
Formerly: Mill Neck Manor Bulletin
Published by: Mill Neck Foundation, Frost Mill Rd, Box 100, Mill Neck, NY 11765. TEL 516-922-4100, FAX 516-922-3759, http://www.millneck.org. Ed., R&P Nancy C Leghart. Circ: 76,000 (controlled). **Subscr. to:** Mill Neck Manor Lutheran School for the Deaf, Frost Mill Rd, PO Box 12, Mill Neck, NY 11765.

371.912 USA ISSN 1059-7506
MISSOURI RECORD. Text in English. 1879. 5/yr. free per issue. **Description:** Dedicated to parents of deaf children, alumni of the Missouri School for the Deaf and professionals in the education of the deaf.
Related titles: Microfilm ed.
Published by: Missouri School for the Deaf, 505 E 5th St, Fulton, MO 65251-1799. TEL 314-592-4000, FAX 314-592-2570. Ed. Peter H Ripley. Circ: 1,029.

MOON RAINBOW. see *HANDICAPPED—Visually Impaired*

362.42 USA ISSN 0887-0004
N D BANNER. Text in English. 1891. 3/yr. USD 2. **Document type:** *Academic/Scholarly.*
Published by: North Dakota School for the Deaf, 1401 College Dr, Devils Lake, ND 58301. TEL 701-662-9001, FAX 701-662-9009, baduncan@sendit.nodak.edu. Ed., R&P Barbara J Duncan. Circ: 600.

362.4 USA
NAT - CENT NEWS. Text in English. 3/yr. USD 10; free to libraries and qualified personnel (effective 2001). *Refereed.* **Description:** Contains articles on legislation, services, aids, devices, human interest, and problems related to deaf-blindness.
Related titles: Braille ed.; Large type ed. 24 pt.
Published by: Helen Keller National Center for Deaf - Blind Youths and Adults, 111 Middle Neck Rd., Sands Point, NY 11050. TEL 516-944-8900, 800-255-0411, FAX 516-944-7302, hkncomed@aol.com, http://www.helenkeller.org/national. Ed. Robert J Smithdas. Circ: 3,700.

362.42 USA ISSN 1046-4417
NATIONAL CONGRESS OF JEWISH DEAF. QUARTERLY✱. Text in English. 1958. q. USD 15. adv. bk.rev., film rev., play rev. **Description:** News, Judaism topics and reports keeping members abreast of new developments in the deaf world.
Published by: National Congress of Jewish Deaf, Temple Beth Solomon, 5429 Lindley Ave, Tarzana, CA 91356-3703. Ed. Jushua Mandelsohn. Circ: 1,000.

155.4512 GBR
NATIONAL DEAF CHILDREN'S SOCIETY. ANNUAL REPORT. Text in English. 1948. a. free per issue. adv. **Document type:** *Corporate.* **Description:** Report of the Society's activities for the previous year.
Formerly: National Deaf Children's Society. Yearbook and Annual Accounts
Published by: National Deaf Children's Society, 15 Dufferin St, London EC1Y 8UR, United Kingdom. TEL 44-2074-908656, FAX 44-20-7251-5020, ndcs@ndcs.org.uk, http://www.ndcs.org.uk. Ed. Emma Kelly. Circ: 2,000.

DIE NEUE SONDERSCHULE. see *EDUCATION*

371.912 DEU
NEUES HOEREN; Hauszeitschrift Ihres Hoergeraete-Akustikers. Text in German. bi-m. **Document type:** *Magazine, Consumer.*
Published by: Median-Verlag von Killisch-Horn GmbH, Hauptstr 64, Heidelberg 69117, Germany. TEL 49-6221-90509-0, FAX 49-6221-9050920, median-verlag@t-online.de, http://www.median-verlag.de.

NEW JERSEY SPEECH AND HEARING ASSOCIATION. JOURNAL. see *MEDICAL SCIENCES*

371.913 USA ISSN 0896-6478
HV2561
NEW MEXICO PROGRESS. Text in English. 1909. bi-m. free per issue. illus. **Document type:** *Newsletter.* **Description:** News and activities of the school. Recognizes outstanding students.
Published by: New Mexico School for the Deaf, 1060 Cerrillos Rd, Santa Fe, NM 87503. TEL 505-827-6747. Ed. Lester D Graham. Circ: 900.

362.4 USA
NEWS FROM ADVOCATES FOR DEAF - BLIND. Text in English. 3/yr. free to members (effective 2001). *Refereed.* **Document type:** *Newsletter.* **Description:** For and by parents and families with individuals who are deaf-blind.
Former titles: National Family Association for the Deaf-Blind; National Parent Network
Related titles: Braille ed.; Large type ed. 24 pt.
Published by: Helen Keller National Center for Deaf - Blind Youths and Adults, 111 Middle Neck Rd., Sands Point, NY 11050. TEL 516-944-8900, 800-255-0411, FAX 516-944-7302, hkncomed@aol.com, http://www.helenkeller.org/national/.

305.908162 USA ISSN 1091-9457
NEWSWAVES FOR DEAF AND HARD-OF-HEARING PEOPLE. Text in English. 1997. m. (except Aug.). USD 20; USD 20 foreign. adv. 36 p./no. 4 cols./p. **Document type:** *Newspaper.* **Description:** Features articles for and about the deaf and hard-of-hearing people and those who live or work with them.
Published by: Willard Publications, 47 Edmonds St, Rochester, NY 14607. TEL 716-461-2263, 800-421-1220, FAX 716-461-4091, newswaves@aol.com. Ed., Pub., Adv. contact Tom Willard. page USD 625; trim 15 x 11. Wire service: AP.

NOISE & HEALTH; an inter-disciplinary journal. see *MEDICAL SCIENCES—Otorhinolaryngology*

362.42 USA
NORCAL CENTER ON DEAFNESS NEWSLINE. Text in English. 1978. q. USD 15 (effective 2000). adv. bk.rev. **Document type:** *Newsletter.* **Description:** Covers deaf awareness, community news and items of interest to the deaf and hard of hearing communities, including community events.
Former titles: NorCal Community Forum; Deaf Community News; Deaf Community Newsletter
Related titles: Braille ed.
Published by: NorCal Center on Deafness, 1820 Tribute Rd, Ste A, Sacramento, CA 95815-4307. TEL 916-921-1045, FAX 916-921-1177. Ed., R&P Leslie Birchell. Adv. contact Don Varley. Circ: 1,200.

371.912 SWE ISSN 0029-1471
NORDISK TIDSKRIFT FOER DOEVUNDERVISNINGEN. Short title: N T D. Text in Danish, Norwegian, Swedish. 1899. 4/yr. SEK 200 (effective 1991). adv. bk.rev. abstr, charts, illus, stat. index. **Document type:** *Trade.*
Former titles (until 1957): Nordisk Tidskrift foer Doefstumskolan (0347-7991); (until 1956): Tidskrift foer Doefstumskolan
Published by: Nordisk Tidskrift foer Doevundervisningen AB, c/o A Fraendh, Graenv 35 B, Tyresoe 13552, Sweden. TEL 046-142016. Ed. Karin Gustafsson. Circ: 1,200.

ON CUE. see *EDUCATION—Special Education And Rehabilitation*

371.912 GBR ISSN 1460-0811
ONE IN SEVEN. Text in English. 1984. bi-m. GBP 16.50 in United Kingdom to individuals membership; GBP 25 overseas to individuals membership; GBP 10 full-time students, retired, unwaged; GBP 40 to institutions membership (effective 2001). adv. bk.rev., film rev., play rev. 68 p./no. back issues avail. **Document type:** *Consumer.* **Description:** Contains news, interviews with deaf and hard of hearing people, information about deafness and hearing loss, legal advice, reviews on new products and the latest on hearing aids, etc. Aimed at the deaf and hard of hearing people and those concerned about deafness.
Former titles (until Aug. 1997): See Hear! (0968-5529); (until Sep. 1992): Soundbarrier (0267-4300)
Published by: Royal National Institute for Deaf People, 19-23 Featherstone St, London EC1Y 8SL, United Kingdom. TEL 44-20-7296-8000, FAX 44-20-7296-8001, oneinseven@rnid.org.uk, informationline@rnid.org.uk, clive.mills@rnid.org.uk, http://www.rnid.org.uk. Ed. Dawn Egan. Pub. Stephen Iliffe. Adv. contact Daniel Riley TEL 44-20-7312-0470. color page GBP 1,075. Circ: 20,000.

371.912 USA ISSN 0277-8785
HV2350
OREGON OUTLOOK. Text in English. 1910. 6/yr. USD 1.50. adv.
Published by: (Oregon. Department of Education), Oregon School for the Deaf, c/o Alan Yankus, 999 Locust St N E, Salem, OR 97303-5254. TEL 503-378-3825, FAX 503-373-7879. Circ: 500 (paid).

OUR WAY. see *RELIGIONS AND THEOLOGY—Judaic*

R E S N A NEWS. (Rehabilitation Engineering and Assistive Technology Society of North America) see *EDUCATION—Special Education And Rehabilitation*

RAINBOW (PETERBOROUGH). see *HANDICAPPED—Physically Impaired*

REEDUCATION ORTHOPHONIQUE. see *MEDICAL SCIENCES—Otorhinolaryngology*

RING DES WORTES; Seelsorgebrief fuer Hoergeschaedigte, Kranke und Senioren. see *RELIGIONS AND THEOLOGY—Roman Catholic*

362.42 YUG
SAVEZ GLUVIH I NAGLUVIH JUGOSLAVIJE. GLAS. Cover title: Glas S G N J. Text in Serbo-Croatian. 1948. m. free per issue. adv. bk.rev. **Document type:** *Bulletin.*
Former titles: Nas Glas (0352-7557); (until 1985): Revija (Belgrade); (until 1977): Nas Glas (0027-8076)
Published by: Savez Gluvih i Nagluvih Jugoslavije/Federation of the Deaf of Yugoslavia, Svetog Save 16-18, Belgrade, Yugoslavia. TEL 381-11-439523, FAX 381-11-439523, sgnj@eunet.yu. Ed., R&P Nenad Minic. Circ: 1,000.

SCANDINAVIAN AUDIOLOGY. see *MEDICAL SCIENCES—Otorhinolaryngology*

SCANDINAVIAN AUDIOLOGY. SUPPLEMENT. see *MEDICAL SCIENCES—Otorhinolaryngology*

362.42 ITA ISSN 0301-5335
SETTIMANA DEL SORDO; organo di informazione dei minorati dell'udito e della parola. Text in Italian. 1954. m. ITL 50,000 to non-members; ITL 30,000 to members. adv. bk.rev. index. **Document type:** *Bulletin.* **Description:** Includes articles on activities for the deaf, how victims can cope with this handicap and how others can help and live with its victims.
Formerly (until 1973): Settimana del Sordomuto (0037-2919)
Published by: Ente Nazionale Sordomuti, Via Gregorio VII, 120, Rome, RM 00165, Italy. TEL 06-39366697, FAX 06-6380936. Ed. Armando Giuranna. Adv. contact Ida Collu. Circ: 40,000.

371.91 USA
SIGHTS AND SOUNDS. Text in English. 1981. q. free. **Document type:** *Consumer.* **Description:** Gives educators, parents, and friends a better understanding of the institute.
Related titles: Audio cassette/tape ed.; Braille ed.
Indexed: Curr.Cont. (coverage dropped).
Published by: Alabama Institute for Deaf & Blind, PO Box 698, Talladega, AL 35160. TEL 205-761-3206, FAX 205-761-3352. Ed. Lynne Hanner. Circ: 10,000.

371.912 USA ISSN 0037-5187
THE SILENT ADVOCATE. Text in English. 1916. q. free. illus. back issues avail. **Document type:** *Newsletter.* **Description:** News about students and school activities of interest to parents, alumni and supporters.
Published by: St. Rita School for the Deaf, 1720 Glendale Milford Rd, Cincinnati, OH 45215. TEL 513-771-7600, FAX 513-326-8264, http://www.srsdeaf.org. Ed., R&P Jodi Weiser. Circ: 32,000 (controlled).

362.42 ZAF ISSN 0037-5195
SILENT MESSENGER/STILLE BOODSKAPPER. Text in Afrikaans, English. m. free per issue. adv. illus. **Document type:** *Newsletter.* **Description:** Articles and news snippets on deafness, deaf people, as well as information on new technological developments.
Published by: South African National Council for the Deaf, Private Bag X4, Westhoven, Johannesburg 2142, South Africa. TEL 27-11-4821610, FAX 27-11-7265873, deafsa@icon.co.za. Ed. A Botes. R&P K Kellerman. Adv. contact A. Botes. Circ: 3,500.

362.42 USA ISSN 0049-0490
SILENT NEWS. Text in English. 1969. m. USD 30 domestic; USD 40 in Canada & Mexico; USD 50 in South America; USD 60 in Europe; USD 70 in Australasia. adv. bk.rev. back issues avail. **Document type:** *Newspaper.* **Description:** Publishes news and feature articles of interest to deaf and hard-of-hearing persons.
Published by: Silent News, Inc., 133 Gaither Dr., Ste. E, Mt. Laurel, NJ 08054-1710. FAX 609-802-1979, silentnews@aol.com. Pub. Julius Wiggins. R&P Monica Downs. Adv. contact Mike Lachance. Circ: 11,500 (paid).

362.42 USA
SOUNDS OF LEXINGTON. Text in English. 1945. m. (11/yr.). USD 3. bk.rev.
Formerly: Lexington School for the Deaf. Parents' Newsletter. (0031-1928)
Media: Duplicated (not offset). **Related titles:** Cards ed.
Published by: Lexington School for the Deaf, Parents Association, Lexington, NY 11370. Ed. Diane Rosen. Circ: 500.

617.89 USA
SPECTRUM (DENVER). Text in English. 1974. q. USD 10 newsstand/cover to non-members (effective 2001). adv. bk.rev. back issues avail. **Document type:** *Newsletter.* **Description:** Provides up-to-date information on technology, research and practices of hearing conservation; and reports on the continually evolving legal and regulatory activities at state and federal levels which impact hearing conservation practice.
Former titles (until 1988): Hearing Conservation News; (until 1987): National Hearing Conservation Association Newsletter
Published by: National Hearing Conservation Association, 9101 E Kenyon Ave, Ste 3000, Denver, CO 80237-1855. TEL 303-224-9022, FAX 303-770-1812, nhca@gwami.com. Ed. Rena Glaser. Circ: 700.

SPEECH COMMUNICATION. see *LINGUISTICS*

362.42 POL ISSN 0238-9746
SWIAT CISZY* ; czasopismo polskich inwalidow sluchu. Text in Polish. 1959. m. PLZ 18. adv. bk.rev. back issues avail. **Document type:** *Bulletin, Newsletter.*
Formerly (until 1983): Swiat Gluchych (0039-7377)
Published by: Polski Zwiazek Gluchych, Ul Podwale 23, Warsaw 00261, Poland. TEL 48-22-314071, FAX 48-22-6357536. Ed. Wladyslaw Szwedowicz. Circ: 2,500 (paid).

362.42 USA
T C H I UPDATE. Text in English. bi-m. play rev. illus. back issues avail. **Document type:** *Newsletter, Government.* **Description:** Informs persons who are hard of hearing, and their parents, of events that accommodate their needs.
Related titles: Braille ed.; Diskette ed.
Published by: Tennessee Council for the Hearing Impaired, 400 Deaderick St, Ste 1100, Nashville, TN 37248-6300. TEL 615-313-4913. Ed. Sherri Rademacher. **Co-sponsor:** Tennessee. Department of Human Services.

362.42 USA
T D I NATIONAL DIRECTORY OF T T Y NUMBERS (YEAR). Text in English. 1968. a. USD 25 domestic to individuals; USD 30 foreign to individuals; USD 55 to institutions. adv. bk.rev. back issues avail. **Document type:** *Directory.* **Description:** Telephone directory of business, organizations, residential numbers that can be accessed via TTY (telecommunication device for the deaf).
Former titles: National Directory for T T Y Users (Year); International Directory for T T Y Users (Year); Formerly: International Telephone Directory of T D D Users (0160-7472)
Published by: Telecommunications for the Deaf, Inc., 8630 Fenton St Ste 604, Silver Spring, MD 20910. TEL 301-589-3786, 301-589-3006 TTY, FAX 301-589-3797, TDIExDir@aol.com, http://www.tdi-online.org. Ed. Claude Stout. Adv. contact Kenneth Glickman. Circ: 20,000.

TINNITUS TODAY. see *MEDICAL SCIENCES—Otorhinolaryngology*

305.908162 USA
U S TEAM SPOTLIGHT* . Text in English. 1987. q. USD 5. **Description:** Focuses on deaf athletes.
Published by: American Athletic Association of the Deaf, c/o DCARA DAC, 14895 E 14th St, Ste 200, San Leandro, CA 94578-2922. TEL 415-895-2430, FAX 415-895-5108. Eds. Donalda Ammons, Jack Levesque. Circ: 5,000.

USHER AROUND THE WORLD. see *HANDICAPPED—Visually Impaired*

HET VAGGESCHIP. see *HANDICAPPED*

371.912 NLD ISSN 0166-5677
VAN HOREN ZEGGEN. Text in Dutch. 1960. q. NLG 10; USD 25 foreign (effective 2000). adv. bk.rev. **Document type:** *Journal, Academic/Scholarly.*
Published by: Vereniging ter Bevordering van het Onderwijs aan Doven in Nederland (VEDON), Meerkoet 25, Schagen 1742 KM, Netherlands. TEL 31-224-214896, FAX 31-224-298945, wilde@multiweb.nl. Ed., R&P, Adv. contact F.C.M. Mollee. Pub. F C M Mollee. Circ: 1,500. **Co-sponsor:** Nederlandse Vereniging tot Bevordering van het Onderwijs aan Slechthorende Kinderen en Kinderen met Spraak- en Taalmoeilijkheden (VeBOSS).

617.7 CAN
VIBES. Text in English. 1974. q. CND 25 to members (effective 2000). adv. bk.rev. **Document type:** *Consumer.* **Description:** Provides practical and useful information to aid in the understanding of and coping with hearing loss.
Formerly: Vibrations (0227-6755)
Indexed: Sh.& Vib.Dig.
Published by: Canadian Hearing Society, 271 Spadina Rd, Toronto, ON M5R 2V3, Canada. TEL 416-964-9595, FAX 416-968-2506. Ed., R&P Angela Palmer. Adv. contact Jon Reid. B&W page CND 1,500; trim 11.13 x 8.63. Circ: 13,000.

362.42 ITA
VOICE OF SILENCE NEWSLETTER. Text in English, French. 1957. q. membership. adv. bk.rev. **Document type:** *Newsletter.* **Description:** Social rehabilitation of the deaf.
Formerly: Voix du Silence (0042-8388)
Published by: World Federation of the Deaf, Via Gregorio VII, 120, Rome, RM 00165, Italy. Ed. Dr. Cesare Magarotto. Circ: 500 (controlled).

H

371.912 USA ISSN 0042-8639
HV2350 CODEN: VOLRAT
THE VOLTA REVIEW. Text in English. 1898. 5/yr. USD 52 (effective 2000). adv. bk.rev. charts, illus, tr.lit. index. reprint service avail. from PQC,PSC,SCH. **Document type:** *Academic/Scholarly.* **Description:** Publishes articles on issues related to hearing-impairment, speech-therapy, and education of people who are deaf or hard of hearing.
Related titles: Microform ed.: (from PQC); Online - full text ed.: (from Institute for Scientific Information).
Indexed: ASCA, ASSIA, C.I.J.E., CINAHL, Child Devel.Abstr., Curr.Cont., Educ.Ind. (May 1983-), Except.Child Educ.Abstr., Fam.Ind., Lang.& Lang.Behav.Abstr., P C I, PsycInfo, Psychol.Abstr. (1935-), SOPODA, SSCI, Sociol.Abstr., Yrbk.Assoc.Educ.& Rehab.Blind, e-psyche.
—BLDSC (9254.400000), GNLM, IDS, ingenta. **CCC.**
Published by: Alexander Graham Bell Association for the Deaf and Hand of Hearing, Inc., 3417 Volta Place, N W, Washington, DC 20007. TEL 202-337-5220, http://www.agbell.org/publications/publications.html. Ed. Nancy Murray. R&P Michalle Vanderhoff TEL 202-337-5220 ext 125. Adv. contact Elizabeth Quigley. Circ: 6,000.

371.912 USA ISSN 1074-8016
HV2510 CODEN: VOVOE6
VOLTA VOICES. Text in English. 1994. 6/yr. USD 60 to individuals; USD 62 to institutions (effective 2000). adv. back issues avail. **Description:** Contains articles on the latest technological advances in the field of hearing impairment. Includes inspirational stories, creative writings, children's educational issues, government action, and news of the association.
Formed by the merger of (1976-1994): Newsounds (0147-4057); (1982-1994): Our Kids Magazine
Indexed: CINAHL, Lang.& Lang.Behav.Abstr., Rehabil.Lit., SOPODA, Sociol.Abstr.
—BLDSC (9254.405000), GNLM, ingenta.
Published by: Alexander Graham Bell Association for the Deaf and Hand of Hearing, Inc., 3417 Volta Place, N W, Washington, DC 20007. TEL 202-337-5220, FAX 202-337-8314. R&P Michalle Vanderhoff TEL 202-337-5220 ext 125. Adv. contact Elizabeth Quigley. Circ: 5,700.

371.912 NLD ISSN 0042-9139
VRIEND. Text in Dutch. 1906. q. NLG 17.50. bk.rev. illus. **Document type:** *Bulletin.*
Published by: Instituut voor Doven/Institute for the Deaf, Theerestraat 42, St Michielsgestel 5271 GD, Netherlands. TEL 31-73-5588111, FAX 31-73-5512157. Ed. Josee Verstappen. Circ: 2,700.

362.42 CAN
W I D H H NEWS. Text in English. 1967. q. CND 15 to members. adv. bk.rev. **Document type:** *Newsletter.*
Formerly: W I D News (0049-7436)
Published by: Western Institute for the Deaf & Hard of Hearing, 2125 W 7th Ave, Vancouver, BC V6K 1X9, Canada. TEL 604-736-7391, FAX 604-736-4381. Ed., Adv. contact Johanna Nicholson. Circ: 1,050.

371.912 NLD ISSN 0167-8930
WOORD EN GEBAAR* . Text in Dutch. m. NLG 50. adv. back issues avail. **Description:** Examines the world of the deaf, from sign-language, education and sports, to participation in the workforce.
Published by: (Stichting Nederlandse Dovenraad/Dutch Council of the Deaf), St. Woord & Gebaar, Harmoniehof 36 hs, Amsterdam 1071 TD, Netherlands. Circ: 6,000.

WORLD AROUND YOU. see *EDUCATION—Special Education And Rehabilitation*

371.912 USA ISSN 1059-9894
WORLD AROUND YOU. TEACHER'S EDITION. Text in English. bi-m. USD 14 domestic; USD 20 foreign (effective 2000). adv. **Document type:** *Journal, Academic/Scholarly.* **Description:** Teaching materials for use with hearing impaired teenagers.
Related titles: ♦ Special ed. of: World Around You. ISSN 0199-8293.
Published by: Gallaudet University, National Deaf Educ Network & Clearinghouse, 800 Florida Ave, N E, KDES PAS 6, Washington, DC 20002-3695. TEL 202-651-5340, 800-526-9105, FAX 202-651-5708. Ed. Cathryn Carroll. Adv. contact Susan Flanigan.

HANDICAPPED—Physically Impaired

ADDRESS LIST, REGIONAL AND SUBREGIONAL LIBRARIES FOR THE BLIND AND PHYSICALLY HANDICAPPED. see *HANDICAPPED—Visually Impaired*

AMPUTEE GOLFER. see *SPORTS AND GAMES—Ball Games*

362.4 GBR ISSN 0144-6339
ARTHRITIS NEWS; the magazine for people with arthritis. Text in English. 1950. bi-m. GBP 18 domestic includes all Arthritis Care publications; GBP 23 foreign includes all Arthritis Care publications; GBP 2 newsstand/cover (effective 2000). adv. bk.rev. illus. **Document type:** *Consumer.* **Description:** Covers all aspects of life with arthritis.
Formerly (until 1980): B R A Review (0005-3279)
Indexed: Rehabil.Lit.
Published by: Arthritis Care, 18 Stephenson Way, London NW1 2HD, United Kingdom. TEL 44-20-7916-1500, FAX 44-20-7916-1505. Ed. Cathy Debenham. Adv. contact Peter Woodvine. Circ: 100,000. **Dist. by:** Diamond Magazine Distribution, Rye Wharf, Harbour Rd, Rye, E Sussex TN31 7TE, United Kingdom. TEL 44-1797-225229, FAX 44-1797-225657.

362.4 USA ISSN 0007-8808
C O P H BULLETIN✶. Text in English. 1960. q. USD 2. adv. bk.rev. illus.
Indexed: Rehabil.Lit.
Published by: National Congress of Organizations of the Physically Handicapped, Inc., c/o Lowder Frances H, 1698 Old Charlotte Rd, Concord, NC 28027-7093. Ed. Rose A Wilson. Circ: 2,500.

362.4 GBR ISSN 1354-0920
CHESHIRE SMILE INTERNATIONAL. Text in English. 1954. q. adv. bk.rev. illus. **Document type:** *Newsletter.* **Description:** News and features on the Foundation's 325 homes and services worldwide, plus items of general interest on disability.
Formerly (until 1994): Cheshire Smile (0009-3297)
Indexed: Rehabil.Lit.
Published by: Leonard Cheshire Foundation, 26 Maunsel St, London SW1P 2QN, United Kingdom. TEL 44-171-828-1822, FAX 44-171-976-5704. Ed., Adv. contact Jennie Taylor. Circ: 8,000 (controlled).

D P H D NEWSLETTER. (Council for Exceptional Children) see *EDUCATION—Special Education And Rehabilitation*

617.087 616.8 USA
▼ **DISABILITIES SOURCEBOOK.** Text in English. 1999. irreg., latest 1999. USD 78 per issue (effective 2001). charts. Index. **Document type:** *Consumer.* **Description:** Basic consumer health information about physical and psychiatric disabilities. Contains descriptions of major disabilities, their causes, and people who are disabled.
Published by: Omnigraphics, Inc., 615 Griswold St, Detroit, MI 48226. TEL 313-961-1340, 800-234-1340, FAX 313-961-1383, 800-875-1340, info@omnigraphics.com, jjts@sprynet.com, http://www.omnigraphics.com/cgi-bin/loadpage.cgi?user_id=1567&file=0-7808-0389-2.html. Ed. Dawn Dawn D Matthews.

305.90816 GBR ISSN 0968-7599
HV1551 CODEN: DSCIET
DISABILITY & SOCIETY. Text in English. 1986. 7/yr. GBP 114, USD 207 to individuals; GBP 473, USD 782 to institutions (effective 2002). adv. bk.rev. illus, stat. index, cum.index. reprints avail. *Refereed.* **Document type:** *Academic/Scholarly.*
Formerly (until 1993): Disability, Handicap and Society (0267-4645)
Related titles: Microfiche ed.; Online - full text ed.: ISSN 1360-0508 (from CatchWord Ltd., Northern Light Technology, Inc., EBSCO Publishing, O C L C Online Computer Library Center, Inc., RoweCom Information Quest, ProQuest Information & Learning, Swets Blackwell, Institute for Scientific Information).
Indexed: AMED, ASCA, ASSIA, AgeLine, Arts & Hum.Cit.Ind. (coverage dropped), Curr.Adv.Ecol.Sci., Curr.Cont., ERA, Except.Child Educ.Abstr., Fam.Ind., Indian Psychol.Abstr., Intl.Bibl.Soc.Sci., Lang.& Lang.Behav.Abstr., Mult.Ed.Abstr., P C I, PsycInfo, Psychol.Abstr. (1986-), Rel.Ind.One, Rel.Ind.Two, SOPODA, SSCI, Soc.Serv.Abstr., Sociol.Abstr., Sociol.Educ.Abstr., Stud.Wom.Abstr., e-psyche.
—BLDSC (3595.420420), CatchWord, IDS, Infotrieve, ingenta. **CCC.**
Published by: Carfax Publishing Limited (Subsidiary of: Taylor & Francis Group), PO Box 25, Abingdon, Oxon OX14 3UE, United Kingdom. TEL 44-1235-401000, FAX 44-1235-401550, enquiries@carfax.co.uk, enquiry@tandf.co.uk, http://www.carfax.co.uk/dso-ad.htm. Ed. Len Barton.

362.4 GBR ISSN 0958-4676
DISABILITY NOW. Text in English. 1953. m. GBP 16 to individuals; GBP 25 to institutions; GBP 30 foreign to institutions (effective 1999). adv. bk.rev. **Document type:** *Consumer.* **Description:** For disabled people, carers, parents, and professionals with an interest in disability issues. Covers news and information as well as classified and job advertisements.
Formerly (until 1984): Spastics News (0049-1810)
Indexed: Rehabil.Lit., Sp.Ed.Needs Abstr.
—BLDSC (3595.421700).
Published by: Scope, Scope, 6 Market Rd, London N7 9PW, United Kingdom. TEL 44-171-619-7317, FAX 44-171-619-7331, editor@disabilitynow.org.uk, http://www.disabilitynow.org.uk. Ed., R&P Mary Wilkinson. Adv. contact Richard Gresham. Circ: 19,607.

305.908 FRA ISSN 0014-6951
FAIRE FACE. Text in French. 1933. m. (11/yr.). FRF 156. adv. bk.rev. illus. **Document type:** *Newspaper.* **Description:** Features articles on the way of life of the disabled.
Published by: Association des Paralyses de France, 17 bd. Auguste Blanqui, Paris 75013, France. TEL 33-1-40786900, FAX 33-1-40786933. Ed. Jean Marie Creff. Circ: 30,000.

362.4 USA
FAMILY SUPPORT BULLETIN. Text in English. q. free per issue. **Document type:** *Bulletin.* **Description:** Directed to families affected by cerebral palsy and other similar disabilities, consumers, care providers and advocates. Provides local and national information updates on trends in family support.
Indexed: e-psyche.
Published by: United Cerebral Palsy Associations, Inc., Governmental Activities Office, 1660 L St, N W, Ste 700, Washington, DC 20036-5602. TEL 202-776-0406, FAX 202-776-0414.

362.4 JPN ISSN 0017-6605
HAGEMI/ENCOURAGEMENT; a journal for the guidance of the parents with crippled children. Text in Japanese. 1955. bi-m. JPY 3,700. adv. bk.rev. charts, illus, stat. **Description:** Medical and educational facts for parents and rehabilitation workers involved with the disabled.
Published by: Japanese Society for Disabled Children/Nihon Shitai Fujiyuji Kyokai, 1-7 Komone 1-chome, Itabashi-ku, Tokyo 173-0037, Japan. Circ: 10,000.

LIBRARY RESOURCES FOR THE BLIND AND PHYSICALLY HANDICAPPED. see *LIBRARY AND INFORMATION SCIENCES*

617.03 GBR
MUSCULAR DYSTROPHY CAMPAIGN. Text in English. a. free per issue. **Document type:** *Magazine, Corporate, Consumer.*
Formerly: Muscular Dystrophy Group of Great Britain and Northern Ireland. Annual Review
—BLDSC (1520.287000).
Address: 7-11 Prescott Pl, London SW4 6BS, United Kingdom. TEL 44-20-7720-8055, FAX 44-20-7498-0670. Ed. Leigh Chambers. R&P Tom Bishop TEL 44-20-7819-1813.

N A G A NEWSLETTER. see *SPORTS AND GAMES—Ball Games*

617.58 USA ISSN 0031-1766
PARAPLEGIA NEWS. Text in English. 1946. m. USD 23 domestic; USD 32 foreign (effective 2001). adv. bk.rev. illus. Index. reprints avail. **Document type:** *Consumer.*
Related titles: Online - full text ed.: (from Gale Group, Northern Light Technology, Inc., Factiva).
Indexed: Hlth.Ind., Rehabil.Lit., Sportsearch (1983-), e-psyche.
—ingenta.
Published by: (Paralyzed Veterans of America, Inc.), P V A Publications, 2111 E Highland Ave, Ste 180, Phoenix, AZ 85016-4702. TEL 602-224-0500, FAX 602-224-0507, http://www.paraplegianews.com. Ed. Cliff Crase. Adv. contact Sherri Shea. Circ: 27,000.

617.03 DEU ISSN 0723-5070
PARAPLEGIKER; das Nachrichtenmagazin der Querschnittgelaehmten. Text in German. q. EUR 25.20 domestic to institutions; EUR 29.20 in Europe to institutions; EUR 34.60 elsewhere to institutions; EUR 5.40 newsstand/cover (effective 2002). adv. **Document type:** *Journal, Academic/Scholarly.*
—**CCC.**
Published by: Karl F. Haug Verlag, Fritz-Frey-Str 21, Heidelberg 69121, Germany. TEL 49-6221-489445, FAX 49-6221-489584, http://www.haug-verlag.de. Ed. Peter Mand. Adv. contact Martina Urban.

PHYSICAL DISABILITIES - EDUCATION & RELATED SERVICES. see *EDUCATION—Special Education And Rehabilitation*

362.4 AUS ISSN 0158-6637
QUAD WRANGLE. Text in English. 1976. q. AUD 30 domestic; AUD 40 foreign (effective 2001). adv. bk.rev. 24 p./no. back issues avail. **Document type:** *Newsletter, Consumer.* **Description:** Contains articles for and about physical disabilities.
Published by: Australian Quadriplegic Association, Letterbox 40, 184 Bourke Rd, Alexandria, NSW 2015, Australia. TEL 61-296618855, FAX 61-296619598, aqa@aqa.org.au, http://www.aqa.com.au. Ed., R&P Digby Hughes. Adv. contact Greg Killeen. B&W page AUD 957, color page AUD 1,782; 260 x 180. Circ: 5,200.

QUEST (TUCSON). see *MEDICAL SCIENCES—Psychiatry And Neurology*

362.41 GBR
RAINBOW (PETERBOROUGH). Text in English. 1932. q. **Description:** Publishes news geared to and written by readers who are deaf-blind.
Formerly: Braille Rainbow (0006-8888)
Media: Braille. **Related titles:** Audio cassette/tape ed.; Large type ed.
Published by: Deafblind UK, 100 Bridge St, Peterborough, Northants PE1 1DY, United Kingdom. TEL 44-1733-358100, FAX 44-1733-317555. Circ: 339.

S C I PSYCHOSOCIAL PROCESS. (Spinal Cord Injury) see *PSYCHOLOGY*

362.41 USA
SOUND COMPUTING. Text in English. 1998. bi-m. USD 19 domestic; USD 34 foreign (effective 2000). back issues avail. **Document type:** *Newsletter.* **Description:** Offers blind computer users (both novice and experienced) and other interested persons information on adaptive technology, computers, and the Internet.
Media: Audio cassette/tape. **Related titles:** Online - full text ed.
Published by: Top Dot Enterprises, 8930 11th Pl S E, Everett, WA 98205. TEL 425-335-4894, deamar@eskimo.com, http://www.eskimo.com/~deamar. Ed., Pub. Dean Martineau.

617.087 USA
SPINAL CORD INJURY LIFE. Text in English. 1972. q. free (effective 2001). adv. bk.rev., film rev. back issues avail. *Refereed.* **Document type:** *Newsletter.* **Description:** Covers legislation, medical and research issues. Includes editorials, stories and news of interest to those who have sustained spinal cord injuries.
Formerly (until 1985): Paraplegia Life
Indexed: Rehabil.Lit.
Published by: (National Spinal Cord Injury Association), H D I Publishers, PO Box 131401, Houston, TX 77219. TEL 800-321-7037, NSCIA2@aol.com, http://www.spinalcord.org. Ed. Thomas H Countee Jr. Adv. contact Charles Haynes Sr. Circ: 35,000 (paid).

362.4 USA
TAPPING TECHNOLOGY. Text in English. m. USD 15. **Document type:** *Bulletin.* **Description:** Provides information on current products, devices, services, and resources to assist individuals with physical disabilities.
Related titles: Audio cassette/tape ed.: free; Braille ed.: free; Diskette ed.: free; Large type ed. 18 pt.: free.
Published by: Maryland Technology Assistance Program, Maryland Rehabilitation Center, MDTAP, 2301 Argonne Dr, Baltimore, MD 21218. TEL 800-832-4827, http://www.mdtap.org. Ed. Mary Brady.

617.087 GBR
TARGET M D. (Muscular Dystrophy) Text in English. q. 32 p./no. **Document type:** *Magazine.* **Description:** Articles include medical research news, medical management issues, disability issues, fund-raising and publicity events, and personal profiles.
Published by: Muscular Dystrophy Campaign, 7-11 Prescott Pl, London SW4 6BS, United Kingdom. TEL 44-20-7720-8055, FAX 44-20-7498-0670. Eds. Leigh Chambers, Teresa Kelly TEL 44-20-7819-1813. R&P Teresa Kelly TEL 44-20-7819-1813. Adv. contact David Russell. Circ: 10,000 (controlled).

HANDICAPPED—Visually Impaired

362.41 USA
A E R REPORT✱ . Text in English. 1984. bi-m. membership.
Former titles: American Association of Workers for the Blind with Association for Education of the Visually Handicapped. Alliance News; (until 1983): American Association of Workers for the Blind. News and Views (0002-7510)
Published by: Association for Education and Rehabilitation of the Blind and Visually Impaired, PO Box 22397, Alexandria, VA 22304-9239. TEL 703-548-1884. Ed. Lynn Abbott. Circ: (controlled).

362.41 USA ISSN 1067-5833
HV1790
A F B DIRECTORY OF SERVICES FOR BLIND AND VISUALLY IMPAIRED PERSONS IN THE UNITED STATES AND CANADA. Text in English. biennial. USD 74.95 (effective 2000). bibl. **Document type:** *Directory.* **Description:** Lists and describes more than 3000 local, state, regional, and national services that help blind and visually impaired persons of all ages participate fully in the mainstream. All listings include organization name, address, telephone, contact person, and program description.
Former titles: A F B Directory of Services for Blind and Visually Impaired Persons in the United States (0899-2533); A F B Directory of Agencies Serving the Visually Handicapped in the U S (0732-1341)
Related titles: CD-ROM ed.: USD 74.95 (effective 2000).
—CCC.
Published by: American Foundation for the Blind Press, 11 Penn Plaza, Ste 300, New York, NY 10001-2017. TEL 212-502-7651, 800-232-3044, FAX 212-502-7774, newyork@afb.net, http://www.afb.org/.

362.41 USA
A F B NEWS. Text in English. 1966. s-a. free; free. adv. **Document type:** *Newsletter.* **Description:** For general readership about blindness and visual impairment, featuring AFB people, programs, services, and activities.
Former titles: American Foundation for the Blind News; American Foundation for the Blind Newsletter (0002-855X)
Related titles: Audio cassette/tape ed.; Online - full text ed.
Indexed: Rehabil.Lit.
Published by: American Foundation for the Blind Press, 11 Penn Plaza, Ste 300, New York, NY 10001-2017. TEL 212-502-7615, FAX 212-502-7770, afbnews@afb.net, http://www.afb.org. Ed. Liz Greco. Circ: 6,000.

362.41 USA ISSN 0195-363X
A L L-O-GRAMS. Text in English. 1977. bi-m.
Published by: Affiliated Leadership League of and for the Blind of America, 1101 17th St, N W, Ste 803, Washington, DC 20036-4704. TEL 202-775-8261. Ed. James H Johnson. Circ: 7,500.

686.2 USA ISSN 1081-5198
A P H SLATE. Text in English. 1985. s-a. free. adv. illus. reprints avail. **Document type:** *Newsletter.* **Description:** Contains articles about new products and new processes at APH.
Media: Large Type (16 pt.). **Related titles:** Braille ed.: free; Diskette ed.: free.
Published by: American Printing House for the Blind, Inc., 1839 Frankfort Ave, Louisville, KY 40206. TEL 502-895-2405, FAX 502-899-2274, info@aph.org, http://www.aph.org/. Eds. Bernadette Mudd, Scott Blome. Circ: 8,700.

A P H TECHNOLOGY UPDATE; technology for people who are visually impaired. see *COMPUTERS—Personal Computers*

A S; maandblad voor de activiteitensector. (Activiteitensektor) see *SOCIAL SERVICES AND WELFARE*

ABILITIES. see *HANDICAPPED—Hearing Impaired*

027.663 USA ISSN 0163-3805
Z675.B6
ADDRESS LIST, REGIONAL AND SUBREGIONAL LIBRARIES FOR THE BLIND AND PHYSICALLY HANDICAPPED. Text in English. 1971. s-a. free per issue. **Document type:** *Directory, Government.*
Related titles: Online - full text ed.
Published by: U.S. Library of Congress, National Library Service for the Blind and Physically Handicapped, Washington, DC 20542. TEL 202-707-5100, FAX 202-707-0712, nls@loc.gov, http://lcweb.loc.gov/nls.

ALATEEN TALK. see *CHILDREN AND YOUTH—For*

371.911 USA
AMERICAN PRINTING HOUSE FOR THE BLIND. DEPARTMENT OF EDUCATIONAL AND TECHNICAL RESEARCH. REPORT OF RESEARCH AND DEVELOPMENT ACTIVITIES. Text in English. 1958. a. free. **Document type:** *Corporate.*
Former titles: American Printing House for the Blind. Department of Educational Research. Report of Research and Development Activities; American Printing House for the Blind. Department of Educational Research. Annual Report. (0065-9800)
Published by: American Printing House for the Blind, Inc., Department of Educational and Technical Research, PO Box 6085, Louisville, KY 40206-0085. TEL 502-895-2405, FAX 502-895-1509. Ed. William E Lohss. Circ: 1,000.

647.96 DEU
AUGENBLICK. Text in German. 1920. q. illus. back issues avail. *Refereed.* **Document type:** *Newsletter, Consumer.*
Formerly (until 1997): Hildesheimer Blindenmission
Published by: Hildesheimer Blindenmission e.V., Helmerstr 6, Hildesheim 31134, Germany. TEL 49-5121-14054, FAX 49-5121-39911, info@hildesheimerblindenmission.de. Ed. Rev. Gerhard Schulte. Circ: 20,000 (controlled).

362.41 USA ISSN 0005-3430
THE B V A BULLETIN. (Blinded Veterans Association) Text in English. 1946. bi-m. free. bk.rev. illus. stat. **Document type:** *Newsletter, Bulletin.* **Description:** Covers legislation, employment, aids and appliances, and association activities.
Media: Large Type (14 pt.). **Related titles:** Audio cassette/tape ed.; Online - full text ed.
Indexed: Diver.Y.World.
Published by: Blinded Veterans Association, National Board of Directors, 477 H St N W, Washington, DC 20001. TEL 202-371-8880, 800-669-7079, FAX 202-371-8258, bva@bva.org, http://www.bva.org. Ed. Stuart Nelson. Circ: 13,800 (controlled).

028.5 362.41 GBR
BLAST OFF. Text in English. 1964. m. GBP 12 (effective 2000). **Document type:** *Consumer.* **Description:** Takes stories, features, jokes and puzzles from popular children's magazines and makes them accessible to children ages 7-11 who are blind or visually impaired.
Formerly: Roundabout (0048-8666)
Media: Braille. **Related titles:** Diskette ed.
Published by: Royal National Institute for the Blind, PO Box 173, Peterborough, Cambs PE2 6WX, United Kingdom. TEL 44-1733-370-777, FAX 44-1733-371555, webmaster @rnib.org.uk, http://www.rnib.org.uk. Ed. Joan Longstaff. Circ: 94.

371.911 DEU ISSN 0176-7836
BLIND - SEHBEHINDERT; Zeitschrift fuer das Sehgeschaedigten-Bildungswesen. Text in German. 1881. q. DEM 46 (effective 2001). adv. bk.rev. abstr. index. **Document type:** *Magazine, Consumer.*
Former titles: Zeitschrift fuer das Blinden- und Sehbehindertenbildungswesen (0006-4858); Blindenfreund
Published by: Verein zur Foerderung der Blindenbildung e.V., Bleekstr 26, Hannover 30559, Germany. TEL 49-511-954650, FAX 49-511-9546580, vzfb@vzfb.de, http://www.vzfb.de. Ed., Adv. contact Bernd Hamann. Circ: 1,500.

362.41 IND ISSN 0006-4823
BLIND WELFARE. Text in English. 1959. 3/yr. INR 30; USD 15 in Asia; USD 15 in Africa; USD 20 in Europe; USD 25 in US & Canada. adv. bk.rev. illus.
Related titles: CD-ROM ed.; Online - full text ed.
Indexed: ExtraMED.
Published by: National Association for the Blind India, Worli Seaface, 11 Khan Abdul Gaffar Khan Rd., Mumbai, Maharashtra 400 025, India. TEL 91-22-493-6930, FAX 91-22-493-2539. Ed., R&P, Adv. contact Subhash A Datrange. B&W page INR 2,750, color page INR 3,750. Circ: 1,000.

369.4 USA
BOYS' LIFE (BRAILLE EDITION). Text in English. m. free to qualified personnel. adv. bk.rev., film rev., rec.rev. illus, tr.lit. **Document type:** *Consumer.* **Description:** Includes articles on the outdoors, sports and hobbies, with adventure fiction and humor.
Media: Braille.
Indexed: Ind.Child.Mag., Ind.How To Do It (1963-).
Published by: Boy Scouts of America, PO Box 152079, Irving, TX 75015-2079. TEL 972-580-2366. Ed. J D Owen. Pub. J Warren Young. R&P B L Peters. Adv. contact Nick Noyes. Circ: 500. **Orders to:** US Library of Congress, National Library Service for the Blind and Physically Handicapped, Washington, DC 20542. TEL 202-707-5100, FAX 202-707-0712.

027.663 USA ISSN 0006-873X
Z5346.Z9
BRAILLE BOOK REVIEW (LARGE PRINT EDITION). Text in English. 1932. bi-m. free to qualified personnel. bk.rev. illus. index. back issues avail.; reprints avail. **Document type:** *Bibliography, Government.* **Description:** News of developments and activities in library services for blind and physically handicapped individuals and announcements of braille books and magazines recently added to the N L S collection.
Media: Large Type (14 pt.). **Related titles:** Braille ed.; Diskette ed.; Online - full text ed.
Published by: U.S. Library of Congress, National Library Service for the Blind and Physically Handicapped, Washington, DC 20542. TEL 202-707-5100, FAX 202-707-0712, nls@loc.gov, http://www.loc.gov/nls/bbr/bbr.html, http://lcweb.loc.gov/nls. Ed. Jane Caulton. Circ: 32,000.

615.8 GBR ISSN 0006-8780
BRAILLE JOURNAL OF PHYSIOTHERAPY. Text in English. 1947. m. **Document type:** *Academic/Scholarly.*
Media: Braille.
Published by: Royal National Institute for the Blind, PO Box 173, Peterborough, Cambs PE2 6WX, United Kingdom. TEL 44-1733-370-777, FAX 44-1733-238-541, http://www.rnib.org.uk. Circ: 189.

070 JPN
BRAILLE MAINICHI WEEKLY✱ . Text in Japanese. 1922. w. JPY 350 per issue. adv.
Formerly: Braille Mainichi (0006-8799)
Media: Braille.
Published by: Mainichi Newspapers Osaka, Braille Mainichi Section, 2-36 Dojima, Kita-ku, Osaka-shi 530-0003, Japan. TEL 06-3348-8826, FAX 06-3348-8966, TELEX 22324. Ed. Katsuke Makita. Circ: 12,000.

071 USA ISSN 0006-8810
BRAILLE MIRROR; a current topic magazine. Text in English. 1926. 10/yr. free. 100 p./no. **Document type:** *Magazine, Consumer.* **Description:** Presents articles in braille format from various national magazines and newspapers.
Media: Braille. **Related titles:** Audio cassette/tape ed.
Published by: Braille Institute of America, Inc, 741 N Vermont Ave, Los Angeles, CA 90029. TEL 323-663-1111, 800-BRA-ILLE. Ed., R&P Douglas Menville. Circ: 2,500 (free).

362.41 USA ISSN 0006-8829
BRAILLE MONITOR (INKPRINT EDITION). Text in English. 1956. m. USD 25 to non-members. adv. bk.rev. illus. index. back issues avail.; reprints avail. **Description:** Covers blindness and matters affecting the blind from the blind person's point of view. Includes social concerns, legal cases, reports on action by the NFB on current legislative issues, news of aids and appliances, how-to information, and features on blind persons.

H

Related titles: Audio cassette/tape ed.; Braille ed.; Online - full text ed.
Indexed: Except.Child Educ.Abstr.
—ingenta.
Published by: National Federation of the Blind, 1800 Johnson St, Baltimore, MD 21230. TEL 410-659-9314, FAX 410-685-5653, http://www.nfb.org/bralmons.htm, http://www.nfb.org/bralmons.htm. Ed. Mrs. Barbara Pierce. Circ: 30,000.

781.24 780 GBR ISSN 0006-8837
BRAILLE MUSIC MAGAZINE. Text in English. 1910. m. GBP 42 (effective 2000). music rev. **Document type:** *Consumer.* **Description:** Contains topical information of interest to blind musicians, teachers, students and music lovers.
Formerly: Braille Musical Magazine
Media: Braille. **Related titles:** Diskette ed.
Published by: Royal National Institute for the Blind, PO Box 173, Peterborough, Cambs PE2 6WX, United Kingdom. TEL 44-1733-370-777, FAX 44-1733-317555, webmaster@rnib.org.uk, http://www.rnig.org.uk. Ed. Roger Firman. Circ: 346.

791.4 GBR ISSN 0006-887X
BRAILLE RADIO TIMES. Text in English. 1927. w. **Document type:** *Consumer.* **Description:** Provides program information for BBC national radios 1, 2, 3, 4, 5 Live and Virgin 1215.
Media: Braille. **Related titles:** Diskette ed.
Published by: Royal National Institute for the Blind, 224 Great Portland St, London W1N 6AA, United Kingdom. FAX 44-1733-371555, cservices@rnib.org.uk, http://www.rnib.org.uk. Circ: 1,272. **Subcr. to:** RNIB Customer Services, PO Box 173, Peterborough, Cambs PE2 6WS, United Kingdom. TEL 44-1733-370777, FAX 44-1733-317555.

500 600 GBR ISSN 0006-8896
BRAILLE SCIENCE JOURNAL; a record of scientific progress. Text in English. 1936. m. GBP 8 (effective 2000). adv. **Document type:** *Academic/Scholarly.* **Description:** Contains reprints for blind and visually impaired readers and articles from New Scientist.
Media: Braille. **Related titles:** Diskette ed.
Published by: Scottish Braille Press, Craigmillar Park, Edinburgh, Scotland EH16 5NB, United Kingdom. TEL 44-131-662-4445, FAX 44-131-622-1968, http://www.scottish-braille-press.org, http://www.scottish-brialle-press.org. Ed. J H Adams. Circ: 300.

790 362.4 GBR ISSN 0006-890X
BRAILLE SPORTING RECORD. Text in English. 1950. w. GBP 10 (effective 2000). adv. **Document type:** *Bulletin, Consumer.* **Description:** Offers all the latest information on a variety of sports.
Media: Braille. **Related titles:** Diskette ed.
Published by: Scottish Braille Press, Craigmillar Park, Edinburgh, Scotland EH16 5NB, United Kingdom. TEL 44-131-662-4445, FAX 44-131-662-1968, http://www.scottish-braille-press.org. Ed. J H Adams. Circ: 800.

BRAILLE STAR THEOSOPHIST. see *RELIGIONS AND THEOLOGY—Other Denominations And Sects*

052 ZAF
BRAILLORAMA. Text in Afrikaans, English. 1968. m. ZAR 20. bk.rev.
Published by: South Africa Blind Workers Organisation, Private Bag X9005, Crown Mines 2025, South Africa. TEL 27-11-8391793, FAX 27-11-8391217. Ed. Christo J de Klerk. Circ: 354.

052 ZAF
BRAILLORETTE. SUPPLEMENT. Text in English. bi-m.
Published by: South Africa Blind Workers Organisation, Private Bag X9005, Crown Mines 2025, South Africa. TEL 27-11-8391793, FAX 27-11-8391217.

362.41 GBR ISSN 0264-6196
HV1571
BRITISH JOURNAL OF VISUAL IMPAIRMENT. Text in English. 1979. 3/yr. GBP 25. adv. bk.rev. illus. index. **Document type:** *Academic/Scholarly.* **Description:** Provides a focus for scholarship in the field of work with visually impaired people. Articles cover aspects of health, welfare, education and employment insofar as they are affected by a visual disability.
Formerly (until vol.4, 1983): Insight (London, 1979); Which superseded (in 1979): Teacher of the Blind (0040-0440)
Related titles: Audio cassette/tape ed.; Braille ed.; Diskette ed.
Indexed: ASSIA, Br.Educ.Ind., Cont.Pg.Educ., ERA, Except.Child Educ.Abstr., Mult.Ed.Abstr., Sp.Ed.Needs Abstr., Tech.Educ.Abstr., Yrbk.Assoc.Educ.& Rehab.Blind.
—BLDSC (2326.400000), ingenta.
Published by: Royal National Institute for the Blind, PO Box 173, Peterborough, Cambs PE2 6WX, United Kingdom. TEL 44-1733-370-777, FAX 44-1733-371555, webmaster@rnib.org.uk, http://www.rnib.org.uk. Circ: 1,500. **Subscr. to:** R N I B - V I E W, The View Office, York Annex, Exhall Grange, Coventry, W Mids CV7 9HP, United Kingdom. TEL 44-1704-537320.

DAS BRUDERHAUS. see *EDUCATION—Special Education And Rehabilitation*

027.663 ARG ISSN 0007-6015
BURBUJAS. Text in Spanish. 1968. bi-m. free per issue.
Related titles: Braille ed.
Published by: Biblioteca Argentina para Ciegos, Lezica, 3909, Capital Federal, Buenos Aires 1202, Argentina. TEL 54-11-4981-0137, FAX 54-11-4981-0137, bac@bac.org.ar, http://www.bac.org.ar. Circ: 1,400 (paid).

362.41 CAN
CANADIAN NATIONAL INSTITUTE FOR THE BLIND. NATIONAL ANNUAL REVIEW. Text in English, French. 1919. a.
Former titles: Canadian National Institute for the Blind. National Annual Report (0826-838X); Canadian National Institute for the Blind. National Report (0068-9378); Canadian National Institute for the Blind. Annual Report (1191-4882)
Published by: Canadian National Institute for the Blind, National Office, 1929 Bayview Ave, Toronto, ON M4G 3E8, Canada. TEL 416-480-7417. Circ: 1,500.

CHANNELS OF BLESSING. see *RELIGIONS AND THEOLOGY—Protestant*

CHRISTIAN RECORD; for adult blind. see *RELIGIONS AND THEOLOGY*

200 GBR
CHURCH OF SCOTLAND BRAILLE MAGAZINE. Text in English. 1934. m. GBP 0.30 per issue (effective 2000). **Document type:** *Bulletin.*
Published by: (Publications Centre, Church of Scotland), Scottish Braille Press, Craigmillar Park, Edinburgh, Scotland EH16 5NB, United Kingdom. TEL 44-131-662-4445, FAX 44-131-662-1968, http://www.scottish-braille-press.org, http://www.scottish-brialle-press.org. Ed. Gloria Rintoul. Circ: 150.

THE COMPLETE DIRECTORY OF LARGE PRINT BOOKS AND SERIALS. see *HANDICAPPED—Abstracting, Bibliographies, Statistics*

CONNECTIVE ISSUES. see *MEDICAL SCIENCES—Cardiovascular Diseases*

362.41 ITA ISSN 0010-9169
IL CORRIERE DEI CIECHI. Text in Italian. 1946. m. ITL 15,000 (effective 1999). bk.rev. illus. *Refereed.* **Document type:** *Newsletter.* **Description:** Deals with subjects concerning life and social problems of visually impaired in Italy.
Related titles: Braille ed.
Published by: Unione Italiana Ciechi, Via Borgognona, 38, Rome, RM 00187, Italy. TEL 39-06-69988375, FAX 39-06-6786815, ustampa@uiciechi.it, http://www.uiciechi.it/cc/1997/ccidx.htm. Ed. Renato Terrosi. R&P Tommaso Daniele. Circ: 67,000.

DAILY DEVOTIONS FOR THE DEAF. see *HANDICAPPED—Hearing Impaired*

371.91 362.4 USA ISSN 1526-9841
DEAF - BLIND PERSPECTIVES. Text in English. 1993. 3/yr. free. **Document type:** *Newsletter, Academic/Scholarly.* **Description:** Examines and discusses all pertinent issues important to people who are deaf-blind and persons who serve them.
Related titles: Braille ed.; Diskette - 3.5 inch 1.44MB ed.; E-mail ed.; Large type ed. 16 pt.
Published by: (Western Oregon State College, Teaching Research Division), Teaching Research Publications, 345 N. Monmouth Ave., Monmouth, OR 97361. TEL 503-838-8885, dbp@wou.edu, http://www.tr.wou.edu/tr/dbp. Circ: 4,000.

305.42 GBR ISSN 0012-236X
DIANE. Text in English. 1960. m. GBP 24 (effective 2000). **Document type:** *Consumer.* **Description:** Extracts informative articles from print publications such as Bella, Best, Woman's Own, and the Lady.
Published by: Royal National Institute for the Blind, PO Box 173, Peterborough, Cambs PE2 6WX, United Kingdom. TEL 44-1733-370-777, FAX 44-1733-238-541, 44-1733-371555, webmaster @rnib.org.uk, http://www.rnib.org. Ed. Chris James. Circ: 90.

362.41 ZAF
DIENSGIDS VIR GESIGSGESTREMDE SUID-AFRIKANERS. Text in Afrikaans. 1985. irreg. ZAR 25. **Document type:** *Directory.*
Former titles (until 1990): Directory of Services for Visually Handicapped South Africans; Directory of Services Available to Visually Handicapped South Africans
Related titles: English ed.
Published by: South African National Council for the Blind, PO Box 11149, Brooklyn, Pretoria 0011, South Africa. TEL 27-12-346-1171, FAX 27-12-346-1177. Circ: 250.

362.41 USA
DIRECTORY OF RESOURCES FOR THE BLIND AND VISUALLY IMPAIRED. Variant title: Directory of Resources for the Blind and Visually Impaired. Text in English. irreg. free. 150 p./no. **Document type:** *Directory, Catalog.* **Description:** Lists national and regional organizations providing Christian and secular publications, services, and products for the blind.
Media: Large Type (18 pt.). **Related titles:** Online - full text ed.
Published by: John Milton Society for the Blind, 475 Riverside Dr, Rm 455, New York, NY 10115. TEL 212-870-3335, 212-870-3336, FAX 212-870-3229, order@jmsblind.org, http://www.jmsblind.org. Ed. Darcy Quigley. Circ: 300 (free).

371.911 USA
DIVISION ON VISUAL IMPAIRMENTS QUARTERLY. Text in English. 1956. q. membership only. adv. **Document type:** *Newsletter.* **Description:** Provides information on current developments concerning educating children with visual impairments and the activities of the division.
Former titles: Division on Visual Handicaps Quarterly; D V H Quarterly
Published by: Council for Exceptional Children, Division on Visual Impairments, 1920 Association Drive, Reston, VA 22091. TEL 703-620-3660, FAX 703-264-9494. R&P Bob Brasher. Circ: 1,200.

362.42 CAN ISSN 0012-5679
DOTS AND TAPS; Canada's national magazine for the deaf-blind. Text in English. 1952. 4/yr. free per issue. **Document type:** *Government.*
Related titles: Braille ed.
Published by: Canadian National Institute for the Blind, National Office, 1929 Bayview Ave, Toronto, ON M4G 3E8, Canada. TEL 416-480-7417, FAX 416-480-7699. Ed. K G Wadman. Circ: 310 (controlled).

808.068 USA
EXPECTATIONS. Text in English. 1948. a. free. illus. **Document type:** *Magazine, Consumer.* **Description:** Provides an anthology in braille for children in grades 3-6; braille grade II.
Media: Braille.
Published by: Braille Institute of America, Inc, 741 N Vermont Ave, Los Angeles, CA 90029. TEL 323-663-1111, 800-BRA-ILLE. Ed., R&P Douglas Menville. Circ: 5,000 (controlled).

FIGHTING BLINDNESS NEWS. see *MEDICAL SCIENCES—Ophthalmology And Optometry*

FLORIDA SCHOOL HERALD. see *EDUCATION—Special Education And Rehabilitation*

THE FORUM (VIRGINIA BEACH). see *DRUG ABUSE AND ALCOHOLISM*

331.59 DEU
FUNK UND ELEKTRONIK. Text in German. q. EUR 47.60 (effective 2002). **Document type:** *Magazine, Consumer.*
Related titles: Braille ed.; Diskette ed.
Published by: Deutsche Blindenstudienanstalt e.V., Postfach 1160, Marburg 35001, Germany. TEL 49-6421-606-0, FAX 49-6421-606229, info@blista.de, http://www.blista.de. Circ: 85.

362.41 USA ISSN 0883-3419
FUTURE REFLECTIONS. Text in English. 1981. q. USD 15 to non-members; USD 8 to members. bk.rev., film rev. illus. back issues avail. **Document type:** *Consumer.* **Description:** Provides practical guidance in the day-to-day aspects of raising blind children of all ages.
Related titles: Audio cassette/tape ed.
Published by: National Federation of the Blind, 1800 Johnson St, Baltimore, MD 21230. TEL 410-659-9314, FAX 410-685-5653, http://www.nfb.org/futref.htm. Ed. Barbara A Cheadle. Circ: 10,000.

362.41 DEU ISSN 0016-5859
DIE GEGENWART; Magazin fuer Blinde, Sehbehinderte und ihre Freunde. Text in German. 1912. 11/yr. DEM 66 (effective 2000). adv. bk.rev. **Document type:** *Magazine, Consumer.*
Incorporates: Blindenselbsthilfe (0172-0163); Which was formerly (until 1974): Blindenwelt (0006-4866)
Related titles: Audio cassette/tape ed.: DEM 66 (effective 2000); Braille ed.: DEM 66 (effective 2000); Diskette ed.: DEM 66 (effective 2000).
Indexed: Russ.Acad.Sci.Bibl.
Published by: Deutscher Blindenverband e.V., Bismarckallee 30, Bonn 53173, Germany. TEL 49-228-955820, FAX 49-228-357719, dbvbonn@t-online.de, http://www.dbvbonn.de. Ed. Thomas Nicolai. Circ: 1,750.

362.41 POL
GLOS KOBIETY; dwumiesiecznik dla pan. Text in Polish. 1962. bi-m. PLZ 12 (effective 1999). **Document type:** *Newsletter, Consumer.* **Description:** Provides information and guidance for blind and short-sighted women.
Media: Large Type. **Related titles:** Braille ed.: PLZ 6 (effective 1999).
Published by: (Polski Zwiazek Niewidomych, Zarzad Glowny), Zaklad Nagran i Wydawnictw Niewidomych, Ul Konwiktorska 7, Warsaw 00216, Poland. TEL 48-22-312271. Ed. Zofia Krzemkowska. Circ: 1,000.

362.41 GBR
GOOD VIBRATIONS. Text in English. 1960. m. GBP 18 (effective 2000). **Document type:** *Consumer.* **Description:** Features reviews of new hi-fi equipment, along with details on exhibitions and snippets of news from the world of hi-fi.
Former titles (until 1994): Soundings; Tape Record (0039-9531)
Media: Braille. **Related titles:** Diskette ed.
Indexed: Curr.Cont. (coverage dropped), G.Soc.Sci.& Rel.Per.Lit.
Published by: Royal National Institute for the Blind, PO Box 173, Peterborough, Cambs PE2 6WX, United Kingdom. TEL 44-1733-370-777, FAX 44-1733-371555, webmaster @rnib.org.uk, http://www.rnib.org.uk. Ed. Steve Worrall. Circ: 166.

240 USA ISSN 0017-2359
GOSPEL MESSENGER. Text in English. 1966 (vol.19). m. free to the blind. **Document type:** *Newsletter.* **Description:** Includes religious articles, poems, and sermons.
Media: Audio cassette/tape.
Published by: Gospel Association for the Blind, Inc., PO Box 62, Delray Beach, FL 33447. TEL 561-274-9700, FAX 561-274-4288. Ed. Rev. Robert Rathbun. Circ: 1,600.

636.7 362.41 USA
GUIDE DOG NEWS. Text in English. 1950. q. membership. *Refereed.* **Document type:** *Newsletter, Trade.* **Description:** Contains information about Guide Dogs for the Blind Inc.
Related titles: Audio cassette/tape ed.; Braille ed.
Published by: Guide Dogs for the Blind, Inc., PO Box 151200, San Rafael, CA 94915-1200. TEL 415-499-4000, 800-295-4050, FAX 415-499-4023, jritter@guidedogs.com, http://www.guidedogs.com. Ed., R&P Joanne Ritter. Circ: 55,000.

GUIDE LINES (YORKTOWN HEIGHTS). see *PETS*

027.663 ARG ISSN 0017-6478
HACIA LA LUZ. Text in Spanish. 1927. bi-m. free per issue.
Media: Braille.
Published by: Biblioteca Argentina para Ciegos, Lezica, 3909, Capital Federal, Buenos Aires 1202, Argentina. TEL 54-11-4981-0137, FAX 54-11-4981-0137, bac@bac.org.ar, http://www.bac.org.ar. Circ: 1,400 (free).

011 DEU
HOERBUCHVERZEICHNIS. Text in German. a. DEM 6. bibl.
Related titles: Braille ed.
Published by: Zentralbuecherei fuer Blinde, Gustav-Adolf-Str 7, Leipzig 04105, Germany. TELEX 70976.

362.41 GBR
HOME HELP. Text in English. 1958. w. GBP 10 (effective 2000). **Document type:** *Bulletin.*
Media: Braille.
Published by: Scottish Braille Press, Craigmillar Park, Edinburgh, Scotland EH16 5NB, United Kingdom. TEL 44-131-662-4445, FAX 44-131-662-1968, http://www.scottish-braille-press.org, http://www.scottish-brialle-press.org. Ed. Gloria Rintoul.

371.911 DEU ISSN 0724-7389
HORUS; Beitraege zur Integration Sehgeschaedigter. Text in German. 1975 (vol.37). q. DEM 38 (effective 2000). adv. bk.rev. illus. **Document type:** *Academic/Scholarly.* **Description:** For and about the blind and sight-impaired: education, integration, conference information.
Published by: Deutsche Blindenstudienanstalt e.V., Postfach 1160, Marburg 35001, Germany. TEL 49-6421-606-0. Circ: 4,000.

371.9 DEU
HORUS - MARBURGER BEITRAEGE ZUR INTEGRATION BLINDER UND SEHBEHINDERTER. Text in German. bi-m. EUR 46 (effective 2002). adv. bk.rev. **Document type:** *Journal, Academic/Scholarly.*
Former titles: Marburger Beitraege Zur Integration Sehgeschaedigter; Marburger Beitraege zum Blindenbildungswesen
Related titles: Audio cassette/tape ed.; Braille ed.
Published by: Deutsche Blindenstudienanstalt e.V., Postfach 1160, Marburg 35001, Germany. TEL 49-6421-606-0, FAX 49-6421-606229, info@blista.de, http://www.blista.de. Circ: 800. **Co-sponsor:** Deutscher Verein Blinder und Sehbehinderter in Studium und Beruf.

362.41 USA
ILLINOIS BRAILLE MESSENGER (BRAILLE EDITION). Text in English. 1930. q. USD 5 (effective 2000). adv. abstr, tr.lit. **Document type:** *Newsletter.* **Description:** Disseminates material submitted by agencies, organizations and individuals to inform, encourage, and inspire the visually impaired people of Illinois.
Media: Braille.
Published by: Illinois Council of the Blind, PO Box 1336, Springfield, IL 62705. Ed. Laura Booker. Adv. contact Howard Thomas. Circ: 2,000.

362.41 USA ISSN 0019-1906
ILLINOIS BRAILLE MESSENGER (INKPRINT EDITION). Text in English. 1930. q. USD 5 (effective 2000). adv. abstr, tr.lit. **Document type:** *Newsletter.*
Related titles: Braille ed.; Large type ed. 14 pt.
Published by: Illinois Council of the Blind, PO Box 1336, Springfield, IL 62705. TEL 217-523-4967. Ed. Laura Booker. Adv. contact Howard Thomas. Circ: 2,000.

362.41 ZAF
IMFAMA (BRAILLE EDITION). Text in Afrikaans, English. 1962. bi-m. free per issue. **Document type:** *Academic/Scholarly.*
Media: Braille. **Related titles:** Audio cassette/tape ed.
Published by: South African National Council for the Blind, PO Box 11149, Brooklyn, Pretoria 0011, South Africa. TEL 27-12-346-1171, FAX 27-12-346-1177. Ed. William Rowland. Circ: 708.

362.41 ZAF ISSN 0019-2724
IMFAMA (INKPRINT EDITION). Text in Afrikaans, English. 1961. bi-m. ZAR 50. adv. illus. **Document type:** *Academic/Scholarly.*
Related titles: Braille ed.; Magnetic Tape ed.
Published by: South African National Council for the Blind, PO Box 11149, Brooklyn, Pretoria 0011, South Africa. TEL 27-12-346-1171, FAX 27-12-346-1177. Ed. William Rowland. Circ: 1,224.

362.41 ZAF
IMFAMA (TAPE EDITION). Text in Afrikaans, English. 1961. bi-m. free per issue. **Document type:** *Academic/Scholarly.*
Media: Magnetic Tape. **Related titles:** Braille ed.
Published by: South African National Council for the Blind, PO Box 11149, Brooklyn, Pretoria 0011, South Africa. TEL 27-12-346-1171, FAX 27-12-346-1177. Ed. William Rowland. Circ: 370.

362.41 USA
IN FOCUS (MOUNTAIN VIEW)* . Text in English. 1994. q. free per issue. back issues avail. **Document type:** *Newsletter.* **Description:** Offers technological aids serving the low vision and blind community.
Former titles: Focus on Technology; (until 1989): R E News
Related titles: Diskette ed.: 1994; Online - full text ed.: 1994.
Published by: TeleSensory, 520 Almanor Ave, Sunnyvale, CA 94086-3533. TEL 415-335-1800, 800-804-8004, FAX 415-335-1816, bthomlin@telesensory.com, http://www.telesensory.com. Ed. Beth Thomlinson. R&P Shirley Deswarte. Circ: 60,000.

362.41 GBR
▼ **INFORMASIAN.** Text in English. 1999. 3/yr. **Document type:** *Academic/Scholarly.* **Description:** Information for Asian families and professionals working with Asian children with serious sight problems in the West Midlands.
Published by: Royal National Institute for the Blind, Asian Families Project: West Midlands, 224 Great Portland St, London W1N 6AA, United Kingdom. FAX 44-1733-371555, cservices@rnib.org.uk, http://www.rnib.org.uk. **Subscr. to:** RNIB Customer Services, PO Box 173, Peterborough, Cambs PE2 6WS, United Kingdom. FAX 44-1733-371555.

H

INSIDE M S. (Multiple Sclerosis) see *MEDICAL SCIENCES—Psychiatry And Neurology*

INSIGHT (WASHINGTON, 1990). see *MEDICAL SCIENCES—Ophthalmology And Optometry*

371.911 DEU
JAHRBUCH FUER BLINDENFREUNDE. Text in German. a. DEM 5. back issues avail. **Document type:** *Corporate.*
Published by: Deutscher Blindenverband e.V., Bismarckallee 30, Bonn 53173, Germany. TEL 49-228-955820, FAX 49-228-357719. Circ: 40,000.

362.41 USA
JEWISH BRAILLE INSTITUTE OF AMERICA. DIRECTORY OF SERVICES. Text in English. a. free per issue. **Document type:** *Directory.* **Description:** Contains directory that describes Jewish Braille Institute programs, activities and services.
Published by: Jewish Braille Institute of America, Inc., 110 E 30th St, New York, NY 10016. TEL 212-889-2525, FAX 212-689-3692.

296.011 USA ISSN 0021-6321
JEWISH BRAILLE REVIEW. Text in English. 1931. m. free to the blind. bk.rev. bibl. **Description:** Covers articles, stories and poetry from all sources of Judaic content for blind Jewish readers or non-Jewish blind readers interested in Judaica.
Published by: Jewish Braille Institute of America, Inc., 110 E 30th St, New York, NY 10016. TEL 212-889-2525. Ed. Dr. Jacob Freid. Circ: 2,300.

647.9654 USA
JEWISH GUILD FOR THE BLIND. NEWSLETTER. Text in English. 1960. q. free per issue. **Document type:** *Newsletter.* **Description:** Covers events, programs and people at the Guild and its affiliate organizations.
Formerly: Jewish Guild of the Blind. Guild News
Published by: Jewish Guild for the Blind, 15 W 65th St, New York, NY 10023. TEL 212-769-6237, FAX 212-769-6343, JGB.org. Ed. Peter C Williamson. Circ: 22,000.

362.41 AUT ISSN 0021-7174
JOHANN WILHELM KLEIN; literarische Zeitschrift fuer Blinde. Text in German. 1904. m. ATS 470. bk.rev. bibl, charts. **Document type:** *Academic/Scholarly.*
Published by: Bundes-Blindenerziehungsinstitut, Wittelsbachstrasse 5, Vienna, W 1020, Austria. Ed., Pub. Eva Papst. Circ: 180.

JOHN MILTON MAGAZINE. see *RELIGIONS AND THEOLOGY*

371.911 USA ISSN 0892-7758
JOTTINGS. Text in English. 1950. m. free per issue. **Document type:** *Newsletter.*
Published by: Gospel Association for the Blind, Inc., PO Box 62, Delray Beach, FL 33447. TEL 561-274-9700, FAX 561-274-9700. Ed. Bea Montanus. Circ: 5,000.

JOURNAL OF COMMUNITY EYE HEALTH; an international journal to promote eye health worldwide. see *MEDICAL SCIENCES—Ophthalmology And Optometry*

H

362.41 USA ISSN 0145-482X
HV1571
JOURNAL OF VISUAL IMPAIRMENT & BLINDNESS. Text in English. 1977. m. USD 100 domestic to individuals; USD 130 foreign to individuals; USD 140 domestic to institutions; USD 170 foreign to institutions (effective 2001). adv. bk.rev. illus. back issues avail.; reprint service avail. from PQC,PSC,SCH. *Refereed.* **Document type:** *Academic/Scholarly.* **Description:** Interdisciplinary journal of record on blindness and visual impairment that serves as a forum for the exchange of ideas, airing of controversies, and discussion of issues currently facing the blindness field today.
Formed by the merger of (1951-1977): New Outlook for the Blind (0028-6435); (1962-1977): A F B Research Bulletin (0065-8367)
Related titles: Audio cassette/tape ed.: USD 100 (effective 2001); Braille ed.: USD 100 (effective 2001); Diskette ed.: USD 100 (effective 2001); Online - full text ed.: USD 100 (effective 2001) (from H. W. Wilson, Institute for Scientific Information).
Indexed: ASCA, Adol.Ment.Hlth.Abstr., AgeLine, Arts & Hum.Cit.Ind. (coverage dropped), C.I.J.E., CINAHL, Curr.Cont., Educ.Ind. (Sep.1983-), Except.Child Educ.Abstr., Excerp.Med., Fam.Ind., Lang.& Lang.Behav.Abstr., PsycInfo, Psychol.Abstr. (1928-), Rehabil.Lit., SOPODA, SSCI, Soc.Work Res.& Abstr., Sociol.Abstr., Sp.Ed.Needs Abstr., Yrbk.Assoc.Educ.& Rehab.Blind, e-psyche.
—BLDSC (5072.495000), CISTI, GNLM, IDS, ingenta, KNAW.
Published by: American Foundation for the Blind Press, 11 Penn Plaza, Ste 300, New York, NY 10001-2017. TEL 212-502-7655, FAX 212-502-7774, afbinfo@afb.org; pubsvc@tsp.sheridan.com, http://www.afb.org. Ed. Jane Erin. Adv. contact Stephanie Biagioli. Circ: 7,000.

362.41 DEU ISSN 0023-463X
HV1571
DER KRIEGSBLINDE; Zeitschrift fuer Verstaendnis und Verstaendigung. Text in German. 1950. m. DEM 26. adv. illus.
Published by: Bund der Kriegsblinden Deutschlands e.V., Schumannstr 35, Bonn 53113, Germany. Ed. Alfred Lauster.

LIBRARY RESOURCES FOR THE BLIND AND PHYSICALLY HANDICAPPED. see *LIBRARY AND INFORMATION SCIENCES*

LICHTBLICKE; Magazin der Christoffel-Blindenmission. see *SOCIAL SERVICES AND WELFARE*

371.911 USA
LIGHT: ANNUAL REPORT. Text in English. 1929. a. free. charts, illus, stat. **Document type:** *Corporate.*
Published by: Braille Institute of America, Inc, 741 N Vermont Ave, Los Angeles, CA 90029. TEL 323-663-1111, 800-BRA-ILLE. Ed. Nancy Niebrugge. R&P Douglas Menville. Circ: 70,000.

362.41 GBR ISSN 0024-3361
LIGHT OF THE MOON. Text in English. 1939. m. GBP 24 (effective 2000). **Document type:** *Consumer.* **Description:** Extracts articles from popular general-interest magazines and makes them accessible to readers who are blind or visually impaired.
Published by: Royal National Institute for the Blind, PO Box 173, Peterborough, Cambs PE2 6WX, United Kingdom. TEL 44-1733-370-777, FAX 44-1733-371555, webmaster@rnib.org.uk, webmaster @rnib.org.uk, http://www.rnib.org.uk. Ed. Steve Worrall. Circ: 97.

630 360 USA
LIGHT (WHEATON). Text in English. 1978. bi-m. free per issue. stat. **Description:** Overview of the medical rehabilitational and spiritual activities of CBM co-workers in over 98 developing countries.
Published by: Christian Blind Mission International Inc., PO Box 19000, Greenville, SC 29602-9000. TEL 803-239-0065, FAX 803-239-0069. Circ: 38,000 (controlled).

305.908161 USA ISSN 0792-0873
LIKUTIM; a journal of visual impairment and blindness. Text in Hebrew. 1981. s-a. free per issue. back issues avail. **Description:** Covers information on blindness and visual impairment distributed in Israel for Israeli blind persons.
Media: Audio cassette/tape. **Related titles:** Talking Book ed.
Indexed: Ind.Heb.Per. (1987-2000).
Published by: Jewish Braille Institute of America, Inc., 110 E 30th St, New York, NY 10016. TEL 212-889-2525. Ed. Joanne Jahr. Circ: 1,000.

052 200 GBR
LINK (MARKET HARBOROUGH). Text in English. q. free per issue. *Refereed.* **Document type:** *Bulletin.* **Description:** Forum magazine for blind people overseas.
Formerly: Flash
Media: Large Type. **Related titles:** Audio cassette/tape ed.; Braille ed.
Published by: Torch Trust for the Blind, Torch House, North End, Hallaton, Market Harborough, Leics LE16 8UJ, United Kingdom. TEL 44-1858-555301, FAX 44-1858-555371. R&P Rosemary Adams. Circ: 664.

362.41 FRA ISSN 0024-6727
LOUIS BRAILLE. Text in French. 1882. m. FRF 107. adv. **Document type:** *Bulletin.*
Media: Braille.
Published by: Association Valentin Hauey pour le Bien des Aveugles, 5 rue Duroc, Paris Cedex 7 75343, France. TEL 33-1-44492727, FAX 33-1-44492710, avh@world-net.sct.fr. Ed. Jean Pierre Schricke. Pub. Louis Ciccone. R&P Jean-Pierre Schricke. Adv. contact Bernard Demarre. Circ: 1,800.

284.10871 USA ISSN 0024-7480
LUTHERAN MESSENGER FOR THE BLIND. Text in English. 1927. m. free per issue (effective 2000). bk.rev. **Description:** Includes Christian devotionals, Bible studies, poetry and short stories.
Media: Braille. **Related titles:** Audio cassette/tape ed.
Published by: (World Mission, Lutheran Church - Missouri Synod), Lutheran Library for the Blind, 1333 S. Kirkwood Rd., St. Louis, MO 63122-7295. TEL 314-965-9000, 800-433-3954. Ed. Rev. David Andrus. Circ: 900.

362.41 FRA ISSN 0024-7685
LUX VERA. Text in French. 1929. bi-m. FRF 22 per issue. illus.
Published by: Association la Croisade des Aveugles, 15 rue Mayet, Paris 75006, France. Ed. Jacques Dard. Circ: 6,500.

052 GBR ISSN 0024-9351
MADAM. Text in English. 1937. m. GBP 12 (effective 2000). adv. **Document type:** *Bulletin.* **Description:** Contains fiction, topical articles, features on beauty and fashion, and pieces on knitting, crafts, and baking.
Media: Braille. **Related titles:** Diskette ed.
Published by: Scottish Braille Press, Craigmillar Park, Edinburgh, Scotland EH16 5NB, United Kingdom. TEL 44-131-662-4445, FAX 44-131-662-1968, http://www.scottish-braille-press.org. Ed. Gloria Rintoul. Circ: 750.

371.911 DEU
MARBURGER BUECHERLISTEN. Text in German. 3/m. free. adv. bk.rev. **Document type:** *Bibliography.*
Related titles: Braille ed.
Published by: Deutsche Blindenstudienanstalt e.V., Postfach 1160, Marburg 35001, Germany. TEL 49-6421-606-0. Circ: 2,500.

051 362 USA ISSN 0025-5955
MATILDA ZIEGLER MAGAZINE FOR THE BLIND. Text in English. 1907. m. free per issue. bk.rev., film rev., play rev. back issues avail. **Document type:** *Magazine, Consumer.* **Description:** General-interest magazine for blind or visually impaired people.
Media: Braille. **Related titles:** Audio cassette/tape ed.; E-mail ed.
Published by: Matilda Ziegler Publishing Co. for the Blind, Inc., 80 Eighth Ave, 1304, New York, NY 10011. TEL 212-242-0263, FAX 212-633-1601, blind@bellatlantic.net, zieglermag@attglobal.net, http://www.zieglermag.org. Ed. Michael Mellor. Circ: 10,600.

362.41 GBR ISSN 0027-0911
MOON MAGAZINE. Text in English. 1906. m. GBP 24 (effective 2000). **Document type:** *Consumer.* **Description:** Takes topical articles from leading UK national magazines and newspapers, covering all aspects of life, and makes them accessible to readers who are blind or visually impaired.
Published by: Royal National Institute for the Blind, PO Box 173, Peterborough, Cambs PE2 6WX, United Kingdom. TEL 44-1733-370-777, FAX 44-1733-371555, webmaster@rnib.org.ukk, webmaster @rnib.org.uk, http://www.rnib.org.uk. Ed. Chris James. Circ: 147.

362.41 GBR ISSN 0047-8083
MOON RAINBOW. Text in English. 1934. q. free per issue.
Published by: Deafblind UK, 100 Bridge St, Peterborough, Northants PE1 1DY, United Kingdom. TEL 44-1733-358100. Circ: 94.

371.911 USA
N A V H UPDATE. Text in English. 1997. q. free. 2 cols./p. **Document type:** *Newsletter.* **Description:** Contains updated information and helpful suggestions on the optimal use of residual vision.
Media: Large Type (16 pt.).
Published by: National Association for Visually Handicapped, 22 W 21st St, 6th Fl, New York, NY 10010. TEL 212-889-3141, FAX 212-727-2931, staff@navh.org, http://www.navh.org. Ed., R&P Lorraine H Marchi. Circ: 13,000.

362.41 IRL
N C B I NEWS. Text in English. 1923. bi-m. free (effective 2002). bk.rev., dance rev., film rev., music rev., Website rev. **Document type:** *Magazine, Consumer, Internal.*
Formerly (until 1999): The Blind Citizen (0006-4815)
Related titles: Audio cassette/tape ed.; Braille ed.; Online - full content ed.
Published by: National Council for the Blind of Ireland, P V Doyle House, Whitworth Rd., Drumcondra, Dublin 9, Ireland. TEL 353-1-8307033, FAX 353-1-8307787, omegapub@eircom.net, http://www.ncbi.ie. Ed. Patrick Lyons. Circ: 3,000.

NAT - CENT NEWS. see *HANDICAPPED—Hearing Impaired*

647.9654 IND
NATIONAL ASSOCIATION FOR THE BLIND, INDIA. ANNUAL REPORT. Text in English. 1959. a. free per issue. stat. **Description:** Reports on the activities and projects run by the Association for the blind in India.
Published by: National Association for the Blind India, Worli Seaface, 11 Khan Abdul Gaffar Khan Rd., Mumbai, Maharashtra 400 025, India. TEL 91-22-493-6930, FAX 91-22-493-2539. Ed. Subhash A Datrange. Circ: 1,000.

362.41 USA ISSN 0550-5666
HV1788
NATIONAL BRAILLE ASSOCIATION. BULLETIN. Key Title: Bulletin of the National Braille Association, Inc. Text in English. 1946. q., latest vol.37. USD 40 domestic; USD 50 foreign (effective 2001). 30 p./no. 2 cols./p. **Document type:** *Newsletter.* **Description:** Series of articles called "Sharpen Your Skills", a thorough summary of technical advice to keep braille transcribers up-to-date.
Formerly: National Braille Club. Bulletin (0097-6512)
Related titles: Audio cassette/tape ed.; Braille ed.; Diskette ed.
Indexed: C.I.J.E. (coverage dropped), Yrbk.Assoc.Educ.& Rehab.Blind.
Published by: National Braille Association, Inc., 3 Townline Cir, Rochester, NY 14623. TEL 716-427-8260, FAX 716-427-0263, http://www.nationalbraille.org. Circ: 2,000.

362.41 USA
NATIONAL LIBRARY SERVICE. REFERENCE CIRCULAR SERIES. Text in English. irreg., latest 2001, no.01-01. free. **Document type:** *Monographic series, Government.* **Description:** Compiles current information on a specific topic of interest to persons with disabilities or persons who provide them services.
Media: Large Type (14 pt.). **Related titles:** Online - full text ed.
Published by: U.S. Library of Congress, National Library Service for the Blind and Physically Handicapped, Washington, DC 20542. TEL 202-707-5100, FAX 202-707-0712, nls@loc.gov, http://lcweb.loc.gov/nls.

DIE NEUE SONDERSCHULE. see *EDUCATION*

362.41 GBR
NEW BEACON (BRAILLE EDITION); the journal of blind welfare. Text in English. 1951. m. GBP 18.70 (effective 1999). adv. charts. index. **Document type:** *Consumer.* **Description:** Publishes in-depth articles, letters, news reviews, leisure articles, and notices of interest to persons with visual disabilities.
Media: Braille. **Related titles:** Audio cassette/tape ed.; Diskette ed.
Indexed: ASSIA, Yrbk.Assoc.Educ.& Rehab.Blind.
Published by: Royal National Institute for the Blind, Education, Training and Employment Division, 224 Great Portland St, London W1N 6AA, United Kingdom. TEL 44-171-388-1266, FAX 44-171-388-0945, cservices@rnib.org.uk, http://www.rnib.org.uk. Ed. Ann Lee. **Subscr. to:** RNIB Customer Services, PO Box 173, Peterborough, Cambs PE2 6WS, United Kingdom. TEL 44-1733-370777, FAX 44-1733-317555.

362.41 GBR ISSN 0028-4270
NEW BEACON (INKPRINT EDITION); the journal of blind welfare. Text in English. 1917. m. (except Aug.). GBP 29.70 (effective 2000). adv. bk.rev. charts. index. **Document type:** *Journal, Consumer.* **Description:** Publishes in-depth articles, letters, news, reviews, leisure articles, and notices and advertisements of interest to persons with visual impairments.
Related titles: Braille ed.; Diskette ed.
Indexed: ASSIA, Except.Child Educ.Abstr., Sp.Ed.Needs Abstr.
—BLDSC (6082.190000).
Published by: Royal National Institute for the Blind, Education, Training and Employment Division, 224 Great Portland St, London W1N 6AA, United Kingdom. TEL 44-171-388-1266, FAX 44-171-388-2034, alee@rnib.org.uk, http://www.rnib.org.uk. Ed. Ann Lee. Circ: 1,829. **Subscr. to:** RNIB, .PO Box 173, Peterborough, Cambs PE2 6WS, United Kingdom.

NEWS FROM ADVOCATES FOR DEAF - BLIND. see *HANDICAPPED—Hearing Impaired*

362.41 ITA
OFTALMOLOGIA SOCIALE - RIVISTA DI SANITA PUBBLICA. Text in Italian. 1977. q. ITL 30,000. adv.
Formerly: Rivista di Oftalmologia Sociale (0391-3112)
Published by: Agenzia Internazionale per la Prevenzione della Cecita, Sezione Italiana/International Agency for the Prevention of Blindness, Italian Section, Via Borgognona, 38, Rome, RM 00187, Italy. TEL 39-6-699881, FAX 39-6-6786815. Circ: 5,000.

305.42 USA ISSN 0030-6959
OUR SPECIAL; magazine devoted to matters of interest to blind women. Text in English. 1930. bi-m. USD 15. bk.rev.
Media: Braille.
Published by: National Braille Press, Inc., 88 St Stephen St, Boston, MA 02115. TEL 617-266-6160, 800-548-7323, FAX 617-437-0456, orders@nbp.org, http://www.nbp.org. Ed. Jeanne Neale. Circ: 2,559.

PARTNERS (SYLMAR). see *SOCIAL SERVICES AND WELFARE*

PHYSIOTHERAPISTS' QUARTERLY. see *MEDICAL SCIENCES—Physical Medicine And Rehabilitation*

786 GBR ISSN 0048-4105
PIANO-TUNERS QUARTERLY. Text in English. 1954. q. GBP 8 (effective 2000). **Document type:** *Trade.* **Description:** Contains advice for the professional piano tuner who is blind or visually impaired.
Media: Braille. **Related titles:** Audio cassette/tape ed.; Diskette ed.; Large type ed.
Published by: Royal National Institute for the Blind, PO Box 173, Peterborough, Cambs PE2 6WX, United Kingdom. TEL 44-1733-370-777, FAX 44-1733-371555, webmaster @rnib.org.uk, http://www.rnig.org.uk. Circ: 66.

PILOT DOGS. see *PETS*

362.41 GBR ISSN 0048-4881
PORTLAND MAGAZINE. Text in English. 1960. m. GBP 4.
Media: Braille.
Published by: Royal National Institute for the Blind, PO Box 173, Peterborough, Cambs PE2 6WX, United Kingdom. TEL 44-733-370777, FAX 44-733-317555. Ed. Donald Bell. Circ: 309.

PREVENT BLINDNESS AMERICA. ANNUAL REPORT. see *PUBLIC HEALTH AND SAFETY*

PREVENT BLINDNESS NEWS. see *PUBLIC HEALTH AND SAFETY*

362.41 GBR ISSN 0033-0566
PROGRESS. Text in English. 1881. m. GBP 24 (effective 2000). adv. bk.rev. **Document type:** *Consumer.* **Description:** Offers a selection of articles of general interest to readers who are blind or visually impaired. Includes a problem page, announcements, a competition, and a crossword puzzle.
Media: Braille. **Related titles:** Diskette ed.
Published by: Royal National Institute for the Blind, PO Box 173, Peterborough, Cambs PE2 6WX, United Kingdom. TEL 44-1733-370-777, FAX 44-1733-238-541, 44-1733-371555, webmaster@rnib.org.uk, webmaster @rnib.org.uk, http://www.rnib.org.uk. Ed. Chris James. Circ: 689.

R E S N A NEWS. (Rehabilitation Engineering and Assistive Technology Society of North America) see *EDUCATION—Special Education And Rehabilitation*

362.41 USA
R F B & D IMPACT. Text in English. q. free per issue. back issues avail. **Document type:** *Newsletter.* **Description:** Covers news and information about the organization's activities and members.
Former titles: R F B Issues; Recording for the Blind. News
Published by: Recording for the Blind & Dyslexic, Inc., 20 Roszel Rd, Princeton, NJ 08540. TEL 609-452-0606. Ed., Pub. Diane Blaszka. R&P Richard Scribner. Circ: 70,000.

362.41 USA ISSN 1095-3949
HV1553
RAGGED EDGE. Text in English. 1980. bi-m. USD 17.50 domestic to individuals; USD 35 domestic to institutions; USD 42 foreign (effective 2002). adv. bk.rev. back issues avail. **Document type:** *Consumer.* **Description:** Examines current and emerging public issues from a disability perspective: civil rights, politics, culture, humor, sexuality, art, and technology.
Former titles (until 1997): Disability Rag and Resource; Disability Rag (0749-8586)
Related titles: Diskette ed.: USD 17.50 domestic to individuals; USD 35 domestic to institutions; USD 42 foreign (effective 2002); E-mail ed.; Online - full text ed.: USD 17.50 domestic to individuals; USD 35 domestic to institutions; USD 42 foreign (effective 2002).
Indexed: Alt.Press Ind., Diver.Y.World.
Published by: Advocado Press, PO Box 145, Louisville, KY 40201. TEL 502-894-9492, FAX 502-899-9562, editor@ragged-edge-mag.com, http://www.ragged-edge-mag.com, http://www.raggededgemagazine.com. Ed. Mary Johnson. Circ: 3,000 (paid).

RAINBOW (PETERBOROUGH). see *HANDICAPPED—Physically Impaired*

362.41 USA
RECORDING FOR THE BLIND & DYSLEXIC. ANNUAL REPORT. Text in English. 1951. a. back issues avail. **Document type:** *Corporate.* **Description:** Provides news, information and financial reports of the organization.
Formerly: Recording for the Blind. Annual Report
Published by: Recording for the Blind & Dyslexic, Inc., 20 Roszel Rd, Princeton, NJ 08540. TEL 609-452-0606, FAX 609-520-7990. Ed., Pub. Diane Blaszka. R&P Richard Scribner. Circ: 15,000.

RECORDING FOR THE BLIND & DYSLEXIC. CATALOG OF BOOKS. see *HANDICAPPED—Abstracting, Bibliographies, Statistics*

371.911 USA ISSN 0899-1510
HV1571
REVIEW (WASHINGTON); rehabilitation and education for blindness and visual impairment. Text in English. 1951. q., latest vol.34, 2002. USD 40 domestic to individuals; USD 52 foreign to individuals; USD 81 domestic to institutions; USD 93 foreign to institutions; USD 20.25 newsstand/cover (effective 2001 - 2002). adv. bk.rev. bibl, illus. index. reprint service avail. from PSC,SCH. *Refereed.* **Document type:** *Academic/Scholarly.* **Description:** Reports on useful practices, research findings, experiments, professional experiences and controversial issues. For all persons concerned with the education and rehabilitation of children, youth and adults who have visual impairments, including those who are multihandicapped and or deaf-blind.
Former titles: Education of the Visually Handicapped (0013-1458); International Journal for the Education of the Blind
Related titles: CD-ROM ed.: (from ProQuest Information & Learning); Microform ed.; Online - full text ed.: (from H. W. Wilson, ProQuest Information & Learning).
Indexed: C.I.J.E., Cont.Pg.Educ., Curr.Cont. (coverage dropped), ERA, Educ.Ind. (Mar.1989-), Except.Child Educ.Abstr., IBR, IBZ, PsycInfo, Psychol.Abstr. (1969-), Rehabil.Lit., SSCI (coverage dropped), Sp.Ed.Needs Abstr., Yrbk.Assoc.Educ.& Rehab.Blind.
—BLDSC (7300.261500), ingenta. **CCC.**
Published by: (Helen Dwight Reid Educational Foundation), Heldref Publications, 1319 Eighteenth St, N W, Washington, DC 20036-1802. TEL 202-296-6267, http://www.heldref.org. Ed. Helen Strang. Adv. contact Grant Williams. B&W page USD 255. Circ: 500. **Co-sponsor:** Association for the Education and Rehabilitation of the Blind and Visually Impaired.

340 GBR
ROYAL NATIONAL INSTITUTE FOR THE BLIND. BUSY SOLICITORS DIGEST. Text in English. 1949. m. **Document type:** *Trade.* **Description:** Provides visually impaired lawyers with the opportunity to keep up to date with valuable case-related information.
Formerly (until 1996): Royal National Institute for the Blind. Law Notes. Extracts (0023-9291)
Media: Braille. **Related titles:** Diskette ed.
Published by: Royal National Institute for the Blind, PO Box 173, Peterborough, Cambs PE2 6WX, United Kingdom. TEL 44-1733-370-777, FAX 44-1733-238-541, 44-1733-371555, webmaster @rnib.org.uk, http://www.rnib.org.uk. Circ: 36.

362.41 GBR ISSN 0080-4479
ROYAL NATIONAL INSTITUTE FOR THE BLIND. INFORMATION LEAFLETS. Text in English. irreg. free per issue.
Published by: Royal National Institute for the Blind, PO Box 173, Peterborough, Cambs PE2 6WX, United Kingdom. TEL 44-1733-370-777, FAX 44-1733-238-541.

ROYAL NATIONAL INSTITUTE FOR THE BLIND. UPDATE. see *SOCIAL SERVICES AND WELFARE*

052 ZAF
S A B W O NEWS. Text in English. m.
Published by: South Africa Blind Workers Organisation, Private Bag X9005, Crown Mines 2025, South Africa. TEL 27-11-8391793, FAX 27-11-8391217. Ed. Mrs. Hazel Marshall.

362.41 ZAF
S A N C B NEWS. Text in English. 1982. s-a. free per issue. **Document type:** *Newsletter.*
Related titles: Afrikaans ed.: S A N R B Nuus.
Published by: South African National Council for the Blind, PO Box 11149, Brooklyn, Pretoria 0011, South Africa. TEL 27-12-346-1171, FAX 27-12-346-1177. Ed. William Rowland. Circ: 45,000.

362.41 USA
THE SEEING EYE ANNUAL REPORT. Text in English. 1939. a. free per issue. illus. **Document type:** *Corporate.*
Related titles: Online - full text ed.
Published by: The Seeing Eye, Inc., PO Box 375, Morristown, NJ 07963-0375. TEL 973-539-4425, FAX 973-539-0922, http://www.seeingeye.org. Ed. Melissa Cambell. Circ: 30,000.

636.088 362.4 USA ISSN 0037-0819
THE SEEING EYE GUIDE. Text in English. 1935. q. free per issue (effective 2000). illus. back issues avail.
Related titles: Online - full text ed.
Published by: The Seeing Eye, Inc., PO Box 375, Morristown, NJ 07963-0375. TEL 973-539-4425, FAX 973-539-0922, http://www.seeingeye.org. Ed. Melissa Campbell. Circ: 25,000 (controlled).

SHAPING UP. see *PHYSICAL FITNESS AND HYGIENE*

SIBLING INFORMATION NETWORK NEWSLETTER. see *CHILDREN AND YOUTH—About*

SIGHTS AND SOUNDS. see *HANDICAPPED—Hearing Impaired*

362.41 USA
SMITH - KETTLEWELL TECHNICAL FILE; a biannual technical journal for the blind and visually impaired. Text in English. 1980. biennial. USD 18 (effective 2000). back issues avail. **Document type:** *Consumer.* **Description:** Reports clinical work and studies that relate directly to eye diseases and disorders, as well as to the development of devices for the partially sighted, blind and hearing impaired.
Published by: Smith - Kettlewell Eye Research Institute, 2318 Fiumorz St, San Francisco, CA 94115. TEL 415-345-2000, rerc@skirs.ski.org, http://www.ski.org. Ed., R&P Bill Gerrey. Circ: 300 (paid). **Co-sponsor:** National Institute of Disability & Rehabilitation Research.

SOUND COMPUTING. see *HANDICAPPED—Physically Impaired*

362.41 ZAF
SOUTH AFRICAN NATIONAL COUNCIL FOR THE BLIND. BIENNIAL REPORT. Text in English. 1932. biennial. **Document type:** *Corporate.*
Related titles: Braille ed.; Afrikaans ed.
Published by: South African National Council for the Blind, PO Box 11149, Brooklyn, Pretoria 0011, South Africa. TEL 27-12-346-1171, FAX 27-12-346-1177. Circ: 1,500.

SPECTRUM (PETERBOROUGH). see *PHYSICAL FITNESS AND HYGIENE*

H

362.41 USA
SPIRIT OF SERVICE. Text in English. 1985. s-a. free per issue. bk.rev. **Document type:** *Catalog.* **Description:** Provides news on service work of the Nepal Blindness Program at the Aravind Eye Hospital; development projects in Guatemala and Mexico, and community service projects in the U.S. and Canada.
Published by: Seva Foundation, 1786 5th St, Berkeley, CA 94710-1716. TEL 510-845-7382, FAX 510-845-7410, admin@seva.org, http://www.seva.org. Ed. Mirabai Bush. Circ: 30,000. **Co-sponsor:** Seva Service Society.

362.41 GBR
ST. DUNSTAN'S ANNUAL BROCHURE. Text in English. 1916. a. free per issue. illus. **Document type:** *Corporate.*
Former titles: St. Dunstan's Annual Review; St. Dunstan's Annual Report
Published by: St. Dunstan's for Men and Women Blinded in the Services, 12-14 Harcourt St, PO Box 4XB, London W1A 4XB, United Kingdom. TEL 44-171-723-5021, FAX 44-171-262-6199. Ed. Raymond Hazan. Circ: (controlled).

362.41 GBR ISSN 0036-2808
ST. DUNSTAN'S REVIEW. Text in English. 1915. bi-m. GBP 21 (effective 1999). bk.rev. illus. **Document type:** *Newsletter.*
Published by: St. Dunstan's for Men and Women Blinded in the Services, 12-14 Harcourt St, PO Box 4XB, London W1A 4XB, United Kingdom. TEL 44-171-723-5021, FAX 44-171-262-6199. Ed. Raymond Hazan. Circ: 2,500.

THE STUDENT (LINCOLN). see *RELIGIONS AND THEOLOGY*

011.38 USA ISSN 0039-9183
HV1708
TALKING BOOK TOPICS (LARGE PRINT EDITION). Text in English. 1935. bi-m. free to qualified personnel. bk.rev. illus. Index. back issues avail.; reprints avail. **Document type:** *Newsletter, Government.* **Description:** Contains news of developments and activities in library services and announcements of recorded books and magazines recently added to the N.L.S. collection.
Media: Large Type (14 pt.). **Related titles:** Audio cassette/tape ed.; Diskette ed.; Online - full text ed.
Indexed: Rehabil.Lit.
Published by: U.S. Library of Congress, National Library Service for the Blind and Physically Handicapped, Washington, DC 20542. TEL 202-707-5100, FAX 202-707-0712, nls@loc.gov, http://lcweb.loc.gov/nls. Ed. Rita Burnes. Circ: 350,000.

TALKING BOOKS IN THE PUBLIC LIBRARY SYSTEMS OF METROPOLITAN TORONTO. see *LIBRARY AND INFORMATION SCIENCES*

TAPE MEDICAL BULLETIN. see *MEDICAL SCIENCES*

TAPPING TECHNOLOGY. see *HANDICAPPED—Physically Impaired*

379.911 USA ISSN 0040-9928
TOWERS. Text in English. 1947. q. free. charts, illus. **Document type:** *Newsletter.*
Published by: Overbrook School for the Blind, 6333 Malvern Ave, Philadelphia, PA 19151. TEL 215-877-0313, FAX 215-877-2465, dennis@obs.org, http://www.obs.org. Ed., R&P Dennis Brookshire. Circ: 5,000.

284.1 USA ISSN 0041-0357
TRACT MESSENGER. Text in English. 1953. m. free per issue. **Description:** Contains devotional and inspirational articles of the Christian faith.
Media: Braille.
Published by: Lutheran Braille Evangelism Association, 1740 Eugene St., White Bear, MN 55110. TEL 651-426-0469. Ed. Rev. Dennis A Hawkinson. Circ: 500.

U S A B A AGENDA. see *SPORTS AND GAMES*

027.663 362 020 USA ISSN 1046-1663
HV1783
U.S. LIBRARY OF CONGRESS. NATIONAL LIBRARY SERVICE FOR THE BLIND AND PHYSICALLY HANDICAPPED. NEWS. Text in English. 1958. q. free per issue. **Document type:** *Newsletter, Government.* **Description:** Presents information on national and international developments in library services to blind and physically disabled persons.
Former titles: U.S. Library of Congress. National Library for the Blind and Physically Handicapped. News (0160-9211); D B P H News
Related titles: Audio cassette/tape ed.; Braille ed.; Online - full text ed.
Published by: U.S. Library of Congress, National Library Service for the Blind and Physically Handicapped, Washington, DC 20542. TEL 202-707-5100, FAX 202-707-0712, nls@loc.gov. Ed. Vicki Fitzpatrick. Circ: 30,000.

362.41 FRA
UNION DES AVEUGLES DE GUERRE. BULLETIN BIMESTRIEL. Text in French. 1921. bi-m. free per issue to qualified personnel. **Document type:** *Bulletin.*
Formerly: Union des Aveugles de Guerre. Bulletin Mensuel (0041-6843)
Published by: Union des Aveugles de Guerre, 49 rue Blanche, Paris 75009, France. TEL 48-74-56-18, FAX 45-26-24-34. Ed. Pierre Guillernet.

053 AUT ISSN 0042-0492
UNSER SCHAFFEN; Monatsschrift fuer das Blindenwesen. Text in German. 1956. m. ATS 200 (effective 2001). adv. bk.rev. **Document type:** *Newspaper, Consumer.* **Description:** Support of interests of the blind and visually impaired. Topics: news, ophtalmology, health, culture, book reviews, news from the organization Hilfsgemeinschaft.
Media: Talking Book.
Indexed: GeoRef.
Published by: Hilfsgemeinschaft der Blinden und Sehschwachen Oesterreichs, Treustrasse 9, Vienna, W 1200, Austria. TEL 43-1-3303545-0, FAX 43-1-330354511, redaktion@hilfsgemeinschaft.at, info@hilfsgemeinschaft.at, http://www.hilfsgemeinschaft.at. Ed., Adv. contact Silvia Lausmann. B&W page ATS 14,000, color page ATS 23,800; trim 190 x 250. Circ: 20,000.

371.9 DEU
UNTER UNS; Zeitschrift fuer Frauen und Maedchen. Text in German. m. EUR 70.50; EUR 62.60 to students (effective 2002). adv. bk.rev. **Document type:** *Magazine, Consumer.*
Related titles: Braille ed.
Published by: Deutsche Blindenstudienanstalt e.V., Postfach 1160, Marburg 35001, Germany. TEL 49-6421-606-0, FAX 49-6421-606229, info@blista.de, http://www.blista.de. Circ: 225.

UPDATE (OWINGS MILLS). see *MEDICAL SCIENCES—Ophthalmology And Optometry*

THE UPPER ROOM; daily devotional guide, interdenominational, international. see *RELIGIONS AND THEOLOGY—Protestant*

617.8 USA
USHER AROUND THE WORLD. Text in English. q. USD 16; USD 19 in Canada & Mexico; USD 22 elsewhere. **Document type:** *Newsletter.* **Description:** Published by and for people with Usher's Syndrome.
Formerly: About U S
Related titles: Audio cassette/tape ed.; Braille ed.; Large type ed. 17 pt.
Address: PO Box 17318, Minneapolis, MN 55417. TEL 612-729-4630. Ed. Maggie Kinge. Circ: 200.

371.911 USA
V C S RESOURCE LIST. Text in English. a. free. **Document type:** *Consumer.* **Description:** Provides resources for individuals who are blind or visually impaired.
Formerly (until 1998): Vision Resource List
Related titles: Audio cassette/tape ed.; Diskette ed.; Large type ed. 16 pt.
Published by: Vision Community Services, A division of the Massachusetts Association for the Blind, 23A Elm St, Watertown, MA 02472-2821. TEL 617-926-4232, 800-852-3029, FAX 617-926-1412, fweisse@mablind.org, http://www.mablind.org. Ed. Fran Weisse. Circ: 2,000.

HET VAGGESCHIP. see *HANDICAPPED*

371.911 DEU
VEREINSMITTEILUNGEN. Text in German. 1946. bi-m.
Related titles: Audio cassette/tape ed.
Published by: Schleswig - Holsteinischer Blindenverein e.V., Memelstr 4, Luebeck 23554, Germany. TEL 0451-40349, FAX 0451-407530. Circ: 1,600.

362.41 USA ISSN 1094-8635
VISION ENHANCEMENT. Text in English. 1996. q. USD 20 in US & Canada to individuals; USD 45 elsewhere (effective 2001). adv. bk.rev. **Document type:** *Trade.* **Description:** Reports on resources and news for individuals who are visually impaired or blind. Covers computer and adaptive technologies, along with medical research. Provides many resources for professionals working with the vision impaired.
Media: Large Type (16 pt.). **Related titles:** Audio cassette/tape ed.: ISSN 1097-0398; Diskette ed.: ISSN 1097-0401.
Published by: Vision World Wide, Inc., 5707 Brockton Dr, 302, Indianapolis, IN 46220-5481. TEL 317-254-1332, 800-431-1739, FAX 317-251-6588, info@visionww.org, http://www.visionww.org. Ed. Patricia Price.

VISIONARY. see *MEDICAL SCIENCES—Ophthalmology And Optometry*

362.41 NLD ISSN 1388-235X
▼ **VISUAL IMPAIRMENT RESEARCH.** Text in English. 1999. 3/yr. NLG 180, USD 97 to individuals; NLG 388, USD 204 to institutions includes online ed. (effective 2000). *Refereed.* **Document type:** *Academic/Scholarly.* **Description:** Covers the entire field of research and practice in visual rehabilitation assessment in, and rehabilitation of, children, multiple handicaps, cognitive impairments, educational programs for rehabilitation workers, and standardized protocols.
Related titles: Online - full text ed.: (from EBSCO Publishing, O C L C Online Computer Library Center, Inc., RoweCom Information Quest, Swets Blackwell).
—BLDSC (9241.259000).
Published by: Aeolus Press (Subsidiary of: Swets & Zeitlinger BV), PO Box 825, Lisse 2160 SZ, Netherlands. FAX 31-344-572562, orders@swets.nl, http://www.swets.nl/sps/AEolus/vir.html. Eds. Aart Kooijman, Aries Arditi. **Subscr. to:** Swets & Zeitlinger BV, PO Box 825, Lisse 2160 SZ, Netherlands. TEL 31-252-435111, FAX 31-252-415888, orders@swets.nl. **Dist. in N. America by:** Swets & Zeitlinger, PO Box 582, Downingtown, PA 19335-998. TEL 800-447-9387.

362.41 USA ISSN 1041-8490
VOICE OF THE DIABETIC; a support and information network. Text in English. 1986. q. USD 20 to non-members (effective 2001). adv. bk.rev. **Document type:** *Newspaper, Consumer.* **Description:** Contains personal stories and practical guidance, medical news, a resource column, and a recipe corner.
Related titles: Audio cassette/tape ed.
Published by: National Federation of the Blind, Diabetes Action Network, 1412 I70 Dr SW, C, Columbia, MO 65203. TEL 573-875-8911, FAX 573-875-8902, http://www.nfb.org/voice.htm. Ed., R&P Ed Bryant. Adv. contact Eileen Rivera-Ley TEL 410-296-7760. B&W page USD 1,875, color page USD 2,775. Circ: 291,436.

WELCOME TO THE WORLD OF... see *SOCIAL SERVICES AND WELFARE*

HEALTH FACILITIES AND ADMINISTRATION

see also MEDICAL SCIENCES; NUTRITION AND DIETETICS

1199 NEWS. see *LABOR UNIONS*

A A B B NEWS. see *MEDICAL SCIENCES*

658 USA ISSN 0891-6608
A H A NEWS∗. Text in English. 1987. w. USD 65 to members; USD 150 to non-members; USD 2 newsstand/cover to members; USD 4 newsstand/cover to non-members (effective 2001). back issues avail. **Document type:** *Newspaper, Trade.* **Description:** Covers the latest health-policy news from Washington as well as national and state health care news.
Published by: (American Hospital Association), American Hospital Publishing, Inc. (Subsidiary of: American Hospital Association Company), 1 N Franklin St, 27th Fl, Chicago, IL 60606-3421. TEL 312-440-6800, FAX 312-951-8491, 312-422-4799. Circ: 24,700.

A H R A RECORD. see *MEDICAL SCIENCES*

362.1072 USA
A H R Q RESEARCH ACTIVITIES. (Agency for Healthcare Research and Quality) Text in English. m. 32 p./no. 3 cols./p. back issues avail. **Document type:** *Academic/Scholarly, Government.*
Formerly (until Dec. 1999): Agency for Health Care Policy and Research

Related titles: Online - full text ed.
Published by: U.S. Department of Health and Human Services, Agency for Healthcare Research and Quality, P.O. Box 8547, Silver Spring, MD 20907-8547. TEL 800-358-9295, http://www.ahrq.gov. Pub. Randie Siegel. R&P, Adv. contact Mary Grady TEL 301-594-6168.

363.7 USA
A S H E S. Text in English. 1986. bi-m. membership. adv. bk.rev. charts, illus. back issues avail. **Document type:** *Newsletter.* **Description:** Articles on trends and developments in environmental services, housekeeping, laundry, interior design, recycling, and waste management provided by healthcare institutions.
Formerly: Healthcare Environmental Services
Published by: (American Society for Healthcare Environmental Services), American Hospital Association, One North Franklin, Chicago, IL 60606-3421. TEL 312-422-3863, FAX 312-422-4572. Ed. Tara O'Briskie. Circ: 1,400.

628 USA
A S H E S ANNUAL CONFERENCE. PROCEEDINGS MANUAL. Text in English. 1985. a. USD 29.95 to members; USD 39.95 to non-members. **Document type:** *Proceedings.*
Published by: (American Society for Healthcare Environmental Services), American Hospital Association, One North Franklin, Chicago, IL 60606-3421. TEL 312-422-3863, FAX 312-422-4572. Ed. Tara O'Briskie. Circ: 1,500.

368.382 USA
A S H R M FORUM. Text in English. 1987. bi-m. **Document type:** *Newsletter.* **Description:** Presents news about chapters and members of ASHRM.
Published by: (American Society for Healthcare Risk Management), American Hospital Association, One North Franklin, Chicago, IL 60606-3421. TEL 312-422-3989, FAX 312-422-4580. Ed. Margaret S Veach. Circ: 3,000 (controlled).

362.110711 USA
A U P H A EXCHANGE*. Text in English. bi-m. **Document type:** *Newsletter.*
Published by: Association of University Programs in Health Administration, 730 11th St N W, 4th Fl, Washington, DC 20001-4510. TEL 703-524-5500, FAX 703-525-4791. Ed. Mary Louise Giunta.

650 FRA ISSN 1155-3839
ABSTRACT HOPITAL. Text in French. 1989. m.
Formerly (until 1990): Abstract Maladies Infectieuses (0997-1785)
Published by: Abstract Medical International, 25 bis, av. Pierre Grenier, Boulogne 92100, France. TEL 49-10-06-06. Ed. Patricia Thelliez. Circ: 15,000.

658 USA ISSN 1084-354X
ACCREDITATION MANUAL FOR AMBULATORY CARE. Text in English. 1996. biennial. **Document type:** *Monographic series.*
Published by: Joint Commission on Accreditation of Healthcare Organizations, 75 Remittance Dr, Ste 1057, Chicago, IL 60675-1057. TEL 630-792-5800, http://www.jcaho.org.

658 USA ISSN 1077-5560
RA645.35
ACCREDITATION MANUAL FOR HOME CARE. VOL. 1: STANDARDS. Variant title: A M H C Standards. Text in English. 1991. biennial. **Document type:** *Monographic series.*
Published by: Joint Commission on Accreditation of Healthcare Organizations, 75 Remittance Dr, Ste 1057, Chicago, IL 60675-1057. TEL 630-792-5800, http://www.jcaho.org.

658 USA ISSN 1077-5579
RA645.35
ACCREDITATION MANUAL FOR HOME CARE. VOL. 2: SCORING GUIDELINES. Variant title: A M H C Scoring Guidelines. Text in English. 1991. biennial. **Document type:** *Monographic series.*
Published by: Joint Commission on Accreditation of Healthcare Organizations, 75 Remittance Dr, Ste 1057, Chicago, IL 60675-1057. TEL 630-916-5800, http://www.jcaho.org.

658 USA ISSN 1083-1762
RA981.A2
ACCREDITATION MANUAL FOR HOSPITALS. VOL. 1: STANDARDS. Text in English. a. **Document type:** *Monographic series.*
Related titles: Online - full text ed.: (from LexisNexis).
Published by: Joint Commission on Accreditation of Healthcare Organizations, 75 Remittance Dr, Ste 1057, Chicago, IL 60675-1057. TEL 630-792-5800, http://www.jcaho.org.

658 USA ISSN 1083-1770
RA981.A2
ACCREDITATION MANUAL FOR HOSPITALS. VOL. 2: SCORING GUIDELINES. Text in English. a. **Document type:** *Monographic series.*
Published by: Joint Commission on Accreditation of Healthcare Organizations, 75 Remittance Dr, Ste 1057, Chicago, IL 60675-1057. TEL 630-792-5800, http://www.jcaho.org.

658 USA ISSN 1084-4376
RA997
ACCREDITATION MANUAL FOR LONG TERM CARE. Text in English. 1992. biennial. **Document type:** *Monographic series.*
Published by: Joint Commission on Accreditation of Healthcare Organizations, 75 Remittance Dr, Ste 1057, Chicago, IL 60675-1057. TEL 630-792-5800, http://www.jcaho.org.

ACIMED. see *MEDICAL SCIENCES*

362 BEL ISSN 0044-6009
ACTA HOSPITALIA. Text in Dutch, English, French; Summaries in English. 1961. q. BEF 1,700 domestic; BEF 2,000 foreign (effective 2000). adv. bk.rev. bibl. cum.index. **Document type:** *Academic/Scholarly.*
Indexed: Excerp.Med., Hosp.Abstr., Med.Care Rev. —BLDSC (0624.410000), EMDOCS, GNLM.
Published by: Katholieke Universiteit te Leuven, Centrum voor Ziekenhuiswetenschap, Kapucijnenvoer 35, Leuven 3000, Belgium. TEL 32-16-336973, FAX 32-16-336970. Ed. P Quaethoven. Circ: 750.

ACTION KIT FOR HOSPITAL LAW. see *LAW*

658 340 USA
ACTION KIT FOR HOSPITAL TRUSTEES. Text in English. 1971. bi-m. USD 295 (effective 1999). **Document type:** *Newsletter.* **Description:** Helps hospital management and governing board members understand the legal and regulatory changes that affect hospitals.
Published by: Action Kit Publications, 4614 Fifth Ave, Pittsburgh, PA 15213. TEL 412-687-7677, 800-245-1205. Ed. John F Horty. R&P Margaret Barker TEL Margaret/Barker.

ACTIVITIES OF IRISH PSYCHIATRIC SERVICES (YEAR). see *MEDICAL SCIENCES—Psychiatry And Neurology*

ADMINISTRATION & MANAGEMENT SPECIAL INTEREST SECTION QUARTERLY. see *OCCUPATIONAL HEALTH AND SAFETY*

ADMINISTRATIVE OPHTHALMOLOGY. see *MEDICAL SCIENCES—Ophthalmology And Optometry*

ADMINISTRATIVE RADIOLOGY; the journal of medical imaging administration & management. see *MEDICAL SCIENCES—Radiology And Nuclear Medicine*

ADULT DAY SERVICES LETTER. see *GERONTOLOGY AND GERIATRICS*

ADVANCE FOR HEALTH INFORMATION EXECUTIVES. see *COMPUTERS—Data Communications And Data Transmission Systems*

ADVANCES IN THANATOLOGY. see *PSYCHOLOGY*

658 JPN ISSN 0911-1549
AKAHIGE/TAKKO TOWN HOSPITAL. ANNUAL REPORT. Text in Japanese; Summaries in English, Japanese. 1984. a.
Published by: Takko Choritsu Takko Byoin/Takko Town Hospital, 2-17 Maeda-Takko, Sannohe-gun, Takko-machi, Aomori-ken 039-0200, Japan.

362.18 616.02 GBR
AMBULANCE SERVICE JOURNAL; a professional journal for ambulance and first aid personnel. Text in English. q. GBP 1.
Incorporating: Ambulance (0044-7455)
Published by: Institute of Certified Ambulance Personnel, c/o F. Thornley, 64 Pen-y-fro, Dunvant, Wales, United Kingdom. Ed. Nan Berger. Circ: 1,200.

362.18 616.02 GBR
AMBULANCE U K. Text in English. 1986. 6/yr. GBP 18 domestic; GBP 30 foreign (effective 2000). adv. back issues avail. **Document type:** *Trade.* **Description:** Provides information about all matters related to the United Kingdom Ambulance Service, including the production of goods and services, communications and medicine.
Published by: Media Publishing Company, Media House, 41 Crayford Way, Dartford, Kent DA1 4JY, United Kingdom. TEL 44-1322-558029, FAX 44-1332-558524, medipub@aol.com. Ed. G Roberts. Pub. T Gardner. Adv. contact Joan Woodhead. Circ: 5,000.

AMERICAN ANIMAL HOSPITAL ASSOCIATION. ANNUAL MEETING SCIENTIFIC PROCEEDINGS. see *VETERINARY SCIENCE*

AMERICAN ANIMAL HOSPITAL ASSOCIATION. JOURNAL. see *VETERINARY SCIENCE*

AMERICAN ASSOCIATION OF BLOOD BANKS. MEMBERSHIP DIRECTORY. see *MEDICAL SCIENCES*

362 USA ISSN 1061-2262
RA977
AMERICAN COLLEGE OF HEALTHCARE EXECUTIVES. DIRECTORY. Text in English. 1960. biennial. USD 175 to non-members; USD 125 to members. **Document type:** *Directory.* **Description:** Contains complete professional information on affiliates, including education, the college status, past positions and addresses.
Formerly: American College of Hospital Administrators. Directory (0065-7794)
Published by: American College of Healthcare Executives, One N Franklin St, Ste 1700, Chicago, IL 60606-3491. TEL 312-424-2800, FAX 312-424-0023, http//www.ache.org. R&P Ann Bartling. Circ: 2,300.

AMERICAN JOURNAL OF HEALTH-SYSTEM PHARMACY. see *PHARMACY AND PHARMACOLOGY*

AMERICAN SCHOOL AND HOSPITAL MAINTENANCE. see *EDUCATION—School Organization And Administration*

658 621 USA
AMERICAN SOCIETY FOR HOSPITAL ENGINEERING TECHNICAL DOCUMENT SERIES. Text in English. 1982. m. membership. charts, illus. back issues avail. **Document type:** *Bulletin.* **Description:** Detailed study of areas of selected topics written for facilities managers of health care institutions.
Published by: (American Society for Hospital Engineering), American Hospital Association, One North Franklin, Chicago, IL 60606-3421. TEL 312-422-3803, FAX 312-422-4572. Ed. Kerry Hacker. Circ: 6,100.

658 USA
AMERICAN SOCIETY FOR HOSPITAL MATERIALS MANAGEMENT. CONFERENCE PROCEEDINGS. Text in English. a. index. back issues avail. **Description:** Provides materials managers with information on how to track opportunities, develop action plans and implement those plans to improve materials management operations.
Published by: (American Society for Hospital Materials Management), American Hospital Association, 840 North Lake Shore Dr, Chicago, IL 60611. TEL 312-422-3841, FAX 312-422-4571. Ed. Shelly Johnson.

610 FRA ISSN 1288-5517
ANNUAIRE DE L'HOSPITALISATION PRIVEE. Text in French. 1949. a. FRF 795. adv. **Document type:** *Directory.* **Description:** Provides names and adresses of clinics and hospitals with the number of beds, types of specialization and medical equipment.
Former titles (until 1997): Annuaire Medical de l'Hospitalisation Francaise Privee (1154-8630); (until 1989): Annuaire Medical de l'Hospitalisation Privee (0398-4222); (until 1972): L' Annuaire Medical de l'Hospitalisation Francaise (0066-3298)
Published by: (Edi-Publi-France - Rosenwald), Rosenwald, 10 rue Vineuse, Paris 75116, France. TEL 33-1-44308100, FAX 33-1-44308111, rosenwal@wanadoo.fr. Pub. Afif Ben Yedder. Adv. contact Dominique Alexandre.

362.1 ITA
ANNUARIO DEI FORNITORI DELLA SANITA IN ITALIA. Text in Italian. 1984. a. ITL 150,000 domestic; USD 120 foreign; ITL 500,000, USD 500 with CD-ROM or diskette. adv. **Document type:** *Directory.* **Description:** Lists all types of suppliers to hospitals and other health institutions.

Related titles: CD-ROM ed.; Diskette ed.
Published by: Pubblicita Italia s.a.s., Via Taglio, 24, Modena, MO 41100, Italy. TEL 39-059-216688, FAX 39-059-220727, info@pubblicitaitalia, http://www.pubit.it, http://www.pubblicitaitalia.com. Ed., Pub. Onelio Benedetti. Adv. contact Lorenzo Fiorentin. color page ITL 4,000,000; bleed 297 x 210. Circ: 5,000.

658 JPN
AOMORI KENRITSU BYOIN NENPO/AOMORI PREFECTURAL HOSPITALS. ANNUAL REPORTS. Text in Japanese. a.
Published by: Aomoriken Kankyo Hokenbu/Aomori Prefectural Government, Environmental Health Division, 1-1 Nagashima 1-chome, Aomori-shi 030-0861, Japan.

658 JPN ISSN 0387-0138 CODEN: AKCIB5
AOMORI KENRITSU CHUO BYOIN ISHI/AOMORI PREFECTURAL CENTRAL HOSPITAL. MEDICAL JOURNAL. Text in English, Japanese. 1956. q.
Indexed: INIS Atomind.
—CASDDS.
Published by: Aomori Kenritsu Chuo Byoin/Aomori Prefectural Central Hospital, 2-24 Nagashima 1-chome, Aomori-shi 030-0861, Japan.

AOMORIKEN JICHITAI IGAKKAISHI/AOMORI MUNICIPAL HOSPITAL ESTABLISHMENT ASSOCIATION. JOURNAL. see *MEDICAL SCIENCES*

APOTHEKE UND KRANKENHAUS. see *PHARMACY AND PHARMACOLOGY*

362.11 CAN
ARBUTUS SOCIETY FOR CHILDREN. ANNUAL REPORT. Text in English. 1927. a. CND 6. **Document type:** *Corporate.*
Former titles: Queen Alexandra Hospital for Children. Annual Report; Queen Alexandra Solarium for Crippled Children Annual Report (0085-526X)
Media: Duplicated (not offset).
Published by: Arbutus Society for Children, 2400 Arbutus Rd, Victoria, BC V8N 1V7, Canada. TEL 604-477-1826, FAX 604-721-6837. Ed. Joy Spencer Barry. Circ: 1,000.

658 USA
ARKANSAS HOSPITAL ASSOCIATION. PRESIDENT'S LETTER. Text in English. 1973. w. USD 700. back issues avail.
Published by: Arkansas Hospital Association, 419 Natural Resources Dr, Little Rock, AR 72205. TEL 501-224-7878, FAX 501-224-0519. Ed. Roger Busfield. Circ: 190.

362 BRA ISSN 0018-5442
ARQUIVOS DOS HOSPITAIS E DA FACULDADE DE CIENCIAS MEDICAS DA SANTA CASA DE SAO PAULO. Text in Portuguese; Summaries in English. 1954. q. USD 20. adv. bk.rev. abstr, bibl, charts, illus, stat. index.
Published by: Faculdade de Ciencias Medicas da Santa Casa de Sao Paulo/School of Medicine of Santa Casa of Sao Paulo, Rua Dr Cesario Motta Junior, 112, VI Buarque, Sao Paulo, SP 01221-020, Brazil.

658 CAN ISSN 0823-4124
ARTERE. Text in French. 1983. m. (10/yr.). CND 68.37; CND 86 foreign (effective 1998). adv. bk.rev. back issues avail. **Document type:** *Trade.* **Description:** Information for hospital administrators, field personnel. Technical news and operation methods.
Published by: (Quebec Hospital Association), Editions 2000 Neuf, 606 Cathcart, Ste 330, Montreal, PQ H3B 1K9, Canada. TEL 514-868-0383, FAX 514-868-0608, 2009@sympatico.ca, http://www.2009.com. Ed. Michel Bissonnette. R&P Francois Marcil. Adv. contact Michel Lauzier. B&W page CND 2,300, color page CND 3,300; trim 17 x 11.13. Circ: 7,202.

658 340 USA
ARTHUR ANDERSEN WASHINGTON HEALTHCARE NEWSLETTER. Text in English. 11/yr. free per issue. **Document type:** *Newsletter.*
Published by: Andersen, 1666 K St, N W, Washington, DC 20006. TEL 202-862-6732, FAX 202-862-7098. Ed. Don Yesukaitis.

ASAHIKAWA SHIRITSU BYOIN ISHI/ASAHIKAWA CITY HOSPITAL. JOURNAL. see *MEDICAL SCIENCES*

658 HKG ISSN 1011-596X
ASIAN HOSPITAL; Asia's quarterly review for health care industry executives. Text in English. 1987. q. USD 190; includes Asian Hospital NewsFax. adv. bk.rev. **Document type:** *Trade.* **Description:** Covers management, financing, information systems, technology, trends and issues critical to hospital and the healthcare industry.
Indexed: HongKongiana.
Published by: Health Asia Communications Ltd., GPO Box 1099, Hong Kong, Hong Kong. TEL 852-2869-4933, FAX 852-2525-6086. Ed., R&P Laura Tse. Pub. John R Longbotham. adv.: B&W page USD 4,800, color page USD 6,060; 210 x 285. Circ: 38,361 (controlled).

362.11068 GBR
ASIAN HOSPITAL & HEALTHCARE MANAGEMENT. Text in English. a. adv. **Document type:** *Journal, Trade.* **Description:** Provides comprehensive editorial coverage of all prevalent medical issues, product and equipment reports, and reviews of the latest technological developments.
Published by: (Asian Hospital Federation), Cornhill Publications Ltd. (Subsidiary of: Sterling Publishing Group Plc.), Kings Ct, 2-16 Goodge St, London W1P 1FF, United Kingdom. TEL 44-207-240-1515, FAX 44-207-379-7371, info@cornhillpublications.com, http://www.cornhillpublications.com/titles/ahh.html, http://www.cornhillpublications.co.uk. adv.: B&W page GBP 6,500, color page GBP 7,400. Circ: 12,600 (controlled).

658 HKG
ASIAN HOSPITAL NEWSFAX; Asia's newsfax for the healthcare industry. Text in English. m. USD 190; includes Asian Hospital. **Document type:** *Trade.* **Description:** For healthcare industry executives.
Published by: Health Asia Communications Ltd., GPO Box 1099, Hong Kong, Hong Kong. TEL 852-2869-4933, FAX 852-2525-6086. Ed. Laura Tse.

658 GBR ISSN 0958-8167
ASPEL'S GAZETTE. Text in English. 1989. m. GBP 48 to public-sector institutions; GBP 98 to private-sector institutions (effective 2001). back issues avail. **Document type:** *Bulletin, Trade.* **Description:** Lists surplus medical and other technical equipment for sale.
Published by: Aspel Publishing Ltd., Shepherd Ln, Beverley, Yorks HU17 8PH, United Kingdom. TEL 44-1482-887028, FAX 44-1482-887029. Ed., R&P Hilary Ryan. Pub. Derek Norman. Adv. contact Kathleen Turner. Circ: 1,000.

362.6 USA
ASSISTED LIVING BUSINESS REPORT. Text in English. 1997. m. USD 357 domestic; USD 387 foreign; USD 60 newsstand/cover per month (effective 2001). back issues avail.; reprints avail. **Document type:** *Newsletter.* **Description:** Discusses topics in the management of residences for senior citizens.
Published by: American Health Consultants (Subsidiary of: Medical Economics Co., Inc.), P O Box 740056, Atlanta, GA 30374. TEL 404-262-7436, 800-688-2421, FAX 404 262-7837, 800-284-3291, custserv@ahcpub.com, http://www.ahcpub.com.

362.6 649.8 USA
ASSISTED LIVING SUCCESS. Text in English. m. USD 55 in United States; USD 80 in Canada; USD 115 elsewhere (effective 2000). adv. **Document type:** *Magazine, Trade.* **Description:** Contains information and news for owners, developers and administrators of assisted-living facilities.
Formerly: Resident Life
Published by: Virgo Publishing, Inc., 3300 N Central Ave, Ste 2500, Phoenix, AZ 85012. TEL 480-990-1101, FAX 480-990-0819, alsuccess@vpico.com, virgopub@vpico.com, http://www.alsuccess.com, http://www.vpico.com. Pub. Troy Bix. Adv. contact Sherrie Orca. B&W page USD 4,455, color page USD 5,625; trim 8.125 x 10.875. Circ: 15,000.

362.1 AUS ISSN 0156-5788
AUSTRALIAN HEALTH REVIEW. Abbreviated title: A H R. Text in English. 1978. q. AUD 99 domestic; AUD 140 foreign (effective 2001). bk.rev. abstr. index. 220 p./no. back issues avail. *Refereed.* **Document type:** *Academic/Scholarly.* **Description:** Geared towards hospital administrators, medical and nursing directors and students.
Indexed: Aus.P.A.I.S., CINAHL, Excerp.Med., Hosp.Lit.Ind., Int.Nurs.Ind.
—BLDSC (1801.250000), CISTI, GNLM, Infotrieve, ingenta. **CCC.**
Published by: Australian Healthcare Association, PO Box 54, Deakin West, ACT 2600, Australia. TEL 61-2-62851488, FAX 61-2-62822395, admin@aha.asn.au, htp://www.aha.asn.au. Ed., R&P Don Hindle TEL 61-2-62851488. Adv. contact Elizabeth McMullan. Circ: 3,100.

AUSTRALIAN JOURNAL OF HOSPITAL PHARMACY. see *PHARMACY AND PHARMACOLOGY*

362 USA
B M C NEWS. Text in English. 1942. bi-m. free per issue. illus. back issues avail.
Published by: Baptist Medical Centers, PO Box 830605, Birmingham, AL 35283-0605. TEL 205-322-9300. Ed. Ann K Wetzel. Circ: 6,000.

362.11 USA
B N A'S HEALTH CARE DAILY REPORT (E-MAIL). Text in English. 1996. d. USD 1,651 (effective 2001). back issues avail. **Description:** Includes federal and state legislative and regulatory developments in health care policy as well as the activities of business, consumer, and special interest groups.
Formerly: B N A's Health Care Daily Report (Print) (1091-4021)
Media: E-mail. **Related titles:** Fax ed.; Online - full text ed.: (from Bureau of National Affairs, Inc., (BNA), The).
Published by: The Bureau of National Affairs, Inc., 1231 25th St, N W, Washington, DC 20037. TEL 202-452-4200, 800-372-1033, 800-452-7773, FAX 202-822-8092, customercare@bna.com, bnaplus@bna.com, http://www.bna.com/. Ed. Paul Albergo. Pub. Gregory McCaffery.

362.11 USA ISSN 1092-1079
KF3605.A15
B N A'S HEALTH CARE FRAUD REPORT. Text in English. 1997. bi-w. USD 869 (effective 2001). index. 40 p./no. back issues avail. **Description:** Covers health care fraud and abuse issues in the private insurance industry, managed care organizations, and federal health care programs.
Related titles: Online - full text ed.: ISSN 1521-9755 (from LexisNexis, Bureau of National Affairs, Inc., (BNA), The).
—**CCC.**
Published by: The Bureau of National Affairs, Inc., 1231 25th St, N W, Washington, DC 20037. TEL 202-452-4200, 800-372-1033, 800-452-7773, FAX 202-822-8092, customercare@bna.com, bnaplus@bna.com, http://www.bna.com/. Pub. Gregory McCaffery.

362.11 340.5 USA ISSN 1087-7185
KF3821.A73
B N A'S HEALTH LAW & BUSINESS SERIES. Text in English. 1996. m. USD 1,636 per issue (effective 2001); price varies. back issues avail. **Description:** Provides authoritative, in-depth analysis of important legal issues affecting the health care industry.
Related titles: CD-ROM ed.
—**CCC.**
Published by: The Bureau of National Affairs, Inc., 1231 25th St, N W, Washington, DC 20037. TEL 202-452-4200, 800-372-1033, 800-452-7773, FAX 202-822-8092, llempert@bna.com, customercare@bna.com, bnaplus@bna.com, http://www.bna.com. Ed. Larry Lempert. Pub. Gregory McCaffery. R&P Judith Miller TEL 202-452-4471.

362.11 GBR ISSN 1470-2282
▼ **BARTS AND THE LONDON CHRONICLE.** Short title: B L C. Text in English. 1999 (Apr.). s-a. free to members. adv. **Document type:** *Academic/Scholarly.* **Description:** Offers continuing contact with, and education of, alumni of St. Batholomew's and the Royal London School of Medicine and Dentistry, and it's predecessor colleges, through scholarly articles, news, comment and correspondence.
Formed by the merger of (1894-1999): London Hospital Gazette (0024-6050); (1977-1999): Bart's Journal (0264-8040); Which was formerly (1893-1977): St. Bartholomew's Hospital Journal (0036-2778)
Published by: Barts and The London Alumni Association, Alumni Office, Queen Mary and Westfield College, University of London, London E1 4NS, United Kingdom. TEL 44-20-7882-3732, FAX 44-20-7882-3706, alumni@qmw.ac.uk. Ed. Sue Boswell. adv.: B&W page GBP 350. Circ: 3,500.

362 USA
BAYLOR PROGRESS. Text in English. 1948. every 6 wks. free per issue. **Description:** For the employees, volunteers, medical staff and guests of Baylor Health Care System.

Published by: Baylor Health Care System, 3500 Gaston Ave, Dallas, TX 75246. TEL 214-820-2116. Ed. Melinda Matthews. Circ: 9,000.

362 GBR
BELL - U C M S M STUDENTS' MAGAZINE. Text in English. 1897. 3/yr. GBP 3. adv. bk.rev. charts, illus. index.
Formerly: Middlesex Hospital Journal (0026-3222)
Indexed: GeoRef.
Published by: University College and Middlesex School of Medicine, Cleveland St, London W1, United Kingdom. Circ: 1,500.

BENDER'S HEALTH CARE LAW MONTHLY. see *LAW*

658 USA ISSN 1085-0635
RA399.A1
BEST PRACTICES AND BENCHMARKING IN HEALTHCARE; a practical journal for clinical and management applications. Text in English. 1996. bi-m. USD 65 to individuals; USD 128 to institutions (effective 2000); USD 13 newsstand/cover. adv. Supplement avail.; reprints avail. **Document type:** *Trade.* **Description:** A practical guide to organizing and conducting best practice programs in the health care setting.
—GNLM, Infotrieve. **CCC.**
Published by: Mosby, Inc. (Subsidiary of: Elsevier Science), 11830 Westline Industrial Dr, St Louis, MO 63146-3318. TEL 314-453-4300, 800-325-4177, FAX 314-872-9164, http://www.mosby.com/periodicals. Eds. James O Hepner, Dr. Walter F Ballinger. Adv. contact Gale Schlogl TEL 314-453-4337. B&W page USD 700, color page USD 1,420; trim 10.88 x 8.25. Circ: 3,000.

BEST PRACTICES FOR HEALTH-SYSTEM PHARMACY. see *PHARMACY AND PHARMACOLOGY*

610.7365 DEU
BLAETTER AUS DEM HENRIETTENSTIFT. Text in German. 1868. s-a. charts, illus, stat.
Published by: Henriettenstiftung Hannover, Marienstr 80, Hannover 30171, Germany. Ed. Wolfgang Helbig. Circ: 6,500.

658 DEU
BLAUE DATEI DER KRANKENHAUSLIEFERANTEN. Text in German. 1979. a. DEM 45 (effective 2000). adv. **Document type:** *Directory, Trade.*
Formerly: Blaue Datei der Krankenhauslieferanten mit Krankenhausverzeichnis
Published by: Baumann Fachverlag, E C Baumann Str 5, Kulmbach 95326, Germany. TEL 49-9221-949313, FAX 49-9221-949377. Ed. Jutta Lange. adv.: B&W page DEM 4,090, color page DEM 6,370; trim 260 x 175. Circ: 7,000.

BOMBAY HOSPITAL JOURNAL. see *MEDICAL SCIENCES*

362 GBR
BOUNTY HOSPITAL INFORMATION GUIDES. Text in English. 1989. a. adv. **Document type:** *Journal, Consumer.*
Published by: Bounty Publications Ltd., 3 Theobald Ct, Theobald St, Borehamwood, Herts WD6 4RN, United Kingdom. TEL 44-181-207-4040, FAX 44-181-207-6966.

658 613 USA ISSN 1076-5972
BRIEFINGS ON HOSPITAL SAFETY; the newsletter for hospital safety committees. Text in English. 1993. m. USD 237. **Document type:** *Newsletter.* **Description:** Covers safety management issues, including planning, regulations. Offers practical information on how to improve safety.
—CCC.
Published by: Opus Communications, PO Box 1168, Marblehead, MA 01945. TEL 781-639-1872, FAX 781-639-2982, customer_service@opuscomm.com, http://www.opuscomm.com.

658 USA ISSN 1054-6995
BRIEFINGS ON J C A H O. (Joint Commission on Accreditation of Healthcare Organizations) Text in English. 1990. m. USD 327 (effective 1998). bk.rev. index. back issues avail. **Document type:** *Newsletter.* **Description:** Covers issues and procedures in health care accreditation and compliance, quality improvement and related issues.
—CCC.
Published by: Opus Communications, PO Box 1168, Marblehead, MA 01945. TEL 781-639-1872, FAX 781-639-2982, customer_service@opuscomm.com, http://www.opuscomm.com. Ed. Ilene MacDonald.

362.11 USA ISSN 1098-0598
BRIEFINGS ON J C A H O - A A A H C: AMBULATORY CARE. (Joint Commission on Accreditation of Healthcare Organizations - Accreditation Association for Ambula) Variant title: Ambulatory Care. Text in English. 1996. m. USD 187 (effective 1999). adv. bk.rev. **Document type:** *Newsletter.* **Description:** Reports activities of both the JCAHO and AAAHC and illustrates exactly what to do to pass a survey and gain accreditation for organizations.
Formerly (until 1996): Briefings on Ambulatory Care Accrediation (1092-4655)
—CCC.
Published by: Opus Communications, PO Box 1168, Marblehead, MA 01945. TEL 781-639-1872, FAX 781-639-2982. Ed. Dan Landriqan. Pub. Suzanne Perney.

362 610 USA ISSN 1076-6014
BRIEFINGS ON LONG-TERM CARE REGULATIONS. Text in English. 1993. m. USD 197. **Document type:** *Newsletter.* **Description:** Covers news and developments affecting administrators of long-term care facilities, including regulations, reimbursement, management issues and clinical procedures.
Indexed: Ref.Zh.
—CCC.
Published by: Opus Communications, PO Box 1168, Marblehead, MA 01945. TEL 781-639-1872, FAX 781-639-2982, customer_service@opuscomm.com, http://www.opuscomm.com.

362 USA
THE BROOKDALE UNIVERSITY HOSPITAL AND MEDICAL CENTER HEALTHSCOPE. Text in English. 1972. q. free per issue. illus. **Description:** Contains news and information about Brookdale Hospital, physicians, services, and staff. Distributed internally and externally.
Former titles: Brookdale Hospital Medical Center News-Scope; Brookdale Hospital Medical Center News
Published by: The Brookdale University Hospital and Medical Center, One Brookdale Plaza, Brooklyn, NY 11212. TEL 718-240-5345. Ed. Kim C Flodin. R&P Eric Matza. Circ: 28,000.

362.1029 USA
BUYERS GUIDE FOR THE HEALTH CARE MARKET* ; a directory of products and service for health care institutions. Text in English. a. USD 14.95 (effective 1997). **Document type:** *Directory.* **Description:** Lists suppliers of all types of hospital supplies. Includes a list of the top group-purchasing organizations.
Former titles: Buyers Guide for the Health Care Industry; Buyers Guide for the Health Care Institutions
Published by: (American Hospital Association), American Hospital Publishing, Inc. (Subsidiary of: American Hospital Association Company), 1 N Franklin St, 27th Fl, Chicago, IL 60606-3421. TEL 312-440-6800, 800-621-6902, FAX 312-951-8491, http://www.aha.org. Circ: 76,700. **Subscr. to:** A H A Sevices Inc., PO Box 92683, Chicago, IL 92683. TEL 800-AHA-2626, FAX 312-422-4505.

658 JPN ISSN 0385-2377
BYOIN/HOSPITAL. Text in Japanese. 1949. m. JPY 31,200.
Indexed: INIS Atomind.
—CISTI, GNLM.
Published by: Igaku-Shoin Ltd., 5-24-3 Hongo, Bunkyo-ku, Tokyo 113-0033, Japan. TEL 81-3-3817-5719. Circ: 6,500.

BYOIN, CHIIKI SEISHIN IGAKU/JAPANESE JOURNAL OF HOSPITAL AND COMMUNITY PSYCHIATRY. see *MEDICAL SCIENCES—Psychiatry And Neurology*

658 JPN ISSN 0386-9571
BYOIN KANRI/HOSPITAL ADMINISTRATION. Text in Japanese; Summaries in English. 1964. q. JPY 5,200, USD 28. adv. back issues avail.
—CCC.
Published by: Japanese Society on Hospital Administration, c/o National Institute of Health Services Management, 23-1 Toyama, Shinjuku-ku, Tokyo 162, Japan. TEL 03-3203-5327, FAX 03-3203-6853. Circ: 1,300.

658 JPN ISSN 0385-3454
BYOIN KANRI KENKYUJO KIYO/NATIONAL INSTITUTE OF HOSPITAL ADMINISTRATION. BULLETIN. Text in Japanese. 1962. a. **Document type:** *Bulletin.*
Published by: Koseisho, Byoin Kanri Kenkyujo/Ministry of Health and Welfare, National Institute of Hospital Administration, 21-13, Toyama 1-chome, Shinjuku-ku, Tokyo 162, Japan.

658 JPN ISSN 0525-3268
RA971
BYOIN KANRI KENKYUJO NENPO/NATIONAL INSTITUTE OF HOSPITAL ADMINISTRATION. ANNUAL REPORT. Text in Japanese. 1961. a.
Published by: Koseisho, Byoin Kanri Kenkyujo/Ministry of Health and Welfare, National Institute of Hospital Administration, 21-13, Toyama 1-chome, Shinjuku-ku, Tokyo 162, Japan.

362 JPN ISSN 0408-0904
BYOIN YORAN/JAPANESE HOSPITAL DIRECTORY. Text in Japanese. 1952-1964; resumed 1989. irreg. JPY 15,000. **Document type:** *Directory.*
Published by: (Japan. Ministry of Health and Welfare), Igaku-Shoin Ltd., 5-24-3 Hongo, Bunkyo-ku, Tokyo 113-0033, Japan. TEL 81-3-3817-5600. Circ: 5,000.

H

362.11 DNK ISSN 0901-067X
C A S NYT. Text in Danish. 1979. q. free per issue. bk.rev. **Document type:** *Newsletter.*
Published by: Statens Seruminstitut, Centrale Afdeling for Sygehushygiejne, Artillerivej 5, Copenhagen S 2300, Denmark. TEL 32-68-32-68, FAX 32-68-38-77, TELEX 31316 SERUM DK, obj@ssi.dk. Ed. O B Jepsen. Circ: 5,000.

362.16 USA
C C C N. (California Community Care News) Text in English. 1965. m. USD 45 (effective 1999). adv. 24 p./no. 3 cols./p. **Document type:** *Trade.* **Description:** Covers regulations, new legislation; includes information concerning operation, licensure and maintenance of community residential care facilities serving the elderly, mentally ill and developmentally disabled in California.
Formerly (until 1969): C A R C H News (0163-2213)
Published by: C R C C, PO Box 163270, Sacramento, CA 95816-9270. TEL 916-455-0723. Ed. Charles W Skoien Jr. Circ: 5,000.

362.11 CAN ISSN 0822-8426
C H A C INFO/INFO A C C S. Text in English, French. 1983. q. membership. **Document type:** *Newsletter.*
Published by: Catholic Health Association of Canada, 1247 Kilborn Pl, Ottawa, ON K1H 6K9, Canada. TEL 613-731-7148, FAX 613-731-7797, chac@web.ca, http://www.chac.ca. Ed., Adv. contact Sylvie Deliencourt. Circ: 1,240 (controlled).

362.11 CAN ISSN 0226-5923
C H A C REVIEW. Text in English. 1958. 3/yr. CND 30, USD 50 (effective 2001). adv. bk.rev. **Document type:** *Academic/Scholarly.*
Former titles (until 1973): Catholic Hospital (0008-8099); C H A C Bulletin
Related titles: French ed.: Association Catholique Canadienne de la Sante. Revue. ISSN 0226-5931. 1980.
—CISTI. **CCC.**
Published by: Catholic Health Association of Canada, 1247 Kilborn Pl, Ottawa, ON K1H 6K9, Canada. TEL 613-731-7148, FAX 613-731-7797. Ed., Adv. contact Sylvie Deliencourt. Circ: 1,200.

362 USA ISSN 1093-3247
C O B R A ADVISORY. (Consolidated Omnibus Budget Reconciliation Act) Text in English. m. USD 192 to individuals; USD 19 newsstand/cover (effective 2002). **Document type:** *Newsletter, Trade.* **Description:** Dedicated to helping consultants, service providers, employers, and administrators stay current and ensure their COBRA compliance.
Published by: Aspen Publishers, Inc., 200 Orchard Ridge Dr, Ste 200, Gaithersburg, MD 20878. TEL 301-417-7500, 800-638-8437, FAX 301-695-7931, customer.service@aspenpubl.com, http://www.aspenpub.com. Ed. Roberta Casper Watson. **Dist. by:** Aspen Publishers Inc., Distribution Center, 7201 McKinney Circle, Frederick, MD 21701. TEL 301-698-7100, FAX 301-417-7550.

▼ **C O R HEALTHCARE MARKET STRATEGIST.** see *BUSINESS AND ECONOMICS—Marketing And Purchasing*

362 USA
C O R HEALTHCARE STAFFING TREND WATCH. Text in English. w. free (effective 2001). **Document type:** *Newsletter, Trade.* **Description:** Covers recruitment, deployment, retention, scheduling, and other mission-critical staffing issues.
Media: E-mail.
Published by: C O R Health, LLC, PO Box 50507, Santa Barbara, CA 93150. TEL 805-564-2177, FAX 805-564-2146, info@corhealth.com, http://www.corhealth.com.

362 025.04 USA
C O R HEALTHCARE STRATEGIST TREND WATCH. Text and summaries in English. w. free (effective 2001). **Document type:** *Newsletter, Trade.* **Description:** Summaries of strategy-related articles and Web site reviews.
Media: E-mail.
Published by: C O R Health, LLC, PO Box 50507, Santa Barbara, CA 93150. TEL 805-564-2177, FAX 805-564-2146, info@corhealth.com, http://www.corhealth.com.

650 FRA ISSN 0295-4591
CAHIERS HOSPITALIERS. Text in French. 1986. 11/yr. FRF 520 (effective 1997). adv. bk.rev. *Refereed.* **Document type:** *Newsletter.* **Description:** Analyses the laws and decrees relating to hospitals and gives hospital managers and staff all informations about their duties.
Published by: Imprimerie et Librairie Berger-Levrault, 5 rue Auguste Comte, Paris 75006, France. TEL 33-1-40467030, FAX 33-1-44071525. Ed., R&P Frederique Lancien. Adv. contact Francoise Lelouvier. Circ: 1,600 (paid).

CALIFORNIA JOURNAL OF HEALTH - SYSTEM PHARMACY. see *PHARMACY AND PHARMACOLOGY*

362.1 USA ISSN 0272-9164
CALIFORNIA STATE HEALTH PLAN. Text in English. 1980. a. USD 15. stat. **Document type:** *Government.* **Description:** Contains an overview of the health care industry in California, an assessment of the current financial condition of hospitals, and identification of health care issues facing the State over the long-term planning horizon.
Former titles (until 1955): California State Plan for Hospital and Health Center Construction (0098-9983); California State Plan for Hospitals and Related Health Facilities (0526-9288); California State Plan for Hospitals (0575-2221)
Indexed: Ind.Med. (coverage dropped).
Published by: Office of Statewide Health Planning and Development, 1600 Ninth St, Rm 440, Sacramento, CA 95814. TEL 916-654-2080, FAX 916-654-3138. Ed. Larry Meeks. Circ: 5,000.

362.1106 CAN ISSN 1202-9718
CANADIAN HEALTHCARE MANAGER. Text in English. 1993. bi-m. CND 59 (effective 2001). adv. **Document type:** *Magazine, Trade.* **Description:** Provides a forum for information and dialogue on current issues of interest to the healthcare industry.
Related titles: Online - full text ed.
Published by: Rogers Media Publishing Ltd, 777 Bay St, 6th Fl, Toronto, ON M5W 1A7, Canada. TEL 416-596-5000, FAX 416-596-5881, http://www.chmonline.ca, http://www.rogers.com. Ed. Don Bisch. Adv. contact Francesca Gibson.

CANADIAN JOURNAL OF HOSPITAL PHARMACY. see *PHARMACY AND PHARMACOLOGY*

362.15 CAN ISSN 0847-5520
CANADIAN NURSING HOME. Text in English. 1985. q. CND 18, USD 20 (effective 1997). **Document type:** *Trade.*
Formerly (until 1989): Ontario Nursing Home Journal (0829-6340)
Indexed: CINAHL.
—BLDSC (3043.118000). **CCC.**
Published by: Health Media Inc., 14453 29A Ave, White Rock, BC V4A 9K8, Canada. TEL 604-535-7933, FAX 604-535-9000. Ed. Frank Fagan. Circ: 4,000.

CAPITATION MANAGEMENT REPORT. see *PUBLIC HEALTH AND SAFETY*

CAPITATION RATES AND DATA. see *PUBLIC HEALTH AND SAFETY*

362.12 USA
CARDIOLOGY PRACTICE ADVISOR. Text in English. m. USD 169 (effective 2001). **Document type:** *Newsletter, Trade.* **Description:** Provides practical, how-to ideas, information and advice specifically for cardiology practices that help improve practice efficiency, productivity and profitability, all while delivering superior patient care.
Published by: Advisory Publications, 15 E Ridge Pike, Ste 510, Conshohocken, PA 19428. TEL 888-941-4488, FAX 610-941-4499, info@smartpracticemanagement.com, http://www.smartpracticemanagement.com/cgi-bin/order/cardio.html.

362.12 USA ISSN 1526-4114
▼ **CARING FOR THE AGES.** Text in English. 2000. m., latest 2000. USD 109 domestic to individuals; USD 160 foreign to individuals; USD 165 domestic to institutions; USD 212 foreign to institutions; USD 17 newsstand/cover (effective 2002). **Document type:** *Newspaper, Academic/Scholarly, Trade.* **Description:** Monthly newspaper covering important clinical, policy, research, and other professional news relevant to members of the long-term care team. Features such topics as risk management, infection control, and palliation; strategies for improving quality of care and systems management; and articles by opinion leaders on the critical issues confronting long-term care today.
Published by: (American Medical Directors Association), Lippincott Williams & Wilkins (Philadelphia) (Subsidiary of: Wolters Kluwer N.V.), 530 Walnut St, Philadelphia, PA 19106-3621. TEL 215-521-8300, FAX 215-521-8902, Caring@lww.com, custserv@lww.com, http://www.caringfortheages.com, http://www.lww.com/. Ed. Dr. Dan Osterweil. Circ: 47,000. **Subscr. to:** PO Box 1600, Hagerstown, MD 21740-1600. TEL 800-638-3030, FAX 310-223-2400.

362 USA ISSN 0008-8684
CEDARS - SINAI MEDICAL CENTER COMPASS. Variant title: Cedars-Sinai Compass. Text in English. 1957. q. free per issue. charts, illus.
Supersedes (in 1962): Cedars of Lebanon Compass
Published by: Cedars - Sinai Medical Center, Public Relations Department, 8700 Beverly Blvd, Box 48750, Los Angeles, CA 90048. TEL 310-855-4767, FAX 310-657-9614. Ed. Jorian Clair. Circ: 14,000.

658 ESP ISSN 1132-8916
CENTRO DE SALUD. Text in Spanish. 1993. m. **Document type:** *Academic/Scholarly, Trade.* **Description:** Covers various aspects of managing a health center.
Published by: Saned S.A., Capitan Haya, 60, Madrid 28020, Spain. TEL 34-91-749-9507, FAX 34-91-749-9507, saned@meditex.es. Ed. Asuncion Colomer Rosas. adv.: page ESP 240,000. Circ: 10,000.

CHESHIRE SMILE INTERNATIONAL. see *HANDICAPPED—Physically Impaired*

630 USA
▼ **CHICAGO CAREGIVER.** Text in English. 2001. bi-m.
Published by: ComCare Net Inc., 601 Skokie Blvd, 306, Northbrook, IL 60062. TEL 847-480-9400, FAX 847-564-7770, http://www.chicagocaregiver.com/.

CHILDREN'S HOSPICE INTERNATIONAL NEWSLETTER. see *MEDICAL SCIENCES—Pediatrics*

CHUBU BYOIN IGAKU ZASSHI/OKINAWA CHUBU HOSPITAL. BULLETIN. see *MEDICAL SCIENCES*

658 JPN ISSN 0389-4894
CHUSEI SOGO BYOIN ZASSHI/CHUSEI GENERAL HOSPITAL. JOURNAL. Text in Japanese. 1978. biennial.
Published by: Chusei Sogo Byoin, 28-30 Kanbe 8-chome, Suzuka-shi, Mie-ken 513-0801, Japan.

CLINICAL ENGINEERING SECTION NEWSLETTER. see *INSTRUMENTS*

362 GBR ISSN 1470-9023
▼ **CLINICAL GOVERNANCE BULLETIN.** Text in English. 2000. bi-m. GBP 32 in Europe to individuals; USD 56 in United States to individuals; GBP 35 elsewhere to individuals; GBP 55 in Europe to institutions; USD 94 in United States to institutions; GBP 58 elsewhere to institutions (effective 2002). back issues avail. **Document type:** *Bulletin, Journal, Academic/Scholarly.* **Description:** Focuses on a broad range of issues in health management such as risk management, clinical effectiveness, managing resources, and improving communication.
Related titles: Online - full content ed.
Published by: Royal Society of Medicine Press Ltd, 1 Wimpole St, London W1M 8AE, United Kingdom. TEL 44-20-7290-2921, FAX 44-20-7290-2929, elizabeth.fredman@rsm.ac.uk, http://www.roysocmed.ac.uk/pub/cgb.htm. Eds. Gabriel Scally, Myriam Lugon.

CLINICAL LABORATORY PRODUCT COMPARISON SYSTEM. see *MEDICAL SCIENCES—Experimental Medicine, Laboratory Technique*

THE CLINICIAN IN MANAGEMENT. see *MEDICAL SCIENCES*

658 AUT
CLINICUM; das Magazin fuer die Fuehrungskraefte im Krankenhaus. Text and summaries in German. 1990. 10/yr. ATS 410; ATS 420 foreign (effective 2000). adv. bk.rev. illus. **Document type:** *Magazine, Trade.* **Description:** Contains news, reviews and articles in the field of biotechnology, genetics, microbiology, anesthesiology, cardiac diseases, gastroenterology, oncology and internal medicine.
Published by: Manstein Verlag GmbH, Brunner Feldstrasse 45, Perchtoldsdorf, N 2380, Austria. TEL 43-1-86648-0, FAX 43-1-86648-34. Ed. Dr. Birgit Beermann. R&P Thomas Zembacher TEL 43-1-5037166-210. Adv. contact Reinhard Rosenberger. B&W page ATS 29,500, color page ATS 39,400; trim 185 x 247. Circ: 17,500.

642.59 USA ISSN 0742-9800
CODING CLINIC FOR ICD-9-CM. Text in English. 1984. q. USD 210 to non-members; USD 145 to members (effective 2000). back issues avail. **Document type:** *Newsletter.* **Description:** Coding information and advice to assist in improving the quality of ICD-9-CM coding, especially for use in hospital prospective pricing, utilization management, and quality assurance programs.
Published by: American Hospital Association, One North Franklin, Chicago, IL 60606-3421. TEL 312-422-3395, FAX 312-422-4583. Ed. Donna Pickett. Circ: 5,000.

362.11 362.23 362.1 ITA ISSN 1120-639X
COLLETTIVITA - CONVIVENZE. Text in Italian. 1962. 6/yr. ITL 115,000 domestic; ITL 160,000 in Europe. adv. **Document type:** *Trade.* **Description:** For stewards, superintendents, managers of institutes, colleges, boarding schools, national health offices, hospitals, and nursing homes.
Address: Via Alessandro Pestalozza, 31, Milan, MI 20131, Italy. TEL 39-02-7063-0022, FAX 39-02-2668-0516. Ed. Luigi Porro. Circ: 19,000.

658 USA ISSN 1063-1720
COMPARATIVE PERFORMANCE OF U.S. HOSPITALS: THE SOURCEBOOK. Text in English. 1992. a. USD 399. **Description:** Features more than 160 hospital comparison groups, including analysis by state, bond rating, system affiliation, ownership and bed size. Information tables and explanatory analyses cover the 52 most important measures of hospital performance, including occupancy rates, profit margins, staffing levels, and debt service coverage ratios.
Related titles: CD-ROM ed.; Diskette ed.
Published by: H C I A Inc., 300 E Lombard St, Baltimore, MD 21202. TEL 800-568-3282, FAX 410-547-8297. **Co-publisher:** Deloitte & Touche.

COMPETITIVE HEALTHCARE MARKET REPORTER. see *BUSINESS AND ECONOMICS—Marketing And Purchasing*

362 ITA ISSN 0589-3267
CONGRESSO EUROPEO DI STORIA OSPITALIERA. ATTI. Text in Italian. 1960. irreg., latest vol.15. ITL 34,000; ITL 42,000 foreign. **Document type:** *Proceedings.*
Published by: Centro Italiano di Storia Sanitaria e Ospitaliera, Biblioteca, Viale Risorgimento, 30, Reggio Emilia, RE 42100, Italy. TEL 0522-24252.

658 632.15 USA
CONNECTIONS (LARGO). Text in English. 1991. 3/yr. free per issue. **Document type:** *Newsletter.* **Description:** Informs professionals on medical, psychosocial and administrative issues related to terminal illness and hospice care.
Published by: Hospice of the Florida Suncoast, 300 E Bay Dr, Largo, FL 34640. TEL 813-586-4432, FAX 813-586-5213. Ed. Karen Cunningham. Circ: 5,000.

CONSUMERS' GUIDE TO HOSPITALS. see *CONSUMER EDUCATION AND PROTECTION*

658 USA ISSN 1521-3447
CONTEMPORARY LONG-TERM CARE PAYMENT AND REGULATORY ALERT. Text in English. 1988. bi-w. USD 297 domestic; USD 307 foreign (effective 2000). **Document type:** *Newsletter.* **Description:** For administrators, financial executives and owners of nursing facilities, residential care centers, and hospitals with long-term care. Provides current news on US national, state and private pay medical reimbursement policies for the chronically ill.
Formerly: Contemporary Long-Term Care Reimbursement Bulletin
—CCC.

Published by: Harling Communications, Inc., 18 2 E Dundee Rd, Ste 200, Barrington, IL 60010. TEL 847-304-1011, FAX 847-304-1035, postacute@aol.com. Ed. Karen Lusky. Pub., R&P Mark Harling TEL 516-379-7097.

658 USA ISSN 8750-9652
CONTEMPORARY LONGTERM CARE. Text in English. 1978. m. free to qualified personnel. adv. bk.rev. **Document type:** *Journal, Trade.* **Description:** For administrators, directors of nursing, medical directors, pharmacists and other professionals responsible for management and patient care at nursing facilities, residential care centers, and hospitals with long-term care.
Former titles (until 1984): Contemporary Administrator for Long-Term Care (8750-9652); Contemporary Administrator (0191-9873)
Related titles: Online - full text ed.: (from Northern Light Technology, Inc., ProQuest Information & Learning, Gale Group).
Indexed: AgeLine, I.P.A., Int.Nurs.Ind.
—BLDSC (3425.191100), CISTI, Infotrieve. **CCC.**
Published by: Bill Communications, Inc. (Subsidiary of: V N U Tijdschriften), 770 Broadway, New York, NY 10003-9595. TEL 646-654-7540, FAX 646-654-7548, http://www.cltcmag.com, http://www.billcom.com/. Ed. Mark Zacharia TEL 646-654-7545. Adv. contact Margarita Serrano. Circ: 39,000.

658 360 USA ISSN 1057-428X
CONTINUING CARE; supporting the transition into post hospital care. Text in English. 1982. m. USD 99; subscr. includes a. Buyer's Guide. adv. bk.rev. charts, illus, tr.lit. index. back issues avail. **Document type:** *Trade.* **Description:** Provides case management and discharge planning professionals with practical and professional information to ensure quality patient services at a cost-effective price.
Former titles: Continuing Care Coordinator; Coordinator (Los Angeles)
Related titles: Online - full text ed.
Indexed: AgeLine, I.P.A.
—Infotrieve. **CCC.**
Published by: Stevens Publishing Corporation, 5151 Beltline Rd, 10th fl, Dallas, TX 75240. TEL 972-687-6700, FAX 972-687-6770. Ed. Kyle Steinhauser. Pub. Dana Corbin. Adv. contact Randy Dye. Circ: 23,000.

CONTINUING CARE NEWS. see *INSURANCE*

362 USA ISSN 1082-8419
CONTINUUM (CHICAGO); an interdisciplinary journal on continuity of care. Text in English. 1980. bi-m. USD 86 to non-members; USD 66 to members (effective 1999). bk.rev. back issues avail. *Refereed.* **Document type:** *Academic/Scholarly.* **Description:** Takes a multidisciplinary approach to the hospital discharge planning process and the delivery of posthospital care.
Formerly (until Mar. 1995): Discharge Planning Update (0276-4652)
Indexed: CINAHL, Hosp.Lit.Ind.
—BLDSC (3425.719100).
Published by: American Hospital Association, Society for Social Work Leadership in Health Care, 1 N Franklin, 31st Fl, Chicago, IL 60606. TEL 312-445-3999, FAX 312-422-4586, salvinija@aol.com. Ed. Salvinija Kernaghan. R&P Jackie Brody. Circ: 1,000. **Subscr. to:** American Hospital Publishing Inc., PO Box 92567, Chicago, IL 60675.

657.832 616.1 USA ISSN 1087-0644
COST MANAGEMENT IN CARDIAC CARE. Text in English. 1996. m. USD 429; USD 377 foreign (effective 1999). **Document type:** *Newsletter.*
Indexed: CINAHL.
—BLDSC (3477.241500).
Published by: American Health Consultants (Subsidiary of: Medical Economics Co., Inc.), 3525 Piedmont Rd, N E, 6 Piedmont Center, Ste 400, Atlanta, GA 30305. TEL 404-262-5476, custserv@ahcpub.com, http://www.ahcpub.com.

658 610 USA ISSN 1069-482X
D R G HANDBOOK; comparative clinical and financial standards. (Diagnosis Related Group) Text in English. 1992. a. USD 399 (effective 1999). **Description:** Compiles data based on 20 million patients and focuses on clinical and financial measures for 50 highest volume DRGs.
Formerly: Medicare D R G Handbook
Published by: H C I A Inc., 300 E Lombard St, Baltimore, MD 21202. TEL 800-568-3282, FAX 410-752-6309. **Co-publisher:** Ernst & Young.

658 JPN
DAIDO BYOIN NENPO/DAIDO HOSPITAL. ANNUAL REPORT. Text in Japanese. 1982. a.
Published by: Kojunkai Daido Byoin/Kojunkai Daido Hospital, 9 Haku-Sui-cho, Minami-ku, Nagoya-shi, Aichi-ken 457-0818, Japan.

DATA STRATEGIES AND BENCHMARKS. see *PUBLIC HEALTH AND SAFETY*

610 DEU ISSN 0344-3167
DEUTSCHE KRANKENHAUS-GESELLSCHAFT. GESCHAEFTSBERICHT. Text in German. biennial. free per issue.
Former titles (until 1975): Deutsche Krankenhausgesellschaft. Jahresbericht (0344-3159); (until 1967): Deutschen Krankenhausgesellschaft. Geschaeftsbericht (0344-3140)
—GNLM.
Published by: Deutsche Krankenhaus-Gesellschaft, Tersteegenstr 9, Duesseldorf 40474, Germany.

658 DEU ISSN 0420-2066
DEUTSCHES KRANKENHAUS ADRESSBUCH. Text in German. 1962. a. DEM 119 (effective 2000). adv. index. **Document type:** *Directory.* **Description:** Brief editorials, mainly hospital addresses for Germany, Austria and Switzerland; includes supplier's register.
—GNLM.
Published by: Rombach GmbH Verlagshaus, Loerracher Str 3, Freiburg Im Breisgau 79115, Germany. TEL 49-761-45002135, FAX 49-761-4500400. Circ: 11,000.

658 MEX
DICCIONARIO DE TECNOLOGIA E INSUMOS MEDICOS. Text in Spanish. 1991. a.
Published by: Ediciones P L M S.A. de C.V., San BERNADINO 17, Col del Valle, Mexico City, DF 03100, Mexico. TEL 687-1766, FAX 536-5027. Ed. Dr. Jose Luis Gonzalez. Circ: 2,000.

658 USA
DIRECTIONS (COLUMBUS); the technical journal for health care material management. Text in English. 1986. s-a. membership. **Description:** Covers warehousing, purchasing, sterilization and re-use, and inventory control.
Published by: Health Care Material Management Society, 99 E Weber Rd, Columbus, OH 43202. TEL 614-263-5927. Ed. S Anne Sostrom. Circ: 1,400.

362.1 MEX
▼ **DIRECTORIO DE CONSULTORIOS.** Text in Spanish. 2000. irreg., latest vol.1, 2000. USD 290 (effective 2001). **Document type:** *Directory.* **Description:** Lists 6,029 physicians' offices in Mexico City, including name, specialty, address, phones, fax and email.
Published by: Ibcon S.A., Gutemberg 224, Col Anzures, Mexico City, DF 11590, Mexico. TEL 52-5-2554577, FAX 52-5-2554577, ibcon@infosel.net.mx, http://www.incon.com.mx. Ed. Gabriel Zaid.

DIRECTORIO DE PROVEEDORES DE LA SALUD. see *BUSINESS AND ECONOMICS—Trade And Industrial Directories*

614.88 616.02 GBR
DIRECTORY OF EMERGENCY AND SPECIAL CARE UNITS (YEAR). Text in English. a. GBP 80 (effective 1999). adv. **Document type:** *Directory.* **Description:** Contains detailed information on emergency and special care units and services throughout the British Isles.
Published by: C M A Medical Data, Cambridge Research Laboratories, 181A Huntingdon Rd, Cambridge CB3 0DJ, United Kingdom. TEL 44-1223-277709, FAX 44-1223-276444. Ed., Pub. Ruth Allan. R&P David Roberts. Adv. contact Myles Davidson.

610 USA
DIRECTORY OF FEDERAL HEALTH CARE FACILITIES. Text in English. a. adv. **Document type:** *Directory.*
Formerly: V A Medical Center Directory
Related titles: ♦ Supplement to: Federal Practitioner. ISSN 1078-4497.
Published by: Quadrant HealthCom, 26 Main St, Ste A, Chatham, NJ 07928-2402. TEL 973-701-8900, FAX 973-701-8892. Pub. Peter Deyoe. Adv. contact Denise Andrade.

DIRECTORY OF HEALTH CARE PROFESSIONALS. see *BUSINESS AND ECONOMICS—Trade And Industrial Directories*

362.175 GBR ISSN 1353-856X
DIRECTORY OF HOSPICE AND PALLIATIVE CARE SERVICES. Text in English. a. **Document type:** *Directory.*
Formerly (until 1994): Directory of Hospice Services in the U K and Republic of Ireland (0965-1462)
Related titles: Online - full content ed.
—BLDSC (3593.938000).
Published by: Hospice Information Service, St. Christopher's Hospice, 51-59 Lawrie Park Rd, London SE26 6DZ, United Kingdom. TEL 44-20-8778-9252, FAX 44-20-8778-9345, info@his2.freeserve.co.uk, http://www.hospiceinformation.co.uk. Eds. Ann Eve, Avril Jackson. Adv. contact Avril Jackson. Circ: 8,000.

H

658 GBR
DIRECTORY OF HOSPITAL & HEALTH SERVICE ADDRESSES (YEAR). Text in English. a. GBP 35 (effective 1999). adv. **Document type:** *Directory.*
Published by: C M A Medical Data, Cambridge Research Laboratories, 181A Huntingdon Rd, Cambridge CB3 0DJ, United Kingdom. TEL 44-1223-277709, FAX 44-1223-276444. Ed., Pub. Ruth Allan. R&P David Roberts. Adv. contact Myles Davidson.

658 GBR
DIRECTORY OF HOSPITAL MANAGEMENT SUPPLIES & SERVICES (YEAR). Text in English. a. GBP 75 (effective 1999). adv. **Document type:** *Directory.* **Description:** Provides contact details by name, department, job title and addresses for all health authorities and trusts. Also contains names, telephone numbers, and numbers of beds for all hospitals within each trust.
Published by: C M A Medical Data, Cambridge Research Laboratories, 181A Huntingdon Rd, Cambridge CB3 0DJ, United Kingdom. TEL 44-1223-277709, FAX 44-1223-276444. Ed., Pub. Ruth Allan. R&P David Roberts. Adv. contact Myles Davidson.

DIRECTORY OF HOSPITAL PERSONNEL. see *BUSINESS AND ECONOMICS—Trade And Industrial Directories*

658 GBR
DIRECTORY OF HOSPITAL TELEPHONE NUMBERS (YEAR). Text in English. 1991. a. GBP 25 (effective 1999). adv. **Document type:** *Directory.* **Description:** Contains more than 2,000 telephone numbers covering all N.H.S. and independent hospitals. The hospitals are listed alphabetically and include the name of the town and the regional Health Authority in which the hospital is located.
Published by: C M A Medical Data, Cambridge Research Laboratories, 181A Huntingdon Rd, Cambridge CB3 0DJ, United Kingdom. TEL 44-1223-277709, FAX 44-1223-276444. Ed., Pub. Ruth Allan. R&P David Roberts. Adv. contact Myles Davidson.

DIRECTORY OF HOSPITALS AND TRUSTS (YEAR). see *BUSINESS AND ECONOMICS—Trade And Industrial Directories*

610 GBR ISSN 0951-0516
DIRECTORY OF INDEPENDENT HOSPITALS AND HEALTH SERVICES; a comprehensive guide to the independent health care sector in the U.K. Text in English. a. GBP 95 (effective 1998). adv. **Document type:** *Directory.* **Description:** Provides a comprehensive guide to independent health care within the UK. Gives listings of relevant organisations, addresses and key contact names in both the acute and long-term sector.
Formerly: Directory of Private Hospitals and Health Services (0260-8820)
—GNLM.
Published by: Financial Times Healthcare, Maple House, 149 Tottenham Ct Rd, London W1P 9LL, United Kingdom. TEL 44-207-896-2066, FAX 44-20-7896-2213, lizg@pearson-pro.com, http://www.fthealthcare.com. Adv. contact Liz Godden. Circ: 3,250.

658 371.42 AUS ISSN 0157-2784
DIRECTORY OF INTERNSHIPS, RESIDENCIES AND REGISTRARSHIPS AVAILABLE IN VICTORIAN HOSPITALS. Text in English. 1967. a. AUD 17 (effective 1999). **Document type:** *Directory.*
—**CCC.**
Published by: Victorian Medical Postgraduate Foundation Inc., PO Box 27, Parkville, VIC 3052, Australia. TEL 61-3-9347-9633, FAX 61-3-9347-4547, vmpf@vicnet.net.au. Ed. P Wilton. Circ: 900.

617 GBR
DIRECTORY OF OPERATING THEATRES AND DEPARTMENTS OF SURGERY (YEAR). Text in English. a. GBP 80 (effective 1999). adv. **Description:** Contains detailed information on operating theatres and Departments of Surgery in NHS and independent hospitals throughout the U.K.
Published by: C M A Medical Data, Cambridge Research Laboratories, 181A Huntingdon Rd, Cambridge CB3 0DJ, United Kingdom. TEL 44-1223-277709, FAX 44-1223-276444. Ed., Pub. Ruth Allan. R&P David Roberts. Adv. contact Myles Davidson.

362.1 USA
RA977
DIRECTORY OF PRIVATELY-OWNED: COMMUNITY HOSPITALS, HOSPITAL MANAGEMENT COMPANIES AND HEALTH SYSTEMS, RESIDENTIAL TREATMENT FACILITIES AND CENTERS, AND KEY MANAGEMENT PERSONNEL. Text in English. a., latest 2001. USD 125 to non-members; USD 85 to members (effective 2001). adv. 260 p./no. back issues avail. **Document type:** *Directory.*
Former titles: Directory of Investor-Owned Hospitals, Hospital Management Companies and Health Systems, Residential Treatment Facilities and Centers, and Key Management Personnel; Directory of Investor-Owned Hospitals, Residential Treatment Facilities and Centers, Hospital Management Companies and Health Systems (1059-7220); Directory of Investor-Owned Hospitals, Hospital Management Companies and Health Systems; Directory of Investor-Owned Hospitals and Hospital Management Companies (0095-5191)
Related titles: Diskette ed.
Published by: F A H, Inc., 1405 N Pierce St, Ste 311, Little Rock, AR 72207. TEL 501-661-9555, FAX 501-663-4903, http://www.americanhospitals.com. R&P Julie Cawthron. Adv. contact Pearl Jones.

DIRECTORY OF RETIREMENT FACILITIES. see *GERONTOLOGY AND GERIATRICS*

658 614.8 ITA ISSN 0416-024X
DIRITTO SANITARIO MODERNO. Text in Italian. q. USD 100 (effective 2002). **Document type:** *Journal, Academic/Scholarly.*
Published by: Edizioni Luigi Pozzi s.r.l., Via Panama, 68, Rome, RM 00198, Italy. TEL 39-06-8553548, FAX 39-06-8554105, edizioni_pozzi@tin.it. Ed. B Primicerio.

DISEASE MANAGEMENT ADVISOR. see *PUBLIC HEALTH AND SAFETY*

DOAI IGAKU ZASSHI/FRATERNITY MEMORIAL HOSPITAL. MEDICAL JOURNAL. see *MEDICAL SCIENCES*

658 USA
DOME (BALTIMORE). Text in English. q. adv. **Document type:** *Newsletter.* **Description:** Covers news of the renowned medical institution.
Published by: Johns Hopkins Medical Institution, 550 N Broadway, Baltimore, MD 21205-2011. Ed., R&P Mary Ellen Miller. Adv. contact Edith Nichols.

658 USA ISSN 0882-5807
ECONOMIC TRENDS (CHICAGO). Text in English. 1985. q. USD 135 to non-members; USD 85 to members. reprint service avail. from SCH. **Document type:** *Newsletter.* **Description:** Data on and analysis of US hospital finances, utilization, and staffing trends.
Published by: American Hospital Association, One North Franklin, Chicago, IL 60606-3421. TEL 312-422-3527, FAX 312-422-4651. Ed. Mary Gallivan. Circ: 1,000.

362 ECU ISSN 0070-8895
ECUADOR. INSTITUTO NACIONAL DE ESTADISTICA Y CENSOS. ANUARIO DE ESTADISTICAS HOSPITALARIAS. Text in Spanish. 1957. a. USD 22 (effective 2001). stat. **Document type:** *Government.*
Related titles: Diskette ed.; E-mail ed.
Published by: Instituto Nacional de Estadistica y Censos, Juan Larrea N15-36 y Jose Riofrio, Quito, Ecuador. TEL 593-2-529858, FAX 593-2-509836, inec1@ecnet.ec, http://www.inec.gov.ec. Circ: 300.

ECUADOR. INSTITUTO NACIONAL DE ESTADISTICA Y CENSOS. CUENTAS NACIONALES DE LA SALUD. see *BUSINESS AND ECONOMICS—Public Finance, Taxation*

658 HUN ISSN 0013-2276
EGESZSEGUGYI GAZDASAGI SZEMLE; health care management review. Text in Hungarian; Summaries in English, German. 1963. bi-m. HUF 1,200; USD 30 foreign (effective 2000). adv. bk.rev. *Refereed.* **Document type:** *Academic/Scholarly.* **Description:** Covers managerial information for health institutions. Includes health care policy, management, economics, information science, human resources, marketing, law and bioethics, quality assurance.
Indexed: Excerp.Med., Hosp.Abstr.
—GNLM.
Published by: (Hungary. Egeszsegugyi Miniszterium/Ministry of Health), Egeszsegugyi Gazdasagi Vezetok Egyesulete, PO Box 987, Budapest 1245, Hungary. TEL 36-1-3323100, FAX 36-1-3534955. Ed. Ervin Kovesi. Pub. Janos Nemes. Adv. contact Zsuzsanna Szappanos. Circ: 500 (paid).

362 USA ISSN 1526-0593
▼ **EHEALTHCARE STRATEGY & TRENDS.** Text in English. 1999. m. USD 237 domestic; USD 247 in Canada & Mexico; USD 262 elsewhere (effective 2000). bk.rev., Website rev. back issues avail. **Document type:** *Trade.* **Description:** Aims to helping healthcare professionals get the most out of their websites and the Internet. Covers what leading-edge hospitals, managed care companies and physician practices are doing.
Published by: Health Care Communications, 11 Heritage Lane, Box 594, Rye, NY 10580. TEL 914-967-6741, FAX 914-967-3054, healthcomm@aol.com, http://www.strategichealthcare.com. Ed. Mark S Gothberg. Pub. Michele von Dambrowski.

ELDERLY HEALTH SERVICES LETTER. see *GERONTOLOGY AND GERIATRICS*

EMERGENCY DEPARTMENT MANAGEMENT. see *MEDICAL SCIENCES—Orthopedics And Traumatology*

362 CAN
ENSEMBLE (MONTREAL). Text in English. 1960. bi-m. bk.rev. illus. **Document type:** *Newsletter.*
Former titles (until 1995): Generally Speaking; Montreal General Hospital News (0027-0709)
Indexed: Inpharma, Reac.
—CCC.
Published by: Montreal General Hospital, Rm E 6227, 1650 Cedar Ave, Montreal, PQ H3G 1A4, Canada. TEL 514-843-1560, FAX 514-934-8277. Ed. Diane McPeak. Circ: 4,500.

649 362.7 FRA
ETABLISSEMENTS MEDICAUX POUR ENFANTS. Text in French. bi-m.
Published by: Federation Francaise des Etablissements de Soins de Cure et de Prevention pour Enfants, 34 rue Bruneseau, Paris Cedex 13 75629, France. TEL 1-44-24-51-11, FAX 1-44-24-56-45. Ed. Fernand Bitterly. Circ: 3,500.

368.392 GBR
EUROPEAN HEALTHCARE MANAGEMENT; the journal for decision makers. Text in English. 1994. q.
Formerly: European Hospital Management (1357-0099)
—BLDSC (3829.717490).
Published by: Intensive Careworld Ltd, Ste 5, Chelsea Wharf, 15 Lots Rd, London SW10 0QJ, United Kingdom. TEL 44-20-7376-4040, FAX 44-20-7795-0219, ghcgltd@aol.com, http://www.ghcg.com. Ed. Belinda Roman. Pub. David R Campbell.

658 DEU ISSN 0942-9085
EUROPEAN HOSPITAL. Text in German. bi-m. EUR 55.22 for 2 yrs. (effective 2001). adv. **Document type:** *Journal, Trade.*
Published by: Beta Verlag und Marketinggesellschaft mbH, Postfach 140121, Bonn 53056, Germany. TEL 49-228-91937-0, FAX 49-228-252067, info@beta-publishing.com, http://www.beta-publishing.com. Ed. Brenda Marsh. R&P Heike Lange TEL 49-228-919370. Adv. contact Hubert Schulz. B&W page XEU 6,985, color page XEU 8,590; trim 265 x 380. Circ: 32,500.

658 GBR
EUROPEAN HOSPITAL DECISIONS. Text in English. a. adv. **Document type:** *Journal, Trade.* **Description:** Contains articles discussing technical problems and best practice solutions involving hospital management.
Published by: Cornhill Publications Ltd. (Subsidiary of: Sterling Publishing Group Plc.), Kings Ct, 2-16 Goodge St, London W1P 1FF, United Kingdom. TEL 44-207-240-1515, FAX 44-207-379-7371, info@cornhillpublications.com, http://www.cornhillpublications.com/titles/ehd.html. adv.: B&W page GBP 6,700, color page GBP 7,600; trim 210 x 286. Circ: 12,600 (controlled).

362.11029 GBR
THE EUROPEAN HOSPITALS DATABASE ON CD-ROM. Text in English. 1997. a. GBP 2,000. adv. **Description:** Contains contact details for European hospitals, departments, and senior health personnel in Europe.
Media: CD-ROM.
Published by: Financial Times Healthcare, Maple House, 149 Tottenham Ct Rd, London W1P 9LL, United Kingdom. TEL 44-207-896-2066, FAX 44-20-7896-2213, lizg@pearson-pro.com, http://www.fthealthcare.com. Adv. contact Liz Godden.

362 610 NLD ISSN 0920-2153
EUROPEAN NEWSLETTER ON QUALITY ASSURANCE. Text in Dutch. ceased 1993; resumed 1984. q. free per issue. bk.rev. back issues avail. **Document type:** *Newsletter.* **Description:** Supports QA activities in foreign countries through technical assistance and program development.
Published by: C B O/National Organization for Quality Assurance in Health Care, Postbus 20064, Utrecht 3502 LB, Netherlands. TEL 31-30-2960647, FAX 31-30-29436444, cbo@cbo.nl, http://www.cbo.nl. Circ: 3,400. **Co-sponsor:** W H O Collaborating Centre for Quality Assurance in Health Care.

EXCERPTA MEDICA. SECTION 36: HEALTH POLICY, ECONOMICS AND MANAGEMENT. see *HEALTH FACILITIES AND ADMINISTRATION—Abstracting, Bibliographies, Statistics*

EXECUTIVE HOUSEKEEPING TODAY. see *HOTELS AND RESTAURANTS*

368.382 USA ISSN 1068-4557
RA413.5.U5
EXECUTIVE MANAGED CARE DIRECTORY. Text in English. 1988. a. USD 120 (effective 2000). adv. **Document type:** *Directory.* **Description:** Provides comprehensive reference information on managed care suppliers and plans.
Related titles: ♦ Supplement to: Managed Care Interface. ISSN 1096-5645.
—CCC.
Published by: Medicom International, Inc., 66 Palmer Ave, Ste 49, Bronxville, NY 10708. TEL 914-337-7878, FAX 914-337-5023, medicomint@aol.com, http://www.Medicomint.com. Ed., R&P Stan Mehr. Pub. Bob Massa. Adv. contact Charlotte Walsh. B&W page USD 5,789, color page USD 7,715. Circ: 27,219.

362.11068 USA ISSN 1099-193X
EXECUTIVE SOLUTIONS ON HEALTH CARE MANAGEMENT. Text in English. 1994. m. USD 375 to individuals; USD 450 to institutions (effective 2000). **Document type:** *Newsletter.*
Formerly (1994-1998): Health System Leader (1075-1807)
Indexed: CINAHL, Int.Nurs.Ind.
—BLDSC (3836.223810).
Published by: Capitol Publications, Inc. (Subsidiary of: Aspen Publishers, Inc.), 1101 King St, Ste 444, Alexandria, VA 22314. TEL 703-683-4100, FAX 703-739-6501.

658 USA
EYE ON IMPROVEMENT✶ . Text in English. s-m. USD 90 in US & Canada; USD 100 elsewhere. *Refereed.* **Document type:** *Newsletter.* **Description:** Provides a quick, convenient, timely and comprehensive review of information about continual improvement in health care.
Published by: Institute for Healthcare Improvement, PO Box 26444, Prescott Valley, AZ 86312-6444. TEL 216-235-8580, FAX 216-235-2714. Ed. Dr. Donald M Berwick. R&P Connie Koran.

658 DEU ISSN 0175-4548
F & W - FUEHREN UND WIRTSCHAFTEN IM KRANKENHAUS. Text in German. 1984. bi-m. DEM 132, EUR 67.49; DEM 25, EUR 12.78 newsstand/cover (effective 2001). adv. bk.rev. index. **Document type:** *Journal, Academic/Scholarly.*
Indexed: Ref.Zh.
—GNLM.

Published by: Bibliomed - Medizinische Verlagsgesellschaft mbH, Postfach 1150, Melsungen 34201, Germany. TEL 49-5661-7344-0, FAX 49-5661-8360, info@bibliomed.de, http://www.bibliomed.de. Ed., Pub. Uta Meurer. Adv. contact Waltraud Zemke. Circ: 6,000.

355.72 USA
FACILITYCARE; design, operation and maintenance of healthcare facilities. Text in English. 1996. 6/yr. USD 55 in North America; USD 140 elsewhere; USD 10 newsstand/cover domestic; USD 13 newsstand/cover foreign (effective 2001). adv. software rev., Website rev. illus, tr.lit. 32 p./no. 4 cols./p. back issues avail. **Document type:** *Magazine, Trade.* **Description:** Provides information for healthcare facility managers on planning, designing, constructing, maintaining or operating a safe environment for employees, patients and visitors.
formerly: Facility Care (1090-7475)
Published by: Douglas Publications, Inc., 2807 N Parham Rd, Ste 200, Richmond, VA 23294. TEL 804-762-9600, 847-202-1577, FAX 804-217-8999, 847-202-1587, bhintch@douglaspublications.com, info@douglaspublications.com, http://www.facilitycare.com. Ed. Betty Hintch. Pub. Stephanie A Ellis TEL 847-202-1577. Adv. contact Russell Lindsay TEL 254-867-1011. B&W page USD 5,742, color page USD 6,942; trim 10 x 14.75. Circ: 32,000 (controlled). **Subscr. to:** Facility Care, P O Box 816, Winchester, MA 01890.

FAMILY PRACTICE MANAGEMENT. see *MEDICAL SCIENCES*

362.15 USA
FANFARE (PITTSBURGH). Text in English. q.?. bk.rev.
Published by: Hospice and Palliative Nurses Association, Medical Center East, Ste 375, 211 N Whitfield St, Pittsburgh, PA 15206-3031. TEL 412-361-2470, FAX 412-361-2425, hnafan@usa.pipeline.com, http://www.roxane.com/HNA. Ed. Suzanne Lego.

362.12 USA
FINANCIAL MANAGEMENT STRATEGIES FOR MEDICAL OFFICES. Text in English. m. USD 149 (effective 2001). **Document type:** *Newsletter, Trade.* **Description:** Contains ideas and information on how to better analyze, understand and react to financial reports, improve your financial controls and procedures, evaluate the profitability of managed care contracts more effectively, address big-picture issues like how to raise capital for expansion, and handle personnel and overhead more efficiently.
Published by: Advisory Publications, 15 E Ridge Pike, Ste 510, Conshohocken, PA 19428. TEL 888-941-4488, FAX 610-941-4499, info@smartpracticemanagement.com, http://www.smartpracticemanagement.com/cgi-bin/order/financial.html.

THE FITZHUGH DIRECTORY OF INDEPENDENT HEALTHCARE AND LONG TERM CARE. FINANCIAL INFORMATION. see *MEDICAL SCIENCES*

FLORIDA BAR. HEALTH LAW SECTION NEWSLETTER. see *LAW*

FLORIDA JOURNAL OF HEALTH-SYSTEM PHARMACY. see *PHARMACY AND PHARMACOLOGY*

355.72 387.7 AUS
FLYING DOCTOR QUEENSLAND. Text in English. 1976. 3/yr. AUD 5. adv. **Document type:** *Newsletter.*
Former titles: Queensland Flying Doctor; Flying Doctor Yearbook
Published by: Royal Flying Doctor Service of Australia, 12 Casuarina St., Brisbane, QLD 4007, Australia. TEL 61-7-38601100, FAX 61-7-38601122, penbrfds@bigpond.com. Ed. Stephen Penberthy. R&P, Adv. contact Janet England. Circ: 20,000.

658 GBR
FREE PRESS. Text in English. w. free per issue. **Description:** Contains organization news.
Published by: Royal Free Hospital Students Union, Clinical Sciences Building, Pond St, Hampstead, London NW3 2PE, United Kingdom. Ed. Leela Biant. Circ: 180.

613.194 USA ISSN 0748-8157
RA971
FRONTIERS OF HEALTH SERVICES MANAGEMENT. Text in English. 1984. a. USD 20 in US & Canada to individuals; USD 40 in US & Canada to institutions; USD 30 elsewhere to individuals; USD 50 elsewhere to institutions (effective 2000). illus. reprint service avail. from PQC. **Document type:** *Trade.* **Description:** Focuses on directions in health services management and policy. Each issue examines a single topic in depth.
Related titles: Microform ed.: (from PQC); Online - full text ed.: (from ProQuest Information & Learning, Northern Light Technology, Inc., Factiva).
Indexed: ABI Inform. (Win.1987-), Abstr.Health Care Manage.Stud., AgeLine, Excerp.Med.
—BLDSC (4042.023000), GNLM, ingenta. **CCC.**
Published by: (Foundation of the American College of Healthcare Executives), Health Administration Press, 1 North Franklin St, Ste 1700, Chicago, IL 60606-3491. TEL 312-424-2800, FAX 312-424-0014, http://www.ache.org, http://www.hsr.org. Ed. Mary Stefl. R&P Jane Williams TEL 312-424-9473. Circ: 2,500. **Subscr. to:** ACHE Publication Services, 1 N Franklin St, Ste 1700, Chicago, IL 60606-3420.

362.11 USA
G H A TODAY NEWSLETTER. (Georgia Hospital Association) Text in English. m. membership. **Document type:** *Newsletter, Trade.* **Description:** Features articles, news about the association, and a calendar of events.
Media: Online - full text.
Published by: G H A: An Association of Hospitals and Health Systems, 1675 Terrell Mill Rd, Marietta, GA 30067. TEL 770-955-0324, gha@gha.org, http://www.gha.org/todaymap.html. Ed., R&P Kevin M Bloye. Circ: 4,000.

362.1 658.8 NLD ISSN 0921-5077
GEDRAG & ORGANISATIE. Text in Dutch. 1988. bi-m. NLG 175 foreign. back issues avail. **Document type:** *Trade.* **Description:** Covers the latest developments in various health and medical specialties and professions, especially in all areas of management and administration.
Indexed: PsycInfo, e-psyche.
—KNAW.
Published by: Elsevier Gezondheidszorg B.V., Tijdstroom (Subsidiary of: Reed Elsevier plc Group), Planetenbaan 1, Maarssen 3600 AK, Netherlands. TEL 31-346-577577, FAX 31-346-554287, http://www.tijdstroom.nl. **Subscr. to:** Elsevier Den Haag, Postbus 16500, The Hague 2500 BM, Netherlands. TEL 31-70-381-9900, FAX 31-70-333-8399.

GERIATRIC CARE. see *GERONTOLOGY AND GERIATRICS*

658 ESP ISSN 0214-8919
GESTION HOSPITALARIA. Text in Spanish. 1990. q. ESP 8,100 to individuals; ESP 11,470 to institutions; ESP 6,480 to students (effective 2001). adv. *Refereed.* **Document type:** *Journal, Academic/Scholarly.* **Description:** Presents investigative articles and clinical notes in managing hospitals and other health care establishments.
Related titles: Online - full text ed.: 1988.
—CINDOC.
Published by: (Sociedad Espanola de Gestion Hospitalaria), Ediciones Doyma S.A., Traversa de Gracia, 17-21, Barcelona 08021, Spain. TEL 34-93-200-0711, gh@doyma.es, doyma@doyma.es, http://www.doyma.es/gh. Ed. Matilde Cortes. R&P Monica Barnes. Adv. contact Jose Antonio Hernandez. Circ: 6,500 (controlled).

362 FRA ISSN 0016-9218
GESTIONS HOSPITALIERES. (Includes special nos.) Text in French. 1960. m. FRF 600; FRF 725 foreign (effective 1998). adv. bk.rev. **Document type:** *Trade, Corporate.*
Indexed: Excerp.Med.
—CISTI, GNLM, Infotrieve. **CCC.**
Published by: Syndicat National des Cadres Hospitaliers, 44 rue Jules Ferry, Vitry-sur-Seine 94400, France. TEL 33-1-45736920, FAX 33-1-46825515. Ed., Adv. contact Veronique Laloue. R&P Guy Trahienbroit. B&W page FRF 7,700, color page FRF 14,500; trim 180 x 260. Circ: 4,728.

GESUNDHEIT IN DER EINEN WELT; Nachrichten aus der Aerzlichen Mission. see *RELIGIONS AND THEOLOGY*

658 657.832 BEL
GEZONDHEIDSZORG, BELEID EN ORGANIZATIE. Text in Flemish. s-m. BEF 4,134. Supplement avail. **Description:** Provides detailed and professional advice on the organizational, fiscal and personnel aspects of running hospitals, retirement homes, sanitaria and rehabilitation centers.
Published by: C E D Samsom (Subsidiary of: Wolters Samsom Belgie n.v.), Kouterveld 14, Diegem 1831, Belgium. TEL 32-2-7231111.

362.11 GBR ISSN 0952-1054
GREAT BRITAIN. DEPARTMENT OF HEALTH AND SOCIAL SECURITY. HEALTH BUILDING NOTES. Text in English. 1961. irreg. price varies. reprint service avail. from PQC. **Document type:** *Government.*
Formerly: Great Britain. Department of Health and Social Security. Hospital Building Notes (0072-601X)
Published by: (Great Britain. Department of Health and Social Security), Stationery Office, 51 Nine Elms Ln, London SW8 5DA, United Kingdom. TEL 44-20-7873-0011, FAX 44-20-7873-8247, book.orders@theso.co.uk, http://www.national-publishing.co.uk.

362.11 GBR ISSN 0141-1403
GREAT BRITAIN. DEPARTMENT OF HEALTH AND SOCIAL SECURITY. HEALTH EQUIPMENT NOTES. Text in English. 1975. irreg. price varies. reprint service avail. from PQC. **Document type:** *Government.*
Formerly: Great Britain. Department of Health and Social Security. Hospital Equipment Notes (0072-6028)
—**CCC.**
Published by: Stationery Office, 51 Nine Elms Ln, London SW8 5DA, United Kingdom. TEL 44-20-7873-0011, FAX 44-20-7873-8247, book.orders@theso.co.uk, http://www.national-publishing.co.uk.

GROOTKEUKEN; food magazine for care institutions. see *FOOD AND FOOD INDUSTRIES*

GROUP PRACTICE JOURNAL. see *MEDICAL SCIENCES*

362.12 USA
GROUP PRACTICE SOLUTIONS. Text in English. m. USD 169 (effective 2001). **Document type:** *Newsletter, Trade.* **Description:** Provides practical, how-to advice and ideas to help solve partner dilemmas like income division, buy-in and pay-out arrangements, leadership choices and effectiveness, disciplining problem partners (including dismissal), and more.
Published by: Advisory Publications, 15 E Ridge Pike, Ste 510, Conshohocken, PA 19428. TEL 888-941-4488, FAX 610-941-4499, info@smartpracticemanagement.com, http://www.smartpracticemanagement.com/cgi-bin/order/group.html.

▼ **GUIDE TO AUDITING HEALTH CARE BILLING PRACTICES.** see *BUSINESS AND ECONOMICS—Public Finance, Taxation*

362 CAN ISSN 1195-0110
RA978.C2
GUIDE TO CANADIAN HEALTHCARE FACILITIES/GUIDE DES ETABLISSEMENTS DE SANTE DU CANADA. Text in English, French. 1953. a. CND 127.95 (effective 1999). adv. reprint service avail. from PQC. **Document type:** *Directory.* **Description:** Lists regional boards, hospitals and long-term care facilities in Canada; includes key personnel, budgets and numbers of beds.
Formerly (until 1993): Canadian Hospital Directory (0068-8932)
Published by: Canadian Healthcare Association, 17 York St, Ste 100, Ottawa, ON K1N 9J6, Canada. TEL 613-241-8005, FAX 613-241-5055, http://www.canadian-healthcare.org. Ed. Indra Seegobin. Circ: 2,000.

362.1 658 USA ISSN 1081-728X
THE GUIDE TO HOSPITAL PERFORMANCE. Text in English. a. USD 499 (effective 1999). **Description:** Isolates major costs and charges a facility can control, adjusted for severity and cost-of-living.
Formerly (until 1995): H C I A Guide to Hospital Performance (1069-0042)
Related titles: CD-ROM ed.; E-mail ed.
Published by: Health Care Investment Analysts, Inc., 300 E Lombard St, Baltimore, MD 21201. http://www.hcia.com.

658 362.6 USA ISSN 1062-8258
GUIDE TO THE NURSING HOME INDUSTRY. Text in English. 1992. a. USD 249 (effective 1999). **Description:** Provides aggregate financial and operating performance data on more than 10,000 nursing homes state-by-state.

H

Published by: H C I A Inc., 300 E Lombard St, Baltimore, MD 21202. TEL 800-568-3282, FAX 410-752-6309. **Co-publisher:** Arthur Andersen & Co.

GUIDELINES FOR HEALTH SUPERVISION. see *MEDICAL SCIENCES—Pediatrics*

GUIDELINES FOR PERINATAL CARE. see *MEDICAL SCIENCES—Obstetrics And Gynecology*

362 GBR ISSN 0963-6390
GUY'S GAZETTE. Text in English. 1872. m. adv. bk.rev., play rev. illus, stat. index. **Document type:** *Bulletin, Newsletter, Academic/Scholarly, Consumer.*
Formerly (until 1990): Guy's Hospital Gazette (0017-5870)
Indexed: Chem.Abstr.
Published by: Guy's Hospital, Boland House, Guy Hospital, St Thomas St, London SE1 9RT, United Kingdom. TEL 44-171-955-5000. Ed. Nartej Chahal. Circ: 3,000.

H

362 USA
H A N Y S NEWS*. Text in English. 1969. w. USD 500 to non-members; USD 50 to members (effective 1999). **Document type:** *Newsletter.* **Description:** Contains healthcare news.
Formerly: Hospital Association of New York State. News (0018-5574)
Published by: Healthcare Association of New York State, 1 Empire Dr, Rensselaer, NY 12144. TEL 518-431-7600, FAX 518-431-7915, http://www.hanys.org. Circ: 2,000.

H C F A'S LAWS, REGULATIONS, AND MANUALS. see *INSURANCE*

174.24 658 NLD ISSN 0956-2737
R724 CODEN: HEFOE8
H E C FORUM; an interprofessional journal on healthcare institutions' ethical and legal issues. (HealthCare Ethics Committee) Text in English. 1989. q. EUR 211, USD 211 to institutions for print or online ed.; EUR 253.20, USD 253.20 to institutions for print & online eds. combined (effective 2002). reprint service avail. from SWZ. *Refereed.* **Document type:** *Journal, Academic/Scholarly.* **Description:** Focuses on ethical and legal issues as they pertain to hospitals. Responds to the increasingly complex issues addressed by hospital ethics committees, including administrative and policy issues and philosophical dilemmas.
Related titles: Microform ed.: (from PQC); Online - full text ed.: (from EBSCO Publishing, O C L C Online Computer Library Center, Inc., RoweCom Information Quest, Swets Blackwell, Kluwer Online).
Indexed: Excerp.Med. (1997-), Hosp.Lit.Ind., Int.Nurs.Ind., Lang.& Lang.Behav.Abstr., SOPODA, Soc.Serv.Abstr., Sociol.Abstr.
—BLDSC (4275.247788), EMDOCS, GNLM, Infotrieve, KNAW. **CCC.**
Published by: Kluwer Academic Publishers Group (Subsidiary of: Wolters Kluwer N.V.), Spuiboulevard 50, PO Box 17, Dordrecht 3300 AA, Netherlands. TEL 31-78-639-2392, FAX 31-78-654-2254, services@wkap.nl, http://www.wkap.nl/journalhome.htm/0956-2737. Ed. Stuart F Spicker. **Subscr. in the Americas to:** Kluwer Academic - Plenum Publishers, 233 Spring St, New York, NY 10013-1578. TEL 212-620-8468, FAX 212-807-1047; **Subscr. to:** Journals Department, PO Box 322, Dordrecht 3300 AH, Netherlands. TEL 31-78-639-2392, FAX 31-78-654-6474.

H M O - P P O DIRECTORY. (Health Maintenance Organization - Preferred Provider Organization) see *BUSINESS AND ECONOMICS—Trade And Industrial Directories*

658 NOR ISSN 0803-2556
H M T. HELSETJENESTEN - MEDICINSK TEKNIKK. Text in Norwegian. 1928. bi-m. NOK 240. adv. bk.rev.
Formed by the 1991 merger of: Medisinsk Teknikk (0800-5656); Helsetjenesten (0333-3299); Which was formerly (until 1982): Norsk Sykehustidende (0377-1792)
—**CCC.**
Published by: Selvig Publishing A-S, Postboks 9070, Groenland, Oslo 0133, Norway. Ed. P Oivind Selvig. Circ: 2,436.

HACHINOHE SHIRITSU SHIMIN BYOIN ISHI/HACHINOHE CITY HOSPITAL. MEDICAL JOURNAL. see *MEDICAL SCIENCES*

362 658.8 USA ISSN 0891-3242
HAYES DIRECTORY OF MEDICAL SUPPLY HOUSES*. Text in English. 1935. a. USD 200. **Document type:** *Directory.*
Formerly: Hayes Directory of Physician and Hospital Supply Houses (0073-1412)
Published by: Edward N. Hayes, Ed. & Pub., PO Box 3436, Mission Viejo, CA 92690-1436. TEL 714-756-9063.

362 IND ISSN 0970-471X
HEALTH ACTION. Text in English. 1988 (Jan.). m. INR 150 domestic; USD 50 foreign (effective 2000). adv. bk.rev. charts, illus, tr.lit. **Document type:** *Consumer.* **Description:** A complete family guide on health, health activism and community development. Includes alternative systems of therapies, women and child issues, etc.
Formerly (until 1988): Medical Service (0008-8102)
Published by: Catholic Hospital Association of India (C H A I), Health Accessories For All (H A F A), Gunrock Enclave, 157/6 Staff Rd., P O Box 2153, Secunderabad, Andhra Pradesh 500 009, India. TEL 91-40-7848457, FAX 91-40-7811982, TELEX 0425 6674 CHAI IN, chai@pol.net.in. Ed., R&P C M Francis. adv.: page INR 20,000, page USD 500. Circ: 35,000.

362.11068 IND ISSN 0971-5673
HEALTH ADMINISTRATOR. Text in English. 1983. s-a. INR 200; USD 40 foreign. adv. bk.rev. index. back issues avail. *Refereed.* **Document type:** *Trade.* **Description:** Devoted to health issues and managers.
Published by: Indian Society of Health Administrators, 15-37 Cambridge Road Cross, Cambridge Rd., Bangalore, Karnataka 560 008, India. TEL 91-80-557-4297, FAX 91-80-557-4297, ashoksah@blr.vsnl.net.in. Ed., Pub., R&P Ashok Sahni. adv.: B&W page INR 2,000, color page INR 5,000. Circ: 10,000 (paid).

HEALTH AND SYSTEM SCIENCE/SANTE ET SYSTEMIQUE. see *MEDICAL SCIENCES*

HEALTH BULLETIN. see *MEDICAL SCIENCES*

362 USA ISSN 1049-2577
RA407.4.N7
HEALTH CARE ANNUAL; an update on trends and facilities in New York. Text in English. a. USD 20 (effective 2000). charts, stat. **Document type:** *Academic/Scholarly.* **Description:** Covers the use of health facilities in New York City, Long Island, and the northern metropolitan area.
Formed by the merger of: Health and Health Care in New York City (0889-0331); Health Facilities in Southern New York (0888-7039)
Published by: United Hospital Fund of New York, 350 Fifth Ave, Fl 23, New York, NY 10118-2399. TEL 212-494-0700, FAX 212-494-0800, pbrooks@uhfnyc.org, http://www.uhfnyc.org.

658 USA ISSN 1063-5335
THE HEALTH CARE BILLER; the communication network for America's health care billers. Text in English. 1992. m. USD 289 to individual members; USD 29 newsstand/cover (effective 2002). **Document type:** *Newsletter, Trade.* **Description:** For health care billers and billing managers. Contains easy-to-understand information and tips on how to get bills out efficiently and avoid collection problems.
—**CCC.**
Published by: Aspen Publishers, Inc., 200 Orchard Ridge Dr, Ste 200, Gaithersburg, MD 20878. TEL 301-417-7500, 800-638-8437, FAX 301-417-7550, customer.service@aspenpubl.com, http://www.aspenpub.com. **Dist. by:** Aspen Publishers Inc., Distribution Center, 7201 McKinney Circle, Frederick, MD 21701. TEL 301-698-7100, FAX 301-695-7931.

658 USA ISSN 1060-0442
THE HEALTH CARE COLLECTOR. Text in English. 1987. m. USD 310 to individuals; USD 31 newsstand/cover (effective 2002). **Document type:** *Newsletter, Trade.* **Description:** For hospital and health care collections managers and their staff. Includes tips on how to collect faster, successful collection techniques from readers, information on collection problems with specific payer groups, and how to incorporate information systems into collecting.
Related titles: Online - full text ed.: (from ProQuest Information & Learning).
—**CCC.**
Published by: Aspen Publishers, Inc., 200 Orchard Ridge Dr, Ste 200, Gaithersburg, MD 20878. TEL 301-417-7500, 800-638-8437, FAX 301-695-7931, customer.service@aspenpubl.com, http://www.aspenpub.com. Ed. Joann Petaschnick. **Dist. by:** Aspen Publishers Inc., Distribution Center, 7201 McKinney Circle, Frederick, MD 21701. TEL 301-698-7100, FAX 301-417-7550.

658 USA
HEALTH CARE CONSTRUCTION REPORT*. Text in English. m. USD 350. back issues avail. **Document type:** *Bulletin.* **Description:** Report of new and planned construction and renovation projects.
Published by: American Hospital Publishing, Inc. (Subsidiary of: American Hospital Association Company), 1 N Franklin St, 27th Fl, Chicago, IL 60606-3421. TEL 312-440-6800, FAX 312-951-8491. Ed. Jaime Shimkus.

HEALTH CARE COST REENGINEERING REPORT. see *PUBLIC HEALTH AND SAFETY*

HEALTH CARE COSTS. see *BUSINESS AND ECONOMICS—Economic Situation And Conditions*

362 610 USA
HEALTH CARE DAILY REPORT. Text in English. d.
Media: Online - full text.
Published by: The Bureau of National Affairs, Inc., 1231 25th St, N W, Washington, DC 20037. TEL 800-372-1033, http://www.bna.com. **Subscr. to:** 9435 Key West Ave, Rockville, MD 20850.

658 664 USA ISSN 1090-2260
HEALTH CARE FOOD & NUTRITION FOCUS. Text in English. 1984. m. USD 230 to individuals; USD 23 newsstand/cover (effective 2002). **Document type:** *Newsletter, Trade.* **Description:** For practicing food service managers and dietitians. Shares proven success stories and offers hands-on tips and strategies that can be put to immediate use to improve the well-being of patients.
Formerly (until Sep. 1996): Hospital Food and Nutrition Focus (0747-7376)
Indexed: Int.Nurs.Ind.
—Infotrieve. **CCC.**
Published by: Aspen Publishers, Inc., 200 Orchard Ridge Dr, Ste 200, Gaithersburg, MD 20878. TEL 800-638-8437, FAX 301-417-7550, customer.service@aspenpubl.com, http://www.aspenpub.com. **Dist. by:** Aspen Publishers Inc., Distribution Center, 7201 McKinney Circle, Frederick, MD 21701. TEL 301-698-7100, FAX 301-695-7931.

362 610 USA
HEALTH CARE FRAUD REPORT. Text in English. bi-w.
Published by: The Bureau of National Affairs, Inc., 1231 25th St, N W, Washington, DC 20037. TEL 800-372-1033, http://www.bna.com. **Subscr. to:** 9435 Key West Ave, Rockville, MD 20850.

331 USA ISSN 1521-3463
HEALTH CARE HUMAN RESOURCES ALERT. Text in English. 1998. s-m.
Incorporates (1976-1998): Health Labor Relations Reports (0148-4761)
Published by: Opus Communications, PO Box 1168, Marblehead, MA 01945. TEL 800-650-6787, customer_service@opuscomm.com, http://www.opuscomm.com.

610 USA ISSN 0197-3738
KF3580.H4
HEALTH CARE LABOR MANUAL. Text in English. 1974. bi-m. USD 689; USD 827 foreign. **Description:** Keeps up with the most advanced personnel systems, tells about new rulings, regulations, and court decisions.
Formerly: Health Care Labor Review
—**CCC.**
Published by: (Aspen Health Law Center), Aspen Publishers, Inc., 200 Orchard Ridge Dr, Ste 200, Gaithersburg, MD 20878. TEL 800-638-8437, FAX 301-417-7550. Circ: 1,652.

HEALTH CARE LAW: A PRACTICAL GUIDE. see *LAW*

HEALTH CARE LAW SOURCEBOOK. see *LAW*

658.91 614.7 USA ISSN 0361-6274
RA393
HEALTH CARE MANAGEMENT REVIEW. Text in English. 1976. q. USD 195 to individuals; USD 59 newsstand/cover (effective 2002). adv. bk.rev. illus. reprint service avail. from PQC. *Refereed.* **Document type:** *Journal, Trade.* **Description:** Provides in-depth analysis, insight, and practical strategies with solutions to real problems of health care management today.
Related titles: Microform ed.: (from PQC); Online - full text ed.: (from ProQuest Information & Learning, Gale Group, Ovid Technologies, Inc., Factiva, Institute for Scientific Information).

Indexed: ABI Inform. (Spr.1979-), ASCA, Abstr.Health Care Manage.Stud., AgeLine, B.P.I. (Jul.1982-), BPIA, Bus.Ind., CINAHL, Curr.Cont., Emerald, Environ.Sci.Poll.Mgmt., Excerp.Med., Hlth.Ind., I.P.A., Ind.Med. (1976-), Int.Nurs.Ind., Med.Care Rev., Pollut.Abstr., Risk Abstr., SSCI, Saf.Sci.Abstr., Tr.& Indus.Ind.
—BLDSC (4274.943000), EMDOCS, GNLM, IDS, ingenta, KNAW. **CCC.**
Published by: Aspen Publishers, Inc., 200 Orchard Ridge Dr, Ste 200, Gaithersburg, MD 20878. TEL 301-417-7500, 800-638-8437, FAX 301-695-7931, customer.service@aspenpubl.com, http://www.aspenpub.com. Ed. Montague Brown. **Dist. by:** Aspen Publishers Inc., Distribution Center, 7201 McKinney Circle, Frederick, MD 21701. TEL 301-698-7100, FAX 301-417-7550.

658.91 614.7 USA ISSN 1386-9620
HEALTH CARE MANAGEMENT SCIENCE. Short title: H C M S. Text in English. 1998. q. USD 332, EUR 331 to institutions for print or online ed.; USD 398.40, EUR 397.20 to institutions for print & online eds.combined (effective 2002). *Refereed.* **Document type:** *Journal, Academic/Scholarly.* **Description:** Publishes research in the areas of theory, applications, novel ideas, and new tools for investigating and producing solutions to complex health care management problems.
Related titles: Online - full text ed.: (from EBSCO Publishing, O C L C Online Computer Library Center, Inc., Swets Blackwell, Kluwer Online).
Indexed: Ind.Med. (1998-), Int.Abstr.Oper.Res.
—BLDSC (4274.943050).
Published by: Kluwer Academic Publishers Boston, 101 Philip Dr, Assinippi Park, Norwell, MA 02061. TEL 781-871-6600, FAX 781-871-9045, services@wkap.nl, http://www.wkap.nl/journalhome.htm/1386-9620. Eds. Peter C Smith, Yasar A Ozcan. **Subscr. outside the Americas to:** Kluwer Academic Publishers Group, Journals Department, PO Box 322, Dordrecht 3300 AH, Netherlands. TEL 31-78-639-2392, FAX 31-78-654-6474; **Subscr. to:** Kluwer Academic - Plenum Publishers, 233 Spring St, New York, NY 10013-1578. TEL 212-620-8468, FAX 212-807-1047.

658.382 USA ISSN 1525-5794
RA971
THE HEALTH CARE MANAGER. Text in English. 1982. q. USD 172 to individuals; USD 52 newsstand/cover (effective 2002). adv. illus. reprints avail. *Refereed.* **Document type:** *Journal.* **Description:** Includes a wealth of proven formulas for success including financial strategies, hiring, motivation techniques, keeping good people, effective communication.
Former titles: Health Care Supervisor (0731-3381); Health Care Supervisors Journal
Related titles: Online - full text ed.: (from Factiva).
Indexed: ABI Inform. (Jan.1984-), CINAHL, Diar.Dis.Res., Int.Nurs.Ind.
—BLDSC (4274.943070), CISTI, GNLM, Infotrieve, ingenta. **CCC.**
Published by: Aspen Publishers, Inc., 200 Orchard Ridge Dr, Ste 200, Gaithersburg, MD 20878. TEL 301-417-7500, 800-638-8437, FAX 301-695-7931, customer.service@aspenpubl.com, http://www.aspenpub.com. Ed. Charles R McConnell. **Dist. by:** Aspen Publishers Inc., Distribution Center, 7201 McKinney Circle, Frederick, MD 21701. TEL 301-698-7100, FAX 301-417-7550.

362 610 USA
HEALTH CARE POLICY REPORT. Text in English. w.
Published by: The Bureau of National Affairs, Inc., 1231 25th St, N W, Washington, DC 20037. TEL 800-372-1033, http://www.bna.com. **Subscr. to:** 9435 Key West Ave, Rockville, MD 20850.

362 610 USA
HEALTH CARE PROGRAM COMPLIANCE GUIDE. Text in English. m.
Published by: The Bureau of National Affairs, Inc., 1231 25th St, N W, Washington, DC 20037. TEL 800-372-1033, http://www.bna.com. **Subscr. to:** 9435 Key West Ave, Rockville, MD 20850.

THE HEALTH CARE REGISTRATION; the newsletter for health care registration professionals. see *BUSINESS AND ECONOMICS—Management*

368.382 GBR ISSN 1356-0611
HEALTH CARE RISK REPORT. Text in English. 1994. m. (10/yr.). GBP 260; GBP 277 foreign (effective 2000). charts, stat. *Refereed.* **Document type:** *Trade.* **Description:** Addresses the practical implications of managing clinical risk. Covers such areas as medical negligence, risk management, and finance and features case reports and studies.
—BLDSC (4274.947000).
Published by: Eclipse Group Ltd. (Subsidiary of: Reed Elsevier plc), 18-20 Highbury Place, London N5 1QP, United Kingdom. TEL 44-20-7354-5858, FAX 44-20-7226-8106, publications@irseclipse.co.uk, http://www.irseclipse.co.uk. Ed. John Tingle. Pub. Andrew Brode.

658 613.7 USA ISSN 0742-1478
HEALTH CARE STRATEGIC MANAGEMENT; the newsletter for hospital strategists. Text in English. 1983. m. USD 284 (effective 2001). adv. bk.rev. back issues avail.; reprints avail. **Document type:** *Newsletter, Trade.* **Description:** The leading strategy newsletter for hospitals and health systems since 1983.
Related titles: Online - full text ed.: (from NewsNet, ProQuest Information & Learning, Northern Light Technology, Inc., Gale Group, Factiva).
Indexed: ABI Inform. (Jan.1991-), AgeLine, CINAHL, I.P.A., Int.Nurs.Ind.
—BLDSC (4274.949200), GNLM, ingenta, KNAW. **CCC.**
Published by: Business Word Inc., 5350 S. Roslyn St, Ste. 400, Greenwood Village, CO 80111-2145. TEL 303-290-8500, FAX 303-290-9025, sandyc@businessword.com, http://www.businessword.com/2020pubs.htm. Circ: 1,200 (paid).

658 610 CAN ISSN 0828-203X
HEALTH CAREER POST. Text in English. 1987. m. CND 20. adv. back issues avail. **Document type:** *Trade.* **Description:** Lists employment vacancies in Canada for health care professionals.
Published by: Oakwood Publications Ltd., 55 Costain Ct, Kitchener, ON N2N 3A5, Canada. TEL 519-742-1099, FAX 519-745-1289. Ed. John Prno. Circ: 9,800.

362 USA ISSN 1079-9869
HG9386.5
HEALTH DATA MANAGEMENT (NEW YORK). Text in English. 1993. m. USD 98 (effective 2001). adv. back issues avail. **Document type:** *Trade.*
Formerly (until 1994): Medical Claims Management (1069-5699)
Related titles: Online - full text ed.: (from LexisNexis, ProQuest Information & Learning, Gale Group).
Indexed: SoftBase (Aug.1998-).
—BLDSC (4274.961400), Infotrieve. **CCC.**
Published by: Thompson Financial / I M G Media (Subsidiary of: Thompson Publishing Group), 22nd Fl, 11 Penn Plaza, New York, NY 10001. TEL 212-967-7000, FAX 212-564-8879.

HEALTH DEVICES SOURCEBOOK. see *MEDICAL SCIENCES*

HEALTH EMPLOYMENT LAW UPDATE. see *BUSINESS AND ECONOMICS—Labor And Industrial Relations*

362.1 GBR ISSN 0957-7742
HEALTH ESTATE JOURNAL. Text in English. 1946. 10/yr. GBP 55 domestic; GBP 63 foreign (effective 2001). adv. bk.rev. charts, illus. **Document type:** *Journal.*
Former titles (until 1990): Institute of Hospital Engineering. Journal (0953-1211); (until 1987): Hospital Engineering (0309-7498); Hospital Engineer
Indexed: Abstr.Health Care Manage.Stud., INSPEC (Jun.1969, Jan.1970-Oct.1982, dropped), Int.Build.Serv.Abstr., Int.Nurs.Ind., W.R.C.Inf.
—BLDSC (4275.015400), GNLM.
Published by: (Institute of Healthcare Engineering and Estate Management), Step Communications Ltd., Shadwell House, 65 Lower Green Rd, Rusthall, Turnbridge Wells TN4 8TW, United Kingdom. TEL 44-1892-518877, FAX 44-1892-518811, hej@stepex.com, http://www.stepex.com/health_estate/pages/hc_introduction.htm. Ed. Nik Marshall. Pub. Trevor Moon. Adv. contact Josh Taylor. Circ: 3,000.

658 USA ISSN 0899-6210
RA971 CODEN: HFAMEI
HEALTH FACILITIES MANAGEMENT. Text in English. m. USD 40 domestic; USD 70 foreign; USD 5 newsstand/cover (effective 2001). **Document type:** *Trade.* **Description:** Covers the complete scope of responsibilities facing facility management administrators and directors in health care institutions.
Related titles: Online - full text ed.: (from LexisNexis).
Indexed: Int.Nurs.Ind.
—BLDSC (4275.015700).
Published by: American Hospital Publishing, Inc. (Subsidiary of: American Hospital Association Company), 1 N Franklin St, 27th Fl, Chicago, IL 60606-3421. TEL 312-440-6800, FAX 312-951-8491, 312-422-4799, http://www.hfmmagazine.com/hfm-home.html. Ed. Michael Hemmes. Circ: 31,300.

658 USA ISSN 1075-6973
HEALTH FACILITIES REPORT. Text in English. 1992. m. USD 369. **Document type:** *Newsletter.* **Description:** Provides information on hospital and dental office safety, protection technology, medical waste disposal and infection control, worker safety, and ergonomics.
Published by: Stevens Publishing Corporation, 5151 Beltline Rd, 10th fl, Dallas, TX 75240. TEL 972-687-6700, FAX 972-687-6770. Ed. Darla Bean.

362 USA
RA960 CODEN: HHNEE5
HEALTH FORUM. Text in English. 1936. m. USD 80 domestic; USD 150 foreign; USD 9 newsstand/cover (effective 2001). adv. bk.rev. illus. index. reprint service avail. from PQC. **Document type:** *Trade.* **Description:** Contains latest deals, policy changes, and trends affecting health care organizations.
Former titles: Hospitals and Health Networks (1068-8838); (until 1993): Hospitals (0018-5973)
Related titles: Microform ed.: 1936 (from PQC); Online - full text ed.: 1936 (from ProQuest Information & Learning, The Dialog Corporation, Gale Group, Ovid Technologies, Inc., H. W. Wilson, Factiva, Institute for Scientific Information).
Indexed: ABI Inform. (Mar.1988-), AIM, ASCA, Abstr.Health Care Manage.Stud., Account.Ind. (1974-), AgeLine, B.P.I. (Jun.1993-), BPIA, CINAHL, Chem.Abstr., Curr.Cont., Excerp.Med., Hlth.Ind., Hosp.Lit.Ind., INIS Atomind., I.P.A., Ind.Med. (1993-), Int.Nurs.Ind., L.R.I., Med.Care Rev., PSI, Pers.Lit., SRI, SSCI, Sci.Cit.Ind. (coverage dropped), Tr.& Indus.Ind.
—BLDSC (4333.270000), CISTI, EMDOCS, GNLM, IDS, ingenta, KNAW.
Published by: American Hospital Publishing, Inc. (Subsidiary of: American Hospital Association Company), 1 N Franklin St, 27th Fl, Chicago, IL 60606-3421. TEL 312-440-6800, FAX 312-422-4799, 312-422-4500, grayson@aha.org, http://www.hhnmag.com/hhn-home.html. Ed. Mary Grayson. adv.: B&W page USD 6,930, color page USD 8,250. Circ: 100,000.

657.832 USA ISSN 1091-4498
HEALTH GRANTS FUNDING ALERT. Text in English. 1978. 12/yr. USD 237 (effective 2001). adv. charts. index. 10 p./no. 2 cols./p. back issues avail. **Document type:** *Newsletter, Trade.* **Description:** Identifies opportunities for federal, corporate and foundation support of healthcare. Alerts development professionals to requests for proposals and upcoming application deadlines.
Formerly: Health Funds Development Letter (0193-7928)
Related titles: Online - full content ed.
—CCC.
Published by: Health Resources Publishing, 1913 Atlantic Ave, Ste F4, Manasquan, NJ 08736. TEL 732-292-1100, FAX 732-292-1111, hrp@healthrespubs.com, http://www.healthrespubs.com. Ed. Beth-Ann Kerber. Pub. Robert K Jenkins. Adv. contact Judy Granholm.

HEALTH INDUSTRY TODAY; the market letter for health care industry vendors. see *MEDICAL SCIENCES*

362 340 USA
HEALTH LAW & BUSINESS LIBRARY ON CD-ROM. Text in English. m.
Media: CD-ROM.
Published by: The Bureau of National Affairs, Inc., 1231 25th St, N W, Washington, DC 20037. TEL 800-372-1033, http://www.bna.com. **Subscr. to:** 9435 Key West Ave, Rockville, MD 20850.

HEALTH LAW NEWS. see *LAW*

HEALTH LAW WEEK; case digests of judicial decisions affecting all healthcare. see *LAW*

362 GBR ISSN 1461-4588
HEALTH MANAGEMENT. Text in English. 1997. m. GBP 80 domestic to non-members; GBP 105 elsewhere to non-members; GBP 10 newsstand/cover; free to members. **Document type:** *Academic/Scholarly.*
—BLDSC (4275.051750).
Published by: Institute of Healthcare Management, 7-10 Chandos St, London W1M 9DE, United Kingdom. TEL 44-20-7460-7654, FAX 44-20-7460-7655, mailbox@ihsm.co.uk. Ed. Andrew Cole TEL 44-20-7880-6230.

HEALTH MANAGEMENT TECHNOLOGY. see *MEDICAL SCIENCES—Computer Applications*

HEALTH PAGES. see *MEDICAL SCIENCES*

H

362 USA ISSN 0882-1577
RA960
HEALTH PROGRESS. Text in English. 1920. bi-m., latest vol.82. USD 50 (effective 2001). adv. bk.rev. bibl, charts, illus. index. back issues avail.; reprint service avail. from PQC. *Refereed.* **Document type:** *Trade.* **Description:** Coverage of management, ethical, administrative, and legal issues among others for administrators, religious sponsors, department heads, trustees, physicians, nurses and other personnel in US Catholic health facilities.
Formerly (until 1984): Hospital Progress (0018-5817)
Related titles: Microform ed.: (from PQC); Online - full text ed.: (from Northern Light Technology, Inc., ProQuest Information & Learning).
Indexed: Abstr.Health Care Manage.Stud., Abstr.Soc.Geront., AgeLine, CERDIC, CINAHL, Cath.Ind., Excerp.Med., Hosp.Lit.Ind., I.P.A., Ind.Med. (coverage dropped), Int.Nurs.Ind., MEDSOC, Med.Care Rev., Rehabil.Lit., Soc.Work Res.& Abstr.
—BLDSC (4275.105150), CISTI, GNLM, ingenta.
Published by: Catholic Health Association of the United States, 4455 Woodson Rd., St. Louis, MO 63134-3797. TEL 314-427-2500, FAX 314-427-0029, hpeditor@chausa.org, http://chausa.org. Ed. Terry Van Schaik. R&P Carrie Stetz TEL 314-253-3454. Adv. contact Donna Troy TEL 314-253-3450. Circ: 12,000.

362 GBR ISSN 0952-2271
RA427 CODEN: HSJOEO
THE HEALTH SERVICE JOURNAL; for people involved in NHS management. Text in English. 1892. w. GBP 59.50 to individuals; GBP 85 domestic to institutions; GBP 152 foreign to institutions (effective 2000). adv. bk.rev. abstr, charts, illus, stat. **Document type:** *Trade.* **Description:** Provides news and information to health care managers to help them manage more effectively.
Formerly: Health and Social Service Journal (0300-8347); Which incorporates: Medical Officer (0025-7400); Community Medicine
Indexed: AMED, ASSIA, Abstr.Health Care Manage.Stud., Abstr.Hyg., Brit.Nur.Ind., Build.Manage.Abstr., CINAHL, Excerp.Med., Hosp.Lit.Ind., INSPEC (Sep.1983-), Ind.Med. (coverage dropped), Nutr.Abstr., Trop.Dis.Bull.
—BLDSC (4275.107200), AskIEEE, GNLM, Infotrieve. **CCC.**
Published by: Emap Healthcare Ltd. (Subsidiary of: Emap Business Communications Ltd.), Greater London House, Hampstead Rd, London NW1 7EJ, United Kingdom. TEL 44-20-7874-0200, FAX 44-20-7874-0201, http://www.hsj.co.uk. Ed. Peter Davies. R&P Josie Cunn. Adv. contact Caroline Ridley-Barker. Circ: 21,067.

658 GBR ISSN 1352-3449
HEALTH SERVICE REPORT; the quarterly journal of health service pay and employment practice. Text in English. 1993. q. GBP 165; GBP 170 foreign. charts, stat. **Document type:** *Newsletter.* **Description:** Covers topics in managing health service organizations. Surveys pay and working conditions, details of collective agreements, and developments.
Indexed: AgeLine.
—BLDSC (4275.107450).
Published by: (Great Britain. National Health Service), Eclipse Group Ltd., Industrial Relations Services, 18 Highbury Park, London N5 2AB, United Kingdom. TEL 44-20-7354-5858, FAX 44-207-226-8618. Ed. Sarah Silcox. Pub. Andrew Brode.

613.194 614 USA ISSN 0017-9124
RA960 CODEN: HESRA
HEALTH SERVICES RESEARCH. Text in English. 1965. bi-m. GBP 219 to institutions in UK & Europe; USD 310 to institutions in the Americas & Caribbean; GBP 219 elsewhere to institutions (effective 2002). back issues avail.; reprint service avail. from PQC. *Refereed.* **Document type:** *Academic/Scholarly.* **Description:** Provides those engaged in research, public policy formulation, healthcare administration, education, and practice with advance information on new trends and the latest techniques of research and evaluation, enabling them to take advantage of current and significant research.
Related titles: Microform ed.: (from PQC); Online - full text ed.: (from ProQuest Information & Learning, Gale Group, Northern Light Technology, Inc., Factiva, Institute for Scientific Information).
Indexed: ABI Inform. (Spr.1983-), ASCA, Abstr.Health Care Manage.Stud., Abstr.Hyg., AgeLine, BPIA, Bus.Ind., CINAHL, Curr.Cont., Diar.Dis.Res., Environ.Sci.Poll.Mgmt., Excerp.Med., Fam.Ind., Hosp.Lit.Ind., I.P.A., Ind.Med. (1966-), Int.Nurs.Ind., J.of Econ.Lit., Lang.& Lang.Behav.Abstr., MEDSOC, Manage.Cont., Med.Care Rev., Pollut.Abstr., Risk Abstr., SOPODA, SSCI, Saf.Sci.Abstr., Sage Race Rel.Abstr., Sci.Cit.Ind., Soc.Serv.Abstr., Sociol.Abstr., Tr.& Indus.Ind., Trop.Dis.Bull.
—BLDSC (4275.120000), GNLM, IDS, ingenta, KNAW.
Published by: (Hospital Research and Educational Trust), Health Administration Press, 1 North Franklin St, Ste 1700, Chicago, IL 60606-3491. TEL 312-424-2800, 708-450-9952, FAX 312-424-0014, 708-450-1618, info@hsr.org, http://www.hsr.org. Ed. Stephen M Shortell. R&P Jane Williams TEL 312-424-9473. Circ: 3,500. **Subscr. to:** ACHE Publication Services. **Co-sponsor:** Association for Health Services Research, Foundation of the American College of Healthcare Executives.

HEALTH SYSTEMS MANAGEMENT. see *PUBLIC HEALTH AND SAFETY*

362 USA ISSN 1048-4167
HEALTH TEXAS. Text in English. 1944. m. USD 36 to non-members; USD 26 to members. adv. bk.rev. charts, illus, tr.lit. index. reprints avail. **Document type:** *Trade.*
Formerly (until 1989): Texas Hospitals (0040-4357)
Related titles: Microform ed.: (from PQC).
Indexed: Abstr.Health Care Manage.Stud., AgeLine.
—CISTI, GNLM.
Published by: Texas Hospital Association, 6225 U S Hwy 290 East, Box 15587, Austin, TX 78761-5587. TEL 512-465-1050, FAX 512-465-1090. Ed. Margaret Harrist. Circ: 7,000.

362 USA ISSN 1091-6768
HEALTHCARE BENCHMARKS. Text in English. 1994. m. USD 499 domestic; USD 529 foreign; USD 83 newsstand/cover (effective 2001). **Document type:** *Newsletter.*
Formerly (until 1996): Hospital Benchmarks (1087-0628); Which incorporated (1992-1995): Idea Letter for Health Care Managers (1068-5286)
Related titles: Online - full text ed.: (from Northern Light Technology, Inc.).
Indexed: CINAHL, Int.Nurs.Ind.
—BLDSC (4275.247740).
Published by: American Health Consultants (Subsidiary of: Medical Economics Co., Inc.), 3525 Piedmont Rd, N E, 6 Piedmont Center, Ste 400, Atlanta, GA 30305. TEL 404-262-5476, 404-262-7436, 800-688-2421, FAX 404-262-7837, 800-284-3291, custserv@ahcpub.com, http://www.ahcpub.com.

362.1 AUS
HEALTHCARE BRIEF. Text in English. 1968. bi-m. membership only. adv. 15 p./no. back issues avail. **Document type:** *Newsletter.* **Description:** Contains information relevant to health care providers and administrators.
Former titles: Hospital Brief (0817-5675); Australian Hospital Newsletter (0084-7410)
—**CCC.**
Published by: Australian Healthcare Association, PO Box 54, Deakin West, ACT 2600, Australia. TEL 61-2-62851488, FAX 61-2-62822395, admin@aha.asn.au, htp://www.aha.asn.au. Eds. Crag Southon, Mark Cormack. Adv. contact Elizabeth McMullan. Circ: 3,500.

362.1 GBR ISSN 0967-3881
HEALTHCARE BUYERS' GUIDE. Text in English. 1966. a. GBP 86 domestic; GBP 97 in Europe; GBP 107 elsewhere (effective 1999). adv. **Document type:** *Directory, Trade.* **Description:** Covers health care products, equipment, and supplies.
Former titles: Health Service Buyers Guide (0140-5748); Sell's Health Service Buyers Guide (0308-7107); Sell's Hospital and Surgical Supplies (0073-3458)
Published by: C M P Information (Subsidiary of: United Business Media), Sovereign House, Sovereign Way, Tonbridge, Kent TN9 1RW, United Kingdom. TEL 44-1732-362666, FAX 44-1732-367301, enquiries@cmpinformation.com, http://www.cmpinformation.com. Ed. Gwen Young. R&P Sarah Walker. Adv. contact Elaine Soni TEL 44-1732-377423.

005.8 USA
HEALTHCARE DATA SECURITY MANUAL. Text in English. 1997. a. USD 269; USD 229 foreign (effective 1999). **Document type:** *Trade.*
Published by: American Health Consultants (Subsidiary of: Medical Economics Co., Inc.), 3525 Piedmont Rd, N E, 6 Piedmont Center, Ste 400, Atlanta, GA 30305. TEL 404-688-2421, custserv@ahcpub.com, http://www.ahcpub.com.

658 USA
HEALTHCARE EDUCATION DATELINE. Text in English. 1991. q. membership. **Document type:** *Newsletter.*
Published by: American Hospital Association, One North Franklin, Chicago, IL 60606-3421. TEL 312-422-3724, FAX 312-422-4580. Ed. Mary Hudson. Circ: 1,700.

362 USA ISSN 0883-5381
RA971 CODEN: HEEXEU
HEALTHCARE EXECUTIVE. Text in English. 1985. 6/yr. USD 65 (effective 2001). adv. back issues avail.; reprint service avail. from PQC. **Document type:** *Trade.* **Description:** Focuses on a single critical management issue, such as human resources, physician roles, governance, technology, information systems, and career planning.
Related titles: Online - full text ed.: (from Northern Light Technology, Inc., ProQuest Information & Learning, Factiva).
Indexed: ABI Inform. (Jan.1991-), Int.Nurs.Ind.
—BLDSC (4275.247790), GNLM, Infotrieve, ingenta. **CCC.**
Published by: American College of Healthcare Executives, One N Franklin St, Ste 1700, Chicago, IL 60606-3491. TEL 312-424-2800, FAX 312-424-0023. Ed. Deborah Labb. Pub. Ann Bartling. Adv. contact Karla Alzona. Circ: 31,000 (paid and controlled).

657.832 USA ISSN 0735-0732
HF5686.H7 CODEN: HFMAD7
HEALTHCARE FINANCIAL MANAGEMENT. Text in English. 1946. m. USD 102 domestic; USD 170 foreign (effective 2002). adv. bk.rev. illus. index. back issues avail.; reprint service avail. from PQC,SCH,PSC. *Refereed.* **Document type:** *Magazine, Trade.* **Description:** Covers management and finance of health care organizations and integrated delivery systems, application of new procedures and systems in accounting, managed care, information systems, patient accounts management groups, practice management, financing of alternative delivery systems, reimbursement issues and legislation.
Former titles (until 1982): Hospital Financial Management; (until 1968): Hospital Accounting (0018-5639)
Related titles: CD-ROM ed.; Microform ed.: (from PQC); Online - full text ed.: (from The Dialog Corporation, Gale Group, ProQuest Information & Learning, Northern Light Technology, Inc., H. W. Wilson, Factiva).
Indexed: ABI Inform. (Mar.1973-), Abstr.Health Care Manage.Stud., Account.& Data Proc.Abstr., Account.Ind. (1974-), AgeLine, B.P.I. (Jan.1982-Jun.1982), BPIA, Bus.& Indus. (Jul.1998-), Bus.Ind., CINAHL, Excerp.Med., Hosp.Lit.Ind., INSPEC (Sep.1972-May 1982, Jul.1982-), I.P.A., Int.Nurs.Ind., L.R.I., Manage.Cont., Tr.& Indus.Ind.
—BLDSC (4275.247800), AskIEEE, EMDOCS, GNLM, ingenta, KNAW. **CCC.**
Published by: Healthcare Financial Management Association, Two Westbrook Corporate Center, Ste 700, Westchester, IL 60154. TEL 708-531-9600, FAX 708-531-0032, http://www.hfma.org/. Ed. Marilyn Ferdinand. Pub. Cheryl T Stachura. R&P Sharon Malik. Adv. contact Julie Ellinger. Circ: 34,000 (paid and controlled).

HEALTHCARE FOODSERVICE MAGAZINE. see *FOOD AND FOOD INDUSTRIES*

HEALTHCARE FOODSERVICE WHO'S WHO. see *FOOD AND FOOD INDUSTRIES*

362 USA ISSN 0899-9287
RA410.A1 CODEN: HFJOEZ
HEALTHCARE FORUM JOURNAL; leadership strategies for healthcare executives. Text in English. 1958. bi-m. USD 65 domestic; USD 80 foreign; USD 13 newsstand/cover (effective 2001). adv. bk.rev. charts, illus, tr.lit. index. reprint service avail. from PQC. **Document type:** *Trade.* **Description:** Presents commentary and critical analysis of key healthcare issues.
Former titles: Healthcare Forum (0885-257X); Hospital Forum (0018-5663)
Related titles: Microform ed.: (from PQC); Online - full text ed.: (from Northern Light Technology, Inc., Institute for Scientific Information).
Indexed: ABI Inform. (Jan.1984-), Abstr.Health Care Manage.Stud., AgeLine, CINAHL, Excerp.Med., Hosp.Lit.Ind., I.P.A., Int.Nurs.Ind.
—GNLM, IDS, ingenta.
Published by: Healthcare Forum, 425 Market St, 16th Fl, San Francisco, CA 94105. TEL 415-356-4300, FAX 415-356-9300, http://www.healthonline.com/thf.htm. Ed. Susan Anthony. Pub. Kathryn Johnson. Adv. contact Cindy Parra. B&W page USD 2,876; trim 10.88 x 8.38. Circ: 24,766.

HEALTHCARE GROUP PURCHASING ORGANIZATIONS. see *BUSINESS AND ECONOMICS—Trade And Industrial Directories*

362 610.285 GBR ISSN 1366-7491
HEALTHCARE I T; the magazine for health sector IT decision makers. (Information Technology) Text in English. 1997. 3/yr. GBP 24; GBP 43 foreign. adv. **Document type:** *Trade.* **Description:** Covers such healthcare information and technology topics as NHS systems, patient records, telemedicine and administration in hospitals.
Published by: Mitre House Publishing Ltd., The Clifton Centre, 110 Clifton St, London, Mddx EC2A 4HD, United Kingdom. TEL 44-20-7729-6644. Ed., Pub. Richard Blausten. Adv. contact Ian Holdom.

HEALTHCARE INSURANCE REPORT. see *INSURANCE*

658 USA ISSN 1082-6718
HEALTHCARE LEADERSHIP REVIEW. Text in English. 1982. m. (except July). USD 187 (effective 2001). bk.rev., Website rev. abstr, bibl, charts, illus, stat. back issues avail. **Document type:** *Newsletter, Trade.* **Description:** Contains informative summaries of articles selected from more than 150 healthcare management periodicals.
Formerly (until 1995): Hospital Management Review (0737-903X)
Related titles: E-mail ed.; Online - full content ed.
—CCC.
Published by: COR Healthcare Resources, PO Box 40959, Santa Barbara, CA 93140. TEL 805-564-2177. Ed., Pub. Dean H Anderson.

362.1106 CAN ISSN 0840-4704
CODEN: HMFOEU
HEALTHCARE MANAGEMENT FORUM. Text in English. 1988. q. CND 74.90, USD 90 domestic; CND 100 foreign. adv. *Refereed.* **Document type:** *Academic/Scholarly.* **Description:** Encourage rigorous analysis of issues related to recent advances in health service management theory and practice in a Canadian context.
Indexed: Emerald, Excerp.Med. (until 1993), Int.Nurs.Ind.
—BLDSC (4275.247880), CISTI, Infotrieve. **CCC.**
Published by: Canadian College of Health Service Executives, 350 Sparks St, Ste 402, Ottawa, ON K1R 7S8, Canada. TEL 613-235-7218, 800-363-9056, FAX 613-235-5451, http://www.canlisks.com/cchse/. Ed. Patricia Alexander. R&P, Adv. contact Michelle Garneau. Circ: 3,362.

658 USA ISSN 0749-6672
HEALTHCARE MATERIALS MANAGEMENT NEWS. Text in English. 1974. q. membership. bk.rev. index. back issues avail. **Document type:** *Newsletter.*
Formerly: American Society for Hospital Materials Management. Perspectives
Published by: (American Society for Hospital Materials Management), American Hospital Association, One North Franklin, Chicago, IL 60606-3421. TEL 312-422-3841, FAX 312-422-4571. Ed. Shelly Johnson. Circ: 2,300.

658.8 USA ISSN 0279-4799
HEALTHCARE PURCHASING NEWS. Text in English. 1977. m. USD 47.95 in United States; USD 57.95 in Canada; USD 62.95 elsewhere; USD 5 newsstand/cover (effective 2001). adv. charts, stat, tr.lit. back issues avail. **Description:** Delivers the latest industry news and trends to purchasing decision-makers at hospitals, multi-hospital systems, integrated networks and alternate site locations nationwide.
Former titles: Hospital Purchasing News; Purchasing Administration (0192-4311)
Related titles: Online - full text ed.: (from Gale Group).
—Infotrieve. **CCC.**
Published by: McKnight Medical Communications (Subsidiary of: Medical Economics Publishing Co., Inc.), Two Northfield Plaza, Ste. 300, Northfield, IL 60093. TEL 847-441-3700, FAX 847-441-3701, hpn@medec.com, http://www.hpnonline.com/. Ed. Jim Berklan. Pubs. John O'Connor, Stephanie A Ellis. Circ: 31,000 (paid and controlled).

658 340 USA
HEALTHCARE RISK CONTROL SYSTEM; an information and consultation system. Text in English. 1981. m. (in 4 vols.). USD 1,404.60 domestic; USD 1,473.60 in Canada; USD 1,602 elsewhere (effective 2002). bk.rev., film rev. abstr. index. *Refereed.* **Document type:** *Newsletter.* **Description:** Covers hospital risk management and quality of care, safety, law and regulations.
Formerly: Hospital Risk Control
Related titles: Online - full text ed.
Published by: (Emergency Care Research Institute), E C R I, 5200 Butler Pike, Plymouth, PA 19462. TEL 610-825-6000, FAX 610-834-1275, info@ecri.org, http://www.ecri.org. Ed. Andrea Zarod.

368.392 USA ISSN 1081-6534
HEALTHCARE RISK MANAGEMENT. Text in English. 1979. m. USD 499 domestic; USD 529 foreign; USD 83 newsstand/cover (effective 2001). bk.rev. back issues avail.; reprints avail. **Document type:** *Newsletter.*
Formerly (until 1995): Hospital Risk Management (0199-6312)
Related titles: Microfilm ed.: (from PQC); Online - full text ed.: (from Northern Light Technology, Inc.).
Indexed: CINAHL.
—BLDSC (4275.247948). **CCC.**
Published by: American Health Consultants (Subsidiary of: Medical Economics Co., Inc.), 3525 Piedmont Rd, N E, 6 Piedmont Center, Ste 400, Atlanta, GA 30305. TEL 404-262-5476, 404-262-7436, 800-688-2421, FAX 404-262-7837, 800-284-3291, custserv@ahcpub.com, http://www.ahcpub.com. Circ: 2,260.

HEALTHCARE TRENDS REPORT; the monthly digest of business and public policy news. see *MEDICAL SCIENCES*

362 USA
HEALTHLEADERS. Text in English. m. USD 49.95 (effective 2001). **Document type:** *Trade.* **Description:** Covers the healthcare industry, the stories behind the trends, practical management advice, technology strategies, in-depth roundtable discussions, career guidance and expert opinion.
Formerly (until 2001): Healthcare Business
Related titles: Online - full content ed.
Published by: HealthLeaders, Inc., 66 Music Sq W, Nashville, TN 37203. TEL 615-385-4131, 888-293-9675, FAX 615-385-4979, magazine@healthleaders.com, http://www.healthleaders.com/.

▼ **HEALTHY TRAVELER.** see *TRAVEL AND TOURISM*

362 USA
HEARTBEAT OF ST. JOSEPH'S MEDICAL CENTER. Text in English. 1968. q. free per issue. illus.
Formerly: Heartbeat of St. Joseph's Hospital (0017-9272)
Published by: St. Joseph's Medical Center, 523 N Third St, Brainerd, MN 56401. TEL 218-828-7373, FAX 218-828-3103, melody@uslink.net. Ed. Melody L Banks. Circ: 85,000.

610 USA ISSN 0018-0416
R11 CODEN: HFHJA6
HENRY FORD HOSPITAL MEDICAL JOURNAL. Text in English. 1953. q. free per issue. bk.rev. abstr, charts, illus. index. 20-yr. cum. index, 1972. back issues avail.; reprint service avail. from PQC.
Formerly: Henry Ford Hospital Medical Bulletin (0096-1868)
Related titles: Microfilm ed.: (from PQC).
Indexed: Biol.Abstr., C.I.S. Abstr., Chem.Abstr., Curr.Cont. (coverage dropped), Excerp.Med., INIS Atomind., Ind.Med. (coverage dropped).
—CASDDS, CISTI, GNLM, ingenta.
Published by: Henry Ford Hospital, Editorial Office, 2799 W Grand Blvd, Detroit, MI 48202. TEL 313-876-2028. Ed. Dr. Raymond C Mellinger. Circ: 10,000.

362 USA
HIGHLIGHTS (FALLS CHURCH). Text in English. q. **Document type:** *Newsletter.* **Description:** Provides information for friends and supporters on the events and information related to the organization.
Published by: Hospice of Northern Virginia, Communications Department, 6565 Arlington Blvd, Ste 501, Falls Church, VA 22042. TEL 703-538-9222, FAX 703- 538-2163, webmaster@allenwayne.com, http://www.hospiceonline.org/.

658 JPN ISSN 0914-8019
HIMEJI SEKIJUJI BYOINSHI/HIMEJI RED CROSS HOSPITAL. JOURNAL. Text in English, Japanese; Summaries in English. 1977. a.
Published by: Himeji Sekijui Byoin, 30-1 Tatsuno-Machi 5-chome, Himeji-shi, Hyogo-ken 670-0032, Japan.

658 JPN ISSN 0912-7089
HIRATA SHIRITSU BYOIN NENPO/HIRATA MUNICIPAL HOSPITAL. JOURNAL. Text in Japanese. 1984. a. *Refereed.* **Document type:** *Academic/Scholarly.*
Published by: Hirata Shiritsu Byoin, 613 Nada-Bun-cho, Hirata-shi, Shimane-ken 691-0003, Japan. TEL 81-853-63-5111, FAX 81-853-63-4228. Ed. Hiroyuki Naniwa. Circ: 700.

HIROSHIMA KENRITSU BYOIN ISHI/HIROSHIMA PREFECTURAL HOSPITAL. MEDICAL JOURNAL. see *MEDICAL SCIENCES*

900 DEU ISSN 0440-9043
HISTORIA HOSPITALIUM. Text in German. 1966. a. DEM 60 (effective 2000). bk.rev. *Refereed.* **Document type:** *Monographic series, Academic/Scholarly.* **Description:** Studies of the history of hospitals and nursing and clinical developments.
Indexed: Amer.Hist.& Life, BHA, Hist.Abstr. (1983-).
—GNLM.
Published by: Deutsche Gesellschaft fuer Krankenhausgeschichte e.V., c/o Institut fuer Geschichte der Medizin und des Krankenhauswesens, R W T H Aachen, Wendlingweg, Aachen 52074, Germany. TEL 49-241-8088095, FAX 49-241-8888466, amurken@post.klinikum.rwth-aachen.de. Ed. Axel Hinrich Murken. Circ: 600.

658 JPN ISSN 0916-9547
HOKKAIDORITSU MIDORIGAOKA BYOIN NENPO/HOKKAIDO PREFECTURAL MIDORIGAOKA HOSPITAL. ANNUAL REPORT. Text in Japanese. 1991. a. free per issue. **Document type:** *Government.*
Published by: Hokkaidoritsu Midorigaoka, 1 Midorigaoka, Kato-gun, Otofuke-cho, Hokkaido 080-0334, Japan. TEL 81-155-42-3377, FAX 81-155-42-4233. Ed. Tanaka Yasuo. Pub. Tetsuhiro Ito.

658 338.476 USA ISSN 1073-9572
HOME HEALTH BUSINESS REPORT; news trends & strategies for the home healthcare executive. Text in English. 1994. s-m. USD 356; USD 386 foreign (effective 1998). bk.rev. back issues avail. **Document type:** *Newsletter.* **Description:** Contains home care business news regarding company and industry trends, including public company financial data, stock indexes, and company and payor profiles.
Incorporates (in Dec. 1995): Home Health Incomes & Outcomes
Related titles: Online - full text ed.: (from Northern Light Technology, Inc.).
Published by: American Health Consultants (Subsidiary of: Medical Economics Co., Inc.), 3525 Piedmont Rd, N E, 6 Piedmont Center, Ste 400, Atlanta, GA 30305. TEL 404-262-5476, custserv@ahcpub.com, http://www.ahcpub.com. Ed. Caralyn Davis. Pub. David Wilson. R&P Lauren Dryfuss TEL 404-262-5476. Circ: 1,300 (paid).

362.15 USA
HOME HEALTH CARE DEALER - PROVIDER. Text in English. 1989. bi-m. adv. **Document type:** *Newsletter, Trade.* **Description:** For home care dealers and home care pharmacies.
Former titles: Home Health Care Dealer - Supplier (1076-0946); (until 1994): Home Health Care Dealer (1041-1720)
Related titles: Online - full text ed.
Published by: Curant Communications, Inc. (Subsidiary of: Medical World Communications), 6701 Center Drive W #450, Los Angeles, CA 90045-1556. TEL 310-306-2206, FAX 310-306-9548. Ed. Kristin Trompeter. Circ: 14,000.

362.15 USA ISSN 1084-8223
RA645.3
HOME HEALTH CARE MANAGEMENT AND PRACTICE. Text in English. 1988. bi-m. USD 95 to individuals; USD 240 to institutions; USD 25 newsstand/cover to individuals; USD 60 newsstand/cover to institutions (effective 2001). **Document type:** *Trade.* **Description:** Practical resource guide that provides home health care professionals with high-level clinical information applicable to everyday situations.
Formerly: Journal of Home Health Care Practice (0897-8018)
Indexed: AMED, AgeLine, CINAHL, IMFL, Nurs.Abstr.
—CISTI, Infotrieve. **CCC.**
Published by: Aspen Publishers, Inc., 200 Orchard Ridge Dr, Ste 200, Gaithersburg, MD 20878. TEL 301-417-7500, 800-638-8437, FAX 301-695-7931, customer.service@aspenpubl.com, http://www.aspenpub.com. Eds. Barbara Stover Gingerich, Deborah Anne Ondeck. **Dist. by:** Aspen Publishers Inc., Distribution Center, 7201 McKinney Circle, Frederick, MD 21701. TEL 301-698-7100, FAX 301-417-7550.

658 USA ISSN 0162-1424
RA645.3
HOME HEALTH CARE SERVICES QUARTERLY; the journal of community care. Text in English. 1980. q. USD 75 to individuals; USD 101 in Canada to individuals; USD 109 elsewhere to individuals; USD 160 to institutions; USD 216 in Canada to institutions; USD 232 elsewhere to institutions; USD 450 to libraries; USD 608 in Canada to libraries; USD 653 elsewhere to libraries (effective Aug. 2001). adv. bk.rev. stat. back issues avail.; reprint service avail. from HAW. *Refereed.* **Document type:** *Journal, Academic/Scholarly.* **Description:** Covers major areas of concern to policy makers, planners, and providers of home health care and related services. Focuses on research and policy issues.
Related titles: Microfiche ed.: (from PQC); Microform ed.
Indexed: Abstr.Health Care Manage.Stud., Abstr.Soc.Geront., AgeLine, CINAHL, Environ.Sci.Poll.Mgmt., Excerp.Med., Fam.Ind., Hosp.Lit.Ind., IMFL, I.P.A., Int.Nurs.Ind., Lang.& Lang.Behav.Abstr., Pollut.Abstr., Psychol.Abstr., Rehabil.Lit., Risk Abstr., SOPODA, Saf.Sci.Abstr., Sage Fam.Stud.Abstr., Soc.Serv.Abstr., Soc.Work Res.& Abstr., Sociol.Abstr.
—BLDSC (4326.053000), GNLM, Haworth, ingenta.
Published by: Haworth Press, Inc., 10 Alice St, Binghamton, NY 13904-1580. TEL 607-722-5857, 800-429-6784, FAX 607-722-6362, 800-895-0582, getinfo@haworthpressinc.com, http://www.haworthpress.com/journals/journallist.asp. Ed. W June Simmons. Pub. William Cohen. R&P Ruthann Heath TEL 607-723-5857 ext 316. Adv. contact Jackie Blakeslee TEL 607-722-5857 ext 346. B&W page USD 315, color page USD 550; trim 6 x 8.5. Circ: 575.

362.15 338.476 USA
HOME HEALTH EXECUTIVE COMPENSATION REPORT. Text in English. 1996. a. USD 227; USD 257 foreign (effective 1999). **Document type:** *Trade.*
Published by: American Health Consultants (Subsidiary of: Medical Economics Co., Inc.), 3525 Piedmont Rd, N E, 6 Piedmont Center, Ste 400, Atlanta, GA 30305. TEL 404-262-5476, custserv@ahcpub.com, http://www.ahcpub.com.

362.1 GBR ISSN 1465-0436
▼ **HOME HEALTHCARE MAGAZINE.** Text in English. 1999. bi-m. GBP 10; GBP 1.95 newsstand/cover (effective 2000). adv. **Description:** Includes lively practical health information for the consumer.
Published by: Phase IV Communications, Westmead Rd, 123 Westmed House, Sutton, Surrey SM1 4JH, United Kingdom. TEL 44-20-8288-0444, FAX 44-20-8288-04445, editor@pahseiv.co.uk. Ed. Valeries Southgate. Pub. Mike Livesey. adv.: page GBP 5,000.

658 BEL ISSN 0439-5476
L'HOPITAL BELGE/BELGISCH ZIEKENHUIS. Text in Flemish, French. 1923. q. BEF 2,600. adv. bk.rev. charts, illus. **Document type:** *Trade.* **Description:** Serves to improve Belgian hospitals and hospital management.
Indexed: Excerp.Med.
—GNLM.
Published by: Association Belge des Hopitaux/Belgische Vereniging der Ziekenhuizen, c/o MA Greven, Sec-Gen, CPAS de Bruxelles, Rue Haute 298A, Brussels 1000, Belgium. TEL 32-2-5333268, FAX 32-2-5383745, TELEX 65123. Circ: 1,000.

610 JPN ISSN 0915-7344
HOSHI SOGO BYOIN NENPO/HOSHI GENERAL HOSPITAL. ANNUAL REPORT. Text in Japanese. 1988. a.
Published by: Hoshi Sogo Byoin, 1-16 Omachi 2-chome, Koriyama-shi, Fukushima-ken 963-0000, Japan.

362 ZAF
HOSPERSA UPDATE. Text in Afrikaans, English. 1962. q. ZAR 0.50. adv. reprints avail. **Document type:** *Newsletter.*
Formerly: Hospital R.S.A. (0018-5833)
Published by: Hospital Personnel Trade Union of S A, PO Box 3284, Pretoria 0001, South Africa. TEL 27-12-333-6252, FAX 27-12-333-9248. Ed. Rod McFarquhar. R&P, Adv. contact Thariza Steyn. Circ: 20,000.

362.15 610.73 GBR ISSN 0965-1470
HOSPICE BULLETIN. Text in English. q. GBP 6; GBP 12 foreign. **Document type:** *Newsletter.* **Description:** Reports on hospice services worldwide and publishes articles of interest to hospice personnel.
Published by: Saint Christopher's Hospice, Hospice Information Service, Saint Christophers Hospice, 51-59, Lawrie Park Rd, London SE26 6DZ, United Kingdom. TEL 44-181-778-9252, FAX 44-181-776-9345.

362 USA ISSN 0913-6681
HOSPICE LETTER. Text in English. 1979. 12/yr. USD 197 (effective 2001). adv. charts. index. 10 p./no. 2 cols./p. back issues avail. **Document type:** *Newsletter, Trade.* **Description:** Covers issues pertaining to the management and administration of hospice services, including financing strategies, staffing, fund raising and marketing.
Related titles: Online - full content ed.
—CCC.
Published by: Health Resources Publishing, 1913 Atlantic Ave, Ste F4, Manasquan, NJ 08736. TEL 732-292-1100, 800-516-4343, FAX 732-292-1111, hrp@healthrespubs.com, info@healthrespubs.com, http://www.healthrespubs.com. Ed. Beth-Ann Kerber. Pub. Robert K Jenkins. Adv. contact Judy Granholm.

658 362.14 USA ISSN 1087-0288
HOSPICE MANAGEMENT ADVISOR. Text in English. 1996. m. USD 319 domestic; USD 349 foreign; USD 53 newsstand/cover (effective 2001). **Document type:** *Newsletter.* **Description:** Offers directors advice on running their hospices.
Related titles: Online - full text ed.: (from Northern Light Technology, Inc.).
Published by: American Health Consultants (Subsidiary of: Medical Economics Co., Inc.), 3525 Piedmont Rd, N E, 6 Piedmont Center, Ste 400, Atlanta, GA 30305. TEL 404-262-5476, 404-262-7436, 800-688-2421, FAX 404-262-7837, 800-284-3291, custserv@ahcpub.com, http://www.ahcpub.com.

HOSPITAIS CIVIS DE LISBOA. BOLETIM CLINICO. see *MEDICAL SCIENCES*

658 BEL
HOSPITAL. Text in English, French, German. bi-m. EUR 45 in Europe; EUR 75 elsewhere. adv.
Related titles: French ed.: EUR 45 in Europe; EUR 75 elsewhere (effective 2000); German ed.: EUR 45 in Europe; EUR 75 elsewhere (effective 2000).
Published by: (European Association of Hospital Managers), Euromedical Communications, Sq Marie Louise 16, Brussels 1000, Belgium. TEL 32-2-2800560, FAX 32-2-2311688, editorial@hospital.be, http://www.hospital.be. adv.: B&W page XEU 2,890; bleed 210 x 276. Circ: 20,000.

642.59 USA ISSN 1079-0365
HOSPITAL ACCESS MANAGEMENT. Text in English. 1982. m. USD 399 domestic; USD 429 foreign; USD 67 newsstand/cover (effective 2001). back issues avail.; reprints avail. **Document type:** *Newsletter.*
Formerly (until 1994): Hospital Admitting Monthly (0745-1466)
Related titles: Online - full text ed.: (from Northern Light Technology, Inc.).
Published by: American Health Consultants (Subsidiary of: Medical Economics Co., Inc.), 3525 Piedmont Rd, N E, 6 Piedmont Center, Ste 400, Atlanta, GA 30305. TEL 404-262-5476, 404-262-7436, 800-688-2421, FAX 404-262-7837, 800-284-3291, custserv@ahcpub.com, http://www.ahcpub.com. Circ: 1,400.

658 USA ISSN 1078-8123
THE HOSPITAL ACCOUNTS RECEIVABLE ANALYSIS. Text in English. 1994. q. USD 489 to individuals; USD 147 newsstand/cover (effective 2002). **Document type:** *Journal, Trade.* **Description:** Synopsis of statistical data related to hospital receivables. Contains easy-to-read charts and tables of statistics and also includes analysis and forecasting of trends.
Published by: Aspen Publishers, Inc., 200 Orchard Ridge Dr, Ste 200, Gaithersburg, MD 20878. TEL 301-417-7500, 800-638-8437, FAX 301-695-7931, customer.service@aspenpubl.com, http://www.aspenpub.com. Ed. Gene Lass. **Dist. by:** Aspen Publishers Inc., Distribution Center, 7201 McKinney Circle, Frederick, MD 21701. TEL 301-698-7100, FAX 301-417-7550.

362 IND ISSN 0018-5531
HOSPITAL ADMINISTRATION. Text in English. 1964. q. INR 160, USD 100 (effective 2001). adv. bk.rev. abstr, charts, illus. 100 p./no. back issues avail.; reprints avail. **Document type:** *Journal, Academic/Scholarly, Internal.*
Related titles: CD-ROM ed.: 1964. USD 100 (effective 2001).
Indexed: Excerp.Med., ExtraMED, Hosp.Lit.Ind.
Published by: Indian Hospital Association, B-401 Sarita, New Delhi 110 044, India. TEL 91-11-6835648, 91-11-6941267, kinpy'smail@vsnl.com. Ed. Dr. P Ghej. Circ: 1,000.

658 USA ISSN 0146-7360
RA981.A2
HOSPITAL AND HEALTH CARE REPORT. Text in English. a. USD 840. charts. **Document type:** *Trade.* **Description:** Provides a wide variety of analyses to compare rates to other facilities in the area of size and type.
Published by: (Executive Compensation Service (ECS)), Wyatt Data Services, 218 Rte 17 N, Rochelle Park, NJ 07622-9832. TEL 201-843-1177, FAX 201-843-0101.

658 AUS ISSN 1320-1263
HOSPITAL AND HEALTHCARE. Text in English. 1932. 11/yr. AUD 63 domestic (effective 2000); AUD 175 foreign (effective 2001). adv. bk.rev. **Document type:** *Trade.* **Description:** Publication of interest to public and private hospital and nursing home executives throughout Australia.
Former titles (until 1993): Hospital and Healthcare Australia (0813-7471); (until 1983): Hospital Journal of Australia (0312-8490); Incorporates (in 1998): Asia Pacific Hospital (1328-0155); Which was formerly (until 1996): Australian Hospital (1328-0147); (until 1991): Health Professional (1328-0139); (until 1990): Australian Hospital (0314-0024); (until 1976): National Hospital and Health Care (0312-794X); Which was formed by the merger of (1949-1975): National Hospital (0470-1046); Which was formerly (until 1957): Australian Modern Hospital (0312-7982); (1969-1975): Hospitals and Health Care and Administration (0301-2182); Which was formerly (until 1972): Hospital and Health Administration (0301-2190); (until 1971): Hospital and Health Care (0018-5515)
Indexed: ABIX (Oct.1994-Mar.1998).
—ingenta.
Published by: Yaffa Publishing Group, 17-21 Bellevue St, Surry Hills, NSW 2010, Australia. TEL 61-2-9281-2333, FAX 61-2-9281-2750, yaffa@yaffa.com.au, http://www.yaffa.com.au/. Ed. Georgina Kenyon. Pub. Michael Merrick. Adv. contact Bea Blanks. B&W page AUD 2,315, color page AUD 3,180; trim 210 x 297. Circ: 9,672.

658 610.73 USA
HOSPITAL & HEALTHCARE NEWS. Text in English. 1986. m. USD 36. adv. **Description:** General interest healthcare journal focused on hospital-based regional healthcare issues and practitioners.
Former titles: Hospital News Delaware Valley; Hospital News
Published by: H. Robert Jacobs Publishing Co., Inc., 2022 E Allegheny Ave, Philadelphia, PA 19134. TEL 215-739-2033, FAX 215-426-4438. Ed. Jane E Emrick. Circ: 46,700 (controlled).

658 USA ISSN 1047-6903
RA981.A2
HOSPITAL BLUE BOOK (OFFICIAL NATIONAL EDITION). Text in English. a. USD 249 (effective 1998). adv. **Description:** Lists over 6,873 U.S. hospitals with over 221,000 key hospital personnel.
Published by: Billian Publishing, Inc., 2100 Powers Ferry Rd, Ste 300, Atlanta, GA 30339. TEL 800-533-8484, FAX 770-955-8485. Ed. Joyce Metzer. Pub. C Jay Perkins. Adv. contact Connie Twiggs.

658 USA ISSN 1047-6911
HOSPITAL BLUE BOOK (OFFICIAL SOUTHERN EDITION). Text in English. 1934. a. USD 134 (effective 1998).
Formerly: Clarks' Directory of Southern Hospitals
Indexed: CINAHL.
Published by: Billian Publishing, Inc., 2100 Powers Ferry Rd, Ste 300, Atlanta, GA 30339. TEL 800-533-8484, FAX 770-955-8485. Circ: 10,654 (controlled).

658 CAN
HOSPITAL BUSINESS. Text in English. 1996. bi-m. **Document type:** *Trade.* **Description:** Covers business, facility management and administrative issues for all Canadian hospitals, nursing homes, clinics and healthcare officials, managers, administrators, executives, and department heads.
Published by: Momentum Media Management, 4040 Creditview Rd, Unit 11, P O Box 1800, Mississauga, ON L5C 3Y8, Canada. TEL 905-813-7100, FAX 905-813-7117. Ed. Jay Barwell. adv.: B&W page CND 1,915, color page CND 2,750; trim 11 x 8. Circ: 8,700 (controlled).

658 USA ISSN 1087-0652
HOSPITAL CASE MANAGEMENT; the monthly update on hospital-based care planning and critical paths. (Includes: Critical Path Network) Text in English. 1993. m. USD 399 domestic; USD 429 foreign; USD 67 newsstand/cover (effective 2001). back issues avail. **Document type:** *Newsletter.*
Incorporates (1996-1997): Oncology Cost Management (1087-0342)
Related titles: Online - full text ed.: (from Northern Light Technology, Inc.).
Indexed: CINAHL, Int.Nurs.Ind.
—BLDSC (4333.137900).
Published by: American Health Consultants (Subsidiary of: Medical Economics Co., Inc.), 3525 Piedmont Rd, N E, 6 Piedmont Center, Ste 400, Atlanta, GA 30305. TEL 404-262-5476, 404-262-7436, 800-688-2421, FAX 404-262-7837, 800-284-3291, custserv@ahcpub.com, http://www.ahcpub.com. Circ: 2,310.

EL HOSPITAL (CINCINNATI). see *MEDICAL SCIENCES*

658 USA ISSN 0734-0028
HOSPITAL CONTRACTS MANUAL. Text in English. 1982. a. Supplement avail.
—CCC.
Published by: Aspen Publishers, Inc., 200 Orchard Ridge Dr, Ste 200, Gaithersburg, MD 20878. TEL 301-417-7500, FAX 301-417-7550.

HOSPITAL DE NINOS. REVISTA. see *MEDICAL SCIENCES—Pediatrics*

690.55 GBR ISSN 0300-5720
HOSPITAL DEVELOPMENT. Text in English. 1968. m. (11/yr.). GBP 68; GBP 87 in Europe; USD 178 in US & Canada; USD 118 elsewhere (effective 1999). adv. charts, illus, stat. **Document type:** *Trade.*
Formerly: Hospital Building and Engineering (0018-5582)
Related titles: Online - full text ed.: (from Northern Light Technology, Inc., ProQuest Information & Learning).
Indexed: Archit.Per.Ind., Brit.Nur.Ind., Build.Manage.Abstr., Excerp.Med., Int.Build.Serv.Abstr.
—GNLM.
Published by: Wilmington Publishing Ltd., Wilmington House, Church Hill, Wilmington, Dartford, Kent DA2 7EF, United Kingdom. TEL 44-1322-277788, FAX 44-1322-276474, wbp@wilmington.co.uk. Ed. James Parker. Circ: 8,635 (controlled).

HOSPITAL DOCTOR. see *MEDICAL SCIENCES*

362.11 DNK ISSN 1397-1492
HOSPITAL DRIFT & TEKNOLOGI/HOSPITAL MANAGEMENT & TECHNOLOGY. Text in Danish. 1997. 6/yr. DKK 360; DKK 68 newsstand/cover (effective 1998). adv. **Document type:** *Trade.* **Description:** Seeks to update on the development and in the debate about hospitals production planning and administration.
Published by: Scanpublishers A-S, Emiliekildevej 35, Klampenborg 2930, Denmark. TEL 45-39-90-80-00, FAX 45-39-90-82-80, vaboej@ibm.net. Ed. Paul Erik Ree. Adv. contact John Vaboe. B&W page DKK 10,475, color page DKK 16,400; trim 184 x 268. Circ: 5,600.

658 USA ISSN 0744-6470
HOSPITAL EMPLOYEE HEALTH. Text in English. 1982. m. USD 399 domestic; USD 429 foreign; USD 67 newsstand/cover (effective 2001). 12 p./no. back issues avail.; reprints avail. **Document type:** *Newsletter.*
Related titles: Online - full text ed.: (from Northern Light Technology, Inc.).
Indexed: CINAHL.
—BLDSC (4333.148800).
Published by: American Health Consultants (Subsidiary of: Medical Economics Co., Inc.), 3525 Piedmont Rd, N E, 6 Piedmont Center, Ste 400, Atlanta, GA 30305. TEL 404-262-5476, 404-262-7436, 800-688-2421, FAX 800-284-3291, custserv@ahcpub.com, http://www.ahcpub.com. Ed. Michele Marill. Circ: 2,535 (paid).

362 JPN
HOSPITAL ENGINEERING ASSOCIATION OF JAPAN. JOURNAL/BYOIN SETSUBI. Text in Japanese. 1959. bi-m. JPY 1,000. adv. bk.rev. abstr, charts. index.
Formerly: Hospital Equipment (0007-764X)
Media: Duplicated (not offset).
Indexed: Excerp.Med.
Published by: Hospital Engineering Association of Japan/Nihon Byoin Setsubi Kyokai, Hongo Kasuga Mansion 403, 30-16 Hongo 1-chome, Bunkyo-ku, Tokyo 113-0033, Japan. Circ: 2,000.

362 GBR ISSN 0018-5620
CODEN: HEQSA3
HOSPITAL EQUIPMENT & SUPPLIES. Text in English. 1955. m. GBP 59; GBP 78 in Europe; USD 241 in US & Canada; GBP 131 elsewhere (effective 1999). adv. charts, illus. **Document type:** *Trade.*
—BLDSC (4333.158000).
Published by: Wilmington Publishing Ltd., Apex House, London Rd, Northfleet, Gravesend, Kent DA11 9JA, United Kingdom. TEL 44-1474-534944, FAX 44-1322-276474, wbp@wilmington.co.uk. Ed. Alan Cork. Circ: 10,490. **Subscr. to:** WDIS, PO Box 200, Ruislip, Mddx HA4 0SY, United Kingdom. TEL 44-20-8841-8545, FAX 44-20-8841-9676.

658 BRA
HOSPITAL-ESCOLA SAO CAMILO E SAO LUIS. BOLETIM. Text in Portuguese. a.
Published by: Hospital-Escola Sao Camilo e Sao Luis, Macapa, AP, Brazil.

657.832 170 USA ISSN 8756-8519
HOSPITAL ETHICS. Text in English. 1985. bi-m. USD 135 to non-members; USD 85 to members. back issues avail. **Document type:** *Newsletter.* **Description:** Review of the latest information in the field of hospital ethics, which reports news and opinions, defines their implications, and provides suggestions and strategies for resolving specific ethical concerns.
Published by: American Hospital Association, One North Franklin, Chicago, IL 60606-3421. TEL 312-422-3996, FAX 312-422-4575. Ed. Donald F Phillips. Circ: 1,800.

THE HOSPITAL FOR SICK CHILDREN JOURNAL. see *MEDICAL SCIENCES—Pediatrics*

618.92 CAN ISSN 0082-5034
HOSPITAL FOR SICK CHILDREN, TORONTO. RESEARCH INSTITUTE. ANNUAL REPORT. Text in English. 1969. a.
Published by: Hospital for Sick Children, 555 University Ave, Toronto, ON M5G 1X8, Canada. TEL 416-813-1500, FAX 416-813-5328, http://www.sickkids.on.ca. Ed. Elizabeth Leake. Circ: 500.

362.11 DNK ISSN 1397-1484
HOSPITAL HEALTH CARE. Text in English. 1997. q. DKK 240; DKK 68 newsstand/cover (effective 1998). adv. **Document type:** *Trade.* **Description:** Nordic, independent and unpolitical journal for professional administrative leadership in the health and social sectors.
Published by: Scanpublishers A-S, Emiliekildevej 35, Klampenborg 2930, Denmark. TEL 45-39-90-80-00, FAX 45-39-90-82-80, vaboej@ibm.net. Eds. Helge Laybourn, John Vaboe. Adv. contact Kirsten Waaben. B&W page DKK 10,475, color page DKK 16,400; trim 184 x 268. Circ: 3,600.

362.15 USA ISSN 0884-8521
HOSPITAL HOME HEALTH; the monthly update for executives and health care professionals. Text in English. 1983. m. USD 399 domestic; USD 429 foreign; USD 67 newsstand/cover (effective 2001). back issues avail.; reprints avail. **Document type:** *Newsletter.*
Related titles: Online - full text ed.: (from Northern Light Technology, Inc.); Supplement: Salary Survey; Home Health Business Quarterly.
Indexed: CINAHL.
—BLDSC (4333.189940).
Published by: American Health Consultants (Subsidiary of: Medical Economics Co., Inc.), 3525 Piedmont Rd, N E, 6 Piedmont Center, Ste 400, Atlanta, GA 30305. TEL 404-262-5476, 404-262-7436, 800-688-2421, FAX 404-262-7837, 800-284-3291, http://www.ahcpub.com. Pub. Brenda L Mooney. Circ: 1,010.

658 USA
THE HOSPITAL INDUSTRY AND ITS ENVIRONMENT. Text in English. 1990. irreg., latest vol.5, 1992. USD 395. **Description:** Provides information on the hospital industry, including performance trends, third-party payers, demographic trends, national health expenditures, history, financial analysis and the outlook for the 1990's.
Published by: Dun & Bradstreet Information Services (Murray Hill) (Subsidiary of: Dun & Bradstreet, Inc.), One Diamond Hill Rd., Murray Hill, NJ 07974. TEL 908-665-5224, FAX 908-771-7599. Ed. Paulette Roberts.

618.92 MEX ISSN 0539-6115
CODEN: BMHIAK
HOSPITAL INFANTIL DE MEXICO. BOLETIN MEDICO. Text and summaries in English, Spanish. 1944. m. MXP 250, USD 50 (effective 1998). adv. bk.rev. index, cum.index: 1959-1973. back issues avail. **Document type:** *Bulletin, Academic/Scholarly.* **Description:** Covers pediatrics and health services.
Indexed: Biol.Abstr., Child Devel.Abstr., Curr.Adv.Ecol.Sci., Dairy Sci.Abstr., Excerp.Med., Ind.Med. (coverage dropped), Nutr.Abstr., Protozool.Abstr.
—BLDSC (2207.540000), CASDDS, EMDOCS, GNLM, KNAW.
Published by: Hospital Infantil de Mexico Federico Gomez, Departamento de Ediciones Medicas, Calle DR MARQUEZ 162, Col. Doctores, Deleg. Cuauhtemoc, Mexico City, DF 06720, Mexico. TEL 228-99-17 ext. 1486, FAX 7610270. Ed. Dr. Luis Velasquez Jones. Circ: 3,500 (paid).

HOSPITAL LAW MANUAL. ADMINISTRATORS. see *LAW*

HOSPITAL LAW MANUAL. ATTORNEYS. see *LAW*

658 340 USA ISSN 0738-0984
KF3825.A15
HOSPITAL LAW NEWSLETTER. Text in English. 1984. m. USD 515 to individuals; USD 52 newsstand/cover (effective 2002). **Document type:** *Newsletter.* **Description:** Updates on issues confronting the health care industry. Covers the latest about malpractice, credential requirements, hospital-physician relationships, financial issues, employee relations, and contracting.
Related titles: Online - full text ed.: (from ProQuest Information & Learning).
Indexed: Int.Nurs.Ind.
—CCC.
Published by: Aspen Publishers, Inc., 200 Orchard Ridge Dr, Ste 200, Gaithersburg, MD 20878. TEL 301-417-7500, 800-638-8437, FAX 301-417-7550, customer.service@aspenpubl.com, http://www.aspenpub.com. Ed. Nathan Hershey. **Dist. by:** Aspen Publishers Inc., Distribution Center, 7201 McKinney Circle, Frederick, MD 21701. TEL 301-698-7100, FAX 301-417-7550.

362 340 USA
HOSPITAL LAW'S REGAN REPORT. Text in English. 1960. m. USD 52 domestic; USD 64 foreign (effective 2000). stat. reprints avail. **Document type:** *Newsletter.* **Description:** Reports the latest appellate court decisions on hospital law in a case and comment format.
Formerly: Regan Report on Hospital Law (0034-317X)
Related titles: Microform ed.: (from PQC); Online - full text ed.: (from Gale Group).
Indexed: CINAHL.
—Infotrieve. **CCC.**
Published by: Medica Press Inc., 10 Dorrance St, Ste 500, Providence, RI 02903-2018. TEL 401-421-4747, FAX 401-521-9226. Ed., R&P, Adv. contact A David Tammelleo. Circ: 5,000.

658 USA ISSN 1048-5201
KF3825.A15
HOSPITAL LITIGATION REPORTER. Text in English. 1990. m., latest vol.12, 2001. USD 367 domestic; USD 397 in Canada; USD 422 elsewhere (effective Jun. 2001). index. back issues avail. **Document type:** *Newsletter.* **Description:** Digest of judicial decisions that specifically concern or affect the hospital environment. For hospital attorneys and administrators, as well as risk-management professionals.
Published by: Strafford Publications, Inc., Specialized Information Services, 590 Dutch Valley Rd, N E, Postal Drawer 13729, Atlanta, GA 30324-0729. TEL 404-881-1141, 800-926-7926, FAX 404-881-0074, 404-881-0041, editors@straffordpub.com, custserv@straffordpub.com, http://www.straffordpub.com. Ed. Jennifer F Vaughan. Pub. Richard M Ossoff.

658 681 GBR
HOSPITAL MAGAZINE. Text in English. bi-m. GBP 34; GBP 44 foreign. adv. **Document type:** *Trade.*
Published by: Mark Allen Publishing Ltd., Croxted Mews, 286-288a Croxted Rd, London SE24 9BY, United Kingdom. TEL 44-208-671-7521, FAX 44-208-971-1722. Ed. Faith Dunne. Pub. Mark Allen. Adv. contact Roger Allen.

658 ITA
HOSPITAL MANAGEMENT. Text in Italian. 1981. m. adv. **Document type:** *Trade.*

H

Published by: Systems Comunicazioni, Via Olanda, 6, Gaggiano, MI 20083, Italy. TEL 02-90841814, FAX 02-90841682. Ed. Michele Di Pisa. Adv. contact Agostina Ronchetti. B&W page ITL 3,160,000, color page ITL 4,500,000; trim 240 x 180. Circ: 20,888.

658 GBR ISSN 0953-9743
HOSPITAL MANAGEMENT INTERNATIONAL. Text in English. 1984. a. GBP 55 to non-members. adv. **Document type:** *Journal, Trade.* **Description:** Offers information on technology and clinical procedure assessment in hospital management, along with planning for health care, hospital supplies, hospital design, surgical and laboratory equipment and supplies, and emergency services.
Formerly (until 1989): International Hospital Federation. Official Handbook (0265-1874)
—BLDSC (4333.204800), CISTI, GNLM.
Published by: (International Hospital Federation), Sterling Publications Ltd. (Subsidiary of: Sterling Publishing Group Plc.), Brunel House, 55-57 North Wharf Rd, London W2 1LA, United Kingdom. TEL 44-20-7915-9660, FAX 44-20-7724-2089, ih@sterlingpublications.com, info@sterlingpublications.com, http://www.sterlingpublications.com/publications/hospitalmgmt.html. Ed. Leslie Paine. R&P Sandy Tucker. Adv. contact Simon Oldfield. Circ: 10,000 (controlled).

362.11 USA ISSN 0888-3068
HOSPITAL MATERIALS MANAGEMENT; the newsletter for materials management and group purchasing. Text in English. 1976. m. USD 269 (effective 2001). adv. bk.rev. illus. **Document type:** *Newsletter, Trade.* **Description:** Contains news about hospital group purchasing organizations; articles on materials management issues.
Formerly: Hospital Purchasing Management (0163-1322)
Related titles: Online - full text ed.: (from Gale Group, NewsNet, ProQuest Information & Learning, Northern Light Technology, Inc., Factiva).
Indexed: ABI Inform. (Jul.1991-), Excerp.Med., I.P.A., Int.Nurs.Ind.
—BLDSC (4333.205180), IDS, Infotrieve. **CCC.**
Published by: Business Word Inc., 5350 S. Roslyn St, Ste. 400, Greenwood Village, CO 80111-2145. TEL 303-290-8500, FAX 303-290-9025, paulad@businessword.com, http://www.businessword.com/2050pubs.htm. Ed. Paula Dejohn. Circ: 2,226.

658 USA ISSN 0192-2262
RA971.33
HOSPITAL MATERIEL MANAGEMENT QUARTERLY. Text in English. 1979. q. USD 135 domestic; USD 162 foreign (effective 2000). reprint service avail. from PQC. **Document type:** *Academic/Scholarly.* **Description:** Presents effective strategies for use in inventory control, purchasing, new technology, staff management, receiving, assessing material utilization, and automation.
Formerly: Topics in Health Care Materiel Management
Related titles: Microform ed.: (from PQC); Online - full text ed.: (from ProQuest Information & Learning, Gale Group, Factiva).
Indexed: ABI Inform. (Nov.1980-), Abstr.Health Care Manage.Stud., BPIA, Bus.Ind., Excerp.Med., Manage.Cont.
—CISTI, GNLM, ingenta, KNAW. **CCC.**
Published by: Aspen Publishers, Inc., 200 Orchard Ridge Dr, Ste 200, Gaithersburg, MD 20878. TEL 301-417-7500, 800-638-8437, FAX 301-695-7931, customer.service@aspenpubl.com, http://www.aspenpub.com. Ed. Charles E Housley. **Dist. by:** Aspen Publishers Inc., Distribution Center, 7201 McKinney Circle, Frederick, MD 21701. TEL 301-698-7100, FAX 301-417-7550.

HOSPITAL MEDICINE (LONDON, 1998). see *MEDICAL SCIENCES*

362 USA
HOSPITAL NEWS. Text in English. 1976. m. USD 22 (effective 1999). adv. tr.lit. 48 p./no. back issues avail. **Document type:** *Trade.* **Description:** Provides healthcare news on hospitals, nursing homes, assisted living, rehabilitation, physicians, nurses, managed care, home care, human resources, and other areas.
Address: 14 Crestview Dr, PO Box 1018, Westborough, MA 01581-6018. TEL 508-366-2225, 800-555-7477, FAX 508-366-5030, hospnews@ultranet.com. Ed. Mike Federman. Pub., R&P, Adv. contact Richard Lesperance TEL 508-366-2225. page USD 1,486; trim 14 x 11. Circ: 28,000 (controlled).

658 CAN
HOSPITAL NEWS - S W ONTARIO*. Text in English. m.
Address: 123 Pleasant Dr, Stratford, ON N5A 4X5, Canada. TEL 519-425-0957, FAX 519-425-0958. Ed. Carl Page. Circ: 20,000.

658 CAN
HOSPITAL NEWS - TORONTO AND REGION. Text in English. 1987. m. CND 26.50. adv. back issues avail. **Document type:** *Newspaper.*
Formed by merger of: Hospital News Downtown Toronto; Hospital News Greater Toronto
Published by: Auto Mart Magazine Ltd., 23 Apex Rd, Toronto, ON M6A 2V6, Canada. TEL 416-781-5516, FAX 416-781-5499. Ed. Connie Michalsky. Adv. contact Esther Dalys. Circ: 50,000.

657.832 338.476 USA ISSN 1074-8334
HOSPITAL PAYMENT AND INFORMATION MANAGEMENT. Text in English. 1983. m. USD 547 domestic; USD 577 foreign; USD 91 newsstand/cover (effective 2001). reprints avail. **Document type:** *Trade.*
Incorporates (1994-1998): Outpatient Reimbursement Management (1087-0369); Former titles (until 1994): Hospital's Medicare Policy and Payment Report (1060-7838); (until 1992): Prospective Payment Survival (0746-4703)
Related titles: Online - full text ed.: (from NewsNet).
Published by: American Health Consultants (Subsidiary of: Medical Economics Co., Inc.), 3525 Piedmont Rd, N E, 6 Piedmont Center, Ste 400, Atlanta, GA 30305. TEL 404-262-5476, 404-262-7436, 800-688-2421, FAX 404-262-7837, 800-284-3291, custserv@ahcpub.com, http://www.ahcpub.com. Circ: 2,100.

362.11 USA ISSN 0149-2632
HOSPITAL PEER REVIEW. Text in English. 1976. m. USD 399 domestic; USD 429 foreign; USD 67 newsstand/cover (effective 2001). bk.rev. reprints avail. **Document type:** *Newsletter.*
Related titles: Microform ed.: (from PQC); Online - full text ed.: (from Northern Light Technology, Inc.); Supplement: Discharge Planning Advisor.
Indexed: Hosp.Lit.Ind., Ind.Med. (coverage dropped), Int.Nurs.Ind.
Published by: American Health Consultants (Subsidiary of: Medical Economics Co., Inc.), 3525 Piedmont Rd, N E, 6 Piedmont Center, Ste 400, Atlanta, GA 30305. TEL 404-262-5476, 404-262-7436, 800-688-2421, FAX 404-262-7837, 800-284-3291, custserv@ahcpub.com, http://www.ahcpub.com. Pub. Brenda L Mooney. R&P Richard Jarvis TEL 404-262-5425.

HOSPITAL PHARMACIST REPORT. see *PHARMACY AND PHARMACOLOGY*

HOSPITAL PHARMACY. see *PHARMACY AND PHARMACOLOGY*

HOSPITAL PHARMACY IN ONTARIO. see *PHARMACY AND PHARMACOLOGY*

HOSPITAL PHARMACY SERVICE INSTANT UP-DATE. see *PHARMACY AND PHARMACOLOGY*

HOSPITAL PHYSICIAN; medical practice for staff & resident. see *MEDICAL SCIENCES*

HOSPITAL PODIATRIST. see *MEDICAL SCIENCES—Orthopedics And Traumatology*

HOSPITAL PRACTICE. see *MEDICAL SCIENCES*

658 USA
HOSPITAL PRODUCT COMPARISON SYSTEM. Variant title: Healthcare Product Comparison System: Hospital Edition. Text in English. 1982. m. USD 1,049.60 domestic; USD 1,149.80 in Canada; USD 1,295 elsewhere (effective 2002). *Refereed.* **Description:** Designed for overall hospital technology purchasing and capital equipment planning. Topics covered range from anesthesia units to wheelchairs.
Related titles: CD-ROM ed.
Published by: (Emergency Care Research Institute), E C R I, 5200 Butler Pike, Plymouth, PA 19462. TEL 610-825-6000, FAX 610-834-1275, info@ecri.org, http://www.ecri.org. Ed. Nanette Bross.

HOSPITAL PRODUCTS ASIA. see *MEDICAL SCIENCES—Experimental Medicine, Laboratory Technique*

HOSPITAL SECURITY AND SAFETY MANAGEMENT. see *CRIMINOLOGY AND LAW ENFORCEMENT—Security*

658 600 USA ISSN 0888-711X
HOSPITAL TECHNOLOGY SERIES. (Three-part Series: Technology Scanner, Feature Reports, Special Report) Text in English. 1981. m. USD 325 to non-members; USD 225 to members. **Document type:** *Newsletter.* **Description:** Covers trends and developments in medical technology and technology management that have strategic planning implications.
Formerly (until 1982): A H A Hospital Technology Series (0735-4681)
Indexed: Int.Nurs.Ind.
—CISTI.
Published by: American Hospital Association, One North Franklin, Chicago, IL 60606-3421. TEL 312-422-3830, FAX 312-422-4571. Ed. Suzanna Hoppszallern.

658 USA ISSN 0018-5868
RA960
HOSPITAL TOPICS. Text in English. 1922. q., latest vol.80, 2002. USD 41 domestic to individuals; USD 54 foreign to individuals; USD 76 domestic to institutions; USD 89 foreign to institutions; USD 19 newsstand/cover (effective 2001 - 2002). adv. bk.rev. reprints avail. *Refereed.* **Document type:** *Academic/Scholarly.*
Formerly: Hospital Topics and Buyer's Guide (0093-173X)
Related titles: CD-ROM ed.: (from ProQuest Information & Learning); Microform ed.: (from PQC); Online - full text ed.: (from Ovid Technologies, Inc., Northern Light Technology, Inc., ProQuest Information & Learning, Gale Group, LexisNexis).
Indexed: ASSIA, Abstr.Health Care Manage.Stud., AgeLine, CINAHL, Excerp.Med., Hosp.Lit.Ind., I.P.A., Ind.Med. (coverage dropped), Int.Nurs.Ind.
—BLDSC (4333.210000), CISTI, GNLM, ingenta. **CCC.**
Published by: Heldref Publications, 1319 Eighteenth St, N W, Washington, DC 20036-1802. TEL 202-296-6267, FAX 202-296-5149, http://www.heldref.org. Ed. Julia Goodwin. Adv. contact Ali Mayhew. Circ: 1,000.

HOSPITAL VARGAS. ARCHIVOS. see *MEDICAL SCIENCES*

362 USA ISSN 1049-3662
HOSPITAL WATCH; a quarterly report on hospitals in New York City. Text in English. 1990. q. free per issue. **Document type:** *Newsletter.* **Description:** Discusses trends in use, operations, and financial performance of voluntary and municipal hospitals in New York City.
Related titles: Online - full content ed.
Published by: United Hospital Fund of New York, 350 Fifth Ave, Fl 23, New York, NY 10118-2399. TEL 212-494-0700, FAX 212-494-0800, pbrooks@uhfnyc.org, http://www.uhfnyc.org.

362 BEL ISSN 0018-5914
HOSPITALIA. Text in Flemish. 1956. q. BEF 1,000. adv. bk.rev. bibl, charts, illus.
Indexed: Excerp.Med.
—GNLM.
Published by: Verbond der Verzorgingsinstellingen, Guimardstraat 1, Brussels 1040, Belgium. FAX 02-513-52-69. Ed. A Aernoudt. Circ: 2,000.

362 CHE ISSN 0018-5930
HOSPITALIS. Text in French, German. 1930. 10/yr. CHF 118.30 (effective 2001). adv. illus. **Document type:** *Magazine, Trade.*
Related titles: Online - full text ed.: (from The Dialog Corporation).
Indexed: Archit.Per.Ind., Med.Care Rev.
—GNLM.
Published by: Hospitalis Verlag AG, Poststr 5, Postfach 4876, Zuerich 8022, Switzerland. TEL 41-1-2221380, FAX 41-1-2221381, hospital@active.ch, http://www.hospitalis.ch. Ed. Dr. Norbert Satz. Pub. Carlo Reimann. Adv. contact Ernst Muerner. B&W page CHF 2,100, color page CHF 3,870; trim 185 x 260. Circ: 11,200 (controlled).

658 FRA ISSN 0751-5766
HOSPITALISATION NOUVELLE. Text in French. 1971. m. (10/yr.). FRF 620 (effective 1998). adv. bk.rev. **Document type:** *Newspaper.*
Published by: Union Hospitaliere Privee, 17 bis bd. Pasteur, Paris 75015, France. TEL 33-1-44385252, http://www.uhp.tm.fr. Ed. Alain Coulomb. Adv. contact Sylvie Petit. Circ: 5,000.

658 FRA ISSN 0439-6162
HOSPITALISATION PRIVEE; revue d'information hospitaliere. Text in French. 1962. bi-m. FRF 640. adv. bk.rev. illus, stat. **Document type:** *Bulletin.*
Published by: Federation Intersyndicale des Etablissements d'Hospitalisation Privee, 81 rue de Monceau, Paris 75008, France. TEL 33-1-53837757, FAX 33-1-43599180. Ed. Dr. Louis Serfaty. Adv. contact Alexandre Savy. Circ: 4,300.

H

362.1 AUS
HOSPITALS AND HEALTH SERVICES BUYERS GUIDE. Text in English. 1973. a. AUD 175 comes with Hospital and Health Services Year Book (effective 2000). **Document type:** *Directory.* **Description:** Contains information on companies supplying health-related products and services. Companies are classified according to their specific activity.
Supersedes in part: Hospitals and Health Services Yearbook and Buyers Guide (0817-5004); Former titles: Hospitals and Health Services Yearbook and Equipment Catalogue (0817-5004); (until 1987): Hospitals and Health Services Yearbook (0810-7513); Hospitals and Health Services Yearbook, Australia (0156-3718); (until 1977): Australian Hospitals and Health Services Yearbook (0312-5599); (until 1975): Australian and New Zealand Hospitals and Health Services Yearbook (0084-7208)
Related titles: CD-ROM ed.: AUD 1,500 comes with Hospitals and Health Services Year Book (effective 2000).
Published by: (School of Health Administration, University of New South Wales), A P N Business Information Group (Subsidiary of: A P N News & Media Ltd), 46-48 Porter St Prahran, Melburne, VIC 3181, Australia. TEL 61-3-9245-7777, FAX 61-3-9245-7840, info@kompass.com.au, http://www.kompass.com. Circ: 5,000.

362.1 AUS
HOSPITALS AND HEALTH SERVICES YEAR BOOK. Text in English. 1973. a. AUD 175 includes Buyers Guide; download facility extra cost (effective 2000). **Document type:** *Directory, Trade.* **Description:** Details hospitals and health service establishments in Australia.
Supersedes in part: Hospitals and Health Services Yearbook and Buyers Guide; Former titles: Hospitals and Health Services Yearbook and Equipment Catalogue (0817-5004); (until 1987): Hospitals and Health Services Yearbook (0810-7513); Hospitals and Health Services Yearbook, Australia (0156-3718); (until 1977): Australian Hospitals and Health Services Yearbook (0312-5599); (until 1975): Australian and New Zealand Hospitals and Health Services Yearbook (0084-7208)
Related titles: CD-ROM ed.: AUD 1,500 (effective 2000).
Published by: A P N Business Information Group (Subsidiary of: A P N News & Media Ltd), 46-48 Porter St Prahran, Melburne, VIC 3181, Australia. TEL 61-3-9245-7777, FAX 61-3-9245-7840, info@kompass.com.au, http://www.kompass.com.

658 JPN ISSN 0389-696X
HOSUPITARU/FUKUOKA HOSPITAL ASSOCIATION. JOURNAL. Text in Japanese. 1973. m. JPY 5,000.
Published by: Fukuokaken Byoin Kyokai, 14-5 Akasaka 1-chome, Chuo-ku, Fukuoka-shi 810-0042, Japan.

610 658 USA ISSN 1066-1565
HOW TO GET PAID. Text in English. 1989. m. USD 99 (effective 2000). adv. **Document type:** *Newsletter, Trade.* **Description:** Helps patient-accounts managers in physicians offices collect accounts payable more effectively.
Formerly (until 1992): Professional Collections Manager (1045-0181)
Published by: Opus Communications, PO Box 1168, Marblehead, MA 01945. TEL 800-331-5196, FAX 781-639-7857, bhawksley@hcpro.com, http://www.hcmarketplace.com. Ed. Ann Mead-Ash. Pub. Jennifer Cofer. R&P Bethany Hawksley. Circ: 24,000.

362.11 614 FRA
HYGIENES. Text in French; Summaries in English, French. 1993. q. FRF 270; FRF 325 foreign (effective 1999). adv. Supplement avail.; back issues avail. *Refereed.* **Description:** Publishes original peer-reviewed articles on hospital infections, health care quality and safety, and related subjects. For professionals involved in infection control and epidemiology.
Published by: (Societe Francaise d'Hygiene Hospitaliere), SePres, 119 rue de Crequi, PO Box 6141, Lyon Cedex 6 69466, France. TEL 33-4-72830830, http://www.pgpromotion.fr. Ed. B Grynfogel. Pub. J Fabry. Adv. contact J Courret. Circ: 3,000 (paid); 500 (controlled).

658 JPN ISSN 0913-7262
HYOGO KENRITSU KODOMO BYOIN NENPO/HYOGO PREFECTURAL KOBE CHILDREN'S HOSPITAL. ANNUAL REPORT. Text in Japanese. a.
Published by: Hyogo Kenritsu Kodomo Byoin, 1-1 Takakuradai 1-chome, Suma-ku, Kobe-shi, Hyogo-ken 654-0081, Japan.

658 362.6 GBR
I H A FOCUS. Text in English. q. membership. **Document type:** *Newsletter.*
Formerly: I H A Bulletin
Published by: Independent Healthcare Association, 22 Little Russell St, London WC1A 2HT, United Kingdom. TEL 44-171-430-0537, FAX 44-171-242-2681. Ed. Barry Hassell. Circ: (controlled).

362 658 GBR
I H F MANAGEMENT HANDBOOKS. Text in English. irreg. GBP 9.50. back issues avail. **Document type:** *Monographic series, Trade.* **Description:** Explores various aspects of hospital management.
Published by: International Hospital Federation, 4 Abbots Pl, London NW6 4NP, United Kingdom. TEL 44-207-372-7181, FAX 44-207-328-7433. R&P Carl Richmond.

I H S M HEALTH & SOCIAL SERVICES YEARBOOK. see *PUBLIC HEALTH AND SAFETY*

362.11068 USA ISSN 1520-8591
I T HEALTH CARE STRATEGIST. Text in English. m. USD 446 to individuals; USD 45 newsstand/cover (effective 2002). **Document type:** *Newsletter, Trade.* **Description:** Delivers practical information to prepare CIOs and CEOs for their daily challenges. Covers topics such as: staff recruiting and retention; integrating systems in a multi-vendor environment; computer-based patient records; Y2K conversion; data mining; legal issues; information technology (IT) interrelationships; the Health Insurance Portability and Accountability Act (HIPAA); and confidentiality.
Related titles: Online - full text ed.: (from ProQuest Information & Learning).
—CCC.
Published by: Aspen Publishers, Inc., 200 Orchard Ridge Dr, Ste 200, Gaithersburg, MD 20878. TEL 301-417-7500, 800-638-8437, FAX 301-695-7931, customer.service@aspenpubl.com, http://www.aspenpub.com. Ed. Jeannie Mjoseth. **Dist. by:** Aspen Publishers Inc., Distribution Center, 7201 McKinney Circle, Frederick, MD 21701. TEL 301-698-7100, FAX 301-417-7550.

IBARAKI KENRITSU BYOIN IGAKU ZASSHI/IBARAKI PREFECTURAL HOSPITAL. MEDICAL JOURNAL. see *MEDICAL SCIENCES*

INCITAMENT/INCENTIVE; foer en haelso och sjukvaard i foervandling. see *MEDICAL SCIENCES*

362.4 GBR
INDEPENDENT HEALTHCARE ASSOCIATION. INITIAL DISCUSSION PAPER. Text in English. irreg. GBP 5 per issue. **Document type:** *Monographic series.* **Description:** Discusses issues in U.K. health care.
Published by: Independent Healthcare Association, 22 Little Russell St, London WC1A 2HT, United Kingdom. TEL 44-171-430-0537, FAX 44-171-242-2681.

658 GBR
INDEPENDENT HEALTHCARE DECISIONS. Text in English. 1997. a. GBP 55. adv. **Document type:** *Journal, Trade.* **Description:** Contains technical papers and case studies that discuss the success of many worldwide projects and developments in the healthcare sector.
Formerly: Independent Health Facilities (1365-8794)
Published by: Sterling Publications Ltd. (Subsidiary of: Sterling Publishing Group Plc.), Brunel House, 55-57 North Wharf Rd, London W2 1LA, United Kingdom. TEL 44-20-7915-9660, FAX 44-20-7724-2089, ihf@sterlingpublications.com, info@sterlingpublications.com, http://www.sterlingpublications.com/publications/healthcaredecisions.html. Pub. Sarah Woddis. Circ: 10,000 (controlled).

INFECTION CONTROL TODAY. see *MEDICAL SCIENCES—Communicable Diseases*

658 FRA ISSN 0180-2224
INFIRMIERS* . Text in French. 1977. m. FRF 280. adv. **Description:** Information for black African French-speaking nurses.
Published by: Sopepharm, 15 rue du Nord, Argenteuil 95100, France. TEL 39-82-02-02, FAX 39-80-84-60. Ed. Dr. Claude Richir. Circ: 5,000.

658 610.73 DEU ISSN 0341-0595
INFORMATIONSDIENST KRANKENHAUSWESEN/ HEALTH CARE INFORMATION SERVICE. Text and summaries in English, German. 1969. bi-m. DEM 195 (effective 2000). bk.rev. cum.index. back issues avail. **Document type:** *Abstract/Index.*
Related titles: Online - full text ed.: (from DIMDI).
—GNLM.
Published by: Technische Universitaet Berlin, Institut fuer Gesundheitswesen, Str des 17 Juni 135, Berlin 10623, Germany. TEL 49-30-31423980, FAX 49-30-31424743, heclinet@tu-berlin.de, http://www.heclinet.tu-berlin.de. Ed. Ruediger Schneemann. Circ: 400.

658 CHE
DER INSELBOTE. Text in German. q.
Published by: Inselspital Bern, Bern 3010, Switzerland. TEL 031-642974. Circ: 5,750.

H

362 USA ISSN 1073-6506
INSIDE AMBULATORY CARE. Text in English. 1994. m. USD 226 domestic; USD 271 foreign (effective 2000). **Document type:** *Trade.* **Description:** Focuses on the day-to-day management concerns of all ambulatory care and outpatient services managers. Covers innovations and trends in ambulatory care at hospitals and freestanding centers nationwide.
Related titles: Online - full text ed.: (from ProQuest Information & Learning).
Indexed: CINAHL.
—BLDSC (4518.151630), Infotrieve. **CCC.**
Published by: Aspen Publishers, Inc., 200 Orchard Ridge Dr, Ste 200, Gaithersburg, MD 20878. TEL 301-417-7500, 800-638-8437, FAX 301-417-7550, customer.service@aspenpubl.com, http://www.aspenpub.com. Ed. Linda Chitwood. **Dist. by:** Aspen Publishers Inc., Distribution Center, 7201 McKinney Circle, Frederick, MD 21701. TEL 301-698-7100, FAX 301-695-7931.

362.1 USA
INSIDE C M S. (Inside Centers Medicare/Medicine Services) Text in English. 1998. bi-w. USD 545 in US & Canada; USD 595 elsewhere (effective 2001). **Document type:** *Newsletter.*
Formerly (until 2001): Inside H C F A
Related titles: E-mail ed.
Published by: Inside Washington Publishers, PO Box 7167, Ben Franklin Sta, Washington, DC 20044-7167. TEL 703-416-8500, FAX 703-416-8543. Eds. Bob Cusack, John Grano.

362 USA
INSIDE INFORMATION. Text in English. 1995. m. **Document type:** *Newsletter.*
Related titles: Online - full text ed.
Published by: University of Virginia Health System, PO Box 800722, Charlottesville, VA 22908. TEL 804-924-0054, inside.info@virginia.edu, http://www.med.virginia.ed/hs-library/newsletter/. Ed. Mike Wilson.

658 616.8 362.2 USA
INSIGHTS (BELLE MEAD). Text in English. q. free per issue. adv. **Document type:** *Newsletter.* **Description:** Discusses the in and outpatient services this psychiatric hospital offers and covers topics in psychiatric and psychological therapy and treatment.
Indexed: e-psyche.
Published by: Carrier Foundation, Marketing and Community Relations Department, Belle Mead, NJ 08502. TEL 908-281-1518, FAX 908-874-4818, http://www.carrier.org. Ed. Jennifer Weston. Adv. contact Kelly Griffin.

INSTITUTE OF HEALTH RECORD INFORMATION & MANAGEMENT. JOURNAL. see *MEDICAL SCIENCES*

INTERNATIONAL CENTER FOR THE DISABLED. ANNUAL REPORT. see *HANDICAPPED*

362 AUS ISSN 1443-4636
INTERNATIONAL HOSPITAL & AGED CARE JOURNAL. Text in English. 1989. bi-m. AUD 124 domestic; AUD 186 foreign (effective 2000); AUD 20 newsstand/cover. adv. bk.rev. charts, illus, stat. back issues avail. **Document type:** *Academic/Scholarly.* **Description:** Provides information for management personnel on the crusade for world's best practice in hospitals, nursing homes and retirement villages.
Former titles (until 1999): Australian Health and Aged Care Journal (1325-5991); (until 1994): The Retirement Industry Journal (1038-1589)

Published by: Australian Health & Aged Care Journal, PO Box 513, Mudgeeraba, QLD 4213, Australia. TEL 61-7-5530-2888, FAX 61-7-5530-3944, ihacj@onthenet.com.au. Ed. Susan Hook. Pub. Karen Linnell. adv.: color page AUD 3,250. Circ: 6,900.

362 GBR ISSN 1366-0756
INTERNATIONAL JOURNAL OF HEALTH CARE QUALITY ASSURANCE INCORPORATING LEADERSHIP IN HEALTH SERVICES. Text in English. 1997. q. (Published quarterly as a center section to International Journal of Health Care Quality Assurance.). EUR 879 in Europe; USD 839 in North America in the UK & rest of the world; AUD 1,039 in Australasia; GBP 519 in the UK & rest of the world (effective 2002). **Document type:** *Journal, Academic/Scholarly.*
Incorporates (in 1996): Leadership in Health Services (1188-3669); Which was formed by the merger of (1977-1992): Hospital Trustee (0704-0407); (1974-1992): Dimensions in Health Service (0317-7645); Which was formerly (1924-1973): Canadian Hospital (0008-3798)
Related titles: Online - full text ed.: (from RoweCom Information Quest); ♦ Supplement to: International Journal of Health Care Quality Assurance. ISSN 0952-6862.
Published by: Emerald, 60-62 Toller Ln, Bradford, W Yorks BD8 9BY, United Kingdom. http://www.emeraldinsight.com/lhs.htm. Eds. Ardelle Harrison, Robin Gourlay.

▼ **INTERNATIONAL JOURNAL OF HEALTHCARE TECHNOLOGY AND MANAGEMENT.** see *MEDICAL SCIENCES—Computer Applications*

658 IRL
IRISH HOSPITAL. Text in English. 6/yr. bk.rev.
Published by: McCann - McGuirk Presentations, 7 Greenmount House, Harold's Cross Rd, Dublin 6W, Ireland. TEL 532497, FAX 544179. Ed. Lindie Naughton. Circ: 3,005.

IRYO KIKI GYOSHA NENKAN/JAPANESE MEDICAL INDUSTRY DIRECTORY. see *BUSINESS AND ECONOMICS—Trade And Industrial Directories*

ISHIKAWA KENRITSU CHUO BYOIN IGAKUSHI/ ISHIKAWA PREFECTURAL CENTRAL HOSPITAL. MEDICAL JOURNAL. see *MEDICAL SCIENCES*

658 JPN ISSN 0916-3387
IWAKI KYORITSU BYOIN IHO/IWAKI KYORITSU GENERAL HOSPITAL. JOURNAL. Text in English, Japanese. 1978. irreg.
Published by: Iwaki Shiritsu Sogo Iwaki Kyoritsu Byoin, 16, Kusehara, Uchigomimayamachi, Iwaki-shi, Fukushima-ken 973, Japan.

658 JPN ISSN 0289-1484
IWAMIZAWA SHIRITSU SOGO BYOIN ISHI/IWAMIZAWA MUNICIPAL GENERAL HOSPITAL. JOURNAL. Text in Japanese. 1975. a.
Published by: Iwamizawa Shiritsu Sogo Byoin, Nishi 7-chome, 9-jo, Iwamizawa-shi, Hokkaido 068, Japan.

IWATE KENRITSU BYOIN IGAKKAI ZASSHI/IWATE PREFECTURAL HOSPITAL. MEDICAL JOURNAL. see *MEDICAL SCIENCES*

IWATE KENRITSU MIYAKO BYOIN IGAKU ZASSHI/IWATE PREFECTURAL MIYAKO HOSPITAL. MEDICAL JOURNAL. see *MEDICAL SCIENCES*

IYAKUHIN SOGO SAYO KENKYU/RESEARCH ON DRUG ACTIONS AND INTERACTIONS. see *PHARMACY AND PHARMACOLOGY*

362.11 USA ISSN 1065-0881
JENKS HEALTHCARE BUSINESS REPORT. Text in English. 1988. s-m., latest vol.11, no.11, June 13, 2000. USD 325 domestic; USD 325 in Canada; USD 325 foreign; USD 550 for 2 yrs. domestic; USD 260 to institutions (effective Jan. 2002). **Document type:** *Newsletter, Trade.* **Description:** Reports on the growth strategies of managed care providers, hospitals, drug companies, medical device manufacturers and other healthcare organizations.
Related titles: Alternate Frequency ed.: s-m.
Published by: Irving Levin Associates, Inc., 237 Elm St. 2nd Floor, New Canaan, CT 06840. TEL 800-248-1668, monroe@levinassociates.com, meredith@levinassociates.com, http://www.jenkshealthcare.com.

362.1 USA ISSN 1070-3241
RA399.A3
THE JOINT COMMISSION JOURNAL ON QUALITY IMPROVEMENT. Text in English. 1974-1996; resumed. m. USD 175 domestic; USD 200 in Canada; USD 215 elsewhere (effective 2000). adv. bk.rev. abstr, bibl, illus. Index. reprints avail. *Refereed.* **Document type:** *Academic/Scholarly.* **Description:** Provides current information on measuring, assessing, and improving the performance of health care organizations.
Formerly (until 1993): Q R B - Quality Review Bulletin (0097-5990)
Indexed: ASCA, Abstr.Health Care Manage.Stud., AgeLine, CINAHL, Curr.Cont. (coverage dropped), Excerp.Med. (until 1993), Hosp.Abstr., Hosp.Lit.Ind., I.P.A., Ind.Med. (1993-), Int.Nurs.Ind., Med.Care Rev., Rehabil.Lit., SSCI (coverage dropped), Soc.Work Res.& Abstr., Sociol.Abstr.
—BLDSC (4672.252450), CISTI, GNLM, IDS, ingenta, KNAW.
Published by: Joint Commission on Accreditation of Healthcare Organizations, 75 Remittance Dr, Ste 1057, Chicago, IL 60675-1057. http://www.jcaho.org. Ed. G Jake Jaquet. Adv. contact Jo Ann Anzalone. B&W page USD 805; trim 11 x 8.25. Circ: 7,955.

658 USA ISSN 1062-2551
JOURNAL FOR HEALTHCARE QUALITY. Text in English. 1979. bi-m., latest vol.23. USD 105 domestic to individuals; USD 150 domestic to institutions; USD 175 foreign (effective 2001). adv. bk.rev. back issues avail. *Refereed.* **Document type:** *Academic/Scholarly.* **Description:** Provides information on state-of-the art technology, management techniques, practical applications of systems, improvement innovations and other specialties in the field of healthcare quality.
Formerly (until 1992): Journal of Quality Assurance (1062-0273)
Indexed: CINAHL, Int.Nurs.Ind.
—BLDSC (4996.872300), CISTI, GNLM.
Published by: National Association for Healthcare Quality, 4700 W Lake Ave, Glenview, IL 60025-1485. TEL 847-375-4720, 800-966-9392, FAX 847-375-4777, info@nahq.org, http://www.nahq.org. Ed. Luc R Pelletier. R&P Barbara Simmons. Adv. contact Noreen Rosdahl. B&W page USD 1,145; trim 11 x 8.5. Circ: 7,750.

610 USA ISSN 0148-9917
RA411
JOURNAL OF AMBULATORY CARE MANAGEMENT. Text in English. 1978. q. USD 172 to individuals; USD 52 newsstand/cover (effective 2002). reprint service avail. from PQC. **Document type:** *Journal, Trade.* **Description:** Provides tips on enhancing productivity to effective accounting systems that can be implemented now. Includes actual case studies, practical guidance and proven hands-on management techniques of leading practitioners in health care settings across the country.
Related titles: Microform ed.: (from PQC); Online - full text ed.: (from Ovid Technologies, Inc., ProQuest Information & Learning).
Indexed: Abstr.Health Care Manage.Stud., AgeLine, CINAHL, Excerp.Med., Int.Nurs.Ind., Med.Care Rev.
—BLDSC (4927.220000), CISTI, GNLM, ingenta, KNAW. **CCC.**
Published by: Aspen Publishers, Inc., 200 Orchard Ridge Dr, Ste 200, Gaithersburg, MD 20878. TEL 301-417-7500, 800-638-8437, FAX 301-695-7931, customer.service@aspenpubl.com, http://www.aspenpub.com. Ed. Norbert Goldfield. **Dist. by:** Aspen Publishers Inc., Distribution Center, 7201 McKinney Circle, Frederick, MD 21701. TEL 301-698-7100, FAX 301-417-7550.

362.11068 610 USA ISSN 1079-6533
JOURNAL OF CLINICAL OUTCOMES MANAGEMENT. Abbreviated title: J C O M. Text in English. 1994. m., latest vol.8. USD 100 domestic; USD 115 in Canada (effective 2000). adv. index. reprint service avail. from PQC. *Refereed.* **Document type:** *Academic/Scholarly.* **Description:** Covers clinical outcomes, outcomes research, clinical reviews and outcomes in practices, for physicians in managed-care practices and executives of managed-care organizations.
Related titles: Microfilm ed.
Indexed: Inpharma, Pharm.&Out.News, Reac.
—BLDSC (4663.443150).
Published by: Turner White Communications, Inc., 125 Strafford Ave, Ste 220, Wayne, PA 19087-3391. TEL 610-975-4541, FAX 610-975-4564, webmaster@turner-white.com, brucewhite@turner-white.com, http://www.turner-white.com. Ed. Bobbie Lewis. Pub., Adv. contact Bruce White. R&P Lisa Hollister. color page USD 5,510; trim 10.75 x 7.88. Circ: 70,192.

362.110711 USA ISSN 0735-6722
RA440.6
JOURNAL OF HEALTH ADMINISTRATION EDUCATION✱ Text in English; Summaries in Spanish. 1983. q. USD 85; USD 70 foreign. bk.rev. bibl, charts, illus, stat. back issues avail.; reprints avail. **Document type:** *Academic/Scholarly.*
Indexed: Abstr.Anthropol., Abstr.Health Care Manage.Stud., Hosp.Lit.Ind., Int.Nurs.Ind.
—BLDSC (4996.690000), GNLM, ingenta.
Published by: Association of University Programs in Health Administration, 730 11th St N W, 4th Fl, Washington, DC 20001-4510. TEL 202-822-8550, FAX 202-822-8555, http://www.aupha.org. Ed. Cindy Liedtke. Circ: 1,600.

658 614.8 USA ISSN 1079-3739
RA1 CODEN: JHHAEJ
JOURNAL OF HEALTH AND HUMAN SERVICES ADMINISTRATION. Text in English. 1978. q. USD 65 to individuals; USD 90 to libraries (effective 2001). bk.rev. index. back issues avail. *Refereed.* **Document type:** *Academic/Scholarly.*
Formerly (until 1995): Journal of Health and Human Resources Administration (0160-4198)
Indexed: Abstr.Health Care Manage.Stud., Abstr.Soc.Geront., AgeLine, BPIA, CINAHL, Environ.Sci.Poll.Mgmt., Excerp.Med., Fam.Ind., Int.Nurs.Ind., Manage.Cont., Med.Care Rev., P.A.I.S., Pollut.Abstr., Rehabil.Lit., Risk Abstr., Soc.Work Res.& Abstr., Viol.& Abuse Abstr.
—BLDSC (4996.704000), GNLM, ingenta.
Published by: Southern Public Administration Education Foundation, Inc., c/o Jack Rabin, 2103 Fairway Ln, Harrisburg, PA 17112. TEL 717-540-1383, FAX 717-893-1763, spaef@prodigy.net, http://www.spaef.com. Eds. Jack Rabin, Thomas Vocino. Circ: 800.

657.832 330 USA ISSN 1078-6767
RA410.A1 CODEN: JHCFFA
JOURNAL OF HEALTH CARE FINANCE. Text in English. 1974. q. USD 185 to individuals; USD 56 newsstand/cover (effective 2002). adv. illus. reprints avail. *Refereed.* **Document type:** *Journal, Trade.* **Description:** Presents strategies for controlling costs, boosting revenues, eliminating waste, maximizing utilization, evaluating pricing, managing investments, and improving productivity.
Formerly: Topics in Health Care Financing (0095-3814)
Related titles: Microform ed.: (from PQC); Online - full text ed.: (from ProQuest Information & Learning, Gale Group, Ovid Technologies, Inc., Factiva).
Indexed: ABI Inform. (Fall 1983-), Abstr.Health Care Manage.Stud., AgeLine, B.P.I. (Jan.1982-Sep.1994), BPIA, Bus.Ind., CINAHL, Excerp.Med., Hlth.Ind., Ind.Med. (1994-), Int.Nurs.Ind., L.R.I., Med.Care Rev., Tr.& Indus.Ind.
—BLDSC (4996.736000), GNLM, ingenta, KNAW. **CCC.**
Published by: Aspen Publishers, Inc., 200 Orchard Ridge Dr, Ste 200, Gaithersburg, MD 20878. TEL 301-417-7500, 800-638-8437, FAX 301-695-7931, customer.service@aspenpubl.com, http://www.aspenpub.com. Ed. James J Unland. **Dist. by:** Aspen Publishers Inc., Distribution Center, 7201 McKinney Circle, Frederick, MD 21701. TEL 301-698-7100, FAX 301-417-7550.

JOURNAL OF HEALTH ECONOMICS. see *PUBLIC HEALTH AND SAFETY*

▼ **JOURNAL OF HEALTH MANAGEMENT.** see *MEDICAL SCIENCES*

JOURNAL OF HEALTH POLITICS, POLICY AND LAW. see *MEDICAL SCIENCES*

362 USA ISSN 1068-1124
RA967
JOURNAL OF HEALTHCARE DESIGN✱ . Text in English. 1989. a. USD 40; USD 45 foreign (effective 1998). **Document type:** *Proceedings.* **Description:** Covers how design can contribute to quality healthcare.
Formerly (until 1992): Journal of Health Care Interior Design (1068-1132)
Indexed: Int.Nurs.Ind.
Published by: Center for Health Design, Inc., 3470 Mt Diablo Blvd, No A150, Lafayette, CA 94549-3977. TEL 510-370-0345, FAX 510-228-4018, ctr4hd@aol.com, http://www.healthdesign.org. Ed. Sara Marberry. R&P Debra Levin. Circ: 1,500.

362 USA ISSN 1096-9012
RA971 CODEN: JHMAFB
JOURNAL OF HEALTHCARE MANAGEMENT. Text in English. 1956. q. USD 65; USD 75 foreign (effective 1998). bk.rev. illus. reprint service avail. from PQC. *Refereed.* **Document type:** *Academic/Scholarly.* **Description:** Provides information on the latest trends, developments, and innovations in the health services field.
Former titles: Hospital and Health Services Administration (8750-3735); Hospital Administration (0018-5523)
Related titles: Microform ed.: (from PQC); Online - full text ed.: (from Gale Group, ProQuest Information & Learning, Ovid Technologies, Inc., Factiva, Institute for Scientific Information).
Indexed: ABI Inform. (Jan.1984-), ASCA, Abstr.Health Care Manage.Stud., Account.Ind. (1974-), AgeLine, BPIA, Bus.Ind., CINAHL, Curr.Cont., Excerp.Med., Hlth.Ind., Hosp.Lit.Ind., I.P.A., Int.Nurs.Ind., L.R.I., Med.Care Rev., Rehabil.Lit., SSCI, Tr.& Indus.Ind.
—BLDSC (4996.870900), CISTI, EMDOCS, GNLM, IDS, Infotrieve, ingenta. **CCC.**
Published by: (Foundation of the American College of Healthcare Executives), Health Administration Press, 1 North Franklin St, Ste 1700, Chicago, IL 60606-3491. TEL 312-424-2800, FAX 312-424-0014, http://www.ache.org, http://www.hsr.org. Ed. James A Johnson. Circ: 28,000. **Subscr. to:** ACHE Publication Services, 1 N Franklin St, Ste 1700, Chicago, IL 60606-3420.

364.4 USA ISSN 0891-7930
JOURNAL OF HEALTHCARE PROTECTION MANAGEMENT. Text in English. 1985. 2/yr. USD 25 domestic; USD 45 foreign (effective 2001). **Document type:** *Trade.*
Indexed: Int.Nurs.Ind.
—BLDSC (4996.872000), CISTI.
Published by: Rusting Publications, PO Box 190, Port Washington, NY 11050. TEL 516-883-1440, FAX 516-883-1683. Ed., R&P Susan Krivin. Pub. Robert R Rusting. Circ: 1,500.

368.392 USA ISSN 1074-4797
RA971.38
JOURNAL OF HEALTHCARE RISK MANAGEMENT. Text in English. 1981. q. membership only. charts, illus. index, cum.index every 5 yrs. back issues avail. *Refereed.* **Document type:** *Trade.* **Description:** Information on quality assurance, professional liability claims management, loss prevention, risk financing, risk management program development, workers' compensation, and risk management legislation and legal issues.
Former titles: Perspectives in Healthcare Risk Management (0899-1073); (until 1987): Perspectives in Hospital Risk Management
Indexed: Int.Nurs.Ind.
Published by: (American Society for Healthcare Risk Management), American Hospital Association, One North Franklin, Chicago, IL 60606-3421. TEL 312-422-3989, FAX 312-422-4580. Ed. Trudy Goldman. Circ: 2,900.

▼ **JOURNAL OF HOSPITAL LIBRARIANSHIP.** see *LIBRARY AND INFORMATION SCIENCES*

JOURNAL OF HOSPITAL MARKETING & PUBLIC RELATIONS. see *BUSINESS AND ECONOMICS—Marketing And Purchasing*

JOURNAL OF J.J. GROUP OF HOSPITALS AND GRANT MEDICAL COLLEGE. see *MEDICAL SCIENCES*

JOURNAL OF MEDICAL ECONOMICS. see *MEDICAL SCIENCES*

JOURNAL OF MEDICAL SYSTEMS. see *MEDICAL SCIENCES—Computer Applications*

JOURNAL OF OUTCOMES RESEARCH. see *PHARMACY AND PHARMACOLOGY*

JOURNAL OF PALLIATIVE CARE. see *MEDICAL SCIENCES*

JOURNAL OF PUBLIC HEALTH POLICY. see *PUBLIC HEALTH AND SAFETY*

362 USA ISSN 1525-8610
▼ **JOURNAL OF THE AMERICAN MEDICAL DIRECTORS ASSOCIATION.** Text in English. 2000. bi-m., latest 2000. USD 120 domestic to individuals; USD 149 domestic to institutions; USD 143 foreign to individuals; USD 179 foreign to institutions (effective 2002). *Refereed.* **Document type:** *Journal, Trade.*
Related titles: Online - full text ed.: USD 193.70 domestic academic site license; USD 216.05 domestic corporate site license; USD 223.70 foreign academic site license; USD 246.05 foreign corporate site license (effective 2002).
Published by: (American Medical Directors Association), Lippincott Williams & Wilkins (Philadelphia) (Subsidiary of: Wolters Kluwer N.V.), 530 Walnut St, Philadelphia, PA 19106-3621. TEL 215-521-8300, FAX 215-521-8902, custserv@lww.com, http://www.lww.com/. Ed. Dr. Dan Osterweil. **Subscr. to:** PO Box 1600, Hagerstown, MD 21740-1600. TEL 800-638-3030, FAX 310-223-2400.

658 USA
JUST FOR YOU. Text in English. 1986. q. free per issue. adv. bk.rev.
Published by: Kase Publications, Inc., 83 N Central Ave, Ramsey, NJ 07446. TEL 201-818-9507. Ed. John E Baer. Circ: 190,000.

658 JPN
KAWASAKI SHIRITSU IDA BYOIN NENPO/KAWASAKI MUNICIPAL IDA HOSPITAL. ANNUAL REPORT. Text in Japanese. 1971. a.
Published by: Kawasaki Shiritsu Ida Byoin, 1272 Ida, Nakahara-ku, Kawasaki-shi, Kanagawa-ken 211-0035, Japan.

658 JPN
KAWASAKI SHIRITSU KAWASAKI BYOIN NENPO/KAWASAKI MUNICIPAL HOSPITAL. ANNUAL REPORT. Text in Japanese. 1965. a.
Published by: Kawasaki Shiritsu Kawasaki Byoin, 12-1 Shinkawa-Dori, Kawasaki-ku, Kawasaki-shi, Kanagawa-ken 210-0013, Japan.

KING'S GAZETTE; the journal of King's College Hospital. see *MEDICAL SCIENCES*

362 DEU ISSN 0023-4486
KRANKENDIENST; Zeitschrift fuer kath. Krankenhaeuser, Sozialstationen und Pflegeberufe. Text in German. 1920. 11/yr. EUR 36; EUR 4.10 newsstand/cover (effective 2002). adv. bk.rev. index. **Document type:** *Journal, Trade.*
—GNLM, Infotrieve. **CCC.**
Published by: (Katholischer Krankenhausverband Deutschlands e.V.), Lambertus-Verlag GmbH, Mitscherlichstr 56, Freiburg Im Breisgau 79108, Germany. TEL 49-761-36825-0, FAX 49-761-3682533, info@lambertus.de, http://www.lambertus.de. Ed. Werner Lauer. Circ: 4,000.

658 DEU ISSN 0340-3602
DAS KRANKENHAUS. Text in German. 1909. m. EUR 169.20, CHF 331; EUR 17.50, CHF 34.25 newsstand/cover (effective 2002). back issues avail.; reprints avail. **Document type:** *Journal, Trade.*
—GNLM. **CCC.**
Published by: (Deutsche Krankenhaus-Gesellschaft), W. Kohlhammer GmbH, Hessbruehlstr 69, Stuttgart 70565, Germany. TEL 49-711-7863-1, FAX 49-711-7863263, info@kohlhammer-katalog.de, http://www.kohlhammer.de. Ed. Peter Ossen.

658 DEU ISSN 0935-977X
KRANKENHAUS-FINANZIERUNGSRECHT. Text in German. 1981. irreg. DEM 148 (effective 2000). **Document type:** *Bulletin, Trade.*
Published by: Erich Schmidt Verlag GmbH & Co. (Berlin), Genthiner Str 30G, Berlin 10785, Germany. TEL 49-30-250085-0, FAX 49-30-25008521, vertrieb@esvmedien.de, http://www.erich-schmidt-verlag.de.

658 DEU ISSN 0720-3373
KRANKENHAUS-HYGIENE & INFEKTIONSVERHUETUNG. Text in German. 1978. 6/yr. EUR 87 (effective 2002). **Document type:** *Journal, Academic/Scholarly.*
Indexed: Abstr.Hyg., Nutr.Abstr.
—BLDSC (5118.141000), GNLM.
Published by: Urban & Fischer Verlag, Loebdergraben 14A, Jena 07743, Germany. TEL 49-3641-626444, FAX 49-3641-626421, info@urbanfischer.de, http://www.urbanfischer.de/journals. Eds. B Wille, Dr. Gerhard Schmidt-Burbach. Circ: 5,500.

658 DEU ISSN 0935-2112
KRANKENHAUS-RECHTSPRECHUNG. Text in German. 1983. irreg. (in 2 vols.). DEM 386 (effective 2000). **Document type:** *Bulletin.*
Published by: Erich Schmidt Verlag GmbH & Co. (Berlin), Genthiner Str 30G, Berlin 10785, Germany. TEL 49-30-250085-0, FAX 49-30-25008521, vertrieb@esvmedien.de, http://www.erich-schmidt-verlag.de.

658 DEU ISSN 0720-3977
KRANKENHAUS TECHNIK. Text in German. 1976. m. DEM 120 domestic; DEM 144 foreign; DEM 15 newsstand/cover (effective 2001). adv. index. back issues avail. **Document type:** *Magazine, Trade.*
—GNLM.
Published by: (Fachvereinigung Krankenhaustechnik e.V.), Ecomed Verlagsgesellschaft AG & Co. KG, Justus-von-Liebig-Str 1, Landsberg 86899, Germany. TEL 49-8191-125-0, FAX 49-8191-125513, info@ecomed.de, http://www.krankenhaus-technik.de, http://www.ecomed.de. adv.: B&W page DEM 4,300; trim 188 x 270. Circ: 9,000.

362 DEU ISSN 0023-4508
KRANKENHAUS UMSCHAU; das Hospital Management Magazin. Text in German. 1927. m. DEM 312 (effective 2000). adv. bk.rev. charts, illus, tr.lit. index, cum.index: 1949-1962. **Document type:** *Magazine, Trade.*
Indexed: Excerp.Med.
—GNLM, Infotrieve. **CCC.**
Published by: (Verband der Krankenhausdirektoren Deutschland e.V.), Baumann Fachverlag, E C Baumann Str 5, Kulmbach 95326, Germany. TEL 49-9221-949393, FAX 49-9221-949377. Ed. Angelika Beyer Rehfeld. Adv. contact Manfred Geist. B&W page DEM 3,560, color page DEM 5,930; trim 186 x 260. Circ: 6,000.

362.110 340 DEU ISSN 1434-2618
KRANKENHAUS UND RECHT. Text in German. 1997. bi-m. DEM 280 (effective 1999). **Document type:** *Academic/Scholarly.*
—GNLM.
Published by: P M I Verlag AG, August-Schanz-Str 8, Frankfurt Am Main 60433, Germany. TEL 49-69-548000-0, FAX 49-69-548000-77, pmiverlag@aol.com.

362 DEU ISSN 0023-4516
KRANKENHAUSARZT. Text in German. 1927. bi-m. DEM 74 domestic; DEM 82 in Europe; DEM 88 elsewhere (effective 1999). adv. bk.rev. abstr, bibl, charts, illus. index. **Document type:** *Bulletin.*
Indexed: Dok.Arbeitsmed., Excerp.Med. (1994-).
—GNLM, Infotrieve, KNAW. **CCC.**
Published by: G. Braun Buchverlag, Karl-Friedrich-Str 14-18, Karlsruhe 76133, Germany. TEL 49-721-165392, FAX 49-721-165103. Ed. H Spaeth. Circ: 20,000.

KUECHE IN KRANKENHAUS UND ALTENHEIM. see *FOOD AND FOOD INDUSTRIES*

362.1 658.8 NLD ISSN 0927-1449
KWALITEIT IN BEELD. Text in Dutch. 1991. bi-m. NLG 110 foreign. charts, illus. **Document type:** *Newsletter, Trade.* **Description:** Covers quality management in all areas of healthcare.
Published by: Elsevier Gezondheidszorg B.V., Tijdstroom (Subsidiary of: Reed Elsevier plc Group), Planetenbaan 1, Maarssen 3600 AK, Netherlands. TEL 31-346-577577, FAX 31-346-554287, http://www.tijdstroom.nl. **Subscr. to:** Elsevier Den Haag, Postbus 16500, The Hague 2500 BM, Netherlands. TEL 31-70-381-9900, FAX 31-70-333-8399.

LABORATORY COMPLIANCE INSIDER. see *LAW*

362.11 DNK ISSN 0107-1165
LAEGESTILLINGER OG SENGEPLADSER PAA INSTITUTIONER. Text in Danish. 1974. a. DKK 75.
Formerly: Normerede og Besatte Laegestillinger Samt Sengepladser paa Institutioner
Published by: Sundhedsstyrelsen, Amaliegade 13, PO Box 2020, Copenhagen K 1012, Denmark. **Subscr. to:** Statens Informationstjeneste, PO Box 1103, Copenhagen K 1009, Denmark.

THE LATEST WORD. see *MEDICAL SCIENCES*

LENGTH OF STAY BY D R G AND PAYMENT SOURCE. (Diagnosis Related Group) see *HEALTH FACILITIES AND ADMINISTRATION—Abstracting, Bibliographies, Statistics*

H

362 USA ISSN 1536-7517
▼ **LONG TERM CARE LITIGATION.** Text in English. 2001. m. USD 475 to individuals; USD 48 newsstand/cover (effective 2002). **Document type:** *Newsletter.* **Description:** Provides analysis of the legal and medical issues. Includes case summaries, jury awards, settlements, legislative and regulatory activity reports, trial tips and techniques, insurance reviews, news, and advice.
Published by: Aspen Publishers, Inc., 1185 Avenue of the Americas, New York, NY 10036. TEL 212-597-0200, FAX 212-597-0338, http://www.aspenpublishers.com.

618.97005 GBR ISSN 1467-6311
LONG-TERM HEALTH MANAGEMENT. Text in English. 1998. a. adv. **Document type:** *Journal, Trade.* **Description:** Provides analyses of the latest developments and trends as well as specific management, technology and drug developments that are essential to quality health care.
Formerly (until 1999): Future Care (1464-5505)
Published by: Sterling Publications Ltd. (Subsidiary of: Sterling Publishing Group Plc.), Brunel House, 55-57 North Wharf Rd, London W2 1LA, United Kingdom. TEL 44-20-7915-9660, FAX 44-20-7724-2089, lth@sterlingpublications.com, info@sterlingpublications.com, http://www.sterlingpublications.com/publications/longtermhealthmgmt.html. Pub. Sarah Woddis. Circ: 10,000 (controlled).

M G M A CONNEXION. (Medical Group Management Association) see *MEDICAL SCIENCES*

012 AUS
M I M S HOSPITAL EQUIPMENT & SUPPLIES DIRECTORY. Text in English. 1978. biennial. AUD 50 domestic; AUD 78 in New Zealand; AUD 90 in PNG, Asia & Pacific Region; AUD 90 in US & Middle East; AUD 111 elsewhere (effective 2000). adv. back issues avail. **Document type:** *Directory.* **Description:** Purchasing reference for equipment officers in hospitals and nursing homes.
Formerly: Hospital Equipment and Supplies (Year) (0159-9100)
Published by: M I M S Australia (Subsidiary of: Medimedia Australia), PO Box 3000, St Leonards, NSW 2065, Australia. TEL 61-2-9902-7700, FAX 61-2-99027701. Ed. Virginia Gagic. Pub. Chris Wills. R&P Amanda Caswell. Adv. contact Brian Parker. Circ: 4,500.

658 659.2 USA
M P R EXCHANGE. Text in English. 1974. bi-m. membership. **Document type:** *Newsletter.* **Description:** Information on public relations and marketing for hospitals.
Former titles: Hospital Marketing and Public Relations; Hospital Public Relations
Published by: (American Society for Health Care Marketing and Public Relations), American Hospital Association, One North Franklin, Chicago, IL 60606-3421. TEL 312-422-3740, FAX 312-422-4579. Ed. Lauren Barnett. Circ: 3,000.

MANAGED CARE; a guide for physicians. see *INSURANCE*

MANAGED CARE AND MEDICAL COST CONTAINMENT IN WORKER'S COMPENSATION: A NATIONAL INVENTORY (YEAR). see *INSURANCE*

362.1 USA ISSN 1096-5645
MANAGED CARE INTERFACE; today's experts tomorrow's health care. Text in English. 1988. m. USD 80 domestic to individuals; USD 100 foreign to individuals; USD 100 domestic to institutions; USD 120 foreign to institutions; USD 15 newsstand/cover domestic; USD 20 newsstand/cover foreign (effective 2001). adv. **Document type:** *Trade.* **Description:** Open forum for the managed health-care industry.
Formerly (until 1997): Medical Interface (0896-4831)
Related titles: ♦ Supplement: Executive Managed Care Directory. ISSN 1068-4557.
Indexed: CINAHL, I.P.A., Int.Nurs.Ind.
—BLDSC (5358.614500), Infotrieve. **CCC.**
Published by: Medicom International, Inc., 66 Palmer Ave, Ste 49, Bronxville, NY 10708. TEL 914-337-7878, FAX 914-337-5023, http://www.Medicomint.com. Ed. Stanton R Mehr. Pub. Raymond B Hargreaves. Adv. contact Charlotte Walsh. B&W page USD 5,294, color page USD 7,220; trim 10.88 x 8.13. Circ: 40,250 (controlled).

▼ **MANAGED CARE LAW STRATEGIST.** see *LAW*

362 USA ISSN 1093-5061
THE MANAGED CARE PAYMENT ADVISOR; capitation & alternative compensation methods. Text in English. 1997. m. USD 220 domestic; USD 264 foreign (effective 2000). **Document type:** *Trade.* **Description:** Provides how-to information to health care providers to improve their operations and help them to succeed in a managed care environment.
Related titles: Online - full text ed.: (from ProQuest Information & Learning).
—CCC.
Published by: Aspen Publishers, Inc., 200 Orchard Ridge Dr, Ste 200, Gaithersburg, MD 20878. TEL 301-417-7500, 800-638-8437, FAX 301-695-7931, customer.service@aspenpubl.com, http://www.aspenpub.com. Ed. Laura J Merisalo. **Dist. by:** Aspen Publishers Inc., Distribution Center, 7201 McKinney Circle, Frederick, MD 21701. TEL 301-698-7100, FAX 301-417-7550.

658 610 USA ISSN 1064-5454
RA413
MANAGED CARE QUARTERLY. Text in English. 1993. q. USD 175 to individuals; USD 53 newsstand/cover (effective 2002). adv. illus. reprint service avail. from PQC. **Document type:** *Journal, Trade.* **Description:** Provides current information to health care executives who require in-depth material on specific managed care issues.
Related titles: Microform ed.: (from PQC); Online - full text ed.: (from ProQuest Information & Learning).
Indexed: CINAHL, Inpharma, Int.Nurs.Ind., Pharm.&Out.News, Reac., Soc.Work Res.& Abstr.
—BLDSC (5358.630000), GNLM, Infotrieve, ingenta, KNAW. **CCC.**
Published by: Aspen Publishers, Inc., 200 Orchard Ridge Dr, Ste 200, Gaithersburg, MD 20878. TEL 301-417-7500, 800-638-8437, customer.service@aspenpubl.com, http://www.aspenpublishers.com. Ed. Allan Fine. Pub. Jane Coyle Garwood. Circ: 2,000 (paid). **Dist. by:** Aspen Publishers Inc., Distribution Center, 7201 McKinney Circle, Frederick, MD 21701. TEL 301-698-7100, FAX 301-417-7550.

362.1029 USA ISSN 1072-2815
RA413.5.U5
MANAGED HEALTH CARE DIRECTORY✶ **.** Text in English. 1991. a. USD 250. index. **Document type:** *Directory.* **Description:** Lists HMOs, PPOs, UROs, POS Plans, FMCs, addresses, phone and fax numbers, service, enrollment, provider contracts, and more.
Formed by the merger of (1985-1991): P P O Directory (Directory of Preferred Provider Organizations and the Industry Report on P P O Development) (0894-9891); (1986-1991): H M O Directory (Directory of Health Maintenance Organizations) (0894-9905)
Published by: American Managed Care and Review Association, 1129 20th St, N W, Ste 600, Washington, DC 20036-3403. TEL 202-728-0506, FAX 202-728-0609. Circ: 1,000.

362.104258 USA ISSN 1060-1392
RA413.5.U5
MANAGED HEALTHCARE; the news magazine for managers of health care costs and quality. Text in English. 1990. m. USD 64 domestic; USD 84 in Canada & Mexico; USD 124 elsewhere; USD 12 newsstand/cover (effective 2001). adv. back issues avail. **Document type:** *Trade.* **Description:** Delivers news and analysis editorial that addresses innovation in health care management and the many business, legal, and technical issues facing the world of managed health care.
Formerly: Managed Healthcare News (1060-1392)
Related titles: Online - full text ed.: (from H. W. Wilson).
Indexed: ABI Inform. (Sep.1994-), B.P.I. (Jan.2001-), I.P.A., Inpharma, Pharm.&Out.News, Reac.
—Infotrieve. **CCC.**
Published by: Advanstar Communications Inc., 201 E Sandpointe Ave Ste 600, Santa Ana, CA 92707. TEL 216-891-2615, FAX 216-891-2383, mhc-pce@en.com, fulfill@superfill.com, http://www.managedhcare.com. Ed. Timothy N Troy. Pub., Adv. contact Jennifer J Day. Circ: 40,000.

658 DEU ISSN 0176-053X
MANAGEMENT UND KRANKENHAUS; Informationsdienst fuer alle Fuehrungskraefte im Krankenhaus. Text in German. 1982. m. DEM 164 (effective 1999). adv. **Document type:** *Trade.*
Indexed: Anal.Abstr.
—GNLM.
Published by: G I T Verlag GmbH, Roesslerstr 90, Darmstadt 64293, Germany. TEL 49-6151-8090-0, FAX 49-6151-809044, gitverlaggmbh@gitverlag.com, http://www.gitverlag.com. Ed. Joerg Peter Matthes. Adv. contact Brigitte Pfeiff. B&W page DEM 9,115, color page DEM 12,705; trim 260 x 185. Circ: 40,000.

362.1108 658 USA ISSN 1099-3916
MARKET PROFILES FOR MEDICARE RISK CONTRACTING. Text in English. 1994. a. **Document type:** *Trade.* **Description:** Investigates regional market potential and risks associated with care for Medicare populations.
Related titles: CD-ROM ed.; E-mail ed.
Published by: Health Care Investment Analysts, Inc., 300 E Lombard St, Baltimore, MD 21201. TEL 410-752-6309, 800-568-3282, http://www.hcia.com.

658 USA ISSN 1059-4531
MATERIALS MANAGEMENT IN HEALTH CARE. Text in English. 1992. m. USD 40 domestic; USD 70 foreign; USD 5 newsstand/cover (effective 2001). **Document type:** *Trade.* **Description:** Covers the selection, purchase and distribution of healthcare supplies, materials, and services.
Related titles: Online - full text ed.: 1992 (from LexisNexis).
—BLDSC (5396.011000).
Published by: (American Society for Healthcare Materials Management), American Hospital Publishing, Inc. (Subsidiary of: American Hospital Association Company), 1 N Franklin St, 27th Fl, Chicago, IL 60606-3421. TEL 312-440-6800, FAX 312-951-8491, http://www.matmanmag.com/mat-home.html. Ed. Laura Souhrada. Circ: 23,300. **Co-sponsor:** American Society for Hospital Central Service Personnel.

MEALEY'S MANAGED CARE LIABILITY REPORT. see *LAW*

658 FRA ISSN 0025-6765
MEDECINE HOSPITALIERE/HOSPITAL MEDICINE. Text in French. 1964. bi-m. adv. **Document type:** *Trade.* **Description:** Information on trade-unionism.
Related titles: Microform ed.: (from PQC).
Indexed: Excerp.Med.
Published by: Syndicat National des Medecins, 56 rue de Vouille, Paris 75015, France. TEL 33-1-45-33-01-71, FAX 33-1-45-33-42-09. Ed. Dr. Etienne Weill. Circ: 3,500.

362 USA
MEDFAX. Text in English. w. (Monday Morning). USD 159 to individuals; USD 289 to institutions (effective 2001). **Document type:** *Trade.*
Media: Fax.
Published by: HealthLeaders, Inc., 66 Music Sq W, Nashville, TN 37203. TEL 615-385-4131, 888-293-9675, FAX 615-385-4979, medfax@healthleaders.com, http://www.healthleaders.com/.

MEDICAID MANAGED CARE CURRENTS. see *INSURANCE*

610 GBR ISSN 0305-3342
MEDICAL DIRECTORY; an alphabetical listing of medical practitioners registered in Britain. Text in English. a. GBP 175. adv. **Document type:** *Directory.* **Description:** Provides details of over 135,000 Medical Practitioners registered to practice in the UK and the Republic of Ireland. It also provides access to the whole range of health services and medical organisations in the UK.
Related titles: CD-ROM ed.: Medical Directory Database CD-ROM (Years). GBP 175.
—BLDSC (5527.070000), GNLM.
Published by: Financial Times Healthcare, Maple House, 149 Tottenham Ct Rd, London W1P 9LL, United Kingdom. TEL 44-20-7896-2424, FAX 44-20-7896-2449, lizg@pearson-pro.com, http://www.fthealthcare.com. Adv. contact Liz Godden. B&W page GBP 395.

657.832 USA ISSN 1078-1285
THE MEDICAL OFFICE BILLER; the communication network exclusively for billers in medical offices. Text in English. 1994. m. USD 175 domestic; USD 210 foreign (effective 2000). **Document type:** *Newsletter, Trade.* **Description:** For billers and billing managers in the medical office. Provides easy-to-understand information and tips on how to get bills out efficiently and avoid collection problems.
—CCC.

Published by: Aspen Publishers, Inc., 200 Orchard Ridge Dr, Ste 200, Gaithersburg, MD 20878. TEL 301-417-7500, 800-638-8437, FAX 301-695-7931, customer.service@aspenpul.com, http://www.aspenpub.com. Ed. Cheryl Sobun. **Dist. by:** Aspen Publishers Inc., Distribution Center, 7201 McKinney Circle, Frederick, MD 21701. TEL 301-698-7100, FAX 301-417-7550.

362.12 USA
MEDICAL OFFICE STAFF MANAGEMENT STRATEGIES. Text in English. m. USD 149 (effective 2001). **Document type:** *Newsletter, Trade.* **Description:** Dedicated to providing physicians practical how-to advice and ideas to hire, train, compensate, motivate, evaluate, manage and develop superior staff who work to grow and improve practice performance.
Published by: Advisory Publications, 15 E Ridge Pike, Ste 510, Conshohocken, PA 19428. TEL 888-941-4488, FAX 610-941-4499, info@smartpracticemanagement.com, http://www.smartpracticemanagement.com/cgi-bin/order/medical.html.

658 USA ISSN 1052-4924
MEDICAL RECORDS BRIEFING. Text in English. 1986. m. USD 197 (effective 1998). bk.rev. charts, stat. index. back issues avail. **Document type:** *Newsletter.* **Description:** Covers issues, procedures and regulations affecting medical records management.
—Infotrieve. **CCC.**
Published by: Opus Communications, PO Box 1168, Marblehead, MA 01945. TEL 781-639-1872, FAX 781-639-2982, customer_service@opuscomm.com, http://www.opuscomm.com. Ed. Claudia Hoffacker. Circ: 3,200.

MEDICAL STAFF BRIEFING; the newsletter for volunteer/elected medical staff leaders. see *MEDICAL SCIENCES*

362 USA
THE MEDICARE ADVISORY CAPSULE. Text in English. 1961. q. free per issue. **Document type:** *Newsletter.* **Description:** News and human interest articles on health, profiles of patients and descriptions of hospital programs.
Former titles (until 1998): Capsule; (until 1974): Capsule Comments
Published by: Wyandotte Hospital and Medical Center, 2333 Biddle Ave, Wyandotte, MI 48192. TEL 313-284-2400. Ed. Mary Ellen McLeod. Circ: 20,000.

MEDICO OSPEDALIERO. see *MEDICAL SCIENCES*

MEDIKAMENT. see *MEDICAL SCIENCES*

MEDITSINSKI PREGLED. PRAKTICHESKA MEDITSINA. see *PUBLIC HEALTH AND SAFETY*

658 DEU ISSN 0721-6076
MEDIZIN IN BERLIN (WEST); aktuelle Anschriften und Telefonnummern des Berliner Gesundheitswesens. Text in German. 1936. a. DEM 32.64. adv.
—GNLM.
Published by: Verlag Joachim Kugler, Machnower Str 7a, Berlin 14133, Germany. Circ: 4,200.

MEMORIAL SLOAN-KETTERING CANCER CENTER. ANNUAL REPORT. see *MEDICAL SCIENCES—Oncology*

658 USA ISSN 0160-7480
RA960
MODERN HEALTHCARE (YEAR); the newsmagazine for administrators and managers in hospitals, and other healthcare institutions. Text in English. 1974. w. USD 135 domestic; USD 226 in Canada; USD 189 elsewhere; USD 63 to students; USD 4 newsstand/cover (effective 2001). adv. illus. Index. back issues avail.; reprints avail. **Document type:** *Magazine, Trade.* **Description:** Contains information on healthcare management. Regular columns include news, technology, financial and legal briefs, new products, literature and a professional exchange.
Incorporates: Modern Healthcare (Long-Term Care) (0093-7053); Modern Healthcare (Short-Term Care) (0093-7061); Modern Hospital (0026-783X); Modern Nursing Home (0026-8178)
Related titles: Online - full text ed.: (from Gale Group, LexisNexis, H. W. Wilson, ProQuest Information & Learning).
Indexed: ABI Inform. (Jul.1985-), Abstr.Health Care Manage.Stud., Account.Ind. (1974-), AgeLine, Archit.Per.Ind., Avery Ind.Archit.Per., B.P.I. (Sep.1998-), BPIA, Bus.& Indus. (Jan.1995-), CINAHL, Excerp.Med., Hlth.Ind., Hosp.Lit.Ind., I.P.A., Ind.Med. (coverage dropped), Int.Nurs.Ind., L.R.I., PROMT, PSI, Tr.& Indus.Ind.
—BLDSC (5886.798000), CISTI, GNLM, IDS, Infotrieve, ingenta, Linda Hall. **CCC.**
Published by: Crain Communications, Inc. (Chicago), 740 Rush St, Chicago, IL 60611. TEL 312-649-5341, FAX 312-280-3183, http://www.modernhealthcare.com, http://www.modernhealthcare.com/, http://www.crain.com. Ed. David Burda. Pub. Charles S Lauer. adv.: B&W page USD 9,990, color page USD 11,415; trim 10 x 7. Circ: 79,371 (controlled).

MODERNA LAEKARE. see *LABOR UNIONS*

MONITOR (WASHINGTON, 1970). see *INSURANCE*

362.11 PHL
▼ **THE MONTHLY D O S E.** (Development through Organization and Solidarity towards Excellence) Text in English. 1999. m. adv. 12 p./no. 4 cols./p. **Document type:** *Newsletter, Academic/Scholarly.*
Published by: University of Santo Tomas Publishing House, Beato Angelico Bldg, UST Compound, Espana, Sampaloc, Manila, Philippines. TEL 632-731-3101 ext. 252, themonthlydose@usthospital.com.ph, publish@ust.edu.ph. Ed. Dr. Grace de la Calzada. adv.: page PHP 30,000; 5 x 7.

MOUNT SINAI JOURNAL OF MEDICINE. see *MEDICAL SCIENCES*

362 USA ISSN 1057-3526
N A H A M MANAGEMENT JOURNAL. Text in English. 1975. q. USD 140. adv. bk.rev. **Description:** Information on hospital admissions and patient access services management, including systems and personnel.
Former titles (until 1991): Admitting Management Journal (0894-1068); Journal for Hospital Admitting Management
Indexed: Ind.Med. (coverage dropped).
Published by: National Association of Healthcare Access Management, 1200 19th St, N W, Ste 300, Washington, DC 20036. TEL 202-857-1125, FAX 202-857-1115, http://www.naham.org. Ed. Dale Konrad. R&P Steve Kemp. Circ: 1,400.

N H O NEWSLINE. see *ALTERNATIVE MEDICINE*

362.11068 GBR
N H S INFORMATION AUTHORITY. OCCASIONAL PAPER. (National Health Service) Text in English. irreg. **Document type:** *Academic/Scholarly.*
Formerly: Northampton General Hospital Trust. Occasional Paper
—BLDSC (6219.138050).
Published by: National Health Service Information Authority (Casemix Programme), High Croft, Romsey Rd, Winchester SO22 DH, United Kingdom. TEL 44-1962-844588, FAX 44-1962-844711, http://www.nhsia.nhs.uk/.

658 USA
THE NATIONAL HOSPITAL PANEL SURVEY REPORTS✱ Text in English. m. **Document type:** *Trade.* **Description:** Delivers a snapshot view of critical hospital performance measures.
Published by: (American Hospital Association), American Hospital Publishing, Inc. (Subsidiary of: American Hospital Association Company), 1 N Franklin St, 27th Fl, Chicago, IL 60606-3421. TEL 312-422-6800, 800-621-6902, http://www.aha.org. **Subscr. to:** A H A Sevices Inc., PO Box 92683, Chicago, IL 92683. TEL 800-AHA-2626, FAX 312-422-1405.

NATIONAL REPORT ON SUBACUTE CARE; the bi-weekly newsletter for strategic issues, trends and management. see *MEDICAL SCIENCES*

362.1 340 USA
NEW JERSEY STATE BAR ASSOCIATION. HEALTH AND HOSPITAL LAW SECTION. NEWSLETTER. Text in English. 1987. irreg. membership only. **Document type:** *Newsletter.*
Published by: New Jersey State Bar Association, Health and Hospital Law Section, 1 Constitution Sq, New Brunswick, NJ 08901. TEL 732-249-5000, FAX 732-828-0034. Ed. Cheryl Baisden TEL 732-937-7521. Circ: 400.

THE NEW YORK HEALTH SYSTEM PHARMACIST. see *PHARMACY AND PHARMACOLOGY*

658 362.2 USA
NEW YORK (STATE). COMMISSION ON QUALITY OF CARE FOR THE MENTALLY DISABLED. ANNUAL REPORT. Text in English. 1979. a. free per issue. **Document type:** *Government.*
Indexed: e-psyche.
Published by: Commission on Quality of Care for the Mentally Disabled, 401 State St, Schenectady, NY 12305-2397. TEL 518-381-7102, FAX 518-381-7101, gigliotm@emi.com, http://www.cqc.state.ny.us. Ed., R&P Marcus A Gigliotti. Circ: 14,000.

362 NZL ISSN 0114-3727
NEW ZEALAND HEALTH & HOSPITAL. Text in English. 1948. bi-m. USD 60 (effective 2001). adv. bk.rev. charts, illus. back issues avail. **Document type:** *Trade.* **Description:** Content ranges widely over the hospital and health field in New Zealand with information of importance and interest to senior and key hospital staff - medical, nursing and administrative.
Formerly: New Zealand Hospital (0028-8217)
Indexed: Excerp.Med., I.P.A., Ind.N.Z.Per., Int.Nurs.Ind.
—BLDSC (6092.263000), GNLM. **CCC.**
Published by: Debbie Monigatti Communications, 11 Vautier Ave, Wadestown, Wellington, New Zealand. TEL 64-4-4721-630, FAX 64-4-4721-621, dmonigatti@xtra.co.nz. Ed., Pub., R&P Deborah Monigatti. Adv. contact Vanessa Clegg TEL 64-9-634-4982. Circ: 1,500 (paid).

H

362.11068 NLD ISSN 1384-4199
NIEUWSBRIEF ZORGVISIE. Text in Dutch. 1996. w. (47/yr.). included with ZorgVisie. **Document type:** *Newsletter.* **Description:** Includes information on hospital management and nursing homes.
Related titles: ♦ Supplement to: ZorgVisie. ISSN 1384-4202.
—GNLM.
Published by: Elsevier Gezondheidszorg B.V., Tijdstroom (Subsidiary of: Reed Elsevier plc Group), Planetenbaan 1, Maarssen 3600 AK, Netherlands. TEL 31-346-577577, FAX 31-346-554287, http://www.tijdstroom.nl. **Subscr. to:** Elsevier Den Haag, Postbus 16500, The Hague 2500 BM, Netherlands. TEL 31-70-381-9900, FAX 31-70-333-8399.

658 610 JPN ISSN 0915-4191
NIKKEI HEALTHCARE. Text in Japanese. 1989. m. JPY 22,000 (effective 2000). adv. **Document type:** *Trade.* **Description:** Provides guidelines for healthcare management. Includes extensive coverage of technological, sociological, and demographic trends.
Published by: Nikkei Business Publications Inc. (Subsidiary of: Nihon Keizai Shimbun, Inc.), 2-7-6 Hirakawa-cho, Chiyoda-ku, Tokyo 102-8622, Japan. TEL 81-3-5210-8311, FAX 81-3-5210-8530, info@nikkeibpnyc.com, info@nikkeibp-america.com, http://www.nikkeibp.com. Ed. Toshiyuki Senda. Pub. Hitoshi Sawai. Adv. contact Kiyoshi Sudo. B&W page JPY 351,000, color page JPY 516; trim 210 x 280. Circ: 15,364. **Dist. in America by:** Nikkei Business Publications America Inc., 575 Fifth Ave, 20th Fl, New York, NY 10017.

658 JPN ISSN 0914-8574
NISHINOMIYA SHIRITSU CHUO BYOIN KIYO/NISHINOMIYA MUNICIPAL CENTRAL HOSPITAL. BULLETIN. Text in Japanese. 1986. irreg.
Published by: Nishinomiya Shiritsu Chuo Byoin, 8-24 Hayashida-cho, Nishinomiya-shi, Hyogo-ken 663-8014, Japan.

362.11 NLD
NOORDERNIEUWS. Text in Dutch. 1987. m. (11/yr.). free. adv. bk.rev. illus. **Document type:** *Newsletter, Trade.* **Description:** For employees and others concerned with Zorggroep Noorderbreedte.
Formerly (until 1997): M C L Nieuws
Published by: Zorggroep Noorderbreedte, Henri Dunantweg 2, Postbus 888, Leeuwarden 8901 BR, Netherlands. TEL 31-58-286-6576, FAX 31-58-286-7353, redactie@znb.nl. Ed. Frits J Mostert. Adv. contact A de Vries. Circ: 6,200.

362 FRA ISSN 1150-8116
NOUVEL HOSPITALIER. Text in French. 1947. bi-m. membership. adv. bibl, charts, stat. index, cum.index.
Formerly (until 1990): Hospitalier (0754-5134)
Published by: Syndicat National des Cadres Hospitaliers, 44 rue Jules Ferry, Vitry-sur-Seine 94400, France. TEL 33-1-45736920, FAX 33-1-46825515. Ed. Veronique Lecomte. Circ: 2,500.

642.54 ESP ISSN 0212-1611 CODEN: NUHOEQ
NUTRICION HOSPITALARIA. Contents page in English, Spanish. 7/yr. ESP 10,500 domestic; ESP 19,000 foreign (effective 2000).
Indexed: Ind.Med. (1986-).
—BLDSC (6187.660000), CINDOC, EMDOCS, Infotrieve. **CCC.**
Published by: (Sociedad Espanola de Nutricion Parenteral y Enteral), Grupo Aula Medica S.A., I. Colbrand 10-12 C.I. Venecia 2 Alfa III, Madrid 28028, Spain. TEL 1-314-43-38, FAX 1-314-44-99. Ed. J A Ruiz.

O H L A NEWSLINE. see *LIBRARY AND INFORMATION SCIENCES*

658 USA ISSN 8756-8047
O R MANAGER. (Operating Room) Text in English. 1985. m. USD 86 in United States; USD 98 in Canada; USD 108 elsewhere (effective 2001). adv. bk.rev. 36 p./no. 3 cols./p. back issues avail. **Document type:** *Trade.* **Description:** Covers management of the operating room, including personnel, budgeting and financial, equipment and supplies, new technology, OR nursing issues, and professional development.
Related titles: Online - full text ed.: (from ProQuest Information & Learning).
Indexed: CINAHL, Int.Nurs.Ind.
—BLDSC (6277.375000), CISTI, Infotrieve. **CCC.**
Published by: O R Manager, Inc., 1807 Second St, Ste 61, Santa Fe, NM 87505. TEL 800-442-9918, FAX 505-983-0790, ormanager@compuserve.com, http://www.ormanager.com/. Ed. Pat Patterson. Pub., R&P Elinor S Schrader. Adv. contact John Schumus TEL 856-256-2315. Circ: 3,200 (paid).

362.12 USA
OB-GYN PRACTICE ADVISOR. Text in English. m. USD 169 (effective 2001). **Document type:** *Newsletter, Trade.* **Description:** Provides practical, how-to ideas, information and advice specifically for ob-gyn practices that help improve practice efficiency, productivity and profitability, all while delivering superior patient care.
Published by: Advisory Publications, 15 E Ridge Pike, Ste 510, Conshohocken, PA 19428. TEL 888-941-4488, FAX 610-941-4499, info@smartpracticemanagement.com, http://www.smartpracticemanagement.com/cgi-bin/order/obgyn.html.

657.832 DNK ISSN 0901-4691
OEKONOMAEN. Text in Danish. 1936. 22/yr. free per issue. adv.
Published by: Oekonomaforeningen, Norre Voldgade 90, Copenhagen K 1358, Denmark. Circ: 6,500.

362 USA ISSN 1091-1472
ON MANAGED CARE. Text in English. 1996. m. USD 201 to individuals; USD 20 newsstand/cover (effective 2002). **Document type:** *Newsletter, Trade.* **Description:** Provides current information on such areas as behavioral health care, competition, consumer health issues, health care costs, health care delivery, legal and regulatory issues, Medicare and Medicaid, pharmaceuticals, quality measure and guidelines, risk contracting and capitation, state developments and technology, and workers' compensation.
Published by: Panel Publishers, Inc. (Subsidiary of: Aspen Publishers, Inc.), 1185 Ave of the Americas, 37th Fl, New York, NY 10036. TEL 212-597-0200, 800-638-8437, FAX 212-597-0338, customer.service@aspenpubl.com, http://www.aspenpub.com. **Dist. by:** Aspen Publishers Inc., Distribution Center, 7201 McKinney Circle, Frederick, MD 21701. TEL 301-698-7100, FAX 301-695-7931.

617.09489 DNK ISSN 1395-2293
RD27.44.D4
OPERATIONSMOENSTERET VED DANSKE SYGEHUSE. Text in Danish. 1984. biennial. DKK 100.
Former titles (until 1994): Operationsmoensteret og Ventetider ved Danske Sygehuse (0906-0316); (until 1990): Operationsmoensteret paa Danske Sygehuse (0109-9957)
Published by: Sundhedsstyrelsen, Amaliegade 13, PO Box 2020, Copenhagen K 1012, Denmark. **Subscr. to:** Statens Informationstjeneste, PO Box 1103, Copenhagen K 1009, Denmark.

362.12 USA
OPHTHALMOLOGY PRACTICE ADVISOR. Text in English. m. USD 169 (effective 2001). **Document type:** *Newsletter, Trade.* **Description:** Provides practical, how-to ideas, information and advice specifically for ophthalmology practices that help improve practice efficiency, productivity and profitability, all while delivering superior patient care.
Published by: Advisory Publications, 15 E Ridge Pike, Ste 510, Conshohocken, PA 19428. TEL 888-941-4488, FAX 610-941-4499, info@smartpracticemanagement.com, http://www.smartpracticemanagement.com/cgi-bin/order/ophth.html.

362.12 USA
ORTHOPEDIC PRACTICE ADVISOR. Text in English. m. USD 169 (effective 2001). **Document type:** *Newsletter, Trade.* **Description:** Provides practical, how-to ideas, information and advice specifically for orthopedic practices that help improve practice efficiency, productivity and profitability, all while delivering superior patient care.
Published by: Advisory Publications, 15 E Ridge Pike, Ste 510, Conshohocken, PA 19428. TEL 888-941-4488, FAX 610-941-4499, info@smartpracticemanagement.com, http://www.smartpracticemanagement.com/cgi-bin/order/ortho.html.

362 ITA ISSN 0030-6231
OSPEDALE. Text in Italian. 1948. m. ITL 36,000. adv. bk.rev.
Published by: Associazione Nazionale Medici Direttori di Ospedali, Istituto di Igiene, Via Santena, 5-Bis, Turin, TO 10126, Italy. Circ: 1,000.

658 610 ITA ISSN 0030-624X
OSPEDALE AL MARE. ARCHIVIO✶. Text in Italian. 1970 (vol.22). q. ITL 3,000. adv. bk.rev. bibl, charts, illus. index.
Indexed: Biol.Abstr., Excerp.Med.
—CISTI.
Published by: Ospedale al Mare, Lido Di Venezia, VE 30126, Italy.

362 USA
OSTEOPATHIC PROGRESS. Text in English. 1957. m. USD 50 (effective 1999). adv. bk.rev. charts, illus, stat. *Refereed.* **Document type:** *Newsletter.*
Former titles (until 1995): A O H A Progress; (until 1992): A O H A (1058-6385); (until 1991): A O H A Today (1044-1980); (until 1989): Osteopathic Hospital Leadership; (until 1985): Osteopathic Hospitals; O H Osteopathic Hospitals (0161-0007); Osteopathic Hospital (0048-2293)
Indexed: Abstr.Health Care Manage.Stud., CINAHL, Hosp.Lit.Ind., MEDSOC.
Published by: American Osteopathic Healthcare Association, 5550 Friendship Blvd, Ste 300, Chevy Chase, MD 20815-7201. TEL 202-686-1700, FAX 202-686-7615. Ed. David Kushner. R&P, Adv. contact Carrie Ayers TEL 301-968-2642. Circ: 2,300.

658 USA
OUTPATIENT CARE TECHNOLOGY. Text in English. 1985. bi-m. USD 50 domestic; USD 80 foreign. **Document type:** *Trade.* **Description:** Trade magazine serving physician specialists, chief medical officers, administrators, business managers and others concerned with product evaluation and procurement in freestanding ambulatory, diagnostic and surgical centers, group practices, HMOs and PPOs.
Formerly: I C C N - Outpatient Care (0897-6198)
Published by: Reilly Publishing Co., 16 E Schaumburg Rd, Schaumburg, IL 60194-3536. TEL 847-882-6336, FAX 847-519-0166, rcgroup@flash.net. Ed. Andrea Donner. Pub. John S O'Neil. Circ: 35,500.

658 617 USA ISSN 0270-207X
OUTREACH (CHICAGO). Text in English. 1980. bi-m. USD 85 to non-members; USD 65 to members. bk.rev. charts, stat. index. back issues avail. **Document type:** *Newsletter.* **Description:** Provides information on ambulatory care, ambulatory surgery, emergency services, freestanding facilities, group practice, health maintenance organizations, preventive care, occupational health, home care, hospices, and primary care.
Indexed: Abstr.Health Care Manage.Stud.
Published by: (Society for Ambulatory Care Professionals), American Hospital Association, One North Franklin, Chicago, IL 60606-3421. TEL 312-422-3907, FAX 312-422-4579. Ed. Ronald Salmela. Circ: 10,000.

657.832 USA ISSN 0195-7775
PATIENT ACCOUNTS. Text in English. 1978. m. USD 119 to non-members; USD 66 to members. adv. **Document type:** *Newsletter.* **Description:** For healthcare professionals who are responsible for patient financial services in hospitals and other provider settings in the U.S.
—CCC.
Published by: Healthcare Financial Management Association, 2 Westbrook Corporate Center, Ste 700, Westchester, IL 60154-5700. TEL 708-531-9600, FAX 708-531-0032. Ed. Marilyn Ferdinand. Pub. Cheryl T Stachura. R&P Sharon Malik. Adv. contact Dianne Lach. Circ: 2,000.

658 USA
PATIENT & NURSING CARE PRODUCTS. Text in English. 1987. q. **Description:** For healthcare professionals who evaluate and purchase products for hospitals, nursing homes, and home healthcare environments.
Former titles: Patient Care Products; Limited Mobility and Immobilized Patient Products
Published by: Card-Zine Communications, Inc., 8912 Ewing Ave Ste A, Evanston, IL 60203-1907. TEL 708-933-0407, FAX 708-933-0217. adv.: B&W page USD 6,171; trim 10.88 x 6. Circ: 75,115.

353.68 USA ISSN 1082-8672
PATIENT-FOCUSED CARE. Text in English. 1993. m. USD 469; USD 449 foreign (effective 1999). **Document type:** *Newsletter.* **Description:** Presents strategies for organizational restructuring, team dynamics, staffing, training and change management.
Incorporates (in 1997): Hospital Food Service Management; Which was formerly (1967-1993): Hospital Food Service (0046-7979)
Published by: American Health Consultants (Subsidiary of: Medical Economics Co., Inc.), 3525 Piedmont Rd, N E, 6 Piedmont Center, Ste 400, Atlanta, GA 30305. TEL 404-262-5476, custserv@ahcpub.com, http://www.ahcpub.com. Circ: 330.

642.59 IND
PATIENT HOSPITAL RELATIONS. Text in English. 1991. bi-m. INR 570, USD 38 (effective 2000). adv. abstr, bibl. index.
Published by: K.K. Roy (Private) Ltd., 55 Gariahat Rd., P O Box 10210, Kolkata, West Bengal 700 019, India. Ed. K K Roy. R&P M Misra TEL 91-33-475-4872. Circ: 1,990.

362.11 USA
PATIENT MANAGEMENT. Text in English. 1982. 9/yr. USD 24 domestic; USD 24 in Canada; USD 34 elsewhere (effective 1999). **Document type:** *Trade.* **Description:** Serves the hospital, nursing home, extended care facility, clinic and emergency, surgi-center market, as well as group purchasing associations across the country.
Formerly (until 1998): Medical Care Products (1066-825X)
Indexed: Inpharma, Reac.
—CCC.
Published by: New Product Information, Part of Cahners Publishing Company, 301 Gibraltar Dr, Box 650, Morris Plains, NJ 07950-0650. TEL 973-292-5100 x224, FAX 973-539-3476, dransdell@cahners.com, http://www.patientmanagement.com. Ed. John Lannon TEL 973-292-5100 x267. Pub. Donald P Ransdell. Circ: 60,100.

658 USA
PATIENT REPRESENTATION AND CONSUMER AFFAIRS. Text in English. 1973. bi-m. membership. **Document type:** *Newsletter.*
Published by: American Hospital Association, One North Franklin, Chicago, IL 60606-3421. TEL 312-422-3996, FAX 312-422-4575. Ed. Donald Phillips. Circ: 1,100.

658 USA
PATIENT SATISFACTION & OUTCOMES MANAGEMENT. Text in English. 1995. m. USD 319; USD 319 foreign (effective 1999). **Document type:** *Newsletter.*
Published by: American Health Consultants (Subsidiary of: Medical Economics Co., Inc.), 3525 Piedmont Rd, N E, 6 Piedmont Center, Ste 400, Atlanta, GA 30305. TEL 404-262-5476, custserv@ahcpub.com, http://www.ahcpub.com.

658 340 USA
PATIENTS' RIGHTS REPORTER. Text in English. 1983. m. **Description:** Keeps patients, their families and those providing pastoral care in health care settings aware of legislative and court decisions affecting patients' rights.
Formerly: Patients' Rights in California (0736-2544)
Media: Online - full text.
Published by: Cox Publications, 1908 Colton Blvd, Billings, MT 59102-2316. TEL 406-256-2248, FAX 406-256-7550. Ed. Meridith B Cox. Circ: 255.

PEDIATRIC CLINICS OF INDIA. see *MEDICAL SCIENCES—Pediatrics*

362.12 USA
PEDIATRIC PRACTICE ADVISOR. Text in English. m. USD 169 (effective 2001). **Document type:** *Newsletter, Trade.* **Description:** Contains practical, how-to ideas, information and advice specifically for pediatric practices that help improve practice efficiency, productivity and profitability, all while delivering superior patient care.
Published by: Advisory Publications, 15 E Ridge Pike, Ste 510, Conshohocken, PA 19428. TEL 888-941-4488, FAX 610-941-4499, info@smartpracticemanagement.com, http://www.smartpracticemanagement.com/cgi-bin/order/pediatric.html.

362.15 FRA ISSN 0757-0481
PERSPECTIVES SANITAIRE ET SOCIALES✱ . Text in French. 1975. 6/yr. **Document type:** *Trade.*
Formerly (until 1982): Perspectives Hospitalieres (0336-1810)
Published by: F E H A P, 10 rue de la Rosiere, Paris 75015, France. TEL 33-1-45786559. Ed. Jean Savy. Circ: 5,000.

PFLEGE- UND KRANKENHAUSRECHT. see *LAW—Civil Law*

▼ **PFLEGEMAGAZIN**; Zeitschrift fuer den gesamten Pflegebereich. see *PUBLIC HEALTH AND SAFETY*

PHARMACIEN HOSPITALIER. see *PHARMACY AND PHARMACOLOGY*

PHARMACY IN PRACTICE. see *PHARMACY AND PHARMACOLOGY*

658 USA ISSN 0898-2759
PHYSICIAN EXECUTIVE; journal of management. Text in English. bi-m. USD 80 domestic to non-members; USD 96 foreign to non-members (effective 2000). adv. *Refereed.* **Document type:** *Trade.* **Description:** Contains timely updates on health economics, clinical technology, health law, health services research, career management, health and business relations, and health policy reform.
Related titles: Online - full text ed.: (from Gale Group, Northern Light Technology, Inc.).
Indexed: Int.Nurs.Ind.
—BLDSC (6476.361540), GNLM.
Published by: American College of Physician Executives, Two Urban Centre, Ste 200, 4890 W Kennedy Blvd, Tampa, FL 33609. TEL 813-287-2000, FAX 813-287-8993. Ed. Susan Sasenick. Adv. contact Tina Ramsey.

362.12 USA ISSN 1088-5218
THE PHYSICIAN'S ADVISORY. Text in English. m. USD 169 (effective 2001). **Document type:** *Newsletter, Trade.* **Description:** Provides practical, expert ideas and advice to boost medical practice performance and profitability.
Published by: Advisory Publications, 15 E Ridge Pike, Ste 510, Conshohocken, PA 19428. TEL 888-941-4488, FAX 610-941-4499, info@smartpracticemanagement.com, http://www.smartpracticemanagement.com/cgi-bin/order/phy_advisory.html.

PHYSICIAN'S MANAGED CARE REPORT. see *INSURANCE*

658 USA ISSN 1042-2625
PHYSICIANS MARKETING & MANAGEMENT. Text in English. m. USD 299 domestic to individuals; USD 293 foreign to individuals; USD 323 domestic to institutions; USD 353 foreign to institutions (effective 1999). charts, illus, tr.lit. index. back issues avail. **Document type:** *Newsletter.* **Description:** Covers all aspects of private practice management, including personnel, capital and risk management, and how-to marketing methods.
Incorporates (1986-1992): Practice Personnel Bulletin (0888-9066); Formerly (until 1988): Physician's Marketing (0883-1459)
Published by: American Health Consultants (Subsidiary of: Medical Economics Co., Inc.), 3525 Piedmont Rd, N E, 6 Piedmont Center, Ste 400, Atlanta, GA 30305. TEL 404-262-5476, custserv@ahcpub.com, http://www.ahcpub.com. Circ: 1,230.

368.382 USA ISSN 1050-8791
PHYSICIAN'S PAYMENT UPDATE. Text in English. 1989. m. USD 437 domestic; USD 467 foreign; USD 73 newsstand/cover (effective 2001). **Document type:** *Newsletter.*
Related titles: Online - full text ed.: (from Northern Light Technology, Inc.).
Published by: American Health Consultants (Subsidiary of: Medical Economics Co., Inc.), 3525 Piedmont Rd, N E, 6 Piedmont Center, Ste 400, Atlanta, GA 30305. TEL 404-262-5476, 404-262-7436, 800-688-2421, FAX 404-262-7837, 800-284-3291, custserv@ahcpub.com, http://www.ahcpub.com. Circ: 2,220.

362.12 USA ISSN 1088-520X
THE PHYSICIAN'S PERSONAL ADVISORY. Text in English. m. USD 149 (effective 2001). **Document type:** *Newsletter, Trade.* **Description:** Dedicated to providing doctors sound, independent, physician-specific advice to better oversee their personal finances and their lives outside of medicine.
Published by: Advisory Publications, 15 E Ridge Pike, Ste 510, Conshohocken, PA 19428. TEL 888-941-4488, FAX 610-941-4499, info@smartpracticemanagement.com, http://www.smartpracticemanagement.com/cgi-bin/order/personal.html.

POST-ACUTE PAYMENT REPORT. see *PUBLIC HEALTH AND SAFETY*

362.11 642.5 USA ISSN 1523-4665
▼ **PREMIER HOSPITAL SERVICES REPORT.** Text in English. 1999. m. USD 495 domestic; USD 595 foreign (effective 2001). **Document type:** *Newsletter, Trade.* **Description:** Deals with premier hospital suites and other innovative patient services, including such issues as amenities, pricing, marketing, staffing, training, facilities design management, billing, fund-raising, and development.
Previously announced as: Hospital Hotelier and Premier Service Report
Published by: Mary Ann Liebert, Inc. Publishers, 2 Madison Ave, Larchmont, NY 10538. TEL 914—834-3100, FAX 914-834-1388, info@liebertpub.com, http://www.liebertpub.com.

658 USA
PROFILES OF U S HOSPITALS. Text in English. 1992. a. USD 299 (effective 1999). **Document type:** *Directory.* **Description:** Provides hospital-specific data for 30 key measures of descriptive, financial and clinical information for every U.S. hospital.
Formerly: Directory of U S Hospitals (1062-1946)
Published by: H C I A Inc., 300 E Lombard St, Baltimore, MD 21202. TEL 800-568-3282, FAX 410-539-5220.

PSYCHIATRIC SERVICES. see *MEDICAL SCIENCES—Psychiatry And Neurology*

PUBLIC HEALTH - STATE CAPITALS. see *LAW*

PUBLIC SECTOR CONTRACTING REPORT. see *PUBLIC HEALTH AND SAFETY*

800 613 PRI
PUERTO RICO. DEPARTMENT OF HEALTH. INFORME ESTADISTICO DE FACILIDADES DE SALUD. Text in Spanish. 1979. a. free per issue. **Document type:** *Government.* **Description:** Contains information on public and private hospitals' resources and services.
Formerly: Puerto Rico. Department of Health. Informe Anual de Facilidades de Salud
Published by: Department of Health, Auxiliary Secretariat for Planning, Evaluation, Statistics and Information Systems, Division of Statistics, P O Box 70184, San Juan, PR 00936. TEL 787-274-7875, FAX 787-274-7877. Circ: 500.

362 PRI
PUERTO RICO. DIVISION OF HEALTH FACILITIES. PLAN FOR HOSPITAL AND MEDICAL FACILITIES. Text and summaries in English. 1949. a.
Media: Duplicated (not offset).
Published by: Department of Health, Division of Health Facilities, PO Box 70184, San Juan, PR 00936. Circ: 250.

658 USA ISSN 1075-0541
Q I - T Q M. (Quality Improvement - Total Quality Management) Text in English. 1991. m. USD 497 domestic; USD 527 foreign; USD 83 newsstand/cover (effective 2001). **Document type:** *Newsletter.* **Description:** Provides practical advice to hospital executives on implementation of the various continuous quality-improvement models.
Incorporates (1995-1996): Managed Care Quality (1087-0636); (1996-1997): Patient Satisfaction Management (1087-3716)
Published by: American Health Consultants (Subsidiary of: Medical Economics Co., Inc.), 3525 Piedmont Rd, N E, 6 Piedmont Center, Ste 400, Atlanta, GA 30305. TEL 404-262-5476, 404-262-7436, 800-688-2421, FAX 404-262-7837, 800-284-3291, custserv@ahcpub.com, http://www.ahcpub.com. Circ: 2,300.

658 USA ISSN 0747-7384
Q R C ADVISOR; managing hospital quality, risk & cost. (Quality, Risk & Cost) Text in English. 1984. m. USD 240 domestic; USD 288 foreign (effective 2000). **Document type:** *Newsletter.* **Description:** Offers sound, authorative advice for effectively handling quality assurance, risk management, and cost control issues.
Related titles: Online - full text ed.: (from ProQuest Information & Learning).
Indexed: Int.Nurs.Ind.
—BLDSC, Infotrieve. **CCC.**
Published by: Aspen Publishers, Inc., 200 Orchard Ridge Dr, Ste 200, Gaithersburg, MD 20878. TEL 301-417-7500, 800-638-8437, FAX 301-417-7550, customer.service@aspenpubl.com, http://www.aspenpub.com. Ed. Barbara J Youngberg. **Dist. by:** Aspen Publishers Inc., Distribution Center, 7201 McKinney Circle, Frederick, MD 21701. TEL 301-698-7100, FAX 301-417-7550.

H

362.6 USA ISSN 0892-6174
QUALITY CARE ADVOCATE. Text in English. 1986. bi-m. USD 45 to non-members. bk.rev. **Document type:** *Newsletter.* **Description:** Reports on federal legislation and regulatory developments, policy implementation and other current events affecting quality of care in nursing homes.
Published by: National Citizens Coalition for Nursing Home Reform, 1424 16th St, N W, 202, Washington, DC 20036-2211. FAX 202-332-2949. Ed., R&P Nicole Gudzowsky. Circ: 6,000.

362 USA ISSN 1047-5311
THE QUALITY LETTER FOR HEALTHCARE LEADERS. Text in English. 1989. m. USD 400 to individuals; USD 40 newsstand/cover (effective 2002). **Document type:** *Newsletter, Trade.* **Description:** Devoted to healthcare quality improvement, providing practical tips on the latest proven strategies.
Indexed: Int.Nurs.Ind.
—BLDSC (7168.152350), Infotrieve. **CCC.**
Published by: Aspen Publishers, Inc., 200 Orchard Ridge Dr, Ste 200, Gaithersburg, MD 20878. TEL 301-417-7500, 800-638-8437, FAX 301-695-7931, customer.service@aspenpubl.com, http://www.aspenpub.com. Ed. Jane Lowers. **Dist. by:** Aspen Publishers Inc., Distribution Center, 7201 McKinney Circle, Frederick, MD 21701. TEL 301-698-7100, FAX 301-417-7550.

658 USA ISSN 1063-8628
RA399.A1
QUALITY MANAGEMENT IN HEALTH CARE; an information service. Abbreviated title: Q M H C. Text in English. 1990. q. USD 172 to individuals; USD 52 newsstand/cover (effective 2002). **Document type:** *Journal.* **Description:** Covers new techniques, laws, regulations, program models, and guidelines from the discipline.
Formerly (until 1992): Quality and Risk Management in Health Care
Related titles: Online - full text ed.: (from ProQuest Information & Learning).
Indexed: Brit.Nur.Ind., CINAHL, Int.Nurs.Ind.
—BLDSC (7168.152550), CISTI, GNLM, Infotrieve, ingenta. **CCC.**
Published by: Aspen Publishers, Inc., 200 Orchard Ridge Dr, Ste 200, Gaithersburg, MD 20878. TEL 301-417-7500, 800-638-8437, FAX 301-417-7550, http://www.aspenpublishers.com. Ed. Glenn Laffar. Circ: 1,500 (paid).

658 615.842 USA ISSN 0198-7097
RA975.5.R3
RADIOLOGY MANAGEMENT. Text in English. 1979. bi-m. USD 54 domestic; USD 67 in Canada; USD 100 elsewhere (effective 2000). adv. bk.rev. back issues avail. **Document type:** *Trade.* **Description:** Publishes articles relating to the management of the nonmedical aspects of radiology.
—BLDSC (7238.160000), CISTI, GNLM.
Published by: American Healthcare Radiology Administrators, 111 Boston Post Rd, Box 334, Sudbury, MA 01776-0003. TEL 978-443-7591, FAX 978-443-8046, publications@ahraonline.org, http://www.ahraonline.org. Ed. Gary Boyd. Circ: 4,200.

H

362 USA
▼ **REAL HEALTHCARE.** Text in English. 2001. bi-m. USD 29 to membership (effective 2001). **Document type:** *Magazine, Consumer.* **Description:** Contains satire, stories, editorial articles on the cost and effectiveness of current healthcare system.
Formed by the merger of (in 2001): N H C Q A Bulletin; C Q; Which was formerly: Cost & Quality; Cost & Quality Quarterly Journal (1079-5057)
Published by: National Healthcare Cost & Quality Association, 11313 Weddington St, 1st Fl, North Hollywood, CA 91601 . TEL 818-761-6546, 888-761-3600, FAX 818-761-5568, Info@nhcqa.org, http://www.realhealthcare.com/, http://www.nhcqa.org/index.html. Ed. Bruce Gipe.

THE RECEIVABLES REPORT; the monthly newsletter for America's health care financial manager. see *BUSINESS AND ECONOMICS—Accounting*

362 ZAF
RECOMMENDED SCALES OF BENEFITS. PRIVATE HOSPITALS & UNATTACHED OPERATING THEATRE UNITS. Text in English. 1994. a.
Published by: Representative Association of Medical Schemes, PO Box 2324, Parklands, Johannesburg 2121, South Africa.

REHAB & COMMUNITY CARE MANAGEMENT. see *MEDICAL SCIENCES—Physical Medicine And Rehabilitation*

658 USA ISSN 0884-2795
REIMBURSEMENT ADVISOR. Variant title: Dennis Barry's Reimbursement Advisor. Text in English. 1985. m. USD 310 to individuals; USD 31 newsstand/cover (effective 2002). **Document type:** *Newsletter, Trade.* **Description:** Provides practical up-to-date information, in-depth analyses of key developments in prospective payments, case studies, recommended courses of action, legislative updates, practical management strategies, legal advice, and sound financial planning tips.
Related titles: Online - full text ed.: (from ProQuest Information & Learning).
—CCC.
Published by: Aspen Publishers, Inc., 200 Orchard Ridge Dr, Ste 200, Gaithersburg, MD 20878. TEL 301-417-7500, 800-638-8437, FAX 301-695-7931, customer.service@aspenpubl.com, http://www.aspenpub.com. Ed. Dennis Barry. Circ: 1,200. **Dist. by:** Aspen Publishers Inc., Distribution Center, 7201 McKinney Circle, Frederick, MD 21701. TEL 301-698-7100, FAX 301-417-7550.

REIMBURSEMENT UPDATE. see *BUSINESS AND ECONOMICS—Economic Situation And Conditions*

362.15 200 FRA ISSN 1146-3759
RELIGIEUSES DANS LES PROFESSIONS DE SANTE✶ . Text in French. 1938. q. FRF 240 domestic; FRF 265 foreign (effective 2000). bk.rev. index. back issues avail. **Document type:** *Bulletin.* **Description:** For religious readers and nuns in the health care profession. Features articles of a religious nature to inspire the reader to reflect on the church and society.
Formerly: Religieuses d'Action Hospitaliere et Social
Published by: R E P S A, 106 rue du Bac, Paris Cedex 7 75341, France. TEL 145-48-05-82, FAX 145-44-83-75. Ed., Pub., R&P Micheline Bougon. Circ: 1,100 (paid); 100 (controlled).

658 USA ISSN 1050-5636
REPORT ON MEDICAL GUIDELINES & OUTCOMES RESEARCH. Text in English. s-m. USD 575; USD 27 newsstand/cover (effective 2001). **Document type:** *Newsletter.* **Description:** For healthcare executives. Covers ways to improve the quality of patient care, cut costs and implement cost-effective treatment methods.
Published by: Medical Care Management Corp., 5272 River Rd., Ste. 650, Bethesda, MD 20816-1405. TEL 301-652-1818, 301-652-1250, m, mcman@mcman.cpm, http://www.mcman.com/default.htm.

658 USA
REPORT ON PATIENT PRIVACY. Text in English. **Document type:** *Newsletter.* **Description:** Focuses on the confidentiality of patient information, HIPAA compliance, telemedicine and internet health.
Published by: Atlantic Information Services, Inc., 1100 17th St, N W, Ste 300, Washington, DC 20036. TEL 202-775-9008, FAX 202-331-9542, http://www.aishealth.com. Pub. Richard Biehl.

362 USA ISSN 0034-5555
RESIDENT AND STAFF PHYSICIAN. Text in English. 1955. m. USD 62 (effective 2000). adv. illus, tr.lit. index. back issues avail.; reprints avail. **Document type:** *Magazine, Trade.*
Formerly: Resident Physician
Related titles: Microform ed.: (from PQC).
Indexed: AgeLine, Curr.Lit.Fam.Plan.
—BLDSC (7777.243000), GNLM, ingenta.
Published by: Romaine Pierson Publishing Co. (Subsidiary of: Medical World Communications), 1065 Old Country Rd, Ste 213, Westbury, NY 11590-5628. TEL 516-883-6350, FAX 516-883-6609. Ed. Dr. Alfred Bollet. Pub. Robert Grant. Adv. contact Grace Cass. Circ: 101,292.

RESPIRATORY CARE MANAGER. see *MEDICAL SCIENCES—Respiratory Diseases*

362.18 616.02 AUS
RESPONSE (FORTITUDE VALLEY)✶ . Text in English. bi-m. AUD 20. adv. **Document type:** *Trade.* **Description:** For ambulance industry and emergency services.
Published by: Institute of Ambulance Officers, M I A O (Australia), P O Box 227, Caringbah, NSW 2229, Australia. TEL 61-2-9580-3106. Ed. John Hall. Adv. contact Trevor Kirk. B&W page AUD 1,782, color page AUD 2,827; trim 210 x 275. Circ: 3,500.

658 FRA ISSN 0397-4626
REVUE HOSPITALIERE DE FRANCE. Text in French. bi-m. FRF 457; FRF 640 foreign. adv. **Document type:** *Trade.*
Indexed: C.I.S. Abstr., Excerp.Med.
—GNLM.
Published by: Federation Hospitaliere de France, 33 av. d'Italie, Paris 75013, France. TEL 33-1-44-06-84-44, FAX 33-1-44-06-84-45. Ed. M Philippe Cadene. Circ: 4,500.

658 USA ISSN 1079-7726
RA971.3
RUSS COILE'S HEALTH TRENDS. Text in English. 1985. m. USD 335 to individuals; USD 34 newsstand/cover (effective 2002). **Document type:** *Newsletter.* **Description:** Aims to help reduce costs and risk, make a hospital more competitive and profitable, attract and keep the best staff, improve the quality of patient care, and attract more patients.
Former titles: Hospital Strategy Report (1040-6263); (until 1988): Hospital Entrepreneur's Newsletter (8756-7253)
Indexed: Int.Nurs.Ind.
—BLDSC (8052.649620). **CCC.**
Published by: Aspen Publishers, Inc., 200 Orchard Ridge Dr, Ste 200, Gaithersburg, MD 20878. TEL 301-417-7500, 800-638-8437, FAX 301-417-7931, customer.service@aspenpubl.com, http://www.aspenpub.com. Ed. Russell C Coile. **Dist. by:** Aspen Publishers Inc., Distribution Center, 7201 McKinney Circle, Frederick, MD 21701. TEL 301-698-7100, FAX 301-417-7550.

362 CAN
S A H O NEWS. Text in English. 1976. bi-m. free per issue. back issues avail. **Document type:** *Newsletter.* **Description:** Covers health care news and innovations in health care delivery.
Formerly (until 1993): Continuum of Care
Published by: Saskatchewan Association of Health Organizations, 1445 Park St, Regina, SK S4N 4C5, Canada. TEL 306-347-5526, FAX 306-525-1960, anoy@regina.saho.org. Ed. Loretta Fritz. R&P Andrew Caswell. Circ: 3,000.

658 USA
S S M NETWORK. Text in English. 1984. q. free per issue. back issues avail. **Document type:** *Newsletter.* **Description:** Communicates the goals, vision, philosophy and mission of the S S M Health Care System.
Published by: S S M Health Care System, 477 N. Lindbergh Blvd., St. Louis, MO 63141. TEL 314-994-7800, FAX 314-994-7900. Ed. Carol Bales. Circ: 15,000.

610 GBR ISSN 0036-2840
SAINT GEORGE'S HOSPITAL GAZETTE. Text in English. 1893. a. GBP 1.50. adv. bk.rev. charts, illus. cum.index.
Formerly: New St. George Hospital Gazette
Published by: St. George's Hospital Medical School, Cranmer Terr, London SW17 0RE, United Kingdom. TEL 44-181-672-9944, FAX 44-181-767-4696. Circ: 750.

362 FIN ISSN 0036-326X
SAIRAALA✶ . Text in Finnish; Summaries in Swedish. 1928. 10/yr. FIM 160. adv. bk.rev. bibl, charts, illus.
—GNLM.
Published by: Infoteam Oy, Nervanderinkatu 5 D 41, Helsinki 00100, Finland. Ed. Pentti Vaananen. Circ: 4,500.

658 CHE
DIE SANITAET. Text in German. m.
Published by: Sanitaet, Wankdorffeldstr 109, Bern 3014, Switzerland. TEL 031-412342. Circ: 4,000.

SCANDINAVIAN JOURNAL OF PRIMARY HEALTH CARE. see *MEDICAL SCIENCES*

SCANDINAVIAN JOURNAL OF PRIMARY HEALTH CARE. SUPPLEMENT. see *MEDICAL SCIENCES*

362 CHE ISSN 0304-4432
SCHWEIZER SPITAL/HOPITAL SUISSE/OSPEDALE SVIZZERO. Text in French, German, Italian. 1937. m. CHF 90; CHF 105 foreign (effective 1999). bk.rev. *Refereed.* **Document type:** *Academic/Scholarly, Trade.* **Description:** Monthly scholarly publication for hospital staff.
Former titles: Schweizer Spital-Veska; Veska
Indexed: Dok.Arbeitsmed., Excerp.Med.
—CISTI, GNLM.
Published by: H Plus Die Spitaeler der Schweiz, Postfach, Aarau 5001, Switzerland. TEL 41-62-8241222, FAX 41-62-8223335, geschaeftsstelle@hplus.ch, http://www.hplus.ch. Ed. Christian Schar. R&P R Blaettler. adv.: B&W page CHF 1,570, color page CHF 3,130; trim 258 x 182. Circ: 3,500.

SCOPE (YORK). see *PHYSICS*

LA SEMAINE DES HOPITAUX. see *MEDICAL SCIENCES*

▼ **SEMINARS IN INFECTION CONTROL.** see *MEDICAL SCIENCES—Communicable Diseases*

SENIOR CARE MANAGEMENT. see *PUBLIC HEALTH AND SAFETY*

658 617.7 616.21 AUS
SIGHT AND SOUND NEWS. Text in English. 1950. q. free per issue. bk.rev. **Document type:** *Newsletter.*
Published by: Royal Victorian Eye and Ear Hospital, c/o Public Relations Dept., 32 Gisborne St, East Melbourne, VIC 3002, Australia. TEL 61-3-99298666, FAX 61-3-96637203. Ed. Joan Pritchard. Circ: 10,000.

SINGAPORE JOURNAL OF OBSTETRICS & GYNAECOLOGY. see *MEDICAL SCIENCES—Obstetrics And Gynecology*

SJUKHUSFARMACI. see *PHARMACY AND PHARMACOLOGY*

658 USA
SMALL OR RURAL HOSPITALS UPDATE. Text in English. 1977. irreg. free per issue. back issues avail. **Document type:** *Bulletin.*
Formerly (until 1989): Small or Rural Hospital Report
Published by: American Hospital Association, Section for Small or Rural Hospitals, One North Franklin, Chicago, IL 60606-3421. TEL 312-422-3305, FAX 312-422-4590. Eds. Jane Gibson, John Supplitt. Circ: 3,500.

SNAKEROOT EXTRACT. see *HISTORY*

SOCIEDAD ESPANOLA DE FARMACIA HOSPITALARIA. BOLETIN INFORMATIVO. see *PHARMACY AND PHARMACOLOGY*

362 USA
SPACE COAST C I L NEWS. Text in English. q. tr.lit. **Document type:** *Newsletter.*
Published by: Space Coast Center for Independent Living, 331 Ramp Rd., Coco Beach, FL 32931. TEL 321-784-9008, FAX 321-784-3702, sccil@digital.org. Ed. Anna Grau.

658 USA
ST. AGNES NEWS. Text in English. 1961. bi-m. free per issue to qualified personnel. **Description:** Covers articles relating to the hospital's events, programs, and employees.
Published by: St. Agnes Hospital, 900 Caton Ave, Baltimore, MD 21229. TEL 410-368-2170, FAX 410-368-2947. Ed. Helen Becker. Circ: 6,000.

658 USA
ST. PATRICK HOSPITAL. ANNUAL REPORT. Text in English. a. free per issue. **Document type:** *Newsletter, Corporate.* **Description:** Reports hospital news and current issues in health care.
Published by: St. Patrick Hospital, 500 W Broadway, Box 4587, Missoula, MT 59806.

362 GBR
ST. THOMAS'S HOSPITAL GAZETTE. Text in English. 1891. 3/yr. USD 25. adv. bk.rev. bibl, illus. **Document type:** *Newsletter.*
Former titles: St. Thomas's Gazette (0306-3860); St. Thomas's Hospital Gazette (0036-3200)
Published by: St. Thomas's Hospital Medical School, c/o Medical School Library, London SE1 7EH, United Kingdom. TEL 44-171-928-9292, gazette@umds.ac.uk, http://www.umds.ac.uk/sth-gazette/. Ed. I Phillips. Circ: 1,500.

362.11 340 USA ISSN 1073-8886
STATE HEALTH CARE REGULATORY DEVELOPMENTS. Text in English. 1994. 26/yr. USD 689 (effective 2001). 40 p./no. back issues avail. **Description:** Contains summaries of health care regulatory developments for all 50 states and the District of Columbia. Covers proposed and final regulations from state registers, published notices, and information supplied by BNA sources. Subscribers get summaries of regulations, notices, and hearings along with citations to the state administrative code, date of publication, hearing schedules, effective dates, comment deadlines and names and telephone numbers of state regulatory contacts.
Related titles: Online - full text ed.: (from Bureau of National Affairs, Inc., (BNA), The).
—CCC.
Published by: The Bureau of National Affairs, Inc., 1231 25th St, N W, Washington, DC 20037. TEL 202-452-4200, 800-372-1033, 800-452-7773, FAX 202-822-8092, customercare@bna.com, bnaplus@bna.com, http://www.bna.com/. Pub. Gregory McCaffery.

362 USA ISSN 0895-688X
RA982.N49
STATE OF NEW YORK CITY'S MUNICIPAL HOSPITAL SYSTEM; report of the City Hospital Visiting Committee. Text in English. a. USD 10 (effective 2000). **Document type:** *Academic/Scholarly.* **Description:** Reports findings that are based on a century-old citizens' group on the conditions affecting patient care in New York City's public hospitals. Includes overview of management, financial conditions, staffing, and individual facilities.
Published by: United Hospital Fund of New York, 350 Fifth Ave, Fl 23, New York, NY 10118-2399. TEL 212-494-0700, FAX 212-494-0800, pbrooks@uhfnyc.org, http://www.uhfnyc.org. **Co-sponsor:** City Hospital Visiting Committee.

STERILIZATION IN AUSTRALIA. see *PUBLIC HEALTH AND SAFETY*

STRATEGIC HEALTH CARE MARKETING. see *BUSINESS AND ECONOMICS—Marketing And Purchasing*

658 USA
STRATEGY FOR SUCCESSFUL J C A H O HOMECARE ACCREDITATION. (Joint Commission on Accreditation of Healthcare Organizations) Text in English. 1997. a. USD 299; USD 317 foreign (effective 1999). **Document type:** *Trade.*
Published by: American Health Consultants (Subsidiary of: Medical Economics Co., Inc.), 3525 Piedmont Rd, N E, 6 Piedmont Center, Ste 400, Atlanta, GA 30305. TEL 404-262-5476, custserv@ahcpub.com, http://www.ahcpub.com.

SURGICAL SERVICES MANAGEMENT. see *MEDICAL SCIENCES—Surgery*

362.11 DNK ISSN 0904-9878
RA989.D4
SYGDOMSMOENSTERET FOR INDLAGTE PATIENTER. Text in Danish. 1979. biennial. DKK 100.
Formerly (until 1989): Sygdomsmoensteret ved Somatiske Sygehusafdelinger (0107-8380)
Published by: Sundhedsstyrelsen, Amaliegade 13, PO Box 2020, Copenhagen K 1012, Denmark. **Subscr. to:** Statens Informationstjeneste, PO Box 1103, Copenhagen K 1009, Denmark.

362.11 DNK ISSN 0107-508X
SYGEHUSKLASSIFIKATION OG KOMMUNEKODER. Text in Danish. 1974. a. DKK 70.
Published by: Sundhedsstyrelsen, Amaliegade 13, PO Box 2020, Copenhagen K 1012, Denmark. **Subscr. to:** Statens Informationstjeneste, PO Box 1103, Copenhagen K 1009, Denmark.

362 ZAF
T L C: THE WAITING ROOM MAGAZINE. Text in English. q. USD 20 foreign (effective 2000). illus. **Document type:** *Trade.*
Published by: South African Medical Association, Health and Medical Publishing Group, 14 Central Sq, Pinelands 7430, South Africa. TEL 27-21-531-3081, FAX 27-21-531-4126, annp@samedical.org, publishing@samedical.org, http://www.samedical.org. **Subscr. to:** PO Box 74789, Lynnwood Ridge, Pretoria 0040, South Africa. TEL 27-12-481-2010, FAX 27-12-481-2061, ann@samedical.org. **Dist. by:** Private Bag X1, Pinelands 7430, South Africa. TEL 27-21-531-3081, FAX 27-21-531-4126.

TECHNOLOGIE & SANTE. see *TECHNOLOGY: COMPREHENSIVE WORKS*

362 ITA ISSN 0392-4831
TECNICA OSPEDALIERA. Text in Italian. 1971. m. ITL 85,000; ITL 160,000 in Europe; ITL 220,000 elsewhere (effective 1999). adv. charts, illus. **Description:** Covers hospital management and technical matters.
Formerly: Nuova Tecnica Ospedaliera (0029-6252)
Indexed: Archit.Per.Ind.
—GNLM.
Published by: Tecniche Nuove s.p.a., Via Ciro Menotti, 14, Milan, MI 20129, Italy. TEL 39-027570232, FAX 39-027570331, abbonamenti@tecnet.it; tecosp@tecnet.it, http://tecnet.it/index1.html. Ed. Enzo Guaglione. adv.: B&W page ITL 1,980,000, color page ITL 3,168,000; trim 297 x 210. Circ: 6,000.

362.1 USA
TELEMEDICINE. Text in English. 1993. m. USD 397. back issues avail. **Document type:** *Trade.* **Description:** Covers the growing telemedicine industry for implementers, end-users, strategic planners and vendors.
Published by: Miller Freeman, Inc. (Subsidiary of: United Newspapers), 600 Harrison St, San Francisco, CA 94107. TEL 415-905-2550, FAX 415-905-2235. Ed. Deborah Dakins.

TEXAS HOSPITAL LAW. see *LAW*

362 GBR ISSN 0308-7808
THERAPY WEEKLY; the newspaper for the remedial professions. Text in English. 1974. w. GBP 35 to individuals; GBP 49 domestic to institutions; GBP 89 foreign to institutions; GBP 20 to students (effective 2000). adv. bk.rev. reprint service avail. from PQC. **Document type:** *Newspaper, Trade.*
Incorporates: Remedial Therapist
Related titles: Microform ed.: (from PQC).
Indexed: CINAHL.
—BLDSC (8814.768000). **CCC.**
Published by: Emap Healthcare Ltd. (Subsidiary of: Emap Business Communications Ltd.), Greater London House, Hampstead Rd, London NW1 7EJ, United Kingdom. TEL 44-20-7874-0200, FAX 44-20-7874-0201, http://www.emap.com. Ed. Melissa Daries. Pub. Andrew Sumner. Adv. contact Ross Talbot. Circ: 9,500.

362.11 DNK
TIDSSKRIFT FOR DANSK SUNDHEDSVAESEN. Text in Danish, Norwegian, Swedish. 1924. 10/yr. DKK 740. adv. bk.rev. bibl, charts, illus, stat.
Formerly (until 1994): Tidsskrift for Danske Sygehuse (0040-702X)
Indexed: Excerp.Med.
Published by: Dansk Selskab for Sygehusledelse, c/o Forlaget John Vaboe AS, Emiliekildevej 35, Klampenborg 2930, Denmark. Ed. Preben Hansen. Circ: 2,278.

TIJDSCHRIFT VOOR HYGIENE EN INFEKTIEPREVENTIE. see *MEDICAL SCIENCES—Communicable Diseases*

TIJDSCHRIFT VOOR VERPLEEGHUISGENEESKUNDE. see *MEDICAL SCIENCES*

658 USA ISSN 1065-0989
TOPICS IN HEALTH INFORMATION MANAGEMENT. Text in English. 1980. q. USD 172 to individuals; USD 52 newsstand/cover (effective 2002). **Document type:** *Journal.* **Description:** Focuses on the unique information needs of the medical information practitioner. Provides a practical look at DRGs, cost control, quality control, ambulatory care, legal responsibilities, patient privacy, computer operations, etc.
Formerly (until 1991): Topics in Health Record Management (0270-5230)
Related titles: Online - full text ed.: (from Ovid Technologies, Inc., ProQuest Information & Learning).
Indexed: Abstr.Health Care Manage.Stud., BPIA, Bus.Ind., CINAHL, Comput.Cont., Int.Nurs.Ind.
—BLDSC (8867.443200), CISTI, GNLM, ingenta. **CCC.**
Published by: Aspen Publishers, Inc., 200 Orchard Ridge Dr, Ste 200, Gaithersburg, MD 20878. TEL 301-417-7500, 800-638-8437, FAX 301-417-7550, http://www.aspenpublishers.com. Ed. Melanie S Brodnik. Circ: 3,000.

TREATISE ON HEALTH CARE LAW. see *LAW*

H

362 USA ISSN 0041-3674
RA960 CODEN: TRSTB
TRUSTEE. Text in English. 1947. 10/yr. USD 40 domestic; USD 70 foreign; USD 5 newsstand/cover (effective 2001). adv. bk.rev. index. back issues avail. **Document type:** *Trade.* **Description:** Provides boards and advisory councils of health care providers with the information they need to improve their institutions' operations and the health of their communities.
Related titles: Microform ed.: 1947 (from PQC); Online - full text ed.: 1947 (from ProQuest Information & Learning, Northern Light Technology, Inc., Factiva).
Indexed: ABI Inform. (Jan.1988-), Abstr.Health Care Manage.Stud., Excerp.Med., Hosp.Lit.Ind., Int.Nurs.Ind.
Published by: American Hospital Publishing, Inc. (Subsidiary of: American Hospital Association Company), 1 N Franklin St, 27th Fl, Chicago, IL 60606-3421. TEL 312-440-6800, FAX 312-951-8491, 312-422-4799, http://www.trusteemag.com/trustee-home.html. Ed. Karen Gardner. Circ: 36,100.

362.1 USA ISSN 1091-1626
24 X 7. Text in English. 1996. m. free to qualified personnel. adv. **Document type:** *Journal, Trade.* **Description:** Aimed at professionals involved in the maintenance and repair of medical, computer and telecommunications technology within a healthcare facility.
Published by: Medical World Communications, Allied Healthcare Group, 295 Promenade St, Ste 2, Providence, RI 02908-5720. TEL 401-455-0555, FAX 401-455-1555, info@healthtechnet.com, http://www.healthtechnet.com. Ed. Bob Larkin. Pub., R&P Jack Spears. Adv. contact Leonora Crook. B&W page USD 1,995, color page USD 2,590; trim 10.88 x 8.13. Circ: 12,900 (controlled).

U.S. NATIONAL CENTER FOR HEALTH STATISTICS. VITAL AND HEALTH STATISTICS. SERIES 13. DATA ON HEALTH RESOURCES UTILIZATION. see *PUBLIC HEALTH AND SAFETY*

362 614 BEL ISSN 0777-9364
U Z MAGAZINE. (Universitaire Ziekenhuis) Text in Dutch. 1985. q. free. adv. bk.rev. illus. back issues avail. **Document type:** *Journal, Trade.* **Description:** Presents news and information for patients, visitors and families.
Published by: U Z Gasthuisberg Organisatie- Ontwikkeling, Herestraat 49, Leuven 3000, Belgium. TEL 32-16-346750, FAX 32-16-345500, roland.vermeylen@uz.kuleuven.ac.be. Ed. Roland Vermeylen. Circ: 55,000.

THE UNIVERSAL HEALTHCARE ALMANAC. see *STATISTICS*

UNIVERSIDADE DE SAO PAULO. HOSPITAL DAS CLINICAS. REVISTA. see *MEDICAL SCIENCES*

362.15 610 ITA ISSN 0391-1470
VITA OSPEDALIERA. Summaries in English. 1946. irreg. ITL 30,000, USD 22.50. adv.
Published by: Fatebenefratelli della Provincia Romana, Via Lucio Cassio, 600, Rome, RM 00189, Italy. TEL 39-06-33553571, cdossegr@melograto.it. Ed. Giuseppe Magliozzi. Adv. contact Marina Stizza. Circ: 5,000.

362 USA ISSN 0005-1861
VOLUNTEER LEADER*. Text in English. 1960. q. USD 10; USD 15 foreign (effective 2000). adv. bk.rev. index. **Document type:** *Bulletin.*
Formerly: Auxiliary Leader

Related titles: Microform ed.: 1960 (from PQC).
Indexed: Hosp.Lit.Ind.
Published by: American Hospital Publishing, Inc. (Subsidiary of: American Hospital Association Company), 1 N Franklin St, 27th Fl, Chicago, IL 60606-3421. TEL 312-440-6800, FAX 312-951-8491. Ed. Mary Grayson. Circ: 6,000.

WESTERN JOURNAL OF NURSING RESEARCH; an international forum for communicating nursing research. see *MEDICAL SCIENCES—Nurses And Nursing*

WHO'S WHO IN THE EMERGENCY & RESCUE SERVICES (YEAR). see *PUBLIC HEALTH AND SAFETY*

362 GBR ISSN 0512-3135
WORLD HOSPITALS AND HEALTH SERVICES. Text mainly in English; Text occasionally in French, Spanish; Summaries in English, French, Spanish. 1929. 3/yr. GBP 70 to non-members. adv. bk.rev. index, cum.index every 3 yrs. *Refereed.* **Document type:** *Academic/Scholarly.* **Description:** Apprises readers of developments in hospitals and health services, quality assurance, ethical issues, hospital architecture and design, national health systems, and strategic planning.
Formerly (until 1964): Nosokomeion; Incorporates (in 1994): World Hospitals. Suplemento Espanol (0308-6062); And: World Hospitals. Supplement Francais (0308-6070)
Related titles: Microform ed.: (from PQC); Online - full text ed.
Indexed: ASSIA, Br.Hum.Ind., CINAHL, Dok.Arbeitsmed., Excerp.Med., I.P.A., Int.Nurs.Ind., Med.Care Rev.
—BLDSC, CISTI, GNLM, ingenta, Linda Hall.
Published by: International Hospital Federation, 4 Abbots Pl, London NW6 4NP, United Kingdom. TEL 44-207-372-7181, FAX 44-207-328-7433, 101662.1262@compuserve.com, http://www.powertek.co.uk/ihf. Ed. Dr. Errol Pickering. R&P Carl Richmond. Circ: 2,500.

WORLD MEDICAL JOURNAL. see *MEDICAL SCIENCES*

658 JPN
YOKOHAMA MINAMI KYOSAI BYOIN NENPO/ YOKOHAMA MINAMI MUTUAL AID ASSOCIATION HOSPITAL. ANNUAL REPORT. Text in Japanese. 1979. a.
Published by: Yokohama Minami Kyosai Byoin, 500 Mutsura-cho, Kanazawa-ku, Yokohama-shi, Kanagawa-ken 236-0032, Japan.

658 362 NLD ISSN 1381-0901
Z M MAGAZINE. (Zorg Management) Text in Dutch. 1985. m. (11/yr.). NLG 155; NLG 205 foreign. adv. **Document type:** *Trade.*
Former titles (until 1994): Ziekenhuismanagement Magazine (0923-1900); (until 1988): Z M Magazine (0169-3026)
Published by: Wyt Uitgeefgroep B.V., Postbus 6438, Rotterdam 3002 AK, Netherlands. TEL 31-10-425-5944, FAX 31-10-478-0904.

368 CZE ISSN 1212-2904
ZDRAVOTNI POJISTENI A REVIZNI LEKARSTVI/HEALTH INSURANCE AND MEDICAL REVIEW. Text in Czech; Summaries in Czech, English. 1997. q. EUR 56, USD 72 (effective 2001). adv. bk.rev. bibl, charts, illus. index. *Refereed.* **Document type:** *Academic/Scholarly.* **Description:** Includes papers, articles, reviews, case studies, and other current information on health insurance and medicine.
Formerly (until 1998): Zdravotnictvi a Zdravotni Pojisteni (1211-6289)
Related titles: E-mail ed.
—BLDSC (9438.797000).
Published by: (Ceska Lekarska Spolecnost J.E. Purkyne/Czech Medical Association), Nakladatelske Stredisko C L S J.E. Purkyne, Sokolska 31, Prague 12026, Czech Republic. TEL 42-2-24911420, FAX 42-2-24911420, nts@iol.cz, http://www.clsjep.cz, http://www.medical.cz. Ed. Jaroslav Gebhart. R&P A Leblova TEL 42-2-71747230. adv.: B&W page CZK 24,500, color page CZK 43,000; 250 x 170. Circ: 1,000.

658 CHN ISSN 1001-5329
ZHONGGUO YIYUAN GUANLI/CHINESE HOSPITAL MANAGEMENT. Text in Chinese. m.
Published by: Heilongjiang Sheng Weishengting/ Heilongjiang Provincial Bureau of Health, 27, Xiangshun Jie, Xiangfang-qu, Harbin, Heilongjiang 150036, China. TEL 53359. Ed. Li Yihe.

ZHONGGUO YIYUAN YAOXUE ZAZHI/CHINESE JOURNAL OF HOSPITAL PHARMACY. see *PHARMACY AND PHARMACOLOGY*

362 CHN ISSN 1000-6672
ZHONGHUA YIYUAN GUANLI ZAZHI/CHINESE JOURNAL OF HOSPITAL ADMINISTRATION. Text in Chinese. 1985. bi-m. CNY 96 domestic; USD 17.40 foreign; CNY 8 newsstand/cover domestic; USD 2.90 newsstand/cover foreign (effective 2001). **Document type:** *Academic/Scholarly.*
Related titles: Online - full content ed.: (from WanFang Data Corp.).
Published by: Zhonghua Yixuehui (Beijing Fenhui)/Chinese Medical Association (Beijing Branch), Dongdan 3 Tiaojia 7 Hao, Beijing 0253-9713, China. TEL 86-1-65257767. Ed. Ying-qi Gu. **Dist. by:** China International Book Trading Corp, 35, Chegongzhuang Xilu, Haidian District, Beijing 100044, China. TEL 86-1-68413849, FAX 86-1-68412048, cibtc@mail.cibtc.com.cn, http://www.cibtc.com.cn.

ZORG & VERZEKERING; actuele informatie in de gezondheidszorg. see *INSURANCE*

362.11068 NLD ISSN 1384-4202
ZORGVISIE. Text in Dutch. 1971. 16/yr. NLG 502.50; includes Newsletter. adv. **Document type:** *Trade.* **Description:** Includes information on hospital management and nursing homes.
Supersedes (in 1996): Ziekenhuis (0044-4715); Incorporates (1993-1997): Gezondheidszorg en Management (0928-5202)
Related titles: ♦ Supplement: Nieuwsbrief ZorgVisie. ISSN 1384-4199.
—GNLM.
Published by: Elsevier Gezondheidszorg B.V., Tijdstroom (Subsidiary of: Reed Elsevier plc Group), Planetenbaan 1, Maarssen 3600 AK, Netherlands. TEL 31-364-577577, FAX 31-346-554287, http://www.tijdstroom.nl. Adv. contact Cor Vannek. B&W page NLG 2,488, color page NLG 4,813; trim 297 x 210. Circ: 4,370. **Subscr. to:** Elsevier Den Haag, Postbus 16500, The Hague 2500 BM, Netherlands. TEL 31-70-381-9900, FAX 31-70-333-8399.

HEALTH FACILITIES AND ADMINISTRATION—Abstracting, Bibliographies, Statistics

362.025 USA ISSN 0094-8969
RA977.A1
A H A GUIDE TO THE HEALTH CARE FIELD✶. Text in English. 1945. a. USD 195 to non-members; USD 75 to members. adv. stat, tr.lit. **Document type:** *Directory.* **Description:** Directory listing registered hospitals, with selected data: health care systems; American Hospital Association institutional members; international, national, and regional organizations; and state organizations and agencies.
Related titles: CD-ROM ed.: 1945; Diskette ed.: 1945.
Indexed: SRI.
Published by: (American Hospital Association), American Hospital Publishing, Inc. (Subsidiary of: American Hospital Association Company), 1 N Franklin St, 27th Fl, Chicago, IL 60606-3421. TEL 312-422-3541, 800-621-6902, FAX 312-422-4651, http://www.aha.org. Ed. Jane Olson. Circ: 30,000. **Orders to:** A H A Sevices Inc., PO Box 92683, Chicago, IL 92683. TEL 800-AHA-2626, FAX 312-422-4505.

362 USA
A H A HOSPITAL STATISTICS (YEAR)✶. Text in English. 1946. a. USD 139 to non-members; USD 59 to members. charts, stat. index. **Document type:** *Directory.* **Description:** Compilation of detailed statistical data on US hospitals, including data on utilization, personnel, finances, facilities and services, approvals, affiliations, and revenue.
Former titles: Hospital Statistics; Data from American Hospital Association Annual Survey (0090-6662); Survey of Hospital Charges (0360-9316)
Related titles: Microfiche ed.: 1946 (from CIS).
Indexed: SRI.
Published by: (American Hospital Association), American Hospital Publishing, Inc. (Subsidiary of: American Hospital Association Company), 1 N Franklin St, 27th Fl, Chicago, IL 60606-3421. TEL 312-422-3541, 800-621-6902, FAX 312-422-4651, http://www.aha.org. Circ: 15,000. **Orders to:** A H A Sevices Inc., PO Box 92683, Chicago, IL 92683. TEL 800-AHA-2626, FAX 312-422-4505.

362.021 AUS ISSN 1036-613X
AUSTRALIA. BUREAU OF STATISTICS. AUSTRALIAN HOSPITAL STATISTICS. Text in English. 1996. a. price varies. **Document type:** *Government.*
Published by: Australian Bureau of Statistics, PO Box 10, Belconnen, ACT 2616, Australia. TEL 61-2-6252-5249, FAX 61-2-6252-6778, http://www.abs.gov.au.

362.021 AUS
AUSTRALIA. BUREAU OF STATISTICS. HOSPITALS, AUSTRALIA. Text in English. 1992. a. AUD 22 (effective 1998). **Document type:** *Government.*
Published by: Australian Bureau of Statistics, PO Box 10, Belconnen, ACT 2616, Australia. TEL 61-2-6252-5249, FAX 61-2-6252-6778, http://www.abs.gov.au.

362.021 AUS
▼ **AUSTRALIA. BUREAU OF STATISTICS. OCCASIONAL PAPER: HOSPITAL STATISTICS, ABORIGINAL AND TORRES STRAIT ISLANDER AUSTRALIANS.** Text in English. 2000. irreg. AUD 23 (effective 2001).
Published by: Australian Bureau of Statistics, PO Box 10, Belconnen, ACT 2616, Australia. TEL 61-2-6252-5249, FAX 61-2-6252-6778, http://www.abs.gov.au.

658.021 AUS ISSN 1039-3005
AUSTRALIA. BUREAU OF STATISTICS. PRIVATE HOSPITALS, AUSTRALIA. Text in English. 1991. a., latest 1998. AUD 20 (effective 2001). **Document type:** *Government.* **Description:** Provides details of the operation of private, acute, psychiatric and day hospitals.
Related titles: Diskette ed.
Published by: Australian Bureau of Statistics, PO Box 10, Belconnen, ACT 2616, Australia. TEL 61-2-6252-5249, FAX 61-2-6252-6778, http://www.abs.gov.au.

658 JPN
BYOIN KANRI KENKYUJO KENKYU SHUDANKAI ENDAI SHOROKU/NATIONAL INSTITUTE OF HOSPITAL ADMINISTRATION. ABSTRACTS OF THE MEETING. Text in Japanese. a. **Document type:** *Abstract/Index.*
Published by: Koseisho, Byoin Kanri Kenkyujo/Ministry of Health and Welfare, National Institute of Hospital Administration, 21-13, Toyama 1-chome, Shinjuku-ku, Tokyo 162, Japan.

658 CHL
CHILE. INSTITUTO NACIONAL DE ESTADISTICAS. ESTADISTICAS DE SALUD. EGRESOS HOSPITALARIOS. Text in Spanish. 1971. a. CLP 1,450; USD 9.50 in United States; USD 10.20 elsewhere.
Published by: Instituto Nacional de Estadisticas, Casilla 498, Correo 3, Ave. Bulnes, 418, Santiago, Chile. TEL 56-2-6991441, FAX 56-2-6712169.

016.614 NLD ISSN 0921-8068
RA410.A1
EXCERPTA MEDICA. SECTION 36: HEALTH POLICY, ECONOMICS AND MANAGEMENT. Text in English. 1971. bi-m. EUR 276 in Europe to qualified personnel; JPY 37,375 in Japan to qualified personnel; USD 308 elsewhere to qualified personnel; EUR 1,293 in Europe to institutions; JPY 171,418 in Japan to institutions; USD 1,447 elsewhere to institutions (effective 2002). adv. charts. index, cum.index. **Document type:** *Abstract/Index, Academic/Scholarly, Trade.* **Description:** Provides a comprehensive current-awareness service for trade and academic articles covering the economic, social, and political aspects of health care and its organization and includes hospital management, health care marketing, hospital automation, and the assessment of new technology for the health care industry.
Former titles: Excerpta Medica. Section 36: Health Economics and Hospital Management (0300-5321); Excerpta Medica. Section 36: Health Economics
Related titles: CD-ROM ed.: (from SilverPlatter Information, Inc.); Online - full text ed.: (from DIMDI, Data-Star, The Dialog Corporation, JICST).
—GNLM, Infotrieve, Linda Hall. **CCC.**
Published by: Excerpta Medica Medical Communications BV (Subsidiary of: Reed Elsevier plc), Rooseveltweg 15, Almere-Stad 1314 SJ, Netherlands. TEL 31-36-538-5600, FAX 31-36-538-5650, http://www.elsevier.com/locate/hlthpolecoman, http://www.excerptamedica.com. **Subscr. in Australasia and the Far East to:** Elsevier Science (Singapore) Pte Ltd, No.1 Temasek Ave, 17-01 Millenia Tower, Singapore 039192, Singapore. TEL 65-434-3727, FAX 65-337-2230; **Subscr. in Japan to:** Elsevier Science Inc - Japan Regional Office, 9-15 Higashi-Azabu 1-chome, Minato-ku, Tokyo 106-0044, Japan. TEL 81-3-5561-5033, FAX 81-3-5561-5047; **Subscr. in the Americas to:** Elsevier Science, PO Box 2129, Marion, OH 43305-2129. usinfo-f@elsevier.com. **Dist. by:** Elsevier Science (Brazil).; Elsevier Science BV, PO Box 211, Amsterdam 1000 AE, Netherlands. TEL 31-20-485-3757, FAX 31-20-485-3432.

658.2 GBR
GREAT BRITAIN. GOVERNMENT STATISTICAL SERVICE. SUMMARY OF BED AVAILABILITY. ENGLAND - FINANCIAL YEAR (YEAR). Text in English. a. GBP 5. **Document type:** *Government.*
Published by: (Puerto Rico. Department of Health USA, Great Britain. Statistics Division), Government Statistical Service, SD2, Rm 804, Hannibal House, Elephant and Castle, London SE1 6TE, United Kingdom. TEL 0171-972-2193. **Orders to:** Department of Health and Social Security (Leaflets), PO Box 21, Stanmore, Mddx HA7 1AY, United Kingdom.

ISRAEL. CENTRAL BUREAU OF STATISTICS. DIAGNOSTIC STATISTICS OF HOSPITALIZATIONS. see *SOCIAL SERVICES AND WELFARE—Abstracting, Bibliographies, Statistics*

658 USA ISSN 1043-9285
LENGTH OF STAY BY D R G AND PAYMENT SOURCE. (Diagnosis Related Group) Text in English. 1988. a. price varies. back issues avail.
Related titles: Diskette ed.; Regional ed.: Length of Stay by D R G and Payment Source (Western Region Edition); Length of Stay by D R G and Payment Source (Southern Region Editon); Length of Stay by D R G and Payment Source (Northcentral Region Edition); Length of Stay by D R G and Payment Source (Northeastern Region Edition).
Indexed: SRI.
Published by: H C I A Inc., 300 E Lombard St, Baltimore, MD 21202. TEL 800-568-3282, FAX 410-752-6309.

658 310 USA ISSN 0895-982X
RA407.3
LENGTH OF STAY BY DIAGNOSIS & OPERATION, UNITED STATES. Text in English. 1964. a. price varies. stat.
Formerly: Length of Stay by Diagnosis, United States (0891-2149); Incorporates: Length of Stay by Operation, United States (0891-2203)
Related titles: Diskette ed.
Indexed: SRI.
Published by: H C I A Inc., 300 E Lombard St, Baltimore, MD 21202. TEL 800-568-3282, FAX 410-752-6309.

658 310 USA ISSN 0895-9846
RA981.M52
LENGTH OF STAY BY DIAGNOSIS & OPERATION, UNITED STATES, NORTH CENTRAL REGION. Text in English. 1964. a. price varies. stat.
Formerly: Length of Stay by Diagnosis, United States, North Central Region (0891-2165); Incorporates: Length of Stay by Operation, United States, North Central Region (0891-222X)
Related titles: Diskette ed.
Published by: H C I A Inc., 300 E Lombard St, Baltimore, MD 21202. TEL 800-568-3282, FAX 410-752-6309.

658 310 USA ISSN 0895-9838
RA981.N86
LENGTH OF STAY BY DIAGNOSIS & OPERATION, UNITED STATES, NORTHEASTERN REGION. Text in English. 1964. a. price varies. stat. back issues avail.
Formerly: Length of Stay by Diagnosis, United States, Northeastern Region (0891-2122); Incorporates: Length of Stay by Operation, United States, Northeastern Region (0888-2673)
Related titles: Diskette ed.; Magnetic Tape ed.; Microfiche ed.
Published by: H C I A Inc., 300 E Lombard St, Baltimore, MD 21202. TEL 800-568-3282, FAX 410-752-6309.

658 310 USA ISSN 0895-9854
RA981.S63
LENGTH OF STAY BY DIAGNOSIS & OPERATION, UNITED STATES, SOUTHERN REGION. Text in English. 1964. a. price varies. stat.
Formerly: Length of Stay by Diagnosis, United States, Southern Region (0891-2130); Incorporates: Length of Stay by Operation, United States, Southern Region (0891-219X)
Related titles: Diskette ed.
Published by: H C I A Inc., 300 E Lombard St, Baltimore, MD 21202. TEL 800-568-3282, FAX 410-752-6309.

658 310 USA ISSN 0895-9862
RA981.W36
LENGTH OF STAY BY DIAGNOSIS & OPERATION, UNITED STATES, WESTERN REGION. Text in English. 1964. a. price varies. stat.
Formerly: Length of Stay by Diagnosis, United States, Western Region (0891-2157); Incorporates: Length of Stay by Operation, United States, Western Region (0891-2211)
Published by: H C I A Inc., 300 E Lombard St, Baltimore, MD 21202. TEL 800-568-3280, FAX 410-539-5220.

362.021 NZL
RA407.5.N4
NEW ZEALAND HEALTH INFORMATION SERVICE. SELECTED MORBIDITY FOR PUBLICLY FUNDED HOSPITALS. Key Title: Hospital and Selected Morbidity Data. Text in English. a., latest 1998/1999. NZD 30 (effective 2001). **Document type:** *Government.*
Formerly: New Zealand. Health Statistical Services. Hospital and Selected Morbidity Data (0548-9938)
Published by: New Zealand Health Information Service, Ministry of Health, Level 11, Ballantrae House, 192-194 Willis St, P.O. Box 5013, Wellington, New Zealand. TEL 64-4-8012700, FAX 64-4-8012769, nzhis-pubs@web1.health.govt.nz, http://www.health.govt.nz/NZHIS/home/thml.

300 NOR ISSN 0806-0711
HA1503
NORWAY. STATISTISK SENTRALBYRAA. PASIENTSTATISTIKK. Key Title: Pasientstatistikk (Kongsvinger). Text in Norwegian. 1965. irreg. NOK 140 (effective 1999). **Document type:** *Government.*
Supersedes (in 1994): Norway. Statistisk Sentralbyraa. Rapporter - R A P P (0806-2056); Which was formerly (until 1993): Norway. Statistisk Sentralbyraa. Rapporter fra Statistisk Sentralbyraa (0332-8422); (until 1979): Norway. Statistisk Sentralbyraa. Aktuelle Skattetall (0301-8970)
Indexed: World Ag.Econ.& Rur.Soc.Abstr.
Published by: Statistisk Sentralbyraa, Postboks 8134, Dep, Oslo 0033, Norway. TEL 47-22-11-67-70, FAX 47-22-42-05-51, http://www.ssb.no. Circ: 23,760.

617 362 USA ISSN 1065-8173
O R REPORTS. (Operating Room) Text in English. 1992. m. USD 88 in United States; USD 98 in Canada; USD 108 elsewhere (effective 2001). index. 6 p./no. 3 cols./p. back issues avail.; reprints avail. **Document type:** *Trade.* **Description:** Abstracts of scientific articles relating to the operating room environment and relevant standards and regulations.
Related titles: Online - full content ed.
Published by: O R Manager, Inc., 1807 Second St, Ste 61, Santa Fe, NM 87505. TEL 800-442-9918, FAX 505-983-0790, ormanager@compuserve.com, http://www.ormanager.com/. Ed. Pat Patterson. Pub., R&P Elinor S Schrader. Circ: 700 (paid).

658 310 USA ISSN 0891-1223
RJ27.2
PEDIATRIC LENGTH OF STAY BY DIAGNOSIS AND OPERATION, UNITED STATES. Text in English. 1964. a. price varies. stat. back issues avail.
Related titles: Diskette ed.
Indexed: SRI.
Published by: H C I A Inc., 300 E Lombard St, Baltimore, MD 21202. TEL 800-568-3280, FAX 410-539-5220.

658 DNK ISSN 0107-1173
RA989.D4
PERSONALE- OG OEKONOMISTATISTIK FOR SYGEHUSVAESENET. Text in Danish. 1976. a. DKK 60.
Formerly: Personale og Sengepladser ved de Sygedomsbehandlende Institutioner
Published by: Sundhedsstyrelsen, Amaliegade 13, PO Box 2020, Copenhagen K 1012, Denmark. **Subscr. to:** Statens Informationstjeneste, PO Box 1103, Copenhagen K 1009, Denmark.

362.1 316.8 ZAF
SOUTH AFRICA. STATISTICS SOUTH AFRICA. CENSUS OF HOSPITALS, CLINICS AND OTHER HEALTH SERVICE ESTABLISHMENTS. Text in English. triennial, latest 1998. ZAR 20 (effective 2000). **Document type:** *Government.*
Formerly (until Aug. 1998): South Africa. Central Statistical Service. Census of Hospitals, Clinics and Other Health Service Establishments
Published by: Statistics South Africa/Statistieke Suid-Afrika, Private Bag X44, Pretoria 0001, South Africa. TEL 27-12-310-8911, FAX 27-12-310-8500, info@statssa.pwv.gov.za, http://www.statssa.gov.za.

SOUTH AFRICA. STATISTICS SOUTH AFRICA. STATISTICAL RELEASE. CENSUS OF AUXILIARY, HEALTH SERVICES AND DENTAL TECHNICIANS (YEAR). see *MEDICAL SCIENCES—Abstracting, Bibliographies, Statistics*

SOUTH AFRICA. STATISTICS SOUTH AFRICA. STATISTICAL RELEASE. CENSUS OF DOCTORS (YEAR). see *MEDICAL SCIENCES—Abstracting, Bibliographies, Statistics*

362.1 316.8 ZAF
SOUTH AFRICA. STATISTICS SOUTH AFRICA. STATISTICAL RELEASE. CENSUS OF HOSPITALS, CLINICS AND OTHER HEALTH SERVICE ESTABLISHMENTS (YEAR). Text in English. irreg., latest 1990. **Document type:** *Government.*
Formerly (until Aug. 1998): South Africa. Central Statistical Service. Statistical Release. Census of Hospitals, Clinics and Other Health Service. Establishments (Year)
Published by: Statistics South Africa/Statistieke Suid-Afrika, Private Bag X44, Pretoria 0001, South Africa. TEL 27-12-310-8911, FAX 27-12-310-8500, info@statssa.pwv.gov.za, http://www.statssa.gov.za.

362.109489 DNK ISSN 0909-4156
SUNDHEDSSTATISTIKKEN (YEAR). Key Title: Sundhedsstatistikken (Koebenhavn). Text in Danish. 1981. irreg. (6-7/yr.). free (effective 2001).
Formed by the merger of (1981-1993): Sygehusstatistik (0107-6434); (1983-1993): Primaer Sundhedstjenestestatistik (0107-7503); (1982-1993): Vitalstatistik (0107-749X)
Published by: Sundhedsstyrelsen, Afd. Medicinalstatistik, Amaliegade 13, PO Box 2020, Copenhagen K 1012, Denmark. TEL 45-33-93-16-36, FAX 45-33-91-16-01.

H

362 URY ISSN 0041-8455
UNIVERSIDAD DE LA REPUBLICA. HOSPITAL DE CLINICAS. INFORME ESTATISTICO. Text in Spanish. 1962. a. USD 1.
Published by: Hospital de Clinicas "Dr. Manuel Quintela", Universidad de la Republica, Avda. Italia s-n, Montevideo, Uruguay. Circ: 400.

362.1109489 DNK ISSN 0903-8086
RA989.D4
VIRKSOMHEDEN VED SYGEHUSE. Text in Danish. 1986. a. DKK 100.
Published by: Sundhedsstyrelsen, Amaliegade 13, PO Box 2020, Copenhagen K 1012, Denmark. **Subscr. to:** Statens Informationstjeneste, PO Box 1103, Copenhagen K 1009, Denmark.

HEARING IMPAIRED

see HANDICAPPED—Hearing Impaired

HEAT

see PHYSICS—Heat

HEATING, PLUMBING AND REFRIGERATION

see also BUILDING AND CONSTRUCTION; ENGINEERING—Mechanical Engineering

628 USA ISSN 0066-068X
AMERICAN SOCIETY OF SANITARY ENGINEERING. YEAR BOOK. Text in English. 1906. a. USD 15. adv. cum.index: 1906-1950, 1951-1963, 1963-1970. **Document type:** *Proceedings, Trade.*
—CISTI.
Published by: American Society of Sanitary Engineering, 901 Canterbury, Ste A, Westlake, OH 44145. TEL 440-835-3040, FAX 440-835-3488, info@asse-plumbing.org, http://www.asse-plumbing.org. Ed., Pub., R&P, Adv. contact Shannon Corcoran TEL 440-835-3040. Circ: 2,700.

▼ **INDOOR ENVIRONMENT CONNECTIONS**; the newspaper for the iaq marketplace. (indoor air quality) see *ENVIRONMENTAL STUDIES*

697 331.8 USA ISSN 0569-4043
TH7392.M6
INDUSTRIAL VENTILATION; A MANUAL OF RECOMMENDED PRACTICE. Text in English. 1951. biennial, latest vol.22, 1995. USD 55 domestic; USD 66 in Canada; USD 77 elsewhere. adv. **Document type:** *Academic/Scholarly.* **Description:** Features a compilation of research data and information on the design, maintenance, and evaluation of industrial exhaust ventilation systems.
—BLDSC (4462.880000).
Published by: American Conference of Governmental Industrial Hygienists, Inc., 1330 Kemper Meadow Dr, Ste 600, Cincinnati, OH 45240-1634. TEL 513-742-2020, FAX 513-742-3355. Ed., R&P Sharon E Ziegler. Pub. Richard A Strano. Adv. contact Mary Ruth Stimmel. Circ: 25,000.

KUKI CHOWA EISEI KOGAKU/HEATING, AIR-CONDITIONING AND SANITARY ENGINEERING. see *PUBLIC HEALTH AND SAFETY*

697 648 NOR ISSN 0029-2265
NORSK V V S. Text in Norwegian. 1957. 12/yr. NOK 620 (effective 2000). adv. bk.rev. illus, stat. index.
Document type: *Journal, Trade.*
Indexed: INIS Atomind., Int.Build.Serv.Abstr., Ref.Zh.
Published by: (Norsk V.V.S. Energi- og Miljoeteknisk Forening/Norwegian Society of Heating, Air-Conditioning and Sanitary Engineers), Skarland Press A-S, Postboks 5042, Majorstua, Oslo 0301, Norway. TEL 47-22-59-88-oo, FAX 47-22-69-36-50, norskvvs@skarland.no. Ed. Per Erik Holm. Adv. contact Aase Rostad. Circ: 5,060 (controlled).

697 628 DEU ISSN 0342-8184
S B Z - SANITAER, HEIZUNGS- UND KLIMATECHNIK. Text in German. 1945. fortn. DEM 264; DEM 292.80 foreign (effective 2000). adv. bk.rev. charts, illus, pat, tr.lit. index. **Document type:** *Trade.*
Former titles: S B Z - Sanitaer-Technik, Heizungs-, und Lueftungsbau (0036-1070); Sanitaer-Installation
Indexed: Int.Build.Serv.Abstr.
—Linda Hall.
Published by: (Zentralverband Sanitaer-, Heizungs- und Klimatechnik), Gentner Verlag Stuttgart, Forststr 131, Stuttgart 70193, Germany. TEL 49-711-63672-0, FAX 49-711-63672-11. Eds. D Schlattmann, E F Reisch. R&P E F Reisch. Adv. contact Walter Eder. Circ: 30,175.

697 628 DEU ISSN 0344-9122
SANITAER UND HEIZUNGS REPORT. Short title: S und H Report. Text in German. 10/yr. DEM 40; DEM 50 foreign (effective 1999). adv. bk.rev. **Document type:** *Trade.* **Description:** Trade publication for the bath and plumbing technicals. Information on new technology, latest trends and design, and new products.
Published by: Krammer Verlag Duesseldorf AG, Hermannstr 3, Duesseldorf 40233, Germany. TEL 49-211-91493, FAX 49-211-9149450, krammer@krammerag.de, http://www.krammerag.de. Eds. Friedrich Neeracher, Knut Siebrasse. Adv. contact Katrin Muckelberg. B&W page DEM 7,500; trim 257 x 185. Circ: 36,000.

HEMATOLOGY

see MEDICAL SCIENCES—Hematology

HIGHER EDUCATION

see EDUCATION—Higher Education

HINDUISM

see RELIGIONS AND THEOLOGY—Hindu

HISTORY

see also ANTHROPOLOGY; ARCHAEOLOGY; BIOGRAPHY; FOLKLORE; HISTORY—History Of Asia; HISTORY—History Of North And South America; and also specific subjects

BRANDSCHUTZ; Deutsche Feuerwehr-Zeitung. see *FIRE PREVENTION*

CHIROPRACTIC HISTORY. see *MEDICAL SCIENCES—Chiropractic, Homeopathy, Osteopathy*

EARLY SCIENCE AND MEDICINE; a journal for the study of science, technology and medicine in the pre-modern period. see *MEDICAL SCIENCES*

FLORIDA MUSEUM OF NATURAL HISTORY. BULLETIN. see *BIOLOGY*

900 500 610 BRA ISSN 0104-5970
R482.B8 CODEN: HCSMFK
HISTORIA, CIENCIAS, SAUDE - MANGUINHOS. Text in English, French, Portuguese, Spanish. 1994. 3/yr. adv. bk.rev. *Refereed.* **Document type:** *Academic/Scholarly.* **Description:** Publishes original papers, interviews, biographies and short notes on social and biological sciences.
Related titles: Online - full text ed.: (from SciELO).
Indexed: Amer.Hist.& Life, Hist.Abstr. (1995-), Lang.& Lang.Behav.Abstr., Rev.Appl.Entomol., SOPODA, Soc.Serv.Abstr., Sociol.Abstr.
Published by: Fundacao Oswaldo Cruz, Rua Nova Brasilia, 4365, Bonsucesso, Rio De Janeiro, RJ 21061-060, Brazil. TEL 55-21-280-9241, FAX 55-21-598-4437, gjben@@dcc001.cict.fiocruz.br. Ed. Jaime L Benchimol. R&P Ruth B Martins. Circ: 1,000.

HISTORIA HOSPITALIUM. see *HEALTH FACILITIES AND ADMINISTRATION*

INTERNATIONAL HISTORY OF NURSING JOURNAL. see *MEDICAL SCIENCES—Nurses And Nursing*

JOURNAL OF PSYCHOHISTORY. see *PSYCHOLOGY*

JOURNAL OF THE HISTORY OF BIOLOGY. see *BIOLOGY*

JOURNAL OF THE HISTORY OF MEDICINE AND ALLIED SCIENCES. see *MEDICAL SCIENCES*

JOURNAL OF THE HISTORY OF THE BEHAVIORAL SCIENCES. see *PSYCHOLOGY*

LESBIAN AND GAY ARCHIVIST. see *HOMOSEXUALITY*

MEDIZINHISTORISCHES JOURNAL. see *MEDICAL SCIENCES*

900 150 CAN ISSN 0111-8854
AP7.5
MENTALITIES/MENTALITES; an interdisciplinary journal. Text in English, French, German. 1982. 2/yr. USD 40 to individuals; USD 60 to institutions. adv. bk.rev. *Refereed.* **Document type:** *Academic/Scholarly.*
Indexed: Bibl.Engl.Lang.& Lit., Hist.Abstr. (1982-1991, 1993-1997, dropped), e-psyche.
—Infotrieve. **CCC.**
Address: 1532 Hillside Dr, London, ON N6G 4M4, Canada. TEL 519-858-0023, 800-395-1216, FAX 519-858-0023, ssusman@julian.uwo.ca. Ed. Dr. Norman Simms. R&P, Adv. contact Sam Sussman. Circ: 500.

THE NATURALIST. see *BIOLOGY*

NIEUWE NEDERLANDSE BIJDRAGEN TOT DE GESCHIEDENIS DER GENEESKUNDE EN DER NATUURWETENSCHAPPEN. see *MEDICAL SCIENCES*

ORVOSTORTENETI KOZLEMENYEK/COMMUNICATION DE HISTORIA ARTIS MEDICINAE. see *MEDICAL SCIENCES*

PRATIQUE; newsletter of the disinfected mail study circle. see *COMMUNICATIONS—Postal Affairs*

901 150.19 GBR ISSN 1460-8235
PSYCHOANALYSIS AND HISTORY. Text in English. 1998. s-a. GBP 18 domestic to individuals; GBP 22 foreign to individuals; GBP 50 domestic to institutions; GBP 54 foreign to institutions (effective 2000). adv. bk.rev. back issues avail. *Refereed.* **Document type:** *Journal, Academic/Scholarly.* **Description:** Devoted to both the study of the history of psychoanalysis and the application of psychoanalytic ideas to historiography.
Indexed: Amer.Hist.& Life, Hist.Abstr., PsycInfo, Psychoanal.Abstr., e-psyche.
—BLDSC (6946.264900).
Published by: Artesian Books Ltd., 18 Artesian Rd, London W2 5AR, United Kingdom. TEL 0208-287-1128, FAX 0208-287-1128, artesianbooks@fsmail.com, http://www.artesianbooks.co.uk. Ed. Andrea Sabbadini.

▼ **REVUE DE L'HISTOIRE DE BIOLOGIE.** see *BIOLOGY*

900 610 USA ISSN 0743-6033
SNAKEROOT EXTRACT. Text in English. 1984. q. USD 20. cum.index. back issues avail. **Document type:** *Bulletin, Newsletter, Academic/Scholarly.* **Description:** Covers the history of the health sciences of the late nineteenth and early twentieth centuries with an emphasis on pathology and psychology.
Published by: Indiana Medical History Museum, 3045 W Vermont St, Indianapolis, IN 46222-4943. TEL 317-635-7329. Ed. Oren S Cooley. Circ: 14,000.

STUDIES IN ANCIENT MEDICINE. see *MEDICAL SCIENCES*

TREASURES. see *MEDICAL SCIENCES*

HISTORY—History Of Asia

see also ORIENTAL STUDIES

ASIAN JOURNAL OF SOCIAL PSYCHOLOGY. see *PSYCHOLOGY*

HISTORY—History Of North And South America

A I H P NOTES. see *PHARMACY AND PHARMACOLOGY*

972.9 VIR
CARIBBEAN RESEARCH INSTITUTE. REPORT. Text in English. 1965. irreg., latest 1975, 10th anniv. issue. free per issue.
Formerly: Caribbean Islands Research Institute. Annual Report (0069-0503)
Published by: Caribbean Research Institute, University of the Virgin Islands, St Thomas, VI 00801. Ed. Clara Wimbro Mitchell Lewis. Circ: 750.

ILLINOIS. NATURAL HISTORY SURVEY. REPORTS. see *CONSERVATION*

ILLINOIS. STATE MUSEUM. SCIENTIFIC PAPERS SERIES. see *SCIENCES: COMPREHENSIVE WORKS*

980 574 CHL ISSN 0716-6478
F3186 CODEN: APSOE5
INSTITUTO DE LA PATAGONIA. ANALES. CIENCIAS SOCIALES. Text in Spanish; Summaries in English. 1970. a. CLP 3,500, USD 15. adv. bk.rev. bibl, charts, illus. *Refereed.* **Document type:** *Academic/Scholarly.* **Description:** Publishes original papers by researchers of the institute in the area of social sciences referring to Patagonia, Tierra del Fuego, Antarctica, adjacent islands and the southeastern Pacific Ocean.
Supersedes in part (vol.25, 1984): Instituto de la Patagonia. Anales (0085-1922)
Indexed: Aqua.Sci.& Fish.Abstr., Aquacult.Abstr., Environ.Sci.Poll.Mgmt., Sport Fish.Abstr.
Published by: Universidad de Magallanes, Instituto de la Patagonia, Casilla de Correos 113 D, Punta Arenas, Magallanes, Chile. TEL 56-61-212913, FAX 56-61-212973, TELEX 380004 UMAG-CK. Ed. Mateo Martinic. Circ: 500.

HOBBIES

see also PHILATELY; SPORTS AND GAMES

SWIMMING POOLS TODAY. see *SPORTS AND GAMES—Outdoor Life*

HOME ECONOMICS

see also NUTRITION AND DIETETICS

613.2 USA ISSN 0886-4446
COOKING LIGHT; the magazine of food and fitness. Text in English. 1987. 11/yr. USD 22 domestic; USD 3.95 newsstand/cover (effective 2001). bk.rev. illus. Index. reprints avail. **Document type:** *Magazine, Consumer.* **Description:** Presents articles on food, nutrition, and exercise, implementing a positive approach to a healthier lifestyle. Moderation, variety, and balance are emphasized.
Related titles: Braille ed.; Online - full text ed.: (from Northern Light Technology, Inc., ProQuest Information & Learning).
—ingenta.
Published by: Southern Progress Corp. (Subsidiary of: Time Warner, Inc.), 2100 Lakeshore Dr, Birmingham, AL 35209. TEL 205-877-6000, cookinglight@spc.com, http://www.cookinglight.com., http://cookinglight.com. Ed. Mary Kay Culpepper. Circ: 1,425,000 (paid). **Subscr. to:** PO Box 830549, Birmingham, AL 35283.

640 362.1 IND
CURRENT RESEARCH IN FAMILY & COMMUNITY SCIENCES. Text in English. 1993. 2/yr. **Document type:** *Academic/Scholarly.* **Description:** Covers family resources management, human nutrition, human development, textiles and clothing, education, public health, epidemiological research and community development.
Published by: S N D T Women's University, Department of Postgraduate Studies and Research in Home Science, Santacruz, Mumbai, Maharashtra 400 049, India. Eds. Ravikala Kamath, S A Udipi.

▼ **DIABETIC COOKING.** see *MEDICAL SCIENCES—Endocrinology*

ENVIRONMENTAL NUTRITION; the newsletter of food, nutrition and health. see *NUTRITION AND DIETETICS*

613.2 USA
TX326.A1
FAMILY ECONOMICS AND NUTRITION REVIEW. Text in English. 1943. q. USD 19 (effective 2001). bk.rev. illus. Index. back issues avail.; reprint service avail. from CIS,PQC. *Refereed.* **Document type:** *Government.*
Description: Features articles on nutrition research and promotion, family financial planning in such areas as food costs, consumer prices, child care services, housing, nutrition, and employment, with practical statistics and data from government research reports and surveys.
Formerly: Family Economics Review (0425-676X); Supersedes: Wartime Family Living and Rural Family Living
Related titles: Microfiche ed.: (from CIS); Microform ed.: (from PQC).
Indexed: AgeLine, Agricola, Amer.Stat.Ind. (1972-), C.I.J.E. (coverage dropped), Fam.Ind., IMFL, Ind.U.S.Gov.Per., J.of Econ.Lit., Lang.& Lang.Behav.Abstr., P.A.I.S., Ref.Pt.Food Indus.Abstr., Russ.Acad.Sci.Bibl., SOPODA, Sociol.Abstr.
—CISTI, ingenta.
Published by: U.S. Department of Agriculture, Center for Nutrition Policy and Promotion, 1120 20th St, N W, Ste 200, North Lobby, Washington, DC 20036. TEL 202-418-2312, FAX 202-208-2321, cnpp-web@www.usda.gov, http://www.usda.gov/cnpp/. Ed. Julia Dinkins. Circ: 5,000. **Subscr. to:** U.S. Government Printing Office, Superintendent of Documents, PO Box 371954, Pittsburgh, PA 15250-7954. TEL 202-512-1800, FAX 202-512-2250, orders@gpo.gov, http://www.access.gpo.gov.

FAMILY SAFETY & HEALTH. see *PUBLIC HEALTH AND SAFETY*

613.2 AUT
FRISCH GEKOCHT; ist halb gewonnen. Text in German. 5/yr. ATS 10 newsstand/cover (effective 2001). adv. **Document type:** *Magazine, Consumer.*
Published by: D und R Verlagsgesellschaft mbH, Leberstr 122, Vienna 1110, Austria. TEL 43-1-740770, FAX 43-1-74077841, office@d-r.at. Ed. Peter Haemmerle. Adv. contact Michael Scharnagl. color page XEU 9,738.16; trim 210 x 297. Circ: 250,000 (paid and controlled).

641.013 DEU ISSN 0323-4762
GASTRONOMIE; Fachmagazin fuer Hotel, Restaurant und Kueche. Text in German. 1970. 10/yr. EUR 55.50 domestic; EUR 70 foreign; EUR 8 newsstand/cover (effective 2002). adv. bk.rev. 120 p./no. **Document type:** *Magazine, Trade.*
Published by: Huss-Medien GmbH, Am Friedrichshain 22, Berlin 10407, Germany. TEL 49-30-42151381, FAX 49-30-42151421, gastro.vertrieb@hussberlin.de, verlag.wirtschaft@hussberlin.de, http://www.gastronomie-mag.de, http://www.hussberlin.de. Ed. Barbara Boehme. Adv. contact Ines Neumann. B&W page DEM 7,080, color page DEM 9,780; trim 184 x 266. Circ: 21,500 (controlled).

613.2 USA
▼ **GUSTO!.** Text in English. 2001 (Apr.). 2/yr. USD 2.99 newsstand/cover (effective 2001). adv. **Document type:** *Magazine, Consumer.* **Description:** Presents articles and features on all aspects of Latino lifestyles, cultures and cuisines, with an emphasis on nutrition and flavor.
Published by: Southern Progress Corp. (Subsidiary of: Time Warner, Inc.), 2100 Lakeshore Dr, Birmingham, AL 35209. TEL 205-877-6000, FAX 205-877-6422. Ed. Viviana Carballo. adv.: color page USD 9,100. Circ: 350,000 (paid and controlled).

JOURNAL OF FAMILY ECOLOGY AND CONSUMER SCIENCE/TYDSKRIF VIR GESINEKOLOGIE EN VERBRUIKERSWETENSKAPPE. see *NUTRITION AND DIETETICS*

641.5 613.2 POL ISSN 1233-2976
KUCHNIA; magazyn dla smakoszy. Text in Polish. 1995. m. PLZ 2.90 per issue; PLZ 3.90 newsstand/cover (effective 1999). adv. illus. **Document type:** *Consumer.*
Description: Includes recipes from all over the world, articles on different culinary cultures, and tips on healthy eating.
Indexed: AgroLibrex.
Published by: Proszynski i S-ka S.A., Ul Garazowa 7, Warsaw 02651, Poland. TEL 48-22-6077700, FAX 48-22-6077704, kuchnia@proszyanki.com.pl, http://www.proszynski.com.pl. Adv. contact Beata Polaczynska.

LOW-FAT & FAST. see *NUTRITION AND DIETETICS*

613.2 USA
NEW CUISINE ALTERNATIVE SERIES. Text in English. bi-m. USD 9.95 newsstand/cover (effective 2001). **Document type:** *Magazine, Consumer.*
Published by: Buckaroo Communications, L.L.C., 12434 Prescilla Rd, Camarillo, CA 93012. TEL 805-523-0990, 877-267-0388, FAX 805-523-0169.

NUTRITION AND FOOD SCIENCE. see *NUTRITION AND DIETETICS*

641.5 USA ISSN 0886-2338
QUICK & HEALTHY COOKING. Key Title: Prevention's Quick & Healthy Cooking. Text in English. 1986. s-a. USD 3.95 newsstand/cover. adv. **Document type:** *Consumer.*
Published by: Rodale, 33 E Minor St, Emmaus, PA 18098. TEL 610-967-5171, FAX 610-967-7725, customer_service@rodale.com, http://www.rodale.com.

SCHOLASTIC CHOICES; personal development & living skills. see *EDUCATION—Teaching Methods And Curriculum*

HOMOSEXUALITY

AFFINITY. see *RELIGIONS AND THEOLOGY—Other Denominations And Sects*

306.7 305.868 USA
AIDSIDA INFO. Text in English, Spanish. quadrennial. USD 35 to membership (effective 2000). **Document type:** *Newsletter.* **Description:** Provides Latina and Latino lesbian, gay, bisexual, and transgendered persons with up-to-date information on AIDS and available services.
Published by: National Latino -a Lesbian, Gay, Bisexual & Transgender Organization, 1612 K St, NW, Ste 500, Washington, DC 20006. TEL 202-466-8240, FAX 202-466-8530, http://www.lledo.org, http://www.llego.org.

306.76 USA
AMERICAN CROSSDRESSER. Text in English. 1990. q. USD 7.50 (effective 1998). back issues avail.
Description: Covers heterosexual crossdressing.
Indexed: e-psyche.
Published by: Chevalier Publications, PO Box 194, Tulare, CA 93275. TEL 209-688-6386. Ed. Carol Beecroft. Circ: 1,500.

306.766 USA
ASSOCIATION OF GAY AND LESBIAN PSYCHIATRISTS. NEWSLETTER. Text in English. 1978. q. USD 20 to non-members (effective 2000). adv. bk.rev. **Document type:** *Newsletter.*
Formerly: American Psychiatric Association Gay Caucus. Newsletter
Published by: Association of Gay and Lesbian Psychiatrists, 4514 Chester Ave, Philadelphia, PA 19143-3707. aglp@aglp.org, http://www.aglp.orgl. Ed. Guy Glass. Pub., R&P, Adv. contact Roy Harker TEL 215-222-2800. Circ: 600.

306.7662 GBR ISSN 1368-4728
AXIOM; living life to the full. Text in English. 1997. m. GBP 18 to individuals; GBP 36 to institutions; GBP 2 newsstand/cover. adv. film rev., music rev., rec.rev. **Document type:** *Consumer.* **Description:** Publishes articles of interest to gay men on a variety of health, fitness, and lifestyle topics.
—BLDSC (1840.978700).
Address: 73 Collier St, London N1 9BE, United Kingdom. TEL 44-171-833-3399, FAX 44-171-837-2707. Ed. Paul Disney. Adv. contact Maria Figgins. **Dist. by:** Portman Distribution, Gadoline House, 2 Godstone Rd, Whyteleafe, Surrey CR3 0EA, United Kingdom. TEL 44-20-8645-8200, FAX 44-20-8645-8239.

306.766 USA
BEAU. Text in English. 1989. 4/yr. USD 17.97; USD 4.95 newsstand/cover. adv. bk.rev., film rev. back issues avail. **Document type:** *Consumer.* **Description:** Covers sexual relations between gay men.
Published by: Sportomatic Ltd., PO Box 170, Irvington, NY 10533. dianaeditr@aol.com. Ed. Dan Maxwell. Pub., Adv. contact Wayne Shuster. R&P Diana Sheridan. Circ: 50,000.

306.766 USA ISSN 1045-2346
ECHO MAGAZINE; the magazine of the Southwest. Text in English. 1989. bi-w. USD 46; USD 1.95 newsstand/cover (effective 1999). adv. bk.rev., film rev., music rev., play rev., tel.rev., video rev. charts, illus. back issues avail. **Document type:** *Consumer.*
Description: Targeted to gay and lesbian community. Contains local and national news, editorials, AIDS treatment news, features, lifestyles, advice column, classified ads, and social calendars.
Related titles: Online - full text ed.
Published by: Ace Publishing, Inc., PO Box 16630, Phoenix, AZ 85011-6630. TEL 602-266-0550, FAX 602-266-0773, jeff4echo@aol.com, http://www.echomag.com/. Ed. Bruce Christian. Pub., R&P William Osovan. Adv. contact Leo Gonzales. page USD 575; trim 10.75 x 8. Circ: 48,000.

305.906 360 USA
EQUAL TIME: OUTREACH NEWSLETTER. Text in English. 1984. s-a. adv. back issues avail. **Document type:** *Newsletter.* **Description:** Covers important issues affecting Madison's lesbian, gay, bisexual and transgender communities.
Former titles: Unity: United Newsletter; United Newsletter
Related titles: Fax ed.
Published by: OutReach, Inc., PO Box 310, Madison, WI 53701-0310. TEL 608-255-8582, FAX 608-255-0018, outreach@outreachinc.com, http://www.outreach.com. Ed., Pub. Joseph Bednarowski.

305.9066 USA
F T M NEWSLETTER. (Female to Male) Text in English. 1987. q. USD 25 domestic; USD 35 foreign; USD 7.50 newsstand/cover. adv. bk.rev., tel.rev., video rev. illus. back issues avail. **Document type:** *Newsletter.*
Description: Dedicated to the issues and voices of female-to-male transsexuals and transgendered people.
Published by: F T M International, Inc., 1360 Mission St, 200, San Francisco, CA 94103. TEL 415-553-5987, tstgmen@aol.com, http://www.ftm-int.org. Ed., R&P Jed Rosenthal Bell. Adv. contact Dion Manley. B&W page USD 1,000; trim 11 x 8.5. Circ: 1,000 (paid).

GAY AND LESBIAN MEDICAL ASSOCIATION. JOURNAL. see *MEDICAL SCIENCES*

305.90664 USA
HAWAII'S NATIONAL GAY COMMUNITY NEWS; Hawaii and Western States. Text in English. 1973. q. USD 25; per issue contribution. adv. bk.rev. **Document type:** *Newspaper.* **Description:** Centers on gay and AIDS issues, task force work, upcoming events. Includes a state community services directory, classifieds, announcements, and news from western states.
Former titles: Gay Community News (Honolulu) (1044-3002); Gay Community Center Newsletter; (until 1987): Sexual Identity Center Newsletter
Published by: Gay Community News, PO Box 37083, Honolulu, HI 96837-0083. TEL 808-532-9000. Ed. William E Woods. Circ: 20,000.

155.34 USA ISSN 1083-4095
IN THE FAMILY; the magazine for lesbians, gays, bisexuals and their relations. Text in English. 1995. q., latest vol.7. USD 22; USD 5.50 newsstand/cover (effective 2001). adv. bk.rev., film rev. illus, stat, tr.lit. 32 p./no. back issues avail. **Document type:** *Magazine, Consumer.* **Description:** Explores family relationships when a member is gay, lesbian or bisexual; examines same-sex couple and family concerns.
Indexed: Alt.Press Ind., e-psyche.
Published by: Family Magazine, Inc., PO Box 5387, Takoma Park, MD 20913. TEL 301-270-4771, FAX 301-270-4660, http://inthefamily.com. Ed., Pub., R&P Laura Markowitz. Adv. contact Lauren Ackerman TEL 516-524-5949. page USD 500; trim 11 x 8.5. Circ: 1,800 (paid).

306.76 USA ISSN 1566-1768
HQ75 CODEN: JGLIFN
INTERNATIONAL JOURNAL OF SEXUALITY AND GENDER STUDIES. Text in English. 1996. q. USD 223, EUR 223 to institutions for print or online ed.; USD 267.60, EUR 267.60 to institutions for print & online eds. combined (effective 2002). adv. bk.rev. illus. back issues avail.; reprints avail. *Refereed.* **Document type:** *Journal, Academic/Scholarly.* **Description:** Promotes knowledge and ideas under the general categories of sexuality and gender studies, and every major aspects of lesbian, gay, bisexual and transgender life.
Formerly (until 2000): Journal of Gay, Lesbian and Bisexual Identity (1083-8147)
Related titles: Online - full text ed.: USD 180 domestic; USD 210 foreign (effective 2000) (from Swets Blackwell, Kluwer Online, RoweCom Information Quest).

H

Indexed: PsycInfo, Sage Fam.Stud.Abstr., Soc.Serv.Abstr., Sociol.Abstr., e-psyche.
—BLDSC (4542.545000), Infotrieve, ingenta. **CCC.**
Published by: Kluwer Academic - Plenum Publishers (Subsidiary of: Wolters Kluwer N.V.), 233 Spring St, New York, NY 10013-1578. TEL 212-620-8000, 800-221-9369, FAX 212-463-0742, info@plenum.com, http://www.wkap.nl/journalhome.htm/1566-1768. Ed. Warren J Blumenfeld. **Subscr. outside the Americas to:** Kluwer Academic Publishers Group, Journals Department, PO Box 322, Dordrecht 3300 AH, Netherlands. TEL 31-78-639-2392, FAX 31-78-654-6474.

306.766 USA ISSN 1529-9716
▼ **JOURNAL OF BISEXUALITY.** Text in English. 2000 (Spring). q. USD 48 domestic to individuals; USD 65 in Canada to individuals; USD 70 elsewhere to individuals; USD 85 domestic to institutions; USD 115 in Canada to institutions; USD 123 elsewhere to institutions; USD 125 domestic to libraries; USD 169 in Canada to libraries; USD 181 elsewhere to libraries (effective Aug. 2001). adv. back issues avail.; reprints avail. *Refereed.* **Document type:** *Journal, Academic/Scholarly.* **Description:** Covers both professional articles and serious essays on bisexuality and its meaning for the individual, the community and society.
Related titles: Online - full content ed.: ISSN 1529-9724.
Indexed: P.A.I.S.
Published by: Haworth Press, Inc., 10 Alice St, Binghamton, NY 13904-1580. TEL 607-722-5857, 800-429-6784, FAX 607-722-6362, 800-895-0582, getinfo@haworthpressinc.com, http://www.haworthpressinc.com, http://www.haworthpress.com. Ed. Fritz Klein. Pub. William Cohen. R&P Ruth Ann Heath. Adv. contact Jackie Blakeslee TEL 607-722-5857 ext 346. B&W page USD 315, color page USD 550; trim 6 x 8.5.

JOURNAL OF GAY & LESBIAN PSYCHOTHERAPY. see *PSYCHOLOGY*

JOURNAL OF GAY & LESBIAN SOCIAL SERVICES; issues in practice, policy & research. see *SOCIAL SERVICES AND WELFARE*

306.766 USA ISSN 0091-8369
HQ75 CODEN: JOHOD7
JOURNAL OF HOMOSEXUALITY. Text in English. 1974. q. (in 2 vols.). USD 60 domestic to individuals; USD 81 in Canada to individuals; USD 87 elsewhere to individuals; USD 125 domestic to institutions; USD 169 in Canada to institutions; USD 181 elsewhere to institutions; USD 385 domestic to libraries; USD 520 in Canada to libraries; USD 558 elsewhere to libraries (effective Aug. 2001). adv. bk.rev. abstr, bibl, charts, illus. index. back issues avail.; reprint service avail. from HAW,PSC,SCH. *Refereed.* **Document type:** *Journal, Academic/Scholarly.* **Description:** Covers theoretical, empirical, and historical research on homosexuality, heterosexuality, sexual identity, social sex roles, and the sexual relationships of both men and women.
Related titles: Microfiche ed.: (from PQC); Microform ed.; Online - full text ed.: (from Gale Group, Factiva, Institute for Scientific Information).
Indexed: ASCA, ASSIA, Abstr.Anthropol., Abstr.Crim.& Pen., Adol.Ment.Hlth.Abstr., AgeLine, Alt.Press Ind., Arts & Hum.Cit.Ind. (coverage dropped), Biol.Abstr., CERDIC, CWI, Crim.Just.Abstr., Curr.Cont., Environ.Sci.Poll.Mgmt., Excerp.Med., Fam.Ind., Gend.Watch, High.Educ.Abstr., Human Resour.Abstr., IMFL, Ind.Med. (1974-), Ind.Per.Art.Relat.Law, Ind.Philos., L.R.I., Lang.& Lang.Behav.Abstr., Mag.Ind., Mid.East: Abstr.& Ind., P C I, P.A.I.S., Packag.Sci.Tech., Past.Care & Couns.Abstr., Polit.Sci.Abstr., Pollut.Abstr., PsycInfo, Psychol.Abstr. (1974-), Psychol.R.G., Rel.Ind.One, Rel.Ind.Two, Risk Abstr., Russ.Acad.Sci.Bibl., SOPODA, SSCI, Saf.Sci.Abstr., Sage Fam.Stud.Abstr., Soc.Sci.Ind. (Sep.1987-), Soc.Serv.Abstr., Soc.Work Res.& Abstr., Sociol.Abstr., Stud.Wom.Abstr., Viol.& Abuse Abstr., Wom.Stud.Abstr., e-psyche.
—BLDSC (5002.970000), GNLM, Haworth, IDS, ingenta.
Published by: (San Francisco State University, Center for Research and Education in Sexuality), Haworth Press, Inc., 10 Alice St, Binghamton, NY 13904-1580. TEL 607-722-5857, 800-429-6784, FAX 607-722-6362, 800-895-0582, getinfo@haworthpressinc.com, http://www.haworthpressinc.com, http://www.haworthpress.com. Ed. John P De Cecco. Pub. William Cohen. R&P Ruthann Heath TEL 607-723-5857 ext 316. Adv. contact Jackie Blakeslee TEL 607-722-5857 ext 346. B&W page USD 375, color page USD 650; trim 6 x 8.5. Circ: 1,115.

363.49 USA ISSN 1089-4160
JOURNAL OF LESBIAN STUDIES. Text in English. 1997. q. USD 60 domestic to individuals; USD 81 in Canada to individuals; USD 87 elsewhere to individuals; USD 95 domestic to institutions; USD 128 in Canada to institutions; USD 138 elsewhere to institutions; USD 125 domestic to libraries; USD 169 in Canada to libraries; USD 181 elsewhere to libraries (effective Aug. 2001). adv. bk.rev. illus. reprint service avail. from HAW. *Refereed.* **Document type:** *Journal, Academic/Scholarly.*
Related titles: Microform ed.: (from PQC); Online - full text ed.: (from LexisNexis).
Indexed: Crim.Just.Abstr., Fem.Per. (1997-), Gend.Watch, P.A.I.S., Ref.Zh., Stud.Wom.Abstr., e-psyche.
—BLDSC (5010.295000), Haworth.
Published by: Haworth Press, Inc., 10 Alice St, Binghamton, NY 13904-1580. TEL 607-722-5857, 800-429-6784, FAX 607-722-6362, 800-895-0582, getinfo@haworthpressinc.com, http://www.haworthpress.com/journals/journallist.asp. Ed. Esther D Rothblum. Pub. William Cohen. R&P Ruthann Heath TEL 607-723-5857 ext 316. Adv. contact Jackie Blakeslee TEL 607-722-5857 ext 346. B&W page USD 315, color page USD 550; trim 6 x 8.5.

306.7663 CAN
LESBIAN AND GAY ARCHIVIST. Text in English. 1977. a. free per issue. adv. bk.rev. back issues avail. **Document type:** *Newsletter.* **Description:** Offers articles about activities and holdings of CLGA, information about other lesbian and gay archives, bibliographical listings.
Formerly: Gay Archivist (0714-3605)
Published by: Canadian Lesbian and Gay Archives, PO Box 639, Sta A, Toronto, ON M5W 1G2, Canada. TEL 416-777-2755, queeries@clga.ca, http://www.clga.ca. Circ: 1,200.

306.7663 AUS
LESBIAN AND GAY COUNSELLING NEWS. Text in English. 1980. a. AUD 30, USD 3. bk.rev. back issues avail. **Document type:** *Newsletter.*
Formerly: Gay Counselling (0705-5935)
Indexed: e-psyche.
Published by: Gay and Lesbian Counselling Service of N.S.W., GPO Box 334, Darlinghurst, NSW 2010, Australia. TEL 02-360-3063. Ed. Larry Singer. Circ: 350.

306.766 USA
LOVING BROTHERHOOD NEWSLETTER; a journal for personal and planetary transformation. Text in English. 1977. m. USD 15 domestic to non-members; USD 20 foreign to non-members (effective 2001). adv. bk.rev. illus. back issues avail. **Document type:** *Newsletter.* **Description:** Directed to gay men; keeps members posted on the growing process and expanding impact of love worldwide. Includes information about members, letters from readers, news of workshops and editorials.
Indexed: e-psyche.
Published by: (Loving Brotherhood, Inc.), Lightning Press, PO Box 556, Sussex, NJ 07461. TEL 973-875-4710, RWalker398@aol.com. Eds. Ralph Walker, Scott Humphries. Circ: 250 (paid and free); 250 (controlled); 150 (paid); 100 (free).

306.766 DEU ISSN 0935-8838
MAENNER AKTUELL. Text in German. 1987. m. DEM 14.80 (effective 2001). adv. bk.rev. back issues avail. **Document type:** *Magazine, Consumer.*
Formerly: Maenner
Published by: Bruno Gmuender Verlag, Leuschnerdamm 31, Berlin 10999, Germany. TEL 49-30-615003-0, FAX 49-30-6159007. Ed. Andreas Toelz. Adv. contact Frank Sperling. B&W page DEM 3,320, color page DEM 4,980. Circ: 22,633.

305.90664 USA ISSN 1529-935X
METRO SOURCE; a celebration and exploration of urban gay life. Text in English. 1990. 5/yr. USD 16.95 (effective 2001). adv. bk.rev., film rev., music rev., play rev., video rev., dance rev., tel.rev. illus. back issues avail. **Document type:** *Magazine, Consumer.* **Description:** National publication serves as a lifestyle magazine for the gay and lesbian community. NY Edition contains a business directory for the metropolitan New York and the tri-state area.
Related titles: Regional ed.: Metro Source N Y.
Published by: Metrosource Publishing, Inc., 180 Varick St, 5th Fl, New York, NY 10014-4606. TEL 212-691-5127, FAX 212-741-2978, metrosourc@aol.com, http://www.metrosource.com/. Ed. Richard Walsh. Pub., R&P Rob Davis. Adv. contact Daryl Hair. color page USD 6,600; trim 10.88 x 8.13. Circ: 15,018 (paid); 65,046 (controlled).

306.766 USA ISSN 0895-5239
NINTH STREET CENTER JOURNAL. Text in English. 1974. irreg. bk.rev. back issues avail. **Document type:** *Academic/Scholarly.* **Description:** Forum for ideas on social progress and human development, with emphasis on psychological polarity.
Indexed: e-psyche.
Published by: Ninth Street Center, Inc., 151 First Ave, Ste 25, New York, NY 10003. TEL 212-228-5153, http://www.geocities.com/~nscenter/pubs.htm. Ed. Dean Hannotte. R&P Dean Hannote.

306.766 DNK ISSN 0902-347X
PAN - BLADET. Text in Danish. 1954. 10/yr. DKK 200 to individuals; DKK 350 to institutions (effective 2001). adv. bk.rev. 35 p./no. back issues avail. **Document type:** *Newspaper.* **Description:** Focuses on the homosexual situation in Denmark as well as internationally. Features interviews, questions on civil rights, culture and health.
Formerly (until 1989): Pan (0906-3439)
Related titles: Online - full text ed.
Published by: Landsforeningen for Boesser og Lesbiske, Teglgaardsstraede 13, PO Box 1023, Copenhagen K 1007, Denmark. TEL 45-33-13-19-48, FAX 45-33-36-00-83, panblad@bl.dk, http://www.panbladet.dk. Ed. Nanna Sylvest. Adv. contact Bert Svaleboelle. Circ: 9,000.

363.49 155.3 USA ISSN 1072-7841
PSYCHOLOGICAL PERSPECTIVES ON LESBIAN AND GAY ISSUES. Text in English. 1994. irreg., latest vol.2, 1995. **Document type:** *Monographic series.*
Related titles: Online - full text ed.: (from ingenta).
Indexed: e-psyche.
—BLDSC (6946.510500).
Published by: Sage Publications, Inc., Books, 2455 Teller Rd, Thousand Oaks, CA 91320. TEL 805-499-0721, FAX 805-499-0871. **Subscr. outside N. America to:** Sage Publications Ltd., 6 Bonhill St, London EC2A 4PU, United Kingdom; Sage Publications India Pvt. Ltd., 32-m Market, Greater Kailash-I, New Delhi 110 048, India.

305 NLD
DE REGENBOOGGIDS. Text in Dutch, English. 1994. a. USD 10. adv. **Document type:** *Consumer.*
Published by: Best Publishing Group, Postbus 10, Best 5680 AA, Netherlands. TEL 31-499-391000, FAX 31-499-390603, bpg@gaykrant.nl. Ed., Pub. Henk Krol. Adv. contact Gert Jan Vangrol. page USD 1,000. Circ: 40,000.

305.235353 USA
TEEN FAG. Text in English. 1993. irreg. USD 3; USD 5 foreign. adv. illus. **Document type:** *Newsletter.*
Published by: Chow Chow Productions, PO Box 20204, Seattle, WA 98102. TEL 206-322-6862. Ed., Pub., Adv. contact Gordon Ornelas. page USD 120. Circ: 1,000.

306.766 USA
THE TEXAS TRIANGLE. Text in English. 1992. w. adv. bk.rev., dance rev., film rev., play rev., tel.rev., video rev. back issues avail. **Document type:** *Newspaper, Consumer.* **Description:** Targeted towards the gay, lesbian, bisexual, and transgendered market. Aims to inform, educate, and entertain both gay-friendly and anti-gay readers in a thoroughly professional way.
Related titles: Online - full text ed.: 1992.
Published by: Texas Triangle, 611 W 6th St, Austin, TX 78701-2705. TEL 214-946-0401, FAX 214-946-0402, http://www.txtriangle.com. Ed. Matt Lum. Pub. Todd Cunningham. Adv. contact James Bengfort. page USD 595. Circ: 25,000.

TRANSGENDER TAPESTRY; the journal for persons interested in crossdressing & transsexualism. see *PSYCHOLOGY*
Published by: XY Media, Ltd., 4104 24th St, Ste 900, San Francisco, CA 94114-3615. TEL 415-552-6668, 877-996-0930, FAX 415-552-6664, xypost@xy.com, http://www.xymag.com, http://www.xy.com. Ed., Pub. Peter Ian Cummings. Adv. contact Benjie Nycum. **Dist. by:** International Publishers Direct, 674 Via de la Valle, Ste 200, Solana Beach, CA 92075. TEL 619-481-5928, FAX 619-259-7580.

HA-YONAH/DOVE. see *ETHNIC INTERESTS*

HORSES AND HORSEMANSHIP

see SPORTS AND GAMES—Horses And Horsemanship

HOTELS AND RESTAURANTS

see also NUTRITION AND DIETETICS; TRAVEL AND TOURISM

613.62 USA ISSN 0738-6583
EXECUTIVE HOUSEKEEPING TODAY. Text in English. 1980. m. USD 40 domestic; USD 50 foreign (effective 2000). adv. bk.rev. index. *Refereed.* **Document type:** *Trade.* **Description:** Geared to management professionals responsible for institutional housekeeping.
Indexed: Hospit.Ind.
—ingenta.
Published by: International Executive Housekeepers Association, 1001 Eastwind Dr, Ste 301, Westerville, OH 43081. TEL 614-895-7166, 800-200-6342, FAX 614-895-1248, excel@ieha.org, http://www.ieha.org. Ed., Adv. contact Cindi Leeman. Pub., R&P Beth B Risinger. B&W page USD 1,016, color page USD 1,816. Circ: 8,000 (paid).

HOUSING AND URBAN PLANNING

see also BUILDING AND CONSTRUCTION; PUBLIC ADMINISTRATION; REAL ESTATE

HEALTH & ENVIRONMENT IN AMERICA'S TOP-RATED CITIES: A STATISTICAL PROFILE (YEARS). see *HOUSING AND URBAN PLANNING—Abstracting, Bibliographies, Statistics*

HEALTH & HOUSING INSIGHT. see *PUBLIC HEALTH AND SAFETY*

649.8 USA ISSN 1050-3234
HD7287.92.U54
HOUSING THE ELDERLY REPORT. Text in English. 1982. m. USD 249 domestic (effective 2001); USD 259 in Canada; USD 289 elsewhere (2001). index. 12 p./no. 2 cols./p. **Document type:** *Newsletter.* **Description:** News and advice for sponsors, managers of retirement homes, projects and nursing homes.
Published by: (Community Development Services, Inc.), C D Publications, 8204 Fenton St, Silver Spring, MD 20910-2889. TEL 301-588-6380, FAX 301-588-6385, her@cdpublications.com, info@cdpublications.com, http://www.cdpublications.com. Ed. Brian Geller. R&P Mike Gerecht.

353.55 CHE
RAUMPLANUNG UND UMWELTSCHUTZ IM KANTON ZURICH. Text in German. 1964. irreg., latest vol.18, 1992. CHF 20. bibl, charts, illus. **Document type:** *Government.*
Formerly (until no.7, 1971): Regionalplanung in Kanton Zurich
Published by: Amt fuer Raumplanung, Stampfenbachstr 14, Zuerich 8090, Switzerland. TEL 01-2593046. Circ: 5,000.

HOUSING AND URBAN PLANNING—Abstracting, Bibliographies, Statistics

363.5021 USA ISSN 1080-4161
RA566.3
HEALTH & ENVIRONMENT IN AMERICA'S TOP-RATED CITIES: A STATISTICAL PROFILE (YEARS). Text in English. 1994. biennial, latest 2001. USD 125 (effective 2000). **Document type:** *Monographic series.*
Published by: Grey House Publishing, 185 Millerton Rd, PO Box 860, Millerton, NY 12546. TEL 518-789-8700, 800-562-2139, FAX 860-435-0867, dg@citystats.com, books@greyhouse.com, http://citystats.com, http://www.greyhouse.com.

HUMANITIES: COMPREHENSIVE WORKS

ANIMA. see *PSYCHOLOGY*

L'ARCO DI GIANO; rivista di medical humanities. see *MEDICAL SCIENCES*

174.2 301 170 001.3 USA ISSN 1065-7274
BIOETHICS FORUM. Text in English. 1988. q. USD 50 to individuals and libraries; USD 30 to students (effective 2001). bk.rev., Website rev. abstr. *Refereed.* **Document type:** *Journal, Academic/Scholarly.* **Description:** Explores contemporary ethical issues in health care.
Formerly (until 1992): Midwest Medical Ethics (1054-4119)
Indexed: AgeLine, Phil.Ind.
—BLDSC (2072.120500).
Published by: Midwest Bioethics Center, 1021 1025 Jefferson St, Kansas City, MO 64105. TEL 816-221-1100, 800-344-3829, FAX 816-221-2002, bioethic@midbio.org, http://www.midbio.org. Ed. Rachel Reeder. Circ: 3,000.

001.3 JPN ISSN 0386-8133
CODEN: BIDKDF
BOEI IKA DAIGAKKO SHINGAKU KATEI KENKYU KIYO/NATIONAL DEFENSE MEDICAL COLLEGE. BULLETIN OF LIBERAL ARTS AND SCIENCES. Text in English, Japanese. 1978. a. **Document type:** *Bulletin.*
Indexed: Intl.Bibl.Soc.Sci.
—BLDSC (2865.890000), CASDDS.
Published by: Boeicho, Boei Ika Daigakko/Defense Agency, National Defense Medical College, 3-2 Namiki, Tokorozawa-shi, Saitama-ken 359-8513, Japan. Ed. Yoshio Ogawa.

001.3 KWT ISSN 1560-5248
HAWLIYAT KULLIYAT AL-A'DAAB/ANNALS OF THE FACULTY OF ARTS. Text and summaries in Arabic, English. 1980. 8/yr. KWD 3,000, USD 15. abstr, charts, illus, maps, stat. back issues avail. *Refereed.* **Document type:** *Monographic series, Academic/Scholarly.* **Description:** Publishes articles on topics relevant to the scientific concerns of the various departments in the faculty of arts.
Indexed: Bibl.Ling., Lang.& Lang.Behav.Abstr., SOPODA, Sociol.Abstr.
Published by: Academic Publication Council, Kuwait University/Majliss an-Nushir al-Elmi, P O Box 17370, El-khaldiah, Kuwait. Ed. Dr. Abdullah Al Omar. Circ: 2,000.

HEBREW UNIVERSITY OF JERUSALEM. AUTHORITY FOR RESEARCH AND DEVELOPMENT. CURRENT RESEARCH. see *MEDICAL SCIENCES*

610 001.3 USA ISSN 0892-2772
MEDICAL HUMANITIES REVIEW. Text in English. 1987. s-a. USD 45; USD 65 foreign (effective 1999). adv. bk.rev. *Refereed.* **Document type:** *Academic/Scholarly.*
Indexed: Bk.Rev.Ind. (1990-), Child.Bk.Rev.Ind. (1990-).
—BLDSC (5527.517000).
Published by: University of Texas Medical Branch, Institute for the Medical Humanities, 301 University Blvd, Galveston, TX 77555-1311. TEL 409-772-2376, FAX 409-772-5640, dpfeil@utmb.edu. Eds. Ronald A Carson, Thomas H Murray. R&P, Adv. contact Diane Pfeil. B&W page USD 125; trim 9 x 6. Circ: 800 (paid).

001 SWE ISSN 0078-0901
NOBEL SYMPOSIUM SERIES. Text in Swedish. 1966. irreg., latest vol.104, 1997. price varies. **Document type:** *Proceedings.*
Indexed: Biol.Abstr., Chem.Abstr., Chem.Indus.Notes, Chem.Titles, GeoRef.
Published by: Nobel Foundation, Sturegatan 14, Fack 5232, Stockholm 10245, Sweden. TEL 46-8-663-09-20, FAX 46-8-660-38-47, TELEX 12382 NOBHAUS S. **US and Canada subscr. to:** Cambridge University Press, 32 E 57 St, New York, NY 10022.

PSICOTERAPIA E SCIENZE UMANE. see *MEDICAL SCIENCES—Psychiatry And Neurology*

UNIVERSITY OF SANTO TOMAS. GRADUATE SCHOOL. JOURNAL OF GRADUATE RESEARCH. see *SOCIAL SCIENCES: COMPREHENSIVE WORKS*

WIEDZA I ZYCIE. see *SCIENCES: COMPREHENSIVE WORKS*

HYDRAULIC ENGINEERING

see ENGINEERING—Hydraulic Engineering

HYDROLOGY

see EARTH SCIENCES—Hydrology

HYPNOSIS

see MEDICAL SCIENCES—Hypnosis

INDUSTRIAL ENGINEERING

see ENGINEERING—Industrial Engineering

INFORMATION SCIENCE AND INFORMATION THEORY

see COMPUTERS—Information Science And Information Theory

INORGANIC CHEMISTRY

see CHEMISTRY—Inorganic Chemistry

INSTRUMENTS

see also JEWELRY, CLOCKS AND WATCHES; METROLOGY AND STANDARDIZATION

681 USA ISSN 0739-0270
A A M I NEWS*. Text in English. m. USD 130; USD 170 foreign (effective 1999). adv. back issues avail. **Document type:** *Newsletter.* **Description:** Keeps readers informed of government standards and AAMI activities regarding medical instrumentation.
Published by: Association for the Advancement of Medical Instrumentation, 1110 N Glebe Rd #220, Arlington, VA 22201-5707. TEL 703-525-4890. Ed. Ann Fishman. Adv. contact Cameron Nyhen. Circ: 6,000.

BIOMEDICAL SCIENCES INSTRUMENTATION. see *MEDICAL SCIENCES*

615 USA
BIORESEARCH MONITORING ALERT. Text in English. 1992. m. 14 p./no. back issues avail.; reprints avail. **Document type:** *Newsletter, Trade.*
Formerly (until 2001): Validation Times
Related titles: E-mail ed.
Published by: Washington Information Source, 6506 Old Stage Rd, Ste 100, Rockville, MD 20852-4326. TEL 301-770-5553, FAX 301-468-0475, wis@fdainfo.com, http://www.fdainfo.com. Ed., Pub. Ken Reid.

BIOTECH EQUIPMENT UPDATE. see *BIOLOGY—Biotechnology*

C L R. (Clinical Laboratory Reference) see *MEDICAL SCIENCES—Experimental Medicine, Laboratory Technique*

681 USA
CLINICAL ENGINEERING SECTION NEWSLETTER. Text in English. 1987. bi-m. membership. charts, illus. back issues avail. **Document type:** *Newsletter.* **Description:** Information on the maintenance and upkeep of diagnostic equipment in hospitals. Geared toward clinical engineers and biomedical equipment technicians.
Published by: (American Society for Hospital Engineering), American Hospital Association, One North Franklin, Chicago, IL 60606-3421. TEL 312-422-3803, FAX 312-422-4572. Ed. Kerry Hacker. Circ: 6,100.

610 USA ISSN 0098-7573
DEVICES & DIAGNOSTICS LETTER. Text in English. 1974. w., latest vol.29, 2002. USD 857 in North America; USD 907 elsewhere (effective Nov. 2001). bk.rev. 8 p./no. Supplement avail.; back issues avail. **Document type:** *Newsletter, Trade.* **Description:** For business leaders concerned with government regulation of medical devices and in vitro diagnostics. Covers compliance and inspection programs, defect reporting, labeling, and testing rules.
Incorporates: M D R Watch (0890-7587)
Related titles: E-mail ed.: (from The Dialog Corporation).
—CCC.
Published by: Washington Business Information, Inc., 300 N Washington St, Ste 200, Falls Church, Arlington, VA 22046. TEL 703-538-7660, FAX 703 538-7676, rcrider@fdanews.com, http://www.fdanews.com. Ed. David Douglass.

DICKINSON'S F D A REVIEW; human & animal drugs - biologics - medical devices. (U.S. Food and Drug Administration) see *PHARMACY AND PHARMACOLOGY*

DRUG AND DEVICE PRODUCT APPROVAL LIST. see *MEDICAL SCIENCES—Experimental Medicine, Laboratory Technique*

EQUIPOS MEDICOS. see *MEDICAL SCIENCES*

681 USA
EUROPEAN MEDICAL DEVICE MANUFACTURER. Text in English. 1990. 7/yr. USD 150 (effective 2001). **Document type:** *Trade.* **Description:** Written exclusively for the European medical device and diagnostic industry. Provides timely and concise information on the latest materials, components, equipment, and services of interest to designers of medical products in Europe.
Formerly: International Medical Device and Diagnostic Industry
Published by: Canon Communications LLC, 11444 W Olympic Blvd, Ste 900, Los Angeles, CA 90064-1549. TEL 310-445-4200, feedback@devicelink.com, norbert.sparrow@cancom.com, http://www.devicelink.com/emdm. Ed. Norbert Sparrow. Pub. William F Cobert. Adv. contact Diana Fisk. Circ: 15,040 (controlled).

681 USA ISSN 0196-626X
KF3827.M4
THE G M P LETTER. (Good Manufacturing Practice) Text in English. 1980. m. USD 477 in North America; USD 492 elsewhere (effective Nov. 2001). bk.rev. 8 p./no. back issues avail. **Document type:** *Newsletter.* **Description:** Covers the FDA's Good Manufacturing Practices and QS regulations for medical devices. Also reports on FDA rules dictating controls on production and quality control.
Related titles: E-mail ed.: (from The Dialog Corporation).
—CCC.
Published by: Washington Business Information, Inc., 300 N Washington St, Ste 200, Falls Church, Arlington, VA 22046. TEL 703-538-7600, 703-538-7660, FAX 703 538-7676, ddouglass@fdanews.com, http://www.fdanews.com. Ed. Samuel Gilston.

610.284 USA
HOME CARE MAGAZINE; for business leaders in home health care. Text in English. 1979. m. **Document type:** *Trade.*
Published by: Primedia Business Magazines & Media, Inc. (Subsidiary of: Primedia Inc.), 23815 Stuart Ranch Rd, Box 8987, Malibu, CA 90265-8987. inquiries@primediabusiness.com, http://www.industryclick.com/, http://www.primediabusiness.com. Pub. Paisley Stevens. Circ: 17,000. **Subscr. to:** PO Box 12914, Overland Park, KS 66282-2914. TEL 800-441-0294, FAX 913-967-1903.

HOSPITAL MAGAZINE. see *HEALTH FACILITIES AND ADMINISTRATION*

681 610 JPN ISSN 0019-1736
IKAKIKAI GAKU ZASSHI/JOURNAL OF MEDICAL INSTRUMENTS. Text in Japanese. 1923. m. JPY 6,000.
Indexed: INIS Atomind.
—CISTI.
Published by: Medical Instrument Society of Japan/Nihon Ikakikai Gakkai, 3-39-15 Hongo, Bunkyo-ku, Tokyo 113-0033, Japan. Ed. Muramatsu Atsuyoshi.

INTERNATIONAL LABMATE. see *MEDICAL SCIENCES—Experimental Medicine, Laboratory Technique*

681 JPN ISSN 0385-4418
CODEN: JNAIDF
J E O L NEWS: ANALYTICAL INSTRUMENTATION. Text in English. 1963. 2/yr. per issue exchange basis. **Document type:** *Academic/Scholarly.*
Formerly: J E O L News - Analytical Instruments: Application
Indexed: Chem.Abstr., INIS Atomind., INSPEC (1984-Oct.1992, dropped), Mass Spectr.Bull.
—AskIEEE, CASDDS.
Published by: Japan Electron Optics Laboratory News/Nihon Denshi K.K., 1-2 Musashino 3-chome, Akishima-shi, Tokyo-to 196-0021, Japan. TEL 0425-42-2161, FAX 0425-46-3353, TELEX 0-2842-135. Ed. Shunichi Enomoto. Circ: 12,000.

629 JPN ISSN 0385-4426
CODEN: JNEIDZ
J E O L NEWS: ELECTRON OPTICS INSTRUMENTATION. Text in English. 1963. 2/yr. per issue exchange basis. **Document type:** *Academic/Scholarly.*
Formerly: J E O L News - Electron Optics Instruments - Application
Indexed: INSPEC (Aug.1983-Aug.1992, dropped), Mass Spectr.Bull.
—AskIEEE, CASDDS.
Published by: J E O L Ltd./Nihon Denshi K.K., 1-2 Musashino 3-chome, Akishima-shi, Tokyo-to 196-0021, Japan. TEL 0425-42-2161, FAX 0425-46-3353, TELEX 0-2842-135. Ed. Shunichi Enomoto. Circ: 18,000.

681 USA ISSN 1079-6630
R856.6
JOURNAL OF VALIDATION TECHNOLOGY; serving the pharmaceutical, medical device, biotechnology and diagnostics industries. Text in English. 1994. q. USD 296; USD 318 in Canada & Mexico; USD 340 elsewhere. reprints avail. *Refereed.* **Document type:** *Academic/Scholarly.*
—BLDSC (5072.230000).
Published by: Institute of Validation Technology, 200 Business Pkwy, Ste F, Royal, Palm Beach, FL 33411-1742. TEL 561-790-2025, 800-276-4242, FAX 561-790-2065, info@ivthome.com, http://www.ivthome.com. Ed. Mike Kennedy. Pub. Glenn Melvin.

LAB SOUTH AMERICA. see *MEDICAL SCIENCES—Experimental Medicine, Laboratory Technique*

LABORATORIUM PRAKTIJK. see *MEDICAL SCIENCES—Experimental Medicine, Laboratory Technique*

681 USA ISSN 0194-844X
HD9994 CODEN: MDIIDI
MEDICAL DEVICE & DIAGNOSTIC INDUSTRY. Text in English. 1979. m. USD 150 (effective 2001); free to qualified personnel. adv. charts, illus, pat, tr.lit. index. back issues avail. **Document type:** *Trade.* **Description:** Emphasizes applied technology in product design, manufacturing and marketing. Covers market trends, business news, regulatory and legal issues and management for manufacturers of medical devices and medical electronics.
Indexed: ASCA, Bioeng.Abstr., Chem.Abstr., Comput.& Info.Sys., Curr.Adv.Ecol.Sci., Curr.Pack.Abstr., Eng.Ind., Environ.Eng.Abstr., Environ.Sci.Poll.Mgmt., RAPRA (1999-), SSCI (coverage dropped), Telegen.
—BLDSC (5527.055000), CASDDS, Ei, GNLM.
Published by: Canon Communications LLC, 11444 W Olympic Blvd, Ste 900, Los Angeles, CA 90064-1549. TEL 310-445-4200, FAX 310-445-4299, feedback@devicelink.com, http://www.devicelink.com/mddi. Ed. John Bethune. Pub. William Cobert. Adv. contact Howard Revitch. B&W page USD 6,735, color page USD 8,330. Circ: 50,540 (controlled).

MEDICAL DEVICE APPROVAL LETTER WITH G M P - DESIGN CONTROLS REVIEWS. see *MEDICAL SCIENCES—Experimental Medicine, Laboratory Technique*

681 610 GBR ISSN 1352-4402
MEDICAL DEVICE COMPANIES ANALYSIS PROFILES. Text in English. 1992. m. GBP 995, USD 1,790; GBP 1,195 cd-rom; GBP 1,395 combined (effective 2000). adv. back issues avail. **Document type:** *Directory.*
Related titles: CD-ROM ed.; Diskette ed.; Online - full text ed.
Published by: Espicom Business Intelligence, Lincoln House, City Fields Business Park, City Fields Way, Tangmere, Chichester, W Sussex PO20 6FS, United Kingdom. TEL 44-1243-533322, FAX 44-1243-533418, sales_desk@espicom.com, http://www.espicom.com. Ed. Tessa Neighbour. R&P Nigel Chivers. adv.: page GBP 250; trim 170 x 247.

MEDICAL DEVICES, DIAGNOSTICS & INSTRUMENTATION REPORTS: THE GRAY SHEET. see *MEDICAL SCIENCES*

610.284 USA ISSN 1055-4262
R856.A1
MEDICAL EQUIPMENT DESIGNER; the digest of medical engineering news. Text in English. bi-m. free per issue to qualified personnel. adv. back issues avail.
Related titles: Online - full text ed.
Published by: Adams Business Media, 6001 Cochran Rd, Ste 300, Solon, OH 44139. TEL 440-248-1125, FAX 440-248-0187, kchapple@mail.aip.com, http://www.mfg-net.com/med/current/default.asp. Ed. Kimberly Chapple. Pub. Thomas V Corcoran. Adv. contact Vivien Gow. Circ: 15,000.

681 610 GBR
MEDICAL INDUSTRY WEEK. Text in English. w. GBP 395, USD 710 (effective 2000). **Document type:** *Newsletter, Trade.* **Description:** Reports the latest device business, product and company news.
Formerly: Medical Device Companies Analysis Newsletter (1357-0471)
Related titles: CD-ROM ed.; Online - full text ed.
Published by: Espicom Business Intelligence, Lincoln House, City Fields Business Park, City Fields Way, Tangmere, Chichester, W Sussex PO20 6FS, United Kingdom. TEL 44-1243-533322, FAX 44-1243-533418, sales_desk@espicom.com, http://www.espicom.com. Ed. Lawrence Miller. R&P Nigel Chivers.

MEDICAL PRODUCTS SALES. see *MEDICAL SCIENCES*

681.2 GBR
MEDINDEX ELECTRONIC ONLINE DIRECTORY. Text in English. a. free per issue. **Document type:** *Directory.* **Description:** Lists suppliers of health care services and equipment, primarily in the UK.
Supersedes: Medindex
Media: Online - full text.
Published by: Chanterelle Publishing Ltd., 34 Florian Ave, Sutton, Surrey SM1 3QH, United Kingdom. TEL 44-870-740-1043, http://www.medindex.com; http://www.chanterelle.co.uk/; http://www.medindex.co.uk.

681 658 GBR ISSN 1352-1179
MEDISTAT. Text in English. 1987. m. GBP 995, USD 1,790; GBP 1,195 cd-rom; GBP 1,395 combined (effective 2000). adv. back issues avail. **Document type:** *Directory, Trade.* **Description:** Contains market data for executives in the international medical device, equipment and supplies markets.
Related titles: CD-ROM ed.: GBP 1,195; Diskette ed.; Online - full text ed.
—CCC.
Published by: Espicom Business Intelligence, Lincoln House, City Fields Business Park, City Fields Way, Tangmere, Chichester, W Sussex PO20 6FS, United Kingdom. TEL 44-1243-533322, FAX 44-1243-532124, sales_desk@espicom.com, http://www.espicom.com. Ed. Ian Taylor. R&P Nigel Chivers. Adv. contact Faye Munn. page GBP 250; trim 170 x 240.

681 GBR
MOVING AND HANDLING. Variant title: M D A Moving and Handling. Text in English. 1974. irreg. GBP 35. **Document type:** *Government.*
Formerly (until 1998): M D A Evaluation Report (0960-5843)
—BLDSC (3830.561500).
Published by: Department of Health, Medical Devices Agency, Crown Bldgs, Rm 2-F05, Kingston By-Pass, Surbiton, Surrey KT6 5QN, United Kingdom. TEL 44-181-268-4488, FAX 44-181-268-4496, dts2@medicl-devices.gov.uk, http://www.open.gov.uk/mda/mdahome.htm.

NEW WORLD HEALTH (YEAR). see *MEDICAL SCIENCES*

SOLID STATE NUCLEAR MAGNETIC RESONANCE; an international journal. see *CHEMISTRY—Analytical Chemistry*

INSURANCE

A A P P O JOURNAL. see *BUSINESS AND ECONOMICS*

A S H R M FORUM. see *HEALTH FACILITIES AND ADMINISTRATION*

368.382 USA ISSN 1044-9426
RA395.A3
ALL ABOUT MEDICARE. Text in English. 1987. a. USD 12.25. **Description:** Provides comprehensive information on Medicare benefits and costs in a question and answer format.
Published by: The National Underwriter Co., 505 Gest St, Cincinnati, OH 45203-1716. TEL 513-721-2140, FAX 513-721-0126.

AMERISURE SAFETY NEWS. see *PUBLIC HEALTH AND SAFETY*

368.3822 USA
THE APPEAL LETTER; your one stop resource for insurance recovery. Text in English. m. **Description:** Publishes articles focusing on effective insurance appeal techniques. Meant to give both hospitals and physicians a source for ongoing information on how to resolve denied insurance claims in the medical provides' favor.
Media: Online - full text.
Published by: Appeal Solutions, PO Box 293403, Lewisville, TX 75029. TEL 972-219-7666, 888-399-4625, tt@integsoft.com, http://www.integsoft.com/appeals. Ed. Tammy Tipton.

616.89 USA
BEHAVIORAL HEALTH BUSINESS NEWS. Text in English. 1995. 24/yr. USD 421 (effective 2001). 8 p./no. **Document type:** *Newsletter, Trade.* **Description:** Provides news of how health plans and managed behavioral firms are structuring delivery of mental health and substance abuse services.
Formerly (until 2000): Managed Behavioral Health News (1089-6821)
Indexed: e-psyche.
Published by: Atlantic Information Services, Inc., 1100 17th St, N W, Ste 300, Washington, DC 20036. TEL 202-775-9008, FAX 202-331-9542, http://www.aishealth.com/Products/newsmbh.htm. Ed. Terry Rudd. Pub. Richard Biehl.

368 DEU ISSN 1435-8492
BERUFSGENOSSENSCHAFT FUER GESUNDHEITSDIENST UND WOHLFAHRTSPFLEGE. MITTEILUNGEN. Text in German. 1970. q. **Document type:** *Newsletter, Trade.*
Former titles (until 1997): B G W Mitteilungen (0937-0811); (until 1988): B G W Mitteilungsblatt (0178-8574)
Published by: Berufsgenossenschaft fuer Gesundheitsdienst und Wohlfahrtspflege, Pappelallee 35-37, Hamburg 22089, Germany. TEL 49-40-20207-0, FAX 49-40-20207-525. Ed. Gerhard Mehrtens.

368.382 USA
HD7102.U4
BUSINESS AND HEALTH; keys to workforce productivity. Text in English. 10/yr. USD 99 domestic; USD 136 foreign; USD 10 newsstand/cover (effective 2001). adv. bk.rev. illus. Index. back issues avail.; reprints avail. **Document type:** *Magazine, Trade.* **Description:** Examines the full range of managed health care concerns affecting purchasers and providers, including cost management, quality assurance, health promotion and wellness, disability, workers' compensation, utilization review, pharmacy benefits, dental and vision care.
Media: Online - full content. **Related titles:** Microform ed.: (from PQC); Online - full text ed.: (from H. W. Wilson).
Indexed: ABI Inform. (Jan.1986-), Abstr.Health Care Manage.Stud., Abstr.Soc.Geront., AgeLine, B.P.I. (Jul.1989-, dropped), CINAHL, I.P.A., Int.Nurs.Ind., L.R.I., P.A.I.S.
—BLDSC (2933.205000), GNLM, ingenta, KNAW. **CCC.**
Published by: Medical Economics Co., Inc., 5 Paragon Dr, Montvale, NJ 07645-1742. TEL 201-358-7200, rick.service@medec.com, http://bnh.pdr.net/be_core/b/index.jsp. Ed. Richard Service. Circ: 5,000 (paid); 38,000 (controlled).

C O B R A ADVISORY. (Consolidated Omnibus Budget Reconciliation Act) see *HEALTH FACILITIES AND ADMINISTRATION*

CANADIAN HEALTH CARE MANAGEMENT. see *MEDICAL SCIENCES*

THE CASE MANAGER. see *MEDICAL SCIENCES*

COMPETITIVE HEALTHCARE MARKET REPORTER. see *BUSINESS AND ECONOMICS—Marketing And Purchasing*

362.11 368.382 USA
CONTINUING CARE NEWS. Text in English. m. USD 77 (effective 2001). **Document type:** *Newsletter, Trade.* **Description:** Covers news and issues about the managed care industry.
Published by: Stevens Publishing Corporation, 5151 Beltline Rd, 10th fl, Dallas, TX 75240. TEL 972-687-6700, FAX 972-687-6770, custserv@stevenspublishing.com, http://www.stevenspublishing.com/. Pub. Ralph Jensen.

DEVELOPMENTS IN HEALTH ECONOMICS AND PUBLIC POLICY. see *PUBLIC HEALTH AND SAFETY*

DIRECTORY OF WORKERS' COMPENSATION MANAGED CARE ORGANIZATIONS. see *LAW—Corporate Law*

EN MARCHE; journal bimensuel d'information pour les beneficiaires des soins de sante. see *PHYSICAL FITNESS AND HYGIENE*

ENVIRONMENTAL COMPLIANCE & LITIGATION STRATEGY. see *LAW*

368.382 USA
ESSENTIALS OF MANAGED HEALTH CARE. Text in English. 1995. irreg. **Document type:** *Academic/Scholarly, Trade.* **Description:** Addresses the many critical concepts of managed care and the various types of managed-care organizations.
Published by: Aspen Publishers, Inc., 200 Orchard Ridge Dr, Ste 200, Gaithersburg, MD 20878. TEL 301-417-7500, FAX 301-417-7550.

EUROPEAN HEALTHCARE MANAGEMENT; the journal for decision makers. see *HEALTH FACILITIES AND ADMINISTRATION*

EXECUTIVE MANAGED CARE DIRECTORY. see *HEALTH FACILITIES AND ADMINISTRATION*

368.382 USA ISSN 0898-9753
THE EXECUTIVE REPORT ON MANAGED CARE. Text in English. 1988. 24/yr. USD 437 (effective 2000). adv. index. back issues avail. **Document type:** *Newsletter.* **Description:** Reports on current trends and issues affecting managed care plans, providers, employers and consumers. Specific areas include: Medicare - Medicaid, legislation, innovative strategies and programs for managed care plans, and quality assurance issues.
—**CCC.**
Published by: Managed Care Information Center, 1913 Atlantic Ave, Ste F4, Manasquan, NJ 08736. TEL 888-843-6242, FAX 888-329-6242, mcic@themcic.com, http://www.themcic.com. Ed. Joseph Schmidt. Pub. Robert K Jenkins. R&P Catherine Casavillo. Adv. contact Suzanne Baker.

362.1 USA ISSN 1097-7309
EXECUTIVE REPORT ON PHYSICIAN ORGANIZATIONS. Text in English. 1998. 12/yr. USD 257 (effective 2000). index. back issues avail. **Document type:** *Newsletter.* **Description:** Covers mergers, acquisitions, practice management agreements and strategic plans being implemented in the physician marketplace, as well as information about how managed care and government regulations influence the physician organization marketplace.
Published by: Managed Care Information Center, 1913 Atlantic Ave, Ste F4, Manasquan, NJ 08736. TEL 888-843-6242, FAX 888-329-6242, mcic@themcic.com, http://www.themcic.com. Pub. Robert K Jenkins.

368 DEU ISSN 1433-7800
FAKTOR ARBEITSSCHUTZ. Text in German. 1949. bi-m. DEM 21 (effective 2001). adv. bk.rev. abstr. **Document type:** *Magazine, Trade.*
Former titles (until 1997): Sicherheit im Oeffentlichen Dienst (0170-6985); (until 1973): Gemeindeunfallversicherung (0016-6162)
Indexed: Dok.Arbeitsmed.
Published by: Universum Verlagsanstalt GmbH KG, Taunusstr 54, Wiesbaden 65183, Germany. TEL 49-611-9030-0, FAX 49-611-9030382, uv@universum.de, http://www.universum.de. Circ: 65,900.

FEDERAL BENEFITS FOR VETERANS AND DEPENDENTS. see *MILITARY*

FRAT. see *HANDICAPPED—Hearing Impaired*

368.382 USA
HG9395
GUIDE TO H M O'S AND HEALTH INSURERS. Text in English. 1995. q., latest 2001. USD 438. Website rev. charts, stat. 477 p./no. back issues avail. **Document type:** *Directory, Consumer.* **Description:** Guide to the financial strength and safety of health insurance companies.
Former titles: Weiss Ratings' Guide to H M O's and Health Insurers; (until 1998): Weiss H M O and Health Insurance Directory (1081-2318)
Published by: Weiss Ratings, Inc., 4176 Burns Rd, Palm Beach, FL 33410. TEL 561-627-3300, FAX 561-625-6685, wr@weissinc.com, http://www.weissratings.com. Pub. Martin Weiss. R&P Shelley Klovsky.

368.382 USA
GUIDE TO HEALTH INSURANCE FOR PEOPLE WITH MEDICARE. Text in English. a. **Document type:** *Directory, Government.*
Published by: U.S. Health Care Financing Administration (Subsidiary of: U.S. Department of Health and Human Services), Department of Health and Human Services, C 3 11 07, 7500 Security Blvd, Baltimore, MD 21244-1850. **Co-sponsor:** National Association of Insurance Commissioners.

368.382 USA ISSN 1070-7158
RA413.5.U5
GUIDE TO THE MANAGED CARE INDUSTRY. Text in English. 1992. a. USD 245 (effective 1999). **Description:** Provides comparative financial information on HMOs and PPOs in the U.S..
Formerly (until 1993): H M O Performance Almanac (1063-1704)
Published by: H C I A Inc., 300 E Lombard St, Baltimore, MD 21202. TEL 800-568-3282, FAX 410-752-6309.

368.382 USA
H C F A'S LAWS, REGULATIONS, AND MANUALS. Text in English. m. USD 254 (effective 2001). back issues avail. **Document type:** *Government.* **Description:** Includes over 20 HCFA program manuals, and related publications and memoranda on Medicare and Medicaid, Titles 52 and 45 of the Code of Federal Regulations, and Titles 11, 18, and 19 of the Social Security Act.
Media: CD-ROM.
Indexed: Russ.Acad.Sci.Bibl.
Published by: U.S. Health Care Financing Administration (Subsidiary of: U.S. Department of Health and Human Services), 7500 Security Blvd, Baltimore, MD 21244. TEL 301-597-3000, http://www.hcfa.gov/. **Subscr. to:** U.S. Government Printing Office, Superintendent of Documents, PO Box 371954, Pittsburgh, PA 15250-7954. TEL 202-512-1800, FAX 202-512-2250, orders@gpo.gov, http://www.access.gpo.gov.

368.382 USA ISSN 1050-9038
H M O MAGAZINE. (Health Maintenance Organization) Text in English. 1959. bi-m. USD 75. bk.rev. **Document type:** *Trade.* **Description:** Provides analysis and news on HMO market trends and legislative and regulatory issues. Includes ideas on management information systems, pharmacy benefits, and health care finances.
Former titles (until vol.31, no.2, 1990): G H A A News (0887-9087); (until Dec. 1986): Group Health News (0164-0542); (until Dec. 1975): Group Health and Welfare News (0017-470X)
Indexed: AgeLine, Med.Care Rev.
Published by: Group Health Association of America, Inc., 1129 Twentieth St, N W, Ste 600, Washington, DC 20036. TEL 202-778-3247, FAX 202-331-7487. Ed. Diana Madden. Circ: 7,000.

368.382 ISR
HADSHOT KUPPOT HOLIM. Text in Hebrew. m.
Published by: (General Labor Federation of Israel), Kupot Holim, 101 Arlozorof St, Tel Aviv 62098, Israel. TEL 03-433340. Ed. David Tagar.

HEALTH AFFAIRS; the policy journal of the health sphere. see *PUBLIC HEALTH AND SAFETY*

368.382 USA
HEALTH CARE FRAUD AND ABUSE NEWSLETTER. Text in English. 1998. m. USD 225 (effective 2001). back issues avail. **Document type:** *Newsletter.* **Description:** Provides developments, strategies, and techniques on the business and legal aspects of health care fraud.
Published by: American Lawyer Media, Inc., D B A Leader Publications, 345 Park Ave S, New York, NY 10010. TEL 212-313-9018, FAX 212-481-8161, http://www.americanlawyermedia.com. Ed. Michael E Clark. R&P Stuart M Wise TEL 917-256-2001.

HEALTH CARE RISK REPORT. see *HEALTH FACILITIES AND ADMINISTRATION*

368.382 GBR ISSN 1460-4884
HEALTH INSURANCE MONITOR. Text in English. 1994. m. **Document type:** *Trade.*
Published by: Emap Finance (Subsidiary of: Emap Business Communications Ltd.), 33-39 Bowling Green Ln, London EC1R 0DA, United Kingdom. TEL 44-171-505-8000, FAX 44-171-505-8185, http://www.emap.com.

HEALTH PLAN & PROVIDER REPORT. see *MEDICAL SCIENCES*

368.382 USA
HEALTH PLAN REQUIREMENTS GUIDE. Text in English. m. USD 577 (effective 2001). **Document type:** *Newsletter.* **Description:** Covers managed care and health plan laws and regulations.
Published by: Atlantic Information Services, Inc., 1100 17th St, N W, Ste 300, Washington, DC 20036. TEL 202-775-9008, FAX 202-331-9542, http://www.aishealth.com. Ed. Frances Fernald. Pub. Richard Biehl.

I

368.382 GBR ISSN 1461-5746
HEALTHCARE INSURANCE REPORT. Text in English. 1998. 10/yr. GBP 315 (effective 2001). software rev., bk.rev. stat. 16 p./no. back issues avail. **Document type:** *Newsletter, Trade.* **Description:** Covers all aspects of health and care insurance in the UK.
Published by: Bank House Communications Ltd., Bank House, Cheltenham, Great Rissington, Glos GL54 2LP, United Kingdom. TEL 44-1451-821982, FAX 44-1451-821972, andycouchman@cs.com, andycouchman @cs.com. Ed., Pub., R&P Andy Couchman.

HEALTHCARE PERSPECTIVE. see *MEDICAL SCIENCES—Computer Applications*

HEALTHCARE RISK MANAGEMENT. see *HEALTH FACILITIES AND ADMINISTRATION*

HEALTHCARE TODAY; journal for NHS boards. see *PUBLIC HEALTH AND SAFETY*

HEALTHCARE TRENDS REPORT; the monthly digest of business and public policy news. see *MEDICAL SCIENCES*

368.382 USA ISSN 1087-3678
HEALTHPLAN; the magazine of trends, insights, and best practices. Text in English. 1959. bi-m. USD 75; USD 155 foreign (effective 1999). bk.rev. charts, illus, tr.lit. back issues avail. **Document type:** *Trade.* **Description:** Provides news analysis and practical information affecting HMO's, PPO's, and similar health care plans to healthcare executives and senior-level administrators.
Indexed: Int.Nurs.Ind.
Published by: American Association of Health Plans, 1129 20th St, N W, Ste 600, Washington, DC 20036. TEL 202-778-3200, FAX 202-331-7487, http://www.aahp.org. Ed. Diane Madden. R&P Jennifer Proctor. adv.: B&W page USD 1,999, color page USD 3,299; trim 10.88 x 8.25. Circ: 8,000.

HOSPITAL PAYMENT AND INFORMATION MANAGEMENT. see *HEALTH FACILITIES AND ADMINISTRATION*

368.382 USA
HG9395
INSURANCE DIRECTORY; nationwide health insurance billing directory. Text in English. 1990. a. USD 59.95 (effective 1997). **Document type:** *Directory.*
Formerly: Insurance Handbook (1062-919X)
Published by: Medicode, Inc., 5225 Wiley Post Way, Ste 500, Salt Lake City, UT 84116-2889. TEL 800-999-4600, FAX 801-536-1009. Ed. Christine Baierschmidt.

▼ **INTERNATIONAL JOURNAL OF HEALTH CARE FINANCE AND ECONOMICS.** see *PUBLIC HEALTH AND SAFETY*

368 NLD ISSN 0924-6479
CODEN: IJMDEM
THE INTERNATIONAL JOURNAL OF RISK AND SAFETY IN MEDICINE; side effects of drugs - devices - surgery - prevention - liability. Text in English. 1990. q. EUR 424, USD 382 to institutions (effective 2002). bk.rev. back issues avail. *Refereed.* **Document type:** *Journal, Academic/Scholarly.* **Description:** Examines the risks involved in the administration of medical attention.
Related titles: Microform ed.: (from PQC); Online - full text ed.: (from EBSCO Publishing, O C L C Online Computer Library Center, Inc., Swets Blackwell, RoweCom Information Quest).
Indexed: ASCA, Chem.Abstr., Curr.Cont. (coverage dropped), Environ.Sci.Poll.Mgmt., Excerp.Med. (1992-), I.P.A., Int.Abstr.Biol.Sci., Mat.Sci.Cit.Ind. (coverage dropped), Pollut.Abstr., Risk Abstr., Saf.Sci.Abstr., Tox.Abstr., Virol.Abstr. (coverage dropped).
—BLDSC (4542.538200), ADONIS, CISTI, EMDOCS, GNLM, Infotrieve, KNAW. **CCC.**
Published by: I O S Press, Nieuwe Hemweg 6B, Amsterdam 1013 BG, Netherlands. TEL 31-20-688-3355, FAX 31-20-620-3419, 100321.2275@compuserve.com, market@iospress.nl, http://www.iospress.nl. Ed. M N G Dukes TEL 47-22-494058. **Subscr. to:** I O S Press, Inc, 5795-G Burke Centre Pkwy, Burke, VA 22015. TEL 703-323-5554, FAX 703-323-3668, iosbooks@iospress.com; Globe Publication Pvt. Ltd., C-62 Inderpuri, New Delhi 100 012, India. TEL 91-11-579-3211, 91-11-579-3212, FAX 91-11-579-8876, custserve@globepub.com, http://www.globepub.com; Kinokuniya Company Ltd, Shinjuku 3-chome, Shinjuku-ku, Tokyo 160-0022, Japan. FAX 81-3-3439-1094, journal@kinokuniya.co.jp, http://www.kinokuniya.co.jp.

JENKS HEALTHCARE BUSINESS REPORT. see *HEALTH FACILITIES AND ADMINISTRATION*

JOURNAL OF CLINICAL OUTCOMES MANAGEMENT. see *HEALTH FACILITIES AND ADMINISTRATION*

JOURNAL OF HEALTHCARE RISK MANAGEMENT. see *HEALTH FACILITIES AND ADMINISTRATION*

368.382 USA ISSN 0743-6661
CODEN: JINNER
JOURNAL OF INSURANCE MEDICINE. Text in English. 1969. q. USD 160 in US & Canada; USD 180 elsewhere (effective 2001). adv. back issues avail. *Refereed.* **Document type:** *Academic/Scholarly.* **Description:** Original articles concerning insurance medicine, including actuariomedical analysis for development of life table, mortality, morbidity, and survival data, underwriting, claims, disability and health insurance issues.
Related titles: Online - full text ed.
—BLDSC (5007.535000).
Published by: American Academy of Insurance Medicine, Attention: Charles S. Jones, MD, ING-Security Life of Denver, 1290 Broadway, 15th Fl, Denver, CO 80203. info@aaimedicine.org, charles-jones@mindspring.com, http://www.aaimedicine.org/. Ed. Dr. Nigel K Roberts. Circ: 1,200.

368.382 GBR ISSN 1473-2297
CODEN: JOICFC
JOURNAL OF INTEGRATED CARE PATHWAYS. Text in English. 1997. 3/yr. GBP 79 in Europe to individuals; USD 142 in United States to individuals; GBP 83 elsewhere to individuals; GBP 150 in Europe to institutions; USD 260 in United States to institutions; GBP 154 elsewhere to institutions (effective 2002). adv. bk.rev. **Document type:** *Academic/Scholarly.* **Description:** Contains case studies of ICP programs, original research articles, debate and commentary, and conference reports.
Former titles (until 2001): Journal of Integrated Care (1462-4567); (until 1998): Journal of Managed Care (1363-9595)
Indexed: Brit.Nur.Ind.
—BLDSC (5007.538300).
Published by: Royal Society of Medicine Press Ltd, 1 Wimpole St, London W1M 8AE, United Kingdom. TEL 44-20-7290-2921, FAX 44-20-7290-2929, rsmjournals@rsm.ac.uk, http://www.roysocmed.ac.uk/pub/jicp.htm. Ed. Sue Johnson.

JOURNAL OF MANAGED CARE PHARMACY. see *PHARMACY AND PHARMACOLOGY*

JOURNAL OF PUBLIC HEALTH MANAGEMENT AND PRACTICE. see *PUBLIC HEALTH AND SAFETY*

368.382 GBR ISSN 0965-7436
KLUWER PERMANENT HEALTH INSURANCE; the city financial review. Variant title: Permanent Health Insurance. Text in English. a. GBP 205.08 (effective 1999). **Document type:** *Trade.*
Incorporates: Health Insurance Briefing (0969-7152)
—BLDSC (4275.019300).
Published by: Croner Publications Ltd. (Subsidiary of: Wolters Kluwer N.V.), Croner Publications Ltd, Croner House, 100 London Rd, Kingston Upon Thames, Surrey KT2 6SR, United Kingdom. TEL 44-20 8547-1175, FAX 44-20-8547-2638, info@croner.co.uk, info@croner.cch.co.uk, http://www.croner.co.uk. Ed. Claire Deacon.

368 DEU ISSN 0939-8104
KRANKENVERSICHERUNG UND UNFALLVERSICHERUNG IN RECHTSPRECHUNG UND SCHRIFTTUM. Text in German. 1959. irreg. DEM 248 (effective 2000). **Document type:** *Monographic series, Trade.*
Formerly (until 1991): Krankenversicherung in Rechtsprechung und Schrifttum (0934-3423)
Published by: Erich Schmidt Verlag GmbH & Co. (Berlin), Genthiner Str 30G, Berlin 10785, Germany. TEL 49-30-250085-0, FAX 49-30-25008511, esv@esvmedien.de, http://www.erich-schmidt-verlag.de.

368.4 USA
LOUISVILLE MEDICINE. Text in English. 1955. m. USD 50 (effective 1997). adv. bk.rev. bibl, charts, illus, stat. *Refereed.* **Document type:** *Bulletin.*
Published by: Jefferson County Medical Society, 101 W Chestnut, Louisville, KY 40202-1805. TEL 502-589-2001, FAX 502-581-9022, profrel@jcmsdocs.org. Ed. Dr. Michael T McFarlane. Adv. contact Cheri K McGuire. B&W page USD 472; trim 9.5 x 7.44. Circ: 3,000.

368.382 USA ISSN 1062-3388
MANAGED CARE; a guide for physicians. Text in English. 1992. m. USD 93 domestic; USD 120 foreign (effective 2001). adv. 2 cols./p. **Document type:** *Trade.* **Description:** Advises physicians and administrators in managed care on the conduct of their business. Informs them of their rapidly changing options and opportunities.
Related titles: Online - full text ed.
Indexed: Int.Nurs.Ind.
—BLDSC (5358.610000).
Published by: MediMedia USA, Inc., 275 Phillips Blvd, Trenton, NJ 08618-1426. TEL 609-882-5700, FAX 609-882-3213, Editors@managedcaremag.com, http://www.managedcaremag.com/. Ed. John Marcille. adv.: B&W page USD 4,752. Circ: 60,000 (controlled).

368.382 USA ISSN 1523-2433
MANAGED CARE AND MEDICAL COST CONTAINMENT IN WORKER'S COMPENSATION: A NATIONAL INVENTORY (YEAR). Text in English. 1998. a. USD 250 (effective 1999). **Document type:** *Trade.*
Published by: Workers Compensation Research Institute, 955 Massachusetts Ave, Cambridge, MA 02139. TEL 617-661-9274, FAX 617-661-9284, astrang@wcrinet.org.

▼ **MANAGED CARE INSIDER ENEWS.** see *PHYSICAL FITNESS AND HYGIENE*

368.382 USA ISSN 0896-6567
RA413.5.U5
MANAGED CARE OUTLOOK; the insider's business briefing on managed health care. Text in English. 50/yr. USD 526 to individuals; USD 13 newsstand/cover (effective 2002). **Document type:** *Newsletter.* **Description:** Includes reports on new business, industry trends, regional happenings, legal and policy news, conference coverage, and case studies.
Incorporates (1988-1990): Managed Care Report (0896-663X)
Related titles: Online - full text ed.: (from Gale Group, NewsNet).
—Infotrieve. **CCC.**
Published by: Aspen Publishers, Inc., 200 Orchard Ridge Dr, Ste 200, Gaithersburg, MD 20878. TEL 301-417-7500, 800-638-8437, FAX 301-695-7931, customer.service@aspenpubl.com, http://www.aspenpub.com. Pub. Marjorie Weiner. R&P Rossette Graham. **Dist. by:** Aspen Publishers Inc., Distribution Center, 7201 McKinney Circle, Frederick, MD 21701. TEL 301-698-7100, FAX 301-417-7550.

THE MANAGED CARE PAYMENT ADVISOR; capitation & alternative compensation methods. see *HEALTH FACILITIES AND ADMINISTRATION*

368.382 USA ISSN 1056-7461
MANAGED CARE WEEK. Text in English. 1991. w. (45/yr.). USD 552 (effective 2001). **Document type:** *Newsletter, Trade.* **Description:** Current news of business affairs and compliance strategies of HMOs, PPOs and other managed care plans and the role of managed care in health care financing reforms.
Related titles: Online - full text ed.: (from Gale Group, Factiva).
—**CCC.**
Published by: Atlantic Information Services, Inc., 1100 17th St, N W, Ste 300, Washington, DC 20036. TEL 202-775-9008, 800-521-4323, FAX 202-331-9542, http://www.aishealth.com/Products/newsmcw.htm. Ed. Jill Brown. Pub. Richard Biehl.

MANAGED HEALTH CARE OVERVIEW. see *INSURANCE—Abstracting, Bibliographies, Statistics*

MEALEY'S LITIGATION REPORT: BREAST IMPLANTS. see *LAW—Civil Law*

MEALEY'S MANAGED CARE LIABILITY REPORT. see *LAW*

368.382 USA ISSN 1088-2642
MEDICAID MANAGED CARE CURRENTS. Text in English. q. free per issue. **Description:** Discusses developments in New York's Medicaid managed care program. Based on research and analytic work at the New York Consortium for Health Services Research.
Related titles: Online - full content ed.
Published by: United Hospital Fund of New York, 350 Fifth Ave, Fl 23, New York, NY 10118-2399. TEL 212-494-0700, FAX 212-494-0800, pbrooks@uhfnyc.org, http://www.uhfnyc.org.

368.382 USA ISSN 0743-8079
HG9371
MEDICAL BENEFITS. Text in English. 1984. s-m. USD 236 to individuals; USD 12 newsstand/cover (effective 2002). charts. **Document type:** *Newsletter, Trade.* **Description:** Gives an executive briefing on the current data, news, and corporate policies shaping the future of health care.
—Infotrieve. **CCC.**
Published by: Panel Publishers, Inc. (Subsidiary of: Aspen Publishers, Inc.), 1185 Ave of the Americas, 37th Fl, New York, NY 10036. TEL 212-597-0200, 800-638-8437, FAX 212-597-0338, customer.service@aspenpubl.com, http://www.aspenpub.com. Ed. Bruce G Carveth. **Dist. by:** Aspen Publishers Inc., Distribution Center, 7201 McKinney Circle, Frederick, MD 21701. TEL 301-698-7100, FAX 301-695-7931.

368.382 USA ISSN 0732-9636
MEDICAL LIABILITY MONITOR; newsletter on professional liability and risk management. Text in English. 1975. m., latest vol.26. USD 200 domestic; USD 225 foreign (effective 2002). bk.rev. mkt. index. 15 p./no. 2 cols./p. Supplement avail.; back issues avail. *Refereed.* **Document type:** *Newsletter, Trade.* **Description:** News updates cover legal, political and market factors affecting medical professional liability insurance.
Formerly (until 1981): Malpractice Lifeline (0361-8412)
Related titles: Supplement: Loss Minimizer.
Published by: Malpractice Lifeline, Inc., PO Box 11147, Chicago, IL 60611-0147. TEL 312-944-7900, FAX 312-944-8845, cptmdgolin@aol.com. Ed., Pub., R&P Carol Brierly Golin. Circ: 1,800 (paid and controlled).

MEDICAL LIABILITY REPORTER; recent decisions of national significance. see *LAW—Civil Law*

MEDICAL OFFICE REPORT. see *MEDICAL SCIENCES*

368.382 USA ISSN 1061-4192
MEDICAL RECORD RISKS: CLAIMS & LITIGATION*. Text in English. 1992. m. USD 250. **Description:** For those who review medical records for claims and litigation.
Published by: Cox Publications, 1908 Colton Blvd, Billings, MT 59102-2316. TEL 406-256-2248, FAX 406-256-7550. Ed. Meridith B Cox. Circ: (controlled).

368.382 USA ISSN 0897-9634
KF3826.N8
MEDICARE ADVISOR. Text in English. 1986. m. USD 155 (effective 2001). back issues avail. **Document type:** *Newsletter.* **Description:** Discusses Medicare coverage and reimbursement for nursing and long-term care facilities. Advises about policy changes from H.C.F.A. and covers subacute trends and health care reform.
Published by: Shannon Publications, Inc., 6380 Lyndon B Johnson Fwy, 286, Dallas, TX 75240-6420. TEL 972-789-1476, FAX 972-503-9760, ellenbl@bradleygroup.com, ellenbl@airmail.net. Ed. Ellen L Bradley. Pub., R&P Ellen Bradley.

368.3 USA ISSN 1068-1019
MEDICARE & MEDICAID LAW BULLETIN. Text in English. 1992. bi-w. USD 245 (effective 1999). back issues avail. **Document type:** *Newsletter.* **Description:** Provides case histories and information on Medicare and Medicaid.
Formerly (until 1994): Medicare & Medicaid Law Reporter (1060-5355)
Related titles: Online - full text ed.: (from LexisNexis).
—CCC.
Published by: L R P Publications, 747 Dresher Rd, Box 980, Horsham, PA 19044. TEL 215-784-0941, 800-341-7874, FAX 215-784-9014, custserve@lrp.com, http://www.lrp.com. Ed. Sandy Johnson.

368.382 USA ISSN 1047-1863
MEDICARE COMPLIANCE ALERT. Text in English. 1989. bi-w. USD 370. Supplement avail. **Description:** Examines enforcement trends in Medicare and Medicaid fraud, abuse law and billing practices. Also gives health care providers and attorneys analysis of administrative law rulings in Civil Money Penalties Reporter.
Formerly: Medicare Compliance Report
—CCC.
Published by: United Communications Group, 1300 Rockville Pike, Ste 1100, Rockville, MD 20852-3030. TEL 301-816-8950, FAX 301-816-8945. Ed. Carol Sardinha.

368.382 USA ISSN 1068-2465
MEDICARE MANAGER. Text in English. 1990. m. USD 145. back issues avail. **Document type:** *Newsletter.* **Description:** Contains tips, solutions, and applications to help clear up the confusion caused by Medicare's constant changes.
Published by: Shannon Publications, Inc., 6380 Lyndon B Johnson Fwy, 286, Dallas, TX 75240-6420. TEL 972-789-1476, FAX 972-503-9760, ellenbl@bradleygroup.com. Ed., Pub., R&P Ellen L Bradley.

368.42600973 USA
MEDICARE. PART A. INTERMEDIARY MANUAL. PART 3. CLAIMS PROCESS. Text in English. base vol. plus irreg. updates. USD 662 for base vol. & indeterminate period of updates (effective 2001). **Document type:** *Government.* **Description:** A ready-reference manual providing informational and procedural material for intermediary claim processors.
Published by: U.S. Health Care Financing Administration (Subsidiary of: U.S. Department of Health and Human Services), 7500 Security Blvd, Baltimore, MD 21244. **Subscr. to:** U.S. Government Printing Office, Superintendent of Documents, PO Box 371954, Pittsburgh, PA 15250-7954. TEL 202-512-1800, FAX 202-512-2250, orders@gpo.gov, http://www.access.gpo.gov.

368.42600973 USA
MEDICARE. PART B. CARRIER MANUAL. PART 3. CLAIMS PROCESS. Text in English. base vol. plus irreg. updates. USD 521 for base vol. & indeterminate period of updates (effective 2001). **Document type:** *Government.* **Description:** Contains informational and procedural material the carrier needs for the efficient processing and payment of claims. Includes instructions dealing with coverage of services, bill review, payment and postpayment actions, reasonable charges, and other pertinent claims procedures.
Published by: U.S. Health Care Financing Administration (Subsidiary of: U.S. Department of Health and Human Services), 7500 Security Blvd, Baltimore, MD 21244. TEL 301-597-3000.

368.382 USA ISSN 0885-0925
KF3608.A4
MEDICARE REVIEW. Text in English. 1984. m. USD 245 (effective 2001). back issues avail. **Document type:** *Newsletter, Trade.* **Description:** Provides in-depth coverage of billing-coding policies, coverage issues, reimbursements, and legislation, as well as updates on health care reform.
Published by: Shannon Publications, Inc., 6380 Lyndon B Johnson Fwy, 286, Dallas, TX 75240-6420. TEL 972-789-1476, FAX 972-503-9760, ellen@bradleygroup.com. Ed. Ellen L Bradley. Pub., R&P Ellen Bradley.

368.0021 310 USA ISSN 0741-9767
HG8963.M5
METROPOLITAN LIFE INSURANCE COMPANY. STATISTICAL BULLETIN S B. Text in English. 1920. q. USD 50 to individuals; USD 60 foreign to individuals (effective 1999 - 2000). charts, illus, maps, stat. index. back issues avail. **Document type:** *Bulletin.* **Description:** Demographic and medical care data on health care coverage, focusing on hospital charges across the nation, mortality trends, life table analyses, and profiles of major population groups.
Former titles (1982-1983): Metropolitan Life Foundation. Statistical Bulletin (0736-4822); (until 1981): Statistical Bulletin - Metropolitan Life (0026-1513)
Related titles: Fax ed.; Microfiche ed.: (from CIS); Microfilm ed.: (from PQC); Online - full text ed.: (from Gale Group, Factiva).
Indexed: AgeLine, B.P.I. (Jan.1982-Apr.1989), BPIA, Biol.Abstr., Bus.Ind., Curr.Cont. (coverage dropped), Ind.Med. (coverage dropped), Nutr.Abstr., P.A.I.S., Popul.Ind., SRI.
—GNLM, ingenta.
Published by: Metropolitan Life Insurance Company, 1 Madison Ave, Area 2 D, New York, NY 10010. TEL 212-578-5014, FAX 212-685-7987, http://www.statbull.com. Ed. Charles G Hertz Dr. R&P Margaret Mushinski. Circ: 3,000 (paid); 1,000 (controlled). **Dist. by:** Sheridan Press, 450 Fame Ave, Hanover, PA 17331. TEL 717-632-3535.

368.382 USA
MONITOR (WASHINGTON, 1970)*. Text in English. 1970. 6/yr. USD 125. bk.rev. back issues avail. **Document type:** *Newsletter.* **Description:** Discusses managed health care trends, delivery of services, and legislative and regulatory initiatives of interest to the industry. Includes special original articles in each issue on particular aspects of managed health care, including state and national updates, legal viewpoint, educational programs, research programs, and technological advances.
Former titles (until Oct. 1992): A M C R A's Managed Care Monitor; (until Dec. 1990): A M C R A Newsletter
Published by: American Managed Care and Review Association, 1129 20th St, N W, Ste 600, Washington, DC 20036-3403. TEL 202-728-0506, FAX 202-728-0609. Ed. Amanda M Orr. Circ: 2,000.

N A R I STETHOSCOPE. see *BUSINESS AND ECONOMICS—Investments*

368.382 USA ISSN 0897-3059
NATIONAL DIRECTORY OF H M OS. Key Title: G H A A's National Directory of H M Os. Text in English. 1986. a. USD 125. **Document type:** *Directory.*
Indexed: SRI.
Published by: Group Health Association of America, Inc., 1129 Twentieth St, N W, Ste 600, Washington, DC 20036. TEL 202-778-3247, FAX 202-331-7487.

368.382 USA ISSN 1089-6589
NEWS AND STRATEGIES FOR MANAGED MEDICARE AND MEDICAID. Text in English. 1995. 24/yr. USD 468 (effective 2001). **Document type:** *Newsletter, Trade.* **Description:** Provides information on managed care opportunities in Medicare and Medicaid.
Published by: Atlantic Information Services, Inc., 1100 17th St, N W, Ste 300, Washington, DC 20036. TEL 202-775-9008, FAX 202-331-9542, customerserv@aispub.com, http://www.aishealth.com/Products/newsmmm.htm. Ed. Chris Gearon. Pub. Richard Biehl.

ON MANAGED CARE. see *HEALTH FACILITIES AND ADMINISTRATION*

368.382 USA ISSN 0893-8121
PART B NEWS. Text in English. 1987. fortn. USD 426. back issues avail. **Description:** Reports on the changes in Medicare insurance reimbursement rules for physicians, plus ways they can get their share of "Part B" dollars.
—CCC.
Published by: United Communications Group, 1300 Rockville Pike, Ste 1100, Rockville, MD 20852-3030. TEL 301-816-8950, FAX 301-816-8945. Ed. Carol Monaco.

PERSONAL INJURY STATE VERDICT SURVEY. see *LAW*

368.382 USA ISSN 1073-9483
PHYSICAL THERAPY REIMBURSEMENT NEWS. Text in English. 1993. bi-m. USD 110 (effective 2001). 12 p./no. 3 cols./p. back issues avail. **Document type:** *Newsletter, Trade.* **Description:** Provides explanations and advice for PTs dealing with third-party payers.
Published by: American Physical Therapy Association, 1111 N Fairfax St, Alexandria, VA 22314-1488. TEL 703-684-2782, FAX 703-684-7343, subscriptions@apta.org, http://www.apta.org. Ed. Jennifer Sdilber. R&P Debra Lansey TEL 703-684-2782. Circ: 1,200 (paid).

368.382 USA ISSN 1087-027X
PHYSICIAN'S MANAGED CARE REPORT. Text in English. 1993. m. USD 457 domestic; USD 487 foreign; USD 76 newsstand/cover (effective 2001). **Document type:** *Newsletter.*
Incorporates (1994-1997): Physician's Capitation Survival (1087-0261); (1996-1997): Patient Cost Management; (in 1998): Managed Care Strategies; Which superseded (in 1997): Hospital Managed Care Strategies (1086-1378); (1993-1996): Hospital Integrated Care Report (1083-284X); Which incorporated (in 1996): Hospital Fundraising; P H O Updates
Related titles: Online - full text ed.: (from Northern Light Technology, Inc.).
Indexed: Int.Nurs.Ind.
Published by: American Health Consultants (Subsidiary of: Medical Economics Co., Inc.), 3525 Piedmont Rd, N E, 6 Piedmont Center, Ste 400, Atlanta, GA 30305. TEL 404-262-5476, 404-262-7436, 800-688-2421, FAX 404-262-7837, 800-284-3291, custserv@ahcpub.com, http://www.ahcpub.com.

I

368 362.1 USA
PHYSICIANS' MEDICARE GUIDE. Text in English. 1992. bi-m. USD 409 (effective 2001). back issues avail. **Document type:** *Trade.* **Description:** Presents the US Medicare program from a physician's point of view.
Related titles: CD-ROM ed.
Published by: C C H Incorporated, 2700 Lake Cook Rd., Riverwoods, IL 60015. TEL 847-627-7000. Pub. Catherine Wolfe.

PHYSICIAN'S PAYMENT UPDATE. see *HEALTH FACILITIES AND ADMINISTRATION*

Q R C ADVISOR; managing hospital quality, risk & cost. (Quality, Risk & Cost) see *HEALTH FACILITIES AND ADMINISTRATION*

368.382 USA
R V S FEE SCHEDULE. (Relative Value Scale) Text in English. base vol. updates 9/yr. USD 370. **Description:** Examines the Medicare payment system for physicians; includes data and worksheet to calculate reimbursement.
Published by: United Communications Group, 1300 Rockville Pike, Ste 1100, Rockville, MD 20852-3030. TEL 301-816-8950, FAX 301-816-8945. Ed. Carol Monaco.

368 NLD ISSN 1382-421X
RECHTSPRAAK ZORGVERZEKERING. Text in Dutch. 1972. 6/yr. NLG 0.53 per page. back issues avail. **Document type:** *Trade.*
Former titles (until 1995): Rechtspraak Z F W, A W B Z en Anderen (0920-9689); (until 1987): Rechtspraak Ziekenfondswet en Algemene Wet Bijzondere Ziektekosten en Aansluitende Wetgeveing (0922-3924); (until 1984): Rechtspraak Ziekenfondswet en Algemene Wet Bijzondere Ziektekosten (0166-9451)
Published by: (Netherlands. Ziekenfondsraad), Uitgeverij Kluwer BV (Subsidiary of: Wolters Kluwer N.V.), Postbus 23, Deventer 7400 GA, Netherlands. TEL 31-570-633155, FAX 31-570-633834.

RECOMMENDED SCALES OF BENEFITS. DENTAL PRACTITIONERS. see *MEDICAL SCIENCES—Dentistry*

RECOMMENDED SCALES OF BENEFITS. MEDICAL PRACTITIONERS. see *MEDICAL SCIENCES*

RECOMMENDED SCALES OF BENEFITS. PHYSIOTHERAPISTS. see *MEDICAL SCIENCES—Physical Medicine And Rehabilitation*

RECOMMENDED SCALES OF BENEFITS. PRIVATE HOSPITALS & UNATTACHED OPERATING THEATRE UNITS. see *HEALTH FACILITIES AND ADMINISTRATION*

368.382 USA
REHAB CONTINUUM REPORT. Text in English. 1992. m. USD 487 domestic; USD 517 foreign; USD 81 newsstand/cover (effective 2001). **Document type:** *Newsletter.* **Description:** Covers reimbursement issues, legal problems, legislative action, regulatory changes, industry trends, and personnel issues.
Formerly: Hospital Rehab (1068-5294)
Published by: American Health Consultants (Subsidiary of: Medical Economics Co., Inc.), 3525 Piedmont Rd, N E, 6 Piedmont Center, Ste 400, Atlanta, GA 30305. TEL 404-262-5476, 404-262-7436, 800-688-2421, FAX 404-262-7837, 800-284-3291, custserv@ahcpub.com, http://www.ahcpub.com. Circ: 845.

REIMBURSEMENT ADVISOR. see *HEALTH FACILITIES AND ADMINISTRATION*

368 USA ISSN 0732-2666
RISK MANAGEMENT FOR EXECUTIVE WOMEN*. Text in English. 1982-1985; resumed 1990. m. USD 100. **Document type:** *Trade.* **Description:** Reports on court decisions affecting insurance, personnel, health records and safety issues which expand liability or set up new areas of risk.
Formerly (until 1983): California Risk Management Report: For the Female Executive
Published by: Cox Publications, 1908 Colton Blvd, Billings, MT 59102-2316. TEL 406-256-8822. Ed. Meridith B Cox. Circ: 470 (controlled).

368.382 CAN ISSN 1195-0307
SASKATCHEWAN. LABORATORY AND DISEASE CONTROL SERVICES BRANCH. ANNUAL STATISTICAL REPORT. Text in English. a.
Related titles: ♦ Supplement to: Saskatchewan Health. Annual Report. ISSN 0822-160X.
Published by: Medical Care Insurance Branch, T C Douglas Bldg, 3475 Albert St, Regina, SK S4S 6X6, Canada. TEL 306-787-3475, FAX 306-787-9000.

SOCIETA LOMBARDA DI MEDICINA LEGALE E DELLE ASSICURAZIONI. ARCHIVIO. see *MEDICAL SCIENCES—Forensic Sciences*

SOZIALGESETZBUCH: GESETZLICHE KRANKENVERSICHERUNG. see *LAW—Civil Law*

ST. ANTHONY'S CODING FOR GENERAL SURGERY REIMBURSEMENT. see *MEDICAL SCIENCES—Surgery*

ST. ANTHONY'S CODING FOR OPHTHALMOLOGY REIMBURSEMENT. see *MEDICAL SCIENCES—Ophthalmology And Optometry*

368.382 USA ISSN 1522-5348
STATE HEALTH MONITOR. Text in English. 1993. 12/yr. USD 258 (effective 2001). **Document type:** *Newsletter.* **Description:** Provides federal news from Congress and the federal agencies on Medicare, Medicaid, health care coverage, and payment policy.
Former titles: Washington Health Week (1089-6864); (until 1995): Inside Health Care Reform (1076-8440)
Related titles: Online - full text ed.: (from Northern Light Technology, Inc., Gale Group).
—CCC.
Published by: Atlantic Information Services, Inc., 1100 17th St, N W, Ste 300, Washington, DC 20036. TEL 202-775-9008, FAX 202-331-9542, http://www.aishealth.com. Pub. Richard Biehl.

SUEDDEUTSCHE METALL-BERUFSGENOSSENSCHAFT. MITTEILUNGEN. see *OCCUPATIONAL HEALTH AND SAFETY*

TIJDSCHRIFT VOOR BEDRIJFS- EN VERZEKERINGSGENEESKUNDE. see *MEDICAL SCIENCES*

TOXIC TORTS; litigation of hazardous substance cases. see *PUBLIC HEALTH AND SAFETY*

368.42600973 USA
U.S. HEALTH CARE FINANCING ADMINISTRATION. MEDICARE COVERAGE ISSUES MANUAL. Text in English. base vol. plus irreg. updates. USD 173 for base vol. & indeterminate period of updates (effective 2001). **Document type:** *Government.* **Description:** Contains appendixes to the following manuals: Medicare Intermediary Manual, Part A, Claims Process, Part 3, HCFA #13-3; and Medicare Carriers Manual, Part B, Claims Process, Part 3, HCFA #14-3.
Related titles: Online - full content ed.
Published by: U.S. Health Care Financing Administration (Subsidiary of: U.S. Department of Health and Human Services), 7500 Security Blvd, Baltimore, MD 21244. TEL 301-597-3000, http://www.hcfa.gov/pubforms/06_cim/ci00.htm. **Subscr. to:** U.S. Government Printing Office, Superintendent of Documents, PO Box 371954, Pittsburgh, PA 15250-7954. TEL 202-512-1800, FAX 202-512-2250, orders@gpo.gov, http://www.access.gpo.gov.

368.42600973 USA
U.S. HEALTH CARE FINANCING ADMINISTRATION. MEDICARE HOME HEALTH AGENCY MANUAL. Text in English. base vol. plus irreg. updates. USD 125 for base vol. & indeterminate period of updates (effective 2001). **Document type:** *Government.* **Description:** Contains information and procedural material needed for filing claims under provisions of the Health Insurance for the Aged Act (Medicare).
Related titles: Online - full content ed.
Published by: U.S. Health Care Financing Administration (Subsidiary of: U.S. Department of Health and Human Services), 7500 Security Blvd, Baltimore, MD 21244. TEL 301-597-3000, http://www.hcfa.gov/pubforms/11_hha/hh00.htm. **Subscr. to:** U.S. Government Printing Office, Superintendent of Documents, PO Box 371954, Pittsburgh, PA 15250-7954. TEL 202-512-1800, FAX 202-512-2250, orders@gpo.gov, http://www.access.gpo.gov.

368.42600973 USA
U.S. HEALTH CARE FINANCING ADMINISTRATION. MEDICARE HOSPITAL MANUAL. Text in English. base vol. plus irreg. updates. USD 735 for base vol. & indeterminate period of updates (effective 2001). **Document type:** *Government.* **Description:** Covers the procedures for filing prompt and accurate claims for services rendered to aged patients under the provisions of the Health Insurance for the Aged Act, Medicare.
Published by: U.S. Health Care Financing Administration (Subsidiary of: U.S. Department of Health and Human Services), 7500 Security Blvd, Baltimore, MD 21244. TEL 301-597-3000, http://www.hcfa.gov/. **Subscr. to:** U.S. Government Printing Office, Superintendent of Documents, PO Box 371954, Pittsburgh, PA 15250-7954. TEL 202-512-1800, FAX 202-512-2250, orders@gpo.gov, http://www.access.gpo.gov.

368.42600973 USA
U.S. HEALTH CARE FINANCING ADMINISTRATION. MEDICARE PROVIDER REIMBURSEMENT MANUAL. Text in English. base vol. plus irreg. updates. USD 327 for base vol. & indeterminate period of updates (effective 2001). **Document type:** *Government.* **Description:** Provides guidelines and policies to implement Medicare regulations which set forth principles for determining the reasonable cost of provider services.
Published by: U.S. Health Care Financing Administration (Subsidiary of: U.S. Department of Health and Human Services), 7500 Security Blvd, Baltimore, MD 21244. http://www.hcfa.gov/. **Subscr. to:** U.S. Government Printing Office, Superintendent of Documents, PO Box 371954, Pittsburgh, PA 15250-7954. TEL 202-512-1800, FAX 202-512-2250, orders@gpo.gov, http://www.access.gpo.gov.

368.42600973 USA
U.S. HEALTH CARE FINANCING ADMINISTRATION. MEDICARE SKILLED NURSING FACILITY MANUAL. Text in English. base vol. plus irreg. updates. USD 136 for base vol. & indeterminate period of updates (effective 2001). **Document type:** *Government.*
Published by: U.S. Health Care Financing Administration (Subsidiary of: U.S. Department of Health and Human Services), 7500 Security Blvd, Baltimore, MD 21244. http://www.hcfa.gov/.

368.382 USA ISSN 1066-2669
WORKERS' COMP MANAGED CARE. Text in English. 1992. m. USD 430; USD 43 newsstand/cover (effective 2002). **Document type:** *Newsletter.* **Description:** Deals with business-related developments and trends on the medical side of workers' compensation as they affect managed health care firms, insurers, providers, employers and government.
—CCC.
Published by: Aspen Publishers, Inc., 200 Orchard Ridge Dr, Ste 200, Gaithersburg, MD 20878. TEL 301-417-7500, 800-638-8437, FAX 301-695-7931, customer.service@aspenpubl.com, http://www.aspenpub.com. Pub. Marjorie Weiner. R&P Rossette Graham. **Dist. by:** Aspen Publishers Inc., Distribution Center, 7201 McKinney Circle, Frederick, MD 21701. TEL 301-698-7100, FAX 301-417-7550.

368.41 USA
WORKERS' COMPENSATION - BUSINESS MANAGEMENT GUIDE. Text in English. 1939. 3 base vols. plus m. updates. USD 545 (effective 2001). back issues avail. **Description:** Provides strategies for preventing workplace injuries, handling accidents and litigations, and bringing employees back to work quickly and cost effectively.
Formerly (until 1993): Workers' Compensation Law Reporter
Published by: C C H Incorporated, 2700 Lake Cook Rd., Riverwoods, IL 60015. TEL 847-267-7000, 800-449-9525, FAX 773-866-3895, http://www.cch.com. Pub. Catherine Wolfe.

368 NLD ISSN 0929-4449
ZORG & VERZEKERING; actuele informatie in de gezondheidszorg. Text in Dutch. 1993. m. (11/yr.). NLG 0.57 per page. adv. **Document type:** *Trade.*
Published by: Uitgeverij Kluwer BV (Subsidiary of: Wolters Kluwer N.V.), Postbus 23, Deventer 7400 GA, Netherlands. TEL 31-570-633155, FAX 31-570-633834. Ed. L Opheikens. Circ: 1,000.

INSURANCE—Abstracting, Bibliographies, Statistics

368.382021 USA ISSN 1074-4444
RA413.5.U5
MANAGED HEALTH CARE OVERVIEW*. Text in English. 1994. a. USD 75. **Document type:** *Monographic series.* **Description:** Presents charts and graphs of statistics on the managed health care industry, including number and types of health plans, enrollments, and services offered.
Published by: American Managed Care and Review Association, 1129 20th St, N W, Ste 600, Washington, DC 20036-3403. TEL 202-728-0506, FAX 202-728-0609.

INSURANCE—Computer Applications

HEALTH DATA MANAGEMENT (CHICAGO); the magazine of electronic health care networking. see *MEDICAL SCIENCES—Computer Applications*

INTERIOR DESIGN AND DECORATION

see also HOME ECONOMICS

INTERNAL MEDICINE

see MEDICAL SCIENCES—Internal Medicine

INTERNATIONAL COMMERCE

see BUSINESS AND ECONOMICS—International Commerce

INTERNATIONAL DEVELOPMENT AND ASSISTANCE

see BUSINESS AND ECONOMICS—International Development And Assistance

INTERNATIONAL EDUCATION PROGRAMS

see EDUCATION—International Education Programs

INTERNATIONAL LAW

see LAW—International Law

INTERNATIONAL RELATIONS

see POLITICAL SCIENCE—International Relations

INTERNET

see COMPUTERS—Internet

▼ **EHEALTHCARE STRATEGY & TRENDS.** see *HEALTH FACILITIES AND ADMINISTRATION*

INVESTMENTS

see BUSINESS AND ECONOMICS—Investments

ISLAM

see RELIGIONS AND THEOLOGY—Islamic

JEWELRY, CLOCKS AND WATCHES

681 617.7 331.881 DNK ISSN 0903-1391
TID OG SYN. Text in Danish. m. (except Aug.). DKK 425 (effective 2001). adv. **Document type:** *Trade.* **Description:** Provides information to members of the trade union for watchmakers and opticians.
Formerly (until 1955): Urmageren
Published by: Urmagernes- og Optikernes Landssammenslutning, Upsalagade 20, 4, Copenhagen Oe 2100, Denmark. TEL 45-35-47-34-00, FAX 45-35-47-34-90, uol@dff-s.dk, http://www.uol.dk. Ed. Anette Pedersen. adv.: B&W page DKK 3,400, color page DKK 7,300; trim. Circ: 2,100.

JOURNALISM

070 617.6 USA
AMERICAN ASSOCIATION OF DENTAL EDITORS. NEWSLETTER✱ . Text in English. 1973. bi-m. USD 25; USD 40 foreign (effective 1998). adv. back issues avail. **Document type:** *Newsletter.*
Formerly: A A D E Editor's Journal (0160-6999)
—GNLM.
Published by: American Association of Dental Editors, 22W054 Stratford Pl, Glen Ellyn, IL 60137-6809. TEL 708-354-2992, FAX 708-354-2914. Ed., Pub., R&P, Adv. contact Joanna Carey. Circ: 325 (controlled).

808.02 617.585 USA
AMERICAN PODIATRIC MEDICAL WRITERS ASSOCIATION. NEWSLETTER. Text in English. 1985. bi-m. USD 12 to non-members (effective 2001); free to members. adv. bk.rev. back issues avail. **Document type:** *Newsletter, Directory.* **Description:** For professional writers of podiatric literature.
Published by: American Podiatric Medical Writers Association, PO Box 750129, Forest Hills, NY 11375. TEL 718-897-9700, FAX 718-896-5747, bblock@prodigy.net. Ed. Barry H Block. Circ: 200.

808.06661 USA ISSN 1054-2353
RT24
NURSE AUTHOR AND EDITOR; a newsletter for nurse authors, editors, and editorial board members. Text in English. 1991. q., latest vol.11, 2001. USD 48 domestic; USD 66 foreign (2000). adv. bk.rev., software rev., Website rev. illus. CINAHL, Yearly Index in Fall issue. back issues avail. **Document type:** *Newsletter, Trade.* **Description:** Offers advice on writing, reviewing and editing articles and books for nursing publications.
Related titles: Online - full text ed.: (from ProQuest Information & Learning).
Indexed: CINAHL, Int.Nurs.Ind.
—BLDSC (6187.028340). **CCC.**
Published by: Hall Johnson Consulting, 9737 W Ohio Ave, Lakewood, CO 80226. TEL 303-988-0056, nurseauthormail@aol.com, http://www.cinahl.com/jrnls/NAED/naed.htm. Ed. Suzanne Hall Johnson.

PROBE; David Zimmerman's newsletter on science, media, policy and health. see *SCIENCES: COMPREHENSIVE WORKS*

JUDAISM

see RELIGIONS AND THEOLOGY—Judaic

JUDICIAL SYSTEMS

see LAW—Judicial Systems

LABOR AND INDUSTRIAL RELATIONS

see BUSINESS AND ECONOMICS—Labor And Industrial Relations

LABOR UNIONS

see also BUSINESS AND ECONOMICS—Labor And Industrial Relations

331.88 615 USA ISSN 1090-3089
1199 NEWS. Text in English. 1965. 10/yr. USD 15 (effective 2000). bk.rev. illus. **Document type:** *Newsletter.*
Formerly (until 1970): 1199 Drug and Hospital News (0742-6003)
Published by: (National Health and Human Service Employees Union), Local 1199, 310 W 43d St, New York, NY 10036. TEL 212-582-1890. Eds. Daniel North, J J Johnson. Circ: 150,000.

331.8 CZE ISSN 0006-0453
BEZPECNOST A HYGIENA PRACE/SAFETY AND HYGIENE OF WORK. Text in Czech. 1951. m. USD 39.20. adv. bk.rev.
Indexed: C.I.S. Abstr.
Published by: Vydavatelstvi a Nakladatelstvi Prace s r.o., Vaclavske nam 17, Prague 11258, Czech Republic. Ed. Jan Drha. Circ: 48,000.

I Z A. (Illustrierte Zeitschrift fuer Arbeitssicherheit) see *OCCUPATIONAL HEALTH AND SAFETY*

LAEGESEKRETAER NYT. see *BUSINESS AND ECONOMICS—Office Equipment And Services*

MEDECINE HOSPITALIERE/HOSPITAL MEDICINE. see *HEALTH FACILITIES AND ADMINISTRATION*

610.6952 331.8 SWE ISSN 1403-5502
MODERNA LAEKARE. Text in Swedish. 1942. 7/yr. SEK 120 to non-members; SEK 68 to members (effective 2001). adv. bk.rev. charts, illus. index. **Document type:** *Magazine, Trade.* **Description:** Provides information and debate about wage negotiations and doctor training, healthcare in general, and the professional life of physicians.
Former titles (until 1998): Tidskrift foer Yngre Laekare (0349-6635); (until 1981): Sylfnytt (0039-7636); (until 1951): Meddelanden fraan Sveriges Yngre Laekares Foerening
Published by: Sveriges Yngre Laekares Foerening/Swedish Junior Hospital Doctors' Association, Box 5610, Stockholm 11486, Sweden. TEL 46-8-790-33-75, FAX 46-8-21-16-68, ml@sylf.se, info@sylf.se, http://www.modernalakare.nu, http://www.sylf.se. Ed., Pub. David Eberhard. Adv. contact Ann Marie Sandstrom. B&W page SEK 14,400, color page SEK 20,000; trim 185 x 270. Circ: 14,100 (paid and controlled).

NOUVEAU CENTRE DE SANTE. see *MEDICAL SCIENCES*

POTRAVINAR. see *FOOD AND FOOD INDUSTRIES*

TANDPLEJEREN. see *MEDICAL SCIENCES—Dentistry*

TID OG SYN. see *JEWELRY, CLOCKS AND WATCHES*

TIDSKRIFTET SYKEPLEIEN. see *MEDICAL SCIENCES—Nurses And Nursing*

331.8 610 USA
U A P D REPORT. Text in English. 1978. m. USD 25 (effective 2000). **Document type:** *Newsletter.* **Description:** Covers news of the labor union.
Related titles: Online - full content ed.
Published by: Union of American Physicians and Dentists, 1330 Broadway, Ste 730, Oakland, CA 94612. TEL 510-839-0193, FAX 510-763-8756, uapd@uapd.com, http://www.uapd.com. Ed. Dr. Robert Weinmann. R&P Gary Robinson. Circ: 3,000 (controlled).

331.8 GBR ISSN 1351-9492
U N I S O N MAGAZINE. Text in English. 1993. m. membership only. adv. bk.rev. illus. **Document type:** *Magazine, Trade.*
Formed by the 1993 merger of: N A L G O Annual Report (0077-4456); (1951-1993): N U P E Journal (0266-8165); C O H S E Journal (0961-3781); Which was formerly (1912-1989): Health Services Journal (0017-9116)
Indexed: ASSIA.
Published by: U N I S O N, 1 Marbledon Pl, London WC1H 9AJ, United Kingdom. TEL 44-207-3882366, FAX 44-207-5511461, unison-focus@unison.org.uk, http://www.unison.org.uk. Ed. Nisa Ali. adv.: color page GBP 12,500; trim 210 x 297. Circ: 1,300,000 (controlled and free).

331.88 305.4 613.62 CAN ISSN 0845-8839
UNION MATTERS. Text in English. 1927. 6/yr. free per issue. charts, illus, stat, tr.lit. back issues avail. **Document type:** *Newsletter.* **Description:** Informs union members about current labor issues and economic and social concerns.
Former titles (until 1989): Common Ground (0838-8032); (until 1986): Dome (0319-8588)
Published by: Saskatchewan Government Employees' Union, 1440 Broadway Ave, Regina, SK S4P 1E2, Canada. TEL 306-522-8571, FAX 306-565-2240. Ed. Trish Elliott. Circ: 15,000 (controlled).

LABORATORY TECHNIQUE

see MEDICAL SCIENCES—Experimental Medicine, Laboratory Technique

LAW

see also CRIMINOLOGY AND LAW ENFORCEMENT; LAW—Civil Law; LAW—Corporate Law; LAW—Criminal Law; LAW—Family And Matrimonial Law; LAW—International Law; LAW—Judicial Systems; LAW—Legal Aid; PATENTS, TRADEMARKS AND COPYRIGHTS

A D A LEGAL ADVISOR. see *MEDICAL SCIENCES—Dentistry*

340 613 USA ISSN 1048-907X
A S H SMOKING AND HEALTH REVIEW. Text in English. 1968 (vol.8). bi-m. USD 15; USD 25 foreign. illus. **Document type:** *Newsletter.* **Description:** Contains news and information about nonsmokers' rights and ASH legal action to protect them.
Formerly: A S H Newsletter

J

Published by: Action on Smoking & Health, 2013 H St, N W, Washington, DC 20006. TEL 202-659-4310, FAX 202-833-3921, http://ash.org/. Ed. John F Banzhaf III. Circ: 32,000.

A V A ADVISOR. see *MEDICAL SCIENCES—Oncology*

340 614.19 USA ISSN 1057-8153
HE5614
ACCIDENT RECONSTRUCTION JOURNAL. Text in English. 1989. bi-m. USD 39 in US & Canada; USD 42 elsewhere. adv. index. back issues avail. **Document type:** *Trade.* **Description:** Covers traffic accident investigation and reconstruction, traffic safety news, safety recalls and related legal developments.
Indexed: HRIS.
—BLDSC (0573.301500).
Address: 3004 Charleton Ct, Waldorf, MD 20602-2527. TEL 301-843-1371, FAX 301-884-5066. Ed., Pub., R&P, Adv. contact Victor T Craig. Circ: 3,600. **Subscr. to:** PO Box 234, Waldorf, MD 20604-0234.

ACTA TECNOLOGIAE ET LEGIS MEDICAMENTI. see *MEDICAL SCIENCES*

658 340 USA
ACTION KIT FOR HOSPITAL LAW. Text in English. 1972. m. USD 495 (effective 1999). **Document type:** *Newsletter.*
Published by: Action Kit Publications, 4614 Fifth Ave, Pittsburgh, PA 15213. TEL 412-687-7677, 800-245-1205. Ed. John F Horty. R&P Margaret Barker TEL Margaret/Barker. Circ: 2,000.

ACTION KIT FOR HOSPITAL TRUSTEES. see *HEALTH FACILITIES AND ADMINISTRATION*

344.04369792 USA
AIDS & FLORIDA LAW. Text in English. 1989. 3 base vols. USD 240. **Description:** Provides an overview of AIDS and Florida law, and gives a systematic analysis of the effect of AIDS on civil rights lawsuits, housing cases, public schools, insurance and other relevant topics.
Published by: Lexis Law Publishing (Subsidiary of: Reed Elsevier plc), PO Box 7587, Charlottesville, VA 22906-7587. TEL 804-972-7600, 800-562-1197, FAX 804-972-7666, llp.customer.support@lexis-nexis.com, http://www.lexislawpublishing.com. Ed. Robert Craig Waters.

AIDS & PUBLIC POLICY JOURNAL. (Acquired Immune Deficiency Syndrome) see *MEDICAL SCIENCES—Communicable Diseases*

610 340 USA
AIDS LAW & LITIGATION REPORTER. Text in English. m. (plus q. updates). USD 575 (effective 2000). **Document type:** *Academic/Scholarly.* **Description:** Presents complete, retrospective, full-text decisions from federal, state, and local courts, surveys proposed and enacted legislation.
Published by: University Publishing Group, Inc., 17100 Cole Rd, Ste 312, Hagerstown, MD 31740. TEL 800-654-8188, FAX 301-582-2406, orders@upgbooks.com.

AIDS LITERATURE & LAW REVIEW. see *MEDICAL SCIENCES—Abstracting, Bibliographies, Statistics*

340 610 USA ISSN 0899-1464
KF3803.A54
AIDS LITIGATION REPORTER; the national journal of record of AIDS-related litigation. (Acquired Immune Deficiency Syndrome) Text in English. 1987. s-m. USD 775 (effective 1999). adv. s-a. index. back issues avail. **Document type:** *Newsletter.*
Related titles: Online - full text ed.: (from LexisNexis).
Published by: Andrews Publications, 175 Strafford Ave, Bldg 4, Ste 140, Wayne, PA 19087. TEL 610-225-0510, FAX 610-225-0501, http://www.andrewspub.com. Ed. Ronald V Baker. Pub., R&P Robert Maroldo. Adv. contact Sofia Pables.

344.043 614 USA ISSN 0887-1493
KF3803.A54
AIDS POLICY AND LAW. (Acquired Immune Deficiency Syndrome) Text in English. 1986. bi-w. USD 487; USD 509 foreign (effective 1999). s-a. index. back issues avail. **Document type:** *Newsletter.* **Description:** Covers legal issues & regulatory aspects of AIDS & HIV. Includes the latest developments on the federal, state and local levels, fair employment practices, litigation, legislation, regulation, policy guidelines, case studies, and interviews.
Related titles: Online - full text ed.: (from Human Resources Information Network).
Indexed: CINAHL.
—Infotrieve. **CCC.**
Published by: L R P Publications, 747 Dresher Rd, Box 980, Horsham, PA 19044. TEL 215-784-0941, 800-341-7874, FAX 215-784-9639, custserve@lrp.com, http://www.lrp.com. Ed. Frank Baran.

ALCOHOL ISSUES INSIGHTS. see *BEVERAGES*

AMERICAN ACADEMY OF PSYCHIATRY AND THE LAW. JOURNAL. see *MEDICAL SCIENCES—Psychiatry And Neurology*

340 616.8 USA ISSN 0896-5633
KF8922
AMERICAN ACADEMY OF PSYCHIATRY AND THE LAW. NEWSLETTER. Text in English. 1975. 3/yr. USD 25 (effective 1998). **Document type:** *Newsletter, Academic/Scholarly.* **Description:** Law and practice in psychiatry and forensic psychiatry.
Indexed: Abstr.Crim.& Pen., e-psyche.
Published by: American Academy of Psychiatry and the Law, PO Box 30, Bloomfield, CT 06002-0030. TEL 860-242-5450, FAX 860-286-0787. Ed. Dr. Robert Miller. Circ: 1,750.

AMERICAN JOURNAL OF FORENSIC PSYCHIATRY. see *MEDICAL SCIENCES—Forensic Sciences*

AMERICAN JOURNAL OF FORENSIC PSYCHOLOGY; interfacing issues of psychology and law. see *PSYCHOLOGY*

340 610 USA ISSN 0098-8588
K1 CODEN: AJLMDN
AMERICAN JOURNAL OF LAW & MEDICINE. Text in English. 1975. q. USD 105 domestic to individuals; USD 140 foreign to individuals; USD 195 domestic to institutions; USD 230 foreign to institutions (effective 2001). adv. bk.rev. bibl, illus. Index. back issues avail.; reprint service avail. from WSH,SCH,PSC. *Refereed.* **Document type:** *Academic/Scholarly.* **Description:** Interdisciplinary law review providing in-depth legal analysis of current medicolegal issues.
Related titles: Microfiche ed.: (from WSH); Microfilm ed.: (from WSH,PMC); Microform ed.: (from WSH); Online - full text ed.: (from Gale Group, LexisNexis, West Group, Northern Light Technology, Inc., H. W. Wilson, ProQuest Information & Learning, Factiva, Institute for Scientific Information).
Indexed: ASCA, Abstr.Bk.Rev.Curr.Leg.Per., Abstr.Health Care Manage.Stud., AgeLine, Biol.Abstr., C.L.I., Curr.Cont., Dok.Arbeitsmed., Environ.Sci.Poll.Mgmt., Excerp.Med., Fam.Ind., Hlth.Ind., Hosp.Lit.Ind., IMFL, INIS Atomind., Ind.Med. (1975-), Int.Nurs.Ind., L.R.I. (Mar.1980-), Lang.& Lang.Behav.Abstr., Leg.Cont., Leg.Per. (Jul.1981-), Med.Care Rev., P C I, Pollut.Abstr., Rel.Ind.One, Rel.Ind.Two, Risk Abstr., SOPODA, SSCI, Saf.Sci.Abstr., Soc.Serv.Abstr., Sociol.Abstr., Telegen.
—BLDSC (0826.880000), EMDOCS, GNLM, IDS, ingenta, KNAW. **CCC.**
Published by: American Society of Law, Medicine & Ethics, 765 Commonwealth Ave, Ste 1634, Boston, MA 02215. TEL 617-262-4990, FAX 617-437-7596, aslme@bu.edu; orders@allenpress.com, http://www.aslme.org. Ed. Frances Miller. R&P, Adv. contact Michael Vasko. page USD 600. Circ: 4,000. **Subscr.to:** Allen Press Inc., PO Box 1897, Lawrence, KS 66044-8897. FAX 875-843-1274, http://www.allenpress.com. **Co-sponsor:** Boston University, School of Law.

AMERICANS WITH DISABILITIES ACT: EMPLOYEE RIGHTS AND EMPLOYER OBLIGATIONS. see *HANDICAPPED*

AMERICANS WITH DISABILITIES ACT: PUBLIC ACCOMMODATIONS AND COMMERCIAL FACILITIES. see *HANDICAPPED*

ANESTHESIA MALPRACTICE PREVENTION. see *MEDICAL SCIENCES—Anaesthesiology*

344.730321 347.3 USA ISSN 1075-2994
ANNALS OF HEALTH LAW. Text in English. 1992. a. USD 20. abstr. *Refereed.* **Document type:** *Academic/Scholarly.* **Description:** Offers original articles of particular relevance to health care practitioners, policymakers, and scholars in the realm of health law and policy.
Related titles: CD-ROM ed.; Online - full text ed.: (from LexisNexis, H. W. Wilson, Gale Group).
Indexed: L.R.I. (Jan.1992-), Leg.Per. (Sep.1994-), P.A.I.S.
Published by: Loyola University Chicago Law Journal, School of Law, Institute for Health Law, One E Pearson St, Chicago, IL 60611. TEL 312-915-6304, FAX 312-915-6212, jblum@luc.edu. Ed. John D Blum. Circ: 800. **Co-sponsor:** American Health Lawyers Association.

ANUARIO DE PSICOLOGIA JURIDICA. see *PSYCHOLOGY*

ARBO BULLETIN. see *OCCUPATIONAL HEALTH AND SAFETY*

ARTHUR ANDERSEN WASHINGTON HEALTHCARE NEWSLETTER. see *HEALTH FACILITIES AND ADMINISTRATION*

DER ARZT UND SEIN RECHT. see *MEDICAL SCIENCES*

ARZTHAFTPFLICHT - RECHTSPRECHUNG. see *MEDICAL SCIENCES*

ARZTHAFTUNGSRECHT. see *MEDICAL SCIENCES*

ARZTRECHT; Kompendium des Gesamten Rechtes der Medizin. see *MEDICAL SCIENCES*

ASSOCIATION OF FOOD AND DRUG OFFICIALS. JOURNAL. see *FOOD AND FOOD INDUSTRIES*

340 610 USA
ATTORNEYS' DICTIONARY OF MEDICINE. Text in English. 1962. irreg. (in 6 vols.).
Related titles: CD-ROM ed.
Published by: Matthew Bender & Co., Inc. (Subsidiary of: Lexis Law Publishing), 2 Park Ave, New York, NY 10016. TEL 212-448-2000, international@bender.com, http://www.bender.com. Ed. B Lieberman.

344.041 USA
ATTORNEY'S MEDICAL ADVANTAGE ON LAWDESK. Text in English. s-a. (in 4 vols.). **Document type:** *Academic/Scholarly.* **Description:** Contains Attorney's Medical Adviser, the Attorney's Medical Atlas, and MEDLINE abstracts; also optional Stedman's Medical Dictionary and Attorneys Medical Deskbook.
Media: CD-ROM. **Related titles:** ♦ Print ed.: Attorney's Medical Advisor - Atlas; ♦ Attorney's Medical Deskbook.
Published by: West Group (Subsidiary of: Thomson Corporation, The), 620 Opperman Dr., Eagan, MN 55123. TEL 651-987-7000, FAX 612-687-7302, http://www.westgroup.com.

ATTORNEY'S MEDICAL ADVISOR - ATLAS. see *MEDICAL SCIENCES*

ATTORNEY'S MEDICAL DESKBOOK. see *MEDICAL SCIENCES*

340 611 USA
ATTORNEYS' TEXTBOOK OF MEDICINE. Text in English. 1934. a. (in 23 vols.) (plus q. updates).
Related titles: CD-ROM ed.
Published by: Matthew Bender & Co., Inc. (Subsidiary of: Lexis Law Publishing), 2 Park Ave, New York, NY 10016. TEL 212-448-2000, international@bender.com, http://www.bender.com.

346.013 USA ISSN 0888-1537
KF390.A4
B I F O C A L. (Bar Associations in Focus on Aging and the Law) Key Title: Bifocal. Text in English. 1979. q., latest vol.22, no.3, 2001. USD 35 (effective 2001). bk.rev. 12 p./no. back issues avail. **Document type:** *Newsletter.*
Published by: American Bar Association, Commission on Legal Problems of the Elderly, 740 15th St, N W, Washington, DC 20005-1022. TEL 202-662-8690, FAX 202-662-8698. Ed. Jamie Philpotts. R&P Rick Vittenson TEL 312-988-6101. Circ: 1,000 (paid).

B N A'S FEDERAL ENVIRONMENT & SAFETY REGULATORY MONITORING REPORT. see *ENVIRONMENTAL STUDIES*

L

610 340 USA ISSN 1064-2137
KF3825.5.A15
B N A'S HEALTH LAW REPORTER; a weekly review of legislative, regulatory, and legal developments. Text in English. 1992. 49/yr. USD 1,385 (effective 2001). s-a. index. 32 p./no. back issues avail. **Description:** Provides comprehensive coverage of the wide range of legal, regulatory, and legislative developments that have an impact on health care attorneys and top-flight health care executives, in such areas as antitrust, tax, professional liability, insurance, fraud and abuse, reimbursement, medical health law, Medicare, Medicaid, and licensure.
Media: E-mail. **Related titles:** Online - full text ed.: ISSN 1521-5350 (from Bureau of National Affairs, Inc., (BNA), The).
—CCC.
Published by: The Bureau of National Affairs, Inc., 1231 25th St, N W, Washington, DC 20037. TEL 202-452-4200, 800-372-1033, 800-452-7773, FAX 202-822-8092, customercare@bna.com, bnaplus@bna.com, http://www.bna.com/. Ed. Susan Webster. Pub. Gregory McCaffery.

B N A'S MEDICARE REPORT. see *MEDICAL SCIENCES*

B N A'S STATE ENVIRONMENT & SAFETY REGULATORY MONITORING REPORT. see *ENVIRONMENTAL STUDIES*

340 610 USA
BARCLAYS HEALTH LAW BULLETIN (CALIFORNIA EDITION). Text in English. 1992. m. USD 245. q. index. **Document type:** *Newsletter.*
Published by: Barclays Law Publishers, PO Box 3066, S San Francisco, CA 94083. TEL 415-588-1155, FAX 415-244-6619.

BEHAVIORAL SCIENCES AND THE LAW. see *PSYCHOLOGY*

344 USA ISSN 1091-5982
KF3821.A15
BENDER'S HEALTH CARE LAW MONTHLY. Text in English. 1985. m. USD 251 (effective 1999). **Document type:** *Newsletter.*
Supersedes (in 1995): Health Care Law Newsletter (0893-6099)
—Infotrieve. **CCC.**
Published by: Matthew Bender & Co., Inc. (Subsidiary of: Lexis Law Publishing), 2 Park Ave, New York, NY 10016. TEL 212-448-2000, international@bender.com, http://www.bender.com. Ed. Kent Frankstone.

BENEFITS GUIDE. see *BUSINESS AND ECONOMICS—Personnel Management*

BIOLAW: A LEGAL AND ETHICAL REPORTER ON MEDICINE, HEALTH CARE, AND BIOENGINEERING. see *BIOLOGY—Bioengineering*

BIORESEARCH MONITORING ALERT. see *INSTRUMENTS*

BIOTECH MARKET NEWS & LEGAL STRATEGIES. see *BIOLOGY—Biotechnology*

BIOTECHNOLOGY LAW REPORT. see *BIOLOGY—Biotechnology*

BRANDEIS UNIVERSITY. INSTITUTE FOR HEALTH POLICY. RESEARCH NEWS. see *MEDICAL SCIENCES*

340 610 USA ISSN 1062-1814
KF1297.M4
BREAST IMPLANT LITIGATION REPORTER; the twice monthly national journal of record on breast implant litigation. Text in English. 1992. s-m. USD 850 (effective 1999). adv. bk.rev. illus. Index. reprints avail. **Document type:** *Newsletter.* **Description:** Provides current information on developments in breast implant lawsuits nationally.
Related titles: Online - full text ed.: (from LexisNexis).
Published by: Andrews Publications, 175 Strafford Ave, Bldg 4, Ste 140, Wayne, PA 19087. TEL 610-255-0510, 800-345-1101, FAX 610-255-0501, http://www.andrewspub.com. Ed. Emily Silva. Pub., R&P Robert Maroldo. Adv. contact Sofia Pables.

THE BULLETIN ON LONG-TERM CARE LAW. see *GERONTOLOGY AND GERIATRICS*

BUREAU OF VOLUNTARY COMPLIANCE NEWSLETTERS. see *PHARMACY AND PHARMACOLOGY*

BUTTERWORTHS FOOD LAW. see *PUBLIC HEALTH AND SAFETY*

C H I L D NEWSLETTER. see *CHILDREN AND YOUTH—About*

CANADIAN EMPLOYMENT SAFETY AND HEALTH GUIDE. see *OCCUPATIONAL HEALTH AND SAFETY*

340 614 CAN
CANADIAN HEALTH FACILITIES LAW GUIDE. Text in English. bi-m. CND 685. index. **Document type:** *Trade.* **Description:** Statutes and commentary related to health care facilities (e.g., hospitals, nursing homes, clinics, chronic care homes) Contains the texts of approximately 70 statutes and selected regulations are reproduced.
Indexed: CBCA Bus. (1996-).
Published by: C C H Canadian Ltd., 90 Sheppard Ave E, Ste 300, North York, ON M2N 6X1, Canada. TEL 416-224-2248, 800-268-4522, FAX 416-224-2243, http://camelot.ca.cch.com.

344.04369792 CAN ISSN 1496-399X
CANADIAN HIV - AIDS POLICY & LAW REVIEW. Key Title: Bulletin Canadien VIH - SIDA et Droit. Text in English, French. 1995. q. CND 36 to individuals; CND 72 to institutions (effective 2000). bk.rev. back issues avail. **Document type:** *Newsletter, Bulletin.* **Description:** Summarizes developments in HIV and AIDS policy and law in Canada and worldwide. Aims to educate readers about policy and legal developments.
Formerly: Canadian HIV - AIDS Policy & Law Newsletter (1195-5252)
Related titles: Online - full text ed.
Indexed: CBCA Ref.
Published by: Canadian HIV - AIDS Legal Network/Reseau Juridique Canadien VIH - SIDA, 417 rue Saint Pierre, bureau 408, Montreal, PQ H2Y 2M4, Canada. TEL 514-397-6828, FAX 514-397-8570, info@aidslaw.ca, http://www.aidslaw.ca. Ed. Ralf Jurgens. R&P, Adv. contact Eric Nolet. Circ: 2,000.

CANADIAN OCCUPATIONAL SAFETY & HEALTH LAW. see *OCCUPATIONAL HEALTH AND SAFETY*

CANADIAN OCCUPATIONAL SAFETY AND HEALTH LAW MONTHLY REPORT. see *OCCUPATIONAL HEALTH AND SAFETY*

CHEMICAL REGULATION REPORTER: HAZARDOUS MATERIALS TRANSPORTATION. see *TRANSPORTATION*

CLINICAL MEDICAL ETHICS. see *MEDICAL SCIENCES*

CLINICAL RISK; incorporating the A V M A Medical & Legal Journal. see *MEDICAL SCIENCES*

CLOSED-HEAD INJURY; a clinical source book. see *MEDICAL SCIENCES*

340 617.3 616.8 USA
COMMON DIAGNOSTIC PROCEDURES: ORTHOPEDICS AND NEUROLOGY. Text in English. 1992. irreg. (in 1 vol.). USD 145 (effective 1999). Supplement avail.
Indexed: e-psyche.
Published by: Matthew Bender & Co., Inc. (Subsidiary of: Lexis Law Publishing), 2 Park Ave, New York, NY 10016. TEL 212-448-2000, international@bender.com, http://www.bender.com. Ed. Menachem Epstein.

COMPLIANCE PROGRAM GUIDANCE MANUALS. see *PUBLIC HEALTH AND SAFETY*

CONFLICT RESOLUTION QUARTERLY. see *PSYCHOLOGY*

CONTEMPORARY DRUG PROBLEMS. see *DRUG ABUSE AND ALCOHOLISM*

340 611 USA
COURTROOM MEDICINE SERIES: ABDOMINAL INJURIES. Text in English. 1973. irreg. (in 2 vols.). USD 365 (effective 1999).
Published by: Matthew Bender & Co., Inc. (Subsidiary of: Lexis Law Publishing), 2 Park Ave, New York, NY 10016. TEL 212-448-2000, international@bender.com, http://www.bender.com. Eds. Harold Williams, Jules Kalisch.

340 616.99 USA
COURTROOM MEDICINE SERIES: CANCER. Text in English. 1978. irreg. (in 3 vols.). USD 590 (effective 1999).
Published by: Matthew Bender & Co., Inc. (Subsidiary of: Lexis Law Publishing), 2 Park Ave, New York, NY 10016. TEL 212-448-2000, international@bender.com, http://www.bender.com. Ed. Arthur Frank.

340 611 USA
COURTROOM MEDICINE SERIES: CHEST, HEART AND LUNGS. Text in English. 1975. irreg. (in 2 vols.). USD 470 (effective 1999).
Published by: Matthew Bender & Co., Inc. (Subsidiary of: Lexis Law Publishing), 2 Park Ave, New York, NY 10016. TEL 212-448-2000, international@bender.com, http://www.bender.com. Eds. Harold Williams, Jules Kalisch.

340 611 USA
COURTROOM MEDICINE SERIES: HEAD AND BRAIN. Text in English. 1972. irreg. (in 3 vols.). USD 660 (effective 1999).
Published by: Matthew Bender & Co., Inc. (Subsidiary of: Lexis Law Publishing), 2 Park Ave, New York, NY 10016. TEL 212-448-2000, international@bender.com, http://www.bender.com. Eds. John Evans, Loring Chapman.

340 611 USA
COURTROOM MEDICINE SERIES: HIP AND THIGH. Text in English. 1972. irreg. (in 2 vols.). USD 365 (effective 1999).
Published by: Matthew Bender & Co., Inc. (Subsidiary of: Lexis Law Publishing), 2 Park Ave, New York, NY 10016. TEL 212-448-2000, international@bender.com, http://www.bender.com. Eds. Harold Williams, Jules Kalisch.

340 610 USA
COURTROOM MEDICINE SERIES: PAIN AND SUFFERING. Text in English. 1965. irreg. (in 4 vols.). USD 780 (effective 1999).
Published by: Matthew Bender & Co., Inc. (Subsidiary of: Lexis Law Publishing), 2 Park Ave, New York, NY 10016. TEL 212-448-2000, international@bender.com, http://www.bender.com. Ed. Loring Chapman.

340 616.89 USA
COURTROOM MEDICINE SERIES: PSYCHIC INJURIES. Text in English. irreg. (in 3 vols.). USD 540 (effective 1999).
Indexed: e-psyche.
Published by: Matthew Bender & Co., Inc. (Subsidiary of: Lexis Law Publishing), 2 Park Ave, New York, NY 10016. TEL 212-448-2000, international@bender.com, http://www.bender.com. Eds. Marvin Lewis, Robert Sadoff.

340 611 USA
COURTROOM MEDICINE SERIES: SHOULDER AND ELBOW. Text in English. 1970. irreg. (in 2 vols.). USD 365 (effective 1999).
Published by: Matthew Bender & Co., Inc. (Subsidiary of: Lexis Law Publishing), 2 Park Ave, New York, NY 10016. TEL 212-448-2000, international@bender.com, http://www.bender.com. Eds. Harold Williams, Jules Kalisch.

340 617.7 USA
COURTROOM MEDICINE SERIES: THE EYE. Text in English. 1981. irreg. (in 2 vols.). USD 435 (effective 1999).
Published by: Matthew Bender & Co., Inc. (Subsidiary of: Lexis Law Publishing), 2 Park Ave, New York, NY 10016. TEL 212-448-2000, international@bender.com, http://www.bender.com.

340 611 USA
COURTROOM MEDICINE SERIES: THE KNEE AND ITS RELATED STRUCTURES. Text in English. 1972. irreg. (in 2 vols.). USD 470 (effective 1999).
Published by: Matthew Bender & Co., Inc. (Subsidiary of: Lexis Law Publishing), 2 Park Ave, New York, NY 10016. TEL 212-448-2000, international@bender.com, http://www.bender.com. Eds. Harold Williams, Jules Kalisch.

340 611 USA
COURTROOM MEDICINE SERIES: THE LOW BACK. Text in English. 1962. irreg. (in 3 vols.). USD 650 (effective 1999).
Published by: Matthew Bender & Co., Inc. (Subsidiary of: Lexis Law Publishing), 2 Park Ave, New York, NY 10016. TEL 212-448-2000, international@bender.com, http://www.bender.com.

L

340 610 USA
COURTROOM MEDICINE SERIES: THE NECK. Text in English. 1965. irreg. (in 3 vols.). USD 590 (effective 1999).
Published by: Matthew Bender & Co., Inc. (Subsidiary of: Lexis Law Publishing), 2 Park Ave, New York, NY 10016. TEL 212-448-2000, international@bender.com, http://www.bender.com.

COURTROOM TOXICOLOGY. see *MEDICAL SCIENCES*

CRONER'S ENVIRONMENTAL MANAGEMENT. see *ENVIRONMENTAL STUDIES*

THE D O; a publication for osteopathic physicians and surgeons. (Doctor of Osteopathy) see *MEDICAL SCIENCES—Chiropractic, Homeopathy, Osteopathy*

D W D NEWSLETTER. see *GERONTOLOGY AND GERIATRICS*

▼ **DEATH & DYING SOURCEBOOK.** see *PHILOSOPHY*

DEFENDING PESTICIDES IN LITIGATION. see *ENVIRONMENTAL STUDIES—Toxicology And Environmental Safety*

344.032 USA
DEPAUL JOURNAL OF HEALTH CARE LAW. Text in English. 1996. q. USD 50. back issues avail.; reprint service avail. from WSH.
Related titles: Microfiche ed.: (from WSH).
Indexed: Leg.Per. (Sep.1997-, dropped).
Published by: DePaul University, College of Law, Health Law Insitute, 25 E Jackson Blvd, Chicago, IL 60604-2287. TEL 312-362-8553, FAX 312-362-5931. Ed. Donald H J Hermann.

348.041 USA
DIABETES EDUCATION REIMBURSEMENTS & POLICY REPORT. Abbreviated title: D E R P. Text in English. m. USD 229 domestic; USD 254 foreign (effective 2000).
Published by: Washington G-2 Reports, 1111 14th St, N W, Ste 500, Washington, DC 20005.

DICTIONNAIRE PERMANENT: BIOETHIQUE ET BIOTECHNOLOGIES. see *BIOLOGY—Biotechnology*

DICTIONNAIRE PERMANENT: SECURITE ET CONDITIONS DE TRAVAIL. see *BUSINESS AND ECONOMICS—Labor And Industrial Relations*

DISABILITY COMPLIANCE BULLETIN. see *HANDICAPPED*

DISABILITY LAW COMPLIANCE REPORT. see *HANDICAPPED*

340 USA
DRINKING DRIVER IN MINNESOTA. Text in English. 1989 (2nd ed.). base vol. plus a. updates. USD 115. Supplement avail. **Description:** Addresses the myriad issues involved in a drunk driving case and provides in-depth discussions of DWI, implied consent, criminal vehicular homicide, and injury laws.
Published by: Lexis Law Publishing (Subsidiary of: Reed Elsevier plc), PO Box 7587, Charlottesville, VA 22906-7587. TEL 804-972-7600, 800-562-1197, FAX 804-972-7666, llp.customer.support@lexis-nexis.com, http://www.lexislawpublishing.com. Ed. Donald H Nichols.

L

340 615.1 USA
DRUG PRODUCT LIABILITY. Text in English. irreg. (in 3 vols.). USD 640 (effective 1999).
Published by: Matthew Bender & Co., Inc. (Subsidiary of: Lexis Law Publishing), 2 Park Ave, New York, NY 10016. TEL 212-448-2000, international@bender.com, http://www.bender.com. Eds. Frank Woodside, Marden Guy Dixon.

DRUGS AND BIOLOGY GUIDANCE MANUAL. see *PUBLIC HEALTH AND SAFETY*

DRUGS AND THE LAW; detection, recognition & investigation. see *DRUG ABUSE AND ALCOHOLISM*

340 615 IND
DRUGS CASES; including narcotics cases. Text in English. m. USD 90 (effective 1998). **Description:** Reports judgments under the Narcotic Drugs and Psychotropic Substances Act, and Drugs and Cosmetics Act, and more.
Published by: International Law Book Co., Nijhawan Bldg., Kashmere Gate, 1562 Church Rd., New Delhi 110 006, India. TEL 91-11-296-7810, lakshmin@giasdla.vsnl.net.in.

DRUGS IN LITIGATION: DAMAGE AWARDS INVOLVING PRESCRIPTION AND NONPRESCRIPTION DRUGS. see *PHARMACY AND PHARMACOLOGY*

340 610 USA ISSN 1087-7347
E D LEGAL LETTER. Text in English. 1990. m. USD 399 domestic; USD 429 foreign; USD 67 newsstand/cover (effective 2001). **Document type:** *Newsletter.*
Formerly (until 1995): Emergency Legal Briefings (1074-8318); Incorporates: Emergency Medicine Reports Legal Briefings
Published by: American Health Consultants (Subsidiary of: Medical Economics Co., Inc.), 3525 Piedmont Rd, N E, 6 Piedmont Center, Ste 400, Atlanta, GA 30305. TEL 404-262-5476, 404-262-7436, 800-688-2421, FAX 404-262-7837, 800-284-3291, custserv@ahcpub.com, http://www.ahcpub.com. Circ: 860.

E-HEALTH & TELEMEDICINE NEWS. see *MEDICAL SCIENCES—Computer Applications*

E S - H W G - ENTSCHEIDUNGSSAMMLUNG HEILMITTELWERBEGESETZ. see *PHARMACY AND PHARMACOLOGY*

ELBOW AND SHOULDER PAIN. see *MEDICAL SCIENCES*

ELECTROMAGNETIC FIELD LITIGATION REPORTER. see *ENERGY—Electrical Energy*

340 610 USA ISSN 1042-2978
KF3826.E5
EMERGENCY DEPARTMENT LAW; the source for comprehensive coverage of legal trends in emergency medicine. Text in English. 1989. m. USD 347; USD 355 out of North America (effective 2000). back issues avail. **Document type:** *Newsletter.* **Description:** Provides coverage of challenges facing emergency care professionals from medical and legal perspectives.
Incorporates (1976-1997): Medical Liability Adisory Service (0199-1272)
—Infotrieve. **CCC.**
Published by: Business Publishers, Inc., 8737 Colesville Rd, 11th Fl, Silver Spring, MD 20910-3928. TEL 301-587-6300, 800-274-6737, FAX 301-589-8493, bpinews@bpinews.com, http://www.bpinews.com. Ed. James Lawlor. Pub. Leonard A Eiserer.

EMERGENCY MEDICAL TECHNICIAN LEGAL BULLETIN. see *MEDICAL SCIENCES*

EMERGENCY NURSE LEGAL BULLETIN. see *MEDICAL SCIENCES—Nurses And Nursing*

EMERGENCY PHYSICIAN LEGAL BULLETIN. see *MEDICAL SCIENCES*

EMPLOYMENT SAFETY AND HEALTH GUIDE. see *OCCUPATIONAL HEALTH AND SAFETY*

ENVIRONMENTAL AND TOXIC TORT TRIALS. see *ENVIRONMENTAL STUDIES—Toxicology And Environmental Safety*

344.0462 USA ISSN 1073-7561
ENVIRONMENTAL COMPLIANCE & LITIGATION STRATEGY. Text in English. 1985. m. USD 169 introductory; USD 249 renewals (effective 2001). back issues avail. **Document type:** *Newsletter.* **Description:** Roundup of significant legislative and regulatory rulings of special interest to manufacturers, insurance companies, trial attorneys, government enforcement agencies, environmental consultants and corporate counsel.
Formerly (until 1993): Hazardous Waste and Toxic Torts Law and Strategy (0884-3775)
Related titles: Online - full text ed.: (from LexisNexis).
Published by: American Lawyer Media, Inc., D B A Leader Publications, 345 Park Ave S, New York, NY 10010. TEL 212-545-6170, FAX 212-481-8161, http://www.ljx.com, http://www.americanlawyermedia.com. Ed. John M Scagnelli. Pub., R&P Stuart M Wise TEL 917-256-2001.

ENVIRONMENTAL LABORATORY WASHINGTON REPORT. see *MEDICAL SCIENCES—Experimental Medicine, Laboratory Technique*

ENVIRONMENTAL REGULATORY ADVISOR. see *ENVIRONMENTAL STUDIES—Waste Management*

ETHICS, LAW, AND AGING REVIEW. see *GERONTOLOGY AND GERIATRICS*

ETHIK IN DER MEDIZIN. see *PHILOSOPHY*

EUROPEAN JOURNAL OF HEALTH LAW. see *MEDICAL SCIENCES*

THE EXCHANGE (SAN FRANCISCO). see *MEDICAL SCIENCES—Communicable Diseases*

347 617.1 USA ISSN 0891-0278
KF2915.E95
EXERCISE STANDARDS AND MALPRACTICE REPORTER. Text in English. 1987. bi-m. USD 39.95 domestic; USD 45.95 in Canada; USD 54.95 elsewhere (effective 2001). adv. index. back issues avail. *Refereed.* **Document type:** *Newsletter.* **Description:** Current standards of practice for exercise, wellness and health promotion programs. Malpractice and professional concerns and developments are examined.
Related titles: Online - full text ed.: (from Institute for Scientific Information).
Indexed: ASCA, Focus on: Sports Sci.& Med.
—IDS.
Published by: P R C Publishing, Inc., 3976 Fulton Dr, N W, Canton, OH 44718-3043. TEL 330-492-6063, 800-336-0083, FAX 330-492-6176. Eds. David L Herbert, William G Herbert. Adv. contact Molly Romig. Circ: 1,500.

346.013 USA ISSN 1054-3473
K5
EXPERIENCE (CHICAGO). Text in English. 1986. q. USD 20 to non-members; USD 23 foreign to non-members (effective 1999). adv. bk.rev. **Document type:** *Trade.* **Description:** Publishes articles on practice problems and aspects of retirement for lawyers 60 and older. Includes news of the division.
Supersedes (in 1990): Senior Lawyer
—ingenta.
Published by: (American Bar Association), A B A Publishing, 750 N Lake Shore Dr, Chicago, IL 60611. TEL 312-988-6063, FAX 312-988-6081, http://www.abanet.org. Ed. Lori King. R&P Richard Vittenson. Circ: 7,500.

340 USA ISSN 0737-8726
KF8961.A15
THE EXPERT AND THE LAW. Text in English. 1979. bi-m. USD 75 domestic; USD 90 foreign (effective 2000). **Document type:** *Newsletter.* **Description:** Devoted to the application of scientific, medical, and technical knowledge to litigation.
Related titles: Online - full text ed.: (from LexisNexis).
Published by: National Forensic Center, 17 Temple Terr., Lawrenceville, NJ 08648. TEL 609-883-0550, 800-526-5177, forenexpts@att.net, http://www.ExpertIndex.com. Ed., Pub., R&P Betty S Lipscher. Adv. contact Mabel Silbery.

F M A TODAY. see *MEDICAL SCIENCES*

F M S FOUNDATION NEWSLETTER. (False Memory Syndrome) see *PSYCHOLOGY*

340 USA ISSN 0364-3581
KF8931.A3
FEDERAL RULES OF EVIDENCE NEWS. Text in English. 1976. m. USD 225. **Document type:** *Newsletter.*
Published by: West Group (Subsidiary of: Thomson Corporation, The), 620 Opperman Dr., Eagan, MN 55123. TEL 651-687-8000, FAX 651-687-7302, http://www.westgroup.com.

340 362.1 USA
FLORIDA BAR. HEALTH LAW SECTION NEWSLETTER. Text in English. 1988. irreg. (2-4/yr.). membership. **Document type:** *Newsletter.*
Published by: Florida Bar, Health Law Section, 650 Apalachee Pkwy, Tallahassee, FL 32399-2300. TEL 850-561-5630. Circ: 1,200.

FOOD AND COSMETICS GUIDANCE MANUAL. see *PUBLIC HEALTH AND SAFETY*

344 615 USA
FOOD AND DRUG ADMINISTRATION. REGULATORY MANUAL. Text in English. 1979. base vol. plus a. updates. USD 260. Supplement avail. **Document type:** *Trade.* **Description:** Provides information for handling FDA cases.
Formerly (until 1993): Food and Drug Administration

Published by: Shepard's (Subsidiary of: Reed Elsevier plc), 555 Middle Creek Pkwy, Colorado Springs, CO 80921. TEL 800-743-7393, customer_service@shepards.com, http://www.shepards.com. Ed. James O'Reilly.

344.04232 USA ISSN 1064-590X
K6 CODEN: FDLJES
FOOD AND DRUG LAW JOURNAL. Text in English. 1946. 3/yr. USD 379 to non-members; USD 299 to members (effective 2001). adv. charts, illus. index. reprint service avail. from WSH. *Refereed.* **Document type:** *Academic/Scholarly.*
Formerly (until 1991): Food Drug Cosmetic Law Journal (0015-6361)
Related titles: Online - full text ed.: (from LexisNexis, Gale Group, Institute for Scientific Information).
Indexed: ASCA, Aqua.Sci.& Fish.Abstr., Aquacult.Abstr., C.L.I., Chem.Abstr., Curr.Cont., Dairy Sci.Abstr., Environ.Sci.Poll.Mgmt., Excerp.Med., Food Sci.& Tech.Abstr., Hlth.Ind., I.P.A., L.R.I. (Jan.1980-Nov.1991, Jan.1992-), Leg.Per. (Jul.1981-Dec.1991), NRN, Nutr.Abstr., Pollut.Abstr., Risk Abstr., SSCI, Saf.Sci.Abstr.
—BLDSC (3977.032300), CISTI, EMDOCS, GNLM, IDS, Infotrieve, ingenta. **CCC.**
Published by: Food and Drug Law Institute, 1000 Vermont Ave, N W, Ste 200, Washington, DC 20005. TEL 202-371-1420, FAX 202-371-0649, comments@fdli.org, http://www.fdli.org/info/journal.htm. Ed. M Cathryn Butler.

340 615 GBR ISSN 1463-0826
FOOD, DRINKS & DRUGS INDUSTRY BULLETIN. Text in English. 1984. 10/yr. GBP 238 in United Kingdom; EUR 409 in Europe; USD 387 elsewhere (effective 2002). back issues avail. **Document type:** *Bulletin.* **Description:** Apprises readers of the main legal and regulatory developments in the UK and EU food and drugs industries.
Formerly: Food and Drugs Industry Bulletin (0266-9366)
Published by: Agra Europe (London) Ltd., 80 Calverley Rd, Tunbridge Wells, Kent TN1 2UN, United Kingdom. TEL 44-1892-533813, FAX 44-1892-544895, marketing@agra-net.com, http://www.agra-net.com.

344 668.55 USA ISSN 1057-2759
KFN5630.A15
FOOD, DRUG, COSMETIC, AND MEDICAL DEVICE LAW DIGEST. Text in English. 1983. 3/yr. (plus index). USD 35 to libraries; USD 45 foreign to libraries. adv. bk.rev. index. **Document type:** *Academic/Scholarly.* **Description:** Articles of interest in the substantive areas of food, drug, cosmetic and medical device law, including information on federal and state legislation and recent administrative decisions and court decisions.
Formerly: Food, Drug and Cosmetic Law Section. Newsletter (0742-4051)
Related titles: Online - full text ed.: (from Gale Group).
Indexed: L.R.I. (Jan.1997-), Leg.Per. (Jul.1992-Mar.1999).
Published by: New York State Bar Association, Food, Drug and Cosmetic Law Section, One Elk St, Albany, NY 12207. TEL 518-463-3200, FAX 518-463-8844. Ed. David S Weinstock. R&P Patricia Betz Stockli. Circ: 400 (controlled).

FOOD DRUG COSMETIC LAW REPORTS (RX EDITION). see *PHARMACY AND PHARMACOLOGY*

FOOD LAW REPORTS. see *FOOD AND FOOD INDUSTRIES*

FOOT AND ANKLE PAIN. see *MEDICAL SCIENCES*

FORENSIC DRUG ABUSE ADVISOR; a monthly digest of information on the forensic aspects of drug abuse. see *DRUG ABUSE AND ALCOHOLISM*

340 USA ISSN 0192-3145
KF195.E96
FORENSIC SERVICES DIRECTORY; national register of experts, engineers, scientific advisors, medical specialists, technical consultants and sources of specialized knowledge. Text in English. 1980. a. USD 139.50 (effective 2000). adv. **Document type:** *Directory.*
Related titles: Online - full text ed.: (from West Group).
Published by: National Forensic Center, 17 Temple Terr., Lawrenceville, NJ 08648. TEL 609-883-0550, 800-526-5177, forenexpts@att.net, http://www.ExpertIndex.com. Ed., Pub., R&P Betty S Lipscher. Adv. contact Mabel Silbery.

G M H C TREATMENT ISSUES; newsletter of experimental AIDS therapies. (Gay Men's Health Crisis) see *MEDICAL SCIENCES—Communicable Diseases*

G M P REGULATIONS OF JAPAN. see *PHARMACY AND PHARMACOLOGY*

HAND AND WRIST PAIN. see *MEDICAL SCIENCES*

340 614.8 USA
HANDGUN CONTROL. SEMI-ANNUAL PROGRESS REPORT. Text in English. 1974. s-a. free per issue to members. **Document type:** *Newsletter.* **Description:** Reports on federal and state legislative efforts toward stronger gun laws. Cites new studies on gun issues.
Formerly (until 1989): Washington Report (Washington, 1974)
Published by: Handgun Control, Inc., 1225 Eye St, N W, Washington, DC 20005. TEL 202-898-0792. Ed. Cheryl Brolin.

HANDHAVINGSZAKBOEKJE. see *ENVIRONMENTAL STUDIES—Toxicology And Environmental Safety*

HANDLING SOFT TISSUE INJURY CASES. see *MEDICAL SCIENCES*

HEALTH ADVOCATE. see *PHYSICAL FITNESS AND HYGIENE*

344.041 USA
HEALTH & LAW TRENDS. Text in English. 1997. irreg. back issues avail. **Document type:** *Newsletter.*
Media: Online - full text.
Published by: Arent Fox Kintner Plotkin & Kahn PLLC, 1050 Connecticut Ave, NW, Washington, DC 20036-5339. TEL 202-827-6000, FAX 202-857-6395, infolaw@arentfox.com, http://www.arentfox.com/.

HEALTH & SAFETY MONITOR. see *OCCUPATIONAL HEALTH AND SAFETY*

HEALTH CARE FRAUD AND ABUSE NEWSLETTER. see *INSURANCE*

HEALTH CARE GUIDE. see *MEDICAL SCIENCES*

HEALTH CARE LABOR MANUAL. see *HEALTH FACILITIES AND ADMINISTRATION*

340 362 USA
HEALTH CARE LAW: A PRACTICAL GUIDE. Text in English. 1985. irreg. USD 305 (effective 1999).
Published by: Matthew Bender & Co., Inc. (Subsidiary of: Lexis Law Publishing), 2 Park Ave, New York, NY 10016. TEL 212-448-2000, international@bender.com, http://www.bender.com.

340 USA
HEALTH CARE LAW SOURCEBOOK. Text in English. 1989. irreg. (in 3 vols.). USD 415 (effective 1999).
Published by: Matthew Bender & Co., Inc. (Subsidiary of: Lexis Law Publishing), 2 Park Ave, New York, NY 10016. TEL 212-448-2000, international@bender.com, http://www.bender.com.

340 610 USA
HEALTH CARE LAWYER. Text in English. 1985. q. USD 68 to non-members; USD 16 to members. bk.rev. back issues avail. **Document type:** *Newsletter.*
Published by: Illinois State Bar Association, Illinois Bar Center, Springfield, IL 62701. TEL 217-525-1760, FAX 217-525-0712. Eds. Ted Leblang, W E Basanta. Circ: 820.

HEALTH EMPLOYMENT LAW UPDATE. see *BUSINESS AND ECONOMICS—Labor And Industrial Relations*

HEALTH LAW & BUSINESS LIBRARY ON CD-ROM. see *HEALTH FACILITIES AND ADMINISTRATION*

HEALTH LAW BULLETIN. see *PUBLIC HEALTH AND SAFETY*

342 614 USA
HEALTH LAW DIGEST. Text in English. 1972. m. USD 250.
Published by: American Health Lawyers Association, 1120 Connecticut Ave, N W, Ste 950, Washington, DC 20036-3921. TEL 202-833-1100. Ed. Elizabeth Turgman. Circ: 10,000.

344.041 GBR ISSN 1363-660X
HEALTH LAW FOR HEALTHCARE PROFESSIONALS. Text in English. 1996. 10/yr. GBP 172; GBP 197, USD 384 foreign (effective 2000). back issues avail. **Document type:** *Newsletter.* **Description:** Provides concise and accessible review of developments in the legal and regulatory environment governing all aspects of health care.
Published by: Monitor Press Ltd. (Subsidiary of: Informa Group PLC), Suffolk House, Church Field Rd, Sudbury, Suffolk CO10 2YA, United Kingdom. TEL 44-1787-378607, FAX 44-1787-880201, http://www.monitorpress.co.uk. Pub. Zoe Turner. R&P Liz Dittner.

340 613.7 CAN ISSN 1192-8336
CODEN: HLJOE9
HEALTH LAW JOURNAL. Text in English. 1993. a. CND 25 (effective 2000). reprint service avail. from WSH. *Refereed.* **Document type:** *Academic/Scholarly.* **Description:** Medical-legal articles addressing emerging issues and suggesting new directions in law and social policy.
Related titles: Online - full text ed.: (from LexisNexis, Gale Group).
Indexed: CBCA Ref., Can.Per.Ind. (Jan.1996-), Ind.Can.L.P.L., Int.Nurs.Ind., L.R.I. (Jan.1993-), Lang.& Lang.Behav.Abstr., Leg.Per. (Sep.1997-), SOPODA, Soc.Serv.Abstr., Sociol.Abstr.
—BLDSC (4275.050075).
Published by: Health Law Institute, 457 Law Centre, University of Alberta, Edmonton, AB T6G 2H5, Canada. TEL 780-492-8343, FAX 780-492-9575, ninahawk@law.ualberta.ca. Ed. Timothy Caulfield. R&P, Adv. contact Nina Hawkins. Circ: 1,000.

340 362.1 USA
HEALTH LAW NEWS. Text in English. 1991. irreg. (2-3/yr.). membership. back issues avail. **Document type:** *Newsletter.*
Formerly: State Bar of Wisconsin. Health Law Section. Newsletter
Published by: (Health Law Section), State Bar of Wisconsin, 5302 Eastpark Blvd, Madison, WI 53718. TEL 608-257-3838, FAX 608-257-5502. Circ: 450.

340 610 USA
HEALTH LAW REPORTER. Text in English. w.
Media: Online - full text.
Published by: The Bureau of National Affairs, Inc., 1231 25th St, N W, Washington, DC 20037. TEL 800-372-1033, http://www.bna.com. **Subscr. to:** 9435 Key West Ave, Rockville, MD 20850.

340 610 CAN ISSN 1188-8725
CODEN: HELRED
HEALTH LAW REVIEW. Text in English. 1991. 3/yr. CND 45 to members (effective 2000). back issues avail. **Document type:** *Academic/Scholarly.* **Description:** Covers issues of interest to lawyers and health care professionals, as well as the general public, in connection to the medical-legal field.
Formerly: Health Law News
Related titles: Online - full text ed.: (from Gale Group).
Indexed: Ind.Can.L.P.L., L.R.I. (Apr.1992-), Lang.& Lang.Behav.Abstr., SOPODA, Sociol.Abstr.
Published by: Health Law Institute, 457 Law Centre, University of Alberta, Edmonton, AB T6G 2H5, Canada. TEL 780-492-8343, FAX 780-492-9575, HLI@law.ualberta.ca. Ed. Timothy Caulfield. R&P, Adv. contact Nina Hawkins. Circ: 1,000 (controlled).

340 362.1 USA ISSN 1063-4061
HEALTH LAW WEEK; case digests of judicial decisions affecting all healthcare. Text in English. 1992. latest vol.11, 2001. USD 697; USD 727 in Canada; USD 752 elsewhere (effective Jun. 2001). index, cum.index. back issues avail. **Document type:** *Newsletter.* **Description:** Summarizes judicial decisions that concern or affect the health care industry. Provides a concise and comprehensive research tool for attorneys and health care administrators and practitioners concerned about trends in health care law.
Related titles: Supplement: Health Law Week Reference Index; Aids Litigation Digest.
Published by: Strafford Publications, Inc., Specialized Information Services, 590 Dutch Valley Rd, N E, Postal Drawer 13729, Atlanta, GA 30324-0729. TEL 404-881-1141, FAX 404-881-0074, editors@straffordpub.com. Ed. Jennifer F Vaughan. Pub. Richard M Ossoff.

340 USA ISSN 0736-3443
KF3821.A15
HEALTH LAWYER. Text in English. bi-m. USD 60 to non-members (effective 2001). reprint service avail. from WSH. **Document type:** *Newsletter.* **Description:** Reports legal trends in health law.
Related titles: Microfiche ed.: (from WSH); Microform ed.
Published by: (Section of Health Law, American Bar Association), A B A Publishing, 750 N Lake Shore Dr, Chicago, IL 60611. TEL 312-988-5000, http://www.abanet.org. Ed. Lawrence Manson. R&P Richard Vittenson. Circ: 3,220.

L

340 614 USA
HEALTH LAWYERS NEWS. Text in English. 1971. m. USD 75.
Former titles: Health Lawyers News Report; N H L A News; Health Lawyers News Report (0145-4129)
Indexed: Med.Care Rev.
Published by: American Health Lawyers Association, 1120 Connecticut Ave, N W, Ste 950, Washington, DC 20036-3921. TEL 202-833-1100. Ed. Kerry B Hoggard. Circ: 10,000.

340 610 USA
HEALTH MATRIX: JOURNAL OF LAW-MEDICINE. Text in English. 1983. s-a. USD 24 (effective 1999 & 2000). adv. bk.rev. reprint service avail. from WSH. *Refereed.* **Document type:** *Academic/Scholarly.* **Description:** Student-edited law journal with focus on the field of law-medicine.
Formerly (until 1990): Health Matrix (0748-383X)
Related titles: Microfiche ed.: (from WSH); Online - full text ed.: (from LexisNexis, H. W. Wilson, Gale Group).
Indexed: L.R.I. (Mar.1991-), Leg.Per. (Sep.1993-), P.A.I.S.
—BLDSC (4275.052870), GNLM, ingenta.
Published by: Case Western Reserve University, School of Law, 11075 East Blvd, Cleveland, OH 44106-7148. TEL 216-368-3304, FAX 216-368-3310, hmatrix@lawwww.cwru.edu. Adv. contact Carolyn L Speaker. Circ: 550.

HEALTH POLICY WEEK. see *PUBLIC HEALTH AND SAFETY*

HEALTHCARE RISK CONTROL SYSTEM; an information and consultation system. see *HEALTH FACILITIES AND ADMINISTRATION*

HEBREW UNIVERSITY OF JERUSALEM. AUTHORITY FOR RESEARCH AND DEVELOPMENT. CURRENT RESEARCH. see *MEDICAL SCIENCES*

HEILMITTELWERBEGESETZ. see *PHARMACY AND PHARMACOLOGY*

HIP AND KNEE PAIN. see *MEDICAL SCIENCES*

340 USA
HOSPITAL LAW MANUAL. ADMINISTRATORS. Text in English. q. USD 699 domestic; USD 839 foreign; USD 875 domestic including Attorneys Section; USD 1,050 foreign including Attorneys Section.
Published by: (Aspen Health Law Center), Aspen Publishers, Inc., 200 Orchard Ridge Dr, Ste 200, Gaithersburg, MD 20878. TEL 800-638-8437, FAX 301-417-7550.

340 USA
HOSPITAL LAW MANUAL. ATTORNEYS. Text in English. 1959. q. USD 799; USD 959 foreign; USD 875 including Administrators Section; USD 1,050 foreign including Administrators Section. charts, illus.
Formerly: Hospital Law Manual and Quarterly Service (0018-5728)
Published by: Aspen Publishers, Inc., 200 Orchard Ridge Dr, Ste 200, Gaithersburg, MD 20878. TEL 800-638-8437, FAX 301-417-7550. Circ: 450.

HOSPITAL LAW NEWSLETTER. see *HEALTH FACILITIES AND ADMINISTRATION*

HOSPITAL LAW'S REGAN REPORT. see *HEALTH FACILITIES AND ADMINISTRATION*

HOSPITAL LITIGATION REPORTER. see *HEALTH FACILITIES AND ADMINISTRATION*

HUMAN RESEARCH REPORT; protecting researchers and research subjects. see *MEDICAL SCIENCES—Experimental Medicine, Laboratory Technique*

INDUSTRIAL HEALTH & HAZARDS UPDATE. see *OCCUPATIONAL HEALTH AND SAFETY*

INDUSTRIAL HEALTH FOUNDATION. LEGAL SERIES BULLETINS. see *OCCUPATIONAL HEALTH AND SAFETY*

344.73 NLD
INTERNATIONAL ENCYCLOPAEDIA OF LAWS. MEDICAL LAW. Text in English. 1993. base vol. (4-6 /yr.). USD 219 (effective 1996). **Document type:** *Monographic series.* **Description:** Covers national and international law relating to the practice of medicine, including discussion of: international and regional bodies such as WHO; the European Code of Medical Ethics; and the law relating to the medical profession, the physician-patient relationship, euthanasia and abortion, and laws and regulation governing health care systems in individual countries.
Published by: Kluwer Law International (Subsidiary of: Wolters Kluwer N.V.), Laan van Meerdervoort 70, PO Box 85889, The Hague 2508 CN, Netherlands. TEL 31-70-308-1500, FAX 31-70-308-1515. Ed. Herman Nys. **Dist. by:** Libresso Distribution Centre, PO Box 23, Deventer 7400 GA, Netherlands. TEL 31-570-633155, FAX 31-570-633834.

INTERNATIONAL JOURNAL OF BIOSCIENCES AND THE LAW. see *BIOLOGY*

340 616.8 GBR ISSN 0160-2527
K9
INTERNATIONAL JOURNAL OF LAW AND PSYCHIATRY. Text in English. 1978. 6/yr. EUR 217 in Europe to qualified personnel; JPY 28,700 in Japan to qualified personnel; USD 243 elsewhere to qualified personnel; EUR 791 in Europe to institutions; JPY 105,000 in Japan to institutions; USD 884 elsewhere to institutions (effective 2002). adv. back issues avail.; reprint service avail. from PQC,WSH. *Refereed.* **Document type:** *Academic/Scholarly.* **Description:** Provides a multi-disciplinary forum for the exchange of ideas and information among professionals concerned with the interface of law and psychiatry.
Related titles: Microfilm ed.: (from PQC); Online - full text ed.: (from ingenta, Gale Group, Swets Blackwell, ScienceDirect, Institute for Scientific Information).
Indexed: ASCA, Abstr.Crim.& Pen., Adol.Ment.Hlth.Abstr., AgeLine, Amer.Bibl.Slavic & E.Eur.Stud., C.L.I., Crim.Just.Abstr., Curr.Cont., Excerp.Med., Ind.Med. (1978-), L.R.I. (Jan.1980-), Lang.& Lang.Behav.Abstr., Leg.Cont., Leg.Per. (Jan.1983-), PsycInfo, Psychol.Abstr. (1978-), SOPODA, SSCI, Sociol.Abstr., e-psyche.
—BLDSC (4542.312500), CISTI, GNLM, IDS, ingenta, KNAW. **CCC.**
Published by: Pergamon (Subsidiary of: Elsevier Science), The Boulevard, Langford Ln, East Park, Kidlington, Oxford OXB 1GB, United Kingdom. FAX 44-1865-843010, http://www.elsevier.com/locate/ijlawpsy. Ed. David N Weisstub. Circ: 1,100. **Subscr. in Australasia and the Far East to:** Elsevier Science (Singapore) Pte Ltd, No.1 Temasek Ave, 17-01 Millenia Tower, Singapore 039192, Singapore. TEL 65-434-3727, FAX 65-337-2230; **Subscr. in the Americas to:** Elsevier Science, PO Box 945, New York, NY 10159-0945. TEL 212-633-3730, FAX 212-633-3680, usinfo-f@elsevier.com; **Subscr. to:** Elsevier Science BV, PO Box 211, Amsterdam 1000 AE, Netherlands. TEL 31-20-485-3757.

INTERNATIONAL MEDICAL DEVICE REGULATORY MONITOR. see *MEDICAL SCIENCES*

ISSUES IN LAW AND MEDICINE. see *MEDICAL SCIENCES*

340 USA
JOURNAL OF C G M P COMPLIANCE. (Current Good Manufacturing Practices) Text in English. 1996. q. USD 219; USD 239 in Canada & Mexico; USD 259 elsewhere. adv. *Refereed.*
Published by: Institute of Validation Technology, 200 Business Pkwy, Ste F, Royal, Palm Beach, FL 33411-1742. TEL 561-790-2025, 800-276-4242, FAX 561-790-2065, info@ivthome.com, http://www.ivthome.com. Ed. Glenn Melvin. Adv. contact Terri Kulesa.

JOURNAL OF CLINICAL ETHICS. see *MEDICAL SCIENCES*

JOURNAL OF CONTEMPORARY HEALTH LAW AND POLICY. see *MEDICAL SCIENCES*

JOURNAL OF CONTROVERSIAL MEDICAL CLAIMS. see *MEDICAL SCIENCES*

JOURNAL OF DISABILITY POLICY STUDIES. see *HANDICAPPED*

JOURNAL OF HEALTH CARE COMPLIANCE. see *MEDICAL SCIENCES*

JOURNAL OF HEALTH LAW. see *MEDICAL SCIENCES*

JOURNAL OF HEALTH POLITICS, POLICY AND LAW. see *MEDICAL SCIENCES*

340 USA ISSN 1044-6419
K10
JOURNAL OF LAW AND HEALTH. Text in English. 1985. s-a. USD 20. reprint service avail. from WSH.
Related titles: Online - full text ed.: (from LexisNexis, Gale Group).
Indexed: C.L.I., Fam.Ind., Hlth.Ind., L.R.I. (Jan.1985-), Leg.Per. (Jun.1905-).
—BLDSC (5010.132500), ingenta.
Published by: Cleveland State University, Cleveland - Marshall College of Law, 1983 E 24th St, Cleveland, OH 44115. TEL 216-687-2336. Ed. Emily Smayda. R&P Holli Goodman.

340 610 AUS
JOURNAL OF LAW AND MEDICINE. Text in English. 1993. q. AUD 265 (effective 2000). reprint service avail. from WSH. **Document type:** *Journal, Academic/Scholarly.* **Description:** Examines legal issues affecting all areas of medicine, both clinical and administrative.
Indexed: Aus.P.A.I.S., Leg.Per. (Sep.1994-, dropped).
—BLDSC (5010.132930).
Published by: L B C Information Services, 100 Harris St, Pyrmont, NSW 2009, Australia. TEL 61-2-8587-7000, FAX 61-2-8587-7100, service@thomson.com.au, http://www.lbc.com.au. Ed. Ian Freckelton.

344 174 USA ISSN 1073-1105
KF3821.A15 CODEN: JLAEEO
THE JOURNAL OF LAW, MEDICINE & ETHICS. Text in English. 1973. q. USD 105 domestic to individuals; USD 140 foreign to individuals; USD 195 domestic to institutions; USD 230 foreign to institutions (effective 2001). adv. bk.rev. illus. index. back issues avail.; reprint service avail. from WSH. *Refereed.* **Document type:** *Academic/Scholarly.* **Description:** Scholarly examination of policy and ethical issues at the intersection of law and medicine.
Formerly: Law, Medicine and Health Care (0277-8459); Formed by the merger of: Medicolegal News (0097-0085); Nursing Law and Ethics (0270-6636)
Related titles: CD-ROM ed.; Microfiche ed.: (from PQC,WSH); Microform ed.: (from WSH); Online - full text ed.: (from Gale Group, West Group, H. W. Wilson, ProQuest Information & Learning, Institute for Scientific Information).
Indexed: ASCA, Abstr.Bk.Rev.Curr.Leg.Per., Acad.Ind., AgeLine, CINAHL, C.L.I., Crim.Just.Abstr., Curr.Cont., Environ.Sci.Poll.Mgmt., Fam.Ind., Hlth.Ind., Hosp.Lit.Ind., I.P.A., Int.Nurs.Ind., L.R.I. (Feb.1982-Dec.1992, Mar.1993-), Lang.& Lang.Behav.Abstr., Leg.Cont., Leg.Per. (Jul.1992-Dec.1992), P.A.I.S., Pollut.Abstr., Psychol.Abstr. (1984-), Rel.Ind.One, Rel.Ind.Two, Risk Abstr., SOPODA, SSCI, Saf.Sci.Abstr., Sci.Cit.Ind., Soc.Serv.Abstr., Sociol.Abstr., Telegen.
—BLDSC (5010.195000), GNLM, IDS, Infotrieve, ingenta. **CCC.**
Published by: American Society of Law, Medicine & Ethics, 765 Commonwealth Ave, Ste 1634, Boston, MA 02215. TEL 617-262-4990, FAX 617-437-7596, mvasko@aslme.org; orders@allenpress.com, http://www.allenpress.com. Eds. Bernard Lo, Ellen Wright Clayton. R&P Michael Vasko. adv.: page USD 800; trim 11 x 8.5. Circ: 5,000. **Subscr. to:** Allen Press Inc., PO Box 1897, Lawrence, KS 66044-8897.

THE JOURNAL OF LEGAL MEDICINE. see *MEDICAL SCIENCES*

THE JOURNAL OF LEGAL NURSE CONSULTING. see *MEDICAL SCIENCES—Nurses And Nursing*

340 620 GBR ISSN 0967-2680
K10 CODEN: JPTLEW
JOURNAL OF PRODUCTS AND TOXICS LIABILITY. Text in English. 1977. q. NLG 733, USD 453 (effective 1997). adv. charts, illus. back issues avail.; reprint service avail. from WSH. *Refereed.* **Document type:** *Academic/Scholarly.* **Description:** Publishes original research papers from the legal as well as from technical fields such as engineering and medicine bearing upon issues of product safety and liability.
Formerly (until vol.14, no.3, 1992): Journal of Products Liability (0363-0404)
Related titles: Microfilm ed.: (from PQC); Online - full text ed.: (from Gale Group).

L

Indexed: ABI Inform. (1978-1995), Aqua.Sci.& Fish.Abstr., BPIA, Bus.Ind., C.L.I., Consum.Ind. (1989-1996), Curr.Cont. (coverage dropped), Environ.Sci.Poll.Mgmt., L.R.I. (Mar.1981-Jun.1992, Jan.1993-), Manage.Cont., Pollut.Abstr., Risk Abstr., Saf.Sci.Abstr., Text.Tech.Dig. (1977-1978, 1981-1987), Tr.& Indus.Ind.
—CISTI, Ei, Infotrieve, Linda Hall. **CCC.**
Published by: Pergamon (Subsidiary of: Elsevier Science), The Boulevard, Langford Ln, East Park, Kidlington, Oxford OXB 1GB, United Kingdom. FAX 44-1865-843010, nlinfo-f@elsevier.nl; usinfo-f@elsevier.com; forinfo-kyf04035@niftyserve.or.jp, nlinfo-f@elsevier/nl; usinfo-f@elsevier.com; forinfo-kyf04035@niftyserve.or.jp, http://www.elsevier.nl, http://www.elsevier.nl/. Eds. Kenneth Ross, Verne L Roberts. Circ: 1,000. **Subscr. in Australasia and the Far East to:** Elsevier Science (Singapore) Pte Ltd, No.1 Temasek Ave, 17-01 Millenia Tower, Singapore 039192, Singapore. TEL 65-434-3727, FAX 65-337-2230; **Subscr. in the Americas to:** Elsevier Science, PO Box 945, New York, NY 10159-0945. TEL 212-633-3730, FAX 212-633-3680, usinfo-f@elsevier.com, http://www.elsevier.com; **Subscr. to:** Elsevier Science BV, PO Box 211, Amsterdam 1000 AE, Netherlands. TEL 31-20-485-3757, FAX 31-20-485-3432, nlinfo-f@elsevier.nl, http://www.elsevier.nl.

340 616.8 USA ISSN 0093-1853
K10 CODEN: JPSLAN
JOURNAL OF PSYCHIATRY AND LAW. Text in English. 1973. q. USD 45 to institutions; USD 48 foreign to institutions (effective 1999). adv. bk.rev. charts, stat. back issues avail.; reprint service avail. from PQC,WSH. **Document type:** *Academic/Scholarly.* **Description:** Discusses issues on law and psychiatry.
Related titles: Microfilm ed.: (from PQC); Online - full text ed.: (from Gale Group).
Indexed: Abstr.Bk.Rev.Curr.Leg.Per., Abstr.Crim.& Pen., Adol.Ment.Hlth.Abstr., C.L.I., Crim.Just.Abstr., Curr.Cont. (coverage dropped), Excerp.Med., Hlth.Ind., Ind.Per.Art.Relat.Law, L.R.I. (Mar.1980-), Leg.Cont., Leg.Per. (Jan.1981-Sep.1986), Mid.East: Abstr.& Ind., PsycInfo, Psychol.Abstr. (1973-), SSCI (coverage dropped), e-psyche.
—BLDSC (5043.260000), GNLM, ingenta, KNAW.
Published by: Federal Legal Publications, Inc., 157 Chambers St, New York, NY 10007. TEL 212-619-4949. Ed. Howard Nashel. Pub. Martin Greenberg. Circ: 1,500.

JURA MEDICA; rivista di medicina legale. see *MEDICAL SCIENCES—Forensic Sciences*

KANSAS PHYSICIAN. see *MEDICAL SCIENCES*

KRANKENHAUS UND RECHT. see *HEALTH FACILITIES AND ADMINISTRATION*

L A B M JURIDIQUE. see *BIOLOGY*

340 USA ISSN 1522-533X
LABORATORY COMPLIANCE INSIDER. Text in English. 1998. m. USD 355 (effective 1999). **Document type:** *Newsletter.* **Description:** Shows medical lab managers how to comply with regulatory requirements set by the Health Care Financing Administration (HCFA). Features ready-to-use compliance plan language, billing and coding guidelines and other model forms.
Published by: Brownstone Publishers, Inc., 149 Fifth Ave, New York, NY 10010-6801. TEL 212-473-8200, FAX 212-473-8786. Ed. Kevin Lamberson. Pub. John M Striker.

LABORATORY REGULATION MANUAL. see *MEDICAL SCIENCES—Experimental Medicine, Laboratory Technique*

340 363.7 FRA ISSN 0999-9973
LAMY ENVIRONNEMENT L'EAU. Text in French. 2 base vols. updates 2/yr. FRF 1,880 print & CD-ROM eds. combined; FRF 2,605 print & CD-ROM & online eds. combined (effective 2000).
Related titles: Abridged ed.: ISSN 1284-1234. FRF 2,370 CD-ROM & online eds. combined (effective 2000); Supplement: Lamy Environnement l'Eau Actualite.
Published by: Lamy S.A., 21 rue des Ardennes, Paris Cedex 19 75935, France. TEL 33-1-44721212, FAX 33-1-44721388, lamy@lamy.fr, http://www.lamy.fr.

340 344.04 FRA
▼ **LAMY HYGIENE ET SECURITE.** Text in French. 1999. 2 base vols. updates 2/yr. FRF 2,750 with CD-ROM & Online ed.; FRF 1,990 with CD-ROM (effective 2001).
Related titles: CD-ROM ed.; Online - full text ed.: FRF 760 (effective 2001); Supplement: Lamy Hygiene et Securite Actualites.
Published by: Lamy S.A., 21 rue des Ardennes, Paris Cedex 19 75935, France. TEL 33-1-44721212, FAX 33-1-44721388, lamy@lamy.fr, http://www.lamy.fr.

LAST RIGHTS. see *MEDICAL SCIENCES*

340 150 USA ISSN 0147-7307
K12 CODEN: LHBEDM
LAW AND HUMAN BEHAVIOR. Text in English. 1977. bi-m. USD 649, EUR 648 to institutions for print or online ed.; USD 778.80, EUR 777.60 to institutions print & online eds.combined (effective 2002). adv. illus. back issues avail.; reprint service avail. from WSH. *Refereed.* **Document type:** *Journal, Academic/Scholarly.* **Description:** Examines issues arising from the relationships between human behavior and the law, the US legal system, and the legal process.
Related titles: Microfilm ed.: (from PQC); Online - full text ed.: (from EBSCO Publishing, O C L C Online Computer Library Center, Inc., RoweCom Information Quest, Gale Group, Swets Blackwell, Kluwer Online, Institute for Scientific Information).
Indexed: ASCA, Abstr.Crim.& Pen., Adol.Ment.Hlth.Abstr., AgeLine, Biol.Abstr., C.L.I., Crim.Just.Abstr., Curr.Cont., Environ.Sci.Poll.Mgmt., Excerp.Med., IMFL, Ind.Med. (1977-), Indian Psychol.Abstr., L.R.I. (Mar.1980-), Lang.& Lang.Behav.Abstr., Leg.Per. (Mar.1987-), PsycInfo, Psychol.Abstr. (1977-), Psycscan A.P., Ref.Zh., Risk Abstr., Russ.Acad.Sci.Bibl., SOPODA, SSCI, Saf.Sci.Abstr., Soc.Serv.Abstr., Sociol.Abstr., e-psyche.
—BLDSC (5161.352500), IDS, ingenta. **CCC.**
Published by: (American Psychological Society, Law Society, Division 41), Kluwer Academic - Plenum Publishers (Subsidiary of: Wolters Kluwer N.V.), 233 Spring St, New York, NY 10013-1578. TEL 212-620-8000, 800-221-9369, FAX 212-463-0742, info@plenum.com, http://www.wkap.nl; http://www.wkap.nl/journalhome.htm/0147-7307. Ed. Richard Wiener. R&P Rose Luongo TEL 781-871-6311. **Subscr. outside the Americas to:** Kluwer Academic Publishers Group, Journals Department, PO Box 322, Dordrecht 3300 AH, Netherlands. TEL 31-78-639-2392, FAX 31-78-654-6474.

344.044 616.8 USA
LAW AND MENTAL DISABILITY. Text in English. 1994. a. USD 47.
Indexed: e-psyche.
Published by: Lexis Law Publishing (Subsidiary of: Reed Elsevier plc), PO Box 7587, Charlottesville, VA 22906-7587. TEL 804-972-7600, 800-562-1197, FAX 804-972-7666, llp.customer.support@lexis-nexis.com, http://www.lexislawpublishing.com. Ed. Michael L Perlin.

340 300 616.8 USA ISSN 0098-5961
K12
LAW AND PSYCHOLOGY REVIEW. Text in English. 1975. a. USD 14 domestic; USD 15 in Canada; USD 16 elsewhere (effective 2001). adv. bk.rev. reprint service avail. from WSH. **Document type:** *Journal, Academic/Scholarly.* **Description:** Combines the discipline of law with the behavioral sciences.
Related titles: Microfiche ed.: (from WSH); Microfilm ed.: (from WSH,PMC); Microform ed.: (from WSH); Online - full text ed.: (from LexisNexis, Gale Group).
Indexed: Abstr.Crim.& Pen., Adol.Ment.Hlth.Abstr., C.L.I., Crim.Just.Abstr., L.R.I. (Mar.1982-), Leg.Per. (Jun.1905-), PsycInfo, Psychol.Abstr. (1975-), Psycscan A.P., e-psyche.
—BLDSC (5161.363800), ingenta.
Published by: University of Alabama, School of Law, PO Box 870382, University, AL 35487-0382. TEL 205-348-4527, http://www.law.ua.edu/lawpsychology. Circ: 400.

LAW OF TOXIC TORTS. see *ENVIRONMENTAL STUDIES—Toxicology And Environmental Safety*

340 610 USA
LAWYERS GUIDE TO MEDICAL PROOF. Text in English. 1967. irreg. (in 7 vols.). USD 940 (effective 1999).
Published by: Matthew Bender & Co., Inc. (Subsidiary of: Lexis Law Publishing), 2 Park Ave, New York, NY 10016. TEL 212-448-2000, international@bender.com, http://www.bender.com. Ed. Marshall Houts.

344.041 USA
LAWYERS' MEDICAL CYCLOPEDIA. Text in English. 1977. 10 base vols. plus a. updates (3rd ed., 1997). USD 550. **Description:** Provides comprehensive coverage on current medicolegal issues. Supplemented annually, it includes all traditional specialities as well as diverse topics such as polygraph, automotive medicine, veterinary medicine and organ transplants.
Published by: Lexis Law Publishing (Subsidiary of: Reed Elsevier plc), PO Box 7587, Charlottesville, VA 22906-7587. TEL 804-972-7600, 800-562-1197, FAX 804-972-7666, llp.customer.support@lexis-nexis.com, http://www.lexislawpublishing.com. Eds. Dr. Charles J Frankel, Dr. James G Zimmerly.

LEGAL QUARTERLY DIGEST OF MINE SAFETY AND HEALTH DECISIONS. see *MINES AND MINING INDUSTRY*

LEGAL RESOURCES FOR THE MENTALLY DISABLED: A DIRECTORY OF LAWYERS AND OTHER SPECIALISTS. see *MEDICAL SCIENCES—Psychiatry And Neurology*

LEGISLATIVE NETWORK FOR NURSES; policy and politics for the nursing profession. see *MEDICAL SCIENCES—Nurses And Nursing*

340 615 HKG
▼ **LIFE SCIENCE LAW REVIEW.** Text in English. 2001 (Nov.). 10/yr. GBP 350, USD 530 (effective 2001). **Document type:** *Academic/Scholarly, Trade.* **Description:** Features case studies of licensing deals, technology transfer, fundraising, including interviews, company profiles, analysis, and opinions.
Published by: Euromoney Publications plc., 5/F Printing House, 6 Duddell Street, Central, Hong Kong. TEL 852-2842-6906, FAX 852-2810-8417, enquiries@alphk.com, http://www.euromoney.com.

▼ **LONG TERM CARE LITIGATION.** see *HEALTH FACILITIES AND ADMINISTRATION*

LOW BACK PAIN. see *MEDICAL SCIENCES*

340 362.11 USA ISSN 1529-4161
▼ **MANAGED CARE LAW STRATEGIST.** Text in English. 2000. m. USD 265 (effective 2001). **Document type:** *Newsletter.*
Published by: American Lawyer Media, Incorporated, 345 Park Ave, S., New York, NY 10010. TEL 212-779-9200, FAX 212-481-8161, catalog@amlaw.com. Ed. Stephanie McEvily. Pub. Stuart M. Wise.

MANAGED HEALTHCARE; the news magazine for managers of health care costs and quality. see *HEALTH FACILITIES AND ADMINISTRATION*

MANUFACTURE OF NARCOTIC DRUGS AND PSYCHOTROPIC SUBSTANCES UNDER INTERNATIONAL CONTROL. see *DRUG ABUSE AND ALCOHOLISM*

346.086382 USA ISSN 1098-173X
KF1184.H4
MEALEY'S MANAGED CARE LIABILITY REPORT. Text in English. 1997. s-m. USD 650; USD 770 foreign (effective 1999). adv. index. **Document type:** *Newsletter.* **Description:** Details legal battles arising from the sweeping and controversial changes in the US health care system. Topics include HMO vicarious liability for medical malpractice, ERISA preemption, antitrust, trade practices, contractual disputes, coverage denials, negligent credentialing, and Medicare and Medicaid fraud and abuse.
Formerly (until Jan. 1998): Mealey's Litigation Report: Managed Care (1092-4671)
Related titles: Online - full text ed.: (from LexisNexis).
Published by: Mealey Publications, Inc., 217 West Church Rd, PO Box 62090, King Of Prussia, PA 19406-0230. TEL 610-768-7800, 800-632-5397, FAX 610-768-0880, news@mealeys.com, http://www.mealeys.com. Ed. Kim Truskowski. Pub., R&P Tom Hagy. Adv. contact Cathy Roach.

MEDECINE ET DROIT; information ethique et juridique du pracicien. see *MEDICAL SCIENCES—Forensic Sciences*

340 610 USA
MEDICAID FRAUD REPORT. Text in English. 1981. 10/yr. USD 150.
Published by: National Association of Medicaid Fraud Control Units, 444 N Capitol St, Washington, DC 20001. TEL 202-434-8020, FAX 202-434-8008. Ed. Barbara L Zelner.

346.032 USA
MEDICAL AND HOSPITAL NEGLIGENCE. Text in English. 1995. 4 base vols. plus a. updates. USD 350.

L

Published by: Lexis Law Publishing (Subsidiary of: Reed Elsevier plc), PO Box 7587, Charlottesville, VA 22906-7587. TEL 804-972-7600, 800-562-1197, FAX 804-972-7666, llp.customer.support@lexis-nexis.com, http://www.lexislawpublishing.com. Eds. Louis S Goldstein, Miles J Zaremski.

MEDICAL AND RADIOLOGICAL DEVICES GUIDANCE MANUAL. see *PUBLIC HEALTH AND SAFETY*

MEDICAL DEVICE ESTABLISHMENT REGISTRATION MASTER FILE. see *PUBLIC HEALTH AND SAFETY*

MEDICAL DEVICE PROBLEMS REPORT FROM THE D E N: REPORTS FROM MEDICAL DEVICE USERS. (Device Experience Network) see *PUBLIC HEALTH AND SAFETY*

MEDICAL DEVICE REPORTING FROM THE D E N: REPORTS FROM MEDICAL DEVICE MANUFACTURERS. (Device Experience Network) see *PUBLIC HEALTH AND SAFETY*

MEDICAL DEVICE TECHNOLOGY. see *MEDICAL SCIENCES*

MEDICAL DEVICES, DIAGNOSTICS & INSTRUMENTATION REPORTS: THE GRAY SHEET. see *MEDICAL SCIENCES*

344.73 GBR ISSN 0968-5332
MEDICAL LAW INTERNATIONAL. Text in English. 1993. 4/yr. GBP 109, USD 199 (effective 2001). adv. bk.rev. back issues avail.; reprint service avail. from WSH. *Refereed.* **Document type:** *Journal, Academic/Scholarly.* **Description:** Covers national and international medicolegal and ethical legal matters.
Formerly (until 1993): International Journal of Medical Practice and the Law (0957-1523)
Indexed: ASSIA, Excerp.Med. (1995-), LJI, Leg.Per. (Sep.1994-).
—BLDSC (5529.460000), GNLM, ingenta.
Published by: A B Academic Publishers, PO Box 42, Bicester, Oxon OX26 6NW, United Kingdom. jrnls@abapubl.demon.co.uk. Eds. Diane Longley, Vivienne Harpwood.

344.73 614 GBR ISSN 1351-6345
MEDICAL LAW MONITOR. Text in English. 1994. m. GBP 226; GBP 502 foreign (effective 2000). adv. back issues avail. *Refereed.* **Document type:** *Newsletter.* **Description:** Targets all professionals in the health and welfare industries.
Related titles: Online - full text ed.
—BLDSC (5529.465000).
Published by: Monitor Press Ltd. (Subsidiary of: Informa Group PLC), Suffolk House, Church Field Rd, Sudbury, Suffolk CO10 2YA, United Kingdom. TEL 44-1787-378607, FAX 44-1787-881147. Ed. Viv Harpwood. Pub. Zoe Turner. Adv. contact Caroline Gasking.

MEDICAL LAW REPORTS. see *MEDICAL SCIENCES*

344.73 614 GBR ISSN 0967-0742
K13
MEDICAL LAW REVIEW. Text in English. 1993. 3/yr. GBP 54, USD 96 to individuals; GBP 145, USD 260 to institutions (effective Mar. 2002). adv. bk.rev. 140 p./no. back issues avail.; reprint service avail. from WSH,SWZ. *Refereed.* **Document type:** *Journal, Academic/Scholarly, Trade.* **Description:** Provides information for academics, lawyers, legal practitioners and all others interested in health care and the law.
Related titles: Online - full text ed.: ISSN 1464-3790. 1999. GBP 130, USD 234 to institutions Online only (effective Mar. 2002) (from EBSCO Publishing, O C L C Online Computer Library Center, Inc., RoweCom Information Quest, ingenta, Swets Blackwell).
Indexed: Euro.LJI, LJI, Leg.Per. (Sep.1994-).
—BLDSC (5529.480000), GNLM, Infotrieve. **CCC.**
Published by: (Centre of Medical Law and Ethics), Oxford University Press, Academic Division, Great Clarendon St, Oxford OX2 6DP, United Kingdom. TEL 44-1865-267907, FAX 44-1865-267835, jnl.info@oup.co.uk, http://www3.oup.co.uk/medlaw/, http://www.oup.co.uk/journals. Eds. A Grubb, Judy Laing, P Fennell. Pub. Clare Morton. R&P Fionna Willis. Adv. contact Helen Pearson TEL 44-1235-201904. page GBP 165, page USD 370; 110 x 129. Circ: 750. **U.S. subscr. to:** Oxford University Press, Journals. TEL 800-852-7323, FAX 919-677-1714, jnlorders@oup-usa.org; **Subscr. to:** Journals Marketing, Great Clarendon St, Oxford OX2 6DP, United Kingdom.

MEDICAL LAW'S REGAN REPORT. see *MEDICAL SCIENCES*

MEDICAL MALPRACTICE: CHECKLISTS AND DISCOVERIES. see *MEDICAL SCIENCES*

340 610 USA
MEDICAL MALPRACTICE: GUIDE TO MEDICAL ISSUES. Text in English. 1986. irreg. (in 7 vols.). USD 1,040 (effective 1999).
Published by: Matthew Bender & Co., Inc. (Subsidiary of: Lexis Law Publishing), 2 Park Ave, New York, NY 10016. TEL 212-448-2000, international@bender.com, http://www.bender.com. Ed. Lee Goldsmith.

MEDICAL WASTE HANDBOOK. see *ENVIRONMENTAL STUDIES—Waste Management*

MEDICARE & MEDICAID LAW BULLETIN. see *INSURANCE*

614.19 340 ISR ISSN 0723-1393
K13 CODEN: MELADG
MEDICINE AND LAW; an international journal. Text in English. 1982. q. USD 150 (effective 1999). adv. back issues avail. *Refereed.* **Document type:** *Academic/Scholarly.* **Description:** Offers an international journal deadline with medico-legal issues such as psychiatry and law, psychology and law, medical ethics, nursing law, dentistry law, pharmaceutical law, clinical criminology, drugs, alcohol, child abuse, medical experimentation, and genetic engineering.
Related titles: Microform ed.: (from PQC).
Indexed: Abstr.Crim.& Pen., BPIA, Ind.Med. (1982-), Leg.Cont., PsycInfo, Psychol.Abstr. (1992-), e-psyche.
—BLDSC (5534.006300), EMDOCS, GNLM, KNAW.
Published by: Yozmot Heiliger (1989) Ltd., 3 Yohanan Hasandlar St., P O Box 56055, Tel Aviv 61560, Israel. TEL 972-3-5284851, FAX 972-3-5285397, books@yozmot.com, http://www.yozmot.com. Ed. Amnon Carm. R&P, Adv. contact Avi Chamo. B&W page USD 450, color page USD 900; trim 175 x 120.

346.013 USA
MENTAL DISABILITY LAW: CIVIL AND CRIMINAL. Text in English. 1989. 3 base vols. plus a. updates. USD 240.
Indexed: e-psyche.
Published by: Lexis Law Publishing (Subsidiary of: Reed Elsevier plc), PO Box 7587, Charlottesville, VA 22906-7587. TEL 804-972-7600, 800-562-1197, FAX 804-972-7666, llp.customer.support@lexis-nexis.com, http://www.lexislawpublishing.com. Ed. Michael L Perlin.

MENTAL HEALTH WEEKLY; news for policy and program decision-makers. see *PSYCHOLOGY*

MESSUNG VON GEFAHRSTOFFEN. see *ENVIRONMENTAL STUDIES—Toxicology And Environmental Safety*

MONASH BIOETHICS REVIEW. see *PHILOSOPHY*

MONTHLY PRESCRIBING REFERENCE. see *PHARMACY AND PHARMACOLOGY*

363.2 USA ISSN 0889-7794
NARC OFFICER. Text in English. 1985. bi-m. USD 40 domestic; USD 70 foreign (effective 2001). adv. illus. **Document type:** *Trade.*
Incorporates (in Sept. 1985): International Narcotic Enforcement Officers Association. Annual Conference Report (0538-8821)
Published by: International Narcotic Enforcement Officers Association, 112 State St, Ste 1200, Albany, NY 12207. TEL 518-463-6232, FAX 518-432-3378. Ed. Celeste Morga. Adv. contact Joe Kirby. Circ: 1,200 (controlled).

NATIONAL MEDICAL-LEGAL JOURNAL. see *MEDICAL SCIENCES—Forensic Sciences*

NATIONAL RIGHT TO LIFE NEWS. see *SOCIAL SERVICES AND WELFARE*

346.013 USA
NATIONAL SENIOR CITIZENS LAW CENTER WASHINGTON WEEKLY. Text in English. 1974. w. USD 275 (effective 2000). bk.rev. **Document type:** *Newsletter.* **Description:** Deals with Medicare, Medicaid, SSI, Social Security, and nursing homes.
Formerly: National Senior Citizens Law Center Weekly (0277-7460)
Published by: National Senior Citizens Law Center, 1101 14th St, N W, Ste 400, Washington, DC 20005-5601. TEL 202-289-6976, FAX 202-289-7224, nsclc@nsclc.org, http://www.nsclc.org. Ed. Christy Ross. Circ: 400.

NECK PAIN. see *MEDICAL SCIENCES*

NEW JERSEY STATE BAR ASSOCIATION. HEALTH AND HOSPITAL LAW SECTION. NEWSLETTER. see *HEALTH FACILITIES AND ADMINISTRATION*

NIEUWSBRIEF W V G; informatie over voorzieningen voor gehandicapten en ouderen. (Wet Voorzieningen Gehandicapten) see *HANDICAPPED*

NORTH CAROLINA MENTAL HEALTH, DEVELOPMENTAL DISABILITIES AND SUBSTANCE ABUSE LAWS. see *MEDICAL SCIENCES—Psychiatry And Neurology*

NOTRE DAME JOURNAL OF LAW, ETHICS & PUBLIC POLICY. see *PUBLIC ADMINISTRATION*

THE NURSE, THE PATIENT AND THE LAW; the journal of nursing law & risk management. see *MEDICAL SCIENCES—Nurses And Nursing*

NURSING LAW'S REGAN REPORT. see *MEDICAL SCIENCES—Nurses And Nursing*

NUTRITION LEGISLATION AND REGULATORY NEWS; a twice-monthly report of United States legislative, executive, and regulatory activities. see *NUTRITION AND DIETETICS*

618 340 USA ISSN 1077-8888
OB-GYN MALPRACTICE PREVENTION. Text in English. 1994. m. USD 245 to individuals; USD 375 to institutions (effective 2002). **Document type:** *Newsletter, Academic/Scholarly, Trade.* **Description:** Provides practical advice and insight on legal risk management for obstetrics and gynecology.
Related titles: Online - full text ed.: USD 487.50 academic site license; USD 543.75 corporate site license (effective 2002).
Published by: Lippincott Williams & Wilkins (Philadelphia) (Subsidiary of: Wolters Kluwer N.V.), 530 Walnut St, Philadelphia, PA 19106-3621. TEL 215-521-8300, FAX 215-521-8902, custserv@lww.com, http://www.lww.com/. Eds. Dr. Julius Piver, Marion Garza.

OBEROENDE. see *DRUG ABUSE AND ALCOHOLISM*

344.7 614 CAN ISSN 0706-5019
OCCUPATIONAL HEALTH AND SAFETY LAW. Text in English. 1977. m. CND 340.
Published by: Business Law Reporting Limited, P O Box 1762, Kingston, ON K7L 5J6, Canada. TEL 613-546-9163.

340 613.62 614.85 AUS
OCCUPATIONAL HEALTH AND SAFETY LAW NEW SOUTH WALES. Text in English. 1995. 2 base vols. plus q. updates. AUD 665 (effective 2000). adv. back issues avail. **Document type:** *Academic/Scholarly.*
Published by: Butterworths, Division of Reed International Books Australia Pty. Ltd. (Subsidiary of: Reed Elsevier Australia Pty. Ltd.), 475-495 Victoria Ave, Chatswood, NSW 2067, Australia. TEL 61-2-9422-2222, FAX 61-2-942-22444. Ed. George A Miller. R&P Deanne Castellino. Adv. contact Mary Greenfield. **Dist. in N. America by:** Wm. W. Gaunt & Sons Inc., Law Book Dealers & Subscription Agents, Gaunt Bldg., 3011 Gulf Dr., Holmes Beach, FL 34217-2199.

OCCUPATIONAL SAFETY & HEALTH DAILY. see *OCCUPATIONAL HEALTH AND SAFETY*

OCCUPATIONAL SAFETY AND HEALTH HANDBOOK; an employer's guide to OSHA laws, regulations, and practices. see *OCCUPATIONAL HEALTH AND SAFETY*

340 610 CAN
ONTARIO HEALTH AND SAFETY LAW; a complete guide to the law and procedures, with digest of cases. Text in English. base vol. plus s-a. updates. CND 320 (2001); includes binder and digest. **Document type:** *Trade.* **Description:** Provides updates of statutory amendments, reviews and analyses of the right to refuse to do unsafe work, and of prosecutions under the Act. Also outlines the regulations covering W.H.M.I.S. and appeals of Ministry of Labour orders.
Published by: Canada Law Book Inc., 240 Edward St, Aurora, ON L4G 3S9, Canada. TEL 905-841-6472, 800-263-2037, FAX 905-841-5085. Ed. Norman A Keith.

PAIN: CAUSE, EFFECT, EVALUATION. see *MEDICAL SCIENCES*

PATIENTS' RIGHTS REPORTER. see *HEALTH FACILITIES AND ADMINISTRATION*

L

340 610 GBR ISSN 0267-3894
PERSONAL AND MEDICAL INJURIES LAW LETTER. Text in English. 1985. 10/yr. GBP 249; GBP 274, USD 548 foreign (effective 2000). bk.rev. index. back issues avail. **Document type:** *Newsletter.* **Description:** Provides information regarding the most significant developments in personal injury law.
Indexed: Euro.LJI, LJI.
—BLDSC (6427.852000).
Published by: Monitor Press Ltd. (Subsidiary of: Informa Group PLC), Suffolk House, Church Field Rd, Sudbury, Suffolk CO10 2YA, United Kingdom. TEL 44-1787-378607, FAX 44-1787-881147, http://www.monitorpress.co.uk. Ed. John Finch. Circ: 1,200.

368.56 USA
PERSONAL INJURY STATE VERDICT SURVEY. (Edition for the 50 U.S. states) Text in English. a. USD 29.50 (effective 1999). back issues avail. **Description:** Analyzes personal-damage verdict trends by state.
Formerly: Personal Injury Verdict Survey
Published by: L R P Publications, 747 Dresher Rd, Box 980, Horsham, PA 19044. TEL 215-784-0941, FAX 215-784-9639, custserve@lrp.com, http://www.lrp.com. Ed. Dave Boxold.

340 150 USA ISSN 0160-4422
PERSPECTIVES IN LAW AND PSYCHOLOGY. Text in English. 1977. irreg., latest vol.11, 1999. price varies. bibl. *Refereed.* **Document type:** *Monographic series.*
Indexed: e-psyche.
Published by: Kluwer Academic - Plenum Publishers (Subsidiary of: Wolters Kluwer N.V.), 233 Spring St, New York, NY 10013-1578. TEL 212-620-8000, 800-221-9369, FAX 212-463-0742, info@plenum.com, http://www.plenum.com. Ed. Ronald Roesch.

PESTICIDE LITIGATION MANUAL. see *ENVIRONMENTAL STUDIES—Toxicology And Environmental Safety*

PHARMA RECHT. see *PHARMACY AND PHARMACOLOGY*

PHARMACEUTICAL ADMINISTRATION IN JAPAN. see *PHARMACY AND PHARMACOLOGY*

PHARMACEUTICAL AND MEDICAL DEVICE LITIGATION BULLETIN. see *PHARMACY AND PHARMACOLOGY*

▼ **PHARMACEUTICALS POLICY AND LAW.** see *PHARMACY AND PHARMACOLOGY*

PHARMACY LAW DIGEST. see *PHARMACY AND PHARMACOLOGY*

340 610 USA
A PRACTICAL GUIDE TO PREVENTING LEGAL MALPRACTICE. Text in English. 1983. base vol. plus a. updates. USD 105. Supplement avail. **Document type:** *Trade.* **Description:** Offers practical ideas that can be incorporated into everyday practice to reduce and eliminate malpractice risk.
Published by: Shepard's (Subsidiary of: Reed Elsevier plc), 555 Middle Creek Pkwy, Colorado Springs, CO 80921. TEL 800-743-7393, customer_service@shepards.com, http://www.shepards.com. Eds. Ann Felix Retzke, Duke Nordlinger Stern.

344.0411 USA
PREPARING AND WINNING MEDICAL NEGLIGENCE CASES. Text in English. 1994 (2nd ed.). 3 base vols. plus a. updates. USD 240. **Description:** Provides information on the complications caused by medical and surgical techniques, and how to present these complications and their results in court.
Published by: Lexis Law Publishing (Subsidiary of: Reed Elsevier plc), PO Box 7587, Charlottesville, VA 22906-7587. TEL 804-972-7600, 800-562-1197, FAX 804-972-7666, llp.customer.support@lexis-nexis.com, http://www.lexislawpublishing.com.

340 IND
PREVENTION OF FOOD ADULTERATION CASES. Text in English. 1972. m. USD 120 (effective 1998). bibl. **Description:** Contains notifications and case on prevention of food adulteration.
Published by: International Law Book Co., Nijhawan Bldg., Kashmere Gate, 1562 Church Rd., New Delhi 110 006, India. TEL 91-11-296-7810, lakshmin@giasdla.vsnl.net.in. Ed. Swarn Bhati Nijhawan.

610 340 USA
PROFESSIONAL LIABILITY NEWSLETTER. Text in English. 1968. m. USD 45. reprints avail. **Document type:** *Newsletter.* **Description:** Analysis of medical malpractice cases for medical doctors and attorneys.
Published by: Professional Liability Newsletter, Inc., PO Box 834, Berkeley, CA 94701. TEL 510-741-8723. Ed. Dr. David S Rubsamen.

614.1 616.075 USA
PROVING MEDICAL DIAGNOSIS AND PROGNOSIS. Text in English. 1970. irreg. (in 14 vols.). USD 1,460 (effective 1999).
Related titles: CD-ROM ed.
Published by: Matthew Bender & Co., Inc. (Subsidiary of: Lexis Law Publishing), 2 Park Ave, New York, NY 10016. TEL 212-448-2000, international@bender.com, http://www.bender.com. Eds. Leonard Marmor, Marshall Houts.

340 150 USA
PSYCHIATRIC & PSYCHOLOGICAL EVIDENCE. Text in English. 1986. base vol. plus a. updates. USD 125. Supplement avail. **Document type:** *Trade.* **Description:** Examines and evaluates evidence from psychiatrists and psychologists in civil and criminal proceedings to provide guidelines for admissibility.
Indexed: e-psyche.
Published by: Shepard's (Subsidiary of: Reed Elsevier plc), 555 Middle Creek Pkwy, Colorado Springs, CO 80921. TEL 800-743-7393, customer_service@shepards.com, http://www.shepards.com. Ed. Daniel W Shuman.

PSYCHIATRY PSYCHOLOGY AND LAW. see *MEDICAL SCIENCES—Psychiatry And Neurology*

PSYCHOLOGY, CRIME AND LAW. see *PSYCHOLOGY*

PSYCHOLOGY, PUBLIC POLICY, AND LAW. see *PSYCHOLOGY*

353.5 USA
PUBLIC ASSISTANCE & WELFARE TRENDS - STATE CAPITALS. Cover title: State Capitals Newsletters. Public Assistance & Welfare Trends. Text in English. 1946. 50/yr. USD 245 in US & Canada; USD 350 in US & Canada Print & Online eds. combined; USD 265 elsewhere; USD 365 elsewhere Print & Online eds. combined; USD 10 newsstand/cover (effective 2001). back issues avail. **Document type:** *Newsletter.* **Description:** Monitors state legislation and activities regarding welfare reform, food stamps, Debit Cards, public housing, assistance to senior citizens, health insurance, Medicaid, services for the disabled, health care, and utility subsidies.
Former titles: From the State Capitals. Public Assistance and Welfare Trends (0734-1601); (until 1983): From the State Capitals. Public Assistance (1062-6689); (until 1982): From the State Capitals. Public Assistance and Welfare Trends (0016-1861)
Media: Duplicated (not offset). **Related titles:** Online - full text ed.: USD 225 (effective 2001).
—CCC.
Published by: Wakeman-Walworth, Inc., PO Box 7376, Alexandria, VA 22307-7376. TEL 703-768-9600, 800-876-2545, FAX 703-768-9690, newsletters@statecapitals.com, http://www.statecapitals.com. Pub. Keyes Walworth.

353.6 USA
PUBLIC HEALTH - STATE CAPITALS. Cover title: State Capitals Newsletters. Public Health. Text in English. 1946. 50/yr. USD 245 in US & Canada; USD 350 in US & Canada Print & online eds. combined; USD 265 elsewhere; USD 365 elsewhere Print & online eds. combined; USD 10 newsstand/cover (effective 2001). **Document type:** *Newsletter.* **Description:** Reports on state laws and other actions regarding health care issues. Covers medical policies such as Medicaid, health care for children, women, and seniors, managed care, drug testing, substance abuse programs, abortion, tobacco issues, mental health and disability programs, and the regulation of hospitals, clinics, and nursing homes.
Formerly: From the State Capitals. Public Health (0734-1156)
Media: Duplicated (not offset). **Related titles:** Online - full text ed.: USD 225 (effective 2001).
—CCC.
Published by: Wakeman-Walworth, Inc., PO Box 7376, Alexandria, VA 22307-7376. TEL 703-768-9600, 800-876-2545, FAX 703-768-9690, newsletters@statecapitals.com, http://www.statecapitals.com. Pub. Keyes Walworth.

353.9 USA
PUBLIC SAFETY AND JUSTICE POLICIES - STATE CAPITALS. Cover title: Public Safety and Justice Policies. Text in English. 1946. 50/yr. USD 245 in US & Canada; USD 350 in US & Canada Print & online eds. combined; USD 265 elsewhere; USD 365 elsewhere Print & online eds. combined; USD 10 newsstand/cover (effective 2001). **Document type:** *Newsletter.* **Description:** Covers laws and regulations on law enforcement, violent crime, domestic violence, drug enforcement, issues relating to the policers, gun control, prisons and jails, juvenile justice, sex crimes, and judicial administration.
Formerly: From the State Capitals. Public Safety and Justice Policies (1061-9704); Which was formed by the merger of: From the State Capitals. Justice Policies (0749-2790); Which was formed by the merger of: From the State Capitals. Prison Administration (0734-0885); From the State Capitals. Judicial Administration (0734-1091); From the State Capitals. Public Safety (0749-2782); Which incorporated: From the State Capitals. Police Administration (0734-1148); Which was formerly: From the State Capitals. Disaster and Emergency Planning (0734-0869); From the State Capitals. Fire Administration (0734-1059); Which incorporated: From the State Capitals. Drug Abuse Control (0734-0877); Which was formerly: From the State Capitals. Drug Abuse Control Report (0097-4862)
Media: Duplicated (not offset). **Related titles:** Online - full text ed.
Indexed: CJPI.
—CCC.
Published by: Wakeman-Walworth, Inc., PO Box 7376, Alexandria, VA 22307-7376. TEL 703-768-9600, 800-876-2545, FAX 703-768-9690, newsletters@statecapitals.com, http://www.statecapitals.com. Pub. Keyes Walworth.

QUALITY MANAGEMENT IN HEALTH CARE; an information service. see *HEALTH FACILITIES AND ADMINISTRATION*

RACHEL'S ENVIRONMENT & HEALTH WEEKLY. see *ENVIRONMENTAL STUDIES*

340 ITA ISSN 0300-3485
RASSEGNA DI DIRITTO, LEGISLAZIONE E MEDICINA LEGALE VETERINARIA. Text in Italian; Summaries in English, French, Italian. 1967. q. ITL 40,000; ITL 45,000 foreign. adv. bk.rev. index.
Published by: Universita degli Studi di Milano, Istituto di Medicina Legale e Legislazione Veterinaria, Via Giovanni Celoria, 10, Milan, MI 20133, Italy. TEL 23-62-724. Ed. Pierluigi Canziani. Circ: 1,000.

344.041 610 AUT ISSN 1022-9434
RECHT DER MEDIZIN. Text in German. 1994. bi-m. ATS 1,060 (effective 2001). **Document type:** *Newsletter, Trade.* **Description:** Covers the latest developments in judiciary, legislation and law for all medical professions.
Published by: (Oesterreichische Aerztekammer), Manzsche Verlags- und Universitaetsbuchhandlung, Kohlmarkt 16, Vienna, W 1014, Austria. TEL 43-1-53161-0, FAX 43-1-53161-181, verlag@manz.at, http://www.manz.at. Ed. Wolfgang Mazal.

RECHT & PSYCHIATRIE. see *PSYCHOLOGY*

RECHTSMEDIZIN. see *MEDICAL SCIENCES—Forensic Sciences*

340 610 DEU
RECHTSMEDIZINISCHE FORSCHUNGSERGEBNISSE. Text in German. 1991. irreg., latest vol.26, 2001. price varies. **Document type:** *Monographic series, Academic/Scholarly.*
Published by: Schmidt-Roemhild Verlag, Mengstr 16, Luebeck 23552, Germany. TEL 49-451-7031-01, FAX 49-451-7031253, msr-luebeck@t-online.de, http://www.schmidt-roemhild.de. Circ: 500 (controlled).

RECHTSPRAAK ZORGVERZEKERING. see *INSURANCE*

340 613.62 USA ISSN 1067-0483
KF1256.A75
REPETITIVE STRESS INJURY LITIGATION REPORTER. Text in English. 1992. m. USD 775 (effective 1999). adv. bibl, stat. cum.index. back issues avail. **Document type:** *Newsletter.* **Description:** Reports information on case developments concerning carpal tunnel injury and cumulative trauma disorders involving product liability and worker compensation issues.
Related titles: Online - full text ed.: (from LexisNexis).

L

Published by: Andrews Publications, 175 Strafford Ave, Bldg 4, Ste 140, Wayne, PA 19087. TEL 610-225-0510, 800-345-1101, FAX 610-225-0501, http://www.andrewspub.com. Ed. Linda Coady. Pub., R&P Robert Maroldo. Adv. contact Sofia Pables.

344.730226 USA ISSN 1089-6872
REPORT ON MEDICARE COMPLIANCE. Text in English. 1991. 45/yr. USD 498 (effective 2001). **Document type:** *Newsletter, Trade.* **Description:** Provides news and analysis on billing problems, reporting errors, documentation, DRG upcoding and other complex compliance issues.
Formerly: Healthcare Business and Legal Strategies
Published by: Atlantic Information Services, Inc., 1100 17th St N W, Ste 300, Washington, DC 20036. TEL 202-775-9008, FAX 202-331-9542, http://www.aishealth.com/Products/newsrmc.htm, http://www.aispub.com. Ed. Nina Youngstrom.

340 USA ISSN 8756-2057
KF3771.A6
REPORTER ON HUMAN REPRODUCTION & THE LAW; cases, statutes and materials on law and life sciences. Text in English. 1971. bi-m. USD 75 (effective 1998). bk.rev. abstr, bibl. back issues avail. **Document type:** *Academic/Scholarly.* **Description:** Court decisions and reports on abortion, artificial insemination, in vitro fertilization, surrogate motherhood and genetic planning.
Published by: Legal-Medical Studies, Inc., PO Box 8219, Boston, MA 02114. TEL 617-742-7959. Circ: (controlled).

340 599.9 ESP ISSN 1134-7198
REVISTA DE DERECHO Y GENOMA HUMANO/LAW AND THE HUMAN GENOME REVIEW. Text in Spanish. s-a. **Document type:** *Academic/Scholarly.*
Indexed: Ind.Med. (coverage dropped).
—BLDSC (5161.352660), CINDOC.
Published by: Universidad del Pais Vasco, Apartado 1397, Bilbao 48080, Spain. TEL 34-94-4139287, FAX 34-94-4455513, catdergenh@genomelaw.deusto.es, http://www.deusto.es/castell/castpags/estuc05/genoma/gen-entr.htm. **Dist. by:** Editorial Comares. S.L., Poligono Juncaril, C A PARCELA, 208, Albolote, Granada 18220, Spain. **Affiliate:** Catedra Interuniversitaria Fundacion BBV. **Co-sponsor:** Universidad de Deusto.

REVISTA DE MEDICINA LEGALA/ROMANIAN JOURNAL OF LEGAL MEDICINE. see *MEDICAL SCIENCES—Forensic Sciences*

RHODE ISLAND FIRE LAW AND RULES ANNOTATED. see *FIRE PREVENTION*

RISK MANAGEMENT FOR EXECUTIVE WOMEN. see *INSURANCE*

ROYAL NATIONAL INSTITUTE FOR THE BLIND. BUSY SOLICITORS DIGEST. see *HANDICAPPED—Visually Impaired*

340 USA ISSN 0894-3486
KFO332.8.P77
S E R B OFFICIAL REPORTER. (State Employment Relations Board) Text in English. 1987. m. USD 400. charts. **Description:** Includes the full text of SERB opinions: new court decisions; relevant statutes and rules; official forms, practice outlines; and research aids.
Published by: Banks - Baldwin Law Publishing Co., PO Box 318063, Cleveland, OH 44131-8063. TEL 216-520-5600, FAX 216-520-5655.

340 DEU ISSN 0945-7097
SCHIEDSAMTSZEITUNG. Text in German. 1926. m. DEM 90 (effective 2000). **Document type:** *Newspaper, Trade.*
Formerly (until 1993): Schiedsmanns Zeitung (0342-7471)
Published by: Carl Heymanns Verlag KG, Luxemburger Str 449, Cologne 50939, Germany. TEL 49-221-94373-0, FAX 49-221-94373901, http://www.heymanns.com. Ed. Ludwig Hans Serwe. Circ: 5,400.

SICHERHEITSVORSCHRIFTEN FUER MEDIZINPRODUKTE. see *PHARMACY AND PHARMACOLOGY*

SOCIAL ACTION AND THE LAW. see *PSYCHOLOGY*

340 610 USA
SOURCEBOOK ON ASBESTOS DISEASES. Text in English. 1980. (in 10 vols.), base vol. plus irreg. updates. USD 400. **Description:** Contains information, insights, and data for trial attorneys and others involved in asbestos litigation or legal research.
—BLDSC.
Published by: Butterworth Legal Publishers (Salem), A Division of Reed Elsevier Inc., Salem, VA 22906-7587. TEL 804-972-7600, 800-562-1197, FAX 804-972-7666, custserv@michie.com, http://www.michie.com. Eds. Barbara J Peters, George A Peters.

SPILL REPORTING PROCEDURES GUIDE. see *ENVIRONMENTAL STUDIES—Waste Management*

340 617.1 USA
SPORTS AND RECREATIONAL INJURIES. Text in English. 1985. base vol. plus a. updates. USD 95. Supplement avail. **Document type:** *Trade.* **Description:** Discusses the liability of sporting goods manufacturers and retailers, governments, schools, commercial recreational facilities and insurance carriers in more than 40 types of sports.
Published by: Shepard's (Subsidiary of: Reed Elsevier plc), 555 Middle Creek Pkwy, Colorado Springs, CO 80921. TEL 800-743-7393, customer_service@shepards.com, http://www.shepards.com. Ed. Jeffrey K Riffer.

340 617.1 USA ISSN 1041-696X
KF2910.S653
SPORTS MEDICINE STANDARDS & MALPRACTICE REPORTER. Text in English. 1989. q. USD 39.95 domestic; USD 43.95 in Canada; USD 49.95 elsewhere (effective 2001). adv. back issues avail. *Refereed.* **Document type:** *Newsletter.* **Description:** Covers legal issues of interest to sports medicine professionals, including current trends in liability, professional standards, drug screening, legal aspects of athletic programs, and more.
Related titles: Online - full text ed.: (from Institute for Scientific Information).
Indexed: ASCA, Focus on: Sports Sci.& Med.
—IDS.
Published by: P R C Publishing, Inc., 3976 Fulton Dr, N W, Canton, OH 44718-3043. TEL 330-492-6063, 800-336-0083, FAX 330-492-6176. Ed., R&P David L Herbert. Circ: 1,500 (paid and free).

SPRINGER SERIES ON ETHICS, LAW, AND AGING. see *GERONTOLOGY AND GERIATRICS*

STATE HEALTH CARE REGULATORY DEVELOPMENTS. see *HEALTH FACILITIES AND ADMINISTRATION*

STATE HEALTH NOTES. see *PUBLIC HEALTH AND SAFETY*

STERILIZATION IN AUSTRALIA. see *PUBLIC HEALTH AND SAFETY*

STREETWIZE COMMUNICATIONS; youth rights comics. see *CHILDREN AND YOUTH—For*

SUEDDEUTSCHE METALL-BERUFSGENOSSENSCHAFT. MITTEILUNGEN. see *OCCUPATIONAL HEALTH AND SAFETY*

SURVEY OF PHARMACY LAW. see *PHARMACY AND PHARMACOLOGY*

SYNTHESIS - REGENERATION: A MAGAZINE OF GREEN SOCIAL THOUGHT. see *ENVIRONMENTAL STUDIES*

346 USA
TENNESSEE MEDICO-LEGAL REPORTER✶ . Text in English. 1983. m. USD 180. **Description:** Reviews trial and appellate cases and developments of interest to Tennessee health care lawyers and managers.
Published by: M. Lee Smith Publishers LLC, 5201 Virginia Way, PO Box 5094, Brentwoood, TN 37024-5094. TEL 615-373-7517, 800-274-6774, FAX 615-373-5183. Ed. Lewis L Laska. Pub. M Lee Smith.

340 USA
TEXAS HOSPITAL LAW. Text in English. 1988. 2 base vols. plus a. updates (2nd ed., 1992). USD 170. **Description:** Case analysis and examination of legal and administrative issues affecting the medical community in Texas.
Published by: Lexis Law Publishing (Subsidiary of: Reed Elsevier plc), PO Box 7587, Charlottesville, VA 22906-7587. TEL 804-972-7600, 800-562-1197, FAX 804-972-7666, llp.customer.support@lexis-nexis.com, http://www.lexislawpublishing.com. Eds. Dewey M Johnston, Richard L Griffith.

TIJDSCHRIFT VOOR GEZONDHEIDSRECHT. see *PUBLIC HEALTH AND SAFETY*

TIMELINES. see *MEDICAL SCIENCES*

TOILETRIES, FRAGRANCES AND SKIN CARE: THE ROSE SHEET. see *BEAUTY CULTURE—Perfumes And Cosmetics*

TOLLEY'S HEALTH AND SAFETY AT WORK HANDBOOK. see *OCCUPATIONAL HEALTH AND SAFETY*

TOXIC TORT AND HAZARDOUS SUBSTANCE LITIGATION. see *ENVIRONMENTAL STUDIES—Toxicology And Environmental Safety*

TRAUMA: PERSONAL INJURY, MEDICINE, AND SURGERY. see *MEDICAL SCIENCES—Orthopedics And Traumatology*

TRAUMATIC BRAIN INJURY; evaluation and litigation. see *MEDICAL SCIENCES—Psychiatry And Neurology*

340 362 USA
TREATISE ON HEALTH CARE LAW. Text in English. 1991. irreg. (in 4 vols.). USD 610 (effective 1999).
Published by: Matthew Bender & Co., Inc. (Subsidiary of: Lexis Law Publishing), 2 Park Ave, New York, NY 10016. TEL 212-448-2000, international@bender.com, http://www.bender.com. Eds. Kenneth McLaughlin, Lisa Sandoz Robinson.

TRINGA PRESS MONOGRAPH SERIES. see *MEDICAL SCIENCES*

U.S. DEPARTMENT OF AGRICULTURE. FOOD SAFETY AND INSPECTION SERVICE. MEAT AND POULTRY INSPECTION DIRECTORY. see *FOOD AND FOOD INDUSTRIES*

U.S. OCCUPATIONAL SAFETY AND HEALTH REVIEW COMMISSION. ADMINISTRATIVE LAW JUDGE AND COMMISSION DECISIONS. see *OCCUPATIONAL HEALTH AND SAFETY*

U S P - D I, VOLUME 3. APPROVED DRUG PRODUCTS AND LEGAL REQUIREMENTS. see *PHARMACY AND PHARMACOLOGY*

UNIVERSITA DI FERRARA. ANNALI. SEZIONE 16: MEDICINA LEGALE. see *MEDICAL SCIENCES*

VETERINARY MEDICINE GUIDANCE MANUAL. see *PUBLIC HEALTH AND SAFETY*

VIRGINIA MENTAL HEALTH, MENTAL RETARDATION, SUBSTANCE ABUSE AND RELATED LAW ANNOTATED. see *MEDICAL SCIENCES—Psychiatry And Neurology*

WIKO - WIESBADENER KOMMENTAR ZUM MEDIZINPRODUKTEGESETZ. see *MEDICAL SCIENCES*

WORKERS' COMP ADVISOR; helping doctors, lawyers, and employers cope with the workers' comp system. see *BUSINESS AND ECONOMICS—Labor And Industrial Relations*

WORKER'S COMPENSATION GUIDE. see *BUSINESS AND ECONOMICS—Personnel Management*

LAW—Abstracting, Bibliographies, Statistics

A R L ACADEMIC LAW AND MEDICAL LIBRARY STATISTICS. see *LIBRARY AND INFORMATION SCIENCES—Abstracting, Bibliographies, Statistics*

362.5 USA
AIDS LEGAL BIBLIOGRAPHY. (Acquired Immune Deficiency Syndrome) Text in English. irreg., latest vol.2, 1993. USD 40. **Document type:** *Bibliography.* **Description:** Identifies articles from the popular and academic presses that deal with the social, political, and legal ramifications of AIDS.

Published by: University of Texas at Austin, Tarlton Law Library, 727 E 26th St, Austin, TX 78705-5799. TEL 512-471-7726, FAX 512-471-0243.

BIOETHICS LITERATURE REVIEW. see *MEDICAL SCIENCES—Abstracting, Bibliographies, Statistics*

C A SELECTS. FOOD, DRUGS, & COSMETICS - LEGISLATIVE & REGULATORY ASPECTS. see *FOOD AND FOOD INDUSTRIES—Abstracting, Bibliographies, Statistics*

VIOLENCE & ABUSE ABSTRACTS; current literature in interpersonal violence. see *SOCIOLOGY—Abstracting, Bibliographies, Statistics*

LAW—Civil Law

A L R A NEWSLETTER. see *BIRTH CONTROL*

340.5 614.85 USA
AMERICANS WITH DISABILITIES ACT LAW AND REGULATIONS. Text in English. 1991. q. USD 95 (effective 2000). **Description:** Provides comprehensive overview of the ADA, complete text of the Americans with Disabilities Act, and all of the ADA implementing regulations.
Published by: L R P Publications, 747 Dresher Rd, Box 980, Horsham, PA 19044. TEL 800-341-7874, FAX 215-784-9639, custserve@lrp.com, http://www.lrp.com. Pub. Kenneth F Kahn.

B N A'S HEALTH LAW & BUSINESS SERIES. see *HEALTH FACILITIES AND ADMINISTRATION*

CRONER'S HEALTH AND SAFETY CASE LAW. see *OCCUPATIONAL HEALTH AND SAFETY*

340.5 618 USA ISSN 1075-0606
KF3821.A59
HEALTH LAW LITIGATION REPORTER; the monthly national journal of record reporting general medical malpractice, obstetrical and gynecological litigation. Text in English. 1985. m. USD 875 (effective 1999). adv. abstr, bibl, stat. cum.index every 12 mos. back issues avail. **Document type:** *Newsletter.* **Description:** Covers litigation involving medical negligence, breach of standard of care, as well as women's health concerns such as contraceptive devices and abortion.
Former tiles (until 1993): Medical Malpractice - Ob-Gyn Litigation Reporter (1056-4098); (until 1991): Medical Malpractice Litigation Reporter (0882-8555)
Related titles: Online - full text ed.: (from LexisNexis).
Published by: Andrews Publications, 175 Strafford Ave, Bldg 4, Ste 140, Wayne, PA 19087. TEL 610-225-0510, 800-345-1101, FAX 610-225-0501, http://www.andrewspub.com. Ed. Damian Carlson. Pub., R&P Robert Maroldo. Adv. contact Sofia Pables. Circ: 92.

340.5 610 JPN
IRYO JIKO JOHO SENTA. SENTA NYUSU/MEDICAL MALPRACTICE INFORMATION CENTER IN JAPAN. NEWSLETTER. Text in Japanese. 1991. m. JPY 3,000.
Published by: Iryo Jiko Joho Senta, 1-1-35 Haiesto-Hisaya Bldg 6F, Izumi, Higashi-ku, Nagoya-shi, Aichi-ken 461-0001, Japan. TEL 052-951-1731, FAX 052-951-1732. Ed. Yoshio Kato.

346.73 USA ISSN 1067-0246
KF1297.B74
MEALEY'S LITIGATION REPORT: BREAST IMPLANTS. Text in English. 1992. s-m. USD 875; USD 995 foreign (effective 1999). index. **Document type:** *Newsletter.* **Description:** Provides detailed coverage of bankruptcy issues, jury verdicts, medical studies, multi-district litigation, discovery coordination, class action updates, settlements, insurance coverage disputes, and other issues relating to breast implant litigation.
Related titles: Diskette ed.; Online - full text ed.: (from LexisNexis, West Group).
Published by: Mealey Publications, Inc., 217 West Church Rd, PO Box 62090, King Of Prussia, PA 19406-0230. TEL 610-768-7800, 800-632-5397, FAX 610-768-0880, news@mealeys.com, http://www.mealeys.com. Ed. Colleen Keenan. Pub. Tom Hagy.

MEALEY'S LITIGATION REPORT: FEN-PHEN - REDUX. see *PHARMACY AND PHARMACOLOGY*

346.086 USA ISSN 0199-1833
KF2905.3.A59
MEDICAL LIABILITY REPORTER; recent decisions of national significance. Text in English. 1979. m. USD 295. bibl. index. back issues avail. **Description:** Summarizes and analyzes all reported and most unreported decisions related to health care law.
Published by: (Litigation Research Group), Shepard's (Subsidiary of: Reed Elsevier plc), 555 Middle Creek Pkwy, Colorado Springs, CO 80921. TEL 800-743-7393, customer_service@shepards.com, http://www.shepards.com. Ed. Kevin Bushnell.

344.041 USA
MEDICAL MALPRACTICE (CHARLOTTESVILLE). Text in English. 1993 (3rd ed.). base vol. plus irreg. updates. USD 95.
Published by: Lexis Law Publishing (Subsidiary of: Reed Elsevier plc), PO Box 7587, Charlottesville, VA 22906-7587. TEL 804-972-7600, 800-562-1197, FAX 804-972-7666, llp.customer.support@lexis-nexis.com, http://www.lexislawpublishing.com. Ed. David M Harney.

340.5 617.6 USA
MEDICAL MALPRACTICE: HANDLING DENTAL CASES. Text in English. 1991. (in 2 vols.), latest 2nd ed., base vol. plus a. updates. USD 200. **Document type:** *Trade.* **Description:** Covers methods of investigating dental malpractice and provides tips on how to trap the defendant and structure the plaintiff's closing argument. Includes sample complaints and interrogations.
Published by: Shepard's (Subsidiary of: Reed Elsevier plc), 555 Middle Creek Pkwy, Colorado Springs, CO 80921. TEL 800-743-7393, customer_service@shepards.com, http://www.shepards.com. Ed. Norman L Schafler.

346.03 USA
MEDICAL MALPRACTICE: HANDLING EMERGENCY CASES. Text in English. 1991. base vol. plus a. updates. USD 125 (effective 1995). Supplement avail. **Document type:** *Trade.* **Description:** Covers medical malpractice cases resulting from emergency care.
Published by: Shepard's (Subsidiary of: Reed Elsevier plc), 555 Middle Creek Pkwy, Colorado Springs, CO 80921. TEL 800-743-7393, customer_service@shepards.com, http://www.shepards.com. Ed. G M Flick.

340.5 610 USA
MEDICAL MALPRACTICE: HANDLING INTERNAL MEDICINE CASES. Text in English. 1992. base vol. plus a. updates. USD 125 (effective 1995). Supplement avail. **Document type:** *Trade.*
Published by: Shepard's (Subsidiary of: Reed Elsevier plc), 555 Middle Creek Pkwy, Colorado Springs, CO 80921. TEL 800-743-7393, customer_service@shepards.com, http://www.shepards.com. Ed. Alvin Lee Block.

340.5 618 USA
MEDICAL MALPRACTICE: HANDLING OBSTETRIC AND NEONATAL CASES. Text in English. 1986. base vol. plus a. updates. USD 125. Supplement avail. **Document type:** *Trade.* **Description:** Answers questions such as whether to accept a case, how to efficiently win a case, and what a case can be worth to a client.
Published by: Shepard's (Subsidiary of: Reed Elsevier plc), 555 Middle Creek Pkwy, Colorado Springs, CO 80921. TEL 800-743-7393, customer_service@shepards.com, http://www.shepards.com. Eds. Melvin D Morgan, Michael D Volk.

340.5 610 USA ISSN 0747-8925
KF2905.3.A15
MEDICAL MALPRACTICE LAW & STRATEGY. Text in English. 1983. m. USD 279 (effective 2001). **Document type:** *Newsletter.* **Description:** Latest court developments, new negotiating techniques, presentation suggestions and changes in the law for malpractice lawyers.
Related titles: Online - full text ed.: (from LexisNexis).
Indexed: CINAHL.
Published by: American Lawyer Media, Inc., 345 Park Ave, S, 8th Fl, New York, NY 10010. TEL 212-313-9018, FAX 212-481-8161, http://www.ljx.com, http://www.americanlawyermedia.com. Ed. Kenneth Mauro. R&P Stuart M Wise TEL 917-256-2001.

340.5 610 USA
MEDICAL MALPRACTICE (NEW YORK). Text in English. 1960. irreg. (in 4 vols.). USD 840 (effective 1999).
Related titles: CD-ROM ed.
Published by: Matthew Bender & Co., Inc. (Subsidiary of: Lexis Law Publishing), 2 Park Ave, New York, NY 10016. TEL 212-448-2000, international@bender.com, http://www.bender.com. Eds. David Louisell, Harold Williams.

340.5 615 USA
MEDICAL MALPRACTICE: PHARMACY LAW. Text in English. 1986. base vol. plus a. updates. USD 125. Supplement avail. **Document type:** *Trade.* **Description:** Presents precedent-setting decisions and explains complicated issues in laymen's terms.
Published by: Shepard's (Subsidiary of: Reed Elsevier plc), 555 Middle Creek Pkwy, Colorado Springs, CO 80921. TEL 800-743-7393, customer_service@shepards.com, http://www.shepards.com. Ed. David B Brushwood.

340.5 616.8 USA
MEDICAL MALPRACTICE: PSYCHIATRIC CARE. Text in English. 1986. base vol. plus a. updates. USD 125. Supplement avail. **Document type:** *Trade.* **Description:** Highlights developing trends in the law that directly affects the standards of care in psychiatric practice.
Indexed: e-psyche.
Published by: Shepard's (Subsidiary of: Reed Elsevier plc), 555 Middle Creek Pkwy, Colorado Springs, CO 80921. TEL 800-743-7393, customer_service@shepards.com, http://www.shepards.com. Ed. Joseph T Smith.

340.5 USA ISSN 1045-960X
KF2905.3.A15
MEDICAL MALPRACTICE REPORTS. Text in English. 1987. m. USD 235 (effective 1999). **Description:** Provides medical malpractice news, abstracts of cases, including text and analysis of the decision, plus discussions of growing trends.
Published by: Matthew Bender & Co., Inc. (Subsidiary of: Lexis Law Publishing), 2 Park Ave, New York, NY 10016. TEL 212-448-2000, international@bender.com, http://www.bender.com. Ed. Leonard J Nelson.

346.73 347.306 USA ISSN 0888-658X
KF2905.3.A59
MEDICAL MALPRACTICE VERDICTS, SETTLEMENTS & EXPERTS. Text in English. 1985. m. USD 247 domestic; USD 297 foreign (effective 2000). index. **Document type:** *Newsletter.* **Description:** Looks at the outcome of medical malpractice cases nationally.
Published by: Lewis L. Laska, Ed. & Pub., 901 Church St, Nashville, TN 37203. TEL 615-255-6288, FAX 615-255-6289, llaska@verdictslaska.com, http://www.verdictslaska.com.

MEDICAL RECORD RISKS: CLAIMS & LITIGATION. see *INSURANCE*

340.5 610 USA
MEDICAL STAFF LEADER HANDBOOK. Text in English. 1984. m. USD 675 (effective 1999). **Document type:** *Newsletter.* **Description:** Helps hospital medical staff leaders understand their legal roles and responsibility, and limit liability.
Formerly: Medical Staff Law Manual
Published by: Action Kit Publications, 4614 Fifth Ave, Pittsburgh, PA 15213. TEL 412-687-7677, 800-245-1205, FAX 412-687-7692. Ed. John F Horty. R&P Margaret Barker TEL Margaret/Barker. Circ: 500.

340.5 610 USA ISSN 0025-7591
MEDICAL TRIAL TECHNIQUE QUARTERLY. Text in English. 1954. q. USD 235. bk.rev. bibl, charts. index. reprint service avail. from WSH. **Description:** Presents articles on contemporary medico-legal issues confronting today's practitioner.
Related titles: Microfiche ed.: (from WSH); Microfilm ed.: (from WSH); Online - full text ed.: (from Gale Group).
Indexed: Abstr.Bk.Rev.Curr.Leg.Per., C.L.I., Hlth.Ind., L.R.I. (Jan.1980-), Leg.Cont., Leg.Per. (Jul.1981-). —GNLM, ingenta.
Published by: West Group (Subsidiary of: Thomson Corporation, The), 620 Opperman Dr., Eagan, MN 55123. TEL 651-687-8000, 800-328-4880, FAX 800-340-9378, http://www.westgroup.com. Ed. Jennifer Guy. Circ: 2,500.

340 610 USA ISSN 0899-0255
RA1001
MEDICO-LEGAL ADVISOR. Text in English. 1985. m. USD 65. **Description:** Reviews the latest medico-legal developments in medicine and product liability.
Formerly (until Apr. 1988): Attorney's Medical Advisory Letter (0887-2015)

L

Published by: Health Law Research Group, Health Law Plaza, 140 E Division Rd, Ste C3, Oak Ridge, TN 37830. TEL 615-482-6600, FAX 615-481-0264. Ed. Dr. Laurence R Dry. Circ: 1,000.

344.041 AUS ISSN 0047-6595
MEDICO-LEGAL SOCIETY OF VICTORIA. PROCEEDINGS. Text in English. 1931. 5/yr. free per issue. **Document type:** *Proceedings.*
Published by: Medico-Legal Society of Victoria, 3 Berkeley St, Hawthorn, VIC 3122, Australia. Ed. Dr. John Silver. Circ: 600 (controlled).

344.73 362.4 USA ISSN 0883-7902
KF480.A15
MENTAL AND PHYSICAL DISABILITY LAW REPORTER; covers all aspects of handicapped law. Text in English. 1976. bi-m. USD 239 to individuals; USD 299 to institutions (effective 1999). adv. bk.rev. illus. index. back issues avail.; reprint service avail. from WSH. **Document type:** *Abstract/Index, Academic/Scholarly.* **Description:** Articles on subjects of interest to practitioners and consumers. Indexes are available by case name and subject matter.
Formerly (until 1984): Mental Disability Law Reporter (0147-3700)
Related titles: Online - full text ed.: (from Gale Group).
Indexed: Adol.Ment.Hlth.Abstr., C.L.I., Crim.Just.Abstr., Hlth.Ind., Ind.Med. (1984-), L.R.I. (Jan.1980-Nov.1983, Jan.1984-), Leg.Cont., Leg.Per. (Nov.1986-Mar.1987), PsycInfo, Psychol.Abstr. (1976-), e-psyche.
—BLDSC (5678.559000), ingenta.
Published by: American Bar Association, Commission on Mental & Physical Disability Law, 740 15th St, N W, Washington, DC 20005-1022. TEL 202-662-1570, FAX 202-662-1032, cmpdl@abanet.org, http://www.lexis-nexis.com/lncc/sources/libcont/aba.html. Ed. John W Parry. R&P Richard Vittenson TEL 312-988-6101. Adv. contact Jamie Philpotts. Circ: 1,000 (paid).

MENTAL CAPACITY: MEDICAL AND LEGAL ASPECTS OF THE AGING. see *GERONTOLOGY AND GERIATRICS*

614.58 340 USA
MENTAL HEALTH LAW BULLETIN. Text in English. irreg., latest vol.6, 2000. **Document type:** *Bulletin, Academic/Scholarly.* **Description:** Addresses mental health law issues of interest to local and state government employees and officials.
Indexed: e-psyche.
Published by: University of North Carolina at Chapel Hill, Institute of Government, Campus Box 3330, Knapp Bldg, Chapel Hill, NC 27599-3330. TEL 919-966-4119, FAX 919-962-2707, sales@iogmail.iog.unc.edu, khunt@iogmail.iog.unc.edu, http://ncinfo.iog.unc.edu. Ed. Mark F Botts. R&P Katrina W Hunt.

614.58 340 USA ISSN 0889-017X
KF2910.P75
MENTAL HEALTH LAW NEWS. Text in English. 1986. m. USD 99 (effective 2002). 6 p./no. 1 cols./p. back issues avail. **Document type:** *Newsletter.* **Description:** Provides case law summaries on mental health malpractice, commitment, appropriate treatment, consent and patient danger to community.
Indexed: e-psyche.
Published by: Interwood Publications, 4 Arnold Rd, Freeport, ME 04032. TEL 207-865-9800. Ed., Pub. Frank J Bardack. R&P Frank Bardack.

614.58 340 USA ISSN 0741-5141
KF480.A15
MENTAL HEALTH LAW REPORTER. Text in English. 1983. m. USD 273; USD 281 out of North America (effective 2000). back issues avail. **Document type:** *Newsletter.* **Description:** Covers the avoidance of mental health lawsuits for mental health professionals, advice on winning suits that are brought.
Related titles: Online - full text ed.
Indexed: e-psyche.
—CCC.
Published by: Business Publishers, Inc., 8737 Colesville Rd, 11th Fl, Silver Spring, MD 20910-3928. TEL 301-587-6300, 800-274-6737, FAX 301-589-8493, bpinews@bpinews.com, http://www.bpinews.com. Ed. Bonnie Becker. Pub. Leonard A Eiserer.

NEUROLAW LETTER. see *MEDICAL SCIENCES—Psychiatry And Neurology*

OFFICIAL DISABILITY GUIDELINES. see *OCCUPATIONAL HEALTH AND SAFETY*

340.5 DEU ISSN 1434-1212
PFLEGE- UND KRANKENHAUSRECHT. Text in German. 1998. 4/yr. DEM 80, EUR 40.90; DEM 20, EUR 10.23 newsstand/cover (effective 2001). **Document type:** *Journal, Academic/Scholarly, Trade.* **Description:** Covers various legal issues involving healthcare and hospitals.
Published by: Bibliomed - Medizinische Verlagsgesellschaft mbH, Postfach 1150, Melsungen 34201, Germany. TEL 49-5661-7344-0, FAX 49-5661-8360, info@bibliomed.de, http://www.bibliomed.de.

349 USA ISSN 0887-7815
KF1297.D7
PHARMACEUTICAL LITIGATION REPORTER; the national journal of record of pharmaceutical litigation. Text in English. 1985. m. USD 775 (effective 1999). adv. abstr, bibl, stat. cum.index every 12 mos. back issues avail. **Document type:** *Newsletter.*
Related titles: Online - full text ed.: (from LexisNexis).
—CCC.
Published by: Andrews Publications, 175 Strafford Ave, Bldg 4, Ste 140, Wayne, PA 19087. TEL 610-225-0510, 800-345-1101, FAX 610-225-0501, http://www.andrewspub.com. Ed. Jodine Mayberry. Pub., R&P Robert Maroldo. Adv. contact Sofia Pables.

PRODUCTS LIABILITY: PHARMACEUTICAL DRUG CASES. see *PHARMACY AND PHARMACOLOGY*

SCIENTIFIC SLEUTHING REVIEW; a quarterly of forensic science in law enforcement. see *MEDICAL SCIENCES—Forensic Sciences*

340.5 DEU ISSN 0936-4773
SOZIALGESETZBUCH: GESETZLICHE KRANKENVERSICHERUNG. Text in German. 1989. irreg. DEM 296 (effective 2000). **Document type:** *Bulletin.*
Published by: Erich Schmidt Verlag GmbH & Co. (Berlin), Genthiner Str 30G, Berlin 10785, Germany. TEL 49-30-250085-0, FAX 49-30-25008511, esv@esvmedien.de, http://www.erich-schmidt-verlag.de.

340.5 614 DEU ISSN 0947-6873
SOZIALGESETZBUCH: PFLEGEVERSICHERUNG. Text in German. 1994. irreg. DEM 186 (effective 2000). **Document type:** *Bulletin.*
Published by: Erich Schmidt Verlag GmbH & Co. (Berlin), Genthiner Str 30G, Berlin 10785, Germany. TEL 49-30-250085-0, FAX 49-30-25008511, esv@esvmedien.de, http://www.erich-schmidt-verlag.de.

LAW—Corporate Law

368.382 USA
DIRECTORY OF WORKERS' COMPENSATION MANAGED CARE ORGANIZATIONS. Text in English. a. USD 179 (effective 1998). **Document type:** *Directory.* **Description:** Provides alphabetical listing of organizations involved in workers' compensation managed care; state-by-state listings of the same organizations; service-by-service listings of 17 categories of activity.
Published by: Capitol Publications, Inc. (Subsidiary of: Aspen Publishers, Inc.), 1101 King St, Ste 444, Alexandria, VA 22314. TEL 703-683-4100, 800-655-5597, FAX 703-739-6517. Pub. Cynthia Carter. R&P Rossette Graham.

346.73 347.3 USA ISSN 1087-1381
KF3885.A59
MEALEY'S LITIGATION REPORT: DRUGS AND MEDICAL DEVICES. Text in English. 1996. s-m. USD 825; USD 945 foreign (effective 1999). index. **Document type:** *Newsletter.* **Description:** Covers cases involving a variety of prescription drugs, implants and devices, and latex sensitization litigation.
Incorporates (1994-1995): Mealey's Litigation Report: Norplant (1080-0557)
Related titles: Diskette ed.; Online - full text ed.: (from West Group, LexisNexis).
Published by: Mealey Publications, Inc., 217 West Church Rd, PO Box 62090, King Of Prussia, PA 19406-0230. TEL 610-768-7800, 800-632-5397, FAX 610-768-0880, news@mealeys.com, http://www.mealeys.com. Ed. Jeff Andrus. Pub. Tom Hagy.

LAW—Criminal Law

see also CRIMINOLOGY AND LAW ENFORCEMENT

FORENSIC DRUG ABUSE ADVISOR; a monthly digest of information on the forensic aspects of drug abuse. see *DRUG ABUSE AND ALCOHOLISM*

INSTITUTO NACIONAL DE MEDICINA LEGAL DE COLOMBIA. REVISTA. see *MEDICAL SCIENCES—Forensic Sciences*

ISSUES IN CHILD ABUSE ACCUSATIONS. see *CHILDREN AND YOUTH—About*

ISSUES IN FORENSIC PSYCHOLOGY. see *PSYCHOLOGY*

▼ **JOURNAL OF FORENSIC PSYCHOLOGY PRACTICE.** see *PSYCHOLOGY*

SCIENTIFIC SLEUTHING REVIEW; a quarterly of forensic science in law enforcement. see *MEDICAL SCIENCES—Forensic Sciences*

LAW—Family And Matrimonial Law

346.01 613.9 USA
HANDLING PREGNANCY AND BIRTH CASES. Text in English. 1983. base vol. plus a. updates. USD 75. Supplement avail. **Document type:** *Trade.* **Description:** Discusses surgical sterilizations, wrongful conception, wrongful pregnancy, artificial insemination, in vitro fertilization, surrogate motherhood, abortion, and prenatal injury actions.
Published by: Shepard's (Subsidiary of: Reed Elsevier plc), 555 Middle Creek Pkwy, Colorado Springs, CO 80921. TEL 800-743-7393, customer_service@shepards.com, http://www.shepards.com.

SAGE SERIES ON VIOLENCE AGAINST WOMEN. see *SOCIOLOGY*

STATE REPRODUCTIVE HEALTH MONITOR; legislative proposals and actions. see *MEDICAL SCIENCES—Obstetrics And Gynecology*

306.85 ITA ISSN 0391-2868
RC488.5
TERAPIA FAMILIARE. Text in Italian. 1977. 3/yr. ITL 60,000 domestic; ITL 100,000 foreign (effective 2000). adv. bk.rev. cum.index: 1977-1986. back issues avail.
Indexed: Lang.& Lang.Behav.Abstr., PsycInfo, Psychol.Abstr. (1977-), SOPODA, Sociol.Abstr., e-psyche.
—BLDSC (8792.075000).
Published by: Accademia di Psicoterapia della Famiglia, Via Giuseppe Antonio Guattani, 15, Rome, RM 00161, Italy. TEL 06-44233030, http://www.francoangeli.it. Ed. Maurizio Andolfi. Circ: 3,000.

VIOLENCE AGAINST WOMEN; an international and interdisciplinary journal. see *SOCIOLOGY*

LAW—International Law

341 636.089 NLD
COMPLETING THE INTERNAL MARKET OF THE EUROPEAN COMMUNITY: 1992 LEGISLATION - VETERINARY & PHYTOSANITARY CONTROLS. Text in Dutch. base vol. plus q. updates. NLG 1,280. Supplement avail. **Document type:** *Trade.* **Description:** Covers the legislation as it affects veterinary and phytosanitary controls.
Published by: (Commission of the European Communities BEL), Kluwer Law International (Subsidiary of: Wolters Kluwer N.V.), Laan van Meerdervoort 70, PO Box 85889, The Hague 2508 CN, Netherlands. TEL 31-70-308-1500, FAX 31-70-308-1515, services@wkap.nl, http://www.wkap.nl. Eds. Conor Quigley, Mark Brealey. **Dist. by:** Libresso Distribution Centre, PO Box 23, Deventer 7400 GA, Netherlands. TEL 31-5700-33155, FAX 31-570-633834.

HEALTH AND SAFETY REGULATIONS; international and national laws. see *PUBLIC HEALTH AND SAFETY*

341 610 USA ISSN 0176-7151
CODEN: MEMEEY
MEDICOLEGAL LIBRARY. Text in English. 1984. irreg. price varies. reprint service avail. from ISI. **Document type:** *Monographic series.*
—CCC.
Published by: Springer-Verlag, Journals (Subsidiary of: BertelsmannSpringer), 175 Fifth Ave, New York, NY 10010. TEL 212-460-1500, FAX 212-473-6272.

L

LAW—Judicial Systems

344.041 USA
JURY INSTRUCTIONS ON MEDICAL ISSUES. Text in English. latest 1992, 4th ed., base vol. plus a. updates. USD 90. Supplement avail. **Description:** Covers the latest medical issues including experimentation on patient, childbirth, anesthesiology, pre-existing conditions, and allergies.
Published by: Lexis Law Publishing (Subsidiary of: Reed Elsevier plc), PO Box 7587, Charlottesville, VA 22906-7587. TEL 804-972-7600, 800-972-7600, FAX 804-972-7666, llp.customer.support@lexis-nexis.com, http://www.lexislawpublishing.com. Ed. Graham Douthwaite.

THE PSYCHOLOGY OF THE AMERICAN JURY. see *PSYCHOLOGY*

SCIENTIFIC EVIDENCE. see *MEDICAL SCIENCES—Forensic Sciences*

347 613.62 614.85 USA
SHEPARD'S O S H A CITATIONS. (Occupational Safety and Health) Text in English. 1992. q. USD 570 (effective 2000). **Description:** Contains citations to Occupational Safety and Health court decisions, law reviews and other legal sources.
Related titles: Online - full text ed.: (from LexisNexis).
Published by: Lexis Publishing, 555 Middle Creek Pkwy, Colorado Springs, CO 80921-3630. TEL 719-488-3000, FAX 719-481-7621, customer_service@shepards.com, http://www.lexis.com.

TRIAL PSYCHOLOGY; communication and persuasion in the courtroom. see *PSYCHOLOGY*

LAW—Legal Aid

AIDS LEGAL BIBLIOGRAPHY. (Acquired Immune Deficiency Syndrome) see *LAW—Abstracting, Bibliographies, Statistics*

LEATHER AND FUR INDUSTRIES

see also CLOTHING TRADE

LEGAL AID

see LAW—Legal Aid

LEISURE AND RECREATION

see also HOBBIES; SPORTS AND GAMES

052 GBR
CLUB NEWS; caring for the carers. Text in English. 1989. 8/yr. adv. **Document type:** *Magazine, Consumer.* **Description:** Covers benefits and leisure and lifestyle issues for employees of the National Health Service.
Published by: (National Health Service, External Communications Unit), C & B Communications, 40 Marsh Wall, Docklands, London E14 9TP, United Kingdom. TEL 44-20-7308-8500, FAX 44-20-7308-8555, info@cbcomm.co.uk, http://www.cbcomm.co.uk. Adv. contact Gaynor Garton. Circ: 700,000 (controlled and free).

306.4 USA ISSN 0149-0400
GV1 CODEN: LESCDC
LEISURE SCIENCES; an interdisciplinary journal. Text in English. 1977. q. GBP 24, USD 40 to individuals; GBP 148, USD 245 to institutions (effective 2002). adv. bk.rev. abstr. index. *Refereed.* **Document type:** *Academic/Scholarly.* **Description:** Presents scientific inquiries into the study of leisure, recreation, and travel and how they affect the physical and social environment.
Related titles: Online - full text ed.: ISSN 1521-0588 (from CatchWord Ltd., EBSCO Publishing, O C L C Online Computer Library Center, Inc., RoweCom Information Quest, Swets Blackwell, Institute for Scientific Information).
Indexed: ASCA, AgeLine, Art.Hosp.& Tour., Arts & Hum.Cit.Ind. (coverage dropped), Commun.Abstr., Curr.Cont., Environ.Per.Bibl. (1992-), Forest.Abstr., Geo.Abstr.H.G., Geo.Abstr.P.G., Human Resour.Abstr., Intl.Bibl.Soc.Sci., P.A.I.S., PsycInfo, Psychol.Abstr. (1980-), Rural Recreat.Tour.Abstr., SSCI, Sage Pub.Admin.Abstr., Sage Urb.Stud.Abstr., Sportsearch (1977-), e-psyche.
—BLDSC (5182.270000), CatchWord, IDS, Infotrieve, ingenta. **CCC.**
Published by: Taylor & Francis Ltd. (Subsidiary of: Taylor & Francis Group), 325 Chestnut St, Suite 800, Philadelphia, PA 19016. TEL 215-625-8900, FAX 215-625-2940, info@taylorandfrancis.com, http://www.taylorandfrancis.com/. Ed. Gary Chick. **Subscr. addr. in Europe:** Taylor & Francis Group, Journals Customer Service, Rankine Rd, Basingstoke, Hants RG24 8PR, United Kingdom. TEL 44-1256-813000, FAX 44-1256-479438, enquiry@tanf.co.uk, http://www.tandf.co.uk/journals.

SUID-AFRIKAANSE TYDSKRIF VIR NAVORSING IN SPORT, LIGGAAMLIKE OPVOEDKUNDE EN ONTSPANNING/SOUTH AFRICAN JOURNAL FOR RESEARCH IN SPORT, PHYSICAL EDUCATION AND RECREATION. see *PHYSICAL FITNESS AND HYGIENE*

LIBRARY AND INFORMATION SCIENCES

see also BIBLIOGRAPHIES; COMPUTERS—Information Science And Information Theory; PUBLISHING AND BOOK TRADE

ADDRESS LIST, REGIONAL AND SUBREGIONAL LIBRARIES FOR THE BLIND AND PHYSICALLY HANDICAPPED. see *HANDICAPPED—Visually Impaired*

ADVANCE FOR HEALTH INFORMATION PROFESSIONALS. see *MEDICAL SCIENCES*

610.91 DNK ISSN 0006-1786
BIBLIOTEK FOR LAEGER. Text in Danish. 1809. 4/yr. DKK 440 (effective 1999). adv. **Document type:** *Trade.*
Indexed: Biol.Abstr., Chem.Abstr., Excerp.Med.
—GNLM.
Published by: Almindelige Danske Laegeforening/Danish Medical Association, Trondhjemsgade 9, Copenhagen Oe 2100, Denmark. TEL 45-35-44-85-00, FAX 45-35-44-85-03. Ed. Henrik R Wulff. Circ: 2,000. **Subscr. to:** Laegeforeningens Forlag, Esplanaden 8 A, Copenhagen K 1263, Denmark. TEL 45-35-44-85-00.

026 CAN ISSN 0707-3674
BIBLIOTHECA MEDICA CANADIANA. Text in English, French. 1979. q. CND 75 to non-members; CND 65 to members; CND 130 to institutions (effective 2001). adv. bk.rev. index. **Document type:** *Academic/Scholarly.* **Description:** Vehicle to increase communication among health libraries and health science librarians in Canada.
Indexed: CINAHL, LISA.
—BLDSC (2019.129420), CISTI, GNLM, Infotrieve, KNAW. **CCC.**
Published by: Canadian Health Libraries Association/Association des Bibliotheques de la Sante du Canada, 3324 Yonge St, P O Box 94038, Toronto, ON M4N 3R1, Canada. TEL 416-485-0377, FAX 416-485-6877. Ed., R&P, Adv. contact Anna Gagliardi. Circ: 450.

BIOFEEDBACK (CINCINNATI). see *BIOLOGY*

BRAILLE BOOK REVIEW (LARGE PRINT EDITION). see *HANDICAPPED—Visually Impaired*

020 USA ISSN 1061-5288
CODEN: CLUPEC
CORPORATE LIBRARY UPDATE; news for information managers and special librarians. Text in English. 1992. 24/yr. USD 95 domestic; USD 109 foreign; USD 5 newsstand/cover domestic; USD 10 newsstand/cover foreign (effective 2001). **Document type:** *Newsletter, Trade.* **Description:** Covers library and information technology and trends for corporate and specialized libraries. Each issue contains management tips, marketing ideas, new product and technological developments, seminar and convention listings, news stories and classifieds.
Related titles: Online - full text ed.
—Infotrieve, Linda Hall. **CCC.**
Published by: Cahners Business Information (New York), Broadcasting & Cable's International Group, 245 W 17th St, New York, NY 10011-5300. TEL 212-463-6813, FAX 212-463-6734. Ed., R&P Susan S DiMattia TEL 212-463-6813. Pub. Fred Ciporen TEL 212-463-6824. Circ: 2,500. **Subscr. to:** PO Box 718, Brewster, NY 10509-0718.

026.6102541 GBR
DIRECTORY OF MEDICAL AND HEALTH CARE LIBRARIES IN THE UNITED KINGDOM AND REPUBLIC OF IRELAND. Text in English. 1957. irreg. USD 70 (effective 2000). **Document type:** *Directory.*
Published by: (Library Association), Library Association Publishing Ltd., 7 Ridgmount St, London WC1E 7AE, United Kingdom. TEL 44-20-7255-0500, FAX 44-20-7255-0501, info@la-hq.org.uk, http://www.la-hq.org.uk/. Ed. William Forrester. **Dist. by:** Bernan Associates, 4611 F Assembly Dr, Lanham, MD 20706. TEL 800-274-4447, FAX 800-865-3450.

DISABILITY RESOURCES MONTHLY; the newsletter that monitors, reviews and reports on resources for independent living. see *HANDICAPPED*

ELSEVIER SCIENCE. DISPATCH LIST FOR JOURNALS, BOOK SERIES AND PROCEEDINGS. see *SCIENCES: COMPREHENSIVE WORKS*

ELSEVIER SCIENCE. NEW AND FORTHCOMING PUBLICATIONS. see *SCIENCES: COMPREHENSIVE WORKS*

020 027.663 USA ISSN 0740-4956
FOCUS: LIBRARY SERVICE TO OLDER ADULTS, PEOPLE WITH DISABILITIES. Text in English. 1983. m. USD 18 domestic; USD 20 in Canada; USD 22 elsewhere. adv. bk.rev. index. back issues avail. **Document type:** *Newsletter.* **Description:** Covers library resources and services pertaining to elderly persons and persons with disabilities.
Published by: Ruth O'Donnell, Ed. & Pub., 3509 Trillium Ct, Tallahassee, FL 32312. TEL 850-668-6911, odonnellr@worldnet.att.net. R&P, Adv. contact Ruth O'Donnell. Circ: 300.

025.3 610 USA
GLOBAL CONNECTIONS (ROCHESTER). Text in English. 1978. irreg. **Document type:** *Newsletter.*
Formerly (until 2001): I F L A Section of Biological and Medical Sciences Libraries. Newsletter (0250-4294)
Related titles: Online - full text ed.: ISSN 1025-5680.
Published by: International Federation of Library Associations and Institutions, Section of Biological and Medical Sciences Libraries, 164 Elmore Rd, Rochester, NY 14618-3651. TEL 716-244-8703, lucretiaru@earthlink.net, http://www.ifla.org. Ed. Lucretia McClure.

GLOWNA BIBLIOTEKA LEKARSKA. BIULETYN. see *MEDICAL SCIENCES*

HEALTH INDUSTRY QUICKSOURCE; a complete descriptive reference to healthcare information resources. see *MEDICAL SCIENCES—Abstracting, Bibliographies, Statistics*

020 610 GBR ISSN 1471-1834
Z675.M4 CODEN: HLREEJ
HEALTH INFORMATION AND LIBRARIES JOURNAL. Text in English. 1984. q., latest vol.19, 2002. GBP 210 in Europe; USD 333 in North America; GBP 231 elsewhere (effective 2002). adv. bk.rev. abstr, bibl, illus. index. back issues avail. *Refereed.* **Document type:** *Journal, Academic/Scholarly.* **Description:** Serves the information, training and continuing education needs of the medical, health and welfare librarians.
Formerly (until 2001): Health Libraries Review (0265-6647)
Related titles: Microform ed.: (from PQC); ♦ Online - full text ed.: Health Information and Libraries Journal Online. ISSN 1471-1842.
Indexed: ASSIA, Brit.Nur.Ind., CINAHL, Int.Nurs.Ind., LISA.
—BLDSC (4275.016950), CISTI, GNLM, Infotrieve. **CCC.**
Published by: (Library Association, Health Libraries Group), Blackwell Science Ltd., PO Box 88, Oxford OX2 0NE, United Kingdom. TEL 44-1865-206180, 44-1865-206002, FAX 44-1865-206219, jnl.orders@blacksci.co.uk, http://www.blackwell-science.com/products/journals/hlr.htm, http://www.blackwellpublishing.com. Ed. Angela Coulter. Pub. Elaine Stott. R&P Sophie Savage. Adv. contact Jenny Applin. B&W page GBP 345; trim 172 x 248. Circ: 580.

020 610 GBR ISSN 1471-1842
▼ **HEALTH INFORMATION AND LIBRARIES JOURNAL ONLINE.** Text in English. 2000. q. GBP 189 in Europe; USD 300 in North America; GBP 189 elsewhere (effective 2002). *Refereed.* **Document type:** *Academic/Scholarly.*
Formerly (until 2001): Health Libraries Review Online (1365-2532)

L

Media: Online - full text (from O C L C Online Computer Library Center, Inc., EBSCO Publishing, RoweCom Information Quest, ingenta, Munksgaard & Blackwell Science's Synergy, Swets Blackwell). **Related titles:** Microform ed.: (from PQC); ♦ Print ed.: Health Information and Libraries Journal. ISSN 1471-1834.
Published by: Blackwell Science Ltd., Osney Mead, Oxford OX2 0EL, United Kingdom. TEL 44-1685-206206, FAX 44-1685-721205, website@blacksci.com, journals.cs@blacksci.co.uk, http://www.blackwell-science.com/uk/journals.htm.

HEALTH INFORMATION MANAGEMENT. see *MEDICAL SCIENCES*

610 026 JPN ISSN 0445-2429
CODEN: IGTODY
IGAKU TOSHOKAN/JAPAN MEDICAL LIBRARY ASSOCIATION. JOURNAL. Text in Japanese. 1954. q. JPY 7,000. adv. bk.rev. **Document type:** *Academic/Scholarly.*
Indexed: LISA.
—BLDSC (4363.387000), CASDDS.
Published by: Nihon Igaku Toshokan Kyokai/Japan Medical Library Association, 5-F, Gakkai Center Bldg, 2-4-16 Yayoi, Bunkyo-ku, Tokyo 113-0032, Japan. FAX 03-3815-1608. Ed. Manabu Aoki. Circ: 1,650.

020 610 ESP
INFORMATICA Y SALUD. Text in Spanish. q. ESP 6,000. adv. *Refereed.* **Document type:** *Academic/Scholarly.*
Related titles: Online - full text ed.
Published by: (Sociedad Espanola de Informatica de la Salud), Editorial M I C, Campanillas 26, Leon 24008, Spain. TEL 34-987-272727, FAX 34-987-271618, mic@editorialmic.com, http://www.seis.es/i_s/index.htm. Ed. Dr. Salvador Arribas Valiente. Pub. Fernando Santos Vicente. Circ: 3,000. **Subscr. to:** CEFIC, C. Olimpio 31, 1o C, Madrid 28043, Spain. TEL 34-91-388-9478, FAX 34-91-388-9479.

INFORMATION SOURCES IN CHEMISTRY. see *CHEMISTRY*

027.663 USA ISSN 0270-6717
Z672
INTERFACE (CHICAGO, 1978). Text in English. 1978. q. USD 20; USD 25 foreign (effective 2001). adv. bk.rev. back issues avail.; reprint service avail. from PQC. **Document type:** *Bulletin.*
Supersedes: A S L A President's Newsletter; H R L S D Journal; Which was formerly (nos.1-2, 1975): Health and Rehabilitative Library Services News (0098-3462); Which superseded: Association of Hospital and Institution Libraries. Quarterly (0090-3116); A H I L Quarterly (0001-1428)
Related titles: Microform ed.: (from PQC).
Indexed: API Abstr., Lib.Lit. (coverage dropped).
Published by: (Association of Specialized and Cooperative Library Agencies), American Library Association, 50 E Huron St, Chicago, IL 60611-2795. TEL 312-944-6780, 800-545-2433, FAX 312-440-9374. Ed. Fred Duda. Circ: 2,000. **Subscr. to:** A L A, Subscription Dept, S&S Computer Services Inc, 434 W Downer Pl, Aurora, IL 60506-9936. TEL 630-892-7465, FAX 630-892-7466.

JOURNAL OF CLASSIFICATION. see *MATHEMATICS*

020 USA ISSN 1532-3269
▼ **JOURNAL OF HOSPITAL LIBRARIANSHIP.** Text in English. 2001 (Spring). q. USD 40 domestic to individuals; USD 54 in Canada to individuals; USD 58 elsewhere to individuals; USD 60 domestic to institutions; USD 81 in Canada to institutions; USD 87 elsewhere to institutions (effective Aug. 2001). adv. *Refereed.* **Document type:** *Trade.* **Description:** Focuses on the technical and administrative issues that most concern you. Medical librarians will find news and reviews of the latest technologies, as well as practical suggestions and innovative strategies that will improve the hospital & clinical work environment.
Related titles: Online - full text ed.: free with subscr. to the print ed.
Indexed: INSPEC.
Published by: Haworth Press, Inc., 10 Alice St, Binghamton, NY 13904-1580. TEL 607-722-5857, 800-429-6784, FAX 607-722-6362, 800-895-0582, getinfo@haworthpressinc.com, http://www.haworthpress.com/journals/journallist.asp. Ed. Carole M Gilbert. Pub. William Cohen. adv.: B&W page USD 315, color page USD 550; trim 6 x 8.5.

JOURNAL OF THE MEDICAL LIBRARY ASSOCIATION. see *MEDICAL SCIENCES*

610 020 IRN
JUNDI SHAPUR UNIVERSITY. FACULTY OF MEDICINE. LIBRARY BULLETIN/DANESHGAH-E JONDISHAPUR. DANESHKADE-YE PEZESAKI. BULTAN-E KETABKHANEH. Text in Persian, Modern. 1972. q. free per issue.
Published by: Jundi Shapur University, Faculty of Medicine, P O Box 339, Ahvaz, Iran.

020 610 GBR
LIBRARIES ASSOCIATION. HEALTH LIBRARIES GROUP. NEWSLETTER. Text in English. 1978. q. membership. adv. bk.rev. **Document type:** *Newsletter.*
Former titles: Medical, Health and Welfare Libraries Group. Newsletter (0266-853X); (until 1984): Library Association. Medical, Health and Libraries Group. Newsletter (0263-2365); (until 1981): Medical, Health and Welfare Libraries Newsletter (0141-6995)
Published by: Libraries Association, Health Libraries Group, 7 Ridgmount St, London WC1E 7AE, United Kingdom. Ed., R&P Margaret Forrest TEL 131-536-5582. Adv. contact Claire Collings.

026.579 USA
LIBRARY NEWS FOR ZOOS AND AQUARIUMS. Text in English. 1982. s-a. free per issue. adv. bk.rev. back issues avail. **Document type:** *Newsletter.* **Description:** Provides information for operation of zoo or aquarium library.
Published by: Indianapolis Zoological Society, Inc., 1200 W Washington St, Indianapolis, IN 46222. TEL 317-630-5110, FAX 317-630-5114. Ed. Suzanne K Braun. Adv. contact Meg Beasley. Circ: 350.

027 USA ISSN 0364-1236
Z675.B6
LIBRARY RESOURCES FOR THE BLIND AND PHYSICALLY HANDICAPPED. Text in English. 1968. a., latest 2000. free per issue to qualified personnel. illus. reprints avail. **Document type:** *Directory, Government.*
Formerly: Directory of Library Resources for the Blind and Physically Handicapped (0278-7857)
Related titles: Online - full text ed.
Indexed: C.I.J.E. (coverage dropped).
Published by: U.S. Library of Congress, National Library Service for the Blind and Physically Handicapped, Washington, DC 20542. TEL 202-707-5100, FAX 202-707-0712, nls@loc.gov, http://lcweb.loc.gov/nls.

026 CAN ISSN 0848-9009
M H L A NEWS. Text in English. 1979. 3/yr. membership. bk.rev.
Formerly (until 1989): M H L A Newsletter (0821-1310)
Published by: Manitoba Health Libraries Association, P O Box 232, Winnipeg, MB R3M 3S7, Canada. Circ: 75.

M L A NEWS (CHICAGO). see *MEDICAL SCIENCES*

026.5107 NLD ISSN 0924-4921
MATHEMATICS EDUCATION LIBRARY. Text in Dutch. 1983. irreg., latest vol.4, 1986. price varies. bibl, illus. back issues avail. *Refereed.* **Document type:** *Monographic series.*
Indexed: C.C.M.J., Zent.Math.
—BLDSC (5405.915000).
Published by: Kluwer Academic Publishers Group (Subsidiary of: Wolters Kluwer N.V.), Spuiboulevard 50, PO Box 17, Dordrecht 3300 AA, Netherlands. FAX 31-78-639-2254, services@wkap.nl, http://www.wkap.nl. Ed. A Bishop. **Dist. by:** Journals Department, PO Box 322, Dordrecht 3300 AH, Netherlands. FAX 31-78-654-6474.

MIDDLE ATLANTIC PERSPECTIVE. see *MEDICAL SCIENCES*

026 610 USA ISSN 1094-5970
CODEN: NLMNFK
N L M NEWSLINE. Text in English. 1945. q. free per issue. illus. back issues avail.; reprint service avail. from PQC. **Document type:** *Catalog, Government.* **Description:** Provides ongoing information about the world's largest medical library's people, programs, projects, and publications.
Formerly: National Library of Medicine News (0027-965X)
Related titles: Microfilm ed.: (from PQC).
Indexed: CINAHL, MEDOC, Ref.Zh.
—BLDSC (6113.842000), CASDDS.
Published by: U.S. National Library of Medicine, Office of Public Information, Bldg 38, 8600 Rockville Pike, Bethesda, MD 20894. TEL 301-496-6308, mm354i@nih.gov, http://www.nlm.gov. Ed. Melanie Modlin. Circ: 6,000.

026 610 USA ISSN 0146-3055
CODEN: NTBUE7
N L M TECHNICAL BULLETIN. (U.S. National Library of Medicine) Text in English. 1977. bi-m. free to registered users. **Document type:** *Bulletin, Government.*
Formed by the merger of (1969-1977): MEDLARS Technical Bulletin (0090-1350); (1974-1977): TOXLINE Technical Bulletin (0093-8793)
Indexed: CINAHL.
—CASDDS, GNLM.
Published by: U.S. National Library of Medicine, Section MEDLARS Management, 8600 Rockville Pike, Bldg 38A Rm 4N421, Bethesda, MD 20894. TEL 301-402-1076. Eds. Mary Herron, Toby Port.

NATIONAL INFORMATION CENTER FOR CHILDREN AND YOUTH WITH DISABILITIES. TRANSITION SUMMARY. see *HANDICAPPED*

020 610 USA
NATIONAL LIBRARY OF MEDICINE CLASSIFICATION; a scheme for the shelf arrangement of library materials in the field of medicine and its related sciences. Text in English. 1951. irreg., latest vol.5, 1994. bibl. **Document type:** *Government.*
Published by: U.S. National Library of Medicine, 8600 Rockville Pike, Bethesda, MD 20894. **Dist. by:** U.S. Government Printing Office, Superintendent of Documents, PO Box 371954, Pittsburgh, PA 15250-7954. TEL 202-512-1800, FAX 202-512-2250, orders@gpo.gov, http://www.access.gpo.gov. **Co-sponsor:** U.S. Department of Health and Human Services, Public Health Service.

NEW ENGLAND SOUNDING LINE. see *MEDICAL SCIENCES—Abstracting, Bibliographies, Statistics*

NEWS ABOUT LIBRARY SERVICES FOR THE BLIND AND PHYSICALLY HANDICAPPED. see *HANDICAPPED*

026 CAN ISSN 0843-5901
O H L A NEWSLINE. Text in English. 1986. q. CND 60 to non-members. adv. bk.rev. back issues avail. **Document type:** *Newsletter.*
Formerly: O H L A Newsletter
Published by: Ontario Hospital Libraries Association, c/o Library Services, London Health Sciences Centre, Victoria Campus, P O Box 5375, London, ON N6A 4G5, Canada. TEL 416-429-2661, FAX 416-429-1363, janice.pividor@lhsc.on.ca. Ed. Jill Campbell. R&P Janice Pividor TEL 519-685-8300. Adv. contact Elizabeth Reid. Circ: 200.

026 610 CAN ISSN 0085-4557
OSLER LIBRARY NEWSLETTER. Text in English. 1969. 3/yr. free per issue. **Document type:** *Newsletter.*
Related titles: Online - full text ed.
Published by: McGill University, Osler Library, 3655 Drummond St, Montreal, PQ H3G 1Y6, Canada. TEL 514-398-4475, FAX 514-398-5747, oslerlib@library.mcgill.ca. Ed. F E Wallis. Circ: 1,300.

026 JPN ISSN 0386-2062
Z675.P48 CODEN: YATODW
PHARMACEUTICAL LIBRARY BULLETIN/YAKUGAKU TOSHOKAN. Text in Japanese. 1956. q. JPY 1,500 per issue (effective 1998). adv. bk.rev. **Document type:** *Bulletin.*
Indexed: Chem.Abstr., Chem.Indus.Notes, LISA.
—BLDSC (6444.007000), CASDDS.
Published by: Japan Pharmaceutical Library Association/Nihon Yakugaku Toshokan Kyogikai, 1091-1 Suwarashi, Tsukui-gun, Sagamiko-machi, Kanagawa-ken 199-0211, Japan. TEL 81-426-85-3710, FAX 81-426-85-1643. Ed. I Horota. Circ: 1,200.

REPORT ON HEALTHCARE INFORMATION MANAGEMENT. see *MEDICAL SCIENCES*

020 616.86 USA
S A L I S DIRECTORY. Text in English. 1981. triennial. **Document type:** *Directory.* **Description:** International listing of nearly 200 alcohol and other drug-specific libraries, clearing houses, resource and information centers.
Published by: Substance Abuse Librarians and Information Specialists, Alcohol Research Group, PO Box 9513, Berkeley, CA 94709-0513. TEL 510-642-5208, FAX 510-642-7175, salis@arg.org, http://www.salis.org. Ed., R&P Andrea Mitchell.

TALKING BOOK TOPICS (LARGE PRINT EDITION). see *HANDICAPPED—Visually Impaired*

L

020 CAN ISSN 0380-2973
TALKING BOOKS IN THE PUBLIC LIBRARY SYSTEMS OF METROPOLITAN TORONTO. Text in English. 1974. a. CND 35. adv. bibl. **Document type:** *Catalog.*
Published by: Metropolitan Toronto Library Board, 789 Yonge St, Toronto, ON M4W 2G8, Canada. TEL 416-393-7018, FAX 416-393-7229. Ed. Pat Burchell. Adv. contact Mario Bernardi.

026.61 GBR ISSN 1368-776X
U H S L NEWSLETTER. (University Health Sciences Librarians) Text in English. 1996. irreg. **Document type:** *Newsletter.* **Description:** Seeks to act as a forum for ideas on issues relating to libraries in the health sciences.
Media: Online - full text.
Published by: University of Portsmouth, Frewen Library, Frewen Library, Cambridge Rd, Portsmouth, Hants PO1 2ST, United Kingdom. TEL 44-1705-843220, FAX 44-1705-843233, roisin.gwyer@port.ac.uk, http://www.sbu.ac.uk/lis.uhsl.news3.html. Ed. Roisin Gwyer.

U.S. LIBRARY OF CONGRESS. NATIONAL LIBRARY SERVICE FOR THE BLIND AND PHYSICALLY HANDICAPPED. NEWS. see *HANDICAPPED—Visually Impaired*

610 020 IRN
UNIVERSITY OF TEHERAN. FACULTY OF MEDICINE. LIBRARY BULLETIN/DANESHGAH-E TEHRAN. DANESHKADE-YE PEZESHKI. NASHRIYE-YE KETABKHANEH. Text in Persian, Modern. 1971. m. bk.rev.
Published by: University of Teheran, Faculty of Medicine, Enghelab Ave., Teheran, Iran.

020 610 USA
THE WATERMARK. Text in English. 1976. q. USD 15; USD 21 foreign (effective 1999). adv. bk.rev. bibl. **Document type:** *Newsletter.* **Description:** Features material of interest to persons working with history of the health sciences collections.
Published by: Archivists and Librarians in the History of the Health Sciences, New York Academy of Medicine, 1216 5th Ave, New York, NY 10029-5293. TEL 212-822-7313, lsentz@nyam.org. Ed., R&P, Adv. contact Lilli Sentz. Circ: 220 (paid).

LIBRARY AND INFORMATION SCIENCES—Abstracting, Bibliographies, Statistics

026 310 USA ISSN 1088-1093
Z675.L2
A R L ACADEMIC LAW AND MEDICAL LIBRARY STATISTICS. Text in English. 1992. a. USD 100 to non-members; USD 44 to members (effective 2001). 83 p./no. back issues avail. **Description:** Provides statistical compilation on academic law and medical libraries, including collection growth materials and operating expenditures, staffing, and public service activities.
Related titles: Diskette ed.
Published by: Association of Research Libraries, 21 Dupont Circle, Ste 800, Washington, DC 20036. TEL 202-296-2296, FAX 202-872-0884, pubs@arl.org, http://www.arl.org/stats/lawmed. Ed. Martha Kyrillidou.

020 610 UGA
MAKERERE UNIVERSITY. ALBERT COOK LIBRARY. LIBRARY BULLETIN AND ACCESSION LIST. Text in English. irreg., latest vol.2, 1977. free per issue. back issues avail. **Description:** Each issue consists of hundreds of bibliographic entries pertaining to monographs only.
Media: Duplicated (not offset).
Published by: Makerere University, Albert Cook Library, PO Box 7072, Kampala, Uganda. Ed. Maria Gioretti Musoke. Circ: (controlled).

PSYCINFO NEWS. see *PSYCHOLOGY—Abstracting, Bibliographies, Statistics*

LIBRARY AND INFORMATION SCIENCES—Computer Applications

ELSEVIER SCIENCE. CATALOGUE ON CD-ROM. see *SCIENCES: COMPREHENSIVE WORKS*

025 610 CAN ISSN 0826-0125
H L A B C FORUM. Text in English. 1976. q. CND 20 (effective 1998). **Document type:** *Newsletter.*
Published by: Health Libraries Association of British Columbia, 1383 W 8th Ave, Vancouver, BC V6H 4C4, Canada. TEL 604-733-6671, FAX 604-737-8582. Ed. Shyann Hiebert. Circ: 80.

LIFESTYLE

AHIMSA. see *NUTRITION AND DIETETICS*

AXIOM; living life to the full. see *HOMOSEXUALITY*

394.14 CAN
CANNABIS CULTURE; marijuana & hemp around the world. Text in English. 1994. bi-m. CND 31.95 domestic; USD 26.95 in United States; USD 47.95 elsewhere; USD 4.95 newsstand/cover (effective 2001). adv. **Document type:** *Magazine, Consumer.* **Description:** Presents cutting edge information on all aspects of marijuana and hemp, including growing tips, legal updates, current and accurate coverage of Canada's exploding hemp industry, and ways to participate in the effort to help end the war on all aspects of cannabis.
Former titles (until 1998): Cannabis Canada; (until 1995): Marijuana and Hemp
Address: Box 15, 199 West Hastings, Vancouver, BC V6B 1H4, Canada. TEL 604-669-9069, tia@cannabisculture.com, http://www.cannabisculture.com. Adv. contact Randy Smith TEL 416-686-2444. Circ: 70,000 (paid).

051 USA
DELICIOUS LIVING. Text in English. m. USD 24 (effective 2001). adv. **Description:** Natural living guide focuses on fitness and diet, centered around natural foods.
Published by: New Hope Natural Media (Subsidiary of: Penton Media, Inc.), 1401 Pearl St, Boulder, CO 80302. TEL 303-939-8440, FAX 303-939-9886. Pub. Maurice Lluch.

ENERGY TIMES; enhancing your life through proper nutrition. see *NUTRITION AND DIETETICS*

FIT FOR FUN. see *PHYSICAL FITNESS AND HYGIENE*

051 USA
▼ **FIT PREGNANCY STYLE.** Text in English. 2001 (Aug.). a. USD 3.99 newsstand/cover; USD 4.99 newsstand/cover in Canada (effective 2001). **Document type:** *Magazine, Consumer.* **Description:** Contains interviews with expectant celebrities as well as articles on the latest styles in maternity wear and baby gear.
Published by: Weider Publications, 21100 Erwin St, Woodland Hills, CA 91367. TEL 818-884-6800, 800-998-0731, FAX 818-716-5626.

THE GREY FOX. see *ALTERNATIVE MEDICINE*

394.14 306.1 DEU
HANF!; das Cannabis-Magazin. Text in German. m. DEM 61.20 domestic; DEM 79.20 foreign; DEM 6 newsstand/cover (effective 2000). adv. **Document type:** *Magazine, Consumer.* **Description:** Contains articles and features on cannabis and alternative lifestyles.
Published by: Hanf! Medien, Dorfstr 8, Vogtsburg 79233, Germany. TEL 49-7662-911990, FAX 49-7662-911995, verlag@hanf.org, http://www.hanf.org.

394.14 306.1 DEU
HANFBLATT; das Magazin fuer Hanfkultur. Text in German. bi-m. DEM 35 domestic; DEM 70 foreign; DEM 6.80 newsstand/cover (effective 2000). adv. **Document type:** *Magazine, Consumer.* **Description:** Provides items of interest to those who include cannabis in their way of life.
Published by: HanfBlatt Verlag Barten & Schwanbeck GbR, Dorfstr 38, Moenkhagen 23619, Germany. TEL 49-4506-1380, FAX 49-4506-1580, verlag@hanfblatt.de, http://www.hanfblatt.de. Adv. contact Oliver Schwanbeck.

394.14 306.1 CAN
HEADS. Text in English. every 6 wks. adv. **Description:** Embodies the passion. spirit, and importance of the independent magazine publisher in an increasingly conglomerate-clustered media culture. It is focusing on a positive, healthy lifestyle theme—one underscored by poignant photography, product reviews, and articles regarding good health.
Published by: Worldwide Heads Inc., 541 Main Rd, Hudson, PQ J0P 1H0, Canada. TEL 450-458-1934, FAX 450-458-2977, boris@headsmagazine.com, http://www.headsmagazine.com. Pub. Jay Roller. Circ: 75,000.

HEALTHY OPTIONS. see *PHYSICAL FITNESS AND HYGIENE*

394.14 306.1 USA ISSN 0362-630X
HV5800
HIGH TIMES; the magazine of the counter-culture. Text in English. 1974. m. USD 29.95 domestic; USD 38.95 in Canada; USD 42.95 elsewhere (effective 2000). adv. bk.rev. abstr, charts, illus, stat, tr.lit. back issues avail. **Document type:** *Consumer.* **Description:** Covers marijuana-related news, legalization issues, humor and adventure stories.
Published by: Trans-High Corp., 235 Park Ave S, 5th Fl, New York, NY 10003-1405. TEL 212-387-0500, 815-734-1104, 800-827-0228, http://www.hightimes.com/ . Ed. Steven Hager. Adv. contact Harry Crossfield Jr. Circ: 250,000.

051 USA
LIFE FORCE NEWS. Text in English. m. USD 10 (effective 1998). **Document type:** *Consumer.* **Description:** Features articles on meditation, yoga, health and nutrition, vegetarianism, social issues, and spiritual insights.
Media: Online - full text.
Address: PO Box 487, Fair Oaks, CA 95628. TEL 916-967-1911, 800-655-9994, http://www.haribol.org.

051 USA
LIFESTYLE AND TRAVEL FOR PHYSICIANS. Text in English. bi-m. adv. **Document type:** *Magazine, Consumer.* **Description:** Provides articles and content on travel, food, wine, electronics, and other consumer goods of interest to physicians and their families.
Published by: American Express Publishing Corp., 1120 Ave of the Americas, New York, NY 10036. TEL 212-382-5600, FAX 212-768-1568, http://www.amexpub.com. Circ: 40,000 (controlled).

051 USA ISSN 1087-5050
NATURAL LIVING TODAY. Text in English. bi-m. USD 13.70; USD 3.95 newsstand/cover (effective 2001). adv. **Document type:** *Consumer.* **Description:** Covers alternative health, vegetarianism, natural beauty, relationships, herbalism, meditation, yoga, massage, aromatherapy, and environmentalism. Targets women between the ages of 18 and 35.
Published by: Tyler Publishing, 175 Varick St, 9th Fl, New York, NY 10014. TEL 212-924-1762, FAX 212-691-7828, naturalliv@aol.com. Ed. Alexis Tannenbaum. Pub. Peter Nussbaum. Adv. contact Grace Saydlowski.

051 USA
PENNSYLVANIA HEALTH & FITNESS. Text in English. 1994. m. adv. back issues avail. **Description:** Helps readers live a healthy lifestyle.
Related titles: Online - full text ed.
Published by: Spence Publishing Group, 101 Emerson Ave, Pittsburgh, PA 15215. TEL 412-784-0750, FAX 412-784-0841, http://www.nauticom.net/www/bfit/. Ed. Nancy Carroll. Pub. Stephanie Spence.

051 AUS ISSN 1038-3514
SIMPLY BETTER. Key Title: Simply Better, Your Choice, Your lifestyle. Text in English. 1992. m. adv. back issues avail. **Document type:** *Newsletter, Consumer.* **Description:** Provides health & lifestyle information, covering many areas of health form physical to mental, personal development and environment. It's purose is to motivate and in effect create a healthy change.
Related titles: CD-ROM ed.
Published by: Strategic Lifestyle Management, Level 2, 695 George St, Haymarket, NSW 2000, Australia. TEL 61-2-9207-6687, FAX 61-2-9281-6660, slm@tradesrv.com.au. Adv. contact Paula De Lellis. B&W page AUD 700, color page AUD 975. Circ: 18,000.

▼ **STRIVE.** see *WOMEN'S HEALTH*

616 USA
SULLY'S LIVING WITHOUT; a lifestyle guide for people with food and chemical sensitivity. Text in English. 1998. q. USD 20 domestic; USD 4.95 newsstand/cover (effective 2001). adv. back issues avail. *Refereed.*
Published by: Sully's Living Without, Inc., PO Box 46, Glencoe, IL 60022-0046. TEL 847-835-9760, 847-480-8810, FAX 847-835-9767, pwagener@livingwithout.com, http://www.livingwithout.com. Ed. Alicia Pitzer. Pub. Peggy Wagener. adv.: B&W page USD 2,250, color page USD 3,000; trim 8 x 10.875. Circ: 10,000 (paid); 5,000 (controlled).

L

▼ **TODAY'S HEALTH AND WELLNESS.** see *PHYSICAL FITNESS AND HYGIENE*

▼ **V O I C E**; victory over incontinence/continence education. see *PUBLIC HEALTH AND SAFETY*

WEED WORLD. see *DRUG ABUSE AND ALCOHOLISM*

ZDRAVIE; fit, krasa, pohoda. see *PHYSICAL FITNESS AND HYGIENE*

LINGUISTICS

see also ORIENTAL STUDIES

AMERICAN JOURNAL OF SPEECH - LANGUAGE PATHOLOGY; a journal of clinical practice. see *HANDICAPPED—Hearing Impaired*

410 150 NLD ISSN 0165-716X
AMSTERDAM STUDIES IN THE THEORY AND HISTORY OF LINGUISTIC SCIENCE. SERIES 2: CLASSICS IN PSYCHOLINGUISTICS. Short title: C I P L. Text in English, German. 1978. irreg., latest vol.5, 1991. price varies. **Document type:** *Monographic series.* **Description:** New editions of seminal works from the nineteenth and twentieth century in the area of psycholinguistics.
Indexed: M.L.A., MLA Intl.Bibl., e-psyche.
Published by: John Benjamins Publishing Co., PO Box 36224, Amsterdam 1020 ME, Netherlands. TEL 31-20-6304747., FAX 31-20-6792956. Ed. E F Konrad Koerner.

ANCHOR POINT MAGAZINE; the practical journal of NLP. see *PSYCHOLOGY*

418 401 616.8 GBR ISSN 0142-7164
P37 CODEN: APPSDZ
APPLIED PSYCHOLINGUISTICS; psychological studies of language processes. Text in English. 1980. q. GBP 81 to individuals; USD 187 to institutions (effective 2002). adv. bk.rev. illus. cum.index. back issues avail.; reprint service avail. from SWZ,PSC,SCH. *Refereed.* **Document type:** *Academic/Scholarly.* **Description:** Presents papers on the psychological processes in language. Articles address the nature, acquisition and impairments of language expression and comprehension, including writing and reading.
Related titles: Microform ed.: (from PQC); Online - full text ed.: (from EBSCO Publishing, O C L C Online Computer Library Center, Inc., RoweCom Information Quest, Swets Blackwell, Institute for Scientific Information).
Indexed: AMED, ASCA, AgeLine, Arts & Hum.Cit.Ind. (coverage dropped), Bibl.Ling., Br.Educ.Ind., C.I.J.E., Child Devel.Abstr., Cont.Pg.Educ., Curr.Cont., ERA, Fam.Ind., Lang.& Lang.Behav.Abstr. (1980-), Lang.Teach.& Ling.Abstr., Ling.Abstr., M.L.A., MLA Intl.Bibl., Mult.Ed.Abstr., P C I, Psyclnfo, Psychol.Abstr. (1980-), Ref.Zh., SOPODA, SSCI, Sociol.Abstr., Sp.Ed.Needs Abstr., e-psyche.
—BLDSC (1576.545000), IDS, ingenta. **CCC.**
Published by: Cambridge University Press, Edinburgh Bldg, Shaftesbury Rd, Cambridge CB2 2RU, United Kingdom. FAX 44-1223-315052, information@cup.cam.ac.uk, information@cambridge.org, http://www.cup.org/journals/CUPJNLS.html. Eds. Catherine E Snow, John L Locke. R&P Linda Nicol. Adv. contact Rebecca Symons.

401 150 USA
APPLIED PSYCHOLINGUISTICS AND COMMUNICATION DISORDERS. Text in English. 1979. irreg., latest 1991. price varies. *Refereed.* **Document type:** *Monographic series.*
Formerly: Studies in Applied Psycholinguistics
Indexed: SSCI (coverage dropped), e-psyche.
Published by: Kluwer Academic - Plenum Publishers (Subsidiary of: Wolters Kluwer N.V.), 233 Spring St, New York, NY 10013-1578. TEL 212-620-8000, 800-221-9369, FAX 212-463-0742, info@plenum.com, http://www.plenum.com. Ed. R W Rieber.

BRAIN AND LANGUAGE. see *PSYCHOLOGY*

CLINICAL LINGUISTICS & PHONETICS. see *MEDICAL SCIENCES—Psychiatry And Neurology*

401 DEU
COGNITIO; Kognitions- und neurowissenschaftliche Beitraege zur natuerlichen Sprachverarbeitung. Text in German. irreg., latest vol.11, 2000. **Document type:** *Monographic series, Academic/Scholarly.*
Published by: Gunter Narr Verlag, Postfach 2567, Tuebingen 72015, Germany. TEL 49-7071-9797-0, FAX 49-7071-75288, narr-francke@t-online.de, http://www.narr.de.

401 USA
COGNITION AND LANGUAGE; a series in psycholinguistics. Text in English. 1979. irreg., latest vol.6, 1999. price varies. back issues avail. *Refereed.* **Document type:** *Monographic series.*
Indexed: e-psyche.
Published by: Kluwer Academic - Plenum Publishers (Subsidiary of: Wolters Kluwer N.V.), 233 Spring St, New York, NY 10013-1578. TEL 212-620-8000, 800-221-9369, FAX 212-463-0742, info@plenum.com, http://www.plenum.com. Ed. R W Rieber.

410 DEU ISSN 0936-5907
P165 CODEN: COGLEJ
COGNITIVE LINGUISTICS. Text in German. 1989. q. EUR 142.60 domestic; EUR 146.20 foreign; EUR 32.95 to students; EUR 34.50 newsstand/cover (effective 2002). adv. illus. Index. reprint service avail. from SCH,PSC. *Refereed.* **Document type:** *Journal, Academic/Scholarly.* **Description:** Covers high-quality research on language from a cognitive perspective - as an instrument for organizing, processing, and conveying information.
Related titles: Online - full text ed.: (from EBSCO Publishing, O C L C Online Computer Library Center, Inc., Swets Blackwell, Institute for Scientific Information).
Indexed: Arts & Hum.Cit.Ind., Bibl.Ling., Curr.Cont., IBZ, INSPEC (1990-1994, dropped), Intl.Bibl.Soc.Sci., Lang.& Lang.Behav.Abstr., MLA Intl.Bibl., Russ.Acad.Sci.Bibl., SOPODA, Sociol.Abstr.
—BLDSC (3292.878000), AskIEEE, IDS, ingenta. **CCC.**
Published by: (International Cognitive Linguistics Association), Walter de Gruyter und Co., Mouton de Gruyter, Genthiner Str 13, Berlin 10785, Germany. TEL 49-30-26005-0, FAX 49-30-26005-251, wdg-info@degruyter.de, http://www.degruyter.de/journals. Ed. Arie Verhagen.

410 DEU
COGNITIVE LINGUISTICS RESEARCH. Text in German. irreg., latest vol.8, 1997. **Document type:** *Monographic series.*
Indexed: Bibl.Ling.
—BLDSC (3292.878200).
Published by: Walter de Gruyter und Co., Genthiner Str 13, Berlin 10785, Germany. TEL 49-30-26005-0, FAX 49-30-26005-251, wdg-info@degruyter.de, http://www.degruyter.de. Ed. Arie Verhagen.

COGNITIVE SCIENCE; a multidisciplinary journal of artificial intelligence, linguistics, neuroscience, philosophy and psychology. see *PSYCHOLOGY*

COGNITIVE SYSTEMS. see *PSYCHOLOGY*

COMMUNICATION OUTLOOK; focusing on communication aids and techniques. see *COMPUTERS—Artificial Intelligence*

410 GBR ISSN 1461-4456
▼ **DISCOURSE STUDIES**; an interdisciplinary journal for the study of text and talk. Text in English. 1999. q. GBP 39 to individuals; GBP 218 to institutions; GBP 11 newsstand/cover to individuals; GBP 56 newsstand/cover to institutions (effective 2002). adv. bk.rev. *Refereed.* **Document type:** *Academic/Scholarly.* **Description:** Publishes notable research on the structures of written and spoken discourse, with emphasis on cross-disciplinary studies of text and talk linguistics, anthropology, ethnomethodology, cognitive and social psychology, communication studies and law.
Related titles: Online - full text ed.: (from EBSCO Publishing, O C L C Online Computer Library Center, Inc., RoweCom Information Quest, ingenta, Swets Blackwell).
Indexed: IBZ, Intl.Bibl.Soc.Sci., MLA Intl.Bibl., Soc.Serv.Abstr., Sociol.Abstr., e-psyche.
—BLDSC (3595.861600).
Published by: Sage Publications Ltd., 6 Bonhill St, London EC2A 4PU, United Kingdom. TEL 44-20-7374-0645, FAX 44-20-7374-8741, market@sagepub.co.uk, http://www.sagepub.co.uk. Ed. Teun van Dijk. Adv. contact Jenny Kirby. page GBP 195; 185 x 114.

HUMAN COMMUNICATION RESEARCH. see *PSYCHOLOGY*

153.7 NLD ISSN 0921-2566
I P O ANNUAL PROGRESS REPORT. (Instituut voor Perceptie Onderzoek) Text in English. 1966. a. free. *Refereed.* **Document type:** *Bulletin, Academic/Scholarly.*
Indexed: Ergon.Abstr., Lang.& Lang.Behav.Abstr., MLA Intl.Bibl., Psychol.Abstr., SOPODA, Sociol.Abstr., e-psyche.
—BLDSC (4567.415000), KNAW.
Published by: I P O Center for User - System Interaction, PO Box 513, Eindhoven 5600 MB, Netherlands. TEL 31-40-247-5200, FAX 31-40-243-1930, secretariaat.ipo@tue.nl, http://www.tue.nl/ipo. Eds. J Pellegrino, U V Amelsfort. Circ: 1,500 (controlled).

420 370.15 610 300 USA
INTERFACES: LINGUISTICS, PSYCHOLOGY AND HEALTH THERAPEUTICS; an international journal of research, notes and commentary. Text in English. 1973. 3/yr. USD 10. bk.rev. abstr, bibl, charts, stat, tr.lit. back issues avail. *Refereed.*
Indexed: C.I.J.E. (coverage dropped), Lang.& Lang.Behav.Abstr., Psychol.Abstr. (dropped), Sociol.Educ.Abstr., e-psyche.
Published by: Providence College Press, Providence, RI 02918. Eds. Elaine Chiaka, Robert E Haskell. Circ: 500.

410 150 JPN ISSN 0165-4055
CODEN: IPLGBV
INTERNATIONAL JOURNAL OF PSYCHOLINGUISTICS. Text in Japanese. 3/yr. USD 120. adv. **Document type:** *Academic/Scholarly.*
Indexed: Ind.Philos., Lang.& Lang.Behav.Abstr., Psyclnfo, Russ.Acad.Sci.Bibl., SOPODA, Sociol.Abstr.
—Infotrieve. **CCC.**
Published by: Center for Academic Societies Osaka, Senri Life Science Center Bldg 14th Fl, 1-4-2 Shinsenri-Higashi-Machi, Toyonaka-shi, Osaka-fu 565-0082, Japan. TEL 81-6-873-2301, FAX 81-6-873-2300, afukuda@bcasj.or.jp. Ed. Tatiana Slama Cazacu. Adv. contact Atsuko Fukuda.

JOURNAL OF CHILD LANGUAGE. see *CHILDREN AND YOUTH—About*

420 USA ISSN 0075-4242
PE1001
JOURNAL OF ENGLISH LINGUISTICS. Text in English. 1967. q. USD 55 to individuals; USD 250 to institutions; USD 20 newsstand/cover to individuals; USD 70 newsstand/cover to institutions (effective 2002). adv. bk.rev. illus. Index. back issues avail.; reprints avail. *Refereed.* **Document type:** *Academic/Scholarly.* **Description:** Publishes articles on the modern and historical periods of the English language, including synchronic and diachronic studies on Old and Middle English, modern English grammar and dialectology, as well as language contact, pidgins and stylistics.
Related titles: Online - full text ed.: (from EBSCO Publishing, O C L C Online Computer Library Center, Inc., RoweCom Information Quest, ingenta, Swets Blackwell).
Indexed: Amer.Hum.Ind., Arts & Hum.Cit.Ind. (coverage dropped), Bibl.Ling., Curr.Cont. (coverage dropped), Educ.Admin.Abstr., IBR, IBZ, Ind.Bk.Rev.Hum., Lang.& Lang.Behav.Abstr. (1973-), Ling.Abstr., M.L.A., MLA Intl.Bibl., SOPODA, Sociol.Abstr.
—Infotrieve, ingenta. **CCC.**
Published by: Sage Publications, Inc., 2455 Teller Rd, Thousand Oaks, CA 91320. TEL 805-499-0721, FAX 805-499-0871, info@sagepub.com, http://www.sagepub.com. Ed. Charles F Meyer Jr. R&P Tanya Udin. Adv. contact DeAnna Vega Hammersley. Circ: 600. **Overseas subscr. to:** Sage Publications Ltd., 6 Bonhill St, London EC2A 4PU, United Kingdom; Sage Publications India Pvt. Ltd., 4215, New Delhi 110 048, India.

410 150 USA ISSN 0749-596X
BF455.A1
JOURNAL OF MEMORY AND LANGUAGE. Text in English. 1962. 8/yr. USD 640 in US & Canada to institutions; USD 650 elsewhere to institutions (effective 2001). adv. charts, illus. index. back issues avail.; reprint service avail. from SCH,PSC. *Refereed.* **Document type:** *Academic/Scholarly.* **Description:** Contributes to the formulation of scientific issues and theories in the areas of memory, language comprehension and production, and cognitive processes.
Formerly: Journal of Verbal Learning and Verbal Behavior (0022-5371)
Related titles: Online - full text ed.: (from EBSCO Publishing, O C L C Online Computer Library Center, Inc., RoweCom Information Quest, ingenta, Swets Blackwell, IDEAL Online Library, Factiva, Institute for Scientific Information).

L

Indexed: ASCA, ASSIA, Abstr.Anthropol., AgeLine, Arts & Hum.Cit.Ind. (coverage dropped), Bibl.Ling., C.I.J.E. (coverage dropped), CINAHL, Child Devel.Abstr., Commun.Abstr., Cont.Pg.Educ., Curr.Cont., Curr.Ind.Stat., Ergon.Abstr., High.Educ.Curr.Aware.Bull., IBR, IBZ, Ind.Philos., Lang.& Lang.Behav.Abstr. (1972-), Lang.Teach.& Ling.Abstr., Ling.Abstr., M.L.A., MLA Intl.Bibl., Mid.East: Abstr.& Ind., Neurosci.Cit.Ind., P C I, PsycInfo, Psychol.Abstr. (1962-), Russ.Acad.Sci.Bibl., SOPODA, SSCI, Soc.Sci.Ind. (Aug.1982-Dec.1984), Sociol.Abstr., e-psyche.

—BLDSC (5017.630000), ADONIS, IDS, ingenta. **CCC.**

Published by: Academic Press, Inc., Journal Division (Subsidiary of: Harcourt Brace & Company), 525 B St, Ste 1900, San Diego, CA 92101-4495. TEL 619-230-1840, FAX 619-699-6800, apsubs@acad.com, http://www.academicpress.com/jml. Ed. Rebecca Treiman.

JOURNAL OF NEUROLINGUISTICS. see *MEDICAL SCIENCES—Psychiatry And Neurology*

401 USA ISSN 0090-6905
P106 CODEN: JPLRB7

JOURNAL OF PSYCHOLINGUISTIC RESEARCH. Text in English. 1971. bi-m. USD 748, EUR 747 to institutions for print or online ed.; USD 897.60, EUR 896.40 to institutions for print & online eds.combined (effective 2002). adv. bk.rev. bibl, charts, illus, stat. back issues avail. *Refereed.* **Document type:** *Journal, Academic/Scholarly.* **Description:** Selects top-quality research in psycholinguistic research from multiple disciplines. Reports on a wide range of approaches to the study of human communication.

Related titles: Microfilm ed.: (from PQC); Online - full text ed.: (from EBSCO Publishing, O C L C Online Computer Library Center, Inc., RoweCom Information Quest, Swets Blackwell, Kluwer Online, Institute for Scientific Information).

Indexed: AMED, ASCA, Abstr.Anthropol., Arts & Hum.Cit.Ind. (coverage dropped), Bibl.Asian Stud. (1983), Bibl.Ling., Biol.Abstr., Child Devel.Abstr., Commun.Abstr., Curr.Cont., IBR, IBZ, Ind.Med. (1971-), Ind.Philos., Indian Psychol.Abstr., Lang.& Lang.Behav.Abstr. (1973-), Lang.Teach.& Ling.Abstr., Ling.Abstr., M.L.A., MLA Intl.Bibl., Mid.East: Abstr.& Ind., P C I, PsycInfo, Psychol.Abstr. (1971-), Ref.Zh., Russ.Acad.Sci.Bibl., SOPODA, SSCI, Sociol.Abstr., Stud.Wom.Abstr., e-psyche.

—BLDSC (5043.285000), GNLM, IDS, ingenta. **CCC.**

Published by: Kluwer Academic - Plenum Publishers (Subsidiary of: Wolters Kluwer N.V.), 233 Spring St, New York, NY 10013-1578. TEL 212-620-8000, 800-221-9369, FAX 212-463-0742, info@plenum.com, http://www.wkap.nl/journalhome.htm/0090-6905. Ed. R W Rieber. R&P Rose Luongo TEL 781-871-6311. **Subscr. outside the Americas to:** Kluwer Academic Publishers Group, Journals Department, PO Box 322, Dordrecht 3300 AH, Netherlands. TEL 31-78-639-2392, FAX 31-78-654-6474.

JOURNAL OF SPEECH, LANGUAGE, AND HEARING RESEARCH. see *HANDICAPPED—Hearing Impaired*

410 GBR ISSN 0169-0965
CODEN: LCPRET

LANGUAGE AND COGNITIVE PROCESSES. Text in English. 1985. bi-m. GBP 107, USD 177 to individuals; GBP 340, USD 561 to institutions (effective 2002). adv. illus. reprints avail. *Refereed.* **Document type:** *Academic/Scholarly.* **Description:** Provides an international forum for the publication of theoretical and experimental research into the mental processes and representations involved in language use.

Related titles: Online - full text ed.: ISSN 1464-0732 (from CatchWord Ltd., EBSCO Publishing, O C L C Online Computer Library Center, Inc., RoweCom Information Quest, Swets Blackwell, Institute for Scientific Information).

Indexed: ASCA, Arts & Hum.Cit.Ind. (coverage dropped), Bibl.Ling., C.I.J.E., Curr.Cont., Eng.Ind., Ergon.Abstr., Lang.& Lang.Behav.Abstr., Ling.Abstr., MLA Intl.Bibl., PsycInfo, Psychol.Abstr. (1986-), Russ.Acad.Sci.Bibl., SOPODA, SSCI, Sociol.Abstr., e-psyche.

—BLDSC (5155.693600), CatchWord, Ei, IDS, Infotrieve, ingenta. **CCC.**

Published by: Psychology Press (Subsidiary of: Taylor & Francis Group), 27 Church Rd, Hove, E Sussex BN3 2FA, United Kingdom. TEL 44-1273-207411, FAX 44-1273-205612, information@psypress.co.uk, http://www.psypress.co.uk. R&P Zoe Peden TEL 44-20-7842-2363. Adv. contact Claire Buckminster. **Subscr. addr. in N America:** Psychology Press, Journals Customer Service, Taylor & Francis Group, 325 Chestnut St, Philadelphia, PA 19106. TEL 800-354-1420, FAX 215-625-8914, info@taylorandfrancis.com, http://www.psypress.com; **Subscr. addr. outside N America:** Journals Customer Service, Taylor & Francis Group, Rankine Rd, Basingstoke, Hants RG24 8PR, United Kingdom. TEL 44-1256-813002, FAX 44-1256-479438, enquiry@tandf.co.uk.

410 USA

LANGUAGE & HEALTHCARE NEWSLETTER. Text in English. bi-m. USD 5 (effective 2000). **Document type:** *Newsletter.*

Supersedes in part (in 2000): Linguistics & Science Fiction (Print Edition)

Media: E-mail.

Published by: Ozark Center for Language Studies, PO Box 1137, Huntsville, AR 72740-1137. TEL 501-559-2273, ocls@madisoncounty.net. Ed., Pub. Suzette Haden Elgin.

410 GBR ISSN 0023-8309
P1

LANGUAGE AND SPEECH. Text in English. 1958. q. GBP 140; GBP 150 foreign (effective 1999 - 2000). adv. bk.rev. bibl, charts, illus. index. reprint service avail. from SCH,PSC. *Refereed.* **Document type:** *Academic/Scholarly.* **Description:** Covers speech transmission and reception.

Related titles: Microform ed.; Online - full text ed.: (from CatchWord Ltd., EBSCO Publishing, ProQuest Information & Learning, Swets Blackwell, Institute for Scientific Information).

Indexed: AMED, ASCA, Arts & Hum.Cit.Ind. (coverage dropped), Bibl.Ling., C.I.J.E. (coverage dropped), CINAHL, Commun.Abstr., Cont.Pg.Educ., Curr.Cont., DSH Abstr., Dent.Ind., IBR, IBZ, Ind.Med. (1958-), Lang.& Lang.Behav.Abstr. (1972-), Lang.Teach.& Ling.Abstr., Ling.Abstr., M.L.A., MLA Intl.Bibl., Mid.East: Abstr.& Ind., Mult.Ed.Abstr., P C I, PsycInfo, Psychol.Abstr. (1958-), Ref.Zh., Russ.Acad.Sci.Bibl., SOPODA, SSCI, Sociol.Abstr., e-psyche.

—BLDSC (5155.700000), GNLM, IDS, ingenta. **CCC.**

Published by: Kingston Press Services Ltd., 43 Derwent Rd, Whitton, Twickenham, Mddx TW2 7HQ, United Kingdom. TEL 44-181-893-3015, FAX 44-181-893-3015, http://www.kingstonpress.com. Eds. D Robert Lado, Ellen Bard. Circ: 1,000.

LOGOPEDIE EN FONIATRIE; vaktijdschrift voor logopedie (stem-, spraak-, taal- en gehoorstoornissen). see *HANDICAPPED—Hearing Impaired*

375.4 800 USA ISSN 1092-6488
PN228.M4 CODEN: MPSBFV

METAPHOR AND SYMBOL. Text in English. 1986. q. USD 45 in US & Canada to individuals; USD 75 elsewhere to individuals; USD 385 in US & Canada to institutions; USD 415 elsewhere to institutions (effective 2002). adv. bk.rev. back issues avail. *Refereed.* **Document type:** *Journal, Academic/Scholarly.* **Description:** Covers the study of figurative language from a wide variety of perspectives.

Formerly (until 1997): Metaphor and Symbolic Activity (0885-7253)

Related titles: Online - full text ed.: ISSN 1532-7868. USD 40.50 to individuals; USD 346.50 to institutions (effective 2002) (from CatchWord Ltd., EBSCO Publishing, O C L C Online Computer Library Center, Inc., RoweCom Information Quest, Swets Blackwell).

Indexed: ASCA, Curr.Cont. (coverage dropped), Lang.& Lang.Behav.Abstr., Ling.Abstr., MLA Intl.Bibl., PsycInfo, Psychol.Abstr. (1986-), SOPODA, SSCI (coverage dropped), Sociol.Abstr., e-psyche.

—BLDSC (5701.630000), CatchWord, ingenta. **CCC.**

Published by: Lawrence Erlbaum Associates, Inc., 10 Industrial Ave, Mahwah, NJ 07430-2262. TEL 201-760-3735, 800-926-6579, FAX 201-236-0072, journals@erlbaum.com, http://www.erlbaum.com/ Journals/journals/MS/ms.htm. Ed. Raymond W Gibbs Jr. adv.: page USD 250; trim 5 x 8.

450 156 ITA ISSN 1120-3854

METHODOLOGIA; pensiero linguaggio modelli - thought language models. Text in English, French, Italian. q. ITL 100,000, USD 150 to individuals; ITL 150,000, USD 250 to institutions. bk.rev. abstr, bibl.

Indexed: e-psyche.

Published by: (Societa di Cultura Metodologico - Operativa/Society of Methodological - Operative Culture), Espansione s.r.l., Via Guido Guinizelli, 56, Rome, RM 00152, Italy. TEL 02-55-181630, FAX 02-5451692. Ed. Felice Accame.

153.6 IND ISSN 0377-3132
P1.A1

PSYCHO-LINGUA; a biannual research journal devoted to communicative behavior. Text in English. 1971. s-a. INR 300; INR 2,800 per vol. back volumes from 1974 to 2000 (effective 2002). adv. bk.rev. abstr, bibl. 75 p./no. 1 cols./p. back issues avail.; reprints avail. *Refereed.* **Document type:** *Proceedings, Journal, Academic/Scholarly.*

Indexed: Indian Psychol.Abstr., Lang.& Lang.Behav.Abstr., Ling.Abstr., PsycInfo, Psychol.Abstr. (1975-), SOPODA, Sociol.Abstr., e-psyche.

—BLDSC (6946.277470).

Published by: Psycholinguistic Association of India, 54/1025 Shanti Vihar Colony Dagnia, Raipur, Chhattisgarh 492 013, India. TEL 91-0771-242980. Ed., R&P, Adv. contact V P Sharma. page INR 1,000, 1/2 page INR 600. Circ: 500. **Dist. by:** National Psychological Corporation, Bhargava Bhavan, 4-230 Kacheri Ghat, Agra, Uttar Pradesh 282 004, India.

418 NLD ISSN 0922-4777
BF456.R2 CODEN: REWRE8

READING AND WRITING; an interdisciplinary journal. Text in English. 1989. bi-m. EUR 494 to institutions for print or online ed.; EUR 592.80 to institutions print & online eds.combined (effective 2002). back issues avail.; reprint service avail. from SWZ. *Refereed.* **Document type:** *Academic/Scholarly.* **Description:** Focuses on the interaction among various fields such as linguistics, information processing, neuropsychology, cognitive psychology, speech and hearing sciences, and education.

Related titles: Microform ed.: (from PQC); Online - full text ed.: (from EBSCO Publishing, O C L C Online Computer Library Center, Inc., RoweCom Information Quest, Swets Blackwell, Kluwer Online, Institute for Scientific Information).

Indexed: ASCA, Bibl.Ling., C.I.J.E., Cont.Pg.Educ., Curr.Cont., ERA, Educ.Ind. (Jul.1992-Jun.1997), Educ.Tech.Abstr., IBR, IBZ, Lang.& Lang.Behav.Abstr., Ling.Abstr., MLA Intl.Bibl., Mult.Ed.Abstr., PsycInfo, Psychol.Abstr. (1989-), Russ.Acad.Sci.Bibl., SOPODA, SSCI, Sci.Cit.Ind. (coverage dropped), Sociol.Abstr., Tech.Educ.Abstr., e-psyche.

—BLDSC (7300.875000), IDS, ingenta. **CCC.**

Published by: Kluwer Academic Publishers Group (Subsidiary of: Wolters Kluwer N.V.), Spuiboulevard 50, PO Box 17, Dordrecht 3300 AA, Netherlands. FAX 31-78-639-2254, services@wkap.nl, http://www.wkap.nl/journalhome.htm.0922-4777. Ed. R Malatesha Joshi. **Dist. by:** Journals Department, PO Box 322, Dordrecht 3300 AH, Netherlands. TEL 781-871-6600, FAX 31-78-654-6474.

418 610 USA

SALUD MEDICAL SPANISH. Text in Spanish. 22/yr. USD 39; USD 60 foreign (effective 1998). illus. **Document type:** *Newsletter.* **Description:** Enables health care providers with an intermediate-level understanding of Spanish to hone on-the-job communication with a Spanish-speaking clientele.

Published by: Educational News Service, PO Box 60478, Florence, MA 01062-0478. TEL 413-586-4490, 800-600-4494, FAX 413-586-3448, info@ednews.com.

SEMIOTIC AND COGNITIVE STUDIES. see *PHILOSOPHY*

419 USA ISSN 0302-1475
HV2350

SIGN LANGUAGE STUDIES. Text in English. 1972. q. USD 40 in US & Canada to individuals; USD 50 elsewhere to individuals; USD 90 to institutions (effective 2001). adv. bk.rev. illus. **Document type:** *Academic/Scholarly.* **Description:** Covers anthropology, linguistics, psychology, sociology as they relate to sign language and the deaf population.

Related titles: Diskette ed.; Online - full text ed.: (from Swets Blackwell, RoweCom Information Quest).

Indexed: A.I.C.P. (1972-1974, 1989-), Bibl.Asian Stud. (1996), Bibl.Ling., C.I.J.E. (coverage dropped), DSH Abstr., Except.Child Educ.Abstr., IBR, Lang.& Lang.Behav.Abstr., Lang.Teach.& Ling.Abstr., M.L.A., MLA Intl.Bibl., P C I, PsycInfo, Psychol.Abstr. (1988-), Russ.Acad.Sci.Bibl., SOPODA, Sociol.Abstr., e-psyche.

—BLDSC (8275.650000), Infotrieve, ingenta. **CCC.**

Published by: Gallaudet University, Department of English, 800 Florida Ave, N E, Washington, DC 20002. TEL 202-651-5580. Ed. David F Armstrong. Circ: 485.

L

SPEECH & LANGUAGE THERAPY IN PRACTICE. see *EDUCATION—Special Education And Rehabilitation*

410 NLD ISSN 0167-6393
BF455 CODEN: SCOMDH
SPEECH COMMUNICATION. Text in Dutch. 1982. m. EUR 95 in Europe to individuals; JPY 12,600 in Japan to individuals; USD 104 elsewhere to individuals; EUR 829 in Europe to institutions; JPY 110,100 in Japan to institutions; USD 927 elsewhere to institutions (effective 2002). back issues avail.; reprint service avail. from SWZ. *Refereed.* **Document type:** *Academic/Scholarly.*
Description: Covers all theoretical and experimental aspects of speech communication processes. Details speech production, transmission and perception, person to machine communication, phonetics, linguistics, as well as speech and hearing defects and aids.
Related titles: Microform ed.: (from PQC); Online - full text ed.: (from EBSCO Publishing, ingenta, Swets Blackwell, Institute for Scientific Information, ScienceDirect).
Indexed: Acoust.Abstr., Bioeng.Abstr., Biotech.& Bioeng.Abstr., Compumath, Comput.& Info.Sys., Comput.Abstr., Curr.Cont., Eng.Ind., Ergon.Abstr., INSPEC (May 1982-), Lang.& Lang.Behav.Abstr., Lang.Teach.& Ling.Abstr., Ling.Abstr., PsycInfo, Psychol.Abstr. (1982-), Russ.Acad.Sci.Bibl., SOPODA, SSCI (coverage dropped), Sci.Cit.Ind., Sociol.Abstr., Tel.Abstr., e-psyche.
—BLDSC (8411.196000), AskIEEE, CISTI, Ei, IDS, ingenta. **CCC.**
Published by: (European Association for Signal Processing), North-Holland (Subsidiary of: Elsevier Science BV), PO Box 211, Amsterdam 1000 AE, Netherlands. TEL 31-20-485-3911, FAX 31-20-485-3598, http://www.elsevier.nl/locate/specom. Ed. Max Wajskop. **Subscr. in Australasia and the Far East to:** Elsevier Science (Singapore) Pte Ltd, No.1 Temasek Ave, 17-01 Millenia Tower, Singapore 039192, Singapore. TEL 65-434-3727, FAX 65-337-2230; **Subscr. in Japan to:** Elsevier Science Inc - Japan Regional Office, 9-15 Higashi-Azabu 1-chome, Minato-ku, Tokyo 106-0044, Japan. TEL 81-3-5561-5033, FAX 81-3-5561-5047; **Subscr. in the Americas to:** Elsevier Science, PO Box 945, New York, NY 10159-0945. TEL 212-633-3730, FAX 212-633-3680. **Co-sponsor:** European Speech Communication Association.

DIE SPRACHHEILARBEIT. see *EDUCATION—Special Education And Rehabilitation*

STUDIES IN LINGUISTICS AND PHILOSOPHY. see *PSYCHOLOGY*

STUDIES IN SPEECH PATHOLOGY AND CLINICAL LINGUISTICS. see *MEDICAL SCIENCES—Psychiatry And Neurology*

410 153 BEL ISSN 0393-8255
P99
VS; quaderni di studi semiotici. Variant title: Versus. Text in Italian. 1971. 3/yr. BEF 1,100 (effective 2001). adv. bk.rev. **Document type:** *Academic/Scholarly.*
Description: Publishes the most recent results of researches carried out in any disciplines in which semiotics manifests itself.
Indexed: Bibl.Ling., MLA Intl.Bibl., e-psyche.
Published by: (Universita di San Marino, International Center for Semiotic and Cognitive Studies), N.V. Brepols, Steenweg op Tielen 68, Turnhout 2300, Belgium. publishers@brepols.com. Eds. P Violi, Umberto Eco.

LINGUISTICS—Computer Applications

401.9 NLD ISSN 1387-6724
HUMAN COGNITIVE PROCESSING. Text in English. 1998. irreg.
—BLDSC (4336.040250).
Published by: John Benjamins Publishing Co., Klaprozenweg 105, Amsterdam 1033 NN, Netherlands. TEL 31-20-6304747, http://www.benjamins.com.

LITERARY AND POLITICAL REVIEWS

see also LITERATURE

AMERICAN IMAGO; studies in psychoanalysis and culture. see *MEDICAL SCIENCES—Psychiatry And Neurology*

ANALYTICAL PSYCHOLOGY CLUB OF NEW YORK. BULLETIN. see *PSYCHOLOGY*

BRAILLE MIRROR; a current topic magazine. see *HANDICAPPED—Visually Impaired*

COMPLEAT NURSE. see *MEDICAL SCIENCES—Nurses And Nursing*

058.7 158 SWE ISSN 1101-1408
DIVAN. Text in Swedish. 1990. q. SEK 300 to individuals; SEK 600 to institutions. reprint service avail. from PSC,SCH.
Indexed: e-psyche.
Published by: Psykoanalytiskt Forum Ideell Foerening, Fack 162, Stockholm 10123, Sweden. TEL 46-8-20-12-15, FAX 46-8-20-12-15, redaktionen@divan.se.

053.931 615.7827 NLD ISSN 0927-5428
HIGHLIFE; tijdschrift voor levensgenieters. Text in Dutch. 1992. bi-m. NLG 49. adv. illus. **Document type:** *Consumer.* **Description:** Lifestyle magazine about marijuana. Covers political, legal and medical issues relating to soft drug use in the Netherlands and internationally.
Published by: Uitgeverij Discover, Huygensweg 7, Shijndel 5482 TH, Netherlands. TEL 31-73-5498112, FAX 31-73-5479732. Ed. Joop Mestrom. Pub. Boy Ramsahai. Circ: 18,000 (paid).

150 616.8 USA ISSN 0737-1195
JOURNAL OF POLYMORPHOUS PERVERSITY. Text in English. 1984. s-a., latest vol.18, 2001. USD 14.95 to individuals; USD 25 to institutions (effective 2000). adv. bk.rev. illus. Index. 24 p./no. back issues avail.; reprints avail. **Document type:** *Journal, Consumer.*
Description: Humorous and satirical look at the fields of psychology, psychiatry, medicine and education.
Indexed: e-psyche.
Published by: Wry-Bred Press, Inc., PO Box 1454, Madison Sq Sta, New York, NY 10159-1454. TEL 212-689-5473, FAX 212-689-6859, info@psychhumor.com, http://www.psychhumor.com. Ed., Pub., R&P, Adv. contact Glenn Ellenbogen. Circ: 4,125.

051 USA
MONOZINE. Text in English. irreg.
Address: PO Box 598, Reisertown, MD 21136. todd@monozine.com, http://www.monozine.com. Ed. Todd Lesser.

LITERATURE

see also LINGUISTICS; LITERARY AND POLITICAL REVIEWS; LITERATURE—Poetry; PUBLISHING AND BOOK TRADE

800 USA ISSN 1075-0320
96 INC. Text in English. 1992. a. USD 15; USD 5 newsstand/cover (effective 2001). adv. bk.rev. illus, tr.lit. back issues avail. *Refereed.* **Document type:** *Trade.*
Description: Publishes fiction and poetry by established and emerging writers.
Indexed: Amer.Hum.Ind. (1992-).
Published by: 96 Inc., PO Box 15559, Boston, MA 02215. TEL 617-267-0543, FAX 617-262-3568, to96inc@ici.net. Ed. Ed Vera Gold. R&P, Adv. contact Nancy Mehegan. B&W page USD 100. Circ: 3,000 (paid and controlled).
Dist. by: Bernhard de Bower, Inc., 113 E Center St, Nutley, NJ 07110. TEL 973-667-9300, FAX 973-667-0086.

800 700 USA ISSN 1074-0872
A & U; America's AIDS magazine. (Art & Understanding) Cover title: A & U. Text in English. 1991. m., latest vol.10, no.7, 2001. USD 24.95 domestic to individuals; USD 30.95 in Canada to individuals; USD 49.95 elsewhere to individuals; USD 80 to institutions; USD 3.95, CND 4.95 newsstand/cover (effective 2001). adv. bk.rev., dance rev., music rev., software rev., tel.rev., video rev., film rev., play rev., rec.rev. illus, stat, tr.lit, charts. 48 p./no. back issues avail.; reprints avail. *Refereed.* **Document type:** *Magazine, Consumer.*
Description: Deals with the cultural response to the AIDS epidemic. Covers the worlds of art and literature, activism, notable events and personalities.
Formerly (until 1996): Art & Understanding
Related titles: E-mail ed.; Fax ed.; Microfiche ed.; Microform ed.; Online - full text ed.
Indexed: Ind.Amer.Per.Verse, P C I.
Published by: Art & Understanding, Inc., 25 Monroe St, Ste 205, Albany, NY 12210-2743. TEL 518-426-9010, 888-245-4333, FAX 518-436-5354, mailbox@aumag.org, http://www.aumag.org. Ed., Pub., R&P David Waggoner TEL 800-824-0366. Adv. contact Harold Burdick Jr. B&W page USD 13,662, color page USD 16,962; trim 8.13 x 10.5. Circ: 205,000. **Dist. by:** Deyco Mag. & Book Dist., 255 Executive Dr, Ste 108, Plainview, NY 11803. TEL 516-576-9400, FAX 516-576-9403.

AMERICAN IMAGO; studies in psychoanalysis and culture. see *MEDICAL SCIENCES—Psychiatry And Neurology*

CONSTRUCTIVE CRITICISM; a journal of construct psychology and the arts. see *PSYCHOLOGY*

DIONYSOS; journal of literature and addiction. see *DRUG ABUSE AND ALCOHOLISM*

▼ **DISCOURSE STUDIES**; an interdisciplinary journal for the study of text and talk. see *LINGUISTICS*

HACIA LA LUZ. see *HANDICAPPED—Visually Impaired*

IMAGERY TODAY. see *PSYCHOLOGY*

JOURNAL OF EVOLUTIONARY PSYCHOLOGY. see *PSYCHOLOGY*

JOURNAL OF MENTAL IMAGERY. see *PSYCHOLOGY*

KALEIDOSCOPE (AKRON); exploring the experience of disability through literature and the fine arts. see *HANDICAPPED*

808 610 USA ISSN 0278-9671
PN56.M38
LITERATURE & MEDICINE. Text in English. 1982. s-a. USD 32 to individuals; USD 76 to institutions (effective 2002). adv. back issues avail. **Document type:** *Academic/Scholarly.* **Description:** Covers medicine in its personal, cultural and moral contexts, with contributions from physician-writers, literary scholars, and medical humanists.
Related titles: Online - full text ed.: ISSN 1080-6571 (from Project MUSE, EBSCO Publishing, O C L C Online Computer Library Center, Inc., RoweCom Information Quest, Swets Blackwell, Institute for Scientific Information).
Indexed: ASCA, Arts & Hum.Cit.Ind., Curr.Cont., Ind.Med. (1982-), M.L.A., MLA Intl.Bibl.
—BLDSC (5276.714500), GNLM, IDS, Infotrieve, ingenta. **CCC.**
Published by: (University of Texas Medical Branch at Galveston), Johns Hopkins University Press, Journals Publishing Division, 2715 N Charles St, Baltimore, MD 21218-4363. TEL 800-548-1784, FAX 410-516-6968, jlorder@jhupress.jhu.edu, http://www.press.jhu.edu/press/journals/lm. Eds. Maura Spiegel, Rita Charon. Adv. contact Anastasia Scherr. Circ: 606. **Co-sponsors:** University of Illinois College of Medicine; Institute for the Medical Humanities.

809 150 USA ISSN 0024-4759
PN49 CODEN: LIPSA
LITERATURE AND PSYCHOLOGY; a quarterly journal of literary criticism as informed by depth psychology. Text in English. 1951-1981; resumed 1984. q. USD 12 to individuals; USD 20 to institutions. bk.rev. bibl. reprint service avail. from PQC,PSC,SCH.
Related titles: Microform ed.: (from PQC); Online - full text ed.: (from H. W. Wilson, ProQuest Information & Learning, Gale Group, Factiva, Institute for Scientific Information).
Indexed: ASCA, Abstr.Engl.Stud., Amer.Bibl.Slavic & E.Eur.Stud., Arts & Hum.Cit.Ind., Curr.Cont., Film Lit.Ind. (1990-), Hum.Ind. (Feb.1984-), Ind.Bk.Rev.Hum., Lang.& Lang.Behav.Abstr., M.L.A., MLA Intl.Bibl., Mid.East: Abstr.& Ind., PsycInfo, Psychol.Abstr. (1967-), SOPODA, Soc.Serv.Abstr., Sociol.Abstr.
—BLDSC (5276.715000), ingenta.
Address: c/o Morton Kaplan and Richard Feldstein, Eds, Department of English, Rhode Island College, Providence, RI 02908. Circ: 1,000.

LOVING BROTHERHOOD NEWSLETTER; a journal for personal and planetary transformation. see *HOMOSEXUALITY*

METAPHOR AND SYMBOL. see *LINGUISTICS*

NURSE AUTHOR AND EDITOR; a newsletter for nurse authors, editors, and editorial board members. see *JOURNALISM*

051 USA ISSN 0897-2648
ORGANICA; a magazine of arts & activism. Cover title: Organica Quarterly. Text in English. 1982. q. USD 10 (effective 1999); free at health food stores. adv. bk.rev., music rev. illus. **Document type:** *Newspaper.* **Description:** Reports on new products and trends in health food and health care. Publishes poetry and articles on artists, musicians and cultural issues.
Published by: (Aubrey Organics), Organica Press, 4419 N Manhattan Ave, Tampa, FL 33614. TEL 813-877-4186, FAX 813-876-8166. Ed. Susan Hussey. Pub. Aubrey Hampton. Adv. contact Anne Knight. Circ: 200,000 (controlled).

PSYCHOANALYSE EN CULTUUR/PSYCHOANALYSIS AND CULTURE. see *PSYCHOLOGY*

REVIEW OF EXISTENTIAL PSYCHOLOGY AND PSYCHIATRY. see *PSYCHOLOGY*

SATURDAY EVENING POST. see *GENERAL INTEREST PERIODICALS—United States*

808.8 152.4 USA
UNHAPPY✶. Text in English. 1996. m. **Description:** Contains short speculative and hallucinatory fiction.
Media: Online - full text.
Indexed: e-psyche.
Published by: Fringeware Inc., P O Box 4858, Austin, TX 78765-4858. weevil@charm.net, http://www.fringeware.com/anathema/unhappy. Eds. Clayton Counts, Wiley Wiggins.

800 ITA ISSN 0042-0646
UOMINI E IDEE. Text in Italian. 1959-1975; resumed 1997. s-a. ITL 40,000; ITL 60,000 foreign (effective 1998). adv. bk.rev. illus. **Description:** Covers philosophy, literature, phenomonology, and experiences of the modified and interior states of consciousness.
Indexed: e-psyche.
Address: Via Poggio Dei Mari, 16, Naples, NA 80129, Italy. TEL 44-81-5490558, FAX 44-81-5564391, laurapi@box1.tin.it, http://www.ricerche-filosofiche.org/uomini-idee; http://space.tin.it/scienza/lpintore. Ed. Corrado Piancastelli. Circ: 5,000.

LITERATURE—Abstracting, Bibliographies, Statistics

800 DEU ISSN 0943-9188
FRITZ-HUESER-INSTITUT FUER DEUTSCHE UND AUSLAENDISCHE ARBEITERLITERATUR. INFORMATIONEN. Text in German. 1967. irreg. **Document type:** *Bibliography.* **Description:** Presents culture and literature of and for the working class from 1848 to the present day.
Published by: Fritz-Hueser-Institut fuer Deutsche und Auslaendische Arbeiterliteratur, Ostwall 64, Dortmund 44122, Germany. TEL 49-231-5023227, FAX 49-231-5023229. Ed. Rainer Noltenius. Circ: 600.

LITERATURE—Poetry

see also LITERARY AND POLITICAL REVIEWS

808.81 616.89 USA ISSN 0889-3675 CODEN: JPTHEK
JOURNAL OF POETRY THERAPY; the interdisciplinary journal of practice, theory, research, and education. Text in English. 1987. q. USD 420, EUR 419 to institutions for print or online ed.; USD 504, EUR 502.80 to institutions for print & online eds.combined (effective 2002). adv. bk.rev. abstr. reprint service avail. from PQC. *Refereed.* **Document type:** *Journal, Academic/Scholarly.* **Description:** Addresses the use of poetics in health, mental health, education, and other human service settings, focusing on the use of language in therapy.
Related titles: Online - full text ed.: (from O C L C Online Computer Library Center, Inc., Swets Blackwell, Kluwer Online, RoweCom Information Quest).
Indexed: C.I.J.E., IBR, IBZ, Ind.Philos., Soc.Work Res.& Abstr., e-psyche.
—BLDSC (5040.820000), Infotrieve, ingenta. **CCC.**
Published by: (National Association for Poetry Therapy, Florida State University, School of Social Work), Kluwer Academic - Plenum Publishers (Subsidiary of: Wolters Kluwer N.V.), 233 Spring St, New York, NY 10013-1578. TEL 212-620-8000, 800-221-9369, FAX 212-463-0742, info@plenum.com, http://www.wkap.nl/journalhome.htm/0889-3675. Ed. Nicholas Mazza. **Subscr. outside the Americas to:** Kluwer Academic Publishers Group, Journals Department, PO Box 322, Dordrecht 3300 AH, Netherlands. TEL 31-78-639-2392, FAX 31-78-654-6474.

LUMBER AND WOOD

see FORESTS AND FORESTRY—Lumber And Wood

MACHINERY

see also ENGINEERING—Mechanical Engineering; TECHNOLOGY: COMPREHENSIVE WORKS

FACULTAD NACIONAL DE AGRONOMIA MEDELLIN. REVISTA. see *AGRICULTURE*

621.9 614.85 JPN
JITSUMU TENBO/SAFETY NEWS ON BOILER AND CRANE ENGINEERING. Text in Japanese. 1967. bi-m. JPY 650 per issue.
Published by: Boira Kuren Anzen Kyokai/Boiler and Crane Safety Association, 41-20, Kameido - chome., Koto-ku, Tokyo 136-0071, Japan.

621.9 ISR ISSN 0792-1322
TA'ASIYOT. Text in Hebrew. 1984. bi-w. ILS 300, USD 75. adv. **Document type:** *Newspaper.*
Published by: Merav Publishing Industries Ltd., 27 Soutine St, Tel Aviv 64684, Israel. TEL 972-3-5211900, FAX 972-3-5211902, merav@trendline.co.il, http://www.merav.co.il. Ed. Sara Skulsky. Adv. contact David Kreizelman. B&W page USD 1,131, color page USD 1,797; trim 36 x 24. Circ: 20,000.

MANAGEMENT

see BUSINESS AND ECONOMICS—Management

MARKETING AND PURCHASING

see BUSINESS AND ECONOMICS—Marketing And Purchasing

MATHEMATICS

BIOMATHEMATICS. see *BIOLOGY*

BIOMETRICS. see *STATISTICS*

BRITISH JOURNAL OF MATHEMATICAL AND STATISTICAL PSYCHOLOGY. see *PSYCHOLOGY*

BULLETIN OF MATHEMATICAL BIOLOGY. see *BIOLOGY*

CAMBRIDGE STUDIES IN MATHEMATICAL BIOLOGY. see *BIOLOGY*

510 CAN ISSN 0731-4043
Z696.A1
CLASSIFICATION LITERATURE AUTOMATED SEARCH SERVICE. Short title: C.L.A.S.S. Text in English. a. USD 100; includes Journal of Classification. *Refereed.* **Document type:** *Bibliography.*
Published by: Classification Society of North America, c/o William H.E. Day, P O Box 17, Port Midland, NS B0W 2V0, Canada. TEL 902-649-2996. **Subscr. in N. America to:** Springer-Verlag Journals Fulfillment Services, 079096 2485, PO Box 2485, Secaucus, NJ. TEL 800-777-4643, FAX 201-348-4505.

COMMENTATIONES PHYSICO-MATHEMATICAE ET CHEMICO-MEDICAE. see *PHYSICS*

510 GBR ISSN 0265-0746
QH323.5 CODEN: IJMBEG
I M A JOURNAL OF MATHEMATICS APPLIED IN MEDICINE & BIOLOGY. Text in English. 1984. q. GBP 189, USD 324 to individuals; GBP 210, USD 360 to institutions (effective Mar. 2002). adv. index. back issues avail. *Refereed.* **Document type:** *Journal, Academic/Scholarly.* **Description:** Covers the uses of mathematics in medical and biological research, with emphasis on the special insights and enhanced understanding that arise from these uses.
Related titles: Online - full text ed.: ISSN 1471-6887. GBP 189, USD 324 to institutions Online only (effective Mar. 2002) (from Institute for Scientific Information).
Indexed: ASCA, Bio-Contr.News & Info., Biol.Abstr., Compumath, Curr.Cont., Eng.Ind., Excerp.Med., INIS Atomind., Ind.Med. (1984-), Inpharma, Math.R., Reac., Rev.Med.& Vet.Mycol., Rev.Plant Path., Sci.Cit.Ind., Zent.Math.
—BLDSC (4368.759000), CISTI, Ei, GNLM, IDS, Infotrieve, ingenta, Linda Hall. **CCC.**
Published by: (Institute of Mathematics and Its Applications), Oxford University Press, Academic Division, Great Clarendon St, Oxford OX2 6DP, United Kingdom. TEL 44-1865-267907, FAX 44-1865-267835, jnl.info@oup.co.uk, http://www3.oup.co.uk/imammb/, http://www.oup.co.uk/journals. Ed. R W Hiorns. Pub. Ian McIntosh. R&P Fionna Willis. adv.: page GBP 200, page USD 360. Circ: 300. **U.S. subscr. to:** Oxford University Press, Journals, 2001 Evans Rd, Cary, NC 27513. TEL 800-852-7323, FAX 919-677-1714, jnlorders@oup-usa.org; **Subscr. to:** Journals Marketing, Great Clarendon St, Oxford OX2 6DP, United Kingdom.

IMAGE ANALYSIS AND STEREOLOGY. see *BIOLOGY*

510 USA ISSN 0176-4268
BD241
JOURNAL OF CLASSIFICATION. Text in English. 1984. s-a. (in 1 vol., 2 nos./vol.). USD 247.40 domestic for Print & Online Eds.; USD 238.60 in Germany for Print & Online Eds.; USD 133.70 newsstand/cover foreign (effective 2002). adv. reprint service avail. from SWZ. *Refereed.* **Document type:** *Academic/Scholarly.* **Description:** Covers a wide range of topics in the fields of classification, taxonomy, scaling and other ordination techniques.
Related titles: Microform ed.: (from PQC); Online - full text ed.: ISSN 1432-1343 (from EBSCO Publishing, RoweCom Information Quest, Swets Blackwell, Springer LINK, Institute for Scientific Information).
Indexed: ASCA, Biol.Abstr., Biostat., C.C.M.J., Compumath, Curr.Cont., Curr.Ind.Stat., IBR, Inform.Sci.Abstr., J.Cont.Quant.Meth., LISA, Math.R., PsycInfo, Psychol.Abstr. (1984-), Russ.Acad.Sci.Bibl., SSCI, Stat.Theor.Meth.Abstr., Zent.Math., Zoo.Rec., e-psyche.
—BLDSC (4958.369550), CISTI, IDS, ingenta. **CCC.**
Published by: (Classification Society of North America CAN), Springer-Verlag, Journals (Subsidiary of: BertelsmannSpringer), 175 Fifth Ave, New York, NY 10010. TEL 212-460-1500, FAX 212-473-6272, journals@springer-ny.com; link@springer-ny.com, http://link.springer.de/link/service/journals/00453/index.htm. Ed. Phipps Arabie. R&P Xian Chuan Lian. Adv. contact Brian Skepton. **N. American subscr. to:** Journal Fulfillment Services, PO Box 2485, Secaucus, NJ 07096-2485. TEL 800-777-4643, FAX 201-348-4505.

JOURNAL OF MATHEMATICAL BIOLOGY. see *BIOLOGY*

JOURNAL OF MATHEMATICAL PSYCHOLOGY. see *PSYCHOLOGY*

JOURNAL OF STRUCTURAL LEARNING AND INTELLIGENT SYSTEMS. see *PSYCHOLOGY*

551.3 USA ISSN 0022-4812
BC1 CODEN: JSYLA6
JOURNAL OF SYMBOLIC LOGIC. Text in English, French, German. 1936. q. USD 365 to institutions (effective 2000); includes q. Bulletin of Symbolic Logic. bk.rev. bibl, abstr, illus. Index. back issues avail.; reprint service avail. from PSC,SCH. *Refereed.* **Document type:** *Academic/Scholarly.* **Description:** Contains scholarly works.
Related titles: Microform ed.: (from PQC,PMC); Online - full text ed.: (from JSTOR (Web-based Journal Archive), Gale Group, Institute for Scientific Information).
Indexed: ASCA, C.C.M.J., Compumath, Curr.Cont., Hum.Ind. (Sep.1983-Sep.1987), INSPEC (Mar.1977-), Ind.Bk.Rev.Hum., Ind.Sci.Rev., Math.R., P C I, Phil.Ind., Ref.Zh., Russ.Acad.Sci.Bibl., SSCI (coverage dropped), Sci.Cit.Ind., Zent.Math.
—BLDSC (5068.000000), AskIEEE, CISTI, IDS, ingenta, Linda Hall. **CCC.**
Published by: Association for Symbolic Logic, Department of Mathematics, University of Illinois at Urbana Champaign, 1409 W Green St, Urbana, IL 61801. TEL 217-244-7902, FAX 217-333-9576, http://www.jstor.org/journals/00224812.html. Ed. Herbert B Enderton. Circ: 2,500. **Subscr. to:** ASL, Journal Dept, UIP, 1325 S Oak St, Champaign, IL 61820.

510 570 USA ISSN 0341-633X CODEN: LNBMAH
LECTURE NOTES IN BIOMATHEMATICS. Text in English. 1974. irreg., latest vol.100, 1995. price varies. reprint service avail. from ISI. **Document type:** *Monographic series.*
Indexed: Biol.Abstr., Chem.Abstr., INSPEC (coverage dropped), Sport Fish.Abstr., Zent.Math.
—CASDDS, CISTI, Linda Hall. **CCC.**
Published by: Springer-Verlag, Journals (Subsidiary of: BertelsmannSpringer), 175 Fifth Ave, New York, NY 10010. TEL 212-460-1500, FAX 212-473-6272. Ed. S Levin.

510 570 USA ISSN 0075-8523
CODEN: LMLSAA
LECTURES ON MATHEMATICS IN THE LIFE SCIENCES. Text in English. 1968. irreg. price varies. **Document type:** *Monographic series.*
Indexed: Biol.Abstr., C.C.M.J., Chem.Abstr., Math.R., Zent.Math., Zoo.Rec.
—BLDSC (5179.980000), CASDDS, Infotrieve. **CCC.**
Published by: American Mathematical Society, 201 Charles St, Providence, RI 02904-2294. TEL 401-455-4000, 800-321-4267, FAX 401-331-3842, cust-serv@ams.org, http://www.ams.org/.

510 576 USA ISSN 0025-5564
QH324 CODEN: MABIAR
MATHEMATICAL BIOSCIENCES; an international journal. Text in English. 1967. m. EUR 120 in Europe to qualified personnel; JPY 16,200 in Japan to qualified personnel; USD 135 elsewhere to qualified personnel; EUR 2,286 in Europe to institutions; JPY 303,600 in Japan to institutions; USD 2,557 elsewhere to institutions (effective 2002). adv. bk.rev. abstr, bibl, charts, illus. index. reprints avail. *Refereed.* **Document type:** *Journal, Academic/Scholarly.* **Description:** Publishes research and expository papers on the formulation, analysis and solution of mathematical models in the biosciences.
Related titles: Microform ed.: (from PQC); Online - full text ed.: (from EBSCO Publishing, ingenta, ScienceDirect, Swets Blackwell, Institute for Scientific Information).
Indexed: ASCA, Abstr.Anthropol., Appl.Ecol.Abstr., Appl.Mech.Rev., Aqua.Sci.& Fish.Abstr., Bibl.Agri., Biol.Abstr., Biostat., C.C.M.J., Cal.Tiss.Abstr., Chem.Abstr., Chem.Indus.Notes, Chem.Titles, Compumath, Comput.Abstr., Curr.Adv.Ecol.Sci., Curr.Cont., Curr.Ind.Stat., Deep Sea Res.& Oceanogr.Abstr., Ecol.Abstr., Eng.Ind., Environ.Sci.Poll.Mgmt., Excerp.Med., Geo.Abstr.H.G., Helminthol.Abstr., IDA, INIS Atomind., INSPEC (pre-1969-), Ind.Med. (1967-), Ind.Sci.Rev., Ind.Vet., Inpharma, Int.Abstr.Biol.Sci., Math.R., Microbiol.Abstr., Pharm.&Out.News, Pollut.Abstr., Reac., Rev.Appl.Entomol., Risk Abstr., SSCI (coverage dropped), Sci.Cit.Ind., Sport Fish.Abstr., Wild.Rev., Zent.Math., Zoo.Rec.
—BLDSC (5401.700000), AskIEEE, CASDDS, CISTI, Ei, GNLM, IDS, ingenta, Linda Hall. **CCC.**
Published by: Elsevier Science, Box 945, New York, NY 10159-0945. TEL 212-989-5800, FAX 212-633-3990, usinfo-f@elsevier.com, http://www.elsevier.nl/locate/mbs, http://www.elsevier.com. Eds. Michael A Savageau, R Bellman. Circ: 1,000. **Subscr. in Australasia and the Far East to:** Elsevier Science (Singapore) Pte Ltd, No.1 Temasek Ave, 17-01 Millenia Tower, Singapore 039192, Singapore. TEL 65-434-3727, FAX 65-337-2230; **Subscr. in Japan to:** Elsevier Science Inc - Japan Regional Office, 9-15 Higashi-Azabu 1-chome, Minato-ku, Tokyo 106-0044, Japan. TEL 81-3-5561-5033; **Subscr. outside the Americas to:** Elsevier Science BV, PO Box 211, Amsterdam 1000 AE, Netherlands. TEL 31-20-485-3757.

MATHEMATICAL COGNITION. see *PSYCHOLOGY*

510 USA ISSN 1098-6065
▼ **MATHEMATICAL THINKING AND LEARNING**; an international journal. Text in English. 1999. q. USD 50 in US & Canada to individuals; USD 80 elsewhere to individuals (effective 2001 & 2002); USD 235 in US & Canada to institutions; USD 265 elsewhere to institutions (effective 2001); USD 280 in US & Canada to institutions; USD 310 elsewhere to institutions (effective 2002). adv. **Document type:** *Journal, Academic/Scholarly.* **Description:** Concentrates on all aspects of mathematical thinking, reasoning, and learning at all ages and stages of development.
Related titles: Online - full text ed.: ISSN 1532-7833. USD 45 to individuals; USD 252 to institutions (effective 2002) (from CatchWord Ltd., EBSCO Publishing, O C L C Online Computer Library Center, Inc., RoweCom Information Quest, Swets Blackwell).
Indexed: Educ.Ind., e-psyche.
—BLDSC (5405.025000), CatchWord. **CCC.**
Published by: Lawrence Erlbaum Associates, Inc., 10 Industrial Ave, Mahwah, NJ 07430-2262. TEL 201-760-3735, 800-926-6579, FAX 201-236-0072, journals@erlbaum.com, http://www.erlbaum.com/ Journals/journals/MTL/mtl.htm. Ed. Lyn D English. adv.: page USD 275; trim 5 x 8.

MATHEMATICS EDUCATION LIBRARY. see *LIBRARY AND INFORMATION SCIENCES*

NONLINEAR DYNAMICS, PSYCHOLOGY, AND LIFE SCIENCES. see *PSYCHOLOGY*

STATISTICAL METHODS IN MEDICAL RESEARCH. see *STATISTICS*

510 530 570 ROM ISSN 1223-964X
AS345.B37 CODEN: BTBSF6
TRANSYLVANIA UNIVERSITY OF BRASOV. BULLETIN. SERIES B; mathematics, economical sciences, philology, medicine, physics, chemistry, sports. Text in English. 1956. a. price varies. bibl, charts, stat. **Document type:** *Bulletin.*
Former titles: Universitatea Transilvania din Brasov. Buletinul. Seria C. Matematica, Fizica, Chimie (1220-9414); (until 1990): Universitatea din Brasov. Buletinul. Seria C. Matematica, Fizica, Chimie; Universitatea din Brasov. Buletinul. Seria C. Stiinte ale Naturri si Pedagogie; Universitatea din Brasov. Buletinul. Seria C. Matematica, Fizica, Chimie
Indexed: C.C.M.J., Chem.Abstr., Chem.Indus.Notes, Chem.Titles, Math.R., Zent.Math.
—CASDDS, CISTI, Linda Hall.
Published by: Universitatea Transilvania din Brasov/Transylvania University of Brasov, Bd. Eroilor 29, Brasov 2200, Romania. TEL 40-921-41580, Libr@vega.unitbv.ro. Ed. Aurel Jula.

UKRAINSKII REFERATIVNYI ZURNAL. SERIA 1. PRIRODNICHI NAUKI, MEDICINA/UKRAINIAN JOURNAL OF ABSTRACTS. SER. 1. PRIRODNICI NAUKI, MEDICINE. see *SCIENCES: COMPREHENSIVE WORKS—Abstracting, Bibliographies, Statistics*

MATHEMATICS—Computer Applications

GAMES AND ECONOMIC BEHAVIOR. see *PSYCHOLOGY*

510 152 NLD ISSN 0169-1015
BF469 CODEN: SPVIEU
SPATIAL VISION. Text in English. 1985. q. EUR 96, USD 110 to individuals includes online ed.; EUR 230, USD 266 to institutions includes online ed. (effective 2002). adv. illus. back issues avail. *Refereed.* **Document type:** *Journal, Academic/Scholarly.* **Description:** Reports international psychophysical, perceptual and cognitive research on the visual processing of spatial information.
Related titles: Online - full content ed.: 2000 (from EBSCO Publishing, Swets Blackwell); Online - full text ed.: (from CatchWord Ltd., Institute for Scientific Information).
Indexed: ASCA, Abstr.Hum.Comp.Inter., Bioeng.Abstr., Biotech.& Bioeng.Abstr., Eng.Ind., INSPEC (1988-), Ind.Med. (1985-), Neurosci.Cit.Ind., PsycInfo, Psychol.Abstr. (1987-), SSCI, e-psyche.
—BLDSC (8361.785700), AskIEEE, CISTI, Ei, GNLM, ingenta.
Published by: V S P (Subsidiary of: Brill Academic Publishers), PO Box 346, Zeist 3700 AH, Netherlands. TEL 31-30-692-5790, FAX 31-30-693-2081, vsppub@compuserve.com, http://www.vsppub.com/ journals/jn-SpaVis.html. Eds. A Reeves, D Sagi.

MATRIMONY

see also HOME ECONOMICS

THE FAMILY JOURNAL; counseling and therapy for couples and families. see *PSYCHOLOGY*

FAMILY THERAPY NEWS. see *PSYCHOLOGY*

301.4157 155.3 AUS ISSN 1322-9400
HQ1 CODEN: JFSTFG
JOURNAL OF FAMILY STUDIES. Text in English. 1980. s-a. AUD 60 in Australia to individuals; AUD 90 in Australia to institutions; AUD 35 in Australia to students; AUD 80 foreign to individuals; AUD 110 foreign to institutions (effective 2002). adv. bk.rev. index. back issues avail. *Refereed.* **Description:** For academics, researchers, administrators, educators and clinicians in the helping professions.
Former titles (until 1995): Australian Journal of Marriage and Family (1034-652X); (until vol.10, 1989): Australian Journal of Sex, Marriage and Family (0159-1487)
Indexed: Abstr.Soc.Geront., Aus.P.A.I.S., Lang.& Lang.Behav.Abstr., PsycInfo, Psychol.Abstr. (1983-), SOPODA, Sage Fam.Stud.Abstr., Soc.Serv.Abstr., Sociol.Abstr., e-psyche.
—BLDSC (4983.738000), ingenta.
Published by: La Trobe University Press, School of Public Health, Bundoora, VIC, VIC 3083, Australia. TEL 61-3-9479-1746, 61-3-9479-1750, FAX 61-3-9479-1783, l.morrison@latrobe.edu.au. Ed., Adv. contact Liz Morrison. Circ: 900.

JOURNAL OF MARITAL AND FAMILY THERAPY. see *PSYCHOLOGY*

MECHANICAL ENGINEERING

see ENGINEERING—Mechanical Engineering

MECHANICS

see PHYSICS—Mechanics

MEDICAL SCIENCES

see also ALTERNATIVE MEDICINE; BIOLOGY; DRUG ABUSE AND ALCOHOLISM; GERONTOLOGY AND GERIATRICS; HEALTH FACILITIES AND ADMINISTRATION; MEDICAL SCIENCES—Allergology And Immunology; MEDICAL SCIENCES—Anaesthesiology; MEDICAL SCIENCES—Cardiovascular Diseases; MEDICAL SCIENCES—Chiropractic, Homeopathy, Osteopathy; MEDICAL SCIENCES—Communicable Diseases; MEDICAL SCIENCES—Computer Applications; MEDICAL SCIENCES—Dentistry; MEDICAL SCIENCES—Dermatology And Venereology; MEDICAL SCIENCES—Endocrinology; MEDICAL SCIENCES—Experimental Medicine, Laboratory Technique; MEDICAL SCIENCES—Forensic Sciences; MEDICAL SCIENCES—Gastroenterology ; MEDICAL SCIENCES—Hematology; MEDICAL SCIENCES—Hypnosis; MEDICAL SCIENCES—Internal Medicine; MEDICAL SCIENCES—Nurses And Nursing; MEDICAL SCIENCES—Obstetrics And Gynecology; MEDICAL SCIENCES—Oncology; MEDICAL SCIENCES—Ophthalmology And Optometry; MEDICAL SCIENCES—Orthopedics And Traumatology; MEDICAL SCIENCES—Otorhinolaryngology; MEDICAL SCIENCES—Pediatrics; MEDICAL SCIENCES—Physical Medicine And Rehabilitation; MEDICAL SCIENCES—Psychiatry And Neurology; MEDICAL SCIENCES—Radiology And Nuclear Medicine; MEDICAL SCIENCES—Respiratory Diseases; MEDICAL SCIENCES—Rheumatology; MEDICAL SCIENCES—Sports Medicine; MEDICAL SCIENCES—Surgery; MEDICAL SCIENCES—Urology And Nephrology; MEN'S HEALTH; NUTRITION AND DIETETICS; OCCUPATIONAL HEALTH AND SAFETY; PHARMACY AND PHARMACOLOGY; PHYSICAL FITNESS AND HYGIENE; PUBLIC HEALTH AND SAFETY; WOMEN'S HEALTH

612 JPN ISSN 0917-5792
CODEN: CIGAEC
13C IGAKU/SOCIETY FOR THE MEDICAL APPLICATION OF CARBON THIRTEEN. BULLETIN. Text in Japanese. 1991. a. JPY 4,000 per issue (effective 2000 - 2001). **Document type:** *Bulletin, Academic/Scholarly.*
Indexed: Chem.Indus.Notes, Chem.Titles.
—BLDSC (2758.564000), CASDDS.
Published by: Society for the Medical Application of Carbon 13, c/o Institute of Life Science, Soka University, 1-236 Tangi-cho, Hachioji-shi, Tokyo 192-8577, Japan. TEL 81-426-91-9382, FAX 81-426-91-9382, kanamatu@t.soka.ac.jp. Ed. Yasuzo Tsukada. Circ: 250.

610 CUB ISSN 0257-7402
16 DE ABRIL; organo cientifico estudiantil de las ciencias medicas de Cuba. Text in Spanish. 1961. q. USD 15 in the Americas; USD 25 in Europe; USD 30 elsewhere. bk.rev. charts, illus. *Refereed.* **Document type:** *Academic/Scholarly.* **Description:** Original papers, research reports, reviews, notes and other medical articles.
Published by: Ministerio de Salud Publica, Instituto Superior de Ciencias Medicas de la Habana, Calle G s-n, e. 25 y 27, Plaza de la Revolucion, Vedado, Havana 10400, Cuba. TEL 537-308942, FAX 537-333063, 16-abril@infomed.sld.cu. Ed. Abel Garcia Valdes. Circ: 5,000. **Dist. by:** Centro Nacional de Informacion de Ciencias Medicas, Calle G No. 110 e. M y N, Vedado, Havana 10400, Cuba.

610 USA
A A B B NEWS. Text in English. 1981. m. (11/yr.). USD 50 to institutional members. **Document type:** *Newsletter.*
Formerly: American Association of Blood Banks. News Briefs (8756-6095)

Published by: American Association of Blood Banks, 8101 Glenbrook Rd, Bethesda, MD 20814. TEL 301-907-6977, FAX 301-907-6895, http://www.aabb.org. Ed. Scott Douglas. Circ: 10,000.

610 USA
A A B B WEEKLY REPORT. Text in English. 1984. w. USD 140 to non-members; USD 190 foreign to non-members; USD 98 to members; USD 130 foreign to members. back issues avail. **Document type:** *Newsletter.*
Formerly: Blood Bank Week (0747-2420)
Published by: American Association of Blood Banks, 8101 Glenbrook Rd, Bethesda, MD 20814. TEL 301-907-6977, FAX 301-907-6895, http://www.aabb.org. Ed. Carmen Phillips. Circ: 3,400.

610.73 362.1 USA ISSN 1079-0713
A A C N CLINICAL ISSUES; advanced practice in acute and critical care. Text in English. 1990. q., latest vol.13. USD 79.95 in North America to individuals; USD 134.95 elsewhere to individuals; USD 201.95 in North America to institutions; USD 240.95 elsewhere to institutions; USD 59 newsstand/cover (effective 2002). adv. *Refereed.* **Document type:** *Academic/Scholarly, Trade.* **Description:** Covers various clinical and research issues in critical-care nursing.
Formerly (until 1995): A A C N Clinical Issues in Critical Care Nursing (1046-7467)
Related titles: Online - full text ed.: (from Ovid Technologies, Inc.).
Indexed: CINAHL, Int.Nurs.Ind., Nurs.Abstr.
—BLDSC (0537.137750), CISTI, GNLM, ingenta.
Published by: (American Association of Critical Care Nurses), Lippincott Williams & Wilkins (Philadelphia) (Subsidiary of: Wolters Kluwer N.V.), 530 Walnut St, Philadelphia, PA 19106-3621. TEL 215-521-8300, FAX 215-521-8902, custserv@lww.com, http://www.lww.com/productdetailresults/1,2265,1079-0713,00.html. **Subscr. to:** Lippincott Williams & Wilkins, Order Dept, 16522 Hunters Green Pkwy, Hagerstown, MD 21740. TEL 301-714-2334, FAX 301-824-7390.

A A C O M ANNUAL STATISTICAL REPORT. see *MEDICAL SCIENCES—Abstracting, Bibliographies, Statistics*

610 614 USA
A A M A EXECUTIVE*. Text in English. bi-m. USD 60; USD 100 foreign (effective 1998). adv. bk.rev. *Refereed.* **Document type:** *Newsletter.*
Former titles: Medical Administration Executive; A A M A Executive (0065-6879)
Published by: American Academy of Medical Administrators, 701 Lee St No.600, Des Plaines, IL 60016-4516. TEL 248-540-4310, FAX 248-645-0590. Ed. Thomas R O'Donovan. R&P, Adv. contact Karen Loughran. Circ: 4,000.

A A M C CURRICULUM DIRECTORY. see *EDUCATION—Teaching Methods And Curriculum*

610.711 USA ISSN 0360-7437
R712.A1
A A M C DIRECTORY OF AMERICAN MEDICAL EDUCATION. Text in English. a. USD 50 to non-members; USD 25 to members (effective 1999). reprint service avail. from PQC. **Document type:** *Directory.* **Description:** Accredited medical schools in the United States, Canada, and Puerto Rico list their administrators and department, division, and section chairs. Each school entry includes enrollment, type of support, clinical facilities, and a brief historical statement.
Published by: Association of American Medical Colleges, 2450 N St N W, Washington, DC 20037-1126. TEL 202-828-0416, FAX 202-828-1123. Ed. Cynthis Bennett. R&P Cynthia Bennett.

610.28 USA ISSN 0146-146X
A A M I ANNUAL MEETING. PROCEEDINGS*. Text in English. 1974. a. USD 40 to non-members; USD 25 to members. adv. **Document type:** *Newsletter, Academic/Scholarly.* **Description:** Papers presented at the association's annual meeting.
Published by: Association for the Advancement of Medical Instrumentation, 1110 N Glebe Rd #220, Arlington, VA 22201-5707. TEL 703-525-4890, FAX 703-276-0793. Ed. Mary Beth Hatem. Adv. contact Cameron Nyhen.

610 USA ISSN 0894-0509
A A P A NEWS. Text in English. 1979. bi-w. membership. adv. **Document type:** *Newsletter.* **Description:** Keeps physician assistants current on academy, legislative, educational and professional issues affecting their practices.
Incorporates (1989-1995): P A Career (Phisician Assistants) (1071-5983)
Published by: American Academy of Physician Assistants, 950 N Washington St, Alexandria, VA 22314-1552. TEL 703-836-2272, FAX 703-684-1924, aapa@aapa.org. Ed., R&P Jane Howard. Adv. contact Russell Johns. Circ: 30,000 (controlled).

610 USA ISSN 8750-9687
A A P S NEWS. Text in English. 1943. m. USD 250 to members (effective 1998). cum.index: 1987-1992. back issues avail. **Description:** Covers socio-economic aspects of medical practice.
Formerly: A A P S News Letter (0001-0170)
Published by: Association of American Physicians & Surgeons, Inc., 1601 N Tucson Blvd, Ste 9, Tucson, AZ 85716-3405. TEL 602-327-4885, FAX 602-290-9674. Ed. Dr. Jane M Orient. Circ: 3,000.

610.29 GBR
A B H I DIRECTORY. Text in English. 1965. a. adv. **Document type:** *Directory.* **Description:** Guide to health care equipment, services and supplies.
Published by: (Association of British Health-Care Industries), Kogan Page Ltd., 120 Pentonville Rd, London N1 9JN, United Kingdom. FAX 44-20-7837-6348. R&P Caroline Gomm. Adv. contact Linda Batham.

610.25 USA
A B M S MEDICAL SPECIALIST PLUS. Text in English. a. (plus s-a. updates). USD 1,210 (effective 1999). **Description:** Provides access to the career and educational histories of over 535,000 board certified medical specialists.
Media: CD-ROM.
Published by: Marquis Who's Who (Subsidiary of: Reed Elsevier plc Group), 121 Chanlon Rd, New Providence, NJ 07964. TEL 800-521-8110, FAX 908-665-6688, info@reedref.com, http://www.reedref.com. **Subscr. to:** Order Dept., PO Box 31, New Providence, NJ 07974-9903.

610 USA
A B M S RECORD. Text in English. 1981. q. **Document type:** *Newsletter.* **Description:** Covers graduate medical education, specialty certification, evaluation of physician performance, and legislation.
Published by: American Board of Medical Specialties, 1007 Church St, Ste 404, Evanston, IL 60201-5913. TEL 847-491-9091, FAX 847-328-3596, http://www.abms.org. Ed. Dr. Stephen H Miller. R&P Alexis Rodgers. Circ: 3,400.

610.7 CAN ISSN 0836-3463
A C M C FORUM. Text in English, French. 1968. q. CND 30 in Canada; CND 35 in United States; CND 40 elsewhere (effective 2000). adv. bk.rev. **Document type:** *Newsletter.* **Description:** Deals primarily with medical education in Canada. Reports on major activities in Canadian medical schools, such as appointments and promotions, and publishes any other news of interest to medical educators.
Formerly (until vol.7, no.2, 1974): A C M C Newsletter (0001-0774)
Media: Duplicated (not offset).
Published by: Association of Canadian Medical Colleges, 774 Echo Dr, Ottawa, ON K1S 5P2, Canada. TEL 613-730-0687, FAX 613-730-1196, dhawkins@acmc.ca. Ed., R&P David Hawkins. Adv. contact Blandine Stringer. B&W page CND 350; trim 11 x 8.5. Circ: 1,200.

A C P JOURNAL CLUB. see *MEDICAL SCIENCES—Abstracting, Bibliographies, Statistics*

610 614.44 USA ISSN 1044-4211
A C P M NEWS. Text in English. 1957. q. USD 25 (effective 1998). adv. bk.rev. charts. **Document type:** *Newsletter.*
Former titles: Preventive Medicine Newsletter (0199-2481); American College of Preventive Medicine Newsletter (0002-8029)
Related titles: Microform ed.: (from PQC).
Published by: American College of Preventive Medicine, 1660 L St, N W, Ste 206, Washington, DC 20036-5603. TEL 202-466-2044, FAX 202-466-2662, info@acpm.org, http://www.acpm.org. Ed. Jennifer Edward. Pub. Jordan Richland. R&P Jennifer Edwards. Circ: 2,000.

610 500 600 FRA
A F P SCIENCES; bulletin information scientifique, technique, medicale. Text in French. 1976. w. FRF 8,568 domestic; FRF 9,384 foreign (effective 2000). adv. bk.rev.
Published by: Agence France Presse, 13 place de la Bourse, Paris 75002, France. TEL 33-1-40414646, Martine.Merle@afp.com. Ed. Eric Givily.

610 658 CAN
A H R A RECORD. Text in English. bi-m. membership. **Document type:** *Newsletter.*
Published by: Alberta Health Records Association, P O Box 1752, Edmonton, AB T5J 2P1, Canada. TEL 780-538-7526. Ed. Holly Tithecott. Circ: 600.

610 USA
A M A ALLIANCE TODAY. (American Medical Association) Text in English. 1939. 5/yr. USD 7 to non-members; USD 3.50 to members (effective 2001). abstr, charts, illus, stat. **Document type:** *Bulletin, Academic/Scholarly.* **Description:** Presents community health issues and project activities of AMA Alliance members (doctor's spouses), plus physician-spouse-family relationships and financial concerns.
Former titles (until 1996): Facets (Chicago) (0163-0512); (until 1978): M D'S Wife (0024-807X); (until 1965): American Medical Association Auxiliary. Bulletin (0098-3748)
—CCC.
Published by: American Medical Association, 515 N State St, P O Box 10946, Chicago, IL 60610-0946. TEL 312-464-4470, FAX 312-464-5020. Ed. Catherine Potts. Circ: 60,000.

610 AUS ISSN 1329-1955
A M A LIST OF MEDICAL SERVICES AND FEES. (Australian Medical Association) Text in English. 1973. a. adv. back issues avail. **Document type:** *Directory, Trade.*
Published by: Australian Medical Association, Level 4, 42 Macquarie St, Barton, ACT 2600, Australia. TEL 61-6-270-5400, FAX 61-6-270-5499. Ed. Michelle Crybaits. adv.: color page AUD 3,390; bleed 226 x 316. Circ: 20,000.

610 AUS ISSN 0813-6394
A M A VICTORIA BRANCH NEWS. (Australian Medical Association) Text in English. m. AUD 20. adv. illus.
Formerly: Australian Medical Association. Victoria Branch. Monthly Paper
—CCC.
Published by: Australian Medical Association, Victoria Branch, 293 Royal Parade, Parkville, VIC 3052, Australia. FAX 03-347-9871. Circ: (controlled).

610.6 USA
▼ **A M D A ADVOCACY IN ACTION.** Text in English. 1999. m. **Document type:** *Newsletter, Trade.* **Description:** Targeted to individuals from industry who have either supported A M D A projects in the past or have expressed an interest in doing so in the future.
Published by: American Medical Directors Association, 10480 Little Patuxent Pkwy, Ste 760, Columbia, MD 21044. TEL 410-740-9743, 301-596-5774, 800-876-2632, FAX 410-740-4572, publications@amda.com, info@amda.com, http://www.amda.com. Ed. Joanne Kaldy.

610 USA
A M I NEWS*. Text in English. 1958. bi-m. USD 25; USD 30 foreign. adv. bk.rev. illus. **Document type:** *Newsletter.*
Formerly: A M I Newsletter (0001-1916)
Indexed: Ind.Med. (coverage dropped).
Published by: Association of Medical Illustrators, 2965 Flowers Rd S, Ste 105, Atlanta, GA 30341-5520. TEL 770-454-7933, FAX 770-458-3314. Ed. Linda Warren. Adv. contact Vernon Lomax. Circ: 950.

070.5 USA
A M P A NEWSLETTER. Text in English. q. USD 50 to non-members. back issues avail. **Document type:** *Newsletter.* **Description:** Provides information on health science publishing industry.
Published by: American Medical Publishers' Association, 14 Fort Hill Rd, Huntington, NY 11743. TEL 516-423-0075. Ed., R&P Jill Rudansky. Circ: 450.

618 USA
RD598.35.A77
A M S E C T TODAY. Text in English. 1973. m. (11/yr.). USD 55 domestic; USD 80 foreign (effective 2000). back issues avail. **Document type:** *Newsletter, Trade.*
Formerly: Perfusion Life (0747-3079)
Published by: American Society of Extra-Corporeal Technology, Inc., 503 Carlisle Dr, Ste 125, Herndon, VA 20170-4838. TEL 703-435-8556, gcate@amsect.org, http://www.amsect.org. Ed. Joe Deptula. Circ: 2,400.

M

610 USA ISSN 0194-004X
A M W A FREELANCE DIRECTORY. Text in English. 1975. biennial. **Document type:** *Directory.* **Description:** Lists freelance writers specializing in any medical or health care topic.
Media: Online - full text.
Published by: American Medical Writers Association, 40 W Gude Dr No.101, Rockville, MD 20850-1192. TEL 301-493-0003, http://www.amwa.org.

610 USA ISSN 1075-6361
A M W A JOURNAL. Text in English. 1972. q. USD 35 (effective 2000). adv. bk.rev. **Document type:** *Bulletin.*
Formerly: Medical Communications (0090-046X); Which supersedes: American Medical Writers Association. Bulletin (0002-9971)
—BLDSC (4689.103000), ingenta.
Published by: American Medical Writers Association, 40 W Gude Dr No.101, Rockville, MD 20850-1192. TEL 301-493-0003, http://www.amwa.org. Circ: 4,500.

A N A D: WORKING TOGETHER. see *PSYCHOLOGY*

610 USA
A P F NEWS. Text in English. 1953. 2/yr. USD 10 (effective 1999). back issues avail. **Document type:** *Newsletter.* **Description:** Committed to advancing the state of medical education, research and care in Israel.
Published by: American Physicians Fellowship for Medicine in Israel, 2001 Beacon St, Ste 210, Boston, MA 02135-7771. TEL 617-232-5382, FAX 617-739-2616, info@apfmed.org; apf@apfmed.org, http://www.apfmed.org. Ed. Geoffrey Brahmer. R&P Geoffery Brahmer. Circ: 5,000.

A P M I S. (Acta Pathologica Microbiologica et Immunologica Scandinavica) see *BIOLOGY*

A P M I S SUPPLEMENTUM. see *BIOLOGY*

610 USA ISSN 1058-2916
RD130 CODEN: AJOUET
A S A I O JOURNAL. Text in English. 1955. 6/yr. USD 354 domestic to individuals; USD 534 foreign to individuals; USD 488 domestic to institutions; USD 668 foreign to institutions; USD 100 newsstand/cover (effective 2002). adv. charts, illus. index. reprint service avail. from PQC. *Refereed.* **Document type:** *Academic/Scholarly.* **Description:** Covers the theory, design, fabrication, in vitro and animal testing, and human application of devices which substitute for, or replace, diseased human organs.
Formerly (until 1992): A S A I O Transactions (0889-7190); Which was formed by the 1986 merger of: American Society for Artificial Internal Organs. Transactions (0066-0078); (1978-1985): A S A I O Journal (0162-1432)
Related titles: Microform ed.; Online - full text ed.: USD 634.40 domestic academic site license; USD 814.40 foreign academic site license; USD 707.60 domestic corporate site license; USD 887.60 foreign corporate site license (2002) (from Ovid Technologies, Inc., Institute for Scientific Information).
Indexed: ASCA, Chem.Abstr., Curr.Cont., Eng.Ind., Environ.Eng.Abstr., Environ.Sci.Poll.Mgmt., Excerp.Med. (1993-), INIS Atomind., Ind.Med. (1992-), Inpharma, Int.Nurs.Ind., Kidney, Pharm.&Out.News, Reac., Sci.Cit.Ind.
—BLDSC (1738.840500), CASDDS, CISTI, Ei, EMDOCS, GNLM, IDS, ingenta, KNAW, Linda Hall.
Published by: (American Society for Artificial Internal Organs, Inc.), Lippincott Williams & Wilkins (Philadelphia) (Subsidiary of: Wolters Kluwer N.V.), 530 Walnut St, Philadelphia, PA 19106-3621. TEL 215-521-8300, FAX 215-521-8902, http://www.Lww.com. Ed. Dr. Eli A Friedman. Pub. Jim Mulligan. R&P Margaret Becker. Adv. contact Ray Thibodeau. B&W page USD 780, color page USD 1,800; trim 8.12 x 11. Circ: 1,796. **Subscr. to:** PO Box 1600, Hagerstown, MD 21740-1600. TEL 800-777-2295, FAX 301-824-7390.

A S H A. see *HANDICAPPED—Hearing Impaired*

A S H A LEADER; building the future of the professions. see *HANDICAPPED—Hearing Impaired*

610 AUS ISSN 0310-8341
ABORIGINAL MEDICAL SERVICE. NEWSLETTER. Text in English. 1973. irreg., latest 1998, Feb. **Document type:** *Newsletter.*
Published by: Aboriginal Medical Service, PO Box 1174, Strawberry Hills, NSW 2012, Australia. TEL 61-2-9319-5823, FAX 61-2-9319-3345, amsredfern@amsredfern.org.au. Ed. Brendon O'Dwyer. R&P Naomi Mayers.

610 CHL ISSN 0716-2588
ACADEMIA CHILENA DE MEDICINA. BOLETIN ANUAL. Text in Spanish. 1967. a. USD 25. index. back issues avail.
Formerly: Academia de Medicina. Boletin
Indexed: Ind.Med. (coverage dropped).
Published by: Academia Chilena de Medicina, Clasificador, 1349, Santiago 1, Chile. Eds. Dr. Alberto Donoso, Dr. Amador Neghme. Circ: 1,000.

610 MEX
ACADEMIA NACIONAL DE MEDICINA. BOLETIN. Text in Spanish. 1993. q. **Document type:** *Bulletin.* **Description:** Presents activities of the organization.
Published by: Academia Nacional de Medicina, Unidad de Congresos, Bloque B, Centro Medico Nacional, Av. Cuauhtemoc 330, Mexico City, DF 06725, Mexico. TEL 52-5-5782044, FAX 52-5-5784271. Ed. Dr. Aquiles Ayala Ruiz.

310.711 USA ISSN 1040-2446
R11 CODEN: ACMEEO
ACADEMIC MEDICINE. Text in English. 1926. m. USD 120 to individuals; USD 180 to institutions; USD 60 to students (effective 2001). adv. bk.rev. bibl, illus, stat. index. back issues avail. *Refereed.* **Document type:** *Academic/Scholarly.* **Description:** Publishes policy papers, analyses, essays, research reports, and other materials covering the full range of issues facing medical schools, teaching hospitals, academic societies, and health policy agencies.
Former titles (until 1988): Journal of Medical Education (0022-2577); (until 1951): Medical Education
Related titles: Microfiche ed.: (from CIS); Microform ed.: (from PMC,PQC); Online - full text ed.: (from HighWire Pr., Institute for Scientific Information); ♦ Supplement: Association of American Medical Colleges. Proceedings of the Annual Conference. Research in Medical Education. ISSN 0892-2543.
Indexed: AIM, ASCA, Abstr.Health Care Manage.Stud., AgeLine, Behav.Med.Abstr., Biol.Abstr., C.I.J.E., CINAHL, Chem.Abstr., Cont.Pg.Educ., Crim.Just.Abstr., Curr.Cont., Curr.Lit.Fam.Plan., ERA, Educ.Tech.Abstr., Environ.Sci.Poll.Mgmt., Excerp.Med., FAMLI, High.Educ.Abstr., Hosp.Lit.Ind., Ind.Med. (1989-), Ind.Sci.Rev., Inpharma, Int.Nurs.Ind., Med.Care Rev., Mult.Ed.Abstr., Pharm.&Out.News, Pollut.Abstr., PsycInfo, Psychol.Abstr. (1967-), Reac., Res.High.Educ.Abstr., Risk Abstr., SRI, SSCI (coverage dropped), Saf.Sci.Abstr., Sci.Cit.Ind., Sp.Ed.Needs Abstr., Stud.Wom.Abstr., Tech.Educ.Abstr., Trop.Dis.Bull., e-psyche.
—BLDSC (0570.513500), CISTI, EMDOCS, GNLM, IDS, ingenta, KNAW.
Published by: Association of American Medical Colleges, 2450 N St N W, Washington, DC 20037-1126. TEL 202-828-0416, FAX 202-828-1123, orders@allenpress.com, http://www.academicmedicine.org/. Ed., R&P Addeane S Caelleigh. Adv. contact Diane Sherel. Circ: 6,000 (paid). **Subscr.to:** Allen Press Inc., PO Box 1897, Lawrence, KS 66044-8897.

610.711 USA ISSN 1093-1139
ACADEMIC PHYSICIAN AND SCIENTIST. Text in English. 1993. bi-m. USD 85 domestic to individuals; USD 114 foreign to individuals; USD 109 domestic to institutions; USD 150 foreign to institutions; USD 25 newsstand/cover (effective 2002). **Document type:** *Journal, Academic/Scholarly.* **Description:** Features news from the world of medical education along with more than 30 pages of listings for open faculty, administrative, and fellowship positions throughout academic medicine.
Published by: (Association of American Medical Colleges), Lippincott Williams & Wilkins (Philadelphia) (Subsidiary of: Wolters Kluwer N.V.), 530 Walnut St, Philadelphia, PA 19106-3621. TEL 215-521-8300, FAX 215-521-8902, custserv@lww.com, http://www.acphysci.com, http://www.lww.com/. Ed. Fay Jarosh. **Subscr. to:** PO Box 1600, Hagerstown, MD 21740-1600. TEL 800-638-3030, FAX 310-223-2400.

610 USA ISSN 1049-7072
ACADEMIC PRACTICE FACULTY COMPENSATION AND PRODUCTION SURVEY. Text in English. 1989. a. USD 300 to non-members; USD 200 to members (effective 2001). stat. **Document type:** *Bulletin.* **Description:** Covers base and total compensation, three productivity measures, and a ratio of compensation to gross charges.
Related titles: CD-ROM ed.
Published by: Medical Group Management Association, 104 Inverness Terrace E, Englewood, CO 80112. TEL 303-799-1111, FAX 303-397-1827, survey@mgma.com, http://www.mgma.com. Circ: 1,000.

610 USA
ACADEMIC PRACTICE MANAGEMENT COMPENSATION SURVEY. Text in English. 1994. a. USD 115 to non-members; USD 75 to members (effective 2001). stat. **Document type:** *Bulletin.* **Description:** Provides data for academic practices to determine fair compensation for clinical department administrators.
Formerly: Academic Practice Management (1076-1586)
Related titles: CD-ROM ed.
Published by: Medical Group Management Association, 104 Inverness Terrace E, Englewood, CO 80112. TEL 303-799-1111, FAX 303-397-1827, survey@mgma.com, http://www.mgma.com. Circ: 1,000.

610 FRA ISSN 0001-4079
CODEN: BANMAC
ACADEMIE NATIONALE DE MEDECINE. BULLETIN. Text in French. 1836. 9/yr. FRF 650 domestic; FRF 700 foreign. bk.rev. charts. *Refereed.* **Document type:** *Bulletin.*
Formerly: Academie de Medicine. Memoirs
Related titles: Microfilm ed.: (from BHP); Microform ed.: (from BHP); Online - full text ed.: (from Institute for Scientific Information).
Indexed: ASCA, Abstr.Hyg., Anim.Breed.Abstr., B.R.I., Biol.Abstr., C.I.S. Abstr., Chem.Abstr., Chem.Indus.Notes, Chem.Titles, Curr.Adv.Ecol.Sci., Curr.Cont., Excerp.Med., GeoRef, Helminthol.Abstr., INIS Atomind., Ind.Med. (1836-), Ind.Vet., Inpharma, Nutr.Abstr., Pharm.&Out.News, Pig News & Info., Reac., Rev.Appl.Entomol., Rev.Med.& Vet.Mycol., Rural Recreat.Tour.Abstr., Trop.Dis.Bull., Vet.Bull.
—BLDSC (2367.300000), CASDDS, CISTI, GNLM, IDS, Infotrieve, KNAW. **CCC.**
Published by: Academie Nationale de Medecine, 16 rue Bonaparte, Paris Cedex 6 75006, France. TEL 33-1-42345770, FAX 33-1-40468755. Ed. R Bastin. Circ: 1,300.

610 BEL ISSN 0377-8231
R41 CODEN: BMABDZ
ACADEMIE ROYALE DE MEDECINE DE BELGIQUE. BULLETIN ET MEMOIRES. Text in French. 1841. m. BEF 3,500 (effective 2000). **Document type:** *Bulletin.*
Formed by the merger of: Academie Royale de Medecine de Belgique. Memoires. (0065-0595); Academie Royale de Medecine de Belgique. Bulletin (0001-4168)
Indexed: Biol.Abstr., Chem.Abstr., Dent.Ind., Excerp.Med., INIS Atomind., Ind.Med. (1975-), Ref.Zh.
—BLDSC (2853.600500), CASDDS, CISTI, GNLM, KNAW.
Published by: Academie Royale de Medecine de Belgique, Palais des Academies, Rue Ducale 1, Brussels 1000, Belgium. TEL 32-2-5502255, academie.de.medecine@beon.be, http://www.acad-roy-med-belg.org.

610 SGP ISSN 0304-4602
CODEN: AAMSCG
ACADEMY OF MEDICINE, SINGAPORE. ANNALS. Text in English. 1972. bi-m. SGD 90, USD 50 domestic; SGD 120 foreign (effective 2000). adv. bk.rev. bibl, charts, illus. *Refereed.* **Document type:** *Academic/Scholarly.* **Description:** Published to help young writers improve in medical and scientific writing.
Related titles: Online - full text ed.
Indexed: AgeLine, Dent.Ind., Excerp.Med., ExtraMED, Ind.Med. (1972-), Inpharma, Int.Nurs.Ind., Reac., So.Pac.Per.Ind.
—BLDSC (1018.300000), CISTI, EMDOCS, GNLM, KNAW.
Published by: Academy of Medicine Singapore, 16 College Rd, 01-01 College Medicine Bldg, Singapore 169854, Singapore. TEL 65-2245166, FAX 65-2255155, anacadsg@pacific.net.sg, annals@academyofmedicine.edu.sg, http://www.annalsmed.org. Ed., R&P Dr. Felix X Sundram. adv.: B&W page SGD 800, color page SGD 1,000; trim 210 x 280.

610 CAN ISSN 0001-4311
ACADEMY OF MEDICINE, TORONTO. BULLETIN. Text in English. 1927. m. CND 12.50. adv. bk.rev. charts. index. **Document type:** *Bulletin.*
—CISTI, GNLM, Infotrieve. **CCC.**
Published by: Academy of Medicine, Toronto, 704 Spadina Rd Sta A, P O Box 549, Toronto, ON M5S 2T1, Canada. TEL 416-922-1134. Ed. Dr. Ted Mullens. Circ: 2,700.

610 ITA ISSN 0394-8811
ACCADEMIA DELLA SCIENZE MEDICHE. ATTI. Text in Italian; Summaries in English, French. 1889. a.
Formerly (1890-1946): Reale Accademia delle Scienze Mediche. Atti (0394-9613)
Published by: Accademia della Scienze Mediche, Via Liborio Giuffre', 5, Palermo, PA 90127, Italy. TEL 091-217938. Ed. Giuseppe Di Gesu.

M

610 ITA ISSN 0390-7783
CODEN: AFISAT
ACCADEMIA DELLE SCIENZE DI SIENA DETTA DE FISIOCRITICI. ATTI. Text in Italian. 1761. a., latest 15th series. ITL 25,000. back issues avail. *Refereed.* **Document type:** *Journal, Academic/Scholarly.* **Description:** Covers medicine, natural sciences, physics and chemistry.
Formerly: Accademia dei Fisiocritici, Siena. Sezione Medico-Fisica (0065-0722)
Indexed: Biol.Abstr., Zoo.Rec.
—CASDDS, CISTI, GNLM.
Published by: Accademia delle Scienze di Siena Detta de Fisiocritici, Piazza S Agostino, 5, Siena, SI 53100, Italy. TEL 39-0577-47002, fisiocritici@unisi.it, fisiocritici@unisi.it. Ed. Baccio Baccetti Niccolini. Circ: 500.

610 AUS ISSN 0817-1351
ACCESS (TOORAK). Text in English. 1976. q. AUD 80 to non-members (effective 1999). adv. **Document type:** *Academic/Scholarly.* **Description:** Diary of postgraduate medical events in Australia and overseas.
Published by: Victorian Medical Postgraduate Foundation Inc., PO Box 27, Parkville, VIC 3052, Australia. TEL 61-3-9347-9633, FAX 61-3-9347-4547, vmpf@vicnet.net.au. Circ: 600.

ACCREDITATION MANUAL FOR AMBULATORY CARE. see *HEALTH FACILITIES AND ADMINISTRATION*

ACCREDITATION MANUAL FOR HOME CARE. VOL. 1: STANDARDS. see *HEALTH FACILITIES AND ADMINISTRATION*

ACCREDITATION MANUAL FOR HOME CARE. VOL. 2: SCORING GUIDELINES. see *HEALTH FACILITIES AND ADMINISTRATION*

ACCREDITATION MANUAL FOR HOSPITALS. VOL. 1: STANDARDS. see *HEALTH FACILITIES AND ADMINISTRATION*

ACCREDITATION MANUAL FOR HOSPITALS. VOL. 2: SCORING GUIDELINES. see *HEALTH FACILITIES AND ADMINISTRATION*

ACCREDITATION MANUAL FOR LONG TERM CARE. see *HEALTH FACILITIES AND ADMINISTRATION*

610 CUB ISSN 1024-9435
ACIMED. Text in Spanish. 1993. q. CUP 9 domestic; USD 30 in North America; USD 32 in South America; USD 34 elsewhere (effective 2001). back issues avail. **Document type:** *Academic/Scholarly.* **Description:** Aims to provide a forum for professionals in the medical and health sciences in Cuba.
Related titles: Online - full text ed.: ISSN 1561-2880.
Published by: Centro Nacional de Informacion de Ciencias Medicas Ed. Illiana Herrera-Lopez. Circ: 1,000.

ACTA ANATOMICA NIPPONICA/KAIBOGAKU ZASSHI. see *BIOLOGY*

ACTA BIOLOGICA ET MEDICA. see *BIOLOGY*

610 BEL
ACTA BIOMEDICA LOVANIENSIA. Text in English. 1988. irreg., latest vol.243, 2001 (8-10/yr.). price varies. back issues avail. **Document type:** *Monographic series, Academic/Scholarly.* **Description:** Research monographs on topics in the bio-medical sciences.
Published by: Leuven University Press, Blijde Inkomststraat 5, Leuven 3000, Belgium. TEL 32-16-325345, FAX 32-16-325352, university.press@upers.kuleuven.ac.be, http://www.lup.be.

610 BEL ISSN 0001-5512
CODEN: ACCBAT
ACTA CLINICA BELGICA. Text in Dutch, French. 1945. bi-m. (6 nos./vol.), latest vol.57. BEF 2,000 domestic; BEF 2,500 foreign; BEF 550 newsstand/cover (effective 2002). adv. bk.rev. abstr, bibl. index. back issues avail.; reprint service avail. from ISI. *Refereed.* **Document type:** *Journal, Academic/Scholarly.*
Formerly (until 1946): Societe Clinique des Hopitaux de Bruxelles. Bulletins et Comptes Rendus
Related titles: Online - full text ed.: (from Institute for Scientific Information).
Indexed: ASCA, Abstr.Hyg., Agri.& Environ.Biotech.Abstr. (coverage dropped), Biol.Abstr., Chem.Abstr., Curr.Adv.Cancer Res., Curr.Adv.Ecol.Sci., Curr.Cont., Derwent Biotech.Abstr., Environ.Sci.Poll.Mgmt., Excerp.Med., Helminthol.Abstr., Ind.Med. (1946-), Ind.Sci.Rev., Inpharma, Int.Abstr.Biol.Sci., Nutr.Abstr., Pharm.&Out.News, Pollut.Abstr., Protozool.Abstr., Reac., Rev.Appl.Entomol., Rev.Med.& Vet.Mycol., Risk Abstr., Saf.Sci.Abstr., Sci.Cit.Ind. (coverage dropped).
—BLDSC (0611.650000), CASDDS, CISTI, EMDOCS, GNLM, IDS, KNAW.
Address: c/o University Hospital Gent, Renal Division, De Pintelaan 185, Ghent 9000, Belgium. TEL 32-9-240-4402, FAX 32-9-240-4403, acb@rug.ac.be, http://www.auserve.rug.ac.be.tf. Ed., R&P Dr. N Lameire. Adv. contact M Goossens. Circ: 1,200.

610 HRV ISSN 0353-9466
CODEN: ABSJAO
ACTA CLINICA CROATICA; journal for clinical medicine and other related fields. Text in English; Summaries in Croatian, English. 1962. q. USD 50 (effective 2001). adv. bk.rev., Website rev. bibl, illus. *Refereed.* **Document type:** *Monographic series, Academic/Scholarly.* **Description:** Publishes original scientific papers, preliminary communications, professional papers, reviews and reports from congresses and symposia from the field of clinical medicine and related fields.
Former titles (until 1991): Anali Klinicke Bolnice "Dr. M. Stojanovic" (0301-2255); Anali Bolnice "Dr. M. Stojanovic"
Related titles: Microform ed.; Online - full text ed.; ♦ Supplement: Acta Clinica Croatica. Supplement. ISSN 0353-9474.
Indexed: Biol.Abstr., Excerp.Med. (1993-).
—BLDSC (0611.650200), CISTI, EMDOCS, KNAW.
Published by: Sestre Milosrdnice University Hospital, Vinogradska 29, Zagreb 10000, Croatia. TEL 385-1-3787173, FAX 385-1-37077, editor@acta-clinica.com, http://www.acta-clinca.com. Eds. Vida Demarin, Zvonko Kusic. Circ: 1,000.

610 HRV ISSN 0353-9474
ACTA CLINICA CROATICA. SUPPLEMENT. Text in English. 1971. irreg.
Formerly (until 1990): Anali Klinicke Bolnice. Suplement (0301-2263)
Related titles: Online - full text ed.; ♦ Supplement to: Acta Clinica Croatica. ISSN 0353-9466.
—BLDSC (0611.650210).
Published by: Sestre Milosrdnice University Hospital, Vinogradska 29, Zagreb 10000, Croatia. TEL 385-1-3787173, FAX 385-1-37077, editor@acta-clinica.com, http://www.acta-clinca.com.

610 HRV ISSN 0065-1206
CODEN: AFMFBB
ACTA FACULTATIS MEDICAE FLUMINENSIS; journal of the faculty of medicine, University of Rijeka. Text in Croatian, English. 1963. s-a. HRK 50 to individuals; HRK 100 to institutions (effective 2000). adv. bk.rev. bibl, charts, illus, mkt, stat. reprints avail. **Document type:** *Academic/Scholarly.* **Description:** Publishes leading articles, original scientific and professional papers, preliminary communications, review articles, reports on scientific meetings and congresses, and other contributions.
Related titles: Fax ed.
Indexed: Biol.Abstr., Chem.Abstr., Excerp.Med. (1988-).
—BLDSC (0580.750000), CASDDS, EMDOCS, GNLM.
Published by: Sveuciliste u Rijeci, Medicinski Fakultet, Branchetta 20-22, Rijeka 51000, Croatia. TEL 385-51-65111, FAX 385-51-651215, dobrila@mamed.medri.hr, http://www.medri.hr/acta.html. Ed. Juraj Sepcic. Pub., R&P Stipan Jonjic TEL 385-51-651100. Adv. contact Mirjana Kunisek. B&W page USD 50, color page USD 500. Circ: 600.

610 CZE ISSN 0521-2561
CODEN: AMUBAJ
ACTA FACULTATIS MEDICAE UNIVERSITATIS BRUNENSIS. Text and summaries in Czech, English, Russian. 1958. irreg. price varies. bk.rev.
Indexed: Apic.Abstr., Biol.Abstr., Excerp.Med.
—CASDDS, KNAW. **CCC.**
Published by: Masarykova Universita, Lekarska Fakulta/Masaryk University, Medical Faculty, Komenskeho nam 2, Brno 66243, Czech Republic. Ed. Dr. Milan Dokladal. Circ: 800.

ACTA GENETICAE MEDICAE ET GEMELLOLOGIAE: TWIN RESEARCH. see *BIOLOGY—Genetics*

ACTA HISTORICA LEOPOLDINA. see *SCIENCES: COMPREHENSIVE WORKS*

ACTA HISTORICA LEOPOLDINA. SUPPLEMENT. see *SCIENCES: COMPREHENSIVE WORKS*

ACTA HISTORICA SCIENTIARUM NATURALIUM ET MEDICINALIUM. see *SCIENCES: COMPREHENSIVE WORKS*

610 CUB ISSN 0864-3210
ACTA MEDICA. Text in Spanish; Summaries in English, Spanish. 1987. s-a. USD 28 in South America; USD 30 in North America; USD 34 elsewhere. **Document type:** *Government.* **Description:** Covers clinical and preventive medicine.
Published by: (Cuba. Hospital Clinico Quirurgico "Hermanos Ameijeiras"), Editorial de Ciencias Medicas, O'Reilly No. 4, Habana, Cuba. TEL 537-628091, FAX 537-338187, ileana@bmn1.sld.cu. Ed. Maura Diaz. Circ: 1,500.

610 CZE ISSN 1211-4286
R95.P7 CODEN: SVLKAO
ACTA MEDICA. Text and summaries in English. 1958. 4/yr. CZK 800 (effective 1999). adv. bk.rev. illus. *Refereed.* **Document type:** *Journal, Academic/Scholarly.* **Description:** Publishes review articles, and original papers from different clinical and theoretical medical disciplines. Includes brief communications, case reports, announcements and notices.
Formerly: Universita Karlova. Lekarska Fakulta. Sbornik Vedeckych Praci (0049-5514)
Related titles: ♦ Supplement: Acta Medica. Supplementum. ISSN 1211-247X.
Indexed: Chem.Abstr., Chem.Indus.Notes, Chem.Titles, INIS Atomind., Ind.Med. (1996-).
—BLDSC (0632.631000), CASDDS, GNLM.
Published by: (Univerzita Karlova, Lekarska Fakulta), Vydavatelstvi Karolinum, Ovocny trh 5, Prague 116 36, Czech Republic. TEL 42-2-24491270, FAX 42-2-24212041, edice@cuni.cz, edice@cuni.cz; gersl@lfhk.cuni.cz. Ed. Vladimir Gersl. Adv. contact Marcela Machackova. Circ: 270. **Subscr. to:** Dlouha 91-92, Hradec Kralove 500 01, Czech Republic.

610 MEX ISSN 0001-5997
R21 CODEN: ACMDBI
ACTA MEDICA. Text in Spanish; Summaries in English, Spanish. 1965. q. MXP 500, USD 20. adv. bk.rev. bibl, charts, illus.
Indexed: Biol.Abstr.
—CASDDS, CISTI.
Published by: Instituto Politecnico Nacional, Escuela Superior de Medicina, Prolongacion de Diaz Miron y Plan de San Luis, 2 piso, Apdos. Postales 42-161 y 42-200 (ZP), Mexico City, 17, DF 11340, Mexico. Ed. Carlos de la Vega Lezama.

610 AUT ISSN 0303-8173
CODEN: AMAUBB
ACTA MEDICA AUSTRIACA. Text in German, English; Summaries in English. 1920. 5/yr. ATS 2,325.20 in Europe; ATS 2,490.30 elsewhere; ATS 2,557.72 in Europe print & online eds. combined; ATS 2,739.33 elsewhere print & online eds. combined (effective 2001). adv. bk.rev. illus, stat. index. reprint service avail. from ISI. *Refereed.* **Document type:** *Journal, Academic/Scholarly.*
Formerly: Wiener Zeitschrift fuer Innere Medizin und ihre Grenzgebiete. (0043-5376)
Related titles: ♦ Online - full text ed.: Acta Medica Austriaca Online. ISSN 1563-2571.
Indexed: ASCA, Biol.Abstr., Chem.Abstr., Curr.Cont., Dent.Ind., Derwent Biotech.Abstr., Dok.Arbeitsmed., Excerp.Med., INIS Atomind., Ind.Med. (1974-), Ind.Sci.Rev., Inpharma, Nutr.Abstr., Pharm.&Out.News, Reac., Ref.Zh., Rev.Appl.Entomol., Sci.Cit.Ind.
—BLDSC (0633.100000), ADONIS, CASDDS, CISTI, EMDOCS, GNLM, IDS, Infotrieve, KNAW. **CCC.**
Published by: (Oesterreichische und Wiener Gesellschaft fuer Innere Medizin), Blackwell Wissenschafts-Verlag Vienna, Firmiangasse 7-1, Vienna, W 1130, Austria. TEL 43-1-8779351-0, FAX 43-1-877935124, verlag@blackwis.at, http://www.blackwell.de/ama.htm. Ed. Dr. M Weissel. Circ: 1,500. **Co-sponsors:** Oesterreichische Gesellschaft fuer Innere Medizin; Oesterreichische Nuklearmedizinische Gesellschaft; Austro-Transplant.

610 AUT ISSN 1563-2571
ACTA MEDICA AUSTRIACA ONLINE. Text in German. 5/yr. ATS 2,093 (effective 2001). **Document type:** *Academic/Scholarly.*
Media: Online - full text (from Munksgaard & Blackwell Science's Synergy, Institute for Scientific Information).
Related titles: ♦ Print ed.: Acta Medica Austriaca. ISSN 0303-8173.

M

Published by: Blackwell Wissenschafts-Verlag Vienna, Firmiangasse 7-1, Vienna, W 1130, Austria. TEL 43-1-8779351-0, FAX 43-1-877935124, verlag@blackwis.at, http://www.blackwell.de/ama.htm.

610 DEU ISSN 0946-3445
ACTA MEDICA BALTICA. Text and summaries in English. 1994. s-a. EUR 30, USD 45 (effective 2001). adv. bk.rev. *Refereed.* **Document type:** *Journal, Academic/Scholarly.*
—GNLM.
Published by: Pabst Science Publishers, Am Eichengrund 28, Lengerich 49525, Germany. TEL 49-5484-308, FAX 49-5484-550, pabst.publishers@t-online.de, http://www.pabst-publishers.de. Ed. Regina Svirska.

610 CRI ISSN 0001-6012
CODEN: ATCTAW
ACTA MEDICA COSTARRICENSE. Text in Spanish; Summaries in English. 1957. 3/yr. CRC 25. adv. abstr, charts, illus. index.
Indexed: Biol.Abstr., Chem.Abstr., Excerp.Med.
—CASDDS, CISTI.
Published by: Colegio de Medicos y Cirujanos, Apdo 4054, San Jose 1000, Costa Rica. Circ: 2,000.

616.07 HRV ISSN 1330-0164
CODEN: AMCREF
ACTA MEDICA CROATICA. Text in English, French, German, Serbo-Croatian; Summaries in English, Serbo-Croatian. 1946. 5/yr. USD 150. adv. index. **Document type:** *Academic/Scholarly.*
Former titles (until 1991): Acta Medica Iugoslavica (0375-8338); Acta Medica Iugoslavica (English Edition) (0375-8346)
Indexed: Biol.Abstr., Chem.Abstr., Dent.Ind., Excerp.Med., INIS Atomind., Ind.Med. (1991-).
—BLDSC (0633.600000), CASDDS, CISTI, EMDOCS, GNLM.
Published by: Hravatska Akademija Medicinskih Znanosti/Croatian Academy of Medical Sciences, Subiceva 29, Zagreb 41000, Croatia. TEL 38-41-419446. Ed. Stojan Knezevic. Circ: 800.

610 DOM ISSN 0379-4857
CODEN: AMDOEB
ACTA MEDICA DOMINICANA; revista cientifica para medicos. Text in Spanish. 1979. bi-m. DOP 125, USD 40. adv. bk.rev. bibl, charts, illus.
Indexed: Excerp.Med.
—BLDSC (0633.750000), EMDOCS.
Address: Apdo. de Correos 20102, Jose Contreras 8, Santo Domingo, Dominican Republic. TEL 809-688-4010. Eds. Dr. Julio M Rodriguez, Dr. Mariano Defillo.

610 570 JPN ISSN 0567-7734
CODEN: AMBNAS
ACTA MEDICA ET BIOLOGICA/IGAKU SEIBUTSUGAKU KENKYU KIYO. Text in English, Multiple languages. 1953. q. JPY 10,000. **Document type:** *Academic/Scholarly.*
Indexed: Abstr.Hyg., Biol.Abstr., Chem.Abstr., Chem.Indus.Notes, Chem.Titles, Excerp.Med., Helminthol.Abstr., INIS Atomind., Ind.Vet., Nutr.Abstr., Pig News & Info., Protozool.Abstr., Rev.Arom.& Med.Plants.
—BLDSC (0634.000000), CASDDS, CISTI, EMDOCS, GNLM, ingenta, KNAW.
Published by: Niigata Daigaku, Igakubu/Niigata University, School of Medicine, Ichiban-cho, Asahimachi-dori, Niigata 951, Japan. Ed. Tsuneo Fujita. Circ: 100 (paid); 600 (controlled).

610 BGR ISSN 0515-2925
ACTA MEDICA ET SOCIOLOGICA. Text in Bulgarian. 1962. irreg., latest vol.9, 1983. **Document type:** *Proceedings.*
Published by: International Medical Association for the Study of Living Conditions and Health, c/o T Tashev, 15 Blvd D Nestorov 15, Sofia 1431, Bulgaria.

610 IRN ISSN 0044-6025
CODEN: AMEIAS
ACTA MEDICA IRANICA. Text in English, French, German; Summaries in English, French. 1960. q. IRR 2,000, USD 20. charts, illus. index. *Refereed.* **Document type:** *Academic/Scholarly.* **Description:** Publishes original research papers, case reports, review articles on all aspects of the medical sciences.
Indexed: Abstr.Hyg., Biol.Abstr., Chem.Abstr., Excerp.Med., Nutr.Abstr., Rev.Med.& Vet.Mycol., Trop.Dis.Bull.
—BLDSC (0635.080000), CASDDS, CISTI, GNLM.
Published by: Tehran University of Medical Sciences, Faculty of Medicine, Poursina St., Tehran 14174, Iran. TEL 98-21-6112743, FAX 98-21-6404377. Ed. Dr. Parviz Jabalameli. Circ: 2,000.

610 JPN ISSN 0386-6092
CODEN: AMKUDT
ACTA MEDICA KINKI UNIVERSITY. Text and summaries in English. 1976. q. JPY 4,000. bk.rev. index. back issues avail. *Refereed.* **Document type:** *Academic/Scholarly.* **Description:** Covers original articles, reviews and case reports of inventive work on medical services.
Indexed: Chem.Abstr., Chem.Indus.Notes, Chem.Titles, Excerp.Med., Ref.Zh.
—BLDSC (0632.684000), CASDDS, GNLM.
Published by: Kinki University Medical Association/Kinki Daigaku Igakkai, 2-377 Ono-Higashi, Osakasayama-shi, Osaka-fu 589-0014, Japan. TEL 81-723-66-0221, FAX 81-723-67-8810. Ed. Takanori Tomura. Circ: 1,300.

610 LTU ISSN 1392-0138
ACTA MEDICA LITUANICA. Text in Lithuanian. 1994. q. USD 145 in United States. adv. **Document type:** *Academic/Scholarly.*
Indexed: INIS Atomind.
—GNLM.
Published by: (Lietuvos Mokslu Akademija), Leidykla Academia, Traku str 15-4, Vilnius 2000, Lithuania. TEL 370-2-625814, FAX 370-2-222832, jurga@mdc.elnet.lt. Ed. A Martsankiavichus. R&P A Garliauskas. Adv. contact A. Garliauskas. Circ: 400. **US dist. addr.:** East View Publications, 3020 Harbor Ln N, Minneapolis, MN 55447. TEL 612-550-0961.

610 YUG ISSN 0365-4478
CODEN: AMMNCH
ACTA MEDICA MEDIANAE✱ . Text in Serbo-Croatian. 1962. 8/yr. YUN 40. adv. bk.rev.
Indexed: Biol.Abstr., Chem.Abstr.
—CASDDS.
Published by: Srpsko Lekarsko Drustvo, Podruznica u Nisu, Nis, Serbia 18000, Yugoslavia. Ed. Radoslav Zivic. Circ: 700.

610 ITA ISSN 0393-6384
ACTA MEDICA MEDITERRANEA. Text in English, French, Italian. 1960. 3/yr. ITL 60,000; ITL 10,000 foreign (effective 1998). adv. abstr, bibl, illus, stat. index. **Document type:** *Proceedings, Academic/Scholarly.* **Description:** Clinical cases are reviewed and discussed.
Formerly: Archivio Siciliano di Medicina e Chirurgia (Sezione Medica)
Indexed: Ref.Zh.
Published by: Carbone Editore, Via Gaetano Daita, 29, Palermo, PA 90139, Italy. TEL 39-91-321-273, FAX 39-91-321782. Ed. Antonino Pennino. Pub. Alfonsa Carbone. R&P Alfonso Carbone. Adv. contact Donatella Donato. Circ: 3,000.

610 JPN ISSN 0001-6055
CODEN: AMNKAB
ACTA MEDICA NAGASAKIENSIA. Text in English. 1939. q. per issue exchange basis. charts, illus. index. *Refereed.* **Document type:** *Academic/Scholarly.* **Description:** Includes original articles, review articles, technical notes, and case reports in medicine.
Indexed: Abstr.Hyg., Biol.Abstr., Chem.Abstr., Chem.Indus.Notes, Chem.Titles, Excerp.Med., INIS Atomind., Ind.Med. (coverage dropped), Nutr.Abstr., Ref.Zh., Trop.Dis.Bull.
—BLDSC (0635.150000), CASDDS, CISTI, EMDOCS, GNLM, KNAW.
Published by: Nagasaki Daigaku, Igakubu/Nagasaki University, School of Medicine, 12-4 Sakamo-To, Nagasaki-shi, Nagasaki-ken 852-8102, Japan. TEL 81-95-849-7353, FAX 81-95-849-7357, http://www.lb.nagasaki-u.ac.jp/kiyo/amn/index.html. Ed., R&P Kuniaki Hayashi. Circ: 350.

610 JPN ISSN 0386-300X
CODEN: AMOKAG
ACTA MEDICA OKAYAMA. Text in English. 1928. bi-m. free per issue or exchange basis. adv. bk.rev. bibl, charts, illus. index, cum.index. back issues avail.; reprint service avail. from ISI. *Refereed.* **Document type:** *Academic/Scholarly, Abstract/Index.* **Description:** Publishes papers from all areas of basic and clinical medicine.
Formerly: Acta Medicinae Okayama (0001-6152)
Related titles: Online - full text ed.: (from Institute for Scientific Information).
Indexed: ASCA, Abstr.Hyg., Biol.Abstr., C.I.S. Abstr., Chem.Abstr., Chem.Indus.Notes, Chem.Titles, Curr.Adv.Cancer Res., Curr.Adv.Cell & Devel.Biol., Curr.Adv.Ecol.Sci., Curr.Cont., Dairy Sci.Abstr., Dent.Ind., Environ.Sci.Poll.Mgmt., Excerp.Med., Helminthol.Abstr., INIS Atomind., Ind.Med. (1973-), Ind.Sci.Rev., Ind.Vet., Inpharma, Int.Nurs.Ind., Nutr.Abstr., Pharm.&Out.News, Pollut.Abstr., Protozool.Abstr., Reac., Ref.Zh., Risk Abstr., SSCI (coverage dropped), Saf.Sci.Abstr., Sci.Cit.Ind., Trop.Dis.Bull., Vet.Bull.
—BLDSC (0635.155000), CASDDS, CISTI, GNLM, IDS, ingenta, KNAW.
Published by: Okayama Daigaku, Igakubu/Okayama University, School of Medicine, 2-5-1 Shikata-cho, Okayama-shi, Okayama-ken 700-0914, Japan. TEL 81-86-235-7057, FAX 81-86-235-7059, actamed@cc.okayama-u.ac.jp. Ed., R&P Tadaatsu Akagi. Adv. contact Takao Tsuji. Circ: 600 (controlled).

610 PER ISSN 1018-8800
ACTA MEDICA PERUANA. Text in Spanish; Summaries in English. 1972. q. USD 6. adv. abstr, charts, illus. index.
Indexed: Biol.Abstr., Curr.Cont. (coverage dropped), INIS Atomind.
Published by: Colegio Medico del Peru, Malecon Armendarir, 791, Miraflores, Lima 18, Peru. Ed. Dr. Fausto Garmendia. Circ: 10,000.

610 PHL ISSN 0001-6071
CODEN: AMPIAF
ACTA MEDICA PHILIPPINA. Text in English. 1938. q. PHP 120, USD 40. adv. bk.rev. abstr, charts, illus. index. **Document type:** *Academic/Scholarly.*
Incorporates: University of the Philippines. College of Medicine. Proceedings
Indexed: Abstr.Hyg., Biol.Abstr., Chem.Abstr., Excerp.Med., INIS Atomind., Ind.Med. (coverage dropped), Ind.Phil.Per.
—CASDDS, CISTI, GNLM.
Published by: University of the Philippines, College of Medicine, P.O. Box 593, Manila, Philippines. Ed. Dr. Romeo R Gutierrez. Circ: 2,000. **Co-sponsor:** College of Public Health.

610 ITA ISSN 0001-6098
CODEN: AMROBA
ACTA MEDICA ROMANA. Text in English. 1963. q. ITL 182,000 domestic; USD 128 foreign (effective 2001); ITL 63,000 newsstand/cover (2001). adv. bk.rev. abstr, bibl, charts, illus, stat. index. **Document type:** *Academic/Scholarly.* **Description:** Publishes original research in psychology, biology, medicine and surgery.
Indexed: Biol.Abstr., Chem.Abstr., Chem.Indus.Notes, Chem.Titles, Excerp.Med. (1994-), e-psyche.
—BLDSC (0635.250000), CASDDS, CISTI, EMDOCS, GNLM.
Published by: (Facolta di Medicina e Chirurgia, Universita Cattolica del Sacro Cuore), Vita e Pensiero, Largo Gemelli 1, Milan, MI 20123, Italy. TEL 39-02-7234-2370, FAX 39-02-7234-2974, TELEX 321033 UCATMI 1, redazione.vp@mi.unicatt.it. Ed. Tommaso Galeotti. Circ: 450.

610 CZE ISSN 1211-247X
CODEN: SVKSA9
ACTA MEDICA. SUPPLEMENTUM. Text in Czech; Summaries in English. 1958. s-a. CZK 600 (effective 1999). adv. bk.rev. illus. *Refereed.* **Document type:** *Academic/Scholarly.* **Description:** Publishes papers from different clinical and theoretical medical disciplines.
Formerly: Universita Karlova. Lekarska Fakulta. Sbornik Vedeckych Praci. Supplementum (0049-5522)
Related titles: ♦ Supplement to: Acta Medica. ISSN 1211-4286.
Indexed: INIS Atomind., Ind.Med. (199?-).
—BLDSC (0632.631100).
Published by: (Universita Karlova, Lekarska Fakulta), Vydavatelstvi Karolinum, Ovocny trh 5, Prague 116 36, Czech Republic. TEL 42-2-24491270, FAX 42-2-24212041, educe@cuni.cz; gersl@lfhk.cuni.cz. Ed. Vladimir Gersl. Adv. contact Marcela Machackova. Circ: 270.

ACTA PHYSIOLOGICA SCANDINAVICA. see *BIOLOGY—Physiology*

ACTA PHYSIOLOGICA SCANDINAVICA. SUPPLEMENTUM. see *BIOLOGY—Physiology*

ACTA REGIAE SOCIETATIS SCIENTIARUM ET LITTERARUM GOTHOBURGENSIS. BIOMEDICA. see *BIOLOGY*

610 340 ITA ISSN 1121-2098
CODEN: ATLMEQ
ACTA TECNOLOGIAE ET LEGIS MEDICAMENTI. Text in Italian. 1990. 3/yr. ITL 90,000; ITL 140,000 foreign (effective 1998). **Document type:** *Academic/Scholarly.*
Indexed: Excerp.Med. (1995-).
—BLDSC (0664.450000), CASDDS, EMDOCS, GNLM.
Published by: Casa Editrice Maccari, Via Palermo, 44, Parma, PR 43100, Italy. TEL 39-521-771268. Circ: 1,000.

ACTA TROPICA; journal of biomedical sciences. see *MEDICAL SCIENCES—Communicable Diseases*

ACTA UNIVERSITARIA. see *SCIENCES: COMPREHENSIVE WORKS*

610 CZE ISSN 0001-7116
CODEN: AUNCA9
ACTA UNIVERSITATIS CAROLINAE: MEDICA. Text in English. a. USD 66 (effective 1999). **Document type:** *Academic/Scholarly.* **Description:** Summarizes results of studies in anatomy.
Indexed: Biol.Abstr., C.I.S. Abstr., Chem.Abstr., Chem.Indus.Notes, Chem.Titles, Dent.Ind., Diar.Dis.Res., Excerp.Med., INIS Atomind., Ind.Med. (1954-).
—BLDSC (0584.520000), CASDDS, CISTI, GNLM, KNAW.
Published by: (Univerzita Karlova, Fakulta Vseobecneho Lekarstvi), Vydavatelstvi Karolinum, Ovocny trh 5, Prague 116 36, Czech Republic. TEL 42-2-24491270, FAX 42-2-24212041, edice@cuni.cz; milan.spala@lfl.cuni.cz. Ed. Milan Spala. **Subscr. to:** 1 LF UK, Katerinska 32, Prague 121 08, Czech Republic.

610 FIN ISSN 0355-3221
CODEN: AUODDK
ACTA UNIVERSITATIS OULUENSIS. SERIES D. MEDICA. Text in English. 1972. irreg. price varies. cum.index. back issues avail. *Refereed.* **Document type:** *Monographic series, Academic/Scholarly.* **Description:** Publishes medical dissertations and monographs.
Related titles: Fax ed.; Online - full text ed.
Indexed: Biol.Abstr., Curr.Adv.Cell & Devel.Biol., Curr.Adv.Ecol.Sci., Curr.Adv.Gen.& Molec.Biol., IBZ, Psychol.Abstr., Ref.Zh.
—BLDSC (0585.290000), CASDDS, KNAW.
Published by: University of Oulu, Publications Committee, PL 5000, Oulu 90401, Finland. FAX 358-81-537-53-20, olli.vuolteenaho@oulu.fi, http://herkules.oulu.fi/ulkaisutoimikunta/hist.html.en. Ed., R&P Olli Vuolteenaho. Circ: 400. **Dist. by:** Oulu University Library, PL 7500, Oulu 90401, Finland. FAX 358-81-5533047.

610 CZE ISSN 0301-2514
CODEN: AUPMAF
ACTA UNIVERSITATIS PALACKIANAE OLOMUCENSIS. FACULTATIS MEDICAE. Text in English. 1955. q. CZK 520 domestic; USD 170 foreign (effective 2000). adv. bk.rev. charts, illus. *Refereed.* **Document type:** *Academic/Scholarly.*
Formerly: Acta Universitatis Palackianae, Facultatis Medicae (0001-7167)
Indexed: Bibl.Ling., Biol.Abstr., C.I.S. Abstr., Chem.Abstr., Chem.Indus.Notes, Chem.Titles, Dent.Ind., Excerp.Med., Helminthol.Abstr., INIS Atomind., Ind.Med. (1960-).
—BLDSC (0585.450000), CASDDS, CISTI, KNAW.
Published by: Universita Palackeho Olomouc, Lekarska Fakulta/Palacky University, Medical Faculty, Olomouc, Hnevotinska 3, Olomouc 77515, Czech Republic. TEL 420-68-5632301, FAX 420-68-5632966, VILIM@RISC.UPOL.CZ. Ed., Adv. contact Vilim Simanek. Circ: 400.

ACTA UNIVERSITATIS UPSALIENSIS. see *SCIENCES: COMPREHENSIVE WORKS*

610 PRT
ACTUALIDADES MEDICAS. Text in Portuguese. 104/yr.
Address: Rua Tristao Vaz, 15-2o D, Lisbon 1400, Portugal.

610 CAN ISSN 0229-9429
L'ACTUALITE MEDICALE. Text in French. 1980. 44/yr. CND 49. **Document type:** *Magazine, Trade.*
Published by: Rogers Media Publishing Ltd, 1001 boul de Maisonneuve Ouest, Rm 1100, Montreal, PQ H3A 3E1, Canada. TEL 514-843-2581, FAX 514-845-7503, http://www.medalliance.ca, http://www.rogers.com. Ed. Michel Legault.

ACUPUNCTURE AND ELECTRO-THERAPEUTICS RESEARCH; the international journal. see *ALTERNATIVE MEDICINE*

ACUPUNCTURE IN MEDICINE. see *ALTERNATIVE MEDICINE*

610.74 ZAF ISSN 0379-6531
ADLER MUSEUM BULLETIN. Text in English. 1975. 3/yr. ZAR 90 domestic to individuals; ZAR 200 domestic to libraries; USD 30 foreign (effective 2001). adv. bk.rev. **Document type:** *Newsletter, Academic/Scholarly.* **Description:** Covers topics relating to the history of medicine.
Indexed: Ind.S.A.Per.
—BLDSC (0681.740000).
Published by: Adler Museum of Medicine, 7 York Rd, Parktown, Johannesburg 2198, South Africa. TEL 27-11-7172081, FAX 27-11-7172067, 178wam@chiron.wits.ac.za, http://www.sunsite.wits.ac.za/museums/adler.html. Ed., R&P Asher Dubb. Adv. contact L Immelman. Circ: 500.

614.58 USA ISSN 0894-587X
RA790.A1 CODEN: APMHEM
ADMINISTRATION AND POLICY IN MENTAL HEALTH. Text in English. 1972. bi-m. USD 88, EUR 88 to individuals For print or online ed.; USD 550, EUR 549 to institutions For print or online ed.; USD 660, EUR 658.80 to institutions for print & online eds. (effective 2002). adv. bk.rev. abstr, bibl. reprint service avail. from PQC,ISI. *Refereed.* **Document type:** *Academic/Scholarly.* **Description:** Examines all applicable issues in administering and setting policy for mental health institutions and related human service programs.
Formerly (until 1988): Administration in Mental Health (0090-1180)
Related titles: Online - full text ed.: (from O C L C Online Computer Library Center, Inc., Swets Blackwell, Kluwer Online, Institute for Scientific Information, RoweCom Information Quest).
Indexed: ASCA, Abstr.Health Care Manage.Stud., AgeLine, C.I.J.E. (coverage dropped), Crim.Just.Abstr., Curr.Cont., Educ.Admin.Abstr., Excerp.Med., Fam.Ind., Hosp.Lit.Ind., Ind.Med. (1988-), Int.Nurs.Ind., Lang.& Lang.Behav.Abstr., PSI, PsycInfo, Psychol.Abstr. (1973-), SOPODA, SSCI, Sage Pub.Admin.Abstr., Soc.Serv.Abstr., Soc.Work Res.& Abstr., Sociol.Abstr., e-psyche.
—BLDSC (0681.956200), EMDOCS, GNLM, IDS, Infotrieve, ingenta, KNAW. **CCC.**
Published by: Kluwer Academic - Plenum Publishers (Subsidiary of: Wolters Kluwer N.V.), 233 Spring St, New York, NY 10013-1578. TEL 212-620-8000, 800-221-9369, FAX 212-463-0742, kluwer@wkap.com; services@wkap.nl, http://www.wkap.nl/journalhome.htm/0894-587X, http://www.plenum.com. Ed. Saul Feldman.

610 USA ISSN 0044-6335
ADOLESCENT MEDICINE (WASHINGTON); report for the health professionals with teenage patients. Text in English. 1972. m. USD 79; USD 89 foreign (effective 2000). bk.rev. stat. back issues avail. **Document type:** *Newsletter.* **Description:** Provides clerical updates based on research for practitioners treating adolescents.
Related titles: E-mail ed.; Fax ed.
Published by: British Trading Company, 860 N DeWitt Pl, no 1704, Chicago, IL 60611. TEL 312-932-0166, FAX 312-640-0339, adomed@worldnet.att.net. Ed., Pub. Natan Polster. R&P Gerlinde Kubitz.

611.85 USA
ADVANCE FOR AUDIOLOGISTS. Text in English. bi-m. Free to qualified subscribers. adv. **Document type:** *Magazine, Trade.* **Description:** Covers business issues, industry news and product information for audiologists.
Related titles: Online - full content ed.
Published by: Merion Publications, Inc., 2900 Horizon Dr, PO Box 61556, King Of Prussia, PA 19406. TEL 800-355-5627, FAX 610-278-1421, 610-278-1425, aobrien@merion.com, http://www.advanceforaud.com, http://www.advanceweb.com.

610 USA
ADVANCE FOR DIRECTORS IN REHABILITATION. Text in English. 1992. m. **Document type:** *Trade.*
Published by: Merion Publications, Inc., 2900 Horizon Dr, PO Box 61556, King Of Prussia, PA 19406. TEL 610-278-1400, 800-355-5627, FAX 610-278-1421, advance@merion.com, http://www.advanceweb.com. Ed. Maria Wolf. adv.: B&W page USD 2,437, color page USD 2,737; trim 10.88 x 8.38. Circ: 25,000.

651 026 USA ISSN 1061-3269
ADVANCE FOR HEALTH INFORMATION PROFESSIONALS. Text in English. 1991. bi-w. *Refereed.* **Document type:** *Trade.*
Formerly (until 1992): Advance for Medical Record Professionals (1061-3188)
Published by: Merion Publications, Inc., 2900 Horizon Dr, PO Box 61556, King Of Prussia, PA 19406. TEL 610-278-1400, 800-355-5627, FAX 610-278-1421, advance@merion.com, http://www.advanceweb.com. Ed. Lisa A Algeo. Pub. Ann Kielinski. adv.: B&W page USD 3,500, color page USD 3,800; trim 10.88 x 8.38. Circ: 48,000.

610.737 USA ISSN 1096-6315
ADVANCE FOR PHYSICIAN ASSISTANTS. Text in English. 1993. m. adv. bk.rev., software rev., video rev. charts, illus, maps, stat, tr.lit. index. back issues avail. *Refereed.*
Published by: Merion Publications, Inc., 2900 Horizon Dr, PO Box 61556, King Of Prussia, PA 19406. TEL 610-278-1400, 800-355-5627, FAX 610-278-1421, advance@merion.com, http://www.advanceweb.com. Ed. Michael Gerchufsky. Pub. Ann Kielinski. Adv. contact Judy Thwaites. B&W page USD 2,109; trim 11.13 x 8.38. Circ: 30,900 (controlled).

ADVANCED TRADITIONAL CHINESE MEDICINE SERIES. see *ALTERNATIVE MEDICINE*

610 USA ISSN 1072-4109
ADVANCES IN ANATOMIC PATHOLOGY. Text in English. 1994. bi-m. USD 166 in North America to individuals; USD 171 elsewhere to individuals; USD 253 in North America to institutions; USD 258 elsewhere to institutions; USD 42 newsstand/cover domestic (effective 2002). adv. back issues avail. *Refereed.* **Document type:** *Academic/Scholarly.* **Description:** Provides specific coverage of the most recent key developments in anatomic and surgical pathology.
Related titles: Online - full text ed.: USD 319.80 academic site license; USD 356.70 corporate site license (2002) (from Institute for Scientific Information).
Indexed: Curr.Cont., Ind.Med. (1994-).
—BLDSC (0698.790000), CISTI, GNLM, KNAW.
Published by: Lippincott Williams & Wilkins (Philadelphia) (Subsidiary of: Wolters Kluwer N.V.), 530 Walnut St, Philadelphia, PA 19106-3621. TEL 215-521-8300, FAX 215-521-8902, http://www.anatomicpathology.com, http://www.Lww.com. Ed. Dr. John G Batsakis. Pub. Shelley Johnson. R&P Margaret Becker. Adv. contact Susan Nangle. B&W page USD 590, color page USD 1,475. Circ: 1,640 (paid). **Subscr. to:** PO Box 1600, Hagerstown, MD 21740-1600. TEL 800-777-2295, FAX 301-824-7390.

612.396 USA ISSN 0065-2318
QD321 CODEN: ACBYAP
ADVANCES IN CARBOHYDRATE CHEMISTRY AND BIOCHEMISTRY. Text in English. 1945. irreg., latest vol.52, 1997. reprint service avail. from ISI. *Refereed.* **Document type:** *Monographic series.*
Formerly (until 1968): Advances in Carbohydrate Chemistry (0096-5332)
Related titles: Online - full text ed.: (from Institute for Scientific Information).
Indexed: ASCA, Abstr.Bull.Inst.Pap.Chem., BBCI, Biol.Abstr., Chem.Abstr., Chem.Cit.Ind., Chem.Indus.Notes, Chem.Infd., Chem.Titles, Curr.Adv.Ecol.Sci., Curr.Chem.React., Excerp.Med., Food Sci.& Tech.Abstr., Ind.Chem. (coverage dropped), Ind.Med. (1969-), Ind.Sci.Rev., Nutr.Abstr., RCI, Sci.Cit.Ind., Trop.Dis.Bull.
—BLDSC (0702.100000), CASDDS, CISTI, EMDOCS, ingenta, Linda Hall. **CCC.**
Published by: Academic Press, Inc., Journal Division (Subsidiary of: Harcourt Brace & Company), 525 B St, Ste 1900, San Diego, CA 92101-4495. TEL 619-231-0926, FAX 619-699-6715. Eds. Melville L Wolfrom, R Stuart Tipson. **Subscr. to:** Order Dept., 6277 Sea Harbor Dr, 4th Fl, Orlando, FL 32887. TEL 800-321-5068.

616.07 ITA ISSN 1125-5552
ADVANCES IN CLINICAL PATHOLOGY; The official journal of the Adriatic Society of Pathology. Text in English. 1997. q., latest vol.4, 2000. ITL 70,000, USD 50 to individuals; ITL 110,000, USD 75 to institutions; ITL 50,000, USD 35 to members. adv. Website rev. abstr. back issues avail. *Refereed.* **Document type:** *Journal, Academic/Scholarly.* **Description:** Contains conference notices and scholarly articles concerning clinical pathology.
Indexed: Ind.Med. (1997-).
—BLDSC (0703.919000), CISTI.
Published by: (Adriatic Society of Pathology), Forum Societa Editrice Universitaria Udinese s.r.l., Via Palladio, 8, Udine, UD 33100, Italy. TEL 39-04-3226001, FAX 39-04-32296756, forum@forumeditrice.it, http://www.forumeditrice.it. Ed. Carlo Alberto Beltrami. Adv. contact Norma Zamparo.

M

ADVANCES IN ELECTROMAGNETIC FIELDS IN LIVING SYSTEMS. see *BIOLOGY—Biophysics*

ADVANCES IN EXPERIMENTAL MEDICINE AND BIOLOGY. see *BIOLOGY*

610 USA ISSN 1054-1888
RA410.A1
ADVANCES IN HEALTH ECONOMICS AND HEALTH SERVICES RESEARCH. SUPPLEMENT. Text in English. 1990. irreg. **Document type:** *Monographic series.*
Published by: J A I Press Inc., 100 Prospect St, Box 811, Stamford, CT 06904-0811. TEL 203-323-9606, FAX 203-357-8446, jai@jaipress.com.

610.711 NLD ISSN 1382-4996
CODEN: AHSEFM
ADVANCES IN HEALTH SCIENCES EDUCATION. Text in English. 1996. 3/yr. EUR 231, USD 231 to institutions for print or online ed.; EUR 65, USD 65 to individuals for print or online ed; EUR 277.20, USD 277.20 to institutions for print & online eds. combined (effective 2002). *Refereed.* **Document type:** *Journal, Academic/Scholarly.* **Description:** Provides an international forum for scholarly and state-of-the-art research and development into all aspects of health sciences education. Includes articles, theoretical discussions, and practical implications.
Related titles: Online - full text ed.: (from EBSCO Publishing, O C L C Online Computer Library Center, Inc., RoweCom Information Quest, Swets Blackwell, Kluwer Online).
Indexed: C.I.J.E., Cont.Pg.Educ., ERA, High.Educ.Abstr., PsycInfo, Res.High.Educ.Abstr.
—BLDSC (0709.008700), GNLM, Infotrieve. **CCC.**
Published by: Kluwer Academic Publishers Group (Subsidiary of: Wolters Kluwer N.V.), Spuiboulevard 50, PO Box 17, Dordrecht 3300 AA, Netherlands. TEL 31-78-639-2392, FAX 31-78-654-2254, services@wkap.nl, http://www.wkap.nl/journalhome.htm/1382-4996. Eds. Geoffrey Norman, Henk G Schmidt. **Subscr to:** Journals Department, PO Box 322, Dordrecht 3300 AH, Netherlands. TEL 31-78-639-2392, FAX 31-78-654-6474; **Subscr. in N America to:** Kluwer Academic - Plenum Publishers, 233 Spring St, New York, NY 10013-1578. TEL 212-620-8468, FAX 212-807-1047.

610 USA ISSN 0197-8322
CODEN: ADIRDF
ADVANCES IN INFLAMMATION RESEARCH. Text in English. 1979. irreg. price varies. reprint service avail. from PQC. *Refereed.* **Document type:** *Monographic series, Academic/Scholarly.*
Indexed: Biol.Abstr., Chem.Abstr., Curr.Adv.Ecol.Sci., Curr.Cont. (coverage dropped).
—CASDDS, CISTI, GNLM, KNAW.
Published by: Lippincott Williams & Wilkins (Philadelphia) (Subsidiary of: Wolters Kluwer N.V.), 530 Walnut St, Philadelphia, PA 19106-3621. TEL 215-521-8300, FAX 215-521-8902, custserv@lww.com, http://www.lww.com/.

ADVANCES IN MEDICAL SOCIAL SCIENCE; health and illness as viewed by anthropology, geography, history, psychology and sociology. see *SOCIAL SCIENCES: COMPREHENSIVE WORKS*

ADVANCES IN MEDICAL SOCIOLOGY. see *SOCIOLOGY*

615 USA ISSN 1067-5698
RS400 CODEN: ADCHEO
ADVANCES IN MEDICINAL CHEMISTRY. Text in English. 1992. irreg., latest vol.4, 1999. USD 109.50. **Document type:** *Monographic series.*
Indexed: Chem.Abstr., Chem.Cit.Ind., Chem.Indus.Notes, Chem.Titles.
—BLDSC (0709.376400), CASDDS, CISTI, GNLM, Infotrieve. **CCC.**
Published by: J A I Press Inc., 100 Prospect St, Box 811, Stamford, CT 06904-0811. TEL 203-323-9606, FAX 203-357-8446, jai@jaipress.com. Eds. Bruce Maryanoff, Cynthia Maryanoff.

M

610 GBR ISSN 1470-3556
RC49
ADVANCES IN MIND - BODY MEDICINE. Text in English. 1983. q. USD 66 in North America to individuals; USD 137 in North America to institutions; GBP 44 to individuals; GBP 91 to institutions (effective 2001). bk.rev. abstr, bibl, charts. back issues avail. **Document type:** *Journal, Academic/Scholarly.* **Description:** Explorations of the developing scientific view that thoughts and feelings can affect physical health.
Formerly (until 1998): Advances (Kalamazoo) (0741-9783)
Related titles: CD-ROM ed.; Online - full text ed.
Indexed: AMED, Ind.Med. (1998-), Int.Nurs.Ind., Lang.& Lang.Behav.Abstr., PsycInfo, Psychol.Abstr. (1983-), SOPODA, Sociol.Abstr., e-psyche.
—BLDSC (0709.431500), GNLM, IDS, Infotrieve, ingenta. **CCC.**
Published by: (Fetzer Institute), Churchill Livingstone (Subsidiary of: Harcourt Publishers Ltd.), Robert Stevenson House, 1-3 Baxter's Pl, Leith Walk, Edinburgh, Midlothian EH1 3AF, United Kingdom. TEL 44-131-556-2424, FAX 44-131-459-1177, cservice@harcourt.com, http://www.harcourt-international.com/journals/ambm/. Ed. Harris Dienstfrey. Circ: 5,000 (paid). **Subscr. to:** Harcourt Publishers Ltd., Foots Cray High St, Sidcup, Kent DA14 5HP, United Kingdom. TEL 44-20-8308-5700, FAX 44-20-8309-0807.

ADVANCES IN PAIN RESEARCH AND THERAPY. see *MEDICAL SCIENCES—Psychiatry And Neurology*

610 USA ISSN 0741-238X
CODEN: ADTHE7
ADVANCES IN THERAPY; the international journal of drug, device and diagnostic research. Text in English. 1984. bi-m. USD 95 domestic to individuals; USD 125 foreign to individuals; USD 150 domestic to institutions; USD 180 foreign to institutions. back issues avail. *Refereed.* **Document type:** *Academic/Scholarly.* **Description:** Publishes studies in clinical medicine and scientific research, case reports, review articles, and other original contributions in the areas of drug therapy, diagnosis, instrumentation, and related fields, as well as proceedings of symposia and special topics.
Related titles: Online - full text ed.: (from Institute for Scientific Information).
Indexed: ASCA, Curr.Cont., I.P.A., Inpharma, Pharm.&Out.News, Reac., Rev.Med.& Vet.Mycol., SSCI (coverage dropped), Sci.Cit.Ind. (coverage dropped).
—BLDSC (0711.622500), CASDDS, CISTI, EMDOCS, GNLM, IDS, Infotrieve, KNAW. **CCC.**
Published by: Health Care Communications, 292 Fernwood Avenue, Edison, NJ 08837. TEL 732-346-0027, FAX 732-346-0442, gshapiro@hcomm.com, http://www.advinther.com. Ed. Dr. James A Schoenberger. Pub. Joel Shapiro. R&P Glenn Shapiro. Circ: 3,500 (controlled).

ADVERSE DRUG REACTION BULLETIN. see *PHARMACY AND PHARMACOLOGY*

610 DEU ISSN 0944-7059
AERZTE-BRIEF KASSENABRECHNUNG AKTUELL. Text in German. m. EUR 114 in Germany; EUR 114 foreign (effective 2002). **Document type:** *Magazine, Trade.*
Published by: (Institut fuer Wirtschaftspublizistik), Vogel Verlag und Druck GmbH & Co. KG, Max-Planck-Str 7-9, Wuerzburg 97064, Germany. TEL 49-931-45353-0, FAX 49-931-4535399, http://www.vogel-medien.de. **Subscr. to:** DataM-Services GmbH, Fichtestr 9, Wuerzburg 97074, Germany. TEL 49-931-417001, FAX 49-931-4170499, swestenberger@datam-services.de, http://www.datam-services.de.

610 AUT
AERZTE WOCHE. Text in German. w. ATS 790 domestic; ATS 1,300 in Europe; ATS 350 to students (effective 2001). adv. **Document type:** *Newspaper, Trade, Academic/Scholarly.* **Description:** Provides current information and news on all aspects of medicine and the medical profession.
Related titles: Online - full text ed.: ISSN 1605-6221.
Published by: Aerzte Woche Zeitungsverlagsgesellschaft mbH (Subsidiary of: BertelsmannSpringer), Wiesingerstr 1, Vienna 1010, Austria. TEL 43-1-5131047, FAX 43-1-5134783, aerzte@aerztewoche.at, http://www.aerztewoche.at. Ed. Herbert Hauser.

610 011 DEU ISSN 0175-5811
AERZTE ZEITUNG. Text in German. 1982. d. (Mon.-Fri.). DEM 149.80. adv. bk.rev. **Document type:** *Newspaper.*
—GNLM. **CCC.**
Published by: Aerzte Zeitung Verlagsgesellschaft mbH (Subsidiary of: BertelsmannSpringer), Am Forsthaus Gravenbruch 5, Neu-Isenburg 63263, Germany. TEL 49-6102-5060, FAX 49-6102-58740, 100316,453@compuserve.com. Ed. Hagen Rudolph. Pub. Gerald Kosaris. Adv. contact Ute Krille. Circ: 65,000 (controlled).

610 DEU ISSN 0720-3489
AERZTEBLATT BADEN-WUERTTEMBERG. Text in German. 1945. m. DEM 205.20; DEM 213.60 foreign (effective 2000). adv. bk.rev. illus. index. back issues avail. **Document type:** *Academic/Scholarly.*
Indexed: Chem.Abstr.
—GNLM.
Published by: (Landesaerztekammer Baden-Wuerttemberg), Gentner Verlag Stuttgart, Forststr 131, Stuttgart 70193, Germany. TEL 49-711-63672-0, FAX 49-711-63672-11. Ed. Juergen Dreher. R&P Gernot Keuchen. Adv. contact Sebastian Vonbeckerath. Circ: 42,000.

610 DEU ISSN 0939-3323
AERZTEBLATT MECKLENBURG-VORPOMMERN. Text in German. 1990. m. EUR 51 domestic; EUR 53 foreign; EUR 4.19 newsstand/cover (effective 2001). adv. **Document type:** *Journal, Trade.*
—GNLM.
Published by: Leipziger Messe-Verlag GmbH, Postfach 901123, Leipzig 04358, Germany. TEL 49-341-678770, FAX 49-341-6787712, info@leipziger-messeverlag.de, http://www.leipziger-messeverlag.de. Circ: 6,900.

610 DEU ISSN 0001-9488
AERZTEBLATT RHEINLAND-PFALZ. Text in German. 1948. m. EUR 86 domestic; EUR 88 foreign; EUR 7.93 newsstand/cover (effective 2001). adv. bk.rev. abstr, illus. index, cum.index. **Document type:** *Journal, Academic/Scholarly, Trade.* **Description:** Publication for physicians and specialists. Covers various medical issues, public health, medical research and news from local medical institutions.
—GNLM, Infotrieve. **CCC.**
Published by: (Landesaerztekammer Rheinland-Pfalz), Leipziger Messe-Verlag GmbH, Postfach 901123, Leipzig 04358, Germany. TEL 49-341-678770, FAX 49-341-6787712, info@leipziger-messeverlag.de, http://www.leipziger-messeverlag.de. Circ: 15,600.

610 DEU ISSN 0938-8478
AERZTEBLATT SACHSEN. Text in German. 1989. m. EUR 71 domestic; EUR 73 foreign; EUR 7.41 newsstand/cover (effective 2001). adv. **Document type:** *Journal, Academic/Scholarly.*
—GNLM.
Published by: (Saechsische Landesaerztekammer), Leipziger Messe-Verlag GmbH, Postfach 901123, Leipzig 04358, Germany. TEL 49-341-678770, FAX 49-341-6787712, info@leipziger-messeverlag.de, http://www.leipziger-messeverlag.de. Ed. Wolfgang Rose. Adv. contact Alain Ducteil. B&W page XEU 1,534, color page XEU 2,557; trim 185 x 252.

610 DEU
AERZTEBLATT SACHSEN-ANHALT. Text in German. 1990. m. DEM 72 (effective 2001). adv. **Document type:** *Newsletter, Academic/Scholarly, Trade.*
Formerly: Offizielles Aerzteblatt fuer Sachsen-Anhalt (0938-9261)
—GNLM.
Published by: Aerztekammer Sachsen-Anhalt, Doctor-Eisenbart-Ring 2, Magdeburg 39120, Germany. TEL 49-391-60546, FAX 49-391-6054700, aeksa@aerztekammer-sa.de. Ed. Dr. Henning Friebel. adv.: B&W page DEM 2,600, color page DEM 4,550; trim 185 x 210. Circ: 8,930.

610 DEU ISSN 0863-5412
AERZTEBLATT THUERINGEN. Text in German. 1872. m. EUR 52 (effective 2002). adv. bk.rev. bibl, charts, illus. index. **Document type:** *Journal, Academic/Scholarly.*
—GNLM.
Published by: Urban & Fischer Verlag, Loebdergraben 14a, Jena 07743, Germany. TEL 49-3641-626444, FAX 49-3641-626500, journals@urbanfischer.de. Ed. Landesartztekammer Thuringen. R&P Martin Huber TEL 49-3641-626430. adv.: page DEM 2,575; trim 240 x 175. Circ: 8,300. **Dist. by:** Nature Publishing Group, Brunel Rd, Basingstoke RG21 6XS, United Kingdom. TEL 44-1256-302629, FAX 44-1256-463570, j.stephens@macmillan.com.

616.98 DEU ISSN 0930-6900
AERZTEBUCH; Fachaddressbuch des gesamten Gesundheitswesens Deutschland. Text in German; Summaries in English, French, German, Italian. 1977. a. DEM 248 (effective 2001). **Document type:** *Directory, Trade.*
Published by: Aerztebuch Verlag GmbH, Flossplatz 24, Leipzig 04107, Germany. TEL 49-341-14938-0, FAX 49-341-1493815, info@aerztebuchverlag.de, http://www.aerztebuchverlag.de. Circ: 8,500.

AERZTEZEITSCHRIFT FUER NATURHEILVERFAHREN. see *ALTERNATIVE MEDICINE*

616.1 DEU ISSN 0001-9534
AERZTLICHE PRAXIS. Text in German. 1948. 2/w. DEM 138 domestic; DEM 160 foreign; DEM 89.65 to students (effective 2001). adv. bk.rev. abstr, bibl, charts, illus, stat. index. **Document type:** *Newspaper, Trade.*

Indexed: C.I.S. Abstr., INIS Atomind.
—CISTI, GNLM. **CCC.**
Published by: Reed Elsevier Deutschland GmbH (Subsidiary of: Reed Elsevier group), Gabrielenstr 9, Munich 80636, Germany. TEL 49-89-89817-0, FAX 49-89-89817400, aepingo@r-e.de, aep-anzeigen@r-e.de, http://www.aerztliche-praxis.de/aktuell. Ed. Hans Juergen Kuntze. Pub., R&P Wolfram Haase. Adv. contact Michael Oeser. B&W page DEM 12,310; trim 281 x 395. Circ: 50,970 (paid).

610 910.202 DEU
AERZTLICHES JOURNAL REISE UND MEDIZIN. Text in German. 1977. m. DEM 90. adv. **Document type:** *Trade.*
Former titles: Aerztliches Reise und Medizin Journal (0946-2945); (until 1994): Aerztliches Reise- und Kultur-Journal (0344-9548)
—GNLM.
Published by: Otto Hoffmanns Verlag GmbH, Arnulfstr 10, Munich 80335, Germany. TEL 49-89-545845-0, FAX 49-89-54584520. Eds. Jan Murken, Konrad Zweyer. Pub. Konrad Zweyer. Adv. contact Ria Lorsbach. Circ: 55,000.

610 DEU ISSN 0723-8010
AERZTLICHES MITTEILUNGSBLATT SCHWABEN*. Text in German. 1980. bi-m. DEM 36. **Document type:** *Academic/Scholarly.*
Address: c/o Rita Botzenhart, Frohsinnstr 2, Augsburg 86150, Germany. Ed. Dr. Klaus Hellmann. Circ: 5,500.

610 FIN ISSN 0400-6747
AESCULAPIUS. Text in Finnish. 1953. bi-m. **Document type:** *Trade.*
Published by: Helsinki Media Company Oy, PL 2, Helsinki 00040, Finland. TEL 358-9-1201, FAX 358-9-120-5988. Ed. Pekka Jarvensivu. Circ: 21,500 (controlled).

610 GBR ISSN 0141-9536
AFRICA HEALTH. Text in English. 1978. bi-m. GBP 54 in Europe; GBP 79, USD 132 foreign (effective 2002). adv. bk.rev. illus. **Document type:** *Academic/Scholarly.* **Description:** Contains review articles, news, and letters for health care working in Africa.
Indexed: ASSIA, Rev.Appl.Entomol., Trop.Dis.Bull.
—BLDSC (0732.157700), GNLM.
Published by: F S G MediMedia Ltd., Vine House, The Barn, Fair Green, Reach, Cambridge CB5 0JD, United Kingdom. TEL 44-1638-743633, FAX 44-1638-743998, info@fsg.co.uk, http://www.fsg.co.uk. Ed. Paul Chinnock. Pub. Bryan Pearson. Adv. contact Stuart Marritt. Circ: 5,000 (controlled).

610 KEN
AFRICA MEDICINE AND HEALTH. Text in English. 1978. m. adv. illus.
Published by: Oryx Publications Ltd., PO Box 40106, Nairobi, Kenya. Circ: 5,000.

610 KEN ISSN 1022-9272
AFRICAN JOURNAL OF HEALTH SCIENCES. Text in English. 1994. q. USD 30 domestic to individuals; USD 52 foreign to individuals; USD 45 domestic to institutions; USD 90 foreign to institutions. adv. bk.rev. *Refereed.* **Document type:** *Journal, Academic/Scholarly.* **Description:** Provides a forum to communicate research results and policy issues in the health sciences and related disciplines.
Indexed: Helminthol.Abstr., Nutr.Abstr., Protozool.Abstr., Rev.Arom.& Med.Plants, Rev.Med.& Vet.Mycol., Rural Devel.Abstr., Triticale Abstr.
—BLDSC (0732.522500), GNLM.
Published by: (Kenya Medical Research Institute (KEMRI)), African Forum for Health Sciences, PO Box 54840, Nairobi, Kenya. TEL 254-2-722541, FAX 254-2-720030, kemrilib@healthnet.or.ke. Ed. Dr. Davy Koech. Adv. contact Bernard Muthaka. Circ: 1,000.

610 KEN ISSN 1023-8190
AFRICAN JOURNAL OF MEDICAL PRACTICE. Text in English. bi-m. KES 2,000 domestic to individuals; USD 50 to individuals rest of Africa; USD 70 elsewhere to individuals; KES 2,500 domestic to institutions; USD 60 to institutions rest of Africa; USD 80 elsewhere to institutions (effective 2000). adv. **Document type:** *Academic/Scholarly.* **Description:** Seeks to promote continued medical education and research in Africa by providing a forum for medical practitioners in the private and primary health care sectors.
Indexed: Abstr.Anthropol., Helminthol.Abstr., Nutr.Abstr., Protozool.Abstr., Rural Devel.Abstr., Trop.Dis.Bull., World Ag.Econ.& Rur.Soc.Abstr.
—BLDSC (0732.524500), GNLM.
Address: PO Box 14798, Nairobi, Kenya. TEL 254-2-884401-5, FAX 254-2-884406, ajmp@arcc.or.ke. Ed. Dr. Tom Mboya. Adv. contact Treazer Oumah. B&W page KES 30,000,500, color page USD 1,500.

610 NGA ISSN 1116-4077
CODEN: AJMMS
AFRICAN JOURNAL OF MEDICINE & MEDICAL SCIENCES (NEW SERIES). Text in English. 1970; N.S. 1991. q. NGN 2,500, USD 80 to individuals; NGN 3,000, USD 160 to institutions (effective 2000). adv. bk.rev. illus. back issues avail.; reprints avail. *Refereed.* **Document type:** *Journal, Academic/Scholarly.* **Description:** Disseminates information about topics and issues in the medical sciences in Africa and throughout the world and provides an international forum to review international conferences in the medical sciences held in Africa.
Supersedes (in 1991): African Journal of Medicine & Medical Sciences (0309-3913); Which was formerly (until 1976): African Journal of Medical Sciences (0002-0028)
Indexed: Abstr.Hyg., Biol.Abstr., Chem.Abstr., Curr.Adv.Ecol.Sci., Curr.Cont. (coverage dropped), Excerp.Med., Helminthol.Abstr., Ind.Med. (1976-), Int.Nurs.Ind., Trop.Dis.Bull.
—BLDSC (0732.530000), CASDDS, CISTI, GNLM, Infotrieve. **CCC.**
Published by: University College Hospital, College of Medicine, PIMRAT College of Medicine, University of Ibadan, Ibadan, Oyo, Nigeria. TEL 234-2-2410088, 234-2-2414578, FAX 234-2-2411768, TELEX 31520 TEACHOS NG. Ed., R&P Babatunde Osotimehin. Adv. contact Bukola Oyejide. page NGN 20,000. Circ: 500.

610 SEN ISSN 0002-0516
AFRIQUE MEDICALE. Text in French. 1958. 11/yr. FRF 300 foreign. adv. charts, illus.
Related titles: CD-ROM ed.
Indexed: Abstr.Hyg., Biol.Abstr., ExtraMED, Nutr.Abstr., Rev.Med.& Vet.Mycol., Trop.Dis.Bull.
—GNLM.
Address: BP 1826, Dakar, Senegal. TEL 23-48-80, FAX 22-56-30, TELEX 1300 ATT AFRICA. Ed. P Correa. Circ: 7,500.

610 KEN ISSN 0378-4851
AFYA. Text in English. 1966. q. KES 75; USD 10 in Africa; USD 13 in Europe; USD 15 in the Americas. bk.rev. **Document type:** *Trade.* **Description:** Contains information for and about medical and health workers.
Published by: African Medical and Research Foundation, PO Box 30125, Nairobi, Kenya. TEL 254-2-501301, FAX 254-2-506112, TELEX 23254. Ed. N O Bwibo. Circ: 7,000.

610 UKR
AGAPIT. Text in Ukrainian, Russian, English. 1995. s-a. USD 95 in the Americas (effective 2000).
Published by: Tsentral'nyi Muzei Meditsini Ukrainy, Ul. B. Khmel'nitskogo, 37, Kiev, Ukraine. TEL 224-29-12, FAX 224-29-02. **Dist. by:** East View Publications, 3020 Harbor Ln N, Minneapolis, MN 55447. TEL 763-550-0961, FAX 763-559-2931.

610 ITA ISSN 0392-9442
AGGIORNAMENTI DI MEDICINA E CHIRURGIA. Text in English, Italian. 1983. bi-m. adv. bk.rev., software rev. bibl, stat. index. back issues avail. **Document type:** *Academic/Scholarly.*
Related titles: Diskette ed.
Published by: A M C Edizioni, Via Latisana, 58, Rome, RM 00177, Italy. TEL 39-06-723950, FAX 39-06-2598085. Ed. Frederico Pezzi. **Subscr. to:** Casella Postale 5501, Rome, RM 00177, Italy.

610 ITA ISSN 0392-3002
AGGIORNAMENTO MEDICO; rivista mensile di cultura e pratica medica. Text in Italian. 1982. m. (10/yr.). EUR 30.99 domestic; USD 60 foreign (effective 2002). **Document type:** *Academic/Scholarly.* **Description:** Presents research papers and articles on a wide variety of topics in modern medicine.
Related titles: Online - full text ed.: EUR 15.49 (effective 2002).
—CISTI.
Published by: Editrice Kurtis s.r.l., Via Luigi Zoja, 30, Milan, MI 20153, Italy. TEL 39-02-48202740, FAX 39-02-4820-1219, info@kurtis.it, http://www.kurtis.it. Circ: 41,000.

AGRI/JOURNAL OF THE TURKISH SOCIETY OF ALGOLOGY; turk algoloji (agri) derneginin yayin organdir. see *MEDICAL SCIENCES—Psychiatry And Neurology*

610 IRN ISSN 1026-8960
AHWAZ UNIVERSITY OF MEDICAL SCIENCES. SCIENTIFIC MEDICAL JOURNAL/MAJALLEH ELMI PESESHKI DANESHGAHE ELOME PEZESHKI AHWAZ. Text in Persian, Modern; Summaries in English. 1971. s-a. free per issue. *Refereed.* **Document type:** *Academic/Scholarly.* **Description:** Publishes original clinical research papers, review articles, case reports and contributions on all subjects relevant to medicine.
Related titles: CD-ROM ed.
Indexed: ExtraMED.
Published by: Ahwaz University of Medical Sciences, P O Box 189, Ahwaz, Iran. TEL 98-61-32036, FAX 98-61-61544. Ed. Dr. S Zahedi. Circ: 1,000.

610 JPN
AICHI IHO/AICHI MEDICAL REPORT. Text in Japanese. 1956. 3/m. JPY 3,600.
Published by: Aichi Ihosha, Aichiken Ishikai, 14-28 Sakae 4-chome, Naka-ku, Nagoya-shi, Aichi-ken 460-0008, Japan.

610 JPN ISSN 0286-9187
AICHI IKA DAIGAKU KISO KAGAKUKA KIYO/AICHI MEDICAL UNIVERSITY. BULLETIN OF THE LIBERAL ARTS AND SCIENCE COURSE. Text in English, Japanese. 1974. a., latest vol.27. **Document type:** *Bulletin, Academic/Scholarly.*
Published by: Aichi Ika Daigaku/Aichi Medical University, Nagakute-cho, Aichi-gun, Aichi-ken 480-1195, Japan.

610 EGY ISSN 0002-2144
CODEN: AIMJA9
AIN SHAMS MEDICAL JOURNAL. Text in Arabic. 1949. bi-m. adv. bk.rev. abstr, charts, illus, stat.
Indexed: Biol.Abstr., C.I.S. Abstr., Chem.Abstr., Excerp.Med., Helminthol.Abstr., Trop.Dis.Bull.
—CASDDS, GNLM.
Published by: Ain Shams University, University Hospital, Abbassia, Cairo, Egypt. Ed. Ahmed Ghareeb. Circ: 2,000. **Co-sponsor:** Ain Shams Clinical and Scientific Society.

616.98 USA ISSN 1067-991X
AIR MEDICAL JOURNAL. Text in English. 1986. bi-m. USD 68 domestic to individuals; USD 89 foreign to individuals; USD 85 domestic to institutions; USD 106 foreign to institutions; USD 18 newsstand/cover (effective 2001). adv. bk.rev. abstr, illus. back issues avail.; reprints avail. *Refereed.* **Document type:** *Journal, Academic/Scholarly.* **Description:** Presents clinical and scientific articles dedicated to advancing the scientific knowledge base of air medical transport professionals.
Formerly (until 1993): Journal of Air Medical Transport (1046-9095); Formed by the 1989 merger of: AeroMedical Journal (0894-8321); Hospital Aviation Journal (0740-8315)
Indexed: CINAHL, Int.Nurs.Ind.
—BLDSC (0776.349990), Infotrieve. **CCC.**
Published by: (Air Medical Physician Association), Mosby, Inc. (Subsidiary of: Elsevier Science), 11830 Westline Industrial Dr, St Louis, MO 63146-3318. TEL 314-872-8370, 800-325-4177, FAX 214-432-1380, periodical.service@mosby.com, http://www.mosby.com/airmed, http://www.mosby.com/periodicals. Eds. Dr. David J Dries, Renee S Holleran, Steve Talbert. Pub. Nathania Sawyer. Adv. contact Carol Kilzer TEL 314-453-4307. B&W page USD 1,585, color page USD 2,410; trim 10.88 x 7.88. Circ: 4,421. **Co-sponsors:** Association of Air Medical Services; Air and Surface Transport Nurses Association; National Flight Paramedics Association; National EMS Pilots Association.

610 JPN ISSN 0917-9267
AIRAGUN ISHIKAI IGAKKAISHI/AIRA COUNTY MEDICAL ASSOCIATION. JOURNAL. Text in Japanese. 1988. a.
Published by: Airagun Ishikai/Aira County Medical Association, 124-1 Uchiyamada, Aira-gun, Hayato-cho, Kagoshima-ken 899-5106, Japan.

610 UKR
AKADEMIYA MEDYCHNYKH NAUK UKRAINY. ZHURNAL. Text in English, Russian, Ukrainian. q. USD 96 foreign (effective 2000). adv. bk.rev. *Refereed.* **Document type:** *Academic/Scholarly.* **Description:** Publishes reviews on issues in current medical science, and brief pieces on the results of original research in the field of experimental, clinical, and preventitive medicine.

M

Published by: Akademiya Medychnykh Nauk Ukrainy, Vul Gertsena 12, Kiev 04050, Ukraine. TEL 380-44-431-0568, FAX 380-44-432-9956, direct@geront.freenet.kiev.ua. Ed. A F Vosianov. **US dist. addr.:** James Beale, Director, Periodicals Division, Victor Kamkin Inc, 4956 Boiling Brook Pkwy, Rockville, MD 20852. TEL 612-559-2931, 612-550-0961.

610 UKR
AKADEMIYA ZDOROV'YA. Text in Ukrainian, Russian. 24/yr. USD 95 in the Americas (effective 2000).
Published by: Dyvosvit, Ul. Entuziastiv, 5, Kiev, Ukraine. TEL 555-54-63, FAX 265-59-29. **Dist. by:** East View Publications, 3020 Harbor Ln N, Minneapolis, MN 55447. TEL 763-550-0961, FAX 763-559-2931.

610 JPN ISSN 0386-6106
CODEN: AKIGDV
AKITA IGAKU/AKITA JOURNAL OF MEDICINE. Text in English, Japanese; Summaries in English. 1974. q. JPY 20,000. adv. *Refereed.* **Document type:** *Academic/Scholarly.*
Indexed: Chem.Abstr., Chem.Indus.Notes, Chem.Titles, INIS Atomind.
—BLDSC (0785.589810), CASDDS.
Published by: Akita Daigaku, Igakubu/Akita University, School of Medicine, 1-1-1 Hondo, Akita 010-8543, Japan. FAX 81-18-884-6443. Ed., R&P, Adv. contact Toshihiro Sugiyama TEL 81-18-884-6074. Circ: 800.

610 JPN ISSN 0002-368X
AKITA JOURNAL OF RURAL MEDICINE/AKITAKEN NOSON IGAKKAI ZASSHI. Text in Japanese. 1954. a. adv. abstr, charts, illus, stat. cum.index.
Published by: Akita Association of Rural Medicine/Akitaken Noson Igakkai, 64-2 Inokawara-Yabase, Akita-shi 010-0000, Japan. Ed. Dr. Masakazu Tatsumi.

610 JPN ISSN 0286-7656
CODEN: AKISAU
AKITAKEN ISHIKAI ZASSHI/AKITA MEDICAL JOURNAL. Text in Japanese. 1949. s-a.
Indexed: Chem.Abstr., INIS Atomind.
—CASDDS.
Published by: Akitaken Ishikai/Akita Medical Association, 6-6 Senshu-Kubota-Machi, Akita-shi 010-0874, Japan.

610 FRA ISSN 1293-2973
AKOS - ENCYCLOPEDIE PRATIQUE DE MEDECINE. Text in French. 1998. 8 base vols. plus q. updates. price varies. bibl, charts, illus. back issues avail. **Document type:** *Academic/Scholarly, Trade.* **Description:** Offers physicians treatment and diagnostic updates in 26 specialty areas.
Related titles: CD-ROM ed.
Published by: Elsevier Paris, Editions Scientifiques et Medicales (Subsidiary of: Reed Elsevier plc. group), 23 rue Linois, Paris 75015, France. TEL 33-1-45589110, FAX 33-1-45589425, redaction-emc@elsevier.fr, redacion-emc@elsevier.fr, http://www.elsevier.fr; http://www.emc.tm.fr; http://www.akos.tm.fr.

AKTUELLE ERNAEHRUNGSMEDIZIN; Zeitschrift fuer Stoffwechselforschung, klinische Ernaehrung und Diaetetik. see *NUTRITION AND DIETETICS*

AKUPUNKTUR: THEORIE UND PRAXIS. see *ALTERNATIVE MEDICINE*

615.89 DEU ISSN 0172-9322
DER AKUPUNKTURARZT - AURIKULOTHERAPEUT. Text in German. 1980. q. EUR 69.68 domestic; EUR 76.68 foreign; EUR 53.79 domestic to students; EUR 60.79 foreign to students; EUR 15.89 newsstand/cover (effective 2002). adv. bk.rev. back issues avail. **Document type:** *Journal, Academic/Scholarly.*
—GNLM, Infotrieve. **CCC.**
Published by: (Deutsche Akademie fuer Akupunktur und Aurikulo-Medizin), Urban und Vogel Medien und Medizin Verlagsgesellschaft mbH (Subsidiary of: BertelsmannSpringer), Neumarkter Str 43, Munich 81673, Germany. TEL 49-89-43721411, FAX 49-89-43721410, verlag@urban-vogel.de, http://www.urban-vogel.de. Ed. Dr. F R Bahr. Adv. contact Barbara Kanters. **Subscr. to:** Springer Auslieferungs Gesellschaft, Postfach 105160, Heidelberg 69041, Germany. TEL 49-6221-345244, FAX 49-6221-345244.

610 USA
ALABAMA EPIC. Text in English. 1981. q. adv. **Document type:** *Newsletter, Trade.* **Description:** Covers emergency medicine.
Published by: American College of Emergency Physicians, Alabama Chapter, PO Box 4629, Montgomery, AL 36103-4629. TEL 334-265-0068. Ed., R&P, Adv. contact J Leland Holman. Circ: 250.

610 USA ISSN 0002-4414
ALAMEDA-CONTRA COSTA MEDICAL ASSOCIATION. BULLETIN. Text in English. 1945. m. membership. adv. **Document type:** *Bulletin.*
Published by: Alameda-Contra Costa Medical Association, 6230 Claremont Ave, Oakland, CA 94618. TEL 510-654-5383, FAX 510-654-8959. Ed. Dr. Donald R Townsend. R&P Donald Waters. Adv. contact Kristen Crapo. Circ: 2,950.

610 USA ISSN 0002-4538
ALASKA MEDICINE. Text in English. 1959. q. USD 30 domestic to individuals; USD 38 in Canada to individuals; USD 50 elsewhere to individuals; USD 75 to institutions (effective 2000). adv. bk.rev. index. reprint service avail. from PQC. *Refereed.* **Document type:** *Trade.*
Indexed: Ind.Med. (1959-).
—BLDSC (0786.528000), CISTI, GNLM, KNAW.
Published by: Alaska State Medical Association, American Society for Circumpolar Health, 4107 Laurel St, Anchorage, AK 99508. TEL 907-562-0304, FAX 907-561-2063, asma@alaska.net. Ed. Dr. William Clark. R&P, Adv. contact Verna Paluba. page USD 400; 8.5 x 11. Circ: 1,000.

610 EGY ISSN 0516-5849
ALEXANDRIA MEDICAL JOURNAL. Text in Arabic, English, French. 1955. q. **Document type:** *Proceedings, Bulletin, Abstract/Index.*
Indexed: Biol.Abstr., C.I.S. Abstr., Excerp.Med., Nutr.Abstr.
—CISTI.
Published by: Alexandria Medical Association, 4 G. Carducci St., Alexandria, Egypt. Ed. Amin Rida. Circ: 1,500.

610 USA ISSN 0098-3772
ALLEGHENY COUNTY MEDICAL SOCIETY. BULLETIN. Text in English. 1911. s-m. (except July and Aug.). USD 45 to institutions; USD 25 to non-profit organizations. adv. bk.rev. charts, illus. index. back issues avail. **Document type:** *Bulletin, Trade.*
Published by: Allegheny County Medical Society, 713 Ridge Ave, Pittsburgh, PA 15212. TEL 412-321-5030, FAX 412-321-5323. Ed. Dr. Jack E Wilberger. Adv. contact Linda L. Smith TEL 412-321-5030 ext. 105. Circ: 3,700 (controlled).

616.07 DEU ISSN 0172-7249
DER ALLGEMEINARZT. Text in German. 1979. q. DEM 91.80; DEM 54.90 to students (effective 1999). adv. charts, illus. **Document type:** *Academic/Scholarly.*
Indexed: Ref.Zh.
—GNLM, Infotrieve. **CCC.**
Published by: (Berufsverband der Allgemeinaerzte Deutschlands - Hausaerzteverband e.V.), Verlag Kirchheim und Co. GmbH, Kaiserstr 41, Mainz 55116, Germany. TEL 49-6131-96070-0, FAX 49-6131-9607070, kirchheim@aol.com. Ed. Dr. Frank Mader. Adv. contact Andreas Goerner. Circ: 29,000.

ALLIANCE (CHARLESTON). see *COLLEGE AND ALUMNI*

613 USA ISSN 0893-5025
ALTERNATIVES (INGRAM). Variant title: Alternatives for the Health Conscious Individual. Text in English. 1985. m. USD 69. back issues avail. **Document type:** *Newsletter.* **Description:** Emphasizes natural therapies and self-help techniques to obtain optimal health without the use of drugs or surgery.
Related titles: Audio cassette/tape ed.
Indexed: CHNI, CINAHL, IDA.
Published by: Mountain Home Publishing, PO Box 829, Ingram, TX 78025. TEL 210-367-4492. Ed. Dr. David Williams. Pub., R&P Brenda Lyman. Circ: 200,000.

610 USA
ALTSCHUL SYMPOSIA SERIES. Text in English. 1991. irreg., latest vol.4, 1997. price varies. back issues avail. **Document type:** *Proceedings.*
Indexed: Chem.Abstr., Chem.Indus.Notes, Chem.Titles.
—BLDSC (0803.902900).
Published by: (Altschul Symposium), Kluwer Academic - Plenum Publishers (Subsidiary of: Wolters Kluwer N.V.), 233 Spring St, New York, NY 10013-1578. TEL 212-620-8000, 800-221-9369, FAX 212-463-0742, info@plenum.com, http://www.plenum.com. Eds. Gary Burkholder, Sergey Fedoroff.

610 658 USA ISSN 1094-6829
AMBULATORY OUTREACH. Text in English. 1997. q. USD 99 (effective 1999). charts, illus, stat. back issues avail. **Document type:** *Trade.* **Description:** Provides high-level articles focusing on all aspects of ambulatory and home management.
Related titles: Fax ed.; Online - full text ed.
Indexed: Int.Nurs.Ind.
Published by: Society for Ambulatory Care Professionals, One N Franklin, Chicago, IL 60606. TEL 312-422-3907, FAX 312-422-4577, gbrown1@aha.org, http://www.sacp-net.org. Ed., R&P Glen Brown. adv.: B&W page USD 600, color page USD 1,100; trim 10 x 7. Circ: 1,500.

610.737 USA ISSN 0893-7400
AMERICAN ACADEMY OF PHYSICIAN ASSISTANTS. JOURNAL. Text in English. 1988. 12/yr. USD 50 domestic; USD 75 foreign; USD 10 newsstand/cover (effective 2001). adv. bk.rev. abstr, charts, illus. back issues avail. *Refereed.* **Document type:** *Academic/Scholarly.* **Description:** Publishes current information and research on clinical care, education, health policy and professional issues for physician assistants.
Related titles: Microform ed.: (from PQC); Online - full text ed.: (from Gale Group).
Indexed: CINAHL.
—BLDSC (4683.732500), CISTI.
Published by: (American Academy of Physician Assistants), Medical Economics Co., Inc., 5 Paragon Dr, Montvale, NJ 07645-1742. TEL 201-358-7200. Ed. John Baranowski. Circ: 38,500.

610.7 USA ISSN 0745-2624
AMERICAN ASSOCIATION FOR MEDICAL TRANSCRIPTION. JOURNAL. Text in English. 1985. bi-m. USD 150 (effective 1999). adv. bk.rev. index. *Refereed.* **Document type:** *Trade.* **Description:** Features medical and non-medical educational articles for the medical transcriptionist as well as medical word lists, updates on medical terminology and discoveries, technology, professional opportunities, and information about products.
Published by: American Association for Medical Transcription, PO Box 576187, Modesto, CA 95357-6187. TEL 209-551-0883, FAX 209-551-9317, aamt@sna.com, http://www.aamt.org. Ed. Claudia Tessier. R&P Janel Heath. Adv. contact Daryl Ochs. B&W page USD 800; trim 11 x 8.5. Circ: 9,000.

362.1784 USA ISSN 1051-0435
AMERICAN ASSOCIATION OF BLOOD BANKS. MEMBERSHIP DIRECTORY. Text in English. biennial. **Document type:** *Directory.*
Published by: American Association of Blood Banks, 8101 Glenbrook Rd, Bethesda, MD 20814. TEL 301-907-6977, FAX 301-907-6895, http://www.aabb.org.

610 USA ISSN 0270-2673
AMERICAN ASSOCIATION OF TISSUE BANKS NEWSLETTER. Text in English. 1976. q. membership. **Document type:** *Newsletter.*
Published by: American Association of Tissue Banks, 1350 Beverly Rd., Ste. 220A, Mclean, VA 22101. TEL 703-827-9582, FAX 703-356-2198. Ed. Jeanne C Mowe. Circ: 1,000 (controlled).

AMERICAN BLOOD RESOURCES ASSOCIATION. JOURNAL. see *BIOLOGY*

610 USA ISSN 0893-8652
CODEN: JABPEJ
AMERICAN BOARD OF FAMILY PRACTICE. JOURNAL. Key Title: Journal of the American Board of Family Practice. Abbreviated title: J A B F P. Text in English. 1988. bi-m. USD 35 domestic to individuals; USD 45 foreign to individuals; USD 60 domestic to institutions; USD 65 foreign to institutions. adv. bk.rev. abstr, bibl, charts, illus. index. back issues avail. *Refereed.* **Document type:** *Academic/Scholarly.* **Description:** Covers clinical studies that have relevance for improved patient care in family medicine.
Related titles: CD-ROM ed.: (from Ovid Technologies, Inc.); Microfiche ed.; Microfilm ed.; Online - full text ed.: (from Ovid Technologies, Inc.).
Indexed: FAMLI, Ind.Med. (1988-), Int.Nurs.Ind.
—BLDSC (4683.950000), EMDOCS, GNLM, ingenta, KNAW.
Published by: American Board of Family Practice, 2228 Young Dr, Lexington, KY 40505. TEL 206-685-3993, FAX 206-543-8911, jabfg@fammed.washington.edu, http://www.abfg.org/abfp/JABFPZ.htm; http://primarycare.medscape.com/ABFP/JABFP/public.journal.JABFP.html. Adv. contact Jane Monaghan. Circ: 54,900.

M

610 USA ISSN 0272-9741
R729.5.S6
AMERICAN BOARD OF MEDICAL SPECIALTIES. ANNUAL REPORT & REFERENCE HANDBOOK. Text in English. 1970. a. USD 5 (effective 1999). **Document type:** *Corporate.*
Formerly: American Board of Medical Specialties. Annual Report (0146-5872)
Published by: American Board of Medical Specialties, 1007 Church St, Ste 404, Evanston, IL 60201-5913. TEL 847-491-9091, FAX 847-328-3596, http://www.abms.org. Ed. Dr. Stephen Miller. R&P Alexis Rodgers. Circ: 6,000.

610 USA
AMERICAN COLLEGE OF MEDICAL QUALITY FOCUS∗. Text in English. 1973. m. USD 70; to libraries; others $75. adv. bk.rev. back issues avail. **Document type:** *Newsletter.* **Description:** Covers quality assurance, utilization review, risk management, cost containment, seminar announcements, and news briefs.
Former titles (until 1993): American College of Medical Quality Newsletter; American College of Utilization Review Physicians Newsletter
Published by: American College of Medical Quality, 4334 Montgomery Ave 2nd Fl, Bethesda, MD 20814-4402. TEL 301-365-3570, FAX 301-365-3202. Ed. Ralph H Rosenblum. Circ: 2,200.

610 USA ISSN 0279-9529
AMERICAN COLLEGE OF PHYSICIANS OBSERVER. Text in English. 1981. m. USD 9 (effective 2000). adv. **Document type:** *Newsletter.* **Description:** Membership newsletter of American College of Physicians.
Related titles: Online - full text ed.: (from EBSCO Publishing).
—CCC.
Published by: American College of Physicians/Co-sponsor: American Society of Internal Medicine, 190 N. Independence Mall W, Philadelphia, PA 19106-1572. TEL 215-351-2600, FAX 215-351-2799, custserv@mail.acponline.org, http://www.acponline.org/journals/acpjc/jcmenu.htm. Ed. Edward Doyle. R&P Joshua Roberts TEL 215-351-2630. Adv. contact Ron Taylor. Circ: 90,000 (paid).

610 USA ISSN 0002-838X
R11
AMERICAN FAMILY PHYSICIAN. Text in English. 1950. 24/yr. USD 95 domestic to individuals; USD 140 foreign to individuals; USD 115 domestic to institutions; USD 160 foreign to institutions (effective 2001). adv. bk.rev. charts, illus, mkt, pat, tr.lit. s-a. index, cum.index. back issues avail.; reprint service avail. from PQC. *Refereed.* **Document type:** *Academic/Scholarly.* **Description:** Aimed at family physicians and others in primary care. Clinical review articles detail the latest daignostic and therapeutic techniques in the medical field.
Formerly (until 1970): G P (0016-3600)
Related titles: CD-ROM ed.; Microfilm ed.: (from PQC,PMC); Online - full text ed.: (from Gale Group, Northern Light Technology, Inc., EBSCO Publishing, ProQuest Information & Learning, LexisNexis, Factiva, Institute for Scientific Information, H. W. Wilson).
Indexed: A.D.& D., AIM, ASCA, Adol.Ment.Hlth.Abstr., AgeLine, Bus.Ind., CHNI, CINAHL, C.I.S. Abstr., Chem.Abstr., Curr.Cont., Dairy Sci.Abstr., Dent.Ind., Dok.Arbeitsmed., Environ.Sci.Poll.Mgmt., Excerp.Med., FAMLI, Fam.Ind., Gen.Sci.Ind. (Nov.1983-), Helminthol.Abstr., Hlth.Ind., INIS Atomind., Ind.Med. (1970-), Ind.Sci.Rev., Inpharma, Int.Nurs.Ind., L.R.I., Med.Care Rev., NRN, Neurosci.Cit.Ind., Nutr.Abstr., Pharm.&Out.News, Pollut.Abstr., Protozool.Abstr., Reac., Rev.Appl.Entomol., Rev.Med.& Vet.Mycol., Risk Abstr., SSCI (coverage dropped), Saf.Sci.Abstr., Sci.Cit.Ind. (coverage dropped), THA, Tr.& Indus.Ind.
—BLDSC (0814.700000), CISTI, EMDOCS, GNLM, IDS, ingenta, KNAW.
Published by: American Academy of Family Physicians, 11400 Tomahawk Creek Pkwy, Leawood, KS 66211-2672. TEL 913-906-6000, 800-274-2237, FAX 913-906-6080, afpedit@aafp.org, http://www.aafp.org. Ed. Jay Siwek. Pub. Joetta Melton. R&P Ariana Reeder. Adv. contact Dan Gowan TEL 201-288-4440. B&W page USD 7,760. Circ: 179,315 (paid and controlled).

610 USA ISSN 1060-5487
RA976 CODEN: JAHIES
AMERICAN HEALTH INFORMATION MANAGEMENT ASSOCIATION. JOURNAL. Text in English. 1929. 10/yr. USD 72 (effective 2001). adv. bk.rev. charts, illus, stat. index. **Document type:** *Journal, Trade.* **Description:** Covers copy and pictorial material of technical, professional and human interest in healthcare information management, activities of national and component organizations of these health professionals.
Former titles (until 1990): American Medical Record Association. Journal (0273-9976); (until 1980): Medical Record News (0025-7486)
Indexed: Abstr.Health Care Manage.Stud., AgeLine, CINAHL, Curr.Cont. (coverage dropped), Curr.Ind.Stat., Excerp.Med., Hosp.Lit.Ind., Int.Nurs.Ind., e-psyche.
—BLDSC (4682.200000), EMDOCS, GNLM, IDS.
Published by: American Health Information Management Association, 233 N Michigan Ave Ste 2150, Chicago, IL 60601. TEL 312-233-1100, FAX 312-233-1090, journal@ahima.org, http://www.ahima.org. Ed., R&P Anne Zender. Adv. contact Jane Jeffries. B&W page USD 1,670, color page USD 3,895. Circ: 40,000 (paid).

AMERICAN INTERNATIONAL JOURNAL OF ARTS, SCIENCES, ENGINEERING AND MEDICINE. see *ART*

AMERICAN JOURNAL OF ACUPUNCTURE. see *ALTERNATIVE MEDICINE*

AMERICAN JOURNAL OF CLINICAL NUTRITION; a journal reporting the practical application of our world-wide knowledge of nutrition. see *NUTRITION AND DIETETICS*

571.9 USA ISSN 0002-9173
RB1 CODEN: AJCPAI
AMERICAN JOURNAL OF CLINICAL PATHOLOGY. Text in English. 1931. m. USD 210 domestic to individuals; USD 330 foreign to individuals; USD 335 domestic to institutions; USD 435 foreign to institutions (effective 2000). adv. illus. index, cum.index. *Refereed.* **Document type:** *Academic/Scholarly.* **Description:** Helps pathologists and other clinical laboratory scientists keep their professional knowledge current. Publishes original investigations and observation in clinical pathology. Articles cover a broad spectrum of subspecialty topics.
Related titles: Microform ed.: (from PQC); Online - full text ed.: (from EBSCO Publishing, Institute for Scientific Information); ♦ Supplement: Pathology Patterns. ISSN 1050-9194.
Indexed: AIDS Abstr., AIM, ASCA, Abstr.Anthropol., Agri.& Environ.Biotech.Abstr. (coverage dropped), Biol.Abstr., C.I.S. Abstr., Chem.Abstr., Chem.Indus.Notes, Chem.Titles, Curr.Adv.Cancer Res., Curr.Adv.Ecol.Sci., Curr.Adv.Gen.& Molec.Biol., Curr.Cont., Dairy Sci.Abstr., Dent.Ind., Derwent Biotech.Abstr., Diar.Dis.Res., Dok.Arbeitsmed., Excerp.Med., Helminthol.Abstr., Hosp.Lit.Ind., INIS Atomind., Ind.Med. (1931-), Ind.Sci.Rev., Ind.Vet., Inpharma, Int.Abstr.Biol.Sci., Lead Abstr., Med.& Surg.Dermat., Nutr.Abstr., Pharm.&Out.News, Protozool.Abstr., Reac., Rev.Appl.Entomol., Rev.Med.& Vet.Mycol., SSCI (coverage dropped), Sci.Cit.Ind., THA, Trop.Dis.Bull., Zincscan.
—BLDSC (0824.000000), CASDDS, CISTI, EMDOCS, GNLM, IDS, ingenta, KNAW.
Published by: American Society of Clinical Pathologists, 2100 W Harrison St, Chicago, IL 60612. TEL 312-738-1336, 800-633-4931, FAX 312-738-0101, http://www.ascp.org/eajcp. Ed. Dr. Mark R Wick. Pub. Joshua Weikersheimer. R&P Nick Watters. Adv. contact Joe Dingee. Circ: 15,323. **Subscr. in Japan to:** Igaku-Shoin, 1-28-36 Hongo, Bunkyo-ku, Tokyo 113-0033, Japan; **Subscr. to:** PO Box 11806, Birmingham, AL 35202-1806.

616.5 USA ISSN 0193-1091
RL95 CODEN: AJODDB
AMERICAN JOURNAL OF DERMATOPATHOLOGY. Text in English. 1979. bi-m. USD 282 domestic to individuals; USD 325 foreign to individuals; USD 511 domestic to institutions; USD 571 foreign to institutions (effective 2002). adv. bk.rev. abstr, charts, illus. index. back issues avail.; reprint service avail. from PQC. *Refereed.* **Document type:** *Journal, Academic/Scholarly.* **Description:** Offers outstanding coverage of the latest diagnostic approaches and laboratory techniques.
Related titles: Microform ed.; Online - full text ed.: USD 664.30 domestic academic site license; USD 724.30 foreign academic site license; USD 740.95 domestic corporate site license; USD 800.95 foreign corporate site license (effective 2002) (from Ovid Technologies, Inc., Institute for Scientific Information).
Indexed: ASCA, Arts & Hum.Cit.Ind. (coverage dropped), Curr.Adv.Cancer Res., Curr.Cont., Dent.Ind., Excerp.Med., INIS Atomind., Ind.Med. (1979-), Ind.Sci.Rev., Ind.Vet., Inpharma, Jrnl.Watch Derm., Med.& Surg.Dermat., Reac., Rev.Appl.Entomol., Rev.Med.& Vet.Mycol., SSCI (coverage dropped), Sci.Cit.Ind., Small Anim.Abstr.
—BLDSC (0824.240000), CASDDS, CISTI, EMDOCS, GNLM, IDS, ingenta, KNAW.
Published by: (International Society of Dermatopathology), Lippincott Williams & Wilkins (Philadelphia) (Subsidiary of: Wolters Kluwer N.V.), 530 Walnut St, Philadelphia, PA 19106-3621. TEL 215-521-8300, FAX 215-521-8902, http://www.Lww.com. Ed. Dr. Philip E Leboit. Pub. Jim Merritt. R&P Margaret Becker. Adv. contact Susan Edison. B&W page USD 830, color page USD 1,785; trim 11 x 8.25. Circ: 1,948. **Subscr. to:** PO Box 1600, Hagerstown, MD 21740-1600. TEL 800-777-2295, FAX 301-824-7390.

610 USA ISSN 0894-8291
AMERICAN JOURNAL OF ELECTROMEDICINE. Text in English. 1957. q. USD 25. adv. bk.rev. bibl, charts, illus, stat. index. back issues avail. *Refereed.* **Document type:** *Academic/Scholarly.* **Description:** International journal devoted to all aspects and applications of electromedicine in biomedical research and medical practice.
Formerly: Nucleus Science Journal
Published by: National Institute of Electromedical Information, 3409 Shelbourne Rd, Baltimore, MD 21208. TEL 410-764-8181, FAX 410-764-8181, ajem@juno.com. Eds. Dr. Mark A Young, Dr. Stanley Kornhauser. Adv. contact Dr. Stanley Kornhauser. Circ: 50,000.

610 USA ISSN 0002-9262
RA421 CODEN: AJEPAS
AMERICAN JOURNAL OF EPIDEMIOLOGY. Text in English. 1921. 24/yr. (2 vols./yr.). GBP 125, USD 185 to individuals Combined rate to the Journal and Epidemiologic Reviews; GBP 250, USD 380 to institutions Combined rate to the Journal and Epidemiologic Reviews (effective 2002). adv. bk.rev. illus. index, cum.index. back issues avail. *Refereed.* **Document type:** *Journal, Academic/Scholarly.* **Description:** Covers empirical research findings, methodological developments in the field of epidemiologic research and opinion pieces. It is aimed at both fellow epidemiologists and those who use epidemiologic data, including public health workers and clinicians.
Former titles: American Journal of Hygiene; Journal of Hygiene (0096-5294)
Related titles: Microfilm ed.: (from WWS); Microform ed.; Online - full text ed.: GBP 112, USD 166 to individuals Online only; Combined rate to the Journal and Epidemiologic Reviews; GBP 225, USD 342 to institutions Online only; Combined rate to the Journal and Epidemiologic Reviews (effective 2002) (from Ovid Technologies, Inc., HighWire Pr., H. W. Wilson, Gale Group, Swets Blackwell, Institute for Scientific Information).
Indexed: AIDS Abstr., ASCA, Abstr.Anthropol., Abstr.Health Care Manage.Stud., Abstr.Hyg., Addic.Abstr., AgeLine, Amer.Bibl.Slavic & E.Eur.Stud., Aqua.Sci.& Fish.Abstr., Behav.Med.Abstr., Bibl.Asian Stud. (1971), Bibl.Dev.Med.& Child Neur., Biol.Abstr., Biol.Dig., Biostat., CINAHL, C.I.S. Abstr., CSNB, Chem.Abstr., Compumath, Crim.Just.Abstr., Curr.Adv.Cancer Res., Curr.Adv.Ecol.Sci., Curr.Cont., Curr.Ind.Stat., Dairy Sci.Abstr., Diab.Cont., Diar.Dis.Res., Dok.Arbeitsmed., Environ.Sci.Poll.Mgmt., Excerp.Med., Fam.Ind., Forest Prod.Abstr., Forest.Abstr., Gen.Sci.Ind. (Jul.1997-), Geo.Abstr.H.G., Helminthol.Abstr., IDA, INIS Atomind., Ind.Med. (1965-), Ind.Sci.Rev., Ind.Vet., Inpharma, Jrnl.Watch Inf.Dis., Jrnl.Watch Wom.Hlth., Lab.Haz.Bull., Med.& Surg.Dermat., NRN, Neurosci.Cit.Ind., Nutr.Abstr., Pharm.&Out.News, Pollut.Abstr., Popul.Ind., Poult.Abstr., Protozool.Abstr., Reac., Rev.Appl.Entomol., Rev.Med.& Vet.Mycol., Rev.Plant Path., Risk Abstr., Rural Devel.Abstr., SSCI (coverage dropped), Saf.Sci.Abstr., Sage Race Rel.Abstr., Sci.Cit.Ind., Sel.Water Res.Abstr., Small Anim.Abstr., So.Pac.Per.Ind., Sport Fish.Abstr., Sugar Ind.Abstr., THA, Trop.Dis.Bull., Vet.Bull., Viol.& Abuse Abstr., W.R.C.Inf., Weed Abstr., Wild.Rev., Zoo.Rec.
—BLDSC (0824.600000), CISTI, EMDOCS, GNLM, IDS, Infotrieve, ingenta, KNAW, Linda Hall. **CCC.**
Published by: (Society for Epidemiologic Research), Oxford University Press, Academic Division, Great Clarendon St, Oxford OX2 6DP, United Kingdom. TEL 44-1865-267907, FAX 44-1865-267835, jnl.info@oup.co.uk, http://aje.oupjournals.org/, http://www.oup.co.uk/journals. Pub. Jackie J Fox. R&P Fionna Willis. Circ: 7,100. **Subscr. outside N. American:** Journals Marketing, Great Clarendon St, Oxford OX2 6DP, United Kingdom.

618.97 USA ISSN 1049-9091
R726.8 CODEN: AJHCF9
THE AMERICAN JOURNAL OF HOSPICE AND PALLIATIVE CARE. Text in English. 1983. bi-m. USD 136 domestic to individuals; USD 172 in Canada to individuals; USD 199 elsewhere to individuals; USD 193 domestic to institutions; USD 245 in Canada to institutions; USD 304 elsewhere to institutions (effective 2002). adv. bk.rev. charts, illus. Index. back issues avail.; reprints avail. *Refereed.* **Document type:** *Academic/Scholarly.* **Description:** Publishes articles and research studies on palliative care and hospice techniques. Features regular columns, articles, and news briefs.
Formerly (until 1990): American Journal of Hospice Care (0749-1565)
Indexed: AMED, AgeLine, CINAHL, Fam.Ind., Int.Nurs.Ind. (1990-), Lang.& Lang.Behav.Abstr., SOPODA, Soc.Work Res.& Abstr., Sociol.Abstr.
—BLDSC (0824.843000), GNLM, Infotrieve, ingenta. **CCC.**
Published by: Prime National Publishing Corp., 470 Boston Post Rd, Weston, MA 02493. TEL 781-899-2702, FAX 781-899-4900, hospice@pnpco.com, http://www.pnpco.com/pn01000.html. Ed. Dr. Robert E Enck. Pub., Adv. contact Richard A DeVito Sr. TEL 781-899-2702 ext. 107. Circ: 2,000.

AMERICAN JOURNAL OF LAW & MEDICINE. see *LAW*

338.476 USA ISSN 1096-1860
RA413.5.U5 CODEN: AJMCFY
THE AMERICAN JOURNAL OF MANAGED CARE; the forum for peer-reviewed literature on healthcare outcomes. Text in English. 1995. m. USD 75 domestic to individuals; USD 135 domestic to institutions; USD 145 in Canada; USD 155 elsewhere; USD 45 to students; USD 15 newsstand/cover (effective 2000). adv. *Refereed.* **Document type:** *Journal, Trade.*
Formerly (until 1996): American Journal of Managed Healthcare (1088-0224)
Related titles: Online - full text ed.: (from Institute for Scientific Information).
Indexed: AgeLine, CINAHL, Curr.Cont., I.P.A., Inpharma, Int.Nurs.Ind., Reac., SSCI.
—BLDSC (0826.920000), IDS.
Published by: American Medical Publishing, LLC (Subsidiary of: Medical World Communications), 241 Forsgate Dr, Ste 102, Jamesburg, NJ 08831. TEL 732-656-1006, FAX 732-656-0818, info@ajmc.com, http://www.ajmc.com. Ed. Dr. J Sanford Schwartz. Pubs. Jack M Ciattarelli, Jeffrey J Hennessy. adv.: page USD 2,800.

AMERICAN JOURNAL OF MEDICAL GENETICS. see *BIOLOGY—Genetics*

AMERICAN JOURNAL OF MEDICAL GENETICS. SUPPLEMENT. see *BIOLOGY—Genetics*

610 USA ISSN 0002-9343
RC60 CODEN: AJMEAZ
THE AMERICAN JOURNAL OF MEDICINE. Text in English. 1946. 18/yr. USD 102 in US & Canada to individuals; USD 249 elsewhere to individuals; USD 252 in US & Canada to institutions; USD 423 elsewhere to institutions (effective 2002). adv. bibl, illus. index. back issues avail. *Refereed.* **Document type:** *Academic/Scholarly.* **Description:** Contains the original output of clinical investigators worldwide. Includes case reports and clinical-pathologic conferences, symposia, and essays and editorials on medicine, science, and society.
Related titles: CD-ROM ed.: (from Ovid Technologies, Inc.); Microform ed.; Online - full text ed.: (from Ovid Technologies, Inc., EBSCO Publishing, ingenta, Gale Group, Swets Blackwell, ScienceDirect, Factiva, Institute for Scientific Information).
Indexed: AIDS Abstr., AIM, ASCA, Abstr.Anthropol., Abstr.Hyg., Abstr.Inter.Med., AgeLine, Agri.& Environ.Biotech.Abstr. (coverage dropped), Behav.Med.Abstr., Biol.Abstr., Biol.Dig., Biostat., CINAHL, C.I.S. Abstr., Chem.Abstr., Chem.Indus.Notes, Chem.Titles, Curr.Adv.Biochem., Curr.Adv.Cancer Res., Curr.Adv.Cell & Devel.Biol., Curr.Adv.Ecol.Sci., Curr.Adv.Gen.& Molec.Biol., Curr.Cont., Curr.Ind.Stat., Dairy Sci.Abstr., Dent.Ind., Derwent Biotech.Abstr., Diab.Cont., Diar.Dis.Res., Dok.Arbeitsmed., Environ.Sci.Poll.Mgmt., Excerp.Med., Helminthol.Abstr., INIS Atomind., I.P.A., Ind.Med. (1946-), Ind.Sci.Rev., Inpharma, Int.Abstr.Biol.Sci., Int.Nurs.Ind., Jrnl.Watch, Jrnl.Watch Gastr., Jrnl.Watch Inf.Dis., Kidney, Lead Abstr., Med.& Surg.Dermat., Nutr.Abstr., Pharm.&Out.News, Pollut.Abstr., Protozool.Abstr., Reac., Rev.Appl.Entomol., Rev.Arom.& Med.Plants, Rev.Med.& Vet.Mycol., Rev.Plant Path., Risk Abstr., SSCI (coverage dropped), Saf.Sci.Abstr., Sci.Cit.Ind., THA, Telegen, Trop.Dis.Bull.
—BLDSC (0828.100000), ADONIS, CASDDS, CISTI, EMDOCS, GNLM, IDS, ingenta, KNAW. **CCC.**
Published by: Excerpta Medica, Inc. (Subsidiary of: Reed Elsevier Medical group), 105 Raider Blvd, Belle Mead, NJ 08502. TEL 908-281-3625, FAX 908-874-8419, d.dionne@elsevier.com, http://www.elsevier.com/locate/ajmselect/. Eds. Dr. Lee Goldman, Warren S Browner. Circ: 53,751. **Subscr. to:** PO Box 7247 7207, Philadelphia, PA 19170-7207.

AMERICAN JOURNAL OF OCCUPATIONAL THERAPY. see *OCCUPATIONAL HEALTH AND SAFETY*

610 USA ISSN 1059-1494
RB127
AMERICAN JOURNAL OF PAIN MANAGEMENT. Text in English. 1991. q. USD 65 (effective 1998). adv. bk.rev. *Refereed.* **Document type:** *Academic/Scholarly.*
Indexed: CINAHL.
—BLDSC (0829.500000), KNAW.
Published by: (American Academy of Pain Management), A J P M Inc., c/o TTUHSC School of Pharmacy, 1300 Coulter, Amarillo, TX 79106. TEL 806-352-0781, supernaw@cortex.ama.ttuhsc.edu, http://www.aapainmanage.org/default.asp. Ed. Robert B Supernaw. R&P Diane McCoy. Circ: 6,300 (paid).

616.07 USA ISSN 0002-9440
RB1 CODEN: AJPAA4
AMERICAN JOURNAL OF PATHOLOGY. Text in English. 1901. m. USD 195 domestic to individuals; USD 270 in Canada & Mexico to individuals; USD 290 elsewhere to individuals; USD 385 domestic to institutions; USD 460 in Canada & Mexico to institutions; USD 480 elsewhere to institutions (effective 2001). adv. index. back issues avail. *Refereed.* **Document type:** *Journal, Academic/Scholarly.* **Description:** Publishes research papers on the cellular and molecular mechanisms of disease, without preference for specific method of analysis.
Formerly: Journal of Medical Research (0097-3599)
Related titles: Microform ed.: (from PQC,PMC); Online - full text ed.: (from HighWire Pr., EBSCO Publishing, ProQuest Information & Learning, Institute for Scientific Information).
Indexed: AIDS Abstr., AIM, ASCA, Agri.& Environ.Biotech.Abstr. (coverage dropped), Biol.Abstr., Biol.Dig., Chem.Abstr., Chem.Indus.Notes, Chem.Titles, Curr.Adv.Cancer Res., Curr.Adv.Cell & Devel.Biol., Curr.Adv.Ecol.Sci., Curr.Adv.Gen.& Molec.Biol., Curr.Cont., Derwent Biotech.Abstr., Diar.Dis.Res., Dok.Arbeitsmed., Excerp.Med., Helminthol.Abstr., INIS Atomind., Ind.Med. (1925-), Ind.Sci.Rev., Ind.Vet., Inpharma, Int.Abstr.Biol.Sci., Kidney, Maize Abstr., Med.& Surg.Dermat., Neurosci.Cit.Ind., Nutr.Abstr., Pharm.&Out.News, Poult.Abstr., Protozool.Abstr., Reac., SSCI (coverage dropped), Sci.Cit.Ind., Sport Fish.Abstr., THA, Vet.Bull., Wild.Rev., Zoo.Rec.
—BLDSC (0829.600000), CASDDS, CISTI, EMDOCS, GNLM, IDS, ingenta, KNAW, Linda Hall. **CCC.**
Published by: American Society for Investigative Pathology, 9650 Rockville Pike, Bethesda, MD 20814. TEL 301-571-0107, FAX 301-571-0108, psmith@pathol.faseb.org, http://www.amjpathol.org/. Ed. Nelson Fausto. Adv. contact Robert McGonnagle. Circ: 5,000. **Subscr. to:** Fulco, PO Box 3000, Denville, NJ 07834. TEL 800-875-2997, FAX 973-627-5872.

AMERICAN JOURNAL OF PHYSIOLOGY (CONSOLIDATED). see *BIOLOGY—Physiology*

610 614.8 USA ISSN 0749-3797
RA421 CODEN: AJPMEA
AMERICAN JOURNAL OF PREVENTIVE MEDICINE. Text in English. 1984. 8/yr. EUR 138 in Europe to individuals; JPY 18,400 in Japan to individuals; USD 155 elsewhere to individuals; EUR 356 in Europe to institutions; JPY 47,200 in Japan to institutions; USD 398 elsewhere to institutions (effective 2002). adv. bk.rev. charts, illus. back issues avail. *Refereed.* **Document type:** *Academic/Scholarly.* **Description:** Contains original articles and correspondence on all aspects of practice, teaching, and research in preventive medicine.
Related titles: Online - full text ed.: (from ingenta, Swets Blackwell, ScienceDirect, Institute for Scientific Information).
Indexed: ASCA, Abstr.Health Care Manage.Stud., AgeLine, Crim.Just.Abstr., Curr.Cont., Environ.Sci.Poll.Mgmt., Excerp.Med., Ind.Med. (1985-), Inpharma, Int.Nurs.Ind., Lang.& Lang.Behav.Abstr., Med.& Surg.Dermat., Microbiol.Abstr., NRN, Nutr.Abstr., Pharm.&Out.News, Pollut.Abstr., PsycInfo, Psychol.Abstr. (1989-), Reac., Risk Abstr., SOPODA, SSCI (coverage dropped), Saf.Sci.Abstr., Soc.Serv.Abstr., Sociol.Abstr., Soyabean Abstr., THA, e-psyche.
—BLDSC (0834.370000), CASDDS, CISTI, EMDOCS, GNLM, IDS, ingenta, KNAW. **CCC.**
Published by: (American College of Preventive Medicine), Elsevier Science, 655 Ave of the Americas, New York, NY 10010. FAX 212-633-3990, ajpmwebmaster@elsevier.com, usinfo-f@elsevier.com, http://www.elsevier.com/locate/amepre. Eds. Dr. F Douglas Scutchfield, Dr. Kevin Patrick. Adv. contact Hank Blaney. B&W page USD 965, color page USD 2,160. Circ: 3,220 (paid). **Subscr. outside N. America to:** Elsevier Science BV, PO Box 211, Amsterdam 1000 AE, Netherlands. TEL 31-20-485-3757. **Co-sponsor:** Association of Teachers of Preventive Medicine.

AMERICAN JOURNAL OF SPEECH - LANGUAGE PATHOLOGY; a journal of clinical practice. see *HANDICAPPED—Hearing Impaired*

616.07 USA ISSN 0147-5185
RD57 CODEN: AJSPDX
AMERICAN JOURNAL OF SURGICAL PATHOLOGY. Text in English. 1977. m. USD 320 domestic to individuals for print & online eds.; USD 413 foreign to individuals for print & online eds.; USD 672 domestic to institutions for print & online eds.; USD 728 foreign to institutions for print & online eds.; USD 56 newsstand/cover (effective 2002). adv. bk.rev. charts, illus, stat. index. back issues avail. *Refereed.* **Document type:** *Academic/Scholarly.* **Description:** Covers diagnostic and prognostic technical advances.
Related titles: Microform ed.; Online - full text ed.: USD 873.60 domestic academic site license; USD 929.60 foreign academic site license; USD 974.40 domestic corporate site license; USD 1,030.40 foreign corporate site license (effective 2002) (from Ovid Technologies, Inc., Swets Blackwell, Institute for Scientific Information); ♦ Supplement to: Diagnostic Molecular Pathology. ISSN 1052-9551.
Indexed: ASCA, Biol.Abstr., Curr.Adv.Cancer Res., Curr.Adv.Ecol.Sci., Curr.Cont., Dent.Ind., Excerp.Med., Helminthol.Abstr., INIS Atomind., Ind.Med. (1977-), Ind.Sci.Rev., Inpharma, Int.Abstr.Biol.Sci., Int.Nurs.Ind., Jrnl.Watch Derm., Kidney, Med.& Surg.Dermat., Neurosci.Cit.Ind., Pharm.&Out.News, Protozool.Abstr., Reac., Rev.Med.& Vet.Mycol., Sci.Cit.Ind.
—BLDSC (0838.520000), CISTI, EMDOCS, GNLM, IDS, ingenta, KNAW.
Published by: (Arthur Purdy Stout Society of Surgical Pathologists), Lippincott Williams & Wilkins (Philadelphia) (Subsidiary of: Wolters Kluwer N.V.), 530 Walnut St, Philadelphia, PA 19106-3621. TEL 215-521-8300, FAX 215-521-8902, http://www.Lww.com. Ed. Dr. Stephen S Sternberg. R&P Alice McElhinney. Adv. contact Susan Eidson. B&W page USD 1,275, color page USD 2,330. Circ: 7,696 (paid). **Subscr. to:** PO Box 1600, Hagerstown, MD 21740-1600. TEL 800-777-2295, FAX 301-824-7390.

610 USA ISSN 0002-9629
R11 CODEN: AJMSA9
AMERICAN JOURNAL OF THE MEDICAL SCIENCES. Text in English. 1820. m. USD 244 domestic to individuals; USD 341 foreign to individuals; USD 478 domestic to institutions; USD 577 foreign to institutions; USD 46 newsstand/cover (effective 2002). adv. bibl, illus. s-a. index. *Refereed.* **Document type:** *Academic/Scholarly.* **Description:** Publishes developments in knowledge and treatment of diseases through clinically relevant original articles, review articles, commentaries, brief reviews, invited editorials and special reports.
Related titles: Microform ed.: (from PQC,PMC); Online - full text ed.: (from Ovid Technologies, Inc., Institute for Scientific Information).
Indexed: AIM, ASCA, Abstr.Hyg., Arts & Hum.Cit.Ind. (coverage dropped), Biol.Abstr., Chem.Abstr., Curr.Adv.Ecol.Sci., Curr.Cont., Dairy Sci.Abstr., Dent.Ind., Derwent Biotech.Abstr., Excerp.Med., GeoRef, Helminthol.Abstr., INIS Atomind., I.P.A., Ind.Med. (1827-), Ind.Sci.Rev., Ind.Vet., Inpharma, Kidney, Med.& Surg.Dermat., NRN, Nutr.Abstr., Pharm.&Out.News, Reac., Rev.Arom.& Med.Plants, Rev.Med.& Vet.Mycol., Rural Recreat.Tour.Abstr., SSCI (coverage dropped), Sci.Cit.Ind., Small Anim.Abstr., Sugar Ind.Abstr., Trop.Dis.Bull., Vet.Bull.
—BLDSC (0828.000000), CASDDS, CISTI, EMDOCS, GNLM, IDS, ingenta, KNAW.
Published by: (Southern Society for Clinical Investigation), Lippincott Williams & Wilkins (Philadelphia) (Subsidiary of: Wolters Kluwer N.V.), 530 Walnut St, Philadelphia, PA 19106-3621. TEL 215-521-8300, FAX 215-521-8902, http://www.Lww.com. Ed. Kent A Kirchner. R&P Alice McElhinney. Adv. contact Danni Monnich. B&W page USD 665, color page USD 985; trim 11 x 8.13. Circ: 1,710. **Subscr. to:** PO Box 1600, Hagerstown, MD 21740-1600. TEL 800-777-2295, FAX 301-824-7390.

615.5 GBR ISSN 1075-2765
RM301.28 CODEN: AJTHFG
AMERICAN JOURNAL OF THERAPEUTICS. Text in English. 1994. bi-m., latest vol.9. USD 215 in North America to individuals; USD 220 elsewhere to individuals; USD 489 per issue in North America to institutions; USD 494 per issue elsewhere to institutions; USD 175 per issue in North America to students; USD 82 newsstand/cover (effective 2002). adv. bk.rev. reprints avail. *Refereed.* **Document type:** *Academic/Scholarly.* **Description:** Assesses pharmacological developments in various medical specialties.
Related titles: Online - full text ed.: USD 626.60 academic site license; USD 698.80 corporate site license (2002) (from EBSCO Publishing).
Indexed: Derwent Biotech.Abstr., Excerp.Med. (1996-), Ind.Med. (1994-), Inpharma, Pharm.&Out.News, Reac., Saf.Sci.Abstr.
—BLDSC (0838.780000), CISTI, EMDOCS, GNLM, KNAW.
Published by: Chapman & Hall, Journals Department (Subsidiary of: International Thomson Publishing Group), Chapman & Hall, 2-6 Boundary Row, London SE1 8HN, United Kingdom. TEL 44-20-7856-0066, FAX 44-20-7522-9623, jhelp@rapidcom.co.uk, http://www.americantherapeutics.com, http://www.Lww.com. Ed. Dr. John C Somberg. **Subscr. to:** International Thompson Publishing Services Ltd.

615.8 USA
AMERICAN JOURNAL OF THERAPY. Text in English. 1974. m. USD 28. back issues avail. *Refereed.*
Published by: McMahon Publishing Co., 83 Peaceable St, West, Redding, CT 06896. TEL 203-544-9343. Ed. Jack Phillips.

610 USA
AMERICAN MEDICAL ASSOCIATION. COUNCIL ON ETHICAL AND JUDICIAL AFFAIRS. CODE OF MEDICAL ETHICS. CURRENT OPINIONS WITH ANNOTATIONS. Text in English. 1981. biennial. USD 35.95 to non-members; USD 14.95 to members (effective 2000). adv. **Document type:** *Academic/Scholarly.* **Description:** Addresses social policy issues, practice matters, professional rights and responsibilities, and other topics important to the practice of medicine.
Former titles (until 1994): American Medical Association. Council on Ethical and Judicial Affairs. Current Opinions; American Medical Association. Judicial Council. Current Opinions
Published by: American Medical Association, Council on Ethical and Judicial Affairs, 515 N State St, P O Box 10946, Chicago, IL 60610-0946. TEL 800-621-8335. Ed. Karine Morin. R&P Benita Ezcrins TEL 312-464-4555. Adv. contact C Benson. Circ: 20,000 (paid).

AMERICAN MEDICAL ASSOCIATION. GRADUATE MEDICAL EDUCATION DIRECTORY (YEARS). see *EDUCATION—Guides To Schools And Colleges*

610 USA
R712.A1
AMERICAN MEDICAL DIRECTORY OF PHYSICIANS IN THE U S. Text in English. 1906. biennial, latest vol.36, 1998. USD 595 (effective 2000). **Document type:** *Directory.*
Former titles: American Medical Directory; American Medical Directory of Physicians; American Medical Directory (0065-9339)
Published by: American Medical Association, 515 N State St, P O Box 10946, Chicago, IL 60610-0946. TEL 312-464-5000, 800-262-8335, FAX 312-464-5600.

610 USA ISSN 0001-1843
AMERICAN MEDICAL NEWS. Text in English. 1958. w. (48/yr.). USD 145 domestic to non-members; GBP 125 foreign to non-members; USD 95 domestic to members; GBP 75 foreign to members; USD 325 domestic to institutions; GBP 275 foreign to institutions (effective 2001). adv. bk.rev. charts, illus. s-a. index. **Document type:** *Academic/Scholarly.*
Formerly: A M A News
Related titles: Microfiche ed.; Microform ed.: (from PQC); Online - full text ed.: (from Gale Group, EBSCO Publishing).
Indexed: Bus.Ind., Chic.Per.Ind., Hlth.Ind., Hosp.Lit.Ind., L.R.I., MEDSOC, Med.Care Rev., Tr.& Indus.Ind.
—GNLM, Infotrieve. **CCC.**
Published by: American Medical Association, 515 N State St, P O Box 10946, Chicago, IL 60610-0946. TEL 312-464-5000, amnews-comments@ama-assn.org, http://www.ama-assn.org. Ed. Kathryn Tirombatore. Pub. Peter Murphy. R&P Ada Jimenez Walker. adv.: B&W page USD 11,552, color page USD 14,032. Circ: 368,300. **Subscr. outside the Americas to:** JAMA Readers Services, PO Box 299, London WC1H 9TD, United Kingdom. TEL 44-171-383-6270.

AMERICAN MEDICAL WOMEN'S ASSOCIATION. JOURNAL. see *WOMEN'S HEALTH*

610 USA ISSN 1045-9901
RC875
AMERICAN SOCIETY OF ANDROLOGY. MEETING PROGRAM AND ABSTRACTS. Text in English. a. USD 225 to institutions; USD 245 foreign to institutions; with Journal of Andrology. adv. abstr. **Document type:** *Proceedings, Academic/Scholarly.*
Published by: (American Society of Andrology), Allen Press Inc., PO Box 1897, Lawrence, KS 66044-8897. TEL 785-843-1235, 800-627-0629, FAX 785-843-1274, asa@hp-assoc.com, http://godot.urol.uic.edu/~androlog. Eds. David W Hamilton, Jon L Pryor. R&P Lonnie Russell TEL 618-453-1596. Adv. contact Onkar S Sandal.

610 USA
AMP. Text in English. 1919. bi-m. USD 25 (effective 2000). adv. bk.rev. **Document type:** *Newsletter.*
Published by: National Amputation Foundation, 38 40 Church St, Malverne, NY 11565. TEL 516-887-3600, FAX 516-887-3667. Ed. Donald Sioss. Circ: 2,000.

616 TUR ISSN 0255-6553
ANADOLU KLINIGI. Text in Turkish. 1933. q.
Published by: Turkish Medical Society/Turk Tip Dernigi, Valikonagi Caddesi 10, Harbiye, Istanbul, Turkey.

610 ESP
ANALES CUIDADOS INTENSIVOS. Text in Spanish. 6/yr.
Address: Nunez de Balboa, 120 2o, Madrid 28006, Spain.

610 ESP ISSN 0003-2530
ANALES DEL INSTITUTO CORACHAN* . Text in Spanish. 1971 (vol.23). q. free per issue. adv. bk.rev. charts, illus, stat.
Indexed: Chem.Abstr., Excerp.Med.
—CCC.
Published by: Instituto Corachan, Buigas, 19, Barcelona 08017, Spain.

THE ANATOMICAL RECORD. see *BIOLOGY*

ANATOMIESE VERENIGING VAN SUIDER-AFRIKA. KONGRESVERRIGTINGE/ANATOMICAL SOCIETY OF SOUTHERN AFRICA. PROCEEDINGS OF ANNUAL CONGRESS. see *BIOLOGY—Physiology*

611 DEU ISSN 0066-1562
QL801 CODEN: VHAGAS
ANATOMISCHE GESELLSCHAFT. VERHANDLUNGEN. Text in German. 1887. a. price varies. reprint service avail. from ISI. **Document type:** *Proceedings, Academic/Scholarly.*
Related titles: ♦ Supplement to: Annals of Anatomy. ISSN 0940-9602.
Indexed: Biol.Abstr., Chem.Abstr., Excerp.Med., Ind.Med. (coverage dropped), Zoo.Rec.
—CASDDS, GNLM, Linda Hall.
Published by: Urban & Fischer Verlag, Loebdergraben 14a, Jena 07743, Germany. TEL 49-3641-626444, FAX 49-3641-626500, journals@urbanfischer.de, http://www.urbanfischer.de. R&P Martin Huber TEL 49-3641-626430. **Dist. by:** Nature Publishing Group, Brunel Rd, Basingstoke RG21 6XS, United Kingdom. TEL 44-1256-302629, FAX 44-1256-463570, j.stephens@macmillan.com.

ANATOMY AND EMBRYOLOGY. see *BIOLOGY—Physiology*

610 ITA
ANCH'IO. Text in Italian. 1978. m. free per issue. illus. **Description:** Covers news and events for and about the handicapped.
Published by: Associazione Laziale Motulesi (A.L.M.), Via Laurentina, 5, Rome, RM 00142, Italy. TEL 5406705. Ed. Carmello Pelle.

ANCIENT SCIENCE OF LIFE. see *ALTERNATIVE MEDICINE*

610 DEU ISSN 0303-4569
CODEN: ANDRDQ
ANDROLOGIA. Text and summaries in English, German. 1969. bi-m. DEM 433 in Europe to individuals; DEM 463 elsewhere to individuals; DEM 643 in Europe to institutions; DEM 673 elsewhere to institutions; DEM 708.01 in Europe to institutions; DEM 455.71 in Europe to individuals; DEM 737.34 elsewhere to institutions; DEM 485.04 elsewhere to individuals; DEM 778.81 in Europe to institutions print & online eds. combined; DEM 501.28 in Europe to individuals print & online eds. combined; DEM 811.07 elsewhere to institutions print & online eds. combined; DEM 533.54 elsewhere to individuals print & online eds. combined (effective 2001). adv. index. reprint service avail. from PQC. *Refereed.* **Document type:** *Journal, Academic/Scholarly.* **Description:** Provides an international forum for original papers on the current clinical, morphological, biochemical, and experimental status of organic male infertility and sexual disorders in men.
Formerly: Andrologie
Related titles: Online - full text ed.: ISSN 1439-0272. DEM 638 to institutions; DEM 411 to individuals (2001) (from EBSCO Publishing, O C L C Online Computer Library Center, Inc., RoweCom Information Quest, ingenta, Munksgaard & Blackwell Science's Synergy, Swets Blackwell, Institute for Scientific Information).
Indexed: ASCA, Agri.& Environ.Biotech.Abstr. (coverage dropped), Anim.Breed.Abstr., Biol.Abstr., Chem.Abstr., Chem.Indus.Notes, Chem.Titles, Curr.Adv.Cell & Devel.Biol., Curr.Adv.Ecol.Sci., Curr.Adv.Gen.& Molec.Biol., Curr.Cont., Derwent Biotech.Abstr., Dok.Arbeitsmed., Excerp.Med., INIS Atomind., Ind.Med. (1974-), Ind.Sci.Rev., Inpharma, Int.Abstr.Biol.Sci., Nutr.Abstr., Pharm.&Out.News, Pig News & Info., Reac., Ref.Zh., Sci.Cit.Ind., Small Anim.Abstr.
—BLDSC (0900.443000), ADONIS, CASDDS, CISTI, EMDOCS, GNLM, IDS, ingenta. **CCC.**
Published by: (Deutsche Gesellschaft fuer Andrologie), Blackwell Wissenschafts Verlag GmbH, Kurfuerstendamm 57, Berlin 10707, Germany. TEL 49-30-32790624, FAX 49-30-32790610, abo@blackwis.de, http://www.blackwell.de. Ed. M Bergmann. adv.: B&W page DEM 1,800; trim 170 x 240. Circ: 1,200.

612 FRA ISSN 1166-2654
CODEN: AROLEO
ANDROLOGIE. Text in French. 1987. 4/yr. FRF 410 in the European Union; FRF 440 elsewhere.
Formerly (until 1991): Societe d'Andrologie de Langue Francaise. Bulletin (1154-3418)
Indexed: Excerp.Med. (1994-).
—BLDSC (0900.445100), CISTI, EMDOCS, GNLM, KNAW.
Published by: (Societe d'Andrologie de Langue Francaise), Andrologie - Med - Editions, 7 bd. Flandrin, Paris 75116, France. TEL 33-1-45033196, FAX 33-1-45047289.

610 CHN ISSN 1000-1492
ANHUI YIKE DAXUE XUEBAO/ACTA UNIVERSITATIS MEDICINALIS ANHUI. Text in Chinese. 1955. bi-m. CNY 8 per issue domestic (effective 2000). **Document type:** *Academic/Scholarly.*
Formerly (until 1984): Anhui Yixueyuan Xuebao (0253-3693)
Related titles: Online - full content ed.: (from WanFang Data Corp.).
Published by: Anhui Yike Daxue/Anhui University of Medical Sciences, Meishan Lu, Hefei, Anhui 230032, China. Ed. Shuyun Xu.

610 CHN ISSN 1000-0399
ANHUI YIXUE/ANHUI MEDICAL SCIENCES. Text in Chinese. 1976. bi-m. CNY 4 (effective 2000). adv. back issues avail. **Document type:** *Academic/Scholarly.*
Published by: Anhui Yixue Qingbao Yanjiusuo/Anhui Institute of Medical Information, 1 Yonghong Lu, Hefei, Anhui 230061, China. TEL 86-551-2827688. Ed. Zhou Keneng.

610 CHN ISSN 1000-2219
CODEN: AZXUEG
ANHUI ZHONGYI XUEYUAN XUEBAO/ANHUI INSTITUTE OF TRADITIONAL CHINESE MEDICINE. JOURNAL. Text in Chinese. q. **Document type:** *Academic/Scholarly.*
Published by: Anhui Zhongyi Xueyuan/Anhui Institute of Traditional Chinese Medicine, Meishan Lu, Hefei, Anhui 230038, China. TEL 331006. Ed. Liu Zhongben.

610 TUR ISSN 1300-5464
ANKARA MEDICAL SCHOOL. JOURNAL. Text in English. 1978. q. TRL 20,000,000 (effective 2001).

M

Published by: Ankara Universitesi, Tip Fakultesi/Anakara University, Faculty of Medicine, Sihhiye, Ankara, Turkey. TEL 90-312-3103333, FAX 90-312-3125251, http://www.ankara.edu.tr. Circ: 500.

610 TUR ISSN 0365-8104
CODEN: AUTFAE

ANKARA UNIVERSITESI. TIP FAKULTESI. MECMUASI/UNIVERSITY OF ANKARA. FACULTY OF MEDICINE. JOURNAL. Text in Turkish; Summaries in English. 1947. q., latest vol.54. TRL 20,000,000 domestic; USD 17, DEM 40 foreign (effective 2001). back issues avail. *Refereed.* **Document type:** *Journal, Academic/Scholarly.* **Description:** This is a general medical journal.
Related titles: Supplement: Ankara Universitesi. Tip Fakultesi. Mecmuasi. Supplementum. ISSN 0365-2238.
Indexed: Biol.Abstr., Chem.Abstr., Helminthol.Abstr., Nutr.Abstr.
—CASDDS, GNLM.
Published by: Ankara Universitesi, Tip Fakultesi/Anakara University, Faculty of Medicine, Sihhiye, Ankara, Turkey. TEL 90-312-3103333, 90-312-3106305, FAX 90-312-3125251, 90-312-3101551, http://www.ankara.edu.tr. Ed. Dr. Cetin Erol. Circ: 1,000.

610 POL ISSN 0303-4135
CODEN: AAMGBD

ANNALES ACADEMIAE MEDICAE GEDANENSIS. Text in English, Polish; Summaries in English. 1971. a. PLZ 10 domestic; USD 20 foreign (effective 2000). index. back issues avail. **Document type:** *Academic/Scholarly.* **Description:** Details medical research and includes historical aspects.
Indexed: Biol.Abstr., Chem.Abstr., Chem.Indus.Notes, Chem.Titles, INIS Atomind., Ind.Med. (coverage dropped), Ref.Zh.
—BLDSC (0914.263100), CASDDS, CISTI, EMDOCS.
Published by: Akademia Medyczna w Gdansku, Ul Marii Sklodowskiej Curie 3 a, Gdansk 80210, Poland. TEL 48-58-3016115, FAX 48-58-316115, TELEX 512997 AMG PL, http://www.amg.gda.pl. Ed. Stefan Raszeja. Circ: 300. **Subscr. to:** Akademia Medyczna w Gdansku, Biblioteka Glowna, ul Debinki 1, Gdansk 80952, Poland. TEL 48-58-3023914, FAX 48-58-3023914.

610 POL ISSN 1427-4930

ANNALES ACADEMIAE MEDICAE STETINENSIS. SUPLEMENT. Text in Polish; Summaries in English. 1967. irreg., latest vol.67. 1 cols./p. *Refereed.* **Document type:** *Monographic series, Academic/Scholarly, Bibliography.*
Related titles: ♦ Supplement to: Pomorska Akademia Medyczna w Szczecinie. Roczniki. ISSN 1427-440X.
Indexed: Ind.Med.
Published by: Pomorska Akademia Medyczna w Szczecinie, Ul Rybacka 1, Szczecin 70204, Poland. TEL 48-91-48-00-860, 48-91-48-00-700, FAX 48-91-48-00-705. Ed. Jreneusz Kojder.

610 BEL ISSN 0003-3863

ANNALES COLLEGII MEDICI ANTVERPIENSIS. Text in French. 1946. m. (10/yr.). BEF 350. adv. bk.rev.
—GNLM.
Published by: Koninklijke Geneeskundige Kring van Antwerpen, Louizastraat 8, Antwerp 2000, Belgium. Circ: 1,000.

ANNALES DE BIOLOGIE CLINIQUE. see *BIOLOGY*

ANNALES DE PATHOLOGIE. see *BIOLOGY*

610 FRA ISSN 0221-3796
CODEN: AMNADI

ANNALES MEDICALES DE NANCY ET DE L'EST. Text in French. 1879. bi-m. FRF 350. adv. abstr. **Document type:** *Academic/Scholarly.*
Former titles (until 1978): Annales Medicales de Nancy (0003-4460); (until 1962): Revue Medicale de Nancy (0370-6354)
Indexed: Biol.Abstr., C.I.S. Abstr., Chem.Abstr., Excerp.Med., Rev.Plant Path.
—CASDDS, CISTI, EMDOCS, GNLM, KNAW.
Published by: Societe de Medecine de Nancy, Centre Hospitalier Regional Universitaire de Nancy, 29 av. de Lattre de Tassigny, Nancy Cedex 54037, France. TEL 33-3-83576161, FAX 33-3-83852622. Ed. A Larcan. Adv. contact M Pierson. Circ: 4,905.

ANNALES MEDICO-PSYCHOLOGIQUES. see *PSYCHOLOGY*

M

610 POL ISSN 0066-2240
B6 CODEN: AUMKAS

ANNALES UNIVERSITATIS MARIAE CURIE-SKLODOWSKA. SECTIO D. MEDICINA. Text in English, Polish; Abstracts and contents page in English. 1946. a. price varies. **Document type:** *Academic/Scholarly.*
Indexed: Biol.Abstr., Chem.Abstr., Curr.Adv.Ecol.Sci., Excerp.Med., Field Crop Abstr., Herb.Abstr., INIS Atomind., Ind.Med. (1946-), Ind.Vet., Rev.Appl.Entomol., Vet.Bull.
—CASDDS, CISTI, GNLM, KNAW, Linda Hall.
Published by: Uniwersytet Marii Curie-Sklodowskiej, Wydawnictwo, Pl M Curie Sklodowskiej 5, Lublin 20031, Poland. TEL 48-81-375304, FAX 48-81-336699. Ed. Stanislaw Bryc. Circ: 600.

616.98 ITA ISSN 0003-4630
CODEN: AMDNA4

ANNALI DI MEDICINA NAVALE. Text in Italian; Summaries in English, Italian. 1895. 3/m. ITL 20,000. bk.rev. **Description:** Features items on military medicine.
Indexed: Abstr.Hyg., Biol.Abstr., C.I.S. Abstr., Chem.Abstr., Excerp.Med., Helminthol.Abstr., INIS Atomind., Ind.Med. (coverage dropped), Trop.Dis.Bull.
—CASDDS, GNLM.
Published by: Ministero Difesa - Marina, Lungotevere Delle Navi, Rome, RM 00196, Italy. Circ: 500.

571.3 611 DEU ISSN 0940-9602
QL801 CODEN: ANANAU

ANNALS OF ANATOMY. Text in English. 1886. irreg. (6 nos./vol.). EUR 218, GBP 180 to individuals; EUR 484 to institutions (effective 2002). adv. bk.rev. bibl, charts, illus. index, cum.index. reprint service avail. from ISI. *Refereed.* **Document type:** *Journal, Academic/Scholarly.*
Formerly: Anatomischer Anzeiger (0003-2786)
Related titles: Microfilm ed.: (from PMC); Online - full text ed.: (from Institute for Scientific Information); ♦ Supplement: Anatomische Gesellschaft. Verhandlungen. ISSN 0066-1562.
Indexed: ASCA, Anim.Breed.Abstr., Biol.Abstr., Chem.Abstr., Curr.Adv.Cell & Devel.Biol., Curr.Adv.Ecol.Sci., Curr.Cont., Dairy Sci.Abstr., Dent.Ind., Excerp.Med., GeoRef, INIS Atomind., Ind.Med. (1992-), Ind.Sci.Rev., Ind.Vet., Inpharma, Int.Abstr.Biol.Sci., Neurosci.Cit.Ind., Nutr.Abstr., Pig News & Info., Poult.Abstr., Reac., Rev.Med.& Vet.Mycol., SSCI (coverage dropped), Sci.Cit.Ind., Sport Fish.Abstr., Vet.Bull., Zoo.Rec.
—BLDSC (1036.200000), CASDDS, CISTI, EMDOCS, GNLM, Infotrieve, KNAW. **CCC.**
Published by: Urban & Fischer Verlag, Loebdergraben 14A, Jena 07743, Germany. TEL 49-3641-626444, FAX 49-3641-626500, journals@urbanfischer.de, http://www.urbanfischer.de. Ed. W Kuehnel. R&P Martin Huber TEL 49-3641-626430. Adv. contact Sabine Schroeter. page DEM 750; trim 280 x 210. Circ: 400.

610.28 USA ISSN 0090-6964
R856.A1 CODEN: ABMECF

ANNALS OF BIOMEDICAL ENGINEERING. Text in English. 1979. bi-m. USD 195 domestic to individuals; USD 215 in Canada & Mexico to individuals; USD 235 elsewhere to individuals; USD 600 domestic to institutions; USD 620 in Canada & Mexico to institutions; USD 640 elsewhere to institutions (effective 2001). adv. illus. index. reprints avail. *Refereed.* **Document type:** *Academic/Scholarly.* **Description:** Comprised of scholarly articles on areas such as bioelectric phenomena and quantitative electrophysiology, biomaterial and biomechanics, biochemical transducers and information systems theory applications.
Incorporates: Journal of Bioengineering (0145-3068)
Related titles: Microfilm ed.: (from PQC); Online - full text ed.: (from EBSCO Publishing, RoweCom Information Quest, Swets Blackwell, Institute for Scientific Information).
Indexed: ASCA, Appl.Mech.Rev., Bioeng.Abstr., Biol.Abstr., Biotech.& Bioeng.Abstr., C.P.I., Chem.Abstr., Compumath, Comput.& Info.Sys., Curr.Adv.Ecol.Sci., Curr.Cont., Electron.& Communic.Abstr.J., Eng.Ind., Excerp.Med., INIS Atomind., INSPEC (Dec.1974-), Ind.Med. (1972-), Ind.Sci.Rev., Inpharma, Int.Abstr.Biol.Sci., METADEX, Pharm.&Out.News, Reac., SPINweb, Sci.Cit.Ind.
—BLDSC (1039.400000), AskIEEE, CASDDS, CISTI, Ei, EMDOCS, GNLM, IDS, ingenta, Linda Hall. **CCC.**
Published by: (Biomedical Engineering Society), American Institute of Physics, One Physics Ellipse, College Park, MD 20740-3843. TEL 516-576-2270, FAX 516-576-2277, abme@nsr.bioeng.washington.edu, http://ojps.aip.org/abme. Ed. James B Bassingthwaighte. adv.: page USD 750. Circ: 2,200.

571.9 HKG ISSN 0219-0753

ANNALS OF CONTEMPORARY DIAGNOSTIC PATHOLOGY. Text in Chinese. 1997. a. USD 25 foreign; USD 25 newsstand/cover (effective 2002). 120 p./no. **Document type:** *Journal, Academic/Scholarly.* **Description:** Aims to provide a synopsis of contemporary diagnostic pathologic classification and criteria to pathologists in China who may not have ready access to western literature.
Published by: (Chinese University of Hong Kong, Department of Anatomical and Cellular Pathology SGP), Springer-Verlag Hong Kong Ltd. (Subsidiary of: BertelsmannSpringer), Unit 1702, Tower 1, Enterprise Square, 9 Sheung Yuet Rd, Kowloon Bay, Kowloon, Hong Kong. TEL 852-2723-9698, FAX 852-2724-2366, springer@springer.com.hk. Ed. H. K. Ng.

616.07 USA ISSN 1092-9134
CODEN: ANDPFM

ANNALS OF DIAGNOSTIC PATHOLOGY. Text in English. 1997. bi-m. USD 135 domestic to individuals; USD 177 foreign to individuals; USD 230 domestic to institutions; USD 274 foreign to institutions; USD 77 domestic to students; USD 107 foreign to students; USD 46 newsstand/cover (effective 2001). **Document type:** *Journal, Academic/Scholarly.* **Description:** Publishes articles dealing with studies based on techniques that are widely available in the general practice of anatomic pathology, stresses traditional morphologic studies, clinciopathologic correlations, and in general, any scientific observation of relevance to the daily practice of pathology.
Related titles: Online - full text ed.: (from IDEAL Online Library).
Indexed: Ind.Med. (1997-).
—BLDSC (1040.352000).
Published by: W.B. Saunders Co. (Subsidiary of: Harcourt Publishers Ltd.), 11830 Westline Industrial Dr, St Louis, MO 63146. TEL 800-325-4177, wbspcs@harcourtbrace.com, http://www.wbsaunders.com. Eds. Cesar A Moran, Saul Suster.

ANNALS OF EPIDEMIOLOGY. see *PUBLIC HEALTH AND SAFETY*

ANNALS OF HEALTH LAW. see *LAW*

616.968 IND ISSN 0971-135X

THE ANNALS OF MEDICAL ENTOMOLOGY. Text in English. 1992. s-a. INR 40, USD 8 (effective 2000). adv. bk.rev. maps, stat, tr.lit. index. back issues avail. *Refereed.* **Document type:** *Bulletin, Academic/Scholarly.*
Indexed: Aqua.Sci.& Fish.Abstr., Environ.Sci.Poll.Mgmt., Protozool.Abstr., Rev.Med.& Vet.Mycol., Zoo.Rec.
Published by: Annals Publishing House, 28 New Panchsheel Nagar, P O Box 62, G P O, Raipur, Madhya Pradesh 492 001, India. TEL 91-7662-56251, anmedent@bom6.vsnl.net.in. Ed., Pub., R&P, Adv. contact S Z Husainy. B&W page USD 200, color page USD 300. Circ: 3,500 (paid).

610 TUR ISSN 1300-0683

ANNALS OF MEDICAL SCIENCES. Text in English. 1992. q. TRL 6,000,000 domestic; USD 60 foreign (effective 2001). adv. *Refereed.* **Document type:** *Academic/Scholarly.* **Description:** Covers medical topics for physicians, researchers, educators, and administrators.
Indexed: Excerp.Med. (1994-).
—BLDSC (1043.110000), EMDOCS, GNLM.
Published by: Cukurova Universitesi, Tip Fakultesi, Yayin ve Dokumentasyon Kurulu, Balcali, Adana 01330, Turkey. TEL 90-322-3386060, FAX 90-322-3386572, ams@mail.cu.edu.tr, http://ams.cu.edu.tr. Ed., R&P Dr. Isik Olcay TEL 90-322-3387095. Adv. contact Nazan Alparslan. Circ: 600.

ANNALS OF MEDICINE. see *MEDICAL SCIENCES—Experimental Medicine, Laboratory Technique*

610 SAU ISSN 0256-4947
CODEN: ANSMEJ

ANNALS OF SAUDI MEDICINE. Text in English; Summaries in Arabic. 1981. bi-m. SAR 25. adv. bk.rev. abstr. back issues avail. *Refereed.* **Document type:** *Academic/Scholarly.* **Description:** A multidisciplinary medical journal dealing with aspects of clinical, academic, investigative medicine and research.
Formerly: King Faisal Specialist Hospital Medical Journal (0253-4770)
Related titles: Online - full text ed.: (from Institute for Scientific Information).

Indexed: ASCA, Abstr.Hyg., CINAHL, Curr.Adv.Ecol.Sci., Curr.Cont., Dairy Sci.Abstr., Diar.Dis.Res., Excerp.Med., Helminthol.Abstr., INIS Atomind., Inpharma, Int.Abstr.Biol.Sci., Neurosci.Cit.Ind., Nutr.Abstr., Pharm.&Out.News, Protozool.Abstr., Reac., Rev.Appl.Entomol., Rev.Med.& Vet.Mycol., SSCI (coverage dropped), THA, Trop.Dis.Bull.
—BLDSC (1043.925000), CISTI, EMDOCS, GNLM, IDS, KNAW.
Published by: King Faisal Specialist Hospital and Research Centre, P O Box 3354, Riyadh 11211, Saudi Arabia. TEL 966-1-4647272, FAX 966-1-4427237, renee@kfshrc.edu.sa, http://www.kfshrc.edu.sa. Ed. Dr. Mohammed Akhtar. R&P Renee Dykeman. adv.: B&W page USD 1,120, color page USD 1,860; trim 220 x 290. Circ: 17,000 (controlled). **Co-sponsors:** King Saud University College of Medicine; King Khalid University Hospital.

ANNUAIRE DE LA RECHERCHE BIO-MEDICALE. see *BIOLOGY*

ANNUAIRE DE L'HOSPITALISATION PRIVEE. see *HEALTH FACILITIES AND ADMINISTRATION*

610 FRA
ANNUAIRE MEDICAL DU DR. PORCHERON ET PROF. G. BELTRAMI. Text in French. 1912. a. FRF 120. adv.
Published by: SO-GE-CO-PRO S.A.R.L, 20-26 rue Caisserie, Marseille Cedex 2 13235, France.

ANNUAL BOOK OF A S T M STANDARDS. VOLUME 13.01. MEDICAL DEVICES; EMERGENCY MEDICAL SERVICES. see *ENGINEERING—Engineering Mechanics And Materials*

610 BRA ISSN 1517-3011
CODEN: RCBIDV
ANNUAL REVIEW OF BIOMEDICAL SCIENCES. Text in Portuguese; Summaries in English, Portuguese. 1980. a., latest vol.2, 2000. USD 30 (effective 2001); or exchange basis. abstr, bibl, charts, illus, stat. back issues avail. *Refereed.* **Document type:** *Journal, Academic/Scholarly.* **Description:** Publishes original review articles surveying recent developments in topical areas of biomedical research.
Formerly (until vol.18, 1997): Revista de Ciencias Biomedicas (0101-322X)
Indexed: Biol.Abstr., Cal.Tiss.Abstr., Chem.Abstr., Excerp.Med. (1994-), Ind.Med. (coverage dropped), Ind.Vet., Protozool.Abstr., Zoo.Rec.
—CASDDS, CISTI, KNAW.
Published by: Universidade Estadual Paulista, Ave. VICENTE FERREIRA, 1278, Centro, Caixa Postal 71, Marilia, SP 17515-901, Brazil. TEL 55-144-222504, FAX 55-144-222504, cgb@marilia.unesp.br. Ed. Dr. Gilson Volpato.

610 USA ISSN 0066-4219
CODEN: ARMCAH
ANNUAL REVIEW OF MEDICINE: SELECTED TOPICS IN THE CLINICAL SCIENCES. Text in English. 1950. a. USD 60 domestic to individuals; USD 65 foreign to individuals; USD 120 domestic to institutions; USD 130 foreign to institutions (effective 1999). adv. bibl, charts. index, cum.index. back issues avail.; reprints avail. *Refereed.* **Document type:** *Academic/Scholarly.* **Description:** Reviews filter and synthesize primary research to identify the principal contributions in the field of medicine.
Related titles: Microfilm ed.: (from PQC); Online - full text ed.: Annual Review of Medicine Online (from HighWire Pr., EBSCO Publishing, Institute for Scientific Information).
Indexed: AESIS, ASCA, Abstr.Hyg., Biol.Abstr., Cal.Tiss.Abstr., Chem.Abstr., Chem.Indus.Notes, Chem.Titles, Curr.Adv.Cancer Res., Curr.Cont., Dent.Ind., Diar.Dis.Res., Environ.Sci.Poll.Mgmt., Excerp.Med., Helminthol.Abstr., INIS Atomind., Ind.Med. (1950-), Ind.Sci.Rev., Ind.Vet., Inpharma, Int.Abstr.Biol.Sci., Int.Nurs.Ind., Media Rev.Dig., Nutr.Abstr., Pharm.&Out.News, Pollut.Abstr., Protozool.Abstr., PsycInfo, Psychol.Abstr. (1969-), Reac., Rev.Appl.Entomol., Risk Abstr., SSCI (coverage dropped), Saf.Sci.Abstr., Sci.Cit.Ind., THA, Vet.Bull., e-psyche.
—BLDSC (1522.700000), ADONIS, CASDDS, CISTI, EMDOCS, GNLM, IDS, ingenta, KNAW. **CCC.**
Published by: Annual Reviews Inc., 4139 El Camino Way, Box 10139, Palo Alto, CA 94303-0139. TEL 650-493-4400, 800-523-8635, FAX 650-424-0910, service@annurev.org; orders@allenpress.com, http://www.annualreviews.org. Ed. Samuel Gubins. R&P, Adv. contact Swati Aneja TEL 650-843-6634. **Subscr.to:** Allen Press Inc., PO Box 1897, Lawrence, KS 66044-8897.

610 ITA ISSN 0365-4621
CODEN: AMSNAB
ANTHOLOGIA MEDICA SANTORIANA. Text in Italian. 1959. a. price varies.
Formed by the merger of: Anthological de Medicina Externa; Archivium de Dermatologia Experimentale et Functionale (0365-1622); Which was formerly (until 1954): Archivi di Dermatologia Sperimentale e Funzionale (0392-9256)
—CASDDS.
Published by: Giardini Editori e Stampatori, Via Santa Bibbiana, 28, Pisa, PI 56127, Italy. TEL 050 502531. Ed. Marcello Comel.

ANTHROPOLOGY & MEDICINE. see *ANTHROPOLOGY*

616.9 GBR ISSN 1366-5146
ANTIBIOTICS CHEMOTHERAPY; newsletter of the international society of chemotherapy. Text in English. 1997. q. free. **Document type:** *Newsletter, Academic/Scholarly.*
Published by: Cambridge Medical Publications Ltd., Wicker House, High St, Worthing, W Sussex BN11 1DJ, United Kingdom. TEL 44-1903-205884, FAX 44-1903-234862, cmp@hbase.com, http://www.cambridge-medical.com. Circ: 20,000.

610 COL ISSN 0044-8389
ANTIOQUIA MEDICA. Text in Spanish; Summaries in English, Spanish. 1950. 10/yr. COP 100, USD 7.50. bk.rev. abstr. index.
Indexed: Biol.Abstr., Chem.Abstr., Excerp.Med., Ind.Vet., Rev.Plant Path., Trop.Dis.Bull., Vet.Bull.
—CISTI, GNLM.
Published by: Universidad de Antioquia, Facultad de Medicina-Academia de Medicina, Apartado Aereo 52278, Medellin, ANT, Colombia. Ed. Jose Luis Ramirez Castro. Circ: 1,200.

612.015 USA ISSN 1523-0864
▼ **ANTIOXIDANTS & REDOX SIGNALING.** Text in English. 1999. bi-m. USD 168 domestic to individuals; USD 199 foreign to individuals; USD 202 domestic to individuals print and online eds. combined; USD 233 foreign to individuals print and online eds. combined; USD 309 domestic to institutions; USD 382 foreign to institutions; USD 371 domestic to institutions print and online eds. combined; USD 444 foreign to institutions print and online eds. combined (effective 2002). adv. back issues avail.; reprints avail. *Refereed.* **Document type:** *Journal, Academic/Scholarly.* **Description:** Encompasses the emerging field of antioxidants and redox biology. Features basic and clinical research papers, brief communications of outstanding interest, reviews, and commentary.
Related titles: Online - full content ed.: USD 168 to individuals; USD 309 to institutions (effective 2002) (from Swets Blackwell); Online - full text ed.: (from CatchWord Ltd., RoweCom Information Quest).
Indexed: Ind.Med.
—BLDSC (1549.525000). **CCC.**
Published by: Mary Ann Liebert, Inc. Publishers, 2 Madison Ave, Larchmont, NY 10538. TEL 914—834-3100, FAX 914-834-1388, info@liebertpub.com, www.liebertpub.com/ars, http://www.liebertpub.com. Eds. Chandan K Sen, Dipak K Das. Adv. contact Harriet Matysko.

610 CHL
ANUARIO ENFERMEDADES DE NOTIFICACION OBLIGATORIA. Text in Spanish. 1947. a. USD 5.
Published by: Ministerio de Salud, Departamento de Control y Evaluacion, Santiago, Chile.

610 JPN ISSN 0918-1369
AOMORI ROSAI BYOIN ISHI/AOMORI ROSAI MEDICAL JOURNAL. Text in Japanese. 1991. s-a.
Published by: Rodo Fukushi Jigyodan, Aomori Rosai Byoin/Labor Welfare Corp., Aomori Rosai Hospital, 1 Minamigaoka-Shiroganecho, Hachinohe-shi, Aomori-ken 031-0000, Japan.

610 JPN ISSN 0914-7500
AOMORI SHIMIN BYOIN ISHI/AOMORI CITY HOSPITAL. MEDICAL JOURNAL. Text in Japanese. 1987. s-a.
Published by: Aomori Shimin Byoin/Aomori City Hospital, 14-20, Katsuta 1-chome, Aomori-shi, Aomori-ken 030, Japan.

610 JPN ISSN 0914-6873
AOMORIKEN ISHIKAIHO/AOMORI MEDICAL ASSOCIATION. JOURNAL. Text in Japanese. 1960. m. JPY 300 per issue.
Published by: Aomoriken Ishikai/Aomori Medical Association, 8-21 Shin-Machi 2-chome, Aomori-shi 030-0801, Japan.

610 658 JPN ISSN 0913-4581
AOMORIKEN JICHITAI IGAKKAISHI/AOMORI MUNICIPAL HOSPITAL ESTABLISHMENT ASSOCIATION. JOURNAL. Text in Japanese. a.
Published by: Aomoriken Jichitai Byoin Kaisetsusha Kyogikai/Aomori Municipal Hospital Establishment Association, Kokuhoren, 4-1 Shin-Machi 2-chome, Aomori-shi 030-0801, Japan.

610 JPN ISSN 0916-0450
AOMORIKEN NOSON IGAKKAI ZASSHI/AOMORI SOCIETY OF RURAL MEDICINE. JOURNAL. Text in Japanese. 1975. irreg. membership.
Published by: Aomoriken Noson Igakkai/Aomori Society of Rural Medicine, Aomoriken Nogyo Kyodo Kumiai Chuokai, 87-11 Maeda Ono, Aomori-shi 038-0053, Japan. TEL 81-177-29-8765, FAX 81-177-62-1085.

APOPTOSIS; an international journal on programmed cell death. see *BIOLOGY—Cytology And Histology*

APOTHEKEN UMSCHAU; das Gesundheits-Magazin. see *PHYSICAL FITNESS AND HYGIENE*

610 USA ISSN 1064-8542
R853.C55 CODEN: ACLTEU
APPLIED CLINICAL TRIALS; the global magazine of applied clinical science. Text in English. 1992. m., latest vol.10. USD 64 domestic; USD 84 in Canada & Mexico; USD 124 elsewhere (effective 2001). adv. back issues avail.; reprints avail. *Refereed.* **Document type:** *Academic/Scholarly, Trade.* **Description:** For clinical research professionals in the United States and Western Europe. Offers practical, hands-on information that helps clinical research scientists develop, execute, and file new drug applications and expedite drug approval.
Indexed: I.P.A., Inpharma, Pharm.&Out.News, Reac., Ref.Zh.
—BLDSC (1571.936450), GNLM, Infotrieve, KNAW. **CCC.**
Published by: Advanstar Communications Inc., 859 Willamette St, Eugene, OR 97401. TEL 541-343-1200, 800-346-0085 ext. 477, fulfill@superfill.com, www.pharma-connections.com. Ed. Jane Ganter. Pub. Ralph Vitaro TEL 732-225-9500. Adv. contact Wayne K Blow. B&W page GBP 2,730, color page GBP 3,210. Circ: 14,000.

610 USA ISSN 1062-3345
RB46.6 CODEN: APIMEH
APPLIED IMMUNOHISTOCHEMISTRY. Text in English. 1993. q. USD 181 domestic to individuals for print & online eds.; USD 181 foreign to individuals for print & online eds.; USD 278 domestic to institutions for print & online eds.; USD 278 newsstand/cover foreign to institutions; USD 71 newsstand/cover (effective 2002). adv. bk.rev. illus. index. back issues avail. *Refereed.* **Document type:** *Academic/Scholarly.* **Description:** Original articles on the diagnostic and prognostic applications of immunohistochemistry to human disease.
Related titles: Microform ed.: (from PQC); Online - full text ed.: USD 361.40 domestic academic site license; USD 361.40 foreign academic site license; USD 403.10 domestic corporate site license; USD 403.10 foreign corporate site license (effective 2002) (from Ovid Technologies, Inc., Institute for Scientific Information).
Indexed: ASCA, Chem.Abstr., Chem.Indus.Notes, Chem.Titles, Curr.Cont., Excerp.Med. (1995-), Ind.Sci.Rev., Inpharma, Reac., Sci.Cit.Ind.
—CASDDS, EMDOCS, GNLM, IDS, KNAW.
Published by: (Society for Applied Immunohistochemistry), Lippincott Williams & Wilkins (Philadelphia) (Subsidiary of: Wolters Kluwer N.V.), 530 Walnut St, Philadelphia, PA 19106-3621. TEL 215-521-8300, FAX 215-521-8902, http://www.appliedimmunohist.com, http://www.Lww.com. Eds. Dr. Clive S Taylor, Dr. Jiang Gu. Pub. Jim Merritt. R&P Margaret Becker. Adv. contact Ray Thiboeau. Circ: 1,324 (paid). **Subscr. to:** PO Box 1600, Hagerstown, MD 21740-1600. TEL 800-777-2295, FAX 301-824-7390.

610 SDN ISSN 0254-9492
ARAB MEDICAL BULLETIN. Text in Arabic, English. 1979. m. USD 200 to individuals; SDP 100 to institutions. adv. bk.rev.
Formerly: Sudan Medical Bulletin
Indexed: Abstr.Hyg., Excerp.Med.
Address: P O Box 1882, Khartoum, Sudan. Ed. T A Rahman. Circ: 1,500.

610 DEU ISSN 0723-5100
ARAB MEDICO; alam al tub wa al-saydallah. Text in Arabic. 1983. q. DEM 74.31, EUR 38 for 2 yrs. (effective 2001). adv. charts, illus. back issues avail. **Document type:** *Journal, Trade.*
Indexed: ExtraMED.

M

—GNLM.
Published by: Beta Verlag und Marketinggesellschaft mbH, Postfach 140121, Bonn 53056, Germany. TEL 49-228-91937-0, FAX 49-228-252067, info@beta-publishing.com, http://www.beta-publishing.com/de/verlag.html?content=medico.html. Ed. Dr. Assassa. R&P Heike Lange TEL 49-228-919370. Adv. contact Birgit Kallusch. B&W page DEM 6,320, color page DEM 8,175; trim 178 x 250. Circ: 17,200.

610 DEU ISSN 0174-268X
ARBEITEN ZUR GESCHICHTE DER MEDIZIN IN GIESSEN. Text in German. 1979. irreg., latest vol.26, 1998. DEM 118. **Document type:** *Monographic series.*
Published by: Wilhelm Schmitz Verlag, Staufenbergerweg 22, Lollar 35457, Germany. TEL 49-6406-2324.

ARBEITSMEDIZIN, SOZIALMEDIZIN, UMWELTMEDIZIN; Zeitschrift fuer Praxis, Klinik, Forschung, Begutachtung. see *PUBLIC HEALTH AND SAFETY*

ARBEITSMEDIZIN, SOZIALMEDIZIN, UMWELTMEDIZIN. SUPPLEMENT. see *PUBLIC HEALTH AND SAFETY*

615.8 SWE ISSN 0345-0988
ARBETSTERAPEUTEN; facklig yrkes- och idetidskrift. Text in Swedish. 1949. 14/yr. (2 double issues). SEK 400; SEK 25 newsstand/cover (effective 2001). adv. bk.rev. **Document type:** *Magazine, Trade.* **Description:** Publishes scientific material on occupational therapy. Reports among other things on good examples from various health services and on developments and achievements within the field of occupational therapy.
Published by: Foerbundet Sveriges Arbetsterapeuter (FSA)/Swedish Association of Occupational Therapists, Fack 760, Nacka 13124, Sweden. TEL 46-8-466-24-40, FAX 46-8-466-24-24, arbetsterapeuten@akademikerhuset.se, mamo.fsa@akademikerhuset.se, http://www.fsa.akadmikerhuset.se. Ed. Tomas Lundenmark. Pub. Inga Britt Lindstroem. adv.: B&W page SEK 11,000, color page SEK 18,500; trim 184 x 265. Circ: 8,500 (controlled).

610 ESP ISSN 0211-2027
ARCANO. Text in Spanish. 1978. 6/yr.
Address: M. Pedrayes 2, 6o, Oviedo 33004, Spain. TEL 85-23-65-10. Ed. B Lozano Llamazares.

610 USA ISSN 0148-5016
QP253 CODEN: ARANDR
ARCHIVES OF ANDROLOGY; an international journal. Text in English. 1978. 6/yr. GBP 262, USD 433 to individuals; GBP 545, USD 899 to institutions (effective 2002). bk.rev. back issues avail.; reprint service avail. from PQC. *Refereed.* **Document type:** *Academic/Scholarly.* **Description:** Covers reproduction, fertility and regulation, and infertility in the human and animal male.
Related titles: Online - full text ed.: ISSN 1521-0375 (from CatchWord Ltd., EBSCO Publishing, O C L C Online Computer Library Center, Inc., RoweCom Information Quest, Swets Blackwell, Institute for Scientific Information).
Indexed: ASCA, AgBiotech, Anim.Breed.Abstr., Biol.Abstr., Chem.Abstr., Curr.Adv.Ecol.Sci., Curr.Cont., Excerp.Med., INIS Atomind., Ind.Med. (1978-), Ind.Sci.Rev., Inpharma, Pharm.&Out.News, Pig News & Info., Reac., Sci.Cit.Ind., THA.
—BLDSC (1631.220000), ADONIS, CASDDS, CatchWord, CISTI, EMDOCS, GNLM, IDS, ingenta. **CCC.**
Published by: Taylor & Francis Ltd. (Subsidiary of: Taylor & Francis Group), 325 Chestnut St, Suite 800, Philadelphia, PA 19016. TEL 215-625-8900, FAX 215-625-2940, info@taylorandfrancis.com, http://www.taylorandfrancis.com/. Ed. E S E Hafez. **Subscr. addr. in Europe:** Taylor & Francis Group, Journals Customer Service, Rankine Rd, Basingstoke, Hants RG24 8PR, United Kingdom. TEL 44-1256-813000, FAX 44-1256-479438, enquiry@tanf.co.uk, http://www.tandf.co.uk/journals.

610 USA ISSN 1063-3987
ARCHIVES OF FAMILY MEDICINE. Text in English. 1992. m. USD 80 domestic to individuals; USD 100 foreign to individuals; USD 110 domestic to institutions; USD 140 foreign to institutions (effective 2000). adv. reprints avail. *Refereed.* **Document type:** *Academic/Scholarly.* **Description:** Provides clinically practical information for family and general physicians.
Related titles: CD-ROM ed.: (from Ovid Technologies, Inc.); Microform ed.: (from PQC); Online - full text ed.: (from The Dialog Corporation, Gale Group, Ovid Technologies, Inc., EBSCO Publishing).
Indexed: Abstr.Hyg., Curr.Cont. (coverage dropped), Dairy Sci.Abstr., Ind.Med. (1992-), Inpharma, Int.Nurs.Ind., NRN, Nutr.Abstr., Pharm.&Out.News, Reac., Rev.Med.& Vet.Mycol.
—CISTI, GNLM, IDS, ingenta, KNAW. **CCC.**
Published by: American Medical Association, 515 N State St, P O Box 10946, Chicago, IL 60610-0946. TEL 312-464-5000, http://www.ama-assn.org/public/journals/fami/famihome.htm. Ed. Dr. Marjorie Bowman. Pub. Peter L Payerli. R&P Ada Jimenez Walker. Adv. contact Phillip B Altamore. Circ: 50,000.

ARCHIVES OF HISTOLOGY AND CYTOLOGY/SOSHIKI SAIBOGAKU KIROKU. see *BIOLOGY—Cytology And Histology*

616.98 ITA ISSN 0003-9934
ARCHIVES OF MEDICAL HYDROLOGY. Text in English, French, German, Italian. 1928. irreg. (3-4/yr.). USD 5. bibl. **Description:** Covers climatological medicine.
Indexed: Chem.Abstr., Ref.Zh.
—CISTI, GNLM.
Published by: International Society of Medical Hydrology and Climatology, Via Rovereto, 11, Rome, RM 00198, Italy. Circ: 550.

610 MEX ISSN 0188-4409
R21
ARCHIVES OF MEDICAL RESEARCH. Text in English. 1970. bi-m. EUR 85 in Europe to individuals; JPY 11,300 in Japan to individuals; USD 95 elsewhere to individuals; EUR 201 in Europe to institutions; JPY 26,700 in Japan to institutions; USD 225 elsewhere to institutions (effective 2002). adv. back issues avail. *Refereed.* **Document type:** *Academic/Scholarly.* **Description:** Includes original articles and brief reports on biomedical issues.
Formerly (until 1991): Archivos de Investigacion Medica (0066-6769)
Related titles: Microform ed.: (from PQC); Online - full text ed.: (from ingenta, Swets Blackwell, ScienceDirect, Institute for Scientific Information); ♦ Supplement: Archivos de Investigacion Medica. Suplemento. ISSN 0365-3293.
Indexed: Abstr.Hyg., Anim.Breed.Abstr., Biol.Abstr., Chem.Abstr. (1992-), Chem.Indus.Notes, Chem.Titles, Curr.Cont., Dairy Sci.Abstr., Excerp.Med., Helminthol.Abstr., Ind.Med. (1992-), Ind.Sci.Rev., Ind.Vet., Inpharma, Int.Nurs.Ind., NRN, Nutr.Abstr., Pharm.&Out.News, Protozool.Abstr., Reac., Rev.Appl.Entomol., Rev.Med.& Vet.Mycol., Sci.Cit.Ind. (coverage dropped), Trop.Dis.Bull.
—BLDSC (1637.630000), CASDDS, CINDOC, CISTI, GNLM.
Published by: (Instituto Mexicano del Seguro Social, Oficina de Bibliotecas y Divulgacion), Elsevier Science, 655 Ave of the Americas, New York, NY 10010. http://www.elsevier.com/locate/arcmed. Ed. Luis Benitez Bribiesca. R&P Maggie Brunner. Adv. contact Fabio Salamanca. Circ: 5,000.

610 FRA ISSN 0750-6244
ARCHIVES OF OTOLARYNGOLOGY* /JOURNAL D'O.R.L. Text in French. 1981. q. FRF 400 foreign. **Document type:** *Academic/Scholarly.*
Indexed: Jrnl.Watch Derm.
Published by: Editions Masson, 120 bd. Saint-Germain, Paris Cedex 6 75280, France. Ed. Michelle Deker.

616.07 USA ISSN 0363-0153
RB1 CODEN: ARPAAQ
ARCHIVES OF PATHOLOGY & LABORATORY MEDICINE. Text in English. 1926. m. USD 160 in US & Canada; USD 230 elsewhere; USD 18 newsstand/cover in US & Canada; USD 22 newsstand/cover elsewhere (effective 2001). adv. bk.rev. charts, illus. index. back issues avail.; reprints avail. *Refereed.* **Document type:** *Journal, Academic/Scholarly.* **Description:** Original, peer-reviewed articles cover every aspect of anatomic and clinical pathology, with emphasis on the evaluation and introduction of new knowledge and new technology in the active clinical arena.
Formerly: Archives of Pathology (0003-9985)
Related titles: Microform ed.: (from PQC,PMC); Online - full text ed.: (from Northern Light Technology, Inc., ProQuest Information & Learning, Institute for Scientific Information).
Indexed: AIDS Abstr., AIM, ASCA, Abstr.Hyg., Biol.Abstr., CINAHL, C.I.S. Abstr., Chem.Abstr., Chem.Indus.Notes, Chem.Titles, Curr.Adv.Cancer Res., Curr.Adv.Ecol.Sci., Curr.Adv.Gen.& Molec.Biol., Curr.Cont., Dairy Sci.Abstr., Dent.Ind., Dok.Arbeitsmed., Excerp.Med., Helminthol.Abstr., INIS Atomind., Ind.Med. (1976-), Ind.Sci.Rev., Ind.Vet., Inpharma, Int.Abstr.Biol.Sci., Int.Nurs.Ind., Neurosci.Cit.Ind., Nutr.Abstr., Pharm.&Out.News, Protozool.Abstr., Reac., Rev.Med.& Vet.Mycol., Rev.Plant Path., SSCI (coverage dropped), Sci.Cit.Ind., Trop.Dis.Bull., Vet.Bull.
—BLDSC (1638.610000), CASDDS, CISTI, EMDOCS, GNLM, IDS, ingenta, KNAW. **CCC.**
Published by: (Archives of Pathology & Laboratory Medicine), College of American Pathologists, 325 Waukegan Rd, Northfield, IL 60093-2750. TEL 847-832-7000, FAX 847-832-8873. Ed. Dr. Kenneth D. McClatchey. Pub. Robert McGonnagle. adv.: B&W page USD 1,280, color page USD 2,160. Circ: 14,500 (paid and controlled).

610 USA ISSN 0004-0002
HQ1 CODEN: ASXBA8
ARCHIVES OF SEXUAL BEHAVIOR; an interdisciplinary research journal. Text in English. 1971. bi-m. USD 123, EUR 122 to individuals for print or online ed.; USD 755, EUR 754 to institutions for print or online ed.; USD 906, EUR 904.80 to institutions for print & online eds. (effective 2002). bk.rev. illus. back issues avail.; reprint service avail. from PSC,SCH. *Refereed.* **Document type:** *Academic/Scholarly.* **Description:** Reports the latest research trends in the area of human sexual behavior, from a multidisciplinary perspective.
Related titles: Online - full text ed.: NLG 1,496, EUR 679 to institutions; NLG 1,795.20, EUR 814.80 to institutions for online & print edition (effective 2001) (from CatchWord Ltd., Gale Group, EBSCO Publishing, O C L C Online Computer Library Center, Inc., RoweCom Information Quest, ProQuest Information & Learning, Swets Blackwell, Kluwer Online, Factiva, Institute for Scientific Information).
Indexed: ASCA, Abstr.Anthropol., Abstr.Crim.& Pen., Adol.Ment.Hlth.Abstr., AgeLine, Arts & Hum.Cit.Ind. (coverage dropped), Behav.Med.Abstr., Biol.Abstr., Chem.Abstr., Crim.Just.Abstr., Curr.Adv.Ecol.Sci., Curr.Cont., Curr.Lit.Fam.Plan., ERA, Environ.Sci.Poll.Mgmt., Excerp.Med., Fam.Ind., High.Educ.Abstr., IMFL, Ind.Med. (1971-), Indian Psychol.Abstr., Lang.& Lang.Behav.Abstr., Mid.East: Abstr.& Ind., Mult.Ed.Abstr., Pollut.Abstr., PsycInfo, Psychol.Abstr. (1971-), Ref.Zh., Rel.Ind.One, Rel.Ind.Two, Risk Abstr., SOPODA, SSCI, Saf.Sci.Abstr., Sage Fam.Stud.Abstr., Soc.Sci.Ind. (Feb.1987-), Soc.Serv.Abstr., Sociol.Abstr., Sp.Ed.Needs Abstr., Stud.Wom.Abstr., Viol.& Abuse Abstr., e-psyche.
—BLDSC (1643.128000), CASDDS, CatchWord, CISTI, EMDOCS, GNLM, IDS, Infotrieve, ingenta. **CCC.**
Published by: (International Academy of Sex Research), Kluwer Academic - Plenum Publishers (Subsidiary of: Wolters Kluwer N.V.), 233 Spring St, New York, NY 10013-1578. TEL 212-620-8000, 800-221-9369, FAX 212-463-0742, http://www.wkap.nl/journalhome.htm/0004-0002. Ed. Dr. Richard Green. Pub. Mariclaire Cloutier TEL 212-620-8013. R&P Rose Luongo TEL 781-871-6311.

ARCHIVIO ITALIANO DI ANATOMIA E DI EMBRIOLOGIA/ITALIAN JOURNAL OF ANATOMY AND EMBRYOLOGY. see *BIOLOGY*

610 BOL ISSN 0004-0525
ARCHIVOS BOLIVIANOS DE MEDICINA. Text in Spanish. 1943. 3/yr. free per issue. adv. bk.rev. bibl, charts, illus.
Published by: Universidad Mayor Real y Pontificia de San Francisco Xavier de Chuquisaca, Facultad de Ciencias de la Salud, Casilla Coreo 460, Calle Colon, 235, Sucre, Bolivia. Eds. Alberto Aquirre, Antonio Dubravcic L. Circ: 650.

ARCHIVOS DE BIOLOGIA ANDINA. see *BIOLOGY*

610 MEX ISSN 0365-3293
ARCHIVOS DE INVESTIGACION MEDICA. SUPLEMENTO. Text in English, Spanish. 1971. irreg.
Related titles: ♦ Supplement to: Archives of Medical Research. ISSN 0188-4409.
Published by: Instituto Mexicano del Seguro Social, Oficina de Bibliotecas y Divulgacion, Apdo. 73-032, Mexico City, DF 06720, Mexico. TEL 52-5-7611503, archives@servidor.unam.mx.

M

616 574.29 POL ISSN 0004-069X CODEN: AITEAT
ARCHIVUM IMMUNOLOGIAE ET THERAPIAE EXPERIMENTALIS. Text in English. 1953. bi-m. USD 186 (effective 2002). charts, illus. index. reprint service avail. from PQC,ISI. **Document type:** *Academic/Scholarly.* **Description:** Publishes papers containing original results of scientific research and experiments that make a contribution to immunology or experimental therapy.
Related titles: Microfilm ed.: (from PMC); Online - full text ed.: (from Institute for Scientific Information).
Indexed: Abstr.Hyg., AgroAgen, C.I.S. Abstr., Chem.Abstr., Chem.Indus.Notes, Chem.Titles, Curr.Adv.Cell & Devel.Biol., Curr.Adv.Ecol.Sci., Curr.Adv.Gen.& Molec.Biol., Curr.Cont. (coverage dropped), Dent.Ind., Excerp.Med., Helminthol.Abstr., INIS Atomind., Ind.Med. (1962-), Ind.Sci.Rev., Ind.Vet., Pollut.Abstr., Sci.Cit.Ind. (coverage dropped), Trop.Dis.Bull.
—BLDSC (1659.500000), CASDDS, CISTI, GNLM, IDS, KNAW.
Published by: (Polska Akademia Nauk/Polish Academy of Sciences, Instytut Immunologii i Terapii Doswiadczalnej), Ossolineum Publishing House of the Polish Academy of Sciences, Pl Solny 14 a, Wroclaw 50062, Poland. TEL 48-71-343-6961, osso_bn@pwr.wroc.pl; krotkiew@immuno.pan.wroc.pl, http://surfer.iitd.pan.wroc.pl. Eds. Andrzej Gorski, Hubert Krotkiewski, Michal Zimecki. Circ: 240.

610 POL ISSN 0860-1844
R131
ARCHIWUM HISTORII I FILOZOFII MEDYCYNY. Text in English, German, Polish; Summaries in English, Polish. 1924. q. PLZ 50 to individuals; PLZ 60 to institutions; PLZ 100 foreign (effective 2000 - 2001). bk.rev. index. reprint service avail. from PQC. *Refereed.* **Document type:** *Academic/Scholarly.* **Description:** Provides papers to Polish scholars in medicine, medical societies, evolution of medical research and results.
Formerly (until 1985): Archiwum Historii Medycyny (0004-0762)
Indexed: Amer.Hist.& Life, Biol.Abstr., Hist.Abstr. (1985-), IBZ, Ind.Med. (coverage dropped).
—CISTI, GNLM, KNAW.
Published by: Polskie Towarzystwo Historii Medycyny i Farmacji/Polish Society of History of Medicine and Pharmacy, Lea 19 a-4, Krakow 30048, Poland. TEL 12-633-2369. Ed., R&P Henryk Gaertner. Circ: 860 (paid). **Dist. by:** Ars Polona, Krakowskie Przedmiescie 7, Warsaw, Poland.

610 001.3 ITA
L'ARCO DI GIANO; rivista di medical humanities. Text in Italian. 1993. 3/yr. ITL 69,000; ITL 90,000 foreign (effective 1993).
Published by: (Istituto per l'Analisi dello Stato Sociale), Franco Angeli Editore, Viale Monza, 106, Milan, MI 20127, Italy. TEL 02-28-27-651. Ed. Sandro Spinsanti.

ARIZONA POISON CONTROL SYSTEM NEWSLETTER. see *PHARMACY AND PHARMACOLOGY*

610 USA ISSN 0004-1858 CODEN: JAMSAB
ARKANSAS MEDICAL SOCIETY. JOURNAL. Text in English. 1890. m. USD 30 domestic; USD 40 foreign; USD 3 newsstand/cover (effective 2001). adv. bk.rev. abstr, bibl, charts, illus, stat. index. 32 p./no. *Refereed.* **Document type:** *Journal, Trade.* **Description:** Contains original scientific articles by members of the medical profession; editorials cover subjects of interest to the medical profession such as legislation, new developments in medicine, etc.
Indexed: AgeLine, Chem.Abstr., Dent.Ind., INIS Atomind., Ind.Med. (1906-), Nutr.Abstr.
—BLDSC (4700.850000), CASDDS, CISTI, GNLM, KNAW.
Published by: Arkansas Medical Society, Communications Coordinator, PO Box 55088, Little Rock, AR 72215-5088. ams@arkmed.org, http://www.arkmed.org/. Ed., R&P Judy Hicks. Adv. contact Stephanie Hopkins. Circ: 4,400 (paid and controlled).

616.07 RUS ISSN 0004-1955 CODEN: ARPTAF
ARKHIV PATOLOGII/ARCHIVES OF PATHOLOGY. Text in Russian; Summaries in English. 1935. bi-m. USD 224 foreign (effective 2000). adv. bk.rev., Website rev. abstr. index. **Document type:** *Journal, Academic/Scholarly.* **Description:** Deals with original investigation on pressing problems of general pathology and pathologic anatomy, performed with the help of the newest research methods and describing major provisions of the theory and practice of different human diseases, as well as problems of experimental, comparative and geographic pathology.
Indexed: Agri.& Environ.Biotech.Abstr. (coverage dropped), Biol.Abstr., Chem.Abstr., Dent.Ind., Derwent Biotech.Abstr., Excerp.Med., Helminthol.Abstr., INIS Atomind., Ind.Med. (1946-), Ind.Vet., Nutr.Abstr., Protozool.Abstr., Ref.Zh., Rev.Med.& Vet.Mycol., Vet.Bull.
—BLDSC (0009.800000), CASDDS, CISTI, East View, GNLM, Infotrieve. **CCC.**
Published by: Izdatel'stvo Meditsina, Petroverigskii per 6-8, Moscow 101000, Russian Federation. TEL 7-095-9248785, FAX 7-095-9211355, 7-095-9286003, TELEX 412282 MEDIZ SU, http://www.medit.ru. Ed. A V Smolyannikov. Pub. A M Stochik. R&P R Chakushkina. Adv. contact O A Fadeeva TEL 7-095-923-51-40. Circ: 1,200. **Dist. by:** Mezhdunarodnaya Kniga, B Yakimanka 39, Moscow 117049, Russian Federation. TEL 7-095-2384967, FAX 7-095-2384634; **US dist. addr.:** East View Publications, 3020 Harbor Ln N, Minneapolis, MN 55447. TEL 612-550-0961.

616.9802305 GBR ISSN 1470-1456
▼ **ARMED FORCES MEDICAL DEVELOPMENTS.** Text in English. 2000. a. **Document type:** *Journal, Trade.* **Description:** Examines all key issues affecting equipment, materials and systems within the healthcare and medical infrastructure for the armed forces.
Published by: (International Committee of Military Medicine), Quasar International Communications Ltd. (Subsidiary of: Sterling Publishing Group Plc.), Brunel House, 55-57 North Wharf Rd, London W2 1LA, United Kingdom. TEL 44-20-7915-9661, FAX 44-20-7915-9662, info@quasar.uk.net, http://www.quasar.uk.net. Circ: 12,000 (controlled).

ARMY MEDICAL SERVICES MAGAZINE. see *MILITARY*

AROGYA; a journal of health sciences. see *PHYSICAL FITNESS AND HYGIENE*

616.07 PRT ISSN 0004-2714 CODEN: APALA4
ARQUIVO DE PATOLOGIA. Text in Portuguese. 1971 (vol.43). 3/yr. PTE 150.
Indexed: Biol.Abstr., Chem.Abstr., Excerp.Med., INIS Atomind., Ind.Med. (coverage dropped).
—CISTI, GNLM.
Published by: Instituto Portugues de Oncologia de Francisco Gentil, Palhava, Lisbon, Portugal. Circ: 800.

610 BRA ISSN 0004-2773
ARQUIVOS CATARINENSES DE MEDICINA∗. Text in Portuguese; Summaries in English. 1967. q. BRL 40, USD 40. adv. bk.rev. bibl, charts. index. back issues avail.
Indexed: Biol.Abstr., INIS Atomind., Ind.Med. (coverage dropped).
Published by: (Associacao Catarinense de Medicina), Artes Graficas Ltda., Av Heitor Dias, 146, P Miudo, Salvador, BA 40317-330, Brazil. Ed. Mario Jose da Conceicao. Circ: 5,000.

610 PRT ISSN 0871-3413 CODEN: ARQME3
ARQUIVOS DE MEDICINA; revista de ciencia e arte medicas. Text in English, Portuguese. 1987. bi-m. PTE 5,000 to doctors; PTE 10,000 foreign; PTE 2,500 to students. adv. **Document type:** *Academic/Scholarly.*
Indexed: Excerp.Med.
—BLDSC (1695.590000), EMDOCS, GNLM, KNAW.
Published by: A E F M U P, Alameda Prof. H. Montiero, Piso 1, Apdo. 4514, Porto Codex 4008, Portugal. TEL 351-2-5509355, FAX 351-2-5509096. Ed. Levi Guerra. Adv. contact Luisa Botelho. B&W page PTE 60,000. Circ: 7,500. **Co-sponsor:** Hospital de Sao Joao, Faculdade de Medicina do Porto, Sociedade Portugesa de Engenharia Biomedica.

ARQUIVOS DOS HOSPITAIS E DA FACULDADE DE CIENCIAS MEDICAS DA SANTA CASA DE SAO PAULO. see *HEALTH FACILITIES AND ADMINISTRATION*

610 CHE ISSN 0004-2897
ARS MEDICI; Schweizer Zeitschrift fuer Allgemeinmedizin. Text in German. 1910. 24/yr. CHF 75; CHF 140 in Europe; CHF 190 elsewhere (effective 2000). adv. bk.rev. index. **Document type:** *Magazine, Academic/Scholarly.*
Related titles: ♦ Supplement: Gynaekologie fuer Hausaerzte. ISSN 1420-6811.
Indexed: Biol.Abstr., Excerp.Med.
—BLDSC (1697.636000), CISTI, EMDOCS, GNLM, KNAW.
Published by: S A E M Verlag AG, Rosenbergstr 115, Neuhausen 8212, Switzerland. TEL 41-52-6727822, FAX 41-52-6727823, info@rosenfluh.ch. Ed., Pub. Dr. Richard Altorfer. Adv. contact Janine Causen. B&W page CHF 2,300, color page CHF 3,820; trim 275 x 190. Circ: 12,500.

610 GBR ISSN 1465-9905
▼ **ARTHRITIS RESEARCH.** Text in English. 1999. bi-m. GBP 200 in United Kingdom; USD 300 elsewhere (effective 2001). illus. **Document type:** *Journal, Academic/Scholarly.* **Description:** Serve as a focus for communication about all aspects of research into arthritis, autoimmune rheumatic diseases and skeletal disorders.
Related titles: Online - full content ed.: ISSN 1465-9913; Online - full text ed.: (from Institute for Scientific Information).
Indexed: Ind.Med.
—BLDSC (1733.876400).
Published by: Current Science Ltd, Middlesex House, 34-42 Cleveland St, London W1P 6LB, United Kingdom. TEL 44-20-7323-0323, FAX 44-20-7580-1938, info@biomedcentral.com, http://www.biomedcentral.com/1465-9905/, http://www.currentsciencegroup.com. Eds. Peter E Lipsky, Ravinder N Naini.

610 DEU ISSN 0933-7946
ARTHROSKOPIE. Text in German. 1988. bi-m. EUR 201.59 domestic; EUR 198.29 in Germany; EUR 57.50 newsstand/cover foreign (effective 2002). *Refereed.* **Document type:** *Journal, Academic/Scholarly.* **Description:** Covers all aspects of arthroscopic examination and surgery.
Related titles: Online - full text ed.: ISSN 1434-3924 (from EBSCO Publishing, RoweCom Information Quest, Swets Blackwell, Springer LINK).
—GNLM.
Published by: (Deutschsprachiger Arbeitsgemeinschaft fuer Arthroskopie), Springer-Verlag (Subsidiary of: BertelsmannSpringer), Tiergartenstr 17, Heidelberg 69121, Germany. TEL 49-6221-345-0, FAX 49-6221-345229, subscriptions@springer.de, http://link.springer.de/link/service/journals/00142/index.htm, http://www.springer.de. **Subscr. in N. America to:** Springer-Verlag New York Inc., PO Box 2485, Secaucus, NJ 07096-2485. TEL 212-460-1500, FAX 212-473-6272.

ARTIFICIAL INTELLIGENCE IN MEDICINE. see *COMPUTERS—Artificial Intelligence*

610 NLD ISSN 0928-611X
ARTS ASSISTENT. Text in Dutch. 1990. q. adv. **Document type:** *Trade.* **Description:** For assistant physicians and doctors.
Published by: (Landelijke Vereniging van Assistent-Geneeskundigen), Elsevier Bedrijfsinformatie BV, Misset (Subsidiary of: Reed Elsevier plc), Postbus 4, Doetinchem 7000 BA, Netherlands. TEL 31-314-349371, FAX 31-314-363638, info@ebi.nl, http://www.ebi.nl. Adv. contact Cor van Nek. B&W page NLG 3,447, color page NLG 5,847; trim 280 x 210. Circ: 5,310.

610 700 780 GBR
▼ **ARTS THERAPIES RESEARCH LIBRARY.** Text in English. 1999. irreg., latest vol.3, 1999. back issues avail. *Refereed.* **Document type:** *Monographic series.* **Description:** Covers the arts therapies and explores themes common to all of them. The volumes are short and thought-provoking, balancing research with case material drawn from practice and developing difference theories.
Published by: Jessica Kingsley Publishers, 116 Pentonville Rd, London N1 9JB, United Kingdom. TEL 44-207-833-2307, FAX 44-20-7837-2917, post@jkp.com, http://www.jkp.com. Ed. Phil Jones. **Dist. by:** Plymbridge Distributors Ltd, Plymbridge House, Estover Rd, Plymouth, Devon PL6 7PY, United Kingdom. TEL 44-1752-202300, FAX 44-1752-202330.

610 NLD ISSN 1387-1870
ARTSENZAKEN. Text in Dutch. 1997. q. free per issue to qualified personnel. adv. bk.rev. **Document type:** *Trade, Academic/Scholarly.* **Description:** Offers practical, professional, to-the-point advice for medical practitioners in all areas and specialties.
Related titles: ♦ Supplement to: Medisch Contact. ISSN 0025-8245.

Published by: (Koninklijke Nederlandse Maatschappij tot Bevordering der Geneeskunst (KNMG)), Elsevier Gezondheidszorg B.V., Tijdstroom (Subsidiary of: Reed Elsevier plc Group), Planetenbaan 1, Maarssen 3600 AK, Netherlands. TEL 31-346-577577, FAX 31-346-554287, http://www.tijdstroom.nl. **Subscr. to:** Elsevier Den Haag, Postbus 16500, The Hague 2500 BM, Netherlands. TEL 31-70-381-9900, FAX 31-70-333-8399.

619 JPN ISSN 0913-7343
ARUMEIDA IHO/OITA CITY MEDICAL ASSOCIATION. JOURNAL. Text in Japanese. 1975. 3/yr.
Published by: Oitashi Ishikai/Oita City Medical Association, 1315 Miyazaki, Oita-shi 870-1133, Japan.

ARUT PERUM JOTHI. see *RELIGIONS AND THEOLOGY—Hindu*

614 AUT ISSN 0004-4180
ARZT IN NIEDEROESTERREICH. Text in German. 1965. m. adv. bk.rev., film rev. abstr, illus, stat.
Published by: Ueberparteilicher Aerzteverband Niederoesterreichs, Klostergasse 6-8, St. Poelten, N 3100, Austria. Ed. Dr. Erich Klier. Circ: 3,000.

610 338.3 DEU ISSN 0341-4434
ARZT UND AUTO; der kraftfahrende Arzt. Text in German. 1924. m. DEM 30 (effective 2000). adv. bk.rev. **Document type:** *Magazine, Academic/Scholarly.*
Formerly (until 1971): Kraftfahrende Arzt
—GNLM, Infotrieve. **CCC.**
Published by: K V D A Verlag, Postfach 940340, Frankfurt Am Main 60461, Germany. TEL 49-69-97843251, FAX 49-69-97843253, kvda.de@t-online.de, http://home.t-online.de/home/kvda.de. Ed. Dr E Wernicke. Circ: 10,000.

610 DEU ISSN 0341-9754
ARZT UND KRANKENHAUS. Text in German. 1976. m. DEM 105; DEM 120 foreign (effective 2000). illus. **Document type:** *Journal, Trade.*
—GNLM.
Published by: (Verband der Leitenden Krankenhausaerzte Deutschlands), Hansisches Verlagskontor, Mengstr 16, Luebeck 23552, Germany. TEL 49-451-7031-01, FAX 49-451-7031281. Ed. K Jeute. Circ: 8,000.

610 AUT ISSN 1026-8421
ARZT UND PRAXIS; der praktische Arzt - der Facharzt in der Praxis. Text in German. 1946. 21/yr. ATS 460 domestic; ATS 700 foreign (effective 2000). adv. bk.rev. **Document type:** *Journal, Trade, Academic/Scholarly.*
Formerly (until 1995): Praktische Arzt (0048-5128)
Indexed: Biol.Abstr.
—GNLM.
Published by: Medizinische Fachzeitschriften GmbH, Rosenbergstrasse 18, Goettlesbrunn, N 2464, Austria. TEL 43-2162-8735, FAX 43-2162-887354. Ed. Monika Dichtl. Adv. contact Karin Schmitt. Circ: 11,000.

610 CHE ISSN 1016-8400
ARZT UND PRAXIS; Magazin fuer Praxismanagement. Text in German. 1989. 10/yr. CHF 48; CHF 65 in Europe; CHF 76 elsewhere (effective 2000). adv. **Document type:** *Magazine, Academic/Scholarly, Trade.*
Published by: Rosenfluh Publikationen, Rosenbergstr 115, Neuhausen 8212, Switzerland. TEL 41-52-6727822, FAX 41-52-6727823. Adv. contact Hans Beusch. B&W page CHF 2,650, color page CHF 4,170; trim 190 x 275. Circ: 10,000 (paid).

610 340 DEU ISSN 0935-5553
DER ARZT UND SEIN RECHT. Text in German. 1989. bi-m. DEM 200 (effective 1999). **Document type:** *Academic/Scholarly.*
—GNLM.
Published by: P M I Verlag AG, August-Schanz-Str 8, Frankfurt Am Main 60433, Germany. TEL 49-69-548000-0, FAX 49-69-548000-77, pmiverlag@aol.com.

610 340 DEU ISSN 0933-1352
ARZTHAFTPFLICHT - RECHTSPRECHUNG. Text in German. 1987. irreg. DEM 386 (effective 2000). **Document type:** *Bulletin, Trade.*
Published by: Erich Schmidt Verlag GmbH & Co. (Berlin), Genthiner Str 30G, Berlin 10785, Germany. TEL 49-30-25005-0, FAX 49-30-25008521, vertrieb@esvmedien.de, http://www.erich-schmidt-verlag.de.

610 340 DEU
ARZTHAFTUNGSRECHT. Text in German. 1987. irreg. DEM 128. **Document type:** *Bulletin.*

Published by: Hermann Luchterhand Verlag GmbH, Heddesdorfer Str 31, Neuwied 56564, Germany. TEL 49-2631-801-0, FAX 49-2631-801204. Ed. Klaus Kuntz.

610 340 DEU ISSN 0343-5733
ARZTRECHT; Kompendium des Gesamten Rechtes der Medizin. Text in German. 1965. m. DEM 60. adv. bk.rev. **Description:** Examines the role of the law in medical practice.
Published by: Verlag fuer Arztrecht, Schinnrainstr 15, Karlsruhe 76227, Germany. TEL 0721-402904. Ed. Dr. Manfred Andreas. Circ: (controlled).

610 JPN ISSN 0285-9017
ASAHI CHUO BYOIN IHO/ASAHI GENERAL HOSPITAL. MEDICAL JOURNAL. Text in English, Japanese. 1979. s-a.
Published by: Asahi Chuo Byoin/Asahi General Hospital, I 1326, Asahi-shi, Chiba-ken 289-25, Japan.

610 JPN ISSN 0913-4603
ASAHIGAWASO KENKYU NENPO/ASAHIGAWASO INSTITUTE OF MEDICAL WELFARE. ANNUAL REPORT. Text in Japanese. 1968. a.
Published by: Asahigawaso/Asahigawaso Institute of Medical Welfare, Chisaki, Gion, Okayama-shi 703-8207, Japan.

610 JPN ISSN 0918-7022
ASAHIKAWA IKA DAIGAKU NENPO/ASAHIKAWA MEDICAL COLLEGE. ANNUAL REPORT. Text in Japanese. 1988. a.
Indexed: Zent.Math.
Published by: Asahikawa Ika Daigaku/Asahikawa Medical College, 5 Go, Nishikagura 4 Sen, Asahikawa-shi, Hokkaido 078, Japan.

610 JPN ISSN 0913-4417
ASAHIKAWA SEKIJUJI BYOIN IGAKU ZASSHI/ASAHIKAWA RED CROSS HOSPITAL. MEDICAL JOURNAL. Text in Japanese. 1987. a.
Published by: Asahikawa Sekijuji Byoin/Asahikawa Red Cross Hospital, 1 Akebono 1-Jo, Asahikawa-shi, Hokkaido 070-0000, Japan.

610 JPN ISSN 0287-024X
ASAHIKAWA SHIRITSU BYOIN ISHI/ASAHIKAWA CITY HOSPITAL. JOURNAL. Text in Japanese. 1968. a.
Published by: Asahikawa Shiritsu Byoin/Asahikawa City Hospital, 1-65 Kinsei-cho 1-chome, Asahikawa-shi, Hokkaido 070-0029, Japan.

306.461 ESP ISSN 0210-4466
R131.A1
ASCLEPIO; archivo iberoamericano de historia de la medicina. Text in Spanish. 1949. s-a. ESP 5,600; ESP 7,700 foreign (effective 1999). bk.rev. bibl. cum.index: 1949-1973. back issues avail.; reprint service avail. from SCH. **Document type:** *Academic/Scholarly.* **Description:** Contains original studies and researches in the fields of medical history, science, and medical anthropology.
Former titles (until 1964): Archivo Iberoamericano de Historia de la Medicina y Antropologia Medica (0210-444X); (until 1954): Archivos Iberoamericanos de Historia de la Medicina (0210-4458)
Indexed: A.I.C.P., Amer.Hist.& Life, Anthropol.Lit. (coverage dropped), Hist.Abstr. (1983-), Ind.Med.Esp.
—BLDSC (1739.250000), CINDOC, CISTI, GNLM.
Published by: (Spain. Consejo Superior de Investigaciones Cientificas), Centro de Estudios Historicos, Departamento de Historia de la Medicina (Subsidiary of: Consejo Superior de Investigaciones Cientificas), Departamento de Publicaciones, Vitruvio 8, Madrid 28006 , Spain. publ@orgc.csic.es, http://www.csic.es/publica. Ed. Dr. D Agustin Albarracin Teulon.

610 USA ISSN 1062-0281
ASEPSIS✱ ; the infection prevention forum. Text in English. 1975. q. free per issue to qualified personnel. adv. **Document type:** *Trade.*
Indexed: CINAHL, Hosp.Lit.Ind.
Published by: (Johnson & Johnson Medical, Inc.), Ad-Com Inc. Publishing, 660 Preston Forest Ctr, 340, Dallas, TX 75230-2718. TEL 800-486-8247, FAX 817-261-1399. Ed. Barbara Gruendemann. Pub. Bill Pierce. Adv. contact Teri Scholtheis. Circ: 30,000 (controlled).

610 AUS ISSN 1444-1683
▼ **ASIA PACIFIC FAMILY MEDICINE.** Text in English. 2001. q. AUD 289 domestic; AUD 262 in New Zealand; USD 160 elsewhere; AUD 318 domestic print & online eds.; AUD 289 in New Zealand print & online eds.; USD 176 elsewhere print & online eds. (effective 2001). adv. **Document type:** *Journal, Academic/Scholarly.*

Related titles: ♦ Online - full text ed.: Asia Pacific Family Medicine Online.
Published by: Blackwell Science Asia Pty Ltd, PO Box 378, Carlton South, VIC 3053, Australia. TEL 61-3-9347-0300, FAX 61-3-9347-5001, info@blacksci-asia.com.au, http://www.blacksci.co.uk/australi. Ed. Zorayda E Leopando.

610 AUS
▼ **ASIA PACIFIC FAMILY MEDICINE ONLINE.** Text in English. 2001. q. AUD 261 domestic; AUD 236 in New Zealand; USD 144 elsewhere (effective 2001). **Document type:** *Academic/Scholarly.*
Media: Online - full text (from Swets Blackwell). **Related titles:** ♦ Print ed.: Asia Pacific Family Medicine. ISSN 1444-1683.
Published by: Blackwell Science Asia Pty Ltd, PO Box 378, Carlton South, VIC 3053, Australia. TEL 61-3-9347-0300, FAX 61-3-9347-3016, info@blacksci-asia.com.au, http://www.blacksci.co.uk/australi/.

ASIAN AMERICAN AND PACIFIC ISLANDER JOURNAL OF HEALTH. see *PUBLIC HEALTH AND SAFETY*

610 CHN
▼ **ASIAN JOURNAL OF ANDROLOGY.** Text in English. 1999 (Jun). q. **Document type:** *Academic/Scholarly.*
Indexed: Curr.Cont.
—BLDSC (1742.471500).
Published by: (Asian Society of Andrology), Shanghai Institute of Materia Medica (Subsidiary of: Chinese Academy of Sciences/Zhongguo Kexueyuan), 294 Taiyuan Rd, Shanghai 200031, China. TEL 86-21-64311833, FAX 86-21-64370269.

610 HKG ISSN 0250-3328
ASIAN MEDICAL NEWS. Text and summaries in English. 1979. m. USD 48 domestic; USD 60 foreign (effective 1999). adv. bk.rev. index. **Document type:** *Newspaper.*
Related titles: ♦ Supplement: Therapeaia. ISSN 0255-8793.
Published by: MediMedia Asia (Subsidiary of: MediMedia Pacific Ltd.), 8-F Pacific Plaza, 410 Des Voeux Rd W, Hong Kong, Hong Kong. TEL 852-2559-5888, FAX 852-2559-6910, amn@medimedia.com.hk, http://www.medimedia.com. Pub. Edgar B Richards. Adv. contact Kristina Lo Kurtz. Circ: 34,635 (controlled).

610 PRI ISSN 0004-4849
ASOCIACION MEDICA DE PUERTO RICO. BOLETIN. Text in English, Spanish. 1903. m. USD 40. adv. bk.rev. bibl, illus. index.
Indexed: Abstr.Hyg., Bio-Contr.News & Info., Biol.Abstr., CINAHL, Chem.Abstr., Dent.Ind., Ind.Med. (1903-), Nutr.Abstr., Sel.Water Res.Abstr., Trop.Dis.Bull.
—CISTI, GNLM.
Published by: Asociacion Medica de Puerto Rico, Avenida Fernandez, Juncos, PR 00908. Circ: 3,500.

610.7 MEX ISSN 0004-4857
ASOCIACION MEXICANA DE FACULTADES Y ESCUELAS DE MEDICINA. BOLETIN. Text in Spanish. 1962. irreg. free per issue. bibl, charts, illus. index.
Published by: Asociacion Mexicana de Facultades y Escuelas de Medicina, Queretaro No. 147, Oficinas 501 y 502, Apdo. Postal 12927, Mexico City, DF 06760, Mexico. Ed. Dr. Manuel Loria Mendez. Circ: 750.

610 MEX ISSN 0004-489X
ASOCIACION PARA EVITAR LA CEGUERA EN MEXICO. ARCHIVOS. Text in Spanish. 1956. q. free per issue. adv. bibl, charts, illus.
Published by: Asociacion para Evitar la Ceguera en Mexico, Vicente Garcia Torres 46, Coyoacan 21, Mexico City, DF 04330, Mexico. Ed. Dr. Teodulo M Agundis.

610 ISR ISSN 0334-3871
ASSIA. Text in Hebrew. 1970. irreg. (4 nos./vol.). USD 25. *Refereed.* **Document type:** *Academic/Scholarly.*
Indexed: Ind.Heb.Per. (1977-).
Published by: Shaare Zadek Medical Center, Falk Schlesinger Institute for Medical Halachic Research, P O Box 3235, Jerusalem 91031, Israel. TEL 972-2-6555266, FAX 972-2-6523295, medhal@szmc.org.il, http://www.szmc.org.il/machon. Ed. Rabbi Dr Mordechai Halperin. Circ: 1,000.

ASSIA - JEWISH MEDICAL ETHICS. see *RELIGIONS AND THEOLOGY—Judaic*

M

610 USA
ASSISTED REPRODUCTIVE TECHNOLOGY - ANDROLOGY; international journal. Abbreviated title: A R T A. Text in English. 1990. q. USD 180 domestic to individuals; USD 190 foreign to individuals; USD 200 domestic to institutions; USD 210 foreign to institutions. *Refereed.* **Document type:** *Academic/Scholarly.*
Published by: Reproductive Health Center, 78 Surfsong Rd., Kiawah Island, SC 29455. TEL 803-768-5556, FAX 803-768-6494.

610 CHE
ASSISTENTI DI STUDIO MEDICO. Text in Italian. 1995. m. **Document type:** *Academic/Scholarly.*
Published by: (Ordine dei Medici del Canton Ticino), Inter Annonces SA, Bellefontaine 2, Lausanne 1003, Switzerland. TEL 41-21-3203251, FAX 41-21-3239737.

ASSISTIVE TECHNOLOGY. see *EDUCATION—Special Education And Rehabilitation*

610 BRA ISSN 0004-5233
ASSOCIACAO MEDICA BRASILEIRA. JORNAL. Text in Portuguese. m. BRL 5, USD 5. adv. bk.rev. charts, illus.
Published by: Associacao Medica Brasileira, Rua Sao Carlos do Pinhal 324, Sao Paulo, SP 01333-903, Brazil. TEL 55-11-289-3511, FAX 55-11-2896002. Ed. Marcia Alves. Circ: 30,000.

610 BRA ISSN 0004-5241
ASSOCIACAO MEDICA BRASILEIRA. REVISTA. Text in Portuguese; Summaries in English. 1954. m. adv. bk.rev. abstr, charts, illus. index.
Related titles: Online - full text ed.: (from SciELO).
Indexed: Biol.Abstr., Chem.Abstr., Excerp.Med., IBZ, INIS Atomind., Ind.Med. (coverage dropped).
—GNLM.
Published by: Associacao Medica Brasileira, Rua Sao Carlos do Pinhal 324, Sao Paulo, SP 01333-903, Brazil. TEL 55-11-289-3511, FAX 55-11-2896002. Ed. Dr. Antonio Carlos Lopes. Circ: 40,000.

610 BRA ISSN 0004-525X
CODEN: RAMMDG
ASSOCIACAO MEDICA DE MINAS GERAIS. REVISTA*. Text in Portuguese; Summaries in English. 1949. q. BRL 400, USD 30. adv. bk.rev. bibl, charts, illus, stat. index. **Document type:** *Academic/Scholarly.*
Related titles: Microfilm ed.: 1949.
Indexed: Biol.Abstr., Nutr.Abstr.
Published by: Associacao Medica de Minas Gerais, Centro, Caixa Postal 260, Belo Horizonte, MG 30000, Brazil. Ed. Jose Netto. Circ: 5,000.

610 CAN ISSN 0004-539X
ASSOCIATION DES MEDECINS DE LANGUE FRANCAISE DU CANADA. BULLETIN. Text in English. 1967. m. membership. bk.rev. illus. reprint service avail. from PQC. **Document type:** *Bulletin.*
—CCC.
Published by: Association des Medecins de Langue Francaise du Canada, 8355 boul St Laurent, Montreal, PQ H2P 2Z6, Canada. TEL 514-388-2228. Ed. Andre de Seve. Circ: 13,446.

ASSOCIATION FOR PSYCHOANALYTIC MEDICINE. BULLETIN. see *PSYCHOLOGY*

388.3 610 USA ISSN 0892-6484
ASSOCIATION FOR THE ADVANCEMENT OF AUTOMOTIVE MEDICINE. PROCEEDINGS*. Text in English. 1959. a. USD 40 in North America; USD 50 in Europe; USD 55 elsewhere. **Document type:** *Proceedings.*
Formerly (until 1987): American Association for Automotive Medicine. Proceedings (0401-6351)
Related titles: Microform ed.: 1959.
Indexed: Ind.Med. (1988-), Psychol.Abstr.
—BLDSC (1090.030000), GNLM.
Published by: Association for the Advancement of Automotive Medicine, c/o Associated Life Ins, 222 Merchandise Mart Plaza, Ste 1450, Chicago, IL 60654-1203. TEL 312-390-8927. Circ: 1,000.

610 970.1 USA
ASSOCIATION OF AMERICAN INDIAN PHYSICIANS NEWSLETTER. Text in English. q. free per issue to qualified personnel. adv. **Document type:** *Newsletter.*
Published by: Association of American Indian Physicians, 1235 Sovereign Row, Ste C 9, Oklahoma City, OK 73108-1833. TEL 405-946-7072, FAX 405-946-7651, aaip@qns.com. Ed. Margaret Knight. Adv. contact Judy McCraw. page USD 1,000.

310.711 USA ISSN 0892-2543
ASSOCIATION OF AMERICAN MEDICAL COLLEGES. PROCEEDINGS OF THE ANNUAL CONFERENCE. RESEARCH IN MEDICAL EDUCATION. Text in English. 1971. a.
Formerly (until 1983): Association of American Medical Colleges. Annual Conference on Research in Medical Education (0190-7255)
Related titles: ♦ Supplement to: Academic Medicine. ISSN 1040-2446.
Published by: Association of American Medical Colleges, 2450 N St N W, Washington, DC 20037-1126.

616.04 USA
ASSOCIATION OF BIRTH DEFECT CHILDREN NEWS. Text in English. 1980. q. USD 30 to individuals; USD 40 to qualified personnel; USD 100 to corporations (effective 2001). adv. bk.rev. back issues avail. **Document type:** *Newsletter.* **Description:** Provides information about birth defects to parents and professionals.
Published by: Association of Birth Defect Children, Inc., 930 Woodcock Rd, 225, Orlando, FL 32803-3752. TEL 407-245-7035, 407-895-0802, 800-313-2232, FAX 407-895-0824, abdc@marketweb.com, abcd@birthdefects.org, http://www.birthdefects.org. Ed., R&P, Adv. contact Betty Mekdeci. Circ: 10,000.

616.07 GBR ISSN 0144-0349
CODEN: JCPPDY
ASSOCIATION OF CLINICAL PATHOLOGISTS. SYMPOSIA. Key Title: Journal of Clinical Pathology. Supplement. Association of Clinical Pathologists. Symposia. Text in English. 1967. irreg., latest 1992. **Document type:** *Proceedings.*
Related titles: ♦ Supplement to: Journal of Clinical Pathology. ISSN 0021-9746.
Indexed: Curr.Cont. (coverage dropped).
—CASDDS, CISTI, Infotrieve. **CCC.**
Published by: (Association of Clinical Pathologists), B M J Publishing Group, B M A House, Tavistock Sq, London WC1H 9JR, United Kingdom. TEL 44-207-383-6270, FAX 44-20-7383-6402, http://www.bmjpg.com/. **Subscr. to:** PO Box 480, Franklin, MA 02038.

610 IND ISSN 0004-5772
CODEN: JPHIAR
ASSOCIATION OF PHYSICIANS OF INDIA. JOURNAL. Text in English. 1952. m. INR 1,500; USD 250 foreign. adv. bk.rev. index. *Refereed.* **Document type:** *Academic/Scholarly.*
Related titles: Online - full text ed.: (from Institute for Scientific Information).
Indexed: Chem.Abstr., Dent.Ind., INIS Atomind., Ind.Med. (1953-), Nutr.Abstr., Trop.Dis.Bull.
—BLDSC (4705.120000), CASDDS, CISTI, GNLM, ingenta, KNAW.
Published by: Association of Physicians of India, Laud Mansion 3rd Fl., 21 M Karve Rd., Mumbai, Maharashtra 400 004, India. TEL 91-22-382-9348, 91-22-261-1719, FAX 91-22-305-1093, 91-22-265-6640, japi@bom5.vsnl.net.in, http://www.japi.org. Ed., Adv. contact S.K. Bichile. Pub. S K Bichile. B&W page INR 10,000, color page INR 35,000; trim 180 x 240. Circ: 9,000.

610 MEX ISSN 0185-6235
ATENCION MEDICA. Text in Spanish. 1970. m. MXP 230, USD 80. adv. *Refereed.* **Document type:** *Trade.*
Published by: Intersistemas S.A. de C.V., Aguiar y Seijas 75,, Lomas de Chapultepec, Mexico City, DF 11000, Mexico. TEL 525-540-0798, FAX 525-540-3764, intersis@data.net.mx. Ed. Pedro Vera Cervera. Pub. Dr. Elvia Espino. Adv. contact Miguel Alberto Gonzalez. Circ: 15,500.

610 ESP ISSN 0212-6567
CODEN: ATEPEY
ATENCION PRIMARIA*. Text in Spanish. 12/yr.
Indexed: FAMLI (1991-1992), Ind.Med. (1983-), Int.Nurs.Ind.
—BLDSC (1765.858500), CINDOC, EMDOCS, GNLM, Infotrieve, KNAW. **CCC.**
Published by: Haymarket, S.A., Travesera Gracia 17-21, 5o 2o, Barcelona 08022, Spain. TEL 3-237-22-66, FAX 3-237-66-88. Ed. Dr. J F Cano Perez.

610 BOL
ATENEO DE MEDICINA. Text in Spanish. 6/yr. adv.
Address: Casilla 549, La Paz, Bolivia.

610 570 ITA ISSN 0392-4203
CODEN: ABPADJ
ATENEO PARMENSE. ACTA BIO-MEDICA. Key Title: Acta Bio-medica de l'Ateneo Parmense. Text and summaries in English, Italian. 1929. bi-m. ITL 25,000; ITL 50,000 foreign (effective 1994). bk.rev. bibl, charts, illus, stat. index, cum.index. **Document type:** *Proceedings, Academic/Scholarly.* **Description:** Research papers covering a variety of medical topics.
Formerly (until 1981): Ateneo Pamense. Acta Biomedica (0004-6531); Which supersedes in part (in 1961): Ateneo Parmense (0376-057X)
Indexed: Biol.Abstr., Chem.Abstr., Excerp.Med. (1996-), GeoRef, INIS Atomind., Ind.Med. (1981-), Nutr.Abstr.
—BLDSC (0603.000000), CASDDS, CISTI, EMDOCS, GNLM.
Published by: (Societa di Medicina e Scienze Naturali di Parma), Ateneo Parmense, Via Gramsci, 14, Parma, PR 43100, Italy. TEL 39-521-983364. Ed. Fulvio Allegra. Pub. Paolo Bobbio. Circ: 550.

301 IDN
ATMA JAYA RESEARCH CENTRE. SOCIO-MEDICAL RESEARCH REPORT/PUSAT PENELITIAN ATMA JAYA. PENELITIAN TENTANG KEBUTUHAN KESEHATAN MASYARAKAT DAN SISTEM PELEYANAN KESEHATAN DI KECAMATAN PENJARINGAN. Text in English. 1978. irreg. **Document type:** *Monographic series.*
Indexed: Abstr.Rural Dev.Trop.
Published by: Atma Jaya Research Centre/Pusat Penelitian Atma Jaya, Jalan Jenderal Sudirman 51, PO Box 2639, Jakarta 10001, Indonesia. Ed. Paul W Kartono.

610 JPN ISSN 0915-6003
ATSUGI BYOIN ISHI/ATSUGI MEDICAL JOURNAL. Text in Japanese. 1981. a.
Published by: Kanagawa Kenritsu Atsugi Byoin/Kanagawa Prefectural Atsugi Hospital, 16-36 Mizuhiki 1-chome, Atsugi-shi, Kanagawa-ken 243-0004, Japan.

ATTORNEYS' DICTIONARY OF MEDICINE. see *LAW*

ATTORNEY'S MEDICAL ADVANTAGE ON LAWDESK. see *LAW*

344.041 USA
ATTORNEY'S MEDICAL ADVISOR - ATLAS. Text in English. 10 base vols. plus s-a. updates. USD 1,850 (effective 2000). **Document type:** *Academic/Scholarly.* **Description:** Contains comprehensive medical information and full-color anatomic illustrations.
Related titles: ♦ CD-ROM ed.: Attorney's Medical Advantage on LawDesk.
Published by: West Group (Subsidiary of: Thomson Corporation, The), 620 Opperman Dr., Eagan, MN 55123. TEL 800-344-5008, FAX 800-340-9378, http://www.westgroup.com. Eds. Bruce F Freeman, Dr. J Stanley Mcquade, Lee R Ross.

344.41 USA
ATTORNEY'S MEDICAL DESKBOOK. Text in English. 3 base vols. plus a. updates. USD 385 (effective 2000). **Document type:** *Academic/Scholarly.* **Description:** Covers the interpretation of medical terminology, records, literature, and evidence.
Related titles: ♦ CD-ROM ed.: Attorney's Medical Advantage on LawDesk.
Published by: West Group (Subsidiary of: Thomson Corporation, The), 620 Opperman Dr., Eagan, MN 55123. TEL 800-344-5008, FAX 800-340-9378, http://www.westgroup.com.

ATTORNEYS' TEXTBOOK OF MEDICINE. see *LAW*

610 USA ISSN 0271-1362
AUDIO-DIGEST FAMILY PRACTICE. Text in English. 1953. w. (& s-m). USD 336 weekly ed.; USD 168 s-monthly ed. (effective 2000). *Refereed.*
Formerly: Audio-Digest General Practice (0571-8619)
Media: Audio cassette/tape.
—ingenta.
Published by: Audio-Digest Foundation (Subsidiary of: California Medical Association), 1577 E Chevy Chase Dr, Glendale, CA 91206. TEL 213-245-8505, 800-423-2308, FAX 818-240-7379, 800-845-4375.

M

617 CAN ISSN 0743-4618
RC429 CODEN: AAACEC
AUGMENTATIVE AND ALTERNATIVE COMMUNICATION. Text in English. q. USD 105 in US & Canada to individuals; USD 135 elsewhere to individuals; USD 175 in US & Canada to institutions; USD 209 elsewhere to institutions (effective 2001). adv. back issues avail. *Refereed.* **Document type:** *Journal, Academic/Scholarly.* **Description:** Articles on systems and devices for speech- and language-impaired individuals for speech-language specialists, special educators, rehabilitation engineers.
Related titles: Online - full text ed.: (from ProQuest Information & Learning).
Indexed: AMED, Bioeng.Abstr., Biotech.& Bioeng.Abstr., CINAHL, Eng.Ind., Except.Child Educ.Abstr., Lang.& Lang.Behav.Abstr., Ling.Abstr., PsycInfo, Psychol.Abstr. (1985-), SOPODA, Sociol.Abstr., e-psyche.
—BLDSC (1791.440000), Ei, ingenta. **CCC.**
Published by: (International Society for Augmentative and Alternative Communication), B.C. Decker Inc., 20 Hughson St S, LCD 1, P O Box 620, Hamilton, ON L8N 3K7, Canada. TEL 905-522-7017, 800-568-7281, FAX 905-522-7839, info@bcdecker.com, http://www.bcdecker.com. Ed. Pat Mirenda. Pub. David LeGallais. R&P Paula Presutti. Adv. contact John Birkby. Circ: 1,600.

610 AUS ISSN 1328-8040
AUSTRALASIAN COLLEGE OF NUTRITIONAL AND ENVIRONMENTAL MEDICINE. JOURNAL. Abbreviated title: A C N E M Journal. Text in English. 1982. 3/yr. adv. bk.rev. Index. back issues avail. *Refereed.* **Document type:** *Academic/Scholarly.* **Description:** Contains original peer reviewed articles on medical research clinical practice in nutritional and environmental medicine; provides up-to-date clinical and scientific information to our members, other health professional and the general public.
Former titles (until 1996): Australian College of Nutritional and Environmental Medicine. Journal (1327-8541); (until 1994): Journal of Nutritional and Environmental Medicine (1035-1620)
Published by: Australasian College of Nutritional and Environmental Medicine, 13 Hilton St, Beaumaris, VIC 3193, Australia. TEL 61-3-9589-6088, FAX 61-3-9589-5158, acnem@mail.austasia.net. Ed., Pub. Dr. Ian E. Brighthope. R&P Mr. Daan Spijer. adv.: B&W page AUD 369, color page AUD 559; trim 205 x 280. Circ: 2,600 (paid); 2,000 (controlled).

610 AUS ISSN 1039-7116
AUSTRALIAN DOCTOR. Text in English. 1984. w. AUD 286.44 (effective 2001). adv. back issues avail. **Document type:** *Trade.* **Description:** Examines the clinical, socioeconomic and leisure aspects of the medical professional.
Former titles (until 1993): Australian Dr Weekly (1033-9221); (until 1987): Australian Dr (0814-6012)
Indexed: INIS Atomind.
Published by: Reed Business Information Pty. Ltd. (Subsidiary of: Reed Elsevier plc), Locked Bag 2999, Chatswood, NSW 2067, Australia. kellie.bisset@reedbusiness.com.au, http://www.reedbusiness.com.au/. Ed. Kellie Bisset. Pub. Russell Norden. Adv. contact Margaret Black. Circ: 25,204.

610 AUS ISSN 0300-8495
CODEN: AFPHCX
AUSTRALIAN FAMILY PHYSICIAN. Text in English. 1956. m., latest vol.29, 2000. AUD 184.80 domestic; AUD 300 foreign (effective 2001 & 2002). adv. bk.rev. abstr, charts, illus. index. back issues avail. **Document type:** *Academic/Scholarly.*
Formerly: Annals of General Practice (0003-4789)
Related titles: Online - full text ed.
Indexed: CINAHL, Curr.Adv.Cancer Res., Curr.Adv.Ecol.Sci., Dent.Ind., Dok.Arbeitsmed., Excerp.Med., FAMLI, Fam.Ind., Ind.Med. (1972-), Inpharma, Int.Nurs.Ind., Pharm.&Out.News, Reac.
—BLDSC (1798.922000), GNLM, ingenta, KNAW. **CCC.**
Published by: Royal Australian College of General Practitioners, 1 Palmerston Crescent, South Melbourne, VIC 3205, Australia. TEL 61-3-92141414, FAX 61-3-92141401, afp@racgp.org.au, http://afp.racgp.org.au/. Ed., R&P Betty Vassiliadis. Adv. contact Tim Young. B&W page AUD 3,485, color page AUD 4,100; trim 210 x 275. Circ: 22,737.

AUSTRALIAN HEALTH AND MEDICAL INDUSTRY GUIDE. see *BUSINESS AND ECONOMICS—Trade And Industrial Directories*

610 616 AUS ISSN 1038-1643
CODEN: AUJMEN
AUSTRALIAN JOURNAL OF MEDICAL SCIENCE. Text in English. q. AUD 75 to non-members; AUD 100 foreign (effective 2000). *Refereed.* **Description:** Scientific and technological papers relating to clinical laboratory practice.
Incorporates (in 1999): A I M S Newsletter (1038-4766); Former titles: Australian Journal of Laboratory Science (0158-4960); (until 1980): Australia Journal of Medical Technology (0312-956X); Medical Technology in Australia
Indexed: Chem.Abstr., Excerp.Med., INIS Atomind.
—BLDSC (1810.270000), CASDDS, CISTI, EMDOCS, GNLM, ingenta, KNAW.
Published by: Australian Institute of Medical Scientists, PO Box 1911, Milton, QLD 4064, Australia. TEL 67-3876-2988, FAX 61-7-3876-2999, aimsnat@medeserv.com.au. Eds. Anthony Woods, John Stirling.

610 AUS ISSN 1324-2296
AUSTRALIAN JOURNAL OF PRIMARY HEALTH - INTERCHANGE. Text in English. 1995. q. AUD 65 domestic to individuals; AUD 90 foreign to individuals; AUD 150 domestic to institutions; AUD 175 foreign to institutions. adv. bk.rev. index. *Refereed.* **Document type:** *Academic/Scholarly.* **Description:** Covers interdisciplinary health sciences relevant to theory and practice of primary health. Contains research articles, policy reports and analyses, case reports, the views of practitioners, consumers, students, and special interest groups.
Indexed: Soc.Serv.Abstr., Sociol.Abstr.
—BLDSC (1811.225000).
Published by: Trobe University, School of Public Health, Primary Health Research and Development Centre, Bundoora, VIC 3083, Australia. TEL 61-3-9479-1750, FAX 61-3-9479-1783, l.paul@latrobe.edu.au, http://www.health.latrobe.edu.au/hs/Health/Schools/PH/sphwebpg/sphfm.html. Ed., R&P Heather Gardner TEL 61-3-9479-1733. Adv. contact Lindsay Paul. Circ: 450.
Co-sponsor: Victorian Community Health Association.

174.2 614 AUS
AUSTRALIAN MEDICINE. Text in English. 1989. 22/yr. AUD 231 domestic; AUD 280 foreign (effective 2001). adv. bk.rev., software rev., video rev. 28 p./no. back issues avail. **Document type:** *Magazine, Trade.* **Description:** Provides information relating to health care politics, medical ethics and legal news.
Related titles: Online - full content ed.
Published by: Australian Medical Association, Level 4, 42 Macquarie St, Barton, ACT 2600, Australia. TEL 61-6-270-5400, FAX 61-6-270-5499, ausmed@ama.com.au, ausmed@ama.con.au, http://www.ama.com.au/publications. Ed., R&P Edwina Light. Adv. contact Julia Horvath. color page AUD 3,390; bleed 316 x 226. Circ: 26,800.

610 AUS ISSN 0817-3834
AUSTRALIAN PRIVATE DOCTOR. Text in English. 1968. bi-m. AUD 90 (effective 1999). adv. bk.rev. illus. back issues avail. **Document type:** *Trade.* **Description:** Designed for private doctors, hospital doctors and pharmaceutical manufacturers.
Formerly (until 1985): Australian G P (0045-0499)
Related titles: Microform ed.
Published by: Private Doctors of Australia Ltd., PO Box 390, Wentworthville, NSW 2145, Australia. TEL 61-47-322977, FAX 61-47-323762, http://pda.org.au. Ed., R&P Ian Tait. Pub., Adv. contact Ron Hill. Circ: 2,500 (controlled).

610.9 AUS ISSN 0816-1860
AUSTRALIAN SOCIETY FOR THE HISTORY OF MEDICINE. OCCASIONAL PAPERS; the impact of the past upon the present. Key Title: Occasional Papers on Medical History Australia. Text in English. 1984. biennial. AUD 40 (effective 2000).
Published by: Australian Society for the History of Medicine, PO Box 130, Northbridge, W.A. 6865, Australia. TEL 61-8-94441677, FAX 61-8-92421201. Circ: 350 (controlled).

610 DNK
AUTORISEREDE LAEGER I DANMARK. Text in Danish. 1982. irreg. DKK 80.
Former titles (until 1992): Autoriserede Laeger, Tandlaeger, Dyrlaeger i Danmark (0108-4739); Fortegnelse over Autoriserede Laeger, Tandlaeger, Dyrlaeger i Danmark (0106-7354)
Published by: Sundhedsstyrelsen, Amaliegade 13, PO Box 2020, Copenhagen K 1012, Denmark. Circ: 900.
Subscr. to: Statens Informationtjeneste, PO Box 1103, Copenhagen K, Denmark.

610 USA
AVENUES (SONORA). Text in English. 1980. 2/yr. USD 7.50. back issues avail. **Document type:** *Newsletter.* **Description:** Publishes research articles, reviews and family experiences to enable families to network on a national and international level.
Published by: National Support Group for Arthrogryposis Multiplex Congenita, PO Box 5192, Sonora, CA 95370. TEL 209-928-3688. Ed. Mary Anne Schmidt. Circ: 1,000.

616.98 RUS ISSN 0233-528X
RC1050 CODEN: AEKME
AVIAKOSMICHESKAYA I EKOLOGICHESKAYA MEDITSINA/AEROSPACE AND ENVIRONMENTAL MEDICINE. Text in Russian; Summaries in English. 1967. bi-m. RUR 156,000; USD 147 foreign. adv. bk.rev. abstr, bibl, charts, illus. index. Supplement avail. **Document type:** *Academic/Scholarly.* **Description:** Articles both of scientific and applied character on a wide range of problems in the field of aerospace medicine and biology. Includes physiology and hygiene of flight, psychophysiological peculiarities of flight activity, psychological screening and medical examination for flight fitness.
Former titles (until 1992): Kosmicheskaya Biologiya i Aviakosmicheskaya Meditsina (0321-5040); Kosmicheskaya Biologiya i Meditsina (0023-4192)
Indexed: Biol.Abstr., Chem.Abstr., Curr.Adv.Ecol.Sci., Curr.Cont. (coverage dropped), Dairy Sci.Abstr., Dent.Ind., Dok.Arbeitsmed., Excerp.Med., Field Crop Abstr., INIS Atomind., Ind.Med. (1992-), Ind.Sci.Rev., Nutr.Abstr., PsycInfo, Psychol.Abstr. (1982-), Ref.Zh., Triticale Abstr., e-psyche.
—BLDSC (0000.230000), CASDDS, CISTI, East View, EMDOCS, GNLM, Infotrieve, Linda Hall. **CCC.**
Published by: (Institut Mediko-biologicheskikh Problem), Slovo Ltd., Khoroshevskoe shosse 76-a, Moscow 123007, Russian Federation. TEL 7-095-1939492, FAX 7-095-1952253, TELEX 411048 VUAL SU, grigoriev@mmcc.ibmp.rssi.ru. Ed. A I Grigoriev. R&P Valentin V Krougovykh. adv.: B&W page USD 200, color page USD 400. **Dist. by:** Mezhdunarodnaya Kniga, B Yakimanka 39, Moscow 117049, Russian Federation. TEL 7-095-2384967, FAX 7-095-2384634.

AVIATION MEDICAL EDUCATION SERIES. see *AERONAUTICS AND SPACE FLIGHT*

616.98 USA ISSN 0095-6562
RC1050 CODEN: ASEMCG
AVIATION, SPACE, AND ENVIRONMENTAL MEDICINE. Text in English. 1930. m., latest vol.73, 2002. USD 160 domestic to individuals; USD 175 in Canada to individuals; USD 200 elsewhere to individuals; USD 175 domestic to institutions; USD 190 in Canada to institutions; USD 225 elsewhere to institutions (effective 2001). adv. bk.rev. illus. index. back issues avail.; reprints avail. *Refereed.* **Document type:** *Academic/Scholarly.* **Description:** It serves and supports all who explore, travel, work, or live in hazardous environments ranging from beneath the sea to the outermost reaches of space.
Formerly (until 1975): Aerospace Medicine (0001-9402)
Related titles: Microfiche ed.: (from PQC); Online - full text ed.: (from Institute for Scientific Information).
Indexed: ASCA, Air Un.Lib.Ind., Biol.Abstr., CINAHL, C.I.S. Abstr., Chem.Abstr., Chem.Indus.Notes, Chem.Titles, Curr.Adv.Ecol.Sci., Curr.Cont., Dent.Ind., Environ.Sci.Poll.Mgmt., Ergon.Abstr., Excerp.Med., Focus on: Sports Sci.& Med., INIS Atomind., Ind.Med. (1975-), Ind.Sci.Rev., Indian Psychol.Abstr., Inpharma, Int.Aerosp.Abstr., NRN, Neurosci.Cit.Ind., Noise Pollut.Publ.Abstr., Nutr.Abstr., Pharm.&Out.News, Pollut.Abstr., PsycInfo, Psychol.Abstr. (1950-), Psycscan A.P., Reac., Rev.Arom.& Med.Plants, Risk Abstr., SSCI (coverage dropped), Saf.Sci.Abstr., Sci.Cit.Ind., THA, e-psyche.
—BLDSC (1838.640000), CASDDS, CISTI, EMDOCS, GNLM, IDS, ingenta, Linda Hall. **CCC.**
Published by: Aerospace Medical Association, 320 S Henry St, Alexandria, VA 22314-3579. TEL 703-739-2240, FAX 703-739-9652, gcarter@asma.org, http://www.asma.org. R&P Pamela Day TEL 703-739-2240. Adv. contact Truby Chiaviello TEL 703-920-1421. Circ: 4,000 (paid).

610 ITA ISSN 0392-6877
L'AVVENIRE MEDICO. Text in Italian. a. price varies.
Published by: Giardini Editori e Stampatori, Via Santa Bibbiana, 28, Pisa, PI 56127, Italy. TEL 050 502531.

610 JPN
AWAJI ISHIKAI NYUSU/AWAJI MEDICAL ASSOCIATION NEWS. Text in Japanese. 1982. q.

Published by: Awaji Ishikai/Awaji Medical Association, 1-12 Sakae-Machi 1-chome, Sumoto-shi, Hyogo-ken 656-0026, Japan.

610 IND ISSN 0005-2469
R606
AYU. Text in English, Gujarati, Hindi, Sanskrit. 1964. m. INR 15. adv. bk.rev. bibl, charts.
Published by: Gujarat Ayurved University, Institute of Post Graduate Teaching and Research, P O Box 511, Jamnagar, Gujarat, India. Circ: 225.

610 IND ISSN 0005-2493
AYURVEDA DOOT. Text in English, Hindi. 1969. w. INR 10.50.
Published by: Rajasthan Ayurvedic Research Laboratories, Ayurveddoot Karyalaya 4, Dhamani Market, Sawai Mansingh Highway, Jaipur, Rajasthan 302 004, India. Ed. Dhan Kumar Jain.

610 AZE ISSN 0005-2523
CODEN: AZMZA6
AZERBAIDZHANSKII MEDITSINSKII ZHURNAL/ AZERBAIDZHAN TIBB ZHURNALY. Text in Azerbaijani, Russian. 1928. m.
Indexed: Biol.Abstr., Chem.Abstr.
—CASDDS, CISTI, GNLM, Infotrieve. **CCC.**
Published by: (Azerbaijan. Ministerstvo Zdravookhraneniya Azerbaijana), Izdatel'stvo Elm, Ul Narimanova 37, Baku 370073, Azerbaijan. **Dist. by:** Mezhdunarodnaya Kniga, B Yakimanka 39, Moscow 117049, Russian Federation.

610 382 USA
B B I N: MEDICAL DEVICE WEEK. (Biomedical Business International Newsletter) Text in English. 1997. w. USD 747 domestic; USD 777 foreign; USD 29 newsstand/cover (effective 2001). **Document type:** *Newsletter.* **Description:** Analyzes healthcare technology and market news and trends.
Media: Fax. **Related titles:** ♦ Print ed.: The B B I Newsletter. ISSN 1049-4316.
Published by: American Health Consultants (Subsidiary of: Medical Economics Co., Inc.), 3525 Piedmont Rd, N E, 6 Piedmont Center, Ste 400, Atlanta, GA 30305. TEL 404-262-7436, 800-688-2421, FAX 404-262-7837, 800-284-3291, custserv@ahcpub.com, http://www.ahcpub.com.

610 382 USA ISSN 1049-4316
CODEN: BBNWEJ
THE B B I NEWSLETTER. Variant title: Biomedical Business International Newsletter. Text in English. 1978. m. USD 827 domestic; USD 857 foreign; USD 138 newsstand/cover (effective 2001). **Document type:** *Newsletter.* **Description:** Includes tracking and analysis of healthcare technology and market trends.
Incorporates in part (in 1997): Healthcare Technology and Business Opportunities (1049-4499); Which was formerly: Medical Product Development
Related titles: ♦ Fax ed.: B B I N: Medical Device Week; Online - full text ed.: (from The Dialog Corporation, Gale Group).
—BLDSC (1871.362500).
Published by: American Health Consultants (Subsidiary of: Medical Economics Co., Inc.), 3525 Piedmont Rd, N E, 6 Piedmont Center, Ste 400, Atlanta, GA 30305. TEL 404-262-7436, 800-688-2421, FAX 404-262-7837, 800-284-3291, custserv@ahcpub.com, http://www.ahcpub.org.

610 GBR
B M A NEWS; the voice of doctors. (In 2 editions: General Practitioner & Hospital) Text in English. 1966. w. GBP 60 (effective 2001). *Refereed.* **Document type:** *Trade.* **Description:** Directed to doctors from all parts of the profession with news and information about a wide range of topics. Includes features on other socio-health-related subjects.
Former titles (until 2001): B M A News Review (The Voice of Doctors) (1463-8975); (until 1998): B M A News Review for Busy Doctors (1463-8959); Which superseded in part (in 1993): B M A News Review (0306-5472); Which was formerly (until 1975): B M A News (0306-2368)
Indexed: Curr.Adv.Ecol.Sci., Sugar Ind.Abstr.
—BLDSC (2116.034900).
Published by: (British Medical Association), B M J Publishing Group, B M A House, Tavistock Sq, London WC1H 9JR, United Kingdom. TEL 44-20-7387-4499, FAX 44-20-7383-6400, bmanews@bma.org.uk, info.norththames@bma.org.uk, http://www.bma.org.uk. Ed. Mark Jessop. Circ: 120,000 (controlled).

610 GBR ISSN 1463-8983
B M A NEWS REVIEW (THE VOICE OF G PS). (British Medical Assciation - General Practitioners) Text in English. 1966. m.
Formerly (until 1998): B M A News Review for Busy G Ps (1463-8967); Which superseded in part (in 1993): B M A News Review (0306-5472); Which was formerly (until 1975): B M A News (0306-2368)
Published by: (British Medical Association), B M J Publishing Group, B M A House, Tavistock Sq, London WC1H 9JR, United Kingdom. TEL 44-20-7387-4499, FAX 44-20-7383-6400, bmanews@bma.org.uk, info.norththames@bma.org.uk, http://www.bma.org.uk.

610 USA
B M E S BULLETIN. Text in English. 1976. q. USD 25 (effective 1999). adv. back issues avail. *Refereed.* **Document type:** *Newsletter.* **Description:** Promotes the increase of biomedical engineering knowledge and its utilization.
Related titles: Online - full text ed.
Indexed: ASCA, METADEX.
Published by: Biomedical Engineering Society, 8401 Corporate Dr., Ste. 110, Landover, MD 20785-2224. TEL 301-459-1999, FAX 301-459-2444, sslack@cc.memphis.edu, http://www.bmes.org. Ed. Jerry Collins. Pub., R&P, Adv. contact Patricia I Horner. Circ: 2,200.

610 GBR ISSN 0959-535X
R31 CODEN: BMJOAE
B M J. (British Medical Journal) Text in English. 1840. w. GBP 132, USD 211 to individuals for print & online eds. combined; GBP 294, USD 469 to institutions for print only (effective 2002). adv. bk.rev. abstr, bibl, charts, illus. index. reprint service avail. from PQC. *Refereed.* **Document type:** *Academic/Scholarly.* **Description:** Covers all branches of medicine for the professional and layperson.
Former titles (until 1980): British Medical Journal (0007-1447); (until 1857): Association Medical Journal
Related titles: Microform ed.: (from PQC,PMC); ♦ Online - full text ed.: bmj.com; ♦ Dutch ed.: British Medical Journal (Dutch Edition); ♦ Polish ed.: British Medical Journal (Wydawnictwo Polskie). ISSN 1231-9775; ♦ Danish ed.: British Medical Journal (Danish Edition); ♦ Chinese ed.: Yingguo Yixue Zazhi (Zhongwen Ban). ISSN 1007-9742; Hungarian ed.: B M J (Magyar Kiady). ISSN 1216-7495. 1992; Greek ed.: B M J (Ellenike Ekdosis). ISSN 1106-4226. 1993; Portuguese ed.: B M J (Edicoe Portuguesa). ISSN 0873-0423. 1992; International ed.: B M J (International Edition). ISSN 0959-8146; ♦ Regional ed.: B M J (South African Edition). ISSN 1019-8350; ♦ Selections from B M J (South Asia Edition); B M J (Nigerian Edition). ISSN 1118-4485. 1996; B M J (Middle East Edition). ISSN 1106-5028. 1993; B M J (West African Edition). ISSN 1119-2984. 1997; ♦ Special ed.: Student B M J. ISSN 0966-6494; B M J - General Practice Edition. ISSN 0959-8154. 1981; ♦ Supplement: Student B M J. ISSN 0966-6494.
Indexed: AIDS Abstr., AIM, ASCA, ASSIA, Abstr.Anthropol., Abstr.Crim.& Pen., Abstr.Health Care Manage.Stud., Abstr.Hyg., Abstr.Inter.Med., Abstr.Soc.Geront., Addic.Abstr., AgeLine, Agri.& Environ.Biotech.Abstr. (coverage dropped), Anal.Abstr., Arts & Hum.Cit.Ind. (coverage dropped), Behav.Med.Abstr., Bibl.Dev.Med.& Child Neur., Biol.Abstr., Biol.Dig., Brit.Nur.Ind., CINAHL, C.I.S. Abstr., Cadscan, Chem.Abstr., Chem.Indus.Notes, Chem.Titles, Curr.Adv.Cancer Res., Curr.Adv.Ecol.Sci., Curr.Adv.Gen.& Molec.Biol., Curr.Cont., Curr.Lit.Fam.Plan., Dairy Sci.Abstr., Dent.Ind., Diab.Cont., Diar.Dis.Res., Dok.Arbeitsmed., Excerp.Med., FAMLI, Food Sci.& Tech.Abstr., HRIS, Helminthol.Abstr., High.Educ.Curr.Aware.Bull., Human Resour.Abstr., INIS Atomind., I.P.A., Ind.Hyg.Dig., Ind.Med. (coverage dropped), Ind.Sci.Rev., Ind.Vet., Inpharma, Int.Nurs.Ind., Jrnl.Watch, Jrnl.Watch Card., Jrnl.Watch Derm., Jrnl.Watch Emer.Med., Jrnl.Watch Gastr., Jrnl.Watch Inf.Dis., Jrnl.Watch Neuro., Jrnl.Watch Psych., Jrnl.Watch Wom.Hlth., Kidney, Lab.Haz.Bull., Lead Abstr., Med.Care Rev., NRN, Neurosci.Cit.Ind., Nutr.Abstr., Pharm.&Out.News, Popul.Ind., Potato Abstr., Protozool.Abstr., Reac., Res.High.Educ.Abstr., Rev.Appl.Entomol., Rev.Arom.& Med.Plants, Rev.Plant Path., Rural Devel.Abstr., SSCI (coverage dropped), Saf.Sci.Abstr., Sage Fam.Stud.Abstr., Sage Race Rel.Abstr., So.Pac.Per.Ind., Soyabean Abstr., Stud.Wom.Abstr., Trop.Dis.Bull., Vet.Bull., Viol.& Abuse Abstr., W.R.C.Inf., Zincscan.
—CASDDS, CISTI, GNLM, ingenta, KNAW. **CCC.**
Published by: (British Medical Association), B M J Publishing Group, B M A House, Tavistock Sq, London WC1H 9JR, United Kingdom. TEL 44-20-7387-4499, FAX 44-20-7383-6400, bmj@bmj.com, info.norththames@bma.org.uk, http://www.bmj.com/, http://www.bma.org.uk. Ed. Richard Smith. Pub. Stella Dutton. R&P Mustak Kothia TEL 44-20-7383-6281. Adv. contact Simon Walker TEL 44-20-7383-6350. B&W page GBP 2,200, color page GBP 3,250; trim 210 x 297. Circ: 117,000 (paid).

610 ZAF ISSN 1019-8350
B M J (SOUTH AFRICAN EDITION). (British Medical Journal) Text in English. 1992. m. ZAR 108.30; ZAR 180 foreign (effective 1997). **Document type:** *Academic/Scholarly, Trade.*
Related titles: ♦ Regional ed.: B M J. ISSN 0959-535X; ♦ Selections from B M J (South Asia Edition); B M J (Nigerian Edition). ISSN 1118-4485. 1996; B M J (Middle East Edition). ISSN 1106-5028. 1993; B M J (West African Edition). ISSN 1119-2984. 1997.
Published by: George Warman Publications (Pty.) Ltd., PO Box 704, Cape Town 8000, South Africa. TEL 27-21-24-5320, FAX 27-21-26-1332. Circ: 5,714.

B N A'S HEALTH LAW REPORTER; a weekly review of legislative, regulatory, and legal developments. see *LAW*

610 340 USA ISSN 1049-7986
B N A'S MEDICARE REPORT. Text in English. 1990. w. USD 877 (effective 2001). 32 p./no. back issues avail. **Description:** Notification service covering legislative, regulatory, and legal developments affecting or pertaining to the Medicare program.
Related titles: Online - full text ed.: ISSN 1521-4699 (from Human Resources Information Network, Bureau of National Affairs, Inc., (BNA), The).
—**CCC.**
Published by: The Bureau of National Affairs, Inc., 1231 25th St, N W, Washington, DC 20037. TEL 202-452-4200, 800-372-1033, 800-452-7773, FAX 202-822-8092, customercare@bna.com, bnaplus@bna.com, http://www.bna.com/. Ed. Mary Davis. Pub. Gregory McCaffery.

610 GBR
B R H S NEWSLETTER. (British Regional Heart Study) Text in English. m. **Document type:** *Newsletter, Academic/Scholarly.* **Description:** Follows progress of the BRHS, which seeks to determine those factors responsible for variation in ischaemic heart disease, hypertension and stroke in Great Britain. Also contains news on recently published articles, papers in press, and upcoming events.
Published by: Royal Free and University College Medical School, Department of Primary Care & Population Sciences, Rowland Hill St, London NW3 2PF, United Kingdom. TEL 44-20-78302335, FAX 44-20-77941224.

610 384 USA ISSN 1520-2674
BACON'S MEDICAL & HEALTH MEDIA DIRECTORY. Text in English. 1998. a. USD 245 (effective 2000). **Document type:** *Directory.*
Published by: Bacon's Information, Inc., 332 S Michigan Ave, Chicago, IL 60604. TEL 312-987-9773, FAX 312-987-9773, directories@baconsinfo.com, http://www.baconsinfo.com. Ed., Pub. Ruth McFarland. Circ: 1,000.

610 BHR ISSN 1012-7666
HC59.8 CODEN: BMBUEU
BAHRAIN MEDICAL BULLETIN. Text in English. 1979. 3/yr. **Document type:** *Bulletin.*
Related titles: CD-ROM ed.
Indexed: Excerp.Med. (until 1992), ExtraMED.
Address: PO Box 32159, Manama, Bahrain. TEL 973-279472. Ed. Jaffar Al Ibriq. Circ: 1,750.

610 BHR ISSN 1015-6321
CODEN: JBSOE
BAHRAIN MEDICAL SOCIETY. JOURNAL. Key Title: Journal of the Bahrain Medical Society. Text in English, Arabic; Summaries in English, Arabic. 1979. q. BHD 8, USD 50 (effective 1999). adv. abstr, bibl, charts, illus, maps, stat. back issues avail. *Refereed.* **Document type:** *Academic/Scholarly.* **Description:** Addresses various medical issues of importance. Encourages research and helps in disseminating information to the medical community.
Related titles: CD-ROM ed.
Indexed: Excerp.Med., ExtraMED.
—BLDSC (4707.637800), EMDOCS, GNLM.

M

Published by: Bahrain Medical Society, PO Box 26136, Manama, Bahrain. TEL 973-742666, FAX 973-715559, fatehamd@usa.net. Ed. Ahmad J Jamal. Adv. contact Ahmed J Jamal. page USD 1,061; trim 10 x 8. Circ: 1,200 (controlled).

614.88 GBR
BAILLIERE'S HANDBOOK OF FIRST AID. Text in English. 1958. irreg., latest vol.7, 1985. GBP 8.95 (effective 1994). back issues avail. *Refereed.* **Document type:** *Academic/Scholarly.*
Published by: Bailliere Tindall (Subsidiary of: Harcourt Publishers Ltd.), 24-28 Oval Rd, London NW1 7DX, United Kingdom. TEL 44-20-7485-4752, FAX 0171-267-4466. **Subscr. in N. America to:** W.B. Saunders Co., Journal Subscription Fulfillment, 6277 Sea Harbor Dr, 4th Fl, Orlando, FL 32887-4800. TEL 800-874-6418; **Subscr. to:** Harcourt Publishers Ltd., Foots Cray High St, Sidcup, Kent DA14 5HP, United Kingdom. TEL 44-20-8300-3322, FAX 44-20-8309-0807.

610 JPN ISSN 0917-4915
BAIOMEDIKARU/JAPANESE BIOMEDICAL FORUM. JOURNAL. Text in Japanese; Summaries in English, Japanese. 1991. a. JPY 2,000.
Published by: Baiomedikaru Foramu/Biomedical Forum, Keisatsu Byoin ICU, 10-41 Fujimi 2-chome, Chiyoda-ku, Tokyo 102-0071, Japan.

610 CHN ISSN 0253-3707
CODEN: PEIPDB
BAIQIUEN YIKE DAXUE XUEBAO/NORMAN BETHUNE UNIVERSITY OF MEDICAL SCIENCES. JOURNAL. Text mainly in Chinese; Text occasionally in English. 1959. bi-m. CNY 6 per issue domestic (effective 2000). **Document type:** *Academic/Scholarly.* **Description:** Contains scientific, clinical and experimental research papers, case reports, and new developments in medical technology and drugs.
Related titles: Online - full content ed.: (from WanFang Data Corp.).
Indexed: Chem.Abstr., Chem.Indus.Notes, Chem.Titles, INIS Atomind., Zoo.Rec.
—BLDSC (4833.735000), CASDDS, CISTI.
Published by: Baiqiu'en Yike Daxue, Xuebao Bianjibu/Norman Bethune University of Medical Sciences, Journal Editorial Department, Xinmin Dajie 8 Hao, Changchun, Jilin 130021, China. TEL 86-431-5645911, FAX 86-431-644739. Ed. Xun Zhu. Circ: 2,500 (paid); 1,000 (controlled). **Dist. overseas by:** China International Book Trading Corp, 35 Chegongzhuang Xilu, Haidian District, Beijing 100044, China.

610 JPN ISSN 0910-5816
BAISHO IGAKU/JOURNAL OF COMPENSATION MEDICINE. Text in Japanese. 1985. s-a. JPY 1,600 per issue.
Published by: (Nihon Baisho Igakkai), Maruzen Co. Ltd./Maruzen Kabushikikaisha, 3-10 Nihonbashi 2-chome, Chuo-ku, Tokyo 103-0027, Japan. TEL 81-3-3272-7211, FAX 81-3-3278-1937.

610 ROM
CODEN: AUBKA7
BALCAN MEDICAL UNION. ARCHIVES. Text in French, English; Summaries in English, French. 1963. q. USD 60 to individuals; USD 100 to institutions (effective 2001). bk.rev. abstr, bibl, charts, illus. index. 60 p./no. *Refereed.* **Document type:** *Journal.*
Formerly (until 1997): Union Medicale Balkanique. Archives (0041-6940)
Indexed: Biol.Abstr., Ind.Med. (coverage dropped), Nutr.Abstr.
—CASDDS.
Published by: Union Medicale Balkanique, G.Clemenceau str.no.1, Bucharest 70148, Romania. Eds. Popescu Buzeu, Dr. Vasile Candea. Circ: 1,000 (controlled). **Subscr. to:** ILEXIM, Str. 13 Decembrie 3, PO Box 136-137, Bucharest 70116, Romania.

615.8 POL ISSN 0005-4402
CODEN: BAPOBT
BALNEOLOGIA POLSKA. Text in Polish; Summaries in English, Polish. 1950. q. USD 5 per issue. adv. bk.rev. illus. index. **Document type:** *Bulletin.*
Formerly: Wiadomosci Uzdrowiskowe
Indexed: Biol.Abstr., Ref.Zh.
—CASDDS.
Published by: Polskie Towarzystwo Balneoklimatologii Bioklimatologii i Medycyny Fizykalnej, Ul Mickiewicza 16, Ciechocinek 87720, Poland. TEL 48-54-833211, FAX 48-54-837220. Ed., R&P, Adv. contact Szymon Kubiak. Circ: 700 (controlled).

BANBU/BAMBOO. see *SOCIAL SERVICES AND WELFARE*

610 GBR ISSN 1353-9906
BANDOLIER; evidence-based health care. Text in English. 1994. m. GBP 36; GBP 72 foreign. bk.rev. **Document type:** *Newsletter, Academic/Scholarly.*
Indexed: Brit.Nur.Ind.
—BLDSC (1861.587800).
Published by: Oxford Anglia N H S Region, Pain Relief Unit, The Churchill, Oxford, Oxon OX3 7LJ, United Kingdom. TEL 44-1865-226132, FAX 44-1865-226978, andrew.moore@pru.ox.ac.uk, http://www.jr2.ox.ac.uk/bandolier. Ed. R A Moore.

610 CHN ISSN 1000-2200
BANGBU YIXUEYUAN XUEBAO/ACTA ACADEMIAE MEDICINAE BENGBU. Text in Chinese. bi-m. CNY 5 per issue domestic (effective 2000). back issues avail. **Document type:** *Academic/Scholarly.*
Related titles: Online - full content ed.: (from WanFang Data Corp.).
Published by: Bangbu Yixueyuan, Yehuai Lu 801 Hao, Bangbu 233003 , China. TEL 86-552-3066412. Ed. Yuxiang Gao.

610 BGD ISSN 0301-035X
BANGLADESH MEDICAL JOURNAL. Short title: B.M.J. Text in English. 1972. q. USD 20. adv. bk.rev. bibl, charts, illus.
Supersedes: East Pakistan Medical Journal (0424-1401)
Indexed: Abstr.Hyg., Diar.Dis.Res., Excerp.Med., Trop.Dis.Bull.
—CISTI, GNLM.
Published by: Bangladesh Medical Association, B.M.A. House, 15-2 Topkhana Rd, Dhaka 2, Bangladesh. Ed. Nazrul Islam. Circ: 6,000.

610 BGD ISSN 0377-9238
CODEN: BMRBDI
BANGLADESH MEDICAL RESEARCH COUNCIL BULLETIN. Text in English. 1976. 3/yr. BDT 300, USD 30 (effective 2000). adv. index. reprint service avail. from IRC. **Document type:** *Bulletin.*
Related titles: CD-ROM ed.
Indexed: Abstr.Hyg., Diar.Dis.Res., Excerp.Med. (until 1993), ExtraMED, Ind.Med. (1975-), Nutr.Abstr., Trop.Dis.Bull.
—BLDSC (1861.717000), GNLM.
Published by: Bangladesh Medical Research Council, Mokakhali, Dhaka 1212, Bangladesh. TEL 880-2-881-1395, bmrc@citechco.net, bmrc@drik.bgd.toolnet.org. Ed. Golam Rabbani. Circ: 1,000.

BARCLAYS HEALTH LAW BULLETIN (CALIFORNIA EDITION). see *LAW*

610 570 CHE
R131.A1
BASLER VEROEFFENTLICHUNGEN ZUR GESCHICHTE DER MEDIZIN UND DER BIOLOGIE. NEUE FOLGE. Text in German. 1953. irreg., latest vol.6, 1994. price varies. index. **Document type:** *Monographic series, Academic/Scholarly.*
Formerly: Basler Veroeffentlichungen zur Geschichte der Medizin und der Biologie (0067-4524)
—GNLM, Infotrieve, KNAW. **CCC.**
Published by: Schwabe und Co. AG, Steinentorstr 13, Basel 4010, Switzerland. TEL 41-61-2789565, FAX 41-61-2789566, verlag@schwabe.ch, http://www.schwabe.ch. Ed. Ulrich Troehler.

610 DEU ISSN 0005-7126
BAYERISCHES AERZTEBLATT. Text in German. 1946. m. DEM 5 per issue (effective 2001). adv. bk.rev. bibl, charts, illus, stat. **Document type:** *Magazine, Trade.*
—GNLM, Infotrieve, KNAW. **CCC.**
Published by: Bayerische Landesaerztekammer, Muehlbaurstr 16, Munich 81677, Germany. TEL 49-89-4147274, FAX 49-89-4147202, aerzteblatt@blaek.de, http://www.blaek.de. Ed., Pub. Dr. Hellmut Koch. R&P Marianne Zadach TEL 49-89-4147274. Circ: 62,000. **Co-sponsor:** Kassenaerztliche Vereinigung Bayerns.

610 USA
BAYLOR MEDICINE. Text in English. 1970. 11/yr. free per issue to qualified personnel. **Document type:** *Newspaper.* **Description:** For the college's friends and supporters, board, alumni, faculty, students, housestaff, and staff.
Published by: Baylor College of Medicine, Office of Publications, One Baylor Plaza, Houston, TX 77030. TEL 713-798-4726, FAX 713-798-3348. Ed. B J Almond. Circ: 28,000.

BAYLOR PROGRESS. see *HEALTH FACILITIES AND ADMINISTRATION*

610 USA ISSN 0899-8280
BAYLOR UNIVERSITY MEDICAL CENTER PROCEEDINGS. Abbreviated title: B U M C Proceedings. Text in English. 1988. q. USD 25 in Canada; USD 50 elsewhere (effective 2001); U.S.A. - Free to interested libraries. adv. abstr, bibl. cum.index. back issues avail. *Refereed.* **Document type:** *Academic/Scholarly.* **Description:** Contains general medical articles related to clinical reviews and conferences, case reports, surgical reports, cardiology, oncology, investigative studies, medical anthropology studies, medical history, and medical ethics.
Related titles: Online - full text ed.
Published by: Baylor University Medical Center, 3500 Gaston Ave, Dallas, TX 75246. TEL 214-820-2815, FAX 214-820-4064, cynthiao@baylordallas.edu, http://www.baylorhealth.com/proceedings. Ed. Dr. William C Roberts. R&P Cynthia Orticio. Circ: 4,000 (controlled).

BEHAVIOR GENETICS; an international journal devoted to research in the inheritance of behavior in animals and man. see *BIOLOGY—Genetics*

610 CHN ISSN 1671-167X
CODEN: BYDXEV
BEIJING DAXUE XUEBAO (YIXUE BAN)/PEKING UNIVERSITY. JOURNAL (HEALTH SCIENCES). Text in Chinese, English. 1959. bi-m. CNY 10 per issue (effective 2000). Index. *Refereed.* **Document type:** *Journal, Academic/Scholarly.* **Description:** Covers clinical medicine, oral medicine, surgery, pharmacology and pharmacy, and public health.
Formerly (until 2001): Beijing Yike Daxue Xuebao (1000-1530)
Related titles: Online - full text ed.: (from WanFang Data Corp.).
Indexed: Chem.Abstr., Chem.Indus.Notes, Chem.Titles, INIS Atomind., Ref.Zh.
—CASDDS, KNAW.
Published by: Peking Daxue Yixuebu/Peking University Health Science Center, Peking Xueyan Lu 38 Hao, Beijing 100083, China. TEL 86-10-62091551, FAX 86-10-62015681, xbbjb2@sun.bjmu.edu.cn, http://www.chinainfo.gov.cn/periodical/bjykdxxx. Ed. Qi-De Han. **Subscr. to:** China International Book Trading Corp, 35 Chegongzhuang Xilu, Haidian District, Beijing 100044, China.

610 CHN ISSN 1002-3208
BEIJING SHENGWU YIXUE GONGCHENG/BEIJING BIOMEDICAL ENGINEERING. Text in Chinese. 1981. q. CNY 40 domestic; CNY 10 per issue domestic (effective 2000). back issues avail. **Document type:** *Academic/Scholarly.*
Related titles: Online - full content ed.: (from WanFang Data Corp.).
Indexed: Eng.Ind.
Published by: Beijing-shi Xinfei Xieguan Jibing Yanjiuyuansuo, Beijing, China. Ed. Yanqing Sun.

630 CHN ISSN 0253-9713
CODEN: PCIHD7
BEIJING YIXUE/BEIJING MEDICAL JOURNAL. Text in Chinese. 1965. bi-m. CNY 5.50 per issue (effective 2000). back issues avail. **Document type:** *Academic/Scholarly.* **Description:** Contains research papers on clinical experiences, and pharmaceutical studies.
Related titles: Online - full content ed.: (from WanFang Data Corp.).
—CASDDS, GNLM.
Published by: Zhonghua Yixuehui (Beijing Fenhui)/Chinese Medical Association (Beijing Branch), Dongdan 3 Tiaojia 7 Hao, Beijing 0253-9713, China. TEL 86-1-6522-3466. Circ: 8,000. **Dist. overseas by:** China International Book Trading Corp, 35 Chegongzhuang Xilu, Haidian District, Beijing 100044, China.

BEIJING ZHONGYI/BEIJING TRADITIONAL CHINESE MEDICINE. see *ALTERNATIVE MEDICINE*

613.7 CHN ISSN 1006-2157
BEIJING ZHONGYI DAXUE XUEBAO/BEIJING UNIVERSITY OF TRADITIONAL CHINESE MEDICINE. JOURNAL. Text in Chinese. 1959. bi-m. CNY 4.50 per issue domestic (effective 2000). **Document type:** *Academic/Scholarly.*
Formerly: Beijing Zhongyi Xueyuan Xuebao (0258-8811)
Indexed: Ref.Zh.
—BLDSC (4707.894100).
Published by: Beijing Zhongyi Daxue/Beijing University of Traditional Chinese Medicine, Beisanhuan Dong Lu 11 Hao, Beijing 100029, China. TEL 86-1-6428-6469. Ed. Wang Yongyan.

M

610 USA ISSN 1064-1424
BEING WELL. Text in English. 1989. q. USD 55 to members. bk.rev. back issues avail. **Document type:** *Bulletin, Newsletter.* **Description:** Covers professional practice from internship through active retirement. Members share useful reprinted articles and information from other publications. Contains membership activities and calendar of events.
Formerly: Professional Well-Being
Published by: Society for Professional Well-Being, 21 W Colony Pl, Ste 150, Durham, NC 27705-5596. TEL 919-419-9167, CPWB@mindspring.com, http://www.cpwb.org. Ed. Dr. John Henry Pfifferling. Circ: 600.

BEITRAEGE ZUR PSYCHOLOGIE UND SOZIOLOGIE DES KRANKEN MENSCHEN. see *PSYCHOLOGY*

BENDER'S HEALTH CARE LAW MONTHLY. see *LAW*

610 IND ISSN 0005-8793
BENGAL MEDICAL JOURNAL. Text in English. 1962. m. INR 12.
Published by: Indian Medical Association, Bengal State Branch, 67 Dharmatola St., Kolkata, West Bengal 700 013, India. Ed. Dr. Amiya Kumar Bose. Circ: 5,500.

610 MYS ISSN 0126-7140
BERITA M M A/MALAYSIAN MEDICAL ASSOCIATION NEWSLETTER. Text in English. 1969. m. free per issue. **Document type:** *Newsletter.*
Published by: Malaysian Medical Association, 4th Fl MMA House, 124 Jalan, Kuala Lumpur, Pahang 53000, Malaysia. TEL 03-4420617, FAX 03-4418187.

610 DEU ISSN 0939-5784
BERLINER AERZTE. Text in German. 1964. m. DEM 84 (effective 2001). illus. **Document type:** *Journal, Academic/Scholarly.*
Formerly: Berliner Aerztekammer (0568-0743)
—CISTI, GNLM, Infotrieve. **CCC.**
Published by: (Aerztekammer Berlin), Quintessenz Verlags GmbH, Ifenpfad 2-4, Berlin 12107, Germany. TEL 49-30-76180646, FAX 49-30-76180680, central@quinline.com, central@quintessenz.de, http://www.quinline.com, http://www.quintessenz.de. Circ: 18,500.

610 DEU ISSN 0172-8490
BERLINER AERZTEBLATT. Text in German. 1887. m. DEM 120 (effective 2000). adv. bk.rev. index, cum.index. back issues avail. **Document type:** *Journal, Academic/Scholarly, Trade.*
—CISTI, Infotrieve. **CCC.**
Published by: C B Verlag Carl Boldt, Baseler Str 80, Berlin 12205, Germany. TEL 49-30-8337087, FAX 49-30-8339125. Ed. Peter Gesellius. Circ: 18,500 (controlled).

610 JPN ISSN 0915-129X
BESSATSU MEDIKARU HYUMANITI* /SUPPLEMENT MEDICAL HUMANITY. Text in Japanese. 1988. irreg. JPY 2,500 per issue.
Related titles: ♦ Supplement to: Medikaru Hyumaniti. ISSN 0911-7075.
Published by: Sokyusha, 3-4-102 Ayamedai, Inoge-ku, Chiba 2630052, Japan. Ed. Kiyoshi Nojima.

BETTER HEALTH. see *PHYSICAL FITNESS AND HYGIENE*

BIBLIOTEK FOR LAEGER. see *LIBRARY AND INFORMATION SCIENCES*

BIBLIOTHECA MEDICA CANADIANA. see *LIBRARY AND INFORMATION SCIENCES*

610 NLD ISSN 0168-9428
BIJBLIJVEN (HOUTEN). Text in Dutch. 1985. m. adv.
Published by: Bohn Stafleu van Loghum B.V. (Subsidiary of: Wolters Kluwer N.V.), Postbus 246, Houten 3990 GA, Netherlands. TEL 31-3403-95711, FAX 31-3403-50903.

579.2 CHN ISSN 1000-8721
BINGDU XUEBAO/CHINESE JOURNAL OF VIROLOGY. Text in Chinese. 1985. q. USD 24.40; CNY 7, USD 6.10 newsstand/cover (effective 2001). **Document type:** *Academic/Scholarly.*
Related titles: Online - full content ed.: (from WanFang Data Corp.).
Indexed: AgBiotech, Bio-Contr.News & Info., Ind.Vet., Pig News & Info., Plant Breed.Abstr., Poult.Abstr., Rev.Appl.Entomol., Rev.Med.& Vet.Mycol., Rev.Plant Path., Rice Abstr., Triticale Abstr., Trop.Dis.Bull., Vet.Bull.
Published by: Zhongguo Weishengwu Xuehui/Chinese Microbiology Society, Xuanwu Qu, 100, Yingxin Jia, Beijing 100052, China. http://www.im.ac.cn/imcas/immain.html. Ed. Demin Lu. **Dist. by:** China International Book Trading Corp, 35, Chegongzhuang Xilu, Haidian District, Beijing 100044, China. TEL 86-1-68413849, FAX 86-1-68412048, cibtc@mail.cibtc.com.cn, http://www.cibtc.com.cn.

610 570 IND
BIO MED. Text in English. 1993. bi-m. USD 70. adv. index. reprints avail. **Document type:** *Trade.* **Description:** Covers the new development of medical world as well as the medical equipment industry.
Related titles: Microfilm ed.
Published by: Industrial Publications (Subsidiary of: Exhibition and Communication Enterprises Pvt. Ltd.), Taj Bldg. 3rd Fl., 210 Dr .D.N. Rd., Fort, Mumbai, Maharashtra 400 001, India. TEL 91-22-207-2044, FAX 91-22-207-0170, pr@excelho.xeebom.xeemail.ems.vsnl.net.in. Ed. Dr. Padam Singhvi. R&P P R Ramesh. Adv. contact P.R. Ramesh. B&W page USD 500, color page USD 700; 190 x 245. Circ: 7,000.

BIO MEDICAL ENGINEERING. see *BIOLOGY—Bioengineering*

BIO-MEDICAL MATERIALS AND ENGINEERING; an international journal. see *BIOLOGY—Bioengineering*

BIOETHICS FORUM. see *HUMANITIES: COMPREHENSIVE WORKS*

BIOETHICS OUTLOOK. see *PHILOSOPHY*

BIOETHICS YEARBOOK. see *RELIGIONS AND THEOLOGY*

615 USA
BIOFEEDBACK CLINICIANS*. Variant title: A A B C Newsletter. Text in English. 1976. q. USD 16. adv.
Formerly: American Association of Biofeedback Clinicians. News
Indexed: Excerp.Med., Psychol.Abstr.
Published by: American Association of Biofeedback Clinicians, P O Box 416, Des Plaines, IL 60016-0416. TEL 312-827-0440. Eds. Charles Sheridan, Joseph Sargent.

BIOLOGICAL THERAPIES IN DENTISTRY. see *MEDICAL SCIENCES—Dentistry*

BIOLOGY OF REPRODUCTION. SUPPLEMENT. see *BIOLOGY—Physiology*

616.01 GBR ISSN 1354-750X
QH438.4.B55 CODEN: BIOMFA
BIOMARKERS. Text in English. 1996. bi-m. GBP 139, USD 231 to individuals; GBP 296, USD 489 to institutions (effective 2002). adv. back issues avail. *Refereed.* **Document type:** *Academic/Scholarly.* **Description:** Brings together work on all aspects of biochemical indicators of exposure, response and susceptibility.
Related titles: Online - full text ed.: ISSN 1366-5804 (from CatchWord Ltd., EBSCO Publishing, O C L C Online Computer Library Center, Inc., RoweCom Information Quest, Swets Blackwell, Institute for Scientific Information).
Indexed: BBCI, Biotech.Cit.Ind., Chem.Abstr., Chem.Indus.Notes, Chem.Titles, Curr.Cont., Inpharma, Int.Abstr.Biol.Sci., Mass Spectr.Bull., Pharm.&Out.News, Reac., Rev.Med.& Vet.Mycol., Sci.Cit.Ind.
—BLDSC (2087.704500), CASDDS, CatchWord, GNLM, IDS, Infotrieve. **CCC.**
Published by: Taylor & Francis Group, Taylor & Francis Ltd., 11 New Fetter Ln, London EC4P 4EE, United Kingdom. TEL 44-20-7583-9855, FAX 44-20-7842-2298, info@tandf.co.uk, http://www.tandf.co.uk. Ed. John A Timbrell. **Subscr. in N. America to:** Taylor & Francis Ltd., 325 Chestnut St, Suite 800, Philadelphia, PA 19016. TEL 800-354-1420, FAX 215-625-8914, info@taylorandfrancis.com, http://www.taylorandfrancis.com/.

610.28 GBR ISSN 0142-9612
R857.M3 CODEN: BIMADU
BIOMATERIALS. Text in English. 1980. s-m. EUR 2,320 in Europe to institutions; JPY 308,100 in Japan to institutions; USD 2,596 elsewhere to institutions (effective 2002). adv. bk.rev. charts, illus, abstr. index. back issues avail. *Refereed.* **Document type:** *Journal, Academic/Scholarly.*
Incorporates (1986-1995): Clinical Materials (0267-6605); Which incorporated (in 1991): Critical Reviews in Biocompatibility (0748-5204)
Related titles: Microform ed.: (from PQC); Online - full text ed.: (from ingenta, Swets Blackwell, ScienceDirect, Institute for Scientific Information).
Indexed: ASCA, Alloys Ind. (1995-), Bioeng.Abstr., Biol.Abstr., Br.Tech.Ind., Cal.Tiss.Abstr., Chem.Abstr., Chem.Cit.Ind., Chem.Indus.Notes, Chem.Titles, Comput.& Info.Sys., Curr.Adv.Ecol.Sci., Curr.Cont., Curr.Leather Lit., Curr.Tit.Dent., Dent.Ind., Eng.Ind., Eng.Mat.Abstr., Environ.Sci.Poll.Mgmt., Excerp.Med., INIS Atomind., INSPEC (Jan.1980-), Ind.Med. (1980-), Ind.Sci.Rev., Ind.Vet., Inpharma, Intl.Polym.Sci.& Tech., METADEX, Mass Spectr.Bull., Mat.Sci.Cit.Ind., Med.& Pharm.Biotech.Abstr., Met.Abstr. (1995-), Met.Abstr.Ind. (1995-), Nonfer.Met.Alert (1995-), PCC Alert (1995-), Pollut.Abstr., Poult.Abstr., RAPRA (1980-), Reac., Ref.Zh., Rev.Med.& Vet.Mycol., Risk Abstr., Saf.Sci.Abstr., Sci.Cit.Ind., Steels Alert (1995-), Sugar Ind.Abstr., Telegen, Vet.Bull., World Alum.Abstr.
—BLDSC (2087.715000), AskIEEE, CASDDS, CINDOC, CISTI, Ei, EMDOCS, GNLM, IDS, Infotrieve, ingenta, Linda Hall. **CCC.**
Published by: Pergamon (Subsidiary of: Elsevier Science), The Boulevard, Langford Ln, East Park, Kidlington, Oxford OXB 1GB, United Kingdom. FAX 44-1865-843010, nlinfo-f@elsevier/nl; usinfo-f@elsevier.com; forinfo-kyf04035@niftyserve.or.jp, http://www.elsevier.com/locate/biomaterials, http://www.elsevier.nl/. Eds. N A Peppas, R S Langer. **Subscr. in Americas to:** Elsevier Science, PO Box 945, New York, NY 10159-0945. TEL 212-633-3730, FAX 212-633-3680, usinfo-f@elsevier.com, http://www.elsevier.com; **Subscr. in Australasia and the Far East to:** Elsevier Science (Singapore) Pte Ltd, No.1 Temasek Ave, 17-01 Millenia Tower, Singapore 039192, Singapore. TEL 65-434-3727, FAX 65-337-2230; **Subscr. to:** Elsevier Science BV, PO Box 211, Amsterdam 1000 AE, Netherlands. TEL 31-20-485-3757, FAX 31-20-485-3432, nlinfo-f@elsevier.nl, http://www.elsevier.nl.

614.49 615.9 CHN ISSN 0895-3988
RA565.A1 CODEN: BESCE5
BIOMEDICAL AND ENVIRONMENTAL SCIENCES. Text in English. 1988. q. CNY 400, USD 160 (effective 2001). 100 p./no. back issues avail.; reprints avail. *Refereed.* **Document type:** *Academic/Scholarly.* **Description:** Provides a forum for the publication of preventive medicine. Covers toxicology, hygiene, environment, health, and health promotion.
Related titles: CD-ROM ed.; Online - full content ed.: (from WanFang Data Corp.); Online - full text ed.: (from Institute for Scientific Information).
Indexed: ASCA, Anim.Breed.Abstr., Apic.Abstr., Crop Physiol.Abstr., Dairy Sci.Abstr., Field Crop Abstr., INIS Atomind., Ind.Med. (1988-), Maize Abstr., NRN, Nutr.Abstr., Plant Grow.Reg.Abstr., Rev.Appl.Entomol., Rice Abstr., Soils & Fert., Weed Abstr., Zoo.Rec.
—BLDSC (2087.753700), CISTI, GNLM, IDS, ingenta, KNAW. **CCC.**
Published by: Zhongguo Yufang Yixue Kexueyuan/Chinese Academy of Preventive Medicine, 27 Nanwei Rd, Beijing 100050, China. info@ccs.capm.ac.cn. Eds. Chunming Chen, Frederick Coulston. Circ: 100 (paid); 200 (controlled). **Dist. overseas by:** Academic Press, Inc., Journal Division. TEL 619-230-1840.

610 BEL ISSN 0778-4910
BIOMEDICAL & HEALTH RESEARCH. Variant title: Newsletter Biomedical & Health Research. Text in English. 1990. 3/yr. free per issue. bk.rev. **Document type:** *Newsletter.*
Indexed: Mass Spectr.Bull.
—BLDSC (2087.753800), GNLM.
Published by: Commission Of The European Communities, Medical Research Division, Rue de la Loi - Wetstraat 200, Brussels 1049, Belgium.

610.28 NLD ISSN 0929-6743
CODEN: BIHREN
BIOMEDICAL AND HEALTH RESEARCH SERIES. Text in English. 1993. irreg., latest vol.43, 2000. price varies. back issues avail. **Document type:** *Monographic series, Academic/Scholarly.* **Description:** Publishes results of the European Union Biomedical & Health Research Programme.
—BLDSC (2087.753740), CASDDS, CISTI. **CCC.**
Published by: (Directorate - General XII, Science, Research and Development BEL, Commission of the European Communities BEL), I O S Press, Van Diemenstraat 94, Amsterdam 1013 CN, Netherlands. TEL 31-20-638-2189, FAX 31-20-620-3419, market@iospress.nl, http://www.iospress.nl. **Subscr. to:** I O S Press, Inc, 5795-G Burke Centre Pkwy, Burke, VA 22015. TEL 703-323-5554, FAX 703-323-3668, iosbooks@iospress.com. **Dist. by:** Ohmsha Ltd, 3-1 Kanda-Nishiki-cho, Chiyoda-ku, Tokyo 101-0054, Japan. TEL 81-3-3233-0641, http://www.ohmsha.co.jp.

M

610.28 NLD ISSN 0006-3398
R856 CODEN: BIOEAF
BIOMEDICAL ENGINEERING. Text in English. 1967. bi-m. EUR 1,801, USD 1,801 to institutions for print or online ed.; EUR 2,161.20, USD 2,164.80 to institutions for print & online eds combined (effective 2002). back issues avail. *Refereed.* **Document type:** *Academic/Scholarly.* **Description:** Disseminates recent advances in the growing field of biomedical technology, instrumentation, and administration, translated from the Russian journal Meditsinskaya Tekhnika. Focuses on theoretical and practical problems associated with the development of medical technology; the introduction of new engineering methods into public health, hospitals and patient care, and the storage and retrieval of biomedical information.
Related titles: Microfilm ed.: (from PQC); Online - full text ed.: (from Swets Blackwell, Kluwer Online, RoweCom Information Quest); ♦ Translation of: Meditsinskaya Tekhnika. ISSN 0025-8075.
Indexed: ASCA, Appl.Mech.Rev., Biol.Abstr., Eng.Ind., Excerp.Med., INIS Atomind., INSPEC (Jan.1972-Dec.1989, dropped), Ind.Med. (coverage dropped), METADEX.
—BLDSC (0406.050000), CISTI, GNLM, ingenta. **CCC.**
Published by: (Russia. Ministerstvo Zdravookhraneniya RUS), Kluwer Academic Publishers Group (Subsidiary of: Wolters Kluwer N.V.), Spuiboulevard 50, PO Box 17, Dordrecht 3300 AA, Netherlands. TEL 31-78-639-2392, FAX 31-78-654-2254, services@wkap.nl, http://www.wkap.nl/journalhome.htm/0006-3398. Ed. V A Viktorov. **Subscr. addr.:** Journals Department, PO Box 322, Dordrecht 3300 AH, Netherlands. TEL 31-78-639-2392, FAX 31-78-654-6474; **Subscr. addr. in N. America:** Kluwer Academic - Plenum Publishers, 233 Spring St, New York, NY 10013-1578. TEL 212-620-8468, 800-221-9369, FAX 212-807-1047.

174.2 USA ISSN 0742-1796
R724
BIOMEDICAL ETHICS REVIEWS. Text in English. 1983. irreg. adv. **Document type:** *Journal, Academic/Scholarly.* **Description:** Dedicated to provide an ethical board of controversial topics in bioethics, such as physician-assisted death, and the allocation of health care resources.
Indexed: P C I.
—BLDSC (2087.816000), GNLM, KNAW. **CCC.**
Published by: Humana Press Inc., 999 Riverview Dr, Ste 208, Totowa, NJ 07512. TEL 973-256-1699, FAX 973-256-8341, humana@humanapr.com, http://humanapress.com. Eds. James M Humber, Robert F Almeder. R&P Richard Hruska. Adv. contact Thomas B Lanigan Jr.

610 JPN ISSN 0915-9274
BIOMEDICAL FUZZY SYSTEMS BULLETIN. Text in English, Japanese. 1990. a.
Published by: Biomedical Fuzzy Systems Association/Baiomedikaru Faji Shisutemu Kenkyukai, 1 Yokota, Iizuka-shi, Fukuoka-ken 820-0044, Japan.

610.28 USA
BIOMEDICAL INFORMATICS. JOURNAL. Text in English. bi-m. USD 455 in US & Canada to institutions; USD 465 elsewhere to institutions (effective 2001).
Published by: Academic Press, Inc., Journal Division (Subsidiary of: Harcourt Brace & Company), 528 B St, Ste 1900, San Diego, CA 92101-4495. TEL 619-230-1840, FAX 619-699-6800, apsubs@acad.com, http://www.academicpress.com.

BIOMEDICAL LETTERS; a prestige international biomedical journal for the rapid publication of biomedical communications. see *BIOLOGY*

BIOMEDICAL MARKET NEWSLETTER. see *BUSINESS AND ECONOMICS—Marketing And Purchasing*

M

610.28 GBR ISSN 0955-7717
CODEN: BMATEM
BIOMEDICAL MATERIALS; an international newsletter. Text in English. 1975. m. GBP 345, USD 567 (effective 2001 - 2002). bk.rev. charts, stat. back issues avail. **Document type:** *Newsletter, Trade.* **Description:** Provides coverage of design, production and research in the biomedical material industry, and in related research departments and institutes. Also provides a survey for senior general management, serving to highlight new trends and possibilities, market gaps and business opportunities.
Formerly (until 1988): Biomedical Polymers (0267-5439)
Related titles: E-mail ed.; Online - full text ed.: (from ingenta, Gale Group, Factiva).
Indexed: Alloys Ind. (1986-), Eng.Mat.Abstr., Intl.Polym.Sci.& Tech., METADEX, Met.Abstr. (1986-), Met.Abstr.Ind. (1986-), Nonfer.Met.Alert (1986-), PCC Alert (1986-), RAPRA (1989-1997), Steels Alert (1986-), Text.Tech.Dig. (May 2000-), World Alum.Abstr., World Text.Abstr.
—BLDSC (2087.838000), CISTI, GNLM, Infotrieve. **CCC.**
Published by: International Newsletters, PO Box 133, Witney, Oxon OX8 6ZH, United Kingdom. TEL 44-199-3824130, FAX 44-199-3824150, in@intnews.com, http://www.intnews.com. Ed. P Read.

BIOMEDICAL MEETINGS INDEX. see *MEETINGS AND CONGRESSES*

610.28 USA ISSN 1387-2176
R856.A1 CODEN: BMICFC
BIOMEDICAL MICRODEVICES; an international journal. Text in English. q. USD 338, EUR 322 to institutions for print or online ed.; USD 405.60, EUR 386.40 to institutions for print & online eds.combined (effective 2002). back issues avail. **Document type:** *Academic/Scholarly.* **Description:** Covers all aspects of research in the diagnostic and therapeutic application of Micro-Electro-Mechanical Systems (MEMS), microfabrication, and nanotechnology.
Related titles: Online - full text ed.: (from EBSCO Publishing, O C L C Online Computer Library Center, Inc., RoweCom Information Quest, Swets Blackwell, Kluwer Online).
Indexed: Biotech.& Bioeng.Abstr., INSPEC (Sep.1998-), Med.& Pharm.Biotech.Abstr., Neurosci.Abstr.
—BLDSC (2087.852000), Infotrieve. **CCC.**
Published by: Kluwer Academic Publishers Boston, 101 Philip Dr, Assinippi Park, Norwell, MA 02061. TEL 781-871-6600, FAX 781-871-9045, services@wkap.nl, http://www.wkap.nl/journalhome.htm/1387-2176. Ed. Mauro Ferrari. R&P Rose Luongo TEL 781-871-6311. **Subscr. in N America:** Kluwer Academic - Plenum Publishers, 233 Spring St, New York, NY 10013-1578. TEL 212-620-8468, FAX 212-807-1047; **Subscr. outside N. America by:** Kluwer Academic Publishers Group, Journals Department, PO Box 322, Dordrecht 3300 AH, Netherlands. TEL 31-78-639-2392, FAX 31-78-654-6474.

610 570 JPN ISSN 0918-6514
BIOMEDICAL PERSPECTIVES. Text in Japanese. 1992. 3/yr. JPY 2,400 per issue (effective 1998).
Published by: Medikaru Rebyusha/Medical Review Co., Ltd., 7-3 Hirano-Machi 1-chome, Chuo-ku, Osaka-shi 541-0046, Japan. TEL 81-6-223-1468, FAX 81-6-223-1245, medrev@osk2.3web.ne.jp.

681.761 610.28 USA ISSN 0192-1266
BIOMEDICAL PRODUCTS. Text in English. 1976. m. USD 12 to non-members (effective 2001). adv. tr.lit. back issues avail. **Document type:** *Trade.* **Description:** Reaches directors, principal investigators, biochemists, chemists, medical researchers, microbiologists, professors and medical school teachers in the life science-biotech research laboratories of universities, medical institutions, pharmaceutical companies, industry, and biotechnology and research centers.
Related titles: Online - full text ed.
Indexed: Curr.Pack.Abstr.
—BLDSC (2087.857000). **CCC.**
Published by: Cahners Business Information, New Product Information Unit (Subsidiary of: Reed Elsevier plc), 301 Gibraltar Dr, P O Box 650, Morris Plains, NJ 07950-0650. TEL 973-292-5100 ext.725, FAX 973-539-3476, mdavis@cahners.com, http://www.bioprodmag.com. Ed. Steve Ernst TEL 973-292-5100 x262. Pub. Darrell White. adv.: color page USD 9,395; trim 11 x 8.19. Circ: 79,000 (controlled).

610 JPN ISSN 0388-6107
CODEN: BRESD5
BIOMEDICAL RESEARCH. Text in English. 1980. bi-m. JPY 23,000; USD 190 foreign. adv. back issues avail. *Refereed.* **Document type:** *Academic/Scholarly.*
Related titles: Fax ed.; Online - full text ed.: (from Institute for Scientific Information).
Indexed: BBCI, Curr.Cont., INIS Atomind., Inpharma, Int.Abstr.Biol.Sci., Pharm.&Out.News, Reac., Sci.Cit.Ind.
—BLDSC (2087.865000), CASDDS, CISTI, GNLM, IDS, ingenta, KNAW.
Published by: (Yanahaira Institute Inc.), Biomedical Research Press Inc., 5 F Kyowa Bldg 2-1-3, Kyobashi, Chuo-ku, Tokyo 104-0031, Japan. FAX 81-3-3275-8018, t-kanno@yanaihara.co.jp. Ed. Tomio Kanno. Pub., R&P Noboru Yanaihara TEL 81-544-22-2771. Circ: 700.

610 AUS ISSN 1442-830X
▼ **BIOMEDICAL RESEARCH**; an interdisciplinary journal for the biomedical sciences. Text in English. 1999. q. *Refereed.* **Document type:** *Journal, Academic/Scholarly.* **Description:** Publishes original research papers and reviews from the leaders in biomedical research.
Media: Online - full text.
Published by: Charles Sturt University, School of Biomedical Sciences, Locked Bag 588, Wagga Wagga, NSW 2678, Australia. hurwin@csu.edu.au, http://www.csu.edu.au/faculty/health/biomed/MHR/journal.htm, http://www.csu.edu.au/faculty/health/bionmed/MHR/journal.htm. Ed. Heather Urwin.

610.2 USA ISSN 1080-9775
BIOMEDICAL SAFETY & STANDARDS NEWSLETTER. Text in English. 1971. 22/yr. USD 435; USD 24 newsstand/cover (effective 2002). bk.rev. index. back issues avail. **Document type:** *Newsletter.* **Description:** Covers medical device safety and standards, hazards, recalls, legal actions, legislation and regulations, BMET and CE activities and meetings.
Formerly: Newsletter of Biomedical Safety and Standards (0048-0282)
Related titles: Online - full text ed.: (from ProQuest Information & Learning).
Indexed: P.N.I.
—GNLM.
Published by: Aspen Publishers, Inc., 200 Orchard Ridge Dr, Ste 200, Gaithersburg, MD 20878. TEL 301-417-7500, 800-638-8437, FAX 301-417-7650, customer.service@aspenpubl.com, http://www.aspenpublishers.com, http://www.aspenpub.com. Pub. Michael Randers Pehrson. R&P Alice McElhinney. **Dist. by:** Aspen Publishers Inc., Distribution Center, 7201 McKinney Circle, Frederick, MD 21701. TEL 301-698-7100, FAX 301-417-7550.

610.28 USA ISSN 0067-8856
R856 CODEN: BMSIA7
BIOMEDICAL SCIENCES INSTRUMENTATION. Text in English. 1963. a. USD 40 to non-members; USD 32 to members. reprint service avail. from PQC,ISI. *Refereed.* **Document type:** *Proceedings.*
Related titles: Microform ed.: (from PQC).
Indexed: Appl.Mech.Rev., Biol.Abstr., Chem.Abstr., Dent.Ind., Eng.Ind., Excerp.Med., Ind.Med. (1968-).
—BLDSC (2087.880000), CASDDS, CISTI, Ei, GNLM, Infotrieve, ingenta, KNAW. **CCC.**
Published by: Instrument Society of America, 67, Alexander, NC 27709. TEL 919-549-8411, FAX 919-549-8288, info@isa.org, http://www.isa.org.

610 USA ISSN 0147-2682
CODEN: BTISE6
BIOMEDICAL TECHNOLOGY INFORMATION SERVICE. Text in English. 1974. s-m. (m. in Jan. & Aug.). USD 335 to individuals; USD 385 foreign to individuals; USD 389 to institutions; USD 399 foreign to institutions (effective 1999). bk.rev. index. back issues avail. **Document type:** *Newsletter.* **Description:** Covers advances in medical device technology and biomedical engineering, including latest biomedical inventions and federal regulations.
Formed by the merger of: Advanced Biomedical Technology (0094-0100); Biomedical Inventions Reporter (0094-0119); Government Documents Review (0094-0127); Health Care Statistics Report (0094-0135)
Related titles: Online - full text ed.: (from ProQuest Information & Learning).
Indexed: P.N.I.
—GNLM.
Published by: Aspen Publishers, Inc., 200 Orchard Ridge Dr, Ste 200, Gaithersburg, MD 20878. TEL 301-417-7500, 800-638-8437, FAX 301-417-7650. Ed. Timothy Bakerger. R&P Alice McElhinney.

610.28025 USA
BIOMEDICAL TECHNOLOGY RESEARCH RESOURCES; a research resources directory. Text in English. 1977. biennial. free per issue. **Document type:** *Directory, Government.* **Description:** Directory of biomedical research technology centers.
Former titles: Biomedical Research Technology Resources (0891-740X); (until 1984): Biomedical Research Technology Program; Biotechnology Resources
Related titles: Online - full text ed.
Published by: U.S. National Institutes of Health, National Center for Research Resources, 6705 Rockledge Dr, Rm 5046, Bethesda, MD 20892. TEL 301-435-0888, ospio@ncrr.nih.gov, http://www.ncrr.nih.gov/ncrrprog/btdir/cont1.htm. Circ: 9,000.

615.532 USA
BIOMEDICAL THERAPY; international journal of integrated medicine. Text in English. 1983. q. USD 18 domestic; USD 35 foreign; USD 5 newsstand/cover (effective 1999). adv. charts, illus. **Description:** Aimed at practitioners of complimentary medicine. Contains English translations of innovative European clinical studies, primarily in homeopathic medicine.
Formerly (until 1997): Biological Therapy (0733-2661)
Related titles: CD-ROM ed.
Published by: Menaco Publishing Co., Inc., PO Box 11280, Albuquerque, NM 87192. TEL 505-292-2225, FAX 505-298-3210, http://www.menaco.com. Ed. Rene Augstburger. Adv. contact Kristen Maass. B&W page USD 1,200, color page USD 1,700; trim 10 x 7.25.

BIOMEDICAS. see *BIOLOGY*

610.285 IND ISSN 0970-2067
BIOMEDICINE. Text in English. 1980. s-a. INR 500 domestic to individuals; USD 30 in developing nations to individuals; USD 50 elsewhere to individuals; INR 2,000 domestic to institutions; USD 80 in developing nations to institutions; USD 100 elsewhere to institutions (effective 2000). **Description:** Publishes original and review articles in the fields of Biomedical Sciences.
—BLDSC (2087.883050).
Published by: Indian Association of Biomedical Scientists, Dept of Physiology, Sri Ramachandra Medical College and Research Institute, Porur, Chennai 600-116, India.

610.285 615 FRA ISSN 0753-3322 CODEN: BIPHEX
BIOMEDICINE AND PHARMACOTHERAPY. Text and summaries in English, French. 1956. 10/yr. EUR 441 in Europe to institutions; USD 526 elsewhere to institutions (effective 2002). adv. bk.rev. bibl, illus. index. back issues avail.; reprint service avail. from ISI. *Refereed.* **Document type:** *Academic/Scholarly.* **Description:** Discusses medical ailments with an emphasis on how they relate to pharmacological drugs and subsequent treatments.
Formed by the merger of (1973-1982): Biomedicine (0300-0893); (1973-1982): Revue Europeenne d'Etudes Cliniques et Biologiques (0035-3019)
Related titles: Microform ed.: (from PQC); Online - full text ed.: (from ingenta, Swets Blackwell, ScienceDirect, Institute for Scientific Information).
Indexed: ASCA, Biol.Abstr., Chem.Abstr., Chem.Indus.Notes, Chem.Titles, Chic.Per.Ind., Curr.Cont., Curr.Ind.Stat., Dairy Sci.Abstr., Derwent Biotech.Abstr., Excerp.Med., Helminthol.Abstr., INIS Atomind., Ind.Med. (1982-), Ind.Sci.Rev., Ind.Vet., Inpharma, Int.Abstr.Biol.Sci., Nutr.Abstr., Pharm.&Out.News, Reac., Rev.Appl.Entomol., Sci.Cit.Ind., Vet.Bull.
—BLDSC (2087.883300), ADONIS, CASDDS, CISTI, EMDOCS, GNLM, IDS, ingenta, KNAW. **CCC.**
Published by: (Hopital Suisses de Paris), Elsevier Paris, Editions Scientifiques et Medicales (Subsidiary of: Reed Elsevier plc. group), 23 rue Linois, Paris 75015, France. TEL 33-1-45589110, FAX 33-1-45589419, biomed@elsevier.fr; academic@elsevier-fr.com, http://www.elsevier.com/locate/biopha. Ed. G Mathe. Circ: 2,000.

610 RUS
BIOMEDITSINSKAYA RADIOELEKTRONIKA. Text in Russian. 1998. 8/yr. USD 195 in the Americas (effective 2000).
Indexed: Ref.Zh.
Published by: Izdatel'skoe Predpriyatie Redakstsii Zhurnala Radiotekhnika, Kuznetskii Most 20-6, Moscow 103031, Russian Federation. TEL 7-095-9214837, FAX 7-095-9259241. **Dist. by:** East View Publications, 3020 Harbor Ln N, Minneapolis, MN 55447. TEL 763-550-0961, FAX 763-559-2931.

610.28 DEU ISSN 0013-5585
R856.A1 CODEN: BMZTA7
BIOMEDIZINISCHE TECHNIK/BIOMEDICAL ENGINEERING. Text in German. 1955. m. (10/yr.). DEM 620 (effective 2000). adv. bk.rev. abstr, bibl, charts. *Refereed.* **Document type:** *Academic/Scholarly.*
Formerly: Elektromedizin
Related titles: Online - full text ed.: (from Institute for Scientific Information).
Indexed: ASCA, Aqua.Sci.& Fish.Abstr., Bioeng.Abstr., Biol.Abstr., C.I.S. Abstr., Cal.Tiss.Abstr., Chem.Abstr., Chem.Indus.Notes, Chem.Titles, Curr.Adv.Ecol.Sci., Curr.Cont., Eng.Ind., Environ.Sci.Poll.Mgmt., Excerp.Med., Helminthol.Abstr., INIS Atomind., INSPEC (Sep.1970, Feb.1971-), Ind.Med. (1971-), Ind.Sci.Rev., Inpharma, Int.Nurs.Ind., Pollut.Abstr., Reac., Risk Abstr., SSCI (coverage dropped), Saf.Sci.Abstr., Sci.Cit.Ind., Vet.Bull.
—BLDSC (2087.890000), AskIEEE, CASDDS, CISTI, Ei, EMDOCS, GNLM, IDS, Infotrieve. **CCC.**
Published by: (Deutsche Gesellschaft fuer Biomedizinische Technik/German Association on Bio-Medical Engineering), Fachverlag Schiele und Schoen GmbH, Markgrafenstr 11, Berlin 10969, Germany. TEL 49-30-253752-0, FAX 49-30-2517248, 0302537520-0001@t-online.de. Eds. M Schaldach, U Boenick. Circ: 1,500.

BIOMETEOROLOGY BULLETIN. see *METEOROLOGY*

BIONYT/BIO-NEWS; populaer forskning. see *BIOLOGY*

BIOORGANIC & MEDICINAL CHEMISTRY. see *CHEMISTRY—Organic Chemistry*

BIOORGANIC & MEDICINAL CHEMISTRY LETTERS; for rapid dissemination of preliminary communications on all aspects of bioorganic chemistry, medicinal chemistry and related disciplines. see *CHEMISTRY—Organic Chemistry*

616.04 330 GBR
BIOPHOENIX DATABASE ON CD-ROM. Text in English. 1997. q. GBP 2,000 (effective 1998). adv. **Description:** Contains profiles of biomedical companies with contact and personnel data, financial data, R&D activities, history, management strategy, and legal proceedings. For pharmaceutical and biotechnology companies, investors, medical device companies, suppliers to biomedical companies, and analysts.
Media: CD-ROM.
Published by: (University of Coventry Biophoenix Group), Financial Times Healthcare, Maple House, 149 Tottenham Ct Rd, London W1P 9LL, United Kingdom. TEL 44-207-896-2066, FAX 44-20-7896-2213, lizg@pearson-pro.com, http://www.fthealthcare.com. Adv. contact Liz Godden.

610.28 USA ISSN 1081-8693
R857.O6 CODEN: BIINFH
BIOPHOTONICS INTERNATIONAL; photonic solutions for biotechnology and medicine. Text in English. 1995. bi-m. USD 58; USD 72 foreign. adv. **Document type:** *Trade.*
Indexed: Bioeng.Abstr., Biotech.& Bioeng.Abstr., Eng.Ind.
—BLDSC (2089.365000).
Published by: Laurin Publishing Co., Inc., Berkshire Common, 2 South Street, Box 4949, Pittsfield, MA 01202-4949. TEL 413-499-0514, FAX 413-442-3180, photonics@laurin.com, http://www.photonicsnet.com. Ed. Roger B Linscott. Pub., R&P Wendy A Laurin. Adv. contact Rebecca Pontier.

616 USA ISSN 0895-2140 CODEN: BINSEM
BIOPSY INTERPRETATION SERIES. Text in English. irreg. price varies. reprint service avail. from PQC. *Refereed.* **Document type:** *Monographic series.*
Indexed: Curr.Cont. (coverage dropped).
Published by: Lippincott Williams & Wilkins (Philadelphia) (Subsidiary of: Wolters Kluwer N.V.), 530 Walnut St, Philadelphia, PA 19106-3621. TEL 301-223-2300, 800-638-3030, FAX 301-223-2400.

BIORESEARCH MONITORING ALERT. see *INSTRUMENTS*

610 GBR ISSN 1465-4644
BIOSTATISTICS. Text in English. 1998. q. GBP 80, USD 110 to individuals; GBP 160, USD 240 to institutions (effective Mar. 2002). adv. 132 p./no. back issues avail. *Refereed.* **Document type:** *Journal, Academic/Scholarly.* **Description:** Aims to publish papers that develop and apply innovative statistical methods to problems of human health and disease including basic biomedical sciences.
Related titles: Online - full text ed.: ISSN 1468-4357. 2000. GBP 144, USD 216 to institutions Online only (effective Mar. 2002) (from RoweCom Information Quest).
—BLDSC (2089.628000).
Published by: Oxford University Press, Academic Division, Great Clarendon St, Oxford OX2 6DP, United Kingdom. TEL 44-1865-267907, FAX 44-1865-267835, jnl.info@oup.co.uk, http://www.biostatistics.oupjournals.org, http://www.oup.co.uk/journals. Eds. Peter J Diggle, Scott L Zegger. Pub. J Boullin. R&P Fionna Willis. adv.: page GBP 230, page USD 415. Circ: 550. **Subscr. in the Americas to:** Oxford University Press, Journals, 2001 Evans Rd, Cary, NC 27513. TEL 800-852-7323, FAX 919-677-1714, jnlorders@oup-usa.org; **Subscr. to:** Journals Marketing, Great Clarendon St, Oxford OX2 6DP, United Kingdom.

BIOTECHNOLOGY ADVANCES; research reviews and patent abstracts. see *BIOLOGY—Biotechnology*

BIOTECHNOLOGY AND GENETIC ENGINEERING REVIEWS. see *BIOLOGY—Biotechnology*

BIOTHERAPY. see *BIOLOGY—Biotechnology*

BLEIKT OG BLATT. see *SOCIOLOGY*

610 DEU ISSN 0944-467X
BLUE PRINT; journal of culture and science. Text in German, English, French. 1997. irreg. **Document type:** *Consumer.* **Description:** Deals with Chinese medicine.
Media: Online - full text.
Address: Postfach 165, Petershausen 85236, Germany. 081397957-1@online.de, http://www.blueprint-magazine.de, http://members.aol.com/bluemagzin/newblue.html. Ed. Dr. Wolfgang Wiesner.

610 GBR
BMJ.COM. Variant title: British Medical Journal.com. Text in English. 1995 (May). w. back issues avail. **Document type:** *Journal, Academic/Scholarly.*
Formerly: eB M J (1468-5833)
Media: Online - full text (from Gale Group, HighWire Pr., Institute for Scientific Information). **Related titles:** Microform ed.: (from PQC,PMC); ♦ Print ed.: B M J. ISSN 0959-535X.
Published by: B M J Publishing Group, B M A House, Tavistock Sq, London WC1H 9JR, United Kingdom. TEL 44-20-7387-4499, FAX 44-20-7383-6400, bmj@bmj.com, info.norththames@bma.org.uk, http://www.bmj.com/, http://www.bma.org.uk.

610 JPN ISSN 0385-1796 CODEN: BIDZDQ
BOEI IKA DAIGAKKO ZASSHI/NATIONAL DEFENSE MEDICAL COLLEGE. JOURNAL. Text in English, Japanese. 1976. q. **Document type:** *Journal, Academic/Scholarly.*
Indexed: Biol.Abstr., Chem.Abstr., Chem.Indus.Notes, Chem.Titles, Excerp.Med., INIS Atomind.
—BLDSC (4830.160000), CASDDS, GNLM.
Published by: Boeicho, Boei Ika Daigakko/Defense Agency, National Defense Medical College, 3-2 Namiki, Tokorozawa-shi, Saitama-ken 359-8513, Japan. Ed. Yoshio Ogawa.

BOLETIN DE BIOTECNOLOGIA. see *BIOLOGY—Biotechnology*

610 MEX
BOLETIN DE INFORMACION PERIODISTICA EN SALUD. Text in Spanish. m. back issues avail.
Related titles: Online - full text ed.
Published by: Universidad Autonoma Metropolitana - Xochimilco, CALZ DEL HUESO 1100, Col Villa Quietud, Mexico City, DF 04960, Mexico. TEL 52-5-7245050, http://www.uam.mx/.

610 CUB
BOLETIN DE MEDICIANA TRADICIONAL GRUPO "JUAN TOMAS ROIG". Text in Spanish. a.
Published by: Academia de Ciencias, Instituto de Documentacion e Informacion Cientifico-Tecnica (I D I C T), Capitolio Nacional, Prado y San Jose, Habana 2, Cuba.

610 MEX
BOLETIN MEDICO FAMILIAR. Text in Spanish. bi-m. **Document type:** *Academic/Scholarly.*
Related titles: Online - full text ed.
Published by: Universidad Nacional Autonoma de Mexico, Facultad de Medicina, Departamento de Medicina Familiar, 3er. Piso, Bloque B, Ciudad Universitaria, Box 70-298, Mexico City, DF 04510, Mexico. TEL 52-5-6232432, liliaar@fournier.facmed.unam.mx, http://www.facmed.unam.mx/bmnd/index.html/. Ed. Juan Jose Mazon. Circ: 10,500.

610 ITA ISSN 0007-5787
BOLLETTINO DELLE SCIENZE MEDICHE. Text in Italian. 1823. 4/yr. ITL 20,000. adv. bk.rev.
Indexed: Biol.Abstr., Chem.Abstr.
—CISTI, GNLM, KNAW.
Published by: Societa Medica Chirurgica di Bologna-Archiginnasio, Piazza Galvani, 1, Bologna, BO 40124, Italy. Ed. Michele Fiorentino.

610 RUS
BOL'NITSA; dlya vrachei i patsientov. Text in Russian. 1996. bi-m. USD 95 in the Americas (effective 2000).

M

Published by: Redaktsiya Bol'nitsa, Ul. Nizhne-Pervomaiskaya, 47, ofis 204, Moscow 105203, Russian Federation. TEL 7-095-4654854, FAX 7-095-4654854. **Dist. by:** East View Publications, 3020 Harbor Ln N, Minneapolis, MN 55447. TEL 763-550-0961, FAX 763-559-2931.

610 IND ISSN 0524-0182
BOMBAY HOSPITAL JOURNAL. Text in English. 1959. q. INR 100. adv. bk.rev. charts, illus. index.
Indexed: Biol.Abstr., INIS Atomind., Indian Sci.Abstr.
—GNLM.
Published by: Bombay Hospital Institute of Medical Sciences, 16th Fl., 12 Marine Lines, Mumbai, Maharashtra 400 020, India. Ed. Dr. O P Kapoor. Circ: 5,000.

610 USA ISSN 0894-4024
RA1190
BOSTON BULLETIN ON CHEMICALS AND DISEASE; objective reports on the health effects of chemicals. Text in English. 1985. q. USD 20 to individuals; USD 30 to libraries; USD 50 to corporations; USD 15 to students. bk.rev. back issues avail. **Description:** Contains summaries, mini-reviews, and brief news items about how chemicals affect our health.
Published by: ChemoPathology ResourCenter, Inc., 30 Worthington St, Boston, MA 02120-1605. TEL 617-731-1350, FAX 617-732-4434. Ed. S Szabo. Circ: 2,000.

610 340 USA
BRANDEIS UNIVERSITY. INSTITUTE FOR HEALTH POLICY. RESEARCH NEWS. Text in English. 1986. s-a. back issues avail. **Document type:** *Newsletter.* **Description:** Includes public policy articles on long-term care, substance abuse, medicare, county health policy, state policy, and home health care.
Published by: Brandeis University, Institute for Health Policy, 415 South St, Waltham, MA 02254. TEL 617-736-3910, FAX 617-736-3905. Ed. Stanley S Wallack. Circ: 1,000.

610 DEU ISSN 0939-3471
BRANDENBURGISCHES AERZTEBLATT. Text in German. 1990. m. DEM 78; DEM 58 to students (effective 2001). adv. Index. **Document type:** *Magazine, Corporate.*
—GNLM.
Published by: Landesaerztekammer Brandenburg, Dreifertstr 12, Cottbus 03044, Germany. TEL 49-355-7801016, FAX 49-355-7801045, http://www.laekb.de. Ed. Erika Kehl. Circ: 9,000 (paid and controlled). **Dist. by:** A V Z GmbH, Am Treptower Park 28-30, Berlin 12435, Germany. TEL 49-30-53210894, FAX 49-30-53210895.

610 BRA ISSN 0006-9205
BRASIL-MEDICO✱ ; revista de medicina e cirurgia. Text in English, French, Portuguese, Spanish. 1887. bi-m. adv. bk.rev. abstr, bibl, illus. index.
Indexed: Biol.Abstr., Chem.Abstr.
—CISTI, GNLM.
Published by: Policlinica Geral do Rio de Janeiro, Av. Nilo Pecanha 38, Rio De Janeiro, RJ, Brazil.

610 BRA ISSN 0524-2053
BRASILIA MEDICA. Text in Portuguese. 1968. s-a. BRL 1,000, USD 30. adv. bk.rev. **Document type:** *Academic/Scholarly.*
Related titles: CD-ROM ed.
Indexed: INIS Atomind., Ind.Med. (coverage dropped).
Published by: Associacao Medica de Brasilia, EQS 713-913, Modulo E, Brasilia, DF 70930, Brazil. TEL 061-245-1408, FAX 061-245-2501. Ed. Dr. Luiz Fernando G Salinas. Circ: 5,000.

610 SVK ISSN 0006-9248
CODEN: BLLIAX
BRATISLAVSKE LEKARSKE LISTY/BRATISLAVA MEDICAL JOURNAL. Text in Slovak; Summaries in English, Slovak. 1921. m. USD 126 (effective 2001 - 2002). bk.rev. charts, illus. s-a. index, cum.index: 1921-1950, 1951-1955. *Refereed.* **Document type:** *Academic/Scholarly.* **Description:** Presents original works written by domestic and foreign authors covering experimental and clinical medicine, public health, therapy and practical spheres as well as reviews and studies of history.
Related titles: Online - full text ed.
Indexed: Biol.Abstr., C.I.S. Abstr., Chem.Abstr., Chem.Indus.Notes, Chem.Titles, Dent.Ind., Dok.Arbeitsmed., Excerp.Med., INIS Atomind., Ind.Med. (1921-), Protozool.Abstr.
—BLDSC (2275.500000), CASDDS, CISTI, GNLM, KNAW.
Published by: Univerzita Komenskeho, Lekarska Fakulta/Comenius University, School of Medicine, Spitalska 24, Bratislava 81372, Slovakia. TEL 421-7-367829, FAX 421-7-365400, bll@fmed.uniba.sk, hulin@fmed.uniba.sk; bernadic@fmed.uniba.sk; bll@fmed.uniba.sk, http://www.elis.sk. Ed. Ivan Hulin. R&P M Berwadic. **Dist. by:** Slovart GTG Ltd., Krupinska 4, PO Box 152, Bratislava 85299, Slovakia.

610 570 BRA ISSN 0100-879X
CODEN: BJMRDK
BRAZILIAN JOURNAL OF MEDICAL AND BIOLOGICAL RESEARCH. Text in English. 1968. m. USD 60 domestic; USD 120 foreign (effective 2001). adv. illus, charts. index. 150 p./no. back issues avail.; reprint service avail. from PQC,ISI. *Refereed.* **Document type:** *Journal, Academic/Scholarly.*
Formerly (until 1981): Revista Brasileira de Pesquisas Medicas e Biologicas (0034-7310)
Related titles: Microform ed.: (from PQC); Online - full text ed.: (from SciELO, Institute for Scientific Information).
Indexed: ASCA, Abstr.Hyg., AgBiotech, Anim.Breed.Abstr., Aqua.Sci.& Fish.Abstr., Bio-Contr.News & Info., Biol.Abstr., Chem.Abstr., Chem.Indus.Notes, Chem.Titles, Crop Physiol.Abstr., Curr.Adv.Biochem., Curr.Adv.Cancer Res., Curr.Adv.Cell & Devel.Biol., Curr.Adv.Ecol.Sci., Curr.Adv.Gen.& Molec.Biol., Curr.Cont., Dairy Sci.Abstr., Dent.Ind., Entomol.Abstr. (coverage dropped), Environ.Sci.Poll.Mgmt., Excerp.Med., Field Crop Abstr., Helminthol.Abstr., Hort.Abstr., INIS Atomind., Ind.Med. (1981-), Ind.Sci.Rev., Ind.Vet., Inpharma, Kidney, Maize Abstr., Neurosci.Cit.Ind., Nutr.Abstr., Pharm.&Out.News, Pollut.Abstr., Postharvest, Protozool.Abstr., Reac., Rev.Appl.Entomol., Rev.Arom.& Med.Plants, Rev.Med.& Vet.Mycol., Risk Abstr., SSCI (coverage dropped), Saf.Sci.Abstr., Sci.Cit.Ind., Seed Abstr., Sugar Ind.Abstr., Trop.Dis.Bull., Vet.Bull., Weed Abstr., Zoo.Rec.
—BLDSC (2277.419500), CASDDS, CISTI, EMDOCS, GNLM, IDS, Infotrieve, KNAW. **CCC.**
Published by: Associacao Brasileira de Divulgacao Cientifica, Av. Bandeirantes 3900, Faculdade de Medicina de Ribeirao Preto, Campus de Ribeirao Preto, Ribeirao Preto, SP 14040904, Brazil. TELEX 0166-354, bjournal@fmrp.usp.br, http://www.scielo.br/bjmbr. Ed., R&P, Adv. contact Lewis Joel Greene. B&W page USD 333; 8.5 x 11. Circ: 2,000.

BREAST IMPLANT LITIGATION REPORTER; the twice monthly national journal of record on breast implant litigation. see *LAW*

610 USA
BRIEFINGS ON J C A H O LONG - TERM AND SUBACUTE CARE. (Joint Commission on Accreditation of Healthcare Organizations) Text in English. 1994. m. USD 177. **Document type:** *Newsletter.* **Description:** Provides news, analysis and advice to develop and operate a subacute care unit.
Formerly: Briefings on Subacute Care (1076-5999)
—CCC.
Published by: Opus Communications, PO Box 1168, Marblehead, MA 01945. TEL 781-639-1872, FAX 781-639-2982, customer_service@opuscomm.com, http://www.opuscomm.com.

BRIEFINGS ON LONG-TERM CARE REGULATIONS. see *HEALTH FACILITIES AND ADMINISTRATION*

BRITISH ACUPUNCTURE ASSOCIATION. NEWSLETTER. see *ALTERNATIVE MEDICINE*

610 CAN ISSN 0007-0556
BRITISH COLUMBIA MEDICAL JOURNAL. Text in English. 1959. 10/yr. CND 50 domestic; CND 65 foreign. adv. bk.rev. charts, illus, stat. index. back issues avail. *Refereed.* **Document type:** *Academic/Scholarly.*
Indexed: Med.Care Rev., Ref.Zh.
—BLDSC (2297.100000), CISTI, Infotrieve. **CCC.**
Published by: British Columbia Medical Association, 115 1665 W Broadway, Vancouver, BC V6J 5A4, Canada. TEL 604-736-5551, FAX 604-733-7317, jdraper@bcma.bc.ca, cupton@bcma.bc.ca. Ed. Dr. James A Wilson. R&P, Adv. contact Kashmira Suraliwalla. Circ: 8,100.

610 658 GBR ISSN 1466-4100
BRITISH JOURNAL OF CLINICAL GOVERNANCE. Text in English. 1991; N.S. 1996. q. USD 309 in North America; EUR 419 in Europe; AUD 599 in Australasia; GBP 249 in United Kingdom & rest of the world (effective 2002). adv. bk.rev. **Document type:** *Journal, Academic/Scholarly.* **Description:** Addresses issues of practical importance in the areas of evidence-based practice, clinical effectiveness, assessment of outcomes of care, and audits. For audit staff and health professionals including doctors, nurse managers, therapists and managers in purchasing and provider organisations.
Former titles (until 1999): Journal of Clinical Effectiveness (1361-5874); (until 1996): Medical Audit News (0959-2903)
Related titles: Online - full text ed.: (from EBSCO Publishing, O C L C Online Computer Library Center, Inc., RoweCom Information Quest, ingenta, Swets Blackwell).
Indexed: ASSIA, CINAHL, Emrld.Intell., Environ.Sci.Poll.Mgmt., Inpharma, Pharm.&Out.News, Pollut.Abstr., Reac., Ref.Zh., Risk Abstr., Saf.Sci.Abstr.
—BLDSC (2307.140000), GNLM, Infotrieve. **CCC.**
Published by: Emerald, 60-62 Toller Ln, Bradford, W Yorks BD8 9BY, United Kingdom. TEL 44-1274-777700, FAX 44-1274-785200, info@emeraldinsight.com, http://www.emeraldinsight.com/bjcg.htm, http://www.mcb.co.uk/, http://www.emeraldinsight.com/journals/. Eds. Jeff Lucas, Dr. John Wright. **Affiliate:** Emerald (North America).

610 GBR ISSN 0960-1643
CODEN: BJGPEJ
BRITISH JOURNAL OF GENERAL PRACTICE. Text in English. 1952. m. GBP 130; GBP 147 foreign (effective 1999). adv. bk.rev. charts, illus, stat. index. back issues avail. *Refereed.* **Document type:** *Academic/Scholarly.*
Former titles (until 1990): Royal College of General Practitioners. Journal (0035-8797); (until 1967): College of General Practitioners. Journal
Related titles: Online - full text ed.: (from Institute for Scientific Information).
Indexed: AMED, ASCA, Abstr.Hyg., Addic.Abstr., Alloys Ind., Brit.Nur.Ind., CINAHL, Curr.Adv.Ecol.Sci., Curr.Cont., Diab.Cont., Dok.Arbeitsmed., FAMLI, Helminthol.Abstr., Ind.Med. (1990-), Ind.Sci.Rev., Inpharma, Int.Nurs.Ind., Med.Care Rev., Met.Abstr., Met.Abstr.Ind., NRN, Nonfer.Met.Alert, Nutr.Abstr., PCC Alert, Pharm.&Out.News, Protozool.Abstr., Reac., SSCI (coverage dropped), Sci.Cit.Ind., Steels Alert, Trop.Dis.Bull.
—BLDSC (2308.360000), CISTI, EMDOCS, GNLM, IDS, ingenta, KNAW.
Published by: Royal College of General Practitioners, Hyde Park, 14 Princes Gate, London SW7 1PU, United Kingdom. TEL 44-171-581-3232, FAX 44-171-225-3047, info@rcgp.org.uk, http://www.rcgp.org.uk. Ed. Dr. A F Wright. Adv. contact Maria Phantis. B&W page GBP 500, color page GBP 1,550; trim 21 x 28. Circ: 18,000. **Subscr. to:** World Wide Subscription Service Ltd., Unit 4, Gibbs Reed Farm, Ticehurst, E Sussex TN5 7HE, United Kingdom.

BRITISH JOURNAL OF HEALTH PSYCHOLOGY. see *PSYCHOLOGY*

614.88 GBR ISSN 0961-7930
CODEN: BJICEO
BRITISH JOURNAL OF INTENSIVE CARE. Text in English. 1991. 10/yr. GBP 60 domestic to individuals; GBP 90 in Europe to individuals; GBP 108 elsewhere to individuals; GBP 84 domestic to institutions; GBP 114 in Europe to institutions; GBP 132 elsewhere to institutions. adv. bk.rev. **Document type:** *Academic/Scholarly.* **Description:** Provides a forum for specialists in critical care, including intensivists, anesthesiologists, nurses, neonatologists, cardiologists, general surgeons, hematologists, and pharmacists.
Indexed: Excerp.Med. (1992-).
—BLDSC (2311.047000), EMDOCS, GNLM, KNAW.
Published by: Greycoat Publishing, 1 Harley St, London W1N 1DA, United Kingdom. TEL 44-20-7637-1828, FAX 44-20-7631-3020. Ed. Michael Rennie. R&P Guy Wallis. Adv. contact Ashley Wallis. Circ: 275 (paid); 13,878 (controlled).

615.85 GBR ISSN 0308-0226
BRITISH JOURNAL OF OCCUPATIONAL THERAPY. Text in English. 1938. m. GBP 84 in the European Union; GBP 120 elsewhere (effective 2000). adv. bk.rev. charts, illus. index. *Refereed.* **Document type:** *Academic/Scholarly.* **Description:** Contains contributions of papers relevant to theory, practice, education, management and research in occupational therapy. These may take the form of articles, opinion pieces, short reports, announcements, editorials, research abstracts, book and media reviews, and letters to the editor.
Indexed: AMED, ASSIA, Abstr.Health Care Manage.Stud., Brit.Nur.Ind., CINAHL, Curr.Adv.Ecol.Sci., PsycInfo, Psychol.Abstr., Rehabil.Lit., e-psyche.
—BLDSC (2312.700000), GNLM, ingenta, KNAW.
Published by: College of Occupational Therapists Ltd., 106-114 Borough High St, London SE1 1LB, United Kingdom. TEL 44-171-450-2338, FAX 44-171-450-2350, bjot.edit@cot.co.uk; bjot.advert@cot.co.uk, http://www.cot.co.uk. Ed. Upma Barnett. Adv. contact Paula Willock. Circ: 20,000.

610 GBR ISSN 0301-5572
CODEN: BJMEDF
BRITISH JOURNAL OF SEXUAL MEDICINE. Abbreviated title: B J S M. Text in English. 1974. bi-m. adv. bk.rev. **Document type:** *Academic/Scholarly.*
Indexed: Biol.Abstr., Curr.Adv.Cancer Res., Curr.Adv.Ecol.Sci., Excerp.Med. (until 1993).
—GNLM, ingenta.
Published by: Hayward Medical Communications Ltd., Covent Garden, Seven Dials Warehouse, 44 Earlham St, London WC2H 9LA, United Kingdom. TEL 44-20-7240-4493, FAX 44-20-7240-4479, admin@hayward.co.uk, http://www.hayward.co.uk. Ed. Dr. Paul Woolley. Circ: 18,000. **Subscr. to:** Rosemary House, Lanwades Park, Kentford, Near, Newmarket, Suffolk CB8 7PW, United Kingdom. TEL 44-1638-751515, FAX 44-163-751517.

610 GBR ISSN 0007-1420
R31 CODEN: BMBUAQ
BRITISH MEDICAL BULLETIN. Text in English. 1943. q. GBP 170, USD 290; GBP 73, USD 115 in developing nations to institutions (effective Mar. 2002). charts, illus. index. 256 p./no. back issues avail.; reprint service avail. from PQC. *Refereed.* **Document type:** *Journal, Academic/Scholarly.* **Description:** Series of expert reviews on selected health topics in fields where significant new developments are occurring.
Related titles: Microform ed.: (from PQC); Online - full text ed.: ISSN 1471-8391. GBP 18, USD 30 in developing nations to institutions (effective Mar. 2002) (from CatchWord Ltd., Ovid Technologies, Inc., HighWire Pr., EBSCO Publishing, O C L C Online Computer Library Center, Inc., RoweCom Information Quest, Swets Blackwell, Institute for Scientific Information).
Indexed: ASCA, Abstr.Hyg., Agri.& Environ.Biotech.Abstr. (coverage dropped), Anim.Breed.Abstr., Bibl.Dev.Med.& Child Neur., Biol.Abstr., C.I.S. Abstr., Chem.Abstr., Chem.Indus.Notes, Chem.Titles, Curr.Adv.Ecol.Sci., Curr.Cont., Dairy Sci.Abstr., Derwent Biotech.Abstr., Diar.Dis.Res., Environ.Sci.Poll.Mgmt., Excerp.Med., Helminthol.Abstr., INIS Atomind., I.P.A., Ind.Med. (1943-), Ind.Sci.Rev., Ind.Vet., Inpharma, Int.Abstr.Biol.Sci., Nutr.Abstr., Pharm.&Out.News, Pollut.Abstr., Protozool.Abstr., Reac., Ref.Zh., Rev.Appl.Entomol., Rev.Plant Path., Risk Abstr., SSCI (coverage dropped), Saf.Sci.Abstr., Sci.Cit.Ind., Vet.Bull., Wild.Rev.
—BLDSC (2329.000000), ADONIS, CASDDS, CatchWord, CISTI, EMDOCS, GNLM, IDS, ingenta, KNAW. **CCC.**
Published by: (Medical Department, British Council), Oxford University Press, Academic Division, Great Clarendon St, Oxford OX2 6DP, United Kingdom. TEL 44-1865-267907, FAX 44-1865-267835, jnl.info@oup.co.uk, http://bmb.oupjournals.org, http://www.oup.co.uk/journals. Eds. L Boysiewicz, M Walport. Pub. Mandy Sketch. R&P Fionna Willis. Circ: 1,550. **Subscr. to:** Oxford University Press, Journals, 2001 Evans Rd, Cary, NC 27513. TEL 800-852-7323, FAX 919-677-1714, jnlorders@oup-usa.org; Journals Marketing, Great Clarendon St, Oxford OX2 6DP, United Kingdom.

610 NLD
BRITISH MEDICAL JOURNAL (DANISH EDITION). Text in Danish. m. NLG 120.
Related titles: ♦ English ed.: B M J. ISSN 0959-535X; ♦ Dutch ed.: British Medical Journal (Dutch Edition); ♦ Chinese ed.: Yingguo Yixue Zazhi (Zhongwen Ban). ISSN 1007-9742; ♦ Polish ed.: British Medical Journal (Wydawnictwo Polskie). ISSN 1231-9775; Hungarian ed.: B M J (Magyar Kiady). ISSN 1216-7495. 1992; Greek ed.: B M J (Ellenike Ekdosis). ISSN 1106-4226. 1993; Portuguese ed.: B M J (Edicoe Portuguesa). ISSN 0873-0423. 1992.
Published by: Medicom Excel, Postbus 151, Bussum 1400 DA, Netherlands. Circ: 2,100.

610 NLD
BRITISH MEDICAL JOURNAL (DUTCH EDITION). Text in Dutch. m. NLG 120.
Related titles: ♦ English ed.: B M J. ISSN 0959-535X; ♦ Danish ed.: British Medical Journal (Danish Edition); ♦ Chinese ed.: Yingguo Yixue Zazhi (Zhongwen Ban). ISSN 1007-9742; ♦ Polish ed.: British Medical Journal (Wydawnictwo Polskie). ISSN 1231-9775; Hungarian ed.: B M J (Magyar Kiady). ISSN 1216-7495. 1992; Greek ed.: B M J (Ellenike Ekdosis). ISSN 1106-4226. 1993; Portuguese ed.: B M J (Edicoe Portuguesa). ISSN 0873-0423. 1992.
Published by: Medicom Excel, Postbus 151, Bussum 1400 DA, Netherlands. Circ: 5,300.

610 POL ISSN 1231-9775
BRITISH MEDICAL JOURNAL (WYDAWNICTWO POLSKIE). Text in Polish. 1994. m. PLZ 60 domestic; PLZ 7.50 newsstand/cover domestic (effective 2000). adv. bk.rev. back issues avail. *Refereed.* **Description:** Reports on important medical research, news and trends.
Related titles: ♦ English ed.: B M J. ISSN 0959-535X; ♦ Dutch ed.: British Medical Journal (Dutch Edition); ♦ Chinese ed.: Yingguo Yixue Zazhi (Zhongwen Ban). ISSN 1007-9742; ♦ Danish ed.: British Medical Journal (Danish Edition); Hungarian ed.: B M J (Magyar Kiady). ISSN 1216-7495. 1992; Greek ed.: B M J (Ellenike Ekdosis). ISSN 1106-4226. 1993; Portuguese ed.: B M J (Edicoe Portuguesa). ISSN 0873-0423. 1992.
Published by: Wydawnictwo Naukowe P W Nowe, Ul Miodowa 10, Warsaw 00251, Poland. TEL 48-22-6954001, FAX 48-22-6954288, http://www.pwn.com.pl. Ed. Pawel Januszewicz. Pub. Grzegorz Boguta. R&P Zbigniew Zawadzki TEL 48-22-6954031. Adv. contact Janusz Kubiak. B&W page PLZ 2,500, color page PLZ 4,000; trim 210 x 297.

610 USA
BRONX MEDICINE. Text in English. 1967 (vol.45). 4/yr. USD 10 (effective 1999). adv. illus. **Document type:** *Bulletin.*
Formerly: Bronx County Medical Society. Bulletin (0007-2257)
Indexed: Med.Care Rev.
Published by: Bronx County Medical Society, 2600 Netherland Ave, Bronx, NY 10463. TEL 718-548-4401, FAX 718-549-6681. Ed. Dr. John P Albanese. Pub., R&P, Adv. contact George Drapeaw TEL 914-631-6088. Circ: 1,800.

610 RUS
BUD'ZDOROV!. Text in Russian. m. **Document type:** *Academic/Scholarly.*
Published by: Shenkman i Synov'ya, Uglovoi per 2, kv 72, Moscow 103055, Russian Federation. TEL 7-095-9288272, FAX 7-095-2673460. Ed. S B Shenkman. **US dist. addr.:** East View Publications, 3020 Harbor Ln N, Minneapolis, MN 55447. TEL 612-550-0961.

410 ALB
BULETINI I SHKENCAVE MJEKESORE/BULLETIN DES SCIENCES MEDICALES. Text in Albanian; Summaries in French. s-a. USD 3.85.
Indexed: Chem.Abstr.
Published by: Enver Hoxha Universitet, Tirana, Albania. Ed. Ylvi Vehbiu.

610 BGR ISSN 0861-9883
BULGARSKA MEDICINA/BULGARIAN MEDICINE. Text in Bulgarian; Summaries in English. 1993. bi-m. USD 54 foreign (effective 2002). **Document type:** *Journal, Academic/Scholarly.* **Description:** Presents scientific publications in different areas of medicine, written by leading Bulgarian medicine scientists.
Indexed: Excerp.Med. (1994-).
—EMDOCS, GNLM.
Published by: Academy of Medicine, 1 Sv Georgi Sofiiski blvd, Sofia 1431, Bulgaria. **Dist. by:** Sofia Books, Ul Silivria 16, Sofia 1404, Bulgaria. TEL 359-2-9586257, sofiabooks@hotmail.com, http://www.sofiabooks.hit.bg.

610 BGR
BULGARSKI LEKAR. Text in Bulgarian. m. USD 48 foreign (effective 2002). **Document type:** *Newspaper, Trade.*
Published by: Natsionalno Izdaniye za Vissheto Meditsinsko Sosloviye, Ul Parizh 3, Sofia 1000, Bulgaria. TEL 359-2-9811033, totkonaidenov@bgekar.com, http://www.bglekar.com/. Ed. Totko Naidenov. **Dist. by:** Sofia Books, Ul Silivria 16, Sofia 1404, Bulgaria. TEL 359-2-9586257, sofiabooks@hotmail.com, http://www.sofiabooks.hit.bg.

BULLETIN OF EXPERIMENTAL BIOLOGY AND MEDICINE. see *BIOLOGY*

610 174.2 GBR ISSN 0962-9564
BULLETIN OF MEDICAL ETHICS. Text in English. 1985. 10/yr. GBP 80 in Europe; USD 125 in United States; GBP 85 elsewhere (effective 2001). **Document type:** *Bulletin, Journal, Academic/Scholarly.* **Description:** Provides an up-to-date, non-partisan source of news, views, official statements, and codes of practice about developments in health care ethics.
Formerly (until 1989): I M E Bulletin (0269-1485)
Indexed: ASSIA, Russ.Acad.Sci.Bibl.
—BLDSC (2870.137000), GNLM.
Published by: Royal Society of Medicine Press Ltd, 1 Wimpole St, London W1M 8AE, United Kingdom. TEL 44-20-7290-2921, FAX 44-20-7290-2929, elizabeth.fredman@rsm.ac.uk, http://www.roysocmed.ac.uk/pub/bme.htm. Ed., Pub. Dr. Richard Nicholson.

610 USA ISSN 0007-5140
R11
BULLETIN OF THE HISTORY OF MEDICINE. Text in English. 1933. q. USD 39 to individuals; USD 110 to institutions; USD 143 to institutions for print & online eds. (effective 2002). adv. bk.rev. bibl, illus. index, cum.index vols.1-56. back issues avail.; reprint service avail. from PQC. *Refereed.* **Document type:** *Academic/Scholarly.* **Description:** Presents articles that analyze advances in medical science, examines changes in clinical practices, and explores how the response of societies to health care needs have varied with times and cultures.
Related titles: Micro Opaque ed.; Microform ed.: (from PQC,PMC); Online - full text ed.: ISSN 1086-3176. 1933. USD 86.40 (effective 2000) (from Project MUSE, EBSCO Publishing, O C L C Online Computer Library Center, Inc., RoweCom Information Quest, Swets Blackwell, Institute for Scientific Information).
Indexed: ASCA, Amer.Bibl.Slavic & E.Eur.Stud., Amer.Hist.& Life, Arts & Hum.Cit.Ind., BHA, Bibl.Asian Stud. (1971-1992), Biol.Abstr., Br.Archaeol.Abstr., Chem.Abstr., Curr.Cont., Excerp.Med., Hist.Abstr. (1963-), IBZ, Ind.Med. (1939-), Ind.Sci.Rev., Inpharma, Int.Nurs.Ind., Numis.Lit., P C I, Protozool.Abstr., Reac., Ref.Zh., Russ.Acad.Sci.Bibl., SSCI, Sci.Cit.Ind., Soc.Serv.Abstr., Sociol.Abstr., Trop.Dis.Bull.
—BLDSC (2856.000000), CISTI, GNLM, IDS, Infotrieve, ingenta. **CCC.**
Published by: (American Association for the History of Medicine), Johns Hopkins University Press, Journals Publishing Division, 2715 N Charles St, Baltimore, MD 21218-4363. TEL 800-548-1784, FAX 410-516-6968, jlorder@jhupress.jhu.edu, http://www.muse.jhu.edu/journals/bulletin_of_the_history_of_medicine/, http://www.press.jhu.edu. Eds. Gert H Brieger, Jerome J Bylebyl. Adv. contact Anastasia Scherr. Circ: 2,394. **Co-sponsor:** Johns Hopkins Institute of the History of Medicine.

610 USA
BULLETIN OF THE MEDICAL SOCIETY OF THE COUNTY OF QUEENS AND THE ACADEMY OF MEDICINE OF QUEENS. Text in English. 1925. 10/yr. USD 10. adv. illus, tr.lit.
Published by: Medical Society of the County of Queens, 112-25 Queens Blvd., Forest Hills, NY 11375. FAX 718-268-6918. Ed. Dr. Lorraine Maria Giordano. Circ: 2,000. **Co-sponsor:** Academy of Medicine of Queens County.

610 570 DEU ISSN 0936-8671
QR180 CODEN: AESBAL
BUNDESAMT FUER SERA UND IMPFSTOFFE. PAUL-EHRLICH-INSTITUT. ARBEITEN. Text in German. a. price varies. **Document type:** *Journal, Academic/Scholarly.*
Formerly (until 1988): Arbeiten aus dem Paul-Ehrlich-Institut, dem Georg-Speyer-Haus und dem Ferdinand-Blum-Institut (0066-5665)
Indexed: Excerp.Med., Ind.Med. (1988-).
—CISTI, GNLM. **CCC.**
Published by: Paul-Ehrlich-Institut (Subsidiary of: Bundesamt fuer Sera und Impfstoffe), Paul-Ehrlich-Str 51-59, Langen 63225, Germany. TEL 49-6103-77-0, FAX 49-6103-771234, pei@pei.de, http://www.pei.de.

610 MMR ISSN 0007-6295
BURMA MEDICAL JOURNAL*. Text in Burmese. 1964 (vol.12). q.
Indexed: Chem.Abstr.
—GNLM.
Published by: Burma Medical Association, 249 Theinbyu Rd., Yangon, Myanmar.

M

610.2 658.8 GBR
BUSINESS RATIO REPORT: THE MEDICAL EQUIPMENT INDUSTRY; an industry sector analysis. Text in English. 1978. a. GBP 275 (effective 2001). charts, stat. **Document type:** *Trade.*
Formerly (until 1992): Business Ratio Report: Medical Equipment Manufacturers (0261-9075)
Published by: The Prospect Shop Ltd., Field House, 72 Oldfield Rd, Hampton, Middx TW12 2HQ, United Kingdom. TEL 44-20-8461-8730, 44-20-8481-8720, FAX 44-20-8783-1940, info@theprospectshop.co.uk.

610 JPN
BYOIN SHINBUN/HOSPITAL NEWS. Text in Japanese. w. JPY 1,300 per month.
Published by: Byoin Shinbunsha, 4-1 Hirakawa-cho 2-chome, Chiyoda-ku, Tokyo 102-0093, Japan.

BYOTAI SEIRI TO SHINDAN CHIRYO/SANWA KAGAKU CO. MEDICAL REPORT. see *BIOLOGY—Physiology*

BYULLETEN' EKSPERIMENTAL'NOI BIOLOGII I MEDITSINY. see *BIOLOGY*

571.9 USA ISSN 0891-1525
C A P TODAY. Text in English. 1987. m. USD 40; USD 60 in Canada & Mexico; USD 95 elsewhere. adv.
Formed by the merger of (1947-1987): Pathologist (0031-3017); (1982-1987): Counterpoints (Skokie) (0740-3275)
Indexed: Excerp.Med., Hosp.Lit.Ind.
—BLDSC (3050.624000), CISTI, GNLM.
Published by: College of American Pathologists, 325 Waukegan Rd, Northfield, IL 60093-2750. TEL 847-832-7000, FAX 847-832-8150.

C A S NYT. see *HEALTH FACILITIES AND ADMINISTRATION*

C A SELECTS. MONOCLONAL ANTIBODIES. see *BIOLOGY—Abstracting, Bibliographies, Statistics*

610.6 USA
C C H MONITOR: THE NEWSLETTER OF MANAGED CARE. (Commerce Clearing House) Text in English. 1993. s-m. USD 399 (effective 2001). **Document type:** *Newsletter.* **Description:** Provides coverage of the issues facing today's managed care providers, with practical advice, how-to tips on compliance, and analyses of legal developments affecting managed care systems.
Published by: C C H Incorporated, 2700 Lake Cook Rd., Riverwoods, IL 60015. TEL 312-583-8500, 800-449-9525, hahns@cch.com, http://www.cch.com. Ed. Susan Hahn Reizner. Pub. Catherine Wolfe.

C H A C INFO/INFO A C C S. see *HEALTH FACILITIES AND ADMINISTRATION*

C H A C REVIEW. see *HEALTH FACILITIES AND ADMINISTRATION*

610 AUS ISSN 0812-9630
C H E C K. (Continuous Home Evaluation of Clinical Knowledge) Key Title: Check. Text in English. 1972. m. **Description:** Provides case histories, background information, diagrams, x-rays and photographs.
Published by: Royal Australian College of General Practitioners, 1 Palmerston Crescent, South Melbourne, VIC 3205, Australia. TEL 03-9214-1414.

614.88 ITA
C I R M RESEARCH; the medical journal of the international radio medical center. Text in English. 1958. s-a., latest vol.4, 2000. free per issue. bk.rev. charts, illus. *Refereed.* **Document type:** *Academic/Scholarly.* **Description:** Publishes scientific papers on seamen pathophysiology. Covers news, activities and services of the medical center.
Formerly (until 1997): C I R M. Atti sezione studi
Published by: Centro Internazionale Radio - Medico, Via Dell' Architettura, 41, Rome, RM 00144, Italy. TEL 39-06-5923331, FAX 39-06-5923333, salastudi@cirm.it, http://www.cirm.it. Ed. Dr. Antonio Dauri. Pub. Dr. F Amenta. Circ: 1,500.

M

610 USA
C I R NEWS. Text in English. 1971. q. USD 12 to individuals; USD 24 to institutions. adv. bk.rev. back issues avail. **Document type:** *Bulletin.*
Former titles: C I R Bulletin; Committee of Interns and Residents Bulletin (0090-1660)
Published by: Committee of Interns and Residents, 386 Park Ave S, New York, NY 10016. TEL 212-725-5500. Ed. Mark Levy. Circ: 15,000.

610 CAN ISSN 0820-3946
CODEN: CMAJAX
C M A J/J A M C (JOURNAL DE L'ASSOCIATION MEDICALE CANADIENNE). (Canadian Medical Association Journal) Text in English, French. 1911. 25/yr. CND 117 domestic; USD 150 foreign (effective 1999). adv. bk.rev. bibl, charts, illus. index. back issues avail.; reprints avail. *Refereed.* **Document type:** *Academic/Scholarly.* **Description:** Includes notices of upcoming conferences, summaries of C.M.A. policies and news and features of interest to members of the association and others in the health care professions.
Formerly (until 1985): Canadian Medical Association Journal (0008-4409)
Media: Microfilm. **Related titles:** CD-ROM ed.: (from Ovid Technologies, Inc.); Microfiche ed.: (from MML); Microform ed.: (from PQC,MML); Online - full text ed.: (from Ovid Technologies, Inc., ProQuest Information & Learning, Institute for Scientific Information).
Indexed: AIM, AMED, ASCA, Abstr.Anthropol., Abstr.Health Care Manage.Stud., Abstr.Hyg., AgeLine, Agri.& Environ.Biotech.Abstr. (coverage dropped), Arts & Hum.Cit.Ind. (coverage dropped), Bibl.Dev.Med.& Child Neur., Biol.Abstr., Biol.Dig., CBCA Ref., CINAHL, C.I.S. Abstr., Can.B.P.I., Can.Per.Ind. (Jan.1988-), Chem.Abstr., Crim.Just.Abstr., Curr.Adv.Biochem., Curr.Adv.Ecol.Sci., Curr.Adv.Gen.& Molec.Biol., Curr.Cont., Dairy Sci.Abstr., Dent.Ind., Derwent Biotech.Abstr., Diar.Dis.Res., Dok.Arbeitsmed., Environ.Sci.Poll.Mgmt., Excerp.Med., FAMLI, Helminthol.Abstr., INIS Atomind., I.P.A., Ind.Med. (1985-), Ind.Sci.Rev., Ind.Vet., Inpharma, Int.Abstr.Biol.Sci., Int.Nurs.Ind., Lab.Haz.Bull., Med.& Surg.Dermat., Med.Care Rev., NRN, Neurosci.Cit.Ind., Nutr.Abstr., Pharm.&Out.News, Pollut.Abstr., Protozool.Abstr., Reac., Rev.Appl.Entomol., Rev.Arom.& Med.Plants, Rev.Med.& Vet.Mycol., Rev.Plant Path., Risk Abstr., Saf.Sci.Abstr., Sage Fam.Stud.Abstr., Sci.Cit.Ind., Sportsearch, Trop.Dis.Bull., Viol.& Abuse Abstr., Weed Abstr.
—BLDSC (3038.000000), ADONIS, CASDDS, CISTI, EMDOCS, GNLM, IDS, ingenta, KNAW. **CCC.**
Published by: Canadian Medical Association, 1867 Alta Vista Dr, Ottawa, ON K1H 5K9, Canada. TEL 613-731-9331, 800-663-7336 ext. 2132, 800-267-9703, FAX 613-565-2382, pubs@cma.ca, rafusj@cma.ca, http://www.cma.ca/cmaj. Ed. Dr. John Hoey. Pub. Peter Milroy. Adv. contact Beverly Kirkpatrick. B&W page CND 2,695, color page CND 4,490; trim 10.88 x 8.13. Circ: 56,103.

610.28 CAN ISSN 0830-8845
C M B E S - S C G B NEWSLETTER. Text in English. 1966. 4/yr. **Document type:** *Newsletter.*
Formerly (until 1984): Canadian Medical and Biological Engineering Society. Newsletter (0384-1820)
—CCC.
Published by: Canadian Medical and Biological Engineering Society Inc./Societe Canadienne de Genie Biomedical, Rm 382, Bldg M 55, National Research Council, Ottawa, ON K1A 0R8, Canada. TEL 613-993-1686, FAX 613-954-2216, societyicmbes@nrc.ca. Ed. Brian Graham. Circ: (controlled).

610 ZAF ISSN 1016-6742
C M E; South Africa's continuing medical education journal. (Continuing Medical Education) Text in English. 1983. 11/yr. USD 126 foreign (effective 2000). adv. bk.rev. index. back issues avail. **Document type:** *Academic/Scholarly.* **Description:** Discusses topics in continuing medical education (CME) for physicians.
Formerly (until 1989): S.A. Journal of Continuing Medical Education (0256-2170)
Related titles: Microfiche ed.
Indexed: INIS Atomind., Ind.S.A.Per.
Published by: South African Medical Association, Health and Medical Publishing Group, 14 Central Sq, Pinelands 7430, South Africa. TEL 27-21-531-3081, FAX 27-21-531-4126, publishing@samedical.org, http://www.samedical.org. Ed. F N Sanders. R&P Peter Roberts. Adv. contact Andre Botes TEL 27-11-706-2088. Circ: 10,500. **Subscr. to:** PO Box 74789, Lynnwood Ridge, Pretoria 0040, South Africa. TEL 27-12-481-2010, FAX 27-12-481-2061, ann@samedical.org. **Dist. by:** Private Bag X1, Pinelands 7430, South Africa. TEL 27-21-531-3081, FAX 27-21-531-4126.

610 610.711 CAN
C M E - CONTINUING MEDICAL EDUCATION. Text in English. m.
Published by: S T A Communications Inc., 955 bd St Jean, bur 306, Pointe Claire, PQ H9R 5K3, Canada. TEL 514-695-7623, FAX 514-695-8554. Ed. Paul Brand. Circ: 30,082.

610 618.97 GBR ISSN 1367-8914
C M E JOURNAL - GERIATRIC MEDICINE. (Continuing Medical Education) Text in English. 1997. 3/yr. (1 volume per annum). GBP 45 domestic to individuals; GBP 60 foreign to individuals; GBP 60 domestic to institutions; GBP 90 foreign to institutions (effective 2001). adv. Website rev. abstr. 24 p./no. 48 cols./p. *Refereed.* **Document type:** *Journal.*
Formerly: C M E Bulletin - Geriatric Medicine
—BLDSC (3287.223045).
Published by: Rila Publications Ltd., 73 Newman St, London W1A 4PG, United Kingdom. TEL 44-20-7631-1299, FAX 44-20-7580-7166, admin@rila.co.uk, http://www.rila.co.uk. Ed. Stephen Allen. Pub., Adv. contact G Da'Cambra. Circ: 4,500 (paid).

610 GBR ISSN 0955-3630
C M S BULLETIN. Text in English. 1987. bi-m. GBP 20 to members. **Document type:** *Bulletin.* **Description:** Promotes individual freedom of choice in health services.
Published by: Conservative Medical Society, 32 Smith Sq, London SW1P 2HH, United Kingdom.

610 GBR ISSN 1464-455X
C N S. Variant title: Central Nervous System. Text in English. q.
—BLDSC (3287.314335).
Published by: Hayward Group, Inc, 44 Earlham St, Convent Garden, London WC2H 9LA, United Kingdom. TEL 44-20-7240-4493, FAX 44-20-7240-4479, edit@hayward.co.uk. Ed. Dr. Jogin Thakore. Pub. John Applegate.

610 USA ISSN 1532-0235
▼ **C O R CLINICAL EXCELLENCE.** Text in English. 2000. m. USD 298 includes online ed. (effective 2001). bk.rev., software rev., Website rev. abstr, bibl, charts, illus, stat. back issues avail.; reprints avail. **Description:** Provides a broad overview of the best clinical management information from hundreds of print and online resources, plus original articles, research, and commentary.
Formed by the merger of (200?): Strategies for Healthcare Excellence (1058-7829); Medical Management Network (1097-0835)
Related titles: Online - full content ed.
Published by: C O R Health, LLC, PO Box 50507, Santa Barbara, CA 93150. TEL 805-564-2177, FAX 805-564-2146, info@corhealth.com, http://www.corhealth.com. Ed. Marilyn Lang. Pub. Dean H. Anderson.

610 025.04 USA
C O R E-HEALTH TREND WATCH. Text in English. w. free (effective 2001). **Document type:** *Newsletter, Trade.* **Description:** Reviews of new Web sites and Internet resources about healthcare.
Media: E-mail.
Published by: C O R Health, LLC, PO Box 50507, Santa Barbara, CA 93150. TEL 805-564-2177, FAX 805-564-2146, info@corhealth.com, http://www.corhealth.com.

610 USA
C O R HEALTHCARE LEADERSHIP TREND WATCH. Text in English. w. free. bk.rev., Website rev. abstr, bibl, charts, illus, stat. back issues avail.; reprints avail. **Document type:** *Newsletter, Trade.* **Description:** Covers the latest strategic information on mission-critical healthcare issues.
Formerly (until 2001): C O R Enterprise Leadership Trend Watch
Media: E-mail.
Published by: C O R Health, LLC, PO Box 50507, Santa Barbara, CA 93150. TEL 805-564-2177, FAX 805-564-2146, info@corhealth.com, http://www.corhealth.com/. Ed. Bridget Meaney. Pub. Dean H. Anderson.

610.711 USA ISSN 0146-2814
C O T H REPORT. Text in English. 1979. q. USD 30 (effective 1998). **Document type:** *Newsletter.*
Published by: (Council of Teaching Hospitals), Association of American Medical Colleges, 2450 N St N W, Washington, DC 20037-1126. TEL 202-828-0497, FAX 202-828-4792, iphilibert@aamc.org, http://www.aamc.org. Ed., R&P Ingrid Philibert.

610 USA ISSN 0276-8283
RB115
C P T. (Physicians' Current Procedural Terminology) Text in English. 1966. a. USD 66.95 (effective 2000). **Document type:** *Academic/Scholarly.*

Formerly (1st & 2nd eds.): Current Procedural Terminology (0065-9312)
Related titles: Diskette ed.: USD 49.95 single user; USD 149.95 2-10 users (effective 2000).
—GNLM.
Published by: American Medical Association, 515 N State St, P O Box 10946, Chicago, IL 60610-0946. TEL 312-464-5000.

610 FRA ISSN 0007-9480
CADUCEE. Text in French. 1961. 13/yr. FRF 170. adv. abstr, bibl, illus, stat. index.
—CCC.
Published by: B.C. Savy, 18 av. de la Marne, Asnieres-sur-Seine 92600, France. TEL 47-93-05-88, FAX 47-93-68-95. Circ: 13,000.

610.28 FRA ISSN 0575-0563
CAHIERS DE BIOTHERAPIE. Text in French. 1964. 6/yr. FRF 450 domestic; FRF 500 foreign (effective 2000). adv. bk.rev. back issues avail.
—CCC.
Published by: (Societe Medicale de Biotherapie), Editions Similia, 71 rue Beaubourg, Paris 75003, France. TEL 33-1-42716866, FAX 33-1-44781147, similia@club-internet. Ed. Max Tetau. Adv. contact Isabelle Regne. Circ: 8,000.

610 FRA
CAHIERS DE GEOGRAPHIE DE LA SANTE/JOURNAL OF GEOGRAPHY OF HEALTH. Short title: GEOS. Text in French. irreg. **Description:** Covers the research done at the university level by geographers, either in the form of excerpts, digests or research positions. Covers the geographical study of illness, health care and health care services.
Published by: Universite de Montpellier III (Universite Paul Valery), Route de Mende, Montpellier Cedex 5 34199 , France. TEL 33-4-67142406, FAX 33-4-67142332, publications.recherche@univ-montp3.fr. Ed. H Picheral.

610 FRA ISSN 0007-9936
CAHIERS DE MEDECINE INTERPROFESSIONNELLE. Text in French. 1961. q. FRF 261. bk.rev.
Indexed: C.I.S. Abstr.
—GNLM.
Published by: (Association Interprofessionnelle des Centres Medicaux et Sociaux de la Region Parisienne), Editions Docis, 10, rue de la Rosiere, Paris 75015, France. TEL 33-01-53953841, FAX 33-01-53953848, docis@cisme.org, http://www.cisme.org/doc/docis. Circ: 1,250.

612 FRA ISSN 0336-5913
CAHIERS DE SEXOLOGIE CLINIQUE* . Text in French. 1975. bi-m. FRF 300; (students 200 F.).
Indexed: Biol.Abstr.
Published by: Nouvelles Editions Medicales Francaises, P.B. 451, Clergy Pontoise Cede 95005, France.

610 FRA ISSN 1157-5999
CODEN: SMOFEX
CAHIERS D'ETUDES ET DE RECHERCHES FRANCOPHONES. SANTE. Key Title: Sante (Montrouge). Variant title: Cahiers Sante. Text in French. 1990. 6/yr. FRF 450 domestic to individuals; EUR 69 in Europe to individuals; FRF 750 domestic to institutions; EUR 114 in Europe to institutions; FRF 300 domestic to students; EUR 45 in Europe to students (effective 2001); FRF 120 newsstand/cover. **Description:** Aims to establish the medical research of the francophone world and expose the research of developing countries.
Indexed: Dairy Sci.Abstr., Excerp.Med. (1994-), Helminthol.Abstr., Ind.Med. (1990-), Nutr.Abstr., Protozool.Abstr., Rev.Appl.Entomol., Rev.Med.& Vet.Mycol., Rice Abstr., Rural Devel.Abstr., Trop.Dis.Bull.
—BLDSC (2952.195550), EMDOCS, GNLM.
Published by: John Libbey Eurotext, 127 av. de la Republique, Montrouge 92120, France. TEL 33-01-46730660, FAX 33-01-40840999, marketing@jle.com, http://www.john-libbey-eurotext.fr/. Ed. Dominique Richard Lenoble. **Subscr. to:** A T E I, 3 av. Pierre Kerautret, Romainville 92230, France. TEL 33-1-48408686, FAX 33-1-48400731, atei@club-internet.fr.

610 CHE ISSN 0409-8757
CAHIERS MEDICO-SOCIAUX. Text in French. 1956. irreg. **Document type:** *Monographic series, Academic/Scholarly.*
—BLDSC (2949.784000). **CCC.**
Published by: Editions Medecine et Hygiene, Case Postale 456, Geneva, 4 1211, Switzerland. TEL 41-22-7029311, FAX 41-22-7029355, abonnements@medhyg.ch, http://www.medhyg.ch. Ed. V Barras.

610 IND ISSN 0008-0667
R97 CODEN: CMJRAY
CALCUTTA MEDICAL JOURNAL. Text in English. 1904. m. INR 12, USD 4. adv. bk.rev. abstr, charts, illus. back issues avail. *Refereed.* **Document type:** *Abstract/Index, Bibliography.*
Indexed: Biol.Abstr., Chem.Abstr., Excerp.Med., Helminthol.Abstr., Ind.Med. (coverage dropped), Nutr.Abstr.
—CASDDS, CISTI, GNLM.
Published by: Calcutta Medical Club, C.M.C. House, 91-B Chittaranjan Ave., Kolkata, West Bengal 700 073, India. TEL 91-33-270171. Ed. Urmila Khanna. Pub. Urmilla Khanna. Circ: 500.

610 ITA ISSN 0394-3291
CALEIDOSCOPIO. Text in Italian. 1983. 10/yr. ITL 20,000 per issue. adv. **Document type:** *Monographic series.*
Published by: Medical Systems S.p.A., Passo Rio Torbido, 40, Genoa, GE 16165, Italy. TEL 39-010-83401, FAX 39-010-804661, rassu@ssnet.it, http:// medicalsystems.editoria.com. Ed. Sergio Rassu. Adv. contact Giusi Cunietti.

610 ITA ISSN 1120-6756
CALEIDOSCOPIO LETTERARIO. Text in Italian. 1990. s-a. free per issue. **Document type:** *Academic/Scholarly.*
Published by: Medical Systems S.p.A., Passo Rio Torbido, 40, Genoa, GE 16165, Italy. TEL 39-010-83401, FAX 39-010-804661, rassu@ssnet.it, http:// medicalsystems.editoria.com. Ed., R&P Sergio Rassu.

CALENDAR OF CONGRESSES OF MEDICAL SCIENCES. see *MEETINGS AND CONGRESSES*

610 CHE
LE CALENDRIER MEDICAL. Text in French. 32/yr. CHF 30, EUR 19.48 (effective 2002). **Document type:** *Bulletin, Trade.*
Published by: Editions Medecine et Hygiene, Case Postale 456, Geneva, 4 1211, Switzerland. TEL 41-22-7029311, FAX 41-22-7029355, abonnements@medhyg.ch, http://www.medhyg.ch.

610 USA ISSN 0410-2894
CALIFORNIA FAMILY PHYSICIAN. Text in English. 1949. q. USD 35 (effective 2001). adv. *Refereed.* **Description:** Covers socioeconomic issues of relevance to family physicians.
Formerly: California G P
Published by: California Academy of Family Physicians, 1520 Pacific Ave, San Francisco, CA 94109. TEL 415-345-8667, FAX 415-345-8668. Ed. Jeffrey Luther. Circ: 7,000 (controlled).

610 USA
CALIFORNIA MEDICINE; the independent healthcare industry newsmagazine. Text in English. 1990. m. USD 48. adv. bk.rev. index. back issues avail. **Document type:** *Trade.*
Formerly: Northern California Medicine (1083-6535)
Published by: California Medicine Publishing, 450 Sansome St, Ste 1100, San Francisco, CA 94111. TEL 415-956-8242, 800-643-7600, FAX 415-956-8333, calmed@aol.com. Ed. Marty Lasden. Pub. David Mack. Adv. contact Denny Riley. page USD 5,000; trim 10.88 x 8.13.

616.98 338.476 USA ISSN 8750-1813
CALIFORNIA PHYSICIAN. Text in English. 1984. m. USD 45 to non-members. adv. back issues avail. **Document type:** *Trade.* **Description:** Non-clinical medical publication. Covers economic, legal, social and political issues affecting medical practice in California.
—CCC.
Published by: California Medical Association, 221 Main St, San Francisco, CA 94105. TEL 415-882-5118, FAX 415-882-5116. Ed., R&P Donna Grubb. Adv. contact Robert Shapiro. Circ: 33,000. **Subscr. to:** PO Box 7690, San Francisco, CA 94120-7690.

610 GBR ISSN 0952-1119
CAMBRIDGE MEDICINE. Text in English. 1981. 3/yr. adv. bk.rev. **Document type:** *Bulletin.*
—BLDSC (3015.962450).
Published by: University of Cambridge, Clinical School, Addenrooke's Hospital, University Of Cambridge, Hills Rd, Cambridge CB2 2SP, United Kingdom. Circ: 1,000.

610 GBR ISSN 0963-1801
R724
CAMBRIDGE QUARTERLY OF HEALTHCARE ETHICS; the international journal for healthcare ethics and ethics committees. Text in English. 1992. q. GBP 65 to individuals; USD 148 to institutions (effective 2002). adv. bk.rev. illus. back issues avail.; reprints avail. *Refereed.* **Document type:** *Academic/Scholarly.* **Description:** Provides an international forum for the wide range of issues faced by members of health care ethics committees. Devoted to the practical application of bioethics in the delivery of health care.
Related titles: Online - full text ed.: (from EBSCO Publishing, O C L C Online Computer Library Center, Inc., RoweCom Information Quest, Swets Blackwell, Institute for Scientific Information).
Indexed: ASCA, ASSIA, AgeLine, CINAHL, Curr.Cont., Fam.Ind., Ind.Med. (1992-), Int.Nurs.Ind., Phil.Ind., SSCI.
—BLDSC (3015.976000), GNLM, IDS, Infotrieve, ingenta. **CCC.**
Published by: Cambridge University Press, Edinburgh Bldg, Shaftesbury Rd, Cambridge CB2 2RU, United Kingdom. FAX 44-1223-315052, information@cup.cam.ac.uk, information@cambridge.org, http://www.cup.org/journals/ CUPJNLS.html. Eds. David C. Thomasma, Steve Heilig, Thomasine Kushner. R&P Linda Nicol. Adv. contact Rebecca Symons.

616.07 CAN ISSN 0703-8372
CANADIAN ASSOCIATION OF PATHOLOGISTS. NEWSLETTER. Text in English, French. 1969. 4/yr. membership. adv. bk.rev. **Document type:** *Newsletter.*
—CCC.
Published by: Canadian Association of Pathologists, 774 Echo Dr, Ottawa, ON K1S 5N8, Canada. TEL 613-730-6230, FAX 613-730-0260, cap@rcpsc.edu, http://www.cap.medical.org. Ed. Dr. Julius Wroblewski. R&P, Adv. contact Daniele Saintonge. Circ: 1,000.

610 CAN ISSN 0823-2105
R461
CANADIAN BULLETIN OF MEDICAL HISTORY/ BULLETIN CANADIEN D'HISTOIRE DE LA MEDECINE. Text and summaries in English, French. 1984. 2/yr. CND 60. bk.rev. back issues avail. *Refereed.* **Document type:** *Academic/Scholarly.* **Description:** Presents articles, notes, review articles and book reviews.
Indexed: Amer.Hist.& Life, CBCA Ref., Can.Per.Ind., Hist.Abstr. (1990-).
—BLDSC (3017.900000), CISTI, GNLM. **CCC.**
Published by: (Canadian Society for the History of Medicine/Societe Canadienne d'Anthropologie), Wilfrid Laurier University Press, 75 University Ave W, Waterloo, ON N2L 3C5, Canada. TEL 519-884-0710, FAX 519-725-1399, press@wlu.ca, http:// www.wlupress.wlu.ca. Ed. Jim Connor.

CANADIAN DIRECTORY OF HEALTH CARE CONFERENCES/REPERTOIRE CANADIEN DES CONFERENCES DE SOINS DE SANTE. see *MEETINGS AND CONGRESSES*

610 CAN ISSN 0008-350X
CANADIAN FAMILY PHYSICIAN/MEDECIN DE FAMILLE CANADIEN. Text in English. 1954. m. CND 78.65 domestic; CND 84 in United States; CND 115 elsewhere. adv. bk.rev. abstr, bibl, charts, illus, stat. index. *Refereed.* **Description:** Aimed at practicing, teaching and research for family physicians and general practitioners.
Formerly: College of General Practice Journal
Related titles: Online - full text ed.: (from Institute for Scientific Information).
Indexed: ASCA, CBCA Ref., Cal.Tiss.Abstr., Can.B.P.I., Curr.Cont., Environ.Sci.Poll.Mgmt., Excerp.Med., FAMLI (1980-1992), Fam.Ind., Helminthol.Abstr., Ind.Med. (1967-), Inpharma, Int.Nurs.Ind., Neurosci.Cit.Ind., Nutr.Abstr., Pharm.&Out.News, Pollut.Abstr., Protozool.Abstr., Reac., Rev.Med.& Vet.Mycol., SSCI (coverage dropped), Saf.Sci.Abstr.
—BLDSC (3022.100000), CISTI, EMDOCS, GNLM, IDS, Infotrieve, KNAW. **CCC.**
Published by: College of Family Physicians of Canada, 2630 Skymark Ave, Mississauga, ON L4W 5A4, Canada. TEL 905-629-0900, FAX 905-629-0893. Ed. Tony Dixon. Adv. contact Gloria C Bowes. Circ: 30,000.

368.382 CAN
CANADIAN HEALTH CARE MANAGEMENT. Text in English. 1986. m. CND 349. **Document type:** *Newsletter.* **Description:** Provides current, need-to-know information for health care administrators, senior personnel.

M

Published by: M P L Communications Inc., 133 Richmond St W, Ste 700, Toronto, ON M5H 3M8, Canada. TEL 416-869-1177, FAX 416-869-0456. Ed. Lynn Wintercorn. Circ: 1,100.

362.1025 CAN ISSN 1201-530X
CANADIAN HEALTHCARE SOURCE BOOK. Text in English. 1995. a. CND 119 (effective 1998-99). adv. **Document type:** *Directory.* **Description:** Direct link to vital and medical support services in Canada.
Related titles: Diskette ed.
Published by: Sherwood Publishing Inc., 18 Sixpenny Court, Thornhill, ON L3T 4E5, Canada. TEL 905-889-8505, FAX 905-889-4117. Ed. Patrick Forrett. Pub., R&P, Adv. contact Garnet Crossman.

610.715 CAN ISSN 0843-994X
CANADIAN JOURNAL OF CONTINUING MEDICAL EDUCATION. Text in English. 1989. m. USD 102 (effective 1997). adv. **Document type:** *Academic/Scholarly.*
—BLDSC (3031.040000).
Published by: S T A Communications Inc., 955 bd St Jean, bur 306, Pointe Claire, PQ H9R 5K3, Canada. TEL 514-695-7623, FAX 514-695-8554. Ed. Paul F Brand. Circ: 34,430.

610 CAN ISSN 0839-1866
CANADIAN JOURNAL OF DIAGNOSIS. Text in English. 1984. m. USD 102 (effective 1997). adv.
Formerly (until 1987): Diagnosis (0825-4656)
—BLDSC (3031.137000).
Published by: S T A Communications Inc., 955 bd St Jean, bur 306, Pointe Claire, PQ H9R 5K3, Canada. TEL 514-695-7623, FAX 514-695-8554. Ed. Paul F Brand. Circ: 34,257.

610 CAN ISSN 1203-7796
THE CANADIAN JOURNAL OF RURAL MEDICINE/JOURNAL CANADIEN DE LA MEDECINE RURALE. Short title: C J R M - J C M R. Text in English. 1996. 4/yr. CND 44; USD 50 foreign. adv. back issues avail.; reprints avail. *Refereed.* **Document type:** *Academic/Scholarly.* **Description:** Aims to promote the health of rural and native communities as well as research into rural health issues.
Related titles: Online - full text ed.: (from ProQuest Information & Learning, LexisNexis).
Indexed: CBCA Ref.
Published by: (Canadian Society of Rural Physicians), Canadian Medical Association, 1867 Alta Vista Dr, Ottawa, ON K1H 5K9, Canada. TEL 613-731-9331, FAX 613-565-2382, pubs@cma.ca; cjrm@fox.nstn.ca, http://www.cma.ca/cjrm. Ed. Dr. John Wootton. Adv. contact Beverley Kirkpatrick. B&W page CND 900, color page CND 2,100; trim 10.88 x 8.13. Circ: 6,100.

CANADIAN JOURNAL OF VETERINARY RESEARCH/REVUE CANADIENNE DE RECHERCHE VETERINAIRE. see *VETERINARY SCIENCE*

610 CAN ISSN 0068-9203
R713.01
CANADIAN MEDICAL DIRECTORY. Text in English. 1954. a. CND 195 (effective 2000). adv. **Document type:** *Directory.* **Description:** Lists doctors both alphabetically and geographically within Canada. Includes addresses, telephone numbers, certifications and specializations, languages spoken.
—GNLM.
Published by: Southam Information Products Ltd., 1450 Don Mills Rd, Don Mills, ON M3B 2X7, Canada. TEL 416-445-6641, 800-668-2374, FAX 416-442-2200. Ed. Christopher Rajan. Pub., Adv. contact Doug Finley.

616.994 FRA ISSN 1292-8658
THE CANCER JOURNAL (ONLINE EDITION)/JOURNAL DU CANCER. Text in French, English. 1995. bi-m.
Formerly (until 1998): The Cancer Journal (Print Edition) (0765-7846)
Media: Online - full content.
Indexed: Int.Abstr.Biol.Sci.
Published by: Association pour le Developpement de la Communication Cancerologique, BP 8, Villejuif Cedex 94801, France. TEL 33-1-49583600, FAX 33-1-49583542, salomon@infobiogen.fr, http://www.infobiogen.fr/agora/journals/cancer/. Ed. Jean-Claude Salomon.

616.04 CAN ISSN 0226-2347
CANDID FACTS/A PROPOS. Text in English, French. 1960. q. free per issue. **Document type:** *Newsletter.*
Published by: Canadian Cystic Fibrosis Foundation, 2221 Yonge St, Ste 601, Toronto, ON M4S 2B4, Canada. TEL 416-485-9149, 800-378-2233, FAX 416-485-0960, info@ccff.ca, postmaster@ccff.ca, http://www.ccff.ca, http://www.ccff.ca/~cfwww/index.html. Ed., R&P June Pierotti. Circ: 12,000.

610 ZAF
THE CAPE DOCTOR. Text in Afrikaans, English. 1959. 4/yr. membership. illus. **Document type:** *Newsletter.*
Former titles (until vol.33, no.1, 1993): M A S A News - Cape Western Branch; (until vol.21, no.1, 1981): Medical Association of South Africa. Cape Western Branch. Newsletter
Published by: Medical Association of South Africa, Cape Western Branch, Private Bag X1, Pinelands 7430, South Africa. TEL 27-21-5313081, FAX 27-21-5314126.

610 ITA ISSN 0576-7202
CARDARELLI; medicina - chirurgia - specialita. Text in Italian. q. free per issue to members. adv. **Description:** Publishes original works on clinical and experimental subjects.
—GNLM.
Published by: Scuola Medica Ospedaliera, Casella Postale 1102, Naples, NA 80100, Italy. Ed. R Sessa.

610 615.89 USA
CARE MAGAZINE; South Carolina's premeir waiting room publication. Text in English. 10/yr. adv. **Description:** Focuses on wellness, new developments in medicine and their effects, new products and individual profiles. Also includes information on low cost medical alternatives and contains a special section for seniors with related lifestyle features.
Published by: Catalyst Media Group, 704 Jane Way, Beaufort, SC 29902. TEL 843-524-8988, FAX 843-524-4113.

610 USA ISSN 1053-5500
CASE MANAGEMENT ADVISOR. Text in English. 1990. m. USD 299 domestic; USD 329 foreign; USD 50 newsstand/cover (effective 2001). **Document type:** *Newsletter.*
Indexed: CINAHL.
—BLDSC (3058.137200).
Published by: American Health Consultants (Subsidiary of: Medical Economics Co., Inc.), 3525 Piedmont Rd, N E, 6 Piedmont Center, Ste 400, Atlanta, GA 30305. TEL 404-262-5476, 404-262-7436, 800-688-2421, FAX 404-262-7837, 800-284-3291, custserv@ahcpub.com, http://www.ahcpub.com. Circ: 1,850.

368.382 USA ISSN 1061-9259
THE CASE MANAGER. Text in English. 1990. bi-m. USD 52 domestic to individuals; USD 72 foreign to individuals; USD 65 domestic to institutions; USD 85 foreign to institutions; USD 20 foreign to students; USD 15 newsstand/cover (effective 2001). adv. bk.rev. index. back issues avail.; reprints avail. **Document type:** *Journal, Trade.* **Description:** Provides education, marketing and networking support to medical case managers who coordinate and manage services involving large or serious claims in the health and compensation industry.
Related titles: Online - full text ed.: (from IDEAL Online Library, RoweCom Information Quest).
Indexed: CINAHL, Inpharma, Pharm.&Out.News, Reac.
—BLDSC (3058.137230), Infotrieve. **CCC.**
Published by: (Case Management Society of America), Mosby, Inc. (Subsidiary of: Elsevier Science), 11830 Westline Industrial Dr, St Louis, MO 63146-3318. TEL 314-872-8370, 800-325-4177, FAX 314-432-1380, periodical.service@mosby.com, http://www.mosby.com/periodicals. Eds. Catherine M Mullahy, Tom Strickland. Pub. Nathania Sawyer. Adv. contact Tracey Schriefer TEL 314-453-4304. B&W page USD 2,065, color page USD 2,595; trim 10.88 x 8.13. Circ: 20,000.

610 CZE ISSN 0008-7335
CODEN: CLCEAL
CASOPIS LEKARU CESKYCH. Text in Czech, Slovak; Summaries in Czech, English. 1862. 24/yr. EUR 120, USD 144 (effective 2001). adv. bk.rev. bibl, charts, illus. index. *Refereed.* **Document type:** *Academic/Scholarly.* **Description:** Publishes original scientific papers from all branches of medicine as well as reviews on selected topics for postgraduate training.
Indexed: Abstr.Hyg., AgBiotech, Anim.Breed.Abstr., Biol.Abstr., C.I.S. Abstr., Chem.Abstr., Curr.Adv.Ecol.Sci., Dent.Ind., Excerp.Med., INIS Atomind., Ind.Med. (1862-), Ind.Vet., Nutr.Abstr., Plant Breed.Abstr., Poult.Abstr., Rev.Appl.Entomol., Soils & Fert.
—BLDSC (3061.400000), CASDDS, CISTI, EMDOCS, GNLM, IDS, Infotrieve, KNAW. **CCC.**
Published by: (Ceska Lekarska Spolecnost J.E. Purkyne/Czech Medical Association), Nakladatelske Stredisko C L S J.E. Purkyne, Sokolska 31, Prague 12026, Czech Republic. TEL 420-2-24911420, FAX 420-2-24911420, http://www.clsjep.cz. Ed. J Petrasek. adv.: B&W page CZK 27,300, color page CZK 41,000; 260 x 177. Circ: 1,500. **Dist. by:** Abont s.r.o., Chlumova 17, Prague, 3 130 00, Czech Republic; **Dist. in Western countries by:** Kubon & Sagner, Hesstr 39-41, Munich 80798, Germany.

610 ESP
CATALOGO DE TRABAJOS DE INVESTIGACION EN SALUD. Text in Spanish. 1990. a.
Published by: (Basque Region. Osasunketa eta Kontsumo Saila/Departamento de Sanidad y Consumo), Eusko Jaurlaritzaren Argitalpen-Zerbitzu Nagusia/Servicio Central de Publicaciones del Gobierno Vasco, Donostia-San Sebastian, 1, Vitoria-gasteiz, Alava 01010, Spain. TEL 34-945-018561, FAX 34-945-018709, hac-sabd@ej-gv.es, http://www.ej-gv.net/publicaciones. Circ: 2,000.

CATHOLIC MEDICAL QUARTERLY. see *RELIGIONS AND THEOLOGY—Roman Catholic*

610 KOR
CATHOLIC UNIVERSITY MEDICAL COLLEGE JOURNAL✱ . Text in English, Korean; Summaries in English. 1957. q. free per issue.
Formerly: Catholic Medical College Journal
Indexed: Biol.Abstr., Chem.Abstr.
Published by: Catholic University, Graduate School, c/o Catholic Medical College, 505 Banpo-dong, Kangnam-gu, Seoul 135, Korea, S.. TEL 02-593-5141, FAX 02-532-3112. Ed. Dr. Yong Whee Bahk. Circ: 1,000 (controlled).

CELL CALCIUM (EDINBURGH). see *BIOLOGY—Cytology And Histology*

616.01 USA ISSN 1355-8145
CODEN: CSCHFG
CELL STRESS & CHAPERONES. Text in English. 1996. q. USD 105 to membership; USD 367 combined subscription domestic to institutions for both print & online eds.; USD 378 combined subscription foreign to institutions for both print & online eds. (effective 2002). adv. back issues avail. *Refereed.* **Document type:** *Academic/Scholarly.* **Description:** Publishes research on stress proteins and molecular chaperones.
Related titles: Online - full text ed.: USD 315 to institutions (effective 2002) (from BioOne, EBSCO Publishing, RoweCom Information Quest, IDEAL Online Library, Institute for Scientific Information).
Indexed: Cal.Tiss.Abstr., Chem.Abstr., Chem.Indus.Notes, Chem.Titles, Curr.Cont., Ind.Med. (1996-), Inpharma, Microbiol.Abstr., Nuc.Acids Abstr., Reac., Ref.Zh., Virol.Abstr. (coverage dropped), Zoo.Rec.
—BLDSC (3097.865000), CASDDS, GNLM, IDS, Infotrieve, KNAW. **CCC.**
Published by: Cell Stress Society International, Dept of Molecular & Cell Biology, 75 N Eagleville Rd, Storrs, CT 06269-3044. TEL 860-486-4257, FAX 860-486-5709, helen.neumann@uconn.edu, http://199.245.200.216/cestonline/?request=index-html, http://www.cellstress.uconn.edu/. Ed. Lawrence E Hightower.

610.28 USA ISSN 1051-6794
R857.M3 CODEN: CEMAEE
CELLS AND MATERIALS. Text in English. 1991. q. USD 75; USD 90 foreign. *Refereed.* **Document type:** *Academic/Scholarly.* **Description:** The scope of topics covered includes cardiovascular, ocular, and orthopedic prostheses, drug delivery systems, and related topics. Emphasis is on morphological aspects of replaceable tissues, and their subsequent fortification or substitution by a biomaterial.
Indexed: ASCA, Alloys Ind., Bioeng.Abstr., Chem.Abstr., Chem.Indus.Notes, Chem.Titles, Curr.Cont. (coverage dropped), Eng.Mat.Abstr., Excerp.Med. (1995-), Ind.Sci.Rev., METADEX, Mat.Sci.Cit.Ind. (coverage dropped), Met.Abstr.Ind., Nonfer.Met.Alert, PCC Alert, Sci.Cit.Ind. (coverage dropped), Steels Alert, World Alum.Abstr.
—BLDSC (3097.913000), CASDDS, CISTI, Ei, EMDOCS, GNLM, IDS, Infotrieve, ingenta, KNAW, Linda Hall. **CCC.**
Published by: Scanning Microscopy International, Inc., 1034 Alabam Dr, Elk Grove Village, IL 60007-2920. TEL 708-529-6677, FAX 708-980-6698. Ed. Dr. A Jay Wasserman.

M

611 CHE ISSN 1422-6405
QL801
CELLS, TISSUES, ORGANS; in vivo, in vitro. Text in English. 1938-1938; N.S. 1945. 8/yr. CHF 2,574 in Europe to institutions; CHF 2,608.80 overseas to institutions; EUR 1,839.60 in Europe to institutions; USD 1,995 overseas to institutions (effective 2002). adv. abstr, illus. index. back issues avail.; reprint service avail. from ISI. *Refereed.* **Document type:** *Journal, Academic/Scholarly.* **Description:** Offers rapid exchange of novel and significant information gained from experimental and theoretical investigations on all aspects that are pertinent to the formation and transformation of biological structure.
Former titles (1945-1998): Acta Anatomica (0001-5180); (in 1938): Bio-morphosis (1421-6582)
Related titles: Microform ed.: (from PMC,RPI); Online - full text ed.: ISSN 1422-6421. CHF 174, EUR 126, USD 135 to institutions (effective 2002) (from EBSCO Publishing, O C L C Online Computer Library Center, Inc., RoweCom Information Quest, Swets Blackwell, Institute for Scientific Information).
Indexed: ASCA, Abstr.Anthropol., Anim.Breed.Abstr., Aqua.Sci.& Fish.Abstr., Biol.Abstr., Cal.Tiss.Abstr., Chem.Abstr., Chem.Indus.Notes, Chem.Titles, Curr.Adv.Ecol.Sci., Curr.Cont., Dairy Sci.Abstr., Dent.Ind., Excerp.Med., GeoRef, Ind.Med. (1999-), Ind.Sci.Rev., Ind.Vet., Inpharma, Int.Abstr.Biol.Sci., Neurosci.Cit.Ind., Pig News & Info., Poult.Abstr., Reac., SSCI (coverage dropped), Sci.Cit.Ind., Small Anim.Abstr., Sport Fish.Abstr., Vet.Bull., Wild.Rev., Zoo.Rec.
—BLDSC (3097.916000), CASDDS, CISTI, EMDOCS, GNLM, IDS, ingenta, KNAW, Linda Hall. **CCC.**
Published by: S. Karger AG, Allschwilerstr 10, PO Box, Basel 4009, Switzerland. TEL 41-61-306-1111, FAX 41-61-306-1234, karger@karger.ch, http://www.online.karger.com/journals/cto, http://www.karger.com. Eds. A W English, H Denker. adv.: page USD 1,185. Circ: 1,200.

616 JPN ISSN 0078-6632
CENTER FOR ADULT DISEASES, OSAKA. ANNUAL REPORT. Text in English. 1961. a. free per issue.
Indexed: Biol.Abstr., Excerp.Med.
Published by: Center for Adult Diseases Osaka, 1-3-3 Naka-Michi, Higashinari-ku, Osaka-shi 537-0025, Japan. Ed. Dr. Nobuyuki Senda.

610 USA
CENTERSCOPE. Text in English. 3/yr. **Description:** Informs alumni and friends of research and events at the School of Medicine.
Published by: Boston University, School of Medicine, Office of Publication Services, 80 E Concord St, Boston, MA 02118. Ed. Owen McNamara. Circ: 13,000.

610 ZWE ISSN 0008-9176
CODEN: CAJMA3
CENTRAL AFRICAN JOURNAL OF MEDICINE. Text in English. 1955. m. ZWD 500 domestic to individuals; USD 210 to individuals in US & Europe; USD 160 in Africa to individuals; ZWD 620 domestic to institutions; ZWD 230 to institutions in US & Europe; ZWD 215 in Africa to institutions (effective 2001). adv. bk.rev. charts, illus. index. reprint service avail. from ISI. **Document type:** *Academic/Scholarly.*
Related titles: CD-ROM ed.
Indexed: Abstr.Anthropol., Abstr.Hyg., Aqua.Sci.& Fish.Abstr., Biol.Abstr., Chem.Abstr., Curr.Adv.Ecol.Sci., Curr.Cont. (coverage dropped), Dairy Sci.Abstr., Dent.Ind., Diar.Dis.Res., Environ.Sci.Poll.Mgmt., Excerp.Med., ExtraMED, Helminthol.Abstr., Ind.Med. (1955-), Ind.S.A.Per., Int.Nurs.Ind., NRN, Nutr.Abstr., Pollut.Abstr., Protozool.Abstr., Rev.Appl.Entomol., Rev.Med.& Vet.Mycol., Rev.Plant Path., Sport Fish.Abstr., Trop.Dis.Bull.
—BLDSC (3105.800000), CISTI, GNLM, IDS, ingenta, KNAW.
Published by: (University of Zimbabwe, Faculty of Medicine), Central African Journal of Medicine Co., Avondale, PO Box A 195, Harare, Zimbabwe. TEL 263-4-791631. Ed. H M Chinyanga. Circ: 1,500.

610 USA ISSN 0008-946X
CENTRAL NEW YORK ACADEMY OF MEDICINE. BULLETIN. Text in English. 1936. s-a. USD 4. adv. charts, illus, stat.
Published by: Central New York Academy of Medicine, 4311 Middle Settlement Rd, New Hartford, NY 13413. TEL 315-735-2204. Ed. Mary Lou Manchester. R&P, Adv. contact Sharon Gulla. Circ: 670. **Co-sponsor:** Medical Societies of the Counties of Oneida, Herkimer, Madison and Chenango.

610 MDG
CENTRE D'INFORMATION ET DE DOCUMENTATION SCIENTIFIQUE ET TECHNIQUE. RECHERCHES POUR LE DEVELOPPEMENT. SERIE MEDECINE. Text in French; Summaries in English, French. 2/yr. MGF 60, USD 10.
Published by: Centre d'Information et de Documentation Scientifique et Technique, BP 6224, Antananarivo 101, Madagascar. TEL 33288.

CENTRE FOR MEDICINES RESEARCH WORKSHOP. see *PHARMACY AND PHARMACOLOGY*

CEREBRAL CORTEX. see *MEDICAL SCIENCES—Psychiatry And Neurology*

610 TUR ISSN 1300-5227
CERRAHPASA TIP DERGISI/CERRAHPASA JOURNAL OF MEDICINE. Text in Turkish; Summaries in English. 1970. q. abstr, bibl, charts, illus. index. **Document type:** *Academic/Scholarly.* **Description:** Contains research studies of the Cerrahpasa Medical Faculty.
Formerly (until vol.26, 1995): Cerrahpasa Tip Fakultesi Dergisi - Cerrahpasa Medical Faculty. Journal (0376-7833)
Indexed: Excerp.Med.
—BLDSC (3120.125700), EMDOCS, GNLM.
Published by: Istanbul Universitesi, Cerrahpasa Tip Fakultesi, Aksaray - Istanbul 34303, Turkey. Ed. Yalcin Tuzun.

616.07 571.9 CZE ISSN 1210-7875
CODEN: CPSLAE
CESKO-SLOVENSKA PATOLOGIE A SOUDNI LEKARSTVI. Text in Czech; Summaries in Czech, English. 1965. q. EUR 60, USD 76 (effective 2001). adv. bk.rev. index. *Refereed.*
Formerly (until 1993): Ceskoslovenska Patologie (0009-0611)
Indexed: Biol.Abstr., Chem.Abstr., Curr.Adv.Ecol.Sci., Curr.Cont. (coverage dropped), Excerp.Med., INIS Atomind., Ind.Med. (1965-).
—CISTI, GNLM, Infotrieve. **CCC.**
Published by: (Ceska Lekarska Spolecnost J.E. Purkyne/Czech Medical Association), Nakladatelske Stredisko C L S J.E. Purkyne, Sokolska 31, Prague 12026, Czech Republic. TEL 42-2-42911420, FAX 42-2-24911420, nts@iol.cz, http://www.clsjep.cz, http://www.medical.cz. Ed. Ivo Steiner. adv.: B&W page CZK 17,700, color page CZK 26,600; 250 x 170. Circ: 1,100. **Dist. by:** Abont s.r.o., Chlumova 17, Prague, 3 130 00, Czech Republic; **Dist. in Western Countries by:** Kubon & Sagner, Hesstr 39-41, Munich 80798, Germany.

610 LKA ISSN 0011-2232
CEYLON JOURNAL OF MEDICAL SCIENCE. Text in English. 1949. 2/yr. USD 10 foreign (effective 2000). bk.rev. charts, illus. back issues avail. *Refereed.* **Document type:** *Academic/Scholarly.* **Description:** Covers all branches of medical, dental, and veterinary sciences.
Indexed: Biol.Abstr., Chem.Abstr., Helminthol.Abstr., Ind.Med. (coverage dropped), Nutr.Abstr., Protozool.Abstr., Rev.Appl.Entomol., Sri Lanka Sci.Ind., Trop.Dis.Bull.
—CISTI.
Published by: University of Colombo, Faculty of Medicine, Kynsey Rd., Colombo 8, Sri Lanka. TEL 94-1-695230, FAX 94-1-695230. Eds. Dr. R L Jayakody, T W Wikramanayake. R&P Dr. R L Jayakody. Circ: 125 (controlled). **Subscr. to:** Librarian, University of Colombo, Colombo, Sri Lanka.

610 LKA ISSN 0009-0875
CEYLON MEDICAL JOURNAL. Text in English. 1887. q. USD 150 (effective 2000). adv. bk.rev. illus, charts. *Refereed.* **Document type:** *Academic/Scholarly.* **Description:** Contains original papers and reviews and case reports.
Related titles: CD-ROM ed.; Online - full text ed.
Indexed: Abstr.Hyg., Biol.Abstr., Chem.Abstr., Dairy Sci.Abstr., Diar.Dis.Res., Excerp.Med., ExtraMED, Helminthol.Abstr., Ind.Med. (1952-), Ind.Vet., Nutr.Abstr., Rev.Appl.Entomol., Rev.Med.& Vet.Mycol., Rural Devel.Abstr., Sri Lanka Sci.Ind., Trop.Dis.Bull., Weed Abstr.
—BLDSC (3128.200000), CISTI, GNLM, ingenta, KNAW.
Published by: Sri Lanka Medical Association, Wijerama House, 6 Wijerama Mawatha, Colombo 7, Sri Lanka. TEL 94-1-693324, FAX 94-1-698802, SLMA@eureka.lk, http://www.medinet.lk/professional/cmj/CMJhome.html, http://www.medianet.lk/professional/cmj/CMJhome.html. Eds. Colvin Goonaratna, Janaka de Silva. adv.: B&W page USD 350, color page USD 500. Circ: 1,300.

610 658 USA
CHANGING MEDICAL MARKETS; the international monthly newsletter for executives in the healthcare and biotechnology industries. Text in English. 1978. m. USD 295 domestic; USD 325 foreign (effective 2000). back issues avail. **Document type:** *Newsletter.* **Description:** Comprehensive coverage of corporate activities, new products and services, emerging opportunities around the world, technology assessment, the impact of legislation and news from healthcare associations and meetings.
Indexed: Nonwov.Abstr.
Published by: Theta Corporation, 2433 Main St., Ste. 4, Rocky Hall, CT 06067-2539. Ed., R&P Phyllis Klaben. Circ: (controlled).

610 USA
CHECK SAMPLE. Text in English. 1949. bi-w. USD 2,140 (effective 2000); for complete series; price varies for individual subject area. **Description:** Each series consists of exercises which present patient cases for continuing medical education study supplemented with kodachromes or specimen glass slides. Each participant receives ICME credit for each exercise completed.
Formerly (until 1958): Institute for Clinical Science. Proficiency Test Service. Report (0073-8638)
Published by: American Society of Clinical Pathologists, 2100 W Harrison St, Chicago, IL 60612. TEL 312-738-1336, FAX 312-738-1619. Ed. Jay L Bock. Pub. Joshua Weikersheimer. R&P Nick Watters. Circ: 1,200.

610 DEU
CHEFAERZTE BRIEF. Text in German. m. DEM 258.17, EUR 132 (effective 2001). **Document type:** *Journal, Trade.*
Published by: (Institut fuer Wirtschaftspublizistik), Vogel Verlag und Druck GmbH & Co. KG, Max-Planck-Str 7-9, Wuerzburg 97064, Germany. TEL 49-931-4535399, FAX 49-931-4535399, http://www.vogel-medien.de.

610 USA
CHEMSCOPE. Text in English. 1995. d. free per issue. **Document type:** *Trade.* **Description:** Covers news relevant to the medical device and diagnostics industry.
Media: Online - full text.
Indexed: Petrol.Energy B.N.I.
Published by: Chemscope, Inc., PO Box 60623, Palo Alto, CA 94306. TEL 415-531-6319, FAX 650-903-1681, info@chemscope.com, http://chemscope.com. Pub. Russell D Beste.

610 THA ISSN 0125-5983
CODEN: CMMBB2
CHIANG MAI MEDICAL BULLETIN. Text in English, Thai. 1961. q. THB 80, USD 40 to individuals; USD 100 to institutions. adv. bk.rev. abstr, charts, illus, stat.
Indexed: Chem.Abstr., Diar.Dis.Res.
Published by: Chiang Mai University, Faculty of Medicine, 110 Intavaroros St, Chiang Mai 50002, Thailand. TEL 52-221122, FAX 53-217144. Ed. Dr. Watana Navacharoen. Circ: 1,000 (controlled).

610 JPN ISSN 0303-5476
CODEN: CIZAAZ
CHIBA IGAKU ZASSHI/CHIBA MEDICAL JOURNAL. Text in Japanese; Summaries in English. 1923. bi-m. JPY 4,000, USD 40. adv. bk.rev. *Refereed.* **Document type:** *Academic/Scholarly.* **Description:** Presents review articles, original papers, case reports, and news of the society.
Formerly: Chiba Medical Society. Journal (0009-3459)
Indexed: Biol.Abstr., Chem.Abstr., Chem.Indus.Notes, Chem.Titles, Excerp.Med., INIS Atomind.
—CASDDS, GNLM.
Published by: Chiba Igakkai/Chiba Medical Society, c/o Chiba Daigaku Igakubu, 1-8-1 Inohana, Chuo-ku, Chiba 260-0856, Japan. TEL 81-43-222-7171, FAX 81-43-226-2005, http://www.m.chiba-u.ac.jp/med-journal. Ed. Yoshio Nakajima. Circ: 3,200.

610 JPN ISSN 0910-7436
CHIBAKEN ISHIKAI ZASSHI/CHIBA MEDICAL ASSOCIATION. JOURNAL. Text in Japanese. 1949. m. JPY 400 per issue.
Published by: Chibaken Ishikai, 5-25 Chibako, Chuo-ku, Chiba-shi 260-0000, Japan.

M

610 USA ISSN 0009-3637
R15
CHICAGO MEDICINE. Text in English. 1902. m. USD 30 to non-members; USD 15 to members (effective 2001). adv. bk.rev. charts, illus. index. *Refereed.* **Document type:** *Trade.* **Description:** Provides a forum for the discussion of medical, ethical, legal, socioeconomic, and other concerns affecting physicians in Chicago and Cook County.
Indexed: Med.Care Rev.
Published by: Chicago Medical Society, 515 N Dearborn, Chicago, IL 60610. TEL 312-670-2550, FAX 312-670-3646. Ed. Liz Sidney. R&P Gary Baldwin. adv.: B&W page USD 500. Circ: 11,000 (controlled).

610 JPN ISSN 0911-5528
CHIGASAKI MEDICUS. Text in English, Japanese. 1985. a.
Published by: Chigasaki Tokushukai Sogo Byoin/Chigasaki Tokushukai Medical Center, 14-1 Saiwai-cho, Chigasaki-shi, Kanagawa-ken 253-0052, Japan.

610 USA ISSN 0069-3685
CHINA MEDICAL BOARD OF NEW YORK. ANNUAL REPORT. Text in English. 1951. a. membership.
Published by: China Medical Board of New York, 750 Third Ave, New York, NY 10003. TEL 212-682-8000, FAX 212-9949-8726. Circ: 300.

610 615 CHN
CHINA PHARMACEUTICAL AND MEDICAL INSTRUMENTS✱ . Text in Chinese, English. q. USD 55.20 (effective 1994). **Description:** Covers Chinese medicine, pharmaceuticals, medical apparatuses and instruments, pharmaceutical production machinery and packaging.
Published by: (State Pharmaceutical Administration of China), China National Publications Import & Export Corporation Ed. Shi Huan. **Dist. by:** 16 Gongti Dong Lu, Chaoyang-qu, PO Box 88, Beijing 100020, China. TEL 01-506-6688.

610 CHN ISSN 1007-8053
CHINESE ACADEMIC JOURNAL. MEDICINE & HYGIENE. Text in Chinese, English. m. USD 120 for the 1st series; USD 6 for each additonal series (effective 2000). **Document type:** *Academic/Scholarly.* **Description:** Covers medicine, hygiene, health care medicine of biology.
Media: CD-ROM (from Chinese Academic Journal (CD), Electronic Journals Publishing House). **Related titles:** Microfiche ed.; Microfilm ed.; Online - full content ed.: 1998 (from WanFang Data Corp.); Online - full text ed.: (from WanFang Data Corp.); ♦ Print ed.: Huaxi Yixue. ISSN 1002-0179; ♦ Zhonghua Shiyan he Linchuang Bingduxue Zazhi. ISSN 1003-9279; ♦ Difangbing Tongbao. ISSN 1000-3711; ♦ Zhonghua Jiehe he Huxi Zazhi. ISSN 1001-0939.
Published by: Chinese Academic Journal (CD), Electronic Journals Publishing House, Tsing Hua University, P.O.BOX 84-48, Beijing 100084, China. TEL 86-1-62781584, 86-10-62396338, FAX 86-1-62771042, 86-10-62396355, caj_cd@tsinghua.edu.cn, http://www.cajcd.edu.cn. **Co-sponsor:** Tsinghua University.

610 CHN ISSN 1006-6497
CHINESE JOURNAL OF INTEGRATED TRADITIONAL AND WESTERN MEDICINE. Text in English. q. USD 43.20; USD 3.60 newsstand/cover (effective 2001). bk.rev. abstr. 80 p./no. reprints avail. *Refereed.* **Document type:** *Journal, Academic/Scholarly.* **Description:** Covers the study of traditional Chinese medicine with modern science and technology.
Related titles: Online - full content ed.: (from WanFang Data Corp.); ♦ Chinese ed.: Zhongguo Zhongxiyi Jiehe Zazhi. ISSN 1003-5370.
Indexed: Ind.Med. (coverage dropped).
Published by: (Zhongyi Yanjiuyuan/Academy of Traditional Chinese Medicine), Zhongguo Zhong-Xiyi Jiehe Yanjiuhui/Chinese Association of the Integration of Traditional and Western Medicine (Subsidiary of: Zhongyi Yanjiuyuan/Academy of Traditional Chinese Medicine), 1 Caochang, Xiyuan, Beijing 100091, China. FAX 86-1-6264-2194, cjim@cjim.net. Circ: 300 (paid); 100 (controlled). **Dist. by:** China International Book Trading Corp, 35 Chegongzhuang Xilu, Haidian District, Beijing 100044, China. yf@mail.cibtc.com.cn, http://www.cibtc.com.cn.

CHINESE JOURNAL OF PHYSIOLOGY/CHUNG-KUO SHENG LI HSUEH TSA CHIH. see *BIOLOGY—Physiology*

610 TWN ISSN 0578-1337
R97.7.C5 CODEN: CIHCDM
CHINESE MEDICAL JOURNAL. Text in English; Summaries in Chinese, English. 1915. m. TWD 1,250, USD 60 domestic to individuals; USD 85 in Asia to individuals; USD 95 elsewhere to individuals; TWD 1,100 domestic medical school staff and students (effective 2000). adv. index. **Document type:** *Journal, Academic/Scholarly.* **Description:** Covers basic, experimental and clinical medical sciences, includes original articles and case reports and review articles.
Indexed: Excerp.Med., Ind.Med. (1954-), Neurosci.Cit.Ind., Nutr.Abstr., Protozool.Abstr., Rev.Med.& Vet.Mycol., Trop.Dis.Bull.
—BLDSC (3181.010000), CISTI, EMDOCS, GNLM.
Published by: (Chinese Medical Association - Taipei), Excerpta Medica Asia Ltd., 17-F 8 Commercial Tower, 9 Sun Yip St, Chai Wan, Hong Kong, Hong Kong. TEL 852-2965-1300, FAX 852-2976-0778, effie@excerptahk.com, http://www.vghtpe.gov.tw/~cmj/. Ed. Mau Song Chang. Pub. Fang Ku Peng.

610 CHN ISSN 0366-6999
CODEN: CMJODS
CHINESE MEDICAL JOURNAL/ZHONGHUA YIXUE ZAZHI YINGWEN BAN. Text in English. 1887-1966; resumed 1975. m. USD 348; USD 29 newsstand/cover (effective 2001). adv. bk.rev. abstr, bibl, charts, illus. back issues avail. *Refereed.* **Document type:** *Academic/Scholarly.* **Description:** Introduces advances and research results in China's medical sciences and technology, serving primarily senior medical clinicians and research personnel of high academic level.
Formerly (until 1932): China Missionary Medical Journal
Related titles: CD-ROM ed.; Microfilm ed.: (from PQC); Online - full content ed.: (from WanFang Data Corp.); Online - full text ed.: (from Institute for Scientific Information); ♦ Chinese ed.: Zhonghua Yixue Zazhi. ISSN 0376-2491.
Indexed: AMED, ASCA, Abstr.Hyg., Biol.Abstr., Chem.Abstr., Curr.Adv.Ecol.Sci., Curr.Cont., Dairy Sci.Abstr., Dent.Abstr., Dent.Ind., Derwent Biotech.Abstr., Diar.Dis.Res., Excerp.Med. (1983-), Helminthol.Abstr., I.P.A., Ind.Med. (1975-), Ind.Sci.Rev., Med.Care Rev., Nutr.Abstr., Protozool.Abstr., Rehabil.Lit., Rev.Appl.Entomol., Rev.Arom.& Med.Plants, Rev.Med.& Vet.Mycol., Rev.Plant Path., SSCI (coverage dropped), Sci.Cit.Ind., Trop.Dis.Bull.
—BLDSC (3180.990000), CASDDS, CISTI, EMDOCS, GNLM, IDS, ingenta, KNAW.
Published by: Zhonghua Yixuehui/Chinese Medical Association, 42 Dongsi Xidajie, Beijing 100710, China. TEL 86-1-6527-1226, FAX 86-1-6400-4231, order@cmj.org, http://www.cmj.org. Ed. Qian Yijian. Pub., R&P Wang De. Adv. contact Wang Ling. Circ: 4,000 (paid); 1,000 (controlled). **Dist. by:** China International Book Trading Corp, 35, Chegongzhuang Xilu, Haidian District, Beijing 100044, China. TEL 86-1-68413849, FAX 86-1-68412048, cibtc@mail.cibtc.com.cn, http://www.cibtc.com.cn.

610 CHN ISSN 1001-9294
CODEN: CMSJEP
CHINESE MEDICAL SCIENCES JOURNAL. Text in English. 1986. q. GBP 153, USD 251 to institutions (effective 2002). adv. bk.rev. bibl, charts. index. back issues avail. *Refereed.* **Document type:** *Academic/Scholarly.* **Description:** Presents recent advances in medical research. Includes information on clinical medicine, pharmacology, as well as traditional Chinese medicine.
Formerly (until 1991): Chinese Academy of Medical Sciences and Peking Union Medical College. Proceedings - Zhongguo Yixue Kexueyuan, Zhongguo Xiehe Yike Daxue Xuebao (0258-8757)
Related titles: CD-ROM ed.; Online - full content ed.: (from WanFang Data Corp.).
Indexed: Chem.Abstr., Chem.Indus.Notes, Chem.Titles, Excerp.Med., Ind.Med. (1991-).
—BLDSC (3181.012000), CASDDS, CISTI, EMDOCS, GNLM, KNAW.
Published by: Chinese Academy of Medical Sciences/Zhongguo Yixue Kexueyuan, 9 Dong Dan San Tiao, Beijing 100730, China. TEL 86-10-5133074, FAX 86-10-6529-5931, TELEX 222689-CAMS-CN, zhongzh@cdm.imicams.ac.cn, http://www.chinainfo.gov.cn/periodical. Ed. Bao Denian. Circ: 1,500. **Subscr. to:** Taylor & Francis Ltd., Rankine Rd, Basingstoke, Hants RG24 0PR, United Kingdom. TEL 44-1256-840366, 800-821-8312, FAX 215—269-0363, 44-1256-479438.

610 FRA ISSN 1240-3156
CHIRURGIE ENDOSCOPIQUE. Text in French. 1992. 4/yr. FRF 665 domestic to individuals; FRF 875 foreign to individuals; FRF 485 to students (effective 2000).
Published by: Meditions Carline, 1 et 3 rue du Depart, Paris 75014, France. TEL 33-1-40640075, FAX 33-1-43222699, groupemeditions@wanadoo.fr.

610 AUS ISSN 1443-3591
CHISHOLM HEALTH ETHICS BULLETIN. Text in English. q. **Document type:** *Bulletin.*
Published by: Caroline Chisholm Centre for Health Ethics, Level 7, 166 Gipps St, East Melbourne, VIC 3002, Australia. TEL 61-3-92702681, FAX 61-3-92702682, ccche@mercy-com.au, http://www.mercyhealth.net/chisholmhealthethics/. Ed. Norman Ford. Circ: 1,100.

CHOICES; sexual and reproductive health and rights in Europe. see *POPULATION STUDIES*

616.07 ITA ISSN 1120-0030
CHOLESTEROL NEWS. Text in Italian. 1989. q. adv. **Document type:** *Newsletter.*
Published by: C I C Edizioni Internazionali s.r.l., Corso Trieste 42, Rome, RM 00198, Italy. TEL 39-06-8412673, FAX 39-06-8412688, info@gruppocic.it, 1160199510. Ed. G Crepaldi. adv.: B&W page ITL 3,100,000, color page ITL 3,900,000; trim 210 x 290.

610 CHN ISSN 1000-7911
CHONGQING YIYAO/CHONGQING MEDICINE. Text in Chinese. bi-m.
Published by: Chongqing Yixue Qingbao Yanjiusuo, 44 Qingnian Lu, Chongqing, Sichuan 630010, China.

CHRIS; Kinderzeitschrift der Christoffel-Blindenmission. see *CHILDREN AND YOUTH—For*

174.2 241.642 NLD ISSN 1380-3603
R725.56 CODEN: CHBIF5
CHRISTIAN BIOETHICS; non-ecumenical studies in medical morality. Text and summaries in English. 1995. 3/yr., latest vol.7, 2001. NLG 109, USD 59 to individuals; NLG 340, USD 174 to institutions (effective 2001). adv. bk.rev. index. back issues avail.; reprint service avail. from SWZ. *Refereed.* **Document type:** *Journal, Academic/Scholarly.* **Description:** Explores the commitments of the Christian faith with regard to the meaning of human life, sexuality, suffering, illness and death within the context of medicine and healthcare.
Related titles: Microfilm ed.: (from SWZ); Online - full text ed.: (from EBSCO Publishing, O C L C Online Computer Library Center, Inc., RoweCom Information Quest, Swets Blackwell).
Indexed: G.Soc.Sci.& Rel.Per.Lit., Phil.Ind.
—CCC.
Published by: Swets & Zeitlinger BV, PO Box 825, Lisse 2160 SZ, Netherlands. TEL 31-252-435111, FAX 31-252-415888, orders@swets.nl, http://www.swets.nl/sps/journals/cb.html. Eds. Andrew B Lustia, H Tristran Engelhardt Jr., Joseph Boyle. R&P J van der Valk. Circ: 500 (paid). **Dist. in N. America by:** Swets & Zeitlinger, PO Box 582, Downingtown, PA 19335-998. TEL 800-477-9387, FAX 610-524-5366.

610 IND ISSN 0009-5451
CHRISTIAN MEDICAL COLLEGE VELLORE ALUMNI JOURNAL. Text in English. 1967. q., latest vol.35. INR 200 domestic; USD 25 foreign; INR 2,000 domestic lifetime subscription; USD 200 foreign lifetime subscription (effective 2001). adv. bk.rev. abstr, bibl, charts, illus. 40 p./no. 2 cols./p. *Refereed.* **Document type:** *Journal, Academic/Scholarly.* **Description:** Provides updated material of scientific interest to doctors.
Related titles: Online - full text ed.
Published by: Christian Medical College, Alumni Association, Vellore, Tamil Nadu 632 002, India. TEL 91-416-262603, FAX 91-416-262788, TELEX 405-202 CMCH IN, alumni@cmcvellore.ac.in, apeedicayil@hotmail.com, http://www.cmch-vellore.edu. Ed., R&P, Adv. contact Abraham Peedicayil. page INR 10,000; trim 15 x 18. Circ: 2,200 (controlled).

610 IND ISSN 0970-5007
CHRISTIAN MEDICAL JOURNAL OF INDIA. Text in English. 1895. q. INR 100; USD 40 foreign. adv. bk.rev. abstr, charts, illus. index. **Description:** Promotes the mission in health and wholeness, focusing on special concerns from a Christian perspective.
Former titles (until 1992): Christian Medical Association of India. Journal (0009-5443); (until 1954): Christian Medical Association of India, Pakistan, Burma and Ceylon (0970-5015); (until 1937): Journal of Medical Missions in India
Indexed: Biol.Abstr.
—GNLM.

M

Published by: Christian Medical Association of India, Plot 2 A-3 Local Shopping Centre, Janakpuri, New Delhi 110 058, India. TEL 91-11-559-9991, cmaidel@giasdl01.vsnl.net.in. Ed. Dr. V K Shah. Pub. C Thomas. Circ: 3,000.

CHRONOBIOLOGY INTERNATIONAL; The Journal of Biological and Medical Rhythm Research. see *BIOLOGY*

610 JPN ISSN 0913-8684
CHUBU BYOIN IGAKU ZASSHI/OKINAWA CHUBU HOSPITAL. BULLETIN. Text in English, Japanese; Summaries in Japanese. 1975. a. **Document type:** *Bulletin.*
Published by: Chubu Byoin, Igaku Zasshi Henshu Iinkai/Okinawa Chubu Hospital, Editorial Committee, Okinawa Kenritsu Chubu Byoin, 208-3 Miyaza-To, Gushikawa-shi, Okinawa-ken 904-2243, Japan. Ed. Takeo Nishihira. Pub. Marumasa Insatsu. **Co-sponsor:** Hawai Daigaku Jimusho - University of Hawaii Postgraduate Medical Education Program.

CHUI RINSHO/CLINICAL JOURNAL OF TRADITIONAL CHINESE MEDICINE. see *ALTERNATIVE MEDICINE*

610 USA ISSN 0163-0075
CINCINNATI MEDICINE. Text in English. 1921. m. USD 25 to members; USD 35 to non-members; USD 60 foreign (effective 2000). adv. bk.rev. bibl, illus. index, cum.index. *Refereed.* **Document type:** *Newsletter, Trade.* **Description:** Provides physicians with information regarding the practice of medicine on the local, regional, and national fronts.
Supersedes (in 1978): Cincinnati Journal of Medicine (0009-6873)
Indexed: Chem.Abstr., Ind.Med. (coverage dropped).
—CISTI, GNLM.
Published by: Academy of Medicine of Cincinnati, 320 Broadway, Cincinnati, OH 45202. TEL 513-421-7010, FAX 513-721-4378, cintimed@usa.net, http://www.academyofmedicine.org. Ed., R&P Pam Fairbanks. Adv. contact Lisa Bentley. Circ: 2,700 (controlled).

610 USA
THE CIVIL ABOLITIONIST. Text in English. 1986. q. USD 5; USD 8 foreign (effective 2001). bk.rev. **Document type:** *Newsletter.* **Description:** Aims to promote better human health care (as opposed to sickness care), by abolishing the practice of vivisection, i.e. animal experimentation and replacing it with science based on human characteristics.
Former titles: C I V I S - Civitas; Civitas Abolitionist; (until vol.3, no.3, 1988): Civitas
Related titles: ♦ Includes: C - Paper; Supplement: C-Paper.
Published by: Coalition to Protect Animals in Parks & Refuges, PO Box 26, Swain, NY 14884. TEL 607-545-6213, FAX 607-545-6213, civitas@linkny.com, http://www.linkny.com/~civitas. Ed. Bina Robinson. Circ: 2,300.

610 USA ISSN 0891-1150
R11 CODEN: CCJMEL
CLEVELAND CLINIC JOURNAL OF MEDICINE. Text in English. 1931. m. USD 90 domestic; USD 113 foreign (effective 2001). adv. charts, illus. index. back issues avail. *Refereed.* **Document type:** *Journal, Academic/Scholarly.* **Description:** Timely reviews on subjects of interest to physicians in clinical practice.
Formerly (until 1987): Cleveland Clinic Quarterly (0009-8787)
Related titles: Microfilm ed.: (from PQC); Online - full text ed.: (from Institute for Scientific Information).
Indexed: ASCA, Biol.Abstr., Curr.Adv.Cancer Res., Curr.Adv.Gen.& Molec.Biol., Curr.Cont., Dok.Arbeitsmed., Excerp.Med., INIS Atomind., Ind.Med. (1987-), Ind.Sci.Rev., Inpharma, Pharm.&Out.News, Reac., SSCI (coverage dropped), Sci.Cit.Ind. (coverage dropped), THA.
—BLDSC (3278.649800), CISTI, EMDOCS, GNLM, IDS, ingenta, KNAW. **CCC.**
Published by: Cleveland Clinic Educational Foundation, 9500 Euclid Ave NA32, Cleveland, OH 44195. TEL 216-444-2661, FAX 216-444-9385, ccjm@ccf.org. Ed. Dr John D Clough. Pub. Linda K Hengstler. R&P Louisa R Paskert. Adv. contact D Joseph Dennehy TEL 516-365-8640. B&W page USD 3,202, color page USD 541; trim 8 x 10.75. Circ: 92,388.

610 USA
CLEVELAND PHYSICIAN. Text in English. 1920. m. USD 24. adv. bk.rev. illus. **Document type:** *Bulletin.*
Formerly: Academy of Medicine of Cleveland. Bulletin (0001-4281)
—CISTI.
Published by: (Academy of Medicine of Cleveland), Academy Graphic Communication, 1000 Brookpark, Cleveland, OH 44109. Ed. George Reitz. Circ: 4,800.

610 AUS ISSN 1328-3359
CLICK IT AT R A C P. Variant title: Click it @ R A C P. Text in English. 1996. m. back issues avail.
Media: Online - full text.
Published by: Royal Australasian College of Physicians, 145 Macquarie St, Sydney, NSW 2000, Australia. TEL 61-2-9256-5444, FAX 61-2-9252-3310, racp@racp.edu.au, http://www.medserv.com.au/racp/clicit/click.htm.

610.28 GBR ISSN 0144-7777
CODEN: CLNCD5
CLINICA; world medical device & diagnostic news. Text in English. 1980. w. GBP 545 in Europe; USD 970 in US & Canada; JPY 156,000 in Japan; GBP 570 rest of world (effective 2001). adv. bk.rev. 2 cols./p. back issues avail.; reprints avail. **Document type:** *Newsletter.* **Description:** News for the medical device and diagnostic industry.
Related titles: Online - full text ed.: (from Data-Star, The Dialog Corporation, S T N International, Gale Group).
Indexed: ABC, P.N.I., PROMT, Psychol.Abstr.
—BLDSC (3286.170000). **CCC.**
Published by: P J B Publications Ltd., 18-20 Hill Rise, Richmond, Surrey TW10 6UA, United Kingdom. TEL 44-20-8948-3262, FAX 44-20-8332-8990, info@pjbpubs.com, http://www.pjbpubs.com/clinica/index.html. Ed. Ashley Yeo. Pub. Philip Brown. R&P Annette Watts TEL 44-20-8332-8961. Adv. contact Tom Jamison TEL 44-20-8332-8871. Circ: 2,373 (paid). **Subscr. addr. in N America:** Pharmabooks Ltd., 1775 Broadway, Ste 511, New York, NY 10019. TEL 212-262-8230, FAX 212-262-8234.

615.19 NLD ISSN 0009-8981
RB1 CODEN: CCATAR
CLINICA CHIMICA ACTA; international journal of clinical chemistry and medical biochemistry. Text in English. 1956. 24/yr. EUR 3,979 in Europe to individuals; JPY 528,000 in Japan to individuals; USD 4,452 elsewhere to individuals (effective 2002). adv. charts, illus. index. reprint service avail. from ISI. *Refereed.* **Document type:** *Academic/Scholarly.* **Description:** Publishes information leading to a better understanding of biological mechanisms of human diseases, their diagnosis and treatment.
Related titles: Microform ed.: (from PQC); Online - full text ed.: (from EBSCO Publishing, ingenta, Swets Blackwell, ScienceDirect, Institute for Scientific Information).
Indexed: ASCA, Agri.& Environ.Biotech.Abstr. (coverage dropped), Anal.Abstr., BBCI, Biol.Abstr., Chem.Abstr., Chem.Cit.Ind., Chem.Indus.Notes, Chem.Titles, Curr.Adv.Biochem., Curr.Adv.Cancer Res., Curr.Adv.Ecol.Sci., Curr.Adv.Gen.& Molec.Biol., Curr.Chem.React., Curr.Cont., Dairy Sci.Abstr., Dent.Ind., Derwent Biotech.Abstr., Excerp.Med., GeoRef, Helminthol.Abstr., INIS Atomind., Ind.Chem., Ind.Med. (1956-), Ind.Sci.Rev., Ind.Vet., Inpharma, Int.Abstr.Biol.Sci., Mass Spectr.Bull., Nutr.Abstr., Pharm.&Out.News, Potato Abstr., RCI, Reac., Sci.Cit.Ind., Sport Fish.Abstr., THA, Triticale Abstr., Vet.Bull., Weed Abstr.
—BLDSC (3286.200000), ADONIS, CASDDS, CISTI, GNLM, IDS, ingenta, Linda Hall. **CCC.**
Published by: Elsevier Science BV, PO Box 211, Amsterdam 1000 AE, Netherlands. TEL 31-20-485-3757, FAX 31-20-485-3432, TELEX 18582 ESPA NL, nlinfo-f@elsevier.nl, http://www.elsevier.com/locate/cca, http://www.elsevier.nl. Eds. A H Wu, D W Moss. **Subscr. in Australasia and the Far East to:** Elsevier Science (Singapore) Pte Ltd, No.1 Temasek Ave, 17-01 Millenia Tower, Singapore 039192, Singapore. TEL 65-434-3727, FAX 65-337-2230, asiainfo@elsevier.com.sg; **Subscr. in Japan to:** Elsevier Science Inc - Japan Regional Office, 9-15 Higashi-Azabu 1-chome, Minato-ku, Tokyo 106-0044, Japan. TEL 81-3-5561-5033, FAX 81-3-5561-5047, info@elsevier.co.jp; **Subscr. in the Americas to:** Elsevier Science, PO Box 945, New York, NY 10159-0945. TEL 212-633-3730, FAX 212-633-3680, usinfo-f@elsevier.com, http://www.elsevier.com, http://www.elsevier.com.

610 ITA ISSN 0393-7585
CLINICA MEDICA DEL NORD AMERICA. Text in Italian. 1968. bi-m. ITL 220,000, USD 180 (effective 1999). reprint service avail. from PQC. **Document type:** *Academic/Scholarly.*
Published by: Piccin Nuova Libreria, Via Altinate, 107, Padua, PD 35121, Italy. TEL 39-049-655566, FAX 39-049-8750693.

610 ESP ISSN 0301-0392
CLINICA; PORTAVOZ DEL INTERNADO. Text in Spanish. 1989. a. ESP 400 (effective 2000). **Document type:** *Academic/Scholarly.*
Published by: Universidad de Valladolid, Secretariado de Publicaciones, Facultad de Medicina, Juan Mambrilla, 14, Valladolid 47003, Spain. TEL 34-983-423000, FAX 34-983-290300.

610 ESP ISSN 0210-7945
CLINICA RURAL. Text in Spanish. s-m.
Address: Ronda De Sant Pere, 22, Barcelona 08010, Spain. TEL 34-93-301-2433. Circ: 17,000.

615.5 ITA ISSN 0009-9074
CODEN: CLTEA4
CLINICA TERAPEUTICA. Text in Italian; Summaries in English, Italian. 1951. s-m. ITL 100,000; ITL 200,000 foreign. adv. bk.rev. abstr, bibl. index. back issues avail. **Document type:** *Academic/Scholarly.*
Indexed: Agri.& Environ.Biotech.Abstr. (coverage dropped), Biol.Abstr., Chem.Abstr., Chem.Indus.Notes, Chem.Titles, Derwent Biotech.Abstr., Excerp.Med., Ind.Med. (1951-), Inpharma, Nutr.Abstr., Reac.
—BLDSC (3286.237000), CASDDS, CISTI, EMDOCS, GNLM, KNAW.
Published by: Societa Editrice Universo, Via Giovanni Battista Morgagni, 1, Rome, RM 00161, Italy. Ed. Michele De Martiis. Circ: 10,000.

CLINICAL ACUPUNCTURE AND ORIENTAL MEDICINE. see *ALTERNATIVE MEDICINE*

571.3 611 USA ISSN 0897-3806
CODEN: CLANE8
CLINICAL ANATOMY. Text in English. 1988. bi-m. USD 1,295 in United States; USD 1,355 in Canada & Mexico; USD 1,406 elsewhere; USD 1,360 combined subscription in United States for print and online eds.; USD 1,420 combined subscription in Canada & Mexico for print and online eds.; USD 1,471 combined subscription elsewhere for print and online eds. (effective 2002). adv. bk.rev. back issues avail. *Refereed.* **Document type:** *Academic/Scholarly.* **Description:** Embraces anatomy in all aspects - gross, histologic, developmental, and neurologic - as applied to medical practice.
Related titles: Microform ed.: (from PQC); Online - full text ed.: ISSN 1098-2353. 1996. USD 1,295 in United States; USD 1,295 in Canada & Mexico; USD 1,295 elsewhere (effective 2002) (from EBSCO Publishing, Wiley InterScience, Institute for Scientific Information).
Indexed: ASCA, Curr.Cont., Ind.Med. (1988-), Sci.Cit.Ind.
—BLDSC (3286.247300), CISTI, EMDOCS, GNLM, IDS, Infotrieve. **CCC.**
Published by: (American Association of Clinical Anatomists), John Wiley & Sons, Inc., Journals (Subsidiary of: Wiley InterScience), 605 Third Ave, New York, NY 10158. TEL 212-850-6645, FAX 212-850-6021, subinfo@jwiley.com, uscs-wis@wiley.com, http://www.interscience.wiley.com/jpages/0897-3806/, http://www.wiley.com. Ed. Donald R Cahill. adv.: B&W page GBP 640, color page GBP 1,515; trim 174 x 254. Circ: 950. **Subscr. outside the Americas to:** John Wiley & Sons Ltd., Baffins Ln, Chichester, Sussex PO19 IUD, United Kingdom. TEL 44-1243-779777, FAX 44-1243-843232, cs-journals@wiley.co.uk, http://www.wiley.co.uk.

610 DEU ISSN 1591-8890
CODEN: ICLREA
▼ **CLINICAL AND EXPERIMENTAL MEDICINE.** Text in English. 2001. q. EUR 624 domestic; EUR 622.80 in Germany; EUR 183 newsstand/cover foreign (effective 2002). adv. bk.rev. abstr, bibl, illus. index. reprint service avail. from PQC. **Document type:** *Journal, Academic/Scholarly.* **Description:** Publishes reports of clinical and experimental work concerned with the following fields: clinical chemistry, hematology, immunology, oncology and virology.
Formed by the merger of (1975-2001): International Journal of Clinical and Laboratory Research (0940-5437); Which was formerly (until 1991): Research in Clinic and Laboratory; Ricerca in Clinica e in Laboratorio (0390-5748); (1913-2001): Research in Experimental Medicine (0300-9130); Which was formerly (until 1972): Zeitschrift fuer die Gesamte Experimentelle Medizin Einschliesslich Experimenteller Chirurgie (0044-2534)
Related titles: Microform ed.: (from PQC); Online - full text ed.: ISSN 1591-9528 (from EBSCO Publishing, RoweCom Information Quest, Swets Blackwell, Springer LINK, Institute for Scientific Information).

Indexed: ASCA, Biol.Abstr., Chem.Abstr., Chem.Indus.Notes, Chem.Titles, Curr.Adv.Ecol.Sci., Curr.Cont., Dent.Ind., Excerp.Med., Ind.Med. (1991-), Ind.Sci.Rev., Inpharma, Pharm.&Out.News, Reac., Sci.Cit.Ind.
—CASDDS, CISTI, EMDOCS, GNLM, IDS, Infotrieve, KNAW. **CCC.**
Published by: Springer-Verlag (Subsidiary of: BertelsmannSpringer), Haber Str 7, Heidelberg 69126, Germany. FAX 49-30-82787448, subscriptions@springer.de, http://link.springer.de/link/service/journals/00599/index.htm. Ed. F Dammacco. Circ: 6,000. **Subscr. in N. America to:** Springer-Verlag New York Inc., PO Box 2485, Secaucus, NJ 07096-2485. TEL 212-460-1500, FAX 212-473-6272.

616.07 FRA ISSN 1292-7953
CODEN: AACPDQ
CLINICAL AND EXPERIMENTAL PATHOLOGY. Text in Multiple languages. 1953. 6/yr. FRF 1,500 domestic to individuals; FRF 1,780 foreign to individuals; FRF 750 domestic to students; FRF 890 foreign to students. **Document type:** *Academic/Scholarly.*
Former titles (until 1999): Archives d'Anatomie et de Cytologie Pathologiques (0395-501X); (until 1976): Archives d'Anatomie Pathologique (0003-9608)
Indexed: Biol.Abstr., C.I.S. Abstr., Chem.Abstr., Curr.Cont. (coverage dropped), Dent.Ind., Excerp.Med., Helminthol.Abstr., Ind.Med. (1999-), Ref.Zh.
—CISTI, EMDOCS, GNLM, Infotrieve, KNAW. **CCC.**
Published by: (Semaine des Hopitaux), Expansion Scientifique Francaise, 31 bd. de la Tour Maubourg, Paris Cedex 7 75343, France. TEL 33-1-40626400, FAX 33-1-45556920. Ed. C Brocheriou. Circ: 1,500. **Subscr. to:** 15 rue St. Benoit, Paris Cedex 6 75278, France.

610 CAN ISSN 0147-958X
CODEN: CNVMDL
CLINICAL AND INVESTIGATIVE MEDICINE/MEDECINE CLINIQUE ET EXPERIMENTALE. Short title: C I M - M C E. Text in English. 1977. 6/yr. CND 187 to institutions; CND 237 foreign to institutions (effective 1999). adv. bk.rev. abstr, bibl, charts, illus, stat. index. back issues avail.; reprints avail. *Refereed.* **Document type:** *Academic/Scholarly.* **Description:** Presents results of research in the areas of clinical investigation, epidemiologic analysis and health services research as well as articles on medical education studies, symposia and clinical conferences.
Related titles: Microform ed.: (from PQC); Online - full text ed.: (from ProQuest Information & Learning, LexisNexis, Institute for Scientific Information).
Indexed: ASCA, Biol.Abstr., CBCA Ref., Chem.Abstr., Chem.Indus.Notes, Chem.Titles, Curr.Adv.Cancer Res., Curr.Adv.Ecol.Sci., Curr.Cont., Dairy Sci.Abstr., Dok.Arbeitsmed., Excerp.Med., Helminthol.Abstr., Ind.Med. (1978-), Ind.Sci.Rev., Inpharma, Int.Abstr.Biol.Sci., Kidney, Nutr.Abstr., Pharm.&Out.News, Reac., Ref.Zh., Rev.Med.& Vet.Mycol., Risk Abstr., SSCI (coverage dropped), Sci.Cit.Ind.
—BLDSC (3286.253000), ADONIS, CASDDS, CISTI, EMDOCS, GNLM, IDS, ingenta, KNAW. **CCC.**
Published by: Canadian Medical Association, 1867 Alta Vista Dr, Ottawa, ON K1H 5K9, Canada. TEL 613-731-9331, FAX 613-565-2382, pubs@cma.ca, http://www.cma.ca/cim. Ed. Dr. George Sweeney. Adv. contact Beverley Kirkpatrick. B&W page CND 765, color page CND 1,565; trim 10.88 x 8.13. Circ: 900. **Co-sponsor:** Canadian Society for Clinical Investigation.

610 USA ISSN 0959-9851
CODEN: CAURE9
CLINICAL AUTONOMIC RESEARCH. Text in English. 1991. bi-m. USD 291 to individuals; USD 665 to institutions; USD 111 newsstand/cover (effective 2001). adv. bk.rev. index. back issues avail.; reprints avail. *Refereed.* **Document type:** *Academic/Scholarly.* **Description:** Aims to draw together and disseminate research work from the various disciplines and specialities dealing with clinical problems resulting from autonomic dysfunction.
Related titles: CD-ROM ed.; Online - full text ed.: (from EBSCO Publishing, Institute for Scientific Information).
Indexed: ASCA, Curr.Cont., Excerp.Med. (1993-), Ind.Med. (1991-), Inpharma, Int.Abstr.Biol.Sci., Neurosci.Abstr. (coverage dropped), Neurosci.Cit.Ind., Pharm.&Out.News, Reac., SSCI (coverage dropped), Sci.Cit.Ind.
—BLDSC (3286.259900), ADONIS, CISTI, EMDOCS, GNLM, IDS, KNAW.
Published by: (Clinical Autonomic Research Society), Lippincott Williams & Wilkins (Philadelphia) (Subsidiary of: Wolters Kluwer N.V.), 530 Walnut St, Philadelphia, PA 19106-3621. TEL 215-521-8300, FAX 215-521-8902, http://www.Lww.com. Eds. C Mathias, R Polinsky. Adv. contact Gemma Heiser. **Subscr. to:** PO Box 1600, Hagerstown, MD 21740-1600. TEL 800-777-2295, FAX 301-824-7390.

CLINICAL BIOCHEMISTRY. see *BIOLOGY—Biochemistry*

610 USA ISSN 0191-7870
CLINICAL BIOMECHANICS. Text in English. 1971. irreg.
Published by: Clinical Biomechanics Corp., PO Box 35185, Los Angeles, CA 90035.

610 011 GBR ISSN 0958-3513
CLINICAL CONGRESS NEWS. Text in English. 1989. irreg. **Document type:** *Proceedings.* **Description:** Covers current topics including conference news, new developments in therapy and the latest infectious disease treatment guidelines.
Published by: Cambridge Medical Publications Ltd., Wicker House, High St, Worthing, W Sussex BN11 1DJ, United Kingdom. TEL 44-1903-205884, FAX 44-1903-234862, http://www.ihmf.org. R&P Kim Leal.

610.28 USA
CLINICAL ENGINEERING SERIES. Text in English. 1972. irreg., latest vol.5, 1981. reprint service avail. from ISI. *Refereed.* **Description:** Details research in the biomedical fields.
Published by: Academic Press, Inc., Journal Division (Subsidiary of: Harcourt Brace & Company), 525 B St, Ste 1900, San Diego, CA 92101-4495. TEL 619-231-0926, FAX 619-699-6715. Ed. Cesar A Caceres. **Subscr. to:** Order Dept., 6277 Sea Harbor Dr, 4th Fl, Orlando, FL 32887. TEL 800-321-5068.

610 613.082 USA ISSN 1527-0289
▼ **THE CLINICAL JOURNAL OF WOMEN'S HEALTH.** Text in English. 2000. q. USD 105 domestic to individuals print and full text on-line; USD 129 foreign to individuals print and full text on-line; USD 158 domestic to institutions print and full text on-line; USD 182 foreign to institutions print and full text on-line; USD 53 domestic to students print and full text on-line; USD 77 foreign to students print and full text on-line; USD 46 newsstand/cover (effective 2001). *Refereed.* **Description:** Offers strategies for preventing and managing medical problems affecting women across the life span.
Related titles: Online - full text ed.
Published by: W.B. Saunders Co. (Subsidiary of: Harcourt Publishers Ltd.), Curtis Center, Independence Sq W, Philadelphia, PA 19106-3399. TEL 215-238-7800, FAX 215-238-6490, http://www.womenshealthjournal.org, http://www.wbsaunders.com. Ed. Susan L Hendrix.

610 USA
CLINICAL LABORATORY NEWS. Text in English. 1978. m. USD 39 domestic; USD 84 foreign (effective 2000); free to qualified personnel. adv. bk.rev. **Description:** Contains top news stories on technology and regulatory issues.
Formerly: Clinical Chemistry News (0161-9640)
Indexed: Chem.Abstr.
—BLDSC (3286.295876), Linda Hall. **CCC.**
Published by: American Association for Clinical Chemistry, Inc., 2101 L St N W, Ste 202, Washington, DC 20037-1526. TEL 800-892-1400, FAX 202-887-5093. Ed. Nancy Sasavage. Pub., R&P Mac Fancher TEL 202-857-0717. Circ: 25,000.

174.2 614.1 NLD ISSN 0926-969X
CLINICAL MEDICAL ETHICS. Text in English. 1991. irreg., latest vol.4, 1993. Price varies. back issues avail. *Refereed.* **Document type:** *Monographic series.* **Description:** In-depth examination of issues at the forefront of the medical ethics debate.
Published by: Kluwer Academic Publishers Group (Subsidiary of: Wolters Kluwer N.V.), Spuiboulevard 50, PO Box 17, Dordrecht 3300 AA, Netherlands. FAX 31-78-639-2254, services@wkap.nl, http://www.wkap.nl/prod/s/CMET. Eds. H Tristam Engelhardt Jr., Stuart F Spicker. **Dist. by:** Journals Department, PO Box 322, Dordrecht 3300 AH, Netherlands. FAX 31-78-654-6474.

610 GBR ISSN 1470-2118
R31 CODEN: RCPJAX
CLINICAL MEDICINE. Text in English. 1966. bi-m. GBP 95 domestic; GBP 130 foreign (effective 2001). adv. bk.rev. charts, illus. index. back issues avail. *Refereed.* **Document type:** *Academic/Scholarly.* **Description:** Seeks to maintain high standards of patient care and medical education.
Formerly (until 2001): Royal College of Physicians of London. Journal (0035-8819)
Related titles: Online - full text ed.: (from CatchWord Ltd., Ovid Technologies, Inc., Institute for Scientific Information).
Indexed: ASCA, Abstr.Health Care Manage.Stud., Abstr.Hyg., Biol.Abstr., CINAHL, C.I.S. Abstr., Curr.Adv.Cancer Res., Curr.Adv.Ecol.Sci., Curr.Cont. (coverage dropped), Diab.Cont., Dok.Arbeitsmed., Environ.Sci.Poll.Mgmt., Excerp.Med., Helminthol.Abstr., Ind.Med. (1966-), Inpharma, Int.Nurs.Ind., Kidney, Microbiol.Abstr., NRN, Nutr.Abstr., Pharm.&Out.News, Pollut.Abstr., Reac., Ref.Zh., Risk Abstr., SSCI (coverage dropped), Saf.Sci.Abstr., Sci.Cit.Ind., THA, Trop.Dis.Bull.
—BLDSC (3286.303100), CISTI, GNLM, IDS, ingenta, KNAW.
Published by: Royal College of Physicians, 11 St Andrews Pl, Regents Park, London NW1 4LE, United Kingdom. TEL 44-20-7935-1174, FAX 44-20-7487-5218, http://www.rcplondon.ac.uk. Ed. Peter Watkins. R&P Bettina Klar. adv.: B&W page GBP 1,180, color page GBP 1,980. Circ: 13,206 (controlled).

610 USA
▼ **CLINICAL MEDICINE AND HEALTH RESEARCH.** Text in English. 1999. d. **Description:** Provides a place for authors to archive their completed studies, before, during or after peer review by other agencies. Includes original research into clinical medicine and health research.
Media: Online - full content.
Published by: B M J Publishing Group, B M A House, Tavistock Sq, London WC1H 9JR, United Kingdom. http://intl-clinmed.netprints.org/home.dtl. Ed. Tony Delamothe.

616.01 GBR ISSN 1198-743X
CODEN: CMINFM
CLINICAL MICROBIOLOGY AND INFECTION. Text in English. 1995. m., latest vol.8, 2002. GBP 67 in Europe to individuals; USD 113 in North America to individuals; GBP 73 elsewhere to individuals; GBP 224 in Europe to institutions; USD 355 in North America to institutions; GBP 246 elsewhere to institutions (effective 2002). adv. bk.rev. back issues avail. *Refereed.* **Document type:** *Academic/Scholarly.* **Description:** Covers the pathogenesis, diagnosis, epidemiology, therapy and prevention of infectious diseases.
Related titles: Online - full text ed.: ISSN 1469-0691. GBP 61 in Europe to individuals; USD 102 in North America to individuals; GBP 61 elsewhere to individuals; GBP 202 in Europe to institutions; USD 320 in North America to institutions; GBP 202 elsewhere to institutions (effective 2002) (from EBSCO Publishing, O C L C Online Computer Library Center, Inc., RoweCom Information Quest, ProQuest Information & Learning, ingenta, Munksgaard & Blackwell Science's Synergy, Swets Blackwell, Institute for Scientific Information).
Indexed: Abstr.Hyg., Chem.Abstr., Chem.Indus.Notes, Chem.Titles, Curr.Cont., Dairy Sci.Abstr., Protozool.Abstr., Rev.Appl.Entomol., Rev.Med.& Vet.Mycol., Trop.Dis.Bull., Vet.Bull.
—BLDSC (3286.305520), CASDDS, GNLM.
Published by: (European Society of Clinical Microbiology and Infectious Diseases), Blackwell Science Ltd., PO Box 88, Oxford OX2 0NE, United Kingdom. TEL 44-1865-206180, 44-1865-206002, FAX 44-1865-206219, jnl.orders@blacksci.co.uk, http://www.blackwell-science.com/~cgilib/jnlpage.asp?Journal=clm&File=clm, http://www.blackwellpublishing.com. Ed. I Phillips. Pub. Allen Stevens. R&P Sophie Savage. Adv. contact Jenny Applin. Circ: 2,650.

CLINICAL ORAL INVESTIGATIONS. see *MEDICAL SCIENCES—Dentistry*

M

610 GBR ISSN 1063-0279
CLINICAL PERFORMANCE AND QUALITY HEALTH CARE. Text in English. 1993. q. USD 165 (effective 2000). *Refereed.* **Document type:** *Academic/Scholarly.* **Description:** Addresses the debate of meeting regulatory requirements without sacrificing the level of patient care and other important issues through its mix of original research articles, case studies and commentaries on the clinical science of quality improvement. Focuses on practical and clinically relevant lessons from national and international work on improving the quality of health care services and is a prime source of information for both academics and practitioners alike.
Related titles: Online - full text ed.: (from EBSCO Publishing, ingenta, Swets Blackwell).
Indexed: Inpharma, Int.Nurs.Ind., Pharm.&Out.News, Reac.
—BLDSC (3286.326300), GNLM, Infotrieve, KNAW. **CCC.**
Published by: Emerald, 60-62 Toller Ln, Bradford, W Yorks BD8 9BY, United Kingdom. TEL 44-1274-777700, FAX 44-1274-785200, customerservices@mcb.co.uk, http://www.mcb.co.uk/cpqhc.htm. Ed. Dr. Mary Nettleman.

612 GBR ISSN 1475-0961
RB113 CODEN: CLPHDU
CLINICAL PHYSIOLOGY AND FUNCTIONAL IMAGING. Text in English. 1981. bi-m., latest vol.22, 2002. GBP 73 in Europe to individuals; USD 117 in North America to individuals; GBP 81 elsewhere to individuals; GBP 525 in Europe to institutions; USD 833 in North America to institutions; GBP 578 elsewhere to institutions (effective 2002). adv. charts, illus. index. back issues avail. *Refereed.* **Document type:** *Academic/Scholarly.* **Description:** Publishes reports on clinical and experimental research pertinent to human physiology in health and disease.
Formerly: Clinical Physiology (0144-5979)
Related titles: Online - full text ed.: ISSN 1365-2281. 1997. GBP 66 in Europe to individuals; USD 106 in North America to individuals; GBP 66 elsewhere to individuals; GBP 473 in Europe to institutions; USD 750 in North America to institutions; GBP 473 elsewhere to institutions (effective 2002) (from EBSCO Publishing, O C L C Online Computer Library Center, Inc., RoweCom Information Quest, ingenta, Munksgaard & Blackwell Science's Synergy, Swets Blackwell, Institute for Scientific Information).
Indexed: ASCA, Biol.Abstr., Chem.Abstr., Chem.Indus.Notes, Chem.Titles, Curr.Adv.Biochem., Curr.Adv.Ecol.Sci., Curr.Cont., Excerp.Med., INIS Atomind., Ind.Med. (1981-), Ind.Sci.Rev., Inpharma, Neurosci.Cit.Ind., Pharm.&Out.News, Reac., Ref.Zh., Sci.Cit.Ind.
—BLDSC (3286.332500), CASDDS, CISTI, GNLM, IDS, ingenta, KNAW. **CCC.**
Published by: (Scandinavian Society of Clinical Physiology), Blackwell Science Ltd., PO Box 88, Oxford OX2 0NE, United Kingdom. TEL 44-1865-206180, 44-1865-206002, FAX 44-1865-206219, jnl.orders@blacksci.co.uk, http://www.blackwell-science.com/~cgilib/ jnlpage.asp?Journal=cphy&File=cphy, http://www.blackwellpublishing.com. Ed. J Bulow. Pub. Allen Stevens. R&P Sophie Savage. Adv. contact Jenny Applin. Circ: 285.

610 USA ISSN 1527-4772
CODEN: JAMEE7
CLINICAL PRACTICE OF ALTERNATIVE MEDICINE. Text in English. 1988. q. USD 55 domestic to individuals; USD 79 foreign to individuals; USD 145 domestic to institutions; USD 195 foreign to institutions (effective 2002). adv. bk.rev. reprint service avail. from PQC. *Refereed.* **Document type:** *Journal, Academic/Scholarly.* **Description:** Presents information about innovative, emerging, and nontraditional advances in preventive medicine, nutrition, risk factors, and modification of harmful life-style.
Formerly (until 2000): Journal of Advancement in Medicine (0894-5888)
—GNLM, Infotrieve, ingenta. **CCC.**
Published by: (American College of Advancement in Medicine), InnoVision Communications, 169 Saxony Rd, Ste 104, Encinitas, CA 92024. TEL 760-633-3910, FAX 760-633-3918, 866-828-2962, info@invcom.com, http://www.acam.org/acamjournal.php. Ed. Derrick Lonsdale.

610 USA
CLINICAL REVIEWS. Text in English. 1997. q. membership only.
Published by: Southern Association for Primary Care, 35 Lakeshore Dr, PO Box 190088, Birmingham, AL 35219-0088. TEL 205-945-1840, FAX 205-945-1548, http://www.sma.org/sapc/sapcapply.htm. Ed. Dr. Ronald C Hamdy. Circ: 7,500.

610 342.441 GBR ISSN 1356-2622
CLINICAL RISK; incorporating the A V M A Medical & Legal Journal. Text in English. 1995. bi-m. GBP 155 in Europe; USD 263 in United States; GBP 160 elsewhere (effective 2002); Subscr. includes online access.. adv. back issues avail. **Document type:** *Journal, Academic/Scholarly.* **Description:** Provides best practice guidelines for doctors and managers through the analysis of key medicolegal issues dealing with the prevention and management of clinical risk.
Incorporates (1990-2000): A V M A Medical & Legal Journal (0959-9304)
Related titles: Online - full text ed.: (from CatchWord Ltd., Swets Blackwell, RoweCom Information Quest); ♦ Supplement: A V M A Medical & Legal Journal. ISSN 0959-9304.
Indexed: ASSIA, Environ.Sci.Poll.Mgmt., Pollut.Abstr., Risk Abstr., Saf.Sci.Abstr., Tox.Abstr.
—BLDSC (3286.374900), CISTI, GNLM, KNAW.
Published by: (Action for Victims of Medical Accidents), Royal Society of Medicine Press Ltd, 1 Wimpole St, London W1M 8AE, United Kingdom. TEL 44-20-7290-2921, FAX 44-20-7290-2929, elizabeth.fredman@rsm.ac.uk, http:// www.roysocmed.ac.uk/pub/cr.htm. Ed. Roger Clements.

610 570 GBR ISSN 0143-5221
CODEN: CSCIAE
CLINICAL SCIENCE. Text in English. 1909. m. USD 175.50 in US & Canada; GBP 110.64 elsewhere; USD 595 in US & Canada for print & online eds.; GBP 330 elsewhere for print & online eds. (effective 2002). adv. bibl, illus. index. back issues avail. *Refereed.* **Document type:** *Journal, Academic/Scholarly.* **Description:** Studies of clinical science with emphasis on biochemical, physiological and metabolic approaches.
Formerly: Heart
Related titles: CD-ROM ed.; Microfilm ed.: (from PMC); Online - full text ed.: ISSN 1470-8736. USD 166 in US & Canada to individuals; GBP 95 elsewhere to individuals; USD 558 in US & Canada to institutions; GBP 309 elsewhere to institutions (effective 2001) (from EBSCO Publishing, RoweCom Information Quest, Swets Blackwell, Institute for Scientific Information).
Indexed: ASCA, Abstr.Hyg., Agri.& Environ.Biotech.Abstr. (coverage dropped), Anim.Breed.Abstr., Biol.Abstr., Chem.Abstr., Chem.Indus.Notes, Chem.Titles, Curr.Adv.Ecol.Sci., Curr.Cont., Dairy Sci.Abstr., Dent.Ind., Derwent Biotech.Abstr., Diar.Dis.Res., Excerp.Med., Helminthol.Abstr., INIS Atomind., Ind.Med. (1979-), Ind.Sci.Rev., Inpharma, Int.Abstr.Biol.Sci., Kidney, NRN, Neurosci.Cit.Ind., Nutr.Abstr., Pharm.&Out.News, Reac., Ref.Zh., SSCI (coverage dropped), Sci.Cit.Ind., Soyabean Abstr., Trop.Dis.Bull.
—BLDSC (3286.375000), ADONIS, CASDDS, CISTI, EMDOCS, GNLM, IDS, ingenta, KNAW. **CCC.**
Published by: (Biochemical Society), Portland Press Ltd., 59 Portland Pl, London W1N 3AJ, United Kingdom. TEL 44-20-7580-5530, FAX 44-20-7323-1136, sales@portland-service.com, http:// cs.portlandpress.com, http://www.cs.portlandpress.com. Ed. K Bartlett. R&P Adam Marshall. Adv. contact Sarah Laflin. Circ: 1,400. **Subscr. to:** Commerce Way, Colchester, Essex CO2 8HP, United Kingdom. TEL 44-1206-796351, FAX 44-1206-799331. **Co-sponsor:** Medical Research Society.

610 USA ISSN 0149-2918
RM260 CODEN: CLTHDG
CLINICAL THERAPEUTICS; the international, peer-reviewed journal of drug therapy. Text in English. 1977. 12/yr. EUR 144 in Europe to institutions; JPY 21,299 in Japan to institutions; USD 142 in United States to institutions; USD 164 elsewhere to institutions; USD 140 to individuals except Europe & Japan (effective 2002). charts, illus. index. back issues avail.; reprints avail. *Refereed.* **Document type:** *Academic/Scholarly.* **Description:** Publishes review articles and results of original clinical and pharmacoeconomic research in the broad field of medical and pharmaceutical therapy and related areas.
Related titles: Online - full text ed.: (from ingenta, Swets Blackwell, ScienceDirect, Institute for Scientific Information).
Indexed: ASCA, Biol.Abstr., Chem.Abstr., Curr.Adv.Cancer Res., Curr.Cont., Derwent Biotech.Abstr., Excerp.Med., Helminthol.Abstr., INIS Atomind., I.P.A., Ind.Med. (1977-), Inpharma, Med.& Surg.Dermat., Nutr.Abstr., Pharm.&Out.News, Protozool.Abstr., PsycInfo, Reac., Rev.Med.& Vet.Mycol., SSCI (coverage dropped), Sci.Cit.Ind., Trop.Dis.Bull., e-psyche.
—BLDSC (3286.399450), ADONIS, CASDDS, CISTI, EMDOCS, GNLM, IDS, ingenta, KNAW. **CCC.**
Published by: Excerpta Medica, Inc. (Subsidiary of: Reed Elsevier Medical group), 105 Raider Blvd, Belle Mead, NJ 08502. TEL 908-281-3625, FAX 908-874-3250, http://www.elsevier.com/locate/clinthera. Eds. Dr. Arthur Krosnick, D A Sclar. Pub. Stan Heimberger. Circ: 3,850.

615 USA
CLINICAL TRIALS MONITOR. Text in English. 1992. m. USD 1,247 (effective 2001). index. back issues avail. **Document type:** *Newsletter.* **Description:** Intelligence service that tracks clinical trials of human pharmaceuticals, in vivo imaging agents and extracorporeal therapies from beginning to end.
Formerly (until Oct. 1993): Clinical Trials (1061-608X)
Media: Online - full text.
—**CCC.**
Published by: C T B International Publishing Inc., PO Box 218, Maplewood, NJ 07040-0218. TEL 973-379-7749, FAX 973-379-1158, info@ctbintl.com, http://www.ctbintl.com. Ed., R&P Christopher Brogna. Pub. Oykue Brogna.

610 IND ISSN 0009-9341
CODEN: CLCNBF
CLINICIAN; monthly journal of medical science and news. Text in English. 1936. m. USD 6. adv. bk.rev.
Indexed: Chem.Abstr., Curr.Cont. (coverage dropped), Excerp.Med., Helminthol.Abstr., INIS Atomind.
—CASDDS, GNLM.
Published by: Cosme Matias Menezes Pvt. Ltd., Rua de Ourem, P O Box 12, Panjim, Goa, India. Circ: 5,000.

610 658 GBR ISSN 0965-5751
CODEN: CLMAFU
THE CLINICIAN IN MANAGEMENT. Text in English. 1992. q. GBP 120 to institutions (effective 2001). adv. bk.rev. illus, stat. **Document type:** *Newsletter, Academic/Scholarly.* **Description:** Publishes material examining various aspects of healthcare delivery and the role of the clinician as manager.
Related titles: Online - full text ed.: (from O C L C Online Computer Library Center, Inc., CatchWord Ltd.).
—BLDSC (3286.512300).
Published by: (British Association of Medical Managers), Radcliffe Medical Press Ltd., 18 Marcham Rd, Abingdon, Oxon OX14 1AA, United Kingdom. TEL 44-1235-528820, FAX 44-1235-528830, contact-us@radcliffemed.com, http://www.radcliffe-oxford.com/. Ed. Jerry Simpson. Pub., R&P Lucy Thomson. Circ: 2,000.

610 USA
CLINICIAN NEWS. Text in English. 1997. 10/yr. back issues avail. **Description:** Dedicated to meeting the needs of primary care and womens health nurse practitioners and physician assistants.
Related titles: Online - full text ed.
Published by: Clinicians Publishing Group, 4 Brighton Rd, Clifton, NJ 07012. TEL 201-916-1000, FAX 201-916-0021, clinnews@clinicianspublishing.com, http://news.medscape.com/CPG/ClinNews/public/ archive/1999/toc-0302.html. Ed. James F Cawley.

610 USA ISSN 1052-0627
R11
CLINICIAN REVIEWS; a journal for physician assistants and nurse practitioners reporting on the latest advances in medicine. Text in English. 1991. m. USD 70 domestic to individuals; USD 100 foreign to individuals; USD 75 domestic to institutions; USD 105 foreign to institutions; USD 50 foreign to students (effective 2000). adv. abstr. *Refereed.* **Document type:** *Trade, Abstract/Index.* **Description:** Reports from medical literature and major medical meetings. Includes review articles of contemporary topics.
Related titles: Online - full text ed.: (from Gale Group).
—BLDSC (3286.512500).
Published by: Clinicians Publishing Group, 4 Brighton Rd, Clifton, NJ 07012. TEL 201-916-1000, FAX 201-916-0021, cpg@aol.com, http:// www.medscape.com/CPG/ClinReviews/public/ journal.ClinReviews.html. Ed. Robert E Dedonato. Pub. David E Mittman. Adv. contact Brian Blitz. B&W page USD 2,260, color page USD 3,135; trim 10.88 x 8.5. Circ: 500 (paid); 52,000 (controlled).

616.07 CAN ISSN 0832-9184
CLINICIEN. Text in English. 1986. 12/yr. adv.
Indexed: Pt.de Rep.
Published by: S T A Communications Inc., 955 bd St Jean, bur 306, Pointe Claire, PQ H9R 5K3, Canada. TEL 514-695-7623, FAX 514-695-8554. Ed. Paul Brand. Circ: 14,896.

M

610 616 USA ISSN 1094-0626
CLINICS ATLAS OF OFFICE PROCEDURES. Text in English. q. USD 146 domestic to individuals; USD 180 foreign to individuals; USD 183 domestic to institutions; USD 221 foreign to institutions; USD 56 per issue (effective 2001). **Description:** Examines medical procedures step-by-step used in family practice and internal medicine. Each issue is devoted to a single issue. Year 2000 issues to include foot and ankle disorders, opthalmologic procedures, dermatologic manifestations of systemic disease, and cardiovascular disease.
Published by: W.B. Saunders Co. (Subsidiary of: Harcourt Publishers Ltd.), 11830 Westline Industrial Dr, St Louis, MO 63146. TEL 800-325-4177, http://www.wbsaunders.com.

610 USA ISSN 1522-5720
CLINICS IN FAMILY PRACTICE. Text in English. q. USD 95 domestic to individuals; USD 108 in Canada to individuals; USD 120 elsewhere to individuals; USD 115 domestic to institutions; USD 140 foreign to institutions (effective 2001); USD 36 per issue (2001). **Description:** Concentrates each month on a single topic related to family medicine. Year 2000 topics to include hepatobiliary disease, preventitive services, trauma, and adolescent health.
Published by: W.B. Saunders Co. (Subsidiary of: Harcourt Publishers Ltd.), 11830 Westline Industrial Dr, St Louis, MO 63146. TEL 800-325-4177, wbspcs@harcourtbrace.com, http://www.wbsaunders.com.

616.98 USA ISSN 1526-0046
▼ **CLINICS IN OCCUPATIONAL AND ENVIRONMENTAL MEDICINE.** Text in English. 2000 (Sep). q. USD 105 domestic to individuals; USD 115 in Canada to individuals; USD 135 elsewhere to individuals; USD 130 domestic to institutions; USD 160 elsewhere to institutions; USD 85 domestic to students; USD 41 per issue (effective 2001). **Description:** Focus on managing health care in the workplace, advise to business on environmental concerns, and current approaches to prevention and treatment of work-related injuries and deceases. Covers regulatory and legal issues and updates on environmental risk management.
Published by: W.B. Saunders Co. (Subsidiary of: Harcourt Publishers Ltd.), 6277 Sea Harbor Dr, Orlando, FL 32887-4800. TEL 407-345-4000, 800-654-2452, FAX 407-363-9661, 800-225-6030, wbspcs@harcourtbrace.com, http://www.wbsaunders.com. Ed. Kenneth H Chase.

610 FRA ISSN 0009-935X
CLINIQUE* ; revue du medecin practicien. Text in French. 1906. m. FRF 100. bibl. index.
Indexed: Ind.Med. (coverage dropped).
—CISTI, GNLM, Infotrieve. **CCC.**
Published by: (Societe Medicale des Praticiens), Editions de Medecine Pratique, 132 av. du General Leclerc, Paris 75014, France.

610 NLD ISSN 0045-7183
R131.A1
CLIO MEDICA. Variant title: Wellcome Institute Series in the History of Medicine. Text in English. 1966. irreg., latest vol.59, 2000. price varies. adv. bk.rev. illus. index. back issues avail. **Document type:** *Monographic series, Academic/Scholarly.* **Description:** Explores all aspects of the history of medicine, including ethical, social and cultural topics.
Related titles: Online - full text ed.: (from CatchWord Ltd., EBSCO Publishing, Swets Blackwell).
Indexed: BHA, Biol.Abstr., Hist.Abstr. (1965-1988, dropped), Ind.Med. (1965-).
—BLDSC (3286.650000), CatchWord, CISTI, GNLM.
Published by: Rodopi, Tijnmuiden 7, Amsterdam 1046 AK, Netherlands. TEL 31-20-611-4821, FAX 31-20-447-2979, F.van.der.Zee@Rodopi.nl, orders-queries@Rodopi.nl, http://www.rodopi.nl. Eds. Chris Lawrence, Roy Porter, Vivian Nutton. Circ: 550. **Dist in France by:** Nordeal; **Dist in N America by:** Rodopi (USA), One Rockefeller Plaza, Ste. 1420, New York, NY 10020. TEL 212-265-6360, 800-225-3998, FAX 212-265-6402.

346.032 617.155 USA
CLOSED-HEAD INJURY; a clinical source book. Text in English. 1994. irreg. USD 95. **Description:** Helps the practitioner understand the physiology and long-term consequences of mild to moderate closed-head injury and postconcussive syndrome. Offers specific guidance in a growing area of plaintiff's personal injury practice.
Published by: Lexis Law Publishing (Subsidiary of: Reed Elsevier plc), PO Box 7587, Charlottesville, VA 22906-7587. TEL 804-972-7600, 800-562-1197, FAX 804-972-7666, llp.customer.support@lexis-nexis.com, http://www.lexislawpublishing.com. Ed. Peter G Bernad.

610 CAN
CMA.CA. Text in English, French. d. **Description:** Designed for physicians and medical students to interact with each other and with the association, and to find the tools and resources to enhance the medical profession.
Media: Online - full content.
Published by: Canadian Medical Association, 1867 ALta Vista Dr., Ottawa, ON K1G 5W8, Canada. TEL 613-236-8864, editor@globalmedic.com, cmamsc@cma.ca, http://www.cma.ca/cma.

610 ESP
COLECCION CIENCIAS MEDICAS DE BOLSILLO. Text in Spanish. 1977. irreg. price varies. **Document type:** *Academic/Scholarly.*
Published by: (Universidad de Navarra, Facultad de Medicina), Ediciones Universidad de Navarra, S.A. (EUNSA), Pza. Los Sauces, 1-2, Baranain, (Navarra) 31010, Spain. TEL 34-948-256850, FAX 34-948-256854, ensaidi@abc.ibernet.com, http://www.unav.es.

610 ESP
COLECCION LIBROS DE MEDICINA. Text in Spanish. 1974. irreg. price varies. **Document type:** *Monographic series.*
Formerly: Coleccion Medicina
Published by: (Universidad de Navarra, Facultad de Medicina), Ediciones Universidad de Navarra, S.A. (EUNSA), Pza. Los Sauces, 1-2, Baranain, (Navarra) 31010, Spain. TEL 34-948-256850, FAX 34-948-256854, eunsaedi@abc.ibernet.com, http://www.unav.es.

610 ESP
COLEGIO MEDICO DE BARCELONA. REVISTA. Abbreviated title: Co M B Revista. Text in Spanish. 12/yr.
Published by: Colegio Medico de Barcelona, Passeig de la Bonanova, 47, Barcelona 08017, Spain. TEL 3-418-88-88.

610 SLV ISSN 0010-0641
COLEGIO MEDICO DE EL SALVADOR. ARCHIVOS. Text in Spanish; Summaries in English. 1947. q. USD 3.50. adv. bibl, charts, illus. index.
Indexed: Biol.Abstr., Ind.Med. (coverage dropped).
Published by: Colegio Medico de El Salvador, Final Pasaje 10, Col. Miramonte, San Salvador, El Salvador. Ed. Dr. Ramon Lucio Fernandez.

610 ZAF
COLIMPEX MEDICAL EXECUPAD. Text in Afrikaans, English. a. free per issue to qualified personnel. adv.
Published by: Colimpex Africa (Pty) Ltd., PO Box 5838, Johannesburg 2000, South Africa.

610 FRA ISSN 1271-9145
COLLECTION PATHOLOGIE, SCIENCES, FORMATION. Cover title: Pathologie, Science, Formation. Text in French. irreg. **Document type:** *Monographic series.* **Description:** Aims to spread the knowledge of well-known and well-regarded specialists on various specializations to keep doctors up to date on the various pathologies from the point of view of research as well as clinical trials. Each issue covers a specific medical topic.
Published by: John Libbey Eurotext, 127 av. de la Republique, Montrouge 92120, France. TEL 33-01-46730660, FAX 33-01-40840999, marketing@jle.com, http://www.john-libbey-eurotext.fr.

610 CAN
COLLEGE DES MEDECINS DU QUEBEC. ANNUAIRE MEDICAL. Text in English, French. a. CND 90.95 (effective 2001). **Document type:** *Directory.* **Description:** List of physicians appearing on the roll of the Corporation Professionnelle des Medecins du Quebec.
Formerly: Corporation Professionnelle des Medecins du Quebec. Annuaire Medical (0315-226X)
Published by: College des Medecins du Quebec, 2170 boul Rene Levesque Ouest, Montreal, PQ H3H 2T8, Canada. TEL 514-933-4441, FAX 514-933-3112. R&P Serge Joly.

610 CAN
COLLEGE DES MEDECINS DU QUEBEC. LE COLLEGE. Text in French. 1961. 3/yr. free per issue. **Document type:** *Bulletin.*
Former titles: College des Medecins du Quebec. Bulletin; (until 1994): Corporation Professionnelle des Medecins du Quebec. Bulletin (0315-2979); (until 1973): College des Medecins et Chirurgiens du Quebec. Bulletin (0069-5599); (until 1967): College des Medecins et Chirurgiens de la Province de Quebec. Journal (0588-2729); (until 1966): College des Medecins et Chirurgiens de la Province de Quebec. Nouvelles. (0315-2960)
Indexed: Pt.de Rep.
Published by: College des Medecins du Quebec, 2170 boul Rene Levesque Ouest, Montreal, PQ H3H 2T8, Canada. TEL 514-933-4441, FAX 514-933-3112. R&P Carole Graveline. Circ: 21,000.

610 CAN
COLLEGE OF PHYSICIANS AND SURGEONS OF BRITISH COLUMBIA. ANNUAL REPORT. Text in English. a. membership. **Document type:** *Directory.*
Published by: College of Physicians and Surgeons of British Columbia, 1807 W 10th Ave, Vancouver, BC V6J 2A9, Canada. TEL 604-736-5551.

610 CAN ISSN 0069-5726
COLLEGE OF PHYSICIANS AND SURGEONS OF BRITISH COLUMBIA. MEDICAL DIRECTORY. Text in English. a. CND 55 (effective 1999). **Document type:** *Directory.*
Published by: College of Physicians and Surgeons of British Columbia, 1807 W 10th Ave, Vancouver, BC V6J 2A9, Canada. TEL 604-733-7758.

610 PAK
COLLEGE OF PHYSICIANS & SURGEONS PAKISTAN. INDEX OF DISSERTATIONS. Text in English. 1998. base vol. plus a. updates. PKR 200 (effective 1999). bibl. cum.index: 1967-1998. **Document type:** *Academic/Scholarly.*
Published by: College of Physicians & Surgeons Pakistan, Defence Housing Authority, 7th Central St., Karachi 75500, Pakistan. TEL 92-21-5892801, FAX 92-21-5887513. Ed. M Sultan Farooqui.

610 PAK ISSN 1022-386X
CODEN: JSPJER
COLLEGE OF PHYSICIANS AND SURGEONS PAKISTAN. JOURNAL. Variant title: J C P S P. Text in English. 1991. m. PKR 1,500 domestic; PKR 2,000 India & Bangladesh; GBP 80 in United Kingdom; USD 120 elsewhere (effective 2001). adv. bk.rev., Website rev. charts, illus, stat. cum.index: 1991-1999. 69 p./no. back issues avail. *Refereed.* **Document type:** *Journal, Academic/Scholarly.* **Description:** Publishes original articles, case reports, review articles, short communications, commentaries and survey reports on medical subjects. Occasionally issues per year are devoted to specific medical health problems and issues of national importance.
Related titles: CD-ROM ed.; Online - full text ed.
Indexed: Dairy Sci.Abstr., Environ.Sci.Poll.Mgmt., Excerp.Med., Helminthol.Abstr., INIS Atomind., Ind.Med. (coverage dropped), Microbiol.Abstr., Nutr.Abstr., Pollut.Abstr., Protozool.Abstr., Rev.Med.& Vet.Mycol., Risk Abstr., Rural Devel.Abstr., Saf.Sci.Abstr., Trop.Dis.Bull.
—BLDSC (4730.440000), GNLM.
Published by: College of Physicians & Surgeons Pakistan, Seventh Central St., Defence Housing Authority, Karachi 75500, Pakistan. TEL 92-21-5892801, FAX 92-21-5887513, jcpsp-pub@usa.net, http://www.cpsp.edu.pk. Eds. Masood Hameed Khan, M Sultan Farooqui, M. Sultan Farooqui. Pub. Saghir Ahmed. R&P M. Sultan Farooqui. Adv. contact M Sultan Farooqui. Circ: 5,500.

610 USA ISSN 0010-1087
R15 CODEN: TSCPAI
COLLEGE OF PHYSICIANS OF PHILADELPHIA. TRANSACTIONS & STUDIES. Text in English. 1793. a. USD 20 domestic; USD 25 foreign (effective 2000). back issues avail. **Document type:** *Academic/Scholarly.*
Related titles: Microfilm ed.: (from BHP).
Indexed: Biol.Abstr., Chem.Abstr., Ind.Med. (1938-).
—BLDSC (9020.210000), CISTI, GNLM, ingenta, KNAW.
Published by: College of Physicians of Philadelphia, 19 S 22nd St, Philadelphia, PA 19103. TEL 215-563-3737, FAX 215-569-0356, cppwi@collphyphil.org, http://www.collphyphil.org. Ed. Marc S Micozzi. R&P Josefa Sereda. Circ: 1,900.

M

610 ZAF ISSN 0375-3220
COLLEGES OF MEDICINE OF SOUTH AFRICA. TRANSACTIONS. Text and summaries in English. 1957. s-a. ZAR 50 to non-members. adv. bk.rev. charts, illus. **Document type:** *Journal, Academic/Scholarly.*
Formerly: College of Physicians, Surgeons and Gynecologists of South Africa. Transactions (0010-1095)
Indexed: Biol.Abstr., Environ.Sci.Poll.Mgmt., INIS Atomind., Ind.S.A.Per.
—BLDSC (8912.800000), CISTI, KNAW.
Published by: Colleges of Medicine of South Africa, 17 Milner Rd, Rondebosch, Cape Town 7700, South Africa. TEL 27-21-689-9533, FAX 27-21-685-3766, cmsa-adm@iafrica.com, http://www.collegemedsa.ac.za. Ed. Dr. Matt Haus. Circ: 6,000.

610 COL ISSN 0120-8322
COLOMBIA MEDICA. Text in Spanish. 1970. 4/yr. COP 20,000, USD 30. adv. bk.rev. illus, stat. **Description:** Includes original papers and clinical case works on medical science.
Formerly (until 1980): Acta Medica del Valle (0044-6017)
Related titles: Microfilm ed.: (from PQC).
Indexed: Chem.Abstr.
—CISTI.
Published by: (Universidad del Valle, Cali, Escuela de Salud Publica, Facultad de Salud), Corporacion Editora Medica del Valle, Calle 4b, 36-00, Cali, VALLE, Colombia. TEL 57-2-558-1939, comedica@mafalda.univalle.edu.co, http://colombiamedica.univalle.edu.co/. Ed. Dr. Pablo Barreto. R&P, Adv. contact Guillermo Llanos. Circ: 2,000. **Co-sponsor:** Academia de Medicina del Valle del Cauca; Asociacion Colombiana de Medicina Interna; Sociedad Colombiana de Epidemiologia.

610 USA ISSN 0199-7343
R11
COLORADO MEDICINE. Text in English. 1903. m. USD 35 (effective 2001). adv. bk.rev. charts, illus, tr.lit. index, cum.index. 40 p./no. 3 cols./p. reprint service avail. from PQC. *Refereed.* **Document type:** *Trade.* **Description:** Reports on society developments, news within the states and national affairs of interest to the profession.
Supersedes in part: Rocky Mountain Medical Journal (0035-760X); Formed by the merger of: Colorado Medicine; Utah State Medical Journal
Related titles: Microform ed.: (from PQC).
Indexed: Biol.Abstr., C.I.S. Abstr., Chem.Abstr., Curr.Cont. (coverage dropped), Dent.Ind., Excerp.Med., INIS Atomind., Ind.Med. (coverage dropped), Med.Care Rev.
—BLDSC (3321.630000), CISTI, GNLM, ingenta, KNAW.
Published by: Colorado Medical Society, PO Box 17550, Denver, CO 80217-0550. TEL 720-859-1001, FAX 720-859-7509, Bill_Pierson@cms.org, http://www.cms.org. R&P, Adv. contact William Pierson. Circ: 5,500 (paid).

610.28 USA
COMMENT; a funding first publication. Text in English. bi-w. **Description:** Offers a concise summary and brief analysis of current issues and events affecting biomedical research.
Media: Online - full text.
Published by: Washington Fax TEL 508-999-6097, FAX 508-994-9366, comment@washingtonfax.com, http://www.fundingfirst.org/comment/. Ed. Shirley Haley. Pub. Bradie Metheny.

COMMENTATIONES PHYSICO-MATHEMATICAE ET CHEMICO-MEDICAE. see *PHYSICS*

COMMENTS ON TOXICOLOGY. see *ENVIRONMENTAL STUDIES—Toxicology And Environmental Safety*

COMMUNITY HEALTH FUNDING REPORT. see *PUBLIC ADMINISTRATION*

360 GBR ISSN 1358-0981
COMMUNITY NURSE. Text in English. 1977. 11/yr. GBP 24 to individuals; GBP 45 to institutions (effective 2000). adv. **Document type:** *Bulletin, Trade.*
Formerly (until 1995): Community Outlook (1351-1416)
Indexed: Art.Hosp.& Tour., Brit.Nur.Ind., CINAHL, Int.Nurs.Ind.
—BLDSC (3363.646595), GNLM, Infotrieve. **CCC.**
Published by: Emap Healthcare Ltd. (Subsidiary of: Emap Business Communications Ltd.), Greater London House, Hampstead Rd, London NW1 7EJ, United Kingdom. TEL 44-20-7874-0200, FAX 44-20-7874-0201, http://www.emap.com. Ed. Funda Suteyman. Pub. Janice Roberts Clark. Adv. contact Chole Goodliffe. Circ: 20,000 (controlled).

610 USA ISSN 1061-5903
COMPARATIVE STUDIES OF HEALTH SYSTEMS & MEDICAL CARE. Text in English. 1978. irreg., latest vol.38, 1994. price varies. back issues avail. *Refereed.* **Document type:** *Monographic series.* **Description:** Discusses the past and present Western and Eastern practice of medicine, as well as sociopolitical, ethical, philosophical, and ecological issues.
Published by: University of California Press, Journals Division, 2000 Center St, Ste 303, Berkeley, CA 94704-1223. TEL 510-642-4247, FAX 510-643-7127. Ed. John M Janzen. **Orders to:** California-Princeton Fulfillment Services, Princeton, NJ 08618. TEL 800-777-4726, FAX 800-999-1958.

COMPETITIVE HEALTHCARE MARKET REPORTER. see *BUSINESS AND ECONOMICS—Marketing And Purchasing*

615.8 USA ISSN 1087-0865
COMPLEMENTARY MEDICINE FOR THE PHYSICIAN*. Text in English. 1996. 10/yr. USD 87 domestic to individuals; USD 112 foreign to individuals; USD 128 domestic to institutions; USD 153 foreign to institutions; USD 16. **Document type:** *Newsletter.*
—**CCC.**
Published by: Churchill Livingstone (Subsidiary of: Harcourt Health Sciences), 15 E 26th St, Fl 15, New York, NY 10010-1505. TEL 212-206-5000, FAX 212-206-7808, http://www.churchillmed.com. **Subscr. in the UK to:** Pearson Professional Ltd., Journals Subscription Department, Fourth Ave., PO Box 77, Harlow, Essex CM19 5AA, United Kingdom. TEL 44-1279-623924, FAX 44-1279-639609.

COMPLEMENTARY MEDICINE INDEX. see *MEDICAL SCIENCES—Abstracting, Bibliographies, Statistics*

615 USA ISSN 0098-8243
R11
COMPREHENSIVE THERAPY. Text in English. 1975. m. USD 169; USD 189 foreign (effective 1999). adv. bk.rev. *Refereed.* **Document type:** *Academic/Scholarly.* **Description:** Contains a collection of articles focusing on cardiovascular disease, arthritis, genitourinary disorders, cancer, pulmonary medicine, nutrition, metabolic disorders, infectious disease, and other major clinical entities.
Related titles: Online - full text ed.: (from Institute for Scientific Information).
Indexed: AgeLine, Biol.Abstr., CINAHL, Dent.Ind., Excerp.Med. (until 1990, 1995-), Fam.Ind., INIS Atomind., Ind.Med. (1975-), Int.Nurs.Ind., Lang.& Lang.Behav.Abstr., NRN.
—BLDSC (3366.390700), CISTI, EMDOCS, GNLM, ingenta, KNAW. **CCC.**
Published by: American Society of Contemporary Medicine, Surgery, and Ophthalmology, 4711 Golf Rd, Ste 408, Skokie, IL 60076-1242. TEL 847-568-1500, 800-621-4002, FAX 847-568-1527, iaos@aol.com. Ed. Dr. Randall T Bellows. R&P Deborah Pinkston. Adv. contact Mike Mason. Circ: 2,000 (paid).

610 USA
CONCERN. Text in English. 1984. 4/yr. USD 15 domestic to non-members; USD 25 foreign to non-members. adv. back issues avail. **Description:** Non-scientific articles and activities of the Society's members.
Published by: Society of Critical Care Medicine, 8101 E Kaiser Blvd, Anaheim, CA 92808-2214. TEL 714-282-6000, FAX 714-282-6050. Ed. Deborah Kincade Branch. Circ: 6,000.

610 FRA ISSN 0010-5309
CODEN: COMEAO
CONCOURS MEDICAL. Text in French. 1879. 40/yr. FRF 715 domestic to qualified personnel; FRF 540 domestic to students; FRF 1,110 foreign to qualified personnel; FRF 930 foreign to students (effective 2001). adv. bk.rev. bibl, charts, illus. index. **Document type:** *Magazine, Trade.*
Indexed: Biol.Abstr., C.I.S. Abstr., Chem.Abstr., Excerp.Med. (until 1993), INIS Atomind., Ind.Med. (coverage dropped), Ref.Zh.
—BLDSC (3399.480000), CISTI, GNLM, Infotrieve, KNAW. **CCC.**
Address: 2, Cite Paradis, Paris 75010, France. TEL 33-1-55-33-68-00, FAX 33-1-55-33-69-12. Ed. Dr. Francois Mignon. Circ: 70,000.

616.043 JPN ISSN 0914-3505
CODEN: CGANE7
CONGENITAL ANOMALIES. Text in English. 1961. q. JPY 8,000, USD 80 (effective 2001). adv. bk.rev. abstr, bibl, charts, illus. index. 100 p./no. back issues avail.; reprints avail. *Refereed.* **Document type:** *Journal, Academic/Scholarly.* **Description:** Publishes research results in clinical and basic sciences related to birth defects and congenital anomalies.
Former titles (until 1987): Senten Ijo (0037-2285); (until 1963): Nihon Senten Ijo Gakkai Kaiho
Indexed: Biol.Abstr., Chem.Abstr., Chem.Indus.Notes, Chem.Titles, Excerp.Med., INIS Atomind.
—BLDSC (3410.683000), CASDDS, CISTI, GNLM, Infotrieve. **CCC.**
Published by: Nihon Senten Ijo Gakkai/Japanese Teratology Society, Dept of Anatomy and Developmental Biology, Faculty of Medicine, Kyoto University, Kyoto-shi 606-8501, Japan. TEL 81-75-753-4670, FAX 81-75-751-7529, kshiota@med.kyoto-y.ac.jp. Ed. Yoshihiro Tsutsui. R&P Kohei Shiota TEL 81-75-753-4341. Circ: 1,700. **Subscr. to:** Japanese Teratology Society, Dept Anat Dev Biol, Kyoto University Fac. Medm, Kyoto-shi 606-8501, Japan. TEL 81-75-753-4670.

610 USA ISSN 0010-6178
CONNECTICUT MEDICINE. Text in English. 1936. m., latest vol.65. USD 25 domestic; USD 40 foreign (effective 2001). adv. bk.rev. bibl, illus. index. back issues avail.; reprints avail. *Refereed.* **Document type:** *Directory, Newsletter, Journal, Academic/Scholarly, Abstract/Index.*
Formerly (1940-1958): Connecticut State Medical Journal (0096-0179)
Related titles: Diskette ed.; Fax ed.; Online - full text ed.
Indexed: AgeLine, Biol.Abstr., CINAHL, C.I.S. Abstr., Chem.Abstr., Curr.Cont. (coverage dropped), Dent.Ind., Excerp.Med., INIS Atomind., Ind.Med. (1958-), Int.Nurs.Ind., Med.Care Rev.
—BLDSC (3417.655000), CISTI, EMDOCS, GNLM, ingenta, KNAW.
Published by: Connecticut State Medical Society, 160 St Ronan St, New Haven, CT 06511. TEL 203-865-0587, FAX 203-492-4112, wjacques-gill@csms.org. Ed. H David Crombie. R&P Wanda E Jacques Gill. Adv. contact Rhonda Hawes. B&W page USD 395, color page USD 1,100; trim 7 x 10. Circ: 7,250.

CONNECTIONS (LARGO). see *HEALTH FACILITIES AND ADMINISTRATION*

610 USA
CONNECTIONS NEWSLETTER (NEW YORK). Text in English. 3/yr. free per issue. **Document type:** *Newsletter.*
Formerly: National Medical Fellowships Newsletter
Published by: National Medical Fellowships Inc., 110 W 32nd St, 8th Fl, New York, NY 10001-3205. Pub. Ruth Conner. Circ: 11,000.

610 JPN ISSN 0916-572X
CODEN: COTIE7
CONNECTIVE TISSUE. Text in English, Japanese; Summaries in English. 1969. q. **Document type:** *Academic/Scholarly.*
Indexed: Chem.Abstr., Chem.Indus.Notes, Chem.Titles, Excerp.Med., Ref.Zh.
—BLDSC (3417.663800), CASDDS, EMDOCS, GNLM. **CCC.**
Published by: Nihon Ketsugo Soshiki Gakkai/Japanese Society for Connective Tissue Research, Ika Daigaku Byorigaku Kyoshitsu, 1-1 Shinjuku 6-chome, Shinjuku-ku, Tokyo 160-0022, Japan.

610 USA ISSN 0010-7069
R11
CONSULTANT (GREENWICH). Text in English. 1961. m. USD 115 domestic; USD 125 foreign (effective 2001). adv. charts, illus. reprint service avail. from PQC. *Refereed.* **Document type:** *Journal, Academic/Scholarly.* **Description:** Provides practical clinical information on diagnosis and therapy of clinical problems in primary care medical practice.
Related titles: Microform ed.: (from PQC); Online - full text ed.: (from Gale Group, Factiva).
Indexed: AgeLine, CINAHL, Hlth.Ind., L.R.I., Tr.& Indus.Ind.
—BLDSC (3423.760000), GNLM, Infotrieve, ingenta. **CCC.**
Published by: Cliggott Publishing Co. (Subsidiary of: S C P Communications, Inc.), 330 Boston Post Rd, Darien, CT 06820. TEL 203-662-6400, FAX 203-662-6420, info.cliggott@scp.com, http://www.ConsultantLive.com. Ed., R&P Susan K Lotstein. Pub., Adv. contact David S March. B&W page USD 8,785, color page USD 10,730. Circ: 223,000.

M

610 JOR ISSN 0254-7147
CONSULTING MEDICAL LABORATORIES. BULLETIN. Text in English. 1983. q. USD 25. back issues avail. **Document type:** *Bulletin.*
Published by: Consulting Medical Laboratories, P O Box 35198, Amman, Jordan. TEL 962-6-644480, FAX 962-6-644414, TELEX 21207 JOR HTL JO. Ed. Yahia F Dajani. Circ: 2,000.

CONTACT; the health & community development magazine of the W C C. see *RELIGIONS AND THEOLOGY*

617.07 USA ISSN 0743-510X
CONTEMPORARY ISSUES IN SURGICAL PATHOLOGY* . Text in English. 1983. irreg., latest vol.19. **Document type:** *Monographic series.*
Indexed: e-psyche.
—BLDSC (3425.187000), CISTI, KNAW.
Published by: Churchill Livingstone (Subsidiary of: Harcourt Health Sciences), 15 E 26th St, Fl 15, New York, NY 10010-1505. TEL 212-206-5040, FAX 212-727-7808.

610.715 USA ISSN 1077-209X
CONTINUING MEDICAL EDUCATION DIRECTORY. Text in English. 1993. biennial. USD 49.95 (effective 2000). **Document type:** *Directory.*
Published by: American Medical Association, 515 N State St, P O Box 10946, Chicago, IL 60610-0946. TEL 312-464-5000, http://www.ama-assn.org.

610 USA ISSN 0886-8220
CONTRIBUTIONS IN MEDICAL STUDIES. Text in English. 1978. irreg., latest vol.36, 1992. price varies.
Formerly: Contributions in Medical History (0147-1058)
—BLDSC (3459.900000), KNAW.
Published by: Greenwood Press, Inc. (Subsidiary of: Greenwood Publishing Group Inc.), 88 Post Rd W, Box 5007, Westport, CT 06881. TEL 203-226-3571, FAX 203-226-1502. Ed. John Burnham.

610 365 USA
CORHEALTH. Text in English. 1975. bi-m. USD 45 (effective 1998). adv. bk.rev. **Description:** Covers health care in correctional institutions.
Published by: American Correctional Health Services Association, PO Box 2307, Dayton, OH 45401-2307. TEL 937-586-3708, FAX 937-586-3699. Ed. Jim Voisard. Circ: 1,700.

610 378 USA
CORNELL MEDICINE. Text in English. 1978 (vol.41). 3/yr. free per issue. adv. bk.rev. illus. **Document type:** *Bulletin.* **Description:** Includes information on medicine and science of Cornell University Medical College.
Former titles (until 1996): Cornell University Medical College Alumni Magazine; (until 1993): Cornell University Medical College Alumni Quarterly (0010-8898); Cornell University Medical College Alumni Bulletin
Published by: Weill Cornell Medical College, 1300 York Ave, New York, NY 10021. TEL 212-821-0560, FAX 212-821-0576, jweil@mail.med.cornell.edu. Eds. C Richard Minick, Thomas McGovern. R&P Jonathan Weil. Circ: 17,000.

610 USA
CORNHUSKER FAMILY PHYSICIAN. Text in English. q. USD 5. adv. **Document type:** *Trade.*
Published by: Nebraska Academy of Family Physicians, 7101 Newport Ave, 201, Omaha, NE 68152-2158. TEL 402-572-3530, FAX 402-572-3532. Ed. Dr. David H Filipi. Circ: 3,000 (controlled).

610 DEU ISSN 0070-0347
R126.A1
CORPUS MEDICORUM GRAECORUM. Text in German. 1958. irreg., latest 1999. price varies. **Document type:** *Monographic series, Academic/Scholarly.*
Published by: Akademie Verlag GmbH, Palisadenstr 40, Berlin 10243, Germany. TEL 49-30-422006-0, FAX 49-30-42200657, info@akademie-verlag.de, http://www.akademie-verlag.de. **Co-sponsors:** Koenigliche Daenische Akademie; Saechsische Akademie der Wissenschaften, Leipzig.

610 ITA
CORRIERE MEDICO. Text in Italian. 104/yr.
Published by: R C S Editoriale Quotidiani S.p.A., Via Solferino, 28, Milan, MI 20121, Italy. TEL 2-63-39. Circ: 75,000.

610 USA ISSN 1048-5791
CORTLANDT FORUM. Text in English. 1988. m. USD 60 domestic; USD 78 foreign; USD 8 newsstand/cover (effective 1999). adv. charts, illus. back issues avail. **Document type:** *Magazine, Trade.* **Description:** Designed for the medical practitioner; includes short clinical vignettes, readers' most unusual cases, question and answer section and authored articles on clinical subjects.
Indexed: Nutr.Abstr.
Published by: Cortlandt Group, 7 Skyline Dr, Hawthorne, NY 10532. TEL 914-347-3800, FAX 914-347-3801, scarleton@cortlandtforum.com. Ed. Ruth Cohen. Adv. contact Leslie Carsman. Circ: 170,000 (controlled).

668.55 USA
COSMETIC SCIENCE AND TECHNOLOGY SERIES. Text in English. 1984. irreg., latest vol.22, 1999. price varies. adv. *Refereed.* **Document type:** *Monographic series.*
Indexed: Chem.Abstr., Chem.Indus.Notes, Chem.Titles, Eng.Ind.
—BLDSC (3477.175650).
Published by: Marcel Dekker, Inc., Attn: Eridania Perrez, 270 Madison Ave, New York, NY 10016-0602. TEL 212-696-9000, 800-228-1160, FAX 212-685-4540, marketing@dekker.com, http://www.dekker.com. Ed. Eric Jungerman. R&P Julia Mulligan. Adv. contact Eridania Perez.

COURTROOM MEDICINE SERIES: ABDOMINAL INJURIES. see *LAW*

COURTROOM MEDICINE SERIES: CHEST, HEART AND LUNGS. see *LAW*

COURTROOM MEDICINE SERIES: HEAD AND BRAIN. see *LAW*

COURTROOM MEDICINE SERIES: HIP AND THIGH. see *LAW*

COURTROOM MEDICINE SERIES: PAIN AND SUFFERING. see *LAW*

COURTROOM MEDICINE SERIES: SHOULDER AND ELBOW. see *LAW*

COURTROOM MEDICINE SERIES: THE KNEE AND ITS RELATED STRUCTURES. see *LAW*

COURTROOM MEDICINE SERIES: THE LOW BACK. see *LAW*

COURTROOM MEDICINE SERIES: THE NECK. see *LAW*

616.07 340 USA
COURTROOM TOXICOLOGY. Text in English. 1981. irreg. (in 8 vols.). USD 1,130 (effective 1999).
Published by: Matthew Bender & Co., Inc. (Subsidiary of: Lexis Law Publishing), 2 Park Ave, New York, NY 10016. TEL 212-448-2000, international@bender.com, http://www.bender.com.

616 USA ISSN 0886-9634
CODEN: CRANEG
CRANIO: JOURNAL OF CRANIOMANDIBULAR PRACTICE. Text in English. 1982. q. USD 90 domestic to individuals; USD 110 foreign to individuals; USD 130 domestic to institutions; USD 150 foreign to institutions (effective 2001). adv. bk.rev. back issues avail.; reprints avail. *Refereed.* **Document type:** *Academic/Scholarly.* **Description:** Discusses diagnosis and treatment of craniomandibular disorders for dentists, physicians and physical therapists.
Formerly (until 1985): Journal of Craniomandibular Practice (0734-5410)
Related titles: Microform ed.: (from PMC); Online - full text ed.: (from Institute for Scientific Information).
Indexed: ASCA, Curr.Cont., Curr.Tit.Dent., Dent.Abstr., Dent.Ind., Excerp.Med., Inpharma, Pharm.&Out.News, Reac.
—BLDSC (3487.046400), CISTI, GNLM, IDS, ingenta.
Published by: Chroma Inc., PO Box 8887, Chattanooga, TN 37414. TEL 800-624-4141, 423-899-1753, FAX 423-490-0791, contact@cranio.com, http://www.cranio.com. Ed. Dr. Riley H Lunn. Adv. contact Cynthia McLeod. Circ: 2,300.

610 USA ISSN 1092-4744
CREDENTIALING ACROSS THE CONTINUUM. Text in English. 1997. m. USD 495 (effective 1999). tr.lit. back issues avail. *Refereed.* **Document type:** *Newsletter.* **Description:** Addresses how to fulfill requirements and standards for credentialing and privileging in-home care, ambulatory care, physicians' offices, long-term care facilities, and management services organizations.
—**CCC.**
Published by: Opus Communications, PO Box 1168, Marblehead, MA 01945. TEL 781-639-1872, customer-service@opuscomm.com, http://www.opuscomm.com. Ed. Jay Kumar. Pub. Suzanne Perney.

610 GBR ISSN 1364-8535
CODEN: CRCAFM
CRITICAL CARE. Text in English. 1997. bi-m. GBP 200 in United Kingdom for both print & online; USD 300 elsewhere for both print & online (effective 2002). back issues avail. **Document type:** *Journal, Academic/Scholarly.* **Description:** Reports the new developments in all areas of critical care and publishes literature reports, reviews, news, commentaries, primary papers and more.
Related titles: Online - full content ed.: Critical Care Forum. ISSN 1466-609X. 1999. GBP 75 in the Americas to individuals; USD 112 elsewhere to individuals (effective 2002); Online - full text ed.: (from Institute for Scientific Information); Supplement: USD 99, GBP 65 (effective 2001); free to online subscribers.
Indexed: Ind.Med.
—BLDSC (3487.450610). **CCC.**
Published by: BioMed Central Ltd. (Subsidiary of: Current Science Ltd), Middlesex House, 34-42 Cleveland St, London W1T 4LB, United Kingdom. TEL 44-20-7323-0323, FAX 44-20-7580-1938, info@biomedcentral.com, http://www.biomedcentral.com/1364-8535/, http://ccforum.com.

610 USA ISSN 0749-0704
RC86 CODEN: CCCLEH
CRITICAL CARE CLINICS. Text in English. 1985. q. USD 139 domestic to individuals; USD 168 in Canada to individuals; USD 187 elsewhere to individuals; USD 195 domestic to institutions; USD 235 foreign to institutions; USD 127 domestic to students; USD 59 per issue (effective 2001). back issues avail. *Refereed.* **Document type:** *Academic/Scholarly.* **Description:** Delivers practical advice from experts in specialty covered as well as information on new developments in a variety of specialties with a fresh perspective on problems and controversies.
Related titles: Microfilm ed.; Online - full text ed.: (from Institute for Scientific Information).
Indexed: ASCA, Brit.Nur.Ind., CINAHL, Chem.Abstr., Chem.Indus.Notes, Chem.Titles, Curr.Cont., Excerp.Med., Ind.Med. (1985-), Inpharma, Int.Nurs.Ind., Nutr.Abstr., Pharm.&Out.News, Reac., SSCI (coverage dropped).
—BLDSC (3487.450700), CASDDS, CISTI, EMDOCS, GNLM, IDS, ingenta, KNAW. **CCC.**
Published by: W.B. Saunders Co. (Subsidiary of: Harcourt Publishers Ltd.), 11830 Westline Industrial Dr, St Louis, MO 63146. TEL 800-325-4177, http://www.wbsaunders.com. Eds. Michael A Geheb, Richard W Carlson. **Subscr. to:** Periodicals Fulfillment, W B Saunders Co, 6277 Sea Harbor Dr, 4th Fl, Orlando, FL 32891-4800.

610 USA ISSN 0090-3493
RC86 CODEN: CCMDC7
CRITICAL CARE MEDICINE. Text in English. 1973. m. USD 213 domestic to individuals for print & online eds.; USD 296 foreign to individuals for print & online eds.; USD 335 domestic to institutions for print & online eds.; USD 419 foreign to institutions for print & online eds.; USD 33 newsstand/cover (effective 2002). adv. illus. *Refereed.* **Document type:** *Academic/Scholarly.* **Description:** Provides multidisciplinary coverage of all aspects of acute and emergency care for hospital-based specialists, including anaesthesiologists and critical-care nurses.
Related titles: CD-ROM ed.: (from Ovid Technologies, Inc.); Microfilm ed.: (from WWS); Online - full text ed.: USD 435.50 domestic academic site license; USD 519.50 foreign academic site license; USD 485.75 domestic corporate site license; USD 569.75 foreign corporate site license (effective 2002) (from Ovid Technologies, Inc., Swets Blackwell, Institute for Scientific Information); ♦ Supplement: New Horizons (Baltimore). ISSN 1063-7389.
Indexed: AIM, ASCA, Abstr.Health Care Manage.Stud., CINAHL, Curr.Adv.Ecol.Sci., Curr.Cont., Environ.Sci.Poll.Mgmt., Excerp.Med., INIS Atomind., Ind.Med. (1973-), Ind.Sci.Rev., Ind.Vet., Inpharma, Int.Nurs.Ind., Jrnl.Watch, Jrnl.Watch Emer.Med., Jrnl.Watch Inf.Dis., Kidney, Neurosci.Cit.Ind., Nutr.Abstr., Pharm.&Out.News, Pollut.Abstr., Reac., Ref.Zh., Rev.Med.& Vet.Mycol., Risk Abstr., SSCI (coverage dropped), Saf.Sci.Abstr., Sci.Cit.Ind., Trop.Dis.Bull., Vet.Bull.
—BLDSC (3487.451000), ADONIS, CISTI, EMDOCS, GNLM, IDS, ingenta, KNAW.

Published by: (Society of Critical Care Medicine), Williams & Wilkins (Subsidiary of: Waverly International), 351 W Camden St, Baltimore, MD 21201-2436. TEL 410-528-4068, 800-222-3790, FAX 410-528-4452, dbaker@wwilkins.com, http://www.wwilkins.com, http://www.Lww.com. Ed. Dr. Joseph E Parrillo. Adv. contact David Baker. Circ: 15,118.

CRITICAL REVIEWS IN BIOMEDICAL ENGINEERING. see *BIOLOGY—Bioengineering*

616.07 610.28 USA ISSN 1040-8363
RB37 CODEN: CRCLBH
CRITICAL REVIEWS IN CLINICAL LABORATORY SCIENCES. Text in English. 1970. bi-m. USD 495 (effective 1998). bibl, charts, illus. back issues avail. *Refereed.* **Document type:** *Academic/Scholarly.* **Description:** Provides critical evaluations of new concepts, methods, and data in the biomedical fields.
Formerly: C R C Critical Reviews in Clinical Laboratory Sciences (0590-8191)
Related titles: Online - full text ed.: (from O C L C Online Computer Library Center, Inc., Swets Blackwell, ScienceDirect, Institute for Scientific Information).
Indexed: ASCA, Biol.Abstr., Chem.Abstr., Chem.Indus.Notes, Chem.Titles, Curr.Cont., Dent.Ind., Helminthol.Abstr., INIS Atomind., Ind.Med. (1980-), Ind.Sci.Rev., Inpharma, Int.Abstr.Biol.Sci., Nutr.Abstr., Pharm.&Out.News, Reac., Sci.Cit.Ind.
—BLDSC (3487.473000), ADONIS, CASDDS, CISTI, EMDOCS, GNLM, IDS, ingenta. **CCC.**
Published by: C R C Press, LLC, 2000 Corporate Blvd, N W, Boca Raton, FL 33431. TEL 561-994-0555, 800-272-7737, FAX 561-998-9784. Eds. David M Goldberg, J Thomas Hindmarsh. Circ: 530.

610 DEU ISSN 0353-9504
CODEN: CMEJE
CROATIAN MEDICAL JOURNAL. Text and summaries in English. 1953-1976 (vol.24); resumed 1984. q. EUR 60, USD 80 (effective 2001). adv. bk.rev. charts, illus. index. *Refereed.* **Document type:** *Journal, Academic/Scholarly.* **Description:** Provides for physicians with interdisciplinary scientific interests.
Formerly (until 1992): Sveuciliste u Zagrebu. Medicinski Fakultet. Radovi (0033-8575)
Related titles: Online - full text ed.: (from Institute for Scientific Information).
Indexed: Abstr.Hyg., Biol.Abstr., Cal.Tiss.Abstr., Chem.Abstr., Curr.Cont., Dairy Sci.Abstr., Environ.Sci.Poll.Mgmt., Excerp.Med., ExtraMED, Ind.Med. (1992-), Nutr.Abstr., Pollut.Abstr., Rev.Med.& Vet.Mycol., Risk Abstr., Saf.Sci.Abstr.
—BLDSC (3487.498200), CISTI, EMDOCS, GNLM, Infotrieve, KNAW. **CCC.**
Published by: (Sveuciliste u Zagrebu HRV, Medicinski Fakultet HRV), Pabst Science Publishers, Am Eichengrund 28, Lengerich 49525, Germany. TEL 49-5484-308, FAX 49-5484-550, pabst.publishers@t-online.de, http://www.pabst-publishers.de/cmj/. Eds. Ana Marusic, Matko Marusic. Circ: 3,800.

610 ESP ISSN 1135-4127
CUADERNOS DE GESTION PARA EL PROFESIONAL DE ATENCION PRIMARIA. Text in Spanish. 1995. q. USD 98. **Document type:** *Academic/Scholarly.*
Published by: Ediciones Doyma S.A., Traversa de Gracia, 17-21, Barcelona 08021, Spain. TEL 34-93-200-0711, FAX 34-93-209-1136. Ed. J Gene Badia. adv.: page ESP 189,000. Circ: 2,000.

610 ECU
CUADERNOS DE SALUD COLECTIVA. Text in Spanish. 1990. q. USD 10. bk.rev. bibl, illus.
Published by: Centro de Estudios y Asesoria en Salud, Dpto. 602, Calle ROCA, 549, Quito, Ecuador. TEL 593-2-506175, FAX 593-2-566714. Ed. Dr. Jose Yepez. **Co-sponsor:** Panamerican Health Organization.

610 500 ESP ISSN 0011-2577
CUADERNOS VALENCIANOS DE HISTORIA DE LA MEDICINA Y DE LA CIENCIA. Text in Spanish, Greek, Latin. 1962. irreg. (2-3/yr.). price varies. charts, illus. reprints avail. **Document type:** *Monographic series.*
—**CCC.**
Published by: Universidad de Valencia, Instituto de Estudios Documentales e Historicos sobre la Ciencias, Avda Blasco Ibanez, 17, Valencia 46010, Spain. FAX 34-6-3313975. Ed. Jose Maria Lopez Pinero. Circ: 500.

CULTURE, ILLNESS AND HEALING; studies in comparative cross-cultural research. see *ANTHROPOLOGY*

CULTURE, MEDICINE AND PSYCHIATRY; an international journal of comparative cross-cultural research. see *ANTHROPOLOGY*

616.97 USA ISSN 0160-1660
CUMITECHS; cumulative techniques and procedures in clinical microbiology. Text in English. 1974. irreg. (2-3/yr.). USD 12 to non-members; USD 9 to members. **Document type:** *Academic/Scholarly.*
Indexed: Diar.Dis.Res., Helminthol.Abstr., Ind.Vet., Protozool.Abstr., Rev.Med.& Vet.Mycol.
—Infotrieve. **CCC.**
Published by: American Society for Microbiology, 1325 Massachusetts Ave, N W, Washington, DC 20005-4171. TEL 703-787-3305. Ed. Steven C Specter.

610 ITA ISSN 0391-8904
CUORE E VASI. Text in Italian. 1979. bi-m. ITL 30,000, USD 30 (effective 2001). adv.
Indexed: Inpharma, Reac.
Published by: C I C Edizioni Internazionali s.r.l., Corso Trieste 42, Rome, RM 00198, Italy. TEL 39-06-8412673, FAX 39-06-8412688, info@gruppocic.it, 1160199510. Ed. A Salvati. adv.: B&W page ITL 4,000,000, color page ITL 5,100,000; trim 300 x 420.

CURARE; Zeitschrift fuer Ethnomedizin - journal for ethnomedicine. see *ANTHROPOLOGY*

CURRENT ADVANCES IN CLINICAL CHEMISTRY. see *CHEMISTRY—Abstracting, Bibliographies, Statistics*

610 570 GBR
CURRENT AWARENESS. S D I SERVICE. Text in English, French, German, Italian. ceased; resumed 1963. w. GBP 20.
Formerly (until 1967): Spectra Index and S D C Bulletin
Published by: Scientific Documentation Centre Ltd., PO Box 314, St Albans, Herts AL1 4ZG, United Kingdom. TEL 44-1727-847322, FAX 44-1727-847323, scilet@scilet.com.

616.07 USA ISSN 0168-6917
CODEN: CCPSEZ
CURRENT CLINICAL PRACTICE. Text in English. 1982. irreg. (lastest 1998). price varies. back issues avail. *Refereed.* **Document type:** *Monographic series, Academic/Scholarly.* **Description:** Discusses treatment protocols in all areas of internal medicine.
—CASDDS, CISTI, KNAW. **CCC.**
Published by: Humana Press Inc., 999 Riverview Dr, Ste 208, Totowa, NJ 07512. TEL 973-256-1699, FAX 973-256-8341, humana@humanapr.com, http://humanapress.com. R&P Richard Hruska.

610 USA ISSN 1071-3964
CURRENT CRITICAL CARE DIAGNOSIS AND TREATMENT. Text in English. 1994. irreg. **Document type:** *Monographic series.*
Published by: Appleton & Lange, Journal Division (Subsidiary of: Simon & Schuster Company), 11 W 19th St, New York, CT 10011-4209. TEL 203-406-4500, FAX 203-406-4600.

CURRENT EMERGENCY DIAGNOSIS AND TREATMENT. see *MEDICAL SCIENCES—Orthopedics And Traumatology*

CURRENT EMERGENCY THERAPY. see *MEDICAL SCIENCES—Orthopedics And Traumatology*

610 USA ISSN 0092-8682
RC71
CURRENT MEDICAL DIAGNOSIS AND TREATMENT* . Text in English. 1962. a. USD 45. **Document type:** *Academic/Scholarly.*
Formerly: Current Diagnosis and Treatment
Related titles: CD-ROM ed.
—BLDSC (3500.220000). **CCC.**
Published by: Appleton & Lange, Journal Division (Subsidiary of: Simon & Schuster Company), 11 W 19th St, New York, CT 10011-4209. TEL 203-406-4500, FAX 203-406-4600.

616.6 616.4 GBR ISSN 0269-185X
CODEN: CMGFEL
CURRENT MEDICAL LITERATURE. G H AND GROWTH FACTORS. Text in English. 1986. q. GBP 25, USD 40 to individuals; GBP 75, USD 120 to institutions. back issues avail. **Document type:** *Abstract/Index.*
—Infotrieve. **CCC.**
Published by: (Royal Society of Medicine), Current Medical Literature Ltd., 40-42 Osnaburgh St, London NW1 3ND, United Kingdom. TEL 44-20-7465-8377, FAX 44-20-7465-8380, enquiries@curmedlit.co.uk. **Dist. by:** Cassis Publishing Ltd., Realpage House, Abingdon Science Park, Barton Ln., Abingdon, Oxon OX13 3NB, United Kingdom. TEL 44-1235-537352, FAX 44-1235-537353.

610 IND ISSN 0011-3700
CODEN: CMDPAW
CURRENT MEDICAL PRACTICE. Text in English. 1956. m. INR 50, USD 15. adv. bk.rev. abstr, illus. reprint service avail. from PQC.
Related titles: Microform ed.: (from PQC).
Indexed: Biol.Abstr., Chem.Abstr., Chem.Indus.Notes, Chem.Titles, INIS Atomind.
—CASDDS, GNLM.
Published by: Current Technical Literature Co. Pvt. Ltd., Malhotra House, P O Box 1374, Mumbai, Maharashtra 400 001, India. Ed. B S Singhal. Circ: 2,500.

610 615 GBR ISSN 0300-7995
CODEN: CMROCX
CURRENT MEDICAL RESEARCH AND OPINION. Text in English. 1972. q. GBP 90, USD 165 (effective 2002). adv. index. back issues avail.; reprint service avail. from PQC. *Refereed.* **Document type:** *Academic/Scholarly.* **Description:** Contains articles concerning current medical research.
Related titles: Microform ed.: (from PQC); Online - full content ed.: (from ProQuest Information & Learning); Online - full text ed.: (from CatchWord Ltd., Institute for Scientific Information).
Indexed: ASCA, Abstr.Hyg., Agri.& Environ.Biotech.Abstr. (coverage dropped), Chem.Abstr., Chem.Indus.Notes, Chem.Titles, Curr.Adv.Ecol.Sci., Curr.Cont., Derwent Biotech.Abstr., Excerp.Med., Helminthol.Abstr., I.P.A., Ind.Med. (1972-), Ind.Sci.Rev., Inpharma, NRN, Nutr.Abstr., Pharm.&Out.News, Reac., Rev.Med.& Vet.Mycol., Rev.Plant Path., Sci.Cit.Ind., Trop.Dis.Bull.
—BLDSC (3500.301000), CASDDS, CatchWord, CISTI, EMDOCS, GNLM, ingenta, KNAW. **CCC.**
Published by: Librapharm Ltd, Gemini House, 162 Craven Rd, Newbury, Berks RG14 5NR, United Kingdom. TEL 44-1635-522651, FAX 44-1635-36294, journals@librapharm.com, http://www.librapharm.com. Pub., R&P P.L. Dr. Clarke. Adv. contact P L Clarke. Circ: 5,500.

610 GBR ISSN 0953-9352
CURRENT MEDICINE. Text in English. 1988. a. **Document type:** *Academic/Scholarly.*
Published by: Royal College of Physicians of Edinburgh, 9 Queen St, Edinburgh EH2 1JQ, United Kingdom. TEL 0131-225-7324, FAX 0131-220-3939.

610 AUT ISSN 1608-2222
▼ **CURRENT NEWS IN MEDICINE.** Text in English, German; Summaries in English. 2001. q. USD 75 domestic; USD 115 foreign; USD 35 newsstand/cover (effective 2001). adv. back issues avail. *Refereed.* **Document type:** *Journal, Consumer.* **Description:** Aims to improve communications and understanding in international medicine.
Related titles: Online - full text ed.
Published by: V I C E R Publishing, PO Box 14, Vienna A-1097, Austria. TEL 43-676-9568085, FAX 43-676-9568086, vicer@vicer.org, http://www.vicer.org. Ed., R&P Roland Hofbauer. adv.: B&W page USD 1,700, color page USD 2,200. Circ: 1,000 (paid and controlled).

610 AUT ISSN 1607-6524
▼ **CURRENT OPINION IN EUROPEAN MEDICINE.** Text in English, French, German, Italian, Spanish; Summaries in English. 2000. q. USD 75 domestic; USD 115 foreign; USD 35 newsstand/cover (effective 2001). adv. back issues avail. *Refereed.* **Document type:** *Journal, Academic/Scholarly.* **Description:** Publishes original articles, reviews, case reports and letters bridging basic science and clinical research in medicine and biomedicine.
Published by: V I C E R Publishing, PO Box 14, Vienna A-1097, Austria. TEL 43-676-9568085, FAX 43-676-9568086, vicer@vicer.org, http://www.vicer.org. Ed., R&P Roland Hofbauer. adv.: B&W page USD 1,700, color page USD 2,200. Circ: 1,000 (paid and controlled).

617.95 USA ISSN 1087-2418
CURRENT OPINION IN ORGAN TRANSPLANTATION. Text in English. q. USD 163 domestic to individuals for print & online eds.; USD 163 foreign to individuals for print & online eds.; USD 365 per issue domestic to institutions; USD 365 per issue foreign to institutions; USD 84 newsstand/cover (effective 2002). adv. bibl. **Document type:** *Academic/Scholarly.*
Related titles: Online - full text ed.: USD 801 site license (effective 2001) (from Ovid Technologies, Inc., Swets Blackwell).
—BLDSC (3500.776520).

M

Published by: Lippincott Williams & Wilkins (Philadelphia) (Subsidiary of: Wolters Kluwer N.V.), 530 Walnut St, Philadelphia, PA 19106-3621. FAX 215-521-8902, 215-521-8902, http://www.Lww.com. Eds. Leonard Makowka, Linda S Sher. Pub. Maria McMichael. R&P Tobias Weschler. Adv. contact Kelly Adamitis. **Subscr. to:** PO Box 1600, Hagerstown, MD 21740-1600.

610 GBR
CURRENT PRACTISE OF MEDICINE. Text in English. 12/yr. USD 295 in North America to individuals; USD 295 in South America to individuals; GBP 189.95 rest of world to individuals; USD 590 in North America to institutions; USD 590 in South America to institutions; GBP 375 rest of world to institutions; USD 153 in North America to students; USD 153 in South America to students; USD 153 rest of world to students (effective 2000).
Published by: Current Science Ltd, Middlesex House, 34-42 Cleveland St, London W1P 6LB, United Kingdom. TEL 44-20-7232-0323, FAX 44-20-7636-6911. **Dist. by:** Turpin Distribution Services Ltd., Blackhorse Rd, Letchworth, Herts SG6 1HN, United Kingdom. TEL 44-1462-488900, FAX 44-1462-483011.

610 USA ISSN 1072-8392
CURRENT REVIEW OF M R I. (Magnetic Resonance Imaging) Text in English. 1995. a. **Document type:** *Academic/Scholarly, Trade.*
Published by: Current Medicine, 400 Market St, Ste 700, Philadelphia, PA 19106. TEL 215-574-2257, 800-427-1796, FAX 215-574-2225. Ed. Lori J Bainbridge. **Subscr. outside N. America to:** Current Science Ltd, Middlesex House, 34-42 Cleveland St, London W1P 6LB, United Kingdom. TEL 44-20-7323-0323.

610 USA ISSN 0011-393X
CODEN: CTCEA9
CURRENT THERAPEUTIC RESEARCH; clinical and experimental. Text in English. 1959. m. EUR 132 in Europe to individuals; JPY 19,489 in Japan to individuals; USD 131 elsewhere to individuals; EUR 132 in Europe to institutions; JPY 19,489 in Japan to institutions; USD 125 elsewhere to institutions (effective 2002). back issues avail.; reprints avail. *Refereed.* **Document type:** *Journal, Academic/Scholarly.* **Description:** Publishes results of original research in the broad field of medical and pharmaceutical therapy and related areas.
Related titles: Online - full text ed.: (from ingenta, Swets Blackwell, ScienceDirect, Institute for Scientific Information).
Indexed: ASCA, AgeLine, Agri.& Environ.Biotech.Abstr. (coverage dropped), Chem.Abstr., Chem.Indus.Notes, Chem.Titles, Curr.Adv.Ecol.Sci., Curr.Cont., Dairy Sci.Abstr., Derwent Biotech.Abstr., Excerp.Med., Helminthol.Abstr., INIS Atomind., I.P.A., Ind.Sci.Rev., Inpharma, Int.Abstr.Biol.Sci., Int.Nurs.Ind., Neurosci.Cit.Ind., Nutr.Abstr., Pharm.&Out.News, PsycInfo, Psychol.Abstr. (1964-), Reac., Rev.Arom.& Med.Plants, Rev.Med.& Vet.Mycol., Rev.Plant Path., SSCI (coverage dropped), Sci.Cit.Ind., Sugar Ind.Abstr., e-psyche.
—BLDSC (3504.600000), ADONIS, CASDDS, CISTI, EMDOCS, GNLM, IDS, ingenta, KNAW. **CCC.**
Published by: Excerpta Medica, Inc. (Subsidiary of: Reed Elsevier Medical group), 105 Raider Blvd, 101, Hillsborough, NJ 08844. TEL 908-281-3625, FAX 908-874-3250, www.currenttherapeutices.com. Eds. C Ream, P Walson. Circ: 2,000.

615.1 AUS ISSN 0311-905X
CURRENT THERAPEUTICS; Australia's journal of disease management and drug treatment. Text in English. 1960. m. AUD 159.50 (effective 2001). adv. abstr, charts, illus. s-a. index. back issues avail.; reprints avail. *Refereed.* **Document type:** *Journal, Academic/Scholarly.*
Formerly: New Ethicals (0028-5064)
Related titles: Online - full text ed.: (from Institute for Scientific Information).
Indexed: Excerp.Med., Inpharma, Pharm.&Out.News, Reac., Rev.Plant Path.
—BLDSC (3504.605000), CISTI, GNLM, IDS, Infotrieve, ingenta. **CCC.**
Published by: Adis International Pty. Ltd. (Subsidiary of: Wolters Kluwer N.V.), Unit E, 5 Skyline Place, Frenchs Forest, NSW 2086, Australia. TEL 61-2-9975-9100, FAX 61-2-9975-9199, current.therapeutics@adis.com.au, http://www.ctonline.com.au. Ed. Dale Seaton. Pub. Chris Mellor. Adv. contact Des Utber. color page AUD 4,010; trim 273 x 207. Circ: 27,205.

610 CHE ISSN 0732-4448
R97 CODEN: CGMSDD
CURRENT TOPICS IN CHINESE SCIENCE. SECTION G: MEDICAL SCIENCE. Text in English. 1982. irreg., latest vol.2, 1984. *Refereed.* **Document type:** *Monographic series.*
—**CCC.**
Published by: Gordon and Breach - Harwood Academic (Subsidiary of: Taylor & Francis Group), PO Box 531, Lausanne 1000, Switzerland. **Subscr. addr. in US:** International Publishers Direct, PO Box 32160, Newark, NJ 07102. FAX 215-750-6343.

571.9 USA ISSN 0070-2188
CODEN: CTPHBG
CURRENT TOPICS IN PATHOLOGY. Text in English. irreg., latest vol.86, 1994. price varies. reprint service avail. from ISI. **Document type:** *Monographic series.*
Formerly: Ergebnisse der Allgemeinen Pathologie und Pathologischen Anatomie
Related titles: Microform ed.: (from PMC).
Indexed: Biol.Abstr., Chem.Abstr., Ind.Med. (1970-), Ind.Vet., Vet.Bull.
—BLDSC (3504.895000), CASDDS, CISTI, GNLM, ingenta, KNAW. **CCC.**
Published by: Springer-Verlag, Journals (Subsidiary of: BertelsmannSpringer), 175 Fifth Ave, New York, NY 10010. TEL 212-460-1500, FAX 212-473-6272.

615.9 ITA
CODEN: CTOTEG
CURRENT TOXICOLOGY AND THERAPY. Text in Italian. 1993. s-a. ITL 50,000; ITL 100,000 foreign (effective 1998). **Description:** Includes monographic studies and original papers concerning observations and experimental clinical research on toxicology and therapy.
Formerly: Currents in Toxicology and Therapy (1122-3804)
Indexed: Chem.Abstr., Chem.Indus.Notes, Chem.Titles, Excerp.Med. (1994-).
—BLDSC (3504.936450).
Published by: Casa Editrice Maccari, Via Palermo, 44, Parma, PR 43100, Italy. TEL 39-521-771268. Ed. Alfonso Cerrati. Circ: 1,200.

616.9 USA ISSN 1523-3820
CURRENT TREATMENT OPTIONS IN INFECTIOUS DISEASES. Text in English. 6/yr. USD 163.95 to individuals; USD 80 to students (effective 2002); Subscr. includes both print & online eds.. **Document type:** *Journal, Academic/Scholarly.*
Related titles: Online - full content ed.: USD 75 (effective 2002).
Published by: Current Science Inc., 400 Market St, Ste 700, Philadelphia, PA 19106. TEL 800-427-1796, FAX 215-574-2225, info@phl.cursci.com, http://www.treatment-options.com/cto_jrnl_home.cfm?JournalID=ID. Ed. Peter A Gross. **Affiliate:** Current Science Ltd.

616.37 DNK ISSN 0901-4500
CYSTISK FIBROSE. Text in Danish. 1980. 4/yr. free per issue. adv. illus. **Document type:** *Newsletter.*
Formerly (until 1985): Hej (0108-5409)
Published by: Landsforeningen til Bekaempelse af Cystisk Fibrose/Danish Cystic Fibrosis Association, Hyrdebakken 246, Viborg 8800, Denmark. TEL 45-86-67-44-22, FAX 45-86-67-66-66. Ed. H W Tybkjaer. Circ: 1,800 (controlled).

610 DEU
D G F MITTEILUNGEN. Text in German. 1976. q. DEM 32, EUR 16 (effective 1999). **Document type:** *Academic/Scholarly.*
Formerly: D G F Mitteilungsblatt
Published by: Deutsche Gesellschaft fuer Fachkrankenpflege e.V., Hermann-Simon-Str 7, Guetersloh 33334, Germany. TEL 49-5241-532203, FAX 49-5241-532205, dgf.guetersloh@t-online.de, http://www.dgf-online.de. Ed. Heiderose Killmer.

610 DNK ISSN 0108-7320
D I M S BULLETIN. Text in Danish. 1981. 3/yr. free per issue. adv. bk.rev.
Published by: Dansk Idraetsmedicinsk Selskab, Idraettens Hus, Broendby Stadion, Brondby 2605, Denmark. Ed. Jens H Kristensen.

D M W DISK-ARCHIV. (Deutsche Medizinische Wochenschrift) see *MEDICAL SCIENCES—Abstracting, Bibliographies, Statistics*

610 DEU ISSN 1617-5964
▼ **D M W PRAXIS PLUS.** (Deutsche Medizinische Wochenschrift) Text in German. 2001. 10/yr. EUR 38.20 domestic to institutions; EUR 46.80 in Europe to institutions; EUR 51.80 elsewhere to institutions; EUR 4 newsstand/cover (effective 2002). **Document type:** *Journal, Academic/Scholarly.*
Published by: Georg Thieme Verlag, Ruedigerstr 14, Stuttgart 70469, Germany. TEL 49-711-8931-0, FAX 49-711-8931298, kunden.service@thieme.de, http://www.thieme.de.

D R G HANDBOOK; comparative clinical and financial standards. (Diagnosis Related Group) see *HEALTH FACILITIES AND ADMINISTRATION*

610 BEL
D. SANTE/D. GEZONDHEID. Text in Flemish, French. 1989. m. BEF 750 (effective 2000). adv. **Document type:** *Consumer.*
Published by: Medi Media Belgium, Horzelstraat 100, Brussels 1180, Belgium. TEL 32-2-333-3411. Adv. contact Jan Bellon. page BEF 265,000. Circ: 270,000.

610 SWE ISSN 1104-7488
DAGENS MEDICIN. Text in Swedish. 1994. 41/yr. SEK 798 (effective 2001). adv. bk.rev. 52 p./no. 5 cols./p. back issues avail. *Refereed.* **Document type:** *Newspaper, Trade.* **Description:** Publishes information for people who work in the Swedish health care sector.
Related titles: Online - full text ed.
—GNLM.
Published by: Dagens Medicin Sverige AB, Fack 3396, Stockholm 10368, Sweden. TEL 46-8-54512300, FAX 46-8-4110102, redaktionen@dagensmedicin.se, http://www.dagensmedicin.se. Ed., Pub. Per Gunnar Holmgren. R&P Karolina Hallgren TEL 46-8-5451-2311. Adv. contact Stefan Hjaerpe TEL 46-8-796-6533. B&W page SEK 28,100, color page SEK 35,200; trim 252 x 365. Circ: 14,600 (paid); 3,200 (controlled).

610 DNK ISSN 1397-3290
DAGENS MEDICIN (COPENHAGEN). Text in Danish. 1997. 35/yr. adv. **Document type:** *Trade.*
Published by: Boersen Magasiner A-S, Christian IX's Gade 3,1, PO Box 194, Copenhagen K 1006, Denmark. TEL 45-33-32-44-00, FAX 45-33-76-96-66, md@dagensmedicin.dk, http://www.dagensmedicin.dk. Eds. Nicolai Doellner TEL 45-33-76-96-51, Marion Hannerup TEL 45-33-76-96-50. Adv. contact Gitte Broholm. Circ: 23,000 (controlled and free).

610 SEN ISSN 0850-797X
DAKAR MEDICAL. Text in French. 1956. s-a. XOF 20,000. adv. bk.rev. illus. **Document type:** *Bulletin.*
Former titles (until 1980): Societe Medicale d'Afrique Noire de Langue Francaise. Bulletin (0049-1101); (until 1959): A.O.F. Bulletin Medical
Related titles: CD-ROM ed.
Indexed: Abstr.Hyg., Biol.Abstr., Dent.Ind., Excerp.Med., ExtraMED, Helminthol.Abstr., Ind.Med. (1979-), Int.Nurs.Ind., Rev.Plant Path., Trop.Dis.Bull.
—CISTI, GNLM.
Published by: Societe Medicale d'Afrique Noire de Langue Francaise/Medical Society of the French Speaking Zone of Black Africa, BP 450, Dakar, Senegal. Ed. Mansour Ndiaye. Circ: 1,300.

610 CHN ISSN 1000-5676
DALIAN YIXUEYUAN XUEBAO/DALIAN MEDICAL COLLEGE. JOURNAL OF MEDICINE. Text in Chinese. 1960. q. USD 20. **Document type:** *Academic/Scholarly.*
Published by: Dalian Yixueyuan/Dalian Medical College, 465 Zhongshan Lu, Dalian, Liaoning 116023, China. TEL 24-0411-491802. Ed. Jin Yongxi.

610 EGY
DALIL AL-AHRAM AL-TIBBI/AL-AHRAM MEDICAL GUIDE. Text in Arabic. 1989. a.
Published by: Mu'assasat al-Ahram, Al-Ahram Building, Al-Galaa St., Cairo, Egypt. TEL 20-2-5747211, FAX 20-2-5747023, TELEX 92001.

610 USA ISSN 0011-586X
DALLAS MEDICAL JOURNAL. Text in English. 1914. m. USD 36; USD 50 foreign. adv. **Document type:** *Academic/Scholarly.*
Indexed: Ind.Med. (coverage dropped).
—CISTI, GNLM.
Published by: Dallas County Medical Society, PO Box 4680, Sta A, Dallas, TX 75208. TEL 214-948-3622, FAX 214-946-5805. Ed. Amy Vanvleck. Circ: 4,000.

610 IRN
DANESHKADE PEZESHKI. Text in Persian, Modern. 1947. 10/yr. adv.

M

Published by: Teheran Medical Sciences University, Faculty of Medicine, Enghelab Ave., Tehran 14714, Iran. TEL 021-6112743. Ed. Hassan Arefi. Circ: 1,500.

610 DNK ISSN 0907-8916
CODEN: DMBUAE

DANISH MEDICAL BULLETIN. Text in Danish. 1954. 5/yr. DKK 375 (effective 1999); (free to medical institutions on request). adv. charts, illus. reprint service avail. from PQC. **Document type:** *Bulletin.*

Former titles (until 1992): D M B (Danish Medical Bulletin) (0011-6092); (until 1975): Danish Medical Bulletin (0901-6929)

Related titles: Microform ed.: (from PQC,PMC); Online - full text ed.: (from Institute for Scientific Information).

Indexed: ASCA, Abstr.Hyg., AgeLine, Biol.Abstr., Chem.Abstr., Chem.Titles, Curr.Adv.Cancer Res., Curr.Adv.Ecol.Sci., Curr.Adv.Gen.& Molec.Biol., Curr.Cont., Dairy Sci.Abstr., Diar.Dis.Res., Excerp.Med., INIS Atomind., Ind.Med. (1954-), Ind.Sci.Rev., Inpharma, Int.Abstr.Biol.Sci., Med.& Surg.Dermat., NAA, NRN, Nutr.Abstr., Pharm.&Out.News, Reac., Rehabil.Lit., Rev.Med.& Vet.Mycol., Risk Abstr., SSCI (coverage dropped), Sci.Cit.Ind., Trop.Dis.Bull.

—BLDSC (3519.400000), CASDDS, CISTI, EMDOCS, GNLM, IDS, ingenta, KNAW.

Published by: Almindelige Danske Laegeforening/Danish Medical Association, Trondhjemsgade 9, Copenhagen Oe 2100, Denmark. TEL 45-35-44-85-00, FAX 45-35-44-85-04. Ed. Svend Schulze. Circ: 5,300. **Subscr. to:** Laegeforeningens Forlag, Esplanaden 8 A, Copenhagen K 1263, Denmark.

610 DNK ISSN 0084-9588
R539

DANSK MEDICIN HISTORISK AARBOG/YEARBOOK OF DANISH MEDICAL HISTORY. Text in Danish; Summaries in English. 1972. a. DKK 120 (effective 2001). adv. bibl, illus, stat. cum.index: 1972-1997. *Refereed.* **Document type:** *Academic/Scholarly.* **Description:** Covers the history of Danish and international medical science; includes larger articles on wide variety of subjects.

Indexed: NAA.

Published by: (Dansk Medicin Historisk Selskab), Odense University Press, Campusvej 55, Odense M 5230, Denmark. TEL 44-6615-79-99, FAX 44-6615-8126, press@forlag.oup.dk, press@forlag.ou.dk, http://www.sdu.dk/press, http://www.ou.dk/press. Ed., Adv. contact Dr. Henrik Permin. Circ: 900.

610 TZA ISSN 0856-0099

DAR ES SALAAM MEDICAL JOURNAL. Text in English. 1969. s-a. adv. bk.rev. bibl, illus. **Document type:** *Academic/Scholarly.*

Indexed: Biol.Abstr.

Published by: University of Dar es Salaam, Faculty of Medicine, Nuhimbili Medical Centre, PO Box 65007, Dar Es Salaam, Tanzania. Ed. Ernest Komba. **Co-sponsor:** Association of Dar es Salaam Medical Students.

610 378 USA

DARTMOUTH MEDICINE. Text in English. 1976. q. free per issue to qualified personnel. adv. bk.rev. charts, illus. back issues avail. **Document type:** *Consumer.*

Formerly: Dartmouth Medical School Alumni Magazine

Published by: Dartmouth Medical School, One Medical Center Dr, HB 7070, Lebanon, NH 03756. TEL 603-650-4039, FAX 603-650-4085, dartmed@dartmouth.edu. Ed. Dana Cook Grossman. Circ: 23,000 (controlled).

610 USA ISSN 0742-7484

DATA CENTRUM* . Text in English. 1984. m. USD 32; free to qualified personnel. adv.

Published by: Whitmore Jenson Publishers, 21 W 38th St, 4th Fl, New York, NY 10018-5506. TEL 212-586-4287. Ed. Stu Chapman. Circ: 127,500 (controlled).

610 CHN ISSN 1000-8470
RC81.A1

DAZHONG YIXUE/POPULAR MEDICINE. Text in Chinese. 1948. m. USD 1 per issue.

Published by: Shanghai Scientific and Technical Publishers, Journal Department, 450 Ruijin Er Rd, Shanghai 200020, China. **Dist. outside China by:** China International Book Trading Corp, 35 Chegongzhuang Xilu, Haidian District, Beijing 100044, China.

610 BEL ISSN 0931-8305

DE NATURA RERUM; international medical review for documentation and information. Text in English, French, German, Italian, Spanish. q. DEM 74 to individuals; DEM 52 to students. **Document type:** *Academic/Scholarly.*

—GNLM. **CCC.**

Published by: (C.E.I.A. Benelux), Editions Haug International, Ch de Ninove 1072, Brussels 1080, Belgium. Ed. Dr. Eric Reymond.

610 016.61 DEU ISSN 0178-3351

DEGUO YIXUE/DEUTSCHE MEDIZIN; an international journal. Text in Chinese. q. EUR 86.40 domestic; EUR 82.60 in Germany; EUR 14.40 newsstand/cover foreign (effective 2002). *Refereed.* **Document type:** *Journal, Academic/Scholarly.* **Description:** Contains selected articles from German medical periodicals.

—**CCC.**

Published by: Springer-Verlag (Subsidiary of: BertelsmannSpringer), Tiergartenstr 17, Heidelberg 69121, Germany. TEL 49-6221-345-0, FAX 49-6221-345229, subscriptions@springer.de, http://link.springer.de/link/service/journals/00364/index.htm, http://www.springer.de. Eds. B R Balda, Qiu Fazu. **Subscr. in N. America to:** Springer-Verlag New York Inc., PO Box 2485, Secaucus, NJ 07096-2485. TEL 212-460-1500, FAX 212-473-6272.

610 USA ISSN 0011-7781

DELAWARE MEDICAL JOURNAL. Text in English. 1929. m. USD 25 domestic; USD 40 foreign (effective 2000). adv. bk.rev. bibl, illus. index. reprint service avail. from PQC. *Refereed.* **Document type:** *Academic/Scholarly, Trade.*

Related titles: Microfilm ed.: (from PQC).

Indexed: AgeLine, Chem.Abstr., Curr.Cont. (coverage dropped), INIS Atomind., Ind.Med. (1960-).

—BLDSC (3547.500000), CISTI, GNLM, KNAW.

Published by: Medical Society of Delaware, 1925 Lovering Ave, Wilmington, DE 19806-2166. TEL 302-658-7596, FAX 302-658-9669, kmr@medsocdel.org, http://www.medsocdel.org. Ed. Dr. G Stephen Decherney. R&P, Adv. contact Kristine Riccardino. B&W page USD 240, color page USD 690; trim 10 x 7. Circ: 1,630.

610 IND ISSN 0011-7854

DELHI MEDICAL JOURNAL. Text in English. 1969 (vol.4). s-a. INR 4. adv. abstr, charts.

Published by: Delhi Medical Association, House Daryaganj, New Delhi 110 006, India. Ed. Dr. Kili Tuli.

DEMETER KONGRESS KALENDER MEDIZIN. see *MEETINGS AND CONGRESSES*

610.711489 DNK ISSN 0108-9781

DENMARK. SUNDHEDSSTYRELSEN. KURSUSOVERSIGT; specialistnaevnets udvalg for den teoretiske videreuddanelse. Text in Danish. 1982. a. DKK 45.

Published by: Sundhedsstyrelsen, Amaliegade 13, PO Box 2020, Copenhagen K 1012, Denmark. **Orders to:** Danske Boghandleres Kommissionsanstalt, Siljangade 6-8, Copenhagen S 2300, Denmark.

DEPAUL JOURNAL OF HEALTH CARE LAW. see *LAW*

610 USA ISSN 0098-471X

DETROIT MEDICAL NEWS. Text in English. w. USD 40. adv. **Document type:** *Newsletter.*

Published by: Wayne County Medical Society, 1010 Antietam, Detroit, MI 48207-2899. TEL 313-567-1640. Ed. Dr. Susan Adelman. Circ: 4,500.

610 DEU ISSN 0027-7460

DEUTSCHE GESELLSCHAFT FUER GESCHICHTE DER MEDIZIN, NATURWISSENSCHAFT UND TECHNIK. NACHRICHTENBLATT. Text in German. 1951. 3/yr. EUR 40 to members (effective 2001). adv. back issues avail. **Document type:** *Newsletter, Academic/Scholarly.*

Indexed: IBZ.

—GNLM, Infotrieve. **CCC.**

Published by: Deutsche Gesellschaft fuer Geschichte der Medizin Naturwissenschaft und Technik e.V., Berggasse 7, Jena 07745, Germany. Ed., Adv. contact Gerhard Wiesenfeldt TEL 49-3641-949510. page XEU 250; trim 140 x 210. Circ: 800.

616.02 USA ISSN 0070-4067
CODEN: VDGIA2

DEUTSCHE GESELLSCHAFT FUER INNERE MEDIZIN. VERHANDLUNGEN. Text in English. 1921. irreg., latest 1994, 94th. price varies. reprint service avail. from ISI. **Document type:** *Monographic series.*

Related titles: Microfiche ed.: (from BHP).

Indexed: Biol.Abstr., Excerp.Med. (until 1995).

—CASDDS, GNLM. **CCC.**

Published by: (Deutsche Gesellschaft fuer Innere Medizin), Springer-Verlag, Journals (Subsidiary of: BertelsmannSpringer), 175 Fifth Ave, New York, NY 10010. TEL 212-460-1500, FAX 212-473-6272. Ed. B Schlegel.

616.07 571.9 DEU ISSN 0070-4113
CODEN: VDGPAN

DEUTSCHE GESELLSCHAFT FUER PATHOLOGIE. VERHANDLUNGEN. Text in German. a. price varies. **Document type:** *Academic/Scholarly.*

Indexed: Biol.Abstr., Chem.Abstr., Chem.Indus.Notes, INIS Atomind., Ind.Med. (1948-).

—BLDSC (9163.310000), CASDDS, CISTI, GNLM, Infotrieve, KNAW. **CCC.**

Published by: (Deutsche Gesellschaft fuer Pathologie), Urban & Fischer Verlag, Loebdergraben 14a, Jena 07743, Germany. TEL 49-3641-626444, FAX 49-3641-626500, marketing.journals@urbanfischer.de, http://www.urbanfischer.de/journals.

610 DEU ISSN 1436-6142

DEUTSCHE GESELLSCHAFT FUER UNFALLCHIRURGIE. MITTEILUNGEN. Text in German. 1978. s-a. EUR 39.70 domestic to institutions; EUR 41.10 in Europe to institutions; EUR 42.80 elsewhere to institutions; EUR 21 newsstand/cover (effective 2002). **Document type:** *Journal, Academic/Scholarly.*

Formerly (until 1991): Deutsche Gesellschaft fuer Unfallheilkunde. Mitteilungen und Nachrichten (0177-3747)

—GNLM.

Published by: (Deutsche Gesellschaft fuer Unfallchirurgie), Demeter Verlag GmbH und Co. KG, Ruedigerstr 14, Stuttgart 70469, Germany. TEL 49-711-8931-0, FAX 49-711-8931322, custserv@thieme.de, http://www.demeter-verlag.de.

610 DEU ISSN 0012-0472
CODEN: DMWOAX

DEUTSCHE MEDIZINISCHE WOCHENSCHRIFT/GERMAN MEDICAL WEEKLY. Summaries in English, German; Text in German. 1875. 46/yr. EUR 230.40 domestic to institutions; EUR 301 in Europe to institutions; EUR 315 elsewhere to institutions; EUR 5.50 newsstand/cover (effective 2002). adv. bk.rev. abstr, bibl, illus, stat. index. reprint service avail. from PQC. *Refereed.* **Document type:** *Journal, Academic/Scholarly.*

Related titles: ♦ CD-ROM ed.: D M W Disk-Archiv. ISSN 3002-1472; Microform ed.: (from PQC,PMC); Online - full text ed.: ISSN 1439-4413 (from Institute for Scientific Information); Japanese ed.

Indexed: Abstr.Hyg., Agri.& Environ.Biotech.Abstr. (coverage dropped), Biol.Abstr., C.I.S. Abstr., Chem.Abstr., Chem.Indus.Notes, Chem.Titles, Curr.Adv.Ecol.Sci., Curr.Adv.Gen.& Molec.Biol., Curr.Cont., Dairy Sci.Abstr., Dent.Ind., Derwent Biotech.Abstr., Excerp.Med., Forest Prod.Abstr., Helminthol.Abstr., INIS Atomind., Ind.Med. (1875-), Ind.Sci.Rev., Inpharma, Int.Nurs.Ind., Med.& Surg.Dermat., Neurosci.Cit.Ind., Nutr.Abstr., Pharm.&Out.News, Protozool.Abstr., Reac., Ref.Zh., Rev.Appl.Entomol., Rev.Arom.& Med.Plants, Rev.Med.& Vet.Mycol., Rev.Plant Path., Risk Abstr., SSCI (coverage dropped), Sci.Cit.Ind., Small Anim.Abstr., Trop.Dis.Bull., Weed Abstr.

—BLDSC (3573.000000), ADONIS, CASDDS, CISTI, EMDOCS, GNLM, IDS, KNAW. **CCC.**

Published by: Georg Thieme Verlag, Ruedigerstr 14, Stuttgart 70469, Germany. TEL 49-711-8931-0, FAX 49-711-8931298, dmw@thieme.de, leser.service@thieme.de, http://www.thieme.de/dmw/index.html. Ed. M Middecke. Circ: 28,000.

615.89 DEU ISSN 0415-6412

DEUTSCHE ZEITSCHRIFT FUER AKUPUNKTUR; Zeitschrift fuer die wissenschaftliche Erforschung und praktische Anwendung der Akupunktur in Klinik und Praxis. Text in German; Summaries in English. q. EUR 59.40 domestic to institutions; EUR 63.40 in Europe to institutions; EUR 72.90 domestic to institutions; EUR 15.90 newsstand/cover (effective 2002). adv. **Document type:** *Journal, Academic/Scholarly.*

Related titles: Online - full text ed.: ISSN 1439-4359.

Indexed: Excerp.Med.

—BLDSC (3575.720000), EMDOCS, GNLM, Infotrieve. **CCC.**

Published by: (Oesterreichische Gesellschaft fuer Akupunktur), Karl F. Haug Verlag, Fritz-Frey-Str 21, Heidelberg 69121, Germany. TEL 49-6221-489445, FAX 49-6221-489584, http://www.haug-verlag.de. Adv. contact Guenter Fecke. **Co-sponsor:** Deutsche Aerztegesellschaft fuer Akupunktur.

610 DEU ISSN 0940-4783
DEUTSCHER FORSCHUNGSDIENST. BERICHTE AUS DER WISSENSCHAFT - AUSWAHL MEDIZIN. Text in German. m. DEM 78. **Document type:** *Academic/Scholarly.*
Published by: Deutscher Forschungsdienst, Ahrstr 45, Bonn 53175, Germany. TEL 0228-302210, FAX 0228-302270.

610 DEU ISSN 0012-1207
DEUTSCHES AERZTEBLATT; aerztliche Mitteilungen. Text in German. 1903. w. DEM 561.20, EUR 286.94; DEM 134.50 to students; DEM 12.20, EUR 6.24 newsstand/cover (effective 2000). adv. bk.rev. **Document type:** *Journal, Trade, Academic/Scholarly.*
Related titles: ♦ Supplement: Praxis Computer. ISSN 0179-1133.
Indexed: Excerp.Med., INIS Atomind., Ref.Zh.
—CINDOC, CISTI, Infotrieve. **CCC.**
Published by: (Bundesaerztekammer), Deutscher Aerzte-Verlag GmbH, Dieselstr 2, Cologne 50859, Germany. TEL 49-2234-7011-0, FAX 49-2234-7011460, verlag@aerzteblatt.de, http://www.aerzteblatt.de. Ed. Norbert Jachertz. Adv. contact Vera Zumbusch. B&W page DEM 23,900, color page DEM 32,000. Circ: 340,000. **Co-sponsor:** Kassenaerztliche Bundesvereinigung.

DEVELOPMENT (CAMBRIDGE). see *BIOLOGY*

DEVELOPMENTAL DYNAMICS. see *BIOLOGY*

DEVELOPMENTS IN BIOTHERAPY. see *BIOLOGY—Biotechnology*

610 FRA ISSN 0396-8014
DEVELOPPEMENT ET SANTE. Text in French. 1975. 6/yr. FRF 300, EUR 46 to individuals; FRF 400, EUR 61 to institutions (effective 2001). **Document type:** *Academic/Scholarly.* **Description:** Pedagogical information for caregivers in developing, tropical areas.
Published by: John Libbey Eurotext, 127 av. de la Republique, Montrouge 92120, France. TEL 33-01-46730660, FAX 33-01-40840999, marketing@jle.com, http://www.john-libbey-eurotext.fr/. Ed. Olivier Isaac Bismuth. **Subscr. to:** A T E I, 3 av. Pierre Kerautret, Romainville 92230, France. TEL 33-1-48408686, FAX 33-1-48400731, atei@club-internet.fr.

610 CHE ISSN 1015-8154
DEVENIR. Text in French. 1989. q. CHF 92, EUR 59.74 to individuals; CHF 139, EUR 90.25 to institutions (effective 2002). **Document type:** *Journal, Academic/Scholarly.*
Published by: Editions Medecine et Hygiene, Case Postale 456, Geneva, 4 1211, Switzerland. TEL 41-22-7029311, FAX 41-22-7029355, abonnements@medhyg.ch, http://www.medhyg.ch.

610 CHN ISSN 1000-2790
CODEN: DJDXEG
DI SI JUNYI DAXUE XUEBAO/FOURTH MILITARY MEDICAL UNIVERSITY. JOURNAL. Text in Chinese; Summaries in English. 1980. m. (1980-1998 Bimonthly). USD 240 (effective 2000). adv. *Refereed.* **Document type:** *Academic/Scholarly.* **Description:** Reports on original results and progress of the key projects undertaken by the scholars of the university and supported by the National Science foundation of China and WHO funds, and at the same time, it also carries contributions by overseas experts and scholars.
Related titles: CD-ROM ed.; E-mail ed.
Indexed: Environ.Sci.Poll.Mgmt., Microbiol.Abstr., Ref.Zh.
Published by: Fourth Military Medical University, 17 Changle Xilu, Xian, Shaanxi 710033, China. TEL 86-29-3373456, edjfmmu@fmmu.edu.cn. Ed. Bo Su. Pub. Liang-Tian Huang. R&P Tian-Feng Yuang. Adv. contact Chang-Tai Xu. Circ: 2,000 (paid); 200 (controlled). **Subscr. to:** China National Publications Import & Export Corp., 16 Gongti Donglu, Chaoyang District, Beijing 1000020, China.

610 ARG ISSN 0012-1762
DIA MEDICO✱ . Text in Spanish. 1928. m. adv. bk.rev. charts, illus. index.
Related titles: Supplement: Boletino. ISSN 0326-9221. 1957.
Indexed: Biol.Abstr., Ind.Med. (coverage dropped).
—GNLM.
Address: Tucuman, 1452, Capital Federal, Buenos Aires 1050, Argentina. Circ: 8,000.

610 CHE
DIABETES JOURNAL. Short title: D Journal. Text in German. 1974. 6/yr. CHF 36; CHF 42 in Europe; CHF 46 overseas (effective 2000). adv. bk.rev. **Document type:** *Journal, Academic/Scholarly.*
Published by: Schweizerische Diabetes Gesellschaft, Postfach 1830, Zuerich 8032, Switzerland. TEL 41-1-3833786, FAX 41-1-4228912. Adv. contact Brigitte Fankhauser. B&W page CHF 1,650, color page CHF 3,370; trim 260 x 195. Circ: 21,000.

616.0754 USA
DIAGNOSTIC IMAGING SCAN. Text in English. 1987. s-m. USD 720; USD 815 foreign (effective 1998). **Document type:** *Newsletter.*
Published by: Miller Freeman, Inc. (Subsidiary of: United Newspapers), 600 Harrison St, San Francisco, CA 94107. TEL 415-905-2200, FAX 415-905-2232. Ed. Brian Casey.

610 USA ISSN 1052-9551
CODEN: DMPAES
DIAGNOSTIC MOLECULAR PATHOLOGY. Text in English. 1991. q. USD 181 domestic to individuals for print & online eds.; USD 181 foreign to individuals for print & online eds.; USD 278 domestic to institutions for print & online eds.; USD 278 per issue foreign to institutions; USD 63 newsstand/cover (effective 2002). adv. bk.rev. charts, illus. reprint service avail. from PQC. *Refereed.* **Document type:** *Academic/Scholarly.* **Description:** Publishes contributions on molecular probes for diagnosis, such as tumor suppressor genes, oncogenes, the polymerase chain reaction, and in situ hybridization.
Related titles: Online - full text ed.: USD 361.40 domestic academic site license; USD 361.40 foreign academic site license; USD 403.10 domestic corporate site license; USD 403.10 foreign corporate site license (effective 2002) (from Ovid Technologies, Inc., Institute for Scientific Information); ♦ Supplement: American Journal of Surgical Pathology. ISSN 0147-5185.
Indexed: Biotech.Cit.Ind., Curr.Cont., Excerp.Med. (1993-), Ind.Med. (1992-), Ind.Sci.Rev., Inpharma, Int.Abstr.Biol.Sci., Reac., Sci.Cit.Ind.
—BLDSC (3579.662500), EMDOCS, GNLM, IDS, ingenta, KNAW.
Published by: Lippincott Williams & Wilkins (Philadelphia) (Subsidiary of: Wolters Kluwer N.V.), 530 Walnut St, Philadelphia, PA 19106-3621. TEL 215-521-8300, FAX 215-521-8902, http://www.Lww.com. Eds. Dr. Hubert J Wolfe, Dr. Ronald A Delellis. Pub. Jim Merritt. R&P Margaret Becker. Adv. contact Ray Thibodeau. B&W page USD 875, color page USD 1,895. Circ: 1,582 (paid). **Subscr. to:** PO Box 1600, Hagerstown, MD 21740-1600. TEL 800-777-2295, FAX 301-824-7390.

DIAGNOSTICS INTELLIGENCE. see *PHARMACY AND PHARMACOLOGY*

616.075 POL ISSN 0012-1932
CODEN: DLJNAQ
DIAGNOSTYKA LABORATORYJNA. Text in Polish. 1964. bi-m. USD 96. adv. bk.rev. **Description:** Examines clinical chemistry, cytomorphology, parasitology and serology.
Indexed: Biol.Abstr., Chem.Abstr., Chem.Indus.Notes, Chem.Titles, Excerp.Med., INIS Atomind.
—GNLM.
Published by: Polskie Towarzystwo Diagnostyki Laboratoryjnej, Ul Kopernika 15, Krakow 31501, Poland. TEL 21-39-76. Ed. Dr. Stefan Angielski. Circ: 1,450. **Dist. by:** Ars Polona, Krakowskie Przedmiescie 7, Warsaw, Poland.

DIARIO DE CONGRESOS MEDICOS. see *MEETINGS AND CONGRESSES*

DICTIONNAIRE PERMANENT: BIOETHIQUE ET BIOTECHNOLOGIES. see *BIOLOGY—Biotechnology*

DIMENSIONE SALUTE. see *PHYSICAL FITNESS AND HYGIENE*

610 570 JOR ISSN 1026-3772
CODEN: DSNJDI
DIRASAT. MEDICAL AND BIOLOGICAL SCIENCES. Text in Arabic, English. 1974. s-a. JOD 9 domestic to individuals; JOD 11 domestic to institutions; USD 30 foreign (effective 2002). illus. index, cum.index. back issues avail. *Refereed.* **Document type:** *Journal, Academic/Scholarly.* **Description:** Presents research papers and articles in biological, medical, nursing, dentistry, and pharmaceutical sciences.
Supersedes in part (in 1996): Dirasat. Series B: Pure and Applied Sciences (0253-424X).
Indexed: Bio-Contr.News & Info., Chem.Abstr., Chem.Indus.Notes, Chem.Titles, INIS Atomind., Ind.Vet., Plant Gen.Res.Abstr., Rev.Arom.& Med.Plants, Rural Devel.Abstr., Trop.Dis.Bull., Zoo.Rec.
—CASDDS, CISTI.
Published by: University of Jordan, Deanship of Academic Research, Dean of Academic Research, Amman, Jordan. TEL 962-6-5355000 ext 3200, FAX 962-6-5355599, dirasatb@ju.edu.jo, http://www.ju.edu.jo/research/dar. Ed. Nabil Shawagfeh. Circ: 1,000 (controlled).

362.1 USA ISSN 1093-6920
DIRECTIONS: LOOKING AHEAD IN HEALTHCARE. Text in English. 1997. 12/yr. USD 89 (effective 2001). abstr, charts. index. 10 p./no. 2 cols./p. back issues avail. **Document type:** *Newsletter, Trade.* **Description:** Publishes management news with a focus on trends, alerts, forecasts, profitable innovations, facts and statistics.
Related titles: Online - full content ed.
—**CCC.**
Published by: Health Resources Publishing, 1913 Atlantic Ave, Ste F4, Manasquan, NJ 08736. TEL 732-292-1100, FAX 732-292-1111, hrp@healthrespubs.com, info@healthrespubs.com, http://www.healthrespubs.com. Ed. Beth-Ann Kerber. Pub. Robert K Jenkins. Adv. contact Judy Granholm.

610 USA ISSN 0891-947X
R835
DIRECTORY OF AUDIO - VISUAL PROGRAMS FOR THE HEALTH SCIENCES AND RELATED FIELDS✱ . Text in English. 1987. a. USD 35. back issues avail. **Document type:** *Directory.*
Published by: Med-Av Publishing Co. Inc., 32 Bellport Pl, Garfield, NJ 07026-1421. TEL 201-423-3330. Ed. Charles M Murtaugh. Circ: 1,000.

DIRECTORY OF BIOMEDICAL AND HEALTH CARE GRANTS. see *EDUCATION—School Organization And Administration*

DIRECTORY OF FEDERAL HEALTH CARE FACILITIES. see *HEALTH FACILITIES AND ADMINISTRATION*

610 ZAF
DIRECTORY OF HEALTH SYSTEMS RESEARCH IN SOUTH AFRICA. Text in English. 1994. a. **Document type:** *Directory.*
Published by: Health Systems Trust, Project for Health Information Dissemination, Smith & Field St, 504 General Bldg, Durban, KwaZulu-Natal 4001, South Africa.

DIRECTORY OF HEALTHCARE GROUP PURCHASING ORGANIZATIONS. see *BUSINESS AND ECONOMICS—Trade And Industrial Directories*

DIRECTORY OF INDEPENDENT HOSPITALS AND HEALTH SERVICES; a comprehensive guide to the independent health care sector in the U.K. see *HEALTH FACILITIES AND ADMINISTRATION*

DIRECTORY OF MEDICAL AND HEALTH CARE LIBRARIES IN THE UNITED KINGDOM AND REPUBLIC OF IRELAND. see *LIBRARY AND INFORMATION SCIENCES*

DIRECTORY OF PATHOLOGY TRAINING PROGRAMS (YEAR). see *EDUCATION—Higher Education*

610 USA ISSN 0011-5029
R11
DISEASE-A-MONTH. Variant title: D M. Text in English. 1954. m. USD 108 domestic to individuals; USD 124 foreign to individuals; USD 179 domestic to institutions; USD 199 foreign to institutions; USD 57 domestic to students; USD 73 foreign to students; USD 17 per issue domestic (effective 2001). charts, illus, stat. cum.index. back issues avail.; reprint service avail. from PQC. *Refereed.* **Description:** For the general internist. Each issue is a single topic discussion that focuses on the integrated management of a particular disease.
Related titles: Microform ed.: (from PQC); Online - full text ed.: (from Institute for Scientific Information).
Indexed: AIM, Curr.Cont., Excerp.Med., Ind.Med. (1954-), Ind.Sci.Rev., Inpharma, NRN, Pharm.&Out.News, Reac., SSCI (coverage dropped), Sci.Cit.Ind., THA.
—BLDSC (3598.100000), CISTI, GNLM, IDS, ingenta, KNAW. **CCC.**
Published by: Mosby, Inc. (Subsidiary of: Elsevier Science), 11830 Westline Industrial Dr, St Louis, MO 63146-3318. TEL 314-872-8370, 800-325-4177, FAX 314-432-1380, http://www.mosby.com/periodicals. Ed. Dr. Erich E Brueschke. Circ: 4,606.

M

362.1 616 USA ISSN 1093-507X CODEN: DMANFR
DISEASE MANAGEMENT. Text in English. 1998. q. USD 119 domestic to individuals; USD 179 foreign to individuals; USD 143 domestic to individuals print and online eds. combined; USD 203 foreign to individuals print and online eds. combined; USD 210 domestic to institutions; USD 265 foreign to institutions; USD 252 domestic to institutions print and online eds. combined; USD 307 foreign to institutions print and online eds. combined (effective 2002). adv. back issues avail.; reprints avail. *Refereed.* **Document type:** *Journal, Academic/Scholarly.* **Description:** Includes clinical and research and case studies, papers on practical aspects involved in implementing disease management initiatives, and perspectives and insights from professionals involved in all aspects of disease management.
Related titles: Online - full text ed.: USD 210 to institutions; USD 119 to individuals (effective 2002) (from EBSCO Publishing, CatchWord Ltd., Swets Blackwell).
—BLDSC (3598.083000). **CCC.**
Published by: Mary Ann Liebert, Inc. Publishers, 2 Madison Ave, Larchmont, NY 10538. TEL 914–834-3100, FAX 914-834-1388, info@liebertpub.com, www.liebertpub.com/dis, http://www.liebertpub.com. Eds. Dr. John Byrnes, Dr. Stan Bernard. Adv. contact Harriet Matysko.

610 USA ISSN 1088-3371
DISEASE MANAGEMENT AND CLINICAL OUTCOMES. Text in English. 1997. bi-m. USD 175 (effective 1999). *Refereed.* **Document type:** *Newsletter, Academic/Scholarly.* **Description:** Reviews all aspects of disease management, clinical outcomes, and health economics.
Related titles: Online - full text ed.: (from ingenta, Swets Blackwell).
Indexed: Inpharma, Reac.
—BLDSC (3598.084000), GNLM, Infotrieve. **CCC.**
Published by: University of Medicine and Dentistry of New Jersey, UMDNJ - Robert Wood Johnson Medical School, One Robert Wood Johnson Pl CN19, New Brunswick, NJ 08903-0019. TEL 732-235-7685, FAX 732-235-7039, 732-235-7039, http://www2.umdnj.edu/dmcocweb/dmcoj.html. Eds. Dr. Clifton R Lacy, Dr. John B Kostis. Pub. Jeanne Dobrzynski.

610 NZL ISSN 1173-8790
DISEASE MANAGEMENT & HEALTH OUTCOMES. Text in English. 1997. m. USD 165 to individuals Print or Online ed.; USD 198 to individuals Print and Online combined eds.; USD 645 to institutions Print or Online ed.; USD 774 to institutions Print and Online combined eds. (effective 2001). back issues avail. *Refereed.* **Document type:** *Academic/Scholarly.* **Description:** Designed as a forum for collating, evaluating and disseminating practical knowledge on the application of components of disease management based on best evidence.
Related titles: Online - full text ed.: (from Ovid Technologies, Inc., EBSCO Publishing, O C L C Online Computer Library Center, Inc., RoweCom Information Quest, ingenta, Swets Blackwell, Institute for Scientific Information).
Indexed: Curr.Cont., I.P.A., Inpharma, Pharm.&Out.News, Reac.
—BLDSC (3598.084500), ADONIS, GNLM, Infotrieve. **CCC.**
Published by: Adis International Limited, Mairangi Bay, Private Bag 65901, Auckland 1010, New Zealand. TEL 64-9-477-0700, FAX 64-9-477-0766, will.charles@adis.co.nz, http://biomednet.com/library/jdmh, http://www.adis.com. Ed. Michelle Wilde. Pub. Paul Chrisp. R&P Will Charles. **Americas subscr. to:** Adis International Inc., Attn: Subscription Dept, 860 Town Center Dr, Langhorne, PA 19047. TEL 877-872-2347.

338.476 610.28 USA ISSN 1084-7146
DISEASE MANAGEMENT NEWS. Text in English. 1995. s-m. USD 387 domestic; USD 397 in Canada; USD 412 elsewhere (effective 2000). charts, mkt, stat. back issues avail. **Document type:** *Newsletter, Trade.* **Description:** Provides competitive business intelligence on disease and demand management with coverage of provider compliance, markets, technology, contracts, acquisitions, and partnerships.
Indexed: Inpharma, Pharm.&Out.News, Reac.
—BLDSC (3598.088000).
Published by: Business Information Services, Inc, 12811 North Point Ln, Laurel, MD 20708. TEL 301-604-4001, FAX 301-604-5126, businfosvc@aol.com. Ed. James H Gutman. R&P Seth Sprecher.

610 USA ISSN 1087-030X
DISEASE STATE MANAGEMENT. Text in English. 1998. m. USD 429 domestic; USD 389 foreign (effective 1999). **Document type:** *Newsletter.*
Indexed: CINAHL.
Published by: American Health Consultants (Subsidiary of: Medical Economics Co., Inc.), 3525 Piedmont Rd, N E, 6 Piedmont Center, Ste 400, Atlanta, GA 30305. TEL 404-688-2421, FAX 404-262-7837, custserv@ahcpub.com, http://www.ahcpub.com.

610 SWE ISSN 0283-9830
DISTRIKTLAEKAREN. Text in Swedish. 1983. 8/yr. **Document type:** *Trade.*
Formerly (until 1987): D L F Informerar
Published by: Svenska Distriktlaekarfoereningen (DLF), Fack 5610, Stockholm 11486, Sweden.

610 JPN ISSN 0288-559X CODEN: DITEDV
DITERUMAN/DETAILMAN INFORMATION. Text in Japanese. 1975. m. JPY 2,900 per issue.
—CASDDS.
Published by: Mikushu/Medical Information Express, 28-2 Kanda-Ogawa-Machi 3-chome, Chiyoda-ku, Tokyo 101-0052, Japan.

610 JPN ISSN 0287-2153
DOAI IGAKU ZASSHI/FRATERNITY MEMORIAL HOSPITAL. MEDICAL JOURNAL. Text in Japanese. 1959. biennial. **Document type:** *Academic/Scholarly.*
Published by: Doai Kinen Byoin/Fraternity Memorial Hospital, 1-11 Yokoami 2-chome, Sumida-ku, Tokyo 130-0015, Japan. Ed. Yasuhiro Saito.

610 GBR ISSN 0046-0451
DOCTOR. Text in English. 1971. w. GBP 91 domestic; GBP 171 for 2 yrs. domestic; USD 256 foreign (effective 2000). adv. bk.rev. abstr. charts, illus. **Document type:** *Trade.* **Description:** Political, financial and clinical news relevant to the day-to-day practice of all general practitioners.
Related titles: Microfilm ed.: (from PQC).
—BLDSC (3606.400000). **CCC.**
Published by: Reed Business Information (Subsidiary of: Reed Elsevier plc), Quadrant House, The Quadrant, Brighton Rd, Sutton, Surrey SM2 5AS, United Kingdom. TEL 44-208-652-3500, FAX 44-208-652-8977, rbp.subscriptions@rbi.co.uk, http://www.reedbusiness.com. Circ: 36,000. **Subscr. to:** Quadrant Subscription Services, PO Box 302, Haywards Heath, W Sussex RH16 3YY, United Kingdom. TEL 44-1444-445566, FAX 44-1444-445447.

610 JPN
DOCTOR. Text in Japanese. 1966. w. JPY 7,300. stat.
Published by: Yakuji Nyususha, 5-5 Dosho-Machi 1-chome, Chuo-ku, Osaka-shi 541-0045, Japan.

613 EGY ISSN 0012-4435
AD-DOCTOR; health education magazine. Text in Arabic. 1947. m. EGP 1, USD 4. bibl. index, cum.index.
Published by: Doctor, 8 Sharia Hoda Shaarawy, Cairo, Egypt. Ed. Dr. Ahmad M Kamal. Circ: 30,000.

610.696 USA
DOCTOR - PATIENT STUDIES. Text in English. 1989. q. free per issue. bk.rev. back issues avail. **Document type:** *Newsletter, Abstract/Index, Bibliography.* **Description:** Describes the activities at the center and provides an abstract service for selected scholars on research concerning the doctor - patient relationship and clinical ethics.
Published by: University of Chicago, Center for Clinical Medical Ethics, MC 6098, 5811 S Maryland, Chicago, IL 60637. TEL 312-702-3742, FAX 312-702-0090. Ed. James J Hughes. Circ: 600 (controlled).

363.347 USA
DOCTORS FOR DISASTER PREPAREDNESS NEWSLETTER. Short title: D D P. Text in English. 1984. bi-m. USD 10. adv. back issues avail.
Formerly: Triage!
Published by: Doctors for Disaster Preparedness, 1601 N Tucson Blvd, Ste 9, Tucson, AZ 85716. TEL 520-325-2689. Ed. Jane Orient. Circ: 1,500.

610 USA
DOCTOR'S FORUM✱; the laypersons guide to modern medicine. Text in English. 1996. bi-m. USD 2.95 newsstand/cover. adv.
Published by: Doctor's Forum, Inc., 3655 Salisbury Hills Dr, Allentown, PA 18103-9629. TEL 800-238-5320. Ed. Robert Oristaglio.

610 USA ISSN 0733-2262
THE DOCTOR'S OFFICE. Text in English. 1982. m. USD 99 (effective 2000). adv. back issues avail. **Document type:** *Newsletter, Trade.* **Description:** Provides information to clarify insurance regulations, collections techniques, marketing ideas and other practice management techniques, as well as dealing with managed care.
Indexed: Hlth.Ind.
Published by: Opus Communications, PO Box 1168, Marblehead, MA 01945. TEL 800-331-5196, FAX 781-639-7857, bhawksley@hcpro.com, http://www.hcmarketplace.com. Ed. Ann Mead-Ash. Pub. Jennifer Cofer. R&P Bethany Hawksley. Circ: 24,000 (paid).

DOCTOR'S REVIEW; leisure-time journal for physicians. see *TRAVEL AND TOURISM*

610 USA
DOCTOR'S SHOPPER. Text in English. 1983. q. USD 5 per issue. adv. bk.rev. illus, pat, stat, tr.lit. **Document type:** *Trade.*
Published by: Marketing Communications, Inc., 1086 Remsen Ave, Brooklyn, NY 11236. TEL 718-257-8484, FAX 718-257-8845. Ed. Ralph Selitzer. Adv. contact Felice Frost. Circ: 208,000 (controlled).

610 NGA ISSN 0046-0508
DOKITA. Text in English. 1960. s-a. NGN 2.40; USD 5 to individuals; USD 3 to students. adv. bk.rev. charts, illus. **Document type:** *Academic/Scholarly.*
Indexed: Biol.Abstr.
Published by: (University of Ibadan Medical Students' Association), Ibadan University Press, University of Ibadan, Ibadan, Oyo, Nigeria. Ed. A Ibe Otuka. Circ: 1,000. **Co-sponsor:** University of Ibadan. Department of Medicine.

610 JPN ISSN 0385-5023 CODEN: DJMSDB
DOKKYO JOURNAL OF MEDICAL SCIENCES. Text in English. 1974. q. JPY 5,000 (effective 1997). bk.rev. *Refereed.* **Document type:** *Academic/Scholarly.* **Description:** Covers basic and clinical medicine.
Related titles: Japanese ed.: Dokkyo Igakukai Zasshi. ISSN 0911-5900.
Indexed: Biol.Abstr., Chem.Abstr., Chem.Indus.Notes, Chem.Titles, Excerp.Med., INIS Atomind., Ind.Med. (coverage dropped).
—CASDDS, CISTI, EMDOCS.
Published by: Dokkyo University School of Medicine, Dokkyo Medical Society/Dokkyo Daigaku Igakubu Dokkyo Igakkai, Mibu, Tochigi 321-02, Japan. TEL 81-282-86-1111, FAX 81-282-86-3276, TELEX 3562118, wakai@dokkyomed.ac.jp. Ed., R&P Susumu Wakai. adv.: page JPY 50,000. Circ: 1,300.

610.69 SWE ISSN 1100-9861
DOKTORAND; en handledning foer dig som taenker doktorera. Text in Swedish. 1988. biennial. SEK 50 (effective 1996).
Published by: S A C O - Sveriges Akademikers Centralorganisation, Fack 2206, Stockholm 10315, Sweden. Ed. Dagmar Bergstroem.

610 JPN ISSN 0389-7303
DOKUTA SARON/DOCTOR SALON. Text in Japanese. 1957. m. JPY 300 per issue.
Published by: Kyorin Medikaru Sapurai/Kyorin Medical Supply, 8-16 Sarugaku-cho 2-chome, Chiyoda-ku, Tokyo 101-0064, Japan.

616.0472 ESP ISSN 0214-0659 CODEN: DOLOFV
DOLOR; investigacion, clinica & terapeutica. Text in Spanish. 1986. q.
Indexed: Excerp.Med.
—BLDSC (3616.613500), CASDDS.
Published by: (Foro para el Estudio del Dolor), Publicaciones Permanyer, Mallorca, 310, Barcelona 08037, Spain. TEL 34-3-2075920, FAX 34-3-4576642, permanyer@bcn.servicom.es. Ed. C de Barutell Farinos.

610 JPN ISSN 0288-1829
DONAN IGAKKAISHI/MEDICAL ASSOCIATION OF SOUTH HOKKAIDO. JOURNAL. Text in Japanese. 1957. a.
Published by: Donan Igakkai, 33-19 Moto-Machi, Hakodate-shi, Hokkaido 040-0054, Japan. Circ: 850.

THE DOOR OPENER; Connecticut's holistic health and metaphysical networking magazine. see *ALTERNATIVE MEDICINE*

610 USA
DORLAND'S PHYSICIAN DIRECTORY & RESOURCE GUIDE - TRISTATE AREA. Text in English. 1952. a. USD 88 (effective 1997). adv. **Document type:** *Directory.* **Description:** Listings of physicians, health care organizations, hospitals and specialists in the greater Philadelphia metropolitan area.
Former titles: Dorland's Medical Directory. Eastern Pennsylvania and Southern New Jersey Edition (1058-9392); Dorland's Medical Directory. Delaware Valley Edition; Dorland's Medical Directory. Philadelphia Metropolitan Area
Published by: Dorland Healthcare Information, 1500 Walnut St Ste 1000, Philadelphia, PA 19102. Circ: 6,500.

610 CHE ISSN 1011-288X
DOULEUR ET ANALGESIE. Text in French. q. CHF 86, EUR 55.84 to individuals; CHF 146, EUR 94.80 to institutions (effective 2002). **Document type:** *Journal, Academic/Scholarly.*
—BLDSC (3619.931800), EMDOCS, GNLM. **CCC.**
Published by: Editions Medecine et Hygiene, Case Postale 456, Geneva, 4 1211, Switzerland. TEL 41-22-7029311, FAX 41-22-7029355, abonnements@medhyg.ch, http://www.medhyg.ch.

610 USA
DR. ALEXANDER GRANT'S HEALTH GAZETTE; a monthly digest of medical facts and news. Text in English. 1978. 10/yr. USD 27 domestic; USD 45 foreign (effective 2001). cum.index. back issues avail. *Refereed.* **Document type:** *Newsletter.* **Description:** Presents a digest of medical facts and news.
Formerly: Healthwise (0740-1086)
Published by: Alexander Grant and Associates, Inc., PO Box 1786, Indianapolis, IN 46206. FAX 317-253-8582. Ed. Dr. Alexander Grant. Circ: 40,000 (paid and controlled).

610 615.19 DEU ISSN 0173-430X
DR. MED. MABUSE; Zeitschrift fuer Gesundheitswesen. Text in German. 1976. 6/yr. DEM 58 domestic; DEM 64 foreign; DEM 9.80 newsstand/cover. adv. bk.rev. back issues avail. **Document type:** *Trade.* **Description:** Publication for those working in the health field. Features a broad variety of health and medical issues worldwide. Includes readers' letters, list of events and positions available.
—GNLM.
Published by: Mabuse Verlag GmbH, Kasseler Str 1A, Frankfurt Am Main 60486, Germany. TEL 49-69-97074071, FAX 49-69-704152, mabuse@oeko-net.de, http://www.oeko-net.de/mabuse/. Ed. Dr. Hermann Loeffler. Adv. contact Ingrid Lang. B&W page DEM 2,300; trim 264 x 185. Circ: 22,000.

610 615 USA ISSN 1053-1564
DRUG AND MARKET DEVELOPMENT NEWSLETTER. Text in English. 1989. m. USD 1,095 domestic; USD 1,120 foreign (effective 2000). adv. charts, stat. back issues avail. *Refereed.* **Document type:** *Newsletter.* **Description:** Covers global business and technology issues facing pharmaceutical and biotech companies during the lengthy and costly drug development process. Significant developments in key therapeutic areas and technologies are covered in-depth.
Related titles: CD-ROM ed.; Online - full text ed.: (from Ovid Technologies, Inc.).
Indexed: Inpharma, Pharm.&Out.News, Reac.
Published by: D & M D Publications, One Research Dr, PO Box 5194, Westborough, MA 01581-5194. TEL 508-616-5566, FAX 508-616-5544, http://www.drugandmarket.com. Eds. Lynn M Savage, Tricia Nagle. Adv. contact Jonathan Gerson. B&W page USD 795, color page USD 1,195; trim 11 x 8.5. Circ: 600 (paid); 100 (controlled). **Co-sponsor:** International Business Communication.

610 USA
DRUG ENFORCEMENT ADMINISTRATION REGISTRATION FILE - ACTIVE. Short title: D E A Registration File - Active. Text in English. q. **Description:** Lists all those registered under the Controlled Substance Act who are doing business registered in their own name.
Media: Magnetic Tape. **Related titles:** CD-ROM ed.: USD 900 domestic; USD 1,800 foreign; Online - full text ed.
Published by: (Department of Treasury, Drug Enforcement Administration), U.S. National Technical Information Service, 5825 Port Royal Rd, Springfield, VA 22161. TEL 703-487-4630, orders@ntis.fedworld.gov, http://www.ntis.gov/dea.

612.39 615 USA ISSN 0360-2532
CODEN: DMTRAR
DRUG METABOLISM REVIEWS. Text in English. 1969. q. USD 95 to individuals print & online eds.; USD 1,495 to institutions print only (effective 2002). adv. *Refereed.* **Document type:** *Journal, Academic/Scholarly.* **Description:** Covers aspects of the development, production, and evaluation of drugs and pharmaceutical products, highlights both the technical and regulatory facets of industrial pharmacy.
Related titles: Microform ed.: (from RPI); Online - full text ed.: (from EBSCO Publishing, O C L C Online Computer Library Center, Inc., RoweCom Information Quest, Swets Blackwell, Institute for Scientific Information).
Indexed: Abstr.Inter.Med., Agri.& Environ.Biotech.Abstr. (coverage dropped), BBCI, Biol.Abstr., Chem.Abstr., Chem.Cit.Ind., Chem.Indus.Notes, Chem.Titles, Curr.Adv.Biochem., Curr.Adv.Ecol.Sci., Curr.Cont., Dairy Sci.Abstr., Derwent Biotech.Abstr., Environ.Sci.Poll.Mgmt., Excerp.Med., INIS Atomind., I.P.A., Ind.Med. (1972-), Ind.Sci.Rev., Ind.Vet., Inpharma, Int.Abstr.Biol.Sci., Pharm.&Out.News, Pig News & Info., Pollut.Abstr., Poult.Abstr., Reac., Ref.Zh., Rev.Med.& Vet.Mycol., Risk Abstr., Saf.Sci.Abstr., Sci.Cit.Ind., Tox.Abstr., Vet.Bull.
—BLDSC (3629.330000), CASDDS, CISTI, EMDOCS, GNLM, IDS, ingenta, KNAW. **CCC.**
Published by: Marcel Dekker Inc., 270 Madison Ave, New York, NY 10016. TEL 212-696-9000, 800-228-1160, FAX 212-685-4540, journals@dekker.com, custserv@dekker.com, http://www.dekker.com/servlet/product/productid/DMR. Ed. Jack A Hinson. R&P Julia Mulligan. Adv. contact Diane Saulon. B&W page USD 800. Circ: 800. **Dist. addr. in Europe, Far East, Middle East & Africa:** Marcel Dekker AG, Hutgasse 4, PO Box 812, Basel 4001, Switzerland. TEL 41-61-261-8482, FAX 41-61-261-8896, intlcustserv@dekker.com.

615 616 GBR ISSN 1368-7646
CODEN: DRUPFW
DRUG RESISTANCE UPDATE. Text in English. 1998. bi-m. GBP 90 to individuals; GBP 234 to institutions (effective 2002). adv. bk.rev. back issues avail.; reprints avail. *Refereed.* **Document type:** *Journal, Academic/Scholarly.* **Description:** Publishes reviews and commentaries on developments in drug resistance in infectious disease and cancer.
Related titles: Online - full text ed.: (from EBSCO Publishing, ingenta, Swets Blackwell, IDEAL Online Library, Institute for Scientific Information).
Indexed: BBCI, Biotech.Cit.Ind., Curr.Cont., Inpharma, Pharm.&Out.News, Protozool.Abstr., Reac., Rev.Med.& Vet.Mycol.
—BLDSC (3629.390500), CASDDS, IDS, Infotrieve. **CCC.**
Published by: Churchill Livingstone (Subsidiary of: Harcourt Publishers Ltd.), Robert Stevenson House, 1-3 Baxter's Pl, Leith Walk, Edinburgh, Midlothian EH1 3AF, United Kingdom. TEL 44-131-556-2424, FAX 44-131-535-1704, http://www.harcourt-international.com/journals/drup. Ed. Nafsika Georgopapadakou. **Subscr. to:** Harcourt Publishers Ltd., Foots Cray High St, Sidcup, Kent DA14 5HP, United Kingdom. TEL 44-20-8308-5700, FAX 44-20-8309-0807.

610 FIN ISSN 0012-7183
CODEN: DUODAG
DUODECIM; laaketieteellinen aikakauskirja. Text in Finnish. 1885. s-m. FIM 710 (effective 1999). adv. bk.rev., film rev. bibl, charts, illus. index, cum.index. **Document type:** *Bulletin.*
Indexed: Biol.Abstr., Chem.Abstr., Curr.Adv.Ecol.Sci., Dent.Ind., Excerp.Med., INIS Atomind., Ind.Med. (1885-).
—BLDSC (3631.195000), CASDDS, CISTI, GNLM.
Published by: Laaketieteellinen Aikakauskirja Duodecim/Finnish Medical Society Duodecim, Kalevankatu 11 A, Helsinki 00100, Finland. TEL 358-0-618-851, FAX 358-0-618-85200. Ed. Hannu Sariola. Circ: 18,500.

610 RUS
DYANOVOSTI. Text in Russian. 1997. m. USD 65 in the Americas (effective 2000).
Published by: Izdatel'stvo Art-Biznes-Tsentr, Ul. Novoslobodskaya, 73-68, Moscow 103055, Russian Federation. TEL 7-095-9733665, FAX 7-095-2850794. Ed. N A Smirnova.

610 CAN
DYNAMICS. Text in English. q. CND 60 domestic to non-members; USD 75 foreign to non-members (effective 2000). adv. **Document type:** *Trade.* **Description:** Represents nurses in clinical practice, education, research and administration within adult, neonatal and pediatric critical care in Canada.
Formerly (until 2000): Canadian Association of Critical Care Nurses. Official Journal
Indexed: Int.Nurs.Ind.
—BLDSC (3637.143083).
Published by: (Canadian Association of Critical Care Nurses), Pappin Communications, The Victoria Centre, 84 Isabella St, Pembroke, ON K8A 5S5, Canada. TEL 613-735-0952, FAX 613-735-7983. Ed. Paula Price. R&P Heather Reid TEL 519-649-5284. Adv. contact C B Pappin. **Subscr. to:** CACCN, P O Box 22006, London, ON N6C 4N0, Canada. TEL 519-649-5284.

610 ESP ISSN 0211-9536
R131.A1
DYNAMIS; acta hispanica ad medicinae scientiarumque historiam illustrandam. Text in Spanish. 1981. a. ESP 3,000 (effective 2001). bk.rev.
Indexed: Amer.Hist.& Life, Hist.Abstr. (1981-), IBZ, Ind.Med.Esp.
—BLDSC (3637.146000), CINDOC, GNLM, Linda Hall.
Published by: (Departamento de Historia de la Medicina, Universidad de Granada), Editorial Universidad de Granada, Antiguo Colegio Maximo, Campus de Cartuja, Granada 18071, Spain. TEL 34-58-243930, FAX 34-58-242827. Eds. Juan Arrizabalaga, Teresa Ortiz. Circ: 150.

610 USA
DYSTONIA DIALOGUE. Text in English. 1976. q. free. adv. **Document type:** *Newsletter.* **Description:** Helps to build awareness of dystonia in the medical and lay communities.
Published by: Dystonia Medical Research Foundation, 1 E Wacker Dr, Ste 2430, Chicago, IL 60601-2001. TEL 312-755-0198, FAX 312-803-0138, dystonia@dystonia-foundation.org, dystfndt@aol.com, http://www.dystonia-foundation.org. Ed. Kimberly Kuman. R&P, Adv. contact Kim Kuman. Circ: 26,000.

610 571.889 USA ISSN 1524-8909
▼ **E-BIOMED**; the journal of regenerative medicine. Text in English. 2000. irreg. USD 495 to institutions (effective 2002). **Document type:** *Academic/Scholarly.* **Description:** Focuses on using the body's own stem cells and growth factors to repair organs, tissues, and cells.
Previously announced as: Regenerative Medicine
Media: Online - full text (from O C L C Online Computer Library Center, Inc., RoweCom Information Quest, CatchWord Ltd.).
Published by: Mary Ann Liebert, Inc. Publishers, 2 Madison Ave, Larchmont, NY 10538. TEL 914—834-3100, FAX 914-834-1388, info@liebertpub.com, www.liebertpub.com/ebi, http://www.liebertpub.com. Ed. William A Haseltine.

E D LEGAL LETTER. see *LAW*

▼ **E-HEALTHCARE MARKET REPORTER.** see *BUSINESS AND ECONOMICS*

▼ **E M B O REPORTS.** (European Molecular Biology Organization) see *BIOLOGY—Genetics*

E M S INSIDER. see *MEDICAL SCIENCES—Orthopedics And Traumatology*

610.285 BEL
E S E M NEWS. Text in English. q. membership. back issues avail. **Document type:** *Bulletin, Academic/Scholarly.* **Description:** Provides a forum for the engineering and medicine research community.
Published by: European Society for Engineering and Medicine, Katholieke Universiteit Leuven, Biomechanica en Grafisch Ontwerpen, Celestijnenlaan 200A, Leuven 3001, Belgium. TEL 32-16-327099, FAX 32-16-327994, P.J.McCullagh@ulst.ac.uk, http://www.esem.org. Ed. P. J. McCullagh.

E-STREAMS (CONTOOCOOK); electronic reviews of science and technology references covering engineering, agriculture, medicine and science. see *AGRICULTURE*

610.09 509 NLD ISSN 1383-7427
EARLY SCIENCE AND MEDICINE; a journal for the study of science, technology and medicine in the pre-modern period. Text in English. 1996. 4/yr. EUR 69, USD 80 to individuals; EUR 128, USD 149 to institutions (effective 2002). bk.rev. back issues avail. *Refereed.* **Document type:** *Academic/Scholarly.* **Description:** Publishes studies dealing with the content and influence of science, medicine and technology from the earliest times through the end of the seventeenth century.
Related titles: Online - full text ed.
Indexed: C.C.M.J., IBZ.

M

—BLDSC (3642.999570), Linda Hall. **CCC.**
Published by: Brill Academic Publishers, PO Box 9000, Leiden 2300 PA, Netherlands. TEL 31-71-535-3500, FAX 31-71-531-7532, TELEX 39692 BRILL NL, cs@brill.nl, http://www.brill.nl. Eds. Anita Guerrini, Christoph Luthy. R&P Elizabeth Venekamp.

610 KEN ISSN 0012-835X
R98 CODEN: EAMJAV
THE EAST AFRICAN MEDICAL JOURNAL. Text in English. 1923. m. KES 60,001, USD 375 (effective 2000). adv. bk.rev. illus. index. reprint service avail. from IRC. *Refereed.* **Document type:** *Journal, Academic/Scholarly, Abstract/Index.* **Description:** Original articles, reviews and case reports. Relevant to medical and para-medical personnel.
Related titles: CD-ROM ed.; Online - full text ed.: (from Institute for Scientific Information).
Indexed: ASCA, Abstr.Hyg., Aqua.Sci.& Fish.Abstr., Biodet.Abstr., Biol.Abstr., Cal.Tiss.Abstr. (coverage dropped), Chem.Abstr., Curr.Cont., Dairy Sci.Abstr., Dent.Ind., Diar.Dis.Res., Dok.Arbeitsmed., ERA, Environ.Sci.Poll.Mgmt., Excerp.Med. (1993-), ExtraMED, Food Sci.& Tech.Abstr., Geo.Abstr.H.G., HRIS, Helminthol.Abstr., IDA, Ind.Med. (1932-), Ind.Sci.Rev., Ind.Vet., Inpharma, Maize Abstr., Med.Abstr., NRN, Neurosci.Cit.Ind., Nutr.Abstr., Pharm.&Out.News, Pollut.Abstr., Poult.Abstr., Protozool.Abstr., Reac., Rev.Appl.Entomol., Rev.Arom.& Med.Plants, Rev.Med.& Vet.Mycol., Rev.Plant Path., Risk Abstr., Rural Devel.Abstr., SSCI (coverage dropped), Saf.Sci.Abstr., Sci.Cit.Ind., Soyabean Abstr., Sp.Ed.Needs Abstr., Trop.Dis.Bull., Vet.Bull.
—BLDSC (3645.000000), CASDDS, CISTI, GNLM, IDS, KNAW.
Published by: Kenya Medical Association, Chyulu Rd., PO Box 41632, Nairobi, Kenya. TEL 254-2-712010, FAX 254-2-724617, eamj@healthnet.or.ke. Ed. W Lore. R&P W. Lore. Adv. contact Silvanus Oriedi. Circ: 4,500 (paid).

EAST ASIAN SCIENCE, TECHNOLOGY, AND MEDICINE. see *SCIENCES: COMPREHENSIVE WORKS*

610 ROM ISSN 1220-8795
EAST EUROPEAN MEDICAL JOURNAL. Text in English. 1992. q. ROL 15,000, USD 15 domestic to individuals; USD 30 foreign to individuals; ROL 20,000, USD 20 domestic to institutions; USD 40 foreign to institutions. adv. bk.rev. abstr. *Refereed.* **Description:** Dedicated to specific health care problems in East Europe and Eurasia.
Related titles: Supplement: East European Medical Journal Supplement. ISSN 1220-8787.
Indexed: Abstr.Anthropol., Ind.Med. (coverage dropped).
Published by: Edit Dan Publishing Co., PO Box 209, Iasi 600, Romania. TEL 40-98-135778, FAX 40-98-117607. Ed. Dr. Traian Mihaescu. Adv. contact Alina Gramescu. B&W page USD 700, color page USD 1,700. Circ: 2,000.

610 USA ISSN 1050-6675
EAST TEXAS MEDICINE*. Text in English. 1989. bi-m. USD 20. adv. **Description:** Forum for physicians in the East Texas area. Presents doctors' case studies and research.
Address: 10702 Hancock Dr, Tyler, TX 75707-9426. TEL 214-592-8533, FAX 903-593-0494. Ed. Dr. Gary D Boyd. Circ: 5,000.

ECONOMICS, MEDICINES, & HEALTH. see *BUSINESS AND ECONOMICS—Production Of Goods And Services*

610 JPN ISSN 0915-9061
EDOGAWA. Text in Japanese. 1965. bi-m.
Published by: Edogawaku Ishikai/Edogawa City Medical Association, 24-14 Chuo 4-chome, Edogawa-ku, Tokyo 132-0021, Japan.

610 JPN ISSN 0915-8693
EDOGAWA IGAKKAISHI/EDOGAWA CITY MEDICAL ASSOCIATION. PROCEEDINGS. Text in Japanese. 1983. a. **Document type:** *Proceedings.*
Published by: Edogawaku Ishikai/Edogawa City Medical Association, 24-14 Chuo 4-chome, Edogawa-ku, Tokyo 132-0021, Japan.

610 PRT ISSN 0871-7958
EDUCACAO MEDICA. Text in English, Portuguese. 1989. 3/yr. free per issue. adv. **Document type:** *Academic/Scholarly.*
—CCC.
Published by: A E F M U P, Alameda Prof. H. Montiero, Piso 1, Apdo. 4514, Porto Codex 4008, Portugal. TEL 351-2-5509355, FAX 351-2-5509096. Ed. Pinto Machado. Adv. contact Luisa Botelho. B&W page PTE 40,000. Circ: 1,250. **Co-sponsor:** Hospital de S. Joao, Faculdade de Medicina do Porto.

610 COL
EDUCACION CONTINUA EN SALUD (YEAR) TEMAS ESCOGIDOS. Text in Spanish. 1989. a. COP 12,000, USD 15. **Document type:** *Academic/Scholarly.* **Description:** Provides updated topics on themes of importance and of interest to general practitioners.
Published by: Corporacion Editora Medica del Valle, Calle 4b, 36-00, Cali, VALLE, Colombia. TEL 57-2-558-1939, comedica@mafalda.univalleedu.co, comedica@mafalda.univalle.edu.co, http://www.icfes.gov.co. Ed. Dr. Pablo Barreto. R&P Guillermo Llanos.

610.71 ESP
EDUCACION MEDICA; aprender y ensenar en las profesiones sanitarias. Text in Spanish. q. **Document type:** *Academic/Scholarly.*
Published by: Ediciones Doyma S.A., Traversa de Gracia, 17-21, Barcelona 08021, Spain. TEL 34-93-200-0711, FAX 34-93-209-1136, comercial@doymanet.es, http://www.doyma.es, http://www.doyma.es/. Ed. Enric Brotons. adv.: page ESP 238,000; trim 28 x 21. Circ: 2,000.

EDUCATION AND HEALTH. see *EDUCATION—School Organization And Administration*

613.07 362.172 GBR ISSN 1357-6283
CODEN: EDHEFH
EDUCATION FOR HEALTH; change in training and practice. Text in English. 1988. 3/yr. GBP 60, USD 98 to individuals; GBP 171, USD 280 to institutions (effective 2001). back issues avail. **Document type:** *Academic/Scholarly.*
Formerly (until vol.9, 1996): Annals of Community - Oriented Education (1016-8745)
Related titles: Online - full text ed.: ISSN 1469-5804 (from CatchWord Ltd., Northern Light Technology, Inc., EBSCO Publishing, O C L C Online Computer Library Center, Inc., RoweCom Information Quest, ProQuest Information & Learning, Swets Blackwell).
Indexed: ASSIA, Br.Educ.Ind., CINAHL, Cont.Pg.Educ., ERA, Educ.Tech.Abstr., Environ.Sci.Poll.Mgmt., Lang.& Lang.Behav.Abstr., Pollut.Abstr., Res.High.Educ.Abstr., Risk Abstr., SOPODA, Saf.Sci.Abstr., Soc.Serv.Abstr., Sociol.Abstr., Tech.Educ.Abstr.
—BLDSC (3661.283150), CatchWord, GNLM, Infotrieve. **CCC.**
Published by: (Network of Community - Oriented Educational Institutions for Health Sciences), Carfax Publishing Limited (Subsidiary of: Taylor & Francis Group), PO Box 25, Abingdon, Oxon OX14 3UE, United Kingdom. TEL 44-1235-401000, FAX 44-1235-401550, enquiries@carfax.co.uk, enquiry@tandf.co.uk, http://www.carfax.co.uk. Ed. Charles Engel.

610.711 GBR ISSN 1473-9879
EDUCATION FOR PRIMARY CARE. Text in English. 1990. 4/yr. GBP 120 domestic; USD 175 in US & Canada (effective 2002). adv. bk.rev. back issues avail. **Document type:** *Journal, Academic/Scholarly.* **Description:** Postgraduate education in family practice, general practice for trainers and all other health care professionals interested.
Former titles (until 2001): Education for General Practice (1367-8523); (until 1993): Postgraduate Education for General Practice (0959-4299)
Related titles: Online - full content ed.; Online - full text ed.: (from CatchWord Ltd.).
Indexed: Cont.Pg.Educ.
—BLDSC (3661.317480), GNLM.
Published by: Radcliffe Medical Press Ltd., 18 Marcham Rd, Abingdon, Oxon OX14 1AA, United Kingdom. TEL 44-1235-528820, FAX 44-1235-528830, contact-us@radcliffemed.com, http://www.radcliffe-oxford.com/epc. Ed. John Pitts. Adv. contact Lucy Thomson. Circ: 1,500.

610.6952 USA ISSN 0145-2037
RA396.A3
EDUCATIONAL COMMISSION FOR FOREIGN MEDICAL GRADUATES. ANNUAL REPORT. Text in English. 1958. a. free per issue. **Description:** Provides information on programs of international medical education, including entry of foreign graduates of medical schools into graduate medical education in the United States, research and development programs.
Formerly: Educational Council for Foreign Medical Graduates. Annual Report (0422-6690)
Published by: Educational Commission for Foreign Medical Graduates, 3624 Market St, 4th Fl, Philadelphia, PA 19104-2685. TEL 215-386-5900, FAX 215-387-9963, http://www.ecfmg.org. Circ: 7,000.

610 USA ISSN 1080-3521
EDUCATIONAL SYNOPSES IN ANESTHESIOLOGY AND CRITICAL CARE MEDICINE; online journal of anesthesiology. Text in English. 1994. m. back issues avail. **Document type:** *Journal.*
Media: Online - full content.
Address: http://gasnet.med.yale.edu/esia/index.html.

610 USA ISSN 1099-8128
EFFECTIVE CLINICAL PRACTICE. Text in English. 1987. bi-m. USD 54 to individuals; USD 70 to institutions (effective 2000). adv. bk.rev. *Refereed.* **Document type:** *Academic/Scholarly.* **Description:** Provides information that encourages continous improvement in the quality of patient care within organized health care delivery systems. Publishes peer-reviewed original research articles, reports, reviews and opinions on topics such as clinical and program innovations, health service research, resource management, new technologies and health policy.
Formerly (until 1998): H M O Practice (0891-6624)
Related titles: Microform ed.: (from PQC); Online - full text ed.
Indexed: Hosp.Lit.Ind., Ind.Med., Int.Nurs.Ind.
—BLDSC (3664.020095), GNLM.
Published by: American College of Physicians/Co-sponsor: American Society of Internal Medicine, 190 N. Independence Mall W, Philadelphia, PA 19106-1572. TEL 215-351-2600, FAX 215-351-2799, custserve@mail.acponline.org, ecpsubs@aol.com, http://www.acponline.org/journals/acpjc/jcmenu.htm. Ed. Gil Welch. R&P Joshua Roberts TEL 215-351-2630. Adv. contact Ron Taylor. B&W page USD 2,195, color page USD 3,840. Circ: 30,000 (controlled). **Subscr. to:** Effective Clinical Practice, PO Box 1055, Ridgefield, CT 06877. TEL 203-894-1704;, FAX 203-438-8232.

362.1 613 GBR ISSN 0965-0288
EFFECTIVE HEALTH CARE; the NHS centre for reviews and dissemination. Text in English. 1992; N.S. 1996. bi-m. USD 82 in United States to individuals; GBP 53 elsewhere to individuals; USD 130 in United States to institutions; GBP 86 elsewhere to institutions (effective 2002). adv. bk.rev. back issues avail. *Refereed.* **Document type:** *Bulletin, Academic/Scholarly.* **Description:** Aims to publish the effectiveness and cost effectiveness of health care interventions. Intends to assist purchasers and providers in identifying actions they can take to improve clinical effectiveness. Each issues deals with one health care topic. Coverage includes background issues surrounding the topic and treatment options.
Related titles: Online - full text ed.: N.S.
Indexed: Brit.Nur.Ind., Inpharma, Pharm.&Out.News, Reac.
—BLDSC (3664.020355), GNLM.
Published by: (N H S Centre for Reviews and Dissemination, University of York), Royal Society of Medicine Press Ltd, 1 Wimpole St, London W1M 8AE, United Kingdom. TEL 44-20-7290-2921, FAX 44-20-7290-2929, elizabeth.fredman@rsm.ac.uk, http://www.roysocmed.ac.uk/pub/ehc.htm, http://www.york.ac.uk/inst/crd/ehcb.htm. Circ: 55,000.

610 EGY ISSN 0013-2411
CODEN: JEMAAJ
EGYPTIAN MEDICAL ASSOCIATION. JOURNAL. Text in Arabic, English. 1917. m. membership. adv. bk.rev. charts, illus. index. **Document type:** *Academic/Scholarly.*
Indexed: Biol.Abstr., C.I.S. Abstr., Chem.Abstr., Excerp.Med. (until 19??), Helminthol.Abstr., Ind.Med. (until 19??, dropped), Nutr.Abstr., Rev.Plant Path., Trop.Dis.Bull., Zoo.Rec.
—CASDDS, GNLM, ingenta.
Published by: Egyptian Medical Association, Dar El-Hekma, 42 Kasr-El Aini St., Cairo, Egypt. Ed. Dr M Ibrahim.

610 JPN ISSN 0286-3677
EHIME IGAKU/EHIME MEDICAL JOURNAL. Text in Japanese; Summaries in English. 1982. q. JPY 1,000 per issue.
Indexed: INIS Atomind.
Published by: Ehime Igakkai/Ehime Medical Association, Ehimeken Ishikai, 5-3 Sanban-cho 4-chome, Matsuyama-shi, Ehime-ken 790-0003, Japan.

610 JPN ISSN 0289-5463
EHIME KENRITSU BYOIN GAKKAI KAISHI/EHIME JOURNAL OF MEDICINE. Text in Japanese. 1961. 2/yr. illus, charts, stat. **Document type:** *Journal, Academic/Scholarly.*

M

—BLDSC (3664.705800).
Published by: Ehime Kenritsu Chuo Byoin/Ehime Central Prefectural Hospital, 83 Kasuga-machi, Matsuyama, Ehime 790-0024 , Japan. TEL 86-899-47-1111.

610 JPN ISSN 0915-3012
EHIME KENRITSU IRYO GIJUTSU TANKI DAIGAKU KIYO/EHIME COLLEGE OF HEALTH SCIENCES. BULLETIN. Text in English, Japanese; Summaries in Japanese. 1988. a. *Refereed.* **Document type:** *Bulletin, Academic/Scholarly.*
Published by: Ehime Kenritsu Iryo Gijutsu Tanki Daigaku, 543 Takoda, Iyo-gun, Tobe-cho, Ehime-ken 791-2103, Japan. TEL 81-89-958-2111, FAX 81-89-958-2177, http://www.ehime-chs.ac.jp. Eds. Ehime Kenritsu, Iryo Gijutsu, Tanki Diagaku. Circ: 300.

610 JPN
EHIMEKEN ISHIKAIHO/MEDICAL ASSOCIATION OF EHIME. JOURNAL. Text in Japanese. 1953. m.
Published by: Ehimeken Ishikai, 5-3 Sanban-cho 4-chome, Matsuyama-shi, Ehime-ken 790-0003, Japan.

THE EINSTEIN QUARTERLY; journal of biology and medicine. see *BIOLOGY*

EIZO JOHO MEDIKARU/IMAGE TECHNOLOGY & INFORMATION DISPLAY, MEDICAL. see *MEDICAL SCIENCES—Radiology And Nuclear Medicine*

610 RUS
EKSTRENNAYA MEDITSINSKAYA POMOSHCH' V MOSKVE. Text in Russian. s-a. USD 75 in the Americas (effective 2000).
Published by: Izdatel'stvo Metafora, Ul. Shchepkina, 24a, Moscow 129090, Russian Federation. TEL 7-095-9258293, FAX 7-095-9235223. Ed. O S Kopylova. **Dist. by:** East View Publications, 3020 Harbor Ln N, Minneapolis, MN 55447. TEL 763-550-0961, FAX 763-559-2931.

616.047 344.041 USA
ELBOW AND SHOULDER PAIN. Text in English. 1989. base vol. plus irreg. updates. USD 65.
Published by: Lexis Law Publishing (Subsidiary of: Reed Elsevier plc), PO Box 7587, Charlottesville, VA 22906-7587. TEL 804-972-7600, 800-562-1197, FAX 804-972-7666, llp.customer.support@lexis-nexis.com, http://www.lexislawpublishing.com.

615.845 621.381 DEU ISSN 0340-5389
ELECTROMEDICA (DEUTSCHE AUSGABE). Text in German. 1932. s-a. **Document type:** *Trade.*
Description: Covers medical electronics.
Formerly: Siemens Electromedica (0037-4660)
Related titles: English ed.: ISSN 0013-4724.
Indexed: Excerp.Med., INIS Atomind., INSPEC (1973-, dropped), Ref.Zh.
—GNLM, Infotrieve. **CCC.**
Published by: Siemens AG, Werner-von-Siemens-Str 50, Erlangen 91050, Germany. TEL 49-9131-746481, FAX 49-9131-725022. **Subscr. in Germany, Austria & Switzerland to:** Med OA, Redaktion "electromedica", Henkestr 127, Erlangen 91052, Germany; **Subscr. in the Americas to:** John Wiley & Sons, Inc., Journals, 605 Third Ave, New York, NY 10158. TEL 212-850-6645, FAX 212-850-6021; **Subscr. outside Germany, Austria & Switzerland to:** John Wiley & Sons Ltd., Baffins Ln, Chichester, Sussex PO19 IUD, United Kingdom. TEL 44-1243-779777, FAX 44-1243-843232.

616.07 GBR ISSN 0948-0382
ELECTRONIC JOURNAL OF PATHOLOGY AND HISTOLOGY. Text in English. irreg. EUR 233 to institutions (effective 2002).
Related titles: Online - full text ed.: (from RoweCom Information Quest).
Published by: I O S Press, Nieuwe Hemweg 6B, Amsterdam 1013 BG, Netherlands. TEL 31-20-688-3355, FAX 31-20-620-3419, elec_j_pathology@lung.de, market@iospress.nl, http://www.iospress.nl.

EMBASE ALERT. see *MEDICAL SCIENCES—Abstracting, Bibliographies, Statistics*

EMBASE LIST OF JOURNALS INDEXED (YEAR). see *MEDICAL SCIENCES—Abstracting, Bibliographies, Statistics*

EMERGENCY DEPARTMENT LAW; the source for comprehensive coverage of legal trends in emergency medicine. see *LAW*

610 340 USA ISSN 0884-4836
EMERGENCY MEDICAL TECHNICIAN LEGAL BULLETIN. Text in English. 1977. q. USD 15. index. back issues avail. **Document type:** *Newsletter, Bulletin.*
Indexed: CINAHL.
Published by: Med-Law Publishers, Inc., PO Box 293, Westville, NJ 08093. Ed. Dr. James E George.

610 340 USA ISSN 0098-1524
EMERGENCY PHYSICIAN LEGAL BULLETIN. Abbreviated title: E P L B. Text in English. 1975. q. USD 25. index. back issues avail. **Document type:** *Newsletter, Bulletin.*
Published by: Med-Law Publishers, Inc., PO Box 293, Westville, NJ 08093. TEL 609-848-3817, FAX 609-848-1431. Ed. Dr. James E George.

610 ARE ISSN 0250-6882
CODEN: EMEJD
EMIRATES MEDICAL JOURNAL. Text in English. 1981. 3/yr. USD 50, AED 150 (effective 2000). bk.rev. *Refereed.* **Document type:** *Journal, Academic/Scholarly, Abstract/Index.*
Related titles: CD-ROM ed.
Indexed: Environ.Sci.Poll.Mgmt., Excerp.Med., ExtraMED, Pollut.Abstr., Risk Abstr., Saf.Sci.Abstr.
—BLDSC (3733.528900), EMDOCS, GNLM.
Published by: Emirates Medical Association, PO Box 6600, Dubai, United Arab Emirates. TEL 971-4-3377377, FAX 971-4-3344082, ema@emirates.net.ae, http://www.emiratesma.org. Ed. Dr. Yousef Mohamed Abdulrazzaq. Circ: 2,000 (paid and controlled).

610 USA
ENCYCLOPEDIA OF MEDICAL MEDIA & COMMUNICATIONS. Text in English. 1996. a. USD 175. **Description:** Lists medical book publishers, medical journals, and electronic databases.
Published by: Aspen Publishers, Inc., 200 Orchard Ridge Dr, Ste 200, Gaithersburg, MD 20878. TEL 800-638-8437, FAX 301-417-7550, http://www.aspenpub.com. Ed. George T Kurian.

610 CZE ISSN 1211-1074
ENDOSKOPIE/ENDOSCOPY. Text in Czech; Summaries in Czech, English. q. EUR 64, USD 80 (effective 2001). adv. bk.rev. bibl, charts, illus, stat. back issues avail. *Refereed.* **Document type:** *Academic/Scholarly.*
Description: Focuses on endoscopic problems of gastroenterology, urology, surgery, orthopedics, gynecology, and pneumology. Includes articles, case reports, review, as well as a congress calendar.
—BLDSC (3743.620000).
Published by: (Ceska Lekarska Spolecnost J.E. Purkyne/Czech Medical Association), Nakladatelske Stredisko C L S J.E. Purkyne, Sokolska 31, Prague 12026, Czech Republic. TEL 420-2-24911420, FAX 420-2-24911420, nts@iol.cz, http://www.clsjep.cz, http://www.medical.cz. Ed. P Fric. R&P A Leblova TEL 42-2-71747230. **Dist. by:** Abont s.r.o., Chlumova 17, Prague, 3 130 00, Czech Republic; Kubon & Sagner, Hesstr 39-41, Munich 80798, Germany.

ENTWICKLUNGSLAENDER-STUDIEN; Bibliographie entwicklungslaenderbezogener Forschungsarbeiten. see *BUSINESS AND ECONOMICS—Abstracting, Bibliographies, Statistics*

ENVIRONMENTAL HEALTH CRITERIA. see *ENVIRONMENTAL STUDIES*

ENVIRONMENTAL MANAGEMENT & HEALTH. see *ENVIRONMENTAL STUDIES*

618.98 JPN ISSN 0287-0517
RA565.A1 CODEN: ENMEE9
ENVIRONMENTAL MEDICINE. Text in English. 1951. s-a. free per issue. *Refereed.* **Document type:** *Academic/Scholarly.*
Formerly (until vol.25, 1980): Nagoya University. Research Institute of Environmental Medicine. Annual Report (0469-4759)
Indexed: Biol.Abstr., Chem.Abstr., Chem.Indus.Notes, Chem.Titles, Excerp.Med., INIS Atomind., Ref.Zh.
—BLDSC (3791.522500), CASDDS, CISTI, GNLM.
Published by: Nagoya Daigaku, Kankyo Igaku Kenkyujo/Nagoya University, Research Institute of Environmental Medicine, Furo-cho, Chikusa-ku, Nagoya-shi, Aichi-ken 464-0814, Japan. TEL 81-52-789-3873, FAX 81-52-789-3876, http://www.riem.nagoya.u.ac.jp/etc/pub/1995env.html. Ed., R&P Hideki Yamamura. Pub. Hideki Yamura. Circ: 400.

610 ITA ISSN 1120-9763
EPIDEMIOLOGIA E PREVENZIONE. Text in Italian. 1977. q. ITL 49,000; ITL 59,000 foreign.
Indexed: Ind.Med. (1976-).
—BLDSC (3793.536000), GNLM.
Published by: Nuova Italia Scientifica, Via Sardegna, 50, Rome, RM 00187, Italy. TEL 06-4742176. Ed. Giuseppe Lojacono.

614.4 USA ISSN 0193-936X
RA648.5 CODEN: EPIRD7
EPIDEMIOLOGIC REVIEWS. Text in English. 1979. s-a. USD 25. *Refereed.*
Related titles: Microfilm ed.: (from WWS); Online - full text ed.: (from Ovid Technologies, Inc., Institute for Scientific Information).
Indexed: ASCA, Abstr.Hyg., AgeLine, Aqua.Sci.& Fish.Abstr., Biol.Dig., Biostat., CINAHL, Curr.Adv.Ecol.Sci., Curr.Cont., Diar.Dis.Res., Environ.Sci.Poll.Mgmt., Excerp.Med., Helminthol.Abstr., INIS Atomind., Ind.Med. (1979-), Ind.Sci.Rev., Ind.Vet., Inpharma, Int.Abstr.Biol.Sci., Microbiol.Abstr., Pharm.&Out.News, Pollut.Abstr., Protozool.Abstr., Reac., Risk Abstr., Saf.Sci.Abstr., Sci.Cit.Ind., THA, Trop.Dis.Bull., Vet.Bull.
—BLDSC (3793.540000), CISTI, GNLM, IDS, ingenta, KNAW. **CCC.**
Published by: Johns Hopkins University, School of Hygiene & Public Health, 111 Market Place, #840, Baeto, MD 21202. TEL 410-223-1600. Ed. Haroutune K Armenian.

610 614 LKA
EPIDEMIOLOGICAL BULLETIN. Text in English. 1960. q. free per issue.
Indexed: IIS, Ind.Med. (coverage dropped), Ind.Vet., Trop.Dis.Bull., Vet.Bull.
—BLDSC (3793.561000).
Published by: Department of Health, Epidemiological Unit, N.T.I. Building, 385 Dean S Rd, Colombo 10, Sri Lanka. Ed. Charles A L Forbes. Circ: 750.

616.853 USA ISSN 1525-5050
▼ **EPILEPSY AND BEHAVIOR.** Text in English. 2000. bi-m. GBP 435 in US & Canada to institutions; GBP 480 elsewhere to institutions (effective 2001). bk.rev. abstr. back issues avail.; reprints avail. *Refereed.*
Description: International journal uniquely devoted to the rapid dissemination of the most current information availble on the behavioral aspects of seizures and epilepsy. Includes original articles based on laboratory and clinical research. Topics covered, but not limited to, will be clinical neurology, neurosurgery, neuropsychiatry, neuropsychology, neurophysiology, neuropharmacology and neuroimaging.
Related titles: Online - full text ed.: ISSN 1525-5069 (from EBSCO Publishing, ingenta, Swets Blackwell, IDEAL Online Library, RoweCom Information Quest).
—BLDSC (3793.800800).
Published by: Academic Press, Inc., Journal Division (Subsidiary of: Harcourt Brace & Company), 525 B St, Ste 1900, San Diego, CA 92101-4495. TEL 619-230-1840, 800-894-3434, FAX 619-699-6742, 619-699-6800, apsubs@acad.com, eb@acad.com, http://www.academicpress.com/ideal-alert.

610 USA
EPISOURCE; a guide to resources in epidemiology. Text in English. 1991. irreg. (1st ed. 1991). USD 149 (effective 1999). adv. **Document type:** *Newsletter.*
Address: 2560 Whisper Wind Ct., Rosewell, GA 30076. TEL 770-594-1613, FAX 770-594-0997. Ed., Pub. Roger H Bernier. Adv. contact Jeanette St Pierre.

EQUILIBRIUM. see *ALTERNATIVE MEDICINE*

610 681 ESP
EQUIPOS MEDICOS. Text in Spanish. 6/yr.
Address: Comercio, 4 bajo C 1a Esc, Madrid 28007, Spain. TEL 1-433-45-23. Ed. A M Blanco Sanchez.

610 CUB
EQUIPOS Y PRODUCTOS. BIOMEDICINA. Text in Spanish. m.
Published by: Academia de Ciencias, Instituto de Documentacion e Informacion Cientifico-Tecnica (I D I C T), Capitolio Nacional, Prado y San Jose, Habana 2, Cuba.

610 JPN ISSN 0913-3887
EREKUTORONIKUSU NO RINSHO/ELECTRONICS IN MEDICAL CLINICS. Text in Japanese. 1971. irreg. JPY 300 per issue.
Published by: Medikaru Erekutoro Taimusu/Medical Electro Times Co., Ltd., 35-8 Hongo 2-chome, Bunkyo-ku, Tokyo 113-0033, Japan.

M

610 DEU ISSN 0014-0082
CODEN: ERFAAK
ERFAHRUNGSHEILKUNDE/ACTA MEDICA EMPIRICA; Zeitschrift fuer die aerztliche Praxis. Text in German; Summaries in English. 1951. 12/yr. EUR 132.80 domestic to institutions; EUR 142.90 in Europe to institutions; EUR 156.90 elsewhere to institutions; EUR 14.90 newsstand/cover (effective 2002). adv. bk.rev. abstr, charts, illus. **Document type:** *Journal, Academic/Scholarly.*
Incorporates (1986-1987; resumed 1991-1995): Hufeland - Journal (0179-7581)
Related titles: Online - full text ed.: ISSN 1439-4294.
Indexed: AMED, Chem.Abstr., Chem.Indus.Notes, Chem.Titles, Dok.Arbeitsmed., INIS Atomind.
—BLDSC (3801.500000), CASDDS, GNLM, Infotrieve, KNAW. **CCC.**
Published by: (Aerztegesellschaft), Karl F. Haug Verlag, Fritz-Frey-Str 21, Heidelberg 69121, Germany. TEL 49-6221-489635, FAX 49-6221-489584, http://www.haug-verlag.de. Eds. Dr. Gyoergy Irmey, Hendrik Bruch. Adv. contact Guenter Fecke. Circ: 7,500.

610 DEU ISSN 0936-9228
ERGEBNISSE DER DIAGNOSTIK, THERAPIE UND NACHSORGE. Text in German. 1989. irreg., latest vol.3, 1995. **Document type:** *Academic/Scholarly.*
Published by: W. Zuckschwerdt Verlag GmbH, Industriestr 1, Germering 82110, Germany. TEL 49-89-894349-0, FAX 49-89-89434950. Ed. H Sauer.

610 DEU ISSN 0170-2327
ERGO-MED; Zeitschrift fuer angewandte Arbeitsmedizin, Arbeitshygiene und Umweltmedizin. Text in German. 1977. bi-m. EUR 51.83 domestic; EUR 61.19 foreign; EUR 9.10 newsstand/cover (effective 2002). **Document type:** *Magazine, Academic/Scholarly.*
Indexed: Ergon.Abstr., IBZ.
—BLDSC (3808.305000), GNLM. **CCC.**
Published by: (Deutsche Gesellschaft fuer Arbeitshygiene e.V.), Dr. Curt Haefner Verlag GmbH, Bachstr 14-16, Heidelberg 69121, Germany. TEL 49-6221-6446-0, FAX 49-6221-644640, info@haefner-verlag.de, http://www.haefner-verlag.de. Ed. Dieter Neumann. Circ: 3,000 (paid).

615.851 DNK ISSN 0105-8282
ERGOTERAPEUTEN. Text in Danish. 1972. 22/yr. DKK 650 domestic; DKK 875 in Europe; DKK 1,025 elsewhere (effective 2001). adv. bk.rev. **Document type:** *Newsletter, Academic/Scholarly.* **Description:** News on occupational therapy.
Formerly (until 1939): Tidsskrift for Ergoterapeuter
Published by: Ergoterapeutforeningen/Danish Organisation of Occupational Therapists, Noerre Voldgade 90, Copenhagen K 1358, Denmark. TEL 45-33-13-82-11, FAX 45-33-13-82-08. Ed. Elisabeth Krogh Mikkelsen. adv.: B&W page DKK 3,250, color page DKK 7,750; trim 154 x 210. Circ: 7,000.

611 USA
ESO MONOGRAPHS. Text in English. 1986. irreg., latest 1995. price varies. reprint service avail. from ISI. **Document type:** *Monographic series.*
Published by: Springer-Verlag, Journals (Subsidiary of: BertelsmannSpringer), 175 Fifth Ave, New York, NY 10010. TEL 212-460-1500, FAX 212-473-6272.

ESSENTIALS OF MANAGED HEALTH CARE. see *INSURANCE*

610 USA ISSN 0014-0937
ESSEX COUNTY MEDICAL SOCIETY. BULLETIN. Text in English. 1970 (vol.314). 9/yr. membership only. adv. illus. **Document type:** *Bulletin, Trade.*
Published by: Essex County Medical Society, 80 Pompton Ave, Verona, NJ 07044. TEL 973-239-9392, FAX 973-239-6083. Ed. Art Ellenberger.

610 ISR ISSN 0334-3928
ETANIM; monthly of health issues. Text in Hebrew. 1948. m. ILS 35, USD 17.50. adv. bk.rev. index.
Indexed: Ind.Heb.Per. (1977-).
Published by: Merkaz Kupat Holim, P O Box 16250, Tel Aviv 62098, Israel. FAX 03-433500. Ed. David Taggar. Circ: 20,000.

174.2 GBR ISSN 0266-688X
ETHICS AND MEDICINE. Text in English. 3/yr. GBP 13.20 domestic; GBP 13.80 foreign (effective 2000). **Document type:** *Academic/Scholarly.* **Description:** Presents an international Christian perspective on bioethics.
Indexed: Phil.Ind., Rel.& Theol.Abstr. (1985-).
—BLDSC (3814.657000), GNLM, Infotrieve. **CCC.**
Published by: The Paternoster Press, Kingstown Broadway, PO Box 300, Carlisle, Cumbria CA3 0QS, United Kingdom. TEL 44-1228-512512, FAX 44-1228-514949, 100526,3434@compuserve.com, 100526.3434@compuserve.com. Ed. Ben Mitchell. **Dist. in U.S. & Canada by:** The Paternoster Press, P O Box 11127, Birmingham, AL 35201-1127.

ETHICS AND MEDICS. see *RELIGIONS AND THEOLOGY—Roman Catholic*

ETHIK IN DER MEDIZIN. see *PHILOSOPHY*

610 ETH ISSN 0014-1755
CODEN: EMDJA2
ETHIOPIAN MEDICAL JOURNAL. Text in English. 1962. 4/yr. ETB 36, USD 40. adv. bk.rev. illus. *Refereed.* **Document type:** *Academic/Scholarly.*
Related titles: CD-ROM ed.; Online - full text ed.: (from Institute for Scientific Information).
Indexed: ASCA, Abstr.Hyg., Biol.Abstr., Curr.Adv.Ecol.Sci., Curr.Adv.Gen.& Molec.Biol., Curr.Cont., Dairy Sci.Abstr., Dent.Ind., Excerp.Med., ExtraMED, Helminthol.Abstr., INIS Atomind., Ind.Med. (1962-), Inpharma, MEDSOC, Nutr.Abstr., Pharm.&Out.News, Protozool.Abstr., Reac., Rev.Appl.Entomol., Rev.Med.& Vet.Mycol., SSCI (coverage dropped), Sci.Cit.Ind. (coverage dropped), Triticale Abstr., Trop.Dis.Bull., Zoo.Rec.
—BLDSC (3814.800000), CISTI, GNLM, IDS, KNAW.
Published by: Ethiopian Medical Association, PO Box 3472, Addis Ababa, Ethiopia. TEL 251-1-158174. Ed., R&P Kebede Oli TEL 251-1-533742. Circ: 500.

616.0089 USA ISSN 1049-510X
RA652 CODEN: ETDIEI
ETHNICITY & DISEASE. Text in English. 1991. q. USD 85 domestic to individuals; USD 115 foreign to individuals; USD 125 domestic to institutions; USD 155 foreign to institutions (effective 2000). adv. bk.rev. back issues avail. *Refereed.* **Document type:** *Academic/Scholarly.* **Description:** Covers population differences in disease patterns and provides a comprehensive source of information on causal relationships in the etiology of common illnesses through the study of ethnic patterns of disease.
Indexed: Cal.Tiss.Abstr., Environ.Sci.Poll.Mgmt., Ind.Med. (1991-), Int.Nurs.Ind., NRN, Pollut.Abstr., Risk Abstr., Saf.Sci.Abstr., THA.
—BLDSC (3814.840500), GNLM, ingenta, KNAW.
Published by: International Society on Hypertension in Blacks, 2045 Manchester St, N E, Atlanta, GA 30324-4110. TEL 404-875-6263, FAX 404-875-6334, orders@allenpress.com, http://www.allenpress.com. Ed. James W Reed. R&P Carrie Hamilton TEL 404-875-6263. Adv. contact Anne Dubois. Circ: 1,700 (paid); 1,500 (controlled). **Subscr. to:** Allen Press Inc., PO Box 1897, Lawrence, KS 66044-8897.

EURO COURSES. HEALTH PHYSICS AND RADIATION PROTECTION. see *ENERGY—Nuclear Energy*

▼ **EUROPEAN JOURNAL OF ACUPUNCTURE.** see *ALTERNATIVE MEDICINE*

610 AUT ISSN 1609-0152
▼ **EUROPEAN JOURNAL OF ALLIED HEALTH.** Text in English. 2000. q. USD 75 domestic; USD 115 foreign; USD 35 newsstand/cover (effective 2001). adv. back issues avail. *Refereed.* **Document type:** *Journal, Academic/Scholarly.* **Description:** Publishes articles, case reports, reviews, and letters that improve communications in understanding the various fields of allied health.
Related titles: Online - full text ed.: ISSN 1609-0160.
Published by: V I C E R Publishing, PO Box 14, Vienna A-1097, Austria. TEL 43-676-9568085, FAX 43-676-9568086, vicer@vicer.org, http://www.vicer.org. Ed., R&P Roland Hofbauer. adv.: B&W page USD 1,700, color page USD 2,200. Circ: 1,000 (paid and controlled).

611 ESP ISSN 1136-4890
CODEN: AANOA7
EUROPEAN JOURNAL OF ANATOMY. Text in English. 1952. 3/yr. ESP 25,000 (effective 2000 - 2001). adv. bk.rev. *Refereed.* **Document type:** *Academic/Scholarly.*
Formerly: Anales de Anatomia (0569-9894)
Indexed: Chem.Abstr., Excerp.Med.
—BLDSC (3829.722230), CASDDS, CISTI, GNLM, Infotrieve. **CCC.**
Published by: Sociedad Anatomica Espanola, c/o Dpto. de Anatomia e Histologia Humanas, Facultad de Medicina, Universidad de Sala, Avda Campo Charro, S/N, Salamanca 37070, Spain. TEL 34-923-294546, FAX 34-923-294559, ejasae@gugu.usal.es, http://www.med.ub.es/sae.htm. Ed. R Vasquez.

EUROPEAN JOURNAL OF APPLIED PHYSIOLOGY. see *BIOLOGY—Physiology*

610 GBR ISSN 0014-2972
R850.A1 CODEN: EJCIB8
EUROPEAN JOURNAL OF CLINICAL INVESTIGATION. Text in English. 1971. m., latest vol.32, 2002. GBP 55 in Europe to individuals; USD 94 in North America to individuals; GBP 60 elsewhere to individuals; GBP 581 in Europe to institutions; USD 931 in North America to institutions; GBP 646 elsewhere to institutions (effective 2002). adv. abstr, bibl, charts, illus. index. back issues avail. *Refereed.* **Document type:** *Academic/Scholarly.* **Description:** Publishes papers in the field of clinical investigation.
Related titles: Microform ed.: (from PQC); Online - full text ed.: ISSN 1365-2362. GBP 50 in Europe to individuals; USD 85 in North America to individuals; GBP 50 elsewhere to individuals; GBP 523 in Europe to institutions; USD 838 in North America to institutions; GBP 523 elsewhere to institutions (effective 2002) (from Ovid Technologies, Inc., EBSCO Publishing, O C L C Online Computer Library Center, Inc., RoweCom Information Quest, ingenta, Munksgaard & Blackwell Science's Synergy, Swets Blackwell, Institute for Scientific Information); ♦ Supplement: European Journal of Clinical Investigation. Supplement. ISSN 0960-135X.
Indexed: ASCA, Agri.& Environ.Biotech.Abstr. (coverage dropped), Biol.Abstr., Chem.Abstr., Chem.Indus.Notes, Chem.Titles, Curr.Adv.Biochem., Curr.Adv.Ecol.Sci., Curr.Cont., Dairy Sci.Abstr., Derwent Biotech.Abstr., Excerp.Med., Helminthol.Abstr., INIS Atomind., Ind.Med. (1970-), Ind.Sci.Rev., Inpharma, Int.Abstr.Biol.Sci., Kidney, Mass Spectr.Bull., NRN, Nutr.Abstr., Pharm.&Out.News, Reac., Ref.Zh., Rev.Med.& Vet.Mycol., SSCI (coverage dropped), Sci.Cit.Ind., Soyabean Abstr., THA, Telegen.
—BLDSC (3829.727100), ADONIS, CASDDS, CISTI, GNLM, IDS, ingenta, KNAW. **CCC.**
Published by: (European Society for Clinical Investigation), Blackwell Science Ltd., PO Box 88, Oxford OX2 0NE, United Kingdom. TEL 44-1865-206180, 44-1865-206002, FAX 44-1865-206219, jnl.orders@blacksci.co.uk, http://www.blackwell-science.com/~cgilib/jnlpage.asp?Journal=ejci&File=ejci, http://www.blackwellpublishing.com. Ed. J J M Marx. Pub. Allen Stevens. R&P Sophie Savage. Adv. contact Jenny Applin. Circ: 1,145.

610 GBR ISSN 0960-135X
EUROPEAN JOURNAL OF CLINICAL INVESTIGATION. SUPPLEMENT. Text in English. 1990. irreg. adv. **Document type:** *Academic/Scholarly.*
Related titles: ♦ Supplement to: European Journal of Clinical Investigation. ISSN 0014-2972.
Indexed: Excerp.Med. (1993-), Int.Abstr.Biol.Sci.
—ADONIS, EMDOCS, Infotrieve, KNAW. **CCC.**
Published by: (European Society for Clinical Investigation), Blackwell Science Ltd., Osney Mead, Oxford OX2 0EL, United Kingdom. TEL 44-1865-206206, FAX 44-1865-721205, TELEX 83355 MEDBOOK G, journals.cs@blacksci.co.uk, http://www.blackwell-science.com. Ed. J J Marx. Pub. Allen Stevens. R&P Sophie Savage. Adv. contact Jenny Applin.

610 614 NLD ISSN 0393-2990
CODEN: EJEPE8
EUROPEAN JOURNAL OF EPIDEMIOLOGY. Text in English. 1985. m. EUR 810, USD 811 to institutions for print or online ed.; EUR 972, USD 973.20 to institutions for print & online eds. combined (effective 2002). bk.rev. index. *Refereed.* **Document type:** *Journal, Academic/Scholarly.* **Description:** Provides forum on the epidemiology of communicable and non-communicable diseases and their control.
Related titles: Online - full text ed.: (from EBSCO Publishing, O C L C Online Computer Library Center, Inc., RoweCom Information Quest, Swets Blackwell, Kluwer Online, Institute for Scientific Information).
Indexed: ASCA, Abstr.Hyg., Aqua.Sci.& Fish.Abstr., Chem.Abstr., Chem.Indus.Notes, Chem.Titles, Curr.Cont., Dairy Sci.Abstr., Environ.Sci.Poll.Mgmt., Excerp.Med., Helminthol.Abstr., Ind.Med. (1985-), Ind.Vet., Inpharma, Int.Abstr.Biol.Sci., Int.Nurs.Ind., Microbiol.Abstr., NRN, Nutr.Abstr., Pharm.&Out.News, Pig News & Info., Pollut.Abstr., Protozool.Abstr., Reac., Ref.Zh., Rev.Appl.Entomol., Rev.Med.& Vet.Mycol., Risk Abstr., SSCI (coverage dropped), Saf.Sci.Abstr., Trop.Dis.Bull., Vet.Bull.
—BLDSC (3829.728900), CASDDS, CISTI, EMDOCS, GNLM, IDS, ingenta, KNAW. **CCC.**

M

Published by: Kluwer Academic Publishers Group (Subsidiary of: Wolters Kluwer N.V.), Spuiboulevard 50, PO Box 17, Dordrecht 3300 AA, Netherlands. TEL 31-78-639-2392, FAX 31-78-654-2254, services@wkap.nl, http://www.wkap.nl/journalhome.htm/0393-2990. Eds. Albert Hofman, Claude Hannoun. **Subscr. to:** Journals Department, PO Box 322, Dordrecht 3300 AH, Netherlands. TEL 31-78-639-2392, FAX 31-78-654-6474; **Subscr. to:** Kluwer Academic - Plenum Publishers, 233 Spring St, New York, NY 10013-1578. TEL 212-620-8468, FAX 212-807-1047.

610 NLD ISSN 1381-4788 CODEN: EJGPFJ

THE EUROPEAN JOURNAL OF GENERAL PRACTICE. Text in English. 1995. q. NLG 13, USD 72 to individuals. adv. *Refereed.* **Document type:** *Academic/Scholarly.* **Description:** Covers general medicine, family practice and related developments in Europe.

—BLDSC (3829.729430), CISTI, GNLM.

Published by: Mediselect B.V., Postbus 63, Leusden 3830 AB, Netherlands. TEL 31-33-4229900, FAX 31-33-4229922, info@mediselect.nl. Ed. M F Sips.

338.476 DEU ISSN 1618-7598

▼ **THE EUROPEAN JOURNAL OF HEALTH ECONOMICS.** Text in English. 2000. 4/yr. EUR 254 domestic; EUR 250.60 in Germany; EUR 72 foreign (effective 2002). *Refereed.* **Document type:** *Journal, Academic/Scholarly.* **Description:** Devoted to original papers and review articles covering all aspects of health economics.

Formerly (until 2001): Health Economics in Prevention and Care (1439-3972)

Related titles: Online - full content ed.: ISSN 1618-7601. 2000 (from EBSCO Publishing, Swets Blackwell); Online - full text ed.: (from RoweCom Information Quest).

Published by: Springer-Verlag (Subsidiary of: BertelsmannSpringer), Tiergartenstr 17, Heidelberg 69121, Germany. TEL 49-6221-345-0, FAX 49-6221-345229, subscriptions@springer.de, http://link.springer.de/link/service/journals/10198/index.htm, http://www.springer.de. Eds. K Lauterbach, M Drummond. **Subscr. to:** Springer-Verlag New York Inc., PO Box 2485, Secaucus, NJ 07096-2485. TEL 212-460-1500, FAX 212-473-6272.

344 610 NLD ISSN 0929-0273
K5 CODEN: EJHLEB

EUROPEAN JOURNAL OF HEALTH LAW. Text in English. 1994. q. EUR 237, USD 237 to institutions for print or online ed.; EUR 284.40, USD 284.40 to institutions for print & online eds.combined (effective 2002). abstr. reprint service avail. from WSH,SWZ. *Refereed.* **Document type:** *Journal, Academic/Scholarly.* **Description:** Discusses the evolution of health law in Europe on a national and international level.

Related titles: Online - full text ed.: (from EBSCO Publishing, O C L C Online Computer Library Center, Inc., RoweCom Information Quest, Swets Blackwell, Kluwer Online).

Indexed: Environ.Sci.Poll.Mgmt., Excerp.Med. (1996-), Pollut.Abstr., Risk Abstr., Saf.Sci.Abstr.

—BLDSC (3829.729850), EMDOCS, GNLM, Infotrieve. **CCC.**

Published by: Kluwer Law International (Subsidiary of: Wolters Kluwer N.V.), Laan van Meerdervoort 70, PO Box 85889, The Hague 2508 CN, Netherlands. TEL 31-70-308-1500, FAX 31-70-308-1515, services@wkap.nl, http://www.wkap.nl/journalhome.htm/0929-0273, http://www.kluwerlaw.com. Eds. H D C Roscam Abbing, J K M Gevers. Pub. Lukas Claerhout. **Subscr. in the Americas to:** Kluwer Academic - Plenum Publishers, 233 Spring St, New York, NY 10013-1578. TEL 212-620-8468, FAX 212-807-1047; **Subscr. to:** Kluwer Academic Publishers Group, Journals Department, PO Box 322, Dordrecht 3300 AH, Netherlands. TEL 31-78-639-2392, FAX 31-78-654-6474.

610 DEU ISSN 0949-2321 CODEN: EJMRFL

EUROPEAN JOURNAL OF MEDICAL RESEARCH. Text in English. 1996. m. DEM 348, USD 218 to individuals; DEM 398, USD 285 to institutions. *Refereed.* **Document type:** *Academic/Scholarly.*

Related titles: Online - full text ed.: (from Institute for Scientific Information).

Indexed: Chem.Abstr., Chem.Indus.Notes, Chem.Titles, Ind.Med. (1995-), Int.Nurs.Ind.

—BLDSC (3829.731313), CASDDS, CISTI, GNLM, Infotrieve, KNAW. **CCC.**

Address: Landshuter Allee 31, Munich 80637, Germany. TEL 49-89-13998732, FAX 49-89-13998731, eurjmedres@t-online.de. Eds. N Zoeller, W Dimpfel. Circ: 1,500 (paid).

EUROPEAN JOURNAL OF ORIENTAL MEDICINE. see *ALTERNATIVE MEDICINE*

610 GBR ISSN 1090-3801 CODEN: EJPAFJ

EUROPEAN JOURNAL OF PAIN. Text in English. 1997. bi-m. GBP 124 to individuals; GBP 192 to institutions (effective 2002). **Document type:** *Academic/Scholarly.* **Description:** Aims to be a global forum on all aspects of pain and its management.

Related titles: Online - full text ed.: (from EBSCO Publishing, O C L C Online Computer Library Center, Inc., Swets Blackwell, IDEAL Online Library, Institute for Scientific Information).

Indexed: Ind.Med. (1997-), Neurosci.Cit.Ind.

—BLDSC (3829.733382), CASDDS, IDS.

Published by: (European Federation of Chapters of the International Association for the Study of Pain), W.B. Saunders Co. Ltd. (Subsidiary of: Harcourt Publishers Ltd.), 24-28 Oval Rd, London NW1 7DX, United Kingdom. TEL 44-20-7424-4200, FAX 44-20-7424-4515, cservice@harcourt.com, http://www.harcourt-international.com/journals/eujp. **Subscr. to:** Harcourt Publishers Ltd., Foots Cray High St, Sidcup, Kent DA14 5HP, United Kingdom. TEL 44-20-8308-5700, FAX 44-20-8309-0807.

EUROPEAN NEWSLETTER ON QUALITY ASSURANCE. see *HEALTH FACILITIES AND ADMINISTRATION*

610.01 174 NLD ISSN 1381-1150

EUROPEAN STUDIES IN PHILOSOPHY OF MEDICINE. Text in English. 1994. irreg. price varies. *Refereed.* **Document type:** *Monographic series.*

Published by: Kluwer Academic Publishers Group (Subsidiary of: Wolters Kluwer N.V.), Spuiboulevard 50, PO Box 17, Dordrecht 3300 AA, Netherlands. FAX 31-78-639-2254, services@wkap.nl, http://www.wkap.nl. **Dist. by:** Journals Department, PO Box 322, Dordrecht 3300 AH, Netherlands. FAX 31-78-654-6474.

610 USA ISSN 0163-2787
RA399.A1

EVALUATION AND THE HEALTH PROFESSIONS. Text in English. 1978. q. USD 75 to individuals; USD 325 to institutions; USD 25 newsstand/cover to individuals; USD 85 newsstand/cover to institutions (effective 2002). adv. bk.rev. bibl, charts, stat. index. back issues avail.; reprints avail. *Refereed.* **Document type:** *Academic/Scholarly.* **Description:** Provides a forum for all health care professionals interested or engaged in the study, design, and control of the physical environment and its interaction with human behavioral systems.

Related titles: Online - full text ed.: (from EBSCO Publishing, O C L C Online Computer Library Center, Inc., RoweCom Information Quest, ProQuest Information & Learning, ingenta, Swets Blackwell, Institute for Scientific Information).

Indexed: ASCA, ASSIA, Abstr.Health Care Manage.Stud., Abstr.Soc.Geront., AgeLine, Biostat., C.I.J.E., CINAHL, Curr.Cont., Curr.Ind.Stat., Excerp.Med., Fam.Ind., Human Resour.Abstr., Inpharma, Lang.& Lang.Behav.Abstr., Med.Care Rev., Mid.East: Abstr.& Ind., Peace Res.Abstr., Pharm.&Out.News, PsycInfo, Psychol.Abstr. (1984-), Reac., Ref.Zh., Risk Abstr., SSCI, Sage Pub.Admin.Abstr., Sociol.Abstr., Viol.& Abuse Abstr., e-psyche.

—BLDSC (3830.564000), GNLM, IDS, ingenta, KNAW. **CCC.**

Published by: Sage Publications, Inc., 2455 Teller Rd, Thousand Oaks, CA 91320. TEL 805-499-0721, FAX 805-499-0871, info@sagepub.com, http://www.sagepub.com. Ed. R Barker Bausell. Pub. Sara Miller McCune. R&P Tanya Udin. Adv. contact DeAnna Vega Hammersley. Circ: 1,100. **Overseas subscr. to:** Sage Publications Ltd., 6 Bonhill St, London EC2A 4PU, United Kingdom; Sage Publications India Pvt. Ltd., 4215, New Delhi 110 048, India.

EVIDENCE - BASED HEALTHCARE; a scientific approach to health policy. see *PUBLIC HEALTH AND SAFETY*

610 GBR ISSN 1356-5524 CODEN: EBMEFS

EVIDENCE - BASED MEDICINE. Text in English. 1995. bi-m. GBP 75, USD 105 combined subscription to individuals includes print & online eds.; GBP 125, USD 175 to institutions for print only (effective 2002). adv. bk.rev. illus, stat. back issues avail. **Document type:** *Academic/Scholarly.* **Description:** Brings the best evidence from clinical and health care research to the bedside, surgery or clinic.

Related titles: CD-ROM ed.: GBP 53 to members; GBP 73 to non-members; GBP 103 to institutions (effective 2001); Online - full text ed.: E M B Online. ISSN 1473-6810. GBP 50, USD 70 to individuals (effective 2002) (from HighWire Pr.).

—BLDSC (3831.037000), GNLM, Infotrieve, ingenta. **CCC.**

Published by: (American College of Physicians/Co-sponsor: American Society of Internal Medicine USA), B M J Publishing Group, B M A House, Tavistock Sq, London WC1H 9JR, United Kingdom. TEL 44-20-7387-4499, FAX 44-20-7383-6400, info.norththames@bma.org.uk, http://www.evidence-basedmedicine.com, http://www.bma.org.uk. Eds. B Haynes, Paul Glasziou.

610 USA

EVIDENCE BASED PRACTICE. Text in English. 1998. m. USD 90 domestic to individuals; USD 110 foreign to individuals; USD 145 domestic to institutions; USD 190 foreign to institutions (effective 2000). back issues avail. **Document type:** *Newsletter.* **Description:** Highlights research articles that investigate important problems in primary care and have the potential to change the way doctors practice medicine.

Published by: Dowden Health Media, Inc, 110 Summit Ave, Montvale, NJ 07645. TEL 201-391-9100, FAX 201-505-5890, http://www.infopoems.com. Pub. Robert Osborn. Circ: 1,000 (paid).

EXPERIMENTAL AND MOLECULAR MEDICINE. see *BIOLOGY—Biochemistry*

616.07 USA ISSN 0014-4800
RB1 CODEN: EXMPA6

EXPERIMENTAL AND MOLECULAR PATHOLOGY. Text in English. 1962. bi-m. USD 685 in US & Canada to institutions; USD 750 elsewhere to institutions (effective 2001). adv. bibl, charts, illus. index. back issues avail. *Refereed.* **Document type:** *Academic/Scholarly.* **Description:** Presents articles on disease processes in relation to structural and biochemical alterations in mammalian tissues and fluids and on the application of the newer techniques of analytical chemistry, histochemistry, pharmacology, toxicology, and electronic microscopy to problems of pathology in humans and animals.

Related titles: Online - full text ed.: (from EBSCO Publishing, O C L C Online Computer Library Center, Inc., RoweCom Information Quest, ingenta, Swets Blackwell, IDEAL Online Library, Institute for Scientific Information).

Indexed: ASCA, Biol.Abstr., Chem.Abstr., Chem.Indus.Notes, Chem.Titles, Curr.Adv.Cancer Res., Curr.Cont. (coverage dropped), Dairy Sci.Abstr., Dent.Ind., Excerp.Med., Helminthol.Abstr., INIS Atomind., Ind.Med. (1962-), Ind.Sci.Rev., Ind.Vet., Inpharma, Int.Abstr.Biol.Sci., Nutr.Abstr., Pharm.&Out.News, Reac., Rev.Med.& Vet.Mycol., Sci.Cit.Ind. (coverage dropped), Vet.Bull., Weed Abstr.

—BLDSC (3838.700000), ADONIS, CASDDS, CISTI, GNLM, IDS, ingenta, Linda Hall. **CCC.**

Published by: Academic Press, Inc., Journal Division (Subsidiary of: Harcourt Brace & Company), 525 B St, Ste 1900, San Diego, CA 92101-4495. TEL 619-230-1840, FAX 619-699-6800, apsubs@acad.com, http://www.academicpress.com/emp. Eds. Frederick Coulston, Wilbur A Thomas.

615.9 DEU ISSN 0940-2993 CODEN: ETPAEK

EXPERIMENTAL AND TOXICOLOGIC PATHOLOGY. Text in English. 1967. 6/yr. EUR 553, GBP 428 (effective 2002). adv. bk.rev. bibl, charts, illus. index. reprint service avail. from ISI. *Refereed.* **Document type:** *Journal, Academic/Scholarly.*

Former titles: Experimental Pathology (0232-1513); Experimentelle Pathologie (0014-4908)

Related titles: Online - full text ed.: (from Institute for Scientific Information).

Indexed: ASCA, Biol.Abstr., Chem.Abstr., Chem.Indus.Notes, Chem.Titles, Curr.Adv.Cancer Res., Curr.Adv.Cell & Devel.Biol., Curr.Adv.Ecol.Sci., Curr.Cont., Dairy Sci.Abstr., Dent.Ind., Excerp.Med., Genet.Abstr., Helminthol.Abstr., INIS Atomind., Ind.Med. (1992-), Ind.Sci.Rev., Inpharma, Int.Abstr.Biol.Sci., Nutr.Abstr., Pharm.&Out.News, Reac., Rev.Appl.Entomol., Rev.Med.& Vet.Mycol., Sci.Cit.Ind.

—BLDSC (3838.720000), CASDDS, CISTI, EMDOCS, GNLM, IDS, Infotrieve, KNAW. **CCC.**

Published by: Urban & Fischer Verlag, Loebdergraben 14a, Jena 07743, Germany. TEL 49-3641-626444, FAX 49-3641-626500, journals@urbanfischer.de, http://www.urbanfischer.de/journals. Eds. Ulrich Deschl, Ulrich Mohr. R&P Martin Huber TEL 49-3641-626430. Adv. contact Sabine Schroeter. page DEM 750; trim 240 x 175. Circ: 550. **Dist. by:** Nature Publishing Group, Brunel Rd, Basingstoke RG21 6XS, United Kingdom. TEL 44-1256-302629, FAX 44-1256-463570, j.stephens@macmillan.com.

610 GBR ISSN 1471-2598
▼ **EXPERT OPINION ON BIOLOGICAL THERAPY.** Text in English. 2001. bi-m. GBP 870, USD 1,480 (effective 2002). abstr. back issues avail. *Refereed.* **Document type:** *Journal, Academic/Scholarly.* **Description:** An essential source of articles focusing on emerging biotherapevtic drugs and technologies.
Related titles: Online - full content ed.
Published by: Ashley Publications Ltd., Unitec House 3rd Fl, 2 Albert Place, Finchley Central, London N3 1QB, United Kingdom. TEL 44-20-8343-3883, FAX 44-20-8343-2313, jdrake@ashley-pub.com, http://www.ashley-pub.com. Ed. Katie Prickett. Pub. James Drake.

EXTRAMED. see *MEDICAL SCIENCES—Abstracting, Bibliographies, Statistics*

610 NLD ISSN 1240-3237
F A C E. (Facial Aesthetic Communication in Europe) Text in Dutch, English. 1992. q. USD 115 (effective 2001). bk.rev. illus. 64 p./no. back issues avail. *Refereed.* **Document type:** *Journal, Academic/Scholarly.*
—BLDSC (3863.151450). **CCC.**
Published by: Kugler Publications (Subsidiary of: S P B Academic Publishing b.v.), PO Box 97747, The Hague 2509 GC, Netherlands. TEL 31-70-330-0253, FAX 31-70-330-0254. Eds. G Nolst Trenite, J Soudant.

610 ESP ISSN 0210-8852
F A C: REVISTA PRACTICA DE MEDICINA. Text in Spanish. 1969. irreg. (4-5/yr.). free per issue to qualified personnel. adv. bk.rev.
Formerly: F A C: Revista Practica del Estudiante de Medicina
—CCC.
Published by: Laboratorio Alonga S.A., Avda Aragon, 18, Madrid 28027, Spain. Ed. Francisco Llagostera Campillo. Circ: 30,000.

610 USA
F M A TODAY. Text in English. 1985. bi-m. USD 15.90. adv. tr.lit. **Document type:** *Newspaper.* **Description:** Covers association news, members' achievements, upcoming and past meetings, health issues, and health-related legislation.
Published by: Florida Medical Association, Inc., 123 South Adams St, Tallahassee, FL 32301. TEL 940-356-1571, FAX 850-222-8030. Ed. Dr. R G Lacsamana. Circ: 18,000. **Subscr. to:** PO Box 2411, Jacksonville, FL 32203.

610 USA
F P REPORT. (Family Physician) Text in English. 1974. m. membership. **Document type:** *Newspaper.* **Description:** News and features covering information specific to family physicians. Covers all medical-socioeconomic matters affecting family medicine.
Formerly (until 1995): A A F P Reporter (0896-6877)
Published by: American Academy of Family Physicians, 11400 Tomahawk Creek Pkwy, Leawood, KS 66211-2672. TEL 913-906-6000, 800-274-2237, FAX 913-906-6089, http://www.aafp.org. Ed. Paula Binder. R&P Renee Anthuis. Circ: 86,000.

610 USA ISSN 0888-5656
RA396.A3
F S M B HANDBOOK. Text in English. a. USD 15 to non-members (effective 1999). **Document type:** *Directory.* **Description:** Covers three areas: history, goals and services; a directory; and articles of incorporation and bylaws.
Published by: Federation of State Medical Boards, 400 Fuller Wiser Rd, Ste 300, Euless, TX 76039-3855. TEL 817-868-4000, FAX 817-868-4098. Ed. Patricia Beatty. R&P Linda Uernale. Circ: 1,000.

610 USA ISSN 1062-5380
F S M B NEWSLINE. Text in English. 1981. m. USD 35 (effective 1999). **Document type:** *Newsletter.* **Description:** Focuses on current issues of interest to medical licensing and disciplinary authorities.
Formerly (until 1991): F S M B Newsletter (0888-5664)
Published by: Federation of State Medical Boards, 400 Fuller Wiser Rd, Ste 300, Euless, TX 76039-3855. TEL 817-868-4000, FAX 817-868-4098. Ed. Patricia Beatty. R&P Linda Uernale. Circ: 2,000.

FACHBUCHVERZEICHNIS MEDIZIN. see *MEDICAL SCIENCES—Abstracting, Bibliographies, Statistics*

610 NLD ISSN 0161-5580
CODEN: FASYDI
FALK SYMPOSIUM. Text in English. irreg., latest vol.85, 1995. price varies. *Refereed.* **Document type:** *Proceedings.*
Indexed: Chem.Abstr., Chem.Indus.Notes, Chem.Titles.
—BLDSC (3865.524000), CASDDS, CISTI, Infotrieve, KNAW. **CCC.**
Published by: Kluwer Academic Publishers Group (Subsidiary of: Wolters Kluwer N.V.), Spuiboulevard 50, PO Box 17, Dordrecht 3300 AA, Netherlands. FAX 31-78-639-2254, services@wkap.nl, http://www.wkap.nl. **Dist. by:** Journals Department, PO Box 322, Dordrecht 3300 AH, Netherlands. FAX 31-78-654-6474.

610 USA ISSN 1091-7527
R729.5.G4 CODEN: FSHEFV
FAMILIES, SYSTEMS & HEALTH; the journal of collaborative family health care. Text in English. 1983. q. USD 47 domestic to individuals; USD 66 foreign to individuals; USD 110 domestic to institutions; USD 132 foreign to institutions (effective 2000). adv. bk.rev. abstr. bibl. charts, illus. stat. back issues avail.; reprint service avail. from SWZ. **Document type:** *Academic/Scholarly.* **Description:** Publishes clinical, research and teaching materials relating to interface between family medicine, healthcare and family therapy.
Formerly (until 1995): Family Systems Medicine (0736-1718)
Related titles: Online - full text ed.: (from Gale Group).
Indexed: Abstr.Soc.Geront., CINAHL, Excerp.Med., FAMLI, Fam.Ind., Lang.& Lang.Behav.Abstr., PsycInfo, Psychol.Abstr., SOPODA, Soc.Serv.Abstr., e-psyche.
—BLDSC (3865.553974), CISTI, EMDOCS, GNLM, Infotrieve, ingenta, KNAW. **CCC.**
Published by: Families, Systems & Health, Inc., PO Box 20838, Rochester, NY 14602-0838. TEL 716-482-1390, FAX 716-482-2901, editors@fsh.org, http://www.fsh.org. Eds. Susan McDaniel, Thomas Campbell. Pub., Adv. contact William Steger. B&W page USD 150; trim 5.5 x 8.5. Circ: 1,500 (paid).

610 USA
FAMILY CARE HEALTH MONITOR. Text in English. bi-m. USD 6.95; USD 1.95 newsstand/cover (effective 2001).
Published by: Data Centrum Communications, Inc., 21 W 38th St, 4th fl, New York, NY 10018. TEL 212-997-9800, FAX 212-997-0078. Eds. Karen Seigal, Anny Queyroy. Pub. Eric Jensen.

610 GBR ISSN 1360-0176
FAMILY MEDICAL PRACTICE ON-LINE; the international journal of family medical practice and primary care. Text in English. 1995. m. free per issue. bk.rev., software rev., video rev. illus. reprints avail. *Refereed.* **Document type:** *Journal, Academic/Scholarly.* **Description:** Contains general information on medical topics of interest to both laypersons and medical professionals.
Media: Online - full text.
Published by: Priory Lodge Education Ltd., 2 Cornflower Way, Moreton, Wirral CH46 1SV, United Kingdom. TEL 44-151-606-1796, FAX 44-151-606-1812, http://www.priory.com/journals/fam.htm, solutions@priory.com, http://www.priory.com/. Ed. Dr. Thomas F Heston. Circ: 30,000 (controlled).

610.7 USA ISSN 0742-3225
FAMILY MEDICINE. Text in English. 1968. 10/yr. USD 85 to individuals; USD 120 to institutions (effective 2000). adv. bk.rev. bibl, charts, illus. cum.index (1981-1986). **Document type:** *Academic/Scholarly.* **Description:** Presents research studies and teaching methods for family physicians, family medicine educators, researchers, residents, and students.
Former titles: Family Medicine Teacher; Family Medicine Times
Related titles: Online - full text ed.: (from Institute for Scientific Information).
Indexed: Behav.Med.Abstr., Curr.Cont., Excerp.Med., FAMLI, Fam.Ind., Ind.Med. (1981-), Int.Nurs.Ind., Sci.Cit.Ind.
—BLDSC (3865.567450), CISTI, EMDOCS, GNLM, ingenta, KNAW.
Published by: Society of Teachers of Family Medicine, 11400 Tomahawk Creek Parkway, Leawood, MO 66211. TEL 913-906-6000, 800-274-2237, FAX 913-906-6096, fmjournal@stfm.org, http://stfm.org. Ed. Dr. Barry D Weiss. Pub., R&P Stacy Brungardt. Adv. contact Jan Cartwright. B&W page USD 870, color page USD 1,125; trim 10.88 x 8.38. Circ: 6,200.

610 USA
▼ **FAMILY MEDICINE NET GUIDE**; your guide to the internet. Text in English. 2000. 4/yr. USD 11.50; USD 4.50 newsstand/cover (effective 2000). **Document type:** *Journal, Consumer.* **Description:** Provides a physician-reviewed resource that presents health care concerns and provides links to online solutions for patients.
Related titles: ♦ E-mail ed.: Family Medicine Net Guide eNewsletter; ♦ Online - full content ed.: Family Medicine Net Guide Online.
Published by: Intellisphere (Subsidiary of: MultiMedia Healthcare Inc.), Office Center at Princeton Meadows, Ste 400, Plainsboro, NJ 08536. TEL 609-275-3800, FAX 609-275-6076, info@mmhc.com, http://www.mdnetguide.com, http://www.fmnetguide.com. Ed. Dr. Amy Helwig.

610 USA
▼ **FAMILY MEDICINE NET GUIDE ENEWSLETTER.** Text in English. 2000. bi-m. **Document type:** *Consumer.* **Description:** Provides updates on health care headlines, upcoming events, and special promotions.
Media: E-mail. **Related titles:** ♦ Online - full content ed.: Family Medicine Net Guide Online; ♦ Print ed.: Family Medicine Net Guide.
Published by: Intellisphere (Subsidiary of: MultiMedia Healthcare Inc.), Office Center at Princeton Meadows, Ste 400, Plainsboro, NJ 08536. TEL 609-275-3800, FAX 609-275-6076, info@mmhc.com, http://www.fmnetguide.com. Ed. Dr. Amy Helwig.

610 USA
▼ **FAMILY MEDICINE NET GUIDE ONLINE.** Text in English. 2000. d. **Document type:** *Consumer.* **Description:** Provides physician-researched links to medical and health care information on the Internet.
Media: Online - full content. **Related titles:** ♦ E-mail ed.: Family Medicine Net Guide eNewsletter; ♦ Print ed.: Family Medicine Net Guide.
Published by: Intellisphere (Subsidiary of: MultiMedia Healthcare Inc.), Office Center at Princeton Meadows, Ste 400, Plainsboro, NJ 08536. TEL 609-275-3800, FAX 609-275-6076, info@mmhc.com, http://www.fmnetguide.com. Ed. Dr. Amy Helwig.

610 USA ISSN 0014-732X
FAMILY PHYSICIAN*. Text in English. 1951. bi-m. USD 30 domestic to members; USD 48 foreign to members. adv. **Document type:** *Newsletter, Bulletin.* **Description:** Includes news of academy programs and articles about issues related to the practice of family medicine in Illinois.
Indexed: Biol.Abstr.
Published by: Illinois Academy of Family Physicians, 4753 Main St, Lisle, IL 60532-1724. TEL 708-240-5522, FAX 708-240-5887. Ed., R&P Christi Emerson. Adv. contact Steve Armetta. B&W page USD 1,490; trim 15.38 x 10. Circ: 5,000.

610 GBR ISSN 0263-2136
FAMILY PRACTICE. Text in English. 1984. bi-m. GBP 190, USD 330 to individuals; GBP 195, USD 340 to institutions (effective Feb. 2002). adv. bk.rev. Supplement avail.; back issues avail. *Refereed.* **Document type:** *Journal, Academic/Scholarly.* **Description:** Intends to serve as a means of broadening the international base of family medicine in general practice. Covers health care delivery, epidemiology, public health and medical sociology.
Related titles: Microform ed.; Online - full text ed.: ISSN 1460-2229. GBP 175, USD 306 to institutions Online only (effective Feb. 2002) (from EBSCO Publishing, O C L C Online Computer Library Center, Inc., RoweCom Information Quest, HighWire Pr., ingenta, Swets Blackwell, Institute for Scientific Information).
Indexed: ASSIA, Curr.Cont., Excerp.Med., Ind.Med. (1984-), Inpharma, Int.Nurs.Ind., Nutr.Abstr., Pharm.&Out.News, PsycInfo, Reac., SSCI (coverage dropped).
—BLDSC (3865.574700), EMDOCS, GNLM, IDS, ingenta, KNAW. **CCC.**

M

Published by: Oxford University Press, Academic Division, Great Clarendon St, Oxford OX2 6DP, United Kingdom. TEL 44-1865-267907, FAX 44-1865-267835, jnl.info@oup.co.uk, http://fampra.oupjournals.org, http://www.oup.co.uk/journals. Ed. R H Jones. Pub. Mandy Sketch. R&P Fionna Willis. adv.: page GBP 260, page USD 470. Circ: 900. **U.S. subscr. to:** Oxford University Press, Journals, 2001 Evans Rd, Cary, NC 27513. TEL 800-852-7323, FAX 919-677-1714, jnlorders@oup-usa.org; **Subscr. to:** Journals Marketing, Great Clarendon St, Oxford OX2 6DP, United Kingdom.

610 CAN
FAMILY PRACTICE. Text in English. 1989. 32/yr. CND 80 domestic; CND 97.85 foreign (effective 2000). adv. bk.rev.
Indexed: CBCA Ref., Curr.Cont. (coverage dropped), Psychol.Abstr. (1991-).
Published by: Maclean Hunter Healthcare, Maclean Hunter Bldg, 777 Bay St, 5th Fl, Toronto, ON M5W 1A7, Canada. TEL 416-596-5000, FAX 416-596-3498. Circ: 24,000.

610 658 USA ISSN 1069-5648
R728
FAMILY PRACTICE MANAGEMENT. Text in English. 1994. 10/yr. USD 48 domestic to individuals; USD 70 foreign to individuals; USD 58 domestic to institutions; USD 80 foreign to institutions; USD 37 to students (effective 2001). adv. **Document type:** *Academic/Scholarly.* **Description:** Advises family physicians on practice management and the socioeconomic aspects of family medicine. It helps remove obstacles to optimal health care and promotes leadership in the health system.
Related titles: Online - full text ed.: (from Northern Light Technology, Inc., ProQuest Information & Learning).
Indexed: CINAHL.
—BLDSC (3865.574725), GNLM, KNAW.
Published by: American Academy of Family Physicians, 11400 Tomahawk Creek Pkwy, Leawood, KS 66211-2672. TEL 913-906-6000, 800-274-2237, FAX 913-906-6080, fpmedit@aafp.org, http://www.aafp.org. Ed. Robert L Edsall. R&P Ariana Reeder. Adv. contact Joe Beck TEL 201-288-4440. B&W page USD 5,490. Circ: 99,954 (controlled); 102,231 (paid and controlled).

610 USA ISSN 0300-7073
FAMILY PRACTICE NEWS. Text in English. 1971. s-m. USD 96. **Document type:** *Newspaper.*
Related titles: Microform ed.: (from PQC); Online - full text ed.: (from Gale Group, Factiva).
Indexed: e-psyche.
—Infotrieve. **CCC.**
Published by: International Medical News Group, 12230 Wilkins Ave, Rockville, MD 20852. TEL 301-816-8700. Ed. Calvin Pierce. Circ: 72,000.

610 USA ISSN 0163-6642
R11
FAMILY PRACTICE RECERTIFICATION. Text in English. 1979. m. USD 66; free to qualified personnel (effective 2000). adv. bk.rev. index. *Refereed.* **Document type:** *Magazine, Trade.* **Description:** Directed towards physicians associated with family medicine; includes articles on new developments in medicine, clinical issues and family practice skills.
Related titles: CD-ROM ed.
Indexed: CINAHL, FAMLI.
—BLDSC (3865.574750).
Published by: (Medical Recertification Associates), M R A Publications, Inc. (Subsidiary of: Medical World Communications), 241 Forsgate Dr, Jamesburg, NJ 08831. TEL 732-656-1140, FAX 732-656-0059. Eds. Jane Monaghan, Paul Dishart. R&P Jane Monaghan. adv.: B&W page USD 4,350, color page USD 6,145; trim 10.75 x 7.88. Circ: 96,500.

610 VEN ISSN 0533-0327
FEDERACION PANAMERICANA DE ASOCIACIONES DE FACULTADES DE MEDICINA. BOLETIN. Text in Spanish. 1963. bi-m. free per issue. bk.rev. bibl. **Document type:** *Bulletin.*
Related titles: English ed.: Panamerican Federation of Associations of Medical Schools. Newsletter.
Indexed: FAMLI.
Published by: Federacion Panamericana de Asociaciones de Facultades y Escuelas de Medicina (FEPAFEM)/Panamerican Federation of Associations of Medical Schools (PAFAMS), Calle el Torreon, Qta. FEPAFEM,, Urb. Sorocaima, La Trinidad, PO Box 60411, Caracas 1060-A, Venezuela. TEL 58-2-945-0857, FAX 58-2-945-4275, fepafempafams@internet.ve, http://www.fepafem.org. Circ: 2,000.

610 USA ISSN 1078-4497
FEDERAL PRACTITIONER; for the health care professionals of the VA, DoD and PHS. Text in English. 1984. m. USD 87 in the Americas to institutions; USD 131 elsewhere to institutions (effective 2000). adv. index. back issues avail. **Document type:** *Trade.* **Description:** An independent journal geared to the needs of the health care professional working in the Federal health care system: the U.S. Public Health Service, Department of Defense, and Department of Veterans Affairs.
Formerly (until vol.11, no.10, 1994): V A Practitioner (0883-5721)
Related titles: Microform ed.: (from PQC); ◆ Supplement: Directory of Federal Health Care Facilities.
Indexed: I.P.A.
—Infotrieve. **CCC.**
Published by: Quadrant HealthCom, 26 Main St, Ste A, Chatham, NJ 07928-2402. TEL 973-701-8900, FAX 973-801-8892. Ed. Maribeth Maher. Pub. Peter Deyoe. Adv. contact Denise Andrade. Circ: 34,000.

610.71 USA ISSN 0014-9306
RA399.A3
FEDERATION BULLETIN; the journal of medical licensure and discipline. Text in English. 1913. q. USD 35 (effective 1999). bk.rev. charts. index. **Description:** Presents study and teaching methods. Devoted exclusively to medical licensure and discipline.
Indexed: Ind.Med. (coverage dropped).
—ingenta.
Published by: Federation of State Medical Boards, 400 Fuller Wiser Rd, Ste 300, Euless, TX 76039-3855. TEL 817-868-4000, FAX 817-868-4098. Ed. Patricia Beatty. R&P Linda Uernale. Circ: 4,400.

610 USA ISSN 0888-5648
RA396.A3
FEDERATION EXCHANGE. Text in English. biennial. USD 60 (effective 1999). **Description:** Contains information on examination and licensing requirements in all US jurisdictions, and on medical board structure and disciplinary function.
Published by: Federation of State Medical Boards, 400 Fuller Wiser Rd, Ste 300, Euless, TX 76039-3855. TEL 817-868-4000, FAX 817-868-4098. Ed. Patricia Beatty. R&P Linda Uernale.

610.6 060 ITA
FEDERAZIONE DELLE SOCIETA MEDICO-SCIENTIFICHE ITALIANE. CONGRESSI (YEAR). Text in English, Italian. 1978. a. adv. charts, illus. **Document type:** *Directory, Academic/Scholarly, Trade.* **Description:** Lists international medical and scientific conferences.
Former titles: Federazione delle Societa Medico-Scientifiche Italiane. Bollettino Congressi (Year); Comitato per la Collaborazione tra Societa Medico-Scientifiche Italiane. Federazione delle Societa Medico-Scientifiche Italiane. Bollettino Congressi (Year); C C S S
Media: Online - full text.
Published by: (Comitato per la Collaborazione tra Societa Medico-Scientifiche Italiane), Centro Trasfusionale e di Immunologia dei Trapianti, Ospedale Policlinico, Via Francesco Sforza, 35, Milan, MI 20122, Italy. TEL 39-02-55194950, FAX 39-02-5458129, gsirchia@mbox.vol.it, http://www.fism.it. Ed., R&P Girolamo Sirchia. Circ: 8,000.

610 ITA ISSN 0014-9659
CODEN: FGTOAW
FEGATO. Text in Italian. 1978 (vol.24). 3/yr. ITL 5,000. bk.rev.
Indexed: Chem.Abstr., Excerp.Med.
—CASDDS, CISTI, GNLM.
Published by: Societa Terme di Chianciano S.p.A., Chianciano Terme, SI 53042, Italy. Ed. Piero Valori.

610 DEU
FIBRIN SEALING IN SURGICAL AND NONSURGICAL FIELDS. Text in German. 1994. irreg. **Document type:** *Monographic series.*
Published by: Springer-Verlag (Subsidiary of: BertelsmannSpringer), Haber Str 7, Heidelberg 69126, Germany. FAX 49-30-82787448, subscriptions@springer.de, http://www.springer.de, http://link.springer-ny.com. Eds. G Schlag, H Redl.

611 USA ISSN 1121-0419
FIDIA RESEARCH SERIES. Text in English. 1986. irreg., latest vol.18, 1989. price varies. reprint service avail. from ISI. **Document type:** *Monographic series.*
—KNAW.
Published by: Springer-Verlag, Journals (Subsidiary of: BertelsmannSpringer), 175 Fifth Ave, New York, NY 10010. TEL 212-460-1500, FAX 212-473-6272.

610 FJI ISSN 0301-1089
FIJI MEDICAL JOURNAL. Text in English. 1960. m. FJD 10. adv. bk.rev.
Indexed: So.Pac.Per.Ind.
Published by: Fiji Medical Association, PO Box 1116, Suva, Fiji. Ed. Dr. K D Sharma. Circ: 1,000.

610 617.6 FIN
FINLAND. LAAKINTOHALLITUS. LAAKARIT - LAKARE/FINLAND. MEDICINALSTYRELSEN. LAEKARE. Text in Finnish, Swedish. 1976. a. FIM 195. **Document type:** *Directory.*
Formerly: Finland. Laakintohallitus. Laakarit, Hammaslaakarit - Laekare, Tandlaekare (0430-5299)
Address: PL 220, Helsinki 00531, Finland. TEL 358-0-39672308, FAX 358-0-39672450.

610 FIN ISSN 0015-2501
FINSKA LAEKARESAELLSKAPET. HANDLINGAR. Text in Swedish; Summaries in English. 1841. 2/yr. adv. charts, illus. **Document type:** *Trade.* **Description:** Covers basic, experimental and clinical medical sciences. Includes original articles, association news, obituaries.
Indexed: Biol.Abstr., Chem.Abstr., Curr.Adv.Ecol.Sci., Excerp.Med.
—BLDSC (4259.000000), CISTI, GNLM, KNAW.
Published by: Finska Laekaresaellskapet/Medical Society of Finland, PL 316, Helsinki 00171, Finland. TEL 358-0-665576, FAX 358-0-1356463. Ed. Per Henrik Groop. Adv. contact Johan Fagerudd. Circ: 2,000.

610.29 GBR
THE FITZHUGH DIRECTORY OF INDEPENDENT HEALTHCARE AND LONG TERM CARE. FINANCIAL INFORMATION. Text in English. 1986. a. GBP 240 (effective 2001). **Document type:** *Directory.* **Description:** Surveys the financial dynamics of this growing market.
Formed by the 1995 merger of: Fitzhugh Directory of Long Term Care (0959-6305); Fitzhugh Directory of Independent Healthcare. Financial Information (1352-8246); Which was formerly (until 1993): Fitzhugh Directory of Independent Healthcare. Financial Information. Acute Sector (0962-130X); (until 1990): Fitzhugh Directory of Independent Hospitals and Provident Associations
—BLDSC (3948.412000).
Published by: Health Care Information Services (Subsidiary of: W A F Health Care Consultant Ltd.), 12 Riverview Grove, London W4 3QJ, United Kingdom. TEL 44-20-8995-1752, FAX 44-20-8742-2418.

FIZIOLOGICHESKII ZHURNAL IM. SECHENOVA/ SECHENOV PHYSIOLOGICAL JOURNAL. see *BIOLOGY—Physiology*

FIZIOLOGICHESKII ZHURNAL (KIEV)/FIZIOLOGICHNYI ZHURNAL; nauchno-teoreticheskii zhurnal. see *BIOLOGY—Physiology*

610 USA
FLIGHT PARAMEDIC NEWS. Text in English. q. **Document type:** *Newsletter.* **Description:** Dedicated to promoting the global development and growth of the flight paramedic profession.
Published by: National Flight Paramedics Association, 383 F St, Salt Lake City, UT 84103-2756. TEL 626-405-9851, 800-381-6372, FAX 626-793-1039. Ed. Donna R Tokh.

616.980213 USA
FLIGHT PHYSICIAN. Text in English. 1955. q. USD 20 (effective 1998). reprints avail. *Refereed.* **Document type:** *Bulletin, Directory, Newsletter.*
Formerly: Civil Aviation Medical Association. Bulletin
Published by: Civil Aviation Medical Association, PO Box 23864, Oklahoma City, OK 73123-2864. TEL 405-840-0199, FAX 405-848-1053, Jimlharris@aol.com. Ed. H Stacy Vereen. Circ: 2,000.

FLORIDA BAR. HEALTH LAW SECTION NEWSLETTER. see *LAW*

610 USA ISSN 0015-4067
FLORIDA FAMILY PHYSICIAN. Text in English. 1953. a. membership. adv. illus. *Refereed.* **Document type:** *Academic/Scholarly.*
Formerly: Florida Academy of General Practice Journal
Published by: Florida Academy of Family Physicians, 6720 Atlantic Blvd, Jacksonville, FL 32211-8730. TEL 904-726-0944, FAX 904-726-0923. Ed. Dr. R Edward Dodge. Adv. contact Linda Keach. Circ: 4,500.

M

610 910.202 DEU ISSN 0947-7616
FLUG- UND REISEMEDIZIN; Tropenmedizin - Tauchmedizin - Bergmedizin - Expeditionsmedizin - Polarmedizin. Text in German. 1992. q. DEM 48 (effective 1998). **Document type:** *Academic/Scholarly.*
Published by: (Deutsche Gesellschaft fuer Luft- und Raumfahrtmedizin e.V.), Kagerer Kommunikation, Koblenzer Str 18, Bonn 53173, Germany. TEL 49-228-95696-0, FAX 49-228-9569640, vasomed@aol.com. Ed. Klaus Held. adv.: B&W page DEM 2,700, color page DEM 4,350; trim 297 x 210. Circ: 5,400 (paid). **Co-sponsor:** Deutsche Gersellschaft fuer Reise- und Touristik-Medizin e.V.

616.98021 USA ISSN 0015-4857
FLYING PHYSICIAN. Text in English. 1955. q. USD 50; USD 60 foreign. adv. bk.rev. illus. **Description:** Discusses aerospace medicine.
Published by: Flying Physician Association, PO Box 677427, Orlando, FL 32867-7427. TEL 407-359-1423, FAX 407-359-1167, 75114.1632@compuserve.com. R&P, Adv. contact Patricia Nodecker. Circ: 5,000.

610 DEU ISSN 0940-9998
FOCUS M U L; Zeitschrift fuer Wissenschaft, Forschung und Lehre an der medizinische Universitaet zu Luebeck. Text in German. q. DEM 76; DEM 79 foreign (effective 2000). adv. **Document type:** *Journal, Academic/Scholarly.*
Indexed: Ref.Zh.
—GNLM.
Published by: (Medizinischen Universitaet zu Luebeck), Hansisches Verlagskontor, Mengstr 16, Luebeck 23552, Germany. TEL 49-451-7031-01, FAX 49-451-7031281. Eds. H F Piper, R Labahn. Adv. contact Christiane Kermel. Circ: 5,000.

610 USA
FOCUS (NEW YORK, 1978). Text in English. 1978. m. (during academic year). free per issue.
Incorporates: State University of New York. Downstate Medical Center. Faculty Briefs (0039-0208); Former titles: Downstate Medical Center; Downstate Examiner; Supersedes (1969-1978): What's News
Published by: State University of New York, Health Science Center at Brooklyn, 450 Clarkson Ave, Brooklyn, NY 11203. Ed. M Ellen Griffin. Circ: (controlled).

610 BRA ISSN 0015-5454
FOLHA MEDICA. Text in Portuguese; Summaries in English, Portuguese. 1920. 3/yr. USD 200. adv. bk.rev. abstr, bibl, charts, illus. index.
Indexed: Biol.Abstr., Chem.Abstr., Excerp.Med., INIS Atomind., Ind.Med. (coverage dropped).
—BLDSC (3965.400000), CISTI, GNLM.
Published by: Cidade - Editora Cientifica Ltda., Rua Mexico, 90-Andar 2, Centro, Rio De Janeiro, RJ 20031-141, Brazil. TEL 55-21-2404578, FAX 55-21-2625462. Ed. Fernando Moyses. Circ: 15,000.

610 BIH ISSN 0352-9657
FOLIA ANATOMICA IUGOSLAVICA. Text in Serbo-Croatian; Summaries in English. 1972. a. USD 14. bk.rev.
Indexed: Excerp.Med. (until 1992).
—GNLM.
Published by: Savez Drustava Anatoma Jugoslavije, Mose Pijade 6, Sarajevo 71000, Bosnia Herzegovina. Ed. M Scepovic. Circ: 600.

610 POL ISSN 0015-5616
CODEN: FMCRAW
FOLIA MEDICA CRACOVIENSIA. Text in Polish; Summaries in English, Russian. 1959. 4/yr. price varies. bibl, charts, illus. index. **Document type:** *Academic/Scholarly.* **Description:** Presents both clinical and experimental research and discusses the mechanisms of pathogenesis of various diseases.
Indexed: Biol.Abstr., Chem.Abstr., Chem.Indus.Notes, Chem.Titles, Excerp.Med. (until 1993), INIS Atomind., Ind.Med. (1959-).
—BLDSC (3971.405000), CASDDS, CISTI, GNLM.
Published by: (Polska Akademia Nauk/Polish Academy of Sciences, Oddzial w Krakowie), Ossolineum Publishing House of the Polish Academy of Sciences, Pl Solny 14 a, Wroclaw 50062, Poland. TEL 48-71-343-6961, FAX 48-71-448-103. Ed. Dr. Zdzislaw Mach.

FOOD AND DRUG LAW JOURNAL. see *LAW*

FOOD, DRUG, COSMETIC, AND MEDICAL DEVICE LAW DIGEST. see *LAW*

616.047 344.041 USA
FOOT AND ANKLE PAIN. Text in English. 1988. a. USD 65.
Published by: Lexis Law Publishing (Subsidiary of: Reed Elsevier plc), PO Box 7587, Charlottesville, VA 22906-7587. TEL 804-972-7600, 800-562-1197, FAX 804-972-7666, llp.customer.support@lexis-nexis.com, http://www.lexislawpublishing.com.

610 USA ISSN 1049-6742
FOR THE RECORD (VALLEY FORGE). Text in English. 1989. w. USD 13 for qualified persons; USD 52 for non-qualified persons. adv. bk.rev. charts, illus. *Refereed.* **Description:** Publishes items of general interest to health information management professionals, including legislation, software, and management issues.
Published by: Great Valley Publishing, PO Box 2224, Valley Forge, PA 19482. TEL 610-917-9300, 800-278-4400, FAX 610-917-9186, edit@gvpub.com, http://www.gvpub.com. Ed. Kate Jackson. Pub., R&P Kathleen Czermanski. Adv. contact Emily Honiker. Circ: 45,000 (controlled).

FORMA. see *BIOLOGY*

610 ESP ISSN 1134-2072
FORMACION MEDICA CONTINUADA EN ATENCION PRIMARIA. Text in Spanish. 1994. 10/yr. USD 176. **Document type:** *Academic/Scholarly.*
Published by: (Sociedad Espanola de Medicina de Familia y Comunitaria), Ediciones Doyma S.A., Traversa de Gracia, 17-21, Barcelona 08021, Spain. TEL 34-93-200-0711, FAX 34-93-209-1136. Ed. A Martin Zurro. adv.: page ESP 295,000. Circ: 10,000.

610 HKG ISSN 0929-6646
CODEN: JFASEO
FORMOSAN MEDICAL ASSOCIATION. JOURNAL. Text in English. 1907. m. USD 60 domestic; USD 90 foreign. adv. charts, illus. Supplement avail.; reprint service avail. from IRC. *Refereed.* **Document type:** *Academic/Scholarly.* **Description:** Covers basic, experimental, and clinical medical sciences. Includes original articles, case reports, brief communications, review articles, association news, and announcements of meetings. Supplement issues include programs and abstracts of meetings.
Former titles (until Nov. 1993): Taiwan I Hsueh Hui Tsa Chih (0371-7682); (until 1946): Taiwan Igakkai Zasshi - Medical Association of Taiwan. Journal (0372-3321)
Related titles: Online - full text ed.: (from Institute for Scientific Information).
Indexed: ASCA, Abstr.Hyg., Aqua.Sci.& Fish.Abstr., Biol.Abstr., Cal.Tiss.Abstr., Chem.Abstr., Chem.Indus.Notes, Chem.Titles, Curr.Cont., Dent.Ind., Environ.Sci.Poll.Mgmt., Excerp.Med., Helminthol.Abstr., Ind.Med. (1991-), Inpharma, Nutr.Abstr., Pharm.&Out.News, Pollut.Abstr., Protozool.Abstr., Reac., Rev.Appl.Entomol., Rev.Arom.& Med.Plants, Rev.Med.& Vet.Mycol., Risk Abstr., Rural Devel.Abstr., Saf.Sci.Abstr., Sci.Cit.Ind., Soyabean Abstr., Trop.Dis.Bull., Weed Abstr.
—BLDSC (4754.900000), CASDDS, CISTI, EMDOCS, GNLM, IDS, ingenta, KNAW.
Published by: (Formosan Medical Association CHN), Excerpta Medica Asia Ltd., Eight Commercial Tower 19th Fl, 8 Sun Yip St, Chai Wan, Hong Kong, Hong Kong. TEL 852-2965-1300. Ed. Dr. Jung Yaw Lin. R&P Sindy Fok TEL 852-2965-1366. Circ: 5,100. **Subscr. to:** Formosan Medical Association, No 1, Chang-Te St, Taipei 10016, Taiwan. TEL 886-2-2381-0367, FAX 866-2-2389-6716.

610 DEU ISSN 0170-3331
FORTSCHRITT UND FORTBILDUNG IN DER MEDIZIN. Text in German. a. **Document type:** *Trade.*
Indexed: Inpharma, Reac.
—BLDSC (4018.610000), GNLM, KNAW.
Published by: Bundesaerztekammer, Herbert-Lewin-Str 1, Cologne 50931, Germany.

610 ESP ISSN 0212-9965
FORUM. Text in Spanish. 1982. 24/yr. free per issue. adv. **Document type:** *Academic/Scholarly.*
—CINDOC.
Published by: Ediciones Mayo S.A., Muntaner, 374-376 4o, Barcelona 08006, Spain. TEL 34-93-2090255, FAX 34-93-2020643. Ed. J M Ferrando. Circ: 10,000.

610 AUT
FORUM DR. MED. Text in German; Summaries in English, German. 1976. 17/yr. ATS 594 (effective 2000). adv. **Document type:** *Journal, Trade.*
Published by: Medizinische Fachzeitschriften GmbH, Rosenbergstrasse 18, Goettlesbrunn, N 2464, Austria. TEL 43-2162-8735, FAX 43-2162-87354. Ed., Adv. contact Gerhard Fillitz. B&W page ATS 31,900, color page ATS 39,900; trim 263 x 185. Circ: 22,500 (controlled).

610 DEU ISSN 0932-0547
FORUM LOGOPAEDIE. Text in German. 1987. 6/yr. DEM 96. adv. bk.rev. index. **Document type:** *Academic/Scholarly.*
Indexed: IBZ.
—GNLM.
Published by: (Deutscher Bundesverband fuer Logopaedie e.V.), Schulz - Kirchner Verlag GmbH, Mollweg 2, Idstein 65510, Germany. TEL 49-6126-9320-0, FAX 49-6126-9320-50. Ed. Michael Wilhelm. Adv. contact Doris Zimmermann. page DEM 1,630; trim 260 x 180. Circ: 7,350.

610 FRA ISSN 0763-7098
FRANCE. INSTITUT NATIONAL DE LA SANTE ET DE LA RECHERCHE MEDICALE. COLLOQUES. Text mainly in English. 1971. irreg. price varies. **Document type:** *Proceedings, Academic/Scholarly.*
Published by: Institut National de la Sante et de la Recherche Medicale, 101 rue de Tolbiac, Paris Cedex 13 75654, France. TEL 44-23-60-00, FAX 44-23-60-99.

610 ITA ISSN 0016-1535
IL FRIULI MEDICO; alpe-adria journal of medicine. Text in English, Italian; Summaries in English, Italian. 1946. q. ITL 75,000; ITL 85,000 foreign. bk.rev. bibl, charts, illus, stat. index, cum.index. *Refereed.* **Document type:** *Proceedings, Academic/Scholarly.* **Description:** Features research papers on a wide variety of topics in medicine. Includes research carried out in northeastern Italy.
Indexed: Biol.Abstr., Chem.Abstr., Excerp.Med., Ind.Med. (coverage dropped).
—CISTI, GNLM.
Published by: (Consorzio per la Costituzione e lo Sviluppo degli Insegnamenti Universitari di Udine), Tipografia Editrice A. Pellegrini, Via della Vigna, 24-A, Udine, UD 33100, Italy. TEL 39-432-559400, FAX 39-432-559420. Ed. Carlos Alberto Beltrami. adv.: page ITL 1,500,000. Circ: 1,500.

610 ITA ISSN 0390-9166
FRONTE SANITARIO* ; quindicinale dei medici italiani. Text in Italian. 1944. 11/yr. ITL 30,000.
Address: Via Di Porta Soprana, 17, Genoa, GE 16123, Italy. TEL 39-20-294500. Ed. Gianfranco de Ferrari. adv.: B&W page ITL 3,200,000. Circ: 12,000.

610 USA ISSN 1062-4767
Q11
FRONTIER PERSPECTIVES. Text in English. s-a. USD 30 to membership (effective 2001). **Description:** Dedicated to open examination of any theory, hypotheses, or model that challenge prevailing scientific views using sound scientific methods or reasoning.
Indexed: CINAHL.
—Linda Hall.
Published by: Temple University, Center for Frontier Sciences, Ritter Hall 003-00, 1301 Cecil B. Moore Ave., Philadelphia, PA 19122. TEL 215-204-8487, FAX 215-204-5553, V2058A@VM.Temple.edu, cfs@blue.temple.edu, http://www.temple.edu/cfs, http://www.temple.edu.cfs.

611 571 USA ISSN 1093-9946
FRONTIERS IN BIOSCIENCE. Text in English. 1996. q. USD 695 to individuals; USD 1,095 to corporations. bk.rev. abstr, bibl, illus. back issues avail. *Refereed.* **Document type:** *Academic/Scholarly.* **Description:** Offers a modern forum to communicate scientific research, reviews, technical notes, reviews, and rare images, videos, and sound files in any discipline in biology and medicine, including biochemistry, microbiology, parasitology, virology, immunology, biotechnology, and bioinformatics.
Related titles: CD-ROM ed.: ISSN 1094-3935; Online - full text ed.: (from Institute for Scientific Information).
Indexed: Curr.Cont., Ind.Med. (coverage dropped), Zoo.Rec.
Address: c/o North Shore University Hospital, Biomedical Research Center, 350 Community Dr, Manhasset, NY 11030. TEL 516-562-1176, FAX 516-365-5090, tabibzadeh@bioscience.org, http://www.bioscience.org/. Ed. S Tabibzadeh.

M

616.072 USA ISSN 1066-8322
CODEN: FHREE3
FRONTIERS IN HEADACHE RESEARCH. Text in English. 1991. irreg. price varies. reprint service avail. from PQC. *Refereed.* **Document type:** *Monographic series.*
Indexed: Chem.Abstr., Chem.Indus.Notes, Chem.Titles.
—BLDSC (4042.022800), CASDDS, CISTI.
Published by: Lippincott Williams & Wilkins (Philadelphia) (Subsidiary of: Wolters Kluwer N.V.), 530 Walnut St, Philadelphia, PA 19106-3621. TEL 301-223-2300, 800-638-3030, FAX 301-223-2400.

FRONTIERS OF HEALTH SERVICES MANAGEMENT. see *HEALTH FACILITIES AND ADMINISTRATION*

FRONTIERS OF MEDICAL AND BIOLOGICAL ENGINEERING. see *BIOLOGY—Bioengineering*

610 JPN ISSN 0288-2744
FUJI MEDIKARU FORAMU/FUJI MEDICAL FORUM. Text in Japanese. 1955. q. JPY 100 per issue.
Published by: Fuji Medikaru Shisutemu K.K./Fuji Medical System Co., Ltd., 13-8 Ginza 7-chome, Chuo-ku, Tokyo 104-0061, Japan.

FUJIAN YIYAO ZAZHI/FUJIAN MEDICAL JOURNAL. see *PHARMACY AND PHARMACOLOGY*

610 CHN ISSN 1004-5627
FUJIAN ZHONGYI XUEYUAN XUEBAO/FUJIAN COLLEGE OF TRADITIONAL CHINESE MEDICINE. JOURNAL. Text in Chinese. 1991. q. CNY 1.50 per issue. adv. bk.rev. **Document type:** *Academic/Scholarly.*
Description: Aims to popularize traditional Chinese medicine. Carries papers, articles that reflect the new developments in Chinese medical science.
Published by: Fujian Zhongyi Xueyuan/Fujian Institute of Traditional Chinese Medicine, 282 Wusi Lu, Fuzhou, Fujian 350003, China. TEL 0591-7841296, FAX 0591-7842524. Ed. Du Jian. Circ: 16,000. **Dist. overseas by:** China International Book Trading Corp, 35 Chegongzhuang Xilu, Haidian District, Beijing 100044, China.

610 JPN ISSN 0288-5441
CODEN: FGIGDO
FUJITA GAKUEN IGAKKAISHI/FUJITA MEDICAL SOCIETY. BULLETIN. Text in Japanese. 1977. s-a. **Document type:** *Bulletin, Academic/Scholarly.*
Indexed: Chem.Abstr., Chem.Indus.Notes, Chem.Titles.
—BLDSC (2523.100800), CASDDS.
Published by: Fujita Gakuen Igakkai, Fujita Hoken Eisei Daigaku, 1-98 Dengakugakubo-kutsukakecho, Toyoake-shi, Aichi-ken 470-1100, Japan. Ed. Katsutaka Torigai.

610 JPN ISSN 0915-423X
FUKUI IKA DAIGAKU KENKYU KATSUDO ICHIRAN/FUKUI MEDICAL SCHOOL. LIST OF RESEARCH ACTIVITIES. Text in English, Japanese. 1989. a.
Published by: Fukui Ika Daigaku, 23-3 Shimo-Aizuki, Yoshida-gun, Matsuoka-cho, Fukui-ken 910-1104, Japan.

610 JPN ISSN 0016-254X
CODEN: FKIZA4
FUKUOKA ACTA MEDICA/FUKUOKA IGAKU ZASSHI. Text in Japanese; Summaries in English. 1907. m. JPY 3,000, USD 6.70 (effective 2000). adv. charts, mkt. index. *Refereed.* **Description:** Contains reviews, original manuscripts and case reports in all of the medical sciences.
Indexed: Biol.Abstr., Chem.Abstr., Curr.Adv.Cancer Res., Curr.Adv.Ecol.Sci., Dent.Ind., Excerp.Med., INIS Atomind., Ind.Med. (1940-), Inpharma, Mass Spectr.Bull., Reac., Ref.Zh.
—BLDSC (4054.896200), CASDDS, CISTI, GNLM, KNAW.
Published by: Fukuoka Medical Society/Fukuoka Igakkai, c/o Graduate School of Medical Sciences, Kyushu University, Kukuoka 812-8582, Japan. FAX 81-92-631-2794. Ed. Yushi Ito. R&P Fukuoka Igakkai TEL 81-92-642-6896. Circ: 1,200 (paid); 150 (controlled).

610 JPN ISSN 0385-9347
CODEN: FIKIDK
FUKUOKA DAIGAKU IGAKU KIYO/FUKUOKA UNIVERSITY. MEDICAL BULLETIN. Text in English, Japanese. 1974. q. **Document type:** *Bulletin, Academic/Scholarly.*
Indexed: INIS Atomind., Zoo.Rec.
Published by: Fukuoka Daigaku, Sogo Kenkyusho/Fukuoka University, Central Research Institute, 19-1 Nanakuma 8-chome, Jonan-ku, Fukuoka-shi 814-0133, Japan. TEL 81-92-871-6631, FAX 81-92-866-2308.

610 JPN ISSN 0285-3418
FUKUOKAKEN IHO/FUKUOKA MEDICAL ASSOCIATION. JOURNAL. Text in Japanese; Summaries in English. 1948. m. JPY 2,400.
Published by: Fukuokaken Ishikai, 9-30 Hakataeki-Minami 2-chome, Hakata-ku, Fukuoka-shi 812-0016, Japan.

610 JPN ISSN 0917-9011
FUKUROI SHIRITSU FUKUROI SHIMIN BYOIN KENKYUSHI/FUKUROI MUNICIPAL HOSPITAL. JOURNAL. Text in Japanese; Abstracts in English, Japanese. 1992. a. JPY 1,000, USD 10. **Document type:** *Academic/Scholarly.*
Published by: Fukuroi Shiritsu Fukuroi Shimin Byoin, 2515-1 Kuno, Fukuroi-shi, Shizuoka-ken 437-0061, Japan. TEL 81-438-43-2511, FAX 81-438-5576. Ed., R&P Ichiro Ito.

610 JPN ISSN 0016-2582
CODEN: FSIZAQ
FUKUSHIMA IGAKU ZASSHI/FUKUSHIMA MEDICAL JOURNAL. Text in Japanese; Summaries in English. 1951. q. membership. charts, illus. index. **Document type:** *Academic/Scholarly.*
Indexed: Biol.Abstr., Chem.Abstr., Chem.Indus.Notes, Chem.Titles, Excerp.Med., INIS Atomind., Ref.Zh.
—BLDSC (4055.200000), CASDDS, CISTI.
Published by: Fukushima Society of Medical Science, Fukushima Medical University, 1 Hikarigaoka, Fukushima-shi 960-1295, Japan. FAX 81-245-48-2535. Ed. Yukihiko Kayama. Circ: 1,330.

610 JPN ISSN 0016-2590
CODEN: FJMSAU
FUKUSHIMA JOURNAL OF MEDICAL SCIENCE. Text in English. 1954. s-a. membership. charts, illus. index. *Refereed.* **Document type:** *Academic/Scholarly.*
Indexed: Abstr.Hyg., Biol.Abstr., Chem.Abstr., Curr.Adv.Ecol.Sci., Excerp.Med., INIS Atomind., Ind.Med. (1954-), Nutr.Abstr., Trop.Dis.Bull.
—BLDSC (4055.000000), CASDDS, CISTI, GNLM, ingenta, KNAW.
Published by: Fukushima Society of Medical Science, Fukushima Medical University, 1 Hikarigaoka, Fukushima-shi 960-1295, Japan. FAX 81-245-48-2535. Ed. Teizo Fujita. Circ: 1,600.

610 JPN ISSN 0913-2864
FUKUSHIMA KENRITSU BYOIN IGAKU KENKYUSHI/FUKUSHIMA MEDICAL BULLETIN. Text in Japanese. 1985. a.
Published by: Fukushima Kenritsu Byoin/Fukushima Prefectural Hospital, 3, Haraguchi, Iizakamachi, Fukushima-shi, Fukushima-ken 960-02, Japan.

610 JPN ISSN 0917-1835
FUKUYAMA IGAKU/FUKUYAMA MEDICAL ASSOCIATION. JOURNAL. Text in Japanese; Summaries in English, Japanese. 1991. a.
Published by: Fukuyamashi Ishikai, Fukuyamashi Ishi Kaikan, 11-25 Miyoshi-cho 2-chome, Fukuyama-shi, Hiroshima-ken 720-0031, Japan.

610 JPN
FURI RAJIKARU NO RINSHO/FREE RADICALS IN CLINICAL MEDICINE. Text in Japanese. 1987. a. JPY 5,150. **Document type:** *Academic/Scholarly.*
Published by: Nihon Igakukan, 9-6-505 Otsuka 3-chome, Bunkyo-ku, Tokyo 112-0012, Japan. TEL 81-3942-7631, FAX 03-3942-2086. Ed. Toshiaki Kikuzawa.

610 DEU ISSN 0179-6372
FUTURA. Text in English, German. 1986. q. Website rev. reprints avail. **Document type:** *Journal, Academic/Scholarly.*
—GNLM, KNAW.
Published by: (Boehringer Ingelheim Fonds, Stiftung fuer Medizinische Grundlagenforschung), Hippokrates Verlag GmbH, Postfach 300504, Stuttgart 70445, Germany. TEL 49-711-8931-0, FAX 49-711-8931453. Eds. Claudia Walther, Hermann Froehlich. Circ: 2,200.

610.69524894 DNK ISSN 0904-6895
FYNSKE LAEGER. Text in Danish. 1981. bi-m. DKK 150 (effective 1999). adv. bk.rev. illus. **Document type:** *Trade.*
Formerly (until 1981): Laegekredsforeningen Fyns Amt (0109-5439)
Published by: Laegekredsforeningen for Fyns Amt, Skt Anne Plads 2, 5 sal, Odense C 5000, Denmark. TEL 45-66-13-32-11. Ed. Erik Himmelstrup. Circ: 2,050.

G H A TODAY NEWSLETTER. (Georgia Hospital Association) see *HEALTH FACILITIES AND ADMINISTRATION*

610 DEU
G I T LABORATORY JOURNAL. Text in English. 1996. q. adv. **Document type:** *Trade.*
Indexed: Anal.Abstr., Mass Spectr.Bull.
—BLDSC (4179.650500).
Published by: G I T Verlag GmbH, Roesslerstr 90, Darmstadt 64293, Germany. TEL 49-6151-8090-0, FAX 49-6151-8090183, gitverlaggmbh@gitverlag.com, http://www.gitverlag.com. Ed. Joerg Peter Matthes. Adv. contact Hubert Schulz TEL 49-6151-8090116. B&W page DEM 7,845, color page DEM 10,755; trim 260 x 185. Circ: 27,000 (paid).

610 GBR ISSN 0268-8417
G P. (General Practitioner) Text in English. 1963. w. GBP 138 in United Kingdom; GBP 140 in Europe; GBP 238 elsewhere (effective 2001). adv. **Document type:** *Trade.*
Former titles (until 1983): General Practitioner (0046-5607); (until 1971): G P (0433-0501)
Related titles: Online - full text ed.: (from Data-Star).
Indexed: AMED.
—BLDSC (4206.305000), Infotrieve. **CCC.**
Published by: Haymarket Medical Ltd., 174 Hammersmith Rd, London W6 7JP, United Kingdom. TEL 44-20-8943-5000, 44-20-8606-7500, FAX 44-20-8606-7301, ed.gp@haynet.com, admin.gp@haynet.com, http://www.haymarketgroup.com. Ed. Colin Cooper. Adv. contact Dave Saunders TEL 44-20-8267-4876. Circ: 43,358.

610 NZL ISSN 1171-347X
G P WEEKLY. (General Practitioners) Text in English. 1984. fortn. NZD 75 (effective 1999). adv. bk.rev. back issues avail. **Document type:** *Newspaper.* **Description:** For general practitioners covering health news and issues, medicopolitical comment and life-style pages.
Former titles (until Dec. 1991): New Zealand General Practice (0114-2550); (until 1988): Journal of General Practice (0112-2541)
Indexed: Ind.N.Z.Per.
—**CCC.**
Published by: Adis International Limited, Mairangi Bay, Private Bag 65901, Auckland 1010, New Zealand. TEL 64-9-477-0700, FAX 64-9-477-0766, chris.lawson@adis.co.nz, http://www.adis.com. Ed. Toni Mason. Pub. Graeme Avery. R&P Gina Still. Adv. contact Gina Stil. Circ: 4,500.

610 COL ISSN 0121-6309
GACETA MEDICA. Text in Spanish. 1991. q. free per issue. adv. *Refereed.* **Document type:** *Newspaper, Academic/Scholarly.*
Published by: (Asociacion Colombiana de Facultades de Medicina), Laboratorios Chalver de Colombia Ltda., Ave. 68, 40-21 Sur, Bogota, CUND, Colombia. TEL 571-7100477, FAX 571-2303573, TELEX 042628 CHACO CO. Ed., R&P, Adv. contact Dr. John R Maynham. Pub. Carlos Morales. Circ: 10,000 (controlled).

610 ESP ISSN 0304-4858
CODEN: GCMBA9
GACETA MEDICA DE BILBAO. Text in Spanish; Summaries in English, Spanish. 1895. q. ESP 1,000, USD 30. adv. back issues avail.
Indexed: Excerp.Med., Ind.Med.Esp., Ref.Zh.
—CASDDS. **CCC.**
Published by: Academia de Ciencias Medicas de Bilbao, Lersundi, 9 1o, Bilbao, Vizcaya 48009, Spain. TEL 4-423-37-68. Ed. Angel Arrien Echevarri. Circ: 5,000.

610 VEN ISSN 0367-4762
GACETA MEDICA DE CARACAS. Text in Spanish. 1893. q. free per issue. bk.rev. bibl, illus. *Refereed.* **Document type:** *Academic/Scholarly.*
Indexed: Abstr.Hyg., Chem.Abstr., Excerp.Med., Trop.Dis.Bull.
—CISTI.
Published by: Academia Nacional de Medicina, Apartado Postal 804, Caracas, DF 1010-A, Venezuela. FAX 582-7811737, ateproca@truenet. Ed. Dr. Oscar Aguero. Circ: 1,000 (paid). **Co-sponsor:** Congreso Venezolano de Ciencias Medicas.

M

610 MEX ISSN 0016-3813
R21 CODEN: GMMEAK
GACETA MEDICA DE MEXICO. Text in Spanish; Summaries in English. 1864. bi-m. USD 100 to individuals; USD 150 to institutions. bk.rev. bibl, illus. index. reprint service avail. from PQC. **Document type:** *Academic/Scholarly.*
Related titles: Microform ed.: (from PQC).
Indexed: Artemisa, Biol.Abstr., Chem.Abstr., Dairy Sci.Abstr., Helminthol.Abstr., Ind.Med. (1864-), Ind.Vet., Int.Nurs.Ind., Nutr.Abstr., Protozool.Abstr., Rev.Med.& Vet.Mycol., Small Anim.Abstr., Soils & Fert., Trop.Dis.Bull.
—BLDSC (4066.080000), CASDDS, CINDOC, CISTI, GNLM, KNAW.
Published by: Academia Nacional de Medicina, Unidad de Congresos, Bloque B, Centro Medico Nacional, Av. Cuauhtemoc 330, Mexico City, DF 06725, Mexico. TEL 52-5-5782044, FAX 52-5-5784271. Eds. Dr. Fabio Salamanca, Dr. Luis Benitez. Circ: 20,000.
Co-sponsor: Instituto Mexicano del Seguro Social.

GACETA SANITARIA. see *PUBLIC HEALTH AND SAFETY*

613.7 NLD ISSN 0966-6362
QP310.W3 CODEN: GAPOFK
GAIT AND POSTURE. Text in English. 1993. bi-m. EUR 474 in Europe to institutions; JPY 62,800 in Japan to institutions; USD 530 elsewhere to institutions (effective 2002). back issues avail. *Refereed.* **Document type:** *Academic/Scholarly.* **Description:** Provides a vehicle for the publication of up-to-date basic and clinical research on all aspects of locomotion and balance.
Related titles: Microform ed.: (from PQC); Online - full text ed.: (from ingenta, Swets Blackwell, ScienceDirect, Institute for Scientific Information).
Indexed: AMED, ASCA, Curr.Cont., Ergon.Abstr., Excerp.Med. (1996-), Focus on: Sports Sci.& Med., Ind.Med. (1993-), Inpharma, Reac., SSCI (coverage dropped), Sci.Cit.Ind.
—BLDSC (4066.386100), CISTI, EMDOCS, GNLM, IDS, Infotrieve, ingenta, KNAW. **CCC.**
Published by: Elsevier Science BV, PO Box 211, Amsterdam 1000 AE, Netherlands. TEL 31-20-485-2911, FAX 31-20-485-2457, http://www.elsevier.com/locate/gaitpost. **Subscr. in Australasia and the Far East to:** Elsevier Science (Singapore) Pte Ltd, No.1 Temasek Ave, 17-01 Millenia Tower, Singapore 039192, Singapore. TEL 65-434-3727, FAX 65-337-2230; **Subscr. in Japan to:** Elsevier Science Inc - Japan Regional Office, 9-15 Higashi-Azabu 1-chome, Minato-ku, Tokyo 106-0044, Japan. TEL 81-3-5561-5033; **Subscr. in the Americas to:** Elsevier Science, PO Box 945, New York, NY 10159-0945. TEL 212-633-3730, FAX 212-633-3680, usinfo-f@elsevier.com.

610 ESP ISSN 0304-4866
GALICIA CLINICA. Text in Spanish. 6/yr.
—EMDOCS.
Address: Juana de Vega, 13 2o, La Coruna 15004, Spain. TEL 81-22-25-96. Ed. Luis G Moyano. Circ: 33,000.

616.04 599.9 371.9 USA ISSN 1077-9965
GATHERED VIEW; national newsletter of the Prader-Willi syndrome Assn. (USA). Text in English. 1975. 6/yr. USD 30 domestic to individuals; USD 40 foreign to individuals (effective 2000). bk.rev. back issues avail. **Document type:** *Newsletter.* **Description:** Intended to educate and/or support anyone involved with persons with Prader-Willi syndrome.
Published by: Prader-Willi Syndrome Association, 5700 Midnight Pass Rd, Ste 6, Sarasota, FL 34242-3000. TEL 941-312-0400, 800-926-4797, FAX 941-312-0142, pwsausa@aol.com, http://www.pwsausa.org. Ed. Linda Keder TEL 301-384-4955. R&P Janalee Heinemann. Circ: 1,950 (paid); 119 (controlled).

610 USA
GAUCHER DISEASE NEWSLETTER. Text in English. 1987. q. USD 35 (effective 1999). back issues avail. **Document type:** *Newsletter.*
Published by: National Gaucher Foundation, 11140 Rockville Pike, 350, Rockville, MD 20852-3106. TEL 301-816-1515, 800-925-8885, FAX 301-816-1516, sadamsngf@aol.com, http:/www.gaucherdisease.org/250. Ed. Rhonda P Buyers. R&P Sharon Adams. Circ: 2,500.

610 306.766 USA ISSN 1090-7173
RA564.9.H65 CODEN: JGLAFX
GAY AND LESBIAN MEDICAL ASSOCIATION. JOURNAL. Text in English. 1997. q. USD 237, EUR 236 to institutions for print or online ed.; USD 284.40, EUR 283.20 to institutions for print & online eds.combined (effective 2002). adv. bk.rev. *Refereed.* **Document type:** *Journal, Academic/Scholarly.* **Description:** Discusses the physical and mental health care needs of the homosexual, bisexual and transgendered populations, along with other issues germane to this community, including homophobia in the medical profession.
Related titles: Online - full text ed.: (from EBSCO Publishing, O C L C Online Computer Library Center, Inc., Swets Blackwell, Kluwer Online, RoweCom Information Quest).
—BLDSC (4755.567000), Infotrieve. **CCC.**
Published by: (Gay and Lesbian Medical Association), Kluwer Academic - Plenum Publishers (Subsidiary of: Wolters Kluwer N.V.), 233 Spring St, New York, NY 10013-1578. TEL 212-620-8000, 800-221-9369, FAX 212-463-0742, info@plenum.com, http://www.wkap.nl; http://www.wkap.nl/journalhome.htm/1090-7173. Eds. Jocelyn C White, Mark H Townsend. R&P Rose Luongo TEL 781-871-6311. **Subscr. outside the americas to:** Kluwer Academic Publishers Group, Journals Department, PO Box 322, Dordrecht 3300 AH, Netherlands. TEL 31-78-639-2392, FAX 31-78-654-6474.

610 POL ISSN 0867-2164
GAZETA LEKARSKA*. Text in Polish. 1990. m. PLZ 42 to members. adv. bk.rev. back issues avail. *Refereed.* **Document type:** *Trade.*
Related titles: Online - full text ed.: 1990.
Published by: Naczelna Izba Lekarska w Warszawie, Ul Grojecka 65 a, Warsaw 02094, Poland. TEL 48-22-6250121, FAX 48-22-6296333, nilgl@ternet.pl. R&P Urszula Bakowska. Adv. contact Andrzej Szelag. page PLZ 6,500; trim 290 x 205. Circ: 125,000 (controlled).

610 MDG
GAZETY MEDIKALY. Text in Malagasy. 1965. m. **Document type:** *Newspaper.*
Address: Lot 12B Ampahibe, Antananarivo 101, Madagascar. TEL 27898. Ed. Paul Ratsimiseta. Circ: 2,000.

610 TUR ISSN 1300-056X
CODEN: GTDEE
GAZI MEDICAL JOURNAL/GAZI TIP DERGISI. Text in English. 1990. q. TRL 20,000,000, USD 40 (effective 2000). back issues avail. *Refereed.* **Document type:** *Academic/Scholarly.* **Description:** Publishes original articles on clinical or experimental investigations and case histories reporting unusual clinical syndromes or diseases.
Related titles: Online - full text ed.
Indexed: Chem.Abstr., Chem.Indus.Notes, Chem.Titles, Excerp.Med. (1992-).
—BLDSC (4094.655800), CASDDS, EMDOCS, GNLM, KNAW.
Published by: Gazi Universitesi, Tip Fakultesi Dekanligi/Gazi University, Faculty of Medicine, Dean's Office, 06500 Besevler, Ankara, Turkey. TEL 90-312-2141000, FAX 90-312-2124647, gmj@tip.gazi.edu.tr, http://tip.gazi.edu.tr/gmj. Ed. Selcuk Boeluekbasi. Circ: 1,000 (controlled).

610 ITA ISSN 0393-3660
CODEN: GMIMES
GAZZETTA MEDICA ITALIANA ARCHIVIO PER LE SCIENZE MEDICHE. Text in Italian. bi-m. USD 105 to individuals; USD 155 to institutions (effective 2000 - 2001). adv. **Document type:** *Academic/Scholarly.* **Description:** Covers clinical and experimental medicine and surgery.
Formed by the merger of: Archivio per le Scienze Mediche (0004-0312); Gazzetta Medica Italiana - Aggiornamenti Clinicoterapeutici (0392-159X); Which was formed by the 1983 merger of: Gazzetta Medica Italiana (0016-5670); Aggiornamenti Clinicoterapeutici (0002-0907)
Indexed: Biol.Abstr., C.I.S. Abstr., Chem.Abstr., Excerp.Med., INIS Atomind., Ind.Med. (coverage dropped), Inpharma, Reac.
—BLDSC (4095.153000), CASDDS, CISTI, EMDOCS, GNLM, KNAW.
Published by: Edizioni Minerva Medica, Corso Bramante, 83-85, Turin, TO 10126, Italy. TEL 39-11-678282, FAX 39-11-674502. Ed. M L Benzo. Pub. Alberto Oliaro. Adv. contact F Filippo. B&W page USD 1,200, color page USD 2,000; trim 270 x 190. Circ: 3,000 (paid).

GEDRAGSTHERAPIE. see *PSYCHOLOGY*

610 JPN ISSN 0914-4277
GEKKAN CHIIKI IGAKU/MONTHLY COMMUNITY MEDICINE. Text in Japanese. 1987. m. JPY 600. adv. bk.rev. *Refereed.* **Description:** Contains scholarly papers, reviews, proceedings of meetings, and activity reports concerning community medicine.
Published by: Chiiki Iryo Shinko Kyokai/Japan Association for Development of Community Medicine, Hibiya-dai Bldg, 13F., 1-2-2 Uchisaiwai-cho, Chiyoda-ku, Tokyo 100-0011, Japan. TEL 81-3-3580-8471, FAX 81-3-3580-8472, hakua@jichi.ac.jp. Ed. Ken Ichi Fumimoto. Adv. contact Tadao Mizuguchi. Circ: 2,900.

610 JPN ISSN 0385-8588
GEKKAN HOKEN SHINRYO/MONTHLY REVIEW OF INSURANCE TREATMENT. Text in Japanese. 1946. m. JPY 2,000.
Formerly (until 1971): Shukan Igaku Tsushin
Published by: Igaku Tsushinsha, 9-4 Uchikanda 1-chome, Chiyoda-ku, Tokyo 101-0047, Japan.

610 JPN ISSN 0917-1061
GEKKAN IGAKU JOHO/CLIPPING MONTHLY REPORT. Text in Japanese. 1989. m. JPY 2,000.
Published by: Koseisha Infomeshon Sabisu/Koseisha Information Service, 2-7 Dojima 3-chome, Kita-ku, Osaka-shi 530-0003, Japan.

610 JPN ISSN 0913-9443
GEKKAN IRYO JOHO/MEDICAL NEWS OF THE MONTH. Text in Japanese. 1987. m. JPY 2,700.
Published by: Nihon Shuppan Koho Senta/Nihon Publishing Center, 10-3 Taito 1-chome, Taito-ku, Tokyo 110-0016, Japan.

610 JPN
GEKKAN MEDIKARU & FAIN/MONTHLY MEDICAL & FINE. Text in Japanese. 1977. m. JPY 60,800.
Published by: Gendai Shuppan Co. Ltd., 30-13 Haccho-Bori 2-chome, Chuo-ku, Tokyo 104-0032, Japan.

610 JPN ISSN 0917-7507
GEKKAN SEKUSHUARU SAIENSU/SEXUAL SCIENCE. Text in Japanese. 1991. m. JPY 1,200 per issue. adv. bk.rev.
Published by: Nihon Akuseru Shupuringa Shuppan K.K./Axel Springer, Japan Publishing Inc., 2-1 Niban-cho, Chiyoda-ku, Tokyo 102-0084, Japan. TEL 81-3-3239-9388.

610 JPN ISSN 0910-7991
GEKKAN SHIN IRYO/NEW MEDICAL TREATMENT. Text in Japanese. 1974. m. JPY 1,500.
Published by: Emu I Shinko Kyokai/Association of Promotion for Medical Engineering, 13-15 Ginza 7-chome, Chuo-ku, Tokyo 104-0061, Japan.

610 JPN ISSN 0386-1791
GEKKAN SOSHIKI BAIYO/TISSUE CULTURE. Text in Japanese. 1975. m. JPY 28,400 (effective 1998). bk.rev. **Document type:** *Academic/Scholarly.* **Description:** Covers the latest development in the study of tissue culture, including reports on techniques, equipments, mediums, base medicines, cells and microscopes.
Published by: Nyu Saiensusha/New Science Co., 3-8-14 Takanawa, Minato-ku, Tokyo 108-0074, Japan. hk-ns@mk1.macnet.or.jp, http://www.macnet.orjp/co/hk-ns, http://www.macnet.or.jp/co/hk-ns. Ed. Hisako Fukuda. Circ: 6,000 (paid).

610 JPN ISSN 0433-3047
CODEN: GEIGAI
GENDAI IGAKU/CURRENT MEDICINE. Text in Japanese. 1950. 3/yr.
Indexed: Chem.Abstr., INIS Atomind., Ref.Zh.
—BLDSC (3500.310000).
Published by: Aichiken Ishikai/Aichi Medical Association, 14-28 Sakae 4-chome, Naka-ku, Nagoya-shi, Aichi-ken 460-0008, Japan.

610 JPN
GENDAI IRYOGAKU/MODERN MEDICAL INTELLIGENCE. Text in Japanese. 1985. bi-m. JPY 2,400 per issue.
Published by: Gendai Shuppan Co. Ltd., 30-13 Haccho-Bori 2-chome, Chuo-ku, Tokyo 104-0032, Japan.

M

616.042 DEU ISSN 1438-7506
GENE FUNCTION AND DISEASE. Text in English. bi-m. EUR 308 in Europe; CHF 518 in Switzerland & Liechtenstein; USD 348 elsewhere; EUR 324 combined subscription in Europe for print and online eds.; CHF 544 combined subscription in Switzerland & Liechtenstein, for print and online eds.; USD 366 combined subscription elsewhere for print and online eds. (effective 2002). *Refereed.* **Document type:** *Journal, Academic/Scholarly.* **Description:** Devoted to the molecular and functional aspects of disease.
Related titles: Online - full text ed.: ISSN 1438-826X. EUR 308 in Europe; CHF 518 in Switzerland & Liechtenstein; USD 348 elsewhere (effective 2002) (from Wiley InterScience).
—BLDSC (4096.402490).
Published by: Wiley - V C H, Postfach 101161, Weinheim 69451, Germany. FAX 49-6201-606-117, 49-6201-606-328, subservice@wiley-vch.de, http://www.wiley-vch.de. Ed. Walter Doerfler. Pub. Karin Dembowsky. R&P Claudia Rutz.

616.042 GBR ISSN 0969-7128
RB155.8 CODEN: GETHEC
GENE THERAPY (BASINGSTOKE). Text in English. 1994. m. GBP 205 in Europe to individuals for print or online ed.; USD 308 elsewhere to individuals for print or online ed.; GBP 226 combined subscription in Europe to individuals print & online; USD 339 combined subscription elsewhere to individuals print & online; GBP 675 in Europe to institutions for print or online ed.; USD 1,013 elsewhere to institutions for print or online ed.; GBP 708 combined subscription in Europe to institutions print & online; USD 1,062 combined subscription elsewhere to institutions print & online (effective 2002). adv. bk.rev. charts, illus, stat. index. back issues avail.; reprints avail. *Refereed.* **Document type:** *Journal, Academic/Scholarly.* **Description:** Publishes papers and reports data on methods and clinical trials for introducing genes into cells for treatment of inherited disease, cancer, the developing of animal models, and all aspects of gene therapy research.
Related titles: Online - full text ed.: (from EBSCO Publishing, O C L C Online Computer Library Center, Inc., RoweCom Information Quest, ingenta, Swets Blackwell, Institute for Scientific Information).
Indexed: ASCA, Biotech.Cit.Ind., Curr.Cont., Derwent Biotech.Abstr., Excerp.Med. (1995-), Focus on: Mol.Med., Genet.Abstr., Hum.Gen.Abstr., Ind.Med. (1994-), Int.Abstr.Biol.Sci., Med.& Pharm.Biotech.Abstr., Nuc.Acids Abstr., Ref.Zh., Sci.Cit.Ind., Virol.Abstr. (coverage dropped).
—BLDSC (4096.402720), CASDDS, CISTI, GNLM, IDS, Infotrieve, KNAW. **CCC.**
Published by: Nature Publishing Group Specialist Journals (Subsidiary of: Holtzbrink Publishers), Houndmills, Basingstoke, Hants RG21 6XS, United Kingdom. TEL 44-1256-329242, FAX 44-1256-328339, subscriptions@nature.com, http://www.nature.com/gt. Eds. Joseph Glorioso, Nicholas Lemoine. Pub. Katy Christomanou. R&P Trace Noel. Adv. contact Robert Sloan TEL 44-20-8882-7199. B&W page GBP 595, color page GBP 1,150; trim 210 x 280.

610 USA ISSN 1078-2842
GENE THERAPY WEEKLY. Text in English. 1994. w. (43/yr.). USD 1,549 in North America; USD 1,649 elsewhere. **Document type:** *Newsletter.*
Related titles: Online - full text ed.: (from Northern Light Technology, Inc., Gale Group, Factiva).
Indexed: Bus.& Indus. (Jan.1995-).
Published by: Charles W. Henderson, Ed. & Pub., PO Box 5528, Atlanta, GA 31107-0528. TEL 770-507-7777, FAX 770-507-7788, cwhender@newsfile.com; info@hendersonnet.atl.ga.us, http://www.newsfile.com.

610 NLD ISSN 0302-864X
R713.49
GENEESKUNDIG ADRESBOEK NEDERLAND. Text in Dutch. a. NLG 276 (effective 2000). adv. **Document type:** *Directory, Academic/Scholarly.*
Supersedes in part: Geneeskundig Jaarboekje
—KNAW.
Published by: Nijgh Periodieken B.V., Postbus 122, Schiedam 3100 AC, Netherlands. TEL 31-10-4274100, FAX 31-10-4739911, gab@nijgh.nl, http://www.nijgh.nl. Ed. G Reek. Pub. M P Vissers. Adv. contact M Jonker. B&W page NLG 4,625, color page NLG 7,305; trim 148 x 210. Circ: 11,024 (paid).

610 NLD ISSN 0302-6752
R101
GENEESKUNDIG JAARBOEK MEDICIJNEN. Text in Dutch. a. NLG 56.13 (effective 2000). adv. **Document type:** *Directory, Academic/Scholarly.*
Supersedes in part: Geneeskundig Jaarboekje
Published by: Nijgh Periodieken B.V., Postbus 122, Schiedam 3100 AC, Netherlands. TEL 31-10-4274100, FAX 31-10-4739911, gjb@nijgh.nl, http://www.nijgh.nl. Ed. B H Graatsma. Pub. M P Vissers. Adv. contact M Jonker. B&W page NLG 3,710, color page NLG 6,390; trim 100 x 150. Circ: 17,045 (paid).

610 GBR
GENERAL MEDICAL COUNCIL. ANNUAL REVIEW. Text in English. 1859. a. **Document type:** *Corporate.*
Formerly: General Medical Council. Annual Report
—BLDSC (1520.213000).
Published by: General Medical Council, 178 Great Portland St, London W1W 5AE, United Kingdom. TEL 44-20-7915-3507, FAX 44-20-7915-3685, publications@gmc-uk.org, http://www.gmc-uk.org. Ed. Stephanie Day.

610.29 GBR ISSN 0072-0763
GENERAL MEDICAL COUNCIL. MEDICAL REGISTER. Text in English. 1859. a. GBP 150 (effective 2001). **Document type:** *Directory.* **Description:** Comprises the UK Register of Medical Practitioners with other information concerning medical registration.
Related titles: CD-ROM ed.: GBP 150 (effective 2001).
Published by: General Medical Council, 178 Great Portland St, London W1W 5AE, United Kingdom. TEL 44-20-7915-3507, FAX 44-20-7915-3685, publications@gmc-uk.org, http://www.gmc-uk.org.

610.6 GBR
GENERAL MEDICAL COUNCIL. MINUTES. Text in English. 1858. a. price varies. **Document type:** *Proceedings.*
Published by: General Medical Council, 178 Great Portland St, London W1W 5AE, United Kingdom. TEL 44-20-7915-3507, FAX 44-20-7915-3685, publications@gmc-uk.org, http://www.gmc-uk.org.

610 GBR ISSN 1359-7639
GENERAL PRACTICE ON-LINE. Variant title: International Journal of General Practice and Primary Care. Text in English. 1994. m. free per issue. bk.rev., software rev., video rev. *Refereed.* **Document type:** *Journal, Academic/Scholarly.* **Description:** Publishes case reports, audits, treatment protocols, review papers and research on general practice and primary care.
Media: Online - full text.
Published by: Priory Lodge Education Ltd., 2 Cornflower Way, Moreton, Wirral CH46 1SV, United Kingdom. TEL 44-151-606-1796, FAX 44-151-606-1812, solutions@priory.com, http://www.priory.com/. Ed. Dr. Ben Green. Circ: 25,000 (controlled).

610 CAN ISSN 0844-1138
GENERAL PRACTITIONER'S SOURCEBOOK. Text in English. 1988. a. CND 109, USD 109 (effective 1998). back issues avail. **Document type:** *Directory.* **Description:** Information resource for healthcare professionals.
Published by: Sherwood Publishing Inc., 18 Sixpenny Court, Thornhill, ON L3T 4E5, Canada. TEL 905-889-8505, FAX 905-889-4117. Ed. Patrick Forrett. Pub., R&P Garnet Crossman. adv.: B&W page CND 9,900; trim 10.88 x 8.13. Circ: 15,000.

▼ **GENESCREEN**; an international journal of medical genomics. see *BIOLOGY—Genetics*

616.07 USA ISSN 1061-2289
GENESIS REPORT - DX; business implications of technology innovation in diagnostic medicine. Text in English. 1991. bi-m. USD 995 domestic; USD 1,050 foreign (effective 2000). **Document type:** *Newsletter.*
Related titles: Online - full text ed.: (from Northern Light Technology, Inc., Gale Group).
Published by: Genesis Group Associates, Inc., 29 Park St, Montclair, NJ 07042. TEL 973-509-7735, FAX 973-509-7745, http://www.genesispov.com. Ed. Charles Galanaugh.

610 USA
GENESIS REPORT - M CX; managed care strategic briefing. Text in English. 1994. 10/yr. USD 995 domestic; USD 1,050 foreign (effective 2000). **Document type:** *Newsletter.*
Related titles: Online - full text ed.
Published by: Genesis Group Associates, Inc., 29 Park St, Montclair, NJ 07042. TEL 973-509-7735, FAX 973-509-7745, http://www.genesispov.com. Ed. Jack Brandner.

610 FRA ISSN 0016-6839
GENIE MEDICAL; symbiose medico-artistique. Text in French. 1949. m. FRF 25. adv. bk.rev., film rev. illus, tr.lit.
Published by: E.S.T.E.C., 127 bd. Saint Michel, Paris 75005, France. Ed. Dr. H Drouin. Circ: 23,500.

610 570 GEO ISSN 1512-0112
GEORGIAN MEDICAL NEWS; monthly scientific bulletin. Text in English, Russian. 1995. m. GEL 220, USD 200 (effective 1999). adv. back issues avail. *Refereed.* **Document type:** *Academic/Scholarly.* **Description:** Contains latest updates on experimental and clinical medical studies for clinical practitioners and medical scientists.
Published by: V I Press Co. Ltd., Asatiani St 7, 5th fl, Tbilisi 380077, Georgia. TEL 995-32-39-31-94, FAX 995-32-29-38-69. Ed., R&P, Adv. contact Nino Mikaberidze. Pub. Vakhtang Maskhulia. B&W page USD 100; trim 7.25 x 10.5. Circ: 660 (paid); 120 (controlled). **Dist. by:** NNP Inc., 62-60 99th St, Ste 403, Rego Park, NY 11374. TEL 718-275-7029, FAX 718-275-7029.

610 615.89 USA
GERSON HEALING NEWSLETTER. Text in English. 1984. bi-m. USD 30 domestic; USD 35 foreign (effective 2000). adv. bk.rev. back issues avail. **Document type:** *Newsletter, Consumer.* **Description:** To educate the public on health and healing through nutrition and lifestyle changes.
Formerly: Healing Newsletter
Published by: Gerson Institute, PO Box 430, Bonita, CA 91908. TEL 619-585-7600, FAX 619-585-7610, info@gerson.org. Ed. Brandon Finucan. R&P Paula Spangenthal. Adv. contact Norma La Madrid. Circ: 2,500 (paid).

610.9 BEL ISSN 0929-6824
GESCHIEDENIS DER GENEESKUNDE. Text in Dutch. 1993. bi-m. NLG 97.50. **Document type:** *Academic/Scholarly.* **Description:** Covers the history of medicine, pharmacy and related disciplines.
—KNAW.
Published by: Garant Uitgevers n.v., Tiensesteenweg 83, Kessel Lo (Leuven) 3010, Belgium. TEL 32-16-253131, FAX 32-16-251314. Eds. Dr. H Beukers, Dr. R Van Mee. Pub. H Van Slambrouck. Circ: 2,000 (paid).

610 CHE ISSN 0016-9161
GESNERUS; Swiss journal of the history of medicine and sciences. Text in English, French, German, Italian. 1943. 2/yr. CHF 120; CHF 68 newsstand/cover (effective 2001). adv. bk.rev. illus. index, cum.index. **Document type:** *Journal, Academic/Scholarly.*
Related titles: ♦ Supplement: Gesnerus. Supplement. ISSN 1017-3293.
Indexed: Amer.Hist.& Life, BHA, Biol.Abstr., Chem.Abstr., Excerp.Med., Hist.Abstr. (1988-), Ind.Med. (1943-), Russ.Acad.Sci.Bibl.
—BLDSC (4163.000000), CISTI, GNLM, Linda Hall. **CCC.**
Published by: (Schweizerische Gesellschaft fuer Geschichte der Medizin und der Naturwissenschaften), Schwabe und Co. AG, Steinentorstr 13, Basel 4010, Switzerland. TEL 41-61-2789565, FAX 41-61-2789566, verlag@schwabe.ch, http://www.schwabe.ch. Ed. Dr. Marcel Bickel. adv.: B&W page CHF 625; trim 170 x 117. Circ: 650.

610 CHE ISSN 1017-3293
GESNERUS. SUPPLEMENT. Text in German. 1922. irreg., latest vol.44, 1995. CHF 45 (effective 2000). **Document type:** *Monographic series, Academic/Scholarly.*
Formerly (until 1990): Schweizerische Gesellschaft fuer Geschichte der Medizin und der Naturwissenschaften. Veroeffentlichungen
Related titles: ♦ Supplement to: Gesnerus. ISSN 0016-9161.
Indexed: Ind.Med. (1990-).
—BLDSC (4163.050000).
Published by: (Schweizerische Gesellschaft fuer Geschichte der Medizin und der Naturwissenschaften), Schwabe und Co. AG, Steinentorstr 13, Basel 4010, Switzerland. TEL 41-61-2789565, FAX 41-61-2789566, verlag@schwabe.ch, http://www.schwabe.ch.

610 AUT
GESUNDES TIROL. Text in German. 1991. 4/yr. adv. **Document type:** *Newsletter, Consumer.*
Published by: (Aerztekammer fuer Tirol), Ablinger und Garber GmbH, Medienturm Saline Hall, Hall In Tirol, T 6060, Austria. TEL 43-5223-513, FAX 43-5223-51330. adv.: page ATS 38,700; trim 210 x 280. Circ: 30,000 (controlled).

GESUNDHEIT (BAIERBRUNN). see *PHYSICAL FITNESS AND HYGIENE*

338.476 DEU ISSN 1432-2625 CODEN: GEQUF3
GESUNDHEITSOEKONOMIE UND QUALITAETSMANAGEMENT; Klinik und Praxis - Wirtschaft und Politik. Text in German; Summaries in English, German. 1996. bi-m. EUR 142 to individuals; EUR 282 to institutions; EUR 84 to students; EUR 58 newsstand/cover (effective 2002). **Document type:** *Journal, Academic/Scholarly.*
Related titles: Online - full text ed.: ISSN 1439-4049.
—BLDSC (4165.060000), GNLM.
Published by: Georg Thieme Verlag, Ruedigerstr 14, Stuttgart 70469, Germany. TEL 49-711-8931-0, FAX 49-711-8931298, leser.service@thieme.de, http://www.thieme.de/gesqm. Ed. R Rychlik. R&P Alessandra Kreibaum. Circ: 1,700 (paid).

610 500 NLD ISSN 0928-303X
GEWINA; tijdschrift voor de geschiedenis der geneeskunde, natuurwetenschappen, wiskunde en techniek. Text in Dutch. 1978. 4/yr. NLG 120 to non-members; NLG 65 to members (effective 1999). adv. bk.rev. *Refereed.* **Document type:** *Journal, Academic/Scholarly.* **Description:** Covers the history of mathematics, physics, engineering, medical and other sciences.
Former titles (until 1992): Tijdschrift voor de Geschiedenis der Geneeskunde, Natuurwetenschappen, Wiskunde en Techniek (0167-2088); (until 1978): GeWina (Leiden) (0928-382X)
Indexed: Amer.Hist.& Life, Hist.Abstr. (1981-87, 1990-90, 1995-).
—CISTI, Linda Hall.
Published by: Erasmus Publishing B.V., Glashaven 14A, Rotterdam 3011XH, Netherlands. TEL 31-10-2800439, FAX 31-10-2800438, info@erasmuspublishing.net; p.verhoef@inter.nl.net, http://www.erasmuspublishing.net. Ed., R&P Peter Verhoef. Circ: 300.

GEZONDHEIDSZORG, BELEID EN ORGANIZATIE. see *HEALTH FACILITIES AND ADMINISTRATION*

610 GHA ISSN 0855-0328
GHANA MEDICAL JOURNAL. Text in English. 1962. q. USD 50. adv. bk.rev. abstr, bibl, charts, illus, stat. reprint service avail. from IRC. **Document type:** *Academic/Scholarly.*
Indexed: Biol.Abstr., Curr.Cont. (coverage dropped), Excerp.Med., INIS Atomind., Ind.Med. (coverage dropped), Nutr.Abstr.
Published by: Ghana Medical Association, PO Box 1596, Accra, Ghana. TEL 233-21-665401. Ed. J H Addy. Adv. contact Dr. Mercy Newman. Circ: 1,000.

610 JPN ISSN 0072-4521 CODEN: GDIKAN
GIFU DAIGAKU IGAKUBU KIYO. Variant title: Acta Scholae Medicinalis Universitatis in Gifu. Text in Japanese. 1953. bi-m.
Formerly (until 1967): Gifu Ika Daigaku Kiyo - Acta Scholae Medicinalis in Gifu (0376-0340)
Indexed: Biol.Abstr., Chem.Abstr., Chem.Indus.Notes, Chem.Titles, Dairy Sci.Abstr., Excerp.Med., INIS Atomind.
—CASDDS, GNLM.
Published by: Gifu Daigaku, Igakubu/Gifu University, School of Medicine, 40 Tsukasa-Machi, Gifu-shi 500-8705, Japan. TEL 81-58-265-1241 ext 2300, FAX 81-58-267-2954. Circ: 350.

610 JPN ISSN 0912-0513
GIFU IRYO GIJUTSU TANKI DAIGAKU KIYO/GIFU COLLEGE OF MEDICAL TECHNOLOGY. BULLETIN. Text in English, Japanese; Summaries in English. 1985. a.
Published by: Gifu Iryo Gijutsu Tanki Daigaku, 795-1 Nagamine-Hiraga, Seki-shi, Gifu-ken 501-3200, Japan.

610 JPN ISSN 0914-9538
GIFUKEN ISHIKAI IGAKU ZASSHI/GIFU MEDICAL ASSOCIATION. JOURNAL. Text in Japanese. 1988. a.
Published by: Gifuken Ishikai, 30-1 Yabuta 10-chome, Gifu-shi 500-0000, Japan.

GIFUKEN KOSEIREN IGAKU ZASSHI/GIFU WELFARE FEDERATION. JOURNAL. see *SOCIAL SERVICES AND WELFARE*

610 JPN ISSN 0385-6259
GINKYO GAKUEN KIYO/GINKYO COLLEGE OF MEDICAL SCIENCE. BULLETIN. Text in English, Japanese. 1976. a.
Published by: Ginkyo Gakuen Tanki Daigaku/Ginkyo College of Medical Science, 819, Okubo, Shimizucho, Kumamoto-shi, Kumamoto-ken 860, Japan.

610 ITA ISSN 0391-8866
GIORNALE DEI CONGRESSI MEDICI. Text in English, French, German, Italian, Spanish. suspended 2000; resumed. bi-m., latest 2000. ITL 90,000, USD 80 (effective 2000).
Published by: C I C Edizioni Internazionali s.r.l., Corso Trieste 42, Rome, RM 00198, Italy. TEL 39-06-8412673, FAX 39-06-8412688, info@gruppocic.it, 1160199510. Ed. A Salvati.

610 ITA ISSN 0393-8492
GIORNALE DEL MEDICO; settimanale di informazione. Text in Italian. 1985. 30/yr. ITL 38,000 (effective 1999).
Published by: Masson S.p.A., Divisione Periodici, Via F.lli Bressan 2, Milan, MI 20126, Italy. TEL 39-2-270741, FAX 39-2-27074210. Ed. Carlo Grassi. adv.: B&W page ITL 12,950,000, color page ITL 16,500,000; trim 285 x 222. Circ: 48,000.

616.98 ITA ISSN 0017-0364 CODEN: GMMIAW
GIORNALE DI MEDICINA MILITARE. Text in Italian. 1851. bi-m. ITL 60,000, USD 75 (effective 1998). adv. bk.rev. abstr, illus. index. **Document type:** *Academic/Scholarly.*
Related titles: Online - full text ed.
Indexed: C.I.S. Abstr., Chem.Abstr., Chem.Indus.Notes, Chem.Titles, Excerp.Med., Ind.Med. (coverage dropped).
—BLDSC (4178.380000), CASDDS, CISTI, GNLM.
Published by: Direzione Generale della Sanita Militare, Via Di Santo Stefano Rotondo, 4, Rome, RM 00184, Italy. TEL 39-4735-7939. Ed. Domenico Mario Monaco. Circ: 3,000.

612.6 ITA
GIORNALE ITALIANO DI ANDROLOGIA. Text in Italian. 1994. q. ITL 85,000; USD 100 foreign.
Published by: Pacini Editore, Via Alessandro Gherardesca, 1, Ospedaletto, PI 56121, Italy. TEL 39-050-313011, FAX 39-050-3130300, pacini@cibernet.it, http://www.cibernet.it/pacini, http://www.pacinieditore.it. Ed. F Menchini Fabris.

616.07 ITA ISSN 0394-459X
GIORNALE ITALIANO DI PATOLOGIA CLINICA. Text in Italian. 1994. q. ITL 60,000; ITL 90,000 foreign (effective 1996).
Published by: Pacini Editore, Via Alessandro Gherardesca, 1, Ospedaletto, PI 56121, Italy. TEL 39-50-982439, FAX 39-50-983906, pacini@cibernet.it, http://www.cibernet.it/pacini. Ed. A Capri.

616.07 ITA ISSN 0393-5957
GIORNALE ITALIANO DI RICERCHE CLINICHE E TERAPEUTICHE. Text and summaries in English, Italian. 1979. bi-m. ITL 25,000. adv. bk.rev. back issues avail. **Description:** Covers clinical medicine.
—EMDOCS, GNLM.
Published by: E S I Stampa Medica s.r.l., Largo Volontari Del Sangue, 10, Casella Postale 42, San Donato, MI 20133, Italy. TEL 39-2-5274241, FAX 39-2-55600670. Adv. contact Ornella Galbiati. Circ: 25,000.

610 UKR
GIPOKRAT DAIDZHEST. Text in Ukrainian, Russian. m. USD 120 in North America (effective 2000).
Published by: Redaktsiya Gipokrat Daidzhest, Ul Degtyarevskaya 38-44, Kiev, Ukraine. TEL 213-34-36. **Dist. by:** East View Publications, 3020 Harbor Ln N, Minneapolis, MN 55447. TEL 763-550-0961, FAX 763-559-2931.

GLOBAL CONNECTIONS (ROCHESTER). see *LIBRARY AND INFORMATION SCIENCES*

613.7 USA
GLOBAL HEALTH DIRECTORY. Text in English. 1980. irreg., latest 2001. USD 150 to non-members; USD 25 to members (effective 2001). adv. bk.rev. **Document type:** *Directory, Trade.* **Description:** Provides a comprehensive list of all major organizations supporting global health.
Former titles: Directory of U.S. International Health Organizations; Directory of U.S. Based Agencies Involved in International Health Assistance
Published by: Global Health Council, 20 Palmer Ct, White River Junction, VT 05001. TEL 802-649-1340, FAX 802-649-1396, ghc@globalhealth.org, http://www.globalhealth.org. Ed., R&P, Adv. contact Annmarie Christensen. Circ: 1,500.

610 POL ISSN 0373-174X
GLOWNA BIBLIOTEKA LEKARSKA. BIULETYN. Text in Polish. 1952. s-a. PLZ 8; USD 30 foreign (effective 1999). adv. bk.rev. bibl, illus. index. back issues avail. **Document type:** *Bulletin, Proceedings.*
Indexed: Excerp.Med.
—CISTI, GNLM.
Published by: Glowna Biblioteka Lekarska/Central Medical Library, Ul Chocimska 22, Warsaw 00791, Poland. TEL 48-22-8497404, FAX 48-22-8497802, gbl@gbl.waw.pl, http://www.gbl.waw.pl. Circ: 180 (paid). **Dist. by:** Ars Polona, Krakowskie Przedmiescie 7, Warsaw, Poland.

GOLD INSTITUTE. INTERNATIONAL CONFERENCE ON GOLD & SILVER IN MEDICINE. PROCEEDINGS. see *MINES AND MINING INDUSTRY*

GOLFER'S COMPANION. see *SPORTS AND GAMES—Ball Games*

610 CHN ISSN 1001-814X
GONGQI YIKAN/ENTERPRISE MEDICAL JOURNAL. Text in Chinese. q.
Published by: Harbin Gongchang Qiye Yiyuan Guanli Weiyuanhui/Harbin Enterprise-owned Hospital Management Committee, 34, Siwu Daojie, Daoli-qu, Harbin, Heilongjiang 150010, China. TEL 413165. Ed. Mu Rui.

610 GBR ISSN 1350-0961
GOOD CLINICAL PRACTICE JOURNAL. Text in English. 1994. m. GBP 115 in Europe; USD 220 in US & Canada; JPY 24,200 in Japan; GBP 130 rest of world (effective 2001). adv. bk.rev. 36 p./no. 2 cols./p. back issues avail.; reprints avail. **Document type:** *Magazine, Academic/Scholarly.* **Description:** Provides up-to-date and authoritative information on the principles of global Good Clinical Practice. It's essential reading for all professionals involved in clinical trials and drug development. As well as the latest news, it features interviews with key figures in government and industry, regulatory updates, meeting reports, and provides a forum for topical, guideline debate.
Incorporates (1991-199?): European Journal of Clinical Research (0961-3692)
Indexed: Excerp.Med. (1996-), Inpharma, Reac.
—BLDSC (4201.318100), EMDOCS, GNLM, Infotrieve. **CCC.**
Published by: Brookwood Medical Publications (Subsidiary of: P J B Publications Ltd.), 18-20 Hill Rise, Richmond, Surrey TW10 6UA, United Kingdom. TEL 44-20-8332-4600, FAX 44-20-8332-4610, maria@brookwd.demon.co.uk, http://www.pjbpubs.com/brookwood/. Ed. Dr. Paula Hensler. Pub. Dr. Philip J Brown. R&P Theresa Saklatvala TEL 44-20-8332-6404. Adv. contact Jenefer Trevena TEL 44-20-8332-4605.

610.6 LKA
GOVERNMENT MEDICAL OFFICERS' ASSOCIATION. NEWSLETTER. Text in English. q. **Document type:** *Newsletter, Government, Trade.*
Published by: Government Medical Officers' Association, 6 Wijerama Mawatha, Colombo 7, Sri Lanka.

GOZZLE NIPPER. see *COLLEGE AND ALUMNI*

610 GBR ISSN 0141-2256
GREAT BRITAIN. MEDICAL RESEARCH COUNCIL. ANNUAL REPORT (YEAR). Text in English. a. GBP 20 (effective 1999). **Document type:** *Corporate.* **Description:** Provides a record of the MRC's activities and financial accounts.
Formerly (until 1965): Great Britain. Medical Research Council. Report (0072-6567)
—BLDSC (1340.190000), GNLM, KNAW.
Published by: Medical Research Council, 20 Park Crescent, London W1N 4AL, United Kingdom. TEL 44-171-636-5422, FAX 44-171-436-6179. Ed. Trevor Dooley.

GREAT BRITAIN. STUDIES ON MEDICAL AND POPULATION SUBJECTS. see *POPULATION STUDIES*

610 USA ISSN 0894-508X
GREATER KANSAS CITY MEDICAL BULLETIN. Text in English. 1907. m. USD 7 to non-members; USD 5 to members. adv. bk.rev.
Published by: Metropolitan Medical Society of Greater Kansas City, Metropolitan Medical Society, 3036 Gillham Rd, Kansas City, MO 64108. TEL 816-531-8432. Ed. Dr. John H Renner. Circ: 3,100.

610 USA
GREENE COUNTY MEDICAL SOCIETY BULLETIN. Text in English. 1942. m. USD 35 (effective 1999). adv. 40 p./no. **Document type:** *Magazine, Academic/Scholarly, Internal, Trade.* **Description:** Contains human-interest and member-oriented articles, news on local and state medical activities and politics.

M

Published by: Greene County Medical Society, 1200 E Woodhurst, Ste D 200, Springfield, MO 65804. TEL 417-887-1017, FAX 417-887-7738, gcms@mailsocket.net, http://www.gcmsonline.com. Ed. Dr. Arthur Hawes. Pub., R&P Lois Hayes. adv.: page USD 450; trim 9.75 x 7.25. Circ: 1,000.

362 610 USA ISSN 0199-5103
GROUP PRACTICE JOURNAL. Text in English. 1951. 10/yr. USD 75 domestic to institutions; USD 125 foreign to institutions (effective 2001). adv. bk.rev. bibl, stat, tr.lit, charts, illus, maps. index. 3 cols./p. back issues avail.; reprints avail. **Document type:** *Journal, Trade.* **Description:** Contains exclusive articles written for, by and about physician executives and other specialists in healthcare. Provides analytical and enlightening reports on current issues and trends in medical care delivery systems.
Formerly (until 1980): Group Practice (0017-4726)
Indexed: Abstr.Health Care Manage.Stud., AgeLine, Excerp.Med., Hosp.Lit.Ind., MEDSOC, Med.Care Rev. —BLDSC (4220.182100), GNLM, ingenta.
Published by: American Medical Group Association, 1422 Duke St, Alexandria, VA 22314-3430. TEL 703-838-0033, FAX 703-548-1890, http://www.amga.org. Ed. Tom Flatt. Pub. Donald W Fisher. R&P, Adv. contact Fred Haag TEL 703-838-0033 ext 329. B&W page USD 3,665. Circ: 60,000 (paid and controlled).

610 BEL ISSN 0771-0313
GROUPE D'ETUDE POUR UNE REFORME DE LA MEDICINE. CAHIERS. Key Title: Cahiers du G.E.R.M. Text in French. 1951. q. **Document type:** *Newsletter.*
Formerly (until 1981): Groupe d'Etude pour une Reforme de la Medicine. Lettre d'Information (0771-0267)
Published by: Groupe d'Etudes pour une Reforme de la Medicine asbl, Rue du Gouvernement Provisoire 29, Brussels 1000, Belgium. TEL 32-2-2196766. Ed. Thierry Poucet.

GROWTH, DEVELOPMENT & AGING. see *BIOLOGY*

610 CHN ISSN 1001-9448
CODEN: GUYIEG
GUANGDONG YIXUE/GUANGDONG MEDICAL JOURNAL. Text in Chinese. 1963. bi-m. CNY 1.60 per issue (effective 1994). adv. **Description:** General medical science periodical reflecting the latest progress in medical sciences, technology and practices.
Indexed: Chem.Abstr., Chem.Indus.Notes, Chem.Titles. —BLDSC (4223.858170), CASDDS.
Published by: Guangdong Yixue Qingbao Yanjiusuo/Guangdong Medical Information Institute, No 2, Jinbuli, Huifu Xilu, Guangzhou, Guangdong 510180, China. TEL 884610. Ed. Zhu Fumin. Adv. contact Su Huanqun.

610 CHN ISSN 1003-8914
GUANGMING ZHONGYI/GUANGMING TRADITIONAL CHINESE MEDICINE. Text in Chinese. 1985. bi-m. USD 9.60; USD 1.60 newsstand/cover (effective 2001). **Document type:** *Academic/Scholarly.*
Published by: Zhongguo Zhongyiyao Xuehui, 18, Bei-Xincang, Dongzhimen, Beijing 100700, China. **Dist. by:** China International Book Trading Corp, 35, Chegongzhuang Xilu, Haidian District, Beijing 100044, China. TEL 86-1-68413849, FAX 86-1-68412048, cibtc@mail.cibtc.com.cn, http://www.cibtc.com.cn.

610 CHN
GUANGXI YIXUE/GUANGXI MEDICAL JOURNAL. Text in Chinese. 1975. bi-m. USD 10.80. **Document type:** *Academic/Scholarly.*
Published by: Guangxi Yixue Qibaosuo/Guangxi Institute of Medical Science Information, 20 Gucheng Lu, Nanning, Guangxi 530022, China. TEL 86-771-5864744. Ed. Yu Zhifang.

GUANGXI ZHONGYI YAO/GUANGXI TRADITIONAL CHINESE MEDICINE. see *ALTERNATIVE MEDICINE*

610 CHN
GUANGZHOU ZHONGYIYAO DAXUE XUEBAO/ GUANGZHOU UNIVERSITY OF TRADITIONAL CHINESE MEDICINE. JOURNAL. Text in Chinese. 1986. q. CNY 32; USD 30 foreign. adv. **Document type:** *Academic/Scholarly.*
Formerly (until 1996): Guangzhou Zhongyi Xueyuan Xuebao - Guangzhou College of Traditional Chinese Medicine. Journal (1000-5056)
Indexed: Cal.Tiss.Abstr., Ref.Zh. —BLDSC (4757.659000).
Published by: Guangzhou Zhongyiyao Daxue/Guangzhou University of Traditional Chinese Medicine, 12, Jichang Lu, Guangzhou, Guangdong 510405, China. TEL 86-20-86591233, FAX 86-20-8659-4735, xbgutcm@ihw.com.cn. Ed. Ou Ming. adv.: page CNY 4,500. Circ: 1,500.

GUIA DE FORNECEDORES HOSPITALARES. see *GERONTOLOGY AND GERIATRICS*

338.7 610.28 USA
GUIDE TO BIOMEDICAL PRODUCT DEVELOPMENT SUPPORT SERVICES*. Text in English. a. USD 594 (effective 1997).
Published by: Dorland Healthcare Information, 1500 Walnut St Ste 1000, Philadelphia, PA 19102.

GUIDE TO HEALTH INSURANCE FOR PEOPLE WITH MEDICARE. see *INSURANCE*

610 JPN
GUIDE TO MEDICAL DEVICE REGISTRATION IN JAPAN. Text in English. irreg., latest 2001, 7th Ed. JPY 18,000; USD 190 in United States (effective 2001). **Document type:** *Government.* **Description:** Covers the Japanese medical device registration systems.
Related titles: Japanese ed.
Published by: Yakuji Nippo Ltd., 1 Kanda-Izumi-cho, Chiyoda-ku, Tokyo 101-8648, Japan. TEL 81-3-3862-2141, FAX 81-3-5821-8757, shuppan@yakuji.co.jp, http://www.yakuji.co.jp/.

610.711 GBR ISSN 0265-2730
GUIDE TO POSTGRADUATE DEGREES, DIPLOMAS AND COURSES IN MEDICINE. Text in English. 1975. a. GBP 18 (effective 2001). adv. **Document type:** *Directory.* **Description:** Contains information on degrees and diplomas awarded by medical educational establishments in the United Kingdom, courses of study and degree requirements. Arranged by medical specialty.
Formerly: Summary of Postgraduate Diplomas and Courses in Medicine (0302-3494)
Published by: (National Advice Center for Postgraduate Medical Education, British Council), IntelliGene, Woodlands, Ford, Pathhead, Midlothian EH37 5RE, United Kingdom. TEL 44-1875-320063, FAX 44-1875-320276, 100741.1374@compuserve.com. Ed., Adv. contact G.M. Haddock. R&P G M Haddock.

610 USA ISSN 0888-6768
RA396.A3
GUIDE TO THE ESSENTIALS OF A MODERN MEDICAL PRACTICE ACT. Text in English. triennial. USD 10 (effective 1999). **Description:** Contains basic recommendations for use in the development, evaluation, or revision of state statutes governing the practice of medicine.
Published by: Federation of State Medical Boards, 400 Fuller Wiser Rd, Ste 300, Euless, TX 76039-3855. TEL 817-868-4000, FAX 817-868-4098. Ed. Patricia Beatty. R&P Linda Uernale.

GUIDE TO THE MANAGED CARE INDUSTRY. see *INSURANCE*

GUIDELINES FOR HEALTH SUPERVISION. see *MEDICAL SCIENCES—Pediatrics*

616.98023 TUR ISSN 1302-0471
CODEN: GATBD
GULHANE MEDICAL JOURNAL. Text in Turkish; Summaries in English. 1956. q., latest vol.41, no.4, 1999. TRL 4,000,000 domestic; USD 80 foreign (effective 2000 - 2001). adv. bk.rev. index. back issues avail. *Refereed.* **Document type:** *Bulletin, Academic/Scholarly.* **Description:** Publishes review articles, original research, case reports and letters on topics relating to medical science.
Formerly (until Sep.1998): Gulhane Askeri Tip Akademisi Bulten (1300-0543)
Related titles: Online - full text ed.
Indexed: Excerp.Med. —EMDOCS, GNLM.
Published by: Gulhane Askeri Tip Akademisi/Gulhane Military Medical Academy, Gata Yayin Kurulu, Etlik - Ankara 06018, Turkey. TEL 90-312-3044101, FAX 90-312-3234923, journal@obs.gata-edu.tr, journal@abs.gata-edu.tr, mozata@obs.gata.edu.tr, http://www.obs.gata.edu.tr/journal. Ed., R&P, Adv. contact Dr. Atilla Yalcin. Pub. Cetin Harmankaya. B&W page USD 200. Circ: 1,000 (paid).

610 JPN ISSN 0389-7540
GUNMA DAIGAKU IRYO GIJUTSU TANKI DAIGAKUBU KIYO/GUNMA UNIVERSITY. COLLEGE OF MEDICAL CARE AND TECHNOLOGY. ANNUAL REPORTS. Text in English, Japanese; Summaries in English. 1980. a. **Document type:** *Academic/Scholarly.*
Published by: Gunma Daigaku, Iryo Gijutsu Tanki Daigakubu, 39-15 Showa-Machi 3-chome, Maebashi-shi, Gunma-ken 371-0034, Japan. Ed. Yoshikazu Ito.

610 JPN ISSN 0285-0656
GUNMA IGAKU/GUNMA MEDICAL ASSOCIATION. JOURNAL. Text in Japanese. 1953. a.
Published by: Gunmaken Ishikai/Gunma Medical Association, 7-4 Chiyoda-Machi 1-chome, Maebashi-shi, Gunma-ken 371-0022, Japan.

610 JPN ISSN 0386-0760
CODEN: GRMSBU
GUNMA REPORTS ON MEDICAL SCIENCES/GUNMA REPOTO. Text in English, Multiple languages. 1952. s-a. illus.
Supersedes (in Jan. 1970): Gunma Journal of Medical Sciences (0017-565X)
Indexed: Biol.Abstr., Chem.Abstr., INIS Atomind. —CISTI.
Published by: Gunma University, School of Medicine/Gunma Daigaku Igakubu, 39-22 Showa-Machi, Maebashi-shi, Gunma-ken 371-0034, Japan. Circ: 700.

612.015 CHN
GUOWAI YIXUE (LINCHUANG SHENGWU HUAXUE YU JIANYAN FENCE)/FOREIGN MEDICAL SCIENCES (CLINIC BIOCHEMISTRY AND MEDICAL TEST). Text in Chinese. bi-m. USD 10.20; USD 1.70 newsstand/cover (effective 2001). **Document type:** *Academic/Scholarly.*
Published by: Chongqing Yixue Qingbao Yanjiusuo, 44 Qingnian Lu, Chongqing, Sichuan 630010, China. **Dist. by:** China International Book Trading Corp, 35, Chegongzhuang Xilu, Haidian District, Beijing 100044, China. TEL 86-1-68413849, FAX 86-1-68412048, cibtc@mail.cibtc.com.cn, http://www.cibtc.com.cn.

GUOWAI YIXUE (SHENGWU YIXUE GONGCHENG FENCE)/FOREIGN MEDICAL SCIENCES (BIOMEDICAL ENGINEERING). see *BIOLOGY—Bioengineering*

610 CHN
GUOWAI YIXUE (ZHONGYI ZHONGYAO FENCE)/FOREIGN MEDICAL SCIENCES (TRADITIONAL CHINESE MEDICINE). Text in Chinese. bi-m. USD 30; USD 5 newsstand/cover (effective 2001). **Document type:** *Academic/Scholarly.*
Published by: China International Book Trading Corp/Zhongguo Guoji Tushu Maoyi Zonggongsi cibtc@mail.cibtc.com.cn, http://www.cibtc.com.cn. **Dist. by:** 35, Chegongzhuang Xilu, Haidian District, Beijing 100044, China.

610 USA ISSN 0882-696X
GUTHRIE JOURNAL. Text in English. 1970 (vol.40). q. free per issue. adv. bk.rev. charts, illus. index. **Document type:** *Academic/Scholarly.*
Former titles (until vol.55, 1985): Guthrie Bulletin (0735-4592); Guthrie Clinic Bulletin (0017-5838)
Indexed: C.I.S. Abstr., Chem.Abstr., Excerp.Med. —BLDSC (4232.650000), CISTI, GNLM, ingenta, KNAW.
Published by: Donald Guthrie Foundation for Medical Research, Sayre, PA 18840. TEL 717-882-2487, FAX 717-882-5151, kmeyer@inet.guthrie.org. Ed. Ralph D Zehr. Adv. contact Kenneth Meyer. Circ: 6,400.

H C E A ASSOCIATION ALERT; The newsletter for the healthcare exhibition & meeting organizer. see *MEETINGS AND CONGRESSES*

H C E A DIRECTORY; a directory of healthcare meetings and conventions. see *MEETINGS AND CONGRESSES*

612 FRA ISSN 1026-9819
H F S P WORKSHOP. Key Title: Human Frontier. Workshop. Text in English. 1996. irreg. **Document type:** *Academic/Scholarly.* —BLDSC (4303.437000).
Published by: Human Frontier Science Program, 20 Place des Halles, Strasbourg 67080, France. TEL 33-3-8821-5121, FAX 33-3-8832-8897, info@hfsp.org, http://www.hfsp.org. Eds. Jennifer S Altman, Michael S Gazzaniga.

M

670.29 USA ISSN 1045-6058
HD9994.U5
H I D A MANUFACTURERS DIRECTORY. Text in English. a. USD 80; USD 85 in Canada; USD 90 elsewhere. **Document type:** *Directory, Trade.* **Description:** Lists more than 9,000 medical products distributed. Contains a company name section, a product index section and a trade name section.
Formerly (until 1989): Directory of Health Care Manufacturers, Products and Supplies (0888-2797)
Related titles: Microform ed.: (from PQC).
Published by: (Health Industry Distributors Association), Medical Economics Co., Inc., 5 Paragon Dr, Montvale, NJ 07645-1742. TEL 201-358-7200, FAX 201-573-8979.

H L A B C FORUM. see *LIBRARY AND INFORMATION SCIENCES—Computer Applications*

H M O MAGAZINE. (Health Maintenance Organization) see *INSURANCE*

610 ISR ISSN 0017-7768
CODEN: HAREA6
HA-REFUAH✶ . Text in Hebrew; Summaries in English. 1920. fortn. USD 350. adv. bk.rev. abstr, bibl, charts, illus, stat. index.
Indexed: Biol.Abstr., Chem.Abstr., Curr.Cont. (coverage dropped), Dent.Ind., Excerp.Med., INIS Atomind., Ind.Heb.Per. (1993-), Ind.Med. (1924-), Psychol.Abstr.
—BLDSC (4264.000000), CASDDS, CISTI, GNLM, KNAW.
Published by: Israel Medical Association, P.O. Box 33003, Tel Aviv 61330, Israel. TEL 972-3-6100444, FAX 972-3-5751616. Ed. Y Rotem.

610 TUR ISSN 0259-2282
CODEN: HMJOEG
HACETTEPE MEDICAL JOURNAL✶ . Text in English. 1968. q. USD 30. adv. bibl, charts, illus. index. **Description:** Contains papers on original research, case reports, reviews, short communications for practical applications, letters, editorials, and announcements concerning the medical sciences.
Formerly (until 1983): Hacettepe Bulletin of Medicine-Surgery - Hacettepe Tip Cerrahi Bulteni (0017-6451)
Related titles: Turkish ed.: Hacettepe Tip Dergisi.
Indexed: Biol.Abstr., Excerp.Med.
—CISTI, EMDOCS, GNLM, KNAW.
Published by: (University of Hacettepe/Hacettepe Universitesi, Faculty of Medicine/Tip Fakultesi), Hacettepe University Press, Edebiyat Fak, Sanat Tarihi Bol, Baheevievler, Ankara 06532, Turkey. TELEX 42-237 HKT TR. Ed. Dr. Dogan Taner. Circ: 980.

610 658 JPN ISSN 0389-5122
HACHINOHE SHIRITSU SHIMIN BYOIN ISHI/HACHINOHE CITY HOSPITAL. MEDICAL JOURNAL. Text in Japanese. 1976. 2/yr.
Published by: Hachinohe Shiritsu Shimin Byoin, Nukazuka, Hachinohe-shi, Aomori-ken 031-0022, Japan.

HADSHOT KUPPOT HOLIM. see *INSURANCE*

614.44 CHN ISSN 1007-2705
HAIXIA YUFANG YIXUE ZAZHI/STRAIT JOURNAL OF PREVENTIVE MEDICINE. Text in Chinese; Summaries in Chinese, English. 1995. bi-m. CNY 24 domestic; USD 6 foreign; CNY 4 newsstand/cover domestic; USD 1 newsstand/cover foreign (effective 2001 & 2002). **Document type:** *Journal, Academic/Scholarly.* **Description:** Reports on the study of progress and achievements in the preventive medicine fields.
Published by: Fujian-sheng Weisheng Fangyi Zhan, Jintai Lu 76, Fuzhou, Fujian 350001, China. TEL 86-591-7519605, FAX 86-591-7533291, hxyfyxzz@pub5.fz.fj.cn, http://www.fjcdc.com.cn. Pub. Longsan Xu.

610 JPN ISSN 0910-0725
HAKODATE IGAKUSHI/HOKODATE MEDICAL JOURNAL. Text in Japanese. 1977. a.
Published by: Shiritsu Hokodate Byoin/Hakodate Municipal Hospital, 2-23 Yayoi-cho, Hakodate-shi, Hokkaido 040-0056, Japan.

610 DEU ISSN 0017-6915
HAMBURGER AERZTEBLATT. Text in German. 1947. m. DEM 130. adv. bk.rev. charts, illus, stat, tr.lit. index. **Document type:** *Academic/Scholarly.*
Published by: Hamburger Aerzteverlag GmbH, Humboldtstr 57-59, Hamburg 22083, Germany. TEL 49-40-22802307, FAX 49-40-2277381. Ed. Dr. Ulrich Lamparter. Adv. contact Donald Horn. Circ: 11,100.

610 PAK ISSN 0250-7188
HAMDARD MEDICUS; journal of science and medicine. Text in English. 1957. q. PKR 400, USD 60 (effective 2000). adv. bk.rev. charts. back issues avail. **Document type:** *Academic/Scholarly.*
Former titles: Hamdard; Hamdard Medical Digest (0017-7024)
Related titles: CD-ROM ed.
Indexed: Abstr.Hyg., Agroforest.Abstr., Biol.Abstr., Curr.Adv.Ecol.Sci., ExtraMED, Forest Prod.Abstr., Forest.Abstr., Helminthol.Abstr., Herb.Abstr., Hort.Abstr., Irr.& Drain.Abstr., Nutr.Abstr., Ornam.Hort., Per.Islam. (1991-), Plant Breed.Abstr., Plant Gen.Res.Abstr., Plant Grow.Reg.Abstr., Postharvest, Poult.Abstr., Protozool.Abstr., Rev.Appl.Entomol., Rev.Arom.& Med.Plants, Rev.Med.& Vet.Mycol., Rev.Plant Path., Rural Devel.Abstr., Seed Abstr., Soils & Fert., Sugar Ind.Abstr., Trop.Dis.Bull., Weed Abstr., World Ag.Econ.& Rur.Soc.Abstr.
—BLDSC (4241.443000).
Published by: Hamdard Foundation, Nazimabad No.3, Karachi 74600, Pakistan. TEL 92-21-6616001, FAX 92-21-6611755, TELEX 29370 HAMD PK. Ed. Sadia Rashid. Circ: 2,000.

610 USA
HAMPDEN HIPPOCRAT. Text in English. 1942. 4/yr. membership. adv. **Document type:** *Academic/Scholarly.*
Published by: Hampden District Medical Society, 1111 Elm St W, Ste 22, Springfield, MA 01089-1540. TEL 413-736-0661. R&P Carol Nystrom. Adv. contact Michael Barnes. Circ: 1,800 (paid).

617.57 USA
THE HAND AND UPPER EXTREMITY✶ . Text in English. 1987. irreg., latest vol.12, 1995. **Document type:** *Monographic series.*
Formerly (until 1995): Hand and Upper Limb (0269-4743)
Published by: Churchill Livingstone (Subsidiary of: Harcourt Health Sciences), 15 E 26th St, Fl 15, New York, NY 10010-1505. TEL 212-206-5040, FAX 212-727-7808, http://www.churchillmed.com. Ed. K M Chan.

616.047 344.041 USA
HAND AND WRIST PAIN. Text in English. 1987. a. USD 65. **Description:** Offers information on the anatomy, epidemiology and patho-physiology of the hand and wrist.
Published by: Lexis Law Publishing (Subsidiary of: Reed Elsevier plc), PO Box 7587, Charlottesville, VA 22906-7587. TEL 804-972-7600, 800-562-1197, FAX 804-972-7666, llp.customer.support@lexis-nexis.com, http://www.lexislawpublishing.com.

610 USA
THE HANDBOOK OF HEALTH ASSESSMENT TOOLS. Text in English. a. USD 149.95 (effective 2001).
Published by: Institute for Health & Productivity Management, 4435 Waterfront Drive, Ste 101, Glen Allen, VA 23060. TEL 540-456-4747, FAX 540-456-6669, ihpm1@aol.com, http://www.ihpm.org.

610.711 IND ISSN 0253-7621
R814.A6
HANDBOOK OF MEDICAL EDUCATION (YEAR). Text in English. irreg., latest 1996. USD 15 (effective 1999). **Document type:** *Newsletter.*
Published by: Association of Indian Universities, A.I.U. House, 16 Kotla Marg, New Delhi 110 002, India. TEL 91-11-3310059, FAX 91-11-3315105, aiu@del2.vsnl.net.in, http://www.aiuweb.org. Circ: 1,600.

616.02 USA ISSN 0072-9841
RM121
HANDBOOK OF MEDICAL TREATMENT✶ . Text in English. 1949. biennial. USD 7.50.
Published by: Jones Medical Publications, 355 Los Cerros Dr, Greenbrae, CA 94904. Ed. Milton J Chatton.

610 615.9 USA
HANDBOOK OF NATURAL TOXINS. Text in English. 1983. irreg., latest vol.8, 1995. adv. *Refereed.* **Document type:** *Monographic series.*
Indexed: Chem.Abstr., Chem.Indus.Notes, Chem.Titles, Nutr.Abstr.
Published by: Marcel Dekker, Inc., Attn: Eridania Perrez, 270 Madison Ave, New York, NY 10016-0602. TEL 212-696-9000, 800-228-1160, FAX 212-685-4540, marketing@dekker.com, http://www.dekker.com. Pub. Russell Dekker. R&P Julia Mulligan. Adv. contact Eridania Perez.

610 GBR ISSN 0962-144X
HANDBOOK OF PRACTICE MANAGEMENT. Text in English. 1991. q., base vol. plus q. updates. GBP 78 per vol. in Europe; USD 127 per vol. in United States; GBP 83 updates elsewhere (effective 2002). adv. **Document type:** *Academic/Scholarly.* **Description:** Provides updates to help practice managers and partners cope with the demands of general practice.
Related titles: CD-ROM ed.: (from RoweCom Information Quest); Online - full content ed.: (from Swets Blackwell).
—BLDSC (4250.968500).
Published by: Royal Society of Medicine Press Ltd, 1 Wimpole St, London W1M 8AE, United Kingdom. TEL 44-20-7290-2921, FAX 44-20-7290-2929, elizabeth.fredman@rsm.ac.uk, http://www.roysocmed.ac.uk/pub/hpm.htm. Eds. John Hasler, Lynne Hobden-Clarke, Philippa Moreston.

613.029 DEU
HANDBUCH FUER DAS GESUNDHEITSWESEN IN SCHLESWIG-HOLSTEIN. Text in German. 1948. a. DEM 49.50. adv. **Document type:** *Directory.* **Description:** Listing of doctors, dentists, hospitals, etc. in Schleswig-Holstein.
Published by: Hallenbetriebe Neumuenster GmbH, Justus-von-Liebig-Str 2-4, Neumuenster 24537, Germany. TEL 49-4321-910190, FAX 49-4321-910199. Circ: 5,500.

610.73 AUT ISSN 0073-0181
R500
HANDBUCH FUER DIE SANITAETSBERUFE OESTERREICH. Text in German. 1950. a. ATS 840; ATS 1,070 foreign (effective 2000). adv. index. **Document type:** *Journal, Trade.*
Related titles: ♦ CD-ROM ed.: Sanitaetshandbuch CD.
—GNLM.
Published by: Verlag Dieter Goeschl GmbH, Hernalser Hauptstrasse 213, Vienna, W 1170, Austria. TEL 43-1-4864240, FAX 43-1-4854902. Ed. K H Kux. Circ: 7,000.

617.13 344.047 USA
HANDLING SOFT TISSUE INJURY CASES. Text in English. 1993 (2nd ed.). base vol. updates 3/yr. USD 240. **Description:** Covers the legal and medical aspects of handling cases involving any soft tissue injury, from simple neck and back sprain cases to serious burns and brain damage.
Published by: Lexis Law Publishing (Subsidiary of: Reed Elsevier plc), PO Box 7587, Charlottesville, VA 22906-7587. TEL 804-972-7600, 800-562-1197, FAX 804-972-7666, llp.customer.support@lexis-nexis.com, http://www.lexislawpublishing.com.

HANGTIAN YIXUE YU YIXUE GONGCHENG/SPACE MEDICINE & MEDICAL ENGINEERING. see *AERONAUTICS AND SPACE FLIGHT*

610 KOR ISSN 0254-5942
HANNYAN NUI-DAI HAGSUR JI/HANYANG MEDICAL COLLEGE. JOURNAL. Text in Korean. 1981. s-a. **Document type:** *Academic/Scholarly.*
Published by: Hannyan Daihaggyo Nigwa Daihag/Hanyang Medical College, Haengdang-dong 17, Sundong-ku, Seoul 133-791, Korea, S.. TEL 82-2-290-8195, 82-2-290-8190, FAX 82-2-292-7737.

610 DEU ISSN 0944-7369
HARTMANNBUND MAGAZIN. Text in German. 1951. 10/yr. DEM 24; DEM 2 newsstand/cover (effective 2001). adv. bk.rev. **Document type:** *Magazine, Trade.* **Description:** Contains news and information of interest to all German physicians. Features new medical research, public health issues, political and economical issues. Includes readers' comments.
Formerly: Deutsche Arzt (0011-9873)
Indexed: Excerp.Med.
—GNLM, Infotrieve. **CCC.**
Published by: Hartmannbund - Verband der Aerzte Deutschlands e.V., Godesberger Allee 54, Bonn 53175, Germany. TEL 49-228-8104-0, FAX 49-228-8104155, hb-info@hartmannbund.de, http://www.hartmannbund.de. Ed. Friedrich Georg Wendl. Adv. contact Gabriele Falkenberg. B&W page DEM 6,825; trim 175 x 233. Circ: 45,000 (paid and controlled).

HARVARD MEDICAL ALUMNI BULLETIN. see *COLLEGE AND ALUMNI*

HARVARD MEDICAL SCHOOL. CENTER FOR HEALTH AND THE GLOBAL ENVIRONMENT. NEWSLETTER. see *PUBLIC HEALTH AND SAFETY*

M

610 100 USA ISSN 0093-0334
R724 CODEN: HSCRAS
HASTINGS CENTER REPORT. Key Title: Report - Hastings Center. Text in English. 1971. bi-m. USD 72 in United States to individuals; USD 89 rest of world to individuals; USD 95 in United States to institutions & libraries; USD 108 rest of world to institutions & libraries; USD 48 in United States to students & seniors; USD 68 rest of world to students & seniors (effective 2001). bk.rev. bibl, illus. index. reprint service avail. from PQC. *Refereed.* **Document type:** *Journal, Trade.*
Formerly: Hastings Center Studies (0093-3252)
Related titles: Microfilm ed.: 1971 (from PQC); Online - full text ed.: 1971 (from Gale Group, ProQuest Information & Learning, Northern Light Technology, Inc., H. W. Wilson, Factiva, Institute for Scientific Information).
Indexed: AMED, ASCA, Acad.Ind., AgeLine, Amer.Bibl.Slavic & E.Eur.Stud., Arts & Hum.Cit.Ind. (coverage dropped), Biol.Abstr., CINAHL, Curr.Cont., Curr.Lit.Fam.Plan., Fam.Ind., Fut.Surv., Gen.Sci.Ind. (Jun.1984-), Hlth.Ind., IMFL, Ind.Med. (1971-), Ind.Per.Art.Relat.Law, Int.Nurs.Ind., L.R.I., Lang.& Lang.Behav.Abstr., Med.Care Rev., NRN, P.A.I.S., Per.Islam. (1991-), Phil.Ind., Rel.Ind.One, Rel.Ind.Two, SOPODA, SSCI, Sage Race Rel.Abstr., Soc.Sci.Ind. (Nov.1982-), Soc.Serv.Abstr., Soc.Work Res.& Abstr., Sociol.Abstr.
—BLDSC (4273.019000), GNLM, IDS, ingenta.
Published by: Hastings Center, Rte 9D, Garrison, NY 10524. TEL 845-424-4040, FAX 845-424-4545, mail@thehastingscenter.org, http://www.thehastingscenter.org/. Ed. Gregory Kaebnick. Circ: 11,000.

610 DEU ISSN 1434-8950
DER HAUSARZT. Text in German. 195?. 20/yr. EUR 79.94 domestic; EUR 95.94 foreign; EUR 49.10 domestic to students; EUR 65.10 foreign to students; EUR 4.67 newsstand/cover (effective 2002). **Document type:** *Journal, Trade, Academic/Scholarly.*
Former titles (until 1997): Zeitschrift fuer den Hausarzt (1434-887X); (until 1995): Der Praktische Arzt (0172-150X); (until 1964): Der Praktische Arzt und Medizin Heute (0551-8849); (until 1961): Der Praktische Arzt Heute (0551-8830); (until 1958): Der Praktische Arzt (0172-1615)
Published by: Urban und Vogel Medien und Medizin Verlagsgesellschaft mbH (Subsidiary of: BertelsmannSpringer), Neumarkter Str 43, Munich 81673, Germany. TEL 49-89-43721300, FAX 49-89-43721399, verlag@urban-vogel.de, http://www.urban-vogel.de.

610 USA ISSN 0017-8594
CODEN: HWMJAE
HAWAII MEDICAL JOURNAL. Text in English. 1941. m. USD 25 (effective 2001). adv. bk.rev. Supplement avail.; back issues avail.; reprint service avail. from PQC,ISI. *Refereed.* **Document type:** *Trade, Academic/Scholarly.* **Description:** Discusses health, diagnosis, case studies, research.
Related titles: Microform ed.: (from PQC).
Indexed: Abstr.Hyg., Biol.Abstr., Chem.Abstr., Curr.Adv.Cancer Res., Curr.Adv.Ecol.Sci., Curr.Cont. (coverage dropped), Excerp.Med., INIS Atomind., Ind.Med. (1962-), Int.Nurs.Ind., Soc.Work Res.& Abstr., Trop.Dis.Bull.
—BLDSC (4273.903000), CISTI, GNLM, ingenta, KNAW.
Published by: Hawaii Medical Association, c/o Norman Goldstein, Historic Tan Sing Building, 1128 Smith St, Honolulu, HI 90817. FAX 808-523-6842, skinyouluv@aol.com. Ed. Dr. Norman Goldstein. Circ: 1,800 (paid and controlled).

610 ARM
CODEN: EKMEEM
HAYASTANI BZHSHKAGITUTYUN/ARMENIAN MEDICAL JOURNAL/MEDITSINSKAYA NAUKA ARMENII. Text in Armenian, English, Russian. 1952. 4/yr. AMD 400. **Document type:** *Academic/Scholarly.*
Formerly: Eksperimental ev Klinikakam Bzhshkut'yun (0514-7484)
Indexed: Biol.Abstr., Chem.Abstr., Ind.Med. (coverage dropped), Ind.Vet., Vet.Bull.
—CASDDS, CISTI, East View, GNLM.
Published by: Akademiya Nauk Armenii, Pr Marshala Bagramayana 24, Erevan 375019, Armenia. TEL 78852-524580.

610 USA
HEADACHE AND MIGRAINE MANAGEMENT JOURNAL. Text in English. **Document type:** *Journal.* **Description:** Helps doctors and patients better assess headaches and migraines by allowing readers to log headache histories.
Address: info@hmmj.com, comments@hmmj.com, http://www.hmmj.com.

610 USA
HEADLINES✱. Text in English. 1990. q. USD 18. adv. **Document type:** *Academic/Scholarly.* **Description:** Studies the many facets of neurologic injury and presents new research.
Indexed: Except.Child Educ.Abstr.
Published by: J R Publishing, Inc. (Boston), 13432 Third Ave., N.E., Brandenton, FL 34202-2729. Ed. Beverly Lucas. Adv. contact Randi Kashnig. Circ: 135,000 (controlled).

610 USA
HEALTH A TO Z NEWS. Text in English. 1995. bi-w. **Description:** Offers a comprehensive information resource in health and medicine.
Media: Online - full text.
Published by: Medical Network info@HealthAtoZ.com, http://www.HealthAtoZ.com.

HEALTH ACTION. see *HEALTH FACILITIES AND ADMINISTRATION*

HEALTH & HEALING. see *PHYSICAL FITNESS AND HYGIENE*

HEALTH & LAW TRENDS. see *LAW*

HEALTH & PLACE; an international journal. see *GEOGRAPHY*

610 USA
HEALTH & PRODUCTIVITY MANAGEMENT. Text in English. q.
Published by: Institute for Health & Productivity Management, 4435 Waterfront Drive, Ste 101, Glen Allen, VA 23060. TEL 540-456-4747, FAX 540-456-6669, ihpm1@aol.com, http://www.ihpm.org.

HEALTH AND SAFETY REGULATIONS; international and national laws. see *PUBLIC HEALTH AND SAFETY*

613.081 618.082 USA
HEALTH AND STRESS; the newsletter of the American Institute of Stress. Text in English. 1985. m. USD 35 domestic; USD 45 foreign (effective 2001). bk.rev. 8 p./no. 2 cols./p. back issues avail.; reprints avail. *Refereed.* **Document type:** *Newsletter.* **Description:** Covers all stress related subjects - stress and cancer, cardiovascular, GI, and skin disease, job stress, stress reduction techniques, psychological stress, stress of retirement, post traumatic stress disorder, and stress assessment and measurement.
Formerly: American Institute of Stress. Newsletter (1047-2517)
Published by: American Institute of Stress, 124 Park Ave, Yonkers, NY 10703. TEL 914-963-1200, FAX 914-965-6267, stress124@earthlink.net, http://www.stress.org. Ed. Dr. Paul J Rosch. R&P PaulJ Rosch. Circ: 2,000.

610 658 FRA ISSN 1280-7834
HEALTH AND SYSTEM SCIENCE/SANTE ET SYSTEMIQUE. Text in English, French. 1997. q. *Refereed.* **Description:** Publishes original studies on: the models and methods stemming from the systems analysis, health applied econometrics, epidemiology and operations research; the methods of multicriteria decision making and those of decisions under uncertainty in relationship with pharmacy-economic evaluations, or collective choices in health care.
Published by: Editions Hermes, 8 quai du Marche Neuf, Paris 75004, France. TEL 33-1-53101520, FAX 33-1-53101521, hermes@iway.fr, http://www.editions-hermes.fr/rev_accueil.asp?id=14. Ed. Sami Menasce.

610 362 GBR ISSN 0374-8014
RA421 CODEN: HBHSA5
HEALTH BULLETIN. Text in English. 1941. bi-m. GBP 6. bk.rev. bibl. index. back issues avail. **Document type:** *Bulletin, Government.*
Indexed: AMED, ASSIA, Abstr.Health Care Manage.Stud., Abstr.Hyg., Addic.Abstr., Biol.Abstr., Brit.Nur.Ind., CINAHL, Curr.Adv.Ecol.Sci., Dairy Sci.Abstr., Dent.Ind., Excerp.Med., Ind.Med. (1941-), LISA, Med.Care Rev., Nutr.Abstr., Rural Devel.Abstr., Trop.Dis.Bull.
—BLDSC (4274.935350), GNLM.
Published by: Scottish Office, Home and Health Department, Scottish Office, St Andrews House, Regent Rd, Edinburgh EH1 3DG, United Kingdom. FAX 0131-244-2835, TELEX 72202. Ed. Dr. Patrick Brooks. Circ: 15,200.

610.6 USA
HEALTH CARE ALMANAC; a resource guide to the medical field. Text in English. irreg., latest 1995. USD 29.95 (effective 2000).
Formerly: Healthcare Resource and Reference Guide
Published by: American Medical Association, 515 N State St, P O Box 10946, Chicago, IL 60610-0946. TEL 312-464-5000.

610 NLD ISSN 1065-3058
RA394 CODEN: HCAVEO
HEALTH CARE ANALYSIS; an international journal of health care philosophy and policy. Text in English. 1992. q. EUR 368, USD 369 to institutions for print or online ed.; EUR 441.60, USD 442.80 to institutions for print & online eds. combined (effective 2002). adv. back issues avail.; reprints avail. *Refereed.* **Document type:** *Journal, Academic/Scholarly.* **Description:** Encourages structures dialogue about central issues in health care among all groups working for health, combining academic rigor with accessible, relevant regular features.
Related titles: Microform ed.: (from PQC); Online - full text ed.: (from EBSCO Publishing, O C L C Online Computer Library Center, Inc., RoweCom Information Quest, Swets Blackwell, Kluwer Online, Institute for Scientific Information).
Indexed: ASCA, ASSIA, Brit.Nur.Ind., Curr.Cont., Excerp.Med. (1997-), Int.Nurs.Ind., SSCI.
—CISTI, EMDOCS, GNLM, IDS, Infotrieve. **CCC.**
Published by: Kluwer Academic Publishers Group (Subsidiary of: Wolters Kluwer N.V.), Spuiboulevard 50, PO Box 17, Dordrecht 3300 AA, Netherlands. TEL 31-78-639-2392, FAX 31-78-654-2254, services@wkap.nl, http://www.wkap.nl/journalhome.htm/1065-3058. Ed. Alan Cribb. **Subscr. in the Americas to:** Kluwer Academic - Plenum Publishers, 233 Spring St, New York, NY 10013-1578. TEL 212-620-8468, FAX 212-807-1047; **Subscr. to:** Journals Department, PO Box 322, Dordrecht 3300 AH, Netherlands. TEL 31-78-639-2392, FAX 31-78-654-6474.

610 USA ISSN 1093-0957
HEALTH CARE BUSINESS DIGEST. Text in English. 1996. m. **Document type:** *Magazine, Trade.* **Description:** Reports on breaking stories and key health care business trends with in-depth analysis and commentary on economics, legal and regulatory issues, legislation, consumer trends, and technology.
Published by: MultiMedia Healthcare Inc., Office Center of Princeton Meadows, Bldg 300, Plainsboro, NJ 08536. TEL 609-275-7355, FAX 609-275-7369, info@mmhc.com, http://www.mmhc.com. Eds. Dr. George Grossberg, Dr. Jeffrey Cummings.

HEALTH CARE DAILY REPORT. see *HEALTH FACILITIES AND ADMINISTRATION*

362.1 USA ISSN 0195-8631
RA410.53
HEALTH CARE FINANCING REVIEW. Text in English. 1979. q. USD 26 (effective 2001). bk.rev. charts, stat, illus. back issues avail.; reprint service avail. from CIS. *Refereed.* **Document type:** *Government.* **Description:** Contains articles that seek to contribute to an improved understanding of the Medicare and Medicaid programs and the U.S. health care system by presenting information and analyses on a broad range of health care financing and delivery issues.
Related titles: Microfiche ed.: (from CIS); Microform ed.: (from PQC); Online - full text ed.: (from Gale Group, ProQuest Information & Learning, Northern Light Technology, Inc., H. W. Wilson, Factiva, Institute for Scientific Information); ♦ Supplement: Health Care Financing Review. Supplement. ISSN 1057-9389.
Indexed: ABI Inform. (Sum.1985-), ASCA, Abstr.Health Care Manage.Stud., Abstr.Soc.Geront., AgeLine, Amer.Stat.Ind. (1979-), B.P.I. (Jul.1999-), Curr.Cont., Excerp.Med., Hosp.Lit.Ind., Ind.U.S.Gov.Per., Inpharma, Int.Nurs.Ind., MEDOC, Med.Care Rev., P.A.I.S., PROMT, Pharm.&Out.News, Reac., SSCI, Sci.Cit.Ind., Soc.Sci.Ind. (Dec.1986-), Soc.Work Res.& Abstr., World Bibl.Soc.Sec.
—BLDSC (4274.941800), GNLM, ingenta, KNAW.
Published by: U.S. Health Care Financing Administration (Subsidiary of: U.S. Department of Health and Human Services), 7500 Security Blvd, Baltimore, MD 21244. TEL 410-786-6577, FAX 410-786-5768, lwolf@hcfa.gov, http://www.hcfa.gov/pubforms/ordpub.htm. Ed. Linda F Wolf. **Subscr. to:** U.S. Government Printing Office, Superintendent of Documents, PO Box 371954, Pittsburgh, PA 15250-7954. TEL 202-512-1800, FAX 202-512-2250, orders@gpo.gov, http://www.access.gpo.gov. **Affiliate:** U.S. Health Care Financing Administration.

HEALTH CARE FRAUD REPORT. see *HEALTH FACILITIES AND ADMINISTRATION*

344.0321 USA
HEALTH CARE GUIDE. Text in English. base vol. plus q. updates. USD 297. Supplement avail. **Description:** Informs readers of legal developments in health care and health insurance.
Published by: Warren, Gorham and Lamont, 395 Hudson St, New York, NY 10014. TEL 212-367-6300, FAX 212-367-6718. Ed. Jeffrey D Mamorsky. **Subscr. to:** Warren, Gorham & Lamont, Park Square Bldg, 31 St James Ave, Boston, MA 02116-4112. TEL 800-950-1207.

HEALTH CARE LAW SOURCEBOOK. see *LAW*

HEALTH CARE LAWYER. see *LAW*

610 GBR
HEALTH CARE MANAGEMENT HANDBOOK (YEAR). Text in English. a. GBP 22.50. adv. **Document type:** *Directory, Trade.*
Formerly: Health Practice Management Handbook (Year) (1351-4679)
Published by: Kogan Page Ltd., 120 Pentonville Rd, London N1 9JN, United Kingdom. FAX 44-20-7837-6348. Ed. Helen Kogan. R&P Caroline Gromm. Adv. contact Linda Batham.

HEALTH CARE POLICY REPORT. see *HEALTH FACILITIES AND ADMINISTRATION*

HEALTH CARE PROGRAM COMPLIANCE GUIDE. see *HEALTH FACILITIES AND ADMINISTRATION*

330 610 USA ISSN 1090-4395
HEALTH CARE STRATEGIST. Text in English. a. (in 2 vols.), latest 16th ed. USD 525 per vol. domestic for vol.1; USD 850 per vol. domestic for vol.2; USD 600 per vol. foreign for vol.1; USD 925 per vol. foreign for vol.2 (effective 2002). **Description:** Provides information on health care deal activity.
Published by: Windhover Information, Inc., 10 Hoyt St, Norwalk, CT 06851 . TEL 203-838 4401, FAX 203-838 3214, custserv@windhoverinfo.com, http://www.windhoverinfo.com.

HEALTH CAREER POST. see *HEALTH FACILITIES AND ADMINISTRATION*

610 USA ISSN 0046-7022
R856.A1
HEALTH DEVICES. Text in English. 1971. m. bk.rev. illus. index. back issues avail. *Refereed.* **Document type:** *Directory.* **Description:** Contains evaluation and ratings of medical devices used by hospitals. Reports on hazardous devices, access to ECRI's online computer network, technical assistance, help with SMDA, and other device-related information.
Indexed: INIS Atomind., Ind.Med. (1971-), P.N.I.
—BLDSC (4274.963000), GNLM. **CCC.**
Published by: (Emergency Care Research Institute), E C R I, 5200 Butler Pike, Plymouth, PA 19462. TEL 610-825-6000, FAX 610-834-1275, info@ecri.org, http://www.ecri.org. Ed. Garry Hayner.

610 USA ISSN 8756-8713
HEALTH DEVICES INSPECTION & PREVENTIVE MAINTENANCE SYSTEM. Text in English. 1990. a. USD 795; USD 595 for Health Devices System members. *Refereed.* **Description:** Includes complete inspection and preventive maintenance forms, how-to's and background information.
—**CCC.**
Published by: (Emergency Care Research Institute), E C R I, 5200 Butler Pike, Plymouth, PA 19462. TEL 610-825-6000, FAX 610-834-1275. Ed. Tim Ritter.

681 USA ISSN 0278-3452
R856.48
HEALTH DEVICES SOURCEBOOK. Text in English. 1979. a. USD 450.80 domestic; USD 466 in Canada; USD 550 elsewhere (effective 2002). *Refereed.* **Document type:** *Directory.* **Description:** Directory of medical device manufacturers and their product lines. Includes service firms which lease or repair equipment, and which buy and sell used equipment.
Related titles: Online - full text ed.: (from The Dialog Corporation).
—GNLM, Infotrieve. **CCC.**
Published by: (Emergency Care Research Institute), E C R I, 5200 Butler Pike, Plymouth, PA 19462. TEL 610-825-6000, FAX 610-834-1275, info@ecri.org, http://www.ecri.org. Ed. Eileen Sykes.

610 USA
(YEAR) HEALTH DIRECTORY. Text in English. a. USD 99. **Description:** Lists state health agencies and congressional, federal, state, and local contacts with addresses and phone numbers.
Published by: Aspen Publishers, Inc., 200 Orchard Ridge Dr, Ste 200, Gaithersburg, MD 20878. TEL 800-678-8437, FAX 301-417-7550, http://www.aspenpub.com.

338.476 GBR ISSN 1057-9230
RA410.A1 CODEN: HEECEZ
HEALTH ECONOMICS. Text in English. 1992. 8/yr. USD 690 in United States; USD 690 in Canada & Mexico; USD 690 elsewhere; USD 725 combined subscription in United States for print and online eds.; USD 725 combined subscription in Canada & Mexico for print and online eds.; USD 725 combined subscription elsewhere for print and online eds. (effective 2002). adv. back issues avail.; reprint service avail. from SWZ. *Refereed.* **Document type:** *Academic/Scholarly.* **Description:** Contains articles on all aspects of health economics: theoretical contributions, empirical studies, economic evaluations and analyses of health policy from the economic perspective.
Related titles: Microform ed.: (from PQC); Online - full text ed.: ISSN 1099-1050. USD 690 in United States; USD 690 in Canada & Mexico; USD 690 elsewhere (effective 2002) (from EBSCO Publishing, Wiley InterScience, Institute for Scientific Information).
Indexed: AgeLine, Curr.Cont., Ind.Med. (1992-), Inpharma, Int.Nurs.Ind., J.of Econ.Lit., Reac., SSCI, Sci.Cit.Ind.
—BLDSC (4274.966900), CISTI, IDS, Infotrieve. **CCC.**
Published by: Wiley Europe Ltd., Baffins Ln, Chichester, W Sussex PO19 1UD, United Kingdom. TEL 44-1243-779777, FAX 44-1243-775878, cs-journals@wiley.co.uk, customer@wiley.co.uk, http://www.wiley.co.uk. adv.: B&W page GBP 650, color page GBP 1,550; trim 200 x 260. Circ: 1,100. **Subscr. to:** John Wiley & Sons, Inc., Journals, 605 Third Ave, New York, NY 10158. TEL 212-850-6021, 212-850-6645, subinfo@jwiley.com.

610 614 CAN
HEALTH ECONOMICS. Text in English. 1993. bi-m. CND 55; CND 75 foreign. adv.
Indexed: CBCA Ref.
Published by: Thomson Healthcare Communications, 1120 Birchmount Rd, Ste 200, Scarborough, ON M1K 5G4, Canada. TEL 416-750-8900, FAX 416-751-8126. Adv. contact Suzanne Stone. B&W page CND 2,850, color page CND 3,245; trim 10.75 x 8.13. Circ: 10,305.

HEALTH EDUCATION RESEARCH; theory and practice. see *SOCIAL SERVICES AND WELFARE*

610 USA
HEALTH HOTLINES. Text in English. a. **Document type:** *Directory, Government.* **Description:** Lists toll-free phone numbers of public and private organizations that provide health information on specific diseases and conditions.
Published by: U.S. National Library of Medicine, 8600 Rockville Pike, Bethesda, MD 20894. **Subscr. to:** U.S. Government Printing Office, Superintendent of Documents. TEL 202-783-3238, FAX 202-512-2233.

610 ARG ISSN 1514-3538
HEALTH I.G. NEWS. Text in English, Spanish. 1997. m. free per issue. **Description:** Designed for the medical community and all interested in health issues.
Media: Online - full text.
Published by: Consultora Periodistica, Diaz Velez, 1425 2o C, Olivos, Buenos Aires 1636, Argentina. TEL 54-114-7942739, healthig@impasat1.com.ar, http://www.healthig.com. Ed. Juan Carlos Guri. Pub. Gabriela Ilczyszyn.

610 USA ISSN 0892-7731
HEALTH INDUSTRY BUYERS GUIDE✶ . Text in English. 1940. a. USD 105. adv.
Formerly: Surgical Trade Buyers Guide (0081-9654)
Related titles: Microform ed.: 1940 (from PQC).
Published by: S - N Publications, Inc., PO Box 908, Spring House, PA 19477-0903. TEL 708-426-6100, FAX 708-426-6416. Ed. Mike Kennedy. Circ: 4,000.

610 USA ISSN 0745-4678
CODEN: HITOD3
HEALTH INDUSTRY TODAY; the market letter for health care industry vendors. Text in English. 1938. m. USD 360 print ed.; USD 420 online ed. (effective 2001). adv. bk.rev. illus. stat. index. reprint service avail. from PQC. **Document type:** *Journal, Trade.* **Description:** Provides market news and reports on the strategies and tactics medical device manufacturers and distributors use to reach health care providers.
Formerly (until 1982): Surgical Business (0039-6095)
Related titles: Microform ed.: (from PQC); Online - full text ed.: (from Gale Group, NewsNet, ProQuest Information & Learning, Northern Light Technology, Inc., Factiva).
Indexed: ABI Inform. (Oct.1991-), PROMT.
—BLDSC (4275.016700), Infotrieve. **CCC.**
Published by: Business Word Inc., 5350 S. Roslyn St, Ste. 400, Greenwood Village, CO 80111-2145. TEL 303-290-8500, FAX 303-290-9025, curthit@businessword.com, http://www.businessword.com/2030pubs.htm. Ed. Curt Werner. Circ: 1,132.

HEALTH INFORMATION AND LIBRARIES JOURNAL. see *LIBRARY AND INFORMATION SCIENCES*

▼ **HEALTH INFORMATION AND LIBRARIES JOURNAL ONLINE.** see *LIBRARY AND INFORMATION SCIENCES*

651.504261 AUS ISSN 1322-4913
HEALTH INFORMATION MANAGEMENT. Text in English. 1971. q. AUD 120 domestic to non-members; USD 150 foreign to non-members (effective 2000). adv. bk.rev., software rev. charts, illus, stat. index. back issues avail. *Refereed.* **Document type:** *Academic/Scholarly.* **Description:** Designed to promote the discipline of health information management by providing a forum for presentation of original research, short communications, reviews and commentaries.
Former titles: Australian Medical Record Journal (0817-3907); (until 1983): Australian Medical Record (0155-4441)
Indexed: CINAHL, Ind.Med. (coverage dropped).
—BLDSC (4275.017500), ingenta.
Published by: Health Information Management Association of Australia, Locked Bag 2045, North Ryde, NSW 2113, Australia. TEL 61-2-98875003, FAX 61-2-98875895, himaa@himaa.org.au, annj@himaa.org.au. Ed. Ann Jones. Adv. contact Kay Watts. Circ: 1,300.

610 025.04 GBR ISSN 1460-4140
HEALTH INFORMATION ON THE INTERNET. Text in English. 1998. bi-m. GBP 34 in Europe to institutions; USD 57 in United States to institutions; GBP 36 elsewhere to institutions; GBP 10 in United Kingdom to students (effective 2002); Subscr. includes free online access.. back issues avail. **Document type:** *Newsletter, Academic/Scholarly.* **Description:** Aims to meet the growing demand from health professionals for information about health resources available on the Internet.
Related titles: Online - full text ed.: (from CatchWord Ltd.).
Indexed: Brit.Nur.Ind.
—BLDSC (4275.017400), GNLM.
Published by: (Wellcome Trust), Royal Society of Medicine Press Ltd, 1 Wimpole St, London W1M 8AE, United Kingdom. TEL 44-20-7290-2921, FAX 44-20-7290-2929, rsmjournals@rsm.ac.uk, http://www.roysocmed.ac.uk/pub/hii.htm. Ed. Sue Childs.

HEALTH LAW BULLETIN. see *PUBLIC HEALTH AND SAFETY*

HEALTH LAW FOR HEALTHCARE PROFESSIONALS. see *LAW*

HEALTH LAW NEWS. see *LAW*

HEALTH LAW REPORTER. see *LAW*

HEALTH LAW REVIEW. see *LAW*

HEALTH LAW WEEK; case digests of judicial decisions affecting all healthcare. see *LAW*

HEALTH LAWYER. see *LAW*

HEALTH LAWYERS NEWS. see *LAW*

610 USA ISSN 1078-2907
HEALTH LETTER ON THE C D C. Text in English. 1994. w. (43/yr.). USD 495 in North America; USD 545 elsewhere. **Document type:** *Newsletter.*
Related titles: Online - full text ed.: (from Gale Group, Factiva).
Indexed: Bus.& Indus. (Jan.1995-), CINAHL.
Published by: (Center for Disease Control), Charles W. Henderson, Ed. & Pub., PO Box 5528, Atlanta, GA 31107-0528. TEL 770-507-7777, FAX 770-507-7788, cwhender@newsfile.com; info@hendersonnet@atl.ga.us, cwhender@newsfile.com; info@hendersonnet.atl.ga.us, http://www.newsfile.com.

M

610 650 USA ISSN 0882-598X
RA421
HEALTH LETTER (WASHINGTON). Text in English. 1985. m. USD 18. bk.rev. **Document type:** *Newsletter.* **Description:** Information on common health problems as well as information pried from tightly sealed government and industry files.
Related titles: Microform ed.: (from PQC); Online - full text ed.: (from ProQuest Information & Learning, Factiva).
Indexed: CHNI, Consum.Ind. (1990-).
Published by: Public Citizen, Inc., 1600 20th St, N W, Washington, DC 20009. TEL 202-588-1000, FAX 202-785-3584. Ed. Sidney M Wolfe. R&P Phyllis McCarthy. Circ: 35,000.

HEALTH MATRIX: JOURNAL OF LAW-MEDICINE. see *LAW*

610 GBR ISSN 0954-903X
HEALTH MATTERS. Text in English. 1988. q. GBP 19 domestic to individuals; GBP 24 foreign to individuals; GBP 29 domestic to institutions; GBP 34 foreign to institutions (effective 2001 - 2002). bk.rev. 28 p./no. back issues avail. **Document type:** *Magazine, Consumer.* **Description:** Covers health policy, environmental issues, the NHS, and related topics.
Published by: Health Matters Publications Ltd., PO Box 459, Sheffield, S Yorks S1 2UP, United Kingdom. TEL 44-114-263-4711, FAX 44-114-263-4711, info@healthmatters.org.uk, http://www.healthmatters.org.uk. Ed. James F Munro. Adv. contact Paul Adams. Circ: 2,000 (paid).

610 USA ISSN 1042-2781
HEALTH NEWS DAILY. Text in English. 1989. d. USD 1,395 (effective 2001). adv. back issues avail.; reprints avail. **Document type:** *Newsletter, Trade.* **Description:** Information service for executives and decision-makers in the health industries. Coverage includes healthcare reform, pharmaceuticals, medical devices and diagnostics, biomedical research, federal health policy, Medicare-Medicaid, and cost containment.
Media: Fax. **Related titles:** E-mail ed.; Online - full text ed.: (from Data-Star, The Dialog Corporation, NewsNet).
—Infotrieve. **CCC.**
Published by: F-D-C Reports, Inc., 5550 Friendship Blvd, Ste One, Chevy Chase, MD 20815-7278. TEL 800-332-2181, FAX 301-664-7238, http://www.fdcreports.com. Ed. Anne Petruska. R&P Laurea Desimio. Adv. contact Michael Keville.

610 GBR ISSN 1363-0393
HEALTH ON THE INTERNET. Text in English. 1996. m. adv. **Document type:** *Newsletter, Trade.* **Description:** Publishes health and medical information.
Related titles: E-mail ed.: ISSN 1367-2258.
Published by: Medecal Ltd. - Healthworks, Unit 8 Riverside Court, Don Rd, Sheffield S9 2TJ, United Kingdom. TEL 44-114- 2619011, FAX 44-114- 2431597, newsletters@medecal.com, info@medecal.com, info@medecal.com, http://www.healthworks.co.uk/.

HEALTH - P A C BULLETIN. see *PUBLIC HEALTH AND SAFETY*

610 USA
HEALTH PAGES*. Text in English. 1993. 3/yr. USD 9.95. adv. **Document type:** *Consumer.*
Address: 821 Broadway, 9th Fl, New York, NY 10003-4708. TEL 212-505-0103. Ed. Martin Schneider. Circ: 90,000.

610 CAN ISSN 0837-7251
HEALTH PERSONNEL IN CANADA/PERSONNEL DE LA SANTE AU CANADA. Text in English, French. 1969. a. free per issue. stat. **Document type:** *Government.* **Description:** Provides year-end statistics for 31 occupational groups of health care practitioners over an 11-year period.
Formerly (until 1988): Canada Health Manpower Inventory (0381-2561)
—CISTI.
Published by: Canadian Institute for Health Information, 377 Dalhousie St, Ste 200, Ottawa, ON K1N 9N8, Canada. TEL 613-241-7860, FAX 613-241-8120, jstrachan@cihi.ca. R&P Jill Strachan. Circ: 1,200.

610 USA ISSN 0017-9078
QH505.A1 CODEN: HLTPAO
HEALTH PHYSICS; the radiation protection journal. Text in English. 1932. m. (2 vols./yr.). USD 310 domestic to individuals; USD 344 foreign to individuals; USD 1,088 domestic to institutions; USD 1,122 foreign to institutions; USD 90 newsstand/cover (effective 2002). adv. bk.rev. abstr, charts, illus, stat. index. back issues avail.; reprint service avail. from PQC. *Refereed.* **Document type:** *Academic/Scholarly.* **Description:** Reports on theoretical and applied disciplines of radiation protection.
Related titles: Microfilm ed.: (from PQC,WWS); Online - full text ed.: (from Ovid Technologies, Inc., Institute for Scientific Information); Supplement: Operation Radiation Safety.
Indexed: AESIS, ASCA, Abstr.Health Care Manage.Stud., Abstr.Hyg., Apic.Abstr., Appl.Mech.Rev., Aqua.Sci.& Fish.Abstr., Biol.Abstr., C.I.S. Abstr., Chem.Abstr., Chem.Indus.Notes, Chem.Titles, Curr.Adv.Ecol.Sci., Curr.Cont. (coverage dropped), Dairy Sci.Abstr., Deep Sea Res.& Oceanogr.Abstr., Dent.Ind., Dok.Arbeitsmed., Energy Info.Abstr., Energy Rev., Environ.Abstr., Environ.Per.Bibl. (1972-), Environ.Sci.Poll.Mgmt., Excerp.Med., Food Sci.& Tech.Abstr., Forest.Abstr., GeoRef, Hort.Abstr., INIS Atomind., INSPEC (Apr.1971-), Ind.Med. (1958-), Ind.Sci.Rev., Ind.Vet., Inpharma, Int.Abstr.Biol.Sci., Int.Aerosp.Abstr., Lab.Haz.Bull., Nutr.Abstr., Ocean.Abstr. (coverage dropped), Pollut.Abstr., Poult.Abstr., Reac., Risk Abstr., SSCI (coverage dropped), Saf.Sci.Abstr., Sci.Cit.Ind., Sel.Water Res.Abstr., So.Pac.Per.Ind., Soils & Fert., Tox.Abstr., Vet.Bull., W.R.C.Inf.
—BLDSC (4275.100000), AskIEEE, CASDDS, CISTI, GNLM, IDS, ingenta.
Published by: (Health Physics Society), Williams & Wilkins (Subsidiary of: Waverly International), 351 W Camden St, Baltimore, MD 21201-2436. TEL 410-528-4068, 800-222-3790, FAX 410-528-4452, sisaacson@wwilkins.com, http://www.health-physic.com/, http://www.Lww.com. Ed. Kenneth L Miller. Adv. contact Sharlene Isaacson. B&W page USD 975; 10.88 x 8.13. Circ: 7,901; 7,781 (paid).

HEALTH PHYSICS SOCIETY. NEWSLETTER. see *MEDICAL SCIENCES—Radiology And Nuclear Medicine*

368.382 USA ISSN 1528-2953
HEALTH PLAN & PROVIDER REPORT. Text in English. 1995. w. USD 878 (effective 2001). Index. back issues avail. **Document type:** *Newsletter, Trade.* **Description:** Covers commercial, legal, legislative, and regulatory activities and news at the federal, state and local levels that have on impact on managed care. Offers analysis of government actions and policies, marketplace trends, mergers, acquisitions and alliances. Includes case studies, surveys and statistics.
Formerly (until 2000): B N A's Managed Care Reporter (1083-1622)
Related titles: Online - full text ed.: ISSN 1528-9435.
—CCC.
Published by: The Bureau of National Affairs, Inc., 1231 25th St, N W, Washington, DC 20037. TEL 800-372-1033, 800-452-7773, FAX 800-253-0332, customercare@bna.com, bnaplus@bna.com, http://www.bna.com/products/health/hppr.htm. Ed. Deborah Spiegelman. Pub. Gregory McCaffery. **Subscr. to:** 9435 Key West Ave, Rockville, MD 20850.

610 USA ISSN 0162-3605
CODEN: DRRSAL
HEALTH POLICY & BIOMEDICAL RESEARCH: THE BLUE SHEET. Text in English. 1957. 51/yr. USD 619 (effective 2001). back issues avail.; reprints avail. **Document type:** *Newsletter, Trade.* **Description:** Covers developments among the major governmental, academic and private biomedical research institutions.
Formerly: Drug Research Reports: The Blue Sheet (0012-6608)
Related titles: Online - full text ed.: (from Data-Star, The Dialog Corporation).
Indexed: Inpharma, P.N.I., Reac., Rehabil.Lit.
—CCC.
Published by: F-D-C Reports, Inc., 5550 Friendship Blvd, Ste One, Chevy Chase, MD 20815-7278. TEL 800-332-2181, FAX 301-664-7238, http://www.fdcreports.com. Ed. Nielsen Hobbs. R&P Laura Desimio.

610.71025 USA
R847
HEALTH PROFESSIONS CAREER AND EDUCATION DIRECTORY. Text in English. 1968. a. USD 60 (effective 2000 - 2001). **Document type:** *Directory.*
Former titles (until 199?): Allied Health and Rehabilitation Professions Education Directory; (until 1996): Allied Health Education Directory (0194-3766); (until 1978): Allied Medical Education Directory (0163-2590)
—GNLM.
Published by: American Medical Association, 515 N State St, P O Box 10946, Chicago, IL 60610-0946. TEL 312-464-5000. Ed. Gloria C Gupta.

610 360 ZAF
HEALTH PROFESSIONS COUNCIL OF SOUTH AFRICA. REGISTER OF SUPPLEMENTARY HEALTH SERVICES PROFESSIONS. Text in English. a. ZAR 400; ZAR 20 supplement. Supplement avail. **Document type:** *Directory.* **Description:** Provides names and addresses of all supplementary health services personnel registered with the council.
Formerly: South African Medical and Dental Council. Register of Supplementary Health Services Professions
Published by: Health Professions Council of South Africa, PO Box 205, Pretoria 0001, South Africa. TEL 27-12-3286680, FAX 27-12-3285120, hpcsa@samdc.co.za.

610.73 USA ISSN 0888-9465
HEALTH PROFESSIONS REPORT; the independent bi-weekly newsletter on the education & training of medical, nursing and health professionals. Text in English. 1971. bi-w. USD 270 (effective 2000). charts, stat. back issues avail. **Document type:** *Newsletter.* **Description:** Reports on the education and training of doctors, nurses and allied health professionals. Includes pending legislation, information on public and private funding sources, cost-cutting measures, new medical breakthroughs, curriculum ideas, and admissions policies.
Former titles: Health Planning and Manpower Report (0362-3165); Health Manpower Report (0161-6781)
—CCC.
Published by: Manisses Communications Group, Inc., PO Box 9758, Providence, RI 02906-9758. TEL 401-861-6020, 800-333-7771, FAX 401-861-6370. Ed. Anne Bittner.

▼ **HEALTH PROMOTION PRACTICE.** see *PUBLIC HEALTH AND SAFETY*

HEALTH PSYCHOLOGY. see *PSYCHOLOGY*

▼ **HEALTH, RISK & SOCIETY.** see *PUBLIC HEALTH AND SAFETY*

610 USA ISSN 1387-3741
▼ **HEALTH SERVICES AND OUTCOMES RESEARCH METHODOLOGY**; an international journal devoted to quantitative methods for the study of utilization, quality, cost and outcomes of health. Text in English. 1999. q. USD 290, EUR 289 to institutions for print or online ed.; USD 348, EUR 346.80 to institutions for print & online eds. combined (effective 2002). **Document type:** *Journal, Academic/Scholarly.* **Description:** Reflects the multidisciplinary nature of the field of health services and outcomes research. It addresses the needs of multiple, interlocking communities, including methodologists in statistics, econometrics, social and behavioral sciences; designers and analysts of health policy and health services research projects; and health care providers and policy makers who need to properly understand and evaluate the results of published research.
Related titles: Online - full text ed.: (from EBSCO Publishing, O C L C Online Computer Library Center, Inc., RoweCom Information Quest, Swets Blackwell, Kluwer Online).
—BLDSC (4275.107805). **CCC.**
Published by: Kluwer Academic Publishers Boston, 101 Philip Dr, Assinippi Park, Norwell, MA 02061. TEL 781-871-6600, FAX 781-871-9045, services@wkap.nl, http://www.wkap.nl/journalhome.htm/1387-3741. Eds. Emmett B Keeler, Frank E Harrell Jr., Constantine A Gatsonis. R&P Rose Luongo TEL 781-871-6311. **Subscr. outside the Americas to:** Kluwer Academic Publishers Group, Journals Department, PO Box 322, Dordrecht 3300 AH, Netherlands. TEL 31-78-639-2392, FAX 31-78-654-6474; **Subscr. to:** Kluwer Academic - Plenum Publishers, 233 Spring St, New York, NY 10013-1578. TEL 212-620-8468, FAX 212-807-1047.

610.6 GBR ISSN 0951-4848
RA440.6 CODEN: HSRMEO
HEALTH SERVICES MANAGEMENT RESEARCH. Text in English. 1988. q. GBP 122 in Europe to institutions; USD 207 in United States to institutions; GBP 126 elsewhere to institutions (effective 2002); Subscr. includes free online access.. adv. bk.rev. index. *Refereed.* **Document type:** *Journal, Academic/Scholarly.* **Description:** Publishes original and review articles on all aspects of healthcare management for improved management of health services.
Related titles: Microfiche ed.; Microfilm ed.; Online - full text ed.: (from CatchWord Ltd., RoweCom Information Quest).
Indexed: ASSIA, Brit.Nur.Ind., Diar.Dis.Res., Int.Nurs.Ind., Ref.Zh.
—BLDSC (4275.108200), EMDOCS, GNLM, Infotrieve. **CCC.**
Published by: (University of Birmingham, Health Services Management Centre), Royal Society of Medicine Press Ltd, 1 Wimpole St, London W1M 8AE, United Kingdom. TEL 44-20-7290-2921, FAX 44-20-7290-2929, rsmjournals@rsm.ac.uk, http://www.roysocmed.ac.uk/pub/hsmr.htm. Ed. Peter Spurgeon. Circ: 700. **Co-sponsor:** Association of University Programs in Health Administration.

HEALTH SERVICES RESEARCH. see *HEALTH FACILITIES AND ADMINISTRATION*

610 600 USA
HEALTH TECHNOLOGY MANAGEMENT. Text in English. a. USD 450. *Refereed.* **Description:** Reference material for handling technology related issues including planning, legal & regulatory responsibilities and procedures, plus special reports.
—BLDSC (4275.225700).
Published by: (Emergency Care Research Institute), E C R I, 5200 Butler Pike, Plymouth, PA 19462. TEL 610-825-6000, FAX 610-834-1275. Ed. Jim Keller.

610 USA ISSN 1041-6072
HEALTH TECHNOLOGY TRENDS; for health care executives. Text in English. 1989. m. USD 420.80 domestic; USD 436 in Canada; USD 485 elsewhere (effective 2002). *Refereed.* **Description:** Covers economic, legal, and product news related to health care technology for executives.
—Infotrieve. **CCC.**
Published by: (Emergency Care Research Institute), E C R I, 5200 Butler Pike, Plymouth, PA 19462. TEL 610-825-6000, FAX 610-834-1275, info@ecri.org, http://www.ecri.org. Ed. Cynthia Wallace.

HEALTH TRANSITION REVIEW. see *SOCIAL SERVICES AND WELFARE*

610 614 GBR ISSN 0017-9132
RA485 CODEN: HETBAT
HEALTH TRENDS. Text in English. 1969. q. GBP 28 (effective 1998). **Document type:** *Government.*
Indexed: ASSIA, Abstr.Health Care Manage.Stud., Abstr.Hyg., Addic.Abstr., Biol.Abstr., Brit.Nur.Ind., Curr.Adv.Ecol.Sci., Excerp.Med., Inpharma, Reac., Trop.Dis.Bull.
—CISTI, GNLM.
Published by: (Great Britain. Departments of Health and Social Security), Stationery Office, 51 Nine Elms Ln, London SW8 5DA, United Kingdom. TEL 44-20-7873-0011, FAX 44-20-7873-8247. Ed. Valerie M Willcocks.

HEALTH WHICH?. see *PHYSICAL FITNESS AND HYGIENE*

610 USA
HEALTHBEAT* . Text in English. 1989. q. free per issue. adv. **Document type:** *Newsletter.* **Description:** Covers various aspects of preventative health, pediatrics, geriatrics, and women's health.
Published by: Write Ideas, 15 Pierson St, Mahwah, NJ 07430-3506. Ed. Suzanne Ordas Curry. Adv. contact Suzanne Ordas-Curry. Circ: 7,500.

HEALTHCARE 1500. see *PUBLIC HEALTH AND SAFETY*

610 371.42 USA
HEALTHCARE EMPLOYMENT JOURNAL; serving healthcare professionals. Text in English. 1991. m. USD 21. **Description:** Focuses on employment opportunities for healthcare professionals.
Formerly (until 1993): Employment Journal of Ohio
Published by: Employment Journals of America, 1614 Lancaster Ave, Reynoldsburg, OH 43068. TEL 614-861-4600, FAX 614-861-5558. Ed. Susan Erwin. adv.: B&W page USD 4,100; trim 13.75 x 11.5. Circ: 65,000.

610 USA
HEALTHCARE HAZARD CONTROL SYSTEM. Text in English. a. (plus m. updates). USD 1,038 domestic; USD 1,075.40 in Canada; USD 1,211 elsewhere (effective 2002); includes access to online and Healthcare Hazard Management Monitor. *Refereed.* **Description:** Provides articles on management plans, compliance directions for environmental and occupational health, safety and security.
Formerly: Healthcare Environmental Management System
Related titles: Online - full content ed.
Published by: (Emergency Care Research Institute), E C R I, 5200 Butler Pike, Plymouth, PA 19462. TEL 610-825-6000, FAX 610-834-1275, info@ecri.org, http://www.ecri.org. Ed. Shanna Halpern. **Co-sponsor:** C H E M - Center for Healthcare Environmental Management.

658 USA
HEALTHCARE HAZARD MANAGEMENT MONITOR. Text in English. 1987. m. USD 335.80 domestic; USD 351 in Canada; USD 400 elsewhere (effective 2002). *Refereed.* **Document type:** *Newsletter.* **Description:** Highlights current information for hazardous materials, and environmental and occupational health safety.
Former titles: Healthcare Hazardous Materials Management (1050-575X); Hospital Hazardous Materials Management (0895-7169)
—Infotrieve. **CCC.**
Published by: (Emergency Care Research Institute), E C R I, 5200 Butler Pike, Plymouth, PA 19462. TEL 610-834-1275, FAX 610-834-1275, info@ecri.org, http://www.ecri.org. Ed. Shanna Halpern. **Co-sponsor:** C H E M - Center for Healthcare Environmental Management.

610 658.8 USA
HEALTHCARE MARKETER'S EXECUTIVE BRIEFING. Text in English. 1987. 12/yr. USD 197 domestic; USD 147 domestic for introductory subscription (effective 2001). adv. index. back issues avail. **Document type:** *Newsletter, Trade.* **Description:** Covers news of interest to healthcare marketing practitioners, including new business opportunities, marketing success stories, solutions to management challenges, how to build a system identity, and the latest market trends.
Formerly: Healthcare Community Relations and Marketing Letter (0894-9980)
Related titles: Online - full content ed.
—CCC.
Published by: Health Resources Publishing, 1913 Atlantic Ave, Ste F4, Manasquan, NJ 08736. TEL 732-292-1100, FAX 732-292-1111, hrp@healthrespubs.com, info@healthrespubs.com, http://www.healthrespubs.com. Ed. Rebeckah McCallister. Pub. Robert K Jenkins. Adv. contact Judy Granholm.

610 USA ISSN 1044-4076
RA399.A3
HEALTHCARE STANDARDS DIRECTORY. Text in English. 1989. a. USD 450.80 domestic; USD 466 in Canada; USD 550 elsewhere (effective 2002). **Document type:** *Directory.* **Description:** Covers published standards, clinical practice guidelines and regulations for the delivery of healthcare services.
Related titles: ♦ Supplement: Healthcare Standards Update. ISSN 1048-8103.
—CCC.
Published by: (Emergency Care Research Institute), E C R I, 5200 Butler Pike, Plymouth, PA 19462. TEL 610-825-6000, FAX 610-834-1275, info@ecri.org, http://www.ecri.org. Ed. Beth Richardson.

610 USA ISSN 1048-8103
HEALTHCARE STANDARDS UPDATE. Text in English. 1990. q.
Related titles: ♦ Supplement to: Healthcare Standards Directory. ISSN 1044-4076.
Published by: (Emergency Care Research Institute), E C R I, 5200 Butler Pike, Plymouth, PA 19462. TEL 610-825-6000, FAX 610-834-1275.

HEALTHCARE TRENDS AND TRANSITION. see *OCCUPATIONS AND CAREERS*

362.1 USA ISSN 0894-7961
HEALTHCARE TRENDS REPORT; the monthly digest of business and public policy news. Text in English. 1987. m. USD 259; USD 279 in Canada; USD 339 elsewhere (effective 2000). **Document type:** *Newsletter, Consumer.*
Indexed: CINAHL.
Published by: Health Trends, 4405 East West Hwy, Ste 406, Bethesda, MD 20814. TEL 301-652-8937, FAX 301-907-6790, http://www.healthtrends.net. Ed., Pub. Sylvia Fubini.

614 USA ISSN 0738-811X
HEALTHFACTS. Text in English. 1976. m. USD 25 domestic; USD 29 in Canada & Mexico; USD 36 in Europe. bk.rev. illus. index, cum.index. back issues avail.; reprints avail. **Document type:** *Trade.* **Description:** Designed for informed medical decision-making.
Related titles: Online - full text ed.: (from Gale Group, Northern Light Technology, Inc., ProQuest Information & Learning, Factiva).
Indexed: CHNI, CINAHL, Hlth.Ind.
—BLDSC (4275.247975).
Published by: Center for Medical Consumers, 237 Thompson St, New York, NY 10012. TEL 212-674-7105, FAX 212-674-7100. Ed. Maryann Napoli. Circ: 12,000.

HEALTHSERVE. see *RELIGIONS AND THEOLOGY—Protestant*

610 617.6 USA
HEALTHSTATE. Text in English. 1982. 3/yr. USD 10 (effective 2000). adv. bk.rev. **Document type:** *Academic/Scholarly, Consumer.*
Published by: University of Medicine and Dentistry of New Jersey, 30 Bergen St, ADMC 114, Newark, NJ 07107-3000. FAX 973-972-7261, hseditor@umdnj.edu, http://www.umdnj.edu/umcweb/hstate. Ed. Barbara Hurley. R&P Eve Jacobs TEL 973-972-5521. Adv. contact Carole Walker. Circ: 55,000; 52,000 (controlled).

610 USA ISSN 1099-8667
HEALTHY TIMES. Text in English. irreg. free per issue. back issues avail. **Document type:** *Newsletter.* **Description:** Devoted to providing information on current health news and resources.
Media: Online - full text.
Published by: Health Press, PO Box 1388, Santa Fe, NM 87504. TEL 505-474-0303, ri@trail.com, goodbooks@healthpress.com, http://www.healthpress.com/newsletter.html. Ed. Corie Conwell.

▼ **HEALTHY TRAVELER.** see *TRAVEL AND TOURISM*

610 CHN ISSN 1007-3205
CODEN: HYXUEI
HEBEI YIKE DAXUE XUEBAO/HEBEI MEDICAL UNIVERSITY. JOURNAL. Text in Chinese; Abstracts in English. bi-m. CNY 12 (effective 1999). 64 p./no. *Refereed.* **Document type:** *Academic/Scholarly.* **Description:** Covers the latest developments in basic and clinical medicines.
Formerly: Hebei Yixue Yuan Xuebao - Hebei Academy of Medical Sciences. Journal (1000-1581)
Related titles: CD-ROM ed.
—BLDSC (4757.984100), CASDDS, KNAW.
Published by: (Hebei Yixue Yuan/Hebei Academy of Medical Sciences), Hebei Yike Daxue/Hebei Medical University, 361 Zhongshan Donglu, Shijiazhuang, Hebei 050017, China. TEL 86-311-6059153, FAX 86-311-6059153, hebydqks@public.sj.he.cn, WL@hebmu.edu.cn. Ed. Wen Jink. adv.: page CNY 2,500. Circ: 5,000. **Dist. overseas by:** China International Book Trading Corp, 35 Chegongzhuang Xilu, Haidian District, Beijing 100044, China.

HEBEI ZHONGYI/HEBEI TRADITIONAL MEDICINE. see *ALTERNATIVE MEDICINE*

610 CHN ISSN 1007-5615
HEBEI ZHONGYIYAO XUEBAO/JOURNAL OF HEBEI TRADITIONAL CHINESE MEDICINE AND PHARMACOLOGY. Text in Chinese. 1986. q. CNY 2.50 per issue domestic (effective 2000). back issues avail. **Document type:** *Academic/Scholarly.*
Related titles: Online - full content ed.: (from WanFang Data Corp.).
Published by: Hebei Yike Daxue/Hebei Medical University, Xinshi Nan Lu 326 Hao, Shijiazhuang 050091, China. Ed. Quanhe Zhong.

M

610 300 ISR ISSN 0333-6964
Q180.I78
HEBREW UNIVERSITY OF JERUSALEM. AUTHORITY FOR RESEARCH AND DEVELOPMENT. CURRENT RESEARCH. Text in English. 1964. a., latest 2000. free. name index. **Document type:** *Catalog, Directory, Abstract/Index, Academic/Scholarly.*
Formed by the merger of: Hebrew University of Jerusalem. Authority for Research and Development. Research Report: Humanities, Social Sciences, Law, Education, Social Work, Library (0075-3645); Hebrew University of Jerusalem. Authority for Research and Development. Research Report. Science and Agriculture (0075-3653); Hebrew University of Jerusalem. Authority for Research Report. Medicine, Pharmacy, Dental Medicine (0075-3637)
—BLDSC (7714.110200), Linda Hall.
Published by: Hebrew University of Jerusalem, Authority for Research and Development, Jerusalem 91904, Israel. TEL 972-2-6586633, FAX 972-2-5664740, moph@vms.huji.ac.il, http://www.ard.huji.ac.il. Ed. S. Glatzer. R&P Shoshana Glatzer TEL 972-2-658-6633. Circ: (controlled).

613 DEU ISSN 0017-9604
HEILBERUFE; Fortbildung fuer Pflege- und Assistenzberufe in stationaeren und ambulanten Bereich. Text in German. 1949. m. EUR 36.45; EUR 28.97 to students (effective 2002). adv. bk.rev. charts, illus. index. **Document type:** *Journal, Academic/Scholarly.*
Indexed: Excerp.Med., INIS Atomind.
—GNLM, Infotrieve. **CCC.**
Published by: Urban und Vogel Medien und Medizin Verlagsgesellschaft mbH (Subsidiary of: BertelsmannSpringer), Neumarkter Str 43, Munich 81673, Germany. TEL 49-89-43721411, FAX 49-89-43721410, verlag@urban-vogel.de, http://www.urban-vogel.de. Ed. Andreas Gericke. R&P Friederik Klein. Adv. contact Paul Berger. Circ: 30,000.

610 CHN ISSN 1000-9906
R97.7.C5
HEILONGJIANG ZHONGYIYAO/HEILONGJIANG TRADITIONAL CHINESE MEDICAL SCIENCE. Text in Chinese. bi-m.
Published by: Heilongjiang Zhongyi Yanjiuyuan/ Heilongjiang Institute of Traditional Chinese Medicine, 72, Sanfu Jie, Xiangfang-qu, Harbin, Heilongjiang 150036, China. TEL 53086. Ed. Zhang Qi.

610 IND ISSN 0017-9922
HELAN MEDICAL MAGAZINE. Text in Tamil. 1960. m. INR 6. adv. pat.
Published by: Thilaga Medical Publications, 28 Melaponnagaram, 8th St., Chennai, Tamil Nadu 600 010, India. Ed. Dr. N Thankaraj. Circ: 1,000.

610 305.8893 GBR ISSN 1365-7291
HELLENIC MEDICAL JOURNAL. Text in English. 1997. s-a. GBP 15, USD 27.50 to individuals; GBP 20, USD 35 to institutions. bk.rev. **Document type:** *Academic/Scholarly.*
—BLDSC (4285.437000).
Published by: (Hellenic Medical Society), Smith-Gordon and Co. Ltd., 13 Shalcomb St, London SW10 0HZ, United Kingdom. TEL 44-171-351-7042, FAX 44-171-351-1250. Ed. D P Mikhailidis. **Subscr. to:** 47 Worthington Rd, East Preston, Nr. Worthing, W Sussex BN16 1DE, United Kingdom.

610 FIN ISSN 0437-2468
HELSINGIN LAAKARILEHTI. Text in Finnish. 1954. 7/yr. FIM 120 (effective 1998). adv. bk.rev. **Document type:** *Academic/Scholarly.* **Description:** Explores doctors' jobs, relations with the government, free time, education and pensions.
Published by: Helsingin Laakariyhdistys ry/Helsinki Medical Society, Museokatu 13 A 2, Helsinki 00100, Finland. TEL 358-9-490403, FAX 358-9-408170. Ed. Dr. Ari Kinnunen. R&P, Adv. contact Tuomo Tennilae. Circ: 15,200.

M

HEMOCHROMATOSIS AWARENESS; a quarterly update on hereditary and acquired iron-overload. see *MEDICAL SCIENCES—Abstracting, Bibliographies, Statistics*

HENRY FORD HOSPITAL MEDICAL JOURNAL. see *HEALTH FACILITIES AND ADMINISTRATION*

616.07 DEU ISSN 0171-9661
HESSISCHES AERZTEBLATT. Text in German. m. DEM 160.80 (effective 1999). adv. charts, illus. **Document type:** *Academic/Scholarly.*
—GNLM.
Published by: Verlag Kirchheim und Co. GmbH, Kaiserstr 41, Mainz 55116, Germany. TEL 49-6131-96070-0, FAX 49-6131-9607070, kirchheim@aol.com. Ed. Angelika Kob. Circ: 26,000.

571.49 USA ISSN 1527-0297
▼ **HIGH ALTITUDE MEDICINE AND BIOLOGY.** Text in English. 2000. q. USD 159 domestic to individuals; USD 200 foreign to individuals; USD 191 domestic to individuals print and online eds. combined; USD 232 foreign to individuals print and online eds. combined; USD 250 domestic to institutions; USD 305 foreign to institutions; USD 300 domestic to institutions print and online eds. combined; USD 355 foreign to institutions print and online eds. combined (effective 2002). back issues avail.; reprints avail. *Refereed.* **Document type:** *Journal, Academic/Scholarly.* **Description:** Covers both clinical high altitude diseases and other high altitude life sciences. Reports on advances in the general area of high altitude medicine, and also in high altitude physiology, pathology, comparative biology, anthropology, evolutionary biology, and human and animal ecology.
Related titles: Online - full content ed.: USD 159 to individuals; USD 258 to institutions (effective 2002) (from EBSCO Publishing, O C L C Online Computer Library Center, Inc., Swets Blackwell); Online - full text ed.: (from CatchWord Ltd., Institute for Scientific Information, RoweCom Information Quest).
—BLDSC (4307.283470), CatchWord.
Published by: Mary Ann Liebert, Inc. Publishers, 2 Madison Ave, Larchmont, NY 10538. TEL 914—834-3100, FAX 914-834-1388, info@liebertpub.com, http://www.liebertpub.com/HAM. Ed. Dr. John B. West TEL 858-534-4192.

616.047 344.041 USA
HIP AND KNEE PAIN. Text in English. 1990. a. USD 65. **Description:** Offers a standardized approach to the diagnosis and treatment of hip and knee pain, and clarifies complex disability issues with clear language, useful charts, tables, and illustrations.
Published by: Lexis Law Publishing (Subsidiary of: Reed Elsevier plc), PO Box 7587, Charlottesville, VA 22906-7587. TEL 804-972-7600, 800-562-1197, FAX 804-972-7666, llp.customer.support@lexis-nexis.com, http://www.lexislawpublishing.com.

616.07 615.8 ITA ISSN 1120-7000
CODEN: HIINFF
HIP INTERNATIONAL; the journal of clinical and experimental research on hip pathology and therapy. Text in English. 1991. q. EUR 151 in Europe to individuals; USD 151 elsewhere to individuals; EUR 195 in Europe to institutions; USD 210 elsewhere to institutions (effective 2001). adv. abstr, bibl, charts, illus. Index. 64 p./no. back issues avail.; reprints avail. *Refereed.* **Document type:** *Journal, Academic/Scholarly.* **Description:** Publishes original contributions, editorial and current reviews dealing with basic and applied research in the field of hip pathology.
Related titles: Online - full text ed.
—BLDSC (4315.201000), GNLM, Infotrieve. **CCC.**
Published by: Wichtig Editore s.r.l., Via Friuli, 72, Milan, MI 20135, Italy. TEL 39-02-55195443, FAX 39-02-55195971, info@wichtig-publisher.com, http://www.hip-int.com. Eds. Dr. Aldo Toni, Dr. I D Learmonth. Pub. Dr. Diego Brancaccio. R&P, Adv. contact Lucia Steele. color page USD 1,350; trim 21 x 28. Circ: 1,500 (controlled).

610 USA ISSN 1050-9631
QP383.25 CODEN: HIPPEL
THE HIPPOCAMPUS. Text in English. 1991. bi-m. USD 895 in United States; USD 955 in Canada & Mexico; USD 1,006 elsewhere; USD 940 combined subscription in United States for print and online eds.; USD 1,000 combined subscription in Canada & Mexico for print and online eds.; USD 1,051 combined subscription elsewhere for print and online eds. (effective 2002). adv. back issues avail. *Refereed.* **Document type:** *Academic/Scholarly.*
Related titles: Microform ed.: (from PQC); Online - full text ed.: ISSN 1098-1063. 1996. USD 895 in United States; USD 895 in Canada & Mexico; USD 895 elsewhere (effective 2002) (from EBSCO Publishing, Wiley InterScience, Institute for Scientific Information).
Indexed: ASCA, Chem.Abstr., Chem.Indus.Notes, Chem.Titles, Curr.Cont., Excerp.Med. (1993-), Ind.Med. (1991-), Ind.Sci.Rev., Inpharma, Int.Abstr.Biol.Sci., Neurosci.Cit.Ind., Pharm.&Out.News, PsycInfo, Reac., SSCI (coverage dropped), Sci.Cit.Ind., e-psyche.
—BLDSC (4315.255000), CASDDS, EMDOCS, GNLM, IDS, Infotrieve, KNAW. **CCC.**
Published by: John Wiley & Sons, Inc., Journals (Subsidiary of: Wiley InterScience), 605 Third Ave, New York, NY 10158. TEL 212-850-6645, FAX 212-850-6021, subinfo@wiley.com, uscs-wis@wiley.com, http://www.wiley.com. Eds. Dr. David Amaral, Dr. Menno Witter. adv.: B&W page GBP 640, color page GBP 1,515; trim 210 x 279. Circ: 650. **Subscr. outside the Americas to:** John Wiley & Sons Ltd., Baffins Ln, Chichester, Sussex PO19 IUD, United Kingdom. TEL 44-1243-779777, FAX 44-1243-843232, cs-journals@wiley.co.uk, http://www.wiley.co.uk.

610 616.1 JPN ISSN 0910-0377
HIROSAKI DAIGAKU IGAKUBU EISEIGAKU KYOSHITSU GYOSEKISHU. Text in Japanese; Summaries in English. 1954. irreg.
Published by: Hirosaki Daigaku, Igakubu/Hirosaki University, School of Medicine, 5 Zaifu-cho, Hirosaki-shi, Aomori-ken 036-8216, Japan. Ed. Naosuke Sasaki. Circ: 90.

610 JPN ISSN 0385-793X
HIROSAKI DAIGAKU IRYO GIJUTSU TANKI DAIGAKUBU KIYO/HIROSAKI UNIVERSITY. SCHOOL OF ALLIED MEDICAL SCIENCES. BULLETIN. Text in English, Japanese. 1976. a. **Document type:** *Bulletin.*
Published by: Hirosaki Dagaku, Iryo Gijutsu Tanki Daigakubu, 66-1 Hon-cho, Hirosaki-shi, Aomori-ken 036-8203, Japan.

610 570 JPN ISSN 0439-1721
CODEN: HIRIA6
HIROSAKI IGAKU/HIROSAKI MEDICAL JOURNAL. Text in English, Japanese; Summaries in English. 1950. q.
Indexed: Biol.Abstr., Chem.Abstr., Chem.Indus.Notes, Chem.Titles, Excerp.Med., INIS Atomind.
—BLDSC (4315.570000), CASDDS, CISTI, EMDOCS, GNLM.
Published by: Hirosaki Daigaku, Igakubu/Hirosaki University, School of Medicine, 5 Zaifu-cho, Hirosaki-shi, Aomori-ken 036-8216, Japan. Circ: 400.

610 JPN ISSN 0912-5930
HIROSAKISHI ISHIKAIHO/HIROSAKI CITY MEDICAL ASSOCIATION. JOURNAL. Text in Japanese. 1966. bi-m.
Published by: Hirosakishi Ishikai, 7-1 Noda 2-chome, Hirosaki-shi, Aomori-ken 036-8045, Japan.

610 JPN ISSN 0018-2087
CODEN: HDIZAB
HIROSHIMA DAIGAKU IGAKU ZASSHI. Text in Japanese; Summaries in English. 1952. bi-m. JPY 5,000. bibl, charts, illus. index.
Former titles (until 1962): Gencho Hiroshima Igaku (0375-8982); (until 1956): Hiroshima Igaku, Gencho Go
Related titles: ♦ English ed.: Hiroshima University. Medical Journal.
Indexed: Biol.Abstr., Chem.Abstr., INIS Atomind., Ref.Zh.
—BLDSC (5527.820000), CASDDS.
Published by: Hiroshima University, School of Medicine/Hiroshima Daigaku Igakubu, 1-2-3 Kasumi, Minami-ku, Hiroshima-shi 734-0037, Japan. Ed. Yoshiyasu Matsuo. Circ: 450.

610 JPN ISSN 0367-5904
CODEN: HIRGAY
HIROSHIMA IGAKU/HIROSHIMA MEDICAL ASSOCIATION. JOURNAL. Text in Japanese. 1896. m. JPY 1,700, USD 13 (effective 1992). adv. bibl, charts, illus. index.
Formerly (until 1948): Geibi-Iji
Indexed: C.I.S. Abstr., Chem.Abstr., INIS Atomind.
—BLDSC (4758.300000), CASDDS.
Published by: Hiroshima Igakkai/Hiroshima Medical Association, 1-1-1 Kanonhon-Machi, Nishi-ku, Hiroshima-shi 733-0033, Japan. TEL 082-232-7211, FAX 082-293-3363. Ed. Dr. Teruaki Fukuhara. Circ: 5,800 (controlled).

610 JPN ISSN 0387-6454
CODEN: HBISDD
HIROSHIMA KENRITSU BYOIN ISHI/HIROSHIMA PREFECTURAL HOSPITAL. MEDICAL JOURNAL. Text in English, Japanese. 1969. a.
Indexed: INIS Atomind.
—CASDDS.
Published by: Hiroshima Kenritsu Byoin, 5-54 Ujina-Kanda 1-chome, Minami-ku, Hiroshima-shi 734-0004, Japan.

HIROSHIMA SHUDO DAIGAKU RINSHO SHINRIGAKU KENKYU/HIROSHIMA SHUDO UNIVERSITY. BULLETIN OF CLINICAL PSYCHOLOGY. see *PSYCHOLOGY*

610 JPN CODEN: HIJMAC
HIROSHIMA UNIVERSITY. MEDICAL JOURNAL. Text in English. 1951. q. USD 20. bibl, charts, illus. index. reprint service avail. from PQC.
Formerly: Hiroshima Journal of Medical Sciences (0018-2052)
Related titles: Microform ed.: (from PQC); ♦ Japanese ed.: Hiroshima Daigaku Igaku Zasshi. ISSN 0018-2087.
Indexed: Biol.Abstr., Chem.Abstr., Chem.Indus.Notes, Chem.Titles, Curr.Adv.Ecol.Sci., Curr.Cont. (coverage dropped), Dairy Sci.Abstr., Dent.Ind., Excerp.Med., Helminthol.Abstr., INIS Atomind., Ind.Med. (1951-), Ind.Sci.Rev., Ref.Zh., Sci.Cit.Ind. (coverage dropped).
—BLDSC (4315.600000), CASDDS, CISTI, GNLM, ingenta, KNAW.
Published by: Hiroshima University, School of Medicine/Hiroshima Daigaku Igakubu, 1-2-3 Kasumi, Minami-ku, Hiroshima-shi 734-0037, Japan. Ed. Yoshiyasu Matsuo. Circ: 600.

610 JPN
HIROSHIMASHI ISHIKAI DAYORI/HIROSHIMA CITY MEDICAL ASSOCIATION. JOURNAL. Text in Japanese. m.
Published by: Hiroshimashi Ishikai, 1-1 Kanonhon-Machi 1-chome, Nishi-ku, Hiroshima-shi 733-0033, Japan.

610 JPN
HIROSHIMASHI ISHIKAI RINSHO KENSA SENTA DAYORI/HIROSHIMA CITY MEDICAL ASSOCIATION. MEDICAL LABORATORY CENTER. NEWS. Text in Japanese. 1970. m.
Published by: Hiroshimashi Ishikai, Rinsho Kensa Senta, 8-6 Senda-Machi 3-chome, Naka-ku, Hiroshima-shi 730-0052, Japan.

610 ESP ISSN 0018-2125
HISPALIS MEDICA; revista sevillana de medicina y cirugia. Text in Spanish. 1944. m. USD 50. adv. bk.rev. abstr, bibl, illus. index, cum.index.
Indexed: Chem.Abstr., Dent.Ind., Ind.Med.Esp., Nutr.Abstr.
—CISTI, Infotrieve. **CCC.**
Published by: Miguel y Rafael Rios Mozo Eds. & Pubs., Gravina, 29, Sevilla 41001, Spain. TEL 54-422-17-51. Circ: 1,000.

HISTOLOGY AND HISTOPATHOLOGY; cellular and molecular biology. see *BIOLOGY—Cytology And Histology*

HISTORIA, CIENCIAS, SAUDE - MANGUINHOS. see *HISTORY*

610 JPN ISSN 0286-0171
HITACHI IGAKKAISHI/HITACHI MEDICAL JOURNAL. Text in Japanese. 1962. s-a.
Published by: Hitachi Igakkai/Hitachi Medical Association, Hitachi Sogo Byoin, 1-1 Jonan-cho 2-chome, Hitachi-shi, Ibaraki-ken 317-0077, Japan.

610 JPN
HITO TO IRYO/HUMAN BEING AND MEDICAL CARE. Text in Japanese. bi-m.
Published by: Jitchi Ika no Tameno Kai/Medical Practitioner's Society, Kyowa Kikaku, 2-20 Shinbashi, Minato-ku, Tokyo 105-0004, Japan.

HOITOTIEDE/NURSING SCIENCE; journal of Nurshing Science. see *MEDICAL SCIENCES—Nurses And Nursing*

610 JPN
HOKEN SANGYO JIHO/MEDICAL INSTRUMENT NEWS. Text in Japanese. 1956. 3/m. JPY 6,000.
Published by: Hoken Sangyo Jihosha, 14-5 Minami-Ikebukuro 3-chome, Toshima-ku, Tokyo 171-0022, Japan.

610 JPN ISSN 0915-2083
HOKKAIDO DAIGAKU IRYO GIJUTSU TANKI DAIGAKUBU KIYO/HOKKAIDO UNIVERSITY. COLLEGE OF MEDICAL TECHNOLOGY. ANNUAL REPORTS. Text in English, Japanese. 1988. a.
Published by: Hokkaido Daigaku, Iryo Gijutsu Tanki Daigakubu, Nishi 5-chome, Kita 12-jo, Kita-ku, Sapporo-shi, Hokkaido 060-0812, Japan.

610 JPN ISSN 0913-0217
HOKKAIDO IHO/HOKKAIDO MEDICAL ASSOCIATION. NEWS. Text in Japanese. s-m. JPY 250 per issue.
Published by: Hokkaido Ishikai, Ishi Kaikan, Nishi 6-chome, Odori, Chuo-ku, Sapporo-shi, Hokkaido 060, Japan.

610 JPN ISSN 0367-6102 CODEN: HOIZAK
HOKKAIDO JOURNAL OF MEDICAL SCIENCE/ HOKKAIDO IGAKU ZASSHI. Text in English, Japanese. 1923. bi-m. JPY 3,000. adv. back issues avail. *Refereed.* **Document type:** *Academic/Scholarly.*
Indexed: Biol.Abstr., Chem.Abstr., INIS Atomind., Ind.Med. (1923-).
—BLDSC (4322.261000), CISTI, GNLM.
Published by: Hokkaido Medical Society/Hokkaido Igakkai, Hokkaido Daigaku Igakubu, Nishi 7-chome, Kita 15-jo, Kita-ku, Sapporo-shi, Hokkaido 060, Japan. TEL 81-11-706-5007, FAX 81-11-706-7866. Ed. Masuo Hosokawa. Circ: 1,200.

610 JPN ISSN 0285-0664
HOKKAIDO KINROSHA IRYO KYOKAI IGAKU ZASSHI/HOKKAIDO ASSOCIATION OF MEDICAL SERVICE FOR WORKERS. MEDICAL JOURNAL. Text in Japanese. 1973. s-a.
Published by: Hokkaido Kinrosha Iryo Kyokai, 5 Kikusui 3-chome 3-Jo, Shiroishi-ku, Sapporo-shi, Hokkaido 003-0000, Japan.

610 JPN
HOKKAIDO NOSON IGAKKAI ZASSHI/HOKKAIDO ASSOCIATION OF RURAL MEDICINE. JOURNAL. Text in Japanese. s-a.
Published by: Hokkaido Noson Igakkai, Hokkaido Nosangyoson Kenko Kanri Senta, Nishi 7-chome, Kita 4-jo, Chuo-ku, Sapporo-shi, Hokkaido 060, Japan.

610 JPN
HOKKAIDO PURAIMARI KEA KENKYUKAI KAIHO/HOKKAIDO JOURNAL OF PRIMARY CARE. Text in English, Japanese. 1985. a.
Published by: Hokkaido Puraimari Kea Kenkyukai/Hokkaido Association of Primary Care, Hokkaido Ishikai, Nishi 6-chome, Odori, Chuo-ku, Sapporo-shi, Hokkaido 060, Japan.

610 JPN ISSN 0389-3928
HOKURIKU ISHI/HOKURIKU MEDICAL HISTORY. Text in Japanese. 1979. a.
Published by: Hokuriku Ishigaku Dokokai/Hokuriku Medical History Society, Fukuiken Ishikaikan, 4-10 Daigan-Ji 3-chome, Fukui-shi 910-0001, Japan.

HOME CARE MAGAZINE; for business leaders in home health care. see *INSTRUMENTS*

610 USA ISSN 1070-2431
HOME HEALTH PRODUCTS. Text in English. 1992. 10/yr. USD 99 (effective 2000). adv. **Document type:** *Trade.* **Description:** Provides information on new products and services for the home medical equipment provider.
Related titles: Online - full text ed.
Published by: Stevens Publishing Corporation, 5151 Beltline Rd, 10th fl, Dallas, TX 75240. TEL 972-687-6700, FAX 972-687-6769. Ed. Kyle Steinhauser. Pub. Dana Corbin. Adv. contact Randy Dye. Circ: 24,000.

610 USA
HOME INFUSION THERAPY MANAGEMENT. Text in English. 1993. m. USD 369 domestic; USD 513 foreign (effective 1999). **Document type:** *Newsletter.*
Published by: American Health Consultants (Subsidiary of: Medical Economics Co., Inc.), 3525 Piedmont Rd, N E, 6 Piedmont Center, Ste 400, Atlanta, GA 30305. TEL 404-262-5476, 800-688-2421, custserv@ahcpub.com, http://www.ahcpub.com.

610 HKG ISSN 1024-2708
HONG KONG MEDICAL JOURNAL. Text in English; Abstracts in Chinese. 1948. q. HKD 550 domestic to non-members; USD 145 foreign to non-members (effective 2000). adv. bk.rev. illus. back issues avail. *Refereed.* **Document type:** *Journal, Academic/Scholarly.* **Description:** Provides a general medical journal containing a mix of original and review articles, case reports.
Former titles (until Mar. 1995): Hong Kong Medical Association. Journal (1010-8424); (until 1985): Hong Kong Medical Association. Bulletin
Indexed: Excerp.Med., ExtraMED, HongKongiana, Ind.Med.
—BLDSC (4326.392000), EMDOCS, GNLM, KNAW.
Published by: (Hong Kong Academy of Medicine), Scientific Communications (Hong Kong) Ltd, 4/F, 11 Queen Victoria St, Central, Hong Kong, Hong Kong. hkmj@hkam.org.hk, http://www.hkmj.org.hk. Ed. Joseph Lee. R&P, Adv. contact Dr. Trevor Lane. B&W page HKD 9,000, color page HKD 12,000; trim 210 x 297. Circ: 6,600. **Co-sponsor:** Hong Kong Medical Association.

610 FRA ISSN 1293-9005
HORIZON; le magazine du monde hospitalier public et prive. Text in French. 1989. m. (10/yr.). FRF 490 domestic; FRF 525 foreign (effective 2000). adv.
Formerly (until 1999): Horizon Clinique (1141-5452)
Published by: Editions S I M, 11-13 rue des Arquebusiers, Paris 75003, France. Ed. Charles Morel. adv.: page FRF 15,500; trim 220 x 300. Circ: 5,500.

HOSPICE TODAY. see *SOCIAL SERVICES AND WELFARE*

610 PRT ISSN 0046-8037
HOSPITAIS CIVIS DE LISBOA. BOLETIM CLINICO. Text in Portuguese. 1974 (vol.35). 4/yr. PTE 150. bibl, charts, illus.
Published by: Livraria Sa da Costa Editora, Praca Luis de Camoes, 22-4, Lisbon 1294, Portugal. TEL 3607215, TELEX 15574 SACOST. Ed. Dr. Fernando Nogueira.

658 USA ISSN 0018-5485
EL HOSPITAL (CINCINNATI). Text in Spanish. 1944. bi-m. free per issue to qualified personnel. adv. bk.rev., film rev. charts, illus, stat, tr.lit. index, cum.index. Supplement avail.; back issues avail. *Refereed.* **Document type:** *Trade.* **Description:** Reports on latest developments in medical technology, equipment and supplies.
Published by: Salud Publications International Inc., 2724 Erie Ave, Ste B, Cincinnati, OH 45208-2125. TEL 513-533-5470, FAX 513-533-5474. Ed. Gregory Loomis. Pub. Greg Loomis. Adv. contact Norrie Loomis. B&W page USD 2,945, color page USD 4,145. Circ: 15,500 (controlled).

610 GBR ISSN 0262-3145
HOSPITAL DOCTOR. Text in English. 1967. w. GBP 80 domestic; GBP 149, USD 224 elsewhere (effective 2000). adv. bk.rev. **Document type:** *Trade.* **Description:** Serves the hospital sector with medical news, views and education in both the medico-political and clinical arenas.
Incorporates (in 1981): On Call
—BLDSC (4333.148000).
Published by: Reed Business Information (Subsidiary of: Reed Elsevier plc), Quadrant House, The Quadrant, Brighton Rd, Sutton, Surrey SM2 5AS, United Kingdom. TEL 44-208-652-3500, FAX 44-208-652-8977, rbp.subscriptions@rbi.co.uk, http://www.reedbusiness.com. Ed. Tim Burrowes TEL 44-20-8652-8849. Circ: 34,000. **Subscr. to:** Quadrant Subscription Services, PO Box 302, Haywards Heath, W Sussex RH16 3YY, United Kingdom. TEL 44-1444-445566, FAX 44-1444-445447.

610 GBR ISSN 1462-3935 CODEN: BJHMAB
HOSPITAL MEDICINE (LONDON, 1998). Text in English. 1966. fortn. GBP 74 domestic; GBP 120 foreign. adv. bk.rev. bibl, charts, illus, stat. index. reprint service avail. from PQC. *Refereed.* **Document type:** *Academic/Scholarly.*
Former titles (until 1997): British Journal of Hospital Medicine (0007-1064); Hospital Medicine
Related titles: Microform ed.: (from PQC); Online - full text ed.: (from Institute for Scientific Information); Spanish ed.: British Journal of Hospital Medicine (Edicion Espanola). ISSN 0210-0258. 1970.
Indexed: ASCA, Abstr.Hyg., Biol.Abstr., Brit.Nur.Ind., Chem.Abstr., Curr.Adv.Cancer Res., Curr.Adv.Ecol.Sci., Curr.Cont., Dent.Ind., Excerp.Med., Helminthol.Abstr., INIS Atomind., INSPEC (1980-1984, dropped), Ind.Med. (1998-), Ind.Sci.Rev., Ind.Vet., Inpharma, Int.Nurs.Ind., NRN, Neurosci.Cit.Ind., Nutr.Abstr., Pharm.&Out.News, Pig News & Info., Protozool.Abstr., Reac., Rev.Appl.Entomol., Rev.Med.& Vet.Mycol., Rural Recreat.Tour.Abstr., SSCI (coverage dropped), Sci.Cit.Ind., Trop.Dis.Bull., Vet.Bull.
—BLDSC (4333.205600), CASDDS, CISTI, GNLM, IDS, ingenta, KNAW.
Published by: Mark Allen Publishing Ltd., Croxted Mews, 286-288a Croxted Rd, London SE24 9BY, United Kingdom. TEL 44-20-8671-7521, FAX 44-20-8671-1722. Ed. Jack Tinker. Pub. Mark Allen. Adv. contact Ian White.

HOSPITAL NEWS. see *HEALTH FACILITIES AND ADMINISTRATION*

M

610 USA ISSN 0888-241X
CODEN: HOPYA

HOSPITAL PHYSICIAN; medical practice for staff & resident. Text in English. 1957. m., latest vol.37. USD 80 domestic to individuals; USD 95 in Canada to individuals; USD 160 elsewhere to individuals; USD 55 to students; USD 20 newsstand/cover (effective 2001). adv. index. back issues avail. *Refereed.* **Document type:** *Trade, Academic/Scholarly.* **Description:** Covers issues concerning or of interest to residents and staff physicians, including epidemiology, diagnosis, and treatment; new prescription drugs; clinical outcomes.
Former titles: Hospital Physician: Internal and Family Medicine Edition (0888-241X); (until 1985): Hospital Physician: Resident - Staff Edition (8750-7560); Hospital Physician (0018-5795); (until 1965): R I S S - National Magazine for Residents, Interns, and Senior Students (0485-8182)
Related titles: Microfiche ed.; Microform ed.: (from PQC); Online - full text ed.
Indexed: Med.Care Rev.
—BLDSC (4333.207700), CISTI, GNLM, ingenta.
Published by: (Association for Hospital Medical Education), Turner White Communications, Inc., 125 Strafford Ave, Ste 220, Wayne, PA 19087-3391. TEL 610-975-4541, FAX 610-975-4564, webmaster@turner.white.com, brucewhite@turner-white.com, http://www.turner-white.com. Ed. Becky Krumm. Pub. Bruce White. R&P Jean Gaul. Adv. contact Patti Castle. B&W page USD 6,020; trim 10.75 x 7.88. Circ: 118,000 (controlled).

610 USA ISSN 8750-2836
R11 CODEN: HOPRBW

HOSPITAL PRACTICE. Text in English. 1966. m. USD 90 domestic; CND 95 in Canada; USD 130 elsewhere; USD 10 newsstand/cover domestic; CND 12 newsstand/cover in Canada; USD 18 newsstand/cover elsewhere (effective 2001); free to qualified physicians. adv. bk.rev. charts, illus. index. reprint service avail. from PQC. *Refereed.* **Document type:** *Academic/Scholarly.* **Description:** Reviews articles with information on problem areas in medicine and clinical research.
Incorporates: Clinical Experience
Related titles: Microfilm ed.: (from PQC); Online - full text ed.: (from ProQuest Information & Learning, Gale Group, Institute for Scientific Information).
Indexed: AIM, ASCA, Abstr.Hyg., AgeLine, Biol.Abstr., CINAHL, Curr.Adv.Cancer Res., Curr.Adv.Ecol.Sci., Curr.Cont., Curr.Lit.Fam.Plan., Dent.Ind., Environ.Sci.Poll.Mgmt., Excerp.Med., Hosp.Lit.Ind., INIS Atomind., I.P.A., Ind.Med. (1981-), Ind.Sci.Rev., Inpharma, Int.Nurs.Ind., Med.Care Rev., Nutr.Abstr., Pharm.&Out.News, Pollut.Abstr., Reac., Rev.Arom.& Med.Plants, Rev.Med.& Vet.Mycol., SSCI (coverage dropped), Sci.Cit.Ind. (coverage dropped).
—BLDSC (4333.208300), CISTI, EMDOCS, GNLM, IDS, Infotrieve, ingenta, KNAW. **CCC.**
Published by: McGraw-Hill Companies, 4530 W 77th St Ste 350, Minneapolis, MN 55435. TEL 952-835-3222, FAX 952-835-3460, http://www.hosppsact.com. Ed. Dr. Leland Powers. Adv. contact Penny Godden. B&W page USD 5,796, color page USD 7,706. Circ: 141,770. **Subscr. to:** PO Box 461, Highstown, NJ 08520-9203.

HOSPITAL PRODUCTS ASIA. see *MEDICAL SCIENCES—Experimental Medicine, Laboratory Technique*

610 VEN ISSN 0018-5884

HOSPITAL VARGAS. ARCHIVOS✱ . Text in Spanish. 1967 (vol.9). q. illus.
Indexed: Abstr.Hyg., Biol.Abstr., Chem.Abstr., IBR, Trop.Dis.Bull.
—BLDSC (1650.900000), CISTI, GNLM.
Published by: Hospital Vargas, Caracas, Venezuela.

610 612 AUS

HOWARD FLOREY INSTITUTE OF EXPERIMENTAL PHYSIOLOGY & MEDICINE. ANNUAL REPORT. Text in English. 1974. a. illus. back issues avail. **Document type:** *Academic/Scholarly.*
Formerly: Howard Florey Institute of Experimental Physiology and Medicine. Annual Report and Notice of Meeting (0314-6162)
Published by: Howard Florey Institute of Experimental Physiology & Medicine, c/o Univeristy of Melbourne, Melbourne, VIC 3010, Australia. TEL 61-3-93447286, 61-3-8344-5654, FAX 61-3-93481707, 61-3-9348-1707, info@hfi.unimelb.edu.au, http://www.hfi.unimelb.edu.au. Ed., R&P Graeme Chandler TEL 61-3-8344-7267. Circ: 3,000.

HUANJING YU JIANKANG ZAZHI/JOURNAL OF ENVIRONMENT AND HEALTH. see *ENVIRONMENTAL STUDIES*

610 570 CHN ISSN 0257-7712
CODEN: HYDXET

HUAXI YIKE DAXUE XUEBAO/WEST CHINA UNIVERSITY OF MEDICAL SCIENCES. JOURNAL. Text in Chinese; Abstracts and contents page in English. 1959. q. CNY 16 domestic; CNY 80 foreign. abstr, bibl, charts, illus, stat. index. back issues avail.
Formerly (until 1985): Sichuan Yixueyuan Xuebao - Acta Academiae Medicinae Sichuan (0253-4290)
Indexed: Biol.Abstr., Chem.Abstr., Chem.Indus.Notes, Chem.Titles, Dairy Sci.Abstr., Excerp.Med., Food Sci.& Tech.Abstr., Ind.Med. (1986-), Nutr.Abstr., Ref.Zh.
—BLDSC (4915.650000), CASDDS, EMDOCS, GNLM, Linda Hall.
Published by: Huaxi Yike Daxue/West China University of Medical Sciences, 17 Renmin Nanlu 3 Duan, Chengdu, Sichuan 610041, China. FAX 583252, TELEX 60251-WCUMS-CN. Ed. Yang Guanghua. Circ: 2,500. **Dist. overseas by:** China International Book Trading Corp, 35 Chegongzhuang Xilu, Haidian District, Beijing 100044, China.

610 CHN ISSN 1002-0179

HUAXI YIXUE/WEST CHINA MEDICAL JOURNAL. Text in Chinese; Summaries in Chinese, English. 1986. q. CNY 24 domestic; USD 24 foreign; CNY 6 newsstand/cover domestic; USD 6 newsstand/cover foreign (effective 2000). adv. abstr, bibl, charts, illus, stat. index. 128 p./no. back issues avail. **Document type:** *Academic/Scholarly.* **Description:** Contains two sections: medicine and surgery.
Related titles: ♦ CD-ROM ed.: Chinese Academic Journal. Medicine & Hygiene. ISSN 1007-8053; Microfiche ed.; Microfilm ed.
Published by: Huaxi Yike Daxue, Fushu Diyi Yiyuan/West China University of Medical Sciences, First University Hospital, 37 Guoxue Xiang, Wuhou-qu, Chengdu 610041, China. TEL 86-28-5422071, FAX 86-28-5582944, hxyx@mcwcums.com, http://www.mcwcums.com. Ed. Yinkang Shi. Adv. contact Huasong Rao. Circ: 4,000 (paid). **Dist. overseas by:** China International Book Trading Corp, 35 Chegongzhuang Xilu, Haidian District, Beijing 100044, China.

610 NLD ISSN 0018-7070

HUISARTS EN WETENSCHAP. Text in Dutch; Summaries in Dutch, English. 1950. m. NLG 157.50; NLG 89.75 to students. adv. bk.rev. *Refereed.*
Indexed: Excerp.Med., FAMLI.
—CISTI, GNLM, KNAW.
Published by: (Nederlands Huisartsengenootschap), Bohn Stafleu van Loghum B.V. (Subsidiary of: Wolters Kluwer N.V.), Postbus 246, Houten 3990 GA, Netherlands. TEL 31-3403-95711, FAX 31-3403-50903. Ed. F J Meyman. Circ: 5,075.

612 CHE ISSN 0018-716X
CODEN: HUDEA8

HUMAN DEVELOPMENT. Text in English. 1958. bi-m. CHF 487, EUR 347.80 in Europe to institutions; CHF 504.40, USD 383 elsewhere to institutions (effective 2002). adv. bk.rev. bibl, charts, illus. index. back issues avail.; reprint service avail. from SWZ. *Refereed.* **Document type:** *Journal, Academic/Scholarly.* **Description:** Scholarly articles on psychological development over an entire lifespan, from infancy through aging.
Formerly: Vita Humana
Related titles: Microform ed.; Online - full text ed.: ISSN 1423-0054. CHF 58 to institutional members with print edition; EUR 42, USD 45 to institutions with print edition (effective 2002) (from EBSCO Publishing, O C L C Online Computer Library Center, Inc., RoweCom Information Quest, Gale Group, Swets Blackwell, Factiva, Institute for Scientific Information).
Indexed: Abstr.Soc.Geront., Adol.Ment.Hlth.Abstr., AgeLine, Arts & Hum.Cit.Ind. (coverage dropped), Bibl.Asian Stud. (1975-1990), Biol.Abstr., C.I.J.E., Cath.Ind., Child Devel.Abstr., Curr.Adv.Ecol.Sci., Curr.Cont., Educ.Ind. (May 1983-), Excerp.Med., IBR, IBZ, Ind.Med. (coverage dropped), Ind.Philos., M.L.A., MLA Intl.Bibl., Mid.East: Abstr.& Ind., PsycInfo, Psychol.Abstr. (1958-), Psycscan D.P., Rehabil.Lit., SSCI, e-psyche.
—BLDSC (4336.050000), GNLM, IDS, Infotrieve, ingenta, KNAW. **CCC.**
Published by: S. Karger AG, Allschwilerstr 10, PO Box, Basel 4009, Switzerland. TEL 41-61-306-1111, FAX 41-61-306-1234, karger@karger.ch, http://www.online.karger.com/journals/hde, http://www.karger.com. Ed. B Rogoff. adv.: page USD 1,205. Circ: 2,200.

HUMAN FACTORS & AVIATION MEDICINE. see *AERONAUTICS AND SPACE FLIGHT*

HUMAN HEREDITY; international journal of human and medical genetics. see *BIOLOGY—Genetics*

HUMAN MOLECULAR GENETICS. see *BIOLOGY—Genetics*

615.8 NLD ISSN 0167-9457
QP303 CODEN: HMSCDO

HUMAN MOVEMENT SCIENCE; journal devoted to pure and applied research on human movement. Text in English. 1982. bi-m. EUR 209 in Europe to individuals; JPY 27,800 in Japan to individuals; USD 234 elsewhere to individuals; EUR 523 in Europe to institutions; JPY 69,400 in Japan to institutions; USD 585 elsewhere to institutions (effective 2002). bk.rev. back issues avail. *Refereed.* **Document type:** *Academic/Scholarly.* **Description:** Consists of empirical reports, overviews, methodologies as well as announcements of seminars, conferences and research programs relevant to the study of human movement.
Related titles: Online - full text ed.: (from ingenta, Swets Blackwell, ScienceDirect, Institute for Scientific Information).
Indexed: ASCA, Curr.Cont., Ergon.Abstr., Focus on: Sports Sci.& Med., INSPEC (Feb.1991-), Neurosci.Cit.Ind., PsycInfo, Psychol.Abstr. (1990-), SSCI, Sci.Cit.Ind., Sportsearch (1987-), e-psyche.
—BLDSC (4336.210000), AskIEEE, CISTI, GNLM, IDS, ingenta, KNAW. **CCC.**
Published by: North-Holland (Subsidiary of: Elsevier Science BV), PO Box 211, Amsterdam 1000 AE, Netherlands. TEL 31-20-485-3911, FAX 31-20-485-3598, http://www.elsevier.com/locate/humov. Eds. H T A Whitting, P Beek. **Subscr. in Australasia and the Far East to:** Elsevier Science (Singapore) Pte Ltd, No.1 Temasek Ave, 17-01 Millenia Tower, Singapore 039192, Singapore. TEL 65-434-3727, FAX 65-337-2230; **Subscr. in Japan to:** Elsevier Science Inc - Japan Regional Office, 9-15 Higashi-Azabu 1-chome, Minato-ku, Tokyo 106-0044, Japan. TEL 81-3-5561-5033; **Subscr. in the Americas to:** Elsevier Science, PO Box 945, New York, NY 10159-0945. TEL 212-633-3730, FAX 212-633-3680.

616.07 USA ISSN 0046-8177
CODEN: HPCQA4

HUMAN PATHOLOGY. Text in English. 1970. m. USD 176 domestic to individuals Full text online included; USD 269 foreign to individuals Full text online included; USD 284 domestic to institutions Full text online included; USD 359 foreign to institutions Full text online included; USD 107 domestic to students Full text online included; USD 208 foreign to students Full text online included; USD 30 per issue (effective 2001). adv. bk.rev. reprint service avail. from PQC,ISI. *Refereed.* **Document type:** *Journal, Academic/Scholarly.* **Description:** Contains original contributions, news items, case studies, and special notices in the field of human pathology.
Related titles: Microform ed.: (from MIM,PQC); Online - full text ed.: (from IDEAL Online Library, Institute for Scientific Information).
Indexed: ASCA, Abstr.Hyg., Biol.Abstr., Chem.Abstr., Chem.Indus.Notes, Chem.Titles, Curr.Adv.Cancer Res., Curr.Adv.Ecol.Sci., Curr.Cont., Excerp.Med., Helminthol.Abstr., INIS Atomind., Ind.Med. (1970-), Ind.Sci.Rev., Inpharma, Int.Abstr.Biol.Sci., Med.& Surg.Dermat., Neurosci.Cit.Ind., Pharm.&Out.News, Protozool.Abstr., Reac., Rev.Med.& Vet.Mycol., Rev.Plant Path., Sci.Cit.Ind., Trop.Dis.Bull.
—BLDSC (4336.260000), CASDDS, CISTI, GNLM, IDS, ingenta, KNAW. **CCC.**
Published by: W.B. Saunders Co. (Subsidiary of: Harcourt Publishers Ltd.), 11830 Westline Industrial Dr, St Louis, MO 63146. TEL 800-325-4177, http://www.harcourthealth.com/humpath, http://www.wbsaunders.com. Ed. Dr. Fred Gorstein. Adv. contact Steve Gray. B&W page USD 1,055, color page USD 2,005; trim 10 x 7. Circ: 6,018. **Subscr. to:** Periodicals Fulfillment, W B Saunders Co, 6277 Sea Harbor Dr, 4th Fl, Orlando, FL 32891-4800.

612 RUS ISSN 0362-1197
QP34.5 CODEN: HUPHDC

HUMAN PHYSIOLOGY. Text in English. 1975. bi-m. EUR 1,991 to institutions for print or online ed.; EUR 2,389.20 to institutions print & online eds.combined (effective 2002). back issues avail. *Refereed.* **Document type:** *Academic/Scholarly.* **Description:** Publishes studies on the physiology of work, speech, and sport, emphasizing their relationship to the physiology of the brain and the neurophysiology of psychological activity.
Related titles: Microfilm ed.: (from PQC); Online - full text ed.: (from Swets Blackwell, Kluwer Online, RoweCom Information Quest); ♦ Translation of: Fiziologiya Cheloveka. ISSN 0131-1646.
Indexed: Biol.Abstr., Curr.Adv.Ecol.Sci., Ergon.Abstr., Excerp.Med., Ind.Med. (coverage dropped), Int.Abstr.Biol.Sci., PsycInfo, Psychol.Abstr. (1979-), e-psyche.

M

—BLDSC (0412.087700), CASDDS, CISTI, GNLM, Infotrieve, ingenta. **CCC.**
Published by: (Rossiiskaya Akademiya Nauk/Russian Academy of Sciences), M A I K Nauka - Interperiodica, Mezhdunarodnyi Otdel, Profsoyuznaya ul 90, Moscow 117864, Russian Federation. TEL 7-095-336-1600, FAX 7-095-336-0666, compmg@maik.ru, http://www.maik.rssi.ru/journals/humphys.htm. Ed. Vsevolod I Medvedev. **Dist. by:** Kluwer Academic Publishers, PO Box 17, Dordrecht 3300 AH, Netherlands. TEL 31-78-392392, FAX 31-78-546474, http://www.wkap.nl.

HUMAN REPRODUCTION UPDATE. see *BIOLOGY—Abstracting, Bibliographies, Statistics*

174.2 DEU ISSN 0938-9717
HUMANES LEBEN - HUMANES STERBEN. Text in German; Summaries in English, German. 1981. 4/yr. DEM 33.60 domestic; DEM 32.40 foreign (effective 2001). bk.rev. charts, stat. Supplement avail.; back issues avail. **Document type:** *Newsletter, Academic/Scholarly.* **Description:** Contains essays concerning all aspects of dying with dignity.
—GNLM.
Published by: Gesellschaft fuer Humanes Sterben e.V., Postfach 110529, Augsburg 86030, Germany. TEL 49-821-502350, FAX 49-821-5023555, dghsaugsb@aol.com, info@dghs.de, www.dghs.de, http://www.dghs.de. Ed. Kurt Schobert. Circ: 42,000 (controlled).

▼ **HYGIEA INTERNATIONALIS.** see *PUBLIC HEALTH AND SAFETY*

610 JPN ISSN 0385-7638
CODEN: HIDZDO
HYOGO IKA DAIGAKU IGAKKAI ZASSHI. Text in Japanese; Summaries in English. 1976. 3/yr. JPY 2,000. back issues avail. **Document type:** *Academic/Scholarly.* **Description:** Publishes both experimental and theoretical papers in the field of medical sciences.
Indexed: Chem.Abstr., Excerp.Med., INIS Atomind.
—BLDSC (0635.020000), CASDDS.
Published by: Hyogo Ika Daigaku Igakkai/Medical Society of Hyogo College of Medicine, 1-1 Muko-Gawa-cho, Nishinomiya-shi, Hyogo-ken 663-8131, Japan. TEL 0798-45-6289, FAX 0798-48-8045. Ed. Toshihide Tamura. Circ: 1,400.

610 JPN ISSN 0910-8238
HYOGOKEN ISHIKAI IGAKU ZASSHI/HYOGO MEDICAL ASSOCIATION. JOURNAL. Text in Japanese. q.
Published by: Hyogoken Ishikai, 1-30 Nakayamatedori 6-chome, Chuo-ku, Kobe-shi, Hyogo-ken 650-0004, Japan.

610 JPN ISSN 0388-7561
HYOGOKEN ISHIKAIHO/HYOGO MEDICAL ASSOCIATION. MONTHLY REPORT. Text in Japanese. 1948. m.
Published by: Hyogoken Ishikai, 1-30 Nakayamatedori 6-chome, Chuo-ku, Kobe-shi, Hyogo-ken 650-0004, Japan.

610 AUS ISSN 0819-9558
I A A H NEWSLETTER. Text in English. 1987. q. USD 25. adv. bk.rev. **Document type:** *Newsletter.* **Description:** Contains reports and discussion of all topics relevant to adolescent health, health education and medical care.
Published by: International Association for Adolescent Health, Center for Adolescent Health, William Buckland House, 2 Gatehouse St, Parkville, VIC 3052, Australia. TEL 03-345-5890, FAX 03-345-6502. Ed. John Court. Circ: 450.

I C H P E R - S D CONGRESS PROCEEDINGS. see *PHYSICAL FITNESS AND HYGIENE*

610 IND ISSN 0377-4910
I C M R BULLETIN. (Indian Council of Medical Research) Text in English. 1971. m. abstr. index. back issues avail. **Document type:** *Bulletin.* **Description:** Offers medical research articles, seminar and training program calendars.
—GNLM.
Published by: Indian Council of Medical Research, Division of Publication & Information, Ansari Nagar, P O Box 4911, New Delhi 110 029, India. TEL 91-11-6963980, FAX 91-11-6868662, icmrhqd@ren.nic.in. Ed. Dr. N Medappa. Circ: 7,200 (controlled).

I E E E BIOMEDICAL ENGINEERING DAYS. see *BIOLOGY—Biotechnology*

I E E E - E M B S CONFERENCE ON INFORMATION TECHNOLOGY APPLICATIONS IN BIOMEDICINE. PROCEEDINGS. see *COMPUTERS*

I E E E ENGINEERING IN MEDICINE AND BIOLOGY MAGAZINE. see *BIOLOGY—Bioengineering*

I E E E TRANSACTIONS ON BIOMEDICAL ENGINEERING. see *BIOLOGY—Bioengineering*

I E H ASSESSMENT. see *ENVIRONMENTAL STUDIES*

I E H REPORT. see *ENVIRONMENTAL STUDIES*

I E H REPORT ON THE USE OF BIOMARKERS IN ENVIRONMENTAL EXPOSURE ASSESSMENT. see *ENVIRONMENTAL STUDIES—Pollution*

I E H SPECIAL REPORT. see *ENVIRONMENTAL STUDIES*

I F M B E NEWS. (International Federation for Medical & Biological Engineering) see *BIOLOGY—Bioengineering*

610 ISR ISSN 1565-1088
R97 CODEN: IJMDAI
I M A J. (Israel Medical Association Journal) Text in English. 1965; N.S. 1997. m. ILS 200, USD 200 to non-members; free to members. adv. bk.rev. bibl, charts, illus. index. back issues avail.; reprint service avail. from PQC. *Refereed.* **Document type:** *Academic/Scholarly.* **Description:** Publishes original papers on basic medical sciences, clinical medicine, epidemiology, public health, and relevant topics in biology, and reports on medical news and scientific meetings in Israel for an international audience.
Formerly: Israel Journal of Medical Sciences (0021-2180); Which was formed by the merger of (1963-1965): Israel Journal of Experimental Medicine (0535-806X); Which was formerly (1956-1963): Research Council of Israel, Section E: Experimental Medicine (0376-091X); (1958-1965): Israel Medical Journal (0368-0150); Which was formerly (1941-1958): Acta Medica Orientalia (0365-4540)
Related titles: Online - full text ed.: (from Institute for Scientific Information).
Indexed: ASCA, Abstr.Hyg., Agri.& Environ.Biotech.Abstr. (coverage dropped), Bioeng.Abstr., Biol.Abstr., Chem.Abstr., Curr.Adv.Cancer Res., Curr.Cont., Dairy Sci.Abstr., Dent.Ind., Derwent Biotech.Abstr., Dok.Arbeitsmed., Eng.Ind., Excerp.Med., Fam.Ind., Helminthol.Abstr., INIS Atomind., Ind.Med. (1999-), Ind.Sci.Rev., Ind.Vet., Inpharma, Int.Abstr.Biol.Sci., Int.Nurs.Ind., Med.& Surg.Dermat., NRN, Neurosci.Cit.Ind., Nutr.Abstr., Pharm.&Out.News, Pig News & Info., Poult.Abstr., Protozool.Abstr., Reac., Rev.Med.& Vet.Mycol., Rev.Plant Path., SSCI (coverage dropped), Sci.Cit.Ind. (coverage dropped), Small Anim.Abstr., Soyabean Abstr., Trop.Dis.Bull., Vet.Bull.
—BLDSC (4369.015200), CASDDS, CISTI, Ei, EMDOCS, GNLM, IDS, ingenta.
Published by: Israel Medical Association, 2 Twin Towers, 11th Fl, 35 Jabotinsky St, PO Box 3604, Ramat Gan 52136, Israel. TEL 972-3-610-0418, FAX 972-3-575-1616, imaj@ima.org.il. Ed. Yehuda Shoenfeld. adv.: B&W page USD 400, color page USD 1,000. Circ: 5,000.

I M A JOURNAL OF MATHEMATICS APPLIED IN MEDICINE & BIOLOGY. see *MATHEMATICS*

610 GBR
I N A S P HEALTH DIRECTORY (YEAR). Text in English. irreg., latest 1999. GBP 15 per vol. for 1999 Vol. (effective 2001). **Document type:** *Directory, Academic/Scholarly.* **Description:** Aims to assist the health workers in developing countries in building professional relationships and improve information distribution among organizations, and to provide a reference for health librarians and others in resource-poor countries who are seeking help to improve local resources.
Published by: International Network for the Availability of Scientific Publications, 27 Park End St, Oxford, Oxon OX1 1HU, United Kingdom. TEL 44-1865-249-909, FAX 44-1865-251-060, inasp@inasp.org.uk, http://www.inasp.org.uk world.org/inasp/newslet/.

616.02 FRA ISSN 0378-0546
CODEN: INSSDM
I N S E R M SYMPOSIA. Text in French. 1975. irreg. price varies. **Document type:** *Proceedings.*
Indexed: Biol.Abstr., Chem.Abstr. (1975-1985), Dairy Sci.Abstr.
—CASDDS, CISTI.
Published by: Institut National de la Sante et de la Recherche Medicale, 101 rue de Tolbiac, Paris Cedex 13 75654, France. TEL 44-23-60-00, FAX 44-23-60-99.

I P P F ANNUAL REPORT. see *BIRTH CONTROL*

I P P F MEDICAL BULLETIN. see *BIRTH CONTROL*

610 USA ISSN 1016-2216
I S S X NEWSLETTER. Text in English. 1981. q. USD 55 to members (effective 2001). adv. bk.rev. **Document type:** *Newsletter.* **Description:** Contains news and views about xenobiotic research and development from around the world.
Published by: International Society for the Study of Xenobiotics, 9650 Rockville Pike, Bethesda, MD 20814. TEL 301-983-2434, FAX 301-983-5357, http://www.issx.org. Ed. Jo Cato. R&P, Adv. contact Nancy Holahan. Circ: 2,500.

▼ **I T B M - R B M.** (Innovation et Technologie en Biologie et Medecine - Revue Europeenne de Biotechnologie Medicale) see *BIOLOGY—Biotechnology*

I T B M - R B M NEWS. (Innovation et Technologie en Biologie et Medecine - Revue Europeene de Biotechnologie Medicale) see *BIOLOGY—Biotechnology*

610 USA ISSN 1093-5207
I V D TECHNOLOGY. (In Vitro Diagnostic) Text in English. 1995. 9/yr. USD 150; free to qualified personnel (effective 2001). adv. **Document type:** *Magazine, Trade.* **Description:** Focuses on the development and manufacturing of in vitro diagnostics.
Indexed: METADEX.
—BLDSC (4589.038500).
Published by: Canon Communications LLC, 11444 W Olympic Blvd, Ste 900, Los Angeles, CA 90064-1549. TEL 310-445-4200, FAX 310-445-4299, feedback@devicelink.com, http://www.devicelink.com/ivdt. Ed. Steve Halasey. Pub. William F Cobert. Adv. contact Robert Truncali. B&W page USD 3,255, color page USD 4,980. Circ: 15,000 (controlled).

610 USA ISSN 1066-534X
I V U N NEWS. Text in English. 1987. q., latest vol.15. USD 17 domestic to individuals; USD 27 foreign to individuals (effective 2001). bk.rev. 8 p./no. 3 cols./p. back issues avail. **Document type:** *Newsletter, Consumer.* **Description:** Shares information of ventilator users and health care professionals experienced in home mechanical ventilation. Discusses topics such as equipment, breathing techniques, travel and family life.
Published by: (International Ventilator Users Network), Gazette International Networking Institute, 4207 Lindell Blvd., Ste. 110, St. Louis, MO 63108-2915. TEL 314-534-0475, FAX 314-534-5070, gini_intl@msn.com, http://www.post-polio.org/ivun.html. Eds. Joan Headley, Judith Raymond Fischer. Circ: 2,500.

IAN RAMSEY CENTRE. PUBLICATIONS. see *PHILOSOPHY*

610 COL ISSN 0121-0793
IATREIA. Text in Spanish. 1988. q. USD 30 (effective 2000). **Document type:** *Journal, Academic/Scholarly.*
—BLDSC (4359.555000).
Published by: Universidad de Antioquia, Facultad de Medicina-Academia de Medicina, Apartado Aereo 1226, Medellin, Colombia. TEL 57-4-510-6919, FAX 57-4-262-0253.

610 GRC ISSN 0303-4925
IATRIKA CHRONIKA/MEDICAL ANNALS. Text in English. 1961. m. GRD 15,000 (effective 1999). adv. **Document type:** *Trade.*
Related titles: Diskette ed.
Address: 77 Aspasias St, Cholargos 155 61, Greece. TEL 30-1-6546-645, FAX 30-1-6546-477, http://www.edipt.qr.members.med.annals.current.htm. Ed. Tzigounis Basilios. Pub. E M Moraitou Sideridi. Adv. contact Sideridis Demetrious. Circ: 11,000.

610 GRC ISSN 0019-0950
IATRIKI. Text in Greek; Summaries in English. 1962. m. GRD 16,500. adv. bk.rev. abstr, bibl, stat. index. cum.index. back issues avail. **Document type:** *Academic/Scholarly.*
Published by: (Society for Medical Studies), Beta Medical Arts, 3 Sisini St, Athens 115 25, Greece. Ed. Galanakis Nearchos. Adv. contact Palamidas Dimitris. Circ: 6,000.

610 NGA
IBADAN TROPICAL MEDICINE SERIES. Text in English. irreg. **Document type:** *Monographic series.*

Published by: (University of Ibadan), Ibadan University Press, Ibadan, Oyo, Nigeria. TEL 234-22-400550, TELEX UNIVPRESS IBADAN NG. **Dist. outside Africa by:** African Books Collective Ltd., The Jam Factory, 27 Park End St, Oxford, Oxon OX1 1HU, United Kingdom. TEL 44-1865-726686, FAX 44-1865-793298.

610 JPN ISSN 0912-9952
IBARAKI KENRITSU BYOIN IGAKU ZASSHI/IBARAKI PREFECTURAL HOSPITAL. MEDICAL JOURNAL. Text in Japanese. 1983. q.
Published by: Ibaraki Kenritsu Chuo Byoin/Ibaraki Prefectural Central Hospital, 6528 Koibuchi, Nishiibaraki-gun, Tomobe-machi, Ibaraki-ken 309-1703, Japan.

610 JPN ISSN 0914-4501
IBARAKIKEN ISHIKAIHO/IBARAKI MEDICAL ASSOCIATION. JOURNAL. Text in Japanese. m. JPY 200 per issue.
Published by: Ibarakiken Ishikai, 489 Kasahara-cho, Mito-shi, Ibaraki-ken 310-0852, Japan.

610 JPN ISSN 0915-1982
IBARAKIKEN NOSON IGAKKAI ZASSHI/IBARAKI SOCIETY OF RURAL MEDICINE. JOURNAL. Text in Japanese. 1988. a.
Published by: Ibarakiken Noson Igakkai, Ibarakiken Kosei Nogyo Kyodo Kumiai Rengokai, 1-4 Baiko 1-chome, Mito-shi, Ibaraki-ken 310-0022, Japan.

IDO NO NIPPON/JOURNAL OF JAPANESE ACUPUNCTURE & MOXIBUSTION. see *ALTERNATIVE MEDICINE*

610 JPN ISSN 0387-0006
IGAKU CHUO ZASSHI/JAPANA CENTRA REVUO MEDICINA. Text in Japanese. 1903. m. JPY 328,860 (effective 2000). *Refereed.* **Document type:** *Abstract/Index.* **Description:** Provides abstracting and indexing database, covering medical, dental, pharmaceutic, nursing and related journals which are published in Japan.
Related titles: CD-ROM ed.: 1987. JPY 546,000 (effective 2000) (from Dai Nippon Printing Co. Ltd.); Online - full content ed.: Igaku Chuo Zasshi Personal Web; Igaku Chuo Zasshi Web (Corporate Ed.). 1994. JPY 367,500 to corporations (effective 2000).
Published by: Igaku Chuo Zasshi Kankokai/Japan Medical Abstracts Society, 5-18 Takaido-Higashi 2-chome, Suginami-ku, Tokyo 168-0072, Japan. TEL 81-3-3334-7575, FAX 81-3-3334-0497, info@jamas.gr.jp, http://www.jamas.gr.jp. Ed., Pub. Tsuneki Shinohara. Circ: 500 (paid).

610 JPN ISSN 0019-1574
IGAKU HYORON/JAPANA MEDICINA REVUO. Text in Japanese. 1950. s-a. JPY 1,350.
Published by: Shin Nihon Ishi Kyokai/New Japanese Doctors' Association, Hidaka Bldg, 1-10-2 Nishi-Ikebukuro, Toshima-ku, Tokyo 171-0021, Japan. Ed. Sadatoshi Yoshida. Circ: 1,200.

610 JPN ISSN 0076-597X
CODEN: IGKEAO
IGAKU KENKYU/ACTA MEDICA. Text in English, Japanese. 1927. irreg.
Indexed: Chem.Abstr., Excerp.Med., INIS Atomind., Ind.Med. (coverage dropped).
—CASDDS, CISTI, GNLM.
Published by: Daido Gakkan Shuppan-bu, c/o Kyushu Daigaku Igakubu Hoigaku Kyoshitsu, 1-1 Maidashi 3-chome, Higashi-ku, Fukuoka-shi 812-0054, Japan.

610.7 JPN ISSN 0386-9644
IGAKU KYOIKU/MEDICAL EDUCATION. Text in Japanese; Summaries in English. 1970. bi-m. JPY 1,600. adv. bk.rev. **Document type:** *Academic/Scholarly.* **Description:** Publishes original reports on current medical education.
Published by: Nihon Igaku Kyoiku Gakkai/Japan Society for Medical Education, 11-7 Hongo 2-chome, Bunkyo-ku, Tokyo 113-0033, Japan. TEL 03-3816-5311, FAX 03-3816-5314. Ed. Takashi Yamada. Adv. contact Hideo Ito.

610 JPN ISSN 0039-2359
CODEN: IGAYAY
IGAKU NO AYUMI/JOURNAL OF CLINICAL AND EXPERIMENTAL MEDICINE. Text in English, Japanese. 1946. w. JPY 61,600. adv. bk.rev. charts, illus. index every 3 mos. **Document type:** *Consumer.*
Indexed: C.I.S. Abstr., Chem.Abstr., Chem.Indus.Notes, Chem.Titles, INIS Atomind., Jap.Per.Ind.
—BLDSC (4363.381000), CASDDS, GNLM.

Published by: Ishiyaku Shuppan K.K./Ishiyaku Publishers, Inc., 7-10 Honkomagome 1-chome, Bunkyo-ku, Tokyo 113-0021, Japan. TEL 81-3-5395-7622, FAX 81-3-5395-7624, KYB01177@miftyserve.or.jp, http://www.so-net.or.jp/medipro/isyk. Ed. Hiroshi Miura. Adv. contact Yoshihisa Ishida. Circ: 8,800 (paid).

610 JPN ISSN 0019-1582
IGAKU TO FUKUIN/MEDICINE AND THE GOSPEL. Text in Japanese. 1949. m. JPY 440, USD 4. bk.rev. **Document type:** *Academic/Scholarly.*
Published by: Japan Christian Medical Association/Nihon Kirisutosha Ika Renmei, 2-3-18-23 Nishi-Waseda, Shinjuku-ku, Tokyo 162-0051, Japan. FAX 03-3232-6922, ifukushi@jocs.mxe.mesh.ne.jp, http://www1.mesh.ne.jp/~jocs-os/jcma. Ed., R&P Kiyosumi Nakamura. Circ: 1,000.

610 JPN ISSN 0287-5950
IGAKU TO KIKAI/MEDICINE AND INSTRUMENTS. Text in Japanese. 1955. m. JPY 360 per issue. adv.
Published by: Igaku Janarusha/Medical Journal Co., Ltd., 12-3 Minami-Senba 1-chome, Chuo-ku, Osaka-shi 542-0081, Japan. Ed. Kosaku Maeda. Pub. Taka Akagi. Adv. contact Ichihiko Akagi.

610 574 JPN ISSN 0019-1604
CODEN: IGSBAL
IGAKU TO SEIBUTSUGAKU/MEDICINE AND BIOLOGY. Text in Japanese. 1942. m. JPY 15,000. adv. abstr, charts, illus. index.
Indexed: C.I.S. Abstr., Chem.Abstr., Chem.Indus.Notes, Chem.Titles, Dairy Sci.Abstr., Food Sci.& Tech.Abstr., INIS Atomind., Ind.Med. (coverage dropped).
—BLDSC (5534.005000), CASDDS, CISTI, GNLM, KNAW.
Published by: Ogata Institute for Medical and Chemical Research, 2-10-14 Higashi-Kanda, Chiyoda-ku, Tokyo 101-0031, Japan. FAX 81-3-3865-7510. Ed. Masahide Abe. Circ: 1,200.

IGAKU TOSHOKAN/JAPAN MEDICAL LIBRARY ASSOCIATION. JOURNAL. see *LIBRARY AND INFORMATION SCIENCES*

610 JPN ISSN 0019-1612
IGAKUSHI KENKYU/STUDIUM HISTORIAE MEDICAE. Text in Japanese. 1961. a. JPY 1,500. adv. bk.rev. abstr, bibl, illus. cum.index: 1961-1968.
Indexed: Curr.Cont. (coverage dropped), Jap.Per.Ind.
Published by: Igakushi Kenkyukai/Collegium ad Studium Historiae Medicae, Osaka Daigaku Igakubu Kankyo Igaku Kyoshitsu, 2-2 Yamada-Oka, Suita-shi, Osaka-fu 565-0871, Japan. Ed. Hiroshi Maruyama. Circ: 700.

610 ITA ISSN 0391-8068
IGEA MEDICA. Text in Italian. 1978. q. ITL 15,000. adv.
Published by: Casa Editrice Menna, Via Corso Vittorio Emanuele, 123, Avellino, AV 83100, Italy. Ed. Luigi Tulimiero. Circ: 3,000.

▼ **IHEALTHCARE WEEKLY.** see *COMPUTERS—Internet*

610 JPN
IHO HANAMAKI/HANAMAKI CITY MEDICAL ASSOCIATION. NEWS. Text in Japanese. 1980. m.
Published by: Hanamakishi Ishikai, Hanamaki Shoko Kaigisho Kaikan, 10-27 Kajo-Machi, Hanamaki-shi, Iwate-ken 025-0075, Japan.

610 JPN ISSN 0912-6597
IJIGAKU KENKYU/JOURNAL OF INTERDISCIPLINARY HUMANISTIC MEDICAL RESEARCH. Text in Japanese. 1986. a.
Published by: Iwate Ika Daigaku, Ijigaku Kenkyukai/Iwate Medical University, Society for Interdisciplinary Humanistic Medical Research, 16-1 Honchi-Yodori 3-chome, Morioka-shi, Iwate-ken 020-0015, Japan.

610 JPN ISSN 0385-440X
IKA KIKAIGAKU/JAPANESE JOURNAL OF MEDICAL INSTRUMENTATION. Text in Japanese; Summaries in English. 1923. m. JPY 500 per issue.
Indexed: INIS Atomind.
—BLDSC (4656.217000), CISTI.
Published by: Nihon Ika Kikai Gakkai/Medical Instruments Society of Japan, 39-15 Hongo 3-chome, Bunkyo-ku, Tokyo 113-0033, Japan.

610 JPN ISSN 0914-5117
CODEN: IOKHEP
IKAGAKU OYO KENKYU ZAIDAN KENKYU HOKOKU/SUZUKEN MEMORIAL FOUNDATION. RESEARCH PAPERS. Text in English, Japanese; Summaries in English. 1982. a. **Description:** Reports the pharmaceutical research and human health achievements supported by the foundation.
Indexed: Chem.Abstr.
Published by: Ikagaku Oyo Kenkyu Zaidan, Suzuken Honsha, 8 Higashi-Kataha-Machi, Higashi-ku, Nagoya-shi, Aichi-ken 461-0015, Japan. TEL 81-52-951-2139, FAX 81-52-951-2166. Pub. Ikagaku Oyo Kenkyu Zaidan.

610 JPN ISSN 0019-1728
IKAI JIHO. Text in Japanese. 1957. 3/m. JPY 10, USD 1.66. adv. bk.rev.
Published by: Kanehara & Co. Ltd., 2-31-14 Yushima, Bunkyo-ku, Tokyo 113-0034, Japan. Ed. Hideo Kanehara. Circ: 100,000.

IKAKIKAI GAKU ZASSHI/JOURNAL OF MEDICAL INSTRUMENTS. see *INSTRUMENTS*

ILLNESS, CRISIS, AND LOSS. see *SOCIOLOGY*

ILLUSTRERAD VETENSKAP. see *SCIENCES: COMPREHENSIVE WORKS*

614.88 DEU ISSN 1617-4283
IM EINSATZ; Zeitschrift fuer Helfer und Fuehrungskraefte. Text in German. 1994. bi-m. DEM 37.50, EUR 20 (effective 2001). adv. software rev., video rev., Website rev. illus, maps, stat. 52 p./no. back issues avail. **Document type:** *Magazine, Academic/Scholarly.*
Formerly (until 2001): S E G - Zeitschrift fuer Schnell - Einsatz - Gruppen (1431-1216)
Published by: Stumpf und Kossendey Verlags GmbH, Postfach 1361, Edewecht 26183, Germany. TEL 49-4405-9181-0, FAX 49-4405-918133, einsatz@skverlag.de, buecher@skverlag.de, anzeigen@skverlag.de, http://www.skverlag.de. Ed. Klaus Smit. R&P Doortje Cramer Scharnagl TEL 49-4405-918120. Adv. contact Bianca Frey TEL 49-4405-918114. B&W page XEU 767, color page XEU 1,342; trim 210 x 297. Circ: 5,000.

IMAGE ANALYSIS AND STEREOLOGY. see *BIOLOGY*

IMPACT MEDECIN; les dossiers de F M C du praticien. see *BUSINESS AND ECONOMICS—Management*

610.711 USA
IMPACT (OMAHA). Text in English. ceased; resumed 1983. q. **Document type:** *Consumer.* **Description:** Covers issues associated with education, research, and medical care at the center.
Published by: University of Nebraska Medical Center, 985230 Nebraska Medical Center, Omaha, NE 68198-5230. TEL 402-559-4353, FAX 402-559-4103, ekumru@unmc.edu, http://www.unmc.edu. Ed., R&P Elizabeth Kumru TEL 402-559-4691. Circ: 9,000.

618.178059 USA ISSN 1071-2690
QH585 CODEN: IVCAED
IN VITRO CELLULAR & DEVELOPMENTAL BIOLOGY - ANIMAL. Text in English. 1965. 11/yr. USD 318 in North America; USD 351 elsewhere; USD 426 in North America Animal & Plant Parts; USD 495 elsewhere Animal & Plant Parts (effective 2001). adv. bk.rev. abstr. back issues avail. *Refereed.* **Document type:** *Academic/Scholarly.* **Description:** Publishes papers dealing with in vitro cultivation of cells, tissues, organs or tumors from multicellular animals.
Supersedes in part (in 1991): In Vitro Cellular and Developmental Biology (0883-8364); Which was formerly: In Vitro (0073-5655)
Related titles: Microform ed.: (from PQC); Online - full text ed.: (from Northern Light Technology, Inc., ProQuest Information & Learning, BioOne, Institute for Scientific Information).
Indexed: ASCA, Abstr.Bull.Inst.Pap.Chem., AgBiotech, Agri.& Environ.Biotech.Abstr., Agricola (coverage dropped), Anim.Breed.Abstr., BBCI, Bio-Contr.News & Info., Biol.Abstr., Chem.Abstr., Chem.Indus.Notes, Chem.Titles, Curr.Adv.Biochem., Curr.Adv.Cancer Res., Curr.Adv.Cell & Devel.Biol., Curr.Biotech.Abstr., Curr.Cont., Dairy Sci.Abstr., Dent.Ind., Derwent Biotech.Abstr., Environ.Sci.Poll.Mgmt., Excerp.Med., Helminthol.Abstr., Hort.Abstr., INIS Atomind., Ind.Med. (1993-), Ind.Sci.Rev., Ind.Vet., Inpharma, Int.Abstr.Biol.Sci., Med.& Pharm.Biotech.Abstr., Neurosci.Cit.Ind., Plant Grow.Reg.Abstr., Reac., Rev.Appl.Entomol., Sci.Cit.Ind., Small Anim.Abstr., Sorghum & Millets Abstr., Soyabean Abstr., Vet.Bull., Weed Abstr., Wild.Rev.

M

—BLDSC (4372.500520), CASDDS, CISTI, EMDOCS, GNLM, IDS, ingenta, Linda Hall. **CCC.**
Published by: Society for In Vitro Biology, Payment Processing Center, P O Box 73230, Baltimore, MD 21273. TEL 301-324-5054, FAX 301-324-5057, sivb@sivb.org, http://www.sivb.org. Ed. Dr. Wallace L McKeehan. Pub. Marietta Ellis. Adv. contact Denise McCall. Circ: 2,300 (paid). **Subscr. to:** Allen Press Inc., PO Box 1897, Lawrence, KS 66044-8897. TEL 785-3-1235.

IN VITRO REPORT. see *BIOLOGY—Physiology*

610 SWE ISSN 1103-503X
INCITAMENT/INCENTIVE; foer en haelso och sjukvaard i foervandling. Text in Swedish. 1992. bi-m. SEK 390 (effective 1999). adv. bk.rev. *Refereed.* **Document type:** *Journal, Trade.* **Description:** Publishes medical news and science for doctors, nurses, dentists and pharmacists.
Related titles: Online - full text ed.
Published by: Bra Mediafoerlag / Sverige AB, Fack 734, Arsta 12002, Sweden. red@incitement.com, http://www.incitament.com. Ed. Staffan Waplan Olsson. Pub. Ove Ernstroem. R&P, Adv. contact Annika Bergkvist. B&W page SEK 17,050, color page SEK 21,010; trim 255 x 173. Circ: 12,000.

616.98 IND ISSN 0970-6666
INDIAN JOURNAL OF AEROSPACE MEDICINE. Text in English. 1954. s-a. INR 200 domestic; USD 25 foreign; INR 100 newsstand/cover domestic; USD 15 newsstand/cover foreign (effective 1999). adv. bk.rev. back issues avail. **Document type:** *Academic/Scholarly.* **Description:** Includes original articles, topical reviews and other scientific information in the field of aerospace medicine and allied sciences.
Former titles (until 1988): Aviation Medicine (0250-5045); (until 1975): Journal of Aeromedical Society of India (0515-5207)
Related titles: Online - full text ed.
—CISTI.
Published by: Indian Society of Aerospace Medicine, Institute of Aerospace Medicine, Indian Air Force, Vimanapura PO, Bangalore, Karnataka 560 017, India. TEL 91-80-5273458, FAX 91-80-5274659, ijam@iam.kar.nic.in, http://www.indmed.delhi.nic.in. Ed. A K Sengupta. adv.: B&W page INR 2,500, color page INR 5,000. Circ: 800.

613.62 IND ISSN 0019-5278
CODEN: IJIDAW
INDIAN JOURNAL OF INDUSTRIAL MEDICINE. Variant title: Indian Association of Occupational Medicine. Journal. Text in English. 1949. q. INR 20, USD 5. bk.rev. abstr, bibl, charts, illus, stat. index, cum.index.
Indexed: Biol.Abstr., C.I.S. Abstr.
—CISTI, GNLM.
Published by: Indian Association of Occupational Health, 82-B Shakespeare Sarani, Kolkata, West Bengal 700 017, India. Ed. Dr. B B Chatterjee. Circ: 1,000.

INDIAN JOURNAL OF MEDICAL PHOTOGRAPHY. see *PHOTOGRAPHY*

616 IND ISSN 0971-5916
THE INDIAN JOURNAL OF MEDICAL RESEARCH. Text in English. 1913. m. USD 90; USD 9 newsstand/cover (effective 2001). *Refereed.*
Formed by the merger of: Indian Journal of Medical Research. Section A, Infectious Diseases (0970-955X); Indian Journal of Medical Research. Section B, Biomedical Research other than Infectious Diseases (0970-9568); Which superseded in part (in 1989): Indian Journal of Medical Research (0019-5340)
Related titles: Online - full text ed.: (from Institute for Scientific Information).
Indexed: Bibl.Asian Stud. (1971-1972), Curr.Cont., INIS Atomind., Ind.Med., Sci.Cit.Ind., Trop.Dis.Bull., Zoo.Rec.
—BLDSC (4416.500000).
Published by: Indian Council of Medical Research, Ansari Nagar, New Delhi 110 029, India. Ed. C S Chellaney.

610 IND ISSN 0367-9012
INDIAN JOURNAL OF MEDICAL RESEARCH. SUPPLEMENT. Text in English. 1922. irreg. INR 1,500, USD 90; subscr. includes Journal. bk.rev. bibl, charts. reprint service avail. from PQC,ISI. **Document type:** *Academic/Scholarly.* **Description:** Features original communications on a specific topic of biomedical research.
Indexed: Biol.Abstr., Chem.Abstr., Curr.Cont. (coverage dropped), Ind.Med. (coverage dropped), Nutr.Abstr., Sci.Cit.Ind. (coverage dropped), Trop.Dis.Bull.
—GNLM.
Published by: Indian Council of Medical Research, Division of Publication & Information, Ansari Nagar, P O Box 4911, New Delhi 110 029, India. TEL 91-11-6963980, FAX 91-11-6868662, icmrhqd@ren.nic.in. Ed. Dr. N Medappa. Circ: 700.

610 IND ISSN 0019-5359
CODEN: INJMAO
INDIAN JOURNAL OF MEDICAL SCIENCES. Text in English. 1947. m. INR 250 domestic; INR 750 foreign (effective 1999). adv. bk.rev. abstr, charts, illus. index. reprint service avail. from IRC. **Document type:** *Academic/Scholarly.*
Incorporates: Medical Bulletin
Indexed: Abstr.Hyg., Biol.Abstr., Chem.Abstr., Curr.Adv.Cancer Res., Curr.Adv.Ecol.Sci., Excerp.Med., INIS Atomind., Ind.Med. (1947-), Ind.Vet., NRN, Nutr.Abstr., Rev.Plant Path., Trop.Dis.Bull.
—BLDSC (4416.550000), CASDDS, CISTI, GNLM, ingenta, KNAW.
Published by: Indian Journal of Medical Sciences Trust, c/o J.C. Patel, Back Bay View, New Queen's Rd., Mumbai, Maharashtra 400 004, India. Ed. J.C. Patel. Pub. J C Patel. Circ: 3,000.

INDIAN JOURNAL OF PATHOLOGY & MICROBIOLOGY. see *BIOLOGY—Microbiology*

INDIAN JOURNAL OF VETERINARY ANATOMY. see *VETERINARY SCIENCE*

610 IND ISSN 0019-5847
CODEN: JIMAAD
INDIAN MEDICAL ASSOCIATION. JOURNAL. Text in English. 1931. m. INR 455, USD 60. bk.rev. abstr, charts, illus. reprint service avail. from PQC.
Indexed: Abstr.Hyg., Biol.Abstr., Chem.Abstr., Dent.Ind., Diar.Dis.Res., Excerp.Med., Helminthol.Abstr., INIS Atomind., Ind.Med. (1931-), Ind.Vet., Nutr.Abstr., Protozool.Abstr., Rev.Appl.Entomol., Rev.Med.& Vet.Mycol., Rev.Plant Path., Rural Devel.Abstr., Rural Recreat.Tour.Abstr., Trop.Dis.Bull., Vet.Bull.
—BLDSC (4767.400000), CASDDS, CISTI, GNLM, ingenta, KNAW.
Published by: Indian Medical Association, I.M.A House, 53 Creek Row, Kolkata, West Bengal 700 014, India. TEL 26-3598. adv.: B&W page INR 6,250; 260 x 220. Circ: 4,055.

INDIAN MEDICAL GAZETTE. see *MEDICAL SCIENCES—Surgery*

610 IND ISSN 0019-6169
THE INDIAN PRACTITIONER; a monthly journal of medicine, surgery & public health. Text in English. 1947. m. INR 200, USD 30. adv. bk.rev. reprint service avail. from IRC. **Document type:** *Trade.*
Related titles: ♦ Supplement to: Journal of General Medicine. ISSN 0970-566X.
Indexed: Biol.Abstr., Chem.Abstr., Dent.Ind., INIS Atomind., Ind.Med. (coverage dropped).
—CISTI, GNLM.
Published by: Indian Practitioner Group, 101, Lawrence Apartments-2, 1st Fl., Vidyanagari Marg, Opp. Lakhbir Petrol Pump, Kalina, Santa Cruz (E), Mumbai, Maharashtra 400 098, India. TEL 91-22-6116170. Ed. M E Yeolekar. Pub. A Peters. R&P Vincent Godinho. Circ: 43,967.

INDUSTRIAL HEALTH FOUNDATION. MEDICAL SERIES. BULLETINS. see *OCCUPATIONAL HEALTH AND SAFETY*

610 DEU ISSN 0300-8126
CODEN: IFTNAL
INFECTION; journal of infectious disease. Text in English, German. 1973. 6/yr. EUR 149.12 domestic; EUR 156.12 foreign; EUR 21.50 newsstand/cover (effective 2002). adv. bk.rev. back issues avail. *Refereed.* **Document type:** *Journal, Academic/Scholarly.*
Related titles: Online - full text ed.: ISSN 1439-0973 (from RoweCom Information Quest, Swets Blackwell, Springer LINK, Institute for Scientific Information).
Indexed: ASCA, Abstr.Hyg., Agri.& Environ.Biotech.Abstr. (coverage dropped), Aqua.Sci.& Fish.Abstr., Biol.Abstr., Chem.Abstr., Chem.Indus.Notes, Chem.Titles, Curr.Adv.Ecol.Sci., Curr.Cont., Dent.Ind., Derwent Biotech.Abstr., Environ.Sci.Poll.Mgmt., Excerp.Med., Helminthol.Abstr., INIS Atomind., Ind.Med. (1973-), Ind.Sci.Rev., Ind.Vet., Inpharma, Int.Abstr.Biol.Sci., Jrnl.Watch Inf.Dis., Med.& Surg.Dermat., Microbiol.Abstr., Nutr.Abstr., Pharm.&Out.News, Pollut.Abstr., Protozool.Abstr., Reac., Rev.Appl.Entomol., Rev.Med.& Vet.Mycol., Risk Abstr., SSCI (coverage dropped), Saf.Sci.Abstr., Sci.Cit.Ind., Trop.Dis.Bull., Vet.Bull., Virol.Abstr.
—BLDSC (4478.710000), ADONIS, CASDDS, CISTI, EMDOCS, GNLM, IDS, ingenta, KNAW. **CCC.**
Published by: (Deutsche Gesellschaft fuer Infektiologie), Urban und Vogel Medien und Medizin Verlagsgesellschaft mbH (Subsidiary of: BertelsmannSpringer), Neumarkter Str 43, Munich 81673, Germany. TEL 49-89-43721411, FAX 49-89-43721410, verlag@urban-vogel.de, http://www.urban-vogel.de. Ed. C Ruef. Pub., R&P Oliver Renn. Adv. contact Christiane Loichinger. **Subscr. to:** Springer Auslieferungs Gesellschaft, Postfach 105160, Heidelberg 69041, Germany. TEL 49-6221-345244, FAX 49-6221-345244.

610 576.5 NLD ISSN 1567-1348
▼ **INFECTION, GENETICS AND EVOLUTION.** Key Title: MEEGID. Variant title: Journal of Molecular Epidemiology and Evolutionary Genetics and Infectious Diseases. Text in English. 2001. q. EUR 313 in Europe to institutions; JPY 41,600 in Japan to institutions; USD 351 elsewhere to institutions (effective 2002). **Document type:** *Journal, Academic/Scholarly.* **Description:** Presents evaluations of the respective impact of genetic diversity of hosts, pathogens and vectors on the transmission and severity of infectious diseases, as well as their coevolutionary interactions.
Related titles: ♦ Online - full text ed.: Infection, Genetics and Evolution Online. ISSN 1567-7257.
Published by: Elsevier Science BV, Sara Burgerhartstraat 25, Amsterdam 1055 KV, Netherlands. TEL 31-20-485-2911, FAX 31-20-485-2457, nlinfo-f@elsevier.nl, http://www.elsevier.com/locate/meegid, http://www.elsevier.nl. Eds. M Achtman, Michael Tibayrenc.

INFECTIOUS DISEASE NEWS. see *MEDICAL SCIENCES—Communicable Diseases*

616.9 USA
INFECTIOUS DISEASE SPECIAL EDITION. Text and summaries in English. a. USD 30 domestic; USD 35 foreign (effective 2001); Free to qualified subscribers. adv. **Document type:** *Trade.* **Description:** Publishes a compendium of infection-related educational reviews, which cover a wide range of populations, from pediatric to immunocompromised patients — and topics, from respiratory infections to antifungal therapies.
Published by: McMahon Group, 545 W 45th St, 8th Fl, New York, NY 10036. TEL 212-957-5300, FAX 212-957-7230, cdeluca@mcmahonmed.com, http://www.mcmahonmed.com/se/indexse.htm. adv.: B&W page USD 3,300, color page USD 1,200.

610 USA ISSN 1056-9103
CODEN: IDCPEY
INFECTIOUS DISEASES IN CLINICAL PRACTICE. Text in English. 1991. 9/yr. USD 164 domestic to individuals; USD 206 foreign to individuals; USD 257 domestic to institutions; USD 304 foreign to institutions; USD 32 newsstand/cover (effective 2002). adv. *Refereed.* **Document type:** *Academic/Scholarly.* **Description:** For physicians who treat patients with infectious diseases.
Related titles: Microfilm ed.: (from WWS).
Indexed: ASCA, Curr.Cont., Dairy Sci.Abstr., Excerp.Med. (1994-), Helminthol.Abstr., Ind.Sci.Rev., Ind.Vet., Inpharma, Jrnl.Watch Inf.Dis., Nutr.Abstr., Pharm.&Out.News, Protozool.Abstr., Reac., Rev.Appl.Entomol., Rev.Med.& Vet.Mycol., SSCI (coverage dropped), Sci.Cit.Ind., Trop.Dis.Bull.
—BLDSC (4478.727950), CISTI, EMDOCS, GNLM, IDS, KNAW.
Published by: Williams & Wilkins (Subsidiary of: Waverly International), 351 W Camden St, Baltimore, MD 21201-2436. TEL 410-528-4068, 800-222-3790, FAX 410-528-4452, dbaker@wwilkins.com, http://www.wwilkins.com, http://www.Lww.com. Ed. Sherwood Gorbach. Adv. contact David Baker. B&W page USD 770; trim 10.88 x 8.13. Circ: 3,194; 2,935 (paid).

INFECTIOUS WASTES NEWS. see *ENVIRONMENTAL STUDIES—Waste Management*

610 FRA ISSN 0981-0560
L'INFIRMIERE MAGAZINE. Text in French. 1923. 11/yr. FRF 390 to individuals; FRF 490 to institutions; FRF 260 to students (effective 1999). adv. illus.
Formerly: Infirmiere Francaise (0019-9613)
Indexed: Int.Nurs.Ind.
—CISTI, GNLM, Infotrieve. **CCC.**
Published by: Initiatives Sante, 26 av. de l'Europe, BP 60, Velizy Villacoublay Cedex 78141, France. TEL 33-1-34633333, FAX 33-1-34653540. Ed. Marie-France Guerel. Pub. Marie France Guerel. Circ: 70,000.

M

610 USA ISSN 0360-3997
RB131 CODEN: INFLD4
INFLAMMATION. Text in English. 1975. bi-m. USD 710, EUR 709 to institutions for print or online ed.; USD 852, EUR 850.80 to institutions for print & online eds. combined (effective 2002). adv. illus. back issues avail. *Refereed.* **Document type:** *Journal, Academic/Scholarly.* **Description:** Reports the latest international advances in experimental and clinical research on the physiology, biochemistry, cell biology, and pharmacology of inflammation.
Related titles: Microfilm ed.: (from PQC); Online - full text ed.: EUR 110.50, USD 111 to individuals; EUR 639, USD 640 to institutions (effective 2001) (from EBSCO Publishing, O C L C Online Computer Library Center, Inc., RoweCom Information Quest, Swets Blackwell, Kluwer Online, Institute for Scientific Information).
Indexed: AIDS & Cancer Res., ASCA, Agri.& Environ.Biotech.Abstr. (coverage dropped), Biol.Abstr., Chem.Abstr., Chem.Indus.Notes, Chem.Titles, Curr.Adv.Biochem., Curr.Adv.Ecol.Sci., Curr.Cont., Derwent Biotech.Abstr., Excerp.Med., INIS Atomind., Immun.Abstr., Ind.Med. (1975-), Ind.Sci.Rev., Ind.Vet., Inpharma, Int.Abstr.Biol.Sci., Nutr.Abstr., Pharm.&Out.News, Protozool.Abstr., Reac., Ref.Zh., Rev.Med.& Vet.Mycol., Sci.Cit.Ind., THA, Vet.Bull.
—BLDSC (4478.845000), ADONIS, CASDDS, CISTI, EMDOCS, GNLM, IDS, ingenta, KNAW. **CCC.**
Published by: Kluwer Academic - Plenum Publishers (Subsidiary of: Wolters Kluwer N.V.), 233 Spring St, New York, NY 10013-1578. TEL 212-620-8000, 800-221-9369, FAX 212-463-0742, info@plenum.com, http://www.wkap.nl/journalhome.htm/0360-3997'. Ed. Bruce N Cronstein. R&P Rose Luongo TEL 781-871-6311. **Subscr. outside the Americas to:** Kluwer Academic Publishers Group, Journals Department, PO Box 322, Dordrecht 3300 AH, Netherlands. TEL 31-78-639-2392, FAX 31-78-654-6474.

INFLAMMOPHARMACOLOGY; experimental and clinical studies. see *PHARMACY AND PHARMACOLOGY*

610 ZAF
INFODOC DIARY; pure reading pleasure for health care professionals. Text in English. 1994. m. adv. illus. **Document type:** *Trade.*
Published by: Infodoc, PO Box 4168, Edenvale 1610, South Africa. TEL 27-11-6094536.

616 CHE ISSN 1021-9056
INFOKARA. Text in French. 1985. q. CHF 40, EUR 25.97 domestic to individuals; CHF 70, EUR 45.45 domestic to institutions; CHF 45, EUR 29.22 foreign to individuals; CHF 75, EUR 48.70 foreign to institutions (effective 2002). **Document type:** *Journal, Academic/Scholarly.*
Related titles: German ed.: ISSN 1422-3740. 1994.
Published by: Editions Medecine et Hygiene, Case Postale 456, Geneva, 4 1211, Switzerland. TEL 41-22-7029311, FAX 41-22-7029355, abonnements@medhyg.ch, http://www.medhyg.ch.

610 CHE ISSN 1422-0059
INFOMED SCREEN. Text in German. 10/yr. CHF 79, EUR 56 (effective 2000). **Document type:** *Newsletter, Trade.* **Description:** Presents articles on all aspects of evidence-based medicine.
Related titles: ♦ CD-ROM ed.: Infomed Screen (Year); ♦ Online - full text ed.: Infomed Screen Online.
Published by: Infomed-Verlag, Bergliweg 17, Wil 9500, Switzerland. TEL 41-71-9100866, FAX 41-71-9100877, infomed@infomed.org, http://www.infomed.org, http://www.infomed.org/pharma-kritik/. Ed., Pub. Dr. Etzel Gysling. Circ: 3,000 (controlled).

610 CHE
INFOMED SCREEN ONLINE. Text in German. 10/yr. **Document type:** *Trade.*
Media: Online - full text. **Related titles:** ♦ CD-ROM ed.: Infomed Screen (Year); ♦ Print ed.: Infomed Screen. ISSN 1422-0059.
Published by: Infomed-Verlag, Bergliweg 17, Wil 9500, Switzerland. TEL 41-71-9100866, FAX 41-71-9100877, infomed@infomed.org, http://www.infomed.org/screen/index.html, http://www.infomed.org/pharma-kritik/. Ed., Pub. Dr. Etzel Gysling.

610 CHE
INFOMED SCREEN (YEAR). Text in German. a. **Document type:** *Trade.*
Media: CD-ROM. **Related titles:** ♦ Online - full text ed.: Infomed Screen Online; ♦ Print ed.: Infomed Screen. ISSN 1422-0059.
Published by: Infomed-Verlag, Bergliweg 17, Wil 9500, Switzerland. TEL 41-71-9100866, FAX 41-71-9100877, infomed@infomed.org, http://www.infomed.org, http://www.infomed.org/pharma-kritik/. Ed., Pub. Dr. Etzel Gysling.

610 USA
INFONET GAZETTE. Text in English. m. **Document type:** *Newsletter.* **Description:** Dedicated to educate and inform health information professionals about the role of the Internet in healthcare and the technology and process of utilizing the sources of the Internet in their lives.
Media: Online - full text.
Published by: Health Net Services, Inc., 4636 S W, Loop, TX 76109. TEL 817-314-7337, FAX 817-314-7338, kmunn@infonetgazette.com, http://www.infonetgazette.com.

INFORMATICA Y SALUD. see *LIBRARY AND INFORMATION SCIENCES*

004 610 USA
INFORMATICS AND MEDICAL COMPUTING NEWS. Text in English. q. **Document type:** *Newsletter.*
Address: http://www.gasnet.org/journals/imcn/, http://gasnet.med.yale.edu/journals.html.

INFORMATIE & ZORG. see *MEDICAL SCIENCES—Computer Applications*

610 570 DEU ISSN 0943-5581
INFORMATIK, BIOMETRIE UND EPIDEMIOLOGIE; in Medizin und Biologie. Text in German. 1969. q. EUR 219 (effective 2002). **Document type:** *Journal, Academic/Scholarly.*
Former titles (until 1993): Biometrie und Informatik (0934-9235); E D V in Medizin und Biologie - E D V in Medicine and Biology (0300-8282)
Indexed: Biol.Abstr., Comput.Rev., Curr.Ind.Stat., Forest.Abstr., VITIS.
—CISTI, GNLM. **CCC.**
Published by: Urban & Fischer Verlag, Loebdergraben 14A, Jena 07743, Germany. TEL 49-3641-626430, FAX 49-3641-626421, info@urbanfischer.de, http://www.urbanfischer.de. Ed. Markus Loeffler. R&P Martin Huber TEL 49-3641-626430. Circ: 1,000. **Subscr. to:** Nature Publishing Group Specialist Journals.

610.6 ESP ISSN 0210-5365
INFORMATIVO MEDICO. Text in Spanish. 1974 (no.131). m. adv. bk.rev.
Formerly: Colegios Medicos de Espana. Consejo General. Boletin Informativo
Published by: Colegios Medicos de Espana, Consejo General, Villanueva, 11, Madrid 28001, Spain. Circ: 108,000.

610 RUS
INFORMATSIONNYI UKAZATEL' NORMATIVNYKH I METODICHESKIKH DOKUMENTOV MINZDRAVA ROSSII. Text in Russian. 1998. q. USD 155 in North America (effective 2000).
Published by: Informatsionno-Izdatel'skii Tsentr Goskomsanepidnadzora, Pr Aeroporta 11, Moscow 125167, Russian Federation. TEL 7-095-1986101. Ed. N E Akopova. **Dist. by:** East View Publications, 3020 Harbor Ln N, Minneapolis, MN 55447. TEL 763-550-0961, FAX 763-559-2931.

610 VEN ISSN 1316-9688
▼ **INFORME MEDICO.** Text in Spanish; Summaries in English. 1999. m. USD 130 (effective 2000 & 2001). adv. **Document type:** *Academic/Scholarly.* **Description:** A continuous medical education journal which considers articles from all medical subjects.
Published by: Publicidad Informe Medico de Venezuela/Informe Medico Publisher Group, Centro Empresarial los Ruices, Piso 5, Of. 514, Av Principal de los Ruices, Caracas 1050, Venezuela. TEL 58-2-2325293, 58-2-2390031, FAX 58-2-2397129, informed@telcel.net.ve. Ed., R&P Dr. Eduardo Romero Vecchione. Pub. Garcia Khatyuska. Adv. contact Luis Martinez. page USD 400;.

610 CHE ISSN 1424-5485
CODEN: IRANEE
INFUSION THERAPY AND TRANSFUSION MEDICINE. Text in English, German. 1974. bi-m. CHF 214, EUR 139 in Europe to institutions; CHF 231.40, USD 173 elsewhere to institutions (effective 2002). adv. illus. index. *Refereed.* **Document type:** *Journal, Academic/Scholarly.*
Former titles: Infusionstherapie und Transfusionsmedizin (1019-8466); (until 1992): Infusionstherapie (1011-6966); Internationale Zeitschrift fuer Infusionstherapie, Klinische Ernaehrung und Transfusionsmedizin; Infusionstherapie und Klinische Ernaehrung - Forschung und Praxis (0378-0791); Infusionstherapie und Klinische Ernaehrung (0301-3243); Infusionstherapie
Related titles: Microform ed.: (from PQC); Online - full text ed.: ISSN 1424-5493. CHF 58, EUR 42, USD 45 to institutions (effective 2002) (from EBSCO Publishing, O C L C Online Computer Library Center, Inc., RoweCom Information Quest, Swets Blackwell, Institute for Scientific Information); ♦ Supplement: Infusionstherapie und Transfusionsmedizin. Supplement. ISSN 1421-5799.
Indexed: ASCA, Biol.Abstr., Chem.Abstr., Curr.Cont., Excerp.Med., Ind.Med. (coverage dropped), Ind.Sci.Rev., Inpharma, Nutr.Abstr., Pharm.&Out.News, Reac., Rev.Med.& Vet.Mycol., Sci.Cit.Ind.
—BLDSC (4499.547000), CASDDS, CISTI, EMDOCS, GNLM, IDS, KNAW. **CCC.**
Published by: (Deutsche Arbeitsgemeinschaft fuer Kuenstliche Ernaehrung), S. Karger AG, Allschwilerstr 10, PO Box, Basel 4009, Switzerland. TEL 41-61-306-1111, FAX 41-61-306-1234, karger@karger.ch, http://www.online.karger.com/journals/iut, http://www.karger.com. Ed. V Kretschmer. Circ: 11,000. **Co-sponsor:** Deutsche Gesellschaft fuer Transfusionsmedizin und Immunhaematologie.

610 CHE ISSN 1421-5799
INFUSIONSTHERAPIE UND TRANSFUSIONSMEDIZIN. SUPPLEMENT. Text in English, German. 1993. irreg.
Related titles: ♦ Supplement to: Infusion Therapy and Transfusion Medicine. ISSN 1424-5485.
Published by: S. Karger AG, Allschwilerstr 10, PO Box, Basel 4009, Switzerland. TEL 41-61-306-1111, FAX 41-61-306-1234.

INNOVATIVE LEADER (ONLINE); monthly tool to increase creativity and productivity. see *BUSINESS AND ECONOMICS—Management*

614 362 USA ISSN 0046-9580
RA410.A1 CODEN: INQYA
INQUIRY (ROCHESTER); the journal of health care organization, provision and financing. Text in English. 1963. q. USD 53 in US & Canada to individuals (effective 2001); USD 75 elsewhere to individuals; USD 75 to institutions (effective 2001 & 2002); USD 60 in US & Canada to individuals (effective 2002). bk.rev. charts, illus. index, cum.index: 1963-1973, 1974-1978. back issues avail.; reprint service avail. from PQC. *Refereed.* **Document type:** *Academic/Scholarly.*
Related titles: Microform ed.: (from PQC); Online - full text ed.: (from ProQuest Information & Learning, Gale Group, Factiva, Institute for Scientific Information).
Indexed: ABI Inform. (Spr.1988-), Abstr.Health Care Manage.Stud., Abstr.Hyg., Acad.Ind., AgeLine, B.P.I. (Jan.1982-), BPIA, Bus.Ind., CINAHL, Curr.Cont., Excerp.Med., Hosp.Abstr., Hosp.Lit.Ind., Human Resour.Abstr., I.P.A., Ind.Med. (1963-), Inpharma, J.of Econ.Lit., Med.Care Rev., Mid.East: Abstr.& Ind., P.A.I.S., Pharm.&Out.News, Reac., SSCI, Sci.Cit.Ind., Soc.Sci.Ind. (coverage dropped), Tr.& Indus.Ind., Trop.Dis.Bull.
—BLDSC (4516.100000), GNLM, IDS, ingenta, KNAW. **CCC.**
Published by: Blue Cross and Blue Shield of the Rochester Area, PO Box 25399, Rochester, NY 14625. TEL 716-264-9122, FAX 716-264-9122, 716-264-9122, http://www.inquiryjournal.org. Eds. Katherine Swartz, Philip J. Puchalski. Pub. David J. Mack. R&P Ronny Frishman. Circ: 2,500. **Subscr. to:** PO Box 527, Glenview, IL 60025. TEL 847-724-9280, FAX 847-729-2199.

610 JPN ISSN 0288-7908
INSATSUKYOKU IHO/JAPAN. MINISTRY OF FINANCE. PRINTING BUREAU. MEDICAL JOURNAL. Text in English, Japanese; Summaries in English. 1955. s-a.
Indexed: Eng.Ind.
Published by: Insatsukyoku Igakkai/Ministry of Finance, Medical Association of the Printing Bureau, Okurasho Insatsukyoku Byoin, 3-6 Nishigahara 2-chome, Kita-ku, Tokyo 114-0024, Japan.

▼ **INSIDE THE HUMAN BODY.** see *BIOLOGY—Physiology*

INSIGHT (ATLANTA). see *MEETINGS AND CONGRESSES*

INSTITUT NATIONAL DE LA SANTE ET DE LA RECHERCHE MEDICALE. ACTUALITES. see *PUBLIC HEALTH AND SAFETY*

610 CAF
INSTITUT PASTEUR DE BANGUI. RAPPORT ANNUEL. Text in French. 1961. a. free per issue. adv. **Document type:** *Corporate.*
Former titles: Institut Pasteur de Bangui. Rapport Bisannuel; (until 1984): Institut Pasteur de Bangui. Rapport Annuel
Indexed: Biol.Abstr.
Published by: Institut Pasteur de Bangui, BP 923, Bangui, Central African Republic. FAX 236-610109. Circ: 200.

610 570 TUN ISSN 0020-2509 CODEN: APTUAO
INSTITUT PASTEUR DE TUNIS. ARCHIVES. Text in French. 1906. q. USD 25 (effective 1994). adv. bk.rev. **Document type:** *Academic/Scholarly.* **Description:** Publishes research in biology and medicine.
Related titles: CD-ROM ed.
Indexed: Abstr.Hyg., Bio-Contr.News & Info., Biol.Abstr., Chem.Abstr., Chem.Indus.Notes, Chem.Titles, Cott.& Trop.Fibr.Abstr., Curr.Adv.Ecol.Sci., Excerp.Med., ExtraMED, Helminthol.Abstr., Ind.Med. (1906-), Ind.Vet., Protozool.Abstr., Rev.Appl.Entomol., Rev.Med.& Vet.Mycol., Small Anim.Abstr., Trop.Dis.Bull., Vet.Bull.
—CASDDS, CISTI, GNLM, KNAW, Linda Hall.
Published by: Institut Pasteur de Tunis, 13 Place Pasteur, B P 74, Tunis Belvedere 1002, Tunisia. TEL 216-1-283022, FAX 216-1-791833, TELEX 14391 PAS TU. Ed. Koussay Dellagi. Circ: 700.

610 GBR ISSN 1364-6974
INSTITUTE OF HEALTH RECORD INFORMATION & MANAGEMENT. JOURNAL. Abbreviated title: I H R I M. Text in English. 1948. q. GBP 25 in United Kingdom to non-members; GBP 30 elsewhere to non-members (effective 2002); free to members. adv. bk.rev. charts, illus, stat. index, cum.index: 1965-1972. 48 p./no. **Document type:** *Newsletter, Academic/Scholarly.* **Description:** Contains articles and papers relevant to health records, informatics, and computing. Reports changes in government policy affecting members and includes member communications.
Former titles (until 1994): A M R O: The Journal for Health Care Information and Medical Records (1352-2329); (until 1988): Medical Records and Health Care Information Journal (0950-5539); (until 1977): Medical Record (0025-7478)
Related titles: Special ed.
Indexed: Excerp.Med., Hosp.Lit.Ind.
—GNLM.
Published by: Institute of Health Record Information & Management, c/o Kim Broom, AHRIM, 45 Cornubia Close, Tregurra Parc, Truro, Cornwall TR1 1SA, United Kingdom. TEL 44-1872-254644, FAX 44-1872-254989, broom@bellisb.freeserve.co.uk. adv.: page GBP 200. Circ: 1,000.

610 OMN
INSTITUTE OF HEALTH SCIENCES. QUARTERLY MEDICAL NEWS BULLETIN. Text in English. q.
Published by: Ministry of Health, Institute of Health Sciences, Ruwi, P O Box 6720, Muscat, Oman. TEL 560066, TELEX 5465.

636.089 610 AUS ISSN 0065-1907
INSTITUTE OF MEDICAL AND VETERINARY SCIENCE. ANNUAL REPORT OF THE COUNCIL. Text in English. 1937. a. free per issue. **Document type:** *Government.*
Published by: Institute of Medical and Veterinary Science, Frome Rd., Adelaide, SA, Australia. TEL 61-8-2287317, FAX 61-8-2287538. Ed. Dr. R J Kimber. Circ: 500.

610 NPL ISSN 0259-0972 CODEN: JIMEET
INSTITUTE OF MEDICINE. JOURNAL. Text in English. 1979. q. USD 12 per issue. adv. bk.rev. charts, illus.
Indexed: Abstr.Hyg., Diar.Dis.Res., Excerp.Med., Protozool.Abstr.
—EMDOCS, GNLM.
Published by: Institute of Medicine, P O Box 2533, Kathmandu, Nepal. Ed. Hemang Dixit. Circ: 500.

610 USA ISSN 0091-746X CODEN: PMICAP
INSTITUTE OF MEDICINE OF CHICAGO. PROCEEDINGS. Text in English. 1916. 2/yr. USD 25. adv. bk.rev. *Refereed.* **Document type:** *Proceedings, Academic/Scholarly.*
Indexed: Biol.Abstr., INIS Atomind.
—CISTI, GNLM.
Published by: Institute of Medicine of Chicago, 332 S Michigan Ave, Chicago, IL 60604-4022. TEL 312-663-0040, FAX 312-663-9058. Ed. Margaret Hastings. Adv. contact David Cugell. Circ: 4,000.

610 BGD ISSN 1017-9216 CODEN: JIPREF
INSTITUTE OF POSTGRADUATE MEDICINE AND RESEARCH. JOURNAL. Text in English. 1986. s-a. BDT 30 domestic; USD 10 foreign. **Document type:** *Academic/Scholarly.* **Description:** Publishes original articles, reviews, practical procedures, case reports on the latest developments in the field of medicine.
Indexed: Excerp.Med.
—BLDSC (4786.020000), EMDOCS.
Published by: Institute of Postgraduate Medicine and Research, Dhaka 1000, Bangladesh. Ed. T A Chowdhury.

INSTITUTION OF MECHANICAL ENGINEERS. PROCEEDINGS. PART H: JOURNAL OF ENGINEERING IN MEDICINE. see *BIOLOGY—Bioengineering*

610 BOL
INSTITUTO MEDICO "SUCRE". REVISTA. Text in Spanish. 1905. a. free per issue. adv. bk.rev. **Document type:** *Monographic series.* **Description:** Information on all aspects of health and medicine in Bolivia.
Published by: Instituto Medico "Sucre", Calle San Alberto, 30, Casilla de Correos 82, Sucre, Bolivia. TEL 591-64-21956, FAX 591-64-25559. Ed. Dr. Antonio Dubravcic Luksic. Adv. contact Gonzalo Virreira Reyes.

INSTITUTO OSWALDO CRUZ, RIO DE JANEIRO. MEMORIAS. see *BIOLOGY*

610 DEU ISSN 0942-6035
INTENSIV; Fachzeitschrift fuer Intensivpflege und Anaesthesie. Text in German. 1993. 6/yr. EUR 83.80 domestic to institutions; EUR 89.60 in Europe to institutions; EUR 93.80 elsewhere to institutions; EUR 16 newsstand/cover (effective 2002). adv. bk.rev. index. back issues avail.; reprints avail. *Refereed.* **Document type:** *Journal, Academic/Scholarly.*
Related titles: Diskette ed.; Online - full text ed.: ISSN 1439-3840.
—GNLM.
Published by: Georg Thieme Verlag, Ruedigerstr 14, Stuttgart 70469, Germany. TEL 49-711-8931-0, FAX 49-711-8931298, leser.service@thieme.de, http://www.thieme.de/intensiv. Ed. Angelika Stockinger. R&P Peter Eich. adv.: page DEM 2,200; trim 175 x 250. Circ: 3,400 (paid).

610 DEU ISSN 0947-5362 CODEN: NTNSDQ
INTENSIV- UND NOTFALLBEHANDLUNG. Text in German. 1976. q. DEM 108, EUR 55.22; DEM 28, EUR 14.32 newsstand/cover (effective 2001). adv. **Document type:** *Journal, Academic/Scholarly.*
Formerly: Intensivbehandlung (0341-3063)
Indexed: Biol.Abstr., Curr.Adv.Ecol.Sci., Curr.Cont. (coverage dropped), Excerp.Med., INIS Atomind., Ref.Zh.
—BLDSC (4531.833000), CISTI, EMDOCS, GNLM, Infotrieve, KNAW. **CCC.**
Published by: Dustri-Verlag Dr. Karl Feistle, Bajuwarenring 4, Oberhaching 82041, Germany. TEL 49-89-613861-0, FAX 49-89-613-5412, info@dustri.de, http://www.dustri.de. Ed. Dr. K Werdan. R&P Renate Lehmann. Adv. contact Joerg Feistle. B&W page DEM 1,720, B&W page XEU 879.72; trim 167 x 242. Circ: 1,500.

614.88 GBR ISSN 0967-5728
INTENSIVE CARE BRITAIN (YEAR). Text in English. 1992. a. GBP 35 in United Kingdom to individuals; GBP 60 in Europe to individuals; GBP 75 elsewhere to individuals; GBP 50 in United Kingdom to institutions; GBP 75 in Europe to institutions; GBP 90 elsewhere to institutions. adv. **Document type:** *Trade.*
—GNLM.
Published by: Greycoat Publishing, 1 Harley St, London W1N 1DA, United Kingdom. TEL 44-20-7637-1828, FAX 44-20-7631-3020. Ed. Michael Rennie. Pub., Adv. contact Ashley Wallis. R&P Guy Wallis.

610 DEU ISSN 0342-4642 CODEN: ICMED9
INTENSIVE CARE MEDICINE. Text in English. 1974. m. EUR 595.90 domestic; EUR 576.70 in Germany; EUR 55 newsstand/cover foreign (effective 2002). back issues avail.; reprint service avail. from ISI. *Refereed.* **Document type:** *Journal, Academic/Scholarly.* **Description:** Provides information for those concerned with pre-clinical subjects and medical sciences basic to intensive care, critical care, internal medicine, bioengineering, surgery and anaesthesiology.
Formerly: European Journal of Intensive Care Medicine
Related titles: Microform ed.: (from PQC); Online - full text ed.: ISSN 1432-1238 (from EBSCO Publishing, RoweCom Information Quest, Swets Blackwell, Springer LINK, Institute for Scientific Information).
Indexed: AIDS Abstr., ASCA, Abstr.Hyg., Curr.Cont., Excerp.Med., INIS Atomind., Ind.Med. (1977-), Ind.Sci.Rev., Inpharma, Int.Nurs.Ind., Neurosci.Cit.Ind., Nutr.Abstr., Pharm.&Out.News, Protozool.Abstr., Reac., Rev.Med.& Vet.Mycol., SSCI (coverage dropped), Sci.Cit.Ind., Sugar Ind.Abstr., Trop.Dis.Bull.
—BLDSC (4531.837000), ADONIS, CASDDS, CISTI, EMDOCS, GNLM, IDS, ingenta, KNAW. **CCC.**
Published by: (European Society of Intensive Care Medicine), Springer-Verlag (Subsidiary of: BertelsmannSpringer), Tiergartenstr 17, Heidelberg 69121, Germany. TEL 49-6221-345-0, FAX 49-6221-345229, subscriptions@springer.de, http://link.springer.de/link/service/journals/00134/index.htm, http://www.springer.de. Ed. K J Falke. **Subscr. in N. America to:** Springer-Verlag New York Inc., PO Box 2485, Secaucus, NJ 07096-2485. TEL 212-460-1500, FAX 212-473-6272. **Co-sponsor:** European Society for Pediatric Intensive Care.

610 GBR ISSN 1360-306X
INTENSIVE CARE MONITOR. Text in English. bi-m. GBP 60; GBP 12 newsstand/cover (effective 2001 & 2002). **Document type:** *Academic/Scholarly.* **Description:** For those specializing in intensive care.
Formerly (until 1994): Intensive Care World Monitor (1353-5625)
Published by: D W L Ltd., 14 Temple Fortune Ln, London NW11 7UD, United Kingdom. TEL 44-20-8455-0760, FAX 44-20-8201-8955, wirth.icm@btinternet.com, http://www.intensive-care-monitor.com. Ed. Dr. Mark Smithies. Pub. Lynda A Wirth.

610 542 GBR ISSN 0266-7037
INTENSIVE CARE WORLD. Text in English. 1984. q. GBP 33, USD 40. adv. bk.rev. abstr, bibl, illus. *Refereed.* **Document type:** *Academic/Scholarly.* **Description:** Articles about state-of-the-art intensive and critical care medicine.
Indexed: Curr.Adv.Ecol.Sci.
—GNLM.
Published by: King & Wirth Publishing Co. Ltd., 14 Temple Fortune Ln, London NW11 7UD, United Kingdom. TEL 44-181-455-0760, FAX 44-181-201-8955. Ed. Geoffrey Dobb. R&P, Adv. contact Lynda Wirth. Circ: 26,163. **Subscr. to:** 85 Campden St, London W8 7EN, United Kingdom.

610 DEU ISSN 0175-3851 CODEN: INNOEK
INTENSIVMEDIZIN UND NOTFALLMEDIZIN; German interdisciplinary journal of intensive care medicine. Text in German; Summaries in English. 1961. 8/yr. EUR 424.16 domestic; EUR 438.26 in Germany; EUR 63.10 newsstand/cover foreign (effective 2002). adv. bk.rev. back issues avail.; reprints avail. *Refereed.* **Document type:** *Journal, Academic/Scholarly.*
Former titles: Intensivmedizin (0303-6251); Wiederbelebung-Organersatz-Intensivmedizin (0043-5252)
Related titles: Microform ed.: (from PQC); Online - full text ed.: ISSN 1435-1420 (from EBSCO Publishing, RoweCom Information Quest, Swets Blackwell, Springer LINK).
Indexed: Biol.Abstr., Curr.Cont. (coverage dropped), Excerp.Med.
—BLDSC (4531.845000), CASDDS, CISTI, GNLM, Infotrieve, KNAW. **CCC.**
Published by: Dr. Dietrich Steinkopff Verlag, Poststr 9, Darmstadt 64293, Germany. TEL 49-6151-82899-0, FAX 49-6151-82899-40, frey.steinkopff@springer.de, http://www.steinkopff.springer.de. Adv. contact Cornelia Haenzi TEL 49-30-82787448. Circ: 2,500. **Subscr. in N. America to:** Springer-Verlag, Journals; **Subscr. to:** Springer GmbH Auslieferungsgesellschaft, Haberstr 7, Heidelberg 69126, Germany. FAX 49-6221-345249.

610 NER ISSN 0534-4735
INTER-AFRICAN CONFERENCE ON MEDICAL CO-OPERATION. MEETING*. Text in English, French. irreg., latest vol.3, 1955. **Document type:** *Proceedings.*
Published by: (Commission for Technical Co-Operation in Africa South of the Sahara), Maison de l'Afrique, BP 878, Niamey, Niger.

610 USA
INTERACTIVE MEDICINE. Text in English. 1998. q. USD 98. **Document type:** *Academic/Scholarly.*

M

Published by: Elsevier Science, PO Box 945, New York, NY 10159-0945. TEL 212-989-5800, FAX 212-633-3990, usinfo-f@elsevier.com; nlinfo-f@elsevier.nl, http://www.elsevier.nl/., http://www.elsevier.com. **Subscr. outside the Americas to:** Elsevier Science BV, PO Box 211, Amsterdam 1000 AE, Netherlands. TEL 31-20-485-3757, http://www.elsevier.nl.

610 ESP
INTERCON. Text in Spanish. 1967. a. ESP 6,000 domestic; USD 60 foreign (effective 2001). **Document type:** *Academic/Scholarly.*
Published by: Editores Medicos S.A., Gabriela Mistral, 2, Madrid 28035, Spain. TEL 34-91-3768140, FAX 34-91-3739907. Circ: 30,000.

610 CHE
▼ **INTER@CTIVA**; das multimediale Magazin der Medical Tribune. Text in German. 1999. m. adv. **Document type:** *Journal, Academic/Scholarly.* **Description:** Provides vital and up-to-date information to the medical community through multimedia applications.
Media: Online - full text.
Published by: Medical Tribune AG, Urs-Graf-Str 8, Postfach 368, Basel 4020, Switzerland. TEL 41-61-3125566, FAX 41-61-3125560, pmueller@medical-tribune.ch, http://www.medical-tribune.ch.

INTERFACES: LINGUISTICS, PSYCHOLOGY AND HEALTH THERAPEUTICS; an international journal of research, notes and commentary. see *LINGUISTICS*

610 CHE ISSN 0026-9212
INTERKANTONALE KONTROLLSTELLE FUER HEILMITTEL. MONATSBERICHT/OFFICE INTERCANTONAL DE CONTROLE DE MEDICAMENTS. BULLETIN MENSUEL/UFFICIO INTERCANTONALE DI CONTROLLO DEI MEDICAMENTI. BOLLETTINO MENSILE. Text in French, German, Italian. 1947. m. CHF 110; CHF 130 foreign. adv. index. **Document type:** *Bulletin.*
Published by: Interkantonale Kontrollstelle fuer Heilmittel, Erlachstr 8, Bern, 9 3000, Switzerland. FAX 031-240654. Circ: 3,000.

INTERNATIONAL ACADEMY OF LEGAL MEDICINE AND SOCIAL MEDICINE. CONGRESS REPORTS. see *MEDICAL SCIENCES—Forensic Sciences*

610 GBR
INTERNATIONAL BACK PAIN NEWS. Text in English. 1986. 3/yr. GBP 30.
Published by: (International Back Pain Society), Congress Team International (U.K.) Ltd., 15 Bedford Rd, Northwood, Mddx HA6 2BA, United Kingdom. TEL 081 206 0426, FAX 081-206-0427.

610 GBR ISSN 0962-4570
INTERNATIONAL CLINICAL PRACTICE SERIES. Text in English. irreg. **Document type:** *Monographic series.*
—BLDSC (4538.673700).
Published by: Wells Medical Ltd., Speldhurst Pl, Speldhurst Rd, Royal Tunbridge Wells, Kent TN4 0JB, United Kingdom. TEL 44-1892-511600, FAX 44-1892-511400, info@wellsmed.co.uk.

INTERNATIONAL DIRECTORY OF MEDICAL, HOSPITAL AND SURGICAL EQUIPMENT IMPORTERS. see *BUSINESS AND ECONOMICS—Trade And Industrial Directories*

INTERNATIONAL ENCYCLOPAEDIA OF LAWS. MEDICAL LAW. see *LAW*

610 NLD ISSN 0074-6037
INTERNATIONAL FEDERATION OF MEDICAL STUDENTS' ASSOCIATIONS. MINUTES AND REPORTS OF THE GENERAL ASSEMBLY. Text in Dutch. 1951. a. **Document type:** *Proceedings.*
Published by: International Federation of Medical Students' Associations, c/o W M A, Cedex, B.P. 63, Ferney Voltaire Cedex 01212, France. TEL 33-450404759, FAX 33-450-40-5937, ifmasa@uva.nl. Circ: 150.

610 NLD
INTERNATIONAL FEDERATION OF MEDICAL STUDENTS' ASSOCIATIONS. NEWSLETTER. Text in Dutch. bi-m. membership only. **Document type:** *Newsletter.*
Published by: International Federation of Medical Students' Associations, c/o W M A, Cedex, B.P. 63, Ferney Voltaire Cedex 01212, France. TEL 33-450404759, FAX 33-450-40-5937, ifmsa@amc.uva.nl.

174.2 362.1 USA ISSN 1073-5771
INTERNATIONAL HEALTHCARE ETHICS. Text in English. 1994. irreg., latest vol.2, 1996. CHF 68 domestic; USD 53.95 foreign (effective 2000). **Document type:** *Monographic series, Academic/Scholarly.*
Published by: Peter Lang Publishing, Inc., 275 Seventh Ave, 28th Fl, New York, NY 10001. TEL 212-647-7706, 800-770-5264, FAX 212-475-7707, customerservice@plang.com, http://www.peterlang.com. Ed. Juliet Rothman. Pub. Christopher Myers. R&P Stephanie Archer. Adv. contact Patricia Mulrane.

610 BEL
INTERNATIONAL HOSPITAL EQUIPMENT & SOLUTIONS; The Magazine for Healthcare Decision Makers. Text in English. 1975. 8/yr. BEF 3,000; USD 95 foreign (effective 1999). adv. illus. **Document type:** *Magazine, Trade.* **Description:** Reports on medical technology news & solutions for the modern hospital.
Indexed: Key to Econ.Sci.
Published by: Elsevier Business Information - Belgium (Subsidiary of: Reed Elsevier plc), Rue des Palais 100, Brussels B-1030, Belgium. TEL 603-778-3848, 32-2-240-2611, FAX 603-778-3858, 32-2-242-7111, ebi@ebi.be, http://www.ebi.be. Ed. Poeny Derom. Pub., R&P Dr. Bernard Leger. Adv. contacts Astrid Wydouw, Louise Betton TEL 603-778-3848. Circ: 30,005 (controlled).

610 GBR ISSN 1353-4505
RA399.A1 CODEN: IJQCF6
INTERNATIONAL JOURNAL FOR QUALITY IN HEALTH CARE. Text in English. 1989. bi-m. GBP 60, USD 99 to individuals; GBP 335, USD 570 to institutions (effective Feb. 2002). adv. bk.rev. back issues avail. *Refereed.* **Document type:** *Journal, Academic/Scholarly.* **Description:** Seeks to make more widely available the results of quality assessment studies and quality assurance activities.
Formerly (until 1994): Quality Assurance in Health Care (1040-6166)
Related titles: Microfilm ed.: (from PQC); Online - full text ed.: ISSN 1464-3677. GBP 301, USD 513 to institutions Online only (effective Feb. 2002) (from EBSCO Publishing, O C L C Online Computer Library Center, Inc., RoweCom Information Quest, ingenta, Swets Blackwell, Institute for Scientific Information).
Indexed: ASCA, AgeLine, Brit.Nur.Ind., Curr.Cont., Environ.Sci.Poll.Mgmt., Ind.Med. (1994-), Int.Nurs.Ind., Pollut.Abstr., Risk Abstr., SSCI, Saf.Sci.Abstr.
—BLDSC (4542.510500), GNLM, IDS, ingenta, KNAW. **CCC.**
Published by: Oxford University Press, Academic Division, Great Clarendon St, Oxford OX2 6DP, United Kingdom. TEL 44-1865-267907, FAX 44-1865-267835, ritterc@oup.co.uk, jnl.info@oup.co.uk, http://www.oup.co.uk/journals. Ed. R Heather Palmer. Pub. Mandy Sketch. adv.: B&W page GBP 536, B&W page USD 965; trim 178 x 255. Circ: 1,500. **US Subscr. addr.:** Oxford University Press, Journals. TEL 800-852-7323, FAX 919-677-1714; **Subscr. to:** Journals Marketing, Great Clarendon St, Oxford OX2 6DP, United Kingdom.

INTERNATIONAL JOURNAL OF ANTI-AGING MEDICINE. see *GERONTOLOGY AND GERIATRICS*

610 619 ITA ISSN 0391-3988
RD130 Db .I576 CODEN: IJAODS
INTERNATIONAL JOURNAL OF ARTIFICIAL ORGANS. Text in English. 1978. m. EUR 368 in Europe to individuals; USD 420 elsewhere to individuals; EUR 488, USD 530 in Europe to institutions (effective 2001). adv. abstr, bibl, charts, illus. Index. 64 p./no. back issues avail.; reprints avail. *Refereed.* **Document type:** *Journal, Academic/Scholarly.* **Description:** Provides the most current information available on clinical and experimental developments in the field of artificial organs. Automated therapeutic aids and devices are covered in occasional articles.
Incorporates: Life Support Systems (0261-989X)
Related titles: Online - full text ed.: (from Institute for Scientific Information).
Indexed: ASCA, Chem.Abstr., Chem.Indus.Notes, Chem.Titles, Curr.Cont., Excerp.Med., Ind.Med. (1978-), Ind.Sci.Rev., Inpharma, Int.Nurs.Ind., Kidney, METADEX, Mat.Sci.Cit.Ind., Pharm.&Out.News, Protozool.Abstr., Reac., Ref.Zh., Rev.Med.& Vet.Mycol., SSCI (coverage dropped), Sci.Cit.Ind.
—BLDSC (4542.105000), CASDDS, CISTI, EMDOCS, GNLM, IDS, ingenta, KNAW. **CCC.**
Published by: Wichtig Editore s.r.l., Via Friuli, 72, Milan, MI 20135, Italy. TEL 39-02-55195443, FAX 39-02-55195971, info@wichtig-publisher.com, http://www.artificial-organs.com. Ed. Dr. Diego Brancaccio. R&P, Adv. contact Lucia Steele. color page USD 1,450; trim 21 x 28. Circ: 2,000.

610 700 USA ISSN 1057-4263
R702.5
INTERNATIONAL JOURNAL OF ARTS MEDICINE. Abbreviated title: I J A M. Text in English. 1991. s-a. USD 20 domestic to individuals; USD 25 foreign to individuals; USD 30 domestic to institutions; USD 35 foreign to institutions (effective 2000). adv. bk.rev. charts, illus. back issues avail. *Refereed.* **Document type:** *Academic/Scholarly.* **Description:** Offers a theoretical, clinical, and philosophical exploration of the creative arts and healing. Covers international conferences, presents current research, and contains reviews of media resources and interviews.
Indexed: CINAHL, Int.Ind.Mus.Per., Music Ind., PsycInfo, RILM, e-psyche.
—BLDSC (4542.105500), GNLM.
Published by: I J A M, M M B Music, Inc., Contemporary Arts Bldg, 3526, Washington, MO 63103-1019. TEL 314-531-9635, FAX 314-531-8384, mmmbmusic@mmbmusic.com, http://www.mmmbmusic.com. Ed. Rosalie Rebollo Pratt. Pub. Norman A Goldberg. R&P Norman Goldberg. Adv. contact Marcia Lee Goldberg. Circ: 1,000. **Co-sponsors:** International Arts Medicine Association; International Society for Music in Medicine.

INTERNATIONAL JOURNAL OF BIOMETEOROLOGY; the description, causes, and implications of climatic change. see *METEOROLOGY*

610 236 FIN ISSN 1239-9736
RC955 CODEN: AMRSEP
INTERNATIONAL JOURNAL OF CIRCUMPOLAR HEALTH. Text in English. 1972. q. USD 25, EUR 29 to individuals; USD 75, EUR 87 to institutions (effective 2002). adv. bk.rev. back issues avail. *Refereed.* **Document type:** *Journal, Academic/Scholarly.* **Description:** Research articles related to circumpolar health including medical, anthropological, sociological, and physical subjects.
Former titles (until 1997): Arctic Medical Research (0782-226X); (until 1984): Nordic Countil for Medical Research. Report (0355-9823); (until 1973): Nordiska Samarbetskomitteen foer Arktisk Medicinsk Forskning - Meddelande (0358-7894)
Indexed: GeoRef, Ind.Med. (1997-), Int.Nurs.Ind.
—BLDSC (4542.167250), CISTI, GNLM, ingenta.
Published by: International Union for Circumpolar Health, P O Box 212001, Anchorage, AK 995212001. TEL 907-786-6576, FAX 907-786-6591, juhani.hassi@ou/u.fi. Ed. Peter Bjerregaard. R&P, Adv. contact Juhani Hassi TEL 358-8-553 7550. B&W page USD 950, color page USD 1,930. Circ: 700 (controlled). **Co-sponsor:** Nordic Society for Arctic Medicine.

INTERNATIONAL JOURNAL OF CLINICAL ACUPUNCTURE. see *ALTERNATIVE MEDICINE*

610 GBR ISSN 1368-5031
R11 CODEN: BJCPAT
INTERNATIONAL JOURNAL OF CLINICAL PRACTICE. Text in English. 1947. 10/yr. GBP 75 in United Kingdom; GBP 100, USD 160 overseas (effective 2001); Supplements included in journal subscription rates. adv. bk.rev. bibl, illus. index. *Refereed.* **Document type:** *Journal, Academic/Scholarly.* **Description:** Publishes original papers, reviews, features, case reports and meeting reports.
Formerly: British Journal of Clinical Practice (0007-0947)
Related titles: Online - full text ed.: (from Institute for Scientific Information); ♦ Supplement: International Journal of Clinical Practice. Symposium Supplement. ISSN 1368-504X.
Indexed: ASCA, Abstr.Hyg., Agri.& Environ.Biotech.Abstr. (coverage dropped), Cal.Tiss.Abstr., Chem.Abstr., Chem.Indus.Notes, Chem.Titles, Curr.Adv.Ecol.Sci., Curr.Cont., Derwent Biotech.Abstr., Environ.Sci.Poll.Mgmt., Excerp.Med., Helminthol.Abstr., INIS Atomind., I.P.A., Ind.Med. (1997-), Ind.Sci.Rev., Inpharma, Int.Nurs.Ind., Microbiol.Abstr., NRN, Nutr.Abstr., Pharm.&Out.News, Pollut.Abstr., Reac., Rev.Appl.Entomol., Rev.Med.& Vet.Mycol., Risk Abstr., Saf.Sci.Abstr., Sci.Cit.Ind., Sp.Ed.Needs Abstr., THA, Trop.Dis.Bull.
—BLDSC (4542.172160), CASDDS, CISTI, GNLM, IDS, ingenta, KNAW.

M

Published by: Medicom International Ltd., Churston House, Portsmouth Rd, Esher, Surrey KT10 9AD, United Kingdom. TEL 44-1372-471671, FAX 44-1372-471672. Ed. Graham Jackson. Pub., R&P, Adv. contact Michael Young. Circ: 2,500 (paid). **Subscr. to:** c/o Laura Young, 42 Avondale Ave, Hinchley Wood, Esher, Surrey KT10 0DA, United Kingdom. TEL 44-20-8339-0300, FAX 44-20-8398-3361.

610 GBR ISSN 1368-504X
CODEN: ICPSFY

INTERNATIONAL JOURNAL OF CLINICAL PRACTICE. SYMPOSIUM SUPPLEMENT. Text in English. 1979. irreg., latest vol.90, 1997. GBP 16 per issue For non-subscribers to the journal; USD 32 per issue foreign For non-subscribers to the journal. adv. *Refereed.* **Document type:** *Monographic series.*

Formerly (until 1996): British Journal of Clinical Practice. Symposium Supplement (0262-8767)

Related titles: ♦ Supplement to: International Journal of Clinical Practice. ISSN 1368-5031.

Indexed: Environ.Sci.Poll.Mgmt., Ind.Med. (1997-), Microbiol.Abstr., Pollut.Abstr., Risk Abstr., Saf.Sci.Abstr.

—BLDSC (4542.172165), CASDDS, CISTI, ingenta.

Published by: Medicom International Ltd., Churston House, Portsmouth Rd, Esher, Surrey KT10 9AD, United Kingdom. TEL 44-1372-471671, FAX 44-1372-471672. Ed. Graham Jackson. Pub., R&P, Adv. contact Michael Young. Circ: 2,500 (paid).

INTERNATIONAL JOURNAL OF ENVIRONMENTAL HEALTH RESEARCH. see *ENVIRONMENTAL STUDIES*

614.4 GBR ISSN 0300-5771
RA651 CODEN: IJEPBF

INTERNATIONAL JOURNAL OF EPIDEMIOLOGY. Text in English. 1972. bi-m. GBP 265, USD 485; GBP 150, USD 245 in developing nations to institutions (effective Feb. 2002). adv. bk.rev. illus. index. back issues avail.; reprint service avail. from PQC. *Refereed.* **Document type:** *Journal, Academic/Scholarly.* **Description:** Epidemiology of infectious and non-infectious diseases. Includes research results, new methods, statistical or otherwise, for the analysis of data used by those who practice social and preventive medicine.

Related titles: Microform ed.: (from PQC); Online - full text ed.: ISSN 1464-3685. GBP 238, USD 436 to institutions Online only (effective Feb. 2002) (from HighWire Pr., Northern Light Technology, Inc., EBSCO Publishing, O C L C Online Computer Library Center, Inc., RoweCom Information Quest, ingenta, Swets Blackwell, Institute for Scientific Information).

Indexed: AIDS Abstr., ASCA, Abstr.Hyg., Addic.Abstr., Aqua.Sci.& Fish.Abstr., Bibl.Dev.Med.& Child Neur., Biol.Abstr., Biol.Dig., C.I.S. Abstr., CSNB, Crim.Just.Abstr., Curr.Adv.Cancer Res., Curr.Adv.Ecol.Sci., Curr.Cont., Curr.Ind.Stat., Dairy Sci.Abstr., Dent.Ind., Diar.Dis.Res., Environ.Sci.Poll.Mgmt., Excerp.Med., Geo.Abstr.H.G., Helminthol.Abstr., IDA, INIS Atomind., Ind.Med. (1972-), Ind.Sci.Rev., Ind.Vet., Inpharma, Int.Abstr.Biol.Sci., Int.Nurs.Ind., Lab.Haz.Bull., NRN, Nutr.Abstr., Pharm.&Out.News, Pollut.Abstr., Popul.Ind., Poult.Abstr., Protozool.Abstr., Reac., Rev.Appl.Entomol., Rev.Med.& Vet.Mycol., Risk Abstr., Rural Devel.Abstr., SSCI (coverage dropped), Saf.Sci.Abstr., Sci.Cit.Ind., Sel.Water Res.Abstr., Small Anim.Abstr., THA, Trop.Dis.Bull., Vet.Bull., W.R.C.Inf., World Ag.Econ.& Rur.Soc.Abstr.

—BLDSC (4542.244000), CISTI, EMDOCS, GNLM, IDS, ingenta, KNAW. **CCC.**

Published by: (International Epidemiological Association), Oxford University Press, Academic Division, Great Clarendon St, Oxford OX2 6DP, United Kingdom. TEL 44-1865-267907, FAX 44-1865-267835, jnl.info@oup.co.uk, http://www.ije.oupjournals.org/, http://www.oup.co.uk/journals. Eds. George Davey Smith, Shah Ebrham. Pub. Mandy Sketch. R&P Fionna Willis. adv.: B&W page GBP 400, B&W page USD 720; trim 178 x 255. Circ: 3,350. **Subscr. to:** Journals Marketing, Great Clarendon St, Oxford OX2 6DP, United Kingdom. **Affiliate:** Oxford University Press, Journals.

616.07 GBR ISSN 0959-9673
CODEN: IJEPEI

INTERNATIONAL JOURNAL OF EXPERIMENTAL PATHOLOGY. Text in English. 1920. bi-m., latest vol.83, 2002. GBP 285 in Europe to institutions; USD 451 in North America to institutions; GBP 313 elsewhere to institutions; GBP 313.50 in Europe to institutions for print and online eds.; USD 496.10 in North America to institutions for print and online eds.; GBP 344.30 elsewhere to institutions for print and online eds. (effective 2002). adv. abstr, bibl, illus. index. reprint service avail. from PQC. *Refereed.* **Document type:** *Academic/Scholarly.* **Description:** REports original experimental investigations into the biogenesis and progression of pathologic processes which afford new insights into the basic mechanisms underlying human disease.

Formerly: British Journal of Experimental Pathology (0007-1021)

Related titles: Microform ed.: (from PQC); Online - full text ed.: ISSN 1365-2613. GBP 257 in Europe; USD 406 in North America; GBP 257 elsewhere (effective 2002) (from Ovid Technologies, Inc., EBSCO Publishing, O C L C Online Computer Library Center, Inc., RoweCom Information Quest, ingenta, Munksgaard & Blackwell Science's Synergy, Swets Blackwell, Institute for Scientific Information).

Indexed: ASCA, Abstr.Hyg., AgBiotech, Agri.& Environ.Biotech.Abstr. (coverage dropped), Anim.Breed.Abstr., Biol.Abstr., Chem.Abstr., Chem.Indus.Notes, Chem.Titles, Curr.Adv.Cancer Res., Curr.Adv.Ecol.Sci., Curr.Cont., Dairy Sci.Abstr., Dent.Ind., Derwent Biotech.Abstr., Excerp.Med., Helminthol.Abstr., INIS Atomind., Ind.Med. (1990-), Ind.Sci.Rev., Ind.Vet., Inpharma, Int.Abstr.Biol.Sci., Lab.Haz.Bull., Nutr.Abstr., Pharm.&Out.News, Protozool.Abstr., Reac., Ref.Zh., Rev.Appl.Entomol., Rev.Med.& Vet.Mycol., Rev.Plant Path., Sci.Cit.Ind., Trop.Dis.Bull., Vet.Bull.

—BLDSC (4542.244820), ADONIS, CASDDS, CISTI, EMDOCS, GNLM, IDS, Infotrieve, ingenta. **CCC.**

Published by: Blackwell Science Ltd., PO Box 88, Oxford OX2 0NE, United Kingdom. TEL 44-1865-206180, 44-1865-206002, FAX 44-1865-206219, jnl.orders@blacksci.co.uk, http://www.blackwell-science.com/products/journals/ijep.htm, http://www.blackwellpublishing.com. Ed. D Katz. Pub. Allen Stevens. R&P Sophie Savage. Adv. contact Jenny Applin. Circ: 2,745.

612.6 574.16 USA
QP251 CODEN: IFMEEV

INTERNATIONAL JOURNAL OF FERTILITY AND WOMEN'S MEDICINE. Text in English. 1955. bi-m., latest vol.46, no.6. USD 122 domestic; USD 135 foreign (effective 2001); USD 22 newsstand/cover. adv. bibl, charts, illus. index. reprints avail. *Refereed.* **Document type:** *Academic/Scholarly.* **Description:** Publishes scholarly articles on medical treatments, surgery, and pathology pertaining to human reproduction and general women's health.

Former titles (until 1997): International Journal of Fertility and Menopausal Studies (1069-3130); (until 1993): International Journal of Fertility (0020-725X)

Related titles: Online - full text ed.: (from Institute for Scientific Information).

Indexed: ASCA, Agri.& Environ.Biotech.Abstr. (coverage dropped), Anim.Breed.Abstr., Biol.Abstr., Chem.Abstr., Chem.Indus.Notes, Chem.Titles, Curr.Adv.Ecol.Sci., Curr.Cont., Curr.Lit.Fam.Plan., Dairy Sci.Abstr., Dent.Ind., Derwent Biotech.Abstr., Excerp.Med., Fam.Ind., Helminthol.Abstr., INIS Atomind., Ind.Med. (coverage dropped), Ind.Sci.Rev., Ind.Vet., Inpharma, Pharm.&Out.News, Reac., Rel.Ind.One, Rel.Ind.Two, SSCI (coverage dropped), Sci.Cit.Ind., THA, Vet.Bull.

—BLDSC (4542.250040), CASDDS, CISTI, EMDOCS, GNLM, ingenta, KNAW.

Published by: (U S International Foundation for Studies in Reproduction, Inc.), M S P (Medical Science Publishing) International, Inc., 405 Main St, Port Washington, NY 11050. TEL 516-944-7340, FAX 516-944-8663, mspinter@aol.com. Ed. Dr. Stephen L Corson. Pub. Michael L Fried. R&P, Adv. contact Joe Zimbardi. Circ: 7,000 (paid). **Co-sponsors:** Scandinavian Association for Studies in Fertility; Fallopius International Society; International Society of Reproductive Medicine; World Foundation for Medical Studies in Female Health.

INTERNATIONAL JOURNAL OF GYNECOLOGICAL PATHOLOGY. see *MEDICAL SCIENCES—Obstetrics And Gynecology*

610 GBR ISSN 0952-6862

INTERNATIONAL JOURNAL OF HEALTH CARE QUALITY ASSURANCE. Text in English. 1988. 7/yr. USD 4,499 in North America; EUR 4,809 in Europe; AUD 5,459 in Australasia; GBP 2,829 in the UK & the rest of the world (effective 2002). reprint service avail. from SWZ. **Document type:** *Academic/Scholarly.* **Description:** Theory and practice of quality assurance: measuring quality and customer satisfaction, alternative methodologies for implementing programs.

Incorporates (1986-1989): Health Care Management (0269-2104)

Related titles: Online - full text ed.: (from EBSCO Publishing, O C L C Online Computer Library Center, Inc., RoweCom Information Quest, ingenta, Swets Blackwell); ♦ Supplement: International Journal of Health Care Quality Assurance Incorporating Leadership in Health Services. ISSN 1366-0756.

Indexed: ABI Inform. (1992-1995), ASSIA, CINAHL, Emerald, Emrld.Intell., Hosp.Abstr., I.P.A., Int.Nurs.Ind.

—BLDSC (4542.275600), GNLM. **CCC.**

Published by: Emerald, 60-62 Toller Ln, Bradford, W Yorks BD8 9BY, United Kingdom. TEL 44-1274-777700, FAX 44-1274-785200, info@emeraldinsight.com, http://www.emeraldinsight.com/ijhcqa.htm, http://www.emeraldinsight.com/journals/. Ed. Robin Gourlay. **Affiliate:** Emerald (North America).

INTERNATIONAL JOURNAL OF HEALTH PLANNING AND MANAGEMENT. see *SOCIAL SERVICES AND WELFARE*

614.88 GBR ISSN 1350-2794
CODEN: IJICFY

INTERNATIONAL JOURNAL OF INTENSIVE CARE; for a global perspective on critical care. Text in English. 1994. q. GBP 50, USD 80 to individuals; GBP 62, USD 95 to institutions. adv. bk.rev. *Refereed.* **Document type:** *Academic/Scholarly.* **Description:** Embraces original research on all aspects of intensive care therapy from countries around the world.

—BLDSC (4542.310900), CISTI.

Published by: Greycoat Publishing, 1 Harley St, London W1N 1DA, United Kingdom. TEL 44-20-7637-1828, FAX 44-20-7637-3020. Ed. J Dennis Edwards. Pub., Adv. contact Ashley Wallis. R&P Guy Wallis. Circ: 27 (paid); 25,868 (controlled).

610 USA
RA1190 CODEN: CUTOEX

INTERNATIONAL JOURNAL OF MEDICAL AND BIOLOGICAL FRONTIERS. Text in English. 1992. q. USD 900 (effective 1999). **Document type:** *Academic/Scholarly.*

Incorporates: International Journal of Biology and Biochemistry; Formed by the merger of: International Journal of Medicine and Biology; Journal of Microbiology; Incorporates: Current Toxicology (1069-4587); International Journal of Radiation Hygiene (1066-7016)

Indexed: Bio-Contr.News & Info., Chem.Abstr., Chem.Indus.Notes, Chem.Titles, Rev.Appl.Entomol., Rev.Med.& Vet.Mycol., Soils & Fert., Soyabean Abstr., Vet.Bull.

—CASDDS, CISTI, GNLM.

Published by: Nova Science Publishers, Inc., 227 Main St, Ste 100, Huntington, NY 11743-6907. TEL 516-499-3103, FAX 516-499-3103, novasci1@aol.com; novascience@earthlink.net, http://www.nexusworld.com/nova.

616 GRC ISSN 1107-3756
CODEN: IJMMFG

INTERNATIONAL JOURNAL OF MOLECULAR MEDICINE. Text in Greek. m. USD 350 in Europe to individuals; USD 390 elsewhere to individuals; USD 720 in Europe to institutions; USD 770 elsewhere to institutions (effective 2002). *Refereed.* **Document type:** *Journal, Academic/Scholarly.* **Description:** Provides rapid publication in the field of molecular and clinical research on the mechanisms of diseases related to man. Includes studies in vitro or in vivo on experimental model systems relevant to the mechanisms of disease.

Related titles: Online - full text ed.: (from Institute for Scientific Information).

Indexed: AIDS & Cancer Res., Biotech.& Bioeng.Abstr., Curr.Cont., Environ.Sci.Poll.Mgmt., Focus on: Mol.Med., Genet.Abstr., Hum.Gen.Abstr., Ind.Med. (1998-), Inpharma, Mass Spectr.Bull., Microbiol.Abstr., Neurosci.Abstr., Pharm.&Out.News, Reac., Virol.Abstr.

—BLDSC (4542.365450), CASDDS, CISTI, GNLM, IDS.

Published by: Demetrios A. Spandidos Ed. & Pub., PO Box 18179, Athens 116 10, Greece. TEL 30-1-722-7809, FAX 30-1-752-3866.

▼ **INTERNATIONAL JOURNAL OF NANOSCIENCE.** see *COMPUTERS—Microcomputers*

INTERNATIONAL JOURNAL OF ORIENTAL MEDICINE/GUOJI HANFANG YIYAO ZAZHI. see *ALTERNATIVE MEDICINE*

INTERNATIONAL JOURNAL OF PHARMACEUTICAL MEDICINE. see *PHARMACY AND PHARMACOLOGY*

THE INTERNATIONAL JOURNAL OF RISK AND SAFETY IN MEDICINE; side effects of drugs - devices - surgery - prevention - liability. see *INSURANCE*

610 USA ISSN 1072-5245
RA785 CODEN: ISMAE8
INTERNATIONAL JOURNAL OF STRESS MANAGEMENT. Text in English. 1994. q. USD 262, EUR 261 to institutions for print or online ed.; USD 314.40, EUR 313.20 to institutions for print & online eds. combined (effective 2002). adv. bk.rev. *Refereed.* **Document type:** *Journal, Academic/Scholarly.* **Description:** Aims to advance the study of stress management by encouraging sound research and practice. Covers the fields of psychology, psychiatry, psychophysiology, education, medicine, dentistry, physical and speech therapy and business.
Related titles: Online - full text ed.: (from EBSCO Publishing, O C L C Online Computer Library Center, Inc., Swets Blackwell, Kluwer Online, Institute for Scientific Information, RoweCom Information Quest).
Indexed: ASCA, Crim.Just.Abstr., Curr.Cont., PsycInfo, SSCI, Soc.Work Res.& Abstr., e-psyche.
—BLDSC (4542.681480), IDS, Infotrieve, ingenta. **CCC.**
Published by: (International Stress Management Association), Kluwer Academic - Plenum Publishers (Subsidiary of: Wolters Kluwer N.V.), 233 Spring St, New York, NY 10013-1578. TEL 212-620-8000, 800-221-9369, FAX 212-463-0742, info@plenum.com, http://www.wkap.nl/journalhome.htm/1072-5245. Ed. John G Carlson. adv.: B&W page USD 400. **Subscr. outside the Americas to:** Kluwer Academic Publishers Group, Journals Department, PO Box 322, Dordrecht 3300 AH, Netherlands. TEL 31-78-639-2392, FAX 31-78-654-6474.

INTERNATIONAL JOURNAL OF TOXICOLOGY. see *ENVIRONMENTAL STUDIES—Toxicology And Environmental Safety*

362.1029 USA ISSN 1045-3121
INTERNATIONAL MED-TECH DIRECTORY; the international financial guide to over 800 publicly traded healthcare companies. Text in English. 1982-199?; resumed 1993. a. USD 295 (effective 1993). **Document type:** *Directory.* **Description:** Compiles information on public health care firms.
Published by: Westergaard Publishing Corporation, c/o Pamela McLernon, 560 W 43rd St, New York, NY 10036. FAX 212-947-6643. Ed. Emile Westergaard.

344 363.19 USA ISSN 1079-6940
K3611.M45
INTERNATIONAL MEDICAL DEVICE REGULATORY MONITOR. Text in English. 1993. m. USD 525; CND 595 in Canada; USD 595 elsewhere (effective 2000). 50 p./no. **Document type:** *Newsletter.* **Description:** Contains international regulatory news affecting medical device manufacturers. Provides English languge texts of official regulatory documents from around the world.
Supersedes in part (in 1993): International Drug and Device Regulatory Monitor (0888-6393); Which was formerly (until 1982): International Drug Regulatory Monitor (0198-7402)
—**CCC.**
Published by: Omniprint Inc., 9700 Philadelphia Ct, Lanham, MD 20706-4405. TEL 301-731-5202, 800-345-2611, FAX 301-731-5203, editor@omniprint.net. Ed. Joanne Eglovitch. Pub., R&P Michael Nagan.

610 JPN ISSN 1341-2051
CODEN: IMJOFS
INTERNATIONAL MEDICAL JOURNAL. Abbreviated title: I M J. Text in English. 1994. q. JPY 7,400 domestic; USD 80 foreign; JPY 1,900 per issue domestic; USD 20 per issue foreign (effective 2001). bk.rev. *Refereed.* **Document type:** *Journal, Academic/Scholarly.* **Description:** Covers the recent development of indigenous diseases, public health, legal medicine, epidomiology, pharmacology, psychiatry, environmental health, clinical medicine and related disciplines in the world.
Related titles: CD-ROM ed.; Online - full text ed.
Indexed: ASSIA, Environ.Sci.Poll.Mgmt., Excerp.Med., Indian Psychol.Abstr., Pollut.Abstr., PsycInfo, Psychol.Abstr.
—BLDSC (4544.034500), CASDDS, GNLM.
Published by: Japan International Cultural Exchange Foundation, 2-15-5-207 Shoto, Shibuya-ku, Tokyo 150-0046, Japan. TEL 81-3-3467-7316, FAX 81-3-3467-7317, bj7w-ucd@asahi-net.or.jp, jicef@nisiq.net, http://www.asahi-net.or.jpl~bJ7w-ucd1, http://www.asahi-net.or.jp/~ID5k-sri/. Eds. Thomas Stapleton, Tsutomu Sakuta. R&P, Adv. contact Wataru Uchida TEL 81-3-3424-9090. Circ: 5,000 (paid and controlled). **Co-publisher:** Seronjiho Co., Ltd.

610 ISR ISSN 0793-8918
INTERNATIONAL MEDICAL JOURNAL. Text in Russian. 1998. m. USD 60 domestic to individuals; USD 125 foreign to individuals; USD 185 domestic to institutions. **Document type:** *Academic/Scholarly.* **Description:** Covers the recent development of indigenous diseases, public health, legal medicine, epidemiology, pharmacology, psychiatry, environmental health, clinical medicine and related desciplines.
Indexed: Ref.Zh.
Published by: Yozmot Heiliger (1989) Ltd., 3 Yohanan Hasandlar St., P O Box 56055, Tel Aviv 61560, Israel. TEL 972-3-5284851, FAX 972-3-5285397, books@yozmot.com, http://www.yozmot.com.

610 JPN ISSN 0535-1405
INTERNATIONAL MEDICAL NEWS. Text in English, Japanese. 1952. m. per issue exchange basis. **Document type:** *Academic/Scholarly.*
Published by: International Medical Society of Japan/Nihon Kokusai Igaku Kyokai, 4-12 Kami-Uma 1-chome, Setagaya-ku, Tokyo 154-0011, Japan.

610 615 JPN
INTERNATIONAL MOCHIDA MEMORIAL SYMPOSIUM. Text in English. 1988. irreg., latest vol.3, 1993. **Document type:** *Proceedings.*
Published by: Mochida Memorial Foundation for Medical and Pharmaceutical Research/Mochida Kinen Igaku Yakugaku Shinko Zaidan, 1-7 Yotsuya, Shinjuku-ku, Tokyo 160-0004, Japan.

610 BEL
INTERNATIONAL ORGANIZATION FOR COOPERATION IN HEALTH CARE. GENERAL ASSEMBLY. REPORT. Text in English. 1979. a. free per issue. **Document type:** *Newsletter, Proceedings.*
Supersedes: International Organization for Medical Cooperation. General Assembly. Report (0579-3912)
Published by: Medicus Mundi International, Rue des Deux Eglises 64, Brussels 1210, Belgium. TEL 32-2-2310609.

362 USA ISSN 0020-8477
CODEN: IRERB
INTERNATIONAL REHABILITATION REVIEW. Text in English. 1949. 3/yr. USD 30. adv. bk.rev., film rev., play rev. illus. back issues avail. **Document type:** *Newspaper.* **Description:** Issues and developments in disability prevention and rehabilitation worldwide.
Formerly: Rehabilitation International Newsletter
Indexed: CINAHL, Except.Child Educ.Abstr., Excerp.Med., Rehabil.Lit., Soc.Work Res.& Abstr.
—CISTI, GNLM.
Published by: Rehabilitation International, 25 E 21st St, 4th Fl, New York, NY 10010. TEL 212-420-1500, FAX 212-505-0871, TELEX 446412. Ed. Barbara Duncan. Circ: 20,000.

616.07 USA ISSN 0074-7718
RB6 CODEN: IRXPAT
INTERNATIONAL REVIEW OF EXPERIMENTAL PATHOLOGY. Text in English. 1962. irreg., latest vol.36, 1996. index. reprint service avail. from ISI. *Refereed.*
Related titles: Online - full text ed.: (from Institute for Scientific Information).
Indexed: Abstr.Hyg., Biol.Abstr., Chem.Abstr., Chem.Indus.Notes, Chem.Titles, Curr.Adv.Cell & Devel.Biol., Excerp.Med., Ind.Med. (coverage dropped), Ind.Sci.Rev., Ind.Vet., Sci.Cit.Ind., Trop.Dis.Bull., Vet.Bull.
—CASDDS, CISTI, GNLM, ingenta, KNAW, Linda Hall. **CCC.**
Published by: Academic Press, Inc., Journal Division (Subsidiary of: Harcourt Brace & Company), 525 B St, Ste 1900, San Diego, CA 92101-4495. TEL 619-231-0926, FAX 619-699-6715. Ed. G W Richter. **Subscr. to:** Order Dept., 6277 Sea Harbor Dr, 4th Fl, Orlando, FL 32887. TEL 800-321-5068.

610 CAN ISSN 1090-2171
INTERNATIONAL SOCIETY FOR PLASTINATION. JOURNAL. Text in English. 1987. s-a. USD 75 for 2 yrs. to members (effective 2000). adv. *Refereed.* **Description:** Provides an international forum for scientists to discuss applications and developments of the plastination technique.
Published by: International Society for Plastination, Dept de Chimie-Biologie, Universite du Quebec a Trois Rivieres, C P 500, Trois Rivieres, PQ G9A 5H7, Canada. TEL 819-376-5053, FAX 819-376-5084, gilles_grondin@uqtr.uquebec.ca, http://www.kfunigraz.ac.at/anawww/plast/index.html. Ed., R&P, Adv. contact Gilles Grondin. Circ: 500.

610 USA
THE INTERNATIONAL SOCIETY OF ANDROLOGY. NEWSLETTER. Text in English. irreg. back issues avail. **Document type:** *Newsletter.*
Related titles: Online - full content ed.
Published by: The International Society of Andrology, c/o Philip Troen, M.D., Dept of Medicine, University of Pittsburgh Medical Center, 200 Lothrop St, Pittsburgh, PA 15213. TEL 412-648-6470, FAX 412-648-6403, http://andrology.org/. Ed. Philip Troen.

610 CHE
INTERNATIONAL SYMPOSIUM ON CERAMICS IN MEDICINE. PROCEEDINGS. Text in English. a. CHF 440, USD 312, GBP 186 (effective 2001). **Document type:** *Proceedings, Academic/Scholarly.*
Published by: (International Society on Ceramics in Medicine USA), Trans Tech Publications Ltd., Brandrain 6, Uetikon-Zurich CH-8707, Switzerland. TEL 41-1-9221022, FAX 41-1-9221033, http://www.ttp.net.

610 JPN
INTERNATIONAL SYMPOSIUM ON QUALITY CONTROL✶. Text in English. 1974. every 4 yrs.
Published by: Ekuseputa Medika K.K./Excerpta Medica Ltd., Tokyo, Kowa Bldg. 5, 15-23 Nishi-Azabu 4-chome, Minato-ku, Tokyo 106-0031, Japan.

INTERNATIONAL TESLA SOCIETY. BULLETIN. see *PHYSICS—Electricity*

610 USA ISSN 1045-0572
RA783.5
INTERNATIONAL TRAVEL HEALTH GUIDE. Text in English. 1989. a.
Published by: Travel Medicine, Inc., 351 Pleasant St, Ste 312, Northampton, MA 01060.

362.1969 USA
▼ **THE INTERNET JOURNAL OF INFECTIOUS DISEASES.** Text in English. 2000. s-a. free per issue. adv. bk.rev. *Refereed.* **Document type:** *Academic/Scholarly.* **Description:** Provides information from the field of infectious diseases and infection control; contains original articles, reviews, case reports, streaming slide shows, streaming videos, letters to the editor, press releases and meeting information.
Media: Online - full content.
Published by: Internet Scientific Publications, L.L.C., 23 Rippling Creek Dr, Sugar Land, TX 77479. TEL 281-240-1533, FAX 281-240-1533, http://www.ispub.com/. R&P, Adv. contact Hope Morrow TEL 832-754-0335.

616.07 USA
▼ **THE INTERNET JOURNAL OF PATHOLOGY.** Text in English. 2000. s-a. free per issue. adv. bk.rev. back issues avail. *Refereed.* **Document type:** *Academic/Scholarly.* **Description:** Provides information from the field of pathology and cytology; contains original articles, reviews, case reports, streaming slide, shows, streaming videos, letters to the editor, press releases, meeting information.
Media: Online - full content.
Published by: Internet Scientific Publications, L.L.C., 23 Rippling Creek Dr, Sugar Land, TX 77479. TEL 281-240-1533, FAX 281-240-1533, http://www.ispub.com/. Eds. Victor Vietro, Victor Vietro. R&P Hope Morrow TEL 832-754-0335.

610 VEN ISSN 0535-5133
CODEN: ICLIAD
INVESTIGACION CLINICA. Text and summaries in English, Spanish. 1960. q. VEB 2,000; USD 60 in Latin America; USD 75 elsewhere (effective 1999). bibl, charts. *Refereed.* **Document type:** *Academic/Scholarly.*
Related titles: CD-ROM ed.; ♦ Supplement: Investigacion Clinica. Suplemento. ISSN 0259-0395.

Indexed: Abstr.Hyg., Biol.Abstr., Chem.Abstr., Curr.Cont. (coverage dropped), Excerp.Med., Helminthol.Abstr., Ind.Med. (1960-), Ind.Vet., Nutr.Abstr., Protozool.Abstr., Rev.Appl.Entomol., Rev.Med.& Vet.Mycol., Sugar Ind.Abstr., Trop.Dis.Bull.
—BLDSC (4557.720000), CASDDS, CISTI, EMDOCS, GNLM, KNAW.
Published by: Universidad del Zulia, Instituto de Investigaciones Clinicas, Facultad de Medicina, Apdo. Postal 1151, Maracaibo, Venezuela. TEL 5861-597247, FAX 58-61-916053, xraleigh@luz.ve. Ed., R&P Elena Ryder. Circ: 1,000.

610 VEN ISSN 0259-0395
INVESTIGACION CLINICA. SUPLEMENTO. Text and summaries in English, Spanish.
Related titles: ♦ Supplement to: Investigacion Clinica. ISSN 0535-5133.
Published by: Universidad del Zulia, Instituto de Investigaciones Clinicas, Apdo. Postal 1151, Maracaibo, Venezuela. TEL 5861-597247, FAX 58-61-916053.

610 USA ISSN 0746-8709
R15
IOWA MEDICINE. Text in English. 1910. bi-m. USD 30 domestic; USD 32 foreign (effective 2001). adv. charts, illus. index. back issues avail. **Document type:** *Trade.* **Description:** Socioeconomic medical journal. Provides feature stories, managed care news, IMS updates, legislative affairs news, medical economics and practice management information.
Formerly (until 1984): Iowa Medical Society. Journal (0021-0587)
Indexed: AgeLine, Biol.Abstr., Chem.Abstr., INIS Atomind., Ind.Med. (1984-), Int.Nurs.Ind., Med.Care Rev.
—BLDSC (4566.400000), CISTI, GNLM, KNAW.
Published by: Iowa Medical Society, 1001 Grand Ave, West Des Moines, IA 50265. TEL 515-223-1401, FAX 515-223-8420. R&P, Adv. contact Ann Shoemaker. Circ: 4,700 (paid).

610 IRN ISSN 0253-0716
CODEN: IJMSDW
IRANIAN JOURNAL OF MEDICAL SCIENCES. Text and summaries in English. 1970. 4/yr. USD 80 (2000). adv. bk.rev. charts, illus, stat. reprint service avail. from IRC. *Refereed.* **Document type:** *Journal, Academic/Scholarly.* **Description:** Publishes original clinical and research experiences of physicians on prevalent diseases in the region, and analysis of various regional parameters which may modulate the incidence, course and management of diseases and relevant medical problems.
Formerly (until 1979): Pahlavi Medical Journal (0030-9427)
Indexed: Agri.& Environ.Biotech.Abstr. (coverage dropped), Biol.Abstr., Chem.Abstr. (coverage dropped), Curr.Cont. (coverage dropped), Excerp.Med., Helminthol.Abstr., Ind.Med. (coverage dropped), Nutr.Abstr., Trop.Dis.Bull.
—BLDSC (4567.528900), CASDDS, CISTI, EMDOCS, GNLM, KNAW.
Published by: Shiraz University of Medical Sciences, Nemazee Hospital, Shiraz 71934, Iran. TEL 98-71-660134, FAX 98-71-661001, ijms@sums.ac.ir, http://www.sums.ac.ir/IJMS. Ed. Dr. Karim Vessal. Circ: 3,000.

610 IRQ ISSN 0021-0927
IRAQI MEDICAL PROFESSIONS' ASSOCIATION. JOURNAL✶ . Text in Arabic, English. 1965 (vol.13). 3/yr. adv. charts, illus, stat.
Indexed: Biol.Abstr., Ind.Med. (coverage dropped).
Published by: Iraqi Medical Professions' Association, c/o Iragi Medical Soceity, Maari St, Al Mansoor, Baghdad, Iraq. Ed. Dr. F H Ghali.

610 JPN
IRI SANGYO SHINBUN/MEDICAL AND PHYSICAL INSTRUMENTS NEWSPAPER. Text in Japanese. 1975. s-m. JPY 5,000. **Document type:** *Newspaper.*
Published by: Iri Sangyo Shinbunsha, 22-9-401 Sakuragawa 3-chome, Itabashi-ku, Tokyo 174-0075, Japan.

610 IRL ISSN 0374-8405
CODEN: IPSJB7
IRISH COLLEGES OF PHYSICIANS AND SURGEONS. JOURNAL. Text in English. 1971. q. EUR 79 in Ireland and UK; EUR 87 rest of Europe; EUR 96.50 rest of world (effective 2001). adv. bk.rev. charts, illus. index. *Refereed.* **Document type:** *Academic/Scholarly.*
Supersedes: Royal College of Surgeons in Ireland. Journal (0035-8827)
Indexed: Biol.Abstr., Curr.Adv.Ecol.Sci., Curr.Cont. (coverage dropped), INIS Atomind., NRN.
—BLDSC (4802.780000), CISTI, EMDOCS, GNLM, KNAW.
Published by: Royal College of Surgeons in Ireland, Mercer Library, Lower Mercer St., Dublin 2, Ireland. TEL 353-1-4780674, FAX 353-1-4022457, jicps@rcsi.ie, http://www.rcsi.ie. Ed. Austin Leahy. Pub., Adv. contact Beatrice Doran. Circ: 5,000.

610 IRL ISSN 0021-1265
CODEN: IJMSAT
IRISH JOURNAL OF MEDICAL SCIENCES. Text in English. 1832. q. IEP 70 in the European Union; IEP 110 elsewhere (effective 2000). adv. bk.rev. reprint service avail. from PQC. *Refereed.* **Document type:** *Academic/Scholarly.*
Related titles: Microfilm ed.; Online - full text ed.: (from Institute for Scientific Information).
Indexed: ASCA, Biol.Abstr., Chem.Abstr., Chem.Indus.Notes, Chem.Titles, Curr.Adv.Cancer Res., Curr.Cont., Dent.Ind., Derwent Biotech.Abstr., Excerp.Med., Helminthol.Abstr., INIS Atomind., Ind.Med. (1971-), Ind.Sci.Rev., Inpharma, Int.Abstr.Biol.Sci., Int.Nurs.Ind., NRN, Nutr.Abstr., Pharm.&Out.News, Reac., Rev.Med.& Vet.Mycol., Rev.Plant Path., Sci.Cit.Ind. (coverage dropped), THA.
—BLDSC (4572.000000), CASDDS, CISTI, GNLM, IDS, ingenta, KNAW. **CCC.**
Published by: Royal Academy of Medicine in Ireland, 6 Kildare St., Dublin 2, Ireland. TEL 353-1-6767650, FAX 353-1-6611684, secretary@rami.iol.ie, http://www.iol.ie/~rami. Ed. Thomas F Gorey. Adv. contact Daniela Korcel. page IEP 1,000. Circ: 2,000 (controlled).

610 IRL ISSN 0332-3102
CODEN: IMDJBD
IRISH MEDICAL JOURNAL. Text in English. 1937-1987 (Dec.); resumed 1988 (Sep.). 10/yr. IEP 100 in Europe; GBP 150 elsewhere (effective 2001). adv. bk.rev., Website rev. charts, illus. s-a. index. back issues avail. *Refereed.* **Document type:** *Journal, Academic/Scholarly.* **Description:** Forum for all aspects of Irish medicine.
Former titles: Irish Medical Organization; Irish Medical Association. Journal (0021-129X)
Related titles: Online - full content ed.
Indexed: ASCA, Abstr.Hyg., Biol.Abstr., Chem.Abstr., Curr.Cont., Dairy Sci.Abstr., Dent.Ind., Dok.Arbeitsmed., Excerp.Med., Helminthol.Abstr., INIS Atomind., Ind.Med. (1974-), Inpharma, Int.Nurs.Ind., NRN, Nutr.Abstr., Pharm.&Out.News, Protozool.Abstr., Reac., Rev.Med.& Vet.Mycol., SSCI (coverage dropped), THA.
—BLDSC (4572.910000), CASDDS, CISTI, GNLM, IDS, ingenta, KNAW.
Published by: Irish Medical Organization, 10 Fitzwilliam Pl., Dublin 2, Ireland. TEL 353-1-6767273, FAX 353-1-6612758, imj@imj.ie, http://www.imj.ie/, http://www.imo.ie/. Ed. John Murphy. R&P, Adv. contact Susan Byrne. Circ: 7,500.

610 IRL ISSN 0790-2905
IRISH MEDICAL NEWS. Text in English. 1974. w. IEP 50 to non-members. adv. bk.rev.
Formerly (until 1984): I M J Appointments
Published by: Winstone Publishing, 10 Fitzwilliam Pl., Dublin 2, Ireland. TEL 01-767273, FAX 01-612758. Ed. John Gibbons. Circ: 5,000.

610 GBR ISSN 0047-147X
IRISH MEDICAL TIMES. Text in English. 1967. w. GBP 45. adv. bk.rev. reprint service avail. from PQC.
Related titles: Microfilm ed.: (from PQC).
—BLDSC (4572.950000). **CCC.**
Published by: Medical Publications Ltd., 30 Lancaster Gate, London W2 3LP, United Kingdom. Ed. Dr. John F O'Connell. Circ: (controlled). **Subscr. to:** 12-14 Ansdell St, London W8 5TR, United Kingdom.

610 JPN
IRYO FUKUSHI GIJUTSU/MEDICAL AND WELFARE TECHNOLOGY. Text in Japanese. 1980. q.
Published by: Gijutsu Kenkyu Kumiai Iryo Fukushi Kiki Kenkyujo/Technology Research Association of Medical and Welfare Apparatus, 5-8 Shibakoen 3-chome, Minato-ku, Tokyo 105-0011, Japan.

IRYO JIKO JOHO SENTA. SENTA NYUSU/MEDICAL MALPRACTICE INFORMATION CENTER IN JAPAN. NEWSLETTER. see *LAW—Civil Law*

610.285 JPN
IRYO JOHO SHISUTEMU KENKYU KAIHATSU HOKOKUSHO/REPORT OF RESEARCH AND DEVELOPMENT OF MEDICAL INFORMATION SYSTEM. Text in Japanese. a.
Published by: Iryo Joho Shisutemu Kaihatsu Senta/Medical Information System Development Center, 3-4 Akasaka 2-chome, Minato-ku, Tokyo 107-0052, Japan.

610 JPN ISSN 0289-8055
IRYO JOHOGAKU/JAPAN JOURNAL OF MEDICAL INFORMATICS. Text in Japanese; Summaries in English, Japanese. 1980. q. JPY 2,500.
Indexed: Excerp.Med.
—EMDOCS, GNLM.
Published by: Nihon Iryo Joho Gakkai/Japan Association for Medical Informatics, Iryo Joho Shisutemu Kaihatsu Senta, Randikku Akasaka, 3-4 Akasaka 2-chome, Minato-ku, Tokyo 107-0052, Japan.

610 360 JPN ISSN 0287-1521
IRYO TO FUKUSHI/JAPANESE JOURNAL OF MEDICAL SOCIAL WORK. Text in Japanese. 1965. a. JPY 1,000.
Published by: Nihon Iryo Shakai Jigyo Kyokai/Medical Social Worker Society, Zenkoku Shinshin Shogaiji Fukushi Zaidan Biru, 2-8 Nishi-Waseda 2-chome, Shinjuku-ku, Tokyo 162-0051, Japan.

610 JPN ISSN 0916-9202
RA418
IRYO TO SHAKAI/JOURNAL OF HEALTHCARE AND SOCIETY. Text in Japanese. 1991. q. JPY 8,000 (effective 2001). abstr. 100 p./no. back issues avail. *Refereed.* **Document type:** *Journal, Academic/Scholarly.*
—BLDSC (4996.731600).
Published by: Iryo Kagaku Kenkyujo/Health Care Science Institute, Akasaka Noa Bldg, 5th FL, 3-2-12 Akasaka, Minato-ku, Tokyo 112-0052, Japan. TEL 81-3-5563-1791, FAX 81-3-5563-1795, journal@iken.org, http://www.iken.org.

610 JPN
IRYO TO SHISETSU/MEDICAL SERVICE AND FACILITY. Text in Japanese. 1971. q. JPY 1,000.
Published by: Iryo Taimususha/Medical Times, 11-2 Kanda-Ogawa-Machi 3-chome, Chiyoda-ku, Tokyo 101-0052, Japan.

610 617.6 615 JPN ISSN 0911-8470
ISHI SHIKAISHI YAKUZAISHI CHOSA✶ /SURVEY ON PHYSICIANS, DENTISTS AND PHARMACEUTISTS. Text in Japanese. 1955. biennial.
Published by: Koseisho, Daijin Kanbo/Ministry of Health and Welfare, Minister's Secretariat, Statistics and Information Department, Tokei Johobu, 1-2-2 Kasumigaseki, Chiyoda-ku, Tokyo 100, Japan.

610 JPN ISSN 0287-1777
ISHIKAWA KENRITSU CHUO BYOIN IGAKUSHI/ ISHIKAWA PREFECTURAL CENTRAL HOSPITAL. MEDICAL JOURNAL. Text in English, Japanese. 1978. a.
Published by: Ishikawa Kenritsu Chuo Byoin, Nu 153 Minami-Shinbo-Machi, Kanazawa-shi, Ishikawa-ken 920-0064, Japan.

ISLAMIC ACADEMY OF SCIENCES. MEDICAL JOURNAL. see *SCIENCES: COMPREHENSIVE WORKS*

ISLAMIC WORLD MEDICAL JOURNAL. see *RELIGIONS AND THEOLOGY—Islamic*

610 ISR
ISRAEL MEDICAL ASSOCIATION. QUARTERLY MEDICAL REVIEW. Text in English. q. membership. adv. illus.
Formerly: Israel Medical Association. Quarterly Review. (0021-2253)
Related titles: French ed.; Spanish ed.
Published by: Fraser, 17 Bugrashov St., Tel Aviv, Israel. Ed. Yehuda Shoefeld.

610 USA ISSN 1531-5150
▼ **ISSUES IN INTERDISCIPLINARY CARE.** Text in English. 1999. q. USD 80 to individuals; USD 360 to institutions; USD 30 newsstand/cover to individuals; USD 95 newsstand/cover to institutions (effective 2002). *Refereed.* **Document type:** *Academic/Scholarly.* **Description:** Devoted to providing innovations and practices that transcend interdisciplinary boundaries in health care.
Formerly (until 2000): National Academies of Practice Forum (1097-5357)
Related titles: Online - full text ed.: (from EBSCO Publishing, O C L C Online Computer Library Center, Inc., RoweCom Information Quest, ingenta, Swets Blackwell).
—BLDSC (6015.752000).

M

Published by: (National Academies of Practice), Sage Publications, Inc., 2455 Teller Rd, Thousand Oaks, CA 91320. TEL 800-818-7243, FAX 800-583-2665, info@sagepub.com, http://www.sagepub.com/. Ed. Judith A Lewis. Pub. Sara Miller McCune. R&P Tanya Udin. Adv. contact DeAnna Vega Hammersley. **Addr. in India:** Sage Publications India Pvt. Ltd., M-32 Market, Greater Kailash-1, PO Box 4215, New Delhi 110 024, India. TEL 91-11-6419884, 91-11-6444958, FAX 91-11-6472426, sageindia@sagepub.com, http://indiasage.com/; **Addr. in the UK:** Sage Publications Ltd., 6 Bonhill St, London EC2A 4PU, United Kingdom. TEL 44-20-7374-0645, FAX 44-20-7374-8741, info@sagepub.co.uk, http://www.sageltd.co.uk/.

362.4 174.2 USA ISSN 8756-8160
KF480.A15 CODEN: ILAME3

ISSUES IN LAW AND MEDICINE. Text in English. 1985. 3/yr., latest 2001, Spr. USD 59 domestic to individuals; USD 74 in Canada to individuals; USD 79 elsewhere to individuals; USD 79 domestic to institutions; USD 94 in Canada to institutions; USD 99 elsewhere to institutions (effective 2001). adv. bk.rev. illus. back issues avail.; reprint service avail. from WSH. *Refereed.* **Document type:** *Academic/Scholarly.* **Description:** Provides technical and informational assistance to attorneys, health care professionals, educators and administrators concerned with the legal, medical and ethical issues arising from the provision of health services.
Related titles: Microfiche ed.: (from WSH); Online - full text ed.: (from Gale Group, National Library of Medicine, West Group, LexisNexis, H. W. Wilson, ProQuest Information & Learning, Factiva, Institute for Scientific Information).
Indexed: AMED, ASCA, AgeLine, Arts & Hum.Cit.Ind. (coverage dropped), C.L.I., Crim.Just.Abstr., Curr.Cont., Except.Child Educ.Abstr., Hlth.Ind., Hosp.Lit.Ind., Human Resour.Abstr., Ind.Med. (1985-), Int.Nurs.Ind., L.R.I. (Mar.1989-), Leg.Per. (Mar.1986-), Peace Res.Abstr., Psychol.Abstr., Rel.Ind.One, Rel.Ind.Two, SSCI, Sage Pub.Admin.Abstr., Sage Urb.Stud.Abstr., Viol.& Abuse Abstr.
—BLDSC (4584.302000), GNLM, ingenta.
Published by: National Legal Center for the Medically Dependent and Disabled, Inc., 3 S 6th St, Terre Haute, IN 47807-3510. TEL 812-232-0103, http://www.elibrary.com. Eds. Barry A. Bostrom, James Bopp Jr., Larry Ligget. Adv. contact Larry Ligget. Circ: 1,000. **Co-sponsor:** Horatio R. Storer Foundation, Inc.

610 TUR ISSN 0374-1656
R97.7.T8 CODEN: TFMEAC

ISTANBUL MEDICAL FACULTY. MEDICAL BULLETIN/ISTANBUL TIP FAKULTESI. MECMUASI. Cover title: Istanbul Universitesi. Istanbul Tip Fakultesi. Mecmuasi. Text in English; Summaries in English, French, German. 1919; N.S. 1938. biennial. USD 50. illus. *Refereed.* **Document type:** *Academic/Scholarly.*
Formerly: Istanbul Universitesi. Tip Fakultesi. Tip Fakultesi Mecmuasi (0047-1623)
Indexed: Biol.Abstr., Chem.Abstr., Excerp.Med. (1992-), Foreign Leg.Per., Ind.Med. (coverage dropped), Nutr.Abstr.
Published by: Istanbul Universitesi, Tip Fakultesi Dekanligi/Istanbul University, Istanbul Medical Faculty, Capa, Istanbul 34390, Turkey. TEL 90-212-5340050, FAX 90-212-6358522, medbulis@istanbul.edu.tr, http://www.istanbul.edu.tr. Circ: 1,000.

ISTITUTO SUPERIORE DI SANITA. ANNALI. see *PUBLIC HEALTH AND SAFETY*

610 JPN ISSN 0536-0307

ITAN/JAPAN SOCIETY OF MEDICAL HISTORY. KANSAI BRANCH. JOURNAL. Variant title: History of Medicine. Text in Japanese. 1938. 2/yr.
Indexed: Jap.Per.Ind.
Published by: Nihon Ishi Gakkai, Kansai Shibu, c/o Mr Yoji Nagatoya, 1-12-308 Shinka-Naoka-cho 3-chome, Sakai-shi, Osaka-fu 591-8021, Japan.

610 RUS ISSN 0202-7135

ITOGI NAUKI I TEKHNIKI. PATOLOGICHESKAYA ANATOMIYA. Text in Russian. irreg.
—Linda Hall.
Published by: Vserossiiskii Institut Nauchnoi i Tekhnicheskoi Informatsii (VINITI), Usievicha ul 20-a, Moscow 125315, Russian Federation. TEL 7-095-1526441, FAX 7-095-943-0060. **US dist. addr.:** East View Publications, 3020 Harbor Ln N, Minneapolis, MN 55447. TEL 612-550-0961.

610 JPN ISSN 0021-3284
CODEN: IIZAAX

IWATE IGAKU ZASSHI/IWATE MEDICAL ASSOCIATION. JOURNAL. Text in Japanese; Text occasionally in English; Abstracts in English. 1945. bi-m. JPY 8,000 (effective 2001). adv. bk.rev. abstr, bibl, charts, illus. index. **Document type:** *Journal, Academic/Scholarly.* **Description:** Publishes original medical research reports.
Formerly: Iwate Igaku Semmongakko Zashi
Indexed: Biol.Abstr., Chem.Abstr., Chem.Indus.Notes, Chem.Titles, Excerp.Med., INIS Atomind., Ref.Zh.
—BLDSC (4803.200000), CASDDS.
Published by: Iwate Igakkai/Iwate Medical Association, c/o Iwate Medical University, 19-1 Uchimaru, Morioka-shi, Iwate-ken 020-8505, Japan. TEL 81-19-651-5111 ext 2224, FAX 81-19-625-0547, mmeterui@lib.iwate-med.ac.jp. Ed., R&P Saburo Horiuchi. Pub. Toryo Insatsu. Circ: 1,550.

610 JPN ISSN 0286-9543

IWATE IHO/IWATE MEDICAL SOCIETY. NEWS. Text in Japanese. m. JPY 500 per issue.
Published by: Iwateken Ishikai, 8-20 Saien 2-chome, Morioka-shi, Iwate-ken 020-0024, Japan.

610 JPN ISSN 0385-9320

IWATE KENRITSU BYOIN IGAKKAI ZASSHI/IWATE PREFECTURAL HOSPITAL. MEDICAL JOURNAL. Text in Japanese. 1961. s-a.
Indexed: INIS Atomind.
Published by: Iwate Kenritsu Byoin Igakkai, Iwate Kenritsu Chuo Byoin, 4-1 Ueda 1-chome, Morioka-shi, Iwate-ken 020-0066, Japan.

610 JPN ISSN 0917-1177

IWATE KENRITSU MIYAKO BYOIN IGAKU ZASSHI/IWATE PREFECTURAL MIYAKO HOSPITAL. MEDICAL JOURNAL. Text in English, Japanese. 1990. a.
Published by: Iwate Kenritsu Miyako Byoin, 1-6 Sakae-cho, Miyako-shi, Iwate-ken 027-0076, Japan.

610 JPN ISSN 0287-0894
CODEN: IYKEDH

IYAKUHIN KENKYU/STUDY OF MEDICAL SUPPLIES. Text in English, Japanese; Summaries in English. 1970. m. USD 600 (effective 2000). *Refereed.*
Indexed: Chem.Abstr., Chem.Indus.Notes, Chem.Titles.
—BLDSC (4589.220000), CASDDS, GNLM. **CCC.**
Published by: Nihon Koteisho Kyokai/Society of Japanese Pharmacopoeia, 12-15 Shibuya 2-chome, Shibuya-ku, Tokyo 150-0002, Japan. TEL 81-3-3400-5634, FAX 81-3-3400-3158, http://www.sjp.or.jp. Ed. Dr. Alcira Takanaka.

615.845 610.28 JPN ISSN 0021-3292
CODEN: IYSEAK

IYO DENSHI TO SEITAI KOGAKU/JAPANESE JOURNAL OF MEDICAL ELECTRONICS AND BIOLOGICAL ENGINEERING. Text in Japanese; Summaries in English. 1963. q. JPY 10,000. adv. bk.rev. bibl, charts, illus, stat. index. *Refereed.* **Document type:** *Academic/Scholarly.*
Indexed: Biol.Abstr., Chem.Abstr., Chem.Indus.Notes, Chem.Titles, Crop Physiol.Abstr., Dent.Ind., Eng.Ind., Excerp.Med., INIS Atomind., INSPEC (Apr.1971-), Ind.Med. (coverage dropped), JCT, JTA, Jap.Per.Ind.
—BLDSC (4656.215000), AskIEEE, CASDDS, CISTI, GNLM, Linda Hall.
Published by: (Japan Society of Medical Electronics and Biological Engineering/Nihon me Gakkai), Gakkaishi Kanko Senta/Center for Academic Publications (Subsidiary of: Japan Society of Medical Electronics and Biological Engineering/Nihon me Gakkai), 4-16 Yayoi 2-chome, Bunkyo-ku, Tokyo 113-0032, Japan. Ed. Dr. Shogo Ueno. R&P Shigeyoshi Kanda. Adv. contact Shingo Mochizuki.

610 JPN

IYO KIKI/MEDICAL APPLIANCE. Text in Japanese. 1974. m.
Published by: Nihon Iyo Kiki Kogyokai/Japan Association of Medical Equipment Industries, 39-15 Hongo 3-chome, Bunkyo-ku, Tokyo 113-0033, Japan.

IYO KOGAKU KENKYU SHISETSU HOKOKU/TOKYO WOMEN'S MEDICAL COLLEGE. INSTITUTE OF BIOMEDICAL ENGINEERING. REPORTS. see *BIOLOGY—Bioengineering*

610 JPN ISSN 0911-0852

IZAI TO MEKKIN/STUDIES ON MEDICAL IMPLEMENTS AND THEIR DISINFECTION. Text in Japanese. 1978. 3/yr.
Published by: Chuzai Gyomu Kenkyukai/Research Group of Central Sterile Supply Department, c/o Ms. Kazue Hayashi, Kokuritsu Byoin, 1-2 Tsubaki-Mori 4-chome, Chuo-ku, Chiba-shi 260-0042, Japan.

610 BRA ISSN 1415-4544

J A M A BRASIL. (Journal of the American Medical Association) Key Title: Jamabrazil. Text in Portuguese. 1997. m. BRL 120, USD 145.20 (effective 2000). adv. bibl, charts, illus. back issues avail. **Document type:** *Academic/Scholarly.* **Description:** Translates clinical and research articles printed in the Journal of the American Medical Association into Portuguese.
Related titles: ♦ Regional ed.: J A M A: The Journal of the American Medical Association. ISSN 0098-7484; ♦ J A M A en Espanol. ISSN 0211-4445; ♦ J A M A en Argentina; ♦ J A M A en Centroamerica; ♦ J A M A en Mexico. ISSN 0185-1160; ♦ J A M A en Venezuela. ISSN 0210-9921; ♦ J A M A en Colombia. ISSN 0210-9913; ♦ J A M A: The Journal of the American Medical Association (Italian Edition). ISSN 0393-554X; ♦ J A M A: The Journal of the American Medical Association (Swiss Edition).
Published by: (American Medical Association USA), Elea Ciencia Editorial Ltda., Rua Haddock Lobo, 86 Andar 6, Estacio, Rio De Janeiro, RJ 20260-132, Brazil. TEL 55-21-293-2112, FAX 55-21-293-7818, elea@openlink.com.br. Ed. Luiz Augusto Rodrigues. Adv. contact Alexandre Augusto Rodrigues. Circ: 100,000.

610 USA ISSN 0098-7484
R15 CODEN: JAMAAP

J A M A: THE JOURNAL OF THE AMERICAN MEDICAL ASSOCIATION. Text in English. 1848. w. (48/yr.). USD 325 in North America to institutions; USD 425 to institutions Central & S. America; GBP 275 elsewhere to institutions (effective 2001). adv. bk.rev. abstr, bibl, charts, illus. s-a. index. reprint service avail. from PQC. *Refereed.* **Document type:** *Academic/Scholarly.* **Description:** Keeps physicians abreast of current events, current therapies and research in progress. Covers virtually every specialty and aspects of medicine.
Former titles (until 1960): American Medical Association. Journal (0002-9955); (until 1883): American Medical Association. Transactions (1050-2793)
Related titles: CD-ROM ed.: (from Ovid Technologies, Inc.); Microform ed.: (from PQC,PMC); Online - full text ed.: (from The Dialog Corporation, Gale Group, Ovid Technologies, Inc., EBSCO Publishing, Institute for Scientific Information); ♦ Chinese ed.: Meiguo Yixuehui Zazhi (Zhongwen Ban). ISSN 1000-842X; ♦ Regional ed.: J A M A en Espanol. ISSN 0211-4445; ♦ J A M A en Argentina; ♦ J A M A en Centroamerica; ♦ J A M A en Mexico. ISSN 0185-1160; ♦ J A M A en Venezuela. ISSN 0210-9921; ♦ J A M A en Colombia. ISSN 0210-9913; ♦ J A M A: The Journal of the American Medical Association (Italian Edition). ISSN 0393-554X; ♦ J A M A: The Journal of the American Medical Association (Swiss Edition); ♦ J A M A Brasil. ISSN 1415-4544.
Indexed: AIDS Abstr., AMED, Abstr.Anthropol., Abstr.Hyg., Addic.Abstr., AgeLine, Amer.Bibl.Slavic & E.Eur.Stud., Biol.Dig., CINAHL, Cal.Tiss.Abstr., Crim.Just.Abstr., Curr.Cont., Dairy Sci.Abstr., Derwent Biotech.Abstr., Environ.Abstr., Environ.Sci.Poll.Mgmt., Food Sci.& Tech.Abstr., Gen.Sci.Ind. (Aug.1984-), Genet.Abstr., Hosp.Abstr., Hum.Gen.Abstr., INIS Atomind., I.P.A., Ind.Med. (1960-), Inpharma, Int.Abstr.Biol.Sci., Int.Nurs.Ind., Jrnl.Watch, Jrnl.Watch Card., Jrnl.Watch Derm., Jrnl.Watch Emer.Med., Jrnl.Watch Gastr., Jrnl.Watch Inf.Dis., Jrnl.Watch Neuro., Jrnl.Watch Psych., Jrnl.Watch Wom.Hlth., L.R.I., MLA Intl.Bibl., NRN, Neurosci.Abstr., Nuc.Acids Abstr., Nutr.Abstr., Peace Res.Abstr., Pharm.&Out.News, Pollut.Abstr., PsycInfo, Reac., Rev.Appl.Entomol., Rev.Arom.& Med.Plants, Rev.Med.& Vet.Mycol., Risk Abstr., Saf.Sci.Abstr., Sci.Cit.Ind., Trop.Dis.Bull., Viol.& Abuse Abstr., e-psyche.
—BLDSC (4689.000000), CASDDS, CIS, CISTI, GNLM, IDS, Infotrieve, ingenta, KNAW. **CCC.**
Published by: American Medical Association, 515 N State St, P O Box 10946, Chicago, IL 60610-0946. TEL 312-464-5000, FAX 312-464-4184, http://jama.ama-assn.org. Eds. Dr. Phil Fontanarosa, Dr. Richard Glass. Pub. Peter Murphy. adv.: B&W page USD 8,939, color page USD 11,414. Circ: 332,337 (paid). **Subscr. outside the Americas to:** JAMA Readers Services, PO Box 299, London WC1H 9TD, United Kingdom.

610 ITA ISSN 0393-554X

J A M A: THE JOURNAL OF THE AMERICAN MEDICAL ASSOCIATION (ITALIAN EDITION). Text in Italian. 1989. m. (10/yr.). ITL 50,000. adv. bk.rev.

M

Related titles: ♦ Regional ed.: J A M A: The Journal of the American Medical Association. ISSN 0098-7484; ♦ J A M A en Espanol. ISSN 0211-4445; ♦ J A M A en Argentina; ♦ J A M A en Centroamerica; ♦ J A M A en Mexico. ISSN 0185-1160; ♦ J A M A en Venezuela. ISSN 0210-9921; ♦ J A M A en Colombia. ISSN 0210-9913; ♦ J A M A: The Journal of the American Medical Association (Swiss Edition); ♦ J A M A Brasil. ISSN 1415-4544.
Published by: E S I Stampa Medica s.r.l., Largo Volontari Del Sangue, 10, Casella Postale 42, San Donato, MI 20133, Italy. TEL 02-5274241, FAX 02-55600670. Ed. Diego Onestinghel. Adv. contact Ornella Galbiati. B&W page ITL 11,000,000, color page ITL 14,500,000; trim 237 x 175. Circ: 56,000.

610 FRA ISSN 0299-3953
J A M I F. (Journal Association des Medecins Israelites de France) Text in French. 1952. 10/yr. FRF 100, USD 75. adv. bk.rev., film rev., play rev. abstr.
Former titles: Association des Medecins Israelites de France. Revue Medicale (0298-2900); A M I F (0400-132X)
—CISTI.
Published by: Association des Medecins Israelites de France, 11 avenue de la Republique, Fresnes 94260, France. Ed. Dr. D Bellaiche. Circ: 8,500 (controlled).

610 530 JPN
J A M P NEWS. Text in Japanese. 1985. s-a.
Published by: Japanese Association of Medical Physics/Nihon Igaku Butsuri Gakkai, Hoshasen Igaku Sogo Kenkyujo Butsuri Kenkyubu, 9-1 Anagawa 4-chome, Inage-ku, Chiba-shi 263-0024, Japan.

616.89 JPN
J A S C T NEWSLETTER. Text in Japanese. 1982. q. membership. **Document type:** *Newsletter.*
Indexed: e-psyche.
Published by: Japanese Association of Sex Counselors and Therapists/Nihon Sei Kagakkai, c/o Hase Kurinikku, Shin'aoyama biru Nishikan, 3f 1-1 Minami-Aoyama 1-chome, Minato-ku, Tokyo 107-0062, Japan. Ed. Takao Osada.

610 USA ISSN 0197-2510
RA645.5 CODEN: JJESF5
J E M S. (Journal of Emergency Medical Services) Text in English. 1980. m. USD 27.97 domestic; USD 45.97 in Canada; USD 47.97 foreign; USD 4 newsstand/cover foreign (effective 2001). adv. bk.rev. charts, illus, stat. back issues avail. **Document type:** *Journal, Trade.* **Description:** Aimed at emergency technicians (EMTs), paramedics, instructors, administrators, nurses and physicians, the journal reports on the issues that most affect the EMS work environment.
Related titles: Microform ed.
Indexed: CINAHL.
—BLDSC (4663.525000), CISTI, GNLM, ingenta.
Published by: J E M S Communications, PO Box 2789, Carlsbad, CA 92018. TEL 800-266-JEMS, http://www.jems.com/jems. Eds. A J Heightmann, Lisa Dionne. Adv. contact Lisa Tucker. Circ: 37,000 (paid and controlled).

J O P S O M. (Journal of Preventive and Social Medicine) see *PUBLIC HEALTH AND SAFETY*

601 USA
JACKSON LABORATORY SCIENTIFIC REPORT. Text in English. a. free per issue.
Formerly: Jackson Laboratory Annual Report
Published by: Jackson Laboratory, 600 Main St, Bar Harbor, ME 04609. TEL 207-288-6051. Ed. Luther Young. Circ: 2,000.

610 USA
JACKSONVILLE MEDICINE; the journal of the Duval County Medical Society. Text in English. m. USD 40. adv. back issues avail. *Refereed.* **Document type:** *Academic/Scholarly.*
Formerly: Jacksonville Medicine Bulletin
Published by: Duval County Medical Society, 1045 Riverside Ave, Ste 190, Jacksonville, FL 32204. TEL 904-355-6561, FAX 904-353-5848, duvalems-phil-gilbert@ibm.net. Ed., R&P, Adv. contact Marigrace Doran. page USD 440; trim 7.25 x 9.5. Circ: 1,800 (controlled).

610 LKA ISSN 0379-3877
JAFFNA MEDICAL JOURNAL. Text in English. 1953. s-a. LKR 1,000, USD 20. adv. bk.rev. **Document type:** *Academic/Scholarly.*
Indexed: Sri Lanka Sci.Ind.
Published by: Jaffna Medical Association, General Hospital, Jaffna, Sri Lanka. TEL 222661. Ed. Dr. N Sivarajah. Circ: 700.

610 614.8 DEU
JAHRBUCH KRITISCHE MEDIZIN. Text in German. 1976. a. DEM 39 to individuals (effective 1999). **Document type:** *Academic/Scholarly.* **Description:** Discusses economic and world politics, peace research, feminism, critical studies of medicine and psychology, international socialism, Marxism, culture, racism, and literary studies.
Formerly: Kritische Medizin im Argument (0341-0943)
—GNLM.
Published by: Argument-Verlag GmbH, Eppendorfer Weg 95A, Hamburg 20259, Germany. TEL 49-40-401800-0, FAX 49-40-40180020. Circ: 2,000.

610 ESP ISSN 0210-220X
JANO "MEDICINA Y HUMANIDADES". Text in Spanish. 1971. w. (45/yr..). USD 154. adv. reprint service avail. from PQC. **Document type:** *Academic/Scholarly.* **Description:** Covers topics in clinical medicine, diagnosis and treatment, to support the continuing education of postgraduates. Includes cultural topics in history, the arts, literature, music, films and theater.
—CINDOC. **CCC.**
Published by: Ediciones Doyma S.A., Traversa de Gracia, 17-21, Barcelona 08021, Spain. TEL 34-93-200-0711, FAX 34-93-209-1136. Ed. Celia Ribera Banus. Adv. contact Cristina Garrote. color page ESP 567,000; trim 295 x 230. Circ: 35,000.

610 572.8 JPN
JAPAN MATRIX (COLLAGEN) CLUB. PROCEEDINGS OF THE ANNUAL MEETING OF JAPAN MARIX CLUB. Text in Japanese; Summaries in English. 1959. a. JPY 3,000 (effective 2001). adv. back issues avail. **Document type:** *Proceedings.* **Description:** Investigates the structure, function and metabolism of extracellular matrix macromolecules, especially collagen.
Formerly: Japanese Collagen Club. Proceedings of the Annual Meeting
Related titles: Fax ed.
Published by: Japan Matrix (Collagen) Club, c/o Kiji Kiwata, Institute for Molecular Science of Medicine, Aichi Medical University, Nagakute, Aichi 480-1195, Japan. TEL 81-561-62-3311 ext 2088, FAX 81-561-63-3532, mbb@aichi-mcd-u.ac.jp, http://www2.aichi-med-u.ac.jp/matrix/index.html. Ed., Pub., R&P, Adv. contact Koji Kimata. Circ: 300.

610 JPN ISSN 0385-9215
JAPAN MEDICAL JOURNAL. Text in Japanese. 1921. w. JPY 693 per issue. back issues avail. **Description:** Published mainly for family physicians.
Published by: Nihon Iji Shimposha, 2-9 Kanda-Surugadai, Chiyoda-ku, Tokyo 101-0062, Japan. FAX 81-3-3292-1550. Ed. Shinji Umezawa. Circ: 46,200.

610 615.329 JPN ISSN 0368-2781
CODEN: JJANAX
JAPANESE JOURNAL OF ANTIBIOTICS. Text in Japanese; Summaries in English. 1947. m. USD 130 (effective 2000). adv. bibl, charts. index. back issues avail.; reprint service avail. from PQC. **Document type:** *Academic/Scholarly.*
Formerly: Journal of Antibiotics. Series B (0447-8991); Which superseded in part: Journal of Antibiotics
Related titles: Microform ed.: (from PQC); ♦ English ed.: Journal of Antibiotics. ISSN 0021-8820.
Indexed: Agri.& Environ.Biotech.Abstr. (coverage dropped), Aqua.Sci.& Fish.Abstr., Chem.Abstr., Chem.Indus.Notes, Chem.Titles, Curr.Chem.React. (coverage dropped), Curr.Cont. (coverage dropped), Dent.Ind., Derwent Biotech.Abstr., Environ.Sci.Poll.Mgmt., Excerp.Med., Ind.Chem. (coverage dropped), Ind.Med. (1968-), Inpharma, Mass Spectr.Bull., Pharm.&Out.News, Reac., Ref.Zh.
—BLDSC (4650.845000), CASDDS, CISTI, EMDOCS, GNLM, IDS, KNAW, Linda Hall.
Published by: Japan Antibiotics Research Association/Nihon Koseibusshitsu Gakujutsu Kyogikai, 2-20-8 Kami-Osaki, Shinagawa-ku, Tokyo 141-0021, Japan. TEL 81-3-3491-0181, FAX 81-3-3491-0179. Ed., R&P Kihachiro Shimizu. Adv. contact Morimasa Yagisawa. Circ: 1,500.

610 JPN ISSN 0047-1852
JAPANESE JOURNAL OF CLINICAL MEDICINE/NIPPON RINSHO. Text in Japanese; Summaries in English. 1943. m. JPY 30,000; JPY 2,500 newsstand/cover (effective 2001). adv. illus. Index. back issues avail. **Document type:** *Academic/Scholarly.*
Indexed: Curr.Cont. (coverage dropped), INIS Atomind., Ind.Med. (1943-), Inpharma, Reac.
—BLDSC (4651.375000), CISTI, GNLM, KNAW.
Published by: Nipponrinsho Co. Inc., 2-3-8 Dosho-Machi, Chuo-ku, Osaka-shi 541-0045, Japan. TEL 81-6-6204-2381, FAX 81-6-6204-2948, info@nippon-rinsho.co.jp, http://www.jcls.co.jp, http://www.nippon.rinsho.co.jp. Ed. Yasuo Suwa. Pub. Yoshio Kozai. Adv. contact Kazushige Ikeuchi. B&W page JPY 77,000, color page JPY 230,000. Circ: 8,000.

610 570 JPN ISSN 1344-6304
CODEN: JJMCAQ
JAPANESE JOURNAL OF INFECTIOUS DISEASES. Abbreviated title: J J I D. Text in English. 1948. bi-m. on exchange or gift basis. bk.rev. charts, illus. *Refereed.* **Document type:** *Journal, Academic/Scholarly, Government.* **Description:** Publishes full and short communications, reviews, epidemiological reports and methods dealing with infectious diseases.
Former titles (until 1998): Japanese Journal of Medical Science and Biology (0021-5112); (until 1952): Japanese Medical Journal (0368-3095)
Related titles: Microform ed.: (from PMC); Online - full content ed.; Online - full text ed.: (from Institute for Scientific Information).
Indexed: ASCA, Abstr.Hyg., Apic.Abstr., Biol.Abstr., Chem.Abstr., Chem.Indus.Notes, Chem.Titles, Curr.Cont. (coverage dropped), Dairy Sci.Abstr., Dent.Ind., Diar.Dis.Res., Excerp.Med., Helminthol.Abstr., INIS Atomind., Ind.Med. (1999-), Ind.Sci.Rev., Ind.Vet., Inpharma, NRN, Nutr.Abstr., Pharm.&Out.News, Pig News & Info., Poult.Abstr., Protozool.Abstr., Reac., Rev.Appl.Entomol., Rev.Arom.& Med.Plants, Rev.Med.& Vet.Mycol., SSCI (coverage dropped), Sci.Cit.Ind. (coverage dropped), THA, Trop.Dis.Bull., Vet.Bull., Zoo.Rec.
—BLDSC (4655.540000), CASDDS, CISTI, GNLM, IDS, ingenta, KNAW.
Published by: National Institute of Infectious Diseases, 23-1, Toyama 1-chome, Shinjuku-ku, Tokyo 162-8640, Japan. TEL 81-3-5285-1111, FAX 81-3-5285-1192, jjid@nih.go.jp, http://www.nih.go.jp/jjid/jjid.html. Ed. Tatsuo Miyamura. Circ: 1,100.

JAPANESE JOURNAL OF MEDICAL MYCOLOGY/NIHON ISHINKIN GAKKAI ZASSHI. see *BIOLOGY—Microbiology*

JAPANESE JOURNAL OF PHYSIOLOGY. see *BIOLOGY—Physiology*

610 JPN ISSN 0536-3489
JAPANESE MEDICAL RESEARCHERS DIRECTORY. Text in English, Japanese. 1959. a. JPY 38,000.
Indexed: Biol.Abstr.
Published by: Igaku-Shoin Ltd., 5-24-3 Hongo, Bunkyo-ku, Tokyo 113-0033, Japan. Ed. Hiromasa Kita. Circ: 4,000.

610 IND ISSN 0379-1653
JASLOK HOSPITAL & RESEARCH CENTRE. BULLETIN. Text in English. 1976. q. INR 25 (effective 2001). adv. bk.rev. 40 p./no. 2 cols./p. *Refereed.* **Document type:** *Bulletin, Academic/Scholarly.* **Description:** Contains research papers published in Jaslok Hospital and Research center.
Published by: Jaslok Hospital & Research Centre, 15 Dr. G. Deshmukh Marg, Mumbai, Maharashtra 400 026, India. TEL 91-22-4933333, FAX 91-22-4950508, TELEX 011-75743-JASH-IN, jaslok@vsnl.com. Ed. S Sadikot. Adv. contact K Dhunjibhoy. B&W page INR 6,800; trim 150 x 210. Circ: 500.

JAWETZ, MELNICK & ADELBERG'S MEDICAL MICROBIOLOGY. see *BIOLOGY—Microbiology*

610 IND
JEEVAK. Text in English, Hindi, Sanskrit. q. INR 41. adv. bk.rev. abstr, tr.lit. index.
Related titles: Microform ed.; Record ed.
Published by: Jeevak Anshathlya, Sahitya Marg, Barnalla, India. Circ: 1,500.

610 USA ISSN 0021-5821
JEFFERSON MEDICAL COLLEGE ALUMNI BULLETIN. Text in English. 1922. q. free per issue. **Document type:** *Bulletin.*
Published by: Jefferson Medical College, 1020 Locust St, Ste M-41, Philadelphia, PA 19107-6799. TEL 215-955-7920, FAX 215-923-9916, Malcolm.Clendenin@mail.tju.edu, jeffline.tju.edu/CWIS/JMC/alumni/bulletin.html. Ed., R&P, Adv. contact Malcolm Clendenin. Circ: 20,000.

610 CHN ISSN 1001-7321
JIAMUSI YIXUEYUAN XUEBAO/JIAMUSI MEDICAL INSTITUTE. JOURNAL. Text in Chinese. q.

M

Published by: Jiamusi Yixueyuan, Xuebao Bianjibu, Jiamusi, Heilongjiang 154002, China. TEL 32949. Ed. Liu Fangzhen.

610 CHN ISSN 0253-3685
JIANGSU YIYAO/JIANGSU MEDICAL JORUNAL. Text in Chinese; Contents page in English. 1975. m. CNY 81.60; CNY 6.80 per month (effective 2000). **Document type:** *Academic/Scholarly.*
Related titles: Online - full content ed.: (from WanFang Data Corp.).
—BLDSC (4668.462000).
Published by: Jiangsu Provincial Bureau of Public Health, 42 Zhongyang Rd, Nanjing 210008, China. TEL 86-25-7711507, FAX 86-25-3616370. Ed. Weixin Tang. **Dist. by:** China International Book Trading Corp, 35, Chegongzhuang Xilu, Haidian District, Beijing 100044, China. TEL 86-1-68413849, FAX 86-1-68412048, cibtc@mail.cibtc.com.cn, http://www.cibtc.com.cn.

JIANGSU ZHONGYI/JIANGSU TRADITIONAL CHINESE MEDICINE. see *ALTERNATIVE MEDICINE*

JIANKANG BAO/HEALTH NEWS. see *PHYSICAL FITNESS AND HYGIENE*

610 CHN
JIATING YISHENG BAO/FAMILY'S DOCTOR WEEKLY. Text in Chinese. w. CNY 20.16. **Document type:** *Newspaper.*
Published by: China International Book Trading Corp/Zhongguo Guoji Tushu Maoyi Zonggongsi cibtc@mail.cibtc.com.cn, http://www.cibtc.com.cn. **Dist. by:** 35, Chegongzhuang Xilu, Haidian District, Beijing 100044, China.

610 CHN ISSN 1001-0203
JIATING YIXUE/FAMILY MEDICINE. Text in Chinese. 1985. m. USD 30; USD 2.50 newsstand/cover (effective 2001).
Published by: China International Book Trading Corp/Zhongguo Guoji Tushu Maoyi Zonggongsi cibtc@mail.cibtc.com.cn, http://www.cibtc.com.cn. Ed. Wang Jian. **Dist. by:** 35, Chegongzhuang Xilu, Haidian District, Beijing 100044, China.

610 CHN ISSN 1005-3743
JIATING ZHONGYIYAO/FAMILY TRADITIONAL CHINESE MEDICINE. Text in Chinese. 1993. m. USD 28.80; USD 2.40 newsstand/cover (effective 2001). **Document type:** *Academic/Scholarly.*
Published by: China International Book Trading Corp/Zhongguo Guoji Tushu Maoyi Zonggongsi cibtc@mail.cibtc.com.cn, http://www.cibtc.com.cn. **Dist. by:** 35, Chegongzhuang Xilu, Haidian District, Beijing 100044, China. **Co-sponsor:** Zhongguo Zhongyi Yanjiuyuan.

610 CHN ISSN 1001-6325
JICHU YIXUE YU LINCHUANG/BASIC MEDICAL SCIENCE AND CLINICS. Text in Chinese. 1990. bi-m.
Published by: Zhongguo Yixue Kexueyuan, Jichu Yixue Yanjiusuo/Chinese Academy of Medical Sciences, Institute of Basic Medical Science, 5 Dongdan Santiao, Beijing 100730, China. TEL 5127733. Ed. Cheng Mengqin.

610 CHN ISSN 0577-7402
JIEFANGJUN YIXUE ZAZHI/MEDICAL JOURNAL OF CHINESE PEOPLE'S LIBERATION ARMY. Text in Chinese. 1964. bi-m. USD 15; CNY 5, USD 2.50 newsstand/cover (effective 2001). **Document type:** *Academic/Scholarly.*
Related titles: Online - full content ed.: (from WanFang Data Corp.).
Published by: Renminjun Yichubanshi, Fuxin Lu 22-Hao Jia 3-Hao, Beijing 100842, China. **Dist. by:** China International Book Trading Corp, 35, Chegongzhuang Xilu, Haidian District, Beijing 100044, China. TEL 86-1-68413849, FAX 86-1-68412048, cibtc@mail.cibtc.com.cn, http://www.cibtc.com.cn.

610 JPN ISSN 0021-6968
CODEN: JMEJAS
JIKEIKAI MEDICAL JOURNAL. Text in English. 1954. q. per issue exchange basis. charts, illus, stat. index.
Indexed: Abstr.Hyg., Biol.Abstr., Chem.Abstr., Chem.Indus.Notes, Chem.Titles, Excerp.Med., INIS Atomind., Trop.Dis.Bull.
—BLDSC (4669.000000), CASDDS, CISTI, GNLM, ingenta, KNAW. **CCC.**
Published by: Jikei University School of Medicine/Tokyo Jikeikai Ika Daigaku, 3-25-8 Nishi-Shinbashi, Minato-ku, Tokyo 105-0003, Japan. Ed., R&P Tsuneya Ohno. Circ: 1,000.

JILIN ZHONGYIYAO/JILIN TRADITIONAL CHINESE MEDICINE. see *ALTERNATIVE MEDICINE*

610 616.6 JPN ISSN 0385-2156
JIN TO TOSEKI/KIDNEY AND DIALYSIS. Text in Japanese. 1976. m. JPY 38,000; JPY 2,400 newsstand/cover (effective 1999).
—BLDSC (5094.210000).
Published by: Tokyo Igakusha Ltd., 35-4 Hongo 3-chome, Bunkyo-ku, Tokyo 113-0033, Japan. TEL 81-3-3811-4119, FAX 81-3-3811-6135. Circ: 6,000.

JINAN DAXUE XUEBAO (ZIRAN KEXUE YU YIXUE BAN)/JOURNAL OF JINAN UNIVERSITY(NATURAL SCIENCE AND MEDICINE EDITION). see *SCIENCES: COMPREHENSIVE WORKS*

610 CHN
JINGYAOTONG ZAZHI/JOURNAL OF CERVICODYNIA AND LUMBODYNIA. Text in Chinese. q. **Document type:** *Academic/Scholarly.*
Published by: China International Book Trading Corp/Zhongguo Guoji Tushu Maoyi Zonggongsi cibtc@mail.cibtc.com.cn, http://www.cibtc.com.cn. **Dist. by:** 35, Chegongzhuang Xilu, Haidian District, Beijing 100044, China.

610 JPN ISSN 0300-0818
CODEN: JNZKA7
JINKO ZOKI/JAPANESE JOURNAL OF ARTIFICIAL ORGANS. Text in Japanese. 1964. bi-m. JPY 1,500 per issue.
Indexed: Biol.Abstr., Excerp.Med., INIS Atomind.
—BLDSC (4650.920000), CASDDS, CISTI, EMDOCS, GNLM, KNAW.
Published by: Nihon Jinko Zoki Gakkai/Japanese Society for Artificial Organs and Tissues, Nihon Gakkai Jimu Senta, 16-9 Honkomagome 5-chome, Bunkyo-ku, Tokyo 113-0021, Japan.

610 BRA ISSN 0047-2077
CODEN: JBRMAP
JORNAL BRASILEIRO DE MEDICINA. Cover title: J B M. Text in Portuguese; Summaries in English. 1959. m. USD 450 (effective 2000 - 2001). adv. bk.rev. abstr, bibl, charts, illus. cum.index.
Indexed: Biol.Abstr., Chem.Abstr., INIS Atomind.
Published by: Editora de Publicacoes Cientificas Ltda., Rua Major Suckow, 30, Rocha, Rio De Janeiro, RJ 20911-160, Brazil. TEL 55-21-2013722, 55-21-5010057, FAX 55-21-2613749. Eds. Ismar C de Silveira, J M Melo. R&P, Adv. contact Ana Paula. Circ: 40,000.

616.07 BRA ISSN 0104-8090
CODEN: RBPTBN
JORNAL BRASILEIRO DE PATOLOGIA. Text in Portuguese; Abstracts in English. 1950. q. BRL 160 to individuals; BRL 240 to institutions. adv. bk.rev. abstr, bibl, charts, illus, stat. index. back issues avail.; reprint service avail. from IRC. **Description:** Contains original review and update papers in laboratory medicine.
Formerly (until 1995): Revista Brasileira de Patologia Clinica (0034-7302)
Related titles: CD-ROM ed.
Indexed: Biol.Abstr., Chem.Abstr., Chem.Indus.Notes, Chem.Titles, INIS Atomind., Ind.Med. (coverage dropped), Ref.Zh.
—CASDDS, GNLM, KNAW.
Published by: Sociedade Brasileira de Patologia Clinica/Brazilian Clinical Pathology Society, Rua Dois de Dezembro, 78 Andar 10, Rio De Janeiro, RJ 22220-040, Brazil. TEL 55-21-5581024, FAX 55-21-2053386. Ed. Octavio Fernandes. Adv. contact Cristina Morgado. B&W page USD 430, color page USD 640; 280 x 210. Circ: 3,000. **Co-sponsor:** Sociedade Brasileira de Patologia, Sociedade Brasileira de Citopatologia.

610 PRT ISSN 0871-8822
CODEN: JCMEE
JORNAL DAS CIENCIAS MEDICAS. Text in Portuguese. 1834. m. PTE 3,500.
Formerly (until 1988): Sociedade das Ciencias Medicas de Lisboa. Jornal
Indexed: Excerp.Med.
—EMDOCS, GNLM, KNAW.
Published by: (Sociedade das Ciencias Medicas de Lisboa), Edicoes Recipe, Calcada do Monte, 23 r-c, Lisbon 1100, Portugal. TEL 1-874847.

610 PRT
JORNAL POLICLINICO. Text in Portuguese. 11/yr.
Address: Rua Tristao Vaz, 15-2o D, Lisbon 1400, Portugal. TEL 3011989, FAX 3015539. Ed. Jose Reis Jr. Circ: 12,500.

610 FRA ISSN 0021-7883
CODEN: JMLYA6
JOURNAL DE MEDECINE DE LYON; organe de professeurs, agreges, medecins des hopitaux et medecins practiciens de Lyon. Text in French; Summaries in English. 1920. m. FRF 365 to institutions; FRF 170 to students (effective 2000). adv. bk.rev. illus. index.
Indexed: Biol.Abstr., Chem.Abstr., Excerp.Med. (until 1993), INIS Atomind., Ind.Med. (coverage dropped), Nutr.Abstr.
—CASDDS, CISTI.
Published by: Sedip Medical, 75 Cours Albert Thomas, Lyon Cedex 3 69447, France. TEL 33-4-72352372, FAX 33-4-72352375.

610 FRA ISSN 0021-7905
CODEN: JMSTBR
JOURNAL DE MEDECINE DE STRASBOURG. Text in French. 1970. 5/yr. FRF 390 domestic to individuals; FRF 555 foreign to individuals; FRF 195 domestic to students; FRF 330 foreign to students (effective 1999). adv. bk.rev. **Document type:** *Academic/Scholarly.*
Related titles: Microform ed.
Indexed: Biol.Abstr., Chem.Abstr., Curr.Cont. (coverage dropped), Excerp.Med., Helminthol.Abstr., INIS Atomind., Inpharma, Nutr.Abstr., Reac.
—CASDDS, CISTI, GNLM, Infotrieve. **CCC.**
Published by: (Faculte de Medecine et de la Communaute Medicale d'Alsace et de Moselle), Expansion Scientifique Francaise, 31 bd. de la Tour Maubourg, Paris Cedex 7 75343, France. TEL 33-1-40626400, FAX 33-1-45556920. Ed. J L Schlienger. Circ: 5,000.

618.92 FRA ISSN 0987-7983
JOURNAL DE PEDIATRIE ET DE PUERICULTURE. Text in French. 1972; N.S. 1988. 8/yr. EUR 120 in Europe to institutions; USD 138 elsewhere to institutions (effective 2002). *Refereed.* **Document type:** *Academic/Scholarly.* **Description:** Publishes in-depth articles on all aspects of child care, including general pediatrics, fetal and neonatal medicine, nutrition, psychiatry and psychology, practical child care and issues relating to children and society.
Formerly (until 1988): Jonctions (0300-0478)
Related titles: Microfilm ed.: N.S. (from PQC); Online - full text ed.: N.S. (from ingenta, Swets Blackwell, ScienceDirect).
Indexed: Excerp.Med. (1996-).
—BLDSC (5030.310000), CISTI.
Published by: Elsevier Paris, Editions Scientifiques et Medicales (Subsidiary of: Reed Elsevier plc. group), 23 rue Linois, Paris 75015, France. TEL 33-1-45589110, FAX 33-1-45589419, jpp@elsevier.fr; academic@elsevier-fr.com, http://www.elsevier.com/locate/pedpeu. Eds. C Turberg Romain, C Turberg-Romain.

610 USA ISSN 1074-5807
R693
JOURNAL FOR MINORITY MEDICAL STUDENTS. Text in English. 1972. q. USD 20. adv. bk.rev. charts, illus, stat. back issues avail. **Document type:** *Academic/Scholarly.* **Description:** Discusses social legal, financial, and academic issues.
Former titles (until 1993): Student National Medical Association. Journal (1044-1654); (until 1989): Black Bag (0196-1594)
Published by: Spectrum Unlimited, 4203 Canal St, New Orleans, LA 70019. TEL 504-488-5100, FAX 504-488-7072, jmmsmag@aol.com, http://gnofn.org/~spectrum. Ed. Valerie J Andrews. Pub., Adv. contact Bill Bowers. Circ: 10,000.

610 DEU
JOURNAL FUER AESTHETISCHE MEDIZIN. Text in German. 17/yr. DEM 75 (effective 2000). **Document type:** *Journal, Academic/Scholarly.*
Published by: B M V - Berliner Medizinische Verlagsanstalt GmbH, Lietzenburger Str 97, Berlin 10719, Germany. TEL 49-30-886749-0, FAX 49-30-88674999, info@bmv-berlin.com, http://www.bmv-berlin.de. Ed. Dr. H G Bull. Circ: 4,000.

▼ **JOURNAL FUER ERNAEHRUNGSMEDIZIN;** interdisziplinaeres Organ fuer Praevention und Therapie von Krankheiten durch Ernaehrung. see *NUTRITION AND DIETETICS*

610 FRA ISSN 0241-0109
JOURNAL INTERNATIONAL DE MEDECINE✱ . Text in French. 1979. 28/yr. FRF 180. adv.
—CISTI.
Published by: Societe d'Edition et de Presse Internationale Medicale, 25 bis, av. Pierre-Grenier, Boulogne 92100, France. TEL 49-10-06-06. Ed. J Haroche. Circ: 35,000.

M

610 IND ISSN 0971-071X
JOURNAL INTERNATIONAL MEDICAL SCIENCES ACADEMY. Cover title: J I M S A. Text in English. 1987. q. INR 200. adv. *Refereed.* **Document type:** *Academic/Scholarly.*
—BLDSC (4802.317000), EMDOCS, GNLM, KNAW.
Published by: International Medical Sciences Academy, National Medical Library Bldg. 2nd Fl., Ansari Nagar Ring Rd., New Delhi 110 029, India. TEL 91-11-696-4660. Ed. P S Gupta. Pub. P.S. Gupta. R&P P D Gulati. Adv. contact S N A Rizvi. Circ: 700.

610 USA ISSN 1054-139X
RJ550 CODEN: JADHE5
JOURNAL OF ADOLESCENT HEALTH. Text in English. 1980. m. EUR 246 in Europe to individuals; JPY 32,600 in Japan to individuals; USD 274 elsewhere to individuals; EUR 605 in Europe to institutions; JPY 80,200 in Japan to institutions; USD 676 elsewhere to institutions; EUR 84 in Europe Residents price; JPY 11,200 in Japan Residents price; USD 95 elsewhere Residents price (effective 2002). back issues avail. *Refereed.* **Document type:** *Academic/Scholarly.* **Description:** Devoted to the unique health care problems of the adolescent.
Formerly (until 1991): Journal of Adolescent Health Care (0197-0070)
Related titles: Microform ed.: (from PQC); Online - full text ed.: J A H Online (from ingenta, Swets Blackwell, ScienceDirect, Institute for Scientific Information).
Indexed: ASCA, ASSIA, Adol.Ment.Hlth.Abstr., Behav.Med.Abstr., Biol.Abstr., CINAHL, Chic.Per.Ind., Crim.Just.Abstr., Curr.Cont., Curr.Lit.Fam.Plan., Dairy Sci.Abstr., Energy Ind., Energy Info.Abstr., Environ.Sci.Poll.Mgmt., Excerp.Med., Fam.Ind., Ind.Med. (1991-), Inpharma, Jrnl.Watch Wom.Hlth., Lang.& Lang.Behav.Abstr., NRN, Nutr.Abstr., Pharm.&Out.News, Pollut.Abstr., Protozool.Abstr., PsycInfo, Psychol.Abstr. (1980-), Reac., Risk Abstr., SOPODA, SSCI, Saf.Sci.Abstr., Sage Fam.Stud.Abstr., Soc.Sci.Ind. (coverage dropped), Soc.Serv.Abstr., Sociol.Abstr., THA, Trop.Dis.Bull., Viol.& Abuse Abstr., e-psyche.
—BLDSC (4918.942800), CISTI, EMDOCS, GNLM, IDS, ingenta, KNAW. **CCC.**
Published by: (Society for Adolescent Medicine), Elsevier Science, 655 Ave of the Americas, New York, NY 10010. TEL 212-989-5800, FAX 212-633-3990, usinfo-f@elsevier.com, http://www.elsevier.com/locate/jadohea. Eds. Dr. Iris F Litt, R Brookman. **Subscr. in Australasia and the Far East to:** Elsevier Science (Singapore) Pte Ltd, No.1 Temasek Ave, 17-01 Millenia Tower, Singapore 039192, Singapore. TEL 65-434-3727, FAX 65-337-2230; **Subscr. in Japan to:** Elsevier Science Inc - Japan Regional Office, 9-15 Higashi-Azabu 1-chome, Minato-ku, Tokyo 106-0044, Japan. TEL 81-3-5561-5033; **Subscr. outside the Americas to:** Elsevier Science BV, PO Box 211, Amsterdam 1000 AE, Netherlands. TEL 31-20-485-3757.

JOURNAL OF AGROMEDICINE; interface of human health & agriculture. see *OCCUPATIONAL HEALTH AND SAFETY*

612 IND ISSN 0970-1842
CODEN: JAS
JOURNAL OF ANATOMICAL SCIENCES. Text in English. 1979. s-a. USD 60. **Document type:** *Academic/Scholarly.*
Indexed: Biol.Abstr., Curr.Cont. (coverage dropped), Excerp.Med., Indian Sci.Abstr.
—EMDOCS.
Published by: Anatomical Society of India, Uttar Pradesh Chapter, c/o Dept. of Anatomy, G.S.V.M. Medical College, Kanpur, Uttar Pradesh 208 002, India. TEL 91-512-214667. Ed. Vinod Kumar. Circ: 500.

JOURNAL OF ANATOMY; molecular, cellular and experimental morphology. see *BIOLOGY*

616.6 USA ISSN 0196-3635
QP253 CODEN: JOAND3
JOURNAL OF ANDROLOGY. Text in English. 1980. bi-m. USD 264 domestic to institutions; USD 287 foreign to institutions (effective 2001). adv. bk.rev. charts, illus, stat. index. back issues avail. *Refereed.* **Document type:** *Academic/Scholarly.* **Description:** Publishes significant new findings of basic and clinical research on human and animal male reproductive tracts.
Related titles: E-mail ed.; Fax ed.; Microform ed.: (from PQC); Online - full text ed.: (from Institute for Scientific Information).
Indexed: ASCA, Anim.Breed.Abstr., Biol.Abstr., Chem.Abstr., Chem.Indus.Notes, Chem.Titles, Curr.Adv.Cell & Devel.Biol., Curr.Cont., Excerp.Med., INIS Atomind., Ind.Med. (1980-), Ind.Sci.Rev., Inpharma, Pharm.&Out.News, Reac., SSCI (coverage dropped), Sci.Cit.Ind., THA.
—BLDSC (4935.340000), CASDDS, CISTI, GNLM, ingenta, KNAW.
Published by: (American Society of Andrology), Allen Press Inc., PO Box 1897, Lawrence, KS 66044-8897. TEL 785-843-1235, 800-627-0629, FAX 785-843-1274, asa@allenpress.com, http://godot.urol.uic.edu/~androlog. Eds. David W Hammilton, Jon L Pryor. Pub. Marissa Barlow. R&P Lonnie Russell TEL 618-453-1596. Adv. contact Onkar S Sandal. B&W page USD 570, color page USD 980; trim 11 x 8.5. Circ: 1,200 (paid).

JOURNAL OF ANTI-AGING MEDICINE. see *GERONTOLOGY AND GERIATRICS*

615.329 JPN ISSN 0021-8820
CODEN: JANTAJ
JOURNAL OF ANTIBIOTICS; an international journal devoted to research on bioactive microbial products. Text in English. 1947. m. USD 300 (effective 2001). bibl, charts. index. reprint service avail. from PQC. *Refereed.* **Document type:** *Academic/Scholarly.*
Formerly (1953-1967): Journal of Antibiotics. Series A (0368-1173); Which superseded in part: Journal of Antibiotics
Related titles: Microform ed.: (from PQC,PMC); Online - full text ed.: (from Institute for Scientific Information); ♦ Japanese ed.: Japanese Journal of Antibiotics. ISSN 0368-2781.
Indexed: ASCA, Agri.& Environ.Biotech.Abstr. (coverage dropped), Aqua.Sci.& Fish.Abstr., Bio-Contr.News & Info., Biol.Abstr., Biotech.Cit.Ind., Chem.Abstr., Chem.Cit.Ind., Chem.Indus.Notes, Chem.Titles, Curr.Adv.Gen.& Molec.Biol., Curr.Biotech.Abstr., Curr.Chem.React., Curr.Cont., Derwent Biotech.Abstr., Environ.Sci.Poll.Mgmt., Excerp.Med., Helminthol.Abstr., INIS Atomind., Ind.Chem., Ind.Med. (1953-), Ind.Sci.Rev., Ind.Vet., Inpharma, Int.Abstr.Biol.Sci., Mass Spectr.Bull., Med.& Pharm.Biotech.Abstr., Microbiol.Abstr., NPU, Nutr.Abstr., Pharm.&Out.News, Pig News & Info., Plant Grow.Reg.Abstr., Pollut.Abstr., Protozool.Abstr., RCI, Reac., Rev.Appl.Entomol., Rev.Arom.& Med.Plants, Rev.Med.& Vet.Mycol., Rev.Plant Path., Risk Abstr., Saf.Sci.Abstr., Sci.Cit.Ind., Sugar Ind.Abstr., Vet.Bull., Weed Abstr.
—BLDSC (4937.900000), CASDDS, CINDOC, CISTI, GNLM, IDS, ingenta, KNAW, Linda Hall.
Published by: Japan Antibiotics Research Association/Nihon Koseibusshitsu Gakujutsu Kyogikai, 2-20-8 Kami-Osaki, Shinagawa-ku, Tokyo 141-0021, Japan. TEL 81-3-3491-0181, FAX 81-3-3491-0179. Ed., R&P Kihachiro Shimizu. Adv. contact Morimasa Yagisawa. Circ: 2,000.

610 JPN
JOURNAL OF APPLIED MEDICINE/OYO IGAKU. Text in English, Japanese, Multiple languages. 1960. q. membership. abstr.
Indexed: Chem.Abstr.
Published by: Society of Applied Medicine/Nihon Oyo Igakkai, 108 Shimo-Gamomiyazaki-cho, Sakyo-ku, Kyoto-shi 606-0802, Japan.

610 IND ISSN 0377-0400
CODEN: JAMED6
JOURNAL OF APPLIED MEDICINE. Text in English. 1975. m. INR 144. adv. bk.rev. bibl, illus.
Indexed: AgeLine, INIS Atomind.
—CASDDS, CISTI.
Published by: Living Media India Pvt. Ltd., F-14-15 Connaught Place, New Delhi 110 001, India. TEL 3313076, FAX 91-11-3712998, TELEX 031-62634 INTO IN. Ed. G S Sainani.

JOURNAL OF APPLIED PHYSIOLOGY. see *BIOLOGY—Physiology*

371.335 GBR ISSN 0140-511X
CODEN: JAUMD2
JOURNAL OF AUDIO VISUAL MEDIA IN MEDICINE. Text in English. 1951. q. GBP 81, USD 133 to individuals; GBP 243, USD 402 to institutions (effective 2002). adv. bk.rev., film rev. abstr, charts, illus. index. back issues avail.; reprints avail. *Refereed.* **Document type:** *Academic/Scholarly.* **Description:** Presents information and ideas on the development, implementation and use of audiovisual media for education, recording and research purposes in all areas of the health sciences.
Formerly: Medical and Biological Illustration (0025-6978)
Related titles: Microform ed.: (from PQC); Online - full text ed.: ISSN 1465-3494 (from CatchWord Ltd., EBSCO Publishing, O C L C Online Computer Library Center, Inc., RoweCom Information Quest, ProQuest Information & Learning, Swets Blackwell).
Indexed: Abstr.Hyg., Biol.Abstr., Chem.Abstr., Curr.Cont. (coverage dropped), Dent.Ind., ERA, Educ.Tech.Abstr., Ind.Med. (1978-), Ind.Vet., LISA, Photo.Abstr., Res.High.Educ.Abstr., Sci.Cit.Ind. (coverage dropped), Trop.Dis.Bull., Vet.Bull.
—BLDSC (4949.350000), CatchWord, CISTI, GNLM, Infotrieve, Linda Hall. **CCC.**
Published by: (Institute of Medical & Biological Illustration), Carfax Publishing Limited (Subsidiary of: Taylor & Francis Group), PO Box 25, Abingdon, Oxon OX14 3UE, United Kingdom. TEL 44-1235-401000, FAX 44-1235-401550, enquiries@carfax.co.uk, enquiry@tandf.co.uk, http://www.carfax.co.uk. Ed. K P Duguid.

174.2 220 USA ISSN 1050-3404
JOURNAL OF BIBLICAL ETHICS IN MEDICINE. Text in English. 1987. q. USD 18. bk.rev. cum.index: 1987-1991. back issues avail.; reprints avail. *Refereed.* **Document type:** *Academic/Scholarly.* **Description:** Focuses on medical-ethical issues from a conservative evangelical worldview.
Indexed: Chr.Per.Ind., Rel.& Theol.Abstr.
Published by: Biblical Medical Ethics, Inc., PO Box 13231, Florence, SC 29504. TEL 803-665-6853. Ed. Hilton P Terrel. Circ: 1,500.

610.78 USA ISSN 0094-2499
R118
THE JOURNAL OF BIOCOMMUNICATION. Text in English. 1974. 4/yr. USD 45 domestic to individuals; USD 48 in Canada to individuals; USD 59 in Mexico to individuals; USD 63 elsewhere to individuals (effective 2000). bk.rev., film rev. illus. back issues avail.; reprint service avail. from PQC.
Incorporates (in 2000): Journal of Biological Photography (0274-497X); Supersedes: Medical Art (0076-5902); Which was formerly (1953-1964): Association of Medical Illustrators. Journal (0098-8456); Graphics
Related titles: Microform ed.: (from PQC).
Indexed: B.R.I., Biol.Abstr., C.I.J.E., Dent.Abstr., Hosp.Lit.Ind., Ind.Med. (1974-), Mid.East: Abstr.& Ind.
—BLDSC (4952.300000), CISTI, GNLM, ingenta.
Published by: BioCommunications Association, 115 Stoneridge Drive, Chapel Hill, NC 27514-9737. bcaoffice@aol.com, http://www.bca.org/docs. Circ: 2,000 (paid). **Co-sponsors:** Association of Biomedical Communications Directors; Health Sciences Communications Association; Association of Medical Illustrators.

610.28 USA ISSN 0148-0731
R856.A1 CODEN: JBENDY
JOURNAL OF BIOMECHANICAL ENGINEERING. Text in English. 1977. q. USD 260 to non-members; USD 300 foreign to non-members; USD 60 to members; USD 100 foreign to members (effective 2001). adv. bk.rev. illus. Index. reprint service avail. from PQC. *Refereed.* **Document type:** *Academic/Scholarly.* **Description:** Reports research results involving the application of mechanical engineering knowledge, skills and principles to the conception, design, development, analysis and operation of biomechanical systems.
Related titles: Microform ed.: (from PQC); Online - full text ed.: (from EBSCO Publishing, Gale Group, Swets Blackwell, Institute for Scientific Information).
Indexed: AMED, A.S.& T.Ind. (Nov.1983-), ASCA, Agri.& Environ.Biotech.Abstr. (coverage dropped), Appl.Mech.Rev., BBCI, Bioeng.Abstr., Biotech.& Bioeng.Abstr., CAD CAM Abstr., Chem.Abstr., Chem.Eng.Abstr., Curr.Cont., Eng.Ind., Excerp.Med., Fluidex, INSPEC (Feb.1977-Oct.1977, Feb.1978-), Ind.Med. (1977-), Ind.Sci.Rev., Inpharma, METADEX, Mass Spectr.Bull., Mat.Sci.Cit.Ind., Reac., Ref.Zh., Sci.Cit.Ind., T.C.E.A.
—BLDSC (8896.700000), AskIEEE, CISTI, Ei, EMDOCS, GNLM, IDS, ingenta, Linda Hall. **CCC.**
Published by: A S M E International, 22 Law Dr, PO Box 2900, Fairfield, NJ 07007-2900. TEL 973-882-1167, FAX 973-882-1717, infocentral@asme.org, http://asme.org. Ed. Kenneth Diller.

610.28 GBR ISSN 0021-9290
QP303 CODEN: JBMCBS
THE JOURNAL OF BIOMECHANICS. Text in English. 1968. m. EUR 266 in Europe to individuals; JPY 35,200 in Japan to individuals; USD 297 elsewhere to individuals; EUR 2,070 in Europe to institutions; JPY 274,900 in Japan to institutions; USD 2,316 elsewhere to institutions (effective 2002). adv. bk.rev. charts, illus, stat. index. back issues avail.; reprint service avail. from PQC. *Refereed.* **Document type:** *Academic/Scholarly.* **Description:** Publishes original research concerning the application of mechanics to medical and biological problems.
Related titles: Microfilm ed.: (from PQC); Online - full text ed.: (from ingenta, Swets Blackwell, ScienceDirect, Institute for Scientific Information).

M

Indexed: AMED, ASCA, Abstr.Anthropol., Appl.Mech.Rev., Aqua.Sci.& Fish.Abstr., BBCI, Bioeng.Abstr., Biol.Abstr., Cal.Tiss.Abstr., Comput.& Info.Sys., Curr.Cont., Dent.Ind., Electron.& Communic.Abstr.J., Eng.Ind., Environ.Sci.Poll.Mgmt., Ergon.Abstr., Excerp.Med., Focus on: Sports Sci.& Med., INIS Atomind., INSPEC (May 1970-), ISMEC, Ind.Med. (1968-), Ind.Sci.Rev., Inpharma, Int.Aerosp.Abstr., Mat.Sci.Cit.Ind., Pollut.Abstr., Reac., Risk Abstr., SSCI (coverage dropped), Saf.Sci.Abstr., Sci.Cit.Ind., Tox.Abstr. (coverage dropped).
—BLDSC (4953.600000), AskIEEE, CISTI, Ei, GNLM, IDS, ingenta, Linda Hall. **CCC.**
Published by: (American Society of Biomechanics), Pergamon (Subsidiary of: Elsevier Science), The Boulevard, Langford Ln, East Park, Kidlington, Oxford OXB 1GB, United Kingdom. FAX 44-1865-843010, http://www.elsevier.nl/locate/jbiomech. Eds. Richard A Brand, Rik Huiskes. Circ: 1,600. **Subscr. in Australasia and the Far East to:** Elsevier Science (Singapore) Pte Ltd, No.1 Temasek Ave, 17-01 Millenia Tower, Singapore 039192, Singapore. TEL 65-434-3727, FAX 65-337-2230; **Subscr. in the Americas to:** Elsevier Science, PO Box 945, New York, NY 10159-0945. TEL 212-633-3730, FAX 212-633-3680, usinfo-f@elsevier.com; **Subscr. to:** Elsevier Science BV, PO Box 211, Amsterdam 1000 AE, Netherlands. TEL 31-20-485-3757. **Co-sponsor:** European Society of Biomechanics.

JOURNAL OF BIOMEDICAL MATERIALS RESEARCH. see *BIOLOGY—Biotechnology*

610 570 CHE ISSN 1021-7770
CODEN: JBCIEA
JOURNAL OF BIOMEDICAL SCIENCE. Text in English. 1994. bi-m. CHF 557, EUR 397.80 in Europe to institutions; CHF 574.40, USD 436 elsewhere to institutions (effective 2002). adv. back issues avail. *Refereed.* **Document type:** *Journal, Academic/Scholarly.* **Description:** Provides a forum devoted to the promotion of basic medical science and its significance for human welfare.
Related titles: Microform ed.: (from PQC); Online - full text ed.: ISSN 1423-0127. CHF 58, EUR 42, USD 45 to institutions with print edition (effective 2002) (from EBSCO Publishing, O C L C Online Computer Library Center, Inc., RoweCom Information Quest, Swets Blackwell, Institute for Scientific Information).
Indexed: Abstr.Hyg., Cal.Tiss.Abstr., Chem.Abstr., Chem.Indus.Notes, Chem.Titles, Curr.Cont., Excerp.Med. (1995-), Ind.Med. (1994-), Inpharma, Pharm.&Out.News, Reac., Rev.Arom.& Med.Plants, Trop.Dis.Bull.
—BLDSC (4953.769000), CASDDS, GNLM, IDS, Infotrieve, ingenta, KNAW. **CCC.**
Published by: (National Science Council CHN), S. Karger AG, Allschwilerstr 10, PO Box, Basel 4009, Switzerland. TEL 41-61-306-1111, FAX 41-61-306-1234, karger@karger.ch, http://www.online.karger.com/journals/jbs, http://www.karger.com. Ed. Samuel H H Chan. adv.: page USD 1,195. Circ: 1,500.

610.285 USA ISSN 1110-7243
▼ **JOURNAL OF BIOMEDICINE AND BIOTECHNOLOGY.** Text in English. 2001. 4/yr., latest vol.1, no.2. USD 195 print & online eds. (effective 2002). adv. 47 p./no. reprints avail. *Refereed.* **Document type:** *Journal, Academic/Scholarly.* **Description:** Publishes original work in all areas of biomedicine and biotechnology, including carcinogenesis, epidemiology, gene therapy, mutagenesis, pathology, pharmacology, toxicology, and microbial, animal and plant biotechnology.
Related titles: Online - full text ed.: USD 156 (effective 2002).
Published by: Hindawi Publishing Corporation, PO Box 3079, Cuyahoga Falls, OH 44223. FAX 866-446-3294, hindawi@hindawi.com, adv@hindawi.com, http://jbb.hindawi.com, http://www.hindawi.com. Ed. Abdelali Haoudi. Pub. Ahmed Hindawi. R&P, Adv. contact Dalia Mokhtar. B&W page USD 195, color page USD 795; 8.33 x 11.

M

614.88 USA ISSN 0273-8481
CODEN: JBCRD2
JOURNAL OF BURN CARE & REHABILITATION. Text in English. 1980. bi-m. USD 106 domestic to individuals; USD 122 foreign to individuals; USD 164 domestic to institutions; USD 180 foreign to institutions; USD 29 newsstand/cover (effective 2002). adv. bk.rev. index. back issues avail.; reprints avail. *Refereed.* **Document type:** *Academic/Scholarly.*
Related titles: Microform ed.: (from PQC); Online - full text ed.: USD 213.20 domestic academic site license; USD 229.20 foreign academic site license; USD 237.80 domestic corporate site license; USD 253.80 foreign corporate site license (2002); (from Institute for Scientific Information).
Indexed: AMED, CINAHL, Chem.Abstr., Curr.Cont., Excerp.Med., INIS Atomind., Ind.Med. (1980-), Inpharma, Int.Nurs.Ind., Pharm.&Out.News, Reac., Rev.Med.& Vet.Mycol.
—BLDSC (4954.640000), CASDDS, CISTI, EMDOCS, GNLM, IDS, ingenta, KNAW. **CCC.**
Published by: (American Burn Association), Lippincott Williams & Wilkins (Baltimore) (Subsidiary of: Wolters Kluwer N.V.), 351 W Camden St, Baltimore, MD 21201-2436. TEL 800-787-8984, custserv@wwilkins.com, http://www.lww.com/productdetailresults/1,2265,34264705,00.html, htt://www.Lww.com. Ed. Dr. Glenn D Warden. adv.: B&W page USD 1,475, color page USD 2,575; trim 10.88 x 8.25. Circ: 3,176.

JOURNAL OF C G M P COMPLIANCE. (Current Good Manufacturing Practices) see *LAW*

610 ROM ISSN 1582-1838
JOURNAL OF CELLULAR AND MOLECULAR MEDICINE. Text in English. 1997. q. ROL 1,100,000, USD 85 to individuals; ROL 2,900,000, USD 130 to institutions (effective 2001). back issues avail. **Document type:** *Academic/Scholarly.* **Description:** Broad spectrum journal focusing on molecular and cellular aspects of medical sciences.
Formerly (until June 2000): Journal of Medicine and Biochemistry (1453-1321)
Indexed: Cal.Tiss.Abstr.
—BLDSC (4955.005000).
Address: Encymology & Biotechnology Research Center, 93-95 Spl. Independentei, Bucharest 7000, Romania. TEL 40-312-0419, editors@univermed-cdgm.ro, http://www.jcmm.org/. Ed. L. M. Popescu.

JOURNAL OF CELLULAR PATHOLOGY. see *BIOLOGY—Cytology And Histology*

JOURNAL OF CHINESE MEDICINE. see *ALTERNATIVE MEDICINE*

610 USA ISSN 1057-3321
JOURNAL OF CHRONIC FATIGUE SYNDROME; multidisciplinary innovations in research, theory & clinical practice. Text in English. 1995. q. USD 60 to individuals; USD 81 in Canada to individuals; USD 87 elsewhere to individuals; USD 125 to institutions; USD 169 in Canada to institutions; USD 181 elsewhere to institutions; USD 200 to libraries; USD 270 in Canada to libraries; USD 290 elsewhere to libraries (effective Aug. 2001). adv. bk.rev. back issues avail.; reprint service avail. from HAW. *Refereed.* **Document type:** *Journal, Academic/Scholarly.* **Description:** Covers all aspects of chronic fatigue syndromes and what are considered to be related immune deficiency disorders (CFIDS).
Related titles: Microfiche ed.: (from PQC); Microform ed.
Indexed: AMED, Abstr.Anthropol., CINAHL, DNP, Dent.Abstr., Environ.Sci.Poll.Mgmt., Excerp.Med. (1996-), Human Resour.Abstr., IMFL, Lang.& Lang.Behav.Abstr., Past.Care & Couns.Abstr., SOPODA, Saf.Sci.Abstr., Sociol.Abstr.
—BLDSC (4958.362000), EMDOCS, GNLM, Haworth.
Published by: Haworth Press, Inc., 10 Alice St, Binghamton, NY 13904-1580. TEL 607-722-5857, 800-429-6784, FAX 607-722-6362, 800-895-0582, getinfo@haworthpressinc.com, http://www.haworthpress.com/journals/journallist.asp. Ed. Roberto Patarca-Montero. Pub. William Cohen. R&P Ruthann Heath TEL 607-723-5857 ext 316. Adv. contact Jackie Blakeslee TEL 607-722-5857 ext 346. B&W page USD 315, color page USD 550; trim 6 x 8.5.

610 USA ISSN 1094-6950
CODEN: JCDTFM
JOURNAL OF CLINICAL DENSITOMETRY. Text in English. 1998. q. USD 235 domestic; USD 250 foreign (effective 2000). adv. *Refereed.* **Document type:** *Journal, Academic/Scholarly.* **Description:** Contains the latest clinical research on the uses of bone mass and denisity measurements in medical practice.
Related titles: Online - full text ed.: (from Institute for Scientific Information).
Indexed: Curr.Cont., Ind.Med. (1998-), Inpharma, Pharm.&Out.News, Reac.
—BLDSC (4958.388300), ADONIS, IDS, Infotrieve. **CCC.**
Published by: (International Society for Clinical Densitometry), Humana Press Inc., 999 Riverview Dr, Ste 208, Totowa, NJ 07512. TEL 973-256-1699, FAX 973-256-8341, humana@humanapr.com, http://humanapress.com. Ed. Dr. Clifford J Rosen. Adv. contact Richard Hruska. Circ: 2,800. **Dist. in Japan by:** Maruzen Co., Ltd., International Division, Export Dept, P.O. Box 5050, Tokyo International 100-3191, Japan. TEL 03-3275-8591, 03-3278-1937.

JOURNAL OF CLINICAL ENGINEERING. see *BIOLOGY—Bioengineering*

616.9 614.4 USA ISSN 0895-4356
RB156 CODEN: JCEPEE
THE JOURNAL OF CLINICAL EPIDEMIOLOGY; including pharmacoepidemiology reports; devoted to the problems and management of chronic illness in all age groups. Text in English. 1955. m. EUR 213 in Europe to individuals; JPY 28,200 in Japan to individuals; USD 238 elsewhere to individuals; EUR 1,420 in Europe to institutions; JPY 188,500 in Japan to institutions; USD 1,587 elsewhere to institutions (effective 2002). adv. bk.rev. bibl, charts, illus. index. reprint service avail. from PQC. *Refereed.* **Document type:** *Academic/Scholarly.* **Description:** Publishes authoritative research and clinical studies developed from the interplay of clinical medicine, epidemiology, biostatistics, and pharmacoepidemiology.
Formerly: Journal of Chronic Diseases (0021-9681)
Related titles: Microfilm ed.: (from PQC); Online - full text ed.: (from ingenta, ScienceDirect, Swets Blackwell, Institute for Scientific Information).
Indexed: ASCA, Abstr.Health Care Manage.Stud., Abstr.Hyg., Addic.Abstr., AgeLine, Behav.Med.Abstr., Biol.Abstr., CINAHL, C.I.S. Abstr., Cal.Tiss.Abstr., Chem.Abstr., Curr.Cont., Curr.Ind.Stat., Dairy Sci.Abstr., Dent.Ind., Diar.Dis.Res., Dok.Arbeitsmed., Environ.Sci.Poll.Mgmt., Excerp.Med., Helminthol.Abstr., Hosp.Lit.Ind., INIS Atomind., I.P.A., Ind.Med. (1988-), Ind.Sci.Rev., Inpharma, Int.Abstr.Biol.Sci., Int.Nurs.Ind., Med.Care Rev., NRN, Nutr.Abstr., Pharm.&Out.News, Pollut.Abstr., Psychol.Abstr., Reac., Rev.Appl.Entomol., Rev.Med.& Vet.Mycol., Risk Abstr., Rural Devel.Abstr., SSCI (coverage dropped), Saf.Sci.Abstr., Sci.Cit.Ind., THA, Trop.Dis.Bull.
—BLDSC (4958.435000), CASDDS, CISTI, EMDOCS, GNLM, IDS, ingenta, KNAW. **CCC.**
Published by: Elsevier Science, 655 Ave of the Americas, New York, NY 10010. FAX 212-633-3990, nlinfo-f@elsevier.nl; usinfo-f@elsevier.com; forinfo-kyf04035@niftyserve.or.jp, http://www.elsevier.nl/locate/jclinepi. Eds. Alvan R Feinstein, Andre J Knotnerus. Adv. contact Hank Blaney. B&W page USD 985, color page USD 2,160. Circ: 1,390 (paid and free). **Subscr. in Australasia and the Far East to:** Elsevier Science (Singapore) Pte Ltd, No.1 Temasek Ave, 17-01 Millenia Tower, Singapore 039192, Singapore. TEL 65-434-3727, FAX 65-337-2230; **Subscr. in Japan to:** Elsevier Science Inc - Japan Regional Office, 9-15 Higashi-Azabu 1-chome, Minato-ku, Tokyo 106-0044, Japan. TEL 81-3-5561-5033; **Subscr. outside the Americas to:** Elsevier Science BV, PO Box 211, Amsterdam 1000 AE, Netherlands. TEL 31-20-485-3757, nlinfo-f@elsevier.nl.

610 340 USA ISSN 1046-7890
R724 CODEN: JCLEEG
JOURNAL OF CLINICAL ETHICS. Text in English. 1990. q. USD 64 domestic to individuals; USD 74 foreign to individuals; USD 127 domestic to institutions; USD 137 foreign to institutions (effective 2001). bk.rev. illus. Index. back issues avail.; reprints avail. *Refereed.* **Document type:** *Academic/Scholarly, Trade.* **Description:** Addresses the complex ethical, legal, and social issues in clinical medicine, biomedicine, ethics consultation, and direct patient care.
Related titles: Online - full text ed.: (from Institute for Scientific Information).
Indexed: AMED, ASCA, AgeLine, Arts & Hum.Cit.Ind. (coverage dropped), CINAHL, Curr.Cont., Ind.Med. (1990-), Int.Nurs.Ind., Lang.& Lang.Behav.Abstr., Phil.Ind., SOPODA, SSCI, Soc.Serv.Abstr., Sociol.Abstr.
—BLDSC (4958.440000), GNLM, IDS, ingenta, KNAW.
Published by: The Journal of Clinical Ethics, Inc., University Publishing Group, 17100 Cole Rd, Ste 312, Hagerstown, MD 21740. TEL 301-582-2200, FAX 301-582-2406, http://www.clinicalethics.com. Ed. Dr. Edmund G Howe. Pub. Norman Quist. R&P April Startzman.

610 GBR ISSN 1465-9883
▼ **JOURNAL OF CLINICAL EXCELLENCE.** Text in English. 1999. q. GBP 120 (effective 2001). *Refereed.* **Document type:** *Journal, Academic/Scholarly, Trade.* **Description:** Examines research into excellence in clinical medical practice.
Related titles: Online - full text ed.: (from CatchWord Ltd.).
Indexed: Brit.Nur.Ind.
—BLDSC (4958.445000). **CCC.**
Published by: Radcliffe Medical Press Ltd., 18 Marcham Rd, Abingdon, Oxon OX14 1AA, United Kingdom. TEL 44-1235-528820, FAX 44-1235-528830, contact-us@radcliffemed.com, http://www.radcliffe-oxford.com/. Eds. Gifford Batstone, Mary Edwards. Adv. contact Lucy Thomson. Circ: 250.

610 GBR ISSN 1467-5277

JOURNAL OF CLINICAL GOVERNANCE. Text in English. 1993. q. GBP 120 (effective 2001). **Document type:** *Journal, Academic/Scholarly.* **Description:** Covers issues of interest to those involved in the development, implementation and support of clinical governance and audit in the setting of primary care, and at the interface between community and acute care.

Formerly (until 1999): Audit Trends (1352-7797)

Related titles: Online - full content ed.; Online - full text ed.: (from CatchWord Ltd.).

Indexed: Brit.Nur.Ind.

—BLDSC (4958.478000).

Published by: (University of Leicester, Department of General Practice and Primary Health Care), Radcliffe Medical Press Ltd., 18 Marcham Rd, Abingdon, Oxon OX14 1AA, United Kingdom. TEL 44-1235-528820, FAX 44-1235-528830, contact.us@radcliffemed.com, http://www.radcliffe-oxford.com/. Eds. Mayur Lakhani, Richard Baker. Pub., Adv. contact Lucy Thomson. Circ: 400.

610 USA ISSN 0021-9738
R11 CODEN: JCINAO

JOURNAL OF CLINICAL INVESTIGATION. Text in English. 1924. s-m., latest vol.108. USD 155 in US & Canada to individuals; USD 300 elsewhere to individuals; USD 590 in US & Canada to institutions; USD 735 elsewhere to institutions; USD 75 in US & Canada to students; USD 220 elsewhere to students (effective 2002). bibl, charts, illus. index. 130 p./no. back issues avail.; reprint service avail. from PQC,ISI. *Refereed.* **Document type:** *Journal, Academic/Scholarly.* **Description:** x-letter sent 7/99.

Related titles: CD-ROM ed.: (from Ovid Technologies, Inc.); Microform ed.: 1924 (from PQC,PMC); Online - full text ed.: 1924 (from HighWire Pr., Ovid Technologies, Inc., EBSCO Publishing, RoweCom Information Quest, Institute for Scientific Information).

Indexed: AIM, ASCA, Abstr.Hyg., AgBiotech, Agri.& Environ.Biotech.Abstr. (coverage dropped), Anim.Breed.Abstr., BBCI, Biol.Abstr., C.I.S. Abstr., Chem.Abstr., Chem.Cit.Ind., Chem.Indus.Notes, Chem.Titles, Curr.Adv.Cancer Res., Curr.Adv.Cell & Devel.Biol., Curr.Adv.Gen.& Molec.Biol., Curr.Cont., Dairy Sci.Abstr., Derwent Biotech.Abstr., Diab.Cont., Diar.Dis.Res., Environ.Sci.Poll.Mgmt., Excerp.Med., Food Sci.& Tech.Abstr., Genet.Abstr., Helminthol.Abstr., Hum.Gen.Abstr., INIS Atomind., Immun.Abstr. (coverage dropped), Ind.Med. (1924-), Ind.Sci.Rev., Ind.Vet., Inpharma, Int.Abstr.Biol.Sci., Jrnl.Watch Inf.Dis., Kidney, Med.& Surg.Dermat., NRN, Neurosci.Cit.Ind., Nuc.Acids Abstr., Nutr.Abstr., Pharm.&Out.News, Pollut.Abstr., Poult.Abstr., Protozool.Abstr., Reac., Rev.Appl.Entomol., Rev.Med.& Vet.Mycol., Rev.Plant Path., Risk Abstr., Saf.Sci.Abstr., Sci.Cit.Ind., Small Anim.Abstr., Soyabean Abstr., THA, Trop.Dis.Bull., Vet.Bull.

—BLDSC (4958.500000), CASDDS, CISTI, GNLM, IDS, ingenta, KNAW, Linda Hall. **CCC.**

Published by: American Society for Clinical Investigation, 35 Research Dr, 300, Ann Arbor, MI 48103. TEL 734-222-6050, FAX 734-222-6058, editor@the-jci.org, jcistaff@the-jci.org, http://www.jci.org. Ed. Stephen J Weiss. R&P Mark Livingston TEL 734-222-6050 ext 112. Circ: 5,577.

616.01 USA ISSN 0095-1137
QR46 CODEN: JCMIDW

JOURNAL OF CLINICAL MICROBIOLOGY. Text in English. 1975. m. USD 386 domestic to non-members; USD 412 in Canada to non-members; USD 442 in Europe to non-members; USD 445 in Latin America to non-members; USD 448 elsewhere to non-members (effective 2001). adv. s-a. index. back issues avail.; reprint service avail. from PQC. *Refereed.* **Document type:** *Academic/Scholarly.* **Description:** Concerns the microbiological aspects of human and animal infections and infestations, with emphasis given to their etiological agents, diagnosis, and epidemiology.

Related titles: CD-ROM ed.: USD 500 in North America; USD 524 elsewhere (effective 1999); Microform ed.: (from PQC); Online - full text ed.: ISSN 1098-660X (from HighWire Pr., EBSCO Publishing, Institute for Scientific Information).

Indexed: AIDS Abstr., ASCA, Abstr.Hyg., AgBiotech, Agricola, Aqua.Sci.& Fish.Abstr., Biol.Abstr., Biotech.Cit.Ind., Chem.Abstr., Chem.Indus.Notes, Chem.Titles, Curr.Adv.Gen.& Molec.Biol., Curr.Cont., Dairy Sci.Abstr., Deep Sea Res.& Oceanogr.Abstr., Dent.Ind., Derwent Biotech.Abstr., Diar.Dis.Res., Environ.Sci.Poll.Mgmt., Excerp.Med., Food Sci.& Tech.Abstr., Helminthol.Abstr., INIS Atomind., Immun.Abstr. (coverage dropped), Ind.Med. (1975-), Ind.Sci.Rev., Ind.Vet., Inpharma, Int.Abstr.Biol.Sci., Jrnl.Watch Inf.Dis., Kidney, Med.& Surg.Dermat., Microbiol.Abstr., Nutr.Abstr., Pharm.&Out.News, Pig News & Info., Pollut.Abstr., Poult.Abstr., Protozool.Abstr., Reac., Rev.Appl.Entomol., Rev.Med.& Vet.Mycol., Rev.Plant Path., Risk Abstr., Saf.Sci.Abstr., Sci.Cit.Ind., Small Anim.Abstr., Sport Fish.Abstr., Telegen, Trop.Dis.Bull., Vet.Bull., Virol.Abstr. (coverage dropped), Wild.Rev., Zoo.Rec.

—BLDSC (4958.570000), CASDDS, CISTI, GNLM, IDS, ingenta, KNAW. **CCC.**

Published by: American Society for Microbiology, 1752 N St N W, Washington, DC 20036-2904. TEL 202-737-3600, 800-633-4931, subscriptions@asmusa.org, http://jcm.asm.org/, http://www.asmusa.org. Eds. Richard C Tilton, Andrew B Orderdonk. Circ: 9,900 (paid).

616.07 NLD ISSN 1387-1307
CODEN: JCMCFG

JOURNAL OF CLINICAL MONITORING AND COMPUTING. Text in English. 1985. 8/yr. EUR 697.50, USD 697.50 to institutions for print or online ed.; EUR 837.60, USD 837.60 to institutions for print & online eds. combined (effective 2002). adv. bk.rev. abstr, charts, illus, stat. index. reprint service avail. from PQC. *Refereed.* **Document type:** *Journal, Academic/Scholarly.* **Description:** Contains original articles on the latest monitoring techniques, research findings, new developments, updates on monitoring equipment, analyses of monitoring procedures, case reports and clinical controversies.

Formerly: Journal of Clinical Monitoring (0748-1977); Incorporates: International Journal of Clinical Monitoring and Computing (0167-9945)

Related titles: Microform ed.: (from PQC); Online - full text ed.: (from EBSCO Publishing, O C L C Online Computer Library Center, Inc., RoweCom Information Quest, Swets Blackwell, Kluwer Online).

Indexed: ASCA, Bioeng.Abstr., Biotech.& Bioeng.Abstr., Comput.& Info.Sys., Curr.Cont., Electron.& Communic.Abstr.J., Eng.Ind., Excerp.Med., INIS Atomind., INSPEC (1987-Nov.1997, Feb.1999-, dropped), Ind.Med. (1998-), Inpharma, Int.Nurs.Ind., Neurosci.Cit.Ind., Pharm.&Out.News, Reac., Solid St.Abstr.

—BLDSC (4958.573000), CISTI, Ei, EMDOCS, GNLM, IDS, Infotrieve, ingenta, KNAW. **CCC.**

Published by: (Society for Technology in Anesthesia), Kluwer Academic Publishers Group (Subsidiary of: Wolters Kluwer N.V.), Spuiboulevard 50, PO Box 17, Dordrecht 3300 AA, Netherlands. TEL 31-78-639-2392, FAX 31-78-654-2254, services@wkap.nl, http://www.wkap.nl/journalhome.htm/1387-1307. Eds. Ilkka Kalli, J S Gravenstein, Jeffrey M Feldman. Circ: 1,312. **Subscr. in the Americas to:** Kluwer Academic - Plenum Publishers, 233 Spring St, New York, NY 10013-1578. TEL 212-620-8468, FAX 212-807-1047; **Subscr. to:** Journals Department, PO Box 322, Dordrecht 3300 AH, Netherlands. TEL 31-78-639-2392, FAX 31-78-654-6474.

616.744 USA ISSN 1522-0443

JOURNAL OF CLINICAL NEUROMUSCULAR DISEASE. Text in English. q. USD 113 domestic to individuals for print & online eds.; USD 113 foreign to individuals for print & online eds.; USD 170 per issue domestic to institutions; USD 170 per issue foreign to institutions; USD 39 newsstand/cover (effective 2002). **Document type:** *Academic/Scholarly.*

Related titles: Online - full content ed.: USD 221 domestic academic site license; USD 221 foreign academic site license; USD 246.50 domestic corporate site license; USD 246.50 foreign corporate site license (effective 2002).

—BLDSC (4958.574500).

Published by: Lippincott Williams & Wilkins (Philadelphia) (Subsidiary of: Wolters Kluwer N.V.), 530 Walnut St, Philadelphia, PA 19106-3621. TEL 301-824-7390, http://www.Lww.com.

JOURNAL OF CLINICAL OUTCOMES MANAGEMENT. see *HEALTH FACILITIES AND ADMINISTRATION*

616.07 GBR ISSN 0021-9746
CODEN: JCPAAK

JOURNAL OF CLINICAL PATHOLOGY. Text in English. 1947. m. GBP 217, USD 349 combined subscription to individuals includes print & online eds.; GBP 419, USD 671 to institutions for print only (effective 2002). adv. bk.rev. abstr, charts, illus. index. back issues avail.; reprint service avail. from PQC. *Refereed.* **Document type:** *Journal, Academic/Scholarly.* **Description:** Core publication for professionals in all disciplines of clinical pathology.

Related titles: CD-ROM ed.: (from Ovid Technologies, Inc.); Microform ed.: (from PQC); Online - full text ed.: J C P Online. ISSN 1472-4146. GBP 80, USD 125 to individuals (effective 2002); Institutions contact publisher for online rates. (from Ovid Technologies, Inc., Northern Light Technology, Inc., EBSCO Publishing, O C L C Online Computer Library Center, Inc., RoweCom Information Quest, ProQuest Information & Learning, ingenta, HighWire Pr., Swets Blackwell, Institute for Scientific Information); ♦ Supplement: Molecular Pathology. ISSN 1366-8714; ♦ Association of Clinical Pathologists. Symposia. ISSN 0144-0349; ♦ Royal College of Pathologists. Symposia. ISSN 0144-0330.

Indexed: AIDS Abstr., AIM, ASCA, Abstr.Hyg., Agri.& Environ.Biotech.Abstr. (coverage dropped), Biol.Abstr., CINAHL, C.I.S. Abstr., Chem.Abstr., Curr.Adv.Biochem., Curr.Adv.Cancer Res., Curr.Adv.Gen.& Molec.Biol., Curr.Cont., Dent.Ind., Derwent Biotech.Abstr., Diar.Dis.Res., Dok.Arbeitsmed., Excerp.Med., Helminthol.Abstr., INIS Atomind., Ind.Med. (1947-), Ind.Sci.Rev., Inpharma, Int.Abstr.Biol.Sci., Int.Nurs.Ind., Jrnl.Watch Derm., Lab.Haz.Bull., Med.& Surg.Dermat., Neurosci.Cit.Ind., Nutr.Abstr., Protozool.Abstr., Reac., Rev.Appl.Entomol., Rev.Med.& Vet.Mycol., Rev.Plant Path., SSCI (coverage dropped), Sci.Cit.Ind., THA, Trop.Dis.Bull., Vet.Bull., W.R.C.Inf.

—BLDSC (4958.650000), ADONIS, CASDDS, CISTI, GNLM, IDS, ingenta, KNAW. **CCC.**

Published by: (Association of Clinical Pathologists), B M J Publishing Group, B M A House, Tavistock Sq, London WC1H 9JR, United Kingdom. TEL 44-20-7387-4499, FAX 44-20-7383-6400, http://www.jclinpath.com, http://www.bma.org.uk. Ed. H Holzel. Adv. contact Euan Currer TEL 44-20-7383-6181.

610 USA ISSN 0898-7386

JOURNAL OF CLINICAL PRACTICE IN SEXUALITY*. Text in English. 1985. m.

Published by: Gordon L. Deal, Inc., 50 Richfield Way, Hilton Head Island, SC 29926-2232. Ed. Dr. Alan J Wabrek.

JOURNAL OF CLINICAL PSYCHOLOGY IN MEDICAL SETTINGS. see *PSYCHOLOGY*

JOURNAL OF CLINICAL RESEARCH. see *PHARMACY AND PHARMACOLOGY*

610 614 USA ISSN 0094-5145
RA421 CODEN: JCMHB

JOURNAL OF COMMUNITY HEALTH; the publication for health promotion and disease prevention. Text in English. 1975. bi-m. USD 572, EUR 571 to institutions for print or online ed.; USD 686.40, EUR 685.20 to institutions for print & online eds.combined (effective 2002). adv. bk.rev. index. back issues avail.; reprint service avail. from PQC,ISI. *Refereed.* **Document type:** *Journal, Academic/Scholarly.* **Description:** Covers new community health information, including the areas of preventive medicine, new forms of health manpower, analysis of environmental factors, delivery of health care services, and the study of health maintenance and health insurance programs.

Related titles: Microform ed.: (from PQC); Online - full text ed.: (from CatchWord Ltd., Gale Group, Northern Light Technology, Inc., EBSCO Publishing, O C L C Online Computer Library Center, Inc., RoweCom Information Quest, ProQuest Information & Learning, Swets Blackwell, Kluwer Online, Factiva, Institute for Scientific Information).

Indexed: ASCA, Abstr.Crim.& Pen., Abstr.Health Care Manage.Stud., Abstr.Hyg., Abstr.Soc.Geront., Acad.Ind., Adol.Ment.Hlth.Abstr., AgeLine, C.I.J.E. (coverage dropped), CINAHL, Chic.Per.Ind., Community Ment.Health Rev., Crim.Just.Abstr., Curr.Cont., Environ.Sci.Poll.Mgmt., Except.Child Educ.Abstr., Excerp.Med., FAMLI, Fam.Ind., Gen.Sci.Ind. (Jul.1984-), Hlth.Ind., Hosp.Lit.Ind., Human Resour.Abstr., IBZ, INIS Atomind., Ind.Med. (1975-), Int.Nurs.Ind., Lang.& Lang.Behav.Abstr., Med.Care Rev., Nurs.Abstr., Nutr.Abstr., P.A.I.S., Pollut.Abstr., PsycInfo, Risk Abstr., SOPODA, SSCI, Saf.Sci.Abstr., Sage Urb.Stud.Abstr., Sel.Water Res.Abstr., Soc.Sci.Ind. (Mar.1987-), Soc.Serv.Abstr., Soc.Work Res.& Abstr., Sociol.Abstr., THA, Trop.Dis.Bull., e-psyche.

—BLDSC (4961.720000), CatchWord, GNLM, IDS, ingenta, KNAW. **CCC.**

Published by: Kluwer Academic - Plenum Publishers (Subsidiary of: Wolters Kluwer N.V.), 233 Spring St, New York, NY 10013-1578. TEL 212-620-8000, 800-221-9369, FAX 212-463-0742, info@plenum.com, http://www.wkap.nl/journalhome.htm/0094-5145. Ed. Pascal J Imperato. **Subscr. outside the Americas to:** Kluwer Academic Publishers Group, Journals Department, PO Box 322, Dordrecht 3300 AH, Netherlands. TEL 31-78-639-2392, FAX 31-78-654-6474.

JOURNAL OF COMPARATIVE PATHOLOGY. see *BIOLOGY*

610 340 USA ISSN 0882-1046
K10 CODEN: JCLPEF
JOURNAL OF CONTEMPORARY HEALTH LAW AND POLICY. Text in English. 1985. 2/yr. USD 15; USD 17 foreign. adv. reprint service avail. from WSH. *Refereed.* **Document type:** *Academic/Scholarly.* **Description:** Dedicated to the analysis of a wide range of issues including trends in modern health care, bioethics, environmental law, constitutional law, family law, labor law, torts, medical practice, social policy and philosophy.
Related titles: Microfiche ed.: (from WSH); Microform ed.: (from WSH); Online - full text ed.: (from LexisNexis, Gale Group).
Indexed: C.L.I., Fam.Ind., Ind.Med. (1985-), L.R.I. (Mar.1985-), Leg.Per. (Apr.1985-).
—BLDSC (4965.228500), GNLM, ingenta.
Published by: Catholic University of America, Columbus School of Law, Washington, DC 20064. TEL 202-319-5732, FAX 202-319-4313. Ed. Gregory J Lahr. R&P J Gregory Lahr. Adv. contact Gregory J Ossi. Circ: 500.

610.715 CAN ISSN 0894-1912
R845 CODEN: JCHPET
JOURNAL OF CONTINUING EDUCATION IN THE HEALTH PROFESSIONS. Text in English. 1981. q. USD 70 in US & Canada to individuals; USD 95 elsewhere to individuals; USD 109 in US & Canada to institutions; USD 139 elsewhere to institutions (effective 2001). adv. bk.rev. index. back issues avail. *Refereed.* **Document type:** *Journal, Academic/Scholarly.* **Description:** Covers development, conduct and evaluation of continuing health education programs.
Formerly (until 1987): Mobius (0272-3425)
Related titles: Microfilm ed.; Online - full text ed.: (from ProQuest Information & Learning).
Indexed: Abstr.Health Care Manage.Stud., AgeLine, C.I.J.E., CINAHL, Curr.Cont. (coverage dropped), Ind.Med.
—BLDSC (4965.245800), CISTI, GNLM, Infotrieve. **CCC.**
Published by: B.C. Decker Inc., 20 Hughson St S, LCD 1, P O Box 620, Hamilton, ON L8N 3K7, Canada. TEL 905-522-7017, 800-568-7281, FAX 905-522-7839, info@bcdecker.com, http://www.bcdecker.com. Pub. David LeGallais. R&P Paula Presutti. Adv. contact John Birkby. Circ: 2,598 (paid). **Co-sponsors:** Alliance for Continuing Medical Education; Society for Academic Continuing Medical Education.

610 USA ISSN 1522-8606
JOURNAL OF CONTINUING EDUCATION TOPICS & ISSUES. Text in English. 1940. 3/yr. USD 50 domestic; USD 60 foreign (effective 2001). adv. bk.rev. back issues avail. **Document type:** *Trade.* **Description:** Technical and industry news for clinical laboratory and allied health professionals.
Formerly ((until 1999): A M T Events (0746-9217); Which superseded in part (in 1984): American Medical Technologists. Journal (0002-9963); Which was formerly (until 1966): American Medical Technologists. Official Journal (0092-6485); (until 1959): American Medical Technologists. Journal (0360-0645)
Media: Microfilm.
Indexed: CINAHL.
—GNLM.
Published by: American Medical Technologists, 710 Higgins Rd, Park Ridge, IL 60068-5765. TEL 847-823-5169, FAX 847-823-0458, http://www.amt1.com. Ed. Dr. Gerard P Boe. adv.: B&W page USD 975. Circ: 25,000 (paid).

610 362 USA
JOURNAL OF CONTROVERSIAL MEDICAL CLAIMS. Text in English. 1991. q. USD 195 to individuals; USD 59 newsstand/cover (effective 2002). *Refereed.* **Document type:** *Journal, Trade.* **Description:** Provides clinical, well-referenced articles on controversial medical conditions, diagnostic methods, and treatments commonly encountered in connection with personal injury claims.
Formerly: Hippocrates' Lantern (1520-8176)

Published by: Aspen Publishers, Inc., 200 Orchard Ridge Dr, Ste 200, Gaithersburg, MD 20878. TEL 301-417-7500, 800-638-8437, FAX 301-695-7931, customer.service@aspenpubl.com, http://www.aspenpub.com. **Dist. by:** Aspen Publishers Inc., Distribution Center, 7201 McKinney Circle, Frederick, MD 21701. TEL 301-698-7100, FAX 301-417-7550.

610 USA ISSN 1078-3458
HV8843 CODEN: JPJHD3
JOURNAL OF CORRECTIONAL HEALTH CARE. Text in English. 1980; N.S. 1994. s-a., latest vol.7. USD 30 domestic to individuals (effective 2001); USD 65 foreign to individuals; USD 65 domestic to institutions (2001). adv. 200 p./no. back issues avail. *Refereed.* **Document type:** *Academic/Scholarly.* **Description:** Provides a forum for professionals to share information on improving health services in correctional settings. Addresses issues such as administration, personnel and staffing, clinical and support services, national policy and medical-legal questions.
Supersedes (in 1994): Journal of Prison and Jail Health (0731-8332); Which was formerly (until 1981): Journal of Prison Health (0192-7051)
Related titles: Microform ed.: N.S. (from PQC).
Indexed: Abstr.Crim.& Pen., Crim.Just.Abstr., Excerp.Med., IMFL, Lang.& Lang.Behav.Abstr., Med.Care Rev., P.A.I.S., Psychol.Abstr. (1982-), SOPODA, Sociol.Abstr.
—BLDSC (4965.370000), EMDOCS, Infotrieve. **CCC.**
Published by: National Commission on Correctional Health Care, 1300 W Belmont Ave, Chicago, IL 60657. TEL 773-880-1460, FAX 773-880-2424, ncchc@ncchc.org, http://www.ncchc.org. Ed. John Miles. R&P, Adv. contact Jaime Shimkus TEL 773-880-1460 ext 292.

610 USA ISSN 1040-0257
CODEN: JCILFN
THE JOURNAL OF CRITICAL ILLNESS. Text in English. 1986. m. USD 95 domestic; USD 105 foreign; USD 10 newsstand/cover domestic; USD 15 newsstand/cover foreign (effective 2001). adv. charts, illus. Index. back issues avail.; reprints avail. *Refereed.* **Document type:** *Journal, Trade.* **Description:** Provides information designed to help clinicians stay up to date on the latest clinical developments enabling them to provide better patient care during acute events and better ongoing management to improve long-term patient care.
Related titles: Online - full text ed.: (from Gale Group, Factiva).
Indexed: CINAHL.
—BLDSC (4965.635000), GNLM, Infotrieve. **CCC.**
Published by: Cliggott Publishing Co. (Subsidiary of: S C P Communications, Inc.), 330 Boston Post Rd, Darien, CT 06820. TEL 203-661-0600. Ed., R&P Sarah Williams. Pub. Alan Imhoff. Circ: 86,335.

JOURNAL OF DRUG ASSESSMENT. see *PHARMACY AND PHARMACOLOGY*

615.9 GBR ISSN 1095-1539
JOURNAL OF ENVIRONMENTAL MEDICINE. Text in English. 1998. q. USD 295 worldwide to institutions (effective 2000). **Document type:** *Academic/Scholarly.* **Description:** Provides a scientific forum for medical doctors and health professionals who are interested or involved in the identification, medical diagnosis, management and prevention of human health disorders related to hazardous environmental exposures.
Related titles: Online - full text ed.: ISSN 1099-1301. 1999 (from Wiley InterScience).
Indexed: Agri.& Environ.Biotech.Abstr., Aqua.Sci.& Fish.Abstr., Biotech.& Bioeng.Abstr., Environ.Sci.Poll.Mgmt., Pollut.Abstr., Risk Abstr., Saf.Sci.Abstr., Tox.Abstr.
Published by: Wiley Europe Ltd., Baffins Ln, Chichester, W Sussex PO19 1UD, United Kingdom. TEL 44-1243-779777, FAX 44-1243-843232, customer@wiley.co.uk, http://www.wiley.co.uk. Ed. Jacques Descotes. R&P Di Southern TEL 44-1243-770347. **Subscr. addr. in the Americas:** John Wiley & Sons, Inc., Journals, 605 Third Ave, New York, NY 10158. TEL 212-850-6645, FAX 212-850-6021, uscs-wis@wiley.com; **Subscr. to:** John Wiley & Sons Ltd., Baffins Ln, Chichester, Sussex PO19 IUD, United Kingdom. cs-journals@wiley.co.uk.

610 JPN ISSN 0917-5040
JOURNAL OF EPIDEMIOLOGY. Text in Japanese. 1991. q. bk.rev. **Document type:** *Academic/Scholarly.* **Description:** Provides a forum for the presentation of scientific investigation in the field of epidemiology.
Indexed: INIS Atomind., Ind.Med. (1991-).
—BLDSC (4979.470000), GNLM.

Published by: Tokyo University of Agriculture, Japan Epidemiological Association, Faculty of Applied Bioscience, F1-1-1 Sakuragaoka, Setagaya, Tokyo 156-8502, Japan. TEL 81-3-5477-2670, FAX 81-3-5477-7222, swatanab@nodai.ac.jp. Ed. Shaw Watanabe.

614.44 GBR ISSN 0143-005X
CODEN: JECHDR
JOURNAL OF EPIDEMIOLOGY & COMMUNITY HEALTH. Text in English. 1947. m. GBP 123, USD 196 combined subscription to individuals includes print & online eds.; GBP 254, USD 407 to institutions for print only (effective 2002). adv. bk.rev. bibl, charts, illus. index. back issues avail.; reprint service avail. from PQC. *Refereed.* **Document type:** *Academic/Scholarly.* **Description:** Presents original work in the field of epidemiology and community health that relates to a total defined population, numerically rated.
Former titles (in 1979): Epidemiology and Community Health (0142-467X); (until 1978): Journal of Epidemiology and Community Medicine (0141-7681); (until Dec. 1977): British Journal of Preventive and Social Medicine (0007-1242)
Related titles: Microform ed.: (from PQC); Online - full text ed.: J E C H Online. 2000. GBP 50, USD 75 to individuals (effective 2002); Institutions call publisher for online rates. (from HighWire Pr., Northern Light Technology, Inc., EBSCO Publishing, O C L C Online Computer Library Center, Inc., RoweCom Information Quest, ProQuest Information & Learning, ingenta, Swets Blackwell, Ovid Technologies, Inc., Institute for Scientific Information).
Indexed: ASCA, Abstr.Hyg., Addic.Abstr., Behav.Med.Abstr., Biol.Abstr., Biostat., Brit.Nur.Ind., C.I.S. Abstr., Chem.Abstr., Curr.Adv.Cancer Res., Curr.Cont., Curr.Ind.Stat., Curr.Lit.Fam.Plan., Dairy Sci.Abstr., Dent.Ind., Dok.Arbeitsmed., Environ.Sci.Poll.Mgmt., Excerp.Med., Food Sci.& Tech.Abstr., Geo.Abstr.H.G., Geo.Abstr.P.G., Helminthol.Abstr., Hosp.Abstr., Hosp.Lit.Ind., IDA, INIS Atomind., Ind.Med. (1979-), Ind.Sci.Rev., Inpharma, Int.Abstr.Biol.Sci., Int.Nurs.Ind., Lab.Haz.Bull., NRN, Nutr.Abstr., Pharm.&Out.News, Pollut.Abstr., Popul.Ind., Protozool.Abstr., PsycInfo, Psychol.Abstr. (1972-), Reac., Ref.Zh., Rev.Med.& Vet.Mycol., Risk Abstr., Rural Devel.Abstr., SSCI (coverage dropped), Saf.Sci.Abstr., Sci.Cit.Ind., Stud.Wom.Abstr., THA, Trop.Dis.Bull., e-psyche.
—BLDSC (4979.475000), ADONIS, CISTI, GNLM, IDS, Infotrieve, ingenta, KNAW. **CCC.**
Published by: B M J Publishing Group, B M A House, Tavistock Sq, London WC1H 9JR, United Kingdom. TEL 44-20-7387-4499, FAX 44-20-7383-6400, info.norththames@bma.org.uk, http://www.jech.com, http://www.bma.org.uk. Ed. C Alvarez Dardet. Adv. contact Euan Currer TEL 44-20-7383-6181.

610 GBR ISSN 1356-1294
CODEN: JECPFJ
JOURNAL OF EVALUATION IN CLINICAL PRACTICE. Text in English. 1995. q., latest vol.8, 2002. GBP 107 in Europe to individuals; USD 170 in North America to individuals; GBP 118 elsewhere to individuals; GBP 349 in Europe to institutions; USD 553 in North America to institutions; GBP 384 elsewhere to institutions (effective 2002). adv. back issues avail. **Document type:** *Journal, Academic/Scholarly.* **Description:** Publishes critical evaluations of clinical effectiveness, clinical appropriateness, and clinical efficiency.
Related titles: ♦ Online - full text ed.: Journal of Evaluation in Clinical Practice Online. ISSN 1365-2753.
Indexed: Curr.Cont., Ind.Med. (1995-), Int.Nurs.Ind.
—BLDSC (4979.640800), CISTI, GNLM, IDS, Infotrieve, KNAW. **CCC.**
Published by: Blackwell Science Ltd., PO Box 88, Oxford OX2 0NE, United Kingdom. TEL 44-1865-206180, 44-1865-206002, FAX 44-1865-206219, jnl.orders@blacksci.co.uk, http://www.blackwell-science.com/~cgilib/jnlpage.asp?Journal=jecp&File=jecp, http://www.blackwellpublishing.com. Ed. Andrew Miles. Pub. Elaine Stott. R&P Sophie Savage. Adv. contact Jenny Applin. Circ: 210.

610 GBR ISSN 1365-2753
▼ **JOURNAL OF EVALUATION IN CLINICAL PRACTICE ONLINE.** Text in English. 1999. q. GBP 97 in Europe to individuals; USD 153 in North America to individuals; GBP 97 elsewhere to individuals; GBP 315 in Europe to institutions; USD 498 in North America to institutions; GBP 315 elsewhere to institutions (effective 2002). **Document type:** *Academic/Scholarly.*
Media: Online - full text (from EBSCO Publishing, O C L C Online Computer Library Center, Inc., RoweCom Information Quest, ingenta, Munksgaard & Blackwell Science's Synergy, Swets Blackwell, Institute for Scientific Information). **Related titles:** ♦ Print ed.: Journal of Evaluation in Clinical Practice. ISSN 1356-1294.

M

Published by: Blackwell Science Ltd., Osney Mead, Oxford OX2 0EL, United Kingdom. TEL 44-1685-206206, FAX 44-1685-721205, website@blacksci.com, journals.cs@blacksci.co.uk, http://www.blackwell-science.com/~cgilib/jnlpage.bin?Journal=jecp&File=jecp.

JOURNAL OF EXPOSURE ANALYSIS AND ENVIRONMENTAL EPIDEMIOLOGY. see *ENVIRONMENTAL STUDIES*

610 USA ISSN 0022-1058
QP110.A7 CODEN: JEXCBD
JOURNAL OF EXTRA-CORPOREAL TECHNOLOGY. Text in English. 1968. q. USD 70 (effective 2000). bk.rev. back issues avail. **Document type:** *Trade.*
Indexed: CINAHL, Excerp.Med.
—BLDSC (4983.300000), CISTI, GNLM, ingenta, KNAW.
Published by: American Society of Extra-Corporeal Technology, Inc., 503 Carlisle Dr, Ste 125, Herndon, VA 20170-4838. TEL 703-435-8556. Ed. Phyllis Palmer Stark. Circ: 2,800.

610 USA ISSN 0094-3509
R11
JOURNAL OF FAMILY PRACTICE. Text in English. 1974. m. USD 105 domestic to individuals; USD 141 foreign to individuals; USD 176 domestic to institutions; USD 237 foreign to institutions; USD 81 domestic to students; USD 109 foreign to students. adv. bk.rev. charts, illus, stat. s-a. index. back issues avail.; reprints avail. *Refereed.* **Document type:** *Journal, Academic/Scholarly.* **Description:** Contains original research articles, clinical reviews, case reports, editorials, journal club and technology reviews that have clinical applications in family medicine.
Related titles: Microform ed.: (from PQC); Online - full text ed.: (from Gale Group, Ovid Technologies, Inc., Northern Light Technology, Inc., Factiva, Institute for Scientific Information).
Indexed: AIM, ASCA, Abstr.Health Care Manage.Stud., Adol.Ment.Hlth.Abstr., AgeLine, Biol.Abstr., CINAHL, Cal.Tiss.Abstr., Curr.Adv.Cancer Res., Curr.Cont., Dairy Sci.Abstr., Dent.Ind., Dok.Arbeitsmed., Environ.Sci.Poll.Mgmt., Excerp.Med., FAMLI, Fam.Ind., HRIS, Helminthol.Abstr., INIS Atomind., I.P.A., Ind.Med. (1974-), Ind.Sci.Rev., Ind.Vet., Inpharma, Int.Nurs.Ind., Jrnl.Watch, Med.Care Rev., Neurosci.Cit.Ind., Nutr.Abstr., Pharm.&Out.News, Pollut.Abstr., PsycInfo, Psychol.Abstr. (1974-), Reac., Rev.Med.& Vet.Mycol., Risk Abstr., SSCI (coverage dropped), Saf.Sci.Abstr., Sci.Cit.Ind., Small Anim.Abstr., THA, e-psyche.
—BLDSC (4983.730000), CISTI, GNLM, IDS, ingenta, KNAW. **CCC.**
Published by: Dowden Health Media, Inc, 110 Summit Ave, Montvale, NJ 07645. TEL 201-391-2778, 201-391-9100. Ed. Dr. Mark Ebell. Circ: 76,000.

610 USA ISSN 1523-7036
THE JOURNAL OF GENDER-SPECIFIC MEDICINE. Abbreviated title: J G S M. Text in English. 1998. bi-m. USD 140 domestic to individuals; USD 150 foreign to individuals; USD 225 to institutions; USD 40 newsstand/cover (effective 2002). **Document type:** *Magazine, Academic/Scholarly.* **Description:** Specifically geared toward exploring the impact of gender on normal physiology and on the pathophysiology of disease.
Related titles: Online - full content ed.
Indexed: Environ.Sci.Poll.Mgmt., Tox.Abstr.
Published by: (Partnership for Women's Health), MultiMedia Healthcare Inc., Office Center of Princeton Meadows, Bldg 300, Plainsboro, NJ 08536. TEL 609-275-7355, FAX 609-275-7369, info@mmhc.com, http://www.mmhc.com/jgsm. Ed. Dr. Marianne Legato. Pub. Ann Marie Flory.

▼ **JOURNAL OF GENE MEDICINE.** see *BIOLOGY—Genetics*

610 IND ISSN 0970-566X
JOURNAL OF GENERAL MEDICINE; a quarterly for the family physician. Text in English. 1988. q. INR 120, USD 35. adv. abstr, bibl, charts, illus, stat. reprint service avail. from IRC. **Document type:** *Academic/Scholarly.*
Related titles: ♦ Supplement: The Indian Practitioner. ISSN 0019-6169.
—BLDSC (4987.950000).
Published by: Indian Practitioner Group, 101, Lawrence Apartments-2, 1st Fl., Vidyanagari Marg, Opp. Lakhbir Petrol Pump, Kalina, Santa Cruz (E), Mumbai, Maharashtra 400 098, India. TEL 91-22-273809. Ed. M E Yoelekar. Pub. A Peters. R&P Vincent Godinho. Circ: 33,413.

JOURNAL OF GENERAL PHYSIOLOGY. see *BIOLOGY—Physiology*

JOURNAL OF HEALTH & HEALING. see *PHYSICAL FITNESS AND HYGIENE*

610 USA ISSN 1520-8303
KF3608.A4
JOURNAL OF HEALTH CARE COMPLIANCE. Text in English. bi-m. USD 209 to individuals; USD 42 newsstand/cover (effective 2002). **Document type:** *Journal, Trade.* **Description:** Provides current information to health care professionals involved in or concerned about compliance.
—**CCC.**
Published by: Aspen Publishers, Inc., 200 Orchard Ridge Dr, Ste 200, Gaithersburg, MD 20878. TEL 301-417-7500, 800-638-8437, FAX 301-695-7931, customer.service@aspenpubl.com, http://www.aspenpub.com. Ed. Roy Snell. **Dist. by:** Aspen Publishers Inc., Distribution Center, 7201 McKinney Circle, Frederick, MD 21701. TEL 301-698-7100, FAX 301-417-7550.

610 362.5 USA ISSN 1049-2089
RA418.5.P6 CODEN: JHCUEK
JOURNAL OF HEALTH CARE FOR THE POOR AND UNDERSERVED. Text in English. 1990. q. USD 60 to individuals; USD 250 to institutions; USD 20 newsstand/cover to individuals; USD 70 newsstand/cover to institutions (effective 2002). adv. bk.rev. illus. Index. back issues avail.; reprints avail. *Refereed.* **Document type:** *Academic/Scholarly.* **Description:** Focuses on the health of underserved communities. Explores health problems of the poor, elderly, rural and inner-city residents, and the uninsured and underinsured. Also addresses issues on accessibility and quality of health care among this population.
Related titles: Microfiche ed.: (from PQC); Online - full text ed.: (from ProQuest Information & Learning, ingenta, Institute for Scientific Information).
Indexed: ASCA, ASSIA, AgeLine, CINAHL, Crim.Just.Abstr., Curr.Cont., Fam.Ind., Hosp.Lit.Ind., Human Resour.Abstr., Ind.Med. (1990-), Ind.Per.Blacks, Int.Nurs.Ind., Lang.& Lang.Behav.Abstr., Past.Care & Couns.Abstr., Peace Res.Abstr., PsycInfo, Psychol.Abstr. (1990-), SOPODA, SSCI, Sage Fam.Stud.Abstr., Sage Pub.Admin.Abstr., Sage Urb.Stud.Abstr., Soc.Serv.Abstr., Soc.Work Res.& Abstr., Sociol.Abstr., Viol.& Abuse Abstr., e-psyche.
—BLDSC (4996.739000), GNLM, IDS, ingenta. **CCC.**
Published by: (Meharry Medical College, Institute on Health Care for the Poor and Underserved), Sage Publications, Inc., 2455 Teller Rd, Thousand Oaks, CA 91320. TEL 805-499-0721, 805-499-9774, FAX 805-499-0721, 805-499-0871, order@sagepub.com, info@sagepub.com, http://www.sagepub.com. Ed. Srila Sen. Pub. Sara Miller McCune. R&P Tanya Udin. Adv. contact DeAnna Vega Hammersley. Circ: 2,000. **Overseas subscr. to:** Sage Publications Ltd., 6 Bonhill St, London EC2A 4PU, United Kingdom. TEL 44-20-7374-0645, FAX 44-20-7374-8741; Sage Publications India Pvt. Ltd., 4215, New Delhi 110 048, India. TEL 91-11-641-9884, FAX 91-11-647-2426

610 USA ISSN 1081-0730
R118 CODEN: JHCOF3
JOURNAL OF HEALTH COMMUNICATION. Text in English. 1996. 5/yr. GBP 46, USD 76 to individuals; GBP 150, USD 247 to institutions (effective 2002). back issues avail. *Refereed.* **Document type:** *Academic/Scholarly.* **Description:** Publishes qualitative and quantitative studies, ethical essays and case studies in the field of health communication, including research in social marketing, decision-making, communication, psychology, government, and health education.
Related titles: Online - full text ed.: ISSN 1087-0415 (from CatchWord Ltd., EBSCO Publishing, O C L C Online Computer Library Center, Inc., RoweCom Information Quest, Swets Blackwell, Institute for Scientific Information).
Indexed: Curr.Cont., Inform.Sci.Abstr., SSCI.
—BLDSC (4996.745000), CatchWord, IDS, Infotrieve, ingenta. **CCC.**
Published by: Taylor & Francis Ltd. (Subsidiary of: Taylor & Francis Group), 325 Chestnut St, Suite 800, Philadelphia, PA 19016. TEL 215-625-8900, FAX 215-625-2940, info@taylorandfrancis.com, http://www.taylorandfrancis.com/. Ed. Scott C Ratzan. **Subscr. addr. in Europe:** Taylor & Francis Group, Journals Customer Service, Rankine Rd, Basingstoke, Hants RG24 8PR, United Kingdom. TEL 44-1256-813000, FAX 44-1256-479438, enquiry@tanf.co.uk, http://www.tandf.co.uk/journals.

610 340 USA
KF3825.A59
JOURNAL OF HEALTH LAW. Variant title: Health and Hospital Law. Text in English. 1969. q. USD 150. charts, illus, stat, tr.lit. index. back issues avail. **Document type:** *Trade.* **Description:** News for physicians, attorneys, hospitals on long and short-term care facilities and current court decisions.
Former titles: Journal of Health and Hospital Law (1046-4360); (until 1988): Hospital Law (0193-9246)
Related titles: Online - full text ed.: (from LexisNexis).
Indexed: L.R.I. (Jan.1993-Jun.1998, Sep.1998-), Leg.Per. (Jan.1999-).
Published by: American Health Lawyers Association, 1120 Connecticut Ave NW Ste 950, Washington, DC 20036. TEL 202-833-1100, FAX 202-833-1105, info@healthlawyers.org, http://www.healthlawyers.org. R&P Stuart Lilly. Circ: 3,000 (paid). **Subscr. to:** DePaul University, College of Law, 25 E Jackson Blvd, Chicago, IL 60604-2287. TEL 312-362-5634.

610 IND ISSN 0972-0634
▼ **JOURNAL OF HEALTH MANAGEMENT.** Text in English. 1999. biennial. INR 275 to individuals; INR 500 to institutions; USD 13 SAARC to individuals; USD 20 SAARC to institutions; INR 160 newsstand/cover to individuals; INR 290 newsstand/cover to institutions; USD 9 newsstand/cover SAARC to individuals; USD 12 newsstand/cover SAARC to institutions (effective 2002). bk.rev. *Refereed.* **Document type:** *Journal, Academic/Scholarly.* **Description:** Explores major issues of health policy and health management in developing countries in order to assist the better implementation of desired changes.
Related titles: Online - full text ed.
Indexed: Human Resour.Abstr., Nutr.Abstr., Rural Devel.Abstr., Sage Pub.Admin.Abstr.
—BLDSC (4996.785000).
Published by: Sage Publications India Pvt. Ltd., M-32 Market, Greater Kailash-1, PO Box 4215, New Delhi 110 024, India. TEL 91-11-6419884, 91-11-6444958, FAX 91-11-6472426, sageindia@sagepub.com, http://indiasage.com/jdisp.asp?id=09720634. Ed. Udai Pareek. **Affiliates:** Sage Publications, Inc.; Sage Publications Ltd.

320.6 USA ISSN 0361-6878
RA395.A3 CODEN: JHPLDN
JOURNAL OF HEALTH POLITICS, POLICY AND LAW. Text in English. 1976. bi-m. USD 54 to individuals; USD 198 to institutions; USD 27 to students (effective 2001). adv. bk.rev. illus. back issues avail.; reprint service avail. from WSH,PSC,SCH. *Refereed.* **Document type:** *Academic/Scholarly.* **Description:** Focuses on the initiation, formulation, and implementation of health policy and analyzes the relations between government and health—past, present, and future. Each issue includes an extensive "Books" section, which helps to make JHPPL the primary source of communication across the many disciplines it serves. The journal is read by scholars, policy makers, and practitioners in political science, economics, public administration, law, medicine, public health, and medical ethics.
Related titles: Microfiche ed.: (from WSH); Microfilm ed.: (from PQC,WSH,PMC); Online - full text ed.: (from Project MUSE, EBSCO Publishing, O C L C Online Computer Library Center, Inc., RoweCom Information Quest, ProQuest Information & Learning, Gale Group, Swets Blackwell, Factiva, Institute for Scientific Information).
Indexed: ABI Inform. (Spr.1986-), ASCA, Abstr.Bk.Rev.Curr.Leg.Per., Abstr.Health Care Manage.Stud., Abstr.Hyg., Abstr.Soc.Geront., Adol.Ment.Hlth.Abstr., AgeLine, Biol.Abstr., CINAHL, C.L.I., Curr.Cont., Dent.Ind., Environ.Sci.Poll.Mgmt., Excerp.Med., Fam.Ind., Fut.Surv., Hlth.Ind., Hosp.Abstr., Hosp.Lit.Ind., Human Resour.Abstr., INIS Atomind., Ind.Med. (1976-), Int.Nurs.Ind., Int.Polit.Sci.Abstr., Intl.Bibl.Soc.Sci., J.of Econ.Lit., L.R.I. (Jan.1980-), Lang.& Lang.Behav.Abstr., Leg.Per. (coverage dropped), Med.Care Rev., P.A.I.S., PSI, Peace Res.Abstr., Polit.Sci.Abstr., Pollut.Abstr., Risk Abstr., SOPODA, SSCI, Saf.Sci.Abstr., Sage Pub.Admin.Abstr., Soc.Serv.Abstr., Sociol.Abstr., Trop.Dis.Bull.
—BLDSC (4996.870000), CISTI, EMDOCS, GNLM, IDS, ingenta. **CCC.**
Published by: (Department of Health Administration, Duke University), Duke University Press, Journals Marketing, 905 W Main St Ste 18B, Durham, NC 27701. TEL 919-687-3600, 888-651-0122, FAX 919-687-3524, dukepress@duke.edu, http://www.duke.edu/web/dupress/, http://www.dukeupress.edu. Ed. Mark A Peterson. R&P Kay Robin Alexander. Adv. contact Amy Hartzler. page USD 300; trim 4.5 x 7.25. Circ: 2,100.

JOURNAL OF HEALTH PSYCHOLOGY; an interdisciplinary, international journal. see *PSYCHOLOGY*

614 362 GBR ISSN 1355-8196
JOURNAL OF HEALTH SERVICES RESEARCH & POLICY. Text in English. 1996. q. GBP 92 in Europe to individuals; USD 163 in United States to individuals; GBP 96 elsewhere to individuals; GBP 155 in Europe to institutions; USD 266 in United States to institutions; GBP 160 elsewhere to institutions (effective 2002). adv. back issues avail. **Document type:** *Journal, Academic/Scholarly.*
Formerly (until 1998): Journal of Health Services Research
Related titles: Online - full text ed.: (from CatchWord Ltd., RoweCom Information Quest).
Indexed: ASSIA, Brit.Nur.Ind., CINAHL, Environ.Sci.Poll.Mgmt., Geo.Abstr.H.G., Inpharma, Int.Nurs.Ind., Pharm.&Out.News, Pollut.Abstr., Reac., Ref.Zh., Risk Abstr., Saf.Sci.Abstr.
—BLDSC (4996.870400), CISTI, EMDOCS, GNLM, Infotrieve. **CCC.**
Published by: Royal Society of Medicine Press Ltd, 1 Wimpole St, London W1M 8AE, United Kingdom. TEL 44-20-7290-2921, FAX 44-20-7290-2929, rsmjournals@rsm.ac.uk, http://www.roysocmed.ac.uk/pub/jhsrp.htm. Eds. Nicholas Mays, Nick Black.

612.2 615.8512 USA ISSN 1520-5495
JOURNAL OF HEART-CENTERED THERAPIES. Text in English. 1998. s-a. USD 35 domestic to individuals; USD 45 foreign to individuals; USD 85 domestic to institutions; USD 110 foreign to institutions. *Refereed.* **Document type:** *Academic/Scholarly.* **Description:** Publishes the research findings and clinical experience of practitioners of Heart-Centered Hypnotherapy and Heart-Centered Breath Therapy. Provides a forum for clinicians around the world who are utilizing the Heart-Centered Therapies modality in their healing work, and for those who want more information about it.
Indexed: AMED.
—BLDSC (4996.874200).
Published by: Heart-Centered Therapies Association, 3716 274th Ave, S E, Issaquah, WA 98029. TEL 425-391-9716, FAX 425-391-9737, diane@wellness-institute.org; orders@allenpress.com, http://www.wellness-institute.org/; http://www.allenpress.com. **Subscr. to:** Allen Press Inc., PO Box 1897, Lawrence, KS 66044-8897.

612.042 JPN ISSN 0300-8134
QP301 CODEN: JHEGAI
JOURNAL OF HUMAN ERGOLOGY. Text in English. 1972. s-a. USD 74. adv. illus. **Document type:** *Academic/Scholarly.*
Indexed: AMED, Abstr.Anthropol., Abstr.Hyg., Agri.Eng.Abstr., Biol.Abstr., C.I.S. Abstr., Curr.Adv.Ecol.Sci., Ergon.Abstr., Excerp.Med., Ind.Med. (1972-), Indian Psychol.Abstr., PsycInfo, Psychol.Abstr. (1972-), Psycscan A.P., e-psyche.
—BLDSC (5003.414000), CISTI, GNLM, KNAW, Linda Hall.
Published by: (Human Ergology Society), Center for Academic Publications Japan, 2-4-16 Yayoi, Bunkyo-ku, Tokyo 113-0032, Japan. TEL 03-3817-5821, FAX 03-3817-5820. Circ: 500. **Dist. by:** Business Center for Academic Societies Japan, 5-16-9 Honkomagome, Bunkyo-ku, Tokyo 113-0021, Japan. TEL 81-3-3475-0824, FAX 81-3-3475-5287.

JOURNAL OF HUMAN MOVEMENT STUDIES. see *PSYCHOLOGY*

610 USA ISSN 1096-4045
RA448.5.I44 CODEN: JIHEF5
▼ **JOURNAL OF IMMIGRANT HEALTH.** Text in English. 1999. q. USD 231, EUR 230 to institutions for print or online ed.; USD 277.20, EUR 276 to institutions for print & online eds. combined (effective 2002). bk.rev. *Refereed.* **Document type:** *Journal, Academic/Scholarly.* **Description:** Studies aspects of the emotional and physical health of immigrants and refugees, the processes that affect their health and health care, and related anthropological, public health, epidemiological, legal, and ethical issues.
Related titles: Online - full text ed.: (from EBSCO Publishing, O C L C Online Computer Library Center, Inc., RoweCom Information Quest, Swets Blackwell, Kluwer Online).
Indexed: AgeLine.
—BLDSC (5004.559000). **CCC.**
Published by: Kluwer Academic - Plenum Publishers (Subsidiary of: Wolters Kluwer N.V.), 233 Spring St, New York, NY 10013-1578. TEL 212-620-8000, 800-221-9369, FAX 212-463-0742, info@plenum.com, http://www.wkap.nl/journalhome.htm/1096-4045. Ed. Sana Loue. Pub. Mariclaire Cloutier TEL 212-620-8013. R&P Rose Luongo TEL 781-871-6311. **Subscr. outside the Americas to:** Kluwer Academic Publishers Group, Journals Department, PO Box 322, Dordrecht 3300 AH, Netherlands. TEL 31-78-639-2392, FAX 31-78-654-6474.

JOURNAL OF INFECTION AND CHEMOTHERAPY. see *PHARMACY AND PHARMACOLOGY*

JOURNAL OF INSURANCE MEDICINE. see *INSURANCE*

610 USA ISSN 0885-0666
JOURNAL OF INTENSIVE CARE MEDICINE. Text in English. 1986. bi-m. USD 165 domestic to individuals; USD 175 in Canada & Mexico to individuals; USD 195 elsewhere to individuals; USD 395 domestic to institutions; USD 410 in Canada & Mexico to institutions; USD 425 elsewhere to institutions; USD 181.50 to individuals print & online eds. combined; USD 434.50 to institutions print & online eds. combined (effective 2001). adv. bk.rev. charts, illus. index. back issues avail.; reprints avail. *Refereed.* **Document type:** *Academic/Scholarly.* **Description:** Keeps physicians informed of the rapidly changing world of intensive care, with papers and reviews on the latest advances in anesthesiology, cardiology, neonatology, nephrology, psychiatry, pulmonology, surgery, and other areas related to ICU practice.
Related titles: Online - full text ed.: ISSN 1525-1489. USD 149 to individuals; USD 356 to institutions (effective 2001) (from EBSCO Publishing, O C L C Online Computer Library Center, Inc., RoweCom Information Quest, ingenta, Munksgaard & Blackwell Science's Synergy, Swets Blackwell, Institute for Scientific Information).
Indexed: Curr.Cont., Excerp.Med., Inpharma, Int.Abstr.Biol.Sci., Pharm.&Out.News, Reac., Sci.Cit.Ind.
—BLDSC (5007.539000), EMDOCS, GNLM, IDS, ingenta, KNAW. **CCC.**
Published by: Blackwell Science Inc., Commerce Pl, 350 Main St, Malden, MA 02148-5018. TEL 781-388-8250, 800-759-6102, FAX 781-388-8255, journals@blacksci.com, http://www.blackwell-science.com. Eds. James M Rippe, Dr. Richard S Irwin. R&P Tracey Davies. Adv. contact Jenny Applin. Circ: 1,300.

610 GBR ISSN 0300-0605
CODEN: JIMRBV
JOURNAL OF INTERNATIONAL MEDICAL RESEARCH. Text in English. 1972. bi-m. GBP 79 in United Kingdom; USD 145 foreign (effective 2000). *Refereed.* **Document type:** *Academic/Scholarly.* **Description:** Presents original papers and reviews in clinical and medical research. Topics include animal and clinical pharmacology, pharmacokinetics and drug metabolism, toxicology, teratology, and clinical trials.
Related titles: Microfiche ed.: (from PQC); Online - full text ed.: (from Institute for Scientific Information); ♦ Supplement: Journal of International Medical Research. Supplement. ISSN 0142-2596.
Indexed: ASCA, Abstr.Hyg., Agri.& Environ.Biotech.Abstr. (coverage dropped), Biol.Abstr., Chem.Abstr., Chem.Titles, Curr.Adv.Ecol.Sci., Curr.Cont., Dent.Ind., Derwent Biotech.Abstr., Diar.Dis.Res., Excerp.Med., HRIS, Helminthol.Abstr., Ind.Med. (1972-), Ind.Sci.Rev., Inpharma, Int.Abstr.Biol.Sci., Int.Sci.Rev., NRN, Nutr.Abstr., Pharm.&Out.News, Reac., Ref.Zh., Rev.Plant Path., Sci.Cit.Ind., Trop.Dis.Bull.
—BLDSC (5007.674000), CASDDS, CISTI, EMDOCS, GNLM, IDS, ingenta, KNAW. **CCC.**
Published by: Cambridge Medical Publications Ltd., Wicker House, High St, Worthing, W Sussex BN11 1DJ, United Kingdom. TEL 44-1903-205884, FAX 44-1903-234862, cmp@hbase.com, http://www.cambridge-medical.com. Circ: 2,500.

610 GBR ISSN 0142-2596
JOURNAL OF INTERNATIONAL MEDICAL RESEARCH. SUPPLEMENT. Text in English. 1974. irreg.
Related titles: ♦ Supplement to: Journal of International Medical Research. ISSN 0300-0605.
Published by: Cambridge Medical Publications Ltd., Wicker House, High St, Worthing, W Sussex BN11 1DJ, United Kingdom. TEL 44-1903-205884, FAX 44-1903-234862.

613 GBR ISSN 1356-1820
CODEN: HOMEEF
JOURNAL OF INTERPROFESSIONAL CARE. Text in English. 1984. q. GBP 85, USD 167 to individuals; GBP 354, USD 592 to institutions (effective 2002). *Refereed.* **Document type:** *Academic/Scholarly.* **Description:** Covers issues in personal care within the community, in primary health, hospital and other institutional settings.
Former titles (until 1990): Holistic Medicine (0884-3988); (until 1984): British Journal of Holistic Medicine (0266-1330)
Related titles: Online - full text ed.: ISSN 1469-9567 (from CatchWord Ltd., Northern Light Technology, Inc., EBSCO Publishing, O C L C Online Computer Library Center, Inc., RoweCom Information Quest, ProQuest Information & Learning, Swets Blackwell).
Indexed: AMED, ASSIA, Brit.Nur.Ind., CINAHL, Curr.Adv.Ecol.Sci., Curr.Cont. (coverage dropped), ERA, Excerp.Med., Lang.& Lang.Behav.Abstr., PsycInfo, Res.High.Educ.Abstr., SOPODA, Soc.Serv.Abstr., Sociol.Abstr., e-psyche.
—BLDSC (5007.695000), CatchWord, CISTI, GNLM, Infotrieve. **CCC.**
Published by: (British Holistic Medical Association), Carfax Publishing Limited (Subsidiary of: Taylor & Francis Group), PO Box 25, Abingdon, Oxon OX14 3UE, United Kingdom. TEL 44-1235-401000, FAX 44-1235-401550, enquiries@carfax.co.uk, enquiry@tandf.co.uk, http://www.carfax.co.uk. Ed. Dr. Hugh Barr. **Co-sponsor:** Marylebone Centre Trust.

610 IND ISSN 0022-2054
JOURNAL OF J.J. GROUP OF HOSPITALS AND GRANT MEDICAL COLLEGE. Text in English. 1956. a. INR 40. adv. bk.rev. abstr, bibl, charts, illus. index. **Document type:** *Academic/Scholarly.*
Indexed: Chem.Abstr., Ind.Med. (coverage dropped), Nutr.Abstr.
Published by: Research Society, Grant Medical College and J.J. Group of Hospitals, 2nd Fl., Front Wing Skin & S.T.D. Bldg., J.J. Hospital Campus, Byculla, Mumbai, Maharashtra 400 008, India. TEL 91-22-376-7949. Ed. Dr. H B Chandalia. Circ: 600.

JOURNAL OF LAW AND HEALTH. see *LAW*

JOURNAL OF LAW AND MEDICINE. see *LAW*

THE JOURNAL OF LAW, MEDICINE & ETHICS. see *LAW*

JOURNAL OF LEARNING DISABILITIES. see *EDUCATION—Special Education And Rehabilitation*

610 340 USA ISSN 0194-7648
K10
THE JOURNAL OF LEGAL MEDICINE. Text in English. 1979. q. GBP 82, USD 135 to individuals; GBP 153, USD 253 to institutions (effective 2002). bk.rev. back issues avail.; reprint service avail. from WSH. *Refereed.* **Document type:** *Academic/Scholarly.* **Description:** Publishes articles, comments and essays on topics of interest in legal medicine: health law and policy, professional liability, hospital law, food and drug law, medicolegal research and education, and the history of legal medicine.
Related titles: Microfiche ed.: (from WSH); Microfilm ed.: (from PQC,WSH); Microform ed.: (from WSH); Online - full text ed.: ISSN 1521-057X (from CatchWord Ltd., EBSCO Publishing, O C L C Online Computer Library Center, Inc., RoweCom Information Quest, Gale Group, LexisNexis, Swets Blackwell, Institute for Scientific Information).
Indexed: ASCA, Abstr.Bk.Rev.Curr.Leg.Per., AgeLine, Arts & Hum.Cit.Ind. (coverage dropped), C.L.I., Crim.Just.Abstr., Curr.Cont., Environ.Sci.Poll.Mgmt., Excerp.Med., Fam.Ind., Hlth.Ind., INIS Atomind., Ind.Med. (1979-), Int.Nurs.Ind., L.R.I. (Jun.1981-), Leg.Cont., Leg.Per. (Jun.1982-), PsycInfo, Psychol.Abstr. (1991-), Risk Abstr., SSCI, Saf.Sci.Abstr., e-psyche.
—BLDSC (5010.270300), ADONIS, CatchWord, CISTI, GNLM, IDS, ingenta. **CCC.**
Published by: (American College of Legal Medicine), Taylor & Francis Ltd. (Subsidiary of: Taylor & Francis Group), 325 Chestnut St, Suite 800, Philadelphia, PA 19016. TEL 215-625-8900, FAX 215-625-2940, info@tandf.co.uk, info@taylorandfrancis.com, http://www.tandf.co.uk/, http://www.taylorandfrancis.com/. Ed. Theodore R LeBlang. **Subscr. addr. in Europe:** Taylor & Francis Group, Journals Customer Service, Rankine Rd, Basingstoke, Hants RG24 8PR, United Kingdom. TEL 44-1256-813000, FAX 44-1256-479438, enquiry@tanf.co.uk, http://www.tandf.co.uk/journals.

JOURNAL OF MAMMARY GLAND BIOLOGY AND NEOPLASIA. see *BIOLOGY—Physiology*

610 GBR ISSN 0268-9235
RA971
JOURNAL OF MANAGEMENT IN MEDICINE. Text in English. 1986. bi-m. USD 3,149 in North America; EUR 3,349 in Europe; AUD 3,779 in Australasia; GBP 1,969 in the UK & the rest of the world (effective 2002). adv. bk.rev. reprint service avail. from SWZ. **Document type:** *Journal, Academic/Scholarly.*
Incorporates (in Nov. 1998): Health Manpower Management (0955-2065); Which superseded (1859-1988): Health Services Manpower Review (0306-0233)
Related titles: CD-ROM ed.; Online - full text ed.: (from EBSCO Publishing, O C L C Online Computer Library Center, Inc., RoweCom Information Quest, ingenta, Swets Blackwell).

M

Indexed: ABI Inform. (1992-1995), ASSIA, Brit.Nur.Ind., Diar.Dis.Res., Emerald, Emrld.Intell., Int.Nurs.Ind. —BLDSC (5011.370000), GNLM, Infotrieve. **CCC.**
Published by: Emerald, 60-62 Toller Ln, Bradford, W Yorks BD8 9BY, United Kingdom. TEL 44-1274-777700, FAX 44-1274-785200, info@emeraldinsight.com, http://www.emeraldinsight.com/jmm.htm, http://www.emeraldinsight.com/journals/. Eds. Jackie Ford, Nancy Harding.

JOURNAL OF MATERIALS SCIENCE: MATERIALS IN MEDICINE. see *ENGINEERING—Engineering Mechanics And Materials*

▼ **JOURNAL OF MECHANICS IN MEDICINE AND BIOLOGY.** see *BIOLOGY*

610 JPN ISSN 1342-8810
CODEN: BTMDAB
JOURNAL OF MEDICAL AND DENTAL SCIENCES. Text in English. 1954. q. per issue exchange basis. abstr, charts, illus. *Refereed.* **Document type:** *Academic/Scholarly.*
Formerly (until vol.43, no.4, 1996): Tokyo Medical and Dental University. Bulletin (0040-8921)
Indexed: Abstr.Hyg., Biol.Abstr., Chem.Abstr., Chem.Indus.Notes, Chem.Titles, Curr.Adv.Ecol.Sci., Dairy Sci.Abstr., Dent.Ind., Excerp.Med., INIS Atomind., Ind.Med. (1997-), NRN, Nutr.Abstr., Trop.Dis.Bull. —BLDSC (5017.047600), CASDDS, CISTI, GNLM, ingenta.
Published by: Tokyo Medical and Dental University/Tokyo Ika Shika Daigaku, 1-5-45 Yushima, Bunkyo-ku, Tokyo 113-0034, Japan. Ed. Sunao Nomoto. Circ: 1,000.

JOURNAL OF MEDICAL AND PHARMACEUTICAL MARKETING. see *BUSINESS AND ECONOMICS—Marketing And Purchasing*

JOURNAL OF MEDICAL BIOGRAPHY. see *BIOGRAPHY*

610 657.832 GBR ISSN 1369-6998
CODEN: BJMEEG
JOURNAL OF MEDICAL ECONOMICS. Text in English. 1991. irreg., latest vol.4 (Each paper is published within 21 days of acceptance.). Avail. with subscr. to Journal of Drug Assessment. abstr. 2 cols./p. Supplement avail.; back issues avail.; reprints avail. *Refereed.* **Document type:** *Journal, Academic/Scholarly.* **Description:** Publishes papers on cost-effectiveness evaluations and aspects of health economics.
Formerly (until 1998): British Journal of Medical Economics (0962-1423)
Indexed: Excerp.Med. (1993-), I.P.A., Inpharma, Reac. —EMDOCS, GNLM, Infotrieve. **CCC.**
Published by: Brookwood Medical Publications (Subsidiary of: P J B Publications Ltd.), 18-20 Hill Rise, Richmond, Surrey TW10 6UA, United Kingdom. TEL 44-20-8332-4600, FAX 44-20-8332-4610, maria@brookwd.demon.co.uk, http://www.pjbpubs.com/brookwood/. Ed., R&P Wendy Kimleer TEL 44-20-8332-4601. Pub. Dr. Philip J Brown. Adv. contact Jenefer Trevena TEL 44-20-8332-4605.

610.28 GBR ISSN 0309-1902
R856.A1 CODEN: JMTEDN
JOURNAL OF MEDICAL ENGINEERING & TECHNOLOGY. Text in English. 1965. bi-m. GBP 128, USD 209 to individuals; GBP 280, USD 463 to institutions (effective 2002). adv. bk.rev. abstr, illus, pat, tr.lit, tr.mk. index. *Refereed.* **Document type:** *Academic/Scholarly.* **Description:** Provides information on the application of engineering and technology in medical research and clinical medicine. Articles from around the world cover treatment techniques, instrument design and development, and evaluation of equipment.
Incorporates (1988-1997): Journal of Ambulatory Monitoring (0951-1830); Formerly: Biomedical Engineering (0006-2898)
Related titles: Online - full text ed.: ISSN 1464-522X (from CatchWord Ltd., EBSCO Publishing, O C L C Online Computer Library Center, Inc., RoweCom Information Quest, Swets Blackwell, Institute for Scientific Information).
Indexed: ASCA, Agri.Eng.Abstr., Appl.Mech.Rev., Bioeng.Abstr., Biol.Abstr., Br.Tech.Ind., Chem.Abstr., Comput.& Info.Sys., Curr.Adv.Ecol.Sci., Curr.Cont., Eng.Ind., Environ.Sci.Poll.Mgmt., Ergon.Abstr., Excerp.Med., INIS Atomind., INSPEC (pre-1969-), Ind.Med. (1977-), Ind.Sci.Rev., Ind.Vet., Inpharma, Pharm.&Out.News, Pollut.Abstr., Reac., Sci.Cit.Ind., Vet.Bull. —BLDSC (5017.057000), ADONIS, AskIEEE, CatchWord, CISTI, Ei, EMDOCS, GNLM, IDS, Infotrieve, ingenta, Linda Hall. **CCC.**

Published by: Taylor & Francis Group, Taylor & Francis Ltd., 11 New Fetter Ln, London EC4P 4EE, United Kingdom. TEL 44-20-7583-9855, FAX 44-20-7842-2298, info@tandf.co.uk, http://www.tandf.co.uk. Ed. Martin Black. **Subscr. in N. America to:** Taylor & Francis Ltd., 325 Chestnut St, Suite 800, Philadelphia, PA 19016. TEL 800-354-1420, FAX 215-625-8914, info@taylorandfrancis.com, http://www.taylorandfrancis.com/.

JOURNAL OF MEDICAL ENTOMOLOGY. see *BIOLOGY—Entomology*

JOURNAL OF MEDICAL ENTOMOLOGY ONLINE. see *BIOLOGY—Entomology*

610 174.2 GBR ISSN 0306-6800
CODEN: JMETDR
JOURNAL OF MEDICAL ETHICS. Text in English. 1975. bi-m. GBP 107, USD 173 combined subscription to individuals includes print & online eds.; GBP 165, USD 266 to institutions for print only (effective 2002). bk.rev. illus. index. Supplement avail.; back issues avail.; reprints avail. *Refereed.* **Document type:** *Academic/Scholarly.* **Description:** Presents interdisciplinary articles on ethical aspects of health care.
Related titles: Online - full text ed.: J M E Online. ISSN 1473-4257. GBP 65, USD 99 to individuals (effective 2001); Institutions contact publisher for online rates. (from ProQuest Information & Learning, HighWire Pr., Northern Light Technology, Inc., EBSCO Publishing, O C L C Online Computer Library Center, Inc., RoweCom Information Quest, ingenta, Gale Group, Swets Blackwell, Ovid Technologies, Inc., Factiva, Institute for Scientific Information); ♦ Supplement: Medical Humanities. ISSN 1468-215X; Journal of Medical Ethics. Supplement. ISSN 1359-5857.
Indexed: AMED, ASCA, AgeLine, Arts & Hum.Cit.Ind. (coverage dropped), Biol.Abstr., CERDIC, CINAHL, Crim.Just.Abstr., Curr.Adv.Ecol.Sci., Curr.Cont., Environ.Sci.Poll.Mgmt., Excerp.Med., Fam.Ind., IBR, INIS Atomind., Ind.Med. (1975-), Ind.Sci.Rev., Inpharma, Int.Nurs.Ind., P C I, Pharm.&Out.News, Phil.Ind., Pollut.Abstr., Reac., Rel.Ind.One, Rel.Ind.Two, Risk Abstr., SSCI, Saf.Sci.Abstr., Sci.Cit.Ind., Soc.Sci.Ind. (Mar.1987-). —BLDSC (5017.062000), CISTI, EMDOCS, GNLM, IDS, ingenta, KNAW.
Published by: (Institute of Medical Ethics), B M J Publishing Group, B M A House, Tavistock Sq, London WC1H 9JR, United Kingdom. TEL 44-20-7387-4499, FAX 44-20-7383-6400, info.norththames@bma.org.uk, http://jme.bmjjournals.com/, http://www.bma.org.uk. Ed. J Savalescu. Adv. contact Euan Currer TEL 44-20-7383-6181.

JOURNAL OF MEDICAL GENETICS. see *BIOLOGY—Genetics*

100 174 USA ISSN 1041-3545
R724 CODEN: JMHBEN
JOURNAL OF MEDICAL HUMANITIES. Text in English. 1976. q. USD 409, EUR 408 to institutions for print or online ed.; EUR 489.60, USD 490.80 to institutions for print & online eds. combined (effective 2002). adv. bk.rev. reprint service avail. from PQC,ISI. *Refereed.* **Document type:** *Journal, Academic/Scholarly.* **Description:** Highlights the relationship among medicine and art, ethics, history, literature, philosophy, sociology, economics, and jurisprudence.
Former titles (until 1991): Journal of Medical Humanities and Bioethics (0882-6498); (until vol.6, 1985): Journal of Bioethics (0278-9523); (until 1982): Bioethics Quarterly (0163-9803); Bioethics Northwest (0362-0824)
Related titles: Microform ed.: (from PQC); Online - full text ed.: (from EBSCO Publishing, O C L C Online Computer Library Center, Inc., RoweCom Information Quest, Swets Blackwell, Kluwer Online).
Indexed: Curr.Adv.Ecol.Sci., Ind.Per.Art.Relat.Law, Lang.& Lang.Behav.Abstr., Phil.Ind., Psychol.Abstr., Russ.Acad.Sci.Bibl., SOPODA, Sociol.Abstr. —BLDSC (5017.070500), CISTI, Infotrieve, ingenta. **CCC.**
Published by: (Northeastern Ohio Universities, College of Medicine), Kluwer Academic - Plenum Publishers (Subsidiary of: Wolters Kluwer N.V.), 233 Spring St, New York, NY 10013-1578. TEL 212-620-8000, 800-221-9369, FAX 212-463-0742, info@plenum.com, http://www.wkap.nl/journalhome.htm/1041-3545. Ed. Delese Wear. Circ: 400. **Subscr. outside the Americas to:** Kluwer Academic Publishers Group, Journals Department, PO Box 322, Dordrecht 3300 AH, Netherlands. TEL 31-78-639-2392, FAX 31-78-654-6474.

616.01 USA ISSN 0022-2615
QR46 CODEN: JMMIAV
JOURNAL OF MEDICAL MICROBIOLOGY. Text in English. 1968. m. USD 356 domestic to individuals; USD 356 foreign to individuals; USD 853 newsstand/cover domestic to institutions; USD 853 newsstand/cover foreign to institutions (effective 2002). adv. bk.rev. bibl, charts, illus. back issues avail. *Refereed.* **Document type:** *Academic/Scholarly.* **Description:** Publishes original articles covering medical, dental, veterinary and food microbiology, including bacteriology, virology, mycology and parasitology.
Related titles: Microform ed.: (from PQC); Online - full text ed.: (from Ovid Technologies, Inc., EBSCO Publishing, Institute for Scientific Information).
Indexed: ASCA, Abstr.Hyg., AgBiotech, Agri.& Environ.Biotech.Abstr. (coverage dropped), Aqua.Sci.& Fish.Abstr., Biol.Abstr., Chem.Abstr., Chem.Titles, Curr.Adv.Ecol.Sci., Curr.Adv.Gen.& Molec.Biol., Curr.Cont., Dairy Sci.Abstr., Derwent Biotech.Abstr., Diar.Dis.Res., Environ.Sci.Poll.Mgmt., Excerp.Med., Food Sci.& Tech.Abstr., Helminthol.Abstr., INIS Atomind., Ind.Med. (1968-), Ind.Sci.Rev., Ind.Vet., Inpharma, Int.Abstr.Biol.Sci., Microbiol.Abstr., Nutr.Abstr., Pharm.&Out.News, Pig News & Info., Pollut.Abstr., Poult.Abstr., Protozool.Abstr., Reac., Rev.Appl.Entomol., Rev.Med.& Vet.Mycol., Rev.Plant Path., Risk Abstr., Saf.Sci.Abstr., Sci.Cit.Ind., Trop.Dis.Bull., Vet.Bull. —BLDSC (5017.079000), ADONIS, CASDDS, CISTI, GNLM, IDS, ingenta, KNAW.
Published by: (Pathological Society of Great Britain and Ireland), Lippincott Williams & Wilkins (Philadelphia) (Subsidiary of: Wolters Kluwer N.V.), 530 Walnut St, Philadelphia, PA 19106-3621. TEL 215-521-8300, FAX 215-521-8902, http://www.lww.com. Ed. B I Duerden. Adv. contact Gemma Heiser. Circ: 1,500. **Subscr. to:** PO Box 1600, Hagerstown, MD 21740-1600. TEL 800-777-2295, FAX 301-824-7390.

610 USA ISSN 8755-0229
JOURNAL OF MEDICAL PRACTICE MANAGEMENT. Text in English. 1985. bi-m. USD 169 to individuals; USD 213 to institutions (effective 2001); to individuals (foreign $199); institutions $199 (foreign $220) (effective 1999). adv. **Document type:** *Academic/Scholarly.* **Description:** Offers perspectives on legislation, litigation, office management and other issues that affect the medical practice of office-based physicians and health care professionals.
Related titles: Microfilm ed.: 1985 (from WWS). —BLDSC (5017.081500), CISTI, EMDOCS, GNLM.
Published by: Greenbranch Publishing, P O Box 208, Phoenix, MD 21131. TEL 410-329-9788, FAX 410-329-1510, ncollins@greenbranch.com. Ed. Marcel Frenkel. Pub. Nancy Collins. Adv. contact Kim Kleinberg. B&W page USD 1,150; trim 10.88 x 8.13. Circ: 2,150 (paid).

616.01 USA ISSN 0146-6615
RC114.5 CODEN: JMVIDB
JOURNAL OF MEDICAL VIROLOGY. Text in English. 1977. m. USD 3,050 in United States; USD 3,170 in Canada & Mexico; USD 3,272 elsewhere; USD 3,203 combined subscription in United States for print and online eds.; USD 3,323 combined subscription in Canada & Mexico for print and online eds.; USD 3,425 combined subscription elsewhere for print and online eds. (effective 2002). adv. charts, illus. back issues avail.; reprint service avail. from ISI. *Refereed.* **Document type:** *Academic/Scholarly.* **Description:** Covers the structure and composition of viruses, epidemiology, humoral and cell-mediated immune responses, and clinical features of infection.
Related titles: Online - full text ed.: ISSN 1096-9071. USD 3,050 in United States; USD 3,050 in Canada & Mexico; USD 3,050 elsewhere (effective 2002) (from EBSCO Publishing, Wiley InterScience, Institute for Scientific Information).
Indexed: AIDS & Cancer Res., AIDS Abstr., ASCA, Abstr.Hyg., Aqua.Sci.& Fish.Abstr., Biol.Abstr., Chem.Abstr., Chem.Titles, Curr.Adv.Ecol.Sci., Curr.Adv.Gen.& Molec.Biol., Curr.Cont., Dairy Sci.Abstr., Dent.Ind., Environ.Sci.Poll.Mgmt., Excerp.Med., INIS Atomind., Ind.Med. (1977-), Ind.Sci.Rev., Ind.Vet., Inpharma, Med.& Surg.Dermat., Pharm.&Out.News, Pig News & Info., Pollut.Abstr., Poult.Abstr., Reac., Ref.Zh., Rev.Appl.Entomol., Rev.Arom.& Med.Plants, Rev.Med.& Vet.Mycol., Risk Abstr., SSCI (coverage dropped), Saf.Sci.Abstr., Sci.Cit.Ind., Trop.Dis.Bull., Vet.Bull., Virol.Abstr. —BLDSC (5017.095000), CASDDS, CISTI, GNLM, IDS, ingenta, KNAW. **CCC.**

M

Published by: John Wiley & Sons, Inc., Journals (Subsidiary of: Wiley InterScience), 605 Third Ave, New York, NY 10158. TEL 212-850-6645, FAX 212-850-6021, subinfo@wiley.com, uscs-wis@wiley.com, http://www.wiley.com. Ed. Arie J Zuckerman. adv.: B&W page GBP 640, color page GBP 1,515; trim 210 x 279. Circ: 1,000. **Subscr. outside the Americas to:** John Wiley & Sons Ltd., Baffins Ln, Chichester, Sussex PO19 IUD, United Kingdom. TEL 44-1243-779777, FAX 44-1243-843232, cs-journals@wiley.co.uk.

615.854 362.176 USA ISSN 1096-620X
RM214 CODEN: JMFOFJ

JOURNAL OF MEDICINAL FOOD. Text in English. 1998. q. USD 169 domestic to individuals; USD 239 foreign to individuals; USD 203 domestic to individuals print and online eds. combined; USD 273 foreign to individuals print and online eds. combined; USD 333 domestic to institutions; USD 445 foreign to institutions; USD 400 domestic to institutions print and online eds. combined; USD 511 foreign to institutions print and online eds. combined (effective 2002). adv. back issues avail.; reprints avail. *Refereed.* **Document type:** *Journal, Academic/Scholarly.* **Description:** Presents rigorous scientific research on disease prevention and therapeutic benefits of foods (e.g., soy, teas, and crucifers) and on the substances they contain (e.g, antioxidants and protease inhibitors). Also researches on the medical uses of foods such as for delivery of vaccines and pharmaceutical and on the development of future foods.
Related titles: Online - full content ed.: USD 333 to institutions; USD 169 to individuals (effective 2002) (from EBSCO Publishing, Swets Blackwell); Online - full text ed.: (from CatchWord Ltd., RoweCom Information Quest).
Indexed: AMED, Agricola, Excerp.Med., Food Sci.& Tech.Abstr., I.P.A.
—BLDSC (5017.250000), CASDDS, CatchWord. **CCC.**
Published by: Mary Ann Liebert, Inc. Publishers, 2 Madison Ave, Larchmont, NY 10538. TEL 914—834-3100, FAX 914-834-1388, info@liebertpub.com, www.liebertpub.com/jmf, http://www.liebertpub.com. Ed. Dr. Sheldon S Hendler.

610 USA ISSN 0025-7850
R11 CODEN: JNMDBO

JOURNAL OF MEDICINE; clinical, experimental, molecular. Text in English. 1970. bi-m. USD 150; USD 185 foreign (effective 1998). adv. bk.rev. charts, illus, stat. index. reprints avail. *Refereed.* **Document type:** *Academic/Scholarly.* **Description:** Presents articles on all areas of medicine and medical science.
Indexed: ASCA, Agri.& Environ.Biotech.Abstr. (coverage dropped), Biol.Abstr., CINAHL, C.I.S. Abstr., Chem.Abstr., Chem.Titles, Curr.Adv.Ecol.Sci., Curr.Cont. (coverage dropped), Curr.Lit.Fam.Plan., Derwent Biotech.Abstr., Excerp.Med., Helminthol.Abstr., INIS Atomind., Ind.Med. (1970-), Inpharma, L.R.I., NRN, Nutr.Abstr., Pharm.&Out.News, Reac., Rev.Med.& Vet.Mycol., Sci.Cit.Ind. (coverage dropped).
—BLDSC (5017.300000), CASDDS, CISTI, GNLM, IDS, ingenta, KNAW. **CCC.**
Published by: P J D Publications Ltd, PO Box 966, Westbury, NY 11590. TEL 516-626-0650, FAX 516-626-5546. Ed. Dr. Julian L Ambrus. Pub., R&P, Adv. contact Siva Sankar.

610 174.24 NLD ISSN 0360-5310
R723 CODEN: JMPHDC

THE JOURNAL OF MEDICINE AND PHILOSOPHY; a forum for bioethics and philosophy of medicine. Text in English. 1976. bi-m., latest vol.26, 2001. NLG 115 to non-members (effective (No. 2001); USD 52 to non-members; NLG 599, USD 309 to institutions (effective 2001). adv. bk.rev. bibl, illus. index. reprint service avail. from SWZ. *Refereed.* **Document type:** *Journal, Academic/Scholarly.* **Description:** Explores issues in bioethics and other topics in the philosophy of medicine.
Related titles: Microform ed.: (from PQC); Online - full text ed.: (from EBSCO Publishing, O C L C Online Computer Library Center, Inc., RoweCom Information Quest, Gale Group, Swets Blackwell, Institute for Scientific Information).
Indexed: ASCA, Abstr.Crim.& Pen., AgeLine, Arts & Hum.Cit.Ind. (coverage dropped), Biol.Abstr., Curr.Cont., Dent.Ind., Excerp.Med., Fam.Ind., G.Soc.Sci.& Rel.Per.Lit., Hum.Ind. (Nov.1983-), IBR, IBZ, Ind.Med. (1976-), Ind.Per.Art.Relat.Law, Ind.Philos., Intl.Bibl.Soc.Sci., Lang.& Lang.Behav.Abstr., P C I, Phil.Ind., Rel.Ind.One, Rel.Ind.Two, SOPODA, SSCI, Soc.Serv.Abstr., Sociol.Abstr.
—BLDSC (5017.385000), CISTI, GNLM, IDS, ingenta, KNAW. **CCC.**
Published by: (Baylor College of Medicine USA, Center for Ethics, Medicine and Public Issues USA), Swets & Zeitlinger BV, PO Box 825, Lisse 2160 SZ, Netherlands. TEL 31-252-435111, FAX 31-252-415888, orders@swets.nl, http://www.swets.nl/sps/journals/jmp.html. Ed. H Tristram Englehardt Jr. **Dist. in N. America by:** Swets & Zeitlinger, PO Box 582, Downingtown, PA 19335-998. TEL 800-477-9387, FAX 610-524-5366. **Co-sponsors:** Society for Health and Human Values, US; Association for Philosophical and Ethical Research in Medicine, JA; European Society for Philosophy of Medicine and Health Care.

JOURNAL OF MICROENCAPSULATION. see *PHARMACY AND PHARMACOLOGY*

616.07 USA ISSN 1525-1578

▼ **THE JOURNAL OF MOLECULAR DIAGNOSTICS.** Text in English. 1999. q. USD 120 domestic to individuals; USD 155 foreign to individuals; USD 385 domestic to institutions; USD 460 in Canada & Mexico to institutions; USD 480 elsewhere to institutions (effective 2001). back issues avail. *Refereed.* **Document type:** *Journal, Academic/Scholarly.* **Description:** Publishes high-quality original papers on scientific advances in the translation and validation of molecular discoveries in medicine into the clinical diagnostic setting, and the description and application of technological advances in the field of molecular diagnostic medicine.
Related titles: Online - full text ed.: (from Institute for Scientific Information).
Indexed: Biotech.Cit.Ind., Curr.Cont., Ind.Med.
—BLDSC (5020.706000), Linda Hall.
Published by: (Association for Molecular Pathology), American Society for Investigative Pathology, 9650 Rockville Pike, Bethesda, MD 20814. TEL 301-571-0107, FAX 301-571-0108, ajp@pathol.faseb.org, http://jmd.amjpathol.org, http://www.amjpathol.org/. Ed. Dr. James L Madara.

610 DEU ISSN 0946-2716
CODEN: JMLME8

JOURNAL OF MOLECULAR MEDICINE. Text in English. 1922. m. EUR 571.10 domestic; EUR 560.70 in Germany; EUR 54 newsstand/cover foreign (effective 2002). adv. bibl, charts, illus. index. back issues avail.; reprint service avail. from ISI. *Refereed.* **Document type:** *Journal, Academic/Scholarly.* **Description:** Publishes original papers and reviews in all fields of clinical research, including case reports, with emphasis on molecular medicine and clinical pharmacology.
Former titles: Clinical Investigator (0941-0198); (until 1993): Clinical Investigation; (until 1991): Klinische Wochenschrift (0023-2173)
Related titles: Microform ed.: (from PQC,PMC); Online - full text ed.: ISSN 1432-1440 (from EBSCO Publishing, RoweCom Information Quest, Swets Blackwell, Springer LINK, Institute for Scientific Information).
Indexed: ASCA, Agri.& Environ.Biotech.Abstr. (coverage dropped), Biol.Abstr., Chem.Abstr., Chem.Indus.Notes, Chem.Titles, Curr.Adv.Cancer Res., Curr.Adv.Ecol.Sci., Curr.Cont., Dairy Sci.Abstr., Dent.Ind., Derwent Biotech.Abstr., Excerp.Med., Focus on: Mol.Med., Helminthol.Abstr., INIS Atomind., Ind.Med. (1995-), Ind.Sci.Rev., Inpharma, Med.& Surg.Dermat., NRN, Neurosci.Cit.Ind., Nutr.Abstr., Pharm.&Out.News, Protozool.Abstr., Reac., Rev.Med.& Vet.Mycol., Risk Abstr., SSCI (coverage dropped), Sci.Cit.Ind., Trop.Oil Seeds Abstr.
—BLDSC (5020.716000), ADONIS, CASDDS, CISTI, EMDOCS, GNLM, IDS, ingenta, KNAW. **CCC.**
Published by: (German Working Group for Gene Therapy), Springer-Verlag (Subsidiary of: BertelsmannSpringer), Tiergartenstr 17, Heidelberg 69121, Germany. TEL 49-6221-345-0, FAX 49-6221-345229, subscriptions@springer.de, http://link.springer.de/link/service/journals/00109/index.htm, http://www.springer.de. Ed. D Ganten. **U.S. subscr. to:** Springer-Verlag New York Inc., PO Box 2485, Secaucus, NJ 07096-2485. TEL 212-460-1500, FAX 212-473-6272.

JOURNAL OF MORPHOLOGY. see *BIOLOGY*

▼ **JOURNAL OF NANOSCIENCE AND NANOTECHNOLOGY.** see *COMPUTERS—Microcomputers*

610 JPN ISSN 1345-0069
CODEN: JNMAFJ

JOURNAL OF NARA MEDICAL ASSOCIATION. Text in Japanese, Multiple languages. 1950. bi-m. JPY 4,000 (effective 2001). index. *Refereed.* **Document type:** *Journal, Academic/Scholarly.*
Formerly (until 1998): Nara Igaku Zasshi (0469-5550)
Indexed: Biol.Abstr., C.I.S. Abstr., Chem.Abstr., Chem.Indus.Notes, Chem.Titles, Dairy Sci.Abstr., Excerp.Med., INIS Atomind., Ind.Med. (coverage dropped), Nutr.Abstr., Rev.Med.& Vet.Mycol.
—BLDSC (4828.700000), CASDDS, EMDOCS, GNLM, KNAW.
Published by: Nara Igakkai/Nara Medical Association, Nara Medical University, Kashihara 634-8521, Nara 634-8521, Japan. TEL 81-744-22-3051, FAX 81-744-25-7308. Ed., Pub. Koichiro Yoshihara. Circ: 1,200 (controlled).

616.98 USA ISSN 1076-2752
RC963 CODEN: JOEMFM

JOURNAL OF OCCUPATIONAL AND ENVIRONMENTAL MEDICINE. Text in English. 1959. m. USD 220 domestic to individuals; USD 284 foreign to individuals; USD 283 domestic to institutions; USD 347 foreign to institutions; USD 30 newsstand/cover (effective 2002). adv. bk.rev. abstr, bibl, charts. index, cum.index. reprint service avail. from PQC. *Refereed.* **Document type:** *Academic/Scholarly.* **Description:** Contains original articles on occupational medical practice, including epidemiology, toxicology, health screening, ergonomics, assessment, rehabilitation, health education, and administration.
Former titles: Journal of Environmental Medicine (0096-1736); J O M: Journal of Occupational Medicine (0022-3212); (until 1968): Journal of Occupational Medicine
Related titles: Microfilm ed.: (from PQC,WWS); Online - full text ed.: (from Ovid Technologies, Inc., Gale Group, Factiva, Institute for Scientific Information).
Indexed: ASCA, Abstr.Hyg., AgeLine, Agri.Eng.Abstr., Alloys Ind., Aqua.Sci.& Fish.Abstr., Biol.Abstr., Br.Tech.Ind., Bus.Ind., CINAHL, C.I.S. Abstr., CSNB, Cadscan, Chem.Abstr., Chem.Indus.Notes, Chem.Titles, Crim.Just.Abstr., Curr.Cont., Dent.Ind., Environ.Per.Bibl. (1990-), Environ.Sci.Poll.Mgmt., Ergon.Abstr., Excerp.Med., Helminthol.Abstr., Hlth.Ind., INIS Atomind., Ind.Hyg.Dig., Ind.Med. (1995-), Ind.Sci.Rev., Ind.Vet., Inpharma, Int.Nurs.Ind., Intl.Polym.Sci.& Tech., Lab.Haz.Bull., Lead Abstr., Med.& Surg.Dermat., Met.Abstr., Met.Abstr.Ind., NRN, Noise Pollut.Publ.Abstr., Nonfer.Met.Alert, PCC Alert, Pharm.&Out.News, RAPRA (1977-), Reac., Risk Abstr., Saf.Sci.Abstr., Sci.Cit.Ind., Steels Alert, Stud.Wom.Abstr., THA, Tr.& Indus.Ind., Trop.Dis.Bull., World Surf.Coat., Zincscan.
—BLDSC (5026.081000), CASDDS, CISTI, GNLM, IDS, ingenta.
Published by: (American College of Occupational and Environmental Medicine), Williams & Wilkins (Subsidiary of: Waverly International), 351 W Camden St, Baltimore, MD 21201-2436. TEL 410-528-4068, 800-222-3790, FAX 410-528-4452, mricks@wwilkins.com, http://www.wwilkins.com/JOEM/, http://www.Lww.com. Ed. Paul W Brandt Rauf. Adv. contact Melanie Ricks. B&W page USD 1,250; trim 10.88 x 8.13. Circ: 9,200 (paid).

616.0472 GBR ISSN 1526-5900

THE JOURNAL OF PAIN. Text in English. bi-m. USD 172 domestic to individuals Full text online included; USD 222 foreign to individuals Full text online included; USD 246 domestic to institutions Full text online included; USD 299 foreign to institutions Full text online included; USD 74 domestic to students Full text online included; USD 106 foreign to students Full text online included; USD 50 per issue (effective 2001); Free for members of American Pain Society. *Refereed.* **Document type:** *Academic/Scholarly.* **Description:** Focuses on issues related to pain, including clinical and basic research, patient care, education and health policy; highlights the application of current research to pain management and the need for further investigation.
Related titles: Online - full text ed.: (from IDEAL Online Library, Institute for Scientific Information).
Indexed: Curr.Cont.
—BLDSC (5027.785000).
Published by: (American Pain Society USA), Churchill Livingstone (Subsidiary of: Harcourt Publishers Ltd.), Robert Stevenson House, 1-3 Baxter's Pl, Leith Walk, Edinburgh, Midlothian EH1 3AF, United Kingdom. TEL 44-131-556-2424, FAX 44-131-489-1177, http://www.jpain.org, http://www.churchilmed.com. Ed. G F Gebhart.

610 362.1 CAN ISSN 0825-8597

JOURNAL OF PALLIATIVE CARE. Text in English. 1985. q. CND 80 domestic to individuals; CND 90 foreign to individuals; CND 120 domestic to institutions; CND 130 foreign to institutions (effective 2001). bk.rev. illus. back issues avail.; reprints avail. *Refereed.* **Document type:** *Academic/Scholarly.* **Description:** Publishes up-to-date scientific research in the field of palliative-hospice care, combining scientific validation with humanistic concerns.
Related titles: Microfiche ed.: (from MML); Microfilm ed.: (from MML); Microform ed.: (from MML); Online - full text ed.: (from Northern Light Technology, Inc., ProQuest Information & Learning, Institute for Scientific Information).

M

Indexed: AMED, ASCA, AgeLine, Brit.Nur.Ind., CBCA Ref., CINAHL, Can.B.P.I., Can.Per.Ind. (Jan.1988-), Curr.Cont., Fam.Ind., Ind.Med. (1985-), Indian Psychol.Abstr., Int.Nurs.Ind., PSI, PsycInfo, Psychol.Abstr. (1985-), Ref.Zh., SSCI, Sci.Cit.Ind., e-psyche.

—BLDSC (5028.260000), CISTI, GNLM, IDS, ingenta. **CCC.**

Published by: Center for Bioethics, Clinical Research Institute of Montreal, 110 Pine Ave W, Montreal, PQ H2W 1R7, Canada. TEL 514-987-5617, FAX 514-987-5695, marcotc@ircm.qc.ca, http://www.ircm.qc.ca/bioethique/english/publications/journal_of_palliative_care.html. Ed. Dr. David J Roy. R&P Electa Baril. Circ: 1,000. **Subscr. in US to:** Allen Press Inc., PO Box 1897, Lawrence, KS 66044-8897.

362.175 615.5 USA ISSN 1096-6218
R726.8 CODEN: JPAMF9

JOURNAL OF PALLIATIVE MEDICINE. Text in English. 1998. bi-m. USD 157 domestic to individuals; USD 240 foreign to individuals; USD 188 domestic to individuals print and online eds. combined; USD 271 foreign to individuals print and online eds. combined; USD 308 domestic to institutions; USD 397 foreign to institutions; USD 369 domestic to institutions print and online eds. combined; USD 458 foreign to institutions print and online eds. combined (effective 2002). adv. illus. reprints avail. *Refereed.* **Document type:** *Journal.* **Description:** Covers the latest developments in drug and non-drug therapies for symptoms and syndromes that affect patients with life-threatening diseases.

Related titles: Online - full text ed.: USD 308 to institutions; USD 157 to individuals (effective 2002) (from EBSCO Publishing, CatchWord Ltd., Swets Blackwell, RoweCom Information Quest).

Indexed: AMED, I.P.A.

—BLDSC (5028.280000), Infotrieve. **CCC.**

Published by: Mary Ann Liebert, Inc. Publishers, 2 Madison Ave, Larchmont, NY 10538. TEL 914—834-3100, FAX 914-834-1388, info@liebertpub.com, http://www.liebertpub.com/jpm. Ed. Dr. David E Weissman.

616.07 CHE ISSN 1024-5359
CODEN: PATHFG

JOURNAL OF PATHOGENESIS; mechanisms in disease processes. Text in English. 1997. 6/yr. EUR 246 to institutions; EUR 396 to corporations (effective 2000). **Document type:** *Academic/Scholarly.* **Description:** Elucidates the fundamental mechanisms of disease processes.

Related titles: CD-ROM ed.; Online - full text ed.: (from EBSCO Publishing, RoweCom Information Quest).

—CASDDS.

Published by: Gordon and Breach - Harwood Academic (Subsidiary of: Taylor & Francis Group), PO Box 531, Lausanne 1000, Switzerland. http://www.gbhap.com/Pathogenesis/. Ed. Joe Lunec. **Subscr. addr. in US:** International Publishers Direct, PO Box 32160, Newark, NJ 07102. FAX 215-750-6343.

616.07 GBR ISSN 0022-3417
CODEN: JPTLAS

JOURNAL OF PATHOLOGY. Text in English. 1892. m. (13/yr.). USD 1,150 in United States; USD 1,150 in Canada & Mexico; USD 1,150 elsewhere; USD 1,208 combined subscription in United States for print and online eds.; USD 1,208 combined subscription in Canada & Mexico for print and online eds.; USD 1,208 combined subscription elsewhere for print and online eds. (effective 2002). adv. bibl, charts, illus. cum.index: vols.1-90. back issues avail. *Refereed.* **Document type:** *Academic/Scholarly.* **Description:** Covers the field of experimental pathology, relevant to the understanding of human disease, and includes papers on the use of techniques such as immunology and molecular biology to elucidate disease mechanisms.

Incorporates (in Jan. 1984): Diagnostic Histopathology (0272-7749); Which was formerly: Investigative and Cell Pathology (0146-7611)

Related titles: Microform ed.: (from PMC,PQC); Online - full text ed.: ISSN 1096-9896. USD 1,150 in United States; USD 1,150 in Canada & Mexico; USD 1,150 elsewhere (effective 2002) (from EBSCO Publishing, Wiley InterScience, Institute for Scientific Information).

Indexed: ASCA, Abstr.Hyg., Aqua.Sci.& Fish.Abstr., Aquacult.Abstr., Biol.Abstr., C.I.S. Abstr., Chem.Abstr., Chem.Indus.Notes, Chem.Titles, Curr.Adv.Cancer Res., Curr.Adv.Cell & Devel.Biol., Curr.Adv.Ecol.Sci., Curr.Adv.Gen.& Molec.Biol., Curr.Cont., Dairy Sci.Abstr., Dent.Ind., Diar.Dis.Res., Environ.Sci.Poll.Mgmt., Excerp.Med., Genet.Abstr. (coverage dropped), Hum.Gen.Abstr., INIS Atomind., Ind.Med. (1969-), Ind.Sci.Rev., Ind.Vet., Inpharma, Int.Abstr.Biol.Sci., Kidney, Med.& Surg.Dermat., Nutr.Abstr., Oncog.G.F.Abstr., Pharm.&Out.News, Pig News & Info., Protozool.Abstr., Reac., Ref.Zh., Rev.Med.& Vet.Mycol., Rev.Plant Path., Sci.Cit.Ind., Trop.Dis.Bull., Vet.Bull.

—BLDSC (5029.900000), CASDDS, CISTI, GNLM, IDS, ingenta, KNAW, Linda Hall. **CCC.**

Published by: (Pathological Society of Great Britain and Ireland USA), Wiley Europe Ltd., Baffins Ln, Chichester, W Sussex PO19 1UD, United Kingdom. TEL 44-1243-779777, FAX 44-1243-775878, customer@wiley.co.uk, http://www.wiley.co.uk. adv.: B&W page GBP 750, color page GBP 1,650; trim 210 x 297. **Subscr. in the Americas to:** John Wiley & Sons, Inc., Journals, 605 Third Ave, New York, NY 10158. TEL 212-850-6021, 212-850-6645, subinfo@jwiley.com.

JOURNAL OF PHARMACEUTICAL AND MEDICAL SCIENCES. see *PHARMACY AND PHARMACOLOGY*

612 ESP ISSN 1138-7548
QP1 CODEN: JPBIF2

JOURNAL OF PHYSIOLOGY AND BIOCHEMISTRY. Text in English, Spanish. 1945. q. ESP 14,500; ESP 18,000 foreign (effective 1999). bk.rev. abstr, bibl, illus, mkt. index. *Refereed.* **Document type:** *Academic/Scholarly.* **Description:** Publishes articles on human normal and pathological physiology, comparative physiology, biochemistry and molecular biology, and related fields.

Formerly (until 1998): Revista Espanola de Fisiologia (0034-9402)

Related titles: Online - full text ed.: (from Institute for Scientific Information).

Indexed: ASCA, Anim.Breed.Abstr., BBCI, Biol.Abstr., Chem.Abstr., Chem.Indus.Notes, Chem.Titles, Curr.Adv.Ecol.Sci., Curr.Cont., Dairy Sci.Abstr., Excerp.Med., Fababean Abstr., Field Crop Abstr., Herb.Abstr., INIS Atomind., Ind.Med. (1998-), Ind.Med.Esp., Ind.SST, Ind.Vet., Inpharma, Neurosci.Cit.Ind., Nutr.Abstr., Pharm.&Out.News, Poult.Abstr., Reac., Sci.Cit.Ind. (coverage dropped), Soyabean Abstr., Vet.Bull., Weed Abstr., Zoo.Rec.

—BLDSC (5039.300000), CASDDS, CINDOC, CISTI, GNLM, IDS, KNAW, Linda Hall. **CCC.**

Address: Apartado 177, Pamplona, Navarra 31080, Spain. TEL 34-48-105600 ext. 6259, FAX 34-48-105649, jpbif2@unav.es. Ed. Francisco Ponz. Circ: 1,000.

610 IND ISSN 0022-3859
CODEN: JPMDA3

JOURNAL OF POSTGRADUATE MEDICINE. Text in English. 1955. q. INR 250, USD 50 to individuals; INR 500, USD 100 to institutions; INR 75, USD 15 newsstand/cover to individuals; INR 150, USD 30 newsstand/cover to institutions (effective 1999). adv. bk.rev. charts, illus, stat. index. **Document type:** *Academic/Scholarly.*

Related titles: CD-ROM ed.; Online - full text ed.

Indexed: Biol.Abstr., Chem.Abstr., Dent.Ind., ExtraMED, Ind.Med. (1955-), Nutr.Abstr.

—BLDSC (5041.150000), CASDDS, CISTI, GNLM, ingenta, KNAW.

Published by: (Seth G.S. Medical College and K.E.M. Hospital, Staff Society), Scientific Publishers, 5-A New Pali Rd., P O Box 91, Jodhpur, Rajasthan 342 001, India. TEL 91-291-433323, FAX 91-291-512580, scienti@sancharnet.in, http://www.scientificpub.com. Ed. K Radhakrishna Murthy. Adv. contact D.K. Sahu. B&W page INR 2,500, B&W page USD 500. Circ: 2,500 (paid and controlled).

JOURNAL OF PRODUCTS AND TOXICS LIABILITY. see *LAW*

616.07 AUS ISSN 1320-5455
CODEN: JQCPE

JOURNAL OF QUALITY IN CLINICAL PRACTICE. Text in English. 1981. q. AUD 329 domestic to institutions; AUD 299 in New Zealand to institutions; USD 308 elsewhere to institutions; AUD 362 domestic to institutions paper & online eds.combined; AUD 329 in New Zealand to institutions paper & online eds. combined; USD 339 elsewhere to institutions paper & online eds. combined (effective 2001). adv. bk.rev. illus. index. *Refereed.* **Document type:** *Academic/Scholarly.* **Description:** Provides reference data designed to keep health professionals informed about quality assurance developments in Australia and abroad.

Formerly (until 1993): Australian Clinical Review (0726-3139)

Related titles: Online - full text ed.: ISSN 1440-1762. AUD 297 domestic to institutions; AUD 270 in New Zealand to institutions; USD 278 elsewhere to institutions (effective 2001) (from EBSCO Publishing, O C L C Online Computer Library Center, Inc., RoweCom Information Quest, ingenta, Munksgaard & Blackwell Science's Synergy, Swets Blackwell).

Indexed: ASSIA, CINAHL, Environ.Sci.Poll.Mgmt., Excerp.Med. (1994-), Ind.Med. (1994-), Int.Nurs.Ind., Pollut.Abstr., Risk Abstr., Saf.Sci.Abstr.

—BLDSC (5043.684700), CISTI, EMDOCS, GNLM, ingenta, KNAW. **CCC.**

Published by: (Australian Council on Healthcare Standards), Blackwell Science Asia Pty Ltd, PO Box 378, Carlton South, VIC 3053, Australia. TEL 61-3-9347-0300, FAX 61-3-9347-5001, info@blacksci-asia.com.au, http://www.blacksci.co.uk. Ed. John Duggan. R&P Sharon Liseek. Adv. contact Kathryn O'Brien. B&W page AUD 935, color page AUD 1,950; trim 210 x 275. Circ: 600. **Co-sponsor:** Australian Medical Association.

JOURNAL OF REHABILITATION MEDICINE. see *SOCIAL SERVICES AND WELFARE*

JOURNAL OF REHABILITATION MEDICINE. SUPPLEMENT. see *SOCIAL SERVICES AND WELFARE*

JOURNAL OF RELIGION AND HEALTH. see *RELIGIONS AND THEOLOGY*

JOURNAL OF REPRODUCTION AND FERTILITY. see *BIOLOGY*

616.07 USA ISSN 0890-765X
RA771.A1

THE JOURNAL OF RURAL HEALTH. Text in English. 1985. q. USD 45 domestic to individuals; USD 60 foreign to individuals; USD 110 domestic to institutions; USD 125 foreign to institutions; USD 35 domestic to students; USD 50 foreign to students (effective 2001). adv. bk.rev. abstr, charts, illus, stat. index. back issues avail. *Refereed.* **Document type:** *Academic/Scholarly.* **Description:** Advances professional practice, research, theory development and public policy relating to rural health.

Related titles: Online - full text ed.: (from Institute for Scientific Information).

Indexed: AgeLine, Agricola, CINAHL, Curr.Cont., Ind.Med. (1985-), Int.Nurs.Ind., Lang.& Lang.Behav.Abstr., SOPODA, SSCI, Soc.Serv.Abstr., Sociol.Abstr.

—BLDSC (5052.128850), EMDOCS, GNLM, IDS, Infotrieve, ingenta. **CCC.**

Published by: (University of North Carolina), National Rural Health Association, 1 W Armour Blvd, Ste 203, Kansas City, MO 64111. TEL 816-756-3140, 800-627-0932, FAX 816-756-3144, pubs@nrharural.org, http://www.NRHArural.org. Ed. Dr. Thomas C. Rosenthal. Pub. Tammy Houck Talbott. R&P Gregory Rieger. Adv. contact Rod Lawrenz. B&W page USD 300. Circ: 2,500.

JOURNAL OF SCIENTIFIC RESEARCH IN PLANTS & MEDICINES. see *PHARMACY AND PHARMACOLOGY*

JOURNAL OF SEX RESEARCH. see *PSYCHOLOGY*

610 150 GBR ISSN 0962-1105
QP425 CODEN: JSRSEU

JOURNAL OF SLEEP RESEARCH. Text in English. 1992. q., latest vol.11, 2002. GBP 209 in Europe; USD 332 in North America; USD 230 elsewhere (effective 2002). adv. bibl, illus. index. back issues avail. *Refereed.* **Document type:** *Journal, Academic/Scholarly.* **Description:** Provides a forum for research papers presenting new findings in the field of sleep and wakefulness, including biological rhythms and dreaming.

Related titles: Microform ed.: (from PQC); ♦ Online - full text ed.: Journal of Sleep Research Online. ISSN 1365-2869; ♦ Supplement: Journal of Sleep Research. Supplement. ISSN 0966-6826.

Indexed: ASCA, Curr.Cont., Excerp.Med. (1993-), Ind.Med. (1992-), Ind.Sci.Rev., Inpharma, Int.Abstr.Biol.Sci., Neurosci.Cit.Ind., Pharm.&Out.News, Reac., SSCI (coverage dropped), Sci.Cit.Ind., e-psyche.

—BLDSC (5064.680000), ADONIS, CISTI, EMDOCS, GNLM, IDS, Infotrieve, KNAW. **CCC.**

Published by: (European Sleep Research Society), Blackwell Science Ltd., PO Box 88, Oxford OX2 0NE, United Kingdom. TEL 44-1865-206180, 44-1865-206002, FAX 44-1865-206219, jnl.orders@blacksci.co.uk, http://www.blackwell-science.com/~cgilib/jnlpage.asp?Journal=jsr&File=jsr, http://www.blackwellpublishing.com. Ed. J A Horne. Pub. Allen Stevens. R&P Sophie Savage. Adv. contact Jenny Applin. Circ: 800.

M

610 150 GBR ISSN 1365-2869
▼ **JOURNAL OF SLEEP RESEARCH ONLINE.** Text in English. 1999. q. GBP 189 in Europe; USD 299 in North America; GBP 189 elsewhere (effective 2002). *Refereed.* **Document type:** *Academic/Scholarly.*
Media: Online - full text (from EBSCO Publishing, ingenta, Munksgaard & Blackwell Science's Synergy, Swets Blackwell, Institute for Scientific Information, RoweCom Information Quest). **Related titles:** Microform ed.: (from PQC); ♦ Print ed.: Journal of Sleep Research. ISSN 0962-1105.
Published by: Blackwell Science Ltd., Osney Mead, Oxford OX2 0EL, United Kingdom. TEL 44-1685-206206, FAX 44-1685-721205, website@blacksci.com, journals.cs@blacksci.co.uk, http://www.blackwell-science.com/~cgilib/jnlpage.bin?Journal=jsr&File=jsr&Page=aims.

610 GBR ISSN 0966-6826
JOURNAL OF SLEEP RESEARCH. SUPPLEMENT. Text in English. 1992. irreg. adv. **Document type:** *Academic/Scholarly.*
Related titles: ♦ Supplement to: Journal of Sleep Research. ISSN 0962-1105.
Indexed: Excerp.Med. (1993-), Int.Abstr.Biol.Sci., e-psyche.
—ADONIS, EMDOCS, KNAW.
Published by: Blackwell Science Ltd., Osney Mead, Oxford OX2 0EL, United Kingdom. TEL 44-1865-206206, FAX 44-1865-721205, journals.cs@blacksci.co.uk, http://www.blackwell-science.com. Pub. Allen Stevens. R&P Sophie Savage. Adv. contact Jenny Applin.

610 JPN ISSN 0916-8737
CODEN: JSMRE2
JOURNAL OF SMOOTH MUSCLE RESEARCH/NIHON HEIKATSUKIN GAKKAI KIKANSHI. Text in English. 1965. q. adv. bk.rev. abstr, charts, illus. index.
Formerly (until 1991): Nihon Heikatsukin Gakkai Zasshi/Japanese Journal of Smooth Muscle Research (0374-3527)
Indexed: Biol.Abstr., Chem.Titles, Excerp.Med., INIS Atomind., INSPEC (Mar.1971-Sep.1973, dropped), Ind.Med. (1991-).
—BLDSC (5064.711500), CASDDS, CISTI, EMDOCS, GNLM, Infotrieve, KNAW. **CCC.**
Published by: (Nihon Heikatsukin Gakkai/Japanese Society of Smooth Muscle Research), Journal of Smooth Muscle Research, 5 Zaifu-cho, Hirosaki-shi, Aomori-ken 036-8216, Japan. TEL 03-3272-7981, FAX 03-3273-2445. Circ: 950.

617.07 GBR ISSN 1078-9553
JOURNAL OF SURGICAL PATHOLOGY. Text in English. 1995. q. USD 95 to individuals; USD 195 to institutions. adv. reprints avail. *Refereed.* **Document type:** *Academic/Scholarly.* **Description:** Covers developments in all the disciplines relevant to surgical pathology.
Related titles: Online - full text ed.: (from Swets Blackwell).
—CISTI, KNAW.
Published by: Chapman & Hall, Journals Department (Subsidiary of: International Thomson Publishing Group), Chapman & Hall, 2-6 Boundary Row, London SE1 8HN, United Kingdom. TEL 44-20-7865-0066, FAX 44-20-7522-9623, jhrlp@chall.co.uk, http://www.chaphall.com/chaphall/journals.html. Eds. Geraldine S Pinkus, Michael J Warhol. Adv. contact Nancy Fogarty. **Subscr. to:** International Thompson Publishing Services Ltd.

362 649.8 GBR ISSN 1357-633X
JOURNAL OF TELEMEDICINE AND TELECARE. Text in English. 1995. bi-m. GBP 99 in Europe to individuals; USD 173 in United States to individuals; GBP 105 elsewhere to individuals; GBP 152 in Europe to institutions; USD 258 in United States to institutions; GBP 158 elsewhere to institutions (effective 2002). **Document type:** *Academic/Scholarly.* **Description:** Publishes papers on all aspects of both telemedicine and telecare, the latter covering distance nursing and community support.
Related titles: Online - full text ed.: (from CatchWord Ltd., EBSCO Publishing, O C L C Online Computer Library Center, Inc., RoweCom Information Quest, Swets Blackwell, Institute for Scientific Information).
Indexed: AMED, Curr.Cont., INSPEC (1999-), Ind.Med. (1995-), Int.Nurs.Ind.
—BLDSC (5069.027000), CatchWord, CISTI, GNLM, IDS, Infotrieve. **CCC.**
Published by: Royal Society of Medicine Press Ltd, 1 Wimpole St, London W1M 8AE, United Kingdom. TEL 44-20-7290-2921, FAX 44-20-7290-2929, rsmjournals@rsm.ac.uk, http://www.roysocmed.ac.uk/pub/jtt.htm. Ed. Richard Wootton. R&P Caroline McLaughlin.

JOURNAL OF THE ANATOMICAL SOCIETY OF INDIA. see *BIOLOGY*

610 USA ISSN 0022-5045
R131.A1 CODEN: JHMAA6
JOURNAL OF THE HISTORY OF MEDICINE AND ALLIED SCIENCES. Text in English. 1946. q. GBP 37, USD 55 to individuals; GBP 81, USD 122 to institutions (effective 2002). adv. bk.rev. charts, illus. cum.index: vols.1-30 (1946-1975). back issues avail.; reprint service avail. from PQC,SWZ. *Refereed.* **Document type:** *Academic/Scholarly.* **Description:** Publishes the latest original research on the written beginnings of medicine in all its aspects.
Related titles: Microform ed.: (from PQC,PMC); Online - full text ed.: (from Project MUSE, EBSCO Publishing, O C L C Online Computer Library Center, Inc., RoweCom Information Quest, Swets Blackwell, Institute for Scientific Information).
Indexed: ASCA, Amer.Hist.& Life, Arts & Hum.Cit.Ind., Bibl.Asian Stud. (1976-1993), Bibl.Engl.Lang.& Lit., Biol.Abstr., Chem.Abstr., Curr.Adv.Ecol.Sci., Curr.Cont., Dent.Ind., Excerp.Med., Hist.Abstr. (1954-), IBZ, Ind.Med. (1946-), Ind.Sci.Rev., Inpharma, MLA Intl.Bibl., Mid.East: Abstr.& Ind., P C I, Reac., Ref.Zh., SSCI, Sci.Cit.Ind. (coverage dropped).
—BLDSC (5001.000000), CISTI, GNLM, IDS, ingenta, Linda Hall. **CCC.**
Published by: Oxford University Press, Academic Division, Great Clarendon St, Oxford OX2 6DP, United Kingdom. TEL 44-1865-267907, FAX 44-1865-267835, jnlorders@oup-usa.org, jnl.info@oup.co.uk, http://www3.oup.co.uk/jalsci/, http://www.oup.co.uk/journals. Ed. Margaret Humphreys. Pub. Erich Staib. R&P Fionna Willis. Adv. contact Helen Pearson TEL 44-1235-201904. B&W page GBP 130, B&W page USD 220. Circ: 1,250.

▼ **JOURNAL OF THE I C R U.** see *PHYSICS—Nuclear Physics*

610 GBR ISSN 1474-3655
JOURNAL OF THE INDIAN MEDICAL ASSOCIATION. Text in English. q. GBP 40 domestic to individuals; GBP 50 foreign to individuals; GBP 80 domestic to institutions; GBP 78 foreign to institutions (effective 2002). bk.rev. index. back issues avail.; reprints avail. *Refereed.* **Description:** Publishes scientific papers, reviews, case reports of particular relevance to the Indian community in the UK.
Published by: Librapharm Ltd, Gemini House, 162 Craven Rd, Newbury, Berks RG14 5NR, United Kingdom. TEL 44-1635-522651, FAX 44-1635-36294, journals@librapharm.com, http://www.librapharm.com. Ed. Dr. Devaki Nair. Pub. P.L. Dr. Clarke. R&P P.L. Clarke. Circ: 1,000 (paid); 4,000 (controlled).

610 IND
JOURNAL OF THE INDIAN MEDICAL PROFESSION. Text in English. 1954. m. INR 15, USD 4.50. adv. charts, illus.
Indexed: Chem.Abstr., Ind.Med. (coverage dropped), Nutr.Abstr., Saf.Sci.Abstr.
Published by: United Asia Publications Pvt. Ltd., 12 Rampart Row, Mumbai, Maharashtra 400 001, India. Ed. Dr. R M Rajpal.

610 617.6 GBR
JOURNAL OF THE MEDICAL AND DENTAL DEFENCE UNIONS. Text in English. 1985. bi-m. **Document type:** *Bulletin.*
Formerly (until 1995): Journal of the Medical Defence Union (0952-9934)
Published by: Medical Defence Union Ltd., 3 Devonshire Pl, London W5 4TR, United Kingdom. TEL 44-171-486-6181, FAX 44-171-935-5503.

610 026 USA
Z675.M4 CODEN: BMLAAG
JOURNAL OF THE MEDICAL LIBRARY ASSOCIATION. Short title: J M L A. Text in English. 1911. q., latest vol.89, no.3. USD 136 in North America; USD 174 elsewhere (effective 2001). adv. bk.rev., software rev. bibl, abstr. index, cum.index. 100 p./no. back issues avail.; reprint service avail. from PQC,PSC,ISI. *Refereed.* **Document type:** *Journal, Academic/Scholarly, Trade.* **Description:** Contains features and articles of interest to information management professionals, particularly those in the health information field.
Formerly: Medical Library Association. Bulletin (0025-7338)
Related titles: Microform ed.: (from PQC); Online - full content ed.; Online - full text ed.: (from Institute for Scientific Information).
Indexed: ASCA, Abstr.Health Care Manage.Stud., Abstr.Hyg., AgeLine, Biol.Abstr., CINAHL, Curr.Adv.Ecol.Sci., Curr.Cont., Dent.Ind., Excerp.Med., INSPEC (Jan.1982-), I.P.A., Ind.Med. (1911-), Inform.Sci.Abstr., Int.Nurs.Ind., LHTB, LISA, Lib.Lit. (Oct.1984-), Nutr.Abstr., Ocean.Abstr. (coverage dropped), SSCI, Sci.Cit.Ind. (coverage dropped), Telegen, Trop.Dis.Bull.
—BLDSC (2612.090000), AskIEEE, CASDDS, GNLM, IDS, ingenta, KNAW.
Published by: Medical Library Association, 65 E Wacker Pl, Ste 1900, Chicago, IL 60601-7298. TEL 312-419-9094, FAX 312-419-8950, info@mlahq.org, http://www.mlahq.org/publications/bmla, http://www.mlanet.org, http://www.mlanet.org/publications. Ed. T Scott Plotchak. R&P Lynanne Feilen TEL 312-419-9094 ext 26. Adv. contact Barbara Redmond TEL 312-419-9094 ext 26. B&W page USD 1,261, color page USD 2,221; 8 x 10.5. Circ: 5,685.

610 IDN ISSN 0126-1312
JOURNAL OF THE MEDICAL SCIENCES/BERKALA ILMU KEDOKTERAN. Text and summaries in English, Indonesian. 1969. q. IDR 8,000, USD 20. adv. bk.rev. charts, illus, stat.
Formerly: Gadjah Mada Journal of the Medical Sciences
Indexed: Chem.Abstr.
—CCC.
Published by: Gadjah Mada University, College of Medicine/Universitas Gadjah Mada, Fakultas Kedokteran, Department of Physical Anthropology, Sekip, Yogyakarta, Indonesia. Ed. Teuku Jacob. Circ: 1,200.

610 GBR ISSN 1470-3203
▼ **JOURNAL OF THE RENIN-ANGIOTENSIN-ALDOSTERONE SYSTEM.** Variant title: J R A A S. Text in English. 2000. q. GBP 80 in Europe to individuals; GBP 110 elsewhere to institutions; GBP 125 in Europe to institutions; GBP 175 elsewhere to institutions; GBP 55 in Europe to students; GBP 75 elsewhere to students (effective 2001). **Document type:** *Journal, Academic/Scholarly.* **Description:** Provides a unique platform for the publication of research and clinical trials in the rapidly developing field of renin-angiotensin-aldosterone system and related peptidergic systems.
—BLDSC (5049.465000).
Published by: J R A A S Ltd, Edgbaston House, 3 Duchess Pl, Edgbaston, Brirmingham B16 8NH, United Kingdom. TEL 44-121-454-4114, FAX 44-121-454-1190, ngibbs@sherbornegibbs.co.uk, production@jraas.co.uk, http://www.jraas.com. Eds. Graham A MacGregor, Peter Sever. Pub., R&P Nina Gibbs. Adv. contact Michael Young.

610 CHE ISSN 1027-3662
▼ **JOURNAL OF THEORETICAL MEDICINE.** Text in English. 1999. q. GBP 60, USD 88, EUR 80 to individuals; GBP 146, USD 218, EUR 240 to institutions; GBP 263, USD 340, EUR 374 to corporations (effective 2002). **Document type:** *Academic/Scholarly.*
Related titles: Online - full text ed.: (from EBSCO Publishing, RoweCom Information Quest).
Published by: Gordon and Breach - Harwood Academic (Subsidiary of: Taylor & Francis Group), PO Box 531, Lausanne 1000, Switzerland. http://www.gbhap.com. Ed. Brian Sleeman. **Subscr. addr. in US:** International Publishers Direct, PO Box 32160, Newark, NJ 07102. FAX 215-750-6343.

610 JPN ISSN 0022-5207
JOURNAL OF THERAPY/CHIRYO. Text in Japanese. 1920. m. JPY 35,280 (effective 2000). adv. **Document type:** *Academic/Scholarly.*
Formed by the merger of: Chiryo Oyobi Shono; Naika Oyobi Shonika
Indexed: Chem.Abstr., INIS Atomind., Jap.Per.Ind.
—GNLM.
Published by: Nanzando Co. Ltd., 4-1-11 Yushima, Bunkyo-ku, Tokyo 113-0034, Japan. TEL 81-3-5689-7868, FAX 81-3-5689-7869, chr@nanzando.com, http://nanzando.com. Ed., Adv. contact Masahiko Kubota. Pub., R&P Hajime Suzuki. Circ: 12,000.

JOURNAL OF TOXICOLOGIC PATHOLOGY. see *ENVIRONMENTAL STUDIES—Toxicology And Environmental Safety*

JOURNAL OF TRACE ELEMENTS IN MEDICINE AND BIOLOGY. see *BIOLOGY*

M

610 CAN ISSN 1195-1982 CODEN: JTRMFK
JOURNAL OF TRAVEL MEDICINE. Text in English. 1994. bi-m. USD 105 in US & Canada to individuals; USD 140 elsewhere to individuals; USD 145 in US & Canada to institutions; USD 195 elsewhere to institutions (effective 2001). adv. back issues avail. *Refereed.* **Document type:** *Academic/Scholarly.* **Description:** Publishes articles for both the investigator and the practitioner in the field of travel medicine.
Related titles: Online - full text ed.: (from Northern Light Technology, Inc., ProQuest Information & Learning, Institute for Scientific Information).
Indexed: Abstr.Hyg., Curr.Cont., Environ.Sci.Poll.Mgmt., Ind.Med. (1994-), Inpharma, Jrnl.Watch Inf.Dis., Pharm.&Out.News, Pollut.Abstr., Protozool.Abstr., Reac., Rev.Appl.Entomol., Rev.Med.& Vet.Mycol., Risk Abstr., Rural Recreat.Tour.Abstr., Saf.Sci.Abstr., Trop.Dis.Bull.
—BLDSC (5070.547000), GNLM, Infotrieve, KNAW. **CCC.**
Published by: (International Society of Travel Medicine), B.C. Decker Inc., 20 Hughson St S, LCD 1, P O Box 620, Hamilton, ON L8N 3K7, Canada. TEL 905-522-7017, 800-568-7281, FAX 905-522-7839, info@bcdecker.com, http://www.bcdecker.com. Ed. Dr. Charles D Ericsson. Pub. David LeGallais. R&P Paula Presutti. Adv. contact John Birkby. Circ: 2,106. **Co-sponsor:** Asia Pacific Travel Health Association.

610 USA ISSN 1099-3460
R15 CODEN: JUHEFL
JOURNAL OF URBAN HEALTH. Text in English. 1925. q. GBP 55, USD 65 to individuals; GBP 70, USD 95 to institutions (effective Mar. 2002). bk.rev. charts, illus, stat. index. back issues avail.; reprint service avail. from PQC. *Refereed.* **Document type:** *Journal, Academic/Scholarly.* **Description:** Serves as a vehicle for publishing articles relevant to urban health; the journal addresses issues from both a clinical and policy perspectives.
Formerly: New York Academy of Medicine. Bulletin (0028-7091)
Related titles: Microform ed.: (from PQC,PMC); Online - full content ed.: GBP 63, USD 85 to institutions Online only (effective Mar. 2002); free with subscr. to the Print Edition (from Oxford University Press Online Journals); Online - full text ed.: (from Institute for Scientific Information).
Indexed: ASCA, Abstr.Anthropol., Abstr.Health Care Manage.Stud., Abstr.Hyg., AgeLine, Agri.& Environ.Biotech.Abstr. (coverage dropped), Biol.Abstr., CINAHL, Chem.Abstr., Curr.Adv.Ecol.Sci., Curr.Cont., Dairy Sci.Abstr., Derwent Biotech.Abstr., Environ.Sci.Poll.Mgmt., Excerp.Med., Helminthol.Abstr., Hosp.Lit.Ind., INIS Atomind., Ind.Med. (1998-), Inpharma, Int.Nurs.Ind., NRN, Numis.Lit., Nutr.Abstr., Pollut.Abstr., Reac., Rel.Ind.One, Rel.Ind.Two, Risk Abstr., SSCI (coverage dropped), Saf.Sci.Abstr., Sci.Cit.Ind., THA, Trop.Dis.Bull.
—BLDSC (5071.555000), CASDDS, CISTI, GNLM, IDS, ingenta, KNAW. **CCC.**
Published by: (New York Academy of Medicine GBR), Oxford University Press, Academic Division, Great Clarendon St, Oxford OX2 6DP, United Kingdom. TEL 44-1865-267907, FAX 44-1865-267835, dvlahov@nyam.org, jnl.info@oup.co.uk, http://www.jurban.oupjournals.org/, http://www.oup.co.uk/journals. Pub. J Fox. Circ: 3,500 (paid).

JOURNAL OF VALIDATION TECHNOLOGY; serving the pharmaceutical, medical device, biotechnology and diagnostics industries. see *INSTRUMENTS*

JOURNALS OF GERONTOLOGY. SERIES A: BIOLOGICAL SCIENCES & MEDICAL SCIENCES. see *GERONTOLOGY AND GERIATRICS*

JUNDI SHAPUR UNIVERSITY. FACULTY OF MEDICINE. LIBRARY BULLETIN/DANESHGAH-E JONDISHAPUR. DANESHKADE-YE PEZESAKI. BULTAN-E KETABKHANEH. see *LIBRARY AND INFORMATION SCIENCES*

610 CHN ISSN 1000-5501 CODEN: JYKYEL
JUNSHI YIXUE KEXUEYUAN YUANKAN/ACADEMY OF MILITARY MEDICAL SCIENCES. BULLETIN. Text in Chinese. 1983. bi-m. USD 16.80; CNY 8, USD 5.20 newsstand/cover (effective 2001). **Document type:** *Academic/Scholarly.*
Related titles: Online - full content ed.: (from WanFang Data Corp.).
Indexed: INIS Atomind.
—BLDSC (2378.395200), CASDDS.
Published by: Zhongguo Renmin Jiefangjun Junshi Yixue Kexueyuan/People's Liberation Army Academy of Military Medical Sciences, 27 Taiping Lu, Beijing 100850, China. Ed. Wu Zuze. **Dist. by:** China International Book Trading Corp, 35, Chegongzhuang Xilu, Haidian District, Beijing 100044, China. TEL 86-1-68413849, FAX 86-1-68412048, cibtc@mail.cibtc.com.cn, http://www.cibtc.com.cn.

610 JPN ISSN 0022-6769 CODEN: JUIZAG
JUNTENDO MEDICAL JOURNAL/JUNTENDO IGAKU. Text in Japanese. 1887. q. JPY 5,000 (effective 2000). adv. abstr. index. *Refereed.* **Document type:** *Academic/Scholarly.*
Indexed: Chem.Abstr., Chem.Indus.Notes, Chem.Titles, INIS Atomind.
—CASDDS.
Published by: Juntendo Medical Society/Juntendo Igakkai, 2-1-1 Hongo, Bunkyo-ku, Tokyo 113-0033, Japan. FAX 81-3-3814-9100. Ed. Yutaka Inaba. Circ: 3,700 (controlled).

610 MYS ISSN 0127-1075
JURNAL PERUBATAN U K M. Text in English, Malay. 1979. s-a. USD 15 per issue.
Published by: Penerbit Universiti Kebangsaan Malaysia, Ukm Bangi, Selangor 43600, Malaysia.

JURY INSTRUCTIONS ON MEDICAL ISSUES. see *LAW—Judicial Systems*

610 JPN ISSN 0022-7226 CODEN: JUZIAG
JUZEN IGAKKAI ZASSHI/JUZEN MEDICAL SOCIETY. JOURNAL. Text in English, Japanese. 1896. 6/yr. JPY 3,000, USD 20. adv. abstr, bibl, illus.
Indexed: Biol.Abstr., C.I.S. Abstr., Chem.Abstr., INIS Atomind.
—BLDSC (4810.100000), CASDDS, CISTI, GNLM.
Published by: Kanazawa Daigaku Igakubu, Juzen Igakkai/Kanazawa University, School of Medicine, Juzen Medical Society, 13-1 Takara-Machi, Kanazawa-shi, Ishikawa-ken 920-0934, Japan.

616 USA ISSN 0090-5089
K A F P JOURNAL. Text in English. 1956. q. membership. adv. **Document type:** *Academic/Scholarly.* **Description:** Articles and essays focusing on the practical issues that affect the health and welfare of families, and on conferences, activities, and issues relevant to contemporary family physicians.
Formerly: K A G P Journal (0022-7250)
Published by: Kentucky Academy of Family Physicians, Medical Arts Bldg, Ste 3323, 1169 Eastern Pkwy, Louisville, KY 40217. TEL 502-451-0370, FAX 502-451-5914. Eds. John A Patterson, Dr. Walter Zukof. Adv. contact Margaret Roberts. Circ: 1,200.

610 USA ISSN 0886-4772
K C M S BULLETIN. Text in English. 1921. bi-m. USD 15 to non-members; USD 2.50 to members. adv. bk.rev. charts, tr.lit. index. back issues avail. **Document type:** *Bulletin.*
Formerly: Medical Society of the County of Kings and Academy of Medicine of Brooklyn. Bulletin (0025-7532)
Published by: Medical Society County of Kings, Inc., 165 Cadman Plaza E, Brooklyn, NY 11201-1402. TEL 718-467-9000, FAX 718-778-0380. Ed. Randall D Bloomfield. Circ: 2,800 (controlled). **Co-publisher:** Academy of Medicine of Brooklyn.

610 JPN ISSN 0368-5063 CODEN: KDIZAA
KAGOSHIMA DAIGAKU IGAKU ZASSHI/MEDICAL JOURNAL OF KAGOSHIMA UNIVERSITY. Text in Japanese. 1945. q. **Document type:** *Academic/Scholarly.*
Indexed: INIS Atomind.
—BLDSC (5527.830000), GNLM.
Published by: Kagoshima Daigaku, Igakubu/Kagoshima University, Faculty of Medicine, 8-35-1 Sakuragaoka, Kagoshima-shi 890-0075, Japan. TEL 81-922-75-5188, FAX 81-992-75-1124.

610 JPN ISSN 0913-5073
KAGOSHIMA KYUKYU IGAKKAISHI/KAGOSHIMA ASSOCIATION FOR ACUTE MEDICINE. JOURNAL. Text in Japanese. 1978. irreg.
Published by: Kagoshima Kyukyu Igakkai, 8-1 Chuo-cho, Kagoshima-shi 890-0053, Japan.

610 JPN
KANAZAWA DAIGAKU IGAKUBU HOKENGAKKA SAGYO RYOHOGAKKA SOTSUGYO KENKYU RONBUNSHU/KANAZAWA UNIVERSITY. SCHOOL OF HEALTH SCIENCES. DEPARTMENT OF OCCUPATIONAL THERAPY. COLLECTION OF PAPERS. Text in Japanese. 1982. a., latest vol.18, 2000. free per issue. *Refereed.* **Document type:** *Academic/Scholarly.* **Description:** Collection of graduate thesis of the Department of Occupational Therapy.
Formerly (until vol.17, 1998): Kanazawa Daigaku Iryou Gijutsu Tanki Daigakubu Sagyo Ryohogakka Sotsugyo Kenkyu Ronbunshu (0917-4796)
Published by: Kanazawa Daigaku, Igakubu Kokengakka, Sagyo Ryohogakusenko/Kanazawa University, School of Health Sciences, Department of Occupational Therapy, 11-80 Kodatsuno 5-chome, Kanazawa-shi, Ishikawa-ken 920-0942, Japan. TEL 81-76-265-2500, FAX 81-76-234-4375. Ed. Fujiko Someya. Circ: 250.

610.7 JPN CODEN: KIDZAK
KANSAI MEDICAL UNIVERSITY. JOURNAL/KANSAI IKA DAIGAKU. ZASSHI. Text and summaries in English, German, Japanese. 1948. q. JPY 1,000, USD 2.80. adv. abstr, bibl, charts, illus. index.
Formerly: Kansai Medical School. Journal (0022-8400)
Indexed: Biol.Abstr., Chem.Abstr., Excerp.Med., INIS Atomind.
—CASDDS, GNLM.
Published by: Kansai Medical University, 1 Fumizono-cho, Moriguchi-shi, Osaka-fu 570-0074, Japan.

344.041 USA
KANSAS PHYSICIAN. Text in English. 1995. m. USD 50 (effective 1999). adv. back issues avail. **Document type:** *Newsletter, Trade.*
Published by: Kansas Medical Society, 623 S W 10th Ave, Topeka, KS 66612. TEL 913-235-2383, FAX 913-235-5114. Ed. Allison Peterson. Adv. contact Christine Schieferecke. page USD 950; trim 14 x 11. Circ: 4,600.

610 TWN ISSN 0257-5655 CODEN: KHHCE2
KAOHSIUNG JOURNAL OF MEDICAL SCIENCES. Key Title: Gaoxiong Yixue Kexue Zazhi. Text in Chinese, English. 1985. m. USD 60. adv. charts, illus. index. back issues avail. **Document type:** *Academic/Scholarly.* **Description:** Contains scientific papers in all fields of medicine, review articles, original articles, and case reports.
Indexed: Abstr.Hyg., Br.Archaeol.Abstr., Chem.Abstr., Chem.Indus.Notes, Chem.Titles, Dairy Sci.Abstr., Excerp.Med., Ind.Med. (coverage dropped), Nutr.Abstr., Protozool.Abstr., Rev.Appl.Entomol., Rev.Med.& Vet.Mycol., Soyabean Abstr., Trop.Dis.Bull.
—BLDSC (5085.674500), CASDDS, EMDOCS, GNLM, KNAW.
Published by: Kaohsiung Medical College, no.100 Shih-Chuan 1st Rd, Kaohsiung 80708, Taiwan. TEL 886-7-3121101, FAX 886-7-3215842, m835003@kmu.edu.tw, http://kjms.kmu.edu.tw/index.html. Ed. Hong Wen Liu. Pub. Juei Hsiung Tsai. Circ: 1,500.

610 IND ISSN 0377-9378
KARNATAKA MEDICAL JOURNAL. Text in English. 1939. q. INR 75 to individuals; INR 100 to institutions. adv. bk.rev.
Formerly (until 1974): Mysore Medical Association. Journal
Indexed: Biol.Abstr.
Published by: Indian Medical Association Karnataka State Branch, IMA House, Alur Venkata Rao Rd., Bangalore, Karnataka 560 018, India. Ed. D Somasekharaiah. Circ: 5,000.

610 USA ISSN 1040-3353 CODEN: KINSEJ
KAROLINSKA INSTITUTE NOBEL CONFERENCE SERIES. Text in English. 1980. irreg. price varies. reprint service avail. from PQC. *Refereed.* **Document type:** *Proceedings.*
Published by: (Karolinska Institute), Lippincott Williams & Wilkins (Philadelphia) (Subsidiary of: Wolters Kluwer N.V.), 530 Walnut St, Philadelphia, PA 19106-3621. TEL 301-223-2300, 800-638-3030, FAX 301-223-2400, http://www.lww.com.

610 VEN ISSN 0075-5222
KASMERA. Text in Spanish; Abstracts in English, Spanish. 1962. 3/yr. per issue exchange basis. bibl, charts, illus, stat. *Refereed.* **Description:** Publishes research by the Faculty of Medicine in areas of bacteriology, immunology, parasitology and other topics.
Related titles: Microform ed.

M

Indexed: Abstr.Hyg., Biol.Abstr., Poult.Abstr., Trop.Dis.Bull. —CISTI.
Published by: Universidad del Zulia, Departamento de Enfermedades Infecciosas y Tropicales, Apdo. 526, Maracaibo 4001A, Venezuela. TEL 61-517717, bcalvo@telcel.net.ve. Ed. Dr. Ricardo Soto Urribarri. Circ: 1,000.

610 DEU
KATHOLISCHER BERUFSVERBAND FUER PFLEGEBERUFE. MITTEILUNGSBLATT. Text in German. bi-m.
Published by: Katholischer Berufsverband fuer Pflegeberufe e.V., Kaiserstr 42, Mainz 55116, Germany. TEL 06131-232340.

610 JPN ISSN 0386-5924
CODEN: KAIGD3
KAWASAKI IGAKKAI SHI. Text in Japanese; Summaries in English, Japanese. 1975. q. JPY 10,000 (effective 2001). bk.rev. illus. **Document type:** *Academic/Scholarly.*
Indexed: INIS Atomind., Zoo.Rec.
—BLDSC (5088.096000), CASDDS, KNAW.
Published by: Kawasaki Medical Society, 577 Matsushima, Kurashiki-shi, Okayama-ken 701-0114, Japan. FAX 81-462-1199. Ed. Shinichiro Yamamoto. Circ: 1,150.

610 JPN ISSN 0385-0234
CODEN: KAMJDW
KAWASAKI MEDICAL JOURNAL. Text in English; Summaries in Japanese. 1975. q. JPY 20,000 (effective 2001). bk.rev. illus. **Document type:** *Academic/Scholarly.*
Indexed: Abstr.Hyg., Biol.Abstr., Chem.Abstr., Chem.Indus.Notes, Chem.Titles, Excerp.Med., Helminthol.Abstr., INIS Atomind., Ind.Vet., NRN, Ref.Zh., Rev.Appl.Entomol., Trop.Dis.Bull., Vet.Bull.
—BLDSC (5088.097000), CASDDS, CISTI, EMDOCS, GNLM.
Published by: Kawasaki Medical Society, 577 Matsushima, Kurashiki-shi, Okayama-ken 701-0114, Japan. FAX 81-86-462-1199. Ed., R&P Seitaro Ohkuma. Circ: 1,350.

610 RUS ISSN 0368-4814
CODEN: KAMZA9
KAZANSKII MEDITSINSKII ZHURNAL. Text in Russian. bi-m. USD 129 in United States.
Indexed: INIS Atomind., Ref.Zh.
—BLDSC (0088.240000), CASDDS, CISTI, East View, GNLM.
Published by: Kazanskii Medistinskii Zhurnal, Ul Dekabristov 2, Kazan 420066, Russian Federation. TEL 8432-437074, redacia@kmj.kcn.ru. Ed. D M Zubairov. **US dist. addr.:** East View Publications, 3020 Harbor Ln N, Minneapolis, MN 55447. TEL 612-550-0961.

610 JPN ISSN 0022-9717
CODEN: KJMEA9
KEIO JOURNAL OF MEDICINE. Text in English. 1952. q. JPY 5,000 domestic; USD 90 foreign (effective 2001). 50 p./no. *Refereed.* **Document type:** *Academic/Scholarly.*
Related titles: Online - full content ed.
Indexed: Abstr.Hyg., Biol.Abstr., Chem.Abstr., Chem.Titles, Diar.Dis.Res., Excerp.Med., INIS Atomind., Ind.Med. (1952-), Int.Nurs.Ind., Nutr.Abstr., Rev.Med.& Vet.Mycol., THA, Trop.Dis.Bull.
—BLDSC (5089.000000), CASDDS, CISTI, GNLM, ingenta, KNAW.
Published by: Keio Gijuku Daigaku, Igakubu/Keio University, School of Medicine, 35 Shinano-Machi, Shinjuku-ku, Tokyo 160-0016, Japan. TEL 81-3-3353-1211, FAX 81-3-5379-6059, http://www.kjm.keio.ac.jp. Ed. Dr. Naoki Aikawa. Circ: 500 (paid); 450 (controlled).

174.2 362 USA ISSN 1054-6863
QH332 CODEN: KIEJEF
KENNEDY INSTITUTE OF ETHICS. JOURNAL. Text in English. 1991. q. USD 55 to individuals; USD 125 to institutions (effective 2002). adv. illus. back issues avail.; reprint service avail. from WSH. *Refereed.* **Document type:** *Academic/Scholarly.* **Description:** Forum for discussion of major issues in bioethics, including such topics as active euthanasia, fetal tissue research, human embryo cloning, genetics, health care reform, and organ transplantation.
Related titles: Online - full text ed.: ISSN 1086-3249. USD 96.30 (effective 2000) (from Project MUSE, EBSCO Publishing, O C L C Online Computer Library Center, Inc., RoweCom Information Quest, Swets Blackwell, Institute for Scientific Information).
Indexed: ASCA, Arts & Hum.Cit.Ind., Curr.Cont., P.A.I.S., Phil.Ind., Rel.Ind.One, Rel.Ind.Two, SSCI.
—BLDSC (5089.517000), GNLM, IDS, Infotrieve, ingenta. CCC.
Published by: (Joseph and Rose Kennedy Institute of Ethics), Johns Hopkins University Press, Journals Publishing Division, 2715 N Charles St, Baltimore, MD 21218-4363. TEL 800-548-1784, FAX 410-516-6968, jlorder@jhupress.jhu.edu, http://www.press.jhu.edu/press/journals/ken/, http://muse.jhu.edu. Ed. Carol Mason Spicer. Adv. contact Anastasia Scherr. page USD 325; trim 5.5 x 9. Circ: 1,948 (paid).

170 610 USA
KENNEDY INSTITUTE OF ETHICS. SCOPE NOTE. Text in English. 1982. irreg., latest vol.40. USD 5 in US, Canada & Mexico; USD 8 elsewhere (effective 2001). **Document type:** *Monographic series.* **Description:** Presents current viewpoints related to specific topics in biomedical ethics. Intended specifically for scholars, journalists, medical and legal practitioners, students and interested laypersons.
Formerly: Kennedy Institute of Bioethics. Scope Note
Indexed: Vert.File Ind.
Published by: Kennedy Institute of Ethics, National Reference Center for Bioethics Literature, Georgetown University, Box 571212, Washington, DC 20057-1212. TEL 202-687-6689, FAX 202-687-6770, medethx@georgetown.edu, http://bioethics.georgetown.edu. Ed. Doris Goldstein. Circ: 2,000.

616 USA ISSN 0023-0294
CODEN: JKMAB5
KENTUCKY MEDICAL ASSOCIATION. JOURNAL. Text in English. 1903. m. USD 40 domestic; USD 60 foreign; USD 5 newsstand/cover (effective 2001). adv. bk.rev. bibl, illus. index. reprints avail. *Refereed.* **Document type:** *Academic/Scholarly.*
Related titles: Microform ed.: (from PQC).
Indexed: Biol.Abstr., Chem.Abstr., Curr.Cont. (coverage dropped), Excerp.Med., Helminthol.Abstr., INIS Atomind., Ind.Med. (1950-), Int.Nurs.Ind., Rev.Plant Path.
—BLDSC (4810.740000), CISTI, GNLM, KNAW.
Published by: Kentucky Medical Association, 4965 US Hwy 42, 2000, Louisville, KY 40222-6372. TEL 502-426-6200, FAX 502-426-6877. Ed. Stephen Z Smith. R&P, Adv. contact Sharon Heckel. Circ: 6,000.

610 USA
KENTUCKY MEDICAL NEWS; the best healthcare news in the business. Text in English. 1994. m. USD 25; USD 2.50 newsstand/cover (effective 1999). adv. illus. **Document type:** *Trade.* **Description:** Contains news for physicians and other medical professionals in Kentucky.
Address: Idle Hour Shopping Center, 2121 Richmond Rd, Ste 204, Lexington, KY 40502. TEL 606-266-6016, FAX 606-266-4490, kymednews@worldnet.att.net, http://mednews.com. Ed. Sandy Wensley. R&P Susan Wensley. Adv. contact Susan Harris. Circ: 30,000.

610 KEN ISSN 0076-5988
KENYA MEDICAL RESEARCH INSTITUTE. ANNUAL REPORT. Text in English. 1966. a. free. adv. **Document type:** *Corporate.*
Indexed: Biol.Abstr.
Published by: (Kenya Medical Research Institute), African Forum for Health Sciences, PO Box 54840, Nairobi, Kenya. TEL 254-2-722541, FAX 254-2-720030, kemrilib@healthnet.or.ke. Ed. Dr. Davy Koech. Adv. contact Bernard Muthaka.

610 KEN
KENYA. MINISTRY OF HEALTH. ANNUAL REPORT. Text in English. a. **Document type:** *Government.*
Published by: Ministry of Health, P.O. Box 20781, Nairobi, Kenya.

610 KEN
KENYA. MINISTRY OF HEALTH. HEALTH INFORMATION SYSTEM. Text in English. 1977. q. **Document type:** *Government.*
Published by: Ministry of Health, Division of Health Information System, P O Box 20781, Nairobi, Kenya. TEL 254-2-501341.

610 IND ISSN 0301-4827
KERALA MEDICAL JOURNAL. Text in English. 1959. m. membership. adv. bk.rev., film rev. bibl, charts, illus.
Published by: Indian Medical Association, Kerala State Branch, Cochin, Kerala 682 016, India. Ed. I S Menon. Circ: 4,500.

610 GBR
KEY NOTE MARKET REPORT: MEDICAL EQUIPMENT. Variant title: Medical Equipment. Text in English. irreg., latest vol.12, 1998. GBP 265 (effective 1999). **Document type:** *Trade.*
Formerly: Key Note Report: Medical Equipment (0961-1665)
Related titles: CD-ROM ed.; Online - full text ed.
Published by: Key Note Ltd., Field House, 72 Oldfield Rd, Hampton, Mddx TW12 2HQ, United Kingdom. TEL 44-20-8481-8750, FAX 44-20-8783-0049, http://www.keynote.co.uk.

610 GBR
KEY NOTE MARKET REPORT: PRIVATE HEALTHCARE. Variant title: Private Healthcare. Text in English. irreg., latest vol.14, 1998. GBP 265 (effective 1999). **Document type:** *Trade.*
Formerly (until 1995): Key Note Report: Private Healthcare (0950-3196)
Related titles: CD-ROM ed.; Online - full text ed.
Published by: Key Note Ltd., Field House, 72 Oldfield Rd, Hampton, Mddx TW12 2HQ, United Kingdom. TEL 44-20-8481-8750, FAX 44-20-8783-0049, http://www.keynote.co.uk. Ed. Donna Jones.

610 GBR ISSN 1356-6113
KEY NOTE MARKET REVIEW: U K HEALTHCARE. Variant title: U K Healthcare. Text in English. 1994. irreg., latest vol.6, 1997. GBP 465 (effective 1999). **Document type:** *Trade.*
Related titles: CD-ROM ed.; Online - full text ed.
Published by: Key Note Ltd., Field House, 72 Oldfield Rd, Hampton, Mddx TW12 2HQ, United Kingdom. TEL 44-20-8481-8750, FAX 44-20-8783-0049, http://www.keynote.co.uk.

610 SAU ISSN 0254-413X
CODEN: KAMJEX
KING ABDUL AZIZ MEDICAL JOURNAL. Text in English. 1981. q. **Document type:** *Academic/Scholarly.*
Related titles: CD-ROM ed.
Indexed: Chem.Abstr., ExtraMED.
—CASDDS, GNLM.
Published by: King Abdul Aziz University, College of Medicine and Allied Sciences, P O Box 1540, Jeddah 21441, Saudi Arabia.

610 USA
KING COUNTY MEDICAL SOCIETY. BULLETIN. Text in English. 1916. m. USD 17.30 in state; USD 21.62 elsewhere. adv.
Published by: (King County Medical Society), Journal and Bulletin Agency, PO Box 10249, Bainbridge Island, WA 98110. TEL 206-682-7813. adv.: B&W page USD 350; trim 7.5 x 9.75. Circ: 4,400.

610 GBR ISSN 0085-2546
KING'S GAZETTE; the journal of King's College Hospital. Text in English. 1921. s-a. GBP 2.75. adv. bk.rev. illus.
Published by: Kings College Hospital Medical School, 124-126 Denmark Hill, London SE5 8RX, United Kingdom. Ed. Sarah Hawxwell. Circ: 1,500.

612.76 CAN ISSN 0823-0536
KINNECTION. Text in English. 1983. bi-m. membership. adv. bk.rev. **Document type:** *Newsletter.* **Description:** Contains information on legislation, association business, continuing education opportunities, employment opportunities and new advances in the science of kinesiology.
Published by: Ontario Kinesiology Association, 6519 B Mississauga Rd, Mississauga, ON L5N 1A6, Canada. TEL 905-567-7194, FAX 905-567-7191, info@oka.on.ca. Ed., R&P Karen de Vaal. Adv. contact Nikki Wright. B&W page CND 500; trim 10.5 x 8. Circ: 1,400.

610 JPN ISSN 0913-6452
KINSEI KAGAKU/KINSEI SCIENCE - A SCIENTIFIC APPROACH TO POSTURES. Text in Japanese; Summaries in English, German. 1986. a.
Published by: Shisei Hoken Igakkai/Medical Association of Posture and Health, 4-22 Ohashi 2-chome, Meguro-ku, Tokyo 153-0044, Japan.

610 JPN ISSN 0023-1908
CODEN: KKAIA2
KITAKANTO MEDICAL JOURNAL/KITAKANTO IGAKU. Text in Japanese; Summaries in English. 1951. bi-m. JPY 6,000. abstr, charts, illus. *Refereed.* **Document type:** *Academic/Scholarly.*
Indexed: Biol.Abstr., Chem.Abstr., Excerp.Med., INIS Atomind.
—BLDSC (5098.100000), CASDDS, GNLM.
Published by: Kitakanto Medical Society/Kitakanto Igakkai, c/o Gumma University, School of Medicine, 3-39-22 Showa-Machi, Maebashi-shi, Gunma-ken 371-0034, Japan. TEL 81-272-20-7111. Ed. Hidetoshi Yamanaka. Circ: 1,000.

610 JPN ISSN 0023-1916
CODEN: KBYKAV
KITANO HOSPITAL JOURNAL OF MEDICINE. Text in Japanese; Abstracts and contents page in English. 1955. q. free. charts, illus, stat. 150 p./no. back issues avail. *Refereed.* **Document type:** *Journal, Academic/Scholarly.*
Indexed: Biol.Abstr., Excerp.Med., Ref.Zh.
—BLDSC (5098.150000), CASDDS, CISTI.
Published by: Tazuke Kofukai, Medical Research Institute, 2-4-20 Ohgimachi, Kita-ku, Osaka-shi 530-8480, Japan. TEL 81-6-6312-1221, FAX 81-6-6361-0588. Ed. Kiyoshi Takatsuki. Circ: 450.

610 JPN ISSN 0385-2024
KITASATO INSTITUTE. ANNUAL REPORT. Text in English, Japanese. 1964. a. back issues avail. **Document type:** *Corporate.*
—BLDSC (1318.680000), KNAW.
Published by: Kitasato Institute, 5-9-1 Shirokane, Minato-ku, Tokyo 1080072, Japan. TEL 81-3-3444-6161, FAX 81-3-5791-6120, http://www.kitasato.or.jp, http://www.kitasato.or.jp.

610 RUS ISSN 0023-2149
R91 CODEN: KLMIAZ
KLINICHESKAYA MEDITSINA/CLINICAL MEDICINE. Text in Russian; Summaries in English. 1920. m. USD 202 foreign (effective 2000). adv. bk.rev., Website rev. abstr. index. reprints avail. **Document type:** *Journal, Academic/Scholarly.* **Description:** Discusses principal issues of clinical medicine, dealing mainly with matters of diagnosis, pathogenesis, prophylaxis, treatment and clinical course. Includes original essays on the scientific developments of Russian medicine and surveys of modern theoretical medicine abroad.
Indexed: Agri.& Environ.Biotech.Abstr. (coverage dropped), Biol.Abstr., Chem.Abstr., Chem.Indus.Notes, Chem.Titles, Dent.Ind., Derwent Biotech.Abstr., Excerp.Med., Helminthol.Abstr., INIS Atomind., Ind.Med. (1920-), Ind.Sci.Rev., Neurosci.Cit.Ind., Nutr.Abstr., Ref.Zh., SSCI (coverage dropped), Sci.Cit.Ind. (coverage dropped).
—BLDSC (0089.240000), CASDDS, CISTI, East View, GNLM, IDS, Infotrieve, KNAW. **CCC.**
Published by: Izdatel'stvo Meditsina, Petroverigskii per 6-8, Moscow 101000, Russian Federation. TEL 7-095-9248785, 7-095-928-86-48, FAX 7-095-9211355, 7-095-9286003, http://www.medit.ru. Ed. F I Komarov. Pub. A M Stochik. R&P O Platova. Adv. contact O A Fadeeva TEL 7-095-923-51-40. Circ: 7,000. **Dist. by:** Mezhdunarodnaya Kniga, B Yakimanka 39, Moscow 117049, Russian Federation. TEL 7-095-2384967, FAX 7-095-2384634; **US dist. addr.:** East View Publications, 3020 Harbor Ln N, Minneapolis, MN 55447. TEL 612-550-0961.

610 TUR ISSN 1300-0675
KLINIK GELISIM. Text in Turkish. 1987. q.
Indexed: Excerp.Med. (1993-).
—EMDOCS.
Published by: Istanbul Tabip Odasi/Istanbul Chamber of Medicine, Turkocagi Caddesi No. 17, Cagaloglu, Istanbul, Turkey.

610 DEU ISSN 0341-2350
CODEN: KLINF
KLINIKARZT; Medizin im Krankenhaus. Text in German. 1972. m. EUR 78.50 domestic to institutions; EUR 92.90 in Europe to institutions; EUR 119.30 elsewhere to institutions; EUR 9 newsstand/cover (effective 2002). adv. bk.rev. index. **Document type:** *Journal, Academic/Scholarly.*
Related titles: Online - full text ed.: ISSN 1439-3859.
Indexed: Excerp.Med. (1996-).
—BLDSC (5099.284900), EMDOCS, GNLM, Infotrieve. **CCC.**
Published by: Demeter Verlag GmbH und Co. KG, Ruedigerstr 14, Stuttgart 70469, Germany. TEL 49-711-8931-0, FAX 49-711-8931322, custserv@thieme.de, http://www.demeter-verlag.de. Circ: 24,000.

610 DEU ISSN 0176-1765
KLINISCHE UND EXPERIMENTELLE NOTFALLMEDIZIN. Text in German. 1984. irreg., latest vol.18, 1997. **Document type:** *Academic/Scholarly.*
Published by: W. Zuckschwerdt Verlag GmbH, Industriestr 1, Germering 82110, Germany. TEL 49-89-894349-0, FAX 49-89-89434950.

616.075 SWE ISSN 0282-440X
KLINISK KEMI; medlemsblad foer S F K K. Text in Swedish. 1975. bi-m. SEK 200 to members (effective 1993).
Formerly (until vol.4, 1985): Svensk Foerening foer Klinisk Kemi - Medlemsblad
Published by: Svensk Foerening foer Klinisk Kemi, c/o K Hellsing, Avdeling foer Klinisk Kemi, Uppsala 75185, Sweden.

616.0756 SWE ISSN 1101-2013
KLINISK KEMI I NORDEN. Text in Swedish. 1989. irreg. (3-4/yr.).
Published by: Nordisk Foerening foer Klinisk Kemi, c/o K Hellsing, Avdelingen foer Klinisk Kemi, Uppsala 75185, Sweden.

616.3 DEU
KLOPFZEICHEN; eine Informationszeitschrift rund um CF. Text in German. 1981. 4/yr. free per issue. adv. bk.rev. **Document type:** *Journal, Academic/Scholarly.*
Published by: Cystic Fibrosis Selbsthilfe Bundesverband e.V., Meyerholz 3, Achim 28832, Germany. TEL 49-4202-82280, FAX 49-4202-6073, cf-selbsthilfe-bv@t-online.de, http://cf-bv.de. Ed. Thomas Malowke. Pub. Thomas Malenke. Circ: 13,500.

KLUWER PERMANENT HEALTH INSURANCE; the city financial review. see *INSURANCE*

610 JPN ISSN 0075-6431
CODEN: KDIKAX
KOBE DAIGAKU IGAKUBU KIYO/KOBE UNIVERSITY. MEDICAL JOURNAL. Abstracts and contents page in English. 1949. q. free per issue. **Document type:** *Academic/Scholarly.*
Formerly (until 1968): Kobe Ika Daigaku. Kiyo
Indexed: Biol.Abstr., Excerp.Med., INIS Atomind., Ind.Med. (coverage dropped).
—BLDSC (5527.840000), CISTI, GNLM.
Published by: (Kobe Daigaku Igakkai), Kobe Daigaku, Igakubu/Kobe University, School of Medicine, 5-1 Kusunoki-cho 7-chome, Chuo-ku, Kobe-shi, Hyogo-ken 650-0017, Japan. TEL 81-78-382-5880, FAX 81-78-382-5898. Ed. Dr. Kazuo Chihara.

610 JPN ISSN 0023-2513
CODEN: KJMDA6
KOBE JOURNAL OF MEDICAL SCIENCES. Text and summaries in English, French, German. 1951. bi-m. JPY 6,000 (effective 1999). abstr, charts, illus. index. back issues avail. **Document type:** *Academic/Scholarly.*
Indexed: Abstr.Hyg., Biol.Abstr., Chem.Abstr., Chem.Indus.Notes, Chem.Titles, Excerp.Med., INIS Atomind., Ind.Med. (1951-), Ref.Zh., Rev.Appl.Entomol., Trop.Dis.Bull.
—BLDSC (5100.580000), CASDDS, CISTI, GNLM, ingenta, KNAW.
Published by: Kobe Daigaku, Igakubu/Kobe University, School of Medicine, 5-1 Kusunoki-cho 7-chome, Chuo-ku, Kobe-shi, Hyogo-ken 650-0017, Japan. TEL 81-78-382-5443. Ed. Dr. Takayoshi Kuno. Circ: 650.

610 JPN ISSN 0911-9531
KOBE UNIVERSITY. BULLETIN OF ALLIED MEDICAL SCIENCES. Text in English. 1985. a.
Published by: Kobe University, School of Allied Medical Sciences/Kobe Daigaku Iryo Gijutsu Tanki Daigakubu, 10-2 Tomogaoka 7-chome, Suma-ku, Kobe-shi, Hyogo-ken 654-0142, Japan.

610 JPN ISSN 0914-4250
KOCHI IRYO GAKUIN DOSOKAISHI/KOCHI SCHOOL OF ALLIED HEALTH AND MEDICAL PROFESSIONS. ALUMNI ASSOCIATION JOURNAL. Text in Japanese. 1983. irreg.
Published by: Kochi Iryo Gakuin Dosokai, 6012-1, Higashinamimatsu, Nagahama, Kochi-shi, Kochi-ken 781-02, Japan.

610 EST
KODUTOKHTER. Text in Estonian. bi-m. USD 149 in North America.
Address: Narva Mnt 63, Tallin, Estonia. TEL 370-630-70-98. Ed. Tiina Kanarbik. **Dist. by:** East View Publications, 3020 Harbor Ln N, Minneapolis, MN 55447. TEL 763-550-0961, FAX 763-559-2931.

616.98 JPN ISSN 0023-2858
KOKU IGAKU JIKKENTAI HOKOKU/JAPAN AIR SELF DEFENSE FORCE. AEROMEDICAL LABORATORY. REPORTS. Text in Japanese; Summaries in English. 1958. q. per issue exchange basis. bibl, charts, illus. *Refereed.* **Description:** Presents the results of research and usability tests for pilots' personnel equipments.
Indexed: Biol.Abstr., INIS Atomind., Int.Aerosp.Abstr., PsycInfo, Psychol.Abstr. (1969-), e-psyche.
—BLDSC (7368.740000), GNLM.
Published by: Japan Air Self Defense Force, Aeromedical Laboratory/Kokujieitai Koku Igaku Jikkentai, 2-10 Sakae-cho 1-chome, Tachikawa-shi, Tokyo-to 190-0003, Japan. TEL 0245-24-4131. Circ: 500.

610 JPN
KOKU KAIBO KENKYU/JOURNAL OF ORAL ANATOMY. Text in Japanese; Summaries in English. irreg. **Document type:** *Academic/Scholarly.*
Published by: Tokyo Dental College, Department of Anatomy, 2-2 Masago 1-chome, Mihama-ku, Chiba-shi 261-0011, Japan.

KOKURITSU KENKO EIYO KENKYUJO HOKOKU/NATIONAL INSTITUTE OF HEALTH AND NUTRITION. ANNUAL REPORT. see *NUTRITION AND DIETETICS*

KOKUTETSU CHUO HOKEN KANRIJOHO; health control. see *PUBLIC HEALTH AND SAFETY*

610 ITA ISSN 0393-2095
KOS. Text in Italian. 1983. m. ITL 70,000, EUR 36.20 domestic; ITL 125,000, EUR 100.70 foreign (effective 1999). adv.
Indexed: Russ.Acad.Sci.Bibl.
Published by: Europa Scienze Umane Editrice s.r.l., Via Olgettina, 60, Milan, MI 20132, Italy. TEL 39-2-26433024, FAX 39-02-26417386, kos@hsr.it. Ed. Luigi Maria Verze. adv.: page ITL 7,000,000. Circ: 15,000.

610 DEU ISSN 1430-4031
KOSMETISCHE MEDIZIN. Text in German, English. 1952. bi-m. DEM 138 (effective 2001). adv. bk.rev. 56 p./no. back issues avail. *Refereed.* **Document type:** *Journal, Academic/Scholarly.*
Former titles (until 1996): Cosmetologica (0070-055X); (until 1970): Aesthetische Medizin (0400-6755); (until 1960): Medizinische Kosmetik (0368-9247); (until 1956): Journal fuer Medizinische Kosmetik (0177-6622); (until 1953): Journal fuer Medizinische Kosmetik und Sexologie (0177-6649)
—GNLM.
Published by: B M V - Berliner Medizinische Verlagsanstalt GmbH, Lietzenburger Str 97, Berlin 10719, Germany. TEL 49-30-886749-0, FAX 49-30-88674999, info@bmv-berlin.com, http://www.bmv-berlin.de. Eds. Klaus Fritz, Uwe Wollina. Adv. contact Caridad Nyari TEL 49-30-88674970. B&W page DEM 3,105, color page DEM 4,305; trim 210 x 280. Circ: 3,392 (controlled).

610 JPN ISSN 0300-919X
CODEN: KUIZAR
KUMAMOTO IGAKKAI ZASSHI/KUMAMOTO MEDICAL SOCIETY. JOURNAL. Text in Japanese; Summaries in English. 1926. 3/yr. JPY 2,000, USD 20. index. back issues avail. *Refereed.* **Document type:** *Academic/Scholarly.* **Description:** Articles cover all fields within the medical sciences, mainly for Society members.
Indexed: INIS Atomind.
—CISTI, GNLM.
Published by: Kumamoto Igakkai/Kumamoto Medical Society, c/o Kumamoto Daigaku Igakubu, 2-1 Honjo-Machi 2-chome, Kumamoto-shi 860-0816, Japan. TEL 81-96-373-5122, FAX 81-96-373-5123, tsune@gpo.kumamoto-u.ac.jp. Ed. Shigeyuki Tsunenari. adv.: page JPY 5,000. Circ: 800 (controlled).

610 JPN ISSN 0023-5326
CODEN: KUMJAX
KUMAMOTO MEDICAL JOURNAL. Text in English. 1938-1942; resumed 1951. q. free per issue. bk.rev. abstr, charts, illus. index. **Document type:** *Academic/Scholarly.* **Description:** Contains original papers from the medical school.
Indexed: Biol.Abstr., Chem.Abstr., Chem.Indus.Notes, Chem.Titles, Excerp.Med., INIS Atomind., Ind.Med. (coverage dropped), Nutr.Abstr.
—CASDDS, CISTI, GNLM, ingenta.
Published by: (Japan. Ministry of Education, Science, Sports and Culture), Kumamoto University School of Medicine, 2-1 Honjo 2-chome, Kumamoto-shi 860-0811, Japan. TEL 81-96-344-2111, FAX 81-96-344-2111, mi-noguchi@jimu.kumamoto-u.ac.jp. Ed., R&P Yasuharu Nishimura TEL 81-96-372-6140. Circ: 440.

610 JPN ISSN 0389-7451
KURINIKKU MAGAJIN/CLINIC MAGAZINE. Text in Japanese. 1974. m. JPY 1,130.
Address: 3-15 Nihonbashihoncho 2-chome, Chuo-ku, Tokyo 103-0023, Japan.

610 JPN ISSN 0387-1541
KURINISHIAN/CLINICIAN. Text in Japanese. 1953. m. JPY 300 per issue. **Document type:** *Academic/Scholarly.*
—CCC.

M

Published by: Ezai K.K./Eisai Co., Ltd., 6-10 Koishi-Kawa 4-chome, Bunkyo-ku, Tokyo 112-0002, Japan. TEL 81-3-3817-3877. Ed. Masaaki Tamura.

610 JPN ISSN 0368-5810
CODEN: KIZAAL

KURUME MEDICAL ASSOCIATION. JOURNAL/KURUME IGAKKAI ZASSHI. Text in Japanese; Summaries in Multiple languages. 1936. m.
Indexed: Biol.Abstr., C.I.S. Abstr., INIS Atomind.
—BLDSC (4812.700000), GNLM.
Published by: Kurume Medical Association/Kurume Igakkai, c/o Kurume University School of Medicine, 67 Asahi-Machi, Kurume-shi, Fukuoka-ken 830-0011, Japan.

610 JPN ISSN 0023-5679
CODEN: KRMJAC

KURUME MEDICAL JOURNAL. Text in English. 1954. q. per issue exchange basis. adv. charts, illus. back issues avail. *Refereed.* **Document type:** *Journal, Academic/Scholarly.*
Indexed: Abstr.Hyg., Biol.Abstr., Chem.Abstr., Chem.Indus.Notes, Chem.Titles, Excerp.Med., INIS Atomind., Ind.Med. (1954-), Nutr.Abstr., Protozool.Abstr., Rural Devel.Abstr., Trop.Dis.Bull.
—BLDSC (5131.420000), CASDDS, CISTI, GNLM, ingenta, KNAW.
Published by: Kurume University School of Medicine/Kurume Daigaku Igakubu, 67 Asahi-Machi, Kurume-shi, Fukuoka-ken 830-0011, Japan. TEL 81-942-35-3311, FAX 81-942-32-1665, kmjedit@med.kurume-u.ac.jp. Ed. Dr. Takashi Akasu. Pub. Dr. Masatoshi Tanaka. Circ: 550.

610 JPN ISSN 0915-5015

KUTSU NO IGAKU/MEDICAL FOOTWEAR. Text in Japanese. 1987. a. JPY 5,100.
Published by: Nihon Kutsu Igakkai/Japanese Society for Study of Medical Footwear, c/o Jonan Byoin, 19-8 Shimo-Meguro 3-chome, Meguro-ku, Tokyo 153-0064, Japan.

610 KWT
CODEN: KMAJAJ

THE KUWAIT MEDICAL JOURNAL. Text in English. 1967. q. adv. bk.rev. abstr, bibl, charts, illus. index. **Document type:** *Academic/Scholarly.* **Description:** Features a collection of review articles, original articles, case reports in all areas within the medical sciences as well as general information concerning the Association.
Formerly (until vol.29, no.4, 1997): Kuwait Medical Association. Journal (0023-5776)
Indexed: Abstr.Hyg., Biol.Abstr., Curr.Adv.Ecol.Sci., Curr.Cont. (coverage dropped), Excerp.Med. (until 1992), Helminthol.Abstr., Nutr.Abstr., Rev.Plant Path., Trop.Dis.Bull.
—BLDSC (5131.934700), CASDDS, GNLM.
Published by: Kuwait Medical Association, P O Box 1202, Safat 13013, Kuwait. TEL 5317972, FAX 5312630, Kmj@kma.arg.kw. Circ: 4,000.

618.97 JPN ISSN 0368-5829
CODEN: KIZSB8

KYORIN IGAKKAI ZASSHI/KYORIN MEDICAL SOCIETY. JOURNAL. Text in Japanese; Summaries in English. 1970. q. JPY 5,000 (effective 2001). adv. index. back issues avail. *Refereed.* **Document type:** *Academic/Scholarly.*
Indexed: Chem.Abstr., Chem.Indus.Notes, Chem.Titles, INIS Atomind., Ref.Zh.
—CASDDS.
Published by: Kyorin Medical Society, Kyorin University, 6-20-2 Shinkawa, Mitaka City, Tokyo- 181-8611, Japan. TEL 81-422-47-5511, FAX 81-422-40-7281, medsoc@lib.kyorin-u.ac.jp. Ed. Akira Wakizaka. Pub. Toshihiko Nagasawa. R&P, Adv. contact Shinichi Kurihara. Circ: 1,800.

M

KYOTO DAIGAKU. REICHORUI KENKYUJO NENPO/KYOTO UNIVERSITY. PRIMATE RESEARCH INSTITUTE. ANNUAL REPORTS. see *ANTHROPOLOGY*

610 JPN ISSN 0023-6012
CODEN: KFIZAO

KYOTO PREFECTURAL UNIVERSITY OF MEDICINE. MEDICAL SOCIETY. JOURNAL/KYOTO-FURITSU IKA DAIGAKU ZASSHI. Text in Japanese, English; Summaries in English. 1927. m. JPY 7,200, USD 50 (effective 2000). adv. abstr. index. *Refereed.* **Document type:** *Academic/Scholarly.*
Indexed: Biol.Abstr., Chem.Abstr., Chem.Indus.Notes, Chem.Titles, INIS Atomind.
—CASDDS, GNLM.
Published by: Kyoto Prefectural University of Medicine, Kyoto Foundations for the Promotion of Medical Science/Kyoto-furitsu Ika Daigaku, Hirokoji, Kawara-machi, Kamigyo-ku, Kyoto-shi 602-8566, Japan. TEL 81-75-212-5466, FAX 81-75-212-5467, morimoto@phys.kpu-m.ac.jp, http://www.kpu-m.ac.jp. Ed. Jiro Imanishi. Circ: 1,400.

610 JPN ISSN 0385-8162

KYUKYU IGAKU/JAPANESE JOURNAL OF ACUTE MEDICINE. Text in Japanese. 1977. m. JPY 1,800 per issue.
Indexed: INIS Atomind., Jap.Per.Ind.
—BLDSC (4650.778600).
Published by: Herusu Shuppan, 2-3 Nakano 2-chome, Nakano-ku, Tokyo 164-0001, Japan.

610 JPN ISSN 0913-9958

KYUMEI KYUKYU IRYO KENKYUKAI ZASSHI/ JAPANESE ASSOCIATION FOR CRITICAL CARE MEDICINE. JOURNAL. Text in Japanese. 1987. a. JPY 2,500.
Published by: Kyumei Kyukyu Iryo Kenkyukai, Nihon Ika Daigaku Kyukyu Igaku Kyoshitsu, 1-5 Sendagi 1-chome, Bunkyo-ku, Tokyo 113-0022, Japan.

610 USA ISSN 0162-7163

L A C M A PHYSICIAN. Text in English. 1871. m. USD 30 to non-members; USD 15 to members (effective 1999). adv. bk.rev. *Refereed.* **Document type:** *Trade.* **Description:** Informs on pertinent trends in the world of medicine, from a socioeconomic and political standpoint. Covers state laws and regulations, trends affecting physicians, and societal events which impact upon physicians.
Formerly: Los Angeles County Medical Association. Bulletin (0047-5076)
Media: Duplicated (not offset).
Indexed: CINAHL.
Published by: Los Angeles County Medical Association, PO Box 513465, Los Angeles, CA 90051-1465. TEL 213-683-9900, FAX 213-630-1152, bfeiner@lacmanet.org, http://www.lacmanet.org. Ed., R&P Barbara Feiner TEL 213-630-1123. Adv. contact Roosevelt Christmas. Circ: 10,000.

610 USA ISSN 0742-3896
CODEN: LMSED6

L E R S MONOGRAPH SERIES. Text in English. 1983. irreg., latest vol.8. price varies. reprint service avail. from PQC. *Refereed.* **Document type:** *Monographic series.*
Indexed: Chem.Abstr., Chem.Indus.Notes, Chem.Titles.
—CASDDS, CISTI, KNAW.
Published by: (Laboratoires d'Etudes et de Recherches Synthelabo FRA), Raven Publishers (Subsidiary of: Wolters Kluwer N.V.), 227 E Washington Sq, Philadelphia, PA 19106. TEL 215-238-4200, FAX 215-238-4235.

LABOR JAHRBUCH. see *MEDICAL SCIENCES—Experimental Medicine, Laboratory Technique*

610.9489 DNK ISSN 0105-1830

LAEGEFORENINGENS VEJVISER. Text in Danish. 1965. a. DKK 400 (effective 2000).
Former titles (until 1976): Vejviser (0105-0427); (until 1973): Laegeforeningens Vejviser (0458-6158)
Published by: (Almindelige Danske Laegeforening/Danish Medical Association), Laegeforeningens Forlag, Esplanaden 8 A, Copenhagen K 1263, Denmark. TEL 45-35-44-85-00, FAX 45-35-44-81-99.

610 DNK ISSN 0902-1787

LAEGEMAGASINET/DOCTORS MAGAZINE; professional journal on medical practice. Text in Danish. 1987. 8/yr. DKK 480; DKK 68 newsstand/cover (effective 1998). adv. **Description:** Aimed primarily at the ordinary and specialty medical practitioners, private hospitals and drugstores.
Formerly: Laegen
Related titles: ♦ Supplement: Dit Laegemagasin. ISSN 0904-2369.
Published by: Scanpublishers A-S, Emiliekildevej 35, Klampenborg 2930, Denmark. TEL 45-39-90-80-00, FAX 45-39-90-82-80, vaboej@ibm.net. Ed. Jannie P Helle. Adv. contact Kirsten Waaben. B&W page DKK 10,100, color page DKK 16,025; trim 180 x 250. Circ: 4,800.

LAEGESEKRETAER NYT. see *BUSINESS AND ECONOMICS—Office Equipment And Services*

LAEKARSEKRETERAREN. see *BUSINESS AND ECONOMICS—Office Equipment And Services*

610 SWE ISSN 0023-7205

LAEKARTIDNINGEN. Text in Swedish; Summaries in English. 1904. w. SEK 870 (effective 2001). adv. bk.rev. bibl, charts, illus. index. back issues avail.; reprints avail. *Refereed.* **Document type:** *Magazine, Academic/Scholarly.*
Former titles (until 1965): Svenska Laekartidningen; (until 1965): Almaenna Svenska Laekartidningen
Related titles: Online - full text ed.: (from Institute for Scientific Information).
Indexed: C.I.S. Abstr., Chem.Abstr., Dok.Arbeitsmed., INIS Atomind., Ind.Med. (1965-), Protozool.Abstr., Rev.Med.& Vet.Mycol.
—BLDSC (5143.920000), CISTI, GNLM, KNAW.
Published by: Sveriges Laekarfoerbund/Swedish Medical Association, Box 5603, Stockholm 11486, Sweden. TEL 46-8-7903300, FAX 46-8-207619, redaktionen@lakartidningen.se, annonser@lakartidningen.se, http://www.lakartidningen.se. Eds. Joseph Milerad, Marianne Kronberg. Pub. Marianne Kronberg. Adv. contact Britt-Marie Aronsson. B&W page SEK 20,900, color page SEK 31,200; trim 178 x 260. Circ: 30,000.

610 ISL ISSN 0023-7213

LAEKNABLADID/ICELANDIC MEDICAL JOURNAL. Text in Icelandic. 1915. m. USD 95 (effective 1999). adv. **Document type:** *Academic/Scholarly.*
—KNAW.
Published by: Icelandic Medical Association, Hlidasmari 8, Kopavogur 200, Iceland. TEL 354-564-4104, FAX 354-564-4106, journal@icemed.is, http://www.icemed.is/laeknabladid. Ed. Dr. Vilhjalmur Rafnsson. R&P Birna Thordardottir. Adv. contact Asta Jensdottir. Circ: 1,600.

610 GBR ISSN 0140-6736
R31 CODEN: LANCAO

THE LANCET. Text in English. 1823. 51/yr. GBP 389 in Europe to institutions print with single access; GBP 469 in Europe to institutions print with multiple access; GBP 421 foreign to institutions print with single access; USD 635 in United States to institutions print with multiple access; USD 528 in United States to institutions print with single access; GBP 501 foreign to institutions print with multiple access (effective 2002). adv. bk.rev. abstr. s-a. index. back issues avail. *Refereed.* **Document type:** *Academic/Scholarly.* **Description:** For doctors who need to know what's happening in medicine and to understand how developments affect their practice. Publishes clinical papers, state-of-the-art reviews, letters and news.
Related titles: Microfiche ed.: (from IDC); Microform ed.: (from PQC); Online - full text ed.: (from Gale Group, ProQuest Information & Learning, Northern Light Technology, Inc., ScienceDirect, Swets Blackwell, Factiva, Institute for Scientific Information); ♦ Spanish ed.: The Lancet (Edicion Espanola). ISSN 0212-0151; ♦ Regional ed.: The Lancet (North American Edition). ISSN 0099-5355.
Indexed: AIDS Abstr., AIM, AMED, ASCA, ASSIA, Abstr.Anthropol., Abstr.Crim.& Pen., Abstr.Health Care Manage.Stud., Abstr.Hyg., Acad.Ind., Addic.Abstr., AgBiotech, Agri.& Environ.Biotech.Abstr. (coverage dropped), Apic.Abstr., Art.Hosp.& Tour., Arts & Hum.Cit.Ind. (coverage dropped), Bibl.Agri., Bibl.Dev.Med.& Child Neur., Biol.Abstr., Biol.Dig., Brit.Nur.Ind., CAD CAM Abstr., C.I.S. Abstr., Cadscan, Chem.Abstr., Chem.Titles, Curr.Adv.Cancer Res., Curr.Adv.Ecol.Sci., Curr.Adv.Gen.& Molec.Biol., Curr.Cont., Curr.Ind.Stat., Curr.Lit.Fam.Plan., Curr.Tit.Dent., Dairy Sci.Abstr., Deep Sea Res.& Oceanogr.Abstr., Dent.Ind., Derwent Biotech.Abstr., Diab.Cont., Diar.Dis.Res., Dok.Arbeitsmed., Environ.Abstr., Excerp.Med., FAMLI, Food Sci.& Tech.Abstr., Forest.Abstr., Gen.Sci.Ind. (1992-, dropped), Genet.Abstr. (coverage dropped), HRIS, Helminthol.Abstr., High.Educ.Curr.Aware.Bull., Hlth.Ind., Hosp.Lit.Ind., INIS Atomind., I.P.A., Ind.Hyg.Dig., Ind.Med. (1823-), Ind.Sci.Rev., Ind.Vet., Inpharma, Int.Nurs.Ind., Jrnl.Watch, Jrnl.Watch Card., Jrnl.Watch Derm., Jrnl.Watch Emer.Med., Jrnl.Watch Gastr., Jrnl.Watch Inf.Dis., Jrnl.Watch Neuro., Jrnl.Watch Psych., Jrnl.Watch Wom.Hlth., Kidney, Lab.Haz.Bull., Lead Abstr., Med.& Surg.Dermat., Med.Care Rev., Microbiol.Abstr., NRN, Neurosci.Abstr. (coverage dropped), Neurosci.Cit.Ind., Nutr.Abstr., Pharm.&Out.News, Pig News & Info., Popul.Ind., Potato Abstr., Poult.Abstr., Protozool.Abstr., Reac., Ref.Zh., Res.High.Educ.Abstr., Rev.Appl.Entomol., Rev.Arom.& Med.Plants, Rev.Med.& Vet.Mycol., Rev.Plant Path., Risk Abstr., Rural Devel.Abstr., SSCI (coverage dropped), Sage Race Rel.Abstr., Sci.Cit.Ind., Small Anim.Abstr., Soils & Fert., Stud.Wom.Abstr., Sugar Ind.Abstr., Telegen, Triticale Abstr., Trop.Dis.Bull., Vet.Bull., W.R.C.Inf., Zincscan.
—BLDSC (5146.000000), ADONIS, CASDDS, CISTI, IDS, KNAW. **CCC.**

Published by: The Lancet Publishing Group (Subsidiary of: Reed Elsevier plc), 84 Theobald's Rd, London WC1X 8RR, United Kingdom. TEL 44-20-7611-4246, FAX 44-20-7611-4479, lanceteditorial@elsevier.co.uk, editorial@lancet.com, http://www.elsevier.com/locate/lancet, http://www.thelancet.com. Ed. Dr. Richard Horton. Pub. Rita Scheman. R&P Sarah Downes. Adv. contact Natalie Maas. B&W page GBP 1,800; trim 10 x 7. Circ: 45,000.

610 ESP ISSN 0212-0151
THE LANCET (EDICION ESPANOLA). Text in Spanish. 1982. m. (2 vols./yr..). USD 114. adv. reprint service avail. from PQC. **Document type:** *Academic/Scholarly.* **Description:** Publishes clinical observations, physiopathological interpretations, descriptions of new syndromes, diagnostic methodology, and other developments in the medical sciences.
Related titles: ♦ English ed.: The Lancet. ISSN 0140-6736.
Indexed: Virol.Abstr. (coverage dropped).
Published by: Ediciones Doyma S.A., Traversa de Gracia, 17-21, Barcelona 08021, Spain. TEL 34-93-200-0711, FAX 34-93-209-1136. Ed. M Foz I Sala. Adv. contact Anna Pahissa. color page ESP 346,000; trim 280 x 210. Circ: 6,000.

610 USA ISSN 0099-5355
R31
THE LANCET (NORTH AMERICAN EDITION). Text in English. 1966. w. USD 112 to individuals; USD 207 to institutions. adv. illus. index. reprints avail. *Refereed.* **Document type:** *Academic/Scholarly.* **Description:** Covers major developments in general medicine and clinical research worldwide.
Related titles: CD-ROM ed.; Microfilm ed.: (from PQC); Microform ed.: (from PQC); Online - full text ed.: (from EBSCO Publishing, Gale Group); ♦ Regional ed.: The Lancet. ISSN 0140-6736.
Indexed: AgeLine, Aqua.Sci.& Fish.Abstr., CINAHL, Cal.Tiss.Abstr., Dairy Sci.Abstr., Environ.Sci.Poll.Mgmt., Gen.Sci.Ind. (Jun.1992-), Genet.Abstr., Hum.Gen.Abstr., INIS Atomind., Ind.Vet., Int.Abstr.Biol.Sci., L.R.I., Microbiol.Abstr., Nuc.Acids Abstr., Pollut.Abstr., Popul.Ind., Risk Abstr., Saf.Sci.Abstr., WMB.
—ingenta. **CCC.**
Published by: The Lancet Ltd. (Subsidiary of: Reed Elsevier plc), 655 Ave of the Americas, New York, NY 10010. TEL 212-633-3800, 800-462-6198, FAX 212-633-3850. Ed. Dr. Richard Horton. Adv. contact Louise Young. Circ: 18,000.

352.14 SWE ISSN 0282-4485
LANDSTINGSVAERLDEN. Text in Swedish. 1914. 36/yr. SEK 825 to non-members; SEK 660 to members (effective 2001). adv. bk.rev. illus. index. **Document type:** *Newspaper, Trade.*
Former titles (until 1985): Landstingens Tidskrift (0023-8074); (until 1966): Sveriges Landstings Tidskrift
Published by: Landstingsfoerbundet/Federation of Swedish County Councils, Hornsgatan 20, Stockholm 11882, Sweden. TEL 46-8-452-72-00, FAX 46-8-452-72-10, redaktionen.lv@lf.se, landstingsforbundet@lf.se, http://www.landstingsvarlden.lf.se, http://www.lf.se. Ed., Pub. Lars-G Holmstroem. Adv. contact Dan Olsson. B&W page SEK 18,900, color page SEK 24,800; trim 185 x 249. Circ: 9,400 (paid and controlled).

LANGUAGE & HEALTHCARE NEWSLETTER. see *LINGUISTICS*

LANGUAGE AND SPEECH. see *LINGUISTICS*

610 300 ITA ISSN 0393-7445
LANTERNINO; trimestrale di storia della medicina e studi sociali. Text in Italian. 1978. q. free per issue. bibl.
Published by: Dr. Claudio Bevilacqua Ed. & Pub., Via Domenico Rossetti, 25, Trieste, TS 34125, Italy. TEL 39-40-360332. Circ: 2,000.

610 JPN ISSN 0898-5901
CODEN: LATHE7
LASER THERAPY; an international journal of low level laser therapy and photobioactivation. Text in Japanese. 1989. q. USD 200 (effective 1996). bk.rev. reprint service avail. from SWZ. *Refereed.* **Document type:** *Academic/Scholarly.* **Description:** Links an international outlook in the field of laser therapy with academic contents; contains clinical and basic scientific studies in the use of low level laser therapy.
Indexed: AMED, INSPEC (Jul.1989-Dec.1993, dropped).
—BLDSC (5156.651000), AskIEEE, CISTI, EMDOCS, GNLM, KNAW. **CCC.**
Published by: International Laser Therapy Association, c/o 14-18 Iwaicho, Tochigi City, Tochigi 328-0052, Japan. TEL 81-282-24-0313, FAX 81-282-22-5019. Eds. C Enwemeka, O Kemmotsu.

610 535.58 GBR ISSN 0268-8921
CODEN: LMSCEZ
LASERS IN MEDICAL SCIENCE. Text in English. 1986. q. EUR 291.30 domestic; EUR 288.70 in Germany; EUR 84 newsstand/cover foreign (effective 2002). back issues avail.; reprint service avail. from SWZ. *Refereed.* **Document type:** *Academic/Scholarly.* **Description:** Brings together the work of clinicians and basic scientists on the use of lasers in medicine and also non-laser light applications in the form of research papers and review articles.
Related titles: Online - full text ed.: ISSN 1435-604X (from EBSCO Publishing, RoweCom Information Quest, Swets Blackwell, Springer LINK, Institute for Scientific Information).
Indexed: ASCA, Curr.Adv.Ecol.Sci., Curr.Cont., Eng.Ind., Inpharma, Med.& Surg.Dermat., Reac., Rev.Med.& Vet.Mycol., Sci.Cit.Ind.
—BLDSC (5156.680800), CISTI, Ei, EMDOCS, GNLM, IDS, ingenta, KNAW. **CCC.**
Published by: (European Laser Association), Springer-Verlag London Ltd. (Subsidiary of: BertelsmannSpringer), Sweetapple House, Catteshall Rd, Godalming, Surrey GU7 3DJ, United Kingdom. TEL 44-1483-418800, FAX 44-1483-415144, http://link.springer-ny.com/link/service/journals/10103/index.htm.

174.24 179.7 CAN ISSN 1198-3922
LAST RIGHTS. Text in English. q. **Description:** Specializes in international coverage of right to die issues and original research in methods of self-deliverance.
Published by: Right to Die Society of Canada, P O Box 39018, Victoria, BC V8V 4X8, Canada. TEL 604-380-1112, FAX 604-386-3800, rights@islandnet.com. Ed. John Hofsess.

610 658 USA ISSN 1067-716X
THE LATEST WORD. Text in English. 1993. bi-m. USD 51 domestic to individuals Full text on-line included; USD 86 foreign to individuals Full text on-line included; USD 67 domestic to institutions Full text on-line included; USD 91 foreign to institutions Full text on-line included; USD 47 domestic to students Full text on-line included; USD 52 foreign to students Full text on-line included; USD 16 newsstand/cover (effective 2001). adv. **Document type:** *Newsletter, Academic/Scholarly.* **Description:** Ensures that medical transcriptionists and medical records administrators and technicians keep abreast of advances in medicine and new terminology.
Indexed: Can.Mus.Per.Ind. (1980-1985).
—CCC.
Published by: W.B. Saunders Co. (Subsidiary of: Harcourt Publishers Ltd.), 11830 Westline Industrial Dr, St Louis, MO 63146. TEL 800-325-4177, www.harcourthealth.com/tlw, http://www.wbsaunders.com. Ed. Barbara E Grow. **Subscr. to:** Periodicals Fulfillment, W B Saunders Co, 6277 Sea Harbor Dr, 4th Fl, Orlando, FL 32891-4800.

610 LVA ISSN 1019-5068
LATVIJAS ARSTS. Text in Latvian. m. USD 149 in North America.
Published by: Latvijas Arstu Biedriba, Skolas str 3, Riga LV-1050, Latvia. TEL 371-7282281. Ed. Vita Vitola. **Dist. by:** East View Publications, 3020 Harbor Ln N, Minneapolis, MN 55447. TEL 763-550-0961, FAX 763-559-2931.

LAWYERS GUIDE TO MEDICAL PROOF. see *LAW*

LAWYERS' MEDICAL CYCLOPEDIA. see *LAW*

610 ITA
LEADERSHIP MEDICA; mensile di medicina, economia, attualita e cultura per opinion leaders. Text in English; Summaries in Italian. 1985. m. USD 186. adv. *Refereed.*
Published by: Ce.S.I.L. srl, Via Olmetto, 5, Milan, MI 20123, Italy. TEL 39-2-878397, FAX 39-2-866576. Ed. Genina Jacoboni. Circ: 85,000.

THE LEANING TREE. see *MEDICAL SCIENCES—Allergology And Immunology*

610 LBN ISSN 0023-9852
R97.5.F8 CODEN: LMJJA7
LEBANESE MEDICAL JOURNAL/JOURNAL MEDICAL LIBANAIS. Text in English, French. 1948. 6/yr., latest vol.48. USD 100 domestic; USD 180 foreign (effective 2002). adv. bk.rev. abstr, bibl, charts, illus. index. 64 p./no. 2 cols./p. back issues avail. *Refereed.* **Document type:** *Journal, Academic/Scholarly.* **Description:** Publishes original articles and research, news from the Order of Physicians, and contributions on the history of medicine in Lebanon.
Indexed: Biol.Abstr., Chem.Abstr., Curr.Cont. (coverage dropped), Excerp.Med., Ind.Med. (1950-), Int.Nurs.Ind.
—CISTI, GNLM.
Published by: Order of Physicians in Lebanon, P O Box 640, Beirut, Lebanon. TEL 961-1-959959, FAX 961-1-451480, jml@lb.refer.org, http://www.lb.refer.org/jml. Ed., R&P Dr. Adel E Berbari TEL 03-347358. Pub. Lucien Georges. Circ: 5,500.

610.7 ZAF ISSN 0377-9696
CODEN: LECHAC
THE LEECH. Text in English. 1929. 3/yr. ZAR 15; ZAR 45 foreign. adv. bk.rev. *Refereed.* **Document type:** *Academic/Scholarly.* **Description:** Contains research articles, drug reviews, conference information, coverage of changing trends in health care, and departmental news for students and graduates of the University of the Witwatersrand Medical School.
Supersedes: Auricle (0004-8070)
—CASDDS.
Published by: University of the Witwatersrand Medical School, 7 York Rd, Parktown, Johannesburg 2193, South Africa. TEL 27-11-647-2451, FAX 27-11-643-4318. Ed. Manfred Spanger. R&P Liron Pantanowitz. Circ: 7,000.

610.28 CZE ISSN 0301-5491
LEKAR A TECHNIKA. Text in Czech. 1970. 6/yr. EUR 48, USD 60 (effective 2001). adv.
Indexed: INIS Atomind.
—CCC.
Published by: (Ceska Lekarska Spolecnost J.E. Purkyne/Czech Medical Association), Nakladatelske Stredisko C L S J.E. Purkyne, Sokolska 31, Prague 12026, Czech Republic. TEL 42-2-24911420, FAX 42-2-24911420, nts@iol.cz, http://www.clsjep.cz, http://www.medical.cz. adv.: B&W page CZK 21,900, color page CZK 30,900; 168 x 230. Circ: 800. **Dist. by:** Abont s.r.o., Chlumova 17, Prague, 3 130 00, Czech Republic; **Dist. in Western Countries by:** Kubon & Sagner, Hesstr 39-41, Munich 80798, Germany.

610 SVK ISSN 0075-8736
LEKARSKE PRACE. Text occasionally in English, German, Russian; Text mainly in Slovak. 1961. irreg., latest vol.10, no.2, 1973 (approx. s-a.).
Indexed: Biol.Abstr., Ind.Med. (coverage dropped).
—CISTI.
Published by: (Slovenska Akademia Vied/Slovak Academy of Sciences), Veda Publishing House of the Slovak Academy of Sciences, Bradacova 7, Bratislava 85286, Slovakia. **Dist. by:** Slovart, Nam Slobody 6, Bratislava 81764, Slovakia.

610 615.19 SVK ISSN 0457-4214
CODEN: LEOBAK
LEKARSKY OBZOR. Text in Czech, Slovak; Summaries in English. 1951. m. USD 78 (effective 2001 - 2002). adv. bk.rev., Website rev. abstr, bibl, charts, illus. 32 p./no. reprint service avail. from IRC. *Refereed.* **Document type:** *Journal, Academic/Scholarly.* **Description:** Medical journal of the Ministry of Health and Slovak Post-graduate Academy of Medicine.
Indexed: C.I.S. Abstr., Chem.Abstr., Chem.Indus.Notes, Chem.Titles, INIS Atomind.
—BLDSC (5182.330000), CASDDS, EMDOCS, GNLM.
Published by: Institut pre Dalsie Vzdelavanie Pracovnikov v Zdravotnictve/Slovak Postgraduate Academy of Medicine, Limbova 12, Bratislava 83305, Slovakia. sasinkam@stonline.sk. Ed. Miroslav Sasinka. Adv. contact Stefan Hrusovsky.

610 POL ISSN 0867-8235
LEKARZ KOLEJOWY. Text in Polish. 1965. s-a. USD 5. adv. bk.rev. charts, illus. **Document type:** *Monographic series, Newsletter, Newspaper, Proceedings, Abstract/Index, Academic/Scholarly.* **Description:** Original papers on medicine of transport, reviews in occupational medicine, conferences and symposia reports, organizational topics in railway health service.
Formerly (until 1989): Medycyna Komunikacyjna (0025-861X)
Indexed: C.I.S. Abstr.
Published by: Centrum Naukowe Medycyny Kolejowej, Ul Grojecka 17 a, PO Box 214, Warsaw 00973, Poland. TEL 48-22-225397, FAX 48-225397. Ed. Jacek A Piatkiewicz. Circ: 1,000.

616.98 POL ISSN 0024-0745
CODEN: LEKWAT
LEKARZ WOJSKOWY. Text in Polish. m. USD 8.40.
Indexed: Chem.Abstr., Chem.Indus.Notes, Chem.Titles, Excerp.Med., INIS Atomind.
—BLDSC (5182.380000), CASDDS.
Published by: Szefostwo Sluzby Zdrowia SG WP, Al. Niepodleglosci 243 A, Warsaw 009-09, Poland. TEL 48-2-6844750. Ed. Piotr Kobylecki.

M

610 FRA ISSN 1243-7581
LA LETTRE DE L'INTERNAT. Text in French. 1989. q. FRF 600 domestic; FRF 700 elsewhere (effective 2001). **Description:** Keeps interns up to date with the latest professional developments in medicine.
Published by: John Libbey Eurotext, 127 av. de la Republique, Montrouge 92120, France. TEL 33-01-46730660, FAX 33-01-40840999, http://www.john-libbey-eurotext.fr/. Ed. Laurence Strompf.

610 FRA ISSN 0398-1436
LETTRE DU MEDECIN✱ . Text in French. 1976. w.
Address: 60 bd. de la Tour Maubourg, Paris 75007, France. TEL 33-1-43-70-97-20. Ed. Joel Haroche. Circ: 10,000.

610 FRA ISSN 0153-4742
LETTRE MEDICALE. Text in French. 1975. 10/yr. USD 31.
Address: 27 rue du Fg. Saint-Jacques, Paris Cedex 14 75674, France. TEL 42341684. Ed. M Detilleux. Circ: 3,000.

LIAONING ZHONGYI ZAZHI/LIAONING JOURNAL OF TRADITIONAL CHINESE MEDICINE. see *ALTERNATIVE MEDICINE*

LIBRARIES ASSOCIATION. HEALTH LIBRARIES GROUP. NEWSLETTER. see *LIBRARY AND INFORMATION SCIENCES*

LIFESTYLE AND TRAVEL FOR PHYSICIANS. see *LIFESTYLE*

610 HRV ISSN 0024-3477
CODEN: LIVJA5
LIJECNICKI VJESNIK. Text in Croatian; Abstracts and contents page in English. 1878. m. USD 120. adv. bk.rev. abstr, bibl, charts, illus. index. *Refereed.* **Document type:** *Academic/Scholarly.*
Indexed: Biol.Abstr., C.I.S. Abstr., Chem.Abstr., Dent.Ind., Excerp.Med., Ind.Med. (1877-), Int.Nurs.Ind.
—BLDSC (5215.800000), CASDDS, CISTI, GNLM.
Published by: Hrvatski Lijecnicki Zbor/Croatian Dental Society, Subiceva 9, Zagreb 10000, Croatia. TEL 385-1-4655446. Ed. Goran Knezevic. R&P Zdenka Glamocak. Circ: 7,000 (controlled).

610 UKR ISSN 1019-5297
R91 CODEN: LISPEC
LIKARSKA SPRAVA/VRACHEBNOE DELO. Text in Russian, Ukrainian. 1918. 8/yr. USD 175 in United States. adv. bk.rev. **Description:** Publishes articles relating to the different fields of medicine.
Formerly (until 1991): Vrachebnoe Delo (0049-6804)
Indexed: Biol.Abstr., Chem.Abstr., Dent.Ind., Excerp.Med., INIS Atomind., Ind.Med. (1992-), Int.Nurs.Ind., SSCI (coverage dropped).
—BLDSC (0097.666500), CASDDS, CISTI, East View, GNLM, IDS, Infotrieve. **CCC.**
Address: Ul Podvysotskogo 4-a, Kiev 252103, Ukraine. TEL 269-75-56. Circ: 5,000 (paid). **US dist. addr.:** East View Publications, 3020 Harbor Ln N, Minneapolis, MN 55447. TEL 612-550-0961.

610 FRA ISSN 0981-1095
CODEN: LIMEEH
LILLE MEDICAL. Summaries in English, French. 1966 (vol.11). 10/yr. FRF 375. adv. abstr, charts, illus, stat, tr.lit.
Former titles: L A R C Medical; Lille Medical (0024-3507); Echo Medical du Nord
Indexed: Biol.Abstr., C.I.S. Abstr., Chem.Abstr., Curr.Cont. (coverage dropped), Dent.Ind., Dok.Arbeitsmed., Excerp.Med., Helminthol.Abstr., INIS Atomind., Ind.Med. (coverage dropped), Nutr.Abstr.
—CASDDS, CISTI, GNLM.
Published by: (Facultes de Medecine de Lille), Medi-Presse, 1 Place de Verdun, Lille Cedex 59045, France.

610 USA ISSN 0024-3639
R15
LINACRE QUARTERLY✱ . Text in English. 1932. q. USD 24. adv. bk.rev. abstr, bibl. index. back issues avail. **Description:** Journal of the philosophy and ethics of medical practice.
Related titles: Microfilm ed.: 1932 (from PQC).
Indexed: CERDIC, Cath.Ind.
—BLDSC (5220.170000), GNLM.
Published by: National Federation of Catholic Physicians Guilds, PO Box 757, Pewaukee, WI 53072-0757. TEL 414-784-3435, FAX 414-523-6211. Ed. Dr. John P Mullooly. Circ: 11,150.

610 CHN
LINCHUANG HUICUI/CLINICAL FOCUS; daneike. Text in Chinese. 1986. s-m. CNY 62.40 (effective 1999). 48 p./no. *Refereed.* **Document type:** *Academic/Scholarly.* **Description:** Focuses on the theories and practices in the field of internal medicine.
Published by: Hebei Yike Daxue/Hebei Medical University, 361 Zhongshan Donglu, Shijiazhuang, Hebei 050017, China. TEL 86-311-6059153, FAX 86-311-6059153, hebydqks@public.sj.he.cn, WL@hebmu.edu.cn. Ed. Du Benfa. adv.: B&W page CNY 7,000, color page CNY 10,000. Circ: 50,000. **Dist. overseas by:** China International Book Trading Corp, 35 Chegongzhuang Xilu, Haidian District, Beijing 100044, China.

610 CHN ISSN 1002-3429
LINCHUANG WUZHEN WUZHI/CLINCIAL MISDIAGNOSIS & MISTHERAPY. Text in Chinese. bi-m. USD 22.20; USD 3.70 newsstand/cover (effective 2001). **Document type:** *Academic/Scholarly.*
Published by: Zhonghua Yiyuan Guanli Xuehui, 398, Zhongshan Xi Lu, Shijiazhuang, Hebei 050082, China. TEL 86-311-3658278, 86-311-7998462, lcwzwz@public.sj.he.cn, http://www.mmm.ac.cn. **Dist. by:** China International Book Trading Corp, 35, Chegongzhuang Xilu, Haidian District, Beijing 100044, China. TEL 86-1-68413849, FAX 86-1-68412048, cibtc@mail.cibtc.com.cn, http://www.cibtc.com.cn.

610 CHN ISSN 1001-7399
LINCHUANG YU SHIYAN BINGLIXUE ZAZHI/JOURNAL OF CLINICAL AND EXPERIMENTAL PATHOLOGY. Text in Chinese. q.
Published by: Anhui Yike Daxue/Anhui University of Medical Sciences, Meishan Lu, Hefei, Anhui 230032, China. TEL 336600. Ed. Zheng Guohao.

610 GBR
▼ **LIPIDS AND ATHEROSCLEROSIS ANNUAL.** Text in English. 2001. a.
Published by: Martin Dunitz Ltd., The Livery House, 7-9 Pratt St., London NW1 0AE, United Kingdom. TEL 44-20-74822202, FAX 44-20-72670159, indo.dunitz@tandf.co.uk, http://www.dunitz.co.uk. Eds. Allan Gaw, James Shepherd.

LITERATURE & MEDICINE. see *LITERATURE*

610 RUS
LITMED. Text in Russian. 1995. q. RUR 10; USD 85 foreign. *Refereed.* **Document type:** *Newsletter.* **Description:** Covers literature on medicine currently published in Russia.
Published by: Rossiiskii Registr Potentsyal'no Opasnykh Khimicheskikh i Biologicheskikh Veshchestv, Vadkovskii per 18-20, Moscow 101479, Russian Federation. TEL 7-095-9733021, FAX 7-095-9732657, root@regdang.msk.ru. Ed. B A Kurlyandskii. Circ: 5,000. **US dist. addr.:** East View Publications, 3020 Harbor Ln N, Minneapolis, MN 55447. TEL 612-550-0961.

LONGITUDINAL RESEARCH IN THE BEHAVIORAL, SOCIAL AND MEDICAL SCIENCES. see *SOCIAL SCIENCES: COMPREHENSIVE WORKS*

610 USA ISSN 0024-6921
CODEN: JLSMAW
LOUISIANA STATE MEDICAL SOCIETY. JOURNAL. Text in English. 1844. m. USD 35; USD 50 foreign (effective 1999). adv. bk.rev. bibl, illus. index. reprint service avail. from PQC. *Refereed.* **Document type:** *Trade, Academic/Scholarly.* **Description:** Published for the benefit of the members of the Society.
Related titles: Microform ed.: (from PQC).
Indexed: Biol.Abstr., C.I.S. Abstr., Chem.Abstr., Dent.Ind., INIS Atomind., Ind.Med. (1953-), Int.Nurs.Ind., Rev.Med.& Vet.Mycol.
—BLDSC (4818.700000), CISTI, GNLM, ingenta, KNAW.
Published by: Journal of the Louisiana State Medical Society, Inc., 6767 Perkins Rd, Baton Rouge, LA 70808-4263. TEL 225-763-8500, FAX 225-763-2332, publicaffairs@lsms.org, http://www.lsms.org. Ed. Dr. Conway S Magee. R&P Charlotte Cavell TEL 225-763-2310. Adv. contact Anne Gooch. Circ: 6,300 (paid).

LOUISVILLE MEDICINE. see *INSURANCE*

610 BEL ISSN 0024-6956
CODEN: LOMEAL
LOUVAIN MEDICAL. Text in French; Summaries in English, French. 1966. m. (10/yr.). BEF 2,250 domestic to individuals; BEF 3,200 foreign to individuals; BEF 5,000 to institutions; BEF 700 to students. adv. bk.rev. abstr. index. back issues avail.
Formerly: Revue Medicale de Louvain et Recipe
Indexed: Biol.Abstr., Chem.Abstr., Curr.Adv.Ecol.Sci., Curr.Cont. (coverage dropped), Excerp.Med., Helminthol.Abstr., Nutr.Abstr.
—BLDSC (5296.350000), CASDDS, GNLM, KNAW.
Address: Av E Mounier 52, Brussels 1200, Belgium. TEL 2-7645265. Ed. M Buysschaert. Circ: 3,000.

616.047 344.041 USA
LOW BACK PAIN. Text in English. 1989. latest 1989, 2nd. ed., base vol. plus irreg. updates. USD 65. Supplement avail.
Published by: Lexis Law Publishing (Subsidiary of: Reed Elsevier plc), PO Box 7587, Charlottesville, VA 22906-7587. TEL 804-972-7600, 800-562-1197, FAX 804-972-7666, llp.customer.support@lexis-nexis.com, http://www.lexislawpublishing.com.

617.58 USA ISSN 1068-6991
CODEN: LOEXF9
LOWER EXTREMITY. Text in English. 1994-1996; resumed 1997 (Oct.). q. USD 85 domestic to individuals; USD 115 foreign to individuals; USD 128 domestic to institutions; USD 158 foreign to institutions. adv. bk.rev. back issues avail. *Refereed.* **Document type:** *Academic/Scholarly.* **Description:** Forum for the scholarly presentation of investigative research and the discussion of issues of interest to practitioners of podiatric orthopedics and the medical specialties of podiatric medicine.
Indexed: Excerp.Med. (1995-).
—GNLM, Infotrieve. **CCC.**
Published by: (American College of Foot and Ankle Orthopedics and Medicine), Churchill Livingstone (Subsidiary of: Harcourt Health Sciences), 15 E 26th St, Fl 15, New York, NY 10010-1505. TEL 212-206-5040, 800-553-5426, FAX 212-727-7808, http://www.churchillmed.com. Ed. Gerald Webur. Pub. Jane Grochowski. R&P Winnie Cha. Adv. contact Lynette Conto. Circ: 1,500 (paid).

LOYOLA MEDICINE. see *COLLEGE AND ALUMNI*

610 RUS
LUCHSHIE MEDITSINSKIE TSENTRY MOSKVY. Text in Russian. s-a. USD 79.95 in United States.
Address: Ul Shchepkina 24-a, Moscow 129090, Russian Federation. TEL 7-095-9258293, FAX 7-095-9235223. Ed. O S Kopylova. **US dist. addr.:** East View Publications, 3020 Harbor Ln N, Minneapolis, MN 55447. TEL 612-550-0961.

610 USA
LYCOMING MEDICINE. Text in English. 1910. m. USD 20. adv. bk.rev.
Published by: Lycoming County Medical Society, 777 Rural Ave, Williamsport, PA 17701-3198. TEL 717-321-2171. Ed. Dr. Judith A Gouldin. Circ: 325.

610 FRA ISSN 0766-5466
LYON MEDITERRANEE MEDICAL - MEDECINE DU SUD EST. Text in French. q. FRF 480 domestic; FRF 700, EUR 106.71 foreign; FRF 335 to students (effective 2001).
Formerly: Lyon Mediterranee Medical (0399-032X)
—BLDSC (5311.980000), EMDOCS, GNLM, KNAW.
Published by: Galliena Promotion, 62 rue Amelot, Paris 75011, France. TEL 45-84-97-66, FAX 45-84-92-56.

M A P NEWS. see *SOCIAL SERVICES AND WELFARE*

610 USA ISSN 1092-1850
M A S A REVIEW. Text in English. 18??. m. USD 30 to non-members; USD 15 to members (effective 1999). adv. bk.rev. bibl, illus. index.
Former titles (until 1996): Alabama Medicine (0738-4947); (until 1983): Medical Association of the State of Alabama. Journal (0025-7044); (until 1930): Medical Association of the State of Alabama. Transactions (1060-0175)
Indexed: Chem.Abstr., Excerp.Med., INIS Atomind., Ind.Med. (1996-), Rev.Med.& Vet.Mycol.
—BLDSC (5383.627000), GNLM, KNAW.
Published by: Medical Association of the State of Alabama, 19 S, Jackson, AL 36102-1900. TEL 334-263-6441. Ed. Dr. William A Curry. Circ: 6,300.

610 BGR ISSN 0324-119X
RM1
M B I. (Medico-Biologic Information) Text in English. 1967. bi-m. free per issue. adv. illus.
Related titles: Russian ed.
Indexed: Biol.Abstr., Curr.Adv.Ecol.Sci., Excerp.Med. (until 1993).
—CISTI, GNLM.
Published by: Pharmachim, 16 Iliensko shose, Sofia 1220, Bulgaria. Ed. A Damyanov. Circ: 2,000.

610 USA ISSN 0047-6471
M C G TODAY. Text in English. 1970. q. free to alumni and donors. **Document type:** *Academic/Scholarly.*
Published by: Medical College of Georgia Foundation, Inc., Alumni Center, 919 15th St, Augusta, GA 30912. TEL 706-721-2124. Ed. Christine Deriso. Circ: 20,000.

610 MEX ISSN 0024-8002
M D EN ESPANOL. (Medical Doctor) Text in Spanish. 1963. m. MXP 400; USD 345 foreign (effective 1999). adv.
Indexed: Bibl.Asian Stud. (1970).
Published by: Mundo Medico S.A., Ejercito Nacional 381, Mexico City, DF 11520, Mexico. TEL 525-545-17-98, FAX 525-203-64-18. Ed. Joaquin Armando Chacon. Adv. contact Oscar Bagnarelli. Circ: 15,000.

658 USA
R729.5.G6 CODEN: MGMJET
M G M A CONNEXION. (Medical Group Management Association) Text in English. 1953. 10/yr. USD 95 to individuals; USD 175 to institutions (effective 2001 - 2002). adv. charts, illus, stat. index. reprints avail. *Refereed.* **Document type:** *Journal.*
Former titles: Medical Group Management Journal (0899-8949); Medical Group Management (0025-7257)
Related titles: Microform ed.: (from PQC).
Indexed: Abstr.Health Care Manage.Stud., Hosp.Lit.Ind., Med.Care Rev.
—BLDSC (5527.432000), GNLM, ingenta.
Published by: Medical Group Management Association, 104 Inverness Terrace E, Englewood, CO 80112. TEL 888-608-5601, FAX 303-397-1824, beh@mgma.com, http://www.mgma.com. Ed. Brenda Hull. Adv. contact Michael Campo. Circ: 32,000.

M G Z. (Maatschappelijke Gezondheidszorg) see *MEDICAL SCIENCES—Nurses And Nursing*

M H H - INFO. see *COLLEGE AND ALUMNI*

M H L A NEWS. see *LIBRARY AND INFORMATION SCIENCES*

M I M S. (Monthly Index of Medical Specialties) see *PHARMACY AND PHARMACOLOGY*

610 AUS
M I M S CD. Text in English. AUD 165.90 per issue (effective 2000). **Document type:** *Academic/Scholarly.*
Description: Provides the complete MIMS reference system, including the full MIMS Drug Database, MIMS Disease Index, MIMS Companion diagnostic reference and MIMS Interact.
Media: CD-ROM. **Related titles:** ♦ Print ed.: M I M S Disease Index. ISSN 1035-5693; ♦ M I M S Companion.
Published by: M I M S Australia (Subsidiary of: Medimedia Australia), PO Box 3000, St Leonards, NSW 2065, Australia. TEL 61-2-9902-7700, FAX 61-2-99027701.

610 AUS
M I M S COMPANION. Text in English. biennial, latest 1998, 5th Ed. AUD 19.25 in New Zealand; AUD 22.25 in PNG, Asia & Pacific Region; AUD 25.25 in US & Middle East; AUD 27.50 elsewhere (effective 2000). adv. **Description:** Guide to symptoms, clinical signs, investigations, pathology, diagnosis, treatment and prognosis.
Related titles: ♦ CD-ROM ed.: M I M S CD.
Published by: M I M S Australia (Subsidiary of: Medimedia Australia), PO Box 3000, St Leonards, NSW 2065, Australia. TEL 02-99027700, FAX 02-99027701. Pub. Chris Wills. R&P Amanda Caswell. Adv. contact Sue McElroy.

610 IRL ISSN 0300-8223
M I M S IRELAND. Text in English. 1960. m. IEP 146.67 (effective 1999). adv. *Refereed.* **Document type:** *Academic/Scholarly.*
Published by: Medical Publications (Ireland) Ltd., 15 Harcourt St., Dublin 2, Ireland. TEL 353-1-4757461, FAX 353-1-757467, office@imt.ie, http://www.imt.ie. Ed. Dr. Andrea Letoha. Pub. Aisling O'Connell. Adv. contact Clodagh Lenehan. Circ: 3,460.

610 026 USA ISSN 0541-5489
Z675.M4
M L A NEWS (CHICAGO). Text in English. 1961. 10/yr., latest no.337. USD 48.50 to non-members; USD 61.50 foreign to non-members (effective 1999). adv. 24 p./no. back issues avail.; reprint service avail. from PQC,ISI. **Document type:** *Newsletter, Internal, Trade.*
Description: Features industry and association news and events, including reports and analysis of current issues, upcoming meetings and employment opportunities.
Related titles: Online - full text ed.: (from Institute for Scientific Information).
Indexed: CINAHL.
—BLDSC (5879.715400), GNLM, IDS.
Published by: Medical Library Association, 65 E Wacker Pl, Ste 1900, Chicago, IL 60601-7298. TEL 312-419-9094, FAX 312-419-8950, info@mlahq.org, http://www.mlanet.org/publications. Ed. Beverly Murphy. R&P Lynanne Feilen TEL 312-419-9094 ext 26. Adv. contact Barbara Redmond TEL 312-419-9094 ext 26. B&W page USD 1,498. Circ: 5,000.

610 USA
M M NEWS. Text in English. 6/yr. USD 15. adv. **Document type:** *Newsletter.*
Formerly: New York County Medical Society Newsletter
Published by: New York County Medical Society, 15 E 26th St, New York, NY 10010. TEL 212-684-4670, FAX 212-684-4741. Ed. Cheryl Malone. R&P Gary A Gatza. Adv. contact Loretta Lewis. Circ: 6,200.

610 DEU ISSN 1438-3276
CODEN: MMMWD7
▼ **M M W - FORTSCHRITTE DER MEDIZIN.** (Muenchener Medizinische Wochenschrift) Text in German; Summaries in English, German. 1999. w. EUR 153.30 domestic; EUR 171.30 foreign; EUR 99.09 domestic to students; EUR 117.09 foreign to students; EUR 7.48 newsstand/cover (effective 2002). adv. bk.rev. bibl, illus. index. back issues avail. *Refereed.* **Document type:** *Journal, Academic/Scholarly.*
Formed by the merger of (1853-1999): Muenchener Medizinische Wochenschrift (0341-3098); (1882-1999): Fortschritte der Medizin (0015-8178)
Related titles: Microform ed.: (from PMC); Online - full text ed.: (from Institute for Scientific Information).
Indexed: Abstr.Hyg., Agri.& Environ.Biotech.Abstr. (coverage dropped), Biol.Abstr., C.I.S. Abstr., Chem.Abstr., Curr.Cont. (coverage dropped), Derwent Biotech.Abstr., Helminthol.Abstr., INIS Atomind., Ind.Med. (1999-), Ind.Vet., Inpharma, Nutr.Abstr., Protozool.Abstr., Reac., Rev.Arom.& Med.Plants, Rev.Med.& Vet.Mycol., Rev.Plant Path., Rural Recreat.Tour.Abstr., Trop.Dis.Bull., Weed Abstr.
—BLDSC (5879.802000), CASDDS, CISTI, EMDOCS, IDS, KNAW. **CCC.**
Published by: Urban und Vogel Medien und Medizin Verlagsgesellschaft mbH (Subsidiary of: BertelsmannSpringer), Neumarkter Str 43, Munich 81673, Germany. TEL 49-89-43721411, FAX 49-89-43721410, verlag@urban-vogel.de, http://www.mmw.de. Ed. Dr. Dirk Einecke. Adv. contact Renate Huesmann. Circ: 55,000. **Subscr. to:** Springer Auslieferungs Gesellschaft, Postfach 105160, Heidelberg 69041, Germany. TEL 49-6221-345244, FAX 49-6221-345244.

610 ZAF
M R C NEWS. Text in English. 1972. bi-m. free per issue. **Document type:** *Newsletter.*
Formerly: M N R Nuus (1017-611X)
Published by: Medical Research Council, PO Box 19070, Tygerberg 7505, South Africa. TEL 27-21-938-0293, FAX 27-21-938-0395, http://www.mrc.ac.za/startnew.htm. R&P Izelle Theunissen. Circ: 1,400.

610 GBR ISSN 0143-0130
M R C NEWS. Text in English. q. free per issue. **Document type:** *Consumer.* **Description:** Discusses the centers research.
Indexed: Ref.Zh.
—KNAW.
Published by: Medical Research Council, 20 Park Crescent, London W1N 4AL, United Kingdom. TEL 44-171-636-5422, FAX 44-171-436-6179, http://www.mrc.ac.uk/. Ed. Trevor Dooley.

610 GBR
M R C STRATEGIC PLAN 1999 - 2003. Text in English. a. **Document type:** *Corporate.*
Formerly (until 1999): M R C Corporate Plan
—BLDSC (5980.749800).
Published by: Medical Research Council, 20 Park Crescent, London W1N 4AL, United Kingdom. TEL 44-171-636-5422, FAX 44-171-436-6179, http://www.mrc.ac.uk/.

610 CAN
M S N S NEWS✱. Text in English. 1994. bi-m. adv. **Document type:** *Newsletter.*
Published by: Medical Society of Nova Scotia, 5 Spectacle Lake Dr, Dartmouth, NS B3B 1X7, Canada. TEL 902-468-1866, FAX 905-278-4850. Ed. Donna Christopher. Adv. contact Kelly Stoddard. B&W page CND 724, color page CND 1,378; trim 11.25 x 8.75.

618 DEU ISSN 0930-4622
CODEN: MTAAEX
M T A - FACHZEITSCHRIFT DER TECHNISCHE ASSISTENTEN DER MEDIZIN; Monatszeitschrift fuer MTA's, Labormediziner, Fachleute Radio-Diagnostik, Lehrer und Studenten. (Medizinisch-Technische Assistenten) Text in German. m. DEM 126; DEM 93.60 to students (effective 2000). adv. **Document type:** *Trade.*
Formerly: M T A - Journal (0171-8037)
Related titles: ♦ Supplement: M T A - Repetitorium. ISSN 0930-4614.
Indexed: Ref.Zh.
—CASDDS, GNLM, Infotrieve. **CCC.**
Published by: Umschau Zeitschriftenverlag Breidenstein GmbH, Stuttgarter Str 18-24, Frankfurt Am Main 60329, Germany. TEL 49-69-2600-670, FAX 49-69-2600-619. Ed. Sabine Paeuser. Adv. contact Barbara Eckert. B&W page DEM 5,600, color page DEM 9,539; trim 176 x 257. Circ: 25,103.

618 DEU ISSN 0930-4614
M T A - REPETITORIUM. (Medizinisch- Technische Assistenten) Text in German. 1979. m.
Formerly (until 1985): Gelernt, Vergessen (0930-4606)
Related titles: ♦ Supplement to: M T A - Fachzeitschrift der Technische Assistenten der Medizin. ISSN 0930-4622.
Published by: Umschau Zeitschriftenverlag Breidenstein GmbH, Stuttgarter Str 18-24, Frankfurt Am Main 60329, Germany. TEL 49-69-2600-621, FAX 49-69-2600-609.

610 DEU ISSN 0935-137X
M T DIALOG. (Medizin-Technischer) Text in German. 1975. m. DEM 262 (effective 2000). adv. **Document type:** *Trade.*
Published by: M T D Verlag GmbH und Co., Wangenerstr 12, Amtzell 88279, Germany. TEL 49-7520-958-0, FAX 49-7520-95899. Ed. Rolf Schmid. Adv. contact Christl Morgen.

610 DEU
CODEN: MDZNDG
M T - MEDIZINTECHNIK. Text in German. 1880. bi-m. DEM 128 domestic; DEM 138 foreign (effective 2000). adv. bk.rev., rec.rev. charts, illus, pat. index. **Document type:** *Trade.*
Former titles: Medizintechnik (0344-9416); Medizinische Technik (0025-8504)
Indexed: Chem.Abstr., Excerp.Med., INIS Atomind.
—CASDDS, CISTI, EMDOCS, GNLM, Infotrieve. **CCC.**
Published by: T Ue V Verlag GmbH, Am Grauen Stein 1, Cologne 51105, Germany. TEL 49-221-8063535, FAX 49-221-8063510, verlag@tuev-rheinland.de, http://www.tuev-rheinland.de. Ed. R D Boeckmann. Adv. contact Gudrun Karafiol. B&W page DEM 2,095; trim 255 x 172. Circ: 3,200.

M X; business strategies for medical technology executives. see *BUSINESS AND ECONOMICS*

610 DNK ISSN 0373-2746
MAANEDSSKRIFT FOR PRAKTISK LAEGEGERNING. Text in Danish. 1922. m. DKK 384 (effective 2000). adv.
Indexed: Chem.Abstr.
Published by: (Koebenhavn Praktiserende Laeger), Laegeforeningens Forlag, PO Box 93, Copenhagen K 1003, Denmark. Ed. Dr. Niels Noekkslund.

610 ISR
MABAT LA-MIRPA'OT. Text in Hebrew. 1987. q.
Published by: Association of Kupat Cholim Doctors, 6 Tel Hai St., Tel Aviv, Israel. TEL 03-280118. Ed. Dr. Dor Michael.

610 RUS
MAFUSAILOV VEK. Text in Russian. 1997. w. USD 65 in North America.
Published by: Redaktsiya Mafusailov Vek, A-ya 77, Moscow 127273, Russian Federation. TEL 7-095-9037070. Ed. V A Tuev. **Dist. by:** East View Publications, 3020 Harbor Ln N, Minneapolis, MN 55447. TEL 763-550-0961, FAX 763-559-2931.

M

616 POL ISSN 0867-1818
MAGAZYN MEDYCZNY; miesiecznik dla lekarzy. Text in Polish. 1990. m. USD 45 (effective 1998). adv. bk.rev. index. back issues avail. **Document type:** *Academic/Scholarly.* **Description:** Medical journal addressed to medical doctors and students.
Published by: Wydawnictwo Medyczne Sanmedica Sp. z o.o., Ul Nowy Zjazd 1, Warsaw 00301, Poland. TEL 48-22-8262287, FAX 48-22-8263182. Ed. Barbara Dworak Bator. Adv. contact Ewa Dabrowska. B&W page USD 800, color page USD 1,000. Circ: 4,500.

669.723 615.328 GBR ISSN 0953-1424
CODEN: MAGREF
MAGNESIUM RESEARCH. Text in English; Summaries in French. 1988. 4/yr. GBP 80 to individuals; GBP 150 to institutions (effective 2001). *Refereed.* **Document type:** *Academic/Scholarly.*
Related titles: Online - full text ed.: (from Institute for Scientific Information).
Indexed: ASCA, Chem.Abstr., Chem.Indus.Notes, Chem.Titles, Curr.Cont., Ind.Med. (1988-), Inpharma, Mass Spectr.Bull., Pharm.&Out.News, Reac.
—BLDSC (5334.930000), CASDDS, CISTI, GNLM, IDS, KNAW.
Published by: (International Development of Research on Magnesium), John Libbey & Co. Ltd., PO Box 276, Eastleigh SO50 5YS, United Kingdom. TEL 44-2380-650208, FAX 44-2380-650259, johnlibbey@aol.com, http://www.johnlibbey.com. Ed. Jean Durlach.

610 GBR
MAINSTREAM RESEARCH PROJECTS HANDBOOK. Text in English. biennial. **Document type:** *Monographic series.*
—BLDSC (5352.384500).
Published by: H S E, Research Strategy Unit, PO Box 1064, Sheffield S3 7YB, United Kingdom. TEL 44-114-289-2321, FAX 44-114-289-2400, fiona.garner@hse.gsi.gov.uk.

610 IDN ISSN 0377-1121
MAJALAH KEDOKTERAN INDONESIA; the journal of the Indonesian Medical Association. Text in English. 1950. m. IDR 35,000, USD 17.75. adv. back issues avail.
Published by: Indonesian Medical Association, Yayasan penerbitan IDI, Jl Dr Samratulangi 29, Jakarta 10350, Indonesia. TEL 62-021-337910. Ed. Chicf Tjokronegoro. Circ: 18,000.

610 IDN ISSN 0303-7932
R97.7.I5
MAJALAH KEDOKTERAN SURABAYA. Text in Indonesian; Summaries in English. 1964. q. IDR 1,000. adv. bk.rev.
Former titles: Madjalah Kedokteran Surabaja (0024-9564); Madjalah Research Kedokteran, Surabaja
Published by: Airlangga University, School of Medicine, Jalan Dharmahusada No. 47, Surabaya, Indonesia. Ed. Soedarso Djojonegoro. Circ: 4,000.

610 SYR
AL-MAJALLA AL-TOUBIYA AL-ARABIYA. Text in Arabic. m.
Published by: Arab Medical Commission, Al-Jala St., Damascus, Syria. Ed. Adnan Takriti.

610 EGY
AL-MAJALLAH AT-TIBBIYYAH AL-MISRIYYAH AL-JADIDAH✱ /NEW EGYPTIAN JOURNAL OF MEDICINE. Text in Arabic. 1988 (vol.2). q. **Document type:** *Academic/Scholarly.*
Related titles: CD-ROM ed.: 1988 (vol.2).
Indexed: ExtraMED.
Published by: Egyptian Junior Medical Doctors Association, Medical Information and Publishing Center, c/o Egyptian Medical Association, 42 Sharia Kasr El-Aini, Cairo, Egypt.

MAKEDONSKA AKADEMIJA NA NAUKITE I UMETNOSTITE. ODDELENIE ZA BIOLOSKI I MEDICINSKI NAUKI. PRILOZI/MACEDONIAN ACADEMY OF SCIENCES AND ARTS. SECTION OF BIOLOGICAL AND MEDICAL SCIENCES. CONTRIBUTIONS. see *BIOLOGY*

610 UGA ISSN 0025-1119
MAKERERE MEDICAL JOURNAL. Abbreviated title: M M J. Text in English. 1957. s-a. USD 6.25. bk.rev. bibl, charts, illus. **Document type:** *Proceedings, Academic/Scholarly.* **Description:** Publishes the research of Makerere University medical students and contains news of the medical school.
Related titles: CD-ROM ed.
Indexed: Biol.Abstr., Chem.Abstr., ExtraMED, Trop.Dis.Bull. —GNLM.
Published by: Makerere University Medical Students' Association (MUMSA), PO Box 7072, Kampala, Uganda. adv.: page USD 85. Circ: 600.

610 UGA
MAKERERE MEDICAL NEWSLETTER. Text in English. 1993. m. USD 5.60. **Document type:** *Consumer.* **Description:** Informs the public about health matters with the aim to improve health and hygiene and to prevent disease.
Published by: Makerere University Students Association (MUMSA), PO Box 7072, Kampala, Uganda. TEL 256-41-531350. Ed. Haumba Samson Malwa. adv.: page USD 50. Circ: 1,000. **Co-sponsor:** World Health Organization.

616.07 MYS ISSN 0126-8635
MALAYSIAN JOURNAL OF PATHOLOGY. Text in English. 1978. 2/yr. MYR 30 domestic; USD 30 overseas. adv. bk.rev. **Document type:** *Academic/Scholarly.* **Description:** Publishes results of study and research in pathology, especially those relating to human disease occurring in Malaysia.
Indexed: Ind.Med. (1978-), Trop.Dis.Bull.
—BLDSC (5356.068500), GNLM.
Published by: Malaysian Society of Pathologists, University of Malaysia, Faculty of Medicine, Department of Pathology, Kuala Lumpur 59100, Malaysia. TEL 603-7502064, FAX 306-755-6845, lmlooi@medicine.med.um.edu.my, http://www.geocities.com/HotSpring/4688/msphome.htm. Ed. Lai-Meng Looi. Adv. contact Phaik Phaik-Leng. Circ: 500 (paid and controlled).

MANAGED CARE INTERFACE; today's experts tomorrow's health care. see *HEALTH FACILITIES AND ADMINISTRATION*

610 330 USA ISSN 1073-1520
MANAGED CARE MEDICINE. Text in English. 1994. 10/yr. USD 90 domestic; USD 120 foreign; USD 15 newsstand/cover. adv. back issues avail. **Document type:** *Trade.* **Description:** Focuses on the business side of medicine.
Published by: (National Association of Managed Care Physicians), Health Care Communications, One Bridge Plaza, Ste 350, Fort Lee, NJ 07024. TEL 201-947-5545, FAX 201-947-8406. Ed. R Stephen Venable. Pub., Adv. contact Bradley D Kalish. B&W page USD 2,925. Circ: 25,000.

MANAGED CARE QUARTERLY. see *HEALTH FACILITIES AND ADMINISTRATION*

MANAGED CARE WEEK. see *INSURANCE*

MANAGED HEALTH CARE OVERVIEW. see *INSURANCE—Abstracting, Bibliographies, Statistics*

610 USA
MANAGED HEALTHCARE NEWS. Text in English. 1986. m. USD 107 to individuals; USD 204 to institutions (effective 2000). adv. bk.rev. abstr. **Document type:** *Newspaper, Trade.* **Description:** Provides useful information for physicians, administrators, pharmacists, and key HMO/PPO professionals in group practice or managed health care settings.
Former titles (until Oct. 1995): Group Practice Managed Healthcare News; Group Practice News
Related titles: Online - full text ed.
Published by: Quadrant HealthCom, 26 Main St, Ste A, Chatham, NJ 07928-2402. TEL 973-701-8900, FAX 973-701-8892, http://www.managedhealthcarenews.com/. Ed. Bill Schu. Pub. Dominic Barone. Adv. contact Denise Andrade. Circ: 69,000.

610 USA ISSN 1076-1594
MANAGEMENT COMPENSATION SURVEY. Text in English. a. USD 115 to non-members; USD 75 to members (effective 2001). **Description:** Includes data pertaining to managerial compensation.
Related titles: Cards ed.
Published by: Medical Group Management Association, 104 Inverness Terrace E, Englewood, CO 80112. TEL 303-799-1111, FAX 303-397-1827, survey@mgma.com, http://www.mgma.com. Circ: 10,000 (paid).

610 JPN ISSN 0913-2899
MANIPYURESHON/MANIPULATION. Variant title: Japanese Journal of Manipulative Therapeutics. Text in Japanese. 1986. q. JPY 2,500 per issue.
Published by: Enterprise Co. Ltd., 1-3 Honkomagome 2-chome, Bunkyo-ku, Tokyo 113-0021, Japan.

610 TUR ISSN 1019-1941
CODEN: MMJOF
MARMARA MEDICAL JOURNAL. Text in English. 1988. q. TRL 6,000,000, USD 50; USD 20 newsstand/cover (effective 1999). adv. *Refereed.* **Document type:** *Academic/Scholarly.* **Description:** Contains orginal articles, case reports, review articles, photo quiz, medicine elsewhere, meetings and annuncements.
Indexed: Excerp.Med. (1996-).
—BLDSC (5381.839000), EMDOCS.
Published by: Marmara University, Faculty of Medicine, Haydarpasa, Istanbul, Turkey. TEL 90-216-414-4734, FAX 90-216-414-4731, nudantozun@hotmail.com. Ed. Dr. Nurdan Tozun. R&P Sea Arbay. Adv. contact Seza Arbay. Circ: 500.

610 USA ISSN 0886-0572
R11 CODEN: MMJRA8
MARYLAND MEDICAL JOURNAL. Text in English. 1952. m. (exc. Jun., Dec.). USD 45 to non-members; USD 57 foreign to non-members. adv. bk.rev. bibl, charts, illus. index. reprint service avail. from ISI. *Refereed.* **Document type:** *Academic/Scholarly.* **Description:** Contains original research, case studies and articles related to clinical medicine; information on medical practice and the art of medicine; legislative updates on medicine-related topics; and member information.
Formerly (until 1985): Maryland State Medical Journal (0025-4363)
Related titles: Microform ed.: (from PQC).
Indexed: AgeLine, Biol.Abstr., CINAHL, Chem.Abstr., Curr.Cont. (coverage dropped), Excerp.Med. (until 1995), INIS Atomind., Ind.Med. (coverage dropped), Med.Care Rev.
—CISTI, GNLM, ingenta, KNAW.
Published by: Medical and Chirurgical Faculty of Maryland, 1211 Cathedral St, Baltimore, MD 21201. TEL 410-539-0872, FAX 410-547-0915. Ed. Dr. Marion Friedman. R&P Vivian Smith. Adv. contact Jeffrey Furniss. Circ: 7,500 (controlled).

▼ **MAST CELLS.** see *BIOLOGY—Cytology And Histology*

610 POL ISSN 0025-5246
CODEN: MMDPA6
MATERIA MEDICA POLONA; the Polish journal of medicine and pharmacy. Text in English, French. 1969. q. USD 60. adv. bk.rev. index.
Indexed: Abstr.Hyg., Biol.Abstr., Chem.Abstr., Chem.Titles, Dent.Ind., Excerp.Med., Ind.Med. (1969-), Nutr.Abstr., Trop.Dis.Bull.
—BLDSC (5392.600000), CASDDS, CISTI, GNLM, KNAW.
Published by: Centrum Medyczne Ksztalcenia Podyplomowego, Ul Marymoncka 99, Warsaw 01813, Poland. TELEX 813567 AGPOL PL. Ed. Edward Ruzyllo. Circ: 3,000.

610 RUS
MATERINSTVO. Text in Russian. 1996. 11/yr. USD 135 in North America.
Published by: Izdatel'skii Dom Pasport Interneishnl, Leningradskii pr-t 80-2 k 5a, Moscow 125178, Russian Federation. TEL 7-095-9433797. **Dist. by:** East View Publications, 3020 Harbor Ln N, Minneapolis, MN 55447. TEL 763-550-0961, FAX 763-559-2931.

610 NLD ISSN 0945-053X
QP552.C6 CODEN: MTBOEC
MATRIX BIOLOGY; clinical and experimental. Text in English. 8/yr. EUR 145 in Europe to individuals; JPY 19,200 in Japan to individuals; USD 163 elsewhere to individuals; EUR 556 in Europe to institutions; JPY 73,900 in Japan to institutions; USD 622 elsewhere to institutions (effective 2002). adv. reprints avail. *Refereed.* **Document type:** *Academic/Scholarly.* **Description:** Examines experiments using the most scientific technologies, including molecular biology, cell biology, immunochemistry, structural biology, computational biology, theoretical biology, and macromolecular chemistry, whereby the subject is extracellular matrix or related to the matrix and its biological role.
Former titles (until 1993): Matrix (0934-8832); (until 1988): Collagen and Related Research (0174-173X)
Related titles: Online - full text ed.: (from ingenta, ScienceDirect, Swets Blackwell, Institute for Scientific Information).
Indexed: ASCA, BBCI, Biol.Abstr., Chem.Abstr., Chem.Indus.Notes, Chem.Titles, Curr.Adv.Ecol.Sci., Curr.Cont., Curr.Leather Lit., Dent.Ind., Excerp.Med., Ind.Med. (1994-), Ind.Sci.Rev., Inpharma, Int.Abstr.Biol.Sci., Reac., Sci.Cit.Ind.
—BLDSC (5412.050000), CASDDS, CISTI, EMDOCS, GNLM, IDS, ingenta, KNAW. **CCC.**

M

Published by: Elsevier Science BV, Regional Sales Office, PO Box 211, Amsterdam 1000 AE, Netherlands. TEL 31-20-485-2911, nlinfo-f@elsevier.nl, http://www.elsevier.nl/locate/matbio. Ed. Karl Piez. R&P Kerstin Schumann TEL 49-3641-626430. **Subscr. in Australasia and the Far East to:** Elsevier Science (Singapore) Pte Ltd, No.1 Temasek Ave, 17-01 Millenia Tower, Singapore 039192, Singapore. TEL 65-434-3727, FAX 65-337-2230; **Subscr. in Japan to:** Elsevier Science Inc - Japan Regional Office, 9-15 Higashi-Azabu 1-chome, Minato-ku, Tokyo 106-0044, Japan. TEL 81-3-5561-5033; **Subscr. in the Americas to:** Elsevier Science, PO Box 945, New York, NY 10159-0945. TEL 212-633-3730, FAX 212-633-3680.

610 USA
MAYO ALUMNI. Text in English. 1965. q. free per issue to qualified personnel. **Description:** Directed to the physicians, scientists and medical educators who trained at Mayo.
Formerly (until 1992): Mayo Alumnus
Published by: Mayo Foundation, Mayo Clinic, Rochester, MN 55905. Ed. Rosemary Cashman. Circ: 14,000 (controlled).

610 DEU ISSN 0946-3704
MAYO CLINIC GESUNDHEITS-BRIEF. Text in German. m. DEM 293.10 (effective 1999). index. back issues avail. *Refereed.* **Document type:** *Newsletter, Consumer.* **Description:** Contains useful, reliable, and easy to understand health information.
Formerly (until 1994): Mayo Clinic Health Letter. German Edition (0933-9914)
Related titles: Online - full text ed.
Published by: F I D Verlag GmbH, Koblenzer Str 99, Bonn 53177, Germany. TEL 49-228-359585, FAX 49-228-361992, http://www.mayo-clinic-gesundheits-brief.de. Ed. Rudolf Juchems. Pub. Helmut Graf. R&P Karin Schott. **Subscr. to:** Leser-Service, Postfach 1327, Neckarsulm 74150, Germany. TEL 49-7132-959205, FAX 49-7132-959209.

362.1 613 610.69 USA ISSN 0741-6245
CODEN: MCHLEG
MAYO CLINIC HEALTH LETTER; reliable information for a healthier life. Text in English. 1983. 24/yr. USD 24 domestic; USD 31 in Canada & Mexico; USD 39 elsewhere (effective 2000). illus. index,cum.index. Supplement avail.; reprints avail. **Document type:** *Newsletter.* **Description:** Presents timely facts and findings on a broad variety of health issues.
Related titles: Online - full text ed.: (from Gale Group, Factiva).
Indexed: Biol.Dig., CHNI, CINAHL, Consum.Ind. (1989-), Hlth.Ind., R.G.
—BLDSC (5413.347000), ingenta.
Published by: (Mayo Foundation for Medical Education and Research), Mayo Medical Ventures, 200 First St, S W, Rochester, MN 55905. TEL 507-284-0773, FAX 507-284-8018, http://www.mayohealth.com. Ed. Christopher C Frye. Circ: 760,000. **Subscr. to:** PO Box 53886, Boulder, CO 80323-3886.

610 USA ISSN 0025-6196
R11 CODEN: MACPAJ
MAYO CLINIC PROCEEDINGS. Text in English. 1926. m. USD 79 to individuals; USD 97 to institutions (effective 2000). adv. bk.rev. abstr, charts, illus. index. *Refereed.* **Document type:** *Proceedings, Academic/Scholarly.* **Description:** Articles on the results of medical research and technology, including abstracts, editorials, subject reviews, case reports and announcements for the medical community.
Related titles: CD-ROM ed.: (from Ovid Technologies, Inc.); Microform ed.: (from PMC); Online - full text ed.: (from Ovid Technologies, Inc., Northern Light Technology, Inc., ProQuest Information & Learning, Factiva, Institute for Scientific Information).
Indexed: AIM, ASCA, Abstr.Hyg., AgeLine, Biol.Abstr., CINAHL, Chem.Abstr., Chem.Titles, Child Devel.Abstr., Curr.Adv.Biochem., Curr.Adv.Cancer Res., Curr.Adv.Ecol.Sci., Curr.Cont., Diar.Dis.Res., Excerp.Med., Helminthol.Abstr., INIS Atomind., Ind.Hyg.Dig., Ind.Med. (1964-), Ind.Sci.Rev., Inpharma, Kidney, Med.& Surg.Dermat., NRN, Neurosci.Cit.Ind., Nutr.Abstr., Pharm.&Out.News, Reac., Rehabil.Lit., Rev.Appl.Entomol., Rev.Med.& Vet.Mycol., Rev.Plant Path., Risk Abstr., SSCI (coverage dropped), Sci.Cit.Ind., THA, Trop.Dis.Bull.
—BLDSC (5413.350000), CASDDS, CISTI, GNLM, IDS, ingenta, KNAW. **CCC.**
Published by: (Mayo Clinic), Dowden Health Media, Inc, 110 Summit Ave, Montvale, NJ 07645. TEL 201-782-5735, FAX 201-505-5890, mayo@dowdenpub.com, http://www.mayo.edu/proceedings. Ed. Dr. William L Lanier. Pub. Pamela M Poppalardo. Adv. contact Pamela Poppalardo. Circ: 113,200.

610 USA ISSN 0882-6617
MAYO CLINICAL UPDATE. Text in English. 1985. q. free per issue to qualified personnel. **Document type:** *Newsletter.* **Description:** Information for physicians.
Published by: Mayo Foundation, Mayo Clinic, 200 First St S W, Rochester, MN 55905.

610 USA
▼ **MD NET GUIDE**; physician's internet directory. Text in English. 1999. m. adv. **Document type:** *Journal, Trade, Consumer.* **Description:** Provides links to medical information and continuing medical education sites.
Related titles: ♦ E-mail ed.: MD Net Guide eNewsletter; ♦ Online - full content ed.: MD Net Guide Online.
Published by: Intellisphere (Subsidiary of: MultiMedia Healthcare Inc.), Office Center at Princeton Meadows, Ste 400, Plainsboro, NJ 08536. TEL 609-275-3800, FAX 609-275-6076, info@mdnetguide.com, http://www.mdnetguide.com.

610 USA
▼ **MD NET GUIDE ENEWSLETTER.** Text in English. 1999. bi-w. **Document type:** *Trade, Consumer.* **Description:** Provides information on pertinent health care topics.
Media: E-mail. **Related titles:** ♦ Online - full content ed.: MD Net Guide Online; ♦ Print ed.: MD Net Guide.
Published by: Intellisphere (Subsidiary of: MultiMedia Healthcare Inc.), Office Center at Princeton Meadows, Ste 400, Plainsboro, NJ 08536. TEL 609-275-3800, FAX 609-275-6076, info@mdnetguide.com, http://www.mdnetguide.com.

610 USA
▼ **MD NET GUIDE ONLINE**; physician's internet directory. Text in English. 1999. d. adv. **Document type:** *Trade, Consumer.* **Description:** Provides physicians with user-friendly access to online medical content.
Media: Online - full content. **Related titles:** ♦ E-mail ed.: MD Net Guide eNewsletter; ♦ Print ed.: MD Net Guide.
Published by: Intellisphere (Subsidiary of: MultiMedia Healthcare Inc.), Office Center at Princeton Meadows, Ste 400, Plainsboro, NJ 08536. TEL 609-275-3800, FAX 609-275-6076, info@mdnetguide.com, http://www.mdnetguide.com.

MEALEY'S LITIGATION REPORT: BREAST IMPLANTS. see *LAW—Civil Law*

MEALEY'S MANAGED CARE LIABILITY REPORT. see *LAW*

610 USA
MECKLENBURG MEDICINE. Text in English. 1970. m. USD 30 (effective 2000). adv. back issues avail. **Document type:** *Bulletin, Trade, Academic/Scholarly.* **Description:** Updates area physicians on health care and medical practice issues.
Formerly: Mecklenburg County Medical Society. Bulletin
Published by: Mecklenburg County Medical Society, 1112 Harding Pl, Ste 200, Charlotte, NC 28204-2825. TEL 704-376-3688, FAX 704-376-3173, meckmed@mindspring.com, http://www.meckmed.org. Ed. Kelli McBride. Adv. contact Leslie Shinn TEL 704-344-1980. Circ: 1,500.

610 DEU ISSN 0934-3148
MED-REPORT. Text in German. 1977. 34/yr. DEM 277.72 in Europe; DEM 336.40 elsewhere; DEM 305.49 in Europe print & online eds. combined; DEM 370.04 elsewhere print & online eds. combined (effective 2001). **Document type:** *Journal, Academic/Scholarly.*
Related titles: Online - full text ed.: ISSN 1439-0493.
—GNLM. **CCC.**
Published by: Blackwell Wissenschafts Verlag GmbH, Kurfuerstendamm 57, Berlin 10707, Germany. TEL 49-30-327906-0, FAX 49-30-32790610, abo@blackwis.de, http://www.blackwell.de. Ed. Dr. Beata Duemde.

610 DEU ISSN 1615-777X
▼ **MED REVIEW**; die Zeitschrift fuer aerztliche Fortbildungskongresse. Text in German. 2000. 10/yr. DEM 269.90 in Europe; DEM 328.58 elsewhere; DEM 296.89 in Europe paper & online eds. combined; DEM 361.44 elsewhere paper & online eds. combined (effective 2001). adv. **Document type:** *Journal, Academic/Scholarly.* **Description:** Contains research articles and papers presented at various medical meetings and congresses.
Related titles: ♦ Online - full text ed.: Med Review Online.
Published by: Blackwell Wissenschafts Verlag GmbH, Kurfuerstendamm 57, Berlin 10707, Germany. TEL 49-30-327906-0, FAX 49-30-32790610, medreview@blackwis.de, abo@blackwis.de, anzeigen@blackwis.de, http://www.blackwell.de/jmr.htm. Ed. Dr. Beata Duemde. Adv. contact Jutta Weber-Pianka.

610 DEU
▼ **MED REVIEW ONLINE.** Text in German. 2000. 10/yr. DEM 243 (effective 2001). **Document type:** *Academic/Scholarly.*
Media: Online - full text. **Related titles:** ♦ Print ed.: Med Review. ISSN 1615-777X.
Published by: Blackwell Wissenschafts Verlag GmbH, Kurfuerstendamm 57, Berlin 10707, Germany. TEL 49-30-327906-0, FAX 49-30-32790610, medreview@blackwis.de, abo@blackwis.de, anzeigen@blackwis.de, http://www.blackwell.de/jmr.htm.

610 CAN ISSN 1496-9289
MEDACTUEL F M C. Text in French. 1993. 6/yr. CND 48.50 domestic; CND 60 in United States; CND 75 elsewhere. **Document type:** *Magazine, Trade.*
Formerly (until 2001): Omnipraticien (1195-0242)
Published by: Rogers Media Publishing Ltd, 1001 boul de Maisonneuve Ouest, Rm 1100, Montreal, PQ H3A 3E1, Canada. TEL 514-843-2581, FAX 514-845-7503, http://www.medalliance.ca, http://www.rogers.com. Ed. Michel Legault. Circ: 10,500.

MEDDELELSER OM GROENLAND. MAN & SOCIETY. see *ANTHROPOLOGY*

610 FRA ISSN 0399-385X
MEDECIN DE FRANCE. Text in French. 1929. 44/yr.
Address: 60 bd. de la Tour Maubourg, Paris 75007, France. TEL 45-55-20-20, FAX 45-51-82-13. Ed. Dr. Jacques Beaupere. Circ: 35,799.

610 FRA ISSN 0397-9172
MEDECIN DE RESERVE. Text in French. 1960. 6/yr. FRF 290; FRF 375 foreign (effective 1998). adv. **Document type:** *Bulletin.*
—CISTI.
Published by: Union Nationale des Medecins de Reserve, 65-67 av. des Champs Elysees, Paris 75008, France. TEL 33-1-45632145. Ed. Jean Pierre Moulinie. Adv. contact Jean-Pierre Moulinie. Circ: 2,600.

610 CAN ISSN 0025-6692
LE MEDECIN DU QUEBEC. Text in French; Summaries in English. 1965. m. CND 75 domestic; USD 100 foreign (effective 2000). adv. bk.rev. bibl. index. back issues avail. *Refereed.* **Document type:** *Trade.*
Indexed: Anim.Breed.Abstr., Pt.de Rep. (1983-).
—CISTI. **CCC.**
Published by: Federation des Medecins Omnipraticiens du Quebec/Federation of General Practitioners of Quebec, 1440 rue St Catherine Ouest, Ste 1000, Montreal, PQ H3G 1R8, Canada. TEL 514-878-1911, FAX 514-878-4455, medque@fmoq.org. Ed. Dr. J Maurice Turgeon. R&P Dr. J. Maurice Turgeon. Adv. contact Helene Brassard TEL 514-624-6979. Circ: 15,823 (controlled).

610 FRA ISSN 1286-1197
LE MEDECIN GENERALISTE. Text in French. 1975. 89/yr. adv. bk.rev. **Document type:** *Newspaper, Trade.*
Formerly (until 1990): Generaliste (0183-4568)
—CCC.
Published by: Editions du Medecin Generaliste, 11 bd. de Sebastopol, Paris 75001, France. TEL 44-82-33-33, FAX 42-21-05-98. Ed. Edouard Bourreau. Circ: 60,000.

616.98 FRA ISSN 0294-0817
RC1050 CODEN: MSMHD4
MEDECINE AERONAUTIQUE ET SPATIALE. Summaries in English, French. 1962. 4/yr. USD 30; FRF 450 foreign. adv. bk.rev. abstr, bibl, charts, illus. index. **Document type:** *Academic/Scholarly.*
Former titles: Medecine Aeronautique et Spatiale - Medecine Subaquatique et Hyperbare (0399-6417); (until 1976): Revue de Medecine Aeronautique et Spatiale (0035-1520); (until 1965): Revue de Medecine Aeronautique
Indexed: Chem.Abstr., Excerp.Med., INIS Atomind.
—CASDDS, CISTI, GNLM, Linda Hall.
Published by: I.M.A.S.S.A., 26 bd Victor, Armees 00460, France. TEL 1-45-52-67-91, FAX 1-45-52-65-90. Ed. J R Galle Tessonneau.

610 FRA
MEDECINE AU FEMININ. Text in French. 1987. bi-m. FRF 350 domestic to individuals; FRF 500, EUR 76.22 foreign to individuals; FRF 220 to students (effective 2001).
Published by: Meditions Carline, 1 et 3 rue du Depart, Paris 75014, France. TEL 33-1-40640075, FAX 33-1-43222699, groupemeditions@wanadoo.fr.

610 FRA ISSN 0543-2243
MEDECINE DE L'HOMME. Text in French. 1968. 4/yr. FRF 350 domestic; FRF 370 foreign (effective 1998). adv. bk.rev.
Indexed: Ref.Zh.
Published by: Centre Catholique des Medecins Francais, 5 av. de l'Observatoire, Paris 75006, France. TEL 33-1-46345915, FAX 33-1-43541007. Ed. Claude Laroche. Circ: 4,376.

610 613 CHE ISSN 0025-6749 CODEN: MEHGAB
MEDECINE ET HYGIENE. Text in French. 1943. w. CHF 115, EUR 74.67 domestic to individuals; CHF 190, EUR 123.37 foreign to individuals; CHF 135, EUR 87.66 domestic to institutions; CHF 210, EUR 136.36 foreign to institutions (effective 2002). adv. bk.rev. bibl, charts, illus. index. reprint service avail. from PQC. **Document type:** *Journal, Academic/Scholarly.*
Related titles: Online - full text ed.: (from Institute for Scientific Information).
Indexed: Biol.Abstr., C.I.S. Abstr., Chem.Abstr., Dent.Ind., Excerp.Med., INIS Atomind., Inpharma, Reac.
—BLDSC (5487.730000), CASDDS, CISTI, GNLM, IDS, Infotrieve, KNAW. **CCC.**
Published by: Editions Medecine et Hygiene, Case Postale 456, Geneva, 4 1211, Switzerland. TEL 41-22-7029311, FAX 41-22-7029355, abonnements@medhyg.ch, http://www.medhyg.ch. Ed. Dr. Bertrand Kiefer. Circ: 7,500.

MEDECINE ET NUTRITION. see *NUTRITION AND DIETETICS*

610 FRA ISSN 0767-0974 CODEN: MSMSE4
MEDECINE - SCIENCES. Text in French. 1985. 10/yr. FRF 620 domestic to individuals; FRF 752 foreign to individuals; FRF 1,600 domestic to institutions; FRF 1,680 foreign to institutions (effective 2000). *Refereed.* **Document type:** *Academic/Scholarly.* **Description:** Focuses on the latest developments and future perspectives in medicine and biology.
Related titles: Online - full text ed.: (from Institute for Scientific Information, RoweCom Information Quest).
Indexed: Curr.Cont., Inpharma, Med.& Surg.Dermat., Neurosci.Cit.Ind., Protozool.Abstr., Reac., Ref.Zh., SSCI (coverage dropped).
—BLDSC (5980.840100), CISTI, EMDOCS, GNLM, IDS, KNAW.
Published by: Masson - Periodiques, 120 bd. St. Germain, Paris 75006, France. TEL 33-1-40466200, FAX 33-1-40466201, s.mathot@masson.fr, http://www.e2med.com/. Ed. Axel Khan.

610 FRA ISSN 1264-6520
MEDECINE THERAPEUTIQUE. Text in French. 1995. 10/yr. FRF 710 domestic to individuals; FRF 900 domestic to individuals with online ed.; EUR 127 in Europe to individuals; EUR 155 in Europe to individuals with online ed.; FRF 880 elsewhere to individuals; FRF 1,070 elsewhere to individuals with online ed.; FRF 1,420 domestic to institutions; EUR 235 in Europe to institutions; FRF 1,590 elsewhere to institutions; FRF 430 domestic to students; EUR 84 in Europe to students (effective 2001). adv. illus. *Refereed.* **Document type:** *Academic/Scholarly.* **Description:** Covers all aspects of modern medicine. Serves as a link between basic research and medical practice.
Related titles: Online - full text ed.: FRF 710 to individuals; FRF 1,420 to institutions; FRF 430 to students (effective 2001).
Indexed: Inpharma, Reac., Ref.Zh.
—BLDSC (5487.960000), GNLM.
Published by: John Libbey Eurotext, 127 av. de la Republique, Montrouge 92120, France. TEL 33-01-46730660, FAX 33-01-40840999, marketing@jle.com, http://www.john-libbey-eurotext.fr/. Eds. Christian Boitard, Pierre Bougneres. **Subscr. to:** A T E I, 3 av. Pierre Keraurtret, Romainville 92230, France. TEL 33-1-48408686, FAX 33-1-48400731, atei@club-internet.fr.

610 FRA
MEDECINS DES HOPITAUX PUBLICS✶. Text in French. bi-m. adv.
Published by: Union Nationale des Syndicats de Medecins des Hopitaux Publics, 15 rue Beaugrenelle, Paris 75015, France. TEL 40-59-48-27. Ed. Jean Cordebar.

610 FRA ISSN 0183-5734
MEDECINS DU VAL-DE-MARNE. Text in French. 1977. 4/yr.
Published by: Medecins du, 4 rue Octave Dumesnil, Creteil 94000, France. TEL 42-07-78-66. Ed. Dr. Vergeylen. Circ: 4,500.

610 GBR ISSN 0144-4271
MEDECONOMICS. Text in English. 1980. m. GBP 75 in United Kingdom; GBP 102 in Europe; GBP 153 in the Middle East; GBP 163 in Asia (effective 2001). adv. **Document type:** *Trade.*
Related titles: Online - full text ed.: (from Data-Star).
—BLDSC (5488.060000). **CCC.**
Published by: Haymarket Medical Ltd., 174 Hammersmith Rd, London W6 7JP, United Kingdom. TEL 44-20-8943-5000, 44-20-8606-7500, FAX 44-20-8606-7301, admin.medeconomics@haynet.com, http://www.haymarketgroup.com. Ed. Beonagh Miskelly. Pub. Helen Morgan. Adv. contact Paul Mann TEL 44-20-8267-4876. Circ: 43,399.

610 GBR ISSN 0962-9351 CODEN: MNFLEF
MEDIATORS OF INFLAMMATION. Text in English. 1992. bi-m. GBP 81, USD 107 to individuals; GBP 533, USD 880 to institutions (effective 2002). reprints avail. *Refereed.* **Document type:** *Academic/Scholarly.* **Description:** Promotes the rapid publication of original and fundamental research articles on all aspects of cellular mediators.
Related titles: CD-ROM ed.; Online - full text ed.: ISSN 1466-1861 (from CatchWord Ltd., EBSCO Publishing, O C L C Online Computer Library Center, Inc., RoweCom Information Quest, Swets Blackwell, Institute for Scientific Information).
Indexed: ASCA, BBCI, Chem.Abstr., Chem.Titles, Curr.Cont., Dairy Sci.Abstr., Excerp.Med. (1993-), Ind.Med. (1992-), Ind.Sci.Rev., Inpharma, Int.Abstr.Biol.Sci., Nutr.Abstr., Pharm.&Out.News, Reac., Rev.Arom.& Med.Plants, Sci.Cit.Ind.
—BLDSC (5525.385100), ADONIS, CASDDS, CatchWord, EMDOCS, GNLM, IDS, Infotrieve, KNAW. **CCC.**
Published by: Carfax Publishing Limited (Subsidiary of: Taylor & Francis Group), PO Box 25, Abingdon, Oxon OX14 3UE, United Kingdom. TEL 44-1235-401000, FAX 44-1235-401550, enquiries@carfax.co.uk, enquiry@tandf.co.uk, http://www.carfax.co.uk. Ed. Ivan Bonta.

610 ITA ISSN 1122-1909
MEDIC. METODOLOGIA E DIDATTICA CLINICA/CLINICAL METHODOLOGY AND DIDACTICS. Text in Italian. 1993. q. USD 107 (effective 2000). adv. **Document type:** *Academic/Scholarly.*
Published by: Il Pensiero Scientifico Editore s.r.l., Via Bradano, 3-C, Rome, RM 00199, Italy. TEL 39-06-862821, FAX 39-06-86282250, pensiero@pensiero.it, http://www.pensiero.it. Ed. Aldo Torsoli. Adv. contact Luciano De Fiore. Circ: 2,000.

610 HRV ISSN 0351-0093 CODEN: MEJAD6
MEDICA JADERTINA. Text in Croatian. 1969. q. HRK 20 newsstand/cover (effective 1999). adv. bk.rev. bibl. index. back issues avail. *Refereed.* **Document type:** *Academic/Scholarly.* **Description:** Features Education of Physicians, publishing original and scientific papers, reviews and book reviews.
Related titles: CD-ROM ed.
Indexed: Excerp.Med., Ref.Zh.
—EMDOCS.
Published by: General Hospital Zadar, Scientific Unit, Boze Pericica 5, Zadar 23000, Croatia. TEL 00385-23-315-677, FAX 000385-23-312-724. Ed., R&P, Adv. contact Josip Dujella TEL 385-23-212493. Pub. Mile Gveric. B&W page HRK 1,500, color page HRK 3,000; trim 240 x 170. Circ: 650.

MEDICAID FRAUD REPORT. see *LAW*

MEDICAID RECIPIENT CHARACTERISTICS AND UNITS OF SELECTED MEDICAL SERVICES. see *SOCIAL SERVICES AND WELFARE*

MEDICAL AND BIOMEDICAL ENGINEERING REPORTS. see *ENGINEERING*

610 BWA
MEDICAL AND DENTAL ASSOCIATION OF BOTSWANA. JOURNAL. Text in English. 1971. q. USD 11. adv. charts. back issues avail.
Indexed: Ind.S.A.Per.
Published by: Medical and Dental Association of Botswana, PO Box 798, Gaborone, Botswana. Circ: 200.

610 USA ISSN 0363-0366
R5
MEDICAL AND HEALTH ANNUAL. Text in English. 1976. a. USD 33.95 (effective 1995). index. **Description:** For lay readers, covers broad areas of medicine and health including in-depth articles. Reviews important developments in the medical specialties.
—GNLM.
Published by: Encyclopaedia Britannica, Inc., 310 S Michigan Ave, Chicago, IL 60604. TEL 312-347-7000, FAX 312-347-7914. Ed. Ellen Bernstein.

MEDICAL & HEALTH EQUIPMENT BUYERS' GUIDE. see *BUSINESS AND ECONOMICS—Trade And Industrial Directories*

MEDICAL AND HEALTHCARE MARKETPLACE GUIDE. see *BUSINESS AND ECONOMICS—Trade And Industrial Directories*

MEDICAL AND HOSPITAL NEGLIGENCE. see *LAW*

MEDICAL AND NUTRITIONAL RESEARCH COMMUNICATIONS. see *NUTRITION AND DIETETICS*

632.7 GBR ISSN 0269-283X CODEN: MVENE4
MEDICAL & VETERINARY ENTOMOLOGY. Text in English. 1987. q., latest vol.16, 2002. GBP 67 in Europe to individuals; USD 107 in North America to individuals; GBP 74 elsewhere to individuals; GBP 290 in Europe to individuals; USD 460 in North America to individuals; GBP 319 elsewhere to individuals (effective 2002). adv. bk.rev. illus. index. back issues avail. *Refereed.* **Document type:** *Journal, Academic/Scholarly.* **Description:** Covers all aspects of the biology and control of insects, ticks, mites and other arthropods of medical and veterinary importance.
Related titles: ♦ Online - full text ed.: Medical & Veterinary Entomology Online. ISSN 1365-2915.
Indexed: ASCA, Abstr.Hyg., AgBiotech, Agricola, Anim.Behav.Abstr., Apic.Abstr., Aqua.Sci.& Fish.Abstr., Aquacult.Abstr., Bibl.Agri., Bio-Contr.News & Info., Curr.Cont., Dairy Sci.Abstr., Derwent Biotech.Abstr., Ecol.Abstr., Entomol.Abstr., Environ.Sci.Poll.Mgmt., Focus on: Vet.Sci.& Med., Genet.Abstr., Helminthol.Abstr., Hum.Gen.Abstr., IDA, Ind.Med. (1987-), Ind.Vet., Int.Abstr.Biol.Sci., Poult.Abstr., Protozool.Abstr., Ref.Zh., Rev.Appl.Entomol., Rev.Arom.& Med.Plants, Rev.Med.& Vet.Mycol., Sci.Cit.Ind., Sport Fish.Abstr., Trop.Dis.Bull., Vet.Bull., Wild.Rev., Zoo.Rec.
—BLDSC (5526.085000), EMDOCS, GNLM, IDS, Infotrieve, ingenta, Linda Hall. **CCC.**
Published by: (Royal Entomological Society), Blackwell Science Ltd., PO Box 88, Oxford OX2 0NE, United Kingdom. TEL 44-1865-206180, 44-1865-206002, FAX 44-1865-206219, jnl.orders@blacksci.co.uk, http://www.blackwell-science.com/products/journals/mve.htm, http://www.blackwellpublishing.com. Eds. G B White, R Nall. Pub. Sue Hewitt. R&P Sophie Savage. Adv. contact Jenny Applin. Circ: 430.

632.7 GBR ISSN 1365-2915
▼ **MEDICAL & VETERINARY ENTOMOLOGY ONLINE.** Text in English. 1999. q. GBP 61 in Europe to individuals; USD 97 in North America to individuals; GBP 61 elsewhere to individuals; GBP 261 in Europe to institutions; USD 414 in North America to institutions; GBP 261 elsewhere to institutions (effective 2002). *Refereed.* **Document type:** *Academic/Scholarly.*
Media: Online - full text (from EBSCO Publishing, O C L C Online Computer Library Center, Inc., RoweCom Information Quest, ingenta, Munksgaard & Blackwell Science's Synergy, Swets Blackwell, Institute for Scientific Information). **Related titles:** ♦ Print ed.: Medical & Veterinary Entomology. ISSN 0269-283X.
Published by: Blackwell Science Ltd., Osney Mead, Oxford OX2 0EL, United Kingdom. TEL 44-1685-206206, FAX 44-1685-721205, website@blacksci.com, journals.cs@blacksci.co.uk, http://www.blackwell-science.com/~cgilib/jnlpage.bin?Journal=mve.

MEDICAL ANTHROPOLOGY; cross-cultural studies in health and illness. see *ANTHROPOLOGY*

MEDICAL ANTHROPOLOGY QUARTERLY; international journal for the cultural and social analysis of health. see *ANTHROPOLOGY*

610 USA ISSN 0025-7028
R15
MEDICAL ASSOCIATION OF GEORGIA. JOURNAL. Text in English. 1911. q. USD 60 domestic; USD 120 foreign (effective 2000). adv. bk.rev. bibl, charts, illus. index. *Refereed.* **Document type:** *Academic/Scholarly.* **Description:** Articles and features are primarily medical or related to every day political and socio-economic interests of physicians.
Related titles: Microform ed.
Indexed: Chem.Abstr., Dent.Ind., Environ.Sci.Poll.Mgmt., INIS Atomind., Ind.Med. (1911-), Pollut.Abstr., Risk Abstr., Saf.Sci.Abstr.
—BLDSC (4824.130000), CISTI, GNLM, ingenta, KNAW.
Published by: Medical Association of Georgia, 1330 W Peachtree St, 500, Atlanta, GA 30309. TEL 404-876-7535, FAX 404-881-5021, plusone@mindspring.com. Ed. Dr. John Cantwell. R&P Melissa Connor. Adv. contact Tina Williams. Circ: 7,000 (paid).

610 THA ISSN 0125-2208
CODEN: JMTHBU
MEDICAL ASSOCIATION OF THAILAND. JOURNAL. Key Title: Chot Mai Het Thang Phaet. Text in English; Summaries in Thai. 1917. m. USD 40. adv. abstr, charts, illus. index. **Document type:** *Academic/Scholarly.*
Related titles: ♦ Supplement: Medical Association of Thailand. Journal. Supplement. ISSN 0025-7036.
Indexed: Abstr.Hyg., Biol.Abstr., Chem.Abstr., Curr.Adv.Ecol.Sci., Curr.Cont. (coverage dropped), Dairy Sci.Abstr., Diar.Dis.Res., Excerp.Med., Helminthol.Abstr., Ind.Med. (1967-), Inpharma, Maize Abstr., Protozool.Abstr., Reac., Rev.Med.& Vet.Mycol., Rev.Plant Path., Seed Abstr., Soyabean Abstr., Trop.Dis.Bull.
—BLDSC (4824.200000), CASDDS, CISTI, GNLM, KNAW.
Published by: Medical Association of Thailand, 67-9 Soi Soonvichai, New Pechburi Rd, Bangkok, 10, Thailand. TEL 66-2-314-4333, FAX 66-2-314-4333. Ed. Dr. Prasert Thongcharoen. Circ: 3,500.

610 THA ISSN 0025-7036
CODEN: JMTHBU
MEDICAL ASSOCIATION OF THAILAND. JOURNAL. SUPPLEMENT. Text in Thai. 1918. m. **Document type:** *Academic/Scholarly.*
Related titles: ♦ Supplement to: Medical Association of Thailand. Journal. ISSN 0125-2208.
Published by: Medical Association of Thailand, 67-9 Soi Soonvichai, New Pechburi Rd, Bangkok, 10, Thailand. TEL 66-2-314-4333, FAX 66-2-314-4333.

610 GBR
THE MEDICAL BOOK (YEAR). Text in English. a. **Document type:** *Monographic series, Academic/Scholarly.* **Description:** Covers wide-range of medical and clinical subjects, and also information on healthcare systems.
—BLDSC (5526.530000).
Published by: Medilink Press, 22 St Albans Ln, London NW11 7QE, United Kingdom. TEL 44-181-455-0607, FAX 44-181-455-6616, medlink@cwcom.net. Pubs. Barry Edson, Richard Ansell.

338.473621 USA
MEDICAL BUSINESS; South Florida edition. Text in English. bi-w. USD 85.20 in US & Canada; USD 175 elsewhere; USD 3.25 newsstand/cover. adv. illus. **Description:** Focuses on the financial, commercial and economic aspects of healthcare delivery in South Florida.
Published by: Industry Publishers, Inc., 1450 Northeast 123 St, N, Miami, FL 33161-6051. TEL 305-893-8771, FAX 305-893-8783. Ed. Brian Elliot Foster. Adv. contact Jennifer Wechsler.

338.473621 USA
MEDICAL BUSINESS GULF COAST EDITION✱. Text in English. 1985. bi-w. USD 85.20; USD 4 newsstand/cover (effective 1998). software rev. charts, illus, stat, tr.lit. back issues avail. **Document type:** *Newspaper.*
Published by: M.B.W.C., Inc., 1450 N E 123rd St, North Miami, FL 33161-6051. TEL 813-289-3551, FAX 813-288-8268. Ed. Linda Gibson. Pub. Brian Foster. adv.: B&W page USD 2,374; trim 15.5 x 10.

MEDICAL BUSINESS REVIEW; medical business analysis for the doctor-executive. see *BUSINESS AND ECONOMICS—Management*

362.10973 USA ISSN 0025-7079
RA1 CODEN: MDLCBD
MEDICAL CARE. Text in English. 1963. m., latest vol.39. USD 255 domestic to individuals Print & Online eds.; USD 322 foreign to individuals Print & Online eds.; USD 535 domestic to institutions Print & Online eds.; USD 577 foreign to institutions Print & Online eds.; USD 45 newsstand/cover (effective 2002). adv. index. *Refereed.* **Document type:** *Academic/Scholarly.*
Related titles: Microform ed.: (from PQC); Online - full text ed.: USD 695.50 domestic academic site license; USD 737.50 foreign academic site license; USD 775.75 domestic corporate site license; USD 817.75 foreign corporate site license (2002) (from Ovid Technologies, Inc., Swets Blackwell, Institute for Scientific Information).
Indexed: Abstr.Health Care Manage.Stud., AgeLine, CINAHL, Curr.Cont., Curr.Ind.Stat., Dent.Ind., Dok.Arbeitsmed., Excerp.Med., FAMLI, Hosp.Lit.Ind., Ind.Med. (1963-), Ind.Sci.Rev., Inpharma, Int.Nurs.Ind., Pharm.&Out.News, PsycInfo, Psychol.Abstr. (1986-), Reac., Risk Abstr., SSCI, Sci.Cit.Ind., e-psyche.
—BLDSC (5526.900000), GNLM, IDS, ingenta, KNAW.
Published by: (Medical Care Section, American Public Health Association), Lippincott Williams & Wilkins (Philadelphia) (Subsidiary of: Wolters Kluwer N.V.), 530 Walnut St, Philadelphia, PA 19106-3621. TEL 215-521-8300, FAX 215-521-8902, www.lww-medicalcare.com, http://www.lww.com. Eds. Dr. Morris Weinberger, Dr. William M. Tierney. Pub. Karen Phillips. R&P Margaret Becker. Adv. contact Ray Thibodeau. B&W page USD 570, color page USD 1,590. Circ: 2,269 (paid). **Subscr. to:** PO Box 1600, Hagerstown, MD 21740-1600. TEL 800-777-2295, FAX 301-824-7390.

610 GBR ISSN 0025-7095
MEDICAL CENTRE JOURNAL. Text in English. 1967. 3/yr. free per issue.
Published by: (Bedfordshire District Health Authority), Luton & Dunstable Hospital, Medical Centre, Luton, Beds, United Kingdom. Ed. D I M Siegler. Circ: 600.

MEDICAL CLIENT NEWSLETTER. see *BUSINESS AND ECONOMICS—Accounting*

610 USA ISSN 0025-7125
RC60 CODEN: MCNAA9
MEDICAL CLINICS OF NORTH AMERICA. Text in English. 1916. bi-m. USD 152 in Canada to individuals; USD 178 elsewhere to individuals; USD 179 domestic to institutions; USD 229 foreign to institutions; USD 81 domestic to students; USD 39 per issue (effective 2001). bibl, charts, illus. index, cum.index. reprint service avail. from PQC,ISI. *Refereed.* **Document type:** *Academic/Scholarly.*
Formerly: Medical Clinics
Related titles: Microform ed.: (from PQC,PMC); Online - full text ed.: (from Institute for Scientific Information); ♦ Spanish Translation: Clinicas Medicas de Norteamerica; Supplement: Continuing Medical Education Supplement to Medical Clinics of North America. USD 176 (effective 2000).
Indexed: AIM, ASCA, AgeLine, Agri.& Environ.Biotech.Abstr. (coverage dropped), Biol.Abstr., CINAHL, Chem.Abstr., Chem.Titles, Curr.Adv.Ecol.Sci., Curr.Cont., Dairy Sci.Abstr., Derwent Biotech.Abstr., Diar.Dis.Res., Excerp.Med., Helminthol.Abstr., INIS Atomind., I.P.A., Ind.Med. (1917-), Ind.Sci.Rev., Inpharma, Int.Nurs.Ind., Neurosci.Cit.Ind., Nutr.Abstr., Pharm.&Out.News, Protozool.Abstr., Reac., Rev.Med.& Vet.Mycol., Risk Abstr., SSCI (coverage dropped), Sci.Cit.Ind., Sugar Ind.Abstr.
—BLDSC (5527.000000), CASDDS, CISTI, GNLM, IDS, ingenta, KNAW. **CCC.**
Published by: W.B. Saunders Co. (Subsidiary of: Harcourt Publishers Ltd.), Curtis Center, Independence Sq W, Philadelphia, PA 19106-3399. TEL 215-238-7800, FAX 215-238-6445, http://www.wbsaunders.com. **Subscr. to:** Periodicals Fulfillment, W B Saunders Co, 6277 Sea Harbor Dr, 4th Fl, Orlando, FL 32891-4800. TEL 800-874-6418, FAX 800-874-6418.

610 IND ISSN 0025-7133
MEDICAL COLLEGE AND HOSPITAL, CALCUTTA. BULLETIN. Text in English. 1967. INR 12. adv. charts, illus.
Published by: Medical College and Hospital, Department of Medicine, 88 College St., Calcutta, West Bengal 700 012, India. Ed. Dr. Nalini Ranjan Konar. Circ: 600.

610 JPN ISSN 0465-4978
MEDICAL CORNER. Text in Japanese. 1967. bi-m.
Published by: Meiji Seika Kaisha Ltd., 4-16 Kyobashi 2-chome, Chuo-ku, Tokyo 104-0031, Japan.

610 USA ISSN 0272-989X
CODEN: MDMADE
MEDICAL DECISION MAKING; an international journal. Text in English. 1980. 6/yr. USD 253 domestic UK, Europe, Middle East & Africa; USD 278 foreign (effective 2002). adv. illus, charts, stat. index. 112 p./no. back issues avail.; reprints avail. *Refereed.* **Document type:** *Journal, Academic/Scholarly.* **Description:** Concerned with the quantitative science of decision-making in medicine.
Related titles: Online - full text ed.: (from Northern Light Technology, Inc., ProQuest Information & Learning, ingenta, Swets Blackwell, Institute for Scientific Information).
Indexed: ASCA, Abstr.Health Care Manage.Stud., Abstr.Hyg., Compumath, Curr.Cont., Curr.Ind.Stat., Excerp.Med., INIS Atomind., Ind.Med. (1981-), Ind.Sci.Rev., Inpharma, Pharm.&Out.News, Reac., Rel.Ind.One, Rel.Ind.Two, Sci.Cit.Ind.
—BLDSC (5527.053500), CISTI, EMDOCS, GNLM, IDS, ingenta, KNAW. **CCC.**
Published by: (Society for Medical Decision Making, Inc.), Sage Publications, Inc., Sage Science Press, 2455 Teller Rd, Thousand Oaks, CA 91320. TEL 805-499-0721, FAX 805-499-0871, info@sagepub.com, http://www.sagesciencepress.com/. Ed. Frank Sonnenberg. Pub. Susan Hanscom. R&P Peter Marino. Adv. contact Robert Vrooman. B&W page USD 651, color page USD 1,622; bleed 8.375 x 11.125. Circ: 2,000.

▼ **MEDICAL DESIGN NEWS.** see *ENGINEERING*

610.28 USA ISSN 1096-1801
MEDICAL DESIGN TECHNOLOGY; new products, materials & components for medical device designers. Text in English. 1997. 10/yr. (plus annual directory). USD 76.90 domestic; USD 86.90 in Canada; USD 80.90 in Mexico; USD 92.90 elsewhere; USD 8 newsstand/cover domestic; USD 12 newsstand/cover foreign (effective 2001). adv. **Document type:** *Trade.* **Description:** Includes information about new products, services, and applications for design engineers and technical personnel.
Related titles: Online - full text ed.: (from Gale Group); Supplement:.
Published by: Cahners Business Information, New Product Information Unit (Subsidiary of: Reed Elsevier plc), 301 Gibraltar Dr, P O Box 650, Morris Plains, NJ 07950-0650. TEL 203-326-5161 x227, FAX 203-326-5160, jcolford@cahners.com, http://www.mdtmag.com. Ed. Sean Fenske TEL 973-292-5100 x271. Pub. Jim Colford. adv.: B&W page USD 4,670, color page USD 5,550; trim 11 x 8.19. Circ: 35,440.

MEDICAL DEVICE COMPANIES ANALYSIS PROFILES. see *INSTRUMENTS*

610 GBR ISSN 1048-6690
MEDICAL DEVICE TECHNOLOGY. Text in English. 1990. 10/yr., latest vol.12. GBP 70 in Europe; GBP 100 elsewhere; free to qualified personnel (effective 2001). adv. tr.lit. back issues avail.; reprints avail. **Document type:** *Magazine, Trade.* **Description:** Features technological articles giving the latest news and views on medical device manufacturing technology for research and development and for QA-QC professionals in the European medical device manufacturing industry.
Related titles: Online - full text ed.: (from LexisNexis).
Indexed: ASCA, Bus.& Indus. (Jan.1997-), I.P.A., Int.Packag.Abstr., Intl.Polym.Sci.& Tech., Mat.Sci.Cit.Ind. (coverage dropped), RAPRA (1991-).
—BLDSC (5527.055380), GNLM, IDS. **CCC.**
Published by: Advanstar Communications, Lamb House, Church St, London CH1 4RN, United Kingdom. TEL 44-208-987-0900, FAX 44-208-987-0901, aellerton@advanstar.com, http://www.medicaldevicesonline.com, http://www.mdtlive.com. Ed. Annie Ellerton. Pub. Mike Clancy. Adv. contact Katie Lay. B&W page GBP 3,255, color page GBP 4,235; trim 8.85 x 11.22. Circ: 18,000 (paid and controlled).

615 USA ISSN 0163-2426
CODEN: MDDIDR
MEDICAL DEVICES, DIAGNOSTICS & INSTRUMENTATION REPORTS: THE GRAY SHEET. Short title: M D D I Reports. Text in English. 1975. w. USD 1,065 domestic; USD 1,190 foreign (effective 2001). adv. back issues avail.; reprints avail. **Document type:** *Newsletter, Trade.* **Description:** Provides coverage of the medical devices, diagnostics and instrumentation industries. Includes regulatory agency and congressional activities, industry developments, investor and financial news.
Related titles: Online - full text ed.: (from Data-Star, The Dialog Corporation, LexisNexis).

M

Indexed: P.N.I.
—BLDSC (5413.519050). **CCC.**
Published by: F-D-C Reports, Inc., 5550 Friendship Blvd, Ste One, Chevy Chase, MD 20815-7278. TEL 800-332-2181, FAX 301-664-7238, http://www.fdcreports.com. Ed. John Zakotnik. R&P Laura Desimio. Adv. contact Michael Keville.

610 USA
MEDICAL DEVICES REPORTS. Text in English. 1976. m. USD 759 (effective 2001).
Formerly: Medical Devices Reporter
Related titles: CD-ROM ed.
Published by: C C H Incorporated, 2700 Lake Cook Rd., Riverwoods, IL 60015. TEL 847-627-7000, 800-449-9525, FAX 773-866-3895, http://www.cch.com. Pub. Catherine Wolfe.

610 JPN ISSN 0543-2618
MEDICAL DIGEST. Text in Japanese. 1952. bi-m. JPY 300 per issue.
Published by: Daiichi Seiyaku Co. Ltd., 14-10 Nihonbashi 3-chome, Chuo-ku, Tokyo 103-0027, Japan.

MEDICAL DIRECTORY; an alphabetical listing of medical practitioners registered in Britain. see *HEALTH FACILITIES AND ADMINISTRATION*

610 USA ISSN 0273-0561
MEDICAL DIRECTORY OF NEW YORK STATE. Text in English. 1950. biennial. USD 125 (effective 2000). **Document type:** *Directory.*
Published by: Medical Society of the State of New York, 420, Lakeville, NY 11040. Eds. Christine Dillard, Frances Martino.

610 USA ISSN 0025-7206
R723.5
MEDICAL ECONOMICS. Text in English. 1923. s-m. USD 109 domestic; USD 175 foreign; USD 10 newsstand/cover (effective 2001). adv. charts, illus, stat. index. reprints avail. **Document type:** *Trade.* **Description:** Publishes original articles designed to help the private practice physician with practice management, professional and patient relations, health insurance issues, relevant legislation, and personal and financial affairs.
Related titles: Microform ed.: (from RPI,PQC); Online - full text ed.: (from The Dialog Corporation, Gale Group, Northern Light Technology, Inc., ProQuest Information & Learning, Factiva).
Indexed: ABI Inform. (Apr.11,1994-), Abstr.Health Care Manage.Stud., Account.Ind. (1974-), AgeLine, B.P.I. (Jul.1995-), BPIA, Bus.Ind., CINAHL, Curr.Lit.Fam.Plan., Hlth.Ind., Inpharma, Int.Nurs.Ind., L.R.I., Med.Care Rev., P.A.I.S., Pharm.&Out.News, Reac., Tr.& Indus.Ind.
—BLDSC (5527.160000), GNLM, ingenta. **CCC.**
Published by: Medical Economics Co., Inc., 5 Paragon Dr, Montvale, NJ 07645-1742. TEL 201-358-7200, customer_service@medec.com. Ed. Jeff Forster. adv.: B&W page USD 8,570, color page USD 11,290; trim 10 x 7. Circ: 154,515. **Subscr. to:** Medical Economics Co, Inc, P D R, PO Box 162, Montvale, NJ 07645-1742. FAX 201-722-2680.

MEDICAL ECONOMICS MAGAZINE; the business magazine of the medical profession. see *BUSINESS AND ECONOMICS*

610.711 GBR ISSN 0308-0110
R735.A1
MEDICAL EDUCATION. Text in English. 1966. 12/yr., latest vol.36, 2002. GBP 85 in Europe to individuals; USD 142 in North America to individuals; GBP 93 elsewhere to individuals; GBP 517 in Europe to individuals; USD 818 in North America to individuals; GBP 568 elsewhere to individuals (effective 2002). adv. bk.rev. bibl. index. back issues avail.; reprint service avail. from ISI. *Refereed.* **Document type:** *Academic/Scholarly.* **Description:** Covers medical school issues pertaining to students and instructors alike.
Formerly: British Journal of Medical Education (0007-1110)
Related titles: Microform ed.: (from PQC); Online - full text ed.: ISSN 1365-2923. GBP 77 in Europe to individuals; USD 128 in North America to individuals; GBP 77 elsewhere to individuals; GBP 466 in Europe to institutions; USD 737 in North America to institutions; GBP 466 elsewhere to institutions (effective 2002) (from Ovid Technologies, Inc., EBSCO Publishing, O C L C Online Computer Library Center, Inc., RoweCom Information Quest, ingenta, Munksgaard & Blackwell Science's Synergy, Swets Blackwell, Institute for Scientific Information).
Indexed: ASCA, Abstr.Health Care Manage.Stud., Abstr.Hyg., Biol.Abstr., CINAHL, Cont.Pg.Educ., Curr.Adv.Ecol.Sci., Curr.Cont., Dent.Ind., Educ.Tech.Abstr., Excerp.Med., FAMLI, High.Educ.Curr.Aware.Bull., Hosp.Abstr., Ind.Med. (1976-), Ind.Sci.Rev., Inpharma, Int.Nurs.Ind., Mid.East: Abstr.& Ind., Mult.Ed.Abstr., Pharm.&Out.News, PsycInfo, Psychol.Abstr. (1986-), Reac., Res.High.Educ.Abstr., SSCI (coverage dropped), Sci.Cit.Ind., Sociol.Educ.Abstr., Tech.Educ.Abstr., Trop.Dis.Bull., e-psyche.
—BLDSC (5527.166000), ADONIS, CISTI, EMDOCS, GNLM, IDS, Infotrieve, ingenta, KNAW. **CCC.**
Published by: (Association for the Study of Medical Education), Blackwell Science Ltd., PO Box 88, Oxford OX2 0NE, United Kingdom. TEL 44-1865-206180, 44-1865-206002, FAX 44-1865-206219, jnl.orders@blacksci.co.uk, http://www.blackwell-science.com/~cgilib/jnlpage.asp?Journal=meded&File=meded, http://www.blackwellpublishing.com. Ed. J Bligh. Pub. Allen Stevens. R&P Sophie Savage. Adv. contact Jenny Applin. Circ: 1,565.

610.7 USA ISSN 1087-2981
MEDICAL EDUCATION ONLINE. Text in English. 1996. q. *Refereed.* **Description:** Covers health science education.
Media: Online - full text.
Address: meo@utmb.edu, http://www.utmb.edu/meo/. Ed. David Solomon.

610.711 GBR ISSN 1352-3929
MEDICAL EDUCATION. SUPPLEMENT. Text in English. irreg.
—ADONIS.
Published by: Blackwell Science Ltd., Osney Mead, Oxford OX2 0EL, United Kingdom. TEL 44-1865-206206, FAX 44-1865-721205, journals.cs@blacksci.co.uk, http://www.blackwell-science.com/.

MEDICAL ELECTRONICS MANUFACTURING. see *ELECTRONICS*

610.28 GBR ISSN 1350-4533
CODEN: MEPHEO
MEDICAL ENGINEERING & PHYSICS. Text in English. 1979. 10/yr. EUR 177 in Europe to individuals; JPY 23,500 in Japan to individuals; USD 198 elsewhere to individuals; EUR 1,162 in Europe to institutions; JPY 154,300 in Japan to institutions; USD 1,300 elsewhere to institutions (effective 2002). adv. bk.rev. abstr, illus. index. back issues avail.; reprints avail. *Refereed.* **Document type:** *Academic/Scholarly.* **Description:** Provides a forum in which developments in health care can be described and analyzed critically. Covers advances in instrumentation, solutions to particular patient problems, biomedical computing, clinical engineering, biological systems, and function replacement.
Formerly (until 1994): Journal of Biomedical Engineering (0141-5425)
Related titles: Microform ed.: (from PQC); Online - full text ed.: (from ingenta, ScienceDirect, Swets Blackwell, Institute for Scientific Information).
Indexed: AMED, ASCA, Appl.Mech.Rev., Bioeng.Abstr., Biol.Abstr., Biotech.& Bioeng.Abstr., Chem.Abstr., Compumath, Curr.Cont., Cyb.Abstr., Dent.Ind., Eng.Ind., Excerp.Med., INSPEC (Oct.1979-Nov.1993, Jan.1994-), Ind.Med. (1994-), Ind.Sci.Rev., Inpharma, Int.Abstr.Biol.Sci., Neurosci.Cit.Ind., Reac., SSCI (coverage dropped), Sci.Cit.Ind.
—BLDSC (5527.323000), ADONIS, AskIEEE, CASDDS, CISTI, Ei, EMDOCS, GNLM, IDS, ingenta, Linda Hall. **CCC.**
Published by: (Biological Engineering Society), Pergamon (Subsidiary of: Elsevier Science), The Boulevard, Langford Ln, East Park, Kidlington, Oxford OXB 1GB, United Kingdom. FAX 44-1865-843010, http://www.elsevier.nl/locate/medengphy. Eds. G H Byford, Robert Allen. **Subscr. in Australasia and the Far East to:** Elsevier Science (Singapore) Pte Ltd, No.1 Temasek Ave, 17-01 Millenia Tower, Singapore 039192, Singapore. TEL 65-434-3727, FAX 65-337-2230; **Subscr. in the Americas to:** Elsevier Science, PO Box 945, New York, NY 10159-0945. TEL 212-633-3730, FAX 212-633-3680, usinfo-f@elsevier.com; **Subscr. to:** Elsevier Science BV, PO Box 211, Amsterdam 1000 AE, Netherlands. TEL 31-20-485-3757.

610 DEU ISSN 0946-5200
MEDICAL EQUIPMENT AND SUPPLY GUIDE. Variant title: Made for Export - Medical Equipment and Supply Guide. Text in English. 1981. a. USD 50 (effective 2001). adv. index. back issues avail. **Document type:** *Catalog, Trade.*
Formerly: Made in Europe - Medical Equipment and Supply Guide (0720-597X)
Related titles: CD-ROM ed.
—GNLM.
Published by: Made in Europe Marketing Organisation GmbH, Unterhainstr 50, Aschaffenburg 63743, Germany. TEL 49-6021-391850, FAX 49-6021-3918525, mie@miesys.com, http://www.miesys.com. Ed., Pub., R&P Martin Romer. Adv. contact Franziska Bastanier. Circ: 20,200.

MEDICAL EQUIPMENT DESIGNER; the digest of medical engineering news. see *INSTRUMENTS*

174.2 USA ISSN 0886-0653
MEDICAL ETHICS ADVISOR. Text in English. 1985. m. USD 399 domestic (effective 2001); USD 389 foreign (effective 1999). reprints avail. **Document type:** *Newsletter.*
Related titles: Online - full text ed.: (from Northern Light Technology, Inc.).
Published by: American Health Consultants (Subsidiary of: Medical Economics Co., Inc.), 3525 Piedmont Rd, N E, 6 Piedmont Center, Ste 400, Atlanta, GA 30305. TEL 404-262-5476, 800-688-2421, FAX 404-262-5447, customerservice@ahcpub.com, http://www.ahcpub.com. Ed. Kevin New. Circ: 4,500 (paid).

610 011 GBR ISSN 0956-8298
MEDICAL EXPRESS REPORTS. Text in English. 1989. irreg. **Document type:** *Proceedings.* **Description:** Provides fast news coverage of specific medical meetings.
Published by: Cambridge Medical Publications Ltd., Wicker House, High St, Worthing, W Sussex BN11 1DJ, United Kingdom. TEL 44-1903-205884, FAX 44-1903-234862, cmp@hbase.com, http://www.cambridge-medical.com.

610 011 GBR ISSN 0958-3505
MEDICAL FORUM REPORTER. Text in English. 1989. irreg. **Document type:** *Proceedings.* **Description:** Provides close reporting of symposia and specific congress and conference sessions.
Published by: Cambridge Medical Publications Ltd., Wicker House, High St, Worthing, W Sussex BN11 1DJ, United Kingdom. TEL 44-1903-205884, FAX 44-1903-234862, cmp@hbase.com, http://www.cambridge-medical.com.

610 PAK
MEDICAL GAZETTE. Text in English. 1971 (vol.2). s-m. PKR 200.
Published by: Pakistan Medical Association, P.M.A. House, Aga Khan III Rd., Karachi 74400, Pakistan. TEL 92-21-7214632, FAX 92-21-7226443. Circ: 12,000.

610 USA ISSN 0277-805X
CODEN: MGRODY
MEDICAL GRAND ROUNDS. Text in English. 1982. w. USD 150 (effective 1996). adv. bibl, illus. back issues avail. *Refereed.* **Document type:** *Academic/Scholarly.*
Indexed: Excerp.Med.
—CISTI, GNLM. **CCC.**
Published by: University of Texas, Southwestern Medical Center, 5323 Harry Hines Blvd, Dallas, TX 75235-9030. TEL 214-648-2635, FAX 214-648-9100. Ed. Patrick Wong.

610 USA ISSN 0891-799X
THE MEDICAL HERALD. Text in English. 1991. m. USD 18. **Document type:** *Newspaper.* **Description:** Reports on subjects of concern to attending physicians who practice in the urban centers of America, including the impact of the current fiscal crisis on health care, AIDS, hypertension, cancer and other diseases.
Published by: Medical Herald Publishing Co., Inc., 211 E 43rd St, Ste 908, New York, NY 10017. TEL 212-983-3525, FAX 212-922-9211. Ed. Hugh W Wyatt. adv.: B&W page USD 3,440, color page USD 4,600; trim 11.5 x 8.19. Circ: 50,000.

610 GBR ISSN 0025-7273
R131.A1 CODEN: MDHIAA
MEDICAL HISTORY; devoted to the history and bibliography of medicine and the related sciences. Text in English. 1957. q. GBP 69. adv. bk.rev. bibl, illus. index. *Refereed.* **Document type:** *Academic/Scholarly.*
Related titles: Online - full text ed.: (from Northern Light Technology, Inc., ProQuest Information & Learning, Institute for Scientific Information).

M

Indexed: ASCA, Abstr.Hyg., Amer.Hist.& Life, Arts & Hum.Cit.Ind., Bibl.Ling., Biol.Abstr., Br.Archaeol.Abstr., Curr.Adv.Ecol.Sci., Curr.Cont., Dairy Sci.Abstr., Excerp.Med., Fam.Ind., Hist.Abstr. (1967-), IBZ, Ind.Med. (1957-), Ind.Sci.Rev., Ind.Vet., Inpharma, Numis.Lit., Nutr.Abstr., P C I, Protozool.Abstr., Reac., Rev.Appl.Entomol., Russ.Acad.Sci.Bibl., SSCI, Sci.Cit.Ind., Trop.Dis.Bull., Vet.Bull.
—BLDSC (5527.500000), CISTI, GNLM, ingenta, Linda Hall.
Published by: (Wellcome Institute for the History of Medicine), Professional & Scientific Publications, BMA House, Tavistock St, London WC2E 7PH, United Kingdom. TEL 0171-383-6640, FAX 0171-383-6662. Eds. V Nutton, W F Bynum. Circ: 1,000.

610 174.2 GBR ISSN 1468-215X
▼ **MEDICAL HUMANITIES.** Text in English. 2000. 2/yr. GBP 22, USD 34 combined subscription to individuals includes print & online eds. (effective 2002). adv. *Refereed.* **Document type:** *Journal, Academic/Scholarly.* **Description:** Explores the integration of the scientific understanding of physical nature and the humanistic understanding of experience.
Related titles: Online - full text ed.: ISSN 1473-4265. GBP 20, USD 30 to individuals (effective 2002) (from ingenta, HighWire Pr., RoweCom Information Quest); ♦ Supplement to: Journal of Medical Ethics. ISSN 0306-6800.
Published by: (Institute of Medical Ethics), B M J Publishing Group, B M A House, Tavistock Sq, London WC1H 9JR, United Kingdom. TEL 44-20-7387-4499, FAX 44-20-7383-6400, info.norththames@bma.org.uk, http://mh.bmjjournals.com/, http://www.bma.org.uk. Eds. David Greaves, Martyn Evans. Adv. contact Euan Currer TEL 44-20-7383-6181.

MEDICAL HUMANITIES REVIEW. see *HUMANITIES: COMPREHENSIVE WORKS*

610 GBR ISSN 0306-9877
R5 CODEN: MEHYDY
MEDICAL HYPOTHESES. Text in English. 1975. m. GBP 123 to individuals; GBP 776 to institutions (effective 2002). adv. bk.rev. back issues avail. *Refereed.* **Document type:** *Academic/Scholarly.* **Description:** Provides a forum for the presentation and criticism of ideas in medicine and the related biomedical sciences.
Related titles: Microform ed.: (from PQC); Online - full text ed.: (from EBSCO Publishing, RoweCom Information Quest, ingenta, Swets Blackwell, IDEAL Online Library, Institute for Scientific Information).
Indexed: ASCA, Anim.Breed.Abstr., Biol.Abstr., C.I.S. Abstr., Chem.Abstr., Chem.Titles, Chic.Per.Ind., Crim.Just.Abstr., Curr.Adv.Cancer Res., Curr.Adv.Cell & Devel.Biol., Curr.Adv.Ecol.Sci., Curr.Adv.Gen.& Molec.Biol., Curr.Cont., Dairy Sci.Abstr., Dok.Arbeitsmed., Excerp.Med., Helminthol.Abstr., Ind.Med. (1975-), Ind.Sci.Rev., Ind.Vet., Inpharma, NRN, Neurosci.Cit.Ind., Nutr.Abstr., Pharm.&Out.News, Protozool.Abstr., Psychol.Abstr., Reac., Ref.Zh., Rev.Appl.Entomol., Rev.Med.& Vet.Mycol., SSCI (coverage dropped), Sci.Cit.Ind., Small Anim.Abstr., Vet.Bull., Weed Abstr.
—BLDSC (5527.530000), ADONIS, CASDDS, CISTI, EMDOCS, GNLM, IDS, ingenta, KNAW. **CCC.**
Published by: Churchill Livingstone (Subsidiary of: Harcourt Publishers Ltd.), Robert Stevenson House, 1-3 Baxter's Pl, Leith Walk, Edinburgh, Midlothian EH1 3AF, United Kingdom. TEL 44-131-556-2424, FAX 44-131-459-1177, cservice@harcourt, http://www.harcourt-international.com/journals/mehy. Ed. Dr. David F Horrobin. Pub. Gillian Griffith. R&P Catherine John TEL 212-424-4200. Adv. contact David Dunnachie. Circ: 300. **Subscr. to:** Harcourt Publishers Ltd., Foots Cray High St, Sidcup, Kent DA14 5HP, United Kingdom. TEL 44-20-8308-5700, FAX 44-20-8309-0807.

610 USA ISSN 1073-1202
MEDICAL IMAGING. Text in English. 1986. m. USD 60 domestic; USD 20 newsstand/cover foreign; USD 140, USD 40 foreign (2002). adv. **Document type:** *Newsletter, Trade.* **Description:** Provides health care professionals with the latest business news and information for the cost-effective management of medical imaging equipment and technology.
Formerly (until 1994): Second Source Imaging (1053-6876); Which superseded in part (in 1990): Second Source (0892-3426)
Published by: Medical World Communications, Allied Healthcare Group, 295 Promenade St, Ste 2, Providence, RI 02908-5720. TEL 401-455-0555, FAX 401-455-1555, info@healthtechnet.com, http://www.healthtechnet.com. Ed. Mary C Tierney. Pub. Jack Spears. adv.: B&W page USD 2,595, color page USD 3,490. Circ: 17,000 (controlled).

610 USA
MEDICAL IMAGING INTERNATIONAL. Text in English; Summaries in French, German, Italian, Spanish. 1991. bi-m. USD 80 to non-members. adv. **Document type:** *Trade.*
Formerly: Medical Care International (1068-1779)
Published by: Globetech Publishing, 8 Cannon Rd, Wilton, CT 06897. TEL 203-762-3432, FAX 203-762-8640. Ed. Jill Quigley Roberge. Pub. Marc Gueron. Adv. contact Patricia Walsh. Circ: 26,000 (controlled).

610 USA ISSN 1074-4819
MEDICAL IMAGING NEWS. Text in English. 1992. w. USD 699 domestic; USD 799 foreign (effective 2000). **Document type:** *Newsletter, Trade.* **Description:** Provides objective coverage of all the breaking news in medical imaging.
Formerly (until 1994): Imaging Newsource (1067-1838)
Published by: Medical World Communications, Allied Healthcare Group, 295 Promenade St, Ste 2, Providence, RI 02908-5720. TEL 401-455-0555, FAX 401-455-1555, info@healthtechnet.com, http://www.healthtechnet.com. Ed. Mary C Tierney.

MEDICAL INDUSTRY EMPLOYMENT OPPORTUNITIES. see *OCCUPATIONS AND CAREERS*

MEDICAL INDUSTRY WEEK. see *INSTRUMENTS*

616.98 IND ISSN 0377-1237
MEDICAL JOURNAL ARMED FORCES INDIA. Text in English. 1945. q. INR 200, USD 60 (effective 2000). adv. bk.rev. charts, illus, stat. *Refereed.* **Document type:** *Academic/Scholarly.* **Description:** Contains original work and case reports.
Formerly (until 1974): Armed Forces Medical Journal, India (0004-2218)
Related titles: CD-ROM ed.
Indexed: Abstr.Hyg., Bio-Contr.News & Info., Biol.Abstr., Excerp.Med. (until 19??), ExtraMED, Helminthol.Abstr., INIS Atomind., Nutr.Abstr., Protozool.Abstr., Rev.Appl.Entomol., Rev.Med.& Vet.Mycol., Trop.Dis.Bull.
Published by: Armed Forces Medical Services, c/o Armed Forces Medical College, Pune, Maharashtra 411 040, India. TEL 91-20-673290, FAX 91-20-674759. Ed., Adv. contact Capt. H Subramanya. page INR 5,000. Circ: 5,000 (paid).

610 AUS ISSN 0025-729X
CODEN: MJAUAJ
MEDICAL JOURNAL OF AUSTRALIA. Text in English. 1914. s-m. AUD 235 domestic; AUD 335 foreign (effective 2000). adv. bk.rev. abstr, bibl, illus. s-a. index. reprint service avail. from PQC. *Refereed.* **Document type:** *Academic/Scholarly.*
Related titles: Microform ed.: (from PQC,PMC); Online - full text ed.: (from Gale Group, Institute for Scientific Information).
Indexed: A.D.& D., AESIS, AIDS Abstr., AMED, ASCA, Abstr.Hyg., AgeLine, Agri.& Environ.Biotech.Abstr. (coverage dropped), Aqua.Sci.& Fish.Abstr., Aus.P.A.I.S. (Coverage Dropped), Aus.Rd.Ind., Bibl.Dev.Med.& Child Neur., Biol.Abstr., CINAHL, C.I.S. Abstr., Chem.Abstr., Curr.Adv.Cancer Res., Curr.Adv.Ecol.Sci., Curr.Cont., Dairy Sci.Abstr., Dent.Ind., Derwent Biotech.Abstr., Diar.Dis.Res., Dok.Arbeitsmed., Environ.Sci.Poll.Mgmt., Excerp.Med., Fam.Ind., Forest Prod.Abstr., HRIS, Helminthol.Abstr., INIS Atomind., I.P.A., Ind.Med. (1914-), Ind.Sci.Rev., Ind.Vet., Inpharma, Int.Nurs.Ind., Kidney, Lab.Haz.Bull., Med.& Surg.Dermat., Med.Care Rev., NRN, Neurosci.Cit.Ind., Nutr.Abstr., Pharm.&Out.News, Pollut.Abstr., Protozool.Abstr., Reac., Rev.Appl.Entomol., Rev.Arom.& Med.Plants, Rev.Med.& Vet.Mycol., Rev.Plant Path., Risk Abstr., Rural Devel.Abstr., Rural Recreat.Tour.Abstr., SSCI (coverage dropped), Saf.Sci.Abstr., Sci.Cit.Ind., Soyabean Abstr., THA, Trop.Dis.Bull., Vet.Bull., Wild.Rev.
—BLDSC (5529.000000), CASDDS, CISTI, GNLM, IDS, ingenta, KNAW. **CCC.**
Published by: Australian Medical Association, Locked Bag 2045, North Ryde, NSW 2113, Australia. TEL 61-2-98875003, FAX 61-2-98875895, ampco@ampco.com.au, http://www.mja.com.au. Ed. Martin Van Der Weyden. R&P Jo Elliot. Adv. contact Peter Butterfield. B&W page AUD 1,475, color page AUD 2,310. Circ: 23,000.

610 MYS ISSN 0300-5283
CODEN: MJMLAI
MEDICAL JOURNAL OF MALAYSIA. Text in English. q. MYR 280. adv. bk.rev. charts, illus, stat.
Formerly: Medical Journal of Malaya (0025-7303)
Indexed: Abstr.Hyg., Bibl.Asian Stud. (1976-1987), Biol.Abstr., CINAHL, Chem.Abstr., Dent.Ind., Excerp.Med., Helminthol.Abstr., Ind.Med. (1972-), Ind.Vet., Nutr.Abstr., Protozool.Abstr., Rev.Appl.Entomol., Rev.Med.& Vet.Mycol., Rural Devel.Abstr., Soyabean Abstr., Trop.Dis.Bull.
—BLDSC (5529.151000), CASDDS, EMDOCS, GNLM, ingenta.
Published by: Malaysian Medical Association, 4th Fl MMA House, 124 Jalan, Kuala Lumpur, Pahang 53000, Malaysia. TEL 03-4420617, FAX 03-4418187. Ed. Victor Lim.

610 IRN ISSN 1016-1430
MEDICAL JOURNAL OF THE ISLAMIC REPUBLIC OF IRAN. Text in English. 1987. q. USD 50 to individuals; USD 80 to institutions. *Refereed.* **Document type:** *Academic/Scholarly.* **Description:** Publishes original articles in clinical science and basic science in medicine, case reports, review articles, and articles on medicine in Islamic culture.
Related titles: CD-ROM ed.
Indexed: Excerp.Med. (1996-), ExtraMED, Per.Islam. (1992-).
—BLDSC (5529.100000), EMDOCS, GNLM.
Published by: National Center for Scientific Research, Enghelab Ave 1188, P O Box 13145-478, Tehran 13158, Iran. TEL 98-21-6462778, FAX 98-21-6468180. Ed. Dr. N Simforoosh. R&P H Sanagouy.

610 ZMB ISSN 0047-651X
CODEN: MJZAAG
MEDICAL JOURNAL OF ZAMBIA* . Text in English. 1967. bi-m. adv. bk.rev. index. **Document type:** *Academic/Scholarly.*
Indexed: Abstr.Hyg., Biol.Abstr., Curr.Cont. (coverage dropped), Excerp.Med., Helminthol.Abstr., Ind.Med. (coverage dropped), Ind.Vet., Nutr.Abstr., Protozool.Abstr., Trop.Dis.Bull., Vet.Bull.
—GNLM.
Published by: Zambia Medical Association, PO Box RW 148, Lusaka, Zambia. Ed. M N Lowenthal. Circ: 1,700.

MEDICAL LASER INSIGHT. see *PHYSICS—Optics*

MEDICAL LASER REPORT. see *PHYSICS—Optics*

MEDICAL LAW INTERNATIONAL. see *LAW*

MEDICAL LAW MONITOR. see *LAW*

342.441 610 GBR ISSN 0957-9346
MEDICAL LAW REPORTS. Text in English. 1989. 10/yr. (plus a. cumulation). GBP 178, USD 274; includes cumulation. **Document type:** *Academic/Scholarly.*
Published by: Lloyds of London Press Ltd., Sheepen Pl, Cochester, Essex C03 3LP, United Kingdom.

MEDICAL LAW REVIEW. see *LAW*

610 344.041 USA
MEDICAL LAW'S REGAN REPORT. Text in English. 1968. m. USD 52 domestic; USD 64 foreign (effective 2000). stat. reprints avail. **Description:** Reports the latest appellate court decisions on medical law.
Formerly: Regan Report on Medical Law (0034-3188)
Related titles: Microform ed.: (from PQC); Online - full text ed.: (from Gale Group).
Indexed: CINAHL.
—CCC.
Published by: Medica Press Inc., 10 Dorrance St, Ste 500, Providence, RI 02903-2018. TEL 401-421-4747, FAX 401-521-9226. Ed., R&P, Adv. contact A David Tammelleo. Circ: 5,000.

MEDICAL MALPRACTICE (CHARLOTTESVILLE). see *LAW—Civil Law*

344.041 USA
MEDICAL MALPRACTICE: CHECKLISTS AND DISCOVERIES. Text in English. a. (in 3 vols.). USD 420 (effective 2000). **Document type:** *Academic/Scholarly.*
Published by: West Group (Subsidiary of: Thomson Corporation, The), 620 Opperman Dr., Eagan, MN 55123. TEL 800-344-5008, FAX 800-340-9378, http://www.westgroup.com. Eds. Douglas Danner, Larry L Varn, Susan J Mathias.

MEDICAL MALPRACTICE: GUIDE TO MEDICAL ISSUES. see *LAW*

MEDICAL MALPRACTICE: HANDLING EMERGENCY CASES. see *LAW—Civil Law*

MEDICAL MALPRACTICE: HANDLING INTERNAL MEDICINE CASES. see *LAW—Civil Law*

MEDICAL MALPRACTICE LAW & STRATEGY. see *LAW—Civil Law*

MEDICAL MALPRACTICE (NEW YORK). see *LAW—Civil Law*

MEDICAL MALPRACTICE REPORTS. see *LAW—Civil Law*

MEDICAL MALPRACTICE VERDICTS, SETTLEMENTS & EXPERTS. see *LAW—Civil Law*

610 USA ISSN 1077-3436
MEDICAL MATERIALS UPDATE. Text in English. 1977. m. USD 395 (effective 1999). **Document type:** *Newsletter.*
Related titles: Online - full text ed.: (from LexisNexis, Northern Light Technology, Inc., Gale Group, Factiva).
Published by: Business Communications Co., Inc. (Norwalk), 25 Van Zant St, Ste 13, Norwalk, CT 06855-1781. TEL 203-853-4266, FAX 203-853-0348. Ed. Melvin Schlechter.

616.01 GBR
MEDICAL MICROBIOLOGIST. Abbreviated title: Med Micro. Text in English. 1996. 2/yr. bk.rev. **Document type:** *Academic/Scholarly.*
Published by: Hayward Medical Communications Ltd., Covent Garden, Seven Dials Warehouse, 44 Earlham St, London WC2H 9LA, United Kingdom. TEL 44-20-7240-4493, FAX 44-20-7240-4479, admin@hayward.co.uk, http://www.hayward.co.uk. Ed. Dr. Paul Wright. Circ: 1,000. **Subscr. to:** Rosemary Huse, Lanades Park, Kentford, Near Newmarket, Suffolk CB8 7PW, United Kingdom. TEL 44-1638-751515, FAX 44-4638-751517.

MEDICAL MISSION NEWS. see *RELIGIONS AND THEOLOGY—Roman Catholic*

610 GBR
MEDICAL MONITOR. Text in English. 1987. fortn. GBP 70 domestic; USD 120 foreign (effective 2000). **Document type:** *Trade.*
Former titles: Medical Monitor Weekly (1350-6897); (until 1993): Medical Monitor (0953-1408)
Published by: Medicom Publishing, Churston House, Portsmouth Rd, Esher, Surrey KT10 9AD, United Kingdom. TEL 44-1372-471671, FAX 44-1372-471672. Ed. Louise Wright. Pub. Stephen Townsend.

MEDICAL NEWS REPORT. see *BUSINESS AND ECONOMICS—Marketing And Purchasing*

MEDICAL OFFICE MANAGER; the newsletter for physician office administrators. see *BUSINESS AND ECONOMICS—Management*

368.382 USA ISSN 0895-4313
MEDICAL OFFICE REPORT. Text in English. 1988. m. USD 168. charts, stat. back issues avail. **Description:** Offers the latest Medicare reimbursement and policy information for the office physician.
Published by: Washington G - 2 Reports, 1111 14th St N W, Ste 500, Washington, DC 20005. TEL 202-789-1034, 800-LAB-REGS, FAX 202-289-4062. Ed. D J Curren. Pub. Dennis W Weissman. Circ: 16,000 (paid).

610 USA ISSN 1067-4195
MEDICAL OUTCOMES AND GUIDELINES ALERT. Text in English. 1993. s-m. USD 395 (effective 1999). **Document type:** *Trade.* **Description:** Covers medical outcomes research and clinical guidelines development.
Related titles: Online - full text ed.: (from Gale Group, NewsNet, ProQuest Information & Learning).
Indexed: Inpharma, Reac.
—CCC.
Published by: Thompson Financial / I M G Media, Healthcare Information Center (Subsidiary of: Thompson Publishing Group), 11 Penn Plaza, 17th Fl, New York, NY 10001-2006. TEL 212-967-7000, 800-535-8403. Ed. Laura Newman.

530 610 USA ISSN 0094-2405
R895.A1 CODEN: MPHYA6
MEDICAL PHYSICS. Text in English. 1974. m. USD 230 to members; USD 725 to non-members (effective 2001). adv. bk.rev. abstr. cum.index: vols. 1-10, 1985; vols. 11-20, 1994. back issues avail. *Refereed.* **Document type:** *Academic/Scholarly.* **Description:** Presents research concerned with the application of physics and mathematics to the solution of problems in medicine and human biology.
Formerly: A.A.P.M. Quarterly Bulletin (0001-0162)
Related titles: Microfiche ed.: (from AIP); Microform ed.: (from AIP); Online - full text ed.: (from EBSCO Publishing, RoweCom Information Quest, Swets Blackwell, Institute for Scientific Information).
Indexed: ASCA, Abstr.Health Care Manage.Stud., Appl.Mech.Rev., Biol.Abstr., C.P.I., Chem.Abstr., Chem.Indus.Notes, Chem.Titles, Compumath, Curr.Cont., Dent.Ind., Excerp.Med., Gen.Phys.Adv.Abstr., INIS Atomind., INSPEC (1974-), Ind.Med. (1974-), Ind.Sci.Rev., Inpharma, Phys.Ber., Reac., SPINweb, Sci.Cit.Ind.
—BLDSC (5531.130000), AskIEEE, CASDDS, CISTI, GNLM, IDS, ingenta. **CCC.**
Published by: (American Association of Physicists in Medicine), American Institute of Physics, 2 Huntington Quadrangle, Suite 1NO1, Melville, NY 11747-4502. TEL 516-576-2270, FAX 516-349-9704, subs@aip.org, http://ojps.aip.org/medphys. Ed. Colin Orton. Adv. contact Richard Kobel. **Subscr. to:** AIP Member and Subscriber Service.

610 CAN ISSN 0025-7435
THE MEDICAL POST. Text in English. 1965. fortn. CND 41. adv. bk.rev. abstr, charts, illus. **Document type:** *Magazine, Trade.* **Description:** Covers clinical, political and social news for physicians.
Related titles: Microfilm ed.: (from MML); Microform ed.: (from MML); Online - full text ed.: (from LexisNexis).
Indexed: CBCA Bus. (1996-), CBCA Ref., Can.B.P.I.
—CISTI, Infotrieve. **CCC.**
Published by: Rogers Media Publishing Ltd, 777 Bay St, 6th Fl, Toronto, ON M5W 1A7, Canada. TEL 416-596-5000, FAX 416-596-5881, medpost@rmpublishing.com, http://www.medicalpost.com, http://www.rogers.com. Circ: 37,000.

610 JPN ISSN 0910-1551
MEDICAL PRACTICE. Variant title: M.P. Medical Practice. Text in Japanese. 1984. m. JPY 2,100 per issue.
Published by: Bunkodo Co. Ltd., 2-7 Hongo 7-chome, Bunkyo-ku, Tokyo 113-0033, Japan.

610 USA ISSN 1074-1321
MEDICAL PRACTICE COMMUNICATOR. Text in English. 1994. 6/yr. USD 195 domestic; USD 235 foreign (effective 2000). adv. bk.rev. **Document type:** *Newsletter.* **Description:** Aimed at enhancing physician communication with patients, peers, and staff. Provides articles on such topics as writing clearly, computerizing medical records, and preventing lawsuits against your practice.
Related titles: Online - full text ed.
Published by: Healthcare Media International (HMI), Inc., 113 Naudain St, Philadelphia, PA 19147-2406. HMI3000@aol.com, http://www.healthpublishing.com. Ed. Dr. John Garland. Circ: 26,000 (paid).

610 GBR
MEDICAL PRACTICES COMMITTEE. RECRUITMENT SURVEY (YEAR). Text in English. a. **Document type:** *Government.* **Description:** Covers membership, surveys, GP vacancies, summary of findings, and more.
Formerly (until 1998): Medical Practices Committee. Survey of G P Recruitment in England and Wales
—BLDSC.
Published by: Medical Practices Committee, 1st Fl Eileen House, 80-94 Newington Causeway, London SE1 6EF, United Kingdom. TEL 44-20-7972-2930, FAX 44-20-7972-2985, http://www.open.gov.uk/doh/mpc/mpch.htm.

▼ **MEDICAL PRESCRIPTION OF NARCOTICS.** see *PHARMACY AND PHARMACOLOGY*

610 CHE ISSN 1011-7571
MEDICAL PRINCIPLES AND PRACTICE. Text in English. 1989. q. CHF 621, EUR 444.20 in Europe to institutions; CHF 632.60, USD 483 elsewhere to institutions (effective 2002). adv. bk.rev. back issues avail. *Refereed.* **Document type:** *Journal, Academic/Scholarly.* **Description:** Concentrates on the recent advances made in basic medical sciences, clinical practice and associated disciplines within human medicine.
Related titles: Microform ed.: (from PQC); Online - full text ed.: ISSN 1423-0151. CHF 58, EUR 42, USD 45 to institutions with print edition (effective 2002) (from EBSCO Publishing, O C L C Online Computer Library Center, Inc., RoweCom Information Quest, Swets Blackwell, Institute for Scientific Information).
Indexed: ASCA, Excerp.Med. (until 1993).
—BLDSC (5531.260000), GNLM, IDS, Infotrieve, KNAW. **CCC.**
Published by: (Kuwait University, Health Science Centre KWT), S. Karger AG, Allschwilerstr 10, PO Box, Basel 4009, Switzerland. TEL 41-61-3061111, http://www.online.karger.com/journals/mpp, http://www.karger.com. Ed. Farida Al-Awadi. adv.: page USD 1,195.

610 780 USA ISSN 0885-1158
CODEN: MPPAEC
MEDICAL PROBLEMS OF PERFORMING ARTISTS. Text in English. 1986. q., latest vol.16, 2001. USD 56 domestic to individuals; USD 66 foreign to individuals; USD 76 domestic to institutions; USD 86 foreign to institutions; USD 20 newsstand/cover (effective 2001). adv. bk.rev. illus. index. back issues avail.; reprints avail. *Refereed.* **Document type:** *Journal, Academic/Scholarly.* **Description:** Concerned with medical and surgical problems deriving from artistic performance in dance, music and theater.
Related titles: Online - full text ed.: (from Institute for Scientific Information).
Indexed: ASCA, Arts & Hum.Cit.Ind., Curr.Cont., Excerp.Med. (1996-), Focus on: Sports Sci.& Med., IIPA (1993-1996, 1999), Ind.Dance Per., Int.Ind.Mus.Per., Music Ind., SSCI (coverage dropped).
—BLDSC (5531.280000), EMDOCS, GNLM, IDS, ingenta. **CCC.**
Published by: Hanley & Belfus, Inc., 210 S 13th St, Philadelphia, PA 19107. TEL 215-546-7293, FAX 215-790-9330, http://www.hanleyandbelfus.com/journals/mppa.html. Ed. Alice Brand fonbrener. Circ: 1,000.

610.29 JPN ISSN 1341-6146
MEDICAL PRODUCTS OF JAPAN; medical equipment directory. Text in English. 1993 (no.15). a. USD 120 (effective 2001). adv. illus. 380 p./no. **Document type:** *Directory.* **Description:** Covers more than 1,900 products from some 250 companies, ranging from small diagnostic tools to large systems like computer tomography unit.
Published by: Genyosha Publications Inc., 4-7 Shibuya 2-chome, Shibuya-ku, Tokyo 150-0002, Japan. TEL 81-3-3407-7521, FAX 81-3-3407-7902, info@genyosha.co.jp, http://www.genyosha.com. Circ: 7,500.

610 681 USA ISSN 0279-4802
MEDICAL PRODUCTS SALES. Variant title: M P S. Text in English. 1970. m. USD 49.95 domestic; USD 55.95 in Canada & Mexico; USD 69.95 elsewhere; USD 9 newsstand/cover domestic (effective 2001). adv. bk.rev. illus, mkt, pat, stat, tr.mk, tr.lit. back issues avail.; reprints avail. **Document type:** *Magazine, Trade.* **Description:** Covers sale and distribution of health care products to the hospital, physician's office and clinic, long-term care and home health care markets.
Incorporates (1995-1999): Infection Control and Sterilization Technology (1078-8972); Formerly (until 1981): Medical Products Salesman (0192-432X)
—Infotrieve. **CCC.**
Published by: (Health Industry Distributors Association), Douglas Publications, Inc., 2807 N Parham Rd, Ste 200, Richmond, VA 23294. TEL 804-762-9600, FAX 804-217-8999, info@douglaspublications.com, http://www.medicalproductssales.com. Ed. Susan Helmer. Pub., Adv. contact Stephanie A Ellis TEL 847-202-1577. B&W page USD 4,210, color page USD 5,670; trim 10.875 x 14. Circ: 30,000 (controlled). **Subscr. to:** Medical Products Sales, P O Box 383, Winchester, MA 01890. FAX 781-729-4862.

610 HKG ISSN 1015-4256
MEDICAL PROGRESS (INDONESIA EDITION). Text and summaries in English. 1973. m. adv. *Refereed.* **Document type:** *Academic/Scholarly, Trade.*
Related titles: ♦ Regional ed.: Medical Progress (Southeast Asia Editions). ISSN 0377-9963; ♦ Medical Progress (Taiwan Edition). ISSN 1015-4310; ♦ Medical Progress (Singapore Edition). ISSN 1015-4302; ♦ Medical Progress (Philippines Edition). ISSN 1015-4299; ♦ Medical Progress (Malaysia Edition). ISSN 1015-4272; ♦ Medical Progress (Korea Edition); ♦ Medical Progress (Thailand Edition). ISSN 1015-4329; ♦ Medical Progress (Pakistan Edition). ISSN 1015-4280.
Published by: MediMedia Asia (Subsidiary of: MediMedia Pacific Ltd.), 8-F Pacific Plaza, 410 Des Voeux Rd W, Hong Kong, Hong Kong. TEL 852-2559-5888, FAX 852-2559-6910, mmp@medimedia.com.hk, http://www.medimedia.com.

610 HKG
MEDICAL PROGRESS (KOREA EDITION). Text and summaries in English. m. adv. *Refereed.* **Document type:** *Academic/Scholarly, Trade.*

M

Related titles: ♦ Regional ed.: Medical Progress (Southeast Asia Editions). ISSN 0377-9963; ♦ Medical Progress (Taiwan Edition). ISSN 1015-4310; ♦ Medical Progress (Singapore Edition). ISSN 1015-4302; ♦ Medical Progress (Philippines Edition). ISSN 1015-4299; ♦ Medical Progress (Malaysia Edition). ISSN 1015-4272; ♦ Medical Progress (Indonesia Edition). ISSN 1015-4256; ♦ Medical Progress (Thailand Edition). ISSN 1015-4329; ♦ Medical Progress (Pakistan Edition). ISSN 1015-4280.
Indexed: Inpharma, Reac.
Published by: MediMedia Asia (Subsidiary of: MediMedia Pacific Ltd.), 8-F Pacific Plaza, 410 Des Voeux Rd W, Hong Kong, Hong Kong. TEL 852-2559-5888, FAX 852-2559-6910, mmp@medimedia.com.hk, http://www.medimedia.com.

610 HKG ISSN 1015-4272
MEDICAL PROGRESS (MALAYSIA EDITION). Text and summaries in English. 1974. m. adv. *Refereed.* **Document type:** *Academic/Scholarly, Trade.*
Related titles: ♦ Regional ed.: Medical Progress (Southeast Asia Editions). ISSN 0377-9963; ♦ Medical Progress (Taiwan Edition). ISSN 1015-4310; ♦ Medical Progress (Singapore Edition). ISSN 1015-4302; ♦ Medical Progress (Philippines Edition). ISSN 1015-4299; ♦ Medical Progress (Korea Edition); ♦ Medical Progress (Indonesia Edition). ISSN 1015-4256; ♦ Medical Progress (Thailand Edition). ISSN 1015-4329; ♦ Medical Progress (Pakistan Edition). ISSN 1015-4280.
Published by: MediMedia Asia (Subsidiary of: MediMedia Pacific Ltd.), 8-F Pacific Plaza, 410 Des Voeux Rd W, Hong Kong, Hong Kong. TEL 852-2559-5888, FAX 852-2559-6910, mmp@medimedia.com.hk, http://www.medimedia.com.

610 HKG ISSN 1015-4280
MEDICAL PROGRESS (PAKISTAN EDITION). Text in Chinese. 1985. m. adv. *Refereed.* **Document type:** *Academic/Scholarly, Trade.*
Related titles: ♦ Regional ed.: Medical Progress (Southeast Asia Editions). ISSN 0377-9963; ♦ Medical Progress (Taiwan Edition). ISSN 1015-4310; ♦ Medical Progress (Singapore Edition). ISSN 1015-4302; ♦ Medical Progress (Philippines Edition). ISSN 1015-4299; ♦ Medical Progress (Malaysia Edition). ISSN 1015-4272; ♦ Medical Progress (Korea Edition); ♦ Medical Progress (Indonesia Edition). ISSN 1015-4256; ♦ Medical Progress (Thailand Edition). ISSN 1015-4329.
Published by: MediMedia Asia (Subsidiary of: MediMedia Pacific Ltd.), 8-F Pacific Plaza, 410 Des Voeux Rd W, Hong Kong, Hong Kong. TEL 852-2559-5888, FAX 852-2559-6910, mmp@medimedia.com.hk, http://www.medimedia.com.

610 HKG ISSN 1015-4299
MEDICAL PROGRESS (PHILIPPINES EDITION). Text and summaries in English. 1973. m. adv. *Refereed.* **Document type:** *Academic/Scholarly, Trade.*
Related titles: ♦ Regional ed.: Medical Progress (Southeast Asia Editions). ISSN 0377-9963; ♦ Medical Progress (Taiwan Edition). ISSN 1015-4310; ♦ Medical Progress (Singapore Edition). ISSN 1015-4302; ♦ Medical Progress (Malaysia Edition). ISSN 1015-4272; ♦ Medical Progress (Korea Edition); ♦ Medical Progress (Indonesia Edition). ISSN 1015-4256; ♦ Medical Progress (Thailand Edition). ISSN 1015-4329; ♦ Medical Progress (Pakistan Edition). ISSN 1015-4280.
Published by: MediMedia Asia (Subsidiary of: MediMedia Pacific Ltd.), 8-F Pacific Plaza, 410 Des Voeux Rd W, Hong Kong, Hong Kong. TEL 852-2559-5888, FAX 852-2559-6910, mmp@medimedia.com.hk, http://www.medimedia.com.

610 HKG ISSN 1015-4302
MEDICAL PROGRESS (SINGAPORE EDITION). Text and summaries in English. 1973. m. adv. *Refereed.* **Document type:** *Academic/Scholarly, Trade.*
Related titles: ♦ Regional ed.: Medical Progress (Southeast Asia Editions). ISSN 0377-9963; ♦ Medical Progress (Taiwan Edition). ISSN 1015-4310; ♦ Medical Progress (Philippines Edition). ISSN 1015-4299; ♦ Medical Progress (Malaysia Edition). ISSN 1015-4272; ♦ Medical Progress (Korea Edition); ♦ Medical Progress (Indonesia Edition). ISSN 1015-4256; ♦ Medical Progress (Thailand Edition). ISSN 1015-4329; ♦ Medical Progress (Pakistan Edition). ISSN 1015-4280.
Published by: MediMedia Asia (Subsidiary of: MediMedia Pacific Ltd.), 8-F Pacific Plaza, 410 Des Voeux Rd W, Hong Kong, Hong Kong. TEL 852-2559-5888, FAX 852-2559-6910, mmp@medimedia.com.hk, http://www.medimedia.com.

610 HKG ISSN 0377-9963
CODEN: MEPRDJ
MEDICAL PROGRESS (SOUTHEAST ASIA EDITIONS). Variant title: Medical Progress - Hong Kong Edition. Text and summaries in English. 1974. m. USD 60; USD 72 foreign. adv. back issues avail. *Refereed.* **Document type:** *Academic/Scholarly, Trade.*
Related titles: ♦ Regional ed.: Medical Progress (Taiwan Edition). ISSN 1015-4310; ♦ Medical Progress (Singapore Edition). ISSN 1015-4302; ♦ Medical Progress (Philippines Edition). ISSN 1015-4299; ♦ Medical Progress (Malaysia Edition). ISSN 1015-4272; ♦ Medical Progress (Korea Edition); ♦ Medical Progress (Indonesia Edition). ISSN 1015-4256; ♦ Medical Progress (Thailand Edition). ISSN 1015-4329; ♦ Medical Progress (Pakistan Edition). ISSN 1015-4280.
—CASDDS, CISTI, GNLM.
Published by: MediMedia Asia (Subsidiary of: MediMedia Pacific Ltd.), 8-F Pacific Plaza, 410 Des Voeux Rd W, Hong Kong, Hong Kong. TEL 852-2559-5888, FAX 852-2559-6910, mmp@medimedia.com.hk, http://www.medimedia.com. Ed. Sarah Aglionby. Pub. Edgar B Richards. Circ: 30,900 (controlled).

610 HKG ISSN 1015-4310
MEDICAL PROGRESS (TAIWAN EDITION). Text and summaries in English. 1973. m. adv. *Refereed.* **Document type:** *Academic/Scholarly, Trade.*
Related titles: ♦ Regional ed.: Medical Progress (Southeast Asia Editions). ISSN 0377-9963; ♦ Medical Progress (Singapore Edition). ISSN 1015-4302; ♦ Medical Progress (Philippines Edition). ISSN 1015-4299; ♦ Medical Progress (Malaysia Edition). ISSN 1015-4272; ♦ Medical Progress (Korea Edition); ♦ Medical Progress (Indonesia Edition). ISSN 1015-4256; ♦ Medical Progress (Thailand Edition). ISSN 1015-4329; ♦ Medical Progress (Pakistan Edition). ISSN 1015-4280.
Published by: MediMedia Asia (Subsidiary of: MediMedia Pacific Ltd.), 8-F Pacific Plaza, 410 Des Voeux Rd W, Hong Kong, Hong Kong. TEL 852-2559-5888, FAX 852-2559-6910, mmp@medimedia.com.hk, http://www.medimedia.com.

610 HKG ISSN 1015-4329
MEDICAL PROGRESS (THAILAND EDITION). Text in Chinese. 1973. m. adv. *Refereed.* **Document type:** *Academic/Scholarly, Trade.*
Related titles: ♦ Regional ed.: Medical Progress (Southeast Asia Editions). ISSN 0377-9963; ♦ Medical Progress (Taiwan Edition). ISSN 1015-4310; ♦ Medical Progress (Singapore Edition). ISSN 1015-4302; ♦ Medical Progress (Philippines Edition). ISSN 1015-4299; ♦ Medical Progress (Malaysia Edition). ISSN 1015-4272; ♦ Medical Progress (Korea Edition); ♦ Medical Progress (Indonesia Edition). ISSN 1015-4256; ♦ Medical Progress (Pakistan Edition). ISSN 1015-4280.
Published by: MediMedia Asia (Subsidiary of: MediMedia Pacific Ltd.), 8-F Pacific Plaza, 410 Des Voeux Rd W, Hong Kong, Hong Kong. TEL 852-2559-5888, FAX 852-2559-6910, mmp@medimedia.com.hk, http://www.medimedia.com.

610 GBR ISSN 0076-5961
MEDICAL PROTECTION SOCIETY. ANNUAL REPORT. Text in English. 1892. a. membership. adv. **Document type:** *Corporate.*
Published by: Medical Protection Society Ltd., 50 Hallam St, London W1N 6DE, United Kingdom. TEL 44-171-637-0541, FAX 44-171-636-0690, TELEX 8952848 MEDPRO G. Ed. Lynne Richmond. Adv. contact Steven Grundy. Circ: 135,000 (controlled).

610 MWI ISSN 1017-2920
MEDICAL QUARTERLY. Text in English. 1980. q. **Document type:** *Academic/Scholarly.*
Indexed: Rural Devel.Abstr., Rural Ext.Educ.& Tr.Abstr.
Published by: (Medical Association of Malawi), Centraf Associates Ltd., Chichiri, PO Box 30462, Blantyre, Malawi.

MEDICAL RECORD RISKS: CLAIMS & LITIGATION. see *INSURANCE*

MEDICAL RECORDS BRIEFING. see *HEALTH FACILITIES AND ADMINISTRATION*

610 CAN
MEDICAL REFORM. Text in English. 1979. q. CND 25 domestic; USD 20 foreign. adv. bk.rev. back issues avail. **Document type:** *Newsletter.* **Description:** Covers the social, economic and political dimensions of health care provision.
Published by: Medical Reform Group, RPO Marlee, P O Box 40074, Toronto, ON M6B 4K4, Canada. TEL 416-588-9167, FAX 416-782-9054, mrg@web.net, http://www.medicalreform/web.net.mrg. Ed. Janet Maher. Circ: 500 (paid).

610 GBR
MEDICAL RESEARCH CENTRES; a world directory of organizations and programmes. Text in English. irreg., latest vol.12, 1997. GBP 325 domestic; GBP 535 in US & Canada (effective 2000). adv. **Document type:** *Directory.* **Description:** Contains essential information on over 9000 medical organizations active in all aspects of medical research worldwide. Covers government laboratories, academic institutes, research centers in hospitals, private sector laboratories, contract research organizations and the R&D units within pharmaceutical and medical device companies.
Formerly: Medical Research Index (0076-6003)
—CISTI.
Published by: John Harper Publishing, 27 Palace Gates Rd, London N22 7BW, United Kingdom. TEL 44-20-8881-4779, jhpublish@aol.com. Adv. contact Anita Monaghan. **Dist. addr.:** Turpin Distribution Services Ltd., Blackhorse Rd, Letchworth, Herts SG6 1HN, United Kingdom. TEL 44-1462-488900, FAX 44-1462-483011.

610 GHA
MEDICAL RESEARCH CENTRES IN GHANA: CURRENT RESEARCH PROJECTS. Text in English. 1973. irreg. free per issue. back issues avail. **Document type:** *Monographic series, Academic/Scholarly.*
Published by: Council for Scientific and Industrial Research, PO Box M 32, Accra, Ghana. Ed. D K Opare Sem.

610 CAN ISSN 0047-6560
MEDICAL RESEARCH COUNCIL NEWSLETTER/ CONSEIL DE RECHERCHES MEDICALES. COMMUNIQUE. Text in English, French. 1970. q. free per issue. **Document type:** *Newsletter.*
—Infotrieve. **CCC.**
Published by: Medical Research Council of Canada, 1600 Scott St, Tower B, Ottawa, ON K1A 0W9, Canada. TEL 613-946-0927, FAX 613-954-6653, fkert@hpb.hwc.ca. R&P Faye Kert. Circ: 4,500 (controlled).

610 CAN ISSN 0839-8283
MEDICAL RESEARCH COUNCIL OF CANADA. GRANTS AND AWARDS GUIDE/GUIDE DE SUBVENTIONS ET BOURSES. Key Title: University - Industry Grants and Awards Guide. Text and summaries in English, French. 1988. a. charts. **Document type:** *Bulletin.*
Media: Online - full text.
Published by: Medical Research Council of Canada, 1600 Scott St, Tower B, Ottawa, ON K1A 0W9, Canada. TEL 613-946-1951, FAX 613-954-6653, fkert@hpb.hwc.ca, http://www.mrc.hc-sc.gc.ca. R&P Faye Kert.

610 CAN ISSN 0384-2029
R854.C2
MEDICAL RESEARCH COUNCIL OF CANADA. REPORT OF THE PRESIDENT. Text in English, French. 1960. a. free per issue. charts, illus, stat. index. **Document type:** *Corporate.*
—CISTI.
Published by: Medical Research Council of Canada, 1600 Scott St, Tower B, Ottawa, ON K1A 0W9, Canada. TEL 613-954-1806, FAX 613-954-6653, fkert@hpb.hwc.ca, http://www.mrc.hc-sc.gc.ca. R&P Faye Kert. Circ: 2,300 (controlled).

610 USA
MEDICAL RESEARCH FUNDING BULLETIN. Text in English. 1972. 2/m. USD 75 (effective 2001). adv. bk.rev. tr.lit. back issues avail. **Document type:** *Newsletter.*
Media: E-mail.
Published by: Science Support Center, PO Box 7507, New York, NY 10150. TEL 212-371-3398, FAX 801-761-4200, grants@attglobal.net, grants1@attglobal.net. Ed. Carroll Jordon. R&P John Connolly. adv.: page USD 5,000; 7.5 x 10. Circ: 28,000 (controlled).

610.711 USA ISSN 0066-9423
R745
MEDICAL SCHOOL ADMISSION REQUIREMENTS, UNITED STATES AND CANADA. Text in English. 1955. a. USD 25 (effective 1999). reprint service avail. from PQC. **Document type:** *Directory.* **Description:** Describes US and Canadian medical schools, including details of entrance requirements of each school, selection factors, curriculum features, current first-year expenses, financial aid information, application and acceptance procedures, and applicant statistics.
Formerly (until 1964): Admission Requirements of American Medical Colleges, Including Canada (0271-6518)
Related titles: Microfiche ed.: (from CIS).
Indexed: SRI.
Published by: Association of American Medical Colleges, 2450 N St N W, Washington, DC 20037-1126. TEL 202-828-0416, FAX 202-828-1123. Ed. Laverne Alexander.

610 JPN ISSN 0019-1590
MEDICAL SCIENCE AND MEDICAL CARE/GEKKAN IGAKU TO IRYO. Text in Japanese. 1969. m. JPY 600.
Published by: Nippon Medical Association/Nippon Igaku Kyokai, 7-2-8 Hongo, Bunkyo-ku, Tokyo 113-0033, Japan. Ed. Tomoyuki Horikoshi. Pub. Takeshi Oda.

610 POL ISSN 1234-1010
MEDICAL SCIENCE MONITOR; international medical journal for clinical and experimental research. Text in English. 1995. bi-m. PLZ 250 domestic; USD 200 foreign; USD 30 newsstand/cover (effective 2002). adv. charts, illus. index. back issues avail. *Refereed.* **Document type:** *Journal, Academic/Scholarly.* **Description:** Publishes original articles in experimental and clinical medicine and related disciplines such as molecular biology, biochemistry, genetics, biophysics, bio- and medical technology.
Related titles: Online - full text ed.
Indexed: Ind.Med.
—BLDSC (5531.890700).
Published by: (International Medical Association for Experimental and Clinical Research USA), Medical Science International Publishing, ul. Ustrzycka 11, Warsaw 02-141, Poland. http://www.msi.com.pl. Eds. John C McGiff, Ryszard Gryglewski. R&P Marek R. Graczynski. adv.: page USD 1,800. Circ: 1,150 (paid).

610 530 USA
MEDICAL SCIENCE SERIES. Text in English. irreg. price varies. **Document type:** *Monographic series.* **Description:** Describes the application of the physical sciences, engineering, and mathematics in medicine and biology.
Published by: (Institute of Physics GBR), I O P Publishing, c/o A I D C, 2 Wintersport Ln, Box 20, Williston, VT 05495-0020. TEL 800-632-0880, FAX 802-862-0095. **Orders outside the U.S. to:** I O P Publishing Ltd., Techno House, Redcliffe Way, Bristol, Avon BS1 6NX, United Kingdom. TEL 44-117-929-7481.

610 NLD ISSN 0928-9550
CODEN: MSSYEI
MEDICAL SCIENCE SYMPOSIA SERIES. Text in English. 1992. irreg., latest vol.8, 1995. price varies. back issues avail. *Refereed.* **Document type:** *Proceedings.*
Indexed: Chem.Abstr., Chem.Indus.Notes, Chem.Titles.
—BLDSC (5531.892380), CASDDS, CISTI, Infotrieve, KNAW. **CCC.**
Published by: Kluwer Academic Publishers Group (Subsidiary of: Wolters Kluwer N.V.), Spuiboulevard 50, PO Box 17, Dordrecht 3300 AA, Netherlands. FAX 31-78-639-2254, services@wkap.nl, http://www.wkap.nl. **Dist. by:** Journals Department, PO Box 322, Dordrecht 3300 AH, Netherlands. FAX 31-78-654-6474.

616.98 USA ISSN 0041-7491
RC1050
MEDICAL SERVICE DIGEST. Variant title: U.S. Air Force Medical Service Digest. Text in English. 1950. q. USD 5; USD 6.25 foreign. back issues avail. **Document type:** *Government.* **Description:** Presents information about the people, programs and activities of the Air Force Medical Service.
Published by: U.S. Air Force, Office of the Surgeon General, HQ USAF SGI, Bldg 5681 Bolling AFB, Washington, DC 20332-6188. TEL 202-767-5046, FAX 202-767-1456. Ed. Elizabeth Taber. Circ: 8,000. **Subscr. to:** U.S. Government Printing Office, Superintendent of Documents. TEL 202-783-3238, FAX 202-512-2233.

610 GBR ISSN 0076-6011
MEDICAL SOCIETY OF LONDON. TRANSACTIONS. Text in English. 1773. a. GBP 15. bk.rev. **Document type:** *Proceedings.*
Indexed: Excerp.Med., Ind.Med. (1810-).
—BLDSC (8982.500000), CISTI, GNLM, ingenta, KNAW.
Published by: Medical Society of London, 11 Chandos St, Cavendish Sq, London W1N OEB, United Kingdom. TEL 44-171-580-1043, FAX 44-171-580-5793. Ed. P S London. Circ: 550 (controlled).

610 USA
MEDICAL SOCIETY OF MILWAUKEE COUNTY. MEMBERSHIP NEWSLETTER. Text in English. 1975. bi-m. USD 30 (effective 1999). adv. **Document type:** *Newsletter.*
Published by: Medical Society of Milwaukee County, 1126 S 70th St, Ste S 507, Milwaukee, WI 53214. TEL 414-475-4750, FAX 414-475-4799, bialekf@execpc.com, http://www.district-l.org. Ed. Frank Bialek. Circ: 2,400.

610 USA ISSN 1076-6022
MEDICAL STAFF BRIEFING; the newsletter for volunteer/elected medical staff leaders. Text in English. 1991. m. USD 327 (effective 1998). bk.rev. index. back issues avail. **Document type:** *Newsletter.* **Description:** Covers issues affecting medical staff administration, staff relations, and physician-patient relations.
Related titles: Supplement: M S B Credentialing.
—CCC.
Published by: Opus Communications, PO Box 1168, Marblehead, MA 01945. TEL 781-639-1872, FAX 781-639-2982, customer_service@opuscomm.com, http://www.opuscomm.com. Ed. Jay Kumar. Circ: 1,500.

MEDICAL STAFF LEADER HANDBOOK. see *LAW—Civil Law*

610 NLD
MEDICAL STUDENT INTERNATIONAL. Text in Dutch. 1995. s-a.
Published by: International Federation of Medical Students' Associations, c/o W M A, Cedex, B.P. 63, Ferney Voltaire Cedex 01212, France. TEL 33-450404759, FAX 33-450-40-5937, ifmsa@amc.uva.nl. Ed. Michel Torbey.

610 USA ISSN 0565-811X
Z695.1.M48 CODEN: MSHEE5
MEDICAL SUBJECT HEADINGS (BLACK BOOK). Text in English. 1960. a. USD 66; USD 82.50 foreign (effective 1998). **Document type:** *Directory, Government.* **Description:** Provides an alphabetized and categorized list of all the subject descriptors used to analyze the biomedical literature in the National Library of Medicine.
—CASDDS.
Published by: U.S. National Library of Medicine, 8600 Rockville Pike, Bethesda, MD 20894. httpf://www.nlm.nih.gov/mesh. Circ: 8,000. **Orders to:** U.S. Government Printing Office, Superintendent of Documents. **Dist. in UK by:** Turpin Distribution Services Ltd., Blackhorse Rd, Letchworth, Herts SG6 1HN, United Kingdom. FAX 44-1462-480947.; **Dist. in US by:** Bernan Associates, 4611 F Assembly Dr, Lanham, MD 20706. TEL 301-459-0056, 301-459-7666.

610.71 GBR ISSN 0142-159X
MEDICAL TEACHER. Text in English. 1979. bi-m. GBP 163, USD 267 to individuals; GBP 581, USD 964 to institutions (effective 2002). adv. bk.rev. charts. cum.index. back issues avail. *Refereed.* **Document type:** *Academic/Scholarly.* **Description:** Examines pedagogy and its relevance to the study and teaching of medicine.
Related titles: Microfiche ed.; Online - full text ed.: ISSN 1466-187X. 1998 (from CatchWord Ltd., Northern Light Technology, Inc., EBSCO Publishing, O C L C Online Computer Library Center, Inc., RoweCom Information Quest, ProQuest Information & Learning, Swets Blackwell, Institute for Scientific Information).
Indexed: AMED, ASCA, ASSIA, Br.Educ.Ind., C.I.J.E., Cont.Pg.Educ., Curr.Adv.Ecol.Sci., Curr.Cont., ERA, Educ.Tech.Abstr., Inpharma, Lang.& Lang.Behav.Abstr., Mult.Ed.Abstr., Reac., Res.High.Educ.Abstr., SOPODA, SSCI (coverage dropped), Sociol.Abstr., Tech.Educ.Abstr.
—BLDSC (5531.965000), CatchWord, GNLM, IDS, Infotrieve, ingenta. **CCC.**
Published by: Carfax Publishing Limited (Subsidiary of: Taylor & Francis Group), PO Box 25, Abingdon, Oxon OX14 3UE, United Kingdom. TEL 44-1235-401000, FAX 44-1235-401550, enquiries@carfax.co.uk, enquiry@tandf.co.uk, http://www.carfax.co.uk/journals. Ed. R M Harden.

610.28 GBR
MEDICAL TECHNOLOGY INTERNATIONAL (YEAR). Text in English. a. GBP 29.95, USD 48 (effective 1998). **Document type:** *Trade.*
Published by: Cornhill Publications Ltd. (Subsidiary of: Sterling Publishing Group Plc.), Kings Ct, 2-16 Goodge St, London W1P 1FF, United Kingdom. TEL 44-207-240-1515, FAX 44-207-379-7371, cornhill@aol.com, info@cornhillpublications.com, http://www.cornhillpublications.co.uk. Ed. Simone Kessler.

MEDICAL TECHNOLOGY STOCK LETTER. see *BUSINESS AND ECONOMICS—Investments*

610 677 GBR ISSN 0266-2078
MEDICAL TEXTILES; an international newsletter. Text in English. 1984. m. GBP 345, USD 567 (effective 2001 - 2002). bk.rev. charts, stat. back issues avail. **Document type:** *Newsletter, Trade.* **Description:** Provides coverage of design, production and industrial research into the use of textiles in medicine. Also provides a survey of the area for senior general management to highlight new trends and possibilities, market gaps and business opportunities.
Related titles: E-mail ed.; Online - full text ed.: (from Gale Group, Northern Light Technology, Inc., Factiva).
Indexed: Nonwov.Abstr., Text.Tech.Dig. (1984-), World Text.Abstr.
—BLDSC (5532.028700), EMDOCS, GNLM, Infotrieve. **CCC.**
Published by: International Newsletters, PO Box 133, Witney, Oxon OX8 6ZH, United Kingdom. TEL 44-199-3824130, FAX 44-199-3824150, in@intnews.com, http://www.intnews.com. Ed. Geoff Fisher.

MEDICAL TRIAL TECHNIQUE QUARTERLY. see *LAW—Civil Law*

610 USA ISSN 0279-9340
R5
MEDICAL TRIBUNE* . Text in English. 1960. fortn. USD 95; free to qualified personnel. adv. bk.rev. charts, illus, stat. Supplement avail. **Document type:** *Trade.* **Description:** Aimed at physicians in family practice.
Former titles (until vol.21, 1980): Medical Tribune and Medical News (0098-6240); (until vol.3, 1963): Medical Tribune (0025-7605)
Related titles: Online - full text ed.
Indexed: Curr.Lit.Fam.Plan., Per.Islam. (1993-).
—GNLM, IDS.
Published by: PressCorps, Inc., 201 West 21st St Apt 10E, New York, NY 10011-3135. TEL 212-686-9080, FAX 212-686-5310. Ed. Jason Kahn. Pub., Adv. contact Jim Kelly. R&P Merritt McKihney TEL 212-219-7807. Circ: 140,000 (controlled).

610 ITA ISSN 0392-7199
MEDICAL TRIBUNE. Text in Italian. 1982. w. (42/yr.). ITL 35,000. adv. bk.rev.
Published by: E S I Stampa Medica s.r.l., Largo Volontari Del Sangue, 10, Casella Postale 42, San Donato, MI 20133, Italy. TEL 39-2-5274241, FAX 39-2-55600670, TELEX 3248944. Ed. Diego Onestinghel. Adv. contact Ornella Galbiati. B&W page ITL 14,500,000, color page ITL 17,500,000; trim 364 x 268. Circ: 56,000.

610 CHE ISSN 0170-1894
MEDICAL TRIBUNE. Text in German. 1968. 46/yr. **Document type:** *Journal, Trade.*
Related titles: ♦ Online - full text ed.: Medical Tribune Online.
Published by: Medical Tribune AG, Urs-Graf-Str 8, Postfach 368, Basel 4020, Switzerland. TEL 41-61-3125566, FAX 41-61-3125560, http://www.medical-tribune.ch. Ed. Klaus Nuernberger. Circ: 10,000.

610 CHE ISSN 1420-6862
MEDICAL TRIBUNE KOLLOQUIUM. Text in German. 1995. 8/yr. adv. **Document type:** *Journal, Academic/Scholarly.*
Published by: Medical Tribune AG, Urs-Graf-Str 8, Postfach 368, Basel 4020, Switzerland. TEL 41-61-3125566, FAX 41-61-3125560, http://www.medical-tribune.ch. Ed. Winfried Powollik. adv.: B&W page CHF 3,260, color page CHF 4,700; 190 x 280.

610 CHE
▼ **MEDICAL TRIBUNE ONLINE.** Text in German. 1999. d. adv. **Document type:** *Journal, Academic/Scholarly.*
Media: Online - full text. **Related titles:** ♦ Print ed.: Medical Tribune. ISSN 0170-1894.
Published by: Medical Tribune AG, Urs-Graf-Str 8, Postfach 368, Basel 4020, Switzerland. TEL 41-61-3125566, FAX 41-61-3125560, http://www.medical-tribune.ch. Ed. Winfried Powollik.

M

610 ZAF
MEDICAL UNIVERSITY OF SOUTH AFRICA. YEARBOOK. Variant title: Medunsa Yearbook. Text in English. 1994. a. illus. **Document type:** *Academic/Scholarly.*
Published by: Medical University of South Africa, Bureau for Public Relations, PO Box 200, Medunsa 0204, South Africa.

MEDICAL UPDATE FOR PSYCHIATRISTS. see *MEDICAL SCIENCES—Psychiatry And Neurology*

610 USA
RA972
MEDICAL UTILIZATION MANAGEMENT. Text in English. 1973. bi-w. USD 395 (effective 1999). back issues avail.; reprints avail. **Document type:** *Trade.* **Description:** Covers operational, financial, governmental and legal issues of the utilization review industry.
Former titles (until 1994): Medical Utilization Review; MacGraw-Hill's Medical Utilization Review (0734-1970); (until 1982): P S R O Letter (Professional Standards Review Organizations) (0149-5844)
Related titles: Online - full text ed.: (from Gale Group, NewsNet).
—Infotrieve. **CCC.**
Published by: Thompson Financial / I M G Media, Healthcare Information Center (Subsidiary of: Thompson Publishing Group), 11 Penn Plaza, 17th Fl, New York, NY 10001-2006. TEL 212-967-7000, 800-535-8403. Ed. Melissa Glim.

610 ITA
MEDICAL VIDEO FLASH. Text in Italian. 1976. 8/yr. adv.
Published by: Editoriale Dumas S.p.A., Via Grandi, 5-7, Rozzano, MI 20089, Italy. Ed. Gianni Mazzocchi. Circ: 108,000.

MEDICAL WASTE HANDBOOK. see *ENVIRONMENTAL STUDIES—Waste Management*

MEDICARE ADVISOR. see *INSURANCE*

MEDICARE COMPLIANCE ALERT. see *INSURANCE*

MEDICARE MANAGER. see *INSURANCE*

MEDICARE REVIEW. see *INSURANCE*

610 BRA ISSN 0076-6046
MEDICINA. Text in Portuguese; Summaries in English, Portuguese. 1961. q. BRL 40, USD 50 (effective 1998). adv. bk.rev. bibl, charts, illus. *Refereed.* **Document type:** *Academic/Scholarly.*
Indexed: Biol.Abstr., Curr.Adv.Gen.& Molec.Biol., Excerp.Med. (1992-), INIS Atomind., Ind.Med. (coverage dropped), Ref.Zh.
—GNLM.
Published by: Universidade de Sao Paulo, Faculdade de Medicina de Ribeirao Preto, Hospital das Clinicas, Campus Universitario, Av Bandeirantes, 3900, VI Mte Alegre, Ribeirao Preto, SP 14040-030, Brazil. FAX 55-16-6331144, TELEX 016-583, jcvoltar@fmvp.usp.br. Ed. Dr. Julio C Voltarelli. R&P Julio Voltarelli. Adv. contact Rudi Madureira. Circ: 2,500.

610 HRV ISSN 0025-7729
MEDICINA. Text in Croatian; Summaries in English. 1964. q. USD 30 (effective 2000). adv. bk.rev. **Document type:** *Academic/Scholarly.* **Description:** Publishes original scientific papers, professional papers on all aspects of medicine.
Indexed: Abstr.Hyg., Biol.Abstr., Chem.Abstr., Excerp.Med., Trop.Dis.Bull.
—GNLM.
Published by: Hrvatski Lijecnicki Zbor, Podruznica Rijeka, Kresimirova 52-a, pp 227, Rijeka 51001, Croatia. TEL 385-51-334542, FAX 385-51-334542. Ed. Ante Skrobonja. Circ: 1,200.

610 ARG ISSN 0025-7680
R21 CODEN: MEDCAD
MEDICINA; Buenos Aires. Text and summaries in English, Spanish. 1939. bi-m. ARS 70 domestic; USD 70 in Latin America; USD 100 elsewhere; ARS 15 newsstand/cover (effective 2000 - 2001). adv. bk.rev. abstr, bibl, illus. index. back issues avail. *Refereed.* **Document type:** *Academic/Scholarly.* **Description:** Covers clinical research, clinical epidemiology and immunology, infectious emergent and re-emergent diseases.
Related titles: Microfilm ed.: (from PQC); Online - full text ed.: (from Institute for Scientific Information); ♦ Supplement: Medicina. Suplemento. ISSN 0325-951X.
Indexed: ASCA, Abstr.Hyg., Anim.Breed.Abstr., Biol.Abstr., Chem.Abstr., Chem.Titles, Curr.Cont., Dairy Sci.Abstr., Dent.Ind., Excerp.Med., Helminthol.Abstr., INIS Atomind., Ind.Med. (1940-), Ind.Sci.Rev., Inpharma, Nutr.Abstr., Pharm.&Out.News, Protozool.Abstr., Reac., Rev.Appl.Entomol., Rev.Med.& Vet.Mycol., Sci.Cit.Ind., Soyabean Abstr., Trop.Dis.Bull.
—BLDSC (5532.390000), CASDDS, CISTI, GNLM, IDS, KNAW.
Published by: Fundacion Revista Medica Argentina, Combatientes de Malvinas 3150, Buenos Aires 1427, Argentina. TEL 54-114-5236619, FAX 54-114-5236619, revmed@intramed.net.ar, http://www.revmed.intramed.net.ar. Ed., Pub. Amadeo Pedro Barousse. Adv. contact Ethel Mabel Divita. color page USD 1,056; trim 20 x 27.5. Circ: 5,000. **Co-sponsor:** Sociedad Argentina de Investigacion Clinica.

610 ESP ISSN 0025-7753
CODEN: MCLBA2
MEDICINA CLINICA. Text in Spanish; Summaries in English. 1943. w. (40/yr.). USD 163. adv. bk.rev. abstr, charts, illus. reprint service avail. from PQC. *Refereed.* **Document type:** *Academic/Scholarly.* **Description:** Contains works of original research and articles for the continuing education of practicing professionals in clinical medicine.
Related titles: Online - full text ed.: (from Institute for Scientific Information).
Indexed: ASCA, Abstr.Hyg., Biol.Abstr., Chem.Abstr., Curr.Cont., Dairy Sci.Abstr., Dent.Ind., Dok.Arbeitsmed., Excerp.Med., Helminthol.Abstr., Ind.Med. (1943-), Ind.Med.Esp., Ind.Sci.Rev., Ind.Vet., Inpharma, Int.Nurs.Ind., Nutr.Abstr., Pharm.&Out.News, Pig News & Info., Postharvest, Poult.Abstr., Protozool.Abstr., Reac., Ref.Zh., Rev.Appl.Entomol., Rev.Med.& Vet.Mycol., SSCI (coverage dropped), Sci.Cit.Ind.
—BLDSC (5532.600000), CASDDS, CINDOC, GNLM, IDS, Infotrieve, KNAW. **CCC.**
Published by: Ediciones Doyma S.A., Traversa de Gracia, 17-21, Barcelona 08021, Spain. TEL 34-93-200-0711, FAX 34-93-209-1136, TELEX 51694 INK-E. Ed. C Rozman Borstnar. Adv. contact Enric Brotons. color page ESP 292,000; trim 280 x 210. Circ: 8,500. **Co-sponsor:** Hospitales y Sociedades Medicas de Barcelona.

610 ITA ISSN 0391-3619
MEDICINA ESTETICA. Text in Italian; Summaries in English, French, German, Italian, Spanish. 1977. q. ITL 80,000, USD 84 (effective 1999). bk.rev. abstr, bibl. back issues avail. **Document type:** *Academic/Scholarly.*
Published by: (Societa Italiana di Medicina Estetica), Editrice Salus Internazionale s.r.l., Via Severo Carmignano, 41, Rome, RM 00151, Italy. TEL 39-06-3217314.

610 ESP ISSN 0210-9433
MEDICINA INTEGRAL; medicina preventiva y asistencial en el medio rural. Text in Spanish. 1980. bi-w. (20/yr.). USD 85 (effective 1996). adv.
Indexed: Ind.Med.Esp.
Published by: Editorial Idepsa S.A., Principe de Vergara, 112 1o F, Madrid 28002, Spain. TEL 34-1-5637306, FAX 34-1-5632393. Ed. J M Sanchez Tapias. Circ: 20,000.

610 ESP ISSN 0210-5691
CODEN: MDINE
MEDICINA INTENSIVA. Text in Spanish; Summaries in English. m. (10/yr.). USD 80 (effective 1996). **Description:** Covers intensive care medicine.
Indexed: Excerp.Med., Ind.Med.Esp.
—BLDSC (5533.420000), CINDOC, GNLM, Infotrieve, KNAW. **CCC.**
Published by: (Sociedad Espanola de Medicina Intensiva y Unidades Coronarias), Editorial Idepsa S.A., Principe de Vergara, 112 1o F, Madrid 28002, Spain. TEL 34-1-5637306, FAX 34-1-5632393. Ed. Dr J Ibanez Juve. Circ: 4,683.

610 ITA ISSN 0394-2627
MEDICINA MODERNA OGGI/MODERN MEDICINE TODAY. Text in English, Italian. 1985. s-a. ITL 10,000, USD 6.
Published by: Amorosino Editore Roma, Via Francesco Salata, 18, Rome, RM 00177, Italy. TEL 06-274040.

610 ROM
MEDICINA MUNCII SI MEDICINA SOCIALA. Text in Romanian. 1990 (vol.38). bi-m.
Published by: Uniunea Societatilor de Stiinte Medicale din Rumania, Str. Progresului 8, Bucharest 70754, Romania. TEL 13-89-73. **Subscr. to:** Rompresfilatelia, Calea Grivitei 64-66, PO Box 12-201, Bucharest 78104, Romania.

610 ITA ISSN 0394-9001
R5 CODEN: MDSCAD
MEDICINA NEI SECOLI: ARTE E SCIENZA; rivista storico medica. Text in English, Italian. 1964; N.S. 1989. 3/yr. ITL 100,000 domestic to individuals; ITL 120,000 foreign to individuals; ITL 130,000 domestic to institutions; ITL 150,000 foreign to institutions (effective 2000). bk.rev. *Refereed.* **Document type:** *Proceedings, Academic/Scholarly.* **Description:** Devoted to dealing with all topics about history of medicine.
Formerly: Medicina nei Secoli (0025-7877); Superseded: Pagine di Storia della Medicina (0030-9400)
Related titles: Microfiche ed.: N.S.
Indexed: Amer.Hist.& Life, Biol.Abstr., Hist.Abstr. (1989-), Ind.Med. (coverage dropped).
—CASDDS, GNLM.
Published by: Universita degli Studi di Roma, Dipartimento di Medicina Sperimentale e Patologia, Sezione di Storia della Medicina, Viale Dell' Universita', 34-A, Rome, RM 00185, Italy. TEL 39-06-4451721, FAX 39-06-4451721, langeletti@axrma.uniroma1.it, vgazzaniga@axrma.uniroma1.it. Ed. Luciana Angeletti. Pub. Antonio Delfino. R&P Valentina Gazzaniga. Adv. contact Carla Terarcangeli. Circ: 500.

610 ITA ISSN 0392-4548
MEDICINA OGGI; periodico di attualita in medicina e chirurgia. Text in Italian; Summaries in English. 1980. q. ITL 55,000, USD 95 (effective 1999). bibl. Supplement avail.; back issues avail. **Description:** Includes a wide variety of topics in medicine, current trends in surgery, and extensive research.
Indexed: Excerp.Med.
—EMDOCS.
Published by: Casa Editrice Idelson, Via A. DeGasperi, 55, Naples, NA 80138, Italy. TEL 39-81-5524733, FAX 39-81-5518295, idelgno@tin.it, http://www.idelson-gnocchi.com. Ed. Lucio Zarrilli.

610 ARG ISSN 0325-951X
MEDICINA. SUPLEMENTO. Text in Spanish. 1968. irreg. adv.
Related titles: ♦ Supplement to: Medicina. ISSN 0025-7680.
Published by: Fundacion Revista Medica Argentina, Combatientes de Malvinas 3150, Buenos Aires 1427, Argentina. TEL 54-114-5236619, FAX 54-114-5236619, revmed@intramed.net.ar. Ed. Amadeo Pedro Barousse. Adv. contact Ethel Mabel Divita. **Co-sponsor:** Sociedad Argentina de Investigacion Clinica.

610 917.106 USA
MEDICINA Y CULTURA* . (Editions avail. for U.S. and Puerto Rico) Text in Spanish. 1992. m. **Document type:** *Consumer.*
Published by: Mundo Medico USA, Inc., 158 Danbury Rd, Ste 8, Ridgefield, CT 06877-3200. adv.: B&W page USD 2,880, color page USD 4,470; trim 10.63 x 8.25. Circ: 32,000.

610 540 USA ISSN 1054-2523
RS400 CODEN: MCREEB
MEDICINAL CHEMISTRY RESEARCH; an international journal for rapid communications on design and mechanisms of action of biologically active agents. Text in English. 1991. 9/yr. CHF 327 to individuals; CHF 998 to institutions; USD 198 to individuals; USD 534 to institutions; CHF 138, USD 73.40 newsstand/cover (effective 2002). adv. *Refereed.* **Document type:** *Journal, Academic/Scholarly.* **Description:** Provides prompt disclosure on novel experimental achievements in the many facets of drug design, drug discovery, and the elucidation of mechanisms of action of biologically active compounds.
Related titles: Online - full text ed.: (from Institute for Scientific Information).
Indexed: ASCA, Arts & Hum.Cit.Ind. (coverage dropped), BBCI, Chem.Abstr., Chem.Cit.Ind., Chem.Indus.Notes, Chem.Titles, Curr.Cont., Derwent Biotech.Abstr., Inpharma, Neurosci.Cit.Ind., Pharm.&Out.News, Reac., Rev.Med.& Vet.Mycol.
—BLDSC (5533.983000), ADONIS, CASDDS, CISTI, GNLM, IDS, Infotrieve, KNAW. **CCC.**
Published by: Birkhaeuser Boston, 675 Massachusetts Ave, Cambridge, MA 02139-3309. TEL 617-876-2333, FAX 617-876-1272, info@birkhauser.com, http://www.birkhauser.com/journals/mcr. Ed. Richard A Glennon. Pub. William Curtis. R&Ps William Curtis, Xiao Chun Lian. Adv. contact Bruce Lyons. **Subscr. to:** Birkhaeuser Verlag AG, Klosterberg, Postfach 133, Basel 4010, Switzerland. TEL 41-61-205-0707, FAX 41-61-205-0792, subscriptions@birkhauser.ch, http://www.birkhauser.ch. **Dist. by:** Springer-Verlag, Journals, Journals Fulfillment, Box 2485, Secaucus, NJ 07096-2485. TEL 212-348-4033, 800-777-4643, FAX 201-348-4505.

610 ESP
MEDICINE. Text in Spanish. 35/yr. USD 120 (effective 1996).
Indexed: Curr.Cont. (coverage dropped), Ind.Sci.Rev.
Published by: Editorial Idepsa S.A., Principe de Vergara, 112 1o F, Madrid 28002, Spain. TEL 34-1-5637306, FAX 34-1-5632393. Ed. A Garcia de la Fuente.

610 USA ISSN 1086-5462
MEDICINE AND HEALTH - RHODE ISLAND. Text in English. 1878. m. USD 50 domestic; USD 100 foreign (effective 2000). bk.rev. bibl, illus. index. reprint service avail. from PQC. *Refereed.* **Document type:** *Academic/Scholarly.*
Former titles (until 1996): Rhode Island Medicine (1061-222X); (until 1992): Rhode Island Medical Journal (0363-7913); (until 1976): R.I. Medical Journal (0360-067X); (until 1974): Rhode Island Medical Journal (0035-4627); (until 1917): Providence Medical Journal (0898-1361); (until 1900): Rhode Island Medical Society. Transactions (0898-137X)
Related titles: Microform ed.: (from PQC).
Indexed: A.D.& D., AgeLine, Apic.Abstr., CINAHL, Chem.Abstr., Chic.Per.Ind., Curr.Cont. (coverage dropped), Dent.Ind., Excerp.Med., Helminthol.Abstr., INIS Atomind., Ind.Med. (1996-), Int.Nurs.Ind.
—BLDSC (5534.005830), CISTI, GNLM, ingenta, KNAW.
Published by: Rhode Island Medical Society, 106 Francis St, Providence, RI 02903. TEL 401-331-3207, FAX 401-751-8050, rims@ids.net. Ed. Dr. Joseph H Friedman. R&P Joan Retsinas TEL 401-272-0422. Adv. contact Eli Panichas. Circ: 2,100.

MEDICINE AND LAW; an international journal. see *LAW*

610 AUS
MEDICINE AUSTRALIA. Text in English. 1996. irreg. *Refereed.* **Document type:** *Trade.* **Description:** Medical journal for doctors and other health care professionals.
Media: Online - full text.
Published by: N R D G P, 186 Molesworth St, Lismore, NSW 2480, Australia. tlembke@om.com.au, http://www.om.com.au/MedicineAu. Ed. Trny Lemke.

610 USA ISSN 0025-7974
R11 CODEN: MEDIAV
MEDICINE (BALTIMORE); analytical reviews of general medicine, neurology, psychiatry, dermatology and pediatrics. Text in English. 1922. bi-m., latest vol.80. USD 169 domestic to individuals Print & Online eds.; USD 189 foreign to individuals Print & Online eds.; USD 319 domestic to institutions Print & Online eds.; USD 319 foreign to institutions Print & Online eds.; USD 50 newsstand/cover (effective 2002). adv. bibl, charts, illus. *Refereed.* **Document type:** *Academic/Scholarly.*
Related titles: CD-ROM ed.: (from Ovid Technologies, Inc.); Microfilm ed.: (from WWS); Online - full text ed.: USD 414.70 domestic academic site license; USD 414.70 foreign academic site license; USD 462.55 foreign corporate site license (2002) (from Ovid Technologies, Inc., Gale Group, Factiva, Institute for Scientific Information).
Indexed: AIM, Biol.Abstr., Chem.Abstr., Curr.Adv.Ecol.Sci., Curr.Adv.Gen.& Molec.Biol., Curr.Cont., Dairy Sci.Abstr., Diar.Dis.Res., Excerp.Med., Helminthol.Abstr., INIS Atomind., Ind.Med. (1922-), Ind.Sci.Rev., Inpharma, Jrnl.Watch Neuro., Kidney, Med.& Surg.Dermat., Nutr.Abstr., Pharm.&Out.News, Reac., Rev.Med.& Vet.Mycol., Rev.Plant Path., Sci.Cit.Ind., THA.
—BLDSC (5534.000000), CASDDS, CISTI, GNLM, IDS, ingenta, KNAW.
Published by: Lippincott Williams & Wilkins (Baltimore) (Subsidiary of: Wolters Kluwer N.V.), 351 W Camden St, Baltimore, MD 21201-2436. TEL 410-528-4068, 800-222-3790, FAX 410-528-4452, TELEX 87669, rezell@wwilkins.com, http://www.md-journal.com, http://www.wwilkins.com/MD/. Ed. Dr. Victor A McKusick. Adv. contact Randy Ezell. B&W page USD 665; trim 10.88 x 8.13. Circ: 3,287; 3,154 (paid).

327.172 GBR ISSN 1362-3699
RC970 CODEN: MEWAE4
MEDICINE, CONFLICT AND SURVIVAL; international medical concerns on global security issues. Text in English. 1965. q. GBP 42, USD 60 to individuals; GBP 155, USD 215 to institutions (effective 2002). adv. bk.rev. stat. index, cum.index: 1965-1969. back issues avail.; reprints avail. *Refereed.* **Document type:** *Journal, Academic/Scholarly.* **Description:** Intended for medical health care professionals and peace researchers. It covers the causes and effects of wars and other forms of social violence, the medical and environmental effects of war, the abuse of human rights, and medical and humanitarian aid in conflict situations.
Former titles (until 1996): Medicine and War (0748-8009); (until 1985): Medical Association for Prevention of War. Journal (0265-2196); (until Autumn 1982): Medical Association for Prevention of War. Proceedings (0025-701X)
Related titles: Microfilm ed.: (from PQC).
Indexed: Abstr.Hyg., Curr.Adv.Ecol.Sci., Curr.Cont. (coverage dropped), IBZ, INIS Atomind., Ind.Med. (1996-), Intl.Bibl.Soc.Sci., Lanc.Ind., Nutr.Abstr., P.A.I.S., Peace Res.Abstr., Protozool.Abstr., Ref.Zh., Rev.Appl.Entomol., Rural Devel.Abstr., Russ.Acad.Sci.Bibl., World Ag.Econ.& Rur.Soc.Abstr.
—BLDSC (5534.008900), GNLM, Infotrieve, ingenta. **CCC.**
Published by: Frank Cass Publishers, Crown House, 47 Chase Side, Southgate, London N14 5BP, United Kingdom. TEL 44-20-8920-2100, FAX 44-20-8447-8548, info@frankcass.com, editors@frankcass.com, http://www.frankcass.com. Eds. Douglas Holdstock, Nevin Hughes Jones. R&P Anna Whiston. Adv. contact Anne Kidson. B&W page GBP 195, B&W page USD 285; trim 110 x 178. **Dist. & Subscr. addr. in N. America:** Frank Cass Publishers, 5824 N E Hassalo St, Portland, OR 97213-3644. TEL 800-944-6190, FAX 503-280-8832, cass@isbs.com.

610 GBR ISSN 0140-9158
MEDICINE DIGEST. Text in English. 1974. m. USD 48; USD 48 in Francophone Africa; USD 18 in Pakistan; USD 60 in China (effective 2000). adv. bk.rev. reprint service avail. from IRC. **Document type:** *Abstract/Index.*
Related titles: French ed.
Indexed: Abstr.Hyg., Diar.Dis.Res., Inpharma, Reac., Trop.Dis.Bull.
Published by: F S G MediMedia Ltd., Vine House, The Barn, Fair Green, Reach, Cambridge CB5 0JD, United Kingdom. TEL 44-1638-743633, FAX 44-1638-743998, mmp@medimedia.com.hk. Circ: 88,785.

610 174.24 NLD ISSN 1386-7423
CODEN: MHCPF5
MEDICINE, HEALTH CARE AND PHILOSOPHY. Text in English. 1998. 3/yr. EUR 197.50 to institutions for print or online ed.; EUR 237 to institutions print & online eds.combined (effective 2002). **Document type:** *Academic/Scholarly.* **Description:** Provides forum for international exchange of research data, theories, reports and opinions in the discipline of bioethics, and the philosophy of medicine and health care in general.
Related titles: Online - full text ed.: (from EBSCO Publishing, O C L C Online Computer Library Center, Inc., RoweCom Information Quest, Swets Blackwell, Kluwer Online).
Indexed: Ind.Med.
—BLDSC (5534.035000). **CCC.**
Published by: (European Society for Philosophy of Medicine and Health Care), Kluwer Academic Publishers Group (Subsidiary of: Wolters Kluwer N.V.), Spuiboulevard 50, PO Box 17, Dordrecht 3300 AA, Netherlands. FAX 31-78-939-2254, 31-78-639-2254, services@wkap.nl, http://www.wkap.nl. Ed. Henk A M J Ten Have. **Dist. by:** Journals Department, PO Box 322, Dordrecht 3300 AH, Netherlands. TEL 781-871-6600, FAX 31-78-654-6474.

610 GBR ISSN 0144-0438
MEDICINE INTERNATIONAL (MIDDLE EASTERN EDITION). Text in English. 1980. m. GBP 54. adv. charts, illus. **Document type:** *Academic/Scholarly.* **Description:** Covers all aspects of medicine.
Published by: The Medicine Group (Journals) Ltd., Publishing House, 62 Stert St, Abingdon, Oxon OX14 3UQ, United Kingdom. TEL 44-1235-555770, FAX 44-1235-554691. Ed. Jill McFarland. Pub. Simon Campbell Smith. Adv. contact John Allardice. Circ: 20,000 (controlled).

610 GBR ISSN 0144-0411
MEDICINE INTERNATIONAL (QUARTERLY EDITION). Text in English. 1981; N.S. 1984; N.S. 1988. q. adv. illus. **Document type:** *Academic/Scholarly.* **Description:** Covers all aspects of medicine.
—GNLM.
Published by: The Medicine Group (Journals) Ltd., Publishing House, 62 Stert St, Abingdon, Oxon OX14 3UQ, United Kingdom. TEL 44-1235-555770, FAX 44-1235-554691.

610 ZAF ISSN 0260-2334
MEDICINE INTERNATIONAL (SOUTHERN AFRICAN EDITION)✶ . Text in English. m. adv. **Document type:** *Trade.*
Formerly (until 1981): Medicine S.A.
Published by: Medicine Group (S A) (Pty) Ltd., PO Box 51930, Randburg, Gauteng 2125, South Africa. TEL 011-789-4010, FAX 011-789-4028. Ed. W Buechner. R&P A Carstens. Adv. contact A. Carstens. B&W page ZAR 3,080, color page ZAR 5,060. Circ: 5,500.

610.711 USA
MEDICINE NORTHWEST. Text in English. 1984. s-a. back issues avail. **Description:** Informs constituents of the University of Washington School of Medicine about its activities in education, instruction, patient care, and community service.
Published by: University of Washington, School of Medicine, Mail Stop SC 60, Seattle, WA 98195. TEL 206-685-0381. Ed. Leila Gray. Pub. Dr. Philip J Fialkow. Circ: 17,000 (controlled).

610 GBR ISSN 1360-0168
MEDICINE ON-LINE. Variant title: International Journal of Medicine. Text in English. 1995. m. free per issue. bk.rev., software rev., video rev. *Refereed.* **Document type:** *Journal, Academic/Scholarly.*
Media: Online - full text.
Published by: Priory Lodge Education Ltd., 2 Cornflower Way, Moreton, Wirral CH46 1SV, United Kingdom. TEL 44-151-606-1796, FAX 44-151-606-1812, solutions@priory.com, http://www.priory.com/med.htm. Ed. Dr. Ben Green. Circ: 40,000 (controlled).

MEDICINE ON THE MIDWAY. see *COLLEGE AND ALUMNI*

610 220 GBR
MEDICINE, RELIGION TOGETHER. Text in English. 1982. 3/yr. GBP 15 (effective 2000); includes membership to The Medical Forum. **Description:** Encourages links between doctors and clergy in the context of healing.
Published by: Churches' Council for Health and Healing, St Luke's Hospital, 12 Fitzroy Square, London W1P 5HQ, United Kingdom. TEL 44-171-486-9644. Ed. Denis Duncan.

610 GBR ISSN 1365-4357
MEDICINE: THE CONTINUOUSLY UPDATED TEXTBOOK OF MEDICINE. Variant title: Medicine. Text in English. 1997. s-a. GBP 199; GBP 75 renewals. **Description:** Covers all major medical disorders. Includes self-assessment tests, color images and graphics, along with video clips and animation, making it fully interactive.
Media: CD-ROM.
Published by: Chapman & Hall, Electronic Publishing Division, Chapman & Hall, 2-6 Boundary Row, London SE1 8HN, United Kingdom. TEL 44-20-7865-0066, FAX 44-20-7522-0101, cust.serv@chall.co.uk, http://epd.chapmanhall.com. **Dist. by:** Cheriton House, North Way, Andover, Hamps SP10 5BE, United Kingdom. TEL 44-1264-332424, FAX 44-1264-342787.

610 ZAF
MEDICINE TODAY. Text in English. m. ZAR 60. adv. **Document type:** *Trade.*
Published by: Complete Publishing (Pty.) Ltd., PO Box 87745, Houghton, Johannesburg 2041, South Africa. TEL 27-11-7892112, FAX 27-11-789-5347. Ed. Ray Watson. Circ: 10,000.

610 AUS ISSN 1443-430X
▼ **MEDICINE TODAY**; the peer reviewed journal of clinical practice. Text in English. 2000. m. AUD 150 in Australia; AUD 190 in Australasia; AUD 220 in United States & Europe (effective 2000). back issues avail. *Refereed.* **Document type:** *Journal, Academic/Scholarly.* **Description:** A journal of continuing medical education and review, it provides authoritative clinical information that is useful and relevant to doctors in their day-to-day practice and to expand their medical knowledge.
—BLDSC (5534.106300).
Published by: Medicine Today Pty Ltd, PO Box 1473, Neutral Bay, NSW 2089, Australia. TEL 61-2-9908-8577, FAX 61-2-9908-7488. Ed. John Ellard. Pubs. Judy Passlow, Tony Scott.

610 GBR ISSN 1357-3039
MEDICINE - U K EDITION. Text in English. 1972; N.S. 1984; N.S. 1988. m. GBP 79.20 domestic; GBP 74 foreign. adv. charts, illus, stat. **Document type:** *Academic/Scholarly.* **Description:** Covers all aspects of medicine.
Formerly (until 1995): Medicine International (U K Edition) (0144-0403)
Indexed: Brit.Nur.Ind., Curr.Adv.Ecol.Sci., Diar.Dis.Res., Helminthol.Abstr., INIS Atomind.
—BLDSC (5533.998000), GNLM.

Published by: The Medicine Group (Journals) Ltd., Publishing House, 62 Stert St, Abingdon, Oxon OX14 3UQ, United Kingdom. TEL 44-1235-555770, FAX 44-1235-554691. Adv. contact Christian Benzing. Circ: 20,000.

610 DNK ISSN 0461-6308
MEDICINSK AARBOG. Text in Danish, Norwegian, Swedish. 1957. a. price varies. illus. **Document type:** *Academic/Scholarly.*
Published by: Blackwell Munksgaard, Book Division, Noerre Soegade 35, PO Box 2148, Copenhagen K 1016, Denmark. FAX 45-77-33-33-77. Ed. Lotte Murmand.

610 MKD ISSN 0065-1214 CODEN: GZMSAH
MEDICINSKA MISLA/ACTA FACULTATIS MEDICINAE SKOPIENSIS; godisen zbornik na medicinskiot fakultet vo Skopje. Text in Macedonian, English. 1954. s-a. USD 30 to institutions.
Indexed: Biol.Abstr., Ind.Med. (coverage dropped).
—CASDDS, GNLM, Infotrieve, KNAW. **CCC.**
Published by: Univerzitet vo Skoplje, Medicinski Fakultet, Central Library, Vodnjanska bb, Skopje 91000, Macedonia. Ed. Avram Sadikario.

610 YUG ISSN 0025-8091
MEDICINSKI GLASNIK* . Text in Serbo-Croatian. 1966 (vol.20). m. YUN 50, USD 5.75.
Indexed: Biol.Abstr., C.I.S. Abstr., Dent.Ind., Ind.Med. (coverage dropped).
—GNLM.
Published by: Savez Lekarskih Drustava SFR Jugoslavije, Zeleni Venac 1-I, Belgrade, Yugoslavia. Ed. Lazar Stanojevic.

610 YUG ISSN 0025-8105 CODEN: MEPEAB
MEDICINSKI PREGLED. Text in Serbian; Abstracts in English. 1948. bi-m., latest vol.54. YUN 250 domestic; USD 60 foreign (effective 2001). adv. bk.rev. reprints avail. *Refereed.* **Document type:** *Journal, Academic/Scholarly.* **Description:** Covers clinical medicine of all specialities.
Indexed: Biol.Abstr., Chem.Abstr., Dent.Ind., Ind.Med. (1948-), Nutr.Abstr.
—BLDSC (0106.400000), CISTI, GNLM.
Published by: Drustvo Lekara Vojvodine/Serbian Medical Society of Vojvodina, Vase Stajica 9, Novi Sad, Vojvodina, Yugoslavia. TEL 021-28767. Ed. Danka Filipovic. Circ: 550.

610 SVN ISSN 0025-8121 CODEN: MRAZAM
MEDICINSKI RAZGLEDI. Text in Slovenian; Abstracts and contents page in English. 1961. q. SIT 900 to individuals; SIT 1,800 to institutions; SIT 500 to students (effective 1999). adv. bk.rev. index. *Refereed.* **Document type:** *Academic/Scholarly.* **Description:** Includes articles on medical practice, research, and reviews.
Indexed: Biol.Abstr., Chem.Abstr., Chem.Titles, Nutr.Abstr.
—CASDDS.
Published by: Drusto Medicinski Razgledi, Korytkova 2, Ljubljana 1000, Slovenia. TEL 386-61-442356, info@medrazgl.org, http://www.medrazgl.org. Ed. Vesna Tlaker. R&P Borut Jug. Adv. contact Andrej Repez. Circ: 3,200. **Co-sponsor:** Ministrstvo za Solstvo, Znanost in Sport/Ministry of Education, Science and Sport of the Republic of Slovenia.

610 SWE ISSN 1104-2370
MEDICINSKT FORUM; tidskrift foer allmaenmedicin. Text in Swedish. 1993. 10/yr.
Published by: Astra - Draco - Tica, Fack 2, Lund 22100, Sweden.

610 USA
MEDICO DE FAMILIA. Text in Spanish. m. **Description:** Provides practical advice to Hispanic-Americans on common health problems. Focuses on family-oriented health issues and lifestyle. Contains separate sections for men and women's health care issues.
Published by: (Interamerican College of Physicians & Surgeons (ICPS)), Interamerican Medical Publications, 40 Galesi Dr, Wayne, NJ 07470. TEL 973-812-8098, FAX 973-812-9140, icps@icps.org, http://www.icps.org/Medico_de_Familia/.

610 ITA ISSN 0025-8148
MEDICO D'ITALIA. Text in Italian. 1964. d. free per issue. adv. bk.rev. charts, illus, stat.
Published by: Federazione Nazionale degli Ordini dei Medici - Chirurghi e degli Odontoiatri, Via G.B. De Rossi, n.9, Rome, RM 00161, Italy. TEL 39-6-44242625, FAX 39-6-44242515, http://www.fnomceo.it. Circ: 313,000.

610 ITA ISSN 0390-0347
MEDICO E PAZIENTE. Text in Italian. 1975. m. ITL 30,000 (effective 2000); (includes suppl.). adv.
Related titles: Supplement: Medico e Adolescente.
Published by: (A C S), Edifarm S.p.A., Via P. Palagi 4, Milan, MI 20129, Italy. TEL 39-02-29520315, FAX 39-02-29520449, http://www.edifarm.com. Adv. contact Carla Tognoni. B&W page ITL 8,400,000, color page ITL 13,500,000; trim 250 x 185. Circ: 75,000.

616.07 USA ISSN 0278-9779
MEDICO INTERAMERICANO. Text in English. 1981. m. USD 25. adv.
Published by: Interamerican College of Physicians and Surgeons, 915 Broadway, Suite 1105, New York, NY 10010-7108. TEL 212-777-3642, FAX 212-505-7984, icps@icps.org, http://www.icps.org. Ed. Charles H Messina. Circ: 32,500.

MEDICO-LEGAL ADVISOR. see *LAW—Civil Law*

MEDICO-LEGAL SOCIETY OF VICTORIA. PROCEEDINGS. see *LAW—Civil Law*

610 658 ITA
MEDICO OSPEDALIERO. Text in Italian. 10/yr.
Address: Via Caminadella, 21, Milan, MI 20123, Italy. TEL 2-870946. Ed. Umberto Marini. Circ: 30,000.

610 ESP
EL MEDICO, PROFESION Y HUMANIDADES. Text in Spanish. w. **Document type:** *Academic/Scholarly.* **Description:** Takes a multidisciplinary approach to discussing various aspects of the medical profession.
Indexed: Excerp.Med.
Published by: Saned S.A., Capitan Haya, 60, Madrid 28020, Spain. TEL 34-91-749-9507, FAX 34-91-749-9507, saned@meditex.es. Ed. Jenaro Bascuas. adv.: B&W page ESP 300,000, color page ESP 325,000. Circ: 35,000.

MEDICOLEGAL LIBRARY. see *LAW—International Law*

610 KEN ISSN 0253-0961
MEDICOM; African journal of hospital medicine. Text in English. 1979. bi-m. adv. bk.rev. back issues avail. **Document type:** *Academic/Scholarly.*
Published by: Update Publishers Ltd., PO Box 73824, Nairobi, Kenya. Circ: 1,000.

610 DEU ISSN 1437-7373
▼ **MEDICUS PLUS**; unabhaengiger Informationsdienst fuer den erfolgreichen Arzt. Text in German. 1999. m. EUR 113.80 domestic to institutions; EUR 123.90 in Europe to institutions; EUR 137.90 elsewhere to institutions; EUR 12.80 newsstand/cover (effective 2002). **Document type:** *Journal, Academic/Scholarly.*
Published by: Hippokrates Verlag GmbH, Postfach 300504, Stuttgart 70445, Germany. TEL 49-711-8931-0, FAX 49-711-8931706, http://www.hippokrates.de/fachzeitschriften/fz_medicusplus.html, http://www.thieme.de.

610 ITA ISSN 1121-2810
MEDIFAX; la rivista del medico che legge. Text in Italian. 1991. q. bk.rev. illus, tr.lit. back issues avail. **Document type:** *Newsletter.* **Description:** Reviews in the medical field to give a broader perspective on medicine to doctors.
Published by: Il Pensiero Scientifico Editore s.r.l., Via Bradano, 3-C, Rome, RM 00199, Italy. TEL 39-06-862821, FAX 39-06-86282250, pensiero@pensiero.it, http://www.pensiero.it. Ed. Luca De Fiore. Adv. contact Luciano De Fiore. Circ: 10,000.

610 TUR ISSN 1301-0034
MEDIKAL & TEKNIK. Text in Turkish; Section in English. 1985. m. USD 100 (effective 2001). 150 p./no. 3 cols./p. **Document type:** *Trade.*
Published by: Ihlas Magazine Group, Ihlas Holding Mrk. Binasi, 29 Ekim Cad. 23, Yenibosna - Istanbul 34530, Turkey. TEL 90-212-4542530, FAX 90-212-4542555, bsensoz@img.com.tr, imga@img.com.tr, http://www.img.com.tr. Ed. Ahmet Kizil. Pub. Ferruh Isik. R&P Muhsin Yilmaz. Adv. contact Ms. Bahar Sensoz. Circ: 17,210.

610 SWE ISSN 1402-3881
MEDIKAMENT. Text in Swedish. 1996. 7/yr. SEK 360 (effective 2001). adv. bk.rev. back issues avail. **Document type:** *Magazine, Trade.* **Description:** Medical art written by the profession, for the profession and other interested audience.
Published by: Ljusnandalens Media AB, Kulthammar, Box 3, Jaervsoe 82040, Sweden. TEL 46-651-76-76-78, FAX 46-651-475-80, redax@medikament.nu, http://www.medikament.nu. Ed. Bo Zackrisson. Pub. Haakan Hedin. R&P, Adv. contact Tord Amre TEL 46-651-475-85. B&W page SEK 19,900, color page SEK 24,900; trim 178 x 262. Circ: 22,900 (paid).

610 JPN ISSN 0911-7075
MEDIKARU HYUMANITI* /MEDICAL HUMANITY. Text in Japanese. 1985. q. JPY 1,602 per issue.
Related titles: ♦ Supplement: Bessatsu Medikaru Hyumaniti. ISSN 0915-129X.
Published by: Sokyusha, 3-4-102 Ayamedai, Inoge-ku, Chiba 2630052, Japan. Ed. Kiyoshi Nojima.

MEDINDEX ELECTRONIC ONLINE DIRECTORY. see *INSTRUMENTS*

MEDIPHARM. see *PHARMACY AND PHARMACOLOGY*

610 NGA ISSN 0794-3733 CODEN: MEMJEF
MEDIPHARM MEDICAL JOURNAL. Text in English. q. USD 50 to individuals; USD 60 to institutions (effective 2000). adv. **Document type:** *Academic/Scholarly.*
—CASDDS.
Published by: Literamed Nigeria Ltd., Oregun Village, PMB 21068, Ikeja, Lagos, Nigeria. Ed. Oladapo A Ashiru. Circ: 2,000.

610 NLD ISSN 0025-8245
MEDISCH CONTACT. Text in Dutch. 1945. w. NLG 378 foreign to members. adv. illus. **Document type:** *Trade.* **Description:** Bridges the gap between doctors and other professionals in health care with articles and commentary, along with opinion.
Related titles: ♦ Supplement: Geneesmiddelenbulletin. ISSN 0304-4629; ♦ ArtsenZaken. ISSN 1387-1870.
Indexed: Abstr.Crim.& Pen., Excerp.Med., Key to Econ.Sci.
—GNLM, KNAW.
Published by: (Koninklijke Nederlandsche Maatschappij tot Bevordering der Geneeskunst (KNMG)), Elsevier Gezondheidszorg B.V., Tijdstroom (Subsidiary of: Reed Elsevier plc Group), Planetenbaan 1, Maarssen 3600 AK, Netherlands. TEL 31-346-577577, FAX 31-346-554287, http://www.tijdstroom.nl. Ed. Dr. C Spreeuwenberg. Adv. contact Cor Vannek. Circ: 26,500 (controlled). **Subscr. to:** Elsevier Den Haag, Postbus 16500, The Hague 2500 BM, Netherlands. TEL 31-70-381-9900, FAX 31-70-381-8399.

610 NLD ISSN 1385-6103
MEDISCH NIEUWS. Text in Dutch. 1981. m. (11/yr.). NLG 110.20. adv. illus. **Document type:** *Trade.* **Description:** Reports medical news in the health care industry.
Published by: Elsevier Gezondheidszorg B.V., Tijdstroom (Subsidiary of: Reed Elsevier plc Group), Planetenbaan 1, Maarssen 3600 AK, Netherlands. TEL 31-346-577577, FAX 31-346-544287, http://www.tijdstroom.nl. **Subscr. to:** Elsevier Den Haag, Postbus 16500, The Hague 2500 BM, Netherlands. TEL 31-70-381-9900, FAX 31-70-333-8399.

610 GBR ISSN 0261-7099
MEDISCOPE. Text in English. 1898. 3/yr. GBP 5 to individuals; GBP 7 foreign to individuals; GBP 6 to libraries; GBP 9 foreign to libraries. adv. bk.rev. charts, illus. **Document type:** *Academic/Scholarly.*
Formerly: Manchester Medical Gazette (0025-2018)
Indexed: Ind.Med. (coverage dropped).
—CISTI, GNLM.
Published by: University of Manchester, Medical School, Stopford Bldg, University Of Manchester, Oxford Rd, Manchester, Lancs M13 9PT, United Kingdom. TEL 44-161-275-5532, mediscope@fs2.scg.man.ac.uk. Ed., R&P Sheraz Ahmad. Adv. contact Amanda Law. Circ: 1,500.

610 RUS
MEDITSINA DLYA VAS. Text in Russian. 24/yr. USD 145 in United States.
Published by: Izdatel'skaya Korporatsiya Meditsina dlya Vas, Novyi Arbat 2, Moscow 121019, Russian Federation. TEL 7-095-2022518, FAX 7-095-2415320. Ed. N G Ignatov. **US dist. addr.:** East View Publications, 3020 Harbor Ln N, Minneapolis, MN 55447. TEL 612-550-0961.

M

610 RUS
MEDITSINA I ZDRAVOOKHRANENIE: AVTORSKII UKAZATEL' NAUCHNYKH STATEI OT A DO YA. Text in Russian. s-a. USD 239.95 in United States.
Published by: Tsentral'naya Meditsinskaya Biblioteka, Ul Krasikova 30, Moscow 117418, Russian Federation. TEL 7-095-1282701. **US dist. addr.:** East View Publications, 3020 Harbor Ln N, Minneapolis, MN 55447. TEL 612-550-0961.

610 RUS
MEDITSINA I ZDRAVOOKHRANENIE: PREDMETNYI UKAZATEL' NAUCHNYKH STATEI. Text in Russian. s-a. USD 69.95 in United States.
Published by: Tsentral'naya Meditsinskaya Biblioteka, Ul Krasikova 30, Moscow 117418, Russian Federation. TEL 7-095-1282701. **US dist. addr.:** East View Publications, 3020 Harbor Ln N, Minneapolis, MN 55447. TEL 612-550-0961.

610 RUS ISSN 0025-8318
MEDITSINSKAYA GAZETA. Text in Russian. 1938. s-w. RUR 387 for 6 mos. (effective 2000). index. **Document type:** *Magazine, Consumer.*
Related titles: Microfilm ed.: (from EVP); Microform ed.: (from PQC).
Indexed: Biol.Abstr., Curr.Dig.Sov.Press.
—CCC.
Published by: (Medical Workers' Union), Meditsinskaya Gazeta, Sukharevskaya pl 1-2, Moscow 129010, Russian Federation. TEL 7-095-2088695, FAX 7-095-2088204, medgazeta@glasnet.ru, http://www.medgazeta.rusmedserv.com. Ed. A Poltorak. Circ: 50,000. **Dist. by:** Mezhdunarodnaya Kniga, B Yakimanka 39, Moscow 117049, Russian Federation. TEL 7-095-2384967, FAX 7-095-2384634; **Dist. in U.S. by:** Victor Kamkin Inc., 4956 Boiling Brook Pkwy, Rockville, MD 20852.

610 RUS
MEDITSINSKAYA KONSUL'TATSIYA. Text in Russian. q. USD 85 in United States.
Indexed: Ref.Zh.
Published by: Tsentr Mediko-Sotsyal'noi i Proizvodstvennoi Adaptatsii, A-ya 389, Moscow 117334, Russian Federation. TEL 7-095-1370629, FAX 7-095-3166812. Ed. Yu D Sharets. **US dist. addr.:** East View Publications, 3020 Harbor Ln N, Minneapolis, MN 55447. TEL 612-550-0961.

610 RUS ISSN 0025-8075
CODEN: MEDTBV
MEDITSINSKAYA TEKHNIKA/MEDICAL ENGINEERING. Text in Russian; Summaries in English. 1967. bi-m. USD 184 foreign (effective 2000). adv. bk.rev., Website rev. abstr. reprints avail. **Document type:** *Journal, Academic/Scholarly.* **Description:** Deals with theoretical and practical problems of the development of medical engineering and its application in public health practice.
Related titles: ♦ English Translation: Biomedical Engineering. ISSN 0006-3398.
Indexed: Bibl.Asian Stud. (1970-1990), Biol.Abstr., Chem.Abstr., Dent.Ind., Eng.Ind., INIS Atomind., INSPEC (Jan.1972-, dropped), Ind.Med. (1967-), Ref.Zh.
—CASDDS, CISTI, East View, GNLM, Infotrieve. **CCC.**
Published by: Izdatel'stvo Meditsina, Petroverigskii per 6-8, Moscow 101000, Russian Federation. TEL 7-095-9248785, 7-095-928-86-48, FAX 7-095-9211355, 7-095-9286003, meditsina@iname.com, http://www.medit.ru. Ed. V A Viktorov. Pub. A M Stochik. R&P G Scherbakova. Adv. contact O A Fadeeva TEL 7-095-923-51-40. Circ: 1,500. **Dist. by:** Mezhdunarodnaya Kniga, B Yakimanka 39, Moscow 117049, Russian Federation. TEL 7-095-2384967, FAX 7-095-2384634; **US dist. addr.:** East View Publications, 3020 Harbor Ln N, Minneapolis, MN 55447. TEL 612-550-0961.

610 RUS
MEDITSINSKIE NOVOSTI. Text in Russian. m. USD 99 in United States.
Address: Krovokolennyi per 12, Moscow 101000, Russian Federation. TEL 7-095-9252370, FAX 7-095-9230407. Ed. N V Gogol'. **US dist. addr.:** East View Publications, 3020 Harbor Ln N, Minneapolis, MN 55447. TEL 612-550-0961.

610 UKR
MEDITSINSKIE VESTI. Text in Ukrainian. q. USD 110 in United States.
Indexed: Ref.Zh.
Published by: Izdatel'stvo Meditsina Ukrainy, A-ya 385, Kiev 253222, Ukraine. TEL 517-23-83, FAX 532-43-85. **US dist. addr.:** East View Publications, 3020 Harbor Ln N, Minneapolis, MN 55447. TEL 612-550-0961.

610 RUS
MEDITSINSKII BIZNES. Text in Russian. m. USD 125 in United States.
Published by: Izdatel'stvo Meditsinskii Biznes, A-ya 12, Moscow 111020, Russian Federation. TEL 7-095-3684703, FAX 7-095-3603441. Ed. M A Kushnareva. **US dist. addr.:** East View Publications, 3020 Harbor Ln N, Minneapolis, MN 55447. TEL 612-550-0961.

610 RUS
MEDITSINSKII VESTNIK. Text in Russian. 24/yr. USD 159.95 in United States.
Published by: Izdatel'skii Dom Meditsinskii Vestnik, A-ya 36, Moscow 103009, Russian Federation. TEL 7-095-2458664, FAX 7-095-1257623. Ed. N N Simonova. **US dist. addr.:** East View Publications, 3020 Harbor Ln N, Minneapolis, MN 55447. TEL 612-550-0961.

610 UZB ISSN 0025-830X
R97.5.R8 CODEN: MZUZA8
MEDITSINSKII ZHURNAL UZBEKISTANA. Text in Uzbek. 1948. m. USD 9.20.
Indexed: Biol.Abstr., Chem.Abstr., Chem.Indus.Notes, Chem.Titles, Nutr.Abstr.
—BLDSC (0106.500000), CASDDS, CISTI, GNLM, Infotrieve. **CCC.**
Published by: Izdatel'stvo Meditsina, Otdelenie v Uzbekistane, Ul Alishera Navoi 30, Tashkent, Uzbekistan. Ed. K C Zaupoe.

610 DEU ISSN 0939-351X
MEDIZIN, GESELLSCHAFT UND GESCHICHTE. Text in English, German. 1985. a. EUR 28.26 domestic; EUR 30.66 in Europe; EUR 35.32 elsewhere; EUR 20.80 to students (effective 2002). **Document type:** *Monographic series, Academic/Scholarly.*
Formerly: Institut fuer Geschichte der Medizin der Robert Bosch Stiftung. Jahrbuch
Indexed: IBZ.
—GNLM.
Published by: (Institut fuer Geschichte der Medizin der Robert Bosch Stiftung), Franz Steiner Verlag Stuttgart GmbH, Birkenwaldstr 44, Stuttgart 70191, Germany. TEL 49-711-2582-0, FAX 49-711-2582390, service@steiner-verlag.de, http://www.steiner-verlag.de. Ed. Robert Juette. R&P Sabine Koerner.

610 DEU ISSN 0941-5033
MEDIZIN, GESELLSCHAFT UND GESCHICHTE. BEIHEFTE. Text in German. 1992. irreg., latest vol.13, 2000. **Document type:** *Monographic series, Academic/Scholarly.*
Published by: Franz Steiner Verlag Stuttgart GmbH, Birkenwaldstr 44, Stuttgart 70191, Germany. TEL 49-711-2582-0, FAX 49-711-2582390, franz.steiner.verlag@t-online.de, http://www.steiner-verlag.de. Ed. Robert Juette. R&P Sabine Koerner.

610 AUT
MEDIZIN POPULAER. Text in German. bi-m. free. adv. **Document type:** *Bulletin.*
Published by: Oesterreichische Aerztekammer, Pressestelle und Verlag, Weihburggasse 9, Vienna, W 1010, Austria. TEL 43-1-5124486, FAX 43-1-512448624.

610 DEU ISSN 1435-1900
MEDIZIN REPORT. Text in German. 1998. q. back issues avail. **Document type:** *Academic/Scholarly, Consumer.*
Media: E-mail. **Related titles:** Online - full text ed.
Published by: (Muenchner Collegium fuer Therapieforschung e.V.), Wort und Bild Verlag Konradshoehe GmbH, Konradshoehe, Baierbrunn 82065, Germany. TEL 49-89-74433-0, FAX 49-89-74433150, red.mr@wortundbildverlag.de.

610 600 DEU ISSN 0943-5131
MEDIZIN, TECHNIK UND GESELLSCHAFT. Text in German. 1993. irreg. **Document type:** *Monographic series.*
—CISTI.
Published by: (Gesellschaft fuer Innovation und Technologietransfer Biomedizin), Peter Lang GmbH Europaeischer Verlag der Wissenschaften, Eschborner Landstr 42-50, Frankfurt Am Main 60489, Germany. TEL 49-69-780705-0, FAX 49-69-78070543, 101622.27@compuserve.com, zentrale.frankfurt@peterlang.com, http://www.peterlang.de. R&P Ruediger Brunsch.

610 170 AUT ISSN 0948-065X
MEDIZIN UND ETHIK. Text in German. 1995. irreg. price varies. **Document type:** *Monographic series, Academic/Scholarly.*
Published by: (Institut fuer Medizinische Anthropologie und Bioethik), Springer-Verlag Wien (Subsidiary of: BertelsmannSpringer), Sachsenplatz 4-6, PO Box 89, Vienna, W 1201, Austria. TEL 43-1-3302415-0, FAX 43-1-330242665, books@springer.at, http://www.springer.at. Eds. J Bonelli, M Schwarz. R&P Angela Foessl TEL 43-1-3302415517. **Dist. in N. America by:** Springer-Verlag, Journals. books@springer.at, http://www.springer-ny.com.

MEDIZIN UND PHILOSOPHIE; Beitraege aus der Forschung. see *PHILOSOPHY*

610 USA
MEDIZINE. Text in English. q. adv. **Document type:** *Magazine, Consumer.* **Description:** Aims to educate consumers about ailments and available treatments in order to initiate intelligent discussions with health care providers.
Related titles: ♦ Online - full content ed.: MediZine.com.
Published by: MediZine, Inc., 298 Fifth Ave, 2nd Fl, New York, NY 10001. TEL 212-695-2223, FAX 212-695-2936, info@medizine.com, http://www.medizine.com. Ed. Diane Umansky. Pub. Traver Hutchins. Circ: 3,500,000.

610 USA
MEDIZINE.COM. Text in English. d. adv. **Document type:** *Consumer.* **Description:** Allows consumers to access up-to-the-minute health news.
Media: Online - full content. **Related titles:** ♦ Print ed.: MediZine.
Published by: MediZine, Inc., 298 Fifth Ave, 2nd Fl, New York, NY 10001. TEL 212-695-2223, FAX 212-695-2936, info@medizine.com, http://www.medizine.com. Ed. Diane Umansky. Pub. Traver Hutchins.

610 USA
▼ **MEDIZINE GUIDEBOOK.** Text in English. 2000. q. adv. **Document type:** *Magazine, Consumer.*
Published by: MediZine, Inc., 298 Fifth Ave, 2nd Fl, New York, NY 10001. TEL 212-695-2223, FAX 212-695-2936, info@medizine.com, http://www.medizine.com.

610 DEU ISSN 0025-8431
R131.A1 CODEN: MEDJE4
MEDIZINHISTORISCHES JOURNAL. Text in English, French, German. 1966. 4/yr. EUR 93, GBP 80 (effective 2002). adv. bk.rev. index. *Refereed.* **Document type:** *Journal, Academic/Scholarly.* **Description:** Provides a forum for research into the history of medicine and health in their scientific, social, political, and cultural contexts.
Indexed: Amer.Hist.& Life, BHA, Biol.Abstr., Chem.Abstr., Hist.Abstr. (1988-), IBZ, Ind.Med. (1966-), P C I.
—GNLM. **CCC.**
Published by: (Akademie der Wissenschaften und der Literatur, Mainz, Kommission fuer Geschichte der Medizin und der Naturwissenschaften), Urban & Fischer Verlag, Loebdergraben 14a, Jena 07743, Germany. TEL 49-3641-626444, FAX 49-3641-626500, journals@urbanfischer.de, http://www.urbanfischer.de/journals. R&P Martin Huber TEL 49-3641-626430. Circ: 1,000. **Subscr. to:** Nature Publishing Group, Brunel Rd, Basingstoke RG21 6XS, United Kingdom. TEL 44-1256-302629, FAX 44-1256-463570, j.stephens@macmillan.com.

610 USA ISSN 0342-4103
MEDIZINISCHE INFORMATIK UND STATISTIK. Text in German. 1976. irreg., latest vol.68, 1988. price varies. reprint service avail. from ISI. **Document type:** *Academic/Scholarly.*
—CISTI, GNLM.
Published by: Springer-Verlag, Journals (Subsidiary of: BertelsmannSpringer), 175 Fifth Ave, New York, NY 10010. TEL 212-460-1500, FAX 212-473-6272.

610 DEU ISSN 0723-5003
CODEN: MEKLA7
MEDIZINISCHE KLINIK. Text in German. 1906. m. EUR 178.62 domestic; EUR 191.62 foreign; EUR 77.68 domestic to students; EUR 90.68 foreign to students; EUR 14.95 newsstand/cover (effective 2002). *Refereed.* **Document type:** *Journal, Academic/Scholarly.*
Related titles: Online - full text ed.: ISSN 1615-6722 (from EBSCO Publishing, RoweCom Information Quest, Swets Blackwell, Springer LINK, Institute for Scientific Information).

M

Indexed: ASCA, Abstr.Hyg., Agri.& Environ.Biotech.Abstr. (coverage dropped), Aqua.Sci.& Fish.Abstr., Biol.Abstr., C.I.S. Abstr., Cal.Tiss.Abstr., Chem.Abstr., Chem.Titles, Curr.Cont., Derwent Biotech.Abstr., Environ.Sci.Poll.Mgmt., Excerp.Med., Helminthol.Abstr., INIS Atomind., Ind.Med. (1983-), Ind.Sci.Rev., Inpharma, Int.Abstr.Biol.Sci., Int.Nurs.Ind., Nutr.Abstr., Pollut.Abstr., Reac., Rev.Med.& Vet.Mycol., Risk Abstr., SSCI (coverage dropped), Saf.Sci.Abstr.
—BLDSC (5535.080000), CASDDS, CISTI, EMDOCS, GNLM, IDS, Infotrieve, KNAW. **CCC.**
Published by: (Deutsche Gesellschaft fuer Innere Medizin), Urban und Vogel Medien und Medizin Verlagsgesellschaft mbH (Subsidiary of: BertelsmannSpringer), Neumarkter Str 43, Munich 81673, Germany. TEL 49-89-43721411, FAX 49-89-43721410, verlag@urban-vogel.de, http://www.urban-vogel.de. Ed. J Koebberling. R&P Oliver Renn. Adv. contact Sibylle Schurr TEL 49-89-43721353. Circ: 10,000 (controlled). **Subscr. to:** Springer Auslieferungs Gesellschaft, Postfach 105160, Heidelberg 69041, Germany. TEL 49-6221-345244, FAX 49-6221-345244.

MEDIZINISCHE KONGRESSE; national - international. see *MEETINGS AND CONGRESSES*

610 USA ISSN 0076-6151
MEDIZINISCHE LAENDERKUNDE. GEOMEDICAL MONOGRAPH SERIES. Short title: Geomedical Monograph Series. Text in German. 1967. irreg., latest vol.5, 1978. price varies. reprint service avail. from ISI. **Document type:** *Monographic series.*
—CISTI.
Published by: Springer-Verlag, Journals (Subsidiary of: BertelsmannSpringer), 175 Fifth Ave, New York, NY 10010. TEL 212-460-1500, FAX 212-473-6272.

610 DEU ISSN 0342-9601
CODEN: MMPHDB
MEDIZINISCHE MONATSSCHRIFT FUER PHARMAZEUTEN. Text and summaries in German. 1947. m. EUR 101.88 domestic; EUR 113.52 foreign; EUR 64.08 to students; EUR 11 newsstand/cover (effective 2002). adv. bk.rev. illus, tr.lit. **Document type:** *Journal, Trade.*
Formerly: Medizinische Monatsschrift (0025-8474)
Indexed: Agri.& Environ.Biotech.Abstr. (coverage dropped), Biol.Abstr., Chem.Abstr., Chem.Indus.Notes, Chem.Titles, Derwent Biotech.Abstr., Excerp.Med., I.P.A., Ind.Med. (1978-), Inpharma, Reac.
—BLDSC (5535.108000), CASDDS, CISTI, EMDOCS, GNLM, Infotrieve, KNAW. **CCC.**
Published by: Deutscher Apotheker Verlag, Postfach 101061, Stuttgart 70009, Germany. TEL 49-711-2582234, FAX 49-711-2582283, mmp@wissenschaftliche-verlagsgesellschaft.de, service@deutscher-apotheker-verlag.de, http://www.deutscher-apotheker-verlag.de/MMP/MMP.HTM. Ed. Susanne Heinzl. Adv. contact Klaus Graef TEL 49-711-2582245. Circ: 12,700. **Co-publisher:** Wissenschaftliche Verlagsgesellschaft mbH.

610 DEU ISSN 0025-8490
DER MEDIZINISCHE SACHVERSTAENDIGE. Text in German. 1904. bi-m. DEM 240.30 domestic; DEM 249.90 foreign (effective 2000). adv. bk.rev. abstr, charts, illus. index. **Document type:** *Academic/Scholarly.*
Indexed: C.I.S. Abstr., Chem.Abstr.
—GNLM. **CCC.**
Published by: Gentner Verlag Stuttgart, Forststr 131, Stuttgart 70193, Germany. TEL 49-711-63672-0, FAX 49-711-63672-11. Ed. Norbert Roesner. R&P Gernot Keuchen. Adv. contact Sebastian Vonbeckerath. Circ: 1,298.

610 DEU ISSN 0025-8512
CODEN: MEWEAC
DIE MEDIZINISCHE WELT. Text in German. 1950. m. DEM 292 to individuals; DEM 353 to institutions; DEM 100 to students (effective 2001). adv. bk.rev. bibl, charts, illus. index. *Refereed.* **Document type:** *Journal, Academic/Scholarly.*
Related titles: Microform ed.: (from PMC); Online - full text ed.: (from Institute for Scientific Information).
Indexed: ASCA, Agri.& Environ.Biotech.Abstr. (coverage dropped), Biol.Abstr., C.I.S. Abstr., Chem.Abstr., Curr.Adv.Ecol.Sci., Curr.Cont. (coverage dropped), Dent.Ind., Derwent Biotech.Abstr., Excerp.Med., Helminthol.Abstr., INIS Atomind., Ind.Med. (coverage dropped), Inpharma, Nutr.Abstr., Reac., SSCI (coverage dropped).
—BLDSC (5535.200000), CASDDS, CISTI, GNLM, IDS, Infotrieve, KNAW. **CCC.**
Published by: Schattauer GmbH, Hoelderlinstr 3, Stuttgart 70174, Germany. TEL 49-711-22987-0, FAX 49-711-2298750, info@schattauer.de, http://www.schattauer.com. Pub. Dieter Bergemann. R&P Annika Schmidt TEL 49-711-2298713. Adv. contact Thomas Christ. B&W page XEU 2,633.15, color page XEU 3,963.94; 184 x 243. Circ: 32,000. **Subscr. to:** CSJ, Postfach 140220, Munich 80452, Germany. TEL 49-89-20959129, schattauer@csj.de.

610 DEU ISSN 0944-1123
MEDIZINLAND; Zeitschrift fuer Patienten und Praxis. Text in German. 1993. m. **Document type:** *Trade.*
Published by: Hoffmann und Hoffmann GmbH, August-Schanz-Str 8-II, Frankfurt A.m. 60433, Germany. TEL 49-69-5400015, FAX 49-69-54800080, huhgmbh@aol.com.

610 DEU ISSN 0944-6885
MEDIZINPRODUKTE JOURNAL; Journal fuer Wissenschaft und Praxis, Handel und Anwender. Abbreviated title: M P J. Text in German. 1994. q. EUR 84.36 domestic; EUR 88.08 foreign; EUR 25 newsstand/cover (effective 2002). **Document type:** *Journal, Trade.*
—GNLM.
Published by: Wissenschaftliche Verlagsgesellschaft mbH, Postfach 101061, Stuttgart 70009, Germany. TEL 49-711-2582-0, FAX 49-711-2582-290, service@wissenschaftliche-verlagsgesellschaft.de, http://www.wissenschaftliche-verlagsgesellschaft.de. Ed. Gert Schorn. Adv. contact Klaus Graef TEL 49-711-2582245.

MEDIZINSOZIOLOGIE. see *SOCIAL SCIENCES: COMPREHENSIVE WORKS*

610 CHE
MEDKALENDER. Text in German. 1878. a. CHF 65 (effective 2001). index. **Document type:** *Trade.*
Description: Provides information for medical doctors and pharmacists on drugs and preparations with notes on pharmacology and dosages, as well as information on emergency treatment of poisoning.
Former titles: Schweizerischer Medizinalkalender; Schweizerischer Medizinalkalender und Arzneimitteluebersicht; Schweizerischer Medizinalkalender (0251-1762)
—GNLM, Infotrieve. **CCC.**
Published by: Schwabe und Co. AG, Steinentorstr 13, Basel 4010, Switzerland. TEL 41-61-2789565, FAX 41-61-2789566, verlag@schwabe.ch, http://www.schwabe.ch.

610.284 USA
MEDPRO MONTH* . Text in English. 1990. m. USD 995; USD 895 renewals. **Document type:** *Newsletter.*
Description: Provides an insight into how the medical device marketplace is unfolding, identifying markets at risk, as well as those with opportunities for growth.
Incorporates (in Mar. 1996): Inside Surgery
Related titles: Online - full text ed.: 1990.
Published by: Medical Data International, 5 Hutton Centre Dr, Ste 1100, Santa Ana, CA 92707-8714. TEL 949-251-2180, FAX 949-251-2781, http://www.medicaldata.com. Ed. Pieter Walter. Circ: 800 (paid).

610 USA
MEDSUPPORT F S F NEWSLETTER. (Friends Supporting Friends) Text in English. 1995. bi-m. *Refereed.* **Document type:** *Newsletter.* **Description:** Offers medical and diet tips, as well as medical news to those with disabilities or medical problems by others with the same.
Media: Online - full text.
Address: http://www.medsupport.org/news.html. Eds. Allen Flores, Peggy Pitkin.

610.72 CAN ISSN 0972-267X
▼ **MEDUCATOR.** Text in English. 2000. q. INR 600 in India to individuals; USD 40 rest of world to individuals; INR 1,200 in India to institutions; USD 120 rest of world to institutions; INR 750 in India to individuals combined Print & Online eds.; USD 60 rest of world to individuals combined Print & Online eds.; INR 1,600 in India to institutions combined Print & Online eds.; USD 200 rest of world to institutions combined Print & Online eds. (effective 2001). **Description:** Aims to provide an outlet for the opinions, communications and original research papers which have a particular interest to healthcare professionals in emerging countries. Seeks to promote interaction in medical education and serve as a meeting place for the global village of medical educators.
Related titles: Online - full text ed.: ISSN 1496-3671. INR 300 in India to individuals; USD 30 rest of world to individuals; INR 600 in India to institutions; USD 100 rest of world to institutions (effective 2001).
Published by: Meducational Skills, Tools and Technology, Inc., 182 Tuscarona Circle NW, Calgary, AB T3L 2B9, Canada. TEL 403-220-9377, FAX 403-220-9387, subscriptinfo@meducational.com, http://www.meducatinal.com/journal. Eds. John S Baumber, Kalyani Premkumar.

MEDYCYNA DOSWIADCZALNA I MIKROBIOLOGIA. see *BIOLOGY—Microbiology*

610.9 POL ISSN 1231-1960
R131.A1
MEDYCYNA NOWOZYTNA/MODERN MEDICINE - STUDY ON HISTORY OF MEDICINE; studia nad historia medycyny. Text in Polish; Summaries in English, German. 1994. s-a. PLZ 15 newsstand/cover. adv. bibl, illus. **Document type:** *Newspaper, Academic/Scholarly, Trade.*
Published by: Polska Akademia Nauk, Instytut Historii Nauki, Palac Staszica, Ul Nowy Swiat 72, Warsaw 00330, Poland. TEL 48-22-6472746, FAX 48-22-82666137, ihn@ihnpan.waw.pl. Ed. Zofia Podgorska Klawe. Adv. contact Bozena Plonka Syroka. Circ: 300 (controlled). **Dist. by:** Ars Polona, Krakowskie Przedmiescie 7, Warsaw, Poland.

610 613.62 POL ISSN 0465-5893
CODEN: MEPAAX
MEDYCYNA PRACY. Text in Polish. 1950. bi-m., latest vol.52. USD 90 (effective 2002). adv. index. 80 p./no. 2 cols./p. **Document type:** *Journal, Academic/Scholarly.*
Description: Explores occupational hygiene, pathologies, epidemiology, physiology and psychology of health care organizations.
Related titles: CD-ROM ed.
Indexed: Abstr.Hyg., Biol.Abstr., C.I.S. Abstr., Chem.Abstr., Chem.Indus.Notes, Chem.Titles, Dent.Ind., Excerp.Med., Forest Prod.Abstr., Forest.Abstr., Fuel & Energy Abstr., INIS Atomind., Ind.Med. (1948-), Nutr.Abstr., PsycInfo, Psychol.Abstr. (1990-), Rev.Appl.Entomol., Rev.Med.& Vet.Mycol., Soyabean Abstr., Trop.Dis.Bull., e-psyche.
—BLDSC (5536.020000), CASDDS, CISTI, GNLM.
Published by: Instytut Medycyny Pracy im. Jerzego Nofera/Nofer Institute of Occupational Medicine, Ul Sw. Teresy 8, PO Box 199, Lodz 90950, Poland. TEL 48-42-6314566, FAX 48-42-6314719, redakcja@porta.imp.lodz.pl. Ed., R&P, Adv. contact Irena Szadkowska Stanczyk. Circ: 650.

610 POL ISSN 0867-499X
MEDYCYNA PRAKTYCZNA. Text in Polish. 1991. m. PLZ 78 (effective 2000). adv. back issues avail. **Document type:** *Academic/Scholarly.* **Description:** Covers all fields of medicine, intended for practising physicians.
Address: Ul Skawinska 8, Krakow 31066, Poland. TEL 48-12-4305520, FAX 48-12-4305536. Ed. Piotr Gajewski. Circ: 12,000 (paid).

610 POL ISSN 0025-8636
MEDYCYNA WIEJSKA/RURAL MEDICINE. Text in English, Polish. 1953. q. USD 60. adv. bk.rev. index. back issues avail.; reprints avail. **Description:** For the rural physicians from the village health centers and the physicians employed in regional outpatient clinics in the towns. Contains publications concerning the evaluation of the living and working environment in rural areas.
Indexed: Apic.Abstr., C.I.S. Abstr.
—GNLM.
Published by: Instytut Medycyny Wsi, Ul Jaczewskiego 2, Lublin 20950, Poland. TEL 48-81-778027, FAX 48-81-778646. Ed. Maciej Latalski. Circ: 1,000. **Dist. by:** Ars Polona, Krakowskie Przedmiescie 7, Warsaw, Poland.

610 POL ISSN 0867-3055
MEDYK/PHYSICIAN. Text in Polish. 1953. m. PLZ 36; PLZ 50 foreign (effective 2002). adv. bk.rev. 48 p./no. 2 cols./p. back issues avail. **Document type:** *Newspaper.*
Formerly: Nowy Medyk (0137-7175)
Published by: Medyk Ltd. Co., Ul Skierniewicka 16-20, Warsaw 01230, Poland. TEL 48-22-6311392, FAX 48-22-6311392, medyk@medyk.com.pl. Ed. Justyna Hofman-Wisniewska. Pub., R&P Andrzej Doroba. Adv. contact Sylwia Bielska. B&W page PLZ 800; trim 205 x 290. Circ: 4,500. **Dist. by:** RUCH S.A., ul Jana Kazimierza 31/33, Warsaw 00958, Poland. TEL 48-22-5328731, FAX 48-22-5238732.

M

610 CHN ISSN 1000-842X
MEIGUO YIXUEHUI ZAZHI (ZHONGWEN BAN)/J A M A: THE JOURNAL OF THE AMERICAN MEDICAL ASSOCIATION (CHINESE EDITION). Text in Chinese. 1982. bi-m. USD 15; USD 2.50, CNY 5 newsstand/cover (effective 2001). **Document type:** *Academic/Scholarly.*
Related titles: Online - full content ed.: (from WanFang Data Corp.); ♦ English ed.: J A M A: The Journal of the American Medical Association. ISSN 0098-7484.
Published by: Zhonghua Yixuehui Zazhishe, 42 Dongsi Xidajie, Beijing 100710, China. cmazzs@public.sti.ac.cn. **Dist. by:** China International Book Trading Corp, 35, Chegongzhuang Xilu, Haidian District, Beijing 100044, China. TEL 86-1-68413849, FAX 86-1-68412048, cibtc@mail.cibtc.com.cn, http://www.cibtc.com.cn.

MEIKAI DAIGAKU SHIGAKU ZASSHI/MEIKAI UNIVERSITY DENTAL JOURNAL/MEIKAI UNIVERSITY SCHOOL OF DENTISTRY. JOURNAL. see *MEDICAL SCIENCES—Dentistry*

610 JPN ISSN 0287-9085
MEJIKARU NYUSU/MEDICAL NEWS. Text in Japanese. 1960. bi-m. JPY 100 per issue.
Published by: (Kyowa Kikaku Tsushin), Dainippon Seiyaku K.K./Dainippon Pharmaceutical Co., Ltd., 3-25, Doshomachi, Higashi-ku, Osaka-shi 541, Japan.

616.988 NLD ISSN 1381-3412
MEMISA MEDISCH. Text in Dutch, English. 1934. bi-m. NLG 40 (effective 1999 - 2000); free to qualified personnel. bk.rev. abstr, bibl, charts, illus, stat. index. back issues avail. *Refereed.* **Document type:** *Bulletin, Academic/Scholarly.* **Description:** Covers tropical medicine.
Formerly: Memisa Nieuws (0025-9063)
Related titles: Online - full text ed.
Published by: Memisa Medicus Mundi, Eendrachtsweg 48, Rotterdam 3012 LD, Netherlands. TEL 31-10-2064646, FAX 31-10-2064647, kok@memisa.nl, postmaster@memisa.nl. Ed. Jos Poels. R&P P W Kok. Circ: 4,000 (controlled).

610 USA
MENDOCINO MEDICINE & GAZETTEER. Text in English. q.
Published by: Mendocino Academy of Science, PO Box 165, Mendocino, CA 95460. Ed. Dr Richard White.

615.58 USA ISSN 0076-6526
RC55
MERCK MANUAL: A HANDBOOK OF DIAGNOSIS AND THERAPY. Text in English. 1899. irreg., latest vol.17, 1999. USD 35 (effective 2000). **Document type:** *Directory.*
Related titles: CD-ROM ed.
—CISTI, Linda Hall.
Published by: Merck Publishing Group, RY-7-220, P.O. Box 2000, Rahway, NJ 07065. TEL 732-594-4600, FAX 732-388-9778. Ed. Dr. Robert Berkow.

615.58 USA
THE MERCK MANUAL OF MEDICAL INFORMATION - HOME. Text in English. 1997. irreg. USD 29.95 (effective 2000). **Document type:** *Monographic series.*
Published by: Merck Publishing Group, 126 E Lincoln Ave, PO Box 2000, Rahway, NJ 07065. TEL 732-594-4600, FAX 732-388-9778.

MERIDIANS (COLUMBIA); redefining health. see *ALTERNATIVE MEDICINE*

DER MERKURSTAB. see *RELIGIONS AND THEOLOGY—Other Denominations And Sects*

610 USA ISSN 0885-7490
RC394.M48 CODEN: MBDIEE
METABOLIC BRAIN DISEASE. Text in English. 1986. q. EUR 658 to institutions for print or online ed.; USD 659, EUR 789.60 to institutions print & online eds.combined (effective 2002). adv. charts, illus. back issues avail. *Refereed.* **Document type:** *Academic/Scholarly.* **Description:** Publishes research and clinical papers dealing with all aspects of metabolic brain disease, including both human and animal studies.
Related titles: Microfilm ed.: (from PQC); Online - full text ed.: (from O C L C Online Computer Library Center, Inc., Swets Blackwell, Kluwer Online, Institute for Scientific Information).
Indexed: ASCA, Chem.Abstr., Chem.Titles, Curr.Adv.Biochem., Curr.Adv.Cell & Devel.Biol., Curr.Cont., INIS Atomind., Ind.Med. (1986-), Ind.Sci.Rev., Inpharma, Int.Abstr.Biol.Sci., Neurosci.Abstr., Neurosci.Cit.Ind., Pharm.&Out.News, Reac., Sci.Cit.Ind.
—BLDSC (5683.266500), CASDDS, CISTI, EMDOCS, GNLM, IDS, ingenta, KNAW. **CCC.**
Published by: Kluwer Academic - Plenum Publishers (Subsidiary of: Wolters Kluwer N.V.), 233 Spring St, New York, NY 10013-1578. TEL 212-620-8000, 800-221-9369, FAX 212-463-0742, services@wkap.nl, http://www.wkap.nl/journalhome.htm/0885-7490. Ed. Roger F Butterworth. R&P Rose Luongo TEL 781-871-6311.

615.19 DEU
METHODS AND PRINCIPLES IN MEDICINAL CHEMISTRY. Text in German. 1993. irreg., latest vol.3, 1994. DEM 158. **Document type:** *Monographic series, Academic/Scholarly.*
Indexed: Chem.Abstr., Chem.Titles.
—BLDSC (5746.690000).
Published by: Wiley - V C H, Postfach 101161, Weinheim 69451, Germany. TEL 49-6201-606-0, FAX 49-6201-606-328, subservice@wiley-vch.de, http://www.wiley-vch.de.

610 029 DEU ISSN 0026-1270
R51 CODEN: MIMCAI
METHODS OF INFORMATION IN MEDICINE; journal of methodology in medical research, information and documentation. Text in English. 1962. 5/yr. DEM 315 in Europe to individuals; DEM 498 in Europe to institutions; USD 206 elsewhere to individuals; USD 316 elsewhere to institutions (effective 2001). adv. bibl, charts, illus. index. *Refereed.* **Document type:** *Journal, Academic/Scholarly.* **Description:** Covers methodology of medical research, documentation, information science and medical informatics.
Related titles: Online - full text ed.: (from Institute for Scientific Information).
Indexed: ASCA, Abstr.Health Care Manage.Stud., Biol.Abstr., Compumath, Curr.Cont., Curr.Ind.Stat., Cyb.Abstr., Excerp.Med., INIS Atomind., INSPEC (Apr.1970-), Ind.Med. (1962-), Ind.Sci.Rev., Inpharma, Int.Nurs.Ind., LISA, Reac., Rev.Appl.Entomol., SSCI (coverage dropped), Sci.Cit.Ind., Telegen.
—BLDSC (5748.100000), AskIEEE, CISTI, GNLM, IDS, ingenta, KNAW. **CCC.**
Published by: Schattauer GmbH, Hoelderlinstr 3, Stuttgart 70174, Germany. TEL 49-711-22987-0, FAX 49-711-2298750, info@schattauer.de, http://www.schattauer.com. Ed. J H van Bemmel. Pub. Dieter Bergemann. R&P Annika Schmidt TEL 49-711-2298713. Adv. contact Claudia Hartmann TEL 49-711-2298727. B&W page DEM 1,880, color page DEM 3,730; 184 x 243. Circ: 1,300. **Subscr. to:** CSJ, Postfach 140220, Munich 80452, Germany. TEL 49-89-20959129, schattauer@csj.de.

610 USA ISSN 1526-4262
▼ **METRODOCTORS;** journal of the Hennepin and Ramsey medical societies. Text in English. 1999. bi-m. USD 15; USD 3 newsstand/cover (effective 2001). 36 p./no. **Document type:** *Journal, Trade.* **Description:** Articles, editorials, and advertising representing the interests of physicians in the Minneapolis - St. Paul, Minnesota communities.
Formed by the 1999 merger of: Hennepin Medical Society. Bulletin; Ramsey Medical Society. Bulletin
Published by: Hennepin Medical Society, 3433 Broadway St., NE, Ste. 325, Minneapolis, MN 55413-1761. TEL 612-623-3030, FAX 612-623-2888. Ed. Sheila Hatcher. Adv. contact Doreen Hines. **Co-sponsor:** Ramsey Medical Society.

610 NLD ISSN 0167-5885
RC90 CODEN: MPDID9
MEYLER AND PECK'S DRUG-INDUCED DISEASES. Variant title: Symposium on Drug-Induced Diseases. Proceedings. Text in Dutch. 1980 (vol 5). irreg. **Document type:** *Proceedings.*
Formerly (until 1980): Drug-Induced Diseases (0586-2779)
Indexed: Chem.Abstr.
—CASDDS, CISTI.
Published by: Elsevier Science BV, PO Box 211, Amsterdam 1000 AE, Netherlands. TEL 31-20-485-3911, FAX 31-20-485-3598, nlinfo-f@elsevier.nl, http://www.elsevier.nl. Eds. H M Peck, L Meyler.

MEYLER'S SIDE EFFECTS OF DRUGS; the encyclopedia of adverse reactions. see *PHARMACY AND PHARMACOLOGY*

610 RUS ISSN 1027-8265
MEZHDUNARODNYI ZHURNAL MEDITSINSKOI PRAKTIKI. Text in Russian. m. RUR 360 for 6 mos. to individuals; RUR 1,080 for 6 mos. to institutions (effective 2000).
Related titles: CD-ROM ed.: RUR 500 for 6 mos. to individuals; RUR 1,000 for 6 mos. to institutions (effective 2002).
Indexed: Ref.Zh.
Published by: Media Sfera, Dmitrovskoe shosse 46, korp 2, etazh 4, P.O. Box 54, Moscow 127238, Russian Federation. TEL 7-095-4824329, FAX 7-095-4824312, mediashp@mediasphera.ru. Ed. Yuriy Belousov. **US dist. addr.:** East View Publications, 3020 Harbor Ln N, Minneapolis, MN 55447. TEL 612-550-0961.

610 USA
MIAMI MEDICINE. Text in English. 1929. m. USD 53.25. adv. back issues avail. *Refereed.* **Description:** Covers legislative updates, computer articles and news of interest to the medical association members.
Indexed: Sport Fish.Abstr.
Published by: Dade County Medical Association, 1501 N W North River Dr, Miami, FL 33125. TEL 305-324-8717, FAX 305-325-1316. Ed. Stephen Vernon. R&P, Adv. contact Karen Cochrane. B&W page USD 490; trim 11 x 8.5. Circ: 3,000.

616.97 CHN ISSN 1000-8861
MIANYIXUE ZAZHI/JOURNAL OF IMMUNOLOGY. Text in Chinese. 1985. bi-m. USD 37.80; USD 6.30 newsstand/cover (effective 2001). **Document type:** *Academic/Scholarly.*
Indexed: AgBiotech, Anim.Breed.Abstr., Protozool.Abstr., Rev.Med.& Vet.Mycol., Trop.Dis.Bull.
Published by: China International Book Trading Corp/Zhongguo Guoji Tushu Maoyi Zonggongsi cibtc@mail.cibtc.com.cn, http://www.cibtc.com.cn. **Dist. by:** 35, Chegongzhuang Xilu, Haidian District, Beijing 100044, China.

610 USA ISSN 0026-2293
R15
MICHIGAN MEDICINE; journal of the Michigan State Medical Society. Text in English. 1902. bi-m. USD 100; USD 5 newsstand/cover (effective 1999). adv. bk.rev. illus, tr.lit. index. back issues avail.; reprint service avail. from PQC. *Refereed.* **Document type:** *Proceedings, Government, Academic/Scholarly.* **Description:** Dedicated to providing information for Michigan physicians about actions of the Michigan State Medical Society. Covers contemporary issues, with special emphasis on socio-economics legislation and news about medicine.
Formerly (until 1964): Michigan State Medical Society. Journal (0098-7522); Incorporates: Michigan State Medical Society. Transactions
Related titles: Microfilm ed.: (from PQC); Online - full text ed.
Indexed: CINAHL, C.I.S. Abstr., INIS Atomind., Ind.Med. (1964-), Int.Nurs.Ind., Med.Care Rev., Mich.Mag.Ind.
—BLDSC (5755.400000), CISTI, GNLM, KNAW.
Published by: Michigan State Medical Society, 120 W Saginau St, P O Box 950, East Lansing, MI 48910. TEL 517-337-1351, FAX 517-336-5797, msms@msms.org, http://msm.org. Ed., R&P Kristen M Lare. Adv. contact Judith Hudson. B&W page USD 639, color page USD 1,412; trim 10.88 x 8.25. Circ: 14,000 (paid).

616.01 USA ISSN 1076-6294
QR177 CODEN: MDREFJ
MICROBIAL DRUG RESISTANCE; mechanism, epidemiology, and disease. Text in English. 1995. q. USD 168 domestic to individuals; USD 309 foreign to individuals; USD 202 domestic to individuals print and online eds. combined; USD 343 foreign to individuals print and online eds. combined; USD 393 domestic to institutions; USD 498 foreign to institutions; USD 472 domestic to institutions print and online eds. combined; USD 577 foreign to institutions print and online eds. combined (effective 2002). adv. back issues avail.; reprints avail. *Refereed.* **Document type:** *Journal, Academic/Scholarly.* **Description:** Focuses on the emergence and spread of antibiotic-resistant microbial pathogens and resistance genes, along with the challenges they present to a wide variety of disciplines.
Related titles: Online - full content ed.: USD 393 to institutions; USD 168 to individuals (effective 2002) (from Swets Blackwell); Online - full text ed.: (from CatchWord Ltd., Institute for Scientific Information, RoweCom Information Quest).
Indexed: ASCA, Agri.& Environ.Biotech.Abstr., Chem.Abstr., Chem.Titles, Curr.Cont., Environ.Sci.Poll.Mgmt., Ind.Med. (1995-), Ind.Vet., Inpharma, Int.Abstr.Biol.Sci., Med.& Pharm.Biotech.Abstr., Microbiol.Abstr., Pharm.&Out.News, Pig News & Info., Poult.Abstr., Reac., Sci.Cit.Ind., Vet.Bull.

M

—BLDSC (5756.914900), CASDDS, CatchWord, CISTI, GNLM, IDS, Infotrieve. **CCC.**
Published by: Mary Ann Liebert, Inc. Publishers, 2 Madison Ave, Larchmont, NY 10538. TEL 914—834-3100, FAX 914-834-1388, info@liebertpub.com, www.liebertpub.com/mdr, http://www.liebertpub.com. Ed. Alexander Tomasz.

616.01 ITA ISSN 1120-0146
MICROBIOLOGIA MEDICA. Text in Italian. 1979. q. ITL 50,000 (effective 1997). Supplement avail. **Document type:** *Academic/Scholarly.*
Indexed: Excerp.Med. (1995-).
—BLDSC (5757.200000), GNLM.
Published by: Associazione Microbiologici Clinici Italiani, Via Carlo Farini, 70, Milan, MI 20159, Italy. TEL 39-2-66801190.

616.01 GBR ISSN 1073-9688
CODEN: MROCER
MICROCIRCULATION. Text in English. 1994. 6/yr. GBP 153 in Europe to individuals for print or online; USD 230 elsewhere to individuals for print or online; GBP 169 combined subscription in Europe to individuals print & online; USD 254 combined subscription elsewhere to individuals print & online; GBP 413 in Europe to institutions for print or online; USD 620 elsewhere to institutions for print or online; GBP 455 combined subscription in Europe to institutions print & online; USD 683 combined subscription elsewhere to institutions print & online (effective 2002). bk.rev. charts, illus, stat. back issues avail.; reprints avail. *Refereed.* **Document type:** *Journal, Academic/Scholarly.* **Description:** Covers applications of the methods of physiology, biophysics, bioengineering, genetics, cell biology, biochemistry, and molecular biology to microcirculation.
Related titles: Online - full text ed.: (from EBSCO Publishing, O C L C Online Computer Library Center, Inc., RoweCom Information Quest, ingenta, Swets Blackwell, Institute for Scientific Information).
Indexed: Aqua.Sci.& Fish.Abstr., Curr.Cont., Ind.Med. (1994-), Sci.Cit.Ind.
—BLDSC (5758.460000), CASDDS, CISTI, GNLM, IDS, Infotrieve. **CCC.**
Published by: (Microcirulatory Society), Nature Publishing Group Specialist Journals (Subsidiary of: Holtzbrink Publishers), Houndmills, Basingstoke, Hants RG21 6XS, United Kingdom. TEL 44-1256-329242, FAX 44-1256-328339, subscriptions@nature.com, http://www.nature.com/mn. Ed. D Neil Granger. Pub. Julia Schulhof. R&P Trace Noel. Adv. contact Robert Sloan TEL 44-20-8882-7199.

610 026 USA
MIDDLE ATLANTIC PERSPECTIVE. Text in English. 1983. bi-m. free per issue to qualified personnel. **Document type:** *Newsletter.* **Description:** News items, information, and announcements pertaining to the Network of Libraries of Medicine serving New York, New Jersey, Pennsylvania and Delaware, as well as the National Online Training Center.
Supersedes in part (in 1991): Greater Northeastern Regional Medical Library Program Newsletter; Formerly (until 1983): New York and New Jersey Regional Medical Library News
Published by: N N - L M Middle Atlantic Region, New York Academy of Medicine, 1216 Fifth Ave, New York, NY 10029. TEL 212-822-7396, FAX 212-534-7042, nlm@nyam.org, http://www.nnlm.nlm.hih.gov/mar/. Ed. Mary Mylenki. Circ: 1,500 (controlled).

610 JPN ISSN 0026-3532
CODEN: MMJJAI
MIE MEDICAL JOURNAL. Text in Multiple languages. 1950. 3/yr. free per issue. charts, illus, stat. index. **Description:** Multidisciplinary papers on medicine.
Indexed: Abstr.Hyg., Biol.Abstr., Chem.Abstr., Chem.Titles, Dent.Abstr., Dent.Ind., Excerp.Med., INIS Atomind., Ind.Med. (coverage dropped), Nutr.Abstr., Protozool.Abstr., Rev.Appl.Entomol., Rev.Med.& Vet.Mycol., Trop.Dis.Bull.
—CASDDS, CISTI, GNLM, ingenta.
Published by: Mie Daigaku, Igakubu/Mie University, School of Medicine, 2-174 Edobashi, Tsu-shi, Mie-ken 514-0001, Japan. Ed. Toshio Tanaka. Circ: 850.

610 ISR ISSN 0026-363X
MIKHTAV LEHAVER✶ **.** Text in Hebrew. 1940. m. USD 300. adv. charts, illus. **Description:** Contains organization news.
Published by: Israel Medical Association, P.O. Box 33003, Tel Aviv 61330, Israel. TEL 972-3-6100444, FAX 972-3-5751616. Ed. Dr. Yoram Blachar.

MIKROBIOLOGI-NYT. see *BIOLOGY—Microbiology*

616.98 USA ISSN 0026-4075
RD1 CODEN: MMEDA9
MILITARY MEDICINE. Text in English. 1891. m. USD 55; USD 60 foreign (effective 1998). adv. bk.rev. bibl, charts, illus, stat. index, cum.index. back issues avail.; reprint service avail. from PQC. *Refereed.* **Document type:** *Academic/Scholarly.* **Description:** Supports knowledge concerning medical activities of the Federal Medical Services, including developments in medical technology, education, management and research.
Related titles: Microfilm ed.; Online - full text ed.: (from Northern Light Technology, Inc., ProQuest Information & Learning, Institute for Scientific Information).
Indexed: ASCA, Abstr.Health Care Manage.Stud., Abstr.Hyg., Aqua.Sci.& Fish.Abstr., Biol.Abstr., CINAHL, C.I.S. Abstr., Chem.Abstr., Crim.Just.Abstr., Curr.Cont., Dent.Ind., Environ.Sci.Poll.Mgmt., Excerp.Med., Helminthol.Abstr., Hosp.Lit.Ind., INIS Atomind., Ind.Med. (1955-), Ind.Vet., Inpharma, Int.Nurs.Ind., Lanc.Ind., Nutr.Abstr., Pollut.Abstr., Protozool.Abstr., PsycInfo, Psychol.Abstr. (1955-), Reac., Rev.Appl.Entomol., Rev.Med.& Vet.Mycol., Risk Abstr., SSCI (coverage dropped), Saf.Sci.Abstr., Small Anim.Abstr., THA, Trop.Dis.Bull., Vet.Bull., e-psyche.
—BLDSC (5768.150000), CASDDS, CISTI, GNLM, IDS, ingenta, KNAW. **CCC.**
Published by: Association of Military Surgeons of the U S, 9320 Old Georgetown Rd, Bethesda, MD 20814. TEL 301-897-8800, FAX 301-530-5446. Ed. Dr. John C Duffy. R&P Mark Shute. Adv. contact Bill Bride. Circ: 16,755.

MILJOEMEDICIN/ENVIRONMENTAL MEDICINE. see *ENVIRONMENTAL STUDIES*

615.8 GBR ISSN 1364-5706
MINIMALLY INVASIVE THERAPY AND ALLIED TECHNOLOGIES. Text in English. 1992. bi-m. GBP 175, USD 285 to individuals; GBP 320, USD 490 to institutions (effective 2002). adv. bibl, illus. index. Supplement avail.; back issues avail. *Refereed.* **Document type:** *Academic/Scholarly.*
Formerly: Minimally Invasive Therapy (0961-625X)
Related titles: Microform ed.: 1992 (from PQC); Online - full text ed.: (from EBSCO Publishing, ingenta, Swets Blackwell, CatchWord Ltd., Institute for Scientific Information).
Indexed: ASCA, Curr.Cont., Excerp.Med. (1993-), Inpharma, Reac.
—BLDSC (5797.714000), CISTI, EMDOCS, GNLM, IDS, Infotrieve, KNAW. **CCC.**
Published by: (Society for Minimally Invasive Therapy DEU), Martin Dunitz Publishers (Subsidiary of: Taylor & Francis Group), The Livery House, 7-9 Pratt St, London NW1 0AE, United Kingdom. TEL 44-20-7482-2202, FAX 44-20-7267-0159, info@dunitz.co.uk, http://www.dunitz.co.uk, http://www.tandf.co.uk. Eds. Gerhard Buess, John Wickham. Circ: 735.

610.5 USA ISSN 0026-556X
R15 CODEN: MIMDAL
MINNESOTA MEDICINE. Text in English. 1918. m., latest vol.84. USD 45 domestic; USD 80 foreign; USD 5 newsstand/cover (effective 2001). adv. bk.rev. abstr, bibl, charts, illus. index. 64 p./no. Supplement avail.; reprint service avail. from PQC. **Document type:** *Magazine, Academic/Scholarly, Trade.* **Description:** Covers clinical, ethical, legal, socioeconomic, and other issues relating to how medicine is practiced in Minnesota.
Related titles: Microform ed.: (from PQC); Online - full text ed.
Indexed: AgeLine, Biol.Abstr., Chem.Abstr., Curr.Adv.Cancer Res., Curr.Cont. (coverage dropped), Dent.Ind., Excerp.Med., Helminthol.Abstr., Hosp.Lit.Ind., INIS Atomind., Ind.Med. (1918-).
—BLDSC (5810.400000), CISTI, GNLM, ingenta, KNAW. **CCC.**
Published by: Minnesota Medical Association, 3433 Broadway St, N E, Ste 300, Minneapolis, MN 55413-1761. TEL 612-378-1875, FAX 612-378-3875, mm@mnmed.org, mma@mnmed.org, http://www.mnmed.org. Ed. Dr. Charles R Meyer. R&P Carmen Peota TEL 612-362-3724. Adv. contact Michele Holzwarth. Circ: 9,000 (paid).

610.711 USA ISSN 0085-3488
R745
MINORITY STUDENT OPPORTUNITIES IN UNITED STATES MEDICAL SCHOOLS. Text in English. 1970. biennial. USD 12 (effective 1999). reprint service avail. from PQC. **Document type:** *Directory.* **Description:** Provides information to underrepresented minorities - Black Americans, American Indians, Mexican Americans - Chicanos, and mainland Puerto Ricans - applying to medical school. Contains descriptive entries of US medical schools with information on recruitment programs, admission policies and procedures, academic support programs, and financial aid for underrepresented minority students.
Published by: Association of American Medical Colleges, 2450 N St N W, Washington, DC 20037-1126. TEL 202-828-0572, FAX 202-828-1123. R&P Lily Mae Johnson.

MIRKACHTON. see *PHARMACY AND PHARMACOLOGY*

610 USA ISSN 0026-6396
CODEN: MSMJB8
MISSISSIPPI STATE MEDICAL ASSOCIATION. JOURNAL✶ **.** Text in English. 1960. m. USD 54 domestic; USD 66 foreign (effective 2001). adv. bk.rev. charts, illus, stat, tr.lit. index. reprint service avail. from PQC. *Refereed.* **Document type:** *Academic/Scholarly.* **Description:** Provides up-to-date material on recent medical discoveries, pertinent legislation, and medical news. Scientific articles by physicians and others in the field.
Related titles: Microform ed.: (from PQC).
Indexed: INIS Atomind., Ind.Med. (1960-), Int.Nurs.Ind.
—BLDSC (4828.210000), CISTI, GNLM, ingenta, KNAW.
Published by: Mississippi State Medical Association, 408 W Pkwy Pl, Ridgeland, MS 39157-6010. TEL 601-354-5433, 601-853-6733, FAX 601-853-6746. Ed. Leslie E England. Adv. contact Karen Evers. B&W page USD 225, color page USD 775. Circ: 3,400 (paid and controlled).

610 USA ISSN 0026-6620
MISSOURI MEDICINE. Text in English. 1904. m. USD 60 (effective 2001). adv. charts, illus. index. back issues avail.; reprints avail. **Document type:** *Academic/Scholarly.* **Description:** Prints scientific articles, editorials on medical issues. Includes medical school news, classifieds, and information on new members, deaths, continuing medical education courses, and practice management.
Related titles: Microfilm ed.
Indexed: Biol.Abstr., Chem.Abstr., Curr.Cont. (coverage dropped), Dent.Ind., Excerp.Med., Helminthol.Abstr., INIS Atomind., Ind.Med. (1953-).
—BLDSC (5829.080000), CISTI, GNLM, ingenta, KNAW.
Published by: Missouri State Medical Association, 113 Madison St, Jefferson City, MO 65102. TEL 573-636-5151, FAX 573-636-8552. Ed. Dr. John Hagan. R&P, Adv. contact Michelle Poire. Circ: 7,000 (paid and free).

610 360 DEU
MITEINANDER. Text in German. 1977. 3/yr. bk.rev. back issues avail. **Description:** Leprosy aid and health problems in developing countries.
Published by: Deutsches Aussaetzigen Hilfswerk e.V., Postfach 110462, Wuerzburg 97031, Germany. TEL 0931-50784, FAX 0931-51358, TELEX 68583-DAHW-D. Ed. Peter Schweiger. Circ: 80,000.

610 AUT
MITTEILUNGEN DER AERZTEKAMMER FUER WIEN - WIENER ARZT. Text in German. 1948. m. ATS 429. adv. bk.rev. back issues avail. **Document type:** *Newsletter.*
Former titles (until 1992): Ae K W M (Aerztekammer fuer Wien Mitteilungen) (0377-9874); (until 1975): Aerztekammer fuer Wien. Mitteilungen (0377-9866); (until 1967): Aerztekammer fuer Wien. Mitteilungsblatt (0377-9858); (until 1956): Aerztekammer fuer Wien. Mitteilungen
Published by: Aerztekammer fuer Wien, Weihburggasse 10-12, Vienna, W 1010, Austria. TEL 43-1-51501223, FAX 43-1-51501289. Ed. Dr. Guenther Knogler. Adv. contact Nina Chalupsky. page ATS 13,350; trim 256 x 186. Circ: 12,000 (controlled).

610 USA ISSN 0888-6792
MODEL FOR THE PREPARATION OF A GUIDEBOOK ON MEDICAL DISCIPLINE. Text in English. triennial. USD 8 (effective 1999). **Description:** Detailed example booklet to help state medical boards to develop guidebooks.

Published by: Federation of State Medical Boards, 400 Fuller Wiser Rd, Ste 300, Euless, TX 76039-3855. TEL 817-868-4000, FAX 817-868-4098. Ed. Patricia Beatty. R&P Linda Uernale.

MODELL'S DRUGS IN CURRENT USE AND NEW DRUGS. see *PHARMACY AND PHARMACOLOGY*

610 AUS ISSN 1030-3782
MODERN MEDICINE OF AUSTRALIA. Text in English. 1957. m. AUD 150; USD 220 foreign. adv. bk.rev. charts, illus, stat. cum.index: 1995-1997. *Refereed.* **Document type:** *Academic/Scholarly.*
Former titles: Modern Medicine (0312-875X); Modern Medicine of Australia (0026-8089)
Indexed: Curr.Adv.Ecol.Sci., Excerp.Med. (1993-), Helminthol.Abstr., Nutr.Abstr.
—BLDSC (5889.880000), EMDOCS, GNLM, ingenta, KNAW.
Published by: Modern Medicine of Australia Pty. Ltd., Level 1, 57 Grosvenor St, Neutral Bay, NSW 2089, Australia. TEL 61-2-99082155, FAX 61-2-99081961. Ed. Dr. John Ellard. Pubs. Judy Passlow, Tony Scott. Adv. contact Paul Mathew. color page AUD 3,660; trim 207 x 273. Circ: 23,610.

610 ZAF ISSN 0259-9333
MODERN MEDICINE OF SOUTH AFRICA. Text in English. 1976. 12/yr. ZAR 333.68 (effective 1999). adv. abstr, illus. index. **Document type:** *Trade.*
Published by: National Publishing (Pty) Ltd., PO Box 2271, Clareinch 7740, South Africa. TEL 27-21-611140, FAX 27-21-611389, accirc@natpub.co.za. Ed. Dr. Pete Vincent. Circ: 7,500.

616.07 571.9 USA ISSN 0893-3952
RB37.A1 CODEN: MODPEO
MODERN PATHOLOGY. Text in English. 1988. m., latest vol.14. USD 305 domestic to individuals Print & Online eds.; USD 379 foreign to individuals Print & Online eds.; USD 512 domestic to institutions Print & Online eds.; USD 585 foreign to institutions Print & Online eds.; USD 48 newsstand/cover (effective 2002). adv. bk.rev. index, cum.index. back issues avail. *Refereed.* **Document type:** *Academic/Scholarly.* **Description:** Provides a forum for the presentation of advances in the understanding of pathological processes. It is practice-oriented and concentrates on diagnostic human pathology.
Related titles: E-mail ed.; Microfilm ed.: (from WWS); Online - full text ed.: ISSN 1530-0285. USD 665.60 domestic academic site license; USD 738.60 foreign academic site license; USD 742.40 domestic corporate site license; USD 815.40 foreign corporate site license (2002) (from Ovid Technologies, Inc., HighWire Pr., Institute for Scientific Information).
Indexed: ASCA, Curr.Cont., Excerp.Med. (1995-), INIS Atomind., Ind.Med. (1988-), Ind.Sci.Rev., Inpharma, Kidney, Med.& Surg.Dermat., Neurosci.Cit.Ind., Pharm.&Out.News, Protozool.Abstr., Reac., Rev.Med.& Vet.Mycol., SSCI (coverage dropped), Sci.Cit.Ind.
—BLDSC (5890.767000), CISTI, GNLM, IDS, ingenta, KNAW.
Published by: (U S and Canadian Academy of Pathology), Williams & Wilkins (Subsidiary of: Waverly International), 351 W Camden St, Baltimore, MD 21201-2436. TEL 410-528-4068, 800-222-3790, FAX 410-528-4452, sisaacson@wwilkins.com, http://modpath.uscapjournals.org/, http://www.wwilkins.com/MP/. Ed. Dr. Stacey E Mills. Adv. contact Sharlene Isaacson. B&W page USD 925; trim 10.88 x 8.13. Circ: 5,136; 5,048 (paid).

610 USA
MODERN PHYSICIAN; essential business news for the executive physician. Text in English. m. USD 45; USD 6 newsstand/cover (effective 2001). adv. **Document type:** *Trade.* **Description:** Provides up-to-date news and information on management, legal, labor, regulatory, socio-economic and financial issues as they impact physician executives with management responsibilities.
Related titles: Online - full text ed.
Published by: Crain Communications, Inc. (Chicago), 740 Rush St, Chicago, IL 60611. TEL 312-649-5350, FAX 312-649-5393, moderndoc@mindspring.com, http://www.modernphysician.com. Ed. Karen Petitte. Pub. Charles S Lauer. Adv. contact Frank H Nobile. Circ: 32,400 (controlled). **Subscr. to:** Modern Physician, 965 E Jefferson, Detroit, MI 48207-3185. TEL 888-446-1422.

MODERNA LAEKARE. see *LABOR UNIONS*

610 USA
CODEN: MOANE
MOLECULAR ANDROLOGY; an international journal. Text in English. 4/yr. USD 180 domestic to individuals; USD 190 foreign to individuals; USD 200 domestic to institutions; USD 210 foreign to institutions. **Document type:** *Academic/Scholarly.*
Indexed: Chem.Abstr., Chem.Indus.Notes, Chem.Titles, Excerp.Med.
Published by: Reproductive Health Center, 78 Surfsong Rd., Kiawah Island, SC 29455. TEL 803-768-5556, FAX 803-768-6494.

610 GBR ISSN 0098-2997
RB112 CODEN: MAMED5
MOLECULAR ASPECTS OF MEDICINE; an interdisciplinary review journal. Text in English. 1975. bi-m. EUR 904 in Europe to institutions; JPY 120,000 in Japan to institutions; USD 1,011 elsewhere to institutions (effective 2002). adv. bk.rev. illus, stat. abstr. index. back issues avail. *Refereed.* **Document type:** *Academic/Scholarly.* **Description:** Integrates molecular biochemistry and clinical medicine, focusing on the application of molecular insights to medical problems.
Related titles: Microfilm ed.: (from PQC); Online - full text ed.: (from ingenta, ScienceDirect, Swets Blackwell).
Indexed: ASCA, BBCI (coverage dropped), Biol.Abstr., Chem.Abstr., Chem.Indus.Notes, Chem.Titles, Curr.Adv.Biochem., Curr.Adv.Cell & Devel.Biol., Curr.Adv.Ecol.Sci., Curr.Cont. (coverage dropped), Excerp.Med., Ind.Med. (1975-), Ind.Sci.Rev., Int.Abstr.Biol.Sci., Sci.Cit.Ind. (coverage dropped).
—BLDSC (5900.768000), CASDDS, CISTI, GNLM, IDS, ingenta. **CCC.**
Published by: Pergamon (Subsidiary of: Elsevier Science), The Boulevard, Langford Ln, East Park, Kidlington, Oxford OXB 1GB, United Kingdom. FAX 44-1865-843010, http://www.elsevier.com/locate/mam. Ed. A Azzi. **Subscr. in Australasia and the Far East to:** Elsevier Science (Singapore) Pte Ltd, No.1 Temasek Ave, 17-01 Millenia Tower, Singapore 039192, Singapore. TEL 65-434-3727, FAX 65-337-2230; **Subscr. in the Americas to:** Elsevier Science, PO Box 945, New York, NY 10159-0945. TEL 212-633-3730, FAX 212-633-3680, usinfo-f@elsevier.com; **Subscr. to:** Elsevier Science BV, PO Box 211, Amsterdam 1000 AE, Netherlands. TEL 31-20-485-3757.

MOLECULAR BIOTECHNOLOGY. see *BIOLOGY—Biotechnology*

616.01 USA ISSN 1084-8592
CODEN: MDIAFU
MOLECULAR DIAGNOSIS; a journal devoted to the understanding of human disease through the clinical application of molecular biology. Text in English. 1996. q. USD 125 domestic to individuals; USD 165 foreign to individuals; USD 208 domestic to institutions; USD 248 foreign to institutions; USD 65 domestic to students; USD 99 foreign to students; USD 63 newsstand/cover (effective 2001). *Refereed.* **Document type:** *Academic/Scholarly.* **Description:** Research and clinical data on understanding of human disease through the application of molecular biology.
Related titles: Online - full text ed.: (from IDEAL Online Library, Institute for Scientific Information).
Indexed: Biotech.Cit.Ind., Curr.Cont., Ind.Med. (1996-), Inpharma, Pharm.&Out.News, Reac., Sci.Cit.Ind.
—BLDSC (5900.817353), CASDDS, IDS. **CCC.**
Published by: Churchill Livingstone (Subsidiary of: Harcourt Health Sciences), The Curtis Center, Independence Square West, Philadelphia, PA 19106-3399. TEL 212-206-5000, FAX 212-206-7808, http://www.churchillmed.com. Ed. David L Cooper. **Subscr. in the UK to:** Pearson Professional Ltd., Journals Subscription Department, Fourth Ave., PO Box 77, Harlow, Essex CM19 5AA, United Kingdom. TEL 44-1279-623924, FAX 44-1279-639609.

612.015 USA ISSN 1096-7192
QP501 CODEN: MGMEFF
MOLECULAR GENETICS AND METABOLISM; an international journal. Text in English. 1969. m. USD 780 in US & Canada to institutions; USD 875 elsewhere to institutions (effective 2001). adv. index. back issues avail. *Refereed.* **Document type:** *Academic/Scholarly.* **Description:** Publishes papers describing original research in biochemistry, physiological chemistry, and metabolic biology. Emphasis is on the determination of the interrelations among reactions, sequences, and formed elements of the cell.
Former title: Biochemical and Molecular Medicine (1077-3150); (until 1995): Biochemical Medicine and Metabolic Biology (0885-4505); Biochemical Medicine (0006-2944)
Related titles: Online - full text ed.: (from EBSCO Publishing, O C L C Online Computer Library Center, Inc., RoweCom Information Quest, ingenta, Swets Blackwell, IDEAL Online Library, Institute for Scientific Information).
Indexed: ASCA, Agri.& Environ.Biotech.Abstr. (coverage dropped), Agricola, Anal.Abstr., BBCI, Biol.Abstr., Chem.Abstr., Chem.Indus.Notes, Chem.Titles, Curr.Adv.Ecol.Sci., Curr.Cont., Dairy Sci.Abstr., Dent.Ind., Derwent Biotech.Abstr., Excerp.Med., Helminthol.Abstr., INIS Atomind., Ind.Med. (1998-), Ind.Sci.Rev., Inpharma, Int.Abstr.Biol.Sci., Mass Spectr.Bull., Nutr.Abstr., Pharm.&Out.News, Poult.Abstr., Reac., Rev.Med.& Vet.Mycol., SSCI (coverage dropped), Sci.Cit.Ind., Trop.Dis.Bull., Trop.Oil Seeds Abstr.
—BLDSC (5900.817540), ADONIS, CASDDS, CISTI, EMDOCS, GNLM, IDS, ingenta, Linda Hall. **CCC.**
Published by: Academic Press, Inc., Journal Division (Subsidiary of: Harcourt Brace & Company), 525 B St, Ste 1900, San Diego, CA 92101-4495. TEL 619-230-1840, FAX 619-699-6800, apsubs@acad.com, http://www.apnet.com/mgm, http://www.academicpress.com/mgm. Ed. Edward R B McCabe.

▼ **MOLECULAR PLANT PATHOLOGY.** see *BIOLOGY—Botany*

MONASH BIOETHICS REVIEW. see *PHILOSOPHY*

630 MNG
MONGOLYN ANAGAAKH UKHAAN/MONGOLIAN MEDICAL SCIENCES. Text in Mongol; Summaries in English. 1970. q. MNT 200. **Document type:** *Academic/Scholarly, Government.*
Published by: Ministry of Health, Ulan Bator, Mongolia. TEL 976-1-321307, FAX 976-1-321278, TELEX 247 MINHE MH. Ed. P Nymadawa. Circ: 3,000.
Co-sponsor: Scientific Society of Physicians.

MONITOR (WASHINGTON, 1970). see *INSURANCE*

610 ESP
MONOGRAFIAS DE SALUD RURAL. Text in Spanish. 20/yr. back issues avail.; reprints avail. **Document type:** *Journal.*
Published by: Jarpyo Editores S.A., Antonio Lopez Aguado, 4, Madrid 28029, Spain. TEL 34-913-144338, FAX 34-913-144499, editorial@jarpyo.es, http://www.jarpyo.es. Ed. Jose Mora. Adv. contact Juan Torres.

610 571.6 CHE ISSN 0077-0809
MONOGRAPHS IN CLINICAL CYTOLOGY. Text in English. 1965. irreg., latest vol.15. CHF 200 in Europe; DEM 240 in Germany; USD 160 in United States (2001). *Refereed.* **Document type:** *Monographic series, Academic/Scholarly.* **Description:** Instructive texts that guide the introduction of improved diagnostic techniques and procedures.
Indexed: Biol.Abstr., Chem.Abstr., Curr.Cont. (coverage dropped), Ind.Med. (1969-).
—BLDSC (5915.410000), GNLM, KNAW. **CCC.**
Published by: S. Karger AG, Allschwilerstr 10, PO Box, Basel 4009, Switzerland. TEL 41-61-306-1111, FAX 41-61-306-1234, karger@karger.ch, http://www.karger.com/bookseries/MOCLC. Ed. S Orell.

MONOZINE. see *LITERARY AND POLITICAL REVIEWS*

610 USA
MONROE COUNTY MEDICAL SOCIETY. BULLETIN. Text in English. 1934. q. USD 25 (effective 1999). back issues avail. *Refereed.* **Document type:** *Trade.*
Published by: Monroe County Medical Society, 1441 East Ave, Rochester, NY 14610. TEL 716-473-7573, FAX 716-473-7641. Ed. Karyn S Runkle. R&P Lisa Brubaker. adv.: B&W page USD 475; trim 10.25 x 7.75. Circ: 1,800.

MONTHLY PRESCRIBING REFERENCE. see *PHARMACY AND PHARMACOLOGY*

MORFOLOGIYA. see *BIOLOGY*

611 571.3 FRA ISSN 1286-0115
MORPHOLOGIE. Variant title: Association des Morphologistes. Bulletin. Text in French. 1899. q. FRF 680; FRF 800 foreign (effective 2000). adv. **Document type:** *Bulletin.*
Former titles (until 1997): Association des Anatomistes. Bulletin (0376-6160); (until 1972): Association des Anatomistes. Comptes Rendus (0066-8915)
Indexed: Biol.Abstr., Dent.Ind., Excerp.Med., GeoRef, Ind.Med. (1997-).

M

—CISTI, GNLM.
Published by: Association des Morphologistes, Faculte Medecine, B.P. 184, Vandoeuvre-les-Nancy Cedex 54505, France. TEL 33-3-83592833, FAX 33-3-83446065, grignon@facmed.u-nancy.fr. Ed. Georges Grignon. Circ: 1,100.

MORTALITY. see *PUBLIC HEALTH AND SAFETY*

611.7 PRT
MOTRICIDADE HUMANA. Text in Portuguese.
—BLDSC (5978.705000).
Published by: Universidade Tecnica de Lisboa, c/o Francisco Sobral, Dir., I.S.E.F., Estrada da Costa - Cruz Quebrada, Lisbon 1499, Portugal.

362 610 USA ISSN 0027-2507
R11 CODEN: MSJMAZ
MOUNT SINAI JOURNAL OF MEDICINE. Text in English. 1934. 6/yr. USD 115; USD 140 foreign (effective 1999). adv. bk.rev. charts, illus, stat. index. back issues avail. *Refereed.* **Document type:** *Academic/Scholarly.* **Description:** Contains wide variety of clinical papers about medical specialties and topical single theme medical issues.
Formerly (until 1970): Mount Sinai Hospital. Journal
Related titles: Microform ed.: (from PQC); Online - full text ed.: (from The Dialog Corporation, Institute for Scientific Information).
Indexed: ASCA, AgeLine, Biol.Abstr., Chem.Abstr., Curr.Cont., Curr.Lit.Fam.Plan., Dent.Ind., Excerp.Med., Helminthol.Abstr., INIS Atomind., Ind.Med. (1970-), Ind.Sci.Rev., Inpharma, Int.Nurs.Ind., NRN, Nutr.Abstr., Pharm.&Out.News, Reac., Ref.Zh., Rev.Med.& Vet.Mycol., SSCI (coverage dropped), Sci.Cit.Ind., THA.
—BLDSC (5978.750000), CASDDS, CISTI, GNLM, IDS, ingenta, KNAW.
Published by: Mount Sinai Hospital, One East 100 St, New York, NY 10029-6574. TEL 212-241-6108, FAX 212-722-6386, msjournal@msvax.mssm.edu, http://www.mssm.edu/msjournal. Ed., Pub. Dr. Sherman Kupfer. R&P Shermam Kupfer. Adv. contact Dr. Julius Wolf. B&W page USD 750, color page USD 1,950; trim 11 x 8.25. Circ: 2,000.

610 ITA ISSN 0393-9405
MOVIMENTO. Text in Italian. 1985. 4/m. USD 50 (effective 2002).
Indexed: Psychol.Abstr.
Published by: Edizioni Luigi Pozzi s.r.l., Via Panama, 68, Rome, RM 00198, Italy. TEL 39-06-8553548, FAX 39-06-8554105, edizioni_pozzi@tin.it.

610 CHN ISSN 1001-7550
MUDANJIANG YIXUEYUAN XUEBAO/MUDANJIANG MEDICAL INSTITUTE. JOURNAL. Text in Chinese. q.
Published by: Mudanjiang Yixueyuan, Xuebao Bianjibu, Tongxiang Lu, Aimin-qu, Mudanjiang, Heilongjiang 157011, China. TEL 26156.

610 CHE ISSN 0251-0111
MUNAZZAMAT AL-SIHHAH AL-'ALAMIYYAH. SILSILAT AL-TAQARIR AL-FANNIYYAH. Text in Arabic. 1950. irreg.
Related titles: ♦ English ed.: W H O Technical Report Series. ISSN 0512-3054; ♦ Spanish ed.: Organizacion Mundial de la Salud. Serie de Informes Tecnicos. ISSN 0509-2507; ♦ French ed.: Organisation Mondiale de la Sante. Serie de Rapports Techniques. ISSN 0373-3998; ♦ Russian ed.: Vsemirnaya Organizatsiya Zdravookhraneniya. Seriya Tekhnicheskikh Dokladov. ISSN 0250-8737.
Published by: World Health Organization, Marketing and Dissemination, Geneva, 27 1211, Switzerland.

610 MEX ISSN 0185-2302
MUNDO MEDICO. Text in Spanish. 1973. m. MXP 400; USD 345 foreign (effective 1999). adv. bk.rev.
Published by: Mundo Medico S.A., Ejercito Nacional 381, Mexico City, DF 11520, Mexico. TEL 525-545-17-98, FAX 525-203-64-18. Ed. Beatriz Elizalde. Adv. contact Oscar Bagnarelli. Circ: 15,000.

616.4 GBR ISSN 0047-8385
MURMUR. Text in English. 1922. 3/yr. GBP 15; GBP 20 foreign. adv. bk.rev. **Document type:** *Academic/Scholarly.* **Description:** Publishes features, news and reviews of interest to preclinical students at Cambridge University.
Published by: Cambridge University Medical Society, Department of Anatomy, Cambridge University, Cambridge CB2 9DT, United Kingdom. TEL 44-1223-60160. Ed. Mark Radon. R&P, Adv. contact Jane Freeston. Circ: 750 (controlled).

610 USA ISSN 0148-639X
RC925.A1 CODEN: MUNEDE
MUSCLE & NERVE. Text in English. 1979. m. USD 1,565 in United States; USD 1,685 in Canada & Mexico; USD 1,787 elsewhere; USD 1,644 combined subscription in United States for print and online eds.; USD 1,764 combined subscription in Canada & Mexico for print and online eds.; USD 1,866 combined subscription elsewhere for print and online eds. (effective 2002). adv. Supplement avail.; back issues avail. *Refereed.* **Document type:** *Academic/Scholarly.* **Description:** Covers muscle, the peripheral motor and sensory neurons, and the neuromuscular junction in both health and disease.
Related titles: Microform ed.: (from PQC); Online - full text ed.: ISSN 1097-4598. 1996. USD 1,565 in United States; USD 1,565 in Canada & Mexico; USD 1,565 elsewhere (effective 2002) (from EBSCO Publishing, Wiley InterScience, Institute for Scientific Information).
Indexed: AMED, ASCA, Arts & Hum.Cit.Ind. (coverage dropped), Bibl.Dev.Med.& Child Neur., Biol.Abstr., Chem.Abstr., Chem.Indus.Notes, Chem.Titles, Curr.Adv.Biochem., Curr.Adv.Ecol.Sci., Curr.Adv.Gen.& Molec.Biol., Curr.Cont., Dent.Ind., Excerp.Med., INIS Atomind., Ind.Med. (1978-), Ind.Sci.Rev., Inpharma, Int.Abstr.Biol.Sci., Jrnl.Watch Neuro., Neurosci.Cit.Ind., Pharm.&Out.News, Poult.Abstr., Reac., Risk Abstr., Sci.Cit.Ind.
—BLDSC (5986.493000), CASDDS, CISTI, GNLM, IDS, ingenta, KNAW. **CCC.**
Published by: John Wiley & Sons, Inc., Journals (Subsidiary of: Wiley InterScience), 605 Third Ave, New York, NY 10158. TEL 212-850-6645, FAX 212-850-6021, subinfo@wiley.com, uscs-wis@wiley.com, http://www.wiley.com. Ed. Jun Kimura. adv.: B&W page GBP 640, color page GBP 1,515; trim 210 x 279. Circ: 5,200. **Subscr. outside the Americas to:** John Wiley & Sons Ltd., Baffins Ln, Chichester, Sussex PO19 IUD, United Kingdom. TEL 44-1243-779777, FAX 44-1243-843232, cs-journals@wiley.co.uk.

610 616.891 DEU ISSN 0933-6885
MUSIK-, TANZ- UND KUNSTTHERAPIE; Zeitschrift fuer kuenstlerische Therapien im Bildungs-, Sozial- und Gesundheitswesen. Text in German; Summaries in English, German. 1990. q. DEM 98 (effective 2001). adv. bk.rev. abstr, bibl, illus. **Document type:** *Journal, Academic/Scholarly.*
Indexed: IBZ, Ind.Philos., e-psyche.
—GNLM.
Published by: (Verlag fuer Angewandte Psychologie), Hogrefe Verlag GmbH und Co. KG, Rohnsweg 25, Goettingen 37085, Germany. TEL 49-551-496090, FAX 49-551-4960988, verlag@hogrefe.de, http://www.hogrefe.de. Ed. Karl Hoermann. Circ: 2,000.

610 JPN ISSN 0454-7586
CODEN: KYIHAZ
MUTUAL AID ASSOCIATION. MEDICAL JOURNAL*. Text and summaries in English, Japanese. 1951. q. index. back issues avail.
Indexed: INIS Atomind.
—CASDDS, CISTI, GNLM.
Published by: Kokka Komuin Kyosai Kumiai Rengokai, Toranomon Hospital, 2-2-2, Minato-ku, Tokyo 105, Japan. Ed. Kinori Kosaka. Circ: 1,550.

MYAKKANGAKU/JAPANESE COLLEGE OF ANGIOLOGY. JOURNAL. see *MEDICAL SCIENCES—Cardiovascular Diseases*

610 DEU ISSN 0933-7407
CODEN: MYCSEU
MYCOSES. Text in English; Summaries in English, German. 1957. 6/yr. DEM 391.17 in Europe to individuals; DEM 434.19 elsewhere to individuals; DEM 430.29 in Europe to individuals print & online eds. combined; DEM 477.61 elsewhere to individuals print & online eds. combined; DEM 735.40 in Europe to institutions; DEM 778.42 elsewhere to institutions; DEM 808.94 in Europe to institutions print & online eds. combined; DEM 856.26 elsewhere to institutions print & online eds. combined (effective 2001). adv. bk.rev. charts, illus, tr.lit. index. *Refereed.* **Document type:** *Journal, Academic/Scholarly.* **Description:** Provides an international forum for papers on the pathogenesis, diagnosis, therapy, prophylaxis, and epidemiology of fungal infectious diseases in humans and animals.
Formerly (until 1987): Mykosen (0027-5557)
Related titles: Online - full text ed.: ISSN 1439-0507. DEM 662 to institutions; DEM 353 to individuals (2001) (from EBSCO Publishing, O C L C Online Computer Library Center, Inc., RoweCom Information Quest, ingenta, Munksgaard & Blackwell Science's Synergy, Swets Blackwell, Institute for Scientific Information); ♦ Supplement: Mycoses. Supplement. ISSN 0943-7312.
Indexed: ASCA, Abstr.Hyg., Agri.& Environ.Biotech.Abstr. (coverage dropped), Aqua.Sci.& Fish.Abstr., Biol.Abstr., Chem.Abstr., Chem.Indus.Notes, Chem.Titles, Curr.Adv.Ecol.Sci., Curr.Cont., Dairy Sci.Abstr., Derwent Biotech.Abstr., Environ.Sci.Poll.Mgmt., Excerp.Med., Hort.Abstr., Ind.Med. (1988-), Ind.Sci.Rev., Ind.Vet., Inpharma, Int.Abstr.Biol.Sci., Med.& Surg.Dermat., Microbiol.Abstr., NRN, Pharm.&Out.News, Pig News & Info., Poult.Abstr., Protozool.Abstr., Reac., Ref.Zh., Rev.Arom.& Med.Plants, Rev.Med.& Vet.Mycol., Rev.Plant Path., Rice Abstr., Rural Devel.Abstr., Sci.Cit.Ind., Soils & Fert., Trop.Dis.Bull., Vet.Bull.
—BLDSC (5995.753000), ADONIS, CASDDS, CISTI, EMDOCS, GNLM, IDS, ingenta, KNAW. **CCC.**
Published by: (Deutschsprachige Mykologische Gesellschaft e.V.), Blackwell Wissenschafts Verlag GmbH, Kurfuerstendamm 57, Berlin 10707, Germany. TEL 49-30-32790624, FAX 49-30-32790610, abo@blackwis.de, http://www.blackwell.de. Ed. J Mueller. adv.: B&W page DEM 1,800, color page DEM 3,270; trim 170 x 240. Circ: 1,200.

610 DEU ISSN 0943-7312
CODEN: MYSUE
MYCOSES. SUPPLEMENT. Text in German. 1988. irreg. **Document type:** *Monographic series, Academic/Scholarly.*
Related titles: Online - full text ed.; ♦ Supplement to: Mycoses. ISSN 0933-7407.
Indexed: Excerp.Med. (1994-), Int.Abstr.Biol.Sci.
—ADONIS, KNAW.
Published by: Blackwell Wissenschafts Verlag GmbH, Kurfuerstendamm 57, Berlin 10707, Germany. TEL 49-30-32790624, FAX 49-30-32790610, aboverwalt@blackwis.de, abo@blackwis.de, http://www.blackwell.de. Ed. Wolfgang Boettuw.

610 USA
N A A C L S NEWS. Text in English. 1970. 3/yr. USD 25; (includes Agency's Annual Report). adv. back issues avail. **Document type:** *Newsletter.* **Description:** Current industry news in allied health education, accreditation, and approval, NAACLS news of interest to clinical laboratory program officials in the U.S.
Published by: National Accrediting Agency for Clinical Laboratory Sciences, 8410 W Bryn Mawr Ave, Ste 670, Chicago, IL 60631-3415. TEL 773-714-8880, FAX 773-714-8886, naacls@mcs.net, http://www.mcs.net/~naacls. Ed. Megan Hennessy Eggert. Circ: 1,000.

610 USA
N A E M T NEWS. Text in English. 1980. bi-m. USD 40 (effective 2000). adv. **Document type:** *Newsletter.*
Formerly: N A E M T Newsletter
Published by: National Association of Emergency Medical Technicians, 102 W Leake St, Clinton, MS 39056-4252. TEL 601-924-7744, 800-346-2368, FAX 601-924-7325. Ed., R&P, Adv. contact Heather D Palmer. Circ: 5,000.

610.6 USA
N A H C REPORT. Text in English. 1983. w. USD 325 (effective 2000). adv. **Document type:** *Newsletter.* **Description:** Covers legislative, regulatory, operational, and financial developments affecting the home care industry.
Published by: National Association for Home Care, 228 Seventh St, S E, Washington, DC 20003-4306. TEL 202-547-7424, FAX 202-547-3540. Ed., R&P Nicholas Caggia. Pub. Val Halamandaris. Adv. contact Cathrine Wolden. Circ: 3,300.

N A R I STETHOSCOPE. see *BUSINESS AND ECONOMICS—Investments*

362.1 613 USA ISSN 1096-231X
N B E R - FRONTIERS IN HEALTH POLICY. Text in English. 1997. a. USD 24 domestic; USD 34 foreign (effective 2001). **Document type:** *Academic/Scholarly.* **Description:** Covers economic research on health care and health policy issues, focusing on papers targeting a policy audience.
Related titles: Online - full text ed.: (from CatchWord Ltd.).
Indexed: P.A.I.S.
—BLDSC (4042.022900).
Published by: (National Bureau of Economic Research), M I T Press, 5 Cambridge Center, Cambridge, MA 02142-1407. TEL 617-253-2866, FAX 617-577-1545, journals-orders@mit.edu, http://mitpress.mit.edu/NBER, http://mit.edu. Ed. Alan M Garber.

M

610 USA ISSN 1057-9400
R850.A1
N C R R REPORTER. (National Center for Research Resources) Text in English. 1977. q. USD 10; USD 1.50 newsstand/cover for cum.index issue (effective 2001). cum.index. back issues avail. **Document type:** *Government, Academic/Scholarly.* **Description:** Describes current biomedical research studies.
Formerly: Research Resources Reporter (0160-807X)
Related titles: Online - full text ed.
Indexed: Ind.U.S.Gov.Per., MEDOC, Ref.Zh.
Published by: U.S. National Institutes of Health, National Center for Research Resources, 6705 Rockledge Dr, Rm 5046, Bethesda, MD 20892. TEL 301-435-0888, info@ncrr.nih.gov, ospio@ncrr.nih.gov, http://www.ncrr.nih.gov/newspub/publica.htm. Ed. Dr. Ole Henriksen. Circ: 16,000. **Subscr. to:** U.S. Government Printing Office, Superintendent of Documents, PO Box 371954, Pittsburgh, PA 15250-7954. TEL 202-512-1800, FAX 202-512-2250, orders@gpo.gov, http://www.access.gpo.gov.

610 FRA ISSN 0301-6374
N G M. (Nouveau Genie Medical) Text in French. 1974. bi-m. FRF 25. adv. bk.rev.
Published by: E.S.T.E.C., 127 bd. Saint Michel, Paris 75005, France. Ed. Christian Damois. Circ: 15,250.

610.6 USA ISSN 1057-5871
RA11
N I H RECORD. Text in English. fortn.
Published by: National Institutes of Health, Bldg 31, Rm 2B03, Bethesda, MD 20892. TEL 301-496-2125. Ed. Richard McManus. Circ: 16,000.

610 RUS
N.I.I. SOTSYAL'NOI GIGIENY I UPRAVLENIYA ZDRAVOOKHRANENIEM. BYULLETEN'. Text in Russian. 1993. q. USD 145 in the Americas (effective 2000).
Published by: N.I.I. Sotsyal'noi Gigieny, Ekonomiki i Upravleniyazdravookhraneniem, Vorontsovo pole, 12, Moscow 121069, Russian Federation. TEL 7-095-9175054. Ed. N A Semashko. **Dist. by:** East View Publications, 3020 Harbor Ln N, Minneapolis, MN 55447. TEL 763-550-0961, FAX 763-559-2931.

N L M NEWSLINE. see *LIBRARY AND INFORMATION SCIENCES*

N L M TECHNICAL BULLETIN. (U.S. National Library of Medicine) see *LIBRARY AND INFORMATION SCIENCES*

N R H A ENEWS. see *PUBLIC HEALTH AND SAFETY*

610 NZL ISSN 0110-022X
CODEN: NZFPDJ
N Z FAMILY PHYSICIAN. Text in English. 1974. s-m. NZD 60 (effective 2000). adv. bk.rev. *Refereed.* **Document type:** *Academic/Scholarly.* **Description:** Contains original papers, news, academic commentary and College reports of interest to NZ and international general practitioners, trainees and students.
Indexed: Ind.N.Z.Per., Inpharma, Pharm.&Out.News, Reac.
—BLDSC (6091.400000), CASDDS, CISTI, Infotrieve. **CCC.**
Published by: Royal New Zealand College of General Practitioners, c/o Dr. Tessa Turnbull, Ed., 62 Park Rd, Katikati, New Zealand. TEL 64-7-54904112, FAX 64-7-5490166. Ed., R&P Dr. Tessa Turnbull. Circ: 4,000.

NAGANOKEN SAGYO RYOHOSHIKAI GAKUJUTSUSHI/NAGANO ASSOCIATION OF OCCUPATIONAL THERAPISTS. JOURNAL. see *OCCUPATIONAL HEALTH AND SAFETY*

610 IND ISSN 0027-7576
NAGARJUN. Text and summaries in English. 1957. m. INR 150. **Description:** Covers medicine and health.
Published by: O. N. Pandeya Ed. & Pub., 105-C Block F, New Alipore, Kolkata, West Bengal 700 053, India. Ed. L K Pandeya.

610 JPN ISSN 0369-3228
CODEN: NAGZAC
NAGASAKI IGAKKAI ZASSHI/NAGASAKI MEDICAL JOURNAL. Text in Japanese; Summaries in English. 1923. q. JPY 2,000, USD 20 (effective 2000). adv. index. back issues avail. *Refereed.* **Document type:** *Academic/Scholarly.* **Description:** Contains papers on the specific diseases of the district and abstracts of local scientific meetings.
Indexed: Biol.Abstr., Chem.Abstr., Chem.Indus.Notes, Chem.Titles, INIS Atomind., Ref.Zh.
—CASDDS, CISTI.
Published by: (Nagasaki Medical Association), Fujiki Publishing Co., 5-13 Yorozuya-Machi, Nagasaki-shi 850-0852, Japan. TEL 095-821-2146, FAX 095-821-2148. Ed. Ichiro Nakasono. Pub. C Fujiki. Circ: 900. **Subscr. to:** Nagasaki University School of Medicine, Department of Pathology, 12-4 Sakamo-to, Nagasaki-shi 852-8102, Japan.

610 JPN ISSN 0027-7622
R97 CODEN: NJMSAG
NAGOYA JOURNAL OF MEDICAL SCIENCE. Text in Multiple languages. 1923. q. free per issue. **Document type:** *Bulletin, Academic/Scholarly.*
Indexed: Abstr.Hyg., Biol.Abstr., Chem.Abstr., Chem.Indus.Notes, Chem.Titles, Curr.Adv.Ecol.Sci., Excerp.Med., INIS Atomind., Ind.Med. (1927-), Nutr.Abstr., Rev.Med.& Vet.Mycol., Trop.Dis.Bull.
—BLDSC (6014.000000), CASDDS, CISTI, GNLM, ingenta, KNAW.
Published by: Nagoya Daigaku, Igakubu/Nagoya University, School of Medicine, 65 Tsurumai-cho, Showa-ku, Nagoya-shi, Aichi-ken 466-0065, Japan. FAX 81-52-744-2511. Ed., R&P Yukihiro Nishiyama TEL 81-52-744-2450. Circ: 750.

610 JPN ISSN 0027-7649
CODEN: NMJOAA
NAGOYA MEDICAL JOURNAL. Text in Multiple languages. 1953. q. free per issue. bk.rev. bibl, charts, illus. index. *Refereed.* **Document type:** *Academic/Scholarly.* **Description:** Presents original articles and reviews in all branches of the medical sciences.
Indexed: Abstr.Hyg., Biol.Abstr., C.I.S. Abstr., Chem.Abstr., Chem.Indus.Notes, Chem.Titles, Curr.Adv.Ecol.Sci., Excerp.Med., INIS Atomind., Ind.Med. (coverage dropped), Nutr.Abstr., Rev.Appl.Entomol., Rev.Med.& Vet.Mycol., Trop.Dis.Bull.
—CASDDS, CISTI, GNLM, ingenta, KNAW.
Published by: Nagoya-shiritsu Daigaku, Igakubu/Nagoya City University, Medical School, Kawasumi 1, Mizuho-cho, Mizuho-ku, Nagoya-shi, Aichi-ken 467-0001, Japan. TEL 81-52-853-8140, FAX 81-52-841-3480. Ed., R&P Shinji Yokoyama. Circ: 800.

610 JPN ISSN 0027-7606
CODEN: NASDA6
NAGOYA SHIRITSU DAIGAKU IGAKKAI ZASSHI/NAGOYA CITY UNIVERSITY. MEDICAL ASSOCIATION. JOURNAL. Text in Japanese. 1950. q. JPY 4,000 to membership. adv. charts, illus. index. *Refereed.* **Document type:** *Academic/Scholarly.* **Description:** Publishes review articles, original papers and case reports.
Indexed: Chem.Abstr., Chem.Indus.Notes, Chem.Titles, Excerp.Med., INIS Atomind.
—CASDDS, GNLM.
Published by: Nagoya-shiritsu Daigaku, Igakkai/Nagoya City University, Medical Association, 1 Kawasumi-Mizuho-cho, Mizuho-ku, Nagoya-shi, Aichi-ken 467-0000, Japan. TEL 81-52-853-8084, FAX 81-52-842-0863. Eds. Hitoo Nishino, Kazuo Yamada. R&P, Adv. contact Shunkichi Baba. Circ: 1,200.

610 CHN ISSN 1001-7275
CODEN: NTYXET
NANJING TIEDAO YIXUEYUAN XUEBAO/NANJING RAILWAY MEDICAL COLLEGE. JOURNAL. Text in Chinese; Abstracts in English. 1960-1963; resumed 1982. q. USD 60. *Refereed.* **Document type:** *Proceedings.* **Description:** Publishes articles on experimental research of modern medical sciences, traditional Chinese medicine, preventive medicine and clinical experiences.
Published by: Nanjing Tiedao Yixueyuan/Nanjing Railway Medical College, 87 Dingjiaqiao, Nanjing, Jiangsu 210009, China. TEL 301509, FAX 3317073. Ed. Liu Yongyan. adv.: page USD 2,000. Circ: 1,000.

610 CHN ISSN 1000-5331
CODEN: NAYXEW
NANJING YIXUEYUAN XUEBAO/NANJING INSTITUTE OF MEDICAL SCIENCES. JOURNAL. Text in Chinese. q.
Indexed: Chem.Abstr., Chem.Indus.Notes, Chem.Titles.
—CASDDS.
Published by: Nanjing Yixueyuan/Nanjing Institute of Medical Sciences, 140 Hanzhong Lu, Nanjing, Jiangsu 210029, China. TEL 649141. Ed. Wang Jingliang.

610 CHN ISSN 1000-5005
NANJING ZHONGYI XUEYUAN XUEBAO/NANJING INSTITUTE OF TRADITIONAL CHINESE MEDICINE. JOURNAL. Text in Chinese. 1959. bi-m. CNY 5 domestic; USD 5 foreign (effective 2000). *Refereed.*
Published by: Nanjing Zhongyi Xueyuan/Nanjing Institute of Traditional Chinese Medicine, 282 Hanzhong Lu, Nanjing, Jiangsu 210029, China. TEL 86-25-6798051, weidong@njutcm.edu.cn. Ed. XinSheng Fan. Circ: 3,000.

610 CHN ISSN 1000-2057
NANTONG YIXUEYUAN XUEBAO/NANTONG INSTITUTE OF MEDICAL SCIENCES. JOURNAL. Text in Chinese. q.
Published by: Nantong Yixueyuan/Nantong Institute of Medical Sciences, 19 Qixiu Lu, Nantong, Jiangsu 216001, China. TEL 517191. Ed. Meng Xianyong.

NAPRALERT ON CD-ROM. see *PHARMACY AND PHARMACOLOGY*

NASE LIECIVE RASTLINY. see *BIOLOGY—Botany*

610 RUS
NASH MALYSH. Text in Russian. 1995. m. USD 95 in North America (effective 2000).
Published by: Mezhdunarodnyi Izdatel'skii Dom, Oktyabr'skaya ul 72, ofis 405-406, Moscow 127521, Russian Federation. TEL 7-095-2186676. **Dist. by:** East View Publications, 3020 Harbor Ln N, Minneapolis, MN 55447. TEL 763-550-0961, FAX 763-559-2931.

630 AZE
NASHE ZDOROV'E. Text in Russian. s-m.
Published by: Quero Ltd, PO Box 7, Baku 370000, Azerbaijan. TEL 994-12-989413, telmed@dyndat.baku.az, http://www.az/dd/newspaper/newspaper.htm. Ed. Akhverdiev Gakhraman.

610 IND
NATIONAL ACADEMY OF INDIAN MEDICINE. ANNALS. Text in English. s-a. INR 100, USD 100.
Published by: National Academy of Indian Medicine, Department of Shalya-Shalakya, Institute of Medical Sciences, Banaras Hindu University, Varanasi, Uttar Pradesh 221 005, India.

610 IND ISSN 0379-038X
CODEN: ANAIDI
NATIONAL ACADEMY OF MEDICAL SCIENCES. ANNALS. Text and summaries in English. 1965. q. INR 50, USD 10. adv. bk.rev. charts. **Description:** Technical articles on many aspects of medical science; news of the Academy.
Formerly: Indian Academy of Medical Sciences. Annals (0019-4263)
Indexed: Biol.Abstr., Chem.Abstr., Curr.Cont. (coverage dropped), Excerp.Med., Nutr.Abstr.
—CASDDS, CISTI, GNLM.
Published by: National Academy of Medical Sciences, Nams House Ansari Nagar, Mahatma Gandhi Marg, New Delhi 110 029, India. Ed. Dr. Somnath Roy. Circ: 755.

612 USA
NATIONAL COMMITTEE ON THE TREATMENT OF INTRACTABLE PAIN. NEWSLETTER✱. Text in English. 1978. 2/yr. donation.
Published by: National Committee on the Treatment of Intractable Pain, c/o Carol Rilley, 5500 Beech Ave, Bethesda, MD 20814. Ed. Jeffrey Finn. Circ: 6,500.

362.175 GBR ISSN 1351-9441
NATIONAL COUNCIL FOR HOSPICE AND SPECIALIST PALLIATIVE CARE SERVICES. OCCASIONAL PAPER. Text in English. 1992. irreg., latest vol.13, 1997. price varies. bk.rev. **Document type:** *Monographic series.*
—BLDSC (6218.560000).
Published by: National Council for Hospice and Specialist Palliative Care Services, First Floor, 33-34 Britannia St, London WC1X 9JG, United Kingdom. TEL 44-20-7520-8299, FAX 44-20-7520-8298, enquiries@hospice-spc-council.org.uk, http://www.hospice-spc-council.org.uk. Ed., R&P Jean Gaffin.

NATIONAL DIRECTORY OF H M OS. see *INSURANCE*

610.92 USA
NATIONAL FEDERATION OF CATHOLIC PHYSICIANS' GUILDS. NEWSLETTER✱. Text in English. q. **Document type:** *Newsletter.*
Published by: National Federation of Catholic Physicians Guilds, PO Box 757, Pewaukee, WI 53072-0757. TEL 414-784-3435, FAX 414-523-6211.

M

610 USA ISSN 1071-1201
R853.R46
NATIONAL GUIDE TO FUNDING IN HEALTH. Text in English. 1990. biennial. USD 150 (effective 1997). **Document type:** *Directory.* **Description:** Contains facts on over 3300 foundations and corporate direct-giving programs interested in funding health and health-related organization, programs and services.
Published by: Foundation Center, 79 Fifth Ave, New York, NY 10003. TEL 212-807-3690, 800-424-9836, FAX 212-807-3677, http://www.fdncenter.org. Ed. James Danmgartner.

NATIONAL INSTITUTE OF POLAR RESEARCH. MEMOIRS. SERIES E: BIOLOGY AND MEDICAL SCIENCE. see *BIOLOGY*

NATIONAL INTELLIGENCE REPORT; the biweekly on Medicare policy for laboratories, blood banks & physician services. see *PUBLIC ADMINISTRATION*

NATIONAL LIBRARY OF MEDICINE CLASSIFICATION; a scheme for the shelf arrangement of library materials in the field of medicine and its related sciences. see *LIBRARY AND INFORMATION SCIENCES*

610 617.6 USA ISSN 0027-9676
NATIONAL MEDICAL AND DENTAL ASSOCIATION. BULLETIN. Text mainly in English; Text occasionally in Polish. 1926. a. USD 15. adv. bk.rev. illus. **Document type:** *Bulletin.*
Published by: (National Medical and Dental Association of America), Polstar Publishing Corp., c/o Raymond S. Dziejma, Ed., 72-41 Grand Ave., Maspeth, NY 11378. TEL 718-478-3333. Circ: 3,000.

610 USA ISSN 0027-9684
R15 CODEN: JNMAAE
NATIONAL MEDICAL ASSOCIATION. JOURNAL. Variant title: National Medical Association. Journal(J N M A). Text in English. 1908. m. USD 110 domestic to individuals; USD 133 in Canada to individuals (effective 2001); USD 156 elsewhere to individuals; USD 129 domestic to institutions; USD 152 in Canada to institutions; USD 175 elsewhere to institutions; USD 13 newsstand/cover domestic; USD 19 newsstand/cover foreign (effective 2002). adv. bk.rev. abstr, bibl, charts, illus, stat. index. 40 p./no. back issues avail.; reprints avail. *Refereed.* **Document type:** *Journal, Academic/Scholarly.* **Description:** Covers all fields of medical research and practice, with emphasis on topics vital to African-American physicians and medical professionals serving the African-American population.
Related titles: Online - full text ed.: (from ProQuest Information & Learning, Institute for Scientific Information).
Indexed: ASCA, AgeLine, Biol.Abstr., Chem.Abstr., Chic.Per.Ind., Crim.Just.Abstr., Curr.Adv.Cancer Res., Curr.Cont., Dairy Sci.Abstr., Dent.Ind., Environ.Sci.Poll.Mgmt., Excerp.Med., Hosp.Lit.Ind., INIS Atomind., I.P.A., Ind.Med. (1909-), Inpharma, Int.Nurs.Ind., Med.Care Rev., Nutr.Abstr., Pharm.&Out.News, Pollut.Abstr., Protozool.Abstr., PsycInfo, Psychol.Abstr. (1977-), Reac., Rev.Med.& Vet.Mycol., Risk Abstr., Saf.Sci.Abstr., Sage Race Rel.Abstr., THA, Trop.Dis.Bull., e-psyche.
—BLDSC (4831.114000), CASDDS, CISTI, GNLM, IDS, ingenta, KNAW.
Published by: National Medical Association, 1012 Tenth St, NW, Washington, DC 20001. TEL 202-347-1895, FAX 202-842-3293, ktaylor@nmanet.org, http://www.NMAnet.org, http://www.nmanet.org. Ed. A. Paul Kelly. Pub., Adv. contact Kim Taylor. Circ: 28,000 (controlled).

610 IND ISSN 0970-258X
R97 CODEN: NMJIEU
NATIONAL MEDICAL JOURNAL OF INDIA. Text in English. 1988. 6/yr. INR 250 domestic to individuals; USD 40 foreign to individuals; INR 500 domestic to institutions; USD 80 foreign to institutions (effective 2001). adv. bk.rev. index. *Refereed.* **Document type:** *Academic/Scholarly.* **Description:** Provides a forum for Indian doctors in India or abroad. Publishes original and review articles relevant to clinical practice. Also encourages discussion of social and political problems.
Related titles: Online - full text ed.: (from Institute for Scientific Information).
Indexed: Abstr.Hyg., Curr.Cont., Dairy Sci.Abstr., Excerp.Med., ExtraMED, Helminthol.Abstr., Ind.Med. (1988-), Inpharma, Nutr.Abstr., Pharm.&Out.News, Protozool.Abstr., Reac., Rev.Appl.Entomol., Rev.Med.& Vet.Mycol., Rural Devel.Abstr., Sci.Cit.Ind., Trop.Dis.Bull.
—BLDSC (6027.090000), EMDOCS, GNLM, IDS, Infotrieve, KNAW. **CCC.**
Published by: All India Institute of Medical Sciences, Ansari Nagar, New Delhi 110 029, India. TEL 91-11-6863002, FAX 91-11-6862663, TELEX 31-73042 AIMS IN, nmji@aiims.aiims.ac.in. Ed., Pub. K S Reddy. R&P, Adv. contact P Sahni. Circ: 3,500 (paid).

362.1 USA ISSN 1073-2551
NATIONAL REPORT ON SUBACUTE CARE; the bi-weekly newsletter for strategic issues, trends and management. Text in English. 1993. s-m. USD 357 (effective 2000). charts, stat. back issues avail. **Document type:** *Newsletter.* **Description:** Designed to give subacute care administrators, nursing staff and company executives insight into business and management strategies. Contains regulatory news and news of mergers and acquisitions in the subacute care industry.
Indexed: Int.Nurs.Ind.
—Infotrieve. **CCC.**
Published by: Harling Communications, Inc., 18 2 E Dundee Rd, Ste 200, Barrington, IL 60010. TEL 847-304-1011, FAX 847-304-1035, postacute@aol.com. Ed. Marjorie Lellis. Pub., R&P Mark Harling TEL 516-379-7097.

610 TWN ISSN 0028-0275
NATIONAL TAIWAN UNIVERSITY. COLLEGE OF MEDICINE. MEMOIRS. Key Title: Guoli Taiwan Daxue Yixueyuan Yanjiu Lunwen Zhaiyaoji. Text in Chinese. 1947. a. bibl, charts, illus, stat. *Refereed.* **Document type:** *Academic/Scholarly.* **Description:** Contains original articles and reviews published by the faculties.
Indexed: Abstr.Hyg., Anim.Breed.Abstr., Biol.Abstr., Trop.Dis.Bull.
Published by: National Taiwan University, College of Medicine, No 1 Jen-Ai Rd Sec 1, Taipei, Taiwan. TEL 02-3970800. Ed. Wen Pin Chen. Circ: 1,500.

NATUR UND KOSMOS. see *ENVIRONMENTAL STUDIES*

610 DEU ISSN 0931-1513
NATURAMED; die Aerztzeitschrift. Text in German. 1986. 11/yr. DEM 78; DEM 45 to students (effective 1999). adv. bk.rev. illus, charts. back issues avail. **Document type:** *Academic/Scholarly.* **Description:** New therapies for general practitioners.
Indexed: AMED.
—BLDSC (6036.580000), GNLM.
Published by: (Deutsche Gesellschaft fuer Akupunktur und Neuraltherapie), Verlag Kirchheim und Co. GmbH, Kaiserstr 41, Mainz 55116, Germany. TEL 49-6131-96070-0, FAX 49-6131-9607070, kirchheim@aol.com. Ed. Marcela Ullmann. Circ: 16,500.

NATURE BIOTECHNOLOGY. see *BIOLOGY—Biotechnology*

610 GBR ISSN 1078-8956
RB113 CODEN: NAMEFI
NATURE MEDICINE. Text in English. 1995. m. USD 169 domestic to individuals; GBP 135 foreign to individuals; USD 710 domestic to institutions; GBP 520 foreign to institutions (effective 2001). adv. bk.rev. illus. back issues avail. *Refereed.* **Document type:** *Academic/Scholarly.* **Description:** Publishes papers at the cutting edge of biomedical research and provides the proper clinical context. Also reports on biomedical news and related issues of interest to scientists, researchers and academic clinicians.
Related titles: Online - full text ed.: (from EBSCO Publishing, ingenta, Gale Group, Institute for Scientific Information).
Indexed: AIDS & Cancer Res., ASCA, Agri.& Environ.Biotech.Abstr., Aqua.Sci.& Fish.Abstr., BBCI, Biol.Dig., Cal.Tiss.Abstr., Chemorec.Abstr., Curr.Cont., Derwent Biotech.Abstr., Diab.Cont., Environ.Sci.Poll.Mgmt., Excerp.Med. (1995-), Focus on: Mol.Med., Gen.Sci.Ind. (Jul.1997-), Genet.Abstr., Hum.Gen.Abstr., Immun.Abstr., Ind.Med. (1995-), Ind.Sci.Rev., Inpharma, Int.Abstr.Biol.Sci., Jrnl.Watch Derm., Jrnl.Watch Inf.Dis., Jrnl.Watch Neuro., Jrnl.Watch Psych., Med.& Pharm.Biotech.Abstr., NRN, Neurosci.Abstr., Nuc.Acids Abstr., Nutr.Abstr., Oncog.G.F.Abstr., Pharm.&Out.News, Protozool.Abstr., Reac., Ref.Zh., Rev.Appl.Entomol., Rev.Med.& Vet.Mycol., Sci.Cit.Ind., Trop.Dis.Bull., Wild.Rev.
—BLDSC (6047.030000), CASDDS, CISTI, GNLM, IDS, Infotrieve, ingenta, KNAW. **CCC.**
Published by: Macmillan Magazines Ltd, Porters South, 4 Crinan Street, London N1 9XW, United Kingdom. TEL 44-171-843-4962, subscriptions@natureny.com, http://www.medicine.nature.com. Ed. Adrian Ivinson. Adv. contact Karen O'Neill. B&W page GBP 2,288, color page GBP 3,088. Circ: 15,000. **Subscr.in US to:** Allen Press Inc., PO Box 1897, Lawrence, KS 66044-8897. TEL 800-524-0384, FAX 615-377-0525, http://www.medicine.nature.com.

NATURHEILPRAXIS MIT NATURMEDIZIN; Fachzeitschrift fuer Naturheilkunde, Erfahrungsheilkunde und biologische Heilverfahren. see *ALTERNATIVE MEDICINE*

NATURWISSENSCHAFTLICH - MEDIZINISCHEN VEREINS IN INNSBRUCK. BERICHTE. see *BIOLOGY*

610 YUG ISSN 0352-5856
NAUCNI PODMLADAK. SVESKA ZA MEDICINKS NAUKE*; strucni casopis studenata Univerziteta u Nisu. Text in Serbo-Croatian; Summaries in English. 1969. q. YUN 4,000, USD 5. adv.
Former titles (until 1984): Naucni Podmladak. Medicinska Sveska (0352-1613); (until 1982): Naucni Podmladak. Medicinske Nauke (0350-6576); Supersedes in part (in 1971): Naucni Podmladak: Tehnicka Nauke. Drustvene Nauki
Published by: Univerzitet u Nisu, Trg Univerzitetski 2, Nis, Serbia 18000, Yugoslavia. Ed. Milorad Pavlovic. Circ: 1,300.

NAUKOVE TOVARYSTVO IMENI SHEVCHENKA. PROCEEDINGS OF THE SECTION OF CHEMISTRY, BIOLOGY AND MEDICINE. see *CHEMISTRY*

616.98 USA ISSN 0895-8211
R11
NAVY MEDICINE. Text in English. 1943. bi-m. USD 13 (effective 2001). bk.rev. s-a. index. back issues avail. **Document type:** *Trade, Government.* **Description:** Contains professional information on medicine, dentistry, and the allied health sciences primarily for U.S. Navy Medical Department personnel.
Former titles (until Mar. 1987): U.S. Navy Medicine (0364-6807); U.S. Navy Medical Newsletter (0041-7998); B U Med Newsletter
Related titles: Microfiche ed.; Online - full text ed.: (from Northern Light Technology, Inc., ProQuest Information & Learning).
Indexed: Curr.Cont. (coverage dropped), Dent.Abstr., Dent.Ind., Ind.U.S.Gov.Per., MEDOC.
—BLDSC (6067.592000), GNLM, ingenta, KNAW.
Published by: U.S. Navy, Bureau of Medicine and Surgery, Attn: MED-09H, 2300 E St NW, Washington, DC 20372. TEL 202-762-3248, http://navymedicine.med.navy.mil/med09H/interest.htm. Ed. Jan Kenneth Herman. Circ: 175,000. **Subscr. to:** U.S. Government Printing Office, Superintendent of Documents, PO Box 371954, Pittsburgh, PA 15250-7954. TEL 202-512-1800, FAX 202-512-2250, orders@gpo.gov, http://www.access.gpo.gov.

616.047 344.041 USA
NECK PAIN. Text in English. 1992 (2nd ed.). base vol. plus a. updates. USD 65. illus.
Published by: Lexis Law Publishing (Subsidiary of: Reed Elsevier plc), PO Box 7587, Charlottesville, VA 22906-7587. TEL 804-972-7600, 800-562-1197, FAX 804-972-7666, llp.customer.support@lexis-nexis.com, http://www.lexislawpublishing.com.

610 NLD ISSN 0028-2103
NEDERLANDS MILITAIR GENEESKUNDIG TIJDSCHRIFT. Text in Dutch; Summaries in English. 1947. bi-m. free per issue to qualified personnel. adv. bk.rev. bibl, charts, illus. index. back issues avail. *Refereed.* **Document type:** *Journal, Government, Academic/Scholarly.* **Description:** Publishes original research and reports on issues relating to health in the military.
Related titles: Diskette ed.; E-mail ed.; Fax ed.; English ed.: Netherlands Military Medical Review. ISSN 0369-4844.
Indexed: Chem.Abstr., Excerp.Med.
Published by: Ministerie van Defensie, Militair Geneeskundig Facilitair Bedrijf, PO Box 20701, The Hague 2500 ES, Netherlands. TEL 31-70-318-7159, FAX 31-70-318-7701, nmgt.mgfbstaf.mgfb@mlis.mindef.nl. Ed. Col. Joseph de Lange. Adv. contact Frank Oudman. B&W page NLG 1,640, color page NLG 2,655; trim 265 x 180. Circ: 11,000 (controlled).

610 NLD ISSN 0028-2162
CODEN: NETJAN
NEDERLANDS TIJDSCHRIFT VOOR GENEESKUNDE. Text in Dutch. 1856. w. NLG 224 to individuals; NLG 99.50 to students. adv. bk.rev. abstr, bibl, charts, illus. index.
Related titles: Microform ed.: (from PMC); Online - full text ed.: (from Institute for Scientific Information).

M

Indexed: Abstr.Crim.& Pen., Abstr.Hyg., Agri.& Environ.Biotech.Abstr. (coverage dropped), Aqua.Sci.& Fish.Abstr., Aquacult.Abstr., Biol.Abstr., Chem.Abstr., Dairy Sci.Abstr., Dent.Ind., Derwent Biotech.Abstr., Environ.Sci.Poll.Mgmt., Excerp.Med., INIS Atomind., Ind.Med. (1957-), Ind.Vet., Int.Nurs.Ind., Nutr.Abstr., Ornam.Hort., Potato Abstr., Protozool.Abstr., Rev.Appl.Entomol., Rev.Arom.& Med.Plants, Rev.Med.& Vet.Mycol., Sugar Ind.Abstr., Trop.Dis.Bull.
—BLDSC (6071.850000), CASDDS, CISTI, GNLM, IDS, KNAW.
Published by: Bohn Stafleu van Loghum B.V. (Subsidiary of: Wolters Kluwer N.V.), Postbus 246, Houten 3990 GA, Netherlands. TEL 31-3403-95711, FAX 31-3403-50903. Circ: 30,000.

610 NLD ISSN 0926-7522
NEDERLANDS TIJDSCHRIFT VOOR HEELKUNDE. Text in Dutch. 1992. bi-m. adv. **Document type:** *Academic/Scholarly.*
—KNAW.
Published by: (Nederlandse Vereniging voor Heelkunde), Mediselect B.V., Postbus 63, Leusden 3830 AB, Netherlands. TEL 31-33-4229900, FAX 31-33-4229922, info@mediselect.nl. **Co-sponsor:** Vereniging voor Assistent-Geneeskundigen in de Heelkunde.

616.01 NLD ISSN 0929-0176
CODEN: NMMIE
NEDERLANDS TIJDSCHRIFT VOOR MEDISCHE MICROBIOLOGIE. Text in Dutch. 1993. 5/yr. NLG 90. adv. Supplement avail. *Refereed.* **Document type:** *Academic/Scholarly, Trade.* **Description:** Informs association members about developments in their profession.
Indexed: Excerp.Med. (1995-).
—BLDSC (6071.990000), GNLM, KNAW.
Published by: (Nederlandse Vereniging voor Medische Microbiologie), Elsevier Gezondheidszorg B.V., Tijdstroom (Subsidiary of: Reed Elsevier plc Group), Planetenbaan 1, Maarssen 3600 AK, Netherlands. TEL 31-346-577577, FAX 31-546-554287, c.vogel@ebi.nl, http://www.tijdstroom. Ed. Dr. J A Kaan. Adv. contact C Mieuwlands. Circ: 630. **Subscr. to:** Elsevier Den Haag, Postbus 16500, The Hague 2500 BM, Netherlands. TEL 31-70-381-9900, FAX 31-70-333-8399.

610 NLD ISSN 1386-1565
NEDERLANDS TIJDSCHRIFT VOOR OSTEOPOROSE EN ANDERE BOTZIEKTEN. Text in Dutch. 1997. q.
Published by: Mediselect B.V., Postbus 63, Leusden 3830 AB, Netherlands. TEL 31-33-4229900, FAX 31-33-4229922, info@mediselect.nl.

610 CHN
NEI JING. Text in Chinese. q.
Published by: Zhonghua Yixuehui (Nanjing Fenhui)/Chinese Medical Association (Nanjing Branch), 291 Zhongshan Lu, Nanjing, Jiangsu 210008, China. TEL 303848.

610 NPL ISSN 0028-2715
NEPAL MEDICAL ASSOCIATION. JOURNAL. Variant title: J N M A. Text in English. 1963. q. USD 18 domestic; USD 55 foreign (effective 2001). adv. bk.rev. abstr, charts, illus. index. back issues avail. *Refereed.* **Document type:** *Journal, Academic/Scholarly.*
Indexed: Diar.Dis.Res., Protozool.Abstr., Rev.Appl.Entomol., Rev.Arom.& Med.Plants, Rev.Med.& Vet.Mycol., Rural Devel.Abstr., Trop.Dis.Bull.
—BLDSC (4831.750000).
Published by: Nepal Medical Association, Siddhi Sadan, Exhibition Rd., G P O Box 189, Kathmandu, Nepal. TEL 977-1225860, FAX 977-1-225300, nma@healthnet.org.np, http://www.nma.org.np. Eds. Dr. Ramesh Prasad Aacharya, Sudha Sharma. R&P Dr. Ramesh Prasad Aacharya. Adv. contact Gopi Krishna Shrestha. Circ: 1,500.

NETHERLANDS JOURNAL OF MEDICINE. see *MEDICAL SCIENCES—Internal Medicine*

M

610 CAN
NEUTROPENIA SUPPORT ASSOC. INC. Text in English. q. free per issue. **Document type:** *Newsletter.*
Published by: Neutropenia Support Association, Inc., 905 Corydon Ave, P O Box 243, Winnipeg, MB R3M 3S7, Canada. TEL 204-489-8454, 800-663-8876, stevensl@neutropenia.ca, http://www.neutropenia.ca. Ed. Mike Carlson. **Co-sponsor:** Neutropenia News Network.

610 USA
NEVADA STATE MEDICAL ASSOCIATION. BULLETIN. Text in English. 1973. bi-m. USD 30. adv. **Document type:** *Bulletin.*
Published by: Nevada State Medical Association, 3660 Baker Ln, Reno, NV 89509. Circ: 1,250.

610 CAN ISSN 0836-2688
NEW BRUNSWICK MEDICAL SOCIETY. NEWSLETTER. Text in English. m. membership. **Document type:** *Newsletter.*
Published by: New Brunswick Medical Society, 176 York St, Fredericton, NB E3B 3N8, Canada. TEL 506-458-8860. Circ: 800.

610 570 DEU ISSN 0935-1906
CODEN: NDBIET
NEW DEVELOPMENTS IN BIOSCIENCES. Text in English. 1985. irreg., latest vol.7, 1992. price varies. back issues avail. **Document type:** *Monographic series.*
—CASDDS, CISTI, KNAW.
Published by: Walter de Gruyter und Co., Genthiner Str 13, Berlin 10785, Germany. TEL 49-30-26005-0, FAX 49-30-26005-251, wdg-info@degruyter.de, http://www.degruyter.de.

610.73 AUS ISSN 0313-2153
NEW DOCTOR. Text in English. 1976. s-a. AUD 30 (effective 1998). adv. bk.rev. back issues avail. **Document type:** *Academic/Scholarly.* **Description:** Concerned with the wider sociological, political and environmental issues of health care provision and medical practice in modern society.
Indexed: Aus.P.A.I.S., INIS Atomind.
—BLDSC (6083.498000).
Published by: Doctors' Reform Society, 4 Goulburn St, PO Box 14, Sydney, NSW 2000, Australia. TEL 61-2-2649084, FAX 61-2-2674393, drs@nlc.net.au, http://www.drs.org.au. Ed. Dr. Theo Van Lieshout. R&P, Adv. contact Carol Zarkesh. page AUD 1,600. Circ: 2,000.

610 USA ISSN 0028-4793
R11 CODEN: NEJMAG
NEW ENGLAND JOURNAL OF MEDICINE. Text in English. 1812. w., latest vol.345. USD 135 domestic to individuals; CND 199 in Canada to individuals; USD 349 domestic to institutions; CND 365 in Canada to institutions; USD 370 elsewhere; USD 5.60 newsstand/cover domestic; CND 9.50 newsstand/cover in Canada; USD 10.50 newsstand/cover elsewhere; USD 63 to students (effective 2001); $69 - residents & interns. adv. bk.rev. bibl, charts, illus, stat. s-a. index. reprints avail. *Refereed.* **Document type:** *Trade.* **Description:** Presents original articles and interpretive reviews of a variety of developments in the major aspects of medicine, its science, its art and practice and its position in today's society.
Related titles: CD-ROM ed.: (from Ovid Technologies, Inc.); Microform ed.: (from PQC,PMC); Online - full text ed.: (from Ovid Technologies, Inc., EBSCO Publishing, Gale Group, Factiva, Institute for Scientific Information, RoweCom Information Quest).
Indexed: AIDS & Cancer Res., AIDS Abstr., AIM, AMED, ASCA, Abstr.Anthropol., Abstr.Crim.& Pen., Abstr.Health Care Manage.Stud., Abstr.Hyg., Abstr.Soc.Geront., Acad.Ind., Addic.Abstr., AgeLine, Agri.& Environ.Biotech.Abstr. (coverage dropped), Behav.Med.Abstr., Bibl.Agri., Bibl.Dev.Med.& Child Neur., Biol.Abstr., Biol.Dig., CHNI, CINAHL, C.I.S. Abstr., Cadscan, Cal.Tiss.Abstr., Chem.Abstr., Chem.Indus.Notes, Chem.Titles, Crim.Just.Abstr., Curr.Adv.Cancer Res., Curr.Adv.Ecol.Sci., Curr.Cont., Curr.Ind.Stat., Curr.Lit.Fam.Plan., Dairy Sci.Abstr., Deep Sea Res.& Oceanogr.Abstr., Dent.Abstr., Dent.Ind., Derwent Biotech.Abstr., Diab.Cont., Diar.Dis.Res., Environ.Abstr., Environ.Ind., Environ.Sci.Poll.Mgmt., Excerp.Med., FAMLI, Focus on: Sports Sci.& Med., Food Sci.& Tech.Abstr., Fut.Surv., Gen.Sci.Ind. (Jun.1984-), Genet.Abstr., Helminthol.Abstr., Hlth.Ind., Hosp.Lit.Ind., Hum.Gen.Abstr., INIS Atomind., I.P.A., Immun.Abstr., Ind.Hyg.Dig., Ind.Med. (1928-), Ind.Sci.Rev., Ind.Vet., Inpharma, Int.Abstr.Biol.Sci., Int.Nurs.Ind., Jrnl.Watch, Jrnl.Watch Card., Jrnl.Watch Derm., Jrnl.Watch Emer.Med., Jrnl.Watch Gastr., Jrnl.Watch Inf.Dis., Jrnl.Watch Neuro., Jrnl.Watch Psych., Jrnl.Watch Wom.Hlth., Kidney, L.R.I., Lang.& Lang.Behav.Abstr., Lead Abstr., Mag.Ind., Med.& Surg.Dermat., Med.Care Rev., Microbiol.Abstr., NRN, Neurosci.Abstr., Neurosci.Cit.Ind., Nurs.Abstr., Nutr.Abstr., Pharm.&Out.News, Pollut.Abstr., Popul.Ind., Protozool.Abstr., PsycInfo, Psychol.Abstr. (1928-), Reac., Rehabil.Lit., Rev.Appl.Entomol., Rev.Arom.& Med.Plants, Rev.Med.& Vet.Mycol., Rev.Plant Path., Risk Abstr., SSCI (coverage dropped), Saf.Sci.Abstr., Sci.Cit.Ind., Soc.Work Res.& Abstr., THA, Telegen, Tox.Abstr., Tr.& Indus.Ind., Triticale Abstr., Trop.Dis.Bull., Vet.Bull., Virol.Abstr., WMB, W.R.C.Inf., Weed Abstr., Yrbk.Assoc.Educ.& Rehab.Blind, Zincscan, e-psyche.
—BLDSC (6084.000000), CASDDS, CIS, CISTI, GNLM, IDS, ingenta, KNAW. **CCC.**
Published by: Massachusetts Medical Society, Publishing Division, 10 Shattuck St, Boston, MA 02115. TEL 617-734-9800, 781-893-3800, FAX 617-739-9864, http://www.nejm.org. Ed. Dr. Jeffrey M Drazen. Adv. contact Art Wilshek. B&W page USD 4,530, color page USD 6,345; trim 10 x 7. Circ: 231,126 (paid).

610 USA
NEW ENGLAND JOURNAL OF MEDICINE (INTERNATIONAL EDITION). Text in English. w. adv. bk.rev. abstr, bibl, charts, illus, stat. reprints avail. **Document type:** *Journal, Academic/Scholarly.* **Description:** Presents original articles and reviews of developments in medical science and art, medical practices and the position of medicine in today's sociopolitical structure.
Related titles: Online - full content ed.
Indexed: Curr.Cont. (coverage dropped), Diar.Dis.Res.
Published by: Massachusetts Medical Society, Publishing Division, 10 Shattuck St, Boston, MA 02115. TEL 617-734-9800, http://www.nejm.org. Ed. Dr. Jeffrey M Drazen. Circ: 55,588.

616 USA
NEW HORIZONS IN THERAPEUTICS: SMITH, KLINE & FRENCH LABORATORIES RESEARCH SYMPOSIA SERIES. Text in English. 1984. irreg., latest 1994. price varies. *Refereed.* **Document type:** *Proceedings.*
Formerly: New Horizons in Therapeutics
Published by: Kluwer Academic - Plenum Publishers (Subsidiary of: Wolters Kluwer N.V.), 233 Spring St, New York, NY 10013-1578. TEL 212-620-8000, 800-221-9369, FAX 212-463-0742, info@plenum.com, http://www.plenum.com. Eds. George Poste, Stanley T Crooke.

617.8 USA ISSN 0028-5935
NEW JERSEY SPEECH AND HEARING ASSOCIATION. JOURNAL✶. Text in English. 1963. s-a. USD 10. adv. bk.rev.
Published by: New Jersey Speech and Hearing Association, c/o Auriemma, 6 Crest Ln, Warren, NJ 07059-5110. Circ: 1,100 (controlled).

610.711 GBR
THE NEW LEARNING MEDICINE. Text in English. 1983. a.
Formerly: Learning Medicine
—BLDSC (5179.328100).
Published by: B M J Publishing Group, B M A House, Tavistock Sq, London WC1H 9JR, United Kingdom. TEL 44-207-383-6270, FAX 44-20-7383-6402. Eds. Peter Richards, Simon Stockill.

610 USA ISSN 1089-2524
R728
NEW MEDICINE. Text in English. 1997. q. USD 125 in North America to individuals; GBP 119 elsewhere to individuals; USD 375 in North America to institutions; GBP 319 elsewhere to institutions. **Document type:** *Academic/Scholarly.*
Related titles: Online - full text ed.
Indexed: Nutr.Abstr.
—**CCC.**
Published by: Current Science Inc., 400 Market St, Ste 700, Philadelphia, PA 19106. Ed. Elena Coler. R&P Lori Holland. **Subscr. to:** Turpin Distribution Services Ltd., Blackhorse Rd, Letchworth, Herts SG6 1HN, United Kingdom. TEL 44-1462-672555, FAX 44-1462-680947.

610 USA ISSN 0028-6451
THE NEW PHYSICIAN. Text in English. 1952. 9/yr. USD 25 to non-members; USD 41 foreign to non-members. adv. bk.rev. reprint service avail. from PQC. **Document type:** *Trade.* **Description:** Examines all aspects of medicine, health policy and medical education through news and feature articles.
Related titles: Microform ed.: (from PQC); Includes: A M S A Focus.
Indexed: AgeLine, Biol.Abstr., Hosp.Lit.Ind., I.P.A., Med.Care Rev., Phys.Ber.
—BLDSC (6084.980000), GNLM, ingenta.
Published by: American Medical Student Association, 1902 Association Dr, Reston, VA 20191-1502. TEL 703-620-6600, FAX 703-620-5873, amsatnp@aol.com, http://www.amsa.org/tnp/tnp.htm. Ed. Amy Myers Payne. R&P Amy Myers-Payne. Adv. contact Lisa Adams. Circ: 25,000.

▼ **THE NEW REVIEW OF HEALTH INFORMATICS.** see *PHYSICAL FITNESS AND HYGIENE*

610 540 DEU
NEW TRENDS IN SYNTHETIC MEDICINAL CHEMISTRY. Text in English. irreg. MRK 248, EUR 126.80, CHF 220 (effective 2001). **Document type:** *Monographic series, Academic/Scholarly.*

—BLDSC (5746.690000).
Published by: Wiley - V C H Verlag GmbH, P. O. Box 101161, Weinheim D-69451 , Germany. TEL 49-6201-606-0, 49-6201-606152, FAX 49-6201-606-328, 49-6201-606184, TELEX 467 155 vchwh d, info@wiley-vch.de, sales-books@wiley-vch.de. Eds. H Kubinyi, H Timmerman, R Mannhold, Dr. Fulvio Gualtieri.

610 681 GBR ISSN 1350-2220
NEW WORLD HEALTH (YEAR). Text in English. a. adv. **Document type:** *Journal, Trade.* **Description:** Provides a means of communication exchange between senior healthcare professionals, enabling them to attain higher standards of patient care in the world's developing and emerging markets.
Published by: Sterling Publications Ltd. (Subsidiary of: Sterling Publishing Group Plc.), Brunel House, 55-57 North Wharf Rd, London W2 1LA, United Kingdom. FAX 44-20-7724-2089, nh@sterlingpublications.com, http://www.sterlingpublications.com/publications/newworldhealth.html. R&P Sandy Tucker. Circ: 10,000 (controlled).

610.6 USA
NEW YORK ACADEMY OF MEDICINE. ANNUAL REPORT. Text in English. a. **Document type:** *Corporate.*
Published by: New York Academy of Medicine, 2 E 103rd St, New York, NY 10029. TEL 212-876-8200, FAX 212-876-6620.

610 USA ISSN 1074-0996
RA421
NEW YORK HEALTH SCIENCES JOURNAL. Text in English. 1994. s-a. USD 80; USD 100 foreign (effective 1999). adv. back issues avail. *Refereed.* **Description:** Provides insight into timely issues, provokes discussion and reflection, and poses solutions that are both theoretical and practical.
—CISTI.
Published by: New York Medical College, Graduate School of Health Sciences, New York, NY 10595. TEL 914-594-4531, FAX 914-594-4292, donna_clark@nymc.edu; orders@allenpresss.com, http://www.allenpress.com. Ed., Adv. contact Esther Dyer. Pub., R&P Sheila M Smythe. **Subscr. to:** Allen Press Inc., PO Box 1897, Lawrence, KS 66044-8897.

610.28 USA
NEW YORK UNIVERSITY BIOMEDICAL ENGINEERING SERIES. Text in English. 1987. irreg. price varies. **Document type:** *Monographic series.*
Published by: New York University Press, 70 Washington Square So, New York, NY 10012. TEL 212-998-2575, 800-996-3833, FAX 212-995-3833. Ed. Walter Welkowitz. R&P Susan Conn.

NEW ZEALAND HEALTH INFORMATION SERVICE. CANCER: NEW REGISTRATIONS AND DEATHS. see *MEDICAL SCIENCES—Abstracting, Bibliographies, Statistics*

610 NZL ISSN 0028-8446
CODEN: NZMJAX
NEW ZEALAND MEDICAL JOURNAL. Text in English. 1887. s-m. USD 135. adv. bk.rev. charts, illus. index, cum.index. reprint service avail. from PQC. *Refereed.* **Document type:** *Academic/Scholarly.*
Related titles: Microform ed.: (from PQC); Online - full text ed.: (from Institute for Scientific Information).
Indexed: ASCA, Abstr.Hyg., Agri.& Environ.Biotech.Abstr. (coverage dropped), Aqua.Sci.& Fish.Abstr., Bibl.Dev.Med.& Child Neur., Biol.Abstr., CINAHL, C.I.S. Abstr., Chem.Abstr., Crim.Just.Abstr., Curr.Adv.Cancer Res., Curr.Adv.Ecol.Sci., Curr.Cont., Dairy Sci.Abstr., Dent.Ind., Derwent Biotech.Abstr., Environ.Sci.Poll.Mgmt., Excerp.Med., HRIS, Helminthol.Abstr., INIS Atomind., Ind.Med. (1887-), Ind.N.Z.Per., Ind.Sci.Rev., Ind.Vet., Inpharma, Int.Nurs.Ind., NRN, Neurosci.Cit.Ind., Nutr.Abstr., Pharm.&Out.News, Pig News & Info., Pollut.Abstr., Protozool.Abstr., Reac., Rev.Appl.Entomol., Rev.Arom.& Med.Plants, Rev.Med.& Vet.Mycol., Rev.Plant Path., Risk Abstr., SSCI (coverage dropped), Saf.Sci.Abstr., Sci.Cit.Ind., So.Pac.Per.Ind., Soyabean Abstr., THA, Trop.Dis.Bull., Vet.Bull.
—BLDSC (6096.100000), CASDDS, CISTI, GNLM, IDS, ingenta, KNAW. **CCC.**
Published by: (New Zealand Medical Association), Southern Colour Print, PO Box 920, Dunedin, New Zealand. TEL 64-3-4550554, FAX 64-3-4550303. Ed. R G Robinson. R&P R.G. Robinson TEL 64-3-4741060. Adv. contact Jill Wood. Circ: 5,000 (paid).

610 CAN ISSN 0078-0316
NEWFOUNDLAND MEDICAL DIRECTORY. Text in English. 1961. a. (plus q. updates). CND 35; free to qualified personnel. **Document type:** *Directory.*
Published by: Newfoundland Medical Board, Registrar, 139 Water St., St. John's, NF A1C 1B2, Canada. TEL 709-726-8546. Circ: 2,000.

NEWS AND STRATEGIES FOR MANAGED MEDICARE AND MEDICAID. see *INSURANCE*

610 USA
NEWS CAPSULE✶. Text in English. 1990 (vol.37, no.9). 6/yr. USD 12 to non-members. adv. **Document type:** *Bulletin.* **Description:** Contains capsulized information for practicing physicians.
Published by: Fairfield County Medical Association, 12 Cambridge Dr, Trumbull, CT 06611-4764. TEL 203-372-4543, FAX 203-372-5293. Ed., R&P Mark S Thompson. Adv. contact Mary Beth Henry. B&W page USD 250. Circ: 2,000.

610.6 USA ISSN 0028-9264
NEWS OF NEW YORK. Text in English. 1945. m. USD 36 (effective 2000). adv. charts, illus. **Document type:** *Trade.* **Description:** Focuses on regulatory, legislative and economic issues that have immediate impact on the daily practice of New York physicians.
Formerly: Medical Society of the State of New York. News Letter
Published by: Medical Society of the State of New York, 420, Lakeville, NY 11040. TEL 516-488-6100, FAX 516-328-1982, http://www.mssny.org. Ed. Christina Cronin Southard. Pub. Thomas M Donoghue. Adv. contact Ann Tierno. Circ: 29,000.

610 JPN ISSN 0029-0424
CODEN: NICHAS
NICHIDAI IGAKU ZASSHI/NIHON UNIVERSITY. JOURNAL OF MEDICINE. Text in Japanese; Summaries in English. 1937. m. JPY 5,000. adv. bk.rev. illus. index. Supplement avail.; reprint service avail. from IRC.
Indexed: Biol.Abstr., C.I.S. Abstr., Chem.Abstr., Chem.Indus.Notes, Chem.Titles, Excerp.Med., INIS Atomind.
—BLDSC (4833.390000), CASDDS, GNLM.
Published by: Nihon Daigaku Igakkai/Nihon University Medical Association, 30 Oyaguchi Kami-cho, Itabashi-ku, Tokyo 173, Japan. Ed. Dr. Yukiyasu Sezai. Circ: 500. **Co-sponsor:** Nihon University School of Medicine.

▼ **NICOTINE & TOBACCO RESEARCH.** see *TOBACCO*

610 DEU ISSN 0468-1746
DER NIEDERGELASSENE ARZT. Text in German. 1952. m. DEM 102. adv. bk.rev.
—GNLM, Infotrieve. **CCC.**
Published by: N A V - Verband der Niedergelassenen Aertze Deutschlands e.V., Belfortstr 9V, Cologne 50668, Germany. TEL 0221-727072, FAX 0221-7391239. Circ: 50,000.

610 DEU ISSN 0028-9795
NIEDERSAECHSISCHES AERZTEBLATT. Text in German. 1927. m. EUR 46.02; EUR 30.68 to students; EUR 5.37 newsstand/cover (effective 2001). adv. bk.rev. abstr, stat. index. 100 p./no. **Document type:** *Magazine, Trade.* **Description:** Publishes information on physician conferences and congresses and discusses questions concerning medical sciences, health and environmental policy.
—GNLM, Infotrieve. **CCC.**
Published by: (Aerztekammer Niedersachsen), Hannoversche Aerzte Verlags Union GmbH, Berliner Allee 20, Hannover 30175, Germany. TEL 49-511-3802282, FAX 49-511-3802281, info@haeverlag.de, http://www.haeverlag.de. Ed. Rolf Heyde. Adv. contact Ulrike Evers. B&W page XEU 2,014.49, color page XEU 3,855.14; trim 171 x 243. Circ: 32,500.

610 NLD ISSN 0168-9827
NIEUWE NEDERLANDSE BIJDRAGEN TOT DE GESCHIEDENIS DER GENEESKUNDE EN DER NATUURWETENSCHAPPEN. Text in Dutch, English, French, German. 1978. irreg., latest vol.33, 1989. price varies. *Refereed.* **Document type:** *Monographic series, Academic/Scholarly.*
Formerly (until 1979): Nieuwe Nederlandse Bijdragen tot de Geschiedenis der Geneeskunde (0167-4404)
—CISTI, KNAW.
Published by: Erasmus Publishing B.V., Glashaven 14A, Rotterdam 3011XH, Netherlands. TEL 31-10-2800439, FAX 31-10-2800438, info@erasmuspublishing.net; p.verhoef@inter.nl.net, http://www.erasmuspublishing.net. Circ: 508.

610 NGA ISSN 0300-1652
CODEN: NGMDAI
NIGERIAN MEDICAL JOURNAL. Text in English. 1964. q. USD 275. adv. bk.rev. **Document type:** *Academic/Scholarly.*
Formerly: Nigerian Medical Association. Journal
Related titles: CD-ROM ed.
Indexed: Biol.Abstr., ExtraMED, Helminthol.Abstr., Ind.Med. (coverage dropped), Nutr.Abstr., Trop.Dis.Bull.
—CISTI, GNLM.
Published by: Nigerian Medical Association, PO Box 1108, Lagos, Nigeria. TEL 234-1-801500, FAX 231-1-837630, TELEX 002763NG. Ed. A E Ohwovoriole. Circ: 4,500.

615.8 JPN ISSN 0029-0343
NIHON ONSEN KIKO BUTSURI IGAKKAI ZASSHI/JAPANESE ASSOCIATION OF PHYSICAL MEDICINE, BALNEOLOGY, AND CLIMATOLOGY. JOURNAL. Text in Japanese; Summaries in English. 1935. q. JPY 2,500, USD 25 (effective 2000). adv. bk.rev. bibl, charts, illus. index, cum.index. **Description:** Includes physiotherapy techniques.
Indexed: Excerp.Med., INIS Atomind.
—BLDSC (4809.050000).
Published by: Nihon Onsen Kiko Butsuri Igakkai/Japanese Association of Physical Medicine, Balneology, and Climatology, c/o Health and Research Institute, 1-5-20 Ishizuka Yaesu Bldg., Yaesu, Chuo-ku, Tokyo, Japan. TEL 81-3-3517-1180, FAX 81-3-3517-1180. Ed. Katsuro Tamizaki. Circ: 1,800.

NIHON SEIRIGAKU ZASSHI/PHYSIOLOGICAL SOCIETY OF JAPAN. JOURNAL. see *BIOLOGY—Physiology*

NIHON SHIKKAN MODERU DOBUTSU KENKYUKAI KIROKU/JAPANESE ASSOCIATION OF ANIMAL MODELS FOR HUMAN DISEASES. PROCEEDINGS. see *BIOLOGY—Physiology*

NIHON TAISHITSUGAKU ZASSHI/JAPANESE JOURNAL OF CONSTITUTIONAL MEDICINE. see *BIOLOGY—Physiology*

610 JPN ISSN 0911-2588
CODEN: NTKKEM
NIHON TEITAION KENKYUKAI KAISHI/JAPANESE SOCIETY OF HYPOTHERMIA. JOURNAL. Text in Japanese; Summaries in English. 1981. a.
Indexed: Chem.Abstr.
—CASDDS.
Published by: Nihon Teitaion Kenkyukai, Kinki University School of Medicine, 377-2 Ono-Higashi, Osakasayama-shi, Osaka-fu 589-0014, Japan.

610 JPN ISSN 0029-0440
CODEN: NIGZAY
NIIGATA IGAKKAI ZASSHI/NIIGATA MEDICAL JOURNAL. Text in Japanese. 1887. m. JPY 6,500. adv. bibl, charts, illus, mkt, stat. index. reprint service avail. from IRC. **Document type:** *Academic/Scholarly.*
Related titles: Microform ed.
Indexed: C.I.S. Abstr., Chem.Abstr., Chem.Indus.Notes, Chem.Titles, INIS Atomind.
—BLDSC (6113.170000), CASDDS, CISTI, GNLM.
Published by: Niigata Igakkai/Niigata Medical Society, c/o Niigata Daigaku Igakubu, 1 Asahi-cho, Niigata 951-8122, Japan. Ed. K Kumaki. Circ: 1,000.

610 JPN
NIIGATAKEN KANKYO HOKENBU KETSUEKI JIGYO NO GENKYO. Text in Japanese. 1865. a. free per issue.
Published by: Niigataken Kankyo Hokenbu/Niigata Prefectural Government, Health and Environment Department, 4-1 Shinko-cho, Niigata-shi 950-0965, Japan.

NIKKEI HEALTHCARE. see *HEALTH FACILITIES AND ADMINISTRATION*

610 JPN ISSN 0385-1699
NIKKEI MEDICAL/NIKKEI MEDIKARU. Text in Japanese. 1972. m. adv. **Document type:** *Trade.* **Description:** Contains specialized reports for clinicians, offering insight into both clinical and economic aspects of medicine.
Indexed: JTA.

M

Published by: Nikkei Business Publications Inc. (Subsidiary of: Nihon Keizai Shimbun, Inc.), 2-7-6 Hirakawa-cho, Chiyoda-ku, Tokyo 102-8622, Japan. TEL 81-3-5210-8311, FAX 81-3-5210-8530, info@nikkeibp-america.com, http://www.nikkeibp.com. Ed. Tatsuya Kawaguchi. Pub. Hitoshi Sawai. Adv. contact Yarada Harada. B&W page JPY 1,116,000, color page JPY 1,564,000; trim 208 x 280. Circ: 103,684.

610 JPN ISSN 0048-0444 CODEN: NIDZAJ
NIPPON MEDICAL SCHOOL. JOURNAL/NIPPON IKA DAIGAKU ZASSHI. Text in English, Japanese. 1927. 6/yr. USD 60. adv. bk.rev. *Refereed.* **Document type:** *Journal, Academic/Scholarly.* **Description:** Covers developments in medical science from the association.
Related titles: Online - full text ed.: (from JICST).
Indexed: Biol.Abstr., C.I.S. Abstr., Chem.Abstr., Chem.Indus.Notes, Chem.Titles, Dent.Ind., Excerp.Med., INIS Atomind., Ind.Med. (coverage dropped).
—BLDSC (4833.600000), CASDDS, CISTI, GNLM, KNAW.
Published by: Nippon Medical School, Medical Association/Nippon Ika Daigaku Igakkai, 1-1-5 Sendagi, Bunkyo-ku, Tokyo 113-0022, Japan. TEL 81-3-3822-2131, FAX 81-3-3822-3759, TELEX 03-3822-2131-314, http://httpmac.ipc.nms.ac.jp/jnms/. Ed., R&P Tsutomu Araki. Circ: 2,850 (controlled).

616.026 DEU ISSN 0029-1609
NORDWESTDEUTSCHE GESELLSCHAFT FUER INNERE MEDIZIN. KONGRESSBERICHT. Text in German. 1953. s-a. DEM 10, USD 6 (effective 2000). adv. illus. **Document type:** *Academic/Scholarly.* **Description:** Covers internal medicine.
—GNLM, Infotrieve. **CCC.**
Published by: (Nortwestdeutsche Gesellschaft fuer Innere Medizin), Hansisches Verlagskontor, Mengstr 16, Luebeck 23552, Germany. TEL 49-451-7031-01. Ed. Dr. A Doenhardt. Circ: 1,800.

610 USA ISSN 0029-2559
R11
NORTH CAROLINA MEDICAL JOURNAL. Text in English. 1940. bi-m. USD 20. adv. bk.rev. illus. index. *Refereed.* **Document type:** *Academic/Scholarly.* **Description:** Contains information on medicine and medical practice in North Carolina written by North Carolina physicians.
Related titles: Microfilm ed.: (from PQC).
Indexed: CINAHL, C.I.S. Abstr., Chem.Abstr., Curr.Cont. (coverage dropped), Dent.Ind., Excerp.Med., Helminthol.Abstr., INIS Atomind., Ind.Med. (1940-), Int.Nurs.Ind., Rev.Med.& Vet.Mycol.
—BLDSC (6149.080000), CISTI, GNLM, KNAW.
Published by: North Carolina Medical Society, PO Box 3910, DUMC, Durham, NC 27710. TEL 919-286-6410, FAX 919-286-9219, nash0004@mc.duke.edu, http://www.ncmedicaljournal.com. Ed. Dr. Francis A Neelon. R&P Florence Nash. Adv. contact Donald R French. Circ: 9,500 (controlled).

610 IND
NORTH EASTERN DOCTORS CALLING✱. Text in English. 1984. bi-m. INR 35; to individuals (foreign Rs.80); institutions Rs.60 (foreign Rs.130). adv. bk.rev. abstr, bibl, charts, stat. *Refereed.* **Description:** Examines current professional, academic and related trends of interest to those in medical professions.
Published by: Indian Medical Association, I.M.A. House, Indraprastha Marg, New Delhi 110 002, India.

610 DEU ISSN 0340-5486
NOTABENE MEDICI. Text in German. 1971. m. DEM 60 (effective 1999). adv. **Document type:** *Academic/Scholarly, Trade.*
Indexed: Ref.Zh.
—GNLM.
Published by: Notamed Verlag GmbH, Buerstoss 2, Melsungen 34212, Germany. TEL 49-5661-8076, FAX 49-5661-1450. Ed. Horst Dehmel. Adv. contact Hannelore Goebel.

610 DEU ISSN 0177-2309
DER NOTARZT; Notfallmedizinische Informationen. Text in German. 1985. bi-m. EUR 91.40 domestic to institutions; EUR 97.80 in Europe to institutions; EUR 99.40 elsewhere to institutions; EUR 18 newsstand/cover (effective 2002). **Document type:** *Journal, Academic/Scholarly.*
Related titles: Online - full text ed.: ISSN 1438-8693.
—GNLM.
Published by: (Bundesuereinigung des Atbeitsgemanschaft Notaerzte Deutschlands), Georg Thieme Verlag, Ruedigerstr 14, Stuttgart 70469, Germany. TEL 49-711-8931-0, FAX 49-711-8931298, notarzt@thieme.de, leser.service@thieme.de, http://www.thieme.de/notarzt, http://www.thieme-connect.de. Ed. P Sefrin. R&P Alessandra Kreibaum. Circ: 10,500.

610 PRT ISSN 0870-2055
NOTICIAS MEDICAS. Text in Portuguese. 1971. s-w. free per issue to qualified personnel. adv. back issues avail. **Document type:** *Newspaper.*
Published by: Citecnica - Publicacoes Tecnicas e Cientificas Lda., Rua Tristao Vaz, 15-2o Dt, Lisbon 1400, Portugal. TEL 351-1-3011989, FAX 351-1-3016636. Ed. Rafael Reis. Pub. Jose Reis Jr. Adv. contact Graca Reis. Circ: 29,000.

610 ESP ISSN 0029-4225
NOTICIAS MEDICAS; el periodico de la medicina espanola. Text in Spanish. 1967. 35/yr. ESP 10,000 domestic; USD 120 foreign; USD 60 Supplement (effective 2001). adv. bk.rev. charts, illus. **Document type:** *Newspaper.*
—CCC.
Published by: Editores Medicos S.A., Gabriela Mistral, 2, Madrid 28035, Spain. TEL 34-91-3768140, FAX 34-91-3739907. Ed. Adolfo Berzosa Blanco. Circ: 35,000.

610 FRA ISSN 0292-384X
NOUVEAU CENTRE DE SANTE. Text in French. 1977 (vol.21). 10/yr. FRF 275; FRF 350 foreign.
Formerly: Revue de Medecine Moderne (0035-1539)
Published by: Union des Syndicats de Medecins de Centres de Sante, Centre de Sante, 23 rue de Leningrad, Paris 75008, France. TEL 45-22-21-40.

610 CHE ISSN 0254-8712
B785.P24
NOVA ACTA PARACELSICA. Text in German. a. **Document type:** *Academic/Scholarly.*
Indexed: IBZ.
Published by: (Schweizerische Paracelsus Gesellschaft), Peter Lang AG, Jupiterstr 15, Bern, 15 3000, Switzerland. TEL 41-31-9402121, FAX 41-31-9402131, langwerbung@datacomm.ch, http://www.peterlang.ch. Ed. Alois Haas.

NOVOSTI FARMATSII I MEDITSINY/NEWS IN PHARMACOLOGY AND MEDICINE. see *PHARMACY AND PHARMACOLOGY*

610 570 JPN ISSN 0469-2071
NUKADA INSTITUTE FOR MEDICAL AND BIOLOGICAL RESEARCH. REPORTS. Text in English. irreg. per issue exchange basis.
Published by: Nukada Institute for Medical and Biological Research/Nukada Igaku Seibutsugaku Kenkyujo, 5-18 Inage-cho, Inage-ku, Chiba-shi 263-0035, Japan.

610 ITA ISSN 0394-8889
NUOVI ARGOMENTI DI MEDICINA. Text in Italian. 12/yr.
Address: Via Napo Torriani 30, Milan, MI 20124, Italy. TEL 2-66-94-767. Ed. Enrico Bollero. Circ: 42,000.

NURSE PRACTITIONERS' PRESCRIBING REFERENCE. see *PHARMACY AND PHARMACOLOGY*

NUTRITION & THE M.D.; a continuing education service for physicians and nutritionists. see *NUTRITION AND DIETETICS*

613.2 CAN
NUTRITION REVIEW. Text in English. a.
Published by: M P I Publishing Inc., 14 Ronan Ave, Toronto, ON M4N 2X9, Canada. TEL 416-481-6384.

610 DNK ISSN 1397-4114
NYE TAL FRA SUNDHEDSSTYRELSEN. Text in Danish. 1997. 10/yr. free (effective 2001). **Description:** Articles on health news using collected statistics.
Published by: Sundhedsstyrelsen, Amaliegade 13, PO Box 2020, Copenhagen K 1012, Denmark. TEL 45-33-93-16-36, FAX 45-33-91-16-01.

610 USA
O H S U VIEWS. Text in English. 1979. 3/yr. USD 25. charts, illus, stat. **Document type:** *Academic/Scholarly.*
Formerly (until Nov. 1988): Oregon Health Sciences University News
Published by: Oregon Health Sciences University, 3181 S W Sam Jackson Park Rd, Portland, OR 97201. TEL 503-494-8231, FAX 503-494-8246. Ed. Marlys Levin Pierson. Circ: 35,000.

O T PRACTICE. (Occupational Therapy) see *OCCUPATIONAL HEALTH AND SAFETY*

610 USA
OAK RIDGE ASSOCIATED UNIVERSITIES. MEDICAL SCIENCES DIVISION. RESEARCH REPORT. Text in English. 1951. a. free per issue. reprint service avail. from NTI.
Formerly: Oak Ridge Institute for Nuclear Studies. Medical Division. Research Report (0078-2890)
Related titles: Microform ed.: (from NTI).
Published by: Oak Ridge Associated Universities, Inc., Office of Information Services, Box 117, Oak Ridge, TN 37831-0117. TEL 615-576-3146. Ed. Fred L Snyder. Circ: 2,500.

616.5 613.7 GBR ISSN 1469-3259
▼ **OBESITY.** Text in English. 2000. s-a. GBP 120 for print ed. or e-mail (effective 2001).
Related titles: E-mail ed.; Online - full text ed.: GBP 108 (effective 2001).
Published by: S U B I S (Subsidiary of: Sheffield Academic Press Ltd), Mansion House, 19 Kingfield Rd, Sheffield, S Yorks S11 9AS, United Kingdom. TEL 44-114-255-4433, FAX 44-114-255-4626, subis@sheffac.demon.co.uk, http://www.shef-ac-press.co.uk/subis.

610 GBR ISSN 0955-6389
OBESITY IN EUROPE. Text in English. 1989. irreg. **Document type:** *Monographic series.*
Published by: John Libbey & Co. Ltd., PO Box 276, Eastleigh SO50 5YS, United Kingdom. TEL 44-2380-650208, FAX 44-2380-650259, johnlibbey@aol.com, http://www.johnlibbey.com.

616.3 USA ISSN 1071-7323
RC628 CODEN: OBREFR
OBESITY RESEARCH. Text in English. 1993. m. USD 135 in North America to individuals; USD 160 elsewhere to individuals; USD 215 in North America to institutions; USD 240 elsewhere to institutions; USD 125 in North America to members; USD 135 elsewhere to members; USD 30 in North America to students; USD 35 elsewhere to students (effective 2000). adv. bibl, abstr. index. Supplement avail.; back issues avail. *Refereed.* **Document type:** *Academic/Scholarly.* **Description:** Publishes original scientific research and review articles in clinical and basic research related to obesity.
Related titles: Online - full text ed.: (from HighWire Pr., EBSCO Publishing, Institute for Scientific Information).
Indexed: ASCA, Agricola, Bibl.Agri., Chem.Abstr., Chem.Titles, Curr.Cont., Dairy Sci.Abstr., Fam.Ind., Food Sci.& Tech.Abstr., Ind.Med. (1993-), Inpharma, Nutr.Abstr., Pig News & Info., Reac., Sci.Cit.Ind.
—BLDSC (6196.952500), CASDDS, CISTI, GNLM, IDS, Infotrieve, KNAW. **CCC.**
Published by: North American Association for the Study of Obesity, 1090 Amsterdam Ave, Ste 14K, New York, NY 10025. TEL 212-523-2049, FAX 212-523-2098, helener@mindspring.com, http://www.obesityresearch.org/, http://www.naaso.org. Ed. F Xavier Pi Sunyer. R&P Helene Rosenhouse Romeo. Adv. contact Helene Rosenhouse Raneo. page USD 920. Circ: 910 (paid). **Subscr. to:** NAASO, 8630 Fenton Street, Suite 412, Silver Spring, MD 20910. TEL 507-255-6768, FAX 507-255-4828.

OCCUPATIONAL MEDICINE. see *OCCUPATIONAL HEALTH AND SAFETY*

615.8 USA ISSN 0738-0577 CODEN: OTHCES
OCCUPATIONAL THERAPY IN HEALTH CARE; a journal of contemporary practice. Text in English. 1984. q. USD 50 to individuals; USD 68 in Canada to individuals; USD 73 elsewhere to individuals; USD 75 to institutions; USD 101 in Canada to institutions; USD 109 elsewhere to institutions; USD 150 to libraries; USD 203 in Canada to libraries; USD 218 elsewhere to libraries (effective Aug. 2001). adv. bk.rev. reprint service avail. from HAW. *Refereed.* **Document type:** *Journal, Academic/Scholarly.* **Description:** Provides answers to clinical questions of current concern to occupational therapy practitioners.
Related titles: Microfiche ed.: (from PQC); Microform ed.
Indexed: AMED, Abstr.Soc.Geront., AgeLine, Arts & Hum.Cit.Ind. (coverage dropped), CINAHL, Curr.Cont. (coverage dropped), Environ.Sci.Poll.Mgmt., Except.Child Educ.Abstr., Excerp.Med., Hosp.Abstr., Human Resour.Abstr., Pollut.Abstr., Soc.Work Res.& Abstr., Viol.& Abuse Abstr.

—BLDSC (6231.254000), EMDOCS, GNLM, Haworth, ingenta, KNAW.
Published by: Haworth Press, Inc., 10 Alice St, Binghamton, NY 13904-1580. TEL 607-722-5857, 800-429-6784, FAX 607-722-6362, 800-895-0582, getinfo@haworthpressinc.com, http://www.haworthpress.com/journals/journallist.asp. Eds. Anne Dickerson, Susan Heling Kaplan. Pub. William Cohen. R&P Ruthann Heath TEL 607-723-5857 ext 316. Adv. contact Jackie Blakeslee TEL 607-722-5857 ext 346. B&W page USD 315, color page USD 550; trim 6 x 8.5. Circ: 650.

OCCUPATIONAL THERAPY IN MENTAL HEALTH; a journal of psychosocial practice and research. see *MEDICAL SCIENCES—Psychiatry And Neurology*

610 USA ISSN 0276-1599
RM735.A1 CODEN: OTJRDE
OCCUPATIONAL THERAPY JOURNAL OF RESEARCH. Abbreviated title: O T J R. Text in English. 1981. q. USD 48 domestic; USD 68 in Canada; USD 88 elsewhere. adv. bk.rev. abstr, charts, bibl, illus. index. back issues avail.; reprints avail. *Refereed.* **Document type:** *Academic/Scholarly.* **Description:** Offers original research articles of professional interest to the occupational therapist.
Related titles: Online - full text ed.: (from ProQuest Information & Learning, Institute for Scientific Information).
Indexed: AMED, ASCA, AgeLine, C.I.J.E., CINAHL, Curr.Cont., Excerp.Med., Fam.Ind., PsycInfo, Psychol.Abstr. (1981-), SSCI, e-psyche.
—BLDSC (6231.255000), EMDOCS, GNLM, IDS, ingenta, KNAW.
Published by: (American Occupational Therapy Foundation, Inc.), Slack, Inc., 6900 Grove Rd, Thorofare, NJ 08086-9447. TEL 856-848-1000, 800-257-8290, FAX 856-853-5991, http://www.slackinc.com/allied/otjr/otjrhome.htm, http://www.slackinc.com/jrs.htm. Ed. Dr. Margaret Short Degraff. Circ: 900.

610.73 AUT
OE M P CD. Text in German. a. ATS 340 (effective 2000). **Document type:** *Trade.*
Media: CD-ROM. **Related titles:** ♦ Print ed.: Oesterreichisches Medizinprodukte Handbuch.
Published by: Verlag Dieter Goeschl GmbH, Hernalser Hauptstrasse 213, Vienna, W 1170, Austria. TEL 43-1-4864240, FAX 43-1-4854902.

610 AUT ISSN 0029-8786
OESTERREICHISCHE AERZTEZEITUNG. Text in German. 1945. s-m. ATS 870 (effective 2000). adv. bk.rev. illus. index. **Document type:** *Newspaper, Trade.* **Description:** Covers politics, laws and regulations, medical news, economics, educational material in all fields of medicine, and culture. Includes announcements of events, foreign news, reports and letters.
Indexed: C.I.S. Abstr., Excerp.Med., INIS Atomind.
—BLDSC (6304.400000), GNLM, KNAW.
Published by: Oesterreichische Aerztekammer, Pressestelle und Verlag, Weihburggasse 9, Vienna, W 1010, Austria. TEL 43-1-5124486, FAX 43-1-512448624. Ed. Martin Stickler. Adv. contact Burghilde Hunger. B&W page ATS 29,900, color page ATS 41,200; trim 260 x 171. Circ: 35,000.

615.1 AUT
OESTERREICHISCHES MEDIZINPRODUKTE HANDBUCH; Lieferfirmen- und Bezugsquellennachweis. Text in German. 1974. a. ATS 340 (effective 2000). adv. **Document type:** *Catalog.*
Formerly: Lieferkatalog fuer Krankenhaus, Arzt, Apotheke und Labor
Related titles: ♦ CD-ROM ed.: Oe M P CD.
Published by: Verlag Dieter Goeschl GmbH, Hernalser Hauptstrasse 213, Vienna, W 1170, Austria. TEL 43-1-4864240, FAX 43-1-4854902. Circ: 10,000.

610.69 SWE ISSN 1100-2913
OEVERLAEKAREN. Variant title: Tidskriften Oeverlaekaren. Text in Swedish. 1989. q. SEK 100 domestic; SEK 150 in Scandinavia; SEK 200 elsewhere. *Refereed.* **Document type:** *Magazine, Academic/Scholarly.*
Published by: Svenska Oeverlaekarfoereningen, Fack 5610, Stockholm 11486, Sweden. TEL 46-8-7903300, FAX 46-8-4115667, svof@overlakaren.se, http://www.overlakaren.se. Ed. Ulf Knutsson. Circ: 17,300.

610 USA ISSN 0000-1406
R712.A1
OFFICIAL A B M S DIRECTORY OF BOARD CERTIFIED MEDICAL SPECIALISTS. Text in English. 1940. a., latest vol.31, 1999. USD 499.95. **Document type:** *Directory.* **Description:** Presents current professional and biographical information on more than 535,000 board-certified specialists, as well as profiles of nearly 35,000 newly board-certified physicians.
Incorporates (in 1992): Directory of Medical Specialists (0070-5829); (1987-1992): A B M S Compendium of Certified Medical Specialists (0884-1543)
Related titles: CD-ROM ed.: A B M S Medical Specialists Plus; Magnetic Tape ed.
—GNLM, Infotrieve. **CCC.**
Published by: Marquis Who's Who (Subsidiary of: Reed Elsevier plc Group), 121 Chanlon Rd, New Providence, NJ 07964. TEL 908-464-6800, FAX 908-665-6688, TELEX 138 755, info@marquiswhoswho.com, http://www.marquiswhoswho.com. Ed. Fred Marks. **Subscr. to:** Order Dept., PO Box 31, New Providence, NJ 07974-9903. TEL 800-521-8110.

610 USA
THE OHIO FAMILY PHYSICIAN. Text in English. 1955. q., latest vol.53, 2001. USD 15 (effective 2001). adv. 28 p./no. 3 cols./p. back issues avail. **Document type:** *Magazine, Trade.* **Description:** Procvided as a membership sercvice to OAFP members, news on F.P. in Ohio.
Formerly: Ohio Family Physician News (0030-0888)
Published by: Ohio Academy of Family Physicians, 4075 N High St, Columbus, OH 43214. TEL 614-267-7867, mail@ohioafp.org, http://www.ohioafp.org. Ed. Edward T Bope. Pub. Ann M Spicer. R&P, Adv. contact Karen Rife Weller. B&W page USD 454; 9.63 x 7.5. Circ: 4,600 (controlled).

610 USA ISSN 0892-2454
CODEN: OHMEE
OHIO MEDICINE* . Text in English. 1905. m. USD 35 to non-members. adv. bk.rev. bibl, illus. index. **Document type:** *Newspaper.* **Description:** Covers legislative, legal and reimbursement issues for Ohio physicians, with association news and reports on Ohio trends in science and medical education.
Formerly: Ohio State Medical Journal (0030-1124)
Indexed: Biol.Abstr., Dent.Ind., Excerp.Med. (until 1993), INIS Atomind., Ind.Med. (until 1992, dropped).
—BLDSC (6247.117000), CISTI, GNLM, KNAW.
Published by: Ohio State Medical Association, 3401 Mill Run Dr, Hilliard, OH 43026-9078. TEL 614-486-2401, FAX 614-486-3130. Ed. Karen Edwards. Adv. contact George Quigley. Circ: 12,000.

610 USA
OHIO STATE UNIVERSITY. COLLEGE OF MEDICINE AND PUBLIC HEALTH. JOURNAL. Text in English. 1947. q. free per issue to qualified personnel. bk.rev. bibl, charts, illus, stat. *Refereed.* **Document type:** *Newsletter, Academic/Scholarly.* **Description:** Includes news and features about faculty, staff, research, and researchers at the Ohio State University College of Medicine and Public Health and OSU Medical Center thatis of interest to faculty, friends, and alumni of OSU health sciences college.
Formerly: Ohio State University. College of Medicine. Journal (0030-1132)
Published by: Ohio State University, College of Medicine and Public Health, 370 W 9th Ave, Columbus, OH 43210-1238. TEL 614-292-5671, FAX 614-292-1544, shaull.2@osu.edu, http://www.med.ohio-state.edu. Ed. Dr. Ernest W Johnson. R&P Ron Shaull TEL 614-293-3661. Circ: 19,000 (controlled).

610 JPN ISSN 0030-1558
CODEN: OIZAAV
OKAYAMA IGAKKAI ZASSHI/MEDICAL ASSOCIATION OF OKAYAMA. JOURNAL. Text in Japanese; Summaries in English. 1975 (vol.87). m. adv. abstr, charts, illus, stat. index.
Indexed: Biol.Abstr., C.I.S. Abstr., Chem.Abstr., INIS Atomind.
—BLDSC (6252.830000), GNLM, KNAW.
Published by: Okayama Igakkai/Medical Association of Okayama, c/o Okayama University Medical School, 5-1 Shikata-cho 2-chome, Okayama 700-0914, Japan. Ed. Isamu Nisida. Circ: 500.

610 JPN ISSN 0917-2424
OKAYAMA KOTSUSOSHOSHO KANFARENSU KIROKUSHU/OSTEOPOROSIS. Text in Japanese. 1989. a.
—BLDSC (6303.873550).
Published by: Okayama Kotsusoshosho Kanfarensu/Okayama Conference on Osteoporosis, c/o Okayama Daigaku Igakubu Seikei Gekagaku Kyoshitsu, 5-1 Shikata-cho 2-chome, Okayama-shi 700-0914, Japan.

610 USA
OKLAHOMA MEDICAL RESEARCH FOUNDATION. FINDINGS. Cover title: O M R F Findings. Text in English. 1991. 6/yr. (5-6/yr.). illus. **Document type:** *Newsletter.* **Description:** Publishes news of research projects, activities and programs sponsored by the foundation.
Published by: Oklahoma Medical Research Foundation, 825 N E 13th St, Oklahoma City, OK 73104. TEL 405-271-8537, shari_hawkins@omrf.ouhsc.edu. Ed. Shari Hawkins. Circ: 62,000.

610 USA ISSN 0030-1876
OKLAHOMA STATE MEDICAL ASSOCIATION. JOURNAL. Text in English. 1908. m. USD 45 (effective 1999). adv. bk.rev. abstr, bibl, illus, stat. index.
Related titles: Microfilm ed.: (from PQC).
Indexed: Biol.Abstr., Chem.Abstr., Dent.Ind., INIS Atomind., Ind.Med. (1908-), Int.Nurs.Ind., Nutr.Abstr.
—BLDSC (4835.300000), CISTI, GNLM, ingenta, KNAW.
Published by: Oklahoma State Medical Association, 601 W I 44 Service Rd, Oklahoma City, OK 73118. TEL 405-843-9571, FAX 405-842-1834, osma@osmaonline.org, http://www.osmaonline.org. Ed. Dr. Michael Pontious. Circ: 5,300.

610 POL ISSN 1233-5037
OKREGOWA IZBA LEKARSKA W KOSZALINIE. BIULETYN. Text in Polish. 1991. bi-m. free per issue. back issues avail. **Document type:** *Bulletin.* **Description:** Contains medical information, local information about medical environment, short articles on medical history.
Formerly: Okregowa Izba Lekarska w Koszalinie. Biuletyn Informacyjny (1233-5215)
Published by: Okregowa Izba Lekarska w Koszalinie, Ul A Lampego 34, Koszalin 75950, Poland. TEL 48-94-423591, FAX 48-94-423591. adv.: page PLZ 500. Circ: 1,500.

610 USA
OMNIGRAPHICS HEALTH REFERENCE SERIES. Variant title: Health Reference Series. Text in English. 1990. irreg. USD 78 per issue (effective 2000). charts, illus. back issues avail. **Document type:** *Monographic series, Consumer.* **Description:** Offers concise information on various medical conditions and diseases, highly accessible to the general reader and academics alike.
Published by: Omnigraphics, Inc., 615 Griswold St, Detroit, MI 48226. TEL 313-961-1340, 800-234-1340, FAX 313-961-1383, 800-875-1340, info@omnigraphics.com, http://www.omnigraphics.com. Pub. Frederick G Ruffner Jr. R&P Laurie Lanzen Harris.

616.9 USA ISSN 0740-218X
ON THE BEAM; newsletter of the Lowe Syndrome Association. Text in English. 1982. 3/yr. USD 15 (effective 2001). bk.rev. back issues avail. **Document type:** *Newsletter.* **Description:** Medical and educational articles about Lowe syndrome, letters from parents and news.
Published by: Lowe Syndrome Association, Inc., 222 Lincoln St, W, Lafayette, IN 47906. TEL 765-743-3634, info@lowesyndrome.org, http://www.lowesyndrome.org. Ed. Kathy Schroerlucke. Circ: 500.

610 NLD ISSN 0920-8100
ONDERWIJS EN GEZONDHEIDSZORG. Text in Dutch. 1977. 10/yr. NLG 87.75. adv. **Document type:** *Trade.*
Published by: (Vereniging van Opleidingsinstituten voor Verplegende en Verzorgende Beroepen), Bohn Stafleu van Loghum B.V. (Subsidiary of: Wolters Kluwer N.V.), Postbus 246, Houten 3990 GA, Netherlands. TEL 31-3403-95711, FAX 31-3403-50903. Circ: 1,285.

610 TUR ISSN 1300-2996
CODEN: OMUDF
ONDOKUZ MAYIS UNIVERSITESI TIP DERGISI/UNIVERSITY OF ONDOKUZ MAYIS JOURNAL OF MEDICINE. Text in Turkish. 1981. q. USD 20. *Refereed.* **Document type:** *Academic/Scholarly.*
Indexed: Excerp.Med. (1996-), Hort.Abstr., Weed Abstr.
—BLDSC (6260.213000), EMDOCS.
Published by: Ondokuz Mayis Universitesi, Tip Fakultesi Dekanligi, Kurupelit, Samsun 55139, Turkey. TEL 90-362-4576070, FAX 90-362-4576041. Ed. Yucel Tanyeri. R&P Cemil Rakunt. Circ: 675 (paid).

M

362 USA ISSN 0258-610X
ONE-IN-TEN. Text in Arabic, English, French, Spanish. 1980. q. free per issue. **Document type:** *Newsletter.* **Description:** Covers childhood disabilities, their prevention and rehabilitation.
Published by: Rehabilitation International, 25 E 21st St, New York, NY 10010. TEL 212-420-1500, FAX 212-505-0871. Ed. Susan Hammerman. Circ: 10,000. **Co-sponsor:** U N I C E F.

610 USA ISSN 1059-2725
CODEN: OJCTEI
THE ONLINE JOURNAL OF CURRENT CLINICAL TRIALS. Text in English. 1992. irreg. USD 120 to individuals; USD 220 to institutions (effective 2000); includes cumulative CD-ROM. abstr, charts, illus. back issues avail.; reprints avail. *Refereed.* **Document type:** *Academic/Scholarly.* **Description:** Publishes studies of current therapies, procedures, and developments relevant to patient care in oncology, infectious disease, cardiology, pediatrics, gynecology, dermatology, psychology, and surgery.
Media: Online - full content (from EBSCO Publishing). **Related titles:** CD-ROM ed.; Microfiche ed.
Indexed: Ind.Med. (1994-, dropped).
—GNLM, Infotrieve. **CCC.**
Published by: Lippincott Williams & Wilkins (Philadelphia) (Subsidiary of: Wolters Kluwer N.V.), 530 Walnut St, Philadelphia, PA 19106-3621. TEL 215-521-8300, FAX 215-521-8902, http://www.lww.com. **Subscr. to:** PO Box 1600, Hagerstown, MD 21740-1600. TEL 800-777-2295, FAX 301-824-7390.

612 AUS ISSN 1443-2374
▼ **ONLINE JOURNAL OF PHYSIOLOGY.** Text in English. 1999. irreg. **Description:** Publishes original work dealing with functional and molecular physiological processes.
Media: Online - full text.
Published by: Pestsearch International Pty. Ltd., 173 Chatswood Rd, Daisy Hill, QLD 4127, Australia. http://www.uq.edu.au/~csvguerr/ojp.htm, http://www.cpb.uokhsc.edu/ojvr/jvet196a.htm. Ed. L J Filippich.

▼ **ONLINE PUBLISHING IN MEDICINE.** see *PUBLISHING AND BOOK TRADE—Computer Applications*

610 CAN ISSN 0030-302X
ONTARIO MEDICAL REVIEW. Text in English. 1922. m. (11/yr). CND 55 to non-members; CND 62 in United States to non-members; CND 79 elsewhere to non-members (effective 1999). adv. bibl, charts, illus. index. back issues avail. **Document type:** *Trade.* **Description:** For all members of the OMA, including physicians, interns, residents and medical students, as well as physicians residing outside Ontario who are members of OMA.
Indexed: Chem.Abstr., INIS Atomind.
—CISTI, GNLM, Infotrieve. **CCC.**
Published by: Ontario Medical Association, 525 University Ave, Ste 300, Toronto, ON M5G 2K7, Canada. TEL 416-599-2580, FAX 416-599-9309, kim_secord@oma.org, http://www.oma.org. Ed. Jeff Henry. R&P Kim Secord. Adv. contact Marg Churchill. B&W page CND 1,160, color page CND 2,345; trim 10.88 x 8.13. Circ: 22,800.

610 CAN ISSN 0712-6689
ONTARIO MEDICINE. Text in English. 24/yr. CND 49.
Related titles: Microfilm ed.: (from MML); Microform ed.: (from MML).
Published by: Maclean Hunter Ltd., Maclean Hunter Bldg, 777 Bay St, Ste 405, Toronto, ON M5W 1A7, Canada.

618.97 GBR
OPINION: SPECIALIST REVIEWS OF KEY PAPERS IN GENERAL & ELDERLY MEDICINE. Abbreviated title: O G E N. Text in English. 1997. 3/yr.
Published by: Hayward Medical Communications Ltd., Covent Garden, Seven Dials Warehouse, 44 Earlham St, London WC2H 9LA, United Kingdom. TEL 44-20-7240-4493, FAX 44-20-7240-4479, admin@hayward.co.uk, http://www.hayward.co.uk. Ed. David Black. Circ: 10,000. **Subscr. to:** Rosemary House, Lanwades Park, Kentford, Near, Newmarket, Suffolk CB8 7PW, United Kingdom. TEL 44-1638-751515, FAX 44-1638-751517.

OPINION: SPECIALIST REVIEWS OF KEY PAPERS IN MICROBIOLOGY. see *BIOLOGY—Microbiology*

610 CHE
OPTIMA. Text in French, German. 1974. m. CHF 39 domestic; CHF 75 foreign (effective 2000). adv. **Document type:** *Magazine, Consumer.*
Published by: Editions Optima SA, Av de Chillon 90, Montreux 1820, Switzerland. TEL 41-21-9635161, FAX 41-21-9631874, e-optima@bluewin.ch, http://www.edicom.ch/optima/index.html. Ed. Gerard Geiger. Adv. contact Lutz Wiedemann. B&W page CHF 11,798, color page CHF 18,995. Circ: 293,094 (paid).

610 FRA ISSN 0030-4565
ORDRE NATIONAL DES MEDECINS. BULLETIN. Text in French. 1941. 11/yr. FRF 153; FRF 225 foreign (effective 1997). reprint service avail. from ISI. **Document type:** *Bulletin.* **Description:** Presents the activity of the national council, and the regional and departamental councils. Deals with the professional organization of medicine.
—CCC.
Published by: (Conseil National de l'Ordre National des Medecins), Masson - Periodiques, 120 bd. St. Germain, Paris 75006, France. TEL 33-1-40466200, FAX 33-1-40466201. Ed. O Dubois. Circ: 70,000. **Subscr. to:** Societe de Periodiques Specialises, BP 22, Vineuil Cedex 41354, France. TEL 33-2-54504612, FAX 33-2-54504611.

610 CHE ISSN 0373-3998
ORGANISATION MONDIALE DE LA SANTE. SERIE DE RAPPORTS TECHNIQUES. Text in French. 1950. irreg.
Related titles: ♦ English ed.: W H O Technical Report Series. ISSN 0512-3054; ♦ Spanish ed.: Organizacion Mundial de la Salud. Serie de Informes Tecnicos. ISSN 0509-2507; ♦ Russian ed.: Vsemirnaya Organizatsiya Zdravookhraneniya. Seriya Tekhnicheskikh Dokladov. ISSN 0250-8737; ♦ Arabic ed.: Munazzamat al-Sihhah al-'Alamiyyah. Silsilat al-Taqarir al-Fanniyyah. ISSN 0251-0111.
Published by: World Health Organization, Marketing and Dissemination, Geneva, 27 1211, Switzerland.

610 CHE ISSN 0509-2507
ORGANIZACION MUNDIAL DE LA SALUD. SERIE DE INFORMES TECNICOS. Text in Spanish. 1950. irreg.
Related titles: ♦ English ed.: W H O Technical Report Series. ISSN 0512-3054; ♦ French ed.: Organisation Mondiale de la Sante. Serie de Rapports Techniques. ISSN 0373-3998; ♦ Russian ed.: Vsemirnaya Organizatsiya Zdravookhraneniya. Seriya Tekhnicheskikh Dokladov. ISSN 0250-8737; ♦ Arabic ed.: Munazzamat al-Sihhah al-'Alamiyyah. Silsilat al-Taqarir al-Fanniyyah. ISSN 0251-0111.
Published by: World Health Organization, Marketing and Dissemination, Geneva, 27 1211, Switzerland.

610 USA
ORGANIZATION OF TEACHERS OF ORAL DIAGNOSIS. NEWSLETTER. Variant title: Organization of Teachers of Oral Diagnosis. News. Text in English. 1963. q. membership. bk.rev. illus. **Document type:** *Newsletter.*
Published by: (Organization of Teachers of Oral Diagnosis), University of Texas Dental School, 7703 Floyd Curl Dr, San Antonio, TX 78284. TEL 512-567-3333. Ed. James A Cottone. Circ: 150.

ORIENTAL MEDICINE. see *ALTERNATIVE MEDICINE*

610 ITA ISSN 0394-2678
ORIS MEDICINA; monthly of cultural, scientific and technical information. Text in English, Italian. 1987. m. USD 95 in Europe; USD 110 in Africa; USD 120 in Asia; USD 120 in the Americas (effective 2000). adv. bk.rev. *Refereed.* **Description:** Publishes original articles, research results and clinical experiments from Italian university professors, researchers and hospital specialists. Also deals with subjects concerning sanitary economy and policy and culture.
Published by: Diade s.r.l., Via Ausonio, 5, Milan, MI 20123, Italy. TEL 39-2-8372407, FAX 39-2-58100311. Ed. Franco Marelli Coppola. Adv. contact Paola Pirogalli. Circ: 23,000.

616 619 USA ISSN 0887-0306
ORPHAN DISEASE UPDATE. Text in English. 1983. 3/yr. USD 25. bk.rev. charts, illus. back issues avail. **Document type:** *Newsletter, Consumer.* **Description:** Information on orphan drugs and diseases. Covers medical advances, biomedical research, patient coping strategies, and legislative issues related to the field.
Related titles: Online - full text ed.
Published by: National Organization for Rare Disorders, Inc. (NORD), PO Box 8923, New Fairfield, CT 06812-8923. TEL 203-746-6518, FAX 203-746-6481, http://www.nord-rdb.com/~orphan. Ed. Abbey S Meyers. R&P Joseph P Gatto. Circ: 80,000.

DE ORTHOMOLECULAIRE KOERIER; Nederlands - Vlaams tijdschrift voor nutritionele geneeskunde. see *NUTRITION AND DIETETICS*

610 HUN ISSN 0030-6002
R96.H8 CODEN: ORHEAG
ORVOSI HETILAP/HUNGARIAN MEDICAL JOURNAL. Text in Hungarian; Summaries in English. 1857. w. DEM 100, USD 232; USD 8.89 newsstand/cover (effective 2001). adv. bk.rev. illus. index. *Refereed.* **Document type:** *Academic/Scholarly.*
Indexed: Biol.Abstr., Chem.Abstr., Dent.Ind., Dok.Arbeitsmed., Excerp.Med., INIS Atomind., Ind.Med. (1857-), Int.Nurs.Ind., Nutr.Abstr., Protozool.Abstr., Sugar Ind.Abstr.
—BLDSC (6296.500000), CASDDS, CISTI, GNLM.
Published by: (Markusovszky Lajos Foundation), Springer Hungarica Kiado Ltd., Csanyi Laszlo utca 36, Budapest 1043, Hungary. TEL 36-1-3709074, FAX 36-1-3909075, http://www.pro-patiente.hu. Ed., R&P Janos Feher. Circ: 8,000.

610.7 HUN ISSN 0030-6037
R91 CODEN: ORVOAE
ORVOSKEPZES. Text in Hungarian; Summaries in English, Russian. 1911. 6/yr. adv. index. **Description:** Covers medical training.
Indexed: Biol.Abstr., Excerp.Med., INIS Atomind.
—BLDSC (6296.520000), CISTI, GNLM.
Address: Szabolcs utca 33-35, Budapest 1389, Hungary. TEL 1-1208588. Ed. Dr. Frigyes Kulka. Circ: 3,200. **Subscr. to:** Kultura, PO Box 149, Budapest 1389, Hungary.

610 HUN ISSN 0010-3551
ORVOSTORTENETI KOZLEMENYEK/COMMUNICATION DE HISTORIA ARTIS MEDICINAE. Text occasionally in English, French, German. 1955. q., latest vol.169, 1999. HUF 2,000, USD 10 (effective 2000). adv. bk.rev. cum.index. 250 p./no. *Refereed.* **Document type:** *Journal, Academic/Scholarly.*
Indexed: Amer.Hist.& Life, Artbibl.Mod., BHA, Hist.Abstr. (1985-87, 1993-), Numis.Lit.
—GNLM, KNAW.
Published by: Semmelweis Orvostorteneti Muzeum Konyvtar es Leveltar, Torok utca 12, Budapest 1023, Hungary. TEL 36-1-2125421, FAX 36-1-2125438, orvostortenet@axelero.hu. Eds. Karoly Kapronczay, Laszlo A Magyar. R&P, Adv. contact Karoly Kapronczay. Circ: 1,000 (paid and controlled). **Co-sponsor:** Magyar Orvostortenelmi Tarsasag.

610 HUN ISSN 1218-2583
ORVOSTOVABBKEPZO SZEMLE/POSTGRADUATE MEDICINE HUNGARY. Text in Hungarian. 1994. m. HUF 300 newsstand/cover.
Related titles: ♦ Translation of: Postgraduate Medicine. ISSN 0032-5481.
Published by: Richard Mills & Co. Inc., Moricz Zs Korter 3-b, Budapest 1117, Hungary. TEL 36-1-1655126, FAX 617-451-6182. Pub. Richard P Mills.

610 JPN ISSN 0386-4103
CODEN: OIGZDE
OSAKA CITY MEDICAL JOURNAL. Text in Multiple languages. 1951. 2/yr. JPY 7,000, USD 35. charts, illus, stat. back issues avail. *Refereed.* **Document type:** *Academic/Scholarly.*
Indexed: Biol.Abstr., C.I.S. Abstr., Chem.Abstr., Chem.Indus.Notes, Chem.Titles, Dairy Sci.Abstr., Diar.Dis.Res., Excerp.Med., INIS Atomind., Ind.Med. (coverage dropped), Nutr.Abstr.
—BLDSC (6297.000000), CASDDS, CISTI, EMDOCS, GNLM.
Published by: Osaka City Medical Center/Osaka-shi Igakkai, Osaka City University Medical School, Asahi-machi, Abeno-ku, Osaka-shi 545, Japan. TEL 81-6-645-3782. Ed. Yano Ikuya. Circ: 1,200.

610 JPN ISSN 0387-446X
OSAKA DAIGAKU IRYO GIJUTSU TANKI DAIGAKUBU KENKYU KIYO. SHIZEN KAGAKU IRYO KAGAKU HEN/OSAKA UNIVERSITY. COLLEGE OF BIO-MEDICAL TECHNOLOGY AND NURSING. STUDIES IN NATURAL SCIENCE AND HEALTH TECHNOLOGY. Text in Japanese; Summaries in English, Japanese. 1968. a.
Published by: Osaka Daigaku, Iryo Gijutsu Tanki Daigakubu/Osaka University. College of Bio-Medical Technology and Nursing, 1-1 Machikaneyama-cho, Toyonaka-shi, Osaka-fu 560-0043, Japan.

610 JPN ISSN 0030-6118
CODEN: OIDZAU
OSAKA IKA DAIGAKU ZASSHI/OSAKA MEDICAL COLLEGE. JOURNAL. Text in Japanese; Summaries in English. 1933. q. JPY 3,000. bk.rev. *Refereed.* **Document type:** *Academic/Scholarly.*
Indexed: Biol.Abstr., Chem.Abstr., Chem.Indus.Notes, Chem.Titles, INIS Atomind.
—BLDSC (4839.200000), CASDDS.

M

Published by: Osaka Medical College/Osaka Ika Daigaku, 2-7 Daigaku-Machi, Takatsuki-shi, Osaka 569-8686, Japan. TEL 81-726-84-6244, FAX 81-726-83-2155, med001@art.osaka.med.ac.jp. Ed. Muneaki Abe. Pub. Hiroyuki Kagamiyama.

610 JPN ISSN 0916-2844 CODEN: BOMCEB
OSAKA MEDICAL COLLEGE. BULLETIN. Text in English. 1954. irreg. (1-2/yr.). free to medical institutions; exchange basis. index. *Refereed.* **Document type:** *Bulletin, Academic/Scholarly.* **Description:** Contains original reports, case reports, and reviews.
Formerly (until 1988): Osaka Medical School. Bulletin (0030-6142)
Indexed: Biol.Abstr., Excerp.Med., INIS Atomind., Ind.Med. (until 1992, dropped).
—BLDSC (2674.520000), CASDDS, CISTI, GNLM.
Published by: Osaka Medical College/Osaka Ika Daigaku, 2-7 Daigaku-Machi, Takatsuki-shi, Osaka 569-8686, Japan. TEL 81-726-84-6244, FAX 81-726-83-2155, ph1004@art.osaka-med.ac.jp. Ed. Yusuke Imai.

OSLER LIBRARY NEWSLETTER. see *LIBRARY AND INFORMATION SCIENCES*

610 USA
THE OSLER MEDICAL JOURNAL. Text in English. 1996. q. free per issue. **Document type:** *Journal, Academic/Scholarly, Trade.* **Description:** Highlights original and reviewed topics in the clinical and basic sciences.
Media: Online - full text.
Published by: Johns Hopkins Department of Medicine, 1830 E Monument St, Baltimore, MD 21218. OMJEeditor@welchlink.welch.jhu.edu, http://omj.med.jhu.edu, http://www.omj.med.jhu.edu/. Ed. Dr. Alan Cheng.

OSPEDALE AL MARE. ARCHIVIO. see *HEALTH FACILITIES AND ADMINISTRATION*

610 ITA ISSN 0369-7843 CODEN: OSMAA
L'OSPEDALE MAGGIORE. Text in Italian. 1906. 4/yr. ITL 79,000 (effective 1999).
Indexed: Excerp.Med. (1995-).
—BLDSC (6301.570000), CISTI, GNLM.
Published by: Masson S.p.A., Divisione Periodici, Via F.lli Bressan 2, Milan, MI 20126, Italy. TEL 39-2-270741, FAX 39-2-27074210. Ed. Luciano Gattinoni. adv.: B&W page ITL 2,950,000, color page ITL 4,200,000. Circ: 3,000.

610 GBR ISSN 0937-941X CODEN: OSINEP
OSTEOPOROSIS INTERNATIONAL. Text in English. 1990. 12/yr. EUR 698.70 domestic; EUR 666.10 in Germany; EUR 64 newsstand/cover foreign (effective 2002). *Refereed.* **Document type:** *Academic/Scholarly.*
Related titles: Microform ed.: (from PQC); Online - full text ed.: ISSN 1433-2965 (from EBSCO Publishing, RoweCom Information Quest, Swets Blackwell, Springer LINK, Institute for Scientific Information).
Indexed: AMED, ASCA, Cal.Tiss.Abstr., Chem.Abstr., Chem.Titles, Curr.Cont., Dairy Sci.Abstr., Excerp.Med. (1992-), Ind.Med. (1990-), Ind.Sci.Rev., Inpharma, Int.Nurs.Ind., Nutr.Abstr., Pharm.&Out.News, Reac., SSCI (coverage dropped), Sci.Cit.Ind.
—BLDSC (6303.873500), CASDDS, CISTI, EMDOCS, GNLM, IDS, KNAW. **CCC.**
Published by: (European Foundation for Osteoporosis), Springer-Verlag London Ltd. (Subsidiary of: BertelsmannSpringer), Sweetapple House, Catteshall Rd, Godalming, Surrey GU7 3DJ, United Kingdom. TEL 44-1483-418800, FAX 44-1483-415144. Eds. Pierre J Meunier, Robert Lindsay. **Co-sponsor:** National Osteoporosis Foundation, US.

612 ITA ISSN 1121-0028
OSTEOPOROSIS NEWS. Text in Italian. 1990. bi-m. adv. **Document type:** *Newsletter.*
Published by: C I C Edizioni Internazionali s.r.l., Corso Trieste 42, Rome, RM 00198, Italy. TEL 39-06-8412673, FAX 39-06-8412688, info@gruppocic.it, 1160199510. Ed. G Mazzuoli. adv.: B&W page XEU 1,601.02, color page XEU 2,014.18; 210 x 290.

616.7 USA
OSTEOPOROSIS REPORT∗. Text in English. 1985. q. USD 10 to individuals; USD 25 foreign to individuals; USD 95 to institutions (effective 1999). *Refereed.* **Document type:** *Newsletter.* **Description:** Covers osteoporosis health issues, reports on activities, programs, and consumer information.
Published by: National Osteoporosis Foundation, 1232 22nd St NW, Washington, DC 20037-1202. TEL 202-223-2226, FAX 202-223-2237, nofmail@nof.org, http://www.nof.org. Ed. Molly Natchipolsky. R&P Tom Damic. Circ: 110,000.

610 USA ISSN 0030-6517
OSTOMY QUARTERLY. Text in English. 1963. q. USD 25 domestic; USD 30 in Canada; USD 40 elsewhere (effective 2001). adv. bk.rev. illus. index. back issues avail.; reprints avail. *Refereed.* **Description:** Features stories of triumph over diseases resulting in ostomy surgery. Contains articles and updates of medical treatment for ostomates.
Related titles: Microform ed.: 1963 (from PQC); Online - full text ed.: 1963 (from Gale Group, Northern Light Technology, Inc., Factiva).
Indexed: Hlth.Ind., Rehabil.Lit.
—CISTI.
Published by: United Ostomy Association, Inc., 19772 MacArthur Blvd, Ste 200, Irvine, CA 92612-2405. TEL 949-660-8624, 800-826-0826, FAX 949-660-9262, editor@uoa.org, http://www.uoa.org. Ed., R&P Thomas Kimball. Circ: 29,000.

610 FRA ISSN 0048-2366
OUEST MEDICAL. Text in French. 1948. 20/yr. FRF 50 (effective 2000). adv. bk.rev. illus.
Related titles: Microform ed.
Indexed: Biol.Abstr., C.I.S. Abstr., Chem.Abstr., Curr.Cont. (coverage dropped), Excerp.Med., Nutr.Abstr.
—CISTI, GNLM, Infotrieve. **CCC.**
Published by: Expansion Scientifique, 15 rue St. Benoit, Paris Cedex 6 75278, France. Circ: 8,500.

610 GBR ISSN 0030-7661
OXFORD MEDICAL SCHOOL GAZETTE. Text in English. 1949. 2/yr. GBP 6; GBP 9 overseas (effective 2000). adv. bk.rev. charts, illus, stat. **Document type:** *Academic/Scholarly.*
—CISTI.
Published by: University of Oxford Medical School, John Radcliffe Hospital, Headington, Oxford OX3 9DU, United Kingdom. TEL 44-1865-221689, FAX 44-1865-750750, caroline.morley@merton.ox.ac.uk. Eds. Matthew Williams-Gray, Patrick Gibson. Adv. contact Caroline Morley. Circ: 3,000.

OXFORD MONOGRAPHS ON MOLECULAR GENETICS. see *BIOLOGY—Genetics*

OXFORD REVIEWS OF REPRODUCTIVE BIOLOGY. see *BIOLOGY—Physiology*

610 USA ISSN 0743-507X
P & S JOURNAL; the journal of the College of Physicians & Surgeons of Columbia University. (Physicians and Surgeons) Text in English. 1955. 3/yr. free per issue to qualified personnel. bk.rev. illus. 48 p./no. reprint service avail. from PQC. **Document type:** *Academic/Scholarly.* **Description:** Profiles of legendary faculty, research reports, news of clinical advances, student programs, college news and information, alumni profiles and obituaries.
Formerly (until 1981): P and S Quarterly (0030-7831)
Related titles: Microfilm ed.: (from PQC); Online - full text ed.
Published by: Columbia University, College of Physicians and Surgeons, 630 W 168th St, New York, NY 10032. TEL 212-305-3877, FAX 212-305-4521, psjournal@columbia.edu, http://cpmcnet.columbia.edu/news/journal. Ed., R&P Bonita Eaton Enochs. Circ: 18,000 (free).

P H R RECORD. see *POLITICAL SCIENCE—Civil Rights*

610 DEU ISSN 0722-477X
P M D - PRAXIS MEDIZINISCHER DOKUMENTATION. Text in German. 1980. q. DEM 60; DEM 70 foreign. adv. bk.rev. back issues avail. *Refereed.* **Document type:** *Academic/Scholarly.* **Description:** Contains articles about medical documentation and record keeping. Also includes health care information, association news and reports, international news, events, and positions available.
—GNLM.
Published by: Deutscher Verband Medizinischer Dokumentare e.V., Haselbuehl 52, Ulm 89075, Germany. FAX 49-731-187390. Ed. Ulli Hoffmann. Pub. Jens Hinrichsen. Adv. contact Christa Boerke. page DEM 2,067; trim 254 x 184. Circ: 2,000.

616.0472 344.041 USA
PAIN: CAUSE, EFFECT, EVALUATION. Text in English. 1987. 6 base vols. plus a. updates. USD 295. illus. **Description:** This medicolegal collection covers the six major areas of musculoskeletal pain and injury resulting in loss of work or diminished earning capacity: neck pain; hand and wrist pain; foot and ankle pain; elbow and shoulder pain; hip and knee pain; and low back pain.
Published by: Lexis Law Publishing (Subsidiary of: Reed Elsevier plc), PO Box 7587, Charlottesville, VA 22906-7587. TEL 804-972-7600, 800-562-1197, FAX 804-972-7666, llp.customer.support@lexis-nexis.com, http://www.lexislawpublishing.com.

616 NLD ISSN 0921-3287
PAIN RESEARCH AND CLINICAL MANAGEMENT. Variant title: World Congress of Pain. Proceedings. Text in English. 1987. irreg., latest vol.10, 1999. price varies. back issues avail. *Refereed.* **Document type:** *Monographic series, Proceedings, Academic/Scholarly, Trade.* **Description:** Covers all aspects of the study of every type of pain and analgesic or anesthetic treatment.
—BLDSC (6333.810000), CISTI, Infotrieve, KNAW. **CCC.**
Published by: Elsevier Science BV, PO Box 211, Amsterdam 1000 AE, Netherlands. TEL 31-20-485-3757, 31-20-485-3911, FAX 31-20-485-3432, 31-20-485-3598, nlinfo-f@elsevier.nl; usinfo-f@elsevier.com; forinfo-kyf04035@niftyserve.or.jp, http://www.elsevier.nl/. **Subscr. in Australasia and the Far East to:** Elsevier Science (Singapore) Pte Ltd, No.1 Temasek Ave, 17-01 Millenia Tower, Singapore 039192, Singapore. TEL 65-434-3727, FAX 65-337-2230, asiainfo@elsevier.com.sg; **Subscr. in Japan to:** Elsevier Science Inc - Japan Regional Office, 9-15 Higashi-Azabu 1-chome, Minato-ku, Tokyo 106-0044, Japan. TEL 81-3-5561-5033, FAX 81-3-5561-5047, info@elsevier.co.jp; **Subscr. in the Americas to:** Elsevier Science, PO Box 945, New York, NY 10159-0945. TEL 212-633-3730, 888-437-4636, FAX 212-633-3680, usinfo-f@elsevier.com, http://www.elsevier.com

610 GBR ISSN 0968-1302 CODEN: PAREFV
PAIN REVIEWS. Text in English. 1994. q. GBP 68 in Europe to individuals; USD 132 in North America to individuals; GBP 88 rest of world to individuals; GBP 148 in Europe to institutions; USD 274 in North America to institutions; GBP 170 rest of world to institutions; GBP 62 in Europe to members Pain Society of UK and Ireland, European Society of Anaesthesiologists (ESA), Australian Pain Society and German Pain Society; USD 109 in North America to members Pain Society of UK and Ireland, European Society of Anaesthesiologists (ESA), Australian Pain Society and German Pain Society; GBP 76 rest of world to members Pain Society of UK and Ireland, European Society of Anaesthesiologists (ESA), Australian Pain Society and German Pain Society; GBP 85 in developing nations; GBP 51 newsstand/cover in Europe; USD 97 newsstand/cover in North America; GBP 55 newsstand/cover rest of world (effective 2002). adv. back issues avail.; reprints avail. *Refereed.* **Document type:** *Journal, Academic/Scholarly.* **Description:** Publishes review articles encompassing the spectrum of pain research, its basis, and its management for an international audience.
Related titles: Online - full text ed.: (from EBSCO Publishing, O C L C Online Computer Library Center, Inc., RoweCom Information Quest, ingenta, Swets Blackwell, Institute for Scientific Information).
Indexed: Brit.Nur.Ind., CINAHL, Environ.Sci.Poll.Mgmt., Excerp.Med. (1995-), Neurosci.Abstr., Neurosci.Cit.Ind., Pollut.Abstr., PsycInfo, Risk Abstr., Saf.Sci.Abstr., e-psyche.
—BLDSC (6333.830000), CASDDS, GNLM, IDS, KNAW.
Published by: Arnold Publishers (Subsidiary of: Hodder Headline plc.), 338 Euston Rd, London NW1 3BH, United Kingdom. TEL 44-20-7873-6337, FAX 44-20-7873-6325, arnoldjournals@hodder.co.uk, http://www.arnoldpublishers.com/jourals/journtitles.htm. Eds. Per Hansson, Wolfgang Hamann. Adv. contact Mary Attree. **Subscr. to:** Turpin Distribution Services Ltd., Blackhorse Rd, Letchworth, Herts SG6 1HN, United Kingdom. TEL 44-1462-488900, FAX 44-1462-483011.

616.0472 USA
THE PAIN SERIES. Text in English. USD 166.84 (effective 2000). **Document type:** *Monographic series.* **Description:** Provides common-sense guidance in diagnosing and treating painful and disabling conditions.
Published by: F.A. Davis Company, 1915 Arch St, Philadelphia, PA 19103. TEL 800-323-3555, FAX 215-440-3016, orders@fadavis.com, http://www.fadavis.com. Ed. Rene Cailliet.

M

610 PAK ISSN 0030-9842
PAKISTAN JOURNAL OF MEDICAL RESEARCH. Text in English. 1958. q. PKR 400, USD 50 (effective 2001). adv. bk.rev. charts, illus, stat. index. reprint service avail. from PQC. *Refereed.* **Document type:** *Journal, Academic/Scholarly.* **Description:** Publishes results of clinical and biomedical research.
Related titles: Microform ed.: (from PQC).
Indexed: Abstr.Hyg., Biol.Abstr., INIS Atomind., Nutr.Abstr. —CISTI, GNLM.
Published by: Pakistan Medical Research Council, Shahrah-e-Jumhuriat G-5-2, P O Box 2598, Islamabad, Pakistan. TEL 92-51-9207386, FAX 92-51-9216774, mak@pmrc2.isb.brain.com.pk, pmrc@isb.comsats.net.pk, www.pakmedinet.com/pjmr. Ed. Jahangir A Khan. Circ: 1,000.

610 PAK CODEN: SPCAE
PAKISTAN JOURNAL OF MEDICAL SCIENCES. Text in English. 1984. q. PKR 800 domestic; GBP 45 in Europe; USD 75 elsewhere (effective 2001). adv. bk.rev. 75 p./no. 2 cols./p. *Refereed.* **Document type:** *Academic/Scholarly.* **Description:** Publishes original research articles, case reports of interesting and rare diseases, and review articles.
Formerly (until 2000): Specialist (1017-4699)
Related titles: CD-ROM ed.
Indexed: Excerp.Med. (1992-), ExtraMED, INIS Atomind. —BLDSC (6341.570000), EMDOCS, GNLM, KNAW.
Published by: Professional Medical Publications, 522, 5th Fl., Panorama Centre-II, Raja Ghazanfar Ali Rd., Saddar, Karachi, Pakistan. TEL 92-21-5688791, FAX 92-21-5689860, pakjmedsciences@pulsepakistan.com, http://www.pulsepakistan.com/pakjmedsciences. Ed. Maqbool H Jafary. Pub., R&P Shaukat Ali Jawaid. Adv. contact Mubarak Ali. Circ: 2,000.

616.07 PAK
PAKISTAN JOURNAL OF PATHOLOGY✶ . Text in English. 1990. 2/yr. **Document type:** *Academic/Scholarly.*
Published by: Pakistan Association of Pathologists, c/o Medical Association, P M A House, Garden Rd., P O Box 7267, Karachi, 3, Pakistan.

610 PAK ISSN 0030-9982 CODEN: JJPAD4
PAKISTAN MEDICAL ASSOCIATION. JOURNAL. Abbreviated title: J P M A. Text in English. 1950. m. PKR 200, USD 75. adv. bk.rev. charts, illus, stat. reprint service avail. from PQC. **Document type:** *Academic/Scholarly.*
Related titles: CD-ROM ed.; Microform ed.: (from PQC).
Indexed: Abstr.Hyg., Dairy Sci.Abstr., Diar.Dis.Res., Excerp.Med., ExtraMED, Helminthol.Abstr., INIS Atomind., Ind.Med. (1974-), Nutr.Abstr., Protozool.Abstr., Rev.Med.& Vet.Mycol., Rural Devel.Abstr., Trop.Dis.Bull. —BLDSC (4839.497000), CASDDS, CISTI, GNLM.
Published by: Pakistan Medical Association, P.M.A. House, Aga Khan III Rd., Karachi 74400, Pakistan. TEL 92-21-7214632, FAX 92-21-7226443. Ed. Dr. S J Zuberi. Circ: 6,000.

610 GBR ISSN 0269-2163 CODEN: PAMDE2
PALLIATIVE MEDICINE; a multiprofessional journal. Text in English. 1987. bi-m. GBP 129 in Europe to individuals; USD 227 in North America to individuals; GBP 140 rest of world to individuals; GBP 394 in Europe to institutions; USD 689 in North America to institutions; GBP 422 rest of world to institutions; GBP 103 in Europe to members qualified associations; USD 181 in North America to members qualified associations; GBP 114 rest of world to members qualified associations; GBP 211 in developing nations; GBP 140 rest of world to qualified personnel sponsored; GBP 78 newsstand/cover in Europe; USD 140 newsstand/cover in North America; GBP 84 newsstand/cover rest of world (effective 2002). adv. bk.rev. illus. back issues avail.; reprints avail. *Refereed.* **Document type:** *Journal, Academic/Scholarly.* **Description:** Dedicated to improving knowledge and clinical practice in the care of patients with advanced diseases.
Related titles: Online - full text ed.: (from EBSCO Publishing, O C L C Online Computer Library Center, Inc., RoweCom Information Quest, ingenta, Swets Blackwell, Institute for Scientific Information).
Indexed: AMED, ASCA, ASSIA, Brit.Nur.Ind., CINAHL, Curr.Cont., Excerp.Med. (1993-), IMFL, Ind.Med. (1987-), Inpharma, Int.Nurs.Ind., Pharm.&Out.News, PsycInfo, Reac., Sci.Cit.Ind., e-psyche. —BLDSC (6345.562060), EMDOCS, GNLM, IDS, Infotrieve, ingenta, KNAW. **CCC.**
Published by: Arnold Publishers (Subsidiary of: Hodder Headline plc.), 338 Euston Rd, London NW1 3BH, United Kingdom. TEL 44-20-7873-6337, FAX 44-20-7873-6325, arnoldjournals@hodder.co.uk, http://www.palliativemedjournal.com. Ed. Dr. Stephen Kirkham. Adv. contact Mary Attree. **Subscr. to:** Turpin Distribution Services Ltd., Blackhorse Rd, Letchworth, Herts SG6 1HN, United Kingdom. TEL 44-1462-488900, FAX 44-1462-483011.

610 ITA ISSN 1120-303X
PANDORA; giornale di ricerca clinica e diagnostica. Text in Italian. 1989. 3/yr. free per issue. adv. back issues avail. **Document type:** *Academic/Scholarly.* **Description:** reports on clinical and diagnostic research.
Related titles: Online - full text ed.
Published by: Medical Systems S.p.A., Passo Rio Torbido, 40, Genoa, GE 16165, Italy. TEL 39-10-83401, FAX 39-10-804661, rassu@ssnet.it, http://medicalsystems.editoria.com. Ed. G C Mazzocchi. Adv. contact Giusi Cunietti.

610 ITA CODEN: PMMDAE
PANMINERVA MEDICA. Text in English. 1959. q. USD 105 to individuals; USD 155 to institutions (effective 2000 - 2001). adv. bk.rev. abstr, bibl, charts, illus. reprint service avail. from PQC. *Refereed.* **Document type:** *Academic/Scholarly.* **Description:** Covers clinical and experimental medicine and surgery.
Formerly: Panminerva Medica - Europa Medica; Which was formed by the merger of: Panminerva Medica (0031-0808); Europa Medica (0014-2557)
Related titles: Microfilm ed.: (from PQC); Online - full text ed.: (from Institute for Scientific Information).
Indexed: ASCA, Biol.Abstr., Chem.Abstr., Curr.Cont., Dairy Sci.Abstr., Dent.Ind., Helminthol.Abstr., INIS Atomind., Ind.Med. (1959-), Inpharma, Nutr.Abstr., Pharm.&Out.News, Reac., Ref.Zh., Sci.Cit.Ind. (coverage dropped). —BLDSC (6357.380000), CASDDS, CISTI, GNLM, IDS.
Published by: Edizioni Minerva Medica, Corso Bramante, 83-85, Turin, TO 10126, Italy. TEL 39-11-678282, FAX 39-11-674502. Ed. M L Benzo. Pub. Alberto Oliaro. Adv. contact F Filippo. B&W page USD 1,200, color page USD 2,000; trim 280 x 215. Circ: 5,000 (paid).

610 MEX
PANORAMA MEDICO. Text in Spanish. 1971. m. free to doctors in Mexico. adv.
Published by: Dr. Javier Aranda Apellaniz, Ed. & Pub., Avda. Coyoacan 1025, Edificio A no. 2, Condominio Jardin del Valle, Mexico City, 12, DF, Mexico. Circ: 15,000.

610 PNG ISSN 0256-2901 CODEN: MSPREG
PAPUA NEW GUINEA INSTITUTE OF MEDICAL RESEARCH. MONOGRAPH SERIES. Text in English. 1970. irreg. price varies. bibl, charts, illus. **Document type:** *Monographic series.* **Description:** A series of monographs on topics related to health and medical science in Papua New Guinea and elsewhere.
Published by: Papua New Guinea Institute of Medical Research, PO Box 60, Goroka, Papua New Guinea. TEL 675-7321469, FAX 675-7321998. Ed. Dr. M P Alpers. R&P Michael Alpers TEL 675-7322013. Circ: 1,000.

610 PNG ISSN 0031-1480 CODEN: PGMJBP
PAPUA NEW GUINEA MEDICAL JOURNAL. Text in English. 1955. q. PGK 150 (effective 2001). adv. bk.rev. abstr, bibl, charts, illus, maps. index every 3 yrs. back issues avail.; reprint service avail. from PQC. *Refereed.* **Document type:** *Journal, Academic/Scholarly.*
Related titles: Microfilm ed.: (from PQC).
Indexed: ASCA, Abstr.Hyg., Biol.Abstr., Curr.Cont. (coverage dropped), Dairy Sci.Abstr., Helminthol.Abstr., Ind.Med. (1955-), Ind.Vet., Inpharma, Int.Nurs.Ind., Nutr.Abstr., Protozool.Abstr., Reac., Rev.Appl.Entomol., Rev.Med.& Vet.Mycol., Rural Devel.Abstr., Rural Ext.Educ.& Tr.Abstr., SSCI (coverage dropped), So.Pac.Per.Ind., Trop.Dis.Bull., Vet.Bull. —BLDSC (6404.514000), CISTI, GNLM, IDS, ingenta.
Published by: Medical Society of Papua New Guinea, PO Box 60, Goroka, EHP 441, Papua New Guinea. TEL 675-7321469, FAX 675-7321998. Eds. C Mgone, P Siba. R&P C Mgone. Adv. contact Cynthea Leahy. Circ: 500.

610 USA
PARK-NICOLLET INSTITUTE FOR RESEARCH AND EDUCATION BULLETIN. Text in English. 1956. q. free per issue to qualified personnel. charts, illus. cum.index. *Refereed.* **Document type:** *Bulletin, Academic/Scholarly.* **Description:** Articles on diseases and treatment for physicians in primary care.
Former titles: Park-Nicollet Medical Foundation Bulletin; St. Louis Park Medical Center. Bulletin (0036-2980)
Indexed: Ind.Med. (coverage dropped).
Published by: (Park Nicollet Institute for Research and Education), Park Nicollet Medical Center, 5000 W 39th St, Minneapolis, MN 55416. TEL 612-993-3123. Ed. Heather Gantzer. R&P Jean Kisson TEL 612-993-3454. Circ: 11,000 (controlled).

291.5642 USA
THE PARK RIDGE CENTER. BULLETIN. Text in English. bi-m. free. bk.rev. charts, illus. back issues avail. **Document type:** *Newsletter, Academic/Scholarly.* **Description:** Covers health, faith, and ethics.
Published by: The Park Ridge Center, 211 E Ontario St, Ste 800, Chicago, IL 60611-3215. TEL 312-266-2222, FAX 312-266-6082, bmc@prchfe.org, http://www.parkridgecenter.org/. Ed., R&P Dan Perreter. Pub. Laurence J O'Connell. Circ: 13,000 (controlled).

610 ITA ISSN 0031-2312
PARMAMEDICA✶ ; bollettino dell'ordine dei medici. Text in Italian. 1967 (vol.15). m. ITL 2,000. adv.
Published by: Ordine dei Medici della Provincia di Parma, Borgo al Collegio Maria Luigia, 17, Parma, PR 43100, Italy. Ed. Carlo Molinari.

PART B NEWS. see *INSURANCE*

616.07 DEU ISSN 0172-8113
DER PATHOLOGE; pathologie und klinik. Text in German. 1979. bi-m. EUR 311.82 domestic; EUR 302.62 in Germany; EUR 57.90 newsstand/cover foreign (effective 2002). reprint service avail. from ISI. *Refereed.* **Document type:** *Journal, Academic/Scholarly.* **Description:** Provides information, news, and discussion in the discipline of pathology.
Related titles: Microform ed.: (from PQC); Online - full text ed.: ISSN 1432-1963 (from EBSCO Publishing, RoweCom Information Quest, Swets Blackwell, Springer LINK, Institute for Scientific Information).
Indexed: ASCA, Curr.Adv.Cell & Devel.Biol., Curr.Adv.Ecol.Sci., Curr.Cont., Excerp.Med., INIS Atomind., Ind.Med. (1979-), Ind.Sci.Rev., Inpharma, Int.Nurs.Ind., Pharm.&Out.News, Reac., Rev.Med.& Vet.Mycol., Sci.Cit.Ind. —BLDSC (6412.747000), CISTI, GNLM, IDS, Infotrieve, KNAW. **CCC.**
Published by: (Deutsche Gesellschaft fuer Pathologie), Springer-Verlag (Subsidiary of: BertelsmannSpringer), Tiergartenstr 17, Heidelberg 69121, Germany. TEL 49-6221-345-0, FAX 49-6221-345229, subscriptions@springer.de, http://link.springer.de/link/service/journals/00292/index.htm, http://www.springer.de. Eds. K M Mueller, W Boecker. **Subscr. in N. America to:** Springer-Verlag New York Inc., PO Box 2485, Secaucus, NJ 07096-2485. TEL 212-460-1500, FAX 212-473-6272. **Co-sponsors:** Internationalen Akademie fuer Pathologie; Oesterreichische Gesellschaft fuer Pathologie; Schweizerische Gesellschaft fuer Pathologie.

616.07 ITA ISSN 0031-2983 CODEN: PATHAB
PATHOLOGICA. Text in English, French, Italian; Summaries in English, Italian. 1908. bi-m. EUR 110 domestic; EUR 22 newsstand/cover foreign (effective 2002). adv. bk.rev. index. back issues avail. **Document type:** *Journal, Academic/Scholarly.*
Related titles: Online - full text ed.: ISSN 1591-951X (from Springer LINK).
Indexed: Excerp.Med., Ind.Med. (1908-). —BLDSC (6412.780000), CISTI, GNLM, KNAW.
Published by: Springer-Verlag Italia Srl (Subsidiary of: BertelsmannSpringer), Via Podgora, 4, Milan, MI 20122, Italy. TEL 39-2-55194656, FAX 39-2-55193360, springer@springer.it, http://link.springer.de. Ed. V Eusebi. Circ: 850.

616.07 571.9 FRA ISSN 0369-8114 CODEN: PTBIAN
PATHOLOGIE ET BIOLOGIE. Text in French. 1958. 10/yr. EUR 284, USD 338 elsewhere to individuals; FRF 1,882 domestic to institutions; EUR 309 in Europe to institutions; USD 380 in United States to institutions; FRF 2,079 elsewhere to institutions (effective 2002). adv. back issues avail. *Refereed.* **Document type:** *Academic/Scholarly.*

M

Formerly (until 1959): Archives de Biologie Medicale, Annales de la Recherche Medicale (0150-7265); Which was formed by the 1958 merger of: Annales de la Recherche Medicale (0997-4415); Societe Francaise de Biologie Medicale. Archives (0997-4423)
Related titles: Online - full text ed.: (from Institute for Scientific Information); ♦ Supplement to: La Semaine des Hopitaux. ISSN 0037-1777.
Indexed: ASCA, Aqua.Sci.& Fish.Abstr., Biol.Abstr., Chem.Abstr., Chem.Titles, Curr.Adv.Ecol.Sci., Curr.Cont., Dairy Sci.Abstr., Environ.Sci.Poll.Mgmt., Excerp.Med., Helminthol.Abstr., INIS Atomind., Ind.Med. (1969-), Ind.Sci.Rev., Ind.Vet., Inpharma, Int.Abstr.Biol.Sci., Int.Nurs.Ind., Microbiol.Abstr., Nutr.Abstr., Pharm.&Out.News, Protozool.Abstr., Reac., Ref.Zh., Rev.Plant Path., Risk Abstr., Sci.Cit.Ind., Vet.Bull.
—BLDSC (6412.798000), CASDDS, Infotrieve, KNAW. **CCC.**
Published by: (Semaine des Hopitaux), Elsevier Paris, Editions Scientifiques et Medicales (Subsidiary of: Reed Elsevier plc. group), 23 rue Linois, Paris 75015, France. TEL 33-1-45589110, FAX 33-1-45589419, http://www.elsevier.com/locate/patbio. Circ: 4,000.

616.07 571.9 GBR ISSN 0031-3025
CODEN: PTLGAX
PATHOLOGY. Text in English. 1969. q. GBP 198, USD 324 to individuals; GBP 362, USD 598 to institutions (effective 2002). adv. bk.rev. charts, illus. index. *Refereed.* **Document type:** *Academic/Scholarly.*
Incorporates (in 1995): Royal College of Pathologists of Australasia. Broadsheet (1036-157X); Which was formerly (1967-198?): Royal College of Pathologists of Australia. Broadsheets (0156-983X)
Related titles: Online - full text ed.: ISSN 1465-3931 (from CatchWord Ltd., EBSCO Publishing, O C L C Online Computer Library Center, Inc., RoweCom Information Quest, Swets Blackwell, Institute for Scientific Information).
Indexed: AESIS, ASCA, Abstr.Hyg., Biol.Abstr., Chem.Abstr., Chem.Titles, Curr.Adv.Ecol.Sci., Curr.Cont., Dairy Sci.Abstr., Excerp.Med., Helminthol.Abstr., INIS Atomind., Ind.Med. (1969-), Ind.Sci.Rev., Ind.Vet., Inpharma, Med.& Surg.Dermat., Nutr.Abstr., Pharm.&Out.News, Reac., Rev.Appl.Entomol., Rev.Med.& Vet.Mycol., Rev.Plant Path., Risk Abstr., Sci.Cit.Ind., So.Pac.Per.Ind., Trop.Dis.Bull., Vet.Bull.
—BLDSC (6412.810000), ADONIS, CASDDS, CatchWord, CISTI, GNLM, IDS, ingenta, KNAW. **CCC.**
Published by: (Royal College of Pathologists of Australasia AUS), Carfax Publishing Limited (Subsidiary of: Taylor & Francis Group), PO Box 25, Abingdon, Oxon OX14 3UE, United Kingdom. TEL 44-1235-401000, FAX 44-1235-401550, enquiries@carfax.co.uk, enquiry@tandf.co.uk, http://www.carfax.co.uk. Circ: 1,800.

610 USA ISSN 1082-9784
PATHOLOGY CASE REVIEWS. Text in English. 1996. bi-m., latest vol.6. USD 155 domestic to individuals; USD 196 foreign to individuals; USD 227 domestic to institutions; USD 269 foreign to institutions; USD 41 newsstand/cover (effective 2002). adv. **Document type:** *Academic/Scholarly.* **Description:** Each issue examines one vital theme in the field with peer-reviewed, clinically oriented case reports that focus on diagnosis, specimen handling and reports generation.
Related titles: Online - full text ed.: USD 295.10 domestic for academic site license; USD 337.10 foreign for academic site license; USD 329.15 domestic for corporate site license; USD 371.15 foreign for corporate site license (effective 2002).
—BLDSC (6412.821000).
Published by: Lippincott Williams & Wilkins (Philadelphia) (Subsidiary of: Wolters Kluwer N.V.), 530 Walnut St, Philadelphia, PA 19106-3621. TEL 215-521-8300, FAX 215-521-8902, www.pathologycasereviews.com, http://www.lww.com. Ed. Dr. Steven G Silverberg. Pub. Jim Merritt. R&P Margaret Becker. adv.: B&W page USD 825, color page USD 1,730; trim 11 x 8.13. Circ: 1,358. **Subscr. to:** PO Box 1600, Hagerstown, MD 21740-1600. TEL 800-777-2295, FAX 301-824-7390.

610 GBR ISSN 1465-9131
▼ **PATHOLOGY IN PRACTICE.** Text in English. 1999. s-a. **Document type:** *Academic/Scholarly.*
Related titles: ♦ Supplement to: Biomedical Scientist. ISSN 1352-7673.
—BLDSC (6412.826000).
Published by: Step Publishing Ltd., Lower Green Rd, Rusthall, Turnbridge Wells TN4 8TT, United Kingdom. TEL 44-1892-518877, mail@stepex.co.uk, http://www.stepex.co.uk.

616.07 574.2 AUS ISSN 1320-5463
CODEN: PITEES
PATHOLOGY INTERNATIONAL. Text in English. 1951. m. AUD 377 domestic to individuals; AUD 343 in New Zealand to individuals; USD 209 elsewhere to individuals; AUD 1,152 domestic to institutions; AUD 1,048 in New Zealand to institutions; JPY 66,600 in Japan to institutions; USD 639 elsewhere to institutions; AUD 415 domestic to individuals paper & online eds. combined; AUD 378 in New Zealand to individuals paper & online eds. combined; USD 230 elsewhere to individuals paper & online eds. combined; AUD 1,268 domestic to institutions paper & online eds. combined; AUD 1,153 in New Zealand to institutions paper & online eds. combined; JPY 73,260 in Japan to institutions paper & online eds. combined; USD 703 elsewhere to institutions paper & online eds. combined (effective 2001). adv. bk.rev. charts, illus. reprint service avail. from ISI. *Refereed.* **Document type:** *Academic/Scholarly.* **Description:** Presents original papers on human and experimental pathology.
Formerly (until 1994): Acta Pathologica Japonica (0001-6632)
Related titles: Online - full text ed.: ISSN 1440-1827. AUD 340 domestic to individuals; AUD 309 in New Zealand to individuals; USD 189 elsewhere to individuals; AUD 1,037 domestic to institutions; AUD 944 in New Zealand to institutions; JPY 59,940 in Japan to institutions; USD 576 elsewhere to institutions (effective 2001) (from Ovid Technologies, Inc., EBSCO Publishing, O C L C Online Computer Library Center, Inc., RoweCom Information Quest, ingenta, Munksgaard & Blackwell Science's Synergy, Swets Blackwell, Institute for Scientific Information).
Indexed: ASCA, Biol.Abstr., Chem.Abstr., Chem.Titles, Curr.Adv.Cell & Devel.Biol., Curr.Adv.Ecol.Sci., Curr.Adv.Gen.& Molec.Biol., Curr.Cont., Excerp.Med., Helminthol.Abstr., INIS Atomind., Ind.Med. (1994-), Ind.Sci.Rev., Inpharma, Int.Abstr.Biol.Sci., Neurosci.Cit.Ind., Pharm.&Out.News, Reac., Rev.Med.& Vet.Mycol., Sci.Cit.Ind.
—BLDSC (6412.823000), ADONIS, CASDDS, CISTI, EMDOCS, GNLM, IDS, Infotrieve, ingenta, KNAW. **CCC.**
Published by: (Japanese Society of Pathology JPN), Blackwell Science Asia Pty Ltd, PO Box 378, Carlton South, VIC 3053, Australia. TEL 61-3-9347-0300, FAX 61-3-9347-5001, info@blacksci-asia.com.au, http://www.blacksci.co.uk. Ed. Kiyoshi Mukai. Adv. contact Kathryn O'Brien. B&W page AUD 1,000, color page AUD 1,950; trim 210 x 275. Circ: 4,200.

616.07 571.9 USA ISSN 1050-9194
PATHOLOGY PATTERNS. Text in English. s-a. **Description:** Provides commentaries on current developments in the field of pathology and laboratory medicine.
Related titles: ♦ Supplement to: American Journal of Clinical Pathology. ISSN 0002-9173.
—CISTI, KNAW.
Published by: (American Society of Clinical Pathologists), J B Lippincott Co, E Washington Sq, Philadelphia, PA 19106. TEL 800-777-2295. Ed. Dr. William T Lockard Jr.

616.07 DEU ISSN 0344-0338
CODEN: PARPDS
PATHOLOGY, RESEARCH AND PRACTICE. Text in English. 1886. m. EUR 399, GBP 294 to individuals; EUR 1,065, GBP 811 to institutions (effective 2002). adv. bk.rev. *Refereed.* **Document type:** *Journal, Academic/Scholarly.* **Description:** Focuses on recent progress and comments on current problems and hypotheses about future developments in pathology.
Former titles: Pathology and Practice; Beitraege zur Pathologie (0005-8165)
Related titles: Online - full text ed.: (from Swets Blackwell, Institute for Scientific Information).
Indexed: ASCA, Biol.Abstr., Chem.Abstr., Chem.Indus.Notes, Chem.Titles, Curr.Adv.Cancer Res., Curr.Adv.Cell & Devel.Biol., Curr.Adv.Ecol.Sci., Curr.Cont., Dent.Ind., Dok.Arbeitsmed., Helminthol.Abstr., INIS Atomind., Ind.Med. (1978-), Ind.Sci.Rev., Ind.Vet., Inpharma, Int.Abstr.Biol.Sci., Neurosci.Cit.Ind., Nutr.Abstr., Pharm.&Out.News, Protozool.Abstr., Reac., Rev.Med.& Vet.Mycol., Sci.Cit.Ind., Vet.Bull.
—BLDSC (6412.827000), CASDDS, CISTI, EMDOCS, GNLM, IDS, ingenta, KNAW. **CCC.**
Published by: (American Registry of Pathology USA), Urban & Fischer Verlag, Loebdergraben 14A, Jena 07743, Germany. TEL 49-3641-626444, FAX 49-3641-626421, info@urbanfischer.de, http://www.urbanfischer.de. Ed. H E Schaefer. R&P Martin Huber TEL 49-3641-626430. Adv. contact Sabine Schroeter. **Co-sponsors:** Japanese Society of Pathology; Canadian Association of Pathologists.

PATHOPHYSIOLOGY. see *BIOLOGY—Physiology*

PATHWAYS TO HEALTH. see *ALTERNATIVE MEDICINE*

610 CHE
PATIENT CARE. Text in English. 10/yr.
Published by: Medon AG, Haltenrain 4, Horw 6048, Switzerland. TEL 41-41-3480035, FAX 41-41-3480039. Circ: 3,000.

610 CAN ISSN 0845-065X
PATIENT CARE. Text in English. 1990. 12/yr. CND 56.50; CND 92.70 foreign (effective 2000). adv. **Document type:** *Magazine, Trade.*
Related titles: Online - full text ed.: (from Northern Light Technology, Inc.).
—CCC.
Published by: Rogers Media Publishing Ltd, 777 Bay St, 6th Fl, Toronto, ON M5W 1A7, Canada. TEL 416-596-5000, FAX 416-596-5881, http://www.rogers.com. adv.: B&W page CND 1,550; trim 10.75 x 8.13. Circ: 25,546.

610.5 USA ISSN 0031-305X
R11
PATIENT CARE. Text in English. 1967. 24/yr. USD 99 domestic; USD 124 foreign; USD 10 newsstand/cover (effective 2001). adv. charts, illus. cum.index. reprint service avail. from RPI. **Document type:** *Trade.* **Description:** Focuses on the diagnosis and treatment of problems encountered by the office-based, primary care physician.
Related titles: Microform ed.: (from RPI,PQC); Online - full text ed.: (from Gale Group, ProQuest Information & Learning, Northern Light Technology, Inc., Factiva, Institute for Scientific Information).
Indexed: AgeLine, Bus.Ind., CHNI, CINAHL, Cal.Tiss.Abstr., Environ.Sci.Poll.Mgmt., FAMLI, Hlth.Ind., Pollut.Abstr., Risk Abstr., Saf.Sci.Abstr., Tr.& Indus.Ind., Virol.Abstr. (coverage dropped).
—BLDSC (6412.861200), CISTI, GNLM, IDS, ingenta, KNAW. **CCC.**
Published by: Medical Economics Co., Inc., 5 Paragon Dr, Montvale, NJ 07645-1742. customer_service@medec.com. Ed. Deborah Kaplan. adv.: B&W page USD 6,875, color page USD 8,965. Circ: 135,000. **Subscr. to:** Medical Economics Co, Inc, P D R, PO Box 162, Montvale, NJ 07645-1742. TEL 800-232-7379, FAX 201-722-2680.

610.6 USA
PATIENT EDUCATION MANAGEMENT. Text in English. 1994. m. USD 365 domestic; USD 395 foreign; USD 61 newsstand/cover (effective 2001). back issues avail. **Document type:** *Newsletter.* **Description:** Designed for nurse managers, education directors, case managers, and discharge planners.
Indexed: CINAHL.
—BLDSC (6412.864600).
Published by: American Health Consultants, Inc. (Subsidiary of: Medical Economics), 3523 Piedmont Rd, N E, Bldg 6, Ste 400, Atlanta, GA 30305. TEL 404-262-7436, FAX 800-284-3291, custserv@ahcpub.com, http://www.ahcpub.com. Ed. Susan Cort Johnson.

610 GBR
PATIENTS' VOICES. Text in English. 1976. q. GBP 1 newsstand/cover. adv. bk.rev. **Document type:** *Newsletter, Consumer.*
Formerly: Patient Voice (1367-1146)
—BLDSC (6412.867500).
Published by: Patients Association, PO Box 935, Harrow, Middlesex HA1 3YJ, United Kingdom. TEL 44-20-8423-9111, FAX 44-20-8423-9119, mailbox@patients-association.com. Ed. Mike Hyde. Adv. contact Stephen Pickles. Circ: 2,000.

610 IND ISSN 0031-3084
CODEN: PAJMAA
PATNA JOURNAL OF MEDICINE. Text in English. 1925. m. INR 215. adv. bk.rev. charts, illus, stat. index. reprint service avail. from IRC. **Document type:** *Academic/Scholarly.* **Description:** Aims to promote and advance medical and allied sciences, and the improvement of public health and medical education in Bihar and India.
Related titles: Microform ed.
Indexed: Biol.Abstr.
—CISTI, GNLM.
Published by: Indian Medical Association Bihar State Branch, Medical Association Bldg., Patna, Bihar 800 004, India. TEL 655542. Ed. Dr. I B Sinha. Circ: 8,500. **Co-sponsor:** Patna Medical Association.

PATOLOGIA; revista latinoamericana. see *BIOLOGY*

M

616.07 571.9 RUS ISSN 0031-2991
RB1 CODEN: PAFEAY
PATOLOGICHESKAYA FIZIOLOGIYA I EKSPERIMENTAL'NAYA TERAPIYA/PATHOLOGICAL PHYSIOLOGY AND EXPERIMENTAL THERAPY. Text in Russian; Summaries in English. 1957. q. USD 132 foreign (effective 2000). adv. bk.rev., Website rev. illus, abstr. index. **Document type:** *Journal, Academic/Scholarly.* **Description:** Publishes materials on pressing problems of modern theoretical medicine: the etiology, pathogenesis of disease processes, and individual nosological forms of the disease.
Indexed: Biol.Abstr., Chem.Abstr., Chem.Titles, Dent.Ind., Derwent Biotech.Abstr., Excerp.Med., INIS Atomind., Ind.Med. (1957-), Int.Aerosp.Abstr., Nutr.Abstr., Ref.Zh.
—BLDSC (0129.200000), CASDDS, CISTI, East View, GNLM, Infotrieve. **CCC.**
Published by: Izdatel'stvo Meditsina, Petroverigskii per 6-8, Moscow 101000, Russian Federation. TEL 7-095-9248785, 7-095-928-86-48, FAX 7-095-9211355, 7-095-9286003, meditsina@iname.com, http://www.medit.ru. Ed. B B Moroz. Pub. A M Stochik. R&P V Ivannikova. Adv. contact O A Fadeeva TEL 7-095-923-51-40. Circ: 500. **Dist. by:** Mezhdunarodnaya Kniga, B Yakimanka 39, Moscow 117049, Russian Federation. TEL 7-095-2384967, FAX 7-095-2384634; **Dist. in US by:** Victor Kamkin Inc., 4956 Boiling Brook Pkwy, Rockville, MD 20852.

616.07 ITA ISSN 0391-0377
PATOLOGO CLINICO. Text in Italian. 1970. bi-m., latest vol.6, 2001. ITL 300,000 in Europe to non-members; ITL 350,000 elsewhere to non-members. adv. bk.rev. *Refereed.* **Description:** Contains clinical pathology lectures and professional articles.
—CCC.
Published by: A I P A C Service s.r.l., Via Luigi Ungarelli, 23, Rome, RM 00162, Italy. TEL 39-6-8600007, FAX 39-6-8600042. Ed. Dr. Luigi Gatta. Adv. contact Vincenzo Massa.

PEDIATRIC AND DEVELOPMENTAL PATHOLOGY. see *MEDICAL SCIENCES—Pediatrics*

610 USA ISSN 0031-4595
R11 CODEN: PNMDAL
PENNSYLVANIA MEDICINE. Text in English. 1897. q. USD 35. adv. abstr, bibl, illus. **Document type:** *Trade.* **Description:** Covers issues related to the practice of medicine, including public health topics, government regulations and policies, medical economics, and other concerns.
Formerly: Pennsylvania Medical Journal
Related titles: Microfilm ed.
Indexed: Biol.Abstr., CINAHL, C.I.S. Abstr., Chem.Abstr., Curr.Cont. (coverage dropped), Excerp.Med., Helminthol.Abstr., INIS Atomind., Ind.Med. (1966-), Int.Nurs.Ind., Med.Care Rev.
—BLDSC (6421.745000), CISTI, GNLM, KNAW.
Published by: Pennsylvania Medical Society, PO Box 8820, Harrisburg, PA 17105-8820. TEL 717-558-7750, FAX 717-558-7740, stat@pamedsoc.org. Ed. Elaine S Herrmann. R&P Elaine Herrman. Circ: 20,000.

615.53 USA ISSN 0479-9534
PENNSYLVANIA OSTEOPATHIC MEDICAL ASSOCIATION. JOURNAL. Key Title: Journal of the Pennsylvania Osteopathic Medical Association. Text in English. 1945. 5/yr. membership only. adv. *Refereed.* **Document type:** *Academic/Scholarly.* **Description:** Publishes articles on topics relating to the practice of osteopathic medicine and osteopathic medical issues.
Published by: Pennsylvania Osteopathic Medical Association, 1330 Eisenhower Blvd, Harrisburg, PA 17111. TEL 717-939-9318, FAX 717-939-7255, publa@poma.org, http://www.poma.org. Ed. Dr. Gerald Scharf. R&P Marce Monroe-Ward TEL 717-939-9318 ext 14. Adv. contact Marce Monroe Ward. Circ: 4,000 (controlled).

M

PEOPLE PLANT CONNECTION. see *PUBLIC HEALTH AND SAFETY*

PEOPLE'S MEDICAL SOCIETY NEWSLETTER. see *CONSUMER EDUCATION AND PROTECTION*

610 USA ISSN 1523-0465
PERFORMANCE AND PRACTICES OF SUCCESSFUL MEDICAL GROUPS. Text in English. 1998. a. USD 350 to non-members; USD 225 to members (effective 2001). stat. **Document type:** *Bulletin.* **Description:** Helps benchmark business practices against MGMA's better performers.
Related titles: CD-ROM ed.
Published by: Medical Group Management Association, 104 Inverness Terrace E, Englewood, CO 80112. TEL 303-799-1111, FAX 303-397-1827, survey@mgma.com, http://www.mgma.com. Circ: 5,000 (paid).

PERIODICUM BIOLOGORUM. see *BIOLOGY*

610 616.6 CAN ISSN 0896-8608
PERITONEAL DIALYSIS INTERNATIONAL. Text in English. 1980. bi-m. USD 110 in US & Canada to resident/nurses; USD 190 rest of world to resident/nurses; USD 175 in US & Canada to medical doctors; USD 255 rest of world to medical doctors; USD 265 in US & Canada to institutions; USD 345 rest of world to institutions (effective 2001). index. back issues avail. *Refeeed.* **Document type:** *Journal, Academic/Scholarly.*
Formerly: Peritoneal Dialysis Bulletin
Related titles: Microform ed.: 1980 (from PQC); Online - full text ed.: (from Institute for Scientific Information).
Indexed: ASCA, Curr.Cont., Excerp.Med., Ind.Med. (1988-), Inpharma, Int.Nurs.Ind., Kidney, Nutr.Abstr., Pharm.&Out.News, Reac., Rev.Med.& Vet.Mycol., Sci.Cit.Ind.
—BLDSC (6426.459000), CISTI, EMDOCS, GNLM, IDS, Infotrieve, KNAW. **CCC.**
Published by: (International Society for Peritoneal Dialysis), Multimed, Inc., 66 Martin St, Milton, ON L9T R2R, Canada. TEL 905-875-2456, 888-834-1001, FAX 905-875-2864, multimed@inforamp.net, http://www.multi-med.com/pdi/winpubmed.html. Ed. Dimitrios G Oreopoulos.

PERSONAL AND MEDICAL INJURIES LAW LETTER. see *LAW*

610 USA ISSN 1061-4125
RC81.A1
PERSONAL HEALTH REPORTER. Text in English. every 8 yrs. (1st ed.). USD 105 (effective 1999). **Document type:** *Trade.* **Description:** Provides excerpts of significant articles concerning physical and mental health.
Published by: Gale Group (Subsidiary of: The Thomson Corporation), 27500 Drake Rd, Farmington Hills, MI 48331-3535. TEL 248-699-4253, 800-877-4253, FAX 248-699-8061, galeord@gale.com, http://www.gale.com. Eds. Alan Rees, Charlene Willey.

610 USA
PERSPECTIVE (SILVER SPRING). Text in English. 1975. q., latest vol.93. USD 30 to members; includes Tuberous Sclerosis Resources. bk.rev. back issues avail. **Document type:** *Newsletter, Internal.* **Description:** Includes current research developments, fund raising efforts and other Association news.
Formerly (until Dec. 2000): N T S A Newsletter
Published by: Tuberous Sclerosis Alliance, 801 Roeder Rd, 750, Landover, MD 20912. TEL 800-225-6872, FAX 301-562-9870, info@tsalliance.org, http:// www.tsalliance.org. Ed. Beth H Michaels. Circ: 14,000.

610 570 USA ISSN 0031-5982
QH301 CODEN: PBMEA8
PERSPECTIVES IN BIOLOGY AND MEDICINE. Text in English. 1957. q. USD 40 domestic to individuals; USD 43.50 in Canada to individuals; USD 48.50 elsewhere to individuals; USD 96 domestic to institutions; USD 89.50 in Canada to institutions; USD 94.50 elsewhere to institutions; USD 34 domestic to students; USD 38.50 in Canada to students; USD 43.50 elsewhere to students; USD 12 newsstand/cover to individuals; USD 25 newsstand/cover to institutions (effective 2002). adv. bk.rev. bibl, illus. index. back issues avail.; reprint service avail. from PQC,ISI. *Refereed.* **Document type:** *Journal, Academic/Scholarly.* **Description:** Communicates insight and stimulates original thought in a broad range of biological and medical topics.
Related titles: Microform ed.: (from PQC); Online - full content ed.: ISSN 1529-8795 (from Project MUSE, EBSCO Publishing, O C L C Online Computer Library Center, Inc., Gale Group, Swets Blackwell); Online - full text ed.: (from Factiva, Institute for Scientific Information, RoweCom Information Quest).
Indexed: ASCA, Biol.& Agr.Ind. (Jul.1983-), Biol.Abstr., Biol.Dig., Chem.Abstr., Chem.Titles, Curr.Adv.Cancer Res., Curr.Adv.Ecol.Sci., Curr.Cont., Deep Sea Res.& Oceanogr.Abstr., Dent.Abstr., Dent.Ind., Excerp.Med., Gen.Sci.Ind. (Jul.1997-), Helminthol.Abstr., INIS Atomind., Ind.Med. (1957-), Ind.Sci.Rev., Ind.Vet., Inpharma, Lang.& Lang.Behav.Abstr., Pharm.&Out.News, Protozool.Abstr., Psychol.Abstr., Reac., Rev.Appl.Entomol., SOPODA, SSCI (coverage dropped), Sci.Cit.Ind., Small Anim.Abstr., Soc.Serv.Abstr., Sociol.Abstr., Sport Fish.Abstr., Vet.Bull., Wild.Rev., Zoo.Rec.
—BLDSC (6428.138200), CASDDS, CISTI, GNLM, IDS, ingenta, KNAW, Linda Hall. **CCC.**
Published by: Johns Hopkins University Press, Journals Publishing Division, 2715 N Charles St, Baltimore, MD 21218-4363. TEL 410-516-6900, FAX 410-516-6968, http://www.press.jhu.edu/press/journals/pbm/pbm.html. Eds. Richard L Landau, Robert L Perlman. adv.: B&W page USD 325; trim 6 x 8.5. Circ: 1,620.

610.09 300 NLD
PERSPECTIVES ON CULTURE AND MEDICINE. Text in English. irreg. price varies. **Document type:** *Monographic series.*
Published by: Kluwer Academic Publishers Group (Subsidiary of: Wolters Kluwer N.V.), Spuiboulevard 50, PO Box 17, Dordrecht 3300 AA, Netherlands. FAX 31-78-639-2254, services@wkap.nl, http://www.wkap.nl. **Dist. by:** Journals Department, PO Box 322, Dordrecht 3300 AH, Netherlands. FAX 31-78-654-6474.

610 614.8 PER ISSN 1018-6212
PERU. POLICIA NACIONAL. REVISTA DE LA SANIDAD. Key Title: Revista de la Sanidad Policia Nacional del Peru. Text in Spanish; Abstracts in English, Spanish. 1940. s-a. USD 60. adv. bk.rev. abstr, bibl, charts, illus. index.
Former titles (until 1988): Peru. Fuerzas Policiales. Revista de la Sanidad (0254-3435); Peru. Direccion de Sanidad. Revista de la Sanidad; Instituto de Investigaciones Medicas de la Fuerza Armada y Fuerzas Policiales del Peru; Revista de la Sanidad de las Fuerzas Policiales del Peru; Revista de la Sanidad de Policia (0034-8430)
Indexed: Chem.Abstr., Excerp.Med., INIS Atomind.
—EMDOCS, GNLM.
Published by: Ministerio del Interior, Direccion de Sanidad de las Fuerzas Policiales, Casilla 1683, Lima 100, Peru. Ed. Oscar Guillermo Quiroz Jara. Circ: 3,000. **Subscr. to:** Ave. Arequipa, 4849, Miraflores, Lima 18, Peru.

610 BRA ISSN 0048-3567
PESQUISA MEDICA. Text in Portuguese; Summaries in English. 1965. s-a. BRL 10, USD 10 (effective 1997). adv. bibl, illus. index. **Document type:** *Academic/Scholarly.*
Indexed: Biol.Abstr., Chem.Abstr.
Published by: Fundacao Faculdade Federal de Ciencias Medicas de Porto Alegre, Centro Academico XXII de Marco, Rua Sarmento Leite, 245, Porto Alegre, RGS 90050-170, Brazil. TEL 55-512-2248822, FAX 55-512-2267913, stangler@pro.via-rs.com.br. Ed. Cliber Alvares Da Silva. Circ: 1,000 (controlled).

PETERSON'S JOB OPPORTUNITIES IN HEALTH CARE. see *OCCUPATIONS AND CAREERS*

PFLEGEN AMBULANT; das Magazin fuer Pflege - Organisation - Betriebsfuehrung. see *PUBLIC HEALTH AND SAFETY*

612 DEU ISSN 0031-6768
QP1 CODEN: PFLABK
PFLUEGERS ARCHIV/EUROPEAN JOURNAL OF PHYSIOLOGY; european journal of physiology. Text mainly in English; Text occasionally in French, German. 1868. m. EUR 2,755.90 domestic; EUR 2,736.70 in Germany; EUR 271 newsstand/cover foreign (effective 2002). adv. charts, illus. back issues avail.; reprint service avail. from ISI. *Refereed.* **Document type:** *Journal, Academic/Scholarly.* **Description:** Covers original research on the most current developments in areas of specialization, in interdisciplinary work, and in the physiological sciences as a whole.
Formerly: Pfluegers Archiv fuer die Gesamte Physiologie des Menschen und der Tiere
Related titles: Microfilm ed.: (from BHP); Microform ed.: (from PQC,BHP,PMC); Online - full text ed.: ISSN 1432-2013 (from EBSCO Publishing, RoweCom Information Quest, Swets Blackwell, Springer LINK, Institute for Scientific Information).
Indexed: ASCA, Anim.Behav.Abstr. (coverage dropped), Aqua.Sci.& Fish.Abstr., BBCI, Biol.Abstr., C.I.S. Abstr., Chem.Abstr., Chem.Titles, Curr.Adv.Ecol.Sci., Curr.Cont., Dairy Sci.Abstr., Derwent Biotech.Abstr., Excerp.Med., INIS Atomind., Ind.Med. (1968-), Ind.Sci.Rev., Ind.Vet., Inpharma, Int.Abstr.Biol.Sci., Neurosci.Abstr. (coverage dropped), Phys.Ber., Reac., Rev.Appl.Entomol., Rev.Med.& Vet.Mycol., Sci.Cit.Ind., Sport Fish.Abstr., THA, Vet.Bull., Wild.Rev., Zoo.Rec.
—BLDSC (6440.999000), ADONIS, CASDDS, CISTI, GNLM, IDS, ingenta, Linda Hall. **CCC.**

Published by: (Federation of Physiological Societies), Springer-Verlag (Subsidiary of: BertelsmannSpringer), Tiergartenstr 17, Heidelberg 69121, Germany. TEL 49-6221-345-0, FAX 49-6221-345229, subscriptions@springer.de, http://link.springer.de/link/service/journals/00424/index.htm, http://www.springer.de. Ed. K Thurau. **Subscr. in N. America to:** Springer-Verlag New York Inc., PO Box 2485, Secaucus, NJ 07096-2485. TEL 212-460-1500, FAX 212-473-6272.

610 615 GBR ISSN 0142-1581
PHARMACEUTICAL MEDICINE (WORTHING); symposium proceedings. Text in English. 1979. irreg. **Document type:** *Proceedings.* **Description:** Book series for rapid publication of symposium proceedings.
Indexed: Curr.Adv.Ecol.Sci., Inpharma, Reac.
Published by: Cambridge Medical Publications Ltd., Wicker House, High St, Worthing, W Sussex BN11 1DJ, United Kingdom. TEL 44-1903-205884, FAX 44-1903-234862, cmp@hbase.com, http://www.parexel-mms.com/cmp, http://www.cambridge-medical.com.

610 USA ISSN 0031-7179
LJ105.A6
PHAROS (MENLO PARK). Text in English. 1938. q. membership. bk.rev. bibl, charts. *Refereed.* **Document type:** *Academic/Scholarly.*
Indexed: BHA, Ind.Med. (coverage dropped).
—BLDSC (6449.120000), GNLM, ingenta.
Published by: Alpha Omega Alpha Honor Medical Society, 525 Middlefield Rd, 130, Menlo Park, CA 94025. TEL 650-329-0291, FAX 650-329-1618. Ed. Dr. Edward D Harris Jr. R&P Carolyn L Kuckein. Circ: 70,000.

610 USA ISSN 0031-7306
CODEN: PHMEBH
PHILADELPHIA MEDICINE. Text in English. 1906. m. USD 15. adv. *Refereed.* **Document type:** *Academic/Scholarly.*
Indexed: AgeLine.
Published by: Philadelphia County Medical Society, 2100 Spring Garden St, Philadelphia, PA 19130. TEL 215-563-5343, FAX 215-563-3627. Ed., R&P Dr. William Weiss. Adv. contact Anne Hlwyiak. Circ: 4,300 (controlled).

610 PHL ISSN 0031-7748
CODEN: JPMEA6
PHILIPPINE MEDICAL ASSOCIATION. JOURNAL. Text in English. 1928. q. USD 20. adv. bk.rev. charts, illus, stat. index.
Indexed: Biol.Abstr., C.I.S. Abstr., Chem.Abstr., Diar.Dis.Res., INIS Atomind., Ind.Phil.Per., Trop.Dis.Bull.
—CASDDS, CISTI, GNLM.
Published by: (Philippine Medical Association), P M A Press, P M A House, North Ave, Diliman, Quezon City Mm 1128, Philippines. Ed. Conrado Dayrit. Circ: 13,000.

610 PHL ISSN 0031-7799
PHILIPPINE SCIENTIFIC JOURNAL. Text in English. 1955. s-a. PHP 125. bk.rev. abstr, charts. index. reprints avail. **Document type:** *Academic/Scholarly.* **Description:** Contains research papers by medical students, interns, residents and consultants.
Indexed: INIS Atomind.
Published by: Manila Central University, F D T Medical Foundation, EDSA, Kaloocan City, Philippines. TEL 632-361-10-46, FAX 632-361-46-64. Ed. Esperanza F Rivera. adv.: B&W page PHP 5,000; 7 x 10. Circ: 2,500.

PHILOSOPHY AND MEDICINE. see *PHILOSOPHY*

616.20 DEU ISSN 0939-978X
CODEN: PHLBE
PHLEBOLOGIE. Text in English, French, German. 1972. 6/yr. DEM 218 to individuals; DEM 284 to institutions; DEM 130 to students (effective 2001). adv. bk.rev. **Document type:** *Journal, Academic/Scholarly.*
Formerly (until 1991): Phlebologie und Proktologie (0340-305X)
Related titles: Online - full text ed.: (from Institute for Scientific Information).
Indexed: Curr.Cont., Excerp.Med.
—BLDSC (6465.100100), EMDOCS, GNLM, Infotrieve, KNAW. **CCC.**
Published by: (German and Swiss Society of Phlebology), Schattauer GmbH, Hoelderlinstr 3, Stuttgart 70174, Germany. TEL 49-711-22987-0, FAX 49-711-2298750, info@schattauer.de, http://www.schattauer.com. Ed. U Schultz Ehrenburg. Pub. Dieter Bergemann. R&P Annika Schmidt TEL 49-711-2298713. Adv. contact Hans-Georg Schwarz. B&W page XEU 1,221.99, color page XEU 2,186.8; 183 x 227. Circ: 3,600. **Subscr. to:** CSJ, Postfach 140220, Munich 80452, Germany. TEL 49-89-20959129, schattauer@csj.de. **Co-sponsor:** Berufsverband der Phlebologen e.V.

PHOTOCHEMISTRY AND PHOTOBIOLOGY. see *CHEMISTRY*

610 530 ITA ISSN 1120-1797
PHYSICA MEDICA. Text in Italian. 1985. q. ITL 264,000; ITL 300,000 foreign (effective 1998). adv. bk.rev. *Refereed.* **Description:** Research and reviews in medical physics and biomedical engineering.
Incorporates: Fisica in Medicina
Related titles: Online - full text ed.: (from Institute for Scientific Information).
Indexed: ASCA, BBCI, INSPEC (Jan.1991-), Neurosci.Cit.Ind.
—BLDSC (6475.070000), AskIEEE, CISTI, EMDOCS, GNLM, IDS.
Published by: (Associazione Italiana di Fisica Biomedica), Istituti Editoriali e Poligrafici Internazionali, Via Giosue' Carducci, 60, Ghezzano La Fontina, PI 56010, Italy. TEL 39-50-878066, FAX 39-050-878732, TELEX 522027, iepi@sirius.pisa.it. Ed. Alberto Del Guerra. Circ: 700.

371.88 613.17 USA
▼ **PHYSICAL & MENTAL ISSUES IN AGING SOURCEBOOK.** Text in English. 1999 (Mar.). irreg. USD 78 per issue (effective 2001). charts. master index. **Description:** Contains basic information about maintaining health through the post-reproductive years. Including a description of the aging process, physical changes, preventive medicine, and mental health issues for seniors, along with statistical and demographic data, recommended lifestyle modifications, a glossary, and a list of resources for additional help and information.
Published by: Omnigraphics, Inc., 615 Griswold St, Detroit, MI 48226. TEL 313-961-1340, 800-234-1340, FAX 313-961-1383, 800-875-1340, info@omnigraphics.com, http://www.omnigraphics.com. Ed. Jenifer Swanson.

610 USA ISSN 1084-6905
PHYSICIAN. Text in English. 1989. bi-m. free to qualified personnel. illus. **Document type:** *Trade.* **Description:** Offers information and support regarding the unique challenges, issues and circumstances that face those who work in the medical field.
Indexed: CCR.
Published by: Focus on the Family, Inc., 8605 Explorer Dr, Colorado Springs, CO 80920-1051. TEL 719-531-3400, 800-232-6459, FAX 719-531-3499. Ed. Susan Stevens. R&P Christine McDonald. Circ: 84,000 (controlled).

610 USA ISSN 1051-600X
R847.5
PHYSICIAN ASSISTANT PROGRAMS DIRECTORY. Text in English. 1975. a. USD 35 (effective 2000). adv. **Document type:** *Directory.* **Description:** Contains full-page program listings and summary charts detailing PA program and postgraduate PA program entrance requirements, fees, deadlines, program length, credentials awarded, selection criteria, and housing and funding information.
Former titles (until 1989): Physician Assistant Programs, A National Directory; National Health Practitioner Program Profile (0277-3376); National New Health Practitioner Program Profile (0145-3793)
Related titles: Online - full text ed.
Published by: Association of Physician Assistant Programs, 950 N Washington St, Alexandria, VA 22314-1534. TEL 703-548-5538, FAX 703-684-1924, http://www.apap.org. Ed., Adv. contact Steven Lane. Circ: 4,500 (paid).

610 USA ISSN 8750-7544
R697.P45
PHYSICIAN ASSISTANT (SPRINGHOUSE). Text in English. 1979. m. USD 58 domestic to individuals; USD 89 in Canada to individuals; USD 95 elsewhere to individuals; USD 70 domestic to institutions; USD 95 in Canada to institutions; USD 105 elsewhere to institutions; USD 10 newsstand/cover (effective 2001). illus. reprint service avail. from PQC. *Refereed.* **Document type:** *Trade.* **Description:** Publishes primary care, clinical articles and profession-oriented material for physician assistants.
Former titles (until 1982): Physician Assistant - Health Practitioner (0197-713X); (until 1979): Health Practitioner, Physician Assistant (0192-7310); Which was formed by the merger of (1976-1979): Physician Assistant; (1977-1979): Health Practitioner (0149-6549)
Related titles: Microfilm ed.: (from PQC); Online - full text ed.: (from ProQuest Information & Learning, Gale Group).
Indexed: CINAHL.
—BLDSC (6476.361500), GNLM, Infotrieve, ingenta. **CCC.**
Published by: Springhouse Corporation (Subsidiary of: Lippincott Williams & Wilkins (Philadelphia)), 1111 Bethlehem Tpk, Springhouse, PA 19477. TEL 215-646-8700, FAX 215-646-4399, 800-783-4903, http://www.pajournal.com/, http://www.springnet.com. Ed. J Dennis Blessing. Circ: 40,261. **Subscr. to:** 30 Broad St, PO Box 3000, Denville, NJ 07834.

PHYSICIAN ASSISTANTS' PRESCRIBING REFERENCE. see *PHARMACY AND PHARMACOLOGY*

PHYSICIAN COMPENSATION REPORT. see *BUSINESS AND ECONOMICS—Management*

PHYSICIAN EXECUTIVE; journal of management. see *HEALTH FACILITIES AND ADMINISTRATION*

610 USA
PHYSICIAN NEWSLETTER. Text in English. 1962. m. USD 24 to non-members (effective 1999). **Document type:** *Newsletter.*
Former titles (until 1998): Wyoming Physicians Newsletter; Medical Wire; Pulse (0043-9797)
Published by: Wyoming State Medical Society, PO Box 4009, Cheyenne, WY 82001. TEL 307-635-2424, FAX 307-632-1973. Ed. Susie P Wacker. Circ: 800.

362.1 USA
PHYSICIAN PROFILING AND BEHAVIOR CHANGE REPORT. Text in English. 1998. m. USD 289; USD 299 in Canada & Mexico; USD 309 elsewhere. **Document type:** *Trade.*
Published by: National Health Information, LLC, PO Box 15429, Atlanta, GA 30333. TEL 404-607-9500.

PHYSICIANS & SURGEONS DIRECTORY. see *BUSINESS AND ECONOMICS—Trade And Industrial Directories*

610 USA ISSN 0093-4461
RS75 CODEN: PDPSBC
PHYSICIANS' DESK REFERENCE. Text in English. 1947. a. USD 82.95 (effective 2000). **Document type:** *Directory, Trade.* **Description:** Provides detailed information on the composition, dosing, indications and contraindications, side effects, and drug interactions for prescription medicines.
Formerly (until 1974): Physicians' Desk Reference to Pharmaceutical Specialties and Biologicals (0093-447X)
Related titles: CD-ROM ed.; Online - full text ed.
—BLDSC (6476.375500), CASDDS, GNLM. **CCC.**
Published by: Medical Economics Co., Inc., 5 Paragon Dr, Montvale, NJ 07645-1742. Circ: 950,000 (controlled). **Subscr. to:** P D R, PO Box 10689, Des Moines, IA 50336. TEL 201-358-7200, 800-232-7379, FAX 201-722-2680.

610 USA
RM671.A1
PHYSICIANS' DESK REFERENCE FOR NONPRESCRIPTION DRUGS AND DIETARY SUPPLEMENTS. Text in English. 1980. a. USD 49.95 (effective 2000). **Document type:** *Directory, Trade.* **Description:** Provides detailed information on dosing, indications and contraindications, side effects, and drug interaction on over-the-counter drugs.
Formerly (until 1999): Physicians' Desk Reference for Nonprescription Drugs (1044-1395)
Related titles: CD-ROM ed.; Online - full text ed.
—GNLM, Linda Hall.
Published by: Medical Economics Co., Inc., 5 Paragon Dr, Montvale, NJ 07645-1742. TEL 201-358-7200. Circ: 300,000 (controlled). **Subscr. to:** P D R, PO Box 10689, Des Moines, IA 50336. FAX 201-722-2680.

PHYSICIANS FINANCIAL NEWS. see *BUSINESS AND ECONOMICS—Banking And Finance*

610 USA
PHYSICIANS FORUM BULLETIN. Text in English. 1985. 3/yr. USD 75. back issues avail. **Document type:** *Newsletter.*
Published by: Physicians Forum, 1507 53rd St, Ste 155, Chicago, IL 60615. TEL 312-922-1968, FAX 312-633-6442. Ed. Barbara Linn.

PHYSICIANS LIFESTYLE MAGAZINE. see *GENERAL INTEREST PERIODICALS—United States*

610 658 CAN ISSN 0705-6311
PHYSICIAN'S MANAGEMENT MANUALS. Text in English. 1976. m. CND 81. adv. **Description:** Information for Canadian doctors on practice management and investment.
Related titles: Microfiche ed.: (from MML); Microform ed.: (from MML).
Indexed: Can.B.P.I.
—CCC.
Published by: Healthcare and Financial Publishing (Subsidiary of: Rogers Media Publishing Ltd), 777 Bay Street, 5th Fl, Toronto, ON M5W 1A7, Canada. TEL 416-596-5724. Ed. Will Koteff. Circ: 41,500.

610 USA ISSN 1079-6312
PHYSICIAN'S NEWS DIGEST; a local forum for physicians to receive information and exchange views. Text in English. 1987. m. USD 35 (effective 2000). adv. charts, illus, stat. back issues avail. **Document type:** *Newspaper.* **Description:** Provides news and information on issues of interest to physicians.
Published by: Physician's News Digest, Inc., 230 Windsor Ave, Narberth, PA 19072. TEL 610-668-1040, FAX 610-668-9177, phyweb@physiciansnews.com, http://www.physiciansnews.com. Ed., Pub., R&P Jeffrey Barg. Adv. contact Peter Heiman. Circ: 29,704 (paid and controlled).

610 USA
PHYSICIAN'S PATIENT NEWSLETTER. Text in English. 1983. q. USD 645 per quarter for 1000 copies (effective 2001). index. 4 p./no. 3 cols./p. **Document type:** *Newsletter, Consumer.* **Description:** For family practice physicians and general practitioners to use to market their practice by providing health information.
Published by: Newsletters Ink, PO Box 2019, Lancaster, PA 17608-2019. TEL 717-393-1000, 800-379-5585, FAX 717-393-4702, http://www.newslettersink.com. Ed. Ann Mead Ash. Pub. Gregory A Gilson.

610 USA ISSN 1072-2912
PHYSICIAN'S PRACTICE DIGEST. Text in English. 1993. bi-m. **Document type:** *Magazine, Trade.* **Description:** Provides timely, practical information on practice management, remaining competitive in the face of managed care, legal and legislative issues, and personal finance.
Published by: Medical Communications Network, 4800 Roland Ave, Ste 201, Baltimore, MD 21210. TEL 410-662-1500, FAX 410-662-4100, info@ppdnet.com, http://www.ppdnet.com. Circ: 174,125 (controlled).

PHYSICIANS' TRAVEL & MEETING GUIDE. see *TRAVEL AND TOURISM*

610 USA ISSN 1047-3793
PHYSICIAN'S WEEKLY. Text in English. 198?. w. free to qualified personnel (effective 2001). **Document type:** *Academic/Scholarly.* **Description:** Offers highlights and analyses of medical news about a wide range of specialties.
Related titles: Online - full text ed.
Address: 529 Fifth Ave, New York, NY 10017. TEL 212-376-2930, editor@physweekly.com, http://www.physweekly.com. Eds. Joyce Frieden, Katherine Wandersee. Pub. Patrice Culligan. R&P Howard Larsen. Adv. contact Tracy Murray.

PHYSICS IN MEDICINE AND BIOLOGY. see *BIOLOGY—Biophysics*

615.8 DEU ISSN 0940-6689
CODEN: PMRKEU
PHYSIKALISCHE MEDIZIN REHABILITATIONSMEDIZIN KURORTMEDIZIN. Text in German; Summaries in English, German. 1949. 6/yr. EUR 121.80 domestic to institutions; EUR 125.80 in Europe to institutions; EUR 130.80 elsewhere to institutions; EUR 24 newsstand/cover (effective 2002). adv. bk.rev. abstr, charts, illus. *Refereed.* **Document type:** *Journal, Academic/Scholarly.*
Former titles (until 1991): Zeitschrift fuer Physiotherapie (0003-9357); Archiv fuer Physikalische Therapie, Balneologie und Klimatologie
Related titles: Online - full text ed.: ISSN 1439-085X (from Institute for Scientific Information).
Indexed: ASCA, Biol.Abstr., Chem.Abstr., Excerp.Med., Focus on: Sports Sci.& Med., INIS Atomind., Ind.Med. (coverage dropped).
—BLDSC (6482.280000), CISTI, EMDOCS, GNLM, IDS, Infotrieve. **CCC.**
Published by: (Deutsche Gesellschaft fuer Physikalische Medizin und Rehabilitation), Georg Thieme Verlag, Ruedigerstr 14, Stuttgart 70469, Germany. TEL 49-711-8931-0, FAX 49-711-8931298, physmed@thieme.de, leser.service@thieme.de, http://www.thieme.de/physmed, http://www.thieme-connect.de. Ed. U Smolenszi. R&P Alessandra Kreibaum. Circ: 3,100. **Subscr. to:** Postfach 301120, Stuttgart 70451, Germany.

615.8 CAN ISSN 0706-4284
PHYSIO-QUEBEC. Text in French. 1975. 4/yr. CND 37 domestic to non-members; CND 48 foreign to non-members (effective 2000). adv. bk.rev. illus. **Document type:** *Trade.*
Published by: Ordre Professionnel des Physiotherapeutes du Quebec/Professional Corporation of Physiotherapists of Quebec, 7101 rue Jean Talon Est, bureau 1120, Anjou, PQ H1M 3N7, Canada. TEL 514-351-2770, FAX 514-351-2658. Ed. Odette Trepanier. adv.: B&W page CND 1,050, color page CND 1,575; 9.5 x 7. Circ: 4,000.

610 530 GBR ISSN 0967-3334
CODEN: PMEAE3
PHYSIOLOGICAL MEASUREMENT. Text in English. 1980. q. USD 467 to institutions (effective 2000). adv. bk.rev. bibl, illus, charts. index. back issues avail.; reprints avail. *Refereed.* **Description:** Covers the applications of physics and physical measurement to clinical practice and investigation.
Formerly: Clinical Physics and Physiological Measurement (0143-0815)
Related titles: Microfiche ed.: USD 351; Microfilm ed.: (from AIP); Online - full text ed.: (from EBSCO Publishing, RoweCom Information Quest, Swets Blackwell, Institute for Scientific Information).
Indexed: ASCA, Aqua.Sci.& Fish.Abstr., BBCI, Biol.Abstr., Cal.Tiss.Abstr., Curr.Adv.Ecol.Sci., Curr.Cont., Dent.Ind., Environ.Sci.Poll.Mgmt., Excerp.Med., INSPEC (Feb.1980-Nov.1992, Feb.1993-), Ind.Med. (1993-), Ind.Sci.Rev., Inpharma, Int.Abstr.Biol.Sci., Neurosci.Cit.Ind., Pharm.&Out.News, Pollut.Abstr., Reac., Risk Abstr., Saf.Sci.Abstr., Sci.Cit.Ind.
—BLDSC (6484.760000), AskIEEE, CISTI, Ei, EMDOCS, GNLM, IDS, ingenta, Linda Hall. **CCC.**
Published by: (Institute of Physics), I O P Publishing Ltd., Dirac House, Temple Back, Bristol BS1 6BE, United Kingdom. TEL 44-117-929-7481, FAX 44-117-929-4318, custserv@iopublishing.co.uk, http://www.iop.org, http:/www.iop.org. Ed. S J Meldrum. Adv. contact Chris Manning. Circ: 214. **Subscr. addr. in US:** American Institute of Physics, Subscriber Service, Ste 1N01, 2 Huntingdon Quadrangle, Melville, NY 11747-4502. TEL 516-576-2200. **Co-sponsor:** Institute of Physical Sciences in Medicine.

PHYSIOLOGICAL REVIEWS. see *BIOLOGY—Physiology*

THE PHYSIOLOGIST. see *BIOLOGY—Physiology*

612 CAN ISSN 0822-9058
PHYSIOLOGY CANADA. Text in English, French. 1969. 3/yr. CND 12 domestic to non-members; CND 15 in United States to non-members; CND 18 foreign to non-members (effective 1999). adv. bk.rev. **Document type:** *Academic/Scholarly.*
Indexed: Biol.Abstr.
—CISTI, GNLM.
Published by: Institute for Biological Sciences, National Research Council Canada, Building M 54, Montreal Rd Campus, Ottawa, ON K1A 0R6, Canada. TEL 613-990-0829, philip.hicks@nrc.ca. Ed. T Philip Hicks. R&P, Adv. contact T. Philip Hicks. Circ: 700.

610 DEU ISSN 0944-7113
RM666.H33
PHYTOMEDICINE. Text in German. 1994. 8/yr. EUR 165 to individuals; DEM 384 to institutions; GBP 103 to individuals; GBP 225 to institutions (effective 2002). *Refereed.* **Document type:** *Journal, Academic/Scholarly.* **Description:** Publishes results of research on phytotherapy, phytopharmacology and phytotoxicology obtained with plant extracts, as well as isolated compounds from these extracts.
Related titles: Online - full text ed.: (from Swets Blackwell, Institute for Scientific Information).
Indexed: Abstr.Hyg., Aqua.Sci.& Fish.Abstr., Aquacult.Abstr., BBCI, Chem.Abstr., Chem.Titles, Curr.Cont. (coverage dropped), Derwent Biotech.Abstr., Environ.Sci.Poll.Mgmt., Forest Prod.Abstr., Forest.Abstr., Hort.Abstr., Ind.Med. (1994-), Inpharma, Nutr.Abstr., Ocean.Abstr., Plant Breed.Abstr., Plant Gen.Res.Abstr., Protozool.Abstr., Reac., Rev.Appl.Entomol., Rev.Arom.& Med.Plants, Rev.Med.& Vet.Mycol., Rev.Plant Path., Seed Abstr., Weed Abstr.
—CASDDS, CISTI, GNLM, IDS, Infotrieve. **CCC.**
Published by: Urban & Fischer Verlag, Loebdergraben 14A, Jena 07743, Germany. TEL 49-3641-626430, FAX 49-3641-626421, info@urbanfischer.de, http://www.urbanfischer.de. Eds. H Wagner, N R Farnsworth.

PHYTOTHERAPY RESEARCH; an international journal devoted to medical and scientific research on plants and plant products. see *BIOLOGY—Botany*

610 ITA
PIANETA MEDICO. Text in Italian. 3/yr. ITL 20,000 (effective 1995).
Published by: Casa Editrice Scientifica Internazionale Periodici s.a.s., Via Cremona, 19, Rome, RM 00161, Italy. TEL 39-6-55490783, FAX 39-6-44241-598.

610 615 USA ISSN 1088-3460
PICTORIAL DIRECTORY OF SPOKANE PHYSICIANS. Text in English. 1977. a. USD 75 (effective 1998 & 1999). adv. bibl. **Document type:** *Directory.* **Description:** For physicians, medical personnel, businesses and community members.
Published by: Spokane County Medical Society, 1101 College Ave, Ste 355, Spokane, WA 99201. TEL 509-325-5010, FAX 509-325-5409, scms@iea.com. Ed. Rod Trytko. Adv. contact Shelley Jeffers. page USD 985; trim 10 x 7.5. Circ: 3,700.

610 ITA
PIEMONTE MEDICO. Text in Italian. 1953. m. free per issue. adv.
Formerly: Ordine dei Medici. Bollettino (0471-7708)
Published by: Federazione Regionale Ordini dei Medici Chirurghi e degli Odontoiatri, Via Sebastiano Caboto, 35, Turin, TO 10129, Italy. Ed. Luigi Triberti. Circ: 20,150.

PILLS-A-GO-GO; journal of pills. see *PHARMACY AND PHARMACOLOGY*

PITTSBURGH SERIES IN PHILOSOPHY & HISTORY OF SCIENCE. see *PHILOSOPHY*

610 BEL ISSN 0774-7950
PLACE DE LA SANTE. Text in French. 1986. m.
Address: Rue du Gouvernement Provisoire 29, Brussels 1000, Belgium. Ed. Christine Peers.

610.69 CAN ISSN 1200-0701
PLACE OF GRADUATION; a status report on the place of graduation for selected health personnel in the province of British Columbia. Text in English. 1975. biennial. free per issue. **Document type:** *Bulletin.* **Description:** Provides an analysis by province or country of graduation for each of the groups represented.
Formerly: Place of Graduation for Selected Health Occupations
Published by: University of British Columbia, Centre for Health Services and Policy Research, 429 2194 Health Sciences Mall, Vancouver, BC V6T 1Z3, Canada. TEL 604-822-4810, FAX 604-822-5690, hhru@chspr.ubc.ca, http://www.chspr.ubc.ca. Circ: 200 (controlled).

612.63 GBR ISSN 0143-4004
QP281 CODEN: PLACDF
PLACENTA. Text in English. 1980. 11/yr. GBP 182 to individuals; GBP 377 to institutions (effective 2002). adv. bk.rev. bibl, charts, illus, stat. index. back issues avail.; reprint service avail. from SWZ. *Refereed.* **Document type:** *Academic/Scholarly.* **Description:** Examines relevant areas of placental morphology, physiology, endocrinology, immunology, pharmacology, cell biology, placental microbiology, pathology, and toxicology.
Related titles: Online - full text ed.: (from EBSCO Publishing, RoweCom Information Quest, Swets Blackwell, IDEAL Online Library, Institute for Scientific Information).
Indexed: ASCA, Abstr.Hyg., Biol.Abstr., Chem.Abstr., Chem.Titles, Curr.Adv.Cell & Devel.Biol., Curr.Adv.Ecol.Sci., Curr.Cont., Excerp.Med., Ind.Med. (1980-), Ind.Sci.Rev., Inpharma, Int.Abstr.Biol.Sci., Nutr.Abstr., Pharm.&Out.News, Protozool.Abstr., Reac., Sci.Cit.Ind., THA.
—BLDSC (6506.800000), CASDDS, CISTI, GNLM, IDS, ingenta, KNAW. **CCC.**
Published by: W.B. Saunders Co. Ltd. (Subsidiary of: Harcourt Publishers Ltd.), 24-28 Oval Rd, London NW1 7DX, United Kingdom. TEL 44-20-7424-4200, FAX 44-20-7424-4515, cservice@harcourt.com, http://www.harcourt-international.com/journals/plac. Eds. C P Sibley, L Myatt. **Subcr. to:** Harcourt Publishers Ltd., Foots Cray High St, Sidcup, Kent DA14 5HP, United Kingdom. TEL 44-20-8308-5700, FAX 44-20-8309-0807.

PLUNKETT'S HEALTH CARE INDUSTRY ALMANAC. see *BUSINESS AND ECONOMICS—Trade And Industrial Directories*

610 CZE ISSN 0551-1038
PLZENSKY LEKARSKY SBORNIK/PLZEN MEDICAL REPORT. Text in Czech; Summaries in English. 1956. a. CZK 60 per issue (effective 1999). *Refereed.* **Document type:** *Academic/Scholarly.* **Description:** Contains original research papers on theoretical and clinical medicine.
Related titles: ♦ Supplement: Plzensky Lekarsky Sbornik. Supplementum. ISSN 0139-603X.
Indexed: INIS Atomind.
—CISTI, GNLM.
Published by: (Univerzita Karlova, Lekarska Fakulta), Vydavatelstvi Karolinum, Ovocny trh 5, Prague 116 36, Czech Republic. TEL 42-2-24491270, FAX 42-2-24212041, edice@cuni.cz; sobotka@lfp.cuni.cz. Ed., Pub. Pavel Sobotka. Circ: 180. **Subscr. addr.:** Ustav Patologicke Fyziologie Lekarske Fakulty UK v Plzni, Lidicka 1, Plzen 30166, Czech Republic. TEL 42-019-557209, FAX 42-019-521943.

610 CZE ISSN 0139-603X
PLZENSKY LEKARSKY SBORNIK. SUPPLEMENTUM. Text in Czech. 1956. irreg.
Related titles: ♦ Supplement to: Plzensky Lekarsky Sbornik. ISSN 0551-1038.
Published by: (Univerzita Karlova), Vydavatelstvi Karolinum, Ovocny trh 5, Prague 116 36, Czech Republic. TEL 42-2-24491270, FAX 42-2-24212041.

616 USA ISSN 1533-029X
▼ **POINT OF CARE**; the journal of near-patient testing and technology. Text in English. forthcoming 2002. q. USD 89 to individuals; USD 150 to institutions (effective 2002). *Refereed.* **Document type:** *Journal, Academic/Scholarly.* **Description:** Provides a guide to the latest technologies, trends, issues, and research in near-patient testing worldwide.
Related titles: Online - full text ed.: USD 195 academic site license; USD 217.50 corporate site license (effective 2002).
Published by: Lippincott Williams & Wilkins (Philadelphia) (Subsidiary of: Wolters Kluwer N.V.), 530 Walnut St, Philadelphia, PA 19106-3621. TEL 215-521-8300, FAX 215-521-8902, custserv@lww.com, http://www.poctjournal.com, http://www.lww.com/. Ed. Dr. Kent B. Lewandrowski. **Subscr. to:** PO Box 1600, Hagerstown, MD 21740-1600. TEL 800-638-3030, FAX 310-223-2400.

POLARFRONTEN. see *EARTH SCIENCES*

610 ITA ISSN 0048-4717
POLICLINICO. SEZIONE MEDICA. Text in English, Italian; Summaries in English. 1893. q. USD 80 (effective 2002). adv. illus.
Indexed: Chem.Abstr., Excerp.Med., Ind.Med. (coverage dropped).
—BLDSC (6543.302000), CISTI.
Published by: Edizioni Luigi Pozzi s.r.l., Via Panama, 68, Rome, RM 00198, Italy. TEL 39-06-8553548, FAX 39-06-8554105, edizioni_pozzi@tin.it. Circ: 1,500.

610 ITA ISSN 0032-2644
POLICLINICO. SEZIONE PRATICA. Text in Italian; Summaries in English, Italian. 1893. m. USD 150 (effective 2002). adv. bk.rev. charts, illus, stat. index. **Description:** Covers internal medicine.
Indexed: Chem.Abstr., Dent.Ind., Excerp.Med.
—BLDSC (6543.304000), CISTI.
Published by: Edizioni Luigi Pozzi s.r.l., Via Panama, 68, Rome, RM 00198, Italy. TEL 39-06-8553548, FAX 39-06-8554105, edizioni_pozzi@tin.it. Circ: 10,300.

POLIMERY W MEDYCYNIE. see *CHEMISTRY—Organic Chemistry*

610 USA ISSN 1066-5331
POLIO NETWORK NEWS. Text in English. q. USD 20 domestic to individuals; USD 30 foreign to individuals (effective 2001). 12 p./no. 3 cols./p. back issues avail. **Document type:** *Newsletter, Consumer.* **Description:** Serves as a communications network for polio survivors, support groups and health professionals. Highlights the late effects of polio (post-polio syndrome): its cause, treatment, and current research.
Published by: (International Polio Network), Gazette International Networking Institute, 4207 Lindell Blvd., Ste. 110, St. Louis, MO 63108-2915. TEL 314-534-0475, FAX 314-534-5070, gini_intl@msn.com, http://www.post-polio.org/ivun.html. Ed. Joan Headley. Circ: 6,000.

610 POL ISSN 1426-9686
CODEN: POLEAQ
POLSKI MERKURIUSZ LEKARSKI. Text in Polish; Summaries in English. 1946. m. PLZ 120 domestic; USD 100 foreign (effective 2002). adv. bk.rev., Website rev. abstr, charts, illus, bibl, tr.lit. s-a. index. reprints avail. *Refereed.* **Document type:** *Journal, Academic/Scholarly.* **Description:** Presents papers, editorials and case reports on radiodiagnosis, nuclear medicine, medical disciplines, social hygiene, deontology and ethics.
Supersedes (in July 1996): Polski Tygodnik Lekarski (0032-3756)
Related titles: E-mail ed.
Indexed: Biol.Abstr., C.I.S. Abstr., Chem.Abstr., Chem.Titles, Dent.Ind., Dok.Arbeitsmed., Excerp.Med. (until 1993), INIS Atomind., Ind.Med. (1996-), Nutr.Abstr., Protozool.Abstr., Rev.Plant Path.
—BLDSC (6545.710000), CASDDS, CISTI, GNLM, KNAW.
Published by: MedPress, Ul Slonki 67, Warsaw 02814, Poland. TEL 48-22-6252420, FAX 48-22-6252420, medpress@waw.pdi.net. Ed. Tadeusz Plusa. Circ: 9,200.

610 RUS
POMOGI SEBE SAM; netraditsionnye metody fizicheskogo i dukhovnogo ozdorovleniya cheloveka. Text in Russian. 1995. m., latest vol.83, 2001. RUR 220 domestic; USD 99 foreign; USD 15 newsstand/cover (effective 2001). adv. 16 p./no. back issues avail. **Document type:** *Newspaper.*
Published by: Mezhdunarodnyi Fond/Pomogi Sebe Sam, Volgogradskii prosp 46-15, Moscow 109125, Russian Federation. TEL 7-095-1734519, FAX 7-095-1789864, fond@pss.ru, fond@fpss.ru, http://www.fpss.ru. Ed. L K Kazar'yan. adv.: page USD 700; 260 x 375. **Dist. by:** East View Publications, 3020 Harbor Ln N, Minneapolis, MN 55447. TEL 763-550-0961, FAX 763-559-2931.

610 POL ISSN 1427-440X
CODEN: RPMKAA
POMORSKA AKADEMIA MEDYCZNA W SZCZECINIE. ROCZNIKI/ANNALES ACADEMIAE MEDICAE STETINENSIS. Text in Polish; Summaries in English. 1951. a. price varies. bibl, illus. **Document type:** *Monographic series, Academic/Scholarly.*
Formerly (until 1991): Pomorska Akademia Medyczna im. Gen. Karola Swierczewskiego. Roczniki (0066-1945)
Related titles: ♦ Supplement: Annales Academiae Medicae Stetinensis. Suplement. ISSN 1427-4930.
Indexed: Chem.Abstr., Chem.Indus.Notes, Chem.Titles, Dent.Ind., Excerp.Med. (until 1995), Ind.Med. (coverage dropped), Int.Nurs.Ind.
—BLDSC, CASDDS, CISTI, GNLM.
Published by: (Pomorska Akademia Medyczna w Szczecinie), Wydawnictwo Lekarskie PZWL, ul Dluga 38/40, Warsaw 00-950, Poland. TEL 48-22-8314281, FAX 48-22-8310054, krystyna.regulska@pzwl.pl, http://www.pzwl.pl. Circ: 400. **Dist. by:** Ars Polona, Krakowskie Przedmiescie 7, Warsaw, Poland. TEL 48-22-9263914, FAX 48-22-9265334, arspolona@arspolona.com.pl.

610 BRA ISSN 0103-2690
PONTIFICIA UNIVERSIDADE CATOLICA DO RIO GRANDE DO SUL. REVISTA DE MEDICINA. Text in Portuguese. 1988. 4/yr. BRL 15, USD 19.
Indexed: INIS Atomind.
Published by: (Pontificia Universidade Catolica do Rio Grande do Sul), Editora da P U C R S, c/o Antoninho M. Naime, Partenon, Caixa Postal 12001, Porto Alegre, RGS 90651-970, Brazil. Ed. Leonel Lerner. Circ: 3,000.

610 USA
POST-POLIO DIRECTORY. Text in English. a. USD 5 domestic to individuals; USD 7 foreign to individuals (effective 2001). 22 p./no. 4 cols./p. **Document type:** *Directory, Consumer, Corporate.* **Description:** Lists self-identified clinics, health professionals, and support groups knowledgeable about the late effects of polio.
Related titles: Online - full text ed.
Published by: (International Polio Network), Gazette International Networking Institute, 4207 Lindell Blvd., Ste. 110, St. Louis, MO 63108-2915. TEL 314-534-0475, FAX 314-534-5070, gini_intl@msn.com, http://www.post-polio.org/ivun.html.

POSTEPY BIOLOGII KOMORKI/ADVANCES IN CELL BIOLOGY. see *BIOLOGY—Cytology And Histology*

610 POL ISSN 0032-5449
CODEN: PHMDAD
POSTEPY HIGIENY I MEDYCYNY DOSWIADCZALNEJ. Text in Polish; Summaries in English, Russian. 1949. bi-m. USD 72. charts, illus. index. reprint service avail. from ISI. **Document type:** *Academic/Scholarly.* **Description:** Reports of experimental medical research, proceedings of scientific conferences on immunology and experimental medicine.
Indexed: Abstr.Hyg., Biol.Abstr., Chem.Abstr., Chem.Indus.Notes, Chem.Titles, Curr.Adv.Ecol.Sci., INIS Atomind., Ind.Med. (1949-), Nutr.Abstr., Rev.Plant Path., Trop.Dis.Bull.
—CASDDS, CISTI, GNLM.
Published by: (Polska Akademia Nauk/Polish Academy of Sciences, Instytut Immunologii i Terapii Doswiadczalnej), Ossolineum Publishing House of the Polish Academy of Sciences, Pl Solny 14 a, Wroclaw 50062, Poland. TEL 48-71-343-6961, FAX 48-71-448-103. Ed. M Mordarski. Circ: 980.

610.711 POL ISSN 0860-6196
POSTEPY NAUK MEDYCZNYCH. Text in Polish. 1988. 6/yr.
Indexed: Nutr.Abstr., Protozool.Abstr., Rev.Med.& Vet.Mycol.
—GNLM.
Published by: Centrum Medyczne Ksztalcenia Podyplomowego, Ul Marymoncka 99, Warsaw 01813, Poland. TEL 48-22-346847, FAX 48-22-340470, TELEX 816826. Ed. Ryszard Brzozowski.

610 CZE ISSN 1212-4184
▼ **POSTGRADUALNI MEDICINA.** Text in Czech. 1999. bi-m. **Document type:** *Magazine, Trade, Academic/Scholarly.*
Published by: Strategie Praha s.r.o., Drtinova 8, Prague, 5 150 00, Czech Republic. TEL 420-2-57323578, FAX 420-2-57018362, strategie.praha@istrategie.cz, http://www.istrategie.cz.

610 GBR ISSN 0267-0275
POSTGRADUATE DOCTOR: CARIBBEAN; the journal of prevention, diagnosis and treatment. Text in English. 1984. bi-m. GBP 45 domestic to individuals; GBP 49 in Europe to individuals; GBP 54 rest of world to individuals; GBP 67.50 domestic to institutions; GBP 71.50 in Europe to institutions; GBP 74.50 rest of world to institutions (effective 2002). adv. bk.rev. charts, illus. index. back issues avail. *Refereed.* **Document type:** *Academic/Scholarly.* **Description:** Contains specially commissioned review articles of general medicine at the postgraduate level for practicing physicians throughout the English-speaking Caribbean.
Indexed: Abstr.Hyg., Nutr.Abstr., Protozool.Abstr., Rev.Med.& Vet.Mycol., Trop.Dis.Bull.
—ingenta. **CCC.**
Published by: P M H Publications Ltd., PO Box 100, Chichester, W Sussex PO18 8HD, United Kingdom. TEL 44-1243-576444, FAX 44-1243-576456, doctor@pmh.uk.com, http://www.pmh.uk.com. Ed. David Harvey. Pub. Peter Harkness. Adv. contact Ryszard Holowenko. Circ: 3,100 (controlled).

610 GBR ISSN 0140-7724
POSTGRADUATE DOCTOR: MIDDLE EAST; the journal of prevention, diagnosis & treatment. Text in English. 1978. bi-m. GBP 28 to individuals; GBP 31 in Europe to individuals; GBP 35 rest of world to individuals; GBP 42 to institutions; GBP 45 in Europe to institutions; GBP 50 rest of world to institutions (effective 2002). adv. bk.rev. charts, illus. back issues avail. **Document type:** *Academic/Scholarly.* **Description:** Contains specially commissioned graduate-level review clinical articles aimed at practicing physicians in the Middle East.
Indexed: Abstr.Hyg., Nutr.Abstr., Trop.Dis.Bull.
—BLDSC (6563.852000), ingenta. **CCC.**
Published by: P M H Publications Ltd., PO Box 100, Chichester, W Sussex PO18 8HD, United Kingdom. TEL 44-1243-576444, FAX 44-1243-576456, doctor@pmh.uk.com, http://www.pmh.uk.com. Ed. David Harvey. Pub., R&P Peter Harkness. Adv. contact Ryszard Holowenko.

610.71 IND ISSN 0302-2404
CODEN: BPIRD8
POSTGRADUATE INSTITUTE OF MEDICAL EDUCATION AND RESEARCH, CHANDIGARH. BULLETIN. Text in English. 1967. q. INR 50 to individuals; USD 25 to institutions. adv. bk.rev. bibl, illus. **Document type:** *Bulletin.* **Description:** Contains articles contributed by faculty and students of the Institute. Includes editorial and research articles, case reports, and a Clinico-Pathological Conference report.

Indexed: Abstr.Hyg., Biol.Abstr., Chem.Abstr., Chem.Indus.Notes, Chem.Titles, Excerp.Med., INIS Atomind., Ind.Sci.Rev., Nutr.Abstr., Rev.Appl.Entomol., Rural Devel.Abstr., Trop.Dis.Bull.
—CASDDS, CISTI, EMDOCS, GNLM, KNAW.
Published by: Postgraduate Institute of Medical Education and Research Chandigarh, Chandigarh, Haryana 160 012, India. TEL 45157, TELEX 395-315 PGI IN. Ed. N K Gangauly. Circ: 550.

610 GBR ISSN 0032-5473
CODEN: PGMJAO

POSTGRADUATE MEDICAL JOURNAL. Text in English. m. GBP 105, USD 169 combined subscription to individuals includes print & online eds.; GBP 231, USD 370 to institutions print only (effective 2002). adv. bk.rev. bibl, charts, illus, stat. index. back issues avail.; reprint service avail. from ISI. *Refereed.* **Document type:** *Journal, Academic/Scholarly.* **Description:** Contains current clinical research and practice, surveys and case reports.
Former titles (until 1925): Fellowship of Medicine and Post-graduate Medical Association. Bulletin (0951-4341); (until 1919): Fellowship of Medicine. Emergency Post-graduate Scheme. Weekly Programme
Related titles: Microfilm ed.: (from PQC,SWZ); Online - full text ed.: GBP 65, USD 99 to individuals (effective 2002) (from HighWire Pr., Northern Light Technology, Inc., EBSCO Publishing, O C L C Online Computer Library Center, Inc., RoweCom Information Quest, ProQuest Information & Learning, ingenta, Swets Blackwell, Ovid Technologies, Inc., Institute for Scientific Information); ♦ Supplement: Postgraduate Medical Journal. Supplement. ISSN 0370-0593.
Indexed: ASCA, Abstr.Health Care Manage.Stud., Abstr.Hyg., Agri.& Environ.Biotech.Abstr. (coverage dropped), Biol.Abstr., CINAHL, Chem.Abstr., Chem.Indus.Notes, Chem.Titles, Curr.Adv.Cancer Res., Curr.Adv.Ecol.Sci., Curr.Cont., Dent.Ind., Derwent Biotech.Abstr., Excerp.Med., Fam.Ind., Food Sci.& Tech.Abstr., Helminthol.Abstr., INIS Atomind., I.P.A., Ind.Med. (1925-), Ind.Sci.Rev., Inpharma, Int.Nurs.Ind., NRN, Neurosci.Cit.Ind., Nutr.Abstr., Pharm.&Out.News, Protozool.Abstr., Reac., Rev.Appl.Entomol., Rev.Med.& Vet.Mycol., SSCI (coverage dropped), Sci.Cit.Ind., THA, Trop.Dis.Bull.
—BLDSC (6563.860000), ADONIS, CASDDS, CISTI, GNLM, IDS, ingenta, KNAW. **CCC.**
Published by: (Fellowship of Postgraduate Medicine), B M J Publishing Group, B M A House, Tavistock Sq, London WC1H 9JR, United Kingdom. TEL 44-20-7387-4499, FAX 44-20-7383-6400, info.norththames@bma.org.uk, http://www.postgradmedj.com, http://www.bma.org.uk. Ed. C Hind.

610 GBR ISSN 0370-0593
CODEN: PMESAJ

POSTGRADUATE MEDICAL JOURNAL. SUPPLEMENT. Text in English. 1949. irreg. **Document type:** *Academic/Scholarly.*
Related titles: ♦ Supplement to: Postgraduate Medical Journal. ISSN 0032-5473.
Indexed: Chem.Abstr., Chem.Indus.Notes, Chem.Titles, Curr.Cont. (coverage dropped).
—CASDDS, KNAW. **CCC.**
Published by: (Fellowship of Postgraduate Medicine), B M J Publishing Group, B M A House, Tavistock Sq, London WC1H 9JR, United Kingdom. TEL 44-20-7387-4499, FAX 44-20-7383-6400, info.norththames@bma.org.uk, http://www.postgradmedj.com, http://www.bma.org.uk.

610 USA ISSN 0032-5481
R11 CODEN: POMDAS

POSTGRADUATE MEDICINE; the journal of applied medicine for physicians providing primary care. Text in English. 1947. m. USD 54 domestic; USD 56 in Canada & Mexico; USD 130 elsewhere; USD 10 newsstand/cover (effective 2000). adv. bk.rev. charts, illus. s-a. index. reprint service avail. from PQC. *Refereed.* **Document type:** *Academic/Scholarly, Trade.* **Description:** Presents original clinical articles stressing the diagnosis and treatment of problems encountered in general medical practice.
Related titles: Microfilm ed.: (from PQC,PMC); Online - full text ed.: (from The Dialog Corporation, Dow Jones Interactive, Gale Group, NewsNet, Northern Light Technology, Inc., LexisNexis, Institute for Scientific Information); ♦ Hungarian Translation: Orvostovabbkepzo Szemle. ISSN 1218-2583.
Indexed: AIDS Abstr., AIM, ASCA, AgeLine, Biol.Abstr., CHNI, CINAHL, C.I.S. Abstr., Chem.Abstr., Curr.Adv.Cancer Res., Curr.Adv.Ecol.Sci., Curr.Cont., Dent.Ind., Diar.Dis.Res., Excerp.Med., FAMLI, Helminthol.Abstr., INIS Atomind., Ind.Med. (1947-), Inpharma, Int.Nurs.Ind., Med.& Surg.Dermat., NRN, Nutr.Abstr., Pharm.&Out.News, Reac., Rev.Med.& Vet.Mycol., SSCI (coverage dropped), Sci.Cit.Ind., THA.
—BLDSC (6563.900000), CISTI, GNLM, IDS, ingenta, KNAW. **CCC.**
Published by: McGraw-Hill Companies, 4530 W 77th St Ste 350, Minneapolis, MN 55435. TEL 952-832-7848, FAX 952-835-3460, http://www.postgradmed.com. Ed. Peter Setness. Pub. Gary Gyss. Adv. contact Debra Watson. B&W page USD 9,640, color page USD 11,900. Circ: 130,000. **Subscr. to:** PO Box 459, Hightstown, NJ 08520-9201.

610 POL ISSN 0137-5350
CODEN: POMDDV

POZNANSKIE ROCZNIKI MEDYCZNE. Text in Polish. 1964. a. **Document type:** *Academic/Scholarly.*
Formerly (until 1977): Roczniki Akademii Medycznej w Poznaniu (0137-5369)
Indexed: Chem.Abstr., Chem.Indus.Notes, Chem.Titles, INIS Atomind., Zoo.Rec.
—CASDDS, GNLM.
Published by: (Akademia Medyczna im. Karola Marcinkowskiego w Poznaniu), Wydawnictwo Naukowe P W Nowe, Ul Miodowa 10, Warsaw 00251, Poland. TEL 48-22-6954321, FAX 48-22-6954288. **Co-sponsors:** Polska Akademia Nauk, Oddzial w Poznaniu; Poznanskie Towarzystwo Przyjaciol Nauk.

613.62 616.9803 CZE ISSN 0032-6291
CODEN: PRLFAG

PRACOVNI LEKARSTVI. Text in Czech, Slovak; Summaries in Czech, English. 1948. q. EUR 56, USD 72 (effective 2001). adv. bk.rev. abstr. index. *Refereed.* **Description:** Covers industrial medicine.
Indexed: Abstr.Hyg., C.I.S. Abstr., Chem.Abstr., Chem.Indus.Notes, Chem.Titles, Ergon.Abstr., Excerp.Med., INIS Atomind., Ind.Med. (coverage dropped), Trop.Dis.Bull.
—BLDSC (6593.500000), CASDDS, CISTI, GNLM, Infotrieve. **CCC.**
Published by: (Ceska Lekarska Spolecnost J.E. Purkyne/Czech Medical Association), Nakladatelske Stredisko C L S J.E. Purkyne, Sokolska 31, Prague 12026, Czech Republic. TEL 420-2-24911420, FAX 420-2-24911420, nts@iol.cz, http://www.clsjep.cz, http://www.medical.cz. Ed. E Hrncit. adv.: B&W page CZK 19,600, color page CZK 27,700; 250 x 170. Circ: 550. **Dist. by:** Abont s.r.o., Chlumova 17, Prague, 3 130 00, Czech Republic; **Dist. in Western Countries by:** Kubon & Sagner, Hesstr 39-41, Munich 80798, Germany. **Co-sponsor:** Ceska Spolecnost pro Pracovni Lekarstvi.

A PRACTICAL GUIDE TO PREVENTING LEGAL MALPRACTICE. see *LAW*

610 GBR ISSN 0032-6518

THE PRACTITIONER. Text in English. 1868. 12/yr. GBP 69, USD 163 (effective 2000). adv. bk.rev. illus, pat. index. back issues avail.; reprint service avail. from PQC. *Refereed.* **Document type:** *Magazine, Trade.*
Related titles: Microform ed.: (from PQC,PMC); Online - full text ed.: (from ProQuest Information & Learning, Institute for Scientific Information).
Indexed: AMED, Abstr.Anthropol., Abstr.Health Care Manage.Stud., Addic.Abstr., Agri.& Environ.Biotech.Abstr. (coverage dropped), Biol.Abstr., Brit.Nur.Ind., CINAHL, Chem.Abstr., Curr.Adv.Cancer Res., Curr.Adv.Ecol.Sci., Dent.Ind., Derwent Biotech.Abstr., Dok.Arbeitsmed., Excerp.Med. (until 1993), Helminthol.Abstr., INIS Atomind., Ind.Med. (1868-), Int.Nurs.Ind., Nutr.Abstr., Rev.Plant Path., Trop.Dis.Bull.
—BLDSC (6598.000000), CISTI, GNLM, IDS, ingenta, KNAW. **CCC.**
Published by: C M P Information (Subsidiary of: United Business Media), City Reach, 5 Greenwich View Pl, Millharbour, London E14 9NN, United Kingdom. TEL 44-20-78616472, FAX 44-20-7861-6259, http://www.cmpinformation.com. Ed. Harvey Jones. R&P E Ravi. Adv. contact Peter Higgins. Circ: 39,342.

DER PRAEPARATOR. see *CONSERVATION*

610 DEU ISSN 0937-552X

PRAEVENTION UND REHABILITATION. Text in German. 1989. q. DEM 108, EUR 55.22; DEM 28, EUR 14.32 newsstand/cover (effective 2001). adv. abstr. **Document type:** *Journal, Academic/Scholarly.*
Indexed: AMED, Excerp.Med. (1993-).
—BLDSC (6603.024700), GNLM.
Published by: Dustri-Verlag Dr. Karl Feistle, Bajuwarenring 4, Oberhaching 82041, Germany. TEL 49-89-613861-0, FAX 49-89-613-5412, info@dustri.de, http://www.dustri.de. Ed. J Lecheler. R&P Renate Lehmann. Adv. contact Joerg Feistle. B&W page DEM 1,600; trim 167 x 242. Circ: 1,500.

610 CZE ISSN 0032-6739
CODEN: PRLEAD

PRAKTICKY LEKAR. Text in Czech, Slovak; Summaries in Czech, English. 1920. m. EUR 72, USD 84 (effective 2001). adv. bk.rev. abstr, bibl, illus, stat. index, cum.index. *Refereed.*
Indexed: Biol.Abstr., C.I.S. Abstr., Chem.Abstr., INIS Atomind.
—BLDSC (6598.700000), CASDDS, EMDOCS, GNLM, Infotrieve. **CCC.**
Published by: (Ceska Lekarska Spolecnost J.E. Purkyne/Czech Medical Association), Nakladatelske Stredisko C L S J.E. Purkyne, Sokolska 31, Prague 12026, Czech Republic. TEL 42-2-24911420, FAX 42-2-24911420, nts@iol.cz, http://www.clsjep.cz, http://www.medical.cz. Ed. R Honzak. adv.: B&W page CZK 56,500, color page CZK 80,300; 253 x 185. Circ: 5,500. **Dist. by:** Abont s.r.o., Chlumova 17, Prague, 3 130 00, Czech Republic; **Dist. in Western countries by:** Kubon & Sagner, Hesstr 39-41, Munich 80798, Germany.

610 NLD ISSN 0169-1910

PRAKTIJKMANAGEMENT. Text in Dutch. 1985. m. adv. **Document type:** *Trade.*
Published by: Mediselect B.V., Postbus 63, Leusden 3830 AB, Netherlands. TEL 31-33-4229900, FAX 31-33-4229922, info@mediselect.nl.

610 DEU ISSN 0948-8596

PRAXIS - DEPESCHE. Text in German. 1987. bi-m. DEM 45 domestic; DEM 72 foreign (effective 2001). adv. bk.rev. abstr. 48 p./no. 3 cols./p. reprints avail. **Document type:** *Newsletter, Academic/Scholarly.*
Published by: Gesellschaft fuer Medizinische Information, Baumkirchner Str 53A, Munich 81673, Germany. TEL 49-89-4366300, FAX 49-89-43670971, info@gfi.online.de, http://www.gfi.online.de. Eds., Pubs. Hans Spude, Hartmut Ley. Adv. contact Hartmut Ley. Circ: 53,000.

610 USA

▼ **PRAXIS POST.** Text in English. 2000 (Jun.). d. **Document type:** *Magazine, Academic/Scholarly.* **Description:** Covers medicine and culture geared toward physicians in general practice, and contains news, views, featured articles and columns.
Media: Online - full content.
Published by: Praxis Press Inc., 30 W 25th St, New York, NY 10010. TEL 212-366-4900, FAX 212-366-5400, info@praxispress.com, http://praxispress.com/. Ed. Dr. Ivan Oransky.

610 BOL

PRENSA MEDICA. Text in Spanish. 6/yr. adv.
Address: Casilla 891, La Paz, Bolivia. Ed. Dr. Santiago Medeiros.

610 VEN

PRENSA MEDICA. Text in Spanish. 1975. m.
Published by: Editorial Terseg C.A., Edif. San Jose 1o, Avda Principal Mariperez, Caracas, DF 1050, Venezuela. Circ: 8,000.

610 ARG ISSN 0032-745X
CODEN: PMARAU

PRENSA MEDICA ARGENTINA. Text in Spanish; Summaries in English. 1914. m. (10/yr.). USD 120 (effective 2000). adv. bk.rev. charts, illus. index. back issues avail.; reprint service avail. from PQC. *Refereed.* **Document type:** *Trade.* **Description:** Covers current medicine and medical practice.
Related titles: Microform ed.: (from PQC).
Indexed: Biol.Abstr., Curr.Cont. (coverage dropped), Environ.Sci.Poll.Mgmt., Excerp.Med., Helminthol.Abstr., Inpharma, Nutr.Abstr., Pollut.Abstr., Reac.
—BLDSC (6607.700000), CASDDS, CISTI, EMDOCS, GNLM, IDS, KNAW.
Published by: Prensa Medica Argentina s.r.l., Junin, 845, Capital Federal, Buenos Aires 1113, Argentina. TEL 54-114-9619793, FAX 54-114-9619494. Ed. Pablo A Lopez. R&P, Adv. contact Nestor Bonanomi. page USD 1,200; trim 280 x 200. Circ: 5,000 (paid).

PREPARING AND WINNING MEDICAL NEGLIGENCE CASES. see *LAW*

M

PRESCRIBING REFERENCE FOR OBSTETRICIANS AND GYNECOLOGISTS. see *PHARMACY AND PHARMACOLOGY*

PRESCRIBING REFERENCE FOR PEDIATRICIANS. see *PHARMACY AND PHARMACOLOGY*

PRESCRIRE INTERNATIONAL. see *PHARMACY AND PHARMACOLOGY*

610 FRA ISSN 0755-4982
CODEN: PRMEEM
LA PRESSE MEDICALE. Text in English, French. 1893. 40/yr. FRF 1,498; FRF 2,007 foreign (effective 2000). adv. bk.rev. abstr, illus. reprint service avail. from ISI. *Refereed.* **Document type:** *Academic/Scholarly.* **Description:** Publishes leading work in all the clinical specialties of medicine. Includes editorials, original articles, authoritative reviews, and correspondence.
Former titles (until 1982): Nouvelle Presse Medicale (0301-1518); (until 1972): Presse Medicale (0032-7867)
Related titles: Microfiche ed.: (from BHP); Microform ed.: (from PQC,PMC); Online - full text ed.: (from Institute for Scientific Information, RoweCom Information Quest).
Indexed: ASCA, Abstr.Hyg., Agri.& Environ.Biotech.Abstr. (coverage dropped), Aqua.Sci.& Fish.Abstr., Biol.Abstr., C.I.S. Abstr., Cal.Tiss.Abstr., Chem.Abstr., Curr.Adv.Cancer Res., Curr.Adv.Ecol.Sci., Curr.Cont., Dairy Sci.Abstr., Dent.Ind., Derwent Biotech.Abstr., Dok.Arbeitsmed., Environ.Sci.Poll.Mgmt., Excerp.Med., Helminthol.Abstr., INIS Atomind., Ind.Med. (1983-), Ind.Sci.Rev., Inpharma, Int.Nurs.Ind., Med.& Surg.Dermat., Microbiol.Abstr., Neurosci.Cit.Ind., Nutr.Abstr., Pharm.&Out.News, Pollut.Abstr., Protozool.Abstr., Reac., Rev.Appl.Entomol., Rev.Med.& Vet.Mycol., Rev.Plant Path., Risk Abstr., SSCI (coverage dropped), Saf.Sci.Abstr., Sci.Cit.Ind., Tox.Abstr. (coverage dropped), Trop.Dis.Bull., Virol.Abstr. (coverage dropped).
—BLDSC (6612.500000), CASDDS, CISTI, EMDOCS, GNLM, IDS, KNAW. **CCC.**
Published by: Masson - Periodiques, 120 bd. St. Germain, Paris 75006, France. TEL 33-1-40466200, FAX 33-1-40466201. Eds. J C Patel, Dr. Ph Letonturier. Adv. contact M J Leroy. Circ: 16,000. **Subscr. to:** Societe de Periodiques Specialises, BP 22, Vineuil Cedex 41354, France. TEL 33-2-54504612, FAX 33-2-54504611.

610 ITA ISSN 0393-0653
LA PRESSE MEDICALE (EDIZIONE ITALIANA). Text in Italian. 1984. 8/yr. ITL 45,000 (effective 1999). **Document type:** *Academic/Scholarly.*
Indexed: Dairy Sci.Abstr.
Published by: Masson S.p.A., Divisione Periodici, Via F.lli Bressan 2, Milan, MI 20126, Italy. TEL 39-2-270741, FAX 39-2-27074210. Ed. Claudio Ortolani. adv.: B&W page ITL 4,750,000, color page ITL 6,800,000; trim 270 x 210. Circ: 7,000.

615.8 FRA ISSN 0032-7875
CODEN: PTCLA3
PRESSE THERMALE ET CLIMATIQUE. Text in French. 1864. 4/yr. FRF 500 domestic to individuals; FRF 650 foreign to individuals; FRF 250 domestic to students; FRF 325 foreign to students (effective 1999). adv. bk.rev.
Related titles: Microform ed.
Indexed: Biol.Abstr., Chem.Abstr., Dent.Ind., Excerp.Med., GeoRef, INIS Atomind., Ref.Zh.
—CASDDS, CISTI, GNLM, Infotrieve. **CCC.**
Published by: (Societe Francaise d'Hydrologie), Expansion Scientifique Francaise, 31 bd. de la Tour Maubourg, Paris Cedex 7 75343, France. TEL 33-1-40626400, FAX 33-1-45556920. Ed. J Francon. Circ: 2,000.

610 USA ISSN 0889-0242
PRESSURE (BETHESDA). Text in English. 1972. bi-m. USD 30 (effective 2000). bk.rev. abstr, bibl. **Document type:** *Newsletter, Academic/Scholarly.*
Formerly: Hyperbaric Medicine Newsletter (0018-831X)
—CISTI.
Published by: Undersea and Hyperbaric Medical Society, Inc., 10531 Metropolitan Ave, Kensington, MD 20895. TEL 301-942-2980, FAX 301-942-7804, uhms@uhms.org, http://www.uhms.org. Ed. N R Schandelmeier. Circ: 3,000.

610 USA
PREVENTION IN PRACTICE LIBRARY. Text in English. 1996. irreg., latest 2000. price varies. **Document type:** *Monographic series.* **Description:** Illustrates practical applications of prevention techniques, focusing on education, social competence enhancement, natural caregiving, and systems change.
Indexed: e-psyche.
Published by: Kluwer Academic - Plenum Publishers (Subsidiary of: Wolters Kluwer N.V.), 233 Spring St, New York, NY 10013-1578. TEL 212-620-8000, 800-221-9369, FAX 212-463-0742, info@plenum.com, http://www.plenum.com. Ed. Thomas Gullotta.

614 610 USA ISSN 0091-7435
RA421 CODEN: PVTMA3
PREVENTIVE MEDICINE; an international journal devoted to practice and theory. Text in English. 1972. m. USD 636 in US & Canada to institutions; USD 730 elsewhere to institutions (effective 2001). index. back issues avail. *Refereed.* **Document type:** *Academic/Scholarly.*
Related titles: Online - full text ed.: (from EBSCO Publishing, O C L C Online Computer Library Center, Inc., RoweCom Information Quest, ingenta, Swets Blackwell, IDEAL Online Library, Institute for Scientific Information).
Indexed: ASCA, Abstr.Hyg., Addic.Abstr., AgeLine, Bibl.Agri., Biol.Abstr., CINAHL, C.I.S. Abstr., Chem.Abstr., Chem.Indus.Notes, Chem.Titles, Crim.Just.Abstr., Curr.Adv.Cancer Res., Curr.Adv.Ecol.Sci., Curr.Cont., Dairy Sci.Abstr., Dent.Ind., Excerp.Med., Helminthol.Abstr., INIS Atomind., Ind.Med. (1972-), Ind.Sci.Rev., Inpharma, NRN, Nutr.Abstr., Pharm.&Out.News, PsycInfo, Psychol.Abstr. (1993-), Reac., Rural Recreat.Tour.Abstr., SSCI (coverage dropped), Sci.Cit.Ind., THA, Trop.Dis.Bull., e-psyche.
—BLDSC (6612.790000), ADONIS, CASDDS, CISTI, GNLM, IDS, ingenta, KNAW. **CCC.**
Published by: (American Society of Preventive Oncology), Academic Press, Inc., Journal Division (Subsidiary of: Harcourt Brace & Company), 525 B St, Ste 1900, San Diego, CA 92101-4495. TEL 619-230-1840, FAX 619-699-6800, apsubs@acad.com, http:// www.academicpress.com/pm. Ed. Ernst L Wynder.

338.476 USA
▼ **PREVENTIVE MEDICINE IN MANAGED CARE.** Text in English. 2000. q. adv. **Document type:** *Magazine, Trade.* **Description:** Features research, reviews, and opinions that examine real-world experiences in applying prevention and heath promotion practices in today's healthcare delivery systems.
Published by: American Medical Publishing, LLC (Subsidiary of: Medical World Communications), 241 Forsgate Dr, Ste 102, Jamesburg, NJ 08831. TEL 732-656-1006, FAX 732-656-0818, info@pmimc.com, http://www.pmimc.com. Ed. Dr. Cary Sennett. Circ: 54,619.

PREVISIONS GLISSANTES DETAILLEES EN PERSPECTIVES SECTORIELLES (VOL.38): PHARMACIE - SANTE. see *BUSINESS AND ECONOMICS—Economic Situation And Conditions*

610 JPN ISSN 0914-8426
PRIMARY CARE. Text in Japanese; Summaries in English, Japanese. 1977. q. JPY 6,000, USD 48. adv. bk.rev. index. back issues avail.
Formerly (until vol.11, no.1): Japanese Journal of Primary Care (0387-3501)
Published by: (Japanese Medical Society of Primary Care), Kyowa Kikaku Tsushin, 2-20 Shinbashi, Minato-ku, Tokyo 105-0004, Japan. FAX 03-3575-4748. Ed. Dr. Katsumi Iijima. Circ: 2,500.

610 USA ISSN 0095-4543
R11
PRIMARY CARE; clinics in office practice. Text in English. 1974. q. USD 116 domestic to individuals; USD 137 in Canada to individuals; USD 162 elsewhere to individuals; USD 163 domestic to institutions; USD 189 foreign to institutions; USD 48 per issue (effective 2001). reprint service avail. from PQC,ISI. *Refereed.* **Document type:** *Journal, Academic/Scholarly.* **Description:** Contains articles to help primary-care physicians in their practices.
Related titles: Microform ed.: (from MIM,PQC); Online - full text ed.: (from Institute for Scientific Information).
Indexed: CINAHL, Curr.Cont., Dent.Ind., Excerp.Med., FAMLI, INIS Atomind., Ind.Med. (1974-), Inpharma, Pharm.&Out.News, Reac.
—BLDSC (6612.908000), CISTI, GNLM, IDS, ingenta, KNAW. **CCC.**
Published by: W.B. Saunders Co. (Subsidiary of: Harcourt Publishers Ltd.), 11830 Westline Industrial Dr, St Louis, MO 63146. TEL 800-325-4177, http:// www.wbsaunders.com. **Subscr. to:** Periodicals Fulfillment, W B Saunders Co, 6277 Sea Harbor Dr, 4th Fl, Orlando, FL 32891-4800.

610 362.1 USA ISSN 1096-8954
PRIMARY CARE CASE REVIEWS. Text in English. q., latest vol.4. USD 103 domestic to individuals; USD 113 foreign to individuals; USD 144 domestic to institutions; USD 172 foreign to institutions; USD 41 newsstand/cover (effective 2002). adv. **Document type:** *Academic/Scholarly.*
Indexed: Inpharma, Pharm.&Out.News, Reac.
—BLDSC (6612.908150).
Published by: Lippincott Williams & Wilkins (Philadelphia) (Subsidiary of: Wolters Kluwer N.V.), 530 Walnut St, Philadelphia, PA 19106-3621. TEL 215-521-8300, FAX 215-521-8902, www.primarycarecasereviews.com, http://www.lww.com. Ed. Dr. Robert W Schrier. Pub. Christine Rullo. Adv. contact Ray Thibodeau. Circ: 1,000 (paid). **Subscr. to:** PO Box 1600, Hagerstown, MD 21740-1600. TEL 800-777-2295, FAX 301-824-7390.

PRIMARY CARE MEDICINE DRUG ALERTS. see *PHARMACY AND PHARMACOLOGY*

610 362.1 USA
PRIMARY CARE MEDICINE ON CD-ROM. Text in English. 1997. q. USD 99 to individuals (effective 2000). **Document type:** *Academic/Scholarly.*
Media: CD-ROM.
Published by: Lippincott Williams & Wilkins (Philadelphia) (Subsidiary of: Wolters Kluwer N.V.), 530 Walnut St, Philadelphia, PA 19106-3621. TEL 301-223-2300, 800-638-3030, FAX 301-223-2400, http://www.lww.com.

610 USA
PRIMARY CARE SPECIAL EDITION. Text in English. s-a. USD 50 domestic; USD 60 foreign (effective 2001); Free to qualified subscribers. adv. **Document type:** *Trade.* **Description:** Publishes a clinical reference of current information to the primary care physician.
Published by: McMahon Group, 545 W 45th St, 8th Fl, New York, NY 10036. TEL 212-957-5300, FAX 212-957-7230, lrichards@mcmahonmed.com, http://www.mcmahonmed.com/se/indexse.htm. adv.: B&W page USD 4,650, color page USD 1,500.

PRIMARY HEALTH CARE NEWS. see *PUBLIC HEALTH AND SAFETY*

362.1 GBR ISSN 1463-4236
▼ **PRIMARY HEALTH CARE RESEARCH AND DEVELOPMENT.** Text in English. 2000. 4/yr., latest vol.1. GBP 38 in Europe to individuals; USD 62 in North America to individuals; GBP 40 rest of world to individuals; GBP 92 in Europe to institutions; USD 153 in North America to institutions; GBP 99 rest of world to institutions; GBP 29 in Europe to members network members; GBP 48 in developing nations; GBP 37 newsstand/cover in Europe; USD 57 newsstand/cover in North America; GBP 39 newsstand/cover rest of world (effective 2002). adv. back issues avail.; reprints avail. *Refereed.* **Document type:** *Journal, Academic/Scholarly.* **Description:** Aimed specifically at both researchers and practitioners in primary health care, thereby,bridging the gap between the two areas.
Related titles: Online - full text ed.: (from EBSCO Publishing, O C L C Online Computer Library Center, Inc., RoweCom Information Quest, ingenta, Swets Blackwell).
Indexed: Brit.Nur.Ind.
—BLDSC (6612.908982).
Published by: Arnold Publishers (Subsidiary of: Hodder Headline plc.), 338 Euston Rd, London NW1 3BH, United Kingdom. TEL 44-20-7873-6337, FAX 44-20-7873-6325, arnoldjournals@hodder.co.uk, http://www.palliativemedjournal.com. Eds. Rosamund Bryar, Sally Kendall. **Dist. by:** Turpin Distribution Services Ltd., Blackhorse Rd, Letchworth, Herts SG6 1HN, United Kingdom. FAX 44-1462-480947.

610 CHE ISSN 1424-3776
▼ **PRIMARYCARE.** Text in German, French, English. 2000. fortn. CHF 115 domestic; CHF 130 in Europe; CHF 150 elsewhere; CHF 20 newsstand/cover (effective 2001). back issues avail. *Refereed.* **Document type:** *Journal, Trade.*
Related titles: Online - full text ed.: ISSN 1424-3806.
Published by: (Schweizerische Gesellschaft fuer Allgemeinmedizin), E M H Swiss Medical Publishers Ltd., Steinentorstr 13, Basel, Switzerland. TEL 41-61-4678555, FAX 41-61-4678556, primary-care@emh.ch, verlag@emh.ch, http://www.primary-care.ch, http://www.emh.ch.

610 USA ISSN 0032-891X
R11
PRIVATE PRACTICE*. Text in English. 1969. m. USD 18. adv. bk.rev. index. reprint service avail. from PQC.
Related titles: Microform ed.: 1969 (from PQC).

M

Published by: Congress of County Medical Societies (CCMS) Publishing Co., PO Box 1485, Shawnee, OK 74802-1485. Ed. Karen Murphy. Circ: 190,000.

610 ESP ISSN 0212-8837
PROFESION MEDICA; guia de congresos medicos. Text in Spanish. q. bk.rev. illus. **Document type:** *Academic/Scholarly.* **Description:** Covers various medical conferences.
Published by: Saned S.A., Capitan Haya, 60, Madrid 28020, Spain. TEL 34-91-749-9507, FAX 34-91-749-9507, saned@meditex.es. Ed. A Martinez Magro. adv.: page ESP 250,000. Circ: 10,000.

PROFESSIONAL LIABILITY NEWSLETTER. see *LAW*

610 ITA
PROFESSIONE MEDICA. Text in Italian. 1921. m. (13/yr.). ITL 86,000. adv. bk.rev. charts, illus, bibl. index. Supplement avail. **Document type:** *Trade.*
Former titles (until 1992): Federazione Medica (1122-3243); (until 1943): Forze Sanitarie (1122-326X); (until 1932): Federazione Medica (0014-9500)
Indexed: C.I.S. Abstr.
Published by: (Federazione Nazionale degli Ordini dei Medici), C G Edizioni Medico Scientifiche, Via Candido Viberti, 7, Turin, TO 10141, Italy. TEL 39-11-338507, FAX 39-11-3852750, cgems1@uol.it, http://www.cgems.com. Ed. Giorgio Cavallo. Circ: 52,000.

PROFILES IN HEALTHCARE MARKETING; idea exchange for the people who plan and create healthcare marketing and PR campaigns. see *ADVERTISING AND PUBLIC RELATIONS*

PROGRESS IN BIOMEDICAL RESEARCH. see *BIOLOGY—Bioengineering*

610 USA ISSN 0361-7742
CODEN: PCBRD2
PROGRESS IN CLINICAL AND BIOLOGICAL RESEARCH. Text in English. 1975. irreg., latest vol.373, 1992. price varies. reprint service avail. from ISI. *Refereed.*
Related titles: Online - full text ed.: (from Institute for Scientific Information).
Indexed: ASCA, Biol.Abstr., Chem.Abstr., Chem.Indus.Notes, Chem.Titles, Chic.Per.Ind., Dent.Ind., Dok.Arbeitsmed., Excerp.Med., INIS Atomind., Ind.Med. (1975-), Ind.Vet., Vet.Bull., Zoo.Rec.
—BLDSC (6867.400000), CASDDS, CISTI, GNLM, ingenta, KNAW.
Published by: John Wiley & Sons, Inc., Journals (Subsidiary of: Wiley InterScience), 605 Third Ave, New York, NY 10158. TEL 212-475-7700.

PROGRESS IN MEDICINAL CHEMISTRY. see *CHEMISTRY*

613 GBR ISSN 0962-7936
CODEN: POBREJ
PROGRESS IN OBESITY RESEARCH (YEAR). Text in English. 1977. irreg., latest vol.8. price varies. illus. *Refereed.* **Document type:** *Academic/Scholarly.*
Formerly (until 1990): Recent Advances in Obesity Research (0306-7548)
Indexed: Chem.Abstr., Chem.Indus.Notes, Chem.Titles.
—BLDSC (6871.240000), CASDDS, GNLM, KNAW.
Published by: John Libbey & Co. Ltd., PO Box 276, Eastleigh SO50 5YS, United Kingdom. TEL 44-2380-650208, FAX 44-2380-650259, http://www.johnlibbey.com.

610 GBR ISSN 1615-4959
▼ **PROGRESS IN OSTEOPOROSIS.** Text in English. 2000. q. EUR 123.30 domestic; EUR 120.70 in Germany; EUR 33.60 newsstand/cover foreign (effective 2002). *Refereed.* **Document type:** *Journal, Academic/Scholarly.* **Description:** Provides a timely update of the most recent articles on scientific advances in the field of osteoporosis and bone metabolism.
Published by: Springer-Verlag London Ltd. (Subsidiary of: BertelsmannSpringer), Sweetapple House, Catteshall Rd, Godalming, Surrey GU7 3DJ, United Kingdom. TEL 44-1483-418800, FAX 44-1483-415144, postmaster@svl.co.uk. Ed. E Seemann.

616.07 GBR ISSN 0968-896X
CODEN: PRPAFQ
PROGRESS IN PATHOLOGY. Text in English. 1995. a. illus. **Document type:** *Academic/Scholarly.* **Description:** Reviews the latest developments in pathology, describing issues of everyday diagnostic relevance and the molecular mechanisms underlying development and metastasis.
Indexed: Chem.Abstr., Chem.Titles.
—BLDSC (6872.415000), CASDDS, GNLM, Infotrieve. **CCC.**
Published by: Churchill Livingstone (Subsidiary of: Harcourt Publishers Ltd.), Robert Stevenson House, 1-3 Baxter's Pl, Leith Walk, Edinburgh, Midlothian EH1 3AF, United Kingdom. TEL 44-131-556-2424, FAX 44-131-459-1177, http://www.churchillmed.com. Eds. Dr. Nigel Kirkham, Dr. Peter A Hall. **Subscr. to:** Harcourt Publishers Ltd., Foots Cray High St, Sidcup, Kent DA14 5HP, United Kingdom. TEL 44-20-8308-5700, FAX 44-20-8309-0807.

612 USA ISSN 0721-9156
QP431 CODEN: PSPYDZ
PROGRESS IN SENSORY PHYSIOLOGY. Text in English. 1981. irreg., latest vol.9, 1989. price varies. reprint service avail. from ISI. **Document type:** *Monographic series.*
—CASDDS, CISTI, Infotrieve, Linda Hall. **CCC.**
Published by: Springer-Verlag, Journals (Subsidiary of: BertelsmannSpringer), 175 Fifth Ave, New York, NY 10010. TEL 212-460-1500, FAX 212-473-6272.

617.07 USA ISSN 0271-2350
RD57
PROGRESS IN SURGICAL PATHOLOGY. Text in English. 1980. irreg., latest vol.13, 1993. USD 135 to individuals; USD 175 to institutions. *Refereed.* **Document type:** *Academic/Scholarly.*
—CISTI, GNLM.
Published by: Field & Wood, Medical Periodicals, Inc., PO Box 975, Blue Bell, PA 19422. TEL 610-828-4010, FAX 215-482-0226.

610 ITA ISSN 0370-1514
CODEN: PRMOAE
IL PROGRESSO MEDICO. Text in Italian; Summaries in English. 1944. bi-m. ITL 150,000 (effective 1998). adv. index. **Document type:** *Academic/Scholarly.* **Description:** Covers internal medicine and surgery.
Related titles: Microform ed.
Indexed: Excerp.Med.
—BLDSC (6924.672000), CISTI, EMDOCS, GNLM.
Published by: Lombardo Editore, Via Verona, 22, Rome, RM 00161, Italy. TEL 39-6-44290974, FAX 39-6-44238543. Ed. Dr. Claudio Puoti. R&P, Adv. contact Giorgio Lombardo.

610 AUT ISSN 0944-6125
PROMED; das Praxismagazin fuer Aerztliche Fortbildung. Text in German. 1993. m. EUR 81 domestic; EUR 75.40 in Germany; EUR 6 newsstand/cover foreign (effective 2002). adv. **Document type:** *Journal, Academic/Scholarly.*
Related titles: Online - full text ed.: (from Springer LINK).
Published by: Springer-Verlag Wien (Subsidiary of: BertelsmannSpringer), Sachsenplatz 4-6, PO Box 89, Vienna, W 1201, Austria. TEL 43-1-3302415-0, FAX 43-1-330242665, journals@springer.at, http://www.springer.at/promed. Ed. A Furrer. R&P Angela Foessl TEL 43-1-3302415517. Adv. contact Michael Katzenberger TEL 43-1-3302415220. B&W page XEU 2,190, color page XEU 2,847; 180 x 260.

610 FRA ISSN 0033-1392
PROPOS UTILES AUX MEDECINS. Text in French. 1950. 50/yr. FRF 490. adv. index.
Address: 6 rue Montalivet, Paris 75008, France. TEL 42-65-84-33, FAX 42-68-05-86, TELEX 290 144. Ed. Roland Lesage. Circ: 11,000.

616.99 USA ISSN 0270-4137
RC899 CODEN: PRSTDS
THE PROSTATE. Text in English. 1980. 16/yr. (in 4 vols., 4 nos./vol.). USD 2,355 in United States; USD 2,515 in Canada & Mexico; USD 2,651 elsewhere; USD 2,473 combined subscription in United States for print and online eds.; USD 2,633 combined subscription in Canada & Mexico for print and online eds.; USD 2,769 combined subscription elsewhere for print and online eds. (effective 2002). adv. bibl, charts, illus. index. back issues avail. *Refereed.* **Document type:** *Academic/Scholarly.* **Description:** Serves as an international medium presenting comprehensive coverage of clinical, anatomic, embryologic, physiologic, endocrinologic, and biochemical studies.
Related titles: Microform ed.: (from PQC); Online - full text ed.: ISSN 1097-0045. 1996. USD 2,355 in United States; USD 2,355 in Canada & Mexico; USD 2,355 elsewhere (effective 2002) (from EBSCO Publishing, Wiley InterScience, Institute for Scientific Information).
Indexed: ASCA, Biol.Abstr., Chem.Abstr., Chem.Indus.Notes, Chem.Titles, Curr.Cont., Excerp.Med., INIS Atomind., Ind.Med. (1980-), Ind.Sci.Rev., Inpharma, Nutr.Abstr., Pharm.&Out.News, Reac., Ref.Zh., Sci.Cit.Ind.
—BLDSC (6935.194000), CASDDS, CISTI, EMDOCS, GNLM, IDS, ingenta, KNAW. **CCC.**
Published by: John Wiley & Sons, Inc., Journals (Subsidiary of: Wiley InterScience), 605 Third Ave, New York, NY 10158. TEL 212-850-6645, FAX 212-850-6021, subinfo@wiley.com, uscs-wis@wiley.com, http://www.wiley.com. Eds. Avery A Sandberg, Gerald P Murphy. adv.: B&W page GBP 640, color page GBP 1,515; trim 174 x 254. Circ: 350. **Subscr. outside the Americas to:** John Wiley & Sons Ltd., Baffins Ln, Chichester, Sussex PO19 IUD, United Kingdom. TEL 44-1243-779777, FAX 44-1243-843232, cs-journals@wiley.co.uk.

616.99 USA ISSN 1095-5100
▼ **THE PROSTATE JOURNAL.** Text in English. 1999. bi-m. USD 80 domestic to individuals; USD 95 in Canada & Mexico to individuals; USD 105 elsewhere to individuals; USD 165 domestic to institutions; USD 180 in Canada & Mexico to institutions; USD 190 elsewhere to institutions; USD 88 domestic to individuals print & online eds. combined; USD 104.50 in Canada & Mexico to individuals print & online eds. combined; USD 115.50 elsewhere to individuals print & online eds. combined; USD 181.50 domestic to institutions print & online eds. combined; USD 198 in Canada & Mexico to institutions print & online eds. combined; USD 209 elsewhere to institutions print & online eds. combined (effective 2001). adv. bk.rev. back issues avail.; reprints avail. *Refereed.* **Document type:** *Academic/Scholarly.* **Description:** Publishes research from variety of clinical and research specialties dealing with the prevention, diagnosis, and treatment of malignant and nonmalignant prostate disorders.
Related titles: ♦ Online - full text ed.: The Prostate Journal Online. ISSN 1525-1411.
—BLDSC (6935.194700). **CCC.**
Published by: Blackwell Science Inc., Commerce Pl, 350 Main St, Malden, MA 02148-5018. TEL 781-388-8250, 800-759-6102, FAX 781-388-8255, journals@blacksci.com, http://www.blackwell-science.com. Ed. Dr. Philip W Kantoff. R&P Tracey Davies. Adv. contact Jenny Applin.

616.99 USA ISSN 1525-1411
THE PROSTATE JOURNAL ONLINE. Text in English. q. USD 72 to individuals; USD 149 to institutions (effective 2001). **Document type:** *Academic/Scholarly.*
Media: Online - full text (from EBSCO Publishing, O C L C Online Computer Library Center, Inc., RoweCom Information Quest, ingenta, Munksgaard & Blackwell Science's Synergy, Swets Blackwell). **Related titles:** ♦ Print ed.: The Prostate Journal. ISSN 1095-5100.
Published by: Blackwell Science Inc., Commerce Pl, 350 Main St, Malden, MA 02148-5018. TEL 781-388-8250, 800-759-6102, FAX 781-388-8255, website@blacksci.com, journals@blacksci.com, http://www.blackwell-science.com/~cgilib/bsinc.bin?Journal=prostate.

610 382 IND
PROVEN TRADE CONTACTS. Text in English. 1992. m. INR 200, USD 40 (effective 2001). adv. tr.lit. 36 p./no. 2 cols./p. back issues avail. **Document type:** *Magazine, Trade.* **Description:** Promotes International trade of medical, surgical, hospital, laboratory, veterinary goods & pharmaceuticals. It has its circulation among exporters, importers, hospitals, health organisations, trade promotion councils, embassies, chambers of commerce, agencies of UNO etc. in more than 125 countries.
Related titles: Online - full content ed.
Published by: Trade Contacts, Narang Tower, 46 Community Center, Naraina Ph-I, New Delhi 28, India. TEL 91-11-5892020, FAX 91-11-5892026, TC@narang.com, tc@narang.com, http://narang.com/ptc. Ed. R V Narang. Adv. contact Mr. Vivek Narang. Circ: 10,000.

PROVING MEDICAL DIAGNOSIS AND PROGNOSIS. see *LAW*

610 POL ISSN 0033-2240
CODEN: PRLKAV
PRZEGLAD LEKARSKI✱. Text in Polish; Summaries in English, Russian. 1862. m. USD 180. index. **Document type:** *Academic/Scholarly.*

M

Indexed: Abstr.Hyg., Biol.Abstr., C.I.S. Abstr., Chem.Abstr., Dairy Sci.Abstr., Dok.Arbeitsmed., Excerp.Med. (until 1993), Helminthol.Abstr., INIS Atomind., Ind.Med. (1945-), Int.Nurs.Ind., Nutr.Abstr., Protozool.Abstr., Rev.Appl.Entomol., Trop.Dis.Bull., Weed Abstr.
—BLDSC (6942.800000), CASDDS, CISTI, GNLM.
Published by: Fundacja Lekarzy Polskich - Pro Medica, c/o Ars Polona, Krakowskie Przedmiescie 7, PO Box 1001, Warsaw 00068, Poland. Ed. Dr. Jan Sznajd. **Dist. by:** Ars Polona, Krakowskie Przedmiescie 7, Warsaw, Poland.

PSYCHOLOGIA A PATOPSYCHOLOGIA DIETATA. see *PSYCHOLOGY*

PSYCHOLOGY, HEALTH & MEDICINE. see *PSYCHOLOGY*

614 610 GBR ISSN 0033-3506
CODEN: PUHEAE
PUBLIC HEALTH (BASINGSTOKE). Text in English. 1888. bi-m. GBP 180 in Europe to institutions for print or online; USD 270 elsewhere to institutions for print or online; GBP 198 combined subscription in Europe to institutions print & online; USD 297 combined subscription elsewhere to institutions print & online (effective 2002). adv. bk.rev. charts, illus, stat. index. back issues avail.; reprints avail. *Refereed.* **Document type:** *Journal, Academic/Scholarly.* **Description:** Covers all aspects of community health and medicine, including preventive medicine and epidemiology.
Related titles: Online - full text ed.: (from EBSCO Publishing, O C L C Online Computer Library Center, Inc., RoweCom Information Quest, ingenta, Swets Blackwell, Institute for Scientific Information).
Indexed: AIDS Abstr., ASSIA, Abstr.Hyg., AgeLine, Aqua.Sci.& Fish.Abstr., Biol.Abstr., Brit.Nur.Ind., C.I.S. Abstr., Chem.Abstr., Curr.Adv.Cancer Res., Curr.Adv.Ecol.Sci., Curr.Cont., Dent.Ind., Diar.Dis.Res., Environ.Sci.Poll.Mgmt., Excerp.Med., Helminthol.Abstr., IDA, IMFL, Ind.Med. (1888-), Ind.Vet., Int.Nurs.Ind., NRN, Nutr.Abstr., Pollut.Abstr., Poult.Abstr., Risk Abstr., SSCI, Saf.Sci.Abstr., Sel.Water Res.Abstr., Sport Fish.Abstr., Stud.Wom.Abstr., Trop.Dis.Bull., Vet.Bull.
—BLDSC (6963.850000), GNLM, IDS, ingenta. **CCC.**
Published by: (Society of Public Health, The Royal Institute of Public Health & Hygiene), Nature Publishing Group Specialist Journals (Subsidiary of: Holtzbrink Publishers), Houndmills, Basingstoke, Hants RG21 6XS, United Kingdom. TEL 44-1256-329242, FAX 44-1256-328339, subscriptions@nature.com, http://www.nature.com/ph. Eds. F Sim, P Mackie. Pub. Sue Deeley. R&P Trace Noel. Adv. contact Robert Sloan TEL 44-20-8882-7199.

610 570 PRI ISSN 0738-0658
CODEN: PRHJDB
PUERTO RICO HEALTH SCIENCES JOURNAL. Text in English, Spanish. 1982. 4/yr. USD 40 to individuals; USD 50 to institutions (effective 1999). bk.rev. index. back issues avail. **Document type:** *Academic/Scholarly.* **Description:** Covers medical, dental, pharmaceutical and biosocial sciences. Discusses historical, philosophical and ethical matters of health sciences.
Related titles: CD-ROM ed.
Indexed: Chem.Abstr., Ind.Med. (1982-), Rev.Med.& Vet.Mycol.
—BLDSC (7156.225000), CASDDS, CISTI, GNLM, KNAW.
Published by: University of Puerto Rico, Office of the Dean for Academic Affairs, Medical Sciences Campus, Box 365067, San Juan, PR 00936-5067. TEL 787-758-2525, FAX 787-764-2470. Ed., R&P Dr. Rafael Villavicencio. Circ: 600.

610 GBR ISSN 0048-6000
PULSE. Text in English. 1959. w. GBP 118, USD 249 (effective 2000). adv. bk.rev. illus. **Document type:** *Newsletter, Trade.*
Related titles: Online - full text ed.: (from ProQuest Information & Learning, LexisNexis).
—BLDSC (7160.070000). **CCC.**
Published by: C M P Information (Subsidiary of: United Business Media), City Reach, 5 Greenwich View Pl, Millharbour, London E14 9NN, United Kingdom. TEL 44-20-78616424, FAX 44-20-7861-6255, pulse@ubminternational.com, http://www.cmpinformation.com. Ed. Howard Griffiths. Adv. contact Fergus Wilson. Circ: 42,382.

610 PAK
PULSE INTERNATIONAL. Variant title: Fortnightly Pulse International. Text in English. 1978. fortn. PKR 700 domestic; USD 70 foreign (effective 2001). adv. bk.rev., Website rev. 8 p./no. 6 cols./p. back issues avail. *Refereed.* **Document type:** *Newspaper.* **Description:** Covers news and views in the health sector.
Formerly: Doctor International (1026-6828)
Related titles: Fax ed.
Published by: Professional Medical Publications, 522, 5th Fl., Panorama Centre-II, Raja Ghazanfar Ali Rd., Saddar, Karachi, Pakistan. TEL 92-21-5688791, FAX 92-21-5689860, pulse@pulsepakistan.com, http://www.pulsepakistan.com. Ed., Pub. Shaukat Ali Jawaid. R&P, Adv. contact Mubarak Ali. B&W page PKR 30,000, color page PKR 45,000; trim 33 x 45. Circ: 8,000.

610 IND ISSN 0033-4340
PUNJAB MEDICAL JOURNAL. Text in English. 1951. m. INR 10, USD 4. adv. bk.rev. abstr, charts, illus. index.
Indexed: Biol.Abstr., Chem.Abstr., Excerp.Med., INIS Atomind.
Address: 590, Sector 10, Punchkula 134 109, India. Ed. Dr. R R Laroia.

610 GBR ISSN 1460-2725
R31 CODEN: QMJPFH
Q J M; monthly journal of the association of physicians. Text in English. 1907. m. GBP 130, USD 230 to individuals; GBP 290, USD 495 to institutions (effective 2002). adv. bk.rev. bibl, charts, illus. cum.index every 20 vols. 84 p./no. back issues avail. *Refereed.* **Document type:** *Journal, Academic/Scholarly.* **Description:** Covers the whole field of medicine with emphasis on internal medicine.
Formerly: Quarterly Journal of Medicine (0033-5622)
Related titles: CD-ROM ed.: (from Ovid Technologies, Inc.); Microform ed.: (from PQC,PMC); Online - full text ed.: ISSN 1460-2393. GBP 260, USD 445 to institutions online only (effective 2002) (from Ovid Technologies, Inc., HighWire Pr., EBSCO Publishing, O C L C Online Computer Library Center, Inc., RoweCom Information Quest, ingenta, Swets Blackwell, Institute for Scientific Information).
Indexed: Abstr.Anthropol., Abstr.Hyg., Adol.Ment.Hlth.Abstr., Anim.Breed.Abstr., Biol.Abstr., Chem.Abstr., Curr.Adv.Ecol.Sci., Curr.Cont., Dairy Sci.Abstr., Diab.Cont., Environ.Sci.Poll.Mgmt., Excerp.Med., INIS Atomind., I.P.A., Ind.Med. (1994-), Ind.Sci.Rev., Ind.Vet., Inpharma, Int.Abstr.Biol.Sci., Med.& Surg.Dermat., NRN, Neurosci.Cit.Ind., Nutr.Abstr., Pharm.&Out.News, Pollut.Abstr., Protozool.Abstr., Reac., Ref.Zh., Rev.Appl.Entomol., Rev.Med.& Vet.Mycol., Risk Abstr., Saf.Sci.Abstr., Sci.Cit.Ind., Trop.Dis.Bull., Weed Abstr.
—BLDSC (7163.731000), CASDDS, CISTI, EMDOCS, GNLM, IDS, ingenta, KNAW. **CCC.**
Published by: (Association of Physicians of Great Britain and Ireland), Oxford University Press, Academic Division, Great Clarendon St, Oxford OX2 6DP, United Kingdom. TEL 44-1865-267907, FAX 44-1865-267835, jnl.info@oup.co.uk, http://www.oup.co.uk/journals. Ed. Dr. Christopher Martyn. Pub. Mandy Sketch. R&P Fionna Willis. adv.: page GBP 350, page USD 630. Circ: 2,000. **U.S. subscr. to:** Oxford University Press, Journals, 2001 Evans Rd, Cary, NC 27513. TEL 800-852-7323, FAX 919-677-1714, jnlorders@oup-usa.org; **Subscr. to:** Journals Marketing, Great Clarendon St, Oxford OX2 6DP, United Kingdom.

610 QAT ISSN 0253-8253
QATAR MEDICAL JOURNAL. Text in English. 1980. a. *Refereed.*
—BLDSC (7163.585040).
Published by: Ministry of Public Health, P O Box 3050, Doha, Qatar. TEL 974-4314-564, FAX 974-4392-132, editros@qmj.net, http://www.qmj.net. Ed. Hajar A Hajar.

610 CHN ISSN 1001-4047
CODEN: QYXUEF
QINGDAO YIXUEYUAN XUEBAO/QINGDAO MEDICAL INSTITUTE. JOURNAL. Text in Chinese. m.
Indexed: Eng.Ind.
—CASDDS.
Published by: Qingdao Yixueyuan, No 10 Huangtai Lu, Qingdao, Shandong 266012, China. TEL 228106. Ed. Li Juesheng.

610.9 ISR ISSN 0023-4109
QOROT; the Israel journal of the history of medicine and science. Text in English, Hebrew. 1952. a., latest vol.13, 1999. USD 25 (effective 2001). adv. bk.rev. abstr, bibl, illus. index. **Document type:** *Academic/Scholarly.*
Formerly: Jerusalem Historical Medical Publications (0449-4881)
Indexed: Hist.Abstr. (1963-1975, dropped), Ind.Heb.Per. (1977-1997).
Published by: (Israel Institute of the History of Medicine), Magnes Press (Subsidiary of: Hebrew University of Jerusalem), Hebrew University, Jerusalem, 39099, Jerusalem 91390, Israel. TEL 972-2-5660341, FAX 972-2-5633370, magnes@vms.huji.ac.il. Ed. Samuel Kottek. Circ: 250.

610 ITA
CODEN: FRACAC
QUADERNI DE IL FRACASTORO. Text in Italian; Summaries in English. 1907. 3/yr. ITL 20,000 (effective 1999). adv. bk.rev. back issues avail. *Refereed.* **Document type:** *Monographic series, Academic/Scholarly.*
Formerly (until 199?): Fracastoro (0015-9271)
Related titles: Fax ed.
Indexed: Biol.Abstr., Chem.Abstr., Curr.Adv.Ecol.Sci., Excerp.Med. (until 1993), Ind.Med. (coverage dropped).
—CISTI, GNLM.
Published by: Azienda Ospitaliera Verona, Piazzale Aristide Stefani, 1, Verona, VR 37126, Italy. TEL 39-45-8071752, FAX 39-45-8071756. Ed. Gianni Mastella. Pub. Michele Romanc. Adv. contact Enzo Fabietti. Circ: 2,000 (controlled).

610 617 ITA ISSN 0393-5930
CODEN: QMCHE
QUADERNI DI MEDICINA E CHIRURGIA. Text in Italian. 1985. 4/yr. free per issue. bk.rev. abstr, bibl, illus. index. **Document type:** *Academic/Scholarly.* **Description:** Contains scientific articles on all medical subjects. For leaders at hospitals, universities, institutes and libraries.
Indexed: Excerp.Med. (1994-).
—BLDSC (7166.369800), EMDOCS, GNLM, KNAW.
Published by: Comitato Progetto Cultura Medica Q M C, Via Massimo Stanzione, 18, Naples, NA 80129, Italy. TEL 39-81-5565285, FAX 39-81-7875500. Circ: 2,500.

610 ITA ISSN 1122-2654
QUADERNI INTERNAZIONALI DI STORIA DELLA MEDICINA E DELLA SANITA. Text in Italian. 1992. s-a. **Document type:** *Academic/Scholarly.*
—GNLM.
Published by: C I S O Toscano, Istituto di Patologia Speciale Medica, Ospedale S. Maria della Scala, Piazza Duomo, 2, Siena, SI 53100, Italy. TEL 0577-43247. Ed. Francesca Vannozzi.

338.476 DEU ISSN 0949-9253
QUALITAETSMANAGEMENT IN KLINIK UND PRAXIS. Text in German. 1993. bi-m. DEM 250 (effective 1999). **Document type:** *Academic/Scholarly.*
Formerly (until 1996): Qualitaets-Sicherung und -Management in der Medizin (0945-7038)
—GNLM.
Published by: P M I Verlag AG, August-Schanz-Str 8, Frankfurt Am Main 60433, Germany. TEL 49-69-548000-0, FAX 49-69-548000-77, pmiverlag@aol.com.

610 USA ISSN 1049-7323
RA440.85 CODEN: QHREEM
QUALITATIVE HEALTH RESEARCH. Text in English. 1991. bi-m. USD 85 to individuals; USD 385 to institutions; USD 20 newsstand/cover to individuals; USD 70 newsstand/cover to institutions (effective 2002). adv. bk.rev. back issues avail.; reprints avail. *Refereed.* **Document type:** *Academic/Scholarly.* **Description:** Provides an interdisciplinary forum that will enhance health care and further the development and understanding of qualitative research methods in health care settings.
Related titles: Online - full text ed.: (from Northern Light Technology, Inc., EBSCO Publishing, O C L C Online Computer Library Center, Inc., RoweCom Information Quest, ProQuest Information & Learning, ingenta, Swets Blackwell, Institute for Scientific Information).
Indexed: ASCA, ASSIA, AgeLine, Brit.Nur.Ind., CINAHL, Curr.Cont., Fam.Ind., Lang.& Lang.Behav.Abstr., PsycInfo, Psychol.Abstr. (1991-), SOPODA, SSCI, Soc.Serv.Abstr., Sociol.Abstr., Viol.& Abuse Abstr., e-psyche.
—BLDSC (7168.124200), GNLM, IDS, Infotrieve, ingenta. **CCC.**
Published by: Sage Publications, Inc., 2455 Teller Rd, Thousand Oaks, CA 91320. TEL 805-499-0721, FAX 805-499-0871, info@sagepub.com, http://www.sagepub.com. Ed. Janice M Morse. Pub. Sara Miller McCune. R&P Tanya Udin. Adv. contact DeAnna Vega Hammersley. Circ: 1,250. **Overseas subscr. to:** Sage Publications Ltd., 6 Bonhill St, London EC2A 4PU, United Kingdom. TEL 44-20-7374-0645, FAX 44-20-7374-8741; Sage Publications India Pvt. Ltd., 4215, New Delhi 110 048, India. TEL 91-11-641-9884, FAX 91-11-647-2426.

610 USA
QUALITY ADVOCATE. Text in English. 1984. bi-m. USD 75 to non-members (effective 1998). back issues avail.
Formerly: A M P R A Review (American Medical Peer Review Association)

M

Published by: American Health Quality Association, 1140 Connecticut Ave, N W, Ste 1050, Washington, DC 20036. TEL 202-331-5790, FAX 202-833-2047. Ed. Michelle Myers. Circ: 900.

610 615 GBR ISSN 1087-8378
RS192 CODEN: QAJOFW
QUALITY ASSURANCE JOURNAL. Text in English. 1996. q. USD 425 in United States; USD 425 in Canada & Mexico; USD 425 elsewhere; USD 447 combined subscription in United States for print and online eds.; USD 447 combined subscription in Canada & Mexico for print and online eds.; USD 447 combined subscription elsewhere for print and online eds. (effective 2002). adv. bk.rev. **Document type:** *Academic/Scholarly.* **Description:** Provides an international forum for quality assurance professionals working within the pharmaceutical, health and environmental industries.
Related titles: Online - full text ed.: ISSN 1099-1786. 1997. USD 425 in United States; USD 425 in Canada & Mexico; USD 425 elsewhere (effective 2002) (from EBSCO Publishing, Wiley InterScience).
Indexed: I.P.A.
—BLDSC (7168.139370).
Published by: Wiley Europe Ltd., Baffins Ln, Chichester, W Sussex PO19 1UD, United Kingdom. TEL 44-1243-779777, FAX 44-1243-843232, customer@wiley.co.uk, http://www.wiley.co.uk. Ed. Dr. Joseph J Trautlein. Pub. Richard Edelstein. R&P Diane Southern TEL 44-1243-770347. adv.: B&W page GBP 650, color page GBP 1,550; trim 210 x 297. Circ: 700. **Subscr. in the Americas to:** John Wiley & Sons, Inc., Journals, 605 Third Ave, New York, NY 10158. TEL 212-850-6645, FAX 212-850-6021, uscs-wis@wiley.com; **Subscr. to:** John Wiley & Sons Ltd., Baffins Ln, Chichester, Sussex PO19 IUD, United Kingdom. cs-journals@wiley.co.uk.

610 GBR ISSN 0963-8172
CODEN: QHCAF4
QUALITY IN HEALTH CARE. Text in English. 1992. q. GBP 94, USD 151 combined subscription to individuals includes print & online eds.; GBP 148, USD 236 to institutions print only (effective 2002). adv. bk.rev. illus, stat. back issues avail. *Refereed.* **Description:** Presents information relevant to any aspect of health care that identifies problems in practice quality or health care delivery, suggests indications for practice change, or helps define standards and outcome of care.
Related titles: Online - full content ed.: GBP 50, USD 75 to individuals (effective 2002) (from HighWire Pr., EBSCO Publishing, O C L C Online Computer Library Center, Inc., ingenta, Swets Blackwell); Online - full text ed.: (from Institute for Scientific Information, RoweCom Information Quest).
Indexed: Brit.Nur.Ind., CINAHL, Curr.Cont., Hosp.Abstr., Inpharma, Int.Nurs.Ind., Pharm.&Out.News, Reac., Sci.Cit.Ind.
—BLDSC (7168.152260), ADONIS, GNLM, IDS, Infotrieve, KNAW. **CCC.**
Published by: B M J Publishing Group http://www.qualityhealthcare.com.

QUALITY MANAGEMENT IN HEALTH CARE; an information service. see *HEALTH FACILITIES AND ADMINISTRATION*

610 USA
QUALITY MATTERS✶ . Text in English. 1985. q. free per issue. **Document type:** *Newsletter.*
Formerly (until Apr. 1995): M F M C Review
Published by: Mississippi Foundation for Medical Care, 385 Highland Colony Pkwy, Ste 120, Ridgeland, MS 39157-6040. TEL 601-354-0304, FAX 601-948-8917, mssdps.PO1.ckelly@sdps.org. Ed. Carole Kelly. Circ: 5,000 (controlled).

610.73 USA ISSN 1064-7988
QUALITY OF LIFE✶ ; a nursing challenge. Text in English. 1992. q. free per issue. **Document type:** *Trade.* **Description:** An educational publication presented to nurses as a service by Glaxo Wellcome Healthcare.
Published by: (Glaxo Wellcome Healthcare), Meniscus Educational Institute (Subsidiary of: Meniscus Ltd.), 18 Elizabeth St, West Conshohocken, PA 19428-2935. TEL 610-660-8080, FAX 610-660-9583, email@meniscus.com, http://www.meniscus.com. Ed. Marie Bakitas Whedon.

610 150 FRA ISSN 1161-6407
QUALITY OF LIFE NEWSLETTER. Abbreviated title: Q O L Newsletter. Text in English. 1991. 21/yr. free per issue. bk.rev. *Refereed.* **Document type:** *Newsletter.* **Description:** Provides a basis for communication among those involved in health-related quality-of-life issues including epidemiologists, psychologists, economists, pharmaceutical industry managers, regulatory authorities, insurance companies and physicians.
Indexed: e-psyche.
—BLDSC (7168.152460).
Published by: M A P I Research Institute, 27 rue de la Villette, Lyon 69003, France. TEL 33-4-72136667, FAX 33-4-72136668, instdoc@mapi.fr. Ed. Catherine Acquadro. Pub. Bernard Jambon. R&P Caroline Anfray. Circ: 7,800.

610 NLD ISSN 0962-9343
CODEN: QLREEG
QUALITY OF LIFE RESEARCH. Text in Dutch. 1992. 8/yr. EUR 1,112 to institutions for print or online ed.; EUR 1,334.40 to institutions print & online eds.combined (effective 2002). adv. reprints avail. *Refereed.* **Document type:** *Academic/Scholarly.* **Description:** Aims specifically at researchers involved with any aspect of quality of life research in theory, methodology and clinical practice.
Related titles: CD-ROM ed.; Online - full text ed.: (from EBSCO Publishing, O C L C Online Computer Library Center, Inc., RoweCom Information Quest, Swets Blackwell, Kluwer Online, Institute for Scientific Information).
Indexed: AMED, ASCA, Abstr.Hyg., AgeLine, Curr.Cont., Excerp.Med. (1993-), Ind.Med. (1992-), Indian Psychol.Abstr., Inpharma, Int.Nurs.Ind., Nutr.Abstr., Pharm.&Out.News, PsycInfo, Psychol.Abstr. (1992-), Reac., Rev.Med.& Vet.Mycol., SSCI (coverage dropped), Sci.Cit.Ind., e-psyche.
—BLDSC (7168.152470), ADONIS, EMDOCS, GNLM, IDS, KNAW. **CCC.**
Published by: Kluwer Academic & Lippincott-Raven (Subsidiary of: Wolters Kluwer N.V.), Postbus 17, Dordrecht 3300 AA, Netherlands. TEL 31-78-639-2392, FAX 31-78-639-2254, services@wkap.nl, http://www.wkap.nl. Ed. Neil K Aaronson. Adv. contact Gemma Heiser. **Dist. by:** Kluwer Academic Publishers Group, Journals Department, PO Box 322, Dordrecht 3300 AH, Netherlands. TEL 781-871-6600, FAX 31-78-639-2254, 31-78-654-6474.

610 USA
QUALITY RESOURCE. Text in English. 1983. bi-m. USD 35 to membership (effective 1999). bk.rev., software rev. charts, stat, tr.lit. index. back issues avail. *Refereed.* **Document type:** *Newsletter, Trade.* **Description:** Contains articles helpful to quality management professionals working in inpatient and outpatient health care facilities.
Formerly (until 1993): Q A Section Connection (1040-2950)
Published by: (Quality Assurance Section, American Health Information Management Association), AAIMA, 919 N Michigan Ave, Ste 1400, Chicago, IL 60611-1601. TEL 312-573-8515, FAX 312-787-9793. Ed. Patrice Spath. Circ: 1,850.

610 IND ISSN 0481-2158
QUARTERLY MEDICAL REVIEW. Text in English. 1949. q. free per issue to qualified personnel. adv.
Indexed: Ind.Med. (coverage dropped).
—CISTI, GNLM.
Published by: Raptakos Brett & Co. Ltd, Dr. Annie Besant Rd., Worli, Mumbai, Maharashtra 400 025, India. Ed. Dr. G B Ramasarma. Circ: 70,000.

610 GBR ISSN 0033-6033
QUEENS MEDICAL MAGAZINE. Text in English. 1970 (vol.62). 3/yr. GBP 5. adv. bk.rev. charts, illus, stat, tr.lit. **Document type:** *Academic/Scholarly.*
Published by: (Birmingham Medical Society), Birmingham Medical and Dental Schools, Birmingham 15, United Kingdom. Ed. Matt Williams. Adv. contact Seema Quasim. Circ: 1,500 (controlled).

610 CAN ISSN 0079-8789
QUEEN'S MEDICAL REVIEW. Text in English. 1951. a. adv.
Published by: Aesculapian Society, Queen s University, Kingston, ON, Canada. TEL 613-545-2542. Circ: 1,000.

610 ARG ISSN 0325-2345
QUIRON. Text in Spanish; Summaries in English, French. 1970. q. USD 25 domestic; USD 45 foreign (effective 2000). adv. bk.rev. charts, bibl, illus. index. reprint service avail. from IRC. *Refereed.* **Document type:** *Academic/Scholarly.* **Description:** Covers various topics on medicine.
Indexed: Ind.Med. (coverage dropped).
Published by: (Fundacion Dr. Jose Maria Mainetti para el Progreso de la Medicina, Centro Oncologico de Excelencia), Editorial Quiron, Calle 508, Entre 16 Y 18, Manuel B. Gonnet, Buenos Aires 1897, Argentina. TEL 54-114-711160, FAX 54-114-712222, coe@netverk.com.ar, http://www.netverk.com.ar/instituciones/coe. Ed. Juan Carlos Secchi. Adv. contact Manuel Lencina. Circ: 3,000.

610 FRA
LE QUOTIDIEN DU MEDECIN. Text in French. d. FRF 300 (effective 1999).
Published by: Societe d'Editions Scientifiques & Culturelles, 140 rue Jules Guesde, Levallois-Perret Cedex 92593, France. TEL 33-1-41407500, FAX 33-1-41407575. Pub. Marie Claude Tesson Millet. Circ: 83,000.

610 AUS
R A C G P TRAINING PROGRAM VICTORIA NEWSLETTER. Text in English. 1977. m. adv. bk.rev. **Document type:** *Newsletter.*
Formerly: Family Medicine Programme. R A C G P Victoria Newsletter
Published by: Royal Australian College of General Practitioners, Private Bag 2000, Hartwell, VIC 3124, Australia. TEL 61-3-98090566, FAX 61-3-98090611. Eds. Dr. Steven Wilkinson, Ms. Sue Harris. Circ: 2,800.

R V S FEE SCHEDULE. (Relative Value Scale) see *INSURANCE*

RADIATION PROTECTION DOSIMETRY. see *PHYSICS—Nuclear Physics*

610 GBR ISSN 1362-3958
RADIONIC JOURNAL; an approach to health and harmony. Text in English. 1954. 2/yr. GBP 16 to members (effective 1999). adv. bk.rev. *Refereed.* **Document type:** *Newsletter.* **Description:** Discusses distant healing practice using instruments and radiesthesia.
Former titles (until 1994): Radionic Quarterly (0481-6722); Formerly (until 1957): Radionic Therapy
Published by: Radionic Association Ltd., Baerlein House, Goose Green, Deddington, Banbury, Oxon OX15 0SZ, United Kingdom. TEL 44-1869-338852, FAX 44-1869-338852. Ed. S Micham. Circ: 400.

616.6 ITA ISSN 0033-992X
RASSEGNA DI UROLOGIA E NEFROLOGIA. Text in Italian; Summaries in English. 1963. s-a. ITL 50,000; ITL 100,000 foreign (effective 1998). adv. bk.rev. **Document type:** *Academic/Scholarly.*
Indexed: Excerp.Med.
—GNLM.
Published by: C E M Casa Editrice Maccari, Via Palermo, 44, Parma, PR 43100, Italy. FAX 039-521-771268. Circ: 1,000.

610 ITA ISSN 1123-9166
RASSEGNA MEDICO-CHIRURGICA. Text in Italian; Summaries in English. 1978. q. ITL 12,000 domestic; USD 10 foreign; ITL 4,000 newsstand/cover domestic; USD 5 newsstand/cover foreign (effective 2000). bk.rev. *Refereed.* **Document type:** *Academic/Scholarly.*
Published by: (Associazione Rassegna Medico Chirurgica Benevento), M & S S Management and Scientific Service, Viale Mellusi, 134, Benevento, BN 82100, Italy. TEL 39-8-24311311, FAX 39-8-24355840, ninorosa@tiscalinet.it, http://web.tiscalinet.it/rmc, http://www.rassegna.org. Ed. A. Rosa. Pub. Nico de Vincentiis. R&P A Rosa.

616.98 DEU ISSN 0722-7949
RAUM UND ZEIT; die neue Dimension der Wissenschaft. Text in German. 1981. bi-m. EUR 48 domestic; EUR 54 foreign (effective 2002). adv. bk.rev. 116 p./no. back issues avail. **Document type:** *Magazine, Consumer.* **Description:** Reports on new developments in live energy, biophysical medicine, and other sorts of non-invasive alternative therapies.
Indexed: Ref.Zh.
Published by: Ehlers Verlag GmbH, Geitlinger Str 14e, Wolfratshausen 82515, Germany. TEL 49-8171-418461, FAX 49-8171-418466, redaktion@ehlersverlag.de, http://www.raum-und-zeit.com. Ed., R&P Hans-Joachim Ehlers. Adv. contact Michaela Markert-Kaeser. B&W page DEM 3,000, color page DEM 5,400; trim 188 x 270. Circ: 20,000.

M

610 PAK ISSN 0303-5212
CODEN: RMEJEI
RAWAL MEDICAL JOURNAL. Text in English. 1976. q. PKR 60, USD 60. adv. bk.rev. **Document type:** *Academic/Scholarly.*
Related titles: CD-ROM ed.
Indexed: ExtraMED, INIS Atomind.
—GNLM.
Published by: Pakistan Medical Association, Rawalpindi-Islamabad Branch, Rawalpindi, Pakistan. Circ: 1,500.

610 AUS
REACH OUT. Text in English. 1982. q. AUD 20 to members. back issues avail. **Document type:** *Newsletter.* **Description:** Covers tuberous sclerosis and related subjects.
Former titles: T S Today; Lynn's Letter
Published by: Australasian Tuberous Sclerosis Society Inc., 39 Speers Rd, North Rocks, NSW 2151, Australia. atss@eagles.com.au, http://www.eagles.com.au/~atss. Eds. Beth Wilson, Sue Pinkerton. Circ: 380.

REACHING OUT. see *HANDICAPPED*

610 ESP ISSN 0034-0634
CODEN: ARANAO
REAL ACADEMIA NACIONAL DE MEDICINA. ANALES. Text in Spanish. 1879. q. ESP 7,200, USD 60. illus. **Document type:** *Academic/Scholarly.*
Indexed: Biol.Abstr., Chem.Abstr., Ind.Med. (1879-).
—BLDSC (0882.150000), CASDDS, CINDOC, CISTI, GNLM, Infotrieve, KNAW. **CCC.**
Published by: Real Academia Nacional de Medicina, c/o Prof. Dr. D Valentin Matilla y Gomez, Arrieta, 12, Madrid 28013, Spain. TEL 34-1-5470320, FAX 34-1-5470318. Circ: 600.

▼ **REAL HEALTHCARE.** see *HEALTH FACILITIES AND ADMINISTRATION*

610 FRA ISSN 0765-5290
CODEN: RMDUA8
REANIMATION, SOINS INTENSIFS, MEDECINE D'URGENCE. Text in French. 1968. 4/yr. FRF 1,210 domestic to individuals; FRF 1,560 foreign to individuals; FRF 245 domestic to students; FRF 310 foreign to students. **Document type:** *Academic/Scholarly.*
Formerly: Reanimation et Medecine d'Urgence (0246-1234)
—CASDDS, CISTI, EMDOCS, GNLM, Infotrieve, KNAW. **CCC.**
Published by: (Societe de Reanimation de Langue Francaise), Expansion Scientifique Francaise, 31 bd. de la Tour Maubourg, Paris Cedex 7 75343, France. TEL 33-1-40626400, FAX 33-1-45556920. Ed. G Barrier. Circ: 3,000.

610 GBR ISSN 0144-1256
RECENT ADVANCES IN COMMUNITY MEDICINE. Text in English. 1978. irreg., latest vol.3. **Document type:** *Monographic series, Academic/Scholarly.*
—GNLM.
Published by: Churchill Livingstone (Subsidiary of: Harcourt Publishers Ltd.), Robert Stevenson House, 1-3 Baxter's Pl, Leith Walk, Edinburgh, Midlothian EH1 3AF, United Kingdom. TEL 44-131-556-2424, FAX 44-131-459-1177, http://www.churchillmed.com. **US subscr. to:** Churchill Livingstone, 650 Ave of the Americas, New York, NY 10011. TEL 212-206-5000.

610 GBR ISSN 0952-1089
RECENT ADVANCES IN CRITICAL CARE MEDICINE. Text in English. 1977. irreg. **Document type:** *Monographic series, Academic/Scholarly.*
Formerly (until 1983): Recent Advances in Intensive Therapy (0143-344X)
—BLDSC (7303.814300), CISTI.
Published by: Churchill Livingstone (Subsidiary of: Harcourt Publishers Ltd.), Robert Stevenson House, 1-3 Baxter's Pl, Leith Walk, Edinburgh, Midlothian EH1 3AF, United Kingdom. TEL 44-131-556-2424, FAX 44-131-459-1177, http://www.churchillmed.com. Eds. C Hinds, T Evans. Pub. Gill Haddock. R&P Moira Trotter.

616.07 571.9 GBR ISSN 0143-6953
RECENT ADVANCES IN HISTOPATHOLOGY. Text in English. irreg. **Document type:** *Monographic series, Academic/Scholarly.*
Formerly (until 1978): Recent Advances in Pathology (0141-3384)
—BLDSC (7303.842300), GNLM, KNAW.
Published by: Churchill Livingstone (Subsidiary of: Harcourt Publishers Ltd.), Robert Stevenson House, 1-3 Baxter's Pl, Leith Walk, Edinburgh, Midlothian EH1 3AF, United Kingdom. TEL 44-131-556-2424, FAX 44-131-459-1177, http://www.churchillmed.com. **US subscr. to:** Churchill Livingstone, 650 Ave of the Americas, New York, NY 10011. TEL 212-206-5000.

610 GBR ISSN 0143-6791
RECENT ADVANCES IN MEDICINE. Text in English. 1924. irreg., latest vol.20. **Document type:** *Monographic series, Academic/Scholarly.*
—GNLM.
Published by: Churchill Livingstone (Subsidiary of: Harcourt Publishers Ltd.), Robert Stevenson House, 1-3 Baxter's Pl, Leith Walk, Edinburgh, Midlothian EH1 3AF, United Kingdom. TEL 44-131-556-2424, FAX 44-131-459-1177, http://www.churchillmed.com. **US subscr. to:** Churchill Livingstone, 650 Ave of the Americas, New York, NY 10011. TEL 212-206-5000.

RECENT ADVANCES IN PHYSIOLOGY. see *BIOLOGY—Physiology*

610 USA ISSN 1073-7251
RD120.7
RECENT DEVELOPMENTS IN TRANSPLANTATION MEDICINE. Text in English. 1994. irreg.
Published by: (University of Wisconsin - Madison. Medical School), Physicians & Scientists Publishing Co., PO Box 435, Glenview, IL 60025. TEL 847-559-0605, FAX 847-559-0699, info@medpub.com, http://www.medpub.com. Ed. Hans Sollinger.

610 ITA ISSN 0034-1193
CODEN: RPMDAN
RECENTI PROGRESSI IN MEDICINA. Text in Italian; Summaries in English. 1946. m. (11/yr.). USD 145 (effective 2000). adv. bk.rev. abstr, bibl, illus. index. **Document type:** *Academic/Scholarly.*
Indexed: Biol.Abstr., Chem.Abstr., Dent.Ind., Dok.Arbeitsmed., Excerp.Med., Ind.Med. (1946-), Inpharma, Reac.
—BLDSC (7305.100000), CASDDS, CISTI, GNLM, KNAW.
Published by: Il Pensiero Scientifico Editore s.r.l., Via Bradano, 3-C, Rome, RM 00199, Italy. TEL 39-06-862821, FAX 39-06-86282250, pensiero@pensiero.it, http://www.pensiero.it. Ed. Lorenzo Bonomo. Adv. contact Luciano De Fiore. Circ: 1,000.

RECHT DER MEDIZIN. see *LAW*

RECHTSMEDIZIN. see *MEDICAL SCIENCES—Forensic Sciences*

RECHTSMEDIZINISCHE FORSCHUNGSERGEBNISSE. see *LAW*

RECOMMENDED SCALES OF BENEFITS. DENTAL PRACTITIONERS. see *MEDICAL SCIENCES—Dentistry*

368.382 ZAF
RECOMMENDED SCALES OF BENEFITS. MEDICAL PRACTITIONERS. Text in English. 1994. a.
Published by: Representative Association of Medical Schemes, PO Box 2324, Parklands, Johannesburg 2121, South Africa.

RECOMMENDED SCALES OF BENEFITS. PHYSIOTHERAPISTS. see *MEDICAL SCIENCES—Physical Medicine And Rehabilitation*

RECOMMENDED SCALES OF BENEFITS. PRIVATE HOSPITALS & UNATTACHED OPERATING THEATRE UNITS. see *HEALTH FACILITIES AND ADMINISTRATION*

REFERATIVNYI ZHURNAL. OBSHCHIE VOPROSY PATOLOGICHESKOI ANATOMII. see *BIOLOGY—Abstracting, Bibliographies, Statistics*

610 ZAF
REGISTER OF MEDICAL PRACTITIONERS, INTERNS AND DENTISTS FOR THE REPUBLIC OF SOUTH AFRICA. Text and summaries in Afrikaans, English. a. ZAR 110. Supplement avail. **Document type:** *Directory.*
Published by: Health Professions Council of South Africa, PO Box 205, Pretoria 0001, South Africa. TEL 27-12-3286680, FAX 27-12-3285120, hpcsa@samdc.co.za.

615.89 DEU ISSN 1430-7561
REGULATIONSMEDIZIN; Zeitschrift fuer medizinische Regulationsdiagnostik und -therapie. Text in German. 1990. q. DEM 52 domestic; DEM 68 foreign (effective 2001). bk.rev. **Document type:** *Magazine, Academic/Scholarly.*
Formerly (until 1996): Panta (0937-2512)
Published by: Medizinisch Literarische Verlagsgesellschaft mbH, Postfach 1151-1152, Uelzen 29501, Germany. TEL 49-581-808151, FAX 49-581-808158, mlverlag@mlverlag.de, http://www.mlverlag.de. Circ: 2,000 (paid).

610 351 USA ISSN 1097-2668
REGULATORY AFFAIRS FOCUS. Text in English. 1996. m. free to members; USD 60 domestic to non-members; USD 75 foreign to non-members (effective 2001). **Document type:** *Trade.*
Related titles: Online - full text ed.
—BLDSC (7349.610000).
Published by: Regulatory Affairs Professionals Society, 11300 Rockville Pike, Ste 1000, Rockville, MD 20852. TEL 301-770-2920, FAX 301-770-2924, raps@raps.org, http://www.raps.org. Ed. Jeff Schomisch. Pub. Sherry Keramidas.

REHAB CONTINUUM REPORT. see *INSURANCE*

615.8 USA ISSN 0899-6237
REHAB MANAGEMENT; the interdisciplinary journal of rehabilitation. Text in English. 1988. bi-m. USD 100 foreign (effective 2000). adv. *Refereed.* **Document type:** *Journal, Trade.* **Description:** Directed toward physical therapists, directors and managers of rehabilitation hospitals, and occupational therapists. Features the business aspects of rehabilitation, plus case histories.
Related titles: Online - full text ed.
Indexed: CINAHL.
—BLDSC (7350.045000).
Published by: Curant Communications, Inc. (Subsidiary of: Medical World Communications), 6701 Center Drive W #450, Los Angeles, CA 90045-1556. TEL 310-306-2206, FAX 310-306-9548, jrich@medpubs.com, http://www.rehabpub.com. Ed. Kristin Trompeter. Pubs. Curtis Pickelle, Tony Ramos. Adv. contact Sharon Marsee. page USD 2,560; trim 9.88 x 7.5. Circ: 20,000 (controlled).

615.8 USA ISSN 1056-6201
REHAB MANAGEMENT INTERNATIONAL. Text in English. 1991. q. adv. **Document type:** *Journal, Trade.* **Description:** Covers topics of rehabilitation on an international level as well as the latest technology advancements for physiotherapists, occupational therapists, and directors/managers of rehabilitation centers.
Indexed: CINAHL.
—BLDSC (7350.045050).
Published by: Curant Communications, Inc. (Subsidiary of: Medical World Communications), 6701 Center Drive W #450, Los Angeles, CA 90045-1556. TEL 310-306-2206, FAX 310-306-9548, http://www.rehabpub.com. Pub. Tony Ramos.

362 DEU ISSN 0034-3536
DIE REHABILITATION; Zeitschrift fuer Praxis und Forschung in der Rehabilitation. Text in German; Summaries in English, German. 1961. bi-m. EUR 151.80 domestic to institutions; EUR 157.80 in Europe to institutions; EUR 162.20 elsewhere to institutions; EUR 30 newsstand/cover (effective 2002). adv. bk.rev. bibl, charts, illus, stat. index. back issues avail.; reprint service avail. from PQC. *Refereed.* **Document type:** *Journal, Academic/Scholarly.*
Related titles: Microform ed.: (from PQC); Online - full text ed.: ISSN 1439-1309.
Indexed: AMED, CINAHL, Curr.Cont. (coverage dropped), Excerp.Med., Ind.Med. (1962-).
—BLDSC (7350.210000), CISTI, GNLM, KNAW. **CCC.**
Published by: (Deutsche Vereinigung fuer die Rehabilitation Behinderter), Georg Thieme Verlag, Ruedigerstr 14, Stuttgart 70469, Germany. TEL 49-711-8931-0, FAX 49-711-8931298, kunden.service@thieme.de, http://www.thieme.de/reha. Eds. F Schliehe, K A Jochheim. R&P Peter Eich. adv.: page DEM 1,850; 175 x 250. Circ: 1,400.

362 USA ISSN 0172-6412
REHABILITATION UND PRAEVENTION. Text in English. 1977. irreg., latest 1995. price varies. reprint service avail. from ISI.
—KNAW.
Published by: Springer-Verlag, Journals (Subsidiary of: BertelsmannSpringer), 175 Fifth Ave, New York, NY 10010. TEL 212-460-1500, FAX 212-473-6272.

M

610 338 USA ISSN 1065-7681
R728.5
RELATIVE VALUES FOR PHYSICIANS. Text in English. 1984. q. USD 239. **Document type:** *Trade.* **Description:** Fee scheduling system for physicians, medical groups and insurers to determine physicians' charges and reimbursement.
Related titles: Diskette ed.; Magnetic Tape ed.
Published by: McGraw-Hill Companies, 1221 Ave of the Americas, New York, NY 10020. TEL 212-512-2995, FAX 212-512-4138.

612.015 ITA ISSN 0048-7198
RELAZIONI CLINICO SCIENTIFICHE*. Text in Italian; Summaries in English. 1948. bi-m. free to medical doctors. adv. bk.rev. abstr, bibl, illus. index, cum.index.
Indexed: Chem.Abstr.
Published by: Istituto Ganassini di Ricerche Biochimiche, Via Pietro Gaggia, 16, Milan, MI 20139, Italy. Circ: 13,000.

RELEVANT. see *PHILOSOPHY*

REMEDIA. see *BIBLIOGRAPHIES*

REMEDY MAGAZINE; prescriptions for a healthy life. see *PHYSICAL FITNESS AND HYGIENE*

610 USA ISSN 1070-3411
THE REMINGTON REPORT. Text in English. 1993. bi-m. USD 44 domestic; USD 55 foreign (effective 2001). adv. back issues avail. **Document type:** *Magazine, Trade.*
Indexed: CINAHL.
Published by: The Remington Report, Inc, 30100 Town Center Dr, Ste 241, Laguna Niguel, CA 62677. TEL 800-247-4781, FAX 949-495-2708, remrptedit@aol.com. Ed., Pub. Lisa Remington. Adv. contact Bob Heiman TEL 856-768-9360. B&W page USD 3,000, color page USD 3,900; trim 10.88 x 8.5. Circ: 26,253.

610 FRA ISSN 1164-8961
REPONSE A TOUT SANTE. Text in French. 1991. m. FRF 160; FRF 16 newsstand/cover (effective 2000). adv. **Document type:** *Magazine, Consumer.* **Description:** Addresses every day health issues.
Published by: Alain Ayache Developpement, 117 rue de la Tour, Paris 75116, France. TEL 33-1-45038000, FAX 33-1-45038023, ham@groupe-ayache.com, http://www.reponseatout.com/shop/polegp.htm. Ed. Caroline Ayache. Pub. Alain Ayache. adv.: B&W page FRF 74,000, color page FRF 87,000; trim 205 x 280. Circ: 250,000 (paid).

610 020 USA
REPORT ON HEALTHCARE INFORMATION MANAGEMENT. Text in English. m. USD 358; USD 378 foreign (effective 1998). **Document type:** *Newsletter.* **Description:** Keeps executives on top of what's working in information systems and what's in store. Reports on standards for claims submission and EDI and what those developments mean.
Indexed: CINAHL.
Published by: Capitol Publications, Inc. (Subsidiary of: Aspen Publishers, Inc.), 1101 King St, Ste 444, Alexandria, VA 22314. TEL 703-683-4100, FAX 703-739-6501. Ed. Bert Latamore. Pub. Marjorie Weiner. R&P Rossette Graham.

REPORT ON MEDICARE COMPLIANCE. see *LAW*

610 ARG
REPORTERO MEDICO. Text in Spanish. m. adv.
Published by: Editorial Artes y Ciencias, Santa Fe 2436, segundo, Buenos Aires, Argentina. Ed. Dr. Rufino J Flores Belaunde.

▼ **REPRODUCTION.** see *BIOLOGY*

REPRODUCTION. SUPPLEMENT. see *BIOLOGY—Physiology*

610 570 TWN ISSN 0255-6596
Q72.5 CODEN: PNBSEF
REPUBLIC OF CHINA. NATIONAL SCIENCE COUNCIL. PROCEEDINGS. PART B: LIFE SCIENCES. Text in English. 1965. q. TWD 280, USD 16 (effective 2001). 60 p./no. back issues avail.; reprints avail. *Refereed.* **Document type:** *Academic/Scholarly.* **Description:** Publishes research papers in biology, agriculture and medical sciences.
Fomerly (until 1983): National Science Council, Republic of China. Proceedings. Part B, Basic Science (0253-6870); Which supersedes in part (1977-1980): National Science Council, Republic of China. Proceedings (0253-6870); Which was formed by the merger of (1969-1977): National Science Council. Proceedings. Proceedings. Part One, Natural and Mathematical Sciences (0378-2727); (1969-1977): National Science Council. Proceedings. Part Two, Biological, Medical and Agricultural Sciences (0377-7677); (1972-1977): National Science Council. Proceedings. Part Three: Engineering and Applied Sciences (0377-9297); Which were formerly (1965-1968): National Council on Science Development. Proceedings (0454-6725)
Related titles: Microfiche ed.; Online - full content ed.
Indexed: AgBiotech, Anim.Breed.Abstr., Aqua.Sci.& Fish.Abstr., Cal.Tiss.Abstr., Chem.Abstr., Chem.Indus.Notes, Chem.Titles, Dairy Sci.Abstr., Field Crop Abstr., Food Sci.& Tech.Abstr., Ind.Med. (1984-), Ind.Vet., Irr.& Drain.Abstr., Nutr.Abstr., Ocean.Abstr., Pig News & Info., Plant Grow.Reg.Abstr., Rev.Arom.& Med.Plants, Rev.Med.& Vet.Mycol., Rev.Plant Path., Rice Abstr., Seed Abstr., Soils & Fert., Sport Fish.Abstr., Vet.Bull., Wild.Rev., Zoo.Rec.
—BLDSC (6769.884600), CASDDS, CISTI, Infotrieve, ingenta, KNAW, Linda Hall. **CCC.**
Published by: National Science Council, Rm 1701, 106 Ho-Ping E. Rd, Sec 2, Taipei, Taiwan. TEL 886-2-27377594, FAX 886-2-27377248, chenlee@nsc.gov.tw, http://www.nsc.gov.tw. Ed. Chia-Yin Tsai. Circ: 2,600.

610 200 ITA ISSN 0014-8784
RES MEDICAE. Text in Italian. 1935. bi-m. ITL 6,000. adv. bk.rev. bibl, charts, illus, stat. index.
Published by: (Ordine Ospedaliero di S. Giovanni di Dio), Fatebenefratelli, Via San Vittore, 12, Milan, MI 20123, Italy. Circ: 6,000.

RESEARCH AND CLINICAL CENTER FOR CHILD DEVELOPMENT. ANNUAL REPORT. see *CHILDREN AND YOUTH—About*

610 GBR ISSN 0143-3083
CODEN: RCLFD4
RESEARCH AND CLINICAL FORUMS. Text in English. 1979. irreg., latest vol.19, no.5, 1997. **Document type:** *Proceedings.* **Description:** Presents materials discussed at medico-scientific and medico-therapeutic congresses and symposia.
Indexed: Chem.Abstr., Curr.Adv.Ecol.Sci., Inpharma, Pharm.&Out.News, Reac.
—BLDSC (7714.445000), CASDDS, CISTI, EMDOCS, GNLM, Infotrieve, KNAW. **CCC.**
Published by: Wells Medical Ltd., Speldhurst Pl, Speldhurst Rd, Royal Tunbridge Wells, Kent TN4 0JB, United Kingdom. TEL 44-1892-511600, FAX 44-1892-511400, info@wellsmed.co.uk. Circ: 50,000.

616.07 615 USA ISSN 1078-0297
IRN1 CODEN: RCMPE6
RESEARCH COMMUNICATIONS IN MOLECULAR PATHOLOGY AND PHARMACOLOGY. Text in English. 1970. m. USD 250; USD 295 foreign (effective 1998). adv. bk.rev. abstr, charts, illus. index. reprint service avail. from ISI. *Refereed.* **Document type:** *Journal, Academic/Scholarly.* **Description:** Articles on all areas of pathology, pharmacology, toxicology in their basic and clinical aspects.
Formerly (until 1994): Research Communications in Chemical Pathology and Pharmacology (0034-5164)
Related titles: Microform ed.: (from PMC); Online - full text ed.: (from Institute for Scientific Information).
Indexed: ASCA, Agri.& Environ.Biotech.Abstr. (coverage dropped), Aqua.Sci.& Fish.Abstr., BBCI, Biol.Abstr., Chem.Abstr., Chem.Indus.Notes, Chem.Titles, Curr.Adv.Biochem., Curr.Adv.Ecol.Sci., Curr.Cont., Dairy Sci.Abstr., Dent.Ind., Derwent Biotech.Abstr., Excerp.Med., INIS Atomind., Ind.Med. (1994-), Ind.Sci.Rev., Ind.Vet., Inpharma, Int.Abstr.Biol.Sci., Neurosci.Cit.Ind., Nutr.Abstr., Pharm.&Out.News, Poult.Abstr., Reac., Rev.Plant Path., Sci.Cit.Ind., THA, Vet.Bull.
—BLDSC (7736.540000), CASDDS, CISTI, EMDOCS, GNLM, IDS, ingenta, KNAW, Linda Hall. **CCC.**
Published by: P J D Publications Ltd, PO Box 966, Westbury, NY 11590. TEL 516-626-0650, FAX 516-626-5546. Ed. D B Sankar. Pub. Barbara Sankar. Circ: 1,000.

301 USA ISSN 0275-4959
RA418
RESEARCH IN THE SOCIOLOGY OF HEALTH CARE. Text in English. 1980. irreg., latest vol.15, 1998. USD 78.50. **Document type:** *Academic/Scholarly.*
Indexed: Lang.& Lang.Behav.Abstr., SOPODA, Soc.Serv.Abstr., Sociol.Abstr. (1980-).
—BLDSC (7770.720000), CISTI. **CCC.**
Published by: J A I Press Inc., 100 Prospect St, Box 811, Stamford, CT 06904-0811. TEL 203-323-9606, FAX 203-357-8446, jai@jaipress.com. Ed. Jennie Kronenfeld.

▼ **RESEARCH NEWS & OPPORTUNITIES IN SCIENCE AND THEOLOGY.** see *SCIENCES: COMPREHENSIVE WORKS*

RESIDENT AND STAFF PHYSICIAN. see *HEALTH FACILITIES AND ADMINISTRATION*

RESIDENTS' PRESCRIBING REFERENCE. see *PHARMACY AND PHARMACOLOGY*

614.88 DEU ISSN 0178-2525
RETTUNGSDIENST; Zeitschrift fuer praeklinische Notfallmedizin. Text in German. 1978. m. DEM 87, EUR 45 (effective 2001). adv. software rev., video rev., Website rev. illus, maps, stat. 104 p./no. back issues avail. **Document type:** *Magazine, Academic/Scholarly.*
—GNLM.
Published by: Stumpf und Kossendey Verlags GmbH, Postfach 1361, Edewecht 26183, Germany. TEL 49-4405-9181-0, FAX 49-4405-918133, rettungsdienst@skverlag.de, buecher@skverlag.de, anzeigen@skverlag.de, http://www.skverlag.de. Eds. Detlef Dahlstrom, Klaus Smit. R&P Doortje Cramer Scharnagl TEL 49-4405-918120. Adv. contact Bianca Frey TEL 49-4405-918114. B&W page XEU 1,600, color page XEU 2,800; trim 210 x 297. Circ: 23,000.

REVIEW OF MEDICAL PHYSIOLOGY. see *BIOLOGY—Physiology*

616.01 USA ISSN 0954-139X
QR46 CODEN: RMEMER
REVIEWS IN MEDICAL MICROBIOLOGY. Text in English. 1990. q., latest vol.12. USD 194 domestic to individuals; USD 194 foreign to individuals; USD 124 newsstand/cover; USD 544 per issue domestic to institutions; USD 544 per issue foreign to institutions (effective 2002). adv. reprints avail. *Refereed.* **Document type:** *Academic/Scholarly.* **Description:** Provides balanced coverage of the entire field of medical microbiology, publishing state-of-the-art reviews of the latest techniques and developments in medical microbiology, virology, mycology, parasitology, clinical microbiology, and nosocomial infection.
Related titles: Online - full text ed.: USD 707.20 domestic academic site license; USD 707.20 foreign academic site license; USD 788.80 domestic corporate site license; USD 788.80 foreign corporate site license (2002) (from EBSCO Publishing, Institute for Scientific Information).
Indexed: Abstr.Hyg., Aqua.Sci.& Fish.Abstr., Curr.Cont., Diar.Dis.Res., Environ.Sci.Poll.Mgmt., Excerp.Med., Ind.Vet., Inpharma, Int.Abstr.Biol.Sci., Microbiol.Abstr., Nutr.Abstr., Pharm.&Out.News, Protozool.Abstr., Reac., Rev.Appl.Entomol., Rev.Med.& Vet.Mycol., Sci.Cit.Ind., Trop.Dis.Bull.
—BLDSC (7792.210000), EMDOCS, GNLM, IDS, KNAW.
Published by: (Pathological Society of Great Britain and Ireland), Lippincott Williams & Wilkins (Philadelphia) (Subsidiary of: Wolters Kluwer N.V.), 530 Walnut St, Philadelphia, PA 19106-3621. TEL 215-521-8300, FAX 215-521-8902, http://www.revmedmicrobiol.com, http://www.lww.com. Ed. Ian Poxton. Adv. contact Gemma Heiser. **Subscr. to:** PO Box 1600, Hagerstown, MD 21740-1600. TEL 800-777-2295, FAX 301-824-7390.

610 BRA ISSN 0102-2105
CODEN: RAMRAS
REVISTA A M R I G S. Text in Portuguese; Summaries in English, Portuguese. 1957. q. USD 60. adv. bk.rev. illus. *Refereed.* **Document type:** *Bulletin, Proceedings.* **Description:** Presents original and review articles and case studies.
Formerly (until 1975): Associacao Medica do Rio Grande do Sul. Revista (0004-5268)
Indexed: Biol.Abstr., Excerp.Med., INIS Atomind., Ind.Med. (coverage dropped).
Published by: Associacao Medica do Rio Grande do Sul, Av Ipiranga, 5311, Porto Alegre, RS 90620, Brazil. TEL 55-51-3392899, FAX 55-51-3392998, prfontes@santacasa.tche-br. Ed. Dr. Roberto Ott Fontes. Circ: 7,000.

M

610 BRA ISSN 0034-7264
CODEN: RBMEAU
REVISTA BRASILEIRA DE MEDICINA. Short title: R B M. Abstracts and contents page in English, Portuguese. 1943. m. BRL 135, USD 250 (effective 2001). adv. bk.rev. abstr, bibl, charts, illus, stat. index. back issues avail. *Refereed.* **Document type:** *Journal, Academic/Scholarly.* **Description:** Presents studies in all fields of medicine.
Indexed: Abstr.Hyg., Biol.Abstr., Chem.Abstr., Curr.Cont. (coverage dropped), Dairy Sci.Abstr., Excerp.Med., Helminthol.Abstr., INIS Atomind., Inpharma, Microbiol.Abstr., Nutr.Abstr., Pharm.&Out.News, Protozool.Abstr., Reac., Rev.Arom.& Med.Plants, Rev.Med.& Vet.Mycol., Trop.Dis.Bull., Weed Abstr.
—BLDSC (7845.275000), CASDDS, GNLM, KNAW.
Published by: Grupo Editorial Moreira Jr., Rua Henrique Martins, 493, Jd Paulista, Sao Paulo, SP 04504-000, Brazil. TEL 55-11-38849911, FAX 55-11-38849993, comercial@moreirajr.com.br, http://www.morelrajr.com.br/. Ed. Joaquim Prado P. de Moraes. Pub. Americo Moreira. Adv. contact Maria Rachel Bellusci. Circ: 40,000.

611 571.3 CHL ISSN 0716-9868
REVISTA CHILENA DE ANATOMIA. Text in Spanish. 1983. s-a. USD 60 in Latin America; USD 80 elsewhere. abstr. back issues avail. *Refereed.* **Document type:** *Journal, Academic/Scholarly.* **Description:** Publishes articles on original research in the area of morphological sciences and related fields.
Formerly (until 1990): Anales de Anatomia Normal (0716-7296)
Related titles: Online - full text ed.: ISSN 0717-6244. 1997 (from SciELO).
Published by: Sociedad Chilena de Anatomia, Casilla 54-D, Temuco, Cautin, Chile. TEL 56-45-325571, FAX 56-45-284343, mdelsol@ufo.cl. Ed. Mariano del Sol C. **Co-sponsor:** Sociedad Panamericana de Anatomia.

610 ESP ISSN 0014-2565
CODEN: RCESA5
REVISTA CLINICA ESPANOLA. Text in Spanish; Summaries in English. 1940. 16/yr. USD 85 (effective 1996). adv. bk.rev. illus. *Refereed.*
Incorporates: Europa Medica (0375-8869)
Related titles: Online - full text ed.: (from Institute for Scientific Information).
Indexed: ASCA, Abstr.Hyg., Biol.Abstr., Chem.Abstr., Chem.Titles, Curr.Cont., Dent.Ind., Excerp.Med., Helminthol.Abstr., INIS Atomind., Ind.Med. (1940-), Ind.Med.Esp., Inpharma, Neurosci.Cit.Ind., Nutr.Abstr., Pharm.&Out.News, Protozool.Abstr., Reac., Rev.Appl.Entomol., Rev.Med.& Vet.Mycol., Rev.Plant Path., SSCI (coverage dropped).
—BLDSC (7851.170500), CASDDS, CINDOC, CISTI, GNLM, IDS, Infotrieve, KNAW. **CCC.**
Published by: Editorial Idepsa S.A., Principe de Vergara, 112 1o F, Madrid 28002, Spain. TEL 34-1-5637306, FAX 34-1-5632393. Ed. E Bouza Santiago. Circ: 7,514.

610 CRI ISSN 0253-2948
CODEN: RCCMEF
REVISTA COSTARRICENSE DE CIENCIAS MEDICAS. Text in Spanish; Abstracts in English. 1979. 4/yr. USD 40. adv. bk.rev. *Refereed.* **Document type:** *Academic/Scholarly.*
Related titles: CD-ROM ed.
Indexed: Biol.Abstr., Excerp.Med., INIS Atomind., Ind.Med. (coverage dropped).
—BLDSC (7852.070000), GNLM.
Published by: Caja Costarricense de Seguro Social, Apdo. 402, Centro Colon 1007, Costa Rica. TEL 506-2905744, FAX 506-2316915, cendeisss@info.ccss.sa.cr. Ed. Dr. Oliva Brenes. Pub. Gerardo Campos. Circ: 2,000.

610.711 CUB ISSN 0864-2141
REVISTA CUBANA DE EDUCACION MEDICA SUPERIOR. Text in Spanish; Summaries in English, Spanish. 1987. s-a. USD 34 in North America; USD 42 in Europe; USD 50 elsewhere. **Description:** Covers pedagogical science and its applications in medicine.
Published by: (Cuba. Ministerio de Salud Publica, Centro Nacional de Informacion de Ciencias Medicas), Editorial de Ciencias Medicas, O'Reilly No. 4, Habana, Cuba. TEL 62-8091, FAX 62338187. Ed. Maria Julia Zamorano. Circ: 1,000. **Co-sponsor:** Sociedad Cubana de Educacion Medica Superior.

REVISTA CUBANA DE INVESTIGACIONES BIOMEDICAS. see *BIOLOGY*

610 CUB ISSN 0034-7523
CODEN: RCBMA6
REVISTA CUBANA DE MEDICINA. Text in Spanish; Summaries in English, Spanish. 1962. bi-m. USD 48 in the Americas; USD 58 in Europe; USD 66 elsewhere. bibl, charts, illus. index.
Indexed: Abstr.Hyg., Bio-Contr.News & Info., Biol.Abstr., Chem.Abstr., Curr.Adv.Ecol.Sci., Excerp.Med., INIS Atomind., Trop.Dis.Bull.
—CASDDS, CISTI, GNLM.
Published by: (Cuba. Ministerio de Salud Publica, Centro Nacional de Informacion de Ciencias Medicas), Editorial de Ciencias Medicas, O'Reilly No. 4, Habana, Cuba. TEL 809-62-8091. Ed. Milagros de los Reyes. Circ: 3,000. **Co-sponsor:** Sociedad Cubana de Medicina Interna.

610 CUB ISSN 0864-2125
REVISTA CUBANA DE MEDICINA GENERAL INTEGRAL. Text in Spanish; Summaries in English. 1985. bi-m. USD 65 in the Americas; USD 75 in Europe; USD 83 elsewhere. abstr, bibl, charts, illus. index. **Description:** Covers preventive medicine, primary health care, diabetes mellitus, community medicine, emergency medical service, and the family physician.
Formerly (until no.3, 1985): Medicina General Integral
Related titles: Online - full text ed.
Published by: (Cuba. Ministerio de Salud Publica, Centro Nacional de Informacion de Ciencias Medicas), Editorial de Ciencias Medicas, O'Reilly No. 4, Habana, Cuba. TEL 809-62-8091. Ed. Elibel Atala. Circ: 6,000. **Co-sponsor:** Sociedad Cubana de Medicina General Integral.

616.98023 CUB ISSN 0138-6557
REVISTA CUBANA DE MEDICINA MILITAR. Text in Spanish. 1971. 2/yr. USD 3.
Published by: (Cuba. Ministerio de Salud Publica, Centro Nacional de Informacion de Ciencias Medicas), Editorial de Ciencias Medicas, O'Reilly No. 4, Habana, Cuba. TEL 809-62-8091. Ed. Milagros de los Reyes. Circ: 1,000. **Co-sponsor:** Instituto de Medicina Militar "Luis Diaz Soto".

616.08 BRA ISSN 1414-3410
CODEN: RBMPFY
REVISTA DA ASSOCIACAO BRASILEIRA DE MEDICINA PSICOSSOMATICA. Text in Portuguese; Abstracts in English, Portuguese. 1997. q. BRL 48 (effective 2000). adv. bk.rev. bibl. index, cum.index. back issues avail. **Document type:** *Academic/Scholarly.*
Indexed: Int.Nurs.Ind., Ref.Zh.
—KNAW.
Published by: (Associacao Brasileira de Medicina Psicossomatica), E C N - Editora Cientifica Nacional Ltda., Rua da Gloria, 366 Andar 3, Gloria, Rio De Janeiro, RJ 20241-180, Brazil. TEL 55-21-2213235, FAX 55-21-2213235, ecn@rj.sol.com.br. Ed. Lorete Kotze. R&P, Adv. contact Maria Luiza Carvalho. Circ: 3,000.

610 BRA ISSN 1415-5796
REVISTA DE CIENCIAS MEDICAS. Text in Portuguese, English, Spanish; Summaries in Portuguese, English. 1992. every 4 mos. BRL 30 domestic; BRL 40 foreign (effective 2001). bk.rev. abstr, bibl. Index. back issues avail. *Refereed.* **Document type:** *Magazine, Academic/Scholarly.* **Description:** Provides information regarding several fields of health and medicine for professionals and academics.
Supersedes (in 1997): Revista de Ciencias Medicas PUCCAMP (0104-0057)
Related titles: E-mail ed.; Fax ed.
Published by: Pontificia Universidade Catolica de Campinas, Faculdade de Ciencias Medicas, Av. John Boyd Dunlop, s/n, Bloco C, Jd. Ipaussurama, Campinas, SP 13020-904, Brazil. TEL 55-19-37298349, FAX 55-19-37298576, femrev@puc-campinas.br, http://www.puccamp.br. Ed., Pub. Luiz Maria Pinto. Circ: 1,000.

REVISTA DE IGIENA, BACTERIOLOGIE, VIRUSOLOGIE, PARAZITOLOGIE, PNEUMOFTIZIOLOGIE. IGIENA. see *PHYSICAL FITNESS AND HYGIENE*

613.2 MEX ISSN 0034-8376
CODEN: RICLAG
REVISTA DE INVESTIGACION CLINICA. Text and summaries in English, Spanish. 1948. bi-m. MXP 75, USD 30 (effective 1997). adv. bk.rev. bibl, charts, illus, stat. index. *Refereed.* **Document type:** *Academic/Scholarly.*
Related titles: CD-ROM ed.; Online - full text ed.: (from Institute for Scientific Information).
Indexed: ASCA, Artemisa, Biol.Abstr., Chem.Abstr., Chem.Titles, Curr.Cont., Dairy Sci.Abstr., Excerp.Med., Helminthol.Abstr., Ind.Med. (1948-), Inpharma, Nutr.Abstr., Pharm.&Out.News, Protozool.Abstr., Reac., Ref.Zh., Rev.Med.& Vet.Mycol., SSCI (coverage dropped).
—BLDSC (7862.010000), CASDDS, CISTI, GNLM, IDS, KNAW.
Published by: Instituto Nacional de la Nutricion "Salvador Zubiran", Av. San Fernando y Viaducto Tlalpan, Mexico City, 22, DF, Mexico. TEL 915-573-1200, FAX 915-655-1076, alvar@cenids.ssa.gob.mx. Eds. Alvar Loria, Ruben Lisker. Circ: 1,800.

610 BRA ISSN 0034-8554
REVISTA DE MEDICINA. Text in Portuguese; Summaries in English. 1916. q. free per issue. adv. bk.rev. bibl, charts, illus, tr.lit, tr.mk. index. reprint service avail. from PQC.
Media: Duplicated (not offset). **Related titles:** Microform ed.: (from PQC).
Indexed: Biol.Abstr., Excerp.Med., INIS Atomind., Ind.Med. (coverage dropped), Trop.Dis.Bull.
Published by: Universidade de Sao Paulo, Faculdade de Filosofia, Letras e Ciencias Humanas, Centro Academico "Oswaldo Cruz", Av Dr Arnaldo, 455, Pacaembu, Caixa Postal 8100, Sao Paulo, SP 01246-000, Brazil. Ed. Sylvia Massue Iriya. Circ: 2,000.

610 ESP ISSN 0556-6177
REVISTA DE MEDICINA. Text in Spanish; Summaries in English, Spanish. 1957. 4/yr. free per issue. adv. bk.rev. bibl, charts, illus, stat. back issues avail.
Indexed: Biol.Abstr., Chem.Abstr., Excerp.Med., Ind.Med. (1963-), Psychol.Abstr.
—CISTI, GNLM, Infotrieve. **CCC.**
Published by: (Universidad de Navarra, Facultad de Medicina), Servicio de Publicaciones de la Universidad de Navarra S.A., Apartado 177, Pamplona, Navarra 31080, Spain. TEL 48-25-2700, FAX 48-17-55-00. Eds. Diego Martinez Caro, Eduardo Alegria. Circ: 12,000.

610 ESP ISSN 1131-5768
CODEN: RMFCF3
REVISTA DE MEDICINA FAMILIAR Y COMUNITARIA. Short title: Medifam. Text in Spanish; Abstracts in Spanish, English. 1991. bi-m. ESP 8,000, EUR 48.08 to individuals; ESP 12,000, EUR 72.12 to institutions; ESP 5,000, EUR 30.05 to students (effective 2000). adv. abstr, bibl, illus, stat. back issues avail. *Refereed.*
—BLDSC (5534.267360).
Published by: Aran Ediciones S.A., Castello, 128 1o, Madrid 28006, Spain. TEL 34-91-782-0030, FAX 34-91-561-5787, edita@grupoaran.com, http://www.grupoaran.com. Ed. J. Morera Montes. Pub. Jose Jimenez. R&P Maria Dolores Linares TEL 34-1-7820035. Circ: 3,000.

616.98023 ROM ISSN 1221-7018
REVISTA DE MEDICINA MILITARA. Text in Romanian. q.?.
Formerly (until 1989): Revista Sanitara Militara (1221-700X)
Address: Calea Plevnei 134, Bucharest 77103, Romania.

610 ROM ISSN 1221-2229
CODEN: REMTAS
REVISTA DE MEDICINA SI FARMACIE/ORVOSI ES GYOGYSZERESZETI SZEMLE. Text in English, French, German, Hungarian, Romanian; Abstracts in English. 1955. q. ROL 250,000, USD 20 (effective 2000). adv. bk.rev. abstr, bibl, charts, illus. reprint service avail. from PQC. *Refereed.* **Document type:** *Academic/Scholarly.* **Description:** For medical and pharmaceutical practitioners and researchers. Includes general reports, clinical studies, experimental studies, medical, dental and pharmaceutical issues.
Formerly (until 1991): Revista Medicala - Medical Review (0034-995X)
Related titles: Microfilm ed.: (from PQC).
Indexed: Chem.Abstr., Excerp.Med.
—CASDDS, GNLM, KNAW.
Published by: Universitatea de Medicina si Farmacie din Targu Mures, Str. Gh. Marinescu 38, Targu-Mures 4300, Romania. TEL 40-65-215551, FAX 40-65-210407, rectorat@umftgm.ro. Ed. Ion Pascu. R&P, Adv. contact Alexandru Botianu TEL 40-65-215133. color page ROL 2,000,000. Circ: 500. **Subscr. to:** Rodipet S.A.

610 ESP ISSN 1136-7342
REVISTA DE MEDICINA Y PRACTICA CLINICA. Text in Spanish. 1996. q. **Document type:** *Academic/Scholarly.*
Published by: Ediciones Doyma S.A., Traversa de Gracia, 17-21, Barcelona 08021, Spain. TEL 34-93-200-0711, FAX 34-93-209-1136, comercial@doymanet.es, http://www.doyma.es, http://www.doyma.es/. Ed. Anna Pahissa. adv.: color page ESP 238,000; trim 280 x 210. Circ: 3,000.

610 ESP
LA REVISTA DIGITAL DE MEDICINA Y SALUD. Text in Spanish. 1998. bi-m. back issues avail.
Media: Online - full text.
Published by: MedSpain, Spain. director@medspain.com, http://www.medspain.com/. Ed. Jose Eduardo Gonzalez Diaz.

610 570 ECU ISSN 0034-9313 CODEN: REMBA8
REVISTA ECUATORIANA DE MEDICINA Y CIENCIAS BIOLOGICAS. Text in Spanish; Summaries in English. 1963. q. USD 20. adv. bk.rev. charts, illus. index.
Indexed: Biol.Abstr., C.I.S. Abstr., Chem.Abstr.
Published by: Casa de la Cultura Ecuatoriana, Casilla 67, Ave. 6de Diciembre, 794, Quito, Ecuador. Ed. Dr. Plutarco Naranjo. Circ: 2,500.

610 BRA ISSN 0034-9585
REVISTA GOIANA DE MEDICINA. Text in Portuguese; Abstracts and contents page in English, Portuguese. 1955. irreg. BRL 10,000 to non-members. adv. bk.rev. abstr, bibl, charts, illus. cum.index. reprint service avail. from PQC. **Document type:** *Academic/Scholarly.*
Description: Original papers and research in all branches of medicine, with emphasis on surgery.
Related titles: Microform ed.: (from PQC).
Indexed: Abstr.Hyg., Chem.Abstr., Excerp.Med., Helminthol.Abstr., Ind.Med. (coverage dropped), Protozool.Abstr., Trop.Dis.Bull.
—KNAW.
Published by: (Associacao Medica de Goias), Imprensa da Universidade Federal de Goias, Ave. PORTUGAL, Esq. Av. Mutirao Sector Bueno, St Central, Caixa Postal 254, Goiania, GO 74001-970, Brazil. TEL 55-62-2051616, FAX 55-62-2051015, caia@recitoria.ufg.br, http://www.ufg.br. Ed. Helio Moreira. Circ: 3,000.
Co-sponsor: Faculdade de Medicina da Universidade Federal de Goias.

616.015 ESP ISSN 1130-1406 CODEN: RIBMEI
REVISTA IBEROAMERICANA DE MICOLOGIA. Text in English, Portuguese, Spanish; Summaries in English, Spanish. 1984. q. EUR 75 in Europe to individuals and Latin America; EUR 150 rest of world to individuals; EUR 100 in Europe to institutions and Latin America; EUR 200 rest of world to institutions (effective 2000). adv. bk.rev. Supplement avail. *Refereed.* **Document type:** *Monographic series, Academic/Scholarly.*
Description: Publishes original articles, clinical notes and reviews of research in general, medical and veterinary mycology.
Formerly (until 1990): Revista Iberica de Micologia (0212-9523)
Related titles: Online - full content ed.: EUR 60 (effective 2000).
Indexed: Abstr.Hyg., Aqua.Sci.& Fish.Abstr., Bio-Contr.News & Info., Dairy Sci.Abstr., Environ.Sci.Poll.Mgmt., Forest.Abstr., Hort.Abstr., Ind.SST, Ind.Vet., Maize Abstr., Microbiol.Abstr., Nutr.Abstr., Postharvest, Rev.Appl.Entomol., Rev.Arom.& Med.Plants, Rev.Med.& Vet.Mycol., Rev.Plant Path., Sugar Ind.Abstr., Triticale Abstr., Trop.Dis.Bull., Vet.Bull.
—BLDSC (7858.825000), CINDOC.
Published by: Asociacion Espanola de Micologia, Depto. Inmunologia Microbiologia y Parasitologia, Universidad del Pais Vasco, Apartado 699, Bilbao, Vizcaya 48080, Spain. TEL 34-94-6012853, FAX 34-94-4649266, oipquang@lg.ehu.es, http://www.RevIberoamMicol.com. Ed., R&P Guillermo Quindos Andres. Adv. contact Pilar Ezkurra. B&W page ESP 60,000, color page ESP 130,000. Circ: 1,200 (paid); 1,000 (controlled).

616 MEX ISSN 1405-101X
REVISTA IBEROLATINOAMERICANA DE CUIDADOS INTENSIVOS. Text in Spanish; Summaries in English. 1992. bi-m. MXP 210, USD 55 (effective 1996 & 1997). **Document type:** *Academic/Scholarly.* **Description:** Contains original articles, research reports, review articles, clinical cases and notices, related to critical medicine.
Published by: Obsidiana Editores S.A., CZDA DE TLALPAN 2365, Col Ciudad Jardin, Mexico City, DF 04370, Mexico. TEL 52-5-689-9133. Eds. Dr. Jose Benitez, Dr. Jose Elizalde. Pub. Jorge Godoy-Gutierrez. Circ: 2,000. **Dist. by:** Distribuidora Editorial de Mexico SA de CV, P.O. Box 76-026, Mexico City, DF 04201, Mexico. TEL 52-5-544-7953, FAX 52-5-689-6545.

616.9802 BRA CODEN: RMABE8
REVISTA MEDICA DA AERONAUTICA DO BRASIL. Text in Portuguese. 1949. s-a. bibl, charts, illus, stat.
Formerly (until 1971): Revista Medica da Aeronautica (0370-6141)
Indexed: Excerp.Med., Ind.Med. (coverage dropped).
Published by: Servico de Saude da Aeronautica, Av Marechal Camara, 223 9o, Centro, Rio De Janeiro, RJ 20020-080, Brazil.

610 CHL ISSN 0034-9887 CODEN: RMCHAW
REVISTA MEDICA DE CHILE. Text in Spanish. 1872. m. USD 200 (effective 1997). adv. bk.rev. abstr, bibl, charts, illus, stat. index. *Refereed.* **Document type:** *Academic/Scholarly.*
Related titles: Online - full text ed.: (from SciELO, Institute for Scientific Information).
Indexed: ASCA, Abstr.Hyg., Aqua.Sci.& Fish.Abstr., Biol.Abstr., Cal.Tiss.Abstr., Chem.Abstr., Chem.Titles, Curr.Cont., Dairy Sci.Abstr., Dent.Ind., Environ.Sci.Poll.Mgmt., Helminthol.Abstr., Ind.Med. (1872-), Ind.Sci.Rev., Ind.Vet., Inpharma, Neurosci.Cit.Ind., Nutr.Abstr., Pharm.&Out.News, Protozool.Abstr., Reac., Rev.Appl.Entomol., Rev.Med.& Vet.Mycol., Rev.Plant Path., Risk Abstr., SSCI (coverage dropped), Saf.Sci.Abstr., Sci.Cit.Ind., Trop.Dis.Bull., Vet.Bull.
—BLDSC (7864.250000), CASDDS, CISTI, GNLM, IDS.
Published by: Sociedad Medica de Santiago, Casilla 168, 9, Correo, 55, Santiago, Chile. TEL 56-2-2748985, FAX 56-2-3651724, revmedchile@entel.chile.net, revmedchile@entelchile.net, http://www.entelchile.net/socmed. Ed. Dr. Humberto Reyes B. Circ: 2,000.

610 CRI
REVISTA MEDICA DE COSTA RICA Y CENTROAMERICA. Text in Spanish. 1933. q. USD 16 in Central America; USD 28 elsewhere (effective 2000). adv. bk.rev. charts, illus. reprint service avail. from PQC. **Document type:** *Academic/Scholarly.*
Formerly (until 1994): Revista Medica de Costa Rica (0034-9909)
Indexed: Biol.Abstr., Excerp.Med. (until 1993).
—GNLM.
Published by: Dr. Manuel Zeledon Perez Ed. & Pub., Apdo 978, San Jose 1000, Costa Rica. TEL 506-255-29-69. adv.: B&W page USD 350, color page USD 400. Circ: 5,000.

610 CHL ISSN 0034-9917
REVISTA MEDICA DE VALPARAISO. Text in Spanish; Summaries in English. 1948. q. USD 15. adv. bibl, charts, illus.
Indexed: Chem.Abstr.
—CISTI.
Published by: Sociedad Medica de Valparaiso, Ave. Brazil, 1689, Valparaiso, Chile. Ed. Dr. Antonio Barbera. Circ: 1,000.

610 MEX ISSN 0185-1063
REVISTA MEDICA DEL HOSPITAL GENERAL DE MEXICO S.S.A. Text in Spanish. 1925. m. USD 45 (effective 1999). adv. bk.rev. illus. back issues avail. **Document type:** *Abstract/Index, Academic/Scholarly.*
Formerly (until 1933): Hospital General (0186-2448)
Related titles: CD-ROM ed.; Online - full text ed.
Indexed: Chem.Abstr., Excerp.Med., Ind.Med. (coverage dropped).
—GNLM.
Published by: Sociedad Medica del Hospital General de Mexico, S.S.A., Dr. Balmis 148, Auditorio Abraham Ayala Gonzalez, Mexico City, DF 06726, Mexico. TEL 52-5-5780506, FAX 52-5-5780505, http://www.facmed.unam.mx/gea/revista/revista.htm. Ed. Guadalupe Tenorio Guajardo. Circ: 1,700 (paid); 1,300 (controlled).

610 PRY ISSN 0034-9933
REVISTA MEDICA DEL PARAGUAY. Text in Spanish; Summaries in Spanish, English. 1955. q. PYG 500, USD 5. adv. bibl, charts, illus, stat. index.
Indexed: Biol.Abstr.
Published by: Sociedad de Pediatria y Puericultura del Paraguay, 25 de Mayo y Tacuai, Asuncion, Paraguay. Circ: 800.

610 BRA ISSN 0100-0195
REVISTA MEDICA DO ESTADO DO RIO DE JANEIRO. Text in English, French, Portuguese. 1941; N.S. 1977. 3/yr. free per issue. bk.rev. abstr. index.
Formerly (until vol.42, no.2, 1975): Revista Medica do Estado da Guanabara (0034-9941)
Indexed: Biol.Abstr., Chem.Abstr., Excerp.Med.
—CISTI.
Published by: Secretaria de Estado de Saude, Centro de Informacao Cientifica para a Saude, Secao de Editoracao, Rua Moncorvo Filho, 100-Andar 2, Centro, Rio De Janeiro, RJ 20211-340, Brazil. Ed. Henrique Antunes Franco. Circ: 3,000.

610 BOL ISSN 0482-6760
REVISTA MEDICA (LA PAZ). Text in Spanish. 1977. q. illus.
Published by: Caja Nacional de Seguridad Social, Casilla 697, Plaza Murillo Esquina Ingavi, La Paz, Bolivia.

610 ROM ISSN 1220-5478
REVISTA MEDICALA ROMANA. Text in Romanian; Summaries in English, French, German, Russian. 1954. m. USD 25. adv. bk.rev. abstr.
Former titles (until 1991): Viata Medicala - pentru Medici; Viata Medicala - pentru Cadre Superioare
Indexed: Biol.Abstr., C.I.S. Abstr., Chem.Abstr., Chem.Indus.Notes, Chem.Titles, Ind.Med. (coverage dropped).
Published by: Uniunea Societatilor de Stiinte Medicale din Rumania, Societatea Nationala de Medicina Generala, Str. Progresului 8, Bucharest 70754, Romania. **Subscr. to:** ILEXIM, Str. 13 Decembrie 3, PO Box 136-137, Bucharest 70116, Romania.

610 617 ROM ISSN 0048-7848
REVISTA MEDICO-CHIRURGICALA. Text mainly in Romanian; Text occasionally in English, French, German; Summaries in English. 1887. q. ROL 4,000, USD 20. adv. bk.rev. illus.
Related titles: Microform ed.: (from PQC).
Indexed: Biol.Abstr., Chem.Abstr., Chem.Titles, Dent.Ind., Environ.Sci.Poll.Mgmt., Excerp.Med., Ind.Med. (coverage dropped), Risk Abstr., Saf.Sci.Abstr.
—CISTI, KNAW.
Published by: Societatea de Medici si Naturalisti din Iasi/Society of Physicians and Natural Scientists, Bd. Independentei 16, PO Box 25, Iasi 6600, Romania. TEL 98-142980. Ed. Gr Scripcaru. Circ: 1,500.

610 ALB ISSN 0255-6790 CODEN: REMJE2
REVISTA MJEKESORE. Text in Albanian. bi-m.
—CASDDS.
Published by: Ministria e Shendetesise/Ministry of Health, Tirana, Albania. TELEX 4205.

616.98 PRT ISSN 0482-7171 CODEN: RPMMAG
REVISTA PORTUGUESA DE MEDICINA MILITAR; orgao dos servicos de saude do exercito, marinha e forca aerea. Text in English, French, Portuguese. 1953. q. PTE 2.20, USD 40. adv. index. back issues avail.
Document type: *Government.*
—CASDDS, GNLM.
Published by: Escola do Servico de Saude Militar, Rua Infantaria, 16, n. 30, Lisbon 1200, Portugal. TEL 3887869, FAX 3874991. Ed. Carlos Manuel Vieira Reis. Circ: 2,000.

610 614.86 FRA
REVUE AUTOMOBILE MEDICALE. Text in French. 6/yr.
Published by: Automobile - Club Medical de France, 74 av. Kleber, Paris 75116, France. TEL 47-04-31-30, FAX 47-55-43-97. Ed. Bruno Soubizan. Circ: 17,201.

610 FRA ISSN 1247-0163
REVUE DE MEDECINE DE TOURS ET DU CENTRE-OUEST. Text in French. 1960. 6/yr. FRF 280, EUR 42.69 domestic; FRF 290, EUR 44.21 foreign (effective 2000).
Former titles (until 1984): Revue de Medicine de Tours (0557-7721); (until 1967): Revue Medicale de Tours (0484-8926)
—EMDOCS, GNLM, KNAW.
Published by: Editions la Simarre, Z.I. No. 2 - rue Joseph-Cugnot, Joue-les-Tours 37300, France. TEL 33-2-47535366, FAX 33-2-47674505.

610 615 FRA ISSN 1240-9782
REVUE DE MEDECINES ET PHARMACOPEES AFRICAINES. Text in French. 1987. s-a. FRF 100; FRF 150 foreign.
Formerly (until 1992): Medecine Traditionnelle et Pharmacopee (1015-0382)
Published by: Agence de Cooperation Culturelle et Technique, 38 rue du Bois Gramond, Eysines 33320, France. TEL 56-28-38-67, FAX 56-16-06-66.
Co-sponsor: Groupe de Recherche et d'Information sur la Pharmacopee et l'Environnement Tropical.

610 FRA
REVUE DE PHYTOTHERAPY PRATIQUE. Text in French. q. FRF 300 foreign. adv.
Formerly: Phytotherapy (0292-9406)
Published by: (Institut National de Phytotherapie), Groupe des Revues Associees, 25 rue Dagorno, Paris 75012, France. FAX 43-47-30-80. **Co-sponsor:** College Francais des Medecines de Terrain et Science Appliquees.

M

610 FRA ISSN 0035-2640
REVUE DU PRATICIEN✱. Text in French. 1951. 20/yr. FRF 850; FRF 1,050 foreign. adv. bk.rev. charts, illus, pat. index.
Related titles: Online - full text ed.: (from Institute for Scientific Information).
Indexed: Biol.Abstr., C.I.S. Abstr., Curr.Cont. (coverage dropped), Dent.Ind., Dok.Arbeitsmed., Excerp.Med., Helminthol.Abstr., INIS Atomind., Ind.Med. (1951-), Int.Nurs.Ind., Nutr.Abstr.
—BLDSC (7942.600000), CISTI, GNLM, IDS, Infotrieve, KNAW. **CCC.**
Published by: Editions J.B. Bailliere, 46 rue la Boetie -Elysees, Paris Cedex 8 75379, France. TEL 33-1-49536900, FAX 33-1-45631016. Ed. Pierre Louis Fagniez. Adv. contact Marianne Bouilloux Lafont. Circ: 59,000.

610 BEL ISSN 0035-3639
CODEN: RMBRDQ
REVUE MEDICALE DE BRUXELLES. Text in French. 1944. 6/yr. BEF 1,272; BEF 2,120 foreign. adv. bk.rev. abstr, bibl, charts, illus, stat, tr.lit. *Refereed.* **Document type:** *Academic/Scholarly.*
Indexed: Biol.Abstr., C.I.S. Abstr., Dent.Ind., Excerp.Med., Ind.Med. (1944-), Int.Nurs.Ind., Ref.Zh.
—BLDSC (7932.037000), CISTI, GNLM, KNAW.
Published by: Association des Medecins Anciens Etudiants de l'Universite Libre de Bruxelles (A.M.U.B.), Rte de Lennik 808, Bte 612, Brussels 1070, Belgium. TEL 32-2-555-6062, FAX 32-2-555-6117. Ed. Jacques Sternon. Pub. Gregory Ezersky. Circ: 2,900 (controlled).

610 CHE ISSN 0035-3655
CODEN: RMSRA6
REVUE MEDICALE DE LA SUISSE ROMANDE. Text in French. 1880. m. CHF 70; CHF 140 foreign (effective 1999). adv. bk.rev. charts, illus, stat. index. **Document type:** *Academic/Scholarly.*
Indexed: Biol.Abstr., C.I.S. Abstr., Chem.Abstr., Dent.Ind., Excerp.Med., Ind.Med. (1881-), Int.Nurs.Ind.
—BLDSC (7932.300000), CISTI, GNLM, KNAW.
Published by: Societe Medicale de la Suisse Romande, Case Postale 3093, Lausanne 1002, Switzerland. TEL 41-21-3417175, FAX 41-21-3417179. Ed. E C Bonard. R&P Francis Pachond. Circ: 5,100.

610 BEL ISSN 0035-3663
REVUE MEDICALE DE LIEGE; journal du praticien. Text in French. 1946. m. BEF 2,000; BEF 2,800 foreign. adv. bk.rev. abstr, bibl, charts, illus. index. reprint service avail. from PQC. *Refereed.* **Description:** Technical journal of interest to physicians; covers all aspects of the medical profession.
Related titles: Microform ed.: (from PQC).
Indexed: Biol.Abstr., C.I.S. Abstr., Chem.Abstr., Chem.Titles, Dent.Ind., Excerp.Med., Ind.Med. (coverage dropped), Ind.Vet., Int.Nurs.Ind., Protozool.Abstr.
—BLDSC (7932.080000), EMDOCS, GNLM.
Published by: (Universite de Liege), Institut de Medecine, Rue Alex Bouvy 13, Liege 4020, Belgium. TEL 32-41-437572, FAX 32-41-437572. Ed. H Kulbertus. Circ: 3,000.

610 614 RWA ISSN 0557-8590
REVUE MEDICALE RWANDAISE. Text in French. 1968. q. adv.
Published by: Ministere de la Sante Publique, BP 84, Kigali, Rwanda. Ed. Dr. Butera.

LA REVUE PRESCRIRE. see *PHARMACY AND PHARMACOLOGY*

610 JPN ISSN 0915-700X
RIGAKU SHINRYO/JOURNAL OF PHYSICAL MEDICINE. Text in Japanese. 1990. a. JPY 2,000.
Published by: Nihon Rigaku Shinryo Igakkai/Japanese Society for Physical Medicine, Nihon Daigaku Igakubu Seikei Gekagaku Kyoshitsu, 30-1, Oyaguchi Kamicho, Itabashi-ku, Tokyo 173, Japan.

610 JPN
RINSHO KENSA NO SHINPO TO TOMONI. Text in Japanese. 1980. 4/yr.
Published by: Kokusai Shiyaku K.K./International Reagents Corp., 1-30 Hamabedori 2-chome, Chuo-ku, Kobe-shi, Hyogo-ken 651-0083, Japan.

610 JPN ISSN 0389-1887
CODEN: METCDS
RINSHO KENSAGAKU ZASSHI/MEDICAL TECHNOLOGY. Text in Japanese. 1973. m. JPY 650 per issue.
Indexed: Chem.Abstr., Chem.Titles.
—CASDDS.

Published by: Ishiyaku Publishers Inc., 7-10 Honkomagome 1-chome, Bunkyo-ku, Tokyo 113-0021, Japan. Ed. Hiroshi Miura. Circ: 14,500.

610 ITA ISSN 0392-4858
RIVISTA DEL MEDICO PRATICO. Text in Italian. 1981. 18/yr. ITL 49,000 (effective 1999). **Document type:** *Academic/Scholarly.*
—CISTI.
Published by: Masson S.p.A., Divisione Periodici, Via F.lli Bressan 2, Milan, MI 20126, Italy. TEL 39-2-270741, FAX 39-2-27074210. Ed. Carlo Grassi. adv.: B&W page ITL 9,000,000, color page ITL 12,900,000; trim 285 x 210. Circ: 25,000.

616.98 ITA ISSN 0035-631X
CODEN: RMDSA2
RIVISTA DI MEDICINA AERONAUTICA E SPAZIALE. Text in Italian. 1938. q. ITL 30,000; ITL 45,000 foreign. adv. bk.rev. abstr, bibl, charts, illus, stat. index. **Description:** Covers aerospace medicine.
Indexed: Biol.Abstr., C.I.S. Abstr., Chem.Abstr., Excerp.Med., INIS Atomind., Ind.Med. (coverage dropped).
—CASDDS, CISTI.
Published by: Corps Sanitario Aeronautico, Viale Piero Gobetti, 2, Rome, RM 00185, Italy. FAX 06-49865611. Ed. L Spuri. Circ: 1,300.

610 616 ITA
RIVISTA DI MEDICINA E CHIRURGIA. Text in Italian. 1979. q.
Published by: Giardini Editori e Stampatori, Via Santa Bibbiana, 28, Pisa, PI 56127, Italy. TEL 050 502531.

616.07 ITA ISSN 0035-6417
RIVISTA DI PATOLOGIA E CLINICA. Text in Italian; Summaries in English, Italian. 1946. bi-m. ITL 80,000; ITL 160,000 foreign (effective 1998). adv. charts, illus, stat. index.
Indexed: Chem.Abstr., Excerp.Med.
—BLDSC (7992.325000), CISTI, GNLM.
Published by: Casa Editrice Maccari, Via Palermo, 44, Parma, PR 43100, Italy. TEL 39-521-771268. Circ: 1,200.

155.3 610 ITA ISSN 0392-1670
RIVISTA DI SESSUOLOGIA. Text in Italian; Summaries in English, Italian. 1960. q. ITL 64,000; ITL 90,000 foreign (effective 1996). adv. bk.rev. bibl, charts, illus. index.
Formerly: Sessuologia (0037-2838)
Indexed: Excerp.Med., Ind.Philos.
—CCC.
Published by: (Centro Italiano di Sessuologia), Cooperativa Libraria Universitaria Editrice Bologna, Via Marsala, 24, Bologna, BO 40126, Italy. TEL 39-051-220736, FAX 39-051-237758, clueb@clueb.com, http://www.clueb.com. Ed. R Forleo. Circ: 1,000.

610 ITA ISSN 0393-1129
RIVISTA ITALIANA DI AGOPUNTURA✱. Text in Italian. 1973. 3/yr. ITL 9,000. adv. bk.rev. bibl, charts, illus.
Published by: Societa Italiana di Agopuntura, Via Diaz, 5, Saronno, VA 21047, Italy. Ed. Dr. U Lanza. Circ: 1,000.

610 570 ITA ISSN 0393-1137
RIVISTA ITALIANA DI BIOLOGIA E MEDICINA. Text in Italian. q. USD 105 to individuals; USD 155 to institutions (effective 1999). **Document type:** *Academic/Scholarly.* **Description:** Devoted to the biological and medical aspects of man.
Indexed: Excerp.Med.
—BLDSC (7987.291500), CISTI, EMDOCS, GNLM.
Published by: Edizioni Minerva Medica, Corso Bramante, 83-85, Turin, TO 10126, Italy. TEL 39-11-678282, FAX 39-11-674502. Ed. P A Vertova. Pub. Alberto Oliaro. Circ: 5,000.

610 ITA ISSN 0394-9109
RIVISTA ITALIANA DI COLON-PROCTOLOGIA. Text and summaries in English. 1982. q. ITL 90,000; includes supplement. bk.rev. **Description:** Covers both psychological and psychological aspects of colorectal disorders, scientific studies of the latest advances, and also include international symposium.
—EMDOCS, GNLM.
Published by: (Italian Society of Coloproctology), Promo Leader Service s.r.l., Via Jacopo Nardi, 60, Florence, FI 50132, Italy. TEL 39-55-243755, FAX 39-55-2342929, plseditoria@dada.it. Ed. Mario Lise. R&P Manela Bertelli.

616.08 ITA ISSN 0394-9982
RIZA PSICOSOMATICA. Text in Italian. 1980. m. ITL 78,000. adv. **Document type:** *Academic/Scholarly.* **Description:** Reports on psychosomatic illnesses and conditions.
Published by: Edizioni Riza, Via Luigi Anelli, 1, Milan, MI 20122, Italy. TEL 39-02-5830-1022, FAX 39-02-5831-8162. Ed. Dr. Raffaele Morelli. adv.: color page ITL 10,800,000. Circ: 57,500.

610 613 USA ISSN 0091-3472
RA440.6
ROBERT WOOD JOHNSON FOUNDATION. ANNUAL REPORT. Key Title: Annual Report - Robert Wood Johnson Foundation. Text in English. 1971. a. free per issue. illus. **Document type:** *Corporate.*
Indexed: Med.Care Rev.
Published by: Robert Wood Johnson Foundation, PO Box 2316, Princeton, NJ 08543-2316. TEL 609-452-8701, http://www.rwjf.org. Ed. Jeanne Weber. Circ: 30,000.

610 GBR ISSN 0305-0688
ROCK CARLING FELLOWSHIP. Text in English. 1971. a. **Document type:** *Bulletin.*
—BLDSC (8001.450000).
Published by: Nuffield Trust, 59 New Cavendish St, London W1M 7RD, United Kingdom.

610 USA
ROCKEFELLER UNIVERSITY, NEW YORK. SCIENTIFIC AND EDUCATIONAL PROGRAMS. Text in English. 1979. a. free per issue. reprint service avail. from PQC,ISI.
Supersedes (1955-1979): Rockefeller University, New York. Annual Report (0080-3405)
Related titles: Online - full text ed.
—CCC.
Published by: (Rockefeller University), Rockefeller University Press, 1114 First Ave, New York, NY 10021. TEL 212-327-7938, FAX 212-327-8513, rupress@mail.rockefeller.edu, http://www.rockefeller.edu/rupress. Circ: 9,000.

610.69 CAN ISSN 0707-3542
ROLLCALL; a status report of selected health personnel in the province of British Columbia. Text in English. 1974. biennial. free per issue. illus. **Document type:** *Bulletin.* **Description:** Describes the distribution of health personnel in British Columbia by health region.
Published by: University of British Columbia, Centre for Health Services and Policy Research, 429 2194 Health Sciences Mall, Vancouver, BC V6T 1Z3, Canada. TEL 604-822-4810, FAX 604-822-5690, hhru@chspr.ubc.ca, http://www.chspr.ubc.ca. Circ: 350.

ROMANIAN JOURNAL OF MORPHOLOGY AND EMBRYOLOGY/REVUE ROUMAINE DE MORPHOLOGIE ET EMBRYOLOGIE. see *BIOLOGY*

610 FRA ISSN 1286-210X
ROSENWALD: L'ANNUAIRE DU MEDECIN. Text in French. 1887. a. FRF 1,190, USD 200. adv.
Formerly: Guide Rosenwald: Annuaire Medical (0992-3993)
Published by: Guide Rosenwald, 10 rue Vineuse, Paris 75116, France. TEL 33-1-44308100, FAX 33-1-44308111, rosenwal@wanadoo.fr. Circ: 10,000.

610 RUS ISSN 0869-6047
CODEN: VAMEE3
ROSSIISKAYA AKADEMIYA MEDITSINSKIKH NAUK. VESTNIK/ACADEMY OF MEDICAL SCIENCES OF RUSSIA. ANNALS. Text in Russian; Summaries in English. 1944. m. USD 408 foreign (effective 1999). adv. bk.rev. charts, illus. index. **Document type:** *Journal, Academic/Scholarly.* **Description:** Publishes original scientific papers and review articles on the important problems of medical science and public health practice.
Formerly: Akademiya Meditsinskikh Nauk S.S.S.R. Vestnik (0002-3027)
Indexed: Biol.Abstr., Chem.Abstr., Chem.Indus.Notes, Dent.Ind., INIS Atomind., Ind.Med. (1992-), Int.Nurs.Ind., Ref.Zh., Russ.Acad.Sci.Bibl.
—BLDSC (0032.753000), CASDDS, CISTI, East View, GNLM, IDS, Infotrieve, KNAW. **CCC.**
Published by: (Rossiiskaya Akademiya Meditsinskikh Nauk), Izdatel'stvo Meditsina, Petroverigskii per 6-8, Moscow 101000, Russian Federation. TEL 7-095-2982052, 7-095-928-86-48, FAX 7-095-9211355, meditsina@iname.com, http://www.medit.ru. Ed. N P Bochkov. Pub. A M Stochik. R&P A Ukhanova. Adv. contact O A Fadeeva TEL 7-095-923-51-40. Circ: 950.
Dist. by: Mezhdunarodnaya Kniga, B Yakimanka 39, Moscow 117049, Russian Federation. TEL 7-095-2384967, FAX 7-095-2384634.

M

610 RUS ISSN 0869-2106
R91 CODEN: RMZHEF
ROSSIISKII MEDITSINSKII ZHURNAL. Text in Russian; Summaries in English. 1937. bi-m. USD 150 foreign (effective 2000). adv. bk.rev. **Document type:** *Journal, Trade.* **Description:** Addressed to practicing physicians of all specialities. Deals with practical problems in the diagnosis and treatment of most common diseases, social hygiene and public health organization.
Formerly (until 1992): Sovetskaya Meditsina (0038-5077)
Indexed: ASCA, Biol.Abstr., C.I.S. Abstr., Dairy Sci.Abstr., Dent.Ind., Helminthol.Abstr., INIS Atomind., Ind.Med. (coverage dropped), Int.Aerosp.Abstr., Nutr.Abstr., Ref.Zh., World Bibl.Soc.Sec.
—CASDDS, CISTI, EMDOCS, GNLM, Infotrieve. **CCC.**
Published by: Izdatel'stvo Meditsina, Petroverigskii per 6-8, Moscow 101000, Russian Federation. TEL 7-095-9248785, 7-095-928-86-48, FAX 7-095-9286003, meditsina@iname.com, http://www.medit.ru. Ed. O V Aleksandrov. Pub. A M Stochik. R&P L Shestakova. Adv. contact O A Fadeeva TEL 7-095-923-51-40. Circ: 3,500. **Dist. by:** Mezhdunarodnaya Kniga, B Yakimanka 39, Moscow 117049, Russian Federation. TEL 7-095-2384967, FAX 7-095-2384634.

616.98 GBR ISSN 0035-8665
UH201 CODEN: JRAMAI
ROYAL ARMY MEDICAL CORPS. JOURNAL. Text in English. 1903. 3/yr. GBP 12. adv. bk.rev. charts, illus. index. **Document type:** *Bulletin.*
Indexed: Abstr.Hyg., Biol.Abstr., Chem.Abstr., Curr.Adv.Ecol.Sci., Ergon.Abstr., Excerp.Med., Helminthol.Abstr., Ind.Med. (1903-), Int.Nurs.Ind., Nutr.Abstr., Trop.Dis.Bull.
—BLDSC (4853.000000), CISTI, GNLM, KNAW.
Published by: Royal Army Medical Corps, RAMC RHQ, Keogh Barracks, Ash Vale, Aldershot, Hants GU12 5RQ, United Kingdom. TEL 44-1252-340250, FAX 44-1252-340224. Ed. Brig G O Hopkins. R&P Brig. G.O. Hopkins. Circ: 1,500.

610 GBR ISSN 1352-2450
ROYAL COLLEGE OF GENERAL PRACTITIONERS. OCCASIONAL PAPER. Text in English. 1976. irreg., latest vol.77, 1998. GBP 12. adv. bk.rev. **Document type:** *Monographic series, Academic/Scholarly.*
Formerly (until 1991): Royal College of General Practitioners. Journal. Occasional Paper (0309-6300)
Indexed: Excerp.Med., Ind.Med. (coverage dropped).
—BLDSC (6219.836000).
Published by: Royal College of General Practitioners, Hyde Park, 14 Princes Gate, London SW7 1PU, United Kingdom. TEL 44-171-823-9698, FAX 44-171-225-0629, sales@rcgp.org.uk, http://www.rcgp.org.uk. Ed. D Pereira Gray. Circ: 1,500.

610 GBR
ROYAL COLLEGE OF GENERAL PRACTITIONERS. PRACTICE ORGANISATION SERIES. Text in English. 1995. irreg. **Document type:** *Monographic series.*
Published by: Royal College of General Practitioners, Hyde Park, 14 Princes Gate, London SW7 1PU, United Kingdom. TEL 44-171-823-9698, FAX 44-171-225-0629, sales@rcgp.org.uk, http://www.rcgp.org.uk. Ed. Dr. Bruce Lervy.

610 CAN ISSN 0035-8800
R15
ROYAL COLLEGE OF PHYSICIANS AND SURGEONS OF CANADA. ANNALS/COLLEGE ROYAL DES MEDECINS ET CHIRURGIENS DU CANADA. ANNALES. Text in English, French. 1968. 8/yr. CND 40 domestic; USD 50 in United States; CND 60 foreign (effective 2000). adv. bk.rev. bibl, charts, illus, stat. index. back issues avail. *Refereed.* **Document type:** *Academic/Scholarly.* **Description:** Covers continuing medical education, medical history, biomedical ethics, health policy, internal medicine and surgery.
Indexed: Biol.Abstr., Curr.Cont. (coverage dropped), Excerp.Med., THA.
—BLDSC (1031.530000), CISTI, EMDOCS, GNLM, Infotrieve, KNAW. **CCC.**
Published by: Royal College of Physicians & Surgeons of Canada/College Royal des Medecins et Chirurgiens du Canada, 774 Echo Dr, Ottawa, ON K1S 5N8, Canada. TEL 613-730-6200, FAX 613-730-8830, lynne.quon-mak@rcpsc.edu. Eds. Lynne Quon Mak, William Feldman. Pub. William Feldman. R&P, Adv. contact Lynne Quon-Mak. Circ: 31,000 (paid and controlled).

610 GBR ISSN 0953-0932
ROYAL COLLEGE OF PHYSICIANS OF EDINBURGH. PROCEEDINGS. Text in English. 1910. 4/yr. GBP 20. adv. *Refereed.* **Document type:** *Proceedings.* **Description:** Editorials on topical medical issues, basic science and current practice of medicine, medical philosophy, history and ethics, and Royal College affairs.
Former titles: Royal College of Physicians of Edinburgh. Directory; Royal College of Physicians of Edinburgh. Yearbook and Calendar
—BLDSC (6793.100000), GNLM.
Published by: Royal College of Physicians of Edinburgh, 9 Queen St, Edinburgh EH2 1JQ, United Kingdom. TEL 0131-225-7324, FAX 0131-220-3939. Ed. W Sircus. Circ: 6,100 (controlled).

616.98 GBR ISSN 0035-9033
CODEN: JRNMAF
ROYAL NAVAL MEDICAL SERVICE. JOURNAL. Text in English. 1915. 3/yr. GBP 15. adv. bk.rev. bibl, illus. index. reprint service avail. from PQC. *Refereed.* **Document type:** *Academic/Scholarly.*
Related titles: Microform ed.: (from PQC).
Indexed: Abstr.Hyg., Biol.Abstr., C.I.S. Abstr., Curr.Adv.Ecol.Sci., Dairy Sci.Abstr., Excerp.Med., INIS Atomind., Ind.Med. (1915-), Ind.Vet., Int.Nurs.Ind., Trop.Dis.Bull.
—BLDSC (4862.150000), CISTI, GNLM, ingenta, KNAW.
Published by: Institute of Naval Medicine, Alverstoke, Gosport, Hants PO12 2DL, United Kingdom. TEL 44-1705-768110, FAX 44-1705-504823. Ed. Surgeon Commodore G H G Mcmillan. R&P Geoff Marshall. Circ: 800.

ROYAL SOCIETY OF LONDON. PHILOSOPHICAL TRANSACTIONS. BIOLOGICAL SCIENCES. see *BIOLOGY*

610 GBR ISSN 0144-8676
R35
ROYAL SOCIETY OF MEDICINE. ANNUAL REPORT OF THE COUNCIL. Text in English. 1959. a. free per issue. reprint service avail. from PQC,ISI. **Document type:** *Proceedings.*
—BLDSC (1423.500000).
Published by: Royal Society of Medicine Press Ltd, 1 Wimpole St, London W1M 8AE, United Kingdom. FAX 44-207-290-2929. R&P Caroline McLaughlin. Circ: 17,500.

610.6 GBR ISSN 0142-2367
CODEN: RMISDU
ROYAL SOCIETY OF MEDICINE. INTERNATIONAL CONGRESS AND SYMPOSIUM SERIES. Text in English. 1978. irreg., latest vol.220, 1997. **Document type:** *Monographic series.*
Related titles: Online - full text ed.: (from Institute for Scientific Information).
Indexed: Chem.Abstr., Chem.Indus.Notes, Chem.Titles, Int.Abstr.Biol.Sci.
—BLDSC (4538.996000), CASDDS, CISTI, IDS, KNAW. **CCC.**
Published by: Royal Society of Medicine Press Ltd, 1 Wimpole St, London W1M 8AE, United Kingdom. FAX 44-207-290-2929. Ed. Walton. R&P Caroline McLaughlin.

610 GBR ISSN 0141-0768
R35 CODEN: JRSMD9
ROYAL SOCIETY OF MEDICINE. JOURNAL. Variant title: Journal of the Royal Society of Medicine. Text in English. 1907. m. GBP 154 in Europe to institutions; USD 275 in United States to institutions; GBP 166 elsewhere to institutions (effective 2002). adv. bk.rev. bibl, charts, illus. index. reprint service avail. from PQC,ISI. *Refereed.* **Document type:** *Academic/Scholarly.* **Description:** Publishes clinical research and reviews across the range of specialties for general medicine.
Formerly (until vol.70, 1978): Royal Society of Medicine. Proceedings (0035-9157)
Related titles: Microform ed.: (from PQC); Online - full text ed.: (from Ovid Technologies, Inc., HighWire Pr., Institute for Scientific Information).
Indexed: ASCA, Abstr.Hyg., Addic.Abstr., Agri.& Environ.Biotech.Abstr. (coverage dropped), Anim.Breed.Abstr., Apic.Abstr., Biol.Abstr., Brit.Nur.Ind., CINAHL, C.I.S. Abstr., Chem.Abstr., Chem.Indus.Notes, Chem.Titles, Curr.Adv.Cancer Res., Curr.Adv.Ecol.Sci., Curr.Cont., Curr.Tit.Dent., Dairy Sci.Abstr., Dent.Abstr., Dent.Ind., Derwent Biotech.Abstr., Diar.Dis.Res., Ergon.Abstr., Excerp.Med., Food Sci.& Tech.Abstr., Helminthol.Abstr., Hort.Abstr., INIS Atomind., I.P.A., Ind.Med. (1978-), Ind.Vet., Inpharma, Int.Nurs.Ind., Lab.Haz.Bull., Med.& Surg.Dermat., NRN, Nutr.Abstr., Pharm.&Out.News, Protozool.Abstr., Reac., Res.High.Educ.Abstr., Rev.Appl.Entomol., Rev.Arom.& Med.Plants, Rev.Med.& Vet.Mycol., Risk Abstr., SSCI (coverage dropped), Sci.Cit.Ind., Sugar Ind.Abstr., THA, Trop.Dis.Bull., Vet.Bull.
—BLDSC (4864.550000), ADONIS, CASDDS, CISTI, GNLM, IDS, ingenta, KNAW. **CCC.**
Published by: Royal Society of Medicine Press Ltd, 1 Wimpole St, London W1M 8AE, United Kingdom. TEL 44-20-7290-2921, FAX 44-20-7290-2929, rsmjournals@rsm.ac.uk, http://www.roysocmed.ac.uk/pub/jrsm.htm. Ed. Robin Fox. R&P Caroline McLaughlin. Circ: 18,000.

610 GBR ISSN 0267-5331
CODEN: JRMSEW
ROYAL SOCIETY OF MEDICINE. JOURNAL. SUPPLEMENT. Text in English. 1982. irreg. **Document type:** *Monographic series.*
Related titles: Online - full text ed.: (from Ovid Technologies, Inc.).
Indexed: Aqua.Sci.& Fish.Abstr., Dairy Sci.Abstr., Environ.Sci.Poll.Mgmt., Nutr.Abstr., Pollut.Abstr., Risk Abstr., Saf.Sci.Abstr., Soyabean Abstr.
—BLDSC (4864.560000), ADONIS, CISTI, EMDOCS, Infotrieve, KNAW. **CCC.**
Published by: Royal Society of Medicine Press Ltd, 1 Wimpole St, London W1M 8AE, United Kingdom. FAX 44-207-290-2929. R&P Caroline McLaughlin.

610 GBR ISSN 0268-3091
CODEN: RTSSES
ROYAL SOCIETY OF MEDICINE. ROUND TABLE SERIES. Text in English. 1980. irreg. **Document type:** *Monographic series.*
Formerly: Royal Society of Medicine. Forum Series (0144-5618)
Indexed: Chem.Abstr., Chem.Indus.Notes, Chem.Titles.
—BLDSC (8025.870000), CASDDS, CISTI, EMDOCS, KNAW. **CCC.**
Published by: Royal Society of Medicine Press Ltd, 1 Wimpole St, London W1M 8AE, United Kingdom. FAX 44-207-290-2929. R&P Caroline McLaughlin.

610 USA
RX T V PRESCRIPTION FOR GOOD HEALTH. Text in English. irreg. **Description:** Presents articles on health related issues.
Media: Online - full text.
Address: cnovack@tribune.com, http://www.rxtv.com. Ed., Pub. Chris Novack.

610 USA
RYPINS' MEDICAL BOARDS REVIEW: CLINICAL SCIENCES. Text in English. 1933. a. index.
Former titles (until 1987): Rypins' Medical Licensure Examinations; (until 1939): Medical State Board Examinations
Published by: J B Lippincott Co, E Washington Sq, Philadelphia, PA 19106. TEL 215-238-4200. Ed. Edward D Frohlich.

610 CHE
S A B INFORMATION. Text in German. 1910. 4/yr. CHF 15 (effective 2000). **Document type:** *Consumer.*
Address: Holenackerstr 85 C - 20, Bern 3027, Switzerland. TEL 41-31-9910949. Ed. Werner Thuerig. Circ: 1,500.

610 ZAF ISSN 0256-9574
R98 CODEN: SAMJAF
S A M J SOUTH AFRICAN MEDICAL JOURNAL. Text in English. 1884. m. ZAR 365 domestic; USD 120 foreign (effective 2001). adv. bk.rev. bibl, illus, stat. index. back issues avail. *Refereed.* **Document type:** *Journal, Academic/Scholarly.* **Description:** Discusses topics and research in all areas of medicine and health care, including medicopolitical news and health policy.

M

Supersedes (in 1985): South African Medical Journal (0038-2469); Which was formed by the merger of (1903-1926): South African Medical Journal (0255-8947); (1913-1926): South African Medical Record (0255-8947); Which was formerly (1903-1913): Transvaal Medical Journal (1012-7283); Incorporated (in 1964): South African Journal of Laboratory and Clinical Medicine (0038-2299); Which was formerly (until 1955): South African Journal of Clinical Science (0560-9747); (1942-1950): Clinical Proceedings (0366-7782)
Related titles: Online - full text ed.: (from Institute for Scientific Information); ♦ Supplement: Cardiovascular Journal of Southern Africa. ISSN 1015-9657; ♦ South African Journal of Obstetrics and Gynaecology. ISSN 0038-2329.
Indexed: ASCA, Abstr.Anthropol., Abstr.Hyg., Agri.& Environ.Biotech.Abstr. (coverage dropped), Aqua.Sci.& Fish.Abstr., Bibl.Dev.Med.& Child Neur., Biol.Abstr., CINAHL, C.I.S. Abstr., Chem.Abstr., Chem.Indus.Notes, Chem.Titles, Curr.Adv.Cancer Res., Curr.Adv.Ecol.Sci., Curr.Cont., Dairy Sci.Abstr., Dent.Ind., Derwent Biotech.Abstr., Diar.Dis.Res., Dok.Arbeitsmed., Environ.Sci.Poll.Mgmt., Excerp.Med., Food Sci.& Tech.Abstr., Helminthol.Abstr., INIS Atomind., Ind.Med. (1932-), Ind.S.A.Per., Ind.Sci.Rev., Ind.Vet., Inpharma, Int.Nurs.Ind., NRN, Neurosci.Cit.Ind., Nutr.Abstr., Pharm.&Out.News, Pollut.Abstr., Protozool.Abstr., Reac., Rev.Appl.Entomol., Rev.Med.& Vet.Mycol., Rev.Plant Path., Risk Abstr., Rural Devel.Abstr., SSCI (coverage dropped), Saf.Sci.Abstr., Sci.Cit.Ind., Sport Fish.Abstr., Trop.Dis.Bull., Vet.Bull., Virol.Abstr., W.R.C.Inf., World Ag.Econ.& Rur.Soc.Abstr., Zoo.Rec.
—BLDSC (8341.700000), CASDDS, CISTI, GNLM, IDS, ingenta, KNAW.
Published by: South African Medical Association, Health and Medical Publishing Group, 14 Central Sq, Pinelands 7430, South Africa. TEL 27-21-531-3081, FAX 27-21-531-4126, publishing@samedical.org, http://www.samedical.org. Ed. Daniel J Ncayayana. R&P Peter Roberts. Adv. contact Andre Botes TEL 27-11-706-2088. B&W page ZAR 5,243, color page ZAR 7,998; trim 210 x 297. Circ: 14,400 (controlled). **Subscr. to:** PO Box 74789, Lynnwood Ridge, Pretoria 0040, South Africa. TEL 27-12-481-2010, FAX 27-12-481-2061, ann@samedical.org. **Dist. by:** Private Bag X1, Pinelands 7430, South Africa. TEL 27-21-531-3081, FAX 27-21-531-4126.

610 AUS
S A MEDICAL REVIEW; official publication of the Australian Medical Association. (South Australia) Text in English. m. adv. charts, illus. *Refereed.* **Document type:** *Academic/Scholarly.* **Description:** Provides information for medical professionals in South Australia; contains medical, clinical, medical-legal and medical-industrial information for members.
Published by: Australian Medical Association (South Australia), Inc, Newland House, 80 Broughan Pl, North Adelaide, SA 5006, Australia. TEL 61-8-8267-4255, FAX 61-8-8267-5349, trisha@amasa.org.au, http://www.amasa.org.au. Ed. Dr. Mark Coleman. R&P Ms. Trisha Helbers TEL 61-8-8267-4355. adv.: B&W page AUD 900, color page AUD 1,200; trim 297 x 210. Circ: 2,000.

610 ESP ISSN 1138-3593
CODEN: SEMRE3
S E M E R G E N. Text in Spanish. 1977. m. (11/yr.). back issues avail. **Document type:** *Academic/Scholarly.* **Description:** Covers a variety of topics in medical practice in rural areas.
Formerly (until 1996): S E M E R (0214-1450)
Published by: (Sociedad Espanola de Medicina Rural y Generalista), Saned S.A., Capitan Haya, 60, Madrid 28020, Spain. TEL 34-91-749-9507, FAX 34-91-749-9507, semergen@medynet.com, http://www.semergen.es/sociedad.htm. Ed. Dr. Jose A Martinez. adv.: page ESP 255,000. Circ: 12,000.

S I E C U S REPORT. see *SOCIOLOGY*

616.07 GBR
S I G N GUIDELINES. Text in English. 1995. irreg., latest vol.3, 1996. price varies. *Refereed.* **Document type:** *Monographic series.* **Description:** Presents evidence-basedclinical practice guidelines on specific subjects.
Formerly: S I G N Publication
—BLDSC.
Published by: Scottish Intercollegiate Guidelines Network, 9 Queen St, Edinburgh, Midlothian EH2 1JQ, United Kingdom. TEL 44-131-225-7324, FAX 44-131-225-1769, a.allman@rcpe.ac.uk, sign@rcpe.ac.uk, http://www.show.scot.nhs.uk/sign/lane.ltm, http://www.sign.ac.uk. Eds. J. C. Petrie, J.F. Miller. Circ: 12,000.

610 PHL
S L U JOURNAL OF MEDICINE. Text in English. 1979. q. free per issue.
Published by: Saint Louis University, PO Box 71, Baguio City, Benguet 2600, Philippines. TEL 442-3043. Ed. Robert Legaspi. Circ: 500.

610 AUS ISSN 0813-1988
S P U M S JOURNAL; South Pacific Underwater Medicine Society Journal. Text in English. 1971. q., latest vol.31, 2001. AUD 121 to qualified personnel; AUD 60.50 to individuals; AUD 121 to institutions (effective 2001 - 2002). adv. bk.rev. index, cum.index 1971-2000. 60 p./no. 2 cols./p. back issues avail. *Refereed.* **Document type:** *Academic/Scholarly.* **Description:** Contains original papers, meeting information, and selections from other medical journals.
—BLDSC (8425.050700), CISTI, GNLM, ingenta.
Published by: South Pacific Underwater Medicine Society Incorporated, c/o Australian and New Zealand College of Anaesthetists, 630 St. Kilda Rd., Melbourne, VIC 3004, Australia. TEL 61-3-98194898, FAX 61-3-98195298, spumsj@labyrinth.net.au, http://www.spums.org.au. Ed., Adv. contact Dr. John Knight. Circ: 1,000 (paid).

610.71 USA
S T F M MESSENGER. Text in English. 1968. bi-m. USD 20 to members (effective 2000). adv. **Document type:** *Newsletter.* **Description:** Contains news of concern to family medicine educators, society meetings and organizational information.
Formerly: S T F M Newsletter
Published by: Society of Teachers of Family Medicine, 11400 Tomahawk Creek Parkway, Leawood, MO 66211. TEL 913-906-6000. Ed. Stacy Brungardt. Adv. contact Jan Cartwright. Circ: 5,400.

SAINT GEORGE'S HOSPITAL GAZETTE. see *HEALTH FACILITIES AND ADMINISTRATION*

610 ESP
SALUD. Text in Spanish. w. back issues avail.
Media: Online - full text. **Related titles:** ♦ Supplement to: El Mundo. ISSN 1576-6969.
—CINDOC.
Address: Pradillo, 42, Madrid 28002, Spain. TEL 34-91-5864800, FAX 34-91-5864848, internet@el-mundo.es, http://www.el-mundo.es/salud/345/index.html.

SALUD MEDICAL SPANISH. see *LINGUISTICS*

616.98 VEN ISSN 0036-3642
SALUS MILITIAE. Text in Spanish. 1965. s-a. free per issue. abstr, bibl, charts, illus.
Published by: Hospital Central de las Fuerzas Armadas, San Martin, Caracas, DF 1060, Venezuela. Ed. Luis Martinez Iturriza. Circ: 1,000 (controlled). **Subscr. to:** Apdo. Postal 16.297, Caracas, Venezuela.

570 610 BRA ISSN 0101-9910
SALUSVITA; revista da area de ciencias biologicas e da saude. Text mainly in Portuguese, English. 1982. a. BRL 20, USD 10 per issue (effective 2000). bk.rev. abstr, bibl, charts, illus, maps. back issues avail. *Refereed.* **Document type:** *Journal, Academic/Scholarly.* **Description:** Contains original works of technical, didactic and scientific character in the area of medical sciences and biology. Promotes research directed to the academic community in general.
Published by: (Universidade do Sagrado Coracao), Editora da Universidade do Sagrado Coracao, Rua Irma Arminda, 10-50, Bauru, SP 17044-160, Brazil. TEL 55-14-2357112, FAX 55-14-2357254, npu@usc.br, edusc@usc.br, http://www.usc.br. Ed. Mari lene Cabello Di Flora. Pub. Lina Ana Santarosa. R&P Luis Eugenio Vescio TEL 55-14-2357378. Circ: 500.

610 CHE
SAMARITER. Text in German. 26/yr.
Published by: Schweizerischer Samariterbund, Postfach, Olten 4601, Switzerland. TEL 062-261818, FAX 062-262141. Ed. Eugen Kiener. Circ: 30,639.

610 BEL ISSN 0775-7905
SAMSOM ARTSENPRAKTIJK. Text in Flemish. 1986. s-m. BEF 3,286. index. Supplement avail. **Description:** Provides fiscal and administrative advice for doctors in regards to their practices.
Published by: C E D Samsom (Subsidiary of: Wolters Samsom Belgie n.v.), Kouterveld 14, Diegem 1831, Belgium. TEL 32-2-7231111.

610 USA ISSN 0036-4061
SAN DIEGO PHYSICIAN. Text in English. 1915. m. USD 25. adv. bk.rev. charts, illus, tr.lit. **Document type:** *Trade.*
Formerly: San Diego County Medical Society. Bulletin
Published by: San Diego County Medical Society, 3702 Ruffin Rd, Box 23581, San Diego, CA 92193. TEL 619-565-8888, FAX 619-569-1334. Ed. Kevin P Glynn. Adv. contact Katrina S Strathmann. Circ: 3,200.

610 USA ISSN 0361-705X
SAN FRANCISCO MEDICINE. Text in English. 1928. 10/yr., latest vol.74, no.10. USD 45 (effective 2001). adv. bk.rev. **Document type:** *Trade.* **Description:** Contains material of interest to physicians residing and practicing in San Francisco County, CA.
Formerly: San Francisco Medical Society. Bulletin (0036-4142)
Published by: San Francisco Medical Society, 1409 Sutter St, San Francisco, CA 94109. TEL 415-561-0861, 415-561-0850, FAX 415-561-0833, sfm@sirius.com, http://www.sfms.org. Ed., R&P Edare K Carroll. adv.: B&W page USD 650; 9.13 x 7. Circ: 3,500.

610.73 AUT
SANITAETSHANDBUCH CD. Text in German. a. ATS 880 (effective 2000).
Media: CD-ROM. **Related titles:** ♦ Print ed.: Handbuch fuer die Sanitaetsberufe Oesterreich. ISSN 0073-0181.
Published by: Verlag Dieter Goeschl GmbH, Hernalser Hauptstrasse 213, Vienna, W 1170, Austria. TEL 43-1-4864240, FAX 43-1-4854902.

610 FRA ISSN 0151-1998
SANTE DE L'HOMME. Text in French. 1941. 6/yr. FRF 165 domestic to individuals; FRF 220 foreign to individuals; FRF 110 domestic to students (effective 2000). adv. bk.rev. bibl, stat.
Published by: Comite Francais d'Education pour la Sante, 2 rue d'Auguste Comte, BP 51, Vanves Cedex 92174, France. TEL 33-1-41333333, FAX 33-1-41333390, cfes@imaginet.fr. Eds. Dr. Francois Baudier, Jacques Draussin. Adv. contact Bernadette Roussille. Circ: 12,000.

610 PHL ISSN 0115-1126
SANTO TOMAS JOURNAL OF MEDICINE. Text in English. 1955. q., latest vol.50, no.1. PHP 400; USD 60 foreign (effective 2001). adv. bk.rev. abstr. 60 p./no. 3 cols./p. back issues avail.; reprints avail. *Refereed.* **Document type:** *Journal, Academic/Scholarly.*
Related titles: CD-ROM ed.; E-mail ed.; Fax ed.; Supplement: Medical Gazette. 1986. Free with the Santo Tomas Journal of Medicine.
Indexed: Biol.Abstr., Chem.Abstr., Excerp.Med. (until 19??), ExtraMED.
Published by: (University Of Santo Tomas, Faculty of Medicine and Surgery), Santo Tomas University Press, Espana St, Manila 1008, Philippines. TEL 02-731-3101, FAX 632-731-3126, 63-2-749-9712, benjigco@info.com.ph. Ed. Benjamin G Co. Adv. contact Noemi T Salazar. Circ: 3,500.

610 BRA ISSN 1516-3180
SAO PAULO MEDICAL JOURNAL. Text in English; Summaries in Portuguese. 1932. bi-m. USD 50 to individuals; USD 70 to institutions (effective 2001 - 2002). adv. bk.rev. bibl, charts, illus. back issues avail. *Refereed.* **Document type:** *Academic/Scholarly.* **Description:** Publishes original articles in the fields of basic health science and clinical health science.
Former titles (until 1994): Revista Paulista de Medicina (0035-0362); (until 1941): Associacao Paulista de Medicina. Revista (0370-3487)
Related titles: Online - full text ed.: 1997 (from SciELO).
Indexed: Biol.Abstr., Chem.Abstr., Dent.Ind., Excerp.Med., INIS Atomind., Ind.Med. (1994-), Int.Nurs.Ind.
—BLDSC (8075.416000), CISTI, GNLM, KNAW.
Published by: Associacao Paulista de Medicina, Av Brigadeiro Luiz Antonio 278, Andar 7, Sao Paulo SP 01318-901, Brazil. TEL 55-11-3188-4200, FAX 55-11-3106-0773, revistas@apm.org.br, http://www.scielo.br/spm1, http://www.apm.org.br/. Ed. Paulo Andrade Lotufo. Circ: 6,100.

M

610 JPN ISSN 0036-472X
CODEN: SIZSAR
SAPPORO IGAKU ZASSHI/SAPPORO MEDICAL JOURNAL. Text in English, Japanese; Abstracts and contents page in English. 1950. bi-m. per issue exchange basis. bibl, charts, illus, stat. index.
Indexed: Biol.Abstr., C.I.S. Abstr., Chem.Abstr., Chem.Titles, Curr.Adv.Ecol.Sci., Excerp.Med., INIS Atomind., Ref.Zh.
—BLDSC (8075.800000), CASDDS, CISTI, GNLM, KNAW.

Published by: Sapporo Ika Daigaku/Sapporo Medical University, Nishi-17-chome, Minami-1-jo, Chuo-ku, Sapporo-shi, Hokkaido 060-8556, Japan. Circ: 500.

610 CAN ISSN 1486-1682
SASKATCHEWANAN. MEDICAL SERVICES AND HEALTH REGISTRATION BRANCH. ANNUAL STATISTICAL REPORT. Text in English. 1997. a.
Related titles: ♦ Supplement to: Saskatchewan Health. Annual Report. ISSN 0822-160X.
Published by: Medical Care Insurance Branch, T C Douglas Bldg, 3475 Albert St, Regina, SK S4S 6X6, Canada. TEL 306-787-3475, FAX 306-787-9000.

610 SAU ISSN 0379-5284
CODEN: SAMJDI
SAUDI MEDICAL JOURNAL. Text in English; Summaries in Arabic, English. 1979. bi-m. GBP 30. adv. bk.rev. index. back issues avail. *Refereed.* **Document type:** *Academic/Scholarly.* **Description:** Covers a broad range of medical problems with emphasis on Saudi Arabia and the Middle East.
Related titles: CD-ROM ed.; Microform ed.: (from PQC); Online - full text ed.: (from Institute for Scientific Information).
Indexed: ASCA, Abstr.Hyg., Curr.Cont., Dairy Sci.Abstr., Diar.Dis.Res., Excerp.Med., ExtraMED, Helminthol.Abstr., Herb.Abstr., Ind.Vet., Inpharma, Nutr.Abstr., Pharm.&Out.News, Protozool.Abstr., Reac., Rev.Appl.Entomol., Rev.Med.& Vet.Mycol., SSCI (coverage dropped), Trop.Dis.Bull.
—BLDSC (8076.975000), CISTI, EMDOCS, GNLM, IDS, Infotrieve, KNAW. **CCC.**
Published by: Saudi Arabian Armed Forces Ministry of Defence and Aviation, Medical Services Department, P O Box 7897, Riyadh 11159, Saudi Arabia. TEL 966-1-4777714, FAX 966-1-4777194, TELEX 401645 RKHPA SJ. Ed. Dr. Saleh Al Deeb. Circ: 24,000.

610 CZE ISSN 0036-5327
CODEN: SBLEA2
SBORNIK LEKARSKY. Text in Czech; Summaries in English, Russian. 1898. m. CZK 60, USD 28.60 (effective 1999). bibl, charts, illus. index. **Document type:** *Academic/Scholarly.*
Indexed: ASCA, Biol.Abstr., Chem.Abstr., Chem.Titles, Curr.Adv.Ecol.Sci., Curr.Cont. (coverage dropped), Dent.Ind., Excerp.Med. (until 1993), Helminthol.Abstr., INIS Atomind., Ind.Med. (coverage dropped), Nutr.Abstr.
—CASDDS, CISTI, GNLM.
Published by: (Univerzita Karlova, Fakulta Vseobecneho Lekarstvi), Vydavatelstvi Karolinum, Ovocny trh 3, Prague 116 36, Czech Republic. TEL 42-2-24491270, FAX 42-2-24212041, edice@cuni.cz; milan.spala@lfl.cuni.cz. Ed. Milan Spala. Circ: 400. **Subscr. to:** Bibliograficko-informacni Oddeleni Ustavu Vedeckych Informaci 1.LF UK, Salmovska 3, Prague, 2 120 00, Czech Republic. **Dist. by:** Artia, Ve Smeckach 30, Prague, 1 111 27, Czechoslovakia.

SCALPEL AND TONGS; medical philately. see *PHILATELY*

610 GBR ISSN 0283-9318
CODEN: SJSCEN
SCANDINAVIAN JOURNAL OF CARING SCIENCES. Text in English. 1987. q., latest vol.16, 2002. GBP 55 in Europe to individuals; USD 88 in North America to individuals; GBP 61 elsewhere to individuals; GBP 179 in Europe to institutions; USD 284 in North America to institutions; GBP 197 elsewhere to institutions (effective 2002). *Refereed.* **Document type:** *Journal, Academic/Scholarly.* **Description:** Strives to communicate scientific knowledge and research findings to different groups within the health field such as nurses, occupational therapists, physiotherapists, physicians, social workers and others with an interest in patient care.
Related titles: Online - full text ed.: ISSN 1471-6712. GBP 50 in Europe to individuals; USD 80 in North America to individuals; GBP 50 elsewhere to individuals; GBP 162 in Europe to institutions; USD 256 in North America to institutions; GBP 162 elsewhere to institutions (effective 2002) (from EBSCO Publishing, O C L C Online Computer Library Center, Inc., RoweCom Information Quest, CatchWord Ltd., ingenta, Swets Blackwell, Institute for Scientific Information).
Indexed: AMED, ASCA, ASSIA, AgeLine, CINAHL, Curr.Cont., Excerp.Med. (until 1993, 1994-), Fam.Ind., Int.Nurs.Ind., NRN, PsycInfo, Psychol.Abstr. (1990-), SSCI, Soc.Serv.Abstr., Sociol.Abstr., e-psyche.
—BLDSC (8087.495000), ADONIS, EMDOCS, GNLM, IDS, Infotrieve. **CCC.**
Published by: (Nordic College of Caring Sciences NOR), Blackwell Science Ltd., Osney Mead, Oxford OX2 0EL, United Kingdom. TEL 44-1685-206206, FAX 44-1685-721205, journals.cs@blacksci.co.uk, http://www.blackwell-science.com. Ed. Agnes Bjoern.

SCANDINAVIAN JOURNAL OF CLINICAL & LABORATORY INVESTIGATION. see *MEDICAL SCIENCES—Experimental Medicine, Laboratory Technique*

SCANDINAVIAN JOURNAL OF CLINICAL AND LABORATORY INVESTIGATION. SUPPLEMENT. see *MEDICAL SCIENCES—Experimental Medicine, Laboratory Technique*

615.8515 613.62 NOR ISSN 1103-8128
SCANDINAVIAN JOURNAL OF OCCUPATIONAL THERAPY. Text in English. 1994. 4/yr. GBP 42, USD 69 to individuals; GBP 64, USD 105 to institutions (effective 2002). adv. *Refereed.* **Document type:** *Academic/Scholarly.* **Description:** Publishes original articles from all branches of occupational therapy.
Related titles: Online - full text ed.: (from EBSCO Publishing, O C L C Online Computer Library Center, Inc., RoweCom Information Quest, CatchWord Ltd., ingenta, Swets Blackwell).
Indexed: AMED, ASSIA, CINAHL, Ergon.Abstr.
—BLDSC (8087.517650), KNAW. **CCC.**
Published by: Taylor & Francis AS (Subsidiary of: Taylor & Francis Group), Cort Adelersgt. 17, Solli, PO Box 2562, Oslo 0202, Norway. TEL 47-22-12-98-80, FAX 47-22-12-98-90, journals@tandf.no, http://www.tandf.co.uk/tfas. Ed. Inga-Britt Braenholm.

362.1 NOR ISSN 0281-3432
CODEN: SJPCD7
SCANDINAVIAN JOURNAL OF PRIMARY HEALTH CARE. Text in English. 1983. q. GBP 58, USD 95 to individuals; GBP 112, USD 185 to institutions (effective 2002). adv. bk.rev. *Refereed.* **Document type:** *Academic/Scholarly.*
Related titles: Online - full text ed.: (from EBSCO Publishing, O C L C Online Computer Library Center, Inc., RoweCom Information Quest, CatchWord Ltd., ingenta, Swets Blackwell, Institute for Scientific Information); ♦ Supplement: Scandinavian Journal of Primary Health Care. Supplement. ISSN 0284-6020.
Indexed: ASCA, ASSIA, Biol.Abstr., Curr.Cont., Excerp.Med., FAMLI, Fam.Ind., IMFL, Ind.Med. (1988-), Inpharma, Int.Nurs.Ind., NRN, Pharm.&Out.News, PsycInfo, Reac., Ref.Zh., THA, e-psyche.
—BLDSC (8087.519500), CISTI, EMDOCS, GNLM, IDS, KNAW. **CCC.**
Published by: Taylor & Francis AS (Subsidiary of: Taylor & Francis Group), Cort Adelersgt. 17, Solli, PO Box 2562, Oslo 0202, Norway. TEL 47-22-12-98-80, FAX 47-22-12-98-90, journals@tandf.no, http://www.tandf.co.uk/tfas. Ed. Calle Bengtsson. Circ: 6,500.

362.1 NOR ISSN 0284-6020
SCANDINAVIAN JOURNAL OF PRIMARY HEALTH CARE. SUPPLEMENT. Text in English. 1988. irreg. **Document type:** *Academic/Scholarly.*
Related titles: ♦ Supplement to: Scandinavian Journal of Primary Health Care. ISSN 0281-3432.
Indexed: Excerp.Med. (1995-), Ind.Med. (coverage dropped).
—CISTI, EMDOCS, KNAW.
Published by: Scandinavian University Press (Subsidiary of: Taylor & Francis Ltd.), Postboks 2959, Toeyen, Oslo 0608, Norway. TEL 47-22-575400, FAX 47-22-57-53-53, journals@scup.no, http://www.scup.no/primhealth.

362.1042 NOR ISSN 1403-4948
CODEN: SJSMAF
SCANDINAVIAN JOURNAL OF PUBLIC HEALTH. Text in English. 1969. 4/yr. GBP 72, USD 118 to individuals; GBP 162, USD 267 to institutions (effective 2002). adv. charts. Supplement avail. *Refereed.* **Document type:** *Academic/Scholarly.*
Former titles (until 1999): Scandinavian Journal of Social Medicine (0300-8037); (until 1973): Acta Socio-Medica Scandinavica (0044-6041)
Related titles: Online - full text ed.: (from EBSCO Publishing, CatchWord Ltd., Swets Blackwell, Institute for Scientific Information, RoweCom Information Quest).
Indexed: ASCA, ASSIA, Abstr.Hyg., AgeLine, Arts & Hum.Cit.Ind. (coverage dropped), Biol.Abstr., CINAHL, C.I.S. Abstr., Curr.Cont., Dairy Sci.Abstr., Dent.Ind., Environ.Sci.Poll.Mgmt., Excerp.Med., Fam.Ind., INIS Atomind., Ind.Med. (1999-), Inpharma, Int.Nurs.Ind., Nutr.Abstr., Pharm.&Out.News, Reac., Risk Abstr., SSCI, THA, Tox.Abstr., Trop.Dis.Bull., Virol.Abstr.
—BLDSC (8087.525000), CISTI, EMDOCS, GNLM, IDS, Infotrieve, ingenta. **CCC.**
Published by: (Nordisk Socialmedicinsk Foerening), Taylor & Francis AS (Subsidiary of: Taylor & Francis Group), Cort Adelersgt. 17, Solli, PO Box 2562, Oslo 0202, Norway. TEL 47-22-12-98-80, FAX 47-22-12-98-90, journals@tandf.no, http://www.tandf.co.uk.tfas. Ed. Stig Wall. Circ: 900.

362.1042 NOR
CODEN: SJSSD2
SCANDINAVIAN JOURNAL OF PUBLIC HEALTH. SUPPLEMENT. Text in English. 1973. irreg. **Document type:** *Academic/Scholarly.*
Indexed: Excerp.Med., Ind.Med. (coverage dropped), THA.
—EMDOCS.
Published by: (Nordisk Socialmedicinsk Foerening), Scandinavian University Press (Subsidiary of: Taylor & Francis Ltd.), Postboks 2959, Toeyen, Oslo 0608, Norway. FAX 47-22-57-53-53, journals@scup.no, http://www.scup.no/sjpublic.

612.6 306.7 DNK ISSN 1398-2966
SCANDINAVIAN JOURNAL OF SEXOLOGY. Text in English. 1983. 4/yr. DKK 495 domestic to individuals; DKK 396 foreign to individuals; DKK 375 domestic to students (effective 2001). adv. bk.rev. abstr, charts, illus. 80 p./no. *Refereed.* **Document type:** *Journal, Academic/Scholarly.* **Description:** Contains scientific communications, review articles, dissertation abstracts, and conference information.
Formerly: Nordisk Sexologi (0108-271X)
Indexed: PsycInfo, Psychol.Abstr. (1986-), e-psyche.
—BLDSC (8087.547000), GNLM, ingenta.
Published by: Dansk Psykologisk Forlag/Danish Psychological Publishers, Stockholmsgade 29, Copenhagen Oe 2100, Denmark. TEL 45-35-38-16-55, FAX 45-35-38-16-65, dk-psych@dpf.dk, http://www.dpf.dk/defSCANSEX.htm. Ed. P O Lundberg. Circ: 900.

616.98 DEU ISSN 0080-679X
SCHIFFAHRTMEDIZINISCHES INSTITUT DER MARINE, KIEL. VEROEFFENTLICHUNGEN. Text in German. 1969. irreg. free per issue. adv. bk.rev. **Document type:** *Proceedings.*
Published by: Schiffahrtmedizinisches Institut der Marine, Kiel, Kopperpahler Allee 120, Kronshagen 24119, Germany. Ed. B Greiner. Circ: 2,000.

610 DEU ISSN 0341-8707
SCHLESWIG-HOLSTEINISCHES AERZTEBLATT. Text in German. 1947. m. DEM 90 (effective 2001). adv. **Document type:** *Newsletter, Trade.*
—GNLM, Infotrieve. **CCC.**
Published by: Quintessenz Verlags GmbH, Ifenpfad 2-4, Berlin 12107, Germany. TEL 49-30-76180646, FAX 49-30-76180680, central@quinline.com, central@quintessenz.de, http://www.quinline.com, http://www.quintessenz.de. Circ: 11,767.

610 DEU ISSN 0932-433X
CODEN: SCMZA
DER SCHMERZ; Konzepte, Klinik und Forschung. Text in German. bi-m. DEM 452 domestic; DEM 467 foreign (effective 2001). *Refereed.* **Document type:** *Academic/Scholarly.* **Description:** Contains research and studies on pain and pain management in all fields of medicine.
Related titles: Online - full text ed.: ISSN 1432-2129 (from EBSCO Publishing, RoweCom Information Quest, Swets Blackwell, Springer LINK, Institute for Scientific Information).
Indexed: ASCA, Curr.Cont., Excerp.Med. (1995-), Inpharma, Neurosci.Cit.Ind., Pharm.&Out.News, Reac., Sci.Cit.Ind.
—BLDSC (8090.965000), GNLM, IDS. **CCC.**
Published by: (Deutsche Gesellschaft zum Studium des Schmerzes), Springer-Verlag (Subsidiary of: BertelsmannSpringer), Tiergartenstr 17, Heidelberg 69121, Germany. TEL 49-6221-345-0, FAX 49-6221-345229, subscriptions@springer.de, http://link.springer.de/link/service/journals/00482/index.htm, http://www.springer.de. Ed. M Zenz. **Subscr. in N. America to:** Springer-Verlag New York Inc., PO Box 2485, Secaucus, NJ 07096-2485. TEL 212-460-1500, FAX 212-473-6272. **Co-sponsors:** Oesterreichische Schmerzgesellschaft; Deutsche Interdisziplinaer Vereinigung fuer Schmerztherapie und Schmerztherapeutisches Kolloquium.

SCHOOL SCIENCE REVIEW. see *SCIENCES: COMPREHENSIVE WORKS*

610 CHE ISSN 0036-7486
SCHWEIZERISCHE AERZTEZEITUNG/BOLLETTINO DEI MEDICI SVIZZERI/BULLETIN DES MEDECINS SUISSES. Text in French, German, Italian. 1919. w. CHF 360 domestic; CHF 418 foreign; CHF 20 newsstand/cover (effective 2001). adv. bk.rev. bibl, charts, stat. index. back issues avail. *Refereed.* **Document type:** *Newspaper, Trade.*
Related titles: Online - full text ed.: ISSN 1424-4004.
Indexed: Biol.Abstr., C.I.S. Abstr.
—GNLM, Infotrieve. **CCC.**

M

Published by: (Schweizerische Aerzteorganisation), E M H Swiss Medical Publishers Ltd., Steinentorstr 13, Basel, Switzerland. TEL 41-61-4678555, FAX 41-61-4678556, redaktion.saez@emh.ch, verlag@emh.ch, http://www.saez.ch, http://www.emh.ch. Circ: 28,500.

610 CHE ISSN 0250-5525
CODEN: SMWSD9

SCHWEIZERISCHE MEDIZINISCHE WOCHENSCHRIFT (SUPPLEMENTUM). Text in French, German; Summaries in English. 1975. irreg., latest vol.85, 1997. CHF 5. adv. back issues avail. **Document type:** *Academic/Scholarly.*
Indexed: Curr.Cont. (coverage dropped), Ind.Med. (1976-), SSCI (coverage dropped).
—BLDSC (8118.571000), CASDDS, CISTI, KNAW. **CCC.**
Published by: Schwabe und Co. AG, Steinentorstr 13, Basel 4010, Switzerland. TEL 41-61-2789565, FAX 41-61-2789565, verlag@schwabe.ch. Circ: 4,500.

610 CHE ISSN 1013-2058
CODEN: SRMPDJ

SCHWEIZERISCHE RUNDSCHAU FUER MEDIZIN PRAXIS/REVUE SUISSE DE MEDECINE. Text in French, German; Summaries in English, French, German. 1912. w. CHF 220 domestic; CHF 281 foreign (effective 2001). adv. bk.rev. abstr, bibl, illus. 64 p./no. **Document type:** *Journal, Academic/Scholarly.*
Formerly (until 1970): Praxis (0369-8394)
Related titles: Online - full text ed.: (from Institute for Scientific Information).
Indexed: Agri.& Environ.Biotech.Abstr. (coverage dropped), C.I.S. Abstr., Curr.Cont. (coverage dropped), Dent.Ind., Derwent Biotech.Abstr., Excerp.Med., INIS Atomind., Ind.Med. (1970-), Inpharma, Int.Nurs.Ind., Reac.
—BLDSC (6603.170000), CASDDS, CISTI, EMDOCS, GNLM, IDS, Infotrieve, KNAW. **CCC.**
Published by: Hans Huber AG, Laengassstr 76, Bern, 9 3000, Switzerland. TEL 41-31-3004500, FAX 41-31-3004591, zeitschriften@hanshuber.com, http://www.hanshuber.com. Adv. contact Rene Waelchli. color page CHF 2,852; trim 216 x 303. Circ: 3,500.

610 CHE ISSN 0080-7400

SCHWEIZERISCHES MEDIZINISCHES JAHRBUCH/ANNUAIRE MEDICAL SUISSE. Text in French, German. 1968. a. CHF 145 (effective 2001). adv. index. **Document type:** *Directory, Trade.* **Description:** Comprised of, in part, a directory of personnel and institutions.
—GNLM, Infotrieve. **CCC.**
Published by: (Schweizerische Aerzteorganisation), E M H Swiss Medical Publishers Ltd., Steinentorstr 13, Basel, Switzerland. TEL 41-61-4678555, FAX 41-61-4678556, verlag@emh.ch, http://www.emh.ch. Ed. Dr. Markus Trutmann. Circ: 2,400.

SCIENCE AS CULTURE. see *SCIENCES: COMPREHENSIVE WORKS*

610 FRA ISSN 0048-9727

SCIENCES MEDICALES✱ ; revue des universites nouvelles. Text in French. 1972 (vol.3). bi-m. reprint service avail. from PQC.
Related titles: Microform ed.: 1972 (vol.3) (from PQC).
Indexed: Chem.Abstr., Excerp.Med.
Published by: L E N Medical, 15 rue des Sablons, Paris 75116, France.

SCIENCES ORGONOMIQUES; revue des lois de la vie. see *BIOLOGY*

610 USA ISSN 0194-9063

SCIENTIFIC AMERICAN MEDICINE. Text in English. 1978. base vol. plus m. updates. USD 245 to individuals; USD 299 to institutions. adv. *Refereed.* **Document type:** *Academic/Scholarly.* **Description:** Contains current medical information for physicians, with reports on the latest developments in medicine.
Related titles: Online - full text ed.
Published by: Scientific American, Inc., 415 Madison Ave, New York, NY 10017-1111. TEL 212-754-0550, FAX 212-754-1138. Eds. Daniel Federman, David C Dale. Circ: 30,000.

610 GBR ISSN 0036-9330
CODEN: SMDJAK

SCOTTISH MEDICAL JOURNAL. Text in English. 1956. bi-m. GBP 65, USD 120 (effective 2001). bk.rev. abstr. a.index. 32 p./no. 2 cols./p. back issues avail. *Refereed.* **Document type:** *Journal, Academic/Scholarly.* **Description:** Publishes papers on original investigations in all branches of medicine. Publishes review articles and clinical memoranda, as well as papers on historical subjects of medical interest.
Related titles: Microform ed.: (from PMC); Online - full text ed.: (from Institute for Scientific Information).
Indexed: ASCA, ASSIA, Abstr.Hyg., Addic.Abstr., Agri.& Environ.Biotech.Abstr. (coverage dropped), Biol.Abstr., Chem.Abstr., Curr.Adv.Ecol.Sci., Curr.Cont., Derwent Biotech.Abstr., Excerp.Med., Helminthol.Abstr., INIS Atomind., Ind.Med. (1956-), Inpharma, Int.Nurs.Ind., NRN, Nutr.Abstr., Pharm.&Out.News, Potato Abstr., Protozool.Abstr., Reac., Rev.Appl.Entomol., Rev.Arom.& Med.Plants, SSCI (coverage dropped), Sci.Cit.Ind., Trop.Dis.Bull.
—BLDSC (8210.900000), CASDDS, CISTI, GNLM, IDS, ingenta, KNAW. **CCC.**
Published by: Hermiston Publications Ltd., 9 Stonelaws, E. Linton, E Lothian EH40 3DX, United Kingdom. TEL 44-1620-870612, FAX 44-1620-870313, http://www.smj.org.uk. Ed., R&P Professor C D Forbes.

610 USA ISSN 1049-5614

SCRIPPS CLINIC PERSONAL HEALTH LETTER. Text in English. 1990. m. USD 29. **Description:** Promotes good health and ways to overcome and solve medical problems.
—**CCC.**
Published by: Phillips Publishing, Inc., Consumer Publishing, 7811 Montrose Rd, Potomac, MD 20854. TEL 301-340-2100, FAX 301-309-3847. Ed. Dr. Donald J Dalessio.

610 USA

SCRIPPS RESEARCH INSTITUTE. SCIENTIFIC REPORT. Text in English. 1974. a. free per issue. **Document type:** *Academic/Scholarly.*
Former titles (until 1990): Research Institute of Scripps Clinic. Scientific Report; Scripps Clinic and Research Foundation. Research Institute. Scientific Report; (until 1977): Scripps Clinic and Research Foundation. Scientific Report (0361-3054)
—GNLM.
Published by: Scripps Research Institute, Office of Communications, 10550 N Torrey Pines Rd, La Jolla, CA 92037. TEL 858-784-8134, FAX 858-784-8118, http://www.scripps.edu/. Ed. Robin Goldsmith. Circ: 5,000 (controlled).

610 CZE ISSN 0036-9721
CODEN: SCMEBF

SCRIPTA MEDICA. Text mainly in English; Text occasionally in German, Russian; Summaries in English. 1922. 8/yr. CZK 80. bk.rev. charts, illus. index. **Description:** Examines scientific research in medical fields.
Indexed: Biol.Abstr., C.I.S. Abstr., Chem.Abstr., Excerp.Med., Ind.Med. (coverage dropped), Nutr.Abstr.
—BLDSC, CASDDS, GNLM.
Published by: Masarykova Universita, Lekarska Fakulta/Masaryk University, Medical Faculty, Komenskeho nam 2, Brno 66243, Czech Republic. Ed. Dr. Milan Dokladal. Circ: 900.

610 SAU ISSN 1319-4607

SEHHATUK ALYOUM; health magazine. Key Title: Sihatak. Text and summaries in Arabic. 1996. q. SAR 112 (effective 1999); USD 30. adv. charts, illus, stat. back issues avail. *Refereed.*
Published by: (Makkah Advertising), Communications Enterprises, P O Box 4288, Jeddah 21491, Saudi Arabia. TEL 966-2-464-7894, FAX 966-2-653-0693, info@makkahadv.com, www.makkahadv.com. Ed. Osama Qandil. R&P, Adv. contact Mohammed Mousa. B&W page USD 4,000, color page USD 5,200; trim 210 x 275. **Dist. by:** Saudi Distribution Co., P O Box 13195, Jeddah 21493, Saudi Arabia. TEL 966-2-653-0909, FAX 966-2-653-3191.

610.71025 JPN ISSN 1341-674X

SEI MARIANNA IKA DAIGAKU KIYO/ST. MARIANNA UNIVERSITY SCHOOL OF MEDICINE. BULLETIN. Text in English, Japanese. 1972. a. back issues avail. *Refereed.* **Document type:** *Bulletin, Academic/Scholarly.*
Formerly (until 1996): Sei Marianna Ika Daigaku Kiyo. Ippan Kyoiku (0286-4932)
Indexed: Chem.Abstr.
Published by: St. Marianna University School of Medicine, 2-16-1 Sugao, Miyamae-ku, Kawasaki-shi, Kanagawa-ken 216-0015, Japan. TEL 81-44-977-8111, FAX 81-44-977-9835. Ed. Tetsuro Asao. Circ: 1,000 (controlled).

610 DEU ISSN 0940-9270

SEIBT MEDIZINISCHE TECHNIK. Text in English, German. 1955. a. DEM 37 (effective 2000). adv. **Document type:** *Directory, Trade.*
Related titles: CD-ROM ed.; Online - full text ed.: (from G B I).
—GNLM.
Published by: Seibt Verlag GmbH, Leopoldstr 208, Munich 80804, Germany. TEL 49-89-360903-0, FAX 49-89-364317, http://www.seibt.com. Adv. contact Brita Graef. Circ: 10,000.

618.1 FRA
CODEN: SENSE

LE SEIN. Text in French. 1991. 4/yr. FRF 820; FRF 986 foreign (effective 2000). adv. bk.rev. abstr, illus. **Document type:** *Academic/Scholarly.* **Description:** Includes 3 sections: original articles, post-graduate teaching and updates, and radio-clinical case reports.
Related titles: Online - full text ed.
Indexed: Excerp.Med. (1994-).
—BLDSC (8219.751500), EMDOCS, GNLM.
Published by: (Societe Francaise de Mastologie et d'Imagerie du Sein), Masson - Periodiques, 120 bd. St. Germain, Paris 75006, France. TEL 33-1-40466200, FAX 33-1-40466201, s.mathot@masson.fr, http://www.e2med.com/revues/index.asp?Journal=ls&Population=im. Ed. J L Lamarque. Circ: 2,000. **Subscr. to:** Societe de Periodiques Specialises, BP 22, Vineuil Cedex 41354, France. TEL 33-2-54504612, FAX 33-2-54504611.

610 IND

SELECTIONS FROM B M J (SOUTH ASIA EDITION). (British Medical Journal) Abbreviated title: B M J (South Asia Edition). Text in English. 1985. m. INR 450 (effective 2001). adv. 100 p./no. back issues avail. **Document type:** *Journal, Academic/Scholarly.* **Description:** Reports on important medical research, news, and trends.
Formerly until (1998): Selections from B M J (Indian Edition) (0971-3646)
Related titles: ♦ Regional ed.: B M J. ISSN 0959-535X; ♦ B M J (South African Edition). ISSN 1019-8350; B M J (Nigerian Edition). ISSN 1118-4485. 1996; B M J (Middle East Edition). ISSN 1106-5028. 1993; B M J (West African Edition). ISSN 1119-2984. 1997.
Published by: Manipal Centre for Media Research & Training, C T C Bldg., Manipal 576 119, India. TEL 91-8252-71201, FAX 91-8252-70062, bmj@manipal.edu, http://www.manipal.edu. Ed. Dr. Ramdas M Pai. adv.: B&W page INR 10,000, color page INR 16,500; trim 250 x 175. Circ: 32,000 (paid).

610 FRA ISSN 0037-1777
CODEN: SHPAAI

LA SEMAINE DES HOPITAUX. Key Title: Semaine des Hopitaux de Paris. Text in French. 1925. bi-m. FRF 500 domestic to individuals; FRF 800 foreign to individuals; FRF 1,940 domestic to institutions; FRF 2,490 foreign to institutions. adv. *Refereed.*
Related titles: Online - full text ed.: (from Institute for Scientific Information); ♦ Supplement: Pathologie et Biologie. ISSN 0369-8114.
Indexed: ASCA, Agri.& Environ.Biotech.Abstr. (coverage dropped), Biol.Abstr., C.I.S. Abstr., Chem.Abstr., Curr.Adv.Cancer Res., Curr.Cont. (coverage dropped), Dent.Ind., Dok.Arbeitsmed., Excerp.Med., Helminthol.Abstr., INIS Atomind., Inpharma, Neurosci.Cit.Ind., Nutr.Abstr., Pharm.&Out.News, Protozool.Abstr., Reac., Rev.Appl.Entomol., Rev.Med.& Vet.Mycol., SSCI (coverage dropped), Trop.Dis.Bull.
—CASDDS, CISTI, GNLM, IDS, Infotrieve, KNAW. **CCC.**
Published by: (Semaine des Hopitaux), Expansion Scientifique Francaise, 31 bd. de la Tour Maubourg, Paris Cedex 7 75343, France. TEL 33-1-40626400, FAX 33-1-45556920. Ed. J Guerre. Circ: 10,000.

610 PRT

SEMANA MEDICA. Text in Portuguese. w. (48/yr.). PTE 8,740. **Document type:** *Trade.*
Published by: Ferreira e Bento Lda., Rua D. Estefania 32-1o, Lisbon 1000, Portugal. TEL 351-1-791-2500, http://www.fbento.pt/FB/.

610 RUS

SEMEINYI DOKTOR; prakticheskie sovety po meditsine. Text in Russian. 1993. m. USD 51 (effective 1999). adv. illus. back issues avail. **Document type:** *Consumer.* **Description:** Provides practical medical advice.
Published by: Arabesque, Planeta Business Centre, Marksistkaya ul 3-1, ofis 52, Moscow 109147, Russian Federation. TEL 7-095-2365417, FAX 7-095-2370821, arabesque@cityline.ru. Ed. Natalia Sharakshane. R&P Alexei Vetrov. Adv. contact Yuri Balushkin. page USD 5,000; trim 280 x 217. Circ: 97,000. **Dist. by:** Mezhdunarodnaya Kniga, B Yakimanka 39, Moscow 117049, Russian Federation. TEL 7-095-2384967, FAX 7-095-2384634.

610 DEU ISSN 1430-4023
SEMINAR HAUSARZTPRAXIS. Text in German. 1996. bi-m. EUR 37.97 domestic; EUR 43.97 foreign; EUR 5.61 newsstand/cover (effective 2002). **Document type:** *Journal, Academic/Scholarly.*
Incorporates (1990-1999): Hausarzt Bayern (0943-6863); (1978-1999): Hausarzt Hessen (0934-3164); (199?-1999): Hausarzt Nordrhein (0943-6855); (1993-1999): Hausarzt Praxis Sachsen (0944-890X); (1996-1999): Hausarzt Sachsen-Anhalt (1430-9882); (199?-1999): Hausarzt Thueringen (0943-6847)
Published by: B M V - Berliner Medizinische Verlagsanstalt GmbH, Lietzenburger Str 97, Berlin 10719, Germany. TEL 49-30-886749-0, FAX 49-30-88674999, bmvberlin@t-online.de, info@bmv-berlin.com, http://www.bmv-berlin.de. Ed. Dr. Dolf Kuenzel. Circ: 27,130 (controlled).

610 616.07 USA ISSN 0740-2570
SEMINARS IN DIAGNOSTIC PATHOLOGY. Text in English. 1983. q. USD 149 domestic to individuals; USD 210 foreign to individuals; USD 256 domestic to institutions; USD 301 foreign to institutions; USD 81 domestic to students; USD 126 foreign to students; USD 76 newsstand/cover (effective 2001). adv. abstr, bibl, charts, illus. index. *Refereed.* **Document type:** *Journal, Academic/Scholarly.* **Description:** Serves as a forum for the dissemination of information in the field; most issues cover a single topic from various viewpoints.
Related titles: Online - full text ed.: (from Institute for Scientific Information).
Indexed: ASCA, Curr.Cont., Ind.Med. (1984-), Inpharma, Reac., Sci.Cit.Ind.
—BLDSC (8239.448900), CISTI, EMDOCS, GNLM, IDS, ingenta, KNAW. **CCC.**
Published by: W.B. Saunders Co. (Subsidiary of: Harcourt Publishers Ltd.), 11830 Westline Industrial Dr, St Louis, MO 63146. TEL 800-325-4177, http://www.wbsaunders.com. Ed. Dr. Daniel J Santa Cruz. Adv. contact Steve Gray. B&W page USD 695, color page USD 1,645; trim 10 x 7. Circ: 2,521. **Subscr. to:** Periodicals Fulfillment, W B Saunders Co, 6277 Sea Harbor Dr, 4th Fl, Orlando, FL 32891-4800.

610 TUR ISSN 1016-5134 CODEN: SENDE
SENDROM. Text in Turkish; Summaries in English. 1988. m. USD 90 (effective 2001). adv. **Document type:** *Journal, Academic/Scholarly.*
Indexed: Excerp.Med. (1993-).
—BLDSC (8241.212000), EMDOCS, GNLM.
Published by: Logos Yayincilik Ticaret A.S., Yildiz Posta Cad., Sinan Apt. No. 36 D 66-67, Gayrettepe, Istanbul 80280, Turkey. TEL 90-212-2880541, FAX 90-212-2116185, info@logos.com.tr, http://logos.com.tr. Ed. Dr. Aydemir Yalman. Adv. contact Sukran Oznalga.

610 615 KOR
SEOUL NATIONAL UNIVERSITY. FACULTY PAPERS*. Text in English; Summaries in Korean. 1972. a. **Document type:** *Academic/Scholarly.*
Indexed: Bibl.Asian Stud. (1971-1975).
Published by: Seoul National University, San 56-1 Sinlim-dong, Kwanak-ku, Seoul 151742, Korea, S.. Ed. Byong Seol Seo.

SEPSIS. see *MEDICAL SCIENCES—Communicable Diseases*

613 USA
SEX WEEKLY PLUS. Text in English. 1997. w. (43/yr.). USD 1,895 in North America; USD 2,095 elsewhere. **Document type:** *Newsletter.* **Description:** Offers about 50 news briefs on legislative initiatives and gender and sex-related studies.
Related titles: Online - full text ed.
Published by: Charles W. Henderson, Ed. & Pub., PO Box 5528, Atlanta, GA 31107-0528. TEL 770-507-7777, FAX 770-507-7788, cwhender@newsfile.com; info@hendersonnet.atl.ga.us, http://www.newsfile.com.

SEXUAL ABUSE; a journal of research and treatment. see *PSYCHOLOGY*

SEXUAL AND RELATIONSHIP THERAPY. see *PSYCHOLOGY*

610 362.4 USA ISSN 0146-1044
HQ30.5 CODEN: SDISDC
SEXUALITY AND DISABILITY; a journal devoted to the psychological and medical aspects of sexuality in rehabilitation and community settings. Text in English. 1978. q. EUR 425 to institutions for print or online ed.; EUR 510 to institutions Print & Online eds.combined (effective 2002). adv. bk.rev. illus. Index. back issues avail.; reprint service avail. from PQC,ISI. *Refereed.* **Document type:** *Academic/Scholarly.* **Description:** Provides a forum for clinical and research developments in the area of sexuality as it relates to a wide range of physical and mental illnesses and disabling conditions.
Related titles: Microform ed.: (from PQC); Online - full text ed.: (from EBSCO Publishing, O C L C Online Computer Library Center, Inc., Swets Blackwell, Kluwer Online, Institute for Scientific Information, RoweCom Information Quest).
Indexed: ASCA, AgeLine, Biol.Abstr., CINAHL, Curr.Cont., Curr.Lit.Fam.Plan., ERA, Excerp.Med., Fam.Ind., IMFL, Lang.& Lang.Behav.Abstr., Past.Care & Couns.Abstr., PsycInfo, Psychol.Abstr. (1978-), Ref.Zh., Rehabil.Lit., SOPODA, SSCI, Soc.Serv.Abstr., Sociol.Abstr., Sp.Ed.Needs Abstr., Stud.Wom.Abstr., e-psyche.
—BLDSC (8254.485200), CISTI, GNLM, IDS, Infotrieve, ingenta. **CCC.**
Published by: (Boston University Medical Center, Sexuality and Disability Training Center), Kluwer Academic - Plenum Publishers (Subsidiary of: Wolters Kluwer N.V.), 233 Spring St, New York, NY 10013-1578. TEL 212-620-8000, 800-221-9369, FAX 212-463-0742, info@plenum.com; kluwer@wkap.com; services@wkap.nl, http://www.wkap.nl/journalhome.htm/0146-1044, http://www.plenum.com. Ed. Stanley Ducharme.

610 CHE ISSN 0170-1908
SEXUALMEDIZIN. Text in German. 1972. m. CHF 90 (effective 1996). adv. **Document type:** *Journal, Academic/Scholarly.*
Incorporates (1972-1993): Sexualmedizin (0341-4884)
Related titles: English ed.: Sexual Medizin (Ausgabe Oesterreich). ISSN 0344-0346.
—GNLM.
Published by: Medical Tribune AG, Urs-Graf-Str 8, Postfach 368, Basel 4020, Switzerland. TEL 41-61-3125566, FAX 41-61-3125560, 41-61-3125560, TELEX 4186160-MTWI-D, http://www.medical-tribune.ch. Ed. Alexander Schulz. Circ: 10,000.

610 DEU ISSN 0944-7105 CODEN: SEXUEX
SEXUOLOGIE; Zeitschrift fuer sexualmedizinische Fortbildung und Forschung. Text in German; Abstracts in English. 1994. irreg. (4 nos./vol.). EUR 60 to individuals; EUR 119 to institutions (effective 2002). **Document type:** *Journal, Academic/Scholarly.*
—BLDSC (8254.489300), GNLM.
Published by: (Akademie fuer Sexualmedizin), Urban & Fischer Verlag, Loebdergraben 14A, Jena 07743, Germany. TEL 49-3641-626444, FAX 49-3641-626421, info@urbanfischer.de, http://www.urbanfischer.de. Eds. H Bosinski, Klaus Beier, Kurt Loewit.

610 CHN ISSN 1002-168X
SHAANXI ZHONGYI XUEYUAN XUEBAO/SHAANXI INSTITUTE OF TRADITIONAL CHINESE MEDICINE. JOURNAL. Text in Chinese. 197?. q. CNY 3. **Document type:** *Academic/Scholarly.* **Description:** Presents theoretical research, emphasizing clinical applications. Also covers clinical medicine, pharmacy, experimental research, and education.
Published by: Shaanxi Zhongyi Xueyuan/Shaanxi Institute of Traditional Chinese Medicine, Xianyang, Shaanxi 712083, China.

SHAFTESBURY PEOPLE. see *SOCIAL SERVICES AND WELFARE*

610 CHN ISSN 1000-0496 CODEN: SYXBEE
SHANDONG YIKE DAXUE XUEBAO/SHANDONG UNIVERSITY OF MEDICAL SCIENCES. JOURNAL. Text in Chinese; Abstracts in Chinese, English. 1956. q. CNY 48 (effective 2001). abstr. index. 96 p./no. **Document type:** *Academic/Scholarly.* **Description:** Presents research reports on clinical medicine, preventive medicine, and traditional Chinese and Western medicine.
Indexed: Chem.Abstr., Chem.Titles, INIS Atomind.
—BLDSC (0579.722600), CASDDS.
Published by: Shandong Yike Daxue, Xuebao Bianjibu, No 44 Wenhua Xilu, Jinan, Shandong 250012, China. TEL 86-531-2942144, FAX 86-531-2953813. Ed. Ma Chunyin. Circ: 8,000. **Dist. overseas by:** China International Book Trading Corp, 35 Chegongzhuang Xilu, Haidian District, Beijing 100044, China.

610 615 CHN ISSN 1002-266X
SHANDONG YIYAO/SHANDONG MEDICAL JOURNAL. Text in Chinese. 1957. s-m. CNY 3 per issue domestic (effective 2000). adv. bk.rev. back issues avail. **Document type:** *Academic/Scholarly.* **Description:** Covers the latest developments in medical research, and serves as a forum to exchange information and ideas.
Formerly: Shandong Medical Periodical
Related titles: Online - full content ed.: (from WanFang Data Corp.).
Published by: Shandong-sheng Weisheng Ting/Shandong Public Health Bureau, Lishan Lu 146 Hao, Shandong 250014 , China. TEL 2956921, FAX 2950172. Eds. Juan Ying Xu, Shu Wen Guo. Circ: 6,800.

610 CHN
SHANGHAI TIEDAO DAXUE XUEBAO YIXUE BAN/SHANGHAI TIEDAO UNIVERSITY. MEDICAL SCIENCE EDITION. Text in Chinese. 2/yr.?. **Document type:** *Academic/Scholarly.*
Supersedes in part (in 1996): Shanghai Tiedao Daxue Xuebao - Shanghai Tiedao University. Journal (1007-2039); Which was formerly: Shanghai Tiedao Xueyuan Xuebao - Shanghai Railway Institute. Journal (1000-1913)
Published by: Shanghai Tiedao Daxue, 450 Zhennan Rd, Shanghai 200333, China. TEL 86-21-5622-0063, FAX 86-21-6250-6812.

610 CHN ISSN 0257-8131 CODEN: SYDXEE
SHANGHAI YIKE DAXUE XUEBAO/SHANGHAI UNIVERSITY OF MEDICAL SCIENCES. JOURNAL. Text in Chinese; Abstracts in English. 1956. bi-m. USD 13.32. **Document type:** *Academic/Scholarly.* **Description:** Covers original contributions in experimental, clinical studies in general medicine, public health, pharmacy and the related fields.
Indexed: Chem.Abstr., Chem.Titles, INIS Atomind., Ref.Zh.
—CASDDS, EMDOCS, GNLM, KNAW.
Published by: (Shanghai Yike Daxue/Shanghai University of Medical Sciences), Shanghai Keji Chubanshe, 450 Ruijin 2 Lu, Shanghai 200020, China. TEL 86-21-4041900. Ed. Wu Jue. **Dist. overseas by:** China International Book Trading Corp, 35 Chegongzhuang Xilu, Haidian District, Beijing 100044, China.

610 CHN ISSN 0253-9934
R97.7.C5 CODEN: SIHSD8
SHANGHAI YIXUE/SHANGHAI MEDICAL JOURNAL. Text in Chinese; Abstracts in Chinese, English. m. USD 16.44.
Indexed: Chem.Abstr., Chem.Indus.Notes, Chem.Titles.
—BLDSC (8254.589900), CASDDS.
Published by: Zhonghua Yixuehui (Shanghai Fenhui)/Chinese Medical Association (Shanghai Branch), 1623 Beijing Xilu, Shanghai 200040, China. TEL 86-21-62531885, FAX 86-21-62550842. Ed. Wu Mengchao. Circ: 5,000.

SHANGHAI ZHONGYIYAO ZAZHI/REVISTA DE MEDICINA TRADICIONAL CHINA DE SHANGHAI/REVUE DE MEDECINE TRADITIONNELLE CHINOISE/SHANGHAI JOURNAL OF TRADITIONAL CHINESE MEDICINE. see *ALTERNATIVE MEDICINE*

SHANXI ZHONGYI/SHANXI JOURNAL OF TRADITIONAL CHINESE MEDICINE. see *ALTERNATIVE MEDICINE*

615.942 CHN ISSN 1001-5639
SHE ZHI/JOURNAL OF SNAKE. Text in Chinese. 1989. q. USD 10; USD 2.50 newsstand/cover (effective 2001). **Document type:** *Academic/Scholarly.*
Published by: China International Book Trading Corp/Zhongguo Guoji Tushu Maoyi Zonggongsi cibtc@mail.cibtc.com.cn, http://www.cibtc.com.cn. **Dist. by:** 35, Chegongzhuang Xilu, Haidian District, Beijing 100044, China.

SHENGLI KEXUE JINZHAN/PROGRESS IN PHYSIOLOGICAL SCIENCES. see *BIOLOGY—Physiology*

610.28 CHN ISSN 1001-5515 CODEN: SYGZF2
SHENGWU YIXUE GONGCHENGXUE ZAZHI/JOURNAL OF BIOMEDICAL ENGINEERING. Text in Chinese, English. 1984. q. USD 80 (effective 2000). adv. **Document type:** *Academic/Scholarly.* **Description:** Covers original research papaers, review articles, and brief notes on biomaterials, artificial organs, biomechanics and computer applications to medical systems.
Indexed: Ind.Med. (1984-).
—CASDDS.
Published by: Sichuan Society for Biomedical Engineering, West China University of Medical Sciences, Chengdu, Sichuan 610041, China. TEL 86-28-5501507. Ed. Huai Qing Chen. R&P, Adv. contact Jing Yang. **Dist. outside China by:** China International Book Trading Corp, 35 Chegongzhuang Xilu, Haidian District, Beijing 100044, China. TEL 86-1-8414284. **Co-sponsors:** West China University of Medical Sciences; Chengdu University of Science and Technology; Sichuan Biomedical Engineering Research and Development Center.

610 TJK
SHIFO. Text in Tajik. bi-m.
Published by: Redaktsiya Shifo, Ul Tegeran 12, Dushanbe, Tajikistan. TEL 27-61-02. Ed. M Tohiri. **Dist. by:** East View Publications, 3020 Harbor Ln N, Minneapolis, MN 55447. TEL 763-550-0961, FAX 763-559-2931.

610 JPN ISSN 0037-3699 CODEN: SKIZAB
SHIKOKU IGAKU ZASSHI/SHIKOKU ACTA MEDICA. Text in Japanese; Summaries in English. 1950. bi-m. JPY 3,000 (effective 2001); exchange basis. adv. tr.lit. index. **Document type:** *Government, Academic/Scholarly.*
Indexed: Abstr.Hyg., Bio-Contr.News & Info., Biol.Abstr., Chem.Abstr., Chem.Titles, Excerp.Med., Nutr.Abstr., Protozool.Abstr., Ref.Zh., Trop.Dis.Bull., Weed Abstr.
—BLDSC (8256.600000), CASDDS, CISTI, GNLM.
Published by: Tokushima Igakkai/Tokushima Medical Association, c/o Tokushima Daigaku Igakubu, 18-15 kuramoto-cho 3-chome, Tokushima-shi 770-8503, Japan. TEL 81-88-633-7104, FAX 81-88-633-7115, shikoku@basic.med.tukushima-u.ac.jp. Pub. Yoshinari Ohnishi. R&P, Adv. contact Shin-ichi Kubo. Circ: 800.

500 JPN ISSN 0387-9097
SHIMANE IKA DAIGAKU KIYO/SHIMANE MEDICAL UNIVERSITY. BULLETIN. Text mainly in Japanese; Abstracts in English. 1978. a. *Refereed.* **Document type:** *Academic/Scholarly.* **Description:** Contains research articles on medicine, as well as articles on anthropology, computers, linguistics, history, and translations of literature.
Related titles: Online - full content ed.
—CCC.
Published by: Shimane Ika Daigaku/Shimane Medical University, 89-1 Enya-cho, Izumo-shi, Shimane-ken 693-8501, Japan. FAX 81-583-21-1731, http://lib.shimane-med.ac.jp/home/kiyo.htm. Ed. Kouske Furuse.

610 JPN ISSN 0386-5959 CODEN: SJSCDM
SHIMANE JOURNAL OF MEDICAL SCIENCE; an official journal of Shimane Medical University. Text and summaries in English. 1977. s-a. charts, illus. back issues avail. *Refereed.* **Document type:** *Academic/Scholarly.*
Indexed: Biol.Abstr., Chem.Abstr.
—BLDSC (8256.716000), CASDDS, CISTI, GNLM.
Published by: Shimane Ika Daigaku/Shimane Medical University, 89-1 Enya-cho, Izumo-shi, Shimane-ken 693-8501, Japan. http://lib.shimane-med.ac.jp/home/shimanej.htm. Ed. Hideki Okunishi.

610 JPN ISSN 0037-3826 CODEN: SIZAA7
SHINSHU MEDICAL JOURNAL/SHINSHU IGAKU ZASSHI. Text in Japanese; Abstracts in English. 1952. bi-m. JPY 9,000, USD 90. adv. charts, illus. *Refereed.* **Document type:** *Academic/Scholarly.*
Indexed: Biol.Abstr., Chem.Abstr., Chem.Titles, Excerp.Med., INIS Atomind., Ind.Med. (coverage dropped).
—BLDSC (8256.870000), CASDDS, GNLM.
Published by: Shinshu University, School of Medicine, 3-1-1 Asahi, Matsumoto-shi, Nagano-ken 390-0802, Japan. FAX 81-263-33-5701. Ed. Fumitaka Ikomi. Circ: 2,000.

610.73 JPN ISSN 0385-1982
SHINSHU UNIVERSITY. SCHOOL OF ALLIED MEDICAL SCIENCES. TREATISES AND STUDIES. Text in Japanese; Summaries in English. 1975. a. free per issue. back issues avail. **Document type:** *Academic/Scholarly.*
Published by: Shinshu Daigaku, Iryo Gijutsu Tanki Daigakubu, 3-1-1 Asahi, Matsumoto-shi, Nagano-ken 390-0802, Japan. Circ: 450.

630 CHN
SHIYONG ZHONGXIYI JIEHE ZAZHI. Text in Chinese. m. **Description:** Discusses the combined application of traditional Chinese medicine and Western medicine.
Published by: Changzhi Yixueyuan/Changzhi Medical Institute, 46, Yan'an Lu, Changzhi, Shanxi 046000, China. TEL 33322. Ed. Wong Weiliang.

SHKOLA ZDOROV'YA. see *EDUCATION*

616 USA ISSN 1073-2322
SHOCK; molecular, cellular and systemic pathobiological aspects and therapeutic approaches. Text in English. 1994. m. USD 215 domestic to individuals; USD 260 foreign to individuals; USD 795 domestic to institutions; USD 895 foreign to institutions (effective 2001). adv. bk.rev. abstr, bibl. Supplement avail.; back issues avail. *Refereed.* **Document type:** *Academic/Scholarly.* **Description:** Publishes original research, short communications, review articles and letters on topics relating to circulatory shock, sepsis, trauma and related disorders.
Related titles: Online - full text ed.: USD 315 domestic to individuals; USD 360 foreign to individuals; USD 895 domestic to institutions; USD 995 foreign to institutions (effective 2001) (from Institute for Scientific Information).
Indexed: ASCA, BBCI, Curr.Cont., Dairy Sci.Abstr., Ind.Med. (1994-), Inpharma, Pharm.&Out.News, Reac., Rev.Med.& Vet.Mycol., Sci.Cit.Ind.
—BLDSC (8267.443000), CISTI, GNLM, IDS, Infotrieve, KNAW. **CCC.**
Published by: BioMedical Press, 1021 15th St, Ste 9, Augusta, GA 30901. TEL 706-722-7511, FAX 706-722-7515, info@biomedicalpress.com, http://www.shocksocieties.org. Ed. Irshad H Chaudry. R&P Sherwood Reichard. Adv. contact Lorrie Griffin. **Subscr. to:** Allen Press Inc., PO Box 1897, Lawrence, KS 66044-8897. **Co-sponsors:** Shock Society; International Federation of Shock Societies; European Shock Society; Brazilian Shock Society; Japan Shock Society.

610 JPN ISSN 0388-9734 CODEN: SHIGE5
SHOJINKAI IGAKUSHI/MATSUSHITA MEDICAL JOURNAL. Text in Japanese. 1980. a.
Indexed: Chem.Abstr., Chem.Indus.Notes, Chem.Titles.
—BLDSC (5413.255700), CASDDS.
Published by: Shohjinkai Medical Society, 2-35 Sotojima-cho, Moriguchi-shi, Osaka-fu 570-0096, Japan. TEL 06-992-5131.

630 CHN CODEN: JCMDEI
SHOUDU YIKE DAXUE/CAPITAL UNIVERSITY OF MEDICAL SCIENCES. JOURNAL. Text in Chinese. 1980. q. CNY 14, USD 10 (effective 2000). *Refereed.* **Document type:** *Academic/Scholarly.*
Former titles (until 1996): Shoudu Yixueyuan Xuebao/Capital Institute of Medicine. Journal (1001-2389); (until 1987): Beijing Di'er Yixueyuan Xuebao (1000-0291)
—CASDDS.
Address: You'anmenwai, Beijing 100054, China. TEL 86-10-6305-1258, FAX 86-10-6329-1972. Ed. Qunyuan Xu. Adv. contact Laiying Zhu.

610 JPN
SHUKAN IGAKKAI SHINBUN/NEW MEDICAL WORLD WEEKLY. Text in Japanese. 1950. w. JPY 5,000.
Published by: Igaku-Shoin Ltd., 5-24-3 Hongo, Bunkyo-ku, Tokyo 113-0033, Japan. TEL 91-3-3817-5694. Circ: 50,000.

SICHUAN ZHONGYI/SICHUAN JOURNAL OF TRADITIONAL CHINESE MEDICINE. see *ALTERNATIVE MEDICINE*

SIDE EFFECTS OF DRUGS ANNUAL; a yearly critical survey of the world's literature on adverse reactions to drugs. see *PHARMACY AND PHARMACOLOGY*

610 ESP ISSN 0214-3011
SIETE DIAS MEDICOS. Text in Spanish. 1988. 44/yr. ESP 10,000 domestic; EUR 60.25 in Europe; USD 60 elsewhere (effective 2001). adv. bk.rev. **Document type:** *Journal, Academic/Scholarly.* **Description:** Covers medical topics and literature. Addressed to the general practitioners and specialists.
Published by: Ediciones Mayo S.A., Muntaner, 374-376 4o, Barcelona 08006, Spain. TEL 34-93-2090255, FAX 34-93-2020643. Ed. Josep M Ferrando. R&P Mercedes Mayoral. Adv. contact Jose Mayoral. Circ: 30,000 (controlled).

610 USA
SIGLETTER. Text in English. 3/yr. free. back issues avail. **Description:** Presents news about the services and supporters of the Al Sigl Center and it's eight partner agencies, which together serve 49,000 people with disabilities in the Rochester area. Audience: Supporters of the Al Sigl Center, Board members and key staff of the partner agencies. Also business and community leaders and the media.
Media: Online - full text. **Related titles:** E-mail ed.
Published by: Al Sigl Center, 1000 Elmwood Ave, Ste 300, Rochester, NY 14620-3098. TEL 716-442-4100, FAX 716-442-7573, ckearns@alsiglcenter.org, jrogers@alsiglcenter.org, http://www.alsiglcenter.org. Ed. Cindy Kearns. Circ: 24,000 (controlled and free).

610 USA
SILVER SHEET; report on medical device design, compliance and quality controls. Text in English. 1997. m. USD 395 (effective 2001). adv. back issues avail.; reprints avail. **Document type:** *Newsletter, Trade.* **Description:** Includes detailed lists and summaries of GMP and MDR warning letters and profiles of key quality control specialists and government regulators.
Published by: F-D-C Reports, Inc., 5550 Friendship Blvd, Ste One, Chevy Chase, MD 20815-7278. TEL 800-332-2181, FAX 301-664-7238. Ed. Mark Brager. R&P Laura Desimio. Adv. contact Michael Keville.

610 SGP ISSN 0037-5675 CODEN: SIMJA3
SINGAPORE MEDICAL JOURNAL. Text in English. 1960. m. SGD 165 domestic; SGD 300 foreign (effective 2001). adv. bk.rev. 60 p./no. back issues avail. *Refereed.* **Document type:** *Journal, Academic/Scholarly.*
Indexed: Abstr.Hyg., Bibl.Asian Stud. (1972-1974), Biol.Abstr., CINAHL, Chem.Abstr., Dairy Sci.Abstr., Dent.Ind., Diar.Dis.Res., Excerp.Med., ExtraMED, Helminthol.Abstr., Ind.Med. (1960-), Ind.Vet., Inpharma, Int.Nurs.Ind., Nutr.Abstr., Pharm.&Out.News, Pig News & Info., Protozool.Abstr., Reac., Rev.Appl.Entomol., Rev.Arom.& Med.Plants, Rev.Med.& Vet.Mycol., Trop.Dis.Bull., Vet.Bull.
—BLDSC (8285.480000), CISTI, GNLM, KNAW.
Published by: Singapore Medical Association, Level 2 Alumni Medical Centre, 2 College Rd, Singapore 169850, Singapore. TEL 65-223-1264, FAX 65-224-7827, smj@sma.org.sg, http://www.sma.org.sg/smjcurrent.html. Ed. Dr. C Rajasoorya. adv.: B&W page SGD 1,800, color page SGD 2,200. Circ: 4,000.

615.82 SWE ISSN 0037-6019
SJUKGYMNASTEN. Text in Swedish. 1943. 11/yr. SEK 595 (effective 2001). adv. bk.rev. illus. index. 68 p./no. 3 cols./p. **Document type:** *Magazine, Trade.*
Formerly (until 1957): Tidskrift i Sjukgymnastik
Related titles: Audio cassette/tape ed.
Indexed: AMED.
Published by: Legitimerade Sjukgymnasters Riksfoerbund, Box 3196, Stockholm 10363, Sweden. TEL 46-8-567-06-100, FAX 46-8-567-06-198, sjukgymnasten@lsr.se. Ed. Tonie Andersen. Adv. contact Eva Linder. B&W page SEK 12,250, color page SEK 17,850; trim 192 x 276. Circ: 12,000 (paid and controlled).

610.9 920 POL
SLOWNIK BIOGRAFICZNY POLSKICH NAUK MEDYCZNYCH XXX WIEKU. Text in Polish. 1991. irreg., latest vol.4, 1996. price varies. adv. bibl, illus. **Document type:** *Academic/Scholarly.* **Description:** Biographical dictionary of Polish medical sciences.
Published by: Polska Akademia Nauk, Instytut Historii Nauki, Palac Staszica, Ul Nowy Swiat 72, Warsaw 00330, Poland. TEL 48-22-8268754, FAX 48-22-8266137. Ed. Zofia Podgorska Klawe. Adv. contact Bozena Urbanek. Circ: 200.

SNAKEROOT EXTRACT. see *HISTORY*

M

615.89 GBR ISSN 0951-631X
R131.A1
SOCIAL HISTORY OF MEDICINE. Text in English. 1970. 3/yr. GBP 90, USD 157 (effective Apr. 2002). adv. bk.rev. abstr, bibl. cum.index: 1970-1977. 204 p./no. back issues avail. *Refereed.* **Document type:** *Journal, Academic/Scholarly.* **Description:** Covers all aspects of health, illness and medical treatment, as well as biological aspects of normal life.
Formerly (until 1987): Society for the Social History of Medicine. Bulletin (0307-6792)
Related titles: Online - full text ed.: (from Institute for Scientific Information).
Indexed: ASCA, AgeLine, Amer.Hist.& Life, Arts & Hum.Cit.Ind., Curr.Cont., Hist.Abstr. (1989-), Lang.& Lang.Behav.Abstr., P C I, SOPODA, SSCI, Sci.Cit.Ind., Soc.Serv.Abstr., Sociol.Abstr., Stud.Wom.Abstr.
—BLDSC (8318.099000), GNLM, IDS, ingenta. **CCC.**
Published by: (Society for the Social History of Medicine), Oxford University Press, Academic Division, Great Clarendon St, Oxford OX2 6DP, United Kingdom. TEL 44-1865-267907, FAX 44-1865-267835, jnl.info@oup.co.uk, http://www3.oup.co.uk/sochis/, http://www.oup.co.uk/journals. Eds. Helen King, M Jackson, Roger Davidson. Pub. Clare Morton. R&P Fionna Willis. Adv. contact Helen Pearson TEL 44-1235-201904. B&W page GBP 245, B&W page USD 405. Circ: 1,250. **Subscr. in the Americas to:** Oxford University Press, Journals, 2001 Evans Rd, Cary, NC 27513. TEL 800-852-7323, FAX 919-677-1714, jnlorder@oup-usa.org; **Subscr. to:** Journals Marketing, Great Clarendon St, Oxford OX2 6DP, United Kingdom.

610 GBR ISSN 0277-9536
RA418 CODEN: SSMDEP
SOCIAL SCIENCE & MEDICINE. Text in English. 1978. s-m. EUR 269 in Europe to qualified personnel; JPY 35,800 in Japan to qualified personnel; USD 302 elsewhere to qualified personnel; EUR 3,259 in Europe to institutions; JPY 432,800 in Japan to institutions; USD 3,646 elsewhere to institutions (effective 2002). adv. bk.rev. abstr. index. reprints avail. *Refereed.* **Document type:** *Academic/Scholarly.* **Description:** Provides an international forum among social scientists, medical researchers and practitioners, and health administrators and planners.
Formed by the 1982 merger of: Social Science and Medicine. Part A: Medical Sociology (0271-7123); Social Science and Medicine. Part B: Medical Anthropology (0160-7987); Social Science and Medicine. Part C: Medical Economics (0160-7995); Social Science and Medicine. Part D: Medical Geography (0160-8002); Social Science and Medicine. Part E: Medical Psychology (0271-5384); Social Science and Medicine. Part F: Medical Ethics (0271-5392); Which was formerly (until 1980): Ethics in Science and Medicine (0306-4581); (until 1976): Science, Medicine and Man (0300-9955)
Related titles: Microfilm ed.: (from PQC); Online - full text ed.: (from ingenta, Gale Group, Swets Blackwell, Factiva, Institute for Scientific Information, ScienceDirect).
Indexed: AIDS Abstr., AMED, ASCA, ASSIA, Abstr.Anthropol., Abstr.Health Care Manage.Stud., Abstr.Hyg., Abstr.Rural Dev.Trop., Addic.Abstr., Adol.Ment.Hlth.Abstr., AgeLine, Amer.Bibl.Slavic & E.Eur.Stud., Arts & Hum.Cit.Ind. (coverage dropped), Behav.Med.Abstr., Bibl.Asian Stud. (1973-1991), Bibl.Dev.Med.& Child Neur., Biol.Abstr., Brit.Nur.Ind., CINAHL, Chic.Per.Ind., Crim.Just.Abstr., Curr.Adv.Ecol.Sci., Curr.Cont., Curr.Lit.Fam.Plan., Dairy Sci.Abstr., Dent.Ind., Diar.Dis.Res., Documentatieblad, E.I., ERA, Ecol.Abstr., Environ.Sci.Poll.Mgmt., Excerp.Med., FAMLI, Fam.Ind., Forest Prod.Abstr., Forest.Abstr., Geo.Abstr.H.G., Geo.Abstr.P.G., IDA, I.P.A., Ind.Med. (1982-), Indian Psychol.Abstr., Int.Nurs.Ind., Intl.Bibl.Soc.Sci., LISA, Lang.& Lang.Behav.Abstr., Med.Care Rev., Mid.East: Abstr.& Ind., Mult.Ed.Abstr., Nutr.Abstr., P.A.I.S., Pollut.Abstr., Popul.Ind., Potato Abstr., Protozool.Abstr., PsycInfo, Psychol.Abstr. (1969-), Res.High.Educ.Abstr., Rev.Appl.Entomol., Rev.Arom.& Med.Plants, Rice Abstr., Risk Abstr., Rural Devel.Abstr., Rural Ext.Educ.& Tr.Abstr., Russ.Acad.Sci.Bibl., SSCI, Saf.Sci.Abstr., So.Pac.Per.Ind., Soc.Sci.Ind. (Jun.1982-), Soc.Serv.Abstr., Sociol.Abstr., Stud.Wom.Abstr., THA, Tech.Educ.Abstr., Trop.Dis.Bull., Viol.& Abuse Abstr., World Ag.Econ.& Rur.Soc.Abstr., e-psyche.
—BLDSC (8318.157000), CISTI, EMDOCS, GNLM, IDS, Infotrieve, ingenta, KNAW. **CCC.**
Published by: Pergamon (Subsidiary of: Elsevier Science), The Boulevard, Langford Ln, East Park, Kidlington, Oxford OXB 1GB, United Kingdom. FAX 44-1865-843010, http://www.elsevier.nl/locate/issn/02779536. Ed. S Macintyre. Circ: 1,400. **Subscr. in Australasia and the Far East to:** Elsevier Science (Singapore) Pte Ltd, No.1 Temasek Ave, 17-01 Millenia Tower, Singapore 039192, Singapore. TEL 65-434-3727; **Subscr. in the Americas to:** Elsevier Science, PO Box 945, New York, NY 10159-0945; **Subscr. to:** Elsevier Science BV, PO Box 211, Amsterdam 1000 AE, Netherlands.

362.1 610 SWE ISSN 0037-833X
SOCIALMEDICINSK TIDSKRIFT. Text in Swedish. 1924. m. (7/yr.). SEK 300; SEK 335 in Scandinavia; SEK 390 elsewhere. adv. bk.rev. abstr, charts, illus. index. **Document type:** *Academic/Scholarly, Consumer.*
Indexed: C.I.S. Abstr., Excerp.Med., Ind.Med. (coverage dropped).
—CISTI.
Published by: Stiftelsen Socialmedicinsk Tidskrift, Slaattervaegen 38, Ekeroe 17837, Sweden. TEL 46-8-560-346-60, FAX 46-8-560-301-21. Ed. Dr. Claes Goeran Westrin. Adv. contact Ann Appelgren. Circ: 4,500.

610 ESP ISSN 0583-7480
SOCIEDAD ESPANOLA DE HISTORIA DE LA MEDICINA. BOLETIN. Text in Spanish. 1974 (vol.14). a. bibl.
Published by: Sociedad Espanola de Historia de la Medicina, Duque de Medinaceli, 4, Madrid 28014, Spain.

616.07 FRA
CODEN: BSPEAM
SOCIETE DE PATHOLOGIE EXOTIQUE. BULLETIN. Text in French; Summaries in English. 1908. 5/yr. adv. bk.rev. bibl, charts, illus, maps. index. reprint service avail. from ISI. *Refereed.* **Document type:** *Academic/Scholarly.* **Description:** Publishes original articles and monographs on epidemiology, tropical and exotic medicine, human and veterinary parasitology and immunology. Includes minutes of the society's meetings.
Formerly (until 1989): Societe de Pathologie Exotique et de ses Filiales. Bulletin (0037-9085)
Related titles: Microform ed.: 1908 (from PMC); Online - full text ed.: (from Institute for Scientific Information).
Indexed: ASCA, Abstr.Hyg., Bio-Contr.News & Info., Biol.Abstr., Chem.Abstr., Curr.Adv.Ecol.Sci., Curr.Cont., Excerp.Med., GeoRef, Helminthol.Abstr., Ind.Med. (coverage dropped), Ind.Vet., Inpharma, Irr.& Drain.Abstr., Nutr.Abstr., Pharm.&Out.News, Pig News & Info., Protozool.Abstr., Reac., Rev.Appl.Entomol., Rev.Med.& Vet.Mycol., Rev.Plant Path., Rural Devel.Abstr., So.Pac.Per.Ind., Soils & Fert., Trop.Dis.Bull., Vet.Bull., Zoo.Rec.
—BLDSC (2747.370000), CASDDS, CISTI, GNLM, Infotrieve. **CCC.**
Published by: Societe de Pathologie Exotique, Institut Pasteur, 25 Rue du Docteur Roux, Paris Cedex 15 75724, France. TEL 33-1-45668869, FAX 33-1-45664485, socpatex@pasteur.fr. Ed. A Chippaux. Circ: 1,350.

610 LUX ISSN 0037-9247
CODEN: BMGLAO
SOCIETE DES SCIENCES MEDICALES DU GRAND-DUCHE DE LUXEMBOURG. BULLETIN. Text in English, French, German. 1863. 2/yr. free to institutions and individual members. adv. bk.rev. bibl, charts, illus. *Refereed.* **Document type:** *Academic/Scholarly.* **Description:** Collection of research papers covering a variety of topics in medicine.
Indexed: Biol.Abstr., Chem.Abstr., Dent.Ind., Excerp.Med., Ind.Med. (1864-).
—BLDSC (2752.700000), CASDDS, CISTI, GNLM.
Published by: Societe des Sciences Medicales du Grand-Duche de Luxembourg, Centre Hospitalier de Luxembourg, 72, rue de Schoenfels, Bridel 8151, Luxembourg. TEL 352-021282029, FAX 352-339608, berchem.guy@chl.lu, bruck.mark@chl.lu. Ed., R&P, Adv. contact Dr. Guy Berchem. Circ: 1,200.

SOCIETY FOR IN VITRO BIOLOGY. PROCEEDINGS. see *BIOLOGY—Physiology*

610 300 USA ISSN 0742-2709
R729
SOCIOECONOMIC CHARACTERISTICS OF MEDICAL PRACTICE. Text in English. 1983. a. USD 159.95 to non-members; USD 109.95 to members. stat. **Document type:** *Monographic series.* **Description:** Provides data in physician practice valuation, consultation, litigation support and tax planning.
Related titles: Diskette ed.
Published by: American Medical Association, Center for Health Policy Research, 515 N State St, P O Box 10946, Chicago, IL 60610-0946. TEL 312-464-5000, 800-621-8335, FAX 312-464-5600, http://www.ama-assn.org.

610 150 DEU ISSN 1432-9123
SOMNOLOGIE/SOMNOLOGY; Zeitschrift fuer Schlafforschung und Schlafmedizin. Text in German, English. 1997. q. DEM 328.58 in Europe; DEM 350.10 elsewhere; DEM 361.44 in Europe print & online eds,. combined; DEM 385.11 elsewhere print & online eds,. combined (effective 2001). **Document type:** *Journal, Academic/Scholarly.*
Related titles: Online - full text ed.: ISSN 1439-054X (from Munksgaard & Blackwell Science's Synergy).
Indexed: e-psyche.
—BLDSC (8327.846000), GNLM.
Published by: (Deutsche Gesellschaft fuer Schlafforschung und Schlafmedizin), Blackwell Wissenschafts Verlag GmbH, Kurfuerstendamm 57, Berlin 10707, Germany. TEL 49-30-327906-0, FAX 49-30-32790610, abo@blackwis.de, http://www.blackwell.de/somno.htm. Ed. Dr. Marianne E Schlaefke.

610 USA ISSN 1087-8807
SONOMA COUNTY PHYSICIAN. Text in English. 1984. q. USD 19.80 (effective 2000). adv. bk.rev. *Refereed.* **Document type:** *Academic/Scholarly.* **Description:** Provides a forum for physicians; topics include managed care, preventive medicine, and at-risk behavior.
Published by: Sonoma County Medical Association, 3033 Cleveland Ave, Santa Rosa, CA 95403. TEL 707-525-4325, FAX 707-525-4289, scma@scma.org, http://www.scma.org. Ed., R&P Steve Osborn. Adv. contact Susan Gumucio. Circ: 1,000 (paid).

SOURCEBOOK ON ASBESTOS DISEASES. see *LAW*

610 ZAF ISSN 1025-1979
SOUTH AFRICAN FAMILY PRACTICE. Text in English. 1980. bi-m. ZAR 200; ZAR 242 foreign. adv. bk.rev. abstr. *Refereed.* **Document type:** *Academic/Scholarly.* **Description:** Publishes original research contributions from family practitioners and primary health care workers, as well as news of issues, meetings and forthcoming events of interest to members.
Formerly (until Apr. 1994): S A Family Practice - S A Huisartspraktyk
Indexed: Ind.S.A.Per.
Published by: South African Academy of Family Practice - Primary Care/Suid-Afrikaanse Akademie van Huisartspraktyk - Primere Sorg, PO Box 459, Umhlanga Rocks 4320, South Africa. TEL 27-31-5628509, FAX 27-11-527812, http://www.kznsa.co.za/website/safp. Ed. Dr. Roy Jobson. Adv. contact Yvette Thomas.

610 ZAF
SOUTH AFRICAN HEALTH TECHNOLOGY MONITOR. Text in English. bi-m. ZAR 250 (effective 2000).
Indexed: Ind.S.A.Per.
Published by: Medical Research Council, PO Box 19070, Tygerberg 7505, South Africa. TEL 27-21-9380207, FAX 27-21-9380385, http://www.mrc.ac.za/monitor/subscrib.htm. Ed. Niresh Bhagwandin.

610 611 ZAF
SOUTH AFRICAN INSTITUTE FOR MEDICAL RESEARCH. PUBLICATION. Text in English. 1917. irreg. back issues avail.
Published by: South African Institute for Medical Research, PO Box 1038, Johannesburg 2000, South Africa. FAX 27-11-489-9302, TELEX 4-22211. Circ: 150.

610 ZAF
R854.S6
SOUTH AFRICAN MEDICAL RESEARCH COUNCIL. ANNUAL REPORT AND HEALTH IMPACT REPORT. Text in English. 1969. a. free per issue. **Document type:** *Corporate.* **Description:** Summarizes the research activities of the council during the preceding year, lists current research programs and units, and provides financial statements.
Formerly: South African Medical Research Council. Annual Report (0081-248X); Which supersedes in part (in 1989): South African Medical Research Council. Research Report (1015-2377); Which supersedes (in 1985): South African Institute for Medical Research. Annual Report (0375-1880)
—CISTI, GNLM.
Published by: Medical Research Council, PO Box 19070, Tygerberg 7505, South Africa. TEL 27-21-938-0293, FAX 27-21-938-0395, http://www.mrc.ac.za. Ed. Leverne Gething. Circ: 2,500.

SOUTH AFRICAN SOCIETY OF PATHOLOGISTS. CONGRESS BROCHURE. see *MEETINGS AND CONGRESSES*

610 USA ISSN 0038-3139 CODEN: JSCMAZ
SOUTH CAROLINA MEDICAL ASSOCIATION. JOURNAL. Text in English. 1905. m. USD 25 to non-members; USD 15 to members. adv. bk.rev. charts, illus. index. reprint service avail. from PQC. *Refereed.* **Document type:** *Academic/Scholarly.* **Description:** Includes scientific articles, case reports, review articles, editorials, letters to the editor, medical history, medical and association news, state legislation, association calendar, President's Pages, medical history, and financial and investment advice.
Related titles: Microform ed.: (from PQC).
Indexed: Biol.Abstr., Chem.Abstr., INIS Atomind., Ind.Med. (1905-), Int.Nurs.Ind.
—BLDSC (4902.110000), CISTI, GNLM, ingenta, KNAW.
Published by: South Carolina Medical Association, PO Box 11188, Columbia, SC 29211. TEL 803-798-6207, 800-327-1021, FAX 803-772-6783, scmanet.org. Ed. Dr. Charles S Bryan. R&P, Adv. contact Dana D Kickey. page USD 250; trim 11 x 8.25. Circ: 5,300 (controlled).

610 USA ISSN 0038-3317 CODEN: SDMEAL
SOUTH DAKOTA JOURNAL OF MEDICINE. Text in English. 1946. m. USD 23; USD 30 foreign (effective 2001). adv. bk.rev. abstr, charts, illus. index. *Refereed.* **Document type:** *Academic/Scholarly.* **Description:** Presents the medical activities of specialty societies. Scientific articles, unpublished case reports and clinical and investigative articles.
Indexed: Biol.Abstr., Chem.Abstr., INIS Atomind., Ind.Med. (1965-), Int.Nurs.Ind.
—BLDSC (8350.900000), CISTI, GNLM, KNAW.
Published by: South Dakota State Medical Association, 1323 S Minnesota Ave, Sioux Falls, SD 57105. TEL 605-336-1965, FAX 605-336-0270, kachenha@sdsma.org, http://www.med.usd.edu/sdsma, http://www.usd.edu/med/sdma. Eds. Dr. Jerome Freeman, John Barlow. R&P, Adv. contact Kelli Achenbach. Circ: 1,850 (paid and controlled).

610 GBR ISSN 1358-6726
SOUTHAMPTON HEALTH JOURNAL. Abbreviated title: S H J. Text in English. 1983. q. free per issue. adv. bk.rev. **Document type:** *Academic/Scholarly.* **Description:** Acts as a forum for current issues, research, and business.
Formerly (until 1995): Southampton Medical Journal (0266-0342)
Published by: University Medicine at Southampton General Hospital, Shirley, Southampton, Hants SO9 4XY, United Kingdom. TEL 44-1703-796891. Ed., Adv. contact Christine Vincent. Circ: 2,500.

610 USA ISSN 0038-4348
R11 CODEN: SMJOAV
SOUTHERN MEDICAL JOURNAL. Text in English. 1908. m. USD 100 to individuals; USD 137 foreign to individuals; USD 132 to institutions; USD 158 foreign to institutions (effective 2001). adv. bibl, charts, illus. Index. back issues avail.; reprints avail. *Refereed.* **Document type:** *Academic/Scholarly.* **Description:** Geared toward practicing physicians and surgeons. Presents original articles and papers in clinical medicine.
Related titles: CD-ROM ed.; Microform ed.: (from PQC); Online - full text ed.: (from EBSCO Publishing, Institute for Scientific Information).
Indexed: AIM, ASCA, Abstr.Hyg., Adol.Ment.Hlth.Abstr., AgeLine, Agri.& Environ.Biotech.Abstr. (coverage dropped), Biol.Abstr., CINAHL, C.I.S. Abstr., Chem.Abstr., Curr.Adv.Cancer Res., Curr.Cont., Curr.Lit.Fam.Plan., Dairy Sci.Abstr., Dent.Ind., Derwent Biotech.Abstr., Dok.Arbeitsmed., Excerp.Med., HRIS, Helminthol.Abstr., Hosp.Lit.Ind., INIS Atomind., Ind.Med. (1908-), Ind.Sci.Rev., Inpharma, Int.Nurs.Ind., Med.& Surg.Dermat., NRN, Neurosci.Cit.Ind., Nutr.Abstr., Pharm.&Out.News, Protozool.Abstr., Reac., Rehabil.Lit., Rev.Appl.Entomol., Rev.Arom.& Med.Plants, Rev.Med.& Vet.Mycol., Rev.Plant Path., Rural Recreat.Tour.Abstr., SSCI (coverage dropped), Sci.Cit.Ind., THA, Trop.Dis.Bull.
—BLDSC (8354.400000), CASDDS, CISTI, GNLM, IDS, ingenta, KNAW. **CCC.**
Published by: Southern Medical Association, 35 Lakeshore Dr, Box 190088, Birmingham, AL 35219-0088. TEL 205-945-1840, 800-423-4992, FAX 205-945-1548, smj@education.sma.org, pwilliams@sma.org, http://www.sma.org. Ed. Dr. Ronald C. Hamdy Jr. R&P Cathy Galloway. Adv. contact Princess Williams. Circ: 22,000 (controlled).

614.44 CHE ISSN 0303-8408 CODEN: SZPMAA
SOZIAL- UND PRAEVENTIVMEDIZIN/MEDECINE SOCIALE ET PREVENTIVE. Text and summaries in English, French, German. 1955. bi-m. CHF 388; CHF 70 newsstand/cover; USD 289; USD 56.40 newsstand/cover (effective 2002). adv. bk.rev. abstr, bibl, charts, illus. index. *Refereed.* **Document type:** *Journal, Academic/Scholarly.* **Description:** Publishes original scientific papers and review articles in the field of epidemiology, preventive medicine, health services research, environmental health, medical sociology and industrial hygiene.
Formerly: Zeitschrift fuer Praeventivmedizin (0044-3379)
Related titles: Online - full text ed.: (from Institute for Scientific Information).
Indexed: ASCA, Abstr.Hyg., Biol.Abstr., C.I.S. Abstr., Chem.Abstr., Chem.Indus.Notes, Chem.Titles, Curr.Cont., Excerp.Med., Helminthol.Abstr., Ind.Med. (1974-), Inpharma, Int.Nurs.Ind., Nutr.Abstr., Pharm.&Out.News, Reac., SSCI (coverage dropped), Trop.Dis.Bull.
—BLDSC (8361.009000), CASDDS, CISTI, EMDOCS, GNLM, IDS, Infotrieve, KNAW. **CCC.**
Published by: (Schweizerische Gesellschaft fuer Praevention und Gesundheitswesen), Birkhaeuser Verlag AG (Subsidiary of: BertelsmannSpringer), Klosterberg, Postfach 133, Basel 4010, Switzerland. TEL 41-61-2050730, FAX 41-61-2050791, spm@birkhauser.ch, subscriptions@birkhauser.ch, http://www.birkhauser.ch/journals/3800/3800_tit.htm. Ed. R Steffen. **Dist. in N. America by:** Springer-Verlag, 333 Meadowlands Parkway, Secaucus, NJ 07094. TEL 800-777-4643, FAX 201-348-4505.

SOZIALE MEDIZIN. see *PUBLIC HEALTH AND SAFETY*

SOZIALGESETZBUCH: GESETZLICHE KRANKENVERSICHERUNG. see *LAW—Civil Law*

SPECIAL. see *EDUCATION—Special Education And Rehabilitation*

610 ZAF ISSN 1028-4753
SPECIALIST UPDATE. Text in English. 1990. m. ZAR 98.04; ZAR 160 foreign (effective 1997). **Document type:** *Academic/Scholarly.*
Formerly: Hospital Update (1018-1458)
Published by: George Warman Publications (Pty.) Ltd., PO Box 704, Cape Town 8000, South Africa. TEL 27-21-24-5320, FAX 27-21-26-1332. Ed. Tony Walker. Circ: 5,238.

SPECTRA BIOLOGIE. see *BIOLOGY*

616.07 USA ISSN 0081-3699
SPEZIELLE PATHOLOGISCHE ANATOMIE. Text in English. 1966. irreg., latest vol.22, 1993. price varies. reprint service avail. from ISI. **Document type:** *Academic/Scholarly.*
Published by: Springer-Verlag, Journals (Subsidiary of: BertelsmannSpringer), 175 Fifth Ave, New York, NY 10010. TEL 212-460-1500, FAX 212-473-6272.

610 GBR ISSN 0038-741X
SPHINCTER. Text in English. 1937. s-a. GBP 0.50. adv. bk.rev. **Document type:** *Academic/Scholarly.*
Related titles: Supplement: Sphincter Minimi.
Published by: University of Liverpool, Medical School, Royal Liverpool Hospital, University Of Liverpool, Box 147, Liverpool L69 3BX, United Kingdom. Ed. Callum Pearce. Circ: 900 (controlled).

616.04 USA ISSN 0160-9475
SPINA BIFIDA THERAPY* . Text in English. 1978. q. bk.rev.
Indexed: Psychol.Abstr.
—CISTI, GNLM.
Published by: Eterna International, Inc., PO Box 5731, Hauppauge, NY 11788-0154. Ed. Stephen B Parrish.

610 DEU ISSN 0932-0555
SPORTVERLETZUNG - SPORTSCHADEN. Text in German; Summaries in English, German. 1987. q. EUR 124.80, EUR 128.80, EUR 131.80 to institutions; EUR 37 newsstand/cover (effective 2002). **Document type:** *Journal, Academic/Scholarly.*
Related titles: Online - full text ed.: ISSN 1439-1236 (from Institute for Scientific Information).
Indexed: Focus on: Sports Sci.& Med., Ind.Med. (1987-), Int.Nurs.Ind.
—BLDSC (8419.860600), GNLM, KNAW.
Published by: Georg Thieme Verlag, Ruedigerstr 14, Stuttgart 70469, Germany. TEL 49-711-8931-0, FAX 49-711-8931298, sport@thieme.de, leser.service@thieme.de, http://www.thieme.de/sport. Ed. P Scharf. R&P Michael Wachinger. Circ: 2,300 (paid and controlled).

610 CHE
SPRECHSTUNDE. Text in German. 6/yr.
Address: Alpenblickstr 15, Rueti Zh 8630, Switzerland. TEL 055-321934. Ed. Augie Hagmann. Circ: 142,000.

610.711 USA ISSN 0277-4186
SPRINGER SERIES ON MEDICAL EDUCATION. Text in English. 1977. irreg., latest vol.20, 1996. price varies. adv. **Document type:** *Monographic series.* **Description:** Explores various issues in professional training for physicians and nurses.
—BLDSC (8424.766700).
Published by: Springer Publishing Company, 536 Broadway, New York, NY 10012. TEL 212-431-4370, FAX 212-941-7842, springer@springerpub.com, http://www.springerpub.com. Ed. Ursula Springer. R&P Dorothy Kouwenberg. Adv. contact Rafael Ortiz.

610 YUG ISSN 0371-4039 CODEN: SUGMAW
SRPSKA AKADEMIJA NAUKA I UMETNOSTI. ODELJENJE MEDICINSKIH NAUKA. GLAS. Text in Serbo-Croatian; Summaries in English, French, German, Russian. 1949. irreg. price varies.
Related titles: ♦ French ed.: Academie Serbe des Sciences et des Arts. Classe des Sciences Mathematiques et Naturelles. Bulletin Sciences Mathematiques. ISSN 0584-9829.
Indexed: Excerp.Med., Ind.Med. (coverage dropped).
—GNLM.
Published by: Srpska Akademija Nauka i Umetnosti/Serbian Academy of Arts and Sciences, Knez Mihailova 35, Belgrade 11000, Yugoslavia. TEL 381-11-187144, FAX 381-11-182825. Circ: 1,000. **Dist. by:** Prosveta, Terazije 16, Belgrade, Serbia, Yugoslavia.

610 YUG ISSN 0081-4016
SRPSKA AKADEMIJA NAUKA I UMETNOSTI. ODELJENJE MEDICINSKIH NAUKA. POSEBNA IZDANJA. Text in Serbo-Croatian; Summaries in English, French, German, Russian. 1950. irreg. price varies.
Indexed: Chem.Abstr., Excerp.Med., Ind.Med. (coverage dropped).
Published by: Srpska Akademija Nauka i Umetnosti/Serbian Academy of Arts and Sciences, Knez Mihailova 35, Belgrade 11000, Yugoslavia. TEL 381-11-187144, FAX 381-11-182825. Circ: 1,000. **Dist. by:** Prosveta, Terazije 16, Belgrade, Serbia, Yugoslavia.

610 YUG ISSN 0370-8179
SRPSKI ARHIV ZA CELOKUPNO LEKARSTVO* /SERBIAN ARCHIVES OF MEDICINE. Text in Serbian; Summaries in English. 1872. m. YUN 200 domestic; DEM 40 foreign. illus. **Document type:** *Academic/Scholarly.*
Indexed: Biol.Abstr., Dent.Ind., Excerp.Med., INIS Atomind., Ind.Med. (1872-), Nutr.Abstr.
—BLDSC (0166.680000), CISTI, GNLM.
Published by: Srpsko Lekarsko Drustvo/Serbian Medical Association, Vase Stajica 9, Novi Sad 21000, Yugoslavia. TEL 381-11-3246529, kentera@eunet.yu. Ed. Vladimir Slavkovic.

610 GBR
ST. GEORGE'S HOSPITAL MEDICAL SCHOOL. REPORT. Text in English. irreg., latest vol.6, 1993. **Document type:** *Monographic series.*
Published by: St. George's Hospital Medical School, Cranmer Terr, London SW17 0RE, United Kingdom. TEL 44-181-672-9944, FAX 44-181-767-4696.

610 362.1 USA
ST. JOHN HOSPITAL AND MEDICAL CENTER. MEDICAL BULLETIN. Text in English. 1979. a. charts, illus. **Document type:** *Bulletin.*
Published by: St. John Hospital and Medical Center, 22101 Moross Rd, Detroit, MI 48236-2172. TEL 313-343-4000. Ed. Dr. David Peiper. Circ: 800.

610 IND ISSN 0970-4221
ST. JOHN'S JOURNAL OF MEDICINE. Text in English. 1988. q. INR 100, USD 20. adv. bibl, charts, illus. back issues avail. *Refereed.*
Published by: St. John's Medical College, Alumni Association, c/o Dr. S.V. Srikishna, Gen. Sec., Robert Koch Bhavan 1st Fl., St. John's Medical College, Bangalore, Karnataka 560 034, India. TEL 565435. Ed. Dr. Ashley D'Cruz. Circ: 1,500.

M

610 USA ISSN 0892-1334
ST. LOUIS METROPOLITAN MEDICINE. Text in English. 1979. m. USD 30 to non-members (effective 2000). adv. bk.rev. index. back issues avail. *Refereed.* **Document type:** *Trade.*
Published by: St. Louis Medical Service Bureau, 3839 Lindell Blvd., St. Louis, MO 63108. TEL 314-371-5225, FAX 314-533-8601, terrywatson@slmms.com. Ed. Dr. J Gail Neely. R&P, Adv. contact Terry Watson. page USD 410; trim 11 x 8.5. Circ: 2,500 (paid and controlled).

614 ITA ISSN 0038-9323
STAMPA MEDICA. Text in Italian. 1960. s-m. (21/yr.). ITL 35,000. adv. bk.rev.
Published by: E S I Stampa Medica s.r.l., Largo Volontari Del Sangue, 10, Casella Postale 42, San Donato, MI 20133, Italy. TEL 39-2-5274241, FAX 39-2-55600670, TELEX 324-894. Ed. Diego Onestinghel. Adv. contact Ornella Galbiati. B&W page ITL 12,100,000, color page ITL 15,000,000; trim 235 x 171. Circ: 69,000.

330.9 610.6 USA ISSN 1090-4417
START-UP; Windhover's review of emerging medical ventures. Text in English. 1996. m. (11/yr., Jul./Aug. comb.). USD 795 domestic; USD 870 foreign (effective 2002). **Document type:** *Trade.* **Description:** Profiles the most important new product companies, identifies the hottest technology areas, reviews funds flowing into private companies and investment trends, and reports on university tech transfer licensing. Industries covered: pharmaceuticals, biotechnology, hospital supply, medical equipment & devices, and in vitro diagnostics.
Related titles: CD-ROM ed.: Strategic Commentary; Online - full text ed.: Strategic Commentary Online; ♦ Cumulative ed. of: Strategic Commentary.
Published by: Windhover Information, Inc., 10 Hoyt St, Norwalk, CT 06851 . TEL 203-838 4401, FAX 203-838 3214, custserv@windhoverinfo.com, http://www.windhoverinfo.com.

STATE HEALTH MONITOR. see *INSURANCE*

STATE HEALTH NOTES. see *PUBLIC HEALTH AND SAFETY*

STATISTICAL METHODS IN MEDICAL RESEARCH. see *STATISTICS*

STERILIZATION IN AUSTRALIA. see *PUBLIC HEALTH AND SAFETY*

610 336.2 DEU ISSN 0943-1896
STEUER-BRIEF FUER AERZTE UND ZAHNAERZTE. Text in German. 1991. m. DEM 10.50 per issue (effective 1999). **Document type:** *Bulletin.*
Formerly (until 1992): Aerzte-Steuer-Brief (0939-5873)
Published by: Verlag Peter Deubner GmbH, Wolfgang-Mueller-Str 14, Cologne 50968, Germany. TEL 49-221-9370180, FAX 49-221-93701890.

610 CAN ISSN 1199-1747
STITCHES; the journal of medical humour. Text in English. 1990. 12/yr. CND 40 domestic; USD 45 in United States; USD 68 elsewhere (effective 1999). adv. illus. back issues avail. **Document type:** *Trade.* **Description:** A humor and life-style magazine for physicians.
Formerly (until 1993): Punch Digest for Canadian Doctors (1182-5405)
Published by: Stitches Publishing Inc., 16787 Warden Ave, R R 3, Newmarket, ON L3Y 4W1, Canada. TEL 905-853-1884, FAX 905-853-6565, stitches@attglobal.net, http:// www.StitchesExplorerclub.com. Ed. Simon Hally. Pub. Peter Cocker. Adv. contact Don Kirkpatrick. Circ: 36,500 (controlled).

610 330 USA
STRATEGIC COMMENTARY. Text in English. m. **Document type:** *Academic/Scholarly.*
Media: Online - full content. **Related titles:** CD-ROM ed.; ♦ Cumulative ed.: Windhover's IN VIVO. ISSN 1520-4901; ♦ Start-Up. ISSN 1090-4417.
Published by: Windhover Information, Inc., 10 Hoyt St, Norwalk, CT 06851 . TEL 203-838 4401, FAX 203-838 3214, custserv@windhoverinfo.com, http://www.windhoverinfo.com.

610 USA ISSN 1080-5222
STRAUB FOUNDATION. PROCEEDINGS. Text in English. 1952. s-a. free to physicians and librarians. adv. bk.rev. charts, illus. index. reprint service avail. from PQC. **Document type:** *Proceedings, Academic/Scholarly.*
Former titles (until 1995): Straub Pacific Health Foundation Proceedings; (until 1988): Straub Proceedings (0741-8930); (until 1982): Straub Clinic Proceedings (0039-2251); (until 1982): Straub Clinic Staff Meetings. Proceedings (0093-3538)
Related titles: Microfiche ed.
Published by: Straub Foundation, 1100 Ward Ave, Ste 1045, Honolulu, HI 96814. TEL 808-524-6755, FAX 808-531-0123, http://www.straub-foundation.org. Ed. Dr. Bo Eklof. Circ: 2,500.

610 CHE ISSN 1025-3890
CODEN: STRSFZ
STRESS; the international journal on the biology of stress. Text in English. 1997. 4/yr. GBP 72, USD 87, EUR 96 to individuals; GBP 254, USD 327, EUR 338 to institutions; GBP 410, USD 536, USD 547 to corporations (effective 2002). **Document type:** *Journal, Academic/Scholarly.* **Description:** Deals with the basic and clinical aspects of stress in terms of regulation of the stress response and factors affecting such a regulation.
Related titles: CD-ROM ed.; Online - full text ed.: (from Northern Light Technology, Inc., EBSCO Publishing, ingenta, RoweCom Information Quest).
Indexed: Anim.Behav.Abstr., Ind.Med. (1996-), PsycInfo.
—BLDSC (8474.127600).
Published by: Gordon and Breach - Harwood Academic (Subsidiary of: Taylor & Francis Group), PO Box 531, Lausanne 1000, Switzerland. TEL 41-21-6411280, FAX 41-21-6411281, info@gbhap.com, http:// www.gbhap.com/Stress/. Eds. E Ronald de Kloet, J A Russell, Richard McCarty. **Subscr. addr. in US:** International Publishers Direct, PO Box 32160, Newark, NJ 07102. FAX 215-750-6343.

610 DNK ISSN 0039-2634
STUD MED. Variant title: Ugeskrift for Naesten Laeger. Text in Danish. 1936. s-a. DKK 60. bk.rev. illus, pat. **Document type:** *Academic/Scholarly.* **Description:** Written by and for medical students in Denmark on all kinds of medical subjects. Includes short stories and poetry.
Published by: Danish Medical Students Association, Blegdamsvej 3, Copenhagen N 2200, Denmark. Ed. Henrik Herloev. Circ: 5,000 (controlled).

610 GBR ISSN 0966-6494
STUDENT B M J. (British Medical Journal) Text in English. 1992. m. GBP 27, USD 42 combined subscription to individuals includes print & online eds.; GBP 89 to institutions for pirnt only; USD 142 to institutions for print only (effective 2002). adv. bk.rev. **Document type:** *Academic/Scholarly.* **Description:** An international monthly journal for medical students with all the quality of the B M J (British Medical Journal.).
Related titles: Online - full text ed.; ♦ Regional ed.: Student B M J (South African Edition); ♦ Special ed. of: B M J. ISSN 0959-535X; ♦ Supplement to: B M J. ISSN 0959-535X.
Indexed: Addic.Abstr., WMB.
Published by: B M J Publishing Group, B M A House, Tavistock Sq, London WC1H 9JR, United Kingdom. TEL 44-20-7387-4499, FAX 44-20-7383-6400, dkatz@bmj.com, info.norththames@bma.org.uk, http://www.studentbmj.com, http://www.bma.org.uk. Ed. Alison Tonks. R&P Diana Katz. Adv. contact Catherine Harding.

610 ZAF
STUDENT B M J (SOUTH AFRICAN EDITION). (British Medical Journal) Text in English. 1994. bi-m. adv. illus. **Document type:** *Academic/Scholarly.*
Related titles: ♦ Regional ed.: Student B M J. ISSN 0966-6494.
Published by: George Warman Publications (Pty.) Ltd., PO Box 704, Cape Town 8000, South Africa. TEL 27-21-24-5320, FAX 27-21-26-1332. Circ: (controlled).

610 ITA ISSN 0371-3172
CODEN: SSSEAK
STUDI SASSARESI✱. Text in Italian; Summaries in English. 1932. q. ITL 40,000. adv. index. back issues avail.
Indexed: Biol.Abstr., Excerp.Med., Food Sci.& Tech.Abstr.
—CASDDS.
Published by: Societa Sassarese di Scienze Mediche e Naturali, Via de Nicola, Sassari, SS 07100, Italy. Ed. Pierangelo Catalano. Circ: 1,000. **Subscr. to:** Institute of Human Physiology, Via Muroni, 23 A, Sassari, SS 07100, Italy.

610 POL ISSN 0860-9594
STUDIA SOCIETATIS SCIENTIARUM TORUNENSIS. SECTIO H. MEDICINA. Text in Polish. 1989. irreg., latest vol.1, no.2, 1991. price varies. **Document type:** *Monographic series.*
—CISTI, KNAW.
Published by: Towarzystwo Naukowe w Toruniu, Ul Wysoka 16, Torun 81100, Poland. TEL 48-56-23941. Ed. Lech Bieganowski. Circ: 220.

610.09 NLD ISSN 0925-1421
STUDIES IN ANCIENT MEDICINE. Text in Dutch. 1991. irreg., latest vol.19, 1998. price varies. back issues avail. *Refereed.* **Document type:** *Monographic series.* **Description:** Scholarly monographs on historical texts and their authors, materia medica, and related topics in ancient medicine.
—CISTI.
Published by: Brill Academic Publishers, PO Box 9000, Leiden 2300 PA, Netherlands. TEL 31-71-535-3500, FAX 31-71-531-7532, cs@brill.nl. Ed. John Scarborough. R&P Elizabeth Venekamp.

612.6 NLD
STUDIES IN FERTILITY AND STERILITY. Text in English. irreg. price varies. *Refereed.* **Document type:** *Monographic series.*
Published by: Kluwer Academic Publishers Group (Subsidiary of: Wolters Kluwer N.V.), Spuiboulevard 50, PO Box 17, Dordrecht 3300 AA, Netherlands. FAX 31-78-639-2254, services@wkap.nl, http://www.wkap.nl. **Dist. by:** Journals Department, PO Box 322, Dordrecht 3300 AH, Netherlands. FAX 31-78-654-6474.

610.28 NLD ISSN 0926-9630
STUDIES IN HEALTH TECHNOLOGY AND INFORMATICS. Text in English. 1992. irreg., latest vol.76, 2000. price varies. back issues avail. *Refereed.* **Document type:** *Monographic series, Proceedings, Academic/Scholarly.* **Description:** Publishes papers and studies dealing with the impact of technological developments and information sciences on health care and health policy, particularly in Europe.
—BLDSC (8490.628200), CISTI.
Published by: I O S Press, Van Diemenstraat 94, Amsterdam 1013 CN, Netherlands. TEL 31-20-638-2189, FAX 31-20-620-3419, market@iospress.nl, http://www.iospress.nl. **Subscr. to:** I O S Press, Inc. **Dist. by:** Ohmsha Ltd, 3-1 Kanda-Nishiki-cho, Chiyoda-ku, Tokyo 101-0054, Japan. TEL 81-3-3233-0641, FAX 81-3-3233-2426, http://www.ohmsha.co.jp.

610 IND ISSN 0970-5562
STUDIES IN HISTORY OF MEDICINE AND SCIENCE. Text in English. 1977. s-a. INR 150, USD 35 (effective 2000). adv. bk.rev. *Refereed.* **Document type:** *Academic/Scholarly.* **Description:** Publishes original research papers or analytical studies of primary sources of Afro-Asia during the ancient and Medieval periods.
Formerly (until 1984): Studies in History of Medicine (0379-3915)
Indexed: Amer.Hist.& Life, C.C.M.J., Hist.Abstr. (1985-85, 1988-), Per.Islam. (1986-1987), Russ.Acad.Sci.Bibl.
—BLDSC (8490.673300), CISTI, GNLM.
Published by: Jamia Hamdard/Hamdard University, Hamdard Nagar, New Delhi 110 062, India. TEL 91-11-6084685, FAX 91-11-6088874, TELEX 031-70318, libraryl@ndf.vsnl.net.in. Eds. Hakeem Abdul Hameed, S M Razaullah Ansari. R&P, Adv. contact S M Razaullah Ansari. Circ: 500.

610 614 GBR ISSN 0473-8837
STUDIES ON CURRENT HEALTH PROBLEMS. Text in English. 1962. irreg. price varies. charts.
Published by: (Association of the British Pharmaceutical Industry), Office of Health Economics, 12 Whitehall, London SW1, United Kingdom. FAX 071-976-1962. Circ: 15,000.

610 USA ISSN 1060-4251
STURZA'S MEDICAL INVESTMENT LETTER. Text in English. 1991. w. (50/yr.). USD 320; USD 366 in Canada & Mexico; USD 395 elsewhere. index, cum.index. back issues avail. **Document type:** *Newsletter.* **Description:** Assesses the most promising stocks and emerging medical technologies in the healthcare industry. Includes independent research by physicians on staff, and long and short term recommendations with actual price targets.
Related titles: Fax ed.
Published by: Taurus Littrow Publishing, Inc., 156 W 56th St 20th Fl, New York, NY 10019-3800. TEL 212-541-8200, FAX 212-541-8288, info@sturzas.com, http://www.sturzas.com. Ed., Pub., R&P Evan Sturza.

610 SDN ISSN 0491-4481
SUDAN MEDICAL JOURNAL. Text in English. 1974 (vol.12). q. USD 10. adv. charts, illus. index. **Document type:** *Academic/Scholarly.*
Related titles: CD-ROM ed.

M

Indexed: C.I.S. Abstr., ExtraMED, INIS Atomind.
—CISTI, GNLM.
Published by: (Sudan Medical Association), Khartoum University Press, P O Box 321, Khartoum, Sudan. Ed. D M Y Sukkar. Circ: 2,000.

610 IND ISSN 0971-0272
SUDHANIDHI. Text in Hindi. 1973. m. INR 35. adv. bk.rev.
Published by: Dhanvantari Karyalaya, Aligarh, Uttar Pradesh, India. Ed. Sri Raghivir Prasad Trivedi. Circ: 12,000.

SUDHOFFS ARCHIV; Zeitschrift fuer Wissenschaftsgeschichte. see *SCIENCES: COMPREHENSIVE WORKS*

SUDHOFFS ARCHIV. BEIHEFTE. see *SCIENCES: COMPREHENSIVE WORKS*

610 FIN ISSN 0039-5560
SUOMEN LAAKARILEHTI/FINLANDS LAEKARTIDNING/ FINNISH MEDICAL JOURNAL. Text in Finnish. 1946. 52/yr. FIM 900 in Eastern Europe; FIM 1,150 rest of world; FIM 35 newsstand/cover (effective 2001). adv. bk.rev. bibl, illus. index. *Refereed.* **Description:** Disseminates information on new developments in medicine and focuses on the continuing education and professional advancement of doctors. Follows and reports on trends in health-care policy and serves as a forum for professional information and discussion.
Indexed: Biol.Abstr., Ind.Med. (coverage dropped).
—CISTI, GNLM.
Published by: Suomen Laakariliitto/Finnish Medical Association, Maekelaenkatu 2, Helsinki 00500, Finland. TEL 358-9-393-091, FAX 358-93930-794. Ed. Taito Pekkarinen. Adv. contact Kristiina Karjalainen. B&W page FIM 11,300, color page FIM 18,500; trim 230 x 175. Circ: 24,000 (controlled).

611 617 616.07 FRA ISSN 0930-1038
SURGICAL AND RADIOLOGIC ANATOMY. Text in French. 1978. bi-m. FRF 2,700, USD 567; USD 112 newsstand/cover (effective 2001). adv. reprint service avail. from ISI. *Refereed.* **Document type:** *Academic/Scholarly.*
Former titles: Journal of Clinical and Radiological Anatomy. Anatomia Clinica; Anatomia Clinica (0343-6098)
Related titles: Microfilm ed.: (from PQC); Online - full text ed.: ISSN 1279-8517 (from EBSCO Publishing, RoweCom Information Quest, Swets Blackwell, Springer LINK, Institute for Scientific Information); English ed.: ISSN 0930-312X.
Indexed: ASCA, Curr.Cont., Excerp.Med., Ind.Med. (1986-), Ind.Sci.Rev., Inpharma, Reac., Sci.Cit.Ind.
—BLDSC (8548.166500), CISTI, EMDOCS, GNLM, IDS, Infotrieve, ingenta, KNAW. **CCC.**
Published by: (College Medical Francais des Professeurs d'Anatomie), Springer-Verlag France (Subsidiary of: BertelsmannSpringer), 1 rue Paul Cezanne, Paris 75008, France. TEL 33-1-53933644, FAX 33-1-53933683, access@link.springer.de; york@springer-paris.fr, http://link.springer.de/link/service/journals/00590/index.htm. Ed. C Fontaine. adv.: B&W page FRF 5,300, color page FRF 10,200; 275 x 210. **Subscr. in N. America to:** Springer-Verlag New York Inc., 44 Hartz Way, Secaucus, NJ 07096-2491. TEL 201-348-4033, FAX 201-348-4505. **Co-sponsor:** European Association of Clinical Anatomy, French Society of Radiology, Chinese Association of Anatomy, Section of Clinical Anatomy.

617.07 USA ISSN 0899-8175
CODEN: SUPAFC
SURGICAL PATHOLOGY. Text in English. 1988. q. USD 125 to individuals; USD 165 to institutions. *Refereed.* **Document type:** *Academic/Scholarly.*
Incorporates (in 1994): Digestive Disease Pathology (0896-0062)
Related titles: Online - full text ed.: (from Institute for Scientific Information).
Indexed: ASCA.
—GNLM, KNAW.
Published by: Field & Wood, Medical Periodicals, Inc., PO Box 975, Blue Bell, PA 19422. TEL 610-828-4010, FAX 215-482-0226. Eds. Dr. Cecilia Fenoglio Preiser, Virginia Livolsi.

610 USA ISSN 1062-4732
SURGICAL PRODUCTS. Text in English. 1980. m. USD 24 in North America; USD 34 elsewhere; USD 4 newsstand/cover domestic; USD 6 newsstand/cover foreign (effective 2001). **Document type:** *Trade.* **Description:** Focuses on hospitals, surgicenters and emergicenters engaged in surgical procedures.
Formerly: Surgical Product News (0279-4829)
—**CCC.**
Published by: Cahners Business Information, New Product Information Unit (Subsidiary of: Reed Elsevier plc), 301 Gibraltar Dr, P O Box 650, Morris Plains, NJ 07950-0650. FAX 973-539-3476, http://www.surgprodmag.com. Ed. Sean Fenske TEL 973-292-5100 x271. Pub. Noreen Costelloe TEL 631-244-7396. Circ: 80,100.

610 370.1 IND
THE SURVEY KIT. Text in English. (in 9 vols.). USD 132.55 for complete set (effective 2000). **Description:** Provides tools to help decide just what works best in a given situation. It is tool for classroom use for students in the health and allied sciences. It is also a reference library for the practitioner.
Published by: Sage Publications India Pvt. Ltd., P O Box 4215, New Delhi 110 048, India. TEL 91-11-644-4958, FAX 91-11-6472426, http://www.sagepub.com.

610 BGR ISSN 0562-7192
CODEN: SUMEA4
SUVREMENNA MEDICINA/MODERN MEDICINE. Text in Bulgarian; Summaries in Bulgarian, English. 1950. bi-m. BGL 20,000; USD 69 foreign (effective 2002). **Document type:** *Journal, Academic/Scholarly.*
Indexed: Abstr.Bulg.Sci.Med.Lit., BSL Biol., Chem.Abstr., INIS Atomind.
—CASDDS, CISTI, GNLM.
Published by: Meditsinski Universitet - Sofia, Tsentur za Informatsiia po Meditsina/Medical University - Sofia, Medical Information Center, 1 Sv Georgi Sofiiski ul, Sofia 1431, Bulgaria. TEL 359 2-522342, mutafov@sun.medun.acad.bg, http://www.medfac.acad.bg/mj.html, http://www.medun.acad.bg. Ed. Z Krastev. Circ: 500. **Dist. by:** Sofia Books, Ul Silivria 16, Sofia 1404, Bulgaria. TEL 359-2-9586257, sofiabooks@hotmail.com, http://www.sofiabooks.hit.bg.

610 CHN ISSN 1000-5749
SUZHOU YIXUEYUAN XUEBAO/SUZHOU INSTITUTE OF MEDICAL SCIENCES. JOURNAL. Text in Chinese. q. **Document type:** *Academic/Scholarly.*
Indexed: INIS Atomind.
Published by: Suzhou Yixueyuan/Suzhou Institute of Medical Sciences, 48 Renmin Lu, Suzhou, Jiangsu 215007, China. TEL 225696. Ed. Du Ziwei.

610 SWE ISSN 0284-5342
SVENSK MEDICIN. Text in Swedish. 1988. irreg. (approx. 8/yr.). SEK 600.
—GNLM.
Published by: Haelso och Sjukvaardens Utvecklingsinstitut/Swedish Institute for Health Services Development, Fack 70487, Stockholm 10726, Sweden. TEL 08-702-4600, FAX 08-702-4799. **Co-sponsor:** Svenska Laekaresaellskapet.

SVENSK TIDSKRIFT FOER MEDICINSK AKUPUNKTUR. see *ALTERNATIVE MEDICINE*

610 SWE ISSN 0349-1722
R85
SVENSKA LAEKARESAELLSKAPETS HANDLINGAR. Text in Swedish. 1812-1834; resumed 1837-1902; resumed 1907. 5/yr. adv. **Document type:** *Academic/Scholarly.*
Former titles (until 1980): Hygiea; (until 1975): Svenska Laekaresaellskapets Handlingar; (until 1902): Svenska Laekaresaellskapets Nya Handlingar; (until 1834): Svenska Laekaresaellskapets Handlingar
Published by: Svenska Laekaresaellskapet, Fack 738, Stockholm 10135, Sweden. TEL 46-8-24-33-50, FAX 46-8-24-43-48, sls@swedemedsoc.se.

610 362.1 SWE ISSN 0346-6000
SWEDEN. SOCIALSTYRELSEN. FOERFATTNINGSSAMLING: MEDICAL. Variant title: S O S F S (M). Text in Swedish. 1883. irreg. (approx. 30/yr.). SEK 502 (effective 2000). index. **Document type:** *Directory.* **Description:** Directory and general advice on medical welfare.
Supersedes in part (in 1976): Sweden. Medicinalvaesendet. Foerfattningssamling (0346-5837)
Related titles: Online - full text ed.
Published by: Socialstyrelsen/National Institute of Economic Research, Stockholm 10630, Sweden. FAX 48-8-783-33-02, TELEX 16773 NBHWS. Ed. Kristina Widgren. Circ: 8,000. **Subscr. to:** National Board of Health and Welfare, Customer Service, Finspangsgatan 51, Spanga 16353, Sweden. TEL 46-8-795-23-30, FAX 46-8-760-58-95.

610.025485 SWE ISSN 0345-0171
SWEDEN. SOCIALSTYRELSEN. LEGITIMERADE LAEKARE/SWEDEN. NATIONAL BOARD OF HEALTH AND WELFARE. AUTHORIZED PHYSICIANS. Text in Swedish. 1971. a. index. **Document type:** *Directory, Government.*
Published by: (Sweden. Socialstyrelsen/National Institute of Economic Research), Fritzes, Stockholm 10647, Sweden. TEL 46-8-690-9090, FAX 46-8-690-9191. Circ: 10,000.

610 CHE ISSN 1424-3784
▼ **SWISS MEDICAL FORUM.** Text in German, French. 2001. w. CHF 320; CHF 20 newsstand/cover (effective 2001). back issues avail. *Refereed.* **Document type:** *Journal, Trade.*
Related titles: Online - full text ed.: ISSN 1424-4020.
Published by: E M H Swiss Medical Publishers Ltd., Steinentorstr 13, Basel, Switzerland. TEL 41-61-4678555, FAX 41-61-4678556, smf@emh.ch, verlag@emh.ch, http://www.medicalforum.ch, http://www.emh.ch.

610 CHE ISSN 1424-7860
CODEN: SMWOAS
SWISS MEDICAL WEEKLY. Text in English. 1871. fortn. CHF 165 domestic; CHF 180 in Europe; CHF 200 elsewhere; CHF 20 newsstand/cover (effective 2001). adv. bk.rev. abstr, bibl, charts, illus, stat. index. 25 p./no. 2 cols./p. back issues avail. *Refereed.* **Document type:** *Journal, Academic/Scholarly, Trade.* **Description:** Publishes original research from all fields of medicine.
Former titles (until 2000): Schweizerische Medizinische Wochenschrift (0036-7672); (until 1919): Correspondenz-Blatt fur Schweizer Arzte (0366-5461)
Related titles: Microform ed.: (from PMC); Online - full content ed.: ISSN 1424-3997; Online - full text ed.: (from Institute for Scientific Information).
Indexed: ASCA, Abstr.Hyg., Agri.& Environ.Biotech.Abstr. (coverage dropped), Biol.Abstr., C.I.S. Abstr., Chem.Abstr., Chem.Indus.Notes, Chem.Titles, Curr.Adv.Ecol.Sci., Curr.Cont. (coverage dropped), Dairy Sci.Abstr., Dent.Ind., Derwent Biotech.Abstr., Excerp.Med., Helminthol.Abstr., INIS Atomind., Ind.Med. (2001-), Ind.Sci.Rev., Int.Nurs.Ind., Neurosci.Cit.Ind., Nutr.Abstr., Protozool.Abstr., Rev.Appl.Entomol., Rev.Med.& Vet.Mycol., Risk Abstr., Sci.Cit.Ind., Trop.Dis.Bull.
—BLDSC, CASDDS, CISTI, GNLM, IDS, ingenta, KNAW. **CCC.**
Published by: E M H Swiss Medical Publishers Ltd., Steinentorstr 13, Basel, Switzerland. TEL 41-61-4678555, FAX 41-61-4678556, red@smw.ch, verlag@emh.ch, http://www.smw.ch, http://www.emh.ch. Circ: 4,500.

SWITZERLAND. BUNDESAMT FUER SOZIALVERSICHERUNG. SPEZIALITAETENLISTE - LISTE DES SPECIALITES - ELENCO DELLE SPECIALITA. see *PHARMACY AND PHARMACOLOGY*

616.089 NLD ISSN 0167-6407
CODEN: SFOMD4
SYMPOSIA FOUNDATION MERIEUX. Text in Dutch. 1979. irreg. price varies. back issues avail. *Refereed.* **Document type:** *Monographic series, Proceedings, Academic/Scholarly.*
—CASDDS. **CCC.**
Published by: Elsevier Science BV, PO Box 211, Amsterdam 1000 AE, Netherlands. TEL 31-20-485-3757, 31-20-485-3911, FAX 31-20-485-3432, 31-20-485-3598, nlinfo-f@elsevier.nl, http://www.elsevier.nl. **Subscr. in Australasia and the Far East to:** Elsevier Science (Singapore) Pte Ltd, No.1 Temasek Ave, 17-01 Millenia Tower, Singapore 039192, Singapore. TEL 65-434-3727, FAX 65-337-2230, asiainfo@elsevier.com.sg; **Subscr. in Japan to:** Elsevier Science Inc - Japan Regional Office, 9-15 Higashi-Azabu 1-chome, Minato-ku, Tokyo 106-0044, Japan. TEL 81-3-5561-5033, FAX 81-3-5561-5047, info@elsevier.co.jp; **Subscr. in the Americas to:** Elsevier Science, PO Box 945, New York, NY 10159-0945. TEL 212-633-3730, 888-437-4636, FAX 212-633-3680, usinfo-f@elsevier.com, http://www.elsevier.com.

610 DEU ISSN 0943-9250
SYMPOSIUM MEDICAL. Text in German. 1990. 18/yr. DEM 175 (effective 2001). adv. bk.rev. *Refereed.* **Document type:** *Journal, Academic/Scholarly.*
Formerly (until 1992): Charite-Report (0938-7307)

M

Published by: (Aerztliche Fortbildungskongresse), B M V - Berliner Medizinische Verlagsanstalt GmbH, Lietzenburger Str 97, Berlin 10719, Germany. TEL 49-30-886749-0, FAX 49-30-88674999, info@bmv-berlin.com, http://www.bmv-berlin.de. Ed. Bettina Baierl. Adv. contact Caridad Nyari TEL 49-30-88674970. B&W page DEM 4,550, color page DEM 5,750; trim 210 x 280. Circ: 10,500.

610 BEL
SYNDIKALE KAMER. Text in Dutch. 1963. s-a. membership. bk.rev.
Published by: Sindikale Kamer der Geneesheren der Provincies Oost & West Vlaanderen, Henri Beyaertstraet 2, Kortrijk 8500, Belgium. Ed. L van Steenberge. Circ: 5,100.

610 FRA ISSN 0399-2160
SYNTHESE MEDICALE; le journal du dialogue entre practiciens. Text in French. w. FRF 100. adv. charts, illus.
Published by: Editions Techniques et Medicales, 18 rue des Huissiers, Neuilly-sur-Seine 92200, France. TEL 47-47-74-74, FAX 47-47-71-03. Ed. Vincent Heugas. Circ: 55,000.

610 FRA ISSN 0993-3557
SYNTHESE MEDICALE GESTION. Text in French. 10/yr. FRF 150. adv. **Description:** Covers the business end of running a medical practice.
Published by: Editions Techniques et Medicales, 18 rue des Huissiers, Neuilly-sur-Seine 92200, France. TEL 47-47-74-74, FAX 47-47-71-03. Ed. Guy Vincent Heugas.

610 POL
SZCZECINSKIE ROCZNIKI NAUKOWE, NAUKI MEDYCZNE. Text in Polish. irreg., latest vol.10, no.1.
Published by: (Szczecinskie Towarzystwo Naukowe), Ossolineum Publishing House of the Polish Academy of Sciences, Pl Solny 14 a, Wroclaw 50062, Poland. TEL 48-71-343-6961, FAX 48-71-448-103.

610 POL ISSN 0082-125X
CODEN: SZTNBY
SZCZECINSKIE TOWARZYSTWO NAUKOWE. WYDZIAL NAUK LEKARSKICH. PRACE. Text in Polish; Summaries in English, Polish, Russian. 1959. irreg. price varies.
—CASDDS.
Published by: Szczecinskie Towarzystwo Naukowe, Wydzial Nauk Lekarskich, Ul Wojska Polskiego 96, Szczecin 70481, Poland. TEL 48-91-231862. **Dist. by:** Ars Polona, Krakowskie Przedmiescie 7, Warsaw, Poland.

610 ITA
T C. (Terapia del Comportamento) Text in Italian. 1984. q. ITL 50,000.
Published by: Bulzoni Editore, Via Dei Liburni, 14, Rome, RM 00185, Italy. TEL 06-4455207, FAX 06-4450355. Ed. Paolo Meazzini.

610 USA ISSN 0885-9191
T M J UPDATE: A CURRENT REVIEW OF TEMPOROMANDIBULAR JOINT DEVELOPMENTS. Text in English. 1983. bi-m. USD 69 domestic to individuals; USD 79 in Canada & Mexico to individuals; USD 84 elsewhere to individuals; USD 79 domestic to institutions; USD 89 in Canada & Mexico to institutions; USD 94 elsewhere to institutions (effective 2000). index. **Document type:** *Newsletter, Trade, Academic/Scholarly.* **Description:** Summarizes medical and dental journal articles about TMJ disorders and craniofacial pain.
Published by: Anadem Publishing, Inc., 3620 N High St, Columbus, OH 43214. TEL 614-262-2539, 800-633-0055, FAX 614-262-6630, anadem@erinet.com. Ed. Karla Gale. Pub. Will Kuhlmann. R&P Mike Cheadle.

T V B. (Tijdschrift voor Verzorging en Beheer) see *GERONTOLOGY AND GERIATRICS*

610 EGY
TABIBAK AL-KHASS. Text in Arabic. 1969. m. USD 35 in Africa, Asia, Europe, India and North America; USD 45 in South America, Japan and Australia (effective 2001). adv. bk.rev.
Published by: Dar Al-Hilal, 16 Sharia Muhammad Ezz Al-Arab, Cairo, Egypt. TEL 02-362-5450, FAX 02-362-5469, TELEX 92703. Ed. Abdel Rahman Nour Ed-Din. Circ: 133,000.

610 LBN
TABIBOK/YOUR DOCTOR. Text in Arabic. 1956. m. LBP 24,000, USD 55 (effective 2001). adv. bk.rev. back issues avail. **Description:** Provides up-to-date medical and health information and advice for a general audience.
Published by: Scientific Publications Ltd., P O Box 90434, Beirut, Lebanon. TEL 963-11-221-1980, FAX 963-11-3738901, TELEX 411513 MEDEQ SY. Ed. Dr. Sami Kabbani. Adv. contact Rima Rihan. Circ: 30,000.

610 DEU ISSN 0494-464X
TAEGLICHE PRAXIS; Zeitschrift fuer den praktisch taetigen Arzt. Text in German. 4/yr. EUR 132; EUR 37 newsstand/cover (effective 2002). **Document type:** *Journal, Academic/Scholarly.*
Related titles: ♦ Spanish ed.: Practica Diaria.
—GNLM, IDS, Infotrieve. **CCC.**
Published by: Hans Marseille Vertrieb Medizinischer Zeitschriften, Buerkleinstr 12, Munich 80538, Germany. TEL 49-89-227988, FAX 49-89-2904643, marseille-verlag@t-online.de, http://www.marseille-verlag.com. Eds. H Feiereis, R Saller.

610 100 USA
TAKING SIDES: CLASHING VIEWS ON CONTROVERSIAL BIOETHICAL ISSUES. Text in English. irreg., latest vol.7, 1997. USD 13. illus. **Document type:** *Academic/Scholarly.*
Published by: Dushkin - McGraw-Hill, Sluice Dock, Guilford, CT 06437-9989. TEL 203-453-4351, FAX 203-453-6000. Ed. Carol Levine. Pub. David Dean. R&P Cheryl Greenleaf.

610 362.41 GBR
TAPE MEDICAL BULLETIN. Text in English. m. **Document type:** *Academic/Scholarly, Trade.* **Description:** Makes selected articles from British, Canadian, and US medical journals accessible to medical professionals who are blind or visually impaired.
Media: Audio cassette/tape.
Published by: Royal National Institute for the Blind, PO Box 173, Peterborough, Cambs PE2 6WX, United Kingdom. TEL 44-1733-370-777, FAX 44-1733-238-541, http://www.rnib.org.uk. **Co-sponsor:** University of London.

610 NLD ISSN 0924-610X
THE TARDIEU SERIES. Text in English. 1978. irreg. price varies. **Document type:** *Monographic series.*
Published by: Kluwer Academic Publishers Group (Subsidiary of: Wolters Kluwer N.V.), Spuiboulevard 50, PO Box 17, Dordrecht 3300 AA, Netherlands. FAX 31-78-639-2254, services@wkap.nl, http://www.wkap.nl. **Dist. by:** Journals Department, PO Box 322, Dordrecht 3300 AH, Netherlands. FAX 31-78-654-6474.

610 USA
TASK FORCE QUARTERLY. Text in English. 1990. q. USD 16 to non-members; USD 8 to members; USD 20 to institutions. **Description:** Written primarily by and for medical students to inform about activities of the task forces and opportunities for involvement in projects, as well as to provide information about each task force's area of interest.
Published by: American Medical Student Association, 1902 Association Dr, Reston, VA 20191-1502. TEL 703-620-6600, FAX 703-620-5873, http://www.amsa.org. R&P Amy Myers Payne. Circ: 3,500.

610.7 USA ISSN 1040-1334
WMLC 93/4812
TEACHING AND LEARNING IN MEDICINE; an international journal. Text in English. 1989. q. USD 45 in US & Canada to individuals; USD 75 elsewhere to individuals; USD 390 in US & Canada to institutions; USD 420 elsewhere to institutions (effective 2002). adv. bk.rev. *Refereed.* **Document type:** *Journal, Academic/Scholarly.* **Description:** Addresses practical issues in the conduct of medical education, providing the analysis and empirical research needed to facilitate decision-making about the education of medical professionals.
Related titles: Online - full text ed.: ISSN 1532-8015. USD 40.50, USD 351 (effective 2002) (from CatchWord Ltd., EBSCO Publishing, O C L C Online Computer Library Center, Inc., RoweCom Information Quest, Swets Blackwell, Institute for Scientific Information).
Indexed: Behav.Med.Abstr., Cont.Pg.Educ., Curr.Cont., ERA, Educ.Tech.Abstr., Ind.Med., Mult.Ed.Abstr., PsycInfo, Psychol.Abstr. (1989-), Res.High.Educ.Abstr., Sci.Cit.Ind., Tech.Educ.Abstr., e-psyche.
—BLDSC (8614.004000), CatchWord, GNLM, Infotrieve. **CCC.**
Published by: Lawrence Erlbaum Associates, Inc., 10 Industrial Ave, Mahwah, NJ 07430-2262. TEL 201-760-3735, 800-926-6579, FAX 201-236-0072, journals@erlbaum.com, http://www.erlbaum.com. Ed. Paul Feltovich. adv.: page USD 325; trim 7 x 10.

362 JPN ISSN 0040-0734
TEASHI NO FUJIYUUNA KODOMOTACHI/CRIPPLED CHILDREN. Text in Japanese. 1958. m. JPY 750. **Description:** Focuses on rehabilitation practices.
Published by: Japanese Society for Disabled Children/Nihon Shitai Fujiyuji Kyokai, 1-7 Komone 1-chome, Itabashi-ku, Tokyo 173-0037, Japan. Circ: 6,000.

610 USA
TECH SAMPLE. (Subject areas offered include: Clinical Chemistry, Clinical Immunology, Hematology, Immunohematology, MicrobiologyManagement and Education, Histotechnology, Cytotechnology, Plebotomy and Generalist) Text in English. 1979. w. USD 555 for complete series (effective 2000). **Document type:** *Academic/Scholarly.* **Description:** Each series consists of exercises which focus on technical problems encountered in the laboratory, providing helpful information and solutions. Participants earn ICMLE credit for each exercise completed.
Published by: American Society of Clinical Pathologists, 2100 W Harrison St, Chicago, IL 60612. TEL 312-738-1336, FAX 312-738-1619, http://www.ascp.org. Ed. John Snyder. Pub. Joshua Weikersheimer. R&P Nick Watters. Circ: 4,500.

616.07 571.9 GBR ISSN 1066-5072
CODEN: TDIPEF
TECHNIQUES IN DIAGNOSTIC PATHOLOGY. Text in English. 1989. irreg., latest vol.3. **Document type:** *Monographic series, Academic/Scholarly.*
Indexed: Chem.Abstr., Chem.Indus.Notes, Chem.Titles.
—CASDDS, KNAW.
Published by: Academic Press (Subsidiary of: Harcourt Publishers Ltd.), 24 Oval Rd, London NW1 7DX, United Kingdom. TEL 44-20-7267-4466, FAX 44-20-7482-2293.

610 NLD ISSN 1567-861X
TECHNOLOGIE IN DE GEZONDHEIDSZORG; beheer en toepassing. Text in Dutch. 1985. 11/yr. NLG 165 domestic; NLG 270 foreign (effective 2001). adv. index. back issues avail. **Document type:** *Journal, Trade.* **Description:** Covers issues relating to technology in health care.
Formerly (until 2000): Techniek in de Gezondheidszorg (0169-622X)
Published by: Phoenix Publishers, De Haag 5, Houten 3993 AV, Netherlands. TEL 31-30-6342790, FAX 31-30-6342795, phoenixp@worldonline.nl, info@phoenixbu.nl. R&P Marianne Boos. Adv. contact Mennie Determan. Circ: 2,500 (paid and controlled).

610.285 NLD ISSN 0928-7329
TECHNOLOGY AND HEALTH CARE. Text in English. 1993. bi-m. EUR 300, USD 353 to institutions (effective 2002). back issues avail. *Refereed.* **Document type:** *Journal, Academic/Scholarly.* **Description:** Serves as a forum for current research in biomedical engineering, advances in diagnostics, therapeutic procedures and devices, including artificial organs and implants, and for the review of major social, policy or ethical issues relating to new applications of technology in medicine.
Related titles: Online - full text ed.: (from EBSCO Publishing, O C L C Online Computer Library Center, Inc., Swets Blackwell, RoweCom Information Quest).
Indexed: ASCA, Aqua.Sci.& Fish.Abstr., Comput.Lit.Ind., Environ.Sci.Poll.Mgmt., Excerp.Med. (1994-), INSPEC (Apr.1993-), Ind.Med. (1993-), Int.Abstr.Biol.Sci., Pollut.Abstr., Risk Abstr., Saf.Sci.Abstr.
—BLDSC (8758.625000), ADONIS, CISTI, EMDOCS, GNLM, IDS, Infotrieve. **CCC.**
Published by: (European Society for Engineering and Medicine BEL), I O S Press, Nieuwe Hemweg 6B, Amsterdam 1013 BG, Netherlands. TEL 31-20-688-3355, FAX 31-20-620-3419, market@iospress.nl, http://www.iospress.nl. Eds. Ali E Engin TEL 334-460-6168, Peter F Niederer TEL 41-1-632-4568. **Subscr. to:** I O S Press, Inc, 5795-G Burke Centre Pkwy, Burke, VA 22015. TEL 703-323-5554, FAX 703-323-3668, iosbooks@iospress.com; Kinokuniya Company Ltd, Shinjuku 3-chome, Shinjuku-ku, Tokyo 160-0022, Japan. FAX 81-3-3439-1094, journal@kinokuniya.co.jp, http://www.kinokuniya.co.jp; Globe Publication Pvt. Ltd.

610 JPN ISSN 0285-4473
TEION IGAKU/LOW TEMPERATURE MEDICINE. Text in English, Japanese; Summaries in English. 1976. q. JPY 2,000 per issue (effective 2000). **Document type:** *Academic/Scholarly.*

Indexed: INIS Atomind.
—BLDSC (5296.497000).
Published by: Nihon Teion Igaku Kenkyukai/Japan Society for Low Temperature Medicine, Tateishi 5-11-16, Katushika, Tokyo 124-0012, Japan. TEL 81-3-5698-3505, FAX 81-3-5698-3505. Ed. Tohru Tamaki.

610 USA ISSN 1091-7853
R119.9
TELEMEDICINE & TELEHEALTH NETWORK. Text in English. m. USD 50; USD 70 foreign (effective 1997). **Document type:** *Trade.*
Related titles: Online - full text ed.: (from ProQuest Information & Learning).
Indexed: SoftBase (Feb.1999-).
—Infotrieve. **CCC.**
Published by: Miller Freeman, Inc. (Subsidiary of: United Newspapers), 600 Harrison St, San Francisco, CA 94107. TEL 415-905-2200, FAX 415-905-2233. Ed. Deborah R Dakins.

610 USA
TELEMEDICINE BUSINESS NEWSLETTER. Text in English. m. USD 397; USD 35 newsstand/cover (effective 1996). **Document type:** *Newsletter, Trade.*
Published by: Miller Freeman, Inc. (Subsidiary of: United Newspapers), 600 Harrison St, San Francisco, CA 94107. TEL 415-905-2200, FAX 415-905-2233.

610 USA ISSN 1078-0351
TELEMEDICINE TODAY* . Text in English. 1992. bi-m. USD 99; USD 110 in Canada & Mexico; USD 125 elsewhere; includes Telemedicine Buyer's Guide and Directory. adv. bk.rev. back issues avail. **Document type:** *Trade.* **Description:** Provides practical methods of starting or improving a distance healthcare program. Covers teleradiology, telehome healthcare, telepathology, organization and management, the medical Internet, and telemedical legal issues etc.
Related titles: Online - full text ed.
Indexed: INSPEC (Dec.1997-).
—BLDSC (8782.961080).
Published by: Dr. Ace Allen, Ed. & Pub., 660 Hampshire Rd, Ste 200, Westlake Village, CA 91361. TEL 805-371-7877, FAX 805-371-7885, asimon@telemedtoday.com, http://www.telemedtoday.com/. Ed. Ace Allen. R&P Allen Simon. Adv. contact Al Sands. Circ: 10,000.

610 PRT
TEMPO MEDICINA. Text in Portuguese. 1982. 48/yr. PTE 3,000. adv. **Document type:** *Newspaper.*
Related titles: Diskette ed.
Published by: Impremedica, Quinta do Pinheiro, Lote 5, Cave A, Pontinha 1675, Portugal. TEL 351-1-4783075, FAX 351-1-4783081. Ed. Jose Antunes. Adv. contact Ana Paula Monteiro. Circ: 15,000 (paid).

610 ITA ISSN 0492-6749
HC391
TEMPO MEDICO. Text in Italian. 1959. w. ITL 30,000. adv. bk.rev. **Document type:** *Newspaper.*
Indexed: MLA Intl.Bibl.
Published by: Parpinelli Tre srl (Subsidiary of: Medimedia), Via Bressan 2, Milan 20126, Italy. TEL 39-02-270741, FAX 39-02-27074210, parpitre@micronet.it, http://www.tempomedico.it/parpine.htm. Ed. Roberto Satolli. Adv. contact Elisabetta Cozzi. B&W page ITL 13,600,000, color page ITL 16,300,000; trim 384 x 262. Circ: 40,000.

610 USA ISSN 1088-6222
TENNESSEE MEDICINE. Text in English. 1902. m. USD 20 domestic; USD 26 foreign (effective 2001). adv. bk.rev. abstr. bibl. illus. index. **Document type:** *Trade, Academic/Scholarly.* **Description:** Covers such subjects as voluntary health insurance, medical legislation and socio-economic problems related to the practice of medicine.
Former titles (until 1996): Tennessee Medical Association. Journal (0040-3318); (until 1963): Tennessee State Medical Association Journal (0735-7338)
Indexed: Dent.Ind., Excerp.Med., INIS Atomind., Ind.Med. (1996-), Int.Nurs.Ind.
—BLDSC (8790.733300), GNLM, ingenta, KNAW.
Published by: Tennessee Medical Association, 2301 21st Ave S, PO Box 120909, Nashville, TN 37212-0909. TEL 615-385-2100, FAX 615-383-5918, jeanw@tma.medwire.org. Ed. Dr. John B Thomison. R&P, Adv. contact Jean Wishnick. Circ: 6,500 (paid).

TENNESSEE MEDICO-LEGAL REPORTER. see *LAW*

610 RUS ISSN 0040-3660
CODEN: TEARAI
TERAPEVTICHESKII ARKHIV/THERAPEUTIC ARCHIVES. Text in Russian; Summaries in English. 1923. m. USD 210 foreign (effective 2000). adv. bk.rev., Website rev. abstr. reprints avail. *Refereed.* **Document type:** *Journal, Academic/Scholarly.* **Description:** Presents clinical and clinico-experimental studies, as well as reviews and articles on all pressing problems concerning the diseases of the internal organs.
Related titles: Online - full text ed.: (from Institute for Scientific Information).
Indexed: ASCA, Agri.& Environ.Biotech.Abstr. (coverage dropped), Biol.Abstr., Chem.Abstr., Curr.Cont., Dent.Ind., Derwent Biotech.Abstr., Excerp.Med., Helminthol.Abstr., INIS Atomind., Ind.Med. (1923-), Inpharma, Nutr.Abstr., Pharm.&Out.News, Protozool.Abstr., Reac., Ref.Zh., Rev.Appl.Entomol., Rev.Med.& Vet.Mycol., Sugar Ind.Abstr.
—BLDSC (0180.000000), CASDDS, CISTI, East View, GNLM, IDS, Infotrieve, KNAW. **CCC.**
Published by: Izdatel'stvo Meditsina, Petroverigskii per 6-8, Moscow 101000, Russian Federation. TEL 7-095-9241241, 7-095-928-86-48, FAX 7-095-9211355, meditsina/com, http://www.medit.ru. Ed. E I Chazov. Pub. A M Stochik. R&P T Soldatova. Adv. contact O A Fadeeva TEL 7-095-923-51-40. Circ: 7,000. **Dist. by:** Mezhdunarodnaya Kniga, B Yakimanka 39, Moscow 117049, Russian Federation. TEL 7-095-3484967, FAX 7-095-2384634.

610 POL ISSN 1230-3917
TERAPIA. Text in Polish. 1993. m. PLZ 48 (effective 1999). adv. illus. **Document type:** *Trade.* **Description:** Contains opinions and articles written by Polish specialists on relevant medical problems, as well as new medical and pharmaceutical products.
Published by: Warsaw Voice S.A., Ksiecia Janusza 64, Warsaw 01452, Poland. TEL 48-22-366377, FAX 48-22-371995, voice@warsawvoice.com.pl, http://www.warsawvoice.com.pl. Ed. Tadeusz Tolloczko. Adv. contact Joanna Staniszewska. page PLZ 5,600; 261 x 180.

570 USA ISSN 0270-3211
CODEN: TCMUD8
TERATOGENESIS, CARCINOGENESIS, AND MUTAGENESIS. Text in English. 1980. bi-m. USD 1,165 in United States; USD 1,225 in Canada & Mexico; USD 1,276 elsewhere; USD 1,224 combined subscription in United States for print and online eds.; USD 1,284 combined subscription in Canada & Mexico for print and online eds.; USD 1,335 combined subscription elsewhere for print and online eds. (effective 2002). adv. bk.rev. back issues avail. *Refereed.* **Document type:** *Academic/Scholarly.* **Description:** Contains reports of original research and methods concerned with the detection, classification, and evaluation of risks associated with exposure to environmentally induced agents. Serves as a forum for comments on controversial issues in biological risk assessment.
Related titles: Microform ed.: (from PQC); Online - full text ed.: ISSN 1520-6866. 1996. USD 1,165 in United States; USD 1,165 in Canada & Mexico; USD 1,165 elsewhere (effective 2002) (from EBSCO Publishing, Wiley InterScience, Institute for Scientific Information).
Indexed: AIDS & Cancer Res., ASCA, Agri.& Environ.Biotech.Abstr. (coverage dropped), Biol.Abstr., Biotech.& Bioeng.Abstr., C.I.S. Abstr., Chem.Abstr., Chem.Indus.Notes, Chem.Titles, Curr.Adv.Ecol.Sci., Curr.Cont., Dent.Ind., Derwent Biotech.Abstr., Dok.Arbeitsmed., Environ.Sci.Poll.Mgmt., Excerp.Med., Genet.Abstr., Hum.Gen.Abstr., INIS Atomind., Ind.Med. (1980-), Inpharma, Int.Abstr.Biol.Sci., Lab.Haz.Bull., NRN, Oncog.G.F.Abstr., Pollut.Abstr., Reac., Rev.Med.& Vet.Mycol., Risk Abstr., Saf.Sci.Abstr., Sci.Cit.Ind., THA, Tox.Abstr.
—BLDSC (8792.130000), CASDDS, CISTI, EMDOCS, GNLM, IDS, ingenta. **CCC.**
Published by: John Wiley & Sons, Inc., Journals (Subsidiary of: Wiley InterScience), 605 Third Ave, New York, NY 10158. TEL 212-850-6645, FAX 212-850-6021, subinfo@wiley.com, uscs-wis@wiley.com, http://www.wiley.com. Ed. Philippe Shubick. adv.: B&W page GBP 640, color page GBP 1,515; trim 174 x 254. **Subscr. outside the Americas to:** John Wiley & Sons Ltd., Baffins Ln, Chichester, Sussex PO19 IUD, United Kingdom. TEL 44-1243-779777, FAX 44-1243-843232, cs-journals@wiley.co.uk.

TERATOLOGY; the international journal of abnormal development. see *BIOLOGY*

610 EST
TERVISELEHT. Text in Estonian. 1993. w. EEK 239 domestic; EEK 935 foreign (effective 2001). bk.rev. **Document type:** *Newspaper, Consumer.*
Published by: Redaktsiya Terviseleht, Parnu Mnt 67a, Tallin, Estonia. TEL 370-6461056, tervisa@eol.ee, http://www.terviseleht.ee. Ed. Piret Maeniit. Circ: 5,000 (paid); 6,400 (controlled). **Dist. by:** East View Publications, 3020 Harbor Ln N, Minneapolis, MN 55447. TEL 763-550-0961, FAX 763-559-2931.

610 USA ISSN 0040-4470
R11 CODEN: TXMDAX
TEXAS MEDICINE. Text in English. 1905. m. USD 40 to non-members; USD 20 to members. adv. charts, illus. index. **Document type:** *Trade, Academic/Scholarly.*
Formerly: Texas State Journal of Medicine
Related titles: Microform ed.: (from PQC).
Indexed: ASCA, AgeLine, Biol.Abstr., CINAHL, C.I.S. Abstr., Chem.Abstr., Curr.Adv.Cancer Res., Curr.Cont. (coverage dropped), Dent.Ind., Dok.Arbeitsmed., Excerp.Med., Helminthol.Abstr., INIS Atomind., Ind.Med. (1966-), Med.Care Rev., Nutr.Abstr., Rehabil.Lit., THA.
—BLDSC (8799.550000), CISTI, GNLM, KNAW.
Published by: Texas Medical Association, 401 W 15th St, Austin, TX 78701. TEL 512-370-1300, FAX 512-370-1362, http://www.texmed.org. Ed. Jean Pietrobono. R&P Jean Pietrohano TEL 512-370-1385. Adv. contact Melissa McAdoo. Circ: 52,000 (paid).

610 ZAF
CODEN: GENEB4
THE/MEDICINE JOURNAL. Text in Afrikaans. 1957. m., latest vol.43. ZAR 68.40. adv. bk.rev., Website rev. charts, illus. index. 48 p./no. 3 cols./p. back issues avail. *Refereed.* **Document type:** *Journal, Academic/Scholarly.* **Description:** Contains scientific articles written by South African doctors for South Africa.
Formerly (until 1999): Geneeskunde (0016-643X)
Related titles: Online - full content ed.
Indexed: Chem.Abstr., INIS Atomind., Ind.S.A.Per.
—CASDDS.
Published by: Medpharm Publications, PO Box 786, Irene 0062, South Africa. TEL 27-12-6647977, FAX 27-12-6646355, medpharm@shibbolet.co.za, http://www.medpharm.co.za/tmj. Eds. BJ Meyer, Dr. Dgs Greeff, OBW Greeff. Pub., R&P Rene' F S Smulders. Adv. contact Caryl De Meillon. Circ: 5,000.

THEOLOGY AND MEDICINE. see *RELIGIONS AND THEOLOGY*

610 100 NLD ISSN 1386-7415
R723 CODEN: TMBIFN
THEORETICAL MEDICINE AND BIOETHICS; philosophy of medical research and practice. Text in English. 1977. bi-m. EUR 404 to institutions for print or online ed.; EUR 484.80 to institutions print & online eds.combined (effective 2002). adv. bk.rev. index. back issues avail.; reprint service avail. from SWZ. *Refereed.* **Document type:** *Academic/Scholarly.* **Description:** Provides a forum for interdisciplinary studies in the philosophy and methodology of medical practice and research, including such issues as clinical judgement and decision making, knowledge acquisition and theory formation in medicine.
Former titles: Theoretical Medicine (0167-9902); Metamedicine (0166-2031); (until 1980): Metamed (0342-6866)
Related titles: Microform ed.: (from PQC); Online - full text ed.: (from EBSCO Publishing, O C L C Online Computer Library Center, Inc., RoweCom Information Quest, Swets Blackwell, Kluwer Online, Institute for Scientific Information).
Indexed: ASCA, AgeLine, Arts & Hum.Cit.Ind. (coverage dropped), Curr.Cont., Excerp.Med., IBZ, INIS Atomind., Ind.Med. (1998-), Int.Nurs.Ind., Phil.Ind., Ref.Zh., SSCI.
—BLDSC (8814.561600), CISTI, GNLM, IDS, Infotrieve, ingenta, KNAW. **CCC.**
Published by: Kluwer Academic Publishers Group (Subsidiary of: Wolters Kluwer N.V.), Spuiboulevard 50, PO Box 17, Dordrecht 3300 AA, Netherlands. FAX 31-78-639-2254, services@wkap.nl, http://www.wkap.nl/journalhome.htm/1386-7415. Ed. David Thomasma. **Dist. by:** Journals Department, PO Box 322, Dordrecht 3300 AH, Netherlands. TEL 781-871-6600, FAX 31-78-654-6474.

610 HKG ISSN 0255-8793
THERAPEAIA. Text in Chinese. 1982. m.
Related titles: ♦ Supplement to: Asian Medical News. ISSN 0250-3328.

Published by: MediMedia Asia (Subsidiary of: MediMedia Pacific Ltd.), 8-F Pacific Plaza, 410 Des Voeux Rd W, Hong Kong, Hong Kong. TEL 852-2559-5888, FAX 852-2559-6910, amn@medimedia.com.hk, http://www.medimedia.com.

THERAPEUTIC COMMUNITIES. see *PHILOSOPHY*

610 AUS
THERAPEUTIC GUIDELINES. ANTIBIOTIC. Text in English. 1978. biennial, latest version 11. AUD 31.90 newsstand/cover (effective 2001). bk.rev. **Document type:** *Academic/Scholarly.* **Description:** Disease-oriented guide to therapeutic use of anti-microbial agents for doctors, nurses and pharmacists.
Formerly: Antibiotic Guidelines (0729-218X)
Related titles: CD-ROM ed.
—CCC.
Published by: Therapeutic Guidelines Ltd., Chelsea House, Level 2, 55 Flemington Rd, North Melbourne, VIC 3051, Australia. TEL 61-3-9329-1566, FAX 61-3-9326-5632, sales@tg.com.au, http://www.tg.com.au. Ed. Ken Harvey. R&P Mary Hemming. Circ: 50,000.

610 FRA ISSN 0396-7107
THERAPEUTIQUES NATURELLES; revue francaise de vulgarisation. Text in French. 1975. bi-m. FRF 180 domestic (effective 2000). adv. bk.rev.
Formerly: Groupement National pour l'Organisation de la Medecine Auxiliaire. Bulletin de Liaison (0396-7115)
Published by: (Groupement National pour l'Organisation des Medecines Alternatives), Presses de la Vallee, 36 rue Alsace Lorraine, Toulouse 31000, France. TEL 33-5-63955915. Ed. Jean Paul Boye. Pub. Christiane Valette.

610 CHE ISSN 0040-5930
THERAPEUTISCHE UMSCHAU; Monatsschrift fuer praktische Medizin. Text in German; Summaries in English, French. 1943. m. CHF 136 domestic; CHF 168 foreign (effective 2001). adv. bk.rev. abstr, bibl, charts, illus. index. 64 p./no. **Document type:** *Journal, Academic/Scholarly.*
Related titles: Microform ed.: (from PMC); Online - full text ed.: (from Institute for Scientific Information).
Indexed: ASCA, Biol.Abstr., C.I.S. Abstr., Chem.Abstr., Curr.Cont. (coverage dropped), Dent.Ind., Excerp.Med., Helminthol.Abstr., INIS Atomind., Ind.Med. (1961-), Int.Nurs.Ind.
—BLDSC (8814.696000), CISTI, GNLM, IDS, Infotrieve, KNAW. **CCC.**
Published by: Hans Huber AG, Laengassstr 76, Bern, 9 3000, Switzerland. TEL 41-31-3004500, FAX 41-31-3004591, zeitschriften@hanshuber.com, http://www.hanshuber.com. Ed. Dr W Reinhart. Adv. contact Rene Waelchli. color page CHF 3,269; trim 216 x 303. Circ: 4,500.

610 GBR ISSN 0040-5957
CODEN: THERAP
THERAPIE. Text in French; Summaries in English, French. 1866. bi-m. adv. bk.rev. bibl, charts, illus. *Refereed.* **Document type:** *Academic/Scholarly.*
Supersedes (in 1946): Societe de Therapeutique. Bulletins et Memoires (1153-3668)
Related titles: Microform ed.: (from PMC); Online - full text ed.: (from Institute for Scientific Information).
Indexed: ASCA, Agri.& Environ.Biotech.Abstr. (coverage dropped), Biol.Abstr., Chem.Abstr., Chem.Titles, Curr.Adv.Ecol.Sci., Curr.Cont. (coverage dropped), Dairy Sci.Abstr., Dent.Ind., Derwent Biotech.Abstr., Excerp.Med., Helminthol.Abstr., INIS Atomind., Ind.Med. (1946-), Ind.Sci.Rev., Neurosci.Cit.Ind., Nutr.Abstr., Protozool.Abstr., Rev.Med.& Vet.Mycol., SSCI (coverage dropped), Sci.Cit.Ind. (coverage dropped).
—BLDSC (8814.750000), CASDDS, CISTI, GNLM, IDS, Infotrieve, KNAW. **CCC.**
Published by: John Libbey & Co. Ltd., PO Box 276, Eastleigh SO50 5YS, United Kingdom. TEL 44-2380-650208, FAX 44-2380-650259, johnlibbey@aol.com, http://www.johnlibbey.com.

610 DEU ISSN 1433-111X
CODEN: THEWA6
THERAPIE UND ERFOLG. Text in English. 1950. 12/yr. DEM 98; DEM 126 foreign (effective 1998). adv. bk.rev., film rev. abstr, charts, illus. index. **Document type:** *Trade.*
Formerly (until 1997): Therapiewoche (0040-5973)
Related titles: Online - full text ed.: (from Institute for Scientific Information).
Indexed: Agri.& Environ.Biotech.Abstr. (coverage dropped), Biol.Abstr., Chem.Abstr., Excerp.Med., INIS Atomind., Ind.Med. (coverage dropped), Inpharma, Reac.
—CASDDS, CISTI, GNLM, IDS, Infotrieve. **CCC.**
Published by: G. Braun Buchverlag, Karl-Friedrich-Str 14-18, Karlsruhe 76133, Germany. TEL 49-721-165392, FAX 49-721-165103. Ed. Jan Engel. Adv. contact Roswitha Giesinger. Circ: 40,000.

610 CHE
THERAPIEWOCHE. Text in German. 1985. m. CHF 76. **Document type:** *Trade.*
Formerly (until 1998): Therapiewoche Schweiz (0256-6869)
Indexed: Inpharma, Reac., Ref.Zh.
—BLDSC, EMDOCS, GNLM, Infotrieve, KNAW. **CCC.**
Published by: Eskamed AG, Postfach 158, Basel 4011, Switzerland. TEL 41-61-2811046, FAX 41-61-2811038. Ed. Silva Keberle.

610 658 USA
THETA MARKET RESEARCH REPORTS. Text in English. 1970. a. price varies. **Description:** Provides comprehensive coverage of new market research in health care, pharmaceutical and biotech industries.
Published by: Theta Corporation, 2433 Main St, Ste 4, Rocky Hill, CT 06067-2539.

610 GBR ISSN 0040-6376
CODEN: THORA7
THORAX. Text in English. 1946. m. GBP 134, USD 215 combined subscription to individuals includes print & online eds.; GBP 301, GBP 481 to institutions for print only (effective 2002). adv. bk.rev. charts, illus. index. back issues avail.; reprint service avail. from PQC. *Refereed.* **Document type:** *Academic/Scholarly.* **Description:** Covers respiratory medicine with clinical and experimental research articles from various disciplines, including pathology, immunology and surgery. Tracks recent developments in basic biomedical sciences including cellular biochemistry and molecular biology.
Related titles: CD-ROM ed.: (from Ovid Technologies, Inc.); Microform ed.: (from PQC); Online - full text ed.: Thorax Online. ISSN 1468-3296. GBP 80, USD 125 to individuals (effective 2002); Institutions contact publisher for online rates. (from HighWire Pr., Ovid Technologies, Inc., Northern Light Technology, Inc., EBSCO Publishing, O C L C Online Computer Library Center, Inc., RoweCom Information Quest, ProQuest Information & Learning, ingenta, Swets Blackwell, SilverPlatter Information, Inc., Institute for Scientific Information).
Indexed: AIDS Abstr., AMED, ASCA, Abstr.Hyg., Biol.Abstr., C.I.S. Abstr., Chem.Abstr., Curr.Adv.Cancer Res., Curr.Adv.Ecol.Sci., Curr.Cont., Dent.Ind., Dok.Arbeitsmed., Excerp.Med., Helminthol.Abstr., INIS Atomind., Ind.Med. (1946-), Ind.Sci.Rev., Ind.Vet., Inpharma, Int.Abstr.Biol.Sci., Int.Nurs.Ind., Lab.Haz.Bull., METADEX, Neurosci.Cit.Ind., Nutr.Abstr., Pharm.&Out.News, Reac., Rev.Appl.Entomol., Rev.Med.& Vet.Mycol., Rev.Plant Path., SSCI (coverage dropped), Sci.Cit.Ind., THA, Trop.Dis.Bull., Weed Abstr.
—BLDSC (8820.250000), ADONIS, CASDDS, CISTI, GNLM, IDS, ingenta, KNAW. **CCC.**
Published by: (British Thoracic Society), B M J Publishing Group, B M A House, Tavistock Sq, London WC1H 9JR, United Kingdom. TEL 44-20-7387-4499, FAX 44-20-7383-6400, info.norththames@bma.org.uk, http://thorax.bmjjournals.com/, http:/www.thoraxnj.com/, http://www.bma.org.uk. Eds. A Knox, J Britton. Pub. Alex Williamson. R&P Carol Torselli TEL 44-20-7383-6674. Adv. contact Euan Currer TEL 44-20-7383-6181.

610 IND ISSN 0970-1257
TIBETAN MEDICINE. Text in English. 1980. irreg. USD 3 per issue (effective 1999). back issues avail. **Document type:** *Academic/Scholarly.* **Description:** Provides an international forum for the study of Tibetan medicine.
Published by: Library of Tibetan Works and Archives, Dharmsala, Orissa 176 215, India. TEL 91-1892-22467, FAX 91-1892-23723, TELEX TF 22467, itwa@ndf.vsnl.net.in, ltwa@ndf.vsnl.net.in. Ed. Thupten K Rikey.

610 CHN ISSN 1001-0912
TIEDAO YIXUE/RAILWAY MEDICAL JOURNAL. Text in Chinese; Abstracts in English. 1964-1966; resumed 1976. bi-m. USD 60. bk.rev. *Refereed.* **Document type:** *Academic/Scholarly.* **Description:** Publishes articles on clinical experiences, traditional Chinese medicine and herbs, hygiene and nursing.
Published by: Nanjing Tiedao Yixueyuan/Nanjing Railway Medical College, 87 Dingjiaqiao, Nanjing, Jiangsu 210009, China. TEL 3301508, FAX 3317073. Ed. Sun Ziayang. adv.: page USD 2,000. Circ: 2,000.

610 ESP ISSN 0210-9999
TIEMPOS MEDICOS. Text in Spanish. 1973. m. (11/yr.). ESP 10,000 domestic; USD 120 foreign (effective 2001). adv. bk.rev. illus. index, cum.index. back issues avail. **Document type:** *Academic/Scholarly.*
—CCC.
Published by: Editores Medicos S.A., Gabriela Mistral, 2, Madrid 28035, Spain. TEL 34-91-3768140, FAX 34-91-3739907. Ed. Dr. A Chicharro Papiri. Adv. contact Raquel Moran. Circ: 20,000.

368.382 NLD ISSN 0929-600X
TIJDSCHRIFT VOOR BEDRIJFS- EN VERZEKERINGSGENEESKUNDE. Short title: T B V. Text in Dutch. 1963. 6/yr. adv. bk.rev. **Document type:** *Trade.*
Former titles (until 1993): Tijdschrift voor Verzekeringsgeneeskunde (0169-0698); (until 1985): Arts en Sociale Verzekering (0004-3974)
—KNAW.
Published by: (Stichting tot Bevordering der Bedrijfs- en Verzekeringsgeneeskunde), Bohn Stafleu van Loghum B.V. (Subsidiary of: Wolters Kluwer N.V.), Postbus 246, Houten 3990 GA, Netherlands. TEL 31-3403-95711, FAX 31-3403-50903. Ed. N H Th Croon. Circ: 4,000.

610 BEL ISSN 0005-8440
TIJDSCHRIFT VOOR GENEESKUNDE. Variant title: Belgisch Tijdschrift voor Geneeskunde. Text in Dutch. 1945. s-m. BEF 1,650 (effective 2001 - 2002). adv. bk.rev. abstr, illus, bibl. index. 80 p./no. back issues avail.; reprints avail. *Refereed.* **Document type:** *Journal, Academic/Scholarly.*
Formerly (until 1966): Belgisch Tydschrift voor Geneeskunde
Related titles: CD-ROM ed.
Indexed: Agri.& Environ.Biotech.Abstr. (coverage dropped), Chem.Abstr., Excerp.Med., Ind.Med. (coverage dropped), Ref.Zh.
—BLDSC, CISTI, GNLM.
Published by: Tijdschrift voor Geneeskunde A.S.B.L., Minderbroedersstraat 12, Leuven 3000, Belgium. TEL 32-16-336614, FAX 32-16-336624. Eds. B van Camp, J Lauweryns, J L Pannier, W Stevens. Pub. N V Peeters. Adv. contact J P Felix TEL 32-4-3661318. Circ: 9,000 (paid).

610 174 NLD ISSN 0925-2819
TIJDSCHRIFT VOOR GENEESKUNDE EN ETHIEK. Text in Dutch. 1991. q. NLG 60. **Document type:** *Academic/Scholarly.* **Description:** Publishes original scholarship on topics relating to medical ethics.
—GNLM, KNAW.
Published by: (Stichting Geneeskunde en Ethiek), Van Gorcum en Co. B.V., PO Box 43, Assen 9400 AA, Netherlands. TEL 31-592-379555, FAX 31-592-379552, assen@vgorcum.nl, http://www.vgorcum.nl.

TIJDSCHRIFT VOOR GEZONDHEIDSRECHT. see *PUBLIC HEALTH AND SAFETY*

610 NLD ISSN 0928-4672
TIJDSCHRIFT VOOR HUISARTSGENEESKUNDE. Text in Dutch. 1984. s-m. adv. **Document type:** *Trade.*
Formerly (until 1992): Practitioner (0168-3047)
—KNAW.
Published by: Mediselect B.V., Postbus 63, Leusden 3830 AB, Netherlands. TEL 31-33-4229900, FAX 31-33-4229922, info@mediselect.nl.

TIJDSCHRIFT VOOR INTEGRALE GENEESKUNDE. see *ALTERNATIVE MEDICINE*

612 NLD ISSN 0167-5915
TIJDSCHRIFT VOOR SEKSUOLOGIE. Text in Dutch. 1976. q. NLG 70 domestic; NLG 85 foreign (effective 2000). adv. bk.rev. *Refereed.* **Document type:** *Journal, Academic/Scholarly.*
Published by: Stichting Tijdschrift voor Seksuologie, Postbus 1738, Rotterdam 3000 DR, Netherlands. TEL 31-10-4087587, FAX 31-10-4089461, slob@endov.fgg.eur.nl. Ed. A K Slob. Adv. contact A.K. Slob. Circ: 1,000.

610 NLD ISSN 0920-0517
TIJDSCHRIFT VOOR SOCIALE GEZONDHEIDSZORG; gezondheid & samenleving. Short title: T S G. Text mainly in Dutch; Text occasionally in English; Summaries in Dutch, English. 1923. 8/yr. NLG 141.78 to individuals; NLG 247.35 to institutions. adv. bk.rev. abstr, bibl, charts. *Refereed.* **Document type:** *Academic/Scholarly.*
Formerly (until 1983): Tijdschrift voor Sociale Geneeskunde (0040-7607)
Indexed: Chem.Abstr., Ergon.Abstr., Excerp.Med., HRIS, INIS Atomind., World Bibl.Soc.Sec.

M

—CISTI, GNLM, KNAW.
Published by: (Vereniging voor Volksgezondheid en Wetenschap), Stichting Journals for Public Health and Science, Admiraal Helfrichlaan 1, Utrecht 3527 KV, Netherlands. TEL 31-30-291-3252, 31-24-361-3116, FAX 31-30-291-3242, 31-24-354-1790, tsg@hsv.kun.nl. Ed. Dr. J W J van der Gulden. R&P A Goossens. Adv. contact Mrs. D Davidse. B&W page NLG 1,980. Circ: 2,000 (paid).

610 NLD ISSN 1386-1514
CODEN: VOHOE
TIJDSCHRIFT VOOR VERPLEEGHUISGENEESKUNDE. Text in Dutch. 1977. q. adv. *Refereed.* **Description:** For nursing home physicians.
Supersedes (in 1996): Vox Hospitii (0924-3186)
Indexed: Excerp.Med. (1994-).
—EMDOCS.
Published by: (Nederlandse Vereniging van Verpleeghuis Artsen), Elsevier Bedrijfsinformatie BV, Misset (Subsidiary of: Reed Elsevier plc), Postbus 4, Doetinchem 7000 BA, Netherlands. TEL 31-314-349371, FAX 31-314-363638, info@ebi.nl, http://www.ebi.nl. Ed. M AP Verhoeven-Reynders. Adv. contact Cor van Nek. Circ: 1,000.

616.85 362.2 340 USA ISSN 1074-1593
R726
TIMELINES. Text in English. 1980. q. USD 35 (effective 1998). adv. bk.rev. back issues avail. **Document type:** *Newsletter.*
Formerly (until 1994): Hemlock Quarterly (0742-5376)
Related titles: Online - full text ed.
Published by: Hemlock Society U S A, PO Box 101810, Denver, CO 80250-1810. TEL 303-639-1202, 800-247-7421, FAX 303-639-1224, hemlock@hemlock.org, http://www.hemlock.org/newsletter.htm. Ed. Helen Voorhis. Circ: 40,000.

571.964 616.07987 DNK ISSN 0001-2815
QR180 CODEN: TSANA2
TISSUE ANTIGENS. Text in English. 1971. m. USD 516 in the Americas to institutions print & online eds. combined; GBP 358 elsewhere to institutions print and online eds. combined (effective 2002). adv. illus. reprint service avail. from SWZ,ISI. *Refereed.* **Document type:** *Academic/Scholarly.*
Related titles: Online - full text ed.: ISSN 1399-0039. GBP 322 (2001) (from Ovid Technologies, Inc., EBSCO Publishing, O C L C Online Computer Library Center, Inc., RoweCom Information Quest, ingenta, Munksgaard & Blackwell Science's Synergy, Swets Blackwell, Institute for Scientific Information).
Indexed: AIDS & Cancer Res., ASCA, Abstr.Hyg., AgBiotech, Anim.Breed.Abstr., Biol.Abstr., Chem.Abstr., Chem.Titles, Curr.Adv.Cancer Res., Curr.Adv.Ecol.Sci., Curr.Cont., Excerp.Med., Forest.Abstr., Helminthol.Abstr., INIS Atomind., Immun.Abstr., Ind.Med. (1971-), Ind.Sci.Rev., Ind.Vet., Inpharma, Int.Abstr.Biol.Sci., Pharm.&Out.News, Pig News & Info., Protozool.Abstr., Reac., Rev.Med.& Vet.Mycol., Sci.Cit.Ind., So.Pac.Per.Ind., Trop.Dis.Bull., Vet.Bull.
—BLDSC (8858.690000), ADONIS, CASDDS, CISTI, GNLM, IDS, ingenta, KNAW. **CCC.**
Published by: Blackwell Munksgaard, Noerre Soegade 35, PO Box 2148, Copenhagen K 1016, Denmark. TEL 45-77-33-33-33, FAX 45-77-33-33-77, fsub@munksgaard.dk, http://journals.munksgaard.dk/tissueantigens, http://www.munksgaard.dk. Ed. Bo Dupont. Adv. contact Eric Rozario TEL 45-77-33-33-01. Circ: 900.

TOBACCO CONTROL; an international journal. see *TOBACCO*

610 USA ISSN 1054-8521
TODAY IN MEDICINE. FAMILY PRACTICE. Text in English. 1991. bi-m.
Published by: Data Centrum Communications, Inc., 21 W 38th St, 4th fl, New York, NY 10018.

241.642 USA
TODAY'S CHRISTIAN DOCTOR. Text in English. 1949. q. USD 25 domestic; USD 30 foreign (effective 2000). adv. bk.rev. *Refereed.* **Document type:** *Trade.* **Description:** Aims to motivate and equip doctors to practice faith in Jesus Christ in their personal and professional lives.
Formerly (until 1996): Christian Medical and Dental Society Journal; Incorporates (in 1993): C M D S; Formerly: Christian Medical Society Journal (0009-546X)
Indexed: Chr.Per.Ind.
Published by: Christian Medical & Dental Society, 501 Fifth St, King Bldg, 3rd Fl, Bristol, TN 37620. TEL 423-844-1000, FAX 423-844-1005, main@christian-doctors.com, http://www.cmds.org. Ed., Pub. Dave Bieble. R&P, Adv. contact Doug Fox. Circ: 15,000.

610 USA
TODAY'S HEALTH CARE. (Published in several regional editions) Text in English. m. adv. reprints avail. **Document type:** *Trade.* **Description:** Contains articles and features of interest to regional medical professionals and key decision-makers in health care.
Published by: Transcontinental Publishing Inc., PO Box 45454, Phoenix, AZ 85064-5454. TEL 602-331-8900, transpub@aol.com, http://physiciannet.com. Pub. Philip T Zeni Sr. Circ: (controlled).

610 URY
TODOVIDA. Text in Spanish. 1991. q. UYP 4,000 per issue. **Document type:** *Consumer.*
Address: Bartolome Mitre, 1488 Ap 105, Montevideo 11004, Uruguay. TEL 953794. Eds. Mara de Oliveira, Selma Varsi.

610 JPN ISSN 0040-8670
CODEN: TOIZAG
TOHO UNIVERSITY MEDICAL SOCIETY. JOURNAL/TOHO IGAKKAI ZASSHI. Text in English, Japanese, Multiple languages. 1954. bi-m. JPY 6,000. adv. bk.rev. illus, stat. *Refereed.* **Document type:** *Academic/Scholarly.*
Media: Duplicated (not offset). **Related titles:** Online - full text ed.
Indexed: Biol.Abstr., Chem.Abstr., Excerp.Med., INIS Atomind.
—BLDSC (4824.300000), GNLM, KNAW.
Published by: Toho University Medical Society/Toho Daigaku Igakkai, c/o Library, School of Medicine, 5-21-16 Omori-Nishi, Ota-ku, Tokyo 143-0015, Japan. TEL 81-3762-4151, FAX 81-3764-1642. Ed. Yoshio Toshifumi. Adv. contact Yamaguchi Naohiko. Circ: 1,200.

610 JPN ISSN 0040-8700
CODEN: THIZAZ
TOHOKU MEDICAL JOURNAL/TOHOKU IGAKU ZASSHI. Text in Japanese; Summaries in English, Japanese. 1916. s-a. JPY 4,000. adv. bibl, charts, illus, mkt. index, cum.index. **Document type:** *Academic/Scholarly.*
Indexed: Biol.Abstr., Chem.Abstr., Curr.Cont. (coverage dropped), Excerp.Med., INIS Atomind., Ind.Med. (coverage dropped).
—GNLM, Infotrieve. **CCC.**
Published by: Tohoku Medical Society/Tohoku Igakkai, 2-1 Seiryo-cho, Aoba-ku, Sendai-shi, Miyagi-ken 980-0872, Japan. TEL 81-22-274-1111, FAX 81-22-272-7273. Ed. Masao Otsuki. Circ: 1,200.

610 JPN ISSN 0385-0005
CODEN: TJEMDR
TOKAI JOURNAL OF EXPERIMENTAL AND CLINICAL MEDICINE. Text and summaries in English. 1976. bi-m. JPY 3,000, USD 15. back issues avail. **Document type:** *Bulletin.*
Related titles: CD-ROM ed.
Indexed: Chem.Abstr., Chem.Indus.Notes, Chem.Titles, Dairy Sci.Abstr., Helminthol.Abstr., INIS Atomind., Ind.Med. (1976-), Ind.Vet., Nutr.Abstr., Protozool.Abstr., Ref.Zh., Rev.Appl.Entomol., Rev.Med.& Vet.Mycol., Trop.Dis.Bull., Vet.Bull.
—BLDSC (8862.705000), CASDDS, CISTI, EMDOCS, GNLM, ingenta.
Published by: (Tokai Daigaku/Tokai University, Igakubu/School of Medicine), Tokai Daigaku Shuppansha - Tokai University Press (Kanagawa), Boseidai, Isehara, Kanagawa 259-11, Japan. FAX 0463-91-3328, TELEX 3882-413. Ed. Makoto Sakai. Circ: 1,700.

610.28 JPN ISSN 1345-2886
CODEN: IKKHBS
TOKYO IKA SHIKA DAIGAKU SEITAI ZAIRYO KOGAKU KENKYUJO HOKOKU/TOKYO MEDICAL AND DENTAL UNIVERSITY. INSTITUTE OF BIOMATERIALS AND BIOENGINEERING. REPORTS. Text in Japanese; Abstracts and contents page in English. 1967. a. free per issue. **Document type:** *Bulletin, Academic/Scholarly.*
Former titles (until Apr. 1999): Iyo Kizai Kenkyujo Hokoku (0082-4739); (until 1966): Shika Zairyo Kenkyujo Hokoku (0495-8004)
Indexed: Dent.Ind.
Published by: Tokyo Medical and Dental University, Institute of Biomaterials and Bioengineering/Tokyo Ika Shika Daigaku, Seitai Zairyo Kogaku Kenkyujo, 3-10 Surugadai 2-chome, Kanda, Chiyoda-ku, Tokyo 101, Japan. TEL 03-5280-8000, FAX 03-5280-8005. Ed. Akimasa Ishida.

610 JPN ISSN 0040-9022
CODEN: TJIZAF
TOKYO JOSHI IKA DAIGAKU ZASSHI/TOKYO WOMEN'S MEDICAL UNIVERSITY. JOURNAL. Text in Japanese; Summaries in English. 1931. m. JPY 6,000, USD 50. adv. index. *Refereed.* **Document type:** *Academic/Scholarly.*
Indexed: C.I.S. Abstr., Chem.Abstr., Excerp.Med., INIS Atomind.
—GNLM.
Published by: Tokyo Joshi Ika Daigaku Gakkai/Society of Tokyo Women's Medical College, c/o Library, 8-1 Kawada-cho, Shinjuku-ku, Tokyo 162-0054, Japan. TEL 81-3-3353-8111, FAX 81-3-5269-7403, TELEX 2322317-TWMLIB-J, gakkai@hq.twmu.ac.jp. Ed. Toshio Tsushima. Pub. Kintomo Takakura. Adv. contact Takako Itoh. Circ: 1,750 (controlled).

610 JPN ISSN 0040-8956
TOKYO MEDICAL ASSOCIATION. JOURNAL/TOKYOTO ISHIKAI ZASSHI. Text in Japanese. 1947. m. adv. bk.rev.
Published by: Tokyo Medical Association/Tokyoto Ishikai, 2-5 Kanda-Surugadai, Chiyoda-ku, Tokyo 101-0062, Japan.

610 JPN ISSN 0082-4771
RA532.T63 CODEN: TRENAF
TOKYO TORITSU EISEI KENKYUJO KENKYU NENPO/TOKYO METROPOLITAN RESEARCH LABORATORY OF PUBLIC HEALTH. ANNUAL REPORT. Text in Japanese; Abstracts occasionally in English. 1950. a., latest vol.51, 2000. per issue exchange basis. **Document type:** *Government.*
Related titles: Online - full content ed.
Indexed: Biodet.Abstr., Chem.Abstr., Chem.Indus.Notes, Chem.Titles, Dairy Sci.Abstr., Food Sci.& Tech.Abstr., Helminthol.Abstr., INIS Atomind., Mass Spectr.Bull., Nutr.Abstr., Protozool.Abstr., Rev.Appl.Entomol., Rev.Med.& Vet.Mycol., Rev.Plant Path., Rice Abstr., Triticale Abstr., Weed Abstr.
—BLDSC (1471.740000), CASDDS, GNLM.
Published by: Tokyo-toritsu Eisei Kenkyujo/Tokyo Metropolitan Research Laboratory of Public Health, 24-1 Hiyakunin-cho 3-chome, Shinjuku-ku, Tokyo 169-0073, Japan. http://www.tokyo-eiken.go.jp/report/index.html. Circ: 600.

610 USA
TOLEDO MEDICINE. Text in English. 1916. q. USD 15 (effective 1999). adv. illus. *Refereed.* **Document type:** *Bulletin.*
Formerly (until 1987): Academy of Medicine of Toledo and Lucas County. Bulletin (0001-4303)
Published by: Academy of Medicine of Toledo and Lucas County, 4428 Secor Rd, Toledo, OH 43623. TEL 419-473-3200, FAX 419-475-6744. Ed. S Amjad Hussain. R&P Mary S Croak. Adv. contact Janice Schutt. Circ: 1,500 (controlled).

610 CHN ISSN 0257-716X
CODEN: JTMUEI
TONGJI MEDICAL UNIVERSITY. JOURNAL. Text in English, German. 1981. q. USD 36 (effective 1996). *Refereed.* **Document type:** *Academic/Scholarly.* **Description:** Comprehensive journal of medical science. Includes basic and clinical medicine, public health, and forensic medicine.
Incorporates (in 1985): Acta Academiae Medicinae Wuhan (0253-3316); Which was formerly: Wuhan Yixueyuan Xuebao (0510-9752)
Related titles: CD-ROM ed.; Chinese ed.: Tongji Yike Daxue Xuebao. ISSN 0258-2090.
Indexed: Chem.Abstr., Chem.Indus.Notes, Chem.Titles, Eng.Ind., ExtraMED, Ind.Med. (1986-), Math.R.
—BLDSC (4909.158000), CASDDS, CISTI, EMDOCS, GNLM, KNAW. **CCC.**
Published by: Tongji Medical University/Tongji Yike Daxue, c/o Prof. Liu Xunfang, Wuhan, Hubei 430030, China. TEL 01-506-6688, FAX 01-506-3101, TELEX 22313 CPC CN. Ed. Qiu Fazu. Circ: 1,000. **Dist. by:** China National Publications Import & Export Corporation, 16 Gongti Dong Lu, Chaoyang-qu, PO Box 88, Beijing 100020, China. TEL 01-506-6688.

610 RUS ISSN 1019-5580
TOP MEDITSINA. Text in Russian. bi-m. USD 99.95 in United States.
Indexed: Ref.Zh.
—East View.
Address: Dolgorukovskaya ul 4, A-ya 52, Moscow 103006, Russian Federation. TEL 7-095-9730191. **US dist. addr.:** East View Publications, 3020 Harbor Ln N, Minneapolis, MN 55447. TEL 612-550-0961.

610 DEU ISSN 0931-9522
TOP MEDIZIN; Zeitschrift fuer internationale Medizin. Text in German. 1987. w. DEM 140 (effective 1998). adv. bk.rev. back issues avail. **Document type:** *Magazine, Academic/Scholarly.*
—GNLM.
Published by: P M I Verlag AG, August-Schanz-Str 8, Frankfurt Am Main 60433, Germany. TEL 49-69-548000-0, FAX 49-69-548000-77, huhgmbh@aol.com, pmiverlag@aol.com. Circ: 16,000.

610 USA ISSN 0882-5645
TOPICS IN PAIN MANAGEMENT; current concepts and treatment strategies. Text in English. 1985. m., latest vol.17. USD 155 domestic to individuals; USD 155 foreign to individuals; USD 217 per issue domestic to institutions; USD 217 per issue foreign to institutions; USD 18 newsstand/cover (effective 2002). **Document type:** *Newsletter, Academic/Scholarly.* **Description:** Contains reviews and abstracts from the international literature available on pain disorders and management.
Related titles: Online - full text ed.: USD 282.10 domestic academic site license; USD 282.10 foreign academic site license; USD 314.65 domestic corporate site license; USD 314.65 foreign corporate site license (2002).
—GNLM.
Published by: Williams & Wilkins, Newsletters (Subsidiary of: Waverly International), 351 W Camden St, Baltimore, MD 21201-2436. TEL 410-528-4000, FAX 410-528-4312, custserv@wwilkins.com, http://www.wwilkins.com. Ed. Dr. Joel R Saper. Circ: 5,500.

TOXICOLOGIC PATHOLOGY. see *ENVIRONMENTAL STUDIES—Toxicology And Environmental Safety*

TOXICOLOGICAL SCIENCES. see *ENVIRONMENTAL STUDIES—Toxicology And Environmental Safety*

TOXICOLOGY IN VITRO. see *ENVIRONMENTAL STUDIES—Toxicology And Environmental Safety*

610 DEU ISSN 0946-2104
CODEN: TEMDE6
TRACE ELEMENTS AND ELECTROLYTES. Text in English. 1984. q. DEM 210, EUR 107.37, USD 134 to individuals; USD 174 to institutions; DEM 60, EUR 30.68 newsstand/cover (effective 2001). adv. bk.rev. abstr. **Document type:** *Journal, Academic/Scholarly.* **Description:** Covers developments in trace elements; intended for clinicians, as well as theoretical scientists (biologists, pharmacologists, physiologists).
Formerly (until 1994): Trace Elements in Medicine (0174-7371)
Related titles: Online - full text ed.: (from Institute for Scientific Information).
Indexed: ASCA, BBCI, Chem.Abstr., Curr.Adv.Ecol.Sci., Curr.Cont. (coverage dropped), Ind.Sci.Rev., Inpharma, Int.Abstr.Biol.Sci., NRN, Reac., Sci.Cit.Ind. (coverage dropped).
—BLDSC (8876.873000), CASDDS, EMDOCS, GNLM, IDS, Infotrieve. **CCC.**
Published by: Dustri-Verlag Dr. Karl Feistle, Bajuwarenring 4, Oberhaching 82041, Germany. TEL 49-89-613861-0, FAX 49-89-613-5412, info@dustri.de, http://www.dustri.de. Eds. Dr. K H Rahn, Dr. W Zidek. R&P Renate Lehmann. Adv. contact Joerg Feistle.

610 IND ISSN 0970-5031
TRADITIONAL MEDICAL SYSTEMS. Text in English. 1979. q. INR 410, USD 68 (effective 2000). adv. abstr, bibl. index.
Published by: K.K. Roy (Private) Ltd., 55 Gariahat Rd., P O Box 10210, Kolkata, West Bengal 700 019, India. R&P M Misra TEL 91-33-475-4872. Circ: 2,100.

615.65 USA ISSN 0041-1132
RC633.A1 CODEN: TRANAT
TRANSFUSION. Text in English. 1947. m. (11/yr). USD 182 domestic to individuals; USD 239 foreign to individuals; USD 239 domestic to institutions; USD 470 foreign to institutions (effective 2000). adv. illus. index. *Refereed.* **Document type:** *Academic/Scholarly.* **Description:** Reports advances regarding transfusion medicine, discusses opposing viewpoints regarding controversial issues on tissue transpalntation and hemotopoietic.
Supersedes (in 1961): American Association of Blood Banks. Bulletin (0360-9197)
Related titles: Microform ed.: (from PQC); Online - full text ed.: (from HighWire Pr., EBSCO Publishing, Institute for Scientific Information).
Indexed: Biol.Abstr., CINAHL, Chem.Abstr., Chem.Titles, Curr.Adv.Cell & Devel.Biol., Curr.Adv.Ecol.Sci., Curr.Cont., Dent.Ind., Excerp.Med., Helminthol.Abstr., Hosp.Lit.Ind., INIS Atomind., Ind.Med. (1961-), Ind.Sci.Rev., Inpharma, Int.Abstr.Biol.Sci., Int.Nurs.Ind., Pharm.&Out.News, Protozool.Abstr., Reac., Rev.Appl.Entomol., Rev.Med.& Vet.Mycol., SSCI (coverage dropped), Sci.Cit.Ind., Trop.Dis.Bull.
—BLDSC (9020.704000), CASDDS, CISTI, GNLM, ingenta, KNAW.
Published by: American Association of Blood Banks, 8101 Glenbrook Rd, Bethesda, MD 20814. TEL 301-907-6977, FAX 301-907-6895, http://www.aabb.og. Ed. Dr. Jeffrey McCullough. Circ: 13,300.

610 CZE ISSN 1212-9887
TRANSFUZE DNES/TRANSFUSION TODAY. Text in Czech; Summaries in Czech, English. 1993. q. EUR 44, USD 56 (effective 2001). adv. bk.rev. bibl, charts, illus. cum. index. back issues avail. *Refereed.* **Document type:** *Magazine, Academic/Scholarly.* **Description:** Examines special problems in transfusion medicine and related fields for physicians and other medical personnel.
Related titles: E-mail ed.; Online - full text ed.
—BLDSC (9020.712300).
Published by: (Ceska Lekarska Spolecnost J.E. Purkyne/Czech Medical Association), Nakladatelske Stredisko C L S J.E. Purkyne, Sokolska 31, Prague 12026, Czech Republic. TEL 420-2-24911420, FAX 420-2-24911420, nts@iol.cz, http://www.clsjep.cz, http://www.medical.cz. Ed. Jiri Masopust. R&P A Leblova TEL 42-2-71747230. **Dist. by:** Abont s.r.o., Chlumova 17, Prague, 3 130 00, Czech Republic; **Dist. in Western countries by:** Kubon & Sagner, Hesstr 39-41, Munich 80798, Germany.

610 DEU ISSN 0934-0874
RD120.7 CODEN: TRINE5
TRANSPLANT INTERNATIONAL. Text in English. 1989. bi-m. DEM 1,116.60 domestic; DEM 1,124.40 foreign (effective 2001). *Refereed.* **Document type:** *Journal, Academic/Scholarly.* **Description:** Serves as a forum in the field of transplantation.
Related titles: Online - full text ed.: ISSN 1432-2277 (from EBSCO Publishing, RoweCom Information Quest, Swets Blackwell, Springer LINK, Institute for Scientific Information).
Indexed: ASCA, Chem.Abstr., Chem.Titles, Curr.Cont., Immun.Abstr., Ind.Med. (1988-), Inpharma, Int.Nurs.Ind., Kidney, Pharm.&Out.News, Reac., Rev.Med.& Vet.Mycol., SSCI (coverage dropped).
—BLDSC (9024.989000), CASDDS, CISTI, EMDOCS, GNLM, IDS, ingenta, KNAW. **CCC.**
Published by: (European Society of Organ Transplantation), Springer-Verlag (Subsidiary of: BertelsmannSpringer), Tiergartenstr 17, Heidelberg 69121, Germany. TEL 49-6221-345-0, FAX 49-6221-345229, subscriptions@springer.de, http://link.springer.de/link/service/journals/00147/index.htm, http://www.springer.de. Ed. F Muehlbacher. **Subscr. in N. America to:** Springer-Verlag New York Inc., PO Box 2485, Secaucus, NJ 07096-2485. TEL 212-460-1500, FAX 212-473-6272.

TRANSPLANTOLOGY; journal of cell and organ transplantation. see *MEDICAL SCIENCES—Surgery*

TRAUMA, VIOLENCE & ABUSE; a review journal. see *PUBLIC HEALTH AND SAFETY*

610 USA
TRAVEL MEDICINE ADVISOR. Text in English. 1991. bi-m. USD 399 domestic; USD 429 foreign; USD 133 newsstand/cover (effective 2001). **Document type:** *Newsletter.*
Published by: American Health Consultants (Subsidiary of: Medical Economics Co., Inc.), 3525 Piedmont Rd, N E, 6 Piedmont Center, Ste 400, Atlanta, GA 30305. TEL 404-262-5476, 404-262-7436, 800-688-2421, FAX 404-262-7837, 800-284-3291, custserv@ahcpub.com, http://www.ahcpub.com. Circ: 800.

610 616.98 GBR ISSN 0267-3606
TRAVEL MEDICINE INTERNATIONAL. Text in English. 1983. bi-m. GBP 120 domestic; GBP 145 foreign. **Document type:** *Academic/Scholarly.*
Formerly (until 1984): Travel and Traffic Medicine International (0263-8657)
Indexed: Abstr.Hyg.
—CISTI, GNLM.
Published by: Mark Allen Publishing Ltd., Croxted Mews, 286-288a Croxted Rd, London SE24 9BY, United Kingdom. TEL 44-208-671-7521, FAX 44-208-671-1722. Ed. Dr. Hugh L'Etang. Pub. Mark Allen.

TRAVELING HEALTHY. see *TRAVEL AND TOURISM*

610 900 USA
TREASURES. Text in English. 1980. 3/yr. free per issue. illus. back issues avail. **Document type:** *Newsletter.* **Description:** Disseminates news and information about the collection of rare books, manuscripts, letters, and papers concerning the history of medicine.
Published by: University of Alabama at Birmingham, Reynolds Historical Library, 1700 University Blvd, Birmingham, AL 35294-0013. TEL 205-934-4475, FAX 205-975-8313, http://www.uab.edu/historical/. Ed., R&P Stefanie Babinsack. Circ: 2,000.

TRENDS IN GENETICS; DNA, differentiation and development. see *BIOLOGY—Genetics*

616.4 GBR ISSN 1471-4914
CODEN: MMTOFK
TRENDS IN MOLECULAR MEDICINE. Text in English. 1995. m. EUR 115 in Europe to individuals; JPY 14,000 in Japan to individuals; USD 126 elsewhere to individuals; EUR 908 in Europe to institutions; JPY 125,900 in Japan to institutions; USD 1,015 elsewhere to institutions; USD 1,308 print & online eds. combined; EUR 144 in Europe to qualified personnel; JPY 17,500 in Japan to qualified personnel; USD 157 elsewhere to qualified personnel (effective 2002). adv. back issues avail.; reprints avail. *Refereed.* **Document type:** *Academic/Scholarly.* **Description:** Facilitates communication between groups of highly trained professionals with distinct backgrounds and skills whose common goals are to understand and explain the molecular basis of disease.
Formerly: Molecular Medicine Today (1357-4310)
Related titles: Microform ed.: (from PQC); Online - full text ed.: (from ingenta, ScienceDirect, Swets Blackwell, Institute for Scientific Information).
Indexed: AIDS & Cancer Res., ASCA, Abstr.Hyg., AgBiotech, BBCI, Chem.Abstr., Chem.Indus.Notes, Chem.Titles, Curr.Cont., Dairy Sci.Abstr., Focus on: Mol.Med., Genet.Abstr., Hum.Gen.Abstr., INIS Atomind., Immun.Abstr., Ind.Med. (2001-), Ind.Sci.Rev., Ind.Vet., Inpharma, Int.Abstr.Biol.Sci., Med.& Pharm.Biotech.Abstr., Neurosci.Abstr., Nuc.Acids Abstr., Nutr.Abstr., Pharm.&Out.News, Plant Breed.Abstr., Reac., Rev.Plant Path., Sci.Cit.Ind.
—BLDSC (9049.666000), CASDDS, GNLM, IDS, Infotrieve. **CCC.**
Published by: Elsevier Science Ltd., Elsevier Trends Journals, 68 Hills Rd, Cambridge CB2 1LA, United Kingdom. TEL 44-1223-315961, FAX 44-1223-464430, mmt@elsevier.co.uk, http://www.elsevier.nl/inca/publications/store/3/0/7/7/2/, http://www.trends.com. Eds. B Perks, Catherine Brooksbank. Adv. contact Thelma Reid. **Subscr. in Australasia and the Far East to:** Elsevier Science (Singapore) Pte Ltd, No.1 Temasek Ave, 17-01 Millenia Tower, Singapore 039192, Singapore. TEL 65-434-3727, FAX 65-337-2230; **Subscr. in the Americas to:** Elsevier Science, PO Box 945, New York, NY 10159-0945. TEL 212-633-3730, FAX 212-633-3680; **Subscr. to:** Elsevier Current Trends Subscriptions, PO Box 331, Haywards Heath, W Sussex RH16 3FG, United Kingdom. TEL 44-1444-475650, FAX 44-1444-445423.

610 COL ISSN 0120-2529
TRIBUNA MEDICA. Text in Spanish. 1960. m. COP 120,000, USD 120; USD 150 foreign. adv. bk.rev. *Refereed.* **Document type:** *Academic/Scholarly.* **Description:** Contains papers on medical science subjects, predominantly clinical, ethical and bioethical matters, the history of medicine, and medical practice in Colombia.
Related titles: ♦ Regional ed.: Tribuna Medica (Edicion Ecuatoriana); ♦ Tribuna Medica (Edicion Mexicana); ♦ Tribuna Medica (Edicion Peruana); Tribuna Medica (Edicion Venezolana). ISSN 0798-0728.
Published by: Ediciones Lerner, Calle 8a, 68-A-41, Bogota, CUND, Colombia. TEL 57-1-4200650, FAX 57-1-2624459. Ed. Dr. Juan Mendoza-Vega. R&P Juan Mendoza Vega. Adv. contact Jenny Bastidas. Circ: 11,500 (paid).

610 PER
TRIBUNA MEDICA (EDICION PERUANA). Text in Spanish. 1964. s-m. adv.
Related titles: ♦ Regional ed.: Tribuna Medica. ISSN 0120-2529; ♦ Tribuna Medica (Edicion Ecuatoriana); ♦ Tribuna Medica (Edicion Mexicana); Tribuna Medica (Edicion Venezolana). ISSN 0798-0728.
Published by: Tribuna Medica, Apto. 405, Ave. Angamos Oeste, 371, Miraflores, Lima 18, Peru. Ed. Jose Alva Neira. Circ: 6,000.

610 CHE ISSN 1420-4541
TRIBUNE MEDICALE. Text in French. 1994. w. adv. **Document type:** *Journal, Academic/Scholarly.*

Published by: Medical Tribune AG, Urs-Graf-Str 8, Postfach 368, Basel 4020, Switzerland. TEL 41-61-3125566, FAX 41-61-3125560, http://www.medical-tribune.ch. adv.: B&W page CHF 2,160, color page CHF 3,136; 266 x 390.

610 340 USA ISSN 1066-3681
TRINGA PRESS MONOGRAPH SERIES. Text in English. 1992. irreg. USD 5 per issue. index. back issues avail. **Document type:** *Monographic series, Academic/Scholarly.*
Published by: Tringa Press, 2074 Highland Pkwy., St. Paul, MN 55116. TEL 651-699-7184, FAX 651-699-0666, help@tringa.com, http://www.tringa.com. Ed. H J Schmidt.

610 DEU ISSN 1434-3622
TROPHOS - MEDIZIN UND ERNAEHRUNG. Text in German. 1992. bi-m. DEM 120 (effective 1999). **Document type:** *Academic/Scholarly.*
Published by: Trophos Verlags-, Vertriebs- und Beratungs GmbH, August-Schanz-Str 8-II, Frankfurt Am Main 60433, Germany. TEL 49-69-54800020, FAX 49-69-54800021, trophos@aol.com.

TSETSE AND TRYPANOSOMIASIS INFORMATION QUARTERLY. see *MEDICAL SCIENCES—Abstracting, Bibliographies, Statistics*

610 USA
TUBEROUS SCLEROSIS CLINICAL & RESEARCH INFORMATION; for scientists, physicians and other health professionals. Text in English. s-a. USD 30 to membership (effective 2001); includes Perspective. **Document type:** *Trade.* **Description:** News for the medical community.
Formerly: Tuberous Sclerosis Resources
Published by: Tuberous Sclerosis Alliance, 801 Roeder Rd, 750, Landover, MD 20912. TEL 800-225-6872, FAX 301-562-9870, info@tsalliance.org, http://www.tsalliance.org.

610 USA
TUFTS MEDICINE. Text in English. 1941. 3/yr. bk.rev. back issues avail. **Document type:** *Bulletin.*
Formerly: Tufts Medical Alumni Bulletin
Published by: Tufts University, School of Medicine, 136 Harrison Ave, Boston, MA 02111. TEL 617-636-3706, FAX 617-636-4075, b.morgan@infonet.tufts.edu. Ed. Bruce Morgan. Circ: 15,000 (controlled).

610 USA
TULANE MEDICINE. Text in English. 1969. q. free per issue. adv. bk.rev. abstr. **Document type:** *Academic/Scholarly.*
Formerly: Tulane Medicine: Faculty and Alumni (0041-400X); Which superseded: Tulane University Medical Faculty. Bulletin
—GNLM.
Published by: Tulane University, Office of University Publications, 300 Hebert Hall, New Orleans, LA 70118-5698. TEL 504-865-5714, FAX 504-865-5621, medlet@mailhost.tcs.tulane.edu. Ed. Anne Yeoman. Circ: 18,500 (controlled).

610.6 USA
TULSA MEDICINE* . Text in English. 1935. m. USD 10. adv.
Formerly (until Oct. 1977): Tulsa County Medical Society. Bulletin
Published by: Tulsa County Medical Society, 2021 S Lewis, 560, Tulsa, OK 74104-5758. Ed. Jack Spears. Circ: 1,100.

610 TUN ISSN 0041-4131
LA TUNISIE MEDICALE. Text in French; Summaries in Arabic, English, French. 1903. 10/yr. TND 45; USD 70 foreign. adv. bk.rev. charts. index. *Refereed.* **Document type:** *Academic/Scholarly.* **Description:** Scientific journal featuring original papers and clinical cases in the medical sciences as well as updating reviews and state of the art discussions of medical questions.
Formed by the merger of: Revue Tunisienne des Sciences Medicales; Bulletin de l'Hopital Sadiki
Related titles: CD-ROM ed.
Indexed: Abstr.Hyg., Biol.Abstr., Chem.Abstr., Excerp.Med., ExtraMED, INIS Atomind., Ind.Med. (1929-), Nutr.Abstr., P.A.I.S. (coverage dropped), Protozool.Abstr., Rev.Med.& Vet.Mycol., Trop.Dis.Bull.
—BLDSC (9071.150000), CISTI, GNLM.
Published by: Societe Tunisienne des Sciences Medicales, 16 rue Touraine, Tunis - Belvedere 1082, Tunisia. TEL 216-790-924, FAX 216-796-602. Ed. A Chabbou. adv.: color page TND 600. Circ: 2,500. **Co-sponsor:** Conseil de l'Ordre des Medecins.

610 TUR ISSN 0377-2497
TURK TIP DERNEGI DERGISI. Text in Turkish; Abstracts and contents page in English. 1935. m. adv. abstr, bibl, charts, stat. **Document type:** *Academic/Scholarly.*
Former titles (until 1973): Turk Tip Cemiyeti Mecmuasi (0494-2736); Supersedes (1965-1973): Turkish Medical Association. Journal (0041-431X)
—GNLM.
Published by: Turkish Medical Society/Turk Tip Dernigi, Valikonagi Caddesi 10, Harbiye, Istanbul, Turkey. Ed. Dr Kazim Ismail Gurkan.

610 570 TUR ISSN 1016-3611
TURKISH JOURNAL OF MEDICAL & BIOLOGICAL RESEARCH. Text in English. 1990. q. **Document type:** *Academic/Scholarly.*
—GNLM.
Published by: Istanbul University, Beyazit, Istanbul, Turkey.

610 TUR ISSN 1300-0144
CODEN: TJMEEA
TURKISH JOURNAL OF MEDICAL SCIENCES. Text and summaries in English. 1976. bi-m. USD 150 (effective 1999). *Refereed.* **Document type:** *Journal, Academic/Scholarly.*
Former titles (until 1994): Doga Turkish Journal of Medical Sciences; (until 1988): Doga Turkish Journal of Medicine and Pharmacy (1010-7584); Incorporates: Doga Turk Eczacilik Dergisi; Supersedes: Doga Bilim Dergisi. Series C: Medicine
Related titles: Online - full text ed.
Indexed: Biol.Abstr., Chem.Abstr., Eng.Ind., Excerp.Med., INIS Atomind.
—BLDSC (9072.469000), CASDDS, EMDOCS, GNLM, KNAW.
Published by: Scientific and Technical Research Council of Turkey - TUBITAK/Turkiye Bilimsel ve Teknik Arastirma Kurumu, Ataturk Bulvari No. 221, Kavaklidere, Ankara 06100, Turkey. TEL 90-312-468-5300, FAX 90-312-426-8073, bdym@tubitak.gov.tr, http://www.tubitak.gov.tr/journals/medical/. Eds. Emin Kansu, Hasan Yazici, Iskender Sayek, Oktay Ozdemir, Selma Yorucan, Sevket Ruacan.

610 FIN ISSN 0355-9483
CODEN: TYJMDL
TURUN YLIOPISTO. JULKAISUJA. SARJA D. MEDICA - ODONTOLOGICA/ANNALES UNIVERSITATIS TURKUENSIS. Text in English. 1972. irreg. price varies. **Description:** Studies medicine and dentistry.
Indexed: Chem.Abstr.
—BLDSC (0963.354000), CASDDS, CISTI, GNLM.
Published by: Turun Yliopiston Kirjasto/University of Turku, Turku 20500, Finland. FAX 358-21-3335050, http://www.utu.fi/kirjasto.

U A P D REPORT. see *LABOR UNIONS*

610 USA
U C S F MAGAZINE. Text in English. 1978. s-a. free per issue. back issues avail. **Document type:** *Consumer.* **Description:** Showcases people, programs, scientific research and biomedical achievements, and outreach efforts that distinguish U.C.S.F.
Published by: University of California at San Francisco, Public Affairs, 3333 California St, Ste 103, San Francisco, CA 94143. TEL 415-476-2557, FAX 415-476-3541. Ed., R&P Jeff Miller TEL 415-476-8299. Circ: 46,000. **Co-sponsor:** U C S F Schools of Dentistry, Medicine, Nursing and Pharmacy and Graduate Division.

U H S L NEWSLETTER. (University Health Sciences Librarians) see *LIBRARY AND INFORMATION SCIENCES*

610 GBR
U M D S DIVISION OF PUBLIC HEALTH SCIENCES. ANNUAL REPORT. (United Medical and Dental Schools) Text in English. 1963. a. free per issue. **Document type:** *Corporate.*
Formerly (until 1995): U M D S Social Medicine and Health Services. Annual Report
—BLDSC (1472.780000).
Published by: United Medical and Dental Schools, Division of Public Health Sciences, Lambeth Palace Rd, London SE1 7EH, United Kingdom. TEL 44-171-928-9292, FAX 44-171-928-1468, j.oladuti@umds.ac.uk, http://www-phm.umds.ac.uk. Ed. Robert Wood. Circ: 500 (controlled).

610.6 615.1 USA
▼ **U N M C DISCOVER.** Text in English. 1999. 3/yr. charts, illus, maps, stat. back issues avail. **Document type:** *Consumer.* **Description:** Covers issues associated with education, research, patient care and outreach at the medical center.
Related titles: Online - full text ed.
Published by: University of Nebraska Medical Center, 985230 Nebraska Medical Center, Omaha, NE 68198-5230. TEL 402-559-4353, FAX 402-559-4103, ekumru@unmc.edu, http://www.unmc.edu. Ed. Elizabeth Kumru TEL 402-559-4691. Circ: 18,000.

U.S. LIBRARY OF CONGRESS. NATIONAL LIBRARY SERVICE FOR THE BLIND AND PHYSICALLY HANDICAPPED. NEWS. see *HANDICAPPED—Visually Impaired*

610 USA
U.S. MEDICINE. Text in English. 1965. m. USD 150 (effective 2000). adv. **Document type:** *Government.* **Description:** Designed as a source of the U.S. Federal medical news and as a guide to government medical activities worldwide.
Media: Online - full text.
Address: 1155 21st St, N W, Washington, DC 20036. TEL 202-463-6000, usmedicine@usmedicine.com, http://www.usmedicine.com. Ed., Pub. Nancy Tomich. R&P Frank Best. Adv. contact James Breuning.

610 USA ISSN 0191-6246
U S MEDICINE; The Voice of Federal Medicine. Text in English. 1964. m. USD 150 (effective 2001). adv. bk.rev. charts, illus. reprints avail. **Document type:** *Newspaper.* **Description:** Serves the field of medicine for civilian, V.A. and military and hospital professionals on the federal, state, and local levels as well as medical schools and managed-care organizations.
Related titles: Online - full text ed.
—GNLM.
Published by: U S Medicine, Inc., 2021 L St N W, Ste 400, Washington, DC 20036. TEL 202-463-6000, usmedicine@usmedicine.com, http://www.usmedicine.com. Ed., Pub. Nancy Tomich. R&P Frank Best. Adv. contact Jim Breuning. Circ: 41,173 (paid and controlled).

U.S. SURGEON GENERAL. REPORT. see *DRUG ABUSE AND ALCOHOLISM*

610 DNK ISSN 0041-5782
CODEN: UGLAAD
UGESKRIFT FOR LAEGER. Text in Danish; Summaries in English. 1839. w. DKK 2,120 (effective 1999). adv. bk.rev. abstr, bibl, charts, illus, stat. index, cum.index. **Document type:** *Trade.*
Related titles: Online - full text ed.: (from Institute for Scientific Information).
Indexed: Biol.Abstr., C.I.S. Abstr., Chem.Abstr., Dairy Sci.Abstr., Dent.Ind., Dok.Arbeitsmed., Excerp.Med., INIS Atomind., Ind.Med. (1839-), Int.Nurs.Ind., Nutr.Abstr., Protozool.Abstr., Ref.Zh., Rev.Med.& Vet.Mycol., Trop.Oil Seeds Abstr.
—BLDSC (9080.000000), CASDDS, CISTI, GNLM, IDS, KNAW.
Published by: Almindelige Danske Laegeforening/Danish Medical Association, Trondhjemsgade 9, Copenhagen Oe 2100, Denmark. TEL 45-35-44-85-00, FAX 45-35-44-85-04. Ed. Joergen Joergensen. Circ: 22,100. **Subscr. to:** Laegeforeningens Forlag, Esplanaden 8 A, Copenhagen K 1263, Denmark.

610 USA ISSN 0041-607X
UKRAINIAN MEDICAL ASSOCIATION OF NORTH AMERICA. JOURNAL. Text in Ukrainian. 1970 (vol.17). m. USD 20. adv. bk.rev.
—GNLM.
Published by: Ukrainian Medical Association of North America, 2 E 79th St, New York, NY 10027. TEL 212-535-8659. Ed. Dr. Paul J Dzul. Circ: 1,000.

610 UKR ISSN 1562-1146
UKRAINSKII MEDICHNII CASOPYS/UKRAINIAN MEDICAL JOURNAL. Text and summaries in Ukrainian, Russian, English. 1997. bi-m. UAK 25.26 domestic; RUR 465.99 in Russian Federation for 6 months; USD 195 elsewhere for 6 months (effective 2000). bk.rev., film rev., software rev. illus, bibl. *Refereed.* **Document type:** *Journal.* **Description:** Covers clinical medicine, clinical pharmacology, general medical practice, including original research.
Published by: Morion LLC, a/c A-82, Kiev 01001, Ukraine. mic@morion.kiev.ua. Ed. Ivan S Zozulya. Circ: 10,000.

M

610 UKR
UKRAINS'KYI MEDYCHNYI CHASOPYS/UKRAINIAN MEDICAL JOURNAL. Text in Ukrainian, Russian, English. bi-m. USD 195 (effective 2002). **Document type:** *Journal, Academic/Scholarly.*
Published by: Morion LLC TEL 380-44-2386860, FAX 380-44-2351302. Ed. Ivan S Zozulya. **US dist. addr.:** East View Publications, 3020 Harbor Ln N, Minneapolis, MN 55447. TEL 612-550-0961.

610 GBR ISSN 0041-6193
ULSTER MEDICAL JOURNAL. Text in English. 1932. s-a., latest vol.70, 2001. GBP 30. adv. bk.rev. bibl, illus, abstr. index. 2 cols./p. back issues avail.; reprint service avail. from IRC,PQC. *Refereed.* **Document type:** *Journal, Academic/Scholarly.*
Related titles: CD-ROM ed.: (from SilverPlatter Information, Inc.); Microfilm ed.: (from PQC); Online - full text ed.: (from Institute for Scientific Information).
Indexed: ASCA, Abstr.Hyg., Addic.Abstr., Chem.Abstr., Curr.Adv.Ecol.Sci., Curr.Cont., Excerp.Med., Helminthol.Abstr., Ind.Med. (1932-), Inpharma, Int.Nurs.Ind., Pharm.&Out.News, Reac., Ref.Zh., Sci.Cit.Ind. (coverage dropped), Trop.Dis.Bull.
—BLDSC (9082.745000), CISTI, GNLM, IDS, ingenta, KNAW.
Published by: Ulster Medical Society, Whitla Medical Bldg., 97 Lisbyrn Road, Belfast, N Ireland BT9 FBL, United Kingdom. TEL 44-2890-322043, 44-2890-335780, FAX 44-2890-247068, TELEX 747578-QUBMED-G. Ed. Dr. J M Gibson. R&P J.M. Gibson TEL 44-2890-240503. Adv. contact Stewart Black. B&W page GBP 100. Circ: 1,400.

610 DEU ISSN 0172-4614
ULTRASCHALL IN DER MEDIZIN. Text in German; Summaries in English, German. 1980. bi-m. EUR 237.80 domestic to institutions; EUR 243.80 in Europe to institutions; EUR 253.60 elsewhere to institutions; EUR 48 newsstand/cover (effective 2002). adv. bk.rev. abstr, bibl, charts, illus. reprint service avail. from PQC. *Refereed.* **Document type:** *Journal, Academic/Scholarly.*
Related titles: Online - full text ed.: ISSN 1438-8782 (from Institute for Scientific Information).
Indexed: ASCA, Curr.Cont., Excerp.Med., Ind.Med. (1980-), Ind.Sci.Rev., Inpharma, Reac., Sci.Cit.Ind.
—BLDSC (9082.786000), CISTI, GNLM, IDS, Infotrieve, KNAW. **CCC.**
Published by: Georg Thieme Verlag, Ruedigerstr 14, Stuttgart 70469, Germany. TEL 49-711-8931-0, FAX 49-711-8931298, ultraschall@thieme.de, leser.service@thieme.de, http://www.thieme.de/ultraschall. Ed. K Seitz. R&P Michael Wachinger. Circ: 9,700 (paid and controlled).

ULTRASOUND IN MEDICINE & BIOLOGY. see *BIOLOGY*

616.98 DEU ISSN 1430-8681
CODEN: UFPRFE
UMWELTMEDIZIN IN FORSCHUNG UND PRAXIS. Text in German. 1996. q. EUR 178; EUR 195.80 print & online eds. (effective 2001). **Document type:** *Journal, Academic/Scholarly.*
Related titles: Online - full text ed.
Indexed: Abstr.Hyg., Food Sci.& Tech.Abstr., Forest Prod.Abstr., Helminthol.Abstr., INIS Atomind., Nutr.Abstr., Rev.Appl.Entomol., Rev.Med.& Vet.Mycol., Rev.Plant Path., Weed Abstr.
—BLDSC (9083.451000), CASDDS, GNLM, Infotrieve. **CCC.**
Published by: Ecomed Verlagsgesellschaft AG & Co. KG, Justus-von-Liebig-Str 1, Landsberg 86899, Germany. TEL 49-8191-125-0, FAX 49-8191-125492, info@ecomed.de, http://www.ecomed.de/journals/ufp/welcome.htm. Ed. Dr. Thomas Eikmann. R&P Dr. Doarthe Besse.

616.98022 USA ISSN 1066-2936
RC1000 CODEN: UHMEE7
UNDERSEA & HYPERBARIC MEDICINE. Text in English. 1993. q. USD 85 (effective 2000). bk.rev. index. *Refereed.* **Document type:** *Academic/Scholarly.*
Formed by the 1993 merger of: Undersea Biomedical Research (0093-5387); Journal of Hyperbaric Medicine (0884-1225); Which superseded (1980-1985): Hyperbaric Oxygen Review (0195-9263)
Related titles: Online - full text ed.: (from Northern Light Technology, Inc., ProQuest Information & Learning, Institute for Scientific Information).
Indexed: ASCA, Aqua.Sci.& Fish.Abstr., Biol.Abstr., Chem.Abstr., Curr.Adv.Ecol.Sci., Curr.Cont., Deep Sea Res.& Oceanogr.Abstr., Dent.Ind., Environ.Sci.Poll.Mgmt., Excerp.Med., INIS Atomind., Ind.Med. (1993-), Ind.Sci.Rev., Inpharma, Ocean.Abstr., Pharm.&Out.News, Pollut.Abstr., Psychol.Abstr., Reac., Risk Abstr., Saf.Sci.Abstr., Sci.Cit.Ind., Tox.Abstr.
—BLDSC (9088.570000), CASDDS, CISTI, GNLM, IDS, ingenta.
Published by: Undersea and Hyperbaric Medical Society, Inc., 10531 Metropolitan Ave, Kensington, MD 20895. TEL 301-942-2980, FAX 301-942-7804, uhms@uhms.org, http://www.uhms.org. Ed. Tom S Neuman. Circ: 2,000.

UNDO SHOGAI/MOVEMENT DISORDER AND DISABILITY. see *HANDICAPPED*

610 USA
UNIFORMED SERVICES ACADEMY OF FAMILY PHYSICIANS NEWSLETTER*. Text in English. q. membership. adv.
Published by: Uniformed Services Academy of Family Physicians, 2301 N Parham Rd no.4, Richmond, VA 23229-3163. TEL 804-794-2106. Ed. Dr. R Dean Kirkham. Circ: 2,600.

610 371.42 USA ISSN 1059-6100
UNIQUE OPPORTUNITIES; the physician's resource. Text in English. 1991. bi-m. USD 30 domestic; USD 35 in Canada (effective 2001). adv. bk.rev. back issues avail.; reprints avail. **Document type:** *Trade.* **Description:** Aimed at physicians interested in their first or next career opportunity. Offers physicians useful information and first-hand experiences to guide them in making informed decisions about their careers.
Related titles: Online - full text ed.
Published by: Unique Opportunities, Inc., 455 S Fourth Ave, Ste 1236, Louisville, KY 40202-2510. TEL 502-589-8250, FAX 502-587-0848, tellus@uoworks.com. Ed. Mollie Vento Hudson. Pubs. Barbara Barry, Mel Weinberger. R&P Bett Coffman. Adv. contact Mel Weinberger. B&W page USD 4,275, color page USD 5,125; trim 10.88 x 8.13. Circ: 80,000 (controlled).

616.98023 ARE
UNITED ARAB EMIRATES. AL-QIYADAH AL-AAMAH LIL-QUWWAT AL-MUSALLIHAH. MAJALLAH AL-TIBBIYYAH/UNITED ARAB EMIRATES. GENERAL COMMAND FOR THE ARMED FORCES. MEDICAL JOURNAL. Text in Arabic. 1989. q. per issue exchange basis. **Description:** Discusses topics in military medicine and medical concerns of the armed forces.
Published by: General Command for the Armed Forces, Medical Services Administration/Al-Qiyadah al-Aamah lil-Quwwat al-Musallihah, Mudiriyyah al-Khidamat al-Tibbiyyah, PO Box 4224, Abu Dhabi, United Arab Emirates. TEL 447999. Ed. Muhammad Farid. Circ: 1,000.

610 FRA ISSN 1267-6926
UNIVERS SANTE. Text in French. 1995. m. FRF 198; FRF 22 newsstand/cover (effective 1998). adv. **Description:** Offers news and advice on every day health issues.
Published by: Universante Editions, Groupe Valdemars, 25 bis av. Pierre Grenier, Boulogne-Billancourt 92100, France. TEL 33-1-49100606, FAX 33-1-46083539. Ed. Dr. Joelle Le Moal. Pub., Adv. contact Gilles Haroche. Circ: 150,000.

610 ECU ISSN 0041-8412
UNIVERSIDAD DE GUAYAQUIL. FACULTAD DE CIENCIAS MEDICAS. REVISTA*. Text in Spanish. s-a. free per issue. charts, illus.
Published by: Universidad de Guayaquil, Apdo 3637, Guayaquil, Guayas, Ecuador. Ed. Dr. Carlos Palan. Circ: 700.

610 ESP ISSN 0210-5527
UNIVERSIDAD DE OVIEDO. FACULTAD DE MEDICINA. ARCHIVOS. Text in Spanish. 1976. a. price varies. abstr, illus. **Document type:** *Academic/Scholarly.*
—CINDOC.
Published by: Universidad de Oviedo, Facultad de Medicina, Servicio de Publicaciones, Arguelles, 19, Oviedo, Asturias 33003, Spain. TEL 34-85-210160, FAX 34-85-218352. Ed. Bernardo Marin Fernandez. Circ: 500.

610 ESP
CODEN: AUHMDC
UNIVERSIDAD DE SEVILLA. SERIE: MEDICINA. Text in Spanish. 1949. irreg., latest vol.65. charts, illus.
Former titles: Universidad Hispalense. Anales. Serie: Medicina (0586-9919); (Until 1967): Universidad Hispalense. Anales. Facultad de Medicina (0210-7651)
—CASDDS.
Published by: Universidad de Sevilla, Servicio de Publicaciones, Porvenir, 27, Sevilla 41013, Spain. TEL 34-5-4487446, FAX 34-5-4487443.

610 COL ISSN 0121-0807
CODEN: RUIMDY
UNIVERSIDAD INDUSTRIAL DE SANTANDER. REVISTA - SALUD. Text in Spanish; Summaries in English, French, German, Spanish. 1959. 3/yr. COP 10,000, USD 12. adv. bk.rev. bibl, charts, illus, stat. cum.index: 1969-1987. back issues avail. **Document type:** *Academic/Scholarly.* **Description:** Covers research and current issues on various topics in medical science and health.
Formerly (until 1988): Universidad Industrial de Santander. Revista - Medicina (0120-0909); Which superseded in part (in 1969): Universidad Industrial de Santander. Revista (0041-8587)
—GNLM, Linda Hall.
Published by: Universidad Industrial de Santander, Facultad de Salud, Apartado Aereo 678, Bucaramanga, SANT, Colombia. FAX 57-76-351946.

610 MEX ISSN 0026-1742
CODEN: UMRMAJ
UNIVERSIDAD NACIONAL AUTONOMA DE MEXICO. FACULTAD DE MEDICINA. REVISTA. Text in Spanish. 1958. quadrennial. MXP 150, USD 35 (effective 2000). bk.rev. **Description:** Aims to be the distance learning education link for general physicians. Includes original papers and clinical case works on medical topics.
Indexed: Chem.Abstr., Chem.Indus.Notes, Chem.Titles.
—CASDDS.
Published by: Universidad Nacional Autonoma de Mexico, Facultad de Medicina, 3er. Piso, Bloque B, Ciudad Universitaria, Box 70-298, Mexico City, DF 04510, Mexico. TEL 52-5-6232154, FAX 52-5-6161616, http://www.facmed.unam.mx/. Eds. Alejandro Cravioto, Manuel Quijano Narezo. Circ: 20,000.

610 MEX ISSN 0186-2987
UNIVERSIDAD NACIONAL AUTONONA DE MEXICO. FACULTAD DE MEDICINA. GACETA. Variant title: Organo Informativo de la Facultad de Medicina. Text in Spanish. 1970. bi-m.
Related titles: Online - full text ed.
Published by: Universidad Nacional Autonoma de Mexico, Facultad de Medicina, 3er. Piso, Bloque B, Ciudad Universitaria, Box 70-298, Mexico City, DF 04510, Mexico. TEL 52-5-6232432, http://www.facmed.unam.mx/.

610 COL ISSN 0120-0011
UNIVERSIDAD NACIONAL DE COLOMBIA. FACULTAD DE MEDICINA. REVISTA. Text in Spanish. 1932. q. per issue exchange basis. adv. illus.
Indexed: Biol.Abstr.
—GNLM.
Published by: Universidad Nacional de Colombia, Facultad de Medicina, Apartado Aereo 14490, Bogota, DE, Colombia. Ed. Milton Arguello Jimeney. Circ: 5,000.

610 ARG ISSN 0014-6722
UNIVERSIDAD NACIONAL DE CORDOBA. FACULTAD DE CIENCIAS MEDICAS. REVISTA*. Text in Spanish; Summaries in English, French, German, Italian. 1943. q. USD 5. abstr, charts, illus. index.
Indexed: Abstr.Hyg., Biol.Abstr., Dent.Ind., Excerp.Med., Ind.Med. (1977-), Trop.Dis.Bull.
—BLDSC (7811.645000), GNLM.
Published by: Universidad Nacional de Cordoba, Facultad de Ciencias Medicas, Pab. Impr., Ciudad Universitaria, Cordoba 5000, Argentina. Ed. E E Tello.

610 BRA ISSN 0041-8781
CODEN: RHCFAP
UNIVERSIDADE DE SAO PAULO. HOSPITAL DAS CLINICAS. REVISTA. Text in English, Portuguese. 1946. bi-m. USD 35. adv. charts, illus. index, cum.index.
Related titles: Online - full text ed.: (from SciELO).
Indexed: Abstr.Hyg., Excerp.Med., INIS Atomind., Ind.Med. (1946-), Int.Nurs.Ind., Nutr.Abstr., Protozool.Abstr., Trop.Dis.Bull.
—BLDSC (7815.850000), CASDDS, CISTI, GNLM.
Published by: Universidade de Sao Paulo, Faculdade de Medicina, Centro, Caixa Postal 2921, Sao Paulo, SP 01060970, Brazil. Ed. Ruy G Bevilacqua. Circ: 10,000.

610 300 BRA ISSN 0102-8227
UNIVERSIDADE DO SAGRADO CORACAO. CADERNOS DE DIVULGACAO CULTURAL. Text in English, Portuguese. 1983. a., latest 2000. BRL 20 per issue domestic; USD 10 per issue foreign (effective 2000). bk.rev. abstr, bibl, charts, illus, maps. back issues avail. *Refereed.* **Document type:** *Monographic series, Academic/Scholarly.* **Description:** Contains original works from theses, dissertations, and monographs of technical, didactic and scientific character in various medical fields. Promotes research directed to the academic community in general.

M

Published by: (Universidade do Sagrado Coracao), Editora da Universidade do Sagrado Coracao - E D U S C, Rua Irma Arminda, 10-50, Bauru, SP 17011-160, Brazil. TEL 55-014-235-7112, FAX 55-014-235-7254, edusc@usc.br, npu@usc.br, http://www.usc.br. Ed. Marilene Cabello Di Flora. Pub. Lina Ana Santarosa. R&P Luis Eugenio Vescio TEL 55-14-2357378. Circ: 500.

610 BRA ISSN 0100-1302 CODEN: RMUCD8
UNIVERSIDADE FEDERAL DO CEARA. CENTRO DE CIENCIAS DA SAUDE. REVISTA DE MEDICINA/FEDERAL UNIVERSITY OF CEARA. SCHOOL OF MEDICINE. JOURNAL OF MEDICINE. Text in English, Portuguese; Summaries in English, Portuguese. 1961. s-a. free per issue. adv. play rev. charts, illus, stat. **Document type:** *Academic/Scholarly.*
Formerly (until 1973): Universidade Federal do Ceara. Faculdade de Medicina. Revista (0041-8889)
Indexed: Excerp.Med.
—BLDSC (7864.440000), CASDDS.
Published by: Universidade Federal do Ceara, Centro de Ciencias da Saude, Rua Alexandre Barauna, 949, R Teofilo, Caixa Postal 3170, Fortaleza, CE 60430-160, Brazil. TEL 085-243-9002, FAX 085-243-90-10. Ed. Maria Guimaraes Ferreira. Circ: 2,000 (controlled).

610 340 ITA ISSN 1125-0755
UNIVERSITA DI FERRARA. ANNALI. SEZIONE 16: MEDICINA LEGALE. Text in Italian. 1968. a.
Published by: (Universita di Ferrara), Casa Editrice Leo S. Olschki, Viuzzo Del Pozzetto, Florence, FI 50126, Italy. TEL 39-55-6530684, FAX 39-55-6530214.

UNIVERSITA DI FERRARA. ANNALI. SEZIONE 2: PATOLOGIA CHIRURGICA. see *BIOLOGY*

610 CZE ISSN 0457-4206
UNIVERSITA KARLOVA. LEKARSKA FAKULTA. LEKARSKE ZPRAVY. Text in Czech; Summaries in English. 1956. q. CZK 400 (effective 1999). reprints avail. *Refereed.* **Document type:** *Academic/Scholarly.*
Description: Presents clinical papers dealing with preventive, diagnostic, and therapeutic medical problems, as well as review articles intended for undergraduate and postgraduate education.
Indexed: INIS Atomind.
—GNLM.
Published by: (Univerzita Karlova, Lekarska Fakulta), Vydavatelstvi Karolinum, Ovocny trh 5, Prague 116 36, Czech Republic. TEL 42-2-24491270, FAX 42-2-24212041, edice@cuni.cz; gersl@lfhk.cuni.cz. Ed. Vladimir Gersl. Circ: 450.

610 AUT ISSN 0579-7772
UNIVERSITAET INNSBRUCK. MEDIZINISCHE FAKULTAET. ARBEITEN✱. Text in German. 1970. irreg. price varies.
Published by: (Universitaet Innsbruck), Oesterreichische Kommissionsbuchhandlung, Glasmalereistr 6, Innsbruck, T 6020, Austria. TEL 43-512-587039, FAX 43-512-5870394, oekobuch@aon.at, http://www.oekobuch.com. Ed. Hans Schroecksnadel.

610 COL ISSN 0041-9095 CODEN: UNMEBC
UNIVERSITAS MEDICA. Text in Spanish; Summaries in English, Spanish. 1951. q. COP 10,000, USD 30; COP 6,000 to students. adv. bk.rev. abstr, bibl, charts, illus, stat. index. **Document type:** *Academic/Scholarly.*
Description: Covers articles written on research done in medicine.
Indexed: Chem.Abstr., Excerp.Med.
—BLDSC (9101.390000), CASDDS.
Published by: Pontificia Universidad Javeriana, Facultad de Medicina, Hospital San Ignacio, Carrera 7a, 40-62 Piso 5, Bogota, CUND, Colombia. TEL 57-1-2882166, FAX 57-1-2889273. Ed., Adv. contact Dr. Saul Rujeles. Circ: 3,000.

610 CIV ISSN 0253-441X
UNIVERSITE D'ABIDJAN. ANNALES. SERIE B. MEDECINE. Text in French. 1965. biennial. **Document type:** *Journal, Academic/Scholarly.*
Formerly (until 1977): Universite d'Abidjan. Annales. Medecine (0374-2040)
Published by: Universite Nationale de Cote d'Ivoire, 22 BP 535, Abidjan 22, Ivory Coast. TEL 225-439000, FAX 225-353635.

610 EGY ISSN 1110-0834 CODEN: BAFMD9
UNIVERSITY OF ALEXANDRIA. FACULTY OF MEDICINE. BULLETIN. Text in English. 1965. q., latest vol.36, 2000. EGP 120 domestic; USD 80 foreign (effective 2001). charts, illus, abstr, stat. 100 p./no. 2 cols./p. reprints avail. **Document type:** *Journal, Academic/Scholarly.*
Related titles: CD-ROM ed.
Indexed: Biol.Abstr., Chem.Abstr., ExtraMED, Soils & Fert.
—CASDDS, GNLM.
Published by: University of Alexandria, Faculty of Medicine, 22 Sharia al-Gaish, Al-Shatby, Alexandria, Egypt. Eds. Ahmad Abdelwahab Rayan, Gawad Gawad Hamada.

610 IRQ ISSN 0041-9419 CODEN: JFAQAE
UNIVERSITY OF BAGHDAD. FACULTY OF MEDICINE. JOURNAL✱. Text in Arabic. 1936. 4/yr. adv. bk.rev. charts. **Document type:** *Academic/Scholarly.*
Indexed: Biol.Abstr., Chem.Abstr., Helminthol.Abstr., Nutr.Abstr., Protozool.Abstr., Trop.Dis.Bull.
—CASDDS, GNLM.
Published by: University of Baghdad, Medical College, Jadiriyah, P O Box 17635, Baghdad, Iraq. Ed. Dr. Fakhri Al Hadthy. Circ: 1,500.

610 EGY ISSN 0045-3803 CODEN: MJCUDW
UNIVERSITY OF CAIRO. FACULTY OF MEDICINE. MEDICAL JOURNAL. Text in English. 1932. q. EGP 8, USD 40. adv. bk.rev. abstr. index. Supplement avail.; back issues avail. *Refereed.* **Document type:** *Academic/Scholarly.* **Description:** Presents original papers and research activities of medical school personnel. Features review articles, abstracts from current literature and historical notes.
Formerly: University of Cairo. Faculty of Medicine. Gazette; Incorporates: Kasr El-Aini Clinical Society. Faculty of Medicine. Gazette
—CASDDS, CISTI.
Published by: University of Cairo, Faculty of Medicine, Clinical Society Office, Manyal University Hospital, Kasr El-Aini Post, Cairo, Egypt. TEL 726-0595. Eds. Khairy A Samrah, Mahmoud Khairy. Circ: 400.

610 IND ISSN 0008-0705 CODEN: BUYMA3
UNIVERSITY OF CALCUTTA. UNIVERSITY COLLEGE OF MEDICINE. BULLETIN. Text in English. 1963. s-a. free per issue. bibl, charts, illus.
Indexed: Biol.Abstr., Chem.Abstr., Excerp.Med.
Published by: (University of Calcutta, University College of Medicine), Calcutta University Press, Sri Sibendra Nath Kanjilal, 48 Hazra Rd., Kolkata, West Bengal 700 019, India. Ed. S N Sen.

UNIVERSITY OF CALIFORNIA. LAWRENCE BERKELEY LABORATORY. BIOLOGY AND MEDICINE DIVISION. ANNUAL REPORT. see *BIOLOGY*

610 IRN
UNIVERSITY OF FERDOWSI. FACULTY OF MEDICINE. LETTERS/DANESHGAH-E FERDOWSI. DANESHKADE-YE PAZESHKI. NAMEH. Text in Persian, Modern. 1956. bi-m. IRR 200.
Published by: University of Ferdowsi, Faculty of Medicine, Ta'lifat Va Entesharat, Mashhad, Iran. Ed. Manuchehr Radpur.

610 LBR
UNIVERSITY OF LIBERIA. A.M. DOGLIOTTI COLLEGE OF MEDICINE. ANNUAL REPORT OF THE DEAN✱. Text in English. a.
Published by: University of Liberia, A.M. Dogliotti College of Medicine, Monrovia, Liberia.

610 AUS ISSN 1323-7926
R831.N46
UNIVERSITY OF NEW SOUTH WALES. HANDBOOK: MEDICINE. Text in English. 1961. a. AUD 4.
Former titles (until 1993): University of New South Wales. Faculty Handbooks: Medicine (1323-7918); (until 1976): University of New South Wales. Faculty of Medicine. Handbook (0312-6137)
Published by: University of New South Wales, Sydney, NSW 2052, Australia. TEL 61-2-385-2840, FAX 61-2-662-2163.

UNIVERSITY OF OCCUPATIONAL AND ENVIRONMENTAL HEALTH. JOURNAL. see *OCCUPATIONAL HEALTH AND SAFETY*

610 NZL ISSN 0301-6331 CODEN: PUOMA
UNIVERSITY OF OTAGO MEDICAL SCHOOL. PROCEEDINGS. Text in English. 1922. 3/yr. NZD 38 (effective 1999). *Refereed.* **Document type:** *Proceedings, Academic/Scholarly.*
Indexed: Excerp.Med., INIS Atomind.
—BLDSC (6830.400000), EMDOCS, GNLM, Infotrieve, ingenta. **CCC.**
Published by: (University of Otago Medical School), Otago Medical School Research Society, P.O. Box 913, Dunedin, New Zealand. TEL 64-3-4797570, FAX 64-3-4790401. Ed. Heather Brooks.

UNIVERSITY OF SOUTH FLORIDA. INTERNATIONAL BIOMEDICAL SYMPOSIA SERIES. see *BIOLOGY*

UNIVERSITY OF TEHERAN. FACULTY OF MEDICINE. LIBRARY BULLETIN/DANESHGAH-E TEHRAN. DANESHKADE-YE PEZESHKI. NASHRIYE-YE KETABKHANEH. see *LIBRARY AND INFORMATION SCIENCES*

610 CAN ISSN 0833-2207
UNIVERSITY OF TORONTO MEDICAL JOURNAL. Text in English. 1923. 3/yr. USD 25. adv. bk.rev. charts, illus. *Refereed.* **Document type:** *Academic/Scholarly.*
Related titles: Microfiche ed.: (from MML); Microform ed.: (from MML).
Indexed: Biol.Abstr., Excerp.Med.
—CISTI.
Published by: University of Toronto, Medical Society, Medical Sciences Bldg, Toronto, ON M5S 1A1, Canada. TEL 416-978-8730. Eds. Chris Bouliasbrook, Joan Saary. Circ: 2,000.

610 CAN ISSN 0042-0336
UNIVERSITY OF WESTERN ONTARIO MEDICAL JOURNAL✱; an interdisciplinary medical sciences publication. Text in English. 1930. s-a. CND 18. adv. bk.rev. bibl, charts, illus, stat. *Refereed.* **Document type:** *Academic/Scholarly.*
Indexed: Biol.Abstr., Chem.Abstr.
—**CCC.**
Published by: (Faculty of Medicine, University of Western Ontario), Willow Press, Health Sciences Addition, London, ON N6A 5C1, Canada. journal@lrc.med.uwo.ca; jsolmon@lrc.med.uwo.ca. Ed., R&P Jordan B Solmon. Adv. contact Loren Watson. Circ: 2,100.

610 PRT ISSN 0871-620X
UPDATE. Variant title: Revista de Educacao Permanente em Clinica Geral. Text in Portuguese. 1993. m. (11/yr.). PTE 6,080. **Document type:** *Trade.*
Address: Rua D. Estefania 32-1o, Lisbon 1000, Portugal. TEL 351-1-791-2500, TELEX 64198 FERBEN P, http://www.fbento.pt/FB. Circ: 15,000.

610 GBR
UPDATE POSTGRADUATE CENTRE SERIES. Text in English. 1970. irreg. adv. back issues avail.; reprints avail. **Document type:** *Monographic series.*
Description: Comprises booklets written for U.K. general practitioners.
Published by: Reed Elsevier Medical Publishers, Reed Healthcare Communications (Subsidiary of: Reed Elsevier plc), Quadrant House, The Quadrant, Brighton Rd, Sutton, Surrey SM2 5AS, United Kingdom. TEL 0181-652-8439, FAX 0181-652-8946. Ed. Catherine Richards. Circ: 11,500.

610 ZAF ISSN 0258-929X
UPDATE (SOUTH AFRICAN EDITION); the journal of continuing education for general practitioners. Text in English. 1986. m. ZAR 252.45 (effective 2001). adv. bk.rev. illus. index. back issues avail. *Refereed.* **Document type:** *Academic/Scholarly, Trade.*
Description: Publishes clinical articles on developments in all medical specializations of interest to the general practitioner.
Related titles: ♦ Regional ed.: Update (Sutton). ISSN 0301-5718.
Indexed: Ind.S.A.Per.
Published by: Primedia Publishing, 366 Pretoria Ave, Randburg, Transvaal 2194, South Africa. TEL 27-11-293-7400, FAX 27-11-787-5776, http://www.primemags.co.za. Ed. Tony Walker. Circ: 7,050 (controlled).

M

610.7 GBR ISSN 0301-5718
UPDATE (SUTTON); the journal of postgraduate medical education. Text in English. 1968. fortn. GBP 102 domestic; GBP 124, USD 186 in United States; GBP 178, USD 267 elsewhere (effective 2000). adv. bk.rev. charts, illus, stat. index. **Document type:** *Trade.* **Description:** Covers the spectrum of medicine addressing the postgraduate needs of the general practitioner.
Related titles: ♦ Regional ed.: Update (South African Edition). ISSN 0258-929X.
Indexed: Excerp.Med., FAMLI, Helminthol.Abstr., L.R.I., Rehabil.Lit.
—BLDSC (9121.900000), CISTI, GNLM, Infotrieve. **CCC.**
Published by: Reed Business Information (Subsidiary of: Reed Elsevier plc), Quadrant House, The Quadrant, Brighton Rd, Sutton, Surrey SM2 5AS, United Kingdom. TEL 44-20-8652-8878, FAX 44-20-8652-8946, rbp.subscriptions@rbi.co.uk, http://www.reedbusiness.com. Ed. Andrew Baxter TEL 44-20-8652-8877. Circ: 35,000. **Subscr. to:** Quadrant Subscription Services, PO Box 302, Haywards Heath, W Sussex RH16 3YY, United Kingdom. TEL 44-1444-445566, FAX 44-1444-445447.

610 SWE ISSN 0282-8928
UPPSALA DISSERTATIONS FROM THE FACULTY OF MEDICINE. Text in Multiple languages. 1986. irreg. price varies. **Document type:** *Monographic series, Academic/Scholarly.*
Published by: (Uppsala Universitet), Acta Universitatis Upsaliensis (Subsidiary of: Uppsala University), PO Box 256, Uppsala 75105, Sweden. **Dist. by:** Almqvist & Wiksell International.

610 NOR ISSN 0300-9734 CODEN: UJMSAP
UPSALA JOURNAL OF MEDICAL SCIENCES. Text in English. 1865. 3/yr. GBP 61, USD 100 to institutions (effective 2002). charts, illus. index. *Refereed.* **Document type:** *Academic/Scholarly.* **Description:** Publishes clinical and experimental original works in the international medical field.
Former titles (until 1972): Acta Societatis Medicorum Upsaliensis (0001-6985); (until 1950): Upsala Laekarefoerenings Foerhandlingar
Related titles: Online - full text ed.: (from Institute for Scientific Information); ♦ Supplement: Upsala Journal of Medical Sciences. Supplement. ISSN 0300-9726.
Indexed: ASCA, Biol.Abstr., Chem.Abstr., Curr.Adv.Biochem., Curr.Adv.Ecol.Sci., Curr.Cont. (coverage dropped), Environ.Sci.Poll.Mgmt., Excerp.Med., Helminthol.Abstr., INIS Atomind., Ind.Med. (1972-), NRN, Nutr.Abstr., Pollut.Abstr., Ref.Zh., Risk Abstr., Saf.Sci.Abstr., Sci.Cit.Ind. (coverage dropped).
—BLDSC (9122.700000), CASDDS, CISTI, GNLM, IDS, ingenta, KNAW. **CCC.**
Published by: (Uppsala Laekarefoerening SWE), Taylor & Francis AS (Subsidiary of: Taylor & Francis Group), Cort Adelersgt. 17, Solli, PO Box 2562, Oslo 0202, Norway. TEL 47-22-12-98-80, FAX 47-22-12-98-90, journals@tandf.no, http://www.tandf.co.uk.tfas. Ed. Claes Hellerstroem. Circ: 1,350.

610 NOR ISSN 0300-9726 CODEN: UJMSBQ
UPSALA JOURNAL OF MEDICAL SCIENCES. SUPPLEMENT. Text in English. irreg. included with Upsala Journal of Medical Sciences. **Document type:** *Academic/Scholarly.*
Formerly (until 1972): Acta Societatis Medicorum Upsaliensis. Supplementum
Related titles: ♦ Supplement to: Upsala Journal of Medical Sciences. ISSN 0300-9734.
Indexed: Ind.Med. (1972-).
—BLDSC (9122.710000), CASDDS, CISTI, KNAW. **CCC.**
Published by: (Uppsala Laekarefoerening SWE), Scandinavian University Press (Subsidiary of: Taylor & Francis Ltd.), Postboks 2959, Toeyen, Oslo 0608, Norway. FAX 47-22-57-53-53, journals@scup.no, http://www.scup.no/ujms.

URBAN HEALTH AND DEVELOPMENT BULLETIN. see *PUBLIC HEALTH AND SAFETY*

V.E. BULLETIN. (Voluntary Euthanasia) see *PHILOSOPHY*

V E NEWS; the campaign journal of the Voluntary Euthanasia Society. see *PHILOSOPHY*

610 CHE ISSN 1422-2086
V S A O JOURNAL. Text in French, German, Italian. 1981. 8/yr. CHF 50 (effective 2001). **Document type:** *Journal, Academic/Scholarly.*
Published by: (Verband Schweizerischer Assistenz- und Oberaerzte), Schwabe und Co. AG, Steinentorstr 13, Basel 4010, Switzerland. TEL 41-61-2789565, FAX 41-61-2789565, verlag@schwabe.ch, http://www.schwabe.ch. Ed. Bernhard Stricker. Circ: 15,000 (paid).

610 USA ISSN 1530-3667
▼ **VECTOR BORNE AND ZOONOTIC DISEASES.** Text in English. 2000. q. USD 129 domestic to individuals; USD 167 foreign to individuals; USD 155 domestic to individuals for Print & Online eds.; USD 193 foreign to individuals for Print & Online eds.; USD 249 domestic to institutions .; USD 299 foreign to institutions; USD 299 domestic to institutions for Print & Online eds.; USD 349 foreign to institutions for Print & Online eds. (effective 2002). adv. back issues avail.; reprints avail. *Refereed.* **Document type:** *Journal, Academic/Scholarly.* **Description:** Covers both vector and zoonotic borne diseases such as Lyme disease, ehrlichiosis, West Nile virus, hantavirus, bartonellosis, and Ebola.
Related titles: Online - full content ed.: USD 129 to individuals; USD 249 to institutions (effective 2002); Online - full text ed.: (from CatchWord Ltd., RoweCom Information Quest).
Published by: Mary Ann Liebert, Inc. Publishers, 2 Madison Ave, Larchmont, NY 10538. TEL 914—834-3100, FAX 914-834-1388, info@liebertpub.com, http://www.liebertpub.com/vbz. Ed. Durland Fish. R&P Esther Bicovany. Adv. contact Harriet Matysko.

610 VEN
VENEZUELA. HOSPITAL CENTRAL DE LA FUERZAS ARMADAS. BOLETIN MEDICO. Text in Spanish. 1970. q. free per issue. abstr, bibl, illus. **Document type:** *Bulletin, Government.*
Published by: Hospital Central de las Fuerzas Armadas, San Martin, Caracas, DF 1060, Venezuela. Ed. Dr. Leandro Potenza. Circ: 1,500.

610 DEU ISSN 0174-738X CODEN: VERDEJ
VERDAUUNGSKRANKHEITEN; gastroenterologische Zeitschrift fuer Klinik und Praxis. Text in German. 1983. bi-m. DEM 146, EUR 74.65; DEM 28, EUR 14.32 newsstand/cover (effective 2001). adv. **Document type:** *Journal, Academic/Scholarly.*
Indexed: Chem.Abstr., Chem.Indus.Notes, Ref.Zh.
—BLDSC (9155.828000), CASDDS, GNLM, Infotrieve, KNAW. **CCC.**
Published by: Dustri-Verlag Dr. Karl Feistle, Bajuwarenring 4, Oberhaching 82041, Germany. TEL 49-89-613861-0, FAX 49-89-613-5412, info@dustri.de, http://www.dustri.de. Ed. Dr. H Bosseckert. R&P Renate Lehmann. Adv. contact Joerg Feistle. B&W page DEM 2,870, B&W page XEU 1,467.41; trim 167 x 242. Circ: 3,600.

610 USA
VERMONT STATE MEDICAL SOCIETY. REPORTER. Text in English. 1949. m. USD 35. adv. back issues avail. **Document type:** *Newsletter.* **Description:** Provides non-technical information of interest to practicing Vermont physicians.
Formerly: Vermont State Medical Society. Newsletter
Published by: Vermont State Medical Society, 136 Main St, P O Box 1457, Montpelier, VT 05601-1457. TEL 802-223-7898, FAX 802-223-1201, bcody@vtmd.org. Ed. Karen N Meyer. Circ: 1,100.

610 DEU ISSN 0933-4548 CODEN: VERSEU
VERSICHERUNGSMEDIZIN; Prognose Therapie Begutachtung. Text in German. 1949. bi-m. DEM 22.43 (effective 2001). adv. bk.rev. abstr, charts, tr.lit. index. back issues avail. **Document type:** *Journal, Academic/Scholarly.*
Formerly: Lebensversicherungsmedizin (0024-0044)
Indexed: Biol.Abstr., Excerp.Med., Ind.Med. (1988-).
—BLDSC (9195.570000), EMDOCS, GNLM, Infotrieve, KNAW. **CCC.**
Published by: (Gesamtverband GDV e.V.), Verlag Versicherungswirtschaft GmbH, Klosestr 22, Karlsruhe 76137, Germany. TEL 49-721-3509-0, FAX 49-721-31833, kampf@vvw.de, http://www.vvw.de. Ed. Gerd-Marko Ostendorf. Adv. contact Angelika Kampf TEL 49-721-3509119. B&W page DEM 1,700; trim 185 x 268. Circ: 13,000.

610 DEU ISSN 0949-2488
VIA MEDICI; das Magazin fuer junge Mediziner/innen. Text in German. 1995. 5/yr. EUR 17.90 domestic to institutions; EUR 25.90 in Europe to institutions; EUR 28.90 elsewhere to institutions; EUR 4 newsstand/cover (effective 2002). **Document type:** *Magazine, Academic/Scholarly.*
Related titles: Online - full text ed.
—GNLM.
Published by: Georg Thieme Verlag, Ruedigerstr 14, Stuttgart 70469, Germany. TEL 49-711-8931-0, FAX 49-711-8931298, leser.service@thieme.de, http://www.thieme.de.

610 ESP ISSN 0213-5744
VIDEO - MEDICINA PRIMARIA. Text in Spanish. 1986. q. ESP 18,000 (effective 1997). adv. **Document type:** *Trade.*
Media: Video.
Published by: Video Medica S.L., Badal, 102 Bis Loc 1, Barcelona 08014, Spain. TEL 34-3-4319666, FAX 34-3-4219942. Ed. A Ferrer Rodriguez. Adv. contact Angela Ferrer Rodriguez. Circ: 20,000.

VIRCHOWS ARCHIV; an international journal of pathology. see *BIOLOGY*

VITA OSPEDALIERA. see *HEALTH FACILITIES AND ADMINISTRATION*

610 RUS
VITA. TRADITSII, MEDITSINA, ZDOROV'E. Text in Russian. q. USD 85 in United States.
Published by: Vita. Traditsii Meditsina Zdorov'e, Ul Medvedeva 13, str 1, Moscow 103006, Russian Federation. TEL 7-095-9730661, FAX 7-095-9730543. **US dist. addr.:** East View Publications, 3020 Harbor Ln N, Minneapolis, MN 55447. TEL 612-550-0961.

VITAL SIGNS (CAMBRIDGE). see *PUBLIC HEALTH AND SAFETY*

610 USA
VITAL SIGNS (FRESNO). Text in English. 1949. m. USD 24. adv. illus. back issues avail. *Refereed.* **Document type:** *Newsletter.* **Description:** Aimed at physicians.
Formerly: Fresno County Medical Society. Bulletin (0016-1160)
Published by: (Fresno-Madera Medical Society), J P A X Communications, PO Box 36, Sangei, CA 93657. TEL 559-875-6585, FAX 559-224-0276. Ed. Dr. John Bonner. R&P Carol Ran. Circ: 1,200.

610 USA
VITALITY DIGEST. Text in English. m.
Published by: MediMedia USA, Inc., 295 North St, Teterboro, NJ 07608. TEL 201-727-9300, FAX 201-727-0099, http://www.medimedia.com.

VITAMINS AND HORMONES: ADVANCES IN RESEARCH AND APPLICATIONS. see *PHARMACY AND PHARMACOLOGY*

610 RUS
VITAS. Text in Russian. 1991. irreg. (1-2/m.). **Document type:** *Newspaper.*
Published by: Assotsiatsiya "Vitas", Ul Pravdy 9, k 20, Novosibirsk 630090, Russian Federation. Circ: 100,000.
Co-sponsor: Assotsiatsiya Transaktnogo Analiza.

616.026 CZE ISSN 0042-773X CODEN: VNLEAH
VNITRNI LEKARSTVI. Text in Czech, Slovak; Summaries in Czech, English. 1955. m. EUR 144, USD 180 (effective 2001). adv. bk.rev. charts, illus, stat. index. *Refereed.* **Description:** Covers internal medicine.
Indexed: C.I.S. Abstr., Chem.Abstr., Chem.Indus.Notes, Chem.Titles, Excerp.Med., INIS Atomind., Ind.Med. (1955-), Nutr.Abstr.
—BLDSC (9250.300000), CASDDS, CISTI, GNLM, Infotrieve, KNAW. **CCC.**
Published by: (Ceska Lekarska Spolecnost J.E. Purkyne/Czech Medical Association), Nakladatelske Stredisko C L S J.E. Purkyne, Sokolska 31, Prague 12026, Czech Republic. TEL 42-2-24911420, FAX 42-2-24911420, nts@iol.cz, http://www.clsjep.cz, http://www.medical.cz. Ed. Dr. P Svacina. adv.: B&W page CZK 25,500, color page CZK 43,000; 248 x 166. Circ: 2,550. **Dist. by:** Abont s.r.o., Chlumova 17, Prague, 3 130 00, Czech Republic; **Dist. in Western Countries by:** Kubon & Sagner, Hesstr 39-41, Munich 80798, Germany.

VOICES (WASHINGTON). see *CONSUMER EDUCATION AND PROTECTION*

M

616.98 CZE ISSN 0372-7025
VOJENSKE ZDRAVOTNICKE LISTY. Text in Czech; Summaries in English, German. 1925. bi-m., latest vol.70. bk.rev. abstr, illus, charts. index. 48 p./no. Supplement avail.; back issues avail. *Refereed.* **Document type:** *Journal, Consumer.* **Description:** Essays on military science, medical sciences, veterinary sciences and pharmacology.
Indexed: INIS Atomind.
—EMDOCS, GNLM.
Published by: Vojenska Lekarska Akademie J.E. Purkyne, Trebesska 1575, Hradec Kralove 50001, Czech Republic. TEL 42-49-5253007, FAX 42-49-5253278, vzl@pmfhk.cz, paces@pmfhk.cz; vzl@pmfhk.cz, http://www.pmfhk.cz/depart/ui/redakce/vzl.htm. Eds. Eva Stastna, Jaroslav Paces. Circ: 1,000.

616.98 355 YUG ISSN 0042-8450
VOJNOSANITETSKI PREGLED/MILITARY MEDICAL AND PHARMACEUTICAL; casopis lekara i farmaceuta vojske Jugoslavije. Text in English, Serbian; Summaries in English. 1944. bi-m., latest vol.58, 2001. YUN 360,000, USD 60 domestic; YUN 1,800,000 foreign (effective 2002). adv. bk.rev. abstr, charts, illus, stat. index. 110 p./no. 2 cols./p. back issues avail. **Document type:** *Academic/Scholarly.* **Description:** Contains editorials, original articles (scientific and professional), preliminary or short communications, general reviews, meta-analyses, current topics, from the medical history of the Yugoslav Medical Corps.
Related titles: E-mail ed.; Fax ed.
Indexed: Biol.Abstr., C.I.S. Abstr., Chem.Abstr., Dent.Ind., Ergon.Abstr., Excerp.Med., INIS Atomind., I.P.A., Ind.Med. (1944-), Psychol.Abstr.
—BLDSC (9251.652000), CISTI, GNLM.
Published by: Savezno Ministarstvo Odbrane, Sanitetska Uprava, Military Medical Academy INI, Crnotravska 17, Postanski Fah 3335, Belgrade 11040, Yugoslavia. TEL 381-1-661122, FAX 381-1-669689, vmaini1@eunet.yu, vmaini1@eunet.yu; vmaini2@eunet.yu. Ed. Vladimir Tadic. Adv. contact Slavko Lukic. Circ: 500.

VOPROSY BIOLOGICHESKOI, MEDITSINSKOI, I FARMATSEVTICHESKOI KHIMII/PROBLEMS OF BIOLOGICAL, MEDICAL AND PHARMACOLOGICAL. see *BIOLOGY*

610 FRA ISSN 1241-9648
VOUS ET VOTRE SANTE. Text in French. 1963. m. FRF 350. bk.rev. **Document type:** *Consumer.*
Former titles: Vous (1143-4686); Actualite de la Medecine Officielle et Medecine Naturelle (0044-6149)
Published by: Vous sarl, 44 bd. de Magenta, Paris 75010, France. TEL 33-1-40-18-70-50, FAX 33-1-40-18-33-30. Ed. Pierre Andrillon. Circ: 20,000.

VOX ME D A L. see *COLLEGE AND ALUMNI*

610 RUS ISSN 0236-3054
VRACH. Text in Russian. m. USD 159.95 in United States.
Indexed: Ref.Zh.
—East View.
Published by: Izdatel'stvo Russkii Vrach, B Pirogovskaya 2-6, Moscow 119881, Russian Federation. TEL 7-095-2485727, FAX 7-095-2487717. Ed. M A Pal'tsev. **US dist. addr.:** East View Publications, 3020 Harbor Ln N, Minneapolis, MN 55447. TEL 612-550-0961.

610 RUS
VRACHEBNYE TAINY. Text in Russian. m. USD 125 in United States (effective 2001).
Published by: Izdatel'sko-Proizvodsvennoe Ob'edinenie Pisatelei TEL 7-095-2002323, FAX 7-095-2002323, plife@postman.ru, http://www.privatelife.ru. Ed. V I Shvarts. **Dist. by:** East View Publications, 3020 Harbor Ln N, Minneapolis, MN 55447. TEL 612-550-0961.

610 CHE ISSN 0250-8737
VSEMIRNAYA ORGANIZATSIYA ZDRAVOOKHRANENIYA. SERIYA TEKHNICHESKIKH DOKLADOV. Text in Russian. 1950. irreg.
Related titles: ♦ English ed.: W H O Technical Report Series. ISSN 0512-3054; ♦ Spanish ed.: Organizacion Mundial de la Salud. Serie de Informes Tecnicos. ISSN 0509-2507; ♦ French ed.: Organisation Mondiale de la Sante. Serie de Rapports Techniques. ISSN 0373-3998; ♦ Arabic ed.: Munazzamat al-Sihhah al-'Alamiyyah. Silsilat al-Taqarir al-Fanniyyah. ISSN 0251-0111.
Published by: World Health Organization, Marketing and Dissemination, Geneva, 27 1211, Switzerland.

610 CHE ISSN 0512-3054
RA8 CODEN: WHOTAC
W H O TECHNICAL REPORT SERIES. Text in English. 1948. irreg. (approx. 6 reports /yr.). CHF 132 (effective 2001). *Refereed.* **Document type:** *Monographic series.* **Description:** Summarizes current technical knowledge on a given disease, health risk, medical technology or research approach.
Related titles: Online - full text ed.: (from Institute for Scientific Information); ♦ Spanish ed.: Organizacion Mundial de la Salud. Serie de Informes Tecnicos. ISSN 0509-2507; ♦ French ed.: Organisation Mondiale de la Sante. Serie de Rapports Techniques. ISSN 0373-3998; ♦ Russian ed.: Vsemirnaya Organizatsiya Zdravookhraneniya. Seriya Tekhnicheskikh Dokladov. ISSN 0250-8737; ♦ Arabic ed.: Munazzamat al-Sihhah al-'Alamiyyah. Silsilat al-Taqarir al-Fanniyyah. ISSN 0251-0111.
Indexed: ASCA, Abstr.Hyg., Abstr.Rural Dev.Trop., Aqua.Sci.& Fish.Abstr., Aquacult.Abstr., Biol.Abstr., Dent.Ind., Diar.Dis.Res., Environ.Sci.Poll.Mgmt., Excerp.Med., Food Sci.& Tech.Abstr., Helminthol.Abstr., I.M.M.Abstr., INIS Atomind., I.P.A., Ind.Med. (1950-), Ind.Vet., Med.Care Rev., Nutr.Abstr., Protozool.Abstr., Ref.Zh., Rev.Appl.Entomol., Rev.Med.& Vet.Mycol., Rural Ext.Educ.& Tr.Abstr., Rural Recreat.Tour.Abstr., Sci.Cit.Ind., Sport Fish.Abstr., Trop.Dis.Bull., Vet.Bull., Wild.Rev., World Ag.Econ.& Rur.Soc.Abstr., Zoo.Rec.
—BLDSC (8725.000000), CISTI, EMDOCS, GNLM, ingenta, KNAW, Linda Hall.
Published by: World Health Organization, Marketing and Dissemination, Geneva, 27 1211, Switzerland. TEL 41-22-791-2476, FAX 41-22-791-4857, publications@who.ch, http://www.who.cnt.

610 USA
R15 CODEN: WJMDA2
W J M. Text in English. 1856. m. GBP 52, USD 81 combined subscription to individuals includes print & online eds.; GBP 108, USD 173 to institutions for print only (effective 2002). adv. illus. index. reprint service avail. from PQC. *Refereed.* **Document type:** *Journal, Academic/Scholarly.* **Description:** Offers up-to-date infromation for clinicians, including regular debates on key issues in health care today.
Formerly (until May 1999): Western Journal of Medicine (0093-0415); Which incorporated (1944-1985): Arizona Medicine (0004-1556); Former titles (until 1974): California Medicine (0008-1264); (until 1946): California and Western Medicine (0093-4038); (until 1924): California State Journal of Medicine (0093-402X); (until 1902): Medical Society of the State of California. Transactions of the Session (0743-3212)
Related titles: Microfilm ed.: (from PQC); Online - full text ed.: (from Gale Group, HighWire Pr., EBSCO Publishing, ProQuest Information & Learning, Institute for Scientific Information).
Indexed: AIM, AMED, ASCA, Abstr.Health Care Manage.Stud., AgeLine, Arts & Hum.Cit.Ind. (coverage dropped), Biol.Abstr., CINAHL, C.I.S. Abstr., Cal.Tiss.Abstr., Chem.Abstr., Chic.Per.Ind., Crim.Just.Abstr., Curr.Adv.Cancer Res., Curr.Adv.Ecol.Sci., Curr.Cont., Dairy Sci.Abstr., Dent.Ind., Dok.Arbeitsmed., Environ.Sci.Poll.Mgmt., Excerp.Med., Fam.Ind., Helminthol.Abstr., Hlth.Ind., Hosp.Lit.Ind., INIS Atomind., Ind.Med. (1974-), Ind.Sci.Rev., Ind.Vet., Inpharma, Int.Nurs.Ind., Med.& Surg.Dermat., Med.Care Rev., NRN, Neurosci.Cit.Ind., Nutr.Abstr., Pharm.&Out.News, Pollut.Abstr., Protozool.Abstr., Reac., Rev.Appl.Entomol., Rev.Med.& Vet.Mycol., Risk Abstr., SSCI (coverage dropped), Saf.Sci.Abstr., Sage Race Rel.Abstr., Sci.Cit.Ind., Small Anim.Abstr., THA.
—BLDSC (9300.830000), CASDDS, CISTI, GNLM, IDS, ingenta, KNAW. **CCC.**
Published by: B M J Publishing Group, PO Box 7690, San Francisco, CA 94120-7690. TEL 415-974-5977, FAX 415-882-3379, wjm@ewjm.com, wjmsf@pacbell.net, http://www.ewjm.com, http://www.bmjgroup.com. Ed. Michael Wilkes. R&P Auban Haydel. adv.: B&W page USD 750, color page USD 1,250. Circ: 10,000 (paid). **Subscr. to:** PO Box 590A, Kennebunkport, ME 04046. TEL 800-236-6265, FAX 800-232-9265, bjpaige@cybertours.com. **Co-sponsors:** Medical Associations of Arizona, California, Idaho, Nevada State, New Mexico, Utah State, Washington State, and Wyoming; U C S F Stanford Healthcare.

610 574 JPN ISSN 0511-084X
CODEN: WKMRAH
WAKAYAMA MEDICAL REPORTS. Text in English, French, German. 1953. q. per issue exchange basis. bibl, charts, illus. index.
Indexed: Abstr.Hyg., Biol.Abstr., C.I.S. Abstr., Chem.Abstr., Chem.Indus.Notes, Excerp.Med., INIS Atomind., Nutr.Abstr., Trop.Dis.Bull.
—BLDSC (9261.400000), CASDDS, CISTI, GNLM, KNAW.
Published by: Wakayama Medical College, Library/Wakayama-kenritsu Ika Daigaku Toshokan, Wakayama 640, Japan. FAX 0734-26-8333, TELEX 5542-488. Ed. Akira Ooshima. Circ: 800.

610 615 USA ISSN 1069-4218
WARNING LETTER BULLETIN. Text in English. 1993. fortn. USD 558 (effective 2001). 8 p./no. back issues avail.; reprints avail. **Document type:** *Newsletter.*
Related titles: Online - full text ed.: (from Gale Group, Northern Light Technology, Inc., Factiva).
—**CCC.**
Published by: Washington Information Source, 6506 Old Stage Rd, Ste 100, Rockville, MD 20852-4326. TEL 301-770-5553. R&P Ken Reid.

WARY CANARY; a news network for allergics, "sensitive birds," & environmental health advocates. see *ENVIRONMENTAL STUDIES*

THE WATERMARK. see *LIBRARY AND INFORMATION SCIENCES*

616.98 DEU ISSN 0043-2148
WEHRMEDIZIN UND WEHRPHARMAZIE. Text in German. 1963. q. DEM 48.90, EUR 25 domestic; DEM 60.63, EUR 31 foreign (effective 2001). adv. back issues avail. **Document type:** *Journal, Trade.* **Description:** For doctors, pharmacists and scientists in the medical corps of Germany.
Formerly (until 1968): Wehrmedizin (0343-155X)
—GNLM, KNAW.
Published by: Beta Verlag und Marketinggesellschaft mbH, Postfach 140121, Bonn 53056, Germany. TEL 49-228-91937-0, FAX 49-228-252067, info@beta-publishing.com, http://www.wehrmed.de, http://www.beta-publishing.com. R&P Heike Lange TEL 49-228-919370. Adv. contact Barbara Schunck. B&W page XEU 4,361.5, color page XEU 8,263.36; trim 185 x 270. Circ: 8,100.

610 DEU ISSN 0043-2156
CODEN: WEMOBZ
WEHRMEDIZINISCHE MONATSSCHRIFT; Organ des Sanitaetsdienstes der Bundeswehr. Text in German; Summaries in English, German. 1956. 8/yr. DEM 56.72, EUR 29 domestic; DEM 68.48, EUR 35 foreign (effective 2001). adv. bk.rev. abstr, charts, illus, stat. cum.index. **Document type:** *Journal, Academic/Scholarly.*
Formerly: Wehrmedizinische Mitteilungen
Indexed: Biol.Abstr., Chem.Abstr., INIS Atomind.
—CASDDS, CISTI, GNLM, Infotrieve, KNAW. **CCC.**
Published by: (Germany. Bundesministerium der Verteidigung), Beta Verlag und Marketinggesellschaft mbH, Postfach 140121, Bonn 53056, Germany. TEL 49-228-91937-0, FAX 49-228-252067, info@beta-publishing.com, http://www.wehrmed.de, http://www.beta-publishing.com. Ed. Helmut Corterier. Adv. contact Barbara Schunck. B&W page XEU 3,364.03, color page XEU 6,356.44; trim 180 x 260. Circ: 5,200 (controlled). **Co-sponsor:** Deutsche Gesellschaft fuer Wehrmedizin und Wehrpharmazie.

630 CHN
WEISHENG DULIXUE ZAZHI. Text in Chinese. q.
Indexed: Chem.Abstr., Chem.Indus.Notes, Chem.Titles.
Published by: Zhonghua Yufang Yixuehui/China Preventive Medical Society, 16 Hepingli Zhongjie, Beijing 100013, China. TEL 4218457. Ed. Liu Shijie.

610 GBR
WELLCOME TRUST. POLICY REPORT. Text in English. irreg., latest vol.9, 1998. GBP 10. **Document type:** *Academic/Scholarly.*
Published by: Wellcome Trust, 210 Euston Rd, London NW1 2DA, United Kingdom. TEL 44-171-611-8479, FAX 44-171-611-8742, prism@wellcome.ac.uk, http://www.wellcome.ac.uk.

615.89 GBR ISSN 0143-7984
WELLCOME UNIT FOR THE HISTORY OF MEDICINE. RESEARCH PUBLICATIONS. Text in English. 1979. irreg., latest no.12. price varies. bibl. back issues avail. **Document type:** *Academic/Scholarly, Bibliography.* **Description:** Contains bibliographical, documentary and research aids for the social history of medicine and health from the year 1500 to the present.
Published by: Wellcome Unit for the History of Medicine, University of, Wellcome Unit For The History Of Medicine, 45 Banbury Rd, Oxford OX2 6PE, United Kingdom. TEL 44-1865-274600, FAX 44-1865-274605, wuhmo@wuhmo.ox.ac.uk. Ed. Margaret Pelling. Circ: 200.

M

WELLNESS PROGRAM MANAGEMENT ADVISOR. see *PUBLIC HEALTH AND SAFETY*

610 GBR
WELSH MEDICAL GAZETTE. Text in English. 1970. q. free per issue to qualified personnel. adv. bk.rev. illus.
Published by: Welsh Medical Press Ltd., 23 Blenheim Rd, Cardiff CF2 5DS, United Kingdom. Eds. Bernard Knight, Dr. Eric Payne. Circ: 5,000.

WENNER GREN CENTER INTERNATIONAL SYMPOSIUM SERIES. see *SCIENCES: COMPREHENSIVE WORKS*

610 CHN ISSN 1000-2138
WENZHOU YIXUEYUAN XUEBAO/WENZHOU INSTITUTE OF MEDICAL SCIENCES. JOURNAL. Text in Chinese. q. **Document type:** *Academic/Scholarly.*
Published by: Wenzhou Yixueyuan/Wenzhou Institute of Medical Sciences, Wenzhou, Zhejiang 325003, China. TEL 34941.

610 JAM ISSN 0043-3144
CODEN: WIMJAD
WEST INDIAN MEDICAL JOURNAL. Text in English. 1947. q. USD 72 (effective 2000). adv. bk.rev. bibl, charts, illus. index. Supplement avail.; back issues avail.; reprint service avail. from IRC,PQC,ISI. *Refereed.* **Document type:** *Academic/Scholarly.* **Description:** Addresses areas of medical research of the greatest potential benefit to the people of the Commonwealth Caribbean. Contains articles covering those relevant medical topics.
Supersedes (in 1951): Jamaica Medical Review (0368-1238)
Related titles: Microform ed.: 1951; Online - full text ed.: (from Institute for Scientific Information); Supplement: West Indian Medical Journal. Supplement.
Indexed: ASCA, Abstr.Hyg., Biol.Abstr., Chem.Abstr., Curr.Cont., Dairy Sci.Abstr., Dent.Ind., Diar.Dis.Res., Excerp.Med., Helminthol.Abstr., I.P.A., Ind.Med. (1951-), Ind.Vet., Inpharma, Int.Nurs.Ind., Nutr.Abstr., Protozool.Abstr., Reac., Rev.Appl.Entomol., Rev.Arom.& Med.Plants, Rev.Med.& Vet.Mycol., Trop.Dis.Bull.
—BLDSC (9299.100000), CASDDS, CISTI, GNLM, IDS, ingenta, KNAW.
Published by: University of the West Indies, Faculty of Medical Sciences, Mona Campus, Kingston 7, Jamaica. TEL 876-927-1846, FAX 876-977-2289. Ed. Dr. E N Barton. R&P, Adv. contact Molly McGann. B&W page USD 225, color page USD 250. Circ: 2,000.

610 USA ISSN 0043-3284
WEST VIRGINIA MEDICAL JOURNAL. Text in English. 1906. bi-m. USD 60; USD 10 newsstand/cover (effective 2001). adv. bk.rev. bibl, illus. index. *Refereed.* **Document type:** *Academic/Scholarly.*
Related titles: Microform ed.: (from PQC).
Indexed: Biol.Abstr., Chem.Abstr., Curr.Cont. (coverage dropped), Dent.Ind., Excerp.Med., Helminthol.Abstr., INIS Atomind., Ind.Med. (1906-), Int.Nurs.Ind., Med.Care Rev., Nutr.Abstr., Rev.Med.& Vet.Mycol.
—BLDSC (9300.050000), CISTI, GNLM, KNAW.
Published by: West Virginia State Medical Association, 4307 MacCorkle Ave, Box 4106, Charleston, WV 25364. TEL 304-925-0342, FAX 304-925-0345, wvsma@aol.com. Ed. F Thomas Sporck. R&P Nancy Hill. Adv. contact Christina R Dixon. Circ: 3,100.

610 USA
WESTCHESTER BULLETIN✱. Text in English. 1974 (vol.42). 10/yr. USD 2. adv. bk.rev.
Published by: Westchester Academy of Medicine, 555 Theodore Fremd Ave, Ste B100, Rye, NY 10560-1451. TEL 914-948-4100. Circ: 2,000.

340 USA ISSN 0000-1708
R153
WHO'S WHO IN MEDICINE AND HEALTHCARE. Text in English. 1996. biennial, latest vol.2, 1998. USD 249.95 (effective 1999). **Document type:** *Directory.* **Description:** Lists approximately 20,000 successful medical professionals, administrators, educators, researchers, clinicians and industry leaders from across the diverse fields of medicine and healthcare.
Published by: Marquis Who's Who (Subsidiary of: Reed Elsevier plc Group), 121 Chanlon Rd, New Providence, NJ 07964. TEL 908-464-6800, FAX 908-665-6688, info@marquiswhoswho.com, http://www.marquiswhoswho.com. Ed. Fred Marks. **Subscr. to:** Order Dept., PO Box 31, New Providence, NJ 07974-9903. TEL 800-521-8110.

610 POL ISSN 0043-5147
CODEN: WILEAR
WIADOMOSCI LEKARSKIE✱. Text in Polish; Summaries in English, Russian. 1948. bi-w. USD 216. **Document type:** *Academic/Scholarly.* **Description:** Explores clinical medicine and postgraduate education of physicians.
Indexed: Biol.Abstr., Chem.Abstr., Dent.Ind., Dok.Arbeitsmed., Excerp.Med., INIS Atomind., Ind.Med. (1960-), Protozool.Abstr.
—BLDSC (9313.800000), CASDDS, CISTI, GNLM.
Published by: Fundacja Lekarzy Polskich - Pro Medica, c/o Ars Polona, Krakowskie Przedmiescie 7, PO Box 1001, Warsaw 00068, Poland. Ed. Dr. Jan Dzieniszewski.

610 DEU ISSN 0179-3004
WIE GEHT'S HEUTE?; Ratschlaege und Informationen aus Ihrem Sanitaetsfachgeschaeft. Text in German. 1985. 3/yr. DEM 0.98 (effective 2000). adv. back issues avail. **Document type:** *Consumer.*
Published by: M T D Verlag GmbH und Co., Wangenerstr 12, Amtzell 88279, Germany. TEL 49-7520-958-0, FAX 49-7520-95899. Ed. Wolf Dieter Seitz. Adv. contact Christl Morgen.

WIEDZA I ZYCIE. see *SCIENCES: COMPREHENSIVE WORKS*

610 AUT ISSN 0043-5325
CODEN: WKWOAO
WIENER KLINISCHE WOCHENSCHRIFT; the Middle European journal of medicine. Text in German, English. 1887. s-m. EUR 298.30 domestic; EUR 296.20 per issue in Germany; EUR 17 newsstand/cover foreign (effective 2002). adv. bk.rev. charts, illus, abstr. index. back issues avail.; reprint service avail. from ISI. *Refereed.* **Document type:** *Journal, Academic/Scholarly.*
Related titles: Microform ed.: (from PQC); Online - full text ed.: (from Springer LINK, Institute for Scientific Information); ♦ Supplement: Wiener Klinische Wochenschrift. Supplementum. ISSN 0300-5178.
Indexed: ASCA, Abstr.Hyg., Agri.& Environ.Biotech.Abstr. (coverage dropped), Biol.Abstr., C.I.S. Abstr., Chem.Abstr., Chem.Indus.Notes, Chem.Titles, Curr.Adv.Biochem., Curr.Adv.Cell & Devel.Biol., Curr.Cont., Dairy Sci.Abstr., Dent.Ind., Derwent Biotech.Abstr., Excerp.Med., Helminthol.Abstr., INIS Atomind., Ind.Med. (1888-), Ind.Sci.Rev., Inpharma, Int.Nurs.Ind., Kidney, Neurosci.Cit.Ind., Nutr.Abstr., Pharm.&Out.News, Protozool.Abstr., Reac., Rev.Appl.Entomol., Rev.Med.& Vet.Mycol., SSCI (coverage dropped), Sci.Cit.Ind., Soyabean Abstr.
—BLDSC (9315.900000), CASDDS, CISTI, GNLM, IDS, KNAW. **CCC.**
Published by: Springer-Verlag Wien (Subsidiary of: BertelsmannSpringer), Sachsenplatz 4-6, PO Box 89, Vienna, W 1201, Austria. TEL 43-1-3302415-0, FAX 43-1-330242665, journals@springer.at, http://www.springer.at/wkw. Ed. W Druml. R&P Angela Foessl TEL 43-1-3302415517. Adv. contact Michael Katzenberger TEL 43-1-3302415220. B&W page XEU 1,000, color page XEU 1,700; 180 x 260. **N. American subscr. to:** Springer-Verlag, Journals, 175 Fifth Ave, New York, NY 10010. TEL 212-460-1500, FAX 212-473-6272, orders@springer-ny.com, http://www.springer-ny.com.

610 AUT ISSN 1434-6869
WIENER KLINISCHE WOCHENSCHRIFT MAGAZIN. Variant title: W K W Magazin. Text in German. 1998. bi-m. EUR 33.70 domestic; EUR 31.10 in Germany; EUR 5 newsstand/cover foreign (effective 2002). adv. illus. **Document type:** *Journal, Academic/Scholarly.*
Related titles: Online - full text ed.: (from Springer LINK).
—KNAW.
Published by: Springer-Verlag Wien (Subsidiary of: BertelsmannSpringer), Sachsenplatz 4-6, PO Box 89, Vienna, W 1201, Austria. TEL 43-1-3302415-0, FAX 43-1-330242665, journals@springer.at, http://www.springer.at/wkw_magazin. Eds. A Furrer, R Hoehl, V Kienast. R&P Angela Foessl TEL 43-1-3302415517. Adv. contact Michael Katzenberger TEL 43-1-3302415220. B&W page XEU 2,000, color page XEU 2,600; 180 x 260. **Subscr. in N. America to:** Springer-Verlag, Journals. TEL 212-460-1500, FAX 212-473-6272, orders@springer-ny.com, http://www.springer-ny.com.

610 AUT ISSN 0300-5178
CODEN: WKWSA2
WIENER KLINISCHE WOCHENSCHRIFT. SUPPLEMENTUM. Text in German, English. 1972. irreg. **Document type:** *Monographic series, Academic/Scholarly.*
Related titles: ♦ Supplement to: Wiener Klinische Wochenschrift. ISSN 0043-5325.
Indexed: Curr.Cont. (coverage dropped), INIS Atomind., Ind.Med. (1972-).
—BLDSC (9315.901000), CASDDS, CISTI, EMDOCS, Infotrieve, KNAW. **CCC.**
Published by: Springer-Verlag Wien (Subsidiary of: BertelsmannSpringer), Sachsenplatz 4-6, PO Box 89, Vienna, W 1201, Austria. TEL 43-1-3302415-0, FAX 43-1-330242665, journals@springer.at, http://www.springer.at/wkw. **N. American subscr. to:** Springer-Verlag, Journals, 175 Fifth Ave, New York, NY 10010. TEL 212-460-1500, FAX 212-473-6272, orders@springer-ny.com.

610 AUT ISSN 0043-5341
CODEN: WMWOA4
WIENER MEDIZINISCHE WOCHENSCHRIFT. Text in German; Summaries in English. 1851. 24/yr. ATS 3,206.20 in Europe; ATS 3,632.70 elsewhere; ATS 3,526.82 in Europe print & online eds. combined; ATS 3,995.97 elsewhere print & online eds. combined (effective 2001). adv. bk.rev. abstr, bibl, illus. index. reprint service avail. from ISI. **Document type:** *Journal, Academic/Scholarly.*
Related titles: Microform ed.: (from PMC); Online - full text ed.: ISSN 1563-258X.
Indexed: Agri.& Environ.Biotech.Abstr. (coverage dropped), Biol.Abstr., Chem.Abstr., Curr.Cont. (coverage dropped), Derwent Biotech.Abstr., Excerp.Med., Helminthol.Abstr., INIS Atomind., Ind.Med. (1946-), Int.Nurs.Ind., Nutr.Abstr., Ref.Zh.
—BLDSC (9315.925000), ADONIS, CASDDS, CISTI, GNLM, IDS, Infotrieve, KNAW. **CCC.**
Published by: Blackwell Wissenschafts-Verlag Vienna, Firmiangasse 7-1, Vienna, W 1130, Austria. TEL 43-1-8779351-0, FAX 43-1-877935124, verlag@blackwis.at, http://www.blackwell.de/wmw.htm. Ed. Dr. G Hitzenberger. Circ: 4,150.

610 340 DEU
WIKO - WIESBADENER KOMMENTAR ZUM MEDIZINPRODUKTEGESETZ. Text in German. 1995. base vol. plus irreg. updates. DEM 148. **Document type:** *Monographic series.*
Published by: Verlag Chmielorz GmbH und Co., Postfach 2229, Wiesbaden 65012, Germany. TEL 49-611-36098-0, FAX 49-611-301303.

617.1 796.552 USA ISSN 1080-6032
RC1220.M6 CODEN: WEMEF9
WILDERNESS AND ENVIRONMENTAL MEDICINE; official publication of the wilderness medical society. Text in English. 1990. q. USD 216 in US & Canada to institutions; USD 255 elsewhere to institutions (effective 2001). adv. bk.rev. abstr, charts, illus, stat. back issues avail. *Refereed.* **Document type:** *Academic/Scholarly.* **Description:** Publishes research on all aspects of medicine in hostile, natural environments.
Formerly (until 1995): Journal of Wilderness Medicine (0953-9859)
Related titles: Online - full text ed.: (from Swets Blackwell, Institute for Scientific Information).
Indexed: ASCA, Aqua.Sci.& Fish.Abstr., Curr.Cont. (coverage dropped), Energy Rev., Environ.Abstr., Environ.Per.Bibl. (1991-), Environ.Sci.Poll.Mgmt., Excerp.Med., Focus on: Sports Sci.& Med., Ind.Med. (1995-), Ind.Vet., Inpharma, Nutr.Abstr., Pollut.Abstr., Reac., Rev.Appl.Entomol., Rev.Med.& Vet.Mycol., Risk Abstr., Saf.Sci.Abstr., Vet.Bull., Zoo.Rec.
—BLDSC (9317.236000), EMDOCS, GNLM, IDS, ingenta. **CCC.**
Published by: (Wilderness Medical Society), Allen Press, Inc., Division Alliance Communications Group, PO Box 1897, Lawrence, KS 66044. TEL 785-843-1235, FAX 785-843-1274, wms@allenpress.org, http://www.wms.org. Ed. William A Robinson. Pub. Angela Pfeifer. Adv. contact Taresa Walbridge. B&W page USD 400, color page USD 750; trim 10.75 x 8. Circ: 3,500 (paid).

610 USA ISSN 1073-502X
WILDERNESS MEDICINE LETTER. Text in English. 1984. q. USD 33 (effective 2000). adv. bk.rev. back issues avail. *Refereed.* **Document type:** *Newsletter.* **Description:** Covers research on human activities in wilderness environments.
Formerly: Wilderness Medicine
Published by: Wilderness Medical Society, 3595 E Fountain Blvd Ste A1, Colorado Springs, CO 80910-1740. TEL 719-572-9255, FAX 719-572-1514, wms@wms.org, http://www.wms.org. Ed. Karl Neumann. R&P Dian Simpkins. Adv. contact Dian Simkins. Circ: 2,500.

M

610 USA ISSN 1059-6518
WILDERNESS MEDICINE NEWSLETTER. Text in English. 1988. bi-m. USD 24 (effective 2001). bk.rev. tr.lit. 8 p./no. **Document type:** *Newsletter, Trade.* **Description:** Publishes articles written from a variety of perspectives for laypersons practicing and teaching in the wilderness medicine arena. Includes regular guest columns by authors considered to be the founders of this branch of medicine.
Address: PO Box 3150, Conway, NH 03818. TEL 603-447-6711, FAX 603-447-2310. Ed., R&P Holly A Weber. Circ: 600 (paid); 1,000 (controlled).

330 610 USA ISSN 1520-4901 CODEN: IVMRFD
WINDHOVER'S IN VIVO; the business and medicine report. Text in English. 1982. m. (11/yr.). USD 895 domestic; USD 980 foreign (effective 2002). adv. back issues avail.; reprints avail. **Document type:** *Newsletter, Trade.* **Description:** Reports about the medical industry and its effect on business. Features range from industry trends and new products to controversial issues in the medical field as they relate to business.
Formerly: In Vivo (0733-1398)
Related titles: CD-ROM ed.: 1983; Online - full text ed.: 1983 (from Gale Group); ♦ Cumulative ed. of: Strategic Commentary.
Indexed: Chem.Abstr., Chem.Indus.Notes, Chem.Titles.
—BLDSC (4372.510000), CASDDS, Infotrieve. **CCC.**
Published by: Windhover Information, Inc., 10 Hoyt St, Norwalk, CT 06851 . TEL 203-838 4401, FAX 203-838 3214, custserv@windhoverinfo.com, http://www.windhoverinfo.com. Eds. David Cassak, Roger Longman. R&P Terri Smith.

610 USA
WINDOW (NEW YORK). Text in English. 1981. irreg. **Document type:** *Newspaper.*
Published by: New York Hospital - Cornell Medical Center, Office of Public Affairs, 525 E 68th St, New York, NY 10021. TEL 212-821-0560. Ed. Felicia E Narvaez. Circ: 16,000.

610 USA ISSN 0043-6542
R11
WISCONSIN MEDICAL JOURNAL. Text in English. 1903. bi-m. USD 60 domestic to non-members; USD 12.50 domestic to members (effective 2001). bk.rev. bibl, illus. index. *Refereed.* **Document type:** *Academic/Scholarly.* **Description:** Details scientific articles on all phases of medicine and public health.
Indexed: AgeLine, Biol.Abstr., CINAHL, Chem.Abstr., Curr.Cont. (coverage dropped), Dent.Ind., Environ.Sci.Poll.Mgmt., Excerp.Med., Helminthol.Abstr., INIS Atomind., Ind.Med. (coverage dropped), Int.Nurs.Ind., Nutr.Abstr., Pollut.Abstr., Rehabil.Lit., Risk Abstr., Saf.Sci.Abstr.
—CISTI, GNLM, ingenta, KNAW.
Published by: State Medical Society of Wisconsin, 330 E Lakeside St, Box 1109, Madison, WI 53701. TEL 608-257-6781, FAX 608-283-5401, kendip@wismed.org. Ed., R&P Kendi Parvin. Circ: 8,500 (paid).

WOHNUNG & GESUNDHEIT; Fachzeitschrift fuer oekologisches Bauen & Leben. see *ARCHITECTURE*

610 USA ISSN 1055-6370
WORCESTER MEDICINE. Text in English. 1937. bi-m. USD 10. adv. bk.rev. **Document type:** *Academic/Scholarly.*
Formerly: Worcester Medical News (0043-7905)
Published by: (Worcester District Medical Society), * Worcester Publishing, 321 Main St, Worcester, MA 01608. TEL 508-753-1579, FAX 508-754-6246, udms@massmed.org. Ed., R&P J Paul Lock. Adv. contact David Simone. Circ: 1,250.

WORLD BOOK HEALTH AND MEDICAL ANNUAL. see *ENCYCLOPEDIAS AND GENERAL ALMANACS*

610.71025 CHE ISSN 0512-2759
R711
WORLD DIRECTORY OF MEDICAL SCHOOLS. Text in English. 1951. irreg. **Document type:** *Directory.*
Related titles: French ed.: Repertoire Mondial des Ecoles de Medecine. ISSN 1010-0377.
Published by: World Health Organization, Marketing and Dissemination, Geneva, 27 1211, Switzerland. TEL 41-22-791-2476, FAX 41-22-791-4857, publications@who.ch, http://www.who.int.

610 CHE ISSN 0042-9686
R5 CODEN: BWHOA6
WORLD HEALTH ORGANIZATION. BULLETIN. Text in English, French, Spanish. 1947. m. CHF 200 domestic (effective 2001). bibl, charts, illus, abstr. index. back issues avail. *Refereed.* **Document type:** *Academic/Scholarly.* **Description:** Presents original research findings selected on the basis of their immediate or potential relevance to problems of human health.
Formerly (until 1948): League of Nations. Health Organization. Bulletin (0368-7961)
Related titles: Microform ed.: (from PMC,CIS); Online - full text ed.: ISSN 1564-0604 (from Gale Group, ProQuest Information & Learning, Factiva, Institute for Scientific Information); Arabic ed.: Munazzamat al-Sihhiyyah al-'Alamiyyah. Nashrah. ISSN 0257-599X; Chinese ed.: Shijie Weisheng Zuzhi Tongbao. Xuanyi. ISSN 0258-0640; Russian ed.: Vsemirnaya Organizatsiya Zdravookhraneniya. Byulleten'. ISSN 0250-8699.
Indexed: ASCA, ASSIA, Abstr.Anthropol., Abstr.Hyg., Addic.Abstr., Adol.Ment.Hlth.Abstr., Agri.& Environ.Biotech.Abstr. (coverage dropped), Aqua.Sci.& Fish.Abstr., Aquacult.Abstr., Bibl.Asian Stud. (1998), Bio-Contr.News & Info., CINAHL, CWI, Cal.Tiss.Abstr., Curr.Adv.Ecol.Sci., Curr.Cont., Dairy Sci.Abstr., Dent.Abstr., Dent.Ind., Derwent Biotech.Abstr., Diar.Dis.Res., Entomol.Abstr., Environ.Per.Bibl., Environ.Sci.Poll.Mgmt., Excerp.Med., Geo.Abstr.H.G., Helminthol.Abstr., Human Resour.Abstr., IBZ, IDA, IIS, INIS Atomind., I.P.A., Ind.Med. (1947-), Ind.Vet., Inpharma, Int.Nurs.Ind., Med.& Surg.Dermat., Microbiol.Abstr., NRN, Nutr.Abstr., Ocean.Abstr., P.A.I.S., Pharm.&Out.News, Pollut.Abstr., Postharvest, Poult.Abstr., Protozool.Abstr., Psychol.Abstr., Reac., Ref.Zh., Repindex, Rev.Appl.Entomol., Rev.Med.& Vet.Mycol., Rev.Plant Path., Rice Abstr., Risk Abstr., Rural Devel.Abstr., Rural Recreat.Tour.Abstr., Russ.Acad.Sci.Bibl., SSCI (coverage dropped), Saf.Sci.Abstr., Sci.Cit.Ind., Sel.Water Res.Abstr., Soils & Fert., Sport Fish.Abstr., THA, Trop.Dis.Bull., Vet.Bull., Weed Abstr., Wild.Rev., Zoo.Rec.
—BLDSC (2819.000000), CISTI, EMDOCS, GNLM, IDS, ingenta, KNAW, Linda Hall.
Published by: World Health Organization, Marketing and Dissemination, Geneva, 27 1211, Switzerland. TEL 41-22-791-2476, FAX 41-22-791-4857, publications@who.ch, http://www.who.int. Ed. G A Feachom. Circ: 5,500.

658.8029 GBR
WORLD HEALTHCARE MARKETING DIRECTORY. Text in English. irreg., latest 1993. GBP 255, USD 510. **Document type:** *Directory.* **Description:** Contains detailed information on every aspect of the health care industry. Profiles 34 of the world's leading pharmaceutical companies and more than 3,000 worldwide health care organizations.
Published by: Euromonitor, 60-61 Britton St, London EC1M 5UX, United Kingdom. TEL 44-20-7251-8024, info@euromonitor.com, http://www.euromonitor.com.

610 DEU ISSN 0049-8122
R5
WORLD MEDICAL JOURNAL. Text in German; Summaries in English. 1954. bi-m. DEM 42; DEM 31.50 to students (effective 2000). adv. bk.rev. abstr, bibl, charts, illus. index. back issues avail. **Document type:** *Bulletin, Magazine, Academic/Scholarly.* **Description:** For national medical associations around the world who are members of WMA. Delivery of healthcare, medical ethics, medical education, socio-medical affairs, human rights.
Formerly (until 1953): World Medical Association Bulletin (1047-1928)
Indexed: Biol.Abstr., Hosp.Lit.Ind., Med.Care Rev.
—BLDSC (9356.650000), CISTI, GNLM, ingenta.
Published by: (World Medical Association), Deutscher Aerzte-Verlag GmbH, Dieselstr 2, Cologne 50859, Germany. TEL 49-2234-7011-0, FAX 49-2234-7011515, verlag@aerzteblatt.de, http://www.aerzteverlag.de. Ed. Iran M Gillibrand. Circ: 10,000.

WORLD MEETINGS: MEDICINE. see *MEETINGS AND CONGRESSES*

610 364 CHN ISSN 1004-3594
WUJING YIXUE/MEDICAL JOURNAL OF THE CHINESE PEOPLE'S ARMED POLICE FORCES. Text in Chinese; Abstracts in English. 1990. m. USD 19.20; CNY 4, USD 2.20 newsstand/cover (effective 2001). adv. *Refereed.* **Document type:** *Academic/Scholarly.* **Description:** Contains original articles, special reports, clinical experience, military medicine in the field of medical sciences and biology, hospital management, short reports, nursing field.
Published by: Wujing Yixue Bianjibu, 69 Yongding Lu, Haidian-qu, Beijing 100039, China. TEL 86-1-68222686. Ed. Zhang Ruijun. Adv. contact Qiuye Liang. **Dist. overseas by:** China International Book Trading Corp, 35, Chegongzhuang Xilu, Haidian District, Beijing 100044, China. TEL 86-1-68413849, FAX 86-1-68412048, cibtc@mail.cibtc.com.cn, http://www.cibtc.com.cn.

610 CHN ISSN 1000-923X
XIAN MEDICAL UNIVERSITY. JOURNAL. Text in English. 1985. s-a. CNY 5 per issue (effective 2000). back issues avail. **Document type:** *Academic/Scholarly.*
Related titles: Online - full content ed.: (from WanFang Data Corp.).
Indexed: Ref.Zh.
—BLDSC (4917.475500).
Published by: Xian Medical University, Shaanxi, Xian 710061, China. Ed. Huimin Ren.

610 CHN ISSN 1001-8174
XIANDAI ZHENDUAN YU ZHILIAO/MODERN DIAGNOSIS & TREATMENT. Text in Chinese. 1990. bi-m. USD 2.93 (effective 2001 & 2002). bk.rev. 64 p./no. *Refereed.* **Document type:** *Journal, Academic/Scholarly.*
Published by: (Jiangxi Sheng Nanchang Shi Yixue Kexue Yanjiusuo/Jiangxi Province Nanchang Municipal Institute of Medical Science), Xiandai Zhenduan yu Zhiliao Bianjibu, No 90 Bayi Ave. 9th Fl, Nanchang, Jiangxi 330003, China. TEL 86-791-6228412, xdzdyz1@public.nc.jx.cn. Ed. Wang Yanfei. R&P Yanfei Wang. Adv. contact Kangxin Hu. Circ: 4,500 (paid). **Dist. overseas by:** China International Book Trading Corp, 35 Chegongzhuang Xilu, Haidian District, Beijing 100044, China. cibtc@mail.cibtc.com.cn, http://www.cibtc.com.cn.

XIBEI LINXUEYUAN XUEBAO/NORTHWESTERN FORESTRY UNIVERSITY. JOURNAL. see *FORESTS AND FORESTRY*

610 CHN ISSN 0253-9802
R97.7.C5 CODEN: XINYD9
XIN YIXUE/NEW MEDICAL SCIENCE. Text in Chinese. m.
Indexed: Ref.Zh.
—CASDDS.
Published by: Zhongshan Yike Daxue/Sun Yat-sen Medical University, 74 Zhongshan Erlu, Guangzhou, Guangdong 510089, China. TEL 778223.

XINZHONGYI/NEW JOURNAL OF TRADITIONAL CHINESE MEDICINE. see *ALTERNATIVE MEDICINE*

610 CHN ISSN 1000-2065
XUZHOU YIXUEYUAN XUEBAO/XUZHOU INSTITUTE OF MEDICAL SCIENCES. JOURNAL. Text in Chinese. q. **Document type:** *Academic/Scholarly.*
Published by: Xuzhou Yixueyuan/Xuzhou Institute of Medical Sciences, 84 Huihai Xilu, Xuzhou, Jiangsu 221002, China. TEL 34650. Ed. Wang Pingyu.

610 JPN ISSN 0916-1139 CODEN: YADOEL
YAKUBUTSU DOTAI/XENOBIOTIC METABOLISM AND DISPOSITION. Text in Japanese. 1986. 7/yr. JPY 8,000 domestic (effective 2001). adv. bk.rev. 8 p./no. *Refereed.* **Document type:** *Bulletin, Academic/Scholarly.* **Description:** Provides information & articles on drug metabolism and disposition.
Indexed: Chem.Abstr., Chem.Indus.Notes, Chem.Titles, Mass Spectr.Bull.
—BLDSC (9367.019500), CASDDS, GNLM, Infotrieve. **CCC.**
Published by: Yakubutsu Dotai Gakkai/Japanese Society for the Study of Xenobiotics, 2-4-16 Yayoi, Bunkyo-ku, Tokyo 113-0032, Japan. TEL 81-3-3816-4550, FAX 81-3-5814-5820, eisei@mail.pharm.tohoku.ac.jp, http://xenobio.kopas.co.jp. Ed. Tetsuya Suga. Pub. Jun Watanabe. Circ: 2,000.

610 570 USA ISSN 0044-0086
R11 CODEN: YJBMAU
YALE JOURNAL OF BIOLOGY AND MEDICINE. Text in English. 1928. bi-m. USD 45 to individuals; USD 53 foreign to individuals; USD 90 to institutions; USD 98 foreign to institutions. adv. bk.rev. bibl, charts, illus. index. reprint service avail. from PSC. *Refereed.* **Document type:** *Academic/Scholarly.* **Description:** Original contributions and review articles in all fields of medicine and related sciences.
Related titles: Microform ed.: (from PQC,PMC); Online - full text ed.: (from Institute for Scientific Information).

Indexed: ASCA, Biol.Abstr., Biol.Dig., Chem.Abstr., Chem.Indus.Notes, Curr.Adv.Ecol.Sci., Curr.Cont. (coverage dropped), Deep Sea Res.& Oceanogr.Abstr., Excerp.Med., Helminthol.Abstr., INIS Atomind., Ind.Med. (1928-), Ind.Sci.Rev., Inpharma, Int.Aerosp.Abstr., Med.& Surg.Dermat., NRN, Nutr.Abstr., Pharm.&Out.News, Reac., Sci.Cit.Ind. (coverage dropped), Sport Fish.Abstr., Vet.Bull., Wild.Rev., Zoo.Rec.
—BLDSC (9370.000000), CASDDS, CISTI, GNLM, IDS, ingenta, KNAW, Linda Hall. **CCC.**
Published by: Yale Journal of Biology and Medicine, Inc., 333 Cedar St, New Haven, CT 06510. TEL 203-785-4251, FAX 203-785-4251, yjbm@yale.edu, http://info.med.yale.edu/yjbm/welcome.html. Ed., Pub. William C Summers. R&P Valerie Kraemer. Circ: 500.

610 USA
YALE MEDICINE. Text in English. q.
Published by: Yale Medicine Publications, 100 Church St, 212, New Haven, CT 06519. TEL 203-785-5824, FAX 203-785-4327, ymm@yale.edu, http://info.med.yale.edu/ymm.

610 JPN ISSN 0513-1812
CODEN: BYMSAN
YAMAGUCHI UNIVERSITY. SCHOOL OF MEDICINE. BULLETIN/YAMAGUCHI DAIGAKU IGAKUBU KIYO. Key Title: Bulletin of the Yamaguchi Medical School. Text in English, German; Summaries in English. 1953. q. per issue exchange basis. **Document type:** *Bulletin, Journal, Academic/Scholarly.*
Indexed: Abstr.Hyg., Biol.Abstr., Chem.Abstr., Chem.Indus.Notes, Chem.Titles, Excerp.Med., INIS Atomind., Nutr.Abstr., Ref.Zh., Trop.Dis.Bull.
—BLDSC (2822.000000), CASDDS, CISTI, GNLM, KNAW.
Published by: Yamaguchi Daigaku, Igakubu/Yamaguchi University, School of Medicine, Kogushi, Ube-shi, Yamaguchi-ken 755-0085, Japan. Circ: (controlled).

YAMAGUCHIKEN EISEI KOGAI KENKYU SENTA GYOSEKI HOKOKU. see *PUBLIC HEALTH AND SAFETY*

610 USA ISSN 0734-3299
YEAR BOOK OF CRITICAL CARE MEDICINE. Text in English. 1983. a. USD 90 domestic; USD 96 foreign (effective 2001). illus. **Document type:** *Academic/Scholarly, Abstract/Index.* **Description:** Presents abstracts of pertinent literature with commentary by leading experts in the field.
Related titles: CD-ROM ed.
—CISTI, GNLM.
Published by: Mosby, Inc., Continuity Division (Subsidiary of: Harcourt Health Sciences), 11830 Westline Industrial Dr, St Louis, MO 63146-3313. TEL 314-872-8370, 800-325-4177, FAX 314-432-1380, http://www.mosby.com/periodicals. Ed. Dr. J Parrillo.

610 USA ISSN 0147-1996
R101
THE YEAR BOOK OF FAMILY PRACTICE. Text in English. 1977. a. USD 78 domestic; USD 84 foreign (effective 2001). illus. **Document type:** *Abstract/Index, Academic/Scholarly.* **Description:** Presents abstracts of pertinent literature with commentary by leaders in the field.
Related titles: CD-ROM ed.
—CISTI, GNLM.
Published by: Mosby, Inc., Continuity Division (Subsidiary of: Harcourt Health Sciences), 11830 Westline Industrial Dr, St Louis, MO 63146-3313. TEL 314-872-8370, 800-325-4177, FAX 314-432-1380, http://www.mosby.com/periodicals.

610 USA ISSN 0084-3873
R101
THE YEAR BOOK OF MEDICINE. Text in English. 1901. a. USD 87 domestic; USD 93 foreign (effective 2001). **Document type:** *Abstract/Index, Academic/Scholarly.* **Description:** Presents abstracts of pertinent literature with commentary by leading experts in the field.
Former titles (until 1949): Year Book of General Medicine (0093-3635); (until 1933): General Medicine (0093-3562)
Related titles: CD-ROM ed.
Indexed: Curr.Adv.Ecol.Sci., Diar.Dis.Res.
—CISTI, GNLM.
Published by: Mosby, Inc., Continuity Division (Subsidiary of: Harcourt Health Sciences), 11830 Westline Industrial Dr, St Louis, MO 63146-3313. TEL 314-872-8370, 800-325-4177, FAX 314-432-1380, http://www.mosby.com/periodicals.

616.07 USA ISSN 1077-9108
THE YEAR BOOK OF PATHOLOGY AND LABORATORY MEDICINE. Text in English. 1901. a. USD 97 domestic; USD 103 foreign (effective 2001). illus. **Document type:** *Academic/Scholarly, Abstract/Index.* **Description:** Presents abstracts of pertinent literature with commentary by leading experts in the field.
Former titles (until 1995): Year Book of Pathology and Clinical Pathology (0084-3946); (until 1942): Year Book of Pathology and Immunology (0891-3617)
Related titles: CD-ROM ed.
Indexed: Curr.Adv.Ecol.Sci.
—CISTI, GNLM.
Published by: Mosby, Inc., Continuity Division (Subsidiary of: Harcourt Health Sciences), 11830 Westline Industrial Dr, St Louis, MO 63146-3313. TEL 314-872-8370, 800-325-4177, FAX 314-432-1380, http://www.mosby.com/periodicals. Ed. Dr. Stephen S Raab.

610 CHN ISSN 1007-9742
YINGGUO YIXUE ZAZHI (ZHONGWEN BAN)/B M J (CHINESE EDITION). Text in Chinese. q. USD 11.60; USD 2.90 newsstand/cover (effective 2001). back issues avail. **Document type:** *Academic/Scholarly.*
Related titles: Online - full content ed.: (from WanFang Data Corp.); ♦ English ed.: B M J. ISSN 0959-535X; ♦ Dutch ed.: British Medical Journal (Dutch Edition); ♦ Danish ed.: British Medical Journal (Danish Edition); ♦ Polish ed.: British Medical Journal (Wydawnictwo Polskie). ISSN 1231-9775; Hungarian ed.: B M J (Magyar Kiady). ISSN 1216-7495. 1992; Greek ed.: B M J (Ellenike Ekdosis). ISSN 1106-4226. 1993; Portuguese ed.: B M J (Edicoe Portuguesa). ISSN 0873-0423. 1992.
Published by: Zhonghua Yixuehui Zazhishe, 42 Dongsi Xidajie, Beijing 100710, China. TEL 86-1-65273367, FAX 86-1-65232552, cmabmj@public.sti.ac.cn. Ed. Xin Zhi Weng. **Dist. by:** China International Book Trading Corp, 35, Chegongzhuang Xilu, Haidian District, Beijing 100044, China. TEL 86-1-68413849, FAX 86-1-68412048, cibtc@mail.cibtc.com.cn, http://www.cibtc.com.cn.

610 CHN ISSN 1002-0764
YISHI JINXIU ZAZHI/JOURNAL OF POSTGRADUATES OF MEDICINE. Text in Chinese. 1981. m. USD 30; USD 2.50 newsstand/cover (effective 2001). **Document type:** *Academic/Scholarly.*
Published by: China International Book Trading Corp/Zhongguo Guoji Tushu Maoyi Zonggongsi cibtc@mail.cibtc.com.cn, http://www.cibtc.com.cn. **Dist. by:** 35, Chegongzhuang Xilu, Haidian District, Beijing 100044, China.

610 CHN ISSN 1001-7585
YIXUE LILUN YU SHIJIAN/JOURNAL OF MEDICAL THEORY AND PRACTICE. Text in Chinese. 1988. m. CNY 30, USD 24 (effective 1999 & 2000). adv. **Document type:** *Academic/Scholarly.* **Description:** Covers the latest developments in medical science.
Published by: Hebei Langfang Diqu Yixue Qingbaozhan, PO Box 62, Langfang, Hebei 102800, China. TEL 86-316-2083206, FAX 86-316-2030445, hjlfyxll@public.lfptt.he.cn, http://www.chinamtp.com; http://www.mtp.com.cn. Ed., Pub., Adv. contact Zhong Yuhua. Circ: 5,500 (paid).

YIXUE YU ZHEXUE/MEDICINE AND PHILOSOPHY. see *PHILOSOPHY*

571.43 CHN ISSN 1004-7220
YIYONG SHENGWU LIXUE/JOURANL OF MEDICAL BIOMECHANICS. Text in Chinese. q. CNY 6 per issue domestic (effective 2000). back issues avail. **Document type:** *Academic/Scholarly.*
Related titles: Online - full content ed.: (from WanFang Data Corp.).
Published by: Zhongguo Lixue Xuehui/Chinese Mechanics Society, Zhizaoju Lu 639 Hao, Shanghai 200011, China. Ed. Kerong Dai. **Co-sponsors:** Zhongguo Shengwu Yixue Gongcheng Xuehui; Shengwu Lixue Zhuanye Weiyuanhui.

610 JPN ISSN 0044-0531
CODEN: YMBUA7
YOKOHAMA MEDICAL BULLETIN. Text in English, French, German. 1950. a. per issue exchange basis. bk.rev. bibl, charts, illus. **Document type:** *Academic/Scholarly.*
Indexed: Biol.Abstr., C.I.S. Abstr., Chem.Abstr., Chem.Indus.Notes, Chem.Titles, Excerp.Med., Helminthol.Abstr., INIS Atomind., Ind.Vet., Nutr.Abstr., Vet.Bull.
—BLDSC (9420.000000), CASDDS, CISTI, GNLM, ingenta, KNAW.
Published by: Yokohama-shiritsu Daigaku, Igakubu/Yokohama City University, School of Medicine, 3-9 Fukura, Kanazawa-ku, Yokohama-shi, Kanagawa-ken 236-0004, Japan. FAX 81-45-787-2560. Ed. Satoshi Fujiwara. Circ: 1,000.

610 611 614.8 JPN ISSN 0372-7726
CODEN: YKIGAK
YOKOHAMA MEDICAL JOURNAL. Text in Japanese; Summaries in English, French, German. 1948. bi-m. per issue exchange basis. index. **Document type:** *Academic/Scholarly.*
Indexed: Biol.Abstr., INIS Atomind., Rev.Med.& Vet.Mycol.
—BLDSC (9420.100000), CASDDS, EMDOCS, GNLM.
Published by: Yokohama-shiritsu Daigaku, Igakubu/Yokohama City University, School of Medicine, 3-9 Fukura, Kanazawa-ku, Yokohama-shi, Kanagawa-ken 236-0004, Japan. FAX 81-45-787-2560. Ed. Fukuko Tanaka. Circ: 3,500.

610 JPN ISSN 0513-5710
CODEN: YOAMAQ
YONAGO ACTA MEDICA. Text in English, Multiple languages. 1954. 3/yr. per issue exchange basis. **Document type:** *Bulletin.*
Indexed: Abstr.Hyg., Anim.Breed.Abstr., Biol.Abstr., Chem.Abstr., Chem.Indus.Notes, Curr.Cont. (coverage dropped), Dairy Sci.Abstr., Excerp.Med., Helminthol.Abstr., INIS Atomind., Ind.Med. (coverage dropped), Ind.Vet., Nutr.Abstr., Rev.Med.& Vet.Mycol., Vet.Bull.
—BLDSC (9421.000000), CASDDS, CISTI, EMDOCS, GNLM, KNAW.
Published by: Tottori Daigaku, Igakubu/Tottori University, Faculty of Medicine, 86 Nishi-cho, Yonago-shi, Tottori-ken 683-0826, Japan. TEL 81-859-34-8053, FAX 81-859-34-8079, yamed@grape.med.tottori-u.ac.jp, http://160.15.29.42/. Ed. Nobuaki Kaibara. Circ: 700.

610 JPN ISSN 0044-0558
CODEN: YOIZA3
YONAGO MEDICAL ASSOCIATION. JOURNAL/YONAGO IGAKU ZASSHI. Text in Japanese; Summaries in English, Multiple languages. 1948. bi-m. JPY 8,000 (effective 1999). adv. bk.rev. index. **Document type:** *Academic/Scholarly.*
Indexed: Chem.Abstr., Chem.Indus.Notes, Chem.Titles, INIS Atomind.
—BLDSC (4917.730000), CASDDS.
Published by: Yonago Medical Association/Yonago Igakkai, Tottori University Faculty of Medicine, 86 Nishi, Yonago 683, Japan. Ed., R&P Takao Inoue. Adv. contact T Sumida. B&W page JPY 20,000; 250 x 180. Circ: 980.

610 KOR ISSN 0513-5796
CODEN: YOMJA9
YONSEI MEDICAL JOURNAL. Text and summaries in English. 1960. bi-m. USD 60 to institutions (effective 1999). abstr, charts, illus, stat. back issues avail. *Refereed.* **Document type:** *Academic/Scholarly.*
Related titles: Diskette ed.; E-mail ed.; Fax ed.; Magnetic Tape ed.; Online - full text ed.: (from Institute for Scientific Information).
Indexed: Biol.Abstr., Chem.Abstr., Chem.Indus.Notes, Curr.Cont., Excerp.Med., Ind.Med. (1960-), Nutr.Abstr., Protozool.Abstr., Rev.Appl.Entomol., Rev.Med.& Vet.Mycol., Trop.Dis.Bull.
—BLDSC (9421.100000), CASDDS, EMDOCS, GNLM, IDS, KNAW.
Published by: Yonsei University, College of Medicine, C.P.O. Box 8044, Seoul, Korea, S.. TEL 82-2-361-5061, FAX 82-2-393-4945, ymj@yumc.yonsei.ac.kr, http://wwwyumc.yonsei.ac.kr/ymj. Ed. Kyung Il Im. Pub. Kwang Se Paik. Circ: 1,400.

610 CHN ISSN 1001-5817
YOUJIANG MINZU YIXUEYUAN XUEBAO/YOUJIANG MEDICAL COLLEGE FOR NATIONAL MINORITIES. JOURNAL. Text in Chinese. 1979. bi-m. CNY 50 foreign (effective 2001); CNY 5 newsstand/cover domestic (effective 2000). bk.rev., software rev., Website rev. abstr. 168 p./no. back issues avail. **Document type:** *Academic/Scholarly.*
Related titles: Online - full content ed.: (from WanFang Data Corp.).
Published by: Youjiang Minzu Yixueyuan, Chengxiang Lu 98 Hao, Baise, Guangxi 533000, China. TEL 86-776-2843414, FAX 86-776-2822066, yjmz@chinajournal.net.cn, http://www.chinajournal.net/yjmz.html. Ed. Bo Jiao Song.

610 CAN ISSN 0044-104X
YOUR HEALTH. Text in English. 1918. s-a. free per issue. bk.rev. charts, illus.

Published by: British Columbia Lung Association, 2675 Oak St, Vancouver, BC V6H 2K2, Canada. TEL 604-731-5864, FAX 604-731-5810. Ed. Jeff McDonald. Circ: 19,500 (controlled).

YOUR PRIVATE HEALTH OPTION. see *BUSINESS AND ECONOMICS—Investments*

640 CHN ISSN 1000-2723
YUNNAN ZHONGYI XUEYUAN XUEBAO/YUNNAN COLLEGE OF TRADITIONAL CHINESE MEDICINE. JOURNAL. Text in Chinese. 1978. q. CNY 3 per issue domestic (effective 2000). back issues avail. **Document type:** *Academic/Scholarly.*
Related titles: Online - full content ed.: (from WanFang Data Corp.).
Published by: Yunnan Zhongyi Xueyuan, Guanshan Shuangqiao Lu, Kunming 650200, China. Ed. Feng Sheng Ma.

YUNNAN ZHONGYI ZAZHI/YUNNAN JOURNAL OF TRADITIONAL CHINESE MEDICINE. see *ALTERNATIVE MEDICINE*

610 CHN ISSN 1006-9674
YUNYANG YIXUEYUAN XUEBAO/YUNYANG MEDICAL COLLEGE. JOURNAL. Text in Chinese. q. CNY 5 per issue domestic (effective 2000). back issues avail. **Document type:** *Academic/Scholarly.*
Related titles: Online - full content ed.: (from WanFang Data Corp.).
Published by: Yunyang Yixueyuan, Remin Nan Lu 25 Hao, Xi'an, Hubei 442000, China. TEL 86-719-8891120. Ed. Gui Yuan Yang.

610 RUS
ZABOLEVANIYA, PEREDAVAEMYE POLOVYM PUTEM. Text in Russian. 1994. bi-m. USD 129 in United States (effective 2000).
Published by: Bioinformservis, Ul Vavilova 40, Moscow 117333, Russian Federation. **Dist. by:** East View Publications, 3020 Harbor Ln N, Minneapolis, MN 55447. TEL 763-550-0961, FAX 763-559-2931.

617.22 POL ISSN 1428-1287
ZAKAZENIA. Text in Polish. 1997. q. PLZ 28 (effective 2000).
Published by: (Polskie Towarzystwo Zakazen Sztitalnych), Medycyna Praktyczna, Ul Skawinska 8, Krakow 31066, Poland. TEL 48-12-4305520, FAX 48-12-4305536, listy@mp.pl, http://mp.pl/czasop.htm. Ed. Piotr B Heczko.

610 SVN ISSN 1318-0347
CODEN: ZDVEEB
ZDRAVNISKI VESTNIK; journal of slovene medical association. Text in Slovenian; Summaries in English. 1929. m., latest vol.69. SIT 12,000, USD 110 (effective 2001). adv. bk.rev. **Document type:** *Journal, Academic/Scholarly.*
Formerly: Zdravstveni Vestnik (0350-0063)
Indexed: Biol.Abstr., Curr.Cont. (coverage dropped), Excerp.Med.
—BLDSC (9438.790000), CISTI, EMDOCS, GNLM.
Published by: Slovensko Zdravnisko Drustvo/Slovene Medical Association, Komenskega 4, Ljubljana 1000, Slovenia. TEL 386-1-2317868, FAX 386-1-2301955, katarina.jovanovic@guest.arnes.si, http://vestnik.szd.si/. Eds. Dr. Joze Drinovec, Martin Janko. R&P Dr. Joze Drinovec. Circ: 4,100. **Co-sponsors:** Ministrstvo za Zdravje, Zavod za Zdravstveno Zavarovanje R Slovenije/Ministry of Health; Ministrstvo za Solstvo, Znanost in Sport/Ministry of Education, Science and Sport of the Republic of Slovenia.

610 DEU ISSN 1431-7621
ZEITSCHRIFT FUER AERZTLICHE FORTBILDUNG UND QUALITAETSSICHERUNG. Text in German. 1904. 10/yr. EUR 142 (effective 2002). adv. bk.rev. abstr, bibl, charts, illus. index. reprint service avail. from ISI. *Refereed.* **Document type:** *Journal, Academic/Scholarly.*
Formerly (until 1997): Zeitschrift fuer Aerztliche Fortbildung (0044-2178)
Related titles: Online - full text ed.
Indexed: Biol.Abstr., C.I.S. Abstr., Chem.Abstr., Dent.Ind., Excerp.Med., INIS Atomind., Ind.Med. (1997-), Inpharma, Int.Nurs.Ind., Reac.
—BLDSC (9452.825000), CISTI, GNLM, Infotrieve, KNAW. **CCC.**
Published by: Urban & Fischer Verlag, Loebdergraben 14A, Jena 07743, Germany. TEL 49-3641-626444, FAX 49-3641-626500, info@urbanfischer.de, http://www.urbanfischer.de. Ed. Dr. G Ollenschlaeger. R&P Martin Huber TEL 49-3641-626430. Adv. contact Sabine Schroeter. page DEM 1,800; trim 280 x 210. Circ: 1,400.

610 DEU ISSN 1433-6251
ZEITSCHRIFT FUER ALLGEMEINMEDIZIN. AUSGABE A. Text in German. 1987. m. EUR 81.90 domestic to institutions; EUR 112.90 in Europe to institutions; EUR 120 elsewhere to institutions; EUR 7.90 newsstand/cover (effective 2002). adv. bk.rev. bibl, charts, illus. index. **Document type:** *Journal, Academic/Scholarly.*
Supersedes in part (1925-1987): Z F A - Zeitschrift fuer Allgemeinmedizin (0341-9835); Which was formerly (until 1976): Zeitschrift fuer Allgemeinmedizin (0300-8673); (until 1969): Landarzt (0023-7728)
Indexed: Dent.Ind., Excerp.Med., INIS Atomind., Ind.Med. (coverage dropped), Nutr.Abstr.
—CISTI, EMDOCS, GNLM, Infotrieve, KNAW. **CCC.**
Published by: (Vereinigung der Hochschullehrer und Lehrbeauftragten fuer Allgemeinmedizin), Hippokrates Verlag GmbH, Postfach 300504, Stuttgart 70445, Germany. TEL 49-711-8931-0, FAX 49-711-8931453, kunden.service@thieme.de, http://www.hippokrates.de. Circ: 45,000.

610 DEU ISSN 0937-6801
ZEITSCHRIFT FUER ALLGEMEINMEDIZIN. AUSGABE B. Text in German. 1987. m. EUR 141.90 domestic to institutions; EUR 172.90 in Europe to institutions; EUR 180 elsewhere to institutions; EUR 58 to students; EUR 15.80 newsstand/cover (effective 2002). **Document type:** *Journal, Academic/Scholarly.*
Supersedes in part (1925-1987): Z F A - Zeitschrift fuer Allgemeinmedizin (0341-9835); Which was formerly (until 1976): Zeitschrift fuer Allgemeinmedizin (0300-8673); (until 1969): Landarzt (0023-7728)
Published by: Hippokrates Verlag GmbH, Postfach 300504, Stuttgart 70445, Germany. TEL 49-711-8931-0, FAX 49-711-8931706, kunden.service@thieme.de, http://www.hippokrates.de.

610 DEU ISSN 1434-4203
ZEITSCHRIFT FUER ALLGEMEINMEDIZIN. AUSGABE C. Text in German. 1987. m. EUR 141.90 domestic to institutions; EUR 172 in Europe to institutions; EUR 180 elsewhere to institutions; EUR 58 to students (effective 2002). **Document type:** *Journal, Academic/Scholarly.*
Supersedes in part (1925-1987): Z F A - Zeitschrift fuer Allgemeinmedizin (0341-9835); Which was formerly (until 1976): Zeitschrift fuer Allgemeinmedizin (0300-8673); (until 1969): Landarzt (0023-7728)
Published by: Hippokrates Verlag GmbH, Postfach 300504, Stuttgart 70445, Germany. TEL 49-711-8931-0, FAX 49-711-8931706, kunden.service@thieme.de, http://www.hippokrates.de.

ZEITSCHRIFT FUER AUDIOLOGIE/AUDIOLOGICAL ACOUSTICS. see *PHYSICS—Sound*

610 170 DEU ISSN 0944-7652
ZEITSCHRIFT FUER MEDIZINISCHE ETHIK. Abbreviated title: Z M E. Text in German. 1954. q. DEM 89 (effective 2001). adv. bk.rev. abstr. **Document type:** *Journal, Academic/Scholarly.*
Formerly (until 1992): Arzt und Christ (0403-3884)
Indexed: IBZ, Ind.Philos.
—GNLM.
Published by: Schwabenverlag AG, Senefelderstr 12, Ostfildern 73760, Germany. TEL 49-711-4406160, FAX 49-711-4406177, zme@schwabenverlag.de, buchverlag@schwabenverlag.de, http://www.schwabenverlag.de. Adv. contact Sabrina Reusch TEL 49-711-4406168.

ZEITSCHRIFT FUER NATURHEILKUNDE. see *ALTERNATIVE MEDICINE*

610 DEU ISSN 1615-2921
▼ **ZEITSCHRIFT FUER PALLIATIVMEDIZIN.** Text in German. 2000. q. EUR 62.80 domestic to institutions; EUR 65.90 in Europe to institutions; EUR 69.50 elsewhere to institutions; EUR 39 to students; EUR 17 newsstand/cover (effective 2002). **Document type:** *Journal, Academic/Scholarly.*
Published by: Georg Thieme Verlag, Ruedigerstr 14, Stuttgart 70469, Germany. TEL 49-711-8931-0, FAX 49-711-8931298, kunden.service@thieme.de, http://www.thieme.de/palliativmedizin/index.html.

615.321 DEU ISSN 0722-348X
CODEN: ZPHYDG
ZEITSCHRIFT FUER PHYTOTHERAPIE. Text in German; Summaries in English. 1979. bi-m. EUR 70.90 domestic to institutions; EUR 76.90 in Europe to institutions; EUR 78.90 elsewhere to institutions; EUR 32 to students; EUR 14.90 newsstand/cover (effective 2002). adv. bk.rev. illus, charts, abstr. 52 p./no. 3 cols./p. back issues avail. **Document type:** *Journal, Academic/Scholarly.*
Indexed: Agri.Eng.Abstr., Hort.Abstr., Plant Breed.Abstr., Plant Gen.Res.Abstr., Rev.Arom.& Med.Plants, Rev.Plant Path., Trop.Dis.Bull., World Ag.Econ.& Rur.Soc.Abstr.
—BLDSC (9484.130000), CASDDS, EMDOCS, GNLM, Infotrieve, KNAW. **CCC.**
Published by: (Gesellschaft fuer Phytotherapie e.V.), Hippokrates Verlag GmbH, Postfach 300504, Stuttgart 70445, Germany. TEL 49-711-8931-0, FAX 49-711-8931706, http://www.hippokrates.de. Ed. Hanno Kretschmer. Adv. contact Guenter Fecke TEL 49-711-8931714. Circ: 6,000.

610 155.3 DEU ISSN 0932-8114
HQ21
ZEITSCHRIFT FUER SEXUALFORSCHUNG. Text in German. 1988. q. EUR 92.30 domestic to institutions; EUR 93.90 in Europe to institutions; EUR 98.60 elsewhere to institutions; EUR 28 newsstand/cover (effective 2002). adv. reprint service avail. from IRC. **Document type:** *Academic/Scholarly.*
Related titles: Online - full text ed.: ISSN 1438-9460.
Indexed: Abstr.Anthropol., IBR, Intl.Bibl.Soc.Sci., Lang.& Lang.Behav.Abstr., PsycInfo, Psychol.Abstr. (1988-), SOPODA, Soc.Serv.Abstr., Sociol.Abstr., Stud.Wom.Abstr., e-psyche.
—GNLM, Infotrieve. **CCC.**
Published by: (Deutsche Gesellschaft fuer Sexualforschung), Georg Thieme Verlag, Ruedigerstr 14, Stuttgart 70469, Germany. TEL 49-711-8931-0, FAX 49-711-8931298, kunden.service@thieme.de, http://www.thieme.de.

610 DEU ISSN 0942-6086
ZENTRALSTERILISATION - CENTRAL SERVICE; international journal of processing and sterile supply. Text in English, German. 1993. bi-m. DEM 91.25 domestic; DEM 99.95 in Europe; DEM 120.36 elsewhere (effective 2001). adv. bk.rev., Website rev. 72 p./no. 3 cols./p. back issues avail.; reprints avail. *Refereed.* **Document type:** *Journal, Academic/Scholarly.*
—GNLM.
Published by: M H P Verlag GmbH, Ostring 13, Wiesbaden 65205, Germany. TEL 49-6122-7709131, FAX 49-6122-7709101, zentrsteril@mhp-verlag.de, http://www.mhp-verlag.de. Ed. P Heeg. R&P Dr. Gudrun Droop TEL 49-6122-7709135. Adv. contact W Bockemuehl TEL 49-6122-7709132. B&W page DEM 3,195. Circ: 3,800.

610 CHN ISSN 1008-9292
ZHEJIANG DAXUE XUEBAO (YIXUE BAN)/ZHEJIANG UNIVERSITY. JOURNAL (MEDICAL SCIENCES EDITION). Text in Chinese. 1958. bi-m. **Document type:** *Journal, Academic/Scholarly.*
Published by: Zhejiang Daxue, Zheda Lu 38, Hangzhou, Zhejiang 310027, China. TEL 86-571-87952244.

610 CHN ISSN 1008-7664
▼ **ZHEJIANG LINCHUANG YIXUE/ZHEJIANG CLINICAL MEDICAL JOURNAL.** Text in Chinese. 1999. bi-m. CNY 4 per issue domestic (effective 2000). back issues avail. **Document type:** *Academic/Scholarly.*
Related titles: Online - full content ed.: (from WanFang Data Corp.).
Published by: Zhejiang Zhongyi Xueyuan/Zhejiang Traditional Chinese Medical College, Wen 2 Lu 218 Hao 4 Lou, Hangzhou, Zhejiang 310012, China. TEL 86-571-8860070, FAX 86-571-8860070. Ed. Shuyou Ping.

610 CHN ISSN 1000-1743
CODEN: ZYDXDM
ZHEJIANG YIKE DAXUE XUEBAO/ZHEJIANG MEDICAL UNIVERSITY. JOURNAL. Text in Chinese; Summaries in English. 1958. bi-m. USD 18. adv. bibl, illus. **Document type:** *Academic/Scholarly.* **Description:** Covers clinical medicine, preventive medicine, biomedical science and pharmacy.
Indexed: Chem.Abstr., INIS Atomind.
—CASDDS.

Published by: (Xuebao Bianjibu), Zhejiang Yike Daxue/Zhejiang Medical University, Population Research Institute, 353 Yan'an Lu, Hangzhou, Zhejiang 310006, China. TEL 86-571-7217073, FAX 86-571-7217044. Ed. Chen Zhaodian. Adv. contact Zhang Rongian. B&W page USD 500. Circ: 5,000.

610 CHN ISSN 1007-0931
ZHEJIANG YUFANG YIXUE. Text in Chinese. m. CNY 3.50 per issue domestic (effective 2000). back issues avail. **Document type:** *Academic/Scholarly.*
Related titles: Online - full content ed.: (from WanFang Data Corp.).
Published by: Zhejiang Yufang Yixue Zazhishe, Laozhe Dazhi Lu 17 Hao, Hangzhou 310009, China. TEL 86-571-7046224. Ed. Shao Cong Zhou.

610 CHN ISSN 1005-4561
ZHEJIANG ZHONGXIYI JIEHE ZAZHI/ZHEJIANG JOURNAL OF INTEGRATED TRADITIONAL CHINESE AND WESTERN MEDICINE. Text in Chinese. m. CNY 3 per issue domestic (effective 2000). back issues avail. **Document type:** *Academic/Scholarly.*
Related titles: Online - full content ed.: (from WanFang Data Corp.).
Published by: Zhejiang Zhongxiyi Jiehe Zazhi Bianji Weiyuanhui, Huancheng Dong Lu 38 Hao, Hangzhou 310003, China. Ed. Jianjin Zhang. **Co-sponsors:** Zhejiang-sheng Weishangting; Zhejiang-sheng Zhongxiyi Jiehe Xuehui; Zhejiang-sheng Zhongxiyi Jiehe Yiyuan.

615.89 615.328 CHN ISSN 1005-5509
ZHEJIANG ZHONGYI XUEYUAN XUEBAO/ZHEJIANG COLLEGE OF TRADITIONAL CHINESE MEDICINE. JOURNAL. Text in Chinese. 1977. bi-m. USD 3 per issue.
—BLDSC (4918.150010).
Published by: Zhejiang Zhongyi Xueyuan/Zhejiang Traditional Chinese Medical College, Zhejiang, China. TEL 86-571-7044418. Ed. Xiao Luwei. **Dist. by:** China International Book Trading Corp, 35 Chegongzhuang Xilu, Haidian District, Beijing 100044, China. TEL 86-10-68411769, FAX 86-10-68420340, bk@mail.cibtc.com.cn, http://www.cibtc.com.cn/.

ZHEJIANG ZHONGYI ZAZHI/ZHEJIANG JOURNAL OF TRADITIONAL CHINESE MEDICINE. see *ALTERNATIVE MEDICINE*

610 CHN ISSN 1000-6486
ZHIYE YIXUE/OCCUPATIONAL MEDICINE. Text in Chinese. 1978. bi-m. USD 20. adv.
Indexed: INIS Atomind.
Published by: Huanan Qu Laodong Weisheng Zhiyebing Fangzhi Zhongxin/South China Centre of Occupational Health, No 78, Yile Rd, Guangzhou, Guangdong 510260, China. TEL 86-20-4448002. Ed. Tan Bingde. Pub. He Yiping. Adv. contact Chen Zhong Yi.

ZHONG CAO YAO/CHINESE HERBAL MEDICINE. see *PHARMACY AND PHARMACOLOGY*

610 100 NLD ISSN 1386-6354
ZHONG WAI YI XUE ZHE ZUE/CHINESE AND INTERNATIONAL PHILOSOPHY OF MEDICINE. Text in Chinese. 1998. q., latest vol.4, 2001. NLG 123, USD 65 to individuals; NLG 186, USD 99 to institutions (effective 2001). illus. back issues avail. *Refereed.* **Document type:** *Journal, Academic/Scholarly.*
Published by: Swets & Zeitlinger BV, PO Box 825, Lisse 2160 SZ, Netherlands. http://www.szp.swets.nl. **Dist. in N. America by:** Swets & Zeitlinger, PO Box 582, Downingtown, PA 19335-998. TEL 800-447-9387.

615.321 CHN ISSN 0253-2670
ZHONGCAOYAO/CHINESE TRADITIONAL AND HERBAL DRUGS. Text in Chinese. 1970. m. CNY 12.80 per issue domestic (effective 2000). back issues avail. **Document type:** *Academic/Scholarly.*
Related titles: Online - full content ed.: (from WanFang Data Corp.).
Indexed: I.P.A., Mass Spectr.Bull.
—BLDSC (3181.122300), Linda Hall.
Published by: Guojia Yaoping Jiandu Guanli Ju, Nankai-qu, Anshan Xi Dao 308 Hao, Tianjin 300193, China. TEL 86-22-27474913. Ed. Ronghai Nie. **Co-sponsors:** Zhongcaoyao Xinxi Zhongxinzhan; Tianjian Yaowu Yanjiuyuan.

616.13 CHN ISSN 1007-3949
ZHONGGOU DONGMAI YINGHUA ZAZHI/CHINESE JOURNAL OF ARTERIOSCLEROSIS. Text in Chinese. 1993. q. USD 18; CNY 8, USD 4.50 newsstand/cover (effective 2001). back issues avail. **Document type:** *Academic/Scholarly.*
Related titles: Online - full content ed.: (from WanFang Data Corp.).
—BLDSC (3180.295220).
Published by: Hengyang Yixueyuan, Hengyang, Hunan 421001, China. TEL 86-734-8281289. Ed. Bili Hu. **Dist. by:** China International Book Trading Corp, 35, Chegongzhuang Xilu, Haidian District, Beijing 100044, China. TEL 86-1-68413849, FAX 86-1-68412048, cibtc@mail.cibtc.com.cn, http://www.cibtc.com.cn.

610 CHN ISSN 1000-4718
CODEN: ZBSZEB
ZHONGGUO BINGLI SHENGLI ZAZHI/CHINESE JOURNAL OF PATHOPHYSIOLOGY. Text in Chinese, English. 1985. m. CNY 6 per issue domestic; USD 20 (effective 2000). adv. *Refereed.* **Document type:** *Academic/Scholarly.* **Description:** Publishes research papers, short communications, reviews and experimental techniques in the field of clinical and experimental pathophysiology.
Related titles: Online - full content ed.: (from WanFang Data Corp.).
Indexed: Apic.Abstr., Chem.Abstr., Chem.Indus.Notes, Chem.Titles.
—CASDDS.
Published by: Zhongguo Bingli Shengli Xuehui/Chinese Pathophysiological Society, Jinan University, Shipai, Guangzhou, Guangdong 510632, China. TEL 86-20-85220269, FAX 86-20-85221941, lbszb@jnu.edu.cn. Ed. Chujie Li. Pub. Qun Cai. Adv. contact Yi Cao.

610 CHN ISSN 1001-568X
ZHONGGUO CHUJI WEISHENG BAOJIAN/CHINESE PRIMARY HEALTH CARE. Text in Chinese. m. CNY 3.80 per issue domestic (effective 2000).
Related titles: Online - full content ed.: (from WanFang Data Corp.).
Published by: Zhongguo Chuji Weisheng Baojian Zazhishe, Xiangfang-qu, Xiangshun Jie 41 Hao, Ha'erbin 150036, China. TEL 86-451-5664637, 86-451-5664683. Ed. Shiming Li.

610 CHN ISSN 1001-1889
ZHONGGUO DIFANGBING FANGZHI ZAZHI/CHINESE JOURNAL OF CONTROL OF ENDEMIC DISEASES. Text in Chinese. 1987. bi-m. CNY 21.60; CNY 3.60 newsstand/cover (effective 1999). adv. **Document type:** *Academic/Scholarly, Government.* **Description:** Focuses on seven endemic diseases - Keshan disease, keshin-beck disease, iodine deficiency disorders, plague, brucellosis, endemic fluorosis and endemic arsenic poisoning.
Published by: Institute for Endemic Disease Control and Research, 23 Chongqing Jie, Jilin 132001, China. TEL 86-432-2456645. Ed. Wang Zhao. R&P Yukun Wang. Adv. contact Huixin Chen. Circ: 4,000 (paid). **Dist. overseas by:** China International Book Trading Corp, 35 Chegongzhuang Xilu, Haidian District, Beijing 100044, China.

362.1 CHN ISSN 1000-4955
ZHONGGUO DIFANGBINGXUE ZAZHI/CHINESE JOURNAL OF ENDEMIOLOGY. Text in Chinese. 1982. bi-m. CNY 6 per issue domestic (effective 2000). back issues avail. **Document type:** *Academic/Scholarly.*
Published by: Ha'erbin Yike Daxue, Nangang-qu, Baojian Lu 159 Hao, Ha'erbin 150086 , China. TEL 86-451-6675924. Ed. Jian Bo Yang. **Co-sponsor:** Zhonghua Yixuehui, Difangbing Xuehui.

ZHONGGUO DONGWU JIANYI/CHINESE JOURNAL OF ANIMAL QUARANTINE. see *VETERINARY SCIENCE*

ZHONGGUO GONGYE YIXUE ZAZHI/CHINESE JOURNAL OF INDUSTRIAL MEDICINE. see *OCCUPATIONAL HEALTH AND SAFETY*

617.05 CHN ISSN 1003-9430
ZHONGGUO JIGUANG YIXUE ZAZHI/CHINESE JOURNAL OF LASER MEDICINE & SURGERY. Text in Chinese. 1992. q. USD 20.80; USD 5.20 newsstand/cover (effective 2001). **Document type:** *Academic/Scholarly.*
Related titles: Online - full content ed.: (from WanFang Data Corp.).
Published by: Zhongguo Guangxue Xuehui, PO Box 800-211, Shanghai 201800 , China. **Dist. by:** China International Book Trading Corp, 35, Chegongzhuang Xilu, Haidian District, Beijing 100044, China. TEL 86-1-68413849, FAX 86-1-68412048, cibtc@mail.cibtc.com.cn, http://www.cibtc.com.cn.

610 CHN ISSN 1002-1949
ZHONGGUO JIJIU YIXUE/CHINESE JOURNAL OF CRITICAL CARE MEDICINE. Text in Chinese; Abstracts in English. 1981. m. USD 32.40; CNY 4.90, USD 2.70 newsstand/cover (effective 2001). adv. *Refereed.* **Document type:** *Academic/Scholarly.* **Description:** Covers the latest developments in all areas related to critical care medicine. Contains papers on operative procedures, clinical or laboratory case reports, and more.
Related titles: CD-ROM ed.; Online - full content ed.: (from WanFang Data Corp.).
Published by: Heilongjiang Sheng Keji Qingbaosuo/Heilongjiang Institute of Science and Technology Information, 74 Yinhang St, Nangang-qu, Harbin, Heilongjiang 150001, China. TEL 86-451-3643877, FAX 86-451-3643877. Ed., Adv. contact Tan Qiao. Circ: 13,000 (paid); 1,000 (controlled). **Dist. overseas by:** China International Book Trading Corp, 35, Chegongzhuang Xilu, Haidian District, Beijing 100044, China. TEL 86-1-68413849, FAX 86-1-68412048, cibtc@mail.cibtc.com.cn, http://www.cibtc.com.cn.

610 CHN ISSN 1001-1242
ZHONGGUO KANGFU YIXUE ZAZHI/CHINESE JOURNAL OF REHABILITATION MEDICINE. Text in Chinese; Abstracts in English. 1986. bi-m. USD 25.20; CNY 7, USD 4.20 newsstand/cover (effective 2001). adv. *Refereed.* **Document type:** *Academic/Scholarly.* **Description:** Publishes original articles that deal with fundamental and clinical research in the fields of physical therapy, occupational therapy, speech therapy, rehabilitation engineering, and rehabilitation medicine and education.
Related titles: CD-ROM ed.; Online - full content ed.: (from WanFang Data Corp.).
Published by: Zhongguo Kangfu Yixuehui/Chinese Association of Rehabilitation Medicine, Zhongri Youhao Yiyuan, Yinghuayuan East St, Beijing 100029, China. TEL 86-10-6420-6649, FAX 86-10-6421-7749, rehabi@public.sti.ac.cn, http://www.chinainfo.gov.cn/periodical. Ed. Fuzhen Liu. R&P, Adv. contact Shuangjuan Wang. **Dist. by:** China International Book Trading Corp, 35, Chegongzhuang Xilu, Haidian District, Beijing 100044, China. TEL 86-1-68413849, FAX 86-1-68412048, cibtc@mail.cibtc.com.cn, http://www.cibtc.com.cn.

610 CHN ISSN 1000-629X
ZHONGGUO MAFENG ZAZHI/CHINESE JOURNAL OF LEPROSY. Text in Chinese. 1985. q. USD 16. adv. bk.rev. **Document type:** *Academic/Scholarly.*
Published by: Zhongguo Mafeng Fangzhi Xiehui/China Leprosy Association, 87 Hengfu Rd, Guangzhou, Guangdong 510095, China. TEL 020-3584472. Ed., R&P Xiding Zhao. Adv. contact Xuefen Ma. Circ: 3,000.

610 CHN
ZHONGGUO MINZU MINJIAN YIXUE ZAZHI/CHINESE JOURNAL OF ETHNOMEDICINE AND ETHNOPHARMACY. Text in Chinese. bi-m. USD 17.40; USD 2.90 newsstand/cover (effective 2001). **Document type:** *Academic/Scholarly.*
Published by: China International Book Trading Corp/Zhongguo Guoji Tushu Maoyi Zonggongsi cibtc@mail.cibtc.com.cn, http://www.cibtc.com.cn. **Dist. by:** 35, Chegongzhuang Xilu, Haidian District, Beijing 100044, China.

630 CHN
ZHONGGUO NONGCUN YIXUE/MEDICAL SCIENCE IN RURAL CHINA. Text in Chinese. m. USD 2.50. adv. **Document type:** *Academic/Scholarly.*
Published by: Renmin Weisheng Chubanshe, 10 Tiantan Xili, Beijing 100050, China. TEL 7015802. Ed. Ji Fang. Adv. contact Xia Zemin. Circ: 150,000.

610.285 CHN ISSN 0258-8021
R856.A1 CODEN: ZSYXEI
ZHONGGUO SHENGWU YIXUE GONGCHENG XUEBAO/CHINESE JOURNAL OF BIOMEDICAL ENGINEERING. Text in Chinese, English. 1982. q. USD 24; USD 30.70 foreign. adv. **Document type:** *Academic/Scholarly.* **Description:** Covers biomechanics, artificial organs, biomedical materials, biocybernetics, and mass transfers.
Indexed: Bioeng.Abstr., Chem.Indus.Notes, Chem.Titles, Comput.& Info.Sys., Eng.Ind., Excerp.Med., INSPEC (Jun.1985-).
—BLDSC (3180.296500), AskIEEE, CASDDS, CISTI, EMDOCS.

M

Published by: Chinese Society of Biomedical Engineering, 9 Dond Dan San Tiao, Beijing 100730, China. TEL 86-10-6529-5930, FAX 86-10-6512-4876. Ed., R&P Guanglu Zhao. Pub. Guexiang Liu. Adv. contact Lili Yang. **Co-sponsor:** Chinese Academy of Medical Sciences/Zhongguo Yixue Kexueyuan.

610 CHN
RD1
ZHONGGUO WEISHENG NIANJIAN/YEAR BOOK: HEALTH CARE IN CHINA. Text in Chinese, English. 1983. a. USD 47.
Formerly: Zhongguo Waike Nianjian (1002-0136)
Published by: Renmin Weisheng Chubanshe, 10 Tiantan Xili, Beijing 100050, China. Circ: 5,000.

610 CHN ISSN 1003-0603
ZHONGGUO WEIZHONGBING JIJIU YIXUE/CHINESE CRITICAL CARE MEDICINE. Text in Chinese. 1989. m. CNY 46.80. adv. **Document type:** *Monographic series.* **Description:** Covers new advances in critical care medicine, including experimental research and clinical research.
Formerly (until 1991): Weizhongbing Jijiu Yixue - Critical Care Medicine
Published by: Tianjin Weisheng Ju, c/o Tian He Hospital, 122 Mu Nan Rd, Tianjin 300050, China. TEL 86-22-334-9935. Ed. Chinta Wang. R&P Chinda Wang. Adv. contact Yinping Li. page USD 500. **Dist. overseas by:** China International Book Trading Corp, 35 Chegongzhuang Xilu, Haidian District, Beijing 100044, China.

630 CHN
ZHONGGUO XIANGCUN YISHENG/CHINESE RURAL DOCTORS. Text in Chinese. m.
Published by: Jilin Kexue Jishu Chubanshe/Jilin Science and Technology Publishers, 102 Stalin St, Changchun, Jilin 130021, China. TEL 884778. Ed. Shan Shujian.

610 CHN ISSN 1001-7658
CODEN: ZXZAFO
ZHONGGUO XIAODUXUE ZAZHI/CHINESE JOURNAL OF DISINFECTION SCIENCE. Text in Chinese. 1984. q. USD 11.60; USD 2.90 newsstand/cover (effective 2001). adv. bk.rev. *Refereed.* **Document type:** *Academic/Scholarly.* **Description:** Reports research achievements in area of disinfection sterilization in China, including mechanism of germicidal action, experimental techniques, administration and monitoring.
Formerly (until 1990): Disinfection and Sterilization
Indexed: Chem.Abstr., Chem.Indus.Notes, Chem.Titles.
—CASDDS.
Published by: Zhonghua Yufang Yixuehui (Fengtai)/China Preventive Medical Society (Fengtai), 20 Dongdajie, Fengtai, Beijing 100071, China. TEL 86-1-6688-8229, FAX 86-1-6688-8229. Ed. Yujing Liu. R&P Chaosen Yuan. Adv. contact Zhongtian Gao. Circ: 6,000. **Dist. outside China by:** China International Book Trading Corp, 35, Chegongzhuang Xilu, Haidian District, Beijing 100044, China. TEL 86-1-68413849, FAX 86-1-68412048, cibtc@mail.cibtc.com.cn, http://www.cibtc.com.cn.

ZHONGGUO XINYAO YU LINCHUANG ZAZHI/CHINESE JOURNAL OF NEW DRUGS AND CLINICAL REMEDIES. see *PHARMACY AND PHARMACOLOGY*

610 CHN
ZHONGGUO YIKAN/INTERMEDIATE MEDICAL JOURNAL. Text in Chinese. m. USD 32.40; USD 2.70 newsstand/cover (effective 2000). **Document type:** *Academic/Scholarly.*
Related titles: Online - full content ed.: (from WanFang Data Corp.).
Published by: Renmin Weisheng Chubanshe, 10 Tiantan Xili, Beijing 100050, China. **Dist. by:** China International Book Trading Corp, 35, Chegongzhuang Xilu, Haidian District, Beijing 100044, China. TEL 86-1-68413849, FAX 86-1-68412048, cibtc@mail.cibtc.com.cn, http://www.cibtc.com.cn.

610 CHN ISSN 0258-4646
ZHONGGUO YIKE DAXUE XUEBAO/CHINA MEDICAL UNIVERSITY. JOURNAL. Text in English. 1982. bi-m. **Document type:** *Academic/Scholarly.*
—BLDSC (4729.218900).
Published by: Zhongguo Yike Daxue/Chinese University of Medical Sciences, 6, Sanhao Jie 1 Duan, Heping-qu, Shenyang, Liaoning 393501, China. **Dist. by:** China International Book Trading Corp, 35, Chegongzhuang Xilu, Haidian District, Beijing 100044, China. TEL 86-1-68413849, FAX 86-1-68412048, cibtc@mail.cibtc.com.cn, http://www.cibtc.com.cn.

610 CHN ISSN 1000-503X
CODEN: CIHPDR
ZHONGGUO YIXUE KEXUEYUAN XUEBAO/ACTA ACADEMIAE MEDICINAE SINICA. Text in Chinese. bi-m. USD 37.80; USD 6.30 newsstand/cover (effective 2001). bk.rev. abstr. *Refereed.* **Document type:** *Academic/Scholarly.* **Description:** Contains original articles, brief reports review articles, editorials, techniques and methods, experience communications, and case reports.
Related titles: CD-ROM ed.; Online - full content ed.: (from WanFang Data Corp.).
Indexed: Chem.Abstr., Chem.Indus.Notes, Chem.Titles, ExtraMED, Helminthol.Abstr., INIS Atomind., Ind.Med. (1979-).
—BLDSC (0579.723200), CASDDS, GNLM.
Published by: (Chinese Academy of Medical Sciences/Zhongguo Yixue Kexueyuan), China International Book Trading Corp/Zhongguo Guoji Tushu Maoyi Zonggongsi, 35 Chegongzhuang Xilu, Haidian District, Beijing 100044, China. Ed. Bao Denian.

610 CHN
ZHONGGUO YIXUE LUNTAN BAO/CHINA MEDICAL TRIBUNE. Text in Chinese. w. CNY 7.56. **Document type:** *Newspaper, Academic/Scholarly.*
Published by: China International Book Trading Corp/Zhongguo Guoji Tushu Maoyi Zonggongsi cibtc@mail.cibtc.com.cn, http://www.cibtc.com.cn. **Dist. by:** 35, Chegongzhuang Xilu, Haidian District, Beijing 100044, China.

610 CHN
ZHONGGUO YIYUE BAO/CHINESE MEDICINE INFORMATION NEWS. Text in Chinese. 4/w. CNY 78.84. **Document type:** *Newspaper.*
Published by: China International Book Trading Corp/Zhongguo Guoji Tushu Maoyi Zonggongsi cibtc@mail.cibtc.com.cn, http://www.cibtc.com.cn. **Dist. by:** 35, Chegongzhuang Xilu, Haidian District, Beijing 100044, China.

ZHONGGUO ZHENJIU/CHINESE ACUPUNCTURE AND MOXIBUSTION. see *ALTERNATIVE MEDICINE*

610 CHN
ZHONGGUO ZHONGUIYAO BAO/JOURNAL OF CHINESE TRADITIONAL MEDICINE. Text in Chinese. 3/w. CNY 29.52. **Document type:** *Newsletter, Academic/Scholarly.*
Published by: China International Book Trading Corp/Zhongguo Guoji Tushu Maoyi Zonggongsi cibtc@mail.cibtc.com.cn, http://www.cibtc.com.cn. **Dist. by:** 35, Chegongzhuang Xilu, Haidian District, Beijing 100044, China.

615.89 CHN ISSN 1003-5370
R97.7.C5
ZHONGGUO ZHONGXIYI JIEHE ZAZHI. Text in Chinese. 1981. m. USD 43.20; USD 3.60 newsstand/cover (effective 2001).
Formerly (until 1991): Zhong-Xiyi Jiehe Zazhi/Chinese Journal of Modern Developments in Traditional Medicine (0254-9034)
Related titles: Online - full content ed.: (from WanFang Data Corp.); ♦ English ed.: Chinese Journal of Integrated Traditional and Western Medicine. ISSN 1006-6497.
Indexed: Dent.Ind., Ind.Med. (1992-).
—BLDSC (3180.358000), GNLM.
Published by: (Zhongyi Yanjiuyuan/Academy of Traditional Chinese Medicine, Zhongguo Zhong-Xiyi Jiehe Yanjiuhui/Chinese Association of the Integration of Traditional and Western Medicine), China International Book Trading Corp/Zhongguo Guoji Tushu Maoyi Zonggongsi cibtc@mail.cibtc.com.cn, http://www.cibtc.com.cn. Ed. Keji Chen. Circ: 28,000 (paid); 500 (controlled). **Dist. by:** 35, Chegongzhuang Xilu, Haidian District, Beijing 100044, China.

610 CHN ISSN 1006-3250
ZHONGGUO ZHONGYI JICHU YIXUE ZAZHI. Text in Chinese. 1995. m. CNY 72 domestic; USD 50.40 foreign; CNY 6 newsstand/cover domestic; USD 4.20 newsstand/cover foreign (effective 2001). **Document type:** *Academic/Scholarly.*
Related titles: Online - full content ed.: (from WanFang Data Corp.).
Published by: Zhongguo Zhongyi Yanjiuyuan, Jichu Lilun, 18 Bei Xincang, Dongzhimen Nei, Beijing 100070, China. TEL 86-1-64014411 ext 2511, 2525, FAX 86-1-64013896. Ed. Qing-Yun Meng. **Dist. by:** China International Book Trading Corp, 35, Chegongzhuang Xilu, Haidian District, Beijing 100044, China. TEL 86-1-68413849, FAX 86-1-68412048, cibtc@mail.cibtc.com.cn, http://www.cibtc.com.cn.

610 CHN ISSN 1005-7072
ZHONGGUO ZHONGYIYAO KEJI/CHINESE JOURNAL OF TRADITIONAL MEDICAL SCIENCE AND TECHNOLOGY. Text in Chinese. 1994. bi-m. USD 22.20; USD 3.70 newsstand/cover (effective 2001). **Document type:** *Academic/Scholarly.*
Published by: China International Book Trading Corp/Zhongguo Guoji Tushu Maoyi Zonggongsi cibtc@mail.cibtc.com.cn, http://www.cibtc.com.cn. **Dist. by:** 35, Chegongzhuang Xilu, Haidian District, Beijing 100044, China.

610 CHN ISSN 1005-5304
ZHONGGUO ZHONGYIYAO XINXI ZAZHI/CHINESE JOURNAL OF INFORMATION ON TRADITIONAL CHINESE MEDICINE. Text in Chinese. 1994. m. USD 50.40; USD 4.20 newsstand/cover (effective 2001). **Document type:** *Academic/Scholarly.*
Published by: China International Book Trading Corp/Zhongguo Guoji Tushu Maoyi Zonggongsi cibtc@mail.cibtc.com.cn, http://www.cibtc.com.cn. **Dist. by:** 35, Chegongzhuang Xilu, Haidian District, Beijing 100044, China.

571.9 CHN ISSN 0529-5807
ZHONGHUA BINGLIXUE ZAZHI/CHINESE JOURNAL OF PATHOLOGY. Text in Chinese. 1955. bi-m. CNY 120 domestic; USD 58.20 foreign; CNY 20 newsstand/cover domestic; USD 3.60 newsstand/cover foreign (effective 2001). **Document type:** *Academic/Scholarly.*
Related titles: Online - full content ed.: (from WanFang Data Corp.).
Indexed: Ind.Med.
Published by: Zhonghua Yixuehui Zazhishe, 42 Dongsi Xidajie, Beijing 100710, China. TEL 86-1-65273364. **Dist. by:** China International Book Trading Corp, 35, Chegongzhuang Xilu, Haidian District, Beijing 100044, China. TEL 86-1-68413849, FAX 86-1-68412048, cibtc@mail.cibtc.com.cn, http://www.cibtc.com.cn.

610 CHN ISSN 1000-6680
ZHONGHUA CHUANRANBING ZAZHI/CHINESE JOURNAL OF INFECTIOUS DISEASES. Text in Chinese; Abstracts in Chinese, English. q. CNY 6 newsstand/cover domestic; USD 3.90 newsstand/cover foreign; CNY 24 domestic; USD 15.60 foreign (effective 2001). **Document type:** *Academic/Scholarly.*
Related titles: CD-ROM ed.; Online - full content ed.: (from WanFang Data Corp.).
Indexed: ExtraMED.
Published by: Zhonghua Yixuehui (Shanghai Fenhui)/Chinese Medical Association (Shanghai Branch), 1623 Beijing Xilu, Shanghai 200040, China. TEL 86-21-62531885, FAX 86-21-62550842. Ed. Xianghui Wu. Circ: 15,000. **Dist. by:** China International Book Trading Corp, 35, Chegongzhuang Xilu, Haidian District, Beijing 100044, China. TEL 86-1-68413849, FAX 86-1-68412048, cibtc@mail.cibtc.com.cn, http://www.cibtc.com.cn.

616.980213 CHN ISSN 1001-6589
ZHONGHUA HANGKONG YIXUE ZAZHI/CHINESE JOURNAL OF AVIATION MEDICINE. Text in Chinese. 1990. q. USD 20.80; USD 5.20 newsstand/cover (effective 2001). **Document type:** *Academic/Scholarly.*
Published by: Zhonghua Yixuehui Zazhishe, 42 Dongsi Xidajie, Beijing 100710, China. **Dist. by:** China International Book Trading Corp, 35, Chegongzhuang Xilu, Haidian District, Beijing 100044, China. TEL 86-1-68413849, FAX 86-1-68412048, cibtc@mail.cibtc.com.cn, http://www.cibtc.com.cn.

610 CHN ISSN 0254-6450
ZHONGHUA LIUXINGBINGXUE ZAZHI/CHINESE JOURNAL OF EPIDEMIOLOGY. Text in Chinese. 1981. bi-m. CNY 42 domestic; USD 38.20 foreign; CNY 7 newsstand/cover domestic; USD 4.70 newsstand/cover foreign (effective 2001). **Document type:** *Academic/Scholarly.*
Related titles: CD-ROM ed.; Online - full content ed.: (from WanFang Data Corp.).
Indexed: Diar.Dis.Res., ExtraMED, Ind.Med. (1981-).
Published by: Zhonghua Yufang Yixuehui Kexueyuan, Liuxingbingxue Weishengwuxue Yanjiusuo, 5, Changping Liuzi, Beijing 102206, China. TEL 86-1-61739449, cmalxb@public.sti.ac.cn. Ed. Cheng-Yu Wei. **Dist. by:** China International Book Trading Corp, 35, Chegongzhuang Xilu, Haidian District, Beijing 100044, China. TEL 86-1-68413849, FAX 86-1-68412048, cibtc@mail.cibtc.com.cn, http://www.cibtc.com.cn. **Co-sponsor:** Zhonghua Yixuehui/Chinese Medical Association.

610 CHN ISSN 1007-631X
ZHONGHUA PUTONG WAIKE ZAZHI/CHINESE JOURNAL OF GENERAL SURGERY. Text in Chinese. 1985. m. USD 34.80; USD 2.90 newsstand/cover (effective 2001). **Document type:** *Academic/Scholarly.*
Formerly (until 1996): Pu-wai Linchuang (1003-112X)
Published by: Zhonghua Yixuehui Zazhishe, 42 Dongsi Xidajie, Beijing 100710, China. **Dist. by:** China International Book Trading Corp, 35, Chegongzhuang Xilu, Haidian District, Beijing 100044, China. TEL 86-1-68413849, FAX 86-1-68412048, cibtc@mail.cibtc.com.cn, http://www.cibtc.com.cn.

610 CHN ISSN 0255-7053
ZHONGHUA YISHI ZAZHI/CHINESE JOURNAL OF MEDICAL HISTORY. Text in Chinese. q. CNY 28 domestic; USD 16.80 foreign; CNY 7 newsstand/cover domestic; USD 4.20 newsstand/cover foreign (effective 2001). **Document type:** *Academic/Scholarly.*
Related titles: CD-ROM ed.
Indexed: Amer.Hist.& Life, ExtraMED, Hist.Abstr. (1991-).
Published by: Zhonghua Yixuehui Zazhishe, 42 Dongsi Xidajie, Beijing 100710, China. TEL 86-1-64017304, cibtc@mail.cibtc.com.cn, http://www.cibtc.com.cn. Ed. Jing-Wei Li. **Dist. by:** China International Book Trading Corp, 35 Chegongzhuang Xilu, Haidian District, Beijing 100044, China. TEL 86-1-68413849, FAX 86-1-68412048, cibtc@mail.cibtc.com.cn, http://www.cibtc.com.cn.

ZHONGHUA YIXUE MEIRONG ZAZHI/CHINESE JOURNAL OF MEDICAL AETHETICS AND COSMETOLOGY. see *BEAUTY CULTURE—Perfumes And Cosmetics*

ZHONGHUA YIXUE YICHUANXUE ZAZHI/CHINESE JOURNAL OF MEDICAL GENETICS. see *BIOLOGY—Genetics*

610 CHN ISSN 0376-2491
ZHONGHUA YIXUE ZAZHI/CHINESE PHARMACEUTICAL JOURNAL. Text in Chinese. 1915. m. CNY 174; CNY 14.50 newsstand/cover; USD 56.40; USD 4.70 newsstand/cover (effective 2001).
Related titles: Online - full content ed.: (from WanFang Data Corp.); ♦ English ed.: Chinese Medical Journal. ISSN 0366-6999.
Indexed: Chem.Abstr., Ind.Med. (1960-).
—BLDSC (6027.070000).
Published by: Zhongguo Yaoxuehui/Chinese Pharmaceutical Association, 42 Dongsi Xidajie, Beijing 100710, China. TEL 86-1-65273362, cmayx@public.sti.ac.cn. **Dist. outside of China by:** China International Book Trading Corp, 35, Chegongzhuang Xilu, Haidian District, Beijing 100044, China. TEL 86-1-68413849, FAX 86-1-68412048, cibtc@mail.cibtc.com.cn, http://www.cibtc.com.cn.

610 CHN ISSN 0253-9624
ZHONGHUA YUFANG YIXUE ZAZHI/CHINESE JOURNAL OF PREVENTIVE MEDICINE. Text in Chinese. 1953. bi-m. CNY 54 domestic; USD 31.20 foreign; CNY 9 newsstand/cover domestic; USD 5.20 newsstand/cover foreign (effective 2001). **Document type:** *Academic/Scholarly.*
Related titles: CD-ROM ed.
Indexed: Chem.Abstr., ExtraMED, Ind.Med. (1967-), Rev.Med.& Vet.Mycol.
—BLDSC (3180.600000).
Published by: Zhonghua Yixuehui Zazhishe, 42 Dongsi Xidajie, Beijing 100710, China. TEL 86-1-65271218, cmabc@public.sti.ac.cn. Ed. Yude Chen. **Dist. by:** China International Book Trading Corp, 35, Chegongzhuang Xilu, Haidian District, Beijing 100044, China. TEL 86-1-68413849, FAX 86-1-68412048, cibtc@mail.cibtc.com.cn, http://www.cibtc.com.cn.

630 CHN ISSN 1001-0025
ZHONGRI YOUHAO YIYUAN XUEBAO/SINO-JAPANESE FRIENDSHIP HOSPITAL. JOURNAL. Text in Chinese. q.
Published by: Zhongri Youhao Yiyuan, Yinghuayuan Dongjie, Beijing 100029, China. TEL 4221122. Ed. Bian Zhiqiang.

610 CHN ISSN 1000-257X
ZHONGSHAN YIKE DAXUE XUEBAO/SUN YAT-SEN UNIVERSITY OF MEDICAL SCIENCES. ACADEMIC JOURNAL. Text in Chinese. 1980. q. CNY 2.50 per issue.
Formerly (until 1983): Zhongshan Yixueyuan Xuebao (0254-1440)
Indexed: INIS Atomind., Ref.Zh.
—BLDSC (0570.512500).
Published by: Zhongshan Yike Daxue/Sun Yat-sen Medical University, 74 Zhongshan Erlu, Guangzhou, Guangdong 510089, China. Ed. Peng Wenwei.

610 CHN ISSN 1005-9717
ZHONGXIYI JIEHE SHIYONG LINCHUANG JIJIU/INTEGRATED TRADITIONAL CHINESE AND WESTERN MEDICINE IN PRACTICE OF CRITICAL CARE MEDICINE. Text in Chinese; Abstracts in English. 1994. m. USD 5. adv.
Published by: Tianjin Weisheng Ju, c/o Tian He Hospital, 122 Mu Nan Rd, Tianjin 300050, China. TEL 86-22-334-9935. R&P Jinda Wang. Adv. contact Yenping Li. page USD 400.

610 CHN
ZHONGYI HANSHOU TONGXUN/CORRESPONDENCE JOURNAL OF TRADITIONAL CHINESE MEDICINE. Text in Chinese. bi-m. USD 12; USD 2 newsstand/cover (effective 2001). **Document type:** *Academic/Scholarly.*
Published by: China International Book Trading Corp/Zhongguo Guoji Tushu Maoyi Zonggongsi cibtc@mail.cibtc.com.cn, http://www.cibtc.com.cn. **Dist. by:** 35, Chegongzhuang Xilu, Haidian District, Beijing 100044, China. **Co-sponsor:** Guojia Zhongyiyao Quanliju.

610 CHN ISSN 1001-6910
ZHONGYI YANJIU/TRADITIONAL CHINESE MEDICINAL RESEARCH. Text in Chinese; Contents page in English. q. CNY 3.20.
Published by: Zhongyi Yanjiu Bianjibu, 7 Chengbei Lu, Zhengzhou, Henan 450004, China. TEL 22705. **Dist. overseas by:** China International Book Trading Corp, 35 Chegongzhuang Xilu, Haidian District, Beijing 100044, China.

ZHONGYI ZAZHI. see *ALTERNATIVE MEDICINE*

610 UKR
ZHURNAL PRAKTICHESKOGO VRACHA. Text in English, Russian, Ukrainian. bi-m. USD 110 in United States.
Published by: Izdatel'stvo Meditsina Ukrainy, A-ya 385, Kiev 253222, Ukraine. TEL 517-23-83, FAX 532-43-85. **US dist. addr.:** East View Publications, 3020 Harbor Ln N, Minneapolis, MN 55447. TEL 612-550-0961.

613 HRV ISSN 0350-7335
ZIVOT I ZDRAVIJE; obitelski casopis za proucavanje i promicanje prirodnih zdravstvenih nacela. Text in Serbo-Croatian. 1972. q. USD 4 per issue. back issues avail.
Related titles: Croatian ed.; Serbian ed.; Hungarian ed.: Elet es Egeszseg. ISSN 0351-6024; Slovenian ed.: Zivljenje in zdravje. ISSN 0351-6113; Macedonian ed.: ISSN 0351-7209.
Published by: Centar za Proucavanje Prirodnih Zdravstvenih Nacela, Maksimirska 9, Zagreb 41000, Croatia. TEL 041 217-264. Ed. Slavko Cop.

ZYGOTE; the biology of gametes and early embryos. see *BIOLOGY—Genetics*

MEDICAL SCIENCES—Abstracting, Bibliographies, Statistics

610.21 USA ISSN 0738-6230
A A C O M ANNUAL STATISTICAL REPORT. Text in English. 1981. a. USD 18 (effective 1999). back issues avail. **Document type:** *Trade.* **Description:** Statistical data relating to the characteristics of applicants and matriculants in osteopathic medical colleges, faculty, curriculum, sources of grants and loans, and distribution of revenues and expenditures.
Indexed: SRI.
Published by: American Association of Colleges of Osteopathic Medicine, 5550 Friendship Blvd, Ste 310, Chevy Chase, MD 20815-7231. TEL 301-968-4100, FAX 301-968-4101, ckearns@aacom.org, http://www.aacom.org. Ed. Dr. Allen M Singer. Circ: 800.

616.1 USA ISSN 1062-1458
CODEN: ACJREE
A C C CURRENT JOURNAL REVIEW. Text in English. 1992. bi-m. EUR 118 in Europe to individuals; JPY 15,700 in Japan to individuals; USD 132 elsewhere to individuals; EUR 219 in Europe to institutions; JPY 29,100 in Japan to institutions; USD 244 elsewhere to institutions; EUR 70 in Europe to qualified personnel; JPY 9,300 in Japan to qualified personnel; USD 79 elsewhere to qualified personnel (effective 2002). adv. abstr. back issues avail. *Refereed.* **Document type:** *Abstract/Index.* **Description:** Provides information for physicians who care for patients with cardiovascular disease.
Related titles: Online - full text ed.: (from ingenta, Swets Blackwell, ScienceDirect).
Indexed: CINAHL, Excerp.Med. (1995-).
—BLDSC (0570.743000), EMDOCS, GNLM, Infotrieve. **CCC.**
Published by: (American College of Cardiology), Elsevier Science, PO Box 945, New York, NY 10159-0945. TEL 212-989-5800, FAX 212-633-3990, usinfo-f@elsevier.com, http://www.elsevier.com/locate/accreview. Eds. K A Eagle, W F Armstrong. Adv. contact Kathleen Harrison. Circ: 24,648. **Subscr. in Australasia and the Far East to:** Elsevier Science (Singapore) Pte Ltd, No.1 Temasek Ave, 17-01 Millenia Tower, Singapore 039192, Singapore. TEL 65-434-3727, FAX 65-337-2230; **Subscr. in Japan to:** Elsevier Science Inc - Japan Regional Office, 9-15 Higashi-Azabu 1-chome, Minato-ku, Tokyo 106-0044, Japan. TEL 81-3-5561-5033, FAX 81-3-5561-5047; **Subscr. outside the Americas to:** Elsevier Science BV, PO Box 211, Amsterdam 1000 AE, Netherlands. TEL 31-20-485-3757, FAX 31-20-485-3432, nlinfo-f@elsevier.nl.

618 USA ISSN 1085-6862
A C O G CLINICAL REVIEW. Text in English. 1987; N.S. 1996. bi-m. EUR 99 in Europe to individuals; JPY 13,700 in Japan to individuals; USD 112 elsewhere to individuals; EUR 195 in Europe to institutions; JPY 25,900 in Japan to institutions; USD 219 elsewhere to institutions (effective 2002). abstr. back issues avail. *Refereed.* **Document type:** *Newsletter.* **Description:** Provides information to keep the reader up-to-date on issues in obstetrics and gynecology. Includes summaries and commentaries on topics of clinical concern in literature in the field.
Supersedes (in 1996): A C O G Current Journal Review (0897-1471)
Related titles: Microform ed.: N.S. (from PQC); Online - full text ed.: (from ingenta, Swets Blackwell, ScienceDirect).
—BLDSC (0578.687026). **CCC.**
Published by: (American College of Obstetricians and Gynecologists), Elsevier Science, PO Box 945, New York, NY 10159-0945. TEL 212-989-5800, FAX 212-633-3990, usinfo-f@elsevier.com, http://www.elsevier.com/locate/clinrev. Ed. Dr. Ralph W Hale. **Subscr. in Australasia and the Far East to:** Elsevier Science (Singapore) Pte Ltd, No.1 Temasek Ave, 17-01 Millenia Tower, Singapore 039192, Singapore. TEL 65-434-3727, FAX 65-337-2230; **Subscr. in Japan to:** Elsevier Science Inc - Japan Regional Office, 9-15 Higashi-Azabu 1-chome, Minato-ku, Tokyo 106-0044, Japan. TEL 81-3-5561-5033; **Subscr. outside the Americas to:** Elsevier Science BV, PO Box 211, Amsterdam 1000 AE, Netherlands. TEL 31-20-485-3757, nlinfo-f@elsevier.nl.

616.005 USA ISSN 1056-8751
R11 CODEN: AJCLEA
A C P JOURNAL CLUB. Text in English. 1991. bi-m. USD 71 to individuals; USD 97 to institutions; USD 193 to individuals Includes Annals of Internal Medicine; USD 272 to institutions Includes Annals of Internal Medicine (effective 2001). adv. back issues avail. **Document type:** *Abstract/Index.* **Description:** Current awareness publication providing abstracts of current medical research of high scientific merit for clinical practice. Includes commentary and clinical applications.
Related titles: CD-ROM ed.; Online - full text ed.
Indexed: Ind.Med. (1991-).
—BLDSC (0578.698300), CISTI, GNLM, KNAW. **CCC.**
Published by: American College of Physicians/Co-sponsor: American Society of Internal Medicine, 190 N. Independence Mall W, Philadelphia, PA 19106-1572. TEL 215-351-2600, FAX 215-351-2799, custserv@mail.acponline.org, http://www.acponline.org/journals/acpjc/jcmenu.htm. Ed. Dr. Brian Haynes. R&P Joshua Roberts TEL 215-351-2630. Adv. contact Ron Taylor.

A M E D. see *ALTERNATIVE MEDICINE—Abstracting, Bibliographies, Statistics*

A R L ACADEMIC LAW AND MEDICAL LIBRARY STATISTICS. see *LIBRARY AND INFORMATION SCIENCES—Abstracting, Bibliographies, Statistics*

016.61 BGR ISSN 0001-3536
CODEN: ABSMBY
ABSTRACTS OF BULGARIAN SCIENTIFIC MEDICAL LITERATURE. Text in English. 1958. q. free per issue. index. **Document type:** *Abstract/Index.* **Description:** Presents abstracts from Bulgarian medical periodicals.
Media: Online - full text.
—CASDDS, GNLM.
Published by: Tsentralna Meditsinska Biblioteka/Central Medical Library, 1 Sv Georgi Sofiiski ul, Sofia 1431, Bulgaria. TEL 359-2-543134, FAX 358-2-543134, lydia@medun.acad.bg, http://www.medun.acad.bg. Ed. L Tatcheva. Circ: 200.

M

610 011 USA ISSN 1042-4423
ABSTRACTS OF CLINICAL CARE GUIDELINES. Text in English. 1989. 10/yr. USD 110 domestic; USD 130.54 in Canada; USD 122 elsewhere. index. **Description:** Contains summaries of selected clinical practice guidelines. Includes peer commentaries, annotated resources and news on guideline methods and tools and implementation experiences.
Related titles: Microform ed.: (from PQC).
—CCC.
Published by: Joint Commission on Accreditation of Healthcare Organizations, 75 Remittance Dr, Ste 1057, Chicago, IL 60675-1057. TEL 630-792-5800, lkaegi@jcaho.org, http://www.jcaho.org. Ed. Louise Kaegi. Circ: 1,900.

016.61698 GBR ISSN 0260-5511
RA421
ABSTRACTS ON HYGIENE AND COMMUNICABLE DISEASES. Text in English. 1926. m. GBP 460 to institutions; USD 805 in the Americas to institutions; GBP 470 to institutions includes single-site online access; USD 815 in the Americas to institutions includes single-site online access (effective 2002). adv. bk.rev. index. reprint service avail. from IRC. **Document type:** *Abstract/Index.*
Former titles: Abstracts on Hygiene (0001-3692); Bulletin of Hygiene
Related titles: Microform ed.: (from PQC); Online - full text ed.: GBP 410, USD 720 to institutions (effective 2002) (from DIMDI, The Dialog Corporation, S T N International).
Indexed: Ergon.Abstr.
—GNLM.
Published by: CABI Publishing, Wallingford, Oxon OX10 8DE, United Kingdom. TEL 44-1491-832111, FAX 44-1491-829198, publishing@cabi.org, http://www.cabi.org/Publishing/Products/Journals/Abstract/AHCD/Index.asp. Adv. contact S Harris. B&W page GBP 100; 120 x 203. Circ: 450. **U.S. subscr. to:** 10 E 40th St, Ste 3203, New York, NY 10016. TEL 212-481-7018, FAX 212-686-7993.

016.61698 USA ISSN 0001-9410
Z6664.3
AEROSPACE MEDICINE AND BIOLOGY* ; a continuing bibliography. Text in English. 1964. m. index. back issues avail. **Document type:** *Bibliography.* **Description:** Abstracts medical and biological research. Articles cover the biological, physiological, and environmental effects to which humans are subjected during and following space flight.
Formerly: Aerospace References in Medicine and Biology
Media: Online - full text.
Indexed: Noise Pollut.Publ.Abstr.
—GNLM.
Published by: U.S. National Aeronautics and Space Administration, Scientific and Technical Information Office, 7121 Standard Dr, Hanover, MD 21076-1320. help@sti.nasa.gov, http://www.sti.nasa.gov. **Co-sponsor:** Compiled by: U.S. Library of Congress and American Institute of Aeronautics and Astronautics.

610 016.3621 USA
AFRICAN HEALTH ANTHOLOGY. Text in English. q. **Document type:** *Abstract/Index, Bibliography.* **Description:** Comprises a wide variety of bibliographic databases covering African health issues. Features the following databases: African Index Medicus, African subset of CAB Health; Healthlink Worldwide; University of Cape Town Medicines Information Centre Reference; CHID; SAMED; AIDS Consortium Reference Centre; AIDSLINE; African subset of MEDLINE; African Health Subsets of WATERLIT, ISAP, South African Index to Theses and Dissertations; and Bibliography of Filariasis.
Related titles: CD-ROM ed.: (from National Information Services Corp. (NISC)); Online - full text ed.: (from NISC).
Published by: National Information Services Corporation (NISC), Wyman Towers, 3100 St Paul St, Baltimore, MD 28218. TEL 410-243-0797, FAX 410-243-0982, sales@nisc.com, http://www.nisc.com.

610 016 ZWE
AFRICAN INDEX MEDICUS. Text in English. 1993. q. USD 100 (effective 2001). adv. illus. *Refereed.* **Document type:** *Abstract/Index.* **Description:** Covers African health & biomedical information from books, reports and studies from international development agencies, nongovernmental organizations and local institutions.
Related titles: CD-ROM ed.; Online - full content ed.
Published by: (Association for Health Information and Libraries in Africa USA), W H O Regional Office for Africa, The Library & Documentation Centre, The African Index Medicus Coordinating Center, Belvedere, BO Box BE 773, Harare, Zimbabwe. http://whqmomiji.who.ch/RIS/RISWEB.ISA. Ed. Lucilda Hunter.

016.6169792 GBR ISSN 0968-5480
AIDS ABSTRACTS; international literature on acquired immunodeficiency syndrome and related retroviruses. Text in English. 1985. m. GBP 235, USD 399 to individuals; GBP 576, USD 950 to institutions (effective 2002). adv. back issues avail. **Document type:** *Abstract/Index.* **Description:** Provides full details of recently published papers on all aspects of AIDS and related animal and human retroviruses.
Formerly (until 1993): AIDS Information (0953-1580)
Related titles: Online - full text ed.: (from ProQuest Information & Learning).
Published by: (Oncology Information Service, University of Leeds), Carfax Publishing Limited (Subsidiary of: Taylor & Francis Group), PO Box 25, Abingdon, Oxon OX14 3UE, United Kingdom. TEL 44-1235-401000, FAX 44-1235-401550, enquiries@carfax.co.uk, enquiry@tandf.co.uk, http://www.carfax.co.uk. Ed. Arthur W Boylston. Circ: 1,000.

016.6169 USA
AIDS & CANCER RESEARCH. Text in English. m. **Document type:** *Abstract/Index.* **Description:** Covers AIDS-related topics such as molecular and in vitro aspects; immunological, clinical and epidemiological aspects; patterns of disease occurrence and transmission; symptoms, diagnosis and treatment; AIDS-related diseases; and investigational drugs. Cancer-related topics focus on the complex molecular aspects of cancer initiation, promotion, progression and metastasis.
Media: Online - full text (from CSA, O C L C Online Computer Library Center, Inc.).
Published by: Cambridge Scientific Abstracts, 7200 Wisconsin Ave., Suite 601, Bethesda, MD 20814. TEL 301-961-6798, FAX 301-961-6799, http://www.csa.com.

616.9 USA ISSN 1074-2891
AIDS & T B WEEKLY ABSTRACTS FROM CONFERENCE PROCEEDINGS. (Tuberculosis) Text in English. 1994. w. index. **Document type:** *Abstract/Index.* **Description:** Features reports on AIDS and tuberculosis research prior to their publication in journals.
—CCC.
Published by: Charles W. Henderson, Ed. & Pub., PO Box 5528, Atlanta, GA 31107-0528. TEL 404-377-8895, FAX 404-378-5411, cwhender@newsfile.com, http://www.newsfile.com. **Subscr. to:** PO Box 830409, Birmingham, AL 35283-0409.

616.9 USA ISSN 1074-2883
AIDS & T B WEEKLY ARTICLE SUMMARIES. (Tuberculosis) Text in English. 1994. w. index. **Document type:** *Abstract/Index.* **Description:** Features summaries of recent AIDS and tuberculosis journal articles published worldwide. Indexed by author, key word and institution.
—CCC.
Published by: Charles W. Henderson, Ed. & Pub., PO Box 5528, Atlanta, GA 31107-0528. TEL 404-377-8895, FAX 404-378-5411, cwhender@newsfile.com, http://www.newsfile.com.

AIDS LEGAL BIBLIOGRAPHY. (Acquired Immune Deficiency Syndrome) see *LAW—Abstracting, Bibliographies, Statistics*

610 USA ISSN 1083-8589
K1
AIDS LITERATURE & LAW REVIEW. Text in English. m. USD 225 (effective 2000). back issues avail. **Document type:** *Newsletter.* **Description:** Provides monthly coverage of AIDS-related articles, developments, and news from more than 500 journals and periodicals. Serves as a reference tool for physicians, attorneys, scientists, policymakers, researchers, health care professionals, administrators, and managers.
Formerly (until 1995): AIDS Literature and News Review (0893-1526)
Published by: University Publishing Group, Inc., 17100 Cole Rd, Ste 312, Hagerstown, MD 31740. TEL 800-654-8188, FAX 301-582-2406, orders@upgBooks.com.

616.9 GBR ISSN 1350-2840
AIDS (YEAR); a year in review. Text in English. 1988. a. GBP 49.95, USD 74.95 to individuals. adv. bibl, illus. **Document type:** *Academic/Scholarly.* **Description:** Reviews all major developments during the preceding year. Topics include virology; epidemiology; vaccines and immunology; clinical treatment; social, cultural and political aspects; and global statistics.
Related titles: ♦ Supplement to: AIDS. ISSN 0269-9370.
Indexed: ASCA, Excerp.Med. (1996-), Ind.Sci.Rev., NRN, Psychol.Abstr., SSCI (coverage dropped).
—ADONIS, EMDOCS, KNAW.

Published by: Kluwer Academic & Lippencott-Raven (Subsidiary of: Wolters Kluwer N.V.), 2-6 Boundary Row, London SE1 8HN, United Kingdom. TEL 44-171-865-0198, FAX 44-171-928-7876, stmsubs@itps.co.uk. Adv. contact Gemma Heiser.

610 016.3612 USA
AIDSEARCH. Text in English. 1980. m. free. **Document type:** *Abstract/Index, Bibliography.* **Description:** Combines three databases which provide information on AIDS and related issues. Includes AIDSDRUGS, AIDSLINE, and AIDSTRIALS.
Formerly: All About AIDS
Media: Online - full text (from NISC).
Indexed: CWI.
Published by: National Information Services Corporation (NISC), Wyman Towers, 3100 St Paul St, Baltimore, MD 28218. TEL 410-243-0797, FAX 410-243-0982, sales@nisc.com, http://www.nisc.com. Pub. Fred Durr.

016.6161 USA ISSN 0065-8502
AMERICAN HEART ASSOCIATION. SCIENTIFIC SESSIONS. ABSTRACTS. Text in English. 1927. a. USD 236 domestic; USD 418 foreign; USD 20 newsstand/cover (effective 2000). index. reprint service avail. from PQC. *Refereed.* **Document type:** *Abstract/Index, Academic/Scholarly.*
Related titles: Microfiche ed.
Published by: Lippincott Williams & Wilkins (Baltimore) (Subsidiary of: Wolters Kluwer N.V.), 351 W Camden St, Baltimore, MD 21201-2436. TEL 410-528-8565, 800-341-2258, FAX 410-528-4312, cdailead@lww.com, http://www.ahajournals.org. Ed. James T Willerson. R&P Debbie Heise TEL 410-528-4050. Circ: 27,151.

610.9514 615.89 USA ISSN 0192-415X
R601 CODEN: AJCMBA
THE AMERICAN JOURNAL OF CHINESE MEDICINE. Text in English. 1973. 3/yr. USD 130 (effective 2001); SGD 270 in Asia Pacific & Australasia except Hong Kong and China; USD 150 elsewhere (effective 2002). bk.rev. charts, illus. back issues avail. *Refereed.* **Document type:** *Abstract/Index, Academic/Scholarly.* **Description:** Covers basic science and clinical research in indigenous medical techniques and therapeutic procedures, medicinal plants, and traditional medicine.
Former titles (until 1979): Comparative Medicine East and West (0147-2917); (until 1977): American Journal of Chinese Medicine (0090-2942)
Related titles: Microfilm ed.: (from PQC); Online - full text ed.: (from Institute for Scientific Information).
Indexed: AMED, ASCA, Agroforest.Abstr., Bibl.Asian Stud. (1975-1996), Biol.Abstr., Curr.Adv.Ecol.Sci., Curr.Cont., Excerp.Med., Food Sci.& Tech.Abstr., Helminthol.Abstr., Hort.Abstr., INIS Atomind., Ind.Med. (1979-), Ind.Vet., Inpharma, Med.Care Rev., Nutr.Abstr., Pharm.&Out.News, Plant Breed.Abstr., Psychol.Abstr., Reac., Rev.Appl.Entomol., Rev.Arom.& Med.Plants, Rev.Med.& Vet.Mycol., Rice Abstr., Seed Abstr., Triticale Abstr.
—BLDSC (0822.700000), CASDDS, CISTI, GNLM, IDS, ingenta, KNAW.
Published by: Institute for Advanced Research in Asian Science and Medicine, PO Box 555, Garden City, NY 11530. TEL 415-831-4289, FAX 415-831-4248, 617-739-1183, admin@ajcm.org, http://www.ajcm.org. Ed. Dr. John J Kao.

016.61 POL ISSN 1232-9371
ANNALES COLLEGII MEDICI UNIVERSITATIS IAGIELLONICAE CRACOVIENSIS. Text in English, Polish. 1953. a. USD 35 (effective 2000).
Former titles (until 1993): Annales Academiae Medicae Cracoviensis (0066-1937); Akademia Medyczna w Krakowie. Dzialalnosc Naukowa
—CISTI, GNLM, KNAW.
Published by: Uniwersytet Jagiellonski, Collegium Medicum, Ul Sw Anny 12, Krakow 31008, Poland. TEL 48-12-4228759. Eds. Adam Wiernikowski, Jacek Bojarski. **Subscr. to:** Wydawnictwo Uniwersytetu Jagiellonskiego - Jagiellonian University Press, ul Grodzka 26, Krakow 31044, Poland.

016.61607 USA ISSN 0883-6612
R726.5 CODEN: ABMEEH
ANNALS OF BEHAVIORAL MEDICINE. Text in English. 1979. q. USD 50 in US & Canada to individuals; USD 80 elsewhere to individuals; USD 210 in US & Canada to institutions; USD 240 elsewhere to institutions (effective 2002). adv. bk.rev. back issues avail. *Refereed.* **Document type:** *Journal, Academic/Scholarly, Abstract/Index.* **Description:** Covers behavioral advances across the spectrum of health care disciplines.
Incorporates (in 1991): Behavioral Medicine Abstracts (0197-7717); Formerly: Behavioral Medicine Update

Related titles: Microfilm ed.: (from PMC,WWS); Online - full text ed.: USD 45 to individuals; USD 189 to institutions (effective 2002) (from CatchWord Ltd., Institute for Scientific Information, RoweCom Information Quest).
Indexed: Abstr.Anthropol., AgeLine, Curr.Cont., Ind.Med. (1985-), Int.Nurs.Ind., PsycInfo, SSCI, e-psyche.
—BLDSC (1038.700000), CISTI, EMDOCS, GNLM, IDS, Infotrieve, ingenta, KNAW. **CCC.**
Published by: (Society of Behavioral Medicine), Lawrence Erlbaum Associates, Inc., 10 Industrial Ave, Mahwah, NJ 07430-2262. TEL 201-760-3735, 800-926-6579, FAX 201-236-0072, journals@erlbaum.com, http://www.erlbaum.com/Journals/journals/ABM/abm.htm. Ed. Robert M Kaplan. adv.: page USD 325. Circ: 3,000.

617 USA ISSN 0090-1393
ANNUAL BIBLIOGRAPHY OF ORTHOPAEDIC SURGERY. Text in English. 1969. a. **Document type:** *Bibliography.*
Published by: National Research Council, Subcommittee on Orthopedic Information Services, 2101 Constitution Ave, N W, Washington, DC 20418. TEL 202-334-2138.

616.1 GBR ISSN 0952-0562
ANNUAL OF CARDIAC SURGERY. Text in English. 1987. a. GBP 99.95, USD 169.95. bibl, illus. **Document type:** *Academic/Scholarly.* **Description:** For cardiac surgeons, cardiologists and researchers involved with coronary artery disease. Reviews the year's research papers and presents invited reviews in such areas as pediatric and fetal cardiac surgery.
—GNLM.
Published by: Rapid Science Publishers, 2-6 Boundary Row, London SE1 8HN, United Kingdom. TEL 44-207-865-0198, FAX 44-207-410-6600, rapid@rapidcom.co.uk. Ed. Magdi Yacoub. Circ: 3,000.

616.3 GBR ISSN 0952-6293
ANNUAL OF GASTROINTESTINAL ENDOSCOPY. Text in English. 1988. a. GBP 79.95, USD 129.95. bibl, illus. **Document type:** *Academic/Scholarly.* **Description:** For physicians, endoscopists, surgeons, radiologists and others interested in gastroenterology and gastrointestinal imaging or therapy.
Related titles: ♦ Supplement: Slide Atlas of Gastrointestinal Endoscopy (Year).
—GNLM.
Published by: Rapid Science Publishers, 2-6 Boundary Row, London SE1 8HN, United Kingdom. TEL 44-207-865-0198, FAX 44-207-410-6600, rapid@rapidcom.co.uk.

016.61 MEX ISSN 1405-0242
ARTEMISA. Text in Spanish. 1993. a. **Document type:** *Abstract/Index.* **Description:** Provides abstracts and articles related to the fields of medicine and health.
Media: CD-ROM.
Published by: Centro Nacional de Informacion y Documentacion Sobre Salud, Insurgentes Sur No 1397, piso 2, Colonia: Insurgentes Mixcoac, Deleg: Benito Juarez, Mexico City, DF 03920, Mexico. TEL 52-5598-2002, 52-5563-1906, 52-5598-9949, FAX 52-5598-9959, cenids@ssa.gob.mx.

610 016.61 USA ISSN 8756-4734
ASTHMA UPDATE; a newsletter for people with asthma. Text in English. 1985. q. USD 15. back issues avail. **Document type:** *Newsletter, Abstract/Index.* **Description:** Contains annotated abstracts from current medical journals.
Address: 123 Monticello Ave, Annapolis, MD 21401. TEL 410-267-8329, FAX 410-267-0309. Ed. David Jamison.

016.6164 615 GBR ISSN 0268-1641
ATRIAL NATRIURETIC FACTORS. Text in English. 1986. s-m. GBP 120 (effective 2001). adv. **Document type:** *Abstract/Index.* **Description:** Current awareness service for researchers in clinical and life sciences. Covers atrial natriuretic factors: peptides, cardionatrin, atriopeptin, and cardiac endocrinology.
Related titles: E-mail ed.: GBP 120 (effective 2001); Online - full text ed.: GBP 108 (effective 2001).
—**CCC.**
Published by: S U B I S (Subsidiary of: Sheffield Academic Press Ltd), Mansion House, 19 Kingfield Rd, Sheffield, S Yorks S11 9AS, United Kingdom. TEL 44-114-255-4433, FAX 44-114-255-4626, subis@sheffac.demon.co.uk, http://www.shef-ac-press.co.uk/subis. Ed. S Huntridge. Adv. contact C Evans.

AUSTRALIA. BUREAU OF STATISTICS. CANCER IN AUSTRALIA. see *MEDICAL SCIENCES—Oncology*

618.92021 AUS
AUSTRALIA. BUREAU OF STATISTICS. CHILDREN'S HEALTH SCREENING. Text in English. 1979. irreg., latest 1995. AUD 14 (effective 2000). **Document type:** *Government.* **Description:** Contains information about health screening practices. Topics include: testing of sight and hearing; visits to dental professionals and visits to baby health clinics.
Formerly: Sight, Hearing and Dental Health (Persons Aged 2 to 14 Years)
Published by: Australian Bureau of Statistics, PO Box 10, Belconnen, ACT 2616, Australia. TEL 61-2-6252-5249, FAX 61-2-6252-6778, http://www.abs.gov.au.

616.097021 618.92021 AUS
AUSTRALIA. BUREAU OF STATISTICS. CHILDREN'S IMMUNISATION, AUSTRALIA. Text in English. 1983. irreg., latest 1995. AUD 14 (effective 2000). **Document type:** *Government.* **Description:** Contains statistics on coverage and practice regarding the immunization of children against selected preventable diseases.
Formerly: Australia. Bureau of Statistics. Children's Immunisation
Published by: Australian Bureau of Statistics, PO Box 10, Belconnen, ACT 2616, Australia. TEL 61-2-6252-5249, FAX 61-2-6252-6778, http://www.abs.gov.au.

610.021 AUS
AUSTRALIA. BUREAU OF STATISTICS. CHIROPRACTIC AND OSTEOPATHIC SERVICES, AUSTRALIA. Text in English. 1998. irreg. AUD 17 (effective 2001). **Document type:** *Government.*
Published by: Australian Bureau of Statistics, PO Box 10, Belconnen, ACT 2616, Australia. TEL 61-2-6252-5249, FAX 61-2-6252-6778, http://www.abs.gov.au.

616.2021 AUS
AUSTRALIA. BUREAU OF STATISTICS. DEATHS DUE TO DISEASES AND CANCERS OF THE RESPIRATORY SYSTEM, AUSTRALIA. Text in English. 1994. irreg. AUD 15 (effective 2000). **Document type:** *Government.*
Published by: Australian Bureau of Statistics, PO Box 10, Belconnen, ACT 2616, Australia. TEL 61-2-6252-5249, FAX 61-2-6252-6778, http://www.abs.gov.au.

617.6021 AUS
AUSTRALIA. BUREAU OF STATISTICS. DENTAL SERVICES, AUSTRALIA. Text in English. 1998. irreg. AUD 17 (effective 2001). **Document type:** *Government.*
Published by: Australian Bureau of Statistics, PO Box 10, Belconnen, ACT 2616, Australia. TEL 61-2-6252-5249, FAX 61-2-6252-6778, http://www.abs.gov.au.

610.021 AUS
AUSTRALIA. BUREAU OF STATISTICS. INJURIES, AUSTRALIA. Text in English. 1990. irreg., latest 1995. AUD 16 (effective 2001). **Document type:** *Government.*
Published by: Australian Bureau of Statistics, PO Box 10, Belconnen, ACT 2616, Australia. TEL 61-2-6252-5249, FAX 61-2-6252-6778, http://www.abs.gov.au.

610.021 AUS
AUSTRALIA. BUREAU OF STATISTICS. MEDICAL LABOUR FORCE. Text in English. 1995. irreg., latest 2000. price varies. **Document type:** *Government.* **Description:** Includes trend information on medical education and migration, Medicare utilisation and Medicare providers, hospital workforce, rural medical workforce, and Aboriginal health service employment.
Published by: Australian Bureau of Statistics, PO Box 10, Belconnen, ACT 2616, Australia. TEL 61-2-6252-5249, FAX 61-2-6252-6778, http://www.abs.gov.au.

616.2021 AUS
AUSTRALIA. BUREAU OF STATISTICS. NATIONAL HEALTH SURVEY: ASTHMA AND OTHER RESPIRATORY CONDITIONS, AUSTRALIA. Text in English. 1990. irreg., latest 1995. AUD 16 (effective 2001). **Document type:** *Government.*
Published by: Australian Bureau of Statistics, PO Box 10, Belconnen, ACT 2616, Australia. TEL 61-2-6252-5249, FAX 61-2-6252-6778, http://www.abs.gov.au.

616.99021 AUS
AUSTRALIA. BUREAU OF STATISTICS. NATIONAL HEALTH SURVEY: CANCER SCREENING, AUSTRALIA. Text in English. 1990. irreg., latest 1998. AUD 16 (effective 1998). **Document type:** *Government.*
Published by: Australian Bureau of Statistics, PO Box 10, Belconnen, ACT 2616, Australia. TEL 61-2-6252-5249, FAX 61-2-6252-6778, http://www.abs.gov.au.

616.1021 AUS
AUSTRALIA. BUREAU OF STATISTICS. NATIONAL HEALTH SURVEY: CARDIOVASCULAR AND RELATED CONDITIONS, AUSTRALIA. Text in English. 1990. irreg., latest 1995. AUD 15 (effective 2001). **Document type:** *Government.*
Published by: Australian Bureau of Statistics, PO Box 10, Belconnen, ACT 2616, Australia. TEL 61-2-6252-5249, FAX 61-2-6252-6778, http://www.abs.gov.au.

616.4021 AUS
AUSTRALIA. BUREAU OF STATISTICS. NATIONAL HEALTH SURVEY: DIABETES, AUSTRALIA. Text in English. 1990. irreg., latest 1995. AUD 16.50 (effective 2001). **Document type:** *Government.*
Published by: Australian Bureau of Statistics, PO Box 10, Belconnen, ACT 2616, Australia. TEL 61-2-6252-5249, FAX 61-2-6252-6778, http://www.abs.gov.au.

610.021 AUS
AUSTRALIA. BUREAU OF STATISTICS. NATIONAL HEALTH SURVEY: USE OF MEDICATIONS, AUSTRALIA. Text in English. 1990. irreg., latest 1995. AUD 19.50 (effective 2001). **Document type:** *Government.*
Published by: Australian Bureau of Statistics, PO Box 10, Belconnen, ACT 2616, Australia. TEL 61-2-6252-5249, FAX 61-2-6252-6778, http://www.abs.gov.au.

617.7021 AUS
AUSTRALIA. BUREAU OF STATISTICS. OPTOMETRY AND OPTICAL DISPENSING SERVICES, AUSTRALIA. Text in English. 1998. irreg. AUD 16.50 (effective 2001). **Document type:** *Government.*
Published by: Australian Bureau of Statistics, PO Box 10, Belconnen, ACT 2616, Australia. TEL 61-2-6252-5249, FAX 61-2-6252-6778, http://www.abs.gov.au.

615.82021 AUS
AUSTRALIA. BUREAU OF STATISTICS. PHYSIOTHERAPY SERVICES, AUSTRALIA. Text in English. 1998. irreg. AUD 16.50 (effective 2001). **Document type:** *Government.*
Published by: Australian Bureau of Statistics, PO Box 10, Belconnen, ACT 2616, Australia. TEL 61-2-6252-5249, FAX 61-2-6252-6778, http://www.abs.gov.au.

610.021 AUS
AUSTRALIA. BUREAU OF STATISTICS. PRIVATE MEDICAL PRACTICE INDUSTRY, AUSTRALIA. Text in English. 1995. irreg. AUD 17 (effective 2001). **Document type:** *Government.*
Published by: Australian Bureau of Statistics, PO Box 10, Belconnen, ACT 2616, Australia. TEL 61-2-6252-5249, FAX 61-2-6252-6778, http://www.abs.gov.au.

610.021 AUS
AUSTRALIA. BUREAU OF STATISTICS. PRIVATE MEDICAL PRACTITIONERS, AUSTRALIA. Text in English. 1995. irreg. AUD 14 (effective 2000). **Document type:** *Government.*
Published by: Australian Bureau of Statistics, PO Box 10, Belconnen, ACT 2616, Australia. TEL 61-2-6252-5249, FAX 61-2-6252-6778, http://www.abs.gov.au.

016.616978 GBR ISSN 0142-8365
AUTOIMMUNE DISEASES. Text in English. s-m. GBP 120 (effective 2001). adv. back issues avail. **Document type:** *Abstract/Index.* **Description:** Current awareness service for researchers in clinical and life sciences.
Related titles: E-mail ed.: GBP 120 (effective 2001); Online - full text ed.: GBP 108 (effective 2001).
—Infotrieve. **CCC.**
Published by: S U B I S (Subsidiary of: Sheffield Academic Press Ltd), Mansion House, 19 Kingfield Rd, Sheffield, S Yorks S11 9AS, United Kingdom. TEL 44-114-255-4433, FAX 44-114-255-4626, subis@sheffac.demon.co.uk, http://www.shef-ac-press.co.uk/subis. Ed. S Huntridge. Adv. contact C Evans.

610 ESP
BASQUE REGION. OSASUN SAILEKO. AURREKONTUA/BASQUE REGION. DEPARTAMENTO DE SANIDAD. PRESUPUESTO. Text in Spanish. a.
Published by: Eusko Jaurlaritzaren Argitalpen-Zerbitzu Nagusia/Servicio Central de Publicaciones del Gobierno Vasco, Donostia-San Sebastian, 1, Vitoria-gasteiz, Alava 01010, Spain. TEL 34-945-018561, FAX 34-945-018709, hac-sabd@ej-gv.es, http://www.ej-gv.net/publicaciones. Circ: 1,000.

M

618.610 BLZ
BELIZE FAMILY HEALTH SURVEY. Text in English. 1991. irreg. free per issue. **Document type:** *Government.* **Description:** Provides information on fertility, infant morality, family planning and the use of maternal and child health services in Belize.
Published by: Ministry of Finance, Central Statistical Office, Belmopan, Belize. TEL 501-8-22352, FAX 501-8-2306, csogob@btl.net, csogob@blt.net.

016.6176 BRA ISSN 0100-6266
RKZ6668
BIBLIOGRAFIA BRASILEIRA DE ODONTOLOGIA. Text in English, Portuguese. 1966. a. USD 40 to individuals; free to institutions (effective 2000). **Document type:** *Bibliography.* **Description:** Covers Brazilian literature in the area of dentistry.
Related titles: CD-ROM ed.; Online - full text ed.
Published by: Universidade de Sao Paulo, Faculdade de Odontologia, Servico de Documentacao Odontologica, Seccao de Documentacao Odontologica, Centro, Caixa Postal 8216, Sao Paulo, SP 01065970, Brazil. TEL 55-11-8187861, FAX 55-11-8187413, bibfo@siso.fo.usp.br. R&P, Adv. contact Lucia M S V Costa Ramos. Circ: 350.

610 016 HRV ISSN 0067-6799
BIBLIOGRAFIJA MEDICINSKE PERIODIKE JUGOSLAVIJE/INDEX MEDICUS IUGOSLAVICUS. Text in Serbo-Croatian; Summaries in English, French, German, Russian. 1966. a. USD 10.
Published by: Opca Bolnica "Dr. Josip Kajfes", Miskine 64, Zagreb, Croatia.

610 016 CZE ISSN 0067-6802
Z6661.C95
BIBLIOGRAPHIA MEDICA CECHOSLOVACA. Text in Czech. 1949. m. CZK 480. bk.rev. index. **Document type:** *Bibliography.*
Formerly (until 1973): Annual of Czechoslovak Medical Literature. Bibliographia Medica Cechoslovaca (0303-4739); Formed by the merger of (1956-1969): Annual of Czechoslovak Medical Literature (0517-9424)
Related titles: CD-ROM ed.; Diskette ed.; Online - full text ed.
—CISTI, Linda Hall.
Published by: Narodni Lekarska Knihovna, Sokolska 31, Prague 12132, Czech Republic. TEL 420-2-24266870, FAX 420-2-24266051, nml@nlk.anet.cz nml@nlk.anet.cz, http://www.nlk.anet.cz. Ed. M Votipkova. Circ: 90.

610 011 USA ISSN 0896-6591
BIBLIOGRAPHIES AND INDEXES IN MEDICAL STUDIES. Text in English. 1988. irreg. price varies.
Published by: Greenwood Press, Inc. (Subsidiary of: Greenwood Publishing Group Inc.), 88 Post Rd W, Box 5007, Westport, CT 06881. TEL 203-226-3571, FAX 203-226-1502.

610 016 USA ISSN 0363-0161
Z6675.E8
BIBLIOGRAPHY OF BIOETHICS. Text in English. 1975. a., latest vol.26. USD 70 domestic; USD 80 foreign (effective 2001). **Document type:** *Bibliography.*
Related titles: CD-ROM ed.: (from SilverPlatter Information, Inc.); Online - full text ed.: (from The Dialog Corporation, National Library of Medicine, Telesystemes-Questel).
Indexed: CERDIC.
Published by: Kennedy Institute of Ethics, National Reference Center for Bioethics Literature, Georgetown University, Box 571212, Washington, DC 20057-1212. TEL 202-687-6689, FAX 202-687-6770, medethx@georgetown.edu, http://bioethics.georgetown.edu. Eds. Leroy Walters, Tamar Joy Kahn. Circ: 1,500.

610 016 USA ISSN 0067-7280
Z6660
BIBLIOGRAPHY OF THE HISTORY OF MEDICINE. Text in English. 1965. quinquennial, latest 1990-93, no.28. USD 55; USD 68.75 foreign. **Document type:** *Bibliography, Government.* **Description:** Bibliographic listing of citations dealing with the history of medicine and related sciences and professions.
Related titles: Online - full text ed.: (from National Library of Medicine).
—GNLM, Linda Hall.
Published by: U.S. National Library of Medicine, 8600 Rockville Pike, Bethesda, MD 20894. **Orders to:** U.S. Government Printing Office, Superintendent of Documents.

610 174.2 USA ISSN 0886-8913
BIOETHICS LITERATURE REVIEW. Text in English. m. USD 49 to individuals; USD 69 to institutions (effective 2000). **Document type:** *Newsletter.* **Description:** Covers recent literature in bioethics and related subject areas; reviews 500 health, medical, and major law journals each month.
Published by: University Publishing Group, Inc., 17100 Cole Rd, Ste 312, Hagerstown, MD 31740. TEL 800-654-8188, FAX 301-739-6842, Orders@upgbooks.com.

BIOLOGICAL RHYTHMS. see *BIOLOGY—Abstracting, Bibliographies, Statistics*

610 USA
BIOMEDICAL ENGINEERING CITATION INDEX. Text in English. bi-m. USD 1,950. **Document type:** *Abstract/Index.* **Description:** Provides bibliographic data, cited references, related records and English-language author abstracts from international scholarly research journals and conference proceedings.
Related titles: CD-ROM ed.; Magnetic Tape ed.
Published by: Institute for Scientific Information, 3501 Market St., Philadelphia, PA 19104. TEL 215-386-0100, FAX 215-386-2911.

016.61615 GBR ISSN 0266-6294
BLOOD COAGULATION FACTORS; current awareness service for researchers in life sciences. Text in English. 1985. s-m. GBP 120 for print or e-mail eds. (effective 2001). adv. **Document type:** *Abstract/Index.* **Description:** Covers fibrinogen, thrombin, plasminogen activators and other coagulation factors.
Related titles: E-mail ed.; Online - full text ed.: GBP 108 (effective 2001).
—CCC.
Published by: S U B I S (Subsidiary of: Sheffield Academic Press Ltd), Mansion House, 19 Kingfield Rd, Sheffield, S Yorks S11 9AS, United Kingdom. TEL 44-114-255-4433, FAX 44-114-255-4626, subis@sheffac.demon.co.uk, http://www.shef-ac-press.co.uk/subis. Ed. S Huntridge. Adv. contact C Evans.

330.9021 614.021 BWA ISSN 1013-5723
BOTSWANA. CENTRAL STATISTICS OFFICE. HEALTH STATISTICS REPORT. Text in English. a. BWP 5. charts. back issues avail. **Document type:** *Government.* **Description:** Provides statistics on the distribution and utilization of health facilities throughout Botswana.
Related titles: E-mail ed.; Fax ed.
Published by: Central Statistics Office, c/o Government Statistician, Private Bag 0024, Gaborone, Botswana. TEL 267-31-352200, FAX 267-31-352201, csobots@gov.bw. Ed. G M Charumbira. Pub. J G Segwe. **Orders to:** Government Printer, Private Bag 0081, Gaborone, Botswana. TEL 267-353202, FAX 267-312001, http://www.gov.bw.

616.8 USA ISSN 1084-5968
BRAIN INJURY UPDATE. Text in English. 1986. m. USD 78; USD 88 foreign (effective 1999). bk.rev., software rev., video rev. abstr, bibl, charts, stat. back issues avail. **Document type:** *Newsletter, Abstract/Index.* **Description:** Contains abstracts and summaries of major journal articles dealing with brain injury rehabilitation. Also includes news on brain injury research, conferences, grants, people, prevention, and government and legislation issues. Written for medical and rehabilitation professionals.
Formerly (until 1995): Head Injury Update (0887-1779)
Indexed: e-psyche.
Published by: H D I Publishers, PO Box 131401, Houston, TX 77219. TEL 713-526-6900, 800-321-7037, FAX 713-526-7787, hdijch@aol.com. Ed. Linda L Thoi. Pub. J Charles Haynes. Circ: 1,200 (paid).

BREAST DISEASES. see *MEDICAL SCIENCES—Obstetrics And Gynecology*

016.64933 016 USA ISSN 0896-4572
BREASTFEEDING ABSTRACTS. Text in English. 1981. q. USD 12.50 domestic; USD 15.50 foreign (effective 2001). adv. bk.rev. *Refereed.* **Document type:** *Abstract/Index.* **Description:** Abstracts medical journal articles related to breastfeeding.
—BLDSC (2277.494250).
Published by: La Leche League International, Inc., 1400 N Meacham Rd, P O Box 4079, Schaumburg, IL 60168-4079. TEL 847-519-7730, FAX 847-519-0035, lllhq@llli.org, http://www.lalecheleague.org. Ed. Rebecca Sliter Hugh. Adv. contact Maureen Schumar. Circ: 2,000.

016.61073 GBR ISSN 1366-5588
BRITISH NURSING INDEX; index of journal articles of interest to nurses, midwives and community staff. Text in English. 1991. m. GBP 145; GBP 205 foreign (effective 2000). index. back issues avail. *Refereed.* **Document type:** *Abstract/Index.* **Description:** Covers all the major British publications and other English-language titles in nursing and midwifery.
Former titles (until 1997): Nursing and Midwifery Index (0965-3716); (until Dec. 1995): Nursing Bibliography
Related titles: CD-ROM ed.
—BLDSC (2331.350000).
Published by: (Bournemouth University, Library and Information Services), B N I Publications, Fern Barrow, Poole, Dorset BH12 5BB, United Kingdom. TEL 44-1202-595454, FAX 44-1202-595724, bgrindro@bournemouth.ac.uk; info@optology.com, http://www.bni.org.uk; http://www.optology.com. Ed. John Gill. Circ: 220 (paid).

C A S BIOTECH UPDATES. ANTIBODY CONJUGATES. see *CHEMISTRY—Abstracting, Bibliographies, Statistics*

616.7 USA ISSN 1040-7111
CODEN: CAISEK
C A SELECTS. AIDS AND RELATED IMMUNODEFICIENCIES. Text in English. 1989. s-w. USD 275 (effective 2001). **Document type:** *Abstract/Index.* **Description:** Covers etiology, pathophysiology, clinical manifestations, diagnosis, and therapy of AIDS and other immunodeficiencies.
Published by: Chemical Abstracts Service (Subsidiary of: American Chemical Society), 2540 Olentangy River Rd, Box 3012, Columbus, OH 43210-0012. TEL 614-447-3600, 800-753-4227, FAX 614-447-3751.

616.97 USA ISSN 1047-8191
CODEN: CSAGE2
C A SELECTS. ALLERGY AND ANTIALLERGIC AGENTS. Text in English. 1981. s-w. USD 275 (effective 2001). reprints avail. **Document type:** *Abstract/Index.* **Description:** Covers the pathogenesis, diagnosis, and biochemistry of various allergic conditions, including asthma, dermatitis, and allergies of food, drugs, and environmental agents.
Formerly (until 1989): BIOSIS CAS Selects: Allergy and Antiallergy (0276-3095)
Published by: Chemical Abstracts Service (Subsidiary of: American Chemical Society), 2540 Olentangy River Rd, Box 3012, Columbus, OH 43210-0012. TEL 614-447-3600, 800-753-4227, FAX 614-447-3751.

616.8 USA ISSN 1047-8183
CODEN: CSDDE8
C A SELECTS. ALZHEIMER'S DISEASE & RELATED MEMORY DYSFUNCTIONS. Text in English. 1986. s-w. USD 275 (effective 2001). **Document type:** *Abstract/Index.* **Description:** Covers Alzheimer's Disease and related dementias; includes pathogenesis, diagnosis, and biochemistry of the disease as well as studies on drugs that control such dementias.
Formerly (until 1989): BIOSIS CAS Selects: Alzheimer's Disease and Senile Dementias
Published by: Chemical Abstracts Service (Subsidiary of: American Chemical Society), 2540 Olentangy River Rd, Box 3012, Columbus, OH 43210-0012. TEL 614-447-3600, 800-753-4227, FAX 614-447-3751.

616.7 USA ISSN 0148-2394
CODEN: CSARDY
C A SELECTS. ANTI-INFLAMMATORY AGENTS AND ARTHRITIS. Text in English. s-w. USD 275 (effective 2001). **Document type:** *Abstract/Index.* **Description:** Covers biochemistry of arthritis and rheumatism; effects and mechanism of action of inflammation inhibitors; and synthesis and structure-activity relationships of drugs with potential anti-inflammatory activity.
Published by: Chemical Abstracts Service (Subsidiary of: American Chemical Society), 2540 Olentangy River Rd, Box 3012, Columbus, OH 43210-0012. TEL 614-447-3600, 800-753-4227, FAX 614-447-3751.

616.1 USA ISSN 1051-3892
CODEN: CANTEE
C A SELECTS. ANTIARRHYTHMICS. Text in English. 1990. s-w. USD 275 (effective 2001). **Document type:** *Abstract/Index.* **Description:** Covers established and developmental drugs that ameliorate disorders of normal heart rhythms.
Published by: Chemical Abstracts Service (Subsidiary of: American Chemical Society), 2540 Olentangy River Rd, Box 3012, Columbus, OH 43210-0012. TEL 614-447-3600, 800-753-4227, FAX 614-447-3751.

610 USA ISSN 1047-8175
CODEN: CSALEH

C A SELECTS. ANTICONVULSANTS & ANTIEPILEPTICS. Text in English. 1986. s-w. USD 275 (effective 2001). **Document type:** *Abstract/Index.* **Description:** Covers the anticonvulsant and antiepileptic activities of both established and developmental drugs. Includes synthesis, mechanism(s) of action, formulation, and structure-activity relationships.
Formerly (until 1989): BIOSIS CAS Selects: Anticonvulsants
Published by: Chemical Abstracts Service (Subsidiary of: American Chemical Society), 2540 Olentangy River Rd, Box 3012, Columbus, OH 43210-0012. TEL 614-447-3600, 800-753-4227, FAX 614-447-3751.

616.1 USA ISSN 0148-2378
CODEN: CASDDO

C A SELECTS. ATHEROSCLEROSIS & HEART DISEASE. Text in English. s-w. USD 275 (effective 2001). **Document type:** *Abstract/Index.* **Description:** Covers atherosclerosis, arteriosclerosis, heart disease, hypertension, hypotension, embolic and thrombotic disorders, shock, pharmacology and treatment of cardiovascular disease.
Published by: Chemical Abstracts Service (Subsidiary of: American Chemical Society), 2540 Olentangy River Rd, Box 3012, Columbus, OH 43210-0012. TEL 614-447-3600, 800-753-4227, FAX 614-447-3751.

616.8 USA ISSN 0162-7716
CODEN: CBASDK

C A SELECTS. BIOGENIC AMINES & THE NERVOUS SYSTEM. Text in English. s-w. USD 275 (effective 2001). **Document type:** *Abstract/Index.* **Description:** Covers biogenic amines in the nervous system and neurotransmission.
Published by: Chemical Abstracts Service (Subsidiary of: American Chemical Society), 2540 Olentangy River Rd, Box 3012, Columbus, OH 43210-0012. TEL 614-447-3600, 800-753-4227, FAX 614-447-3751.

616.15 USA ISSN 0162-7732
CODEN: CBCODI

C A SELECTS. BLOOD COAGULATION. Text in English. s-w. USD 275 (effective 2001). **Document type:** *Abstract/Index.* **Description:** Covers blood-coagulation factors, vitamin K, anticoagulants; blood preservation and preservatives; and blood platelet biochemistry.
Published by: Chemical Abstracts Service (Subsidiary of: American Chemical Society), 2540 Olentangy River Rd, Box 3012, Columbus, OH 43210-0012. TEL 614-447-3600, 800-753-4227, FAX 614-447-3751.

C A SELECTS. DRUG INTERACTIONS. see *PHARMACY AND PHARMACOLOGY—Abstracting, Bibliographies, Statistics*

C A SELECTS. MONOCLONAL ANTIBODIES. see *BIOLOGY—Abstracting, Bibliographies, Statistics*

616.19 011 USA ISSN 1047-8116
CODEN: CSNCEL

C A SELECTS. NUTRITIONAL ASPECTS OF CANCER. Text in English. 1985. s-w. USD 275 (effective 2001). **Document type:** *Abstract/Index.* **Description:** Covers all aspects of cancer and nutrition; includes the role of nutrition in the development and control of neoplastic diseases.
Formerly: BIOSIS CAS Selects: Cancer and Nutrition
Published by: Chemical Abstracts Service (Subsidiary of: American Chemical Society), 2540 Olentangy River Rd., Box 3012, Columbus, OH 43210-0012. TEL 614-447-3600, 800-753-4227, FAX 614-447-3751.

610 011 USA ISSN 1047-8132
CODEN: CSOLEJ

C A SELECTS. OSTEOPOROSIS & RELATED BONE LOSS. Text in English. 1989. s-w. USD 275 (effective 2001). **Document type:** *Abstract/Index.* **Description:** Covers osteoporosis and related bone losses; includes the etiology, diagnosis, pathophysiology, biochemistry, and pharmacology of osteoporosis.
Formerly (until 1989): BIOSIS CAS Selects: Osteoporosis
Published by: Chemical Abstracts Service (Subsidiary of: American Chemical Society), 2540 Olentangy River Rd, Box 3012, Columbus, OH 43210-0012. TEL 614-447-3600, 800-753-4227, FAX 614-447-3751.

610 USA ISSN 1083-2661
CODEN: CSPNFV

C A SELECTS PLUS. ANTITUMOR AGENTS. Text in English. s-w. USD 275 (effective 2001). **Document type:** *Abstract/Index.* **Description:** Covers cytotoxic agents, antimetabolites, alkylating agents, neoplasm inhibitors; effect and mechanism of action; synthesis and structure-activity relationships of drugs with potential antitumor activity; and pharmacology of most common antitumor agents.
Formerly: C A Selects. Antitumor Agents (0148-2386)
Published by: Chemical Abstracts Service (Subsidiary of: American Chemical Society), 2540 Olentangy River Rd, Box 3012, Columbus, OH 43210-0012. TEL 614-447-3600, 800-753-4227, FAX 614-447-3751.

616.99 USA ISSN 1084-2322
CODEN: CSCTFI

C A SELECTS PLUS. CARCINOGENS, MUTAGENS & TERATOGENS. Text in English. s-w. USD 275 (effective 2001). **Document type:** *Abstract/Index.* **Description:** Covers biological response to carcinogens, mutagens, and teratogens; mechanism of action and structural requirements for activity; detection and quantification in feed and food material; occupational exposure and resulting health hazards and safety requirements.
Formerly: C A Selects. Carcinogens, Mutagens and Teratogens (0148-2408)
Published by: Chemical Abstracts Service (Subsidiary of: American Chemical Society), 2540 Olentangy River Rd, Box 3012, Columbus, OH 43210-0012. TEL 614-447-3600, 800-753-4227, FAX 614-447-3751.

C A SELECTS PLUS. FORENSIC CHEMISTRY. see *CHEMISTRY—Abstracting, Bibliographies, Statistics*

616.07 USA ISSN 1047-8159
CODEN: CSUIE6

C A SELECTS. ULCER INHIBITORS. Text in English. 1986. s-w. USD 275 (effective 2001). **Document type:** *Abstract/Index.* **Description:** Covers the digestive-tract antiulcer inhibitors of both established and developmental drugs; includes synthesis, mechanic(s) of action, formulation, and structure-activity relationship.
Formerly: BIOSIS CAS Selects: Antiulcer Agents
Published by: Chemical Abstracts Service (Subsidiary of: American Chemical Society), 2540 Olentangy River Rd, Box 3012, Columbus, OH 43210-0012. TEL 614-447-3600, 800-753-4227, FAX 614-447-3751.

616.9 USA

C D C HIV-AIDS SURVEILLANCE REPORTS. Text in English. 1988. q. free per issue. **Document type:** *Government.* **Description:** Provides official analysis of AIDS statistics.
Indexed: Abstr.Hyg., IIS.
Published by: U.S. Centers for Disease Control, OD OPS MASO, 1 B49, Mailstop A 22, Atlanta, GA 30333. TEL 404-639-3311.

616.99 GBR

C R C FACTSHEETS. (Cancer Research Campaign) Text in English. q. GBP 20 (effective 1999). bibl, charts, illus. back issues avail. **Document type:** *Academic/Scholarly.* **Description:** Consists of regularly updated statistical reports on key cancer topics for information services, libraries, and individuals. Some issues deal with specific cancers; others address patterns of incidence, survival and risk.
Published by: Cancer Research Campaign, Information Unit, 10 Cambridge Terr, Regent's Park, London NW1 4JL, United Kingdom. TEL 44-171-224-1333, FAX 44-171-486-8317, http://www.crc.org.uk.

616.8 011 USA ISSN 0141-7711
QP351

C S A NEUROSCIENCES ABSTRACTS. Text in English. 1982. bi-m. USD 1,115 for print & online eds. combined (effective 2002). abstr. a. index on CD-ROM. back issues avail. **Document type:** *Abstract/Index.* **Description:** Covers all aspects of vertebrate and invertebrate neuroscience, with special coverage of neuroimaging, dementia, pain, drug addiction, and memory.
Incorporates: Endocrinology Abstracts (0749-8020)
Related titles: Online - full content ed.: USD 835 for online only (effective 2002) (from The Dialog Corporation, S T N International, CSA).
Published by: Cambridge Scientific Abstracts, 7200 Wisconsin Ave., Suite 601, Bethesda, MD 20814. TEL 301-961-6798, FAX 301-961-6799, journals@csa.com, http://www.csa.com/journals. Ed. Fred Spangler. Pub. Ted Caris.

616.1 USA

▼ **C V SURGERY ONLINE.** (Cardiovascular) Text in English. 2000. m. USD 60 to members; USD 100 to non-members (effective 2001). **Document type:** *Abstract/Index.* **Description:** Compiles an online compilation of articles pertinent to the cardiothoracic and vascular surgeon from five American Heart Association journals: Circulation, Circulation Research, Hypertension, Stroke, and Arteriosclerosis, Thrombosis, and Vascular Surgery.
Media: Online - full text (from HighWire Pr.).
Published by: (American Heart Association), Lippincott Williams & Wilkins (Baltimore) (Subsidiary of: Wolters Kluwer N.V.), 351 W Camden St, Baltimore, MD 21201-2436. TEL 410-528-4000, FAX 410-528-4312, ahavj-feedback@forsythe.stanford.edu, custerv@lww.com, http://cvsonline.org, htt://www.Lww.com.

016.61699 GBR ISSN 1365-330X

CANCER EPIDEMIOLOGY. Text in English. 1996. s-m. GBP 120 for print or e-mail eds. (effective 2001). adv. **Document type:** *Abstract/Index.*
Related titles: E-mail ed.; Online - full text ed.: GBP 108 (effective 2001).
Published by: S U B I S (Subsidiary of: Sheffield Academic Press Ltd), Mansion House, 19 Kingfield Rd, Sheffield, S Yorks S11 9AS, United Kingdom. TEL 44-114-255-4433, FAX 44-114-255-4626, subis@sheffac.demon.co.uk, http://www.shef-ac-press.co.uk/subis. Ed. S Huntridge. Adv. contact C Evans.

CANCER INCIDENCE AND MORTALITY MICHIGAN. see *PUBLIC HEALTH AND SAFETY—Abstracting, Bibliographies, Statistics*

616.9 SWE ISSN 0280-7165

CANCER INCIDENCE IN SWEDEN. Text in Swedish. 1960. a. stat. **Document type:** *Government.*
Published by: (Sweden. Statistiska Centralbyraan), Fritzes, Stockholm 10647, Sweden. TEL 46-8-690-9090, FAX 46-8-690-9091. Circ: 2,000.

CELL MEMBRANES. see *BIOLOGY—Abstracting, Bibliographies, Statistics*

616 CHN ISSN 1000-9086

CHINA MEDICAL ABSTRACTS (INTERNAL MEDICINE). Text in English. 1985. q. USD 28.10 (effective 2000). **Document type:** *Abstract/Index.* **Description:** Abstracts of experimental research of modern medical sciences, traditional Chinese medicine, preventive medicine and clinical experiences.
Related titles: ♦ Chinese ed.: Zhongguo Yixue Wenzhai (Neike Xue). ISSN 1001-4136.
Published by: Nanjing Tiedao Yixueyuan/Nanjing Railway Medical College, 87 Dingjiaqiao, Nanjing, Jiangsu 210009, China. TEL 3301509, FAX 3317073. Ed. Sun Zaiyang. adv.: page USD 2,000. Circ: 1,000. **Dist. overseas by:** China International Book Trading Corp, 35 Chegongzhuang Xilu, Haidian District, Beijing 100044, China.

617.3 JPN

CHUBU NIPPON SEIKEI GEKA SAIGAI GEKA GAKKAI SHOROKU/CENTRAL JAPAN ASSOCIATION OF ORTHOPAEDIC AND TRAUMATIC SURGERY. ABSTRACTS. Text in Japanese. s-a. **Document type:** *Abstract/Index.*
Published by: Chubu Nippon Seikei Geka Saigai Geka Gakkai/Central Japan Association of Orthopaedic Surgery and Traumatology, Teramachi, Imadegawa-Sagaru, Kamigyo-ku, Kyoto-shi 602-0848, Japan. TEL 81-75-231-7599, FAX 81-75-231-7499, chubu-seisai@ma7.seikyou.ne.jp. R&P Hiroshi Sawada.

617.1 FRA ISSN 0009-7209

CINESIOLOGIE; la revue internationale des medecins du sport. Text in French; Summaries in English, French. 1962. 6/yr. FRF 500 domestic to individuals (effective 1999); FRF 126.50 newsstand/cover; FRF 600 foreign to individuals; FRF 380 to students (effective 1999). adv. bk.rev. *Refereed.* **Document type:** *Abstract/Index, Academic/Scholarly, Bibliography.* **Description:** Practical and scientific review of sport medicine and stress.
Indexed: Aqua.Sci.& Fish.Abstr., Aquacult.Abstr., Environ.Sci.Poll.Mgmt., Sportsearch (1975-).
—BLDSC (3198.645000), GNLM. **CCC.**
Published by: Syndicat National des Medecins du Sport, 1 rue d'Alsace, Angers 49100, France. TEL 33-1-41870285, FAX 33-1-41881355, monroche@sport-medical.org. Ed., Adv. contact Dr. Andre Monroche. B&W page FRF 6,900, color page FRF 9,200; trim 27 x 21.

619 USA
CLINICAL RESEARCH RESOURCES DIRECTORY. Text in English. 1978. biennial. free per issue. **Document type:** *Directory, Government.* **Description:** Provides a directory of general clinical research resource centers.
Formerly: General Clinical Research Centers
Related titles: Online - full text ed.
Published by: U.S. National Institutes of Health, National Center for Research Resources, 6705 Rockledge Dr, Rm 5046, Bethesda, MD 20892. TEL 301-435-0888, ospio@ncrr.nih.gov, http://www.ncrr.nih.gov/ncrrprog/clindir/contents.htm. Circ: 9,000.

616.1 GBR ISSN 0958-1650
CLINICIAN'S MANUAL ON HYPERLIPIDEMIA (YEAR). Text in English. 1991. a. USD 15.95. illus. **Document type:** *Academic/Scholarly.* **Description:** For the general practitioner. Focuses on hyperlipidemia, including diagnostic, treatment and screening concerns.
Published by: Current Science Ltd, Middlesex House, 34-42 Cleveland St, London W1P 6LB, United Kingdom. FAX 44-20-7580-1958. Ed. A M Gotto.

616.1 GBR ISSN 0964-5969
CLINICIAN'S MANUAL ON HYPERTENSION AND CONCOMITANT HYPERLIPIDAEMIA. Text in English. 1990. a. USD 15.95. illus. **Document type:** *Academic/Scholarly.* **Description:** For the general practitioner. Focuses on all aspects of hypertension treatment in a concise, easy-to-read format.
Formerly (until 1992): Clinician's Manual on Hypertension (Year) (0952-6307)
Published by: Current Science Ltd, Middlesex House, 34-42 Cleveland St, London W1P 6LB, United Kingdom. FAX 44-20-7580-1938.

617 USA ISSN 0894-8062
COLON AND RECTAL SURGERY OUTLOOK. Text in English. 1988. 10/yr. DEM 60 per issue; free with Colon & Rectal Surgery. adv. **Document type:** *Newsletter, Abstract/Index.* **Description:** Encapsulates journal articles, reports on clinical findings, and symposium proceedings dealing with advances and trends in colon and rectal surgery.
Related titles: ♦ Supplement to: Clinics in Colon & Rectal Surgery. ISSN 1531-0043.
—GNLM.
Published by: Thieme Medical Publishers, 333 Seventh Ave, New York, NY 10001. TEL 212-760-0888, 800-782-3488, FAX 212-947-1112, http://www.thieme.com. Ed. Dr. Theodore R Schrock. Adv. contact Sally Khan. **Orders in Europe to:** Thieme International, Georg Thieme Verlag, Postfach 01120, Stuttgart 70451, Germany. TEL 49-711-8931-0, 49-711-8931-298.

016.619 USA
COMPARATIVE MEDICINE RESEARCH RESOURCES. Text in English. 1978. biennial. free per issue. **Document type:** *Directory, Government.* **Description:** Source directory of animals used for research purposes.
Former titles: Resources for Comparative Biomedical Research; Animal Research Resources
Related titles: Online - full text ed.
Published by: U.S. National Institutes of Health, National Center for Research Resources, 6705 Rockledge Dr, Rm 5046, Bethesda, MD 20892. TEL 301-435-0888, ospio@ncrr.nih.gov, http://www.ncrr.nih.gov. Circ: 9,000.

016.61 GBR ISSN 0950-6667
COMPLEMENTARY MEDICINE INDEX. Text in English. m. GBP 71 in Europe; GBP 90 elsewhere (effective 1999). adv. index. **Document type:** *Bulletin, Abstract/Index, Bibliography.* **Description:** Provides a classified list of English language citations from the current literature of alternative and complementary medicine, with author and subject indexes to each issue. Includes some French and German literature and some abstracts.
Related titles: Online - full text ed.
—BLDSC (3364.203720), GNLM.
Published by: British Library, Health Care Information Service, British Library, Boston Spa, Wetherby, W Yorks LS23 7BQ, United Kingdom. TEL 44-1937-546039, FAX 44-1937-546458, phillipa.seaton@bl.uk. Ed., R&P, Adv. contact Phillipa Seaton.

610 011 USA ISSN 1040-4074
COMPREHENSIVE MEDLINE. (Subscription Option A: current & 2 yr. backfile; Option B: current & 5 yr. backfile; Option C: current & 9 yr. backfile; Option D: full file from 1966 to present) Text in English. 1987. m. USD 1,095 for Option A; USD 1,495 for Option B; USD 2,195 for Option C; USD 2,795 for Option D. **Description:** Includes material on all titles in Index Medicus, International Nursing Index and Index to Dental Literature.
Media: CD-ROM.
Published by: (U.S. National Library of Medicine), EBSCO Publishing (Subsidiary of: EBSCO Industries, Inc.), 10 Estes St, Box 682, Ipswich, MA 01938. TEL 508-356-6565, 800-653-2726, ep@epnet.com, http://www.epnet.com. **Co-sponsor:** U.S. Department of Health & Human Services.

617.75 USA ISSN 0885-9264
CONTACT LENS UPDATE. Text in English. 1982. bi-m. USD 69 domestic to individuals; USD 79 in Canada & Mexico to individuals; USD 84 elsewhere to individuals; USD 79 domestic to institutions; USD 89 in Canada & Mexico to institutions; USD 94 elsewhere to institutions (effective 2000). index. **Document type:** *Newsletter.* **Description:** Summarizes medical and optometry journal articles about specialty contact lens practice.
Published by: Anadem Publishing, Inc., 3620 N High St, Columbus, OH 43214. TEL 614-262-2539, 800-633-0055, FAX 614-262-6630, anadem@erinet.com. Ed. Karla Gale. Pub. Will Kuhlmann. R&P Mike Cheadle.

617.7 USA
CONTACTO. Text in English. 1955. 3/yr. USD 85 domestic; USD 135 foreign (effective 2000). adv. bk.rev. charts, illus. index. **Document type:** *Academic/Scholarly.* **Description:** Scientific clinical journal.
Former titles: Contacto: Mini-Abstracts; Contacto (0045-8317)
Indexed: Excerp.Med.
—GNLM.
Published by: National Eye Research Foundation, 910 Skokie Blvd, Ste 207A, Northbrook, IL 60062. TEL 847-564-4652, 800-621-2258, FAX 847-564-0807, info@nerf.org, http://www.nerf.org. Ed., R&P Andrew K Kim TEL 847-564-5642. Circ: 500.

616.12 016 NLD ISSN 0165-9405
CODEN: CJCADW
CORE JOURNALS IN CARDIOLOGY. Text in English. 1980. 11/yr. EUR 305 in Europe to qualified personnel; JPY 41,265 in Japan to qualified personnel; USD 340 elsewhere to qualified personnel; EUR 479 in Europe to institutions; JPY 63,479 in Japan to institutions; USD 536 elsewhere to institutions (effective 2002). **Document type:** *Abstract/Index.* **Description:** Abstracts of relevant articles in cardiology from the principal medical journals.
Related titles: Online - full text ed.
—CCC.
Published by: Elsevier Science BV, PO Box 211, Amsterdam 1000 AE, Netherlands. nlinfo-f@elsevier.nl, http://www.elsevier.com/locate/corecard, http://www.elsevier.nl. **Subscr. in Australasia and the Far East to:** Elsevier Science (Singapore) Pte Ltd, No.1 Temasek Ave, 17-01 Millenia Tower, Singapore 039192, Singapore. TEL 65-434-3727, FAX 65-337-2230; **Subscr. in Japan to:** Elsevier Science Inc - Japan Regional Office, 9-15 Higashi-Azabu 1-chome, Minato-ku, Tokyo 106-0044, Japan. TEL 81-3-5561-5033; **Subscr. in the Americas to:** Elsevier Science, PO Box 945, New York, NY 10159-0945. TEL 212-633-3730, FAX 212-633-3680.

016 616.8 NLD ISSN 0165-1056
CORE JOURNALS IN CLINICAL NEUROLOGY. Text in Dutch. 1978. 11/yr. NLG 639, EUR 289.97 in Europe to individuals; JPY 39,300 in Japan to individuals; USD 324 elsewhere to individuals; NLG 968, EUR 439.26 in Europe to institutions; JPY 59,600 in Japan to institutions; USD 492 elsewhere to institutions (effective 2001). **Document type:** *Abstract/Index.* **Description:** Current awareness service reporting relevant developments in clinical neurology from the principal medical journals.
Related titles: Online - full text ed.
—CCC.
Published by: Elsevier Science BV, PO Box 211, Amsterdam 1000 AE, Netherlands. nlinfo-f@elsevier.nl, http://www.elsevier.com/locate/coreclin, http://www.elsevier.nl. **Subscr. in Australasia and the Far East to:** Elsevier Science (Singapore) Pte Ltd, No.1 Temasek Ave, 17-01 Millenia Tower, Singapore 039192, Singapore. TEL 65-434-3727, FAX 65-337-2230; **Subscr. in Japan to:** Elsevier Science Inc - Japan Regional Office, 9-15 Higashi-Azabu 1-chome, Minato-ku, Tokyo 106-0044, Japan. TEL 81-3-5561-5033; **Subscr. in the Americas to:** Elsevier Science, PO Box 945, New York, NY 10159-0945. TEL 212-633-3730, FAX 212-633-3680.

616.5 016 NLD ISSN 0167-5796
CORE JOURNALS IN DERMATOLOGY. Text in English. 1982. 11/yr. EUR 305 in Europe to qualified personnel; JPY 41,265 in Japan to qualified personnel (effective 2001); USD 340 elsewhere to qualified personnel; EUR 479 in Europe to institutions; JPY 63,479 in Japan to institutions; USD 536 elsewhere to institutions (effective 2002). **Document type:** *Abstract/Index.* **Description:** Current awareness service reporting important developments in dermatology from the principal medical journals.
Related titles: Online - full text ed.
—CCC.
Published by: Elsevier Science BV, PO Box 211, Amsterdam 1000 AE, Netherlands. nlinfo-f@elsevier.nl, http://www.elsevier.com/locate/corederm, http://www.elsevier.nl. **Subscr. in Australasia and the Far East to:** Elsevier Science (Singapore) Pte Ltd, No.1 Temasek Ave, 17-01 Millenia Tower, Singapore 039192, Singapore. TEL 65-434-3727, FAX 65-337-2230; **Subscr. in Japan to:** Elsevier Science Inc - Japan Regional Office, 9-15 Higashi-Azabu 1-chome, Minato-ku, Tokyo 106-0044, Japan. TEL 81-3-5561-5033; **Subscr. in the Americas to:** Elsevier Science, PO Box 945, New York, NY 10159-0945. TEL 212-633-3730, FAX 212-633-3680.

616.3 016 NLD ISSN 0165-8719
CODEN: CJGADI
CORE JOURNALS IN GASTROENTEROLOGY. Text in English. 1980. 11/yr. EUR 305 in Europe to qualified personnel; JPY 41,265 in Japan to qualified personnel (effective 2001); USD 340 elsewhere to qualified personnel; EUR 479 in Europe to institutions; JPY 63,479 in Japan to institutions; USD 536 elsewhere to institutions (effective 2002). **Document type:** *Abstract/Index.* **Description:** Current awareness service providing abstracts of recent papers in gastroenterology from the principal medical journals.
Related titles: Online - full text ed.
—CCC.
Published by: Elsevier Science BV, PO Box 211, Amsterdam 1000 AE, Netherlands. nlinfo-f@elsevier.nl, http://www.elsevier.com/locate/coregast, http://www.elsevier.nl. **Subscr. in Australasia and the Far East to:** Elsevier Science (Singapore) Pte Ltd, No.1 Temasek Ave, 17-01 Millenia Tower, Singapore 039192, Singapore. TEL 65-434-3727, FAX 65-337-2230; **Subscr. in Japan to:** Elsevier Science Inc - Japan Regional Office, 9-15 Higashi-Azabu 1-chome, Minato-ku, Tokyo 106-0044, Japan. TEL 81-3-5561-5033; **Subscr. in the Americas to:** Elsevier Science, PO Box 945, New York, NY 10159-0945. TEL 212-633-3730, FAX 212-633-3680.

618 016 NLD ISSN 0376-5059
CODEN: CJOGD8
CORE JOURNALS IN OBSTETRICS - GYNECOLOGY. Text in Dutch. 1977. 11/yr. EUR 305 in Europe to qualified personnel; JPY 41,265 in Japan to qualified personnel; USD 340 elsewhere to qualified personnel; EUR 479 in Europe to institutions; JPY 63,479 in Japan to institutions; USD 536 elsewhere to institutions (effective 2002). **Document type:** *Abstract/Index.* **Description:** Current awareness service providing abstracts of recent articles relevant to obstetrics and gynecology from the principal medical journals.
Related titles: Online - full text ed.
—CCC.
Published by: Elsevier Science BV, PO Box 211, Amsterdam 1000 AE, Netherlands. nlinfo-f@elsevier.nl, http://www.elsevier.com/locate/coreobstet, http://www.elsevier.nl. **Subscr. in Australasia and the Far East to:** Elsevier Science (Singapore) Pte Ltd, No.1 Temasek Ave, 17-01 Millenia Tower, Singapore 039192, Singapore. TEL 65-434-3727, FAX 65-337-2230; **Subscr. in Japan to:** Elsevier Science Inc - Japan Regional Office, 9-15 Higashi-Azabu 1-chome, Minato-ku, Tokyo 106-0044, Japan. TEL 81-3-5561-5033; **Subscr. in the Americas to:** Elsevier Science, PO Box 945, New York, NY 10159-0945. TEL 212-633-3730, FAX 212-633-3680.

016 617.7 NLD ISSN 0165-1005
CORE JOURNALS IN OPHTHALMOLOGY. Text in Dutch. 1978. 11/yr. EUR 305 in Europe to qualified personnel; JPY 41,265 in Japan to qualified personnel; USD 340 elsewhere to qualified personnel; EUR 479 in Europe to institutions; JPY 63,479 in Japan to institutions; USD 536 elsewhere to institutions (effective 2002). **Document type:** *Abstract/Index.* **Description:** Current awareness service providing abstracts of recent papers in ophthalmology from the principal medical journals.
Related titles: Online - full text ed.
—CCC.

M

Published by: Elsevier Science BV, PO Box 211, Amsterdam 1000 AE, Netherlands. nlinfo-f@elsevier.nl, http://www.elsevier.com/locate/coreoph, http://www.elsevier.nl. **Subscr. in Australasia and the Far East to:** Elsevier Science (Singapore) Pte Ltd, No.1 Temasek Ave, 17-01 Millenia Tower, Singapore 039192, Singapore. TEL 65-434-3727, FAX 65-337-2230; **Subscr. in Japan to:** Elsevier Science Inc - Japan Regional Office, 9-15 Higashi-Azabu 1-chome, Minato-ku, Tokyo 106-0044, Japan. TEL 81-3-5561-5033; **Subscr. in the Americas to:** Elsevier Science, PO Box 945, New York, NY 10159-0945. TEL 212-633-3730, FAX 212-633-3680.

618.92 016 NLD ISSN 0376-5040
CODEN: CJPED7

CORE JOURNALS IN PEDIATRICS. Text in Dutch. 1978. 11/yr. EUR 305 in Europe to qualified personnel; JPY 41,265 in Japan to qualified personnel; USD 340 elsewhere to qualified personnel; EUR 479 in Europe to institutions; JPY 63,479 in Japan to institutions; USD 536 elsewhere to institutions (effective 2002). **Document type:** *Abstract/Index.* **Description:** Current awareness service providing abstracts of current papers from the principal medical journals on topics pertaining to pediatrics.
Related titles: Online - full text ed.
—CCC.
Published by: Elsevier Science BV, PO Box 211, Amsterdam 1000 AE, Netherlands. nlinfo-f@elsevier.nl, http://www.elsevier.com/locate/coreped, http://www.elsevier.nl. **Subscr. in Australasia and the Far East to:** Elsevier Science (Singapore) Pte Ltd, No.1 Temasek Ave, 17-01 Millenia Tower, Singapore 039192, Singapore. TEL 65-434-3727, FAX 65-337-2230; **Subscr. in Japan to:** Elsevier Science Inc - Japan Regional Office, 9-15 Higashi-Azabu 1-chome, Minato-ku, Tokyo 106-0044, Japan. TEL 81-3-5561-5033; **Subscr. in the Americas to:** Elsevier Science, PO Box 945, New York, NY 10159-0945. TEL 212-633-3730, FAX 212-633-3680.

610 011 USA ISSN 1040-4066

CORE MEDLINE. Text in English. 1989. q. USD 795. **Description:** Includes abstracts and indexing for over 560 journals encompassing all titles in the Abridged Index Medicus and all Medline titles from the three Brandon and Hill lists. Clinically oriented and contains most of English-language nursing and psychology titles.
Published by: (U.S. National Library of Medicine), EBSCO Publishing (Subsidiary of: EBSCO Industries, Inc.), 10 Estes St, Box 682, Ipswich, MA 01938. TEL 508-356-6565, 508-356-6500, ep@epnet.com, http://www.epnet.com.

338.4021 610.6021 USA ISSN 1064-4571
R729.5.G6

COST SURVEY. Cover title: Cost Survey Report. Text in English. 1980. a. USD 300 to non-members; USD 200 to members (effective 2001). charts, stat. back issues avail. **Document type:** *Bulletin.*
Supersedes in part (in 1992): Cost and Production Survey Report (0741-9287); Which was formed by the merger of (1975-1980): Cost Survey (0196-2434); Production Survey (0196-9439)
Related titles: CD-ROM ed.
Indexed: SRI.
Published by: Medical Group Management Association, 104 Inverness Terrace E, Englewood, CO 80112. TEL 888-608-5601, FAX 303-397-1827, survey@mgma.com, http://www.mgma.com. Circ: 10,000.

610.73 016 USA ISSN 0146-5554
Z6675.N7

CUMULATIVE INDEX TO NURSING & ALLIED HEALTH LITERATURE. Short title: C I N A H L. Text in English. 1961. q. USD 365 (effective 1999). adv. illus. cum.index: 1956 to date. reprint service avail. from PQC. **Document type:** *Abstract/Index.* **Description:** Contains more than 200,000 citations from 1982 to present with abstracts to articles published in more than 800 nursing and allied health journals, including selected non-English titles. Also covers relevant materials from biomedicine, management, behavioral sciences, health sciences librarianship, education and consumer health and 17 allied health disciplines.
Incorporates: Nursing and Allied Health Index (0744-8732); Which was formerly (1956-1976): Nursing Literature Index; (until 1977): Cumulative Index to Nursing Literature (0011-3018); Incorporates: C I N A H L'S List of Subject Headings; Which was formerly (until 1977): Cumulative Index to Nursing Literature, Nursing Subject Headings (0070-1793)
Related titles: CD-ROM ed.: (from SilverPlatter Information, Inc.); Magnetic Tape ed.; Microform ed.: (from PQC); Online - full text ed.: (from Data-Star, EBSCO Publishing).
—BLDSC (3492.190000).
Published by: C I N A H L Information Systems, 1509 Wilson Terr, Glendale, CA 91209-0871. TEL 818-409-8005, 800-959-7167, FAX 818-546-5679, cinahl@cinahl.com, http://www.cinahl.com/. Ed. Sarah Marcarian. Circ: 2,500.

616.994 GBR ISSN 0895-9803
Z6664.C2

CURRENT ADVANCES IN CANCER RESEARCH. Text in English. 1988. m. EUR 120 in Europe to qualified personnel; JPY 16,275 in Japan to qualified personnel; USD 135 elsewhere to qualified personnel; EUR 1,569 in Europe to institutions; JPY 208,010 in Japan to institutions; USD 1,755 elsewhere to institutions (effective 2002). back issues avail. **Document type:** *Abstract/Index.* **Description:** Provides a current awareness service in the sphere of cancer research. Lists titles of cancer research papers published throughout the world and classified into 38 main areas, with a comprehensive list of review articles.
Related titles: Diskette ed.; Microfilm ed.: (from PQC); Online - full text ed.
—BLDSC (3494.061500), Infotrieve. **CCC.**
Published by: Elsevier Science BV, PO Box 211, Amsterdam 1000 AE, Netherlands. TEL 31-20-485-2911, FAX 31-20-485-2457, http://www.elsevier.com/locate/cacancer, http://www.elsevier.nl. **Subscr. in Australasia and the Far East to:** Elsevier Science (Singapore) Pte Ltd, No.1 Temasek Ave, 17-01 Millenia Tower, Singapore 039192, Singapore. TEL 65-434-3727, FAX 65-337-2230; **Subscr. in Japan to:** Elsevier Science Inc - Japan Regional Office, 9-15 Higashi-Azabu 1-chome, Minato-ku, Tokyo 106-0044, Japan. TEL 81-3-5561-5033; **Subscr. in the Americas to:** Elsevier Science, PO Box 945, New York, NY 10159-0945. TEL 212-633-3730, FAX 212-633-3680, usinfo-f@elsevier.com.

616.97 GBR ISSN 0964-8747
Z6663.I4

CURRENT ADVANCES IN IMMUNOLOGY & INFECTIOUS DISEASES. Text in English. 1984. m. EUR 120 in Europe to qualified personnel; JPY 16,275 in Japan to qualified personnel; USD 135 elsewhere to qualified personnel; EUR 1,581 in Europe to institutions; JPY 209,583 in Japan to institutions; USD 1,769 elsewhere to institutions (effective 2002). adv. **Document type:** *Abstract/Index.* **Description:** Provides a current awareness service in the sphere of immunology and infectious diseases. Gives listings of titles of immunological papers published throughout the world classified into 271 main areas and provides a comprehensive listing of review articles.
Formerly (until 1992): Current Advances in Immunology (0741-1650)
Related titles: Diskette ed.; Microfilm ed.: (from PQC); Online - full text ed.
—BLDSC (3494.064220), Infotrieve. **CCC.**
Published by: Elsevier Science BV, PO Box 211, Amsterdam 1000 AE, Netherlands. FAX 31-20-485-2457, nlinfo-f@elsevier.nl, http://www.elsevier.com/locate/caimm, http://www.elsevier.nl. Ed. H Smith. **Subscr. in Australasia and the Far East to:** Elsevier Science (Singapore) Pte Ltd, No.1 Temasek Ave, 17-01 Millenia Tower, Singapore 039192, Singapore. TEL 65-434-3727, FAX 65-337-2230; **Subscr. in Japan to:** Elsevier Science Inc - Japan Regional Office, 9-15 Higashi-Azabu 1-chome, Minato-ku, Tokyo 106-0044, Japan. TEL 81-3-5561-5033; **Subscr. in the Americas to:** Elsevier Science, PO Box 945, New York, NY 10159-0945. TEL 212-633-3730, FAX 212-633-3680, usinfo-f@elsevier.com, http://www.elsevier.com.

616.8 GBR ISSN 0741-1677
QP351

CURRENT ADVANCES IN NEUROSCIENCE. Text in English. 1984. m. EUR 120 in Europe to qualified personnel; JPY 16,275 in Japan to qualified personnel; USD 135 elsewhere to qualified personnel; EUR 1,975 in Europe to institutions; JPY 261,783 in Japan to institutions; USD 2,209 elsewhere to institutions (effective 2002). adv. **Document type:** *Abstract/Index.* **Description:** Provides a current awareness service in the sphere of neuroscience. Gives listings of titles of neuroscientific papers published throughout the world classified into 28 main areas and provides a comprehensive listing of review articles.
Related titles: Diskette ed.; Microfilm ed.: (from PQC); Online - full text ed.
Indexed: Curr.Cont. (coverage dropped), e-psyche.
—BLDSC (3494.064340), Infotrieve. **CCC.**
Published by: Elsevier Science BV, PO Box 211, Amsterdam 1000 AE, Netherlands. TEL 31-20-485-2911, FAX 31-20-485-2457, http://www.elsevier.com/locate/caneuro, http://www.elsevier.nl. **Subscr. in Australasia and the Far East to:** Elsevier Science (Singapore) Pte Ltd, No.1 Temasek Ave, 17-01 Millenia Tower, Singapore 039192, Singapore. TEL 65-434-3727, FAX 65-337-2230; **Subscr. in Japan to:** Elsevier Science Inc - Japan Regional Office, 9-15 Higashi-Azabu 1-chome, Minato-ku, Tokyo 106-0044, Japan. TEL 81-3-5561-5033; **Subscr. in the Americas to:** Elsevier Science, PO Box 945, New York, NY 10159-0945. TEL 212-633-3730, FAX 212-633-3680, usinfo-f@elsevier.com.

616.99 USA ISSN 1070-9576

CURRENT CLINICAL TRIALS: ONCOLOGY. Text in English. 1994. bi-m. **Document type:** *Journal, Abstract/Index.* **Description:** Comprises over 1,700 active oncology treatment, supportive care, and screening/prevention studies.
Related titles: CD-ROM ed.: 1999; Online - full text ed.
Published by: Pyros Education Group (Subsidiary of: MediMedia USA, Inc.), 295 North St, Teterboro, NJ 07608. TEL 201-727-9700, FAX 201-727-9333, pyros@medimedia.com, http://www.maelstromgrafx.com/pyros/index2.html.

610 016 USA ISSN 0891-3358
CODEN: CCCMEK

CURRENT CONTENTS: CLINICAL MEDICINE. Short title: C C: C M. Text in English. 1973. w. USD 730. author index; title word index. **Document type:** *Academic/Scholarly, Bibliography.* **Description:** Tables of contents of the world's most important publications covering clinical medicine.
Formerly: Current Contents: Clinical Practice (0091-1704)
Related titles: CD-ROM ed.: (from Institute for Scientific Information); Diskette ed.: ISSN 1062-3159; Magnetic Tape ed.; Online - full text ed.: (from The Dialog Corporation).
Indexed: Inpharma, Pharm.&Out.News, Reac.
—BLDSC (3496.162000), CASDDS, GNLM.
Published by: Institute for Scientific Information, 3501 Market St., Philadelphia, PA 19104. TEL 215-386-0100, FAX 215-386-2911.

016.6161 GBR
CODEN: AYSTFG

CURRENT MEDICAL LITERATURE. ADVANCES IN STROKE. Text in English. 1998. a. GBP 25, USD 40 to individuals; GBP 75, USD 120 to institutions (effective 1999). back issues avail. **Document type:** *Abstract/Index.*
Formerly: Current Medical Literature. Year in Stroke (1359-849X)
—CCC.
Published by: Current Medical Literature Ltd., 40-42 Osnaburgh St, London NW1 3ND, United Kingdom. TEL 44-20-7465-8377, FAX 44-20-7465-8380, enquiries@curmedlit.co.uk. **Dist. by:** Cassis Publishing Ltd., Realpage House, Abingdon Science Park, Barton Ln., Abingdon, Oxon OX13 3NB, United Kingdom. TEL 44-1235-537352, FAX 44-1235-537353.

616.97 GBR ISSN 0968-5626
CODEN: AERGEZ

CURRENT MEDICAL LITERATURE. ALLERGY. Text in English. 1993. q. USD 60 to individuals; USD 20 newsstand/cover to individuals; USD 140, USD 40 to institutions (effective 2002). back issues avail. **Document type:** *Abstract/Index.*
—Infotrieve. **CCC.**
Published by: (Royal Society of Medicine), Current Medical Literature Ltd., 40-42 Osnaburgh St, London NW1 3ND, United Kingdom. TEL 44-20-7465-8377, FAX 44-20-7465-8380, enquiries@curmedlit.co.uk. **Dist. by:** Cassis Publishing Ltd., Realpage House, Abingdon Science Park, Barton Ln., Abingdon, Oxon OX13 3NB, United Kingdom. TEL 44-1235-537352, FAX 44-1235-537353.

016.61796 GBR ISSN 0269-6959
CODEN: CMLAEV

CURRENT MEDICAL LITERATURE. ANAESTHESIOLOGY. Text in English. 1986. 3/yr. USD 60 to individuals; USD 140 to institutions; USD 25 newsstand/cover to individuals; USD 50 newsstand/cover to institutions (effective 2002). back issues avail. **Document type:** *Abstract/Index.*
—CCC.

M

Published by: (Royal Society of Medicine), Current Medical Literature Ltd., 40-42 Osnaburgh St, London NW1 3ND, United Kingdom. TEL 44-20-7465-8377, FAX 44-20-7465-8380, enquiries@curmedlit.co.uk. **Dist. by:** Cassis Publishing Ltd., Realpage House, Abingdon Science Park, Barton Ln., Abingdon, Oxon OX13 3NB, United Kingdom. TEL 44-1235-537352, FAX 44-1235-537353.

016.61699449 GBR ISSN 0956-6511 CODEN: CMBCEL

CURRENT MEDICAL LITERATURE. BREAST CANCER. Text in English. 1989. q. USD 60 to individuals; USD 20 newsstand/cover to individuals; USD 140 to institutions; USD 40 newsstand/cover to institutions (effective 2002). back issues avail. **Document type:** *Abstract/Index.*

Incorporates in part (1988-1997): Current Medical Literature. Breast and Prostate Cancer (0953-6787)

—CCC.

Published by: (Royal Society of Medicine), Current Medical Literature Ltd., 40-42 Osnaburgh St, London NW1 3ND, United Kingdom. TEL 44-20-7465-8377, FAX 44-20-7465-8380, enquiries@curmedlit.co.uk. **Dist. by:** Cassis Publishing Ltd., Realpage House, Abingdon Science Park, Barton Ln., Abingdon, Oxon OX13 3NB, United Kingdom. TEL 44-1235-537352, FAX 44-1235-537353.

016.616075 GBR ISSN 1364-4858 CODEN: CIMOFH

CURRENT MEDICAL LITERATURE. CARDIAC IMAGING MONITOR. Text in English. 1997. q. GBP 25, USD 40 to individuals; GBP 75, USD 120 to institutions (effective 1999). back issues avail. **Document type:** *Abstract/Index.*

—CCC.

Published by: (Royal Society of Medicine), Current Medical Literature Ltd., 40-42 Osnaburgh St, London NW1 3ND, United Kingdom. TEL 44-20-7465-8377, FAX 44-20-7465-8380, enquiries@curmedlit.co.uk. **Dist. by:** Cassis Publishing Ltd., Realpage House, Abingdon Science Park, Barton Ln., Abingdon, Oxon OX13 3NB, United Kingdom. TEL 44-1235-537352, FAX 44-1235-537353.

016.61612 GBR ISSN 1354-0122 CODEN: CMLCF4

CURRENT MEDICAL LITERATURE. CARDIOLOGY. Text in English. 1981. q. USD 60 to individuals; USD 20 newsstand/cover to individuals; USD 140, USD 40 to institutions (effective 2002). back issues avail. **Document type:** *Abstract/Index.*

Formerly (until 1994): Current Medical Literature. Cardiovascular Medicine (0261-3352)

—CCC.

Published by: (Royal Society of Medicine), Current Medical Literature Ltd., 40-42 Osnaburgh St, London NW1 3ND, United Kingdom. TEL 44-20-7465-8377, FAX 44-20-7465-8380, enquiries@curmedlit.co.uk. **Dist. by:** Cassis Publishing Ltd., Realpage House, Abingdon Science Park, Barton Ln., Abingdon, Oxon OX13 3NB, United Kingdom. TEL 44-1235-537352, FAX 44-1235-537353.

016.616994347 GBR ISSN 1364-4831 CODEN: CMCCFR

CURRENT MEDICAL LITERATURE. COLORECTAL CANCER. Text in English. 1997. q. USD 60 to individuals; USD 20 newsstand/cover to individual members; USD 140 to institutions; USD 20 newsstand/cover to institutions (effective 2002). back issues avail. **Document type:** *Abstract/Index.*

—CCC.

Published by: (Royal Society of Medicine), Current Medical Literature Ltd., 40-42 Osnaburgh St, London NW1 3ND, United Kingdom. TEL 44-20-7465-8377, FAX 44-20-7465-8380, enquiries@curmedlit.co.uk. **Dist. by:** Cassis Publishing Ltd., Realpage House, Abingdon Science Park, Barton Ln., Abingdon, Oxon OX13 3NB, United Kingdom. TEL 44-1235-537352, FAX 44-1235-537353.

016.617 GBR CODEN: MJDMFF

CURRENT MEDICAL LITERATURE. CRITICAL CARE MONITOR. Text in English. 1996. s-a. GBP 25, USD 40 to individuals; GBP 75, USD 120 to institutions (effective 1999). back issues avail. **Document type:** *Abstract/Index.*

Formerly: Current Medical Literature. Intensive Care Monitor (1359-8406)

—CCC.

Published by: Current Medical Literature Ltd., 40-42 Osnaburgh St, London NW1 3ND, United Kingdom. TEL 44-20-7465-8377, FAX 44-20-7465-8380, enquiries@curmedlit.co.uk. **Dist. by:** Carfax Publishing Limited, c/o Sue Dommett, PO Box 25, Abingdon, Oxford OX14 3UE, United Kingdom. TEL 44-1235-537352, FAX 44-1235-537353.

616.5 GBR ISSN 1361-4215 CODEN: CMLDF7

CURRENT MEDICAL LITERATURE. DERMATOLOGY. Text in English. 1996. q. USD 60 to individuals; USD 20 newsstand/cover to individuals; USD 140, USD 40 to institutions (effective 2002). back issues avail. **Document type:** *Abstract/Index.*

—Infotrieve. **CCC.**

Published by: (Royal Society of Medicine), Current Medical Literature Ltd., 40-42 Osnaburgh St, London NW1 3ND, United Kingdom. TEL 44-20-7465-8377, FAX 44-20-7465-8380, enquiries@curmedlit.co.uk. **Dist. by:** Cassis Publishing Ltd., Realpage House, Abingdon Science Park, Barton Ln., Abingdon, Oxon OX13 3NB, United Kingdom. TEL 44-1235-537352, FAX 44-1235-537353.

016.616462 GBR ISSN 0265-797X CODEN: CMLDE6

CURRENT MEDICAL LITERATURE. DIABETES. Text in English. 1984. q. USD 60 to individuals; USD 20 newsstand/cover to individuals; USD 140 to institutions; USD 40 newsstand/cover to institutions (effective 2002). back issues avail. **Document type:** *Abstract/Index.*

Related titles: Online - full text ed.

—CCC.

Published by: (Royal Society of Medicine), Current Medical Literature Ltd., 40-42 Osnaburgh St, London NW1 3ND, United Kingdom. TEL 44-20-7465-8377, FAX 44-20-7465-8380, enquiries@curmedlit.co.uk. **Dist. by:** Cassis Publishing Ltd., Realpage House, Abingdon Science Park, Barton Ln., Abingdon, Oxon OX13 3NB, United Kingdom. TEL 44-1235-537352, FAX 44-1235-537353.

016.616853 GBR ISSN 1359-8384 CODEN: EPMOFK

CURRENT MEDICAL LITERATURE. EPILEPSY MONITOR. Text in English. 1996. q. USD 60 to individuals; USD 25 newsstand/cover to individuals; USD 140 to institutions; USD 50 newsstand/cover to institutions (effective 2002). back issues avail. **Document type:** *Abstract/Index.*

Indexed: e-psyche.

—CCC.

Published by: Current Medical Literature Ltd., 40-42 Osnaburgh St, London NW1 3ND, United Kingdom. TEL 44-20-7465-8377, FAX 44-20-7465-8380, enquiries@curmedlit.co.uk. **Dist. by:** Cassis Publishing Ltd., Realpage House, Abingdon Science Park, Barton Ln., Abingdon, Oxon OX13 3NB, United Kingdom. TEL 44-1235-537352, FAX 44-1235-537353.

016.6163005 GBR ISSN 0263-2659 CODEN: CMLGDE

CURRENT MEDICAL LITERATURE. GASTROENTEROLOGY. Text in English. 1982. q. USD 60, USD 20 to individuals; USD 140, USD 40 to institutions (effective 2002). back issues avail. **Document type:** *Abstract/Index.*

—CCC.

Published by: (Royal Society of Medicine), Current Medical Literature Ltd., 40-42 Osnaburgh St, London NW1 3ND, United Kingdom. TEL 44-20-7465-8377, FAX 44-20-7465-8380, enquiries@curmedlit.co.uk. **Dist. by:** Cassis Publishing Ltd., Realpage House, Abingdon Science Park, Barton Ln., Abingdon, Oxon OX13 3NB, United Kingdom. TEL 44-1235-537352, FAX 44-1235-537353.

016.617 GBR ISSN 0966-0224 CODEN: CMLSEH

CURRENT MEDICAL LITERATURE. GENERAL SURGERY. Text in English. 1992. q. membership only. back issues avail. **Document type:** *Abstract/Index.*

—CCC.

Published by: (Royal Society of Medicine), Current Medical Literature Ltd., 40-42 Osnaburgh St, London NW1 3ND, United Kingdom. TEL 44-20-7465-8377, FAX 44-20-7465-8380, enquiries@curmedlit.co.uk. **Dist. by:** Cassis Publishing Ltd., Realpage House, Abingdon Science Park, Barton Ln., Abingdon, Oxon OX13 3NB, United Kingdom. TEL 44-1235-537352, FAX 44-1235-537353.

016.6181 GBR ISSN 1356-742X CODEN: CLGOE7

CURRENT MEDICAL LITERATURE. GYNAECOLOGY AND OBSTETRICS. Text in English. 1995. q. USD 60 to individuals; USD 20 newsstand/cover to individuals; USD 140 to institutions; USD 40 newsstand/cover to institutions (effective 2002). back issues avail. **Document type:** *Abstract/Index.*

—CCC.

Published by: (Royal Society of Medicine), Current Medical Literature Ltd., 40-42 Osnaburgh St, London NW1 3ND, United Kingdom. TEL 44-20-7465-8377, FAX 44-20-7465-8380, enquiries@curmedlit.co.uk. **Dist. by:** Cassis Publishing Ltd., Realpage House, Abingdon Science Park, Barton Ln., Abingdon, Oxon OX13 3NB, United Kingdom. TEL 44-1235-537352, FAX 44-1235-537353.

CURRENT MEDICAL LITERATURE. HEALTH CARE OF OLDER PEOPLE. see *GERONTOLOGY AND GERIATRICS—Abstracting, Bibliographies, Statistics*

016.6169 GBR ISSN 0951-9602 CODEN: CLDIEI

CURRENT MEDICAL LITERATURE. INFECTIOUS DISEASES. Text in English. 1988. q. GBP 25, USD 40 to individuals; GBP 75, USD 120 to institutions (effective 1999). back issues avail. **Document type:** *Abstract/Index.*

—CCC.

Published by: (Royal Society of Medicine), Current Medical Literature Ltd., 40-42 Osnaburgh St, London NW1 3ND, United Kingdom. TEL 44-20-7465-8377, FAX 44-20-7465-8380, enquiries@curmedlit.co.uk. **Dist. by:** Cassis Publishing Ltd., Realpage House, Abingdon Science Park, Barton Ln., Abingdon, Oxon OX13 3NB, United Kingdom. TEL 44-1235-537352, FAX 44-1235-537353.

CURRENT MEDICAL LITERATURE. INTERNATIONAL HOSPITAL PHARMACY. see *PHARMACY AND PHARMACOLOGY—Abstracting, Bibliographies, Statistics*

016.6161 GBR ISSN 1352-738X CODEN: ICAME8

CURRENT MEDICAL LITERATURE. INTERVENTIONAL CARDIOLOGY MONITOR. Text in English. 1994. q. USD 100 to individuals; USD 37.50 newsstand/cover to individuals; USD 260 to institutions; USD 75 newsstand/cover to institutions (effective 2002). back issues avail. **Document type:** *Abstract/Index.*

—CCC.

Published by: Current Medical Literature Ltd., 40-42 Osnaburgh St, London NW1 3ND, United Kingdom. TEL 44-20-7465-8377, FAX 44-20-7465-8380, enquiries@curmedlit.co.uk. **Dist. by:** Cassis Publishing Ltd., Realpage House, Abingdon Science Park, Barton Ln., Abingdon, Oxon OX13 3NB, United Kingdom. TEL 44-1235-537352, FAX 44-1235-537353.

016.61699419 GBR ISSN 0969-7063 CODEN: LYMYEJ

CURRENT MEDICAL LITERATURE. LEUKAEMIA AND LYMPHOMA. Text in English. 1993. q. USD 60, USD 20 to individuals; USD 140, USD 40 to institutions (effective 2002). back issues avail. **Document type:** *Abstract/Index.*

—Infotrieve. **CCC.**

Published by: (Royal Society of Medicine), Current Medical Literature Ltd., 40-42 Osnaburgh St, London NW1 3ND, United Kingdom. TEL 44-20-7465-8377, FAX 44-20-7465-8380, enquiries@curmedlit.co.uk. **Dist. by:** Cassis Publishing Ltd., Realpage House, Abingdon Science Park, Barton Ln., Abingdon, Oxon OX13 3NB, United Kingdom. TEL 44-1235-537352, FAX 44-1235-537353.

016.61607 GBR CODEN: CMRAER

CURRENT MEDICAL LITERATURE. MEDICAL IMAGING. Text in English. 1989. q. GBP 25, USD 40 to individuals; GBP 75, USD 120 to institutions (effective 1999). back issues avail. **Document type:** *Abstract/Index.*

Formerly: Current Medical Literature. Radiology (0955-1476)

—CCC.

Published by: (Royal Society of Medicine), Current Medical Literature Ltd., 40-42 Osnaburgh St, London NW1 3ND, United Kingdom. TEL 44-20-7465-8377, FAX 44-20-7465-8380, enquiries@curmedlit.co.uk. **Dist. by:** Cassis Publishing Ltd., Realpage House, Abingdon Science Park, Barton Ln., Abingdon, Oxon OX13 3NB, United Kingdom. TEL 44-1235-537352, FAX 44-1235-537353.

016.6166 GBR ISSN 1357-1540 CODEN: CMNHFT
CURRENT MEDICAL LITERATURE. NEPHROLOGY AND HYPERTENSION. Text in English. 1987; N.S. 1995. q. USD 60 to individuals; USD 20 newsstand/cover to individuals; USD 140 to institutions; USD 40 newsstand/cover to institutions (effective 2002). back issues avail. **Document type:** *Abstract/Index.*
Supersedes in part (in 1995): Current Medical Literature. Nephrology and Urology (0951-9629)
—CCC.
Published by: (Royal Society of Medicine), Current Medical Literature Ltd., 40-42 Osnaburgh St, London NW1 3ND, United Kingdom. TEL 44-20-7465-8377, FAX 44-20-7465-8380, enquiries@curmedlit.co.uk. **Dist. by:** Cassis Publishing Ltd., Realpage House, Abingdon Science Park, Barton Ln., Abingdon, Oxon OX13 3NB, United Kingdom. TEL 44-1235-537352, FAX 44-1235-537353.

016.6168 GBR CODEN: CMLNEZ
CURRENT MEDICAL LITERATURE. NEUROLOGY & NEUROSURGERY. Text in English. 1984. q. GBP 25, USD 40 to individuals; GBP 75, USD 120 to institutions (effective 1999). back issues avail. **Document type:** *Abstract/Index.*
Former titles: Current Medical Literature. Neurology (1356-6237); Current Medical Literature. Neurology and Neurosurgery (1356-6245); (until 1991): Current Medical Literature. Neurology (0267-0445)
Indexed: e-psyche.
—CCC.
Published by: (Royal Society of Medicine), Current Medical Literature Ltd., 40-42 Osnaburgh St, London NW1 3ND, United Kingdom. TEL 44-20-7465-8377, FAX 44-20-7465-8380, enquiries@curmedlit.co.uk. **Dist. by:** Cassis Publishing Ltd., Realpage House, Abingdon Science Park, Barton Ln., Abingdon, Oxon OX13 3NB, United Kingdom. TEL 44-1235-537352, FAX 44-1235-537353.

016.6177 GBR ISSN 0963-0112 CODEN: CMOPEN
CURRENT MEDICAL LITERATURE. OPHTHALMOLOGY. Text in English. 1991. q. USD 60 to individuals; USD 20 newsstand/cover to individuals; USD 140, USD 40 to institutions (effective 2002). back issues avail. **Document type:** *Abstract/Index.*
—CCC.
Published by: (Royal Society of Medicine), Current Medical Literature Ltd., 40-42 Osnaburgh St, London NW1 3ND, United Kingdom. TEL 44-20-7465-8377, FAX 44-20-7465-8380, enquiries@curmedlit.co.uk. **Dist. by:** Cassis Publishing Ltd., Realpage House, Abingdon Science Park, Barton Ln., Abingdon, Oxon OX13 3NB, United Kingdom. TEL 44-1235-537352, FAX 44-1235-537353.

016.61892 GBR ISSN 0951-9610 CODEN: CMLPE8
CURRENT MEDICAL LITERATURE. PAEDIATRICS. Text in English. 1987. q. USD 60, USD 20 to individuals; USD 140, USD 40 to institutions (effective 2002). back issues avail. **Document type:** *Abstract/Index.*
—CCC.
Published by: (Royal Society of Medicine), Current Medical Literature Ltd., 40-42 Osnaburgh St, London NW1 3ND, United Kingdom. TEL 44-20-7465-8377, FAX 44-20-7465-8380, enquiries@curmedlit.co.uk. **Dist. by:** Cassis Publishing Ltd., Realpage House, Abingdon Science Park, Barton Ln., Abingdon, Oxon OX13 3NB, United Kingdom. TEL 44-1235-537352, FAX 44-1235-537353.

016.6168527 GBR ISSN 1361-634X CODEN: CMPDFR
CURRENT MEDICAL LITERATURE. PERSPECTIVES IN DEPRESSION. Text in English. 1993. 3/yr. USD 60 to individuals; USD 25 newsstand/cover to individuals; USD 140 to institutions; USD 50 newsstand/cover to institutions (effective 2002). back issues avail. **Document type:** *Abstract/Index.*
Formerly (until 1996): Current Medical Literature. Focus on Depression (1351-9395)
Indexed: e-psyche.
—BLDSC (6428.141000). **CCC.**
Published by: Current Medical Literature Ltd., 40-42 Osnaburgh St, London NW1 3ND, United Kingdom. TEL 44-20-7465-8377, FAX 44-20-7465-8380, enquiries@curmedlit.co.uk. **Dist. by:** Cassis Publishing Ltd., Realpage House, Abingdon Science Park, Barton Ln., Abingdon, Oxon OX13 3NB, United Kingdom. TEL 44-1235-537352, FAX 44-1235-537353.

016.616 GBR ISSN 1366-8552
CURRENT MEDICAL LITERATURE. PROSTATIC DISEASE. Text in English. 1997. q. GBP 25, USD 40 to individuals; GBP 75, USD 120 to institutions. back issues avail. **Document type:** *Abstract/Index.*
Incorporates in part (1988-1997): Current Medical Literature. Breast and Prostate Cancer (0953-6787)
Published by: (Royal Society of Medicine), Current Medical Literature Ltd., 40-42 Osnaburgh St, London NW1 3ND, United Kingdom. TEL 44-20-7465-8377, FAX 44-20-7465-8380, enquiries@curmedlit.co.uk. **Dist. by:** Cassis Publishing Ltd., Realpage House, Abingdon Science Park, Barton Ln., Abingdon, Oxon OX13 3NB, United Kingdom. TEL 44-1235-537352, FAX 44-1235-537353.

016.61689 GBR ISSN 0957-770X CODEN: CMLPF9
CURRENT MEDICAL LITERATURE. PSYCHIATRY. Text in English. 1990. q. USD 60 to individuals; USD 20 newsstand/cover to individuals; USD 140 to institutions; USD 40 newsstand/cover to institutions (2002). back issues avail. **Document type:** *Abstract/Index.*
Indexed: e-psyche.
—Infotrieve. **CCC.**
Published by: (Royal Society of Medicine), Current Medical Literature Ltd., 40-42 Osnaburgh St, London NW1 3ND, United Kingdom. TEL 44-20-7465-8377, FAX 44-20-7465-8380, enquiries@curmedlit.co.uk. **Dist. by:** Cassis Publishing Ltd., Realpage House, Abingdon Science Park, Barton Ln., Abingdon, Oxon OX13 3NB, United Kingdom. TEL 44-1235-537352, FAX 44-1235-537353.

016.61689 GBR ISSN 1363-7339
CURRENT MEDICAL LITERATURE. PSYCHIATRY REVIEWS; recent developments in psychiatric care for General Practitioners. Key Title: Psychiatry Reviews. Text in English. 1996. q. GBP 25, USD 40 to individuals; GBP 75, USD 120 to institutions (effective 2000). back issues avail. **Document type:** *Abstract/Index.*
Indexed: e-psyche.
—CCC.
Published by: (Royal Society of Medicine), Current Medical Literature Ltd., 40-42 Osnaburgh St, London NW1 3ND, United Kingdom. TEL 44-20-7465-8733, FAX 44-20-7465-8380, enquiries@curmedlit.co.uk. Ed. Dr. Trevor Turner. **Dist. by:** Cassis Publishing Ltd., Realpage House, Abingdon Science Park, Barton Ln., Abingdon, Oxon OX13 3NB, United Kingdom. TEL 44-1235-537352, FAX 44-1235-537353.

016.61624 GBR ISSN 1361-6706 CODEN: CMLRFF
CURRENT MEDICAL LITERATURE. RESPIRATORY MEDICINE. Text in English. 1987. q. USD 60 to individuals; USD 20 newsstand/cover to individuals; USD 140 to institutions; USD 40 newsstand/cover to institutions (2002). back issues avail. **Document type:** *Abstract/Index.*
Formerly (until 1993): Current Medical Literature. Reversible Obstructive Airways Disease (0950-8724)
—CCC.
Published by: (Royal Society of Medicine), Current Medical Literature Ltd., 40-42 Osnaburgh St, London NW1 3ND, United Kingdom. TEL 44-20-7465-8377, FAX 44-20-7465-8380, enquiries@curmedlit.co.uk. **Dist. by:** Cassis Publishing Ltd., Realpage House, Abingdon Science Park, Barton Ln., Abingdon, Oxon OX13 3NB, United Kingdom. TEL 44-1235-537352, FAX 44-1235-537353.

016.6167 GBR ISSN 0261-3360 CODEN: CLRMDL
CURRENT MEDICAL LITERATURE. RHEUMATOLOGY. Text in English. 1982. q. USD 60 to individuals; USD 20 newsstand/cover to individuals; USD 140 to institutions; USD 40 newsstand/cover to institutions (2002). back issues avail. **Document type:** *Abstract/Index.*
—CCC.
Published by: (Royal Society of Medicine), Current Medical Literature Ltd., 40-42 Osnaburgh St, London NW1 3ND, United Kingdom. TEL 44-20-7465-8377, FAX 44-20-7465-8380, enquiries@curmedlit.co.uk. **Dist. by:** Cassis Publishing Ltd., Realpage House, Abingdon Science Park, Barton Ln., Abingdon, Oxon OX13 3NB, United Kingdom. TEL 44-1235-537352, FAX 44-1235-537353.

016.617 GBR ISSN 0969-1537 CODEN: SRNFET
CURRENT MEDICAL LITERATURE. SURGICAL INFECTION. Text in English. 1989. 3/yr. GBP 25, USD 40 to individuals; GBP 75, USD 120 to institutions. **Document type:** *Abstract/Index.*
—CCC.
Published by: (Royal Society of Medicine), Current Medical Literature Ltd., 40-42 Osnaburgh St, London NW1 3ND, United Kingdom. TEL 44-20-7465-8377, FAX 44-20-7465-8380, enquiries@curmedlit.co.uk. **Dist. by:** Cassis Publishing Ltd., Realpage House, Abingdon Science Park, Barton Ln., Abingdon, Oxon OX13 3NB, United Kingdom. TEL 44-1235-537352, FAX 44-1235-537353.

016.6166 GBR ISSN 1357-1532 CODEN: CMLUEN
CURRENT MEDICAL LITERATURE. UROLOGY. Text in English. 1987; N.S. 1995. q. USD 60 to individuals; USD 20 newsstand/cover to individuals; USD 140 to institutions; USD 40 newsstand/cover to institutions (2002). back issues avail. **Document type:** *Abstract/Index.*
Supersedes in part (in 1995): Current Medical Literature. Nephrology and Urology (0951-9629)
—CCC.
Published by: (Royal Society of Medicine), Current Medical Literature Ltd., 40-42 Osnaburgh St, London NW1 3ND, United Kingdom. TEL 44-20-7465-8377, FAX 44-20-7465-8380, enquiries@curmedlit.co.uk. **Dist. by:** Cassis Publishing Ltd., Realpage House, Abingdon Science Park, Barton Ln., Abingdon, Oxon OX13 3NB, United Kingdom. TEL 44-1235-537352, FAX 44-1235-537353.

616.97 GBR ISSN 0952-7915 CODEN: COPIEL
CURRENT OPINION IN IMMUNOLOGY. Text in English. 1988. bi-m. USD 206 in North America to individuals; USD 247 in North America to individuals with online ed; GBP 125 elsewhere to individuals; GBP 150 elsewhere to individuals with online ed; USD 822 in North America to institutions includes online ed; GBP 500 elsewhere to institutions includes online ed; USD 90, GBP 60 elsewhere to students (effective 1999 & 2000). adv. bibl, illus. back issues avail. *Refereed.* **Document type:** *Academic/Scholarly.* **Description:** Directed toward researchers, educators, and students in immunology. Presents review articles, followed by annotated bibliographies of references consulted. Includes a "Paper Alert" section, giving brief summaries of relevant papers recently published in other journals.
Related titles: CD-ROM ed.; Online - full text ed.: USD 227 in North America to individuals; USD 247 in North America to individuals with print ed; GBP 137 elsewhere to individuals; USD 822 elsewhere to institutions includes print ed; GBP 150 elsewhere to individuals includes print ed (effective 1999 & 2000) (from EBSCO Publishing, ingenta, Swets Blackwell, ScienceDirect, Institute for Scientific Information).
Indexed: AIDS & Cancer Res., ASCA, AgBiotech, Anim.Breed.Abstr., Chem.Abstr., Chem.Indus.Notes, Chem.Titles, Curr.Cont., Environ.Sci.Poll.Mgmt., Excerp.Med., Helminthol.Abstr., Immun.Abstr., Ind.Med. (1988-), Ind.Sci.Rev., Ind.Vet., Inpharma, Int.Abstr.Biol.Sci., Microbiol.Abstr., Pharm.&Out.News, Plant Breed.Abstr., Protozool.Abstr., Reac., Rev.Appl.Entomol., Rev.Plant Path., Sci.Cit.Ind., Virol.Abstr. (coverage dropped).
—BLDSC (3500.775300), ADONIS, CASDDS, CISTI, EMDOCS, GNLM, IDS, Infotrieve, ingenta, KNAW. **CCC.**
Published by: Elsevier Science Ltd., Elsevier Trends Journals, 84 Theobald's Rd, London WC1X 8RR, United Kingdom. TEL 44-20-7611-4400, FAX 44-20-7611-4468, cbl@current-biology.com, info@current-opinion.com, http://current-biology.com/info/imminfo.htm, http://www.current-opinion.com. Circ: 3,000. **Subscr. to:** PO Box 331, Haywards Heath, West Sussex RH16 3FG, United Kingdom. TEL 44-1444-475650, FAX 44-1444-445423.

610 016 GBR ISSN 0011-3999
CURRENT WORK IN THE HISTORY OF MEDICINE; an international bibliography. Text in English. 1954. q. GBP 21 to individuals; GBP 31.35 to institutions. bibl. **Document type:** *Bibliography.* **Description:** Covers the history of medicine.
Indexed: A.I.C.P.
—GNLM.
Published by: (Wellcome Institute for the History of Medicine), Professional & Scientific Publications, BMA House, Tavistock St, London WC2E 7PH, United Kingdom. TEL 0171-383-6640, FAX 0171-383-6662. Circ: 750.

016.61637 GBR ISSN 1365-3318
CYSTIC FIBROSIS. Text in English. 1996. s-m. GBP 120 for print or e-mail eds. (effective 2001). adv. **Document type:** *Abstract/Index.*
Related titles: E-mail ed.; Online - full text ed.: GBP 108 (effective 2001).
Indexed: Chem.Abstr., Chem.Indus.Notes, Chem.Titles.

M

Published by: S U B I S (Subsidiary of: Sheffield Academic Press Ltd), Mansion House, 19 Kingfield Rd, Sheffield, S Yorks S11 9AS, United Kingdom. TEL 44-114-255-4433, FAX 44-114-255-4626, subis@sheffac.demon.co.uk, http://www.shef-ac-press.co.uk/subis. Ed. S Huntridge. Adv. contact C Evans.

610 DEU ISSN 3002-1472
D M W DISK-ARCHIV. (Deutsche Medizinische Wochenschrift) Text in German. 1990. s-a. EUR 67.70 domestic to institutions; EUR 81.80 in Europe to institutions; EUR 85 elsewhere to institutions; EUR 29.50 newsstand/cover to institutions (effective 2002). **Document type:** *Abstract/Index.*
Media: CD-ROM. **Related titles:** Microform ed.: (from PQC,PMC); Online - full text ed.: ISSN 1439-4413 (from Institute for Scientific Information); ♦ Print ed.: Deutsche Medizinische Wochenschrift. ISSN 0012-0472.
Published by: Georg Thieme Verlag, Ruedigerstr 14, Stuttgart 70469, Germany. TEL 49-711-8931-0, FAX 49-711-8931298, leser.service@thieme.de, http://www.thieme.de.

DEGUO YIXUE/DEUTSCHE MEDIZIN; an international journal. see *MEDICAL SCIENCES*

DEMOGRAPHIC AND HEALTH SURVEY (YEAR). see *POPULATION STUDIES—Abstracting, Bibliographies, Statistics*

016.6176 USA ISSN 0011-8486
RK1
DENTAL ABSTRACTS. Text in English. 1955. bi-m. USD 60 domestic to individuals; USD 79 foreign to individuals; USD 121 domestic to institutions; USD 141 foreign to institutions; USD 39 domestic to students; USD 57 foreign to students; USD 24 newsstand/cover domestic (effective 2001). reprint service avail. from PQC. **Document type:** *Abstract/Index.* **Description:** Presents articles from more than 100 dental and medical journals; keeps dentists informed of developments and advances in general dentistry and its specialties.
Related titles: Microform ed.: (from PQC).
Indexed: CINAHL.
—BLDSC (3553.240000), CISTI, GNLM. **CCC.**
Published by: (American Dental Association), Mosby, Inc. (Subsidiary of: Elsevier Science), 11830 Westline Industrial Dr, St Louis, MO 63146-3318. TEL 314-872-8370, 800-325-4177, FAX 314-432-1380, TELEX 44-2402, journal.service@mosby.com, http://www.mosby.com/periodicals. Ed. Lawrence H Meskin.

610 USA
DETWILER'S DIRECTORY OF HEALTH AND MEDICAL RESOURCES (YEAR). Text in English. 1992. biennial. USD 195 (effective 2001). **Document type:** *Directory.* **Description:** It's a comprehensive guide to over 2,000 health and medical corporations, associations, state and federal agencies, healthcare market research firms, foundations, institutes and more. Organized for access by service, subject, publication or acronym.
Formerly (until 1997): Detwiler Directory of Medical Market Sources (1058-2797)
Published by: (S.M. Detwiler and Associates), Information Today, Inc., 143 Old Marlton Pike, Medford, NJ 08055-8750. TEL 609-654-6266, 800-300-9868, FAX 609-654-4309, www.infotoday.com, http://www.infotoday.com. Ed. Susan M Detwiler.

016.616462 GBR ISSN 0263-7294
DIABETES MELLITUS. Text in English. s-m. GBP 120 for print or e-mail eds. (effective 2001). adv. back issues avail. **Document type:** *Abstract/Index.* **Description:** Current awareness service for researchers in clinical and life sciences.
Related titles: E-mail ed.; Online - full text ed.: GBP 108 (effective 2001).
—Infotrieve. **CCC.**
Published by: S U B I S (Subsidiary of: Sheffield Academic Press Ltd), Mansion House, 19 Kingfield Rd, Sheffield, S Yorks S11 9AS, United Kingdom. TEL 44-114-255-4433, FAX 44-114-255-4626, subis@sheffac.demon.co.uk, http://www.shef-ac-press.co.uk/subis. Ed. S Huntridge. Adv. contact C Evans.

016.6168 USA ISSN 0012-2769
RC321
DIGEST OF NEUROLOGY & PSYCHIATRY. Text in English. 1932. q. USD 25 domestic; USD 30 foreign (effective 1999). bk.rev. abstr. index. reprint service avail. from PQC.
Related titles: Microfilm ed.: (from PQC).
Published by: Institute of Living, 400 Washington St, Hartford, CT 06106. TEL 860-545-7276, FAX 860-545-7275. Ed. Dr. Harold I Schwartz. Circ: 500.

610 016 GBR ISSN 1352-321X
DIRECTORY OF EUROPEAN MEDICAL ORGANISATIONS. Text in English. 1993. irreg. GBP 90, USD 180 (effective 2001). **Document type:** *Directory.* **Description:** Lists 4,000 national medical organizations based in all countries of Europe.
Published by: C.B.D. Research Ltd., 15 Wickham Rd, Beckenham, Kent BR3 5JS, United Kingdom. TEL 44-20-86507745, FAX 44-20-86500768. **Dist. in the U.S. by:** Gale Research Co., Book Tower, Detroit, MI 48226.

610 620 USA ISSN 1060-1759
DIRECTORY OF PUBLISHED PROCEEDINGS. SERIES M L S - MEDICAL, LIFE SCIENCES. Text in English. 1991. a. USD 135. bibl. index, cum.index. **Document type:** *Directory, Proceedings, Bibliography.* **Description:** Contains an index of conferences and the published proceedings in the fields of medicine and life sciences.
—KNAW.
Published by: InterDok Corp., 173 Halstead Ave, Box 326, Harrison, NY 10528. TEL 914-835-3506, FAX 914-835-6757, http://www.interdok.com. Ed. Jomarie Broccoli. R&P Laurence Baschkin.

610 USA ISSN 1071-7560
R11
DOODY'S HEALTH SCIENCES BOOK REVIEW JOURNAL. Text in English. 1993. bi-m. USD 320 in US & Canada; USD 350 foreign (effective 2000). adv. **Document type:** *Academic/Scholarly.* **Description:** Aimed at health sciences librarians. Provides timely, independent reviews of newly published health sciences books. Includes complete bibliographic information.
Incorporates: Doody's Rating Service (1074-9640)
—GNLM, Infotrieve. **CCC.**
Published by: Doody Publishing, Inc., 1101 Lake St, Ste 306, Oak Park, IL 60301-1047. TEL 708-386-9500, 800-219-9500, FAX 708-386-0860. Eds. Anne Hennissey, Kris Horeis. R&Ps Daniel J Doody, Florence Merkl. Adv. contact Florence Merkl.

016.61 USA
EMBASE ALERT. Text in English. bi-w. **Document type:** *Abstract/Index, Bibliography.* **Description:** Provides updates of citations and abstracts scanned for EMBASE.
Related titles: CD-ROM ed.: (from SilverPlatter Information, Inc.); Online - full text ed.: (from SilverPlatter Information, Inc.).
Published by: SilverPlatter Information, Inc., 100 River Ridge Dr, Norwood, MA 02062-5026. TEL 781-769-2599, 800-343-0064, FAX 781-769-87632, info@silverplatter.com, http://www.silverplatter.com.

016.61 NLD ISSN 0929-3302
EMBASE LIST OF JOURNALS INDEXED (YEAR). Text in English. 1964. a. index. back issues avail. **Document type:** *Abstract/Index, Bibliography.* **Description:** Lists approximately 3,600 biomedical journals screened for items for inclusion in EMBASE and the other Excerpta Medica services. Each entry includes full journal title, EMBASE abbreviation, ISSN and CODEN, publisher's name, address and telephone and frequency.
Former titles (until 1993): List of Journals Abstracted (0923-5582); (until 1989): Excerpta Medica Foundation. List of Journals Abstracted (0167-613X); Excerpta Medica. List of Journals Abstracted (0531-5123)
Related titles: CD-ROM ed.: EMBASE C D (from SilverPlatter Information, Inc.); Online - full text ed.: (from SilverPlatter Information, Inc.).
—BLDSC (3733.004500), GNLM.
Published by: Elsevier Science BV, PO Box 211, Amsterdam 1000 AE, Netherlands. nlinfo-f@elsevier.nl, http://www.elsevier.nl/. **Subscr. in Australasia and the Far East to:** Elsevier Science (Singapore) Pte Ltd, No.1 Temasek Ave, 17-01 Millenia Tower, Singapore 039192, Singapore. TEL 65-434-3727, FAX 65-337-2230; **Subscr. in Japan to:** Elsevier Science Inc - Japan Regional Office, 9-15 Higashi-Azabu 1-chome, Minato-ku, Tokyo 106-0044, Japan. TEL 81-3-5561-5033; **Subscr. in the Americas to:** Elsevier Science, PO Box 945, New York, NY 10159-0945. TEL 212-633-3730, FAX 212-633-3680, http://www.elsevier.com.

016.6165 GBR ISSN 0142-808X
ERYTHROCYTES. Text in English. 1979. s-m. GBP 120 for print or e-mail eds. (effective 2001). adv. bk.rev. **Document type:** *Abstract/Index.* **Description:** Covers red blood cell function, structure, hemoglobin and parasitology.
Related titles: E-mail ed.; Online - full text ed.: GBP 108 (effective 2001).
Published by: S U B I S (Subsidiary of: Sheffield Academic Press Ltd), Mansion House, 19 Kingfield Rd, Sheffield, S Yorks S11 9AS, United Kingdom. TEL 44-114-255-4433, FAX 44-114-255-4626, subis@sheffac.demon.co.uk, http://www.shef-ac-press.co.uk/subis. Ed. S Huntridge. Adv. contact C Evans.

610 BRA ISSN 0101-3033
RA984.B8
ESTATISTICAS DA SAUDE: ASSISTENCIA MEDICO-SANITARIA. Text in Portuguese. 1976. a. USD 70 (effective 1998). charts, stat. **Document type:** *Government.*
Media: Diskette.
Published by: Fundacao Instituto Brasileiro de Geografia e Estatistica, Centro de Documentacao e Disseminacao de Informacoes, Rua General Canabarro, 706 Andar 2, Maracana, Rio De Janeiro, RJ 20271-201, Brazil. TEL 55-21-264-5424, FAX 55-21-2841959, http://www.ibge.gov.br.

616.99 310 GRC ISSN 0302-9697
RC279.G75
ETESIA STATISTIKE. EREVNA TOU KARKINOU/ANNUAL STATISTICAL SURVEY OF CANCER. Text in Greek. 1967. a., latest 1981-82. USD 5. back issues avail. **Document type:** *Government.*
Published by: National Statistical Service of Greece, Statistical Information and Publications Division/Ethniki Statistiki Yperesia tes Ellados, 14-16 Lykourgou St, Athens 101 66, Greece. TEL 30-1-3289-397, FAX 30-1-3241-102. Circ: 1,000.

016.6161 GBR ISSN 0421-7527
EUROPEAN CONGRESS OF CARDIOLOGY. ABSTRACTS OF PAPERS. Text in English. 1952. a. adv. **Document type:** *Abstract/Index.*
Related titles: ♦ Supplement to: European Heart Journal. ISSN 0195-668X.
Published by: (European Society of Cardiology FRA), Academic Press (Subsidiary of: Harcourt Publishers Ltd.), 24 Oval Rd, London NW1 7DX, United Kingdom. TEL 44-20-7267-4466, FAX 44-20-7482-2293. R&P Catherine John. Adv. contact Nik Screen. **Subscr. to:** Harcourt Publishers Ltd., Foots Cray High St, Sidcup, Kent DA14 5HP, United Kingdom. TEL 44-20-8300-3322.

EXCERPTA MEDICA. ABSTRACT JOURNALS. see *BIOLOGY—Abstracting, Bibliographies, Statistics*

016.618 NLD ISSN 0014-4142
CODEN: EMOGAE
EXCERPTA MEDICA. SECTION 10: OBSTETRICS AND GYNECOLOGY. Text in English. 1948. 20/yr. EUR 2,292 in Europe to institutions; JPY 303,883 in Japan to institutions; USD 2,564 elsewhere to institutions (effective 2002). adv. index, cum.index. back issues avail. **Document type:** *Abstract/Index, Academic/Scholarly.* **Description:** Provides a comprehensive current-awareness service for professional and academic journal articles covering human obstetrics and gynecology, including female infertility, fetal monitoring, anticonception in women, and neonatal care of normal infants.
Related titles: CD-ROM ed.: (from SilverPlatter Information, Inc.); Online - full text ed.: (from DIMDI, Data-Star, The Dialog Corporation, JICST).
—GNLM. **CCC.**
Published by: Excerpta Medica Medical Communications BV (Subsidiary of: Reed Elsevier plc), Rooseveltweg 15, Almere-Stad 1314 SJ, Netherlands. nlinfo-f@elsevier.nl, http://www.elsevier.com/locate/obgy. **Subscr. in Australasia and the Far East to:** Elsevier Science (Singapore) Pte Ltd, No.1 Temasek Ave, 17-01 Millenia Tower, Singapore 039192, Singapore. TEL 65-434-3727, FAX 65-337-2230, asiainfo@elsevier.com.sg; **Subscr. in Japan to:** Elsevier Science Inc - Japan Regional Office, 9-15 Higashi-Azabu 1-chome, Minato-ku, Tokyo 106-0044, Japan. TEL 81-3-5561-5033, FAX 81-3-5561-5047, info@elsevier.co.jp; **Subscr. in the Americas to:** Elsevier Science, PO Box 945, New York, NY 10159-0945. TEL 212-633-3730, 888-437-4636, FAX 212-633-3680, usinfo-f@elsevier.com, http://www.elsevier.com. **Dist. by:** Elsevier Science (Brazil).; Elsevier Science BV, PO Box 211, Amsterdam 1000 AE, Netherlands. TEL 31-20-485-3757, FAX 31-20-485-3432, nlinfo-f@elsevier.nl, http://www.elsevier.nl.

M

016.61621 NLD ISSN 0014-4150
RF1 CODEN: ORLGA8

EXCERPTA MEDICA. SECTION 11: OTORHINOLARYNGOLOGY. Text in English. 1948. m. EUR 1,670 in Europe to institutions; JPY 221,322 in Japan to institutions; USD 1,868 elsewhere to institutions (effective 2002). adv. index, cum.index. back issues avail. **Document type:** *Abstract/Index, Academic/Scholarly.* **Description:** Provides a comprehensive current-awareness service of professional and clinical articles covering all aspects of diseases of the ear, nose, and throat. Also covers phonetics and speech disorders, craniofacial disorders, vestibular disorders, surgery, stomatology, and audiology.

Related titles: CD-ROM ed.: (from SilverPlatter Information, Inc.); Online - full text ed.: (from DIMDI, Data-Star, The Dialog Corporation, JICST).

—GNLM, Infotrieve. **CCC.**

Published by: Excerpta Medica Medical Communications BV (Subsidiary of: Reed Elsevier plc), Rooseveltweg 15, Almere-Stad 1314 SJ, Netherlands. TEL 31-36-538-5600, FAX 31-36-538-5650, http://www.elsevier.com/locate/otol, http://www.excerptamedica.com. **Subscr. in Australasia and the Far East to:** Elsevier Science (Singapore) Pte Ltd, No.1 Temasek Ave, 17-01 Millenia Tower, Singapore 039192, Singapore. TEL 65-434-3727, FAX 65-337-2230; **Subscr. in Japan to:** Elsevier Science Inc - Japan Regional Office, 9-15 Higashi-Azabu 1-chome, Minato-ku, Tokyo 106-0044, Japan. TEL 81-3-5561-5033, FAX 81-3-5561-5047; **Subscr. in the Americas to:** Elsevier Science, PO Box 945, New York, NY 10159-0945. TEL 212-633-3730, 888-437-4636, FAX 212-633-3680, usinfo-f@elsevier.com, http://www.elsevier.com. **Dist. by:** Elsevier Science (Brazil).; Elsevier Science BV, PO Box 211, Amsterdam 1000 AE, Netherlands. TEL 31-20-485-3757, FAX 31-20-485-3432.

016.6177 NLD ISSN 0014-4169
CODEN: OPHYAS

EXCERPTA MEDICA. SECTION 12: OPHTHALMOLOGY. Text in English. 1947. m. EUR 1,670 in Europe to institutions; JPY 221,322 in Japan to institutions; USD 1,868 elsewhere to institutions (effective 2002). adv. index, cum.index. back issues avail. **Document type:** *Abstract/Index, Academic/Scholarly.* **Description:** Provides a comprehensive current-awareness service of clinical and academic journal articles covering both the surgical and non-surgical aspects of eye disease and vision disorders and includes articles on the anatomy, physiology and biochemistry of the eye, orbit and visual system.

Related titles: CD-ROM ed.: (from SilverPlatter Information, Inc.); Online - full text ed.: (from DIMDI, Data-Star, The Dialog Corporation, JICST).

—GNLM, Infotrieve. **CCC.**

Published by: Excerpta Medica Medical Communications BV (Subsidiary of: Reed Elsevier plc), Rooseveltweg 15, Almere-Stad 1314 SJ, Netherlands. TEL 31-36-538-5600, FAX 31-36-538-5650, http://www.elsevier.com/locate/opthalmology, http://www.excerptamedica.com. **Subscr. in Australasia and the Far East to:** Elsevier Science (Singapore) Pte Ltd, No.1 Temasek Ave, 17-01 Millenia Tower, Singapore 039192, Singapore. TEL 65-434-3727, FAX 65-337-2230; **Subscr. in Japan to:** Elsevier Science Inc - Japan Regional Office, 9-15 Higashi-Azabu 1-chome, Minato-ku, Tokyo 106-0044, Japan. TEL 81-3-5561-5033, FAX 81-3-5561-5047; **Subscr. in the Americas to:** Elsevier Science, PO Box 945, New York, NY 10159-0945. TEL 212-633-3730, 888-437-4636, FAX 212-633-3680, usinfo-f@elsevier.com, http://www.elsevier.com. **Dist. by:** Elsevier Science (Brazil).; Elsevier Science BV, PO Box 211, Amsterdam 1000 AE, Netherlands. TEL 31-20-485-3757, FAX 31-20-485-3432.

016.6165 NLD ISSN 0014-4177
CODEN: DVENB4

EXCERPTA MEDICA. SECTION 13: DERMATOLOGY AND VENEREOLOGY. Text in English. 1947. m. EUR 1,834 in Europe to institutions; JPY 243,093 in Japan to institutions; USD 2,051 elsewhere to institutions (effective 2002). adv. index, cum.index. **Document type:** *Abstract/Index, Academic/Scholarly.* **Description:** Provides a comprehensive current-awareness service of clinical and academic articles covering all aspects of skin and venereal diseases, and includes microbiology, sexually transmitted diseases, immunology, allergy and skin toxicology, skin physiology and biochemistry.

Related titles: CD-ROM ed.: (from SilverPlatter Information, Inc.); Online - full text ed.: (from DIMDI, Data-Star, The Dialog Corporation, JICST).

—GNLM. **CCC.**

Published by: Excerpta Medica Medical Communications BV (Subsidiary of: Reed Elsevier plc), Rooseveltweg 15, Almere-Stad 1314 SJ, Netherlands. TEL 31-36-538-5600, FAX 31-36-538-5650, http://www.elsevier.com/locate/dermven, http://www.excerptamedica.com. **Subscr. in Australasia and the Far East to:** Elsevier Science (Singapore) Pte Ltd, No.1 Temasek Ave, 17-01 Millenia Tower, Singapore 039192, Singapore. TEL 65-434-3727, FAX 65-337-2230; **Subscr. in Japan to:** Elsevier Science Inc - Japan Regional Office, 9-15 Higashi-Azabu 1-chome, Minato-ku, Tokyo 106-0044, Japan. TEL 81-3-5561-5033, FAX 81-3-5561-5047; **Subscr. in the Americas to:** Elsevier Science, PO Box 945, New York, NY 10159-0945. TEL 212-633-3730, 888-437-4636, FAX 212-633-3680, usinfo-f@elsevier.com, http://www.elsevier.com. **Dist. by:** Elsevier Science (Brazil).; Elsevier Science BV, PO Box 211, Amsterdam 1000 AE, Netherlands. TEL 31-20-485-3757, FAX 31-20-485-3432.

016.615842 NLD ISSN 0014-4185
CODEN: RDGYA6

EXCERPTA MEDICA. SECTION 14: RADIOLOGY. Text in English. 1947. 20/yr. EUR 2,357 in Europe to institutions; JPY 312,408 in Japan to institutions; USD 2,636 elsewhere to institutions (effective 2002). adv. index, cum.index. back issues avail. **Document type:** *Abstract/Index, Academic/Scholarly.* **Description:** Provides a comprehensive current-awareness service of articles covering radiodiagnosis, radiotherapy and radiobiology, including ultrasound diagnosis, thermography, and adverse reactions to radiotherapy, as well as techniques and apparatus.

Related titles: CD-ROM ed.: (from SilverPlatter Information, Inc.); Online - full text ed.: (from DIMDI, Data-Star, The Dialog Corporation, JICST).

—GNLM, Infotrieve. **CCC.**

Published by: Excerpta Medica Medical Communications BV (Subsidiary of: Reed Elsevier plc), Rooseveltweg 15, Almere-Stad 1314 SJ, Netherlands. TEL 31-36-538-5600, FAX 31-36-538-5650, http://www.elsevier.com/locate/radiology, http://www.excerptamedica.com. **Subscr. in Australasia and the Far East to:** Elsevier Science (Singapore) Pte Ltd, No.1 Temasek Ave, 17-01 Millenia Tower, Singapore 039192, Singapore. TEL 65-434-3727, FAX 65-337-2230; **Subscr. in Japan to:** Elsevier Science Inc - Japan Regional Office, 9-15 Higashi-Azabu 1-chome, Minato-ku, Tokyo 106-0044, Japan. TEL 81-3-5561-5033, FAX 81-3-5561-5047; **Subscr. in the Americas to:** Elsevier Science, PO Box 2129, Marion, OH 43305-2129. usinfo-f@elsevier.com, http://www.elsevier.com. **Dist. by:** Elsevier Science (Brazil).; Elsevier Science BV, PO Box 211, Amsterdam 1000 AE, Netherlands. TEL 31-20-485-3757, FAX 31-20-485-3432.

016.6162 NLD ISSN 0014-4193
RC306 CODEN: CDTSA

EXCERPTA MEDICA. SECTION 15: CHEST DISEASES, THORACIC SURGERY AND TUBERCULOSIS. Text in English. 1948. 16/yr. EUR 1,643 in Europe to institutions; JPY 217,780 in Japan to institutions; USD 1,838 elsewhere to institutions (effective 2002). adv. index, cum.index. back issues avail. **Document type:** *Abstract/Index, Academic/Scholarly.* **Description:** Provides a comprehensive current-awareness service of clinical and academic articles covering all aspects of lung and respiratory-tract diseases, thoracic surgery and tuberculosis, including respiratory infections, mediastical and pleural diseases, chronic chest diseases, allergy and bronchial asthma, and neoplastic disease.

Related titles: CD-ROM ed.: (from SilverPlatter Information, Inc.); Online - full text ed.: (from DIMDI, Data-Star, The Dialog Corporation, JICST).

—Infotrieve. **CCC.**

Published by: Excerpta Medica Medical Communications BV (Subsidiary of: Reed Elsevier plc), Rooseveltweg 15, Almere-Stad 1314 SJ, Netherlands. TEL 31-36-538-5600, FAX 31-36-538-5650, http://www.elsevier.nl/locate/chest, http://www.excerptamedica.com. **Subscr. in Australasia and the Far East to:** Elsevier Science (Singapore) Pte Ltd, No.1 Temasek Ave, 17-01 Millenia Tower, Singapore 039192, Singapore. TEL 65-434-3727, FAX 65-337-2230, asiainfo@elsevier.com.sg; **Subscr. in Japan to:** Elsevier Science Inc - Japan Regional Office, 9-15 Higashi-Azabu 1-chome, Minato-ku, Tokyo 106-0044, Japan. TEL 81-3-5561-5033, FAX 81-3-5561-5047, info@elsevier.co.jp; **Subscr. in the Americas to:** Elsevier Science, PO Box 945, New York, NY 10159-0945. TEL 212-633-3730, 888-437-4636, FAX 212-633-3680, usinfo-f@elsevier.com, http://www.elsevier.com. **Dist. by:** Elsevier Science (Brazil).; Elsevier Science BV, PO Box 211, Amsterdam 1000 AE, Netherlands. TEL 31-20-485-3757, FAX 31-20-485-3432, nlinfo-f@elsevier.nl, http://www.elsevier.nl.

016.616994 NLD ISSN 0014-4207
CODEN: CEXCA3

EXCERPTA MEDICA. SECTION 16: CANCER. Text in English. 1953. 32/yr. EUR 3,206 in Europe to institutions; JPY 425,003 in Japan to institutions; USD 3,586 elsewhere to institutions (effective 2001). adv. index, cum.index. back issues avail. **Document type:** *Abstract/Index, Academic/Scholarly.* **Description:** Provides a comprehensive current-awareness service of articles covering both the experimental and clinical aspects of malignant neoplastic disease, including research in cancer immunology, oncogenes, viral and chemical carcinogenesis, and cancer chemotherapeutic agents.

Related titles: CD-ROM ed.: (from SilverPlatter Information, Inc.); Online - full text ed.: (from DIMDI, Data-Star, The Dialog Corporation, JICST).

—GNLM, Infotrieve. **CCC.**

Published by: Excerpta Medica Medical Communications BV (Subsidiary of: Reed Elsevier plc), Rooseveltweg 15, Almere-Stad 1314 SJ, Netherlands. http://www.elsevier.nl/locate/cancer. **Subscr. in Australasia and the Far East to:** Elsevier Science (Singapore) Pte Ltd, No.1 Temasek Ave, 17-01 Millenia Tower, Singapore 039192, Singapore. TEL 65-434-3727, FAX 65-337-2230, asiainfo@elsevier.com.sg; **Subscr. in Japan to:** Elsevier Science Inc - Japan Regional Office, 9-15 Higashi-Azabu 1-chome, Minato-ku, Tokyo 106-0044, Japan. TEL 81-3-5561-5033, FAX 81-3-5561-5047, info@elsevier.co.jp; **Subscr. in the Americas to:** Elsevier Science, PO Box 945, New York, NY 10159-0945. TEL 212-633-3730, 888-437-4636, FAX 212-633-3680, usinfo-f@elsevier.com, http://www.elsevier.com. **Dist. by:** Elsevier Science (Brazil).; Elsevier Science BV, PO Box 211, Amsterdam 1000 AE, Netherlands. TEL 31-20-485-3757, FAX 31-20-485-3432, nlinfo-f@elsevier.nl, http://www.elsevier.nl.

EXCERPTA MEDICA. SECTION 17: PUBLIC HEALTH, SOCIAL MEDICINE AND EPIDEMIOLOGY. see *PUBLIC HEALTH AND SAFETY—Abstracting, Bibliographies, Statistics*

016.6161 NLD ISSN 0014-4223
CODEN: CDCSA

EXCERPTA MEDICA. SECTION 18: CARDIOVASCULAR DISEASES AND CARDIOVASCULAR SURGERY. Text in English. 1957. s-m. EUR 2,503 in Europe to institutions; JPY 331,884 in Japan to institutions; USD 2,801 elsewhere to institutions (effective 2002). adv. index, cum.index. **Document type:** *Abstract/Index, Academic/Scholarly.* **Description:** Provides a comprehensive current-awareness service of clinical and academic articles covering both the surgical and nonsurgical aspects of cardiovascular disease.

Related titles: CD-ROM ed.: (from SilverPlatter Information, Inc.); Online - full text ed.: (from DIMDI, Data-Star, The Dialog Corporation, JICST).

—GNLM, Infotrieve. **CCC.**

M

Published by: Excerpta Medica Medical Communications BV (Subsidiary of: Reed Elsevier plc), Rooseveltweg 15, Almere-Stad 1314 SJ, Netherlands. TEL 31-36-538-5600, FAX 31-36-538-5650, http://www.elsevier.com/locate/cardiscarsur, http://www.excerptamedica.com. **Subscr. in Australasia and the Far East to:** Elsevier Science (Singapore) Pte Ltd, No.1 Temasek Ave, 17-01 Millenia Tower, Singapore 039192, Singapore. TEL 65-434-3727, FAX 65-337-2230, asiainfo@elsevier.com.sg; **Subscr. in Japan to:** Elsevier Science Inc - Japan Regional Office, 9-15 Higashi-Azabu 1-chome, Minato-ku, Tokyo 106-0044, Japan. TEL 81-3-5561-5033, FAX 81-3-5561-5047, info@elsevier.co.jp; **Subscr. in the Americas to:** Elsevier Science, PO Box 945, New York, NY 10159-0945. TEL 212-633-3730, 888-437-4636, FAX 212-633-3680, usinfo-f@elsevier.com, http://www.elsevier.com. **Dist. by:** Elsevier Science (Brazil).; Elsevier Science BV, PO Box 211, Amsterdam 1000 AE, Netherlands. TEL 31-20-485-3757, FAX 31-20-485-3432, nlinfo-f@elsevier.nl, http://www.elsevier.nl.

016.61582 NLD ISSN 0014-4231
CODEN: RHPMA

EXCERPTA MEDICA. SECTION 19: REHABILITATION AND PHYSICAL MEDICINE. Text in English. 1958. 8/yr. EUR 1,087 in Europe to institutions; JPY 144,073 in Japan to institutions; USD 1,216 elsewhere to institutions (effective 2002). adv. index, cum.index. back issues avail. **Document type:** *Abstract/Index, Academic/Scholarly.* **Description:** Provides a comprehensive current-awareness service of clinical and trade articles covering all aspects of the rehabilitation of somatic and mental disorders using physiotherapy and other therapeutic techniques.
Related titles: CD-ROM ed.: (from SilverPlatter Information, Inc.); Online - full text ed.: (from DIMDI, Data-Star, The Dialog Corporation, JICST).
—GNLM, Infotrieve. **CCC.**
Published by: Excerpta Medica Medical Communications BV (Subsidiary of: Reed Elsevier plc), Rooseveltweg 15, Almere-Stad 1314 SJ, Netherlands. TEL 31-36-538-5600, FAX 31-36-538-5650, http://www.elsevier.com/locate/rehphysmed, http://www.excerptamedica.com. **Subscr. in Australasia and the Far East to:** Elsevier Science (Singapore) Pte Ltd, No.1 Temasek Ave, 17-01 Millenia Tower, Singapore 039192, Singapore. TEL 65-434-3727, FAX 65-337-2230; **Subscr. in Japan to:** Elsevier Science Inc - Japan Regional Office, 9-15 Higashi-Azabu 1-chome, Minato-ku, Tokyo 106-0044, Japan. TEL 81-3-5561-5033, FAX 81-3-5561-5047; **Subscr. in the Americas to:** Elsevier Science, PO Box 945, New York, NY 10159-0945. TEL 212-633-3730, 888-437-4636, FAX 212-633-3680, usinfo-f@elsevier.com, http://www.elsevier.com. **Dist. by:** Elsevier Science (Brazil).; Elsevier Science BV, PO Box 211, Amsterdam 1000 AE, Netherlands. TEL 31-20-485-3757, FAX 31-20-485-3432.

016.61 NLD ISSN 0367-1089
CODEN: PHSGA

EXCERPTA MEDICA. SECTION 2: PHYSIOLOGY. Text in English. 1948. 30/yr. EUR 2,973 in Europe to institutions; JPY 394,182 in Japan to institutions; USD 3,326 elsewhere to institutions (effective 2002). adv. charts. index, cum.index. back issues avail. **Document type:** *Abstract/Index, Academic/Scholarly.* **Description:** Provides a comprehensive current-awareness service for academic and professional writings in the field of physiology.
Supersedes in part (in 1964): Excerpta Medica. Section 2: Physiology, Biochemistry and Pharmacology (0014-4061)
Related titles: CD-ROM ed.: (from SilverPlatter Information, Inc.); Online - full text ed.: (from DIMDI, Data-Star, The Dialog Corporation, JICST).
—GNLM, Infotrieve, Linda Hall. **CCC.**
Published by: Excerpta Medica Medical Communications BV (Subsidiary of: Reed Elsevier plc), Rooseveltweg 15, Almere-Stad 1314 SJ, Netherlands. TEL 31-36-538-5600, FAX 31-36-538-5650, nlinfo-f@elsevier.nl, http://www.elsevier.nl/locate/physiology, http://www.excerptamedica.com. Ed. R N Sudan. **Subscr. in Australasia and the Far East to:** Elsevier Science (Singapore) Pte Ltd, No.1 Temasek Ave, 17-01 Millenia Tower, Singapore 039192, Singapore. TEL 65-434-3727, FAX 65-337-2230; **Subscr. in Japan to:** Elsevier Science Inc - Japan Regional Office, 9-15 Higashi-Azabu 1-chome, Minato-ku, Tokyo 106-0044, Japan. TEL 81-3-5561-5033, FAX 81-3-5561-5047; **Subscr. in the Americas to:** Elsevier Science, PO Box 945, New York, NY 10159-0945. TEL 212-633-3730, 888-437-4636, FAX 212-633-3680, usinfo-f@elsevier.com, http://www.elsevier.com. **Dist. by:** Elsevier Science (Brazil).; Elsevier Science BV, PO Box 211, Amsterdam 1000 AE, Netherlands. TEL 31-20-485-3757, FAX 31-20-485-3432.

016.61607575 NLD ISSN 0014-4274
CODEN: NUMEAH

EXCERPTA MEDICA. SECTION 23: NUCLEAR MEDICINE. Text in English. 1964. 10/yr. EUR 1,534 in Europe to institutions; JPY 203,353 in Japan to institutions; USD 1,716 elsewhere to institutions (effective 2002). adv. index, cum.index. back issues avail. **Document type:** *Abstract/Index, Academic/Scholarly.* **Description:** Provides a current-awareness service of academic and clinical articles covering the diagnostic and therapeutic applications of radioisotopes in biomedicine, including the radiobiology of isotopes, aspects of radiohygiene, new labelling techniques and tracer applications.
Related titles: CD-ROM ed.: (from SilverPlatter Information, Inc.); Online - full text ed.: (from DIMDI, Data-Star, The Dialog Corporation, JICST).
—GNLM, Infotrieve. **CCC.**
Published by: Excerpta Medica Medical Communications BV (Subsidiary of: Reed Elsevier plc), Rooseveltweg 15, Almere-Stad 1314 SJ, Netherlands. TEL 31-36-538-5600, FAX 31-36-538-5650, http://www.elsevier.com/locate/nucmed, http://www.excerptamedica.com. **Subscr. in Australasia and the Far East to:** Elsevier Science (Singapore) Pte Ltd, No.1 Temasek Ave, 17-01 Millenia Tower, Singapore 039192, Singapore. TEL 65-434-3727, FAX 65-337-2230; **Subscr. in Japan to:** Elsevier Science Inc - Japan Regional Office, 9-15 Higashi-Azabu 1-chome, Minato-ku, Tokyo 106-0044, Japan. TEL 81-3-5561-5033, FAX 81-3-5561-5047; **Subscr. in the Americas to:** Elsevier Science, PO Box 945, New York, NY 10159-0945. TEL 212-633-3730, 888-437-4636, FAX 212-633-3680, usinfo-f@elsevier.com, http://www.elsevier.com. **Dist. by:** Elsevier Science (Brazil).; Elsevier Science BV, PO Box 211, Amsterdam 1000 AE, Netherlands. TEL 31-20-485-3757, FAX 31-20-485-3432.

016.61796 NLD ISSN 0014-4282
CODEN: ATSYA

EXCERPTA MEDICA. SECTION 24: ANESTHESIOLOGY. Text in English. 1966. 10/yr. EUR 1,340 in Europe to institutions; JPY 177,648 in Japan to institutions; USD 1,499 elsewhere to institutions (effective 2002). adv. index, cum.index. **Document type:** *Abstract/Index, Academic/Scholarly.* **Description:** Provides a current-awareness service for articles covering both the clinical and experimental aspects of anesthesiology and includes resuscitation and intensive care medicine, pharmacology of anesthetic agents, spinal, epidural and caudal anesthesia, and acupuncture used as an anaesthetic procedure.
Related titles: CD-ROM ed.: (from SilverPlatter Information, Inc.); Online - full text ed.: (from DIMDI, Data-Star, The Dialog Corporation, JICST).
—GNLM, Infotrieve. **CCC.**
Published by: Excerpta Medica Medical Communications BV (Subsidiary of: Reed Elsevier plc), Rooseveltweg 15, Almere-Stad 1314 SJ, Netherlands. TEL 31-36-538-5600, FAX 31-36-538-5650, http://www.elsevier.com/anesthesiology, http://www.excerptamedica.com. **Subscr. in Australasia and the Far East to:** Elsevier Science (Singapore) Pte Ltd, No.1 Temasek Ave, 17-01 Millenia Tower, Singapore 039192, Singapore. TEL 65-434-3727, FAX 65-337-2230, asiainfo@elsevier.com.sg; **Subscr. in Japan to:** Elsevier Science Inc - Japan Regional Office, 9-15 Higashi-Azabu 1-chome, Minato-ku, Tokyo 106-0044, Japan. TEL 81-3-5561-5033, FAX 81-3-5561-5047, info@elsevier.co.jp; **Subscr. in the Americas to:** Elsevier Science, PO Box 945, New York, NY 10159-0945. TEL 212-633-3730, 888-437-4636, FAX 212-633-3680, usinfo-f@elsevier.com, http://www.elsevier.com. **Dist. by:** Elsevier Science (Brazil).; Elsevier Science BV, PO Box 211, Amsterdam 1000 AE, Netherlands. TEL 31-20-485-3757, FAX 31-20-485-3432, nlinfo-f@elsevier.nl, http://www.elsevier.nl.

016.61615 NLD ISSN 0014-4290
CODEN: HEMYA

EXCERPTA MEDICA. SECTION 25: HEMATOLOGY. Text in English. 1967. s-m. EUR 2,395 in Europe to institutions; JPY 317,522 in Japan to institutions; USD 2,679 elsewhere to institutions (effective 2002). adv. index, cum.index. **Document type:** *Abstract/Index, Academic/Scholarly.* **Description:** Provides a comprehensive current-awareness service for articles covering all aspects of blood cell biology and disorders of the blood, its cells and the lymphatic tissues.
Related titles: CD-ROM ed.: (from SilverPlatter Information, Inc.); Online - full text ed.: (from DIMDI, Data-Star, The Dialog Corporation, JICST).
—GNLM, Infotrieve. **CCC.**
Published by: Excerpta Medica Medical Communications BV (Subsidiary of: Reed Elsevier plc), Rooseveltweg 15, Almere-Stad 1314 SJ, Netherlands. TEL 31-36-538-5600, FAX 31-36-538-5650, http://www.elsevier.com/locate/hematology, http://www.excerptamedica.com. **Subscr. in Australasia and the Far East to:** Elsevier Science (Singapore) Pte Ltd, No.1 Temasek Ave, 17-01 Millenia Tower, Singapore 039192, Singapore. TEL 65-434-3727, FAX 65-337-2230; **Subscr. in Japan to:** Elsevier Science Inc - Japan Regional Office, 9-15 Higashi-Azabu 1-chome, Minato-ku, Tokyo 106-0044, Japan. TEL 81-3-5561-5033, FAX 81-3-5561-5047; **Subscr. in the Americas to:** Elsevier Science, PO Box 945, New York, NY 10159-0945. TEL 212-633-3730, 888-437-4636, FAX 212-633-3680, usinfo-f@elsevier.com, http://www.elsevier.com. **Dist. by:** Elsevier Science (Brazil).; Elsevier Science BV, PO Box 211, Amsterdam 1000 AE, Netherlands. TEL 31-20-485-3757, FAX 31-20-485-3432.

016.61537 NLD ISSN 0014-4304
CODEN: ISTNB

EXCERPTA MEDICA. SECTION 26: IMMUNOLOGY, SEROLOGY AND TRANSPLANTATION. Text in English. 1967. 32/yr. EUR 2,977 in Europe to institutions; JPY 394,641 in Japan to institutions; USD 3,330 elsewhere to institutions (effective 2002). adv. index, cum.index. back issues avail. **Document type:** *Abstract/Index, Academic/Scholarly.* **Description:** Provides a comprehensive current-awareness service of academic and research articles covering both clinical and experimental immunology and includes humoral immunity and associated factors.

M

Related titles: CD-ROM ed.: (from SilverPlatter Information, Inc.); Online - full text ed.: (from DIMDI, Data-Star, The Dialog Corporation, JICST).
—GNLM, Infotrieve. **CCC.**
Published by: Excerpta Medica Medical Communications BV (Subsidiary of: Reed Elsevier plc), Rooseveltweg 15, Almere-Stad 1314 SJ, Netherlands. TEL 31-36-538-5600, FAX 31-36-538-5650, http://www.elsevier.com/locate/immsertra, http://www.excerptamedica.com. **Subscr. in Australasia and the Far East to:** Elsevier Science (Singapore) Pte Ltd, No.1 Temasek Ave, 17-01 Millenia Tower, Singapore 039192, Singapore. TEL 65-434-3727, FAX 65-337-2230; **Subscr. in Japan to:** Elsevier Science Inc - Japan Regional Office, 9-15 Higashi-Azabu 1-chome, Minato-ku, Tokyo 106-0044, Japan. TEL 81-3-5561-5033, FAX 81-3-5561-5047; **Subscr. in the Americas to:** Elsevier Science, PO Box 945, New York, NY 10159-0945. TEL 212-633-3730, 888-437-4636, FAX 212-633-3680, usinfo-f@elsevier.com, http://www.elsevier.com. **Dist. by:** Elsevier Science (Brazil).; Elsevier Science BV, PO Box 211, Amsterdam 1000 AE, Netherlands. TEL 31-20-485-3757, FAX 31-20-485-3432.

016.6166 NLD ISSN 0014-4320
CODEN: URNLA

EXCERPTA MEDICA. SECTION 28: UROLOGY AND NEPHROLOGY. Text in English. 1967. 16/yr. EUR 2,263 in Europe to institutions; JPY 299,948 in Japan to institutions; USD 2,531 elsewhere to institutions (effective 2002). adv. index, cum.index. back issues avail. **Document type:** *Abstract/Index, Academic/Scholarly.* **Description:** Provides a comprehensive current-awareness service for clinical and academic articles covering both the clinical and experimental aspects of nephrological and urological disorders in either sex, kidney transplantation and dialysis, and the male reproductive system, including male fertility and the prostate.
Related titles: CD-ROM ed.: (from SilverPlatter Information, Inc.); Online - full text ed.: (from DIMDI, Data-Star, The Dialog Corporation, JICST).
—GNLM, Infotrieve. **CCC.**
Published by: Excerpta Medica Medical Communications BV (Subsidiary of: Reed Elsevier plc), Rooseveltweg 15, Almere-Stad 1314 SJ, Netherlands. TEL 31-36-538-5600, FAX 31-36-538-5650, http://www.elsevier.nl/inca/publications/store/5/0/5/9/9/7/, http://www.excerptamedica.com. Eds. Dr. A T Alberda, A Schwimmer, R N Sudan. **Subscr. in Australasia and the Far East to:** Elsevier Science (Singapore) Pte Ltd, No.1 Temasek Ave, 17-01 Millenia Tower, Singapore 039192, Singapore. TEL 65-434-3727, FAX 65-337-2230; **Subscr. in Japan to:** Elsevier Science Inc - Japan Regional Office, 9-15 Higashi-Azabu 1-chome, Minato-ku, Tokyo 106-0044, Japan. TEL 81-3-5561-5033, FAX 81-3-5561-5047; **Subscr. in the Americas to:** Elsevier Science. usinfo-f@elsevier.com. **Dist. by:** Elsevier Science (Brazil).; Elsevier Science BV, PO Box 211, Amsterdam 1000 AE, Netherlands. TEL 31-20-485-3757, FAX 31-20-485-3432, http://www.elsevier.nl.

016.6164 NLD ISSN 0014-407X
CODEN: EEXCA

EXCERPTA MEDICA. SECTION 3: ENDOCRINOLOGY. Text in English. 1947. 24/yr. EUR 2,374 in Europe to institutions; JPY 314,769 in Japan to institutions; USD 2,656 elsewhere to institutions (effective 2002). adv. charts. index, cum.index. **Document type:** *Abstract/Index, Academic/Scholarly.* **Description:** Provides a comprehensive current-awareness service for academic and professional articles on clinical and experimental endocrinology.
Related titles: CD-ROM ed.: (from SilverPlatter Information, Inc.); Online - full text ed.: (from DIMDI, Data-Star, The Dialog Corporation, JICST).
—GNLM. **CCC.**
Published by: Excerpta Medica Medical Communications BV (Subsidiary of: Reed Elsevier plc), Rooseveltweg 15, Almere-Stad 1314 SJ, Netherlands. TEL 31-36-538-5600, FAX 31-36-538-5650, http://www.elsevier.com/locate/endocrinology, http://www.excerptamedica.com. **Subscr. in Australasia and the Far East to:** Elsevier Science (Singapore) Pte Ltd, No.1 Temasek Ave, 17-01 Millenia Tower, Singapore 039192, Singapore. TEL 65-434-3727, FAX 65-337-2230; **Subscr. in Japan to:** Elsevier Science Inc - Japan Regional Office, 9-15 Higashi-Azabu 1-chome, Minato-ku, Tokyo 106-0044, Japan. TEL 81-3-5561-5033, FAX 81-3-5561-5047; **Subscr. in the Americas to:** Elsevier Science. **Dist. by:** Elsevier Science (Brazil).; Elsevier Science BV, PO Box 211, Amsterdam 1000 AE, Netherlands. TEL 31-20-485-3757, FAX 31-20-485-3432.

EXCERPTA MEDICA. SECTION 30: CLINICAL AND EXPERIMENTAL PHARMACOLOGY. see *PHARMACY AND PHARMACOLOGY—Abstracting, Bibliographies, Statistics*

016.616742 NLD ISSN 0014-4355
RC933.A1 CODEN: EXARB

EXCERPTA MEDICA. SECTION 31: ARTHRITIS AND RHEUMATISM. Text in English. 1965. 8/yr. EUR 1,014 in Europe to institutions; JPY 134,368 in Japan to institutions; USD 1,134 elsewhere to institutions (effective 2002). adv. index, cum.index. **Document type:** *Abstract/Index, Academic/Scholarly.* **Description:** Provides a comprehensive current-awareness service for articles covering both the clinical and experimental aspects of arthritis, rheumatism, and bone and joint pathology and includes spinal conditions, connective tissue disorders, and rheumatic fever.
Related titles: CD-ROM ed.: (from SilverPlatter Information, Inc.); Online - full text ed.: (from DIMDI, Data-Star, The Dialog Corporation, JICST).
—GNLM, Linda Hall. **CCC.**
Published by: Excerpta Medica Medical Communications BV (Subsidiary of: Reed Elsevier plc), Rooseveltweg 15, Almere-Stad 1314 SJ, Netherlands. TEL 31-36-538-5600, FAX 31-36-538-5650, http://www.elsevier.com/locate/arth, http:// www.excerptamedica.com. **Subscr. in Australasia and the Far East to:** Elsevier Science (Singapore) Pte Ltd, No.1 Temasek Ave, 17-01 Millenia Tower, Singapore 039192, Singapore. TEL 65-434-3727, FAX 65-337-2230, asiainfo@elsevier.com.sg; **Subscr. in Japan to:** Elsevier Science Inc - Japan Regional Office, 9-15 Higashi-Azabu 1-chome, Minato-ku, Tokyo 106-0044, Japan. TEL 81-3-5561-5033, FAX 81-3-5561-5047, info@elsevier.co.jp; **Subscr. in the Americas to:** Elsevier Science, PO Box 2129, Marion, OH 43305-2129. **Dist. by:** Elsevier Science (Brazil).; Elsevier Science BV, PO Box 211, Amsterdam 1000 AE, Netherlands. TEL 31-20-485-3757, FAX 31-20-485-3432, nlinfo-f@elsevier.nl, http://www.elsevier.nl.

016.61689 NLD ISSN 0014-4363
CODEN: PSCYA

EXCERPTA MEDICA. SECTION 32: PSYCHIATRY. Text in English. 1948. 20/yr. EUR 2,248 in Europe to institutions; JPY 297,981 in Japan to institutions; USD 2,515 elsewhere to institutions (effective 2002). adv. index, cum.index. back issues avail. **Document type:** *Abstract/Index, Academic/Scholarly.* **Description:** Provides a comprehensive current-awareness service of academic, clinical, and professional articles covering all aspects of medical psychology and psychiatry, including the psychological aspects of addiction, alcoholism, sexual behavior, and suicide.
Related titles: CD-ROM ed.: (from SilverPlatter Information, Inc.); Online - full text ed.: (from DIMDI, Data-Star, The Dialog Corporation, JICST).
—GNLM, Infotrieve, Linda Hall. **CCC.**
Published by: Excerpta Medica Medical Communications BV (Subsidiary of: Reed Elsevier plc), Rooseveltweg 15, Almere-Stad 1314 SJ, Netherlands. TEL 31-36-538-5600, FAX 31-36-538-5650, http://www.elsevier.com/locate/psychiatry, http://www.excerptamedica.com. **Subscr. in Australasia and the Far East to:** Elsevier Science (Singapore) Pte Ltd, No.1 Temasek Ave, 17-01 Millenia Tower, Singapore 039192, Singapore. TEL 65-434-3727, FAX 65-337-2230; **Subscr. in Japan to:** Elsevier Science Inc - Japan Regional Office, 9-15 Higashi-Azabu 1-chome, Minato-ku, Tokyo 106-0044, Japan. TEL 81-3-5561-5033, FAX 81-3-5561-5047; **Subscr. in the Americas to:** Elsevier Science, PO Box 945, New York, NY 10159-0945. TEL 212-633-3730, 888-437-4636, FAX 212-633-3680, usinfo-f@elsevier.com, http://www.elsevier.com. **Dist. by:** Elsevier Science (Brazil).; Elsevier Science BV, PO Box 211, Amsterdam 1000 AE, Netherlands. TEL 31-20-485-3757, FAX 31-20-485-3432.

016.6173 NLD ISSN 0014-4371
RD701 CODEN: OSUGA

EXCERPTA MEDICA. SECTION 33: ORTHOPEDIC SURGERY. Text in English. 1956. m. EUR 1,625 in Europe to institutions; JPY 215,420 in Japan to institutions; USD 1,818 elsewhere to institutions (effective 2002). adv. index, cum.index. back issues avail. **Document type:** *Abstract/Index, Academic/Scholarly.* **Description:** Provides a comprehensive current-awareness service of clinical and academic articles covering the general, diagnostic, and surgical aspects of orthopedics and includes surgical aspects of other bone diseases, bone tumors, trauma of the musculoskeletal system, and biomechanics of the musculoskeletal system.
Related titles: CD-ROM ed.: (from SilverPlatter Information, Inc.); Online - full text ed.: (from DIMDI, Data-Star, The Dialog Corporation, JICST).
—GNLM, Linda Hall. **CCC.**
Published by: Excerpta Medica Medical Communications BV (Subsidiary of: Reed Elsevier plc), Rooseveltweg 15, Almere-Stad 1314 SJ, Netherlands. TEL 31-36-538-5600, FAX 31-36-538-5650, http://www.elsevier.com/locate/orthsurg, http://www.excerptamedica.com. **Subscr. in Australasia and the Far East to:** Elsevier Science (Singapore) Pte Ltd, No.1 Temasek Ave, 17-01 Millenia Tower, Singapore 039192, Singapore. TEL 65-434-3727, FAX 65-337-2230; **Subscr. in Japan to:** Elsevier Science Inc - Japan Regional Office, 9-15 Higashi-Azabu 1-chome, Minato-ku, Tokyo 106-0044, Japan. TEL 81-3-5561-5033, FAX 81-3-5561-5047; **Subscr. in the Americas to:** Elsevier Science, PO Box 945, New York, NY 10159-0945. TEL 212-633-3730, 888-437-4636, FAX 212-633-3680, usinfo-f@elsevier.com, http://www.elsevier.com. **Dist. by:** Elsevier Science (Brazil).; Elsevier Science BV, PO Box 211, Amsterdam 1000 AE, Netherlands. TEL 31-20-485-3757, FAX 31-20-485-3432.

016.61362 NLD ISSN 0014-4398
RC963 CODEN: EMOHAH

EXCERPTA MEDICA. SECTION 35: OCCUPATIONAL HEALTH AND INDUSTRIAL MEDICINE. Text in English. 1971. m. EUR 1,787 in Europe to institutions; JPY 236,863 in Japan to institutions; USD 1,999 elsewhere to institutions (effective 2002). adv. index, cum.index. back issues avail. **Document type:** *Abstract/Index, Academic/Scholarly.* **Description:** Provides a comprehensive current-awareness service of professional, trade, and academic articles covering the health aspects of work and the working environment, and includes ergonomics, sports medicine, the influence of life style and psychosocial aspects.
Related titles: CD-ROM ed.: (from SilverPlatter Information, Inc.); Online - full text ed.: (from DIMDI, Data-Star, The Dialog Corporation, JICST, ingenta).
—GNLM, Linda Hall. **CCC.**
Published by: Excerpta Medica Medical Communications BV (Subsidiary of: Reed Elsevier plc), Rooseveltweg 15, Almere-Stad 1314 SJ, Netherlands. TEL 31-36-538-5600, FAX 31-36-538-5650, http://www.elsevier.com/locate/ohim, http://www.excerptamedica.com. **Subscr. in Australasia and the Far East to:** Elsevier Science (Singapore) Pte Ltd, No.1 Temasek Ave, 17-01 Millenia Tower, Singapore 039192, Singapore. TEL 65-434-3727, FAX 65-337-2230; **Subscr. in Japan to:** Elsevier Science Inc - Japan Regional Office, 9-15 Higashi-Azabu 1-chome, Minato-ku, Tokyo 106-0044, Japan. TEL 81-3-5561-5033, FAX 81-3-5561-5047; **Subscr. in the Americas to:** Elsevier Science, PO Box 945, New York, NY 10159-0945. TEL 212-633-3730, 888-437-4636, FAX 212-633-3680, usinfo-f@elsevier.com, http://www.elsevier.com. **Dist. by:** Elsevier Science (Brazil).; Elsevier Science BV, PO Box 211, Amsterdam 1000 AE, Netherlands. TEL 31-20-485-3757, FAX 31-20-485-3432.

EXCERPTA MEDICA. SECTION 36: HEALTH POLICY, ECONOMICS AND MANAGEMENT. see *HEALTH FACILITIES AND ADMINISTRATION—Abstracting, Bibliographies, Statistics*

EXCERPTA MEDICA. SECTION 40: DRUG DEPENDENCE, ALCOHOL ABUSE AND ALCOHOLISM. see *DRUG ABUSE AND ALCOHOLISM—Abstracting, Bibliographies, Statistics*

EXCERPTA MEDICA. SECTION 46: ENVIRONMENTAL HEALTH AND POLLUTION CONTROL. see *ENVIRONMENTAL STUDIES—Abstracting, Bibliographies, Statistics*

016.6163 NLD ISSN 0031-3580
CODEN: EMGSA

EXCERPTA MEDICA. SECTION 48: GASTROENTEROLOGY. Text in English. 1971. 16/yr. EUR 1,696 in Europe to institutions; JPY 224,798 in Japan to institutions; USD 1,897 elsewhere to institutions (effective 2002). adv. bk.rev. index, cum.index. back issues avail. *Refereed.* **Document type:** *Abstract/Index, Academic/Scholarly.* **Description:** Provides a comprehensive current-awareness service of academic and clinical articles covering all aspects of digestive system disease and includes disorders of the mouth and pharynx, hepatobiliary system, exocrine pancreas, peritoneum, mesentery, and omentum.
Related titles: CD-ROM ed.: (from SilverPlatter Information, Inc.); Online - full text ed.: (from DIMDI, Data-Star, The Dialog Corporation, JICST).
—GNLM, Infotrieve, Linda Hall. **CCC.**

M

Published by: Excerpta Medica Medical Communications BV (Subsidiary of: Reed Elsevier plc), Rooseveltweg 15, Almere-Stad 1314 SJ, Netherlands. TEL 31-36-538-5600, FAX 31-36-538-5650, http://www.elsevier.com/locate/gastroenterology, http://www.excerptamedica.com. **Subscr. in Australasia and the Far East to:** Elsevier Science (Singapore) Pte Ltd, No.1 Temasek Ave, 17-01 Millenia Tower, Singapore 039192, Singapore. TEL 65-434-3727, FAX 65-337-2230; **Subscr. in Japan to:** Elsevier Science Inc - Japan Regional Office, 9-15 Higashi-Azabu 1-chome, Minato-ku, Tokyo 106-0044, Japan. TEL 81-3-5561-5033, FAX 81-3-5561-5047; **Subscr. in the Americas to:** Elsevier Science, PO Box 945, New York, NY 10159-0945. TEL 212-633-3730, 888-437-4636, FAX 212-633-3680, usinfo-f@elsevier.com. **Dist. by:** Elsevier Science (Brazil).; Elsevier Science BV, PO Box 211, Amsterdam 1000 AE, Netherlands. TEL 31-20-485-3757, FAX 31-20-485-3432.

016.614 016.3632 NLD ISSN 0303-8459
RA1001 CODEN: FSABD

EXCERPTA MEDICA. SECTION 49: FORENSIC SCIENCE ABSTRACTS. Text in English. 1975. bi-m. NLG 2,133, EUR 967.91 in Europe to institutions; JPY 131,200 in Japan to institutions; USD 1,082 elsewhere to institutions (effective 2001). adv. index, cum.index. back issues avail. **Document type:** *Abstract/Index, Academic/Scholarly, Trade.* **Description:** Provides a comprehensive current-awareness service of trade and scholarly articles covering all aspects of biomedicine and science of relevance to criminal investigators or coroners.
Formerly: Excerpta Medica. Section 49: Forensic Science
Related titles: CD-ROM ed.: (from SilverPlatter Information, Inc.); Online - full text ed.: (from DIMDI, Data-Star, The Dialog Corporation, JICST).
—GNLM, Infotrieve, Linda Hall. **CCC.**
Published by: Excerpta Medica Medical Communications BV (Subsidiary of: Reed Elsevier plc), Rooseveltweg 15, Almere-Stad 1314 SJ, Netherlands. TEL 31-36-538-5600, FAX 31-36-538-5650, http://www.elsevier.com/locate/forsciabs, http://www.excerptamedica.com. **Subscr. in Australasia and the Far East to:** Elsevier Science (Singapore) Pte Ltd, No.1 Temasek Ave, 17-01 Millenia Tower, Singapore 039192, Singapore. TEL 65-434-3727, FAX 65-337-2230, asiainfo@elsevier.com.sg; **Subscr. in Japan to:** Elsevier Science Inc - Japan Regional Office, 9-15 Higashi-Azabu 1-chome, Minato-ku, Tokyo 106-0044, Japan. TEL 81-3-5561-5033, FAX 81-3-5561-5047, info@elsevier.co.jp; **Subscr. in the Americas to:** Elsevier Science. **Dist. by:** Elsevier Science (Brazil).; Elsevier Science BV, PO Box 211, Amsterdam 1000 AE, Netherlands. TEL 31-20-485-3757, FAX 31-20-485-3432, nlinfo-f@elsevier.nl, http://www.elsevier.nl.

EXCERPTA MEDICA. SECTION 52: TOXICOLOGY. see *ENVIRONMENTAL STUDIES—Abstracting, Bibliographies, Statistics*

016.616026 NLD ISSN 0014-410X
R37 CODEN: IMDCBQ

EXCERPTA MEDICA. SECTION 6: INTERNAL MEDICINE. Text in English. 1947. s-m. EUR 2,354 in Europe to institutions; JPY 312,015 in Japan to institutions; USD 2,633 elsewhere to institutions (effective 2002). adv. index, cum.index. back issues avail. **Document type:** *Abstract/Index, Academic/Scholarly.* **Description:** Provides a complete current-awareness service of articles in international biomedical journals covering clinical and experimental issues in internal medicine.
Related titles: CD-ROM ed.: (from SilverPlatter Information, Inc.); Online - full text ed.: (from DIMDI, Data-Star, The Dialog Corporation, JICST).
—GNLM, Infotrieve. **CCC.**
Published by: Elsevier Science BV, PO Box 211, Amsterdam 1000 AE, Netherlands. TEL 31-20-485-3757, http://www.elsevier.com/locate/internalmed. **Subscr. in Australasia and the Far East to:** Elsevier Science (Singapore) Pte Ltd, No.1 Temasek Ave, 17-01 Millenia Tower, Singapore 039192, Singapore. TEL 65-434-3727, FAX 65-337-2230, asiainfo@elsevier.com.sg; **Subscr. in Japan to:** Elsevier Science Inc - Japan Regional Office, 9-15 Higashi-Azabu 1-chome, Minato-ku, Tokyo 106-0044, Japan. TEL 81-3-5561-5033, FAX 81-3-5561-5047, info@elsevier.co.jp; **Subscr. in the Americas to:** Elsevier Science. http://www.elsevier.com. **Dist. by:** Elsevier Science (Brazil).

016.61892 NLD ISSN 0373-6512
RJ1 CODEN: PPSUDH

EXCERPTA MEDICA. SECTION 7: PEDIATRICS AND PEDIATRIC SURGERY. Text in English. 1948. 18/yr. EUR 2,436, JPY 322,966, USD 2,725 to institutions (effective 2002). adv. index, cum.index. **Document type:** *Abstract/Index, Academic/Scholarly.* **Description:** Provides a comprehensive current-awareness service of professional and academic articles covering all aspects of development and organic disease in neonates, children and adolescents, including surgery.
Formerly: Excerpta Medica. Section 7: Pediatrics (0014-4118)
Related titles: CD-ROM ed.: (from SilverPlatter Information, Inc.); Online - full text ed.: (from DIMDI, Data-Star, The Dialog Corporation, JICST).
—GNLM, Infotrieve. **CCC.**
Published by: Excerpta Medica Medical Communications BV (Subsidiary of: Reed Elsevier plc), Rooseveltweg 15, Almere-Stad 1314 SJ, Netherlands. http://www.elsevier.nl/locate/pedsurg. **Subscr. in Australasia and the Far East to:** Elsevier Science (Singapore) Pte Ltd, No.1 Temasek Ave, 17-01 Millenia Tower, Singapore 039192, Singapore. TEL 65-434-3727, FAX 65-337-2230; **Subscr. in Japan to:** Elsevier Science Inc - Japan Regional Office, 9-15 Higashi-Azabu 1-chome, Minato-ku, Tokyo 106-0044, Japan. TEL 81-3-5561-5033, FAX 81-3-5561-5047; **Subscr. in the Americas to:** Elsevier Science. usinfo-f@elsevier.com, http://www.elsevier.com. **Dist. by:** Elsevier Science (Brazil).; Elsevier Science BV, PO Box 211, Amsterdam 1000 AE, Netherlands. TEL 31-20-485-3757, FAX 31-20-485-3432.

016.6168 NLD ISSN 0014-4126
CODEN: NLNSB2

EXCERPTA MEDICA. SECTION 8: NEUROLOGY AND NEUROSURGERY. Text in English. 1948. 32/yr. EUR 3,456 in Europe to institutions; JPY 458,120 in Japan to institutions; USD 3,866 elsewhere to institutions (effective 2002). adv. index, cum.index. back issues avail. **Document type:** *Abstract/Index, Academic/Scholarly.* **Description:** Provides a comprehensive current-awareness service of academic and professional articles covering clinical neurology and neurosurgery, including epilepsy and neuromuscular disorders.
Related titles: CD-ROM ed.: (from SilverPlatter Information, Inc.); Online - full text ed.: (from DIMDI, Data-Star, The Dialog Corporation, JICST).
—GNLM, Infotrieve. **CCC.**
Published by: Excerpta Medica Medical Communications BV (Subsidiary of: Reed Elsevier plc), Rooseveltweg 15, Almere-Stad 1314 SJ, Netherlands. TEL 31-36-538-5600, FAX 31-36-538-5650, http://www.elsevier.com/neuneu, http://www.excerptamedica.com. **Subscr. in Australasia and the Far East to:** Elsevier Science (Singapore) Pte Ltd, No.1 Temasek Ave, 17-01 Millenia Tower, Singapore 039192, Singapore. TEL 65-434-3727, FAX 65-337-2230; **Subscr. in Japan to:** Elsevier Science Inc - Japan Regional Office, 9-15 Higashi-Azabu 1-chome, Minato-ku, Tokyo 106-0044, Japan. TEL 81-3-5561-5033, FAX 81-3-5561-5047; **Subscr. in the Americas to:** Elsevier Science, PO Box 945, New York, NY 10159-0945. TEL 212-633-3730, 888-437-4636, FAX 212-633-3680, usinfo-f@elsevier.com, http://www.elsevier.com. **Dist. by:** Elsevier Science (Brazil).; Elsevier Science BV, PO Box 211, Amsterdam 1000 AE, Netherlands. TEL 31-20-485-3757, FAX 31-20-485-3432.

016.617 NLD ISSN 0014-4134
CODEN: EMSGAY

EXCERPTA MEDICA. SECTION 9: SURGERY. Text in English. 1947. 20/yr. EUR 2,606 in Europe to institutions; JPY 345,525 in Japan to institutions; USD 2,916 elsewhere to institutions (effective 2002). adv. index, cum.index. back issues avail.; reprints avail. *Refereed.* **Document type:** *Abstract/Index, Academic/Scholarly.* **Description:** Provides a comprehensive current-awareness service of professional and academic articles covering general, abdominal, thoracic and peripheral vascular surgery, cosmetic, plastic and reconstructive surgery, microsurgery, pre- and post-operative care, and surgical aspects of intensive care medicine.
Related titles: CD-ROM ed.: (from SilverPlatter Information, Inc.); Online - full text ed.: (from DIMDI, Data-Star, The Dialog Corporation, JICST).
—GNLM, Infotrieve. **CCC.**
Published by: Excerpta Medica Medical Communications BV (Subsidiary of: Reed Elsevier plc), Rooseveltweg 15, Almere-Stad 1314 SJ, Netherlands. http://www.elsevier.nl/locate/surgery. **Subscr. in Australasia and the Far East to:** Elsevier Science (Singapore) Pte Ltd, No.1 Temasek Ave, 17-01 Millenia Tower, Singapore 039192, Singapore. TEL 65-434-3727, FAX 65-337-2230; **Subscr. in Japan to:** Elsevier Science Inc - Japan Regional Office, 9-15 Higashi-Azabu 1-chome, Minato-ku, Tokyo 106-0044, Japan. TEL 81-3-5561-5033, FAX 81-3-5561-5047; **Subscr. in the Americas to:** Elsevier Science, PO Box 945, New York, NY 10159-0945. TEL 212-633-3730, 888-437-4636, FAX 212-633-3680, usinfo-f@elsevier.com, http://www.elsevier.com. **Dist. by:** Elsevier Science (Brazil).; Elsevier Science BV, PO Box 211, Amsterdam 1000 AE, Netherlands. TEL 31-20-485-3757, FAX 31-20-485-3432.

616.5 617 DEU ISSN 0342-2828

EXTRACTA DERMATOLOGICA; weltweit Auserlesen. Text in German. 1977. bi-m. DEM 45. adv. bk.rev. bibl, charts, illus. back issues avail.
—GNLM.
Published by: Media-Derm, Postfach 100745, Hamburg 20005, Germany. Ed. Volker Misgeld. Circ: 3,000.

617.3 DEU ISSN 0344-5046

EXTRACTA ORTHOPAEDICA; Weltweit Auserlesen. Text in German. 1978. bi-m. DEM 99. adv. bk.rev. back issues avail. **Document type:** *Academic/Scholarly.*
—GNLM.
Published by: Selecta Verlagsgesellschaft mbH, Postfach 4240, Wiesbaden 65032, Germany. TEL 0611-1705-0, FAX 0611-1705379. Ed. Dr. Wolfgang Dorn. Circ: 3,200.

016.61 610 GBR

EXTRAMED. Text in English. 1994. m. GBP 1,200, USD 1,800; GBP 600, USD 900 in developing nations (effective 2001). abstr, bibl, illus. back issues avail. *Refereed.* **Document type:** *Catalog, Academic/Scholarly, Abstract/Index.* **Description:** Covers over 300 of the principal Third World biomedical journals. Provides searchable abstracts and bibliographical data with full-text images, including illustrations and graphs.
Media: CD-ROM. **Related titles:** Online - full text ed.
—BLDSC (3854.418500).
Published by: (ExtraMED Consortium), Informania Limited, PO Box 40, Petersfield, Hants GU32 2YH, United Kingdom. TEL 44-1730-301297, FAX 44-1730-265398, dvt@compuserve.com, http://www.extramed.com. Ed. Chris Zielinski.

016.61 DEU

FACHBUCHVERZEICHNIS MEDIZIN. Text in German. a. **Document type:** *Bibliography.* **Description:** Bibliography of available medical books for students.
Formerly: Buecher fuer das Studium - Medizin
Published by: Rossipaul Kommunikation GmbH, Menzinger Str 37, Munich 80638, Germany. TEL 49-89-179106-0, FAX 49-89-179106-22. Ed. Angela Sendlinger. Circ: 25,000.

610 310 USA ISSN 1074-8849
R11

FACTS ABOUT FAMILY PRACTICE. Text in English. 1987. a. USD 60 to non-members; USD 40 to members (effective 2001). **Document type:** *Academic/Scholarly.* **Description:** Provides statistics on family medicine, such as income, patient visits, ratio of physicians to population. Designed for use by the medical community.
Published by: American Academy of Family Physicians, 11400 Tomahawk Creek Pkwy, Leawood, KS 66211-2672. TEL 913-906-6000, 800-274-2237, FAX 913-906-6077, afpedit@aafp.org, http://www.aafp.org. R&P Gordon Schmittling. Circ: 3,500.

FIRE STATISTICS UNITED KINGDOM. see *FIRE PREVENTION—Abstracting, Bibliographies, Statistics*

617.3 616.8 FRA ISSN 1276-356X

FLASH-INFORMATIONS HANDICAP. Text in French. 1978. w. FRF 650 (effective 2000). adv. bk.rev. abstr, bibl. **Document type:** *Bulletin.*
Formerly: Flash-Informations (0223-4696)
Published by: Centre Technique National d'Etudes et de Recherches sur les Handicaps et les Inadaptations, 236 bis rue de Tolbiac, Paris 75013, France. TEL 33-1-45655900, FAX 33-1-45654494, ctnerhi@club-internet.fr. Ed. M Maudinet. R&P A Piquet. Adv. contact Guillaumeau.

M

617.643 NZL ISSN 0015-4725
QP535.F1 CODEN: FLUOA4
FLUORIDE; journal of the international society for fluoride research. Text in English. 1968. q. NZD 40, AUD 40 in Australia & New Zealand to membership; USD 40, JPY 4,000, GBP 25 elsewhere to membership (effective 2000). bk.rev. abstr, bibl, charts, illus, stat. reprint service avail. from PQC,ISI. *Refereed.* **Document type:** *Academic/Scholarly.* **Description:** Reports on biological, chemical, ecological, industrial, toxicological and clinical aspects of inorganic and organic fluoride compounds.
Related titles: Microform ed.: (from PQC); Online - full text ed.: (from Institute for Scientific Information).
Indexed: ASCA, Alloys Ind., Aqua.Sci.& Fish.Abstr., Biol.Abstr., C.I.S. Abstr., Cadscan, Cal.Tiss.Abstr., Chem.Abstr., Crop Physiol.Abstr., Curr.Adv.Ecol.Sci., Curr.Cont., Dairy Sci.Abstr., Eng.Mat.Abstr., Environ.Sci.Poll.Mgmt., Excerp.Med., Field Crop Abstr., Food Sci.& Tech.Abstr., INIS Atomind., Ind.Sci.Rev., Ind.Vet., Lead Abstr., Met.Abstr., Met.Abstr.Ind., Microbiol.Abstr., Nonfer.Met.Alert, Nutr.Abstr., Ocean.Abstr. (coverage dropped), PCC Alert, Pollut.Abstr., Rice Abstr., SSCI (coverage dropped), Sci.Cit.Ind., Sel.Water Res.Abstr., Soils & Fert., Steels Alert, Tox.Abstr., Vet.Bull., World Alum.Abstr., Zincscan.
—BLDSC (3962.262800), CASDDS, CISTI, IDS, Infotrieve, ingenta, KNAW, Linda Hall. **CCC.**
Published by: International Society for Fluoride Research, 727 Brighton Rd, Ocean View, Dunedin 9051, New Zealand. FAX 64-3-4811418, spittle@es.co.nz, http://www.fluoride-journal.com. Circ: 600.

016.610 USA
FOCUS ON: MOLECULAR MEDICINE. Text in English. m. USD 395 (effective 1998). **Document type:** *Abstract/Index.* **Description:** Covers more than 2,500 source items per issue regarding basic research and clinical studies in humans and laboratory animals.
Media: Diskette.
Published by: Institute for Scientific Information, 3501 Market St., Philadelphia, PA 19104. TEL 215-386-0100, 800-336-4474, FAX 215-386-2911, webmaster@isinet.com, http://www.isinet.com. **Dist. in Europe by:** ISI Europe, Brunel Science Park, Kingston Ln, Uxbridge, Mddx UB8 3PQ, United Kingdom. TEL 44-1895-270016, FAX 44-1895-256710.

016.617 USA ISSN 1069-7004
FOCUS ON: SPORTS SCIENCE AND MEDICINE. Text in English. m. USD 240 (effective 1998). **Document type:** *Abstract/Index.* **Description:** Provides bibliographic data and English-language author abstracts from international scholarly research journals and conference proceedings.
Media: Diskette.
Published by: Institute for Scientific Information, 3501 Market St., Philadelphia, PA 19104. TEL 215-386-0100, 800-336-4474, FAX 215-386-2911, webmaster@isinet.com, http://www.isinet.com. **Dist. in Europe by:** ISI Europe, Brunel Science Park, Kingston Ln, Uxbridge, Mddx UB8 3PQ, United Kingdom. TEL 44-1895-270016, FAX 44-1895-256710.

617.0021 FRA
FRANCE. SERVICE D'ETUDE DES STRATEGIES ET DES STATISTIQUES INDUSTRIELLES. RESULTATS TRIMESTRIELS DES ENQUETES DE BRANCHE. FABRICATION DE MATERIEL MEDICO-CHIRURGICAL ET DES PROTHESES. Text in French. q. FRF 180; FRF 210 foreign (effective 1991). stat. **Description:** Provides detailed industry-wide performance statistics for comparative evaluations.
Published by: Service d'Etude des Strategies et des Statistiques Industrielles (SESSI), 85 bd. du Montparnasse, Paris Cedex 6 75270, France. TEL 45-56-42-34, FAX 45-56-40-71.

FRITZ-HUESER-INSTITUT FUER DEUTSCHE UND AUSLAENDISCHE ARBEITERLITERATUR. INFORMATIONEN. see *LITERATURE—Abstracting, Bibliographies, Statistics*

016.6163 GBR ISSN 1461-5118
GASTROINTESTINAL HORMONES AND GASTRIC SECRETION. Text in English. 1998. s-m. GBP 120 for print ed. or e-mail (effective 2001). adv. **Document type:** *Abstract/Index.* **Description:** Current awareness service for researchers. Covers gastrin, bombesin, G-I-polypeptide, secretin, motilin, VIP, pancreatic polypeptide and other hormones. Now includes gastric secretion and stomach motility.
Formed by the merger of (1977-1998): Gastrointestinal Hormones (0142-8101); (1979-1998): Gastric Secretion (0142-8098)
Related titles: E-mail ed.; Online - full text ed.: GBP 108 (effective 2001).
—CCC.
Published by: S U B I S (Subsidiary of: Sheffield Academic Press Ltd), Mansion House, 19 Kingfield Rd, Sheffield, S Yorks S11 9AS, United Kingdom. TEL 44-114-255-4433, FAX 44-114-255-4626, subis@sheffac.demon.co.uk, http://www.shef-ac-press.co.uk/subis. Ed. S Huntridge. Adv. contact C Evans.

617 JPN
GEKA SHUDANKAI SHOROKUSHU/TOKYO SURGICAL SOCIETY. ABSTRACTS. Text in Japanese. 4/yr. **Document type:** *Abstract/Index.*
Published by: Geka Shudankai, Daigaku Igakubu Dai 1 Geka, 3-1 Hongo 7-chome, Bunkyo-ku, Tokyo 113-0033, Japan.

GENE THERAPY (SHEFFIELD). see *BIOLOGY—Abstracting, Bibliographies, Statistics*

GREAT BRITAIN. GOVERNMENT STATISTICAL SERVICE. ABORTION STATISTICS. see *BIRTH CONTROL—Abstracting, Bibliographies, Statistics*

616.99 GBR ISSN 0143-4829
RC279.G7
GREAT BRITAIN. GOVERNMENT STATISTICAL SERVICE. CANCER STATISTICS REGISTRATIONS. ENGLAND AND WALES. Text in English. 1979. a.?. **Document type:** *Government.*
Published by: (Puerto Rico. Department of Health USA, Great Britain. Statistics Division), Government Statistical Service, SD2, Rm 804, Hannibal House, Elephant and Castle, London SE1 6TE, United Kingdom. TEL 0171-972-2193. **Orders to:** Department of Health and Social Security (Leaflets), PO Box 21, Stanmore, Mddx HA7 1AY, United Kingdom.

616.04 GBR ISSN 0265-3567
GREAT BRITAIN. GOVERNMENT STATISTICAL SERVICE. CONGENITAL MALFORMATION STATISTICS NOTIFICATIONS. Text in English. 1983. a.?. **Document type:** *Government.*
Published by: (Puerto Rico. Department of Health USA, Great Britain. Statistics Division), Government Statistical Service, SD2, Rm 804, Hannibal House, Elephant and Castle, London SE1 6TE, United Kingdom. TEL 0171-972-2193. **Orders to:** Department of Health and Social Security (Leaflets), PO Box 21, Stanmore, Mddx HA7 1AY, United Kingdom.

616.863 310 GBR ISSN 0143-1463
HV5840.G7
GREAT BRITAIN. HOME OFFICE. STATISTICS OF THE MISUSE OF DRUGS: SEIZURES AND OFFENDERS DEALT WITH, UNITED KINGDOM (YEAR). Text in English. 1978. a.
Former titles (until 1992): Great Britain. Home Office. Statistics of the Misuse of Drugs in the United Kingdom: Seizures and Offenders Dealt with; (until 1986): Great Britain. Home Office. Statistics of the Misuse of Drugs in the United Kingdom, Supplementary Tables.
Published by: Home Office, 50 Queen Annes Gate, London SW1H 9AT, United Kingdom.

016.616 GBR ISSN 1359-7604
GROWTH FACTORS & CYTOKINES - CLINICAL. Text in English. 1985. s-m. GBP 168 for print ed. or e-mail (effective 2001). adv. **Document type:** *Abstract/Index.* **Description:** Current awareness service for researchers in clinical and life sciences.
Supersedes in part: Growth Factors and Cytokines (0964-7554); Which supersedes: Growth Factors (0268-1595); Cytokines (0960-3212); Which was formerly (until 1990): Lymphokines (0264-9586)
Related titles: E-mail ed.; Online - full text ed.: GBP 108 (effective 2001).
—CCC.
Published by: S U B I S (Subsidiary of: Sheffield Academic Press Ltd), Mansion House, 19 Kingfield Rd, Sheffield, S Yorks S11 9AS, United Kingdom. TEL 44-114-255-4433, FAX 44-114-255-4626, subis@sheffac.demon.co.uk, http://www.shef-ac-press.co.uk/subis. Ed. S Huntridge. Adv. contact C Evans.

016.616 GBR ISSN 1359-7590
GROWTH FACTORS & CYTOKINES - RESEARCH. Text in English. s-m. GBP 120 for print ed. or e-mail (effective 2001). adv. **Document type:** *Abstract/Index.*
Supersedes in part: Growth Factors and Cytokines (0964-7554)
Related titles: E-mail ed.; Online - full text ed.: GBP 108 (effective 2001).
Published by: S U B I S (Subsidiary of: Sheffield Academic Press Ltd), Mansion House, 19 Kingfield Rd, Sheffield, S Yorks S11 9AS, United Kingdom. TEL 44-114-255-4433, FAX 44-114-255-4626, subis@sheffac.demon.co.uk, http://www.shef-ac-press.co.uk/subis. Ed. S Huntridge. Adv. contact C Evans.

616.1 GBR
HANDBOOK OF HYPERLIPIDAEMIA. Text in English. 1990. a. GBP 29.95, USD 59.95. illus. **Document type:** *Academic/Scholarly.* **Description:** For lipid and cardiovascular specialists as well as the general practitioner. Covers all aspects of hyperlipidemia including pathophysiology, classification and clinical practice.
Published by: Rapid Science Publishers, 2-6 Boundary Row, London SE1 8HN, United Kingdom. TEL 44-207-865-0198, FAX 44-20-7865-6600, rapid@rapidcom.co.uk. Ed. G R Thompson.

610 USA ISSN 1059-7565
RC392 CODEN: HQUAEN
HEADACHE QUARTERLY; current treatment and research. Text in English. 1990. q. USD 51.50 domestic to individuals; USD 96 foreign to individuals; USD 77.25 domestic to institutions; USD 122 foreign to institutions (effective 1999). adv. bk.rev. abstr, charts. *Refereed.* **Document type:** *Proceedings, Academic/Scholarly, Abstract/Index.* **Description:** Reports on current research, futuristic therapies and headache theories. Covers histamines, serotonin, prostaglandins, radiological and diagnostic advances and behavioral medicine.
Related titles: Online - full text ed.: (from Institute for Scientific Information).
Indexed: ASCA, CINAHL, Inpharma, Neurosci.Cit.Ind., Pharm.&Out.News, PsycInfo, Psychol.Abstr., Reac., Ref.Zh., SSCI (coverage dropped), e-psyche.
—BLDSC (4274.643000), EMDOCS, GNLM, KNAW.
Published by: H Q, 467 W Demming Pl, Ste 500, Chicago, IL 60614. TEL 773-388-6376. Ed. Dr. Seymour Diamond. R&P Mary Franklin TEL 773-388-6363. Adv. contact Idell Applebaum. **Co-sponsor:** Diamond Headache Foundation, Inpatient Headache Unit of Weiss Memorial Hospital.

HEALTH DEVICES SOURCEBOOK. see *MEDICAL SCIENCES*

016.61 USA
HEALTH DEVICES SYSTEM; a summary of reported problems, hazards, recalls, and updates. Text in English. 1976. w. USD 3,649.40 domestic; USD 3,675.40 in Canada; USD 3,765.20 elsewhere (effective 2002). abstr. back issues avail. *Refereed.* **Description:** Includes over 250,000 reports from international sources, focusing on problems with equipment, disposables, in vitro diagnostics, implants, and other critical devices.
Formerly: Health Devices Alerts (0163-0458)
Related titles: CD-ROM ed.: USD 625 to individuals; USD 1,150 to institutions; USD 3,650 to non-members (effective 2002) (from The Dialog Corporation); Online - full text ed.: (from The Dialog Corporation).
—BLDSC (4274.963500), GNLM, Infotrieve. **CCC.**
Published by: (Emergency Care Research Institute), E C R I, 5200 Butler Pike, Plymouth, PA 19462. TEL 610-825-6000, FAX 610-834-1275, info@ecri.org, http://www.ecri.org.

362.1 016.4 USA ISSN 1077-9469
HEALTH INDUSTRY QUICKSOURCE; a complete descriptive reference to healthcare information resources. Key Title: Health Industry. Text in English. 1994. a. USD 225 (effective 1997). **Document type:** *Directory, Bibliography.*
Related titles: CD-ROM ed.
Published by: Dorland Healthcare Information, 1500 Walnut St Ste 1000, Philadelphia, PA 19102. Circ: 500.

016.3621 GBR ISSN 0268-0459
HEALTH SERVICE ABSTRACTS. Text in English. 1974. m. GBP 40 in United Kingdom; GBP 58 in Europe; GBP 72.30 elsewhere (effective 2001). bibl. **Document type:** *Abstract/Index, Government.* **Description:** Summarizes books, reports, journal articles, and other publications on the nonclinical aspects of health services, with emphasis on the U.K. Covers such topics as health service administration, policy and planning, economics and finance, and ethics.
Incorporates (in May 1985): Hospital Abstracts (0018-5507); Current Literature on Health Services (0141-0571); Current Literature on General Medical Practice
Related titles: Online - full text ed.: (from Data-Star).
—GNLM, Infotrieve. **CCC.**

M

Published by: Department of Health, Library and Information Services, Health and Social Services Information Unit, Rm 5C07, Quarry House, Quarry Hill, Leeds LS2 7UE, United Kingdom. TEL 44-113-254-5072, FAX 44-113-254-5084, health-service-abstracts@doh.gsi.gov.uk. Ed., R&P Jennifer Goodfellow. Circ: 3,500. **Subscr. to:** Dept. of Health, H S A Subscriptions, PO Box 777, London SE1 6XH, United Kingdom.

610 USA ISSN 0361-4468
RA407.3
HEALTH, UNITED STATES. Text in English. a. price varies. **Document type:** *Government.*
—CISTI, GNLM.
Published by: U.S. National Center for Health Statistics, Data Dissemination Branch, 6525 Belcrest Rd, Hyattsville, MD 20782. TEL 301-458-4636, http://www.cdc.gov/nchs/. **Orders to:** U.S. Government Printing Office, Superintendent of Documents.

026 610.73 CAN
HELEN K. MUSSALLEM LIBRARY SELECTED ACQUISITIONS. Text in English, French. m. free per issue. **Document type:** *Catalog.* **Description:** Partial catalogs of the library's collection highlighting some of its holdings. Listed according to subject.
Media: Online - full text.
Published by: Canadian Nurses Association/Association des Infirmieres et Infirmiers du Canada, 50 Drway, Ottawa, ON K2P 1E2, Canada. TEL 613-237-2133, FAX 613-237-3520, pubs@cna-nurses.ca, http://www.cna-nurses.ca.

610.73 CAN
HELEN K. MUSSALLEM. PERIODICAL HOLDINGS LIST. Text in English, French. 1981. a. CND 15 (effective 1997). **Document type:** *Catalog, Bibliography.* **Description:** Provides a complete catalogue of the library periodicals, listed alphabetically. Includes titles, publishers and the extent of the holdings.
Former titles: Canadian Nurses Association. Helen K. Mussallem Library. Periodical Holdings (0710-2437); (until 1981): Canadian Nurses Association. Library. Periodical Holdings (0383-0101)
Published by: Canadian Nurses Association/Association des Infirmieres et Infirmiers du Canada, 50 Drway, Ottawa, ON K2P 1E2, Canada. TEL 613-627-2133, FAX 613-237-3520, pubs@cna-nurses.ca.

016.61 USA ISSN 0883-2285
HEMOCHROMATOSIS AWARENESS; a quarterly update on hereditary and acquired iron-overload. Text in English. 1982. q. USD 35; USD 40 foreign (effective 1999). bk.rev. tr.lit. **Document type:** *Newsletter, Proceedings.* **Description:** Discusses all aspects of hereditary hemochromatosis, a disorder of iron metabolism in which dietary iron absorption exceeds body needs. Reviews relevant literature, public policy and food regulatory issues.
Published by: Hemochromatosis Foundation, Inc., PO Box 8569, Albany, NY 12208. TEL 518-489-0972, FAX 518-489-0227, http://www.hemochromatosis.org. Ed. M A Krikker. Circ: 3,500 (paid).

HIGH PERFORMANCE LIQUID CHROMATOGRAPHY. see *PHARMACY AND PHARMACOLOGY—Abstracting, Bibliographies, Statistics*

016.61697 GBR ISSN 1463-4376
HIV & AIDS. Text in English. 1998. s-m. (diskette m.). GBP 120. adv. **Document type:** *Abstract/Index.* **Description:** Current awareness service for researchers investigating HIV infections and AIDS.
Related titles: Diskette ed.; E-mail ed.; Online - full text ed.
Published by: S U B I S (Subsidiary of: Sheffield Academic Press Ltd), Mansion House, 19 Kingfield Rd, Sheffield, S Yorks S11 9AS, United Kingdom. TEL 44-114-255-4433, FAX 44-114-255-4626, subis@sheffac.demon.co.uk, http://www.shef-ac-press.co.uk/subis. Adv. contact C Evans.

616.6 JPN
HOKKAIDO TOSEKI RYOHO GAKKAI PUROGURAMU ENDAI SHOROKU/HOKKAIDO SOCIETY FOR DIALYSIS THERAPY. PROGRAM AND ABSTRACTS. Text in Japanese. a. **Document type:** *Abstract/Index.*
Published by: Hokkaido Toseki Ryoho Gakkai, 3, Nishi 7-chome, Kita 1-jo, Chuo-ku, Sapporo-shi, Hokkaido 090, Japan.

HUMAN REPRODUCTION UPDATE. see *BIOLOGY—Abstracting, Bibliographies, Statistics*

016.3067 GBR ISSN 0142-811X
HUMAN SEXUALITY. Text in English. 1977. s-m. GBP 96 for print ed. or e-mail (effective 2001). adv. **Document type:** *Abstract/Index.* **Description:** Current awareness service for researchers in the clinical and social sciences investigating all aspects of human sexuality.
Related titles: E-mail ed.; Online - full text ed.: GBP 108 to individuals (effective 2001).
—Infotrieve. **CCC.**
Published by: S U B I S (Subsidiary of: Sheffield Academic Press Ltd), Mansion House, 19 Kingfield Rd, Sheffield, S Yorks S11 9AS, United Kingdom. TEL 44-114-255-4433, FAX 44-114-255-4626, subis@sheffac.demon.co.uk, http://www.shef-ac-press.co.uk/subis. Ed. S Huntridge. Adv. contact C Evans.

610 016 HUN ISSN 0441-4438
HUNGARIAN MEDICAL BIBLIOGRAPHY; abstracts. Text in English. 1961. s-a. HUF 2,400, USD 60 (effective 1997). adv. **Document type:** *Bibliography.* **Description:** Lists selected publications in English on Hungarian medicine and allied fields.
—GNLM.
Published by: Orszagos Orvostudomanyi Informacios Intezet es Konyvtar/National Institute for Medical Information and Library of Medicine, Szentkiralyi utca 21, PO Box 278, Budapest 1444, Hungary. TEL 36-1-117-6352, FAX 36-1-266-9710, konyvtar@nt-ph.medinfo.hu. Ed. Dr. Tivadar Jakab. Pub. Dr. Alexander Fedinecz. Adv. contact Ilona Borbas. B&W page HUF 24,000, color page HUF 36,000. Circ: 320.

016.61697 GBR ISSN 0142-8128
IMMUNOASSAY. Text in English. 1970. s-m. GBP 168 for print ed. or email (effective 2001). adv. abstr. **Document type:** *Abstract/Index.* **Description:** Current awareness service for researchers. Covers radioimmunoassay, fluorescence immunoassay and enzyme immunoassay.
Related titles: E-mail ed.; Online - full text ed.: GBP 108 to individuals (effective 2001).
—Infotrieve. **CCC.**
Published by: S U B I S (Subsidiary of: Sheffield Academic Press Ltd), Mansion House, 19 Kingfield Rd, Sheffield, S Yorks S11 9AS, United Kingdom. TEL 44-114-255-4433, FAX 44-114-255-4626, subis@sheffac.demon.co.uk, http://www.shef-ac-press.co.uk/subis. Ed. S Huntridge. Adv. contact C Evans.

615.37 016 USA ISSN 0307-112X
QR180
IMMUNOLOGY ABSTRACTS. Text in English. 1976. bi-m. USD 1,425 (effective 2002). abstr. index. back issues avail. **Document type:** *Abstract/Index.* **Description:** Covers immune systems in humans and animals, both basic research and clinical applications.
Related titles: Online - full text ed.: USD 1,070 (effective 2002) (from The Dialog Corporation, S T N International).
—BLDSC (4369.701000), GNLM.
Published by: Cambridge Scientific Abstracts, 7200 Wisconsin Ave., Suite 601, Bethesda, MD 20814. TEL 301-961-6798, FAX 301-961-6799, journals@csa.com, http://www.csa.com/journals. Ed. D Whitman. Pub. Ted Caris.

016.61 USA ISSN 0019-3879
Z6660
INDEX MEDICUS. Text in English. 1960. m. USD 505; USD 65 for Medical Subject Headings Section; USD 38 for List of Journals Indexed Section (effective 2001). illus. reprints avail. **Document type:** *Abstract/Index, Bibliography, Government.* **Description:** Compiles and lists articles from 3,000 of the world's leading biomedical journals published in 36 languages.
Related titles: CD-ROM ed.: Medline CD. ISSN 1081-4914 (from The Dialog Corporation, SilverPlatter Information, Inc., CSA); Microform ed.: (from PQC,PMC); Online - full text ed.: Medline (from The Dialog Corporation, National Library of Medicine, S T N International).
—BLDSC (4382.500000), KNAW, Linda Hall.
Published by: U.S. National Library of Medicine, 8600 Rockville Pike, Bethesda, MD 20894. http://www.nlm.nih.gov. Circ: 6,000. **Subscr. to:** U.S. Government Printing Office, Superintendent of Documents, PO Box 371954, Pittsburgh, PA 15250-7954. TEL 202-512-1800, FAX 202-512-2250, orders@gpo.gov, http://www.access.gpo.gov. **Dist. in UK by:** Turpin Distribution Services Ltd., Blackhorse Rd, Letchworth, Herts SG6 1HN, United Kingdom. FAX 44-1462-480947.

610 016 IDN ISSN 0853-9952
INDEX MEDICUS INDONESIA. Text in Indonesian. 1986. a. **Document type:** *Abstract/Index.*
Published by: National Institute of Health Research and Development, Jl. Percetakan Negara No. 23A, Jakarta 10560, Indonesia.

610 RUS
INDEX OF CURRENT MEDICAL LITERATURE IN THE R F. Text in Russian. s-m. **Description:** Covers all publications in the biomedical sciences in the Russian Federation.
Formerly: Index of Current Medical Literature in the U S S R (0206-0515)
Published by: N P O Soyuzmedinform, Moskvoretskaya nab 2-a, Moscow 109240, Russian Federation.

016.6176 ARG ISSN 0325-0679
INDICE DE LA LITERATURA DENTAL EN CASTELLANO. Text in Spanish. 1950. a. USD 40. bibl. **Document type:** *Abstract/Index.*
Supersedes: Indice de la Literatura Dental Periodica en Castellano y Portugues
Media: CD-ROM.
Published by: Asociacion Odontologica Argentina, BIREME,PAHO, WHO, Rua Botucatu 862, Sao Paulo, SP, Brazil. TEL 541-9611062, FAX 541-9611110, biblioteca@aoa.org.ar. Circ: 300.

016.61 ESP ISSN 0019-7068
INDICE MEDICO ESPANOL. Text in Spanish. 1965. 3/yr. ESP 5,000 to individuals; ESP 6,000 to institutions (effective 2000). reprints avail. **Document type:** *Abstract/Index.* **Description:** Two issues each year list Spanish medical bibliographic references and the third lists Spanish authors and their works.
Related titles: CD-ROM ed.; Online - full text ed.
—CINDOC.
Published by: Instituto de Historia de la Ciencia y Documentacion Lopez Pinero, Universidade de Valencia - CSIC, Avda Blasco Ibanez - 17, Valencia 46010, Spain. TEL 34-96-3610654, FAX 34-96-3613975. Circ: 2,000.

016.6176 USA ISSN 0534-669X
INTERNATIONAL ASSOCIATION FOR DENTAL RESEARCH. ABSTRACTS OF THE GENERAL MEETING. Variant title: Program and Abstracts of Papers. Text in English. 1919. a. USD 30 (effective 2000). adv. **Document type:** *Proceedings.*
Related titles: Microform ed.: (from PQC); ♦ Special ed. of: Journal of Dental Research. ISSN 0022-0345.
Indexed: Dent.Abstr.
—**CCC.**
Published by: International Association for Dental Research, 1619 Duke St, Alexandria, VA 22314. TEL 703-548-0066. Ed. Dr. Mark C Herzberg. R&P Thomas Kolstad TEL 703-548-0066 ext 28. Circ: 9,500.
Co-sponsor: American Association for Dental Research.

340.6 016 USA ISSN 0098-2393
INTERNATIONAL BIBLIOGRAPHY OF THE FORENSIC SCIENCES. Text in English. 1975. biennial. USD 25.
Published by: International Reference Organization in Forensic Medicine & Sciences, PO Box 8282, Wichita, KS 67208. TEL 316-685-7612.

016.6163 GBR ISSN 0261-4995
INTESTINAL FUNCTION. Text in English. 1965. s-m. GBP 120 for print ed. or e-mail (effective 2001). adv. **Document type:** *Abstract/Index.* **Description:** Current awareness service for researchers. Covers intestinal transport, structure, physiology, motility and biochemistry.
Former titles (until 1981): Intestinal Absorption (0306-3003); Intestinal Absorption and Related Topics
Related titles: E-mail ed.; Online - full text ed.: USD 108 (effective 2001).
—**CCC.**
Published by: S U B I S (Subsidiary of: Sheffield Academic Press Ltd), Mansion House, 19 Kingfield Rd, Sheffield, S Yorks S11 9AS, United Kingdom. TEL 44-114-255-4433, FAX 44-114-255-4626, subis@sheffac.demon.co.uk, http://www.shef-ac-press.co.uk/subis. Ed. S Huntridge. Adv. contact C Evans.

INVERTEBRATE NEUROBIOLOGY. see *BIOLOGY—Abstracting, Bibliographies, Statistics*

IRON METABOLISM. see *BIOLOGY—Abstracting, Bibliographies, Statistics*

M

610 362 JPN ISSN 0911-8411
JAPAN. MINISTRY OF HEALTH AND WELFARE. STATISTICS AND INFORMATION DEPARTMENT. REPORT ON ACTIVITIES OF PUBLIC HEALTH CENTERS. Key Title: Hokenjo Un'ei Hokoku. Text in Japanese. a. JPY 4,830 (effective 1998). **Document type:** *Government.*
Formerly (until 1960): Hokenjo Un'ei Hokoku Nenpo (0437-6633)
Published by: Ministry of Health and Welfare, Statistics and Information Department/Koseisho Daijin Kanbo Tokei Johobu, 1-2-3 Kasumigaseki, Chiyoda-ku, Tokyo 100-0013, Japan. TEL 81-3-3503-1711, FAX 81-3-3595-1607. R&P Yoke Kanegae. **Subscr. to:** Health & Welfare Statistics Association, 5-13-14 Roppongi, Minato-ku, Tokyo 106-0032, Japan. TEL 81-3-3586-3361, FAX 81-3-3584-4710.

JATROS DERMA. see *MEDICAL SCIENCES—Dermatology And Venereology*

JATROS GYN. see *MEDICAL SCIENCES—Obstetrics And Gynecology*

JATROS NEURO. see *MEDICAL SCIENCES—Psychiatry And Neurology*

JATROS ORTHO. see *MEDICAL SCIENCES—Orthopedics And Traumatology*

JATROS PAED. see *MEDICAL SCIENCES—Pediatrics*

JATROS URO. see *MEDICAL SCIENCES—Urology And Nephrology*

016.6163 BGD ISSN 1606-0997
CODEN: JDDREM
JOURNAL OF HEALTH POPULATION AND NUTRITION. Text in English. 1983. q. BDT 500 domestic; USD 30 in developing nations to individuals; USD 60 in developing nations to institutions; USD 40 elsewhere to individuals; USD 80 elsewhere to institutions (effective 2001). back issues avail. *Refereed.* **Document type:** *Journal, Abstract/Index, Academic/Scholarly.* **Description:** Publishes review articles, original research articles, short communications, preliminary communications, and letters dealing with all aspects of health, population and nutrition.
Supersedes (in 2000): Journal of Diarrhoeal Diseases Research (0253-8768)
Related titles: Online - full text ed.: (from Institute for Scientific Information).
Indexed: Abstr.Hyg., Curr.Cont., Dairy Sci.Abstr., Ind.Med. (2000-), Ind.Vet., Inpharma, Int.Nurs.Ind., NRN, Pharm.&Out.News, Protozool.Abstr., Reac., Rev.Appl.Entomol., Trop.Dis.Bull.
—BLDSC (4996.870050), CISTI, EMDOCS, GNLM, IDS, ingenta, KNAW. **CCC.**
Published by: International Centre for Diarrhoeal Disease Research Bangladesh, GPO Box 128, Dhaka 1000, Bangladesh. TEL 880-2-8811751, FAX 880-2-8823116, 880-2-8826050, TELEX 675612 ICDD BJ, jhph@icddrb.org, http://www.icddrb.org/jhpn. Ed. David A Sack. R&P M S I Khan TEL 880-2-8822467. Adv. contact M.S.I. Khan. Circ: 750.

610 USA ISSN 0896-7210
JOURNAL WATCH. Text in English. 1987. s-m. USD 98 domestic to individuals; USD 181.90 in Canada to individuals; USD 119 elsewhere to individuals; USD 139 domestic to institutions; USD 258.94 in Canada to institutions; USD 169 elsewhere to institutions (effective 2000). Index. 8 p./no. back issues avail. **Document type:** *Newsletter.* **Description:** Each month brings about 30 concise summaries from over 50 infectious disease, general medicine and other specialty journals.
Related titles: Audio cassette/tape ed.: Journal Watch Audio. ISSN 1063-1887. 1992; Online - full text ed.: Journal Watch Online (from HighWire Pr., EBSCO Publishing); Supplement: Journal Watch Direct. USD 69.
Published by: Massachusetts Medical Society, 1440 Main St, Waltham, MA 02254. TEL 781-893-3800, http://www.jwatch.org/gm/current.shtml, http://mms.org. Ed. Alan Brett.

016.61612 USA ISSN 1521-5822
JOURNAL WATCH CARDIOLOGY. Key Title: Journal Watch for Cardiology. Text in English. 1995. m. USD 89. 8 p./no. **Document type:** *Newsletter, Academic/Scholarly.* **Description:** Presents concise summaries of important research appearing in the cardiology literature.
Related titles: Online - full text ed.: (from HighWire Pr.).
Published by: Massachusetts Medical Society, P O Box 9085, Waltham, MA 02254-9085. TEL 617-734-9800, FAX 617-893-8103.

016.6163 USA
▼ **JOURNAL WATCH GASTROENTEROLOGY.** Text in English. 2000 (Feb.). m. USD 98. 8 p./no. **Document type:** *Newsletter.* **Description:** Presents concise summaries of important research appearing in the gastroenterology literature.
Published by: Massachusetts Medical Society, P O Box 9085, Waltham, MA 02254-9085.

016.6169 USA ISSN 1521-3609
JOURNAL WATCH INFECTIOUS DISEASES. Key Title: Journal Watch for Infectious Diseases. Text in English. 1998 (Feb.). m. USD 98. 8 p./no. **Document type:** *Newsletter.* **Description:** Presents concisse summaries of important research appearing in the infectious disease literature.
Published by: Massachusetts Medical Society, P O Box 9085, Waltham, MA 02254-9085.

016.6168 USA
▼ **JOURNAL WATCH NEUROLOGY.** Text in English. 1999 (May). m. USD 98. 8 p./no. **Document type:** *Newsletter.* **Description:** Presents concise summaries of important research appearing in the neurology literature.
Published by: Massachusetts Medical Society, P O Box 9085, Waltham, MA 02254-9085.

106.61689 USA ISSN 1521-3617
JOURNAL WATCH PSYCHIATRY. Key Title: Journal Watch for Psychiatry. Text in English. 1995. m. 8 p./no. **Document type:** *Newsletter.* **Description:** Presents concise summaries of important research appearing in the psychiatry literature.
Published by: Massachusetts Medical Society, P O Box 9085, Waltham, MA 02254-9085. TEL 617-734-9800, FAX 617-893-8103.

610 016 DEU ISSN 0022-9113
KARTEI DER PRAKTISCHEN MEDIZIN✱ ; unabhaengige Referatenzeitschrift des in- und auslaendischen Fachschrifttums. Text in German. 1927. s-m. DEM 58. bk.rev. abstr, illus. index. **Document type:** *Abstract/Index.*
Media: Cards.
Published by: Hippokrates Verlag GmbH, Postfach 300504, Stuttgart 70445, Germany. TEL 0711-8931-0, FAX 0711-8931453.

616.6 USA ISSN 0940-7936
CODEN: KIDEET
KIDNEY (NEW YORK, 1992); a current survey of world literature. Text in English. 1992. bi-m. (in 1 vol., 6 nos./vol.). USD 267.90 domestic for Print & Online Eds.; USD 261.60 in Germany for Print & Online Eds; USD 46.90 newsstand/cover foreign (effective 2002). adv. reprints avail. *Refereed.* **Document type:** *Abstract/Index.* **Description:** Covers over 140 journals. Provides summaries in diagnosis, pathology and pathophysiology, renal disease and failure, hypertension and systemic disease, dialysis, transplantation, clinical renal pharmacology and therapeutics.
Related titles: Online - full content ed.; Online - full text ed.: (from Springer LINK).
—**CCC.**
Published by: Springer-Verlag, Journals (Subsidiary of: BertelsmannSpringer), 175 Fifth Ave, New York, NY 10010. TEL 212-460-1500, FAX 212-473-6272, orders@springer-ny.com, http://www.springer-ny.com. Eds. George Dunea, J A L Arruda. R&P Ian Gross. Adv. contact Jay Feinman. **N. American subscr. to:** Journal Fulfillment Services, PO Box 2485, Secaucus, NJ 07096-2485. TEL 800-777-4643, FAX 201-348-4505.

618.92 016 DEU
KINDER- UND JUGENDARZT. Text in German. 1953. m. DEM 200; DEM 195 foreign (effective 2000). **Document type:** *Journal, Academic/Scholarly.*
Former titles: Kinderarzt (0340-5877); (until 1970): Mitteilungen fuer Kinderaerzte (0462-9345)
Indexed: Dok.Arbeitsmed., INIS Atomind.
—BLDSC (5095.560000), GNLM.
Published by: (Berufsverband der Kinderaerzte Deutschlands e.V.), Hansisches Verlagskontor, Mengstr 16, Luebeck 23552, Germany. TEL 49-451-7031-01, FAX 49-451-7031281. Eds. Dr. H Olbing, Dr. K Gritz.

618.92 JPN
KITA NIHON SHONIKA GAKKAI SHOROKUSHU/ PEDIATRICS SOCIETY OF NORTH JAPAN. ABSTRACTS. Text in Japanese. a.
Published by: Kita Nihon Shonika Gakkai, Asahikawa Ika Daigaku Shonikagaku Kyoshitsu, 3-11, 5 Go, Nihikagura 4 Sen, Asahikawa-shi, Hokkaido 078, Japan.

610 016 KOR ISSN 0047-360X
KOREAN MEDICAL ABSTRACTS. Text in English. 1971. q. USD 25. abstr. index. reprint service avail. from PQC.
Related titles: Microfilm ed.
Published by: Korea Institute for Economics and Technology, 206-9 Cheongryangri-Dong, Dongdaimun-Ku, P.O. Box 205, Seoul, Korea, S.. Circ: 400.

016.61 BRA
Z6661.L29
L I L A C S - CD-ROM. (Literatura Latinoamericana y del Caribe en Ciencias de la Salud) Text in English, Portuguese, Spanish. 1982. 3/yr. USD 180 domestic; USD 500 in Latin America. abstr, bibl. back issues avail. **Document type:** *Bibliography.* **Description:** Contains bibliographic citations and abstracts of articles from 650 Latin American and Caribbean journal titles.
Formerly (until 1992): Index Medicus Latinoamericano (0100-4743)
Media: CD-ROM.
Published by: (Panamerican Health Organization), Latin American and Caribbean Center on Health Sciences Information (BIREME), Rua Botucatu, 862, Vila Clementino, Sao Paulo, SP 04023-901, Brazil. TEL 55-11-5769800, FAX 55-11-5711919, peml@brm.bireme.br. Circ: 500. **Affiliate:** World Health Organization.

616.616135 NZL ISSN 1172-2126
L M S ALERT. ANTITHROMBOTICS. (Literature Monitoring and Evaluation Service) Text in English. 1993. m. charts. *Refereed.* **Document type:** *Abstract/Index.*
Incorporates: L M S Executive Review. Antithrombotics (1172-4250)
Related titles: CD-ROM ed.; Online - full text ed.
Published by: Adis International Limited, Mairangi Bay, Private Bag 65901, Auckland 1010, New Zealand. TEL 64-9-477-0700, FAX 64-9-477-0784, ruth.williams@adis.com, http://www.adis.com. Ed. Christopher J Mellor.

016.6169 NZL ISSN 1170-8182
L M S ALERT. ANTIVIRALS. (Literature Monitoring and Evaluation Service) Text in English. 1989. m. illus. *Refereed.* **Document type:** *Abstract/Index.*
Incorporates (1991-1993): L M S Executive Review. Antivirals (1170-8174); Which was formerly: L M S Antivirals. Executive Review (0114-4650); L M S Antivirals. Monthly Alert (0114-2674)
Related titles: CD-ROM ed.; Online - full text ed.
Published by: Adis International Limited, Mairangi Bay, Private Bag 65901, Auckland 1010, New Zealand. TEL 64-9-477-0700, FAX 64-9-477-0784, rayl.hill@adis.com, http://www.adis.com. Ed. Ray Hill. Pub. Christopher J Mellor.

016.616128 NZL ISSN 1170-8247
L M S ALERT. ARRHYTHMIAS. (Literature Monitoring and Evaluation Service) Text in English. 1983. m. *Refereed.* **Document type:** *Abstract/Index.*
Incorporates (1991-1993): L M S Executive Review. Arrhythmias (1170-8239); Which was formerly: L M S Arrhythmias. Executive Review (0113-8871); L M S Arrhythmias. Monthly Alert (0113-5236); (1983-1987): ADIS Literature Monitoring and Evaluation Service. Antiarrhythmic Drugs in Arrhythmias. Montlhy Alert (0113-5228)
Related titles: CD-ROM ed.; Online - full text ed.
Published by: Adis International Limited, Mairangi Bay, Private Bag 65901, Auckland 1010, New Zealand. TEL 64-9-477-0700, FAX 64-9-477-0784, susan.beasley@adis.com, http://www.adis.com. Ed. Susan Beasley. Pub. Christopher J Mellor.

016.61558 NZL ISSN 1170-8085
L M S ALERT. CANCER CHEMOTHERAPY. (Literature Monitoring and Evaluation Service) Text in English. 1988. m. charts. *Refereed.* **Document type:** *Abstract/Index.*
Incorporates (1991-1993): L M S Executive Review. Cancer Chemotherapy (1170-8077); Which was formerly: L M S Cancer Chemotherapy. Executive Review (0113-888X); L M S Cancer Chemotherapy. Monthly Alert (0113-9274)
Related titles: CD-ROM ed.; Online - full text ed.
Published by: Adis International Limited, Mairangi Bay, Private Bag 65901, Auckland 1010, New Zealand. TEL 64-9-477-0700, FAX 64-9-477-0700, kelley.robinson@adis.com, http://www.adis.com. Ed. Kelley Robinson. Pub. Christopher J Mellor.

016.616462 NZL ISSN 1170-8123
L M S ALERT. DIABETES. (Literature Monitoring and Evaluation Service) Text in English. 1990. m. charts. *Refereed.* **Document type:** *Abstract/Index.*

M

Formerly (until 1991): L M S Diabetes. Monthly Alert (0114-9210)
Related titles: CD-ROM ed.; Online - full text ed.
Published by: Adis International Limited, Mairangi Bay, Private Bag 65901, Auckland 1010, New Zealand. TEL 64-9-477-0700, FAX 64-9-477-0784, monique.curran@adis.com, http://www.adis.com. Ed. Monique Curran. Pub. Christopher J Mellor.

016.61612 NZL ISSN 1170-8298
L M S ALERT. HEART FAILURE. (Literature Monitoring and Evaluation Service) Text in English. 1983. m. charts. *Refereed.* **Document type:** *Abstract/Index.*
Incorporates (in 1987): L M S Heart Failure. Monthly Alert (0113-454X); Which was formerly: L M S Failure. Executive Review (0113-8898); (1983-1987): ADIS Literature Monitoring and Evaluation Service. Heart Failure and Drugs Used in Heart Failure. Monthly Alert (0113-4531)
Related titles: CD-ROM ed.; Online - full text ed.
Published by: Adis International Limited, Mairangi Bay, Private Bag 65901, Auckland 1010, New Zealand. TEL 64-9-477-0700, FAX 64-9-477-0700, susan.beasley@adis.com, http://www.adis.com. Ed. Susan Beasley. Pub. Christopher J Mellor.

016.612397 NZL ISSN 1170-9596
L M S ALERT. HYPERLIPIDAEMIA. (Literature Monitoring and Evaluation Service) Text in English. 1989. m. charts. *Refereed.* **Document type:** *Abstract/Index.*
Formerly (until 1990): L M S Hyperlipidaemia. Bimonthly Alert (0114-2399)
Related titles: CD-ROM ed.; Online - full text ed.
Published by: Adis International Limited, Mairangi Bay, Private Bag 65901, Auckland 1010, New Zealand. TEL 64-9-477-0700, FAX 64-9-477-0784, tracey.earl.@adis.com, http://www.adis.com. Ed. Tracey Earl. Pub. Christopher J Mellor.

016.616132 NZL ISSN 1170-8069
L M S ALERT. HYPERTENSION. (Literature Monitoring and Evaluation Service) Text in English. 1983. m. charts. *Refereed.* **Document type:** *Abstract/Index.*
Incorporates (1991-1993): L M S Executive Review. Hypertension (1170-8050); Which was formerly: L M S Hypertension. Executive Review (0113-6798); L M S Hypertension. Monthly Alert (0113-5198); (1983-1987): ADIS Literature Monitoring and Evaluation Service. Antihypertensive Drugs in Hypertension. Monthly Alert (0113-518X)
Related titles: CD-ROM ed.; Online - full text ed.
Published by: Adis International Limited, Mairangi Bay, Private Bag 65901, Auckland 1010, New Zealand. TEL 64-9-477-0700, FAX 64-9-477-0784, cathy.vanmiert@adis.com, http://www.adis.com. Pub. Christopher J Mellor.

016.617 NZL ISSN 1172-8906
L M S ALERT. IMMUNOTHERAPEUTICS. TRANSPLANT REJECTION. (Literature Monitoring and Evaluation Service) Text in English. 1994. m. charts. *Refereed.* **Document type:** *Abstract/Index.*
Related titles: CD-ROM ed.; Online - full text ed.
Published by: Adis International Limited, Mairangi Bay, Private Bag 65901, Auckland 1010, New Zealand. TEL 64-9-477-0700, FAX 64-9-477-0784, marianne.duston@adis.com, http://www.adis.com. Ed. Marianne Duston. Pub. Christopher J Mellor.

016.616079 NZL ISSN 1172-8914
L M S ALERT. IMMUNOTHERAPEUTICS. VACCINES. (Literature Monitoring and Evaluation Service) Text in English. 1994. m. charts. *Refereed.* **Document type:** *Abstract/Index.*
Related titles: CD-ROM ed.; Online - full text ed.
Published by: Adis International Limited, Mairangi Bay, Private Bag 65901, Auckland 1010, New Zealand. TEL 64-9-477-0700, FAX 64-9-477-0784, ray.hill@adis.com, http://www.adis.com. Ed. Ray Hill. Pub. Christopher J Mellor.

016.61612 NZL ISSN 1170-8220
L M S ALERT. ISCHAEMIC HEART DISORDERS. (Literature Monitoring and Evaluation Service) Text in English. 1983. m. charts. *Refereed.* **Document type:** *Abstract/Index.*
Incorporates (1991-1993): L M S Executive Review. Ischaemic Heart Disease (1170-8212); Which was formerly: L M S Ischaemic Heart Disease. Executive Review (0113-8855); L M S Ichaemic Heart Disease. Monthly Alert (0113-5104); (until 1987): ADIS Literature Monitoring and Evaluation Service. Ischaemic Heart Disease and Drugs Used in Ischaemic Heart Disease. Monthly Alert (0113-5112)
Related titles: CD-ROM ed.; Online - full text ed.
Published by: Adis International Limited, Mairangi Bay, Private Bag 65901, Auckland 1010, New Zealand. TEL 64-9-477-0700, FAX 64-9-477-0784, ruth.williams@adis.com, http://www.adis.com. Pub. Christopher J Mellor.

016.61624 NZL ISSN 1170-8204
L M S ALERT. OBSTRUCTIVE AIRWAYS DISEASE. (Literature Monitoring and Evaluation Service) Text in English. 1987. m. charts. *Refereed.* **Document type:** *Abstract/Index.*
Incorporates (1991-1993): L M S Executive Review. Obstructive Airways Disease (1170-8190); L M S Obstructive Airways Disease. Executive Review (0113-8847); L M S Obstructive Airways Disease. Monthly Alert (0113-5562)
Related titles: CD-ROM ed.; Online - full text ed.
Published by: Adis International Limited, Mairangi Bay, Private Bag 65901, Auckland 1010, New Zealand. TEL 64-9-477-0700, FAX 64-9-477-0748, deborah.cochrane@adis.com, http://www.adis.com. Pub. Christopher J Mellor.

016.616723 NZL ISSN 1173-7123
L M S ALERT. PAIN CONTROL. (Literature Monitoring and Evaluation Service) Text in English. 1996. m. *Refereed.* **Document type:** *Abstract/Index.*
Related titles: CD-ROM ed.; Online - full text ed.
Published by: Adis International Limited, Mairangi Bay, Private Bag 65901, Auckland 1010, New Zealand. TEL 64-9-477-0700, FAX 64-9-477-0784, jenny.thorn@addis.com, http://www.adis.com. Ed. Jenny Thorn. Pub. Christopher J Mellor.

016.616343 NZL ISSN 1170-8263
L M S ALERT. PEPTIC ULCER DISEASE. (Literature Monitoring and Evaluation Service) Text in English. 1987. m. charts. *Refereed.* **Document type:** *Abstract/Index.*
Incorporates (1991-1993): L M S Executive Review. Peptic Ulcer Disease (1170-8255); Which was formerly: L M S Peptic Ulcer Disease. Executive Review (0113-6461); L M S Peptic Ulcer Disease. Monthly Alert (0113-5163); ADIS Literature Monitoring Evaluation Service. Drugs in Peptic Ulcer Disease. Monthly Alert (0113-5171)
Related titles: CD-ROM ed.; Online - full text ed.
Published by: Adis International Limited, Mairangi Bay, Private Bag 65901, Auckland 1010, New Zealand. TEL 64-9-477-0700, FAX 64-9-477-0784, marlene.kendon@adis.com, http://www.adis.com. Ed. Marlene Kendon. Pub. Christopher J Mellon.

016.616723 NZL ISSN 1170-8107
L M S ALERT. RHEUMATIC DISEASE. (Literature Monitoring and Evaluation Service) Text in English. 1982. m. charts. back issues avail. *Refereed.* **Document type:** *Abstract/Index.*
Incorporates (1991-1993): L M S Executive Review. Rheumatic Disease (1170-8093); L M S Rheumatic Disease. Executive Review (0113-8839); L M S Rheumatic Disease. Monthly Alert (0113-5120); (1982-1987): ADIS Literature Monitoring and Evaluation Service. Antirheumatic Drugs in Rheumatic Disease. Monthly Alert (0113-5139)
Related titles: CD-ROM ed.; Online - full text ed.
Published by: Adis International Limited, Mairangi Bay, Private Bag 65901, Auckland 1010, New Zealand. TEL 64-9-477-0700, FAX 64-9-477-0784, matthew.lowe@adis.com, http://www.adis.com. Ed. Matthew Lowe. Pub. Christopher J Mellor.

016.616 016.57116 GBR ISSN 0142-8160
LEUCOCYTES. Text in English. 1976. s-m. GBP 120 for print ed. or e-mail (effective 2001). adv. bk.rev. **Document type:** *Abstract/Index.* **Description:** Current awareness service for researchers. Covers leucocytes: structure, biochemistry, function, granulopoiesis, adherence and migration.
Related titles: E-mail ed.; Online - full text ed.: GBP 108 (effective 2001).
—Infotrieve. **CCC.**
Published by: S U B I S (Subsidiary of: Sheffield Academic Press Ltd), Mansion House, 19 Kingfield Rd, Sheffield, S Yorks S11 9AS, United Kingdom. TEL 44-114-255-4433, FAX 44-114-255-4626, subis@sheffac.demon.co.uk, http://www.shef-ac-press.co.uk/subis. Ed. S Huntridge. Adv. contact C Evans.

610.73 CAN ISSN 0844-0999
LIST OF CANADIAN NURSING-RELATED PERIODICALS. Text in English, French. a. CND 5. **Document type:** *Catalog.* **Description:** Catalog of Canadian periodicals in nursing, listed alphabetically. Information includes titles, the frequency of publication, where the periodicals may be obtained and the approximate cost.
Published by: Canadian Nurses Association/Association des Infirmieres et Infirmiers du Canada, 50 Drway, Ottawa, ON K2P 1E2, Canada. TEL 613-237-2133, FAX 613-237-3520, pubs@cna-nurses.magi.com.

610 USA ISSN 0093-3821
Z6660 CODEN: LJIMDR
LIST OF JOURNALS INDEXED IN INDEX MEDICUS (YEAR). Text in English. 1960. a. USD 23; USD 28.75 foreign (effective 1998). **Document type:** *Bibliography, Government.* **Description:** Lists the 3,000 journals indexed in Index Medicus as of January 1990.
—BLDSC (5233.400000), CASDDS, EMDOCS, KNAW.
Published by: U.S. National Library of Medicine, 8600 Rockville Pike, Bethesda, MD 20894. Circ: 3,500. **Orders to:** U.S. Government Printing Office, Superintendent of Documents. **Dist. in UK by:** Turpin Distribution Services Ltd., Blackhorse Rd, Letchworth, Herts SG6 1HN, United Kingdom. FAX 44-1462-480947.; **Dist. in US by:** Bernan Associates, 4611 F Assembly Dr, Lanham, MD 20706. TEL 301-459-0056, 301-459-7666.

610 AUS
LIST OF MEDICAL SERVICES AND FEES. Text in English. 1973. a. AUD 100 to institutions; AUD 325 to non-members (effective 2000). adv. **Document type:** *Catalog.* **Description:** Used by service providers for billing purposes and by payment centers, such as insurance firms, for processing claims.
Related titles: Diskette ed.
Published by: Australian Medical Association Parkes, PO Box E 115, Kingston, ACT 2604, Australia. TEL 61-2-62705400, FAX 61-2-62705499. Ed., R&P Kirsty Morrison. Adv. contact Bev Porteous.

610 015 USA ISSN 0736-7139
Z6660
LIST OF SERIALS INDEXED FOR ONLINE USERS. Text in English. 1980. a. USD 27.95 in North America; USD 55.90 elsewhere. **Document type:** *Bibliography, Government.* **Description:** Provides complete bibliographic information on serials and congress proceedings. Contains about 8,689 titles listed alphabetically by abbreviated title followed by full title.
Formerly: List of Serials and Monographs Indexed for Online Users (0196-755X)
Related titles: Online - full text ed.: (from National Library of Medicine).
Published by: U.S. National Library of Medicine, 8600 Rockville Pike, Bethesda, MD 20894. TEL 301-496-6308, FAX 301-496-4450. **Orders to:** National Technical Information Service, Government Research Center. FAX 703-321-8547. **Dist. in UK by:** Turpin Distribution Services Ltd., Blackhorse Rd, Letchworth, Herts SG6 1HN, United Kingdom. FAX 44-1462-480947.; **Dist. in US by:** Bernan Associates, 4611 F Assembly Dr, Lanham, MD 20706. TEL 301-459-0056, 301-459-7666.

016.61692 NZL ISSN 1170-8166
LITERATURE MONITORING AND EVALUATION SERVICE ALERT. ANTIBACTERIAL. Key Title: L M S Alert. Antibacterials. Text in English. 1985. m. charts. *Refereed.* **Document type:** *Abstract/Index.*
Former titles: L M S Antibacterial. Monthly Alert (0114-345X); (until 1989): L M S Bacterial Infections. Monthly Alert (0113-5147); (until 1987): ADIS Literature Evaluation and Monitoring Service. Antibacterial Drugs. Monthly Alert (0113-5155)
Related titles: CD-ROM ed.; Online - full text ed.
Published by: Adis International Limited, Mairangi Bay, Private Bag 65901, Auckland 1010, New Zealand. TEL 64-9-477-0700, FAX 64-9-477-0784, marlene.kendon@adis.com, http://www.adis.com. Ed. Marlene Kendon. Pub. Christopher J Mellor.

610 011 AUS ISSN 1035-5693
M I M S DISEASE INDEX. Text in English. biennial, latest 1996, 2nd Ed. AUD 24.75 in New Zealand; AUD 29.75 in PNG, Asia & Pacific Region; AUD 34.75 in US & Middle East; AUD 38.50 elsewhere (effective 2000). adv. **Description:** Presents expert discussion on the diagnosis, management and drug treatment of common diseases, written by Australian consultants for Australian medical practitioners.
Related titles: ♦ CD-ROM ed.: M I M S CD.
Published by: M I M S Australia (Subsidiary of: Medimedia Australia), PO Box 3000, St Leonards, NSW 2065, Australia. Ed., R&P Amanda Caswell. Pub. Chris Wills. Adv. contact Sue McElroy.

016.61 ZAF ISSN 0580-6755
M I M S MEDICAL SPECIALITIES. (Monthly Index of Medical Specialties) Key Title: Mims (Pretoria). Text in English. 1960. m. ZAR 463 domestic; ZAR 1,081 in United States; ZAR 969 in Europe; ZAR 1,188 in Australia & New Zealand (effective 2000). adv. index, cum.index. **Description:** An index containing medicines available in South Africa in pharmacological order, alphabetically.
Formerly: M I M S (0027-0431)
Indexed: Curr.Adv.Ecol.Sci.
—CISTI.
Published by: M I M S, Division of Times Media Limited, PO Box 2059, Pretoria 0001, South Africa. TEL 27-12-3485010, FAX 27-12-3617716. Ed. J R Snyman. R&P Kathy Webb. Adv. contact Peter McGonigle. Circ: 5,603 (paid).

016.61697 016.5716 GBR ISSN 0142-8195
MACROPHAGES. Text in English. 1976. s-m. GBP 120 for print ed. or e-mail (effective 2001). adv. bk.rev. **Document type:** *Abstract/Index.* **Description:** Current awareness service for researchers in clinical and life sciences. Covers the biochemistry, structure and function of monocytopoiesis, macrophages, and monocytes.
Related titles: E-mail ed.; Online - full text ed.: GBP 108 (effective 2001).
—CCC.
Published by: S U B I S (Subsidiary of: Sheffield Academic Press Ltd), Mansion House, 19 Kingfield Rd, Sheffield, S Yorks S11 9AS, United Kingdom. TEL 44-114-255-4433, FAX 44-114-255-4626, subis@sheffac.demon.co.uk, http://www.shef-ac-press.co.uk/subis. Ed. S Huntridge. Adv. contact C Evans.

610 016 HUN ISSN 0025-0252
MAGYAR ORVOSI BIBLIOGRAFIA; bibliographia medica hungarica. Text in Hungarian. 1957. bi-m. HUF 2,450; USD 60 foreign. adv. bibl. index. **Document type:** *Bibliography.* **Description:** Provides data on Hungarian medical publications and those of allied fields.
Published by: Orszagos Orvostudomanyi Informacios Intezet es Konyvtar/National Institute for Medical Information and Library of Medicine, Szentkiralyi utca 21, PO Box 278, Budapest 1444, Hungary. TEL 36-1-117-6352, FAX 36-1-266-9710, konyvtar@nt-ph.medinfo.hu. Ed. Dr. Tivadar Jakab. Pub., R&P Dr. Alexander Fedinecz. Adv. contact Ilona Borbas. B&W page HUF 24,000, color page HUF 36,000. Circ: 350.

MAKERERE UNIVERSITY. ALBERT COOK LIBRARY. LIBRARY BULLETIN AND ACCESSION LIST. see *LIBRARY AND INFORMATION SCIENCES—Abstracting, Bibliographies, Statistics*

MAMMARY GLAND. see *BIOLOGY—Abstracting, Bibliographies, Statistics*

MANAGED HEALTH CARE OVERVIEW. see *INSURANCE—Abstracting, Bibliographies, Statistics*

613.7 614.8 USA ISSN 0730-7810
MEDICAL ABSTRACTS NEWSLETTER; your direct pipeline to the latest breakthroughs in health care. Text in English. 1981. m. USD 24.95. **Document type:** *Newsletter, Consumer.*
Indexed: CHNI.
Published by: Communi-T Publications, 1101 30th St, N W, Ste 130, PO Box 25498, Washington, DC 20007-8498. TEL 201-836-5030, 800-368-0115, FAX 201-836-5030. Ed. Toni L Goldfarb. Pub. Daniel Levinas. Circ: 6,000.

610 016 USA ISSN 0000-085X
Z6658
MEDICAL AND HEALTH CARE BOOKS AND SERIALS IN PRINT; an index to literature in health sciences. Text in English. 1972. a. (in 2 vols.). USD 299 (effective Mar. 2001). **Document type:** *Directory, Bibliography.* **Description:** Provides a comprehensive reference to currently published books and international serials in the biomedical and specialized health sciences, for professionals, students, librarians and others in the health sciences community. Provides bibliographic and ordering information, book classifications by subject, author and title, with an index to publishers and distributors; serial publications are classified by subject and title.
Former titles (until 1985): Medical Books and Serials in Print (0000-0574); (until 1978): Medical Books in Print (0076-5929)
Related titles: CD-ROM ed.; Magnetic Tape ed.; Online - full text ed.: (from The Dialog Corporation).
—BLDSC (5525.955000), CISTI, Infotrieve. **CCC.**
Published by: R.R. Bowker, 630 Central Ave., New Providence, NJ 07974. TEL 908-464-6800, FAX 908-665-3502, info@bowker.com, http://www.bowker.com. **Subscr. to:** Order Dept., PO Box 31, New Providence, NJ 07974-9903. TEL 800-521-8110.

610.285 USA ISSN 1063-1178
MEDICAL & PHARMACEUTICAL BIOTECHNOLOGY ABSTRACTS. Text in English. 1984. q. USD 495 for print & online combined (effective 2002); USD 365 foreign. **Document type:** *Abstract/Index.*
Supersedes in part (in 1993): Biotechnology Research Abstracts (0733-5709)
Related titles: Online - full text ed.: USD 370 (effective 2002) (from The Dialog Corporation, S T N International).
—BLDSC (5525.989000).
Published by: Cambridge Scientific Abstracts, 7200 Wisconsin Ave., Suite 601, Bethesda, MD 20814. TEL 301-961-6798, FAX 301-961-6799, journals@csa.com, http://www.csa.com/journals. Ed. D Whitman. Pub. Ted Caris.

016.61 IND ISSN 0025-7060
MEDICAL BOOK NEWS; a guide to new books. Text in English. 1967. bi-m. INR 200, USD 50. adv. bk.rev. **Description:** To be used by institutions as a basis for selection of books to be purchased.
Published by: Medical Publications, No.6 Owners Court, Near Strand Cinema, Colaba, Mumbai, Maharashtra 400 005, India. TEL 022-233962, FAX 022-202-2267, TELEX 11-2466-5863-KTKIN. Ed. Dr. Champaklal K Parikh. Circ: 3,000.

MEDICAL CARE RESEARCH AND REVIEW. see *PUBLIC HEALTH AND SAFETY—Abstracting, Bibliographies, Statistics*

610 016 IND ISSN 0025-7109
MEDICAL CHECKLIST. Text in English. 1966. bi-m. INR 150, USD 30 (effective 2000). adv. bk.rev. bibl. index.
Published by: K.K. Roy (Private) Ltd., 55 Gariahat Rd., P O Box 10210, Kolkata, West Bengal 700 019, India. Ed. K K Roy. R&P M Misra TEL 91-33-475-4872. Circ: 1,750.

MEDICAL COMPANIES GUIDE TO JAPAN. see *PHARMACY AND PHARMACOLOGY—Abstracting, Bibliographies, Statistics*

016.610 PAK
MEDICAL LITERATURE INDEXING SERVICES IN PAKISTAN. Short title: M E D L I P. Text in English. 1991. a. PKR 300, USD 20 (effective 2001). bibl. bibl 216 cum.index: 1991-1999. reprints avail. **Document type:** *Directory, Abstract/Index, Bibliography.* **Description:** Indexes articles of the major Pakistani medical journals approved by the Medical and Dental council of Pakistan.(PMDC).
Published by: College of Physicians & Surgeons Pakistan, Defence Housing Authority, 7th Central St., Karachi 75500, Pakistan. TEL 92-21-5892801, FAX 92-21-5887513, jcpsp-pub@usa.net. Eds. M. Sultan Farooqui, Masood Hameed Khan. Pub. Saghir Ahmed. R&P M Sultan Farooqui. Circ: 5,000 (controlled).

610 USA ISSN 0147-5711
Z695.1.M48
MEDICAL SUBJECT HEADINGS - ANNOTATED ALPHABETIC LIST. Text in English. a. USD 49.95; USD 99.50 foreign. **Document type:** *Government.*
Related titles: Online - full text ed.
—CISTI.
Published by: U.S. National Library of Medicine, 8600 Rockville Pike, Bethesda, MD 20894. http://www.nlm.nih.gov/mesh/. **Orders to:** National Technical Information Service, Government Research Center. FAX 703-321-8547. **Dist. in UK by:** Turpin Distribution Services Ltd., Blackhorse Rd, Letchworth, Herts SG6 1HN, United Kingdom. FAX 44-1462-480947.; **Dist. in US by:** Bernan Associates, 4611 F Assembly Dr, Lanham, MD 20706. TEL 301-459-0056, 301-459-7666.

610 USA ISSN 0147-099X
Z695.1.M48
MEDICAL SUBJECT HEADINGS - TREE STRUCTURE (YEAR). Text in English. a. USD 44.95; USD 89.90 foreign. **Document type:** *Government.* **Description:** Contains all the Medical Subject Headings currently in use among the National Library of Medicine indexers, catalogers, and searchers.
Related titles: Online - full text ed.
—CISTI.
Published by: U.S. National Library of Medicine, 8600 Rockville Pike, Bethesda, MD 20894. http://www.nlm.nih.gov/mesh/. **Orders to:** National Technical Information Service, Government Research Center. FAX 703-321-8547. **Dist. in UK by:** Turpin Distribution Services Ltd., Blackhorse Rd, Letchworth, Herts SG6 1HN, United Kingdom. TEL 44-1462-893694.; **Dist. in US by:** Bernan Associates, 4611 F Assembly Dr, Lanham, MD 20706. TEL 301-459-0056, 301-459-7666.

016.61 IND ISSN 0250-4367
MEDICINAL AND AROMATIC PLANTS ABSTRACTS. Text in English. 1979. bi-m. INR 500, USD 250 (effective 2001). adv. bk.rev. **Document type:** *Abstract/Index.* **Description:** Reports current world literature on medicinal and aromatic plants. Covers about 600 journals published in 22 languages from 55 countries of the world.
Related titles: CD-ROM ed.; Online - full text ed.
Indexed: Hort.Abstr.
—GNLM.
Published by: (National Institute of Science Communication, Council of Scientific and Industrial Research), Scientific Publishers, 5-A New Pali Rd., P O Box 91, Jodhpur, Rajasthan 342 001, India. TEL 91-291-433323, FAX 91-291-512580, scienti@sancharnet.in, http://www.scientificpub.com. Ed. G.P. Phondke. R&P G P Phondke. **Dist. by:** H P C Publishers Distributors Pvt. Ltd., 1st Fl., Flats 1 & 2, Darya Ganj, 4805-24 Bharat Ram Rd., New Delhi 110 002, India. TEL 91-11-3254401, FAX 91-11-619-3511.

618 DNK ISSN 0904-1966
RG503.2.D4
MEDICINSK FOEDSELSSTATISTIK OG MISDANNELSESSTATISTIK. Text in Danish. 1973. biennial. DKK 60.
Formerly: Medicinsk Foedselsstatistik (0107-7597)
Published by: Sundhedsstyrelsen, Amaliegade 13, PO Box 2020, Copenhagen K 1012, Denmark. **Subscr. to:** Statens Informationstjeneste, PO Box 1103, Copenhagen K 1009, Denmark.

610 JPN
MEDIFAX INDEX. Text in Japanese. 1986. m. membership.
Published by: Yakugyo Jiho Co. Ltd., 2-36 Kanda-Jinbo-cho, Chiyoda-ku, Tokyo 101-0051, Japan.

016.61 BGR ISSN 1311-509X
MEDITSINSKI PREGLED. KLINIKA I PREDKLINIKA. Text in Bulgarian. 1966. bi-m., latest vol.37, 2001. BGL 21 domestic; USD 65 foreign (effective 2001 - 2002). adv. bk.rev. abstr, bibl, illus. index. 48 p./no. back issues avail. *Refereed.* **Document type:** *Journal, Academic/Scholarly, Abstract/Index, Bibliography.* **Description:** Abstracts foreign publications on medical sciences and pharmacology.
Former titles: Biomeditsina; Meditsinski Pregled (0204-7241)
Published by: Meditsinski Universitet - Sofia, Tsentur za Informatsiia po Meditsina/Medical University - Sofia, Medical Information Center, 1 Sv Georgi Sofiiski ul, Sofia 1431, Bulgaria. TEL 359-2-5222342, FAX 359-2-9522393, mutafov@medun.acad.bg, http://www.medun.acad.bg. Ed. V I Ovcharov. R&P, Adv. contact Dr. Christo Mutafov. B&W page USD 70, color page USD 150; trim 220 x 170. Circ: 600. **Dist. by:** Sofia Books, Ul Silivria 16, Sofia 1404, Bulgaria. TEL 359-2-9586257, sofiabooks@hotmail.com, http://www.sofiabooks.hit.bg.

610 011 DEU
MEDIZINISCHER LITERATUR ANZEIGER; bibliographische Zeitschrift fuer medizinische Neuerscheinungen. Text in German. 1950. m. DEM 22.80. adv. **Document type:** *Bibliography.* **Description:** Bibliography of new medical books.
Published by: Dustri-Verlag Dr. Karl Feistle, Bajuwarenring 4, Oberhaching 82041, Germany. TEL 49-89-613861-0, FAX 49-89-613-5412, info@dustri.de, http://www.dustri.de. Ed., Adv. contact Joerg Feistle. Circ: 6,000.

MENTAL HEALTH STATISTICAL NOTES. see *SOCIAL SERVICES AND WELFARE—Abstracting, Bibliographies, Statistics*

M

610.28 016 USA
N T I S ALERTS: BIOMEDICAL TECHNOLOGY & HUMAN FACTORS ENGINEERING. Text in English. s-m. USD 210 in North America; USD 275 elsewhere (effective 1999). abstr. index, cum.index. back issues avail. **Document type:** *Newsletter, Bibliography, Government.* **Description:** Reports on biomedical facilities, instumentation and supplies. Human factors engineering and man-machine relations, bionics and artifical intelligence preservation and storage.
Former titles: Abstract Newsletter: Biomedical Technology and Human Factors Engineering (0163-1497); Weekly Abstract Newsletter: Biomedical Technology and Human Factors Engineering; Weekly Government Abstracts. Biomedical Technology and Human Factors Engineering; Weekly Government Abstracts. Biomedical Technology and Engineering (0364-4952)
Related titles: Microform ed.: (from NTI).
Published by: U.S. National Technical Information Service, 5285 Port Royal Rd, Springfield, VA 22161. TEL 703-605-6060, 800-363-2068, FAX 703-605-6880, subscriptions@aints.fedworld.gov, http://www.ntis.gov/alerts.htm.

016 610 USA ISSN 1052-9063
Z6660
NATIONAL LIBRARY OF MEDICINE. CURRENT BIBLIOGRAPHIES IN MEDICINE. Text in English. 1966. irreg. (approx. 10/yr.). USD 47; USD 58.75 foreign. **Document type:** *Bibliography, Government.* **Description:** Documents approximately 7 bibliographies per year on a variety of biomedical topics, excluding AIDS (see AIDS Bibliography) similar to those found in the N.L.M. Literature Search Series.
Formerly: National Library of Medicine. Literature Search Series (0083-2251)
—CISTI, GNLM.
Published by: U.S. National Library of Medicine, Reference Section, 8600 Rockville Pike, Bethesda, MD 20894. Circ: 1,000. **Orders to:** U.S. Government Printing Office, Superintendent of Documents.

NERVE CELL BIOLOGY. see *BIOLOGY—Abstracting, Bibliographies, Statistics*

NEUROPEPTIDES (SHEFFIELD). see *BIOLOGY—Abstracting, Bibliographies, Statistics*

NEUROPHYSIOLOGY. see *BIOLOGY—Abstracting, Bibliographies, Statistics*

610 USA ISSN 1083-4915
NEUROPSYCHOLOGY ABSTRACTS. Text in English. q. USD 69 domestic to non-members; USD 84 foreign to non-members; USD 39 domestic to members; USD 49 foreign to members; USD 125 domestic to institutions; USD 157 foreign to institutions (effective 2001). adv. **Document type:** *Abstract/Index.* **Description:** Pulls approximately 2,500 news items of information from scholarly books and journals that are reviewed and included in the database.
Formerly: PsychSCAN: Neuropsychology (1058-6660)
Indexed: e-psyche.
Published by: American Psychological Association, 750 First St., N.E., Washington, DC 20002-4242. TEL 202-336-5600, 800-374-2721, FAX 202-336-5568, subscriptions@apa.org, http://www.apa.org/psycinfo/products/scan-neuro.html, http://www.apa.org/journals/psn.html. Circ: 3,000.

616.8 USA ISSN 1057-6096
NEUROSCIENCE CITATION INDEX. Text in English. bi-m. USD 1,725 for CD-ROM. **Document type:** *Academic/Scholarly, Bibliography.* **Description:** Provides bibliographic data, cited references, related records and English-language author abstracts for international scholarly research journals and conference proceedings.
Related titles: CD-ROM ed.: (from Institute for Scientific Information); Magnetic Tape ed.
Published by: Institute for Scientific Information, 3501 Market St., Philadelphia, PA 19104. TEL 215-386-0100, FAX 215-386-2911.

616.8 CHE ISSN 1025-9279
NEUROSCIENCE COMMUNICATIONS. Text in English. bi-m. USD 87 to institutions; USD 135 to corporations. **Document type:** *Abstract/Index.* **Description:** Provides abstracts of the latest submissions to the journal Neuroscience.
Related titles: Online - full text ed.
Indexed: e-psyche.
Published by: Gordon and Breach - Harwood Academic (Subsidiary of: Taylor & Francis Group), PO Box 531, Lausanne 1000, Switzerland. http://www.gbhap.com/Neuroscience_Communications/. Ed. Dr. Sidney Weinstein. **Subscr. addr. in US:** International Publishers Direct, PO Box 32160, Newark, NJ 07102. FAX 215-750-6343.

610 020 USA
NEW ENGLAND SOUNDING LINE. Text in English. 1991. bi-m. free per issue. **Document type:** *Newsletter.* **Description:** Covers activities of the National Network of Libraries of Medicine, New England Region.
Published by: National Network of Libraries of Medicine, New England Region, Univ of Connecticut Health Center, 263 Farmington Ave, Farmington, CT 06030-5370. TEL 860-679-4500, FAX 860-679-1305, http://www.nnlm.nlm.nih.gov/ner/nehsl. Ed. Edward Donnald.

NEW LITERATURE ON VISUAL IMPAIRMENT. see *HANDICAPPED—Abstracting, Bibliographies, Statistics*

610 174 USA ISSN 0361-6347
Z6675.E8
NEW TITLES IN BIOETHICS. Text in English. 1975. q. USD 20 domestic; USD 30 foreign (effective 2001). **Document type:** *Bibliography.* **Description:** Includes the Kampelman Collection of Jewish Ethics, the Shriver Collection of Christian Ethics and updates to the Syllabus Exchange catalog.
Published by: Kennedy Institute of Ethics, National Reference Center for Bioethics Literature, Georgetown University, Box 571212, Washington, DC 20057-1212. TEL 202-687-6689, FAX 202-687-6770, medethx@georgetown.edu, http://bioethics.georgetown.edu. Ed. Lucinda Fitch Huttlinger. Circ: 2,000.

616.021 NZL
NEW ZEALAND HEALTH INFORMATION SERVICE. CANCER: NEW REGISTRATIONS AND DEATHS. Text in English. a., latest 1999, for the year 1995. NZD 30 (effective 2001). stat. **Document type:** *Government.*
Former titles: New Zealand. Health Statistical Services. Cancer Data: New Registrations and Deaths (1171-6509); Cancer Data: Deaths and Cases Reported (0548-9415)
Published by: New Zealand Health Information Service, Ministry of Health, Level 11, Ballantrae House, 192-194 Willis St, P.O. Box 5013, Wellington, New Zealand. TEL 64-4-8012700, FAX 64-4-8012769, nzhis-pubs@web1.halth.govt.nz, http://www.health.govt.nz/NZHIS/home.html. Circ: (controlled).

616.8 NZL ISSN 0548-992X
RC451.N4
NEW ZEALAND HEALTH INFORMATION SERVICE. MENTAL HEALTH DATA. Key Title: Mental Health Data. Text in English. a., latest 1994. NZD 30 (effective 2001). back issues avail. **Document type:** *Government.*
Formerly: New Zealand. Health Statistical Services. Mental Health Data
Published by: New Zealand Health Information Service, Ministry of Health, Level 11, Ballantrae House, 192-194 Willis St, P.O. Box 5013, Wellington, New Zealand. TEL 64-4-8012700, FAX 64-4-8012769, nzhis-pubs@web1.health.govt.nz, http://www.health.govt.nz/NZHIS/home.html. Circ: (controlled).

617 JPN
NIHON GEKAKEI RENGO GAKKAI GAKUJUTSU SHUKAI SHOROKUGO/JAPANESE COLLEGE OF SURGEONS. ABSTRACTS OF MEETING. Text in English, Japanese. 1975. a. membership. **Document type:** *Abstract/Index.*
Published by: Nihon Gekakei Rengo Gakkai, 4-3 Iida-Bashi 3-chome, Chiyoda-ku, Tokyo 102-0072, Japan.

617 JPN ISSN 0385-7883
NIHON GEKAKEI RENGO GAKKAISHI/JAPANESE COLLEGE OF SURGEONS. JOURNAL. Text in English, Japanese. 1976. irreg.
Published by: Nihon Gekakei Rengo Gakkai, 4-3 Iida-Bashi 3-chome, Chiyoda-ku, Tokyo 102-0072, Japan.

610 JPN
NIHON KAIBOGAKU BUNKENSHU/ABSTRACTS OF JAPANESE ANATOMY. Text in Japanese. 1936. every 2 yrs. **Document type:** *Abstract/Index.*
Published by: Nihon Kaibo Gakkai/Japanese Association of Anatomists, c/o Nihon Gakkai Jimu Senta, 16-9 Honkomagome 5-chome, Bunkyo-ku, Tokyo 113-0021, Japan.

617.4 616.89 JPN
NIHON NO SHINKEI GEKA GAKKAI SOKAI SHOROKUSHU/JAPAN NEUROSURGICAL SOCIETY. ABSTRACTS OF THE ANNUAL MEETING. Text in English, Japanese. a.
Indexed: e-psyche.
Published by: Nihon No Shinkei Geka Gakkai, c/o Kyoto Daigaku Igakubu No Shinkei Geka, Yosida Konoecho, Sakyo-ku, Kyoto-shi 606-01, Japan.

016.61621 ITA ISSN 1121-4163
NOTIZIARIO BIBLIOGRAFICO DI AUDIOLOGIA O R L E FONIATRIA. Text in Italian. 1967. s-a. free per issue. adv. bk.rev. back issues avail. **Document type:** *Academic/Scholarly, Abstract/Index.*
Formerly: Notiziario Bibliografico di Audiologia (0392-3711)
Published by: Centro Ricerche e Studi Amplifon, Via Giuseppe Ripamonti, 133, Milan, MI 20141, Italy. TEL 02-57472361, FAX 02-57400384, TELEX 02-57400384. Ed. Isabella Costa. Adv. contact A M Holland. Circ: 2,000.

610 016 CZE ISSN 1212-3862
Z6660
NOVINKY LITERATURY. ZDRAVOTNICTVI-PRIRUSTKY FONDU NARODNI LEKARSKE KNIHOVNY. Text in Czech. 1955. 4/yr. CZK 100, USD 4 (effective 2001). **Document type:** *Bibliography.*
Supersedes (in 1996): Novinky Literatury: Zdravotnictvi (0029-5205)
Published by: Narodni Lekarska Knihovna, Sokolska 31, Prague 12132, Czech Republic. TEL 420-2-24266870, FAX 420-2-24266051, nml@nlk.anet.cz nml@nlk.anet.cz, http://www.nlk.anet.cz. Ed. M Hulovcova. Circ: 200.

618 JPN
NYUSEN HINYU KENKYUKAI KOEN YOSHISHU/ SOCIETY FOR MAMMARY GLANDS AND LACTATION RESEARCH. ABSTRACTS OF THE MEETING. Text in Japanese. a. **Document type:** *Abstract/Index.*
Published by: Nyusen Hinyu Kenkyukai, Daigaku Nogakubu Dobutsu Ikusyu Hanshokugakka, 1-1 Yayoi 1-chome, Bunkyo-ku, Tokyo 113-0032, Japan.

OBSTETRIC ANESTHESIA DIGEST. see *MEDICAL SCIENCES—Anaesthesiology*

615.82 GBR ISSN 0950-6675
OCCUPATIONAL THERAPY INDEX. Text in English. m. GBP 71 in Europe; GBP 90 elsewhere (effective 1999). index. **Document type:** *Bulletin, Abstract/Index, Bibliography.* **Description:** Provides a classified list of English language citations from the current literature of occupational therapy (over 1200 per year). Includes a list of research projects collected by the College of Occupational Therapists. Each issue has detailed author and subject indexes.
Related titles: Online - full text ed.
—BLDSC (6231.254500).
Published by: British Library, Health Care Information Service, British Library, Boston Spa, Wetherby, W Yorks LS23 7BQ, United Kingdom. TEL 44-1937-546039, FAX 44-1937-546458, phillipa.seaton@bl.uk. R&P Phillipa Seaton.

016.61699 GBR ISSN 0950-0561
ONCOGENES. Text in English. 1987. s-m. GBP 120 for print ed. or e-mail (effective 2001). adv. **Document type:** *Abstract/Index.* **Description:** Current awareness service for researchers. Covers oncogenes and neoplastic cell transformation.
Related titles: E-mail ed.; Online - full text ed.: GBP 108 (effective 2001).
—Infotrieve. **CCC.**
Published by: S U B I S (Subsidiary of: Sheffield Academic Press Ltd), Mansion House, 19 Kingfield Rd, Sheffield, S Yorks S11 9AS, United Kingdom. TEL 44-114-255-4433, FAX 44-114-255-4626, subis@sheffac.demon.co.uk, http://www.shef-ac-press.co.uk/subis. Ed. S Huntridge. Adv. contact C Evans.

616.4 011 USA ISSN 1043-8963
RC268.42
ONCOGENES AND GROWTH FACTORS ABSTRACTS. Text in English. 1989. m. abstr. index. back issues avail. **Document type:** *Abstract/Index.* **Description:** Covers worldwide research into the molecular basis of malignant transformation.
Media: Online - full text.
Published by: Cambridge Scientific Abstracts, 7200 Wisconsin Ave., Suite 601, Bethesda, MD 20814. TEL 301-961-6798, FAX 301-961-6799, journals@csa.com, http://www.csa.com/journals. Pub. Ted Caris.

M

ONLINE JOURNAL OF CLINICAL INNOVATIONS. see *MEDICAL SCIENCES—Nurses And Nursing*

617.7 016 GBR ISSN 0030-3720
Z6669
OPHTHALMIC LITERATURE. Text in English. 1947. q. NLG 730, USD 419 (effective 1998). adv. bk.rev. index. reprint service avail. from PQC. **Document type:** *Abstract/Index.* **Description:** Abstracts the world literature on all aspects of ophthalmology and optometry.
Related titles: Microform ed.: (from PQC); Online - full text ed.: (from ingenta).
—GNLM, Infotrieve. **CCC.**
Published by: (Institute of Ophthalmology), Elsevier Science, PO Box 800, Kidlington, Oxon OX5 1XD, United Kingdom. TEL 44-1865-843000, FAX 44-1865-843010, TELEX 83111 BHPOXF G, nlinfo-f@elsevier.nl; usinfo-f@elsevier.com; forinfo-kyf04305@niftyserve.or.jp. **Subscr. in Australasia and the Far East to:** Elsevier Science (Singapore) Pte Ltd, No.1 Temasek Ave, 17-01 Millenia Tower, Singapore 039192, Singapore. TEL 65-434-3727, FAX 65-337-2230; **Subscr. in the Americas to:** Elsevier Science, PO Box 945, New York, NY 10159-0945. TEL 212-633-3730, FAX 212-633-3680; **Subscr. to:** Elsevier Science BV, PO Box 211, Amsterdam 1000 AE, Netherlands. TEL 31-20-485-3757, http://www.elsevier.nl.

ORTHOPAEDIE UND RHEUMA. see *MEDICAL SCIENCES—Orthopedics And Traumatology*

610 JPN ISSN 0913-4751
OSAKA UNIVERSITY. RESEARCH INSTITUTE FOR MICROBIAL DISEASES. ANNUAL REPORTS. Text in Japanese. 1986. a. per issue exchange basis. abstr. **Description:** Provides abstracts of papers published in the previous year from various departments of the institute.
Indexed: Ref.Zh.
—BLDSC (1410.645000), CISTI.
Published by: Osaka Daigaku, Biseibutsubyo Kenkyujo/Osaka University, Research Institute for Microbial Diseases, 3-1 Yamada-Oka, Suita-shi, Osaka-ken 5650871, Japan. TEL 06-879-8359, FAX 06-879-8360. Ed. Akira Hakura.

016.61267 GBR ISSN 1365-3326
OSTEOPOROSIS. Text in English. 1996. s-m. GBP 120 for print ed. or e-mail (effective 2001). adv. **Document type:** *Abstract/Index.*
Related titles: E-mail ed.; Online - full text ed.: GBP 108 (effective 2001).
Published by: S U B I S (Subsidiary of: Sheffield Academic Press Ltd), Mansion House, 19 Kingfield Rd, Sheffield, S Yorks S11 9AS, United Kingdom. TEL 44-114-255-4433, FAX 44-114-255-4626, subis@sheffac.demon.co.uk, http://www.shef-ac-press.co.uk/subis. Ed. S Huntridge. Adv. contact C Evans.

610 GBR ISSN 0961-4591
PALLIATIVE CARE INDEX. Text in English. m. GBP 63 in Europe; GBP 81 elsewhere (effective 1999). index. **Document type:** *Bulletin, Abstract/Index, Bibliography.* **Description:** Provides a classified list of English language citations, many with abstracts, from the current literature on palliative and terminal care, hospices, symptom control bereavement. Includes journal articles and new books. Each issue contains detailed author and subject indexes.
Formerly: Terminal Care Index (0953-6779)
—BLDSC (6345.562055), GNLM.
Published by: British Library, Health Care Information Service, British Library, Boston Spa, Wetherby, W Yorks LS23 7BQ, United Kingdom. TEL 44-1937-546039, FAX 44-1937-546458, phillipa.seaton@bl.uk. R&P Phillipa Seaton.

PANCREATIC AND SALIVARY SECRETION. see *BIOLOGY—Abstracting, Bibliographies, Statistics*

PAPILLOMAVIRUS REPORT. see *MEDICAL SCIENCES—Communicable Diseases*

618.92 USA ISSN 1059-0870
PEDIATRIC EMERGENCY & CRITICAL CARE; a clinical update for those who care for infants and children. Text in English. 1988. m. USD 69 to individuals; USD 110 to institutions; USD 47 residents & nurses (effective 2001). *Refereed.* **Document type:** *Newsletter.* **Description:** Clinical update for those who care for acutely ill or injured infants and children. Digest of clinically useful literature and papers; each abstract has an expert's comment focusing on the clinical point.
Formerly (until vol.5, 1992): Pediatric Trauma and Acute Care (0894-1122)
—**CCC.**
Published by: Riverpress, Inc., PO Box 23, Jersey City, NJ 07303-0023. TEL 201-434-5073, FAX 201-434-7230, riverpress.inc@verizon.net, http://www.riverpress-inc.com/. Ed. Douglas W E Wagner. Pub. Douglas W.E. Wagner. Circ: 1,200 (paid and free).

016.61892 USA ISSN 1071-5711
PEDIATRIC PRIMARY CARE; practical pediatrics for the pediatric practitioner. Text in English. 1987. m., latest vol.15, 2001, Dec. USD 59 domestic to individuals; USD 57 in Canada & Mexico to individuals; USD 67 elsewhere to individuals; USD 110 domestic to institutions; USD 100 in Canada & Mexico to institutions; USD 110 elsewhere to institutions; USD 47 domestic to qualified personnel (effective 2001). 4 p./no. 1 cols./p. back issues avail. *Refereed.* **Document type:** *Newsletter.* **Description:** Digest of clinically useful articles; each abstract has an expert's comment focusing on the clinical point.
Formerly (until vol.7, no.8, 1993): Pediatric Therapeutics and Toxicology (0893-6218)
—**CCC.**
Published by: Riverpress, Inc., PO Box 23, Jersey City, NJ 07303-0023. TEL 201-434-5073, FAX 201-434-7230, riverpress.inc@verizon.net, http://www.riverpress-inc.com/. Ed. Douglas W E Wagner. Circ: 1,020 (paid and free).

610 USA ISSN 1045-2338
Z695.1.M48
PERMUTED MEDICAL SUBJECT HEADINGS (YEAR). Text in English. q. USD 40.95 in North America; USD 81.90 elsewhere. **Document type:** *Government.* **Description:** Displays all terms for the National Library of Medicine's Medical Subject Headings for the year.
—KNAW.
Published by: U.S. National Library of Medicine, 8600 Rockville Pike, Bethesda, MD 20894. http://www.nlm.nih.gov/, http://www.nlm.nih.gov. **Orders to:** National Technical Information Service, Government Research Center. FAX 703-321-8547. **Dist. in UK by:** Turpin Distribution Services Ltd., Blackhorse Rd, Letchworth, Herts SG6 1HN, United Kingdom. FAX 44-1462-480947.; **Dist. in US by:** Bernan Associates, 4611 F Assembly Dr, Lanham, MD 20706. TEL 301-459-0056, 301-459-7666.

610 016 PHL ISSN 0116-6506
PHILIPPINE INDEX MEDICUS. Text in English. 1963. irreg. **Document type:** *Abstract/Index.* **Description:** Contains compilation of articles from Philippine medical & health periodicals to provide information to researchers, health professionals, academics, and government officials.
Published by: University of the Philippines, College of Medicine, P.O. Box 593, Manila, Philippines. http://www.upcm.net/.

610 615 HKG ISSN 0218-4206
PHILIPPINES INDEX OF MEDICAL SPECIALITIES. Short title: P I M S. Text in English. 1972. 3/yr. HKD 60, USD 27 (effective 1999). adv. **Document type:** *Directory, Trade.* **Description:** Indexes brief prescribing information on pharmaceutical products available in Philippines for doctors.
Published by: MediMedia Asia (Subsidiary of: MediMedia Pacific Ltd.), 2102 Tung Sun Commercial Centre, 194-200 Lockhart Rd, Wanchai, Hong Kong, Hong Kong. TEL 852-2511-0765, FAX 852-2507-3817, http://www.medimedia.com.hk/. Ed. Patricia T Kin. Adv. contact Annie T Fuentes. color page HKD 5,711. Circ: 22,000.

331.119161069 USA ISSN 0731-0315
RA410.7
PHYSICIAN CHARACTERISTICS & DISTRIBUTION IN THE U S (YEARS). Text in English. 1943. a. USD 99.95 (effective 2000). **Document type:** *Monographic series.*
Former titles: Physician Characteristics and Distribution; Physician Distribution and Medical Licensure in the U S (0364-6610); Distribution of Physicians in the U S (0146-4558); Distribution of Physicians, Hospital, Hospital Beds in the U S (0419-4357)
Indexed: SRI.
Published by: American Medical Association, 515 N State St, P O Box 10946, Chicago, IL 60610-0946. TEL 312-464-5000, 800-262-8335, FAX 312-464-5600. Ed. G A Roback.

610.21 USA ISSN 1064-4563
PHYSICIAN COMPENSATION AND PRODUCTION SURVEY. Text in English. 1980. a. stat. **Document type:** *Bulletin.* **Description:** Covers issues on direct compensation and retirement benefits for over 30,000 physicians and mid-level providers in 102 specialties.
Supersedes in part (in 1992): Cost and Production Survey Report (0741-9287); Which was formed by the merger of (1975-1980): Cost Survey (0196-2434); Production Survey (0196-9439)
Related titles: CD-ROM ed.
Published by: Medical Group Management Association, 104 Inverness Terrace E, Englewood, CO 80112. TEL 303-799-1111, FAX 303-397-1827, survey@mgma.com, http://www.mgma.com. Circ: 10,000 (paid).

615.82 GBR ISSN 0950-6659
PHYSIOTHERAPY INDEX. Text in English. m. GBP 71 in Europe; GBP 90 elsewhere (effective 1999). index. **Document type:** *Abstract/Index.* **Description:** Provides a classified list of English language citations from the current literature of physical therapy (over 2000 per year). Includes a list of research projects collected by the Chartered Society of Physiotherapy. Each issue has detailed author and subject indexes.
Related titles: Online - full text ed.
—BLDSC (6489.107000).
Published by: British Library, Health Care Information Service, British Library, Boston Spa, Wetherby, W Yorks LS23 7BQ, United Kingdom. TEL 44-1937-546039, FAX 44-1937-546458, phillipa.seaton@bl.uk. R&P Phillipa Seaton.

617 USA ISSN 0892-3965
PLASTIC SURGERY OUTLOOK. Text in English. 1987. 10/yr. DEM 30 per issue (effective 2000); free with Perspectives in Plastic Surgery. adv. index. **Document type:** *Newsletter, Abstract/Index.* **Description:** Encapsulates journal articles, reports on special clinical findings, and symposium proceedings dealing with this medical specialty.
Related titles: ♦ Supplement to: Seminars in Plastic Surgery. ISSN 1535-2188.
Published by: Thieme Medical Publishers, 333 Seventh Ave, New York, NY 10001. TEL 212-760-0888, 800-782-3488, FAX 212-947-1112, http://www.thieme.com. Ed. Dr. Saleh M Shenaq. Adv. contact Sally Kahn. Circ: 1,050 (paid). **Orders in Europe to:** Thieme International, Postfach 301120, Stuttgart 70451, Germany. TEL 49-711-8931-0.

016.617585 GBR ISSN 1354-9979
PODIATRY INDEX. Text in English. 1994. q. GBP 57 in Europe; GBP 78 elsewhere. **Document type:** *Bulletin, Abstract/Index, Bibliography.* **Description:** Provides a classified list of citations from the current literature of podiatry including articles on foot diseases and injuries, deformities, surgery and equipment and methods. Each issue has subject and author indexes.
—BLDSC (6541.498050).
Published by: British Library, Health Care Information Service, British Library, Boston Spa, Wetherby, W Yorks LS23 7BQ, United Kingdom. TEL 44-1937-546039, FAX 44-1937-4546458, phillipa.seaton@bl.uk. R&P Phillipa Seaton.

POHYBOVE USTROJI; pokroky ve vyzkumu diagnostice a terapii. see *MEDICAL SCIENCES—Orthopedics And Traumatology*

PROGRESS IN PALLIATIVE CARE. see *MEDICAL SCIENCES—Oncology*

016.6164 GBR ISSN 0142-8276
PROLACTIN. Text in English. 1992. s-m. GBP 96 for print ed. or email (effective 2001). adv. back issues avail. **Document type:** *Abstract/Index.* **Description:** Current awareness service for researchers in clinical and life sciences.
Related titles: E-mail ed.; Online - full text ed.: GBP 108 to individuals (effective 2001).
—**CCC.**
Published by: S U B I S (Subsidiary of: Sheffield Academic Press Ltd), Mansion House, 19 Kingfield Rd, Sheffield, S Yorks S11 9AS, United Kingdom. TEL 44-114-255-4433, FAX 44-114-255-4626, subis@sheffac.demon.co.uk, http://www.shef-ac-press.co.uk/subis. Ed. S Huntridge. Adv. contact C Evans.

016.6164 GBR ISSN 0142-8284
PROSTAGLANDINS - BIOLOGY. Text in English. 1979. s-m. GBP 120 for print ed. or e-mail (effective 2001). adv. **Document type:** *Abstract/Index.* **Description:** Current awareness service for researchers. Covers prostaglandin precursors, production, release, effects, medical uses and metabolism.

Related titles: E-mail ed.; Online - full text ed.: GBP 108 (effective 2001).
—CCC.
Published by: S U B I S (Subsidiary of: Sheffield Academic Press Ltd), Mansion House, 19 Kingfield Rd, Sheffield, S Yorks S11 9AS, United Kingdom. TEL 44-114-255-4433, FAX 44-114-255-4626, subis@sheffac.demon.co.uk, http://www.shef-ac-press.co.uk/subis. Ed. S Huntridge. Adv. contact C Evans.

016.6167 USA
PSYCSCAN: LEARNING DISORDERS AND MENTAL RETARDATION. Text in English. 1982. q. USD 49 domestic to non-members; USD 64 foreign to non-members; USD 29 domestic to members; USD 39 foreign to members; USD 84 domestic to institutions; USD 116 foreign to institutions (effective 2001). adv. **Document type:** *Abstract/Index.* **Description:** Abstracts articles on learning disorders, communication disorders, and mental retardation, drawn from PsycINFO's annual coverage of more than 1,300 journals.
Former titles: PsycSCAN: Learning and Communication Disorders and Mental Retardation; PsycSCAN: Learning Disabilities - Mental Retardation (0730-1928)
Published by: American Psychological Association, 750 First St., N.E., Washington, DC 20002-4242. TEL 202-336-5600, 800-374-2721, FAX 202-336-5568, subscriptions@apa.org, http://www.apa.org/psycinfo/products/scan-ldmr.html, http:/www.apa.org/journals/psl.html. Circ: 1,800.

610 JPN ISSN 0285-4694
PURASUMIN BUNKEN MOKUROKU/BIBLIOGRAPHY OF PLASMIN. Text in English, Japanese. bi-m. **Document type:** *Bibliography.*
Published by: (Kokusai Igaku Joho Senta), Daiichi Seiyaku Co. Ltd., 14-10 Nihonbashi 3-chome, Chuo-ku, Tokyo 103-0027, Japan.

016.61607 USA
R S N A INDEX TO IMAGING LITERATURE. Text in English. q. **Document type:** *Abstract/Index.*
Related titles: Online - full text ed.: R S N A Index Online (from HighWire Pr.).
Published by: Radiological Society of North America, Inc., 820 Jorie Blvd., Oak Brook, IL 60523. TEL 630-571-2670, FAX 630-571-7837, http://rsnaindex.rsnajnls.org/.

016.61697 RUS ISSN 0869-4087
REFERATIVNYI ZHURNAL. BIOLOGIYA - IMMUNOLOGIYA. Text in Russian. m. USD 1,100 in United States. **Document type:** *Abstract/Index.*
—East View.
Published by: Vserossiiskii Institut Nauchnoi i Tekhnicheskoi Informatsii (VINITI), Usievicha ul 20-a, Moscow 125315, Russian Federation. TEL 7-095-1526441, FAX 7-095-943-0060. **US dist. addr.:** East View Publications, 3020 Harbor Ln N, Minneapolis, MN 55447. TEL 612-550-0961.

016.61697 RUS
REFERATIVNYI ZHURNAL. BRONKHYALNAYA ASTMA I DRUGIE ALLERGICHESKIE ZABOLEVANIYA. Text in Russian. 1997. m. **Document type:** *Abstract/Index.*
Published by: Vserossiiskii Institut Nauchnoi i Tekhnicheskoi Informatsii (VINITI), Usievicha ul 20-a, Moscow 125315, Russian Federation. TEL 7-095-1526441, FAX 7-095-943-0060. **Dist. by:** Mezhdunarodnaya Kniga, B Yakimanka 39, Moscow 117049, Russian Federation. TEL 7-095-2384967, FAX 7-095-2384634.

016.6163 RUS
REFERATIVNYI ZHURNAL. ENDOSKOPIYA. Text in Russian. 1997. 6/yr. **Document type:** *Abstract/Index.*
Published by: Vserossiiskii Institut Nauchnoi i Tekhnicheskoi Informatsii (VINITI), Usievicha ul 20-a, Moscow 125315, Russian Federation. TEL 7-095-1526441, FAX 7-095-943-0060. **Dist. by:** Mezhdunarodnaya Kniga, B Yakimanka 39, Moscow 117049, Russian Federation. TEL 7-095-2384967, FAX 7-095-2384634.

016.61615 RUS
REFERATIVNYI ZHURNAL. GEMATOLOGIYA. Text in Russian. 1997. 6/yr. **Document type:** *Abstract/Index.*
Published by: Vserossiiskii Institut Nauchnoi i Tekhnicheskoi Informatsii (VINITI), Usievicha ul 20-a, Moscow 125315, Russian Federation. TEL 7-095-1526441, FAX 7-095-943-0060. **Dist. by:** Mezhdunarodnaya Kniga, B Yakimanka 39, Moscow 117049, Russian Federation. TEL 7-095-2384967, FAX 7-095-2384634.

016.61697 RUS ISSN 0202-9154
REFERATIVNYI ZHURNAL. IMMUNOLOGIYA - ALLERGOLOGIYA. Text in Russian. 1978. m. USD 487. **Document type:** *Abstract/Index.*
Published by: Vserossiiskii Institut Nauchnoi i Tekhnicheskoi Informatsii (VINITI), Usievicha ul 20-a, Moscow 125315, Russian Federation. TEL 7-095-1526441. **Dist. by:** Mezhdunarodnaya Kniga, B Yakimanka 39, Moscow 117049, Russian Federation. TEL 7-095-2384967, FAX 7-095-2384634.

016.61697 RUS
REFERATIVNYI ZHURNAL. KLINICHESKAYA IMMUNOLOGIYA I ALLERGOLOGIYA. IMMUNOREABILITATSIYA. IMMUNOFARMAKOLOGIYA. Text in Russian. 1998. 6/yr. **Document type:** *Abstract/Index.*
Published by: Vserossiiskii Institut Nauchnoi i Tekhnicheskoi Informatsii (VINITI), Usievicha ul 20-a, Moscow 125315, Russian Federation. TEL 7-095-1526441, FAX 7-095-943-0060. **Dist. by:** Mezhdunarodnaya Kniga, B Yakimanka 39, Moscow 117049, Russian Federation. TEL 7-095-2384967, FAX 7-095-2384634.

016.615842 RUS
REFERATIVNYI ZHURNAL. LUCHEVAYA DIAGNOSTIKA. PART 1: ULTRAZVUKOVAYA DIAGNOSTIKA. Text in Russian. 1997. m. **Document type:** *Abstract/Index.*
Indexed: Ref.Zh.
Published by: Vserossiiskii Institut Nauchnoi i Tekhnicheskoi Informatsii (VINITI), Usievicha ul 20-a, Moscow 125315, Russian Federation. TEL 7-095-1526441, FAX 7-095-943-0060. **Dist. by:** Mezhdunarodnaya Kniga, B Yakimanka 39, Moscow 117049, Russian Federation. TEL 7-095-2384967, FAX 7-095-2384634.

016.615842 RUS
REFERATIVNYI ZHURNAL. LUCHEVAYA DIAGNOSTIKA. PART 2: RENTGENODIAGNOSTIKA. MAGNITNOREZONANSNAYA TOMOGRAFIYA. Text in Russian. 1997. m. **Document type:** *Abstract/Index.*
Published by: Vserossiiskii Institut Nauchnoi i Tekhnicheskoi Informatsii (VINITI), Usievicha ul 20-a, Moscow 125315, Russian Federation. TEL 7-095-1526441, FAX 7-095-943-0060. **Dist. by:** Mezhdunarodnaya Kniga, B Yakimanka 39, Moscow 117049, Russian Federation. TEL 7-095-2384967, FAX 7-095-2384634.

016.615842 RUS
REFERATIVNYI ZHURNAL. LUCHEVAYA DIAGNOSTIKA. PART 3: RADIONUKLIDNAYA DIAGNOSTIKA. Text in Russian. 1997. 6/yr. **Document type:** *Abstract/Index.*
Published by: Vserossiiskii Institut Nauchnoi i Tekhnicheskoi Informatsii (VINITI), Usievicha ul 20-a, Moscow 125315, Russian Federation. TEL 7-095-1526441, FAX 7-095-943-0060. **Dist. by:** Mezhdunarodnaya Kniga, B Yakimanka 39, Moscow 117049, Russian Federation. TEL 7-095-2384967, FAX 7-095-2384634.

016.61 RUS
REFERATIVNYI ZHURNAL. MEDITSINA. Text in Russian. 1997. m. **Document type:** *Abstract/Index.*
Published by: Vserossiiskii Institut Nauchnoi i Tekhnicheskoi Informatsii (VINITI), Usievicha ul 20-a, Moscow 125315, Russian Federation. TEL 7-095-1526441, FAX 7-095-943-0060. **US dist. addr.:** East View Publications, 3020 Harbor Ln N, Minneapolis, MN 55447. TEL 612-550-0961.

016.61 RUS
REFERATIVNYI ZHURNAL. MEDITSINA KATASTROF. SLUZHBA MEDITSINY KATASTROF. Text in Russian. m. USD 175 foreign. **Document type:** *Abstract/Index.*
Published by: Vserossiiskii Institut Nauchnoi i Tekhnicheskoi Informatsii (VINITI), Usievicha ul 20-a, Moscow 125315, Russian Federation. TEL 7-095-1526441, FAX 7-095-943-0060. **US dist. addr.:** East View Publications, 3020 Harbor Ln N, Minneapolis, MN 55447. TEL 612-550-0961.

016.3631 RUS
REFERATIVNYI ZHURNAL. MEDITSINA TRUDA. Text in Russian. m. USD 175 in United States. **Document type:** *Abstract/Index.*
Published by: Vserossiiskii Institut Nauchnoi i Tekhnicheskoi Informatsii (VINITI), Usievicha ul 20-a, Moscow 125315, Russian Federation. TEL 7-095-1526441, FAX 7-095-943-0060. **US dist. addr.:** East View Publications, 3020 Harbor Ln N, Minneapolis, MN 55447. TEL 612-550-0961.

016.61 RUS ISSN 0034-2475
REFERATIVNYI ZHURNAL. MEDITSINSKAYA GEOGRAFIYA. Text in Russian. 1962. m. USD 179. **Document type:** *Abstract/Index.*
—East View.
Published by: Vserossiiskii Institut Nauchnoi i Tekhnicheskoi Informatsii (VINITI), Usievicha ul 20-a, Moscow 125315, Russian Federation. TEL 7-095-1526441, FAX 7-095-943-0060. Ed. Kim Losev. **Dist. by:** Mezhdunarodnaya Kniga, B Yakimanka 39, Moscow 117049, Russian Federation. TEL 7-095-2384967, FAX 7-095-2384634; **US dist. addr.:** East View Publications, 3020 Harbor Ln N, Minneapolis, MN 55447. TEL 612-550-0961.

016.61697 RUS ISSN 0207-8627
REFERATIVNYI ZHURNAL. MOLEKULYARNAYA I KLETOCHNAYA IMMUNOLOGIYA. Text in Russian. m. USD 765 in United States. **Document type:** *Abstract/Index.*
—East View.
Published by: Vserossiiskii Institut Nauchnoi i Tekhnicheskoi Informatsii (VINITI), Usievicha ul 20-a, Moscow 125315, Russian Federation. TEL 7-095-1526441, FAX 7-095-943-0060. **US dist. addr.:** East View Publications, 3020 Harbor Ln N, Minneapolis, MN 55447. TEL 612-550-0961.

REFERATIVNYI ZHURNAL. MORFOLOGIYA CHELOVEKA I ZHIVOTNYKH. ANTROPOLOGIYA. see *BIOLOGY—Abstracting, Bibliographies, Statistics*

REFERATIVNYI ZHURNAL. OBSHCHIE VOPROSY PATOLOGICHESKOI ANATOMII. see *BIOLOGY—Abstracting, Bibliographies, Statistics*

016.61699 RUS ISSN 0202-9197
REFERATIVNYI ZHURNAL. ONKOLOGIYA. Text in Russian. 1961. m. **Document type:** *Abstract/Index.*
Published by: Vserossiiskii Institut Nauchnoi i Tekhnicheskoi Informatsii (VINITI), Usievicha ul 20-a, Moscow 125315, Russian Federation. TEL 7-095-1526441, FAX 7-095-943-0060. **Dist. by:** Mezhdunarodnaya Kniga, B Yakimanka 39, Moscow 117049, Russian Federation. TEL 7-095-2384967, FAX 7-095-2384634.

016.61699 RUS
REFERATIVNYI ZHURNAL. ONKOLOGIYA: EKSPERIMENTALNAYA. Text in Russian. 1961. m. **Document type:** *Abstract/Index.*
Published by: Vserossiiskii Institut Nauchnoi i Tekhnicheskoi Informatsii (VINITI), Usievicha ul 20-a, Moscow 125315, Russian Federation. TEL 7-095-1526441, FAX 7-095-943-0060. **Dist. by:** Mezhdunarodnaya Kniga, B Yakimanka 39, Moscow 117049, Russian Federation. TEL 7-095-2384967, FAX 7-095-2384634.

016.616992 RUS ISSN 0869-4117
REFERATIVNYI ZHURNAL. ONKOLOGIYA: KLINICHESKAYA. Text in Russian. 1961. m. USD 467. **Document type:** *Abstract/Index.*
—East View.
Published by: Vserossiiskii Institut Nauchnoi i Tekhnicheskoi Informatsii (VINITI), Usievicha ul 20-a, Moscow 125315, Russian Federation. TEL 7-095-1526441, FAX 7-095-943-0060. **Dist. by:** Mezhdunarodnaya Kniga, B Yakimanka 39, Moscow 117049, Russian Federation. TEL 7-095-2384967, FAX 7-095-2384634; **US dist. addr.:** East View Publications, 3020 Harbor Ln N, Minneapolis, MN 55447. TEL 612-550-0961.

016.61699 RUS
REFERATIVNYI ZHURNAL. ONKOLOGIYA: TERAPIYA OPUKHOLEI. Text in Russian. 1961. m. **Document type:** *Abstract/Index.*
Published by: Vserossiiskii Institut Nauchnoi i Tekhnicheskoi Informatsii (VINITI), Usievicha ul 20-a, Moscow 125315, Russian Federation. TEL 7-095-1526441, FAX 7-095-943-0060. **Dist. by:** Mezhdunarodnaya Kniga, B Yakimanka 39, Moscow 117049, Russian Federation. TEL 7-095-2384967, FAX 7-095-2384634.

016.61689 RUS
REFERATIVNYI ZHURNAL. PSIKHYATRIYA. Text in Russian. 1997. m. USD 175 foreign. **Document type:** *Abstract/Index.*
Published by: Vserossiiskii Institut Nauchnoi i Tekhnicheskoi Informatsii (VINITI), Usievicha ul 20-a, Moscow 125315, Russian Federation. TEL 7-095-1526441, FAX 7-095-943-0060. **US dist. addr.:** East View Publications, 3020 Harbor Ln N, Minneapolis, MN 55447. TEL 612-550-0961.

M

016.6162 RUS
REFERATIVNYI ZHURNAL. TUBERKULEZ. Text in Russian. 1997. 6/yr. USD 175 foreign. **Document type:** *Abstract/Index.*
Published by: Vserossiiskii Institut Nauchnoi i Tekhnicheskoi Informatsii (VINITI), Usievicha ul 20-a, Moscow 125315, Russian Federation. TEL 7-095-1526441, FAX 7-095-943-0060. **US dist. addr.:** East View Publications, 3020 Harbor Ln N, Minneapolis, MN 55447. TEL 612-550-0961.

616.6 CZE ISSN 1212-320X
REFERATOVY VYBER A AKTUALITY Z UROLOGIE/ABSTRACTS OF UROLOGY. Text in Czech. 1979. q. CZK 100, USD 4 (effective 2001). bk.rev. **Document type:** *Abstract/Index.* **Description:** Abstracts of medical journal articles from around the world.
Supersedes (in 1993): Referatovy Vyber z Urologie (0139-9322)
Published by: Narodni Lekarska Knihovna, Sokolska 31, Prague 12132, Czech Republic. TEL 420-2-24266870, FAX 420-2-24266051, nml@nlkdec.nlk.anet.cz, http://www.nlk.anet.cz/. Ed. P Verner. Circ: 500.

617.96 016 CZE ISSN 1212-3048
REFERATOVY VYBER Z ANESTEZIOLOGIE, RESUSCITACE A INTENZIVNI MEDICINY/ ABSTRACTS OF ANESTHESIOLOGY AND RESUSCITATION. Text in Czech. 1954. bi-m. CZK 150, USD 6 (effective 2001). bk.rev. **Document type:** *Abstract/Index.*
Supersedes (in 1997): Referatovy Vyber z Anestesiologie a Resuscitace (0034-2688)
Published by: Narodni Lekarska Knihovna, Sokolska 31, Prague 12132, Czech Republic. TEL 420-2-24266870, FAX 420-2-24266051, nml@nlk.anet.cz nml@nlk.anet.cz, http://www.nlk.anet.cz. Ed. J Drabkova. Circ: 1,400.

617 016 CZE ISSN 0034-2696
REFERATOVY VYBER Z CHIRURGIE/ABSTRACTS OF SURGERY. Text in Czech. 1969. bi-m. CZK 150, USD 6 (effective 1999). **Document type:** *Abstract/Index.*
Published by: Narodni Lekarska Knihovna, Sokolska 31, Prague 12132, Czech Republic. TEL 420-2-24266870, FAX 420-2-24266051, nml@nlkdec.nlk.anat.cz, nml@nlk.anet.cz nml@nlk.anet.cz, http:// www.nlk.anet.cz. Ed. O Vojtisek. Circ: 590.

616.9 016 CZE ISSN 0034-270X
REFERATOVY VYBER Z CHOROB INFEKCNICH/ ABSTRACTS OF INFECTIOUS DISEASES. Text in Czech. 1960. q. CZK 100, USD 4 (effective 1999). **Document type:** *Abstract/Index.*
Published by: Narodni Lekarska Knihovna, Sokolska 31, Prague 12132, Czech Republic. TEL 420-2-24266870, FAX 420-2-24266051, nml@nlkdec.nlk.anet.cz, http://www.nlk.anet.cz. Ed. J Vanista. Circ: 455.

616.5 616.9 016 CZE ISSN 0139-648X
REFERATOVY VYBER Z DERMATOVENEROLOGIE/ ABSTRACTS OF DERMATOLOGY AND VENEROLOGY. Text in Czech. 1959. q. CZK 100, USD 4 (effective 1999). **Document type:** *Abstract/Index.*
Formerly (until 1976): Referatovy Vyber z Dermatovenerologie a Pribuznych Oboru (0034-2718)
Published by: Narodni Lekarska Knihovna, Sokolska 31, Prague 12132, Czech Republic. TEL 420-2-24266870, FAX 420-2-24266051, nml@nlkdec.nlk.anet.cz, http://www.nlk.anet.cz. Ed. T Frej. Circ: 460.

616.1 016 CZE ISSN 0139-6536
REFERATOVY VYBER Z KARDIOLOGIE/ABSTRACTS OF CARDIOLOGY. Text in Czech. 1960. bi-m. CZK 100, USD 4 (effective 1999). bk.rev. **Document type:** *Abstract/Index.*
Formerly (until 1975): Referatovy Vyber z Kardiologie, Fysiologie a Patologie Obehoveho Ustroji (0034-2769)
Published by: Narodni Lekarska Knihovna, Sokolska 31, Prague 12132, Czech Republic. TEL 420-2-24266870, FAX 420-2-24266051, nml@nlkdec.nlk.anet.cz, http://www.nlk.ant.cz. Ed. J Pokorny. Circ: 620.

616.8 016 CZE ISSN 0034-2793
REFERATOVY VYBER Z NEUROLOGIE/ABSTRACTS OF NEUROLOGY. Text in Czech. 1969. q. CZK 100, USD 4 (effective 1999). **Document type:** *Abstract/Index.*
Indexed: e-psyche.
Published by: Narodni Lekarska Knihovna, Sokolska 31, Prague 12132, Czech Republic. TEL 420-2-24266870, FAX 420-2-24266051, nml@nlkdec.nlk.anet.cz, http://www.nlk.ant.cz. Ed. Josef Simek. Circ: 490.

617.7 016 CZE ISSN 0034-2807
REFERATOVY VYBER Z OFTALMOLOGIE/ABSTRACTS OF OPHTHALMOLOGY. Text in Czech. 1969. q. CZK 100, USD 4 (effective 1999). bk.rev. **Document type:** *Abstract/Index.*
Published by: Narodni Lekarska Knihovna, Sokolska 31, Prague 12132, Czech Republic. TEL 420-2-24266870, FAX 420-2-24266051, nml@nlkdec.nlk.anet.cz, http://www.nlk.ant.cz. Ed. H Kraus. Circ: 360.

618.92 016 CZE ISSN 0034-2858
REFERATOVY VYBER Z PEDIATRIE/ABSTRACTS OF PEDIATRICS. Text in Czech. 1959. bi-m. CZK 150 (effective 1999). **Document type:** *Abstract/Index.*
Published by: Narodni Lekarska Knihovna, Sokolska 31, Prague 12132, Czech Republic. TEL 420-2-24266870, FAX 420-2-24266051, nml@nlkdec.nlk.anet.cz, http://www.nlk.anet.cz. Ed. M Frank. Circ: 400.

618 016 CZE ISSN 0034-2866
REFERATOVY VYBER Z PORODNICTVI A GYNEKOLOGIE/ABSTRACTS OF OBSTETRICS AND GYNECOLOGY. Text in Czech. 1962. bi-m. CZK 150, USD 6 (effective 1999). **Document type:** *Abstract/Index.*
Published by: Narodni Lekarska Knihovna, Sokolska 31, Prague 12132, Czech Republic. TEL 420-2-24266870, FAX 420-2-24266051, nml@nlkdec.nlk.anet.cz, http://www.nlk.anet.cz. Ed. V Trnka. Circ: 500.

615.842 016 CZE ISSN 0862-2183
REFERATOVY VYBER Z RADIODIAGNOSTIKY/ ABSTRACTS OF RADIOLOGY. Text in Czech. 1955. q. CZK 100, USD 4 (effective 2001). **Document type:** *Abstract/Index.*
Formerly (until 1985): Referatovy Vyber z Rentgenologie (0034-2874)
Related titles: Online - full text ed.
Published by: Narodni Lekarska Knihovna, Sokolska 31, Prague 12132, Czech Republic. TEL 420-2-24266870, FAX 420-2-24266051, nml@nlk.anet.cz nml@nlk.anet.cz, http://www.nlk.anet.cz. Ed. S Vesin. Circ: 340.

616.742 016 CZE ISSN 0034-2882
REFERATOVY VYBER Z REVMATOLOGIE/ABSTRACTS OF RHEUMATOLOGY. Text in Czech. 1961. q. CZK 100, USD 3 (effective 2001). bk.rev. **Document type:** *Abstract/Index.*
Related titles: Online - full content ed.
Published by: Narodni Lekarska Knihovna, Sokolska 31, Prague 12132, Czech Republic. TEL 420-2-24266870, FAX 420-2-24266051, nml@nlk.anet.cz nml@nlk.anet.cz, http://www.nlk.anet.cz Ed. R Bardfeld. Circ: 380.

016.61703 GBR ISSN 0955-0984
REHABILITATION INDEX. Text in English. 1988. m. GBP 71 in Europe; GBP 90 elsewhere (effective 1999). index. **Document type:** *Bulletin, Abstract/Index, Bibliography.* **Description:** Provides a classified list of English language citations from the current literature of rehabilitation (over 1,600 per year). Each issue has detailed author and subject indexes.
Related titles: Online - full text ed.
—BLDSC (7350.243000).
Published by: British Library, Health Care Information Service, British Library, Boston Spa, Wetherby, W Yorks LS23 7BQ, United Kingdom. TEL 44-1937-546520, FAX 44-1937-546458, phillipa.seaton@bl.uk. R&P Phillipa Seaton.

RENAL PHYSIOLOGY. see *BIOLOGY—Abstracting, Bibliographies, Statistics*

RENIN, ANGIOTENSIN & KININS. see *BIOLOGY—Abstracting, Bibliographies, Statistics*

REPRODUCTION. ABSTRACT SERIES. see *BIOLOGY—Abstracting, Bibliographies, Statistics*

610 CUB ISSN 0864-2184
RESUMENES MEDICOS. Short title: ResuMed. Text in Spanish; Summaries in English, Spanish. 1987. s-a. USD 26 in South America; USD 28 in North America; USD 30 elsewhere. **Description:** Covers the fields of basic, preventive and clinical medical science and public health and safety.
Published by: Ministerio de Salud Publica, Centro Nacional de Informacion de Ciencias Medicas, Calle E No. 452, e-19 y 21, Plaza de la Revolucion, Apdo. 6520, Havana, Cuba. TEL 809-23-5338. Ed. Sara Perez. Circ: 1,000. **Dist. by:** Ediciones Cubanas, Obispo No. 527, Apdo. 605, Havana, Cuba.

016.5957 016.6327 GBR ISSN 0957-6770
REVIEW OF MEDICAL AND VETERINARY ENTOMOLOGY. Text in English. 1913. m. GBP 395 Includes single site Internet access (effective 2000); USD 710 in the Americas Includes single site Internet access; GBP 355, USD 630 For Internet access only (effective 1999). adv. bk.rev. abstr. index. back issues avail. **Document type:** *Abstract/Index, Academic/Scholarly.* **Description:** Deals with insects and other arthropods that transmit diseases or are otherwise injurious to man and animals of significance to man.
Formerly: Review of Applied Entomology. Series B: Medical and Veterinary (0305-0084)
Related titles: Online - full text ed.: (from DIMDI, The Dialog Corporation, S T N International).
—CISTI, GNLM, Linda Hall. **CCC.**
Published by: CABI Publishing, Wallingford, Oxon OX10 8DE, United Kingdom. TEL 44-1491-832111, FAX 44-1491-829198, publishing@cabi.org, http://www.cabi.org. **U.S. subscr. to:** 10 E 40th St, Ste 3203, New York, NY 10016. TEL 212-481-7018, 800-528-4841, FAX 212-686-7993, cabi-nao@cabi.org.

610 USA
SELECTED PERIODICALS FOR THE MEDICAL LIBRARY. Text in English. 1967. a. free per issue to qualified personnel. adv. tr.lit.
Published by: EBSCO Industries, Inc., Title Information Department, 5724 Hwy 280 E, Birmingham, AL 35242. TEL 205-991-6600, FAX 205-995-1518, tidc%tid@iss.ebsco.com. Ed. Erdeal Moore. Circ: 18,000 (controlled). **Subscr. to:** EBSCO, PO Box 2543, Birmingham, AL 35201. TEL 800-826-3024.

SIGNAL TRANSDUCTION & CYCLIC NUCLEOTIDES. see *BIOLOGY—Abstracting, Bibliographies, Statistics*

616.1 RUS ISSN 0234-9760
SIGNAL'NAYA INFORMATSIYA. ISHIMICHESKAYA BOLEZN' SERDTSA. Text in Russian. 1987. m. **Document type:** *Abstract/Index.*
Published by: Vserossiiskii Institut Nauchnoi i Tekhnicheskoi Informatsii (VINITI), Usievicha ul 20-a, Moscow 125315, Russian Federation. TEL 7-095-1526441.

610 RUS ISSN 0234-9752
SIGNAL'NAYA INFORMATSIYA. NEIROPEPTIDY. Text in Russian. 1987. m. **Document type:** *Abstract/Index.*
Indexed: e-psyche.
Published by: Vserossiiskii Institut Nauchnoi i Tekhnicheskoi Informatsii (VINITI), Usievicha ul 20-a, Moscow 125315, Russian Federation. TEL 7-095-1526441.

SISTER COMMUNITIES HEALTH PROFILES OF THE U S - MEXICO BORDER/PERFILES DE SALUD DE LAS COMUNIDADES HERMANAS DE LA FRONTERA MEXICO - ESTADOS UNIDOS. see *PUBLIC HEALTH AND SAFETY—Abstracting, Bibliographies, Statistics*

615.53 316.8 ZAF
SOUTH AFRICA. STATISTICS SOUTH AFRICA. CENSUS OF MEDICAL, DENTAL AND OTHER HEALTH SERVICES - CHIROPRACTORS, HOMEOPATHS, NATUROPATHS, OSTEOPATHS AND HERBALISTS. Text in English. irreg., latest 1998. ZAR 10 (effective 2000). **Document type:** *Government.*
Formerly (until Aug. 1998): South Africa. Central Statistical Service. Census of Medical, Dental and Other Health Services - Chiropractors, Homeopaths, Naturopaths, Osteopaths and Herbalists
Published by: Statistics South Africa/Statistieke Suid-Afrika, Private Bag X44, Pretoria 0001, South Africa. TEL 27-12-310-8911, FAX 27-12-310-8500, info@statssa.pwv.gov.za, http://www.statssa.gov.za.

617.6 316.8 ZAF
SOUTH AFRICA. STATISTICS SOUTH AFRICA. CENSUS OF MEDICAL, DENTAL AND OTHER HEALTH SERVICES - DENTISTS. Text in English. irreg., latest 1998. ZAR 10 (effective 2000). **Document type:** *Government.*
Formerly (until Aug. 1998): South Africa. Central Statistical Service. Census of Medical, Dental and Other Health Services - Dentists
Published by: Statistics South Africa/Statistieke Suid-Afrika, Private Bag X44, Pretoria 0001, South Africa. TEL 27-12-310-8911, FAX 27-12-310-8500, info@statssa.pwv.gov.za, http://www.statssa.gov.za.

610 316.8 ZAF
SOUTH AFRICA. STATISTICS SOUTH AFRICA. CENSUS OF MEDICAL, DENTAL AND OTHER HEALTH SERVICES - DOCTORS. Text in English. irreg., latest 1998. ZAR 10 (effective 2000). **Document type:** *Government.*
Formerly (until Aug. 1998): South Africa. Central Statistical Service. Census of Medical, Dental and Other Health Services - Doctors
Published by: Statistics South Africa/Statistieke Suid-Afrika, Private Bag X44, Pretoria 0001, South Africa. TEL 27-12-310-8911, FAX 27-12-310-8500, info@statssa.pwv.gov.za, http://www.statssa.gov.za.

610 316.8 ZAF
SOUTH AFRICA. STATISTICS SOUTH AFRICA. CENSUS OF MEDICAL, DENTAL AND OTHER HEALTH SERVICES - SUPPLEMENTARY HEALTH SERVICES AND DENTAL TECHNICIANS. Text in English. irreg., latest 1998. ZAR 10 (effective 2000). **Document type:** *Government.*
Formerly (until Aug. 1998): South Africa. Central Statistical Service. Census of Medical, Dental and Other Health Services - Supplementary Health Services and Dental Technicians
Published by: Statistics South Africa/Statistieke Suid-Afrika, Private Bag X44, Pretoria 0001, South Africa. TEL 27-12-310-8911, FAX 27-12-310-8500, info@statssa.pwv.gov.za, http://www.statssa.gov.za.

610 316.8 ZAF
SOUTH AFRICA. STATISTICS SOUTH AFRICA. STATISTICAL RELEASE. CENSUS OF AUXILIARY, HEALTH SERVICES AND DENTAL TECHNICIANS (YEAR). Text in English. irreg., latest 1987. free per issue. **Document type:** *Government.*
Formerly (until Aug. 1998): South Africa. Central Statistical Service. Statistical Release. Census of Auxiliary, Health Services and Dental Technicians (Year)
Published by: Statistics South Africa/Statistieke Suid-Afrika, Private Bag X44, Pretoria 0001, South Africa. TEL 27-12-310-8911, FAX 27-12-310-8500, info@statssa.pwv.gov.za, http://www.statssa.gov.za.

610 316.8 ZAF
SOUTH AFRICA. STATISTICS SOUTH AFRICA. STATISTICAL RELEASE. CENSUS OF CHIROPRACTORS AND HOMEOPATHS. Text in English. irreg., latest 1987. **Document type:** *Government.*
Formerly (until Aug. 1998): South Africa. Central Statistical Service. Statistical Release. Census of Chiropractors and Homeopaths
Published by: Statistics South Africa/Statistieke Suid-Afrika, Private Bag X44, Pretoria 0001, South Africa. TEL 27-12-310-8911, FAX 27-12-310-8500, info@statssa.pwv.gov.za, http://www.statssa.gov.za.

610 316.81 ZAF
SOUTH AFRICA. STATISTICS SOUTH AFRICA. STATISTICAL RELEASE. CENSUS OF DENTISTS (YEAR). Text in English. irreg., latest 1995. free per issue. **Document type:** *Government.*
Formerly (until Aug. 1998): South Africa. Central Statistical Service. Statistical Release. Census of Dentists (Year)
Published by: Statistics South Africa/Statistieke Suid-Afrika, Private Bag X44, Pretoria 0001, South Africa. TEL 27-12-310-8911, FAX 27-12-310-8500, info@statssa.pwv.gov.za, http://www.statssa.gov.za.

610 316.8 ZAF
SOUTH AFRICA. STATISTICS SOUTH AFRICA. STATISTICAL RELEASE. CENSUS OF DOCTORS (YEAR). Text in English. irreg., latest 1987. free per issue. **Document type:** *Government.*
Formerly (until Aug. 1998): South Africa. Central Statistical Service. Statistical Release. Census of Doctors (Year)
Published by: Statistics South Africa/Statistieke Suid-Afrika, Private Bag X44, Pretoria 0001, South Africa. TEL 27-12-310-8911, FAX 27-12-310-8500, info@statssa.pwv.gov.za, http://www.statssa.gov.za.

610 USA ISSN 1078-6961
RA407.3
STATISTICAL RECORD OF HEALTH AND MEDICINE. Text in English. 1995. biennial. USD 115 (effective 1999).
Published by: Gale Group (Subsidiary of: The Thomson Corporation), 27500 Drake Rd, Farmington Hills, MI 48331-3535. TEL 248-699-4253, 800-877-4253, FAX 248-699-8061, galeord@gale.com, http://www.gale.com. Ed. Arsen Darney.

610 519 GBR ISSN 0277-6715
RA409 CODEN: SMEDDA
STATISTICS IN MEDICINE. Text in English. 1982. 24/yr. USD 2,740 in United States; USD 2,740 in Canada & Mexico; USD 2,740 elsewhere; USD 2,877 combined subscription in United States for print and online eds.; USD 2,877 combined subscription in Canada & Mexico for print and online eds.; USD 2,877 combined subscription elsewhere for print and online eds. (effective 2002). adv. bk.rev. charts, illus, stat. cum.index: vols.1-15. back issues avail.; reprint service avail. from SWZ,PQC. *Refereed.* **Document type:** *Academic/Scholarly.* **Description:** Covers all aspects of the collection, analysis, presentation and interpretation of medical data.
Related titles: Microform ed.: (from PQC); Online - full text ed.: ISSN 1097-0258. 1996. USD 2,740 in United States; USD 2,740 in Canada & Mexico; USD 2,740 elsewhere (effective 2002) (from EBSCO Publishing, Wiley InterScience, Institute for Scientific Information).
Indexed: ASCA, Abstr.Hyg., Biostat., Compumath, Comput.Abstr., Curr.Cont. (1990-), Curr.Ind.Stat., Diar.Dis.Res., Dok.Arbeitsmed., Environ.Sci.Poll.Mgmt., Excerp.Med., INIS Atomind., Ind.Med. (1982-), Ind.Vet., Inpharma, Int.Abstr.Biol.Sci., Nutr.Abstr., Oper.Res.Manage.Sci., Pharm.&Out.News, Protozool.Abstr., Qual.Contr.Appl.Stat., Reac., Ref.Zh., Rev.Med.& Vet.Mycol., Risk Abstr., SSCI (coverage dropped), Saf.Sci.Abstr., Sci.Cit.Ind., Stat.Theor.Meth.Abstr. (1990-), THA, Trop.Dis.Bull.
—BLDSC (8453.576000), CISTI, EMDOCS, GNLM, IDS, ingenta, KNAW. **CCC.**
Published by: Wiley Europe Ltd., Baffins Ln, Chichester, W Sussex PO19 1UD, United Kingdom. TEL 44-1243-779777, FAX 44-1243-843232, customer@wiley.co.uk, http://www.wiley.co.uk. R&P Diane Southern TEL 44-1243-770347. adv.: B&W page GBP 750, color page GBP 1,650; trim 200 x 260. Circ: 1,800. **Subscr. in the Americas to:** John Wiley & Sons, Inc., Journals, 605 Third Ave, New York, NY 10158. TEL 212-850-6645, FAX 212-850-6021, uscs-wis@wiley.com; **Subscr. to:** John Wiley & Sons Ltd., Baffins Ln, Chichester, Sussex PO19 IUD, United Kingdom. cs-journals@wiley.co.uk.

610.73 DNK ISSN 0108-9714
STATISTIK OM SUNDHEDSPLEJERSKERNES VIRKSOMHED. Text in Danish. 1983. irreg. DKK 75. illus.
Published by: Sundhedsstyrelsen, Amaliegade 13, PO Box 2020, Copenhagen K 1012, Denmark. **Subscr. to:** Statens Informationstjeneste, PO Box 1103, Copenhagen K 1009, Denmark.

610.73 CAN ISSN 0843-1167
SUGGESTED LIST OF PERIODICALS FOR NURSES FOR THE CANADIAN HEALTH SCIENCE LIBRARY. Text in English. a. CND 5 (effective 1997). **Document type:** *Catalog, Bibliography.* **Description:** A list of suggested and recommended periodicals in nursing published in Canada, the U.S., Switzerland, England and France. Information includes titles, where periodicals may be obtained and the approximate cost.
Published by: Canadian Nurses Association/Association des Infirmieres et Infirmiers du Canada, 50 Drway, Ottawa, ON K2P 1E2, Canada. TEL 613-237-2133, FAX 613-237-3520, pubs@cna-nurses.ca.

SUNDHEDSSTATISTIKKEN (YEAR). see *HEALTH FACILITIES AND ADMINISTRATION—Abstracting, Bibliographies, Statistics*

617.96 016 USA ISSN 0039-6206
RD81.A1 CODEN: SANEA5
SURVEY OF ANESTHESIOLOGY. Text in English. 1957. bi-m., latest vol.45. USD 154 domestic to individuals; USD 187 foreign to individuals; USD 243 domestic to institutions; USD 288 foreign to institutions; USD 44 newsstand/cover (effective 2002). adv. bk.rev. abstr. **Document type:** *Academic/Scholarly, Abstract/Index.* **Description:** Abstracts anesthesiology-related literature from around the world.
Related titles: Microfilm ed.: (from WWS); Online - full text ed.: USD 315.90 domestic for academic site license; USD 360.90 foreign for academic site license; USD 352.35 domestic for corporate site license; USD 397.35 foreign for corporate site license (effective 2002).
Indexed: Curr.Adv.Ecol.Sci.
—BLDSC (8548.834400), CISTI, GNLM, ingenta.
Published by: Williams & Wilkins (Subsidiary of: Waverly International), 351 W Camden St, Baltimore, MD 21201-2436. TEL 785-843-1235, 410-528-4068, 800-222-3790, FAX 410-528-4452, cbrooks@wwilkins.com, http://www.surveyanesthesiology.com, http://www.wwilkins.com. Ed. Dr. Kathryn E McGoldrick. Adv. contact Carol Brooks. Circ: 2,111.

617.7 016 USA ISSN 0039-6257
CODEN: SUOPAD
SURVEY OF OPHTHALMOLOGY. Text in English. 1956. bi-m. EUR 150 in Europe to individuals; JPY 19,900 in Japan to individuals; USD 97 in United States to individuals; USD 167 elsewhere to individuals; EUR 237 in Europe to institutions; JPY 31,400 in Japan to institutions; USD 165 in United States to institutions; USD 265 elsewhere to institutions (effective 2002). adv. bk.rev. abstr, charts, illus. index. reprint service avail. from PQC. *Refereed.* **Document type:** *Academic/Scholarly.* **Description:** Contains articles in a review format that enables ophthamologists to maintain a critical awareness about the volume of literature in the field. Integrates and interprets the information on subjects selected for their clinical importance.
Related titles: Microform ed.: (from MIM,PQC,WWS); Online - full text ed.: (from ingenta, Swets Blackwell, Institute for Scientific Information, ScienceDirect).
Indexed: ASCA, Biol.Abstr., Chem.Abstr., Curr.Adv.Cancer Res., Curr.Cont., Environ.Sci.Poll.Mgmt., Excerp.Med., INIS Atomind., Ind.Med. (1956-), Ind.Sci.Rev., Inpharma, Neurosci.Cit.Ind., Pharm.&Out.News, Pollut.Abstr., Reac., Ref.Zh., Rev.Med.& Vet.Mycol., Rev.Plant Path., Risk Abstr., Saf.Sci.Abstr., Sci.Cit.Ind.
—BLDSC (8550.770000), ADONIS, CASDDS, CISTI, GNLM, IDS, ingenta, KNAW. **CCC.**
Published by: (Survey of Ophthalmology, Inc.), Elsevier Science, 655 Ave of the Americas, New York, NY 10010. FAX 212-633-3680, usinfo-f@elsevier.com, http://www.elsevier.com/locate/survophthal. Ed. Dr. Bernard Schwartz TEL 617-566-2138. R&P Frances Rothwell. Adv. contact Joan Coffey. Circ: 11,024.

SWEDEN. STATISTISKA CENTRALBYRAAN. STATISTISKA MEDDELANDEN. SUBGROUP HS (PUBLIC HEALTH AND MEDICAL CARE). see *PUBLIC HEALTH AND SAFETY—Abstracting, Bibliographies, Statistics*

016.61 RUS
TABACHNAYA ZAVISIMOST I KURENIE TABAKA. Text in Russian. 1997. q. **Document type:** *Academic/Scholarly.*
Published by: Vserossiiskii Institut Nauchnoi i Tekhnicheskoi Informatsii (VINITI), Usievicha ul 20-a, Moscow 125315, Russian Federation. TEL 7-095-1526441, FAX 7-095-943-0060. **Dist. by:** Mezhdunarodnaya Kniga, B Yakimanka 39, Moscow 117049, Russian Federation. TEL 7-095-2384967, FAX 7-095-2384634.

016.6164 610 GBR ISSN 0142-8349
THYROID HORMONES. Text in English. 1976. s-m. GBP 120 for print ed. or e-mail (effective 2001). adv. **Document type:** *Abstract/Index.* **Description:** Current awareness service for researchers. Covers hormone synthesis and secretion, receptors, effects, and hypothalamic-pituitary control of thyroid function.
Related titles: E-mail ed.; Online - full text ed.: GBP 108 to individuals (effective 2001).
—CCC.
Published by: S U B I S (Subsidiary of: Sheffield Academic Press Ltd), Mansion House, 19 Kingfield Rd, Sheffield, S Yorks S11 9AS, United Kingdom. TEL 44-114-255-4433, FAX 44-114-255-4626, subis@sheffac.demon.co.uk, http://www.shef-ac-press.co.uk/subis. Ed. S Huntridge. Adv. contact C Evans.

TRANSMITTERS, RECEPTORS & SYNAPSES. see *PHARMACY AND PHARMACOLOGY—Abstracting, Bibliographies, Statistics*

016.616988 GBR ISSN 0041-3240
TROPICAL DISEASES BULLETIN. Text in English. 1912. m. GBP 380 to institutions; USD 650 in the Americas to institutions; GBP 390 to institutions Includes single site online access; USD 665 in the Americas to institutions Includes single site online access (effective 2002). adv. bk.rev. abstr. index. **Document type:** *Bulletin, Abstract/Index.*
Related titles: Microform ed.: (from PMC); Online - full text ed.: GBP 335, USD 585 to institutions (effective 2002) (from DIMDI, The Dialog Corporation, S T N International).
—GNLM, Linda Hall.
Published by: CABI Publishing, Wallingford, Oxon OX10 8DE, United Kingdom. TEL 44-1491-832111, FAX 44-1491-829198, publishing@cabi.org, http://www.cabi.org/Publishing/Products/Journals/Abstract/TDB/Index.asp. Adv. contact S Harris. B&W page GBP 200; 120 x 203. **U.S. subscr. to:** 10 E 40th St, Ste 3203, New York, NY 10016. TEL 212-481-7018, 800-528-4841, FAX 212-686-7993, cabi-nao@cabi.org.

016.6169363 ITA ISSN 0142-193X
TSETSE AND TRYPANOSOMIASIS INFORMATION QUARTERLY. Short title: T T I Q. Text in English. 1978. q. free. abstr, bibl. **Document type:** *Abstract/Index.* **Description:** Includes abstracts of scientific articles about tsetse and trypanosomiasis.
Related titles: French ed.
Indexed: Helminthol.Abstr., Ind.Vet., Rev.Appl.Entomol., Vet.Bull.
Published by: Food and Agriculture Organization of the United Nations (Rome), Sales and Marketing Group, Viale delle Terme di Caracalla, Rome 00100, Italy. TEL 39-06-57054350, FAX 39-06-57053360.

TUMOUR MARKER UPDATE. see *MEDICAL SCIENCES—Oncology*

619 USA
R854.U5
U.S. NATIONAL INSTITUTES OF HEALTH. NATIONAL CENTER FOR RESEARCH RESOURCES. SCIENTIFIC HIGHLIGHTS. Text in English. 1978. biennial. free per issue. **Document type:** *Government.* **Description:** Report of the National Center for Research Resources.
Former titles: U.S. National Institutes of Health. National Center for Research Resources. Program Highlights; U.S. National Institutes of Health. Division of Research Resources. Program Highlights (0278-5374)
Related titles: Online - full text ed.
Published by: U.S. National Institutes of Health, National Center for Research Resources, 6705 Rockledge Dr, Rm 5046, Bethesda, MD 20892. TEL 301-435-0888, ospio@ncrr.nih.gov, http://www.ncrr.nih.gov/ncrrpubl.htm. Circ: 11,000.

UKRAINSKII REFERATIVNYI ZURNAL. SERIA 1. PRIRODNICHI NAUKI, MEDICINA/UKRAINIAN JOURNAL OF ABSTRACTS. SER. 1. PRIRODNICI NAUKI, MEDICINE. see *SCIENCES: COMPREHENSIVE WORKS—Abstracting, Bibliographies, Statistics*

610 016 IRN
UNIVERSITY OF TEHERAN. FACULTY OF HEALTH. INSTITUTE OF RESEARCH. LIST OF PUBLICATIONS RECEIVED IN THE LIBRARY∗ /DANESHGAH-E TEHRAN. DANESHKADE-YE BEDASHT VA ANSTITU TAHQIQAT-E BEHDASHTI. AKHBAR-E KETABKHANEH VA SURAT-E NASHRIYAT-E RESIDEH. Text in English, Persian, Modern. 1946. m. free per issue.
Published by: University of Teheran, Faculty of Health, P O Box 1310, Teheran, 5, Iran.

UPPSALA DISSERTATIONS FROM THE FACULTY OF MEDICINE. see *MEDICAL SCIENCES*

610 ZWE ISSN 1021-5549
UTANO - ZIMBABWE; an annotated health information bibliography. Text in English. 1993. 2/yr. USD 20. **Document type:** *Bibliography.*
Published by: University of Zimbabwe Medical Library, Mount Pleasant, PO Box MP45, Harare, Zimbabwe. TEL 263-4-791631, FAX 263-4-795019, edmujera@healthnet.zw. Ed. Edward Mujera. Circ: 500.

617 616.1 USA ISSN 0894-8038
VASCULAR SURGERY OUTLOOK. Text in English. 1988. 10/yr. DEM 73.50 per issue (effective 2000); included with Perspectives in Vascular Surgery. adv. **Document type:** *Abstract/Index.* **Description:** Encapsulates the most important journal articles, reports on special clinical findings, and symposia proceedings dealing with this specialty.
Related titles: ♦ Supplement to: Perspectives in Vascular Surgery and Endovascular Therapy. ISSN 1531-0035.
—GNLM.
Published by: Thieme Medical Publishers, 333 Seventh Ave, New York, NY 10001. TEL 212-760-0888, 800-782-3488, FAX 212-947-1112, http://www.thieme.com. Ed. Dr. Jerry Goldstone. Adv. contact Sally Kahn. **Orders in Europe to:** Thieme International, Postfach 3001120, Stuttgart 70451, Germany. TEL 49-711-8931-0.

M

VIOLENCE & ABUSE ABSTRACTS; current literature in interpersonal violence. see *SOCIOLOGY—Abstracting, Bibliographies, Statistics*

016.6177 GBR ISSN 0142-8543
VISION (SHEFFIELD). Text in English. 1981. s-m. GBP 120 for print ed. or e-mail (effective 2001). adv. **Document type:** *Abstract/Index.* **Description:** Current awareness service for researchers in clinical and life sciences. Studies the structure, function, and pharmacology of the eye and its transmitters.
Related titles: E-mail ed.; Online - full text ed.: GBP 108 to individuals (effective 2001).
—CCC.
Published by: S U B I S (Subsidiary of: Sheffield Academic Press Ltd), Mansion House, 19 Kingfield Rd, Sheffield, S Yorks S11 9AS, United Kingdom. TEL 44-114-255-4433, FAX 44-114-255-4626, subis@sheffac.demon.co.uk, http://www.shef-ac-press.co.uk/subis. Ed. S Huntridge. Adv. contact C Evans.

617.6 USA ISSN 0048-3389
WESTERN SOCIETY OF PERIODONTOLOGY. JOURNAL. PERIODONTAL ABSTRACTS. Text in English. 1957. q. USD 60; USD 70 in Canada & Mexico; USD 75 elsewhere (effective 1999 - 2000). adv. bk.rev. back issues avail. **Document type:** *Trade.*
Indexed: Curr.Tit.Dent., Dent.Ind.
—BLDSC (4917.110000).
Published by: Western Society of Periodontology, 907 Tahoe Blvd, Ste 3, Incline Village, NV 89451-9416. TEL 775-832-9120, FAX 775-832-9128, wsperio@aol.com. Ed. Dr. Richard Nagy. Pub. Esther Marie Bennett. R&P Esther Marie Bennet. Adv. contact Esther-Marie Bennett. Circ: 1,500.

615.53 610 USA ISSN 1066-484X
RZ201
YEAR BOOK OF CHIROPRACTIC. Text in English. 1994. a. USD 88 domestic; USD 94 foreign (effective 2001). **Document type:** *Academic/Scholarly, Abstract/Index.* **Description:** Presents abstracts of pertinent literature with commentary by readers in the field.
Related titles: CD-ROM ed.
Published by: Mosby, Inc. (Subsidiary of: Elsevier Science), 11830 Westline Industrial Dr, St Louis, MO 63146-3313. TEL 314-872-8370, 800-325-4177, FAX 314-432-1380, http://www.mosby.com/periodicals. Ed. Dana J Lawrence.

016.616505 USA
RL26
▼ **THE YEAR BOOK OF DERMATOLOGY AND DERMATOLOGIC SURGERY.** Text in English. 1999. a. USD 93 domestic; USD 99 foreign (effective 2001). illus. **Document type:** *Academic/Scholarly, Abstract/Index.* **Description:** Presents abstracts of pertinent literature with commentary by leading experts in the field.
Formed by the merger of (1992-1999): Year Book of Dermatologic Surgery (1059-0587); (1933-1999): Year Book of Dermatology (0093-3619); Which was formerly (until 1960): Year Book of Dermatology and Syphilology (0093-3627)
Related titles: CD-ROM ed.
Indexed: Biol.Abstr., Curr.Adv.Ecol.Sci.
—BLDSC, CISTI, GNLM.
Published by: Mosby, Inc., Continuity Division (Subsidiary of: Harcourt Health Sciences), 11830 Westline Industrial Dr, St Louis, MO 63146-3313. TEL 314-872-8370, 800-325-4177, FAX 314-432-1380, customer.support@mosby.com, http://www.mosby.com/periodicals. Ed. Dr. Bruce Thiers.

617.305 USA ISSN 0276-1092
RD711
THE YEAR BOOK OF ORTHOPEDICS. Text in English. 1940. a. USD 95 domestic; USD 101 foreign (effective 2001). illus. **Document type:** *Academic/Scholarly, Abstract/Index.* **Description:** Presents abstracts of pertinent literature with commentary by leading experts in the field.
Former titles (until 1980): Year Book of Orthopedics and Traumatic Surgery (0084-3938); (until 1969): Year Book of Orthopedics, traumatic and Plastic Surgery (0190-3713); (until 1963): Year Book of Orthopedics and Traumatic Surgery (0190-3721); (until 1947): Year Book of Industrial and Orthopedic Surgery (1041-1216)
Related titles: CD-ROM ed.
—BLDSC (9414.677000), CISTI, GNLM, ingenta.
Published by: Mosby, Inc., Continuity Division (Subsidiary of: Harcourt Health Sciences), 11830 Westline Industrial Dr, St Louis, MO 63146-3313. TEL 314-872-8370, 800-325-4177, FAX 314-432-1380, http://www.mosby.com/periodicals. Ed. Dr. Bernard F Morrey.

616.7 610 USA ISSN 1070-5406
YEAR BOOK OF RHEUMATOLOGY, ARTHRITIS, AND MUSCULOSKELETAL DISEASE. Text in English. 1994. a. USD 96 domestic; USD 102 foreign (effective 2001). illus. **Document type:** *Academic/Scholarly, Abstract/Index.* **Description:** Presents abstracts of pertinent literature with commentary by leaders in the field.
Formerly (until 1998): Year Book of Rheumatology (1070-5406)
—GNLM.
Published by: Mosby, Inc. (Subsidiary of: Elsevier Science), 11830 Westline Industrial Dr, St Louis, MO 63146-3313. TEL 314-872-8370, 800-325-4177, FAX 314-432-1380, http://www.mosby.com/periodicals. Ed. Dr. Richard S Panush.

610 CHN
YIXUE WENZHAI/MEDICAL ABSTRACTS. Text in Chinese. bi-m. **Document type:** *Abstract/Index.*
Published by: Guangxi Yixue Qingbao Yanjiusuo/Guangxi Institute of Medical Information, 20 Gucheng Lu, Nanning, Guangxi 530022, China. TEL 29823. Ed. Ma Banghai.

610 CHN
ZHONGGUO YIXUE WENZHAI (ERKEXUE)/CHINA MEDICAL ABSTRACTS (PEDIATRICS). Text in Chinese. bi-m. USD 48. **Document type:** *Academic/Scholarly, Abstract/Index.*
Published by: Liaoning Provincial Institute of Medical Information, Information Retrieval Office, 79 Jixian Jie, Heping-qu, Shenyang, Liaoning 110005, China. TEL 362837. Ed. Lin He.

618 CHN ISSN 1001-1315
ZHONGGUO YIXUE WENZHAI (JIHUA SHENGYU, FUCHAN KEXUE)/CHINA MEDICAL ABSTRACTS (BIRTH CONTROL AND GYNECOLOGY). Text in Chinese. q. **Document type:** *Abstract/Index.*
Published by: Sichuan Yixue Qingbao Yanjiusuo/Sichuan Medical Science Information Research Institute, 34, Wangjiaguai Jie, Chengdu, Sichuan 610041, China. TEL 28790. Ed. Song Wenli.

617.6 CHN
ZHONGGUO YIXUE WENZHAI (KOUQIANG YIXUE)/CHINA MEDICAL ABSTRACTS (STOMATOLOGY). Text in Chinese. q. **Document type:** *Abstract/Index.*
Published by: Nanjing Yixueyuan/Nanjing Institute of Medical Sciences, 140 Hanzhong Lu, Nanjing, Jiangsu 210029, China. TEL 649141. Ed. Yin Liqiao.

616 CHN ISSN 1001-4136
ZHONGGUO YIXUE WENZHAI (NEIKE XUE). Text in Chinese. bi-m. USD 22. **Document type:** *Abstract/Index.*
Related titles: ♦ English ed.: China Medical Abstracts (Internal Medicine). ISSN 1000-9086.
Published by: Guangxi Yixue Qibaosuo/Guangxi Institute of Medical Science Information, 20 Gucheng Lu, Nanning, Guangxi 530022, China. TEL 86-771-5864744. Ed. Lin Zhongchang. **Dist. outside China by:** China International Book Trading Corp, 35 Chegongzhuang Xilu, Haidian District, Beijing 100044, China.

610 CHN
ZHONGGUO YIXUE WENZHAI (ZHONGYI)/CHINA MEDICAL ABSTRACTS (TRADITIONAL MEDICINE SCIENCE). Text in Chinese. q. USD 14.40, USD 2.40 (effective 2001). abstr. **Document type:** *Academic/Scholarly.*
Published by: China International Book Trading Corp/Zhongguo Guoji Tushu Maoyi Zonggongsi cibtc@mail.cibtc.com.cn, http://www.cibtc.com.cn. **Dist. by:** 35, Chegongzhuang Xilu, Haidian District, Beijing 100044, China.

MEDICAL SCIENCES—Allergology And Immunology

616.97 USA
A A O A NEWS. Text in English. 1981. q. free per issue. adv. tr.lit. back issues avail. **Document type:** *Newsletter.* **Description:** Developments in otolaryngic allergy for physicians and allied health practitioners.
Published by: American Academy of Otolaryngic Allergy, 1990 M St, NW, Ste 680, Washington, DC 20036. TEL 202-955-5010, FAX 202-955-5016, info@aaoaf.org, http://www.entallergy.org. Ed. Dr. Richard Haydon III. Circ: 12,000.

616.97 USA ISSN 1094-4745
ACADEMY NEWS (MILWAUKEE). Text in English. 1943. m. membership. adv. charts, illus, stat. **Document type:** *Newsletter.* **Description:** Covers membership and educational activities, and news as it affects the allergy, asthma and immunology specialty.
Formerly (until 1995): American Academy of Allergy and Immunology. News and Notes (0899-7489)

Published by: American Academy of Allergy, Asthma & Immunology, 611 E Wells St, Milwaukee, WI 53202. TEL 414-272-6071, FAX 414-272-6070, news@aaaai.org, http://www.aaaai.org. Ed., R&P Rebecca Dinan Schneider. Pub. Rick Iber. Adv. contact Carrie Ann Hoppe. B&W page USD 1,250; trim 14.75 x 10.75. Circ: 8,000 (controlled).

ACTA MICROBIOLOGICA ET IMMUNOLOGICA HUNGARICA. see *BIOLOGY—Microbiology*

ADVANCES IN HOST DEFENSE MECHANISMS. see *MEDICAL SCIENCES—Communicable Diseases*

616.97 USA ISSN 0065-2776
QR180 CODEN: ADIMAV
ADVANCES IN IMMUNOLOGY. Text in English. 1961. irreg., latest vol.68, 1998. index. reprint service avail. from ISI. *Refereed.*
Related titles: Online - full text ed.: (from Institute for Scientific Information).
Indexed: ASCA, Abstr.Hyg., Anim.Breed.Abstr., Biol.& Agr.Ind. (Jan.1996-), Biol.Abstr., Chem.Abstr., Chem.Indus.Notes, Chem.Titles, Curr.Adv.Ecol.Sci., Dairy Sci.Abstr., Diar.Dis.Res., Excerp.Med., Immun.Abstr., Ind.Med. (1961-), Ind.Sci.Rev., Ind.Vet., Int.Abstr.Biol.Sci., Nutr.Abstr., Sci.Cit.Ind., Telegen, Trop.Dis.Bull., Vet.Bull.
—BLDSC (0709.100000), CASDDS, CISTI, EMDOCS, GNLM, ingenta, KNAW, Linda Hall. **CCC.**
Published by: Academic Press, Inc., Journal Division (Subsidiary of: Harcourt Brace & Company), 525 B St, Ste 1900, San Diego, CA 92101-4495. TEL 619-231-0926, FAX 619-699-6715. Eds. J H Humphrey, W H Taliaferro. **Subscr. to:** Order Dept., 6277 Sea Harbor Dr, 4th Fl, Orlando, FL 32887. TEL 800-321-5068.

AIDS ALERT. see *MEDICAL SCIENCES—Communicable Diseases*

616.9 USA ISSN 1090-7165
RA644.A25 CODEN: AIBEFC
AIDS & BEHAVIOR. Text in English. 1997. q. USD 286, EUR 285 to institutions for print or online ed.; USD 64, EUR 64 to individuals for print or online ed.; USD 343.20, EUR 342 to institutions for print & online eds. combined (effective 2002). *Refereed.* **Document type:** *Journal, Academic/Scholarly.* **Description:** Publishes studies of the neurobehavioral factors in the initial spread, behavioral consequences, and social impact and response to HIV infection.
Related titles: Online - full text ed.: (from EBSCO Publishing, O C L C Online Computer Library Center, Inc., RoweCom Information Quest, Swets Blackwell, Kluwer Online).
Indexed: CINAHL, Soc.Serv.Abstr., Sociol.Abstr., e-psyche.
—BLDSC (0773.083087), Infotrieve, ingenta. **CCC.**
Published by: Kluwer Academic - Plenum Publishers (Subsidiary of: Wolters Kluwer N.V.), 233 Spring St, New York, NY 10013-1578. TEL 212-620-8000, 800-221-9369, FAX 212-463-0742, services@wkap.nl, http://www.wkap.nl/journalhome.htm/1090-7165. Ed. Thomas L Patterson. R&P Rose Luongo TEL 781-871-6311.

AIDS RESEARCH AND HUMAN RETROVIRUSES. see *MEDICAL SCIENCES—Communicable Diseases*

616.97 DEU ISSN 0931-2579
AKTUELLE IMMUNOLOGIE. Text in German. 1986. irreg., latest vol.12, 1998. **Document type:** *Academic/Scholarly.*
—CISTI.
Published by: W. Zuckschwerdt Verlag GmbH, Industriestr 1, Germering 82110, Germany. TEL 49-89-894349-0, FAX 49-89-89434950. Ed. G Gross.

616.97 MEX ISSN 0002-5151
CODEN: ALEGAF
ALERGIA. Text in Spanish; Summaries in English. 1953. bi-m. USD 125 (effective 2000). adv. bk.rev. *Refereed.* **Document type:** *Academic/Scholarly.* **Description:** Original research articles in clinical case studies on allergy and immunology.
Indexed: Biol.Abstr., Chem.Abstr., Dent.Ind., Excerp.Med., Ind.Med. (coverage dropped), Ref.Zh.
—BLDSC (7840.857000), CISTI, GNLM, KNAW.
Published by: Sociedad Mexicana de Alergia e Inmunologia, A.C., Fuente Emperador 6, Huixquiliucan, Edo. de Mexico 53950, Mexico. TEL 52-5-2511844, FAX 52-5-2513975. Ed. Jesus Perez Martin. Circ: 3,000 (controlled).

616.97 YUG ISSN 0354-3978
ALERGOLOGIJA I KLINICKA IMUNOLOGIJA* . Variant title: Tumorska Imunologija. Text in Serbo-Croatian. 1995. irreg.
Published by: Udruzenje Alergologa i Klinickih Imunologa Jugoslavije, Belgrade, Yugoslavia. Ed. Jasmina Ljalijevic.

616.97 SWE ISSN 0002-5747
ALLERGIA. Text in Swedish. 1957. 8/yr. SEK 250 (effective 2001). adv. bk.rev. charts, illus. **Document type:** *Magazine, Consumer.*
Published by: Astma- och Allergifoerbundet/Swedish National Federation Against Allergy, St: Eriksgatan 44 5tr, Box 49303, Stockholm 10029, Sweden. TEL 46-8-50628200, FAX 46-8-50628249, allergia@astmaoallergifoerbundet.se, info@astmaoallergifoerbundet.se, http://www.astmaoallergifoerbundet.se. Ed. Annika Olsson. Adv. contact Jan Olson. color page SEK 17,300. Circ: 20,000.

616.97 USA ISSN 1053-1092
CODEN: ADITEM
ALLERGIC DISEASE AND THERAPY. Text in English. 1990. irreg., latest vol.7, 1992. price varies. adv. **Document type:** *Monographic series.*
—BLDSC (0790.500000), CISTI.
Published by: Marcel Dekker, Inc., Attn: Eridania Perrez, 270 Madison Ave, New York, NY 10016-0602. TEL 212-696-9000, 800-228-1160, FAX 212-685-4540, marketing@dekker.com, http://www.dekker.com. Pub. Russell Dekker. R&P Julia Mulligan. Adv. contact Eridania Perez.

615.37 616.97 FRA ISSN 0397-9148
CODEN: ALGIB
ALLERGIE ET IMMUNOLOGIE. Text in French. 1969. 10/yr. FRF 535 domestic to individuals; FRF 655, EUR 99.85 foreign to individuals; FRF 375 to students (effective 2000). adv. bk.rev.
Indexed: Apic.Abstr., Biol.Abstr., Excerp.Med., GeoRef, Ind.Med. (1969-), Nutr.Abstr.
—BLDSC (0790.600000), CISTI, EMDOCS, GNLM, KNAW.
Published by: Meditions Carline, 1 et 3 rue du Depart, Paris 75014, France. TEL 33-1-40640075, FAX 33-1-43222699. Ed. G M Halpern. Circ: 5,000.

616.97 DEU
ALLERGIE KONKRET. Text in German. q. **Document type:** *Bulletin.*
Published by: (Deutsche Allergie- und Asthmabund e.V.), Vereinigte Verlagsanstalten GmbH, Hoeherweg 278, Duesseldorf 40231, Germany. TEL 49-211-7357589, FAX 49-211-7357507, am@vva.de, http://www.vva.de. Circ: 30,000 (controlled).

616.97 DEU ISSN 0941-8849
CODEN: ALJOE
ALLERGO JOURNAL. Text in German. 1992. 8/yr. EUR 67.01 domestic; EUR 75.01 foreign; EUR 53.79 domestic to students; EUR 65.66 foreign to students; EUR 14.02 newsstand/cover (effective 2002). adv. *Refereed.* **Document type:** *Journal, Academic/Scholarly.*
Indexed: Excerp.Med. (1994-).
—BLDSC (0790.925000), EMDOCS, GNLM, Infotrieve, KNAW. **CCC.**
Published by: Urban und Vogel Medien und Medizin Verlagsgesellschaft mbH (Subsidiary of: BertelsmannSpringer), Neumarkter Str 43, Munich 81673, Germany. TEL 49-89-43721411, FAX 49-89-43721410, verlag@urban-vogel.de, http://www.urban-vogel.de. Eds. B Przybilla, G Schulze. Adv. contact Peter Urban. **Subscr. to:** Springer Auslieferungs Gesellschaft, Postfach 105160, Heidelberg 69041, Germany. TEL 49-6221-345244, FAX 49-6221-345244.

616.97 615.37 ESP ISSN 0301-0546
CODEN: AGIMBJ
ALLERGOLOGIA ET IMMUNOPATHOLOGIA/ INTERNATIONAL JOURNAL FOR CLINICAL AND INVESTIGATIVE ALLERGOLOGY AND CLINICAL IMMUNOLOGY. Text in English, Spanish. 1972. bi-m. ESP 14,000 to individuals; ESP 19,500 to institutions; ESP 11,200 to students (effective 2001). adv. back issues avail.; reprints avail. *Refereed.* **Document type:** *Journal, Academic/Scholarly.*
Related titles: Online - full text ed.: 1996.
Indexed: Biol.Abstr., CINAHL, Chem.Abstr., Curr.Adv.Ecol.Sci., Dent.Ind., Excerp.Med., Helminthol.Abstr., Ind.Med. (1973-), Ind.Med.Esp., Int.Nurs.Ind., Nutr.Abstr., Protozool.Abstr., Rev.Med.& Vet.Mycol.
—BLDSC (0790.930000), CASDDS, CISTI, EMDOCS, GNLM, Infotrieve, KNAW. **CCC.**
Published by: (Sociedad Espanola de Inmunologia Clinica y Alergologia Pediatrica), Ediciones Doyma S.A., Traversa de Gracia, 17-21, Barcelona 08021, Spain. TEL 34-93-200-0711, ai@doyma.es, doyma@doyma.es, http://www.doyma.es/ai. Ed. F Munoz Lopez. R&P Monica Barnes. Adv. contact Jose Antonio Hernandez. B&W page ESP 106,000, color page ESP 138,000; 280 x 210. Circ: 3,000.

616.97 DEU ISSN 0344-5062
CODEN: ALLRDI
ALLERGOLOGIE. Text in German. 1978. m. DEM 258, EUR 131.91; DEM 28, EUR 14.32 newsstand/cover (effective 2001). adv. *Refereed.* **Document type:** *Journal, Academic/Scholarly.*
Related titles: Online - full text ed.: (from Institute for Scientific Information).
Indexed: ASCA, Apic.Abstr., Biol.Abstr., Chem.Abstr., Curr.Adv.Ecol.Sci., Curr.Cont., Dairy Sci.Abstr., Derwent Biotech.Abstr., Excerp.Med., Inpharma, Nutr.Abstr., Pharm.&Out.News, Pig News & Info., Reac., Ref.Zh., Rev.Appl.Entomol., Rev.Med.& Vet.Mycol., Triticale Abstr., Weed Abstr.
—BLDSC (0790.940000), CASDDS, CISTI, EMDOCS, GNLM, IDS, Infotrieve, KNAW. **CCC.**
Published by: Dustri-Verlag Dr. Karl Feistle, Bajuwarenring 4, Oberhaching 82041, Germany. TEL 49-89-613861-0, FAX 49-89-613-5412, info@dustri.de, http://www.dustri.de. Ed. Dr. C Bachert. R&P Renate Lehmann. Adv. contact Joerg Feistle. B&W page DEM 3,200, B&W page XEU 1,636.13; trim 167 x 242. Circ: 4,600.

616.97 AUS ISSN 1323-8930
CODEN: ARERAM
ALLERGOLOGY INTERNATIONAL. Text in English. 1952. q. AUD 216 domestic to individuals; AUD 197 in New Zealand to individuals; USD 120 elsewhere to individuals; AUD 586 domestic to institutions; AUD 533 in New Zealand to institutions; JPY 37,600 in Japan to institutions; USD 325 elsewhere to institutions; AUD 238 domestic to individuals paper & online eds. combined; AUD 217 in New Zealand to individuals paper & online eds. combined; USD 132 elsewhere to individuals paper & online eds. combined; AUD 645 domestic to institutions paper & online eds. combined; AUD 587 in New Zealand to institutions paper & online eds. combined; JPY 41,360 in Japan to institutions paper & online eds. combined; USD 358 elsewhere to institutions paper & online eds. combined (effective 2001). adv. bk.rev. *Refereed.* **Document type:** *Journal, Academic/Scholarly.* **Description:** Publishes articles of scientific excellence in human and experimental allergology and related fields of research.
Formerly (until 1996): Japanese Journal of Allergology (0021-4884)
Related titles: Online - full text ed.: ISSN 1440-1592. AUD 195 domestic to individuals; AUD 178 in New Zealand to individuals; USD 108 elsewhere to individuals; AUD 528 domestic to institutions; AUD 480 in New Zealand to institutions; JPY 33,840 in Japan to institutions; USD 293 elsewhere to institutions (effective 2001) (from EBSCO Publishing, O C L C Online Computer Library Center, Inc., RoweCom Information Quest, ingenta, Munksgaard & Blackwell Science's Synergy, Swets Blackwell).
Indexed: Apic.Abstr., Chem.Abstr., Chem.Indus.Notes, Chem.Titles, Dent.Ind., Environ.Sci.Poll.Mgmt., Excerp.Med., INIS Atomind., Ind.Med. (1952-), Nutr.Abstr., Rev.Med.& Vet.Mycol., Risk Abstr., Saf.Sci.Abstr.
—BLDSC (4650.785000), CASDDS, CISTI, GNLM, Infotrieve, KNAW. **CCC.**
Published by: (Japanese Society of Allergology JPN), Blackwell Science Asia Pty Ltd, PO Box 378, Carlton South, VIC 3053, Australia. FAX 61-3-9347-0300, 61-3-9347-5001, info@blacksci-asia.com.au, http://www.blacksci.co.uk. Ed. Takeru Ishikawa. Adv. contact Kathryn O'Brien. B&W page AUD 900, color page AUD 1,960; trim 210 x 275. Circ: 8,000.

616.97 DNK ISSN 0105-4538
RC583 CODEN: LLRGDY
ALLERGY; European journal of allergy and immunology. Text in English. 1948. m. USD 528 in the Americas to institutions print & online eds. combined; GBP 367 elsewhere to institutions print & online eds. combined (effective 2002). adv. bk.rev. bibl, charts, illus. index. reprint service avail. from ISI. *Refereed.* **Document** **type:** *Academic/Scholarly.*
Formerly: Acta Allergologica (0001-5148)
Related titles: Microform ed.: (from SWZ); Online - full text ed.: ISSN 1398-9995. GBP 340 (2002) (from Ovid Technologies, Inc., EBSCO Publishing, O C L C Online Computer Library Center, Inc., RoweCom Information Quest, Munksgaard & Blackwell Science's Synergy, Swets Blackwell, Institute for Scientific Information).

M

Indexed: AIDS & Cancer Res., ASCA, Abstr.Hyg., Agri.& Environ.Biotech.Abstr. (coverage dropped), Aqua.Sci.& Fish.Abstr., Biol.Abstr., C.I.S. Abstr., CSNB, Chem.Abstr., Chem.Indus.Notes, Chem.Titles, Curr.Adv.Ecol.Sci., Curr.Adv.Gen.& Molec.Biol., Curr.Cont., Dairy Sci.Abstr., Dent.Ind., Derwent Biotech.Abstr., Dok.Arbeitsmed., Environ.Sci.Poll.Mgmt., Excerp.Med., Food Sci.& Tech.Abstr., Forest Prod.Abstr., Forest.Abstr., Helminthol.Abstr., INIS Atomind., Immun.Abstr., Ind.Med. (1978-), Ind.Sci.Rev., Inpharma, Int.Abstr.Biol.Sci., Int.Nurs.Ind., Med.& Surg.Dermat., NRN, Nutr.Abstr., Pharm.&Out.News, Reac., Rev.Appl.Entomol., Rev.Med.& Vet.Mycol., Rice Abstr., Risk Abstr., Saf.Sci.Abstr., Sci.Cit.Ind., Seed Abstr., Soyabean Abstr., THA, Triticale Abstr., Trop.Dis.Bull., Weed Abstr.
—BLDSC (0790.945000), ADONIS, CASDDS, CISTI, EMDOCS, GNLM, IDS, ingenta, KNAW. **CCC.**
Published by: (European Academy of Allergology and Clinical Immunology), Blackwell Munksgaard, Noerre Soegade 35, PO Box 2148, Copenhagen K 1016, Denmark. TEL 45-77-33-33-33, FAX 45-77-33-33-77, customerservice@munksgaard.dk, http://journals.munksgaard.dk/allergy, http://www.munksgaard.dk. Ed. S G O Johansson. Adv. contact Eric Rozario TEL 45-77-33-33-01. Circ: 2,800.

616.97 USA
ALLERGY & ASTHMA ADVOCATE. Text in English. 1985. q. USD 6 (effective 2000). illus, stat. **Document type:** *Newsletter.* **Description:** Provides patients with information about topics in allergy, asthma and other allergic disorders.
Formerly: Asthma and Allergy Advocate (0899-7470)
Published by: American Academy of Allergy, Asthma & Immunology, 611 E Wells St, Milwaukee, WI 53202. TEL 414-272-6071, FAX 414-272-6070, advocate@aaaai.org, http://www.aaaai.org. Ed., R&P Rebecca Dinan Schneider. Circ: 112,000 (paid).

616.97 USA
▼ **ALLERGY AND ASTHMA HEALTH**; The official magazine of the Allergy & Asthma Network - Mothers of Asthmatics, Inc. Text in English. 1999. bi-m., latest vol.3, 2002. adv. bk.rev., video rev., Website rev. 72 p./no. 3 cols./p. back issues avail.; reprints avail. **Document type:** *Magazine, Consumer.*
Published by: Signature Health Publications, 11030 Ables Lane, Dallas, TX 75229-4593. TEL 974-406-4664, FAX 972-484-6010, griffiths@aarc.org. Eds. Dale Griffiths, Nancy Sander. Pub. Sam Giordano. Adv. contacts Catalina Mendoza, Ray Coppula TEL 561-243-2001. Circ: 12,000.

616.97 USA ISSN 1088-5412
CODEN: NESPD5
ALLERGY AND ASTHMA PROCEEDINGS. Text in English. 1980. bi-m. USD 120 domestic to individuals; USD 150 foreign to individuals; USD 200 domestic to institutions; USD 230 foreign to institutions; USD 15 newsstand/cover domestic to institutions (effective 2001). adv. back issues avail. *Refereed.* **Document type:** *Proceedings, Academic/Scholarly.*
Former titles (until 1996): Allergy Proceedings (1046-9354); (until 1988): New England and Regional Allergy Proceedings (0742-2814); (until 1983): New England Society of Allergy. Proceedings (0276-7511)
Related titles: Online - full text ed.: (from Institute for Scientific Information).
Indexed: ASCA, Chem.Abstr., Chem.Indus.Notes, Chem.Titles, Curr.Adv.Ecol.Sci., Curr.Cont., Dairy Sci.Abstr., Forest Prod.Abstr., INIS Atomind., Ind.Med. (1996-), Ind.Vet., Inpharma, Int.Abstr.Biol.Sci., Int.Nurs.Ind., NRN, Nutr.Abstr., Pharm.&Out.News, Reac., Ref.Zh., Rev.Appl.Entomol., Rev.Med.& Vet.Mycol., Small Anim.Abstr.
—BLDSC (0791.020000), CASDDS, CISTI, EMDOCS, GNLM, IDS, Infotrieve, KNAW. **CCC.**
Published by: OceanSide Publications, Inc., 95 Pitman St, Providence, RI 02906. TEL 401-331-2510, FAX 401-331-5138, oceanside@oceansidepubl.com. Ed., R&P Dr. Guy A Settipane. Circ: 3,000.

616.97 USA
ALLERGY & CLINICAL IMMUNOLOGY INTERNATIONAL. Short title: A C I International. Text in English. 1989. bi-m. USD 68 to non-members; USD 44 to members; USD 78 to institutions (effective 2001). adv. Website rev. abstr. back issues avail. *Refereed.* **Document type:** *Journal, Academic/Scholarly.* **Description:** Includes clinical trends and practice, research trends and notes, reports on meetings, forum, people and calendar of events.
Formerly: Allergy and Clinical Immunology News (0838-1925)
Related titles: Online - full text ed.
Indexed: Inpharma, Pharm.&Out.News, Reac.
—BLDSC (0791.030000), GNLM, KNAW. **CCC.**

Published by: (International Association of Allergology and Clinical Immunology and Interasma), Hogrefe & Huber Publishers, PO Box 2487, Kirkland, WA 98083. TEL 425-820-1500, FAX 425-823-8324, hh@hhpub.com, http://www.acii.net/index.html, http://www.hhpub.com/journals. Ed. A P Kaplan. Adv. contact Iris Pruegl. Circ: 20,000.

616.9 664 USA
ALLERGY HOTLINE. Text in English. m. USD 39 (effective 1999). adv. bk.rev. **Document type:** *Newsletter.*
Indexed: CINAHL.
Published by: Hotline Printing and Publishing, PO Box 161132, Altamonte Springs, FL 32716. TEL 407-628-1377, FAX 407-628-9935. Ed., R&P, Adv. contact Dennis Blank. Circ: 1,700.

616.97 DNK ISSN 0108-1675
RC583 CODEN: ALSUET
ALLERGY. SUPPLEMENTUM. Text in English. 1950. irreg. free to subscr. of Allergy. adv. reprint service avail. from ISI. **Document type:** *Academic/Scholarly.*
Formerly: Acta Allergologica. Supplementum (0065-096X)
Related titles: Online - full text ed.: (from Ovid Technologies, Inc., ingenta, Swets Blackwell).
Indexed: Biol.Abstr., Curr.Cont. (coverage dropped), Excerp.Med., INIS Atomind., Int.Abstr.Biol.Sci.
—BLDSC (0790.946000), ADONIS, CASDDS, CISTI, EMDOCS, Infotrieve, KNAW. **CCC.**
Published by: (European Academy of Allergology and Clinical Immunology), Blackwell Munksgaard, Noerre Soegade 35, PO Box 2148, Copenhagen K 1016, Denmark. TEL 45-77-33-33-33, FAX 45-77-33-33-77, customerservice@munksgaard.dk, http://www.munksgaard.dk/allergy. Ed. S G O Johansson. Adv. contact Eric Rozario TEL 45-77-33-33-01.

616.97 618 DNK ISSN 1046-7408
QP252.5 CODEN: AJRIE8
AMERICAN JOURNAL OF REPRODUCTIVE IMMUNOLOGY. Text in English. 1980. m. GBP 358 print & online eds. combined (effective 2002). adv. bibl, charts, illus. index. reprints avail. *Refereed.* **Document type:** *Journal, Academic/Scholarly.*
Former titles (until 1989): American Journal of Reproductive Immunology and Microbiology (8755-8920); (until 1985): American Journal of Reproductive Immunology (0271-7352)
Related titles: ♦ Online - full text ed.: American Journal of Reproductive Immunology Online. ISSN 1600-0897.
Indexed: AIDS & Cancer Res., ASCA, AgBiotech, Anim.Breed.Abstr., Biol.Abstr., Chem.Abstr., Curr.Adv.Ecol.Sci., Curr.Cont., Dairy Sci.Abstr., Excerp.Med., INIS Atomind., Immun.Abstr., Ind.Med. (1989-), Ind.Sci.Rev., Ind.Vet., Inpharma, Int.Abstr.Biol.Sci., Kidney, Nutr.Abstr., Pharm.&Out.News, Pig News & Info., Reac., Sci.Cit.Ind., Vet.Bull.
—BLDSC (0836.500000), CASDDS, CISTI, EMDOCS, GNLM, IDS, ingenta, KNAW. **CCC.**
Published by: (American Society of Reproductive Immunology USA), Blackwell Munksgaard, Noerre Soegade 35, PO Box 2148, Copenhagen K 1016, Denmark. TEL 45-77-33-33-33, FAX 45-77-33-33-77, customerservice@munksgaard.dk, http://www.munksgaard.dk/ajri. Ed. Norbert Gleicher. Adv. contact Eric Rozario TEL 45-77-33-33-01. Circ: 700.

616.97 618 DNK ISSN 1600-0897
AMERICAN JOURNAL OF REPRODUCTIVE IMMUNOLOGY ONLINE. Text in English. m. GBP 322 (effective 2002). **Document type:** *Academic/Scholarly.*
Media: Online - full text (from EBSCO Publishing, ingenta, Swets Blackwell, Institute for Scientific Information). **Related titles:** ♦ Print ed.: American Journal of Reproductive Immunology. ISSN 1046-7408.
Published by: Blackwell Munksgaard, Noerre Soegade 35, PO Box 2148, Copenhagen K 1016, Denmark. TEL 45-77-33-33-33, FAX 45-77-33-33-77, fsub@mail.munksgaard.dk, http://www.munksgaard.dk/ajri. Ed. Norbert Gleicher. Adv. contact Eric Rozario TEL 45-77-33-33-01.

▼ **AMERICAN JOURNAL OF TRANSPLANTATION.** see *MEDICAL SCIENCES—Surgery*

▼ **AMERICAN JOURNAL OF TRANSPLANTATION ONLINE.** see *MEDICAL SCIENCES—Surgery*

616.97 USA ISSN 1081-1206
CODEN: ANAEA3
ANNALS OF ALLERGY, ASTHMA, & IMMUNOLOGY. Text in English. 1943. m. USD 60 domestic to individuals; USD 75 foreign to individuals; USD 120 domestic to institutions; USD 130 foreign to institutions (effective 2001). adv. bk.rev. bibl, charts, illus. index. *Refereed.* **Document type:** *Journal, Academic/Scholarly.* **Description:** Contains case reports, reviews, reports of original research, brief abstracts of articles published elsewhere and abstracts presented at the annual meeting of the college.
Formerly (until 1995): Annals of Allergy (0003-4738)
Related titles: Microfilm ed.: (from PQC); Online - full text ed.: (from Ovid Technologies, Inc., ProQuest Information & Learning, Institute for Scientific Information).
Indexed: AIDS & Cancer Res., ASCA, Abstr.Hyg., Abstr.Inter.Med., Agri.& Environ.Biotech.Abstr. (coverage dropped), Apic.Abstr., Aqua.Sci.& Fish.Abstr., Biol.Abstr., CINAHL, C.I.S. Abstr., Chem.Abstr., Chem.Indus.Notes, Chem.Titles, Curr.Adv.Ecol.Sci., Curr.Cont., Dairy Sci.Abstr., Dent.Ind., Derwent Biotech.Abstr., Environ.Sci.Poll.Mgmt., Excerp.Med., Food Sci.& Tech.Abstr., Forest Prod.Abstr., Forest.Abstr., Helminthol.Abstr., INIS Atomind., Immun.Abstr., Ind.Med. (1995-), Ind.Sci.Rev., Inpharma, Med.& Surg.Dermat., NRN, Nutr.Abstr., Pharm.&Out.News, Pollut.Abstr., Potato Abstr., Reac., Rev.Appl.Entomol., Rev.Arom.& Med.Plants, Rev.Med.& Vet.Mycol., Rev.Plant Path., Risk Abstr., SSCI (coverage dropped), Saf.Sci.Abstr., Sci.Cit.Ind., Soyabean Abstr., Sugar Ind.Abstr., THA, Triticale Abstr., Trop.Dis.Bull., Weed Abstr.
—BLDSC (1036.050000), CASDDS, CISTI, EMDOCS, GNLM, IDS, ingenta, KNAW. **CCC.**
Published by: American College of Allergy, Asthma, & Immunology, 85 W Algonquin Rd, Ste 550, Arlington Heights, IL 60005-4425. Ed., R&P Edward O'Connell. Adv. contact Kim Kleinber. Circ: 6,200 (paid).

616.97 USA ISSN 0732-0582
QR180 CODEN: ARIMDU
ANNUAL REVIEW OF IMMUNOLOGY. Text in English. 1983. a. USD 64 domestic to individuals; USD 69 foreign to individuals; USD 128 domestic to institutions; USD 138 foreign to institutions (effective 1999). adv. bibl, charts. index, cum.index. back issues avail.; reprints avail. *Refereed.* **Document type:** *Academic/Scholarly.* **Description:** Reviews synthesize and filter primary research in order to identify the principal contributions in the field of immunology.
Related titles: Microform ed.: (from PQC); Online - full text ed.: (from HighWire Pr., EBSCO Publishing, H. W. Wilson, Institute for Scientific Information).
Indexed: AIDS & Cancer Res., ASCA, Abstr.Hyg., AgBiotech, Anim.Breed.Abstr., Biol.& Agr.Ind. (Jan.1989-), Biol.Abstr., Chem.Abstr., Chem.Indus.Notes, Chem.Titles, Curr.Adv.Ecol.Sci., Curr.Cont., Diar.Dis.Res., Food Sci.& Tech.Abstr., Helminthol.Abstr., INIS Atomind., Immun.Abstr., Ind.Med. (1983-), Ind.Sci.Rev., Ind.Vet., Inpharma, Int.Abstr.Biol.Sci., Nutr.Abstr., Pharm.&Out.News, Protozool.Abstr., Reac., Rev.Appl.Entomol., Sci.Cit.Ind.
—BLDSC (1522.565800), ADONIS, CASDDS, CISTI, EMDOCS, GNLM, IDS, ingenta, KNAW, Linda Hall. **CCC.**
Published by: Annual Reviews Inc., 4139 El Camino Way, Box 10139, Palo Alto, CA 94303-0139. TEL 650-493-4400, 800-523-8635, FAX 650-424-0910, service@annurev.org; orders@allenpress.com, http://www.annualreviews.org. Ed. Samuel Gubins. R&P, Adv. contact Swati Aneja TEL 650-843-6634. **Subscr. to:** Allen Press Inc., PO Box 1897, Lawrence, KS 66044-8897.

616.079 USA ISSN 1086-0207
ANTIVIRAL WEEKLY. Text in English. 199?. w. (43/yr.). USD 1,549 in North America; USD 1,649 elsewhere. **Document type:** *Newsletter.* **Description:** Covers important research and developments in the field.
Related titles: Microform ed.: (from PQC); Online - full text ed.: (from Northern Light Technology, Inc., Gale Group, LexisNexis, Factiva).
Indexed: Bus.& Indus. (Apr.1998-).
Published by: Charles W. Henderson, Ed. & Pub., PO Box 5528, Atlanta, GA 31107-0528. TEL 770-507-7777, FAX 770-507-7788, info@hendersonnet.atl.ga.us, http://www.newsfile.com.

616.97 JPN ISSN 1344-6932
CODEN: ARRYFB
ARERUGI, MEN'EKI/ALLERGOLOGY & IMMUNOLOGY. Text in Japanese. 1994. m. JPY 31,500 (effective 2000). adv. **Document type:** *Academic/Scholarly.*
Formerly (until 1999): Arerugi no Ryoiki (1340-2358)
Indexed: Int.Nurs.Ind.
—BLDSC (0790.943500).

Published by: Iyaku Journal-sha/Medicine & Drug Journal Co., Ltd., 2-8 Hirano-Machi 3-chome, Chuo-ku, Osaka-shi 541-0046, Japan. TEL 81-6-6202-7280, FAX 81-6-6202-5295, iyakujor@skyblue.ocn.ne.jp, http://www.so-net.ne.jp/medipro/iyaku. R&P, Adv. contact Kiriko Numata.

616.97 THA ISSN 0125-877X
ASIAN PACIFIC JOURNAL OF ALLERGY & IMMUNOLOGY. Text in English. 1983. s-a. *Refereed.* **Document type:** *Academic/Scholarly.*
Related titles: Online - full text ed.: (from Institute for Scientific Information).
Indexed: Curr.Cont., Field Crop Abstr., Ind.Med., Nutr.Abstr., Protozool.Abstr., Seed Abstr., Trop.Dis.Bull.
—BLDSC (1742.705250).
Published by: The Allergy and Immunology Society of Thailand, Dept of Immunology, Faculty of Medicine Siriraj Hospital, Mahidol University, 2 Prannok Road, Bangkoknoi, Bangkok 10700, Thailand. TEL 66-2-4180569, FAX 66-2-4181636, sisso@mahidol.ac.th.

616 USA
ASTHMA AND ALLERGY ADVANCE✱ . Text in English. bi-m. USD 25; includes membership. **Document type:** *Consumer.* **Description:** Provides information on the latest treatments, medications, scientific advancements, education-support group news, and ways to make your day-to-day life a little easier.
Published by: Asthma and Allergy Foundation of America, 1233, 20th St N W No 402, Washington, DC 20036-2330. TEL 202-466-7643, 800-727-8462, FAX 202-466-8940, http://www.aafa.org.

616 USA ISSN 1092-7042
ASTHMA AND ALLERGY EXCHANGE✱ . Text in English. 1997. q. free per issue to qualified personnel. **Document type:** *Trade.* **Description:** Provides practical tips and "how-to" based on knowledge gained from working with asthma and allergy patients on a daily basis.
Published by: Asthma and Allergy Foundation of America, 1233, 20th St N W No 402, Washington, DC 20036-2330. TEL 202-466-7643, 800-727-8462, FAX 202-466-8940, http://www.aafa.org.

616.97 USA
ASTHMA MAGAZINE; strategies for taking control. Text in English. 1995. bi-m.
Published by: Lifelong Publications, 3 Bridge St, Newton, MA 02158. TEL 617-964-4910, FAX 617-964-8095, asthmamag@aol.com. Ed. Rachel Butler. Circ: 100,000.

616.97 USA
ASTHMA RESOURCES DIRECTORY. Text in English. 1990. irreg. (every 2-3 yrs.). USD 29.95 (effective 2000). adv. **Document type:** *Directory.* **Description:** Presents information on allergens that may trigger asthma symptoms; organizations and programs that provide support; information, education or products and services to asthma patients, doctors and treatment centers for asthma, and libraries or organizations with allergy specialty departments, databases and publications on asthma.
Published by: Allergy Publications, Inc., 3104 E Camelback No.459, Phoenix, AZ 85016. TEL 415-322-1663. Ed. Carol Rudoff.

616 CAN
ASTHMA SOCIETY OF CANADA QUARTERLY NEWSLETTER. Text in English. q. CND 20; includes membership. **Document type:** *Newsletter, Consumer.* **Description:** Provides current information on asthma issues as well as the society's events.
Published by: Asthma Society of Canada, 425-130 Bridgeland Ave, Toronto, ON M6A 1Z4, Canada. TEL 416-787-4050, FAX 416-787-5807, http://www.asthmasociety.com.

616 AUS
ASTHMA UPDATE NEWSLETTER. Text in English. q. **Document type:** *Newsletter, Consumer.* **Description:** Provides information on asthma research, products, and topical issues.
Published by: Asthma Foundation of Victoria, 69 Flemington Rd, North Melbourne, VIC 3051, Australia. TEL 61-3-9326-7088, FAX 61-3-9326-7055, afv@asthma.org.au, http://www.asthma.org.au.

616.97 NOR ISSN 0801-3799
ASTMA ALLERGI✱ . Text in Norwegian. 1961. 6/yr. NOK 200 (effective 2001). adv. bk.rev. illus, pat. 52 p./no. **Document type:** *Magazine, Consumer.*
Formerly: Astma- og Allergi-Nytt (0004-6086)
—CCC.
Published by: Norges Astma- og Allergiforbund, Hegdehaugsveien 31, Oslo 0352, Norway. TEL 47-22-93-37-30, FAX 47-22-93-37-50, naaf@naaf.no, http://www.naaf.no. Ed. Tonje Waaktaar Gamst. Circ: 25,000.

616.97 DNK ISSN 0900-4262
ASTMA ALLERGI BLADET✱ . Text in Danish. 1971. q. DKK 100. adv. bk.rev.
Published by: Danmarks Astma - Allergiforbund, Hovedvej 9 C, Glostrup 2600, Denmark. Circ: 15,000.

AUSTRALIA. BUREAU OF STATISTICS. CHILDREN'S IMMUNISATION, AUSTRALIA. see *MEDICAL SCIENCES—Abstracting, Bibliographies, Statistics*

AUTOIMMUNE DISEASES. see *MEDICAL SCIENCES—Abstracting, Bibliographies, Statistics*

616.97 CHE ISSN 0891-6934
QR188.3 CODEN: AUIMEI
AUTOIMMUNITY. Text in English. 1988. 8/yr. (in 3 vols., 4 nos./vol.). GBP 276, USD 405, EUR 369 to individuals; GBP 1,205, USD 1,800, EUR 1,950 to institutions; GBP 1,265, USD 2,808, EUR 3,042 to corporations (effective 2002). index. back issues avail. *Refereed.* **Description:** For researchers and clinicians interested in all aspects of autoimmune diseases.
Related titles: CD-ROM ed.; Microform ed.; Online - full text ed.: (from EBSCO Publishing, Institute for Scientific Information, RoweCom Information Quest).
Indexed: AIDS & Cancer Res., ASCA, Curr.Cont., Diab.Cont., Immun.Abstr., Ind.Med. (1988-), Inpharma, Int.Abstr.Biol.Sci., Pharm.&Out.News, Reac.
—BLDSC (1828.345000), CISTI, EMDOCS, GNLM, Infotrieve. **CCC.**
Published by: Gordon and Breach - Harwood Academic (Subsidiary of: Taylor & Francis Group), PO Box 531, Lausanne 1000, Switzerland. http://www.gbhap.com/Autoimmunity/. Ed. Terence J Wilkin. **Subscr. addr. in US:** International Publishers Direct, PO Box 32160, Newark, NJ 07102. FAX 215-750-6343.

616.07 USA ISSN 1568-9972
▼ **AUTOIMMUNITY REVIEWS.** Text in English. 2002. bi-m. EUR 273 in Europe to institutions; JPY 36,100 in Japan to institutions; USD 305 elsewhere to institutions (effective 2002). **Description:** Articles on autoimmunity will include demonstrative illustrations and tables. Includes contributions on the pathophysiology and mechanisms of disorders and genomics and proteomics. Clinical items will focus on the diseases, novel therapies and clinical associations.
Published by: Elsevier Science, 655 Ave of the Americas, New York, NY 10010. TEL 212-989-5800, usinfo-f@elsevier.com, http://www.elsevier.com. Eds. M E Gershwin, Y Shoenfeld.

615.37 CHE ISSN 0301-3782
QR180
BASEL INSTITUTE FOR IMMUNOLOGY. ANNUAL REPORT. Text in English. 1972. a. free to libraries and immunologists. **Document type:** *Academic/Scholarly.* **Description:** Presents research reports on all aspects of basic immunology.
Indexed: Biol.Abstr.
Published by: Basel Institute for Immunology, Grenzacherstr 487, Basel 4058, Switzerland. TEL 061-6051232, FAX 061-6051353, annual.report@bii.ch, http://www.bii.ch. Ed. E Palmer. Circ: 8,000.

616.97 USA ISSN 0891-2076
RC582
BASIC AND CLINICAL IMMUNOLOGY✱ . Text in English. 1976. triennial. **Document type:** *Monographic series.*
Published by: Appleton & Lange, Journal Division (Subsidiary of: Simon & Schuster Company), 11 W 19th St, New York, CT 10011-4209. TEL 203-406-4500, FAX 203-406-4600.

BIODRUGS; clinical immunotherapeutics, biopharmaceuticals and gene therapy. see *PHARMACY AND PHARMACOLOGY*

616 USA
BLUE SKIES NEWSLETTER. Text in English. w. (during peak allergy months; m., during non-peak months). **Document type:** *Newsletter, Consumer.* **Description:** Informative collection of facts and advice for the allergy sufferer.
Media: Online - full text.
Published by: Schering-Plough Corporation, Schering Allergy & Respiratory, One Giralda Farms, Madison, NJ 07940-1010. TEL 973-822-7000, FAX 973-822-7048, http://www.allergy-relief.com/newsletter/.

616.97 USA ISSN 0889-1591
QP356.47 CODEN: BBIMEW
BRAIN, BEHAVIOR, AND IMMUNITY. Text in English. 1987. q. USD 485 in US & Canada to institutions; USD 519 elsewhere to institutions (effective 2001). back issues avail. *Refereed.* **Document type:** *Academic/Scholarly.* **Description:** Concerned with the interaction between the nervous system and the immune system at the molecular, cellular, and organismic levels. Addresses the relationships among behavioral, neural, and immunoregulatory processes.
Related titles: Online - full text ed.: (from EBSCO Publishing, O C L C Online Computer Library Center, Inc., RoweCom Information Quest, ingenta, Swets Blackwell, IDEAL Online Library, Institute for Scientific Information).
Indexed: AIDS & Cancer Res., ASCA, Anim.Behav.Abstr., Chem.Abstr., Chem.Indus.Notes, Chem.Titles, Curr.Cont., INIS Atomind., Immun.Abstr., Ind.Med. (1987-), Ind.Sci.Rev., Inpharma, Int.Nurs.Ind., Neurosci.Abstr., Neurosci.Cit.Ind., PsycInfo, Psychol.Abstr. (1987-), Reac., SSCI (coverage dropped), Sci.Cit.Ind., e-psyche.
—BLDSC (2268.101000), ADONIS, CASDDS, CISTI, EMDOCS, GNLM, IDS, ingenta, KNAW. **CCC.**
Published by: Academic Press, Inc., Journal Division (Subsidiary of: Harcourt Brace & Company), 525 B St, Ste 1900, San Diego, CA 92101-4495. TEL 619-230-1840, FAX 619-699-6800, apsubs@acad.com, http://www.academicpress.com/bbi. Ed. Robert Ader.

616 NZL
BUTEYKO NEWSLETTER. Text in English. m. **Document type:** *Newsletter, Consumer.* **Description:** Contains updates, alerts, practical tips, and advice on managing your asthma, allergies, and medication.
Media: Online - full text.
Published by: Buteyko Online, PO Box 1458, Hastings 4215, New Zealand. TEL 64-6-427-8462, FAX 64-6-878-0103, info@buteyko.co.nz.

C A SELECTS. ALLERGY AND ANTIALLERGIC AGENTS. see *MEDICAL SCIENCES—Abstracting, Bibliographies, Statistics*

616.97 GBR ISSN 1367-8949
C P D BULLETIN. IMMUNOLOGY AND ALLERGY. (Continuing Professional Development) Text in English. 1997. 3/yr. (1 volume per annum). GBP 45 domestic to individuals; GBP 60 foreign to individuals; GBP 60 domestic to institutions; GBP 90 foreign to institutions (effective 2000). adv. Website rev. abstr. 24 p./no. 2 cols./p. *Refereed.* **Document type:** *Journal, Academic/Scholarly.*
—BLDSC (3486.192200).
Published by: Rila Publications Ltd., 73 Newman St, London W1A 4PG, United Kingdom. TEL 44-20-7631-1299, FAX 44-20-7580-7166, admin@rila.co.uk, subscriptions@rila.co.uk, http://www.rila.co.uk. Ed. Dr. David Webster. Pub., Adv. contact G Da'Cambra. Circ: 250 (paid).

616.97 CAN ISSN 1203-844X
CODEN: CJAIFE
CANADIAN JOURNAL OF ALLERGY AND CLINICAL IMMUNOLOGY; practical journal of allergy for the primary care specialist. Text in English. 1986. bi-m. CND 60 domestic; USD 72 in United States; USD 94 elsewhere (effective 1999). adv. bk.rev. illus. index. back issues avail. **Document type:** *Trade.* **Description:** Publishes articles on the diagnosis, causes and treatment of allergies and immunologic disorders.
Formerly (until Mar. 1996): Practical Allergy and Immunology (0831-0998)
—GNLM.
Published by: (Canadian Society of Allergy and Clinical Immunology), Medicopea International Inc., 3333 Cote Vertu Blvd, Ste 300, St Laurent, PQ H4R 2N1, Canada. TEL 514-333-4561, FAX 514-336-1129, Medicopea@netaxis.qc.ca. Ed. Gordon Sussman. Pub. Laurence Golstein. R&P Linda Armitage. Adv. contact Helen Kaplin. Circ: 3,600 (controlled).

615.37 CAN ISSN 0068-9653
CANADIAN SOCIETY FOR IMMUNOLOGY. BULLETIN. Text in English, French. 1967. 3/yr. membership. adv. bk.rev. reprint service avail. from PQC. **Document type:** *Bulletin, Academic/Scholarly.*
Related titles: Microform ed.: (from PQC).
—CISTI.
Published by: Canadian Society for Immunology, c/o Department of Immunology, University of Manitoba, 730 William Ave, Winnipeg, MB R3E 0W3, Canada. TEL 204-789-3793, FAX 204-772-7924. Ed. Dr. Kent T Hayglass. Circ: 500.

M

616.97 USA ISSN 0008-8749
QR185.C4 CODEN: CLIMB8
CELLULAR IMMUNOLOGY. Text in English. 1970. 16/yr. USD 2,999 in US & Canada to institutions; USD 3,350 elsewhere to institutions (effective 2001). index. back issues avail. *Refereed.* **Document type:** *Academic/Scholarly.* **Description:** Publishes original investigations concerned with the immunological activities of cells in experimental or clinical situations.
Related titles: Online - full text ed.: (from EBSCO Publishing, O C L C Online Computer Library Center, Inc., RoweCom Information Quest, ingenta, Swets Blackwell, IDEAL Online Library, Institute for Scientific Information).
Indexed: AIDS & Cancer Res., ASCA, Abstr.Hyg., Anim.Breed.Abstr., BBCI, Biol.Abstr., Chem.Abstr., Curr.Adv.Cancer Res., Curr.Adv.Ecol.Sci., Curr.Cont., Dairy Sci.Abstr., Dent.Ind., Derwent Biotech.Abstr., Excerp.Med., Helminthol.Abstr., INIS Atomind., Immun.Abstr., Ind.Med. (1970-), Ind.Sci.Rev., Ind.Vet., Inpharma, Int.Abstr.Biol.Sci., Neurosci.Cit.Ind., Pharm.&Out.News, Protozool.Abstr., Reac., Rev.Med.& Vet.Mycol., Rev.Plant Path., Sci.Cit.Ind., Small Anim.Abstr., Trop.Dis.Bull., Vet.Bull.
—BLDSC (3097.930000), ADONIS, CASDDS, CISTI, EMDOCS, GNLM, IDS, ingenta, KNAW, Linda Hall. **CCC.**
Published by: Academic Press, Inc., Journal Division (Subsidiary of: Harcourt Brace & Company), 525 B St, Ste 1900, San Diego, CA 92101-4495. TEL 619-230-1840, FAX 619-699-6800, apsubs@acad.com, http://www.academicpress.com/ci. Ed. H Sherwood Lawrence.

615.37 POL ISSN 1426-3912
QR180 CODEN: PJIME4
CENTRAL-EUROPEAN JOURNAL OF IMMUNOLOGY. Text in English; Summaries in English, Polish. 1969. q. PLZ 60 domestic; USD 60 foreign; PLZ 15 newsstand/cover. adv. bk.rev. illus. *Refereed.* **Document type:** *Academic/Scholarly.* **Description:** Publishes original papers from the field of experimental, evolutionary and clinical immunology, including laboratory immunology, immunogenetics, immunology of infectious diseases.
Former titles (until 1996): Polish Journal of Immunology (1233-0167); (until 1992): Immunologia Polska (0324-8534); Annals of Immunology (0044-8338)
Indexed: Agri.& Environ.Biotech.Abstr. (coverage dropped), Biol.Abstr., Chem.Abstr., Chem.Indus.Notes, Chem.Titles, Excerp.Med., INIS Atomind.
—BLDSC (3106.138050), CASDDS, CISTI, EMDOCS, GNLM, KNAW.
Published by: Polskie Towarzystwo Immunologiczne/Polish Society for Immunology, c/o Samodzielna Pracownia Immunologii, Centrum Zdrowia Dziecka, Al Dzieci Polskich 20, Warsaw 04736, Poland. TEL 48-22-8157156, FAX 48-22-8157159, kmadal@czd.waw.pl. Ed., R&P Kazimierz Madalinski. Adv. contact Mariola Piotrowska. Circ: 1,000.

616.97 CHE ISSN 1015-0145
RC583 CODEN: CHMIEP
CHEMICAL IMMUNOLOGY. Text in English. 1939. irreg., latest vol.79. CHF 210 in Europe; DEM 250 in Germany; USD 180 in United States (2001). back issues avail. *Refereed.* **Document type:** *Journal, Academic/Scholarly.*
Formerly (until 1989): Progress in Allergy (0079-6034)
Related titles: Online - full text ed.: (from Institute for Scientific Information).
Indexed: ASCA, BBCI, Biol.Abstr., Chem.Abstr., Chem.Indus.Notes, Chem.Titles, Curr.Adv.Ecol.Sci., Curr.Cont. (coverage dropped), Excerp.Med., INIS Atomind., Ind.Med. (1989-), Ind.Sci.Rev., Sci.Cit.Ind.
—BLDSC (3146.750000), CASDDS, CISTI, EMDOCS, GNLM, IDS, Infotrieve, ingenta, KNAW, Linda Hall. **CCC.**
Published by: S. Karger AG, Allschwilerstr 10, PO Box, Basel 4009, Switzerland. TEL 41-61-306-1111, FAX 41-61-306-1234, karger@karger.ch, http://www.karger.com/bookseries/CHEMI.

616.97 USA ISSN 1075-7910
CODEN: CALMEH
CLINICAL ALLERGY AND IMMUNOLOGY. Text in English. 1994. irreg., latest vol.14, 1999. adv. **Document type:** *Monographic series, Academic/Scholarly.*
Indexed: Chem.Abstr., Chem.Indus.Notes, Chem.Titles, Ind.Med.
—BLDSC (3286.246500), CASDDS, CISTI, Infotrieve. **CCC.**
Published by: Marcel Dekker, Inc., Attn: Eridania Perrez, 270 Madison Ave, New York, NY 10016-0602. TEL 212-696-9000, 800-228-1160, FAX 212-685-4540, marketing@dekker.com, http://www.dekker.com. Pub. Russell Dekker. R&P Julia Mulligan. Adv. contact Eridania Perez.

616.97 USA ISSN 1529-1049
CODEN: CIMNDC
CLINICAL AND APPLIED IMMUNOLOGY REVIEWS. Text in English. 1980. bi-m. EUR 250 in Europe to qualified personnel; JPY 33,200 in Japan to qualified personnel; USD 280 elsewhere to qualified personnel; EUR 457 in Europe to institutions; JPY 60,700 in Japan to institutions; USD 511 elsewhere to institutions (effective 2002). back issues avail. *Refereed.* **Document type:** *Newsletter.* **Description:** Provides information for clinical immunologists, clinical pathologists, microbiologists, and infectious disease physicians.
Formerly (until 2000): Clinical Immunology Newsletter (0197-1859)
Related titles: Online - full text ed.: (from ingenta, Swets Blackwell, ScienceDirect).
Indexed: Abstr.Hyg., Biol.Abstr., Excerp.Med., Immun.Abstr., Ind.Vet., Nutr.Abstr., Virol.Abstr.
—BLDSC (3286.247750), GNLM, Infotrieve. **CCC.**
Published by: Elsevier Science, PO Box 945, New York, NY 10159-0945. TEL 212-989-5800, FAX 212-633-3990, http://www.elsevier.com/locate/cair. Ed. Maurice R G O'Gorman. **Subscr. in Australasia and the Far East to:** Elsevier Science (Singapore) Pte Ltd, No.1 Temasek Ave, 17-01 Millenia Tower, Singapore 039192, Singapore. TEL 65-434-3727, FAX 65-337-2230; **Subscr. in Japan to:** Elsevier Science Inc - Japan Regional Office, 9-15 Higashi-Azabu 1-chome, Minato-ku, Tokyo 106-0044, Japan. TEL 81-3-5561-5033, FAX 81-3-5561-5047; **Subscr. outside the Americas to:** Elsevier Science BV, PO Box 211, Amsterdam 1000 AE, Netherlands. TEL 31-20-485-3757, nlinfo-f@elsevier.nl, http://www.elsevier.nl.

616.079 USA ISSN 1071-412X
RB46.5 CODEN: CDIMEN
CLINICAL AND DIAGNOSTIC LABORATORY IMMUNOLOGY. Text in English. 1994. bi-m. USD 245 domestic; USD 249 in Canada; USD 286 in Europe; USD 287 in Latin America; USD 288 elsewhere (effective 2001). back issues avail.; reprint service avail. from PQC. *Refereed.* **Document type:** *Academic/Scholarly.* **Description:** Covers human immune response assessment, including indication for testing, methods used, and interpretation of the results.
Related titles: CD-ROM ed.; Online - full text ed.: ISSN 1098-6588 (from HighWire Pr., EBSCO Publishing, Institute for Scientific Information).
Indexed: AIDS & Cancer Res., ASCA, Abstr.Hyg., AgBiotech, Chem.Abstr., Chem.Indus.Notes, Chem.Titles, Curr.Cont., Dairy Sci.Abstr., Environ.Sci.Poll.Mgmt., Excerp.Med. (1995-), Helminthol.Abstr., Immun.Abstr., Ind.Med. (1994-), Ind.Sci.Rev., Ind.Vet., Inpharma, Int.Nurs.Ind., Microbiol.Abstr., Nutr.Abstr., Pharm.&Out.News, Pig News & Info., Pollut.Abstr., Poult.Abstr., Protozool.Abstr., Reac., Rev.Appl.Entomol., Rev.Med.& Vet.Mycol., Sci.Cit.Ind., Trop.Dis.Bull., Vet.Bull., Virol.Abstr. (coverage dropped).
—BLDSC (3286.248800), CASDDS, CISTI, GNLM, IDS, Infotrieve, KNAW. **CCC.**
Published by: American Society for Microbiology, 1325 Massachusetts Ave, N W, Washington, DC 20005-4171. TEL 202-737-3600, 800-633-4931, subscriptions@amsusa.org, http://cdli.asm.org/, http://www.asmusa.org. Ed. Steven D Douglas.

616.97 GBR ISSN 0954-7894
CODEN: CLEAEN
CLINICAL AND EXPERIMENTAL ALLERGY. Text in English. 1971. m., latest vol.32, 2002. GBP 860 in Europe; USD 1,363 in North America; GBP 946 elsewhere (effective 2002). adv. bk.rev. illus. index. back issues avail.; reprint service avail. from ISI. *Refereed.* **Document type:** *Academic/Scholarly.* **Description:** Features editorials, letters, special sections, including current abstracts, allergy practice forum and news and commentary.
Formerly (until Jan. 1989): Clinical Allergy (0009-9090)
Related titles: Microform ed.: (from PQC); Online - full text ed.: ISSN 1365-2222. 1997. GBP 774 in Europe; USD 1,227 in North America; GBP 774 elsewhere (effective 2002) (from Ovid Technologies, Inc., EBSCO Publishing, O C L C Online Computer Library Center, Inc., RoweCom Information Quest, ingenta, Munksgaard & Blackwell Science's Synergy, Swets Blackwell, Institute for Scientific Information); ♦ Supplement: Clinical and Experimental Allergy. Supplement. ISSN 0960-2178.
Indexed: ASCA, Abstr.Hyg., Agri.& Environ.Biotech.Abstr. (coverage dropped), Apic.Abstr., Biol.Abstr., C.I.S. Abstr., Chem.Abstr., Curr.Adv.Ecol.Sci., Curr.Cont., Dairy Sci.Abstr., Derwent Biotech.Abstr., Dok.Arbeitsmed., Excerp.Med., Food Sci.& Tech.Abstr., Forest.Abstr., Helminthol.Abstr., Herb.Abstr., Hort.Abstr., INIS Atomind., Immun.Abstr., Ind.Med. (1989-), Ind.Sci.Rev., Ind.Vet., Inpharma, Int.Abstr.Biol.Sci., Lab.Haz.Bull., Med.& Surg.Dermat., NRN, Nutr.Abstr., Pharm.&Out.News, Reac., Rev.Appl.Entomol., Rev.Med.& Vet.Mycol., Sci.Cit.Ind., THA, Trop.Dis.Bull., Weed Abstr.
—BLDSC (3286.249700), ADONIS, CASDDS, CISTI, EMDOCS, GNLM, IDS, ingenta, KNAW. **CCC.**
Published by: (British Society for Allergy & Clinical Immunology), Blackwell Science Ltd., PO Box 88, Oxford OX2 0NE, United Kingdom. TEL 44-1865-206180, 44-1865-206002, FAX 44-1865-206219, jnl.orders@blacksci.co.uk, http://www.blackwell-science.com/products/journals/cea.htm, http://www.blackwellpublishing.com. Eds. A B Kay, S T Holgate. Pub. Allen Stevens. R&P Sophie Savage. Adv. contact Jenny Applin. Circ: 1,455.

616.97 GBR ISSN 0960-2178
CLINICAL AND EXPERIMENTAL ALLERGY. SUPPLEMENT. Text in English. irreg. adv. **Document type:** *Academic/Scholarly.*
Related titles: Online - full text ed.: (from Ovid Technologies, Inc.); ♦ Supplement to: Clinical and Experimental Allergy. ISSN 0954-7894.
Indexed: AIDS & Cancer Res., Curr.Cont. (coverage dropped), Immun.Abstr. (coverage dropped), Int.Abstr.Biol.Sci.
—ADONIS, EMDOCS, Infotrieve, KNAW. **CCC.**
Published by: (British Society for Allergy & Clinical Immunology), Blackwell Science Ltd., Osney Mead, Oxford OX2 0EL, United Kingdom. TEL 44-1865-206206, FAX 44-1865-721205, journals.cs@blacksci.co.uk, http://www.blackwell-science.com. Pub. Allen Stevens. R&P Sophie Savage. Adv. contact Jenny Applin.

615.37 GBR ISSN 0009-9104
RC583 CODEN: CEXIAL
CLINICAL AND EXPERIMENTAL IMMUNOLOGY. Text in English. 1966. m., latest vol.127, 2002. GBP 829 in Europe; USD 1,308 in North America; GBP 908 elsewhere (effective 2002). adv. bibl, charts, illus. index. back issues avail.; reprint service avail. from ISI. *Refereed.* **Document type:** *Academic/Scholarly.* **Description:** Provides an international forum for the publication of original research n all aspects of clinical immunology.
Related titles: CD-ROM ed.; Microform ed.: (from PQC); Online - full text ed.: ISSN 1365-2249. 1987. GBP 747 in Europe; USD 1,178 in North America; GBP 747 elsewhere (effective 2002) (from Ovid Technologies, Inc., EBSCO Publishing, O C L C Online Computer Library Center, Inc., RoweCom Information Quest, ingenta, Munksgaard & Blackwell Science's Synergy, Swets Blackwell, Institute for Scientific Information); ♦ Supplement: Clinical and Experimental Immunology. Supplement. ISSN 0964-2536.
Indexed: AIDS & Cancer Res., AIDS Abstr., ASCA, Abstr.Hyg., Agri.& Environ.Biotech.Abstr. (coverage dropped), Anim.Breed.Abstr., Biol.Abstr., Chem.Abstr., Chem.Indus.Notes, Chem.Titles, Curr.Adv.Cancer Res., Curr.Adv.Ecol.Sci., Curr.Adv.Gen.& Molec.Biol., Curr.Cont., Dairy Sci.Abstr., Dent.Ind., Derwent Biotech.Abstr., Diar.Dis.Res., Excerp.Med., Helminthol.Abstr., INIS Atomind., Immun.Abstr., Ind.Med. (1966-), Ind.Sci.Rev., Ind.Vet., Inpharma, Int.Abstr.Biol.Sci., Nutr.Abstr., Pharm.&Out.News, Protozool.Abstr., Reac., Ref.Zh., Rev.Med.& Vet.Mycol., Rev.Plant Path., SSCI (coverage dropped), Sci.Cit.Ind., Telegen, Trop.Dis.Bull., Vet.Bull., Virol.Abstr. (coverage dropped).
—BLDSC (3286.251000), ADONIS, CASDDS, CISTI, EMDOCS, GNLM, IDS, ingenta, KNAW. **CCC.**
Published by: (British Society for Immunology), Blackwell Science Ltd., PO Box 88, Oxford OX2 0NE, United Kingdom. TEL 44-1865-206180, 44-1865-206002, FAX 44-1865-206219, jnl.orders@blacksci.co.uk, http://www.blackwell-science.com/~cgilib/jnlpage.asp?Journal=cei&File=cei, http://www.blackwellpublishing.com. Ed. M J Walport. Pub. Allen Stevens. R&P Sophie Savage. Adv. contact Jenny Applin. Circ: 1,700.

616.97 GBR ISSN 0964-2536
CLINICAL AND EXPERIMENTAL IMMUNOLOGY. SUPPLEMENT. Text in English. irreg. adv. **Document type:** *Academic/Scholarly.*
Related titles: Online - full text ed.: (from Ovid Technologies, Inc.); ♦ Supplement to: Clinical and Experimental Immunology. ISSN 0009-9104.
Indexed: Excerp.Med. (1992-), Int.Abstr.Biol.Sci.

—ADONIS, EMDOCS, KNAW.
Published by: Blackwell Science Ltd., Osney Mead, Oxford OX2 0EL, United Kingdom. TEL 44-1865-206206, FAX 44-1865-721205, journals.cs@blacksci.co.uk, http://www.blackwell-science.com. Pub. Allen Stevens. R&P Sophie Savage. Adv. contact Jenny Applin.

616.97 USA ISSN 1521-6616
RC583 CODEN: CLIIFY
CLINICAL IMMUNOLOGY. Text in English. 1972. m. USD 1,720 in US & Canada to institutions; USD 1,895 elsewhere to institutions (effective 2001). adv. illus, abstr. index. back issues avail. *Refereed.* **Document type:** *Academic/Scholarly.* **Description:** Publishes original research on the molecular and cellular bases of immunological diseases.
Formerly (until 1999): Clinical Immunology and Immunopathology (0090-1229)
Related titles: Online - full text ed.: ISSN 1521-7035 (from EBSCO Publishing, O C L C Online Computer Library Center, Inc., RoweCom Information Quest, ingenta, Swets Blackwell, IDEAL Online Library, Institute for Scientific Information).
Indexed: AIDS & Cancer Res., ASCA, Abstr.Hyg., Biol.Abstr., Chem.Abstr., Chem.Indus.Notes, Chem.Titles, Curr.Adv.Ecol.Sci., Curr.Adv.Gen.& Molec.Biol., Curr.Cont., Dairy Sci.Abstr., Environ.Sci.Poll.Mgmt., Excerp.Med., Helminthol.Abstr., INIS Atomind., Immun.Abstr., Ind.Med. (1999-), Ind.Sci.Rev., Ind.Vet., Inpharma, Int.Abstr.Biol.Sci., Med.& Surg.Dermat., Microbiol.Abstr., Nutr.Abstr., Pharm.&Out.News, Protozool.Abstr., Reac., Rev.Appl.Entomol., Rev.Arom.& Med.Plants, Rev.Med.& Vet.Mycol., Sci.Cit.Ind., Vet.Bull.
—BLDSC (3286.291550), ADONIS, CASDDS, CISTI, EMDOCS, GNLM, IDS, Infotrieve, ingenta, KNAW. **CCC.**
Published by: (Clinical Immunology Society), Academic Press, Inc., Journal Division (Subsidiary of: Harcourt Brace & Company), 525 B St, Ste 1900, San Diego, CA 92101-4495. TEL 619-230-1840, FAX 619-699-6800, apsubs@acad.com, http://wpnet.com/clinimm, http://www.academicpress.com/clinimm. Ed. Noel Rose.

CLINICAL MICROBIOLOGY REVIEWS. see *BIOLOGY—Microbiology*

616.96 USA ISSN 1080-0549
CODEN: CRVADD
CLINICAL REVIEWS IN ALLERGY & IMMUNOLOGY. Text in English. 1983. bi-m. USD 410 domestic; USD 435 foreign (effective 2000). adv. abstr, bibl, charts, illus. index. back issues avail. *Refereed.* **Document type:** *Journal, Academic/Scholarly.* **Description:** Provides comprehensive coverage of subjects critical to the study of allergy and immunology. Each issue is thematic with the articles designed for immediate clinical use.
Formerly (until vol.13, 1995): Clinical Reviews in Allergy (0731-8235)
Related titles: Microform ed.; Online - full text ed.: (from Institute for Scientific Information).
Indexed: ASCA, Biol.Abstr., Chem.Abstr., Curr.Adv.Ecol.Sci., Curr.Cont., Dok.Arbeitsmed., Excerp.Med., Helminthol.Abstr., INIS Atomind., Ind.Med. (1995-), Ind.Sci.Rev., Inpharma, NRN, Nutr.Abstr., Pharm.&Out.News, Protozool.Abstr., Reac., Rev.Appl.Entomol., Rev.Med.& Vet.Mycol., Sci.Cit.Ind.
—BLDSC (3286.374520), ADONIS, CASDDS, CISTI, GNLM, IDS, Infotrieve, ingenta, KNAW. **CCC.**
Published by: Humana Press Inc., 999 Riverview Dr, Ste 208, Totowa, NJ 07512. TEL 973-256-1699, FAX 973-256-8341, humana@humanapr.com, http://humanapress.com. Ed. Dr. M Eric Gershwin. R&P Richard Hruska. Adv. contact Thomas B Lanigan Jr. **Dist. in Japan by:** Maruzen Co., Ltd., International Division, Export Dept, P.O. Box 5050, Tokyo International 100-3191, Japan. TEL 81-3-3275-8591.

COMPARATIVE HAEMATOLOGY INTERNATIONAL. see *MEDICAL SCIENCES—Hematology*

COMPARATIVE IMMUNOLOGY, MICROBIOLOGY AND INFECTIOUS DISEASES; the international journal for medical and veterinary researchers and practitioners. see *BIOLOGY—Microbiology*

616.97 USA ISSN 0149-1148
CODEN: COIMDV
COMPREHENSIVE IMMUNOLOGY. Text in English. irreg., latest vol.9. price varies. *Refereed.* **Document type:** *Monographic series.*
Indexed: Biol.Abstr., Chem.Abstr.
—CASDDS, CISTI, GNLM.
Published by: Kluwer Academic - Plenum Publishers (Subsidiary of: Wolters Kluwer N.V.), 233 Spring St, New York, NY 10013-1578. TEL 212-620-8000, 800-221-9369, FAX 212-463-0742, info@plenum.com, http://www.plenum.com. Eds. Robert A Good, Stacey B Day.

616.97 USA
CONTEMPORARY IMMUNOLOGY. Text in English. 1981. irreg., latest vol.8, 1999. price varies. illus. back issues avail. *Refereed.* **Document type:** *Monographic series, Academic/Scholarly.* **Description:** Examines issues in immunology, including diseases affecting the immune system.
—BLDSC (3425.182920).
Published by: Humana Press Inc., 999 Riverview Dr, Ste 208, Totowa, NJ 07512. TEL 973-256-1699, FAX 973-256-8341, humana@humanapr.com, http://humanapress.com. R&P Richard Hruska.

616.97 571.9 USA ISSN 0093-4054
QR180 CODEN: CTIBBV
CONTEMPORARY TOPICS IN IMMUNOBIOLOGY. Text in English. 1972. irreg., latest vol.15, 1985. price varies. illus. *Refereed.* **Document type:** *Monographic series.*
Indexed: ASCA, Biol.Abstr., INIS Atomind., Ind.Med. (coverage dropped), Int.Sci.Rev., Sci.Cit.Ind. (coverage dropped).
—CASDDS, CISTI, GNLM, Linda Hall. **CCC.**
Published by: Kluwer Academic - Plenum Publishers (Subsidiary of: Wolters Kluwer N.V.), 233 Spring St, New York, NY 10013-1578. TEL 212-620-8000, 800-221-9369, FAX 212-463-0742, info@plenum.com, http://www.plenum.com.

616.97 USA ISSN 1040-8401
QR180 CODEN: CCRIDE
CRITICAL REVIEWS IN IMMUNOLOGY. Text in English. 1980. bi-m. USD 99.95 to individuals; USD 483 to institutions (effective 2000). adv. back issues avail. *Refereed.* **Document type:** *Academic/Scholarly.* **Description:** Presents a multidisciplinary overview of contemporary immunology, bringing together molecular immunology and immunobiology.
Formerly: C R C Critical Reviews in Immunology (0197-3355)
Related titles: Online - full text ed.: (from Institute for Scientific Information).
Indexed: AIDS & Cancer Res., ASCA, Anim.Breed.Abstr., Biol.Abstr., Chem.Abstr., Chem.Indus.Notes, Chem.Titles, Curr.Adv.Ecol.Sci., Curr.Cont., Excerp.Med., Helminthol.Abstr., Immun.Abstr., Ind.Med. (1980-), Ind.Sci.Rev., Ind.Vet., Inpharma, Int.Abstr.Biol.Sci., Pharm.&Out.News, Reac., Sci.Cit.Ind., Telegen.
—BLDSC (3487.477000), CASDDS, CISTI, EMDOCS, GNLM, IDS, ingenta, KNAW, Linda Hall. **CCC.**
Published by: Begell House Inc., 79 Madison Ave, Ste 1205, New York, NY 10016-7892. TEL 212-725-1999, FAX 212-213-8368, begellhouse@worldnet.att.net, orders@begellhouse.com. Ed. M Z Atassi. Pub. William Begell. R&P, Adv. contact Jung Ra. Circ: 270.

CURRENT ADVANCES IN IMMUNOLOGY & INFECTIOUS DISEASES. see *MEDICAL SCIENCES—Abstracting, Bibliographies, Statistics*

616.97 CHE ISSN 1422-2132
CURRENT DIRECTIONS IN AUTOIMMUNITY. Text in English. 1998. irreg., latest vol.4. CHF 180 in Europe; DEM 215 in Germany; USD 180 in United States (effective 2001). **Document type:** *Monographic series, Academic/Scholarly.* **Description:** Designed to synthesize and consolidate current directions in basic and clinical research on autoimmunity with primary emphasis on relevant genes and genetics.
—BLDSC (3496.353000).
Published by: S. Karger AG, Allschwilerstr 10, PO Box, Basel 4009, Switzerland. TEL 41-61-306-1111, FAX 41-61-306-1234, karger@karger.ch, http://www.karger.com/bookseries/CUDIA. Ed. A N Theofilopoulos.

616.9 USA ISSN 1523-3847
CURRENT INFECTIOUS DISEASE REPORTS. Text in English. 6/yr. USD 163.95, GBP 120 to individuals; USD 327.95 to institutions; USD 85, GBP 60 to students (effective 2002); Subscr. includes both print & online eds..
Related titles: Online - full content ed.: USD 85, GBP 65 (effective 2002).
Published by: Current Science Inc., 400 Market St, Ste 700, Philadelphia, PA 19106. TEL 800-427-1796, FAX 215-574-2225, info@current-reports.com, http://www.current-reports.com/cr_jrnl_home.cfm?JournalID=IR, http://www.current-science.com/, http://www.current-science-group.com/. Ed. Gerald L Mandell. **Affiliate:** Current Science Ltd.

CURRENT MEDICAL LITERATURE. ALLERGY. see *MEDICAL SCIENCES—Abstracting, Bibliographies, Statistics*

616.97 GBR ISSN 1528-4050
▼ **CURRENT OPINION IN ALLERGY AND CLINICAL IMMUNOLOGY.** Text in English. 2001 (Feb.). bi-m. USD 209 domestic to individuals; USD 209 foreign to individuals; USD 465 per issue domestic to institutions; USD 465 per issue foreign to institutions; USD 103 newsstand/cover (effective 2002). bibl. **Document type:** *Academic/Scholarly.* **Description:** Provides expert reviews on the latest development in the research of allergic disorders.
Related titles: Online - full content ed.: (Feb.). USD 604.50 domestic academic site license; USD 604.50 foreign academic site license; USD 674.25 domestic corporate site license; USD 674.25 foreign corporate site license (2002) (from Swets Blackwell).
Published by: Lippincott Williams & Wilkins, Ltd., 241 Borough High St, London SE1 1GB, United Kingdom. TEL 44-20-79407544, FAX 44-20-79407573, cgeorgal@lww.co.uk, http://www.co-allergy.com/, http://www.lww.com/. Eds. G Walter Canonica, Mark Ballow. Pub. Elizabeth Ferguson. **Subscr. in India, Pakistan, Sri Lanka, Bangladesh and Nepal to:** Globe Publication Pvt. Ltd., B-13, 3rd Fl, A Block, Shopping Complex, Naraina Vihar, Ring Rd, New Delhi 110028, India. TEL 91-11-5790212, FAX 91-11-5798876, jaideep.globe@axcess.net.in; **Subscr. in Japan to:** Igaku-Shoin Ltd., 5-24-3 Hongo, Bunkyo-ku, Tokyo 113-0033, Japan.

CURRENT OPINION IN IMMUNOLOGY. see *MEDICAL SCIENCES—Abstracting, Bibliographies, Statistics*

616.079 USA
CURRENT PROTOCOLS IN IMMUNOLOGY. Text in English. 3 base vols. plus q. updates. USD 695 (effective 2001); USD 730 combined subscription for base vol. & update; USD 390 updates for base vol. & update (effective 2002). **Document type:** *Academic/Scholarly.*
Related titles: CD-ROM ed.: USD 675 (effective 2001); USD 705 combined subscription for base vol. & update; USD 375 renewals for base vol. & update (effective 2002).
—BLDSC (3501.535000).
Published by: John Wiley & Sons, Inc., Journals (Subsidiary of: Wiley InterScience), 605 Third Ave, New York, NY 10158. TEL 212-850-6645, FAX 212-850-6021, uscs-wis@wiley.com, http://www.wiley.com. **Subscr. to:** John Wiley & Sons Ltd., Baffins Ln, Chichester, Sussex PO19 IUD, United Kingdom. TEL 44-1243-779777, FAX 44-1243-843232, cs-journals@wiley.co.uk.

CURRENT TOPICS IN MICROBIOLOGY AND IMMUNOLOGY. see *BIOLOGY—Microbiology*

616.079 JPN
CURRENTS IN HEMATOIMMUNOLOGY* . Text in Japanese. 1985. q.
Published by: Ekuseputa Medika K.K./Excerpta Medica Ltd., Tokyo, Kowa Bldg. 5, 15-23 Nishi-Azabu 4-chome, Minato-ku, Tokyo 106-0031, Japan.

CYTOKINE. see *BIOLOGY—Genetics*

616.079 GBR ISSN 0145-305X
QR180 CODEN: DCIMDQ
DEVELOPMENTAL AND COMPARATIVE IMMUNOLOGY; ontogeny - phylogeny - aging. Text in English. 1977. 9/yr. EUR 1,461 in Europe to institutions; JPY 194,000 in Japan to institutions; USD 1,635 elsewhere to institutions (effective 2002). adv. bibl, charts, illus, abstr. index, cum.index. back issues avail.; reprint service avail. from PQC. *Refereed.* **Document type:** *Academic/Scholarly.* **Description:** Publishes original research addressing the development and maturation of the immune system in the broadest sense, emphasizing ontogenetic (including aging) and phylogenetic aspects, including recognition mechanisms, cellular interactions, immunoglobins, and products of T cells and macrophages.
Announced as: Journal of Developmental and Comparative Immunology

M

Related titles: Microfilm ed.: (from PQC); Online - full text ed.: (from ingenta, Swets Blackwell, ScienceDirect, Institute for Scientific Information).
Indexed: AIDS & Cancer Res., ASCA, AgBiotech, Anim.Breed.Abstr., Aqua.Sci.& Fish.Abstr., Aquacult.Abstr., Bio-Contr.News & Info., Biol.Abstr., Chem.Abstr., Chem.Indus.Notes, Chem.Titles, Curr.Adv.Ecol.Sci., Curr.Cont., Dairy Sci.Abstr., Environ.Sci.Poll.Mgmt., Excerp.Med., Focus on: Vet.Sci.& Med., Helminthol.Abstr., INIS Atomind., Immun.Abstr., Ind.Med. (1977-), Ind.Sci.Rev., Ind.Vet., Inpharma, Int.Abstr.Biol.Sci., Pharm.&Out.News, Poult.Abstr., Protozool.Abstr., Reac., Rev.Appl.Entomol., Rev.Med.& Vet.Mycol., Sci.Cit.Ind., Sport Fish.Abstr., Vet.Bull., W.R.C.Inf., Zoo.Rec.
—BLDSC (3579.051000), CASDDS, CISTI, GNLM, IDS, ingenta. **CCC.**
Published by: (International Society of Developmental and Comparative Immunology), Pergamon (Subsidiary of: Elsevier Science), The Boulevard, Langford Ln, East Park, Kidlington, Oxford OXB 1GB, United Kingdom. FAX 44-1865-843010, nlinfo-f@elsevier.nl; usinfo-f@elsevier.com; forinfo-kyf04035@niftyserve.or.jp, nlinfo-f@elsevier/nl; usinfo-f@elsevier.com; forinfo-kyf04035@niftyserve.or.jp, http://www.elsevier.com/locate/devcompimm, http://www.elsevier.nl/. Eds. G W Warr, L W Clem. Circ: 1,020. **Subscr. in U.S. and Canada to:** Elsevier Science, 660 White Plains Rd, Tarrytown, NY 10591-5153. TEL 212-633-3730, FAX 212-633-3680; **Subscr. to:** Elsevier Science BV, PO Box 211, Amsterdam 1000 AE, Netherlands. TEL 31-20-485-3757.

616.97 CHE ISSN 1044-6672
QR184.5 CODEN: DEIME7
DEVELOPMENTAL IMMUNOLOGY. Text in English. 1990. 4/yr. (in 2 vols., 4 nos./vol.). GBP 101, USD 123, EUR 135 to individuals; GBP 355, USD 452, EUR 473 to institutions; GBP 588, USD 741, EUR 784 to corporations (effective 2002). *Refereed.* **Document type:** *Academic/Scholarly.*
Related titles: CD-ROM ed.; Microform ed.; Online - full text ed.: (from EBSCO Publishing, RoweCom Information Quest).
Indexed: AIDS & Cancer Res., ASCA, Aqua.Sci.& Fish.Abstr., Curr.Cont. (coverage dropped), Excerp.Med. (1994-), Immun.Abstr., Ind.Med. (1990-), Inpharma, Int.Abstr.Biol.Sci., Reac.
—BLDSC (3579.054700), CISTI, EMDOCS, GNLM, ingenta, KNAW. **CCC.**
Published by: Gordon and Breach - Harwood Academic (Subsidiary of: Taylor & Francis Group), PO Box 531, Lausanne 1000, Switzerland. http://www.gbhap.com/Developmental_Immunology/. Ed. Richard Boyd. **Subscr. addr. in US:** International Publishers Direct, PO Box 32160, Newark, NJ 07102. FAX 215-750-6343.

DEVELOPMENTS IN HEMATOLOGY AND IMMUNOLOGY. see *MEDICAL SCIENCES—Hematology*

616.97 ITA ISSN 0392-6699
CODEN: EOSSDJ
EOS; rivista di immunologia ed immunofarmacologia. Text and summaries in English, Italian. 1981. q. ITL 120,000 domestic; USD 120 foreign. bk.rev. index. back issues avail. **Document type:** *Academic/Scholarly.*
Indexed: AIDS & Cancer Res., Apic.Abstr., Chem.Abstr., Curr.Cont. (coverage dropped), Excerp.Med., Immun.Abstr., Sci.Cit.Ind. (coverage dropped).
—BLDSC (3793.030000), CASDDS, CISTI, EMDOCS, GNLM, IDS, KNAW.
Published by: Sigma-Tau SpA, Viale Shakespeare, 47, Rome, RM 00144, Italy. FAX 6-9108260. Ed. Claudio De Simone. Circ: 4,100.

EPIDEMIOLOGIE, MIKROBIOLOGIE, IMUNOLOGIE. see *BIOLOGY—Microbiology*

615.37 DEU ISSN 0014-2980
QR180 CODEN: EJIMAF
EUROPEAN JOURNAL OF IMMUNOLOGY. Text in English. 1970. 12/yr. EUR 908 in Europe; CHF 1,688 in Switzerland & Liechtenstein; USD 1,078 elsewhere; EUR 954 combined subscription in Europe for print and online eds.; CHF 1,773 combined subscription in Switzerland & Liechtenstein, for print and online eds.; USD 1,132 combined subscription elsewhere for print and online eds. (effective 2002). reprint service avail. from ISI. *Refereed.* **Document type:** *Journal, Academic/Scholarly.* **Description:** Covers molecular immunology, immunogenetics, cytokines, immunochemistry, cellular immunology and clinical immunology.
Related titles: Microfilm ed.: (from VCI); Online - full text ed.: ISSN 1521-4141. EUR 908 in Europe; CHF 1,688 in Switzerland & Liechtenstein; USD 1,078 elsewhere (effective 2002) (from EBSCO Publishing, Wiley InterScience, Institute for Scientific Information).
Indexed: AIDS & Cancer Res., AIDS Abstr., ASCA, Abstr.Hyg., AgBiotech, Agri.& Environ.Biotech.Abstr. (coverage dropped), Anim.Breed.Abstr., Aqua.Sci.& Fish.Abstr., Biol.Abstr., Chem.Abstr., Chem.Indus.Notes, Chem.Titles, Curr.Adv.Cell & Devel.Biol., Curr.Adv.Ecol.Sci., Curr.Adv.Gen.& Molec.Biol., Curr.Cont., Dairy Sci.Abstr., Derwent Biotech.Abstr., Excerp.Med., Genet.Abstr., Helminthol.Abstr., Hum.Gen.Abstr., INIS Atomind., Immun.Abstr., Ind.Med. (1971-), Ind.Sci.Rev., Ind.Vet., Inpharma, Int.Abstr.Biol.Sci., Microbiol.Abstr., Neurosci.Cit.Ind., Nuc.Acids Abstr., Nutr.Abstr., Pharm.&Out.News, Pig News & Info., Poult.Abstr., Protozool.Abstr., Reac., Rev.Appl.Entomol., Rev.Arom.& Med.Plants, Rev.Med.& Vet.Mycol., Rev.Plant Path., Sci.Cit.Ind., Telegen, Trop.Dis.Bull., Vet.Bull., Virol.Abstr. (coverage dropped).
—BLDSC (3829.730100), CASDDS, CISTI, GNLM, IDS, ingenta, KNAW. **CCC.**
Published by: Wiley - V C H, Postfach 101161, Weinheim 69451, Germany. FAX 49-6201-606-117, subservice@wiley-vch.de, http://www.eji.de, http://www.interscience.wiley.com. Ed. L Leclercq Reth. R&P Claudia Rutz. Adv. contact Simone Tremmel TEL 49-6201-606562. Circ: 2,000. **Subscr. in the Americas to:** John Wiley & Sons, Inc., Journals, PO Box 661, Holmes, PA 19043. TEL 44-1243-779777, 212-850-6645, FAX 212-850-6021; **Subscr. outside Germany, Austria & Switzerland to:** John Wiley & Sons Ltd., Baffins Ln, Chichester, Sussex PO19 IUD, United Kingdom. TEL 44-1243-779777, FAX 44-1243-843232.

EXCERPTA MEDICA. SECTION 26: IMMUNOLOGY, SEROLOGY AND TRANSPLANTATION. see *MEDICAL SCIENCES—Abstracting, Bibliographies, Statistics*

EXERCISE IMMUNOLOGY REVIEW. see *MEDICAL SCIENCES—Sports Medicine*

F E M S IMMUNOLOGY AND MEDICAL MICROBIOLOGY. see *BIOLOGY—Microbiology*

616.97 GBR ISSN 1468-8530
▼ **FOOD ALLERGY AND INTOLERANCE JOURNAL**; a journal for the world food industry. Text in English. 2000. 3/yr. EUR 195; GBP 155 to members (effective 2002). **Document type:** *Journal.* **Description:** Aims to increase awareness within the world food industry of new developments and technology in all areas relating to food allergy and intolerance, and contains articles written by international experts specializing in the area of food allergy and intolerance.
Published by: Leatherhead Food R.A., Randalls Rd, Leatherhead, Surrey KT22 7RY, United Kingdom. TEL 44-1372-376761, FAX 44-1372-386228, hbennett@lfra.co.uk, http://www.ifra.co.uk. Ed. Victoria Emerton.

616 USA ISSN 1075-4318
CODEN: FANEF3
FOOD ALLERGY NEWS. Text in English. bi-m. membership. **Document type:** *Newsletter.*
Published by: Food Allergy Network, 10400 Eaton Pl, Fairfax, VA 22030-2208. TEL 703-691-3179, http://www.foodallergy.org. Ed., Pub. Anne Munoz-Furlong. R&P Mary Jo Widmer.

615.37 DEU ISSN 0016-6006
DIE GELBEN HEFTE. Text in German. 1961. q. DEM 36 (effective 2001). illus. cum.index. **Document type:** *Academic/Scholarly.*
—GNLM.
Published by: Die Medizinische Verlagsgesellschaft Umwelt & Medizin mbH, Scharderhohlweg 35, Koenigstein 61462, Germany. TEL 49-69-638204, FAX 49-69-637109. Ed. Dr. Dietmar Nedde. Circ: 20,000.

GROWTH FACTORS & CYTOKINES - CLINICAL. see *MEDICAL SCIENCES—Abstracting, Bibliographies, Statistics*

GROWTH FACTORS & CYTOKINES - RESEARCH. see *MEDICAL SCIENCES—Abstracting, Bibliographies, Statistics*

H I V COUNSELOR PERSPECTIVES. (Human Immunodeficiency Virus) see *MEDICAL SCIENCES—Communicable Diseases*

▼ **H I V MEDICINE.** (Human Immunodeficiency Virus) see *MEDICAL SCIENCES—Communicable Diseases*

616 USA
HEALTHLINES SAY; support for the asthmatic youth. Text in English. bi-m. free. **Document type:** *Newsletter, Consumer.* **Description:** Written by and for adolescents living with asthma and allergies. Contains tips and a question and answer column written by a physician.
Published by: Asthma and Allergy Foundation of America, 1233, 20th St N W No 402, Washington, DC 20036-2330. TEL 202-466-7643, 800-727-8462, FAX 202-466-8940, info@aafa.org, http://www.aafa.org.

HEMATOLOGIA, CITOQUINAS, INMUNOTERAPIA Y TERAPIA CELULAR. see *MEDICAL SCIENCES—Hematology*

616.97 USA ISSN 1535-2048
▼ **HIV TREATMENT ALERTS!.** Text in English. 2001. 3/yr. back issues avail. *Refereed.* **Document type:** *Newsletter, Consumer.* **Description:** Intended for those affected by HIV/AIDS and their caregivers.
Related titles: Online - full text ed.
Published by: The Center for AIDS, Hope & Remembrance Project, 1407 Hawthorne, Houston, TX 77006. Ed., R&P Thomas Gegeny. Pub. L. Joel Martinez. Circ: 5,000 (controlled).

HOKKAIDO UNIVERSITY. INSTITUTE OF IMMUNOLOGICAL SCIENCE. BULLETIN. see *MEDICAL SCIENCES—Respiratory Diseases*

616.9 NLD ISSN 1093-2607
QR185.8.H93 CODEN: HUANFP
HUMAN ANTIBODIES. Text in English. 1990. q. EUR 324, USD 292 to institutions (effective 2002). adv. bk.rev. abstr, illus. index. back issues avail. *Refereed.* **Document type:** *Academic/Scholarly.* **Description:** Publishes original contributions on all aspects of hybridoma and antibody engineering, science and technology covering basic research, applied science and clinical applications.
Formerly: Human Antibodies and Hybridomas (0956-960X)
Related titles: Microfilm ed.: (from PQC); Online - full text ed.: (from Swets Blackwell, RoweCom Information Quest).
Indexed: AIDS & Cancer Res., Excerp.Med., INIS Atomind., Immun.Abstr., Ind.Med. (1997-).
—ADONIS, CASDDS, EMDOCS, GNLM, Infotrieve, KNAW. **CCC.**
Published by: I O S Press, Nieuwe Hemweg 6B, Amsterdam 1013 BG, Netherlands. TEL 31-20-688-3355, FAX 31-20-620-3419, market@iospress.nl. Ed. Dr. Mark C Glassy TEL 858-566-9490. **Subscr. to:** I O S Press, Inc, 5795-G Burke Centre Pkwy, Burke, VA 22015. TEL 703-323-5554, FAX 703-323-3668, iosbooks@iospress.com; Globe Publication Pvt. Ltd., C-62 Inderpuri, New Delhi 100 012, India. TEL 91-11-579-3211, 91-11-579-3212, FAX 91-11-579-8876, custserve@globepub.com, http://www.globepub.com; Kinokuniya Company Ltd, Shinjuku 3-chome, Shinjuku-ku, Tokyo 160-0022, Japan. FAX 81-3-3439-1094, journal@kinokuniya.co.jp, http://www.kinokuniya.co.jp.

616.97 USA ISSN 0198-8859
QR180 CODEN: HUIMDQ
HUMAN IMMUNOLOGY. Text in English. 1980. 12/yr. EUR 185 in Europe to qualified personnel; JPY 24,600 in Japan to qualified personnel; USD 207 elsewhere to qualified personnel; EUR 1,140 in Europe to institutions; JPY 151,300 in Japan to institutions; USD 1,274 elsewhere to institutions (effective 2002). Supplement avail.; back issues avail.; reprint service avail. from SWZ. *Refereed.* **Document type:** *Academic/Scholarly.* **Description:** Provides information on the immune system of man and the analogous systems of other vertebrates, emphasizing topics in histocompatibility and immunogenetics.
Related titles: Microform ed.: (from PQC); Online - full text ed.: (from EBSCO Publishing, ingenta, Swets Blackwell, ScienceDirect, Institute for Scientific Information).
Indexed: AIDS & Cancer Res., ASCA, Biol.Abstr., Chem.Abstr., Chem.Indus.Notes, Chem.Titles, Curr.Adv.Cancer Res., Curr.Adv.Gen.& Molec.Biol., Curr.Cont., Excerp.Med., Helminthol.Abstr., INIS Atomind., Immun.Abstr., Ind.Med. (1980-), Ind.Sci.Rev., Inpharma, Int.Abstr.Biol.Sci., Neurosci.Cit.Ind., Pharm.&Out.News, Reac., Sci.Cit.Ind., So.Pac.Per.Ind., Weed Abstr.
—BLDSC (4336.160000), CASDDS, CISTI, GNLM, IDS, ingenta, KNAW. **CCC.**

M

Published by: (American Society for Histocompatibility and Immunogenetics), Elsevier Science, 655 Ave of the Americas, New York, NY 10010. TEL 212-989-5800, FAX 212-633-3990, usinfo-f@elsevier.com, http://www.elsevier.com/locate/humimm. Ed. N Suiu Foca. **Subscr. in Australasia and the Far East to:** Elsevier Science (Singapore) Pte Ltd, No.1 Temasek Ave, 17-01 Millenia Tower, Singapore 039192, Singapore. TEL 65-434-3727, FAX 65-337-2230; **Subscr. in Japan to:** Elsevier Science Inc - Japan Regional Office, 9-15 Higashi-Azabu 1-chome, Minato-ku, Tokyo 106-0044, Japan. TEL 81-3-5561-5033; **Subscr. outside the Americas to:** Elsevier Science BV, PO Box 211, Amsterdam 1000 AE, Netherlands. TEL 31-20-485-3757.

616.97 USA ISSN 1074-7613
QR180 CODEN: IUNIEH
IMMUNITY. Text in English. 1994. m. USD 90 domestic to individuals; USD 125 in Canada to individuals; USD 140 elsewhere to individuals; USD 571 domestic to institutions; USD 608 in Canada to institutions; USD 630 elsewhere to institutions; USD 50 newsstand/cover (effective 2001); Individual price includes online access. adv. abstr. *Refereed.* **Document type:** *Academic/Scholarly.* **Description:** Publishes research articles and reviews of broad interest in the entire discipline of immunology.
Related titles: Online - full text ed.: USD 90 (effective 2001) (from HighWire Pr., ingenta, Institute for Scientific Information).
Indexed: AIDS & Cancer Res., ASCA, Aqua.Sci.& Fish.Abstr., Chem.Abstr., Chem.Indus.Notes, Chem.Titles, Curr.Cont., Environ.Sci.Poll.Mgmt., Excerp.Med. (1995-), Genet.Abstr., Hum.Gen.Abstr., Immun.Abstr., Ind.Med. (1994-), Ind.Sci.Rev., Inpharma, Microbiol.Abstr., Neurosci.Abstr., Nuc.Acids Abstr., Pollut.Abstr., Protozool.Abstr., Reac., Saf.Sci.Abstr., Sci.Cit.Ind., Trop.Dis.Bull.
—BLDSC (4369.649000), ADONIS, CASDDS, CISTI, GNLM, ingenta, KNAW.
Published by: Cell Press (Subsidiary of: Reed Elsevier plc), 1100 Massachusetts Ave, Cambridge, MA 02138. TEL 617-661-7057, FAX 617-661-7061, editor@immunity.com, http://www.immunity.com, http://www.cellpress.com. Pub. Lynne Herndon.

IMMUNOANALYSE ET BIOLOGIE SPECIALISEE. see *BIOLOGY*

IMMUNOASSAY. see *MEDICAL SCIENCES—Abstracting, Bibliographies, Statistics*

616.07 NLD ISSN 0926-2067
THE IMMUNOASSAY KIT DIRECTORY. SERIES A: CLINICAL CHEMISTRY. Text in English. 1991. 5/yr. USD 560 in United States to institutions. back issues avail. *Refereed.* **Document type:** *Directory.* **Description:** Comprehensive, independent reference source listing commercially available immunoassay kits, including information on assay and sample type, number of tests, antibodies and antigens used, sensitivity, and limitations.
—GNLM, Infotrieve. **CCC.**
Published by: Kluwer Academic Publishers Group (Subsidiary of: Wolters Kluwer N.V.), Spuiboulevard 50, PO Box 17, Dordrecht 3300 AA, Netherlands. FAX 31-78-639-2254, services@wkap.nl, http://www.wkap.nl. Ed. Dr. John Seth. **Dist. by:** Journals Department, PO Box 322, Dordrecht 3300 AH, Netherlands. FAX 31-78-654-6474.

616 NLD ISSN 1381-5067
THE IMMUNOASSAY KIT DIRECTORY. SERIES B: INFECTIOUS DISEASES. Text in English. 1995. 3/yr. NLG 850 domestic to institutions; USD 486 in United States to institutions. **Document type:** *Directory.* **Description:** Provides an independent reference source on immunoassay kits for the diagnosis of clinically important infectious diseases.
—GNLM.
Published by: Kluwer Academic Publishers Group (Subsidiary of: Wolters Kluwer N.V.), Spuiboulevard 50, PO Box 17, Dordrecht 3300 AA, Netherlands. FAX 31-78-639-2254, services@wkap.nl, http://www.wkap.nl. Ed. Hugh Young. **Dist. by:** Journals Department, PO Box 322, Dordrecht 3300 AH, Netherlands. FAX 31-78-654-6474.

615.37 DEU ISSN 0171-2985
QR180 CODEN: IMMND4
IMMUNOBIOLOGY; experimental and clinical. Text and summaries in English. 1909. 5/yr. EUR 149, GBP 210 to individuals; EUR 711, GBP 540 to institutions (effective 2002). *Refereed.* **Document type:** *Journal, Academic/Scholarly.*
Former titles: Zeitschrift fuer Immunitaetsforschung - Immunologie; Zeitschrift fuer Immunitaetsforschung, Experimentelle und Klinische Immunologie (0300-872X)
Related titles: Microform ed.: (from PMC); Online - full text ed.; (from Institute for Scientific Information); ♦ Supplement: Immunobiology. Supplement. ISSN 0722-6365.
Indexed: AIDS & Cancer Res., ASCA, Anim.Breed.Abstr., Aqua.Sci.& Fish.Abstr., Biol.Abstr., Chem.Abstr., Chem.Indus.Notes, Chem.Titles, Curr.Adv.Gen.& Molec.Biol., Curr.Cont., Environ.Sci.Poll.Mgmt., Excerp.Med., Genet.Abstr., Helminthol.Abstr., Hum.Gen.Abstr., INIS Atomind., Immun.Abstr., Ind.Med. (1979-), Ind.Sci.Rev., Ind.Vet., Inpharma, Int.Abstr.Biol.Sci., Med.& Pharm.Biotech.Abstr., Microbiol.Abstr., Nuc.Acids Abstr., Poult.Abstr., Reac., Sci.Cit.Ind., Vet.Bull.
—BLDSC (4369.656000), CASDDS, CISTI, GNLM, IDS, Infotrieve, ingenta, KNAW. **CCC.**
Published by: Urban & Fischer Verlag, Loebdergraben 14a, Jena 07743, Germany. TEL 49-3641-626444, FAX 49-3641-626500, marketing.journals@urbanfischer.de, http://www.urbanfischer.de/journals. Ed. D Gemsa. R&P Martin Huber TEL 49-3641-626430. Circ: 600. **Subscr. to:** Nature Publishing Group, Brunel Rd, Basingstoke RG21 6XS, United Kingdom. TEL 44-1256-302629, FAX 44-1256-463570, j.stephens@macmillan.com.

615.37 DEU ISSN 0722-6365
IMMUNOBIOLOGY. SUPPLEMENT. Text in English. 1987. irreg. **Document type:** *Monographic series, Academic/Scholarly.*
Related titles: ♦ Supplement to: Immunobiology. ISSN 0171-2985.
Published by: Urban & Fischer Verlag, Loebdergraben 14a, Jena 07743, Germany. TEL 49-721-165123, FAX 49-721-165103.

IMMUNOFACTS VACCINES & IMMUNOLOGIC DRUGS. see *PHARMACY AND PHARMACOLOGY*

IMMUNOGENETICS. see *BIOLOGY—Genetics*

616.97 USA ISSN 0257-277X
CODEN: IMRSEB
IMMUNOLOGIC RESEARCH; a selective reference to current research and practice. Text in English. 1982. bi-m. USD 450 domestic; USD 460 foreign (effective 2000). adv. back issues avail. *Refereed.* **Document type:** *Journal, Academic/Scholarly.* **Description:** Encompasses the immunologic subspecialites including cellular, molecular, genetic and biochemical, as well as clinical and pathological aspects of immunologic research.
Formerly: Survey of Immunologic Research (0252-9564)
Related titles: Microform ed.: (from PQC); Online - full text ed.: (from Institute for Scientific Information).
Indexed: AIDS & Cancer Res., ASCA, Anim.Breed.Abstr., Aqua.Sci.& Fish.Abstr., Chem.Abstr., Chem.Indus.Notes, Chem.Titles, Curr.Adv.Ecol.Sci., Curr.Cont., Dent.Ind., Environ.Sci.Poll.Mgmt., Excerp.Med., Immun.Abstr., Ind.Med. (1986-), Ind.Sci.Rev., Ind.Vet., Inpharma, Microbiol.Abstr., Pig News & Info., Reac., Sci.Cit.Ind., Telegen.
—BLDSC (4369.677800), ADONIS, CASDDS, CISTI, EMDOCS, GNLM, IDS, ingenta. **CCC.**
Published by: Humana Press Inc., 999 Riverview Dr, Ste 208, Totowa, NJ 07512. TEL 973-256-1699, FAX 973-256-8341, humana@humanapr.com, http://humanapress.com. Eds. Dr. Julius M Cruse, Robert E Lewis Jr. R&P Richard Hruska. Adv. contact Thomas B Lanigan Jr. **Dist. in Japan by:** Maruzen Co., Ltd., International Division, Export Dept, P.O. Box 5050, Tokyo International 100-3191, Japan. TEL 81-3-3275-8591.

576 USA ISSN 0882-0139
QR180 CODEN: IMINEJ
IMMUNOLOGICAL INVESTIGATIONS; a journal of molecular and cellular immunology. Text in English. 1972. q. USD 115 to individuals print and online eds.; USD 1,095 to institutions print only (effective 2002). adv. bk.rev. charts, illus. index. *Refereed.* **Document type:** *Academic/Scholarly.* **Description:** Encompasses all facets of fundamental and applied immunology, including immunohematology and the study of allergies.
Formerly: Immunological Communications (0090-0877); Incorporates (1982-1985): Clinical Immunology Reviews (0277-9366)
Related titles: Microform ed.: (from RPI); Online - full content ed.; Online - full text ed.: (from Institute for Scientific Information).
Indexed: AIDS & Cancer Res., ASCA, Anim.Breed.Abstr., Aqua.Sci.& Fish.Abstr., Biol.Abstr., Chem.Abstr., Chem.Indus.Notes, Chem.Titles, Curr.Adv.Cell & Devel.Biol., Curr.Adv.Ecol.Sci., Curr.Cont., Dairy Sci.Abstr., Environ.Sci.Poll.Mgmt., Excerp.Med., Helminthol.Abstr., INIS Atomind., Immun.Abstr., Ind.Med. (1985-), Ind.Sci.Rev., Ind.Vet., Inpharma, Int.Abstr.Biol.Sci., Microbiol.Abstr., Nutr.Abstr., Pharm.&Out.News, Protozool.Abstr., Reac., Ref.Zh., Rev.Arom.& Med.Plants, Sci.Cit.Ind., Telegen, Vet.Bull.
—BLDSC (4369.682500), CASDDS, CISTI, EMDOCS, GNLM, IDS, ingenta, KNAW. **CCC.**
Published by: Marcel Dekker Inc., 270 Madison Ave, New York, NY 10016. TEL 212-696-9000, 800-228-1160, FAX 212-685-4540, http://www.dekker.com/servlet/product/productid/IMM. Ed. Carel J Van Oss. R&P Julia Mulligan. Adv. contact Anne Mullins. B&W page USD 800. Circ: 375.

617 612 DNK ISSN 0105-2896
CODEN: IMRED2
IMMUNOLOGICAL REVIEWS. Text in English. 1969. bi-m. USD 540 in the Americas to institutions print & online eds. combined; GBP 375 elsewhere to institutions print & online eds. combined (effective 2002). adv. illus. reprint service avail. from ISI. *Refereed.* **Document type:** *Academic/Scholarly.*
Formerly: Transplantation Reviews (0082-5948)
Related titles: Online - full text ed.: ISSN 1600-065X. GBP 337 (2002) (from Ovid Technologies, Inc., Swets Blackwell, Institute for Scientific Information).
Indexed: AIDS & Cancer Res., ASCA, Anim.Breed.Abstr., Biol.Abstr., Chem.Abstr., Chem.Indus.Notes, Chem.Titles, Curr.Adv.Ecol.Sci., Curr.Adv.Gen.& Molec.Biol., Curr.Biotech.Abstr., Curr.Cont., Environ.Sci.Poll.Mgmt., Excerp.Med., Helminthol.Abstr., Immun.Abstr., Ind.Med. (1977-), Ind.Sci.Rev., Inpharma, Int.Abstr.Biol.Sci., Microbiol.Abstr., Pharm.&Out.News, Reac., Sci.Cit.Ind., Telegen.
—BLDSC (4369.687000), ADONIS, CASDDS, CISTI, GNLM, IDS, ingenta. **CCC.**
Published by: Blackwell Munksgaard, Noerre Soegade 35, PO Box 2148, Copenhagen K 1016, Denmark. TEL 45-77-33-33-33, FAX 45-77-33-33-77, fsub@munksgaard.dk, http://journals.munksgaard.dk/immunologicalreviews, http://www.munksgaard.dk. Ed. Peter Parnam. Adv. contact Eric Rozario TEL 45-77-33-33-01. Circ: 1,600.

616.97 DEU ISSN 1435-2842
IMMUNOLOGIE UND IMPFEN. Text in German. 1998. q. DEM 157 domestic; DEM 165.60 foreign (effective 2001). *Refereed.* **Document type:** *Journal, Academic/Scholarly.* **Description:** Covers all aspects of immunology and infection.
Related titles: Online - full text ed.: ISSN 1435-862X (from EBSCO Publishing, RoweCom Information Quest, Swets Blackwell, Springer LINK).
Published by: Springer-Verlag (Subsidiary of: BertelsmannSpringer), Tiergartenstr 17, Heidelberg 69121, Germany. TEL 49-6221-345-0, FAX 49-6221-345229, subscriptions@springer.de, http://link.springer.de/link/service/journals/10102/index.htm, http://www.springer.de. Ed. H von Prondzynsji. **Subscr. in N. America to:** Springer-Verlag New York Inc., PO Box 2485, Secaucus, NJ 07096-2485. TEL 212-460-1500, FAX 212-473-6272.

616.97 USA ISSN 1192-5612
CODEN: INOLEG
THE IMMUNOLOGIST. Text in English. 1993. 6/yr. USD 68 to non-members; USD 44 to members; USD 78 to institutions (effective 2001). *Refereed.* **Document type:** *Journal, Academic/Scholarly.* **Description:** Serves as a forum for all matters immunological, including society news and official proposals and discussions, as well as for interesting arguments, critical analyses of products, meeting reports and the latest clinical or research techniques.
Related titles: Online - full text ed.: (from Institute for Scientific Information).
Indexed: Chem.Abstr., Chem.Indus.Notes, Chem.Titles, Curr.Cont., Inpharma, Int.Abstr.Biol.Sci., Pharm.&Out.News, Reac., Ref.Zh.
—BLDSC (4369.688000), CASDDS, EMDOCS, GNLM, IDS, Infotrieve, KNAW. **CCC.**
Published by: (International Union of Immunological Societies), Hogrefe & Huber Publishers, PO Box 2487, Kirkland, WA 98083. TEL 425-820-1500, FAX 425-823-8324. Ed. J B Natvig. Circ: 5,000.
Co-sponsor: Clinical Immunology Society.

M

616.97 RUS ISSN 0206-4952
CODEN: IMUNDA

IMMUNOLOGIYA/IMMUNOLOGY. Text in Russian; Summaries in English. 1980. bi-m. USD 206 foreign (effective 2000). adv. Website rev. abstr. reprints avail. **Document type:** *Journal, Academic/Scholarly.* **Description:** Publishes data on original investigations in immunogenetics, molecular and cellular immunology, immunochemistry, biochemistry of immunogenesis, immunomorphology, functional bases of immunity, immunology of allergic reaction, clinical immunology and immunopathology.
Indexed: Biol.Abstr., Chem.Abstr., Chem.Indus.Notes, Chem.Titles, Excerp.Med., INIS Atomind., Ref.Zh.
—BLDSC (0086.168250), CASDDS, CISTI, East View, GNLM.
Published by: Izdatel'stvo Meditsina, Petroverigskii per 6-8, Moscow 101000, Russian Federation. TEL 7-095-9248785, 7-095-928-86-48, FAX 7-095-9211355, 7-095-9286003, http://www.medit.ru. Ed. R M Khaitov. Pub. A M Stochik. R&P G Gavrikova. Adv. contact O A Fadeeva TEL 7-095-923-51-40. Circ: 1,000. **Dist. by:** Mezhdunarodnaya Kniga, B Yakimanka 39, Moscow 117049, Russian Federation. TEL 7-095-2384967, FAX 7-095-2384634.

576 GBR ISSN 0019-2805
QR180 CODEN: IMMUAM

IMMUNOLOGY. Text in English. 1958. m., latest vol.105, 2002. GBP 589 in Europe; USD 938 in North America; GBP 651 elsewhere (effective 2002). adv. bk.rev. bibl, charts, illus. index. back issues avail.; reprint service avail. from ISI. *Refereed.* **Document type:** *Academic/Scholarly.* **Description:** Publishes articles on subjects of topical interest to immunologists.
Related titles: Microform ed.: (from PQC); Online - full text ed.: ISSN 1365-2567. 1998. GBP 531 in Europe; USD 845 in North America; GBP 531 elsewhere (effective 2002) (from Ovid Technologies, Inc., EBSCO Publishing, O C L C Online Computer Library Center, Inc., RoweCom Information Quest, ingenta, Munksgaard & Blackwell Science's Synergy, Swets Blackwell, Institute for Scientific Information); ♦ Supplement: Immunology. Supplement. ISSN 0953-4954.
Indexed: AIDS & Cancer Res., AIDS Abstr., Abstr.Hyg., AgBiotech, Agri.& Environ.Biotech.Abstr. (coverage dropped), Anim.Breed.Abstr., Aqua.Sci.& Fish.Abstr., Biol.Abstr., Chem.Abstr., Chem.Indus.Notes, Chem.Titles, Curr.Adv.Biochem., Curr.Adv.Ecol.Sci., Curr.Cont., Dairy Sci.Abstr., Dent.Ind., Derwent Biotech.Abstr., Diar.Dis.Res., Environ.Sci.Poll.Mgmt., Excerp.Med., Food Sci.& Tech.Abstr., Helminthol.Abstr., INIS Atomind., Immun.Abstr., Ind.Med. (1958-), Ind.Sci.Rev., Ind.Vet., Inpharma, Int.Abstr.Biol.Sci., Microbiol.Abstr., NRN, Neurosci.Cit.Ind., Nutr.Abstr., Pharm.&Out.News, Pig News & Info., Poult.Abstr., Protozool.Abstr., Reac., Rev.Appl.Entomol., Rev.Med.& Vet.Mycol., Sci.Cit.Ind., Sport Fish.Abstr., Telegen, Triticale Abstr., Trop.Dis.Bull., Vet.Bull., Virol.Abstr. (coverage dropped).
—BLDSC (4369.700000), ADONIS, CASDDS, CISTI, GNLM, IDS, ingenta, KNAW. **CCC.**
Published by: (British Society for Immunology), Blackwell Science Ltd., PO Box 88, Oxford OX2 0NE, United Kingdom. TEL 44-1865-206180, 44-1865-206002, FAX 44-1865-206219, jnl.orders@blacksci.co.uk, http://www.blackwell-science.com/products/journals/imm.htm, http://www.blackwellpublishing.com. Ed. M Kemeny. Pub. Allen Stevens. R&P Sophie Savage. Adv. contact Jenny Applin. Circ: 1,685.

616.97 USA ISSN 0889-8561
CODEN: INCAEP

IMMUNOLOGY AND ALLERGY CLINICS OF NORTH AMERICA. Text in English. 1981. q. USD 140 domestic to individuals; USD 168 in Canada to individuals; USD 188 elsewhere to individuals; USD 195 domestic to institutions; USD 235 foreign to institutions; USD 59 per issue (effective 2001). *Refereed.* **Document type:** *Journal, Academic/Scholarly.*
Formerly: Clinics in Immunology and Allergy (0260-4639)
Related titles: Online - full text ed.: (from Institute for Scientific Information).
Indexed: ASCA, CINAHL, Chem.Abstr., Curr.Adv.Ecol.Sci., Curr.Cont. (coverage dropped), Dairy Sci.Abstr., Excerp.Med., Helminthol.Abstr., Ind.Sci.Rev., Inpharma, Nutr.Abstr., Pharm.&Out.News, Reac., Rev.Med.& Vet.Mycol., SSCI (coverage dropped), Sci.Cit.Ind. (coverage dropped), Sugar Ind.Abstr.
—BLDSC (4369.701500), CASDDS, CISTI, EMDOCS, GNLM, IDS, ingenta, KNAW. **CCC.**
Published by: W.B. Saunders Co. (Subsidiary of: Harcourt Publishers Ltd.), 11830 Westline Industrial Dr, St Louis, MO 63146. TEL 800-325-4177, http://www.wbsaunders.com. **Subscr. to:** Periodicals Fulfillment, W B Saunders Co, 6277 Sea Harbor Dr, 4th Fl, Orlando, FL 32891-4800.

616.97 570 AUS ISSN 0818-9641
QH301 CODEN: ICBIEZ

IMMUNOLOGY AND CELL BIOLOGY. Text in English. 1923. bi-m. AUD 297 domestic to individuals; AUD 270 in New Zealand to individuals; USD 165 elsewhere to individuals; AUD 644 domestic to institutions; AUD 585 in New Zealand to institutions; USD 475 elsewhere to institutions; AUD 327 domestic to individuals paper & online eds. combined; AUD 237 in New Zealand to individuals paper & online eds. combined; USD 182 elsewhere to individuals paper & online eds. combined; AUD 709 domestic to institutions paper & online eds. combined; AUD 644 in New Zealand to institutions paper & online eds. combined; USD 523 elsewhere to institutions paper & online eds. combined (effective 2001). adv. charts, illus. index. *Refereed.* **Document type:** *Academic/Scholarly.* **Description:** Covers original research, methods or concepts in the broad fields of immunology and cell biology.
Formerly (until 1987): Australian Journal of Experimental Biology and Medical Science (0004-945X)
Related titles: Microfilm ed.: (from PQC,PMC); Online - full text ed.: ISSN 1440-1711. AUD 268 domestic to individuals; AUD 243 in New Zealand to individuals; USD 149 elsewhere to individuals; AUD 580 domestic to institutions; AUD 527 in New Zealand to institutions; USD 428 elsewhere to institutions (effective 2001) (from Ovid Technologies, Inc., EBSCO Publishing, O C L C Online Computer Library Center, Inc., RoweCom Information Quest, ingenta, Munksgaard & Blackwell Science's Synergy, Swets Blackwell, Institute for Scientific Information).
Indexed: AIDS & Cancer Res., ASCA, Abstr.Hyg., AgBiotech, Agroforest.Abstr., Anim.Breed.Abstr., Biol.Abstr., Chem.Abstr., Chem.Indus.Notes, Chem.Titles, Curr.Adv.Cancer Res., Curr.Adv.Ecol.Sci., Curr.Biotech.Abstr., Curr.Cont., Dairy Sci.Abstr., Dent.Ind., Diar.Dis.Res., Environ.Sci.Poll.Mgmt., Excerp.Med., Field Crop Abstr., Helminthol.Abstr., Herb.Abstr., INIS Atomind., Immun.Abstr., Ind.Med. (1987-), Ind.Sci.Rev., Ind.Vet., Inpharma, Int.Abstr.Biol.Sci., Microbiol.Abstr., Nutr.Abstr., Pharm.&Out.News, Poult.Abstr., Protozool.Abstr., Reac., Ref.Zh., Rev.Appl.Entomol., Rev.Arom.& Med.Plants, Rev.Med.& Vet.Mycol., Rural Recreat.Tour.Abstr., Sci.Cit.Ind., Trop.Dis.Bull., Vet.Bull.
—BLDSC (4369.702400), ADONIS, CASDDS, CISTI, EMDOCS, GNLM, IDS, ingenta, KNAW, Linda Hall. **CCC.**
Published by: (Australasian Society for Immunology, Australian National University, The John Curtin School of Medical Research), Blackwell Science Asia Pty Ltd, PO Box 378, Carlton South, VIC 3053, Australia. TEL 61-3-9347-0300, FAX 61-3-9347-5001, info@blacksci-asia.com.au; Christopher.Parish@anu.edu.au, http://www.blacksci.co.uk. Ed. Chris R Parish. Adv. contact Kathryn O'Brien. B&W page AUD 902, color page AUD 1,897; trim 210 x 275. Circ: 1,300.

616.97 NLD

IMMUNOLOGY AND MEDICINE. Text in English. irreg., latest vol.21, 1994. price varies. *Refereed.* **Document type:** *Monographic series.*
—BLDSC (4369.704000).
Published by: Kluwer Academic Publishers Group (Subsidiary of: Wolters Kluwer N.V.), Spuiboulevard 50, PO Box 17, Dordrecht 3300 AA, Netherlands. FAX 31-78-639-2254, services@wkap.nl, http://www.wkap.nl. Ed. Keith Whaley. **Dist. by:** Journals Department, PO Box 322, Dordrecht 3300 AH, Netherlands. FAX 31-78-654-6474.

616.97 NLD ISSN 0165-2478
CODEN: IMLED6

IMMUNOLOGY LETTERS; for the rapid publication of short reports in immunology. Text in English. 1979. 15/yr. EUR 2,135 in Europe to institutions; JPY 283,500 in Japan to institutions; USD 2,388 elsewhere to institutions (effective 2002). adv. bk.rev. abstr. back issues avail. *Refereed.* **Document type:** *Academic/Scholarly.* **Description:** Publishes research articles and minireviews on all aspects of immunology.
Related titles: Microform ed.: (from PQC); Online - full text ed.: (from ingenta, Swets Blackwell, ScienceDirect, Institute for Scientific Information).
Indexed: AIDS & Cancer Res., ASCA, Anim.Breed.Abstr., Aqua.Sci.& Fish.Abstr., Biol.Abstr., Chem.Abstr., Chem.Indus.Notes, Chem.Titles, Curr.Adv.Cancer Res., Curr.Adv.Cell & Devel.Biol., Curr.Adv.Ecol.Sci., Curr.Adv.Gen.& Molec.Biol., Curr.Cont., Dairy Sci.Abstr., Environ.Sci.Poll.Mgmt., Excerp.Med., Helminthol.Abstr., INIS Atomind., Immun.Abstr., Ind.Med. (1979-), Ind.Sci.Rev., Ind.Vet., Inpharma, Int.Abstr.Biol.Sci., Microbiol.Abstr., Pharm.&Out.News, Protozool.Abstr., Reac., Rev.Appl.Entomol., Rev.Med.& Vet.Mycol., Sci.Cit.Ind., Telegen, Vet.Bull.
—BLDSC (4369.705000), ADONIS, CASDDS, CISTI, EMDOCS, GNLM, IDS, ingenta, KNAW. **CCC.**
Published by: (European Federation of Immunological Societies (E.F.I.S.)), Elsevier Science BV, PO Box 211, Amsterdam 1000 AE, Netherlands. TEL 31-20-485-2911, FAX 31-20-485-3598, http://www.elsevier.com/locate/immlet. Ed. I Pecht. Circ: 500. **Subscr. in Australasia and the Far East to:** Elsevier Science (Singapore) Pte Ltd, No.1 Temasek Ave, 17-01 Millenia Tower, Singapore 039192, Singapore. TEL 65-434-3727, FAX 65-337-2230; **Subscr. in Japan to:** Elsevier Science Inc - Japan Regional Office, 9-15 Higashi-Azabu 1-chome, Minato-ku, Tokyo 106-0044, Japan. TEL 81-3-5561-5033; **Subscr. in the Americas to:** Elsevier Science, PO Box 945, New York, NY 10159-0945. TEL 212-633-3730, FAX 212-633-3680, usinfo-f@elsevier.com.

616.97 USA

IMMUNOLOGY SERIES. Text in English. 1973. irreg., latest vol.61, 1994. price varies. adv. *Refereed.* **Document type:** *Monographic series.*
Indexed: Chem.Abstr., Chem.Indus.Notes, Chem.Titles, Ind.Med. (coverage dropped).
Published by: Marcel Dekker, Inc., Attn: Eridania Perrez, 270 Madison Ave, New York, NY 10016-0602. TEL 212-696-9000, 800-228-1160, FAX 212-685-4540, marketing@dekker.com, http://www.dekker.com. Pub. Russell Dekker. R&P Julia Mulligan. Adv. contact Eridania Perez.

576 GBR ISSN 0953-4954

IMMUNOLOGY. SUPPLEMENT. Text in English. 1988. irreg. **Document type:** *Journal, Academic/Scholarly.*
Related titles: ♦ Supplement to: Immunology. ISSN 0019-2805.
Indexed: Ind.Med.
—ADONIS.
Published by: Blackwell Science Ltd., Osney Mead, Oxford OX2 0EL, United Kingdom. TEL 44-1685-206206, FAX 44-1685-721205, journals.cs@blacksci.co.uk, http://www.blackwell-science.com.

616.9 660 NLD ISSN 1380-2933
QR184.7 CODEN: IOTEER

IMMUNOTECHNOLOGY; an international journal of immunological engineering. Text in English. 1995. q. NLG 543, USD 312 (effective 1998). back issues avail. *Refereed.* **Document type:** *Academic/Scholarly.* **Description:** Publishes scientific reports on the application of biotechnology to cells and molecules of the immune system.
Related titles: Microform ed.: (from PQC); Online - full text ed.: (from ingenta, Swets Blackwell, ScienceDirect).
Indexed: AIDS & Cancer Res., ASCA, Biotech.Cit.Ind. (coverage dropped), Chem.Abstr., Chem.Indus.Notes, Chem.Titles, Excerp.Med. (1996-), Immun.Abstr., Ind.Med. (until 1999, dropped), Ind.Vet., Int.Abstr.Biol.Sci., Med.& Pharm.Biotech.Abstr., Nuc.Acids Abstr., Ornam.Hort., Rev.Appl.Entomol., Rev.Plant Path.
—CASDDS, CISTI, EMDOCS, GNLM, IDS, Infotrieve, KNAW. **CCC.**
Published by: Elsevier Science BV, PO Box 211, Amsterdam 1000 AE, Netherlands. TEL 31-20-485-2911, FAX 31-20-485-3598, nlinfo-f@elsevier.nl; usinfo-f@elsevier.com, http://www.elsevier.nl/. Ed. Carl A K Borrebaeck. **Subscr. in Australasia and the Far East to:** Elsevier Science (Singapore) Pte Ltd, No.1 Temasek Ave, 17-01 Millenia Tower, Singapore 039192, Singapore. TEL 65-434-3727, FAX 65-337-2230; **Subscr. in Japan to:** Elsevier Science Inc - Japan Regional Office, 9-15 Higashi-Azabu 1-chome, Minato-ku, Tokyo 106-0044, Japan. TEL 81-3-5561-5033; **Subscr. in the Americas to:** Elsevier Science, PO Box 945, New York, NY 10159-0945. TEL 212-633-3730, FAX 212-633-3680.

616.97 USA

IMMUNOTHERAPY WEEKLY. Text in English. 1997. w. (43/yr.). USD 1,549 in North America; USD 1,649 elsewhere. **Document type:** *Newsletter.*
Related titles: Online - full text ed.
Indexed: Bus.& Indus. (May 1998-).
Published by: Charles W. Henderson, Ed. & Pub., PO Box 5528, Atlanta, GA 31107-0528. TEL 770-507-7777, FAX 770-507-7788, cwhender@newsfile.com; info@hendersonnet.atl.ga.us, http://www.newsfile.com.

616 IND ISSN 0255-0857
CODEN: IJMMEF

INDIAN JOURNAL OF MEDICAL MICROBIOLOGY. Text in English. 1983. q. INR 75, USD 20.
Indexed: Chem.Abstr., Chem.Indus.Notes, Chem.Titles, Diar.Dis.Res., Excerp.Med.
—BLDSC (4416.400000), CASDDS, EMDOCS, GNLM.

Published by: Indian Association of Medical Microbiologists, c/o Dept. of Experimental Medicine, Postgraduate Institute of Medical Education and Research, Chandigarh, Haryana 160 012, India. Ed. N K Ganguly.

616.97 CHE ISSN 1420-326X CODEN: IBENFP
INDOOR AND BUILT ENVIRONMENT. Text in English. 1992. 6/yr. CHF 809, EUR 577.80 in Europe to institutions; CHF 826.40, USD 631 elsewhere to institutions (effective 2002). adv. back issues avail. *Refereed.* **Document type:** *Journal, Academic/Scholarly.* **Description:** Publishes original reports on topics pertaining to the quality of indoor air and environment, and how these might affect the health, performance, efficiency and comfort of persons so exposed.
Formerly (until 1996): Indoor Environment (1016-4901)
Related titles: Microform ed.: (from PQC); Online - full text ed.: ISSN 1423-0070. CHF 58, EUR 42, USD 45 to institutions with print edition (effective 2002) (from EBSCO Publishing, O C L C Online Computer Library Center, Inc., RoweCom Information Quest, Swets Blackwell, Institute for Scientific Information).
Indexed: ASCA, Abstr.Hyg., Chem.Abstr., Chem.Indus.Notes, Chem.Titles, Environ.Per.Bibl. (1994-), Environ.Sci.Poll.Mgmt., INIS Atomind., Int.Build.Serv.Abstr., Pollut.Abstr., Risk Abstr., Saf.Sci.Abstr., Tox.Abstr., Trop.Dis.Bull.
—BLDSC (4438.046800), CASDDS, CISTI, GNLM, IDS, Infotrieve, ingenta, KNAW. **CCC.**
Published by: (International Society of the Built Environment), S. Karger AG, Allschwilerstr 10, PO Box, Basel 4009, Switzerland. TEL 41-61-306-1111, FAX 41-61-306-1234, karger@karger.ch, http://www.online.karger.com/journals/ibe, http://www.karger.com. Ed. J A Hoskins. adv.: page USD 1,195. **Subscr. in N. America to:** S. Karger Publishers, Inc., 26 W. Avon Rd., Box 529, Farmington, CT 06085; **Subscr. in UK to:** S. Karger Publishers, 58 Grove Hill Rd, Tunbridge Wells, Kent TN1 1SP, United Kingdom.

INFECTION AND IMMUNITY. see *MEDICAL SCIENCES—Communicable Diseases*

INFECTIOUS DISEASES IN OBSTETRICS AND GYNECOLOGY. see *MEDICAL SCIENCES—Obstetrics And Gynecology*

INSTITUT PASTEUR DE DAKAR. RAPPORT SUR LE FONCTIONNEMENT TECHNIQUE. see *BIOLOGY—Microbiology*

615.37 616.97 CHE ISSN 1018-2438
RC583 CODEN: IAAIEG
INTERNATIONAL ARCHIVES OF ALLERGY AND IMMUNOLOGY. Text in English. 1950. m. (3 vols./yr.). CHF 2,961 in Europe to institutions; CHF 2,995.80 elsewhere to institutions; EUR 2,115.60 in Europe to institutions; USD 2,295 elsewhere to institutions (effective 2002). adv. bk.rev. abstr, bibl, illus. back issues avail. *Refereed.* **Document type:** *Journal, Academic/Scholarly.* **Description:** Provides a forum for all areas of modern molecular and cellular allergology and immunology.
Formerly: International Archives of Allergy and Applied Immunology (0020-5915)
Related titles: Microform ed.: (from PQC); Online - full text ed.: ISSN 1423-0097. CHF 174, EUR 126, USD 135 to institutions with print edition (effective 2002) (from EBSCO Publishing, O C L C Online Computer Library Center, Inc., RoweCom Information Quest, Swets Blackwell, Institute for Scientific Information); ♦ Supplement: Allergologicum; Transactions of the Collegium Internationale. ISSN 0065-6372.
Indexed: AIDS & Cancer Res., ASCA, Abstr.Hyg., AgBiotech, Agri.& Environ.Biotech.Abstr. (coverage dropped), Anim.Breed.Abstr., Aqua.Sci.& Fish.Abstr., Biol.Abstr., C.I.S. Abstr., Chem.Abstr., Chem.Indus.Notes, Chem.Titles, Curr.Adv.Ecol.Sci., Curr.Cont., Dairy Sci.Abstr., Dent.Ind., Derwent Biotech.Abstr., Dok.Arbeitsmed., Environ.Sci.Poll.Mgmt., Excerp.Med., Forest Prod.Abstr., Helminthol.Abstr., Herb.Abstr., INIS Atomind., Immun.Abstr., Ind.Med. (1992-), Ind.Sci.Rev., Ind.Vet., Inpharma, Int.Abstr.Biol.Sci., NRN, Nutr.Abstr., Pharm.&Out.News, Pig News & Info., Plant Breed.Abstr., Reac., Rev.Appl.Entomol., Rev.Med.& Vet.Mycol., Rev.Plant Path., Sci.Cit.Ind., Seed Abstr., THA, Trop.Dis.Bull., Vet.Bull., Weed Abstr.
—BLDSC (4536.050000), CASDDS, CISTI, EMDOCS, GNLM, IDS, ingenta, KNAW. **CCC.**
Published by: S. Karger AG, Allschwilerstr 10, PO Box, Basel 4009, Switzerland. TEL 41-61-306-1111, FAX 41-61-306-1234, karger@karger.ch, http://www.online.karger.com/journals/iaa, http://www.karger.com. Ed. D Kraft. adv.: page USD 1,185. Circ: 1,400.

INTERNATIONAL ASSOCIATION OF PHYSICIANS IN AIDS CARE. JOURNAL. see *MEDICAL SCIENCES—Communicable Diseases*

616.97 GBR ISSN 0953-8178 CODEN: INIMEN
INTERNATIONAL IMMUNOLOGY. Text in English. 1989. m. GBP 215, USD 365 to individuals; GBP 510, USD 905 to institutions (effective 2002). adv. back issues avail. *Refereed.* **Document type:** *Journal, Academic/Scholarly.* **Description:** Publishes a broad range of experimental and theoretical studies in molecular and cellular immunology conducted in laboratories throughout the world.
Related titles: Online - full text ed.: ISSN 1460-2377. GBP 459, USD 814 to institutions Online only (effective 2002) (from HighWire Pr., Northern Light Technology, Inc., EBSCO Publishing, O C L C Online Computer Library Center, Inc., RoweCom Information Quest, ingenta, Swets Blackwell, Institute for Scientific Information).
Indexed: AIDS & Cancer Res., ASCA, AgBiotech, Anim.Breed.Abstr., Aqua.Sci.& Fish.Abstr., Chem.Abstr., Chem.Indus.Notes, Chem.Titles, Curr.Cont., Helminthol.Abstr., Immun.Abstr., Ind.Med. (1989-), Ind.Sci.Rev., Ind.Vet., Inpharma, Int.Abstr.Biol.Sci., Pharm.&Out.News, Protozool.Abstr., Reac., Rev.Appl.Entomol., Rev.Med.& Vet.Mycol., Sci.Cit.Ind.
—BLDSC (4541.038930), CASDDS, CISTI, EMDOCS, GNLM, IDS, ingenta, KNAW. **CCC.**
Published by: (Japanese Society of Immunology), Oxford University Press, Academic Division, Great Clarendon St, Oxford OX2 6DP, United Kingdom. TEL 44-1865-267907, FAX 44-1865-267835, jnl.info@oup.co.uk, http://www.oup.co.uk/intimm/, http://www.oup.co.uk/journals. Ed. Tomio Tada. Pubs. Mandy Sketch, Toyoshi Onji. R&P Fionna Willis. adv.: page GBP 410, page USD 760. Circ: 1,150. **U.S. subscr. to:** Oxford University Press, Journals, 2001 Evans Rd, Cary, NC 27513. TEL 800-852-7323, FAX 919-677-1714, jnl.info@oup.co.uk; **Subscr. to:** Journals Marketing, Great Clarendon St, Oxford OX2 6DP, United Kingdom.

▼ **INTERNATIONAL IMMUNOPHARMACOLOGY.** see *PHARMACY AND PHARMACOLOGY*

INTERNATIONAL JOURNAL OF ALTERNATIVE & COMPLEMENTARY MEDICINE. see *ALTERNATIVE MEDICINE*

616.07 CHE ISSN 1560-4284
INTERNATIONAL JOURNAL OF EXPERIMENTAL DIABETES RESEARCH. Text in English. 4/yr. GBP 61, USD 73, EUR 81 to individuals; GBP 162, USD 242, EUR 218 to institutions; GBP 219, USD 361, EUR 327 to corporations (effective 2002).
Published by: Gordon and Breach - Harwood Academic (Subsidiary of: Taylor & Francis Group), PO Box 531, Lausanne 1000, Switzerland. TEL 41-21-6411280, http://www.gbhap-us.com/. Ed. Anders A F Sima.

616.97 615.19 ITA ISSN 0394-6320 CODEN: IJIPE4
INTERNATIONAL JOURNAL OF IMMUNOPATHOLOGY AND PHARMACOLOGY. Text in Italian. 1988. 3/yr. ITL 49,000, USD 49 to individuals; ITL 190,000, USD 190 to institutions. adv. *Refereed.* **Document type:** *Academic/Scholarly.*
Related titles: Online - full text ed.: (from Institute for Scientific Information).
Indexed: AIDS & Cancer Res., ASCA, Chem.Abstr., Chem.Indus.Notes, Chem.Titles, Curr.Cont. (coverage dropped), Environ.Sci.Poll.Mgmt., Excerp.Med., Immun.Abstr., Int.Abstr.Biol.Sci., Microbiol.Abstr., Sci.Cit.Ind. (coverage dropped).
—BLDSC (4542.300500), CASDDS, EMDOCS, GNLM, IDS, KNAW.
Published by: Biomedical Research Press s.a.s., c/o Universita di Chieti, Depto. di Immunologia, Via dei Vestini, Chieti, CH 66100, Italy. TEL 39-871-355293, FAX 39-871-561635. Ed. Dr. Pio Conti. R&P R C Barbacane. Adv. contact Renato Barbacane. Circ: 600.

616.97 CHE ISSN 0255-9625 CODEN: IJIMET
INTERNATIONAL JOURNAL OF IMMUNOTHERAPY. Short title: Immunotherapy. Text in English. 1985. q. CHF 400 (effective 2002). reprint service avail. from PQC. *Refereed.* **Document type:** *Journal, Academic/Scholarly.*
Related titles: Online - full text ed.: (from Institute for Scientific Information).
Indexed: AIDS & Cancer Res., ASCA, Chem.Abstr., Chem.Indus.Notes, Chem.Titles, Curr.Cont., Dairy Sci.Abstr., Derwent Biotech.Abstr., Environ.Sci.Poll.Mgmt., Excerp.Med., Immun.Abstr., Ind.Sci.Rev., Inpharma, Int.Abstr.Biol.Sci., Microbiol.Abstr., Nutr.Abstr., Pharm.&Out.News, Reac., Ref.Zh., Sci.Cit.Ind., Telegen.
—BLDSC (4542.302000), CASDDS, CISTI, EMDOCS, GNLM, IDS, KNAW. **CCC.**
Published by: Bioscience Ediprint Inc., Rue Alexandre Gavard 16, Carouge 1227, Switzerland. TEL 41-22-3003383, FAX 41-22-3002489, bioscience.smey@gkb.com. Ed. A Bertelli.

616.97 POL ISSN 1232-9142
INTERNATIONAL REVIEW OF ALLERGOLOGY AND CLINICAL IMMUNOLOGY. Text in English; Summaries in Polish. 1994. q. PLZ 40 domestic; USD 100 foreign (effective 2002). Website rev. illus. 80 p./no. 2 cols./p. *Refereed.* **Document type:** *Journal, Academic/Scholarly.* **Description:** Presents original papers, case reports on allergology and clinical immunology.
Related titles: E-mail ed.
—BLDSC (4546.110000), GNLM.
Published by: MedPress, Ul Slonki 67, Warsaw 02814, Poland. TEL 48-22-6252420, FAX 48-22-6252420, medpress@waw.pdi.net. Ed. Tadeusz Plusa.

616.97 CHE ISSN 0883-0185 CODEN: IRIMEH
INTERNATIONAL REVIEWS OF IMMUNOLOGY. Text in English. 1986. bi-m. GBP 137, USD 181, EUR 181 to individuals; GBP 888, USD 1,272, EUR 1,275 to institutions; GBP 1,460, USD 2,109, EUR 1,919 to corporations (effective 2002). back issues avail. *Refereed.* **Document type:** *Journal, Academic/Scholarly.* **Description:** Provides current information on research in immunology.
Related titles: CD-ROM ed.; Online - full text ed.: (from EBSCO Publishing, RoweCom Information Quest).
Indexed: Ind.Med. (1986-), Int.Abstr.Biol.Sci.
—BLDSC (4547.310000), CISTI, GNLM, KNAW. **CCC.**
Published by: Gordon and Breach - Harwood Academic (Subsidiary of: Taylor & Francis Group), PO Box 531, Lausanne 1000, Switzerland. TEL 41-21-6411280, FAX 41-21-6411281, info@gbhap.com, http://www.gbhap.com/IR_Immunology/. Ed. Dr. Constantin Bona. **Subscr. addr. in US:** International Publishers Direct, PO Box 32160, Newark, NJ 07102. FAX 215-750-6343.

616.97 RUS ISSN 0202-7046
ITOGI NAUKI I TEKHNIKI. IMMUNOLOGIYA. Text in Russian. irreg.
—Linda Hall.
Published by: Vserossiiskii Institut Nauchnoi i Tekhnicheskoi Informatsii (VINITI), Usievicha ul 20-a, Moscow 125315, Russian Federation. TEL 7-095-1526441, FAX 7-095-943-0060. **US dist. addr.:** East View Publications, 3020 Harbor Ln N, Minneapolis, MN 55447. TEL 612-550-0961.

616.97 CHE
JA! - WIR ATMEN. Text in German. 1989. 6/yr. CHF 20. bk.rev. **Document type:** *Bulletin.*
Formerly: Band
Published by: Das Band- Selbsthilfe der Asthmatiker, Gryphenhuebeliweg 40, Bern, 6 3000, Switzerland. TEL 41-31-3521138, FAX 41-31-3516185. Ed. Zuzana Fajfr. Circ: 10,000.

589.2 FRA ISSN 1156-5233 CODEN: JMYME
JOURNAL DE MYCOLOGIE MEDICALE. Text in English, French. 1960. 4/yr. FRF 980; FRF 1,234 foreign (effective 2000). adv. bk.rev. illus. *Refereed.* **Document type:** *Academic/Scholarly.* **Description:** Aims to improve understanding of fungal diseases and mycoses that have developed in recent years and unravel the complications they cause.
Formerly (until 1991): Societe Francaise de Mycologie Medicale. Bulletin (0037-9336)
Related titles: Online - full text ed.: (from Institute for Scientific Information, RoweCom Information Quest).

M

Indexed: ASCA, Abstr.Hyg., AgBiotech, Biol.Abstr., Curr.Cont., Dairy Sci.Abstr., Excerp.Med. (1994-), Ind.Vet., Inpharma, Pharm.&Out.News, Protozool.Abstr., Reac., Ref.Zh., Rev.Arom.& Med.Plants, Rev.Med.& Vet.Mycol., Rev.Plant Path., Small Anim.Abstr., Trop.Dis.Bull., Vet.Bull.
—BLDSC (5021.169000), CISTI, EMDOCS, GNLM, IDS, KNAW.
Published by: (Societe Francaise de Mycologie Medicale), Masson - Periodiques, 120 bd. St. Germain, Paris 75006, France. TEL 33-1-40466200, FAX 33-1-40466201. Ed. E Drouhet. Circ: 1,000. **Subscr. to:** Societe de Periodiques Specialises, BP 22, Vineuil Cedex 41354, France. TEL 33-2-54504612, FAX 33-2-54504611.

616.97 615.37 USA ISSN 0091-6749
RC583 CODEN: JACIBY
THE JOURNAL OF ALLERGY AND CLINICAL IMMUNOLOGY. Text in English. 1929. m. USD 172 domestic to individuals; USD 218 foreign to individuals; USD 350 domestic to institutions; USD 395 foreign to institutions; USD 85 domestic to students; USD 127 foreign to students; USD 33 newsstand/cover (effective 2001). adv. abstr, charts, illus. index. Supplement avail.; reprint service avail. from PQC. *Refereed.* **Document type:** *Journal, Academic/Scholarly.* **Description:** Articles on the clinical manifestations of allergies for the clinical allergist and immunologist, dermatologist, general practitioner, pediatrician and otolaryngologist.
Formerly: Journal of Allergy (0021-8707); Which incorporated: Allergy Abstracts
Related titles: CD-ROM ed.; Microfilm ed.: (from PQC,PMC); Online - full text ed.: (from Ovid Technologies, Inc., EBSCO Publishing, IDEAL Online Library, Institute for Scientific Information, RoweCom Information Quest); Alternate Frequency ed.: ISSN 1085-8725.
Indexed: AIDS & Cancer Res., AIM, ASCA, Abstr.Hyg., AgBiotech, Agri.& Environ.Biotech.Abstr. (coverage dropped), Apic.Abstr., Aqua.Sci.& Fish.Abstr., Biol.Abstr., Biol.Dig., Chem.Abstr., Chem.Indus.Notes, Chem.Titles, Curr.Cont., Dairy Sci.Abstr., Derwent Biotech.Abstr., Dok.Arbeitsmed., Entomol.Abstr. (coverage dropped), Environ.Sci.Poll.Mgmt., Excerp.Med., Fababean Abstr., Food Sci.& Tech.Abstr., Forest Prod.Abstr., Forest.Abstr., Helminthol.Abstr., INIS Atomind., I.P.A., Immun.Abstr., Ind.Med. (1971-), Ind.Sci.Rev., Ind.Vet., Inpharma, Int.Abstr.Biol.Sci., Int.Nurs.Ind., Lab.Haz.Bull., Med.& Surg.Dermat., Microbiol.Abstr., NRN, Neurosci.Cit.Ind., Nutr.Abstr., Pharm.&Out.News, Plant Breed.Abstr., Pollut.Abstr., Postharvest, Poult.Abstr., Reac., Ref.Zh., Rev.Appl.Entomol., Rev.Arom.& Med.Plants, Rev.Med.& Vet.Mycol., Rev.Plant Path., Risk Abstr., Rural Recreat.Tour.Abstr., SSCI (coverage dropped), Saf.Sci.Abstr., Sci.Cit.Ind., Seed Abstr., Small Anim.Abstr., Soyabean Abstr., Sugar Ind.Abstr., THA, Triticale Abstr., Trop.Dis.Bull., Weed Abstr.
—BLDSC (4927.100000), ADONIS, CASDDS, CISTI, GNLM, IDS, ingenta, KNAW, Linda Hall. **CCC.**
Published by: (American Academy of Allergy, Asthma & Immunology), Mosby, Inc. (Subsidiary of: Elsevier Science), 11830 Westline Industrial Dr, St Louis, MO 63146-3318. TEL 314-453-4304, 800-325-4177, FAX 314-872-9164, http://www.mosby.com/jaci, http://www.mosby.com/periodicals. Ed. Dr. Donald Y M Leung. Pub. Cheryl A Smart. Adv. contact Tracey Schriefer TEL 314-453-4304. B&W page USD 1,320, color page USD 2,645; trim 10.88 x 8.13. Circ: 9,073 (paid).

616.97 GBR ISSN 0896-8411
QR188.3 CODEN: JOAUEP
JOURNAL OF AUTOIMMUNITY. Text in English. 8/yr. GBP 399 to institutions (effective 2001). adv. index. reprint service avail. from SWZ. *Refereed.* **Document type:** *Academic/Scholarly.* **Description:** Publishes papers on all aspects of autoimmunity and its diverse aspects.
Related titles: Online - full text ed.: (from EBSCO Publishing, O C L C Online Computer Library Center, Inc., RoweCom Information Quest, ingenta, Swets Blackwell, IDEAL Online Library, Institute for Scientific Information).
Indexed: AIDS & Cancer Res., ASCA, Curr.Cont., Immun.Abstr., Ind.Med. (1988-), Ind.Sci.Rev., Inpharma, Int.Abstr.Biol.Sci., Nutr.Abstr., Pharm.&Out.News, Reac., Sci.Cit.Ind.
—BLDSC (4949.555000), ADONIS, CISTI, EMDOCS, GNLM, IDS, ingenta, KNAW. **CCC.**
Published by: Academic Press (Subsidiary of: Harcourt Publishers Ltd.), 24 Oval Rd, London NW1 7DX, United Kingdom. TEL 44-20-7267-4466, FAX 44-20-7482-2293, apsubs@acad.com, http://www.academicpress.com/jautoimmunity; http://www.europe.idealibrary.com/. Ed. J F Bach. R&P Catherine John. Adv. contact Nik Screen. **Subscr. to:** Harcourt Publishers Ltd., Foots Cray High St, Sidcup, Kent DA14 5HP, United Kingdom. TEL 44-20-8300-3322, FAX 44-20-7309-0807.

616.97 GBR ISSN 0141-2760
CODEN: JLIMDJ
JOURNAL OF CLINICAL & LABORATORY IMMUNOLOGY. Text in English. 1978. bi-m. GBP 395; GBP 495 in the European Union; USD 975 in the Americas. adv. bk.rev. **Document type:** *Academic/Scholarly.*
Indexed: AIDS & Cancer Res., ASCA, Chem.Abstr., Chem.Indus.Notes, Chem.Titles, Chemorec.Abstr., Curr.Cont. (coverage dropped), Dairy Sci.Abstr., Excerp.Med., Helminthol.Abstr., Immun.Abstr., Ind.Med. (1978-), Ind.Sci.Rev., Ind.Vet., Rev.Med.& Vet.Mycol., Sci.Cit.Ind. (coverage dropped), Vet.Bull.
—BLDSC (4958.380700), CASDDS, CISTI, GNLM, IDS, ingenta, KNAW. **CCC.**
Published by: Teviot Scientific Publications Ltd., 82 Great King St, Edinburgh EH3 6QU, United Kingdom. TEL 44-131-220-8209, FAX 44-131-226-5435. Ed. W James Irvine.

616.97 USA ISSN 0271-9142
RC581 CODEN: JCIMDO
JOURNAL OF CLINICAL IMMUNOLOGY. Text in English. 1981. bi-m. USD 677, EUR 676 to institutions for print or online ed.; USD 812.40, EUR 811.20 to institutions for print & online eds.combined. (effective 2002). adv. bk.rev. illus. back issues avail. *Refereed.* **Document type:** *Journal, Academic/Scholarly.* **Description:** Features articles on all aspects of research in clinical immunology as it applies to medical practice.
Related titles: Microfilm ed.: (from PQC); Online - full text ed.: (from Ovid Technologies, Inc., EBSCO Publishing, O C L C Online Computer Library Center, Inc., RoweCom Information Quest, Swets Blackwell, Kluwer Online, Institute for Scientific Information).
Indexed: AIDS Abstr., ASCA, Biol.Abstr., Chem.Abstr., Chem.Indus.Notes, Chem.Titles, Curr.Adv.Cancer Res., Curr.Cont., Dairy Sci.Abstr., Dent.Ind., Diar.Dis.Res., Excerp.Med., INIS Atomind., Immun.Abstr., Ind.Med. (1981-), Ind.Sci.Rev., Inpharma, Int.Abstr.Biol.Sci., Nutr.Abstr., Pharm.&Out.News, Reac., SSCI (coverage dropped), Sci.Cit.Ind.
—BLDSC (4958.490000), ADONIS, CASDDS, CISTI, EMDOCS, GNLM, IDS, ingenta, KNAW. **CCC.**
Published by: Kluwer Academic - Plenum Publishers (Subsidiary of: Wolters Kluwer N.V.), 233 Spring St, New York, NY 10013-1578. TEL 212-620-8000, 800-221-9369, FAX 212-463-0742, info@plenum.com, http://www.wkap.nl/journalhome.htm/0271-9142. Ed. Dr. Sudhir Gupta. R&P Rose Luongo TEL 781-871-6311. **Subscr. ourside the Americas to:** Kluwer Academic Publishers Group, Journals Department, PO Box 322, Dordrecht 3300 AH, Netherlands. TEL 31-78-639-2392, FAX 31-78-654-6474.

616.97 USA ISSN 1081-1672
CODEN: JCLIES
JOURNAL OF CLINICAL LIGAND ASSAY✶. Text in English. 1978. q. USD 85 domestic; USD 95 in Canada; USD 105 elsewhere. adv. bk.rev. *Refereed.* **Document type:** *Academic/Scholarly.*
Former titles (until 1995): Journal of Clinical Immunoassay (0736-4393); (until 1983): Ligand Quarterly (0199-4794)
Related titles: Microfiche ed.; Microfilm ed.; Microform ed.: (from PQC); Online - full text ed.: (from Institute for Scientific Information).
Indexed: ASCA, Chem.Abstr., Curr.Cont., Excerp.Med., Inpharma, Int.Abstr.Biol.Sci., Nutr.Abstr., Pharm.&Out.News, Reac., Rev.Appl.Entomol., Rev.Plant Path., SSCI (coverage dropped).
—BLDSC (4958.545000), CASDDS, CISTI, EMDOCS, GNLM, IDS, KNAW.
Published by: (Clinical Ligand Assay Society, Inc.), Kellner-McCaffery Associates, Inc., PO Box 58, Croton on Hudson, NY 10520-0058. TEL 212-741-0280. Ed. George Johnson. Circ: 1,600.

616.97 ITA ISSN 1124-8203
CODEN: JCLAF5
JOURNAL OF CLINICAL LIGAND ASSAY (EDIZIONE ITALIANA). Text in Italian. 1996. q. ITL 120,000 (effective 2000). adv. **Document type:** *Academic/Scholarly.* **Description:** Publishes current research in clinical ligand assays.
Published by: (Clinical Ligand Assay Society), Medical Systems S.p.A., Passo Rio Torbido, 40, Genoa, GE 16165, Italy. TEL 39-010-83401, FAX 39-010-804661, rassu@ssnet.it, http://medicalsystems.editoria.com.

616 576.2 NLD ISSN 0022-1759
QR183 CODEN: JIMMBG
JOURNAL OF IMMUNOLOGICAL METHODS. Text in English. 1971. 24/yr. EUR 3,972 in Europe to institutions; JPY 528,000 in Japan to institutions; USD 4,443 elsewhere to institutions (effective 2002). adv. bk.rev. illus. index. back issues avail.; reprint service avail. from ISI. *Refereed.* **Document type:** *Academic/Scholarly.* **Description:** Devoted to covering techniques for studying items closely related to immunity.
Related titles: Microform ed.: (from PQC); Online - full text ed.: (from ingenta, ScienceDirect, Swets Blackwell, Institute for Scientific Information).
Indexed: AIDS & Cancer Res., AIDS Abstr., ASCA, Abstr.Hyg., AgBiotech, Anal.Abstr., Anim.Breed.Abstr., Apic.Abstr., Biol.Abstr., Biotech.Cit.Ind., Chem.Abstr., Chem.Cit.Ind., Chem.Indus.Notes, Chem.Titles, Curr.Adv.Cancer Res., Curr.Adv.Cell & Devel.Biol., Curr.Adv.Ecol.Sci., Curr.Biotech.Abstr., Curr.Cont., Dairy Sci.Abstr., Dent.Ind., Derwent Biotech.Abstr., Excerp.Med., Helminthol.Abstr., INIS Atomind., Immun.Abstr., Ind.Med. (1971-), Ind.Sci.Rev., Ind.Vet., Inpharma, Int.Abstr.Biol.Sci., Med.& Pharm.Biotech.Abstr., Nutr.Abstr., Pig News & Info., Postharvest, Poult.Abstr., Protozool.Abstr., Reac., Ref.Zh., Rev.Appl.Entomol., Rev.Med.& Vet.Mycol., Rev.Plant Path., Risk Abstr., Sci.Cit.Ind., Telegen, Trop.Dis.Bull., Vet.Bull., Weed Abstr.
—BLDSC (5004.600000), ADONIS, CASDDS, CISTI, GNLM, IDS, ingenta, KNAW. **CCC.**
Published by: Elsevier Science BV, PO Box 211, Amsterdam 1000 AE, Netherlands. TEL 31-20-485-3757, FAX 31-20-485-3432, TELEX 18582 ESPA NL, http://www.elsevier.com/locate/jim, http://www.elsevier.nl. Eds. M C Nussenzweig, M W Turner. Circ: 2,500. **Subscr. in Australasia and the Far East to:** Elsevier Science (Singapore) Pte Ltd, No.1 Temasek Ave, 17-01 Millenia Tower, Singapore 039192, Singapore. TEL 65-434-3727, FAX 65-337-2230; **Subscr. in Japan to:** Elsevier Science Inc - Japan Regional Office, 9-15 Higashi-Azabu 1-chome, Minato-ku, Tokyo 106-0044, Japan. TEL 81-3-5561-5033, FAX 81-3-5561-5047; **Subscr. in the Americas to:** Elsevier Science, PO Box 945, New York, NY 10159-0945. TEL 212-633-3730, FAX 212-633-3680, usinfo-f@elsevier.com.

615.37 USA ISSN 0022-1767
QR180 CODEN: JOIMA3
JOURNAL OF IMMUNOLOGY. Text in English. 1916. 2/m. USD 270 domestic to individuals; USD 410 foreign to individuals; USD 470 domestic to institutions; USD 605 foreign to institutions; USD 20, USD 25 newsstand/cover (effective 2000). adv. bibl, illus. Index. reprints avail. *Refereed.* **Document type:** *Academic/Scholarly.*
Related titles: Microform ed.: (from PQC); Online - full text ed.: (from HighWire Pr., EBSCO Publishing, Institute for Scientific Information).
Indexed: AIDS & Cancer Res., AIDS Abstr., AIM, ASCA, Abstr.Hyg., AgBiotech, Agri.& Environ.Biotech.Abstr. (coverage dropped), Anim.Behav.Abstr. (coverage dropped), Anim.Breed.Abstr., Apic.Abstr., Aqua.Sci.& Fish.Abstr., Behav.Med.Abstr., Biol.& Agr.Ind. (Jan.1990-), Biol.Abstr., Cal.Tiss.Abstr. (coverage dropped), Chem.Abstr., Chem.Indus.Notes, Chem.Titles, Chemorec.Abstr., Curr.Adv.Biochem., Curr.Adv.Cancer Res., Curr.Adv.Cell & Devel.Biol., Curr.Adv.Ecol.Sci., Curr.Adv.Gen.& Molec.Biol., Curr.Biotech.Abstr., Curr.Cont., Dairy Sci.Abstr., Dent.Ind., Derwent Biotech.Abstr., Diar.Dis.Res., Environ.Sci.Poll.Mgmt., Excerp.Med., Forest.Abstr., Genet.Abstr., Helminthol.Abstr., Hum.Gen.Abstr., INIS Atomind., Immun.Abstr., Ind.Med. (1950-), Ind.Sci.Rev., Ind.Vet., Inpharma, Int.Abstr.Biol.Sci., Int.Aerosp.Abstr., Kidney, Med.& Pharm.Biotech.Abstr., Med.& Surg.Dermat., Microbiol.Abstr., Neurosci.Abstr., Neurosci.Cit.Ind., Nuc.Acids Abstr., Nutr.Abstr., Pharm.&Out.News, Pig News & Info., Plant Breed.Abstr., Poult.Abstr., Protozool.Abstr., Reac., Rev.Appl.Entomol., Rev.Arom.& Med.Plants, Rev.Med.& Vet.Mycol., Rev.Plant Path., Sci.Cit.Ind., Telegen, Tox.Abstr. (coverage dropped), Trop.Dis.Bull., Vet.Bull., Virol.Abstr. (coverage dropped), Weed Abstr.
—BLDSC (5005.000000), CASDDS, CISTI, GNLM, IDS, ingenta, KNAW, Linda Hall. **CCC.**
Published by: American Association of Immunologists, 9650 Rockville Pike, Bethesda, MD 20814. TEL 301-530-7197, FAX 301-571-1813, infoji@faseb.org, http://www.jimmunol.org. Ed. Frank W Fitch. R&P Cheryl M Burke. Adv. contact Beth Kallareou. Circ: 8,600 (paid).

616.02 USA ISSN 1524-9557
RM270 CODEN: JIEIEZ
JOURNAL OF IMMUNOTHERAPY. Text in English. 1982. bi-m. USD 336 domestic to individuals; USD 398 foreign to individuals; USD 684 domestic to institutions; USD 789 foreign to institutions (effective 2002). adv. bk.rev. illus. index. back issues avail.; reprint service avail. from PQC. *Refereed.* **Document type:** *Journal, Academic/Scholarly.* **Description:** Publishes laboratory, preclinical, and clinical reports on mechanisms and methods in immunotherapy.
Former titles (until 1997): Journal of Immunotherapy with Emphasis on Tumor Immunology (1067-5582); (until 1993): Journal of Immunotherapy (1053-8550); (until 1991): Journal of Biological Response Modifiers (0732-6580)
Related titles: Online - full text ed.: USD 889.20 domestic academic site license; USD 994.20 foreign academic site license; USD 991.80 domestic corporate site license; USD 1,096.80 foreign corporate site license (effective 2002) (from Ovid Technologies, Inc., Institute for Scientific Information).
Indexed: AIDS & Cancer Res., ASCA, Chem.Abstr., Chem.Indus.Notes, Chem.Titles, Curr.Cont., Derwent Biotech.Abstr., Excerp.Med., INIS Atomind., Immun.Abstr., Ind.Med. (coverage dropped), Ind.Sci.Rev., Inpharma, Int.Abstr.Biol.Sci., Med.& Pharm.Biotech.Abstr., Pharm.&Out.News, Reac., Sci.Cit.Ind.
—BLDSC (5005.040000), CASDDS, CISTI, EMDOCS, GNLM, IDS, ingenta, KNAW.
Published by: (Society for Biological Therapy), Lippincott Williams & Wilkins (Philadelphia) (Subsidiary of: Wolters Kluwer N.V.), 530 Walnut St, Philadelphia, PA 19106-3621. TEL 215-521-8300, FAX 215-521-8902, http://www.immunotherapy-journal.com, http://www.lww.com. Ed. Dr. David R Parkinson. Pub. Terri Monturano. R&P Margaret Becker. Adv. contact Ray Thibodeau. B&W page USD 725, color page USD 1,820. Circ: 887 (paid). **Subscr. to:** PO Box 1600, Hagerstown, MD 21740-1600. TEL 800-777-2295, FAX 301-824-7390.

616.97 USA ISSN 1079-9907
QR187.5 CODEN: JICRFJ
JOURNAL OF INTERFERON & CYTOKINE RESEARCH. Text in English. 1995. m. USD 529 domestic to individuals; USD 768 foreign to individuals; USD 635 domestic to individuals print and online eds. combined; USD 875 foreign to individuals print and online eds. combined; USD 1,144 domestic to institutions; USD 1,404 foreign to institutions; USD 1,373 domestic to institutions print and online eds. combined; USD 1,633 foreign to institutions print and online eds. combined (effective 2002). adv. back issues avail.; reprint service avail. from ISI. *Refereed.* **Document type:** *Journal, Academic/Scholarly.* **Description:** Publishes original articles on varied aspects of interferons and cytokines from basic science to clinical applications.
Formed by the merger of (1980-1995): Journal of Interferon Research (0197-8357); (1991-1995): Lymphokine and Cytokine Research (1056-5477)
Related titles: Online - full text ed.: USD 529 to individuals; USD 1,144 to institutions (effective 2002) (from CatchWord Ltd., EBSCO Publishing, O C L C Online Computer Library Center, Inc., RoweCom Information Quest, Swets Blackwell, Institute for Scientific Information).
Indexed: AIDS & Cancer Res., ASCA, Anim.Breed.Abstr., BBCI, Biol.Abstr., Biotech.Cit.Ind., Chem.Abstr., Chem.Indus.Notes, Chem.Titles, Curr.Adv.Cell & Devel.Biol., Curr.Adv.Ecol.Sci., Curr.Adv.Gen.& Molec.Biol., Curr.Biotech.Abstr., Curr.Cont., Derwent Biotech.Abstr., Excerp.Med., INIS Atomind., Immun.Abstr., Ind.Med. (1995-), Ind.Sci.Rev., Ind.Vet., Inpharma, Int.Abstr.Biol.Sci., Med.& Pharm.Biotech.Abstr., Pharm.&Out.News, Pig News & Info., Poult.Abstr., Protozool.Abstr., Reac., Rev.Med.& Vet.Mycol., Sci.Cit.Ind., Telegen, Vet.Bull.
—BLDSC (5007.548200), ADONIS, CASDDS, CatchWord, CISTI, GNLM, IDS, ingenta, KNAW. **CCC.**
Published by: (International Society for Interferon and Cytokine Research), Mary Ann Liebert, Inc. Publishers, 2 Madison Ave, Larchmont, NY 10538. TEL 914—834-3100, FAX 914-834-1388, info@liebertpub.com, www.liebertpub.com/jir, http://www.liebertpub.com. Eds. Dr. Lawrence B. Lachman, Philip I. Marcus.

616.97 DEU ISSN 1018-9068
CODEN: JIAIEF
JOURNAL OF INVESTIGATIONAL ALLERGOLOGY AND CLINICAL IMMUNOLOGY. Text in English. 1991. q. EUR 134 to individuals; EUR 198 to institutions; EUR 49.50 newsstand/cover (effective 2002). *Refereed.* **Document type:** *Journal, Academic/Scholarly.* **Description:** Provides an international forum for disseminating information on practical allergology in the form of new findings in basic and clinical immunology.
Related titles: Online - full text ed.: (from Institute for Scientific Information).
Indexed: ASCA, Chem.Abstr., Chem.Indus.Notes, Chem.Titles, Curr.Cont., Dairy Sci.Abstr., Excerp.Med. (1993-), Forest.Abstr., Helminthol.Abstr., Ind.Med. (1991-), Inpharma, Nutr.Abstr., Pharm.&Out.News, Postharvest, Protozool.Abstr., Reac., Rev.Appl.Entomol., Rev.Med.& Vet.Mycol., Rev.Plant Path., Soyabean Abstr., Triticale Abstr., Trop.Dis.Bull., Weed Abstr.
—CASDDS, CISTI, EMDOCS, GNLM, IDS, Infotrieve, KNAW. **CCC.**
Published by: (International Association of Asthmology ESP), Hogrefe Verlag GmbH und Co. KG, Rohnsweg 25, Goettingen 37085, Germany. TEL 49-551-496090, FAX 49-551-4960988, verlag@hogrefe.de, http://www.hogrefe.de. Ed. A. Oehling. **Co-sponsor:** Sociedad Latinoamericana de Alergia e Inmunologia.

JOURNAL OF MICROBIOLOGY, IMMUNOLOGY AND INFECTION/WEIMIAN YU GANRAN ZAZHI. see *BIOLOGY—Microbiology*

JOURNAL OF NEUROIMMUNOLOGY. see *MEDICAL SCIENCES—Psychiatry And Neurology*

616.97 618 IRL ISSN 0165-0378
CODEN: JRIMDR
JOURNAL OF REPRODUCTIVE IMMUNOLOGY. Text in English. 1979. 8/yr. EUR 83 in Europe to individuals; JPY 11,200 in Japan to individuals; USD 93 elsewhere to individuals; EUR 788 in Europe to institutions; JPY 104,800 in Japan to institutions; USD 881 elsewhere to institutions (effective 2002). adv. bk.rev. back issues avail.; reprint service avail. from SWZ. *Refereed.* **Document type:** *Academic/Scholarly.* **Description:** Provides a critical forum for the dissemination of results from high quality research in all aspects of experimental, animal and clinical reproductive immunology.
Related titles: Microform ed.: (from PQC); Online - full text ed.: (from ingenta, ScienceDirect, Swets Blackwell, Institute for Scientific Information).
Indexed: AIDS & Cancer Res., ASCA, AgBiotech, Anim.Breed.Abstr., Biol.Abstr., Chem.Abstr., Chem.Indus.Notes, Chem.Titles, Curr.Adv.Ecol.Sci., Curr.Cont., Dairy Sci.Abstr., Excerp.Med., INIS Atomind., Immun.Abstr., Ind.Med. (1979-), Ind.Sci.Rev., Ind.Vet., Inpharma, Int.Abstr.Biol.Sci., Nutr.Abstr., Pharm.&Out.News, Pig News & Info., Reac., Rev.Med.& Vet.Mycol., Sci.Cit.Ind., Vet.Bull.
—BLDSC (5049.670000), CASDDS, CISTI, GNLM, IDS, ingenta, KNAW. **CCC.**
Published by: (International Society for Immunology of Reproduction), Elsevier Science Ireland Ltd, Elsevier House, Brookvale Plaza, E. Park, Shannon, Co. Clare, Ireland. TEL 353-61-471944, FAX 353-61-472144, http://www.elsevier.com/locate/jreprimm. Eds. A E Beer, W D Billington. R&P Annette Moloney. **Subscr. in Australasia and the Far East to:** Elsevier Science (Singapore) Pte Ltd, No.1 Temasek Ave, 17-01 Millenia Tower, Singapore 039192, Singapore. TEL 65-434-3727, FAX 65-337-2230; **Subscr. in the Americas to:** Elsevier Science, PO Box 945, New York, NY 10159-0945. TEL 212-633-3730, FAX 212-633-3680; **Subscr. to:** Elsevier Science BV, PO Box 211, Amsterdam 1000 AE, Netherlands. TEL 31-20-485-3757.

616.97 JPN ISSN 0916-8966
KAFUNSHO KENKYUKAI KAIHO/POLLEN ALLERGY AND PREVENTION. Text in Japanese. 1990. a., latest vol.12. JPY 3,000 (effective 2001). bk.rev. 50 p./no. *Refereed.* **Document type:** *Bulletin, Academic/Scholarly.*
Published by: Kafunsho Kenkyukai/Society of Pollen Allergy and Prevention, Toyama Ika Yakka Daigaku, Igakubu Koshu Eiseigaku Kyoshitsu, 2630 Sugitani, Toyama-shi, Toyama-ken 930-0194, Japan. pollena@ms.toyama-mpu.ac.jp, http://www.toyama-mpu.ac.jp/md/pubhlth/kafunsho.html. Ed. H Teranishi.

L M S ALERT. IMMUNOTHERAPEUTICS. VACCINES. (Literature Monitoring and Evaluation Service) see *MEDICAL SCIENCES—Abstracting, Bibliographies, Statistics*

616.97 USA
THE LEANING TREE. Text in English. w. free per issue. **Document type:** *Newsletter.* **Description:** News, information and support for the sufferers and caregivers of chronic fatigue syndrome, fibromyalgia syndrome, Gulf War syndrome, or multiple chemical sensitivities.
Media: Online - full text.
Published by: The Mining Company, PO Box 6572, New York, NY 10128-0006. TEL 212-876-3512, chronicfatigue.guide@miningco.com, http://chronicfatigue.miningco.com/library/other/blextra.htm. Ed. Donna Yeaw.

LEUCOCYTES. see *MEDICAL SCIENCES—Abstracting, Bibliographies, Statistics*

616.97 USA ISSN 1042-4075
THE M A REPORT. (Mother of Asthmatics) Text in English. 1985. m. USD 25; USD 35 foreign (effective 1999). video rev. stat, tr.lit. back issues avail. *Refereed.* **Description:** Offers information and support for persons who have asthma and allergies.
Published by: Allergy and Asthma Network, Mother of Asthmatics, Inc., 2751 Prosperity Ave, Ste 150, Fairfax, VA 22031. TEL 703-641-9595, FAX 703-573-7794, aanma@aol.com. Ed. Nancy Sander. Circ: 10,000.

MACROPHAGES. see *MEDICAL SCIENCES—Abstracting, Bibliographies, Statistics*

616.97 NLD
MANUAL OF BIOLOGICAL MARKERS OF DISEASE. Text in English. 1994. base vol. plus irreg. updates. USD 69.50. Supplement avail. **Document type:** *Academic/Scholarly.* **Description:** Presents information on recent advances in the study of autoantibodies of interest to immunologists, molecular biologists, and clinicians treating autoimmune disorders.
Published by: Kluwer Academic Publishers Group (Subsidiary of: Wolters Kluwer N.V.), Spuiboulevard 50, PO Box 17, Dordrecht 3300 AA, Netherlands. FAX 31-78-639-2254, services@wkap.nl, http://www.wkap.nl. Eds. R N Maini, W J van Venrooij. **Dist. by:** Journals Department, PO Box 322, Dordrecht 3300 AH, Netherlands. TEL 781-871-6600, FAX 31-78-654-6474.

616 615.37 DEU ISSN 0300-8584
CODEN: MMIYAO
MEDICAL MICROBIOLOGY AND IMMUNOLOGY. Text in English. 1886. q. EUR 909.40 domestic; EUR 906.90 in Germany; EUR 270 newsstand/cover foreign (effective 2002). reprint service avail. from ISI. *Refereed.* **Document type:** *Journal, Academic/Scholarly.* **Description:** Covers a broad spectrum of the interrelationships between micro-organisms and the human host, with special emphasis on medical virology and immunology, and how they relate to the mechanisms of pathogenesis.
Formerly: Zeitschrift fuer Medizinische Mikrobiologie und Immunologie (0044-3077)
Related titles: Microform ed.: (from PQC); Online - full text ed.: ISSN 1432-1831 (from EBSCO Publishing, RoweCom Information Quest, Swets Blackwell, Springer LINK, Institute for Scientific Information).
Indexed: AIDS & Cancer Res., ASCA, Biol.Abstr., Chem.Abstr., Chem.Indus.Notes, Chem.Titles, Curr.Adv.Ecol.Sci., Curr.Cont., Environ.Sci.Poll.Mgmt., Excerp.Med., Helminthol.Abstr., INIS Atomind., Immun.Abstr., Ind.Med. (1971-), Ind.Sci.Rev., Ind.Vet., Inpharma, Int.Abstr.Biol.Sci., Microbiol.Abstr., Pharm.&Out.News, Protozool.Abstr., Reac., Rev.Plant Path., Sci.Cit.Ind., Telegen, Trop.Dis.Bull., Vet.Bull.
—BLDSC (5529.990000), ADONIS, CASDDS, CISTI, EMDOCS, GNLM, IDS, Infotrieve, ingenta, KNAW. **CCC.**
Published by: Springer-Verlag (Subsidiary of: BertelsmannSpringer), Tiergartenstr 17, Heidelberg 69121, Germany. TEL 49-6221-345-0, FAX 49-6221-345229, subscriptions@springer.de, http://link.springer.de/link/service/journals/00430/index.htm, http://www.springer.de. Eds. B Fleischer, S Bhakdi. **Subscr. in N. America to:** Springer-Verlag New York Inc., PO Box 2485, Secaucus, NJ 07096-2485. TEL 212-460-1500, FAX 212-473-6272.

MEDICAL SCIENTIFIC UPDATE. see *MEDICAL SCIENCES—Respiratory Diseases*

M

616.97 BGR ISSN 0204-9724
MEDITSINSKI PREGLED. ALERGOLOGIIA I KLINICHNA IMUNOLOGIIA/MEDICAL REVIEW. ALLERGOLOGY AND IMMUNOLOGY. Text in Bulgarian; Summaries in Bulgarian, English. 1978. q., latest vol.24, 2001. BGL 14 domestic; USD 48 foreign (effective 2001 - 2002). adv. bk.rev. abstr, bibl. index. 48 p./no. back issues avail. **Document type:** *Journal, Academic/Scholarly.* **Description:** Presents original articles and abstracts of foreign publications in the field of allergology and clinical immunology.
Indexed: Abstr.Bulg.Sci.Med.Lit.
Published by: Meditsinski Universitet - Sofia, Tsentur za Informatsiia po Meditsina/Medical University - Sofia, Medical Information Center, 1 Sv Georgi Sofiiski ul, Sofia 1431, Bulgaria. TEL 359-2-9522342, FAX 359-2-9522393, mutafov@sun.medun.acad.bg, http://www.medun.acad.bg. Ed. Dr. G Kosturkov. R&P, Adv. contact Dr. Christo Mutafov. B&W page USD 50, color page USD 150; 12 x 18. Circ: 200.

MEDITSINSKI PREGLED. IMMUNNI DEFITSITI. see *MEDICAL SCIENCES—Communicable Diseases*

616.97 JPN ISSN 0917-0774
CODEN: IMFREG
MEN-EKI IMMUNOLOJI FURONTIA/IMMUNOLOGY FRONTIER. Text in Japanese. 1991. 6/yr. JPY 1,500 per issue (effective 1998).
Indexed: Chem.Abstr., Chem.Indus.Notes, Chem.Titles.
—BLDSC (4369.704800), CASDDS.
Published by: Medikaru Rebyusha/Medical Review Co., Ltd., 7-3 Hirano-Machi 1-chome, Chuo-ku, Osaka-shi 541-0046, Japan. TEL 81-6-223-1667, FAX 81-6-223-1338, meview@osk3.3web.ne.jp.

616.97 JPN ISSN 0914-8639
MEN'EKI KAKU IGAKU/IMMUNONUCLEAR MEDICINE. Text in Japanese. 1986. s-a.
Published by: Men'eki Kaku Igaku Kenkyukai/ Immunonuclear Medicine Study Group, Kitasato Daigaku Igakubu Hoshasenka, 15-1 Kitaza-To 1-chome, Sagamihara-shi, Kanagawa-ken 228-0829, Japan.

MICROBIOLOGY AND IMMUNOLOGY. see *BIOLOGY—Microbiology*

MICROBIOLOGY AND MOLECULAR BIOLOGY REVIEWS. see *BIOLOGY—Microbiology*

MIKROBIOLOGICHNYI ZHURNAL; nauchnyi zhurnal. see *BIOLOGY—Microbiology*

616.97 USA ISSN 0891-3676
MODERN CONCEPTS IN IMMUNOLOGY. Text in English. 1985. irreg. **Document type:** *Monographic series.*
—CISTI.
Published by: John Wiley & Sons, Inc., Journals (Subsidiary of: Wiley InterScience), 605 Third Ave, New York, NY 10158. **Subscr. outside the Americas to:** John Wiley & Sons Ltd., Baffins Ln, Chichester, Sussex PO19 IUD, United Kingdom. FAX 44-1243-776128.

MOLECULAR IMMUNOLOGY. see *BIOLOGY—Biochemistry*

MONOCLONAL ANTIBODIES. see *BIOLOGY—Abstracting, Bibliographies, Statistics*

616.97 CHE ISSN 0077-0760
CODEN: MOALAR
MONOGRAPHS IN ALLERGY. Text in English. 1966. irreg., latest vol.33. CHF 220 in Europe; DEM 260 in Germany; USD 160 in United States (effective 2001). reprint service avail. from ISI. *Refereed.* **Document type:** *Monographic series, Academic/Scholarly.*
Related titles: Online - full text ed.: (from Institute for Scientific Information).
Indexed: ASCA, Apic.Abstr., Biol.Abstr., Chem.Abstr., Chem.Indus.Notes, Chem.Titles, Curr.Cont. (coverage dropped), Dent.Ind., Ind.Med. (1966-), Ind.Sci.Rev., Rev.Med.& Vet.Mycol., Sci.Cit.Ind.
—BLDSC (5914.975000), CASDDS, CISTI, GNLM, IDS, KNAW. **CCC.**
Published by: S. Karger AG, Allschwilerstr 10, PO Box, Basel 4009, Switzerland. TEL 41-61-306-1111, FAX 41-61-306-1234, karger@karger.ch, http://www.karger.com/bookseries/MOALL. Eds. F Shakib, L A Hanson.

616.9 USA ISSN 1068-7629
MUCOSAL IMMUNOLOGY UPDATE. Text in English. 1993. q. USD 60 domestic to individuals; USD 70 foreign to individuals; USD 80 domestic to institutions; USD 100 foreign to institutions; USD 23 newsstand/cover. adv. charts, illus. **Document type:** *Newsletter.* **Description:** Presents mini-reviews, abstracts from meetings and society news.
Published by: Society for Mucosal Immunology, 4340 East West Highway, Ste 401, Bethesda, MD 20814-4411. Eds. Hiroshi Kiyono, Peter B Ernst. Adv. contact Ray Thibodeau. B&W page USD 690, color page USD 1,715. Circ: 887 (paid).

N O H A NEWS. see *NUTRITION AND DIETETICS*

616.97 616.238 GBR ISSN 1363-268X
NATIONAL ASTHMA CAMPAIGN'S ASTHMA JOURNAL. Variant title: Asthma Journal. Text in English. 1995. q. GBP 27 (effective Oct. 1999). adv. charts, illus, stat. back issues avail. *Refereed.* **Document type:** *Magazine.* **Description:** Contains up to date information and reviews on asthma care and management.
—BLDSC (1747.048340).
Published by: (National Asthma Campaign), Reed Business Information (Subsidiary of: Reed Elsevier plc), Quadrant House, The Quadrant, Brighton Rd, Sutton, Surrey SM2 5AS, United Kingdom. TEL 44-20-8652-8878, FAX 44-20-8652-8946. Ed. Dr. Martyn Partridge. Pub. Caley Montgomery. Adv. contact Monica Baghi. Circ: 1,500.

616.97 614.4 USA
NEEDLE TIPS AND THE HEPATITIS B COALITION NEWS. Text in English. s-a. **Document type:** *Bulletin.* **Description:** Features articles and reprintable resources on all aspects of vaccine-preventable diseases in children and adults.
Formed by the merger of: Needle Tips; Hepatitis B Coalition News
Related titles: Online - full text ed.
Published by: Immunization Action Coalition, 1573 Selby Ave., Ste. 234, St. Paul, MN 55104. TEL 651-647-9009, FAX 651-647-9131, admin@immunize.org, http://www.immunize.org. Eds. Dr. Deborah Wexler, Dr. Margaret Vaillancourt. R&P Dr. Deborah Wexler. Circ: 220,000.

616.97 CHE ISSN 1021-7401
CODEN: NROIEM
NEUROIMMUNOMODULATION. Text in English. 1994. 8/yr. CHF 1,037 in Europe to institutions; CHF 1,054.40 elsewhere to institutions; EUR 740.80 in Europe to institutions; USD 806 elsewhere to institutions (effective 2002). adv. back issues avail. *Refereed.* **Document type:** *Journal, Academic/Scholarly.* **Description:** Explores the way in which the nervous system interacts with the immune system via neural, hormonal, and paracrine actions.
Related titles: Microform ed.: (from PQC); Online - full text ed.: ISSN 1423-0216. CHF 58, EUR 42, USD 45 to institutions with print edition (effective 2002) (from EBSCO Publishing, O C L C Online Computer Library Center, Inc., RoweCom Information Quest, Swets Blackwell, Institute for Scientific Information).
Indexed: ASCA, Chem.Abstr., Chem.Indus.Notes, Chem.Titles, Curr.Cont., Excerp.Med. (1995-), Ind.Med. (1994-), Neurosci.Cit.Ind., Sci.Cit.Ind., e-psyche.
—BLDSC (6081.373400), CASDDS, CISTI, GNLM, IDS, Infotrieve, KNAW. **CCC.**
Published by: S. Karger AG, Allschwilerstr 10, PO Box, Basel 4009, Switzerland. TEL 41-61-306-1111, FAX 41-61-306-1234, karger@karger.ch, http://www.online.karger.com/journals/nim, http://www.karger.com. Eds. J M Lipton, S M McCann. adv.: page USD 1,195. Circ: 1,000. **Subscr. in U.S. to:** S Karger Publishers Inc.

NEW DIRECTIONS (DENVER). see *MEDICAL SCIENCES—Respiratory Diseases*

O P A PRATIQUE. (ORL, Pneumo, Allergo) see *MEDICAL SCIENCES—Otorhinolaryngology*

OCULAR IMMUNOLOGY AND INFLAMMATION. see *MEDICAL SCIENCES—Ophthalmology And Optometry*

576 AUS ISSN 1443-265X
▼ **ONLINE JOURNAL OF IMMUNOLOGY.** Text in English. 1999. **Document type:** *Academic/Scholarly.* **Description:** Focuses on original research work either as full-text reports or short communications.
Media: Online - full text.
Published by: Pestsearch International Pty. Ltd., 173 Chatswood Rd, Daisy Hill, QLD 4127, Australia. http://www.uq.edu.au/~csvguerr/immunolo.htm, http://www.cpb.uokhsc.edu/ojvr/jvet196a.htm.

ORAL MICROBIOLOGY AND IMMUNOLOGY. see *BIOLOGY—Microbiology*

616 USA
OUR TOXIC TIMES. Abbreviated title: O T T. Text in English. m. USD 30 to individuals. adv. **Document type:** *Newsletter, Consumer.* **Description:** Covers a wide range of pertinent information for those concerned about Multiple Chemical Sensitivity (MCS), from the technical to the practical.
Published by: Chemical Injury Information Network (CIIN), PO Box 301, White Sulphur Springs, MT 59645. TEL 406-547-2255, FAX 406-547-2455, http://biz-comm.com.

PARASITE IMMUNOLOGY. see *MEDICAL SCIENCES—Communicable Diseases*

616.079 CHE ISSN 1015-2008
RB125 CODEN: PATHEF
PATHOBIOLOGY; journal of immunopathology, molecular and cellular biology. Text in English. 1938. bi-m. CHF 1,156 in Europe to institutions; CHF 1,173.40 elsewhere to institutions; EUR 825.80 in Europe to institutions; USD 898 elsewhere to institutions (effective 2002). adv. bibl, charts, illus. index, cum.index. back issues avail. *Refereed.* **Document type:** *Journal, Academic/Scholarly.* **Description:** Addresses timely topics in pathobiology, immunopathology, cellular and molecular biology, and medicine.
Formed by the merger of: Experimental Cell Biology (0304-3568); Pathology and Immunopathology Research (0257-2761); Experimental Cell Biology; Which was formerly: Pathologia et Microbiologia; Schweizerische Zeitschrift fuer Allgemeine Pathologie und Bakteriologie (0031-2959); Pathology and Immunopathology Research; Which was formerly: Survey and Synthesis of Pathology Research (0253-438X)
Related titles: Microform ed.: (from RPI); Online - full text ed.: ISSN 1423-0291. 199?. CHF 58, EUR 42, USD 45 to institutions print with edition (effective 2002) (from Northern Light Technology, Inc., EBSCO Publishing, O C L C Online Computer Library Center, Inc., RoweCom Information Quest, ProQuest Information & Learning, Swets Blackwell, Institute for Scientific Information).
Indexed: AIDS Abstr., ASCA, Abstr.Hyg., Agri.& Environ.Biotech.Abstr. (coverage dropped), Biol.Abstr., C.I.S. Abstr., Chem.Abstr., Chem.Indus.Notes, Chem.Titles, Curr.Adv.Cancer Res., Curr.Adv.Cell & Devel.Biol., Curr.Adv.Ecol.Sci., Curr.Cont., Dairy Sci.Abstr., Dent.Ind., Derwent Biotech.Abstr., Excerp.Med., Helminthol.Abstr., INIS Atomind., Ind.Med. (1990-), Ind.Sci.Rev., Ind.Vet., Inpharma, Nutr.Abstr., Pharm.&Out.News, Reac., Rev.Plant Path., Sci.Cit.Ind., Trop.Dis.Bull., Vet.Bull.
—BLDSC (6412.738000), CASDDS, CISTI, EMDOCS, GNLM, IDS, Infotrieve, ingenta, KNAW, Linda Hall. **CCC.**
Published by: S. Karger AG, Allschwilerstr 10, PO Box, Basel 4009, Switzerland. TEL 41-61-306-1111, FAX 41-61-306-1234, karger@karger.ch, http://www.online.karger.com/journals/pat, http://www.karger.com. Ed. C Wittekind. adv.: page USD 1,195. Circ: 1,050.

PEDIATRIC ALLERGY AND IMMUNOLOGY. see *MEDICAL SCIENCES—Pediatrics*

PEDIATRIC ALLERGY AND IMMUNOLOGY. SUPPLEMENTUM. see *MEDICAL SCIENCES—Pediatrics*

PEDIATRIC ASTHMA, ALLERGY & IMMUNOLOGY. see *MEDICAL SCIENCES—Pediatrics*

615.37 USA
PERSPECTIVES IN IMMUNOLOGY; a series of publications based on symposia. Text in English. 1969. irreg., latest vol.10, 1981. reprint service avail. from ISI. *Refereed.*
Published by: Academic Press, Inc., Journal Division (Subsidiary of: Harcourt Brace & Company), 525 B St, Ste 1900, San Diego, CA 92101-4495. TEL 619-231-0926, FAX 619-699-6715. **Subscr. to:** Order Dept., 6277 Sea Harbor Dr, 4th Fl, Orlando, FL 32887. TEL 800-321-5068.

PSORI NEWSLETTER. see *MEDICAL SCIENCES—Dermatology And Venereology*

616.97 GBR ISSN 0140-6957
RECENT ADVANCES IN CLINICAL IMMUNOLOGY. Text in English. 1977. irreg., latest vol.4. **Document type:** *Monographic series, Academic/Scholarly.*
—CISTI, GNLM.

M

Published by: Churchill Livingstone (Subsidiary of: Harcourt Publishers Ltd.), Robert Stevenson House, 1-3 Baxter's Pl, Leith Walk, Edinburgh, Midlothian EH1 3AF, United Kingdom. TEL 44-131-556-2424, FAX 44-131-459-1177, http://www.churchillmed.com. **US subscr. to:** Churchill Livingstone, 650 Ave of the Americas, New York, NY 10011. TEL 212-206-5000.

REFERATIVNYI ZHURNAL. BIOLOGIYA - IMMUNOLOGIYA. see *MEDICAL SCIENCES—Abstracting, Bibliographies, Statistics*

REFERATIVNYI ZHURNAL. BRONKHYALNAYA ASTMA I DRUGIE ALLERGICHESKIE ZABOLEVANIYA. see *MEDICAL SCIENCES—Abstracting, Bibliographies, Statistics*

REFERATIVNYI ZHURNAL. KLINICHESKAYA IMMUNOLOGIYA I ALLERGOLOGIYA. IMMUNOREABILITATSIYA. IMMUNOFARMAKOLOGIYA. see *MEDICAL SCIENCES—Abstracting, Bibliographies, Statistics*

REFERATIVNYI ZHURNAL. MOLEKULYARNAYA I KLETOCHNAYA IMMUNOLOGIYA. see *MEDICAL SCIENCES—Abstracting, Bibliographies, Statistics*

616.97 USA ISSN 1520-8745
RESEARCH INITIATIVE, TREATMENT ACTION!. Abbreviated title: R I T A. Text in English. 1995. s-a. free. back issues avail. *Refereed.* **Document type:** *Journal, Academic/Scholarly.* **Description:** Covers issues in HIV/AIDS research and policy, and is intended for the HIV/AIDS medical, research, and professional communities.
Related titles: Online - full text ed.
Published by: The Center for AIDS, Hope & Remembrance Project, 1407 Hawthorne, Houston, TX 77006. Ed., R&P Thomas Gegeny. Pub. L. Joel Martinez. Circ: 3,000 (paid).

REVIEWS IN MEDICAL VIROLOGY. see *BIOLOGY—Microbiology*

616.97 ESP ISSN 0214-1477
CODEN: REACEN
REVISTA ESPANOLA DE ALERGOLOGIA E INMUNOLOGIA CLINICA. Text in Spanish. 1991 (vol.6). bi-m. back issues avail. **Document type:** *Academic/Scholarly.* **Description:** Contains original articles and reviews in allergology and rheumatology.
Related titles: Online - full text ed.
Indexed: Excerp.Med.
—CINDOC, EMDOCS, GNLM, Infotrieve, KNAW. **CCC.**
Published by: (Sociedad Espanola de Alergologia e Inmunologia Clinica), Saned S.A., Capitan Haya, 60, Madrid 28020, Spain. TEL 34-91-749-9507, FAX 34-91-749-9507, saned@meditex.es, http://www.seaic.es/revista. Ed. Dr. Enrique Buendia. adv.: page ESP 250,000. Circ: 2,000.

REVISTA LATINOAMERICANA DE MICROBIOLOGIA. see *BIOLOGY—Microbiology*

616.97 FRA ISSN 0335-7457
REVUE FRANCAISE D'ALLERGOLOGIE ET D'IMMUNOLOGIE CLINIQUE. Text in French. 1961. 8/yr. EUR 173 in Europe to individuals; USD 218 elsewhere to individuals; EUR 220 in Europe to institutions; USD 262 elsewhere to institutions (effective 2002). adv. bk.rev. abstr, bibl, charts. reprint service avail. from PQC. *Refereed.*
Former titles: Revue Francaise d'Allergologie et Immunologie; Revue Francaise d'Allergologie (0035-2845); Revue Francaise d'Allergie
Related titles: Microform ed.: (from PQC); Online - full text ed.: (from Institute for Scientific Information).
Indexed: ASCA, Biol.Abstr., C.I.S. Abstr., Chem.Abstr., Curr.Adv.Ecol.Sci., Curr.Cont., Dairy Sci.Abstr., Forest.Abstr., Ind.Med. (coverage dropped), Inpharma, Nutr.Abstr., Pharm.&Out.News, Reac., Ref.Zh., Rev.Appl.Entomol., Rev.Med.& Vet.Mycol., Rev.Plant Path., Weed Abstr.
—BLDSC (7902.470000), CISTI, EMDOCS, GNLM, IDS, Infotrieve, KNAW. **CCC.**
Published by: (Societe Francaise d'Allergologie), Elsevier Paris, Editions Scientifiques et Medicales (Subsidiary of: Reed Elsevier plc. group), 23 rue Linois, Paris 75015, France. TEL 33-1-45589110, FAX 33-1-45589419, http://www.elsevier.com/locate/allerg. Circ: 3,000.

ROMANIAN ARCHIVES OF MICROBIOLOGY AND IMMUNOLOGY. see *BIOLOGY—Microbiology*

616.97 GBR ISSN 0300-9475
QR180 CODEN: SJIMAX
SCANDINAVIAN JOURNAL OF IMMUNOLOGY. Text in English. 1972. m., latest vol.55, 2002. GBP 477 in Europe; USD 687 in North America; GBP 477 elsewhere (effective 2002). adv. reprint service avail. from ISI. *Refereed.* **Document type:** *Academic/Scholarly.* **Description:** Publishes papers on the results of work of the highest standard on cellular and molecular immunology.
Related titles: Microform ed.: (from PQC); Online - full text ed.: Scandinavian Journal of Immunology Online. ISSN 1365-3083. 1998. GBP 430 in Europe; USD 619 in North America; GBP 430 elsewhere (effective 2002) (from Ovid Technologies, Inc., EBSCO Publishing, O C L C Online Computer Library Center, Inc., RoweCom Information Quest, ingenta, Munksgaard & Blackwell Science's Synergy, Swets Blackwell, Institute for Scientific Information); ♦ Supplement: Scandinavian Journal of Immunology. Supplement. ISSN 0301-6323.
Indexed: AIDS & Cancer Res., ASCA, Anim.Breed.Abstr., Biol.Abstr., Chem.Abstr., Chem.Indus.Notes, Chem.Titles, Curr.Adv.Biochem., Curr.Adv.Cancer Res., Curr.Adv.Cell & Devel.Biol., Curr.Adv.Ecol.Sci., Curr.Adv.Gen.& Molec.Biol., Curr.Cont., Dairy Sci.Abstr., Excerp.Med., Helminthol.Abstr., INIS Atomind., Immun.Abstr., Ind.Med. (1972-), Ind.Vet., Inpharma, Int.Abstr.Biol.Sci., Neurosci.Cit.Ind., Pharm.&Out.News, Protozool.Abstr., Reac., Sci.Cit.Ind., Vet.Bull.
—BLDSC (8087.516800), ADONIS, CASDDS, CISTI, EMDOCS, GNLM, IDS, ingenta, KNAW. **CCC.**
Published by: Blackwell Science Ltd., Osney Mead, Oxford OX2 0EL, United Kingdom. TEL 44-1865-206206, FAX 44-1865-721205, journals.cs@blacksci.co.uk, http://www.blackwell-science.com. Ed. J Natvig. Pub. Allen Stevens. R&P Sophie Savage. Adv. contact Jenny Applin. Circ: 1,265.

616.97 GBR ISSN 0301-6323
CODEN: SJISDK
SCANDINAVIAN JOURNAL OF IMMUNOLOGY. SUPPLEMENT. Text in English. 1973. irreg. adv. **Document type:** *Academic/Scholarly.*
Related titles: ♦ Supplement to: Scandinavian Journal of Immunology. ISSN 0300-9475.
Indexed: Excerp.Med. (1993-), Ind.Med. (1973-), Int.Abstr.Biol.Sci.
—ADONIS, CASDDS, CISTI, EMDOCS, Infotrieve, KNAW. **CCC.**
Published by: Blackwell Science Ltd., Osney Mead, Oxford OX2 0EL, United Kingdom. TEL 44-1865-206206, FAX 44-1865-721205, journals.cs@blacksci.co.uk, http://www.blackwell-science.com. Pub. Allen Stevens. R&P Sophie Savage. Adv. contact Jenny Applin.

SEMINARS IN DIAGNOSTIC PATHOLOGY. see *MEDICAL SCIENCES*

616.97 GBR ISSN 1044-5323
CODEN: SEIME2
SEMINARS IN IMMUNOLOGY. Text in English. 1989. bi-m. GBP 235 to institutions (effective 2001). adv. reprint service avail. from SWZ. **Document type:** *Academic/Scholarly.* **Description:** Reviews the latest news in R&D in studies of the human immune system.
Related titles: Online - full text ed.: (from EBSCO Publishing, O C L C Online Computer Library Center, Inc., RoweCom Information Quest, ingenta, Swets Blackwell, IDEAL Online Library, Institute for Scientific Information).
Indexed: AIDS & Cancer Res., Chem.Abstr., Chem.Indus.Notes, Chem.Titles, Curr.Cont., Immun.Abstr., Ind.Med. (1989-), Inpharma, Pharm.&Out.News, Reac.
—BLDSC (8239.451000), ADONIS, CASDDS, CISTI, GNLM, IDS, ingenta, KNAW. **CCC.**
Published by: Academic Press (Subsidiary of: Harcourt Publishers Ltd.), 24 Oval Rd, London NW1 7DX, United Kingdom. TEL 44-20-7267-4466, FAX 44-20-7482-2293, apsubs@acad.com, http://www.academicpress.com/semimm; http://www.europe.idealibrary.com/. Ed. Michael Julius. R&P Catherine John. Adv. contact Nik Screen. **Subscr. to:** Harcourt Publishers Ltd., Foots Cray High St, Sidcup, Kent DA14 5HP, United Kingdom. TEL 44-20-8300-3322, FAX 44-20-8309-0807.

616.97 AUS
SENSITIVITY MATTERS. Text in English. 1982. q. AUD 25. adv. bk.rev. back issues avail. **Document type:** *Newsletter.* **Description:** Covers the treatment and management of allergy and sensitivity related diseases (asthma, eczema, Multiple Chemical Sensitivity, Chronic Fatigue Syndrome, hayfever, ADHD) as well as local and overseas news and activities.
Formerly (until 1994): A A A News (0817-1300)
Published by: Allergy and Environmental Sensitivity Support and Research Association, PO Box 298, Ringwood, VIC 3134, Australia. TEL 61-3-98881382. Ed., Pub., R&P, Adv. contact Catherine McIver. Circ: 400.

616.97 USA
SJOGREN'S SYNDROME FOUNDATION INC.; the moisture seekers newsletter. Text in English. 1984. 9/yr. USD 25; USD 30 in Canada; USD 35 elsewhere. back issues avail. *Refereed.* **Document type:** *Newsletter.* **Description:** Informs patients and medical professionals about all aspects of Sjogren's syndrome, including the various manifestations of the disorder, treatment modalities, news on research developments, important legislation, and advice on how to live more comfortably and prevent or prolong the onset of major debilitating consequences. Provides information on support groups and on meetings and symposia.
Address: 333 N Broadway, Ste 2000, Jericho, NY 11753-2007. TEL 516-933-6365, 800-475-6473, FAX 516-933-6368, http://www.sjogrens.com. Circ: 11,000.

616.97 DEU ISSN 0344-4325
CODEN: SSIMDV
SPRINGER SEMINARS IN IMMUNOPATHOLOGY. Text in English. 1978. q. DEM 1,183 domestic; DEM 1,188.40 foreign (effective 2001). charts, illus. index. back issues avail.; reprint service avail. from ISI. *Refereed.* **Document type:** *Journal, Academic/Scholarly.* **Description:** Offers up-to-date developments in the field of immunopathology.
Related titles: Microform ed.: (from PQC); Online - full text ed.: (from EBSCO Publishing, RoweCom Information Quest, Swets Blackwell, Springer LINK, Institute for Scientific Information).
Indexed: ASCA, Abstr.Hyg., Anim.Breed.Abstr., Chem.Abstr., Chem.Indus.Notes, Chem.Titles, Curr.Adv.Ecol.Sci., Curr.Adv.Gen.& Molec.Biol., Curr.Cont., Excerp.Med., Helminthol.Abstr., Immun.Abstr., Ind.Med. (coverage dropped), Ind.Sci.Rev., Inpharma, Pharm.&Out.News, Reac., Sci.Cit.Ind., Trop.Dis.Bull.
—BLDSC (8424.730000), ADONIS, CASDDS, CISTI, EMDOCS, GNLM, IDS, ingenta. **CCC.**
Published by: Springer-Verlag (Subsidiary of: BertelsmannSpringer), Tiergartenstr 17, Heidelberg 69121, Germany. TEL 49-6221-345-0, FAX 49-6221-345229, subscriptions@springer.de, http://link.springer.de/link/service/journals/00281/index.htm, http://www.springer.de. Ed. P A Miescher. **Subscr. in N. America to:** Springer-Verlag New York Inc., PO Box 2485, Secaucus, NJ 07096-2485. TEL 212-460-1500, FAX 212-473-6272.

SULLY'S LIVING WITHOUT; a lifestyle guide for people with food and chemical sensitivity. see *LIFESTYLE*

TEXAS HIV - STD UPDATE. see *MEDICAL SCIENCES—Communicable Diseases*

616.97 CHE ISSN 0896-341X
CODEN: THUPEZ
THYMUS UPDATE SERIES. Text in English. irreg., latest vol.4. price varies. *Refereed.* **Document type:** *Monographic series.*
Published by: Gordon and Breach - Harwood Academic (Subsidiary of: Taylor & Francis Group), PO Box 531, Lausanne 1000, Switzerland. Eds. M A Ritter, M D Kendall. **Subscr. addr. in US:** International Publishers Direct, PO Box 32160, Newark, NJ 07102. FAX 215-750-6343.

616.97 NLD ISSN 0966-3274
CODEN: TRIME2
TRANSPLANT IMMUNOLOGY. Text in English. 1993. q. USD 172 in US & Canada to individuals; EUR 154 in Europe to individuals; JPY 20,400 in Japan to individuals; USD 172 elsewhere to individuals; EUR 395 in Europe to institutions; JPY 52,400 in Japan to institutions; USD 442 elsewhere to institutions (effective 2002). adv. *Refereed.* **Document type:** *Academic/Scholarly.* **Description:** Includes original articles and reviews on all aspects of immunology as they relate to clinical and experimental transplants.
Related titles: Online - full text ed.: (from EBSCO Publishing, RoweCom Information Quest, ingenta, Swets Blackwell, Institute for Scientific Information, ScienceDirect).
Indexed: AIDS & Cancer Res., Chem.Abstr., Chem.Indus.Notes, Curr.Cont., Excerp.Med. (1994-), Immun.Abstr., Ind.Med. (1993-), Inpharma, Pharm.&Out.News, Reac., Sci.Cit.Ind.
—BLDSC (9024.988500), CASDDS, CISTI, EMDOCS, GNLM, IDS, Infotrieve, KNAW. **CCC.**

Published by: Elsevier Science BV, Life Sciences Department, Molenwerf 1, Amsterdam 1014 AG, Netherlands. TEL 31-20-485-2911, http://www.elsevier.nl/inca/publications/store/6/2/0/9/2/5/. Eds. Charles G Orosz, Ian V Hutchinson. **Subscr. to:** Turpin Distribution Services Ltd., Blackhorse Rd, Letchworth, Herts SG6 1HN, United Kingdom. TEL 44-1462-488900, FAX 44-1462-483011.

TRANSPLANTATION. see *MEDICAL SCIENCES—Surgery*

616.97 GBR ISSN 1471-4906
CODEN: IMTOD8

TRENDS IN IMMUNOLOGY. Text in English. 1980. m. GBP 88, EUR 115 in Europe to individuals; JPY 14,000 in Japan to individuals; USD 126 elsewhere to individuals; EUR 908 in Europe to institutions; JPY 125,900 in Japan to institutions; USD 1,015 elsewhere to institutions; GBP 44 in Europe to students; JPY 9,500 in Japan to students; USD 73 elsewhere to students; USD 1,308 to institutions Print & online eds. combined; EUR 144 in Europe to qualified personnel; JPY 17,500 in Japan to qualified personnel; USD 157 elsewhere to qualified personnel (effective 2002). adv. bk.rev. charts, illus, abstr. index. back issues avail.; reprint service avail. from SWZ. *Refereed.* **Document type:** *Academic/Scholarly.* **Description:** For immunologists and transplantation researchers, and all other scientists with an interest in the theory, practice, applications and techniques of modern immunology.

Formerly: Immunology Today (0167-5699)

Related titles: Online - full text ed.: Trends in Immunology Online. USD 168 to individuals; USD 965 to institutions (effective 1999) (from EBSCO Publishing, ingenta, Swets Blackwell, ScienceDirect, Institute for Scientific Information).

Indexed: AIDS & Cancer Res., AIDS Abstr., ASCA, Abstr.Hyg., Anim.Breed.Abstr., Aqua.Sci.& Fish.Abstr., Biol.Abstr., Chem.Abstr., Chem.Indus.Notes, Chem.Titles, Curr.Cont., Dairy Sci.Abstr., Diar.Dis.Res., Entomol.Abstr., Environ.Sci.Poll.Mgmt., Excerp.Med., Food Sci.& Tech.Abstr., Helminthol.Abstr., Immun.Abstr., Ind.Med. (2001-), Ind.Sci.Rev., Ind.Vet., Inpharma, Microbiol.Abstr., Nutr.Abstr., Pharm.&Out.News, Protozool.Abstr., Reac., Ref.Zh., Rev.Appl.Entomol., Rev.Med.& Vet.Mycol., SSCI (coverage dropped), Sci.Cit.Ind., Telegen, Vet.Bull.

—BLDSC (9049.630500), ADONIS, CISTI, EMDOCS, IDS, KNAW. **CCC.**

Published by: Elsevier Science Ltd., Elsevier Trends Journals, 68 Hills Rd, Cambridge CB2 1LA, United Kingdom. TEL 44-1223-315961, FAX 44-1223-464430, http://www.elsevier.nl/inca/publications/store/4/0/5/9/1/4/. Eds. Elaine Bell, Kirsty McCormack. Adv. contact Thelma Reid. Circ: 4,000. **Subscr. in Australasia and the Far East to:** Elsevier Science (Singapore) Pte Ltd, No.1 Temasek Ave, 17-01 Millenia Tower, Singapore 039192, Singapore. TEL 65-434-3727, FAX 65-337-2230; **Subscr. in the Americas to:** Elsevier Science, PO Box 945, New York, NY 10159-0945. TEL 212-633-3730, FAX 212-633-3680, http://www.elsevier.com; **Subscr. to:** Elsevier Current Trends Subscriptions, PO Box 331, Haywards Heath, W Sussex RH16 3FG, United Kingdom. TEL 44-1444-475650, FAX 44-1444-445423.

TRENDS IN MICROBIOLOGY. see *BIOLOGY—Microbiology*

616.97 TUR ISSN 1301-109X
CODEN: TJIMFF

TURKISH JOURNAL OF IMMUNOLOGY. Text in Turkish. 1996. s-a. membership. adv. **Document type:** *Academic/Scholarly.*

—BLDSC (9072.468762), CASDDS.

Published by: Turkish Society of Immunology, Cerrahpasa, P K 1, Istanbul 34303, Turkey. TEL 90-212-530-2095, FAX 90-212-586-1595. Ed. Birsen Y Ulku.

616.97 GBR

UNIVERSITY OF DUNDEE. TAYSIDE CENTRE FOR GENERAL PRACTICE. ASTHMA RESEARCH UNIT. PROGRESS REPORT. Text in English. irreg., latest vol.49. **Document type:** *Bulletin.*

Published by: University of Dundee, Tayside Centre for General Practice, Asthma Research Unit, Kirsty Semple Way, Dundee DD2 4BF, United Kingdom.

616.97 GBR ISSN 0264-410X
CODEN: VACCDE

VACCINE. Text in English. 1983. 34/yr. EUR 233 in Europe to individuals; JPY 30,900 in Japan to individuals; USD 261 elsewhere to individuals; EUR 2,013 in Europe to institutions; JPY 267,200 in Japan to institutions; USD 2,252 elsewhere to institutions (effective 2002). adv. bk.rev. abstr, bibl, charts, illus, pat, stat. index. back issues avail. *Refereed.* **Document type:** *Academic/Scholarly.* **Description:** Covers research and development, production and use of both human and veterinary vaccines.

Related titles: Microform ed.: (from PQC); Online - full text ed.: Vaccine Online. ISSN 1358-8745 (from EBSCO Publishing, ingenta, Swets Blackwell, Institute for Scientific Information, ScienceDirect).

Indexed: AIDS & Cancer Res., ASCA, Abstr.Hyg., AgBiotech, Agri.& Environ.Biotech.Abstr., Chem.Abstr., Chem.Indus.Notes, Chem.Titles, Curr.Adv.Ecol.Sci., Curr.Adv.Gen.& Molec.Biol., Curr.Biotech.Abstr., Curr.Cont., Dairy Sci.Abstr., Derwent Biotech.Abstr., Diar.Dis.Res., Dok.Arbeitsmed., Environ.Sci.Poll.Mgmt., Excerp.Med., Helminthol.Abstr., Immun.Abstr., Ind.Med. (1983-), Ind.Sci.Rev., Ind.Vet., Inpharma, Int.Abstr.Biol.Sci., Int.Nurs.Ind., Lab.Haz.Bull., Med.& Pharm.Biotech.Abstr., Microbiol.Abstr., Nutr.Abstr., Pharm.&Out.News, Pig News & Info., Pollut.Abstr., Poult.Abstr., Protozool.Abstr., Reac., Rev.Appl.Entomol., Rev.Arom.& Med.Plants, Rev.Med.& Vet.Mycol., Risk Abstr., Rural Devel.Abstr., SSCI (coverage dropped), Saf.Sci.Abstr., Sci.Cit.Ind., Small Anim.Abstr., Telegen, Trop.Dis.Bull., Vet.Bull., Virol.Abstr. (coverage dropped).

—BLDSC (9138.628000), ADONIS, CASDDS, CISTI, EMDOCS, GNLM, IDS, ingenta, KNAW. **CCC.**

Published by: Pergamon (Subsidiary of: Elsevier Science), The Boulevard, Langford Ln, East Park, Kidlington, Oxford OXB 1GB, United Kingdom. FAX 44-1865-843010, http://www.elsevier.nl/inca/publications/store/3/0/5/2/1/. Eds. J B Campbell, K Yamanishi, R E Spier. **Subscr. in Australasia and the Far East to:** Elsevier Science (Singapore) Pte Ltd, No.1 Temasek Ave, 17-01 Millenia Tower, Singapore 039192, Singapore. TEL 65-434-3727, FAX 65-337-2230; **Subscr. in the Americas to:** Elsevier Science, PO Box 945, New York, NY 10159-0945. TEL 212-633-3730, FAX 212-633-3680; **Subscr. to:** Elsevier Science BV, PO Box 211, Amsterdam 1000 AE, Netherlands. TEL 31-20-485-3757, nlinfo-f@elsevier.nl.

616.96 USA ISSN 0899-4056
QR189 CODEN: VMAVEA

VACCINES (YEAR). Text in English. a. reprints avail. **Document type:** *Monographic series.*

—KNAW. **CCC.**

Published by: Cold Spring Harbor Laboratory Press, Publications Department, 10 Skyline Dr, Plainview, NY 11803. TEL 800-843-4388, FAX 516-349-1946, cshpress@cshl.org, http://www.cshl.org.

VETERINARY IMMUNOLOGY AND IMMUNOPATHOLOGY; an international journal of comparative immunology. see *VETERINARY SCIENCE*

616.925 616.079 USA ISSN 0882-8245
CODEN: VIIMET

VIRAL IMMUNOLOGY. Text in English. 1987. q. USD 179 domestic to individuals; USD 289 foreign to individuals; USD 215 domestic to individuals print and online eds. combined; USD 325 foreign to individuals print and online eds. combined; USD 409 domestic to institutions; USD 523 foreign to institutions; USD 491 domestic to institutions print and online eds. combined; USD 605 foreign to institutions print and online eds. combined (effective 2002). abstr, charts, stat. back issues avail.; reprints avail. *Refereed.* **Document type:** *Journal, Academic/Scholarly.* **Description:** Covers human and animal viral immunology. Includes research and development of viral vaccines. Features regular mini-reviews of all relevant literature.

Related titles: Online - full content ed.: USD 179 to individuals; USD 409 to institutions (effective 2002); Online - full text ed.: (from CatchWord Ltd., Institute for Scientific Information, RoweCom Information Quest).

Indexed: AIDS & Cancer Res., Chem.Abstr., Chem.Indus.Notes, Chem.Titles, Curr.Cont., Excerp.Med., INIS Atomind., Immun.Abstr., Ind.Med. (1987-), Inpharma, Int.Abstr.Biol.Sci., Pharm.&Out.News, Reac., Sci.Cit.Ind., Virol.Abstr.

—BLDSC (9237.876000), CASDDS, CISTI, EMDOCS, GNLM, IDS, ingenta, KNAW. **CCC.**

Published by: Mary Ann Liebert, Inc. Publishers, 2 Madison Ave, Larchmont, NY 10538. TEL 914—834-3100, FAX 914-834-1388, info@liebertpub.com, www.liebertpub.com/vim, http://www.liebertpub.com. Ed. Carol Shoshkes Reiss.

615.65 GBR ISSN 0042-9007
CODEN: VOSAAD

VOX SANGUINIS; international journal of transfusion medicine. Text in English. 1956. 8/yr. (in 2 vols.), latest vol.82, 2002. GBP 75 in Europe to individuals; USD 131 in North America to individuals; GBP 82 elsewhere to individuals; GBP 324 in Europe to institutions; USD 525 in North America to institutions; GBP 356 elsewhere to institutions (effective 2002). adv. bibl, charts, illus. index. back issues avail. *Refereed.* **Document type:** *Journal, Academic/Scholarly.* **Description:** Reports on important developments in transfusion medicine. Original papers and reviews are published on all aspects of blood transfusion, with emphasis on new molecular biological techniques, the detection of viral antigens or antibodies and the activation of transmittable viruses.

Related titles: Microform ed.; Online - full text ed.: ISSN 1423-0410. 199?. GBP 68 in Europe to individuals; USD 118 in North America to individuals; GBP 68 elsewhere to individuals; GBP 292 in Europe to institutions; USD 473 in North America to institutions; GBP 292 elsewhere to institutions (effective 2002) (from Northern Light Technology, Inc., EBSCO Publishing, O C L C Online Computer Library Center, Inc., RoweCom Information Quest, ProQuest Information & Learning, Swets Blackwell, Institute for Scientific Information).

Indexed: ASCA, Abstr.Hyg., Anim.Breed.Abstr., Biol.Abstr., Chem.Abstr., Chem.Indus.Notes, Curr.Adv.Ecol.Sci., Curr.Cont., Dairy Sci.Abstr., Dent.Ind., Environ.Sci.Poll.Mgmt., Excerp.Med., Genet.Abstr., Helminthol.Abstr., INIS Atomind., Ind.Med. (1953-), Ind.Sci.Rev., Ind.Vet., Inpharma, Int.Abstr.Biol.Sci., Int.Nurs.Ind., Nutr.Abstr., Pharm.&Out.News, Pollut.Abstr., Reac., Risk Abstr., SSCI (coverage dropped), Saf.Sci.Abstr., Sci.Cit.Ind., Trop.Dis.Bull., Vet.Bull.

—BLDSC (9258.700000), CASDDS, CISTI, GNLM, IDS, ingenta, KNAW. **CCC.**

Published by: (International Society of Blood Transfusion CHE), Blackwell Science Ltd., Osney Mead, Oxford OX2 0EL, United Kingdom. TEL 44-1685-206206, FAX 44-1685-721205, journals.cs@blacksci.co.uk, http://www.blackwell-science.com. Ed. M Contreras. Circ: 2,900. **Co-sponsor:** League of Red Cross Societies.

616.97 CHN ISSN 1007-8738

XIBAO YU FENZI MIANYIXUE ZAZHI/JOURNAL OF CELLULAR AND MOLECULAR IMMUNOLOGY. Text in Chinese. 1985. bi-m. USD 25.20; CNY 8, USD 4.20 newsstand/cover (effective 2001). **Document type:** *Academic/Scholarly.*

Related titles: Online - full content ed.: (from WanFang Data Corp.).

Published by: Zhongguo Mianyi Xuehui, 169, Changle Xi Lu, Xi'an 710032, China. TEL 86-29-3374550, immuedit@fmmu.edu.cn, http://www.immunology.net/jcmi. Ed. Boquan Jin. **Dist. by:** China International Book Trading Corp, 35, Chegongzhuang Xilu, Haidian District, Beijing 100044, China. TEL 86-1-68413849, FAX 86-1-68412048, cibtc@mail.cibtc.com.cn, http://www.cibtc.com.cn.

616.97 USA ISSN 1082-9776
RC583

YEAR BOOK OF ALLERGY, ASTHMA AND CLINICAL IMMUNOLOGY. Text in English. 1994. a. USD 87 domestic; USD 93 foreign (effective 2001). illus. **Document type:** *Academic/Scholarly.*

Formerly (until 1995): Year Book of Allergy and Clinical Immunology (1074-9225)

Published by: Mosby, Inc. (Subsidiary of: Elsevier Science), 11830 Westline Industrial Dr, St Louis, MO 63146-3318. TEL 314-872-8370, 800-325-4177, FAX 314-43213804, http://www.mosby.com/periodicals. Ed. Lanny J Rosenwasser.

616.97 CHN

ZHONGGUO MEIJIE SHENGWUXUE JI KONGZHI ZAZHI. Text in Chinese. bi-m.

Indexed: Bio-Contr.News & Info., Forest.Abstr., Ind.Vet., Protozool.Abstr., Rev.Appl.Entomol., Rev.Arom.& Med.Plants, Rev.Med.& Vet.Mycol., Trop.Dis.Bull., Vet.Bull., Zoo.Rec.

Published by: Zhonghua Yufang Yixuehui/China Preventive Medical Society, 16 Hepingli Zhongjie, Beijing 100013, China. TEL 4218457. Ed. Wang Chengxin.

616.97 CHN ISSN 1000-484X

ZHONGGUO MIANYIXUE ZAZHI/CHINESE JOURNAL OF IMMUNOLOGY. Text in Chinese. 1985. m. USD 50.40; USD 4.20 newsstand/cover (effective 2001). *Refereed.* **Document type:** *Academic/Scholarly.*

Related titles: Online - full content ed.: (from WanFang Data Corp.).

Indexed: Chem.Abstr., Chem.Indus.Notes, Chem.Titles.

M

Published by: (Zhongguo Mianyi Xuehui), Jilin Sheng Weisheng Ting/Jilin Provincial Bureau of Health, Fu 2, Dong Minzhu Dajie, Changchun, Jilin 130061, China. Ed. Xie Guangwen. **Dist. by:** China International Book Trading Corp, 35, Chegongzhuang Xilu, Haidian District, Beijing 100044, China. TEL 86-1-68413849, FAX 86-1-68412048, cibtc@mail.cibtc.com.cn, http://www.cibtc.com.cn.

616.97 CHN ISSN 0254-5101 CODEN: ZWMZDP
ZHONGHUA WEISHENGWUXUE HE MIANYIXUE ZAZHI/CHINESE JOURNAL OF MICROBIOLOGY AND IMMUNOLOGY. Text in Chinese. 1981. bi-m. CNY 54 domestic; USD 31.20 foreign; CNY 9 newsstand/cover domestic; USD 5.20 newsstand/cover foreign (effective 2001). **Document type:** *Academic/Scholarly.*
Related titles: Online - full content ed.: (from WanFang Data Corp.).
Indexed: Biodet.Abstr., Chem.Abstr., Excerp.Med. (1993-), Food Sci.& Tech.Abstr., INSPEC (1993-, dropped), Rev.Appl.Entomol.
—BLDSC (3180.430500), CASDDS, EMDOCS, Linda Hall.
Published by: Beijing Shengwu Zhipin Yanjiusuo, Zhaoyang-qu, Sanjianfang Nanli 4-hao, Beijing 100024, China. TEL 86-1-65756595. Ed. Hemin Li. **Dist. by:** China International Book Trading Corp, 35, Chegongzhuang Xilu, Haidian District, Beijing 100044, China. TEL 86-1-68413849, FAX 86-1-68412048, cibtc@mail.cibtc.com.cn, http://www.cibtc.com.cn.

MEDICAL SCIENCES—Anaesthesiology

617.96 DEU CODEN: AINNDT
A I N S - ANAESTHESIOLOGIE INTENSIVMEDIZIN NOTFALLMEDIZIN SCHMERZTHERAPIE. Text in German; Summaries in English, German. 1966. m. EUR 294.40 domestic to institutions; EUR 304.80 in Europe to institutions; EUR 322.80 elsewhere to institutions; EUR 29 newsstand/cover (effective 2002). adv. bk.rev. bibl, charts, illus, stat. index. reprint service avail. from PQC. *Refereed.* **Document type:** *Journal, Academic/Scholarly.*
Former titles: Anaesthesie - Intensivtherapie - Notfallmedizin - Schmerztherapie (0939-2661); (until 1990): Anaesthesie - Intensivtherapie - Notfallmedizin (0174-1837); (until 1980): Praktische Anaesthesie (0302-7600); (until 1974): Zeitschrift fuer Praktische Anaesthesie, Wiederbelebung und Intensivtherapie (0044-3387)
Related titles: Online - full text ed.: ISSN 1439-1074 (from Institute for Scientific Information).
Indexed: Curr.Cont. (coverage dropped), Excerp.Med., INIS Atomind., Ind.Med. (1991-), Ref.Zh., Sci.Cit.Ind. (coverage dropped).
—BLDSC (0897.895000), CASDDS, CISTI, EMDOCS, GNLM, IDS, Infotrieve, KNAW. **CCC.**
Published by: (Deutsche Gesellschaft fuer Anaesthesiologie und Intensivmedizin), Georg Thieme Verlag, Ruedigerstr 14, Stuttgart 70469, Germany. TEL 49-711-8931-0, FAX 49-711-8931298, kunden.service@thieme.de, http://www.thieme.de/ains/index.html. adv.: page DEM 3,150; 175 x 250. Circ: 6,100.

612 USA ISSN 1057-1590
A P S BULLETIN. Text in English. 1991. bi-m. membership. adv. bk.rev. charts, illus, stat. **Document type:** *Newsletter, Academic/Scholarly.* **Description:** Covers clinical and scientific research, public policy, epidemiology, and organizational news.
Related titles: Online - full text ed.
Published by: American Pain Society, 4700 W Lake Ave, Glenview, IL 60025-1485. TEL 847-375-4715, FAX 847-375-6315, info@ampainsoc.org, http://www.ampainsoc.org. Ed., R&P Peter J Vicente TEL 513-241-2370. Adv. contact Kathryn Checea. page USD 575; 10 x 7. Circ: 3,400.

617.96 USA ISSN 0363-471X
A S A REFRESHER COURSES IN ANESTHESIOLOGY. Text in English. 1973. a., latest vol.29. USD 29.95 (effective 2000). **Document type:** *Academic/Scholarly.*
Related titles: Microform ed.: (from PQC).
—BLDSC (7333.765000), GNLM.
Published by: (American Society of Anesthesiologists), Lippincott Williams & Wilkins (Philadelphia) (Subsidiary of: Wolters Kluwer N.V.), 530 Walnut St, Philadelphia, PA 19106-3621. TEL 301-223-2300, 800-638-3030, FAX 301-223-2400, http://www.asa-refresher.com/, http://www.Lww.com. Ed. Alan Jay Schwartz.

617.96 BEL ISSN 0001-5164 CODEN: AABEAJ
ACTA ANAESTHESIOLOGICA BELGICA. Text in Flemish. 1966 (vol.17). 4/yr. EUR 64.45 domestic; EUR 74.35 foreign; EUR 16.10 domestic; EUR 18.60 foreign (effective 2002). Supplement avail. **Document type:** *Journal, Academic/Scholarly.*
Indexed: Biol.Abstr., Chem.Abstr., Dent.Ind., Excerp.Med., Ind.Med. (1950-).
—BLDSC (0593.600000), CASDDS, CISTI, EMDOCS, GNLM, ingenta, KNAW.
Published by: (Association des Societes Scientifiques Medicales Belges/Vereiniging van de Belgische Wetenschappelijke Genootschappen), Acta Medica Belgica, Av Circulaire 138A, Brussels 1180, Belgium. TEL 32-2-374-5158, FAX 32-2-3749628, amb@skynet.be, http://www.ulb.ac.be/medecine/loce/amb.htm. Ed. Dr. G Rolly.

617.96 ITA ISSN 1124-8882 CODEN: AANIBO
ACTA ANAESTHESIOLOGICA ITALICA & ANAESTHESIA AND INTENSIVE CARE IN ITALY; rivista di anestesia e cure pre e post-operatorie. Text in Italian, English. 1996. 3/yr. ITL 80,000 domestic; ITL 150,000, EUR 77 foreign (effective 2000). adv. abstr, illus. index. back issues avail.
Formed by the merger of (1989-1995): Anaesthesia and Intensive Care in Italy (1125-0143); (1972-1995): Acta Anaesthesiologica Italica (0374-4965); Which was formerly (until 1971): Acta Anaesthesiologica (0001-5156)
Indexed: Biol.Abstr., Chem.Abstr., Excerp.Med., Ind.Med. (coverage dropped), Ref.Zh.
—BLDSC (0593.635000), CASDDS, CISTI, EMDOCS, GNLM.
Published by: Tipografia Editrice la Garangola, Via Montona, 4, Padua, PD 35137, Italy. FAX 39-49-8751743.

617.96 DNK ISSN 0001-5172 CODEN: AANEAB
ACTA ANAESTHESIOLOGICA SCANDINAVICA. Text and summaries in English. 1957. 11/yr. GBP 183 combined subscription print & online eds. combined (effective 2002). adv. bibl, charts, illus, stat. index. reprint service avail. from ISI. *Refereed.* **Document type:** *Journal, Academic/Scholarly.*
Related titles: Online - full text ed.: ISSN 1399-6576. GBP 165 (effective 2002) (from Ovid Technologies, Inc., EBSCO Publishing, O C L C Online Computer Library Center, Inc., RoweCom Information Quest, ingenta, Munksgaard & Blackwell Science's Synergy, Swets Blackwell, Institute for Scientific Information).
Indexed: ASCA, Agri.& Environ.Biotech.Abstr. (coverage dropped), Biol.Abstr., Chem.Abstr., Chem.Indus.Notes, Chem.Titles, Curr.Adv.Ecol.Sci., Curr.Cont., Curr.Tit.Dent., Dent.Ind., Derwent Biotech.Abstr., Dok.Arbeitsmed., Environ.Sci.Poll.Mgmt., Excerp.Med., INIS Atomind., Ind.Med. (1957-), Ind.Sci.Rev., Inpharma, Int.Abstr.Biol.Sci., Int.Nurs.Ind., Neurosci.Cit.Ind., Pharm.&Out.News, Pollut.Abstr., Reac., Risk Abstr., SSCI (coverage dropped), Saf.Sci.Abstr., Sci.Cit.Ind., THA.
—BLDSC (0593.650000), ADONIS, CASDDS, CISTI, EMDOCS, GNLM, IDS, ingenta, KNAW. **CCC.**
Published by: (Acta Anaesthesiologica Foundation), Blackwell Munksgaard, Noerre Soegade 35, PO Box 2148, Copenhagen K 1016, Denmark. FAX 45-77-33-33-77, customerservice@munksgaard.dk, http://www.acta-anaesth.dk, http://www.munksgaard.dk. Ed. Sven Erik Gisvold. Adv. contact Eric Rozario TEL 45-77-33-33-01. Circ: 4,800.

617.96 DNK ISSN 0515-2720 CODEN: AASXAP
ACTA ANAESTHESIOLOGICA SCANDINAVICA. SUPPLEMENTUM. Text in English. irreg. free with subscription to Acta Anaesthesiologica Scandinavica. **Document type:** *Academic/Scholarly.*
Related titles: Online - full text ed.: ISSN 1600-5430 (from Ovid Technologies, Inc.).
Indexed: Biol.Abstr., Chem.Abstr., Chem.Indus.Notes, Chem.Titles, Curr.Adv.Ecol.Sci., Curr.Cont. (coverage dropped), Excerp.Med., INIS Atomind., Ind.Med. (1959-).
—BLDSC (0593.651000), ADONIS, CASDDS, CISTI, EMDOCS, KNAW. **CCC.**
Published by: (Acta Anaesthesiologica Foundation), Blackwell Munksgaard, Noerre Soegade 35, PO Box 2148, Copenhagen K 1016, Denmark. TEL 45-77-33-33-33, customerservice@munksgaard.dk, http://www.acta-anaesth.dk. Ed. Sven Erik Gisvold. Adv. contact Eric Rozario TEL 45-77-33-33-01.

617.96 ESP ISSN 1132-0095
ACTUALIZACIONES EN ANESTESIOLOGIA Y REANIMACION. Text in Spanish; Abstracts in Spanish, English. 1991. q. ESP 7,000 to individuals; ESP 10,000 to institutions; USD 200 foreign (effective 2000). adv. abstr, bibl, illus, stat. back issues avail. **Document type:** *Academic/Scholarly.*
—BLDSC (0677.605000), GNLM, KNAW.
Published by: Aran Ediciones S.A., Castello, 128 1o, Madrid 28006, Spain. TEL 34-91-782-0030, FAX 34-91-561-5787, edita@grupoaran.com, http://www.grupoaran.com. Ed. F. Gilsanz Rodrigues. Pub. Jose Jimenez. R&P Maria Dolores Linares TEL 34-1-7820035. Circ: 3,000.

617.96 USA ISSN 0737-6146
RD78.3
ADVANCES IN ANESTHESIA. Text in English. 1982. a. USD 93 domestic; USD 99 foreign (effective 2001). **Document type:** *Academic/Scholarly.* **Description:** Presents a collection of original, fully referenced articles from experts in the field.
—BLDSC (0698.850000), CISTI, GNLM, ingenta, KNAW.
Published by: Mosby, Inc. (Subsidiary of: Elsevier Science), 11830 Westline Industrial Dr, St Louis, MO 63146-3313. TEL 314-872-8370, 800-325-4177, FAX 314-432-1380, http://www.mosby.com/periodicals. Ed. Carol L Lake.

617.96 USA ISSN 1078-4500
RD78.3 CODEN: AJANF7
THE AMERICAN JOURNAL OF ANESTHESIOLOGY. Text in English. 1973. 9/yr. USD 132 in the Americas to institutions; USD 170 elsewhere to institutions (effective 2000). adv. bk.rev. charts, illus. **Document type:** *Trade.*
Former titles (until 1995): Anesthesiology Review (0093-4437)
Related titles: Microform ed.: (from PQC).
Indexed: Excerp.Med.
—BLDSC (0821.040000), CISTI, EMDOCS, GNLM, Infotrieve, KNAW. **CCC.**
Published by: Quadrant HealthCom, 26 Main St, Ste A, Chatham, NJ 07928-2402. TEL 973-701-8900, FAX 973-701-8892. Ed. Barbara Ready. Pub. Linda Fox. Adv. contact Denise Andrade. Circ: 18,045 (controlled).

617.96 USA ISSN 0270-5877
AMERICAN SOCIETY OF ANESTHESIOLOGISTS NEWSLETTER. Text in English. 1938. m. USD 25 to non-members (effective 2000 - 2001). index. **Document type:** *Newsletter.* **Description:** Covers subjects of interest to anesthesiologists.
Published by: American Society of Anesthesiologists, 520 N Northwest Hwy, Park Ridge, IL 60068-2573. TEL 847-825-5586, FAX 847-825-5658, mail@asahq.org, http://www.asahq.org. Ed. Dr. Mark Lema. R&P Denise M Jones. Circ: 35,000.

617.96 AUS ISSN 0310-057X
ANAESTHESIA AND INTENSIVE CARE. Text in English. 1972. bi-m. AUD 205 to individuals; AUD 345 to institutions (effective 2001); AUD 230 to individuals; AUD 380 to institutions (effective 2002). adv. bk.rev. bibl, charts, illus. index. 120 p./no. back issues avail. *Refereed.* **Document type:** *Academic/Scholarly.* **Description:** Presents original articles of scientific and clinical interest in the specialties of anaesthesia, intensive care, pain therapy, and related disciplines.
Related titles: CD-ROM ed.: AUD 120 (effective 2001); Microfiche ed.: (from PQC); Online - full text ed.: (from ProQuest Information & Learning, Institute for Scientific Information).
Indexed: ASCA, Biol.Abstr., CINAHL, Curr.Adv.Ecol.Sci., Curr.Cont., Excerp.Med., Ind.Med. (1972-), Ind.Sci.Rev., Inpharma, Int.Nurs.Ind., Nutr.Abstr., Pharm.&Out.News, Protozool.Abstr., Reac., Sci.Cit.Ind.
—BLDSC (0859.901500), CISTI, EMDOCS, GNLM, IDS, ingenta, KNAW.
Published by: Australian Society of Anaesthetists, PO Box 600, Edgecliff, NSW 2027, Australia. TEL 61-2-9327-4022, FAX 61-2-9362-9139, mconolly@fed.asa.org.au, http://www.aaic.net.au. Ed. John G Roberts. R&P Jeanette Thirlwell Jones. Adv. contact Margaret Conolly. Circ: 3,800.

617.96 JOR ISSN 0259-1162 CODEN: AESRE
ANAESTHESIA ESSAYS AND RESEARCHES. Text in Arabic, English. 1985. a. USD 18. adv. bk.rev. **Document type:** *Academic/Scholarly.* **Description:** Specialized research journal published by the Arabic Scientific Committee on anaesthesia and intensive care.
Indexed: Excerp.Med. (until 1993).
Published by: (Pan-Arabic Scientific Committee), Dar Ammar for Publication, Petra Market, P O Box 921691, Amman, Jordan. TEL 01-652437, TELEX 55545 JUST JO. Ed. Dr. M Takrouri. Circ: 3,000.

M

617.96 GBR ISSN 1361-8245
ANAESTHESIA ON-LINE. Variant title: International Journal of Anaesthesia. Text in English. 1995. m. adv. bk.rev., software rev., video rev. *Refereed.* **Document type:** *Journal, Academic/Scholarly.* **Description:** Publishes case reports, audits, treatment protocols, review papers and reseach on anaesthesia.
Media: Online - full text.
Published by: Priory Lodge Education Ltd., 2 Cornflower Way, Moreton, Wirral CH46 1SV, United Kingdom. TEL 44-151-606-1796, FAX 44-151-606-1812, solutions@priory.com, http://www.priory.com/anaes.htm. Ed. Dr. Ben Green. Circ: 20,000 (controlled).

617.96 GBR ISSN 0003-2409
CODEN: ANASAB
ANAESTHESIA (OXFORD). Text in English. 1945. m., latest vol.57, 2002. GBP 99 in Europe to individuals; USD 157 in North America to individuals; GBP 109 elsewhere to individuals; GBP 317 in Europe to institutions; USD 503 in North America to institutions; GBP 349 elsewhere to institutions (effective 2002). adv. bk.rev. bibl, illus. index. back issues avail.; reprint service avail. from SWZ,ISI. *Refereed.* **Document type:** *Academic/Scholarly.* **Description:** Covers practical techniques of general and local anaesthesia, pre- and postoperative management, resuscitation and intensive care, and acute and chronic pain therapy.
Related titles: Online - full text ed.: ISSN 1365-2044. 199?. GBP 90 in Europe to individuals; USD 142 in North America to individuals; GBP 90 elsewhere to individuals; GBP 286 in Europe to institutions; USD 453 in North America to institutions; GBP 286 elsewhere to institutions (effective 2002) (from Ovid Technologies, Inc., EBSCO Publishing, O C L C Online Computer Library Center, Inc., RoweCom Information Quest, ingenta, Munksgaard & Blackwell Science's Synergy, Swets Blackwell, Institute for Scientific Information).
Indexed: AIM, ASCA, Agri.& Environ.Biotech.Abstr. (coverage dropped), Biol.Abstr., Brit.Nur.Ind., Chem.Abstr., Chem.Indus.Notes, Chem.Titles, Curr.Adv.Ecol.Sci., Curr.Cont., Derwent Biotech.Abstr., Environ.Sci.Poll.Mgmt., Excerp.Med., INIS Atomind., Ind.Med. (1946-), Ind.Sci.Rev., Inpharma, Int.Nurs.Ind., Jrnl.Watch Emer.Med., Nutr.Abstr., Pharm.&Out.News, Pollut.Abstr., Reac., Rev.Plant Path., Risk Abstr., SSCI (coverage dropped), Saf.Sci.Abstr., Sci.Cit.Ind.
—BLDSC (0859.900000), CASDDS, CISTI, EMDOCS, GNLM, IDS, ingenta, KNAW. **CCC.**
Published by: (Association of Anaesthetists of Great Britain and Ireland), Blackwell Science Ltd., PO Box 88, Oxford OX2 0NE, United Kingdom. TEL 44-1865-206180, 44-1865-206002, FAX 44-1865-206219, jnl.orders@blacksci.co.uk, http://www.blackwell-science.com/~cgilib/jnlpage.asp?Journal=anae&File=anae, http://www.blackwellpublishing.com. Ed. M Harmer. Pub. Allen Stevens. R&P Sophie Savage. Adv. contact Jenny Applin. Circ: 8,365.

617.96 CHE
ANAESTHESIE JOURNAL. Text in French, German, Italian. 1978. q. CHF 56. adv. bk.rev. **Document type:** *Bulletin.*
Former titles: S B A P - A S I A Bulletin; (until 1992): S F A - A S A Bulletin
Address: Ulimattweg 12, St. Niklaus Vs 3924, Switzerland. TEL 41-32-801279, FAX 071-253321. Ed. D Barthlome. Adv. contact H Wiskerke. Circ: 2,000.

617 DEU ISSN 0170-5334
CODEN: ATIMDA
ANAESTHESIOLOGIE UND INTENSIVMEDIZIN. Text in German. 1970. m. DEM 457.86 in Europe; DEM 516.34 elsewhere; DEM 503.65 in Europe print & online eds. combined; DEM 567.97 elsewhere print & online eds. combined (effective 2001). *Refereed.* **Document type:** *Journal, Academic/Scholarly.*
Formerly: Anaesthesiologische Informationen
Related titles: ♦ Online - full text ed.: Anaesthesiologie und Intensivmedizin Online. ISSN 1439-0256.
Indexed: Biol.Abstr., Chem.Abstr., Curr.Cont., Ref.Zh.
—BLDSC (0897.905000), CASDDS, EMDOCS, GNLM, IDS, KNAW. **CCC.**
Published by: (Deutsche Gesellschaft fuer Anaesthesiologie und Intensivmedizin, Berufsverband Deutscher Anaesthesisten), Blackwell Wissenschafts Verlag GmbH, Kurfuerstendamm 57, Berlin 10707, Germany. TEL 49-30-32790630, FAX 49-30-32790610, abo@blackwis.de, http://www.blackwell.de. Ed. Dr. B Landauer. Circ: 16,500.

617.96 USA ISSN 0171-1814
CODEN: ANIMD2
ANAESTHESIOLOGIE UND INTENSIVMEDIZIN/ ANAESTHESIOLOGY AND INTENSIVE CARE MEDICINE. Text in German, English, French. 1963. irreg., latest vol.212, 1990. price varies. reprint service avail. from ISI. **Document type:** *Monographic series.*
Formerly: Anaesthesiology and Resuscitation (0066-1341)
Indexed: Int.Nurs.Ind.
—CASDDS, CISTI, GNLM, Infotrieve, KNAW. **CCC.**
Published by: Springer-Verlag, Journals (Subsidiary of: BertelsmannSpringer), 175 Fifth Ave, New York, NY 10010. TEL 212-460-1500, FAX 212-473-6272.

617 DEU ISSN 1439-0256
ANAESTHESIOLOGIE UND INTENSIVMEDIZIN ONLINE. Text in German. m. DEM 413 (effective 2001). **Document type:** *Academic/Scholarly.*
Media: Online - full text (from Institute for Scientific Information). **Related titles:** ♦ Print ed.: Anaesthesiologie und Intensivmedizin. ISSN 0170-5334.
Published by: Blackwell Wissenschafts Verlag GmbH, Kurfuerstendamm 57, Berlin 10707, Germany. TEL 49-30-327906-0, FAX 49-30-32790610, abo@blackwis.de, http://www.blackwell.de/ai.htm.

617.96 DEU ISSN 0323-4983
CODEN: ANREDN
ANAESTHESIOLOGIE UND REANIMATION; Zeitschrift fuer Anaesthesiologie, Intensivtherapie, Notfallmedizin und Schmerztherapie. Text in English, German; Summaries in English. 1976. bi-m. DEM 150. **Document type:** *Academic/Scholarly.*
Indexed: Excerp.Med., INIS Atomind., Ind.Med. (1976-), Int.Nurs.Ind.
—BLDSC (0859.904700), CASDDS, CISTI, EMDOCS, GNLM, Infotrieve, KNAW. **CCC.**
Published by: (Gesellschaft fuer Anaesthesiologie und Intensivmedizin), Selecta Verlagsgesellschaft mbH, Postfach 4240, Wiesbaden 65032, Germany. TEL 0611-1705-0. Ed. G Benad. Circ: 1,200.

617.96 DEU ISSN 0003-2417
CODEN: ANATAE
DER ANAESTHESIST. Text in German. 1952. m. EUR 319.62 foreign; EUR 305.32 in Germany; EUR 29 newsstand/cover foreign (effective 2002). adv. bk.rev. abstr, bibl, charts, illus. index. back issues avail.; reprint service avail. from ISI. *Refereed.* **Document type:** *Journal, Academic/Scholarly.* **Description:** Covers all aspects of anaesthesia and pain management.
Related titles: Microform ed.: (from PQC); Online - full text ed.: ISSN 1432-055X (from EBSCO Publishing, RoweCom Information Quest, Swets Blackwell, Springer LINK, Institute for Scientific Information); ♦ Supplement: Der Anaesthesist. Supplement. ISSN 1437-4943.
Indexed: ASCA, Abstr.Health Care Manage.Stud., Agri.& Environ.Biotech.Abstr. (coverage dropped), Biol.Abstr., Chem.Abstr., Chem.Indus.Notes, Chem.Titles, Curr.Cont., Dent.Ind., Derwent Biotech.Abstr., Excerp.Med., INIS Atomind., Ind.Med. (1952-), Ind.Sci.Rev., Inpharma, Int.Nurs.Ind., Pharm.&Out.News, Reac., Sci.Cit.Ind.
—BLDSC (0859.920000), ADONIS, CASDDS, CISTI, EMDOCS, GNLM, IDS, KNAW. **CCC.**
Published by: (Deutschen Gesellschaft fuer Anaesthesiologie und Intensivmedizin), Springer-Verlag (Subsidiary of: BertelsmannSpringer), Tiergartenstr 17, Heidelberg 69121, Germany. TEL 49-6221-345-0, FAX 49-6221-345229, subscriptions@springer.de, http://link.springer.de/link/service/journals/00101/index.htm, http://www.springer.de. Eds. K Peter, R Larsen. **Subscr. in N. America to:** Springer-Verlag New York Inc., PO Box 2485, Secaucus, NJ 07096-2485. TEL 212-460-1500, FAX 212-473-6272. **Co-sponsor:** Oesterreichischen Gesellschaft fuer Anaesthesiologie, Reanimation und Intensivtherapie, Schweizerischen Gesellschaft fuer Anaesthesiologie und Reanimation.

617.96 DEU ISSN 1437-4943
DER ANAESTHESIST. SUPPLEMENT. Text in German. irreg.
Related titles: ♦ Supplement to: Der Anaesthesist. ISSN 0003-2417.
Published by: Springer-Verlag (Subsidiary of: BertelsmannSpringer), Haber Str 7, Heidelberg 69126, Germany. TEL 49-30-8278-7358. Ed. Dr. Beate Fruhstorfer.

617.96 616.8 USA ISSN 1071-569X
CODEN: AALGEB
ANALGESIA. Text in English. 1994. q. USD 200 domestic; USD 220 foreign (effective 2001). adv. *Refereed.* **Document type:** *Academic/Scholarly.* **Description:** Covers preclinical studies that are directed toward an aspect of pain pathways (e.g. anatomical, biochemical, molecular, pharmacological or physiological) and their identification; that involve the study of neurotransmitters of modulators; or that investigate some aspect of known or experimental analgesic-antinociceptive compounds (including side effects).
Indexed: Chem.Abstr., Chem.Indus.Notes, Chem.Titles, Ind.Med. (coverage dropped), Inpharma, Reac., e-psyche.
—BLDSC (0890.239700), CASDDS, GNLM. **CCC.**
Published by: Cognizant Communication Corporation, 3 Hartsdale Rd, Elmsford, NY 10523-3701. TEL 914-592-7720, FAX 914-592-8981, cogcomm@aol.com, http://www.cognizantcommunication.com. Eds. Frank Porreca, Dr. Robert B Raffa. Pub., R&P Robert N Miranda. Adv. contact Lori Miranda.

617.96 MEX ISSN 1405-0056
CODEN: AMEXFA
ANESTESIA EN MEXICO. Text in Spanish; Summaries in English. 1989. bi-m. MXP 300, USD 55 (effective 1996 & 1997). *Refereed.* **Document type:** *Academic/Scholarly.* **Description:** Contains original articles, research reports, review articles, clinical cases, and notices related to anesthesiology.
Published by: (Federacion Mexicana de Sociedades de Anestesiologia), Obsidiana Editores S.A., CZDA DE TLALPAN 2365, Col Ciudad Jardin, Mexico City, DF 04370, Mexico. TEL 52-5-689-9133. Ed. Dr. Orlando Tamariz. Pub. Jorge Godoy-Gutierrez. Circ: 3,000. **Dist. by:** Distribuidora Editorial de Mexico SA de CV, P.O. Box 76-026, Mexico City, DF 04201, Mexico. TEL 52-5-544-7953, FAX 52-5-689-6545.

617.96 ITA ISSN 0392-5854
ANESTESISTA. Text in Italian. 1978. bi-m.
Published by: Associazione Anestesisti Rianimatori Ospedalieri Italiani, Via Angelo Poliziano, 69, Rome, RM 00184, Italy. Ed. Alessandro Pesce.

617.89 616.02 CZE ISSN 0862-4968
ANESTEZIOLOGIE A NEODKLADNA PECE. Text in Czech, Slovak; Summaries in Czech, English. 1990. 6/yr. EUR 66, USD 84 (effective 2001). adv. *Refereed.* **Document type:** *Academic/Scholarly.* **Description:** In addition to anaesthesiology covers problems of resuscitation and intensive (emergency) care, medicine of disasters, treatment of acute and chronic pain and problems of pre-hospital care.
Indexed: INIS Atomind.
—GNLM.
Published by: (Ceska Lekarska Spolecnost J.E. Purkyne/Czech Medical Association), Nakladatelske Stredisko C L S J.E. Purkyne, Sokolska 31, Prague 12026, Czech Republic. TEL 420-2-24911420, FAX 420-2-24911420. Ed. J Pocta. adv.: B&W page CZK 31,000, color page CZK 44,000; 176 x 256. Circ: 2,000. **Dist. by:** Abont s.r.o., Chlumova 17, Prague, 3 130 00, Czech Republic; **Dist. in Western countries by:** Kubon & Sagner, Hesstr 39-41, Munich 80798, Germany. **Co-sponsor:** Czech Society for Anaesthesiology, Resuscitation and Intensive Care.

617.96 616.891 BGR ISSN 1310-4284
ANESTEZIOLOGIIA I INTENSIVNO LECHENIE. Text in Bulgarian; Summaries in Bulgarian, English. 1974. q. USD 52 foreign; BGL 6 newsstand/cover domestic (effective 2002). adv. bk.rev. abstr. index. back issues avail. **Document type:** *Journal, Academic/Scholarly.* **Description:** Publishes original articles in the field of anesthesiology, reanimation and intensive care.
Indexed: Abstr.Bulg.Sci.Med.Lit., Ref.Zh.
Published by: Meditsinski Universitet - Sofia, Tsentur za Informatsiia po Meditsina/Medical University - Sofia, Medical Information Center, 1 Sv Georgi Sofiiski ul, Sofia 1431, Bulgaria. TEL 359-2-9522342, FAX 359-2-9522393, mutafov@sun.medun.acad.bg, http://www.medun.acad.bg. Ed. I Smilov. adv.: B&W page USD 70, color page USD 150; trim 230 x 170. Circ: 300.

617 RUS ISSN 0201-7563
CODEN: AREAD8
ANESTEZIOLOGIYA I REANIMATOLOGIYA/ ANESTHESIOLOGY AND INTENSIVE CARE. Text in Russian; Summaries in English. 1956. bi-m. USD 731 foreign (effective 2000). adv. bk.rev., Website rev. abstr. index. reprints avail. **Document type:** *Journal, Academic/Scholarly.* **Description:** Covers general anesthesiology in surgery, intensive treatment and resuscitation. Promotes progressive methods and new developments in the above and related fields.
Formerly (until 1977): Eksperimental'naya Khirurgiya i Anesteziologiya (0013-3329)
Indexed: Biol.Abstr., Chem.Abstr., Chem.Indus.Notes, Chem.Titles, Excerp.Med., Ind.Med. (1977-), Ref.Zh.
—BLDSC (0006.650000), CASDDS, CISTI, East View, EMDOCS, GNLM, Infotrieve. **CCC.**
Published by: Izdatel'stvo Meditsina, Petroverigskii per 6-8, Moscow 101000, Russian Federation. TEL 7-095-9248785, 7-095-928-86-48, FAX 7-095-9211355, 7-095-9286003, meditisina@iname.com. Ed. A A Bunyatyan. Pub. A M Stochik. R&P O Vlasova. Adv. contact O A Fadeeva TEL 7-095-923-51-40. Circ: 2,700. **Dist. by:** Mezhdunarodnaya Kniga, B Yakimanka 39, Moscow 117049, Russian Federation. TEL 7-095-2384967, FAX 7-095-2384634; **US dist. addr.:** East View Publications, 3020 Harbor Ln N, Minneapolis, MN 55447. TEL 612-550-0961.

617.96 USA ISSN 0003-2999
CODEN: AACRAT
ANESTHESIA AND ANALGESIA. Text in English. 1921. m. USD 343 newsstand/cover domestic to individuals print and online eds. combined; USD 427 foreign to individuals print and online eds. combined; USD 483 domestic to institutions print and online eds. combined; USD 567 foreign to institutions print and online eds. combined; USD 45 newsstand/cover print and online eds. combined (effective 2002). adv. bk.rev. bibl, charts, illus. index. Supplement avail. *Refereed.* **Document type:** *Academic/Scholarly.* **Description:** Publishes original research and clinical articles, providing researchers, practicing physicians, and allied medical personnel in anesthesiology and related fields with a wealth of information to keep them up to date with the latest issues and advances in the field.
Formerly: Current Researches in Anesthesia and Analgesia
Related titles: CD-ROM ed.: (from Ovid Technologies, Inc.); Microfilm ed.: (from PMC,WWS); Online - full text ed.: USD 627.90 domestic academic site license; USD 711.90 foreign academic site license; USD 700.35 domestic corporate site license; USD 784.35 foreign corporate site license (effective 2002) (from Ovid Technologies, Inc., HighWire Pr., EBSCO Publishing, Swets Blackwell, Institute for Scientific Information).
Indexed: AIM, ASCA, Abstr.Health Care Manage.Stud., Agri.& Environ.Biotech.Abstr. (coverage dropped), Aqua.Sci.& Fish.Abstr., Biol.Abstr., CINAHL, C.I.S. Abstr., Chem.Abstr., Chem.Indus.Notes, Chem.Titles, Curr.Adv.Ecol.Sci., Curr.Cont., Dent.Abstr., Dent.Ind., Derwent Biotech.Abstr., Environ.Sci.Poll.Mgmt., Excerp.Med., INIS Atomind., Ind.Med. (1957-), Ind.Sci.Rev., Inpharma, Int.Abstr.Biol.Sci., Int.Nurs.Ind., Jrnl.Watch Emer.Med., Neurosci.Abstr. (coverage dropped), Neurosci.Cit.Ind., Pharm.&Out.News, Pollut.Abstr., Reac., Ref.Zh., Rev.Med.& Vet.Mycol., Risk Abstr., SSCI (coverage dropped), Saf.Sci.Abstr., Sci.Cit.Ind., THA.
—BLDSC (0900.500000), CASDDS, CISTI, EMDOCS, GNLM, IDS, ingenta, KNAW.
Published by: (International Anesthesia Research Society), Williams & Wilkins (Subsidiary of: Waverly International), 351 W Camden St, Baltimore, MD 21201-2436. TEL 410-528-4068, 800-222-3790, FAX 410-528-4452, dbakerv@wwilkins.com, http://www.anesthesia-analgesia.org, http://www.Lww.com. Ed. Dr. Ronald D Miller. Pub. Alma Wills. Adv. contact David Baker. B&W page USD 1,235; trim 10.88 x 8.13. Circ: 21,321 (paid). **Co-sponsor:** Society of Cardiovascular Anesthesiologists.

617.96 USA ISSN 1090-3577
ANESTHESIA AND CRITICAL CARE RESOURCES ON THE INTERNET. Text in English. 1994. m. back issues avail. **Description:** Tracks electronic resources of interest to anesthesiologists, nurse anesthetists and critical care and pain management physicians and other health care personnel.
Related titles: Online - full text ed.
Published by: University of Alabama at Birmingham, Department of Anesthesiology, 619 19th St S JT965, Birmingham, AL 35233-6810. TEL 205-975-5114, FAX 205-975-5963, meds002@uabdpo.dpo.uab.edu, awright@ms.jit.anes.uab.edu, http://www.eur.nl/fgg/anest/wrigh/index.html. Eds. A J Wright, Frank O'Connor. **Co-publisher:** Erasmus University, Department of Anaesthesiology.

617.96 USA ISSN 1085-6897
ANESTHESIA MALPRACTICE PREVENTION. Text in English. 1996. m., latest vol.6. USD 315 domestic to individuals; USD 335 foreign to individuals; USD 455 domestic to institutions; USD 455 newsstand/cover foreign to institutions; USD 37 newsstand/cover (effective 2002). **Document type:** *Newsletter.* **Description:** Features new or vexing threats with medico-legal implications. Presents advice on how to prevent malpractice situations.
Related titles: Online - full text ed.: USD 591.50 domestic for academic site license; USD 591.50 foreign for academic site license; USD 659.75 domestic for corporate site license; USD 659.75 foreign for corporate site license (effective 2002).
Published by: Lippincott Williams & Wilkins (Philadelphia) (Subsidiary of: Wolters Kluwer N.V.), 530 Walnut St, Philadelphia, PA 19106-3621. TEL 800-638-6423, http://www.lww.com. Eds. Dr. A Terry Walman, Norra Macready. **Subscr. to:** TEL 410-528-8572, FAX 410-528-4105.

617.96 USA
ANESTHESIA PATIENT SAFETY FOUNDATION. NEWSLETTER. Text in English. q. back issues avail. **Document type:** *Newsletter.* **Description:** Covers safety and organization activities, and other related topics.
Published by: Anesthesia Patient Safety Foundation, 4246 Colonial Park Dr, Pittsburgh, PA 15227. TEL 412-882-8040, info@apsf.com, http://gasnet.med.yale.edu/societies/apsf/newsletter/newsleter.html.

ANESTHESIA PROGRESS; a journal for pain and anxiety control. see *MEDICAL SCIENCES—Dentistry*

617.96 FRA ISSN 0996-8296
ANESTHESIE - REANIMATION PRATIQUE. Text in French. 1989. m. (10/yr.). FRF 250 domestic; FRF 400 foreign; FRF 175 domestic to libraries; FRF 325 foreign to libraries (effective 2001). **Document type:** *Newspaper.*
Published by: L E N Medical, 15 rue des Sablons, Paris 75116, France. TEL 33-1-47553131, FAX 33-1-47553132, lenmed@club-internet.fr, http://www.webmedguide.com. Ed. Dr. Francois Gaudillat.

617.96 USA ISSN 0003-3022
RD81.A1 CODEN: ANESAV
ANESTHESIOLOGY. Text in English. 1940. m. USD 246 domestic to individuals print and online eds. combined; USD 326 foreign to individuals print and online eds. combined; USD 445 domestic to institutions print and online eds. combined; USD 497 foreign to institutions print and online eds. combined; USD 35 newsstand/cover (effective 2002). adv. bk.rev. illus. cum.index. reprint service avail. from PQC. *Refereed.* **Document type:** *Academic/Scholarly.* **Description:** Publishes original manuscripts featuring clinical investigations, laboratory investigations, case reports, laboratory reports, reviews, medical intelligence, special articles, reports of scientific meetings, Web site reviews, reviews of educational material and correspondence.
Related titles: CD-ROM ed.: (from Ovid Technologies, Inc.); Microform ed.: (from PQC); Online - full text ed.: ISSN 1528-1175. USD 825 domestic academic site license; USD 825 foreign academic site license; USD 948.75 domestic corporate site license; USD 948.75 foreign corporate site license (2002) (from Ovid Technologies, Inc., EBSCO Publishing, Swets Blackwell, Institute for Scientific Information).
Indexed: AIM, ASCA, Agri.& Environ.Biotech.Abstr. (coverage dropped), Biol.Abstr., CINAHL, Chem.Abstr., Chem.Indus.Notes, Chem.Titles, Curr.Adv.Ecol.Sci., Curr.Cont., Derwent Biotech.Abstr., Environ.Sci.Poll.Mgmt., Excerp.Med., INIS Atomind., Ind.Med. (1940-), Ind.Sci.Rev., Ind.Vet., Inpharma, Int.Nurs.Ind., Jrnl.Watch Emer.Med., Med.& Surg.Dermat., Neurosci.Cit.Ind., Pharm.&Out.News, Pig News & Info., Pollut.Abstr., Reac., Risk Abstr., SSCI (coverage dropped), Saf.Sci.Abstr., Sci.Cit.Ind., THA, Tox.Abstr., Vet.Bull.
—BLDSC (0900.600000), CASDDS, CISTI, EMDOCS, GNLM, IDS, ingenta, KNAW, Linda Hall.
Published by: (American Society of Anesthesiologists), Lippincott Williams & Wilkins (Philadelphia) (Subsidiary of: Wolters Kluwer N.V.), 530 Walnut St, Philadelphia, PA 19106-3621. TEL 301-223-2300, 800-638-3030, FAX 301-223-2400, http://www.anesthesiology.org, http://www.Lww.com. adv.: B&W page USD 2,645; trim 10.88 x 8.13. Circ: 37,847 (paid).

617.96 USA ISSN 0889-8537
CODEN: ACNAEH
ANESTHESIOLOGY CLINICS OF NORTH AMERICA. Text in English. 1987. q. USD 145 domestic to individuals; USD 175 in Canada to individuals; USD 205 elsewhere to individuals; USD 197 domestic to institutions; USD 256 foreign to institutions; USD 85 domestic to students; USD 65 per issue (effective 2001). **Document type:** *Academic/Scholarly.* **Description:** Each issue treats a topic on the administration of anesthesia.
Supersedes in part (in 1986): Clinics in Anaesthesiology (0261-9881)
Related titles: Online - full text ed.: (from Institute for Scientific Information); ♦ Spanish Translation: Clinicas de Anestesiologia de Norteamerica.
Indexed: CINAHL, Chem.Abstr., Chem.Indus.Notes, Chem.Titles, Ind.Med.
—BLDSC (0900.725000), CASDDS, EMDOCS, GNLM, IDS, ingenta, KNAW. **CCC.**
Published by: W.B. Saunders Co. (Subsidiary of: Harcourt Publishers Ltd.), 11830 Westline Industrial Dr, St Louis, MO 63146. TEL 215-238-7800, 800-325-4177, FAX 215-238-6445, http://www.wbsaunders.com. Ed. Dr. Jonathan L Benumof.

617.96 USA ISSN 0747-4679
ANESTHESIOLOGY NEWS. Text in English. 1975. m. USD 60; USD 75 foreign (effective 1999).
Formerly: Anesthesia Staff News
Related titles: Online - full text ed.
—BLDSC (0900.750000).
Published by: McMahon Group, 545 W 45th St, 8th Fl, New York, NY 10036. TEL 212-957-5300, FAX 212-957-7230, johnd@mumahonmed.com. Ed. John Henry. adv.: B&W page USD 2,100, color page USD 3,600; trim 11.25 x 8.25. Circ: 17,500.

617.96 FRA ISSN 0750-7658
CODEN: AFAREO
ANNALES FRANCAISES D'ANESTHESIE ET DE REANIMATION. Text and summaries in English, French. 1982. m. EUR 262 in Europe to institutions; USD 332 elsewhere to institutions (effective 2002). adv. bk.rev. abstr, charts, illus. reprint service avail. from ISI. *Refereed.* **Document type:** *Academic/Scholarly.*
Formed by the merger of (1963-1982): Annales de l'Anesthesiologie Francaise (0003-4061); And: Anesthesie, Analgesie, Reanimation (0003-3014); Which superseded (1935-1957): Anesthesie et Analgesie (0301-4452)
Related titles: Online - full text ed.: (from ingenta, ScienceDirect, Institute for Scientific Information).
Indexed: ASCA, Biol.Abstr., Chem.Abstr., Curr.Cont., Dent.Ind., Derwent Biotech.Abstr., Excerp.Med., Ind.Med. (1982-), Inpharma, Int.Nurs.Ind., Neurosci.Cit.Ind., Nutr.Abstr., Pharm.&Out.News, Reac., Weed Abstr.
—BLDSC (0973.800000), CASDDS, CISTI, EMDOCS, GNLM, IDS, Infotrieve, KNAW. **CCC.**
Published by: (Societe Francaise d'Anesthesie et de Reanimation), Elsevier Paris, Editions Scientifiques et Medicales (Subsidiary of: Reed Elsevier plc. group), 23 rue Linois, Paris 75015, France. TEL 33-1-45589110, FAX 33-1-45589419, afar@elsevier.fr; academic@elsevier-fr.com, http://www.elsevier.com/locate/annfar, http://www.elsevier.fr; http://www.sfar.org. Ed. Jean Claude Otteni. Circ: 5,500.

617.96 615.804 IND ISSN 0301-0368
CODEN: AAARDM
ASIAN ARCHIVES OF ANAESTHESIOLOGY AND RESUSCITATION*. Text in English. 1971. q. USD 100. adv. bk.rev. bibl, charts, illus. back issues avail.
Formerly (1973): Archives of Anaesthesiology and Resuscitation
Indexed: Biol.Abstr., Chem.Abstr.
—CASDDS, CISTI, ingenta.
Published by: National Association of Critical Care Medicine, c/o Indian Medical Association, I.M.A. House, Indraprastha Marg., New Delhi 110 002, India. TEL 3014755. Ed. Dr. N P Singh. Circ: 2,000.

617.96 USA ISSN 0271-1265
AUDIO-DIGEST ANESTHESIOLOGY. Text in English. 1958. s-m. USD 168 (effective 2000). *Refereed.*
Media: Audio cassette/tape.
Published by: Audio-Digest Foundation (Subsidiary of: California Medical Association), 1577 E Chevy Chase Dr, Glendale, CA 91206. TEL 213-245-8505, 800-423-2308, FAX 818-240-7379, 800-845-4375.

617.96 ZAF ISSN 1024-6851
B J A: INTERNATIONAL JOURNAL OF ANAESTHESIA (SOUTH AFRICAN EDITION). (British Journal of Anaesthesia) Text in English. 1994. bi-m. adv.
Indexed: Chem.Abstr., Chem.Indus.Notes, Chem.Titles.

M

Published by: (Royal College of Surgeons GBR), George Warman Publications (Pty.) Ltd., PO Box 704, Cape Town 8000, South Africa. TEL 27-21-24-5320, FAX 27-21-26-1332. Circ: 1,843.

617.96 GBR ISSN 1521-6896
CODEN: BBPAFW
BAILLIERE'S BEST PRACTICE & RESEARCH IN CLINICAL ANAESTHESIOLOGY. Text in English. 1986. q. GBP 111 to individuals; GBP 161 to institutions (effective 2002). *Refereed.* **Document type:** *Academic/Scholarly.*
Formerly: Bailliere's Clinical Anaesthesiology (0950-3501); Which supersedes in part (in 1986): Clinics in Anaesthesiology (0261-9881)
Related titles: Microform ed.: (from PQC); Online - full text ed.: (from EBSCO Publishing, O C L C Online Computer Library Center, Inc., Swets Blackwell, IDEAL Online Library, RoweCom Information Quest).
Indexed: ASCA, Abstr.Health Care Manage.Stud., Curr.Adv.Ecol.Sci., Curr.Cont. (coverage dropped), Excerp.Med., Inpharma, Pharm.&Out.News, Reac., Ref.Zh.
—BLDSC (1856.716600), CASDDS, EMDOCS, GNLM, IDS, Infotrieve, KNAW. **CCC.**
Published by: Bailliere Tindall (Subsidiary of: Harcourt Publishers Ltd.), 24-28 Oval Rd, London NW1 7DX, United Kingdom. TEL 44-20-7424-4200, FAX 44-20-7424-4515, cservice@harcourt.com, http://www.harcourt-international.com/journals/bean/, http://www.hbuk.co.uk. Ed. Hugo Van Aken. **Subscr. to:** Harcourt Publishers Ltd., Foots Cray High St, Sidcup, Kent DA14 5HP, United Kingdom. TEL 44-20-8308-5700, FAX 44-20-8309-0807.

617.96 UKR
BIL', ZNEBOLYUVANNYA I INTENSYVNA TERAPIYA. Text in Russian, Ukrainian. q. USD 95 in United States.
Published by: Asotsyatsiya Anesteziologiv Ukrainy, Ul P Zaporozhtsa 26, Kiev, Ukraine. TEL 380-44-514-49-21. **US dist. addr.:** East View Publications, 3020 Harbor Ln N, Minneapolis, MN 55447. TEL 612-550-0961.

617.96 610.73 USA
BREATHLINE✱ . Text in English. bi-m. membership. bk.rev.
Indexed: CINAHL.
Published by: Uniformed Services Academy of Family Physicians, 2301 N Parham Rd no.4, Richmond, VA 23229-3163. TEL 804-379-5516.

617.96 USA
BRISTOL-MYERS SQUIBB SYMPOSIUM ON PAIN RESEARCH SERIES. Text in English. 1991. irreg. price varies. **Document type:** *Proceedings.*
Published by: Lippincott Williams & Wilkins (Philadelphia) (Subsidiary of: Wolters Kluwer N.V.), 530 Walnut St, Philadelphia, PA 19106-3621. TEL 301-223-2300, 800-638-3030, FAX 301-223-2400.

617.96 GBR ISSN 0007-0912
CODEN: BJANAD
BRITISH JOURNAL OF ANAESTHESIA. Short title: B J A. Variant title: B J A: British Journal of Anaesthesia. Text in English. 1923. m. GBP 255, USD 400 to individuals; GBP 255, USD 400 to institutions (effective 2002). adv. bk.rev. bibl, charts, illus. index. back issues avail.; reprint service avail. from SWZ. *Refereed.* **Document type:** *Journal, Academic/Scholarly.* **Description:** Contains original articles in all branches of Anaesthesia. Submitted manuscripts are subject to stringent review to ensure that the journal only contains papers of the highest standard.
Related titles: Microfilm ed.: (from PQC); Online - full text ed.: ISSN 1471-6771. GBP 229, USD 360 to institutions (effective 2002) (from EBSCO Publishing, HighWire Pr., ProQuest Information & Learning, Institute for Scientific Information).
Indexed: ASCA, Agri.& Environ.Biotech.Abstr. (coverage dropped), Biol.Abstr., Chem.Abstr., Curr.Adv.Ecol.Sci., Curr.Cont., Dairy Sci.Abstr., Dent.Ind., Derwent Biotech.Abstr., Dok.Arbeitsmed., Excerp.Med., Helminthol.Abstr., INIS Atomind., Ind.Med. (1923-), Ind.Sci.Rev., Ind.Vet., Inpharma, Int.Nurs.Ind., Neurosci.Cit.Ind., Nutr.Abstr., Pharm.&Out.News, Reac., Rev.Med.& Vet.Mycol., Risk Abstr., Sci.Cit.Ind., Small Anim.Abstr., THA, Vet.Bull.
—BLDSC (2303.900000), CASDDS, CISTI, GNLM, IDS, ingenta, KNAW.
Published by: Oxford University Press, Academic Division, Great Clarendon St, Oxford OX2 6DP, United Kingdom. TEL 44-1865-267907, FAX 44-1865-267835, jnl.info@oup.co.uk, http://bja.oupjournals.org/, http://www.oup.co.uk/journals. Ed. Jenny Hunter. Pub. Janet Boullin. adv.: page GBP 600, page USD 1,188. Circ: 13,500. **Subscri. in the Americas to:** Oxford University Press, Journals, 2001 Evans Rd, Cary, NC 27513. TEL 800-852-7323, FAX 919-677-1714, jnlorders@oup-usa.org; **Subscr. to:** Journals Marketing, Great Clarendon St, Oxford OX2 6DP, United Kingdom.

BUNBEN TO MASUI/JOURNAL OF OBSTETRICS AND ANESTHESIA. see *MEDICAL SCIENCES—Obstetrics And Gynecology*

617.96 GBR ISSN 1466-2922
▼ **C P D ANAESTHESIA.** (Continuing Professional Development) Text in English. 1999. 3/yr. (1volume per annum). GBP 45 domestic to individuals; GBP 60 foreign to individuals; GBP 60 domestic to institutions; GBP 90 foreign to institutions (effective 1999). adv. Website rev. abstr. 24 p./no. 2 cols./p. *Refereed.* **Document type:** *Journal, Academic/Scholarly.*
—BLDSC (3486.190500).
Published by: Rila Publications Ltd., 73 Newman St, London W1A 4PG, United Kingdom. TEL 44-20-7631-1299, FAX 44-20-7580-7166, admin@rila.co.uk, subscriptions@rila.co.uk, http://www.rila.co.uk. Eds. David Greaves, Stephen Bonner. Pub., Adv. contact G Da'Cambra. Circ: 3,600 (paid).

617.96 FRA ISSN 0007-9685
CODEN: CAANBU
CAHIERS D'ANESTHESIOLOGIE. Text in French. 1953. 6/yr. FRF 460 to students; FRF 990 foreign to individuals; FRF 720 domestic to individuals (effective 1999); FRF 175 newsstand/cover. adv. bk.rev. index. **Document type:** *Academic/Scholarly.*
Indexed: Biol.Abstr., Excerp.Med., Ind.Med. (coverage dropped).
—BLDSC (2948.620000), CASDDS, CISTI, EMDOCS, GNLM, Infotrieve, KNAW. **CCC.**
Published by: Initiatives Sante, 26 av. de l'Europe, BP 60, Velizy Villacoublay Cedex 78141, France. TEL 33-1-34633333, FAX 33-1-34659308. Ed. St Maurice. Circ: 3,005.

617.96 CAN ISSN 0832-610X
CODEN: CJOAEP
CANADIAN JOURNAL OF ANAESTHESIA/JOURNAL CANADIEN D'ANESTHESIE. Text in English, French. 1954. m. CND 200 to individuals; CND 226 foreign to individuals; CND 258 to institutions; CND 289 foreign to institutions (effective 2000). adv. bk.rev. bibl, charts, illus. index. back issues avail.; reprint service avail. from PQC. *Refereed.* **Document type:** *Academic/Scholarly.* **Description:** Publishes original papers on subjects related to anesthesia: critical care, pain management, and resuscitation.
Formerly (until 1986): Canadian Anaesthetists' Society. Journal (0008-2856)
Related titles: CD-ROM ed.; Microform ed.: (from PQC); Online - full text ed.: (from Institute for Scientific Information).
Indexed: ASCA, Biol.Abstr., CINAHL, Chem.Abstr., Curr.Adv.Ecol.Sci., Curr.Cont., Dairy Sci.Abstr., Dent.Ind., Environ.Sci.Poll.Mgmt., Excerp.Med., INIS Atomind., Ind.Med. (1987-), Ind.Sci.Rev., Inpharma, Int.Nurs.Ind., Jrnl.Watch Emer.Med., Kidney, Neurosci.Abstr. (coverage dropped), Neurosci.Cit.Ind., Nutr.Abstr., Pharm.&Out.News, Pollut.Abstr., Reac., Risk Abstr., Saf.Sci.Abstr., Sci.Cit.Ind., Soyabean Abstr.
—BLDSC (3028.300000), CASDDS, CISTI, EMDOCS, GNLM, IDS, ingenta, KNAW. **CCC.**
Published by: Canadian Anaesthetists' Society/Societe Canadienne des Anesthesistes, 1 Eglinton Ave E Ste 208, Toronto, ON M4P 3A1, Canada. TEL 416-480-0602, FAX 416-480-0320, cas@multinet.org. Ed. Dr. David R Bevan. R&P Angela Fritsch. Adv. contact Lisa Fleischaker. Circ: 5,040 (paid).

CLINICAL JOURNAL OF PAIN. see *MEDICAL SCIENCES—Psychiatry And Neurology*

617.96 GBR ISSN 0953-7112
CODEN: CCCAEI
CURRENT ANAESTHESIA AND CRITICAL CARE. Text in English. 1989. bi-m. GBP 109 to individuals; GBP 256 to institutions (effective 2002). adv. **Document type:** *Academic/Scholarly.* **Description:** Reviews articles of interest to anesthesiologists.
Related titles: Online - full text ed.: (from EBSCO Publishing, O C L C Online Computer Library Center, Inc., Swets Blackwell, IDEAL Online Library).
Indexed: Ref.Zh.
—BLDSC (3494.128000), EMDOCS, GNLM, Infotrieve, KNAW. **CCC.**
Published by: Churchill Livingstone (Subsidiary of: Harcourt Publishers Ltd.), Robert Stevenson House, 1-3 Baxter's Pl, Leith Walk, Edinburgh, Midlothian EH1 3AF, United Kingdom. TEL 44-131-556-2424, FAX 44-131-459-1177, cservice@harcourt.com, http://www.harcourt-international.com/journals/cacc. Ed. B J Pollard. Pub. Gillian Griffith. R&P Catherine John TEL 212-424-4200. Adv. contact David Dunnachie. Circ: 1,100. **Subscr. to:** Harcourt Publishers Ltd., Foots Cray High St, Sidcup, Kent DA14 5HP, United Kingdom. TEL 44-20-8308-5700, FAX 44-20-8309-0807.

CURRENT MEDICAL LITERATURE. ANAESTHESIOLOGY. see *MEDICAL SCIENCES—Abstracting, Bibliographies, Statistics*

617.96 USA ISSN 0952-7907
CODEN: COAEE2
CURRENT OPINION IN ANAESTHESIOLOGY. Text in English. 1988. bi-m. USD 273 domestic to individuals for print & online eds.; USD 273 foreign to individuals for print & online eds.; USD 665 per issue domestic to institutions; USD 665 per issue foreign to institutions; USD 103 newsstand/cover (effective 2002). adv. bibl, illus. **Document type:** *Academic/Scholarly.* **Description:** Directed toward researchers and practicing anesthesiologists. Presents review articles followed by annotated bibliographies of references consulted. Includes a bibliography of the current world literature published during the previous year.
Related titles: CD-ROM ed.; Diskette ed.; Online - full text ed.: USD 864.50 domestic academic site license; USD 864.50 foreign academic site license; USD 964.25 domestic corporate site license; USD 964.25 foreign corporate site license (2002) (from Ovid Technologies, Inc., EBSCO Publishing, Swets Blackwell).
Indexed: CINAHL, Excerp.Med. (1994-).
—BLDSC (3500.772000), ADONIS, EMDOCS, GNLM, KNAW.
Published by: Lippincott Williams & Wilkins (Philadelphia) (Subsidiary of: Wolters Kluwer N.V.), 530 Walnut St, Philadelphia, PA 19106-3621. TEL 215-521-8300, FAX 215-521-8902, http://www.Lww.com. Eds. Hugo van Aken, Julien Biebuyck. Adv. contact Gemma Heiser. B&W page USD 790, color page USD 1,790; trim 11 x 8.5. Circ: 4,975. **Subscr. to:** PO Box 1600, Hagerstown, MD 21740-1600. TEL 800-777-2295, FAX 301-824-7390.

617.96 USA ISSN 0164-310X
CURRENT REVIEWS FOR NURSE ANESTHETISTS. Text in English. 1978. bi-w. USD 210 (effective 1999 & 2000). adv.
Indexed: CINAHL.
Published by: Current Reviews, 7480 Fairway Dr, Ste 106, Miami, FL 33014-6861. TEL 305-822-1415. Ed., R&P Frank Moya. Pub. Joan McNulty. Adv. contact Barbara McNulty.

617.96 610.736 USA
CURRENT REVIEWS FOR PERIANESTHESIA NURSES. Text in English. bi-w. USD 160 (effective 2000). adv. **Document type:** *Trade.*
Former titles (until 1997): Current Reviews for Post Anesthesia Care Nurses (0896-1182); (until 1987): Current Reviews for Recovery Room Nurses (0164-3118)
Indexed: CINAHL.
Published by: Current Reviews, 7480 Fairway Dr, Ste 106, Miami, FL 33014-6861. TEL 305-822-1415. Ed., R&P Frank Moya. Pub. Joan McNulty. Adv. contact Barbara McNulty.

617.96 NLD ISSN 0924-5294
CODEN: DCCAET
DEVELOPMENTS IN CRITICAL CARE MEDICINE AND ANESTHESIOLOGY. Text in English. 1982. irreg., latest vol.30, 1995. price varies. *Refereed.* **Document type:** *Monographic series.*
—BLDSC (3579.070000), CISTI, KNAW.
Published by: Kluwer Academic Publishers Group (Subsidiary of: Wolters Kluwer N.V.), Spuiboulevard 50, PO Box 17, Dordrecht 3300 AA, Netherlands. FAX 31-78-639-2254, services@wkap.nl, http://www.wkap.nl. **Dist. by:** Journals Department, PO Box 322, Dordrecht 3300 AH, Netherlands. FAX 31-78-654-6474.

617.96 FRA ISSN 1283-0771
ENCYCLOPEDIE MEDICO-CHIRURGICALE. ANESTESIA - RIANIMAZIONE. Cover title: Trattato di Anestesia - Rianimazione. Text in Italian. 1998. 5 base vols. plus q. updates. price varies. bibl, charts, illus. **Document type:** *Academic/Scholarly.* **Description:** Reports advances in anesthesiology in surgery and other medical procedures.

Related titles: ♦ French ed.: Encyclopedie Medico-Chirurgicale. Anesthesie - Reanimation. ISSN 0246-0289.
Published by: Elsevier Paris, Editions Scientifiques et Medicales (Subsidiary of: Reed Elsevier plc. group), 23 rue Linois, Paris 75015, France. TEL 33-1-45589110, FAX 33-1-45589425, redaction-emc@elsevier.fr, http://www.elsevier.fr, http://www.elsevier.com. Ed. Pascal Horay.

617.96 FRA ISSN 0246-0289
ENCYCLOPEDIE MEDICO-CHIRURGICALE. ANESTHESIE - REANIMATION. Cover title: Traite d'Anesthesie - Reanimation. Variant title: Encyclopedie Medico-Chirurgicale, Instantanes Medicaux. Anesthesie - Reanimation. Receuil de l'Encyclopedie Medico-Chirurgicale. Anesthesie - Reanimation. Text in French. 1958. 5 base vols. plus q. updates. price varies. bibl, charts, illus. *Refereed.* **Document type:** *Academic/Scholarly.* **Description:** Reports advances in anesthesiology in surgery and other medical procedures.
Related titles: ♦ Italian ed.: Encyclopedie Medico-Chirurgicale. Anestesia - Rianimazione. ISSN 1283-0771.
Published by: Elsevier Paris, Editions Scientifiques et Medicales (Subsidiary of: Reed Elsevier plc. group), 23 rue Linois, Paris 75015, France. TEL 33-1-45589110, FAX 33-1-45589425, redaction-emc@elsevier.fr, http://www.elsevier.fr, http://www.elsevier.com. Ed. Pascal Horay.

617.96 ESP ISSN 0071-2671
EUROPEAN CONGRESS OF ANAESTHESIOLOGY. PROCEEDINGS. (Proceedings published in host countries) Text in Spanish. 1962. quadrennial, latest 1974, 4th, Madrid. **Document type:** *Proceedings.*
Published by: (World Federation of Societies of Anaesthesiologists NLD), European Congress of Anaesthesiology, c/o Professor Arias, Arapiles, 16, Madrid 28015, Spain.

617.96 GBR ISSN 0265-0215
CODEN: EJANEG
EUROPEAN JOURNAL OF ANAESTHESIOLOGY. Text in English. 1984. m. GBP 63 in Europe to individuals; USD 109 in North America to individuals; GBP 69 elsewhere to individuals; GBP 599 in Europe to institutions; USD 985 in North America to institutions; GBP 639 elsewhere to institutions; GBP 69.30 in Europe to individuals print & online eds.; USD 119.90 in North America to individuals print & online eds.; GBP 75.90 elsewhere to individuals print & online eds.; GBP 658.90 in Europe to institutions print & online eds.; USD 1,083.50 in North America to institutions print & online eds.; GBP 702.90 elsewhere to institutions print & online eds. (effective 2001). adv. bk.rev. abstr, bibl, illus. index. back issues avail. *Refereed.* **Document type:** *Academic/Scholarly.*
Related titles: Microform ed.: (from PQC); Online - full text ed.: ISSN 1365-2346. USD 887 in North America to institutions; USD 99 in North America to individuals; GBP 540 elsewhere to institutions; GBP 57 elsewhere to individuals (effective 2001) (from Ovid Technologies, Inc., EBSCO Publishing, O C L C Online Computer Library Center, Inc., RoweCom Information Quest, ingenta, Munksgaard & Blackwell Science's Synergy, Swets Blackwell, Institute for Scientific Information); ♦ Supplement: European Journal of Anaesthesiology. Supplement. ISSN 0952-1941.
Indexed: ASCA, Chem.Abstr., Chem.Indus.Notes, Chem.Titles, Curr.Adv.Ecol.Sci., Curr.Cont., Excerp.Med., Ind.Med. (1984-), Inpharma, Neurosci.Cit.Ind., Pharm.&Out.News, Reac., Ref.Zh.
—BLDSC (3829.722200), ADONIS, CASDDS, CISTI, EMDOCS, GNLM, IDS, ingenta, KNAW. **CCC.**
Published by: (European Academy of Anaesthesiology), Blackwell Science Ltd., Osney Mead, Oxford OX2 0EL, United Kingdom. TEL 44-1865-206206, FAX 44-1865-721205, journals.cs@blacksci.co.uk, http://www.blackwell-science.com. Ed. A Adams. Pub. Allen Stevens. R&P Sophie Savage. Adv. contact Jenny Applin. Circ: 1,190.

617.96 GBR ISSN 0952-1941
CODEN: EJSUEP
EUROPEAN JOURNAL OF ANAESTHESIOLOGY. SUPPLEMENT. Text in English. 1987. irreg. price varies. adv. **Document type:** *Monographic series, Academic/Scholarly.*
Related titles: Online - full text ed.: (from Ovid Technologies, Inc.); ♦ Supplement to: European Journal of Anaesthesiology. ISSN 0265-0215.
Indexed: Curr.Cont. (coverage dropped), Excerp.Med., Ind.Med. (1987-).
—BLDSC (3829.722202), ADONIS, CISTI, EMDOCS, ingenta, KNAW. **CCC.**
Published by: (European Academy of Anaesthesiology), Blackwell Science Ltd., Osney Mead, Oxford OX2 0EL, United Kingdom. TEL 44-1865-206206, FAX 44-1865-721205, journals.cs@blacksci.co.uk, http://www.blackwell-science.com. Pub. Allen Stevens. R&P Sophie Savage. Adv. contact Jenny Applin.

EUROPEAN JOURNAL OF PAIN. see *MEDICAL SCIENCES*

EXCERPTA MEDICA. SECTION 24: ANESTHESIOLOGY. see *MEDICAL SCIENCES—Abstracting, Bibliographies, Statistics*

617.96 IND ISSN 0019-5049
INDIAN JOURNAL OF ANAESTHESIA✶ . Text in English. 1953. q. USD 35. adv. bk.rev. abstr, bibl, charts, illus, stat. index.
Indexed: Biol.Abstr.
—CISTI, GNLM.
Published by: Indian Society of Anaesthetists, c/o Dr. D. Das Gupta, Department of Anaesthesia, K.E.M. Hospital, Parel, Mumbai, Maharashtra, India. Circ: 2,000.

617.96 USA
INTERFACE (SPRINGFIELD). Text in English. q.
Published by: Society for Technology in Anesthesia, c/o Beverly Anderson, Society Coordinator, 2743 S. Veterans Pkwy, PMB 193, Springfield, IL 62704. TEL 217-787-3281, SocTecAnes@aol.com. Ed. Paul Ting TEL 804-924-5903.

617.96 USA ISSN 0020-5907
RD81.A1 CODEN: IACLAV
INTERNATIONAL ANESTHESIOLOGY CLINICS. Text in English. 1963. q. USD 218 domestic to individuals; USD 242 foreign to individuals; USD 261 domestic to institutions; USD 328 foreign to institutions; USD 74 newsstand/cover (effective 2002). charts, illus, stat. index. back issues avail.; reprint service avail. from PQC. *Refereed.* **Document type:** *Academic/Scholarly.* **Description:** Focuses on a single topic in each issue. Presents discussions of physiology, pharmacology of the agents, clinical application of techniques, and causes and treatments of complications.
Related titles: Microform ed.: (from PQC); Online - full text ed.: USD 339.30 domestic academic site license; USD 406.30 foreign academic site license; USD 378.45 domestic corporate site license; USD 445.45 foreign corporate site license (2002) (from Ovid Technologies, Inc., Institute for Scientific Information).
Indexed: ASCA, Biol.Abstr., CINAHL, Chem.Abstr., Chem.Indus.Notes, Chem.Titles, Curr.Cont. (coverage dropped), Dent.Ind., Excerp.Med., Ind.Med. (1962-), Inpharma, Pharm.&Out.News, Reac., Ref.Zh., SSCI (coverage dropped), Sci.Cit.Ind. (coverage dropped).
—BLDSC (4535.750000), CASDDS, CISTI, GNLM, IDS, ingenta, KNAW.
Published by: Lippincott Williams & Wilkins (Philadelphia) (Subsidiary of: Wolters Kluwer N.V.), 530 Walnut St, Philadelphia, PA 19106-3621. TEL 215-521-8300, FAX 215-521-8902, http://www.Lww.com. Eds. Dr. Thomas W Feeley, Dr. William Hurford. R&P Alice McElhinney. Circ: 1,180. **Subscr. to:** PO Box 1600, Hagerstown, MD 21740-1600. TEL 800-777-2295, FAX 301-824-7390.

INTERNATIONAL JOURNAL OF OBSTETRIC ANESTHESIA. see *MEDICAL SCIENCES—Obstetrics And Gynecology*

617.96 USA ISSN 1092-406X
THE INTERNET JOURNAL OF ANESTHESIOLOGY. Text in English. 1997. q. free per issue. adv. bk.rev. back issues avail. *Refereed.* **Document type:** *Academic/Scholarly.* **Description:** Covers the field of anesthesiology, critical care, and pain management. Original articles, reviews, case reports, streaming slide shows, streaming videos, letters to the editor, press releases, meeting information.
Media: Online - full text.
Published by: (Society of Advanced Telecommunications in Anesthesia), Internet Scientific Publications, L.L.C., 23 Rippling Creek Dr, Sugar Land, TX 77479. TEL 281-240-1533, FAX 281-240-1533, http://www.ispub.com/journals/ija.htm. Pub., R&P, Adv. contact Hope Morrow TEL 832-754-0335.

617.96 616.992 USA
▼ **THE INTERNET JOURNAL OF PAIN, SYMPTOM CONTROL AND PALLIATIVE CARE.** Text in English. 2000. s-a. free per issue. bk.rev. **Document type:** *Academic/Scholarly.* **Description:** Provides information for the field of pain management, symptom control, palliative care, anesthesiology, rehabilitation medicine and oncology. Original articles, reviews, case reports, streaming slide shows, streaming videos, letters to the editor, press releases, meeting information.
Media: Online - full content.
Published by: Internet Scientific Publications, L.L.C., 23 Rippling Creek Dr, Sugar Land, TX 77479. TEL 281-240-1533, FAX 281-240-1533, http://www.ispub.com/. Ed. Peter Lierz. R&P, Adv. contact Hope Morrow TEL 832-754-0335.

▼ **THE INTERNET JOURNAL OF POLISH ANESTHESIOLOGY AND SURGERY.** see *MEDICAL SCIENCES—Surgery*

617.96 JPN ISSN 0021-4892
CODEN: MASUAC
JAPANESE JOURNAL OF ANESTHESIOLOGY/MASUI. Text in Japanese; Summaries in English. 1952. m. JPY 41,740. **Document type:** *Academic/Scholarly.* **Description:** Contains original articles, clinical reports, short communications and announcements.
Related titles: Microform ed.: (from PQC).
Indexed: Dent.Ind., Excerp.Med., INIS Atomind., Ind.Med. (1952-).
—BLDSC (4650.810000), CISTI, GNLM, KNAW.
Published by: (Japan Society of Anesthesiology/Nippon Masui Gakkai), Kokuseido Shuppan K.K./Kokuseido Publishing Co., Ltd., 23-5-202 Hongo 3-chome, Bunkyo-ku, Tokyo 113-0033, Japan. FAX 81-3-3813-1866. Ed. K Hanaoka.

617.96 DEU ISSN 0941-4223
JOURNAL FUER ANAESTHESIE UND INTENSIVBEHANDLUNG. Text and summaries in English, German. 1994. q. EUR 20, USD 20 (effective 2001). adv. bk.rev. *Refereed.* **Document type:** *Journal, Academic/Scholarly.*
—BLDSC (4928.750000), GNLM.
Published by: Pabst Science Publishers, Am Eichengrund 28, Lengerich 49525, Germany. TEL 49-5484-308, FAX 49-5484-550, pabst.publishers@t-online.de, http://www.pabst-publishers.de/jai/. Ed. Wolfgang Pabst. Circ: 12,800.

617.96 PAK ISSN 1021-8009
JOURNAL OF ANAESTHESIA & CRITICAL CARE. Text in English. 1993. q. PKR 200 domestic; PKR 1,000, USD 40 foreign (effective 2001). adv. bk.rev. charts, illus. back issues avail. *Refereed.* **Document type:** *Journal, Academic/Scholarly.* **Description:** Devoted to the research and practice of anaesthesia and critical care medicine.
Related titles: Fax ed.
Published by: Medical Information Services, PO Box 8036, Karachi 75400, Pakistan. TEL 91-21-4554691, FAX 91-21-2434569. Ed. Dr. Ursula Chohan. Pub. Dr. Hasan Tharani. Adv. contact Munawwar Alam. B&W page PKR 8,000, color page PKR 14,000; trim 8.5 x 11. Circ: 1,000 (paid and controlled).

617.96 IND ISSN 0970-9185
JOURNAL OF ANAESTHESIOLOGY - CLINICAL PHARMACOLOGY. Text in English. 1985. q. INR 100, USD 20 to individuals; INR 180 to institutions.
—BLDSC (4927.900000), CISTI, GNLM.
Published by: Research Society of Anaesthesiology - Clinical Pharmacology, All India Institute of Medical Sciences, Dept. of Anaesthesiology, Rm. 5020, Ansari Nagar 11 0029, India. Ed. Dr. H L Kaul.

617.96 JPN ISSN 0913-8668
CODEN: JANEEC
JOURNAL OF ANESTHESIA. Text in English. 1987. q. (in 1 vol., 4 nos./vol.). JPY 20,000 domestic; USD 201 in North America; DEM 358 elsewhere; DEM 388, EUR 198.38 in Germany for Print & Online Eds.; DEM 392.80, EUR 200.83 elsewhere for Print & Online Eds. (effective 2001). **Document type:** *Academic/Scholarly.* **Description:** Publishes original articles, clinical reports, short communications, review articles, and letters to the editor.
Related titles: Online - full content ed.: ISSN 1438-8359 (from EBSCO Publishing, Swets Blackwell); Online - full text ed.: (from Springer LINK, RoweCom Information Quest).
Indexed: Excerp.Med. (1993-).
—BLDSC (4935.360000), CISTI, EMDOCS, GNLM, Infotrieve, KNAW. **CCC.**

Published by: (Japan Society of Anesthesiology/Nippon Masui Gakkai), Springer-Verlag Tokyo, Eastern Book Service, Inc. (Subsidiary of: BertelsmannSpringer), 3-13 Hongo 3-chome, Bunkyo-ku, Tokyo 113-0033, Japan. TEL 81-3-3812-0617, FAX 81-3-3812-4699, orders@svt-ebs.co.jp, http://link.springer-ny.com/link/service/journals/00540/index.htm, http://link.springer.de. Ed. Hidenori Toyooka. **Subscr. in N. America to:** Springer-Verlag New York Inc., PO Box 2485, Secaucus, NJ 07096-2485. TEL 800-777-4643, 201-348-4033, 212-460-1526, FAX 201-348-4505, orders@springer-ny.com; **Subscr. to:** Springer-Verlag, c/o Gabriele Kubitza, Haberstrasse 7, Heidelberg 69126, Germany. TEL 49-6221-345242, FAX 49-6221-345229, subscriptions@springer.de, http://link.springer-ny.com. **Dist. by:** Eastern Book Service, Inc.. TEL 81-3-3818-0861, FAX 81-3-3818-0864, orders@svt-ebs.co.jp.

JOURNAL OF CARDIOTHORACIC AND VASCULAR ANESTHESIA. see *MEDICAL SCIENCES—Cardiovascular Diseases*

617.96 USA ISSN 0952-8180
CODEN: JCLBE7

THE JOURNAL OF CLINICAL ANESTHESIA; an international journal of anesthesia practice. Text in English. 1988. 8/yr. EUR 187 in Europe to individuals; JPY 24,700 in Japan to individuals; USD 209 elsewhere to individuals; EUR 401 in Europe to institutions; JPY 53,300 in Japan to institutions; USD 450 elsewhere to institutions (effective 2002). adv. bk.rev. charts, illus. index. back issues avail. *Refereed.* **Document type:** *Academic/Scholarly.* **Description:** Serves as a forum for practical clinical information for the anesthesiologist from the resident level onward.
Related titles: Microform ed.: (from PQC); Online - full text ed.: (from ingenta, ScienceDirect, Swets Blackwell, Institute for Scientific Information).
Indexed: ASCA, Chem.Abstr., Chem.Indus.Notes, Chem.Titles, Curr.Cont., INIS Atomind., Ind.Med. (1988-), Inpharma, Int.Nurs.Ind., Neurosci.Cit.Ind., Pharm.&Out.News, Reac.
—BLDSC (4958.381070), CASDDS, EMDOCS, GNLM, IDS, Infotrieve, KNAW. **CCC.**
Published by: Elsevier Science, PO Box 945, New York, NY 10159-0945. TEL 212-989-5800, FAX 212-633-3990, usinfo-f@elsevier.com, http://www.elsevier.nl/locate/jclinane. Eds. Dr. David J Cullen, S Gelman. **Subscr. in Australasia and the Far East to:** Elsevier Science (Singapore) Pte Ltd, No.1 Temasek Ave, 17-01 Millenia Tower, Singapore 039192, Singapore. TEL 65-434-3727; **Subscr. in Japan to:** Elsevier Science Inc - Japan Regional Office, 9-15 Higashi-Azabu 1-chome, Minato-ku, Tokyo 106-0044, Japan. TEL 81-3-5561-5033; **Subscr. outside the Americas to:** Elsevier Science BV, PO Box 211, Amsterdam 1000 AE, Netherlands. TEL 31-20-485-3757, FAX 31-20-485-3432.

JOURNAL OF CLINICAL MONITORING AND COMPUTING. see *MEDICAL SCIENCES*

617.96 617 USA ISSN 0898-4921
CODEN: JNANEV

JOURNAL OF NEUROSURGICAL ANESTHESIOLOGY. Text in English. 1989. q. USD 218 domestic to individuals; USD 299 foreign to individuals; USD 399 domestic to institutions; USD 399 per issue foreign to institutions; USD 91 newsstand/cover (effective 2002). adv. charts, illus. *Refereed.* **Document type:** *Academic/Scholarly.* **Description:** Features articles on new drugs, equipment, and procedures, and presents reports of major clinical and laboratory research projects.
Related titles: Online - full text ed.: USD 518.70 domestic academic site license; USD 518.70 foreign academic site license; USD 578.55 domestic corporate site license; USD 578.55 foreign corporate site license (2002) (from Ovid Technologies, Inc., Institute for Scientific Information).
Indexed: ASCA, Curr.Cont., Excerp.Med., Ind.Med. (1989-), Inpharma, Neurosci.Cit.Ind., Pharm.&Out.News, Reac., Sci.Cit.Ind.
—BLDSC (5022.150000), CISTI, EMDOCS, GNLM, IDS, KNAW.
Published by: (Society of Neurosurgical Anesthesiology and Critical Care), Lippincott Williams & Wilkins (Philadelphia) (Subsidiary of: Wolters Kluwer N.V.), 530 Walnut St, Philadelphia, PA 19106-3621. TEL 215-521-8300, FAX 215-521-8902, http://www.lww.com. Ed. Dr. James E Cottrell. Pub. Shelley Johnson. R&P Margaret Becker. Adv. contact Ray Thibodeau. B&W page USD 775, color page USD 1,780. Circ: 1,289 (paid). **Subscr. to:** PO Box 1600, Hagerstown, MD 21740-1600. TEL 800-777-2295, FAX 301-824-7390.

JOURNAL OF PERIANESTHESIA NURSING. see *MEDICAL SCIENCES—Nurses And Nursing*

617.96 CHN

LINCHUANG MAZUIXUE ZAZHI/JOURNAL OF CLINICAL ANESTHESIOLOGY. Text in Chinese; Abstracts in English. 1985. bi-m. CNY 15. **Document type:** *Academic/Scholarly.*
Published by: Zhonghua Yixuehui (Nanjing Fenhui)/Chinese Medical Association (Nanjing Branch), 291 Zhongshan Lu, Nanjing, Jiangsu 210008, China. TEL 303848. Ed. Li Dexin.

617.96 JPN ISSN 0385-1664
CODEN: MASODV

MASUI TO SOSEI/ANESTHESIA AND RESUSCITATION. Text in Japanese. 1965. q. JPY 5,000; JPY 10,000 foreign. **Document type:** *Academic/Scholarly.*
Formerly (until 1970): Hiroshima Masui Igakkai Zasshi - Hiroshima Journal of Anesthesia (0440-8764)
Indexed: Chem.Abstr., Chem.Titles.
—BLDSC, CASDDS, EMDOCS, GNLM, KNAW.
Published by: Hiroshima Masui Igakkai, c/o Hiroshima University, School of Medicine, Dept of Anesthesiology & Critical Care Medicine, Minami-ku, Hiroshima 734, Japan. TEL 81-82-257-5267, FAX 81-82-257-5269, aanests@ue.ipc.hiroshima-u.ac.jp, http://mh.med.hiroshima-u.ac.jp/. Ed. Osafumi Yuge.

617.96 ITA ISSN 0375-9393
CODEN: MIANAP

MINERVA ANESTESIOLOGICA. Variant title: Giornale Italiano di Anestesia e di Analgesia. Text in Italian; Summaries in English, Italian. 1935. m. (10/yr.). USD 125 to individuals; USD 165 to institutions (effective 2000 - 2001). adv. bk.rev. bibl, charts, illus. index. *Refereed.* **Document type:** *Academic/Scholarly.* **Description:** Covers anesthesiology, analgesia, resuscitation and intensive care.
Related titles: Microform ed.: (from PQC).
Indexed: Biol.Abstr., Chem.Abstr., Dent.Ind., Excerp.Med., Ind.Med. (1953-), Int.Nurs.Ind.
—BLDSC (5794.040000), CASDDS, CISTI, GNLM, KNAW.
Published by: (Societa Italiana di Anestesia, Analgesia, Rianimazione e Terapia Intensiva), Edizioni Minerva Medica, Corso Bramante, 83-85, Turin, TO 10126, Italy. TEL 39-11-678282, FAX 39-11-674502. Ed. G Martinelli. Pub. Alberto Oliaro. Adv. contact F Filippo. B&W page USD 1,400, color page USD 2,300; trim 270 x 190.

617.96 NLD ISSN 0303-254X
CODEN: MOAND2

MONOGRAPHS IN ANAESTHESIOLOGY. Text in Dutch. 1974. irreg., latest vol.21, 1991. price varies. back issues avail. *Refereed.* **Document type:** *Monographic series.*
Indexed: Biol.Abstr., Chem.Abstr.
—CASDDS, GNLM.
Published by: Elsevier Science BV, Regional Sales Office, PO Box 211, Amsterdam 1000 AE, Netherlands. nlinfo-f@elsevier.nl, http://www.elsevier.nl. Ed. T E J Healy. **Subscr. in Australasia and the Far East to:** Elsevier Science (Singapore) Pte Ltd, No.1 Temasek Ave, 17-01 Millenia Tower, Singapore 039192, Singapore. TEL 65-434-3727, FAX 65-337-2230; **Subscr. in Japan to:** Elsevier Science Inc - Japan Regional Office, 9-15 Higashi-Azabu 1-chome, Minato-ku, Tokyo 106-0044, Japan. TEL 81-3-5561-5033; **Subscr. in the Americas to:** Elsevier Science, PO Box 945, New York, NY 10159-0945. TEL 212-633-3730, FAX 212-633-3680.

617.96 USA ISSN 0095-2273

N Y S S A SPHERE. Text in English. 1948. q. USD 40. adv. bk.rev. abstr, charts, illus, tr.lit. **Document type:** *Newsletter, Academic/Scholarly.* **Description:** Publishes articles and news relating to the practice of anesthesiology, including case reports, review articles, drug profiles, historical articles and meeting news.
Former titles: N Y S S A Bulletin (0027-7169); New York State Society of Anesthesiologists. Bulletin (0095-2265)
Published by: New York State Society of Anesthesiologists, Inc., 360 Lexington Ave, Ste 1800, New York, NY 10017. TEL 212-867-7140, FAX 212-867-7153, kurt@nyssa-pga.org, http://www.nyssa-pga.org. Ed. Dr. Douglas R Bacon. R&P Dr. Mark J Lema. Circ: 3,200 (controlled).

617.96 NLD ISSN 0921-8769

NEDERLANDS TIJDSCHRIFT VOOR ANESTHESIOLOGIE. Text in Dutch; Summaries in Dutch, English. 1988. q. NLG 90; NLG 146 foreign (effective 1999). adv. abstr. *Refereed.* **Document type:** *Academic/Scholarly, Trade.* **Description:** Contains original articles, reviews, congress calendar and news of the association.
—BLDSC (6071.387000), KNAW.
Published by: (Nederlandse Vereniging voor Anesthesiologie), Elsevier Gezondheidszorg B.V., Tijdstroom (Subsidiary of: Reed Elsevier plc Group), Planetenbaan 1, Maarssen 3600 AK, Netherlands. TEL 31-346-577577, FAX 31-346-554287, gezondheidszorg@ebi.nl, http://www.tijdstroom.nl. Ed. R Stienstra. Adv. contact Johan Ysebrands. **Subscr. to:** Elsevier Den Haag, Postbus 16500, The Hague 2500 BM, Netherlands. TEL 31-70-381-9900, FAX 31-70-333-8399.

617.96 617 GBR ISSN 0963-7974

NEWS REVIEW; a journal for theatre personnel nationwide. Text in English. 1988. m. GBP 17.62 domestic to individuals; GBP 28.20 foreign to individuals; GBP 24.67 domestic to institutions; GBP 35.25 foreign to institutions (effective 2001). adv. bk.rev., Website rev., software rev. charts, illus, pat, stat, tr.lit. 4 cols./p. back issues avail. **Document type:** *Newsletter, Journal, Trade.*
Related titles: Online - full content ed.
Published by: Lawrand Ltd., PO Box 51, Pontyclun, M Glam CF72 9YY, United Kingdom. admin@lawrand.co.uk, http://www.lawrand.co.uk. Ed. Lawrence Aston Evans. R&P Lawrence A Evans. Adv. contact Cleighton Johns. B&W page GBP 425, color page GBP 525; trim 197 x 276. Circ: 35,000 (controlled).

617.6 JPN ISSN 0386-5835
CODEN: NSMZDZ

NIHON SHIKA MASUI GAKKAI ZASSHI/JAPANESE DENTAL SOCIETY OF ANESTHESIOLOGY. JOURNAL. Text in English, Japanese. 1973. 4/yr. JPY 10,000 (effective 2000). adv. *Refereed.* **Document type:** *Proceedings, Bulletin, Academic/Scholarly.* **Description:** Contains scientific articles related to dental anesthesia, fundamentals of anesthesiology and the general management of the dental patients with some underlying systemic diseases.
Related titles: CD-ROM ed.
Indexed: Excerp.Med. (1993-).
—BLDSC (4809.260000), CASDDS, CISTI, EMDOCS, GNLM, Infotrieve, KNAW. **CCC.**
Published by: Nihon Shika Masui Gakkai/Japanese Dental Society of Anesthesiology, Tokyo Dental College, 1-2-2 Masago, Mihama-ku, Chiba 565-0871, Japan. TEL 81-3-3947-8891, FAX 81-3-3947-8341. Ed., R&P Yuzuru Kaneko. Pub. Yutaka Ueda. Circ: 2,050.

618.2 617.96 USA ISSN 0275-665X
CODEN: OADIDS

OBSTETRIC ANESTHESIA DIGEST. Text in English. 1981. q., latest vol.21. USD 153 domestic to individuals; USD 176 foreign to individuals; USD 222 domestic to institutions; USD 255 foreign to institutions; USD 59 newsstand/cover (effective 2002). adv. bk.rev. *Refereed.* **Document type:** *Academic/Scholarly, Abstract/Index.* **Description:** Provides annotated abstracts from world literature pertaining to the administration of anaesthesia during the perinatal period.
Related titles: Microform ed.: (from PQC); Online - full text ed.: USD 288.60 domestic for academic site license; USD 321.60 foreign for academic site license; USD 321.90 domestic for corporate site license; USD 354.90 foreign for corporate site license (effective 2002).
Published by: Lippincott Williams & Wilkins (Philadelphia) (Subsidiary of: Wolters Kluwer N.V.), 530 Walnut St, Philadelphia, PA 19106-3621. TEL 215-521-8300, FAX 215-521-8902, http://www.obstetricanesthesia.com, http://www.lww.com. Eds. Dr. Gerard M Bassell, Dr. Robert S F McKay. R&P Margaret Becker. Adv. contact Ray Thibodeau. B&W page USD 675, color page USD 1,675. Circ: 904 (paid). **Subscr. to:** PO Box 1600, Hagerstown, MD 21740-1600. TEL 800-777-2295, FAX 301-824-7390.

616.99 618.92 GBR ISSN 1155-5645
CODEN: PAANF7

PAEDIATRIC ANAESTHESIA. Text in English. 1991. bi-m., latest vol.12, 2002. GBP 145 in Europe to individuals; USD 222 in North America to individuals; GBP 154 elsewhere to individuals; GBP 336 in Europe to institutions; USD 533 in North America to institutions; GBP 370 elsewhere to institutions (effective 2002). adv. *Refereed.* **Document type:** *Journal, Academic/Scholarly.* **Description:** Devoted to the publication of information of interest and importance to practicing anaesthetists everywhere.
Related titles: ♦ Online - full text ed.: Paediatric Anaesthesia Online. ISSN 1460-9592.
Indexed: ASCA, Curr.Cont., Ind.Med. (1991-), Inpharma, Int.Nurs.Ind., Pharm.&Out.News, Reac.
—BLDSC (6333.399705), ADONIS, CISTI, GNLM, IDS, Infotrieve, KNAW. **CCC.**

M

Published by: Blackwell Science Ltd., PO Box 88, Oxford OX2 0NE, United Kingdom. TEL 44-1865-206180, 44-1865-206002, FAX 44-1865-206219, jnl.orders@blacksci.co.uk, http://www.blackwell-science.com/~cgilib/jnlpage.asp?Journal=pan&File=pan, http://www.blackwellpublishing.com. Ed. E Sumner. Pub. Allen Stevens. R&P Sophie Savage. Adv. contact Jenny Applin. Circ: 920.

616.99 618.92 GBR ISSN 1460-9592
PAEDIATRIC ANAESTHESIA ONLINE. Text in English. 1998. bi-m. GBP 131 in Europe to individuals; USD 200 in North America to individuals; GBP 131 elsewhere to individuals; GBP 303 in Europe to institutions; USD 480 in North America to institutions; GBP 303 elsewhere to institutions (effective 2002). *Refereed.* **Document type:** *Academic/Scholarly.*
Media: Online - full text (from EBSCO Publishing, O C L C Online Computer Library Center, Inc., RoweCom Information Quest, ingenta, Munksgaard & Blackwell Science's Synergy, Swets Blackwell, Institute for Scientific Information). **Related titles:** ♦ Print ed.: Paediatric Anaesthesia. ISSN 1155-5645.
Published by: Blackwell Science Ltd., Osney Mead, Oxford OX2 0EL, United Kingdom. TEL 44-1685-206206, FAX 44-1685-721205, journals.cs@blacksci.co.uk, http://www.blackwell-synergy.com/Journals/issuelist.asp?journal=pan, http://www.blackwell-science.com.

617.96 NLD ISSN 0169-1112
CODEN: PACLEA
THE PAIN CLINIC. Text in English. 1986. q. EUR 112, USD 130 to individuals includes online ed.; EUR 230, USD 266 to institutions includes online ed. (effective 2002). adv. bk.rev. back issues avail. *Refereed.* **Document type:** *Journal, Academic/Scholarly.* **Description:** Focuses on the clinical methods used and the problems involved in the diagnosis and treatment of persistent and recurrent types of pain.
Related titles: Online - full content ed.: 2000 (from EBSCO Publishing, Swets Blackwell); Online - full text ed.: (from CatchWord Ltd., Institute for Scientific Information).
Indexed: AMED, Inpharma, Neurosci.Cit.Ind., Pharm.&Out.News, Reac., SSCI (coverage dropped), e-psyche.
—BLDSC (6333.798800), CISTI, GNLM.
Published by: (World Society of Pain Clinicians USA), V S P (Subsidiary of: Brill Academic Publishers), PO Box 346, Zeist 3700 AH, Netherlands. TEL 31-30-692-5790, FAX 31-30-693-2081, vsppub@compuserve.com, http://www.vsppub.com/journals/jn-ThePaiCli.html. Ed. M Zoppi.

▼ **THE PAIN CLINIC: A MULTIDISCIPLINARY APPROACH TO ACUTE AND CHRONIC PAIN MANAGEMENT.** see *MEDICAL SCIENCES—Orthopedics And Traumatology*

617.96 NLD
THE PAIN CLINIC (PROCEEDINGS). Text in English. 1985. irreg., latest vol.4, 1992. price varies. back issues avail. **Document type:** *Proceedings, Academic/Scholarly.*
Indexed: ASCA, e-psyche.
Published by: (Pain Clinic Symposium), V S P (Subsidiary of: Brill Academic Publishers), PO Box 346, Zeist 3700 AH, Netherlands. TEL 31-30-692-5790, FAX 31-30-693-2081, vsppub@compuserve.com, http://www.vsppub.com. **Dist. in US & Canada by:** Books International, PO Box 605, Herndon, VA 20172. TEL 703-661-1501, 703-661-1500, FAX 703-661-1501.

617.98 USA ISSN 0938-9016
RB127 CODEN: PADIE6
PAIN DIGEST. Text in English. 1991. bi-m. (in 1 vol., 6 nos./vol.). USD 286.40 domestic for Print & Online Eds.; USD 280.10 in Germany for Print & Online Eds.; USD 50.60 newsstand/cover foreign (effective 2002). adv. back issues avail.; reprints avail. *Refereed.* **Document type:** *Academic/Scholarly.* **Description:** Contains up-to-date knowledge of the research, evaluation methods, and techniques of pain management.
Related titles: Microform ed.: (from PQC); Online - full content ed.; Online - full text ed.: (from Springer LINK).
Indexed: Excerp.Med. (1994-), Inpharma, Pharm.&Out.News, Reac.
—BLDSC (6333.799000), CISTI, EMDOCS, GNLM, Infotrieve. **CCC.**
Published by: Springer-Verlag, Journals (Subsidiary of: BertelsmannSpringer), 175 Fifth Ave, New York, NY 10010. TEL 212-460-1575, FAX 212-473-6272, orders@springer-ny.com, http://www.springer-ny.com. R&P Ian Gross. Adv. contact Jay Feinman. **N. American subscr. to:** Journal Fulfillment Services, PO Box 2485, Secaucus, NJ 07096-2485. TEL 800-777-4643, FAX 201-348-4505.

617.96 610.736 USA ISSN 1524-9042
▼ **PAIN MANAGEMENT NURSING.** Text in English. 2000. q. USD 60 domestic to individuals; USD 100 foreign to individuals; USD 88 domestic to institutions; USD 133 foreign to institutions; USD 20 domestic to students; USD 60 foreign to students; USD 34 newsstand/cover (effective 2001). **Document type:** *Journal, Academic/Scholarly.* **Description:** Presents original and review articles from experts in the field offer key insight in the areas of clinical practice, education, administration and research. Additional features include practice guidelines and articles dealing with pharmacologic issues.
Related titles: Online - full text ed.: (from IDEAL Online Library).
—BLDSC (6333.805500).
Published by: (American Society of Pain Management Nursing), W.B. Saunders Co. (Subsidiary of: Harcourt Publishers Ltd.), Curtis Center, Independence Sq W, Philadelphia, PA 19106-3399. TEL 215-238-2800, FAX 215-238-6490, http://www.painmanagementnursing.com, http://www.wbsaunders.com. Ed. Christine Miaskowski.

▼ **PAIN MEDICINE.** see *MEDICAL SCIENCES—Psychiatry And Neurology*

PAIN MEDICINE ONLINE. see *MEDICAL SCIENCES—Psychiatry And Neurology*

▼ **PAIN PRACTICE.** see *MEDICAL SCIENCES—Psychiatry And Neurology*

▼ **PAIN PRACTICE ONLINE.** see *MEDICAL SCIENCES—Psychiatry And Neurology*

POSTGRADUATE SURGERY: MIDDLE EAST. see *MEDICAL SCIENCES—Surgery*

617.96 USA ISSN 0889-4698
RD82.5
PROBLEMS IN ANESTHESIA. Text in English. 1987. q., latest vol.13. USD 151 domestic to individuals; USD 181 foreign to individuals; USD 204 domestic to institutions; USD 251 foreign to institutions; USD 63 newsstand/cover (effective 2001). adv. index. **Document type:** *Academic/Scholarly.*
Related titles: Microform ed.: (from PQC).
—BLDSC (6617.876900), GNLM, KNAW.
Published by: Lippincott Williams & Wilkins (Philadelphia) (Subsidiary of: Wolters Kluwer N.V.), 530 Walnut St, Philadelphia, PA 19106-3621. TEL 215-521-8300, FAX 215-521-8902, http://www.problemsinanes.com, http://www.lww.com. Eds. Dr. Donald S Prough, Dr. Lee Fleisher. Pub. Kathleen Gaffney. R&P Margaret Becker. Adv. contact Ray Thibodeau. Circ: 995. **Subscr. to:** PO Box 1600, Hagerstown, MD 21740-1600. TEL 800-777-2295, FAX 301-824-7390.

617.96 USA ISSN 0891-5784
PROGRESS IN ANESTHESIOLOGY (SAN ANTONIO). Text in English. 1984. m. USD 295 domestic to individuals; USD 360 foreign to individuals; USD 325 domestic to institutions; USD 390 foreign to institutions (effective 2000). *Refereed.* **Document type:** *Academic/Scholarly.* **Description:** Explores a topic in detail and offers clinical advice and information on the latest techniques and technologies. An educational medical journal devoted totally to the multifaceted specialty of anesthesiology.
Formerly (until 1987): Clinical Anesthesiology (0883-0282)
Related titles: Online - full text ed.
—BLDSC (6865.909400).
Published by: Dannemiller Memorial Educational Foundation, 12500 Network Blvd, Ste 101, San Antonio, TX 78249-3302. TEL 210-641-8311, 800-328-2308, FAX 210-641-8329, http://www.pain.com. Ed. Dr. James B Eisenkraft. R&P Barbara Tranbarger. Adv. contact Larry P Vervack.

617.96 617.3 FRA ISSN 1164-6756
CODEN: REURFX
REANIMATION - URGENCES. Text in French; Abstracts in English, French. 1991. 8/yr. EUR 274 in Europe to institutions; USD 330 rest of world to institutions (effective 2002). back issues avail. *Refereed.* **Document type:** *Academic/Scholarly.* **Description:** Publishes articles, reviews, and case studies concerning resuscitation in emergency situations.
Related titles: Online - full text ed.: (from ingenta).
Indexed: Excerp.Med.
—BLDSC, GNLM, Infotrieve. **CCC.**
Published by: (Societe Francophone d'Urgences Medicales), Elsevier Paris, Editions Scientifiques et Medicales (Subsidiary of: Reed Elsevier plc. group), 23 rue Linois, Paris 75015, France. TEL 33-1-45589110, FAX 33-1-45589419, rea-urg@elsevier.fr; academic@elsevier-fr.com, http://www.elsevier.com/locate/reaurg. Ed. Y Castaing. **Co-sponsor:** Societe de Reanimation de Langue Francaise.

617.96 GBR ISSN 0309-2305
CODEN: RAAADM
RECENT ADVANCES IN ANAESTHESIA AND ANALGESIA. Text in English. 1932. irreg. **Document type:** *Monographic series, Academic/Scholarly.*
—BLDSC (7303.755000), CASDDS, KNAW.
Published by: Churchill Livingstone (Subsidiary of: Harcourt Publishers Ltd.), Robert Stevenson House, 1-3 Baxter's Pl, Leith Walk, Edinburgh, Midlothian EH1 3AF, United Kingdom. TEL 44-131-556-2424, FAX 44-131-459-1177, http://www.churchillmed.com. **Subscr. to:** Harourt Brace & Company Ltd., Foots Cray High St, Sidcup, Kent DA 14, United Kingdom. TEL 44-181-308-5700, FAX 44-181-309-0807.

617.96 USA ISSN 1098-7339
RD84 CODEN: RGANDZ
REGIONAL ANESTHESIA AND PAIN MEDICINE. Text in English. 1975. bi-m. USD 169 combined subscription domestic to individuals for print & online eds.; USD 223 combined subscription foreign to individuals for print & online eds.; USD 238 combined subscription domestic to institutions for print & online eds.; USD 283 combined subscription foreign to institutions for print & online eds.; USD 64 combined subscription domestic to students for print & online eds.; USD 113 combined subscription foreign to students for print & online eds.; USD 48 newsstand/cover (effective 2001). adv. illus. index. back issues avail. *Refereed.* **Document type:** *Journal, Academic/Scholarly.* **Description:** Contains original articles, case reports, and other material relevant to practitioners concerned with local anesthetics, regional anesthesia, and pain management.
Formerly (until 1998): Regional Anesthesia (0146-521X)
Related titles: Microform ed.: 1975 (from PQC); Online - full text ed.: (from ProQuest Information & Learning, IDEAL Online Library, Institute for Scientific Information).
Indexed: ASCA, CINAHL, Chem.Abstr., Chem.Indus.Notes, Chem.Titles, Curr.Cont., Excerp.Med. (1993-), Ind.Med. (1998-), Inpharma, Int.Nurs.Ind., Neurosci.Cit.Ind., Pharm.&Out.News, Reac.
—BLDSC (7336.572210), CASDDS, CISTI, GNLM, IDS, ingenta, KNAW. **CCC.**
Published by: (American Society of Regional Anesthesia), W.B. Saunders Co. (Subsidiary of: Harcourt Publishers Ltd.), 11830 Westline Industrial Dr, St Louis, MO 63146. TEL 800-325-4177, http://www.rapm.org, http://www.wbsaunders.com. Ed. Dr. David Brown. Circ: 11,000.

617.96 TUR
REJYONAL ANESTEZI BULTEN. Text in Turkish. 1993. bi-m. USD 50 (effective 1999). adv. bk.rev. abstr. *Refereed.* **Document type:** *Bulletin, Newsletter.* **Description:** Reports on news, medical and technical issues affecting regional anesthesiologists, with summaries in Turkish of recent articles appearing in international literature.
Published by: Rejyonal Anestezi Dernegi, c/o Dr. Serdar Erdine, Ed., Istanbul Tip Fakultesi, Agri Merkezi Capa Klinikleri, Istanbul 34390, Turkey. TEL 90-212-6350135, FAX 90-212-6310541, algotur@ibm.net. Ed., R&P Dr. Serdar Erdine. Adv. contact Suleyman Ozyalcin.

RESUSCITATION; an interdisciplinary journal for the dissemination of clinical and basic science research relating to acute care medicine and cardiopulmonary resuscitation. see *MEDICAL SCIENCES—Respiratory Diseases*

617.96 COL ISSN 0120-3347
REVISTA COLOMBIANA DE ANESTESIOLOGIA. Text in Spanish. 1973. q. USD 20. adv. bk.rev. back issues avail. **Document type:** *Academic/Scholarly.*
Published by: Sociedad Colombiana de Anestesiologia y Reanimacion, Apartado Aereo 11206, Bogota, CUND, Colombia. TEL 57-1-2883985, FAX 57-1-2454481. Ed. Julio Enrique Pena. Circ: 1,000.

M

617.96 ESP ISSN 0034-9356 CODEN: REANBJ
REVISTA ESPANOLA DE ANESTESIOLOGIA Y REANIMACION. Text in Spanish; Summaries in English. 1953. m. (10/yr.). USD 117 to non-members. adv. bk.rev. abstr, charts, illus, stat. reprint service avail. from PQC. **Document type:** *Academic/Scholarly.* **Description:** Diffuses information on the clinical and experimental work of Spanish anesthesiologists.
Formerly: Revista Espanola de Anestesiologia
Indexed: Biol.Abstr., Chem.Abstr., Chem.Indus.Notes, Chem.Titles, Dent.Ind., Excerp.Med., Ind.Med. (1967-), Ind.Med.Esp., Int.Nurs.Ind., Ref.Zh.
—BLDSC (7853.910000), CASDDS, CINDOC, CISTI, GNLM, KNAW. **CCC.**
Published by: (Sociedad Espanola de Anestesiologia - Reanimacion y Terapia del Dolor), Ediciones Doyma S.A., Traversa de Gracia, 17-21, Barcelona 08021, Spain. TEL 34-93-200-0711, FAX 34-93-209-1136, TELEX 51964 INK-E. Ed. R Garcia Guasch. Adv. contact Marte Vidal. color page ESP 259,000; trim 280 x 210. Circ: 5,000.

617.96 MEX ISSN 0185-1012
REVISTA MEXICANA DE ANESTESIOLOGIA. Text in Spanish; Summaries in English, Spanish. 1952. q. MXP 250 domestic to individuals; MXP 280 domestic to institutions; USD 70 foreign (effective 2000). adv. bk.rev. charts, illus, stat. index. back issues avail. *Refereed.* **Document type:** *Academic/Scholarly.*
Related titles: CD-ROM ed.
Indexed: Excerp.Med., Ind.Med. (coverage dropped), Ref.Zh.
—BLDSC (7866.200000), CISTI, GNLM, KNAW.
Published by: Sociedad Mexicana de Anestesiologia A.C., Des. 502, Mexico, Ave. INSURGENTES SUR 636, Del Valle, Mexico City, DF 03100, Mexico. TEL 52-5-6691457, FAX 52-5-6691659, jamj@mail.internet.com.mx, http://www.anestesia.com.mx/rma.html. Ed. Jose de Jesus Jaramillo. R&P, Adv. contact Yolanda Celis Hernandez. Circ: 2,500.

617 GBR
ROYAL COLLEGE OF ANAESTHETISTS. NEWSLETTER. Text in English. 1965. bi-m. membership. **Document type:** *Newsletter.* **Description:** Report to Fellows and Members of College. Covers activities, events, and personalities.
Former titles: Royal College of Surgeons of England. Faculty of Anaesthetists. Dean's Newsletter; Royal College of Surgeons of England. Faculty of Anaesthetists. Newsletter
Published by: Royal College of Anaesthetists, 48-49 Russell Sq, London WC1B 4JY, United Kingdom. TEL 44-171-813-1900, FAX 44-171-813-1876. Ed. R M Jones. R&P A J Kelly. Circ: 10,000 (controlled).

617.96 USA CODEN: SEANDW
SEMINARS IN ANESTHESIA, PERIOPERATIVE MEDICINE AND PAIN. Text in English. 1982 (Mar.). q. USD 116 domestic to individuals; USD 188 foreign to individuals; USD 210 domestic to institutions; USD 257 foreign to institutions; USD 70 domestic to students; USD 113 foreign to students; USD 65 newsstand/cover (effective 2001). adv. bibl, charts, illus. index. **Document type:** *Journal, Academic/Scholarly.* **Description:** Experts discuss a single topic from their clinical experience in each issue.
Formerly: Seminars in Anesthesia (0277-0326)
Related titles: Online - full text ed.: (from Institute for Scientific Information).
Indexed: ASCA, CINAHL, Chem.Abstr., Chem.Titles, Curr.Cont. (coverage dropped), Sci.Cit.Ind. (coverage dropped).
—BLDSC, CASDDS, EMDOCS, GNLM, IDS, ingenta. **CCC.**
Published by: W.B. Saunders Co. (Subsidiary of: Harcourt Publishers Ltd.), 11830 Westline Industrial Dr, St Louis, MO 63146. TEL 800-325-4177, http://www.wbsaunders.com. Ed. Dr. Ronald L Katz. adv.: B&W page USD 910, color page USD 2,060; trim 10 x 7. Circ: 1,616. **Subscr. to:** Periodicals Fulfillment, W B Saunders Co, 6277 Sea Harbor Dr, 4th Fl, Orlando, FL 32891-4800.

SEMINARS IN CARDIOTHORACIC AND VASCULAR ANESTHESIA. see *MEDICAL SCIENCES—Cardiovascular Diseases*

SEMINARS IN HEADACHE MANAGEMENT. see *PSYCHOLOGY*

617.96 ESP ISSN 1134-8046 CODEN: RSEDF9
SOCIEDAD ESPANOLA DEL DOLOR. REVISTA. Text in Spanish; Abstracts in Spanish, English. 1994. bi-m. (8/yr.). ESP 8,000 domestic; USD 200 foreign (effective 2000). adv. abstr, bibl, illus, stat. back issues avail.; reprints avail. *Refereed.* **Document type:** *Academic/Scholarly.*
Related titles: Online - full text ed.
—BLDSC (7831.070000).
Published by: (Sociedad Espanola del Dolor), Aran Ediciones S.A., Castello, 128 1o, Madrid 28006, Spain. TEL 34-91-782-0030, FAX 34-91-561-5787, edita@grupoaran.com, http://www.grupoaran.com. Ed. Luis Miguel Torres Morera. Pub. Jose Jimenez. R&P Maria Dolores Linares TEL 34-1-7820035. adv.: B&W page ESP 120,000, color page ESP 154. Circ: 3,000.

617.96 ITA ISSN 1126-4683
SOCIETA ITALIANA DI ANESTESIA, ANALGESIA, RIANIMAZIONE E TERAPIA INTENSIVA. NOTIZARIO. Key Title: Notiziaro della S I A A R T I. Text in Italian. 1994. 3/yr. adv. **Document type:** *Newsletter.*
Indexed: RAPRA.
Published by: (Societa Italiana di Anestesia, Analgesia, Rianimazione e Terapia Intensiva), C I C Edizioni Internazionali s.r.l., Corso Trieste 42, Rome, RM 00198, Italy. TEL 39-06-8412673, FAX 39-06-8412688, info@gruppocic.it, 1160199510. Ed. V Bruni. adv.: B&W page XEU 1,807.6, color page XEU 2,582.82; 210 x 290.

617.96 ZAF ISSN 1027-9148
SOUTH AFRICAN JOURNAL OF ANAESTHESIOLOGY AND ANALGESIA. Text in English. 1995. q. USD 60 foreign (effective 2001). adv. back issues avail.; reprints avail. *Refereed.* **Document type:** *Journal, Academic/Scholarly.* **Description:** Aimed at anesthesiologists and general practitioners with an interest in anasthesiology.
Related titles: Online - full text ed.
—BLDSC (8338.600000).
Published by: In House Publications, PO Box 412748, Craighall, Johannesburg 2024, South Africa. TEL 27-11-4429759, FAX 27-11-8807898, inhouse@iafrica.com, http://www.inhousepub.co.za. Ed. C Lundgren. Pub., R&P A. Thomas. Adv. contact A Thomas. B&W page USD 887, color page USD 1,200; trim 210 x 297. Circ: 2,000.

▼ **SURGICAL THEATRE EQUIPMENT AND TECHNNOLOGY (S T E T).** see *MEDICAL SCIENCES—Surgery*

SURVEY OF ANESTHESIOLOGY. see *MEDICAL SCIENCES—Abstracting, Bibliographies, Statistics*

617.96 USA ISSN 1084-208X
TECHNIQUES IN REGIONAL ANESTHESIA & PAIN MANAGEMENT. Text in English. 1997. q. USD 135 domestic to individuals; USD 190 foreign to individuals; USD 210 domestic to institutions; USD 270 foreign to institutions; USD 83 domestic to students; USD 114 foreign to students; USD 68 newsstand/cover (effective 2001). adv. *Refereed.* **Document type:** *Journal, Academic/Scholarly.* **Description:** Provides specialized information on common complications of regional anesthesia and pain management procedures and their appropriate treatments.
—BLDSC (8745.332000).
Published by: W.B. Saunders Co. (Subsidiary of: Harcourt Publishers Ltd.), 11830 Westline Industrial Dr, St Louis, MO 63146. TEL 800-325-4177, wbspcs@harcourtbrace.com, http://www.wbsaunders.com. Ed. Dr. William Urmey. adv.: B&W page USD 675, color page USD 1,625. Circ: 1,000 (paid).

617.96 USA ISSN 8756-8578
TECHNOLOGY FOR ANESTHESIA. Text in English. m. USD 205.80 domestic; USD 221 in Canada; USD 249.60 elsewhere (effective 2002). *Refereed.* **Document type:** *Trade.* **Description:** Covers news and development of technology for anesthesia. Summarizes comparative product evaluations, principles of device operation, and reported medical device problems and recalls.
Former titles: Technology of Anesthesiology; Health Devices Update: Anesthesiology
—**CCC.**
Published by: (Emergency Care Research Institute), E C R I, 5200 Butler Pike, Plymouth, PA 19462. TEL 610-825-6000, FAX 610-834-1275, info@ecri.org, http://www.ecri.org. Ed. Beth Richardson.

617.96 AUS
THERAPEUTIC GUIDELINES. ANALGESIC. Text in English. 1988. irreg., latest version 3 (every 3-4 yrs.). **Document type:** *Academic/Scholarly.* **Description:** Covers clinical aspects of the management of pain for doctors, nurses and pharmacists.
Formerly: Analgesic Guidelines (1033-8810)
Related titles: CD-ROM ed.
Published by: Therapeutic Guidelines Ltd., Chelsea House, Level 2, 55 Flemington Rd, North Melbourne, VIC 3051, Australia. TEL 61-3-9329-1566, FAX 61-3-9326-5632, sales@tg.com.au, http://www.tg.com.au. Ed., R&P Mary Hemming. Circ: 18,000.

617.96 GBR ISSN 0969-0166
TODAY'S ANAESTHETIST. Text in English. 1986. q. GBP 18 domestic to individuals; GBP 30 foreign to individuals; GBP 30 domestic to institutions; GBP 50 foreign to institutions (effective 2000). **Document type:** *Trade.*
Published by: Media Publishing Company, Media House, 41 Crayford Way, Dartford, Kent DA1 4JY, United Kingdom. TEL 44-1322-558029, FAX 44-1322-558524, medipub@aol.com. Ed. M Vickers.

617 TUR ISSN 1016-5150 CODEN: TANRE
TURK ANESTEZIYOLOJI VE REANIMASYON CEMIYETI DERGISI. Text in Turkish; Summaries in English. 1972. 10/yr. USD 80 (effective 2001). adv. **Document type:** *Journal.*
Indexed: Excerp.Med.
—BLDSC (9071.888500), EMDOCS, GNLM, KNAW.
Published by: (Turk Anesteziyoloji ve Reanimasyon Cemiyeti), Logos Yayincilik Ticaret A.S., Yildiz Posta Cad., Sinan Apt. No. 36 D 66-67, Gayrettepe, Istanbul 80280, Turkey. TEL 90-212-2880541, info@logos.com.tr, http://logos.com.tr. Ed. Dr. Mois Bahar. Adv. contact Sukran Oznalga.

617.96 SWE ISSN 0348-6257
VENTILEN. Text in Swedish. 1978. q. SEK 170; SEK 50 newsstand/cover (effective 2000 & 2001). **Document type:** *Trade.*
Published by: (Riksfoereningen foer Anestesi och Intensivvaard), Via Media, Fack 640, Landskrona 26125, Sweden. TEL 46-418-10780, FAX 46-418-12394, viamedia@nornemark.com, http://www.nornemark.com/viamedia. Ed. Karin Bjoerkman Bjoerkelund. Circ: 6,200 (paid).

617.96 USA ISSN 1073-5437
THE YEAR BOOK OF ANESTHESIOLOGY AND PAIN MANAGEMENT. Text in English. 1961. a. USD 91 domestic; USD 97 foreign (effective 2001). illus. reprints avail. **Document type:** *Academic/Scholarly, Abstract/Index.* **Description:** Presents abstracts of pertinent literature with commentary by leaders in the field.
Former titles (until 1994): Year Book of Anesthesia and Pain Management (1091-5133); (until 1992): Year Book of Anesthesia (0084-3652); Which incorporated in part (1933-1970): Year Book of General Surgery (0084-3776)
Related titles: CD-ROM ed.
—CISTI, GNLM.
Published by: Mosby, Inc., Continuity Division (Subsidiary of: Harcourt Health Sciences), 11830 Westline Industrial Dr, St Louis, MO 63146-3313. TEL 314-872-8370, 800-325-4177, FAX 314-432-1380, http://www.mosby.com/periodicals. Ed. John H Tinker.

617.96 CHN
ZHONGHUA MAZUIXUE ZAZHI/CHINESE JOURNAL OF ANAESTHESIOLOGY. Text in Chinese. q. USD 1.30 per issue. **Document type:** *Academic/Scholarly.*
Related titles: CD-ROM ed.
Indexed: Chem.Abstr., ExtraMED.
Published by: China International Book Trading Corp/Zhongguo Guoji Tushu Maoyi Zonggongsi, 35 Chegongzhuang Xilu, Haidian District, Beijing 100044, China. TEL 86-1-68413849, FAX 86-1-68412048, cibtc@mail.cibtc.com.cn, http://www.cibtc.com.cn.

MEDICAL SCIENCES—Cardiovascular Diseases

A C C CURRENT JOURNAL REVIEW. see *MEDICAL SCIENCES—Abstracting, Bibliographies, Statistics*

M

616.1 USA
A C C E L; audio journal of clinical cardiology. (American College of Cardiology Extended Learning) Text in English. 1969. m. USD 200 domestic to non-members; USD 230 foreign to non-members; USD 165 domestic to members; USD 195 foreign to members (effective 2000 - 2001). index. **Document type:** *Academic/Scholarly.* **Description:** Presents one-on-one interviews with experts, offering practice-oriented information on cardiology.
Former titles: A C C E L for Physicians; A C C E S S (0001-0626)
Media: Audio cassette/tape.
Indexed: Risk Abstr.
Published by: American College of Cardiology, 9111 Old Georgetown Rd, Bethesda, MD 20814-1699. TEL 301-897-5400, 800-253-4636, FAX 301-897-9745, http://www.acc.org/education/online/accel/. Ed. Dr. Sylvan L Weinberg. R&P Julie Jani Bainbridge. Circ: 7,000. **Subscr. to:** Attn. ACCEL, PO Box 79231, Baltimore, MD 21279-0231.

616.1 BEL ISSN 0001-5385
CODEN: ACCAAQ
ACTA CARDIOLOGICA; international journal of cardiology. Text in English. 1946. bi-m. BEF 3,100. adv. bk.rev. charts, illus. index. *Refereed.* **Document type:** *Academic/Scholarly.* **Description:** Papers on fundamental, clinical, epidemiological and nutritional research in the field of cardiovascular disease.
Related titles: Online - full text ed.: (from Institute for Scientific Information); ♦ Supplement: Acta Cardiologica. Supplementum. ISSN 0373-7934.
Indexed: ASCA, Agri.& Environ.Biotech.Abstr. (coverage dropped), Biol.Abstr., Chem.Abstr., Curr.Cont., Derwent Biotech.Abstr., Environ.Sci.Poll.Mgmt., Excerp.Med., Ind.Med. (1946-), Inpharma, Nutr.Abstr., Pharm.&Out.News, Reac., Ref.Zh., Risk Abstr., Saf.Sci.Abstr., THA.
—BLDSC (0608.400000), CISTI, EMDOCS, GNLM, IDS, ingenta, KNAW.
Published by: Association des Societes Scientifiques Medicales Belges/Vereiniging van de Belgische Wetenschappelijke Genootschappen, Av Circulaire 138A, Brussels 1180, Belgium. TEL 32-2-3755892, FAX 32-2-3749628, acta.cardiologica@tvd.be. Ed. H Kesteloot. Circ: 900.

616.1 ITA ISSN 0392-9698
ACTA CARDIOLOGICA MEDITERANEA. Text in English, Italian. 1960. 3/yr. ITL 60,000; ITL 100,000 foreign (effective 1998). adv. abstr, bibl, illus, stat. index. **Document type:** *Proceedings, Academic/Scholarly.* **Description:** Discusses and reviews clinical cases of cardiovascular diseases.
Published by: Carbone Editore, Via Gaetano Daita, 29, Palermo, PA 90139, Italy. TEL 39-91-321-273, FAX 39-91-321782. Ed. Antonino Pennino. Pub., R&P Alfonsa Carbone. Adv. contact Donatella Donato. Circ: 3,000.

616.1 BEL ISSN 0373-7934
ACTA CARDIOLOGICA. SUPPLEMENTUM. Text in English. 1946. 3/w.
Related titles: ♦ Supplement to: Acta Cardiologica. ISSN 0001-5385.
Published by: Association des Societes Scientifiques Medicales Belges/Vereiniging van de Belgische Wetenschappelijke Genootschappen, Av Circulaire 138A, Brussels 1180, Belgium. TEL 32-2-3755892, FAX 32-2-3749628, acta.cardiologica@tvd.be. Ed. H Kesteloot.

616.1 ITA ISSN 1128-2460
ACTA MYOLOGICA; myopathies and cardiomyopathies. Text in Italian. 1989. 3/yr. USD 55 (effective 1999). bk.rev. back issues avail. *Refereed.* **Document type:** *Academic/Scholarly.*
Formerly (until 1997): Acta Cardiomyologica (1124-8874)
—BLDSC (0639.370000).
Published by: Mediterranean Society of Myology, Viale dei Pimi 101, Naples, NA 80131, Italy. TEL 39-08-17414775, FAX 39-08-15665100, gianigro@cds.unina.it. Circ: 3,000.

616 FRA ISSN 0245-8659
ACTUALITES D'ANGEIOLOGIE. Text in French. 1976. m., latest vol.27, 2002 (10/yr.). EUR 35; EUR 53 foreign (effective 2002). adv. charts, illus. back issues avail.
Formerly (until 1978): Actualites d'Angeiologie et de Pathologie Vasculaire (0397-2003)
—CINDOC.
Published by: P D G Communication, 30 rue d'Armaille, Paris 75017, France. TEL 33-1-40550595, FAX 33-1-45746567.

616.1 FRA ISSN 1169-0682
ACTUALITES VASCULAIRES INTERNATIONALES. Text in French. m. (10/yr). FRF 300 domestic to individuals; FRF 450 foreign to individuals; FRF 210 domestic to libraries; FRF 360 foreign to libraries (effective 2001). **Document type:** *Academic/Scholarly.*
Published by: L E N Medical, 15 rue des Sablons, Paris 75116, France. TEL 33-1-47553131, FAX 33-1-47553132, lenmed@club-internet.fr, http://www.webmedguide.com.

616.1 NLD ISSN 0884-6863
RC685.C6
ACUTE CORONARY CARE. Text in English. 1985. irreg., latest vol.2, 1987. price varies. *Refereed.* **Document type:** *Monographic series.*
Published by: Kluwer Academic Publishers Group (Subsidiary of: Wolters Kluwer N.V.), Spuiboulevard 50, PO Box 17, Dordrecht 3300 AA, Netherlands. FAX 31-78-639-2254, services@wkap.nl, http://www.wkap.nl. **Dist. by:** Journals Department, PO Box 322, Dordrecht 3300 AH, Netherlands. FAX 31-78-654-6474.

616.1 GBR ISSN 1369-5312
CODEN: ACSYFD
ACUTE CORONARY SYNDROMES. Text in English. 1997. q. GBP 50 in Europe; USD 70 in US & Canada; USD 75 elsewhere. **Document type:** *Academic/Scholarly.*
—BLDSC (0678.075000).
Published by: Remedica Publishing Ltd., 32-38 Osnaburgh St, London NW1 3ND, United Kingdom. TEL 44-171-388-7677, FAX 44-171-388-7678, info@remedica.com, http://www.remedica.com. Eds. James Ferguson, Nicolas Chronos.

616.1 USA ISSN 0889-5074
ADVANCES IN CARDIAC SURGERY. Text in English. 1989. a. USD 97 domestic; USD 103 foreign (effective 2001). **Document type:** *Academic/Scholarly.* **Description:** Presents a collection of original and fully referenced articles from experts in the field.
Formerly: Advances in Cardiovascular Surgery
Indexed: Ind.Med. (1990-).
—BLDSC (0702.200000), GNLM, KNAW. **CCC.**
Published by: Mosby, Inc. (Subsidiary of: Elsevier Science), 11830 Westline Industrial Dr, St Louis, MO 63146-3313. TEL 314-872-8370, 800-325-4177, FAX 314-432-1380, http://www.mosby.com/periodicals. Ed. Dr. Robert B Karp.

616.1 CHE ISSN 0065-2326
RC681.A25 CODEN: ACDYB2
ADVANCES IN CARDIOLOGY. Text in English. 1956. irreg., latest vol.38. CHF 190 in Europe; DEM 230 in Germany; USD 150 in United States (2001). reprint service avail. from ISI. *Refereed.* **Document type:** *Monographic series, Academic/Scholarly.*
Related titles: Online - full text ed.: (from Institute for Scientific Information).
Indexed: ASCA, Biol.Abstr., CINAHL, Chem.Abstr., Curr.Adv.Ecol.Sci., Curr.Cont. (coverage dropped), Excerp.Med., Ind.Med. (1970-).
—BLDSC (0702.300000), CASDDS, CISTI, GNLM, KNAW. **CCC.**
Published by: S. Karger AG, Allschwilerstr 10, PO Box, Basel 4009, Switzerland. TEL 41-61-306-1111, FAX 41-61-306-1234, karger@karger.ch, http://www.karger.com/bookseries/ADCAR. Ed. W J Remme.

ADVANCES IN VASCULAR SURGERY. see *MEDICAL SCIENCES—Surgery*

616.10711 USA
AFFILIATES IN TRAINING. Text in English. 1983. bi-m. USD 30 (effective 2000). adv. charts. 8 p./no. back issues avail.; reprints avail. **Document type:** *Newsletter.* **Description:** Covers new directions in managed care, opportunities in subspecialization, positions available, meeting updates, board exams. Aimed at doctors in cardiovascular fellowships and their training directors.
Published by: American College of Cardiology, 9111 Old Georgetown Rd, Bethesda, MD 20814-1699. TEL 301-897-5400, 800-253-4636, FAX 301-897-9745, http://www.acc.org. Ed., R&P Kathy Boyd. Adv. contact Stacy Blume. Circ: 4,000.

ALGOLOGIA. see *MEDICAL SCIENCES—Psychiatry And Neurology*

616.12 USA ISSN 0735-1097
CODEN: JACCDI
AMERICAN COLLEGE OF CARDIOLOGY. JOURNAL. Key Title: Journal of the American College of Cardiology. Text in English. 14/yr. EUR 420 in Europe to individuals; JPY 55,800 in Japan to individuals; USD 469 elsewhere to individuals; USD 194 in United States to individuals; USD 118 to individuals resident price; EUR 429 in Europe to institutions; JPY 57,000 in Japan to institutions; USD 346 in Canada & Mexico to institutions; USD 480 elsewhere to institutions; JPY 76,300 in Japan to institutions air mail; EUR 575 in Europe to institutions air mail (effective 2002). adv. index. back issues avail. *Refereed.* **Document type:** *Academic/Scholarly.* **Description:** Publishes original clinical and experimental reports on all aspects of cardiovascular disease.
Related titles: CD-ROM ed.: J A C C on CD-ROM; Microform ed.: (from PQC); Online - full text ed.: (from ingenta, ScienceDirect, Swets Blackwell, Institute for Scientific Information); ♦ Supplement: American College of Cardiology. Symposia.
Indexed: AIM, ASCA, Biol.Abstr., CINAHL, Cal.Tiss.Abstr., Chem.Abstr., Chem.Indus.Notes, Chem.Titles, Curr.Cont., Dent.Ind., Derwent Biotech.Abstr., Environ.Sci.Poll.Mgmt., Excerp.Med., INIS Atomind., Ind.Med. (1983-), Ind.Sci.Rev., Inpharma, Int.Abstr.Biol.Sci., Jrnl.Watch, Jrnl.Watch Card., Jrnl.Watch Emer.Med., Jrnl.Watch Wom.Hlth., NRN, Nutr.Abstr., Pharm.&Out.News, Pig News & Info., Pollut.Abstr., Reac., Ref.Zh., Risk Abstr., SSCI (coverage dropped), Saf.Sci.Abstr., Sci.Cit.Ind., THA.
—BLDSC (4685.500000), ADONIS, CASDDS, CISTI, EMDOCS, GNLM, IDS, ingenta, KNAW. **CCC.**
Published by: (American College of Cardiology), Elsevier Science, PO Box 945, New York, NY 10159-0945. TEL 212-989-5800, FAX 212-633-3990, usinfo-f@elsevier.com, http://www.elsevier.com/locate/jac. Eds. S Dack, Dr. William W Parmley. **Subscr. in Australasia and the Far East to:** Elsevier Science (Singapore) Pte Ltd, No.1 Temasek Ave, 17-01 Millenia Tower, Singapore 039192, Singapore. TEL 65-434-3727, FAX 65-337-2230; **Subscr. in Japan to:** Elsevier Science Inc - Japan Regional Office, 9-15 Higashi-Azabu 1-chome, Minato-ku, Tokyo 106-0044, Japan. TEL 81-3-5561-5033; **Subscr. outside the Americas to:** Elsevier Science BV, PO Box 211, Amsterdam 1000 AE, Netherlands. TEL 31-20-485-3757.

616.1 ESP ISSN 1133-4304
AMERICAN COLLEGE OF CARDIOLOGY. JOURNAL (EDICION ESPANOLA). Text in Spanish. 1992. bi-m. USD 99 (effective 1996). **Document type:** *Academic/Scholarly.*
Published by: Ediciones Doyma S.A., Traversa de Gracia, 17-21, Barcelona 08021, Spain. TEL 34-93-200-0711, FAX 34-93-209-1136. Ed. F Navarro Lopez. adv.: color page ESP 259,000. Circ: 2,000.

616.1 USA
AMERICAN COLLEGE OF CARDIOLOGY SCIENTIFIC SESSION NEWS. Text in English. 1982. 5/yr. back issues avail. **Document type:** *Newsletter.* **Description:** For attendees of the college's Annual Scientific Session. Highlights clinical presentations, events and activities of the meetings as well as activities within the city.
Formerly: American College of Cardiology Annual Scientific Session News
Published by: American College of Cardiology, 9111 Old Georgetown Rd, Bethesda, MD 20814-1699. TEL 301-897-5400, FAX 301-897-9745, http://www.acc.org. Eds. Kathy Boyd, Melanie Caudron. Adv. contact Keith Dillon TEL 301-897-5400. Circ: 41,000 (controlled).

616.1 USA
AMERICAN COLLEGE OF CARDIOLOGY. SYMPOSIA. Text in English. 1973. a. **Document type:** *Proceedings.*
Related titles: ♦ Supplement to: American College of Cardiology. Journal. ISSN 0735-1097.
Published by: (American College of Cardiology), Elsevier Science, PO Box 945, New York, NY 10159-0945. TEL 212-989-5800, FAX 212-633-3990. **Subscr. in Australasia and the Far East to:** Elsevier Science (Singapore) Pte Ltd, No.1 Temasek Ave, 17-01 Millenia Tower, Singapore 039192, Singapore. TEL 65-434-3727, FAX 65-337-2230; **Subscr. in Japan to:** Elsevier Science Inc - Japan Regional Office, 9-15 Higashi-Azabu 1-chome, Minato-ku, Tokyo 106-0044, Japan. TEL 81-3-5561-5033; **Subscr. outside the Americas to:** Elsevier Science BV, PO Box 211, Amsterdam 1000 AE, Netherlands. TEL 31-20-485-3757, nlinfo-f@elsevier.nl, http://www.elsevier.nl.

AMERICAN HEART ASSOCIATION. SCIENTIFIC SESSIONS. ABSTRACTS. see *MEDICAL SCIENCES—Abstracting, Bibliographies, Statistics*

M

616.1 USA ISSN 0002-8703
RC681.A1 CODEN: AHJOA2
AMERICAN HEART JOURNAL; the international publication for the study of the heart and circulation. Text in English. 1925. m. USD 163 domestic to individuals; USD 201 foreign to individuals; USD 348 domestic to institutions; USD 392 foreign to institutions; USD 82 domestic to students; USD 120 foreign to students; USD 33 newsstand/cover (effective 2001). adv. bibl, charts, illus. s-a. index. reprint service avail. from PQC. *Refereed.* **Document type:** *Journal, Academic/Scholarly.* **Description:** For those concerned with the diagnosis and management of cardiovascular disease.
Related titles: Microfilm ed.: (from PMC,PQC); Online - full text ed.: (from Ovid Technologies, Inc., EBSCO Publishing, Gale Group, IDEAL Online Library, Institute for Scientific Information, RoweCom Information Quest).
Indexed: AIM, ASCA, Abstr.Hyg., Abstr.Inter.Med., Agri.& Environ.Biotech.Abstr. (coverage dropped), Behav.Med.Abstr., Biol.Abstr., Biol.Dig., CINAHL, Chem.Abstr., Chem.Indus.Notes, Chem.Titles, Curr.Adv.Ecol.Sci., Curr.Cont., Dairy Sci.Abstr., Derwent Biotech.Abstr., Diab.Cont., Environ.Sci.Poll.Mgmt., Excerp.Med., Helminthol.Abstr., INIS Atomind., I.P.A., Ind.Med. (1925-), Ind.Sci.Rev., Inpharma, Int.Nurs.Ind., Jrnl.Watch Card., Kidney, NRN, Neurosci.Cit.Ind., Pharm.&Out.News, Pollut.Abstr., Protozool.Abstr., Reac., Rev.Med.& Vet.Mycol., Rev.Plant Path., Risk Abstr., SSCI (coverage dropped), Saf.Sci.Abstr., Sci.Cit.Ind., THA, Trop.Dis.Bull.
—BLDSC (0817.000000), ADONIS, CASDDS, CISTI, EMDOCS, GNLM, IDS, ingenta, KNAW. **CCC.**
Published by: Mosby, Inc. (Subsidiary of: Elsevier Science), 11830 Westline Industrial Dr, St Louis, MO 63146-3318. TEL 314-872-8370, 800-325-4177, FAX 314-432-1380, http://www.mosby.com/ahj, http://www.mosby.com/periodicals. Eds. Daniel B Mark, Dr. Robert M Califf. Pub. Jane Grochowski. Adv. contact Gina Burkert TEL 314-453-4306. B&W page USD 1,385, color page USD 2,535; trim 10.88 x 8.13. Circ: 6,354 (paid).

616.1 USA ISSN 0002-9149
RC681.A1 CODEN: AJCDAG
THE AMERICAN JOURNAL OF CARDIOLOGY. Text in English. 1958. s-m. USD 104 in US & Canada to individuals; USD 249 elsewhere to individuals; USD 301 in US & Canada to institutions; USD 454 elsewhere to institutions (effective 2002). adv. bk.rev. bibl, charts, illus. index. *Refereed.* **Document type:** *Academic/Scholarly.* **Description:** Explores and highlights advances in diagnosis and treatment of cardiovascular disease, stressing a practical, clinical approach to cardiology.
Related titles: CD-ROM ed.: (from Ovid Technologies, Inc.); Microform ed.; Online - full text ed.: (from Ovid Technologies, Inc., ingenta, Swets Blackwell, ScienceDirect, Factiva, Institute for Scientific Information).
Indexed: AIM, ASCA, Abstr.Hyg., Abstr.Inter.Med., Agri.& Environ.Biotech.Abstr. (coverage dropped), Behav.Med.Abstr., Biol.Abstr., Biol.Dig., CINAHL, C.I.S. Abstr., Chem.Abstr., Chem.Indus.Notes, Chem.Titles, Curr.Adv.Ecol.Sci., Curr.Cont., Dent.Ind., Derwent Biotech.Abstr., Dok.Arbeitsmed., Environ.Sci.Poll.Mgmt., Excerp.Med., Helminthol.Abstr., INIS Atomind., I.P.A., Ind.Med. (1958-), Ind.Sci.Rev., Inpharma, Int.Nurs.Ind., Jrnl.Watch Card., Jrnl.Watch Emer.Med., Kidney, NRN, Neurosci.Cit.Ind., Nutr.Abstr., Pharm.&Out.News, Pollut.Abstr., Protozool.Abstr., Reac., Ref.Zh., Risk Abstr., SSCI (coverage dropped), Saf.Sci.Abstr., Sci.Cit.Ind., THA, Trop.Dis.Bull.
—BLDSC (0822.500000), ADONIS, CASDDS, CISTI, EMDOCS, GNLM, IDS, ingenta, KNAW. **CCC.**
Published by: Excerpta Medica, Inc. (Subsidiary of: Reed Elsevier Medical group), 105 Raider Blvd, Belle Mead, NJ 08502. TEL 908-281-3625, FAX 908-874-8419, http://www.elsevier.com/locate/amjcard. Ed. Dr. William C Roberts. Circ: 30,050. **Subscr. to:** PO Box 10670, Riverton, NJ 08076.

616.1 NZL ISSN 1175-3277
▼ **AMERICAN JOURNAL OF CARDIOVASCULAR DRUGS.** Text in English. 2001. 6/yr. USD 150 to individuals Print or Online ed.; USD 180 to individuals Print & Online eds.; USD 495 to institutions Print or Online ed.; USD 594 to institutions Print & Online eds. (effective 2001). abstr. **Document type:** *Academic/Scholarly.* **Description:** Promotes rational therapy and disease management within the discipline of cardiology by providing a regular program of independent review articles covering all aspects of the management of cardiovascular disorders, particularly the place in therapy of newer and established agents and procedures.
Related titles: Online - full text ed.: (from Swets Blackwell, Ovid Technologies, Inc.).
Published by: Adis International Limited, Mairangi Bay, Private Bag 65901, Auckland 1010, New Zealand. TEL 64-9-477-0700, FAX 64-9-477-0766, cardiocasc@adis.co.nz, http://www.adis.com/. Ed. Amitabh Prakash.

616.1 USA ISSN 0887-8005
RC669.9 CODEN: AJCPEM
AMERICAN JOURNAL OF CARDIOVASCULAR PATHOLOGY. Text in English. 1987. q. USD 125 to individuals; USD 175 to institutions. *Refereed.* **Document type:** *Academic/Scholarly.*
Related titles: Online - full text ed.: (from Institute for Scientific Information).
Indexed: ASCA, Excerp.Med., INIS Atomind., Ind.Med. (1987-).
—BLDSC (0822.520000), CASDDS, EMDOCS, GNLM, ingenta, KNAW.
Published by: Field & Wood, Medical Periodicals, Inc., PO Box 975, Blue Bell, PA 19422. TEL 610-828-4010, FAX 215-482-0226. Ed. Dr. Colin M Bloor.

612.67 USA ISSN 1076-7460
CODEN: AJGCE3
AMERICAN JOURNAL OF GERIATRIC CARDIOLOGY. Text in English. 1992. bi-m. USD 90 domestic to individuals; USD 105 foreign to individuals; USD 105 domestic to institutions; USD 120 foreign to institutions (effective 2001). adv. bk.rev. abstr, charts, illus. back issues avail.; reprints avail. *Refereed.* **Document type:** *Journal, Academic/Scholarly.* **Description:** Devoted to the study of heart disease in the elderly.
Indexed: Excerp.Med. (1993-), Inpharma, Pharm.&Out.News, Reac.
—BLDSC (0824.655000), GNLM, KNAW.
Published by: LeJacq Communications, Inc., 777 W Putnam Ave, Greenwich, CT 06830-5014. TEL 203-531-0450, FAX 203-531-0533, showell@lejacq.com. Ed. Nanette Wenger. R&P Andrea Townsend. Adv. contact Joann Kalaka-Adams TEL 732-747-6525. B&W page USD 2,200, color page USD 1,095; trim 10.75 x 8. Circ: 20,000.

616.132 USA ISSN 0895-7061
CODEN: AJHYE6
AMERICAN JOURNAL OF HYPERTENSION. Text in English. 1988. m. EUR 295 in Europe to individuals; JPY 40,950 in Japan to individuals; USD 207 in United States to individuals; USD 331 elsewhere to individuals; EUR 392 in Europe to institutions; JPY 52,100 in Japan to institutions; USD 388 in United States to institutions; USD 439 elsewhere to institutions (effective 2002). adv. *Refereed.* **Document type:** *Academic/Scholarly.* **Description:** Offers wide coverage of experimental and clinical hypertension and related cardiovascular diseases.
Incorporates (1985-1987): Journal of Clinical Hypertension (0748-450X)
Related titles: Microform ed.: (from PQC); Online - full text ed.: (from ingenta, Swets Blackwell, ScienceDirect, Institute for Scientific Information); ♦ Spanish ed.: American Journal of Hypertension. Edicion en Espanol.
Indexed: ASCA, Biol.Dig., Chem.Abstr., Chem.Indus.Notes, Chem.Titles, Curr.Cont., Excerp.Med., INIS Atomind., Ind.Med. (1988-), Inpharma, Int.Abstr.Biol.Sci., Kidney, NRN, Nutr.Abstr., Pharm.&Out.News, Reac., Ref.Zh., Sci.Cit.Ind., THA.
—BLDSC (0826.400000), ADONIS, CASDDS, CISTI, EMDOCS, GNLM, IDS, ingenta, KNAW. **CCC.**
Published by: (American Society of Hypertension), Elsevier Science, 655 Ave of the Americas, New York, NY 10010. FAX 212-633-3990, http://www.elsevier.com/locate/amjhyper. Ed. John H Laragh. Adv. contact Hank Blaney. B&W page USD 1,385, color page USD 2,985. Circ: 4,300 (paid). **Subscr. in Australasia and the Far East to:** Elsevier Science (Singapore) Pte Ltd, No.1 Temasek Ave, 17-01 Millenia Tower, Singapore 039192, Singapore. TEL 65-434-3727, FAX 65-337-2230; **Subscr. in Japan to:** Elsevier Science Inc - Japan Regional Office, 9-15 Higashi-Azabu 1-chome, Minato-ku, Tokyo 106-0044, Japan. TEL 81-3-5561-5033; **Subscr. outside the Americas to:** Elsevier Science BV, PO Box 211, Amsterdam 1000 AE, Netherlands. TEL 31-20-485-3757, nlinfo-f@elsevier.nl.

616.132 ESP
AMERICAN JOURNAL OF HYPERTENSION. EDICION EN ESPANOL. Text in Spanish. 8/yr. **Document type:** *Academic/Scholarly.* **Description:** Offers wide coverage of experimental and clinical hypertension and related cardiovascular diseases.
Related titles: ♦ English ed.: American Journal of Hypertension. ISSN 0895-7061.
Published by: (American Society of Hypertension USA), Saned S.A., Capitan Haya, 60, Madrid 28020, Spain. TEL 34-91-749-9506, FAX 34-91-749-9507, saned@meditex.es. Ed. J L Palma Gamiz. adv.: page ESP 250,000.

AMERICAN JOURNAL OF PHYSIOLOGY: HEART AND CIRCULATORY PHYSIOLOGY. see *BIOLOGY—Physiology*

616.01 USA ISSN 0894-7317
CODEN: JSECEJ
AMERICAN SOCIETY OF ECHOCARDIOGRAPHY. JOURNAL. Text in English. 1988. m. USD 154 domestic to individuals; USD 196 foreign to individuals; USD 217 domestic to institutions; USD 259 foreign to institutions; USD 78 domestic to students; USD 120 foreign to students; USD 22 newsstand/cover (effective 2001). adv. s-a. index. back issues avail.; reprint service avail. from PQC. *Refereed.* **Document type:** *Journal, Academic/Scholarly.* **Description:** Contains the latest clinical, scientific, legal, and economic information regarding the use of cardiac ultrasound.
Related titles: Microform ed.: (from PQC); Online - full text ed.: (from Ovid Technologies, Inc., EBSCO Publishing, IDEAL Online Library, Institute for Scientific Information, RoweCom Information Quest).
Indexed: CINAHL, Curr.Cont., Ind.Med. (1988-), Inpharma, Int.Nurs.Ind., Pharm.&Out.News, Reac., Sci.Cit.Ind.
—BLDSC (4692.680000), CISTI, GNLM, IDS, KNAW. **CCC.**
Published by: (American Society of Echocardiography (ASE)), Mosby, Inc. (Subsidiary of: Elsevier Science), 11830 Westline Industrial Dr, St Louis, MO 63146-3318. TEL 314-872-8370, 800-325-4177, FAX 314-432-1380, http://www.mosby.com/echo, http://www.mosby.com/periodicals. Ed. Dr. Harvey Feigenbaum. Pub. Jane Grochowski. Adv. contact Gale Schlogl TEL 314-453-4337. B&W page USD 1,120, color page USD 2,170; trim 10.88 x 8.25. Circ: 7,354.

616.132 USA ISSN 0898-672X
CODEN: ASHSEH
AMERICAN SOCIETY OF HYPERTENSION. SYMPOSIUM SERIES. Text in English. 1987. irreg. price varies. reprint service avail. from PQC. *Refereed.* **Document type:** *Monographic series.*
—CASDDS, KNAW.
Published by: (American Society of Hypertension), Lippincott Williams & Wilkins (Philadelphia) (Subsidiary of: Wolters Kluwer N.V.), 530 Walnut St, Philadelphia, PA 19106-3621. TEL 301-223-2300, 800-638-3030, FAX 301-223-2400.

616.1 617 ESP ISSN 1135-2760
CODEN: ANGOAT
ANALES DE CIRUGIA CARDIACA Y CIRUGIA VASCULAR. Text in Spanish; Summaries in English. 1949. 5/yr. ESP 6,300, USD 115 (effective 1999). adv. bk.rev. abstr, charts, illus. index. **Document type:** *Trade.*
Formerly (until 1995): Angiologia (0003-3170)
Indexed: Biol.Abstr., Chem.Abstr., Excerp.Med., Ind.Med. (coverage dropped), Ref.Zh.
—BLDSC (0902.650000), CISTI, EMDOCS, GNLM, Infotrieve, KNAW. **CCC.**
Published by: Editorial Dips Rocas, Muntaner, 393 pral. 4, Barcelona 08021, Spain. TEL 39-3-2001389, FAX 39-3-2021958, edipsro@intercom.es. R&P Alvaro Trevino. Adv. contact Carles Martin. color page ESP 105,000. Circ: 3,000.

616.1 USA
ANGINA: DISEASE STATE MANAGEMENT RESOURCE. Text in English. 1997. a. USD 295 domestic; USD 325 foreign (effective 2001). **Document type:** *Trade.*
Published by: American Health Consultants (Subsidiary of: Medical Economics Co., Inc.), 3525 Piedmont Rd, N E, 6 Piedmont Center, Ste 400, Atlanta, GA 30305. TEL 404-262-5476, 404-262-7436, 800-688-2421, FAX 404-262-7837, 800-284-3291, custserv@ahcpub.com, http://www.ahcpub.com.

ANGIOGENESIS. see *MEDICAL SCIENCES—Oncology*

616.12 FRA ISSN 0765-4871
ANGIOLOGIE. Text in French. 1983. m. FRF 460, EUR 70.12 domestic to individuals; FRF 580, USD 105 foreign to individuals; FRF 580, EUR 88.42 domestic to institutions; FRF 700, USD 127 foreign to institutions; FRF 290 domestic to students (effective 2000). adv. *Refereed.* **Document type:** *Academic/Scholarly.*
Published by: Medica-Press International, 62-64 rue Jean-Jaures, Puteaux 92800, France. TEL 33-1-4145800, FAX 33-1-41458025, contact@edimark.fr, http://www.edimark.fr. Ed. Dr. G Megret. Pub. Claudie Damour Terrasson.

M

616.1 USA ISSN 0003-3197
RC691 CODEN: ANGIAB
ANGIOLOGY. Text in English. 1950. m., latest vol.52. USD 189 domestic to individuals; USD 214 foreign to individuals; USD 360 domestic to institutions; USD 385 foreign to institutions (effective 2001). adv. bk.rev. 2 cols./p. back issues avail.; reprints avail. *Refereed.* **Document type:** *Journal, Academic/Scholarly.* **Description:** Contains original papers relating to cerebrovascular, cardiovascular and peripheral vascular diseases.
Related titles: Online - full text ed.: (from Ovid Technologies, Inc., Northern Light Technology, Inc., ProQuest Information & Learning, Institute for Scientific Information).
Indexed: AIDS Abstr., ASCA, Agri.& Environ.Biotech.Abstr. (coverage dropped), Biol.Abstr., Chem.Abstr., Curr.Adv.Ecol.Sci., Curr.Cont., Derwent Biotech.Abstr., Excerp.Med., Helminthol.Abstr., INIS Atomind., Ind.Med. (1950-), Ind.Sci.Rev., Inpharma, Neurosci.Cit.Ind., Nutr.Abstr., Pharm.&Out.News, Reac., Sci.Cit.Ind.
—BLDSC (0902.700000), CASDDS, CISTI, EMDOCS, GNLM, ingenta, KNAW.
Published by: (American College of Angiology), Westminster Publications, Inc., 708 Glen Cove Ave, Glen Head, NY 11545. TEL 516-759-0025, FAX 516-759-5524. Ed. Lawrence Gould, MD. Pub. Timothy R McLaughlin. adv.: B&W page USD 1,050, color page USD 1,035; trim 8.5 x 11. Circ: 6,061.

616.13 FRA ISSN 0003-3928
CODEN: ACAABH
ANNALES DE CARDIOLOGIE ET D'ANGEIOLOGIE. Summaries in English. 1952. 8/yr. EUR 198 in Europe to institutions; USD 247 elsewhere to institutions (effective 2002). adv. bk.rev. abstr, bibl, illus. **Document type:** *Academic/Scholarly.*
Formerly: Actualities Cardiologiques et Angeiologiques Internationales
Related titles: Microform ed.; Online - full text ed.: (from Institute for Scientific Information).
Indexed: ASCA, Biol.Abstr., Chem.Abstr., Curr.Cont. (coverage dropped), Dent.Ind., Excerp.Med., Ind.Med. (1968-), Ind.Sci.Rev., Inpharma, Reac., Ref.Zh., SSCI (coverage dropped), Sci.Cit.Ind. (coverage dropped).
—BLDSC (0969.500000), CASDDS, CISTI, EMDOCS, GNLM, IDS, Infotrieve, KNAW. **CCC.**
Published by: Elsevier Paris, Editions Scientifiques et Medicales (Subsidiary of: Reed Elsevier plc. group), 23 rue Linois, Paris 75015, France. http://www.elsevier.com/locate/ancard. Ed. Pierre Bergeaud. Circ: 3,000. **Subscr. to:** Expansion Scientifique Francaise, 15 rue St. Benoit, Paris Cedex 6 75278, France. TEL 33-1-40626400, FAX 33-1-45556920.

617.41 FRA ISSN 0066-2054
CODEN: ACSSBP
ANNALES DE CHIRURGIE THORACIQUE ET CARDIO-VASCULAIRE. Text in English, French. 1962. 2/yr. adv. bk.rev.
Related titles: ♦ Supplement to: Annales de Chirurgie. ISSN 0003-3944.
Indexed: Biol.Abstr., Curr.Cont. (coverage dropped), Ind.Med. (coverage dropped).
—CISTI, GNLM.
Published by: (Societe de Chirurgie Thoracique de Langue Francaise), Expansion Scientifique, 31 bd. de la Tour Maubourg, Paris 75007, France. TEL 40-62-64-00, FAX 45-55-69-20. Circ: 3,500.

616.1 USA ISSN 1082-720X
CODEN: ANELFF
ANNALS OF NONINVASIVE ELECTROCARDIOLOGY. Text in English. 1996. q. USD 95 domestic; USD 120 foreign; USD 142 to libraries; USD 30 newsstand/cover (effective 2000). adv. back issues avail. *Refereed.* **Document type:** *Trade.* **Description:** Presents advances in the clinical application and technology of noninvasive electrocardiology.
Indexed: CINAHL, INSPEC (Jan.1998-).
—BLDSC (1043.144000), ADONIS, CISTI, GNLM, Infotrieve. **CCC.**
Published by: (International Society for Holter and Noninvasive Electrocardiology, Inc.), Futura Publishing Company, Inc., 135 Bedford Rd, PO Box 418, Armonk, NY 10504-0418. TEL 914-273-1014, FAX 914-273-1016, lisa@futuraco.comuturaco.com. Ed. Dr. Arthur Moss. R&P Joan McLaughlin. Adv. contact Lisa Piedimonte. B&W page USD 800, color page USD 1,735; trim 10.88 x 8.25. Circ: 900 (paid).

ANNALS OF VASCULAR SURGERY; international journal of vascular surgery. see *MEDICAL SCIENCES—Surgery*

ANNUAL OF CARDIAC SURGERY. see *MEDICAL SCIENCES—Abstracting, Bibliographies, Statistics*

616.1 JPN
ANNUAL REVIEW JUNKANKI/ANNUAL REVIEW. CIRCULATORY ORGAN. Text in Japanese. 1988. a. JPY 9,135 (effective 1998). adv. **Document type:** *Academic/Scholarly.*
Published by: Chugai Igakusha, 62 Yarai-cho, Shinjuku-ku, Tokyo 162-0805, Japan. R&P M Takahashi. Adv. contact M. Takahashi.

APPLIED CARDIOPULMONARY PATHOPHYSIOLOGY; the interface between laboratory and clinical practice. see *BIOLOGY—Physiology*

616.1 FRA ISSN 0003-9683
CODEN: AMCVAN
ARCHIVES DES MALADIES DU COEUR ET DES VAISSEAUX. Text in French. 1908. m. FRF 880; FRF 980 foreign (effective 1997). adv. bk.rev. abstr, charts, illus. index. *Refereed.* **Document type:** *Academic/Scholarly.*
Formerly (until 1937): Archives des Maladies du Coeur, des Vaisseaux et du Sang (0301-4525)
Related titles: Microform ed.; Online - full text ed.: (from Institute for Scientific Information).
Indexed: ASCA, Biol.Abstr., C.I.S. Abstr., Chem.Abstr., Curr.Adv.Ecol.Sci., Curr.Cont., Excerp.Med., Helminthol.Abstr., INIS Atomind., Ind.Med. (1937-), Ind.Sci.Rev., Inpharma, Int.Nurs.Ind., Nutr.Abstr., Pharm.&Out.News, Reac., Ref.Zh., SSCI (coverage dropped), Sci.Cit.Ind.
—BLDSC (1637.370000), CISTI, EMDOCS, GNLM, IDS, KNAW. **CCC.**
Published by: Editions J.B. Bailliere, 46 rue la Boetie, Paris Cedex 8 75379, France. TEL 33-1-49536900, FAX 33-1-45631016. Pub. O Fleurot. R&P Arlette Hertig TEL 33-1-49536907. Adv. contact Marika Papageorgiou. Circ: 4,300.

616.1 FRA ISSN 1261-694X
CODEN: AMCVF
ARCHIVES DES MALADIES DU COEUR ET DES VAISSEAUX - PRATIQUE. Text in French. 1995. 20/yr. FRF 300 to students; FRF 400 to doctors; FRF 700 foreign. adv. *Refereed.* **Document type:** *Academic/Scholarly.*
Indexed: Excerp.Med. (1996-), Ref.Zh.
—BLDSC (1637.375000), EMDOCS, GNLM.
Published by: Editions J.B. Bailliere, 46 rue la Boetie, Paris Cedex 8 75379, France. TEL 33-1-49536900, FAX 33-1-45631016. Ed. Dr. Monsuez. Pub. G Brochen. R&P Arlette Hertig TEL 33-1-49536907. Adv. contact Sylvie Kleinhans.

ARCHIVIO DI CHIRURGIA TORACICA E CARDIOVASCOLARE. see *MEDICAL SCIENCES—Surgery*

616.1 MEX ISSN 0020-3785
CODEN: AICMA2
ARCHIVOS DE CARDIOLOGIA DE MEXICO. Text in English, Spanish; Summaries in English, French. 1930. bi-m. MXP 180; USD 75 foreign. adv. bk.rev. charts, illus, stat. index. **Document type:** *Bulletin.*
Related titles: CD-ROM ed.
Indexed: Biol.Abstr., Chem.Abstr., Curr.Adv.Ecol.Sci., Dent.Ind., Excerp.Med., Ind.Med. (1944-), Ref.Zh.
—BLDSC (1654.890500), GNLM, KNAW.
Published by: Instituto Nacional de Cardiologia "Ignacio Chavez"/National Institute of Cardiology "Ignacio Chavez", Oficina de Publicaciones, Juan Badiano No.1, Tlalpan, Mexico City, DF 14080, Mexico. TEL 52-5-5732911 ext. 310, FAX 52-5-5730994, archivos@cardiologia.org.mx, http://www.ssa.gob.mx. Ed. Dr. Eduardo Salazar. Circ: 2,500.

616.12 ITA ISSN 1120-8635
ARGOMENTI DI CARDIOLOGIA. Text in Italian. 1990. 4/yr. ITL 12,000 (effective 1999). **Document type:** *Proceedings.*
Published by: Masson S.p.A., Divisione Periodici, Via F.lli Bressan 2, Milan, MI 20126, Italy. TEL 39-2-270741, FAX 39-2-27074210. Ed. P Pegoraro. adv.: B&W page ITL 4,600,000, color page ITL 6,600,000; trim 265 x 195. Circ: 6,000.

616.1 FRA ISSN 0293-5090
ARTERES ET VEINES. Text in French. 1982. 6/yr. FRF 280 domestic to individuals; FRF 340 foreign to individuals; FRF 180 domestic to students; FRF 300 foreign to students. adv. bk.rev. illus.
—CISTI, GNLM.
Published by: (Arteres et Veines), Publications Medicales, 32-36 av. des Moulins Gemeaux, Saint-Denis Cedex 93207, France. TEL 33-1-49-33-41-08, FAX 33-1-49-33-41-10. Ed. A Castillo Fenoy. Adv. contact A. Castillo Fenoy.

616.136 USA ISSN 1079-5642
RC692 CODEN: ATVBFA
ARTERIOSCLEROSIS, THROMBOSIS, AND VASCULAR BIOLOGY. Text in English. 1981. m. USD 276 domestic to individuals print and online eds.; USD 337 foreign to individuals print and online eds.; USD 475 domestic to institutions print and online eds.; USD 528 foreign to institutions print and online eds. (effective 2002). adv. bk.rev. index. back issues avail. *Refereed.* **Document type:** *Academic/Scholarly.* **Description:** Relates original research and reviews on the biology, prevention, and impact of vascular diseases.
Former titles (until 1994): Arteriosclerosis and Thrombosis (1049-8834); Arteriosclerosis (0276-5047)
Related titles: CD-ROM ed.: (from Ovid Technologies, Inc.); Microform ed.: (from PQC); Online - full text ed.: USD 617.50 domestic academic site license; USD 670.50 foreign academic site license; USD 688.75 domestic corporate site license; USD 741.75 foreign corporate site license (effective 2002) (from HighWire Pr., Ovid Technologies, Inc., EBSCO Publishing, ProQuest Information & Learning, Institute for Scientific Information).
Indexed: ASCA, Biol.Abstr., Chem.Abstr., Chem.Indus.Notes, Chem.Titles, Curr.Adv.Ecol.Sci., Curr.Adv.Gen.& Molec.Biol., Curr.Cont., Dairy Sci.Abstr., Excerp.Med., INIS Atomind., Ind.Med. (1995-), Ind.Sci.Rev., Inpharma, Int.Abstr.Biol.Sci., NRN, Nutr.Abstr., Pharm.&Out.News, Poult.Abstr., Reac., Ref.Zh., Sci.Cit.Ind., Soyabean Abstr., THA.
—BLDSC (1733.670000), CASDDS, CISTI, EMDOCS, GNLM, IDS, ingenta, KNAW.
Published by: (American Heart Association), Lippincott Williams & Wilkins (Baltimore) (Subsidiary of: Wolters Kluwer N.V.), 351 W Camden St, Baltimore, MD 21201-2436. TEL 301-223-2307, 800-787-8984, FAX 301-223-2327, ahaonline@lww.com, http://www.atvb.ahajournals.org. Ed. Dr Donald Heistad. Pub. Cara Kaufman. R&P Debbie Heise TEL 410-528-4050. Adv. contact Angela Hopkins. Circ: 2,900.

616.1 USA ISSN 0098-6127
RC691 CODEN: ARTEDR
ARTERY* ; an international journal for rapid communication of arterial research. Text in English. 1974. 6/yr. adv. bk.rev. illus. *Refereed.* **Document type:** *Academic/Scholarly.*
Related titles: Microfilm ed.: 1974 (from PMC).
Indexed: Biol.Abstr., Chem.Abstr., Chem.Indus.Notes, Chem.Titles, Curr.Adv.Ecol.Sci., Curr.Cont. (coverage dropped), Dairy Sci.Abstr., Excerp.Med., INIS Atomind., Ind.Med. (1974-), Int.Abstr.Biol.Sci., Nutr.Abstr., Sci.Cit.Ind. (coverage dropped).
—BLDSC (1733.703000), CASDDS, CISTI, EMDOCS, GNLM, IDS, ingenta.
Published by: Artery Publishing, 13998 West Ave E, Fulton, MI 49052.

616.1 SGP ISSN 0218-4923
ASIAN CARDIOVASCULAR & THORACIC ANNALS. Text in English. 1993. q. USD 200 (effective 1999). adv. **Document type:** *Academic/Scholarly.* **Description:** Covers Asia-Pacific Rim research and contributions to cardiovascular and thoracic knowledge. Focuses on the Asian patient population and medical facilities.
Related titles: Online - full text ed.: (from HighWire Pr.).
Published by: Springer-Verlag Singapore (Subsidiary of: BertelsmannSpringer), No. 04-01, Cencon I, One Tannery Rd, Singapore 347719, Singapore. TEL 65-84-20-112, FAX 65-84-20-107, springer@cyberway.com.sg, http://asianannals.ctsnetjournals.org/, http://www.springer.com.sg. Ed. Director Sack.

616.1 IDN ISSN 0587-5471
ASIAN PACIFIC CONGRESS OF CARDIOLOGY. SYMPOSIA* . Text in Indonesian. irreg. **Document type:** *Proceedings.*
Indexed: Biol.Abstr.
Published by: Asian-Pacific Society of Cardiology, c/o Cardiac Centre, Jalan Diponegoro 69, Jakarta, Indonesia.

616.1 IRL ISSN 0021-9150
CODEN: ATHSBL
ATHEROSCLEROSIS; international journal for research and investigation on atherosclerosis and related diseases. Text in English. 1961. m. EUR 2,930 in Europe; JPY 389,400 in Japan; USD 3,278 elsewhere (effective 2002). adv. charts, illus. index. back issues avail. *Refereed.* **Document type:** *Academic/Scholarly.* **Description:** Brings together research and clinical papers related to the focal accumulation of collagen, lipids, complex carbohydrates, blood and blood products, fibrous tissue and calcium deposits in the intima of arteries, its medical complications, related phenomena and diseases.

M

Formerly (until 1970): Journal of Atherosclerosis Research
Related titles: Online - full text ed.: (from ingenta, Swets Blackwell, ScienceDirect, Institute for Scientific Information).
Indexed: ASCA, Biol.Abstr., Chem.Abstr., Chem.Indus.Notes, Chem.Titles, Curr.Adv.Biochem., Curr.Cont., Dairy Sci.Abstr., Derwent Biotech.Abstr., Environ.Sci.Poll.Mgmt., Excerp.Med., INIS Atomind., Ind.Med. (1970-), Ind.Sci.Rev., Inpharma, Int.Abstr.Biol.Sci., Mass Spectr.Bull., NRN, Pharm.&Out.News, Pollut.Abstr., Poult.Abstr., Reac., Ref.Zh., Rice Abstr., Russ.Acad.Sci.Bibl., Sci.Cit.Ind., Sugar Ind.Abstr., THA, Vet.Bull.
—BLDSC (1765.874000), ADONIS, CASDDS, CISTI, EMDOCS, GNLM, IDS, ingenta, KNAW. **CCC.**
Published by: (International Atherosclerosis Society), Elsevier Science Ireland Ltd, Elsevier House, Brookvale Plaza, E. Park, Shannon, Co. Clare, Ireland. TEL 353-61-709600, FAX 353-61-709100, http://www.elsevier.com/locate/atherosclerosis. Eds. E J Schaefer, J Shepherd. R&P Annette Moloney. **Subscr. in Australasia and the Far East to:** Elsevier Science (Singapore) Pte Ltd, No.1 Temasek Ave, 17-01 Millenia Tower, Singapore 039192, Singapore. TEL 65-434-3727, FAX 65-337-2230, asiainfo@elsevier.com.sg; **Subscr. in the Americas to:** Elsevier Science, PO Box 945, New York, NY 10159-0945. TEL 212-633-3730, FAX 212-633-3680, usinfo-f@elsevier.com; **Subscr. to:** Elsevier Science Inc - Japan Regional Office, 9-15 Higashi-Azabu 1-chome, Minato-ku, Tokyo 106-0044, Japan. TEL 81-3-5561-5033, FAX 81-3-5561-5047, info@elsevier.co.jp. **Subscr. to:** Elsevier Science BV, PO Box 211, Amsterdam 1000 AE, Netherlands.; **Dist. by:** Elsevier Science (Brazil).

616.136 USA ISSN 0362-1650
RC692 CODEN: ATHEDF
ATHEROSCLEROSIS REVIEWS. Text in English. 1975. irreg. price varies. reprint service avail. from PQC. *Refereed.* **Document type:** *Monographic series.*
Indexed: Biol.Abstr., Chem.Abstr., Curr.Cont. (coverage dropped), Ind.Sci.Rev., Sci.Cit.Ind. (coverage dropped).
—CASDDS, CISTI, GNLM, ingenta, KNAW.
Published by: Lippincott Williams & Wilkins (Philadelphia) (Subsidiary of: Wolters Kluwer N.V.), 530 Walnut St, Philadelphia, PA 19106-3621. TEL 301-223-2300, 800-638-3030, FAX 301-223-2400.

AUSTRALIA. BUREAU OF STATISTICS. NATIONAL HEALTH SURVEY: CARDIOVASCULAR AND RELATED CONDITIONS, AUSTRALIA. see *MEDICAL SCIENCES—Abstracting, Bibliographies, Statistics*

616.1 USA
BASIC AND CLINICAL CARDIOLOGY SERIES. Text in English. 1981. irreg., latest vol.11, 1988. price varies. adv. *Refereed.*
Published by: Marcel Dekker, Inc., Attn: Eridania Perrez, 270 Madison Ave, New York, NY 10016-0602. TEL 212-696-9000, 800-228-1160, FAX 212-685-4540, marketing@dekker.com, http://www.dekker.com. Pub. Russell Dekker. R&P Julia Mulligan. Adv. contact Eridania Perez.

616.1 DEU ISSN 0300-8428
RC633.A1 CODEN: BRCAB7
BASIC RESEARCH IN CARDIOLOGY. Text in English. 1938. bi-m. EUR 935.50 domestic; EUR 930.40 in Germany; EUR 184 newsstand/cover foreign (effective 2002). adv. charts, illus, pat. index. back issues avail.; reprints avail. *Refereed.* **Document type:** *Journal, Academic/Scholarly.* **Description:** Publishes original reports and review articles providing progress in basic research on the cardiovascular system in health and disease, and originating from various disciplines, such as molecular and cell biology.
Related titles: Microform ed.: (from PQC); Online - full text ed.: ISSN 1435-1803 (from EBSCO Publishing, RoweCom Information Quest, Swets Blackwell, Springer LINK, Institute for Scientific Information); ♦ Supplement: Basic Research in Cardiology. Supplement. ISSN 1433-0946.
Indexed: ASCA, Biol.Abstr., Chem.Abstr., Chem.Indus.Notes, Chem.Titles, Curr.Adv.Ecol.Sci., Curr.Cont., Curr.Ind.Stat., Excerp.Med., INIS Atomind., Ind.Med. (1973-), Ind.Sci.Rev., Inpharma, Int.Abstr.Biol.Sci., NRN, Nutr.Abstr., Pharm.&Out.News, Reac., Sci.Cit.Ind.
—BLDSC (1864.080000), CASDDS, CISTI, EMDOCS, GNLM, IDS, ingenta, KNAW. **CCC.**
Published by: (German Cardiac Society), Dr. Dietrich Steinkopff Verlag (Subsidiary of: BertelsmannSpringer), Platz der deutschen Einheit 25, Darmstadt 64293, Germany. TEL 49-6151-82899-0, FAX 49-6151-82899-40, frey.steinkopff@springer.de, http://www.steinkopff.springer.de. Ed. Gerd Heusch. Pub. Dietrich Steinkopff. R&P Sabine Ibkendanz. Circ: 2,000. **Subscr. in Austria to:** Springer-Verlag Wien, Sachsenplatz 4-6, PO Box 89, Vienna, W 1201, Austria; **Subscr. to:** Springer-Verlag, Journals; Eastern Book Service, Inc., 3-13 Hongo 3-chome, Bunkyo-ku, Tokyo 113-8480, Japan.

616.1 DEU ISSN 1433-0946
BASIC RESEARCH IN CARDIOLOGY. SUPPLEMENT. Text in English. 1996. irreg.
Related titles: ♦ Supplement to: Basic Research in Cardiology. ISSN 0300-8428.
Indexed: Int.Abstr.Biol.Sci.
Published by: Dr. Dietrich Steinkopff Verlag (Subsidiary of: BertelsmannSpringer), Platz der deutschen Einheit 25, Darmstadt 64293, Germany. TEL 49-6151-82899-0, FAX 49-6151-82899-40. Ed. H D Esperer H Klein.

BLOOD COAGULATION FACTORS; current awareness service for researchers in life sciences. see *MEDICAL SCIENCES—Abstracting, Bibliographies, Statistics*

616.1 NOR ISSN 0803-7051
CODEN: BLPREG
BLOOD PRESSURE; for the advancement of hypertension research. Text in English. 1991. 6/yr. GBP 97, USD 160 to individuals; GBP 167, USD 275 to institutions (effective 2002). adv. **Document type:** *Academic/Scholarly.* **Description:** Covers essential research from basic science to clinical discipline related to blood pressure research, including the physiology and pathophysiology of cerebrocardiovascular diseases, and renal hypertensive diseases.
Related titles: Online - full text ed.: (from EBSCO Publishing, O C L C Online Computer Library Center, Inc., RoweCom Information Quest, CatchWord Ltd., ingenta, Swets Blackwell, Institute for Scientific Information); ♦ Supplement: Blood Pressure. Supplement. ISSN 0803-8023.
Indexed: Chem.Abstr., Chem.Indus.Notes, Chem.Titles, Curr.Cont., Excerp.Med. (1993-), Ind.Med. (1992-), Inpharma, Pharm.&Out.News, Reac., Sci.Cit.Ind.
—BLDSC (2113.034000), CASDDS, CISTI, EMDOCS, GNLM, Infotrieve, KNAW. **CCC.**
Published by: (Scandinavian Foundation for Cardiovascular Research), Taylor & Francis AS (Subsidiary of: Taylor & Francis Group), Cort Adelersgt. 17, Solli, PO Box 2562, Oslo 0202, Norway. TEL 47-22-12-98-80, FAX 47-22-12-98-90, journals@tandf.no, http://www.tandf.co.uk/tfas. Ed. Lennart Hansson.

616.1 USA ISSN 1359-5237
CODEN: BPMOFL
BLOOD PRESSURE MONITORING. Text in English. 1996. bi-m. USD 230 domestic to individuals; USD 230 foreign to individuals; USD 694 per issue domestic to institutions; USD 694 per issue foreign to institutions; USD 106 newsstand/cover (effective 2002). adv. bk.rev. index. back issues avail. *Refereed.* **Document type:** *Academic/Scholarly.*
Related titles: Online - full text ed.: USD 902.20 domestic academic site license; USD 902.20 foreign academic site license; USD 1,006.30 domestic corporate site license; USD 1,006.30 foreign corporate site license (effective 2002) (from Ovid Technologies, Inc., EBSCO Publishing, Institute for Scientific Information).
Indexed: Curr.Cont., Ind.Med. (1996-).
—BLDSC (2113.035500), ADONIS, GNLM, Infotrieve, KNAW.
Published by: Lippincott Williams & Wilkins (Philadelphia) (Subsidiary of: Wolters Kluwer N.V.), 530 Walnut St, Philadelphia, PA 19106-3621. TEL 215-521-8300, FAX 215-521-8902, http://www.Lww.com. Ed. Dr. William E White. Adv. contact Gemma Heiser. B&W page USD 675, color page USD 1,675; trim 11 x 8.5. Circ: 1,632. **Subscr. to:** PO Box 1600, Hagerstown, MD 21740-1600. TEL 800-777-2295, FAX 301-824-7390.

616.1 NOR ISSN 0803-8023
CODEN: BPSUEY
BLOOD PRESSURE. SUPPLEMENT. Text in English. 1991. irreg. **Document type:** *Academic/Scholarly.*
Related titles: Online - full text ed.; ♦ Supplement to: Blood Pressure. ISSN 0803-7051.
Indexed: Excerp.Med. (1994-), Ind.Med. (1992-).
—BLDSC (2113.034100), CASDDS, CISTI, EMDOCS, Infotrieve, KNAW. **CCC.**
Published by: (Scandinavian Foundation for Cardiovascular Research), Scandinavian University Press (Subsidiary of: Taylor & Francis Ltd.), Postboks 2959, Toeyen, Oslo 0608, Norway. FAX 47-22-57-53-53, journals@scup.no, http://www.scup.no/bp.

616.1 GBR ISSN 0969-6113
CODEN: BJCAEM
THE BRITISH JOURNAL OF CARDIOLOGY. Text in English. 1993. m. GBP 60 in Europe to individuals; GBP 95 elsewhere to individuals; GBP 90 in Europe to institutions; GBP 130 elsewhere to institutions (effective 2002). adv. bk.rev. **Document type:** *Academic/Scholarly.* **Description:** Provides reviews and discussions of current developments in cardiology and other relevant specialities to cardiologists and general practitioners with a stated interest in this field.
Indexed: Excerp.Med. (1995-).
—BLDSC (2307.010000), CISTI, GNLM.
Published by: MediNews (Cardiology) Ltd. (Subsidiary of: J R A A S Ltd), Edgbaston House, 3 Duchess Pl, Birmingham B16 8NH, United Kingdom. TEL 44-121-454-4114, FAX 44-121-454-1190, ngibbs@sherbornegibbs@co.uk, ngibbs@sherbornegibbs.co.uk. Ed. Dr. Henry Purcell. Pub. Michael Gibbs. R&P Nina Gibbs TEL 44-121-456-1466. Adv. contact Michael Young. Circ: 20,000 (paid).

C A SELECTS. ANTIARRHYTHMICS. see *MEDICAL SCIENCES—Abstracting, Bibliographies, Statistics*

616.132 USA ISSN 1051-3922
CODEN: CAHAET
C A SELECTS. HYPERTENSION & ANTIHYPERTENSIVES. Text in English. 1990. s-w. USD 275 (effective 2001). **Document type:** *Abstract/Index.* **Description:** Covers etiology, pathophysiology, clinical manifestations, and diagnosis of hypertension.
Published by: Chemical Abstracts Service (Subsidiary of: American Chemical Society), 2540 Olentangy River Rd, Box 3012, Columbus, OH 43210-0012. TEL 614-447-3600, 800-753-4227, FAX 614-447-3751.

616.1 ITA ISSN 1120-0421
CODEN: CARMED
C I - CARDIOVASCULAR IMAGING. Text in Italian. 1989. q. USD 110. adv. bk.rev. **Document type:** *Academic/Scholarly.*
Indexed: Excerp.Med. (1993-).
—EMDOCS, GNLM, KNAW.
Published by: C E P I - Centro Editoriale Pubblicitario Italiano s.r.l., Via Nicolo' Tartaglia, 3, Rome, RM 00197, Italy. TEL 39-6-8082101, FAX 39-6-8072458. Ed. Armando Dagianti. Adv. contact Marina Buongiorno.

616.1 USA
C P DIGEST*. (Cardiovascular Pulmonary) Text in English. bi-m. USD 35. adv.
Published by: American Society of Cardiovascular Professionals - Society for Cardiovascular Management, 910 Charles St, Ste A, Fredericksburg, VA 22401-5810. TEL 703-891-0079, FAX 703-898-2393. Ed. Peggy McElgunn. Circ: 3,000.

616.1 USA ISSN 1095-4155
C V D PREVENTION. (Cardiovascular Disease) Text in English. 1998. q. *Refereed.* **Document type:** *Journal, Academic/Scholarly.* **Description:** Designed to support the prevention of heart and vascular diseases and stroke throughout the world by global communication of relevant research findings.
Related titles: Supplement:.
Published by: (World Heart Prevention CHE), Futura Publishing Company, Inc., 135 Bedford Rd, PO Box 418, Armonk, NY 10504-0418. TEL 914-273-1014, FAX 914-273-1016, 800-877-8761, jrlinfo@futuraco.com, http://www.futuraco.com/cvd.htm. Ed. Darwin R Labarthe.

616.1 CAN ISSN 0828-282X
CODEN: CJCAEX
CANADIAN JOURNAL OF CARDIOLOGY. Text in English. 1985. m. CND 235 domestic; CND 290 foreign (effective 2000). adv. bk.rev. abstr, bibl, charts, illus. index. back issues avail. *Refereed.* **Document type:** *Trade.* **Description:** Original studies in the area of cardiovascular medicine.
Related titles: Online - full text ed.: (from Institute for Scientific Information).
Indexed: ASCA, Biol.Abstr., Chem.Abstr., Chem.Indus.Notes, Chem.Titles, Curr.Cont., Excerp.Med., Ind.Med. (1985-), Inpharma, NRN, Nutr.Abstr., Pharm.&Out.News, Reac., Sci.Cit.Ind.
—BLDSC (3030.500000), CASDDS, CISTI, EMDOCS, GNLM, IDS, ingenta, KNAW. **CCC.**

M

Published by: (Canadian Cardiovascular Society), Pulsus Group Inc., 2902 S Sheridan Way, Oakville, ON L6J 7L6, Canada. TEL 905-829-4770, FAX 905-829-4799, pulsus@pulsus.com, http://www.pulsus.com. Ed. Dr. E R Smith. Circ: 15,500 (controlled).

CANADIAN JOURNAL OF CARDIOVASCULAR NURSING. see *MEDICAL SCIENCES—Nurses And Nursing*

CARDIAC ALERT. see *PHYSICAL FITNESS AND HYGIENE*

616.1 USA ISSN 1527-7917
▼ **CARDIAC AND VASCULAR REGENERATION**; angiogenesis & myogenesis from basic to therapeutic. Text in English. 2000. q. USD 120 (effective 2001).
—ADONIS.
Published by: Futura Publishing Company, Inc., 135 Bedford Rd, PO Box 418, Armonk, NY 10504-0418. TEL 914-273-1014, FAX 914-273-1016, 800-877-8761, jrlinfo@futuraco.com, http://www.futuraco.com/. Ed. Ray C.-J. Chiu.

616.1 USA ISSN 1385-2264
CODEN: CELRFR
CARDIAC ELECTROPHYSIOLOGY REVIEW. Text in English. 1997. q. USD 120, EUR 120 to individuals for print or online ed.; USD 397, EUR 396 to institutions for print or online ed.; USD 476.40, EUR 475.20 to institutions for print & online eds. combined (effective 2002). adv. **Document type:** *Journal, Academic/Scholarly.* **Description:** Provides information for clinicians who care for patients with arrhythmias and arrhythmia-related disorders.
Related titles: Online - full text ed.: (from EBSCO Publishing, O C L C Online Computer Library Center, Inc., RoweCom Information Quest, Swets Blackwell, Kluwer Online).
—BLDSC (3051.087250), CISTI. **CCC.**
Published by: Kluwer Academic Publishers Boston, 101 Philip Dr, Assinippi Park, Norwell, MA 02061. TEL 781-871-6600, FAX 781-871-9045, services@wkap.nl, http://www.wkap.nl/journalhome.htm/1385-2264. Ed. Kelley P Anderson. R&P Rose Luongo TEL 781-871-6311. **Subscr. outside N America to:** Kluwer Academic Publishers Group, Journals Department, PO Box 322, Dordrecht 3300 AH, Netherlands. TEL 31-78-639-2392, FAX 31-78-654-6474; **Subscr. to:** Kluwer Academic - Plenum Publishers, 233 Spring St, New York, NY 10013-1578. TEL 212-620-8468, FAX 212-807-1047.

616.1 JPN ISSN 0915-874X
CARDIAC PRACTICE. Text in Japanese. 1990. 4/yr. JPY 2,400 (effective 1998).
Published by: Medikaru Rebyusha/Medical Review Co., Ltd., 7-3 Hirano-Machi 1-chome, Chuo-ku, Osaka-shi 541-0046, Japan. TEL 81-6-223-1556, FAX 81-6-223-1414, medrev@osk2.3web.ne.jp.

CARDIAC SURGERY. see *MEDICAL SCIENCES—Surgery*

616.1 USA
CARDIO INTERVENTION. Text in English. 1991. q. **Document type:** *Academic/Scholarly.* **Description:** Covers the field of interventional cardiology: angioplasty, angiography, and other therapeutic and diagnostic lab procedures.
Published by: Miller Freeman, Inc. (Subsidiary of: United Newspapers), 600 Harrison St, San Francisco, CA 94107. TEL 415-905-2200, FAX 415-905-2235. Ed. Steve Stiles. adv.: B&W page USD 2,450, color page USD 3,770; trim 10.88 x 8.13. Circ: 10,000.

616.1 DEU ISSN 1437-1073
CARDIO NEWS. Text in German. 1995. m. DEM 156, USD 208; USD 19.40 newsstand/cover (effective 2001). **Document type:** *Journal, Academic/Scholarly.*
Formerly (until 1998): Cardiovascularia (1430-838X)
Published by: Urban und Vogel Medien und Medizin Verlagsgesellschaft mbH (Subsidiary of: BertelsmannSpringer), Neumarkter Str 43, Munich 81673, Germany. TEL 49-89-43721411, FAX 49-89-43721410, niemann@urban-vogel.de, http://www.urban-vogel.de. Ed. Dr. Jochen Aumiller. Circ: 20,000 (controlled). **Subscr. to:** Springer Auslieferungs Gesellschaft, Postfach 105160, Heidelberg 69041, Germany. TEL 49-6221-345244, FAX 49-6221-345244.

616.1 GBR ISSN 1368-731X
CARDIO-VASCULAR CLINICAL TRIALS. Text in English. 1997. q. USD 270 in North America to individuals; GBP 170 elsewhere to individuals; USD 520 in North America to institutions; GBP 300 elsewhere to institutions. **Document type:** *Academic/Scholarly.*
Published by: Current Science Ltd, Middlesex House, 34-42 Cleveland St, London W1P 6LB, United Kingdom. FAX 44-20-7636-6911. **Dist. by:** Turpin Distribution Services Ltd., Blackhorse Rd, Letchworth, Herts SG6 1HN, United Kingdom. FAX 44-1462-480947.

616.12 ITA ISSN 0945-8298
LA CARDIOLOGIA NELLA PRATICA CLINICA. Text in Italian. 1994. q. ITL 168,000 (effective 1999). *Refereed.* **Document type:** *Academic/Scholarly.* **Description:** Bridges the gap between research and clinical developments in cardiology.
—BLDSC (3051.351000), GNLM.
Published by: Springer-Verlag Italia Srl (Subsidiary of: BertelsmannSpringer), Via Podgora, 4, Milan, MI 20122, Italy. TEL 39-2-55194656, FAX 39-2-55193360, springer@springer.it. Ed. E Ambrosioni.

616.12 NLD ISSN 0929-7456
CARDIOLOGIE. Text in Dutch, English. 1994. 11/yr. NLG 182; USD 111 foreign. adv. **Document type:** *Academic/Scholarly.* **Description:** Publishes articles of interest to cardiologists and specialists in related fields.
Formed by the merger of (1987-1994): Nederlands Tijdschrift voor Cardiologie (0921-4674); (1988-1994): Netherlands Journal of Cardiology (0921-5018)
—KNAW.
Published by: (Nederlandse Vereniging voor Cardiologie), Mediselect B.V., Postbus 63, Leusden 3830 AB, Netherlands. TEL 31-33-4229900, FAX 31-33-4229922, info@mediselect.nl. Ed. E E van der Wall. **Co-sponsor:** Nederlandse Hartstichting.

616.12 FRA ISSN 0983-4532
CARDIOLOGIE. Text in French. 1987. 6/yr. FRF 230. adv. bk.rev.
—GNLM.
Published by: Maloine Editeur, 27 rue de l'Ecole de Medecine, Paris 75006, France. Ed. N Gofstein. **Subscr. to:** Publicite Batard, 38 rue Pascal, Paris 75013, France.

616.1 FRA ISSN 0766-3633
CARDIOLOGIE PRATIQUE. Text in French. 1985. w. (40/yr.). EUR 54 domestic to individuals; EUR 84 foreign to individuals; EUR 38 domestic to libraries; EUR 68 foreign to libraries (effective 2002). **Document type:** *Newspaper.*
Related titles: ♦ Supplement: Cardiologie Pratique. Supplement. ISSN 1240-3318.
Published by: L E N Medical, 15 rue des Sablons, Paris 75116, France. TEL 33-1-47553131, FAX 33-1-47553132, lenmed@club-internet.fr, http://www.webmedguide.com. Ed. Dr. J Chapsal.

616.1 FRA ISSN 1240-3318
CARDIOLOGIE PRATIQUE. SUPPLEMENT. Text in French. 1987. irreg. back issues avail.
Related titles: ♦ Supplement to: Cardiologie Pratique. ISSN 0766-3633.
Published by: L E N Medical, 15 rue des Sablons, Paris 75116, France. TEL 33-1-47550606, FAX 33-1-47553132, http://www.webmedguide.com.

616.12 FRA ISSN 0769-0819
LE CARDIOLOGUE. Text in French. 1965. m., latest vol.25, 2002 (10/yr.). EUR 35; EUR 53 foreign (effective 2002). back issues avail.
Published by: P D G Communication, 30 rue d'Armaille, Paris 75017, France. TEL 33-1-40550595, FAX 33-1-45746567.

616.1 CHE ISSN 0008-6312
RC681.A1 CODEN: CAGYAO
CARDIOLOGY; international journal of cardiovascular medicine, surgery and pathology. Text in English. 1937. 8/yr. (2 vols.). CHF 1,534 in Europe to institutions; CHF 1,557.20 overseas to institutions; EUR 1,096.40 in Europe to institutions; USD 1,192 overseas to institutions (effective 2002). adv. bk.rev. charts, illus. index. back issues avail. *Refereed.* **Document type:** *Journal, Academic/Scholarly.* **Description:** Features papers from all over the world to keep its readers regularly informed of current strategies in the prevention, diagnosis and treatment of heart disease.
Formerly: Cardiologia
Related titles: Microfilm ed.: (from PMC); Online - full text ed.: CHF 116, EUR 84, USD 90 to institutions with print edition (effective 2002) (from EBSCO Publishing, O C L C Online Computer Library Center, Inc., RoweCom Information Quest, Swets Blackwell, Institute for Scientific Information).
Indexed: Agri.& Environ.Biotech.Abstr. (coverage dropped), Biol.Abstr., Chem.Abstr., Chem.Indus.Notes, Chem.Titles, Curr.Adv.Ecol.Sci., Curr.Cont., Derwent Biotech.Abstr., Excerp.Med., Helminthol.Abstr., Ind.Med. (1970-), Ind.Sci.Rev., Nutr.Abstr., Protozool.Abstr., Sci.Cit.Ind.
—BLDSC (3051.410000), CASDDS, CISTI, EMDOCS, GNLM, IDS, ingenta, KNAW. **CCC.**
Published by: S. Karger AG, Allschwilerstr 10, PO Box, Basel 4009, Switzerland. TEL 41-61-306-1111, FAX 41-61-306-1234, karger@karger.ch, http://www.online.karger.com/journals/crd, http://www.karger.com. Ed. J S Alpert. adv.: page USD 1,185. Circ: 1,300.

616.1 USA
CARDIOLOGY (BETHESDA). Text in English. 1972. m. USD 59 (effective 2001). adv. charts. back issues avail.; reprints avail. **Document type:** *Newsletter.* **Description:** Describes the activities, services and products of the American College of Cardiology and provides information of interest to those involved in the practice of cardiovascular medicine.
Indexed: Inpharma, Pharm.&Out.News, Protozool.Abstr., Reac.
Published by: (Communications Department), American College of Cardiology, 9111 Old Georgetown Rd, Bethesda, MD 20814-1699. TEL 301-897-5400, FAX 301-897-9745, http://www.acc.org. Eds. Kathy Boyd, Melanie Caudron. R&P Kathy Boyd. Circ: 27,000.

616.12 USA ISSN 0733-8651
RC681.A1 CODEN: CACLE3
CARDIOLOGY CLINICS. Text in English. 1983. q. USD 139 domestic to individuals; USD 172 in Canada to individuals; USD 199 elsewhere to individuals; USD 198 domestic to institutions; USD 241 elsewhere to institutions; USD 127 domestic to students; USD 172 in Canada to students; USD 199 elsewhere to students; USD 61 per issue (effective 2001). **Document type:** *Journal, Academic/Scholarly.* **Description:** Each issue discusses an aspect of heart disease in detail.
Related titles: Microform ed.: (from PQC); Online - full text ed.
Indexed: CINAHL, Curr.Adv.Ecol.Sci., Excerp.Med., INIS Atomind., Ind.Med. (1983-), Inpharma, Pharm.&Out.News, Reac.
—BLDSC (3051.417000), EMDOCS, GNLM, IDS, ingenta, KNAW. **CCC.**
Published by: W.B. Saunders Co. (Subsidiary of: Harcourt Publishers Ltd.), 11830 Westline Industrial Dr, St Louis, MO 63146. TEL 800-325-4177, http://www.wbsaunders.com. Ed. Dr. Michael H Crawford. **Subscr. to:** Periodicals Fulfillment, W B Saunders Co, 6277 Sea Harbor Dr, 4th Fl, Orlando, FL 32891-4800.

616.12 USA ISSN 1089-408X
RM345
CARDIOLOGY CLINICS: ANNUAL OF DRUG THERAPY. Variant title: Annual of Drug Therapy. Text in English. 1997. a. USD 59 domestic; USD 65 foreign (effective 2000). **Description:** Tracks the progress that has been made in pharmaceutical therapy of cardiovascular diseases.
—GNLM.
Published by: W.B. Saunders Co. (Subsidiary of: Harcourt Publishers Ltd.), 11830 Westline Industrial Dr, St Louis, MO 63146. TEL 800-325-4177, http://www.wbsaunders.com. Ed. Dr. Michael H Crawford. **Subscr. to:** Periodicals Fulfillment, W B Saunders Co, 6277 Sea Harbor Dr, 4th Fl, Orlando, FL 32891-4800.

616.12 USA ISSN 1067-9332
CARDIOLOGY HEALTH MONITOR. Text in English. 1993. m. **Document type:** *Newsletter, Consumer.*
Published by: Data Centrum Communications, Inc., 21 W 38th St, 4th fl, New York, NY 10018.

616.12 CAN ISSN 0844-5575
CARDIOLOGY IN PRACTICE. Text in English. 1989. m. USD 48. adv.
Published by: M P I Medical Publishing Inc., 14 Ronan Ave, Toronto, ON M4N 2X9, Canada. TEL 416-481-6384. Ed. Dr. Harry Rakowski. Circ: 22,028.

M

616.12 USA ISSN 1061-5377
CODEN: CRVIE4
CARDIOLOGY IN REVIEW. Text in English. 1993. bi-m. USD 176 domestic to individuals; USD 218 foreign to individuals; USD 292 domestic to institutions; USD 345 foreign to institutions; USD 52 newsstand/cover (effective 2002). adv. **Document type:** *Academic/Scholarly.* **Description:** Covers the pathogenesis, diagnosis, clinical course, prevention and treatment of cardiovascular disorders.
Related titles: Microfilm ed.: (from WWS); Online - full text ed.: USD 379.60 domestic academic site license; USD 432.60 foreign academic site license; USD 423.40 domestic corporate site license; USD 476.40 foreign corporate site license (2002).
Indexed: Excerp.Med. (1995-), Ind.Med. (1993-).
—BLDSC (3051.433800), CISTI, GNLM, KNAW.
Published by: Williams & Wilkins (Subsidiary of: Waverly International), 351 W Camden St, Baltimore, MD 21201-2436. TEL 410-528-4068, 800-222-3790, FAX 410-528-4452, arossman@wwilkins.com, http://www.wwilkins.com, http://www.Lww.com. Ed. Dr. Douglas P Zipes. Adv. contact Aliza Rossman. B&W page USD 700; trim 8.125 x 10.875. Circ: 2,329; 2,168 (paid).

616.12 GBR ISSN 1047-9511
CARDIOLOGY IN THE YOUNG. Text in English. 1990. q. GBP 137, USD 215. adv. bk.rev. *Refereed.* **Document type:** *Academic/Scholarly.* **Description:** Devoted to cardiovascular issues affecting the young and older patient with sequels of heart disease acquired by childhood. Serves the interest of all professionals concerned with these topics.
Related titles: Online - full text ed.: (from CatchWord Ltd., Institute for Scientific Information).
Indexed: Curr.Cont., Ind.Med. (1991-), Inpharma, Pharm.&Out.News, Reac.
—BLDSC (3051.436300), GNLM, IDS, KNAW.
Published by: Greenwich Medical Media, 219 Linen Hall, Greenwich Medical Media Ltd, Flat 162, 162-168 Regent St, London W1R 5TB, United Kingdom. TEL 44-207-494-1515, FAX 44-207-494-1616, gm@greenwich-medical.co.uk. Ed. Robert H Anderson. Pub., Adv. contact Gavin Jamieson. R&P Justine Santer.

616.12 GBR ISSN 1368-8979
CARDIOLOGY NEWS. Text in English. 1997. bi-m. GBP 25 (effective 2000). adv. software rev. abstr, illus, tr.lit. **Document type:** *Academic/Scholarly.*
Address: Pinpoint Scotland, 9 Gayfield St, Edinburgh EH1 3NR, United Kingdom. TEL 44-131-557-4184, FAX 44-131-557-4701, rachael@pinpoint-scotland.com. Ed. Jim McLenachan. Pub. Cedric Chater. R&P, Adv. contact Rachael Hansford TEL 44-131-478-8403. Circ: 6,300 (controlled).

CARDIOLOGY PRACTICE ADVISOR. see *HEALTH FACILITIES AND ADMINISTRATION*

616.12 USA ISSN 1092-6607
CARDIOLOGY REVIEW. Text in English. 1984. m. USD 86 domestic; USD 90 foreign; free to qualified personnel (effective 2000). adv. bk.rev. bibl, charts, illus. index. back issues avail. *Refereed.* **Document type:** *Magazine, Trade.* **Description:** Designed to help the busy cardiologist and internist keep up with the latest developments in the field of cardiovascular medicine.
Formerly: Cardiology Board Review (0888-8418)
Indexed: Excerp.Med.
—BLDSC (3051.433850), EMDOCS, GNLM, KNAW.
Published by: M R A Publications, Inc. (Subsidiary of: Medical World Communications), 241 Forsgate Dr, Jamesburg, NJ 08831. TEL 732-656-1140, FAX 732-656-0059. Ed. Dr. Peter F Cohn. Pub. David Dempsey. Adv. contact Lisa Greene. B&W page USD 2,845, color page USD 4,640; trim 10.75 x 7.88. Circ: 68,400.

616.1 USA
CARDIOLOGY SPECIAL EDITION. Text in English. 1995. s-a. USD 50 domestic; USD 60 foreign (effective 2001). adv. **Description:** Publishes a clinical reference that takes an in-depth look at various disease states appropriate to the practice of cardiology.
Published by: McMahon Group, 545 W 45th St, 8th Fl, New York, NY 10036. TEL 212-957-5300, FAX 212-957-7230, lrichards@mcmahonmed.com, http://www.mcmahonmed.cohttp:// www.mcmahonmed.com/se/indexse.htm. adv.: B&W page USD 4,450, color page USD 1,900.

616.1 USA
CARDIOLOGY TODAY. Text in English. m. USD 170 domestic to individuals; USD 195 in Canada to individuals; USD 210 elsewhere to individuals; USD 180 domestic to institutions; USD 205 in Canada to institutions; USD 220 elsewhere to institutions. **Document type:** *Academic/Scholarly.*
Published by: Slack, Inc., 6900 Grove Rd, Thorofare, NJ 08086-9447. TEL 856-848-1000, 800-257-8290, FAX 856-853-5991, http://www.slackinc.com.

616.1 USA ISSN 0163-1675
RC681.A1
CARDIOLOGY UPDATE; reviews for physicians. Text in English. 1979. irreg., latest 1990. price varies. *Refereed.* **Document type:** *Academic/Scholarly.*
—CISTI, GNLM.
Published by: Elsevier Science, PO Box 945, New York, NY 10159-0945. TEL 212-989-5800, FAX 212-633-3990. Ed. E Rapaport. **Subscr. in Australasia and the Far East to:** Elsevier Science (Singapore) Pte Ltd, No.1 Temasek Ave, 17-01 Millenia Tower, Singapore 039192, Singapore. TEL 65-434-3727, FAX 65-337-2230; **Subscr. in Japan to:** Elsevier Science Inc - Japan Regional Office, 9-15 Higashi-Azabu 1-chome, Minato-ku, Tokyo 106-0044, Japan. TEL 81-3-5561-5033; **Subscr. outside the Americas to:** Elsevier Science BV, PO Box 211, Amsterdam 1000 AE, Netherlands. TEL 31-20-485-3757, nlinfo-f@elsevier.nl, http://www.elsevier.nl.

616.12 DEU ISSN 1617-4933
▼ **CARDIOVASC.** Text in German. 2001. bi-m. EUR 51.99 domestic; EUR 62.99 foreign; EUR 42.64 domestic to students; EUR 53.64 foreign to students; EUR 10.28 newsstand/cover (effective 2002). adv. *Refereed.* **Document type:** *Journal, Academic/Scholarly.*
Published by: Urban und Vogel Medien und Medizin Verlagsgesellschaft mbH (Subsidiary of: BertelsmannSpringer), Neumarkter Str 43, Munich 81673, Germany. TEL 49-89-43721411, FAX 49-89-43721410, http://www.cardiovasc.de, http://www.urban-vogel.de. Ed. Dr. Dirk Einecke. Adv. contact Christiane Loichinger. B&W page DEM 4,600, color page DEM 7,400. Circ: 20,000 (controlled).

616.1 ESP ISSN 1133-6846
CARDIOVASCULAR* ; actualidad internacional en enfermedades del cardiacas. Text in Spanish. 1980. m. (13/yr.). ESP 4,820, USD 48.
Formerly (until 1993): Cardiovascular Reviews and Reports (Edicion Espanola) (0211-6553)
Published by: Haymarket, S.A., Travesera Gracia 17-21, 5o 2o, Barcelona 08022, Spain. TEL 3-237-22-66, FAX 3-237-66-88. Ed. Dr. F B Ferrer Ruscalleda. Circ: 10,000.

CARDIOVASCULAR AND INTERVENTIONAL RADIOLOGY. see *MEDICAL SCIENCES—Radiology And Nuclear Medicine*

616.1 USA ISSN 1084-3930
CARDIOVASCULAR DEVICE UPDATE. Text in English. 1995. m. USD 497 domestic; USD 527 foreign; USD 83 newsstand/cover (effective 2001). **Document type:** *Newsletter.*
Incorporates in part (in 1997): Healthcare Technology and Business Opportunities (1049-4499); Which was formerly: Medical Product Development
Published by: American Health Consultants (Subsidiary of: Medical Economics Co., Inc.), 3525 Piedmont Rd, N E, 6 Piedmont Center, Ste 400, Atlanta, GA 30305. TEL 404-262-5476, 404-262-7436, 800-688-2421, FAX 404-262-7837, 800-284-3291, custserv@ahcpub.com, http://www.ahcpub.com.

616.1 GBR ISSN 1466-4992
▼ **CARDIOVASCULAR DISEASE IN PRACTICE.** Text in English. 1999. q. **Document type:** *Academic/Scholarly.*
—BLDSC (3051.457000).
Published by: Hayward Group, Inc, 44 Earlham St, Convent Garden, London WC2H 9LA, United Kingdom. TEL 44-20-7240-4493, FAX 44-20-7240-4479, edit@hayward.co.uk. Ed. Richard Hobbs.

616.1 USA ISSN 1086-041X
CARDIOVASCULAR DISEASE MANAGEMENT. Text in English. 1995. m. USD 385 (effective 2001). bk.rev., Website rev. abstr, bibl, charts, illus, stat. back issues avail.; reprints avail. **Document type:** *Newsletter.* **Description:** Features innovative approaches for managing patients with cardiovascular disease.
Related titles: E-mail ed.; Online - full content ed.
—CCC.
Published by: COR Healthcare Resources, PO Box 40959, Santa Barbara, CA 93140. TEL 805-564-2177, info@corhealth.com, www.corhealth.com. Ed. Marilyn Lang. Pub. Dean H Anderson.

CARDIOVASCULAR DRUG REVIEWS. see *PHARMACY AND PHARMACOLOGY*

616.1 USA ISSN 0920-3206
RM345 CODEN: CDTHET
CARDIOVASCULAR DRUGS AND THERAPY. Text in English. 1987. bi-m. USD 276, EUR 276 to individuals for print or online ed.; USD 520, EUR 519 to institutions for print or online ed.; USD 624, EUR 622.80 to institutions for print & online eds. combined (effective 2002). adv. bk.rev. back issues avail.; reprint service avail. from SWZ,PQC. *Refereed.* **Document type:** *Academic/Scholarly.* **Description:** Contains articles on laboratory investigators and clinical studies related to cardiovascular drug therapy.
Related titles: Microform ed.: (from PQC); Online - full text ed.: (from Ovid Technologies, Inc., EBSCO Publishing, O C L C Online Computer Library Center, Inc., RoweCom Information Quest, Swets Blackwell, Kluwer Online, Institute for Scientific Information).
Indexed: ASCA, Biol.Abstr., Curr.Cont., Derwent Biotech.Abstr., Excerp.Med., INIS Atomind., Ind.Med. (1987-), Inpharma, Int.Abstr.Biol.Sci., Nutr.Abstr., Pharm.&Out.News, Reac., Rev.Appl.Entomol., Rev.Arom.& Med.Plants, SSCI (coverage dropped), Sci.Cit.Ind.
—BLDSC (3051.462500), ADONIS, CASDDS, CISTI, EMDOCS, GNLM, IDS, Infotrieve, ingenta, KNAW. **CCC.**
Published by: (International Society of Cardiovascular Pharmacotherapy), Kluwer Academic Publishers Boston, 101 Philip Dr, Assinippi Park, Norwell, MA 02061. TEL 781-871-6600, FAX 781-871-9045, services@wkap.nl, http://www.wkap.nl/journalhome.htm/0920-3206. Eds. Henry N Neufeld, Lionel H Opie, Willem J. Remme. R&P Rose Luongo TEL 781-871-6311. **Subscr. outside N America to:** Kluwer Academic Publishers Group, Journals Department, PO Box 322, Dordrecht 3300 AH, Netherlands. TEL 31-78-639-2392, FAX 31-78-654-6474; **Subscr. to:** Kluwer Academic - Plenum Publishers, 233 Spring St, New York, NY 10013-1578. TEL 212-620-8468, FAX 212-807-1047.

616.1 USA ISSN 1567-8822
▼ **CARDIOVASCULAR ENGINEERING**; an international journal. Text in English. 2001. q. USD 213, EUR 224 to institutions for print or online ed.; USD 255.60, EUR 268.80 to institutions for print & online eds. combined (effective 2002). **Document type:** *Journal, Academic/Scholarly.* **Description:** Aims to promote innovative methods and technological advancements in the basic understanding of the cardiovascular system and in cardiovascular diagnosis and treatment applications.
Related titles: Online - full content ed.; Online - full text ed.: (from Kluwer Online).
—BLDSC (1432.9077).
Published by: Kluwer Academic - Plenum Publishers (Subsidiary of: Wolters Kluwer N.V.), 233 Spring St, New York, NY 10013-1578. TEL 212-620-8000, 800-221-9369, FAX 212-463-0742, info@plenum.com, http://www.wkap.nl/journalhome.htm/1567-8822. Ed. John K-J Li. **Subscr. outside N America to:** Kluwer Academic Publishers Group, Journals Department, PO Box 322, Dordrecht 3300 AH, Netherlands. TEL 31-78-639-2392, FAX 31-78-654-6474.

616.1 ZAF ISSN 1015-9657
CODEN: CJSAE
CARDIOVASCULAR JOURNAL OF SOUTHERN AFRICA. Text in English. 1990. 5/yr. USD 65 (effective 2000). illus. back issues avail. **Document type:** *Journal, Academic/Scholarly.*
Related titles: ♦ Supplement to: S A M J South African Medical Journal. ISSN 0256-9574.
Indexed: Environ.Sci.Poll.Mgmt., Excerp.Med. (1995-), Ind.S.A.Per., Pollut.Abstr., Risk Abstr., Saf.Sci.Abstr.
—BLDSC (3051.464500), GNLM, KNAW.
Published by: (Medical Association of South Africa), South Africans Medical Association, Lynnwood Ridge, Box 74789, Pretoria, South Africa. Ed. Daniel J Ncayayana. R&P A J Brink TEL 27-21-968129. Adv. contact Julia Aalbers TEL 27-21-964378. **Subscr. to:** South African Medical Association, Health and Medical Publishing Group, PO Box 74789, Lynnwood Ridge, Pretoria 0040, South Africa. TEL 27-12-481-2010, FAX 27-12-481-2061, ann@samedical.org. **Co-sponsors:** Southern Africa Cardiac Society; South African Society of Cardiac Practitioners.

M

616.21 USA ISSN 1088-7180
CODEN: CPATFL

CARDIOVASCULAR PATHOBIOLOGY. Text in English. 1996. q. USD 120 to individuals; USD 155 to institutions. adv. index, cum.index. back issues avail. *Refereed.* **Document type:** *Academic/Scholarly.* **Description:** Publishes original papers on the cellular, biochemical, and molecular mechanisms of cardiovascular function and disease.
Indexed: Int.Abstr.Biol.Sci.
—CASDDS.
Published by: Woodland Publications, Inc., 69 Murray St, New York, NY 10007. TEL 212-566-4294, FAX 212-406-6496, woodlpub@pipeline.com. Ed. Dr. Colin Bloor. Adv. contact Sue Cassidy. page USD 750; trim 11 x 8.5.

616.1 USA ISSN 1054-8807
CODEN: CATHE8

CARDIOVASCULAR PATHOLOGY. Text in English. 1992. bi-m. EUR 181 in Europe to individuals; JPY 24,000 in Japan to individuals; USD 202 elsewhere to individuals; EUR 366 in Europe to institutions; JPY 48,600 in Japan to institutions; USD 409 elsewhere to institutions; EUR 99 in Europe to qualified personnel; JPY 13,200 in Japan to qualified personnel; USD 112 elsewhere to qualified personnel (effective 2002). abstr. back issues avail. *Refereed.* **Document type:** *Academic/Scholarly.* **Description:** Papers on disease-oriented morphology and pathobiology from pathologists and investigators in the cardiovascular field.
Related titles: Microform ed.: (from PQC); Online - full text ed.: (from ingenta, Swets Blackwell, ScienceDirect, Institute for Scientific Information).
Indexed: ASCA, Chem.Abstr., Chem.Indus.Notes, Chem.Titles, Curr.Cont., Excerp.Med. (1994-), Ind.Med. (1992-), Ind.Sci.Rev., Inpharma, Mat.Sci.Cit.Ind. (coverage dropped), Pharm.&Out.News, Protozool.Abstr., Reac., Rev.Appl.Entomol., Sci.Cit.Ind.
—BLDSC (3051.470700), CASDDS, CISTI, EMDOCS, GNLM, IDS, Infotrieve, ingenta, KNAW. **CCC.**
Published by: (Society for Cardiovascular Pathology), Elsevier Science, PO Box 945, New York, NY 10159-0945. TEL 212-989-5800, FAX 212-633-3990, TELEX 420643 AEP UI, http://www.elsevier.nl/locate/carpath. Ed. Dr. Stephen M Factor. **Subscr. in Australasia and the Far East to:** Elsevier Science (Singapore) Pte Ltd, No.1 Temasek Ave, 17-01 Millenia Tower, Singapore 039192, Singapore. TEL 65-434-3727, FAX 65-337-2230; **Subscr. in Japan to:** Elsevier Science Inc - Japan Regional Office, 9-15 Higashi-Azabu 1-chome, Minato-ku, Tokyo 106-0044, Japan. TEL 81-3-5561-5033; **Subscr. outside the Americas to:** Elsevier Science BV, PO Box 211, Amsterdam 1000 AE, Netherlands. TEL 31-20-485-3757, nlinfo-f@elsevier.nl, http://www.elsevier.nl.

CARDIOVASCULAR PHARMACOLOGY. see *PHARMACY AND PHARMACOLOGY—Abstracting, Bibliographies, Statistics*

616.1 615.842 USA ISSN 1522-1865

▼ **CARDIOVASCULAR RADIATION MEDICINE.** Text in English. 1999. q. EUR 75 in Europe to individuals; JPY 10,000 in Japan to individuals; USD 84 elsewhere to individuals; EUR 154 in Europe to institutions; JPY 20,500 in Japan to institutions; USD 173 elsewhere to institutions (effective 2002). back issues avail.; reprints avail. *Refereed.* **Document type:** *Academic/Scholarly.* **Description:** Publishes original laboratory and clinical investigations relating to the ability of radiation therapy to prevent or delay arterial restenosis post-angioplasty in hemodialysis access patients and femoral popliteals artery by-pass patients, and in coronary arteries and peripheral arteries in a variety of anatomic sites.
Related titles: Online - full text ed.: (from ingenta, Swets Blackwell, ScienceDirect).
Indexed: Ind.Med.
—BLDSC (3051.483000).
Published by: (American Brachytherpy Society), Elsevier Science, PO Box 945, New York, NY 10159-0945. TEL 212-989-5800, FAX 212-633-3990, usinfo-f@elsevier.com, http://www.elsevier.com/locate/carrad. Eds. P W Serruys, P Rubin, R Waksman. **Subscr. in Australasia and the Far East to:** Elsevier Science (Singapore) Pte Ltd, No.1 Temasek Ave, 17-01 Millenia Tower, Singapore 039192, Singapore. TEL 65-434-3727, FAX 65-337-2230; **Subscr. in Japan to:** Elsevier Science Inc - Japan Regional Office, 9-15 Higashi-Azabu 1-chome, Minato-ku, Tokyo 106-0044, Japan. TEL 81-3-5561-5033; **Subscr. outside the Americas to:** Elsevier Science BV, PO Box 211, Amsterdam 1000 AE, Netherlands. TEL 31-20-485-3757, FAX 31-20-485-3432.

616.1 NLD ISSN 0008-6363
CODEN: CVREAU

CARDIOVASCULAR RESEARCH. Text in English. 1967. 14/yr. EUR 275 in Europe to individuals; JPY 36,400 in Japan to individuals; USD 307 elsewhere to individuals; EUR 775 in Europe to institutions; JPY 102,800 in Japan to institutions; USD 867 elsewhere to institutions (effective 2002). adv. abstr. index. back issues avail.; reprint service avail. from PQC. *Refereed.* **Document type:** *Academic/Scholarly.* **Description:** Strives to promote links between fundamental research and clinical cardiology and to enhance the understanding of the pathophysiology of cardiovascular disease with an international scope.
Incorporates (1990-1995): Cardioscience (1015-5007)
Related titles: Microform ed.: (from PQC); Online - full text ed.: (from ingenta, Swets Blackwell, ScienceDirect, Institute for Scientific Information).
Indexed: ASCA, Agri.& Environ.Biotech.Abstr. (coverage dropped), Biol.Abstr., Chem.Abstr., Chem.Indus.Notes, Chem.Titles, Curr.Adv.Ecol.Sci., Curr.Cont., Dairy Sci.Abstr., Derwent Biotech.Abstr., Excerp.Med., Helminthol.Abstr., INIS Atomind., Ind.Med. (1967-), Ind.Sci.Rev., Ind.Vet., Inpharma, Int.Abstr.Biol.Sci., NRN, Neurosci.Cit.Ind., Nutr.Abstr., Pharm.&Out.News, Pig News & Info., Reac., SSCI (coverage dropped), Sci.Cit.Ind., Soyabean Abstr.
—BLDSC (3051.490000), ADONIS, CASDDS, CISTI, EMDOCS, GNLM, IDS, ingenta, KNAW. **CCC.**
Published by: Elsevier Science BV, PO Box 211, Amsterdam 1000 AE, Netherlands. TEL 31-20-485-2911, FAX 31-20-485-2457, nlinfo-f@elsevier.nl, http://www.elsevier.com/locate/cardiores. Ed. M J Janse. **Subscr. in Australasia and the Far East to:** Elsevier Science (Singapore) Pte Ltd, No.1 Temasek Ave, 17-01 Millenia Tower, Singapore 039192, Singapore. TEL 65-434-3727, FAX 65-337-2230; **Subscr. in Japan to:** Elsevier Science Inc - Japan Regional Office, 9-15 Higashi-Azabu 1-chome, Minato-ku, Tokyo 106-0044, Japan. TEL 81-3-5561-5033; **Subscr. in the Americas to:** Elsevier Science, PO Box 945, New York, NY 10159-0945. TEL 212-633-3730, FAX 212-633-3680. **Co-sponsor:** European Society of Cardiology.

616.1 USA ISSN 0197-3118
CODEN: CRRPD4

CARDIOVASCULAR REVIEWS & REPORTS. Text in English. 1980. m. USD 90 domestic to individuals; USD 105 foreign to individuals; USD 105 domestic to institutions; USD 120 foreign to institutions (effective 2001). adv. bk.rev., software rev. abstr, charts, illus, bibl. back issues avail.; reprints avail. *Refereed.* **Document type:** *Journal, Academic/Scholarly.*
Indexed: Excerp.Med., Inpharma, NRN, Pharm.&Out.News, Reac.
—BLDSC (3051.513000), CISTI, GNLM, KNAW.
Published by: LeJacq Communications, Inc., 777 W Putnam Ave, Greenwich, CT 06830-5014. TEL 203-531-0450, FAX 203-531-0533, showell@lejacq.com. Ed. Stephen Scheidt. Pub. Sarah Howell. R&P Andrea Townsend. Adv. contact Joann Kalaka-Adams TEL 732-747-6525. B&W page USD 3,825, color page USD 1,235; trim 10.75 x 8. Circ: 70,026.

616.12 ESP ISSN 1133-9160

CARDIOVASCULAR RISK FACTORS; an international journal. Text in Spanish. 1991. bi-m. adv. *Refereed.* **Document type:** *Academic/Scholarly.* **Description:** Publishes original research and review articles on factors important to the prevention of coronary heart disease and other diseases of the heart and blood vessels.
Related titles: Online - full text ed.
Indexed: Excerp.Med. (1992-).
—BLDSC (3051.514000), EMDOCS.
Published by: Saned S.A., Capitan Haya, 60, Madrid 28020, Spain. TEL 34-91-749-9506, FAX 34-91-749-9507, saned@medynet.com. Ed. A Fernandez Cruz W Castelli. R&P Alicia Martinez. Adv. contact Ana Martinez. page ESP 250,000.

616.1 617 GBR ISSN 0967-2109

CARDIOVASCULAR SURGERY. Text in English. 1993. bi-m. EUR 112 in Europe to individuals; JPY 14,800 in Japan to individuals; USD 125 elsewhere to individuals; EUR 393 in Europe to institutions; JPY 52,200 in Japan to institutions; USD 440 elsewhere to institutions (effective 2002). back issues avail. *Refereed.* **Document type:** *Academic/Scholarly.* **Description:** Publishes original articles, reviews and case reports relating to the study and surgical management of cardiovascular disease.
Related titles: Microform ed.: (from PQC); Online - full text ed.: (from ingenta, Swets Blackwell, ScienceDirect, Institute for Scientific Information).
Indexed: Curr.Cont., Excerp.Med. (1994-), Ind.Med. (1993-), Ref.Zh.
—BLDSC (3051.515050), CISTI, EMDOCS, GNLM, IDS, Infotrieve, KNAW. **CCC.**
Published by: (International Society for Cardiovascular Surgery), Pergamon (Subsidiary of: Elsevier Science), The Boulevard, Langford Ln, East Park, Kidlington, Oxford OXB 1GB, United Kingdom. FAX 44-1865-843010, nlinfo-f@elsevier/nl; usinfo-f@elsevier.com; forinfo-kyf04035@niftyserve.or.jp, http://www.elsevier.nl/locate/cardiosur. Eds. J M T Bakker, M J Janse. **Subscr. in Australasia and the Far East to:** Elsevier Science (Singapore) Pte Ltd, No.1 Temasek Ave, 17-01 Millenia Tower, Singapore 039192, Singapore. TEL 65-434-3727, FAX 65-337-2230; **Subscr. in the Americas to:** Elsevier Science, PO Box 945, New York, NY 10159-0945. TEL 212-633-3730, FAX 212-633-3680, usinfo-f@elsevier.com, http://www.elsevier.com; **Subscr. to:** Elsevier Science BV, PO Box 211, Amsterdam 1000 AE, Netherlands. TEL 31-20-485-3757, FAX 31-20-485-3432, nlinfo-f@elsevier.nl, http://www.elsevier.nl.

617.41 USA ISSN 0069-0406

CARDIOVASCULAR SURGERY. Text in English. 1962. a. USD 20 domestic; USD 25 foreign (effective 2000). adv. *Refereed.* **Document type:** *Monographic series.*
Indexed: Ind.Med. (coverage dropped), Inpharma, Pharm.&Out.News, Reac.
—Infotrieve. **CCC.**
Published by: Lippincott Williams & Wilkins (Baltimore) (Subsidiary of: Wolters Kluwer N.V.), 351 W Camden St, Baltimore, MD 21201-2436. TEL 410-528-4000, FAX 410-528-4312. Pub. Cara Kaufman. R&P Debbie Heise TEL 410-528-4050. Adv. contact Angela Hopkins. Circ: 23,000.

616.1 GBR ISSN 1465-1327

CAROTID AND NEUROVASCULAR INTERVENTION. Text in English. 3/yr. USD 70 in US & Canada; GBP 50 in Europe; USD 75 elsewhere (effective 2000). **Document type:** *Academic/Scholarly.* **Description:** Provides an up-to-date overview of the recent literature compiled by an international team of practicing physicians; also contains article reviews of new therapeutic techniques and emerging technologies, and news from major international meetings.
Published by: Remedica Publishing Ltd., 32-38 Osnaburgh St, London NW1 3ND, United Kingdom. TEL 44-171-388-7677, FAX 44-171-388-7678, http://www.remedica.com, http://www.remedica.com.

616.1 USA

CATH LAB DIGEST. Text in English. 1992. m. free domestic to qualified personnel; USD 90 foreign (effective 2001). adv. **Description:** A product news periodical providing information on all treatments, procedures, and technological advancement in the Cath Lab. It is the official publication of the Society of Invasive Cardiovascular Professionals.
Published by: H M P Communications, LLC, 950 W Valley Rd, Ste 2800, Wayne, PA 19087. TEL 610-688-8220, FAX 610-688-1060. adv.: B&W page USD 2,599, color page USD 3,899. Circ: 15,000 (controlled).

616.1 USA ISSN 1522-1946
RC683 CODEN: CARIF2

CATHETERIZATION AND CARDIOVASCULAR INTERVENTIONS. Text in English. 1975. m. USD 1,910 in United States; USD 2,030 in Canada & Mexico; USD 2,132 elsewhere; USD 2,006 combined subscription in United States for print and online eds.; USD 2,126 combined subscription in Canada & Mexico for print and online eds.; USD 2,228 combined subscription elsewhere for print and online eds. (effective 2002). adv. bibl, charts, illus. back issues avail.; reprint service avail. from ISI. *Refereed.* **Document type:** *Academic/Scholarly.* **Description:** Devoted to invasive cardiology. Emphasizes angioplasty and the newest techniques of interventional cardiology.
Formerly (until vol.45, no.4, 1998): Catheterization and Cardiovascular Diagnosis (0098-6569)
Related titles: Microform ed.: (from PQC); Online - full text ed.: ISSN 1522-726X. USD 1,910 in United States; USD 1,910 in Canada & Mexico; USD 1,910 elsewhere (effective 2002) (from EBSCO Publishing, Wiley InterScience, Institute for Scientific Information).
Indexed: ASCA, Biol.Abstr., Curr.Cont., Excerp.Med., INIS Atomind., Ind.Med. (1999-), Ind.Sci.Rev., Inpharma, Jrnl.Watch Card., Pharm.&Out.News, Reac., Sci.Cit.Ind.
—BLDSC (3092.992000), CISTI, EMDOCS, GNLM, IDS, ingenta, KNAW. **CCC.**

Published by: (Society for Cardiac Angiography & Interventions), John Wiley & Sons, Inc., Journals (Subsidiary of: Wiley InterScience), 605 Third Ave, New York, NY 10158. TEL 212-850-6645, FAX 212-850-6021, subinfo@jwiley.com, uscs-wis@wiley.com, http://www.interscience.wiley.com/jpages/1522-1946, http://www.wiley.com. adv.: B&W page GBP 640, color page GBP 1,515; trim 210 x 279. Circ: 3,450. **Subscr. outside the Americas to:** John Wiley & Sons Ltd., Baffins Ln, Chichester, Sussex PO19 IUD, United Kingdom. TEL 44-1243-779777, FAX 44-1243-843232, cs-journals@wiley.co.uk, http://www.wiley.co.uk.

CHEST; the cardiopulmonary and critical care journal. see *MEDICAL SCIENCES—Respiratory Diseases*

616.1 USA ISSN 0009-7322
RC681.A1 CODEN: CIRCAZ

CIRCULATION (BALTIMORE). Text in English. 1950. 50/yr. USD 275 domestic to individuals print & online eds.; USD 471 foreign to individuals print & online eds; USD 522 domestic to institutions print & online eds; USD 708 foreign to institutions print & online eds; USD 25 newsstand/cover (effective 2002). adv. abstr, bibl, illus. index. back issues avail.; reprint service avail. from PQC. *Refereed.* **Document type:** *Academic/Scholarly.* **Description:** For cardiologists and internists; presents clinical and laboratory research relevant to cardiovascular diseases.

Related titles: CD-ROM ed.: (from Ovid Technologies, Inc.); Microform ed.: (from PMC,PQC); Online - full text ed.: USD 678.60 domestic academic site license; USD 864.60 foreign academic site license; USD 756.90 domestic corporate site license; USD 942.90 foreign corporate site license (effective 2002) (from HighWire Pr., Ovid Technologies, Inc., EBSCO Publishing, ProQuest Information & Learning, Institute for Scientific Information); ♦ Spanish ed.: Circulation (Edicion Espanola). ISSN 1134-5187; ♦ Supplement: Circulation Research. ISSN 0009-7330; ♦ Circulation. Supplement. ISSN 0069-4193.

Indexed: AIM, Abstr.Hyg., Abstr.Inter.Med., AgeLine, Agri.& Environ.Biotech.Abstr. (coverage dropped), Behav.Med.Abstr., Biol.Abstr., CINAHL, C.I.S. Abstr., Chem.Abstr., Curr.Adv.Ecol.Sci., Curr.Cont., Curr.Ind.Stat., Derwent Biotech.Abstr., Diab.Cont., Excerp.Med., INIS Atomind., Ind.Med. (1950-), Ind.Sci.Rev., Inpharma, Int.Abstr.Biol.Sci., Int.Nurs.Ind., Jrnl.Watch, Jrnl.Watch Card., Jrnl.Watch Emer.Med., Jrnl.Watch Inf.Dis., Jrnl.Watch Wom.Hlth., Kidney, Mat.Sci.Cit.Ind. (coverage dropped), NRN, Nutr.Abstr., Pharm.&Out.News, Pig News & Info., Protozool.Abstr., Reac., Risk Abstr., SSCI (coverage dropped), Sci.Cit.Ind., Trop.Dis.Bull.

—BLDSC (3265.200000), CASDDS, CISTI, EMDOCS, GNLM, IDS, ingenta, KNAW.

Published by: (American Heart Association), Lippincott Williams & Wilkins (Baltimore) (Subsidiary of: Wolters Kluwer N.V.), 351 W Camden St, Baltimore, MD 21201-2436. TEL 410-528-4000, 800-787-8984, 800-787-8984, http://www.circr.ahajournals.org. Pub. Susan Harris. Adv. contact Angela Hopkins. B&W page USD 2,140, color page USD 3,735. Circ: 25,000 (paid).

616.1 ESP ISSN 1134-5187

CIRCULATION (EDICION ESPANOLA)✶. Text in Spanish. 1994. 8/yr. ESP 11,200, USD 123 (effective 1996).

Related titles: ♦ English ed.: Circulation (Baltimore). ISSN 0009-7322.

Indexed: Curr.Cont. (coverage dropped).

Published by: Grupo Masson, Rda General Mitre, 149, Barcelona 08022, Spain. TEL 34-93-2530200, FAX 34-93-2530515, http://www.masson.es, http://masson.es, http://masson.es.

616.1 JPN ISSN 1343-2036

THE CIRCULATION FRONTIER. Text in Japanese. 1997. q. JPY 3,000 per issue (effective 1998). **Document type:** *Academic/Scholarly.*

Published by: Medikaru Rebyusha/Medical Review Co., Ltd., 7-3 Hirano-Machi 1-chome, Chuo-ku, Osaka-shi 541-0046, Japan. TEL 81-6-223-1556, FAX 81-6-223-1414, medrev@osk2.3web.ne.jp.

616.1 USA ISSN 0009-7330
RC681.A1 CODEN: CIRUAL

CIRCULATION RESEARCH. Text in English. 1953. 24/yr. USD 306 domestic to individuals for print & online eds.; USD 377 foreign to individuals for print & online eds; USD 615 domestic to institutions for print & online eds; USD 690 foreign to institutions for print & online eds (effective 2002). adv. bk.rev. charts, illus, stat. index. Supplement avail.; back issues avail.; reprint service avail. from PQC. *Refereed.* **Document type:** *Academic/Scholarly.* **Description:** Documents research advances in basic science, research, and experimental medicine.

Related titles: CD-ROM ed.: (from Ovid Technologies, Inc.); Microform ed.: (from MIM,PMC,PQC); Online - full text ed.: USD 799.50 domestic academic site license; USD 489 foreign academic site license; USD 891.75 domestic corporate site license; USD 966.75 foreign corporate site license (effective 2002) (from HighWire Pr., Ovid Technologies, Inc., Northern Light Technology, Inc., EBSCO Publishing, ProQuest Information & Learning, Institute for Scientific Information); ♦ Supplement to: Circulation (Baltimore). ISSN 0009-7322.

Indexed: ASCA, AgeLine, Agri.& Environ.Biotech.Abstr. (coverage dropped), BBCI, Biol.Abstr., Chem.Abstr., Chem.Indus.Notes, Chem.Titles, Curr.Adv.Biochem., Curr.Adv.Cell & Devel.Biol., Curr.Adv.Ecol.Sci., Curr.Cont., Derwent Biotech.Abstr., Diab.Cont., Excerp.Med., INIS Atomind., INSPEC (Oct.1971-Apr.1976, dropped), Ind.Med. (1953-), Ind.Sci.Rev., Ind.Vet., Inpharma, Int.Abstr.Biol.Sci., NRN, Neurosci.Cit.Ind., Nutr.Abstr., Pharm.&Out.News, Reac., Ref.Zh., Sci.Cit.Ind., THA, Vet.Bull.

—BLDSC (3265.300000), CASDDS, CISTI, EMDOCS, GNLM, IDS, ingenta, KNAW.

Published by: (American Heart Association), Lippincott Williams & Wilkins (Baltimore) (Subsidiary of: Wolters Kluwer N.V.), 351 W Camden St, Baltimore, MD 21201-2436. TEL 410-528-4000, 301-223-2307, 800-787-8984, FAX 410-528-4312, 301-223-2327, ahaonline@lww.com, http://www.circres.ahajournals.org, http://www.circr.ahajournals.org. Ed. Dr. Eduardo Maraban. Pub. Cara Kaufman. R&P Debbie Heise TEL 410-528-4050. Adv. contact Angela Hopkins. Circ: 3,800.

616.1 USA ISSN 0069-4193
CODEN: CISUAQ

CIRCULATION. SUPPLEMENT. Text in English. 1964. s-a., latest 1993. included in subscr. to Circulation. adv. reprint service avail. from PQC. **Document type:** *Academic/Scholarly.*

Related titles: ♦ Supplement to: Circulation (Baltimore). ISSN 0009-7322.

Indexed: Chem.Abstr., Chem.Indus.Notes, Chem.Titles, Ind.Med. (coverage dropped).

—CASDDS, CISTI, Infotrieve, KNAW. **CCC.**

Published by: (American Heart Association), Lippincott Williams & Wilkins (Baltimore) (Subsidiary of: Wolters Kluwer N.V.), 351 W Camden St, Baltimore, MD 21201-2436. TEL 410-528-4000, 800-787-8984, FAX 410-528-4312, http://www.americanheartassociation.org. Pub. Vicki Sullivan. R&P Linda Venable. Adv. contact Bonnie McCabe. Circ: 27,000.

616.1 ESP ISSN 0212-1808
CODEN: CCAREP

CLINICA CARDIOVASCULAR. Text in Spanish. 1982. bi-m. ESP 6,000 domestic; USD 65 in Europe; USD 70 elsewhere (effective 2001). adv. charts. *Refereed.* **Document type:** *Academic/Scholarly.* **Description:** Publishes clinical and research articles in cardiology.

—BLDSC (3286.190000), CINDOC, CISTI, EMDOCS, GNLM, Infotrieve, KNAW. **CCC.**

Published by: Alpe Editores S.A., Pedro Rico, 27, Madrid 28029, Spain. TEL 34-91-733-8811, FAX 34-91-315-9652, alpeeditores@sistelcom.com. Eds. Dr. Leandro Plaza Celemin, Dr. Vincente Tormo Alfonso. Pub. Angeles Alvarez Sanchez. Adv. contact Ana Jurado. color page ESP 160,000; trim 280 x 210. Circ: 5,000 (controlled).

616.136 ESP ISSN 0214-9168

CLINICA E INVESTIGACION EN ARTERIOSCLEROSIS. Text in Spanish. q. USD 74 to non-members. adv. **Document type:** *Academic/Scholarly.* **Description:** Covers basic science aspects such as etiology, epidemiology, physiopathology, and the diagnosis and treatment of arteriosclerosis and related processes.

Related titles: ♦ Supplement: Clinica e Investigacion en Arteriosclerosis. Suplemento. ISSN 0214-9176.

Published by: (Sociedad Espanola de Arteriosclerosis), Ediciones Doyma S.A., Traversa de Gracia, 17-21, Barcelona 08021, Spain. TEL 34-93-200-0711, FAX 34-93-209-1136. Ed. R Carmena Rodriguez. Adv. contact Olga Gomez. color page ESP 238,000; trim 280 x 210. Circ: 2,000.

616.136 ESP ISSN 0214-9176

CLINICA E INVESTIGACION EN ARTERIOSCLEROSIS. SUPLEMENTO. Text in Spanish. 1989. irreg.

Related titles: ♦ Supplement to: Clinica e Investigacion en Arteriosclerosis. ISSN 0214-9168.

Published by: (Sociedad Espanola de Arteriosclerosis), Ediciones Doyma S.A., Traversa de Gracia, 17-21, Barcelona 08021, Spain. TEL 34-1-200-07-11, FAX 34-1-209-11-36.

616.1 USA ISSN 1064-1963
RC685.H8 CODEN: CEHYER

CLINICAL AND EXPERIMENTAL HYPERTENSION. Text in English. 1979. 8/yr. USD 185 to individuals print & online eds.; USD 2,050 to institutions print only (effective 2002). adv. bk.rev. index. back issues avail. *Refereed.* **Document type:** *Academic/Scholarly.* **Description:** Covers all aspects of human and animal hypertension ranging from neurogenic mechanisms to circulatory control and drug development and application.

Formerly: Clinical and Experimental Hypertension. Part A: Theory and Practice (0730-0077); Which supersedes in part: Clinical and Experimental Hypertension (0148-3927)

Related titles: Microform ed.: (from RPI); Online - full text ed.: (from EBSCO Publishing, O C L C Online Computer Library Center, Inc., RoweCom Information Quest, Swets Blackwell, Institute for Scientific Information).

Indexed: ASCA, Agri.& Environ.Biotech.Abstr. (coverage dropped), Biol.Dig., Chem.Abstr., Chem.Indus.Notes, Chem.Titles, Curr.Adv.Cell & Devel.Biol., Curr.Adv.Ecol.Sci., Curr.Adv.Gen.& Molec.Biol., Curr.Cont., Dent.Ind., Derwent Biotech.Abstr., Excerp.Med., INIS Atomind., Ind.Med. (1993-), Ind.Sci.Rev., Inpharma, Int.Abstr.Biol.Sci., NRN, Neurosci.Cit.Ind., Nutr.Abstr., Pharm.&Out.News, Reac., Ref.Zh., Sci.Cit.Ind.

—BLDSC (3286.250500), CASDDS, CISTI, EMDOCS, GNLM, IDS, ingenta, KNAW. **CCC.**

Published by: Marcel Dekker Inc., 270 Madison Ave, New York, NY 10016. TEL 212-696-9000, 800-228-1160, FAX 212-685-4540, http://www.dekker.com/servlet/product/productid/CEH. Ed. Mustafa F Lokhandwala. R&P Julia Mulligan. Adv. contact Anne Mullins. B&W page USD 800. Circ: 425.

616.1 USA

CLINICAL APPROACHES TO TACHYARRHYTHMIAS. Text in English. 1993. irreg., latest vol.5, 1996. price varies. **Document type:** *Monographic series.*

—BLDSC (3286.259100).

Published by: Futura Publishing Company, Inc., 135 Bedford Rd, PO Box 418, Armonk, NY 10504-0418. TEL 914-273-1014, 800-877-8761, FAX 914-973-1016. Ed. Dr. A John Camm.

616.1 USA ISSN 0741-4218

CLINICAL CARDIOLOGY ALERT. Text in English. 1982. m. USD 219 domestic; USD 249 foreign; USD 37 newsstand/cover (effective 2001). index. reprints avail. **Document type:** *Newsletter.* **Description:** Reports on the latest advances and clinical developments in cardiology and cardiovascular disease.

Formerly: Cardiology Alert

Related titles: Audio cassette/tape ed.; Online - full text ed.: (from Gale Group).

Published by: American Health Consultants (Subsidiary of: Medical Economics Co., Inc.), 3525 Piedmont Rd, N E, 6 Piedmont Center, Ste 400, Atlanta, GA 30305. TEL 404-262-5476, custserv@ahcpub.com, http://www.ahcpub.com. Circ: 2,265.

616.1 USA ISSN 0160-9289
CODEN: CLCADC

CLINICAL CARDIOLOGY (MAHWAH); international journal for cardiovascular diseases. Text in English. 1978. m. USD 80; USD 126.50 foreign (effective 2001). adv. bk.rev. December. 104 p./no. 2 cols./p. back issues avail.; reprints avail. *Refereed.* **Document type:** *Journal, Trade.* **Description:** Provides a forum for the coordination of clinical research in cardiology and cardiovascular surgery; also publishes the results of experimental studies closely related to clinical problems.

Related titles: Online - full text ed.: (from Institute for Scientific Information).

Indexed: ASCA, Biol.Abstr., Curr.Cont., Excerp.Med., INIS Atomind., Ind.Med. (1978-), Ind.Sci.Rev., Int.Nurs.Ind., NRN, Nutr.Abstr., Ref.Zh., Sci.Cit.Ind.

—BLDSC (3286.265000), CASDDS, CISTI, EMDOCS, GNLM, IDS, ingenta, KNAW. **CCC.**

Published by: Clinical Cardiology Publishing Company, Inc., PO Box 832, Mahwah, NJ 07430-0832. TEL 201-818-1010, FAX 201-818-0086, clinicalcardiology@fams.org, clinical-cardiology@fams.org, http://www.clinicalcardiology.org. Ed. Dr. C Richard Conti. Pub. Tony Bourgholtzer. R&P Lillian Conly TEL 201-818-1010. Adv. contact John Bourgholtzer TEL 201-818-1010. B&W page USD 2,595, color page USD 4,260; 7 x 10. Circ: 35,000.

616.1 USA ISSN 0891-2092
CLINICAL CARDIOLOGY (STAMFORD)* . Text in English. 1977. triennial. **Document type:** *Monographic series.*
—CISTI. **CCC.**
Published by: Appleton & Lange, Journal Division (Subsidiary of: Simon & Schuster Company), 11 W 19th St, New York, CT 10011-4209. TEL 203-406-4500, FAX 203-406-4600.

CLINICIAN'S MANUAL ON HYPERLIPIDEMIA (YEAR). see *MEDICAL SCIENCES—Abstracting, Bibliographies, Statistics*

CLINICIAN'S MANUAL ON HYPERTENSION AND CONCOMITANT HYPERLIPIDAEMIA. see *MEDICAL SCIENCES—Abstracting, Bibliographies, Statistics*

COEUR ET SANTE. see *PHYSICAL FITNESS AND HYGIENE*

616.1 USA ISSN 1079-7998
CODEN: CHFAFZ
CONGESTIVE HEART FAILURE. Text in English. 1994. bi-m. USD 90 domestic to individuals; USD 105 foreign to individuals; USD 105 domestic to institutions; USD 120 foreign to institutions (effective 2001). adv. bk.rev. abstr, illus. back issues avail.; reprints avail. *Refereed.* **Document type:** *Journal, Academic/Scholarly.*
Related titles: Online - full text ed.: (from Northern Light Technology, Inc.).
—BLDSC (3410.684200), CISTI, EMDOCS, GNLM.
Published by: LeJacq Communications, Inc., 777 W Putnam Ave, Greenwich, CT 06830-5014. TEL 203-531-0450, FAX 203-531-0533, showell@lejacq.com. Eds. John Strobeck, Marc Silver. R&P Andrea Townsend. Adv. contact Joann Kalaka-Adams TEL 732-747-6525. B&W page USD 2,960, color page USD 1,235. Circ: 26,000.

616.1 USA
CONGESTIVE HEART FAILURE: DISEASE STATE MANAGEMENT RESOURCE. Text in English. 1997. a., latest vol.4, 2000. USD 299 domestic; USD 329 foreign (effective 2001). **Document type:** *Trade.*
Published by: American Health Consultants (Subsidiary of: Medical Economics Co., Inc.), 3525 Piedmont Rd, N E, 6 Piedmont Center, Ste 400, Atlanta, GA 30305. TEL 404-262-5476, 404-262-7436, 800-688-2421, FAX 404-262-7837, 800-284-3291, custserv@ahcpub.com, http://www.ahcpub.com.

616.12 USA ISSN 8756-9086
CONNECTIVE ISSUES. Text in English. 1984. q. USD 35 to members. back issues avail. **Document type:** *Newsletter.* **Description:** Provides information on the Marfan syndrome, a genetic disorder of connective tissue that affects the cardiovascular system, the skeletal system and the eyes.
Published by: National Marfan Foundation, 382 Main St., Pt. Washington, NY 11050. TEL 516-883-8712, 800-862-7326, FAX 516-883-8040, staff@marfan.org, http://www.marfan.org. Ed. Eileen Masciale. R&P Carolyn Levering. Circ: 20,000.

616.12 USA
CONTEMPORARY CARDIOLOGY. Text in English. 1998. irreg., latest vol.5, 1999. price varies. illus. *Refereed.* **Document type:** *Monographic series, Academic/Scholarly.* **Description:** Leading physicians provide the latest research, therapies and treatment recommendations for cardiovascular physicians.
Published by: Humana Press Inc., 999 Riverview Dr, Ste 208, Totowa, NJ 07512. TEL 973-256-1699, FAX 973-256-8341, humana@humanapr.com, http://humanapress.com. Ed. Christopher Cannon. R&P Richard Hruska.

616.1 ITA
CONTROVERSIES IN CARDIOLOGY. Text in Italian. 1991 (vol.3, no.3). q.
Published by: Zambon Group S.p.A., Via Lillo del Duca, 10, Bresso, MI 20091, Italy. Ed. Germano Marchetti.

616.1 CZE ISSN 0010-8650
CODEN: COVAAN
COR ET VASA; journal of the Czech Society of Cardiology. Text in Czech, Slovak, English. 1993. 10/yr. CZK 1,600 domestic; CHF 373 foreign (effective 2000). adv. bk.rev. index. back issues avail. *Refereed.* **Document type:** *Academic/Scholarly.*
Related titles: Online - full text ed.
Indexed: Biol.Abstr., Chem.Abstr., Curr.Adv.Ecol.Sci., Curr.Cont. (coverage dropped), Excerp.Med., INIS Atomind., Ind.Med. (coverage dropped), Nutr.Abstr.
—CASDDS, CISTI, EMDOCS, GNLM, KNAW.
Published by: (Ceska Kardiologicka Spolecnost/Czech Cardiological Society), Praha Publishing Ltd., Anglicka 17, Prague, 2 120 00, Czech Republic. TEL 420-2-22518436, 420-2-22512649, FAX 420-2-24247568, publish@bohem-net.cz, http://www.coretvasa.html, http://www.mediclub.cz/coretvasa. Ed. Jirina Kaderavkova. R&P Andrew Benkowitz TEL 420-2-22511042. Adv. contact Ivana Kaderkova. Circ: (controlled).

CORE JOURNALS IN CARDIOLOGY. see *MEDICAL SCIENCES—Abstracting, Bibliographies, Statistics*

616.1 USA ISSN 0954-6928
CODEN: CAELFE
CORONARY ARTERY DISEASE. Text in English. 1990. 8/yr. USD 299 domestic to individuals; USD 299 foreign to individuals; USD 759 per issue domestic to institutions; USD 759 per issue foreign to institutions; USD 84 newsstand/cover (effective 2002). adv. bk.rev. bibl, illus. back issues avail. *Refereed.* **Document type:** *Academic/Scholarly.* **Description:** Presents original research and clinical investigations in the expanding field of coronary artery research; includes reviews with annotated references. Each issue features a bibliography of the current world literature published during the previous quarter of the year.
Incorporates (1993-199?): Cardiology in the Elderly (1058-3661)
Related titles: Online - full text ed.: (from Ovid Technologies, Inc., EBSCO Publishing, Swets Blackwell, Institute for Scientific Information).
Indexed: ASCA, Curr.Cont., Excerp.Med., Ind.Med. (1990-), Ind.Sci.Rev., Inpharma, Nutr.Abstr., Pharm.&Out.News, Reac., SSCI (coverage dropped), Sci.Cit.Ind.
—BLDSC (3472.049000), ADONIS, CISTI, EMDOCS, GNLM, IDS, KNAW.
Published by: Lippincott Williams & Wilkins (Philadelphia) (Subsidiary of: Wolters Kluwer N.V.), 530 Walnut St, Philadelphia, PA 19106-3621. TEL 215-521-8300, FAX 215-521-8902, http://www.Lww.com. Ed. Dr. Burton E Sobel. Adv. contact Gemma Heiser. Circ: 1,897. **Subscr. to:** PO Box 1600, Hagerstown, MD 21740-1600. TEL 800-777-2295, FAX 301-824-7390.

CORONARY HEALTH CARE. see *MEDICAL SCIENCES—Nurses And Nursing*

COST MANAGEMENT IN CARDIAC CARE. see *HEALTH FACILITIES AND ADMINISTRATION*

616.1 GBR ISSN 0956-2257
CODEN: CRISE3
CRITICAL ISCHAEMIA. Text in English. 1990. q. GBP 62 in United Kingdom; GBP 69 overseas (effective 2000). **Document type:** *Academic/Scholarly.* **Description:** Contains review articles and commentary on all aspects of critical limb ischemia and peripheral arterial occlusive disease, including pathophysiology, biochemistry, surgery, and clinical treatment.
Indexed: Excerp.Med. (1993-).
—BLDSC (3487.454100), CISTI, EMDOCS, GNLM, Infotrieve, KNAW. **CCC.**
Published by: Cambridge Medical Publications Ltd., Wicker House, High St, Worthing, W Sussex BN11 1DJ, United Kingdom. TEL 44-1903-205884, FAX 44-1903-234862, cmp@hbase.com, http://www.cambridge-medical.com.

616.12 USA ISSN 1535-282X
▼ **CRITICAL PATHWAYS IN CARDIOLOGY**; a journal of evidence-based medicine. Text in English. forthcoming 2002. q. USD 126 to individuals; USD 183 to institutions (effective 2002). *Refereed.* **Document type:** *Journal, Academic/Scholarly.* **Description:** Provides the latest details on diagnostic and therapeutic protocols for specific cardiac disorders.
Related titles: Online - full text ed.: USD 237.90 academic site license; USD 265.35 corporate site license (effective 2002).

Published by: Lippincott Williams & Wilkins (Philadelphia) (Subsidiary of: Wolters Kluwer N.V.), 530 Walnut St, Philadelphia, PA 19106-3621. TEL 215-521-8300, FAX 215-521-8902, custserv@lww.com, http://www.critpathcardio.com, http://www.lww.com/. Ed. Dr. Christopher P. Cannon. **Subscr. to:** PO Box 1600, Hagerstown, MD 21740-1600. TEL 800-638-3030, FAX 310-223-2400.

616.1 ITA ISSN 1122-7176
CUORE; rivista di cardiochirurgia e cardiologia. Text in Italian. 1994 (vol.11). bi-m. ITL 50,000; USD 50 foreign. *Refereed.*
—EMDOCS, GNLM, KNAW.
Published by: (Mediterranean Association of Cardiology and Cardiac Surgery), Casa Editrice Scientifica Internazionale Periodici s.a.s., Via Cremona, 19, Rome, RM 00161, Italy. TEL 39-6-44290783, FAX 39-6-44241-598.

616.12 ITA
CUORE E SALUTE. Text in Italian. 9/yr. adv. 2 cols./p.
Published by: Centro Lotta contra l'Infarto, Viale Bruno Buozzi, 60, Rome, RM 00197, Italy. TEL 39-6-3218205, FAX 39-6-3221068. Ed. Franco Fontanini. Adv. contact Sandra Delpapa. B&W page ITL 3,000,000, color page ITL 3,850,000; 260 x 190. Circ: 20,000.

616.136 USA ISSN 1523-3804
▼ **CURRENT ATHEROSCLEROSIS REPORTS.** Text in English. 1999. 6/yr. USD 163.95, GBP 120 to individuals; USD 327.95 to institutional members; USD 80, GBP 60 to students (effective 2002); Subscr. includes both print & online eds.. **Document type:** *Journal, Academic/Scholarly.*
Related titles: Online - full content ed.: USD 85, GBP 65 (effective 2002).
Indexed: Ind.Med.
—BLDSC (3494.267000).
Published by: Current Science Inc., 400 Market St, Ste 700, Philadelphia, PA 19106. TEL 800-427-1796, FAX 215-574-2225, info@current-reports.com, http://www.current-reports.com/cr_jrnl_home.cfm?JournalID=AT, http://www.current-science.com/. Ed. Antonio M Gotto. **Affiliate:** Current Science Ltd.

616.12 USA ISSN 1523-3782
CURRENT CARDIOLOGY REPORTS. Text in English. 6/yr. USD 163.95, GBP 120 to individuals; USD 327.95 to institutions; USD 80, GBP 60 to students (effective 2002); Subscr. includes both print & online eds.. **Document type:** *Journal, Academic/Scholarly.*
Related titles: Online - full content ed.: USD 85, GBP 65 (effective 2002).
Indexed: Ind.Med.
—BLDSC (3494.860000).
Published by: Current Science Inc., 400 Market St, Ste 700, Philadelphia, PA 19106. TEL 800-427-1796, FAX 215-574-2225, info@current-reports.com, http://www.current-reports.com/cr_jrnl_home.cfm?JournalID=CR, http://www.current-science.com/, http://www.current-science-group.com/. Ed. Joseph S Alpert. **Affiliate:** Current Science Ltd.

616.1 615 USA ISSN 1070-4345
RM345
CURRENT CARDIOVASCULAR DRUGS (YEAR). Text in English. 1992. biennial. USD 39.95. illus. **Document type:** *Academic/Scholarly, Trade.* **Description:** Guide to cardiovascular drugs; includes introductions to each drug class, and information on all US FDA approved drugs describing dosage guidelines and prescribing information and a full reference list.
Published by: Current Medicine, 400 Market St, Ste 700, Philadelphia, PA 19106. TEL 215-574-2257, 800-427-1796, FAX 215-574-2225. Ed. W H Frishman. **Subscr. outside N. America to:** Current Science Ltd, Middlesex House, 34-42 Cleveland St, London W1P 6LB, United Kingdom. TEL 44-20-7636-6911, 44-20-7323-0323.

616.12 GBR ISSN 1468-6708
▼ **CURRENT CONTROLLED TRIALS IN CARDIO VASCULAR MEDICINE.** Text in English. 2000. bi-m. GBP 200 in United Kingdom; USD 300 elsewhere (effective 2001). **Description:** Publishes commentaries, reviews, reports and original research relevant to cardiovascular controlled trials.
Published by: Current Science Ltd, Middlesex House, 34-42 Cleveland St, London W1P 6LB, United Kingdom. TEL 44-20-7323-0323, FAX 44-20-7580-1938, info@cvm.controlled-trials.com, http://cvm.controlled-trials.com/, http://www.currentsciencegroup.com. Eds. Bertram Pitt, Curt Furberg.

M

CURRENT CRITICAL PROBLEMS IN VASCULAR SURGERY. see *MEDICAL SCIENCES—Surgery*

616.1 USA ISSN 1079-1051
CURRENT DIAGNOSIS AND TREATMENT IN CARDIOLOGY. Text in English. 1995. irreg. **Document type:** *Monographic series.*
Published by: Appleton & Lange, Journal Division (Subsidiary of: Simon & Schuster Company), 11 W 19th St, New York, CT 10011-4209. TEL 203-406-4500, FAX 203-406-4600.

616.132 USA ISSN 1522-6417
CURRENT HYPERTENSION REPORTS. Text in English. 6/yr. USD 163.95, GBP 120 to individuals; USD 327.95 to institutions; USD 85, GBP 60 to students (effective 2002); Subscr. includes both print & online eds..
Related titles: Online - full content ed.: USD 85, GBP 65 (effective 2002).
Indexed: Ind.Med.
—BLDSC (3497.760000).
Published by: Current Science Inc., 400 Market St, Ste 700, Philadelphia, PA 19106. TEL 800-427-1796, FAX 215-574-2225, info@current-reports.com, http://www.current-reports.com/cr_jrnl_home.cfm?JournalID=HR, http://www.current-science.com/, http://www.current-science-group.com/. Ed. Norman K Hollenberg. **Affiliate:** Current Science Ltd.

616.12 USA ISSN 1523-3839
CURRENT INTERVENTIONAL CARDIOLOGY REPORTS. Text in English. 4/yr. USD 163.95, GBP 120 to individuals; USD 327.95 to institutions; USD 85, GBP 60 to students (effective 2002); Subscr. includes both print & online eds..
Related titles: Online - full content ed.: ISSN 1534-3103. USD 85, GBP 65 (effective 2002).
—BLDSC (3498.900000).
Published by: Current Science Inc., 400 Market St, Ste 700, Philadelphia, PA 19106. TEL 800-427-1796, FAX 215-574-2225, info@current-reports.com, http://www.current-reports.com/cr_jrnl_home.cfm?JournalID=IC, http://www.current-science.com/, http://www.current-science-group.com/. Ed. David R Holmes Jr. **Affiliate:** Current Science Ltd.

CURRENT MEDICAL LITERATURE. ADVANCES IN STROKE. see *MEDICAL SCIENCES—Abstracting, Bibliographies, Statistics*

CURRENT MEDICAL LITERATURE. CARDIAC IMAGING MONITOR. see *MEDICAL SCIENCES—Abstracting, Bibliographies, Statistics*

CURRENT MEDICAL LITERATURE. CARDIOLOGY. see *MEDICAL SCIENCES—Abstracting, Bibliographies, Statistics*

CURRENT MEDICAL LITERATURE. INTERVENTIONAL CARDIOLOGY MONITOR. see *MEDICAL SCIENCES—Abstracting, Bibliographies, Statistics*

616.2 USA ISSN 0268-4705
CODEN: COPCE3
CURRENT OPINION IN CARDIOLOGY. Text in English. 1986. bi-m. USD 249 domestic to individuals for print & online eds.; USD 249 foreign to individuals for print & online eds.; USD 585 per issue domestic to institutions; USD 585 per issue foreign to institutions; USD 91 newsstand/cover (effective 2002). adv. bibl. *Refereed.* **Document type:** *Academic/Scholarly.* **Description:** Directed toward clinicians and surgeons in cardiology. Presents review articles followed by annotated bibliographies of references consulted. Includes a bibliography of the current world literature published during the previous year.
Related titles: CD-ROM ed.; Diskette ed.; Online - full text ed.: USD 760.50 domestic academic site license; USD 760.50 foreign academic site license; USD 848.25 domestic corporate site license; USD 848.25 foreign corporate site license (effective 2002) (from Ovid Technologies, Inc., EBSCO Publishing, Swets Blackwell, Institute for Scientific Information); ♦ Supplement: Current Opinion in Cardiology. Supplement. ISSN 1354-7232.
Indexed: ASCA, CINAHL, Curr.Cont., Excerp.Med., Ind.Med. (1986-), Inpharma, Pharm.&Out.News, Reac., Sci.Cit.Ind.
—BLDSC (3500.773000), ADONIS, CISTI, EMDOCS, GNLM, IDS, ingenta, KNAW.
Published by: Lippincott Williams & Wilkins (Philadelphia) (Subsidiary of: Wolters Kluwer N.V.), 530 Walnut St, Philadelphia, PA 19106-3621. TEL 215-521-8300, FAX 215-521-8902, http://www.Lww.com. Ed. Robert Roberts. Pub. Maria McMichael. R&P Tobias Weschler. Adv. contact Kelly Adamitis. Circ: 4,187. **Subscr. to:** PO Box 1600, Hagerstown, MD 21740-1600.

616.12 USA ISSN 1354-7232
CURRENT OPINION IN CARDIOLOGY. SUPPLEMENT. Text in English. irreg.
Related titles: ♦ Supplement to: Current Opinion in Cardiology. ISSN 0268-4705.
Published by: Lippincott Williams & Wilkins (Philadelphia) (Subsidiary of: Wolters Kluwer N.V.), 530 Walnut St, Philadelphia, PA 19106-3621. TEL 215-521-8300, FAX 215-521-8902, custserv@lww.com, http://www.lww.com/.

616.1 GBR ISSN 0957-9672
QP751 CODEN: COPLEU
CURRENT OPINION IN LIPIDOLOGY. Text in English. 1990. bi-m. GBP 273 domestic to individuals for print & online eds.; USD 273 foreign to individuals for print & online eds. (effective 2002); USD 103 newsstand/cover; USD 665 per issue domestic to institutions; USD 665 per issue foreign to institutions (2002). bibl, illus. *Refereed.* **Document type:** *Academic/Scholarly.* **Description:** Directed toward cardiologists involved with lipids in research and clinical practice. Presents reviews and updates on the latest developments in all areas of lipidology. Each issue features a bibliography of the current world literature published during the previous year.
Related titles: CD-ROM ed.; Diskette ed.; Online - full text ed.: USD 864.50 domestic academic site license; USD 864.50 foreign academic site license; USD 964.25 domestic corporate site license; USD 964.25 foreign corporate site license (effective 2002) (from Ovid Technologies, Inc., EBSCO Publishing, Swets Blackwell, Institute for Scientific Information).
Indexed: ASCA, BBCI, Chem.Abstr., Chem.Indus.Notes, Chem.Titles, Curr.Cont., Dairy Sci.Abstr., Excerp.Med., Ind.Med. (1990-), Inpharma, Int.Abstr.Biol.Sci., Nutr.Abstr., Pharm.&Out.News, Reac., SSCI (coverage dropped), Sci.Cit.Ind.
—BLDSC (3500.775800), ADONIS, CASDDS, CISTI, EMDOCS, GNLM, IDS, KNAW.
Published by: Kluwer Academic & Lippencott-Raven (Subsidiary of: Wolters Kluwer N.V.), 2-6 Boundary Row, London SE1 8HN, United Kingdom. TEL 44-171-410-6600, FAX 44-171-410-6600, coinfo@rapidcom.co.uk, http://www.chapmanhall.com/li/default.html, http://www.Lww.com. Ed. Dr. S M Grundy. Circ: 2,954.

616.12 USA ISSN 0146-2806
CURRENT PROBLEMS IN CARDIOLOGY. Short title: C P C. Text in English. 1976. m. USD 115 domestic to individuals; USD 139 foreign to individuals; USD 186 domestic to individuals; USD 210 foreign to institutions; USD 56 domestic to students; USD 80 foreign to students; USD 18 newsstand/cover domestic (effective 2001). cum.index. back issues avail.; reprint service avail. from PQC. *Refereed.* **Description:** A fully referenced monographic journal that consists of original review articles on practical clinical topics.
Related titles: Microform ed.: (from PQC); Online - full text ed.: (from Institute for Scientific Information).
Indexed: ASCA, Curr.Cont., Excerp.Med., Ind.Med. (1976-), Ind.Sci.Rev., Inpharma, Pharm.&Out.News, Reac., SSCI (coverage dropped), Sci.Cit.Ind.
—BLDSC (3501.347000), CISTI, EMDOCS, GNLM, IDS, ingenta, KNAW. **CCC.**
Published by: Mosby, Inc. (Subsidiary of: Elsevier Science), 11830 Westline Industrial Dr, St Louis, MO 63146-3318. TEL 314-872-8370, 800-325-4177, FAX 314-432-1380, http://www.mosby.com/cpcardiol, http://www.mosby.com/periodicals. Ed. Robert A O'Rourke. Circ: 5,564.

616.1 USA ISSN 1068-4115
CURRENT REVIEW OF INTERVENTIONAL CARDIOLOGY. Text in English. 1994. irreg. **Document type:** *Monographic series, Academic/Scholarly.*
Published by: Current Medicine, 400 Market St, Ste 700, Philadelphia, PA 19106. TEL 215-574-2257, 800-427-1796, FAX 215-574-2225. **Subscr. outside N. America to:** Current Science Ltd, Middlesex House, 34-42 Cleveland St, London W1P 6LB, United Kingdom. TEL 44-20-7323-0323.

616.1 NLD
CURRENT STATUS OF CLINICAL CARDIOLOGY. Text in Dutch. 1985. irreg., latest 1990. back issues avail. *Refereed.* **Document type:** *Monographic series.*
Published by: Kluwer Academic Publishers Group (Subsidiary of: Wolters Kluwer N.V.), Spuiboulevard 50, PO Box 17, Dordrecht 3300 AA, Netherlands. FAX 31-78-639-2254, services@wkap.nl, http://www.wkap.nl. **Dist. by:** Journals Department, PO Box 322, Dordrecht 3300 AH, Netherlands. FAX 31-78-654-6474.

616.12 USA ISSN 1092-8464
CURRENT TREATMENT OPTIONS IN CARDIOVASCULAR MEDICINE. Text in English. 6/yr. USD 163.95 to individuals; USD 80 to students (effective 2002); Subscr. includes both print & online eds.. **Document type:** *Journal, Academic/Scholarly.*
Related titles: Online - full content ed.: USD 75 (effective 2002).
Published by: Current Science Inc., 400 Market St, Ste 700, Philadelphia, PA 19106. TEL 800-427-1796, FAX 215-574-2225, info@phl.cursci.com, http://www.treatment-options.com/cto_jrnl_home.cfm?JournalID=CM. Ed. Mark Creager. **Affiliate:** Current Science Ltd.

616.1 USA ISSN 1054-917X
CURRENTS IN EMERGENCY CARDIAC CARE. Text in English. 1990. q. USD 12 to individuals; USD 16 foreign to individuals; USD 20 to institutions; USD 24 foreign to institutions (effective 2000). bk.rev. *Refereed.* **Document type:** *Newsletter.* **Description:** For EMS personnel, healthcare professionals and instructors in CPR and advanced lifesaving. Offers scientific information about ideas, developments, and trends in emergency cardiac care, including stroke.
Related titles: Online - full content ed.
—CCC.
Published by: American Heart Association, Citizen CPR Foundation, 7272 Greenville Ave, Dallas, TX 75231-4596. TEL 214-706-1310, FAX 214-373-3461, fgs@amhrt.org, http://www.proed.net/ecc/currents/curr_menu.htm. Ed. F G Stoddard. R&P Debra Dirden. Circ: 22,000 (paid).

616.1 USA ISSN 1046-6959
DEVELOPMENTS IN CARDIOLOGY. Text in English. m. USD 150 domestic to individuals; USD 215 foreign to individuals; USD 160 domestic to institutions; USD 225 foreign to institutions. **Document type:** *Academic/Scholarly.* **Description:** Keeps readers up to date on the developments in the diagnosis and treatment of heart-related diseases.
Supersedes (in 1989): Progress in Cardiology (Philadelphia) (1041-3375)
—GNLM.
Published by: (Dannemiller Memorial Educational Foundation), W.B. Saunders Co. (Subsidiary of: Harcourt Publishers Ltd.), Curtis Center, Independence Sq W, Philadelphia, PA 19106-3399. TEL 215-238-7800, FAX 215-238-6445, http://www.wbsaunders.com. Ed. Dr. Gregory L Freeman. **Subscr. to:** Periodicals Fulfillment, W B Saunders Co, 6277 Sea Harbor Dr, 4th Fl, Orlando, FL 32891-4800.

616.1 NLD ISSN 0166-9842
CODEN: DCMEDM
DEVELOPMENTS IN CARDIOVASCULAR MEDICINE. Text in English. 1979. irreg., latest vol.156, 1994. price varies. *Refereed.* **Document type:** *Monographic series.*
Indexed: Chem.Abstr., Chem.Indus.Notes, Chem.Titles, INSPEC (coverage dropped).
—BLDSC (3579.067400), CASDDS, CISTI, Infotrieve, KNAW. **CCC.**
Published by: Kluwer Academic Publishers Group (Subsidiary of: Wolters Kluwer N.V.), Spuiboulevard 50, PO Box 17, Dordrecht 3300 AA, Netherlands. FAX 31-78-639-2254, services@wkap.nl, http://www.wkap.nl. **Dist. by:** Journals Department, PO Box 322, Dordrecht 3300 AH, Netherlands. FAX 31-78-654-6474.

615.65 ITA ISSN 0012-544X
DONO. Text in Italian. 1959. m. free per issue. illus, stat. **Description:** Contains health information and news of the organization, which is dedicated to blood donation in the Friuli region.
Published by: Associazione Friulana Donatori di Sangue, Ospedale General Regionale, Piazza della Misericordia, Udine, UD 33100, Italy. TEL 39-432-481818. Ed. Gianpaolo Sbaiz. Circ: 46,000.

616.12 IND
DR. MANI'S HEART SCOUT. Text in English. 1997. m. free per issue. **Document type:** *Newsletter.* **Description:** Includes articles on coronary artery stents, heart failure and heart diseases or defects.
Formerly: Heart Beat
Media: Online - full text.

Published by: Heart Disease Online, 955, 13th Main Rd., Anna Nagar West, Chennai, Tamil Nadu 600 040, India. TEL 91-44-626-7132, drmani@vsnl.com, http://www.dencats.org/heart/nl/nl.htm. Ed. S Sivasubramanian.

616.12 USA
E-CHOCARDIOGRAPHY; journal of cardiac ultrasound. Variant title: Echocardiography Journal. Text in English. 1995. bi-m. free per issue. *Refereed.* **Document type:** *Trade.* **Description:** Covers medical, cardiac ultrasound for physicians and other health care professionals.
Formerly: Echocardiography Journal of Cardiac Ultrasound
Related titles: Online - full text ed.
Published by: (Robert Wood Johnson Medical School, University of Medicine and Dentistry of New Jersey), Daniel Shindler, Ed.& Pub, 1 Gloucester Court, East Brunswick, NJ 08816. TEL 732-937-8727, FAX 732-937-8742, shindler@umdnj.edu, http://www2.umdnj.edu/~shindler. Circ: 50,000.

616.12 USA ISSN 0742-2822
ECHOCARDIOGRAPHY; a journal of cardiovascular ultrasound and allied techniques. Text in English. 1984. 8/yr. USD 195 domestic; USD 235 foreign; USD 292 to libraries; USD 30 newsstand/cover (effective 2000). adv. bk.rev. abstr. *Refereed.* **Document type:** *Academic/Scholarly.* **Description:** Contains articles on specific applications of diagnostic ultrasound and other related techniques. Includes special topics, panel discussions, case reports, bibliographic reviews and news items.
Related titles: Online - full text ed.: (from CatchWord Ltd., Institute for Scientific Information).
Indexed: ASCA, CINAHL, Curr.Cont., INSPEC, Ind.Med. (1984-), Inpharma, Pharm.&Out.News, Reac.
—BLDSC (3647.572500), ADONIS, CISTI, EMDOCS, GNLM, IDS, Infotrieve, ingenta, KNAW. **CCC.**
Published by: Futura Publishing Company, Inc., 135 Bedford Rd, PO Box 418, Armonk, NY 10504-0418. TEL 914-273-1014, 800-877-8761, lisa@futuraco.com. Ed. Dr. Navin C Nanda. R&P Joan McLaughlin. Adv. contact Lisa Piedimonte. B&W page USD 890, color page USD 1,825; trim 8.25 x 10.875. Circ: 2,623.

616.12 FRA
ENCYCLOPEDIE MEDICO-CHIRURGICALE. CARDIOLOGIE. Cover title: Traite de Cardiologie. Variant title: Encyclopedie Medico-Chirurgicale, Instantanes Medicaux. Cardiologie. Text in French. 1936. 4 base vols. plus q. updates. bibl, charts, illus. *Refereed.* **Document type:** *Academic/Scholarly.* **Description:** Offers cardiologists a comprehensive and up-to-date reference for diagnosing and treating cardiovascular diseases and conditions.
Former titles: Encyclopedie Medico-Chirurgicale. Cardiologie - Angeiologie (1166-4568); (until 1991): Encyclopedie Medico-Chirurgicale. Coeur - Vaisseaux (0246-0300)
Published by: Elsevier Paris, Editions Scientifiques et Medicales (Subsidiary of: Reed Elsevier plc. group), 23 rue Linois, Paris 75015, France. TEL 33-1-45589110, FAX 33-1-45589425, redaction-emc@elsevier.fr, redacion-emc@elsevier.fr, http://www.elsevier.fr, http://www.elsevier.com.

ENCYCLOPEDIE MEDICO-CHIRURGICALE. TECHNIQUES CHIRURGICALES. CHIRURGIE VASCULAIRE; la reference du chirurgien - actualisee en permanence. see *MEDICAL SCIENCES—Surgery*

ENCYCLOPEDIE MEDICO-CHIRURGICALE. TECNICHE CHIRURGICHE. CHIRURGIA VASCOLARE. see *MEDICAL SCIENCES—Surgery*

616.11 FRA ISSN 1251-3571
ETUDES & EVALUATIONS CARDIO-VASCULAIRES. Text in French. 1994. m. FRF 420 domestic to individuals; FRF 645, EUR 98.33 foreign to individuals; FRF 265 to students (effective 2001). adv. bk.rev. **Document type:** *Newspaper.* **Description:** For cardiovascular specialists wishing to keep up with the latest studies and opinions.
Published by: Apex, 1 et 3 Rue du Depart, Paris 75014, France. TEL 33-1-40640075, FAX 33-1-43222699, groupemeditions@wanadoo.fr. Ed. Jean Louis Gayet. Adv. contact Rene Michel.

616.1 GBR ISSN 1099-5129
▼ **EUROPACE**; European journal for cardiac pacing arrhythmias and cardiac electrophysiology. Variant title: European Journal for Cardiac Pacing Arrhythmias and Cardiac Electrophysiology. Text in English. 1999. q. GBP 64 to individuals; GBP 190 to institutions (effective 2002). *Refereed.* **Document type:** *Academic/Scholarly.* **Description:** Covers original papers and reviews in the fields of pacing and arrhythmias.
Related titles: Online - full text ed.: (from EBSCO Publishing, O C L C Online Computer Library Center, Inc., Swets Blackwell, IDEAL Online Library, Institute for Scientific Information).
Indexed: Curr.Cont., Ind.Med.
—BLDSC (3829.340450).
Published by: (European Society of Cardiology FRA, Working Group on Cardiac Pacing and Arrhythmias FRA), W.B. Saunders Co. Ltd. (Subsidiary of: Harcourt Publishers Ltd.), 24-28 Oval Rd, London NW1 7DX, United Kingdom. TEL 44-20-7424-4200, FAX 44-20-7424-4515, cservice@harcourt.com, http://www.harcourt-international.com/journals/eupc. Eds. Luc Jordaens, Richard Sutton. **Subscr. to:** Harcourt Publishers Ltd., Foots Cray High St, Sidcup, Kent DA14 5HP, United Kingdom. TEL 44-20-8308-5700, FAX 44-20-8309-0807.

EUROPEAN CONGRESS OF CARDIOLOGY. ABSTRACTS OF PAPERS. see *MEDICAL SCIENCES—Abstracting, Bibliographies, Statistics*

616.1 GBR ISSN 0423-7242
EUROPEAN CONGRESS OF CARDIOLOGY. PROCEEDINGS. Text in English. 1952. a. adv. **Document type:** *Proceedings.*
Published by: (European Society of Cardiology FRA), Academic Press (Subsidiary of: Harcourt Publishers Ltd.), 24 Oval Rd, London NW1 7DX, United Kingdom. TEL 44-20-7267-4466, FAX 44-20-7482-2293. R&P Catherine John. Adv. contact Nik Screen. **Subscr. to:** Harcourt Publishers Ltd., Foots Cray High St, Sidcup, Kent DA14 5HP, United Kingdom. TEL 44-20-8300-3322.

616.1 GBR ISSN 0195-668X
CODEN: EHJODF
EUROPEAN HEART JOURNAL. Text in English. 1980. 24/yr. GBP 148 to individuals; GBP 480 to institutions (effective 2002). adv. illus. index. reprint service avail. from SWZ. *Refereed.* **Document type:** *Journal, Academic/Scholarly.* **Description:** Directed to practicing cardiologists publishing original papers on all aspects of cardiovascular medicine and surgery.
Related titles: Online - full text ed.: (from EBSCO Publishing, O C L C Online Computer Library Center, Inc., RoweCom Information Quest, ingenta, Swets Blackwell, IDEAL Online Library, Institute for Scientific Information); ♦ Supplement: European Congress of Cardiology. Abstracts of Papers. ISSN 0421-7527.
Indexed: ASCA, Agri.& Environ.Biotech.Abstr. (coverage dropped), Chem.Abstr., Chem.Indus.Notes, Chem.Titles, Curr.Cont., Derwent Biotech.Abstr., Dok.Arbeitsmed., Excerp.Med., Helminthol.Abstr., Ind.Med. (1980-), Ind.Sci.Rev., Inpharma, Int.Nurs.Ind., Jrnl.Watch Card., NRN, Neurosci.Cit.Ind., Nutr.Abstr., Pharm.&Out.News, Reac., SSCI (coverage dropped), Sci.Cit.Ind., THA.
—BLDSC (3829.717500), CASDDS, CISTI, GNLM, IDS, Infotrieve, ingenta, KNAW. **CCC.**
Published by: (European Society of Cardiology FRA), W.B. Saunders Co. Ltd. (Subsidiary of: Harcourt Publishers Ltd.), 24-28 Oval Rd, London NW1 7DX, United Kingdom. TEL 44-20-7424-4200, FAX 44-20-7424-4515, cservice@harcourt.com, http://www.harcourt-international.com/journals/euhj. Ed. H E Kulbertus. **Subscr. to:** Harcourt Publishers Ltd., Foots Cray High St, Sidcup, Kent DA14 5HP, United Kingdom. TEL 44-20-8308-5700, FAX 44-20-8309-0807.

616.2 DEU ISSN 0939-6780
CODEN: EJCEEX
EUROPEAN JOURNAL OF CARDIAC PACING AND ELECTROPHYSIOLOGY. Text in English. 1991. q. DEM 195; DEM 255 foreign. adv. **Document type:** *Academic/Scholarly.*
—EMDOCS, GNLM, Infotrieve, KNAW. **CCC.**
Published by: E B M Erdmann-Brenger GmbH, Postfach 810225, Munich 81902, Germany. TEL 089-935779, FAX 089-9301943. Ed. Richard Sutton. Adv. contact K Brenger. B&W page DEM 4,500, color page DEM 7,485; trim 280 x 210.

616.1 NLD ISSN 1010-7940
EUROPEAN JOURNAL OF CARDIO-THORACIC SURGERY. Text in English. 1989. m. EUR 224 in Europe to individuals; JPY 29,800 in Japan to individuals; USD 251 elsewhere to individuals; EUR 510 in Europe to institutions; JPY 67,600 in Japan to institutions; USD 570 elsewhere to institutions (effective 2002). back issues avail. *Refereed.* **Document type:** *Academic/Scholarly.* **Description:** Documents progress made in cardiac and thoracic surgery, reporting on clinical and experimental advances relating to surgery of the heart, great vessels, and the chest.
Related titles: Online - full text ed.: (from HighWire Pr., EBSCO Publishing, ingenta, Swets Blackwell, ScienceDirect, Institute for Scientific Information).
Indexed: ASCA, Curr.Cont., Ind.Med. (1987-), Ind.Vet., Inpharma, Int.Nurs.Ind., Nutr.Abstr., Pharm.&Out.News, Reac., Sci.Cit.Ind.
—BLDSC (3829.725620), CISTI, GNLM, IDS, ingenta, KNAW. **CCC.**
Published by: Elsevier Science BV, PO Box 211, Amsterdam 1000 AE, Netherlands. http://www.elsevier.com/locate/ejcts. Ed. M Turina. **Subscr. in Australasia and the Far East to:** Elsevier Science (Singapore) Pte Ltd, No.1 Temasek Ave, 17-01 Millenia Tower, Singapore 039192, Singapore. TEL 65-434-3727, FAX 65-337-2230; **Subscr. in Japan to:** Elsevier Science Inc - Japan Regional Office, 9-15 Higashi-Azabu 1-chome, Minato-ku, Tokyo 106-0044, Japan. TEL 81-3-5561-5033; **Subscr. in the Americas to:** Elsevier Science, PO Box 945, New York, NY 10159-0945. TEL 212-633-3730, FAX 212-633-3680, usinfo-f@elsevier.com.

616.1 616.075 GBR ISSN 1525-2167
▼ **EUROPEAN JOURNAL OF ECHOCARDIOGRAPHY.** Text in English. 2000. q. GBP 64 to individuals; GBP 190 to institutions (effective 2002). **Document type:** *Academic/Scholarly.* **Description:** Articles on the ultrasonic examination of the cardiovascular system, including ischemic heart disease, valve disease, cardiomyopathy, congenial heart disease, and vascular disease.
Related titles: Online - full text ed.: (from EBSCO Publishing, O C L C Online Computer Library Center, Inc., Swets Blackwell, IDEAL Online Library).
—BLDSC (3829.728330).
Published by: (European Society of Cardiology FRA, Working Group on Echocardiography), Churchill Livingstone (Subsidiary of: Harcourt Publishers Ltd.), Robert Stevenson House, 1-3 Baxter's Pl, Leith Walk, Edinburgh, Midlothian EH1 3AF, United Kingdom. TEL 44-131-556-2424, FAX 44-131-489-1177, cservice@harcourt.com, http://www.harcourt-international.com/journals/euje. **Subscr. to:** Harcourt Publishers Ltd., Foots Cray High St, Sidcup, Kent DA14 5HP, United Kingdom. TEL 44-20-8308-5700, FAX 44-20-8309-0807.

616.12 NLD ISSN 1388-9842
CODEN: EJHF
▼ **THE EUROPEAN JOURNAL OF HEART FAILURE.** Text in English. 1999. bi-m. EUR 70 in Europe to individuals; JPY 9,300 in Japan to individuals; USD 79 elsewhere to individuals; EUR 311 in Europe to institutions; JPY 41,300 in Japan to institutions; USD 79 elsewhere to institutions (effective 2002). adv. bk.rev. charts, illus. *Refereed.* **Document type:** *Academic/Scholarly.* **Description:** Publishes research and reviews that advance knowledge in the field of heart failure in such areas as molecular and cellular biology, pathology, physiology, electrophysiology, pharmacology, and relevant demographics.
Related titles: Online - full text ed.: (from ingenta, Swets Blackwell, ScienceDirect, Institute for Scientific Information).
Indexed: Curr.Cont., Ind.Med., Inpharma, Pharm.&Out.News, Reac.
—BLDSC (3829.729860).
Published by: (European Society of Cardiology FRA), Elsevier Science BV, PO Box 211, Amsterdam 1000 AE, Netherlands. TEL 31-20-485-2911, FAX 31-20-485-2457, nlinfo-f@elsevier.nl. Ed. H Hillen. **Subscr. in Australasia and the Far East to:** Elsevier Science (Singapore) Pte Ltd, No.1 Temasek Ave, 17-01 Millenia Tower, Singapore 039192, Singapore. TEL 65-434-3727, FAX 65-337-2230; **Subscr. in Japan to:** Elsevier Science Inc - Japan Regional Office, 9-15 Higashi-Azabu 1-chome, Minato-ku, Tokyo 106-0044, Japan. TEL 81-3-5561-5033; **Subscr. in the Americas to:** Elsevier Science, PO Box 945, New York, NY 10159-0945. TEL 212-633-3730, FAX 212-633-3680.

616.1 GBR ISSN 1078-5884
CODEN: EJVSFZ
EUROPEAN JOURNAL OF VASCULAR AND ENDOVASCULAR SURGERY. Text in English. m. GBP 148 to individuals; GBP 507 to institutions (effective 2002). adv. bk.rev. reprint service avail. from SWZ. *Refereed.* **Document type:** *Journal, Academic/Scholarly.* **Description:** Covers all aspects of diagnosis, investigation, and management of vascular disorders. Includes papers on technical aspects of vascular surgery.
Formerly: European Journal of Vascular Surgery (0950-821X)
Related titles: Online - full text ed.: (from EBSCO Publishing, RoweCom Information Quest, Swets Blackwell, IDEAL Online Library, Institute for Scientific Information).
Indexed: ASCA, Curr.Cont., Excerp.Med., Ind.Med. (1995-), Inpharma, Int.Nurs.Ind., Neurosci.Cit.Ind., Pharm.&Out.News, Reac.

—BLDSC (3829.747280), CISTI, EMDOCS, GNLM, IDS, Infotrieve, ingenta, KNAW. **CCC.**
Published by: (European Society for Vascular Surgery), W.B. Saunders Co. Ltd. (Subsidiary of: Harcourt Publishers Ltd.), 24-28 Oval Rd, London NW1 7DX, United Kingdom. TEL 44-20-7424-4200, FAX 44-20-7424-4515, cservice@harcourt.com, http://www.harcourt-international.com/journals/ejvs. Ed. Torben Schroeder. Circ: 2,250. **Subscr. to:** Harcourt Publishers Ltd., Foots Cray High St, Sidcup, Kent DA14 5HP, United Kingdom. TEL 44-20-8308-5700, FAX 44-20-8309-0807.

616.1 FRA
EUROPEAN SOCIETY OF CARDIOLOGY. ANNUAL REPORT. Text in English. a. free per issue. **Document type:** *Corporate.* **Description:** Outlines the Society's activities over the past year and plans for the coming year. Discusses relevent issues.
Published by: European Society of Cardiology, Publishing Department, European Heart House, 2035 rte. des Colles, Les Templiers, BP 179, Sophia Antipolis Cedex 06903, France. TEL 33-4-92947600, FAX 33-4-92947601, blefevre@escardio.org, http://www.escardio.org.

616.1 FRA
EUROPEAN SOCIETY OF CARDIOLOGY. NEWSLETTER. Text in English. 1992. q. free per issue. back issues avail. **Document type:** *Newsletter.* **Description:** Informs members and other interested persons about new activities and developments at the Society.
Related titles: Online - full text ed.
Published by: European Society of Cardiology, Publishing Department, European Heart House, 2035 rte. des Colles, Les Templiers, BP 179, Sophia Antipolis Cedex 06903, France. TEL 33-4-92947600, FAX 33-4-92947601, blefevre@escardio.org, http://www.escardio.org.

616.1 GBR ISSN 1361-2611
EVIDENCE - BASED CARDIOVASCULAR MEDICINE. Text in English. 1997. q. GBP 70 to individuals; GBP 185 to institutions (effective 2002). adv. *Refereed.* **Document type:** *Journal, Academic/Scholarly.* **Description:** Helps clinicians to combine the best external evidence from systematic research with individual clinical expertise to make effective decisions about patient treatment and care.
Related titles: Online - full text ed.: (from EBSCO Publishing, O C L C Online Computer Library Center, Inc., Swets Blackwell, IDEAL Online Library).
—BLDSC (3831.036600).
Published by: Churchill Livingstone (Subsidiary of: Harcourt Publishers Ltd.), Robert Stevenson House, 1-3 Baxter's Pl, Leith Walk, Edinburgh, Midlothian EH1 3AF, United Kingdom. TEL 44-131-556-2424, FAX 44-131-459-1177, http://www.harcourt-international.com/journals/ebcm. Ed. Michael Kilborn. Pub. Gillian Griffith. R&P Greg Davies. Adv. contact David Dunnachie. **Subscr. to:** Harcourt Publishers Ltd., Foots Cray High St, Sidcup, Kent DA14 5HP, United Kingdom. TEL 44-20-8308-5700, FAX 44-20-8309-0807.

EXCERPTA MEDICA. SECTION 18: CARDIOVASCULAR DISEASES AND CARDIOVASCULAR SURGERY. see *MEDICAL SCIENCES—Abstracting, Bibliographies, Statistics*

615.65 FRA ISSN 0253-1321
F I O D S REVUE. Text in English. 1967. q. FRF 100. adv. bk.rev. illus.
Formerly (until 1980): Don Universel du Sang (0012-5407)
Related titles: French ed.; Spanish ed.
Published by: (Federation Internationale des Organisations de Donneurs de Sang Benevoles/International Federation of Blood Donors Organizations), F I O D S, c/o Vico Fresia, Dir., 34 Place Raoul Dautry, Paris Cedex 15 75748, France. TEL 45-38-71-93, FAX 43-20-33-87. Ed. Jean Gallard. Circ: 5,000.

616.1 ARG ISSN 0326-646X
FEDERACION ARGENTINA DE CARDIOLOGIA. REVISTA. Text in English, Spanish. 1972. q. back issues avail. **Document type:** *Academic/Scholarly.*
Related titles: Online - full text ed.
—CISTI.
Published by: Federacion Argentina de Cardiologia, 9o. B, Avda. Pueyrredon, 860, Capital Federal, Buenos Aires 1032, Argentina. TEL 54-114-9612557, FAX 54-114-9622765, http://www.fac.com.ar/. Ed. Raul Breglia.

616.1 USA ISSN 1067-5264 CODEN: FCCAEH
FUNDAMENTAL AND CLINICAL CARDIOLOGY. Text in English. 1991. irreg., latest vol.38, 1999. price varies. adv. **Document type:** *Monographic series.*
Indexed: Chem.Abstr., Chem.Indus.Notes, Chem.Titles, Curr.Cont. (coverage dropped).
—BLDSC (4056.031500), CASDDS, CISTI, Infotrieve. **CCC.**
Published by: Marcel Dekker, Inc., Attn: Eridania Perrez, 270 Madison Ave, New York, NY 10016-0602. TEL 212-696-9000, 800-228-1160, FAX 212-685-4540, marketing@dekker.com, http://www.dekker.com. Pub. Russell Dekker. R&P Julia Mulligan. Adv. contact Eridania Perez.

GEFAESSCHIRURGIE; Zeitschrift fuer vaskulaere und endovaskulaere Chirurgie. see *MEDICAL SCIENCES—Surgery*

616.136 ITA ISSN 0017-0224 CODEN: GIARA5
GIORNALE DELLA ARTERIOSCLEROSI. Text in Italian; Summaries in English. 1965. 3/yr. ITL 70,000, USD 60 (effective 2000). adv. **Description:** Features original articles, reviews and letters on topics of physiopathology, clinics and the therapy of arteriosclerosis.
Indexed: Chem.Abstr., Chem.Indus.Notes, Chem.Titles.
—CASDDS, GNLM.
Published by: (Societa Italiana di Gerontologia e Geriatria), C I C Edizioni Internazionali s.r.l., Corso Trieste 42, Rome, RM 00198, Italy. TEL 39-06-8412673, FAX 39-06-8412688, info@gruppocic.it, 1160199510. Pub. A Salvati. adv.: B&W page XEU 1,239.5, color page XEU 1,704.31; 210 x 280.

GLOSSARIUM CARDIOLOGIA. see *PHARMACY AND PHARMACOLOGY*

GUOWAI YIXUE (NAOXIEGUAN JIBING)/FOREIGN MEDICAL SCIENCES (CEREBROVASCULAR DISEASES). see *MEDICAL SCIENCES—Psychiatry And Neurology*

H L B NEWSLETTER; reporting on heart, lung and blood disease research policy development. see *MEDICAL SCIENCES—Experimental Medicine, Laboratory Technique*

HANDBOOK OF HYPERLIPIDAEMIA. see *MEDICAL SCIENCES—Abstracting, Bibliographies, Statistics*

616.132 NLD ISSN 0924-6541 CODEN: HAHYEK
HANDBOOK OF HYPERTENSION. Text in English. 1983. irreg., latest vol.18, 1997. price varies. back issues avail. *Refereed.* **Document type:** *Monographic series.*
Indexed: Chem.Abstr., Chem.Indus.Notes, Chem.Titles.
—BLDSC (4250.528000), CASDDS, CISTI.
Published by: Elsevier Science BV, Regional Sales Office, PO Box 211, Amsterdam 1000 AE, Netherlands. nlinfo-f@elsevier.nl, http://www.elsevier.nl. Eds. J L Reid, W H Birkenhaeger. **Subscr. in Australasia and the Far East to:** Elsevier Science (Singapore) Pte Ltd, No.1 Temasek Ave, 17-01 Millenia Tower, Singapore 039192, Singapore. TEL 65-434-3727, FAX 65-337-2230; **Subscr. in Japan to:** Elsevier Science Inc - Japan Regional Office, 9-15 Higashi-Azabu 1-chome, Minato-ku, Tokyo 106-0044, Japan. TEL 81-3-5561-5033; **Subscr. in the Americas to:** Elsevier Science, PO Box 945, New York, NY 10159-0945. TEL 212-633-3730, FAX 212-633-3680.

616.1 USA ISSN 1051-5313
HARVARD HEART LETTER. Text in English. 1990. m. USD 28 domestic; USD 40 in Canada; USD 47 elsewhere (effective 2000). illus. reprints avail. *Refereed.* **Document type:** *Newsletter, Consumer.* **Description:** Features articles and information on cardiovascular health for the lay reader.
Related titles: Online - full text ed.: (from Gale Group, Northern Light Technology, Inc., Factiva).
Indexed: Biol.Dig., CHNI.
Published by: (Harvard Medical School), Harvard Health Publications Group (Subsidiary of: Harvard Medical School), 164 Longwood Ave, Boston, MA 02115. TEL 617-432-1485, 800-829-9171, FAX 617-432-1506, jrudin@warren.med.edu, hhp@hms.harvard.edu, http://www.health.harvard.edu/newsletters/hrttext.html. Eds. Nancy Ferrari, Dr. Thomas H Lee. Circ: 150,000. **Subscr. to:** PO Box 420300, Palm Coast, FL 32142-0300.

HEALTHY WEIGHT JOURNAL; research, news and commentary across the weight spectrum. see *NUTRITION AND DIETETICS*

616.1 GBR ISSN 1355-6037
RC681.A1 CODEN: HEARFR
HEART. Text in English. 1939. m. GBP 130, USD 201 combined subscription to individuals includes print & online eds.; GBP 309, USD 476 to institutions for print only (effective 2002). adv. bk.rev. abstr, charts, illus. index, cum.index: 1939-1955; 1956-1967. *Refereed.* **Document type:** *Academic/Scholarly.* **Description:** Concentrates on providing current clinical information on cardiac diseases, conditions, and research.
Formerly (until 1996): British Heart Journal (0007-0769)
Related titles: CD-ROM ed.: (from Ovid Technologies, Inc.); Microform ed.: (from PQC); Online - full text ed.: Heart Online. 1997. USD 125, GBP 80 in United States to individuals (effective 2001); Institutions contact publisher for online rates. (from HighWire Pr., Ovid Technologies, Inc., Northern Light Technology, Inc., EBSCO Publishing, O C L C Online Computer Library Center, Inc., RoweCom Information Quest, ProQuest Information & Learning, ingenta, Swets Blackwell, Institute for Scientific Information).
Indexed: AIM, ASCA, Abstr.Hyg., Agri.& Environ.Biotech.Abstr. (coverage dropped), Aqua.Sci.& Fish.Abstr., Behav.Med.Abstr., Biol.Abstr., CINAHL, C.I.S. Abstr., Chem.Abstr., Curr.Adv.Ecol.Sci., Curr.Cont., Dent.Ind., Derwent Biotech.Abstr., Diab.Cont., Excerp.Med., Helminthol.Abstr., INIS Atomind., Ind.Med. (1996-), Ind.Sci.Rev., Inpharma, Int.Abstr.Biol.Sci., Int.Nurs.Ind., Jrnl.Watch Card., NRN, Neurosci.Cit.Ind., Nutr.Abstr., Pharm.&Out.News, Protozool.Abstr., Reac., Rev.Med.& Vet.Mycol., Risk Abstr., SSCI (coverage dropped), Sci.Cit.Ind., THA, Trop.Dis.Bull.
—BLDSC (4275.288900), ADONIS, CISTI, GNLM, IDS, ingenta, KNAW. **CCC.**
Published by: (British Cardiac Society), B M J Publishing Group, B M A House, Tavistock Sq, London WC1H 9JR, United Kingdom. TEL 44-20-7387-4499, FAX 44-20-7383-6400, info.norththames@bma.org.uk, http://www.heartjnl.com, http://www.bma.org.uk. Ed. R J Hall. Adv. contact Euan Currer TEL 44-20-7383-6181.

616.1 USA ISSN 1523-9004
HEART ADVISOR. Text in English. 1972. m. bk.rev. index. back issues avail. **Document type:** *Consumer.* **Description:** Provides current information on heart problems for the lay public.
Former titles: Heartline (8755-5271); (until 1985): Coronary Club Bulletin (8755-6308)
Indexed: Biol.Dig.
Published by: Cleveland Clinic Foundation, Cardia Club, 9500 Euclid Ave E37, Cleveland, OH 44195-5058. TEL 216-444-3690, FAX 216-444-9385, pashkof@cesmtp.ccf.org, http://www.heartcenter.org. Ed. Dr. Fredric J Pashkow. Circ: 10,000.

616.1 CAN
HEART AND STROKE FOUNDATION OF CANADA. ANNUAL REPORT. Text in English, French. 1956. a. free per issue.
Formerly: Canadian Heart Foundation. Annual Report (0068-8851)
Published by: Heart and Stroke Foundation of Canada, 222 Queen St, Ste 1402, Ottawa, ON K1P 5VP, Canada. TEL 613-569-4361, FAX 613-241-3278. Ed. J Fox. Circ: 3,000.

616.1 JPN ISSN 0910-8327 CODEN: HEVEEO
HEART AND VESSELS; an international journal. Text in English. 1985. bi-m. (in 1 vol., 6 nos./vol.). EUR 118 domestic; EUR 118.40 in Germany; EUR 66 newsstand/cover foreign for Print & Online Eds. (effective 2002). adv. bk.rev. index. back issues avail.; reprints avail. *Refereed.* **Document type:** *Academic/Scholarly.* **Description:** Publishes research, ideas, methods, and techniques on cardiovascular diseases.
Related titles: Microform ed.: (from PQC); Online - full content ed.: ISSN 1615-2573; Online - full text ed.: (from Swets Blackwell, Springer LINK, Institute for Scientific Information, RoweCom Information Quest).
Indexed: ASCA, Chem.Abstr., Curr.Cont., Excerp.Med., INIS Atomind., Ind.Med. (1985-), Inpharma, Pharm.&Out.News, Reac.
—BLDSC (4275.297000), CASDDS, CISTI, GNLM, IDS, ingenta, KNAW. **CCC.**

M

Published by: (Heart Institute of Japan, Tokyo), Springer-Verlag Tokyo (Subsidiary of: BertelsmannSpringer), 3-13 Hongo 3-chome, Bunkyo-ku, Tokyo 113-0033, Japan. TEL 81-3-3812-0617, FAX 81-3-3812-4699, orders@svt-ebs.co.jp, http://link.springer-ny.com/link/service/journals/00380/index.htm. Ed. Shigetake Sasayama. adv.: B&W page JPY 70,000. Circ: 1,000. **Subscr. in N. America to:** Springer-Verlag New York Inc., PO Box 2485, Secaucus, NJ 07096-2485. TEL 800-777-4643, 212-460-1526, FAX 201-348-4505, orders@springer-ny.com; **Subscr. to:** Springer-Verlag, c/o Gabriele Kubitza, Haberstrasse 7, Heidelberg 69126, Germany. TEL 49-6221-345242, FAX 49-6221-345229, subscriptions@springer.de, http://link.springer.de, http://link.springer-ny.com. **Co-sponsor:** Tokyo Women's Medical College.

616.1 IND ISSN 0046-7111
HEART CARE. Text in English. 1970. q. INR 10, USD 6. adv. bk.rev. charts, illus.
Published by: (Society for the Prevention of Heart Disease and Rehabilitation), Praga Publications, Churchgate, 43 Sundar Mahal, Mumbai, Maharashtra 400 020, India. Ed. C V Shah. Circ: 3,000.

616.1 USA ISSN 1521-737X
▼ **HEART DISEASE**; a journal of cardiovascular medicine. Text in English. 1999. bi-m. USD 170 domestic to individuals; USD 170 foreign to individuals; USD 256 domestic to institutions; USD 276 foreign to institutions (effective 2002).
Related titles: Online - full text ed.: USD 332.80 domestic for academic site license; USD 352.80 foreign for academic site license; USD 371.20 domestic for corporate site license; USD 391.20 foreign for corporate site license (effective 2002).
—BLDSC (4275.324000).
Published by: Lippincott Williams & Wilkins (Baltimore) (Subsidiary of: Wolters Kluwer N.V.), 12107 Insurance Way, Hagerstown, MD 21740. Ed. William H Frishman.

616.1 ESP
HEART DISEASE AND STROKE (EDICION ESPANOLA). Text in Spanish. bi-m. ESP 6,200, USD 48 (effective 1996).
Published by: Grupo Masson, Rda General Mitre, 149, Barcelona 08022, Spain. TEL 34-93-2530200, FAX 34-93-2530515, masson@masson.es, http://www.masson.es, http://masson.es.

616.1 USA
▼ **HEART DISEASES & DISORDERS SOURCEBOOK.** Text in English. 1999. irreg., latest 1999. USD 78 per issue (effective 2001). charts, bibl. Index. **Document type:** *Consumer.* **Description:** Supplies non-tecnical information to help people maintain healthy hearts.
Published by: Omnigraphics, Inc., 615 Griswold St, Detroit, MI 48226. TEL 313-961-1340, 800-234-1340, FAX 313-961-1383, 800-875-1340, info@omnigraphics.com, jjts@sprynet.com, http://www.omnigraphics.com/cgi-bin/loadpage.cgi?user_id=1567&file=0-7808-0238-1.html. Ed. Karen Bellenir.

▼ **HEART DRUG.** see *PHARMACY AND PHARMACOLOGY*

616.1 USA ISSN 1382-4147
RC685.C53 CODEN: HFREFC
HEART FAILURE REVIEWS. Text in English. 1996. q. USD 366, EUR 366 to institutions for print or online ed.; USD 439.20, EUR 439.20 to institutions for print & online eds. combined (effective 2002). *Refereed.* **Document type:** *Journal, Academic/Scholarly.* **Description:** Develops links between basic scientists and clinical investigators, creating a unique, interdisciplinary dialogue focused on heart failure, its pathogenesis and treatment. Topics covered include clinical and surgical approaches to therapy, basic pharmacology, biochemistry, molecular biology, pathology, and electrophysiology.
Related titles: Online - full text ed.: (from EBSCO Publishing, O C L C Online Computer Library Center, Inc., RoweCom Information Quest, Swets Blackwell, Kluwer Online).
Indexed: Chem.Abstr., Chem.Indus.Notes, Chem.Titles, Inpharma, Pharm.&Out.News, Reac.
—BLDSC (4275.342200), CASDDS, Infotrieve, KNAW. **CCC.**
Published by: Kluwer Academic Publishers Boston, 101 Philip Dr, Assinippi Park, Norwell, MA 02061. TEL 781-871-6600, FAX 781-871-9045, services@wkap.nl, http://www.wkap.nl/journalhome.htm/1382-4147. Eds. Hani N Sabbah, Dr. Sidney Goldstein. R&P Rose Luongo TEL 781-871-6311. **Subscr. to:** Kluwer Academic - Plenum Publishers, 233 Spring St, New York, NY 10013-1578. TEL 212-620-8468, FAX 212-807-1047; **Subscr. to outside the Americas to:** Kluwer Academic Publishers Group, Journals Department, PO Box 322, Dordrecht 3300 AH, Netherlands. TEL 31-78-639-2392, FAX 31-78-654-6474.

616.1 AUS ISSN 1443-9506
HEART, LUNG & CIRCULATION. Text in English. 1991. 3/yr. AUD 138 domestic to individuals; AUD 125 in New Zealand to individuals; USD 125 elsewhere to individuals; AUD 343 domestic to institutions; AUD 311 in New Zealand to institutions; USD 190 elsewhere to institutions; AUD 152 domestic to individuals print & online eds.; AUD 138 in New Zealand to individuals print & online eds.; USD 138 elsewhere to individuals print & online eds.; AUD 378 domestic to institutions print & online eds.; AUD 343 in New Zealand to institutions print & online eds.; USD 209 elsewhere to institutions print & online eds. (effective 2001). adv. bk.rev. abstr. illus. back issues avail. *Refereed.* **Document type:** *Journal, Academic/Scholarly.* **Description:** Provides a forum for scientific articles, technical papers and other communications of interest to cardiologists and cardiac and thoracic surgeons.
Former titles (until 2000): The Asia Pacific Heart Journal (1328-0163); (until 1996): Asia Pacific Journal of Thoracic and Cardiovascular Surgery (1324-2881); (until 1993): Australasian Journal of Cardiac and Thoracic Surgery (1037-2091)
Related titles: ♦ Online - full text ed.: Heart, Lung & Circulation Online. ISSN 1444-2892.
—BLDSC (4275.347000).
Published by: Blackwell Science Asia Pty Ltd, PO Box 378, Carlton South, VIC 3053, Australia. TEL 61-3-9347-0300, FAX 61-3-9347-5001, info@blacksci-asia.com.au, http://www.blackwell-science.com/~cgilib/jnlpage.bin?Journal=hlc&File=hlc&Page=aims, http://www.blacksci.co.uk/australi. Ed. Franklin Rosenfeldt.

616.1 AUS ISSN 1444-2892
HEART, LUNG & CIRCULATION ONLINE. Text in English. 3/yr. AUD 125 domestic to individuals; AUD 113 in New Zealand to individuals; USD 113 elsewhere to individuals; AUD 309 domestic to institutions; AUD 280 in New Zealand to institutions; USD 171 elsewhere to institutions (effective 2001). *Refereed.* **Document type:** *Academic/Scholarly.*
Media: Online - full text (from EBSCO Publishing, O C L C Online Computer Library Center, Inc., ingenta, Munksgaard & Blackwell Science's Synergy, Swets Blackwell, RoweCom Information Quest). **Related titles:** ♦ Print ed.: Heart, Lung & Circulation. ISSN 1443-9506.
Published by: Blackwell Science Asia Pty Ltd, PO Box 378, Carlton South, VIC 3053, Australia. TEL 61-3-9347-0300, FAX 61-3-9347-3016, website@blacksci.com, info@blacksci-asia.com.au, http://www.blackwell-science.com/~cgilib/jnlpage.bin?Journal=hlc&File=hlc&Page=aims, http://www.blacksci.co.uk/australi.

617.412 USA ISSN 1522-6662
THE HEART SURGERY FORUM; A Cardiothoracic Multimedia Journal. Text in English. 1998. q. USD 125 in North America; USD 175 elsewhere (effective 2000). abstr, illus. 98 p./no. 3 cols./p. back issues avail.; reprints avail. *Refereed.* **Document type:** *Journal, Academic/Scholarly.* **Description:** Designed for cardiothoracic surgery personnel, featuring full multimedia sound, video, color stills images and text.
Media: CD-ROM. **Related titles:** Online - full text ed.; Print ed.
Indexed: Curr.Cont.
Published by: The Heart Surgery Forum, 1224 W Main St, Ste 200, Charlottesville, VA 22903. TEL 804-817-2000, gbranch@cjp.com, http://www.hsforum.com/. Ed. Dr. Mark Levinson. Pub. William T jCarden Jr. Adv. contact Marc Weathersby. Circ: 1,379 (paid).

THE HEARTH BEAT. see *PHYSICAL FITNESS AND HYGIENE*

616.12 USA
HEARTLINX. Text in English. d. adv. **Document type:** *Newsletter.* **Description:** Includes medical news and information covering cardiology and heart diseases.
Media: Online - full text.
Published by: MDLinx.com Inc, 316 F St NE Ste 200, Washington, DC 20002. TEL 202-543-6544, FAX 202-543-6674, info@mdlinx.com, http://www.heartlinx.com/. Ed. Dave Rothenberg.

616.1 USA
HEARTROM. Text in English. 1998. irreg. USD 30. **Description:** Offers reviews of topics in cardiology and cardiovascular surgery.
Media: CD-ROM.
Published by: Amadeus Multimedia Technologies, Ltd., One Bridge St Ste 93, Irvington, NY 10533. TEL 914-591-0028, FAX 914-591-0083, amadeus@webaxis.com, http://www.amadeusmultimedia.com.

616.1 GRC ISSN 1011-7970
CODEN: HLKEA
HELLENIC JOURNAL OF CARDIOLOGY/HELLENIKI KARDIOLOGIKI EPITHEORISI. Text in English, Greek. 1960. bi-m. USD 150 (effective 1998). adv. bk.rev. Supplement avail. *Refereed.* **Document type:** *Academic/Scholarly.* **Description:** Disseminates cardiologic research.
Indexed: Excerp.Med.
—BLDSC (4285.435500), GNLM.
Published by: Hellenic Cardiological Society/Hellenikis Kardiologikis Etaireias, 6 Potamianou St, Athens 115 28, Greece. TEL 30-1-7221-633, FAX 30-1-7226-139, TELEX 222408 HE CS, http://www.eexi.gr/hcs. Ed. H Toutouzas. Adv. contact A Daskaloupoulos. Circ: 2,000.

616.15 GBR ISSN 1466-4860
▼ **THE HEMATOLOGY JOURNAL**; the official journal of the European Haematology Association. Text in English. 2000. bi-m. GBP 57 in Europe to individuals; GBP 93 rest of world to individuals; GBP 170 in Europe to institutions; GBP 214 rest of world to institutions (effective 2000). **Document type:** *Journal, Academic/Scholarly.* **Description:** Includes papers concerning all aspects of hematological research.
Related titles: Online - full text ed.: (from ingenta, Swets Blackwell, RoweCom Information Quest).
Indexed: Biotech.& Bioeng.Abstr., Med.& Pharm.Biotech.Abstr.
—BLDSC (4291.605000).
Published by: Nature Publishing Group Specialist Journals (Subsidiary of: Holtzbrink Publishers), Houndmills, Basingstoke, Hants RG21 6XS, United Kingdom. TEL 44-1256-329242, FAX 44-1256-328339, subscriptions@nature.com, http://www.nature.com/thj.

616.12 DEU ISSN 0340-9937
CODEN: HERZDW
HERZ; kardiovaskulaere Erkraenkungen. Text in German, English. 1976. 8/yr. EUR 189.64 domestic; EUR 196.64 foreign; EUR 113.93 domestic to students; EUR 120.93 foreign to students; EUR 37.38 newsstand/cover (effective 2002). *Refereed.* **Document type:** *Journal, Academic/Scholarly.*
Related titles: Online - full text ed.: ISSN 1615-6692 (from EBSCO Publishing, RoweCom Information Quest, Swets Blackwell, Springer LINK, Institute for Scientific Information).
Indexed: ASCA, Curr.Cont., Excerp.Med., INIS Atomind., Ind.Med. (1976-), Ind.Sci.Rev., Inpharma, Int.Nurs.Ind., Pharm.&Out.News, Reac., Ref.Zh., Sci.Cit.Ind.
—BLDSC (4300.396000), CISTI, EMDOCS, GNLM, IDS, ingenta, KNAW. **CCC.**
Published by: Urban und Vogel Medien und Medizin Verlagsgesellschaft mbH (Subsidiary of: BertelsmannSpringer), Neumarkter Str 43, Munich 81673, Germany. TEL 49-89-43721411, FAX 49-89-43721410, verlag@urban-vogel.de, http://www.urban-vogel.de. Pub., R&P Oliver Renn. Adv. contact Sibylle Schurr TEL 49-89-43721353. Circ: 4,000. **Subscr. to:** Springer Auslieferungs Gesellschaft, Postfach 105160, Heidelberg 69041, Germany. TEL 49-6221-345244, FAX 49-6221-345244.

616.1 DEU ISSN 0046-7324
CODEN: HZKLAV
HERZ KREISLAUF; Zeitschrift fuer Kardiologie und Angiologie in Klinik und Praxis. Text in German. 1969. m. DEM 210; DEM 228 in Europe. adv. bk.rev. bibl, charts, illus. *Refereed.* **Document type:** *Academic/Scholarly.*
Indexed: ASCA, Chem.Abstr., Chem.Indus.Notes, Chem.Titles, Curr.Cont. (coverage dropped), Excerp.Med., INIS Atomind., Ind.Sci.Rev., Inpharma, Reac., SSCI (coverage dropped), Sci.Cit.Ind. (coverage dropped).
—CASDDS, CISTI, GNLM, IDS, Infotrieve, KNAW. **CCC.**

M

Published by: (Deutsche Gesellschaft fuer Praevention und Rehabilitation von Herz-Kreislauf-Erkrankungen e.V.), Richard Pflaum Verlag GmbH und Co. KG, Lazarettstr 4, Munich 80636, West Germany. TEL 49-89-12607-0, FAX 49-89-12607202. Ed. K W Westermann. Adv. contact I Brandl. Circ: 20,200.
Subscr. to: Postfach 190737, Munich 80607, Germany.

616.1 DEU ISSN 0720-0730
HERZ UND GEFAESSE; Zeitschrift fuer praktische Kardioangiologie. Text in German. 1981-1993; resumed 199?. q. DEM 30 (effective 1999). adv. bk.rev. index. **Document type:** *Journal, Academic/Scholarly, Trade.*
Indexed: Excerp.Med.
—GNLM.
Published by: Demeter Verlag GmbH und Co. KG, Ruedigerstr 14, Stuttgart 70469, Germany. TEL 49-711-8931-0, FAX 49-711-8931322. Circ: 27,000.

616.1 DEU ISSN 0944-260X
HERZ UND GESUNDHEIT. Text in German. ceased 1986; resumed. 4/yr. DEM 24. **Document type:** *Academic/Scholarly.*
Published by: Deutsche Herzhilfe e.V., Pestalozzistr 3A, Munich 80469, Germany. TEL 49-89-2603636, FAX 49-89-269148, deutsche-herzhilde@e-v.de. Eds. A Kroedel, Peter Mand.

616.1 DEU ISSN 0938-7412
CODEN: HEELFT
HERZSCHRITTMACHERTHERAPIE UND ELEKTROPHYSIOLOGIE; german journal of cardiac pacing and electrophysiology. Text in German; Summaries in English. 1990. q. EUR 206.26 domestic; EUR 203.16 in Germany; USD 255.16 foreign (effective 2002). adv. bk.rev. bibl, charts, illus. back issues avail.; reprints avail. **Document type:** *Journal, Academic/Scholarly.*
Related titles: Online - full text ed.: ISSN 1435-1544 (from EBSCO Publishing, RoweCom Information Quest, Swets Blackwell, Springer LINK).
—GNLM, Infotrieve. **CCC.**
Published by: Dr. Dietrich Steinkopff Verlag (Subsidiary of: BertelsmannSpringer), Poststr 9, Darmstadt 64293, Germany. TEL 49-6151-82899-0, FAX 49-6151-82899-40, frey.steinkopff@springer.de, http://www.steinkopff.springer.de. Ed. H D Esperer H Klein. R&P Sabine Ibkendanz. Circ: 1,500. **Subscr. in N. America to:** Springer-Verlag, Journals; **Subscr. to:** Springer GmbH Auslieferungsgesellschaft, Haberstr 7, Heidelberg 69126, Germany. TEL 49-6221-345239, FAX 49-6221-345249.

616.132 ESP ISSN 0212-8241
HIPERTENSION. Text in Spanish. 1984. 10/yr. USD 70 (effective 1996).
Published by: Editorial Idepsa S.A., Principe de Vergara, 112 1o F, Madrid 28002, Spain. TEL 34-1-5637306, FAX 34-1-4632393.

HIROSAKI DAIGAKU IGAKUBU EISEIGAKU KYOSHITSU GYOSEKISHU. see *MEDICAL SCIENCES*

616.1 616.2 SWE
HJAERT-LUNGFONDENS KVARTALSSKRIFT. Text in Swedish. 1960. q. SEK 22 to members (effective 1998). back issues avail.
Former titles (until 1988): Hjaerta Kaerl Lungor (0280-4638); (until 1982): Svenska Nationalfoereningen Mot Hjaert- och Lungsjukdomar (0373-2665)
Published by: Hjaert-Lungfonden/Swedish Heart Lung Foundation, Riddargatan 18, Stockholm 11451, Sweden. TEL 46-8-56-62-42-004, FAX 46-8-56-62-42-29. Ed. Gunilla Lockne. Circ: 13,000.

616.1 ISL ISSN 1022-4955
HJARTAVERND. Text in Icelandic. 1964. a. ISK 250, USD 3.50 (effective 2000). charts, illus. cum.index. back issues avail. **Document type:** *Academic/Scholarly.* **Description:** Features articles on cardiovascular disease and risk factors in Iceland.
Address: Lagmuli 9, Reykjavik 108, Iceland. TEL 354-535-1800, FAX 354-535-1801, http://www.hjarta.is. Ed., R&P Astros Sverrisdottir. Adv. contact Hjoerdis Kroyer. Circ: 5,000.

616.1 DNK ISSN 0105-9785
HJERTEFORENINGEN. Text in Danish. 1978. a. free per issue. illus.
Address: Hauser Plads 10, Copenhagen K 1127, Denmark.

616.1 DNK ISSN 0108-8904
HJERTENYT; orientering om sundhed og praeventiv medicin. Text in Danish. 1982. irreg. free per issue. adv.
Published by: Hjerteforeningen, Hauser Plads 10, Copenhagen K 1127, Denmark. Ed. Arne Kurdahl. Pub. Arhuus Stiftsbogtrykkerie. R&P Hanne Hauerslev TEL 33931788. Adv. contact Stibo Media.

616.1 USA ISSN 0194-911X
RC685.H8 CODEN: HPRTDN
HYPERTENSION. Text in English. 1979. m. USD 244 domestic to individuals for print & online eds.; USD 322 foreign to individuals for print & online eds.; USD 382 domestic to institutions for print & online eds.; USD 440 foreign to institutions for print & online eds.; USD 40 newsstand/cover (effective 2002). adv. index. back issues avail.; reprint service avail. from PQC. *Refereed.* **Document type:** *Academic/Scholarly.* **Description:** For cardiologists, internists, and researchers; reports clinical and laboratory investigations in hypertension.
Incorporates (1957-1977): Council for High Blood Pressure Research. Proceedings (0073-425X)
Related titles: CD-ROM ed.: (from Ovid Technologies, Inc.); Microform ed.: (from PQC); Online - full text ed.: USD 496.60 domestic academic site license; USD 554.60 foreign academic site license; USD 553.90 domestic corporate site license; USD 611.90 foreign corporate site license (effective 2002) (from HighWire Pr., Ovid Technologies, Inc., Northern Light Technology, Inc., EBSCO Publishing, ProQuest Information & Learning, Institute for Scientific Information).
Indexed: Agri.& Environ.Biotech.Abstr. (coverage dropped), Biol.Abstr., Curr.Adv.Gen.& Molec.Biol., Curr.Cont., Dent.Ind., Derwent Biotech.Abstr., Excerp.Med., INIS Atomind., Ind.Med. (1979-), Ind.Sci.Rev., Int.Abstr.Biol.Sci., Jrnl.Watch Card., Kidney, Ref.Zh., Risk Abstr., Sci.Cit.Ind.
—BLDSC (4352.629000), CASDDS, CISTI, GNLM, IDS, ingenta, KNAW.
Published by: (American Heart Association), Lippincott Williams & Wilkins (Baltimore) (Subsidiary of: Wolters Kluwer N.V.), 351 W Camden St, Baltimore, MD 21201-2436. TEL 410-528-4000, 301-223-2307, 800-787-8984, FAX 410-528-4312, 301-223-2327, http://www.hyper.ahajournals.org. Ed. Dr. Edward D. Pub. Cara Kaufman. R&P Debbie Heise TEL 410-528-4050. Adv. contact Angela Hopkins. Circ: 4,100.

616.12 FRA ISSN 1279-5623
HYPERTENSION ET PREVENTION CARDIOVASCULAIRE. Text in French. 1988. m. FRF 460, EUR 70.12 domestic to individuals; FRF 580, USD 105 foreign to individuals; FRF 580, EUR 88.42 domestic to institutions; FRF 700, USD 127 foreign to institutions; FRF 290 domestic to students; USD 75 foreign to students (effective 2000). adv. Supplement avail. *Refereed.* **Document type:** *Academic/Scholarly.*
Formerly (until 1997): Hypertension (0997-7287)
Published by: Medica-Press International, 62-64 rue Jean-Jaures, Puteaux 92800, France. TEL 33-1-41458000, FAX 33-1-41458025, contact@edimark.fr, http://www.edimark.fr. Ed. X Girerd. Pub. Claudie Damour Terrasson.

616.1 618.2 USA ISSN 1064-1955
RG580.H9 CODEN: HYPPEV
HYPERTENSION IN PREGNANCY. Text in English. 1982. 3/yr. USD 95 to individuals print & online eds.; USD 825 to institutions print only (effective 2002). adv. *Refereed.* **Document type:** *Academic/Scholarly.* **Description:** Publishes data pertaining to human and animal hypertension during gestation.
Formerly: Clinical and Experimental Hypertension. Part B: Hypertension in Pregnancy (0730-0085); Which supersedes in part: Clinical and Experimental Hypertension (0148-3927)
Related titles: Microform ed.: (from RPI); Online - full text ed.: (from EBSCO Publishing, O C L C Online Computer Library Center, Inc., RoweCom Information Quest, Swets Blackwell, Institute for Scientific Information).
Indexed: ASCA, Agri.& Environ.Biotech.Abstr. (coverage dropped), Biol.Dig., Chem.Abstr., Chem.Indus.Notes, Chem.Titles, Curr.Adv.Ecol.Sci., Curr.Cont., Derwent Biotech.Abstr., Excerp.Med., Ind.Med. (1993-), Ind.Sci.Rev., Inpharma, Int.Abstr.Biol.Sci., Kidney, Pharm.&Out.News, Reac., Ref.Zh., Sci.Cit.Ind.
—BLDSC (4352.635260), CASDDS, CISTI, EMDOCS, GNLM, IDS, Infotrieve, ingenta, KNAW. **CCC.**
Published by: (International Society for the Study of Hypertension in Pregnancy), Marcel Dekker Inc., 270 Madison Ave, New York, NY 10016. TEL 212-696-9000, 800-228-1160, FAX 212-685-4540, journals@dekker.com, http://www.dekker.com/servlet/product/productid/PRG. Eds. Fiona Lyall, Michael A Belfort. Adv. contact Anne Mullins. B&W page USD 760. Circ: 800.

616.1 JPN
CODEN: HRESE4
HYPERTENSION RESEARCH. Text in English. 1978. bi-m. USD 120 to individuals (effective 2001). adv. 100 p./no. *Refereed.* **Document type:** *Journal, Academic/Scholarly.* **Description:** Publishes articles on worldwide research topics of hypertension.
Former titles: Hypertension Research - Clinical and Experimental (0916-9636); (until 1991): Koketsuatsu (0288-0032)
Related titles: Online - full text ed.: (from Institute for Scientific Information).
Indexed: Biol.Abstr., Chem.Abstr., Chem.Indus.Notes, Chem.Titles, Curr.Cont., Excerp.Med. (1993-), Ind.Med. (1992-), Inpharma, Reac., Sci.Cit.Ind. (coverage dropped).
—BLDSC (4352.635270), CASDDS, CISTI, EMDOCS, GNLM, IDS, KNAW.
Published by: Japanese Society of Hypertension, Center for Academic Societies Osaka/Nihon Koketsuatsu Gakkai, Senri Life Science Center Bldg 14th Fl, 1-4-2 Shinsenri-Higashi-Machi, Toyonaka-shi, Osaka 565-0082, Japan. TEL 81-6-6873-2301, FAX 81-6-6873-2300, o-edit@bcasj.or.jp. Ed. Kunio Hiwada. Circ: 2,800 (paid and controlled).

616.12 617 JPN
I S C T S - WORLD SOCIETY OF CARDIO - THORACIC SURGEONS. ANNUAL MEETING. Text in English, Japanese. 1988. a. adv. *Refereed.* **Document type:** *Academic/Scholarly.*
Formerly: International Society of Cardio-Thoracic Surgeons. Annual Meeting
Published by: I S C T S - World Society of Cardio-Thoracic Surgeons, I.P.O. Box 5048, Tokyo 100-3191, Japan. TEL 81-3-5800-5090, FAX 81-3-5800-5090. Ed., Adv. contact Susumu Tanaka. Circ: 500 (controlled).

616.1 ESP ISSN 1136-5943
IBEROAMERICAN JOURNAL OF HYPERTENSION. Text in Spanish. 1993. 10/yr. **Document type:** *Academic/Scholarly.* **Description:** Publishes experimental and clinical research into the etiology and cure of hypertension.
Former titles (until 1996): International Journal of Hypertension. Edicion Iberoamericana (1136-4092); (1993-1995): Journal of Hypertension. Edicion Espanola (1133-7354)
Published by: Ediciones Doyma S.A., Traversa de Gracia, 17-21, Barcelona 08021, Spain. TEL 34-93-200-0711, FAX 34-93-209-1136, comercial@doymanet.net, doyma@doyma.es, http://www.doyma.es/. Ed. Carlos Herrera. adv.: color page ESP 238,000; trim 280 x 210. Circ: 3,000.

616.12 FRA ISSN 0220-2476
L'INFORMATION CARDIOLOGIQUE. Text in French. 1978. 11/yr. FRF 420 to individuals; FRF 490 foreign to individuals; FRF 290 to students; FRF 360 foreign to students. adv. bk.rev.
Related titles: English ed.: Editorials in Cardiology. ISSN 1259-492X.
—GNLM.
Published by: (Centre Cardiologique du Nord), Publications Medicales, 32-36 av. des Moulins Gemeaux, Saint-Denis Cedex 93207, France. TEL 33-1-49-33-41-08, FAX 33-1-49-33-41-40. Ed. A Castillo Fenoy. Adv. contact A. Castillo Fenoy. Circ: 2,500.

616.12 ITA
INFORMAZIONE CARDIOLOGICA. Text in Italian. m.
Address: Viale Verdi, 18, Novara, NO 28100, Italy. TEL 39-321-36331. Ed. Dr. Paolo Rossi. Circ: 7,000.

INTERNAL MEDICINE NEWS. see *MEDICAL SCIENCES—Internal Medicine*

616.1 ITA ISSN 0392-9590
CODEN: INANEK
INTERNATIONAL ANGIOLOGY. Text in English. q. USD 105 to individuals; USD 155 to institutions (effective 1999). adv. *Refereed.* **Document type:** *Academic/Scholarly.* **Description:** Addresses latest news concerning the vascular system, vascular pathophysiology and therapy.
Related titles: Online - full text ed.: (from Northern Light Technology, Inc., ProQuest Information & Learning, Institute for Scientific Information).
Indexed: ASCA, Curr.Cont., Excerp.Med., Ind.Med. (1982-), Inpharma, Pharm.&Out.News, Reac., Sci.Cit.Ind. (coverage dropped).
—BLDSC (4535.770000), CISTI, EMDOCS, GNLM, IDS, ingenta, KNAW.

M

Published by: (International Union of Angiology), Edizioni Minerva Medica, Corso Bramante, 83-85, Turin, TO 10126, Italy. TEL 39-11-678282, FAX 39-11-674502. Ed. P Balas. Pub. Alberto Oliaro. Adv. contact F Filippo. B&W page USD 1,200, color page USD 2,000; trim 280 x 215. Circ: 5,000 (paid).

616.12 USA ISSN 0173-0282
INTERNATIONAL BOEHRINGER MANNHEIM. SYMPOSIA. Text in English. 1976. irreg., latest 1983. price varies. reprint service avail. from ISI. **Document type:** *Proceedings.*
Published by: Springer-Verlag, Journals (Subsidiary of: BertelsmannSpringer), 175 Fifth Ave, New York, NY 10010. TEL 212-460-1500, FAX 212-473-6272.

616.13 GRC ISSN 0074-347X
INTERNATIONAL CONGRESS OF ANGIOLOGY. PROCEEDINGS. Text in Greek. 1952. biennial, latest 1992, 16th, Paris. **Document type:** *Proceedings.*
Published by: International Union of Angiology, c/o Prof. Panayotis Balas, 4 Hiraklitou St, Athens 106 73, Greece.

616.1 617 USA ISSN 1061-1711
CODEN: IJAGE5
INTERNATIONAL JOURNAL OF ANGIOLOGY. Text in English. 1992. q. (in 1 vol., 4 nos./vol.). USD 333.40 domestic for Print & Online Eds.; USD 329.10 in Germany for Print & Online Eds.; USD 93.30 newsstand/cover foreign (effective 2002). adv. back issues avail. *Refereed.* **Document type:** *Academic/Scholarly.* **Description:** Dedicated to promoting multidisciplinary approaches to all aspects of vascular diseases aimed at clinicians and scientists in cardiovascular surgery and medicine.
Related titles: Microform ed.: (from PQC); Online - full text ed.: (from EBSCO Publishing, RoweCom Information Quest, Swets Blackwell, Springer LINK).
Indexed: Excerp.Med. (1995-), Inpharma, Pharm.&Out.News, Reac.
—BLDSC (4542.081500), ADONIS, CISTI, GNLM, Infotrieve, KNAW. **CCC.**
Published by: Springer-Verlag, Journals (Subsidiary of: BertelsmannSpringer), 175 Fifth Ave, New York, NY 10010. TEL 212-460-1500, FAX 212-473-6272, link@springer-ny.com, http://link.springer.de/link/service/journals/00547/index.htm. Ed. John B Chang. R&P Ian Gross. Adv. contact Brian Skepton. **Subscr. in N. America to:** Journal Fulfillment Services, PO Box 2485, Secaucus, NJ 07096-2485. TEL 800-777-4643, FAX 201-348-4505; **Subscr. outside N. America to:** Springer-Verlag, Haber Str 7, Heidelberg 69126, Germany. **Co-sponsors:** International College of Angiology; International College of Surgeons; Phlebology Society of America.

616.1 IRL ISSN 0167-5273
CODEN: IJCDD5
INTERNATIONAL JOURNAL OF CARDIOLOGY. Text in English. 1973. 15/yr. EUR 163 in Europe to individuals; JPY 21,500 in Japan to individuals; USD 183 elsewhere to individuals; EUR 1,626 in Europe to institutions; JPY 216,000 in Japan to institutions; USD 1,819 elsewhere to institutions (effective 2002). bk.rev. illus. back issues avail. *Refereed.* **Document type:** *Academic/Scholarly.* **Description:** For clinical practitioners and research workers in cardiovascular research and surgery, clinical cardiology and paediatric cardiology.
Formerly: European Journal of Cardiology (0301-4711); Incorporates: Association of European Paediatric Cardiologists. Proceedings (0066-9547)
Related titles: Microform ed.: (from PQC); Online - full text ed.: (from ingenta, Swets Blackwell, ScienceDirect, Institute for Scientific Information).
Indexed: ASCA, Agri.& Environ.Biotech.Abstr. (coverage dropped), Biol.Abstr., Chem.Abstr., Curr.Adv.Ecol.Sci., Curr.Cont., Dent.Ind., Derwent Biotech.Abstr., Excerp.Med., INIS Atomind., Ind.Med. (1981-), Ind.Sci.Rev., Inpharma, Jrnl.Watch Card., Kidney, NRN, Nutr.Abstr., Pharm.&Out.News, Protozool.Abstr., Reac., Ref.Zh., Rev.Appl.Entomol., Rev.Med.& Vet.Mycol., SSCI (coverage dropped), Sci.Cit.Ind., THA.
—BLDSC (4542.158000), ADONIS, CASDDS, CISTI, GNLM, IDS, ingenta, KNAW. **CCC.**
Published by: Elsevier Science Ireland Ltd, Elsevier House, Brookvale Plaza, E. Park, Shannon, Co. Clare, Ireland. TEL 353-61-471944, FAX 353-61-472144, http://www.elsevier.com/locate/ijcard. Ed. Andrew J S Coats. R&P Annette Moloney. **Subscr. in Australasia and the Far East to:** Elsevier Science (Singapore) Pte Ltd, No.1 Temasek Ave, 17-01 Millenia Tower, Singapore 039192, Singapore. TEL 65-434-3727, FAX 65-337-2230; **Subscr. in the Americas to:** Elsevier Science, PO Box 945, New York, NY 10159-0945. TEL 212-633-3730, FAX 212-633-3680; **Subscr. to:** Elsevier Science BV, PO Box 211, Amsterdam 1000 AE, Netherlands. TEL 31-20-485-3757.

616.1 NLD
CODEN: IJCIEL
INTERNATIONAL JOURNAL OF CARDIOVASCULAR IMAGING. Text in English. 1984. bi-m. EUR 402.50, USD 403 to institutions for print or online ed.; EUR 483.60, USD 483.60 to institutions for print & online eds. combined (effective 2002). adv. bk.rev. reprint service avail. from SWZ. *Refereed.* **Document type:** *Journal, Academic/Scholarly.* **Description:** Provides a forum for communications on the basic and applied technologies relating to video and digital image acquisition and analysis, and the clinical applications of imaging modalities in the diagnosis and treatment of cardiovascular disease.
Formerly: International Journal of Cardiac Imaging (0167-9899)
Related titles: Microform ed.: (from PQC); Online - full text ed.: (from EBSCO Publishing, O C L C Online Computer Library Center, Inc., RoweCom Information Quest, Swets Blackwell, Institute for Scientific Information).
Indexed: ASCA, Compumath, Curr.Cont., Excerp.Med., INIS Atomind., INSPEC (Feb.1999-), Ind.Med. (1985-), Inpharma, Pharm.&Out.News, Reac., Sci.Cit.Ind.
—BLDSC (4542.157000), CISTI, GNLM, IDS, ingenta, KNAW. **CCC.**
Published by: Kluwer Academic Publishers Group (Subsidiary of: Wolters Kluwer N.V.), Spuiboulevard 50, PO Box 17, Dordrecht 3300 AA, Netherlands. TEL 31-78-639-2392, FAX 31-78-654-2254, services@wkap.nl, http://www.wkap.nl/journalhome.htm/0167-9899. Eds. Andre J Duerinckx, Ernst E van der Wall, Johan H C Reiber. **Subscr. in the Americas to:** Kluwer Academic - Plenum Publishers, 233 Spring St, New York, NY 10013-1578. TEL 212-620-8468, FAX 212-807-1047; **Subscr. to:** Journals Department, PO Box 322, Dordrecht 3300 AH, Netherlands. TEL 31-78-639-2392, FAX 31-78-654-6474.

616.12 GBR ISSN 1462-8848
INTERNATIONAL JOURNAL OF CARDIOVASCULAR INTERVENTIONS. Text in English. 1998. q. GBP 83, USD 130 to individuals; GBP 185, USD 300 to institutions (effective 2002). adv. illus. Index. back issues avail. *Refereed.* **Document type:** *Academic/Scholarly.* **Description:** Covers the new developments and practical issues interventional cardiology.
Related titles: Online - full content ed.: ISSN 1471-1796; Online - full text ed.: (from CatchWord Ltd.).
—BLDSC (4542.159100), CatchWord.
Published by: Martin Dunitz Ltd. (Subsidiary of: Taylor & Francis Group), 7-9 Pratt St, London NW1 0AE, United Kingdom. TEL 44-20-7482-2202, FAX 44-20-7482-7088, info@dunitz.co.uk, http://www.dunitz.co.uk. Eds. G. Keren, P W Serruys, R. Beyar. R&P, Adv. contact Ian Mellor. Circ: 1,000 (paid).

616.12 ITA ISSN 0393-6066
CODEN: ISCAE
INTERNATIONAL JOURNAL OF SPORTS CARDIOLOGY. Text in Italian. 1984. q. ITL 60,000, USD 70 (effective 1997). back issues avail.
Indexed: Excerp.Med. (until 1992, 1995-), NRN, Sportsearch (1984-).
—CISTI, GNLM, ingenta.
Published by: (Italian Society of Sports Cardiology), C E P I - Centro Editoriale Pubblicitario Italiano s.r.l., Via Nicolo' Tartaglia, 3, Rome, RM 00197, Italy. TEL 39-6-8077011, FAX 39-6-8072458, cepi.p@micanet.it, http://www.micanet.it/cepi. Ed. Antonio Venerando.

INTERNATIONAL SOCIETY OF BLOOD TRANSFUSION. PROCEEDINGS OF THE CONGRESS. see *MEDICAL SCIENCES—Hematology*

616.1 USA ISSN 0074-8765
INTERNATIONAL SYMPOSIUM ON ATHEROSCLEROSIS. PROCEEDINGS. Text in English. irreg., latest 1982. price varies. **Document type:** *Proceedings.*
Published by: Springer-Verlag, Journals (Subsidiary of: BertelsmannSpringer), 175 Fifth Ave, New York, NY 10010. TEL 212-460-1500, FAX 212-473-6272.

616.1 USA
▼ **THE INTERNET JOURNAL OF CARDIOLOGY.** Text in English. 2000. s-a. free per issue. adv. bk.rev. back issues avail. *Refereed.* **Document type:** *Academic/Scholarly.* **Description:** Provides information from the field of cardiovascular diseases and cardiology; contains original articles, reviews, case reports, streaming slide shows, streaming videos, letters to the editor, press releases, and meeting information.
Media: Online - full content.
Published by: Internet Scientific Publications, L.L.C., 23 Rippling Creek Dr, Sugar Land, TX 77479. TEL 281-240-1533, FAX 281-240-1533, http://www.ispub.com/. R&P, Adv. contact Hope Morrow TEL 832-754-0335.

616.1 USA
▼ **THE INTERNET JOURNAL OF PERFUSIONISTS.** Text in English. 2000. s-a. free per issue. bk.rev. back issues avail. *Refereed.* **Document type:** *Academic/Scholarly.* **Description:** Provides information from the field of cardiac surgery, cardiopulmonary bypass and perfusion technology; contains original articles, reviews, case reports, streaming slide shows, streaming videos, letters to the editor, press releases and meeting information.
Media: Online - full content.
Published by: Internet Scientific Publications, L.L.C., 23 Rippling Creek Dr, Sugar Land, TX 77479. TEL 281-240-1533, FAX 281-240-1533, http://www.ispub.com/. R&P, Adv. contact Hope Morrow TEL 832-754-0335.

THE INTERNET JOURNAL OF PULMONARY MEDICINE. see *MEDICAL SCIENCES—Respiratory Diseases*

THE INTERNET JOURNAL OF THORACIC AND CARDIOVASCULAR SURGERY. see *MEDICAL SCIENCES—Surgery*

616.1 NLD ISSN 0926-9649
INTERVENTIONAL CARDIOLOGY. Text in English. 1991. irreg. price varies. *Refereed.* **Document type:** *Monographic series.*
—KNAW.
Published by: Kluwer Academic Publishers Group (Subsidiary of: Wolters Kluwer N.V.), Spuiboulevard 50, PO Box 17, Dordrecht 3300 AA, Netherlands. FAX 31-78-639-2254, services@wkap.nl, http://www.wkap.nl. Ed. Amar S Kapoor. **Dist. by:** Journals Department, PO Box 322, Dordrecht 3300 AH, Netherlands. FAX 31-78-654-6474.

616.1 USA ISSN 1063-4282
CODEN: ICANEB
INTERVENTIONAL CARDIOLOGY NEWSLETTER. Text in English. 1993. bi-m. NLG 243, USD 150 (effective 1997). back issues avail. **Document type:** *Newsletter.*
Related titles: Microform ed.: (from PQC); Online - full text ed.: (from ingenta, Swets Blackwell, ScienceDirect).
—CCC.
Published by: Elsevier Science, PO Box 945, New York, NY 10159-0945. TEL 212-989-5800, FAX 212-633-3990. **Subscr. in Australasia and the Far East to:** Elsevier Science (Singapore) Pte Ltd, No.1 Temasek Ave, 17-01 Millenia Tower, Singapore 039192, Singapore. TEL 65-434-3727, FAX 65-337-2230; **Subscr. in Japan to:** Elsevier Science Inc - Japan Regional Office, 9-15 Higashi-Azabu 1-chome, Minato-ku, Tokyo 106-0044, Japan. TEL 81-3-5561-5033; **Subscr. outside the Americas to:** Elsevier Science BV, PO Box 211, Amsterdam 1000 AE, Netherlands. TEL 31-20-485-3757, nlinfo-f@elsevier.nl, http://www.elsevier.nl.

616.145 GBR ISSN 1366-7122
INTRAVASCULAR IMAGING; commentary and analysis on progress in vascular investigation. Text in English. 1997. q. GBP 50 in Europe; GBP 70 in US & Canada; GBP 75 elsewhere. **Document type:** *Academic/Scholarly.*
—BLDSC (4557.480540).
Published by: Remedica Publishing Ltd., 32-38 Osnaburgh St, London NW1 3ND, United Kingdom. TEL 44-171-388-7677, FAX 44-171-388-7678, info@remedica.com, http://www.remedica.com. Eds. Anthony De Franco, Neal Uren.

616.1 ITA ISSN 1129-471X
CODEN: CARDDJ
▼ **ITALIAN HEART JOURNAL.** Summaries in English, French, German. 1999. m. USD 25. adv. bk.rev. charts, illus. index.
Formed by the merger of (1982-1999): Cardiologia (0393-1978); Which was formerly (1956-1981): Societa Italiana di Cardiologia. Bollettino (0037-878X); (1971-1999): Giornale Italiano di Cardiologia (0046-5968); Which was formed by the 1971 merger of (1960-1969): Malattie Cardiovascolari (0542-268X); (1924-1970): Cuore e Circolazione (0300-8894); (1940-1969): Folia Cardiologica (0390-5756)
Indexed: Biol.Abstr., Chem.Abstr., Excerp.Med., Ind.Med. (2000-).
—BLDSC (4588.335700), CASDDS, CISTI, GNLM, KNAW.
Published by: Societa Italiana di Cardiologia, Corso Di Francia, 197, Rome, RM 00191, Italy. Ed. Antonio Strano. Circ: 1,600.

M

616.1 JPN ISSN 0912-4837
JAKUNENSHA SHINSHIKKAN TAISAKU KYOGIKAISHI/YOUNGER CARDIAC DISEASE COUNTERMEASURE ASSOCIATION. JOURNAL. Text in Japanese. 1973. s-a.
Published by: Jakunensha Shinshikkan Taisaku Kyogikai, Kyoto Junkankibyo Yobokai, Onmae Higashi, Marutamachi Dori, Nakagyo-ku, Kyoto-shi 604, Japan.

616.1 JPN ISSN 0386-2682
JAPAN ATHEROSCLEROSIS SOCIETY. JOURNAL/DOMYAKU KOKA. Text in English, Japanese. 1973. 9/yr. **Document type:** *Academic/Scholarly.*
Indexed: INIS Atomind.
—BLDSC (4804.615000), CISTI, GNLM.
Published by: Japan Atherosclerosis Society/Nihon Domyaku Koka Gakkai, 3-2-29-401 Shibaura, Minato-ku, Tokyo 108-0023, Japan. TEL 81-3-3455-4439, FAX 81-3-3798-1372. Ed. Yoshiya Hata.

616.1 JPN ISSN 0047-1828
RC681 CODEN: JCIRA2
JAPANESE CIRCULATION JOURNAL. Text in English. 1935. m. USD 295 (effective 2001). adv. *Refereed.* **Document type:** *Academic/Scholarly.*
Related titles: Online - full text ed.: (from Institute for Scientific Information).
Indexed: Biol.Abstr., Chem.Abstr., Chem.Indus.Notes, Chem.Titles, Curr.Cont., Derwent Biotech.Abstr., Excerp.Med., INIS Atomind., Ind.Med. (1960-), Ind.Sci.Rev., Inpharma, Neurosci.Cit.Ind., Nutr.Abstr., Pharm.&Out.News, Reac., Sci.Cit.Ind.
—BLDSC (4650.750000), CASDDS, CISTI, GNLM, IDS, ingenta, KNAW. **CCC.**
Published by: Japanese Circulation Society/Nihon Junkanki Gakkai, Kinki Invention Center, 14 Yoshidakawara-cho, Sakyo-ku, Kyoto-shi 606-8305, Japan. TEL 81-75-751-8643, FAX 81-75-771-3060, jcj@j-circ.or.jp, http://www.j-circ.or.jp. Ed. Masunori Matsuzaki. Circ: 20,000.

616.1 JPN
JAPANESE CIRCULATION JOURNAL SUPPLEMENT. Text in Japanese. irreg. (3/yr.). **Document type:** *Academic/Scholarly.*
Related titles: Online - full content ed.
Published by: Japanese Circulation Society/Nihon Junkanki Gakkai, Kinki Invention Center, 14 Yoshidakawara-cho, Sakyo-ku, Kyoto-shi 606-8305, Japan. TEL 81-75-751-8643, FAX 81-75-771-3060, jcj@j-circ.or.jp, http://ww.j-circ.or.jp. Ed. Yasuro Sugishita.

616.1 JPN ISSN 0021-4868
CODEN: JHEJAR
JAPANESE HEART JOURNAL. Text in English. 1960. bi-m. EUR 375, USD 376 to institutions (effective 2002). adv. bk.rev. charts, illus. index. reprint service avail. from PQC. *Refereed.* **Document type:** *Journal, Academic/Scholarly.* **Description:** Reports original work in the fields of clinical and experimental cardiovascular research.
Related titles: Microfilm ed.: (from PQC); Online - full text ed.: (from Institute for Scientific Information).
Indexed: ASCA, Biol.Abstr., Chem.Abstr., Chem.Indus.Notes, Chem.Titles, Curr.Cont., Derwent Biotech.Abstr., Excerp.Med., INIS Atomind., Ind.Med. (1960-), Ind.Sci.Rev., Inpharma, NRN, Pharm.&Out.News, Protozool.Abstr., Reac., Sci.Cit.Ind. (coverage dropped), THA.
—BLDSC (4650.770000), CASDDS, CISTI, GNLM, IDS, ingenta, KNAW.
Published by: (University of Tokyo/Tokyo Daigaku Soryushi Butsuri Kokusai Kenkyu Senta, Faculty of Medicine, Department of Internal Medicine), Nankodo Co. Ltd., 42-6 Hongo 3-chome, Bunkyo-ku, Tokyo 113-0033, Japan. TEL 81-3-3811-7239, FAX 81-3-3811-7230, TELEX 963475. Ed. Dr. Satoru Murao. Circ: 1,000. **Dist. in the Americas by:** Kluwer Academic - Plenum Publishers, 233 Spring St, New York, NY 10013-1578. TEL 212-620-8000, 800-221-9369, FAX 212-620-8468; **Dist. outside Japan by:** Kluwer Academic Publishers Group, Journals Department, PO Box 322, Dordrecht 3300 AH, Netherlands. TEL 31-78-639-23-92, FAX 31-78-654-64-74, services@wkap.nl, http://www.wkap.nl/journalhome.htm/0021-4868.

617.41 JPN ISSN 0914-8922
CODEN: JJICFB
JAPANESE JOURNAL OF INTERVENTIONAL CARDIOLOGY✱. Text in Japanese. 1988. q.
Supersedes: Nihon Kandomyaku Keiseijutsu Kenkyukaishi
Indexed: Excerp.Med. (1995-).
—BLDSC (4655.700000), GNLM.
Published by: (Nihon Shinkekkan Keiseijutsu Kenkukai), Miwa-Shoten Ltd., 17-9 Hongo, Bunkyo-ku, Tokyo 113-0033, Japan. TEL 3-3816-7796.

610 616.1 DEU ISSN 1432-5136
JATROS KARDIO. Text in German. 1983. 12/yr. DEM 140 (effective 1998). **Document type:** *Journal, Academic/Scholarly.*
Former titles: Jatros Kardiologie - Mit Kardiologische Klinik; Jatros Kardiologie - Hypertonie und Artherosklerose (0943-3341); Kardio (0724-9187)
—GNLM.
Published by: P M I Verlag AG, August-Schanz-Str 8, Frankfurt Am Main 60433, Germany. TEL 49-69-548000-0, FAX 49-69-548000-77, huhgmbh@aol.com, pmiverlag@aol.com. Circ: 4,000.

616.65 JPN ISSN 0915-0188
JIKOKETSU YUKETSU/JAPANESE JOURNAL OF AUTOLOGOUS BLOOD TRANSFUSION. Text in English, Japanese. 1987. s-a. JPY 5,000 to members (effective 2001). **Document type:** *Academic/Scholarly.*
Formerly (until 1987): Kaishushiki Jiko Yuketsu (0914-0204)
Published by: Nihon Jikoketsu Yuketsu Kenkyukai, c/o of Center for Academic Societies Japan, Osaka, 14th Fl, Senri Life Science Center Bldg., 1-4-2 Shinsenrihigashi-machi, Toyonaka 560-0082, Japan. TEL 81-6-6873-2301, FAX 81-6-6873-2300. Ed. Takeshi Fuji. R&P Masuhik Takaori.

616 FRA ISSN 0398-0499
JOURNAL DES MALADIES VASCULAIRES. Text in French. 1976. 5/yr. FRF 1,099; FRF 1,327 foreign (effective 2000). reprint service avail. from ISI. *Refereed.* **Document type:** *Academic/Scholarly.* **Description:** Publishes texts of the annual congress of the college, original work selected by the editorial committee and the best postgraduate courses of the faculty.
Related titles: Microform ed.: (from PQC); Online - full text ed.: (from Institute for Scientific Information, RoweCom Information Quest).
Indexed: ASCA, Curr.Cont., Excerp.Med., Ind.Med. (1976-), Ind.Sci.Rev., Inpharma, Pharm.&Out.News, Reac., Sci.Cit.Ind. (coverage dropped).
—BLDSC (5010.850000), CISTI, EMDOCS, GNLM, IDS, Infotrieve, KNAW. **CCC.**
Published by: (College Francais de Pathologie Vasculaire, Societe d'Angiologie de Langue Francaise et Societe Francaise de Microcirculation), Masson - Periodiques, 120 bd. St. Germain, Paris 75006, France. TEL 33-1-40466200, FAX 33-1-40466201. Ed. Vayssairat. Circ: 2,000. **Subscr. to:** Societe de Periodiques Specialises, BP 22, Vineuil Cedex 41354, France. TEL 33-2-54504612, FAX 33-2-54504611.

616.1 AUT ISSN 1028-2327
JOURNAL FUER HYPERTONIE; Zeitschrift fuer Hochdruckerkrankungen. Text in German. 1997. q. ATS 400 (effective 2001). adv. abstr, bibl. back issues avail. **Document type:** *Journal, Academic/Scholarly.* **Description:** Presents research articles on the effects of hypertension.
—BLDSC (5004.525000).
Published by: (Oesterreichischen Gesellschaft fuer Hypertensiologie), Krause & Pachernegg GmbH, Mozartgasse 10, Gablitz 3003, Austria. TEL 43-2231-61258-0, FAX 43-2231-6125810, k_u_p@eunet.at, http://members.eunet.at/k_u_p/hyp.htm, http://members.eunet.at/k_u_p/verlag.htm.

616.1 AUT ISSN 1024-0098
JOURNAL FUER KARDIOLOGIE; Oesterreichische Zeitschrift fuer Herz-Kreislauf-Erkrankungen. Text in German. 1994. 10/yr. ATS 550 (effective 2001). abstr, bibl. back issues avail. *Refereed.* **Document type:** *Journal, Academic/Scholarly.* **Description:** Contains research articles on various aspects of cardiovascular and circulatory diseases and disorders.
—BLDSC (5009.795000).
Published by: Krause & Pachernegg GmbH, Mozartgasse 10, Gablitz 3003, Austria. TEL 43-2231-61258-0, FAX 43-2231-6125810, k_u_p@eunet.at, http://members.eunet.at/k_u_p/kar.htm, http://members.eunet.at/k_u_p/verlag.htm. Ed. Dr. Bernd Eber.

616.1 JPN ISSN 1340-3478
CODEN: JATHEH
JOURNAL OF ATHEROSCLEROSIS AND THROMBOSIS. Text in English. 1994. q. JPY 12,000. **Document type:** *Academic/Scholarly.* **Description:** Contains original articles, reviews, and information on conferences related to atherosclerosis and thrombosis, and their risk factors.
Indexed: Chem.Abstr., Chem.Indus.Notes, Chem.Titles, Ind.Med. (1994-).
—BLDSC (4947.790000), CASDDS, CISTI.
Published by: Japan Atherosclerosis Society/Nihon Domyaku Koka Gakkai, 3-2-29-401, Shibarura, Minato-ku, Tokyo 108, Japan. TEL 81-3-3455-4439, FAX 81-3-3798-1372. Ed. Yoshiya Hata.

616.12 USA ISSN 1071-9164
CODEN: JCFAF9
JOURNAL OF CARDIAC FAILURE. Text in English. 1994. q. USD 159 combined subscription domestic to individuals for print & online eds.; USD 198 combined subscription foreign to individuals for print & online eds.; USD 229 combined subscription domestic to institutions for print & online eds.; USD 281 combined subscription foreign to institutions for print & online eds.; USD 72 combined subscription domestic to students for print & online eds.; USD 111 combined subscription foreign to students for print & online eds.; USD 71 per issue (effective 2001). adv. *Refereed.* **Document type:** *Academic/Scholarly.* **Description:** Features original and review articles on clinical research, basic human studies, animal studies, and bench research, with potential clinical application to heart failure.
Related titles: Online - full text ed.: (from IDEAL Online Library, Institute for Scientific Information).
Indexed: CINAHL, Curr.Cont., Ind.Med. (1994-), Inpharma, Pharm.&Out.News, Reac.
—BLDSC (4954.862000), CASDDS, GNLM, IDS, Infotrieve, KNAW. **CCC.**
Published by: W.B. Saunders Co. (Subsidiary of: Harcourt Publishers Ltd.), Curtis Center, Independence Sq W, Philadelphia, PA 19106-3399. TEL 215-238-7800, FAX 215-238-6490, kstover@wbsaunders.com, http://www.harcourthealth.com/cardfail, http://www.churchillmed.com. Ed. Jay N Cohn. Pub. Jane Grochowski. adv.: B&W page USD 785, color page USD 1,860. Circ: 2,131. **Subscr. in the UK to:** Pearson Professional Ltd., Journals Subscription Department, Fourth Ave., PO Box 77, Harlow, Essex CM19 5AA, United Kingdom. TEL 44-1279-623924, FAX 44-1279-639609.

616.1 USA ISSN 0886-0440
JOURNAL OF CARDIAC SURGERY. Text in English. 1986. bi-m. USD 130 domestic; USD 165 foreign; USD 195 to libraries; USD 30 newsstand/cover (effective 2000). adv. bk.rev. abstr. back issues avail. *Refereed.* **Document type:** *Academic/Scholarly.* **Description:** Includes technical papers and review articles on a wide variety of cardiac surgical techniques for both congenital and acquired conditions.
Incorporates (1981-199?): Modern Technics in Surgery. Head and Neck Surgery (0271-8219); (1979-199?): Modern Technics in Surgery. Neurosurgery (0163-7037); (1980-199?): Modern Technics in Surgery. Urologic Surgery (0193-8568)
Related titles: Online - full text ed.: (from Institute for Scientific Information).
Indexed: ASCA, Curr.Cont., Excerp.Med., Ind.Med. (1986-), Inpharma, Int.Nurs.Ind., Reac.
—BLDSC (4954.863500), ADONIS, CISTI, EMDOCS, GNLM, IDS, ingenta, KNAW. **CCC.**
Published by: Futura Publishing Company, Inc., 135 Bedford Rd, PO Box 418, Armonk, NY 10504-0418. TEL 914-273-1014, FAX 914-973-1016, lisa@futuraco.com. Ed. Dr. Robert B Karp. Adv. contact Lisa Piedimonte. B&W page USD 810, color page USD 1,745; trim 8.25 x 10.875. Circ: 2,507.

616.1 USA ISSN 0883-9212
RC702
JOURNAL OF CARDIOPULMONARY REHABILITATION. Text in English. bi-m. USD 95 domestic to individuals; USD 157 foreign to individuals; USD 237 domestic to institutions (effective 2002); USD 273 foreign to institutions (effective 2003); USD 45 newsstand/cover (effective 2002). bk.rev. back issues avail. *Refereed.* **Document type:** *Academic/Scholarly.* **Description:** Covers articles in peripheral, vascular, and pulmonary rehabilitation.
Formerly: Journal of Cardiac Rehabilitation (0275-1429)
Related titles: Microform ed.: (from PQC); Online - full text ed.: USD 308.10 domestic academic site license; USD 344.10 foreign academic site license; USD 343.65 domestic corporate site license; USD 379.65 foreign corporate site license (2002) (from Ovid Technologies, Inc.).
Indexed: AMED, CINAHL, Ind.Med. (1985-), Phys.Ed.Ind.
—BLDSC (4954.864500), CISTI, EMDOCS, GNLM, ingenta, KNAW.

Published by: (American Association of Cardiovascular & Pulmonary Rehabilitation), Lippincott Williams & Wilkins (Philadelphia) (Subsidiary of: Wolters Kluwer N.V.), 530 Walnut St, Philadelphia, PA 19106-3621. TEL 301-223-2300, 800-638-3030, FAX 301-223-2400, http://www.Lww.com. Ed. Kathy Berra. Circ: 3,934. **Subscr. to:** PO Box 1600, Hagerstown, MD 21740-1600.

616.1 USA ISSN 1053-0770 CODEN: JCVAEK

JOURNAL OF CARDIOTHORACIC AND VASCULAR ANESTHESIA. Text in English. 1987. bi-m. USD 224 domestic to individuals for print & online eds.; USD 315 combined subscription foreign to individuals for print & online eds.; USD 310 combined subscription domestic to institutions for print & online eds.; USD 377 combined subscription foreign to institutions for print & online eds.; USD 125 combined subscription domestic to students for print & online eds.; USD 189 combined subscription foreign to students for print & online eds.; USD 63 per issue (effective 2001). adv. bk.rev. abstr, bibl, charts, illus. index. back issues avail. *Refereed.* **Document type:** *Journal, Academic/Scholarly.* **Description:** Primarily aimed at anesthesiologists who deal with patients undergoing heart, throat, or blood vessel surgery.
Formerly: Journal of Cardiothoracic Anesthesia (0888-6296)
Related titles: Online - full text ed.: (from IDEAL Online Library, Institute for Scientific Information).
Indexed: ASCA, Curr.Cont., Excerp.Med., INIS Atomind., Ind.Med. (1991-), Ind.Sci.Rev., Inpharma, Int.Nurs.Ind., Pharm.&Out.News, Reac., Ref.Zh., Sci.Cit.Ind.
—BLDSC (4954.864700), CISTI, EMDOCS, GNLM, IDS, ingenta, KNAW. **CCC.**
Published by: W.B. Saunders Co. (Subsidiary of: Harcourt Publishers Ltd.), 11830 Westline Industrial Dr, St Louis, MO 63146. TEL 800-325-4177, http://www.jcardioanesthesia.com, http://www.wbsaunders.com. Ed. Dr. Joel A Kaplan. Pub. Joan W Blumberg. adv.: B&W page USD 1,000, color page USD 2,200; trim 10 x 7. Circ: 2,958. **Subscr. to:** Periodicals Fulfillment, W B Saunders Co, 6277 Sea Harbor Dr, 4th Fl, Orlando, FL 32891-4800.

616.1 USA ISSN 1045-3873 CODEN: JCELE2

JOURNAL OF CARDIOVASCULAR ELECTROPHYSIOLOGY. Text in English. 1990. m. USD 190 domestic; USD 245 foreign; USD 285 to libraries; USD 30 newsstand/cover (effective 2000). adv. bk.rev. abstr. *Refereed.* **Document type:** *Academic/Scholarly.* **Description:** Devoted to the study of the electrophysiology of the heart and its blood vessels.
Formerly (until 1989): Journal of Electrophysiology (0892-1059)
Related titles: CD-ROM ed.; Online - full text ed.: (from CatchWord Ltd., Institute for Scientific Information).
Indexed: ASCA, CINAHL, Curr.Cont., INSPEC (Jan.1998-), Ind.Med. (1990-), Ind.Sci.Rev., Inpharma, Pharm.&Out.News, Reac., Sci.Cit.Ind.
—BLDSC (4954.866000), ADONIS, CISTI, EMDOCS, GNLM, IDS, Infotrieve, ingenta, KNAW. **CCC.**
Published by: Futura Publishing Company, Inc., 135 Bedford Rd, PO Box 418, Armonk, NY 10504-0418. TEL 914-273-1014, 800-877-8761, FAX 914-973-1016, lisa@futuraco.com, msoliz@futuraco.com. Ed. Dr. Douglas P Zipes. Adv. contact Lisa Piedimonte. B&W page USD 950, color page USD 1,915; trim 8.25 x 10.875. Circ: 2,838.

616.1 USA ISSN 1097-6647 CODEN: JCMRFR

▼ **JOURNAL OF CARDIOVASCULAR MAGNETIC RESONANCE.** Text in English. 1999. q. USD 135 to individuals print & online eds.; USD 365 to institutions print only (effective 2002). adv. *Refereed.* **Document type:** *Academic/Scholarly.* **Description:** Provides an international forum for communicating the latest findings and reviews on the burgeoning field of cardiovascular magnetic resonance and imaging and spectroscopy.
Related titles: Online - full content ed.; Online - full text ed.: (from Institute for Scientific Information, RoweCom Information Quest).
Indexed: Curr.Cont., Ref.Zh.
—BLDSC (4954.866600).
Published by: (Society for Cardiovascular Magnetic Resonance), Marcel Dekker Inc., 270 Madison Ave, New York, NY 10016. TEL 212-696-9000, 800-228-1160, FAX 212-685-4540, http://www.dekker.com/servlet/product/productid/JCMR. Ed. Dr. Gerald M Pohost. R&P Julia Milligan. Adv. contact Diane Saulon. B&W page USD 800. Circ: 1,100.

616.12 USA ISSN 1053-5330
RA975.5.C3

JOURNAL OF CARDIOVASCULAR MANAGEMENT✱ **.** Text in English. 1990. bi-m. USD 48 domestic; USD 56 in Canada; USD 66 elsewhere. adv. **Description:** Facilitates the dissemination of information and ideas among those professionals involved with the day-to-day management and administrative duties in hospital cardiovascular departments.
—BLDSC (4954.866900).
Published by: Knolls Publishing Group, Inc., 105 Raider Blvd, Belle Mead, NJ 08502-1510. TEL 201-285-0855, FAX 201-285-1472. Ed. Nancy Salerno Davis. Adv. contact Stuart G Mann. Circ: 11,564.

616.12 610.73 USA ISSN 0889-4655

JOURNAL OF CARDIOVASCULAR NURSING. Text in English. 1986. q. USD 132 to individuals; USD 40 newsstand/cover (effective 2002). **Document type:** *Journal, Trade.* **Description:** Addresses the physiologic, psychologic, and social needs of cardiovascular patients and their families in a variety of environments.
Related titles: Online - full text ed.: (from Ovid Technologies, Inc., ProQuest Information & Learning, Gale Group).
Indexed: CINAHL, Ind.Med. (1986-), Int.Nurs.Ind., Nurs.Abstr.
—BLDSC (4954.867500), CISTI, GNLM, ingenta. **CCC.**
Published by: (American Academy of Nursing), Aspen Publishers, Inc., 200 Orchard Ridge Dr, Ste 200, Gaithersburg, MD 20878. TEL 301-417-7500, 800-638-8437, FAX 301-695-7931, customer.service@aspenpubl.com, http://www.aspenpublishers.com. Ed. Judy Marcus. **Dist. by:** Aspen Publishers Inc., Distribution Center, 7201 McKinney Circle, Frederick, MD 21701. TEL 301-698-7100, FAX 301-417-7550.

JOURNAL OF CARDIOVASCULAR PHARMACOLOGY. see *PHARMACY AND PHARMACOLOGY*

JOURNAL OF CARDIOVASCULAR PHARMACOLOGY AND THERAPEUTICS. see *PHARMACY AND PHARMACOLOGY*

616.1 USA ISSN 1350-6277 CODEN: JCRIEO

JOURNAL OF CARDIOVASCULAR RISK. Text in English. 1994. bi-m. USD 240 domestic to individuals; USD 240 foreign to individuals; USD 661 per issue domestic to institutions; USD 661 per issue foreign to institutions; USD 97 newsstand/cover (effective 2002). adv. back issues avail. *Refereed.* **Document type:** *Academic/Scholarly.* **Description:** Provides a central forum for the dissemination of original research in all fields of cardiovascular disease.
Related titles: Online - full text ed.: USD 859.30 domestic academic site license; USD 859.30 foreign academic site license; USD 958.45 domestic corporate site license; USD 958.45 foreign corporate site license (effective 2002) (from EBSCO Publishing, Institute for Scientific Information).
Indexed: Curr.Cont., Excerp.Med. (1995-), Ind.Med. (1994-), Inpharma, Pharm.&Out.News, Reac.
—BLDSC (4954.869000), ADONIS, CISTI, GNLM, IDS, KNAW.
Published by: Lippincott Williams & Wilkins (Philadelphia) (Subsidiary of: Wolters Kluwer N.V.), 530 Walnut St, Philadelphia, PA 19106-3621. TEL 215-521-8300, FAX 215-521-8902, http://www.Lww.com. Eds. Antonio M Gotto Jr., Peter Sleight. Adv. contact Gemma Heiser. **Subscr. to:** PO Box 1600, Hagerstown, MD 21740-1600. TEL 800-777-2295, FAX 301-824-7390.

616.1 ITA ISSN 0021-9509 CODEN: JCVSA2

THE JOURNAL OF CARDIOVASCULAR SURGERY. Text in English. 1960. bi-m. USD 125 to individuals; USD 165 to institutions (effective 2000 - 2001). adv. bk.rev. bibl, charts, illus. index. back issues avail. *Refereed.* **Document type:** *Academic/Scholarly.* **Description:** Covers pathophysiology and therapy of surgical diseases of the chest and heart, the blood vessels and cardiorespiratory system.
Related titles: Microform ed.: (from SWZ); Online - full text ed.: (from Northern Light Technology, Inc., ProQuest Information & Learning, Institute for Scientific Information).
Indexed: ASCA, Biol.Abstr., Chem.Abstr., Curr.Cont., Environ.Sci.Poll.Mgmt., Excerp.Med., Ind.Med. (1960-), Inpharma, Pharm.&Out.News, Pollut.Abstr., Reac., Ref.Zh., Rev.Med.& Vet.Mycol., Risk Abstr., Saf.Sci.Abstr., Sci.Cit.Ind. (coverage dropped).
—BLDSC (4954.870000), CISTI, GNLM, IDS, ingenta, KNAW.
Published by: (International Society of Cardiothoracic Surgeons), Edizioni Minerva Medica, Corso Bramante, 83-85, Turin, TO 10126, Italy. TEL 39-11-678282, FAX 39-11-674502. Ed. L Castellani. Pub. Alberto Oliaro. Adv. contact F Filippo. B&W page USD 1,200, color page USD 2,000; trim 280 x 215. Circ: 5,000 (paid).

616.1 USA

JOURNAL OF CARDIOVASCULAR TECHNOLOGY✱ **.** Text in English. 1970. s-a. USD 45. adv. index. back issues avail.
Formerly: Journal of Cardiovascular and Pulmonary Technology (0893-2972); Supersedes (in 1985): Analyzer (0146-5449)
—GNLM.
Published by: American Society of Cardiovascular Professionals - Society for Cardiovascular Management, 910 Charles St, Ste A, Fredericksburg, VA 22401-5810. TEL 703-891-0079, FAX 703-898-2393. Ed. Dr. John Cissik. Circ: 3,200.

616.12 AUT ISSN 1561-2775

JOURNAL OF CLINICAL AND BASIC CARDIOLOGY; an independent international scientific journal. Text in English. 1998. q. adv. abstr, bibl. back issues avail. *Refereed.* **Document type:** *Journal, Academic/Scholarly.* **Description:** Publishes original communications of scientific excellence concerned with clinical research on cardiovascular diseases, including observational studies, clinical trials, and advances in applied and basic laboratory cardiovascular research.
—BLDSC (4958.369850).
Published by: Krause & Pachernegg GmbH, Mozartgasse 10, Gablitz 3003, Austria. TEL 43-2231-61258-0, FAX 43-2231-6125810, k_u_p@eunet.at, http://members.eunet.at/k_u_p/cardiol.htm, http://members.eunet.at/k_u_p/verlag.htm. Ed. W Klein.

616.132 USA ISSN 1524-6175 CODEN: JCHYFN

▼ **JOURNAL OF CLINICAL HYPERTENSION.** Text in English. 1999. bi-m., latest vol.3, 2001. USD 90 domestic to individuals; USD 105 foreign to individuals; USD 105 domestic to institutions; USD 120 foreign to institutions (effective 2000). adv. bk.rev. abstr, bibl, charts, illus. 235 p./no. back issues avail.; reprints avail. **Document type:** *Journal, Academic/Scholarly.*
—BLDSC (4958.484100).
Published by: Le Jacq Communications, Inc., 777 W Putnam Ave, Greenwich, CT 06830. TEL 203-531-0450, FAX 203-531-0533, showell@lejacq.com. adv.: B&W page USD 4,208; 7.5 x 10.25. Circ: 60,000 (controlled).

616.1 GBR ISSN 1468-3768

JOURNAL OF CONGESTIVE HEARTH FAILURE & CIRCULATORY SUPPORT. Text in English. 1998. q. GBP 85, USD 145 to individuals; GBP 170, USD 270 to institutions (effective 2000).
Formerly (until 1999): Journal of Circulatory Support (1365-5736)
Related titles: Online - full text ed.: (from ingenta, CatchWord Ltd.).
—BLDSC (4965.136000).
Published by: Isis Medical Media Ltd. (Subsidiary of: Martin Dunitz Ltd.), 59 St Aldates, Oxford, Oxon OX1 1ST, United Kingdom. TEL 44-1865-202939, FAX 44-1865-202940, info@isismedical.com, http://www.isismedical.com. Ed. Maren White.

JOURNAL OF CRITICAL CARE. see *MEDICAL SCIENCES—Orthopedics And Traumatology*

616.1 USA ISSN 0022-0736
RC681.A1 CODEN: JECAB4

JOURNAL OF ELECTROCARDIOLOGY. Text in English. 1968. q. USD 141 domestic to individuals; USD 187 foreign to individuals; USD 226 domestic to institutions; USD 282 foreign to institutions; USD 76 domestic to students; USD 126 foreign to students; USD 71 per issue (effective 2001). adv. bk.rev. charts, illus. index. reprint service avail. from PQC,ISI. *Refereed.* **Document type:** *Journal, Academic/Scholarly.* **Description:** Devoted to the clinical and experimental studies of the electrical activities of the heart.
Related titles: Microfilm ed.: (from PQC); Online - full text ed.: (from Northern Light Technology, Inc., ProQuest Information & Learning, IDEAL Online Library, Institute for Scientific Information).
Indexed: ASCA, Biol.Abstr., Curr.Cont., Excerp.Med., INIS Atomind., Ind.Med. (1968-), Ind.Sci.Rev., Inpharma, Pharm.&Out.News, Reac., Sci.Cit.Ind.
—BLDSC (4974.750000), CISTI, GNLM, IDS, ingenta, KNAW. **CCC.**

M

Published by: W.B. Saunders Co. (Subsidiary of: Harcourt Publishers Ltd.), 11830 Westline Industrial Dr, St Louis, MO 63146. TEL 800-325-4177, http://www.wbsaunders.com. Ed. Dr. Ronald H Selvester. adv.: B&W page USD 780, color page USD 1,855. Circ: 842. **Subscr. in the UK to:** Pearson Professional Ltd., Journals Subscription Department, Fourth Ave., PO Box 77, Harlow, Essex CM19 5AA, United Kingdom. TEL 44-1279-623924, FAX 44-1279-639609

616.129 USA ISSN 1070-3837

JOURNAL OF HEART FAILURE. Text in English. 1993. q. —GNLM.

Published by: (International Society of Heart Failure), K.L.I. Medical Communications, Inc., PO Box 17659, Beverly Hills, CA 90209. TEL 310-275-8922. Eds. Asher Kimichi, Basil S Lewis.

616.125 GBR ISSN 0966-8519 CODEN: JHVDEU

THE JOURNAL OF HEART VALVE DISEASE. Text in English. 1992. bi-m. USD 135 worldwide to individuals; USD 230 worldwide to institutions (effective 2002). Supplement avail.; back issues avail. *Refereed.* **Document type:** *Academic/Scholarly.* **Description:** Covers all topics related to heart valves, and the prevention, pathology, diagnosis, and treatment of heart-valve disease.

Related titles: Online - full text ed.: (from Institute for Scientific Information).

Indexed: Curr.Cont., Excerp.Med. (1994-), Ind.Med. (1992-), Inpharma, Reac., Sci.Cit.Ind.

—BLDSC (4996.876000), CISTI, EMDOCS, GNLM, KNAW.

Published by: I C R Publishers Ltd., Crispin House, 12a South Approach, Moor Pk, Northwood, Mddx HA6 2ET, United Kingdom. TEL 44-1923-836871, FAX 44-1923-836872, eb@icr-heart.com, http://www.icr-heart.com/journal/. Ed. Dr. Endre Bodnar. Circ: 5,200.

616.1 GBR ISSN 0950-9240
RC685.H8

JOURNAL OF HUMAN HYPERTENSION. Text in English. 1987. m. GBP 165 in Europe to individuals for print or online ed.; USD 264 elsewhere to individuals for print or online ed.; GBP 182 combined subscription in Europe to individuals print & online; USD 290 combined subscription elsewhere to individuals print & online; GBP 370 in Europe to institutions for print or online; USD 555 elsewhere to institutions for print or online; GBP 407 combined subscription in Europe to institutions print & online; USD 611 combined subscription elsewhere to institutions print & online (effective 2002). bk.rev. charts, illus, stat. index. back issues avail.; reprints avail. *Refereed.* **Document type:** *Journal, Academic/Scholarly.* **Description:** Covers all clinical aspects of human hypertension. Aims to increase knowlegde of the problem of high blood pressure and improve the standard of patient care worldwide.

Related titles: Online - full text ed.: GBP 156, USD 250 to individuals; GBP 340, USD 544 to institutions (effective 2001) (from EBSCO Publishing, O C L C Online Computer Library Center, Inc., RoweCom Information Quest, ingenta, Swets Blackwell, Institute for Scientific Information).

Indexed: ASCA, Curr.Cont., Excerp.Med., Ind.Med. (1987-), Inpharma, Int.Nurs.Ind., Kidney, Nutr.Abstr., Pharm.&Out.News, Reac., SSCI (coverage dropped), Trop.Dis.Bull.

—BLDSC (5003.416000), CASDDS, CISTI, EMDOCS, GNLM, IDS, ingenta, KNAW. **CCC.**

Published by: Nature Publishing Group Specialist Journals (Subsidiary of: Holtzbrink Publishers), Houndmills, Basingstoke, Hants RG21 6XS, United Kingdom. TEL 44-1256-329242, FAX 44-1256-328339, subscriptions@nature.com, http://www.nature.com/jhh. Eds. Franz Messerli, Gareth Beevers. Pub. Sue Deeley. R&P Trace Noel. Adv. contact Robert Sloan TEL 44-20-8882-7199.

616.132 USA ISSN 0263-6352 CODEN: JOHYD3

JOURNAL OF HYPERTENSION. Text in English. 1982. m. USD 383 domestic to individuals includes print and online eds.; USD 383 foreign to individuals includes print and online eds.; USD 797 per issue domestic to institutions includes print and online eds.; USD 797 per issue foreign to institutions includes print and online eds.; USD 60 newsstand/cover includes print and online eds. (effective 2002). adv. bibl, illus. *Refereed.* **Document type:** *Academic/Scholarly.* **Description:** Presents original papers ranging from studies in clinical care to the investigation of experimental hypertension. Includes review articles, editorials and debates.

Related titles: Online - full text ed.: USD 1,036.10 domestic academic site license; USD 1,036.10 foreign academic site license; USD 1,155.65 domestic corporate site license; USD 1,155.65 foreign corporate site license (effective 2002) (from Ovid Technologies, Inc., EBSCO Publishing, Institute for Scientific Information); ♦ Supplement: Journal of Hypertension. Supplement. ISSN 0952-1178.

Indexed: ASCA, Abstr.Hyg., Behav.Med.Abstr., CINAHL, Chem.Abstr., Chem.Indus.Notes, Chem.Titles, Curr.Adv.Biochem., Curr.Adv.Cancer Res., Curr.Cont., Derwent Biotech.Abstr., Excerp.Med., Ind.Med. (1983-), Ind.Sci.Rev., Inpharma, Int.Abstr.Biol.Sci., Kidney, NRN, Neurosci.Cit.Ind., Nutr.Abstr., Pharm.&Out.News, Reac., SSCI (coverage dropped), Sci.Cit.Ind., THA, Trop.Dis.Bull.

—BLDSC (5004.510000), ADONIS, CASDDS, CISTI, EMDOCS, GNLM, IDS, ingenta, KNAW.

Published by: (International Society of Hypertension), Lippincott Williams & Wilkins (Philadelphia) (Subsidiary of: Wolters Kluwer N.V.), 530 Walnut St, Philadelphia, PA 19106-3621. TEL 215-521-8300, FAX 215-521-8902, http://www.lww.com. Ed. A Zanchetti. Adv. contact Gemma Heiser. B&W page USD 980, color page USD 2,030; trim 11 x 8.5. Circ: 3,575. **Subscr. to:** PO Box 1600, Hagerstown, MD 21740-1600. TEL 800-777-2295, FAX 301-824-7390. **Co-sponsor:** European Society of Hypertension.

616.1 USA ISSN 1383-875X CODEN: JICEFE

JOURNAL OF INTERVENTIONAL CARDIAC ELECTROPHYSIOLOGY; an international journal of arrhythmias and pacing. Text in English. 1997. q. USD 360, EUR 359 to institutions for print or online ed.; USD 432, EUR 430.80 to institutions for print & online eds.combined (effective 2002). *Refereed.* **Document type:** *Journal, Academic/Scholarly.* **Description:** Publishes original research studies, and reviews of applied science and clinical research, in the field of interventional techniques and therapies for the management of cardiac arrhythmias.

Related titles: Online - full text ed.: (from EBSCO Publishing, O C L C Online Computer Library Center, Inc., RoweCom Information Quest, Swets Blackwell, Kluwer Online, Institute for Scientific Information).

Indexed: Curr.Cont., Ind.Med. (1997-), Inpharma, Pharm.&Out.News, Reac.

—BLDSC (5007.695900), IDS, Infotrieve. **CCC.**

Published by: Kluwer Academic Publishers Boston, 101 Philip Dr, Assinippi Park, Norwell, MA 02061. TEL 781-871-6600, FAX 781-871-9045, services@wkap.nl, http://www.wkap.nl/journalhome.htm/1383-875X. Ed. Sanjeev Saksena. **Subscr. in the Americas to:** Kluwer Academic - Plenum Publishers, 233 Spring St, New York, NY 10013-1578. TEL 212-620-8468, FAX 212-807-1047; **Subscr. to:** Kluwer Academic Publishers Group, Journals Department, PO Box 322, Dordrecht 3300 AH, Netherlands. TEL 31-78-639-2392, FAX 31-78-654-6474.

616.1 USA ISSN 0896-4327

JOURNAL OF INTERVENTIONAL CARDIOLOGY. Text in English. 1988. bi-m. USD 135 domestic; USD 170 foreign; USD 203 to libraries; USD 30 newsstand/cover (effective 2000). adv. bk.rev. *Refereed.* **Document type:** *Academic/Scholarly.* **Description:** Provides the latest information on interventional cardiology, including diagnostics, monitoring, therapeutic techniques and equipment.

Indexed: ASCA, Curr.Cont. (coverage dropped), Excerp.Med. (1995-), INSPEC, Inpharma, Pharm.&Out.News, Reac.

—BLDSC (5007.696000), ADONIS, GNLM, IDS, ingenta, KNAW. **CCC.**

Published by: Futura Publishing Company, Inc., 135 Bedford Rd, PO Box 418, Armonk, NY 10504-0418. TEL 914-273-1014, FAX 914-273-1016, lisa@futuraco.com, msoliz@futuraco.com. Ed. Dr. Gerald C Timins. R&P Lisa Piedimonte. Adv. contact Michelle Soliz. B&W page USD 945, color page USD 1,910; trim 8.25 x 10.875. Circ: 2,061.

616.1 USA ISSN 1042-3931 CODEN: JOCAFA

JOURNAL OF INVASIVE CARDIOLOGY. Text in English. 1988. m. USD 109.95; USD 152.95 foreign (effective 2001). adv. back issues avail. *Refereed.* **Document type:** *Trade.* **Description:** Covers cardiac catheterization, coronary and peripheral angioplasty, including thrombolytic and associated therapy.

Related titles: Online - full text ed.

Indexed: ASCA, Curr.Cont. (coverage dropped), Ind.Med. (1988-), Inpharma, Pharm.&Out.News, Reac., SSCI (coverage dropped).

—BLDSC (5007.800000), GNLM, IDS, KNAW.

Published by: H M P Communications, LLC, 950 W Valley Rd, Ste 2800, Wayne, PA 19087. TEL 610-688-8220, 800-237-7285, FAX 610-688-8050, http://cardiology.medscape.com/HMP/JIC/publica/JIC-journal.html. Adv. contact Jeff Martin. B&W page USD 1,953, color page USD 3,303. Circ: 10,000 (controlled).

616.1 GBR ISSN 0022-2828
RC681.A1 CODEN: JMCDAY

JOURNAL OF MOLECULAR AND CELLULAR CARDIOLOGY. Text in English. 1970. m. GBP 1,445 to institutions (effective 2001). adv. index. reprint service avail. from SWZ. *Refereed.* **Document type:** *Academic/Scholarly.* **Description:** Provides a forum for research papers dealing with the molecular biology, physiology, pharmacology, and pathophysiology of the heart and cardiovascular system.

Related titles: Online - full text ed.: (from EBSCO Publishing, O C L C Online Computer Library Center, Inc., RoweCom Information Quest, ingenta, Swets Blackwell, IDEAL Online Library, Institute for Scientific Information).

Indexed: ASCA, Agri.& Environ.Biotech.Abstr. (coverage dropped), Apic.Abstr., BBCI, Biol.Abstr., Chem.Abstr., Chem.Indus.Notes, Chem.Titles, Curr.Adv.Biochem., Curr.Adv.Cell & Devel.Biol., Curr.Adv.Ecol.Sci., Curr.Adv.Gen.& Molec.Biol., Curr.Cont., Dent.Ind., Derwent Biotech.Abstr., Excerp.Med., Helminthol.Abstr., INIS Atomind., Ind.Med. (1970-), Ind.Sci.Rev., Inpharma, Int.Abstr.Biol.Sci., Nutr.Abstr., Pharm.&Out.News, Protozool.Abstr., Reac., Rev.Arom.& Med.Plants, Sci.Cit.Ind.

—BLDSC (5020.690000), ADONIS, CASDDS, CISTI, GNLM, IDS, ingenta, KNAW. **CCC.**

Published by: (International Society for Heart Research), Academic Press (Subsidiary of: Harcourt Publishers Ltd.), 24 Oval Rd, London NW1 7DX, United Kingdom. TEL 44-20-7267-4466, FAX 44-20-7482-2293, apsubs@acad.com, http://www.academicpress.com/jmcc; http://www.europe.idealibrary.com/. Ed. N R Alpert. R&P Catherine John. Adv. contact Nik Screen. **Subscr. to:** Harcourt Publishers Ltd., Foots Cray High St, Sidcup, Kent DA14 5HP, United Kingdom. TEL 44-20-8300-3322, FAX 44-20-8309-0807.

616.13 USA ISSN 1045-7984 CODEN: JMYIER

JOURNAL OF MYOCARDIAL ISCHEMIA✶ . Text in English. 1989. 10/yr. USD 60 to individuals; USD 75 foreign to individuals; USD 90 to institutions. adv. index. **Description:** Forum for reports and reviews on the diagnosis and treatment of angina, silent ischemia, atherosclerosis and acute myocardial infarction.

Indexed: Excerp.Med. (1993-).

—EMDOCS, GNLM, Infotrieve. **CCC.**

Published by: P R R, Inc., 48 S Service Rd, Melville, NY 11747-2335. TEL 516-424-8900, FAX 516-424-8503. Ed. Dr. Carl J Pepine. Pub. Tiberius H Schuldner. adv.: B&W page USD 2,290, color page USD 3,540; trim 10.75 x 7.88. Circ: 27,833 (controlled).

616.1 USA ISSN 1052-3057
RC388.5

JOURNAL OF STROKE AND CEREBROVASCULAR DISEASES. Text in English. 1991. bi-m. USD 143 domestic to individuals Full text online included; USD 178 foreign to individuals Full text online included; USD 229 domestic to institutions Full text online included; USD 265 foreign to institutions Full text online included; USD 81 domestic to students Full text online included; USD 59 foreign to students Full text online included; USD 45 newsstand/cover (effective 2001). adv. bk.rev. *Refereed.* **Document type:** *Academic/Scholarly.* **Description:** Contains original articles, review articles and other features relating to comprehensive diagnosis and management of cerebrovascular disease.

Related titles: Online - full text ed.: (from IDEAL Online Library).

Indexed: CINAHL.

—BLDSC (5066.873900), GNLM.

Published by: (National Stroke Association), W.B. Saunders Co. (Subsidiary of: Harcourt Publishers Ltd.), 11830 Westline Industrial Dr, St Louis, MO 63146. TEL 800-325-4177, http://www.strokejournal.org, http://www.wbsaunders.com. Ed. Dr. K M A Welch. adv.: B&W page USD 700, color page USD 1,775; trim 11 x 8.25. Circ: 4,041. **Subscr. to:** Periodicals Fulfillment, W B Saunders Co, 6277 Sea Harbor Dr, 4th Fl, Orlando, FL 32891-4800.

616.12 AUS ISSN 1027-7811
JOURNAL OF THE HONG KONG COLLEGE OF CARDIOLOGY. Text in English. 1983. q. AUD 238 domestic; AUD 216 in New Zealand; USD 132 elsewhere; AUD 262 domestic print & online eds. combined; AUD 238 in New Zealand print & online eds. combined; USD 146 elsewhere print & online eds. combined (effective 2001). adv. *Refereed.* **Document type:** *Journal, Academic/Scholarly.* **Description:** Publishes articles on all aspects of cardiovascular disease, including original clinical studies, review articles and experimental investigations.
Related titles: ♦ Online - full text ed.: Journal of the Hong Kong College of Cardiology Online.
Published by: (Hong Kong College of Cardiology HKG), Blackwell Science Asia Pty Ltd, PO Box 378, Carlton South, VIC 3053, Australia. TEL 61-3-9347-0300, FAX 61-3-9347-5001, shwan@hkstar.com, info@blacksci-asia.com.au, http://www.medicine.org.hk/hkcc/journal/home.htm, http://www.blacksci.co.uk/australi. Ed. Chu-Pak Lau.

616.12 AUS
JOURNAL OF THE HONG KONG COLLEGE OF CARDIOLOGY ONLINE. Text in English. s-a. AUD 215 domestic; AUD 195 in New Zealand; USD 119 elsewhere (effective 2001). *Refereed.* **Document type:** *Academic/Scholarly.*
Media: Online - full text. **Related titles:** ♦ Print ed.: Journal of the Hong Kong College of Cardiology. ISSN 1027-7811.
Published by: (Hong Kong College of Cardiology HKG), Blackwell Science Asia Pty Ltd, PO Box 378, Carlton South, VIC 3053, Australia. TEL 61-3-9347-0300, FAX 61-3-9347-3016, info@blacksci-asia.com.au, http://www.medicine.org.hk/hkcc/journal/home.htm, http://www.blacksci.co.uk/australi.

616.1 USA ISSN 0929-5305
CODEN: JTTHFF
JOURNAL OF THROMBOSIS AND THROMBOLYSIS; an international journal for clinicians and scientists. Text in English. 1994. bi-m. USD 235 to individuals for print or online ed. (effective 2001); USD 500, EUR 500 to institutions for print or online ed.; USD 600, EUR 600 to institutions for print & online eds.combined (effective 2002). reprint service avail. from SWZ. *Refereed.* **Document type:** *Journal, Academic/Scholarly.* **Description:** Publishes original papers integrating basic science and clinical investigation of thrombotic disorders.
Related titles: Online - full text ed.: (from EBSCO Publishing, O C L C Online Computer Library Center, Inc., RoweCom Information Quest, Swets Blackwell, Kluwer Online, Institute for Scientific Information).
Indexed: Aqua.Sci.& Fish.Abstr., Aquacult.Abstr., Chem.Abstr., Chem.Indus.Notes, Chem.Titles, Curr.Cont., Environ.Sci.Poll.Mgmt., Excerp.Med. (1996-), Ind.Med. (1994-).
—BLDSC (5069.350000), CASDDS, CISTI, EMDOCS, GNLM, IDS, Infotrieve, KNAW. **CCC.**
Published by: Kluwer Academic Publishers Boston, 101 Philip Dr, Assinippi Park, Norwell, MA 02061. TEL 781-871-6600, FAX 781-871-9045, services@wkap.nl, http://www.wkap.nl/journalhome.htm/0929-5305. Ed. Dr. Richard C Becker. R&P Rose Luongo TEL 781-871-6311. **Subscr. outside the Americas to:** Kluwer Academic Publishers Group, Journals Department, PO Box 322, Dordrecht 3300 AH, Netherlands. TEL 31-78-639-2392, FAX 31-78-654-6474; **Subscr. to:** Kluwer Academic - Plenum Publishers, 233 Spring St, New York, NY 10013-1578. TEL 212-620-8468, FAX 212-807-1047.

616.1 ITA ISSN 1129-7298
▼ **THE JOURNAL OF VASCULAR ACCESS.** Text in English. 2000. q. EUR 130 in Europe to individuals; USD 170 elsewhere to individuals; EUR 170 in Europe to institutions; USD 210 elsewhere to institutions (effective 2001). adv. abstr, bibl, charts, illus. 64 p./no. back issues avail.; reprints avail. *Refereed.* **Document type:** *Journal, Academic/Scholarly.* **Description:** Publishes original manuscripts dealing with clinical and laboratory investigations in the fast growing field of vascular access.
Related titles: Online - full text ed.
—BLDSC (5072.261900).
Published by: Wichtig Editore s.r.l., Via Friuli, 72, Milan, MI 20135, Italy. TEL 39-02-55195443, FAX 39-02-55195971, info@wichtig-publisher.com, http://www.wichtig-publisher.com. Ed. Dr. Diego Brancaccio. R&P, Adv. contact Lucia Steele. color page USD 1,450; trim 21 x 28. Circ: 1,500 (controlled). **Subscr. to:** EBSCO, PO Box 1943, Birmingham, AL 35201-1943. TEL 205-991-1234.

JOURNAL OF VASCULAR NURSING. see *MEDICAL SCIENCES—Nurses And Nursing*

611.0186 CHE ISSN 1018-1172
RC691 CODEN: JVREE9
JOURNAL OF VASCULAR RESEARCH. Text in English. 1964. bi-m. CHF 999, EUR 713.80 in Europe to institutions; CHF 1,016.40, USD 777 elsewhere to institutions (effective 2002). adv. bibl, charts, illus. index. back issues avail. *Refereed.* **Document type:** *Journal, Academic/Scholarly.* **Description:** Covers a broad spectrum of vascular and lymphatic research including vascular structure, vascular function, hemodynamics, mechanics, cell signalling, intercellular communication, growth and differentiation.
Incorporates (1982-1997): International Journal of Microcirculation: Clinical and Experimental (0167-6865); Former titles (until 1991): Blood Vessels (0303-6847); Angiologica (0003-3189)
Related titles: Microform ed.: (from RPI); Online - full text ed.: ISSN 1423-0135. CHF 58, EUR 42, USD 45 to institutions with print edition (effective 2002) (from Northern Light Technology, Inc., EBSCO Publishing, O C L C Online Computer Library Center, Inc., RoweCom Information Quest, ProQuest Information & Learning, Swets Blackwell, Institute for Scientific Information).
Indexed: ASCA, Biol.Abstr., Chem.Abstr., Chem.Indus.Notes, Chem.Titles, Curr.Adv.Ecol.Sci., Curr.Cont., Excerp.Med., Ind.Med. (1992-), Ind.Sci.Rev., Inpharma, Kidney, Med.& Surg.Dermat., Nutr.Abstr., Pharm.&Out.News, Reac., Sci.Cit.Ind., THA.
—BLDSC (5072.269000), CASDDS, CISTI, EMDOCS, GNLM, IDS, Infotrieve, ingenta, KNAW. **CCC.**
Published by: (European Society for Microcirculation), S. Karger AG, Allschwilerstr 10, PO Box, Basel 4009, Switzerland. TEL 41-61-306-1111, FAX 41-61-306-1234, karger@karger.ch, http://www.online.karger.com/journals/jvr, http://www.karger.com. Ed. M J Mulvany. adv.: page USD 1,195. Circ: 1,800.

JOURNAL OF VASCULAR SURGERY. see *MEDICAL SCIENCES—Surgery*

616.1 USA ISSN 1044-4122
CODEN: JVTEEJ
JOURNAL OF VASCULAR TECHNOLOGY. Text in English. 1979. q. USD 90 in US & Canada to individuals; USD 110 elsewhere to individuals; USD 110 in US & Canada to institutions; USD 135 elsewhere to institutions (effective 2001). adv. bk.rev. back issues avail. *Refereed.* **Document type:** *Academic/Scholarly.* **Description:** Provides an educational service for practicing noninvasive vascular technologists, technologists involved in supervision and education in a clinical setting, physicians, surgeons, researchers, manufacturers, and other health care professionals. Covers advances in the field, case studies, and opinions.
Formerly (until 1986): Bruit (0739-8670)
Related titles: Online - full text ed.: (from CatchWord Ltd.).
Indexed: Excerp.Med. (1993-).
—BLDSC (5072.271000), EMDOCS, GNLM, KNAW.
Published by: Society of Vascular Technology, 4601 Presidents Dr, Ste 260, Lanham, MD 20706-4831. TEL 301-459-7550, FAX 301-459-5651, orders@allenpress.com; svtnet@msn.com, http://www.svtnet.org. Ed. Barbara A Rhodes. Pub., R&P Patricia Horner. Adv. contact Onkar Sandal. B&W page USD 755, color page USD 1,450; trim 9.38 x 7. Circ: 10,000. **Subscr. to:** Allen Press Inc., PO Box 1897, Lawrence, KS 66044-8897.

JOURNAL WATCH CARDIOLOGY. see *MEDICAL SCIENCES—Abstracting, Bibliographies, Statistics*

616.1 POL ISSN 0022-9032
KARDIOLOGIA POLSKA/POLISH HEART JOURNAL. Text in Polish; Text occasionally in English. 1958. m. PLZ 90 domestic to individuals; USD 90 foreign to individuals; PLZ 220 domestic to institutions; USD 320 foreign to institutions (effective 2001). adv. bk.rev. 90 p./no. reprints avail. *Refereed.* **Document type:** *Journal, Academic/Scholarly.*
Related titles: Online - full text ed.
Indexed: Biol.Abstr., Chem.Abstr., Excerp.Med., INIS Atomind., Ind.Med. (coverage dropped).
—BLDSC (5085.700000), CISTI, GNLM.
Published by: Polskie Towarzystwo Kardiologiczne, Klinika Kardiologii CMKP, Szpital Grochowski, Ul Grenadierow 51-59, Warsaw 04073, Poland. TEL 48-22-8101738, FAX 48-22-8107095. Ed. Leszek Ceremuzynski. Adv. contact Jadwiga Klos. Circ: 3,000.

616.1 DEU ISSN 0938-7293
KARDIOLOGIE ASSISTENZ. Text in German. 1989. q. EUR 54.30 domestic; EUR 45.40 in Germany; EUR 12.60 newsstand/cover foreign (effective 2002). adv. bibl. back issues avail.; reprints avail. **Document type:** *Journal, Academic/Scholarly.* **Description:** Contains articles of interest to physicians' assistance in cardiac medicine.
—GNLM.
Published by: (Bundesarbeitsgemeinschaft des Assistenzpersonals in der Kardiologie e.V.), Dr. Dietrich Steinkopff Verlag (Subsidiary of: BertelsmannSpringer), Poststr 9, Darmstadt 64293, Germany. TEL 49-6151-82899-0, FAX 49-6151-82899-40, subscriptions@springer.de, http://www.steinkopff.springer.de. **Subscr. in N. America to:** Springer-Verlag, Journals. TEL 201-348-4033; **Subscr. to:** Springer Verlag GmbH, Haberstr 7, Heidelberg 69126, Germany. FAX 49-6221-345229.

616.1 RUS ISSN 0022-9040
CODEN: KARDA2
KARDIOLOGIYA/CARDIOLOGY. Text in Russian. 1961. m. RUR 360 for 6 mos. to individuals; ROL 1,080 for 6 mos. to institutions (effective 2002). adv. bk.rev. bibl. index. *Refereed.* **Description:** Deals with the major problems of cardiovascular pathology in the clinical, morphological, biochemical and pathophysiological aspects. Including coronary heart disease, arterial hypertension, atherosclerosis, acquired and congenital disease of the heart, circulatory insufficiency, disorders of the cardiac rhythm.
Related titles: Online - full text ed.: (from Institute for Scientific Information).
Indexed: ASCA, Biol.Abstr., Chem.Abstr., Chem.Titles, Curr.Cont., Dok.Arbeitsmed., Excerp.Med., INIS Atomind., Ind.Med. (coverage dropped), Ind.Sci.Rev., Inpharma, Int.Aerosp.Abstr., Nutr.Abstr., Reac., Ref.Zh.
—CASDDS, CISTI, East View, GNLM, IDS, Infotrieve, KNAW. **CCC.**
Published by: Media Sfera, Dmitrovskoe shosse 46, korp 2, etazh 4, P.O. Box 54, Moscow 127238, Russian Federation. TEL 7-095-4824329, FAX 7-095-4824312, mediashp@mediasphera.ru. Ed. Y N Belenkov. Adv. contact Valery Nemtsov. **Dist. by:** Mezhdunarodnaya Kniga, B Yakimanka 39, Moscow 117049, Russian Federation. TEL 7-095-2384967, FAX 7-095-2384634; **US dist. addr.:** East View Publications, 3020 Harbor Ln N, Minneapolis, MN 55447. TEL 612-550-0961.

616.1 CHE ISSN 1423-5528
KARDIOVASKULAERE MEDIZIN/MEDECINE CARDIOVASCULAIRE. Text in German. 8/yr. CHF 60 (effective 2001). **Document type:** *Journal, Trade.*
Published by: (Schweizerische Gesellschaft fuer Kardiologie), E M H Swiss Medical Publishers Ltd., Steinentorstr 13, Basel, Switzerland. TEL 41-61-4678555, FAX 41-61-4678556, verlag@emh.ch, http://www.emh.ch.

616.1 JPN ISSN 0911-4637
KEKKAN/JAPANESE JOURNAL OF CIRCULATION RESEARCH. Text in Japanese. 1976. 4/yr.
—BLDSC (4651.365000).
Published by: Nihon Myakkan Sado Busshitsu Gakkai/Japanese Society for Circulation Research, Nagoya Daigaku Igakubu Yakuri Kyoshitsu, 65 Tsurumai-cho, Showa-ku, Nagoya-shi, Aichi-ken 466-0065, Japan.

616.1 JPN ISSN 0917-5318
CODEN: KENAE5
KEKKAN TO NAIHI/BLOOD VESSEL & ENDOTHELIUM. Text in Japanese. 1991. 6/yr. JPY 2,200 per issue (effective 1998).
Published by: Medikaru Rebyusha/Medical Review Co., Ltd., 7-3 Hirano-Machi 1-chome, Chuo-ku, Osaka-shi 541-0046, Japan. TEL 81-6-223-1468, FAX 81-6-223-1245, meview@osk3.3web.ne.jp.

L M S ALERT. ANTITHROMBOTICS. (Literature Monitoring and Evaluation Service) see *MEDICAL SCIENCES—Abstracting, Bibliographies, Statistics*

L M S ALERT. ARRHYTHMIAS. (Literature Monitoring and Evaluation Service) see *MEDICAL SCIENCES—Abstracting, Bibliographies, Statistics*

L M S ALERT. HEART FAILURE. (Literature Monitoring and Evaluation Service) see *MEDICAL SCIENCES—Abstracting, Bibliographies, Statistics*

L M S ALERT. HYPERTENSION. (Literature Monitoring and Evaluation Service) see *MEDICAL SCIENCES—Abstracting, Bibliographies, Statistics*

L M S ALERT. ISCHAEMIC HEART DISORDERS. (Literature Monitoring and Evaluation Service) see *MEDICAL SCIENCES—Abstracting, Bibliographies, Statistics*

616.132 ITA ISSN 0394-9559
LA LETTERA DELLA IPERTENSIONE. Text in Italian. 1988. q. adv.

M

Published by: C I C Edizioni Internazionali s.r.l., Corso Trieste 42, Rome, RM 00198, Italy. TEL 39-06-8412673, FAX 39-06-8412688, info@gruppocic.it, 1160199510. Ed. C Dal Palu. adv.: B&W page ITL 3,100,000, color page ITL 3,900,000; trim 210 x 290.

616.12 FRA ISSN 0761-5035
LA LETTRE DU CARDIOLOGUE. Text in French. 1983. bi-m. FRF 460 domestic to individuals; FRF 580, USD 105 foreign to individuals; FRF 580 domestic to institutions; FRF 700, USD 127 foreign to institutions; FRF 290 domestic to students; USD 75 foreign to students (effective 2000). Supplement avail. *Refereed.* **Document type:** *Academic/Scholarly.*
Published by: Edimark S.A., 62-64 rue Jean Jaures, Puteaux 92800, France. TEL 33-1-414-58000, FAX 33-1-41458000, contact@edimark.fr, http://www.edimark.fr. Ed. M Komajda. Pub. Claudie Damour-Terrasson.

LIVEWELL. see *PHYSICAL FITNESS AND HYGIENE*

M E E N CARDIOLOGY - CRITICAL CARE TECHNOLOGY. see *MEDICAL SCIENCES—Radiology And Nuclear Medicine*

616.1 BGR ISSN 0204-6865
MEDICINSKI PREGLED. SARDECHNO-SADOVI ZABOLIAVANIIA. Text in Bulgarian; Summaries in Bulgarian, English. 1970. q., latest vol.32, 2001. BGL 14 domestic; USD 38 foreign (effective 2001 - 2002). adv. bk.rev. abstr, bibl, illus. index. 48 p./no. back issues avail. *Refereed.* **Document type:** *Journal, Academic/Scholarly, Abstract/Index, Bibliography.* **Description:** Presents original articles and abstracts of foreign publications on diagnosis and treatment of cardiovascular diseases, including experimental studies on risk factors, and new drugs.
Indexed: Abstr.Bulg.Sci.Med.Lit.
—GNLM.
Published by: Meditsinski Universitet - Sofia, Tsentur za Informatsiia po Meditsina/Medical University - Sofia, Medical Information Center, 1 Sv Georgi Sofiiski ul, Sofia 1431, Bulgaria. TEL 359-2-9522342, FAX 359-2-9522393, mutafov@sun.medun.acad.bg, http://www.medun.acad.bg. Ed. Dr. Ml Grigorov. R&P, Adv. contact Dr. Christo Mutafov. B&W page USD 50, color page USD 200; 12 x 18. Circ: 400.

616.12 ITA ISSN 1128-4293
▼ **MEDITERRANEAN JOURNAL OF PACING AND ELECTROPHYSIOLOGY.** Text in English. 1999. q. USD 65 (effective 2002). adv. bk.rev. abstr. *Refereed.* **Document type:** *Academic/Scholarly.* **Description:** Contains studies on cardiac pacing and arrhythmology.
Published by: (Mediterranean Society of Pacing and Electrophysiology), Edizioni Luigi Pozzi s.r.l., Via Panama, 68, Rome, RM 00198, Italy. TEL 39-06-8553548, FAX 39-06-8554105, edizioni_pozzi@tin.it. Eds. E Adornato, N El Sherif. Circ: 3,000.

616.12 BGR
MEDITSINSKI PREGLED. SURDECHNO-SUDOVI ZABOLIAVANIA. Text in Bulgarian. q. USD 48 foreign (effective 2002). **Description:** Covers cardiology, inner diseases, children's cardiology and heart surgery.
Published by: Meditsinski Universitet - Sofia, Tsentur za Informatsiia po Meditsina/Medical University - Sofia, Medical Information Center, 1 Sv Georgi Sofiiski ul, Sofia 1431, Bulgaria. TEL 359-2-9522342, FAX 359-2-9522393, http://www.medun.acad.bg. **Dist. by:** Sofia Books, Ul Silivria 16, Sofia 1404, Bulgaria. TEL 359-2-9586257, sofiabooks@hotmail.com, http://www.sofiabooks.hit.bg.

MICROCIRCULATION REVIEWS. see *BIOLOGY—Physiology*

616.1 USA ISSN 0026-2862
RC681.A1 CODEN: MIVRA6
MICROVASCULAR RESEARCH; an international journal. Text in English. 1968. bi-m. USD 847 in US & Canada to institutions; USD 975 rest of world to institutions (effective 2001). adv. charts, illus. index. back issues avail. *Refereed.* **Document type:** *Academic/Scholarly.* **Description:** Disseminates information related to the microvascular field.
Related titles: Online - full text ed.: (from EBSCO Publishing, O C L C Online Computer Library Center, Inc., RoweCom Information Quest, ingenta, Swets Blackwell, IDEAL Online Library, Institute for Scientific Information).
Indexed: ASCA, Biol.Abstr., Chem.Abstr., Chem.Indus.Notes, Chem.Titles, Curr.Adv.Ecol.Sci., Curr.Cont., Dent.Ind., Excerp.Med., INIS Atomind., Ind.Med. (1968-), Ind.Sci.Rev., Ind.Vet., Inpharma, Neurosci.Cit.Ind., Pharm.&Out.News, Pig News & Info., Reac., Sci.Cit.Ind., Vet.Bull.
—BLDSC (5761.060000), ADONIS, CASDDS, CISTI, GNLM, IDS, ingenta, KNAW, Linda Hall. **CCC.**
Published by: Academic Press, Inc., Journal Division (Subsidiary of: Harcourt Brace & Company), 525 B St, Ste 1900, San Diego, CA 92101-4495. TEL 619-230-1840, FAX 619-699-6800, apsubs@acad.com, http://www.academicpress.com/mvr. Ed. David Shepro.

616.1 ITA ISSN 0026-4725
MINERVA CARDIOANGIOLOGICA; rivista mensile di clinica e terapia medica e chirurgica delle malattie del cuore e dei vasi. Text in Italian; Summaries in English, Italian. 1953. m. (10/yr.). USD 125 to individuals; USD 165 to institutions (effective 2000 - 2001). adv. abstr, bibl, illus. *Refereed.* **Document type:** *Academic/Scholarly.* **Description:** Covers pathophysiology, clinical medicine and therapy of heart and vessels.
Incorporates (1976-1996): Minerva Angiologica (0391-3627)
Related titles: Microform ed.: (from PQC).
Indexed: Biol.Abstr., Chem.Abstr., Curr.Adv.Ecol.Sci., Curr.Cont. (coverage dropped), Dent.Ind., Excerp.Med., Ind.Med. (1953-), Inpharma, Nutr.Abstr., Reac.
—CISTI, GNLM, KNAW.
Published by: Edizioni Minerva Medica, Corso Bramante, 83-85, Turin, TO 10126, Italy. TEL 39-11-678282, FAX 39-11-674502. Ed., Pub. Alberto Oliaro. Adv. contact F Filippo. B&W page USD 1,200, color page USD 2,000; trim 270 x 190. Circ: 4,000 (paid). **Co-sponsors:** Italian Society of Vascular Pathology; Italian Group of Vascular Ultrasonics; Italian Society of Clinical and Experimental Phlebology; Italian Society of Lymphangiology.

616.132 GBR ISSN 1465-5691
MODERN HYPERTENSION MANAGEMENT. Text in English. q. **Document type:** *Academic/Scholarly.* **Description:** Covers all aspects of hypertension including diet, diagnosis, diseases, pregnancy and more.
—BLDSC (5886.905000).
Published by: Medical Education Partnership, 1 Chelsea Manor Gardens, London SW3 5PN, United Kingdom. TEL 44-20-7795-0220, FAX 44-20-7351-4053, sbradley@mepuk.com, http://www.mepuk.com/. Ed. A H Barnett. Pub. Jane Jones.

616.1 610 JPN ISSN 0387-1126
MYAKKANGAKU/JAPANESE COLLEGE OF ANGIOLOGY. JOURNAL. Text in Japanese; Summaries in English, Japanese. 1961. m. **Document type:** *Academic/Scholarly.*
Indexed: INIS Atomind.
—CISTI, GNLM.
Published by: (Nihon Myakkan Gakkai/Japanese College of Angiology), Bunkodo Co. Ltd., 2-7 Hongo 7-chome, Bunkyo-ku, Tokyo 113-0033, Japan.

N M C D. (Nutrition, Metabolism and Cardiovascular Diseases) see *NUTRITION AND DIETETICS*

616.1 AUS
NATIONAL HEART FOUNDATION OF AUSTRALIA. ANNUAL REPORT (YEAR). Text in English. 1965. a. free per issue. **Document type:** *Corporate.*
Published by: National Heart Foundation of Australia, PO Box 2, Woden, ACT 2606, Australia. TEL 61-2-6282-2144, FAX 61-2-6282-5147, nhfact@heartfoundation.com.au. R&P Helen Willimott.

616.12 616.8 DEU ISSN 1439-4847
CODEN: EEGLE5
NEUROPHYSIOLOGIE - LABOR. Text in German; Summaries in English, German. 1979. q. EUR 105 (effective 2002). **Document type:** *Journal, Academic/Scholarly.*
Formerly (until 2000): E E G Labor (0170-8287)
Indexed: Excerp.Med.
—BLDSC (6081.517900), CISTI, EMDOCS, GNLM, Infotrieve. **CCC.**
Published by: (Fachvereinigung der Elektrophysiologischen Assistenten e.V.), Urban & Fischer Verlag, Loebdergraben 14a, Jena 07743, Germany. TEL 49-3641-626444, FAX 49-3641-626500, marketing.journals@urbanfischer.de, http://www.urbanfischer.de/journals. Eds. E-J Speckmann, P Rappelsberger, S Kubicki. **Dist. by:** Nature Publishing Group, Brunel Rd, Basingstoke RG21 6XS, United Kingdom. TEL 44-1256-302629, FAX 44-1256-463570, j.stephens@macmillan.com.

616.12 616.07 GBR
▼ **NEW ADVANCES IN NUCLEAR CARDIOLOGY**; current practice and latest developments. Text in English. 1999. q.
Related titles: Online - full text ed.
—BLDSC (6081.724500).
Published by: Current Medical Literature Ltd., 40-42 Osnaburgh St, London NW1 3ND, United Kingdom. TEL 44-20-7465-8380, FAX 44-20-7465-8377, enquiries@curmedlit.co.uk, http://www.curmedlit.com/index.html. Eds. Ernst E van der Wall, Richard Underwood.

616.1 NLD
NEW CLINICAL APPLICATIONS. CARDIOLOGY. Text in English. irreg. price varies. **Document type:** *Monographic series.*
Published by: Kluwer Academic Publishers Group (Subsidiary of: Wolters Kluwer N.V.), Spuiboulevard 50, PO Box 17, Dordrecht 3300 AA, Netherlands. FAX 31-78-639-2254, services@wkap.nl, http://www.wkap.nl. **Dist. by:** Journals Department, PO Box 322, Dordrecht 3300 AH, Netherlands. FAX 31-78-654-6474.

616.1 DEU ISSN 0300-5224
CODEN: NIHOD9
NIEREN- UND HOCHDRUCKKRANKHEITEN. Text in German. 1972. m. DEM 258, EUR 131.91; DEM 28, EUR 14.32 newsstand/cover (effective 2001). adv. abstr. *Refereed.* **Document type:** *Journal, Academic/Scholarly.*
Indexed: ASCA, Biol.Abstr., Chem.Abstr., Chem.Indus.Notes, Chem.Titles, Curr.Adv.Ecol.Sci., Curr.Cont., Excerp.Med., INIS Atomind., Inpharma, Pharm.&Out.News, Reac., Ref.Zh.
—CASDDS, EMDOCS, GNLM, IDS, Infotrieve, KNAW. **CCC.**
Published by: Dustri-Verlag Dr. Karl Feistle, Bajuwarenring 4, Oberhaching 82041, Germany. TEL 49-89-613861-0, FAX 49-89-613-5412, info@dustri.de, http://www.dustri.de. Ed. Dr. H Brass. R&P Renate Lehmann. Adv. contact Joerg Feistle. B&W page DEM 2,870, B&W page XEU 1,467.41; trim 167 x 242. Circ: 3,700.

616.1 MEX ISSN 1405-2229
NUEVA CARDIOLOGIA. Text in Spanish; Summaries in English. 1987. m. MXP 430, USD 90 (effective 1996 & 1997). **Document type:** *Academic/Scholarly.* **Description:** Publishes works presented orally at the general sessions of the institute.
Published by: (Instituto Nacional de Cardiologia), Obsidiana Editores S.A., CZDA DE TLALPAN 2365, Col Ciudad Jardin, Mexico City, DF 04370, Mexico. TEL 52-5-689-9133. Eds. Dr. Fause Attie, Dr. Paris Troyo. Pub. Jorge Godoy-Gutierrez. Circ: 1,430 (paid); 570 (controlled). **Dist. by:** Distribuidora Editorial de Mexico SA de CV, P.O. Box 76-026, Mexico City, DF 04201, Mexico. TEL 52-5-544-7953, FAX 52-5-689-6545.

OPERATIVE TECHNIQUES IN THORACIC AND CARDIOVASCULAR SURGERY. see *MEDICAL SCIENCES—Surgery*

616.132 ESP ISSN 1139-1596
▼ **P A A P PRESION ARTERIAL**; revista de hipertension para la atencion primaria. Text in Spanish. 1999. 6/yr. ESP 5,000 domestic; EUR 30.10 in Europe; USD 67 elsewhere (effective 2001). **Document type:** *Academic/Scholarly.*
Published by: Ediciones Mayo S.A., Muntaner, 374-376 4o, Barcelona 08006, Spain. TEL 34-93-2090255, FAX 34-93-2020643, edmayo@app.es, http://www.edicionesmayo.es. Ed. Dr. Roca-Cusachs Coll.

616.1 USA ISSN 0147-8389
RC684.P3
PACING AND CLINICAL ELECTROPHYSIOLOGY (PACE). Text in English. 1978. m. USD 215 domestic; USD 270 foreign; USD 323 to libraries; USD 30 newsstand/cover (effective 2000). adv. bk.rev. abstr, bibl, charts, illus, pat, stat. index, cum.index. *Refereed.* **Document type:** *Academic/Scholarly.* **Description:** Information regarding the major advances in clinical cardiac pacing, electrophysiology, electrostimulation, biostimulation, and implantable devices.
Related titles: Online - full text ed.: (from CatchWord Ltd., Institute for Scientific Information).
Indexed: Biol.Abstr., CINAHL, Curr.Cont., Excerp.Med., INIS Atomind., INSPEC (Jan.1997-), Ind.Med. (1978-), Ind.Sci.Rev., Inpharma, Int.Nurs.Ind., Jrnl.Watch Card., Pharm.&Out.News, Reac., Rev.Med.& Vet.Mycol., Sci.Cit.Ind.
—BLDSC (6328.210000), ADONIS, CISTI, GNLM, IDS, ingenta, KNAW. **CCC.**

M

Published by: Futura Publishing Company, Inc., 135 Bedford Rd, PO Box 418, Armonk, NY 10504-0418. TEL 914-273-1014, 800-877-8761, FAX 914-273-1016, lisa@futuraco.com. Ed. Dr. Seymour Furman. R&P Joan McLaughlin. Adv. contact Lisa Piedimonte. B&W page USD 1,230, color page USD 2,195; trim 8.25 x 10.875. Circ: 6,891. **Co-sponsors:** North American Society of Pacing and Clinical Electrophysiology; Asian-Pacific Working Group on Cardiac Pacing.

616.1 PAK ISSN 0048-2706
PAKISTAN HEART JOURNAL. Text in English. 1968. q. PKR 200, USD 25 (effective 1998). adv. bk.rev. bibl, charts, illus. **Document type:** *Academic/Scholarly.* **Description:** Covers cardiac science in Pakistan with original papers and review papers.
Indexed: INIS Atomind.
Published by: Pakistan Cardiac Society, c/o National Institute of Cardiovascular Diseases, Jinnah Hospital Rd., Karachi, Pakistan. TEL 92-21-9201286, FAX 92-21-9201287. Ed. Azhar M A Faruqui. Circ: 1,000.

PATHOPHYSIOLOGY OF HAEMOSTASIS AND THROMBOSIS; international journal on haemostasis and thrombosis research. see *MEDICAL SCIENCES—Hematology*

616.1 USA ISSN 1092-9126
PEDIATRIC CARDIAC SURGERY ANNUAL OF THE SEMINARS IN THORACIC AND CARDIOVASCULAR SURGERY. Text in English. a. **Document type:** *Academic/Scholarly.*
—BLDSC (6417.534000).
Published by: (American Association for Thoracic Surgery), W.B. Saunders Co. (Subsidiary of: Harcourt Publishers Ltd.), Curtis Center, Independence Sq W, Philadelphia, PA 19106-3399. TEL 407-345-4000, FAX 800-654-2452. **Subscr. to:** 6277 Sea Harbour Dr, Orlando, FL 32887-4800. TEL 407-345-4000.

618.92 616.12 USA ISSN 0172-0643
RJ421 CODEN: PECAD4
PEDIATRIC CARDIOLOGY. Text in English. 1980. bi-m. (in 1 vol., 6 nos./vol.). EUR 383.30 domestic for Print & Online Eds.; USD 356.60 in Germany for Print & Online Eds.; USD 65.90 newsstand/cover foreign (effective 2002). adv. reprint service avail. from ISI. *Refereed.* **Document type:** *Academic/Scholarly.* **Description:** Devoted exclusively to the diagnosis and management of heart disease in young people. Presents research reports and the latest clinical information from across the entire field.
Related titles: Microform ed.: (from PQC); Online - full text ed.: ISSN 1432-1971 (from EBSCO Publishing, RoweCom Information Quest, Swets Blackwell, Springer LINK, Institute for Scientific Information).
Indexed: ASCA, Curr.Cont., Dent.Ind., Excerp.Med., Helminthol.Abstr., INIS Atomind., Ind.Med. (1979-), Ind.Sci.Rev., Inpharma, Nutr.Abstr., Pharm.&Out.News, Reac., Sci.Cit.Ind.
—BLDSC (6417.535000), CISTI, GNLM, IDS, ingenta, KNAW. **CCC.**
Published by: Springer-Verlag, Journals (Subsidiary of: BertelsmannSpringer), 175 Fifth Ave, New York, NY 10010. FAX 212-473-6272, orders@springer-ny.com, http://www.springer-ny.com. Eds. Ian Carr, James Taylor. R&P Ian Gross. Adv. contact Jay Feinman. **Subscr. in N. America to:** Journal Fulfillment Services, PO Box 2485, Secaucus, NJ 07096-2485. TEL 800-777-4643, FAX 201-348-4505.

616.1 DEU ISSN 0935-0020
PERFUSION; Kreislauferkrankungen in Klinik und Praxis. Text in English, German. 1988. m. DEM 96 (effective 2000). adv. *Refereed.* **Document type:** *Journal, Academic/Scholarly.*
Related titles: Online - full text ed.: (from Institute for Scientific Information).
Indexed: Curr.Cont., Inpharma, Pharm.&Out.News, Reac.
—BLDSC (6425.015000), GNLM, IDS, Infotrieve. **CCC.**
Published by: Verlag Perfusion GmbH, Regensburger Str 44-46, Nuernberg 90478, Germany. TEL 49-911-49108, FAX 49-911-493579. Ed. E Erust. Adv. contact Sibylle Michna. Circ: 20,500.

616.1 GBR ISSN 0267-6591
CODEN: PERFER
PERFUSION. Text in English. 1986. bi-m. GBP 127 in Europe to individuals; USD 219 in North America to individuals; GBP 143 rest of world to individuals; GBP 442 in Europe to institutions; USD 710 in North America to institutions; GBP 467 rest of world to institutions; USD 85 in North America to members aacp; GBP 233 in developing nations; GBP 78 newsstand/cover in Europe; USD 140 newsstand/cover in North America; GBP 83 newsstand/cover rest of world (effective 2002). adv. bk.rev. index. back issues avail.; reprints avail. *Refereed.* **Document type:** *Journal, Academic/Scholarly.* **Description:** Dedicated to the advancement of knowledge and clinical practice in the field of extracorporeal circulation.
Related titles: Online - full text ed.: (from EBSCO Publishing, O C L C Online Computer Library Center, Inc., RoweCom Information Quest, ingenta, Swets Blackwell, Institute for Scientific Information).
Indexed: CINAHL, Curr.Cont., Excerp.Med., Ind.Med. (1986-), Inpharma, Pharm.&Out.News, Reac.
—BLDSC (6425.020000), CISTI, EMDOCS, GNLM, Infotrieve, ingenta, KNAW. **CCC.**
Published by: Arnold Publishers (Subsidiary of: Hodder Headline plc.), 338 Euston Rd, London NW1 3BH, United Kingdom. TEL 44-20-7873-6337, FAX 44-20-7873-6325, arnoldjournals@hodder.co.uk, http://www.palliativemedjournal.com. Ed. K M Taylor. Adv. contact Mary Attree. **Subscr. to:** Turpin Distribution Services Ltd., Blackhorse Rd, Letchworth, Herts SG6 1HN, United Kingdom. TEL 44-1462-488900, FAX 44-1462-483011.

616.12 CAN ISSN 0828-6396
PERSPECTIVES IN CARDIOLOGY. Text in English. 1985. 10/yr. adv.
Published by: S T A Communications Inc., 955 bd St Jean, bur 306, Pointe Claire, PQ H9R 5K3, Canada. TEL 514-695-7623, FAX 514-695-8554. Ed. Paul Brand. Circ: 15,269.

616.132 USA ISSN 0898-6770
PERSPECTIVES IN HYPERTENSION SERIES. Text in English. 1987. irreg. price varies. reprint service avail. from PQC. *Refereed.* **Document type:** *Monographic series.*
—CISTI, KNAW.
Published by: Lippincott Williams & Wilkins (Philadelphia) (Subsidiary of: Wolters Kluwer N.V.), 530 Walnut St, Philadelphia, PA 19106-3621. TEL 301-223-2300, 800-638-3030, FAX 301-223-2400, http://www.lww.com.

616.12 USA ISSN 1044-4157
RJ421
PERSPECTIVES IN PEDIATRIC CARDIOLOGY. Text in English. 1988. irreg.
—BLDSC (6428.147700).
Published by: Futura Publishing Company, Inc., 135 Bedford Rd, PO Box 418, Armonk, NY 10504-0418. TEL 914-273-1014, 800-877-8761, FAX 914-273-1015.

616.1 GBR ISSN 0268-3555
CODEN: PHLEEF
PHLEBOLOGY. Text in English. 1986. q. EUR 231.30 domestic; EUR 228.70 in Germany; USD 66 newsstand/cover foreign (effective 2002). index. back issues avail. *Refereed.* **Document type:** *Academic/Scholarly.*
Related titles: Online - full text ed.: ISSN 1433-3031 (from EBSCO Publishing, RoweCom Information Quest, Swets Blackwell, Springer LINK, Institute for Scientific Information).
Indexed: ASCA, Curr.Cont., Excerp.Med., Ind.Med. (coverage dropped), Inpharma, Pharm.&Out.News, Reac., Sci.Cit.Ind.
—BLDSC (6465.101100), CISTI, EMDOCS, GNLM, IDS, Infotrieve, KNAW. **CCC.**
Published by: (International Union of Phlebology), Springer-Verlag London Ltd. (Subsidiary of: BertelsmannSpringer), Sweetapple House, Catteshall Rd, Godalming, Surrey GU7 3DJ, United Kingdom. TEL 44-1483-418800, FAX 44-1483-415144. Ed. David Negus. Circ: 700. **Subscr. in N. America to:** Springer-Verlag New York Inc., PO Box 2485, Secaucus, NJ 07096-2485.

PLATELETS (SHEFFIELD). see *BIOLOGY—Abstracting, Bibliographies, Statistics*

616.132 DEU
PRESSURE. Text in German. irreg. **Document type:** *Academic/Scholarly.*
—BLDSC (6612.556250).

Published by: (Sanofi Winthrop GmbH), Springer-Verlag Heidelberg (Subsidiary of: BertelsmannSpringer), Tiergartenstr 17, Heidelberg 69121, Germany. TEL 49-6221-487502, FAX 49-6221-413982, subscriptions@springer.de. Ed. Beate Fruhstorfer.

616.12 USA ISSN 1520-037X
CODEN: PCARFX
PREVENTIVE CARDIOLOGY. Text in English. 1998. q. USD 90 domestic to individuals; USD 105 foreign to individuals; USD 105 domestic to institutions; USD 120 foreign to institutions (effective 2001). adv. bk.rev. abstr, charts, illus. back issues avail.; reprints avail. *Refereed.* **Document type:** *Journal, Academic/Scholarly.*
—BLDSC (6612.779700).
Published by: LeJacq Communications, Inc., 777 W Putnam Ave, Greenwich, CT 06830-5014. TEL 203-531-0450, FAX 203-531-0533, showell@lejacq.com. Ed. Ezra Amsterdam. Pub. Louis Lejacq. R&P Andrea Townsend. Adv. contact Joann Kalaka-Adams TEL 732-747-6525. B&W page USD 2,200, color page USD 1,095; trim 10.75 x 8. Circ: 20,000 (controlled).

616.12 ITA ISSN 0393-6139
PRIMARY CARDIOLOGY (EDIZIONE ITALIANA). Text in Italian. 1986. bi-m. adv.
Published by: E S I Stampa Medica s.r.l., Lgo Volontari del Sangue, 10, S Donato Milanese, MI 20097, Italy. TEL 39-2-5274241, FAX 39-2-55600670. Adv. contact Ornella Galbiati. Circ: 37,000.

616.1 CHE ISSN 0254-5195
CODEN: MFKLDH
PROGRESS IN APPLIED MICROCIRCULATION. Text in English. 1983. irreg., latest vol.24. CHF 130 in Europe; DEM 155 in Germany; USD 105 in United States (effective 2001). *Refereed.* **Document type:** *Monographic series, Academic/Scholarly.* **Description:** Series that confronts some of the most challenging problems of microcirculation research and demonstrates how their solutions can alter clinical practice.
Related titles: Online - full text ed.: (from Institute for Scientific Information).
Indexed: Chem.Abstr.
—BLDSC, CASDDS, KNAW. **CCC.**
Published by: S. Karger AG, Allschwilerstr 10, PO Box, Basel 4009, Switzerland. TEL 41-61-306-1111, FAX 41-61-306-1234, karger@karger.ch, http://www.karger.com/bookseries/PRAPM. Ed. K Messmer.

616.1 USA ISSN 0033-0620
CODEN: PCVDAN
PROGRESS IN CARDIOVASCULAR DISEASES. Text in English; Summaries in French, Spanish. 1958. bi-m. USD 159 domestic to individuals Full text online included; USD 243 foreign to individuals Full text online included; USD 276 domestic to institutions Full text online included; USD 355 foreign to institutions Full text online included; USD 73 domestic to students Full text online included; USD 153 foreign to students Full text online included; USD 60 per issue (effective 2001). adv. bibl, charts, illus. index. *Refereed.* **Document type:** *Journal, Academic/Scholarly.* **Description:** Each issue covers a single major topic, which experts discuss from various perspectives.
Related titles: Online - full text ed.: (from Institute for Scientific Information).
Indexed: AIM, Biol.Abstr., CINAHL, Chem.Abstr., Chem.Titles, Curr.Adv.Ecol.Sci., Curr.Cont., Excerp.Med., INIS Atomind., Ind.Med. (1958-), Ind.Sci.Rev., Inpharma, NRN, Nutr.Abstr., Pharm.&Out.News, Reac., Sci.Cit.Ind.
—BLDSC (6866.650000), CASDDS, CISTI, GNLM, IDS, ingenta, KNAW. **CCC.**
Published by: W.B. Saunders Co. (Subsidiary of: Harcourt Publishers Ltd.), 11830 Westline Industrial Dr, St Louis, MO 63146. TEL 800-325-4177, http://www.progcardvascdis.com, http://www.wbsaunders.com. Eds. Edmund H Sonnenblick, Dr. Michael Lesch. adv.: B&W page USD 910, color page USD 1,985; 10 x 7. Circ: 2,728 (paid). **Subscr. to:** Periodicals Fulfillment, W B Saunders Co, 6277 Sea Harbor Dr, 4th Fl, Orlando, FL 32891-4800.

616.12 610.73 USA ISSN 0889-7204
PROGRESS IN CARDIOVASCULAR NURSING. Text in English. 1985. q. USD 60 domestic to individuals; USD 75 foreign to individuals; USD 75 domestic to institutions; USD 95 foreign to institutions (effective 2001). adv. bk.rev. abstr, charts, illus. back issues avail.; reprints avail. *Refereed.* **Document type:** *Journal, Academic/Scholarly.* **Description:** Reflects current practice in caring for the cardiac patient, emphasizing research, new therapies and technologies.
Related titles: Online - full text ed.: (from Northern Light Technology, Inc., ProQuest Information & Learning).

Indexed: CINAHL, Ind.Med. (1986-), Int.Nurs.Ind.
—BLDSC (6866.660000), GNLM, Infotrieve, ingenta.
Published by: LeJacq Communications, Inc., 777 W Putnam Ave, Greenwich, CT 06830-5014. TEL 203-531-0450, FAX 203-531-0533, showell@lejacq.com. Ed. Manguerite Engler. Pub. Louis Lejacq. R&P Andrea Townsend. Adv. contact Joann Kalaka-Adams TEL 732-747-6525. B&W page USD 2,200, color page USD 1,095; trim 8 x 10.75. Circ: 10,000.

616.1 NLD ISSN 0923-4020
PROGRESS IN HYPERTENSION. Text in English. 1988. irreg., latest vol.4, 1999. price varies. illus. back issues avail. **Document type:** *Monographic series, Academic/Scholarly.* **Description:** Reports on all aspects of basic and clinical research of hypertension in its broadest sense.
Indexed: Chem.Abstr., Chem.Titles.
—BLDSC (6868.439000), CISTI, KNAW.
Published by: V S P (Subsidiary of: Brill Academic Publishers), PO Box 346, Zeist 3700 AH, Netherlands. TEL 31-30-692-5790, FAX 31-30-693-2081, vsppub@compuserve.com, http://www.vsppub.com/books/bs16.html. Ed. H Saito. **Dist. in US and Canada by:** Books International, PO Box 605, Herndon, VA 20172. TEL 703-661-1500, FAX 703-661-1501.

616.1 618.92 IRL ISSN 1058-9813
CODEN: PPCAFF
PROGRESS IN PEDIATRIC CARDIOLOGY. Text in English. 1992. q. EUR 197 in Europe to individuals; JPY 29,000 in Japan to individuals; USD 220 elsewhere to individuals; EUR 307 in Europe to institutions; JPY 45,300 in Japan to institutions; USD 343 elsewhere to institutions (effective 2002). *Refereed.* **Document type:** *Academic/Scholarly.* **Description:** Presents information and opinion important to the understanding and management of cardiovascular disease in children.
Related titles: Microform ed.: (from PQC); Online - full text ed.: (from ingenta, Swets Blackwell, ScienceDirect).
Indexed: ASCA, Curr.Cont. (coverage dropped), Inpharma, Pharm.&Out.News, Reac.
—BLDSC (6872.440000), EMDOCS, GNLM, IDS, Infotrieve, KNAW. **CCC.**
Published by: Elsevier Science Ireland Ltd, Elsevier House, Brookvale Plaza, E. Park, Shannon, Co. Clare, Ireland. TEL 353-61-471944, FAX 353-61-472144, http://www.elsevier.com/locate/ppedcard. Ed. Dr. William W Miller. R&P Annette Moloney. **Subscr. in Australasia and the Far East to:** Elsevier Science (Singapore) Pte Ltd, No.1 Temasek Ave, 17-01 Millenia Tower, Singapore 039192, Singapore. TEL 65-434-3727, FAX 65-337-2230; **Subscr. in the Americas to:** Elsevier Science, PO Box 945, New York, NY 10159-0945. TEL 212-633-3730, FAX 212-633-3680, http://www.elsevier.com; **Subscr. to:** Elsevier Science BV, PO Box 211, Amsterdam 1000 AE, Netherlands. TEL 31-20-485-3757, nlinfo-f@elsevier.nl.

616.1 GBR ISSN 0143-2435
RECENT ADVANCES IN CARDIOLOGY. Text in English. 1929. irreg. **Document type:** *Monographic series, Academic/Scholarly.*
—GNLM, KNAW.
Published by: Churchill Livingstone (Subsidiary of: Harcourt Publishers Ltd.), Robert Stevenson House, 1-3 Baxter's Pl, Leith Walk, Edinburgh, Midlothian EH1 3AF, United Kingdom. TEL 44-131-556-2424, FAX 44-131-459-1177, http://www.churchillmed.com. Ed. Derek J Rowlands. Pub. Gill Haddock. R&P Moira Trotter. **Subscr. to:** Harcourt Publishers Ltd., Foots Cray High St, Sidcup, Kent DA14 5HP, United Kingdom. TEL 44-20-8308-5700, FAX 44-20-8309-0807.

REFERATOVY VYBER Z KARDIOLOGIE/ABSTRACTS OF CARDIOLOGY. see *MEDICAL SCIENCES—Abstracting, Bibliographies, Statistics*

616.15 USA ISSN 0272-507X
RB145 CODEN: REHEDT
REVIEWS OF HEMATOLOGY. Text in English. 1980. irreg. USD 69.95. back issues avail. *Refereed.* **Document type:** *Academic/Scholarly.* **Description:** Provides information of value to hematologists, biochemists and other medical scientists.
Indexed: Biol.Abstr., Chem.Abstr., Curr.Cont. (coverage dropped).
—CASDDS, CISTI.
Published by: P J D Publications Ltd, PO Box 966, Westbury, NY 11590. TEL 516-626-0650, FAX 516-626-5546. Ed. Dr. Julian L Ambrus. Pub. Barbara Sankar.

616.1 ARG ISSN 0034-6993
REVISTA ARGENTINA DE ANGIOLOGIA✱. Text in Spanish; Summaries in English. 1967. q. ARS 20, USD 8. adv. bk.rev. abstr, bibl, charts, illus, stat. reprint service avail. from PQC.
Related titles: Microform ed.: 1967 (from PQC).
Indexed: Biol.Abstr.
Published by: (Argentine Society of Angiology), Plantie Talleres Graficos S.A., Avda. Juan Bautista Alberdi, 571, Capital Federal, Buenos Aires 1424, Argentina. Ed. Dr. Miguel Angel Lucas. Circ: 1,500.

617.41 BRA ISSN 0102-7638
REVISTA BRASILEIRA DE CIRURGIA CARDIOVASCULAR. Text in Portuguese. 1986. q. membership. back issues avail. **Document type:** *Academic/Scholarly.*
Related titles: Online - full text ed.: (from SciELO).
Published by: Sociedade Brasileira de Cirurgia Cardiovascular/Brazilian Society for Cardiovascular Surgery, Rua Beira Rio, 45 Andar 7 CONJ 73, VI Olimpia, Sao Paulo, SP 04548-050, Brazil. TEL 55-11-8290341, http://www.scielo.br. Ed. Adib D Jalene.

616.12 CUB ISSN 0864-2168
REVISTA CUBANA DE CARDIOLOGIA Y CIRUGIA CARDIOVASCULAR. Text in Spanish. 1987. s-a. USD 34 in the Americas; USD 42 in Europe; USD 50 elsewhere.
Formerly (until 1987): Boletin de Cardiologia y Cirugia Cardiovascular
—GNLM.
Published by: (Cuba. Ministerio de Salud Publica, Centro Nacional de Informacion de Ciencias Medicas), Editorial de Ciencias Medicas, O'Reilly No. 4, Habana, Cuba. TEL 809-62-8091. Ed. Sara Perez. Circ: 1,300. **Co-sponsors:** Instituto de Cardiologia y Cirugia Cardiovascular de Cuba; Sociedad Cubana de Cardiologia.

616.1 ESP ISSN 0300-8932
CODEN: RCDOAM
REVISTA ESPANOLA DE CARDIOLOGIA. Text in Spanish; Summaries in English, Spanish. 1958. m. USD 132 to non-members. adv. bk.rev. index. *Refereed.* **Document type:** *Academic/Scholarly.* **Description:** Covers cardiac physiopathology and the diagnostic and therapeutic resources applicable to heart disease.
Related titles: Online - full text ed.: (from Institute for Scientific Information); ♦ Supplement: Revista Espanola de Cardiologia. Suplemento. ISSN 1131-3587.
Indexed: Abstr.Hyg., Chem.Abstr., Curr.Cont., Excerp.Med., Ind.Med. (1947-), Ind.Med.Esp., Inpharma, Protozool.Abstr., Reac., Rev.Med.& Vet.Mycol.
—BLDSC (7853.930000), CASDDS, CINDOC, CISTI, EMDOCS, GNLM, Infotrieve, KNAW. **CCC.**
Published by: (Sociedad Espanola de Cardiologia), Ediciones Doyma S.A., Traversa de Gracia, 17-21, Barcelona 08021, Spain. TEL 34-93-200-0711, FAX 34-93-209-1136. Ed. F Fernandez Aviles. Adv. contact Anna Pahissa. color page ESP 259,000; trim 180 x 210. Circ: 4,000.

616.1 ESP ISSN 1131-3587
REVISTA ESPANOLA DE CARDIOLOGIA. SUPLEMENTO. Text in Spanish. 1981. m.
Related titles: ♦ Supplement to: Revista Espanola de Cardiologia. ISSN 0300-8932.
Published by: (Sociedad Espanola de Cardiologia), Ediciones Doyma S.A., Traversa de Gracia, 17-21, Barcelona 08021, Spain. TEL 34-1-200-07-11, FAX 34-1-209-11-36.

616.1 ESP ISSN 0214-3941
REVISTA IBEROAMERICANA DE TROMBOSIS Y HEMOSTASIA. Text in Spanish. 1988. q. ESP 10,300 to individuals; ESP 14,700 to institutions; ESP 8,250 to students (effective 2001). adv. back issues avail.; reprints avail. *Refereed.* **Document type:** *Journal, Academic/Scholarly.*
Related titles: Online - full text ed.: 1996; ♦ Supplement: Revista Iberoamericana de Trombosis y Hemostasia. Suplemento. ISSN 0214-395X.
Published by: (Sociedad Espanola de Trombosis y Hemostasia), Ediciones Doyma S.A., Traversa de Gracia, 17-21, Barcelona 08021, Spain. TEL 34-93-200-0711, rith@doyma.es, doyma@doyma.es, http://www.doyma.es/rith. Ed. Aznar J Lucea. R&P Monica Barnes. Adv. contact Jose Antonio Hernandez. B&W page ESP 122,000, color page ESP 152,000; 280 x 210. Circ: 1,000. **Co-sponsors:** Grupo Cooperativo Latino Americano de Hemostasia y Trombosis (AG); Sociedade Portuguesa de Trombose e Hemostase (PO); Liga del Danubio contra la Trombosis y Enfermedades Hemorragicas (AU); Grupo Espanol de Hemorreologia.

616.1 ESP ISSN 0214-395X
REVISTA IBEROAMERICANA DE TROMBOSIS Y HEMOSTASIA. SUPLEMENTO. Text in Spanish. 1988. irreg. *Refereed.* **Document type:** *Academic/Scholarly.*
Related titles: ♦ Supplement to: Revista Iberoamericana de Trombosis y Hemostasia. ISSN 0214-3941.
Published by: (Sociedad Espanola de Trombosis y Hemostasia), Ediciones Doyma S.A., Traversa de Gracia, 17-21, Barcelona 08021, Spain. TEL 34-93-200-0711, rith@doyma.es, doyma@doyma.es, http://www.doyma.es/riht. R&P Monica Barnes. Adv. contact Jose Antonio Hernandez.

616.12 ESP ISSN 0210-8755
CODEN: RLCEEK
REVISTA LATINA DE CARDIOLOGIA. Text in Spanish. 6/yr. USD 70 (effective 1996).
—BLDSC (7863.250000), GNLM, KNAW.
Published by: Editorial Idepsa S.A., Principe de Vergara, 112 1o F, Madrid 28002, Spain. TEL 34-1-5637306, FAX 34-1-5632393. Ed. Dr. Valles de Lema.

REVUE DE PNEUMOLOGIE CLINIQUE; le poumon et le coeur. see *MEDICAL SCIENCES—Respiratory Diseases*

616.1 SAU ISSN 1018-077X
SAUDI HEART JOURNAL. Text in English. 1989. 2/yr. free per issue. *Refereed.* **Document type:** *Academic/Scholarly.* **Description:** Publishes research articles of interest, case reports, reviews, discussions of new operative techniques and medical matters relating to the human heart.
Formerly (until vol.2, no.1, 1990): Saudi Heart Bulletin
Related titles: CD-ROM ed.
Indexed: Excerp.Med. (1993-), ExtraMED.
—EMDOCS.
Published by: (Saudi Heart Foundation/Jam'iah Asdiqa' al-Qalb al-Khairiyyah), King Abdul Aziz University Hospital, P O Box 6615, Jeddah 21452, Saudi Arabia. TEL 966-2-6697043, FAX 966-2-6697043. Ed. Dr. Hassan Raffa. adv.: B&W page SAR 5,000. Circ: 5,000.

616.145 NLD ISSN 0929-1776
SCRIPTA PHLEBOLOGICA. Text in Dutch, English; Summaries in Dutch, English, French. 1992. 3/yr. NLG 99; NLG 121 foreign (effective 1999). adv. **Document type:** *Academic/Scholarly.* **Description:** Contains original articles, congress reviews, abstracts, congress calendar, etc.
Published by: (Benelux Vereniging voor Flebologie), Elsevier Gezondheidszorg B.V., Tijdstroom (Subsidiary of: Reed Elsevier plc Group), Planetenbaan 1, Maarssen 3600 AK, Netherlands. TEL 31-346-577577, FAX 31-346-556287, gezondheidszorg@ebi.nl, http://www.tijdstroom.nl. Ed. J C J M Veraart. Adv. contact Johan Ysebrands. **Subscr. to:** Elsevier Den Haag, Postbus 16500, The Hague 2500 BM, Netherlands. TEL 31-70-381-9900, FAX 31-70-333-8399.

SCRIPTA SCIENTIFICA MEDICA. see *MEDICAL SCIENCES—Oncology*

616.12 617.96 USA ISSN 1089-2532
SEMINARS IN CARDIOTHORACIC AND VASCULAR ANESTHESIA. Text in English. 1997. q. USD 130 domestic to individuals; USD 178 foreign to individuals; USD 182 domestic to institutions; USD 233 foreign to institutions; USD 87 domestic to students; USD 107 foreign to students; USD 59 newsstand/cover (effective 2001). adv. **Document type:** *Academic/Scholarly.* **Description:** Provides current overview of a clinical, surgical, or physiologic entity, monitoring modality, or pharmacologica advance relevant to cardiac, thoracic, or vascular anesthesia and related areas of critical care medicine.
—BLDSC (8239.448343).
Published by: W.B. Saunders Co. (Subsidiary of: Harcourt Publishers Ltd.), 11830 Westline Industrial Dr, St Louis, MO 63146. TEL 800-325-4177, http://www.wbsaunders.com. Ed. Carol Lake. adv.: B&W page USD 715, color page USD 1,740. Circ: 805. **Subscr. to:** 6277 Sea Harbour Dr, Orlando, FL 32887-4800. TEL 800-654-2452.

SEMINARS IN HEMATOLOGY. see *MEDICAL SCIENCES—Hematology*

616.1 GBR ISSN 1084-2764
SEMINARS IN INTERVENTIONAL CARDIOLOGY. Text in English. ceased; resumed 1996. bi-m. GBP 71 to individuals; USD 109 in North America to individuals; GBP 178 to institutions; USD 274 in North America to institutions (effective 2001). adv. **Document type:** *Academic/Scholarly.* **Description:** Presents a comprehensive view of interventional cardiology, describing new biological challenges, technological innovations and advances in clinical applications through topic-based issues.
Indexed: Ind.Med. (1996-).
—BLDSC (8239.452500), GNLM, Infotrieve. **CCC.**
Published by: W.B. Saunders Co. Ltd. (Subsidiary of: Harcourt Publishers Ltd.), 24-28 Oval Rd, London NW1 7DX, United Kingdom. TEL 44-20-7424-4200, FAX 44-20-7424-4515, cservice@harcourt.com, http://www.harcourt-international.com/journals/siic. Ed. Patrick Serruys. **Subscr. to:** Harcourt Publishers Ltd., Foots Cray High St, Sidcup, Kent DA14 5HP, United Kingdom. TEL 44-20-8308-5700, FAX 44-20-8309-0807.

SEMINARS IN THORACIC AND CARDIOVASCULAR SURGERY. see *MEDICAL SCIENCES—Surgery*

616.1 USA ISSN 1528-9648
▼ **SEMINARS IN VASCULAR MEDICINE.** Text in English. 2001. q. EUR 107 to individuals; EUR 200 to institutions; EUR 43 newsstand/cover (effective 2002). **Document type:** *Journal, Academic/Scholarly.*
Published by: Thieme Medical Publishers, 333 Seventh Ave, New York, NY 10001. TEL 212-760-0888, 800-782-3488, FAX 212-947-1112, custserv@thieme.com, http://www.thieme.com.

SEMINARS IN VASCULAR SURGERY. see *MEDICAL SCIENCES—Surgery*

616.12 JPN ISSN 0911-0836
CODEN: SHPEEY
SHINZO PESHINGU/JAPANESE JOURNAL OF CARDIAC PACING AND ELECTROPHYSIOLOGY. Text in Japanese. 1984. q. JPY 4,000 per issue.
Indexed: Excerp.Med., INIS Atomind.
—EMDOCS.
Published by: Nihon Shinzo Peshingu Gakkai/Japanese Cardiac Pacing Society, Tokyo Joshi Ika Daigaku, Fuzoku Nihon Shinzo Ketsuatsu Kenkyujo, 8-1, Ichigaya Kawadacho, Shinjuku-ku, Tokyo 162, Japan.

SIGNAL'NAYA INFORMATSIYA. ISHIMICHESKAYA BOLEZN' SERDTSA. see *MEDICAL SCIENCES—Abstracting, Bibliographies, Statistics*

610 ESP
SISTOLE; ciencia y medicina. Text in Spanish. m. **Document type:** *Academic/Scholarly.* **Description:** Explores the science and pharmacology of cardiovascular medicine.
Published by: Saned S.A., Capitan Haya, 60, Madrid 28020, Spain. TEL 34-91-749-9507, FAX 34-91-749-9507, saned@meditex.es. Ed. Alicia Martinez Magro. adv.: page ESP 300,000.

616.1 FRA ISSN 0395-403X
SOCIETE FRANCAISE DE CARDIOLOGIE. BULLETIN D'INFORMATIONS. Text in French. q. membership. adv.
Related titles: Online - full text ed.: 1976.
Indexed: I.P.A.
Published by: Societe Francaise de Cardiologie, 15 rue Cels, Paris 75014 , France. Circ: 1,800.

616.1 USA
SPECTRUM (LANHAM). Text in English. q. USD 35 in North America to non-members; USD 40 elsewhere to non-members. adv. **Document type:** *Newsletter.* **Description:** Covers technological, social, economic, and legislative news of interest to medical professionals in the field. Reviews new products, reports chapter news, and lists forthcoming events and educational programs.
Published by: Society of Vascular Technology, 4601 Presidents Dr, Ste 260, Lanham, MD 20706-4831. TEL 301-459-7550, 800-SVT-VEIN, FAX 301-459-5651. Ed. Carol Ann Faull. Pub. Patricia Horner. R&P Teresa Todd. Adv. contact Teresa A Todd. page USD 650; 9.5 x 7.5. Circ: 5,000.

SPORTS MEDICINE REPORTS; a physician-to-physician update on critical issues in sports medicine. see *MEDICAL SCIENCES—Sports Medicine*

616.1 GBR ISSN 1369-5339
CODEN: STENFN
STENT; comment and analysis on progress in coronary stenting. Text in English. 1998. q. GBP 50 in Europe; USD 75 in US & Canada; USD 75 elsewhere. **Document type:** *Academic/Scholarly.*
—BLDSC (8464.207000).
Published by: Remedica Publishing Ltd., 32-38 Osnaburgh St, London NW1 3ND, United Kingdom. TEL 44-171-388-7677, FAX 44-171-388-7678, info@remedica.com, http://www.remedica.com. Eds. Neal Uren, Nicolas Chronos.

616.1 USA ISSN 0039-2499
RC388.5 CODEN: SJCCA7
STROKE; a journal of cerebral circulation. Text in English. 1970. m., latest vol.31. USD 248 domestic to institutions Print & Online eds. combined; USD 334 foreign to institutions Print & Online eds. combined; USD 382 domestic to institutions Print & Online eds. combined; USD 449 foreign to institutions Print & Online eds. combined; USD 40 newsstand/cover (effective 2002). abstr, charts, illus. index. back issues avail.; reprint service avail. from PQC. *Refereed.* **Document type:** *Academic/Scholarly.* **Description:** For neurologists, cardiologists and internists. Includes articles on prevention, diagnosis, treatment and rehabilitation of stroke victims.
Related titles: CD-ROM ed.: (from Ovid Technologies, Inc.); Microform ed.: (from PQC,MIM); Online - full text ed.: USD 496.60 domestic academic site license; USD 563.60 foreign academic site license; USD 553.90 domestic corporate site license; USD 620.90 foreign corporate site license (effective 2002) (from HighWire Pr., Ovid Technologies, Inc., Northern Light Technology, Inc., EBSCO Publishing, ProQuest Information & Learning, Institute for Scientific Information).
Indexed: AMED, ASCA, Agri.& Environ.Biotech.Abstr. (coverage dropped), Biol.Abstr., Brit.Nur.Ind., CINAHL, Chem.Abstr., Chem.Indus.Notes, Chem.Titles, Chic.Per.Ind., Curr.Adv.Ecol.Sci., Curr.Cont., Dent.Ind., Derwent Biotech.Abstr., Excerp.Med., Helminthol.Abstr., INIS Atomind., Ind.Med. (1970-), Ind.Sci.Rev., Inpharma, Int.Abstr.Biol.Sci., Int.Nurs.Ind., Jrnl.Watch Emer.Med., Jrnl.Watch Neuro., NRN, Neurosci.Abstr. (coverage dropped), Neurosci.Cit.Ind., Nutr.Abstr., Pharm.&Out.News, Reac., SSCI (coverage dropped), Sci.Cit.Ind., THA.
—BLDSC (8474.900000), CASDDS, CISTI, GNLM, IDS, ingenta, KNAW.
Published by: (American Heart Association), Lippincott Williams & Wilkins (Baltimore) (Subsidiary of: Wolters Kluwer N.V.), 351 W Camden St, Baltimore, MD 21201-2436. TEL 410-528-4000, 800-787-8984, FAX 410-528-4312, http://www.stroke.ahajournals.org, http://www.strokeaha.org. Ed. Dr. Mark Dyken. Pub. Cara Kaufman. R&P Debbie Heise TEL 410-528-4050. Adv. contact Angela Hopkins. Circ: 7,800.

616.1 USA
STROKE CLUB INTERNATIONAL BULLETIN. Text in English. 1968. a. bibl. **Document type:** *Bulletin.* **Description:** Contains information about the rights of citizens who have suffered from strokes.
Published by: Stroke Clubs International, 805 12th St, Galveston, TX 77550. TEL 409-762-1022. Ed., R&P Ellis Williamson. Circ: 45,000.

616.1 USA ISSN 1047-014X
STROKE CONNECTION MAGAZINE. Text in English. 1980. bi-m. USD 12 domestic; USD 25 foreign (effective 2000 - 2001). adv. bk.rev., Website rev. 28 p./no. back issues avail. **Document type:** *Magazine, Consumer.* **Description:** For stroke survivors, caregivers, and healthcare professionals. Focuses on the lay population's ability to deal with various aspects of stroke-prevention, rehabilitation, and treatments and advances.
Published by: American Heart Association, 7272 Greenville Ave, Dallas, TX 75231-4596. strokeconnection@heart.org, http://www.strokeassociation.org, http://www.amhrt.org. Eds. Debi McGill, Emily Springer, Jon Caswell. Adv. contact Debi McGill. Circ: 14,195 (paid).

616.1 USA
STROKE: DISEASE STATE MANAGEMENT RESOURCE. Text in English. 1997. a. USD 269; USD 229 foreign (effective 1999). **Document type:** *Trade.*
Published by: American Health Consultants (Subsidiary of: Medical Economics Co., Inc.), 3525 Piedmont Rd, N E, 6 Piedmont Center, Ste 400, Atlanta, GA 30305. TEL 404-262-5476, custserv@ahcpub.com, http://www.ahcpub.com.

616.1 FIN ISSN 0039-7571
SYDAN. Text in Finnish, Swedish. 1958. 6/yr. FIM 150 to non-members; FIM 20 to members (effective 1999). adv. bk.rev. 48 p./no. **Document type:** *Magazine, Consumer.* **Description:** Reports on the prevention, treatment and rehabilitation of cardio-vascular diseases and the activities of the association.
Published by: Suomen Sydantautiliitto/Finnish Heart Association, Oltermannintie 8, PL 50, Helsinki 00621, Finland. TEL 358-5430902, FAX 358-5430920, marjatta.karvinen@sydanliitto.fi, http://www.sydanliitto.fi. Ed. Marjatta Karvinen. adv.: B&W page FIM 11,500, color page FIM 16,000. Circ: 60,000.

616.1 FRA ISSN 1143-4171
SYNTHESE MEDICALE CARDIOLOGIE. Text in French. 10/yr. FRF 150. adv. charts. **Description:** Covers current cardiology news.
Published by: Editions Techniques et Medicales, 18 rue des Huissiers, Neuilly-sur-Seine 92200, France. TEL 47-47-74-74, FAX 47-47-71-03. Ed. Guy Vincent Heugas. Circ: 7,000.

616.12 USA ISSN 8756-8586
TECHNOLOGY FOR CARDIOLOGY. Text in English. m. USD 205.80 domestic; USD 221 in Canada; USD 249.60 elsewhere (effective 2002). *Refereed.* **Document type:** *Newsletter.* **Description:** Contains technology-related information about cardiology for healthcare professionals.
Formerly: Health Devices Update: Cardiology
—**CCC.**
Published by: (Emergency Care Research Institute), E C R I, 5200 Butler Pike, Plymouth, PA 19462. TEL 610-825-6000, FAX 610-834-1275, info@ecri.org, http://www.ecri.org. Ed. Beth Richardson.

616.1 USA ISSN 0730-2347
RC681.A1 CODEN: THIJDO
TEXAS HEART INSTITUTE JOURNAL. Text in English. 1974. q. USD 35; USD 45 foreign. adv. bk.rev. illus, stat. back issues avail.; reprints avail. *Refereed.* **Document type:** *Academic/Scholarly.*
Formerly: Cardiovascular Diseases (0093-3546)
Related titles: Online - full text ed.: (from Ovid Technologies, Inc., Institute for Scientific Information).
Indexed: ASCA, Biol.Abstr., Curr.Cont., Environ.Sci.Poll.Mgmt., Excerp.Med., Helminthol.Abstr., Ind.Med. (1982-), Inpharma, Pharm.&Out.News, Reac., Rev.Med.& Vet.Mycol., SSCI (coverage dropped), Saf.Sci.Abstr.
—BLDSC (8798.865000), CISTI, EMDOCS, GNLM, IDS, ingenta, KNAW.
Published by: Texas Heart Institute, Publications & Communications, MC 1 194, Box 20345, Houston, TX 77225-0345. TEL 713-794-6630, FAX 713-791-3714, jmccollum@heart.thi.tmc.edu, http://www.tmc.edu/thi/journal. Ed. Dr. Robert J Hall. R&P James E Bagg Jr. Adv. contact Rod Lawrenz. Circ: 23,000.

616.1 AUS ISSN 1327-9513
THERAPEUTIC GUIDELINES. CARDIOVASCULAR. Text in English. 1991. irreg., latest version 3 (every 3-4 yrs.). AUD 31.90 newsstand/cover (effective 2001). bk.rev. **Document type:** *Academic/Scholarly.* **Description:** Gives concrete recommendations for rational therapy of cardiovascular disease and, where necessary, justifies the choice.
Formerly (until 1999): Cardiovascular Guidelines
Related titles: CD-ROM ed.
Published by: Therapeutic Guidelines Ltd., Chelsea House, Level 2, 55 Flemington Rd, North Melbourne, VIC 3051, Australia. TEL 61-3-9329-1566, FAX 61-3-9326-5632, sales@tg.com.au, http://www.tg.com.au. Ed., R&P Mary Hemming. Circ: 18,000.
Co-sponsor: Victorian Drug Usage Advisory Committee.

616.1 DEU ISSN 0340-6245
CODEN: THHADQ
THROMBOSIS AND HAEMOSTASIS. Text in English. 1957. 12/yr. DEM 590 in Europe to individuals; DEM 834 in Europe to institutions; USD 460 elsewhere to individuals; USD 644 elsewhere to institutions (effective 2001). adv. 180 p./no. 2 cols./p. back issues avail.; reprints avail. *Refereed.* **Document type:** *Journal, Academic/Scholarly.* **Description:** Contains papers, reports, news and inside information about current research and science involving thrombosis and haemostasis.
Formerly: Thrombosis et Diathesis Haemorrhagica (0040-6597)
Related titles: Online - full text ed.: (from EBSCO Publishing, Institute for Scientific Information).

M

Indexed: ASCA, Agri.& Environ.Biotech.Abstr. (coverage dropped), Biol.Abstr., Chem.Abstr., Chem.Indus.Notes, Chem.Titles, Curr.Adv.Cancer Res., Curr.Adv.Ecol.Sci., Curr.Cont., Curr.Ind.Stat., Dairy Sci.Abstr., Dent.Ind., Derwent Biotech.Abstr., Helminthol.Abstr., INIS Atomind., Ind.Med. (1976-), Ind.Sci.Rev., Ind.Vet., Inpharma, Mass Spectr.Bull., Neurosci.Cit.Ind., Nutr.Abstr., Pharm.&Out.News, Reac., Rev.Appl.Entomol., Rev.Med.& Vet.Mycol., Sci.Cit.Ind., Soyabean Abstr., THA, Vet.Bull.
—BLDSC (8820.344000), CASDDS, CISTI, EMDOCS, GNLM, IDS, Infotrieve, ingenta, KNAW. **CCC.**
Published by: (International Society on Thrombosis and Haemostasis), Schattauer GmbH, Hoelderlinstr 3, Stuttgart 70174, Germany. TEL 49-711-2298714, FAX 49-711-2298775, info@schattauer.de, http://www.thrombosis-online.com, http://www.schattauer.com. Ed. P M Manucci. Pub. Dieter Bergemann. R&P, Adv. contact Hannelore Hensen. Circ: 4,000.

616.1 GBR ISSN 0049-3848
CODEN: THBRAA
THROMBOSIS RESEARCH; an international journal on vascular obstruction, hemorrhage and hemostasis. Text in English, French, German, Russian; Summaries in English. 1972. 24/yr. EUR 272 in Europe to individuals; JPY 36,000 in Japan to individuals; USD 305 elsewhere to individuals; EUR 2,637 in Europe to institutions; JPY 350,000 in Japan to institutions; USD 2,950 elsewhere to institutions (effective 2002). adv. bk.rev. charts, illus. index. back issues avail. *Refereed.* **Document type:** *Academic/Scholarly.* **Description:** Forum for the rapid dissemination of original research on thrombosis, hemostasis and fibrinolysis.
Related titles: Microfilm ed.: (from PQC); Online - full text ed.: (from ingenta, Swets Blackwell, Institute for Scientific Information, ScienceDirect).
Indexed: ASCA, Agri.& Environ.Biotech.Abstr. (coverage dropped), Biol.Abstr., Chem.Abstr., Chem.Titles, Curr.Adv.Biochem., Curr.Adv.Cell & Devel.Biol., Curr.Adv.Ecol.Sci., Curr.Cont., Dairy Sci.Abstr., Dent.Ind., Derwent Biotech.Abstr., Excerp.Med., INIS Atomind., Ind.Med. (1972-), Ind.Sci.Rev., Inpharma, Int.Abstr.Biol.Sci., Neurosci.Cit.Ind., Nutr.Abstr., Pharm.&Out.News, Reac., Risk Abstr., Sci.Cit.Ind., THA.
—BLDSC (8820.365000), ADONIS, CASDDS, CISTI, GNLM, IDS, Infotrieve, ingenta, KNAW. **CCC.**
Published by: Pergamon (Subsidiary of: Elsevier Science), The Boulevard, Langford Ln, East Park, Kidlington, Oxford OXB 1GB, United Kingdom. FAX 44-1865-843010, http://www.elsevier.com/locate/inca/369. Eds. Birger Blombak, Calvin M Redman. Circ: 700. **Subscr. in Australasia and the Far East to:** Elsevier Science (Singapore) Pte Ltd, No.1 Temasek Ave, 17-01 Millenia Tower, Singapore 039192, Singapore. TEL 65-434-3727, FAX 65-337-2230; **Subscr. in the Americas to:** Elsevier Science, PO Box 945, New York, NY 10159-0945. TEL 212-633-3730, FAX 212-633-3680, usinfo-f@elsevier.com; **Subscr. to:** Elsevier Science BV, PO Box 211, Amsterdam 1000 AE, Netherlands. TEL 31-20-485-3757.

616.1 GBR ISSN 0896-0569
THROMBOSIS RESEARCH. SUPPLEMENT. Text in English. 1974. irreg. **Document type:** *Monographic series.*
Indexed: Ind.Med. (coverage dropped).
—CISTI, ingenta, KNAW.
Published by: Pergamon (Subsidiary of: Elsevier Science), The Boulevard, Langford Ln, East Park, Kidlington, Oxford OXB 1GB, United Kingdom. FAX 44-1865-843010. **Subscr. in Australasia and the Far East to:** Elsevier Science (Singapore) Pte Ltd, No.1 Temasek Ave, 17-01 Millenia Tower, Singapore 039192, Singapore. TEL 65-434-3727, FAX 65-337-2230; **Subscr. in the Americas to:** Elsevier Science, PO Box 945, New York, NY 10159-0945. TEL 212-633-3730, FAX 212-633-3680; **Subscr. to:** Elsevier Science BV. TEL 31-20-485-3757, FAX 31-20-485-3432.

616.1 USA ISSN 1042-2455
TODAY IN MEDICINE. CARDIOVASCULAR DISEASE. Text in English. 1986. m.
Published by: Data Centrum Communications, Inc., 21 W 38th St, 4th fl, New York, NY 10018.

616.1 615.82 USA ISSN 1074-9357
CODEN: TSREFV
TOPICS IN STROKE REHABILITATION. Text in English. 1994. q. USD 79 to individuals; USD 105 to libraries; USD 43 to students; USD 24 newsstand/cover (effective 2001). back issues avail.; reprint service avail. from PQC. *Refereed.* **Description:** Devoted to the study and dissemination of theoretical and practical information related to the subject of stroke rehabilitation. Reviews and reports common clinical practices, state-of-the-art concepts, and new developments in stroke patient care and research.
Related titles: Microform ed.: (from PQC); Online - full text ed.: (from ProQuest Information & Learning).
Indexed: CINAHL, Excerp.Med. (1996-), PsycInfo, e-psyche.
—BLDSC (8867.490300), GNLM, ingenta.
Published by: Aspen Publishers, Inc., 200 Orchard Ridge Dr, Ste 200, Gaithersburg, MD 20878. TEL 301-417-7500, 800-638-8437, FAX 301-695-7931, customer.service@aspenpubl.com, http://www.aspenpub.com. Eds. Don A Olson, Elliot J Roth. **Dist. by:** Aspen Publishers Inc., Distribution Center, 7201 McKinney Circle, Frederick, MD 21701. TEL 301-698-7100, FAX 301-417-7550.

616.1 GBR ISSN 1464-4460
TRENDS IN CARDIOLOGY & VASCULAR DISEASE. Text in English. 1998. bi-m. **Document type:** *Trade.*
—BLDSC (9049.548700).
Published by: A & M Publishing Ltd., First House, Park Street, Guildford, Surrey GU1 4XB, United Kingdom. TEL 44-1483-534888, FAX 44-1483-533316, cvtrends@am-publishing.co.uk, http://am-publishing.co.uk. Pub. Brian Palphramand.

616.1 USA ISSN 1050-1738
RC666 CODEN: TCMDEQ
TRENDS IN CARDIOVASCULAR MEDICINE. Text in English. 1991. 8/yr. EUR 136 in Europe to individuals; JPY 18,000 in Japan to individuals; USD 151 elsewhere to individuals; EUR 380 in Europe to institutions; JPY 50,400 in Japan to institutions; USD 151 elsewhere to institutions (effective 2002). back issues avail. *Refereed.* **Document type:** *Academic/Scholarly.* **Description:** Designed to help clinical cardiologists and basic researchers keep up with advances in cardiovascular research.
Related titles: Microform ed.: (from PQC); Online - full text ed.: (from ingenta, Swets Blackwell, Institute for Scientific Information, ScienceDirect).
Indexed: ASCA, Chem.Abstr., Chem.Titles, Curr.Cont., Derwent Biotech.Abstr., Excerp.Med. (1992-), Ind.Med. (1991-), Ind.Sci.Rev., Inpharma, Int.Abstr.Biol.Sci., Pharm.&Out.News, Reac., Sci.Cit.Ind.
—BLDSC (9049.549000), CASDDS, CISTI, EMDOCS, GNLM, IDS, Infotrieve, KNAW. **CCC.**
Published by: Elsevier Science, PO Box 945, New York, NY 10159-0945. TEL 212-989-5800, FAX 212-633-3990, usinfo-f@elsevier.com, http://www.elsevier.com/locate/issn/10501738. Eds. A Grace, G A FitzGerald, K R Chien. **Subscr. in Australasia and the Far East to:** Elsevier Science (Singapore) Pte Ltd, No.1 Temasek Ave, 17-01 Millenia Tower, Singapore 039192, Singapore. TEL 65-434-3727, FAX 65-337-2230; **Subscr. in Japan to:** Elsevier Science Inc - Japan Regional Office, 9-15 Higashi-Azabu 1-chome, Minato-ku, Tokyo 106-0044, Japan. TEL 81-3-5561-5033, FAX 81-3-5561-5047; **Subscr. outside the Americas to:** Elsevier Science BV, PO Box 211, Amsterdam 1000 AE, Netherlands. TEL 31-20-485-3757, FAX 31-20-485-3432, nlinfo-f@elsevier.nl.

616.1 UKR
UKRAINS'KYI KARDIOLOGICHNYI ZHURNAL. Text in Russian, Ukrainian. m. USD 165 in United States. **Document type:** *Academic/Scholarly.*
Address: Ul Narodnogo Opolcheniya 5, Kiev, Ukraine. TEL 277-66-22. **US dist. addr.:** East View Publications, 3020 Harbor Ln N, Minneapolis, MN 55447. TEL 612-550-0961.

616.1 CHE ISSN 0301-1526
CODEN: VASAAH
VASA; Zeitschrift fuer Gefaesskrankheiten - journal of vascular diseases. Text in English, German. 1972. q. CHF 151 domestic; CHF 163 foreign (effective 2001). adv. bk.rev. abstr, charts, illus. index. 64 p./no. *Refereed.* **Document type:** *Journal, Academic/Scholarly.* **Description:** Contains case reports, overviews and congress information.
Formerly: Zentralblatt fuer Phlebologie (0044-426X)
Related titles: Online - full text ed.: (from Institute for Scientific Information).
Indexed: ASCA, Biol.Abstr., Curr.Cont., Excerp.Med., INIS Atomind., Ind.Med. (1972-), Ind.Sci.Rev., Inpharma, Pharm.&Out.News, Reac., Sci.Cit.Ind.
—BLDSC (9148.300000), CISTI, EMDOCS, GNLM, IDS, KNAW. **CCC.**
Published by: Hans Huber AG, Laengassstr 76, Bern, 9 3000, Switzerland. TEL 41-31-3004500, FAX 41-31-3004591, zeitschriften@hanshuber.com, http://www.hanshuber.com. Ed. Dr. A Creutzig. Adv. contact Rene Waelchli. color page CHF 2,314; trim 216 x 303. Circ: 2,300.

616.1 GBR
VASCULAR DISEASE. Text in English. 1997. q. GBP 25, USD 40. **Document type:** *Academic/Scholarly.*
Published by: Current Medical Literature Ltd., 40-42 Osnaburgh St, London NW1 3ND, United Kingdom. TEL 44-20-7465-8377, FAX 44-20-7465-8380, enquiries@curmedlit.co.uk. **Dist. by:** Cassis Publishing Ltd., Realpage House, Abingdon Science Park, Barton Ln., Abingdon, Oxon OX13 3NB, United Kingdom. TEL 44-1235-537352, FAX 44-1235-537353.

616.1 GBR ISSN 1358-863X
CODEN: VAMLFP
VASCULAR MEDICINE. Text in English. 1990; N.S. 1996. q. GBP 116 in Europe to individuals; USD 169 in North America to individuals; GBP 129 rest of world to individuals; GBP 234 in Europe to institutions; USD 362 in North America to institutions; GBP 282 rest of world to institutions; GBP 92 in Europe to members Vascular Biology Society Angiology Forum; USD 140 in North America to members Vascular Biology Society Angiology Forum; GBP 102 rest of world to members Vascular Biology Society Angiology Forum; GBP 58 in Europe to members Society for Vascular Medicine and Biology and Royal Society of Medicine Angiology Forum; USD 85 in North America to members Society for Vascular Medicine and Biology and Royal Society of Medicine Angiology Forum; GBP 61 rest of world to members Society for Vascular Medicine and Biology and Royal Society of Medicine Angiology Forum; GBP 141 in developing nations; GBP 66 newsstand/cover in Europe; USD 111 newsstand/cover in North America; GBP 69 newsstand/cover rest of world (effective 2002). adv. back issues avail.; reprints avail. *Refereed.* **Document type:** *Journal, Academic/Scholarly.* **Description:** Brings together the latest related biological findings, emphasizing their bearing on the practice of clinical medicine.
Supersedes (in 1996): Vascular Medicine Review (0954-2582)
Related titles: Online - full text ed.: N.S. (from EBSCO Publishing, O C L C Online Computer Library Center, Inc., RoweCom Information Quest, ingenta, Swets Blackwell, Institute for Scientific Information).
Indexed: Curr.Cont., Excerp.Med. (1992-), Ind.Med. (1996-).
—BLDSC (9148.851000), EMDOCS, GNLM, IDS, Infotrieve, KNAW. **CCC.**
Published by: Arnold Publishers (Subsidiary of: Hodder Headline plc.), 338 Euston Rd, London NW1 3BH, United Kingdom. TEL 44-20-7873-6337, FAX 44-20-7873-6325, arnoldjournals@hodder.co.uk, http://www.arnoldpublishers.com/Journals/Journpages/1358863x.htm, http://www.palliativemedjournal.com. Ed. Mark Creager. Adv. contact Mary Attree. **Subscr. to:** Turpin Distribution Services Ltd., Blackhorse Rd, Letchworth, Herts SG6 1HN, United Kingdom. TEL 44-1462-488900, FAX 44-1462-483011.

VASCULAR SURGERY (GLEN HEAD). see *MEDICAL SCIENCES—Surgery*

VASCULAR SURGERY OUTLOOK. see *MEDICAL SCIENCES—Abstracting, Bibliographies, Statistics*

616.1 DEU ISSN 0942-1181
VASOMED; die Fachzeitschrift fuer Gefaesserkrankungen. Text in German; Summaries in English, French, German. 1989. bi-m. DEM 96 (effective 1998). adv. bk.rev. index. back issues avail. **Document type:** *Trade.*
Formerly (until 1992): Vasomed Aktuell (0935-9729)
Indexed: Excerp.Med.
—BLDSC (9149.521000), GNLM.
Published by: Vasomed Verlag GmbH, Koblenzer Str 18, Bonn 53173, Germany. TEL 49-228-95696-0, FAX 49-228-9569640. Ed. Dr. E Rabe. Adv. contact B Thiemeyer. B&W page DEM 3,980, color page DEM 5,930; trim 280 x 210. Circ: 21,000 (paid).

616.1 USA ISSN 1052-2174
VIDEO JOURNAL OF ECHOCARDIOGRAPHY. Text in English. 1987. q. USD 250; USD 275 in Canada; USD 295 in Japan; USD 335 elsewhere. adv. back issues avail. *Refereed.* **Document type:** *Academic/Scholarly.* **Description:** Covers ultrasound imaging. Consists of tutorials, reviews, case reports and original research.

Supersedes in part (in 1991): Dynamic Cardiovascular Imaging (0891-9313)
—GNLM, Infotrieve. **CCC.**
Published by: Dynamedia, Inc., 2 Fulham Court, Silver Spring, MD 20902. TEL 301-649-6886, FAX 301-649-3447. Ed. George W Lighty Jr. Circ: 1,000.

VOX SANGUINIS; international journal of transfusion medicine. see *MEDICAL SCIENCES—Allergology And Immunology*

616.145 CHE
WORLD DIABETES/DIABETE MONDIAL. Text in English, French. 1995. irreg. back issues avail. **Document type:** *Newsletter.* **Description:** Aims to inform health authorities and interested professionals of activities with which the WHO program is either directly or indirectly involved concerning diabetes prevention and clinical management.
Related titles: Online - full text ed.
Published by: World Health Organization, Marketing and Dissemination, Geneva, 27 1211, Switzerland. TEL 41-22-791-2476, FAX 41-22-791-4857, info@who.ch, http://www.who.org/programmes/ncd/dia/dia_nlet.htm.

616.12 CHN
XINXUEGUANBINGXUE JINZHAN/ADVANCES IN CARDIOVASCULAR DISEASE. Text in Chinese. 1980. bi-m. CNY 4. adv. *Refereed.* **Document type:** *Academic/Scholarly.*
Related titles: CD-ROM ed.
Published by: Chengdu Xingxueguanbing Yanjiusuo/Chengdu Research Institute of Cardiovascular Diseases, 82 Qinglong Jie, Chengdu, Sichuan 610031, China. TEL 86-28-6649831. Ed. Chuanli Du. Pub. Faqiong Wu. R&P Liangjie Wang. Adv. contact Yunde Liu. Circ: 10,000. **Co-sponsor:** Chengdu Disan Renming Yiyuan - Chengdu Third People's Hospital.

616.1005 USA ISSN 0145-4145
RC681.A1
THE YEAR BOOK OF CARDIOLOGY. Text in English. 1968. a. USD 91 domestic; USD 97 foreign (effective 2001). illus. **Document type:** *Academic/Scholarly, Abstract/Index.* **Description:** Presents abstracts of pertinent literature, with commentary by leaders in the field.
Former titles (until 1976): Year Book of Cardiovascular Medicine (0360-6023); (until 1975): Year Book of Cardiovascular Medicine and Surgery (0084-3687); Supersedes in part title issued 1962-1967 as: Year Book of Cardiovascular and Renal Disease
Related titles: CD-ROM ed.: (from SilverPlatter Information, Inc.).
—CISTI, GNLM.
Published by: Mosby, Inc., Continuity Division (Subsidiary of: Harcourt Health Sciences), 11830 Westline Industrial Dr, St Louis, MO 63146-3313. TEL 314-872-8370, 800-325-4177, FAX 314-432-1380, http://www.mosby.com/periodicals. Ed. Dr. Robert C Schlant.

616.1 617 USA ISSN 0749-4041
RD598.5
THE YEAR BOOK OF VASCULAR SURGERY. Text in English. 1987. a. USD 95 domestic; USD 101 foreign (effective 2001). **Document type:** *Abstract/Index, Academic/Scholarly.* **Description:** Presents abstracts of the pertinent literature with commentary by experts in the field.
Related titles: CD-ROM ed.
Indexed: ASCA.
—CISTI, GNLM.
Published by: Mosby, Inc., Continuity Division (Subsidiary of: Harcourt Health Sciences), 11830 Westline Industrial Dr, St Louis, MO 63146-3313. TEL 314-872-8370, 800-325-4177, FAX 314-432-1380, http://www.mosby.com/periodicals. Ed. Dr. John M Porter.

616.12 617 DEU ISSN 0930-9225
CODEN: ZHTGF2
ZEITSCHRIFT FUER HERZ, THORAX- UND GEFAESSCHIRURGIE. Text in German; Summaries in English. 1987. bi-m. EUR 247.84 domestic; EUR 244.04 in Germany; USD 46.70 foreign (effective 2002). abstr. back issues avail.; reprints avail. **Document type:** *Journal, Academic/Scholarly.*
Related titles: Microform ed.: (from PQC); Online - full text ed.: ISSN 1435-1277 (from EBSCO Publishing, RoweCom Information Quest, Swets Blackwell, Springer LINK).
—GNLM, Infotrieve. **CCC.**
Published by: Dr. Dietrich Steinkopff Verlag (Subsidiary of: BertelsmannSpringer), Poststr 9, Darmstadt 64293, Germany. TEL 49-6151-82899-0, FAX 49-6151-82899-40, frey.steinkopff@springer.de, http://www.steinkopff.springer.de. Ed. R Hetzer. **Subscr. in N. America to:** Springer-Verlag, Journals; **Subscr. to:** Springer GmbH Auslieferungsgesellschaft, Haberstr 7, Heidelberg 69126, Germany. TEL 49-6221-345239, FAX 49-6221-345249, subscriptions@springer.de.

616.12 DEU ISSN 0300-5860
CODEN: ZKRDAX
ZEITSCHRIFT FUER KARDIOLOGIE. Text in German; Summaries in English. 1909. m. EUR 555.25 domestic; EUR 536.05 in Germany; EUR 50.90 newsstand/cover foreign (effective 2002). adv. bk.rev. bibl, charts, illus, abstr. index. back issues avail.; reprints avail. *Refereed.* **Document type:** *Journal, Academic/Scholarly.*
Formerly: Zeitschrift fuer Kreislaufforschung (0044-295X)
Related titles: Microform ed.: (from PQC); Online - full text ed.: ISSN 1435-1285 (from EBSCO Publishing, RoweCom Information Quest, Swets Blackwell, Springer LINK, Institute for Scientific Information).
Indexed: ASCA, Agri.& Environ.Biotech.Abstr. (coverage dropped), Biol.Abstr., Chem.Abstr., Chem.Indus.Notes, Chem.Titles, Curr.Adv.Ecol.Sci., Curr.Cont., Derwent Biotech.Abstr., Excerp.Med., INIS Atomind., Ind.Med. (1973-), Ind.Sci.Rev., Inpharma, Int.Nurs.Ind., Nutr.Abstr., Pharm.&Out.News, Reac., Sci.Cit.Ind.
—BLDSC (9467.430000), ADONIS, CASDDS, CISTI, EMDOCS, GNLM, IDS, KNAW. **CCC.**
Published by: (Deutsche Gesellschaft fuer Kardiologie - Herz- und Kreislaufforschung), Dr. Dietrich Steinkopff Verlag (Subsidiary of: BertelsmannSpringer), Poststr 9, Darmstadt 64293, Germany. TEL 49-6151-82899-0, FAX 49-6151-82899-40, frey.steinkopff@springer.de, http://www.steinkopff.springer.de. Eds. T Meinertz, W Kuebler. Circ: 3,000. **Subscr. in N. America to:** Springer-Verlag, Journals, 175 Fifth Ave, New York, NY 10010. **Dist. by:** Springer GmbH Auslieferungsgesellschaft.

616.12 CHN ISSN 0253-3758
CODEN: CHHCDF
ZHONGHUA XIN-XUEGUANBING ZAZHI/CHINESE JOURNAL OF CARDIOLOGY. Text in Chinese, English. q. USD 31.20 foreign; USD 5.20 newsstand/cover foreign; CNY 62.40 domestic; CNY 10.40 newsstand/cover domestic (effective 2001). **Document type:** *Academic/Scholarly.*
Related titles: CD-ROM ed.; Online - full content ed.: (from WanFang Data Corp.).
Indexed: Biol.Abstr., Chem.Abstr., Excerp.Med., ExtraMED, Ind.Med. (coverage dropped).
—BLDSC (3180.298000), CASDDS, CISTI, EMDOCS, GNLM.
Published by: Zhonghua Yixuehui Zazhishe, 42 Dongsi Xidajie, Beijing 100710, China. TEL 86-1-65229209, cmaxxg@public.sti.ac.cn. **Dist. by:** China International Book Trading Corp, 35, Chegongzhuang Xilu, Haidian District, Beijing 100044, China. TEL 86-1-68413849, FAX 86-1-68412048, cibtc@mail.cibtc.com.cn, http://www.cibtc.com.cn.

616.1 CHN
ZHONGHUA XINLU SHICHANGXUE ZAZHI/CHINA JOURNAL OF CARDIAC ARRHYTHMIA. Text in Chinese. bi-m. USD 31.20; USD 5.20 newsstand/cover (effective 2001). **Document type:** *Academic/Scholarly.*
Published by: Zhonghua Yixuehui Zazhishe, 42 Dongsi Xidajie, Beijing 100710, China. **Dist. by:** China International Book Trading Corp, 35, Chegongzhuang Xilu, Haidian District, Beijing 100044, China. TEL 86-1-68413849, FAX 86-1-68412048, cibtc@mail.cibtc.com.cn, http://www.cibtc.com.cn.

616.1 CHN ISSN 1001-4497
ZHONGHUA XIONG-XIN XUEGUAN WAIKE ZAZHI/CHINESE JOURNAL OF THORACIC AND CARDIOVASCULAR SURGERY. Text in Chinese. 1985. q. CNY 90 domestic; USD 43.80 foreign; CNY 15 newsstand/cover domestic; USD 7.30 newsstand/cover foreign (effective 2001). **Document type:** *Academic/Scholarly.*
Formerly (until 1987): Xiong Xinxueguan Waike Zazhi (1000-3533)
Published by: Zhonghua Yixuehui/Chinese Medical Association, Beijing Yiyuan (Beijing Hospital), 1 Dahua Lu, Beijing 100730, China. TEL 86-1-64212431ext 2425, cmaxxx@public.sti.ac.cn. **Dist. by:** China International Book Trading Corp, 35, Chegongzhuang Xilu, Haidian District, Beijing 100044, China. TEL 86-1-68413849, FAX 86-1-68412048, cibtc@mail.cibtc.com.cn, http://www.cibtc.com.cn.

MEDICAL SCIENCES—Chiropractic, Homeopathy, Osteopathy

615.533071 USA
A A C O M ORGANIZATIONAL GUIDE. Text in English. 1980. a. USD 18 (effective 1999). **Document type:** *Directory.* **Description:** Contains information on the organizational structure of the Association; including members of its councils, sections, committees, administrative staff and faculty in the 19 accredited US colleges of osteopathic medicine.
Published by: American Association of Colleges of Osteopathic Medicine, 5550 Friendship Blvd, Ste 310, Chevy Chase, MD 20815-7231. TEL 301-968-4100, FAX 301-968-4101, ckearns@aacom.org, http://www.aacom.org/education/Orgguide.pdf. Ed. Cathleen Kearns. Circ: 250.

615.633 USA
A A O A ACCENTS. Text in English. 1941. q. **Description:** For spouses of osteopathic physicians. Covers issues pertinent to the osteopathic profession.
Published by: (Auxiliary to the American Osteopathic Association), McVey Marketing & Advertising, PO Box 569, Flint, MI 48501-0569. TEL 313-735-7892, FAX 313-735-4226. Ed. Mary M Balog. Circ: 1,900. **Subscr. to:** 142 E Ontario St, Chicago, IL 60611.

615.53 USA
THE A A O JOURNAL. Text in English. 1991. q. USD 60 (effective 2001). adv. back issues avail. **Document type:** *Abstract/Index.* **Description:** Includes clinically related articles that illustrate the art and science of osteopathic practice.
Formerly: A A O Newsletter
Published by: American Academy of Osteopathy, 3500 DePauw Blvd, Ste 1080, Indianapolis, IN 46268. TEL 317-879-1881, FAX 317-879-0563, http://www.aao.medguide.net, http://www.academyofosteopathy.org. Ed. Dr. Anthony G Chila. Adv. contact Diana L Finley. Circ: 4,000 (paid and free).

A F H H A INSIDER. see *MEDICAL SCIENCES—Nurses And Nursing*

615.533 USA
A O A YEARBOOK AND DIRECTORY OF OSTEOPATHIC PHYSICIANS. Text in English. 1908. a. USD 170 (effective 1999). adv. stat. index.
Formerly: Yearbook and Directory of Osteopathic Physicians (0084-358X)
Indexed: SRI.
Published by: American Osteopathic Association, 142 E Ontario St, Chicago, IL 60611. TEL 312-202-8000. Ed. Gilbert E D'Alonzo. Pub. Philip Saigh. Adv. contact Linda Dunn. Circ: 30,000.

ACTA BIOLOGICA; Zeitschrift fuer angewandte Homoeo-Phytotherapie, Ganzheitsbehandlungen und Sondermethoden der Medizin. see *BIOLOGY*

AIDS ANALYSIS ASIA. see *SOCIAL SERVICES AND WELFARE*

615.532 DEU ISSN 0002-5887
ALLGEMEINE HOMOEOPATHISCHE ZEITUNG. Text in German. 1832. 6/yr. EUR 87.90 domestic to institutions; EUR 92.40 in Europe to institutions; EUR 100.90 elsewhere to institutions; EUR 15.90 newsstand/cover (effective 2002). **Document type:** *Newspaper, Trade.*
Indexed: Excerp.Med.
—BLDSC (0791.775000), GNLM, Infotrieve. **CCC.**
Published by: (Deutscher Zentralverein Homoeopathischer Aerzte e.V.), Karl F. Haug Verlag, Fritz-Frey-Str 21, Heidelberg 69121, Germany. TEL 49-6221-489445, FAX 49-6221-489584, http://www.haug-verlag.de. Ed. Karl Heinz Gebhardt. Adv. contact Guenter Fecke. **Subscr. to:** Postfach 102869, Heidelberg 69018, Germany.

ALTERNATIV MEDICIN. see *ALTERNATIVE MEDICINE*

615.533 USA ISSN 0732-703X
AMERICAN ACADEMY OF OSTEOPATHY YEARBOOK. Variant title: Yearbook of Selected Osteopathic Papers. Text in English. 1943. a. USD 50 (effective 2000). illus. cum.index 1972, 1977, 1996. **Document type:** *Monographic series.*
Published by: American Academy of Osteopathy, 3500 DePauw Blvd, Ste 1080, Indianapolis, IN 46268. TEL 317-879-1881, FAX 317-879-0563, http://www.aao.medguide.net, http://www.academyofosteopathy.org. Ed. Myron C Beal. Circ: 1,800 (controlled).

M

615.533 USA
AMERICAN ASSOCIATION OF PHYSICIANS SPECIALISTS. NEWSLETTER. Text in English. 1979. q. USD 150 (effective 2000). adv. *Refereed.* **Document type:** *Newsletter.* **Description:** Offers news about the association of physicians.
Former titles: American Association of Osteopathic Specialists. Newsletter; American Association of Osteopathic Specialists. Journal; A A O S Newsletter
Published by: American Association of Physicians Specialists, Inc., 2296 Henderson Mill Rd N E, Ste 206, Atlanta, GA 30345-2739. TEL 770-939-8555, FAX 770-939-8559, jacqueline.evans@aaps.cobbmail.com, http://www.aapsga.com. Ed., Pub., R&P, Adv. contact Jacqueline Evans. Circ: 2,000.

615.543 USA ISSN 1081-7166
AMERICAN CHIROPRACTIC ASSOCIATION. JOURNAL. Text in English. 1930. m. USD 90 domestic; USD 120 foreign (effective 2001). adv. bk.rev. charts, illus. index. back issues avail.; reprint service avail. from PQC. *Refereed.* **Document type:** *Trade.* **Description:** Discusses current procedures, research and developments in the field of chiropractic and in related fields of interest to chiropractors.
Former titles (until 1995): Journal of Chiropractic (0744-9984); (until 1981): A C A Journal of Chiropractic (0044-7609); Supersedes (in 1964): National Chiropractic Journal
Related titles: Microform ed.: (from PQC); Online - full text ed.: (from ProQuest Information & Learning).
Indexed: AMED.
—BLDSC (4685.150000), GNLM.
Published by: American Chiropractic Association, Council on Sports Injuries and Physical Fitness, 1701 Claredon Blvd., Arlington, VA 22209. Ed., Pub. Carol Kline. Adv. contact Nataliya Schatchikova. B&W page USD 1,460, color page USD 1,960; trim 10.63 x 8.13. Circ: 16,000 (paid).

615.53 USA ISSN 0002-8967
RX1
AMERICAN INSTITUTE OF HOMEOPATHY. JOURNAL✶ . Text in English. 1907. q. USD 45 domestic; USD 48 in Canada & Mexico; USD 55 elsewhere (effective 2000). adv. bk.rev. index. **Document type:** *Academic/Scholarly.* **Description:** Presents articles of historical interest, current research, and case studies. Includes listings of foreign and U.S. homeopathic organizations and upcoming homeopathic conferences and meetings.
Indexed: AMED.
—BLDSC (4686.730000), GNLM, ingenta.
Published by: American Institute of Homeopathy, 801 N Fairfax St, Ste 306, Alexandria, VA 22314-1757. TEL 303-898-5477, FAX 804-295-0798, gguess@igc..apc.org. Ed., R&P George Guess. Adv. contact Dean Crothers. Circ: 550.

ANNALES DE KINESITHERAPIE. see *MEDICAL SCIENCES—Sports Medicine*

615.33 DEU ISSN 0940-9963
ARCHIV FUER HOMOEOPATHIK. Text in German. 1992. q. DEM 63; DEM 72 foreign. adv. bk.rev. **Document type:** *Academic/Scholarly.*
Indexed: AMED.
—GNLM.
Published by: Dynamis-Verlag GbR, Am Vogelherd 18, Oberhausen 46147, Germany. TEL 49-208-676525, FAX 49-208-677047, dynamisrt@aol.com. Eds. Michael Terlinden, Stefan Reis.

ARTHRITIS HOTLINE. see *MEDICAL SCIENCES—Rheumatology*

615.53 USA
BEACON (DAVENPORT). Text in English. 1967. m. USD 20. **Document type:** *Newspaper.*
Published by: Palmer College of Chiropractic, 1000 Brady St, Davenport, IA 52803. Ed. Mark D Laverkvist. Circ: 3,000.

615.53 DEU ISSN 0340-8671
CODEN: BIMEFA
BIOLOGISCHE MEDIZIN. Text in English, German, Italian, Polish, Russian, Spanish. 1962. bi-m. DEM 34; DEM 42 foreign (effective 1999). adv. *Refereed.* **Document type:** *Academic/Scholarly.* **Description:** Aims to support efforts towards natural treatment without side effects.
Indexed: AMED, Ind.Vet., Nutr.Abstr., Rev.Arom.& Med.Plants.
—BLDSC (2083.700000), GNLM.
Published by: Aurelia Verlag GmbH, Dr.-Reckeweg-Str 2-4, Baden-Baden 76532, Germany. TEL 49-7221-50102, FAX 49-7221-501420, info@aurelia-verlag.de, http://www.aurelia-verlag.de. Ed. Bettina Nellen. adv.: B&W page DEM 6,600, B&W page XEU 3,374.53, color page DEM 8,760, color page XEU 4,478.92; trim 185 x 247. Circ: 36,000 (paid).

615.532 GBR ISSN 0007-0785
BRITISH HOMEOPATHIC JOURNAL. (Will be published by W.B. Saunders (Tel. 44-20-8300-3322) from 2002. Title will change to Homeopathy (ISSN 1475-4916); and subscr. prices are as follows, GBP 62 (to individuals); GBP 115 (to institutions) (effective 2002)) Text in English. 1911. q. GBP 56 in Europe to individuals for print or online ed.; USD 90 elsewhere to individuals for print or online ed.; GBP 62 combined subscription in Europe to individuals print & online eds.; USD 99 combined subscription elsewhere to individuals print & online eds.; GBP 105 in Europe to institutions for print or online ed.; USD 168 elsewhere to institutions for print or online ed.; GBP 115 combined subscription in Europe to institutions print & online eds.; USD 184 combined subscription elsewhere to institutions print & online eds. (effective 2001). adv. bk.rev. charts, illus, stat. index. back issues avail.; reprint service avail. from PQC. *Refereed.* **Document type:** *Newsletter, Proceedings, Journal, Academic/Scholarly.* **Description:** Aims at improving the understanding and clinical practice of homeopathy. Promotes debate and reviews homeopathic literature.
Formed by the merger of: British Homeopathy Review; Journal of the British Homeopathic Society
Related titles: Microform ed.: (from PQC); Online - full text ed.: GBP 50 to individuals; GBP 75 to institutions (effective 2000) (from EBSCO Publishing, O C L C Online Computer Library Center, Inc., RoweCom Information Quest, ingenta, Swets Blackwell).
Indexed: AMED, Excerp.Med., Ind.Med. (1911-), Rev.Appl.Entomol.
—BLDSC (2301.340000), GNLM, ingenta.
Published by: (Faculty of Homoeopathy), Nature Publishing Group Specialist Journals (Subsidiary of: Holtzbrink Publishers), Houndmills, Basingstoke, Hants RG21 6XS, United Kingdom. TEL 44-1256-329242, FAX 44-1256-328339, subscriptions@nature.com, http://www.nature.com/bhj. Ed. P Fisher. Pub. Sue Deeley. R&P Trace Noel. Adv. contact Robert Sloan TEL 44-20-8882-7199. Circ: 1,500 (paid).

615.534 GBR ISSN 1466-2108
THE BRITISH JOURNAL OF CHIROPRACTIC. Text in English. 1997. q. GBP 24 in United Kingdom; GBP 28 in Europe; GBP 32 elsewhere; GBP 14 to students (effective 2001). back issues avail. **Document type:** *Journal, Academic/Scholarly.*
Indexed: AMED.
—BLDSC (2307.110000).
Published by: College of Chiropractors, 106 London St, Reading, Berks RG1 4BF, United Kingdom. Ed. Martin Young.

CAHIERS DE KINESITHERAPIE; revue d'enseignement post-scolaire et de documentation technique. see *MEDICAL SCIENCES—Physical Medicine And Rehabilitation*

615.53 USA ISSN 1060-1155
CALIFORNIA CHIROPRACTIC ASSOCIATION JOURNAL✶ . Text in English. 1985. m. USD 50. adv. *Refereed.* **Document type:** *Trade.* **Description:** Promotes chiropractic and general health progress.
Formerly (until 1991): California Chiropractic Journal (0899-0204)
Indexed: CINAHL.
Published by: California Chiropractic Association, 1600 Sacramento Inn Way Ste 106, Sacramento, CA 95815-3450. TEL 916-387-0177, FAX 916-387-6222. Ed. Dawn E Moline.

615.534 CAN ISSN 0008-3194
CANADIAN CHIROPRACTIC ASSOCIATION. JOURNAL. Abbreviated title: J C C A (Journal of the Canadian Chiropractic Association). Text in English. 1957. q. CND 60 domestic; CND 75 foreign (effective 2000). adv. bk.rev. charts, illus, stat. index. reprint service avail. from PQC. *Refereed.* **Document type:** *Academic/Scholarly.* **Description:** Captures the breadth of chiropractic literature, ranging from historical reviews to case studies to original designed research.
Related titles: Online - full text ed.: (from ProQuest Information & Learning).
Indexed: AMED, CINAHL.
—BLDSC (4723.003000), CISTI, Infotrieve. **CCC.**
Published by: Canadian Chiropractic Association, 1396 Eglinton Ave W, Toronto, ON M6C 2E4, Canada. TEL 416-781-5656, FAX 416-781-7344. Ed., R&P, Adv. contact Allan Gotlib. Circ: 4,000.

615.53 USA ISSN 1087-1985
CHIROPRACTIC ECONOMICS. Text in English. 1954. 8/yr. USD 42 domestic; USD 67 in Canada; USD 87 elsewhere. adv. bk.rev. back issues avail. **Document type:** *Trade.* **Description:** Business and practice management for the doctor of chiropractic.
Formerly (until 1995): Digest of Chiropractic Economics (0415-8407)
Published by: Doyle Group, 5150 Palm Valley Rd, Ste 103, Ponte Vedra Beach, FL 32082. TEL 904-285-6020, FAX 904-285-9944, http://www.chiroeco.com. Ed. Tara Stultz. Pub. Douglas Apelian. Circ: 30,000.

615.534 USA
CHIROPRACTIC HEALTH WAYS. Text in English. 1994. 6/w. USD 14 (effective 2001). **Document type:** *Newsletter.*
Formerly (until 1997): Staying Well
Published by: Foundation for Chiropractic Education and Research, 704 E 4th St, Des Moines, IA 50309. TEL 800-622-6309, http://www.fcer.org. Ed. Robin Merrifield.

615.53 920 900 USA ISSN 0736-4377
RZ221
CHIROPRACTIC HISTORY. Text in English. 1981. s-a. USD 50; USD 60 foreign (effective 1999). adv. bk.rev., video rev. abstr, bibl, charts, illus. cum.index every 5 yrs. back issues avail. *Refereed.* **Document type:** *Academic/Scholarly.* **Description:** Contains papers, book reviews, short subjects dealing with the history of chiropractic and - to a lesser extent - other alternative health sciences.
Indexed: AMED, CINAHL.
—BLDSC (3181.144000), GNLM.
Published by: Association for the History of Chiropractic, 1000 Brady St, Davenport, IA 52803. TEL 319-884-5894, FAX 319-884-5897, wieseg@palmer.edu. Ed., R&P, Adv. contact John Willis TEL 540-963-0395. Circ: 400.

615.53 USA
THE CHIROPRACTIC JOURNAL. Text in English. 1986. m. adv. **Document type:** *Newspaper, Trade.* **Description:** Includes information on practice enhancement, legislative developments, insurance regulations, products and other topics of professional interest.
Indexed: CINAHL.
—BLDSC (3181.144020).
Published by: Chiropractic Journal, 2950 N Dobson Rd, Ste 1, Chandler, AZ 85224-1800. TEL 602-786-9235, 800-347-1011, FAX 602-732-9313. Pub. Terry A Rondberg. Adv. contact Linda C Bevel. B&W page USD 2,490, color page USD 2,990. Circ: 60,000 (controlled).

615.534 AUS ISSN 1036-0913
CHIROPRACTIC JOURNAL OF AUSTRALIA. Text in English. 1966. q. AUD 75 domestic to individuals; AUD 90, USD 64 foreign to individuals; AUD 110 domestic to institutions; AUD 125, USD 90 foreign to institutions (effective 2002). adv. bk.rev. 48 p./no. back issues avail. *Refereed.* **Document type:** *Academic/Scholarly.* **Description:** Contains peer-reviewed research, professional and review papers relevant to the practice of chiropractic, history, commentary, abstracts, book reviews and news briefs of interest to chiropractors and allied professionals.
Formerly (until 1991): Australian Chiropractors' Association. Journal (0045-0359)
Related titles: Microform ed.: (from PQC); Online - full text ed.
Indexed: AMED, Aus.P.A.I.S. (Coverage Dropped).
—BLDSC (3181.144050), ingenta.
Published by: Chiropractors' Association of Australia, PO Box 748, Wagga Wagga, NSW 2650, Australia. TEL 61-2-6921-3238, FAX 61-2-6926-2556, chance@wagga.net.au, http://www.caa.com.au. Eds. Mary Ann Chance, Rolf E Peters. R&P, Adv. contact Mary Ann Chance. Circ: 2,000 (paid and controlled).

615.534 USA
CHIROPRACTIC ONLINE TODAY. Text in English. 1995. m. free per issue. adv. Supplement avail. **Description:** Provides current health information and interactive discussion groups.
Media: Online - full text. **Related titles:** E-mail ed.
Address: PO Box 1980, New York, NY 10013-0873. interadcom@aol.com, http://www.chiro-online.com/, http://www.panix.com/~tonto1/dc.html. Ed. Todd D Eglow.

M

615.53 USA ISSN 1041-2360
CHIROPRACTIC PRODUCTS✱ ; business management solutions for chiropractic professionals. Text in English. 1985. 12/yr. free to qualified Chiropractors. adv. bk.rev. charts, illus. **Document type:** *Magazine, Trade.* **Description:** Covers news of product releases, topics of interest to professionals in the field, and special features.
Published by: Novicom, Inc. (Subsidiary of: Medical World Communications), 6701 Center Dr West, Ste 450, Los Angeles, CA 90045-1556. TEL 310-642-4400, FAX 310-641-1511, http://www.chiropub.com, http://www.novicom.com. Ed. Won Seo. Pub. Debra Schmitt. R&P Marvin Rosenfeld. Adv. contact Lisa Chose. B&W page USD 2,194, color page USD 2,894; trim 7 x 10. Circ: 40,000 (controlled).

615.534 CAN ISSN 0836-1444
THE CHIROPRACTIC REPORT; an international review of professional and research issues. Text in English. 1987. bi-m. CND 78 in North America; AUD 98 in Australia; USD 80 elsewhere. **Document type:** *Academic/Scholarly, Trade.*
Related titles: French ed.: Dossier Chiropratique. ISSN 1207-0750.
Indexed: CINAHL.
Published by: Chiropractic Report, 3080 Yonge St, Ste 3002, P O Box 39, Toronto, ON M4N 3N1, Canada. TEL 416-484-9601, FAX 416-484-9665. Ed. David Chapman Smith.

615.534 USA ISSN 0899-6938
CHIROPRACTIC RESEARCH JOURNAL. Text in English. 1988. s-a. USD 30; USD 40 foreign (effective 1999). bk.rev. back issues avail. *Refereed.* **Document type:** *Academic/Scholarly.* **Description:** Dedicated to basic and clinical subluxation-related research. Contains original research, case studies and reviews of the literature.
Indexed: AMED, CINAHL.
Published by: Life University, School of Chiropractic, 1269 Barclay Circle, Marietta, GA 30060. TEL 770-426-2636, 800-543-3201, FAX 770-425-5496, eowens@lifenet.life.edu, http://www.life.edu/newlife/crj/. Ed., R&P Sarah K Webster TEL 318-873-3017. Circ: 1,500.

615.543 USA ISSN 0899-3467
CHIROPRACTIC TECHNIQUE. Text in English. 1989. q. USD 69 domestic to individuals; USD 94 foreign to individuals; USD 99 domestic to institutions; USD 124 foreign to institutions. adv. *Refereed.* **Document type:** *Academic/Scholarly, Trade.* **Description:** Provides practical articles on the latest manipulative techniques.
Related titles: Microfilm ed.: (from WWS).
Indexed: CINAHL.
—BLDSC (3181.144500), CISTI, GNLM.
Published by: (National College of Chiropractic), Williams & Wilkins (Subsidiary of: Waverly International), 351 W Camden St, Baltimore, MD 21201-2436. TEL 410-528-4068, 800-222-3790, FAX 410-528-4452, sisaacson@wwilkins.com, http://www.wwilkins.com. Ed. Dana J Lawrence. Adv. contact Sharlene Isaacson. B&W page USD 460, color page USD 765; trim 10.88 x 8.13. Circ: 858; 766 (paid).

615.53 AUS ISSN 1037-8839
CHIROPRACTORS' ASSOCIATION OF AUSTRALIA. MEMBERSHIP DIRECTORY. Text in English. 1938. a. members only. **Document type:** *Directory.* **Description:** Listing of the Association's members.
Formerly (until 1992): Australian Chiropractor's Association. Membership Directory (0728-7291)
Published by: Chiropractors' Association of Australia, Editorial Office, PO Box 6246, South Penrith DC, NSW 2750, Australia. TEL 61-2-47318011, FAX 61-2-47318088, nhq@caa.asn.au, http://www.caa.com.au. Ed., R&P Gavin Hewton. Circ: 1,700.

615.53 230 USA
CHRISTIAN CHIROPRACTOR. Text in English. 1953. bi-m. membership. back issues avail. **Document type:** *Newsletter.*
Published by: Christian Chiropractors Association, PO Box 9715, Fort Collins, CO 80525-0501. TEL 303-482-1404, 800-999-1970, FAX 303-482-1404. Ed. Ronald Murphy. Circ: 1,300.

615.53 230 USA
CHRISTIAN CHIROPRACTORS ASSOCIATION JOURNAL. Text in English. 1953. bi-m. membership.
Formerly: Christian Chiropractors Association Bulletin
Published by: Christian Chiropractors Association, PO Box 9715, Fort Collins, CO 80525-0501. TEL 800-999-1970, FAX 303-482-1404. Circ: 1,200.

615.533 617.3 GBR ISSN 0268-0033 CODEN: CLBIEW
CLINICAL BIOMECHANICS. Text in English. 1968. 10/yr. EUR 89 in Europe to individuals; JPY 11,800 in Japan to individuals; USD 100 elsewhere to individuals; EUR 720 in Europe to institutions; JPY 95,600 in Japan to institutions; USD 805 elsewhere to institutions (effective 2002). adv. bk.rev. abstr, illus. index. back issues avail. *Refereed.* **Document type:** *Academic/Scholarly.* **Description:** Contains original research papers, reviews and abstracts on clinical aspects of biomechanics related to dysfunction of the musculoskeletal system.
Formerly (until 1986): British Osteopathic Journal
Related titles: Microform ed.: (from PQC); Online - full text ed.: (from ingenta, Swets Blackwell, ScienceDirect, Institute for Scientific Information).
Indexed: AMED, BBCI, Bioeng.Abstr., Biotech.& Bioeng.Abstr., Comput.& Info.Sys., Curr.Adv.Ecol.Sci., Curr.Cont., Electron.& Communic.Abstr.J., Excerp.Med., Focus on: Sports Sci.& Med., ISMEC, Ind.Med. (1986-), Inpharma, Reac., SSCI (coverage dropped).
—BLDSC (3286.262800), CISTI, Ei, EMDOCS, GNLM, IDS, Infotrieve, ingenta, KNAW, Linda Hall. **CCC.**
Published by: Pergamon (Subsidiary of: Elsevier Science), The Boulevard, Langford Ln, East Park, Kidlington, Oxford OXB 1GB, United Kingdom. FAX 44-1865-843010, http://www.elsevier.nl/locate/clinbiomech. Eds. G Andersson, Kim Burton. Circ: 750. **Subscr. in Australasia and the Far East to:** Elsevier Science (Singapore) Pte Ltd, No.1 Temasek Ave, 17-01 Millenia Tower, Singapore 039192, Singapore. TEL 65-434-3727, FAX 65-337-2230; **Subscr. in the Americas to:** Elsevier Science, PO Box 945, New York, NY 10159-0945. TEL 212-633-3730, FAX 212-633-3680; **Subscr. to:** Elsevier Science BV, PO Box 211, Amsterdam 1000 AE, Netherlands. TEL 31-20-485-3757.

CLINICAL CALCIUM. see *MEDICAL SCIENCES—Endocrinology*

610.711 USA
COLLEGE INFORMATION BOOKLET. Text in English. 1977. a. USD 2 (effective 1999). **Document type:** *Directory.* **Description:** Contains information on the 19 accredited osteopathic medical colleges including a brief description of each college, admissions criteria, minimum entrance requirements, supplementary application materials required, an indication of class size or enrollment, application deadlines, and tuition.
Published by: American Association of Colleges of Osteopathic Medicine, 5550 Friendship Blvd, Ste 310, Chevy Chase, MD 20815-7231. TEL 301-968-4100, FAX 301-968-4101, ckearns@aacom.org, http://www.aacom.org. Ed. Carolyn Leedecker.

COMPLEMENTARY HEALTH PRACTICE REVIEW. see *ALTERNATIVE MEDICINE*

615.53 615.89 GBR ISSN 0965-2299 CODEN: CTHMES
COMPLEMENTARY THERAPIES IN MEDICINE. Text in English. 1993. q. GBP 64 to individuals; GBP 164 to institutions (effective 2002). adv. bk.rev. **Document type:** *Journal, Academic/Scholarly.* **Description:** Aimed at general practitioners, nurses, and other medical professionals interested in chiropractics, acupuncture, and homeopathic and osteopathic medicine.
Related titles: Online - full text ed.: (from Swets Blackwell, IDEAL Online Library, Institute for Scientific Information).
Indexed: AMED, Brit.Nur.Ind., CINAHL, Curr.Cont., Excerp.Med. (1994-), Ind.Med. (1993-), Int.Nurs.Ind., Ref.Zh., Rev.Appl.Entomol., Rev.Arom.& Med.Plants, Weed Abstr.
—BLDSC (3364.203750), EMDOCS, GNLM, KNAW. **CCC.**
Published by: Churchill Livingstone (Subsidiary of: Harcourt Publishers Ltd.), Robert Stevenson House, 1-3 Baxter's Pl, Leith Walk, Edinburgh, Midlothian EH1 3AF, United Kingdom. TEL 44-131-556-2424, FAX 44-131-459-1177, cservice@harcourt.com, http://www.harcourt-international.com/journals/ctim. Ed. Dr. Adrian White. Pub. Inta Ozols. R&P Catherine John TEL 212-424-4200. Adv. contact David Dunnachie. Circ: 410. **Subscr. to:** Harcourt Publishers Ltd., Foots Cray High St, Sidcup, Kent DA14 5HP, United Kingdom. TEL 44-20-8308-5700, FAX 44-20-8309-0807.

615.53 GBR
CONTACT MAGAZINE. Text in English. q. adv. bk.rev. tr.lit. back issues avail. **Document type:** *Bulletin.*
Indexed: Can.Per.Ind.
Published by: British Chiropractic Association, Belgrave House, 17 Belgrave St, Reading, Berks RG1 1QB, United Kingdom. TEL 44-118-950-5950, FAX 44-118-958-8946, enquiries@chiropractic-uk.co.uk, http://www.chiropractic-uk.co.uk/. adv.: page GBP 195. Circ: 1,000 (controlled).

615.53 617.3 USA ISSN 1041-469X
D.C. TRACTS. Text in English. 1989. q. USD 195 to individuals; USD 225 to institutions (effective 2000). adv. **Document type:** *Academic/Scholarly.* **Description:** A continuing education program for chiropractors providing condensations of current chiropractic literature. Each issue includes a 90-minute audiotape lecture by experts and a 20-question continuing education exam.
Indexed: CINAHL.
—**CCC.**
Published by: Data Trace Publishing Company, 110 West Rd, Ste 227, Baltimore, MD 21204. TEL 410-494-4994, FAX 410-494-0515, info@datatrace.com, http://www.datatrace.com. Ed. Bruce Gundersen. R&P Cindy Lee Floyd. Adv. contact Frank Tufariello.

615.533 340 USA ISSN 0011-5088
THE D O; a publication for osteopathic physicians and surgeons. (Doctor of Osteopathy) Text in English. 1960. m. USD 65 (effective 1999). adv. bk.rev. stat. **Description:** For practicing physicians. Contains articles on legislative developments and news of the profession and its members.
Supersedes: Forum of Osteopathy
Indexed: Chem.Abstr.
Published by: American Osteopathic Association, 142 E Ontario St, Chicago, IL 60611. TEL 312-202-8000. Ed. Gilbert E D'Alonzo. Pub. Philip Saigh. R&P Michael Fitzgerald. Adv. contact Linda Dunn. Circ: 33,000.

610.711 USA
DEBTS AND CAREER PLANS OF OSTEOPATHIC MEDICAL STUDENTS. Text in English. 1982. a. USD 16 (effective 1999). back issues avail. **Document type:** *Bulletin.* **Description:** Survey examining indebtedness of osteopathic medical students. The situations, characteristics and plans of students are compared at their entrance to osteopathic medical schools and just prior to their graduation.
Indexed: SRI.
Published by: American Association of Colleges of Osteopathic Medicine, 5550 Friendship Blvd, Ste 310, Chevy Chase, MD 20815-7231. TEL 301-968-4100, FAX 301-968-4101, ckearns@aacom.org, http://www.aacom.org. Ed. Dr. Allen M Singer. Circ: 500.

610.711 USA
DIRECTORY OF OSTEOPATHIC POSTDOCTORAL EDUCATION. Text in English. q. **Document type:** *Directory, Trade.*
Media: Online - full text.
Published by: American Osteopathic Association, 142 E Ontario St, Chicago, IL 60611. TEL 312-202-8000, 312-202-8200, FAX 312-280-5893, http://www.aoa-net.orgsn.org. R&P Karen Stipp. Circ: 3,000.

615.53 USA
DYNAMIC CHIROPRACTIC. Text in English. 1983. fortn. USD 18 domestic; USD 43 in Canada & Mexico; USD 115 elsewhere. adv. **Document type:** *Trade.*
Indexed: CINAHL.
Published by: Maxwell Petersen & Associates, Maxwell, CA 92646. TEL 714-960-6577, FAX 714-536-1482. Ed. Steve Kelly. Pub. Donald M Petersen Jr. R&P Elizabeth Auger. Adv. contact Anne Gardner.

615.53 GBR ISSN 0263-9114 CODEN: EJCHE8
EUROPEAN JOURNAL OF CHIROPRACTIC. Text in English. 1932. 3/yr. GBP 37.50 to individuals; GBP 76 to institutions. adv. bk.rev. bibl, charts, illus. back issues avail. *Refereed.* **Document type:** *Academic/Scholarly.*
Related titles: Microform ed.: (from PQC).
Indexed: AMED, CINAHL.
—BLDSC (3829.725900), CISTI, GNLM.
Published by: European Chiropractors' Union, c/o Simon Leyson, Ed, 16 Uplands Crescent, Uplands, Swansea SA2 0PB, United Kingdom. TEL 44-1792-476644, FAX 44-1639-639649. R&P Simon Leyson. Circ: 2,100.

615.532 IND ISSN 0015-0827
FIFTY MILLESIMAL NEWS LETTER; the journal of pure homoeopathy. Text and summaries in English. 1969. q. INR 6, USD 2. adv. bk.rev.
Published by: Hahnemann Homoeopathic Pharmacy, Hahnemann House, College Rd., Kottayam, Kerala, India. Ed. Dr. Ramanial P Patel. Circ: 1,600.

DIE FUNKTIONSKRANKHEITEN DES BEWEGUNGSSYSTEMS; Zeitschrift fuer interdisziplinaere Diagnostik und Therapie. see *MEDICAL SCIENCES—Orthopedics And Traumatology*

GOOD LIFE TIMES; choices in health, education and the arts. see *NEW AGE PUBLICATIONS*

M

610 GBR ISSN 0965-1292
HEALTH AND HOMEOPATHY. Text in English. q. GBP 15; GBP 23 overseas (effective 2002). adv. bk.rev. illus. *Refereed.* **Document type:** *Consumer.* **Description:** Covers informative articles on homoeopathy. Read by homoeopathy doctors and those interested in a holistic approach to their health.
Incorporates (1932-2000): Homoeopathy (1351-4903); Incorporates (1980-19??): Homoeopathy Today (0261-2828)
Published by: British Homeopathic Association, 15 Clerkenwell Close, London EC1R 0AA, United Kingdom. TEL 44-20-7566-7800, FAX 44-20-7566-7815, info@trusthomeopathy.org, http://www.trusthomeopathy.org. Ed., R&P Enid Segall. adv.: page GBP 200; trim 181 x 266. Circ: 7,000.

HEALTH WORLD. see *ALTERNATIVE MEDICINE*

615.532 IND ISSN 0377-4902
HOMEOPATHIC HERALD. Text in English. 1940. m. INR 9.
Address: 73 Netaji Subhas Rd., Kolkata, West Bengal 700 001, India.

615.532 NLD ISSN 1380-5096
HOMEOPATHIE* . Text in Dutch. 1889. bi-m. NLG 39.50. adv. bk.rev. abstr, bibl, illus, stat. index. **Document type:** *Consumer.* **Description:** Publishes articles relating to homeopathic medicine, including case studies and discussions of diagnosis, treatment, health policy.
Former titles (until 1994): Tijdschrift Homeopathie (0920-4113); (until 1986): Homoeopathisch Tijdschrift (0378-6048); (until 1976): Homoeopathisch Maandblad (0018-4489)
Published by: (Koninklijke Vereniging tot Bevordering der Homeopathie in Nederland (KVHN)), Kroon Uitgevers bv, Postbus 30, Olst 8120 AA, Netherlands. TEL 31-313-479570. Ed., Pub. Aad Kroon. Circ: 10,000.

615.532 FRA ISSN 1244-2356
HOMEOPATHIE EUROPEENNE. Text in French; Summaries in English, French. 1993. 6/yr. FRF 615 domestic to individuals; FRF 715, EUR 109 foreign to individuals; FRF 435 to students (effective 2000). adv. bk.rev. bibl. index.
Formed by the merger of (1988-1993): Medecin Homeopathe (0990-7483); (1912-1993): Homeopathie Francaise (0018-4225); (1984-1993): Homeopathie (0762-638X); Which was formerly (1954-1983): Annales Homeopathiques Francaises (0003-4444)
—CISTI, Infotrieve. **CCC.**
Published by: (Centre Homeopathique de France), Meditions Carline, 1 et 3 rue du Depart, Paris 75014, France. TEL 33-1-40640075, FAX 33-1-43222699, groupemeditions@wanadoo.fr. Eds. Dr. Dupre, Dr. Poitevin. Adv. contact Soizyk Brault.

615.53 USA
HOMEOPATHY ONLINE. Text in English. 1996. bi-m. **Document type:** *Academic/Scholarly.* **Description:** Provides a forum for information exchange among homeopaths and students.
Media: Online - full text.
Published by: Homeopathy Mailing List enos@wolfenet.com, http://www.lyghtforce.com/homeopathyonline/. Ed. Chris Kurz. Pub. Jon Haworth.

615.532 SWE ISSN 0280-3356
HOMEOPRAKTIKERN. Text in Swedish. 1979. q. SEK 100 to members.
Published by: Svenska Homeopraktikers Riksfoerbund (SHR), Gladiolusgatan 6 B, Moelndal 43161, Sweden.

615.532 IND ISSN 0971-4839
HOMOEOPATHIC UPDATE. Text in Multiple languages. 1994. s-a.
—BLDSC (4326.341995).
Published by: B. Jain Publishers Pvt. Ltd., 1921 Chuna Mandi, St. 10th, Pahar Ganj, New Delhi 110 055, India. TEL 91-11-7770430, FAX 91-11-3610471, bjain@vsnl.com. Eds. Dr. Kamal Kansal, Dr. Prem Nath Jain.

615.532 IND ISSN 0046-7812
HOMOEOPATHIC WORLD. Text in English. 1964. m. INR 35. adv. bk.rev.
Published by: Sundar Homoeo Sadan, 113 Netaji Subhas Rd., Kolkata, West Bengal 700 001, India. TEL 387632. Ed. Sri Abinash Das. Circ: 1,500.

615.532 IND ISSN 0046-7820
HOMOEOPATHY; for health and life. Text in English, Tamil. 1948. m. INR 5, USD 3.
Published by: Indian Institute of Homoeopaths, c/o Dr. R.J. Murty, Murty Gardens, Srinagar Colony, Kumbakonam, Tamil Nadu, India. Eds. Dr. R J Murty, Sri R Srinivasan. Circ: 2,000.

615.53 IND
HOMOEOPATHY HERITAGE 9. Text in English. 1976. q. INR 140 in India & Nepal; USD 12 in Bangladesh; USD 25 elsewhere (effective 2000). adv. bk.rev. back issues avail. *Refereed.* **Document type:** *Academic/Scholarly.* **Description:** Covers homeopathic research on preventative and curative medicine.
Formerly (until 1993): Homoeopathic Heritage (0970-6038)
Indexed: AMED.
—BLDSC (4326.341910), GNLM.
Published by: B. Jain Publishers Pvt. Ltd., 1921 Chuna Mandi, St. 10th, Pahar Ganj, New Delhi 110 055, India. TEL 91-11-7770430, FAX 91-11-3610471, bjain@vsnl.com. Eds. Dr. Prem Nath Jain, Dr. Farokh J Master. R&P, Adv. contact Kuldeep Jain. Circ: 14,000 (paid). **Subscr. to:** P O Box 5775, New Delhi 110 055, India.

615.532 NZL ISSN 1171-1159
HOMOEOPATHY NEWZ. Text in English. 1991. 10/yr. NZD 25 domestic; NZD 59 foreign (effective 2001). adv. bk.rev. illus, bibl, stat. back issues avail. **Document type:** *Newsletter, Academic/Scholarly.* **Description:** A newsletter for the homeopathic community in New Zealand, containing case reports, book reviews, conference notices.
Address: Tawa, PO Box 51-156, Wellington, New Zealand. TEL 64-4-232-0672, jwinston@actrix.gen.nz, http://www.homeopathic.co.nz/newz.htm. Ed., Pub., Adv. contact Julian Winston. page NZD 120; trim 5.25 x 8.75. Circ: 250.

615.532 NOR ISSN 0333-0044
HOMOOPATISK TIDSSKRIFT. Text in Norwegian. 1963. q. NOK 150; NOK 250 foreign (effective 2001). adv. bk.rev. back issues avail. **Document type:** *Magazine, Consumer, Trade.* **Description:** Presents articles on homeopathy, alternative medicine and nutrition for all people interested in such issues.
Published by: Norsk Homoopatisk Pasientforening, Postboks 412, Trondheim 7001, Norway. TEL 47-73-51-00-44, FAX 47-73-51-00-58, trine.carsten@c2i.net. Ed. Henrich Lysholm. Adv. contact Trine Carstens TEL 47-73-52-23-07.

370 USA ISSN 0899-9260
I C A REVIEW; international review of Chiropractic. Text in English. 1944. bi-m. USD 50. adv. bk.rev. illus. index. **Description:** Scientific and general articles on chiropractic and health-related issues.
Formerly (until 1985): International Review of Chiropractic (0738-6850)
Published by: International Chiropractors Association, 1110 N Glebe Rd, Ste 1000, Arlington, VA 22201. Ed. Molly Rangnath. Circ: 10,000.

615.532 IND ISSN 0019-5243
INDIAN JOURNAL OF HOMOEOPATHIC MEDICINE. Text in English. 1967. q. INR 150, USD 25 (effective 1997). adv. bk.rev. abstr. index. **Document type:** *Academic/Scholarly.* **Description:** Contains detailed discussion on concepts and articles on clinical research, and homoeopathic education.
Incorporates: Indian Journal of Homoeopathy (0537-202X); Journal of Homoeopathic Medicine
Indexed: AMED.
—BLDSC (4414.800000), CISTI, GNLM.
Published by: Homoeopathic Education Society, Gadkari Marg, Vile Parle West, Mumbai, Maharashtra 400 056, India. TEL 91-22-620-1135, FAX 91-22-516-5985. Ed. P M Barvalla. R&P Praful Barvalia. Adv. contact C M Menon. B&W page INR 750. Circ: 2,000.

INTERNATIONAL JOURNAL OF ALTERNATIVE & COMPLEMENTARY MEDICINE. see *ALTERNATIVE MEDICINE*

615.533 USA ISSN 0098-6151
RZ301 CODEN: JAOAAZ
J A O A: JOURNAL OF THE AMERICAN OSTEOPATHIC ASSOCIATION. Text in English. 1901. m. USD 65 (effective 1999). adv. bk.rev. abstr, charts, illus. index, cum.index 1901-1956; 1956-1965. reprint service avail. from PQC. *Refereed.*
Formerly: American Osteopathic Association. Journal (0003-0287)
Related titles: Microfilm ed.: (from PQC).
Indexed: AMED, Biol.Abstr., C.I.S. Abstr., Chem.Abstr., Curr.Cont. (coverage dropped), Dok.Arbeitsmed., Excerp.Med., INIS Atomind., Ind.Med. (1901-), Int.Nurs.Ind., Med.Care Rev., Nutr.Abstr.
—BLDSC (4689.400000), CISTI, GNLM, ingenta, KNAW.
Published by: American Osteopathic Association, 142 E Ontario St, Chicago, IL 60611. TEL 312-202-8000, FAX 312-280-5893. Ed. Gilbert E D'Alonzo. Pub., R&P Philip Saigh. Adv. contact Linda Dunn. Circ: 33,000.

JOURNAL OF BACK AND MUSCULOSKELETAL REHABILITATION. see *MEDICAL SCIENCES—Orthopedics And Traumatology*

615 617.3 USA ISSN 0161-4754
RM724
JOURNAL OF MANIPULATIVE AND PHYSIOLOGICAL THERAPEUTICS. Abbreviated title: J M P T. Text in English. 1978. 9/yr. USD 107 domestic to individuals for both Print & Online eds.; USD 137 foreign to individuals for both Print & Online eds.; USD 162 domestic to institutions for both Print & Online eds.; USD 192 foreign to institutions for both Print & Online eds.; USD 67 domestic to students for both Print & Online eds.; USD 97 foreign to students for both Print & Online eds.; USD 22 newsstand/cover for both Print & Online eds. (effective 2001). adv. bk.rev. back issues avail. *Refereed.* **Document type:** *Journal, Academic/Scholarly.* **Description:** Deals with chiropractic medicine issues such as manipulation, physical therapy and other conservative treatment methods.
Related titles: Microfilm ed.: (from WWS); Online - full text ed.: (from EBSCO Publishing, IDEAL Online Library, Institute for Scientific Information, RoweCom Information Quest).
Indexed: AMED, ASCA, Apic.Abstr., Biol.Abstr., CINAHL, Curr.Cont., Dent.Ind., Excerp.Med., INIS Atomind., Ind.Med. (1978-), Inpharma, Neurosci.Cit.Ind., Pharm.&Out.News, Reac., SSCI (coverage dropped).
—BLDSC (5011.600000), CISTI, GNLM, IDS, ingenta, KNAW. **CCC.**
Published by: (National College of Chiropractic), Mosby, Inc. (Subsidiary of: Elsevier Science), 11830 Westline Industrial Dr, St Louis, MO 63146-3318. TEL 800-453-4351, FAX 314-431-1158, periodical.service@mosby.com, http://www.mosby.com/jmpt. Eds. Chris Baumle, Dana J Lawrence. Adv. contact Carol Kilzer TEL 314-453-4307. B&W page USD 855; trim 10.88 x 8.13. Circ: 1,900.

JOURNAL OF MUSCULOSKELETAL PAIN; innovations in research, theory & clinical practice. see *MEDICAL SCIENCES—Orthopedics And Traumatology*

615.53 617.1 USA ISSN 1084-1288
RZ275.S65 CODEN: JSCRFL
JOURNAL OF SPORTS CHIROPRACTIC AND REHABILITATION. Text in English. 1987. q. USD 98 domestic to individuals; USD 112 foreign to individuals; USD 142 domestic to institutions; USD 153 foreign to institutions (effective 2001). adv. *Refereed.* **Document type:** *Academic/Scholarly.* **Description:** Covers chiropractic advances in sports injury treatment, athletic training and injury prevention.
Formerly (until 1996): Chiropractic Sports Medicine (0889-6976)
Related titles: Microfilm ed.: 1987 (from WWS); Online - full text ed.: (from Institute for Scientific Information).
Indexed: AMED, ASCA, CINAHL, Excerp.Med., Focus on: Sports Sci.& Med.
—BLDSC (5066.189500), EMDOCS, GNLM, IDS, Infotrieve, KNAW.
Published by: (American Chiropractic Association, Council on Sports Injuries and Physical Fitness), Atwood Publishing, LLC (Subsidiary of: Gem Communications), 11600 College Blvd., Overland Park, KS 66210. TEL 913-469-1110, FAX 913-469-0806. Ed. Bart Green. adv.: B&W page USD 555, color page USD 1,380; trim 10.88 x 8.13. Circ: 2,447 (paid).

615.53 616.8 USA ISSN 1067-8239
JOURNAL OF THE NEUROMUSCULOSKELETAL SYSTEM. Short title: J N M S. Text in English. 1993. q. USD 58 to individuals; USD 118 to institutions. adv. *Refereed.* **Document type:** *Academic/Scholarly.* **Description:** Covers all areas reflecting the manifestations of neuromusculoskeletal function and dysfunction, including biomechanics, adjustive and manipulative therapy, neurology, nutrition, orthopedics, radiology and imaging, and physical therapy.
Related titles: Online - full text ed.: (from Institute for Scientific Information).
Indexed: ASCA, CINAHL, Neurosci.Cit.Ind., e-psyche.
—BLDSC (4669.470800), CISTI, IDS, Infotrieve. **CCC.**
Published by: (American Chiropractic Association, Inc.), Data Trace Publishing Company, 110 West Rd, Ste 227, Baltimore, MD 21204. TEL 410-494-4994, FAX 410-494-0515, info@datatrace.com, http://www.datatrace.com/. Ed. Scott Haldeman. R&P Cindy Lee Floyd. Adv. contact Frank Tufariello. Circ: 12,014.

615.534 USA
JOURNAL OF VERTEBRAL SUBLUXATION RESEARCH. Text in English. 1996. q. USD 100 domestic to individuals; USD 140 foreign to individuals; USD 150 domestic to institutions; USD 190 foreign to institutions. *Refereed.* **Document type:** *Academic/Scholarly.*
Description: Disseminates research in this subspecialty.
Indexed: CINAHL.
Published by: Council on Chiropractic Practice, 2950 N Dobson Rd, Ste 1, Chandler, AZ 85224. TEL 800-347-1011, FAX 480-732-9313. Ed. Dr. William R Boone. Pub. Dr. Terry A Rondberg.

615.532 IND ISSN 0300-3957
KERALA HOMOEO JOURNAL. Text and summaries in English. 1971. q. INR 8. adv. bk.rev. abstr, stat.
Published by: All Kerala Homeopathic Physicians Association, Kanjikuzhy, Kottayam, Kerala 4, India. Ed. Dr. T R Sivan Tholoor. Circ: 15,890. **Co-sponsor:** Indian Homoeo Chemists Federation.

615.53 378 USA
LOS ANGELES COLLEGE OF CHIROPRACTIC. NEWS & ALUMNI REPORT. Text in English. 1977. q. free per issue. adv. **Document type:** *Newsletter.* **Description:** News, announcements, and notes on the activities and people associated with the College.
Published by: Los Angeles College of Chiropractic, 16200 E Amber Valley Dr, Box 1166, Whittier, CA 90609-1166. TEL 310-947-8755, FAX 310-947-5724. Ed. Steven E Reifel. Circ: 6,000.

MASSAGE AUSTRALIA. see *MEDICAL SCIENCES—Physical Medicine And Rehabilitation*

615.5 ITA ISSN 1121-5518
MEDICINA NATURALE. Text in Italian. 1990. bi-m. ITL 50,000; ITL 100,000 in Europe; ITL 150,000 elsewhere. adv. **Description:** Covers all aspects of natural medicine: homeopathy, acupuncture, naturopathy, chiropractic, nutrition and more.
Published by: Tecniche Nuove s.p.a., Via Ciro Menotti, 14, Milan, MI 20129, Italy. TEL 39-027570321, FAX 39-027570332, abbonamenti@tecnet.it; medicina@tecnet.it, http://www.tecnet.it/index1.html. adv.: B&W page ITL 3,380,000, color page ITL 4,560,000; trim 297 x 210. Circ: 8,220.

615.533 USA ISSN 0892-0249
N J A O P S JOURNAL. Text in English. 1901. 6/yr. USD 25. adv. bk.rev. illus. *Refereed.* **Document type:** *Directory, Newsletter.*
Formerly: New Jersey Association of Osteopathic Physicians and Surgeons. Journal (0028-5528)
Published by: New Jersey Association of Osteopathic Physicians and Surgeons, 1 Distribution Way, Monmouth Jct., NJ 08852-3001. TEL 732-940-9000, FAX 732-940-8899. Ed., R&P Jeffrey A Kramer. Circ: 2,000. **Affiliate:** American Osteopathic Association.

NATIONAL DIRECTORY OF CHIROPRACTIC. see *BUSINESS AND ECONOMICS—Trade And Industrial Directories*

615.53 JPN ISSN 0912-1110
NIPPON KAIROPURAKUTIKKU GAKKAI ZASSHI/JAPAN JOURNAL OF CHIROPRACTIC SCIENCE. Text in Japanese. 1984. s-a. JPY 4,000 per issue.
Published by: Rinsho Kairopurakutikku Gakkai/Association of Clinical Chiropractic, Nihon Kairopurakutikku Renmei, 5-9 Aoyama 3-chome, Minato-ku, Tokyo 105-0000, Japan.

NURSES IN TRANSITION. see *MEDICAL SCIENCES—Nurses And Nursing*

615.534 616 USA
THE ORIGINAL INTERNIST; Official publication of the AIMA (American Integrative Medical Association). Text in English. 1994. q. USD 50 (effective 2000 - 2001). adv. bk.rev. charts, illus. back issues avail.; reprints avail. *Refereed.* **Document type:** *Bulletin, Journal, Academic/Scholarly.* **Description:** Covers all aspects of natural health care - chiropractic, homeopathy, osteopathy, naturopathy, etc.
Formerly: Internist (1091-3068)
Indexed: AgeLine.
Published by: Clint Publications, 720 Oak Knoll, Rolla, MO 65401. TEL 573-341-8448, FAX 573-341-8494, internis@rollanet.org, http://www.rollanet.org/~internis. Ed. Jack Kessinger. Adv. contact Virginia Kessinger.

615.532 IND ISSN 0048-2242
ORISSA HOMOEOPATHIC BULLETIN; bilingual monthly magazine. Text in English, Oriya. 1969. m. INR 40, USD 20. adv. bk.rev. reprint service avail. from PQC.
Related titles: Microform ed.: (from PQC).
Published by: Natabar Naik Ed. & Pub., Tilottame Homoeo House, P.O. Jagatsinghpur, Cuttack, Orissa 754 103, India. TEL 754103. Circ: 500.

617.3 USA ISSN 0030-591X
ORTHOPOD. Text in English. 1960. 2/yr. free per issue to qualified personnel. adv. illus. **Document type:** *Bulletin, Academic/Scholarly.*
Media: Duplicated (not offset).
Published by: American Osteopathic Academy of Orthopedics, PO Box 291690, Davie, FL 33329-1690. TEL 954-262-1700. Ed. Dr. Daniel L Morrison. Adv. contact Margaret S Moore. Circ: 1,200.

OSTEOPATHIC PROGRESS. see *HEALTH FACILITIES AND ADMINISTRATION*

615.53 DEU ISSN 1615-9071
▼ **OSTEOPATHISCHE MEDIZIN.** Text in German. 2000. 4/yr. EUR 68 (effective 2002). adv. *Refereed.* **Document type:** *Journal, Academic/Scholarly.* **Description:** Covers all aspects of osteopathic medicine.
Published by: Urban & Fischer Verlag, Loebdergraben 14a, Jena 07743, Germany. TEL 49-3641-626430, FAX 49-3641-626421, info@urbanfischer.de, http://www.urbanfischer.de/journals. Ed. Dr. Sabine Schmidt. Adv. contact Sabine Schroeter.

615.333 DEU ISSN 0944-6516
OSTEOSYNTHESE INTERNATIONAL. Text in German. 1993. q. EUR 107.40 domestic to institutions; EUR 110 in Europe to institutions; EUR 112.80 elsewhere to institutions; EUR 49 to students; EUR 29 newsstand/cover (effective 2002). **Document type:** *Journal, Academic/Scholarly.*
Related titles: Online - full text ed.: ISSN 1439-0868.
—GNLM.
Published by: (Verein zur Foerderung von Verfahren zur Knochenbruchbehandlung), Johann Ambrosius Barth Verlag in Medizinverlage Heidelberg GmbH & Co. KG, Ruedigerstr 14, Stuttgart 70469, Germany. TEL 49-711-8931-0, FAX 49-711-8931422, kunden.service@thieme.de, http://www.thieme.de. Ed. Klaus Klemm.

PENNSYLVANIA OSTEOPATHIC MEDICAL ASSOCIATION. JOURNAL. see *MEDICAL SCIENCES*

615.53 ESP ISSN 0212-7393
PODOSCOPIO. Text in Spanish. 1984. 4/yr. ESP 5,000 (effective 1999). adv.
Address: San Bernardo, 74, Madrid 28015, Spain. TEL 34-91-5326006, FAX 34-91-5228763, copoma@mumdivia.es. Ed. Manuel Meneses Garde. Adv. contact A Cros. Circ: 5,000.

615.53 CHE
PRO CHIROPRAKTIK. Text in German. q.
Address: Stampachgasse 6, Bolligen 3065, Switzerland. TEL 031-585210, FAX 031-587246. Ed. Rudolf Weber. Circ: 13,475.

616.7 ESP ISSN 1132-8460
REVISTA ESPANOLA DE ENFERMEDADES METABOLICAS OSEAS. Text in Spanish. 1989. bi-m. USD 55 (effective 1996). **Document type:** *Academic/Scholarly.*
Formerly (until 1992): Enfermedades Metabolicas Oseas (0214-7254)
—BLDSC (7853.971000), CINDOC, GNLM.
Published by: Editorial Idepsa S.A., Principe de Vergara, 112 1o F, Madrid 28002, Spain. TEL 34-1-5637306, FAX 34-1-5632393. Ed. Aurelio Rapado Errazti.

REVMATOLOGIIA. see *MEDICAL SCIENCES—Rheumatology*

615.532 BEL ISSN 0035-0885
CODEN: RBHOD4
REVUE BELGE D'HOMOEOPATHIE. Text in English. 1949. q. BEF 1,800 domestic; BEF 2,000 foreign (effective 1999). adv. bk.rev. bibl, illus. index. **Document type:** *Bulletin, Academic/Scholarly.*
Indexed: AMED.
—BLDSC (7891.930000).
Published by: Societe Royale Belge d'Homoeopathie, Av Cardinal Micara 7, Brussels 1160, Belgium. TEL 32-2-735-35-25, FAX 32-2-242-75-55. Ed. Dr. Ch Schepens. Adv. contact J Alaerts. Circ: 2,000.

615.53 USA ISSN 1068-2953
SECOND OPINION (DUNWOODY). Key Title: Dr. William Campbell Douglass' Second Opinion. Text in English. 1976. m. USD 49. bk.rev. **Document type:** *Newsletter.*
Incorporates: Doctor's People; Which was formerly: People's Doctor
Address: 7100 Peachtree Dunwoody Rd, N E 100, Atlanta, GA 30328-1689. TEL 770-399-5617, 800-728-2288, FAX 770-399-0815. Ed. Dr. William Campbell Douglass. Pub. Wallis W Wood. R&P Garret Wood. Circ: 90,000.

615.533 JPN ISSN 0910-1225
SOGO SEIKOTSU/SYNTHESIS OSTEOPATHY. Text in Japanese. 1984. q. JPY 1,500 per issue.
Published by: Medikaru Puresu/Medical Press Ltd., 43-9 Sakuradai 3-chome, Nerima-ku, Tokyo 176-0002, Japan.

SOUTH AFRICA. STATISTICS SOUTH AFRICA. CENSUS OF MEDICAL, DENTAL AND OTHER HEALTH SERVICES - CHIROPRACTORS, HOMEOPATHS, NATUROPATHS, OSTEOPATHS AND HERBALISTS. see *MEDICAL SCIENCES—Abstracting, Bibliographies, Statistics*

615.53 USA
SPINAL COLUMN. Text in English. 6/yr. USD 10. adv.
Published by: Palmer College of Chiropractic, 1000 Brady St, Davenport, IA 52803. TEL 319-326-9662.

615.53 USA
TEXAS CHIROPRACTIC COLLEGE MAGAZINE. Text in English. 1974. 3/yr. adv. back issues avail. **Document type:** *Academic/Scholarly.* **Description:** Contains articles on pertinent legislation and on supporting alumni.
Former titles: Texas Chiropractic Magazine; Texas Chiropractic Review
Published by: Texas Chiropractic College, 5912 Spencer Hwy, Pasadena, TX 77505-1699. TEL 713-487-1170, 800-TCC-ALUM, FAX 281-991-4981. Ed., R&P, Adv. contact Kathryn Cooper. Circ: 5,000.

615.53 USA ISSN 0275-1453
TEXAS D O. Text in English. 1945. m. USD 35.50. adv. **Document type:** *Trade.*
Formerly (until 1980): Association: Journal of Texas Osteopathic Medical Association (0275-1445)
Published by: Texas Osteopathic Medical Association, 1415 Lavaca St, Austin, TX 78701-1634. TEL 512-708-8662, FAX 512-708-1415. Ed. Terry R Boucher. Circ: 2,650.

615.53 USA
TEXAS JOURNAL OF CHIROPRACTIC. Text in English. 10/yr. free to members; USD 36 (effective 2001). adv. **Document type:** *Trade, Academic/Scholarly.*
Published by: Texas Chiropractic Association, 1601 Rio Grande, Ste 420, Austin, TX 78701. TEL 512-477-9292, FAX 512-477-9296. Eds. John Martin, Nancy Josephson. Adv. contact Christine M Lehmann. B&W page USD 220, color page USD 440; 10 x 7.5. Circ: 3,400.

TIJDSCHRIFT VOOR INTEGRALE GENEESKUNDE. see *ALTERNATIVE MEDICINE*

615.543 USA ISSN 0091-2360
RZ201
TODAY'S CHIROPRACTIC. Text in English. 1972. bi-m. USD 24 in United States; USD 28 in Canada; USD 33 elsewhere. adv. bk.rev. charts, illus. **Document type:** *Trade.*
—BLDSC (8859.727800).
Published by: Life University, 1269 Barclay Circle, Marietta, GA 30060. TEL 770-424-0554, FAX 770-419-0568, http://www.todayschiropractic.com. Ed., R&P James B Panter TEL 770-426-2990. Adv. contact John Schilin. Circ: 70,000.

615.534 USA ISSN 1073-2837
TOPICS IN CLINICAL CHIROPRACTIC. Text in English. 1994. q. USD 135 to individuals; USD 41 newsstand/cover (effective 2002). adv. reprint service avail. from PQC. *Refereed.* **Document type:** *Journal.* **Description:** Addresses the practical concerns of the chiropractic physician. Focuses on assessment and diagnosis, practical treatment and intervention strategies, standards of care, insurance and reimbursement.
Related titles: Microform ed.: (from PQC); Online - full text ed.: (from ProQuest Information & Learning).
Indexed: AMED, CINAHL.
—BLDSC (8867.432660), GNLM, ingenta. **CCC.**

M

Published by: Aspen Publishers, Inc., 200 Orchard Ridge Dr, Ste 200, Gaithersburg, MD 20878. TEL 301-417-7500, 800-638-8437, FAX 301-417-7550, customer.service@aspenpul.com, http://www.aspenpub.com. Eds. Jane Coyle Garwood, Sandra L Lunsford. Pub. Michael B Brown. Adv. contact Frances S Ray. **Dist. by:** Aspen Publishers Inc., Distribution Center, 7201 McKinney Circle, Frederick, MD 21701. TEL 301-698-7100, FAX 301-695-7931.

TOUCH FOR HEALTH. see *PHYSICAL FITNESS AND HYGIENE*

615.533 USA ISSN 1046-4948
TRIAD (OKEMOS). Text in English. 1989. q. USD 50 (effective 1997). adv. bk.rev. charts, illus. Supplement avail. **Document type:** *Trade.* **Description:** Covers activities and topics interesting to the osteopathic community in Michigan.
Formerly (until Aug. 1989): Michigan Osteopathic Journal (0026-2374)
Published by: Michigan Osteopathic Association, 2445 Woodlake Cir, Okemos, MI 48864-5941. TEL 517-347-1555, FAX 517-347-1566. Ed. Maurya Johnston. R&P Mauria Johnston. Adv. contact Patricia Horan. Circ: 3,200.

YEAR BOOK OF CHIROPRACTIC. see *MEDICAL SCIENCES—Abstracting, Bibliographies, Statistics*

YOUR LIFE - YOUR CHOICE. see *ALTERNATIVE MEDICINE*

615.532 DEU ISSN 0935-0853
ZEITSCHRIFT FUER KLASSISCHE HOMOEOPATHIE; kritisches Organ fuer Homoeopathie. Text in German; Summaries in English. 1957. 6/yr. EUR 87.90 domestic to institutions; EUR 92.40 in Europe to institutions; EUR 100.90 elsewhere to institutions; EUR 15.90 newsstand/cover (effective 2002). adv. bk.rev. **Document type:** *Journal, Academic/Scholarly.*
Former titles: Klassische Homeopathie (0301-1402); (until 1971): Acta Homeopathica (0001-5881)
Indexed: AMED.
—BLDSC (9467.719000), GNLM. **CCC.**
Published by: Karl F. Haug Verlag, Fritz-Frey-Str 21, Heidelberg 69121, Germany. TEL 49-6221-489584, FAX 49-6221-489584, http://www.haug-verlag.de. Ed. Dr. U Friedrich. Adv. contact Martina Urban. Circ: 2,800.

MEDICAL SCIENCES—Communicable Diseases

A & U; America's AIDS magazine. (Art & Understanding) see *LITERATURE*

616.9 USA
A F A R ANNUAL REPORT. Abbreviated title: Am F A R Annual Report. Text in English. 1985. a., latest 1998-99. free. **Description:** Highlights the Foundation's program activities and accomplishments, includes FY 98-99 financial statements and features a special article on the search for a safe and effective AIDS vaccine.
Published by: American Foundation for AIDS Research, 120 Wall St, Fl 13, New York, NY 10005-3902. TEL 212-682-7440, FAX 212-806-1601. Circ: 60,000.

A P A I T; HIV - AIDS from another angle. see *ETHNIC INTERESTS*

ABSTRACTS ON HYGIENE AND COMMUNICABLE DISEASES. see *MEDICAL SCIENCES—Abstracting, Bibliographies, Statistics*

619.9 AUS ISSN 1031-4873
ACCENT. Text in English. 1988. q. free per issue. bk.rev. **Document type:** *Newsletter.* **Description:** Provides staff, volunteers, and general members of AIDS Council of South Australia with current information about HIV infection and AIDS, as well as the organization's services and programs.
Published by: A I D S Council of South Australia Inc., PO Box 907, Kent Town, SA 5071, Australia. TEL 61-8-8362-1611, FAX 61-8-8363-1046, aidscouncilsa@bigpond.com, http://www.aidscouncil.org.au. Ed., R&P Stephen Cox. Circ: 500.

616.998 CHE ISSN 0001-5938 CODEN: ALEPA8
ACTA LEPROLOGICA; revue editee par le comite international executif de l'Ordre S.M. de Malte. Text in English, French, Spanish. 1960. s-a. free per issue. adv. bk.rev. bibl. **Document type:** *Academic/Scholarly.* **Description:** Technical journal devoted to leprosy research, its treatment and prevention, drug therapy and health education. Contains articles about survey methodology, and recent technological and medical developments. Also includes reports of events and list of courses.
Indexed: Excerp.Med., Ind.Med. (1960-).
—BLDSC (0629.100000), CASDDS, CISTI, EMDOCS, GNLM, KNAW.
Published by: Ordre de Malte pour l'Assistance aux Lepreux, 3 Place Claparede, Geneva 1205, Switzerland. TEL 41-22-3468687, FAX 41-22-3470861, mission.order-malta@ties.itu.int. Ed. J M Decazes. Circ: 2,000.

616.9 ITA ISSN 0392-9515
ACTA MEDITERRANEA DI PATOLOGIA INFETTIVA E TROPICALE. Text in English, Italian. 1960. 3/yr. ITL 60,000; ITL 100,000 foreign (effective 1998). adv. abstr, bibl, illus, stat. index. **Document type:** *Proceedings, Academic/Scholarly.* **Description:** Reviews clinical cases of communicable and tropical diseases.
Indexed: Helminthol.Abstr., Protozool.Abstr.
Published by: Carbone Editore, Via Gaetano Daita, 29, Palermo, PA 90139, Italy. TEL 39-91-321-273, FAX 39-91-321782. Ed. Antonino Pennino. Pub., R&P Alfonsa Carbone. Adv. contact Donatella Donato. Circ: 3,000.

616.988 NLD ISSN 0001-706X
Q3 CODEN: ACTRAQ
ACTA TROPICA; journal of biomedical sciences. Text in English, French, German; Summaries in English. 1944. m. EUR 1,225 in Europe to institutions; JPY 162,000 in Japan to institutions; USD 1,370 elsewhere to institutions (effective 2002). adv. bk.rev. abstr, charts, illus. index. back issues avail. *Refereed.* **Document type:** *Academic/Scholarly.* **Description:** Details every aspect of biomedical sciences relevant to humans, including veterinary medicine and biology in the tropics.
Related titles: Online - full text ed.: (from ingenta, Swets Blackwell, ScienceDirect, Institute for Scientific Information).
Indexed: ASCA, Abstr.Hyg., AgBiotech, Agri.& Environ.Biotech.Abstr. (coverage dropped), Aqua.Sci.& Fish.Abstr., Bio-Contr.News & Info., Biol.Abstr., Chem.Abstr., Chem.Indus.Notes, Chem.Titles, Curr.Adv.Ecol.Sci., Curr.Cont., Dairy Sci.Abstr., Derwent Biotech.Abstr., Ecol.Abstr., Entomol.Abstr., Environ.Sci.Poll.Mgmt., Excerp.Med., Geo.Abstr.H.G., Helminthol.Abstr., IDA, Ind.Med. (1944-), Ind.Sci.Rev., Ind.Vet., Inpharma, Int.Abstr.Biol.Sci., Key Word Ind.Wildl.Res., Microbiol.Abstr., Nutr.Abstr., Pharm.&Out.News, Pig News & Info., Plant Breed.Abstr., Pollut.Abstr., Protozool.Abstr., Reac., Rev.Appl.Entomol., Rev.Arom.& Med.Plants, Rev.Med.& Vet.Mycol., Rice Abstr., Risk Abstr., Rural Devel.Abstr., SSCI (coverage dropped), Saf.Sci.Abstr., Sci.Cit.Ind., Sport Fish.Abstr., Stud.Wom.Abstr., Trop.Dis.Bull., Vet.Bull., Wild.Rev., Zoo.Rec.
—ADONIS, CASDDS, CISTI, Ei, EMDOCS, GNLM, IDS, ingenta, Linda Hall. **CCC.**
Published by: (Schweizerisches Tropeninstitut), Elsevier Science BV, PO Box 211, Amsterdam 1000 AE, Netherlands. TEL 31-20-485-3757, FAX 31-20-485-3432, TELEX 18582 ESPA NL, nlinfo-f@elsevier.nl, http://www.elsevier.nl/locate/actatropica. Ed. A Bjorkman. **Subscr. in Australasia and the Far East to:** Elsevier Science (Singapore) Pte Ltd, No.1 Temasek Ave, 17-01 Millenia Tower, Singapore 039192, Singapore. TEL 65-434-3727, FAX 65-337-2230, asiainfo@elsevier.com.sg; **Subscr. in Japan to:** Elsevier Science Inc - Japan Regional Office, 9-15 Higashi-Azabu 1-chome, Minato-ku, Tokyo 106-0044, Japan. TEL 81-3-5561-5033, FAX 81-3-5561-5047, info@elsevier.co.jp; **Subscr. in the Americas to:** Elsevier Science, PO Box 945, New York, NY 10159-0945. TEL 212-633-3730, FAX 212-633-3680, usinfo-f@elsevier.com, http://www.elsevier.com.

ACTA VIROLOGICA; international journal. see *BIOLOGY—Microbiology*

610 CHE
ACTION AGAINST INFECTION; a newsletter for WHO and its partners. Text in English. bi-m. back issues avail. **Document type:** *Newsletter.*
Related titles: Online - full content ed.; Spanish ed.; French ed.
Published by: World Health Organization, Marketing and Dissemination, Geneva, 27 1211, Switzerland. TEL 41-22-791-2476, FAX 41-22-791-4857, http://www.who.int/infectious-disease-news/newsletter/index.html.

616.9 USA ISSN 0934-6112
ADVANCES IN DISEASE VECTOR RESEARCH. Text in English. 1983. irreg. **Document type:** *Monographic series, Academic/Scholarly.*
Formerly (until 1988): Current Topics in Vector Research (0737-8491)
—CISTI, GNLM, Infotrieve, ingenta, KNAW, Linda Hall. **CCC.**
Published by: Springer-Verlag, Journals (Subsidiary of: BertelsmannSpringer), 175 Fifth Ave, New York, NY 10010. TEL 212-460-1500, FAX 212-473-6272.

616.3623 NZL ISSN 1530-5767
▼ **ADVANCES IN HEPATITIS C.** Text in English. 2000. irreg. abstr. back issues avail.
Media: Online - full text.
Published by: Adis International Limited, Mairangi Bay, Private Bag 65901, Auckland 1010, New Zealand. TEL 64-9-477-0700, FAX 64-9-477-0766, http://www.adis.com/advances_hepc/issue1/ahcstart.htm. Eds. Alfredo Albert, Ferruccio Bonino.

616.9 USA ISSN 0732-0566 CODEN: AHDMD3
ADVANCES IN HOST DEFENSE MECHANISMS. Text in English. 1983. irreg. price varies. reprint service avail. from PQC. **Document type:** *Monographic series.*
Indexed: Aqua.Sci.& Fish.Abstr.
—CASDDS, CISTI, KNAW.
Published by: Lippincott Williams & Wilkins (Philadelphia) (Subsidiary of: Wolters Kluwer N.V.), 530 Walnut St, Philadelphia, PA 19106-3621. TEL 301-223-2300, 800-638-3030, FAX 301-223-2400.

ADVANCES IN VIRUS RESEARCH. see *BIOLOGY—Microbiology*

616.9 USA ISSN 0269-9370
RC607.A26 CODEN: AIDSET
AIDS; an international monthly journal. (Acquired Immune Deficiency Syndrome) Text in English. 1986. 18/yr. USD 406 in North America to individuals print and online eds. combined; USD 406 in Europe to individuals; USD 442 elsewhere to individuals; USD 1,364 in North America to institutions print and online eds. combined; USD 1,364 per issue in Europe to institutions; USD 1,400 elsewhere to institutions; USD 77 newsstand/cover (effective 2002). adv. bibl, illus. back issues avail. *Refereed.* **Document type:** *Journal, Academic/Scholarly.* **Description:** Publishes original papers on all aspects of acquired immunodeficiency syndrome, AIDS. Features rapid publication of the latest in the clinical and scientific aspects of the disease.
Related titles: Online - full text ed.: USD 1,774.10 in North America academic site license; USD 1,774.10 in Europe academic site license; USD 1,807.10 elsewhere academic site license; USD 1,967.65 domestic corporate site license; USD 1,967.65 foreign corporate site license (effective 2002) (from EBSCO Publishing, Ovid Technologies, Inc., Swets Blackwell, Institute for Scientific Information); ♦ Supplement: AIDS (Year). ISSN 1350-2840.
Indexed: AIDS & Cancer Res., AIDS Abstr., Abstr.Hyg., Chem.Indus.Notes, Chem.Titles, Curr.Cont., Derwent Biotech.Abstr., Environ.Sci.Poll.Mgmt., Excerp.Med., Immun.Abstr., Ind.Med. (1987-), Ind.Sci.Rev., Ind.Vet., Indian Psychol.Abstr., Inpharma, Int.Abstr.Biol.Sci., Int.Nurs.Ind., Jrnl.Watch Inf.Dis., Med.& Surg.Dermat., Microbiol.Abstr., NRN, Neurosci.Abstr., Pharm.&Out.News, Pollut.Abstr., Protozool.Abstr., PsycInfo, Psychol.Abstr. (1988-), Reac., Risk Abstr., Rural Devel.Abstr., Saf.Sci.Abstr., Sci.Cit.Ind., Soc.Serv.Abstr., Sociol.Abstr., THA, Trop.Dis.Bull., Virol.Abstr., e-psyche.
—BLDSC (0773.083000), ADONIS, CASDDS, EMDOCS, GNLM, IDS, ingenta, KNAW.
Published by: Lippincott Williams & Wilkins (Philadelphia) (Subsidiary of: Wolters Kluwer N.V.), 530 Walnut St, Philadelphia, PA 19106-3621. TEL 215-521-8300, FAX 215-521-8902, http://www.AIDSonline.com, http://www.Lww.com. Eds. A M Johnson, J A Levy, J P Phair, M Laga. Adv. contact Gemma Heiser. B&W page USD 1,100, color page USD 2,500; trim 11 x 8.5. Circ: 4,502. **Subscr. to:** PO Box 1600, Hagerstown, MD 21740-1600. TEL 800-777-2295, FAX 301-824-7390.

AIDS ABSTRACTS; international literature on acquired immunodeficiency syndrome and related retroviruses. see *MEDICAL SCIENCES—Abstracting, Bibliographies, Statistics*

M

616.9 USA ISSN 0887-0292
AIDS ALERT. Variant title: Acquired Immune Deficiency Syndrome Alert. Text in English. 1986. m. USD 427 domestic; USD 457 foreign; USD 71 newsstand/cover (effective 2001). reprints avail. *Refereed.* **Document type:** *Newsletter.* **Description:** Information source for frontline health care workers in the AIDS epidemic.
Incorporates: AIDS Medical Report (1042-0762)
Related titles: Online - full text ed.: (from Northern Light Technology, Inc., Gale Group, Factiva).
Indexed: CINAHL.
—BLDSC (0773.083070).
Published by: American Health Consultants (Subsidiary of: Medical Economics Co., Inc.), 3525 Piedmont Rd, N E, 6 Piedmont Center, Ste 400, Atlanta, GA 30305. TEL 404-262-7436, 800-688-2421, FAX 404-262-7837, 800-284-3291, customerservice@ahcpub.com, http://www.ahcpub.com. Circ: 2,130. **Subscr. to:** PO Box 530161, Atlanta, GA 30353-0161.

AIDS ANALYSIS AFRICA. see *SOCIAL SERVICES AND WELFARE*

AIDS & CANCER RESEARCH. see *MEDICAL SCIENCES—Abstracting, Bibliographies, Statistics*

AIDS & FLORIDA LAW. see *LAW*

614 ZMB
AIDS & HEALTH NEWS. Text in English. 1991 (no.5). bi-m. ZMK 5 per issue. **Document type:** *Newspaper.*
Published by: Kara Counseling and Training Trust, PO Box 37559, Lusaka, Zambia. Ed. Oliver Kanene.

616.9 GBR ISSN 1473-012X
AIDS & HEPATITUS DIGEST. (Acquired Immune Deficiency Syndrome) Text in English. 1987. bi-m. GBP 32, USD 54 to institutions (effective 2002). adv. **Document type:** *Journal, Academic/Scholarly.* **Description:** Includes up-to-date information about research and treatment for AIDS; and related political and social issues.
Formerly: The AIDS Letter (0952-7427)
Indexed: Brit.Nur.Ind., Inpharma, Pharm.&Out.News, Reac.
—BLDSC (0773.083490), GNLM.
Published by: Royal Society of Medicine Press Ltd, 1 Wimpole St, London W1M 8AE, United Kingdom. TEL 44-20-7290-2921, FAX 44-20-7290-2929, rsmjournals@rsm.ac.uk, http://www.roysocmed.ac.uk/pub/ahd.htm. Ed. Dr. David R Morgan. Pub. Delia Siedle.

616.9 340 USA ISSN 0887-3852
RA644.A25
AIDS & PUBLIC POLICY JOURNAL. (Acquired Immune Deficiency Syndrome) Text in English. 1986. q. USD 59 to individuals; USD 115 to institutions (effective 2000). bk.rev. illus. reprints avail. *Refereed.* **Document type:** *Academic/Scholarly, Trade.* **Description:** Addresses AIDS related social, political, ethical, educational and legal issues in public health and health policy. Draws from a variety of disciplines and intellectual perspectives, including medicine, law, education, business, and the social sciences.
Related titles: Online - full text ed.: (from Gale Group, Institute for Scientific Information).
Indexed: ASCA, Curr.Cont., Excerp.Med. (1992-), Fam.Ind., Lang.& Lang.Behav.Abstr., P.A.I.S., SOPODA, SSCI, Soc.Sci.Ind. (Jan.1994-), Soc.Serv.Abstr., Sociol.Abstr.
—BLDSC (0773.083090), EMDOCS, GNLM.
Published by: University Publishing Group, Inc., 17100 Cole Rd, Ste 312, Hagerstown, MD 31740. TEL 800-654-8188, FAX 301-582-2406, orders@upgbooks.com. Ed. David Weber.

AIDS & T B WEEKLY ABSTRACTS FROM CONFERENCE PROCEEDINGS. (Tuberculosis) see *MEDICAL SCIENCES—Abstracting, Bibliographies, Statistics*

AIDS & T B WEEKLY ARTICLE SUMMARIES. (Tuberculosis) see *MEDICAL SCIENCES—Abstracting, Bibliographies, Statistics*

616.99 USA ISSN 1068-4174
RA644.A25
AIDS BOOK REVIEW JOURNAL. Text in English. 1993. irreg. (1-2/mo.). free per issue. bk.rev. **Document type:** *Academic/Scholarly.* **Description:** Reviews books and videos on AIDS, STD, and safe sex.
Media: Online - full text.
Published by: University of Illinois at Chicago, Library, PO Box 8198, Chicago, IL 60680-8198. TEL 312-996-2730, FAX 312-413-0424, hrm@uic.edu, http://www.uic.edu/depts/lib/aidsbkrv/. Ed. H. Robert Malinowsky. R&P H Robert Malinowsky. Circ: 2,000 (controlled).

614 ZAF ISSN 1019-8334
AIDS BULLETIN. Text in English. 1992. q. Free. bk.rev. **Document type:** *Bulletin.* **Description:** Provides information on AIDS education, prevention, care and research of interest to policymakers, personnel managers, researchers, education centers and the information industry.
Indexed: Ind.S.A.Per.
Published by: Medical Research Council, PO Box 19070, Tygerberg 7505, South Africa. TEL 27-21-938-0205, FAX 27-21-938-0395, http://www.mrc.ac.za/aids/contents.htm. Ed. Michelle Galloway. Circ: 1,600.

616.9 USA
AIDS BULLETIN. Text in English. irreg., latest vol.4, 1990. USD 15 to non-members; USD 10 to members. **Description:** Discusses CDC classification system for HTLV-III - LAV infections; the case definition of AIDS, CDC AIDS update, sample history and physical examination, guidelines for prevention of transmission of HIV and Hepatitis B virus to healthcare and public-safety workers.
Published by: American Correctional Health Services Association, PO Box 2307, Dayton, OH 45401-2307. TEL 937-586-3708, FAX 937-586-3699. R&P G M Hockaday.

616.9 GBR ISSN 0954-0121
RA644.A25 CODEN: AIDCEF
AIDS CARE; psychological and socio-medical aspects of AIDS-HIV. Text in English. 1989. bi-m. GBP 170, USD 280 to individuals; GBP 560, USD 924 to institutions (effective 2002). adv. bk.rev. *Refereed.* **Document type:** *Academic/Scholarly.* **Description:** Examines the biopsychosocial aspects of AIDS and HIV infection.
Related titles: Microfiche ed.; Online - full text ed.: ISSN 1360-0451 (from CatchWord Ltd., Northern Light Technology, Inc., EBSCO Publishing, O C L C Online Computer Library Center, Inc., RoweCom Information Quest, ProQuest Information & Learning, Swets Blackwell, Institute for Scientific Information).
Indexed: AIDS & Cancer Res., AIDS Abstr., AMED, ASCA, ASSIA, Abstr.Hyg., Addic.Abstr., AgeLine, CINAHL, Curr.Cont., Dairy Sci.Abstr., ERA, Environ.Sci.Poll.Mgmt., Fam.Ind., Ind.Med. (1989-), Indian Psychol.Abstr., Int.Nurs.Ind., Lang.& Lang.Behav.Abstr., Mult.Ed.Abstr., NRN, Pollut.Abstr., PsycInfo, Psychol.Abstr. (1989-), Rev.Appl.Entomol., Risk Abstr., Rural Devel.Abstr., SOPODA, SSCI, Saf.Sci.Abstr., Sage Fam.Stud.Abstr., Soc.Serv.Abstr., Sociol.Abstr., Stud.Wom.Abstr., Trop.Dis.Bull., Virol.Abstr., e-psyche.
—BLDSC (0773.083190), ADONIS, CatchWord, EMDOCS, GNLM, IDS, ingenta, KNAW. **CCC.**
Published by: Carfax Publishing Limited (Subsidiary of: Taylor & Francis Group), PO Box 25, Abingdon, Oxon OX14 3UE, United Kingdom. TEL 44-1235-401000, FAX 44-1235-401550, enquiries@carfax.co.uk, enquiry@tandf.co.uk, http://www.carfax.co.uk.

616.9 USA ISSN 1043-1543
AIDS CLINICAL CARE. Text in English. 1989. m. USD 98; USD 129 foreign (effective 1998). adv. charts, illus, stat. index. back issues avail. **Document type:** *Newsletter, Academic/Scholarly.* **Description:** Brings the latest developments in the diagnosis and treatment of HIV-related diseases to the practicing clinician.
Indexed: Abstr.Hyg., Lab.Haz.Bull.
—BLDSC (0773.083193).
Published by: Massachusetts Medical Society, Publishing Division, 10 Shattuck St, Boston, MA 02115. TEL 617-734-9800, 800-843-6356. Ed. Deborah Cotton. Adv. contact Art Wilshek. Circ: 30,000.

616.9 USA ISSN 1065-6162
RC607.A26
THE AIDS DIRECTORY. Text in English. 1992. a. USD 250 (effective 1999). **Document type:** *Directory.* **Description:** Provides profiles of 1,500 organizations including the first interdisciplinary compilation of leaders in the struggle against AIDS, those who care for people with HIV disease, funding sources, and government agencies (federal, state, and regional).
—Infotrieve. **CCC.**
Published by: L R P Publications, 747 Dresher Rd, Box 980, Horsham, PA 19044. TEL 215-784-0941, 800-341-7874, FAX 215-784-9639, custserve@irp.com, dshadovitz@lrp.com, http://www.lrp.com. Ed. Bill Feldman. Pub. Ken Kahn.

614 616.96 USA ISSN 0891-7426
AIDS INFORMATION EXCHANGE. (Acquired Immune Deficiency Syndrome) Text in English. 1984. q. USD 50 for 2 yrs.. bk.rev. charts, illus. *Refereed.* **Document type:** *Government.* **Description:** Provides information on innovative and effective AIDS-related policies and programs.
Published by: U.S. Conference of Mayors, Office of Public Affairs, 1620 Eye St, N W, Washington, DC 20006. TEL 202-293-7330, FAX 202-293-2352. Ed. J Thomas Cochran. **Co-sponsor:** U.S. Department of Health and Human Services.

616.9 GBR ISSN 1465-5470
▼ **THE AIDS INFORMER.** Text in English. 1999. m. GBP 90 domestic; USD 145 foreign (effective 2000). **Description:** Covers new AIDS information sources, resources and comprehensive reports.
Published by: Modus Operandi, PO Box HP346, Leeds LS6 1UL, United Kingdom. http://www.modus-op.demon.co.uk. Ed. Adam Christie.

616.9 CHE ISSN 1021-321X
AIDS INFOTHEK. Text in German. 1989. bi-m. CHF 41 (effective 2000). bk.rev., video rev. index (1989-). **Document type:** *Bulletin, Consumer.* **Description:** Publishes information on the progress of AIDS research, for the general public.
Related titles: French ed.: Infotheque SIDA. ISSN 1017-8791.
Published by: AIDS Info Docu Schweiz, Schauplatzgasse 26, Bern 3001, Switzerland. TEL 41-31-3121266, FAX 41-31-3116414, info@aid.ch, http://www.aidsnet.ch. Ed. Christa Brunswicker. Circ: 10,000.

AIDS LAW & LITIGATION REPORTER. see *LAW*

THE AIDS LEADER; covering business, economic policy and employment implications of AIDS & HIV. see *PUBLIC HEALTH AND SAFETY*

AIDS LEGAL BIBLIOGRAPHY. (Acquired Immune Deficiency Syndrome) see *LAW—Abstracting, Bibliographies, Statistics*

AIDS LITERATURE & LAW REVIEW. see *MEDICAL SCIENCES—Abstracting, Bibliographies, Statistics*

AIDS LITIGATION REPORTER; the national journal of record of AIDS-related litigation. (Acquired Immune Deficiency Syndrome) see *LAW*

616.97 615.5 GBR
AIDS ORGANISATIONS WORLDWIDE. Text in English, French, Portuguese, Spanish. 1995. a. GBP 19.95 in United Kingdom; GBP 24.95 in Europe; GBP 29.95 elsewhere (effective 2001). **Document type:** *Directory.* **Description:** Information on HIV and AIDS organizations throughout the world.
Formerly (until 1997): International Update (1357-2873)
Published by: N A M Publications, 16a Clapham Common, South Side, London SW4 7AB, United Kingdom. TEL 44-20-7627-3200, FAX 44-20-7627-3101, info@nam.org.uk. Ed. Sylvie Beaumont.

362.1969792 USA ISSN 1087-2914
RC607.A26 CODEN: APCSF6
AIDS PATIENT CARE AND S T DS. Text in English. 1987. m. USD 129 domestic to individuals; USD 257 foreign to individuals; USD 155 domestic to individuals print and online eds. combined; USD 283 foreign to individuals print and online eds. combined; USD 262 domestic to institutions; USD 352 foreign to institutions; USD 314 domestic to institutions print and online eds. combined; USD 405 foreign to institutions print and online eds. combined (effective 2002). adv. illus. back issues avail.; reprints avail. *Refereed.* **Document type:** *Journal, Academic/Scholarly.* **Description:** Covers the spectrum of adult and pediatric HIV disease diagnosis, treatment prevention, and education.
Formerly (until 1996): AIDS Patient Care (0893-5068)
Related titles: Online - full text ed.: USD 129 worldwide to individuals; USD 262 worldwide to institutions (effective 2002) (from CatchWord Ltd., Ovid Technologies, Inc., EBSCO Publishing, O C L C Online Computer Library Center, Inc., RoweCom Information Quest, Gale Group, Swets Blackwell, Factiva, Institute for Scientific Information).
Indexed: AIDS & Cancer Res., AIDS Abstr., AMED, ASCA, CINAHL, Curr.Cont., Environ.Sci.Poll.Mgmt., Excerp.Med., Fam.Ind., Hlth.Ind., Int.Nurs.Ind., Microbiol.Abstr., Pollut.Abstr., Rev.Med.& Vet.Mycol., Risk Abstr., SSCI, Saf.Sci.Abstr., Telegen, Virol.Abstr.
—BLDSC (0773.083873), CatchWord, EMDOCS, GNLM, IDS, ingenta, KNAW.
Published by: Mary Ann Liebert, Inc. Publishers, 2 Madison Ave, Larchmont, NY 10538. TEL 914—834-3100, FAX 914-834-1388, info@liebertpub.com, http://www.liebertpub.com/apc. Ed. Jeffrey Laurence. Adv. contact Harriet Matysko.

AIDS POLICY AND LAW. (Acquired Immune Deficiency Syndrome) see *LAW*

M

616.9 USA
AIDS PREVENTION AND MENTAL HEALTH. Text in English. 1993. irreg., latest 2000. price varies. *Refereed.* **Document type:** *Monographic series.* **Description:** Presents current research and clinical applications dealing with the preventive, social and psychological aspects of HIV and AIDS.
Indexed: e-psyche.
Published by: Kluwer Academic - Plenum Publishers (Subsidiary of: Wolters Kluwer N.V.), 233 Spring St, New York, NY 10013-1578. TEL 212-620-8000, 800-221-9369, FAX 212-463-0742, info@plenum.com, http://www.plenum.com.

616.9 USA ISSN 1053-0894
RC607.A26
THE AIDS READER. Text in English. 1991. m. USD 60 domestic to individuals; USD 40 residents and students; USD 120 to libraries double subscr. only; USD 105 per issue foreign; USD 10 newsstand/cover domestic; USD 15 newsstand/cover foreign (effective 2001). back issues avail. *Refereed.* **Document type:** *Journal, Trade.* **Description:** Provides clinicians with practical, scientifically sound information on the prevention, diagnosis and treatment of HIV disease. Helps clinicians improve the quality of life and treatment options for their patients, by helping to bridge the gap between the specialist and the primary care physician.
Related titles: Online - full text ed.
—BLDSC (0773.083990), Infotrieve. **CCC.**
Published by: Cliggott Publishing Co. (Subsidiary of: S C P Communications, Inc.), 330 Boston Post Rd, Darien, CT 06820. TEL 203-662-6400, FAX 203-662-6776, editor@scp.com, info.cliggott@scp.com, http://hiv.medscape.com/SCP/TAR/public/journal.TAR.html, http://www.scp.com/. Ed. John Hawes. Pub. Alan Imhoff. Circ: 27,000 (controlled).

616.9792 362.196 USA
AIDS REFERENCE GUIDE. Text in English. 1988. m. (in 2 vols. plus 12 updates & 12 newsletters). USD 448 (effective 2001). **Description:** Information source tracking the cost, financing and impact of AIDS by monitoring the experiences and findings of hundreds of AIDS programs and projects.
Published by: Atlantic Information Services, Inc., 1100 17th St, N W, Ste 300, Washington, DC 20036. TEL 202-775-9008, 800-521-4323, FAX 202-331-9542, http://www.aishealth.com. Ed. Frances Fernald. Pub. Richard Biehl.

616.97 615.5 GBR
AIDS REFERENCE MANUAL. Text in English. 1987. a. GBP 46.95 in United Kingdom; GBP 51.95 in Europe; GBP 56.95 elsewhere (effective 2001). **Document type:** *Bulletin.* **Description:** Contains comprehensive information on all nonmedical aspects of HIV and AIDS.
Published by: N A M Publications, 16a Clapham Common, South Side, London SW4 7AB, United Kingdom. TEL 44-20-7627-3200, FAX 44-20-7627-3101, info@nam.org.uk. Ed. Keith Alcorn.

616.979 USA ISSN 0889-2229
RC607.A26 CODEN: ARHRE7
AIDS RESEARCH AND HUMAN RETROVIRUSES. Text in English. 1983. 18/yr., latest vol.18, 2002. USD 668 domestic to individuals; USD 798 foreign to individuals; USD 802 domestic to individuals print and online eds. combined; USD 932 foreign to individuals print and online eds. combined; USD 1,342 domestic to institutions; USD 1,534 foreign to institutions; USD 1,610 domestic to institutions print and online eds. combined; USD 1,803 foreign to institutions print and online eds. combined (effective 2002). adv. back issues avail.; reprints avail. *Refereed.* **Document type:** *Journal, Academic/Scholarly.* **Description:** Provides studies of new viruses pertaining to cancer, degenerative diseases, and the immune system.
Formerly (until 1987): AIDS Research (0737-6006)
Related titles: Online - full text ed.: USD 668 worldwide to individuals; USD 1,342 worldwide to institutions (effective 2002) (from CatchWord Ltd., EBSCO Publishing, O C L C Online Computer Library Center, Inc., RoweCom Information Quest, Swets Blackwell, Institute for Scientific Information).
Indexed: AIDS & Cancer Res., AIDS Abstr., ASCA, Chem.Abstr., Chem.Indus.Notes, Chem.Titles, Curr.Adv.Ecol.Sci., Curr.Cont., Dairy Sci.Abstr., Environ.Sci.Poll.Mgmt., Excerp.Med., IBR, IBZ, INIS Atomind., Immun.Abstr., Ind.Med. (1987-), Ind.Vet., Inpharma, Int.Abstr.Biol.Sci., Med.& Surg.Dermat., Pharm.&Out.News, Pollut.Abstr., Protozool.Abstr., Reac., Rev.Med.& Vet.Mycol., Risk Abstr., SSCI (coverage dropped), Saf.Sci.Abstr., Sci.Cit.Ind., Telegen, Vet.Bull., Virol.Abstr.
—BLDSC (0773.089000), ADONIS, CASDDS, CatchWord, CISTI, EMDOCS, GNLM, IDS, ingenta, KNAW. **CCC.**
Published by: Mary Ann Liebert, Inc. Publishers, 2 Madison Ave, Larchmont, NY 10538. TEL 914—834-3100, FAX 914-834-1388, info@liebertpub.com, http://www.liebertpub.com/aid. Ed. Eric Hunter.

616.9792 USA
AIDS SOURCEBOOK. Text in English. 1995. irreg., latest vol.2, 1999. USD 78 per vol. (effective 2001). charts, illus, stat. Index. **Document type:** *Consumer.* **Description:** Offers laypersons basic information on AIDS and HIV infection, along with advice on treatment options and clinical trials, coping with the disease, and developments in treating AIDS symptoms.
Published by: Omnigraphics, Inc., 615 Griswold St, Detroit, MI 48226. TEL 313-961-1340, 800-234-1340, FAX 313-961-1383, 800-875-1340, info@omnigraphics.com, http://www.omnigraphics.com. Ed. Karen Bellenir. Pub. Frederick G Ruffner Jr.

616.7 USA
AIDS THERAPIES. Text in English. 1987. 11 base vols. plus m. updates. USD 1,549 in North America; USD 1,649 elsewhere. index. **Document type:** *Newsletter.* **Description:** Incorporates in an 800-page notebook service the latest information available on treatment protocols, experimental drugs, clinical trials and advances on the horizon. Includes a guide to opportunistic infections of AIDS.
Related titles: Online - full text ed.
Published by: Charles W. Henderson, Ed. & Pub., PO Box 5528, Atlanta, GA 31107-0528. TEL 770-507-7777, FAX 770-507-7788, cwhender@newsfile.com; info@hendersonnet.atl.ga.us, http://www.newsfile.com.

616.9792 USA
AIDS TREATMENT DATA NETWORK INFORMATION BULLETIN. Text in English. 6/yr.
Media: Online - full text.
Published by: Mediapolis, 307 Seventh Ave 11th Fl, New York, NY 10001. TEL 212-377-3333, FAX 212-377-3334, info@mediapolis.com, http://aidsinfonyc.org/network/trs/trs.html.

616.97 615.5 GBR ISSN 0969-4706
AIDS TREATMENT UPDATE. Text in English. 1992. m. GBP 69 in United Kingdom; GBP 74 in Europe; GBP 79 elsewhere (effective 2001). **Document type:** *Newsletter.* **Description:** Covers all new trials, treatments conferences, newly published research and changes in drugs licensing, as well as offering regular expert opinions.
—BLDSC (0773.096150).
Published by: N A M Publications, 16a Clapham Common, South Side, London SW4 7AB, United Kingdom. TEL 44-20-7627-3200, FAX 44-20-7627-3101, info@nam.org.uk, http://www.aidsmap.com. Ed. Anna Poppa.

616.97 570 330 USA
AIDS WEEKLY PLUS. Text in English. 1985. w. (43/yr.). USD 1,895 in North America; USD 2,095 out of North America (effective 1999). adv. bk.rev. index. back issues avail. **Document type:** *Newsletter.* **Description:** Covers all aspects of AIDS, including research, treatments, psychosocial and prevention issues and politics.
Former titles (until Nov. 1995): AIDS Weekly (1069-1456); (until 1991): C D C - AIDS Weekly (0884-903X); Which incorporated (in 1988): Brown University S T D Update
Related titles: Microform ed.: (from PQC); Online - full text ed.: (from Data-Star, Gale Group, The Dialog Corporation, NewsNet).
Indexed: Bus.& Indus. (Jan.1995-), CWI, WMB.
—BLDSC (0773.096900), Infotrieve. **CCC.**
Published by: Charles W. Henderson, Ed. & Pub., PO Box 830409, Birmingham, AL 35283-0409. TEL 205-995-1567, 800-633-4931, FAX 205-995-1588, TELEX 3762848, 72571.2363@compuserve.com; info@hendersonnet.atl.ga.us, http://www.newsfile.com.

AIDS (YEAR); a year in review. see *MEDICAL SCIENCES—Abstracting, Bibliographies, Statistics*

AIDSIDA INFO. see *HOMOSEXUALITY*

ALPE ADRIA MICROBIOLOGY JOURNAL. see *BIOLOGY—Microbiology*

614.4 USA ISSN 0196-6553
RA969
AMERICAN JOURNAL OF INFECTION CONTROL. Abbreviated title: A J I C. Text in English. 1973. bi-m. USD 76 domestic to individuals; USD 95 foreign to individuals; USD 202 domestic to institutions; USD 221 foreign to institutions; USD 41 domestic to students; USD 60 foreign to students; USD 37 newsstand/cover domestic (effective 2001). adv. bk.rev., film rev. abstr, bibl, charts, illus, stat. index. back issues avail.; reprint service avail. from PQC. *Refereed.* **Document type:** *Journal, Academic/Scholarly.* **Description:** Serves infection-control practitioners and hospital epidemiologists concerned with the control of infection associated with hospitals and extended-care facilities.
Former titles: A P I C Bulletin; A P I C Journal (0161-6005); A P I C Newsletter
Related titles: CD-ROM ed.: (from Ovid Technologies, Inc.); Microfilm ed.: (from PQC); Online - full text ed.: (from Ovid Technologies, Inc., EBSCO Publishing, IDEAL Online Library, Institute for Scientific Information, RoweCom Information Quest).
Indexed: ASCA, Biol.Abstr., CINAHL, Curr.Adv.Ecol.Sci., Curr.Cont., Dok.Arbeitsmed., Excerp.Med., Helminthol.Abstr., INIS Atomind., Ind.Med. (1980-), Inpharma, Int.Abstr.Biol.Sci., Int.Nurs.Ind., Nurs.Abstr., Pharm.&Out.News, Reac., Ref.Zh., Rev.Med.& Vet.Mycol., Sci.Cit.Ind. (coverage dropped), Trop.Dis.Bull.
—BLDSC (0826.761000), ADONIS, CISTI, EMDOCS, GNLM, IDS, ingenta, KNAW. **CCC.**
Published by: (Association for Professionals in Infection Control and Epidemiology, Inc.), Mosby, Inc. (Subsidiary of: Elsevier Science), 11830 Westline Industrial Dr, St Louis, MO 63146-3318. TEL 314-872-8370, 800-325-4177, FAX 314-432-1380-3318, http://www.mosby.com/ajic, http://www.mosby.com/periodicals. Ed. Elaine Larson. Pub. Todd Hummel. Adv. contact Gale Schlogl TEL 314-453-4337. B&W page USD 1,690, color page USD 3,055; trim 10.88 x 8.13. Circ: 14,778 (paid and free).

616.988 USA ISSN 0002-9637
RC960 CODEN: AJTHAB
AMERICAN JOURNAL OF TROPICAL MEDICINE AND HYGIENE. Text in English. 1921. m. USD 400 in the Americas; USD 450 elsewhere (effective 2001). adv. bk.rev. bibl, charts, illus. back issues avail. *Refereed.* **Document type:** *Trade.* **Description:** Serves as a communication bridge between the application of new laboratory science technologies and the control of human disease in the developing tropics.
Supersedes in part (in 1951): American Journal of Tropical Medicine (0096-6746)
Related titles: CD-ROM ed.; Online - full text ed.: (from Institute for Scientific Information).
Indexed: AIM, ASCA, Abstr.Anthropol., Abstr.Hyg., AgBiotech, Agri.& Environ.Biotech.Abstr. (coverage dropped), Anim.Breed.Abstr., Aqua.Sci.& Fish.Abstr., Bio-Contr.News & Info., Biol.Abstr., Chem.Abstr., Chem.Indus.Notes, Chem.Titles, Chic.Per.Ind., Curr.Adv.Ecol.Sci., Curr.Adv.Gen.& Molec.Biol., Curr.Cont., Dairy Sci.Abstr., Dent.Ind., Derwent Biotech.Abstr., Diar.Dis.Res., Entomol.Abstr., Environ.Sci.Poll.Mgmt., Excerp.Med., Helminthol.Abstr., INIS Atomind., I.P.A., Ind.Med. (1952-), Ind.Sci.Rev., Ind.Vet., Inpharma, Jrnl.Watch Inf.Dis., Med.& Surg.Dermat., Microbiol.Abstr., Neurosci.Cit.Ind., Nutr.Abstr., Pharm.&Out.News, Pig News & Info., Pollut.Abstr., Poult.Abstr., Protozool.Abstr., Reac., Rev.Appl.Entomol., Rev.Arom.& Med.Plants, Rev.Med.& Vet.Mycol., Risk Abstr., Rural Devel.Abstr., SSCI (coverage dropped), Saf.Sci.Abstr., Sci.Cit.Ind., Small Anim.Abstr., So.Pac.Per.Ind., Sport Fish.Abstr., Trop.Dis.Bull., Vet.Bull., Virol.Abstr., Wild.Rev., Zoo.Rec.
—BLDSC (0839.000000), CASDDS, CISTI, EMDOCS, GNLM, IDS, ingenta, KNAW, Linda Hall. **CCC.**
Published by: American Society of Tropical Medicine and Hygiene, PO Box 1897, Lawrence, KS 66044-8897. TEL 404-636-3621, http://www.astmh.org, tmed@allenpress.com, tmed@allenpress.com. Ed. Dr. James W Kazura. Adv. contact Susan K Johnson. Circ: 4,400 (paid). **Subscr.to:** Allen Press Inc.. FAX 784-843-1274.

614.8 USA
AMERICAN LEPROSY MISSIONS ANNUAL REPORT. Text in English. a. **Document type:** *Corporate.*
Published by: American Leprosy Missions International, 1 ALM Way, Greenville, SC 29601. TEL 803-271-7040, FAX 803-271-7062, http://www.leprosy.org.

616.998 GBR ISSN 0003-4983
RC960 CODEN: ATMPA2
ANNALS OF TROPICAL MEDICINE AND PARASITOLOGY. Text in English. 1907. 8/yr. GBP 192, USD 342 to individuals; GBP 389, USD 641 to institutions (effective 2001). adv. bibl, illus. index. back issues avail.; reprint service avail. from SWZ. *Refereed.* **Document type:** *Academic/Scholarly.* **Description:** Deals with tropical diseases and medical and veterinary parasitology in their broadest aspects.
Related titles: E-mail ed.; Microform ed.: (from PQC,PMC); Online - full text ed.: ISSN 1364-8594. 199? (from CatchWord Ltd., EBSCO Publishing, O C L C Online Computer Library Center, Inc., RoweCom Information Quest, Swets Blackwell, Institute for Scientific Information).
Indexed: AMED, ASCA, Abstr.Hyg., Agri.& Environ.Biotech.Abstr. (coverage dropped), Aqua.Sci.& Fish.Abstr., Bio-Contr.News & Info., Biol.Abstr., Chem.Abstr., Chem.Indus.Notes, Chem.Titles, Curr.Adv.Ecol.Sci., Curr.Cont., Dent.Ind., Derwent Biotech.Abstr., Diar.Dis.Res., Entomol.Abstr., Environ.Sci.Poll.Mgmt., Excerp.Med., Helminthol.Abstr., INIS Atomind., Ind.Med. (1907-), Ind.Sci.Rev., Ind.Vet., Inpharma, Int.Abstr.Biol.Sci., Microbiol.Abstr., Nutr.Abstr., Pharm.&Out.News, Pig News & Info., Protozool.Abstr., Reac., Ref.Zh., Rev.Appl.Entomol., Rev.Arom.& Med.Plants, Rev.Med.& Vet.Mycol., Rev.Plant Path., SSCI (coverage dropped), Sci.Cit.Ind., Soils & Fert., Sport Fish.Abstr., Trop.Dis.Bull., Vet.Bull., Wild.Rev., Zoo.Rec.
—BLDSC (1045.000000), ADONIS, CASDDS, CatchWord, CISTI, EMDOCS, GNLM, IDS, ingenta, KNAW, Linda Hall. **CCC.**
Published by: (Liverpool School of Tropical Medicine), Carfax Publishing Limited (Subsidiary of: Taylor & Francis Group), PO Box 25, Abingdon, Oxon OX14 3UE, United Kingdom. TEL 44-1235-401000, FAX 44-1235-401550, enquiries@carfax.co.uk, enquiry@tandf.co.uk, http://www.carfax.co.uk/atm-ad.htm.

ANTIBIOTICS CHEMOTHERAPY; newsletter of the international society of chemotherapy. see *MEDICAL SCIENCES*

616.9 USA ISSN 1069-417X
RM265.A68 CODEN: AIDIEX
ANTIMICROBICS AND INFECTIOUS DISEASES NEWSLETTER. Text in English. 1984. m. EUR 189 in Europe to individuals; JPY 26,200 in Japan to individuals; USD 211 elsewhere to individuals; EUR 324 in Europe to institutions; JPY 44,800 in Japan to institutions; USD 362 elsewhere to institutions (effective 2002). *Refereed.* **Document type:** *Newsletter.* **Description:** Provides information for professionals and researchers in clinical microbiology, infectious diseases, clinical pharmacology, and clinical pharmacy.
Formed by the 1993 merger of: Antimicrobic Newsletter (0738-1751); I D N - Infectious Diseases Newsletter (0278-2316)
Related titles: Microform ed.: (from PQC); Online - full text ed.: (from ingenta, ScienceDirect).
Indexed: Abstr.Hyg., Biol.Abstr., Diar.Dis.Res., Excerp.Med., Rev.Med.& Vet.Mycol.
—BLDSC (1549.252000), CASDDS, CISTI, GNLM, Infotrieve. **CCC.**
Published by: Elsevier Science, 655 Ave of the Americas, New York, NY 10010. TEL 212-989-5800, FAX 212-633-3990, http://www.elsevier.com/locate/antimicrobnews. Ed. Dr. Charles W Stratton. **Subscr. in Australasia and the Far East to:** Elsevier Science (Singapore) Pte Ltd, No.1 Temasek Ave, 17-01 Millenia Tower, Singapore 039192, Singapore. TEL 65-434-3727, FAX 65-337-2230; **Subscr. in Japan to:** Elsevier Science Inc - Japan Regional Office, 9-15 Higashi-Azabu 1-chome, Minato-ku, Tokyo 106-0044, Japan. TEL 81-3-5561-5033; **Subscr. outside the Americas to:** Elsevier Science BV, PO Box 211, Amsterdam 1000 AE, Netherlands. TEL 31-20-485-3757, nlinfo-f@elsevier.nl.

ANTIVIRAL AGENTS BULLETIN; antiviral drug and vaccine development information. see *PHARMACY AND PHARMACOLOGY*

ANTIVIRAL CHEMISTRY AND CHEMOTHERAPY. see *BIOLOGY—Biochemistry*

ANTIVIRAL RESEARCH; a multidisciplinary journal of antiviral agents, natural host defence mechanisms, interferons and antiviral vaccines. see *BIOLOGY—Microbiology*

616.9 572 579 GBR ISSN 1359-6535
CODEN: ANTHFA
ANTIVIRAL THERAPY. Text in English. 1996. q. USD 109, GBP 72 to individuals; USD 419, GBP 272 to institutions (effective 2001). adv. back issues avail. *Refereed.* **Document type:** *Academic/Scholarly.* **Description:** Covers clinical development and use of antiviral agents, and the treatment of all virus diseases.
Related titles: Online - full text ed.: (from Institute for Scientific Information).
Indexed: Abstr.Hyg., Chem.Abstr., Chem.Indus.Notes, Chem.Titles, Curr.Cont., Ind.Med. (1996-), Inpharma, Pharm.&Out.News, Reac., Rev.Appl.Entomol.
—BLDSC (1552.832000), CASDDS, CISTI, GNLM.
Published by: International Medical Press, 125 High Holborn, London WC1V 6QA, United Kingdom. TEL 44-20-7398-0700, FAX 44-20-7398-0701, imp@intmedpress.com, http://www.intmedpress.com. Eds. Douglas Richman, Joep Lange. Pub. Stephen Cameron. Adv. contact Simon Gee.

616.9 USA ISSN 1071-0906
CODEN: AARSE9
ARCHIVES OF S T D - HIV RESEARCH; an international journal. Text in English. 1987. 4/yr. USD 180 to individuals; USD 190 foreign to individuals; USD 200 to institutions; USD 210 foreign to institutions. *Refereed.* **Document type:** *Academic/Scholarly.*
Formerly (until 1992): Archives of AIDS Research (0899-4811)
Indexed: Excerp.Med.
—CASDDS, CISTI, EMDOCS, GNLM.
Published by: Reproductive Health Center, 78 Surfsong Rd., Kiawah Island, SC 29455. TEL 803-768-5556, FAX 803-768-6494.

ARCHIVES OF VIROLOGY. SUPPLEMENTUM. see *BIOLOGY—Microbiology*

610.73 USA ISSN 1055-3290
ASSOCIATION OF NURSES IN AIDS CARE. JOURNAL. Key Title: Journal of the Association of Nurses in AIDS Care. Short title: J A N A C. Text in English. 1990. bi-m. USD 240 domestic; USD 264 foreign (effective 2002). adv. bk.rev. 48 p./no. back issues avail.; reprints avail. *Refereed.* **Document type:** *Journal, Academic/Scholarly.* **Description:** Articles focus on clinical practice, health services, education, research, and social issues related to the care of persons with HIV infection or AIDS.
Related titles: Microform ed.: (from PQC); Online - full text ed.: (from ProQuest Information & Learning, Gale Group, ingenta).
Indexed: AIDS & Cancer Res., AMED, CINAHL, Environ.Sci.Poll.Mgmt., IBZ, Ind.Med. (1989-), Int.Nurs.Ind., Pollut.Abstr., Risk Abstr., Saf.Sci.Abstr., Viol.& Abuse Abstr., Virol.Abstr.
—BLDSC (4645.870000), GNLM, ingenta.
Published by: (Association of Nurses in AIDS Care), Sage Publications, Inc., Sage Science Press, 2455 Teller Rd, Thousand Oaks, CA 91320. TEL 805-499-0721, FAX 805-499-0871, info@sagepub.com, sagescience@sagepub.com, http://www.sagepub.com/ssp, http://www.sagesciencepress.com. Ed. Richard L Sowell. Pub. Susan Hanscom. R&P Peter Marino. Adv. contact Kevin Dunn TEL 201-767-4170. B&W page USD 1,040, color page USD 2,440; trim 10.75 x 8.25. Circ: 2,698. **Subscr. to:** Sage Publications Ltd.

AUSTRALIAN AND NEW ZEALAND JOURNAL OF PUBLIC HEALTH. see *PUBLIC HEALTH AND SAFETY*

AUTOIMMUNITY. see *MEDICAL SCIENCES—Allergology And Immunology*

616.85 USA ISSN 1058-708X
B E T A. (Bulletin of Experimental Treatment for AIDS) Text in English. 1989. q. **Document type:** *Bulletin.* **Description:** Contains information for HIV-positive individuals and their care-givers on the latest advancements in the treatment of HIV and AIDS-related illnesses.
Related titles: Spanish ed.: Boletin de Tratamientos Experimentales Contra el SIDA.
—BLDSC (1942.554100).
Published by: San Francisco AIDS Foundation, PO Box 426182, San Francisco, CA 94142-6182. TEL 415-487-8060, 800-833-0159, FAX 415-487-8069, beta@sfaf.org, http://www.sfaf.org/beta.html. Eds. Leslie Hanna, Liz Highleyman.

BACTERIOLOGIA, VIRUSOLOGIA, PARAZITOLOGIA, EPIDEMIOLOGIA. see *BIOLOGY—Microbiology*

616.9 GBR ISSN 1071-6564
RC109 CODEN: BCIDFD
BAILLIERE'S CLINICAL INFECTIOUS DISEASES. Text in English. 1994. 3/yr. GBP 61 to individuals; GBP 82 to institutions. *Refereed.* **Document type:** *Academic/Scholarly.*
Indexed: ASCA, Curr.Cont. (coverage dropped), Excerp.Med. (1995-), Ind.Sci.Rev., Inpharma, Int.Abstr.Biol.Sci., Pharm.&Out.News, Protozool.Abstr., Reac., Rev.Med.& Vet.Mycol., Sci.Cit.Ind. (coverage dropped).
—BLDSC (1856.724200), GNLM, IDS, Infotrieve, KNAW. **CCC.**
Published by: Bailliere Tindall (Subsidiary of: Harcourt Publishers Ltd.), 24-28 Oval Rd, London NW1 7DX, United Kingdom. TEL 44-20-7485-4752, FAX 44—20-7267-4466, http://www.hbuk.co.uk. **Subscr. in N. America to:** W.B. Saunders Co., Journal Subscription Fulfillment, 6277 Sea Harbor Dr, 4th Fl, Orlando, FL 32887-4800. TEL 800-874-6418; **Subscr. to:** Journals Subscription Fulfillment, Foots Cray High St, Sidcup, Kent DA14 5HP, United Kingdom. TEL 44-20-8300-3322, FAX 44-20-8309-0807.

616.9 USA
BEING ALIVE NEWSLETTER*. Text in English, Spanish. m. USD 24 (effective 2000). back issues avail. **Document type:** *Newsletter.* **Description:** Contains articles with information about AIDS and HIV in medical issues, drug trials and developments, etc.
Related titles: Online - full text ed.
Published by: Being Alive, People with HIV - AIDS Action Coalition, 621 N San Vicente Blvd, West Hollywood, CA 90069-5018. TEL 213-667-3262, FAX 213-667-2735, http://www.beingalive.org/newsletter.html. Ed. Jim Stoecker. Circ: 11,000.

BLOOD WEEKLY. see *MEDICAL SCIENCES—Hematology*

616.97 USA ISSN 1048-4396
RC607.A26
BODY POSITIVE. Text in English. 1987. m. USD 35 donation (effective 2000). adv. back issues avail. **Document type:** *Newsletter.* **Description:** Focuses on issues of interest to HIV-positive and HIV-affected people across the country, with features dealing with all aspects of HIV/AIDS, including medical, legal, social services, and financial issues aimed at people with HIV, their friends, families, caregivers, and service providers.
Related titles: Online - full text ed.; Spanish ed.: Cuerpo Positivo.
Published by: Body Positive, Inc, 19 Fulton St, Ste 308B, New York, NY 10038. TEL 212-566-7333, FAX 212-566-4539, bodypos@aol.com, http://www.thebody.com/bp/bp.html. Ed., R&P Laura Engle. adv.: page USD 2,255; 7 x 9. Circ: 16,000 (controlled). **Dist. by:** Contemporary Guidance.

BOTSWANA. MINISTRY OF HEALTH. EPIDEMIOLOGICAL BULLETIN. see *PUBLIC HEALTH AND SAFETY*

616.9 GBR
▼ **THE BRITISH JOURNAL OF INFECTION CONTROL.** Text in English. 1999. q. GBP 25 to individuals; GBP 40 to institutions; GBP 25 foreign (effective 2001). *Refereed.*
Indexed: Brit.Nur.Ind.
—BLDSC (2311.035000).
Published by: Infection Control Nurses Association, Fitwise, Drumcross Hall, Bathgate, West Lothian EH48 4BR, United Kingdom. Ed. Sue Millward.

616.9 GBR ISSN 1356-0832
BULLETIN OF TROPICAL MEDICINE AND INTERNATIONAL HEALTH. Text in English. 3/yr. membership. adv. **Document type:** *Newsletter.*
Formerly (until 1994): Royal Society of Tropical Medicine and Hygiene. Newsletter
Indexed: Ind.Vet., Protozool.Abstr., Rev.Med.& Vet.Mycol.
Published by: Royal Society of Tropical Medicine and Hygiene, Manson House, 26 Portland Pl, London W1N 4EY, United Kingdom. TEL 44-20-7580-2127, FAX 44-20-7436-1389, trans@rstmh.org, http://www.rstmh.org. Eds. D A Evans, G Webbe. adv.: B&W page GBP 500, color page GBP 1,000. Circ: 2,500 (controlled).

C A SELECTS. AIDS AND RELATED IMMUNODEFICIENCIES. see *MEDICAL SCIENCES—Abstracting, Bibliographies, Statistics*

C D C HIV-AIDS SURVEILLANCE REPORTS. see *MEDICAL SCIENCES—Abstracting, Bibliographies, Statistics*

M

614.4241 616.905 GBR
C D R SUPPLEMENT. (Communicable Disease Report) Text in English. 1983. irreg. **Document type:** *Bulletin.*
Related titles: ♦ Supplement to: C D R Weekly. ISSN 1350-9357.
Indexed: Abstr.Hyg., Ind.Med. (1993-, dropped).
Published by: Public Health Laboratory Service, 61 Colindale Ave, London NW9 5HT, United Kingdom. TEL 44-20-8200-6868, FAX 44-20-8200-7868, http://www.phls.co.uk, http://www.phls.co.uk/cdsc.

614.4241 616.9 GBR ISSN 1350-9357
C D R WEEKLY. (Communicable Disease Report) Text in English. 1967. w. GBP 159 domestic; GBP 193 foreign (effective 2000). **Document type:** *Bulletin, Trade.*
Supersedes in part (in 1991): Communicable Disease Report. Weekly Edition (0144-3186)
Related titles: ♦ Supplement: C D R Supplement.
Indexed: Abstr.Hyg., Food Sci.& Tech.Abstr., Ind.Med. (1992-), Protozool.Abstr., Rev.Appl.Entomol., Rural Recreat.Tour.Abstr., Trop.Dis.Bull.
—BLDSC (3096.526850), GNLM, KNAW.
Published by: Public Health Laboratory Service, 61 Colindale Ave, London NW9 5HT, United Kingdom. TEL 44-20-8200-6868, FAX 44-20-8200-7868, http://www.phls.co.uk/cdsc. Ed. Dr. Stuart Handysides. Circ: 4,000.

616.9 USA
CALIFORNIA MORBIDITY; bi-weekly report from the Division of Communicable Disease Control. Text in English. 1968. m. index.
Published by: Department of Health Services, Division of Communicable Disease Control (D C D C), 2151 Berkeley Way, Berkeley, CA 94704-1011. TEL 510-540-2566. Circ: 4,000.

CANADIAN HIV - AIDS POLICY & LAW REVIEW. see *LAW*

616.9792 USA
CLINICAL CARE OPTIONS FOR HIV ONLINE JOURNAL. Text in English. irreg. free per issue. back issues avail. **Description:** Provides information to advancing medical knowledge for practical use by clinicians, patients, and the broader health care industry. Features articles on HIV issues.
Media: Online - full text.
Address: http://www.healthcg.com/hiv/journal. Ed. Stephen Becker.

616.9 USA ISSN 1058-4838
RC110 CODEN: CIDIEL
CLINICAL INFECTIOUS DISEASES. Text in English. 1979. 2/m. (in 2 vols., 12 nos./vol.), latest vol.32, 2001, Jan. 1. USD 119 in United States to individuals; USD 166.33 in Canada to individuals; USD 158 elsewhere to individuals; USD 420 in United States to institutions; USD 488.40 in Canada to institutions; USD 459 elsewhere to institutions; USD 8.95 to individuals; USD 21.50 to institutions (effective 2002). adv. bk.rev. reprint service avail. from PQC,ISI. *Refereed.* **Document type:** *Academic/Scholarly.* **Description:** Features state-of-the-art clinical articles on the diagnosis and treatment of infectious diseases, plus review articles and sections covering medical, legal, and managed care topics.
Formerly (until 1991): Reviews of Infectious Diseases (0162-0886)
Related titles: Microform ed.: (from PQC,PMC); Online - full text ed.: (from EBSCO Publishing, Institute for Scientific Information).
Indexed: AIDS & Cancer Res., AIDS Abstr., ASCA, Abstr.Hyg., Biol.Dig., Chem.Abstr., Chem.Indus.Notes, Chem.Titles, Curr.Cont., Dairy Sci.Abstr., Dent.Ind., Derwent Biotech.Abstr., Diar.Dis.Res., Dok.Arbeitsmed., Environ.Sci.Poll.Mgmt., Excerp.Med., Helminthol.Abstr., INIS Atomind., Immun.Abstr. (coverage dropped), Ind.Med. (1992-), Ind.Sci.Rev., Ind.Vet., Inpharma, Int.Abstr.Biol.Sci., Jrnl.Watch Derm., Jrnl.Watch Emer.Med., Jrnl.Watch Inf.Dis., Kidney, Med.& Surg.Dermat., Microbiol.Abstr., Neurosci.Cit.Ind., Nutr.Abstr., Pharm.&Out.News, Pig News & Info., Pollut.Abstr., Poult.Abstr., Protozool.Abstr., Reac., Ref.Zh., Rev.Appl.Entomol., Rev.Med.& Vet.Mycol., Risk Abstr., SSCI (coverage dropped), Saf.Sci.Abstr., Sci.Cit.Ind., Soyabean Abstr., Sport Fish.Abstr., Tox.Abstr., Trop.Dis.Bull., Vet.Bull., Virol.Abstr., Wild.Rev.
—BLDSC (3286.293860), ADONIS, CASDDS, CISTI, EMDOCS, GNLM, IDS, ingenta, KNAW. **CCC.**
Published by: (Infectious Diseases Society of America), University of Chicago Press, Journals Division, PO Box 37005, Chicago, IL 60637. TEL 773-753-3347, FAX 773-753-0811, subscriptions@journals.uchicago.edu, subscriptions@press.uchicago.edu, http://www.journals.uchicago.edu/CID/. Ed. Sydney M Finegold. Adv. contact Timothy Hill. B&W page USD 505; trim 10.88 x 8.25. Circ: 8,700.

616.9792 USA
COMMON SENSE ABOUT AIDS. Text in English. 1992. a. USD 323; USD 353 foreign (effective 1998). **Document type:** *Trade.*
Published by: American Health Consultants (Subsidiary of: Medical Economics Co., Inc.), 3525 Piedmont Rd, N E, 6 Piedmont Center, Ste 400, Atlanta, GA 30305. TEL 404-262-5476, custserv@ahcpub.com, http://www.ahcpub.com.

COMMUNICABLE DISEASE AND PUBLIC HEALTH. see *BIOLOGY—Microbiology*

610 CHE
COMMUNICABLE DISEASES INFORMATION RESOURCES. Text in English. s-a. back issues avail. **Document type:** *Catalog.*
Related titles: Online - full content ed.
Published by: World Health Organization, Marketing and Dissemination, Geneva, 27 1211, Switzerland. TEL 41-22-791-2476, FAX 41-22-791-4875, http://www.who.int/infectious-disease-news.

614.49 AUS ISSN 0725-3141
COMMUNICABLE DISEASES INTELLIGENCE. Text in English. 1976. 13/yr. free per issue. stat. index. back issues avail. **Document type:** *Bulletin, Government.* **Description:** Communicable disease epidemiology, surveillance and alert for health professionals.
Related titles: Online - full text ed.
Indexed: Abstr.Hyg., Ind.Med. (198?-), Ind.Vet., Protozool.Abstr., Rev.Appl.Entomol., Rev.Med.& Vet.Mycol., Trop.Dis.Bull., Vet.Bull.
—BLDSC (3341.347800).
Published by: Department of Health and Family Services, National Center for Disease Control, GPO Box 9848, Canberra, ACT 2601, Australia. TEL 61-2-6289-7240, FAX 61-2-6289-7791, cdi.editor@health.gov.au, http://www.health.gov.au/pubhlth/cdi/cdihtml.htm. Circ: 4,000.

COMPARATIVE IMMUNOLOGY, MICROBIOLOGY AND INFECTIOUS DISEASES; the international journal for medical and veterinary researchers and practitioners. see *BIOLOGY—Microbiology*

COMPLICATIONS IN SURGERY. see *MEDICAL SCIENCES—Surgery*

616.9 USA ISSN 0888-7756
CODEN: CIIDEV
CONTEMPORARY ISSUES IN INFECTIOUS DISEASES✱ . Text in English. 1984. irreg., latest vol.10. **Document type:** *Monographic series.*
—CASDDS, CISTI, ingenta, KNAW.
Published by: Churchill Livingstone (Subsidiary of: Harcourt Health Sciences), 15 E 26th St, Fl 15, New York, NY 10010-1505. TEL 212-206-5040, FAX 212-727-7808, http://www.churchillmed.com.

616.9 USA ISSN 8755-4046
RA643
CONTROL OF COMMUNICABLE DISEASES IN MAN. Text in English. 1950. irreg. **Document type:** *Monographic series, Academic/Scholarly.*
—CISTI, Infotrieve. **CCC.**
Published by: American Public Health Association, 1015 15th St, N W, Washington, DC 20005. TEL 202-789-5600.

616.9792 USA ISSN 1085-7605
CRITICAL PATH AIDS PROJECT✱ . Text in English. 1981. q. USD 50. illus. reprints avail. **Document type:** *Newsletter.* **Description:** Features in-depth reports on experimental AIDS treatments.
Related titles: Online - full text ed.
Address: 1233 Locust St #5, Philadelphia, PA 1907-5400. kiyoshi@critpath.org, http://www.critpath.org. Ed. Kiyoshi Kuromiya.

CURRENT ADVANCES IN IMMUNOLOGY & INFECTIOUS DISEASES. see *MEDICAL SCIENCES—Abstracting, Bibliographies, Statistics*

616.9 615 USA ISSN 1082-8877
CURRENT INFECTIOUS DISEASE DRUGS✱ . Text in English. 1996. irreg. **Document type:** *Monographic series.*
Published by: Churchill Livingstone (Subsidiary of: Harcourt Health Sciences), 15 E 26th St, Fl 15, New York, NY 10010-1505. TEL 212-206-5040, FAX 212-727-7808, http://www.churchillmed.com.

CURRENT MEDICAL LITERATURE. INFECTIOUS DISEASES. see *MEDICAL SCIENCES—Abstracting, Bibliographies, Statistics*

616.9 USA ISSN 0951-7375
RC109 CODEN: COIDE5
CURRENT OPINION IN INFECTIOUS DISEASES. Text in English. 1987. bi-m. USD 249 domestic to individuals for print & online eds.; USD 249 foreign to individuals for print & online eds.; USD 585 per issue domestic to institutions; USD 585 per issue foreign to institutions; USD 91 newsstand/cover (effective 2002). adv. bibl, illus. back issues avail. *Refereed.* **Document type:** *Academic/Scholarly.* **Description:** Directed toward clinicians and researchers in infectious diseases, both general and specialized. Presents review articles followed by annotated bibliographies of references consulted. Includes a bibliography of the current world literature published during the previous year.
Related titles: CD-ROM ed.; Diskette ed.; Online - full text ed.: USD 760.50 domestic academic site license; USD 760.50 foreign academic site license; USD 848.25 domestic corporate site license; USD 848.25 foreign corporate site license (effective 2002) (from Ovid Technologies, Inc., EBSCO Publishing, Swets Blackwell, Institute for Scientific Information).
Indexed: AIDS & Cancer Res., ASCA, Abstr.Hyg., Aqua.Sci.& Fish.Abstr., CINAHL, Curr.Cont., Diar.Dis.Res., Environ.Sci.Poll.Mgmt., Excerp.Med., Helminthol.Abstr., Immun.Abstr. (coverage dropped), Inpharma, Int.Abstr.Biol.Sci., Microbiol.Abstr., Pharm.&Out.News, Pollut.Abstr., Protozool.Abstr., Reac., Rev.Appl.Entomol., Rev.Med.& Vet.Mycol., Risk Abstr., Rural Recreat.Tour.Abstr., Saf.Sci.Abstr., Virol.Abstr. (coverage dropped).
—BLDSC (3500.775500), ADONIS, CASDDS, CISTI, EMDOCS, GNLM, IDS, KNAW.
Published by: Lippincott Williams & Wilkins (Philadelphia) (Subsidiary of: Wolters Kluwer N.V.), 530 Walnut St, Philadelphia, PA 19106-3621. FAX 215-521-8902, 215-521-8902, http://www.Lww.com. Eds. R G Finch, V T Andriole. Pub. Maria McMichael. R&P Tobias Weschler. Adv. contact Kelly Adamitis. B&W page USD 790, color page USD 1,790; trim 11 x 8.5. Circ: 3,441.
Subscr. to: PO Box 1600, Hagerstown, MD 21740-1600.

616.9 USA
CURRENT OPINION IN INFECTIOUS DISEASES. SUPPLEMENT. Text in English. irreg.
—ADONIS.
Published by: Lippincott Williams & Wilkins (Philadelphia) (Subsidiary of: Wolters Kluwer N.V.), 530 Walnut St, Philadelphia, PA 19106-3621. TEL 215-521-8300, FAX 215-521-8902, custserv@lww.com, http://www.lww.com/.

616.015 USA ISSN 0177-4204
CODEN: CTMMEJ
CURRENT TOPICS IN MEDICAL MYCOLOGY. Text in English. 1985. irreg., latest vol.4, 1992. price varies. **Document type:** *Monographic series.* **Description:** Reports on research and developments in pharmaceutical uses of fungi.
Indexed: Chem.Abstr., Chem.Indus.Notes, Chem.Titles, Ind.Med. (until 1999, dropped).
—CASDDS, CISTI, GNLM, Infotrieve. **CCC.**
Published by: Springer-Verlag, Journals (Subsidiary of: BertelsmannSpringer), 175 Fifth Ave, New York, NY 10010. TEL 212-460-1500, FAX 212-473-6272.

616.0194 NLD ISSN 0924-5367
DEVELOPMENTS IN MEDICAL VIROLOGY. Text in English. 1985. irreg. price varies. *Refereed.* **Document type:** *Monographic series.*
—CISTI, KNAW.
Published by: Kluwer Academic Publishers Group (Subsidiary of: Wolters Kluwer N.V.), Spuiboulevard 50, PO Box 17, Dordrecht 3300 AA, Netherlands. FAX 31-78-639-2254, services@wkap.nl, http://www.wkap.nl. **Dist. by:** Journals Department, PO Box 322, Dordrecht 3300 AH, Netherlands. FAX 31-78-654-6474.

DEVELOPMENTS IN MOLECULAR VIROLOGY. see *BIOLOGY—Microbiology*

DIAGNOSTIC MICROBIOLOGY AND INFECTIOUS DISEASE. see *BIOLOGY—Microbiology*

616.9 CHN ISSN 1000-3711
DIFANGBING TONGBAO/ENDEMIC DISEASES BULLETIN. Text in Chinese; Abstracts in Chinese, English. 1986. q. CNY 28 domestic (effective 2001 & 2002); USD 20 foreign (2001 & 2002). charts, illus. 96 p./no. back issues avail. **Document type:** *Academic/Scholarly.* **Description:** Reports on various communicable diseases, including plague, bruccellosis, IDD, cretinism, Kaschin-Beck disease, Keshan disease, and hyatid disease. Also covers such conditions as endemic fluorosis and arsenic poisoning.
Related titles: ♦ CD-ROM ed.: Chinese Academic Journal. Medicine & Hygiene. ISSN 1007-8053; E-mail ed.; Online - full content ed.
Indexed: Dairy Sci.Abstr., Helminthol.Abstr., Ind.Vet., Nutr.Abstr., Pig News & Info., Protozool.Abstr., Rev.Appl.Entomol., Rev.Arom.& Med.Plants, Rev.Med.& Vet.Mycol., Trop.Dis.Bull., Vet.Bull., Zoo.Rec.
—BLDSC (3740.300000).
Published by: (Xinjiang Difangbing Fangzhi Yanjiusuo/Xinjiang Institute for Endemic Disease Control and Research), Difangbing Tongbao Bianjibu, 4 Jianquan 1st St, Urumqi, Xinjiang 830002, China. TEL 86-991-2642734, FAX 86-991-2625962, xjdfbtb@xj.cninfo.net, xjdfbtb@xj.chinfo.net, http://www.caj-cd.tsinghua.edu.cn. Eds. Juan Wen, Yujiang Zhang. Pub. Haoli Cao. **Dist. overseas by:** China National Publishing Industry Trading Corporation, PO Box 782, Beijing 100011, China.

610 CHE
DISEASE OUTBREAK NEWS. Text in English, French, Spanish. irreg.
Published by: World Health Organization, Marketing and Dissemination, Geneva, 27 1211, Switzerland. TEL 41-22-791-2476, FAX 41-22-791-4875, http://www.who.int.

616.9 USA
DISEASE WEEKLY PLUS. Text in English. 1997. w. (43/yr.). USD 1,895 in North America; USD 2,095 elsewhere. **Document type:** *Newsletter.* **Description:** Concentrates on nosocomial infections, therapeutic drug resistance, and immunology.
Formed by the merger of (1994-1997): Drug Resistance Weekly (1074-2913); (1994-1997): Infection Control Weekly (1074-2905); (1994?-1997): Infectious Disease Weekly (1078-2850)
Related titles: Microform ed.: (from PQC); Online - full text ed.: (from Gale Group).
Indexed: Bus.& Indus. (Jan.1995-).
—CCC.
Published by: Charles W. Henderson, Ed. & Pub., PO Box 5528, Atlanta, GA 31107-0528. TEL 770-507-7777, FAX 770-507-7788, info@hendersonnet.atl.ga.us, http://www.newsfile.com.

616.9792 GBR
DOCTOR FAX. Text in English. 1996. fortn. back issues avail. **Description:** Aims to provide HIV positive people and those involved in the treatment of HIV and AIDS with up-to-date and accurate information.
Media: Fax. **Related titles:** Online - full content ed.
Published by: AIDS Treatment Project, 250 Kennington Lane, London SE11 5RD, United Kingdom. TEL 44-171-793-8300, admin@atp.org.uk, http://www.atp.org.uk/dff.html.

616.9 USA ISSN 1064-1815
THE DOUBLE HELIX. Text in English. 1975. q. free per issue. **Document type:** *Newsletter.* **Description:** Supports research. education, and the prevention of infectious diseases.
Related titles: Online - full content ed.
Published by: National Foundation for Infectious Diseases, 4733 Bethesda Ave, Ste 750, Bethesda, MD 20814-5228. TEL 301-656-0003, FAX 301-907-0878, info@nfid.org, http://www.nfid.org. Ed., R&P Len Novick. Circ: 6,000.

616.9 TZA
EAST AFRICAN INSTITUTE OF MALARIA AND VECTORBORNE DISEASES. ANNUAL REPORT. Text in English. a. **Document type:** *Corporate.*
Indexed: Biol.Abstr., Rev.Appl.Entomol.
Published by: East African Institute of Malaria and Vectorborne Diseases, PO Box 4, Amani, Tanzania.

616.988 EGY ISSN 0301-8849
CODEN: EJBLAB
EGYPTIAN JOURNAL OF BILHARZIASIS. Text in English; Summaries in Arabic, English. 1974. a. USD 42 (effective 2000). adv. charts, illus. reprint service avail. from IRC. **Document type:** *Academic/Scholarly.*
Indexed: Biol.Abstr., Chem.Abstr., Excerp.Med., Helminthol.Abstr., Ind.Med. (coverage dropped).
—BLDSC (3664.280000), CASDDS, CISTI, GNLM.
Published by: (Egyptian Society of Tropical Medicine and Parasitology, Research Department), National Information and Documentation Centre (NIDOC), Tahrir St., Dokki, Awqaf P.O., Cairo, Egypt. TEL 20-2-3371696. Ed. S. S. Aly. Circ: 1,000. **Co-sponsor:** General Society for Combat of Bilharziasis.

616.9 EGY ISSN 0253-5890
CODEN: JESPDT
EGYPTIAN SOCIETY OF PARASITOLOGY. JOURNAL. Text in Arabic. 1972. s-a. **Document type:** *Academic/Scholarly.*
Indexed: Abstr.Hyg., Anim.Breed.Abstr., Bio-Contr.News & Info., Food Sci.& Tech.Abstr., Helminthol.Abstr., Ind.Med. (1970-), Ind.Vet., Irr.& Drain.Abstr., Nutr.Abstr., Poult.Abstr., Protozool.Abstr., Rev.Appl.Entomol., Rev.Arom.& Med.Plants, Rev.Med.& Vet.Mycol., Rural Devel.Abstr., Trop.Dis.Bull., Vet.Bull., Weed Abstr., Zoo.Rec.
—BLDSC (4735.910000), CISTI, GNLM, KNAW.
Published by: Egyptian Society of Parasitology, Tager Bldg, Ozoris St., Garden City, Cairo, Egypt.

616.9 USA
EMERGING INFECTIONS. Text in English.
Indexed: Ind.Vet.
—BLDSC (3733.426020).
Published by: American Society for Microbiology, 1325 Massachusetts Ave, N W, Washington, DC 20005-4171. TEL 703-787-3305, subscriptions@asmusa.org, subscriptions@amsusa.org, http://www.asmusa.org/asm-bin/search. Ed. Michael W Scheld.

EMERGING INFECTIOUS DISEASES (ONLINE EDITION). see *PUBLIC HEALTH AND SAFETY*

EMERGING INFECTIOUS DISEASES (PRINT EDITION). see *PUBLIC HEALTH AND SAFETY*

616.9 FRA ISSN 1166-8598
ENCYCLOPEDIE MEDICO-CHIRURGICALE. TRAITE DES MALADIES INFECTIEUSES. Key Title: Encyclopedie Medico-Chirurgicale. Maladies Infectieuses. Cover title: Traite des Maladies Infectieuses. Text in French. 1935. 4 base vols. plus q. updates. bibl, charts, illus. *Refereed.* **Document type:** *Academic/Scholarly.* **Description:** Offers epidemiologists a comprehensive, up-to-date reference for diagnosing and treating communicable diseases.
Formerly (until 1992): Encyclopedie Medico-Chirurgicale. Maladies Infectieuses et Parasitaires (0246-0637)
Published by: Elsevier Paris, Editions Scientifiques et Medicales (Subsidiary of: Reed Elsevier plc. group), 23 rue Linois, Paris 75015, France. TEL 33-1-45589110, FAX 33-1-45589425, redaction-emc@elsevier.fr, redacion-emc@elsevier.fr, http://www.elsevier.fr, http://www.elsevier.com.

616.9 MEX ISSN 1405-0994
ENFERMEDADES INFECCIOSAS Y MICROBIOLOGIA. Text in Spanish; Summaries in English. 1980. bi-m. MXP 300, USD 55. *Refereed.* **Document type:** *Academic/Scholarly.* **Description:** Contains original articles, research reports, review articles, clinical cases and notices related to infectious diseases.
Published by: Obsidiana Editores S.A., CZDA DE TLALPAN 2365, Col Ciudad Jardin, Mexico City, DF 04370, Mexico. TEL 52-5-689-9133. Eds. Dr. Jose Ruiloba Benitez, Dr. Jose Sifuentes Osornio. Pub. Jorge Godoy-Gutierrez. Circ: 3,000. **Dist. by:** Distribuidora Editorial de Mexico SA de CV, P.O. Box 76-026, Mexico City, DF 04201, Mexico. TEL 52-5-544-7953, FAX 52-5-689-6545. **Co-sponsors:** Asociacion Mexicana de Infectologia; Consejo Nacional de Certificacion en Infectologia.

616.9 ESP ISSN 0213-005X
CODEN: EIMCE2
ENFERMEDADES INFECCIOSAS Y MICROBIOLOGIA CLINICA. Text in Spanish; Summaries in English. 1982. m. (10/yr.). USD 113 to non-members. adv. reprint service avail. from PQC. **Document type:** *Academic/Scholarly.* **Description:** Diffuses investigative works, clinical and microbiological, related to infectious pathology. Contributes to the continuing education of professionals.
Formerly: Enfermedades Infecciosas (0212-5218)
Related titles: Online - full text ed.: (from Institute for Scientific Information).
Indexed: Curr.Cont., Ind.Med. (1984-), Ind.Med.Esp., Inpharma, Reac., Ref.Zh.
—BLDSC (3747.900500), CINDOC, EMDOCS, GNLM, Infotrieve, KNAW. **CCC.**
Published by: (Sociedad Espanola de Enfermedades Infecciosas y Microbiologia Clinica), Ediciones Doyma S.A., Traversa de Gracia, 17-21, Barcelona 08021, Spain. TEL 34-93-200-0711, FAX 34-93-209-1136. Ed. V Ausina Ruiz. Adv. contact Marte Vidal. page ESP 270,000; trim 280 x 210. Circ: 3,700.

616.9 SGP ISSN 0218-0103
RA643.7.S55
EPIDEMIOLOGICAL NEWS BULLETIN. Text in English. 1974. m. free per issue to qualified personnel. stat. *Refereed.* **Document type:** *Bulletin.* **Description:** Provides and updates information on infectious diseases and other public health issues in Singapore for medical practitioners.
Related titles: CD-ROM ed.
Indexed: ExtraMED.
—BLDSC (3793.566000), GNLM.
Published by: Committee on Epidemic Diseases, Quarantine and Epidemiology Department, 40 Scotts Rd, Environment Bldg, Singapore 228231, Singapore. TEL 65-731-9758, FAX 65-734-8287, envqe@cs.gov.sg. Ed., R&P Goh Kee Tai. Circ: 2,500.

616.9 RUS
EPIDEMIOLOGIYA I INFEKTSIONNYE BOLEZNI/EPIDEMIOLOGY AND INFECTIOUS DISEASES. Text in Russian; Summaries in English. 1996. bi-m. USD 138 foreign (effective 2000). adv. Website rev. abstr. reprints avail. **Document type:** *Journal, Academic/Scholarly.* **Description:** Covers problems of diagnosis, treatment and prevention of infectious diseases.
Indexed: Ref.Zh.
Published by: Izdatel'stvo Meditsina, Petroverigskii per 6-8, Moscow 101000, Russian Federation. TEL 7-095-9241241, 7-095-928-86-48, FAX 7-095-9211355, http://www.medit.ru. Ed. V I Pokrovsky. Pub. A M Stochik. R&P N Biyatova. Adv. contact O A Fadeeva TEL 7-095-923-51-40. Circ: 1,500. **Dist. by:** Mezhdunarodnaya Kniga, B Yakimanka 39, Moscow 117049, Russian Federation. TEL 7-095-2384967, FAX 7-095-2384634; **US dist. addr.:** East View Publications, 3020 Harbor Ln N, Minneapolis, MN 55447. TEL 612-550-0961.

EPIDEMIOLOGY AND INFECTION. see *BIOLOGY—Microbiology*

616.9 GBR ISSN 0969-9252
EPSTEIN-BARR VIRUS REPORT. Text in English. 1995. bi-m. GBP 78, USD 138 to individuals; GBP 134, USD 238 to institutions (effective 2002). back issues avail. **Document type:** *Journal, Academic/Scholarly, Abstract/Index.* **Description:** Locates and reports the scientific and research literature on Epstein-Barr Virus internationally.
Indexed: AMED.
—BLDSC (3794.399220).
Published by: Maney Publishing, Hudson Rd, Leeds, W Yorks LS9 7DL, United Kingdom. TEL 44-113-249-7481, FAX 44-113-248-6983, maney@maney.co.uk, http://www.maney.co.uk. Ed. Lawrence Young.

616.97 615.5 GBR
EUROPEAN AIDS DIRECTORY. Text in English, French, German, Italian, Spanish. a. GBP 24.95 in United Kingdom; GBP 29.95 in Europe; GBP 39.95 elsewhere (effective 2001). **Document type:** *Directory.* **Description:** Information on all non-governmental HIV and AIDS services in Europe.
Formerly: European Union AIDS Directory
Related titles: French ed.; German ed.; Italian ed.; Spanish ed.
Published by: N A M Publications, 16a Clapham Common, South Side, London SW4 7AB, United Kingdom. TEL 44-20-7627-3200, FAX 44-20-7627-3101, info@nam.org.uk. Ed. Philip Browning.

EUROPEAN JOURNAL OF CLINICAL MICROBIOLOGY & INFECTIOUS DISEASES; an international journal on pathogenesis, diagnosis, epidemiology, therapy, and prevention of infectious diseases. see *BIOLOGY—Microbiology*

610 CHE
EUROPEAN SCIENTIFIC WORKING GROUP ON INFLUENZA. BULLETIN. Text in English. s-a. **Description:** Covers influenza news worldwide, focusing on vaccination programs and prevention, as well as treatment.
Published by: (European Scientific Working Group on Influenza), Gardiner - Caldwell Communications Ltd., Victoria Mill, Windmill St, Macclesfield, Ches SK11 7HQ, United Kingdom. TEL 44-1625-618507, FAX 44-1625-614161. Eds. A.D.M.E. Osterhaus, A.M. Palache, C Hannoun.

EXCERPTA MEDICA. SECTION 13: DERMATOLOGY AND VENEREOLOGY. see *MEDICAL SCIENCES—Abstracting, Bibliographies, Statistics*

EXCERPTA MEDICA. SECTION 17: PUBLIC HEALTH, SOCIAL MEDICINE AND EPIDEMIOLOGY. see *PUBLIC HEALTH AND SAFETY—Abstracting, Bibliographies, Statistics*

EXCERPTA MEDICA. SECTION 26: IMMUNOLOGY, SEROLOGY AND TRANSPLANTATION. see *MEDICAL SCIENCES—Abstracting, Bibliographies, Statistics*

616.9 340 USA ISSN 1042-4652
KF3803.A54
THE EXCHANGE (SAN FRANCISCO)✶ . Text in English. 1986. 3/yr. USD 35 to membership.
Published by: National Lawyers Guild, AIDS Network, 126 University Pl 4th Fl, New York, NY 10003-4538. Ed. Eileen Hansen.

616.96 USA ISSN 0014-4894
QL757 CODEN: EXPAAA
EXPERIMENTAL PARASITOLOGY. Text in English. 1952. 12/yr. USD 985 in US & Canada to institutions; USD 1,130 elsewhere to institutions (effective 2001). adv. bibl, illus. index. back issues avail. *Refereed.* **Document type:** *Academic/Scholarly.* **Description:** Emphasizes modern approaches to parasitology, including molecular biology and immunology.
Related titles: Online - full text ed.: (from EBSCO Publishing, O C L C Online Computer Library Center, Inc., RoweCom Information Quest, ingenta, Swets Blackwell, IDEAL Online Library, Institute for Scientific Information).
Indexed: ASCA, Abstr.Hyg., AgBiotech, Agri.& Environ.Biotech.Abstr. (coverage dropped), Agricola, Aqua.Sci.& Fish.Abstr., Bio-Contr.News & Info., Biol.Abstr., Chem.Abstr., Chem.Indus.Notes, Chem.Titles, Curr.Adv.Ecol.Sci., Curr.Cont., Dent.Ind., Derwent Biotech.Abstr., Entomol.Abstr., Excerp.Med. (1993-), Focus on: Vet.Sci.& Med., Genet.Abstr., Helminthol.Abstr., Hum.Gen.Abstr., INIS Atomind., Immun.Abstr. (coverage dropped), Ind.Med. (1951-), Ind.Sci.Rev., Ind.Vet., Inpharma, Microbiol.Abstr., Nutr.Abstr., Pharm.&Out.News, Pig News & Info., Poult.Abstr., Protozool.Abstr., Reac., Ref.Zh., Rev.Appl.Entomol., Rev.Arom.& Med.Plants, Rev.Med.& Vet.Mycol., Rev.Plant Path., Sci.Cit.Ind., Small Anim.Abstr., Sport Fish.Abstr., Trop.Dis.Bull., Vet.Bull., Wild.Rev., Zoo.Rec.
—BLDSC (3840.000000), ADONIS, CASDDS, CISTI, GNLM, IDS, ingenta, Linda Hall. **CCC.**
Published by: Academic Press, Inc., Journal Division (Subsidiary of: Harcourt Brace & Company), 525 B St, Ste 1900, San Diego, CA 92101-4495. TEL 619-230-1840, FAX 619-699-6800, apsubs@acad.com, http://www.academicpress.com/ep. Ed. Dyann F Wirth.

610 USA ISSN 1047-0719
FOCUS (SAN FRANCISCO); a guide to AIDS research & counseling. Text in English. 1985. m. USD 48 domestic to individuals; USD 60 foreign to individuals; USD 105 domestic to institutions; USD 125 foreign to institutions (effective 2001 & 2002). bk.rev. back issues avail. **Document type:** *Newsletter.* **Description:** Reviews the mental health and counseling aspects of AIDS and HIV disease. Puts medical, epidemiological, and social aspects of the epidemic in the context of HIV-related counseling and psychotherapy.
Related titles: E-mail ed.: USD 36 to individuals; USD 90 to institutions (effective (No. 2001).
—BLDSC (3964.199500).
Published by: University of California at San Francisco AIDS Health Project, Box 0884, San Francisco, CA 94143-0884. TEL 415-502-7270, info@ucsf.edu, ccrawfo@itsa.ucsf.edu, http://www.ucsf-ahp.org/FOCUS.html. Eds. James W Dilley, Robert Marks. R&P Carrel Crawford TEL 415-502-7270. Circ: 2,000 (paid).

616.96 590 579.65 CZE ISSN 0015-5683
QL757 CODEN: FPARA9
FOLIA PARASITOLOGICA. Text and summaries in English. 1966. q. USD 75 to individuals; USD 195 to institutions (effective 1999). adv. bk.rev. bibl, charts, illus. index. *Refereed.* **Document type:** *Academic/Scholarly.* **Description:** Includes papers on human and veterinary parasitology and on the biology, morphology, ultrastructure, physiology and biochemistry of parasites.
Formerly (until 1965): Ceskoslovenska Parasitologie
Related titles: Online - full text ed.: (from Institute for Scientific Information).
Indexed: ASCA, Abstr.Hyg., Aqua.Sci.& Fish.Abstr., Bio-Contr.News & Info., Biol.Abstr., Chem.Abstr., Chem.Indus.Notes, Chem.Titles, Curr.Adv.Ecol.Sci., Curr.Cont., Curr.Ref.Fish Res., Environ.Sci.Poll.Mgmt., Excerp.Med., Helminthol.Abstr., Ind.Med. (1966-), Ind.Sci.Rev., Ind.Vet., Int.Abstr.Biol.Sci., Pig News & Info., Pollut.Abstr., Poult.Abstr., Protozool.Abstr., Rev.Appl.Entomol., Rev.Med.& Vet.Mycol., Sci.Cit.Ind., Soils & Fert., Sport Fish.Abstr., Trop.Dis.Bull., Vet.Bull., Zoo.Rec.
—BLDSC (3971.850000), CASDDS, CISTI, EMDOCS, GNLM, Linda Hall. **CCC.**
Published by: Ceska Akademie Ved, Parazitologicky Ustav, Branisovska 31, Ceske Budejovice 37005, Czech Republic. TEL 42-38-777-5406, FAX 42-38-47743, folia@paru.cas.cz; bukva@paru.cas.cz, http://www.paru.cas.cz. Ed. Jiri Lom. R&P, Adv. contact Vladimir Bukva. Circ: 850.

616.9 USA ISSN 1535-3141
▼ **FOODBORNE PATHOGENS AND DISEASE.** Text in English. forthcoming 2002. q. USD 119 domestic to individuals; USD 149 foreign to individuals; USD 219 domestic to institutions; USD 265 foreign to institutions; USD 143 combined subscription domestic to individuals for both print & online eds.; USD 173 combined subscription foreign to individuals for both print & online eds.; USD 263 combined subscription domestic to institutions for both print & online eds.; USD 309 combined subscription foreign to institutions for both print & online eds. (effective 2002). adv. back issues avail.; reprints avail. *Refereed.* **Document type:** *Academic/Scholarly.* **Description:** Includes original research papers on diseases caused by foodborne pathogens.
Related titles: Online - full content ed.: forthcoming. USD 119 to individuals; USD 219 to institutions (effective 2002).
Published by: Mary Ann Liebert, Inc. Publishers, 20 W Third St., Ste 200, Media, PA 19063-2824. TEL 610-892-9580, FAX 610-892-9577, info@liebertpub.com, http://www.liebertpub.com/FPD/default1.asp. Ed. Stephen P Oliver. Adv. contact Harriet Matysko.

616.998 CAN
FRONTLINE. Text in English. 1973. q. free per issue. bk.rev., video rev. **Document type:** *Bulletin, Newsletter, Academic/Scholarly.*
Formerly: In Action
Published by: Leprosy Mission Canada, 75 The Donway W, Ste 1410, North York, ON M3C 2E9, Canada. TEL 416-441-3618, FAX 416-441-0203, nhunter@lmcanada.org. Ed. Nicholas Hunter. Circ: 14,000.

616.9 USA ISSN 1077-1824
RC607.A26
G M H C TREATMENT ISSUES; newsletter of experimental AIDS therapies. (Gay Men's Health Crisis) Text in English. 1987. m. USD 55 to individuals; USD 95 to institutions (effective 2001); Contact publisher for special subscr. rates available for low income and individuals with HIV/AIDS.. illus. reprints avail. **Document type:** *Newsletter.* **Description:** Addresses the various medical aspects of AIDS, including experimental treatments, descriptions of opportunistic infections often seen in AIDS, drug licensing issues, and medical articles of general interest to people who are HIV-infected.
Formerly: Treatment Issues (1050-625X)
—BLDSC (4196.430000).
Published by: Gay Men's Health Crisis, Inc., Treatment Education and Advocacy, 119 W 24th St, New York, NY 10011. FAX 212-367-1528, fredg@gmhc.org, http://www.gmhc.org. Ed. David Gilden. R&P Charles Sock. Circ: 18,000.

GAY MEN'S HEALTH CRISIS. see *MEDICAL SCIENCES—Experimental Medicine, Laboratory Technique*

616.96 ITA
CODEN: GMIPAX
GIORNALE ITALIANO DI MALATTIE INFETTIVE. Text in Italian. 1948. m. ITL 120,000; ITL 180,000 foreign (effective 1998). adv. bk.rev. abstr, bibl, charts, illus, stat. index, cum.index. reprint service avail. from IRC.
Formerly: Giornale di Malattie Infettive e Parassitarie (0017-0321)
Indexed: Abstr.Hyg., Biol.Abstr., Chem.Abstr., Curr.Adv.Ecol.Sci., Dent.Ind., Excerp.Med., Helminthol.Abstr., Ind.Vet., Protozool.Abstr., Rev.Med.& Vet.Mycol., Trop.Dis.Bull.
—CASDDS, CISTI, GNLM.
Published by: (Societa Italiana per lo Studio delle Malattie Infettive e Parassitarie), U T E T SpA, Viale Tunisia, 37, Milan, MI 20124, Italy. TEL 39-2-6241171, FAX 39-2-62411748. Ed. Roberto Esposito. Circ: 1,350.

616.998 USA
GLOBAL MISSIONS. Text in English. 1943. 3/yr. **Document type:** *Newsletter.*
Published by: International Christian Leprosy Mission, Inc., PO Box 23353, Portland, OR 97223. TEL 803-285-9098. Ed. Dr. Daniel Pulliam. Circ: 1,650.

616.9792 USA
H I N FAX NEWSLETTER. (HIV Information Network) Text in English. irreg. **Document type:** *Newsletter.* **Description:** Provides timely, relevant information for physicians and allied healthcare professionals who treat or counsel persons living with HIV/AIDS.
Related titles: Fax ed.; Online - full text ed.
Published by: World Health C M E, 41 Madison Ave, 42nd Fl, New York, NY 10010-2202. FAX 205-975-6902, http://www.hivline.com/member/faxnews/faxindex.htm.

616.9 616.97 USA ISSN 1532-026X
H I V COUNSELOR PERSPECTIVES. (Human Immunodeficiency Virus) Text in English. bi-m. USD 24 domestic to individuals; USD 32 foreign to individuals; USD 60 domestic to institutions; USD 72 foreign to institutions (effective 2001). **Document type:** *Newsletter.*
Published by: University of California at San Francisco AIDS Health Project, Box 0884, San Francisco, CA 94143-0884. TEL 415-502-7270, FAX 415-476-7996, ccrawfo@itsa.ucsf.edu, http://www.ucsf-ahp.org/Perspback.html.

616.9 AUS
H I V JOURNAL CLUB. Text in English. m.
Media: Online - full text.
Published by: Australian Society for H I V Medicine, Australia. davidful@ozemail.com.au; davidf@westmed.wh.su.edu.au, http://www.unsw.edu.au/clients/ashm/HIV_JC.html.

616.9792 GBR ISSN 1464-2662
▼ **H I V MEDICINE.** (Human Immunodeficiency Virus) Text in English. 2000. q., latest vol.3, 2002. GBP 63 in Europe to individuals; USD 98 in North America to individuals; GBP 68 elsewhere to individuals; GBP 193 in Europe to institutions; USD 301 in North America to institutions; GBP 209 elsewhere to institutions (effective 2002). adv. *Refereed.* **Document type:** *Journal, Trade.* **Description:** A broad based journal for researchers and clinicians with responsibility for treating HIV seropositive patients. The Journal will feature original articles, case reports and reviews. A regular section addressing ethical issues and their implications for clinical management will also be included.
Related titles: Online - full text ed.: ISSN 1468-1293. GBP 57 in Europe to individuals; USD 89 in North America to individuals; GBP 57 elsewhere to individuals; GBP 174 in Europe to institutions; USD 271 in North America to institutions; GBP 174 elsewhere to institutions (effective 2002) (from EBSCO Publishing, O C L C Online Computer Library Center, Inc., RoweCom Information Quest, ingenta, Munksgaard & Blackwell Science's Synergy, Swets Blackwell).
—BLDSC (4319.045900).
Published by: Blackwell Science Ltd., PO Box 88, Oxford OX2 0NE, United Kingdom. TEL 44-1865-206180, 44-1865-206002, FAX 44-1865-206219, jnl.orders@blacksci.co.uk, http://www.blackwell-science.com/~cgilib/jnlpage.asp?Journal=hiv&File=hiv, http://www.blackwellpublishing.com. Eds. B Gazzard, M Johnson. Pub. Allen Stevens. R&P Sophie Savage. Adv. contact Jenny Applin. B&W page GBP 440, color page GBP 1,100. Circ: 700. **Co-sponsors:** European AIDS Clinical Society; British HIV Association.

616.9 USA
H I V PLUS. (Human Immunodeficiency Virus) Text in English. bi-m. free to qualified personnel. **Document type:** *Magazine.*
Indexed: P.A.I.S.
Published by: H I V plus, Circulation Coordinator, 80 Eight Ave., Ste 305, New York, NY 10011-5126. http://www.hivplusmag.com. Ed. Michael W Elkins. Adv. contact Joe Valentino.

HARVARD AIDS INSTITUTE SERIES ON GENE REGULATION OF HUMAN RETROVIRUSES. see *BIOLOGY—Genetics*

362.196 USA
HEADLINE TREATMENT NEWS. Text in English. m.

M

Published by: San Francisco AIDS Foundation, PO Box 426182, San Francisco, CA 94142-6182. TEL 415-487-8060, 800-833-0159, FAX 415-487-8069, beta@sfaf.org, http://www.sfaf.org.

616.9 USA ISSN 1064-4873
THE HELPER. Text in English. 1979. q. USD 25 (effective 1999). bk.rev. *Refereed.* **Document type:** *Newsletter.* **Description:** Presents emerging issues in the treatment of herpes simplex. Covers both scientific breakthroughs and psychosocial aspects.
Published by: Herpes Resource Center, PO Box 13827, Research Triangle Park, NC 27709. TEL 919-361-8400, FAX 919-361-8425, http://ashastd.org. Ed. Amy Austell. R&P Kelli Edwards TEL 919-361-8498. Circ: 15,000.

616.9 USA
HEPATITIS. Text in English. bi-m. USD 20; USD 25 in Canada (effective 2000). adv. **Document type:** *Magazine, Consumer.* **Description:** Assists hepatitis patients and their families in taking control of their own health care by providing current and comprehensive information.
Published by: Quality Publishing Inc., 523 N Sam Houston Pkwy, Ste 300, Houston, TX 77060. TEL 281-272-2744, FAX 281-847-5368, editor@hepatitismag.com, http://www.hepatitismag.com.

HEPATITIS SOURCEBOOK. see *MEDICAL SCIENCES—Gastroenterology*

616.9 USA ISSN 1086-0223
HEPATITIS WEEKLY. Text in English. 1995. w. (43/yr.). USD 1,549 in North America; USD 1,649 elsewhere. **Document type:** *Newsletter.*
Related titles: Online - full text ed.: (from Northern Light Technology, Inc., Gale Group, Factiva).
Indexed: Bus.& Indus. (Apr.1995-).
Published by: Charles W. Henderson, Ed. & Pub., PO Box 5528, Atlanta, GA 31107-0528. TEL 770-507-7777, FAX 770-507-7788, cwhender@newsfile.com; info@hendersonnet.atl.ga.us, http://www.newsfile.com.

616.9 617.7 GBR ISSN 0969-7667
HERPES; journal of the IHMF. Text in English. 1994. 3/yr. GBP 51, USD 56 (effective 2000). **Document type:** *Academic/Scholarly.* **Description:** Provides reviews on key issues and recommendations relating to patient management of herpes virus infection. Communicates to a broad range of specialists including: virologists, dermatologists, venereologists and others.
—BLDSC (4300.270000).
Published by: Cambridge Medical Publications Ltd., Wicker House, High St, Worthing, W Sussex BN11 1DJ, United Kingdom. TEL 44-1903-205884, FAX 44-1903-234862, cmp@hbase.com, http://www.ihmf.org. Pub. Robert Kasprowicz. R&P Elaine Preece. Circ: 8,800.

669 USA
HERPESVIRUSES WEEKLY. Text in English. w. USD 342; USD 367 foreign. **Document type:** *Newsletter.*
Related titles: Online - full text ed.
Indexed: Bus.& Indus. (May 1998-).
Published by: Charles W. Henderson, Ed. & Pub., PO Box 5528, Atlanta, GA 31107-0528. TEL 404-377-8895, FAX 404-378-5411, cwhender@newsfile.com; info@hendersonnet.atl.ga.us, http://www.newsfile.com.

616.9 FRA
HIV - AIDS SURVEILLANCE IN EUROPE./ SURVEILLANCE DU VIH - SIDA EN EUROPE. Text in English, French. 1984. s-a. **Document type:** *Bulletin, Academic/Scholarly.* **Description:** Statistics on AIDS in Europe.
Former titles (until 1995): AIDS Surveillance in Europe. Quarterly Report; European Centre for the Epidemiological Monitoring of AIDS. Quarterly Report
Published by: European Centre for the Epidemiological Monitoring of AIDS/Centre Europeen pour la Surveillance Epidemiologique du SIDA, Hopital National de Saint-Maurice, 14 rue du Val d'Osne, St Maurice 94410, France. TEL 33-1-41796800, FAX 33-1-41796801, j.alise@ceses.org, http://www.ceses.org/sida.htm. Ed. Francoise Hamers. R&P Ribeiro Laurence TEL 33-1-41796815. Circ: 800.

616.9 USA ISSN 0898-5030
RC607.A26
HIV - AIDS TREATMENT DIRECTORY; experimental and approved agents and methods. Text in English. 1987. s-a. USD 55 in US & Canada to individuals; USD 100 elsewhere to individuals (effective 2000). **Document type:** *Directory.* **Description:** Comprehensive source of information on treatments in development for AIDS-HIV infections and neoplasms.
Published by: American Foundation for AIDS Research, 120 Wall St, Fl 13, New York, NY 10005-3902. TEL 212-806-1600, 800-382-6327, FAX 212-806-1601, txdir@amfar.org, http://www.amfar.org/td. Eds. Dr. Donald I Abrams, Michael H Grieco. R&P Bob Huff TEL 212-806-1631.

HIV & AIDS. see *MEDICAL SCIENCES—Abstracting, Bibliographies, Statistics*

616.9 GBR ISSN 1358-8370
HIV AND AIDS CURRENT TRENDS. Text in English. 1995. q. GBP 27; GBP 29 in Europe; GBP 33 elsewhere. bk.rev. back issues avail. *Refereed.* **Document type:** *Academic/Scholarly.* **Description:** Contains reviews and articles on all aspects of HIV and AIDS.
Published by: Mediscript Ltd., 1 Mountview Ct, 310 Friern Barnet Ln, London N20 0LD, United Kingdom. TEL 44-20-8446-8898, FAX 44-20-8446-9194, 101607.3205@compuserve.com. Ed., R&P, Adv. contact Linda Lazarus. Pub. Fatima Patel. Circ: 5,000 (paid).

616.97 615.6 GBR ISSN 1357-6410
HIV AND AIDS TREATMENTS DIRECTORY. Text in English. 1987. s-a. GBP 64.95 in United Kingdom; GBP 69.95 in Europe; GBP 74.95 elsewhere (effective 2001). **Document type:** *Directory.* **Description:** Comprehensive information on all treatments for HIV and AIDS.
Published by: N A M Publications, 16a Clapham Common, South Side, London SW4 7AB, United Kingdom. TEL 44-20-7627-3200, FAX 44-20-7627-3101, info@nam.org.uk. Ed. Keith Alcorn.

616.9792 USA
HIV FRONTLINE. Text in English. q. **Document type:** *Newsletter.* **Description:** Resource for social workers, treatment educators, case managers, and other allied healthcare professionals who counsel people living with HIV.
Related titles: Online - full text ed.
Published by: World Health C M E, 41 Madison Ave, 42nd Fl, New York, NY 10010-2202. http://www.hivline.com/member/frontline/front_frameset.htm.

HIV POLICY WATCH. see *PUBLIC HEALTH AND SAFETY*

▼ **HIV TREATMENT ALERTS!.** see *MEDICAL SCIENCES—Allergology And Immunology*

616.9 USA
HOPKINS HIV REPORT. Text in English. bi-m. **Document type:** *Newsletter.* **Description:** Publishes for practitioners who care for patients with HIV/AIDS.
Related titles: Online - full text ed.
Published by: Johns Hopkins University, Division of Infectious Diseases, PO Box 5252, Baltimore, MD 21224. http://www.hopkins-aids.edu/publications/report/. Ed. Mary Beth Hansen. R&P Mary Beth Hansen TEL 410-614-0558.

616.9 USA ISSN 0098-180X
HOSPITAL INFECTION CONTROL. Text in English. 1974. m. USD 399 domestic; USD 427 foreign; USD 67 newsstand/cover (effective 2001). bk.rev. bibl. index. back issues avail.; reprints avail. **Document type:** *Newsletter.*
Related titles: Microform ed.: (from PQC); Online - full text ed.: (from Northern Light Technology, Inc., EBSCO Publishing); Supplement: Healthcare Infection Prevention.
Indexed: CINAHL, Hosp.Lit.Ind., Ind.Med. (coverage dropped).
—BLDSC (4333.192000).
Published by: American Health Consultants (Subsidiary of: Medical Economics Co., Inc.), 3525 Piedmont Rd, N E, 6 Piedmont Center, Ste 400, Atlanta, GA 30305. TEL 404-262-7436, 800-688-2421, FAX 404-262-7837, 800-284-3291, customerservice@ahcpub.com, http://www.HIConline.com, http://www.ahcpub.com. Ed. Gary Evans. Pub. Brenda L Mooney. Circ: 2,500 (paid).
Subscr. to: PO Box 71266, Chicago, IL 60691-9986.

016.6 USA ISSN 0197-8160
RB155
HUMAN GENETICS, INFORMATIONAL AND EDUCATIONAL MATERIALS. SUPPLEMENT. Text in English. 1980. a.
Published by: U.S. Public Health Service, 5600 Fishers Ln, Rockville, MD 20857. TEL 301-444-6656.

616.9 DEU
CODEN: HYGMED
HYGIENE & MEDIZIN - INFECTION CONTROL AND HEALTHCARE; international journal for applied hygiene and preventive medicine in hospital and general practice. Text in German; Summaries in English. 1976. m. DEM 148 domestic; DEM 162 foreign (effective 2001). adv. bk.rev. 56 p./no. 3 cols./p. back issues avail.; reprint service avail. from IRC. *Refereed.* **Document type:** *Journal, Academic/Scholarly.* **Description:** Information on all areas of applied hygiene and preventive medicine, especially infection control, nosocomial infections, epidemiology and hospital hygiene.
Formerly: Hygiene und Medizin (0172-3790)
Indexed: Excerp.Med.
—BLDSC (4352.267000), GNLM.
Published by: M H P Verlag GmbH, Ostring 13, Wiesbaden 65205, Germany. TEL 49-6122-7709131, FAX 49-6122-7709101, hygmed@mhp-verlag.de, http://www.mhp-verlag.de. Ed. H P Werner. R&P Susanne Kudicke TEL 49-6122-7709135. Adv. contact W Bockemuehl TEL 49-6122-7709132. B&W page DEM 3,520. Circ: 4,000.

HYGIENES. see *HEALTH FACILITIES AND ADMINISTRATION*

616.9792 USA
I A V I REPORT. (International Aids Vaccine Initiative) Text in English. 1996. bi-m. **Document type:** *Newsletter.* **Description:** Devoted exclusively to HIV vaccine research and development.
Media: Online - full text.
Published by: I A V I, 110 William St, New York, NY 10038. TEL 212-847-1111, FAX 212-847-1112, http://216.150.6.228/. Ed. David Gold.

616.9 GBR
THE I C N A NEWS. Text in English. bi-m. **Description:** Provides local and national information on people, events and items of general interest to members.
Published by: Infection Control Nurses Association, Fitwise, Drumcross Hall, Bathgate, West Lothian EH48 4BR, United Kingdom. Eds. Kathryn Little, Sheila O'Brien.

INDIAN JOURNAL OF DERMATOLOGY, VENEREOLOGY AND LEPROLOGY. see *MEDICAL SCIENCES—Dermatology And Venereology*

616.998 IND ISSN 0254-9395
RC154.7.I6
INDIAN JOURNAL OF LEPROSY. Text in English. 1929. q. INR 60; GBP 12 in Europe; GBP 12 in Africa; GBP 12 in Asia; USD 22 elsewhere. adv. bk.rev. abstr, charts, illus, stat. index.
Formerly (until 1984): Leprosy in India (0024-1024)
Related titles: CD-ROM ed.
Indexed: Abstr.Hyg., Biol.Abstr., Dent.Ind., Environ.Sci.Poll.Mgmt., Excerp.Med., ExtraMED, Ind.Med. (1984-), Indian Sci.Abstr., Microbiol.Abstr., Pollut.Abstr., Ref.Zh., Risk Abstr., Saf.Sci.Abstr., Trop.Dis.Bull.
—BLDSC (4415.850000), CISTI, EMDOCS, GNLM, ingenta, KNAW.
Published by: Indian Leprosy Association/Hind Kusht Nivaran Sangh, 1 Red Cross Rd., New Delhi 110 001, India. TEL 3714748. Ed. Dr. H Srinivasan. Circ: 1,750.

616.9 IND ISSN 0367-8326
RC164.I3 CODEN: IJMAA9
INDIAN JOURNAL OF MALARIOLOGY; Indian J. Malariol. Text in English. 1947-1963; resumed 1981. q. INR 150, USD 40 (effective 2001). adv. bk.rev. 50 p./no. 2 cols./p. back issues avail. *Refereed.* **Document type:** *Journal, Academic/Scholarly, Government.* **Description:** Contains original research articles, short notes and reviews on all fields of malariology.
Indexed: Agroforest.Abstr., Bio-Contr.News & Info., Excerp.Med., ExtraMED, Ind.Med. (1947-), Ind.Sci.Rev., Ind.Vet., Protozool.Abstr., Rev.Appl.Entomol., Rev.Med.& Vet.Mycol., Rice Abstr., Rural Devel.Abstr., Sport Fish.Abstr., Trop.Dis.Bull., Weed Abstr., Zoo.Rec.
—BLDSC (4416.000000), CISTI, EMDOCS, GNLM, ingenta, KNAW.
Published by: Indian Council of Medical Research, Malaria Research Center, 22 Sham Nath Marg, New Delhi 110 054, India. TEL 91-11-3981905, FAX 91-11-2946150, TELEX 31-65518 MRC IN, sks@ndf.vsnl.net.in. Ed., Pub., R&P Sarala K Subbarao. Adv. contact Dr. A Srivastava. Circ: 300.

M

616.9 NLD ISSN 0925-711X
INFECTIEZIEKTEN BULLETIN. Variant title: Bulletin Infectieziekten. Text in Dutch. 1990. m. free per issue. bk.rev. *Refereed.* **Document type:** *Bulletin.*
Description: Includes articles and short news on research, policy, and outbreak management, viral and bacteriological surveillance programs, and information on conferences and courses.
Published by: Rijksinstituut voor Volksgezondheid en Milieu, Postbus 1, Bilthoven 3720 BA, Netherlands. TEL 31-30-2743551, FAX 31-30-2744409, lynette.wijgergangs@rivm.nl, http://www.isis.rivm.nl/inf.bul/home_bul.html. Ed. Dr. Lynette Wijgergangs. Circ: 1,200. **Co-sponsor:** Inspectie voor de Gezondheidszorg.

616.9 CHE ISSN 1420-3448
CODEN: INFEFJ
INFECTIOLOGY. Text in English. 1996. irreg., latest vol.2. CHF 200 in Europe; DEM 240 in Germany; USD 160 in United States (effective 2001). *Refereed.* **Document type:** *Journal, Academic/Scholarly.* **Description:** Presents original data and reviews the latest information on infectious diseases of bacterial, viral, fungal and parasitic origin.
Related titles: Online - full text ed.
—BLDSC (4478.708000), CASDDS, KNAW. **CCC.**
Published by: S. Karger AG, Allschwilerstr 10, PO Box, Basel 4009, Switzerland. TEL 41-61-306-1111, FAX 41-61-306-1234, karger@karger.ch, http://www.karger.com/bookseries/INFEC. Ed. H Zeichhardt.

616.9 USA ISSN 0019-9567
QR1.A47 CODEN: INFIBR
INFECTION AND IMMUNITY. Text in English. 1970. m. USD 575 domestic to non-members; USD 610 in Canada to non-members; USD 650 in Europe to non-members; USD 659 in Latin America to non-members; USD 677 elsewhere to non-members; USD 70 domestic to members (effective 2001). adv. charts, stat. index. back issues avail.; reprint service avail. from PQC. *Refereed.* **Document type:** *Academic/Scholarly.* **Description:** Directed toward immunologists, epidemiologists, pathologists, and clinicians. Areas covered include molecular and cellular pathogenesis, bacterial infections, host-response, inflammation, fungal and parasitic inflammation, microbial immunity, and vaccines.
Related titles: CD-ROM ed.: ISSN 1070-6313. USD 500 in North America; USD 524 elsewhere (effective 1999); Microform ed.: (from PQC); Online - full text ed.: ISSN 1098-5522 (from HighWire Pr., EBSCO Publishing, Institute for Scientific Information).
Indexed: AIDS & Cancer Res., ASCA, Abstr.Hyg., AgBiotech, Agri.& Environ.Biotech.Abstr. (coverage dropped), Agricola, Anim.Breed.Abstr., Aqua.Sci.& Fish.Abstr., Biol.Abstr., Chem.Abstr., Chem.Indus.Notes, Chem.Titles, Chemorec.Abstr., Curr.Adv.Gen.& Molec.Biol., Curr.Cont., Curr.Tit.Dent., Dairy Sci.Abstr., Dent.Ind., Derwent Biotech.Abstr., Diar.Dis.Res., Dok.Arbeitsmed., Environ.Sci.Poll.Mgmt., Excerp.Med., Food Sci.& Tech.Abstr., Genet.Abstr., Helminthol.Abstr., Hum.Gen.Abstr., INIS Atomind., Immun.Abstr., Ind.Med. (1970-), Ind.Sci.Rev., Ind.Vet., Inpharma, Int.Abstr.Biol.Sci., Mass Spectr.Bull., Med.& Pharm.Biotech.Abstr., Med.& Surg.Dermat., Microbiol.Abstr., Nuc.Acids Abstr., Nutr.Abstr., Pharm.&Out.News, Pig News & Info., Plant Grow.Reg.Abstr., Poult.Abstr., Protozool.Abstr., Reac., Rev.Appl.Entomol., Rev.Med.& Vet.Mycol., Rev.Plant Path., Sci.Cit.Ind., Small Anim.Abstr., Soils & Fert., THA, Telegen, Trop.Dis.Bull., Vet.Bull.
—BLDSC (4478.720000), CASDDS, CISTI, GNLM, IDS, ingenta, KNAW, Linda Hall. **CCC.**
Published by: American Society for Microbiology, 1752 N St N W, Washington, DC 20036-2904. TEL 202-737-3600, 800-633-4931, subsubscriptions@amsusa.org, http://asmusa.edoc.com/iai/, http://www.asmusa.org. Eds. Vincent A Fischetti, Alison D O'Brien. Circ: 4,900 (paid).

616.9 USA ISSN 0899-823X
RA969 CODEN: ICEPE3
INFECTION CONTROL & HOSPITAL EPIDEMIOLOGY. Text in English. 1980. m. USD 109 domestic to individuals (effective 2001); USD 118 in Canada to individuals; USD 158 elsewhere to individuals; USD 139 domestic to institutions (effective 2001); USD 140 in Canada to institutions; USD 209 elsewhere to institutions; USD 19 newsstand/cover (effective 2001). adv. 80 p./no. 2 cols./p. back issues avail.; reprints avail. *Refereed.* **Document type:** *Academic/Scholarly.* **Description:** Provides original, peer-reviewed scientific articles for anyone involved with an infection control or epidemiology program with a hospital or health care facility.
Formerly: Infection Control (0195-9417)
Related titles: CD-ROM ed.; Microform ed.: (from PQC); Online - full text ed.: (from Northern Light Technology, Inc., ProQuest Information & Learning, Institute for Scientific Information).
Indexed: ASCA, Abstr.Hyg., Biol.Abstr., CINAHL, Chem.Abstr., Curr.Adv.Ecol.Sci., Curr.Cont., Diar.Dis.Res., Dok.Arbeitsmed., Environ.Sci.Poll.Mgmt., Helminthol.Abstr., INIS Atomind., Ind.Med. (1988-), Ind.Sci.Rev., Inpharma, Int.Nurs.Ind., Jrnl.Watch Inf.Dis., Lab.Haz.Bull., Microbiol.Abstr., Nurs.Abstr., Pharm.&Out.News, Pollut.Abstr., Reac., Rev.Med.& Vet.Mycol., Risk Abstr., SSCI (coverage dropped), Saf.Sci.Abstr., Sci.Cit.Ind., Sugar Ind.Abstr., Virol.Abstr. (coverage dropped).
—BLDSC (4478.721050), CASDDS, CISTI, GNLM, IDS, ingenta, KNAW. **CCC.**
Published by: (Society for Healthcare Epidemiology of America), Slack, Inc., 6900 Grove Rd, Thorofare, NJ 08086-9447. TEL 856-848-1000, 800-257-8290, FAX 856-853-5991, http://www.slackinc.com. Ed. Dr. Michael Decker. Circ: 5,289 (paid).

616.9 GBR ISSN 1464-2891
INFECTION CONTROL AND WOUNDCARE YEARBOOK. Text in English. a. GBP 50 (effective 1999). adv. **Document type:** *Directory.* **Description:** Contains a complete listing of infection-control, woundcare, tissue viability and stoma care nurses, and other members of staff who have control of infection as one of their responsibilities. Hospitals are listed alphabetically by both NHS region and NHS Trust.
Formerly (until 1997): Infection Control Yearbook (0956-9510)
Published by: C M A Medical Data, Cambridge Research Laboratories, 181A Huntingdon Rd, Cambridge CB3 0DJ, United Kingdom. TEL 44-1223-277709, FAX 44-1223-276444. Ed., Pub. Ruth Allan. R&P David Roberts. Adv. contact Myles Davidson.

616.9 USA ISSN 1522-063X
INFECTION CONTROL TODAY. Text in English. m. USD 79 in United States; USD 109 in Canada; USD 175 elsewhere (effective 2000). adv. illus. back issues avail.; reprints avail. **Document type:** *Magazine, Trade.* **Description:** Helps healthcare practitioners responsible for purchasing and administering healthcare products cleanly and safely select and use the best products. Includes best practices for cleaning, disinfecting, decontaminating, and sterilizing medical products and devices.
Published by: Virgo Publishing, Inc., 3300 N Central Ave, Ste 2500, Phoenix, AZ 85012. TEL 480-990-1101, FAX 480-990-0819, ictoday@vpico.com, virgopub@vpico.com, http://www.infectioncontroltoday.com; http://www.vpico.com. adv.: B&W page USD 3,750, color page USD 5,000; trim 10.88 x 8.13. Circ: 25,765.

616.9 USA ISSN 0749-6524
CODEN: INMDEG
INFECTIONS IN MEDICINE; infectious disease in medical and family practice. Text in English. 1983. m. USD 95 domestic; USD 105 foreign; USD 120 to libraries; USD 10 newsstand/cover domestic; USD 15 newsstand/cover foreign (effective 2001). adv. Index. back issues avail. *Refereed.* **Document type:** *Trade.* **Description:** Provides clinician with practical reports on preventing, diagnosing and treating infectious complications.
Related titles: Online - full text ed.: (from Institute for Scientific Information).
Indexed: ASCA.
—BLDSC (4478.721550), CISTI, EMDOCS, GNLM, IDS, Infotrieve, KNAW. **CCC.**
Published by: Cliggott Publishing Co. (Subsidiary of: S C P Communications, Inc.), 330 Boston Post Rd, Darien, CT 06820. TEL 203-662-6400, FAX 203-662-6776, info.cliggott@scp.com, http://www.medscape.com, http://www.scp.com/. Ed., R&P Leo Cristofar. Pub. Jill Bresnick.

669 USA
▼ **INFECTIOUS DISEASE.** Text in English. 2000. irreg. price varies. illus. back issues avail. *Refereed.* **Document type:** *Monographic series, Academic/Scholarly.* **Description:** Contains articles and features on infectious diseases, immunology, internal medicine, microbiology, oncology and hematology.
Published by: Humana Press Inc., 999 Riverview Dr, Ste 208, Totowa, NJ 07512. TEL 973-256-1699, FAX 973-256-8341, humana@humanapr.com, http://humanapress.com. Ed. Vassil St. Georgiev. R&P Wendy A Warren.

616.9 USA ISSN 0739-7348
INFECTIOUS DISEASE ALERT. Text in English. 1981. s-m. USD 229 domestic; USD 259 foreign; USD 19 newsstand/cover (effective 2001). index. reprints avail. **Document type:** *Newsletter.*
Incorporates (1988-1991): A I D S Clinical Digest (0899-0263)
Related titles: Online - full text ed.: (from Northern Light Technology, Inc., Gale Group).
Published by: American Health Consultants (Subsidiary of: Medical Economics Co., Inc.), 3525 Piedmont Rd, N E, 6 Piedmont Center, Ste 400, Atlanta, GA 30305. TEL 404-262-5476, 404-262-7436, 800-688-2421, FAX 404-262-7837, 800-284-3291, custserv@ahcpub.com, http://www.ahcpub.com. Circ: 2,380.

616.9 USA ISSN 1043-2981
CODEN: IDTHER
INFECTIOUS DISEASE AND THERAPY SERIES. Text in English. 1989. irreg., latest vol.22, 1998. price varies. adv. **Document type:** *Monographic series.*
—BLDSC (4478.721800), CASDDS, CISTI, GNLM, Infotrieve, KNAW. **CCC.**
Published by: Marcel Dekker, Inc., Attn: Eridania Perrez, 270 Madison Ave, New York, NY 10016-0602. TEL 212-696-9000, 800-228-1160, FAX 212-685-4540, marketing@dekker.com, http://www.dekker.com. Pub. Russell Dekker. R&P Julia Mulligan. Adv. contact Eridania Perez.

616.9 USA ISSN 0891-5520
RC109 CODEN: IDCAEN
INFECTIOUS DISEASE CLINICS OF NORTH AMERICA. Variant title: Infectious Disease Clinics. Text in English. 1987. q. USD 140 domestic to individuals; USD 164 in Canada to individuals; USD 184 elsewhere to individuals; USD 197 domestic to institutions; USD 238 foreign to institutions; USD 60 per issue (effective 2001). index. back issues avail. *Refereed.* **Document type:** *Academic/Scholarly.* **Description:** Discusses a topic on the diagnosis or treatment of infectious diseases in each issue.
Related titles: Microform ed.: (from PQC); Online - full text ed.: (from Institute for Scientific Information).
Indexed: ASCA, CINAHL, Curr.Cont., Excerp.Med. (1992-), Helminthol.Abstr., INIS Atomind., Ind.Med. (1987-), Ind.Sci.Rev., Inpharma, Int.Nurs.Ind., Pharm.&Out.News, Protozool.Abstr., Reac., Rev.Appl.Entomol., SSCI (coverage dropped), Sci.Cit.Ind.
—BLDSC (4478.722000), CISTI, EMDOCS, GNLM, IDS, ingenta, KNAW. **CCC.**
Published by: W.B. Saunders Co. (Subsidiary of: Harcourt Publishers Ltd.), 11830 Westline Industrial Dr, St Louis, MO 63146. TEL 800-325-4177, http://www.wbsaunders.com. Ed. Robert C Moellering Jr.
Subscr. to: Periodicals Fulfillment, W B Saunders Co, 6277 Sea Harbor Dr, 4th Fl, Orlando, FL 32891-4800.

616.9 610 USA ISSN 1056-9251
INFECTIOUS DISEASE NEWS. Text in English. 1988. m. USD 170 domestic to individuals; USD 195 in Canada to individuals; USD 210 elsewhere to individuals; USD 180 domestic to institutions; USD 205 in Canada to institutions; USD 220 elsewhere to institutions.
Document type: *Academic/Scholarly.* **Description:** Features interviews with infectious disease specialists, reports from medical conferences and research presentations, and the latest information on government legislation affecting the infectious disease practice.
—**CCC.**
Published by: Slack, Inc., 6900 Grove Rd, Thorofare, NJ 08086-9447. TEL 856-848-1000, 800-257-8290, FAX 856-853-5991, http://www.slackinc.com. Ed. Dr. Theodore Eickhoff.

616.9 USA ISSN 0162-6493
INFECTIOUS DISEASE PRACTICE. Text in English. 1977. m. USD 89 domestic; USD 111 foreign (effective 2001). adv. back issues avail. **Description:** For physicians in practice or research. Each issue focuses on a specific disease presenting symptoms, differential diagnosis, clinical course, management, and treatment or prevention.
—**CCC.**
Published by: M B C Publications, Winthrop University Hospital, 222 Station Plaza N, Ste 432, Mineola, NY 11501-3432. TEL 516-663-4435, FAX 513-663-2753. Ed. Dr. Burke A Cunha. Adv. contact Barbara Miller. Circ: 700.

616.9 GBR ISSN 1465-7724
▼ **THE INFECTIOUS DISEASE REVIEW.** Text in English. 1999. q. GBP 35, USD 65 to individuals; GBP 92, USD 148 to institutions (effective 2001). 50 p./no. 2 cols./p. back issues avail. *Refereed.* **Document type:** *Journal, Academic/Scholarly.*

M

Related titles: Online - full text ed.: I D R Online.
—BLDSC (4478.722900).
Published by: Tamurlane Press Ltd, Greenfields 28 Conyngham Ln, Bridge, Canteburbury CT4 5JX, United Kingdom. FAX 44-1227-830-860, zoomed1@aol.com, http://www.idreview.co.uk/. Pub., Adv. contact Chris Furley.

616.9 ARG ISSN 0327-4438
INFECTOLOGIA Y MICROBIOLOGIA CLINICA. Text in Spanish. 1989. q.
Indexed: Abstr.Hyg., Trop.Dis.Bull.
—CISTI.
Published by: Asociacion Argentina de Microbiologia, P.B. B, Bulnes, 44, Capital Federal, Buenos Aires 1176, Argentina. TEL 54-114-85948880, aam@drwebsa.com.ar, http://www.drwebsa.com.ar/aam/.

616.9 BGR ISSN 0861-8259 CODEN: EMIBA3
INFEKTOLOGIIA/INFECTOLOGY. Text in Bulgarian; Summaries in English. 1991. q. USD 48 foreign (effective 2002). adv. *Refereed.* **Document type:** *Journal, Academic/Scholarly.* **Description:** Presents original articles, clinical cases and surveys from Bulgarian medical researchers and specialists in the field of epidemiology, microbiology, virology, parasitology, immunology, and infectious deseases.
Formerly (until 1992): Epidemiologiia, Mikrobiologiia i Infektsiozni Bolesti (0425-1482)
Indexed: Abstr.Bulg.Sci.Med.Lit., BSL Biol., Helminthol.Abstr., INIS Atomind.
—CASDDS, CISTI.
Published by: Natsionalen Tsentar po Zarasni i Parasitni Bolesti/National Center of Infectious and Parasitic Diseases, Yanko Sakazov blvd 26, Sofia 1504, Bulgaria. TEL 395-2-4347399, FAX 359-2-442260, 0473@main.infotel.bg. Ed. Bogdan Petrunov. adv.: B&W page USD 45, color page USD 130. Circ: 1,000. **Dist. by:** Sofia Books, Ul Silivria 16, Sofia 1404, Bulgaria. TEL 359-2-9586257, sofiabooks@hotmail.com, http://www.sofiabooks.hit.bg.

616.9792 USA
INSIGHTS IN H I V DISEASE MANAGEMENT* . Text in English. irreg. (2-4/yr.). free per issue. back issues avail. *Refereed.* **Document type:** *Academic/Scholarly, Trade.* **Description:** Presents articles to health care professionals providing treatment and support to patients with HIV infections and AIDS.
Formerly: Opportunistic Complications
Media: Online - full text.
Published by: (Pharmacia), Meniscus Educational Institute (Subsidiary of: Meniscus Ltd.), 18 Elizabeth St, West Conshohocken, PA 19428-2935. TEL 610-660-8080, FAX 610-660-9634, http://www.meniscus.com/hiv/. Ed. Kristi E Eidsvoog. Pub. Lois Trench Hines.
Co-sponsor: Upjohn.

INSTITUT PASTEUR HELLENIQUE. ARCHIVES. see *BIOLOGY—Microbiology*

616.9 636.089 IRN ISSN 0365-3439
INSTITUT RAZI. ARCHIVES. Key Title: Arshiv-i Mu'assasah-i Razi. Text and summaries in English, French. 1933. a. free per issue. 150 p./no. 1 cols./p. reprints avail. *Refereed.* **Document type:** *Journal, Academic/Scholarly.* **Description:** Covers human and veterinary vaccines and the diagnosis of infectious diseases.
Formerly (until 1963): Institut d'Hessarek. Archives (0365-3196)
Indexed: Biol.Abstr., Dairy Sci.Abstr., Ind.Vet., Poult.Abstr., Protozool.Abstr., Vet.Bull., Zoo.Rec.
Published by: Institut Razi/Razi Vaccine & Serum Research Institute, P O Box 11365-1588, Tehran, Iran. TEL 98-261-452005, FAX 98-261-454658. Ed. Dr. M A Akhavizadegan.

INSTITUTO DE HIGIENE E MEDICINA TROPICAL. ANAIS. see *PUBLIC HEALTH AND SAFETY*

616.988 BRA ISSN 0036-4665 CODEN: RMTSAE
INSTITUTO DE MEDICINA TROPICAL DE SAO PAULO. REVISTA. Text in English; Summaries in English, Portuguese, Spanish. 1959. bi-m. USD 200 (effective 1999). adv. bk.rev. abstr, illus. index. back issues avail. **Document type:** *Academic/Scholarly.*
Related titles: Microform ed.: (from PQC); Online - full text ed.: (from SciELO, ProQuest Information & Learning).
Indexed: Abstr.Hyg., B.R.I., Bio-Contr.News & Info., Biol.Abstr., Curr.Adv.Ecol.Sci., Curr.Cont. (coverage dropped), Dairy Sci.Abstr., Dent.Ind., Excerp.Med., Helminthol.Abstr., INIS Atomind., Ind.Med. (1959-), Ind.Vet., Nutr.Abstr., Pig News & Info., Protozool.Abstr., Ref.Zh., Rev.Appl.Entomol., Rev.Med.& Vet.Mycol., Rev.Plant Path., Rural Devel.Abstr., Sci.Cit.Ind. (coverage dropped), Trop.Dis.Bull., Vet.Bull., Zoo.Rec.
—BLDSC (7819.850000), CASDDS, CISTI, GNLM, ingenta, KNAW.
Published by: Instituto de Medicina Tropical de Sao Paulo, Universidad de Sao Paulo, Av Dr Eneas Carvalho de Aguiar, 470, C Cesar, Sao Paulo, SP 05403-000, Brazil. TEL 55-11-852-2174, FAX 55-11-852-2174, rimtsp@edu.usp.br, http://www.usp.br/geral/noticia/imtsp.html. Ed. Thales F de Brito. Circ: 1,300.

616.9 572 579 GBR ISSN 0965-2310 CODEN: IANWEL
INTERNATIONAL ANTIVIRAL NEWS. Abbreviated title: I A V N. Text in English. 1993. 10/yr. GBP 65 domestic to individuals; USD 105 foreign to individuals; GBP 320 domestic to institutions; USD 515 foreign to institutions (effective 2000). adv. bk.rev. *Refereed.* **Document type:** *Newsletter.* **Description:** Reviews the latest developments in antiviral research.
Indexed: Abstr.Hyg., Excerp.Med. (1994-), Inpharma, Pharm.&Out.News, Reac.
—BLDSC (4535.940000), EMDOCS, GNLM.
Published by: International Medical Press, 125 High Holborn, London WC1V 6QA, United Kingdom. TEL 44-20-7831-3106, FAX 44-20-7831-0036, iavn@intmedpress.com, http://www.intmedpress.com/impweb/journals/iavn/iavnhome.html. Ed. Hugh J Field. Pub. Stephen Cameron. R&P Colin Drummond. Adv. contact Simon Gee. page GBP 1,000. Circ: 150.

616.97 USA ISSN 1081-454X
INTERNATIONAL ASSOCIATION OF PHYSICIANS IN AIDS CARE. JOURNAL. Text in English. 1989. m. USD 60 domestic; USD 100 foreign (effective 2000). adv. bk.rev. *Refereed.* **Document type:** *Trade.* **Description:** Provides insightful updates on the status of promising AIDS research and covers research policy and proposed regulations. Provides a forum for the observations and recommendations of leading researchers.
Former titles (until 1995): Physicians Association for AIDS Care. Journal (1074-2395); P A A C Notes (1059-7913)
Indexed: Abstr.Hyg., CINAHL, Rev.Med.& Vet.Mycol., Rural Devel.Abstr.
Published by: International Association of Physicians in AIDS Care, 33 N La Salle St, Ste 1700, Chicago, IL 60602-2601. TEL 312-795-4934, FAX 312-795-4938, JIAPAC@iapac.org, http://www.iapac.org. Ed. Richard Marlink. Adv. contact Jill Perrigo.

616.96 POL ISSN 0074-3356
INTERNATIONAL COMMISSION ON TRICHINELLOSIS. PROCEEDINGS. Text in Polish. 1962. irreg. price varies. bk.rev. **Document type:** *Proceedings.*
Related titles: ♦ Issued with: Wiadomosci Parazytologiczne. ISSN 0043-5163.
Published by: Polskie Towarzystwo Parazytologiczne/Polish Parasitological Society, Ul Grochowska 272, Warsaw 03849, Poland. TEL 48-22-6089061. Ed. Aleksander Bielecki. Circ: 800.

616.9 USA ISSN 0074-4212
INTERNATIONAL CONGRESSES ON TROPICAL MEDICINE AND MALARIA. (PROCEEDINGS). (Proceedings issued at discretion of host country; none issued for 8th, 1968, Teheran) Text in English. 1948. quadrennial, latest 1992, 13th, Bangkok. **Document type:** *Proceedings.*
Published by: International Federation for Tropical Medicine, c/o Dr Wm A Sodeman, Sec -Gen, Medical College of Ohio, Box 10008, Toledo, OH 43699-0008. Circ: 1,500.

616.96 GBR ISSN 0020-7519
QL757 CODEN: IJPYBT
INTERNATIONAL JOURNAL FOR PARASITOLOGY. Text in English. 1971. 14/yr. EUR 1,321 in Europe to institutions; JPY 175,400 in Japan to institutions; USD 1,477 elsewhere to institutions (effective 2002). adv. bk.rev. back issues avail.; reprint service avail. from PQC. *Refereed.* **Document type:** *Academic/Scholarly.* **Description:** Serves as an international medium for the communication of scientific contributions in the field of parasitology.
Related titles: Microfilm ed.: (from PQC); Online - full text ed.: (from ingenta, Swets Blackwell, ScienceDirect, Institute for Scientific Information).
Indexed: AIDS & Cancer Res., ASCA, Abstr.Hyg., AgBiotech, Agricola, Anim.Breed.Abstr., Appl.Ecol.Abstr., Aqua.Sci.& Fish.Abstr., Aquacult.Abstr., Bibl.Agri., Bio-Contr.News & Info., Biotech.& Bioeng.Abstr., Chem.Abstr., Chem.Indus.Notes, Chem.Titles, Curr.Adv.Ecol.Sci., Curr.Cont., Dairy Sci.Abstr., Dent.Ind., Derwent Biotech.Abstr., Ecol.Abstr., Entomol.Abstr., Environ.Sci.Poll.Mgmt., Excerp.Med., Focus on: Vet.Sci.& Med., Food Sci.& Tech.Abstr., Genet.Abstr., Helminthol.Abstr., Hort.Abstr., Hum.Gen.Abstr., IDA, INIS Atomind., Immun.Abstr., Ind.Med. (1971-), Ind.Sci.Rev., Ind.Vet., Inpharma, Int.Abstr.Biol.Sci., Microbiol.Abstr., Nutr.Abstr., Ocean.Abstr. (coverage dropped), Ornam.Hort., Pig News & Info., Poult.Abstr., Protozool.Abstr., Reac., Rev.Appl.Entomol., Rev.Arom.& Med.Plants, Rev.Med.& Vet.Mycol., Rev.Plant Path., Sci.Cit.Ind., Small Anim.Abstr., Soyabean Abstr., Sport Fish.Abstr., Trop.Dis.Bull., Vet.Bull., Weed Abstr., Wild.Rev., Zoo.Rec.
—BLDSC (4542.449000), ADONIS, CASDDS, CISTI, EMDOCS, GNLM, IDS, ingenta. **CCC.**
Published by: (Australian Society for Parasitology AUS), Pergamon (Subsidiary of: Elsevier Science), The Boulevard, Langford Ln, East Park, Kidlington, Oxford OXB 1GB, United Kingdom. FAX 44-1865-843010, http://www.elsevier.com/locate/ijpara. Ed. A M Johnson. Circ: 1,250. **Subscr. in Australasia and the Far East to:** Elsevier Science (Singapore) Pte Ltd, No.1 Temasek Ave, 17-01 Millenia Tower, Singapore 039192, Singapore. TEL 65-434-3727, FAX 65-337-2230; **Subscr. in the Americas to:** Elsevier Science, PO Box 945, New York, NY 10159-0945. TEL 212-633-3730, FAX 212-633-3680, usinfo-f@elsevier.com; **Subscr. to:** Elsevier Science BV, PO Box 211, Amsterdam 1000 AE, Netherlands. TEL 31-20-485-3757.

616.9 CAN ISSN 1201-9712 CODEN: IJIDF3
INTERNATIONAL JOURNAL OF INFECTIOUS DISEASES. Text in English. 1996. q. USD 95 in US & Canada to individuals; USD 119 elsewhere to individuals; USD 145 in US & Canada to institutions; USD 169 elsewhere to institutions (effective 2001). back issues avail. *Refereed.* **Document type:** *Journal, Academic/Scholarly.* **Description:** Communicates information relevant to the epidemiology, clinical evaluation, diagnosis, treatment, and control of infectious diseases, with an emphasis on those most prevalent in less-developed countries.
Related titles: Online - full text ed.: (from ProQuest Information & Learning).
Indexed: Ind.Med. (1996-), Jrnl.Watch Inf.Dis., Ref.Zh., Rev.Appl.Entomol., Rev.Med.& Vet.Mycol.
—BLDSC (4542.304750), GNLM, Infotrieve, KNAW. **CCC.**
Published by: (International Society of Infectious Diseases), B.C. Decker Inc., 20 Hughson St S, LCD 1, P O Box 620, Hamilton, ON L8N 3K7, Canada. TEL 905-522-7017, 800-568-7281, FAX 905-522-7839, info@bcdecker.com, http://www.bcdecker.com. Ed. Donald Armstrong. Pub. David LeGallais. R&P Paula Presutti. Adv. contact John Birkby. Circ: 3,145.

616.998 USA ISSN 0148-916X CODEN: IJLEAG
INTERNATIONAL JOURNAL OF LEPROSY AND OTHER MYCOBACTERIAL DISEASES. Text in English. 1933. q. USD 80 to individuals; USD 120 to institutions (effective 2001). adv. bk.rev. abstr, bibl, charts, illus. cum.index: 1932-1966. back issues avail. *Refereed.* **Document type:** *Academic/Scholarly.* **Description:** Includes articles on clinical leprosy, diagnosis, management, leprosy control, and research. Functions as the house organ of the International Leprosy Association.
Formerly: International Journal of Leprosy (0020-7349)
Related titles: Online - full text ed.: (from ProQuest Information & Learning, Institute for Scientific Information).
Indexed: ASCA, Abstr.Hyg., Biol.Abstr., Chem.Abstr., Curr.Adv.Ecol.Sci., Curr.Cont., Environ.Sci.Poll.Mgmt., Excerp.Med., Helminthol.Abstr., INIS Atomind., Ind.Med. (1966-), Ind.Sci.Rev., Inpharma, Med.& Surg.Dermat., Microbiol.Abstr., Pharm.&Out.News, Pollut.Abstr., Reac., Ref.Zh., Risk Abstr., SSCI (coverage dropped), Saf.Sci.Abstr., Sci.Cit.Ind., So.Pac.Per.Ind., Trop.Dis.Bull.
—BLDSC (4542.319000), CASDDS, CISTI, GNLM, IDS, ingenta, KNAW.
Published by: International Leprosy Association, One ALM Way, Greenville, SC 29601. TEL 864-271-7040, FAX 864-271-7062, IJL@leprosy.org, http://uncweb.carl.org. Ed., R&P Robert C Hastings. Adv. contact Robert Hastings. Circ: 1,000. **Subscr. to:** Allen Press Inc., PO Box 1897, Lawrence, KS 66044-8897.

M

616.014 DEU ISSN 1438-4221
QR46 CODEN: ZEBAE8
INTERNATIONAL JOURNAL OF MEDICAL MICROBIOLOGY. Text in English. 8/yr. EUR 337, GBP 230 to individuals; EUR 783, GBP 574 to institutions (effective 2002). *Refereed.* **Document type:** *Journal, Academic/Scholarly.* **Description:** Maintains a broad concept of microbiology that includes all aspects of medical as well as veterinary bacteriology, virology, parasitology and infectious diseases.
Former titles (until 2000): Zentralblatt fuer Bakteriologie (0934-8840); Zentralblatt fuer Bakteriologie, Parasitenkunde, Infektionskrankheiten und Hygiene. Series A: Medizinische Mikrobiologie und Parasitologie (0174-3031)
Related titles: Microfilm ed.: (from VCI); Online - full text ed.; (from Institute for Scientific Information).
Indexed: ASCA, Abstr.Hyg., AgBiotech, Aqua.Sci.& Fish.Abstr., Biol.Abstr., Chem.Abstr., Chem.Indus.Notes, Chem.Titles, Curr.Cont., Dairy Sci.Abstr., Dent.Ind., Derwent Biotech.Abstr., Environ.Sci.Poll.Mgmt., Genet.Abstr., Helminthol.Abstr., Ind.Med. (2000-), Ind.Sci.Rev., Ind.Vet., Inpharma, Int.Abstr.Biol.Sci., Microbiol.Abstr., Pharm.&Out.News, Poult.Abstr., Protozool.Abstr., Reac., Rev.Appl.Entomol., Rev.Arom.& Med.Plants, Rev.Med.& Vet.Mycol., Sci.Cit.Ind., Soils & Fert., Trop.Dis.Bull., Vet.Bull., Weed Abstr.
—BLDSC (4542.346000), CASDDS, CISTI, EMDOCS, GNLM, IDS, Infotrieve, ingenta, KNAW. **CCC.**
Published by: Urban & Fischer Verlag, Loebdergraben 14A, Jena 07743, Germany. TEL 49-3641-626444, FAX 49-3641-626421, info@urbanfischer.de, http://www.urbanfischer.de. Ed. Joerg Hacker. Adv. contact Sabine Schroeter.

616.9 GBR ISSN 0956-4624
RC201.A1 CODEN: INSAE3
INTERNATIONAL JOURNAL OF S T D & AIDS. Variant title: International Journal of Sexually Transmitted Diseases and Acquired Immunodeficiency Syndrome. Text in English. 1990. m. GBP 169 in Europe to individuals; USD 304 in United States to individuals; GBP 181 elsewhere to individuals; GBP 260 in Europe to institutions; USD 445 in United States to institutions; GBP 272 elsewhere to institutions (effective 2002). adv. bk.rev. illus. index. *Refereed.* **Document type:** *Journal, Academic/Scholarly.* **Description:** Clinically oriented forum for papers on both the traditional sexually transmissible diseases (STD) and AIDS.
Related titles: Online - full text ed.: (from CatchWord Ltd., Ovid Technologies, Inc., EBSCO Publishing, O C L C Online Computer Library Center, Inc., RoweCom Information Quest, ProQuest Information & Learning, Swets Blackwell, Institute for Scientific Information).
Indexed: AIDS & Cancer Res., AIDS Abstr., Abstr.Hyg., Curr.Cont., Environ.Sci.Poll.Mgmt., Helminthol.Abstr., Ind.Med. (1990-), Inpharma, Int.Abstr.Biol.Sci., Int.Nurs.Ind., Pharm.&Out.News, Protozool.Abstr., PsycInfo, Psychol.Abstr. (1993-), Reac., Rev.Med.& Vet.Mycol., Risk Abstr., SSCI (coverage dropped), Saf.Sci.Abstr., Trop.Dis.Bull., Virol.Abstr., e-psyche.
—BLDSC (4542.681350), ADONIS, CatchWord, CISTI, EMDOCS, GNLM, IDS, ingenta, KNAW. **CCC.**
Published by: Royal Society of Medicine Press Ltd, 1 Wimpole St, London W1M 8AE, United Kingdom. TEL 44-20-7290-2921, FAX 44-20-7290-2929, rsmjournals@rsm.ac.uk, http://www.roysocmed.ac.uk/pub/std.htm. Ed. Wallace Dinsmore. Circ: 900.

616.988 POL
CODEN: BIMGDE
INTERNATIONAL MARITIME HEALTH. Text and summaries in English. 1948. q. USD 50 (effective 2000). adv. bk.rev. *Refereed.* **Document type:** *Bulletin, Academic/Scholarly.* **Description:** Covers occupational diseases and maritime hygiene related to the work of seamen, fishermen and maritime ports personnel; parasitology, bacteriology, sea water control, and travel medicine.
Former titles (until vol.50, 1999): Instytut Medycyny Morskiej i Tropikalnej w Gdyni. Bulletin Institute of Maritime and Tropical Medicine in Gdynia. Bulletin (0324-8542); (until 1974): Instytut Medycyny Morskiej w Gdansku. Biuletyn Institute of Marine Medicine in Gdansk. Bulletin (0020-4463)
Indexed: Abstr.Hyg., Anal.Abstr., Biol.Abstr., C.I.S. Abstr., Chem.Abstr., Excerp.Med., Ind.Med. (coverage dropped), Protozool.Abstr., Rev.Appl.Entomol., Rev.Med.& Vet.Mycol., Rural Devel.Abstr., Rural Recreat.Tour.Abstr., Trop.Dis.Bull.
—BLDSC (2580.890500), CASDDS, CISTI, GNLM.
Published by: Instytut Medycyny Morskiej i Tropikalnej w Gdyni, Ul Powstania Styczniowego 9 B, Gdynia-Radlowo 81-519, Poland. TEL 48-58-223011, FAX 48-58-6223354, root@immt.gdynia.pl. Ed. S Tomaszunas. R&P Stanislaw Tomaszunas. Circ: 700.

616.9 ZAF
INTERNATIONAL STATISTICAL CLASSIFICATION OF DISEASES & RELATED HEALTH PROBLEMS. Text in English. irreg., latest 1996. Free. stat. **Document type:** *Government.*
Published by: Statistics South Africa/Statistieke Suid-Afrika, Private Bag X44, Pretoria 0001, South Africa. TEL 27-12-310-8911, FAX 27-12-310-8500, info@statssa.pwv.gov.za, http://www.statssa.gov.za.

616.9 IRL
IRELAND. NATIONAL DISEASE SURVEILLANCE CENTRE. REPORT ON THE EPIDEMIOLOGY OF TUBERCULOSIS IN IRELAND. Text in English. irreg.
Published by: National Disease Surveillance Centre, Sir Patrick Dun's Hospital, Lower Grand Canal Street, Dublin 2, Ireland. TEL 353-1-6617346, FAX 353-1-6617347, info@ndsc.ie, http://www.ndsc.ie.

616.9792 USA ISSN 1525-4135
RC607.A26 CODEN: JDSRET
J A I D S. (Journal of Acquired Immune Deficiency Syndromes) Text in English. 1988. 15/yr. USD 308 domestic to individuals for print & online eds.; USD 368 foreign to individuals for print & online eds.; USD 791 domestic to institutions for print & online eds.; USD 791 newsstand/cover foreign to institutions (effective 2002). adv. bibl. reprint service avail. from PQC. *Refereed.* **Document type:** *Academic/Scholarly.* **Description:** Provides results of clinical trials, case reports, reviews of current research, discussions of national policy issues and a literature citation index.
Former titles (until 1999): Journal of Acquired Immune Deficiency Syndromes and Human Retrovirology (1077-9450); (until 1995): Journal of Acquired Immune Deficiency Syndromes (0894-9255)
Related titles: Online - full text ed.: USD 1,028.30 domestic academic site license; USD 1,028.30 foreign academic site license; USD 1,146.95 domestic corporate site license; USD 1,146.95 foreign corporate site license (effective 2002) (from Ovid Technologies, Inc., Swets Blackwell, Institute for Scientific Information).
Indexed: AIDS & Cancer Res., AIDS Abstr., ASCA, Abstr.Hyg., Addic.Abstr., Biol.Abstr., CINAHL, Chem.Abstr., Chem.Indus.Notes, Chem.Titles, Curr.Cont., Curr.Ind.Stat., Environ.Sci.Poll.Mgmt., Excerp.Med., Immun.Abstr., Ind.Med. (1999-), Ind.Sci.Rev., Ind.Vet., Inpharma, Int.Nurs.Ind., Jrnl.Watch Inf.Dis., Med.& Surg.Dermat., NRN, Nutr.Abstr., Pharm.&Out.News, Pollut.Abstr., Protozool.Abstr., Reac., Rev.Med.& Vet.Mycol., Risk Abstr., SSCI (coverage dropped), Saf.Sci.Abstr., Sci.Cit.Ind., THA, Trop.Dis.Bull., Vet.Bull., Virol.Abstr.
—BLDSC (4644.422000), CASDDS, EMDOCS, GNLM, IDS, ingenta, KNAW.
Published by: Lippincott Williams & Wilkins (Philadelphia) (Subsidiary of: Wolters Kluwer N.V.), 530 Walnut St, Philadelphia, PA 19106-3621. TEL 215-521-8300, FAX 215-521-8902, http://www.Lww.com. Pub. Terri Monturano. R&P Alice McElhinney. adv.: B&W page USD 1,065, color page USD 2,375; trim 11 x 8.25. Circ: 3,000 (paid). **Subscr. to:** PO Box 1600, Hagerstown, MD 21740-1600. TEL 800-777-2295, FAX 301-824-7390.

616.9792 USA
▼ **J A M A HIV - AIDS NEWSLINE.** (Journal of the American Medical Association) Text in English. 1999. w. back issues avail. *Refereed.*
Media: Online - full text.
Published by: American Medical Association, J A M A Information Centers, 515 N State St, Chicago, IL 60610. TEL 312-464-5000, 800-262-2350, FAX 312-464-4181, hiv-comments@ama-assn.org, http://www.ama-assn.org/special/hiv/hivhome.htm.

616.95 USA
J A M A SEXUALLY TRANSMITTED DISEASE. (Journal of the American Medical Association) Text in English. 1998. w. back issues avail. *Refereed.*
Media: Online - full text.
Published by: American Medical Association, J A M A Information Centers, 515 N State St, Chicago, IL 60610. TEL 312-464-5000, 800-262-2350, FAX 312-464-4181, std@ama-assn.org, http://www.ama-assn.org/special/std/std.htm.

614.49 IND ISSN 0971-8834
J K PRACTITIONER. Text in English. 1994. q. INR 400 to individuals; INR 500 to institutions (effective 2001). adv. abstr, bibl, charts, illus. 100 p./no. 2 cols./p. back issues avail.; reprints avail. *Refereed.* **Document type:** *Journal.* **Description:** International journal of current medical sciences & practice.
—BLDSC (4669.427500).
Address: P O Box 884, Srinagar, Jammu & Kashmir, India. TEL 0194-432060, FAX 0194-479298, jkpractm@vsnl.com. Ed., Pub., R&P, Adv. contact GM Malik. B&W page INR 8,000, color page INR 12,000. Circ: 1,500 (paid); 500 (controlled).

616.9 JPN ISSN 0387-5911
CODEN: KSSZAT
JAPANESE ASSOCIATION FOR INFECTIOUS DISEASES. JOURNAL/KANSENSHOGAKU ZASSHI. Text in Japanese; Summaries in English. 1911. m. membership. adv. charts, illus.
Formerly (until 1970): Nippon Densembyo Gakkai Zasshi (0021-4817)
Indexed: Biol.Abstr., Chem.Abstr., Dent.Ind., Excerp.Med., INIS Atomind., Ind.Med. (1970-), Inpharma, Int.Nurs.Ind., Reac., Ref.Zh., Rev.Med.& Vet.Mycol.
—BLDSC (4808.800000), CASDDS, CISTI, GNLM, KNAW.
Published by: Japanese Association for Infectious Diseases/Nihon Kansensho Gakkai, Sankei 8 Bldg, 6F, 1-8-7 Ebisu, Shibuya-ku, Tokyo 150-0013, Japan.

616.01 JPN ISSN 0021-4930
CODEN: NSKZAM
JAPANESE JOURNAL OF BACTERIOLOGY/NIHON SAIKINGAKU ZASSHI. Text in English. 1944. q. JPY 18,540. adv. bk.rev. bibl, charts. **Document type:** *Academic/Scholarly.*
Indexed: Abstr.Hyg., Biol.Abstr., Chem.Abstr., Dairy Sci.Abstr., Excerp.Med., Food Sci.& Tech.Abstr., Hort.Abstr., INIS Atomind., Ind.Med. (1944-), Jap.Per.Ind., Rev.Med.& Vet.Mycol., Rev.Plant Path., Sugar Ind.Abstr., Trop.Dis.Bull.
—CASDDS, CISTI, GNLM, Infotrieve, Linda Hall. **CCC.**
Published by: (Japanese Society for Bacteriology/Nihon Saikin Gakkai), Business Center for Academic Societies Japan/Nihon Gakkai Jimu Senta, 5-16-9 Honkomagome, Bunkyo-ku, Tokyo 113-0021, Japan. FAX 81-3-5814-5822, 81-3-5814-5822. Circ: 3,700.

616.998 JPN ISSN 0386-3980
CODEN: NRGZDW
JAPANESE JOURNAL OF LEPROSY. Text mainly in Japanese; Summaries in English. 1930. q. JPY 5,000, USD 15. adv. bk.rev. charts, illus. index.
Formerly (until vol.46, no.1): Leppro (0024-1008)
Indexed: Abstr.Hyg., Chem.Abstr., Excerp.Med., INIS Atomind., Ind.Med. (coverage dropped), Trop.Dis.Bull.
—BLDSC (4655.870000), CASDDS, EMDOCS, GNLM.
Published by: Japanese Leprosy Association/Nihon Rai Gakukai, 2-1 Aoba-cho 4-chome, Higashimurayama-shi, Tokyo-to 189-0002, Japan. Ed. Dr. Masahide Abe. Circ: 700.

616.988 JPN ISSN 0304-2146
JAPANESE JOURNAL OF TROPICAL MEDICINE AND HYGIENE. Text in English. 1959. q. JPY 7,000 (effective 2000). abstr. reprints avail.
Formerly (until 1973): Japanese Journal of Tropical Medicine
Indexed: Abstr.Hyg., Diar.Dis.Res., Helminthol.Abstr., Ind.Vet., Protozool.Abstr., Rev.Appl.Entomol., Rev.Arom.& Med.Plants, Rev.Med.& Vet.Mycol., Trop.Dis.Bull., Vet.Bull., Zoo.Rec.
—BLDSC (4658.970000), CISTI, Infotrieve. **CCC.**
Published by: Japanese Society of Tropical Medicine/Nihon Nettai Igakkai, c/o Institute of Tropical Medicine, University, 12-4 Sakamo-To, Nagasaki-shi 852-8523, Japan. http://www.tm.nagasaki-u.ac.jp/society/jstm/gkmain.html. Ed. Dr. Masahiro Takagi TEL 81-95-849-7810. Circ: 700.

616.9 GBR ISSN 0305-7453
CODEN: JACHDX
JOURNAL OF ANTIMICROBIAL CHEMOTHERAPY. Text in English. 1975. m. (in 2 vols.). GBP 260, USD 430 to individuals; GBP 460, USD 810 to institutions (effective 2002). adv. bk.rev. illus, charts. index. back issues avail.; reprint service avail. from SWZ. *Refereed.* **Document type:** *Journal, Academic/Scholarly.* **Description:** Presents original articles about laboratory and clinical aspects of the use of antimicrobials, including antibacterial, antiviral, antifungal, antihelminthic, and antiprotozoal agents; also includes reviews, articles, Working Party reports, and correspondence on related subjects.
Related titles: Online - full text ed.: ISSN 1460-2091. GBP 234, USD 387 to individuals Online only; GBP 414, USD 729 to institutions Online only (effective 2002) (from HighWire Pr., EBSCO Publishing, O C L C Online Computer Library Center, Inc., RoweCom Information Quest, ingenta, Swets Blackwell, Institute for Scientific Information).

M

Indexed: AIDS Abstr., ASCA, Abstr.Hyg., Agri.& Environ.Biotech.Abstr., Biol.Abstr., Chem.Abstr., Chem.Indus.Notes, Chem.Titles, Curr.Cont., Dairy Sci.Abstr., Dent.Ind., Derwent Biotech.Abstr., Diar.Dis.Res., Environ.Sci.Poll.Mgmt., Excerp.Med., Helminthol.Abstr., INIS Atomind., I.P.A., Ind.Med. (1975-), Ind.Sci.Rev., Ind.Vet., Inpharma, Int.Abstr.Biol.Sci., Med.& Pharm.Biotech.Abstr., Med.& Surg.Dermat., Microbiol.Abstr., Pharm.&Out.News, Protozool.Abstr., Reac., Rev.Med.& Vet.Mycol., Rev.Plant Path., Sci.Cit.Ind., Trop.Dis.Bull., Vet.Bull.

—BLDSC (4939.100000), CASDDS, CISTI, EMDOCS, GNLM, IDS, ingenta, KNAW. **CCC.**

Published by: (British Society for Antimicrobial Chemotherapy), Oxford University Press, Academic Division, Great Clarendon St, Oxford OX2 6DP, United Kingdom. TEL 44-1865-267907, FAX 44-1865-267835, jnl.info@oup.co.uk, http://jac.oupjournals.org/, http://www.oup.co.uk/journals. Ed. M J Wood. Pub. Mandy Sketch. R&P Fionna Willis. adv.: B&W page GBP 250, B&W page USD 450; trim 238 x 182. Circ: 2,450. **Subscr. in the US to:** Oxford University Press, Journals. TEL 800-852-7323, FAX 919-677-1714, jnl.info@oup.co.uk; **Subscr. to:** Journals Marketing, Great Clarendon St, Oxford OX2 6DP, United Kingdom.

616.9 NLD ISSN 1386-6532 CODEN: JCVIFB

JOURNAL OF CLINICAL VIROLOGY. Text in English. 1993. 9/yr. EUR 1,048 in Europe to institutions; JPY 139,200 in Japan to institutions; USD 1,172 elsewhere to institutions (effective 2002). adv. bk.rev. index. back issues avail.; reprints avail. *Refereed.* **Document type:** *Academic/Scholarly.* **Description:** Publishes papers on all aspects of human virology directly pertaining to virus-induced clinical conditions, covering epidemiology, pathogenesis, diagnosis and detection, and prevention and treatment.

Formerly: Clinical and Diagnostic Virology (0928-0197)

Related titles: Microform ed.: (from PQC); Online - full text ed.: (from ingenta, Swets Blackwell, ScienceDirect, Institute for Scientific Information).

Indexed: ASCA, Abstr.Hyg., Biotech.& Bioeng.Abstr., Curr.Cont., Environ.Sci.Poll.Mgmt., Excerp.Med. (1994-), Ind.Med. (1998-), Ind.Sci.Rev., Ind.Vet., Inpharma, Int.Abstr.Biol.Sci., Pharm.&Out.News, Reac., Rev.Appl.Entomol., Rev.Med.& Vet.Mycol., Sci.Cit.Ind., Trop.Dis.Bull., Vet.Bull., Virol.Abstr.

—BLDSC (4958.791700), CASDDS, CISTI, EMDOCS, GNLM, IDS, Infotrieve, KNAW. **CCC.**

Published by: Elsevier Science BV, PO Box 211, Amsterdam 1000 AE, Netherlands. TEL 31-20-485-2911, FAX 31-20-485-2457, http://www.elsevier.nl/locate/jcv. Eds. M Chernesky, P Leinikki. **Subscr. in Australasia and the Far East to:** Elsevier Science (Singapore) Pte Ltd, No.1 Temasek Ave, 17-01 Millenia Tower, Singapore 039192, Singapore. TEL 65-434-3727, FAX 65-337-2230; **Subscr. in Japan to:** Elsevier Science Inc - Japan Regional Office, 9-15 Higashi-Azabu 1-chome, Minato-ku, Tokyo 106-0044, Japan. TEL 81-3-5561-5033; **Subscr. in the Americas to:** Elsevier Science, PO Box 945, New York, NY 10159-0945. TEL 212-633-3730, FAX 212-633-3680, usinfo-f@elsevier.com.

610 IND ISSN 0019-5138 CODEN: JCDSBF

JOURNAL OF COMMUNICABLE DISEASES. Text in English. 1969. q. INR 40, USD 10.

Indexed: Abstr.Hyg., Aqua.Sci.& Fish.Abstr., Aquacult.Abstr., Bio-Contr.News & Info., Biol.Abstr., Dairy Sci.Abstr., Diar.Dis.Res., Environ.Sci.Poll.Mgmt., Excerp.Med., Helminthol.Abstr., IDA, Ind.Med. (1969-), Ind.Vet., Int.Nurs.Ind., Pig News & Info., Pollut.Abstr., Protozool.Abstr., Ref.Zh., Rev.Appl.Entomol., Rev.Arom.& Med.Plants, Rev.Med.& Vet.Mycol., Rice Abstr., Trop.Dis.Bull., Vet.Bull., Zoo.Rec.

—BLDSC (4961.450000), CISTI, GNLM, ingenta, KNAW.

Published by: Indian Society for Malaria and Other Communicable Diseases, 22 Alipur Rd., New Delhi 110 006, India.

JOURNAL OF HEALTHCARE SAFETY, COMPLIANCE & INFECTION CONTROL. see *OCCUPATIONAL HEALTH AND SAFETY*

616.96 GBR ISSN 0022-149X CODEN: JOHLAT

JOURNAL OF HELMINTHOLOGY. Text in English. 1923. q. GBP 240 to institutions; USD 420 in the Americas to institutions; GBP 255 to institutions Includes single site online accesss; USD 425 in the Americas to institutions Includes single site online access (effective 2002). adv. bk.rev. charts, illus. back issues avail. *Refereed.* **Document type:** *Academic/Scholarly.* **Description:** Provides an international vehicle for the publication of original papers and review articles on all aspects of pure and applied heminthology, particularly those helmminth parasites of environmental health, medical or veterinary importance.

Related titles: Online - full text ed.: GBP 215 to institutions; USD 375 in the Americas to institutions (effective 2002) (from EBSCO Publishing, RoweCom Information Quest, ingenta, Swets Blackwell, Institute for Scientific Information).

Indexed: ASCA, Abstr.Hyg., Agri.& Environ.Biotech.Abstr. (coverage dropped), Agricola, Bio-Contr.News & Info., Biol.Abstr., Chem.Abstr., Chem.Indus.Notes, Chem.Titles, Curr.Adv.Ecol.Sci., Curr.Cont., Curr.Ref.Fish Res., Derwent Biotech.Abstr., Ecol.Abstr., Excerp.Med., Food Sci.& Tech.Abstr., Helminthol.Abstr., IDA, INIS Atomind., Ind.Med. (1923-), Ind.Sci.Rev., Ind.Vet., Int.Abstr.Biol.Sci., Nutr.Abstr., Pig News & Info., Poult.Abstr., Protozool.Abstr., Rev.Appl.Entomol., Rev.Arom.& Med.Plants, Rev.Med.& Vet.Mycol., Sci.Cit.Ind., Small Anim.Abstr., Sport Fish.Abstr., Trop.Dis.Bull., Vet.Bull., Wild.Rev., Zoo.Rec.

—BLDSC (4997.000000), CASDDS, CISTI, GNLM, IDS, ingenta, Linda Hall. **CCC.**

Published by: CABI Publishing, Wallingford, Oxon OX10 8DE, United Kingdom. TEL 44-1491-832111, FAX 44-1491-829198, publishing@cabi.org, http://www.cabi.org/Publishing/Products/Journals/Primary/JOH/Index.asp. Ed. J W Lewis. Adv. contact S Harris. B&W page GBP 175; 170 x 225. **U.S. subscr. to:** 10 E 40th St, Ste 3203, New York, NY 10016. TEL 212-481-7018, 800-528-4841, FAX 212-686-7993, cabi-nao@cabi.org.

616.988 EGY

JOURNAL OF HEPATOLOGY, GASTROENTEROLOGY, INFECTIOUS DISEASES. Abbreviated title: J H G I D. Text in English. 1991 (vol.1, no.3). irreg. *Refereed.* **Document type:** *Academic/Scholarly.*

Formerly (until 1995): Journal of Tropical Medicine (1110-0796)

—BLDSC (4997.730000), CISTI, GNLM.

Published by: Egyptian Society of Hepatology, Gastroenterology & Infectious Diseases, 41 Talaat Harb St., Cairo, Egypt. TEL 20-2-391-5115, FAX 20-2-393-8723. Ed. S M Kabil. **Co-sponsor:** Royal Society of Tropical Medicine & Hygiene. Egyptian Branch.

616.9792 610.7 USA ISSN 1069-837X RJ387.A25 CODEN: JHACFP

JOURNAL OF HIV - AIDS PREVENTION & EDUCATION FOR ADOLESCENTS & CHILDREN. Text in English. 1997. q. USD 60 to individuals; USD 81 in Canada to individuals; USD 87 elsewhere to individuals; USD 95 to institutions; USD 128 in Canada to institutions; USD 138 elsewhere to institutions; USD 110 to libraries; USD 149 in Canada to libraries; USD 160 elsewhere to libraries (effective Aug. 2001). adv. bk.rev. back issues avail.; reprint service avail. from HAW. *Refereed.* **Document type:** *Journal, Academic/Scholarly.* **Description:** Covers the social and economic implications of AIDS and HIV infection in children and adolescents.

Related titles: Microform ed.: (from PQC).

Indexed: AIDS & Cancer Res., AIDS Abstr., ASSIA, CINAHL, Child Devel.Abstr., ERA, Environ.Sci.Poll.Mgmt., G.Soc.Sci.& Rel.Per.Lit., Lang.& Lang.Behav.Abstr., Mult.Ed.Abstr., Pollut.Abstr., Ref.Zh., Risk Abstr., SOPODA, Saf.Sci.Abstr., Sage Fam.Stud.Abstr., Sociol.Abstr., Sp.Ed.Needs Abstr., Stud.Wom.Abstr., Virol.Abstr.

—BLDSC (5002.450000), GNLM, Haworth.

Published by: Haworth Press, Inc., 10 Alice St, Binghamton, NY 13904-1580. TEL 607-722-5857, 800-429-6784, FAX 607-722-6362, 800-895-0582, getinfo@haworthpressinc.com, http://www.haworthpress.com/journals/journallist.asp. Eds. Julio Morales, Marcia Bok. Pub. William Cohen. R&P Ruthann Heath TEL 607-723-5857 ext 316. Adv. contact Jackie Blakeslee TEL 607-722-5857 ext 346. B&W page USD 315, color page USD 550; trim 6 x 8.5.

616.979 GBR ISSN 1462-0308

JOURNAL OF HIV THERAPY. Text in English. 1996. q. GBP 48; GBP 12.50 newsstand/cover (effective 1999). adv. bk.rev. tr.lit. back issues avail. *Refereed.* **Document type:** *Academic/Scholarly.* **Description:** Contains reviews and articles on HIV therapy research and results.

Formerly (until 1998): Journal of HIV Combination Therapy (1363-8424)

Related titles: Online - full text ed.

—BLDSC (5002.471000).

Published by: (Glaxo Wellcome), Mediscript Ltd., 1 Mountview Ct, 310 Friern Barnet Ln, London N20 0LD, United Kingdom. TEL 44-20-8446-8898, FAX 44-20-8446-9194, 101607.3205@compuserve.com. Ed., Adv. contact Linda Lazarus. Pub. Fatima Patel. Circ: 4,000 (paid).

616.9 GBR ISSN 0195-6701 CODEN: JHINDS

JOURNAL OF HOSPITAL INFECTION. Text in English. 1980. m. (in 3 vols., 4 nos./vol.). GBP 134 to individuals; GBP 404 to institutions (effective 2002). adv. bk.rev. illus. reprint service avail. from SWZ. *Refereed.* **Document type:** *Academic/Scholarly.* **Description:** Provides a forum for original observations of international significance in all aspects of hospital infection.

Related titles: Online - full text ed.: (from EBSCO Publishing, O C L C Online Computer Library Center, Inc., Swets Blackwell, IDEAL Online Library, Institute for Scientific Information).

Indexed: ASCA, Abstr.Health Care Manage.Stud., Abstr.Hyg., Brit.Nur.Ind., CINAHL, Curr.Adv.Ecol.Sci., Curr.Cont., Dairy Sci.Abstr., Dent.Ind., Dok.Arbeitsmed., Environ.Sci.Poll.Mgmt., Excerp.Med., INIS Atomind., Ind.Med. (1980-), Ind.Sci.Rev., Inpharma, Int.Nurs.Ind., Jrnl.Watch Inf.Dis., Microbiol.Abstr., Pharm.&Out.News, Pollut.Abstr., Protozool.Abstr., Reac., Rev.Arom.& Med.Plants, Rev.Med.& Vet.Mycol., Risk Abstr., Saf.Sci.Abstr., Sci.Cit.Ind., Trop.Dis.Bull.

—BLDSC (5003.285000), CISTI, GNLM, IDS, ingenta, KNAW. **CCC.**

Published by: (Hospital Infection Society), W.B. Saunders Co. Ltd. (Subsidiary of: Harcourt Publishers Ltd.), 24-28 Oval Rd, London NW1 7DX, United Kingdom. TEL 44-20-7424-4200, FAX 44-20-7424-4515, cservice@harcourt.com, http://www.harcourt-international.com/journals/jhin. Ed. G L French. **Subscr. to:** Harcourt Publishers Ltd., Foots Cray High St, Sidcup, Kent DA14 5HP, United Kingdom. TEL 44-20-8308-5700, FAX 44-20-8309-0807.

616.0194 USA ISSN 1090-9508 CODEN: JHVIFC

JOURNAL OF HUMAN VIROLOGY. Text in English. 1997. bi-m. USD 117 domestic to individuals; USD 130 foreign to individuals; USD 186 domestic to institutions; USD 206 foreign to institutions; USD 32 newsstand/cover (effective 2002). adv. *Refereed.* **Document type:** *Academic/Scholarly.* **Description:** Provides a clinically relevant forum for disseminating information on human viruses as they relate to chronic diseases.

Related titles: Online - full text ed.: USD 241.80 domestic for academic site license; USD 261.80 foreign for academic site license; USD 269.70 domestic for corporate site license; USD 289.70 foreign for corporate site license (effective 2002) (from Institute for Scientific Information).

Indexed: Biotech.Cit.Ind., Curr.Cont., Ind.Med. (1997-).

—BLDSC (5003.441500), CASDDS.

Published by: (Institute of Human Virology), Lippincott Williams & Wilkins (Philadelphia) (Subsidiary of: Wolters Kluwer N.V.), 530 Walnut St, Philadelphia, PA 19106-3621. TEL 215-521-8300, FAX 215-521-8902, http://www.lww.com. adv.: B&W page USD 520, color page USD 1,445. **Subscr. to:** PO Box 1600, Hagerstown, MD 21740-1600. TEL 800-777-2295, FAX 301-824-7390.

616.9 GBR ISSN 0163-4453 CODEN: JINFD2

JOURNAL OF INFECTION. Text in English. 1979. 8/yr. GBP 111 to individuals; GBP 309 to institutions (effective 2002). adv. bk.rev. illus. index. reprint service avail. from SWZ. *Refereed.* **Document type:** *Academic/Scholarly.* **Description:** Publishes papers that reflect the diverse nature of infection and seeks to brings together the views of clinicians, microbiologists, epidemiologists, molecular biologists, and other researchers in the field.

Related titles: Online - full text ed.: (from EBSCO Publishing, O C L C Online Computer Library Center, Inc., Swets Blackwell, IDEAL Online Library, Institute for Scientific Information).

Indexed: AIDS Abstr., ASCA, Abstr.Hyg., Agri.& Environ.Biotech.Abstr. (coverage dropped), Aqua.Sci.& Fish.Abstr., Chem.Abstr., Curr.Adv.Cancer Res., Curr.Adv.Ecol.Sci., Curr.Cont., Dairy Sci.Abstr., Dent.Ind., Derwent Biotech.Abstr., Dok.Arbeitsmed., Environ.Sci.Poll.Mgmt., Excerp.Med., Food Sci.& Tech.Abstr., Helminthol.Abstr., I.P.A., Ind.Med. (1979-), Ind.Sci.Rev., Ind.Vet., Inpharma, Med.& Surg.Dermat., Microbiol.Abstr., Pharm.&Out.News, Pollut.Abstr., Protozool.Abstr., Reac., Rev.Appl.Entomol., Rev.Med.& Vet.Mycol., Risk Abstr., Russ.Acad.Sci.Bibl., Saf.Sci.Abstr., Sci.Cit.Ind., Trop.Dis.Bull., Vet.Bull.
—BLDSC (5006.690000), CASDDS, CISTI, GNLM, IDS, ingenta, KNAW. **CCC.**
Published by: (British Infection Society), W.B. Saunders Co. Ltd. (Subsidiary of: Harcourt Publishers Ltd.), 24-28 Oval Rd, London NW1 7DX, United Kingdom. TEL 44-20-7424-4200, FAX 44-20-7424-4515, cservice@harcourt.com, http://www.harcourt-international.com/journals/jinf. Ed. A M L Lever. **Subscr. to:** Harcourt Publishers Ltd., Foots Cray High St, Sidcup, Kent DA14 5HP, United Kingdom. TEL 44-20-8308-5700, FAX 44-20-8309-0807.

JOURNAL OF INFECTIOUS DISEASE PHARMACOTHERAPY; antimicrobial evaluation, development & clinical application. see *PHARMACY AND PHARMACOLOGY*

616.9 USA ISSN 0022-1899
CODEN: JIDIAQ
JOURNAL OF INFECTIOUS DISEASES. Text in English. 1904. 2/m. (in 2 vols., 12 nos./vol.), latest vol.183, 2001, Jan. 1. USD 119 in United States to individuals; USD 166.33 in Canada to individuals; USD 158 elsewhere to individuals; USD 420 in United States to institutions; USD 488.40 in Canada to institutions; USD 459 elsewhere to institutions; USD 8.95 newsstand/cover to individuals; USD 21.50 to institutions (effective 2002). adv. bk.rev. bibl, charts, illus. index. reprint service avail. from PQC,ISI. *Refereed.* **Document type:** *Academic/Scholarly.* **Description:** Disseminates original research on the pathogenesis, diagnosis, and treatment of infectious diseases; on the microbes that cause them; and on disorders of host immune mechanisms.
Related titles: Microform ed.: (from PQC,PMC); Online - full text ed.: (from EBSCO Publishing, ProQuest Information & Learning, Institute for Scientific Information).
Indexed: AIDS & Cancer Res., AIDS Abstr., AIM, ASCA, Abstr.Anthropol., Abstr.Health Care Manage.Stud., Abstr.Hyg., Addic.Abstr., AgBiotech, Agri.& Environ.Biotech.Abstr. (coverage dropped), Aqua.Sci.& Fish.Abstr., Biol.Abstr., Biol.Dig., CINAHL, Chem.Abstr., Chem.Indus.Notes, Chem.Titles, Curr.Adv.Ecol.Sci., Curr.Adv.Gen.& Molec.Biol., Curr.Cont., Dairy Sci.Abstr., Dent.Ind., Derwent Biotech.Abstr., Diar.Dis.Res., Dok.Arbeitsmed., Environ.Sci.Poll.Mgmt., Excerp.Med., Food Sci.& Tech.Abstr., Helminthol.Abstr., INIS Atomind., I.P.A., Immun.Abstr., Ind.Med. (1904-), Ind.Sci.Rev., Ind.Vet., Inpharma, Int.Abstr.Biol.Sci., Int.Nurs.Ind., Jrnl.Watch, Jrnl.Watch Inf.Dis., Med.& Surg.Dermat., Microbiol.Abstr., NRN, Neurosci.Cit.Ind., Nutr.Abstr., Pharm.&Out.News, Pig News & Info., Plant Breed.Abstr., Pollut.Abstr., Potato Abstr., Protozool.Abstr., Reac., Rev.Appl.Entomol., Rev.Med.& Vet.Mycol., Risk Abstr., SSCI (coverage dropped), Saf.Sci.Abstr., Sci.Cit.Ind., Small Anim.Abstr., So.Pac.Per.Ind., Sport Fish.Abstr., Trop.Dis.Bull., Vet.Bull., Virol.Abstr., W.R.C.Inf., Wild.Rev., Zoo.Rec.
—BLDSC (5006.700000), ADONIS, CASDDS, CISTI, GNLM, IDS, ingenta, KNAW. **CCC.**
Published by: (Infectious Diseases Society of America), University of Chicago Press, Journals Division, PO Box 37005, Chicago, IL 60637. TEL 773-753-3347, FAX 773-753-0811, subscriptions@journals.uchicago.edu, subscriptions@press.uchicago.edu, http://www.journals.uchicago.edu/JID/. Ed. Marvin Turck. Adv. contact Timothy Hill. page USD 505; trim 9 x 6. Circ: 11,200.

606.9 GBR ISSN 0969-1413
CODEN: JMSCFE
JOURNAL OF MEDICAL SCREENING. Text in English. 1994. q. GBP 85, USD 136 combined subscription to individuals includes print & online eds.; GBP 143, USD 231 to institutions for print only (effective 2002). adv. bk.rev. abstr, charts, illus. index. *Refereed.* **Document type:** *Journal, Academic/Scholarly.* **Description:** Covers all aspects of medical screening. Aims to bring together specialist groups conducting screening research and to establish a liaison with health authorities and policymakers.
Related titles: Online - full text ed.: J M S Online. ISSN 1475-5793. GBP 50, USD 75 to individuals (effective 2002) (from EBSCO Publishing, O C L C Online Computer Library Center, Inc., RoweCom Information Quest, ingenta, HighWire Pr., SilverPlatter Information, Inc., Institute for Scientific Information).
Indexed: Curr.Cont., Ind.Med. (1994-), Inpharma, Int.Nurs.Ind., Pharm.&Out.News, Reac., Sci.Cit.Ind.
—BLDSC (5017.087250), ADONIS, CISTI, GNLM, IDS, Infotrieve, KNAW. **CCC.**
Published by: B M J Publishing Group, B M A House, Tavistock Sq, London WC1H 9JR, United Kingdom. TEL 44-20-7387-4499, FAX 44-20-7383-6400, info.norththames@bma.org.uk, http://www.jmedscreen.com, http://www.bma.org.uk. Ed. N Wald. Pub. Alex Williamson. R&P Carol Torselli TEL 44-20-7383-6674. Adv. contact Euan Currer TEL 44-20-7383-6181.

JOURNAL OF MICROBIOLOGY, IMMUNOLOGY AND INFECTION/WEIMIAN YU GANRAN ZAZHI. see *BIOLOGY—Microbiology*

616.96 USA ISSN 0022-3395
QL757 CODEN: JOPAA2
JOURNAL OF PARASITOLOGY. Text in English. 1914. bi-m. USD 170 domestic; USD 175 foreign (effective 2001). adv. bk.rev. bibl, illus. index, cum.index. back issues avail.; reprint service avail. from PQC. *Refereed.* **Document type:** *Academic/Scholarly.* **Description:** Results of research, primarily on animal parasitology.
Related titles: Microform ed.: (from PQC,PMC); Online - full text ed.: (from H. W. Wilson, BioOne, Institute for Scientific Information).
Indexed: ASCA, Abstr.Hyg., AgBiotech, Agri.& Environ.Biotech.Abstr. (coverage dropped), Agricola, Anim.Behav.Abstr., Appl.Ecol.Abstr., Aqua.Sci.& Fish.Abstr., Bio-Contr.News & Info., Biol.& Agr.Ind. (Nov.1982-), Biol.Abstr., Chem.Abstr., Chem.Indus.Notes, Chem.Titles, Curr.Adv.Ecol.Sci., Curr.Cont., Curr.Ref.Fish Res., Dairy Sci.Abstr., Derwent Biotech.Abstr., Diar.Dis.Res., Ecol.Abstr., Entomol.Abstr., Environ.Sci.Poll.Mgmt., Excerp.Med., Focus on: Vet.Sci.& Med., Helminthol.Abstr., IDA, INIS Atomind., Ind.Med. (1914-), Ind.Sci.Rev., Ind.Vet., Inpharma, Int.Abstr.Biol.Sci., Microbiol.Abstr., Nutr.Abstr., Ocean.Abstr., Pig News & Info., Plant Breed.Abstr., Pollut.Abstr., Poult.Abstr., Protozool.Abstr., Reac., Rev.Appl.Entomol., Rev.Arom.& Med.Plants, Rev.Med.& Vet.Mycol., Risk Abstr., SSCI (coverage dropped), Saf.Sci.Abstr., Sci.Cit.Ind., Small Anim.Abstr., Soils & Fert., Sport Fish.Abstr., Trop.Dis.Bull., Vet.Bull., W.R.C.Inf., Weed Abstr., Wild.Rev., Zoo.Rec.
—BLDSC (5029.000000), CASDDS, CISTI, GNLM, ingenta, Linda Hall.
Published by: American Society of Parasitologists, Dept of Biology, Wake Forest Univ, P O Box 7629, Winston Salem, NC 27109. TEL 910-759-4487, FAX 910-759-6008, asp@allenpress.com, http://www.allenpress.com. Ed., R&P Gerald W Esch TEL 336-758-4487. Circ: 2,800. **Subscr. to:** Allen Press Inc., PO Box 1897, Lawrence, KS 66044-8897.

616.92 USA
JOURNAL OF SPIROCHETAL AND TICKBORNE DISEASES. Text in English. 1994. q. USD 75 domestic to individuals; USD 85 in Canada to individuals; USD 90 elsewhere to individuals; USD 95 domestic to institutions; USD 105 in Canada to institutions; USD 110 elsewhere to institutions. back issues avail. **Document type:** *Academic/Scholarly.* **Description:** Covers topics relating to the understanding of disease mechanisms and the application of better diagnostic techniques and treatment strategies for persons suffering from spirochetal and tick-borne diseases.
Indexed: Rev.Appl.Entomol., Zoo.Rec.
—BLDSC (5066.183300).
Published by: (Lyme Disease Foundation), Slack, Inc., 6900 Grove Rd, Thorofare, NJ 08086-9447. TEL 856-848-1000, 800-257-8290, FAX 856-853-5991, http://www.slackinc.com. Ed. Dr. Edward Bosler.

JOURNAL WATCH INFECTIOUS DISEASES. see *MEDICAL SCIENCES—Abstracting, Bibliographies, Statistics*

KENYA. MINISTRY OF HEALTH. HEALTH INFORMATION BULLETIN. see *PUBLIC HEALTH AND SAFETY*

616.9 JPN ISSN 0915-5007
KISEICHU BUNRUI KEITAI DANWAKAI KAIHO/JAPANESE SOCIETY FOR SYSTEMATIC PARASITOLOGY. CIRCULAR. Text in Japanese. 1983. a. JPY 2,000 per issue (effective 2000). **Document type:** *Academic/Scholarly.*
Indexed: Zoo.Rec.
Published by: Kiseichu Bunrui Keitai Danwakai/Japanese Society for Systematic Parasitology, c/o Toshiaki Kuramochi, Dept. of Zoology, National Science Museum, 3-23-1, Hyakuniu, Shinjuku-Ku, Tokyo 169-0073, Japan. TEL 81-3-3364-7122, FAX 81-3-3364-7104, kuramotr@kahaku.go.jp. Ed. Toshiaki Kuramochi. Circ: 225 (controlled).

614 616.998 JPN ISSN 0454-2029
KOKURITSU TAMA KENKYUJO NENPO/NATIONAL INSTITUTE FOR LEPROSY RESEARCH ANNUAL REPORT. Text in Japanese. 1955. a. free per issue. adv. **Document type:** *Academic/Scholarly.*
Published by: Kokuritsu Tama Kenkyujo/National Institute for Leprosy Research, 2-1 Aoba-cho 4-chome, Higashimurayama-shi, Tokyo-to 189-0002, Japan. TEL 81-423-91-8211, FAX 81-423-94-9092. Ed., Adv. contact Hajime Saito.

616.96 KOR ISSN 0023-4001
QL757 CODEN: KSCHAV
KOREAN JOURNAL OF PARASITOLOGY. Text in English. 1963. q. JPY 3,000, USD 30 to membership (effective 2001). abstr, charts, illus. 100 p./no. back issues avail.; reprints avail. *Refereed.* **Document type:** *Journal, Academic/Scholarly.* **Description:** Contains original papers of research articles, case records, and brief communications on parasites of humans or animals, and host-parasite relations.
Formerly (until 1999): Kisengchunghak Chapji (0368-6809)
Related titles: Online - full text ed.
Indexed: Abstr.Hyg., AgBiotech, Biol.Abstr., Diar.Dis.Res., Excerp.Med., Helminthol.Abstr., Ind.Med. (1993-), Ind.Vet., Poult.Abstr., Protozool.Abstr., Rev.Appl.Entomol., Rev.Med.& Vet.Mycol., Rural Devel.Abstr., Trop.Dis.Bull., Vet.Bull., Zoo.Rec.
—BLDSC (5113.570000), GNLM, Linda Hall.
Published by: Korean Society for Parasitology, c/o Dept. of Parasitology, College of Medicine, Seoul National University, Seoul 110799, Korea, S.. TEL 82-2-740-8348, FAX 82-2-765-6142, hst@snu.ac.kr, http://www.parasitol.or.kr/kjp/, http://www.parasitol.or.kr/engl/. Ed., R&P Sung-Tae Hong TEL 82-2-740-8343. Circ: 1,000.

616.9 JPN ISSN 0910-6073
CODEN: KKZAE5
KOSANKINBYO KENKYUSHO ZASSHI. Text in Japanese. 1949. q. per issue exchange basis. **Document type:** *Academic/Scholarly.*
Formerly (until 1984): Kosankinbyo Kenkyu Zasshi - Journal of Tuberculosis and Leprosy (0368-6078)
Indexed: Excerp.Med. (1992-), INIS Atomind.
—CASDDS, EMDOCS.
Published by: Tohoku Daigaku, Kosankinbyo Kenkyusho Kenyukai/Tohoku University, Research Institute for Tuberculosis, Leprosy, and Cancer, Seiryo-cho, Aoba-ku, Sendai-shi, Miyagi-ken 980-0872, Japan.

616.998 IND
KUSHT VINASHAK. Text in English, Hindi. m. INR 30; USD 8 foreign.
Published by: Indian Leprosy Association/Hind Kusht Nivaran Sangh, 1 Red Cross Rd., New Delhi 110 001, India. TEL 3714748.

L M S ALERT. ANTIVIRALS. (Literature Monitoring and Evaluation Service) see *MEDICAL SCIENCES—Abstracting, Bibliographies, Statistics*

616.9 NZL ISSN 1173-1591
LABLINK. Text in English. 1994. q. free. charts, stat. 8 p./no. back issues avail.; reprints avail. *Refereed.* **Document type:** *Newsletter, Academic/Scholarly.*
Incorporates (in 1994): Antimicrobial Newsletter (1170-8875)
Published by: Institute of Environmental Science & Research, P.O. Box 50 348, Porirua 6215, New Zealand. TEL 64-4-9140700, FAX 64-4-9140770, craig.thornley@esr.cri.nz, http://www.esr.cri.nz. Ed. M Brett. Circ: 450.

616.9 GBR ISSN 1473-3099
▼ **THE LANCET INFECTIOUS DISEASES.** Text in English. 2001 (Aug.). m. GBP 248 foreign to institutions print with multiple access; USD 390 in United States to institutions print with multiple access (effective Aug. 2002). **Description:** Covers scientific discovery, ideas, and treatment against pathogens. Contains strategic reviews, frontline dispatches, interviews with the leading personalities, debate controversial issues, and provide a forum for readers' opinions through personal view articles and lively correspondence.
Related titles: Online - full content ed.

M

Published by: The Lancet Publishing Group (Subsidiary of: Reed Elsevier plc), 84 Theobald's Rd, London WC1X 8RR, United Kingdom. TEL 44-20-7611-4246, FAX 44-20-7611-4479, editorial@lancet.com, http://infection.thelancet.com/, http://www.thelancet.com.

616.9 GBR ISSN 0305-7518
CODEN: LEREAA

LEPROSY REVIEW. Text in English. 1927. q. GBP 34 (effective 2000). adv. bk.rev. *Refereed.* **Document type:** *Academic/Scholarly.*
Related titles: Microform ed.: (from SWZ); Online - full text ed.: (from Institute for Scientific Information).
Indexed: ASCA, Abstr.Hyg., Biol.Abstr., Chem.Abstr., Curr.Adv.Ecol.Sci., Curr.Cont., INIS Atomind., Ind.Med. (1930-), Ind.Sci.Rev., Inpharma, Int.Nurs.Ind., Med.& Surg.Dermat., Pharm.&Out.News, Reac., Ref.Zh., Rev.Med.& Vet.Mycol., SSCI (coverage dropped), Sci.Cit.Ind., Trop.Dis.Bull.
—BLDSC (5183.300000), CASDDS, CISTI, EMDOCS, GNLM, IDS, ingenta, KNAW. **CCC.**
Published by: British Leprosy Relief Association (LEPRA), Fairfax House, Causton Rd, Colchester, Essex CO1 1PU, United Kingdom. TEL 44-1206-562286, FAX 44-1206-762151, irene_allen@lepra.org.uk, http://www.lepra.org.uk. Ed. Dr. Diana Lockwood. R&P Irene Allen. Adv. contact Susan Boobis. Circ: 1,800.

616.9 FRA ISSN 0296-9009

LA LETTRE DE L'INFECTIOLOGUE; de la microbiologie a la clinique. Text in French. 1985. m. FRF 460 domestic to individuals; FRF 580, USD 105 foreign to individuals; FRF 580 domestic to institutions; FRF 700, USD 127 foreign to institutions; FRF 290 domestic to students; USD 75 foreign to students (effective 2000). *Refereed.* **Document type:** *Academic/Scholarly.*
—GNLM.
Published by: Edimark S.A., 62-64 rue Jean Jaures, Puteaux 92800, France. TEL 33-1-414-58000, FAX 33-1-41458025, contact@edimark.fr, http://www.edimark.fr. Eds. M H Nicolas Chanvine, Y Mouton. Pub. Claudie Damour-Terrasson.

LITERATURE MONITORING AND EVALUATION SERVICE ALERT. ANTIBACTERIAL. see *MEDICAL SCIENCES—Abstracting, Bibliographies, Statistics*

616.9 NZL ISSN 1173-1672

M S R A REPORT. Text in English. 1994. w. stat. back issues avail. **Document type:** *Newsletter, Academic/Scholarly.*
Published by: Institute of Environmental Science & Research, P.O. Box 50 348, Porirua 6215, New Zealand. TEL 64-4-9140700, FAX 64-4-9140770, heather.davies@esr.cri.nz, http://www.esr.cri.nz. Circ: 242.

669 USA

MALARIA & TROPICAL DISEASE WEEKLY. Text in English. 1995. w. (43/yr.). USD 1,549 in North America; USD 1,649 elsewhere. **Document type:** *Newsletter.*
Formerly: Malaria Weekly (1086-0231)
Related titles: Online - full text ed.
Indexed: Bus.& Indus. (Apr.1995-).
Published by: Charles W. Henderson, Ed. & Pub., PO Box 5528, Atlanta, GA 31107-0528. TEL 770-507-7777, FAX 770-507-7788, cwhender@newsfile.com; info@hendersonnet.atl.ga.us, http://www.newsfile.com.

614.49 616.96 FRA ISSN 0399-077X

MEDECINE ET MALADIES INFECTIEUSES; revue francaise d'epidemiologie, de pathologie infectieuse et parasitaire. Text in French, English. 1978. 14/yr. EUR 171 in Europe to institutions; USD 235 elsewhere to institutions; EUR 237 in Europe to institutions; USD 302 elsewhere to institutions (effective 2002). bk.rev. bibl, charts, illus. index. back issues avail. *Refereed.* **Document type:** *Academic/Scholarly.* **Description:** Approaches the various infectious pathologies and pathogens through clinical and research articles, general reviews, and short communications.
Related titles: Online - full text ed.: (from ingenta, Institute for Scientific Information); Supplement: Medecine et Maladies Infectieuses. Supplement. ISSN 1166-8237.
Indexed: ASCA, Abstr.Hyg., Curr.Adv.Cancer Res., Curr.Cont., Dairy Sci.Abstr., Excerp.Med., Forest Prod.Abstr., Forest.Abstr., Helminthol.Abstr., Ind.Vet., Inpharma, Nutr.Abstr., Pharm.&Out.News, Pig News & Info., Protozool.Abstr., Reac., Ref.Zh., Rev.Appl.Entomol., Rev.Med.& Vet.Mycol., Trop.Dis.Bull., Vet.Bull.
—BLDSC (5487.732000), CISTI, EMDOCS, GNLM, IDS, Infotrieve, KNAW. **CCC.**
Published by: (Societe de Pathologie Infectieuse de Langue Francaise), Elsevier Paris, Editions Scientifiques et Medicales (Subsidiary of: Reed Elsevier plc. group), 23 rue Linois, Paris 75015, France. TEL 33-1-45589110, FAX 33-1-45589419, mmi@elsevier.fr; academic@elsevier.fr, http://www.elsevier.com/locate/medmal. Eds. J P Stahl, O Patey. Circ: 5,000.

616.988 FRA ISSN 0025-682X
CODEN: METRA2

MEDECINE TROPICALE. Summaries in English, French. 1941. q. FRF 250; FRF 250 foreign (effective 1998). adv. bk.rev. bibl, charts, illus, stat. index. Supplement avail.
Indexed: Abstr.Hyg., Biol.Abstr., Chem.Abstr., Excerp.Med., Helminthol.Abstr., Ind.Med. (1941-), Ind.Vet., Nutr.Abstr., Protozool.Abstr., Ref.Zh., Rev.Appl.Entomol., Rev.Med.& Vet.Mycol., Rev.Plant Path., Rural Devel.Abstr., Trop.Dis.Bull.
—BLDSC (5488.000000), CASDDS, CISTI, GNLM, KNAW.
Published by: Institut de Medecine Tropicale, Le Pharo, B.P. 46, Marseille Armees 13998, France. TEL 33-4-91150120, FAX 33-4-91594477, imtssa@gulliver.fr. Ed. B Maistre. Circ: 1,500.

616.969 GBR ISSN 1369-3786
RC117 CODEN: MEMYFR

MEDICAL MYCOLOGY. Text in English. 1963. bi-m. USD 141 in North America to individuals; GBP 88 rest of world to individuals; GBP 492 in the European Union to institutions; USD 856 in North America to institutions; GBP 539 rest of world to institutions; USD 144 newsstand/cover in North America; GBP 90 newsstand/cover rest of world (effective 2001); Online access free with print subscr.. adv. bk.rev. abstr, bibl, charts, illus. index. back issues avail. *Refereed.* **Document type:** *Academic/Scholarly.* **Description:** Articles on all aspects of research dealing with fungal disease in humans and animals.
Former titles (until 1998): Journal of Medical and Veterinary Mycology (0268-1218); (until 1986): Sabouraudia: Journal of Medical and Veterinary Mycology (0036-2174)
Related titles: Microform ed.: (from PQC); Online - full text ed.: ISSN 1460-2709. GBP 72 in Europe to individuals; USD 115 in North America to individuals; GBP 72 elsewhere to individuals; GBP 399 in Europe to institutions; USD 635 in North America to institutions; GBP 399 elsewhere to institutions (effective 2000) (from EBSCO Publishing, O C L C Online Computer Library Center, Inc., RoweCom Information Quest, CatchWord Ltd., ingenta, Munksgaard & Blackwell Science's Synergy, Swets Blackwell, Institute for Scientific Information).
Indexed: ASCA, Abstr.Hyg., Biol.Abstr., Curr.Adv.Ecol.Sci., Curr.Cont., Dairy Sci.Abstr., Dent.Ind., Derwent Biotech.Abstr., Excerp.Med., Focus on: Vet.Sci.& Med., Ind.Med. (1998-), Ind.Sci.Rev., Ind.Vet., Inpharma, Int.Abstr.Biol.Sci., Microbiol.Abstr., Pharm.&Out.News, Reac., Rev.Arom.& Med.Plants, Rev.Med.& Vet.Mycol., Rev.Plant Path., Sci.Cit.Ind., Small Anim.Abstr., So.Pac.Per.Ind., Soils & Fert., Sport Fish.Abstr., Vet.Bull., Wild.Rev., Zoo.Rec.
—BLDSC (5530.168000), CASDDS, CatchWord, CISTI, EMDOCS, GNLM, IDS, Infotrieve, ingenta, KNAW, Linda Hall. **CCC.**
Published by: (International Society for Human and Animal Mycology), BIOS Scientific Publishers Ltd., 9 Newtec Pl, Magdalen Rd, Oxford, Berks OX4 1RE, United Kingdom. TEL 44-1865-726286, FAX 44-1865-200386, mansell@bios.co.uk, http://www.bios.co.uk/journals/mmy/index.htm. Ed. Dr. Richard Summerbell. R&P Paul Barlais. Circ: 1,037. **Dist. by:** Turpin Distribution Services Ltd., Blackhorse Rd, Letchworth, Herts SG6 1HN, United Kingdom.

616 USA ISSN 1043-1837
CODEN: MEVIEN

MEDICAL VIROLOGY. Variant title: International Symposium on Medical Virology. Proceedings. Text in English. 1982. a., latest vol.10, 1991. price varies. **Document type:** *Proceedings.*
Indexed: Chem.Abstr., Chem.Indus.Notes, Chem.Titles.
—CASDDS, KNAW.
Published by: Kluwer Academic - Plenum Publishers (Subsidiary of: Wolters Kluwer N.V.), 233 Spring St, New York, NY 10013-1578. TEL 212-620-8000, 800-221-9369, FAX 212-463-0742, info@plenum.com, http://www.plenum.com.

616.96 RUS ISSN 0025-8326
RC960 CODEN: MPPBAB

MEDITSINSKAYA PARAZITOLOGIYA I PARAZITARNYE BOLEZNI/MEDICAL PARASITOLOGY AND PARASITIC DISEASES. Text in Russian; Summaries in English. 1923. q. USD 93. bibl, charts, illus. index. **Description:** Covers general and medical parasitology, results of elaborating, testing and introduction into public health practice of scientifically substantiated measures of the control of parasitic and transmissible diseases, as well as bloodsucking insects and ticks.
Indexed: Abstr.Hyg., Agri.& Environ.Biotech.Abstr. (coverage dropped), Bio-Contr.News & Info., Biol.Abstr., Chem.Abstr., Chem.Titles, Derwent Biotech.Abstr., Excerp.Med., Helminthol.Abstr., Ind.Med. (1932-), Ind.Vet., Irr.& Drain.Abstr., Pig News & Info., Poult.Abstr., Protozool.Abstr., Ref.Zh., Rev.Appl.Entomol., Rev.Med.& Vet.Mycol., Trop.Dis.Bull., Vet.Bull., Zoo.Rec.
—BLDSC (0104.000000), CASDDS, CISTI, East View, GNLM. **CCC.**
Published by: Vsesoyuznoe Nauchnoe Meditsinskoe Obshchestvo im. I.I. Mechnikova, Ul Polikarpova 8, Moscow 125284, Russian Federation. TEL 7-095-9460435, FAX 7-095-9456946. Ed. V P Sergiev. **Dist. by:** Mezhdunarodnaya Kniga, B Yakimanka 39, Moscow 117049, Russian Federation. TEL 7-095-2384967, FAX 7-095-2384634; **US dist. addr.:** East View Publications, 3020 Harbor Ln N, Minneapolis, MN 55447. TEL 612-550-0961.

616.97 BGR ISSN 1310-9057

MEDITSINSKI PREGLED. IMMUNNI DEFITSITI. Text in Bulgarian; Summaries in Bulgarian, English. 1988. q., latest vol.14, 2001. BGL 14 domestic; USD 48 foreign (effective 2001 - 2002). adv. bk.rev. illus, abstr, bibl. index. back issues avail. *Refereed.* **Document type:** *Journal, Academic/Scholarly, Abstract/Index, Bibliography.* **Description:** Presents original articles and abstracts of foreign publications on HIV infection, diagnosis, prevention.
Formerly: S P I N (AISA) (0861-0088)
Indexed: Abstr.Bulg.Sci.Med.Lit.
Published by: Meditsinski Universitet - Sofia, Tsentur za Informatsiia po Meditsina/Medical University - Sofia, Medical Information Center, 1 Sv Georgi Sofiiski ul, Sofia 1431, Bulgaria. TEL 359-2-9522342, FAX 359-2-9522393, mutafov@sun.medun.acad.bg, http://www.medun.acad.bg. Ed. Dr. R Argirova. R&P, Adv. contact Dr. Christo Mutafov. B&W page USD 50, color page USD 150; 12 x 18. Circ: 300. **Dist. by:** Sofia Books, Ul Silivria 16, Sofia 1404, Bulgaria. TEL 359-2-9586257, sofiabooks@hotmail.com, http://www.sofiabooks.hit.bg.

616.9 BGR ISSN 0324-1432

MEDITSINSKI PREGLED. INFEKTSIOZNI ZABOLIAVANIIA. Text in Bulgarian. 1970. q. BGL 14 domestic; USD 48 foreign (effective 2002). adv. back issues avail. **Document type:** *Academic/Scholarly.* **Description:** Presents original articles and abstracts of foreign publications on communicable diseases (diagnosis, prevention, treatment, control).
Published by: Meditsinski Universitet - Sofia, Tsentur za Informatsiia po Meditsina/Medical University - Sofia, Medical Information Center, 1 Sv Georgi Sofiiski ul, Sofia 1431, Bulgaria. TEL 359-2-9522342, FAX 359-2-9522393, mutafov@sun.medun.acad.bg, http://www.medun.acad.bg. Ed. M Radev. adv.: B&W page USD 50, color page USD 150; trim 160 x 110. Circ: 250. **Dist. by:** Sofia Books, Ul Silivria 16, Sofia 1404, Bulgaria. TEL 359-2-9586257, sofiabooks@hotmail.com, http://www.sofiabooks.hit.bg.

▼ **MICROBES AND INFECTION**; a journal on infectious agents and host defenses. see *BIOLOGY—Microbiology*

616.9 NOR ISSN 0891-060X
QR171.A1 CODEN: MEHDE6

MICROBIAL ECOLOGY IN HEALTH & DISEASE. Text in Norwegian. 1988. q. GBP 119, USD 197 to individuals; GBP 225, USD 372 to institutions (effective 2002). bk.rev. back issues avail.; reprint service avail. from SWZ. *Refereed.* **Document type:** *Academic/Scholarly.* **Description:** Draws together research on various human microbial ecosystems to increase understanding of their role in health and disease.
Related titles: Microform ed.: (from PQC); Online - full text ed.: (from EBSCO Publishing, O C L C Online Computer Library Center, Inc., RoweCom Information Quest, CatchWord Ltd., ingenta, Swets Blackwell).

M

Indexed: ASCA, AgBiotech, Biotech.& Bioeng.Abstr., Curr.Adv.Cancer Res., Curr.Cont. (coverage dropped), Dairy Sci.Abstr., Diar.Dis.Res., Environ.Sci.Poll.Mgmt., Food Sci.& Tech.Abstr., Ind.Med. (coverage dropped), Ind.Sci.Rev., Ind.Vet., Inpharma, Microbiol.Abstr., Nutr.Abstr., Pollut.Abstr., Poult.Abstr., Reac., Ref.Zh., Rev.Appl.Entomol., Rev.Arom.& Med.Plants, Rev.Med.& Vet.Mycol., Rev.Plant Path., Risk Abstr., Saf.Sci.Abstr., Sci.Cit.Ind. (coverage dropped), Vet.Bull.
—BLDSC (5756.922000), CASDDS, CISTI, EMDOCS, GNLM, IDS, Infotrieve, ingenta. **CCC.**
Published by: Taylor & Francis AS (Subsidiary of: Taylor & Francis Group), Cort Adelersgt. 17, Solli, PO Box 2562, Oslo 0202, Norway. TEL 47-22-12-98-80, FAX 47-22-12-98-90, journals@tandf.no, http://www.tandf.co.uk.tfas. Ed. Tore Midtvedt. Circ: 173.

616.9 GBR ISSN 0882-4010
QR175 CODEN: MIPAEV
MICROBIAL PATHOGENESIS; molecular and cellular biology of infectious disease. Text in English. 1986. m. GBP 369 to institutions (effective 2001). adv. index. back issues avail.; reprint service avail. from SWZ. *Refereed.* **Document type:** *Academic/Scholarly.* **Description:** Publishes original contributions, mini-reviews, and notes on molecular and cellular mechanisms in infectious disease.
Related titles: Online - full text ed.: (from EBSCO Publishing, O C L C Online Computer Library Center, Inc., RoweCom Information Quest, ingenta, Swets Blackwell, IDEAL Online Library, Institute for Scientific Information).
Indexed: ASCA, Abstr.Hyg., AgBiotech, Agricola, Aqua.Sci.& Fish.Abstr., Chem.Abstr., Chem.Titles, Curr.Adv.Ecol.Sci., Curr.Adv.Gen.& Molec.Biol., Curr.Cont., Dairy Sci.Abstr., Diar.Dis.Res., Environ.Sci.Poll.Mgmt., Excerp.Med. (1993-), Food Sci.& Tech.Abstr., Ind.Med. (1986-), Ind.Sci.Rev., Ind.Vet., Inpharma, Int.Abstr.Biol.Sci., Microbiol.Abstr., Nutr.Abstr., Pig News & Info., Poult.Abstr., Protozool.Abstr., Reac., Rev.Appl.Entomol., Rev.Med.& Vet.Mycol., Sci.Cit.Ind., Vet.Bull.
—BLDSC (5756.955000), ADONIS, CASDDS, CISTI, EMDOCS, GNLM, IDS, ingenta, KNAW, Linda Hall. **CCC.**
Published by: Academic Press (Subsidiary of: Harcourt Publishers Ltd.), 24 Oval Rd, London NW1 7DX, United Kingdom. TEL 44-20-7267-4466, FAX 44-20-7482-2293, apsubs@acad.com, http://www.academicpress.com/micpath; http://www.europe.idealibrary.com/. R&P Catherine John. Adv. contact Nik Screen. **Subscr. to:** Harcourt Publishers Ltd., Foots Cray High St, Sidcup, Kent DA14 5HP, United Kingdom. TEL 44-20-8300-3322, FAX 44-20-8309-0807.

MIKROBIOLOGICHNYI ZHURNAL; nauchnyi zhurnal. see *BIOLOGY—Microbiology*

MIKROBIYOLOJI BULTENI/BULLETIN OF MICROBIOLOGY. see *BIOLOGY—Microbiology*

MOLECULAR AND CELL BIOLOGY OF HUMAN DISEASES. see *BIOLOGY—Cytology And Histology*

616.96 ARG ISSN 0524-952X
MUSEO ARGENTINO DE CIENCIAS NATURALES "BERNARDINO RIVADAVIA." INSTITUTO NACIONAL DE INVESTIGACION DE LAS CIENCIAS NATURALES. REVISTA. PARASITOLOGIA. Text in Spanish. 1968. irreg., latest vol.2, no.5, 1980.
—CISTI, Linda Hall.
Published by: Museo Argentino de Ciencias Naturales "Bernardino Rivadavia", Instituto Nacional de Investigacion de las Ciencias Naturales, Avda. Angel Gallardo 470, Casilla de Correo 220-Sucursal 5, Buenos Aires, Argentina.

616.9792 USA
N A T A P REPORTS. Text in English. 1997. irreg. USD 25 to individuals; USD 75 to institutions. back issues avail. **Document type:** *Newsletter.* **Description:** Provides the latest in HIV and AIDS drug development, research, and treatment information.
Related titles: Online - full text ed.
Published by: National Aids Treatment Advocacy Project, 580 Broadway St, Ste 403, New York, NY 10012. TEL 212-219-0106, 800-266-2827, FAX 212-219-8473, info@natap.org, http://www.natap.org. Ed. Jules Levin.

616.9 USA
NATIONAL COUNCIL OF LA RAZA. AIDS NEWSLETTER✶. Text in English. q. free per issue. **Document type:** *Newsletter.* **Description:** Covers medical and legislative news of AIDS with a focus on the Hispanic community. Also disseminates news of the NCLR AIDS Center's activities.
Published by: National Council of La Raza, 1111 19th St, N W, Washington, DC 20036-3603. TEL 202-289-1380, FAX 202-289-8173. Ed. Miguel Serrez.

NEW ZEALAND PUBLIC HEALTH REPORT. see *PUBLIC HEALTH AND SAFETY*

NIHON SANFUJINKA KANSENSHO KENKYUKAI GAKUJUTSU KOENKAI KIROKUSHU/CONFERENCE ON OBSTETRICAL AND GYNECOLOGICAL INFECTION. PROCEEDINGS. see *MEDICAL SCIENCES—Obstetrics And Gynecology*

O I E BULLETIN. see *VETERINARY SCIENCE*

O I E REVUE SCIENTIFIQUE ET TECHNIQUE/O I E SCIENTIFIC AND TECHNICAL REVIEW. see *VETERINARY SCIENCE*

616.9 GBR ISSN 1362-6787
OPINION: SPECIALIST REVIEWS OF KEY PAPERS IN GUM - AIDS. Variant title: Opinion: GUM - AIDS. Text in English. 1996. 3/yr. bk.rev. **Document type:** *Academic/Scholarly.*
Published by: Hayward Medical Communications Ltd., Covent Garden, Seven Dials Warehouse, 44 Earlham St, London WC2H 9LA, United Kingdom. TEL 44-20-7240-4493, FAX 44-20-7240-4479, admin@hayward.co.uk, http://www.hayward.co.uk. Ed. Dr. R Basu Roy. Circ: 2,000. **Subscr. to:** Rosemary House, Lanwades Park, Kentford, Near, Newmarket, Suffolk CB8 7PW, United Kingdom. TEL 44-1638-751515, FAX 44-1638-751517.

616.9 NLD ISSN 1386-2618
CODEN: OPPAFZ
OPPORTUNISTIC PATHOGENS. Text in English. 1987. q. NLG 447, USD 257 (effective 1998). back issues avail. *Refereed.* **Document type:** *Academic/Scholarly.*
Formerly (until 1997): Serodiagnosis and Immunotherapy in Infectious Disease (0888-0786)
Related titles: Microform ed.: (from PQC); Online - full text ed.: (from ingenta, ScienceDirect, Swets Blackwell).
Indexed: ASCA, Curr.Cont. (coverage dropped), Excerp.Med., Int.Abstr.Biol.Sci., Vet.Bull.
—CISTI, EMDOCS, GNLM, Infotrieve, KNAW. **CCC.**
Published by: Elsevier Science BV, PO Box 211, Amsterdam 1000 AE, Netherlands. TEL 31-20-485-2911, FAX 31-20-485-2457. Eds. David A Watson, James P Burnie. **Subscr. in Australasia and the Far East to:** Elsevier Science (Singapore) Pte Ltd, No.1 Temasek Ave, 17-01 Millenia Tower, Singapore 039192, Singapore. TEL 65-434-3727, FAX 65-337-2230; **Subscr. in Japan to:** Elsevier Science Inc - Japan Regional Office, 9-15 Higashi-Azabu 1-chome, Minato-ku, Tokyo 106-0044, Japan. TEL 81-3-5561-5033, FAX 81-3-5561-5047; **Subscr. in the Americas to:** Elsevier Science, PO Box 945, New York, NY 10159-0945. TEL 212-633-3730, FAX 212-633-3680.

362.196 USA
OUTREACH (SAN FRANCISCO). Text in English. bi-m.
Published by: San Francisco AIDS Foundation, PO Box 426182, San Francisco, CA 94142-6182. TEL 415-487-8060, 800-833-0159, FAX 415-487-8069, beta@sfaf.org, http://www.sfaf.org. Ed. Scot Murray.

P H L S DIRECTORY. see *BIOLOGY—Microbiology*

616.9 GBR ISSN 0958-1316
P H L S HIV BULLETIN. Text in English. ceased; resumed 1989. m. GBP 50 in United Kingdom; GBP 65 in Europe; GBP 85 elsewhere (effective 2000). **Document type:** *Bibliography.* **Description:** Covers microbiological and epidemiological aspects of AIDS and HIV.
Published by: Public Health Laboratory Service, 61 Colindale Ave, London NW9 5HT, United Kingdom. TEL 44-20-8200-4400, FAX 44-20-8200-7875. Ed. Margaret Clennett. Circ: 500.

P P O UPDATE. (Principles and Practices of Oncology) see *MEDICAL SCIENCES—Oncology*

616.9 362.1 USA
P W A C RESOURCE DIRECTORY✶. Text in English. irreg. free per issue. **Document type:** *Directory.* **Description:** Lists social service agencies in the greater New York City area.
Published by: People With AIDS Coalition of New York, 50 W 17th St, 8th fl, New York, NY 10011. TEL 212-647-1415.

616.9 362.1 USA ISSN 1069-3637
P W A COALITION NEWSLINE✶. Text in English. 1985. 10/yr. USD 35; free to persons with AIDS or ARC. **Document type:** *Newsletter.* **Description:** Reports new developments dealing with the health crisis, as well as alternative treatments, and personal perspectives of people with AIDS and HIV infection.
Published by: People With AIDS Coalition of New York, 50 W 17th St, 8th fl, New York, NY 10011. TEL 212-647-1415. Circ: 15,000.

616.9 NCL ISSN 1018-2152
RA644.A25
PACIFIC AIDS ALERT BULLETIN. Text in English. 1991. irreg. **Document type:** *Newsletter.*
Related titles: French ed.: Alerte au S I D A Oceanie. ISSN 1023-1730.
Published by: Secretariat of the Pacific Community, PO Box D5, Noumea Cedex 98848, New Caledonia. TEL 687-262000, FAX 687-263818, spc@spc.int, http://www.spc.int.

616.9 GBR ISSN 0957-4190
PAPILLOMAVIRUS REPORT. Text in English. 1990. bi-m. USD 140 in United States to individuals; GBP 72 in the European Union to individuals; USD 238 in United States to institutions; GBP 128 in the European Union to institutions (effective 2002). bibl. back issues avail. **Document type:** *Academic/Scholarly, Abstract/Index.* **Description:** Contains bibliographic information, including abstracts and authors' addresses, for papers on all aspects of papillomavirus infection in humans and animals published worldwide.
—BLDSC (6403.165000), GNLM.
Published by: Maney Publishing, Hudson Rd, Leeds, W Yorks LS9 7DL, United Kingdom. TEL 44-113-249-7481, FAX 44-113-248-6983, maney@maney.co.uk, http://www.maney.co.uk. Ed. Simon Herrington.

PARASITE. see *BIOLOGY—Microbiology*

616.9 570 GBR ISSN 0141-9838
CODEN: PAIMD8
PARASITE IMMUNOLOGY. Text in English. 1979. m., latest vol.24, 2002. GBP 71 in Europe to individuals; USD 110 in North America to individuals; GBP 71 elsewhere to individuals; GBP 607 in Europe to institutions; USD 962 in North America to institutions; GBP 668 elsewhere to institutions (effective 2002). adv. bibl, charts, illus. index. back issues avail.; reprint service avail. from ISI. *Refereed.* **Document type:** *Academic/Scholarly.* **Description:** Devoted to research on parasite immunology in the general sense.
Related titles: Microform ed.: (from PQC); Online - full text ed.: Parasite Immunology Online. ISSN 1365-3024. 1999. USD 98 in North America to individuals; GBP 62 elsewhere to individuals; USD 857 in North America to institutions; GBP 506 elsewhere to institutions (2001) (from EBSCO Publishing, O C L C Online Computer Library Center, Inc., RoweCom Information Quest, ingenta, Munksgaard & Blackwell Science's Synergy, Swets Blackwell, Institute for Scientific Information).
Indexed: AIDS & Cancer Res., ASCA, Abstr.Hyg., AgBiotech, Aqua.Sci.& Fish.Abstr., Biol.Abstr., Chem.Abstr., Chem.Indus.Notes, Chem.Titles, Curr.Adv.Ecol.Sci., Curr.Adv.Gen.& Molec.Biol., Curr.Cont., Dairy Sci.Abstr., Diar.Dis.Res., Excerp.Med., Helminthol.Abstr., Immun.Abstr., Ind.Med. (1979-), Ind.Sci.Rev., Ind.Vet., Inpharma, Int.Abstr.Biol.Sci., Microbiol.Abstr., Nutr.Abstr., Pig News & Info., Poult.Abstr., Protozool.Abstr., Reac., Rev.Appl.Entomol., Rev.Med.& Vet.Mycol., Sci.Cit.Ind., Trop.Dis.Bull., Vet.Bull., Wild.Rev., Zoo.Rec.
—BLDSC (6404.940000), ADONIS, CASDDS, CISTI, GNLM, IDS, Infotrieve, ingenta. **CCC.**
Published by: Blackwell Science Ltd., PO Box 88, Oxford OX2 0NE, United Kingdom. TEL 44-1865-206180, 44-1865-206002, FAX 44-1865-206219, jnl.orders@blacksci.co.uk, http://www.blackwell-science.com/~cgilib/jnlpage.asp?Journal=pimm&File=pimm, http://www.blackwellpublishing.com. Eds. D Wakelin, G A T Targett. Pub. Elizabeth Whelan. R&P Sophie Savage. Adv. contact Jenny Applin. Circ: 470.

616.96 GBR ISSN 0031-1820
CODEN: PARAAE
PARASITOLOGY (CAMBRIDGE). Text in English. 1908. m. (Plus two supplements). USD 760 to institutions (effective 2002). adv. bk.rev. index. back issues avail. *Refereed.* **Document type:** *Academic/Scholarly.* **Description:** Publishes papers on all aspects of pure and applied parasitology, including biochemical, immunological, physiological, and ecological topics, with emphasis on parasites and their control.

Related titles: Microfiche ed.: (from IDC,BHP); Microfilm ed.: (from PQC); Online - full text ed.: ISSN 1469-8161 (from EBSCO Publishing, O C L C Online Computer Library Center, Inc., RoweCom Information Quest, Swets Blackwell, Institute for Scientific Information).
Indexed: AIDS & Cancer Res., Abstr.Hyg., Agri.& Environ.Biotech.Abstr. (coverage dropped), Agricola, Anim.Breed.Abstr., Appl.Ecol.Abstr., Aqua.Sci.& Fish.Abstr., Aquacult.Abstr., Bibl.Agri., Bio-Contr.News & Info., Biol.Abstr., Biotech.& Bioeng.Abstr., Chem.Abstr., Curr.Adv.Ecol.Sci., Curr.Cont., Dairy Sci.Abstr., Derwent Biotech.Abstr., Ecol.Abstr., Entomol.Abstr., Environ.Sci.Poll.Mgmt., Excerp.Med., Genet.Abstr. (coverage dropped), Helminthol.Abstr., Hum.Gen.Abstr., INIS Atomind., Immun.Abstr. (coverage dropped), Ind.Med. (1908-), Ind.Sci.Rev., Ind.Vet., Int.Abstr.Biol.Sci., Microbiol.Abstr., Nutr.Abstr., Pollut.Abstr., Potato Abstr., Rev.Appl.Entomol., SSCI (coverage dropped), Saf.Sci.Abstr., Sci.Cit.Ind., Sport Fish.Abstr., Trop.Dis.Bull., Vet.Bull., Wild.Rev., Zoo.Rec.
—BLDSC (6406.000000), ADONIS, CASDDS, CISTI, GNLM, IDS, ingenta, Linda Hall. **CCC.**
Published by: Cambridge University Press, Edinburgh Bldg, Shaftesbury Rd, Cambridge CB2 2RU, United Kingdom. FAX 44-1223-315052, information@cup.cam.ac.uk, information@cambridge.org, http://www.cup.cam.ac.uk, http://www.uk.cambridge.org/journals/pmu. Eds. C Arme, F E G Cox, R.S. Phillips. R&P Linda Nicol.

616.96 NLD ISSN 1383-5769
CODEN: PAINFD
PARASITOLOGY INTERNATIONAL. Text in English. 1951. q. EUR 287 in Europe to institutions; JPY 38,100 in Japan to institutions; USD 322 elsewhere to institutions (effective 2002). adv. charts, illus. back issues avail.; reprint service avail. from PQC. *Refereed.* **Document type:** *Journal, Academic/Scholarly.* **Description:** Disseminates research in all areas of the field of human and animal parasitology, including immunology, cell biology, biochemistry, and molecular biology.
Formerly (until 1997): Kiseichugaku Zasshi - Japanese Journal of Parasitology (0021-5171)
Related titles: Microform ed.: (from PQC); Online - full text ed.: (from ingenta, ScienceDirect, Swets Blackwell, Institute for Scientific Information).
Indexed: Abstr.Hyg., AgBiotech, Agri.& Environ.Biotech.Abstr. (coverage dropped), Appl.Ecol.Abstr. (coverage dropped), Aqua.Sci.& Fish.Abstr., Biotech.& Bioeng.Abstr., Chem.Abstr., Derwent Biotech.Abstr., Entomol.Abstr., Environ.Sci.Poll.Mgmt., Excerp.Med., Genet.Abstr., Helminthol.Abstr., INIS Atomind., Ind.Med. (1997-), Ind.Vet., Microbiol.Abstr., Nuc.Acids Abstr., Pig News & Info., Poult.Abstr., Protozool.Abstr., Ref.Zh., Rev.Appl.Entomol., Rev.Med.& Vet.Mycol., Trop.Dis.Bull., Vet.Bull., Zoo.Rec.
—BLDSC (6406.115000), CASDDS, CISTI, GNLM, Infotrieve, ingenta. **CCC.**
Published by: (Japanese Society of Parasitology JPN), Elsevier Science BV, PO Box 211, Amsterdam 1000 AE, Netherlands. TEL 31-20-485-3757, FAX 31-20-485-3432, TELEX 18582 ESPA NL, http://www.elsevier.nl/locate/parint. Eds. S L Hajduk, Tsumotu Takeuchi. Circ: 1,250. **Subscr. in Australasia and the Far East to:** Elsevier Science (Singapore) Pte Ltd, No.1 Temasek Ave, 17-01 Millenia Tower, Singapore 039192, Singapore. TEL 65-434-3727, FAX 65-337-2230**; Subscr. in Japan to:** Elsevier Science Inc - Japan Regional Office, 9-15 Higashi-Azabu 1-chome, Minato-ku, Tokyo 106-0044, Japan. TEL 81-3-5561-5033, FAX 81-3-5561-5047**; Subscr. in the Americas to:** Elsevier Science, PO Box 945, New York, NY 10159-0945. TEL 212-633-3730, 888-437-4636, FAX 212-633-3680, usinfo-f@elsevier.com, http://www.elsevier.com. **Dist. by:** Elsevier Science (Brazil).

PARASITOLOGY RESEARCH. see *BIOLOGY—Microbiology*

616.96 574.524 ITA ISSN 0048-2951
QL757 CODEN: PSSGAR
PARASSITOLOGIA. Text in English, French, Italian; Summaries in English. 1959. q. ITL 240,000 (effective 1998). index. **Document type:** *Academic/Scholarly.*
Related titles: Microform ed.
Indexed: Abstr.Hyg., Aqua.Sci.& Fish.Abstr., Aquacult.Abstr., Biol.Abstr., Chem.Abstr., Entomol.Abstr., Environ.Sci.Poll.Mgmt., Excerp.Med., Helminthol.Abstr., Ind.Med. (1959-), Ind.Vet., Microbiol.Abstr., Poult.Abstr., Protozool.Abstr., Rev.Appl.Entomol., Rev.Med.& Vet.Mycol., Rice Abstr., Trop.Dis.Bull., Vet.Bull., Zoo.Rec.
—BLDSC (6406.130000), CASDDS, CISTI, GNLM, ingenta.
Published by: (Societa Italiana di Parassitologia), Lombardo Editore, Via Verona, 22, Rome, RM 00161, Italy. TEL 39-6-44290974, FAX 39-6-44238543. Ed. Mario Coluzzi. R&P Giorgio Lombardo.

616.96 RUS ISSN 0031-1847
QL757 CODEN: PAZGA4
PARAZITOLOGIYA/PARASITOLOGY. Text in Russian. 1966. bi-m. USD 167. index.
Related titles: Microfiche ed.: (from BHP).
Indexed: Abstr.Hyg., Apic.Abstr., Aqua.Sci.& Fish.Abstr., Aquacult.Abstr., Bio-Contr.News & Info., Biol.Abstr., Chem.Abstr., Chem.Indus.Notes, Chem.Titles, Curr.Adv.Ecol.Sci., Curr.Cont. (coverage dropped), Environ.Sci.Poll.Mgmt., Excerp.Med., Genet.Abstr. (coverage dropped), GeoRef, Helminthol.Abstr., Immun.Abstr., Ind.Med. (1967-), Ind.Vet., Microbiol.Abstr., Pig News & Info., Potato Abstr., Poult.Abstr., Protozool.Abstr., Ref.Zh., Rev.Appl.Entomol., Rev.Med.& Vet.Mycol., Risk Abstr., Sci.Cit.Ind. (coverage dropped), Trop.Dis.Bull., Vet.Bull., Weed Abstr., Zoo.Rec.
—BLDSC (0129.130000), CASDDS, CISTI, East View, GNLM, IDS, Infotrieve, KNAW, Linda Hall. **CCC.**
Published by: (Rossiiskaya Akademiya Nauk/Russian Academy of Sciences), M A I K Nauka - Interperiodica, S.-Peterburgskoe Otdelenie, Mendeleevskaya liniya 1, St Petersburg 199034, Russian Federation. TEL 812-2184609. Ed. Yu S Balashov. **US dist. addr.:** East View Publications, 3020 Harbor Ln N, Minneapolis, MN 55447. TEL 612-550-0961.

616.998 GBR ISSN 0308-745X
PARTNERS; magazine for paramedical workers. Text in Bengali, Chinese, English, French, Hindi. 1976. s-a. free per issue. adv. bk.rev. **Document type:** *Bulletin.* **Description:** Provides health information for health workers involved in leprosy and related subjects.
Indexed: Curr.Adv.Ecol.Sci., Rehabil.Lit., Trop.Dis.Bull.
Published by: Leprosy Mission International, 80 Windmill Rd, Brentford, Mddx TW8 0QH, United Kingdom. TEL 44-181-5697292, FAX 44-181-5697808, junen@tlmint.org, http://www.leprosymission.org/. Adv. contact June Nash. Circ: 30,000.

THE PEDIATRIC INFECTIOUS DISEASE JOURNAL. see *MEDICAL SCIENCES—Pediatrics*

PEDIATRIC PATHOLOGY & MOLECULAR MEDICINE. see *MEDICAL SCIENCES—Pediatrics*

616.998 PHL
PHILIPPINE JOURNAL OF DERMATOLOGY AND LEPROSY. Text and summaries in English. 1966. s-a. per issue exchange basis. bk.rev. abstr. illus.
Formerly: Philippine Journal of Leprosy (0031-7632)
Published by: Dermatology Research and Training Center, Ministry of Health, Manila, Philippines. Ed. Perpetua D Reyes Javier. Circ: 500.

PNEUMOLOGIA. see *MEDICAL SCIENCES—Respiratory Diseases*

616.9 362 ZAF ISSN 1022-5277
POSITIVE OUTLOOK; the thinking person's AIDS awareness magazine. Text in English; Text occasionally in Zulu. 1993. q. ZAR 20 to individuals; ZAR 50 to institutions. bk.rev. illus. *Refereed.* **Document type:** *Newsletter.*
Indexed: Ind.S.A.Per.
Published by: AIDS Training Information & Counselling Centre (ATICC), 42 Havelock Rd, Pietermaritzburg, KwaZulu-Natal 3201, South Africa. TEL 27-331-942111, FAX 27-331-423245, aticcpmb@aztec.co.za. Ed. Greg Wood. R&P Toine Vantilburg. Circ: 3,000. **Co-sponsor:** P A A G.

616.9 362.1 USA ISSN 1075-5705
RC607.A26
POZ; health, hope & HIV. Text in English. 1994. m. USD 19.97 domestic; USD 29.97 foreign (effective 2002); free to HIV patients. adv. bk.rev. illus. back issues avail.; reprints avail. **Document type:** *Magazine, Consumer.* **Description:** For anyone living with or affected by HIV. Includes profiles, investigative journalism, celebrity interviews, and the latest treatment information.
Related titles: Online - full text ed.; ♦ Spanish ed.: Poz en Espanol.
Indexed: Ind.Amer.Per.Verse, Soils & Fert.
—ingenta.
Published by: Poz Publishing, LLC, One Little W 12th St, 6th Fl, New York, NY 10014. TEL 212-242-2163, 800-973-2376, FAX 212-675-8505, webmaster@poz.com, poz-editor@poz.com, http://www.poz.com/, http://www.poz.com; http://thebody.com/poz/pozix.html. Eds. Sean Strub, Walter Armstrong. Pub. Megan Whiting. adv.: B&W page USD 7,735, color page USD 11,050; trim 10.5 x 7.88. Circ: 91,000.

362.1 USA
POZ EN ESPANOL. Text in Spanish. q. **Document type:** *Consumer.*
Related titles: ♦ English ed.: Poz. ISSN 1075-5705.
Published by: Poz Publishing, LLC, One Little W 12th St, 6th Fl, New York, NY 10014. TEL 800-973-2376, http://www.poz.com/espanol/. Ed. Alejandro Brito.

616.9 USA ISSN 1389-4986
▼ **PREVENTION SCIENCE.** Text in English. 2000. q. EUR 214 to institutions for print or online ed.; EUR 256.80 to institutions print & online eds.combined (effective 2002). illus. back issues avail. *Refereed.* **Document type:** *Journal, Academic/Scholarly.* **Description:** Disseminates developments in the theory, research, and practice of epidemiologic prevention.
Related titles: Online - full text ed.: (from EBSCO Publishing, O C L C Online Computer Library Center, Inc., RoweCom Information Quest, Swets Blackwell, Kluwer Online); Abridged ed.: USD 195 domestic to institutions; USD 230 foreign to institutions; USD 234 domestic to institutions includes print ed; USD 276 foreign to institutions includes print ed (effective 2000).
—BLDSC (6612.774430).
Published by: (Society for Prevention Research), Kluwer Academic - Plenum Publishers (Subsidiary of: Wolters Kluwer N.V.), 233 Spring St, New York, NY 10013-1578. TEL 212-620-8000, FAX 212-463-0742, http://www.wkap.nl/kaphtml.htm/KODETAILS. Ed. Gilbert J Botvin. Pub. Mariclaire Cloutier TEL 212-620-8013. **Dist. by:** Kluwer Academic Publishers Group, Journals Department, PO Box 322, Dordrecht 3300 AH, Netherlands. services@wkap.nl, http://www.wkap.nl.

616.9 BGR ISSN 0204-9155
PROBLEMS OF INFECTIOUS AND PARASITIC DISEASES. Text in English. 1973. s-a. USD 34 foreign (effective 2002). **Document type:** *Journal, Academic/Scholarly.*
Published by: Meditsinski Universitet - Sofia, Tsentur za Informatsiia po Meditsina/Medical University - Sofia, Medical Information Center, 1 Sv Georgi Sofiiski ul, Sofia 1431, Bulgaria. TEL 359-2-9522342, FAX 359-2-9522393, http://www.medun.acad.bg. **Dist. by:** Sofia Books, Ul Silivria 16, Sofia 1404, Bulgaria. TEL 359-2-9586257, sofiabooks@hotmail.com, http://www.sofiabooks.hit.bg.

PROCEEDINGS OF PARASITOLOGY. see *BIOLOGY—Microbiology*

616.9 USA ISSN 1042-363X
CODEN: PAPAE8
PROGRESS IN AIDS PATHOLOGY. Text in English. 1989. irreg., latest vol.4. USD 125 to individuals; USD 155 to institutions. *Refereed.* **Document type:** *Academic/Scholarly.*
Indexed: Curr.Cont. (coverage dropped), Ind.Med. (coverage dropped).
—GNLM, KNAW.
Published by: Field & Wood, Medical Periodicals, Inc., PO Box 975, Blue Bell, PA 19422. TEL 610-828-4010, FAX 215-482-0226. Eds. Dr. H Rotterdam, M A Greco.

616.0194 CHE ISSN 0079-645X
RC114.5 CODEN: PMVIA6
PROGRESS IN MEDICAL VIROLOGY. Text in English. 1958. irreg., latest vol.40. CHF 220 in Europe; DEM 265 in Germany; USD 175 in United States (2001). reprint service avail. from ISI. *Refereed.* **Document type:** *Monographic series, Academic/Scholarly.*
Related titles: Online - full text ed.: (from Institute for Scientific Information).
Indexed: ASCA, Abstr.Hyg., Biol.Abstr., Chem.Abstr., Chem.Titles, Curr.Adv.Ecol.Sci., Curr.Cont. (coverage dropped), Dent.Ind., INIS Atomind., Ind.Med. (1958-), Ind.Sci.Rev., Ind.Vet., Sci.Cit.Ind., Vet.Bull.
—BLDSC (6868.960000), CASDDS, CISTI, GNLM, IDS, KNAW. **CCC.**
Published by: S. Karger AG, Allschwilerstr 10, PO Box, Basel 4009, Switzerland. TEL 41-61-306-1111, FAX 41-61-306-1234, karger@karger.ch, http://www.karger.com/bookseries/PRMEV.

M

616.9 614 GBR
PUBLIC HEALTH LABORATORY SERVICE BOARD. REPORT. Text in English. 1975. irreg. **Document type:** *Corporate.*
Former titles: Public Health Laboratory Service Board. Annual Report (0142-3517); Public Health Laboratory Service Board. Year Book (0306-1531)
Published by: Public Health Laboratory Service, 61 Colindale Ave, London NW9 5HT, United Kingdom. TEL 44-20-8200-4400, FAX 44-20-8200-7875. Circ: 1,500.

616.998 362.1 ITA ISSN 1121-0435
QUADERNI DI COOPERAZIONE SANITARIA/CAHIERS DE COOPERATION MEDICALE/HEALTH COOPERATION PAPERS. Text in English, French, Italian. 1980. s-a. free per issue. bk.rev. bibl, charts, illus, maps, stat. back issues avail. *Refereed.* **Document type:** *Monographic series.* **Description:** Covers mainly leprosy and tropical diseases and rehabilitation. Focuses on problems in developing countries.
Related titles: E-mail ed.
—GNLM.
Published by: Amici di Raoul Follereau, Via Girolamo Borselli, 4-6, Bologna, BO 40135, Italy. TEL 39-051-433402, FAX 39-051-434046, info@aifo.it, http:www.aifo.it. Ed. Enrico Nunzi. Circ: 2,000 (controlled).

616.998 GBR ISSN 0266-3775
RECENT ADVANCES IN TROPICAL MEDICINE. Text in English. irreg. **Document type:** *Monographic series, Academic/Scholarly.*
Published by: Churchill Livingstone (Subsidiary of: Harcourt Publishers Ltd.), Robert Stevenson House, 1-3 Baxter's Pl, Leith Walk, Edinburgh, Midlothian EH1 3AF, United Kingdom. TEL 44-131-556-2424, FAX 44-131-459-1177, http://www.churchillmed.com. **US subscr. to:** Churchill Livingstone, 650 Ave of the Americas, New York, NY 10011. TEL 212-206-5000.

RESEARCH INITIATIVE, TREATMENT ACTION!. see *MEDICAL SCIENCES—Allergology And Immunology*

616.9 CHL ISSN 0716-1018
REVISTA CHILENA DE INFECTOLOGIA. Text in Spanish. 1984. 3/yr. CLP 30,000 domestic; CLP 60,000 foreign (effective 2001). back issues avail.
Related titles: Online - full text ed.: ISSN 0717-6341.
Published by: Sociedad Chilena de Infectologia, Bernarda Morin 488 Piso 2, Santiago de Chile, Providencia 9, Chile. TEL 56-2-341-3539, revinf@cmet.net, http://www.sochif.web.cl. Ed. Jose Cofre.

616.988 CUB ISSN 0375-0760
RC960 CODEN: RCMTBF
REVISTA CUBANA DE MEDICINA TROPICAL. Text in Spanish; Summaries in English, Spanish. 1945. 3/yr. USD 55 in the Americas; USD 60 in Europe; USD 68 elsewhere. bibl, charts, illus. index.
Formerly (until 1966): Revista Kuba de Medicina Tropical y Parasitologia (0025-794X)
Related titles: Online - full text ed.
Indexed: Abstr.Hyg., Bio-Contr.News & Info., Biol.Abstr., Chem.Abstr., Curr.Adv.Ecol.Sci., Excerp.Med., Helminthol.Abstr., Ind.Med. (1966-), Nutr.Abstr., Protozool.Abstr., Repindex, Rev.Appl.Entomol., Rev.Med.& Vet.Mycol., Trop.Dis.Bull., Zoo.Rec.
—CISTI, GNLM.
Published by: (Cuba. Ministerio de Salud Publica, Centro Nacional de Informacion de Ciencias Medicas), Editorial de Ciencias Medicas, O'Reilly No. 4, Habana, Cuba. TEL 62-8091. Ed. Ivette Cabrera. Circ: 1,000. **Co-sponsor:** Instituto de Medicina Tropical "Pedro Kouri".

616.988 ECU ISSN 0048-7775
CODEN: REHMAG
REVISTA ECUATORIANA DE HIGIENE Y MEDICINA TROPICAL. Text in Spanish. 1944. q. per issue exchange basis. illus. reprint service avail. from ISI.
Indexed: Biol.Abstr., Ind.Med. (coverage dropped), Rev.Appl.Entomol.
—GNLM.
Published by: Instituto Nacional de Higiene y Medicina Tropical "Leopoldo Izquieta Perez", Casilla de Correos 3961, Guayaquil, Guayas, Ecuador. Circ: 3,500.

616.0194 ROM ISSN 1018-0532
CODEN: RRVIEX
REVUE ROUMAINE DE VIROLOGIE/RUMANIAN JOURNAL OF VIROLOGY. Text in English, French, German, Russian. 1964. q. bk.rev. **Document type:** *Academic/Scholarly.*
Former titles: Revue Roumaine de Medecine. Serie Virologie; Revue Roumaine de Virologie; Revue Roumaine d'Inframicrobiologie (0035-4082)
Indexed: Abstr.Hyg., Biol.Abstr., Chem.Abstr., Chem.Indus.Notes, Chem.Titles, Excerp.Med., Ind.Med. (coverage dropped), Ind.Vet., Poult.Abstr., Rev.Appl.Entomol., Trop.Dis.Bull., Vet.Bull., Virol.Abstr. (coverage dropped).
—BLDSC (8019.655000), CASDDS, CISTI, EMDOCS, GNLM, KNAW, Linda Hall.
Published by: (Institutul de Virologie St. Nicolau, Academia Romana), Editura Academiei Romane, Calea 13 Septembrie 13, Bucharest 76117, Romania. TEL 40-0-507680. Ed. N Cajal. Circ: 800. **Dist. by:** Rodipet S.A.. TEL 401-618-5103, FAX 401-222-6407.

RIVISTA DI PARASSITOLOGIA. see *BIOLOGY—Microbiology*

616.9 RUS ISSN 1560-9588
ROSSIISKII ZHURNAL KOZHNYKH I VENERICHESKIKH BOLEZNEI/RUSSIAN JOURNAL OF SKIN AND SEXUALLY TRANSMITTED DISEASES. Text in Russian; Summaries in English. 1998. bi-m. USD 190 foreign (effective 2000). adv. bk.rev. abstr, bibl, illus. reprints avail. **Document type:** *Journal.* **Description:** Covers issues related to sexually transmitted diseases, including new approaches to diagnosis, treatment and prevention of skin and venereal diseases.
Published by: Izdatel'stvo Meditsina, Petroverigskii per 6-8, Moscow 101000, Russian Federation. TEL 7-095-4244044, 7-095-928-86-48, FAX 7-095-4244188, 7-095-9211355, meditsina@iname.com, http://www.medit.ru. Ed. O L Ivanov. Pub. A M Stochik. R&P J N Afanasyeva. Adv. contact O A Fadeeva TEL 7-095-923-51-40. Circ: 660. **Dist. by:** Mezhdunarodnaya Kniga, B Yakimanka 39, Moscow 117049, Russian Federation. TEL 7-095-2384967, FAX 7-095-2384634; **US dist. addr.:** East View Publications, 3020 Harbor Ln N, Minneapolis, MN 55447. TEL 612-550-0961.

616.9 USA
ROYAL COLLEGE OF PHYSICIANS AND SURGEONS OF U S A. JOURNAL. Text in English. 1984. s-a. USD 75 to non-members; USD 50 to members; USD 100 to institutions (effective 1999). adv. bk.rev. back issues avail.; reprints avail. *Refereed.* **Document type:** *Directory, Academic/Scholarly.* **Description:** Offers practical approaches to diagnosis and treatment of tropical diseases as a continuing education to physicians in tropical countries.
Formerly: American Academy of Tropical Medicine and Surgery. Journal (0891-544X)
Published by: Royal College of Physicians and Surgeons of U S A, 16126 E Warren, Box 24224, Detroit, MI 48224. TEL 313-882-0641, FAX 313-882-5110. Ed. Dr. Ben Alli.

616.988 GBR ISSN 1366-9443
ROYAL SOCIETY OF TROPICAL MEDICINE AND HYGIENE, LONDON. YEARBOOK. Text in English. 1908. biennial. GBP 20 to non-members (effective 1999). **Document type:** *Directory.*
Indexed: Curr.Cont. (coverage dropped).
Published by: Royal Society of Tropical Medicine and Hygiene, Manson House, 26 Portland Pl, London W1N 4EY, United Kingdom. TEL 44-20-7580-2127, FAX 44-20-7436-1389, mail@rstmh.org, trans@rstmh.org, http://www.rstmh.org. Ed. C R Guest. Circ: 2,500.

616.988 GBR ISSN 0035-9203
CODEN: TRSTAZ
ROYAL SOCIETY OF TROPICAL MEDICINE AND HYGIENE. TRANSACTIONS. Text in English. 1907. bi-m. GBP 140; GBP 185 Print & CD eds. (effective 1999). adv. bibl, charts, illus. index. *Refereed.* **Document type:** *Proceedings, Academic/Scholarly.*
Related titles: CD-ROM ed.; Online - full text ed.: (from Institute for Scientific Information).
Indexed: ASCA, Abstr.Hyg., Aqua.Sci.& Fish.Abstr., Bio-Contr.News & Info., Biol.Abstr., Chem.Abstr., Chem.Indus.Notes, Curr.Adv.Cancer Res., Curr.Adv.Ecol.Sci., Curr.Adv.Gen.& Molec.Biol., Curr.Cont., Dairy Sci.Abstr., Dent.Ind., Diar.Dis.Res., Entomol.Abstr. (coverage dropped), Environ.Sci.Poll.Mgmt., Excerp.Med., Helminthol.Abstr., INIS Atomind., Ind.Med. (1920-), Ind.Sci.Rev., Ind.Vet., Inpharma, Int.Abstr.Biol.Sci., Med.& Surg.Dermat., Microbiol.Abstr., Nutr.Abstr., Pharm.&Out.News, Pig News & Info., Pollut.Abstr., Protozool.Abstr., Reac., Rev.Appl.Entomol., Rev.Med.& Vet.Mycol., Rev.Plant Path., Risk Abstr., Rural Devel.Abstr., SSCI (coverage dropped), Saf.Sci.Abstr., Sci.Cit.Ind., Sel.Water Res.Abstr., So.Pac.Per.Ind., Soils & Fert., Sport Fish.Abstr., Trop.Dis.Bull., Vet.Bull., Wild.Rev., Zoo.Rec.
—BLDSC (9003.000000), CASDDS, CISTI, GNLM, IDS, ingenta, KNAW. **CCC.**
Published by: Royal Society of Tropical Medicine and Hygiene, Manson House, 26 Portland Pl, London W1N 4EY, United Kingdom. TEL 44-20-7580-2127, FAX 44-20-7436-1389, trans@rstmh.org, http://www.rstmh.org. Ed. Dr. C A Brown. adv.: B&W page GBP 500, color page GBP 1,000. Circ: 3,300.

616.9 ESP
S E I SIDA. Variant title: S E I Sindrome de Inmunologia Deficiente Adquirido. Text in Spanish. 1990. 12/yr. ESP 5,000. adv.
Published by: Sociedad Espanola Interdisciplinaria del SIDA, Principe de Vergara, 112 1o G, Madrid 28002, Spain. TEL 34-1-5637306, FAX 34-1-5632393. Ed. Dr. Najera Morrondo. Circ: 3,500.

616.9792 MEX ISSN 1405-2946
RA644.A25
S I D A - E T S. Text in Spanish; Summaries in English. 1995. q. MXP 210, USD 40 (effective 1996 & 1997). *Refereed.* **Document type:** *Academic/Scholarly.* **Description:** Presents Mexico's current official epidemiological data on HIV. Includes review articles on prevention and notices.
Published by: (Consejo Nacional para la Prevencion y Control del SIDA), Obsidiana Editores S.A., CZDA DE TLALPAN 2365, Col Ciudad Jardin, Mexico City, DF 04370, Mexico. TEL 52-5-689-9133. Eds. Dr. Blanca Rico, Elisa Salame. Pub. Jorge Godoy-Gutierrez. **Dist. by:** Distribuidora Editorial de Mexico SA de CV, P.O. Box 76-026, Mexico City, DF 04201, Mexico. TEL 52-5-544-7953, FAX 52-5-689-6545.

SASKATCHEWAN. LABORATORY AND DISEASE CONTROL SERVICES BRANCH. ANNUAL STATISTICAL REPORT. see *INSURANCE*

616 NOR ISSN 0036-5548
CODEN: SJIDB7
SCANDINAVIAN JOURNAL OF INFECTIOUS DISEASES. Text in English. 1969. 12/yr. GBP 145, USD 240 to individuals; GBP 276, USD 455 to institutions (effective 2002). adv. *Refereed.* **Document type:** *Academic/Scholarly.* **Description:** Publishes original papers on clinical aspects of infectious diseases.
Related titles: Online - full text ed.: (from EBSCO Publishing, O C L C Online Computer Library Center, Inc., RoweCom Information Quest, CatchWord Ltd., ingenta, Swets Blackwell, Institute for Scientific Information); ♦ Supplement: Scandinavian Journal of Infectious Diseases. Supplementum. ISSN 0300-8878.
Indexed: ASCA, Abstr.Hyg., Agri.& Environ.Biotech.Abstr. (coverage dropped), Aqua.Sci.& Fish.Abstr., Biol.Abstr., Biol.Dig., CINAHL, Chem.Abstr., Curr.Adv.Ecol.Sci., Curr.Cont., Dairy Sci.Abstr., Dent.Ind., Derwent Biotech.Abstr., Diar.Dis.Res., Dok.Arbeitsmed., Environ.Sci.Poll.Mgmt., Excerp.Med., Helminthol.Abstr., INIS Atomind., Ind.Med. (1969-), Ind.Sci.Rev., Ind.Vet., Inpharma, Int.Abstr.Biol.Sci., Jrnl.Watch Derm., Jrnl.Watch Inf.Dis., Med.& Surg.Dermat., Microbiol.Abstr., NRN, Neurosci.Cit.Ind., Nutr.Abstr., Pharm.&Out.News, Pollut.Abstr., Protozool.Abstr., Reac., Ref.Zh., Rev.Appl.Entomol., Rev.Med.& Vet.Mycol., Rev.Plant Path., Risk Abstr., SSCI (coverage dropped), Saf.Sci.Abstr., Sci.Cit.Ind., Trop.Dis.Bull., Vet.Bull.
—BLDSC (8087.517000), CASDDS, CISTI, GNLM, IDS, ingenta, KNAW. **CCC.**
Published by: Taylor & Francis AS (Subsidiary of: Taylor & Francis Group), Cort Adelersgt. 17, Solli, PO Box 2562, Oslo 0202, Norway. TEL 47-22-12-98-80, FAX 47-22-12-98-90, journals@tandf.no, http://www.tandf.co.uk/tfas. Ed. Ragnar S Noerreby. Circ: 1,200.

616.9 NOR ISSN 0300-8878
CODEN: SJISAH
SCANDINAVIAN JOURNAL OF INFECTIOUS DISEASES. SUPPLEMENTUM. Text in Norwegian. 1970. irreg. free to Journal subscribers. **Document type:** *Academic/Scholarly.*
Related titles: ♦ Supplement to: Scandinavian Journal of Infectious Diseases. ISSN 0036-5548.
Indexed: Aqua.Sci.& Fish.Abstr., CINAHL, Cal.Tiss.Abstr., Chemorec.Abstr., Environ.Sci.Poll.Mgmt., Excerp.Med. (1988-), Ind.Med. (1970-), Int.Abstr.Biol.Sci., Microbiol.Abstr., Neurosci.Abstr. (coverage dropped), Rev.Med.& Vet.Mycol.
—BLDSC (8087.517100), CASDDS, CISTI, EMDOCS, ingenta, KNAW. **CCC.**
Published by: Scandinavian University Press (Subsidiary of: Taylor & Francis Ltd.), Postboks 2959, Toeyen, Oslo 0608, Norway. FAX 47-22-57-53-53, journals@scup.no, http://www.scup.no/sjid.

SEMINARS IN DIAGNOSTIC PATHOLOGY. see *MEDICAL SCIENCES*

M

616.9 USA ISSN 1531-8192
▼ **SEMINARS IN INFECTION CONTROL.** Text in English. 2001. q. USD 109 domestic to individuals; USD 139 domestic to institutions; USD 75 domestic to students; USD 154 foreign to individuals; USD 189 foreign to institutions; USD 154 foreign to students; USD 48 newsstand/cover (effective 2001). adv. *Refereed.* **Document type:** *Journal, Academic/Scholarly.* **Description:** Contains articles and information on infection control and hospital epidemiology.
Published by: W.B. Saunders Co. (Subsidiary of: Harcourt Publishers Ltd.), 11830 Westline Industrial Dr, St Louis, MO 63146. TEL 800-325-4177, http://www.wbsaunders.com. Eds. Dr. David Weber, Dr. William A Rutala.

SEMINARS IN PEDIATRIC INFECTIOUS DISEASES. see *MEDICAL SCIENCES—Pediatrics*

616.944 USA ISSN 1385-0229 CODEN: SEPSFM
SEPSIS. Text in English. 1997. q. USD 286, EUR 286 to institutions for print or online ed.; USD 343.20, EUR 343.20 to institutions for print & online eds.combined (effective 2002). back issues avail. *Refereed.* **Document type:** *Academic/Scholarly.* **Description:** Promotes the interdisciplinary exchange of knowledge and ideas in the study of Sepsis and brings together the insights and perspectives of acknowledged authorities with the objective of facilitating the creative exchange of ideas and perspectives.
Related titles: Online - full text ed.: (from EBSCO Publishing, O C L C Online Computer Library Center, Inc., RoweCom Information Quest, Swets Blackwell, Kluwer Online).
Indexed: AIDS & Cancer Res., Abstr.Hyg., Environ.Sci.Poll.Mgmt., Microbiol.Abstr., Virol.Abstr.
—BLDSC (8242.272230), Infotrieve. **CCC.**
Published by: Kluwer Academic Publishers Boston, 101 Philip Dr, Assinippi Park, Norwell, MA 02061. TEL 781-871-6600, FAX 781-681-9045, services@wkap.nl, http://www.wkap.nl/journalhome.htm/1385-0229, http//www.wkap.nl. Ed. John C Marshall. R&P Rose Luongo TEL 781-871-6311. **Dist. outside N. America by:** Kluwer Academic Publishers Group, Journals Department, PO Box 322, Dordrecht 3300 AH, Netherlands. FAX 31-78-639-2254, 31-78-654-6474.

▼ **SEX EDUCATION.** see *EDUCATION*

616.9 NLD ISSN 1388-3046
RA644.A25
SEXUAL HEALTH EXCHANGE. Text in English. 1988. q. NLG 50; free in developing nations. back issues avail. *Refereed.* **Document type:** *Newsletter, Consumer.* **Description:** Reports on AIDS and sexually transmitted disease education and prevention activities worldwide, with an emphasis on developing nations.
Former titles (until 1997): AIDS - S T D Health Promotion Exchange (1384-2692); AIDS Health Promotion Exchange (1013-7785)
Related titles: CD-ROM ed.
Indexed: ExtraMED.
—BLDSC (8254.484400), GNLM, ingenta, KNAW.
Published by: Royal Tropical Institute (KIT), Library and Documentation Department, PO Box 95001, Amsterdam 1090 HA, Netherlands. TEL 31-20-568-8311, FAX 31-20-665-4423, acb@kit.nl, http://www.kit.nl/ibd/html/exchange.htm. Ed. Joost Hoppenbrouwer. R&P Dorothy Timmerman. Circ: 12,500. **Co-sponsor:** Southern Africa AIDS Information Dissemination Service (SAfAIDS).

616.9 917.306 USA
SIDA; todo lo que usted debe saber. Variant title: S I D A. Text in Spanish. m. **Description:** Gives preventative measures, medical views and interviews, and news of recent AIDS research and advancements.
Published by: Latin American News and Book Inc., 614 Franklin St, Elizabeth, NJ 07206. TEL 908-355-8835, FAX 908-527-9160. Ed. Jose Tenreiro Napoles. Pub. Jesus M Tenreiro. adv.: B&W page USD 650; trim 9.5 x 6.75. Circ: 45,000.

616.9 362.4 305.89 USA
SIDA AHORA✶ . Variant title: S I D A Ahora. Text in Spanish. 1989. bi-m. USD 20. **Description:** Written for the Latino community; contains original personal stories, legal and medical information about AIDS, editorial observation, and political coverage.
Published by: People With AIDS Coalition of New York, 50 W 17th St, 8th fl, New York, NY 10011. TEL 212-647-1415, FAX 212-647-1419, http://www.aidsinfonyc.org/pwac/.

616.97 USA
SIDAAHORA. Text in Spanish. 1989. bi-m. USD 35 donation (effective 2000). adv. **Description:** Deals with all aspects of HIV/AIDS, including medical, legal, social services, and financial issues aimed at people with HIV, their friends, families, caregivers, and service providers.
Published by: Body Positive, Inc, 19 Fulton St, Ste 308B, New York, NY 10038. TEL 212-566-7333, FAX 212-566-4539, bodypos@aol.com, http://thebody.com/bp/bp.html. R&P Rich Brigandi. adv.: page USD 2,255; 7 x 9. Circ: 13,500 (controlled). **Dist. by:** Contemporary Guidance, 229 West 28th St, New York, NY 10001.

616.9 916 FRA ISSN 1245-060X
SIDAFRIQUE. Text in French. 4/yr. FRF 200; FRF 75 newsstand/cover. **Description:** Analyzes the epidemiology, scientific and clinical research, treatment and care issues, ethical, socio-economic and political issues regarding AIDS.
Related titles: English ed.
Published by: John Libbey Eurotext, 127 av. de la Republique, Montrouge 92120, France. TEL 33-01-46730660, FAX 33-01-40840999, marketing@jle.com, http://www.john-libbey-eurotext.fr. Ed. Gilles Brucker.

616.9792 ESP ISSN 1130-1597
SOCIEDAD ESPANOLA INTERDISCIPLINARIA DE S I D A. PUBLICACION OFICIAL. (Sindrome de Inmunodeficiencia Adquirida) Text in Spanish. 1990. m. (10/yr.). USD 75 (effective 1996).
—CINDOC.
Published by: (Sociedad Espanola Interdisciplinaria de S.I.D.A.), Editorial Idepsa S.A., Principe de Vergara, 112 1o F, Madrid 28002, Spain. TEL 34-1-5637306, FAX 34-1-5632393.

616.988 THA ISSN 0125-1562 CODEN: SJTMAK
SOUTHEAST ASIAN JOURNAL OF TROPICAL MEDICINE AND PUBLIC HEALTH. Text in English. 1970. q. USD 80. adv. bk.rev. abstr, bibl, illus. index. reprint service avail. from PQC. **Document type:** *Academic/Scholarly.*
Related titles: CD-ROM ed.; Microform ed.: (from PQC).
Indexed: Abstr.Hyg., Aqua.Sci.& Fish.Abstr., Aquacult.Abstr., Bio-Contr.News & Info., Biol.Abstr., Chem.Abstr., Chem.Indus.Notes, Chem.Titles, Dairy Sci.Abstr., Diar.Dis.Res., Entomol.Abstr., Environ.Sci.Poll.Mgmt., Excerp.Med., ExtraMED, Food Sci.& Tech.Abstr., Helminthol.Abstr., Ind.Med. (coverage dropped), Ind.Vet., Inpharma, Int.Nurs.Ind., Microbiol.Abstr., Nutr.Abstr., Pharm.&Out.News, Pig News & Info., Pollut.Abstr., Poult.Abstr., Protozool.Abstr., Reac., Rev.Appl.Entomol., Rev.Med.& Vet.Mycol., Rev.Plant Path., Risk Abstr., Rural Devel.Abstr., Saf.Sci.Abstr., Sel.Water Res.Abstr., So.Pac.Per.Ind., Trop.Dis.Bull., Vet.Bull., Zoo.Rec.
—BLDSC, CASDDS, KNAW. **CCC.**
Published by: Southeast Asian Ministers of Education Organisation (SEAMEO), Regional Tropical Medicine & Public Health Project (TROPMED), 420-6 Rajvithi Rd, Bangkok 10400, Thailand. TEL 66-2-2457193, FAX 66-2-2477721. Ed. Chev Kidson. Circ: 1,000.

SPAIN. MINISTERIO DE AGRICULTURA, PESCA Y ALIMENTACION. BOLETIN DE SANIDAD VEGETAL: PLAGAS. see *AGRICULTURE—Crop Production And Soil*

616.9 USA ISSN 0895-755X
SPOTLIGHT ON AIDS✶ . Text in English. 198?. 12/yr. USD 20.
Formerly: Odyssey Institute Journal
Published by: Odyssey Institute Corporation, Concerned Physicians Network, 5 Hedley Rd, Westport, CT 06880.

616.998 USA ISSN 0049-2116 CODEN: STARC
THE STAR (CARVILLE); radiating the light of truth on Hansen's disease. Text in English. 1941. bi-m. USD 2. bk.rev. charts, illus. reprint service avail. from PQC.
Related titles: Microform ed.: (from PQC).
Indexed: Excerp.Med., Rehabil.Lit., Trop.Dis.Bull.
—BLDSC (8434.560000), EMDOCS, GNLM, ingenta.
Published by: Star (Carville), National Hansen s Disease Center, Box 325, Point Clair Br, Carville, LA 70721. TEL 504-642-5559. Ed. Manuel Faris. Circ: 70,000.

616.96 USA
STUDIES IN INFECTIOUS DISEASES RESEARCH. Text in English. 1975. irreg., latest 1989. price varies. *Refereed.*
Published by: University of Chicago Press, 5801 S Ellis Ave, Chicago, IL 60637. TEL 773-702-7899, sales@press.uchicago.edu, http://www.press.uchicago.edu.

▼ **SURGICAL INFECTIONS.** see *MEDICAL SCIENCES—Surgery*

616.979201 USA
THE T E A C H EDUCATOR. (Treatment Education Activists Combating HIV) Text in English. irreg. (2-3/yr.). *Refereed.* **Description:** Provides information on training programs for people living with HIV, focusing on secondary prevention, drug treatment programs and support for families.
Published by: T E A C H Educator, 1233 Locus St, 5th Fl, Philadelphia, PA 19107. TEL 215-985-4448, FAX 215-985-4952, harleyag@critpath.org; jdavids@critpath.org, http://www.fight.org/teach/educator.html. Eds. Agnes Harley, Julie Davids.

616.9 USA
TEXAS HIV - STD UPDATE. Text in English. 1988. q. free per issue. back issues avail. **Document type:** *Newsletter.* **Description:** Statewide news on Sexually Transmitted Diseases (STD), Human Immunodeficiency Virus (HIV) and AIDS, resources for health education and risk reduction.
Former titles: HIV - STD Update; HIV Prevention News
Published by: Texas Department of Health, Bureau of HIV and STD Prevention, 1100 W 49th St, Austin, TX 78756. TEL 512-490-2535, FAX 512-490-2538, gbeets@std.tdh.state.tx.us, http://www.tdh.state.tx.us/hivstd/. Ed. Greg Bees. Circ: 3,000.

616.9 362.1 NLD ISSN 0928-2998
TIJDSCHRIFT VOOR HYGIENE EN INFEKTIEPREVENTIE. Text in Dutch. 1981. bi-m. NLG 67.50 (effective 2001). 36 p./no. 3 cols./p. **Document type:** *Academic/Scholarly.* **Description:** Publishes original papers on all aspects of hospital hygiene and infection prevention, investigations, reviews of the literature, and communications about practical problems in infection prevention.
Formerly (until 1992): Ziekenhuishygiene en Infektiepreventie
Published by: Stichting Tijdschrift Hygiene en Infektiepreventie, Kennedystraat 4A, Duiven 6921 CW, Netherlands. TEL 31-24-6454513. Circ: 800 (paid).

616.9792 CAN
TREATMENT UPDATE. Text in English, French. 1992. 10/yr. back issues avail. **Document type:** *Bulletin.* **Description:** Provides news on current research in treatments for HIV and AIDS in Canada.
Media: Online - full text.
Published by: C A T I E, 555-505 Richmond St W, Toronto, ON M5V 2B1, Canada. TEL 416-203-7122, FAX 416-203-8284, 800-263-1638, http://www.catie.ca/tu.nsf.

TRENDS IN PARASITOLOGY. see *BIOLOGY—Microbiology*

TROPICAL DISEASES BULLETIN. see *MEDICAL SCIENCES—Abstracting, Bibliographies, Statistics*

616.988 GBR ISSN 0049-4755
RC960 CODEN: TPDCAV
TROPICAL DOCTOR; a journal of modern medical practice. Text in English. 1971. q. GBP 52 in Europe to institutions; USD 97 in United States to institutions; GBP 56 elsewhere to institutions (effective 2002). bk.rev. illus. reprint service avail. from ISI. *Refereed.* **Document type:** *Journal, Academic/Scholarly.* **Description:** Publishes contributions on the prevention, management and treatment of prevalent diseases in developing countries and on the promotion of health.
Related titles: Online - full text ed.: (from Institute for Scientific Information).
Indexed: ASCA, Abstr.Hyg., Abstr.Rural Dev.Trop., Biol.Abstr., Curr.Adv.Ecol.Sci., Curr.Cont., Diar.Dis.Res., Excerp.Med., Helminthol.Abstr., Ind.Med. (1971-), Inpharma, Int.Nurs.Ind., Nutr.Abstr., Pharm.&Out.News, Protozool.Abstr., Reac., Rev.Appl.Entomol., Rev.Arom.& Med.Plants, Rev.Med.& Vet.Mycol., Rice Abstr., SSCI (coverage dropped), So.Pac.Per.Ind., Trop.Dis.Bull.
—BLDSC (9056.060000), ADONIS, CISTI, GNLM, IDS, ingenta, KNAW. **CCC.**
Published by: Royal Society of Medicine Press Ltd, 1 Wimpole St, London W1M 8AE, United Kingdom. TEL 44-20-7290-2921, FAX 44-20-7290-2929, rsmjournals@rsm.ac.uk, http://www.roysocmed.ac.uk/pub/td.htm. Ed. Michael E Jones. R&P Caroline McLaughlin. Circ: 2,000.

616.988 JPN ISSN 0041-3267
TROPICAL MEDICINE/NETTAI IGAKU. Text in English. 1959. q. per issue exchange basis only. abstr, charts, illus. index. *Refereed.* **Document type:** *Academic/Scholarly.*

M

Formerly: Endemic Diseases Bulletin of Nagasaki University
Indexed: Abstr.Hyg., Bio-Contr.News & Info., Biol.Abstr., Diar.Dis.Res., Excerp.Med., Helminthol.Abstr., Ind.Vet., Poult.Abstr., Protozool.Abstr., Ref.Zh., Rev.Appl.Entomol., Rev.Med.& Vet.Mycol., Rural Devel.Abstr., Trop.Dis.Bull., Vet.Bull., Zoo.Rec.
—BLDSC, GNLM.
Published by: Nagasaki Daigaku, Nettai Igaku Kenkyujo/Nagasaki University, Institute of Tropical Medicine, 1-12-4 Sakamoto, Nagasaki-shi 852-8523, Japan. Ed. Yoshiki Aoki TEL 81-95-849-7822. Circ: 450.

616.988 USA ISSN 0041-3275
RC960 CODEN: TMHNAT
TROPICAL MEDICINE AND HYGIENE NEWS. Text in English. 1952. bi-m. membership. bk.rev. **Document type:** *Newsletter.*
Indexed: Abstr.Hyg., Biol.Abstr., Helminthol.Abstr., Protozool.Abstr., Trop.Dis.Bull.
—GNLM.
Published by: American Society of Tropical Medicine and Hygiene (Washington), 6436 31st St, N W, Washington, DC 20015. TEL 202-364-5969, FAX 202-369-5969. Eds. Dr. Karl A Western, Kathryn S Aultman. Circ: 3,500 (controlled).

TROPICAL MEDICINE & INTERNATIONAL HEALTH. see *PUBLIC HEALTH AND SAFETY*

616.9 THA
TROPMED SEMINARS ON TROPICAL MEDICINE. PROCEEDINGS. Text in English. irreg., latest vol.29, 1986. USD 10. **Document type:** *Proceedings.*
Former titles: Tropmed Seminars on Parasitology and Tropical Medicine. Proceedings.; Southeast Asian Seminar on Parasitology and Tropical Medicine. Proceedings (0085-6517)
Published by: Southeast Asian Ministers of Education Organisation (SEAMEO), Regional Tropical Medicine & Public Health Project (TROPMED), 420-6 Rajvithi Rd, Bangkok 10400, Thailand. TEL 66-2-2457193, FAX 66-2-2477721. Circ: 500.

616.9 USA
TUBERCULOSIS & AIRBORNE DISEASE WEEKLY. Text in English. 1993. w. (43/yr.). USD 1,549 in North America; USD 1,649 elsewhere. **Document type:** *Newsletter.* **Description:** Concentrates on tuberculosis-related news and research worldwide, with original reporting, reviews of periodicals and journal articles, calendars of forthcoming professional meetings. Topics include TB-control programs, vaccine development, the dual epidemics of AIDS and TB, and government roles and responses.
Formerly: T B Weekly (1065-982X)
Related titles: Microform ed.: (from PQC); Online - full text ed.: (from CompuServe, Inc., Data-Star, The Dialog Corporation, Dow Jones Interactive, Gale Group, NewsNet).
Indexed: Bus.& Indus. (Jan.1995-).
—CCC.
Published by: Charles W. Henderson, Ed. & Pub., PO Box 5528, Atlanta, GA 31107-0528. TEL 770-507-7777, FAX 770-507-7788, cwhender@newsfile.com; info@hendersonnet.atl.ga.us, http://www.newsfile.com.

616.97 615.5 GBR
U K AIDS DIRECTORY. Text in English. 1987. s-a. GBP 54.95 in United Kingdom; GBP 59.95 in Europe; GBP 69.95 elsewhere (effective 2001). **Document type:** *Directory.* **Description:** Information on all HIV and AIDS services in the UK.
Formerly (199?): AIDS Directory (1354-5493)
Published by: N A M Publications, 16a Clapham Common, South Side, London SW4 7AB, United Kingdom. TEL 44-20-7627-3200, FAX 44-20-7627-3101, info@nam.org.uk. Ed. Philip Browning. R&P Colin Nee.

616.9 USA
U.S. CENTERS FOR DISEASE CONTROL. DIPHTHERIA SURVEILLANCE REPORT. Text in English. 1962. irreg. charts, stat. **Document type:** *Government.*
Published by: U.S. Centers for Disease Control, 1600 Clifton Rd, Atlanta, GA 30333. TEL 404-639-3311.

616.998 USA
U.S. CENTERS FOR DISEASE CONTROL. LEPROSY SURVEILLANCE REPORT. Text in English. 1970. irreg., latest vol.2, 1972. charts, stat. **Document type:** *Government.*
Published by: U.S. Centers for Disease Control, 1600 Clifton Rd, Atlanta, GA 30333. TEL 404-639-3311.

616.9 USA ISSN 0501-8390
U.S. CENTERS FOR DISEASE CONTROL. MALARIA SURVEILLANCE REPORT. Text in English. 1955. a. free per issue. **Document type:** *Government.*
Published by: U.S. Centers for Disease Control, 1600 Clifton Rd, Atlanta, GA 30333. TEL 404-488-7760. Ed. Dr. Jane R Zucker. Circ: 2,000.

616.9 GBR
UNLINKED ANONYMOUS PREVALENCE MONITORING PROGRAMME IN THE UNITED KINGDOM. Text in English. irreg. **Document type:** *Monographic series.*
Formerly (until 1999): Unlinked Anonymous HIV Seroprevalence Monitoring Programme in England and Wales
—BLDSC.
Published by: Public Health Laboratory Service, 61 Colindale Ave, London NW9 5HT, United Kingdom. TEL 44-20-8200-6868, FAX 44-20-8200-7868, http://www.phls.co.uk/.

VACCINE WEEKLY. see *PHARMACY AND PHARMACOLOGY*

VIROLOGY. see *BIOLOGY—Microbiology*

VIROLOGY MONOGRAPHS/VIRUSFORSCHUNG IN EINZELDARSTELLUNGEN. see *BIOLOGY—Microbiology*

VIRUS/UIRUSU. see *BIOLOGY—Microbiology*

W O R L D; a newsletter by, for and about women facing HIV disease. (Women Organized to Respond to Life-Threatening Diseases) see *WOMEN'S HEALTH*

WEEKLY EPIDEMIOLOGICAL RECORD. see *PUBLIC HEALTH AND SAFETY*

616.9 USA
WISCONSIN AIDS UPDATE. Text in English. q. free per issue. **Document type:** *Government.*
Published by: Department of Health and Social Services, Division of Health, PO Box 2659, Madison, WI 53701. TEL 608-267-5287, FAX 608-666-2906, risierwd@dhdd.wi.us. Ed. Bill Reiser.

614.8 USA
WORD & DEED. Text in English. 1976. bi-m. free per issue. **Document type:** *Newsletter.* **Description:** Report to donors on how their gifts help people with leprosy.
Formerly: Crossways
Published by: American Leprosy Missions International, 1 ALM Way, Greenville, SC 29601. TEL 803-271-7040, 800-543-3135, FAX 803-271-7062, http://www.leprosy.org. Ed. Susan S Renault. R&P Susan Renault. Circ: 35,000.

610 CHE
WORLD HEALTH ORGANIZATION. TECHNICAL REPORTS. Text in English. 8/yr.
Published by: World Health Organization, Marketing and Dissemination, Geneva, 27 1211, Switzerland. TEL 41-22-791-2476, FAX 41-22-791-4875, http://www.who.int.

617.14 616.025 USA
WOUND CARE. Text in English. 1996. m. USD 299; USD 259 foreign (effective 1999). **Document type:** *Newsletter.*
Published by: American Health Consultants (Subsidiary of: Medical Economics Co., Inc.), 3525 Piedmont Rd, N E, 6 Piedmont Center, Ste 400, Atlanta, GA 30305. TEL 404-262-5476, custserv@ahcpub.com, http://www.ahcpub.com.

610 KOR ISSN 0375-5207
CODEN: YRTMA6
YONSEI REPORTS ON TROPICAL MEDICINE. Text in English. 1970. a. per issue exchange basis. adv. abstr, bibl, charts, stat. **Document type:** *Academic/Scholarly.*
Indexed: Biol.Abstr., Excerp.Med., Protozool.Abstr., Zoo.Rec.
—GNLM.
Published by: Yonsei University, Institute of Tropical Medicine, PO Box 8044, Seoul 120752, Korea, S.. TEL 82-2-361-5290, FAX 82-2-363-8676. Ed. Kyung Il Im.

616.96 CHN
ZHONGGUO JISHENGCHONG YU JISHENGCHONGBING ZAZHI/CHINESE JOURNAL OF PARASITOLOGY AND PARASITIC DISEASES. Text in Chinese. bi-m. USD 28.20; USD 2.40 newsstand/cover (effective 2001). **Document type:** *Academic/Scholarly.*
Published by: Zhongguo Yufang Yixue Kexueyuan, Jishengchongbing Yanjiusuo/Chinese Academy of Preventive Medicine, Institute of Parasitic Diseases, 207 Ruijin 2 Lu, Shanghai 200025, China. **Dist. by:** China International Book Trading Corp, 35, Chegongzhuang Xilu, Haidian District, Beijing 100044, China. TEL 86-1-68413849, FAX 86-1-68412048, cibtc@mail.cibtc.com.cn, http://www.cibtc.com.cn.

616.96 CHN ISSN 1001-6627
ZHONGGUO JISHENGCHONGBING FANGZHI ZAZHI/CHINESE JOURNAL OF PARASITIC DISEASE CONTROL. Text in Chinese. 1988. q. CNY 5 newsstand/cover domestic (effective 2001). **Document type:** *Academic/Scholarly.*
Related titles: Online - full content ed.: (from WanFang Data Corp.).
Indexed: Ind.Vet., Pig News & Info., Postharvest, Poult.Abstr., Protozool.Abstr., Rural Devel.Abstr., Trop.Dis.Bull., Vet.Bull.
—BLDSC (3180.464500).
Published by: Shandong-sheng Jishengchongbing Fangzhi Yanjiusuo, 13, Taibailou Zhong Lu, Jining 272033, China. TEL 86-537-2342934, cjpdc@ji-public.sd.cninfo.net.. Ed. Zhao Wang.

ZHONGGUO RENSHOU GONGHUANBING ZAZHI/CHINESE JOURNAL OF ZOONOSES. see *BIOLOGY—Microbiology*

616.951 CHN ISSN 1007-3523
ZHONGGUO XINGBING AIZIBING FANGZHI/CHINESE JOURNAL OF PREVENTION AND CONTROL OF STD & AIDS. Text in Chinese. 1995. bi-m. USD 31.20; USD 5.20 newsstand/cover (effective 2001). **Document type:** *Academic/Scholarly.*
Published by: China International Book Trading Corp/Zhongguo Guoji Tushu Maoyi Zonggongsi cibtc@mail.cibtc.com.cn, http://www.cibtc.com.cn. **Dist. by:** 35, Chegongzhuang Xilu, Haidian District, Beijing 100044, China.

616.01 CHN ISSN 1003-9279
CODEN: ZSLZFS
ZHONGHUA SHIYAN HE LINCHUANG BINGDUXUE ZAZHI/CHINESE JOURNAL OF EXPERIMENTAL AND CLINICAL VIROLOGY. Text in Chinese; Abstracts in Chinese, English. 1990. q. CNY 40, USD 11.60; CNY 10, USD 2.90 newsstand/cover (effective 2001). adv. bk.rev. illus. 100 p./no. back issues avail.; reprints avail. **Document type:** *Academic/Scholarly.* **Description:** Provides essential methods and techniques as well as updated information in areas of experimental virology, diagnostic virology and infectious diseases important to daily teachings and research works of researchers, practitioners, and educators.
Related titles: ♦ CD-ROM ed.: Chinese Academic Journal. Medicine & Hygiene. ISSN 1007-8053; Online - full text ed.: (from WanFang Data Corp.).
Indexed: AgBiotech, Ind.Med. (1987-), Ind.Vet., Protozool.Abstr., Rev.Appl.Entomol., Rev.Arom.& Med.Plants, Rev.Med.& Vet.Mycol., Rev.Plant Path., Trop.Dis.Bull., Vet.Bull.
—BLDSC (3180.318080), CASDDS, GNLM.
Published by: Zhonghua Yixuehui, Bingdu Xuehui/Chinese Medical Association, Institute of Clinical Virology, 100 Ying Xin Jie, Xuan Wu-qu, Beijing 100052, China. TEL 86-1-63530971, FAX 86-1-63529809, hungt@public3.bta.net.cn, http://www.chinainfo.gov.cn/periodical. Ed., R&P Hung Tao TEL 86-10-63529809. Adv. contact Peili Chen. B&W page USD 800, color page USD 1,400; 21 x 28.5. Circ: 1,500 (paid); 500 (controlled). **Subscr. to:** 35 Che Gong Zhuang Lu, Beijing 100044, China. **Dist. by:** China International Book Trading Corp, 35, Chegongzhuang Xilu, Haidian District, Beijing 100044, China. TEL 86-1-68413849, FAX 86-1-68412048, cibtc@mail.cibtc.com.cn, http://www.cibtc.com.cn.

ZHURNAL MIKROBIOLOGII, EPIDEMIOLOGII I IMMUNOBIOLOGII/JOURNAL OF MICROBIOLOGY, EPIDEMIOLOGY AND IMMUNOBIOLOGY. see *BIOLOGY—Microbiology*

MEDICAL SCIENCES—Computer Applications

610.285 004 USA
R858.A2 CODEN: PCMCDC
A M I A SYMPOSIUM. PROCEEDINGS. Text in English. 1977. a. USD 95 domestic; USD 105 foreign (effective 2001). *Refereed.* **Document type:** *Proceedings.*
Former titles (until 1998): A M I A - Annual Fall Symposium. Proceedings (1091-8280); (until 1996): Symposium on Computer Applications in Medical Care. Proceedings (0195-4210)

Related titles: ♦ Supplement to: American Medical Informatics Association. Journal. ISSN 1067-5027.
Indexed: GeoRef, INSPEC (coverage dropped), Ind.Med. (1992-, dropped), Int.Nurs.Ind.
—BLDSC (0858.760000). **CCC.**
Published by: (American Medical Informatics Association), Hanley & Belfus, Inc., 210 S 13th St, Philadelphia, PA 19107. TEL 215-546-7293, FAX 215-790-9330. Ed. Dr. William W Stead. Circ: 3,000.

616.075 NLD ISSN 0925-5206
CODEN: ADECEJ
ADVANCES IN ECHO-CONTRAST; ultrasound imaging innovations, echo-enhancing agents, clinical impact. Text in English. 1991. q. NLG 155 to institutions; USD 92.50 in United States to institutions. back issues avail. *Refereed.* **Document type:** *Academic/Scholarly.*
Related titles: Microform ed.: (from PQC).
Indexed: Excerp.Med. (1995-).
—CISTI, EMDOCS, GNLM, Infotrieve, KNAW. **CCC.**
Published by: Kluwer Academic Publishers Group (Subsidiary of: Wolters Kluwer N.V.), Spuiboulevard 50, PO Box 17, Dordrecht 3300 AA, Netherlands. FAX 31-78-639-2254, services@wkap.nl, http://www.wkap.nl. **Dist. by:** Journals Department, PO Box 322, Dordrecht 3300 AH, Netherlands. FAX 31-78-654-6474.

ADVANCES IN M R I - CONTRAST; MRI innovations, contrast-enhancing agents, clinical impact. (Magnetic Resonance Imaging) see *MEDICAL SCIENCES—Radiology And Nuclear Medicine*

610 USA ISSN 1067-5027
R858.A1 CODEN: JAMAFU
AMERICAN MEDICAL INFORMATICS ASSOCIATION. JOURNAL. Abbreviated title: J A M I A. Text in English. 1994. bi-m., latest vol.8, 2001. USD 166 domestic to individuals; USD 178 foreign to individuals; USD 250 domestic to institutions; USD 260 foreign to institutions; USD 30 newsstand/cover (effective 2001). adv. 2 cols./p. back issues avail. *Refereed.* **Document type:** *Journal, Academic/Scholarly.* **Description:** Presents state-of-the-art material to assist physicians, informaticians, scientists, nurses and other health care professionals to develop and apply medical informatics to patient care, teaching, research, and health care administration.
Related titles: Online - full text ed.: USD 95 domestic; USD 105 foreign (effective 2001) (from HighWire Pr., EBSCO Publishing, Institute for Scientific Information); ♦ Supplement: A M I A Symposium. Proceedings.
Indexed: ASCA, AgeLine, CINAHL, Compumath, Curr.Cont., Ind.Med. (1994-), Ind.Sci.Rev., Inform.Sci.Abstr., Inpharma, Int.Nurs.Ind., Pharm.&Out.News, Reac., Risk Abstr., SSCI, Sci.Cit.Ind.
—BLDSC (4689.025000), CISTI, GNLM, IDS, Infotrieve, KNAW. **CCC.**
Published by: (American Medical Informatics Association), Hanley & Belfus, Inc., 210 S 13th St, Philadelphia, PA 19107. TEL 215-546-7293, FAX 215-790-9330, http://www.jamia.org/. Ed. Dr. William W Stead. Adv. contact Diane R Sherel. B&W page USD 1,100;. Circ: 5,000 (paid).

610 001.6 CHE ISSN 0095-0963
R858.A1 CODEN: AUMDC9
AUTOMEDICA; an international journal of Biomedical Engineering & Physics, Informatics & Technology. Text in French. 1974. q. EUR 980, USD 1,086 to institutions; EUR 1,530, USD 1,694 to corporations (effective 2000); USD 359 to individuals (effective 2001). adv. bk.rev. abstr, bibl, charts, illus. index, cum.index. *Refereed.* **Document type:** *Journal, Academic/Scholarly.*
Related titles: Microform ed.
Indexed: Bioeng.Abstr., Biol.Abstr., Chem.Abstr., Comput.Cont., Comput.Rev., Eng.Ind., INSPEC (1974-1990, dropped).
—BLDSC (1831.770000), CISTI, GNLM, Infotrieve. **CCC.**
Published by: Gordon and Breach - Harwood Academic (Subsidiary of: Taylor & Francis Group), PO Box 531, Lausanne 1000, Switzerland. TEL 41-21-6411280, FAX 41-21-6411281, info@gbhap.com, http://www.gbhap.com. Ed. Siaw Meng Chou. **Subscr. addr. in US:** International Publishers Direct, PO Box 32160, Newark, NJ 07102. FAX 215-750-6343.

610.285 GBR
BRITISH JOURNAL OF HEALTHCARE COMPUTING & INFORMATION MANAGEMENT. Text in English. 1984. 10/yr. GBP 55 in United Kingdom; GBP 65 in Europe; GBP 70 elsewhere (effective 2001). back issues avail. **Document type:** *Trade.* **Description:** Discusses managing information in a clinical environment. Combines topical news stories, case studies, and product and service directories. Analyzes the impact that information management has on patient care.
Formerly: British Journal of Healthcare Computing (0265-5217)
Indexed: ASCA, Brit.Nur.Ind., CINAHL, INSPEC (Feb.1994-), Ref.Zh., SSCI (coverage dropped).
—BLDSC (2309.150000), AskIEEE, CISTI, IDS.
Published by: B J H C Ltd., 45 Woodland Grove, Weybridge, Surrey KT13 9EQ, United Kingdom. TEL 44-1932-852776, FAX 44-1932-858035, mail@bjhcim.demon.co.uk, http://www.bjhc.co.uk. Ed. Nettie de Glanville. Pub. Dr. Hugh de Glanville. Adv. contact Peter Richardson TEL 44-1932-821723.

610.73 USA ISSN 1098-7126
C I N PLUS. (Computers in Nursing) Text in English. 1998. 3/yr. USD 29 domestic; USD 33 foreign (effective 2002). **Document type:** *Journal, Academic/Scholarly, Trade.* **Description:** Contains articles, software reviews, and quick access material useful to nurses using computers for practice, research, and education.
Related titles: ♦ Supplement to: Computers in Nursing. ISSN 0736-8593.
Published by: Lippincott Williams & Wilkins (Philadelphia) (Subsidiary of: Wolters Kluwer N.V.), 530 Walnut St, Philadelphia, PA 19106-3621. TEL 215-521-8300, FAX 215-521-8902, custserv@lww.com, http://www.lww.com/. Ed. Leslie H Nicoll. **Subscr. to:** PO Box 1600, Hagerstown, MD 21740-1600. TEL 800-638-3030, FAX 310-223-2400.

COGNITIVE BRAIN RESEARCH. see *MEDICAL SCIENCES—Psychiatry And Neurology*

COMPUTER AIDED SURGERY. see *MEDICAL SCIENCES—Surgery*

610.28 616 IRL ISSN 0169-2607
R858.A1 CODEN: CMPBEK
COMPUTER METHODS AND PROGRAMS IN BIOMEDICINE; an international journal devoted to the development, implementation and exchange of computing methodology and software systems in biomedical research and medical practice. Text in English. 1970. 9/yr. EUR 1,156 in Europe to institutions; JPY 153,600 in Japan to institutions; USD 1,293 elsewhere to institutions (effective 2002). bk.rev. charts. *Refereed.* **Document type:** *Academic/Scholarly.* **Description:** For all life science researchers, clinicians, statisticians, health scientists, computer scientists, programmers and bio-engineers, engaged in applying and teaching biomedical information processing.
Incorporates: Journal of Biomedical Measurement Informatics and Control; Formerly (until 1985): Computer Programs in Biomedicine (0010-468X)
Related titles: Microform ed.: (from PQC); Online - full text ed.: (from ingenta, Swets Blackwell, ScienceDirect, Institute for Scientific Information).
Indexed: ASCA, Bioeng.Abstr., Biol.Abstr., Compumath, Comput.& Info.Sys., Comput.Abstr., Curr.Adv.Ecol.Sci., Curr.Cont., Curr.Ind.Stat., Cyb.Abstr., Electron.& Communic.Abstr.J., Eng.Ind., Excerp.Med., INIS Atomind., INSPEC (Jan.1970-), Ind.Med. (1985-), Ind.Sci.Rev., Ind.Vet., Inpharma, Int.Nurs.Ind., Reac., SSCI (coverage dropped), Sci.Cit.Ind., Stat.Theor.Meth.Abstr., Telegen.
—BLDSC (3394.095000), AskIEEE, CISTI, Ei, EMDOCS, GNLM, IDS, ingenta. **CCC.**
Published by: Elsevier Science Ireland Ltd, Elsevier House, Brookvale Plaza, E. Park, Shannon, Co. Clare, Ireland. TEL 353-61-709600, FAX 353-61-709100, http://www.elsevier.com/locate/cmpb, http://www.elsevier.nl. Ed. T Groth. R&P Annette Moloney. **Subscr. in Australasia and the Far East to:** Elsevier Science (Singapore) Pte Ltd, No.1 Temasek Ave, 17-01 Millenia Tower, Singapore 039192, Singapore. TEL 65-434-3727, FAX 65-337-2230, asiainfo@elsevier.com.sg; **Subscr. in the Americas to:** Elsevier Science, PO Box 945, New York, NY 10159-0945. TEL 212-633-3730, FAX 212-633-3680, usinfo-f@elsevier.com; **Subscr. to:** Elsevier Science Inc - Japan Regional Office, 9-15 Higashi-Azabu 1-chome, Minato-ku, Tokyo 106-0044, Japan. **Subscr. to:** Elsevier Science BV, PO Box 211, Amsterdam 1000 AE, Netherlands. TEL 31-20-485-3757, FAX 31-20-485-3432, nlinfo-f@elsevier.nl.

610 GBR ISSN 0895-6111
CODEN: CMIGEY
COMPUTERIZED MEDICAL IMAGING AND GRAPHICS; the international journal on imaging and image archiving in all medical specialties. Text in English. 1977. 6/yr. EUR 151 in Europe to individuals; JPY 20,100 in Japan to individuals; USD 169 elsewhere to individuals; EUR 1,315 in Europe to institutions; JPY 174,600 in Japan to institutions; USD 1,471 elsewhere to institutions (effective 2002). adv. back issues avail. *Refereed.* **Document type:** *Academic/Scholarly.* **Description:** Discusses new developments in computerized medical imaging and graphics and the application of these to patient care. Publishes research results in medical imaging techniques, modalities, analysis and clinical applications of medical images.
Former titles (until 1988): Computerized Radiology (0730-4862); (until 1982): Computerized Tomography (0363-8235)
Related titles: Microfilm ed.: (from PQC); Online - full text ed.: (from ingenta, Swets Blackwell, ScienceDirect, Institute for Scientific Information).
Indexed: ASCA, Aqua.Sci.& Fish.Abstr., Bioeng.Abstr., Biol.Abstr., Cal.Tiss.Abstr., Comput.& Info.Sys., Comput.Cont., Curr.Cont., Dent.Ind., Eng.Ind., Excerp.Med., Helminthol.Abstr., INIS Atomind., INSPEC (Jan.1977-Feb.1983, Jan.1993-), Ind.Imag.Lit., Ind.Med. (1988-), Ind.Sci.Rev., Inpharma, Int.Nurs.Ind., Neurosci.Abstr. (coverage dropped), Neurosci.Cit.Ind., Pharm.&Out.News, Protozool.Abstr., Reac., Ref.Zh., Rev.Med.& Vet.Mycol., Sci.Cit.Ind. (coverage dropped).
—BLDSC (3394.586000), AskIEEE, CISTI, Ei, EMDOCS, GNLM, IDS, Infotrieve, ingenta, KNAW. **CCC.**
Published by: (Computerized Medical Imaging and Graphics Society), Pergamon (Subsidiary of: Elsevier Science), The Boulevard, Langford Ln, East Park, Kidlington, Oxford OXB 1GB, United Kingdom. FAX 44-1865-843010, nlinfo-f@elsevier/nl; usinfo-f@elsevier.com; forinfo-kyf04035@niftyserve.or.jp, http://www.elsevier.com/locate/compmedimag. Ed. Robert S Ledley. Circ: 1,500. **Subscr. in Australasia and the Far East to:** Elsevier Science (Singapore) Pte Ltd, No.1 Temasek Ave, 17-01 Millenia Tower, Singapore 039192, Singapore. TEL 65-434-3727, FAX 65-337-2230; **Subscr. in the Americas to:** Elsevier Science, PO Box 945, New York, NY 10159-0945. TEL 212-633-3730, FAX 212-633-3680; **Subscr. to:** Elsevier Science BV, PO Box 211, Amsterdam 1000 AE, Netherlands. TEL 31-20-485-3757, http://www.elsevier.nl.

610.285 004 USA ISSN 0163-0547
CODEN: CMPMDI
COMPUTERS AND MEDICINE. Text in English. 1972. m. USD 157; USD 177 foreign (effective 2001). adv. bk.rev. charts, illus, pat, stat. cum.index. 18 p./no. back issues avail. **Document type:** *Magazine, Trade.* **Description:** For medical personnel interested in computer applications. Articles cover current computer technology in medicine, medical education, practice management, and hospitals.
Indexed: Comput.Cont., Comput.Lit.Ind., INSPEC (pre-1969-Aug.1983, dropped), LAMP, MEDSOC.
—GNLM, ingenta.
Published by: Computers & Medicine, Inc., PO Box 11147, Chicago, IL 60611. TEL 312-944-7900, FAX 312-944-8845, cptmdgolin@aol.com, http://www.computersandmedicine.com. Ed. Carol Brierly. Pub., R&P, Adv. contact Milton Golin. page USD 550. Circ: 4,000 (paid).

COMPUTERS IN BIOLOGY AND MEDICINE; an international journal. see *BIOLOGY—Computer Applications*

621.3 616 USA ISSN 0276-6574
RC683.5.D36 CODEN: COCADX
COMPUTERS IN CARDIOLOGY. Text in English. 1974. a. USD 182 to institutions (effective 2001). adv. **Document type:** *Proceedings.* **Description:** Presents topics of mutual interest to computer scientists and cardiologists.
Indexed: Bioeng.Abstr., Eng.Ind., Environ.Eng.Abstr., Environ.Sci.Poll.Mgmt., INSPEC (coverage dropped).
—BLDSC (3394.895000), Ei, ingenta. **CCC.**
Published by: (Institute of Electrical and Electronics Engineers, Inc.), I E E E Computer Society Press, 10662 Los Vaqueros Circle, P.O. Box 3014, Los Alamitos, CA 90720-1314. TEL 714-821-8380, FAX 714-821-4641. Ed. Cat Harris. Pub. Matt Loeb. Adv. contact Frieda Koester. **Co-sponsors:** European Society of Cardiology; U.S. National Institutes of Health.

610.73 USA ISSN 0736-8593
COMPUTERS IN NURSING. Abbreviated title: C I N. Text in English. bi-m. USD 79 domestic to individuals; USD 119 foreign to individuals; USD 219 domestic to institutions; USD 269 foreign to institutions; USD 44 newsstand/cover (effective 2002). adv. illus. index. **Document type:** *Academic/Scholarly.*
Related titles: CD-ROM ed.: (from Ovid Technologies, Inc.); Microform ed.: (from PQC); Online - full text ed.: USD 284.70 domestic academic site license; USD 334.70 foreign academic site license; USD 317.55 domestic corporate site license; USD 367.55 foreign corporate site license (2002) (from Ovid Technologies, Inc., Institute for Scientific Information); ♦ Supplement: C I N Plus. ISSN 1098-7126.
Indexed: ASCA, CINAHL, Curr.Ind.Stat., Ind.Med. (1983-), Int.Nurs.Ind., Nurs.Abstr., SSCI (coverage dropped), SoftBase (May 1988-Jun.1989, Jan.1990-).
—BLDSC (3394.925500), GNLM, IDS, ingenta.
Published by: Lippincott Williams & Wilkins (Philadelphia) (Subsidiary of: Wolters Kluwer N.V.), 530 Walnut St, Philadelphia, PA 19106-3621. TEL 301-223-2300, 800-638-3030, FAX 301-223-2400, http://www.Lww.com. Ed. Leslie H Nicoll. Circ: 3,617. **Subscr. to:** PO Box 1600, Hagerstown, MD 21740-1600.

COMPUTERTALK; for contemporary pharmacy management. see *PHARMACY AND PHARMACOLOGY—Computer Applications*

COMPUTERTALK PHARMACY SYSTEMS BUYERS GUIDE. see *PHARMACY AND PHARMACOLOGY—Computer Applications*

CONTEMPORARY ISSUES IN COMPUTED TOMOGRAPHY. see *MEDICAL SCIENCES—Radiology And Nuclear Medicine*

610.285 USA
CYBERLOG; library of applied medical software. Text in English. 1985. q. USD 99.95. **Description:** Library and interactive software for physicians. Each program is devoted to a single topic, presented by prominent experts and organizations.
Published by: Cardinal Health Systems, Inc., 4600 W. 77th St., Ste. 150, Edina, MN 55435. TEL 800-328-0180, FAX 612-835-7141.

617.60285 USA ISSN 0738-9744
DENTAL COMPUTER NEWSLETTER. Text in English. 1978. q. USD 25 domestic; USD 30 foreign (effective 2001). adv. bk.rev. illus. *Refereed.* **Document type:** *Newsletter.* **Description:** For dentists and other medical practitioners interested in office computers. Offers notes on hardware, software, peripherals and integration with dental office personnel.
Indexed: LAMP.
Published by: Andent, Inc., 1000 North Ave, Waukegan, IL 60085. TEL 847-223-5077, eneiburger@cs.com. Ed., Pub., R&P E J Neiburger. Adv. contact S Nye. Circ: 3,000 (paid).

617.6 USA
DENTISTS' COMPUTER NEWS. Text in English. 1981. 12/yr. bk.rev.
Published by: American Newsfeatures Syndicate, 113 Wattenbarger Rd, Sweetwater, TN 37874-6135. TEL 800-484-4074, FAX 423-337-0222. Ed. Ray Burr. Circ: 101,711.

610.28 USA
E-HEALTH & TELEMEDICINE NEWS. Text in English. m. **Document type:** *Newsletter.* **Description:** Focuses on legal issues related to advanced health information systems and telemedicine.
Media: Online - full text.
Published by: Arent Fox Kintner Plotkin & Kahn PLLC, 1050 Connecticut Ave, NW, Washington, DC 20036-5339. TEL 202-827-6000, FAX 202-857-6395, infolaw@arentfox.com, http://www.arentfox.com/telemedicine.html/. Ed. Robert J Waters.

610 USA
GROUP PRACTICE DATA MANAGEMENT; information technology strategies for medical groups. Text in English. 1998. s-a. free subscr. to Health Data Management. software rev. **Document type:** *Trade.* **Description:** Offers in-depth news and analysis on important issues in information technology that medical-practice administrators face.
Published by: Faulkner & Gray, Inc. (Chicago), Health Data Management, 300 S Wacker Dr, Chicago, IL 60606. TEL 312-913-1331, 800-535-8403, FAX 312-913-1959, http://hdm.fgray.com/html/publications/. Pub. Howard J Anderson.

610 USA
GUIDE TO HEALTH DATA SECURITY. Text in English. a. USD 315 (effective 2001). software rev. **Document type:** *Trade.* **Description:** Draws upon the expertise of noted authorities to report on important issues and developments in the field of protecting medical data. Discusses all aspects of the hardware, software, and peripheral tools involved, with functions and benefits. Includes a quick-reference section and a directory of vendors and organizations.
Published by: Faulkner & Gray, Inc. (Chicago), Health Data Management, 300 S Wacker Dr, Chicago, IL 60606. TEL 312-913-1334, 800-535-8403, FAX 312-913-1959, http://hdm.fgray.com/html/publications/. Pub. Howard J Anderson.

610.285 AUS
H I C. (Health Informatics Conference) Text in English. 1993. a. AUD 50 (effective 1999). back issues avail. **Document type:** *Trade, Academic/Scholarly.* **Description:** Covers all sectors of healthcare, industry, information science, research, management and technology.
Related titles: CD-ROM ed.
Published by: Health Informatics Society of Australia, 413 Lygon St, Brunswick East, VIC 3057, Australia. TEL 61-3-9388-0555, FAX 61-3-9388-2086, hisa@hisa.org.au, http://www.his.org.au. Ed. Joan Edgecumbe. Circ: 400.

613.029 USA ISSN 1093-1821
HEALTH DATA DIRECTORY. Text in English. 199?. a. USD 450 (effective 2001). software rev. **Document type:** *Directory.* **Description:** Profiles more than 2,700 providers, payers, claims processors, software companies and other firms involved with health care information technology, along with more than 8,000 executive contacts. Contains articles on developments in this field.
Published by: Faulkner & Gray, Inc. (Chicago), Health Data Management, 300 S Wacker Dr, Chicago, IL 60606. TEL 312-913-1959, 800-535-8403, FAX 312-913-1959, http://hdm.fgray.com/html/publications/. Pub. Howard J Anderson.

362.1 USA
HEALTH DATA MANAGEMENT (CHICAGO); the magazine of electronic health care networking. Text in English. m. USD 98 (effective 2001); includes Resource Guide. adv. **Document type:** *Trade.* **Description:** Offers comprehensive information on every aspect of health care information technology, enabling readers to use this technology to improve the quality of care while controlling costs.
Related titles: Online - full text ed.
Indexed: Comput.Lit.Ind., Int.Nurs.Ind.
Published by: Faulkner & Gray, Inc. (Chicago), Health Data Management, 300 S Wacker Dr, Chicago, IL 60606. TEL 312-913-1334, 800-535-8403, FAX 312-913-1959, http://hdm.fgray.com. Ed., Pub. Howard J Anderson. Adv. contact Chris Ahern.

610 GBR ISSN 1460-4582
HEALTH INFORMATICS JOURNAL. Text in English. 1992. q. GBP 35 to individuals; USD 53, GBP 99, USD 149 to institutions (effective 2001). adv. **Document type:** *Academic/Scholarly.*
Former titles (until 1997): Health Informatics (1355-4743); (until 1995): International Journal of Health Informatics (0965-8335)
Indexed: ASSIA, Brit.Nur.Ind., CINAHL, Hosp.Abstr., LISA.
—BLDSC (4275.016850).
Published by: Sheffield Academic Press Ltd, Mansion House, 19 Kingfield Rd, Sheffield, S Yorks S11 9AS, United Kingdom. TEL 44-114-255-4433, FAX 44-114-255-4626, admin@sheffac.demon.co.uk, http://www.shef.ac.uk/uni/projects/hij/. Ed. M F Smith.

610 658 USA ISSN 1074-4770
R858.A1 CODEN: HMTEE2
HEALTH MANAGEMENT TECHNOLOGY. Text in English. 1980. m. USD 38 domestic; USD 58 in Canada & Mexico; USD 98 elsewhere. adv. bk.rev. charts, illus, stat. reprint service avail. from PQC. **Document type:** *Trade.* **Description:** For healthcare systems professionals. Features articles on systems applications for hospitals and other health facilities.
Former titles (until 1994): Computers in Healthcare (0745-1075); (until 1982): Computers in Hospitals (0274-631X)
Related titles: Microfiche ed.; Online - full text ed.: (from The Dialog Corporation, Gale Group, ProQuest Information & Learning, Northern Light Technology, Inc., H. W. Wilson, LexisNexis, Factiva).
Indexed: ABI Inform. (Jun.1985-), Abstr.Health Care Manage.Stud., B.P.I. (Jul.1999-), CINAHL, Comput.Dtbs., INSPEC (May 1984-Dec.1993, Feb.1994-), I.P.A., Int.Nurs.Ind., SoftBase (Jun.1989-).
—BLDSC (4275.052140), AskIEEE, CISTI, GNLM, Infotrieve, ingenta. **CCC.**
Published by: Nelson Publishing Co., 2500 N Tamiami Trail, Nokomis, FL 34275. TEL 941-966-9521, FAX 941-966-2590. Ed. Damon Braly. Circ: 21,880.

610 GBR ISSN 1366-5278
HEALTH TECHNOLOGY ASSESSMENT. Text in English. 1997. irreg., latest vol.5, no.12. GBP 52 per issue (effective 2001); free to qualified personnel. 2 cols./p. back issues avail. *Refereed.* **Document type:** *Journal, Academic/Scholarly.*
Related titles: Online - full text ed.
Indexed: Brit.Nur.Ind., Ind.Med. (1997-).
—BLDSC (4275.224200).
Published by: National Coordinating Centre for Health Technology Assessment, Mailpoint 728, Boldrewood, University of Southampton, Southhampton SO16 7PX, United Kingdom. TEL 44-2380-595586, FAX 44-2380-595639, hta@soton.ac.uk, http://www.ncchta.org. Eds. Andrew Stevens, John Gabbay, Dr. Ken Stein.

610 GBR
HEALTHCARE COMPUTING CONFERENCE PROCEEDINGS. Text in English. a. GBP 45. **Document type:** *Proceedings.* **Description:** Concentrates on a particular aspect of health care computing.
Published by: British Computer Society, Health Informatics Committee, c/o John Bryant, Chairman, 11 Edensor Rd, Eastbourne BN20 7XR, United Kingdom. TEL 44-1323-430331, FAX 44-1323-430331, jbryant@atlas.co.uk.

610 USA ISSN 1093-6912
HEALTHCARE I S - I T MARKET REPORTER. Text in English. 1997. 24/yr. USD 447 (effective 2000). index. back issues avail. **Document type:** *Trade.* **Description:** Covers the healthcare information technology market: new products, product updates, contracts awarded, contract development, licensing agreements, market partnerships, acquisitions and Internet-Intranet applications.
—**CCC.**
Published by: Managed Care Information Center, 1913 Atlantic Ave, Ste F4, Manasquan, NJ 08736. TEL 888-843-6242, FAX 888-329-6242, mcic@themcic.com, http://www.themcic.com. Ed. Jodi Kastel. Pub. Robert K Jenkins.

HEALTHCARE I T; the magazine for health sector IT decision makers. (Information Technology) see *HEALTH FACILITIES AND ADMINISTRATION*

610 USA ISSN 1050-9135
HEALTHCARE INFORMATICS. Text in English. 1983. m. USD 39.95 domestic; USD 72 in Canada & Mexico; USD 99.95 elsewhere (effective 2000). adv. tr.lit. back issues avail. **Document type:** *Trade.* **Description:** Provides monthly news and coverage of technology in the healthcare industry along with the information technologies of tomorrow.
Former titles (until Jan. 1990): U S Healthcare (1040-3973); (until Aug. 1988): Healthcare Computing and Communications (8750-149X)
Related titles: Online - full text ed.
Indexed: CINAHL, Environ.Sci.Poll.Mgmt., I.P.A., Int.Nurs.Ind., Pollut.Abstr., Risk Abstr., Saf.Sci.Abstr., SoftBase (Jan.1989-Jun.1996).
—BLDSC (4275.247850), ingenta.
Published by: McGraw-Hill Companies, 4530 W 77th St Ste 350, Minneapolis, MN 55435. TEL 952-835-3222, FAX 952-835-3460, tmonahan@mcgraw-hill.com, http://www.healthcare-informatics.com/. Ed. Dr. Terry Monahan. Adv. contact Deb Higgins. B&W page USD 4,750, color page USD 6,000. Circ: 42,000. **Subscr. to:** PO Box 527, Hightstown, NJ 08520-9210.

368.382 USA
HEALTHCARE PERSPECTIVE. Text in English. 1991. every 6 wks. USD 395. back issues avail. **Document type:** *Newsletter.* **Description:** Covers developments in the design and use of computer systems in healthcare organizations.
Former titles (until Mar. 1998): Singer Report on Healthcare Systems and Technology; (until Jan. 1997, vol.45): Singer Report on Managed Care Systems and Technology (1071-1910)
Related titles: CD-ROM ed.; Diskette ed.

M

Published by: Gartner Inc., 56 Top Gallant Rd, Stamford, CT 06904-2212. TEL 781-246-7585, FAX 781-246-8263, sandra.cummings@gartner.com. Ed., R&P Sandy Cummings. Circ: 520 (paid).

610 001.6 USA ISSN 1094-687X
I E E E ENGINEERING IN MEDICINE AND BIOLOGY SOCIETY. INTERNATIONAL CONFERENCE. Text in English. 1979. a. USD 248 to institutions (effective 2001).
Former titles: I E E E Engineering in Medicine and Biology Society. Conference; (until 1984): Frontiers of Engineering and Computing in Health Care; Which was formed by the merger of (1981-1982): I E E E Frontiers of Computers in Medicine; (1979-1982): I E E E Frontiers of Engineering in Health Care
Related titles: CD-ROM ed.; Microfiche ed.
Indexed: ASCA, Eng.Ind.
—BLDSC (6841.187030).
Published by: Institute of Electrical and Electronics Engineers, Inc., 3 Park Ave, 17th Fl, New York, NY 10017. TEL 800-678-4333, customer.service@ieee.org, http://www.ieee.org. **Co-sponsor:** Engineering in Medicine and Biology Society.

610 USA
I E E E SYMPOSIUM ON COMPUTER - BASED MEDICAL SYSTEMS. PROCEEDINGS. Abbreviated title: C B M S. Text in English. 1988. a. USD 130. **Document type:** *Proceedings.* **Description:** Focuses on the use of computers in medicine and presents methods, insights and examples on the engineering development process.
Related titles: Microfiche ed.
Indexed: Biotech.& Bioeng.Abstr., Eng.Ind.
Published by: (Institute of Electrical and Electronics Engineers, Inc.), I E E E Computer Society Press, 3 Park Ave, 17th Fl, New York, NY 10017. TEL 714-821-8380, 800-678-4333, FAX 714-821-4641, customer.service@ieee.org, customer.service.ieee.org, http://www.ieee.org.

I E E E TRANSACTIONS ON INFORMATION TECHNOLOGY IN BIOMEDICINE. see *BIOLOGY—Biotechnology*

I F M B E NEWS. (International Federation for Medical & Biological Engineering) see *BIOLOGY—Bioengineering*

610.285 AUS ISSN 1323-4382
INFORMATICS IN HEATHCARE AUSTRALIA. Text in English. 2/yr. AUD 100 to members; AUD 120 to libraries. adv. back issues avail. **Document type:** *Academic/Scholarly.*
Related titles: CD-ROM ed.
Indexed: CINAHL.
—BLDSC (4481.299850).
Published by: Health Informatics Society of Australia, 413 Lygon St, Brunswick East, VIC 3057, Australia. TEL 61-3-9388-0555, FAX 61-3-9388-2086, hisa@hisa.org.au. Adv. contact Joan Edgecumbe. Circ: 800.

610.285 USA
INFORMATICS REVIEW. Text in English. 1998. m. back issues avail. **Description:** Designed to allow busy medical and information system professionals interested in the latest academic developments in clinical informatics and computing to stay abreast of this rapidly evolving field.
Media: Online - full text.
Published by: Association of Medical Directors of Information Systems, 61 Jordan Rd, Keene, NH 03431. infor@amdis.org, http://www.informatics-review.com/. Ed. Dean F Sittig.

610 NLD
INFORMATIE & ZORG. Short title: T M I. Variant title: Informatie & Zorg(I & Z). Text in Dutch. 1973. q. NLG 125; NLG 150 foreign (effective 2001). adv. bk.rev. bibl, charts, illus. index. back issues avail. *Refereed.* **Document type:** *Journal, Academic/Scholarly, Consumer.* **Description:** Covers healthcare information science and applications.
Formely: Tijdschrift voor Medische Informatica (0920-5144)
Published by: Vereniging voor Medische en Biologische Informatieverwerking, c/o Erasmus University EE 2116, Postbus 1738, Rotterdam 3000 DR, Netherlands. FAX 31-30-6963551, abokaut.@wxs.nl, abokant@wxs.nl, http://www.umbi.nl. Ed. S Groothuis TEL 31-30-6992323. adv.: B&W page NLG 1,500. Circ: 1,000 (paid).

610 USA ISSN 1098-6049
INTERACTIVE HEALTHCARE DIRECTORY ON CD-ROM. Text in English. s-a. USD 199 (effective 2000). adv. software rev. **Document type:** *Directory.* **Description:** Liists nearly 2,000 software titles developed for health-related education and reference.
Formed by the merger of: Healthcare C A I Directory; Healthcare CD-ROM Directory (1074-6064); Healthcare Patient Education
Media: CD-ROM.
Published by: Graphic Education, 903 Old Hwy 63, Columbia, MO 65201. TEL 573-449-1200, 888-354-6600, FAX 573-449-3344, graphiced@graphiced.com, http://www.interactive-healthcare.com.

610 USA
INTERACTIVE HEALTHCARE REPORT. Text in English. 1985. m. USD 199 domestic; USD 219 foreign (effective 2001). adv. **Document type:** *Newsletter, Consumer.* **Description:** Covers the use of multimedia and related technology in the health sciences.
Former titles: Interactive Healthcare Newsletter (1048-0501); (until 1989): MedicalDisc Reporter (0882-4665)
Published by: Graphic Education, 903 Old Hwy 63, Columbia, MO 65201. TEL 573-449-1200, 888-354-6600, FAX 573-449-3344, graphiced@graphiced.com, http://info2.graphiced.com/home.html.

INTERNATIONAL JOURNAL OF COMPUTERIZED DENTISTRY; computer application in clinical treatment. see *MEDICAL SCIENCES—Dentistry*

668.382 CHE ISSN 1368-2156
CODEN: IJHMFP
▼ **INTERNATIONAL JOURNAL OF HEALTHCARE TECHNOLOGY AND MANAGEMENT.** Abbreviated title: I J H C T M. Text in English. 1999. 6/yr., latest vol.4, 2002. USD 400; USD 480 print & online eds. (effective 2001). adv. *Refereed.* **Document type:** *Journal, Academic/Scholarly.* **Description:** Provides an international forum in the fields of management, economics, and the management of technology in healthcare.
Indexed: Environ.Sci.Poll.Mgmt., INSPEC (1999-), Pollut.Abstr., Risk Abstr., Saf.Sci.Abstr.
—BLDSC (4542.278500).
Published by: Inderscience Enterprises Ltd., World Trade Centre Bldg., 29 route de Pre Bois, Case Postale 896, Geneva, 15 1215, Switzerland. FAX 41-22-7910885, 44-1234-240515, ijhtm@inderscience.com, info@inderscience.com, http://www.inderscience.com.

610.285 IRL ISSN 1386-5056
R858.A1 CODEN: IJMIF4
INTERNATIONAL JOURNAL OF MEDICAL INFORMATICS. Text in English. 1971. m. EUR 1,332 in Europe to institutions; JPY 176,800 in Japan to institutions; USD 1,490 elsewhere to institutions (effective 2002). charts, illus. index. back issues avail. *Refereed.* **Document type:** *Academic/Scholarly.* **Description:** Provides an international medium for dissemination of original results and interpretative reviews concerning the field of medical informatics.
Formerly (until 1997): International Journal of Bio-Medical Computing (0020-7101)
Related titles: Online - full text ed.: (from ingenta, Swets Blackwell, ScienceDirect, Institute for Scientific Information).
Indexed: ASCA, Bioeng.Abstr., Biol.Abstr., Biostat., Biotech.& Bioeng.Abstr., Chem.Abstr., Compumath, Comput.Cont., Comput.Rev., Curr.Adv.Ecol.Sci., Curr.Cont., Curr.Ind.Stat., Eng.Ind., Excerp.Med., Helminthol.Abstr., INSPEC (Jan.1974-Dec.1996, Mar.1997-), Ind.Med. (1997-), Inpharma, Int.Nurs.Ind., Math.R., Pharm.&Out.News, Reac., SSCI (coverage dropped), Sci.Cit.Ind.
—BLDSC (4542.345250), AskIEEE, CASDDS, CISTI, Ei, GNLM, IDS, Infotrieve, ingenta, KNAW. **CCC.**
Published by: Elsevier Science Ireland Ltd, Elsevier House, Brookvale Plaza, E. Park, Shannon, Co. Clare, Ireland. TEL 353-61-471944, FAX 353-61-472144, hasman@umi.unimaas.nl, http://www.elsevier.com/locate/ijmedinf. Eds. A Hasman, C Safran. R&P Annette Moloney. **Subscr. in Australasia and the Far East to:** Elsevier Science (Singapore) Pte Ltd, No.1 Temasek Ave, 17-01 Millenia Tower, Singapore 039192, Singapore. TEL 65-434-3727, FAX 65-337-2230; **Subscr. in the Americas to:** Elsevier Science, PO Box 945, New York, NY 10159-0945. TEL 212-633-3730, FAX 212-633-3680; **Subscr. to:** Elsevier Science BV, PO Box 211, Amsterdam 1000 AE, Netherlands. TEL 31-20-485-3757.

610 USA ISSN 1528-7386
INTERNET HEALTHCARE STRATEGIES. Text in English. 1996. q. USD 386 (effective 2001). bk.rev., Website rev. abstr, charts, illus, stat. back issues avail.; reprints avail. **Document type:** *Newsletter, Trade.* **Description:** Contains a comprehensive listing and review of medical internet sites.
Formerly: Healthcare Guide to the Internet (1522-7405)
Related titles: CD-ROM ed.; Online - full content ed.
Published by: C O R Health, LLC, PO Box 50507, Santa Barbara, CA 93150. TEL 805-564-2177, FAX 805-564-2146, info@corhealth.com, http://www.corhealth.com. Ed. Larry Stevens. Pub. Dean H. Anderson.

610 025.04 ESP ISSN 1138-6215
INTERNET - MEDICINA. Text in Spanish. 1998. irreg. (approx. 3/yr.). back issues avail.; reprints avail. *Refereed.* **Document type:** *Trade, Academic/Scholarly.* **Description:** Discusses how the Internet can be used to disseminate all types of medical information and research.
Published by: Ediciones Doyma S.A., Traversa de Gracia, 17-21, Barcelona 08021, Spain. TEL 34-93-200-0711, doyma@doyma.es, http://www.doyma.es/. R&P Monica Barnes. Adv. contact Jose Antonio Hernandez.

610.28 004 USA ISSN 1532-0464
CODEN: CBMRB7
JOURNAL OF BIOMEDICAL INFORMATICS. Text in English. 1969. bi-m. USD 99 in US & Canada to individuals; USD 114 rest of world to individuals; USD 395 in US & Canada to institutions; USD 454 rest of world to institutions (effective 2000). adv. charts, illus. back issues avail. *Refereed.* **Document type:** *Academic/Scholarly.* **Description:** Provides researchers with current information concerning the use of computers in biomedicine.
Formerly (until 2001): Computers and Biomedical Research (0010-4809)
Related titles: Online - full text ed.: ISSN 1532-0480 (from EBSCO Publishing, O C L C Online Computer Library Center, Inc., RoweCom Information Quest, ingenta, Swets Blackwell, IDEAL Online Library, Institute for Scientific Information).
Indexed: ASCA, Abstr.Hyg., Anim.Breed.Abstr., Appl.Mech.Rev., Biol.Abstr., Biostat., Biotech.& Bioeng.Abstr., Chem.Abstr., Chem.Indus.Notes, Chem.Titles, Compumath, Comput.Cont., Comput.Rev., Curr.Adv.Ecol.Sci., Curr.Cont., Curr.Ind.Stat., Eng.Ind., Environ.Sci.Poll.Mgmt., Excerp.Med., INIS Atomind., INSPEC (pre-1969-), Ind.Med. (2001-), Ind.Sci.Rev., Ind.Vet., Inpharma, Med.& Pharm.Biotech.Abstr., Pharm.&Out.News, Pollut.Abstr., Reac., Risk Abstr., SSCI (coverage dropped), Saf.Sci.Abstr., Sci.Cit.Ind., Trop.Dis.Bull., Vet.Bull.
—BLDSC (4953.680000), ADONIS, AskIEEE, CASDDS, CISTI, Ei, EMDOCS, GNLM, IDS, ingenta, Linda Hall. **CCC.**
Published by: (American Medical Informatics Association), Academic Press, Inc., Journal Division (Subsidiary of: Harcourt Brace & Company), 525 B St, Ste 1900, San Diego, CA 92101-4495. TEL 619-230-1840, FAX 619-699-6800, apsubs@acad.com, http://www.academicpress.com/jbi, http://www.academicpress.com/cbr. Ed. T Allan Pryor.

610 USA ISSN 0090-1091
CODEN: JCLCB
JOURNAL OF CLINICAL COMPUTING*. Text in English. 1971. bi-m. USD 30. adv. bk.rev. back issues avail.
Indexed: Comput.Cont., Cyb.Abstr., Eng.Ind., Environ.Sci.Poll.Mgmt., Excerp.Med., INSPEC (1977-Aug.1995, dropped), Pollut.Abstr.
—AskIEEE, CISTI, Ei, GNLM, KNAW.
Published by: Journal of Clinical Computing, Inc., 75 Cambridge Parkway PH 6, Cambridge, MA 02142-1237. Ed. E R Gabrieli. Circ: 700.

JOURNAL OF COMPUTER-ASSISTED TOMOGRAPHY; a radiological journal dedicated to the basic and clinical aspects of reconstructive tomography. see *MEDICAL SCIENCES—Radiology And Nuclear Medicine*

JOURNAL OF DIGITAL IMAGING. see *MEDICAL SCIENCES—Radiology And Nuclear Medicine*

M

610 004 USA ISSN 0148-5598
R858.A1 CODEN: JMSYDA
JOURNAL OF MEDICAL SYSTEMS. Text in English. 1977. bi-m. USD 666, EUR 664 to institutions for print or online ed.; USD 409, EUR 796.80 to institutions for print & online eds.combined (effective 2002). adv. illus. back issues avail.; reprints avail. *Refereed.* **Document type:** *Journal, Academic/Scholarly.* **Description:** Presents and discusses the increasingly extensive applications of new systems techiques and methods in hospital, clinic, and physician's office administration; pathology, radiology, and pharmaceutical delivery systems; medical records storage and retrieval; and ancillary patient-support systems.
Related titles: Microfilm ed.: (from PQC); Online - full text ed.: (from EBSCO Publishing, O C L C Online Computer Library Center, Inc., RoweCom Information Quest, Swets Blackwell, Kluwer Online, Institute for Scientific Information).
Indexed: ASCA, Biol.Abstr., CINAHL, Curr.Cont. (coverage dropped), Environ.Sci.Poll.Mgmt., Excerp.Med., INIS Atomind., INSPEC, Ind.Med. (1977-), Inform.Sci.Abstr., Int.Nurs.Ind., LISA, Med.Care Rev., Microcomp.Ind. (Jun.1998-), Pollut.Abstr., Ref.Zh., Risk Abstr., SSCI (coverage dropped), Saf.Sci.Abstr.
—BLDSC (5017.088000), CISTI, GNLM, IDS, ingenta, KNAW. **CCC.**
Published by: Kluwer Academic - Plenum Publishers (Subsidiary of: Wolters Kluwer N.V.), 233 Spring St, New York, NY 10013-1578. TEL 212-620-8000, 800-221-9369, FAX 212-463-0742, info@plenum.com, http://www.wkap.nl/journalhome.htm/0148-5598. Ed. Dr. Ralph R Grams. R&P Rose Luongo TEL 781-871-6311. **Subscr. outside the Americas to:** Kluwer Academic Publishers Group, Journals Department, PO Box 322, Dordrecht 3300 AH, Netherlands. TEL 31-78-639-2392, FAX 31-78-654-6474.

MEDICAL ARTIFICIAL INTELLIGENCE. see *COMPUTERS—Artificial Intelligence*

610.285 USA
MEDICAL COMPUTING TODAY. Text in English. 1998. irreg. back issues avail. *Refereed.* **Document type:** *Academic/Scholarly, Trade.* **Description:** Publishes original articles, annotated references to Web resources and exchanges on medical computing by and among health care professionals.
Media: Online - full text.
Published by: Healthcare Computing Publications Inc., 462 Second St, Brooklyn, NY 11215. TEL 718-499-5910, FAX 718-768-3260, editor@medicalcomputingtoday.com, http://www.medicalcomputingtoday.com/. Ed. Sue Frisch.

610 GBR ISSN 1463-9238
CODEN: MIIMFX
MEDICAL INFORMATICS AND THE INTERNET IN MEDICINE; an international journal of computing in health care. Text in English. 1976. q. GBP 134, USD 221 to individuals; GBP 429, USD 709 to institutions (effective 2002). adv. bk.rev. back issues avail. *Refereed.* **Document type:** *Academic/Scholarly.* **Description:** Serves as a focus for most aspects of the application of computers to medicine, and promotes the application of analysis, inference and reasoning to medical information.
Former titles (until 1999): Medical Informatics (0959-8316); (until 1985): Medecine et Informatique (0307-7640)
Related titles: Online - full text ed.: ISSN 1464-5238 (from CatchWord Ltd., EBSCO Publishing, O C L C Online Computer Library Center, Inc., RoweCom Information Quest, Swets Blackwell, Institute for Scientific Information).
Indexed: ASCA, Abstr.Hum.Comp.Inter., Art.Int.Abstr., Biol.Abstr., CAD CAM Abstr., CINAHL, Compumath, Comput.Lit.Ind., Curr.Cont., Eng.Ind., Environ.Sci.Poll.Mgmt., Ergon.Abstr., Excerp.Med., Helminthol.Abstr., Hosp.Lit.Ind., INSPEC (Apr.1976-), Ind.Med. (1999-), Inpharma, LISA, Pharm.&Out.News, Pollut.Abstr., Reac., SSCI (coverage dropped).
—BLDSC (5527.554000), AskIEEE, CatchWord, CISTI, Ei, EMDOCS, GNLM, IDS, ingenta. **CCC.**
Published by: Taylor & Francis Group, Taylor & Francis Ltd., 11 New Fetter Ln, London EC4P 4EE, United Kingdom. TEL 44-20-7583-9855, FAX 44-20-7842-2298, info@tandf.co.uk, http://www.tandf.co.uk. Ed. John Bryant. **Subscr. in N. America to:** Taylor & Francis Ltd., 325 Chestnut St, Suite 800, Philadelphia, PA 19016. TEL 800-354-1420, FAX 215-625-8914, info@taylorandfrancis.com, http://www.taylorandfrancis.com/.

610.285 CAN
MEDICAL INFORMATICS NEWSLETTER. Text in English. 4/yr. **Document type:** *Newsletter.* **Description:** Includes articles on informatics in health care.
Related titles: Online - full text ed.
Published by: International Medical Informatics Association, 5782 172th St, Edmonton, AB T6M 1B4, Canada. TEL 403-489-4553, FAX 403-489-3290, haegar@med.uni-goettingen.de, http://www.imia.org. Ed. O Rienhoff.

610 USA
MEDICAL INTELLIGENCE✱. Text in English. 1990. 12/yr. USD 745 in US & Canada; USD 900 elsewhere. **Description:** For investors and researchers exploring the interrelationships between medicine and technology as well as current and future advances in medical therapy.
Published by: Gallifrey Publishing, 1912 Darnell St, Libertyville, IL 60048-4331. Ed. Derek F Stubbs.

610 005.3 USA ISSN 1059-907X
MEDICAL SOFTWARE REVIEWS; the leading resource for objective evaluations of medical software. Text in English. m. USD 117 in North America to individuals; USD 139 elsewhere to individuals; USD 149 in North America to institutions; USD 171 elsewhere to institutions. software rev. index. **Document type:** *Trade.* **Description:** Discusses software evaluated by doctors for a wide variety of practice sizes and settings for functions such as medical records management, patient education, CD-ROM references, voice-activated note-taking, billing and coding, CME and medical education, and drug interaction and prescribing. Also includes ratings and investigations of performance, ease of operation, system requirements, and online help.
Published by: Healthcare Computing Publications Inc., 462 Second St, Brooklyn, NY 11215. TEL 718-499-5910, FAX 718-768-3260, http://www.healthcarecomputing.com.

610 USA ISSN 1085-3502
MEDICINE ON THE NET. Text in English. 1995. m. USD 169 domestic to individuals; USD 229 domestic to institutions; USD 225 foreign (effective 2001). adv. bk.rev., software rev., Website rev. abstr, bibl, charts, illus, stat. Index. 28 p./no. back issues avail.; reprints avail. **Document type:** *Magazine, Trade.* **Description:** Covers medical resources on the internet and how medical professionals are using the internet in patient care.
Related titles: Online - full text ed.
Indexed: LISA.
—BLDSC (5534.090550), Infotrieve. **CCC.**
Published by: COR Healthcare Resources, PO Box 40959, Santa Barbara, CA 93140. TEL 805-564-2177, FAX 805-564-2146, info@corhealth.com, http://www.mednet-i.com. Ed. Bridget Meaney. Pub. Dean H Anderson. adv.: page USD 1,336, color page USD 1,911; 11.25 x 8.75.

610.285 USA
MICRO MEDICAL NEWSLETTER. Text in English. 1981. 12/yr. bk.rev. **Document type:** *Newsletter.*
Published by: American Newsfeatures Syndicate, 113 Wattenbarger, Sweetwater, TN 37874-6135. TEL 800-484-4074, FAX 423-337-5331. Ed. Ray Burr. Circ: 171,214.

610 USA ISSN 0748-2051
MICROPSYCH NETWORK; computer applications in psychology. Text in English. 1985. bi-m. USD 20; USD 30 foreign. adv. bk.rev. back issues avail. **Description:** Publishes computer-related material that psychologists will find useful; articles about using computers in clinical practice, the classroom, and research laboratory, and reviews of software and original programs.
Published by: (Professional Resource Exchange, Inc.), Human Technology Interface, Ink Press, 163 Wood Wedge Way, Sanford, NC 27330. Ed. Emory Sadler. Circ: 500.

610 USA ISSN 0273-4974
NATIONAL REPORT ON COMPUTERS AND HEALTH. Text in English. 1980. 25/yr. USD 427. software rev. back issues avail. **Document type:** *Trade.* **Description:** Features articles pertaining to new software, technologies in the fast changing field of hospital data processing and clinical information systems.
Related titles: Online - full text ed.: (from Data-Star, Gale Group, The Dialog Corporation).
—**CCC.**
Published by: United Communications Group, 1300 Rockville Pike, Ste 1100, Rockville, MD 20852-3030. TEL 301-816-8950, FAX 301-816-8945. Ed. Bob Gough.

610 USA ISSN 0891-8163
PHYSICIANS & COMPUTERS. Text in English. 1982. m. USD 40 domestic; USD 60 foreign (effective 1999). adv. tr.lit. reprints avail. **Document type:** *Trade.* **Description:** For physicians who have little or no computer experience. Articles cover applications to office management and clinical medicine environment.
Published by: Moorhead Publications, Inc., 810 S Waukegan Rd, Ste 200, Lake Forest, IL 60045-2672. TEL 847-615-8333, FAX 847-615-8345. Ed. Rogers H Piercy. Pub. Thomas J Moorhead. adv.: B&W page USD 3,225, color page USD 4,010; trim 10.75 x 8.13. Circ: 90,131.

PROCESS CONTROL; vakblad voor procesbesturing en analysetechniek. see *COMPUTERS—Automation*

RADIOLOGIC TECHNOLOGY. see *MEDICAL SCIENCES—Radiology And Nuclear Medicine*

610 011 FRA ISSN 1169-6176
REPERTOIRE INTERNATIONAL DES BANQUES DE DONNEES BIOMEDICALES. Text in French. 1991. irreg. FRF 370 (effective 1998). adv. **Document type:** *Directory.* **Description:** A directory of worldwide databases in the field of medical, pharmaceutical and biological sciences with a description of each database.
Published by: (Ministere de la Recherche et de l'Espace), Editions F L A Consultants, 27 rue de la Vistule, Paris 75013, France. TEL 33-1-45827575, FAX 33-1-45824604, flabases@iway.fr, http://www.fla-consultants.fr. Ed. Madeleine Wolff Terroine. Adv. contact Beatrice Riou.

651.8 USA
S I G B I O NEWSLETTER. (Special Interest Group on Biomedical Computing) Text in English. 1970. q. USD 30 to non-members; USD 20 to members. bk.rev. **Document type:** *Newsletter.*
Indexed: Abstr.Hum.Comp.Inter., INSPEC (Nov.1979-, dropped).
—BLDSC.
Published by: Association for Computing Machinery, Special Interest Group on Biomedical Computing, One Astor Plaza, 1515 Broadway, New York, NY 10036-5701. TEL 212-869-7440, FAX 212-302-5826. Ed. Cathy Rubens. Circ: 1,000.

STUDIES IN HEALTH TECHNOLOGY AND INFORMATICS. see *MEDICAL SCIENCES*

610.28 USA ISSN 1530-5627
CODEN: TEJOFP
TELEMEDICINE JOURNAL AND E-HEALTH. Text in English. 1995. q. USD 386 domestic to institutions; USD 491 foreign to institutions; USD 463 domestic to institutions print and online; USD 568 foreign to institutions print and online; USD 199 domestic to individuals; USD 269 foreign to individuals; USD 239 domestic to individuals print and online; USD 309 foreign to individuals print and online (effective 2002). *Refereed.* **Document type:** *Journal, Academic/Scholarly.* **Description:** Reviews all aspects of clinical telemedical practice, encompassing videoconferencing and transmission of medical imaging, such as teleradiology, telecardiology, and telepathology.
Formerly: Telemedicine Journal (1078-3024)
Related titles: Online - full text ed.: USD 386 to institutions; USD 199 to individuals (effective 2002) (from CatchWord Ltd., EBSCO Publishing, O C L C Online Computer Library Center, Inc., RoweCom Information Quest, Swets Blackwell, Institute for Scientific Information).
Indexed: Curr.Cont., Eng.Ind., Excerp.Med. (1996-), INSPEC (Jan.1980-), Ind.Med. (2000-), Int.Nurs.Ind., LISA, Sci.Cit.Ind.
—CatchWord, EMDOCS, GNLM, IDS, Infotrieve, ingenta, KNAW. **CCC.**
Published by: (American Telemedicine Association), Mary Ann Liebert, Inc. Publishers, 2 Madison Ave, Larchmont, NY 10538. TEL 914—834-3100, FAX 914-834-1388, info@liebertpub.com, http://www.liebertpub.com/tmj. Ed. Dr. Rashid L Bashshur.

651.8 610.28 USA ISSN 1063-973X
R864
TOWARD AN ELECTRONIC PATIENT RECORD; updates on standards and developments. Text in English. 1992. 10/yr. USD 175; USD 195 foreign (effective 1998). bk.rev. back issues avail. *Refereed.* **Document type:** *Newsletter, Academic/Scholarly.*
—GNLM.

Published by: Medical Records Institute, PO Box 600770, Newtonville, MA 02160. TEL 617-964-3923, FAX 617-964-3926, cust_service@medrecinst.com, http://www.medrecinst.com. Ed. C Peter Waegemann. R&P Jason Glass. Circ: 500 (paid).

610 USA
WINDOWS IN HEALTH CARE. Text in English. q. USD 93.95; USD 119 foreign. software rev. **Document type:** *Trade.* **Description:** Reports on the use of Microsoft Windows technology in health care settings.
Indexed: SoftBase (Jun.1998-).
Published by: Faulkner & Gray, Inc. (Chicago), Health Data Management, 300 S Wacker Dr, Chicago, IL 60606. TEL 312-913-1334, 800-535-8403, FAX 312-913-1959, http://hdm.fgray.com/html/publications, http://hdm.fgray.com/html/publications/. Pub. Howard J Anderson.

MEDICAL SCIENCES—Dentistry

617.6 BRA
A B E S P BOLETIM. Text in Portuguese. 1972. q. BRL 200, USD 13. adv.
Published by: Associacao Brasileira de Endodontia Seccao Sao Paulo, Praca Amadeu Amaral, 47-8, B Vista, Sao Paulo, SP 01327-010, Brazil. Ed. Antonio Elias Makaron. Circ: 2,500 (controlled).

617.6 CAN ISSN 0820-5949
A C F D FORUM. Text mainly in English; Text occasionally in French. 1968. 3/yr. membership. **Document type:** *Newsletter.*
Formerly: Association of Canadian Faculties of Dentistry. Newsletter (0044-9555)
Media: Duplicated (not offset).
Published by: Association of Canadian Faculties of Dentistry, Central Office, Ste 109, 1815 Alta Vista Dr, Ottawa, ON K1G 3Y6, Canada. TEL 604-822-3413, FAX 604-822-6698, rmsh@unixg.ubc.ca. Ed. R M Shah. Circ: 700.

617.6 340 USA
A D A LEGAL ADVISOR. Text in English. m. USD 189 to non-members; USD 129 to members; USD 295 to institutions. **Document type:** *Newsletter.* **Description:** Covers legal issues relating to dental practice.
Published by: American Dental Association, 211 E Chicago Ave, Chicago, IL 60611. TEL 312-440-2867.

617.6 USA ISSN 0895-2930
RK1
A D A NEWS. Text in English. 1970. 22/yr. USD 55 to non-members; USD 66 foreign to non-members; USD 78 to institutions; USD 98 foreign to institutions (effective 2001). adv. **Document type:** *Newspaper.* **Description:** Provides information on social, political and economic developments affecting dentistry and health care in general.
Related titles: Microform ed.: (from PQC).
—CCC.
Published by: American Dental Association, 211 E Chicago Ave, Chicago, IL 60611. FAX 312-440-2790, 312-440-3538, http://www.ada.org. Ed. Judy Jakush. Pub. Laura A Kosden. Adv. contact Carol Krause TEL 312-440-2782. Circ: 140,000 (paid).

617.6 MEX ISSN 0001-0944
A D M. Text in Spanish. 1943. bi-m. USD 100 (effective 1999). bk.rev. abstr, charts, illus. *Refereed.* **Document type:** *Academic/Scholarly.* **Description:** Contains academic and social information related to dentistry. Includes general, domestic and international events.
Related titles: CD-ROM ed.
Indexed: Chem.Abstr., INIS Atomind., Ind.Med. (coverage dropped).
—BLDSC (7802.195000), CISTI, GNLM.
Published by: Asociacion Dental Mexicana, A.C., Ezequiel Montes No. 92, Col. Revolucion, Delegacion Cuauhtemoc, Mexico City, DF 06030, Mexico. TEL 52-5-29400095, FAX 52-5-2945143. Ed., R&P Elias Grego Samra. Circ: 3,000 (paid). **Co-sponsor:** Federacion Nacional de Colegios de Cirujanos Dentistas.

617.6 USA ISSN 0194-729X
A G D IMPACT. Text in English. 1973. m. (11/yr.). USD 30 domestic to individuals; USD 35 in Canada to individuals; USD 50 elsewhere to individuals; USD 48 domestic to institutions; USD 53 in Canada to institutions; USD 68 elsewhere to institutions (effective 2001). adv. illus. **Document type:** *Newsletter.* **Description:** Features issues, controversies, legislation and trends that affect the practice of general dentistry.
—CCC.
Published by: Academy of General Dentistry, 211 E Chicago Ave, Ste 900, Chicago, IL 60611-1999. TEL 312-440-4300, 888-243-3368, FAX 312-440-4261, agdimpact@aol.com, agdimpact@agd.org, http://www.agd.org. Ed. Dr. Roger D Winland. R&P Jo-Ellyn Posselt TEL 312-440-4307. Adv. contact Todd Goldman. B&W page USD 2,005, color page USD 3,155. Circ: 36,000.

617.6 BRA
A P C D JOURNAL. Text in Portuguese. 1957. m. free to members and qualified personnel. adv. illus. *Refereed.*
Formerly (until 1993): Associacao Paulista de Cirurgioes Dentistas. Journal
Related titles: Online - full text ed.: 1997.
Published by: Associacao Paulista de Cirurgioes Dentistas/Sao Paulo State Dental Association, Praca Campos de Bagatelle, 100, Sao Paulo, SP 02012-000, Brazil. TEL 55-11-62213022, FAX 55-11-62213612, directoria@apcd.org.br, http://www.apcd.org.br/. Ed. Luciano Artioli Moreira. R&P Sergio Bueno da Silveria. Circ: 42,000 (controlled).

617.6 USA ISSN 0277-3627
A S D A NEWS (YEAR). Text in English. 1971. m. (Sep.-June). USD 5 to members; USD 20 domestic to non-members; USD 30 foreign (effective 2001). adv. 8 p./no. 4 cols./p. **Document type:** *Newsletter, Trade.* **Description:** Assortment of dental, association and student news, viewpoints, features.
Former titles (until 1981): New Dentist; (until 1979): A S D A News (0161-8431); A S D A Newsletter (0044-8052)
Related titles: Online - full text ed.: Members only.
Indexed: Dent.Abstr., Dent.Ind.
Published by: American Student Dental Association, 211 E Chicago Ave, Ste. 1160, Chicago, IL 60611-2616. TEL 312-440-2795, FAX 312-440-2820, asda@asdanet.org, asda@asdanet.org, http://www.asdanet.org. Pub. Cynthia L Kennedy. R&P Lauren Waggoner. Adv. contact Stephanie Cesna TEL 312-440-2845. B&W page USD 2,048, color page USD 2,948. Circ: 16,000 (paid and free).

617.6 USA
A S D A TODAY. Text in English. 1980. q. membership. adv. **Document type:** *Newsletter.* **Description:** Covers porcelain laminates, bonding, new dental materials and techniques presented on the post graduate level of advanced dentistry.
Formerly: American Association for Dental Aesthetics Newsletter
Published by: American Society for Dental Aesthetics, 635 Madison Ave, New York, NY 10022. TEL 212-371-4575. Ed., R&P, Adv. contact Melvin S Babad. Circ: 3,000 (controlled).

617.6 USA ISSN 1050-0758
ACCESS (CHICAGO). Text in English. 10/yr. USD 48 to non-members (effective 2000). **Document type:** *Trade.*
Formerly (until 1987): A D H A Access (0894-9042)
—CCC.
Published by: American Dental Hygienists' Association, 444 N Michigan Ave, Ste 3400, Chicago, IL 60611. TEL 312-440-8929, FAX 312-440-8900. Ed. Rosetta Gervasi. Pub. Banta Greenfield. Adv. contact Wesley Blaszczynski. Circ: 30,000.

617.6 618.92 DOM ISSN 0252-1032
ACTA DE ODONTOLOGIA PEDIATRICA; una revista internacional para la odontologia pediatrica. Text in English, Spanish. 1979. s-a. USD 30 foreign; free to qualified personnel. adv. bk.rev. **Document type:** *Academic/Scholarly.* **Description:** Dedicated to promoting the practice, education, and research of pediatric and familial dentistry.
Indexed: Dent.Ind., Ind.Med. (coverage dropped).
—GNLM.
Published by: Centro de Odontologia Pediatrica, Jose Joaquin Perez No. 101 - Zona 1, Apartado Postal 2753, Santo Domingo, Dominican Republic. TEL 809-688-8969, FAX 809-221-2041, villagodoy@codetel.net.do. Ed. Dr. Fredrico Garcia Godoy. Adv. contact Altagracia Villalba. B&W page USD 780, color page USD 1,400; 11 x 8.5. Circ: 3,000.

617.6 NOR ISSN 0001-6357
CODEN: AOSCAQ
ACTA ODONTOLOGICA SCANDINAVICA; Scandinavian dental research journal. Text in English. 1939. 6/yr. GBP 185, USD 305 to institutions (effective 2002). adv. bibl, charts, illus. index. back issues avail.; reprints avail. *Refereed.* **Document type:** *Academic/Scholarly.* **Description:** Presents dental research in the Scandinavian countries to an international forum.
Related titles: Microform ed.: (from PQC); Online - full text ed.: (from EBSCO Publishing, O C L C Online Computer Library Center, Inc., RoweCom Information Quest, CatchWord Ltd., ingenta, Swets Blackwell, Institute for Scientific Information).
Indexed: ASCA, Abstr.Health Care Manage.Stud., Biol.Abstr., Chem.Abstr., Chem.Indus.Notes, Curr.Adv.Ecol.Sci., Curr.Cont., Curr.Tit.Dent., Dent.Abstr., Dent.Ind., Energy Res.Abstr., Excerp.Med., IBZ, INIS Atomind., Ind.Med. (1939-), Ind.Sci.Rev., Inpharma, Pharm.&Out.News, Reac., Rev.Med.& Vet.Mycol., Sci.Cit.Ind.
—BLDSC (0641.630000), CASDDS, CISTI, EMDOCS, GNLM, IDS, ingenta, KNAW. **CCC.**
Published by: Taylor & Francis AS (Subsidiary of: Taylor & Francis Group), Cort Adelersgt. 17, Solli, PO Box 2562, Oslo 0202, Norway. TEL 47-22-12-98-80, FAX 47-22-12-98-90, journals@tanf.no, http://www.tandf.co.uk/tfas. Ed. Folke Lagerloef. Circ: 500.

617.6 BEL ISSN 0001-7000
CODEN: ASBEBA
ACTA STOMATOLOGICA BELGICA. Text in Flemish, French; Summaries in English, Flemish, French, German. 1970 (vol.67). q. BEF 1,800; BEF 2,000 foreign (effective 1999). bk.rev. abstr, bibl, illus. index. **Document type:** *Academic/Scholarly.*
Indexed: Biol.Abstr., Dent.Ind., Excerp.Med., Ind.Med. (1960-).
—CISTI, GNLM.
Published by: (Association des Societes Scientifiques Medicales Belges/Vereiniging van de Belgische Wetenschappelijke Genootschappen), Acta Medica Belgica, Av Circulaire 138A, Brussels 1180, Belgium. TEL 32-2-374-5158, FAX 32-2-3749628, amb@skynet.be, http://www.ulb.ac.be/medecine/loce/amb.htm.

617.6 HRV ISSN 0001-7019
ACTA STOMATOLOGICA CROATICA. Text in Croatian, English; Summaries in English. 1966. q. HRK 120; DEM 100 in Europe; DEM 120 elsewhere. adv. bk.rev. abstr, bibl, charts, illus. back issues avail. *Refereed.* **Document type:** *Academic/Scholarly.* **Description:** Covers research in dental, oral, maxillofacial, and periodontic surgery. Contains reviews of congresses and interviews.
Indexed: Biol.Abstr., Chem.Abstr., Dent.Ind., Ref.Zh.
—GNLM.
Published by: Hrvatski Lijecnicki Zbor/Croatian Dental Society, Petrinjska 34, Zagreb 10000, Croatia. TEL 385-1-4819433, FAX 385-1-4819435, ured@znanost.hr, http://www.sfzg.hr. Ed., R&P, Adv. contact Goran Knezevic. B&W page DEM 400, color page DEM 600. Circ: 1,200.

617.6 YUG ISSN 0352-5252
ACTA STOMATOLOGICA NAISSI. Text in Serbo-Croatian. 1984. s-a.
Related titles: ♦ Supplement: Acta Stomatologica Naissi. Supplement. ISSN 0354-7957.
Published by: Stomatoloska Klinika, c/o Univerzitet u Nisu, Izdavacka Jedinica, Trg. Bratstva i Jedinstva 2, Nis 18000, Yugoslavia. Ed. Budimir B Sokolovic.

617.6 FRA ISSN 0001-7817
CODEN: ACOPAR
ACTUALITES ODONTO-STOMATOLOGIQUES. Text in French; Summaries in English, German, Spanish. 1946. q. FRF 950 to individuals; FRF 300 newsstand/cover. adv. **Document type:** *Academic/Scholarly.*
Indexed: Biol.Abstr., Chem.Abstr., Curr.Cont. (coverage dropped), Dent.Ind., Ind.Med. (coverage dropped), Ref.Zh.
—CASDDS, CISTI, GNLM.
Published by: Editions C D P, 1 av. Edward Belin, Rueil Malmaison 92856, France. Ed. Jean-Pierre Ragot. Adv. contact Sybille Barbera.

617.6071 USA ISSN 0091-729X
RK91
ADMISSION REQUIREMENTS OF U S AND CANADIAN DENTAL SCHOOLS. Text in English. 1963. a. USD 25 (effective 2000). **Document type:** *Directory.* **Description:** Contains comprehensive details of requirements for application and admission to all US and Canadian dental schools.
Formerly: Admission Requirements of American Dental Schools (0065-1990)
Published by: American Association of Dental Schools, 1625 Massachusetts Ave, N W, Washington, DC 20036-2212. TEL 202-667-9433. Circ: 3,500.

M

617.6 USA ISSN 0895-9374
ADVANCES IN DENTAL RESEARCH. Text in English. 1987. irreg. (2-6/yr.). included in subscription to Journal of Dental Research. cum.index every 3 yrs. back issues avail.; reprint service avail. from PQC. **Document type:** *Proceedings, Academic/Scholarly.* **Description:** Provides a forum for detailed exploration and timely discussion of significant research developments in the sciences relevant to dentistry and to the chemistry, biology, and function of the oral cavity in health and disease.
Incorporates: International Conference on Oral Biology. Proceedings (0074-3216)
Related titles: Microform ed.: (from PQC); ♦ Supplement to: Journal of Dental Research. ISSN 0022-0345.
Indexed: Alloys Ind. (1987-1996), Biol.Abstr., Chem.Abstr., Curr.Cont. (coverage dropped), Dairy Sci.Abstr., Dent.Abstr., Dent.Ind., Eng.Mat.Abstr., Excerp.Med., INIS Atomind., Ind.Med. (coverage dropped), Ind.Sci.Rev., Met.Abstr. (1987-1996), Met.Abstr.Ind. (1987-1996), Nonfer.Met.Alert (1987-1996), Nutr.Abstr., PCC Alert (1987-1996), Sci.Cit.Ind. (coverage dropped), Steels Alert (1987-1996), World Alum.Abstr.
—BLDSC (0704.242200), CISTI, GNLM, ingenta, KNAW. **CCC.**
Published by: (International and American Associations for Dental Research), American Association for Dental Research, 1619 Duke St, Alexandria, VA 22314-3406. TEL 703-548-0066, FAX 703-548-1883, research@iadr.com, http://www.iadr.com. Ed. Dr. Charles Liebow. Circ: 3,000.

617.6 JPN ISSN 0044-6912
CODEN: AGDSAB
AICHI-GAKUIN JOURNAL OF DENTAL SCIENCE. Text in Japanese; Summaries in English. 1964. q. JPY 5,000, USD 20 per issue. adv. bk.rev. abstr, charts, stat. **Document type:** *Academic/Scholarly.*
Indexed: Biol.Abstr., Dent.Ind., INIS Atomind.
—BLDSC (0773.074200), CASDDS, CISTI, GNLM, Infotrieve. **CCC.**
Published by: Aichi-Gakuin Society of Dental Science, School of Dentistry, Gakuin University, 1-100 kusumoto-cho, Chikusa-ku, Nagoya-shi, Aichi-ken 464-0037, Japan. Ed. Jiro Hasegawa. Pub. Hajime Hanamura. Adv. contact Yoichiro Kameya. Circ: 4,000.

617.6 USA ISSN 0002-3701
AKRON DENTAL SOCIETY. BULLETIN. Text in English. 1970 (vol.29). 8/yr. USD 40; USD 60 foreign. adv. **Document type:** *Bulletin.*
—GNLM.
Published by: Akron Dental Society, 440 Grant St, Akron, OH 44311. TEL 216-376-3551. Ed. Samuel N Pupino. Adv. contact Nancy L Seigfreid. Circ: 450.

617.6 CAN
ALBERTA DENTAL ASSOCIATION. UPDATER. Text in English. 1967. m. membership. adv. **Document type:** *Newsletter.*
Former titles (until 1996): A D A Newsletter (0849-5866); (until 1988): A D A News Information (0383-6355)
Published by: Alberta Dental Association, 8230 105 St, Ste 101, Edmonton, AB T6E 5H9, Canada. Ed. Dr. Wally West. Circ: 1,750.

617.6 EGY
ALEXANDRIA DENTAL JOURNAL/AL-MAGALLAT AL-ISKANDIRIYYAH LI-TIBB AL-ASNAN. Text in Arabic. 1989 (vol.14). q.
Published by: Alexandria University, Faculty of Dentistry, 22 Sharia al-Gaish, Al-Shatby, Alexandria, Egypt.

617.6 USA ISSN 0002-6417
ALPHA OMEGAN✱**.** Text in English. 1908. q. USD 30; USD 40 foreign. adv. bk.rev. back issues avail. **Description:** Scientific and membership information.
—BLDSC (0802.091000), CISTI, GNLM.
Published by: Alpha Omega International Fraternity, 1314 Bedford Ave, Ste 206, Baltimore, MD 21208-3737. TEL 212-683-4155, FAX 212-683-0027. Ed. Dr. Roger Spott. Circ: 8,000.

617.643 USA ISSN 0886-1064
AMERICAN ACADEMY OF GNATHOLOGIC ORTHOPEDICS. JOURNAL. Text in English. 1984. q. USD 90 domestic; USD 115 foreign (effective 2000). adv. back issues avail. **Document type:** *Academic/Scholarly.*
Published by: American Academy of Gnathologic Orthopedics, 2651 Oak Grove Rd, Walnut Creek, CA 94598. TEL 800-510-2246, http://www.aago.com. Ed., Pub., Adv. contact Jack Hockel. Circ: 400.

AMERICAN ASSOCIATION OF DENTAL EDITORS. NEWSLETTER. see *JOURNALISM*

617.6 USA ISSN 0002-7421
AMERICAN ASSOCIATION OF DENTAL EXAMINERS. BOARD BULLETIN. Text in English. 1965. q. USD 10. illus. **Document type:** *Bulletin.*
Published by: American Association of Dental Examiners, 211 E Chicago Ave, Ste 760, Chicago, IL 60611. TEL 312-440-7464, FAX 312-440-3525. Ed. Ronald Maitland. Circ: 1,100 (controlled).

617.6 USA
AMERICAN ASSOCIATION OF WOMEN DENTISTS. CHRONICLE. Text in English. 1964. 6/yr. USD 30 (effective 1999). adv. bk.rev. **Document type:** *Newsletter.*
Former titles (until 1980): American Association of Women Dentists. Journal; (until 1978): Association of American Women Dentists. Newsletter
Published by: American Association of Women Dentists, 645 N Michigan Ave 800, Chicago, IL 60611. TEL 312-280-9296, FAX 312-280-9893, info@womendentists.org, http://www.womendentists.org. Ed., Adv. contact Sharon Gautschy. Circ: 2,200 (controlled).

617.6 USA ISSN 0002-7979
RK1
AMERICAN COLLEGE OF DENTISTS. JOURNAL. Text in English. 1934. q. USD 40; USD 50 foreign (effective 1999). bk.rev. index. reprint service avail. from PQC. *Refereed.* **Document type:** *Academic/Scholarly.*
Related titles: Microform ed.: (from PQC).
Indexed: Curr.Tit.Dent., Dent.Abstr., Dent.Ind., GeoRef, Ind.Med. (1934-).
—BLDSC (4685.700000), CISTI, GNLM, ingenta.
Published by: American College of Dentists, 839 Quince Orchard Blvd, Ste J, Gaithersburg, MD 20878-1614. TEL 301-977-3223, 888-223-1920, FAX 301-977-3330, robyn@acdentists.org. Ed. David W Chambers. R&P Robyn Hulvey. Circ: 5,300.

617.6 USA ISSN 0002-8177
RK1 CODEN: JADSAY
AMERICAN DENTAL ASSOCIATION. JOURNAL. Text in English. 1913. m. USD 100 domestic to individuals; USD 111 in Canada to individuals; USD 126 elsewhere to individuals; USD 121 domestic to institutions; USD 137 in Canada to institutions; USD 153 elsewhere to institutions; USD 12 newsstand/cover domestic; USD 19 newsstand/cover foreign (effective 2001). adv. charts, illus, stat. s-a. index. back issues avail.; reprint service avail. from PQC. *Refereed.* **Document type:** *Academic/Scholarly.* **Description:** Contains news on the latest developments in practice and research: clinical reports, original research, case reports, and editorials on new techniques and improvements. Provides official reports.
Related titles: CD-ROM ed.; Microform ed.: (from PQC); Online - full text ed.: (from Gale Group, Factiva, Institute for Scientific Information); Cumulative ed.: J A D A on CD-ROM (1990-1998). USD 129 per issue to members; USD 199 per issue to non-members; USD 299 per issue to institutions (effective 2001).
Indexed: AIDS Abstr., ASCA, Abstr.Anthropol., Abstr.Health Care Manage.Stud., Behav.Med.Abstr., Biol.Abstr., CINAHL, C.I.S. Abstr., Chem.Abstr., Chem.Indus.Notes, Chem.Titles, Curr.Adv.Ecol.Sci., Curr.Cont., Curr.Tit.Dent., Dent.Abstr., Dent.Ind., Dok.Arbeitsmed., Environ.Sci.Poll.Mgmt., Gen.Sci.Ind. (Jun.1992-), Helminthol.Abstr., Hosp.Lit.Ind., INIS Atomind., Ind.Med. (1922-), Ind.Sci.Rev., Inpharma, Mat.Sci.Cit.Ind. (coverage dropped), Med.Care Rev., NRN, Nutr.Abstr., Pharm.&Out.News, Pollut.Abstr., Reac., SSCI (coverage dropped), Sci.Cit.Ind.
—BLDSC (4686.075000), CASDDS, CISTI, GNLM, IDS, ingenta. **CCC.**
Published by: American Dental Association, 211 E Chicago Ave, Chicago, IL 60611. TEL 312-440-2740, FAX 312-440-3538, jada@ada.org, http://www.ada.org. Ed. Dr. Lawrence Meskin. Pub. Laura A Kosden. Adv. contact Carol Krause TEL 312-440-2782. B&W page USD 9,490, color page USD 9,140. Circ: 150,000 (paid).

617.6 USA
AMERICAN DENTAL ASSOCIATION. TRANSACTION SERIES: ANNUAL REPORTS AND RESOLUTIONS, SUPPLEMENTS ONE AND TWO, TRANSACTIONS. Text in English. a. price varies. **Document type:** *Corporate.*
Formerly: American Dental Association. Annual Reports and Resolutions (0090-3329)
Published by: American Dental Association, 211 E Chicago Ave, Chicago, IL 60611. TEL 312-440-2500, FAX 312-440-3538.

617.6 USA ISSN 0065-8073
RK37
AMERICAN DENTAL DIRECTORY. Text in English. 1947. a. USD 187.50; USD 215.63 foreign. **Document type:** *Directory.*
Published by: American Dental Association, 211 E Chicago Ave, Chicago, IL 60611. TEL 312-440-2500, FAX 312-440-3538.

617.6 USA ISSN 0894-8275
CODEN: AJDEES
AMERICAN JOURNAL OF DENTISTRY. Text in English. 1988. bi-m. USD 70 domestic; USD 95 in Canada & Mexico; USD 115 elsewhere (effective 2000). adv. bk.rev. index. back issues avail. *Refereed.* **Document type:** *Trade.* **Description:** Deals with clinically relevant research in general-practice dentistry.
Related titles: Online - full text ed.: (from Institute for Scientific Information).
Indexed: ASCA, Biol.Dig., Curr.Cont., Dent.Abstr., Inpharma, Nutr.Abstr., Reac., Sci.Cit.Ind., Sugar Ind.Abstr.
—BLDSC (0824.230000), GNLM, IDS, ingenta.
Published by: Mosher & Linder, Inc., 1004 Wurzbach Rd no.368, San Antonio, TX 78230. TEL 210-493-9660, FAX 210-493-4660, amjdent@sprintmail.com, http://www.amjdent.com. Ed. Franklin Garcia Godoy. R&P, Adv. contact Katherine Godoy. B&W page USD 1,000, color page USD 1,600. Circ: 10,000 (paid and controlled).

617.643 USA ISSN 0889-5406
RK1 CODEN: AJOOEB
AMERICAN JOURNAL OF ORTHODONTICS AND DENTOFACIAL ORTHOPEDICS. Abbreviated title: A J O D O. Text in English. 1915. m. USD 147 domestic to individuals; USD 176 foreign to individuals; USD 311 domestic to institutions; USD 340 foreign to institutions; USD 75 domestic to students; USD 104 foreign to students; USD 29 newsstand/cover (effective 2001). adv. s-a. index. reprint service avail. from PQC. *Refereed.* **Document type:** *Journal, Academic/Scholarly.* **Description:** International research covering all phases of orthodontic treatment.
Formerly (until 1986): American Journal of Orthodontics (0096-6347); Which incorporated: International Journal of Orthodontics (0020-7500); (1938-1937): American Journal of Orthodontics and Oral Surgery (0002-9416)
Related titles: Microfilm ed.: (from PQC); Online - full text ed.: (from EBSCO Publishing, IDEAL Online Library, Institute for Scientific Information, RoweCom Information Quest); French ed.: ISSN 1145-0541.
Indexed: ASCA, Abstr.Anthropol., Biol.Abstr., CINAHL, Curr.Cont., Curr.Ind.Stat., Curr.Tit.Dent., Dent.Abstr., Dent.Ind., Excerp.Med., INIS Atomind., Ind.Med. (1986-), Ind.Sci.Rev., Inpharma, Reac., SSCI (coverage dropped), Sci.Cit.Ind.
—BLDSC (0829.152000), CISTI, GNLM, IDS, Infotrieve, ingenta. **CCC.**
Published by: (American Association of Orthodontists), Mosby, Inc. (Subsidiary of: Elsevier Science), 11830 Westline Industrial Dr, St Louis, MO 63146-3318. TEL 314-872-8370, 800-325-4177, FAX 314-432-1380, http://www.mosby.com/ajodo, http://www.mosby.com/periodicals. Ed. David Turpin. Pub. Cynthia Baudendistel. Adv. contact Carol Kilzer TEL 314-453-4307. B&W page USD 1,935, color page USD 3,410; trim 10.88 x 8.13. Circ: 16,243 (paid and controlled). **Co-sponsor:** American Board of Orthodontics.

617.6 USA ISSN 0164-1700
AMERICAN SOCIETY FOR THE ADVANCEMENT OF ANESTHESIA IN DENTISTRY. PROCEEDINGS. Variant title: Pain Control in Dentistry. Text in English. 1972. s-a. USD 85 (effective 2000). adv. bk.rev. **Document type:** *Proceedings.*
Published by: American Society for the Advancement of Anesthesia in Dentistry, 6 East Union Ave, Box 551, Bound Brook, NJ 08805. Ed. Dr. Louis Zall. Circ: 650.

617.6 AUS
ANATOMY; Royal Australiasian College of Dental Surgeons. Lecture notes in anatomy. Text in English. 1998. irreg. AUD 36 newsstand/cover (effective 2001). 96 p./no. **Document type:** *Academic/Scholarly.* **Description:** Covers lecture notes in the basic science subject of anatomy.
Published by: Royal Australasian College of Dental Surgeons, 64 Castlereagh St, Sydney, NSW 2000, Australia. TEL 61-2-9232-3800, FAX 61-2-9221-8108, registrar@racds.org, http://www.racds.org. Ed. John K McGeachie. Circ: 100 (controlled).

M

617.6 USA ISSN 0003-3006
CODEN: ANPRBG
ANESTHESIA PROGRESS; a journal for pain and anxiety control. Text in English. 1957. q. USD 187; USD 220 foreign (effective 1999). adv. bk.rev. abstr, bibl, charts, illus, stat. index. back issues avail. *Refereed.* **Document type:** *Academic/Scholarly.* **Description:** Directed to practicing dentists. Devoted to the management of pain and anxiety in dental outpatients.
Formerly: American Dental Society of Anesthesiology. Journal
Related titles: Microform ed.: (from PQC).
Indexed: Biol.Abstr., Curr.Tit.Dent., Dent.Abstr., Dent.Ind., Excerp.Med., Oral Res.Abstr.
—BLDSC (0900.520000), CISTI, EMDOCS, GNLM, KNAW. **CCC.**
Published by: (American Dental Society of Anesthesiology), Allen Press, Inc., Division Alliance Communications Group, PO Box 1897, Lawrence, KS 66044. TEL 785-843-1235, FAX 785-843-1274, ordes@allenpress.com; adsa@compuserve.com, http://www.adsahome.org, http://www.allenpress.com. Ed. Joel M Weaver. R&P Knight Charlton TEL 312-664-8270. adv.: B&W page USD 570, color page USD 790; trim 11 x 8.25. Circ: 4,000 (paid).

617.6 USA ISSN 0003-3219
CODEN: ANORA
ANGLE ORTHODONTIST. Text in English. 1931. bi-m. USD 95 domestic to individuals; USD 105 foreign to individuals; USD 125 domestic to institutions; USD 135 foreign to institutions (effective 2001). charts, illus. index. back issues avail. *Refereed.* **Document type:** *Academic/Scholarly.* **Description:** Covers all phases of orthodontic treatment as well as the basic sciences related to orthodontics.
Related titles: CD-ROM ed.; Microfiche ed.: (from PQC); Microfilm ed.; Online - full text ed.: (from Institute for Scientific Information).
Indexed: ASCA, Curr.Cont., Curr.Tit.Dent., Dent.Abstr., Dent.Ind., Excerp.Med., INIS Atomind., Ind.Med. (1931-), Ind.Sci.Rev., Inpharma, Nutr.Abstr., Reac., Sci.Cit.Ind.
—CISTI, GNLM, ingenta.
Published by: (Edward H. Angle Society of Orthodontists, Inc.), Angle Orthodontists Research & Education Foundation, Inc., PO Box 2577, Appleton, WI 54913-2577. TEL 920-738-6938, angle@allenpress.com, http://www.angleorthodontist.org. Ed., Pub. David Turpin. R&P John S Kloehn. Circ: 4,000 (paid). **Subscr. to:** Allen Press Inc., PO Box 1897, Lawrence, KS 66044-8897. FAX 785-843-1274.

617.6 USA ISSN 0003-4770
ANNALS OF DENTISTRY. Text in English. 1934. s-a. USD 20; USD 22 foreign. bk.rev. charts, illus. **Document type:** *Academic/Scholarly.*
Indexed: Curr.Tit.Dent., Dent.Abstr., Dent.Ind., Ind.Med. (1936-), NRN.
—BLDSC (1040.350000), CISTI, GNLM, ingenta, KNAW.
Published by: New York Academy of Dentistry, PO Box 522, Hackensack, NJ 07602-0522. TEL 201-440-4498, FAX 201-440-7963. Ed. Murray A Cantor. Circ: 750.

618 USA ISSN 0147-0264
ANNUAL REPORT ON ADVANCED DENTAL EDUCATION. Text in English. 1972. a. USD 20 to non-members; USD 10 to members. **Document type:** *Academic/Scholarly.*
Related titles: Microfiche ed.: (from CIS).
Indexed: SRI.
Published by: American Dental Association, 211 E Chicago Ave, Chicago, IL 60611. TEL 312-440-2674, FAX 312-440-3538.

617.60071 USA
ANNUAL REPORT ON ALLIED DENTAL HEALTH EDUCATION. Text in English. 1967. a. USD 20 to non-members; USD 10 to members. **Document type:** *Academic/Scholarly.*
Formerly: Annual Report on Dental Auxiliary Education (0084-6554)
Related titles: Microfiche ed.: (from CIS).
Indexed: SRI.
Published by: American Dental Association, 211 E Chicago Ave, Chicago, IL 60611. TEL 312-440-2674, FAX 312-440-3538.

617.60071 USA ISSN 0147-0256
ANNUAL REPORT ON DENTAL EDUCATION. Text in English. 1967. a. USD 20 to non-members; USD 10 to members. **Document type:** *Academic/Scholarly.*
Formerly: Dental Students' Register (0065-8049)
Related titles: Microfiche ed.: (from CIS).
Indexed: SRI.
Published by: American Dental Association, 211 E Chicago Ave, Chicago, IL 60611. TEL 312-440-2674, FAX 312-440-3538.

617.6 GBR ISSN 1460-1729
APEX (LEEDS); an information update for dental practitioners. Text in English. 1998. q. GBP 38 domestic to individuals; GBP 64 domestic to institutions (effective 2001). **Document type:** *Journal, Academic/Scholarly.* **Description:** Provides comprehensive selection of the current clinical literature and a forum for discussion and debate.
Published by: Leeds Medical Information, University of Leeds, Leeds, W Yorks LS2 9JT, United Kingdom. TEL 44-113-233-5550, FAX 44-113-233-5568, m.e.j.curzon@leeds.ac.uk, lmi@leeds.ac.uk, http://www.leeds.ac.uk/lmi/apex/apexmain.html, http://www.leeds.ac.uk/lmi/intro.html.

617.6 DEU
ARAB DENTAL/ALAM TIB AL-ASNAN. Text in Arabic. 1989. q. DEM 74.31, EUR 38 for 2 yrs. (effective 2001). adv. charts, illus. **Document type:** *Journal, Trade.*
Indexed: ExtraMED.
Published by: Beta Verlag und Marketinggesellschaft mbH, Postfach 140121, Bonn 53056, Germany. TEL 49-228-91937-0, FAX 49-228-252067, info@beta-publishing.com, http://www.arabdental.com, http://www.beta-publishing.com. Ed. Dr. Rabih Nahas. Adv. contact Heinz Neumann TEL 49-2182-811274. B&W page XEU 2,875, color page XEU 3,720; trim 181 x 250. Circ: 8,700.

ARCHIVES OF ORAL BIOLOGY; a multidisciplinary journal in oral research. see *BIOLOGY—Zoology*

617.6 ESP ISSN 0213-4144
ARCHIVOS DE ODONTOESTOMATOLOGIA*. Text in Spanish; Summaries in English. 1985. m. ESP 6,400. adv. bk.rev. index. back issues avail.
Published by: Ediciones Ergon S.A., Pza. Josep Pallach 10, 1o, Barcelona 08035, Spain. TEL 2010911, FAX 2015911. Ed. Jose Javier Echeverria. Circ: 2,000. **Subscr. to:** Cempro, Plaza Conde Valle Suchil 20, Madrid 28015, Spain.

617.6 ESP
ARCHIVOS DE ODONTOESTOMATOLOGIA PREVENTIVA Y COMUNITARIA*. Text in Spanish; Summaries in English. 1989. s-a. ESP 1,800. adv. bk.rev. index. back issues avail.
Published by: Ediciones Ergon S.A., Pza. Josep Pallach 10, 1o, Barcelona 08035, Spain. TEL 2010911, FAX 2015911. Eds. Dr. Emilio Cuenca, Dr. Carolina. Circ: 1,500. **Subscr. to:** Cempro, Plaza Conde Valle Suchil 20, Madrid 28015, Spain.

617.6 USA ISSN 1056-4764
ARKANSAS DENTISTRY; a quarterly review of dental affairs. Text in English. 1930. 3/yr. USD 16 domestic to non-members; USD 26 foreign to non-members (effective 2000). adv. bk.rev. abstr, illus. **Document type:** *Academic/Scholarly.*
Formerly (until 1991): Arkansas Dental Journal (0004-1769)
Related titles: Microfilm ed.: (from PQC).
Indexed: Dent.Ind.
—BLDSC (1671.085000), GNLM.
Published by: Arkansas State Dental Association, 2501 Crestwood Dr, Ste 205, North Little Rock, AR 72116-7613. TEL 501-771-7650. Circ: 1,100.

617.6 FRA ISSN 0571-1525
ART DENTAIRE LIBERAL. Text in French. 1974. bi-m. FRF 400 (effective 1999). adv. bk.rev. **Document type:** *Trade.*
Published by: Federation des Chirurgiens-Dentistes de France, 15 bis av. Foch, Chelles 77500, France. TEL 33-3-60205345, FAX 33-3-60209983. Ed. Pierre Petit. Adv. contact Herve Parfait. Circ: 36,000.

617.6 FRA ISSN 1146-0717
ART ET TECHNIQUE DENTAIRES. Text in French. 1990. bi-m. FRF 650 to individuals; FRF 285 to students; FRF 193 newsstand/cover. adv. **Document type:** *Trade, Academic/Scholarly.*
Published by: Editions C D P, 1 av. Edward Belin, Rueil Malmaison 92856, France. Ed. Imad Serhan. Adv. contact Sybille Barbera. Circ: 2,500.

617.6 USA ISSN 0272-9067
ARTICULATOR. Text in English. 1971. m. membership. adv. *Refereed.* **Document type:** *Newsletter.*
Published by: North Central Ohio Dental Society, 1604 E Perkins Ave, Ste 209, Sandusky, OH 44870. TEL 419-621-8830, FAX 419-621-8632. Ed., R&P Dr. David M Murphy. Circ: 108.

617.6 DEU ISSN 0720-972X
DER ARTIKULATOR; Zeitschrift fuer Kritische Zahnmedizin. Text in German. 1976. q. DEM 10 (effective 2000). **Document type:** *Journal, Academic/Scholarly.*
—GNLM.
Published by: Vereinigung Demokratische Zahnmedizin e.V., Adenauerallee 58, Bonn 53113, Germany.

617.6 HKG
ASIA - PACIFIC DENTAL NEWS. Text in Chinese, English, Korean. 1987. q. adv.
Published by: MediMedia Asia (Subsidiary of: MediMedia Pacific Ltd.), 2102 Tung Sun Commercial Centre, 194-200 Lockhart Rd, Wanchai, Hong Kong, Hong Kong. TEL 852-2559-5888, FAX 852-2559-6910, http://www.medimedia.com.hk/. Adv. contact Olive Mak. color page USD 7,685. Circ: 52,116.

617.6 SGP
ASIAN DENTIST; a publication for the Asia Pacific region. Text in English. 1993. bi-m. USD 210. adv. **Document type:** *Trade.* **Description:** Provides news and articles on the latest dental equipment and technology for the dental industry and professionals in the Asia-Pacific region.
Published by: First Asia Publishing Pte. Ltd., 6 New Industrial Rd 02-02-04, Singapore 536199, Singapore. TEL 65-858-0040, FAX 65-858-1141, jovankahauer@firstasia.com.sg. Pub. Tan Kay Hui. Adv. contact Louis Lee. B&W page USD 4,995, color page USD 5,895; trim 385 x 275. Circ: 31,100.

617.6 JPN ISSN 0915-6992
CODEN: AJMSFE
ASIAN JOURNAL OF ORAL AND MAXILLOFACIAL SURGERY. Text in English. 1989. s-a.
Published by: Asian Association of Oral and Maxillofacial Surgeons/Ajia Koku Gaku Ganmen Geka Gakkai, Tsurumi Daigaku Shigakubu, Koku Gekagaku Kyoshitsu, 1-3 Tsurumi 2-chome, Tsurumi-ku, Yokohama-shi, Kanagawa-ken 230-0063, Japan.

617.6 ARG ISSN 0004-4881
CODEN: RAOABM
ASOCIACION ODONTOLOGICA ARGENTINA. REVISTA. Text in Spanish. 1898. bi-m. USD 80 (effective 2001). adv. bk.rev. abstr, bibl, charts, illus. index. 112 p./no. *Refereed.* **Document type:** *Academic/Scholarly.*
Indexed: Dent.Ind.
—BLDSC (7804.425000), GNLM.
Published by: Asociacion Odontologica Argentina, Junin, 959, Capital Federal, Buenos Aires 1113, Argentina. TEL 54-114-9616141, FAX 54-114-9611110, aoa@aoa.org.ar, http://www.aoa.org.ar. Ed. Zulema Targovnik. Circ: 9,000.

617.6 FRA
ASSISTANCE ET LE PROTHESISTE DENTAIRES. Text in French. bi-m. adv.
Published by: Syndicat National des Assistantes et Prothesistes Dentaires, 21 rue Defresne Bast, Argenteuil 95100, France. Ed. M Hachmanian.

617.6 BRA ISSN 0004-5276
ASSOCIACAO PAULISTA DE CIRURGIOES DENTISTAS. REVISTA. Text in Portuguese. 1947. bi-m. USD 100 (effective 2002). adv. bk.rev. back issues avail. *Refereed.*
Related titles: Online - full text ed.: 1997.
Indexed: Dent.Ind., INIS Atomind.
—GNLM.
Published by: Associacao Paulista de Cirurgioes Dentistas/Sao Paulo State Dental Association, Praca Campos de Bagatelle, 100, Sao Paulo, SP 02012-000, Brazil. TEL 55-11-62213022, FAX 55-11-62213612, directoria@apcd.org.br, http://www.apcd.org.br/. Ed. Andrea Trajano de mello Ferreira. Circ: 155,000 (controlled).

617.6 617 USA ISSN 1061-3315
ATLAS OF THE ORAL AND MAXILLOFACIAL SURGERY CLINICS OF NORTH AMERICA. Text in English. 1993. s-a. USD 141 domestic; USD 177 foreign; USD 89 per issue (effective 2001). illus. back issues avail. **Document type:** *Journal, Academic/Scholarly.* **Description:** Contains detailed line drawings and photographs, along with articles on various aspects of a single type of surgery or a surgical problem.
—GNLM.

M

Published by: W.B. Saunders Co. (Subsidiary of: Harcourt Publishers Ltd.), 11830 Westline Industrial Dr, St Louis, MO 63146. TEL 800-325-4177, http://www.wbsaunders.com. Ed. Dr. Leon Assael. **Subscr. to:** Periodicals Fulfillment, W B Saunders Co, 6277 Sea Harbor Dr, 4th Fl, Orlando, FL 32891-4800.

AUSTRALIA. BUREAU OF STATISTICS. DENTAL SERVICES, AUSTRALIA. see *MEDICAL SCIENCES—Abstracting, Bibliographies, Statistics*

617.6 AUS ISSN 0810-7440
AUSTRALIAN DENTAL ASSOCIATION. NEWS BULLETIN. Text in English. 11/yr. AUD 88; AUD 130 foreign (effective 1999). adv. bk.rev. **Document type:** *Newsletter.*
Published by: Australian Dental Association Inc., 75 Lithgow St, St Leonards, NSW 2065, Australia. TEL 61-2-9906-4412, FAX 61-2-9906-4917, newsbull@ada.org.au, http://www.ada.org.au. Ed., R&P Dr. Robert Butler. Adv. contact Julie Green. B&W page USD 962, color page USD 1,954; trim 270 x 200. Circ: 8,300 (paid).

617.6 AUS ISSN 0045-0421
CODEN: ADEJA2
AUSTRALIAN DENTAL JOURNAL. Text in English. 1956. q. AUD 90 domestic; USD 120 foreign (effective 1999). adv. bk.rev. abstr, bibl, illus. index. back issues avail.; reprint service avail. from PQC. *Refereed.* **Document type:** *Academic/Scholarly.* **Description:** Contains research, clinical developments, opinions, treatments and other key issues of relevance to dentistry as practised in Australia.
Formed by the merger of (1947-1956): Queensland Dental Journal (1038-703X); (1929-1956): Dental Journal of Australia (0366-9270); (1905-1956): Australian Journal of Dentistry (0365-3595)
Related titles: Microfilm ed.: (from PQC); Online - full text ed.: (from Institute for Scientific Information).
Indexed: ASCA, Biol.Abstr., C.I.S. Abstr., Cal.Tiss.Abstr., Chem.Abstr., Curr.Adv.Cancer Res., Curr.Adv.Ecol.Sci., Curr.Cont., Curr.Tit.Dent., Dent.Abstr., Dent.Ind., Environ.Sci.Poll.Mgmt., Excerp.Med., INIS Atomind., Ind.Med. (1956-), Ind.Sci.Rev., Inpharma, Mat.Sci.Cit.Ind. (coverage dropped), Microbiol.Abstr., NRN, Pharm.&Out.News, Pollut.Abstr., Reac., Risk Abstr., Saf.Sci.Abstr., Sci.Cit.Ind. (coverage dropped), So.Pac.Per.Ind.
—BLDSC (1798.450000), CASDDS, CISTI, EMDOCS, GNLM, ingenta, KNAW.
Published by: Australian Dental Association Inc., PO Box 520, St Leonards, NSW 2065, Australia. TEL 61-2-9906-4412, FAX 61-2-9906-4917, adj@ada.org.au; accounts@ada.org.au. Ed. P M Bartold. R&P, Adv. contact Belinda Neill. B&W page AUD 1,010, color page AUD 1,945; trim 210 x 297. Circ: 8,200.

617.6 658 AUS ISSN 1320-2340
AUSTRALIAN DENTAL PRACTICE MAGAZINE. Text in English. 1980. bi-m. AUD 95. adv. bk.rev. back issues avail. **Document type:** *Trade.* **Description:** Covers news, practice management, tax, team building, issues affecting effective business management.
Formerly (until 1990): Dental Reporter (0727-7261)
Published by: Main Street Publishing Pty. Ltd., PO Box 1481, Sydney, NSW 2001, Australia. TEL 61-2-9438-5333, FAX 61-2-9438-2999, dentist@dentist.aust.com, http://www.dentist.aust.com. Ed. Peter O'Sullivan. Pub., R&P Joseph Allbeury. Circ: 3,000.

617.6 AUS ISSN 1329-1947
RK351
AUSTRALIAN ENDODONTIC JOURNAL. Text in English. 1967. 3/yr. AUD 99.75 domestic; AUD 140 foreign (effective 2000). adv. bk.rev. *Refereed.* **Document type:** *Bulletin, Academic/Scholarly.*
Formerly (until 1998): Australian Society of Endodontology. Newsletter (0313-7384)
Published by: Australian Society of Endodontology, 5th Fl 766 Elizabeth St, Melbourne, VIC 3000, Australia. TEL 61-3-9349-7600, FAX 61-3-9349-7602, parashos@conect.net.au. Ed., R&P Dr. Peter Parashos. Adv. contact Dr. Stephen Harlamb. Circ: 900 (paid and controlled).

617.6 AUS ISSN 0587-3908
AUSTRALIAN ORTHODONTIC JOURNAL. Text in English. 1967. 3/yr. AUD 112 to individuals; AUD 168 to institutions (effective 2000). adv. bk.rev. *Refereed.* **Document type:** *Academic/Scholarly.* **Description:** Includes scientific and clinical articles.
Indexed: Dent.Ind., NRN.
—GNLM, ingenta.

Published by: Australian Society of Orthodontists, PO Box 434, Toorak, VIC 3142, Australia. TEL 61-3-9826-8318, FAX 61-3-9804-7222, aoj@netcon.net.au. Ed. Dr. Brian W Lee. R&P Dee Sansom. Adv. contact Dr. Samar Amari. Circ: 750 (paid).

617.6 USA ISSN 0005-7258
BAYLOR DENTAL JOURNAL. Text in English. 1951. s-a. free per issue to qualified personnel. abstr, illus. **Document type:** *Academic/Scholarly.* **Description:** Alumni publication with dental features, college and alumni news.
Indexed: Dent.Ind.
—BLDSC (1871.240000).
Published by: Baylor College of Dentistry, Office of Institutional Advancement, 3302 Gaston Ave, Dallas, TX 75246. TEL 214-828-8214, FAX 214-828-8906, ccox@tambcd.edu. Ed. Carolyn Cox. Circ: 7,000 (controlled).

617.6 USA ISSN 1079-4476
BERGEN COUNTY DENTAL SOCIETY. NEWSLETTER. Abbreviated title: B C D S Newsletter. Text in English. 1920. m. USD 12 domestic; USD 18 foreign (effective 2001). adv. back issues avail. **Document type:** *Newsletter, Trade.* **Description:** Provides Bergen county dentists with social, societal, political, and legislative information; includes scientific sessions.
Formerly (until 1994): Bergen County Dental Society. Journal (0092-9832)
Indexed: Dent.Ind.
—GNLM.
Published by: Bergen County Dental Society, 1060 Main St, River Edge, NJ 07661. TEL 201-487-1073, FAX 201-487-2513. Ed. Thomas DiLauro. Adv. contact Liana Basceana TEL 201-666-2330. Circ: 700 (controlled).

BIBLIOGRAFIA BRASILEIRA DE ODONTOLOGIA. see *MEDICAL SCIENCES—Abstracting, Bibliographies, Statistics*

617.6 610 CAN ISSN 0882-1852
BIOLOGICAL THERAPIES IN DENTISTRY. Text in English. 1985. bi-m. USD 49 in US & Canada to individuals; USD 85 elsewhere to individuals; USD 85 in Scandinavia to institutions; USD 120 elsewhere to institutions (effective 2000). back issues avail. **Document type:** *Newsletter, Academic/Scholarly.* **Description:** Keeps the dental profession up-to-date with current developments in dental therapeutics.
—GNLM, Infotrieve. **CCC.**
Published by: B.C. Decker Inc., 20 Hughson St S, LCD 1, P O Box 620, Hamilton, ON L8N 3K7, Canada. TEL 905-522-7017, 800-568-7281, FAX 905-522-7839, info@bcdecker.com, http://www.bcdecker.com. Ed. Sebastian G Ciancio. Pub. David LeGallais. R&P Paula Presutti. Circ: 322.

617.6 DEU ISSN 1616-0177
▼ **BIOMATERIALEN;** Organ der Deutschen Gesellschaft fuer Biomaterialen. Text in German; Summaries in English. 2000. 4/yr. DEM 598.48, EUR 306 domestic; DEM 620, EUR 317 foreign (effective 2001). adv. *Refereed.* **Document type:** *Journal, Academic/Scholarly.* **Description:** Covers all aspects of dental implantation and surgical procedures and materials.
Published by: VNM Science Publishing GmbH & Co. KG (Subsidiary of: Verlag Neuer Merkur GmbH), Anton-Ditt-Bogen 23, Munich 80939, Germany. TEL 49-89-31890537, FAX 49-89-31890586, bio.redaktion@vnmonline.de, info@vnmonline.de, http://www.vnmscience.de/BIOmaterialien/index.html. Ed. Angelika Schaller. Pub. Burkhard Bierschenck. Adv. contact Elisabeth Hesse TEL 49-89-318905-25. B&W page DEM 1,700, color page DEM 2,975; trim 185 x 260.

617.6 DNK ISSN 0905-006X
RK55.C5
BOERNE- OG UNGDOMSTANDPLEJEN I DANMARK. Text in Danish. 1983. irreg. DKK 60.
Formerly: Boernetandplejen i Danmark (0108-6618)
Published by: Sundhedsstyrelsen, Amaliegade 13, PO Box 2020, Copenhagen K 1012, Denmark. **Subscr. to:** Statens Informationstjeneste, PO Box 1103, Copenhagen K 1009, Denmark.

617.6 BRA ISSN 0103-6440
BRAZILIAN DENTAL JOURNAL. Text in English. 1990. 3/yr., latest vol.12, 2001. free. adv. charts, illus. *Refereed.* **Document type:** *Journal, Academic/Scholarly.* **Description:** Examines all areas of dental research and case reports.
Related titles: Online - full text ed.
—BLDSC (2277.357000), GNLM.

Published by: Associacao Brasileira de Divulgacao Cientifica, Av. Bandeirantes 3900, Faculdade de Medicina de Ribeirao Preto, Campus de Ribeirao Preto, Ribeirao Preto, SP 14040904, Brazil. TEL 55-16-6333825, FAX 55-16-6333825, bjournal@fmrp.usp.br, wgmsom@universe.com.br, http://www.forp.usp.br/bdj/bdj.htm, http://www.epub.org.br/bjmbr; http://www.forp.usp.br/bdj/bdj.htm. Ed. Jesus Djalma Pecora. R&P Melissa A Marchesan. Adv. contact Sarah O Marchesan. Circ: 1,500.

617.643 FRA
BREF INFO. Text in French. 2/yr. **Document type:** *Corporate.*
Published by: Promo U.N., 80 rue de la Roquette, Paris 75011, France. TEL 33-1-49294619, FAX 33-1-49294626. Ed. Robert Frederic Dumont. Circ: 5,000.

617.6 GBR ISSN 0007-0610
CODEN: BDJOHJ
BRITISH DENTAL JOURNAL. Text in English. 1880. bi-m. GBP 175 in Europe to individuals outside the UK; USD 280 elsewhere to individuals outside the UK; GBP 193 combined subscription in Europe to individuals (print & online eds.) outside the UK; USD 309 combined subscription elsewhere to individuals (print & online eds.) outside the UK; GBP 367, GBP 374 in Europe to institutions; USD 598 elsewhere to institutions; GBP 404 combined subscription in Europe to institutions print & online eds.; GBP 411, USD 658 combined subscription elsewhere to institutions print & online eds. (effective 2001); Individual subscriptions are only avaliable outside the UK. adv. bk.rev. abstr, charts, illus. s-a. index. back issues avail.; reprints avail. *Refereed.* **Document type:** *Journal, Academic/Scholarly.* **Description:** Includes opinions, developments and key issues in clinical, practical and scientific dentistry, stimulating interest, debate and discussion amongst dentists of all disciplines.
Related titles: Microform ed.: (from PQC); Online - full text ed.: GBP 175 in Europe to individuals outside the UK; USD 280 elsewhere to institutions outside the UK; GBP 367 in Europe to institutions; USD 587 elsewhere to institutions (effective 2001) (from EBSCO Publishing, RoweCom Information Quest, Institute for Scientific Information).
Indexed: AIDS Abstr., ASCA, Abstr.Hyg., Alloys Ind. (1968-1982), Biol.Abstr., C.I.S. Abstr., Cal.Tiss.Abstr., Chem.Abstr., Curr.Adv.Cancer Res., Curr.Adv.Ecol.Sci., Curr.Cont., Curr.Tit.Dent., Dairy Sci.Abstr., Dent.Abstr., Dent.Ind., Environ.Sci.Poll.Mgmt., Food Sci.& Tech.Abstr., INIS Atomind., Ind.Med. (1903-), Ind.Sci.Rev., Inpharma, Met.Abstr. (1968-1982), Met.Abstr.Ind. (1968-1982), NRN, Nonfer.Met.Alert (1968-1982), Nutr.Abstr., PCC Alert (1968-1982), Pharm.&Out.News, Pollut.Abstr., Reac., Rev.Med.& Vet.Mycol., Risk Abstr., SSCI (coverage dropped), Saf.Sci.Abstr., Sci.Cit.Ind., Steels Alert (1968-1982), Sugar Ind.Abstr., Tox.Abstr. (coverage dropped), Trop.Dis.Bull., World Alum.Abstr.
—BLDSC (2299.000000), CISTI, GNLM, IDS, ingenta, KNAW. **CCC.**
Published by: (British Dental Association), Nature Publishing Group Specialist Journals (Subsidiary of: Holtzbrink Publishers), Houndmills, Basingstoke, Hants RG21 6XS, United Kingdom. TEL 44-1256-329242, FAX 44-1256-328339, bdj@bda-dentistry.org.uk, subscriptions@nature.com, http://www.bdj.co.uk; http://www.nature.com/bdj. Ed. Mike Grace. Pub. Sue Deeley. R&P Trace Noel. Adv. contact Joe Aspis TEL 44-20-7843-4785. Circ: 18,000.

BRITISH DENTAL NURSES' JOURNAL. see *MEDICAL SCIENCES—Surgery*

BRITISH JOURNAL OF ORAL AND MAXILLOFACIAL SURGERY. see *MEDICAL SCIENCES—Surgery*

617.6 GBR ISSN 0957-7173
BRITISH SOCIETY OF DENTAL AND MAXILLOFACIAL RADIOLOGY. PROCEEDINGS. Text in English. 1978. a. GBP 20. bk.rev.
Formerly (until 1986): British Society of Dental and Maxillofacial Radiology. Newsletter
—GNLM.
Published by: British Society of Dental and Maxillofacial Radiology, University of Dental School, Radiology Dept., Higher Cambridge St, Manchester, Lancs M15 6FH, United Kingdom. TEL 061-275-6690, FAX 061-275-6776. Circ: 200.

M

617.600711 USA ISSN 0007-4837
BULLETIN OF DENTAL EDUCATION. Text in English. 1959. m. USD 18 domestic to non-members; USD 24 foreign to non-members (effective 2000). adv. reprint service avail. from PQC. **Document type:** *Newsletter.* **Description:** Reports on innovations and opportunities in dental education, pertinent federal legislation and regulations, and individual and institutional members.
Indexed: Dent.Ind.
Published by: American Association of Dental Schools, 1625 Massachusetts Ave, N W, Washington, DC 20036-2212. TEL 202-667-9433. Ed. M Sue Sandmeyer. Circ: 3,800.

617.6 USA ISSN 1048-3594
C D A UPDATE. Text in English. 1989. m. USD 24 to non-members; USD 30 foreign to non-members. adv. back issues avail. **Document type:** *Newsletter.*
Published by: California Dental Association, PO Box 13749, Sacramento, CA 95853. TEL 916-443-3382, FAX 916-443-2943. Ed. Brian Blomster. Adv. contact Ingrid Landis. Circ: 20,000.

617.6 BRA ISSN 0104-4923
C E C A D E NEWS. (Centro de Estudios da Carie Dentaria) Text in Portuguese; Summaries in English, Portuguese. 1993. 3/yr. bibl, charts.
Published by: Universidade de Sao Paulo, Faculdade de Odontologia de Bauru, Al. Dr. O.P. Brizolla, 9-75, Bauru, SP 17043101, Brazil. TEL 55-142-234133 ext. 218, FAX 55-142-230415, TELEX 142314 FOBU. Ed. Dr. Maria Francesca T B Bijella.

617.6 FRA ISSN 0397-1643
CAHIERS DE PROTHESE. Text in French. 4/yr. FRF 995; FRF 298 newsstand/cover. adv.
Indexed: Ref.Zh.
—BLDSC (2952.113000), GNLM.
Published by: Editions C D P, 1 av. Edward Belin, Rueil Malmaison 92856, France. Eds. Eric Robbiani, Jean Schittly. Adv. contact Sybille Barbera. Circ: 6,500.

617.6 USA ISSN 0008-0977
CALIFORNIA DENTAL ASSOCIATION. JOURNAL. Text in English. 1918. m. USD 60 to non-members; USD 40 foreign to non-members (effective 1999). adv. bk.rev. charts, illus. **Document type:** *Academic/Scholarly.* **Description:** Provides dentists with scientific, technique-oriented and practice management information.
Incorporates (in 1973): Southern California Dental Association. Journal (0049-156X); Which was formerly (1934-1966): Southern California State Dental Association. Journal (0098-7115); S C D A Newsletter; Composite
Indexed: Curr.Tit.Dent., Dent.Abstr., Dent.Ind., INIS Atomind.
—CISTI, GNLM.
Published by: California Dental Association, PO Box 13749, Sacramento, CA 95853. TEL 916-443-3382, FAX 916-443-2943. Ed. Jack Conley. R&P Jeanne Marie Tokunaga. Adv. contact Ingrid Landis. B&W page USD 1,815, color page USD 2,640. Circ: 20,000.

617.6 CAN ISSN 1199-1666
CANADIAN DENTAL ASSISTANTS ASSOCIATION. JOURNAL. Text in English. 1956. 3/yr. CND 45 domestic; CND 60 foreign (effective 2001). adv. bk.rev. back issues avail. **Document type:** *Trade.* **Description:** Provides up-to-date information on national and provincial initiatives of the dental assisting profession in Canada.
Formerly: Canadian Dental Assistants Association (0833-8264)
Published by: Canadian Dental Assistants' Association, 1750 Courtwood Crescent, Ste 208, Ottawa, ON K2C 2B5, Canada. TEL 613-521-5495, 800-345-5137, FAX 613-521-5572, esaunders@cdaa.ca, http://www.cdaa.ca. Pub. Michael Brennan. Circ: 20,000.

617.6 CAN ISSN 0709-8936
CODEN: JCDAAS
CANADIAN DENTAL ASSOCIATION. JOURNAL/ ASSOCIATION DENTAIRE CANADIENNE. JOURNAL. Text in English, French. 1935. m. (except July-Aug. combined). CND 55 domestic; CND 80 in United States; CND 100 elsewhere (effective 2000). bk.rev. abstr, charts. index. *Refereed.* **Document type:** *Academic/Scholarly.* **Description:** Clinical and scientific articles directed toward general practitioners.
Former titles (until 1979): Dental Journal (0382-8514); Canadian Dental Association. Journal (0008-3372)
Indexed: Biol.Abstr., Chem.Abstr., Curr.Tit.Dent., Dent.Abstr., Dent.Ind., Dok.Arbeitsmed., Environ.Sci.Poll.Mgmt., INIS Atomind., Ind.Med. (1979-), NRN, Nutr.Abstr., Pollut.Abstr., Risk Abstr., Saf.Sci.Abstr.
—BLDSC (4723.010000), CISTI, GNLM, ingenta, KNAW. **CCC.**
Published by: Canadian Dental Association/Association Dentaire Canadienne, 1815 Alta Vista Dr, Ottawa, ON K1G 3Y6, Canada. TEL 613-523-1770, FAX 613-523-7736, reception@cda-adc.ca, http://www.cda-adc.ca. Ed. Dr. John P O'Keefe. Pub. George Weber. R&P Rachel Galipeau. Adv. contact Marg Churchill. Circ: 19,000.

617.6 CAN ISSN 0834-1494
CANADIAN DENTAL HYGIENISTS ASSOCIATION. PROBE. Text in English. 1967. bi-m. CND 69.55; CND 110 foreign. adv. bk.rev. charts, illus. *Refereed.* **Document type:** *Bulletin.* **Description:** Covers scientific, continuing education, reviews and internet information.
Formerly: Canadian Dental Hygienist (0008-3380)
Indexed: Dent.Ind.
—BLDSC (6617.275000), GNLM, Infotrieve. **CCC.**
Published by: Canadian Dental Hygienists Association, 96 Centrepointe Dr, Ottawa, ON K2G 6B1, Canada. TEL 613-224-5515, FAX 613-224-7283, info@cdha.ca, cdha@magi.com, http://www.cdha.ca. adv.: B&W page CND 825, color page CND 1,405; trim 11 x 8.5. Circ: 7,000. **Subscr. to:** Keith Health Care Communications, 1599 Hurontario St, Ste 104, Mississauga, ON L5G 4S1, Canada. TEL 905-278-6700, FAX 905-278-4850.

617.6 CHE ISSN 0008-6568
CODEN: CAREBK
CARIES RESEARCH. Text in English. 1967. bi-m. CHF 956 in Europe to institutions; CHF 973.40 overseas to institutions; EUR 682.80 in Europe to institutions; USD 744 overseas to institutions (effective 2002). adv. bibl, charts, illus. index. back issues avail.; reprint service avail. from ISI. *Refereed.* **Document type:** *Journal, Academic/Scholarly.* **Description:** Coverage of human and animal experimental work for the researcher; clinical trials of interest to the practicing dentist.
Related titles: Microform ed.; Online - full text ed.: ISSN 1421-976X. CHF 58, EUR 42, USD 45 to institutions (effective 2002) (from EBSCO Publishing, O C L C Online Computer Library Center, Inc., RoweCom Information Quest, ProQuest Information & Learning, Swets Blackwell, Institute for Scientific Information).
Indexed: ASCA, Apic.Abstr., Aqua.Sci.& Fish.Abstr., Biol.Abstr., CINAHL, Cal.Tiss.Abstr., Chem.Abstr., Chem.Indus.Notes, Chem.Titles, Curr.Adv.Ecol.Sci., Curr.Cont., Curr.Tit.Dent., Dairy Sci.Abstr., Dent.Abstr., Dent.Ind., Environ.Sci.Poll.Mgmt., Excerp.Med., Food Sci.& Tech.Abstr., INIS Atomind., Ind.Med. (1967-), Ind.Sci.Rev., Inpharma, NRN, Nutr.Abstr., Pharm.&Out.News, Reac., Rev.Med.& Vet.Mycol., Risk Abstr., Saf.Sci.Abstr., Sci.Cit.Ind., So.Pac.Per.Ind., Sugar Ind.Abstr., Tox.Abstr. (coverage dropped).
—BLDSC (3053.200000), CASDDS, CISTI, GNLM, IDS, ingenta, KNAW. **CCC.**
Published by: (European Organization for Caries Research), S. Karger AG, Allschwilerstr 10, PO Box, Basel 4009, Switzerland. TEL 41-61-306-1111, FAX 41-61-306-1234, karger@karger.ch, http://www.online.karger.com/journals/cre, http://www.karger.com. Ed. R P Shellis. adv.: page USD 1,185. Circ: 1,450.

617.6 USA
CASE WESTERN RESERVE UNIVERSITY. SCHOOL OF DENTISTRY. ALUMNI MAGAZINE. Text in English. 1985. s-a. free per issue. adv. bk.rev. illus. **Description:** Covers dental advancement and school status, university and alumni news.
Former titles: Case Western Reserve University. School of Dentistry. Dental Alumni News; Case Western Reserve University. School of Dentistry. Dental Alumni Newsletter; Case Western Reserve University. School of Dentistry. Dental Alumni News; Case Western Reserve University. School of Dentistry. Dental Alumni Bulletin (0043-4140); Western Reserve University Dental Alumni Bulletin
Published by: Case Western Reserve University, School of Dentistry, 2123 Abington Rd, Cleveland, OH 44106. TEL 216-368-3480, FAX 216-368-3204. Ed. Mary Wirtz Juhnke. Circ: 3,500.

617.6 CZE ISSN 1213-0613
CODEN: CKSTF8
CESKA STOMATOLOGIE A PRAKTICKE ZUBNI LEKARSTVI. Text in Czech, Slovak; Summaries in English, Russian. 1996. 6/yr. EUR 72, USD 84 (effective 2001). adv. bk.rev. abstr, charts, illus. index, cum.index. *Refereed.* **Document type:** *Journal, Academic/Scholarly.*
Formed by the merger of (1953-1996): Prakticke Zubni Lekarstvi (0032-6720); (1994-1996): Ceska Stomatologie (1210-7891); Which was formerly (1901-1994): Ceskoslovenska Stomatologie (0009-0654)
Indexed: Chem.Abstr., Dent.Abstr., Dent.Ind., INIS Atomind., Ind.Med. (coverage dropped), Nutr.Abstr., Protozool.Abstr.
—CISTI, GNLM. **CCC.**
Published by: (Ceska Lekarska Spolecnost J.E. Purkyne/Czech Medical Association), Nakladatelske Stredisko C L S J.E. Purkyne, Sokolska 31, Prague 12026, Czech Republic. TEL 42-2-24911420, FAX 42-2-24911420, nts@iol.cz, http://www.clsjep.cz, http://www.medical.cz. Ed. E Jirava. adv.: B&W page CZK 19,900, color page CZK 31,000; 190 x 126. Circ: 1,500. **Dist. by:** Abont s.r.o., Chlumova 17, Prague, 3 130 00, Czech Republic; **Dist. in Western countries by:** Kubon & Sagner, Hesstr 39-41, Munich 80798, Germany.

617.6 USA ISSN 0091-1666
CHICAGO DENTAL SOCIETY REVIEW. Text in English. 1920. m. (11/yr.). USD 25 to non-members; USD 17 to members; USD 30 to institutions; USD 45 foreign to institutions. adv. bk.rev. illus. reprint service avail. from PQC. **Document type:** *Trade.* **Description:** Covers a wide range of topics to assist practicing dentists including: clinical and scientific subjects; local, state and national news and meetings; news and programs of the Chicago Dental Society and its nine branches.
Formerly: Chicago Dental Society Fortnightly Review (0009-353X)
Related titles: Microform ed.: (from PQC).
Indexed: Dent.Abstr., Dent.Ind., INIS Atomind.
—BLDSC (3096.530000), CISTI, GNLM.
Published by: Chicago Dental Society, 401 N Michigan Ave, Ste 300, Chicago, IL 60611-4205. TEL 312-836-7300, FAX 312-836-7337. Ed. Dr. Roger H Scholle. R&P Elizabeth Giangrego. Adv. contact Todd Goldman. B&W page USD 880; trim 10.88 x 8.38. Circ: 8,000.

CHIKEN ISHIYAKU JOHO/INVESTIGATIONAL DRUG INFORMATION. MEDICAL AND DENTAL. see *PHARMACY AND PHARMACOLOGY*

617.6 USA ISSN 1462-6446
THE CHINESE JOURNAL OF DENTAL RESEARCH. Text in English. 1998. 4/yr. USD 68, GBP 60, EUR 78; USD 35, GBP 40, EUR 40 to students (effective 2002). **Document type:** *Journal, Academic/Scholarly.*
—BLDSC (3180.314000).
Published by: Quintessence Publishing Co., Inc., 551 Kimberly Dr, Carol Stream, IL 60188-1881. TEL 630-682-3223, FAX 630-682-3288, quintpub@aol.com, http://www.quintpub.com.

CHIRURGIA MAXILLOFACIALIS ET PLASTICA/ MAXILLOFACIAL AND PLASTIC SURGERY. see *MEDICAL SCIENCES—Surgery*

617.6 FRA ISSN 0009-4838
CHIRURGIEN-DENTISTE DE FRANCE. Text in French. 1976 (vol.46). w. FRF 880 domestic to non-members; FRF 440 domestic to members; FRF 1,440 foreign; FRF 42 newsstand/cover (effective 2002). adv. bk.rev. illus. s-a. index. **Document type:** *Academic/Scholarly, Trade.*
Indexed: Dent.Ind., Dok.Arbeitsmed.
—CISTI, GNLM, Infotrieve. **CCC.**
Published by: Confederation Nationale des Syndicats Dentaires, 22 av. de Villiers, Paris 75017, France. TEL 33-01-56792020, http://www.cnsd.fr. Ed. Claude Boucher. Circ: 21,000.

617.6 USA ISSN 0894-0975
CINCINNATI DENTAL SOCIETY BULLETIN. Text in English. 1930. m. USD 25. adv. **Document type:** *Trade.* **Description:** Contains information about dentistry on the local, state and national levels for member dentists.
Published by: Cincinnati Dental Society, 9200 Montgomery Rd, Ste 21A, Cincinnati, OH 45242. TEL 513-984-3443, FAX 513-984-3047. Ed. John B Bennett. Adv. contact Beverly G Fortner. Circ: 700.

617.6 ARG ISSN 0009-7357
CIRCULO ODONTOLOGICO DE ROSARIO. REVISTA. Text in Spanish; Summaries in English. 1929. q. per issue exchange basis. adv. bk.rev. bibl, illus.
Related titles: Microfiche ed.
Indexed: Dent.Ind.
Published by: Circulo Odontologico de Rosario, Rioja 2471, Rosario, Argentina. Ed. Dr. Natalio Grynberg. Circ: 1,000.

CLEFT PALATE - CRANIOFACIAL JOURNAL; Official Publication of the American Cleft Palate-Craniofacial Association. see *MEDICAL SCIENCES—Surgery*

M

617.6 FRA
CLINIC. Text in French. 1980. 10/yr. FRF 940; FRF 140 newsstand/cover. adv. Supplement avail.
Former titles: Clinic - Odontologia (0998-3392); (until 1988): Odontologia (0244-9331)
Indexed: Ref.Zh.
—GNLM.
Published by: Editions C D P, 1 av. Edward Belin, Rueil Malmaison 92856, France. Ed. Anne Boulanger. Adv. contact Sybille Barbera. Circ: 11,000.

617.6 USA
CLINICAL CONTOURS. Text in English. q. **Document type:** *Magazine, Trade.* **Description:** Serves as an instructional source for the latest innovative products and the most effective application techniques.
Published by: Montage Media Corp., 1000 Wyckoff Ave, Mahwah, NJ 07430. TEL 201-891-3200, FAX 201-891-2626, info@montagemedia.com, http://www.montagemedia.com/bras.html.

617.6 GBR ISSN 0961-253X
CLINICAL DENTISTRY IN HEALTH AND DISEASE. Text in English. 1988. irreg., latest vol.3. **Document type:** *Monographic series, Academic/Scholarly.*
Published by: Butterworth - Heinemann (Subsidiary of: Reed Elsevier Group), Linacre House, Jordan Hill, Oxford OX2 8DP, United Kingdom. TEL 44-1865-310366, 44-1865-888180, FAX 44-1865-310898, 44-1865-314091.

617.6 CAN ISSN 1523-0899
▼ **CLINICAL IMPLANT DENTISTRY AND RELATED RESEARCH.** Text in English. 1999. q. USD 100 domestic to individuals; USD 119 foreign to individuals; USD 125 domestic to institutions; USD 149 foreign to institutions (effective 2000). *Refereed.* **Document type:** *Journal, Academic/Scholarly.*
—BLDSC (3286.293825).
Published by: B.C. Decker Inc., 20 Hughson St S, LCD 1, P O Box 620, Hamilton, ON L8N 3K7, Canada. TEL 905-522-7017, FAX 905-522-7839, info@bcdecker.com, http://www.bcdecker.com. Pub. David LeGallais. R&P Paula Presutti. Circ: 420 (paid); 4,580 (controlled).

617.6 DNK ISSN 0905-7161
CLINICAL ORAL IMPLANTS RESEARCH. Text in English. 1990. bi-m. USD 384 in the Americas to institutions print & online eds. combined; GBP 267 Sat. elsewhere to institutions print & online eds. combined (effective 2002). adv. illus. reprints avail. *Refereed.* **Document type:** *Academic/Scholarly.*
Related titles: Online - full text ed.: DKK 2,250 (2001) (from Ovid Technologies, Inc., EBSCO Publishing, ingenta, Munksgaard & Blackwell Science's Synergy, Swets Blackwell, Institute for Scientific Information).
Indexed: ASCA, Curr.Cont., Inpharma, Mat.Sci.Cit.Ind. (coverage dropped), Reac., Sci.Cit.Ind.
—BLDSC (3286.318000), CISTI, GNLM, IDS, Infotrieve, ingenta. **CCC.**
Published by: (European Association for Osseointegration), Blackwell Munksgaard, Noerre Soegade 35, PO Box 2148, Copenhagen K 1016, Denmark. TEL 45-77-33-33-33, FAX 45-77-33-33-77, customerservice@munksgaard.dk, http://www.munksgaard.dk. Ed. Niklaus P Lang. Circ: 1,700.

617.522 DEU ISSN 1432-6981
CLINICAL ORAL INVESTIGATIONS. Text in English. 1997. q. EUR 194 domestic; EUR 190.40 in Germany; EUR 54 newsstand/cover foreign (effective 2002). *Refereed.* **Document type:** *Journal, Academic/Scholarly.* **Description:** Publishes original scientific articles and invited reviews, providing up-to-date results of basic and clinical studies in oral maxillofacial science and medicine clarifying them for a modern practice.
Related titles: Online - full text ed.: ISSN 1436-3771 (from EBSCO Publishing, RoweCom Information Quest, Swets Blackwell, Springer LINK).
—BLDSC (3286.318500), GNLM.
Published by: (German Society for Oral and Maxillofacial Medicine), Springer-Verlag (Subsidiary of: BertelsmannSpringer), Tiergartenstr 17, Heidelberg 69121, Germany. TEL 49-6221-345-0, FAX 49-6221-345229, subscriptions@springer.de, http://link.springer.de/link/service/journals/00784/index.htm, http://www.springer.de. Ed. G Schmalz. **Subscr. in N. America to:** Springer-Verlag New York Inc., PO Box 2485, Secaucus, NJ 07096-2485. TEL 212-460-1500, FAX 212-473-6272.

617.643 DNK ISSN 1397-5927
CLINICAL ORTHODONTICS AND RESEARCH. Text in Danish. 1998. q. USD 204 in the Americas to institutions print & online eds. combined; GBP 142 elsewhere to institutions print & online eds. combined (effective 2002). **Document type:** *Journal, Academic/Scholarly.*
Related titles: ♦ Online - full text ed.: Clinical Orthodontics and Research Online.
—BLDSC (3286.318700).
Published by: Blackwell Munksgaard, Noerre Soegade 35, PO Box 2148, Copenhagen K 1016, Denmark. TEL 45-77-33-33-33, FAX 45-77-33-33-77, customerservice@munksgaard.dk, http://www.munksgaard.dk.

617.643 DNK
CLINICAL ORTHODONTICS AND RESEARCH ONLINE. Text in English. q. DKK 765 to individuals; DKK 1,395 to institutions (effective 2001). **Document type:** *Academic/Scholarly.*
Media: Online - full text (from EBSCO Publishing, ingenta, Swets Blackwell). **Related titles:** ♦ Print ed.: Clinical Orthodontics and Research. ISSN 1397-5927.
Published by: Blackwell Munksgaard, Noerre Soegade 35, PO Box 2148, Copenhagen K 1016, Denmark. TEL 45-77-33-33-33, FAX 45-77-33-33-77, customerservice@munksgaard.dk, http://www.ingenta.com/journals/browse/mksg/cor, http://www.munksgaard.dk.

617.6 SGP
▼ **CLINICAL PROSTHODONTICS AND IMPLANT DENTISTRY.** Text in English. 1999. s-a. USD 200 (effective 1999). **Document type:** *Academic/Scholarly.*
Published by: Springer-Verlag Singapore (Subsidiary of: BertelsmannSpringer), No. 04-01, Cencon I, One Tannery Rd, Singapore 347719, Singapore. TEL 65-84-20-112, FAX 65-84-20-107, springer@cyberway.com.sg, http://www.springer.com.sg.

617.6 USA ISSN 0010-1559
COLORADO DENTAL ASSOCIATION. JOURNAL. Text in English. 1922. q. USD 35 in North America to individuals; USD 30 in North America to libraries; USD 40 elsewhere to libraries. adv. bk.rev. *Refereed.* **Document type:** *Academic/Scholarly.*
Indexed: Dent.Abstr., Dent.Ind., INIS Atomind.
—BLDSC (4730.800000), GNLM, ingenta.
Published by: Colorado Dental Association, 3690 S Yosemite, Ste 100, Denver, CO 80237-1808. TEL 303-740-6900, FAX 303-740-7989. Ed. Michael Iacoboni. R&P, Adv. contact Pam Vossen. Circ: 3,000 (paid).

617.6 USA
COMMUNICATOR (JOHNSTOWN). Text in English. 1971. q.
Published by: American Academy of Dental Practice Administration, First United Federal Bldg, 227 Franklyn St, Ste 220, Johnstown, PA 15901. Ed. W F Hrin. Circ: 1,100.

617.6 USA
COMMUNIQUE (IOWA CITY). Text in English. q. reprint service avail. from PQC.
Published by: American Association of Public Health, c/o Marsha Cunningham, Ed, College of Dentistry, University of Iowa, Iowa City, IA 52242.

617.6 GBR ISSN 0265-539X
CODEN: CDHEES
COMMUNITY DENTAL HEALTH. Text in English. 1984. q. GBP 88 in Europe to non-members; GBP 95 elsewhere to non-members; GBP 70 in Europe to FDI members; GBP 76 elsewhere to FDI members (effective 2000). adv. bk.rev. abstr. **Document type:** *Academic/Scholarly.* **Description:** Contains papers, articles, abstracts, and news on all aspects of community and public health dentistry.
Related titles: Online - full text ed.: (from Institute for Scientific Information).
Indexed: Curr.Adv.Ecol.Sci., Curr.Cont., Curr.Tit.Dent., Hosp.Abstr., Ind.Med. (1984-).
—BLDSC (3363.608900), GNLM.
Published by: (British Association for the Study of Community Dentistry), F D I World Dental Press Ltd., 7 Carlisle St, London W1V 5RG, United Kingdom. TEL 44-2079-357852, FAX 44-2074-860183. Ed. M C Downer. Circ: 1,200.

617.6 DNK ISSN 0301-5661
CODEN: CDOEAP
COMMUNITY DENTISTRY AND ORAL EPIDEMIOLOGY. Text in English. 1973. bi-m. USD 312 in the Americas to institutions print & online eds. combined; GBP 217 elsewhere to institutions print & online eds. combined (effective 2002). adv. bk.rev. illus. reprint service avail. from SWZ,ISI. *Refereed.* **Document type:** *Journal, Academic/Scholarly.*
Related titles: Microform ed.: (from SWZ); ♦ Online - full text ed.: Community Dentistry and Oral Epidemiology Online.
Indexed: ASCA, Biol.Abstr., Curr.Cont., Curr.Tit.Dent., Dent.Abstr., Dent.Ind., Dok.Arbeitsmed., Environ.Sci.Poll.Mgmt., Excerp.Med., Hosp.Abstr., Ind.Med. (1973-), Ind.Sci.Rev., Inpharma, Int.Abstr.Biol.Sci., NRN, Nutr.Abstr., Pollut.Abstr., Reac., Risk Abstr., SSCI (coverage dropped), Saf.Sci.Abstr., Sci.Cit.Ind.
—BLDSC (3363.609000), CISTI, GNLM, IDS, ingenta, KNAW. **CCC.**
Published by: Blackwell Munksgaard, Noerre Soegade 35, PO Box 2148, Copenhagen K 1016, Denmark. TEL 45-77-33-33-33, FAX 45-77-33-33-77, customerservice@munksgaard.dk, http://www.munksgaard.dk. Ed. Brian A Burt. Circ: 900.

617.643 DNK
COMMUNITY DENTISTRY AND ORAL EPIDEMIOLOGY ONLINE. Text in English. bi-m. DKK 2,070 (effective 2001). **Document type:** *Academic/Scholarly.*
Media: Online - full text (from Swets Blackwell, Institute for Scientific Information). **Related titles:** Microform ed.: (from SWZ); ♦ Print ed.: Community Dentistry and Oral Epidemiology. ISSN 0301-5661.
Published by: Blackwell Munksgaard, Noerre Soegade 35, PO Box 2148, Copenhagen K 1016, Denmark. TEL 45-77-33-33-33, FAX 45-77-33-33-77, fsub@mail.munksgaard.dk, http://www.ingenta.com/journals/browse/mksg/com, http://www.munksgaard.dk.

617.6 USA ISSN 0894-1009
THE COMPENDIUM OF CONTINUING EDUCATION IN DENTISTRY. Variant title: Compendium. Text in English. 1980. m. USD 112 domestic; USD 142 in Canada; USD 153 elsewhere (effective 2001). adv. bk.rev. back issues avail. *Refereed.* **Document type:** *Journal, Academic/Scholarly, Trade.* **Description:** Published for generalists and specialists in private practice who wish to expand their knowledge in a variety of dental specialties.
Former titles (until 1986): Compendium of Continuing Education in Dentistry (0734-0338); (until 1980): Compendium on Continuing Education in General Dentistry (0196-1756)
Indexed: Curr.Tit.Dent., Dent.Abstr., Dent.Ind.
—BLDSC (3363.958000), GNLM.
Published by: (School of Dental Medicine, University of Pennsylvania), Dental Learning Systems Co., Inc. (Subsidiary of: Medical World Communications), 241 Forsgate Dr, Jamesburg, NJ 08831. TEL 732-656-1143, FAX 732-656-1148, http://www.dentallearning.com. Ed. Walter D Cohen. Pub. Daniel Perkins. R&P Allison Walker TEL 732-656-1143. Adv. contact Jeff Gordon TEL 732-656-1143. B&W page USD 6,719, color page USD 8,419; trim 7 x 10. Circ: 120,000. **Co-sponsor:** University of Southern California, Los Angeles.

617.6 USA ISSN 0010-6232
CONNECTICUT STATE DENTAL ASSOCIATION. JOURNAL. Text in English. 1925. a. USD 15 to non-members (effective 1999). adv. bk.rev. charts, illus. back issues avail. **Document type:** *Monographic series, Academic/Scholarly.*
Indexed: Dent.Abstr., Dent.Ind., INIS Atomind.
—CISTI, GNLM.
Published by: Connecticut State Dental Association, 62 Russ St, Hartford, CT 06106. TEL 860-659-2623, FAX 860-244-8287, public@ct2nai.net, http://www.csda.com. Ed. Howard I Mark. R&P, Adv. contact Christine Graichen. Circ: 2,700 (controlled).

617.6 ESP ISSN 1136-4319
CONSEJO GENERAL DE ONDOTOLOGOS Y ESTOMATOLOGOS. REVISTA. Short title: R C O E. Text in Spanish. 1954. bi-m. ESP 11,700, USD 134; free to qualified personnel. adv. bk.rev. bibl. illus. **Description:** Contains original articles, review articles, clinical articles, and an activities calendar.
Supersedes in part (in 1996): Actualidad Odonto Estomatologica Espanola (1136-4386); Which was formerly (until 1994): Revista de Actualidad Estomatologica Espanola (1130-0094); (until 1990): Revista de Actualidades de Estomatologica Espanola (0212-9701); (until 1983): Boletin de Informacion Dental (0006-6311)
Indexed: Dent.Ind., Ind.Med.Esp.
—BLDSC, GNLM.

M

Published by: (Consejo General de Colegios de Odontologos y Estomatologos de Espana), Editorial Siglo S.L., Comunidad Castillo, La Mancha 3, Las Rozas 28230, Spain. TEL 34-91-6360553, FAX 34-91-6406329, siglo@pulso.com. Ed. Alberto Sicilia. Circ: 18,000.

617.6 USA ISSN 0010-7301
RK97
CONTACT POINT. Text in English. 1924. q. free per issue. adv. illus.
Indexed: Chem.Abstr., Dent.Ind.
—GNLM.
Published by: University of the Pacific, School of Dentistry, 2155 Webster St, San Francisco, CA 94115. TEL 415-929-6400. Ed. David W Chambers. Circ: 6,700.

617.6 USA ISSN 1523-2581
CONTEMPORARY ESTHETICS AND RESTORATIVE PRACTICE. Text in English. 1997. 12/yr. CND 106, FKP 175 (effective 2001). adv. back issues avail. **Document type:** *Magazine, Trade.* **Description:** Informs dentists about the latest procedures in esthetic and restorative dentistry through step-by-step clinical technique articles, related features on practice management, and a comprehensive resource guide that lists sources for the various materials needed to complete these procedures.
Published by: (University of Pennsylvania), Dental Learning Systems Co., Inc. (Subsidiary of: Medical World Communications), 241 Forsgate Dr, Jamesburg, NJ 08831. TEL 732-656-1143, FAX 732-656-1148, http://www.dentallearning.com/contemporary. Pub. Daniel Perkins. R&P Allison Walker TEL 732-656-1143. Adv. contact Anthony Angelini. page USD 9,774; trim 10.875 x 14.125. Circ: 105,000.

617.6 USA
▼ **CONTEMPORARY ORAL HYGIENE.** Text in English. 2001 (Aug.). bi-m. (3 issues published in 2001). **Document type:** *Journal, Trade.*
Published by: Medical World Communications, 241 Forsgate Dr, Jamesburg, NJ 08831. TEL 732-656-1140, FAX 732-656-1323, http://www.mwc.com/. Circ: 65,000.

617.6 ARG ISSN 0069-9799
COOPERADOR DENTAL* . Text in Spanish. 1933. irreg. membership. adv. bk.rev.
Published by: Cooperativa Dental Argentina, Marcelo T. De Alvear, 2167, Capital Federal, Buenos Aires 1122, Argentina. Eds. H B Ferreri, Horacio Martinez. Circ: 6,000.

COSMETIC SURGERY TIMES; a magazine for the innovative cosmetic surgery practice. see *MEDICAL SCIENCES—Surgery*

617.6 USA ISSN 1045-4411
CODEN: CROMEF
CRITICAL REVIEWS IN ORAL BIOLOGY AND MEDICINE. Text in English. 1989. q. USD 109 worldwide to individuals; USD 235 worldwide to institutions (effective 2001). adv. back issues avail. *Refereed.* **Document type:** *Academic/Scholarly.* **Description:** Analyzes the field of oral biology and medicine in the form of review articles of interest to a broad base of scientists engaged in dental research.
Related titles: Online - full text ed.: (from Institute for Scientific Information).
Indexed: ASCA, Chem.Abstr., Chem.Indus.Notes, Chem.Titles, Curr.Cont., Excerp.Med., Ind.Med. (1990-), Inpharma, Int.Abstr.Biol.Sci., Pharm.&Out.News, Reac., Sci.Cit.Ind.
—BLDSC (3487.479500), CASDDS, EMDOCS, GNLM, IDS, Infotrieve, KNAW. **CCC.**
Published by: (American Association of Oral Biologists), American Association for Dental Research, 1619 Duke St, Alexandria, VA 22314-3406. TEL 703-548-0066, FAX 703-548-1883, research@iadr.com, http://www.iadr.com, http://www.dentalresearch.com. Ed. Olav F Alvares. **Co-sponsor:** International and American Associations for Dental Research.

617.6 GBR ISSN 1065-626X
CURRENT OPINION IN PERIODONTOLOGY. Text in English. 1991. a. GBP 109.95, USD 175.95 (effective 1996). bibl, illus. *Refereed.* **Document type:** *Academic/Scholarly.* **Description:** Directed toward dentists in clinical and office environments. Presents comprehensive review articles, reporting on new developments in this specialty. Each article contains annotated references and a reference to the current literature available on the subject.
Incorporates (1991-1995): Current Opinion in Orthodontics and Pedodontics; Supersedes in part (in 1993): Current Opinion in Dentistry (1046-0764)
Related titles: CD-ROM ed.; Online - full text ed.
Indexed: ASCA, Environ.Sci.Poll.Mgmt., Risk Abstr.
—GNLM, IDS.
Published by: Rapid Science Publishers, 2-6 Boundary Row, London SE1 8HN, United Kingdom. TEL 44-207-865-0198, FAX 44-207-410-6600, rapid@rapidcom.co.uk; info@hugo.curbio.com, http://BioMedNet.com/cgi-bin/members1/titles.pl. Circ: 2,400.

617.6 USA
D L A N Y NEWSLETTER. Text in English. 1989. 11/yr. USD 15 (effective 2001). **Document type:** *Newsletter, Trade.* **Description:** Designed for owners and operators of commercial dental laboratories and dentists with a general practice including prosthetics.
Published by: Dental Lab Association of the State of New York, One Barstow Rd, Ste P-20, Great Neck, NY 11021. TEL 516-829-1144, FAX 516-829-1988, dlany@aol.com. Ed. Teresa M Sager. Pub. Mark J Polevoy. Circ: 1,500 (paid).

617.6 USA
D.L.A.N.Y. NEWSLETTER. Text in English. 1939. 11/yr. USD 15 domestic; USD 30 foreign (effective 2000). adv. bk.rev. illus, stat. **Document type:** *Newsletter.* **Description:** Contains technical and management articles of interest to dental laboratory owners and technicians.
Formerly (until 1989): Dental Laboratory News (0011-8664)
Published by: Dental Laboratory Association of State of New York, 1 Barstow Rd, Ste P 20, Great Neck, NY 11021. TEL 516-829-1144, FAX 516-829-1988, dlany@aol.com. Ed., R&P, Adv. contact Teresa M Sager. Circ: 3,000 (paid and controlled).

617.6 CAN ISSN 0418-3010
DALHOUSIE DENTAL JOURNAL. Text in English. 1961. a. free per issue. adv. back issues avail.
Published by: Dalhousie Dental Students Society, Dalhousie University, Halifax, NS B3H 4H8, Canada. TEL 902-424-2211. Circ: 1,000.

617.6 RUS
DANTIST. Text in Russian. 1994. m. free. **Document type:** *Newspaper.*
Related titles: Online - full text ed.
Published by: OOO Nordmed, Ul. Tverskaya 12/15, Sankt-Peterburg 193124, Russian Federation. TEL 7-812-2754197, FAX 7-812-1100206, dantist@stom.ru, http://www.stom.ru/dentist/. Circ: 7,000.

617.6 DNK
DENS. Text in Danish. 1910. m. adv.
Published by: Tandteknikenen Foereningen, Upsalagade 20 B, Copenhagen Oe 2100, Denmark. FAX 009-45-35432104. Circ: 800.

617.6 FRA
DENTAIRE - HEBDO. Text in French. 42/yr.
Published by: Union des Jeunes Chirurgiens-Dentistes, 14 rue Etex, Paris 75018, France. TEL 46-27-45-39. Ed. Gilles Drain. Circ: 10,000.

617.6 USA
DENTAL ADMISSION TESTING PROGRAM. Text in English. 1951. a. free per issue. **Document type:** *Academic/Scholarly.*
Published by: American Dental Association, 211 E Chicago Ave, Chicago, IL 60611. TEL 312-440-2500, FAX 312-440-3538. Ed. Dr. Gene A Kramer. Circ: 110,000.

617.6 USA ISSN 0733-9836
DENTAL ASEPSIS REVIEW. Text in English. 1980. m. USD 10 domestic; USD 13 foreign (effective 2001). adv. bk.rev. index. back issues avail. **Document type:** *Monographic series.*
Indexed: CINAHL.
Published by: Indiana University School of Dentistry, Department of Oral Microbiology, 1121 W Michigan St, Indianapolis, IN 46202. TEL 317-274-5427, FAX 317-274-5425, cpalenik@iupui.edu. Ed. Charles J Palenik. Adv. contact Charles John Palenik. Circ: 1,450.

617.6 USA ISSN 1088-3886
CODEN: DEASEJ
THE DENTAL ASSISTANT. Text in English. 1931. bi-m. USD 20 domestic to non-members; USD 25 foreign to non-members (effective 2001). adv. bk.rev. abstr, illus. back issues avail. *Refereed.* **Document type:** *Journal, Trade.* **Description:** Emphasizes dental assistant education in all phases of dentistry. Contains technical and theoretical articles, current technical advances, national organization news, coming events, and information regarding the current status of education in the dental assisting field.
Former titles (until 1993): The Dental Assistant Journal (1072-754X); (until 1992): The Dental Assistant (0011-8508)
Indexed: AgeLine, Curr.Tit.Dent., Dent.Abstr., Dent.Ind., INIS Atomind., Oral Res.Abstr.
—BLDSC (3553.255000), GNLM.
Published by: American Dental Assistants Association, 203 N La Salle St, Ste 1320, Chicago, IL 60601-1225. TEL 312-541-1550, FAX 312-541-1496, AADA1@aol.com, http://dentalassistant.org. Ed., R&P Douglas McDonough. Adv. contact Robert Palmer. Circ: 15,500 (paid).

617.6 THA ISSN 0045-9917
DENTAL ASSOCIATION OF THAILAND. JOURNAL. Text in Thai. 1949. bi-m. USD 180 (effective 2001). illus, abstr. reprint service avail. from IRC. *Refereed.* **Document type:** *Academic/Scholarly.* **Description:** Reports research in dentistry.
Indexed: Dent.Ind.
—BLDSC (4732.750000), GNLM.
Published by: Dental Association of Thailand, 71 Ladprao 95, Wangtonglang, Bangkok 10310, Thailand. TEL 66-2-539-748, FAX 66-2-514-1100. Ed. Paisan Kangvonkit. Adv. contact Poranee Berananda.

617.6 GBR ISSN 1360-5941
DENTAL BUSINESS. Text in English. 1996. s-a. GBP 38, USD 63 to institutions. **Document type:** *Trade.*
Indexed: Cal.Tiss.Abstr., Environ.Sci.Poll.Mgmt., Pollut.Abstr., Risk Abstr., Saf.Sci.Abstr.
—KNAW. **CCC.**
Published by: Nature Publishing Group Specialist Journals (Subsidiary of: Holtzbrink Publishers), Houndmills, Basingstoke, Hants RG21 6XS, United Kingdom. TEL 44-1256-329242, FAX 44-1256-328339, k.remmington@stockton-press.co.uk, subscriptions@nature.com, http://www.stockton-press.co.uk, http://www.nature.com.

617.6 ITA ISSN 0011-8524
DENTAL CADMOS; rivista quindicinale di odontoiatria e tecnica dentaria. Text in Italian. 1933. 20/yr. ITL 190,000 (effective 1999). bk.rev. index. **Document type:** *Academic/Scholarly.*
Indexed: Dent.Ind., Ind.Med. (coverage dropped).
—BLDSC (3553.260000), GNLM.
Published by: Masson S.p.A., Divisione Periodici, Via F.lli Bressan 2, Milan, MI 20126, Italy. TEL 39-2-270741, FAX 39-2-27074210. Ed. Carlo Guastamacchia. adv.: B&W page ITL 2,960,000, color page ITL 4,300,000; trim 265 x 193. Circ: 19,000.

617.6 USA ISSN 0011-8532
RK1 CODEN: DCNAAC
DENTAL CLINICS OF NORTH AMERICA. Variant title: Dental Clinics. Text in English. 1956. q. USD 127 domestic to individuals; USD 150 in Canada to individuals; USD 171 elsewhere to individuals; USD 176 domestic to institutions; USD 220 foreign to institutions; USD 56 per issue (effective 2001). illus. index, cum.index every 3 yr. reprint service avail. from PQC,ISI. **Document type:** *Journal, Academic/Scholarly.* **Description:** Delivers practical advice from experts in specialty covered as well as information on new developments in a variety of specialties with a fresh perspective on problems and controversies.
Related titles: Microform ed.: (from MIM,PQC); ♦ Spanish Translation: Clinicas Odontologicas de Norteamerica.
Indexed: AgeLine, CINAHL, Curr.Cont. (coverage dropped), Dent.Ind., Excerp.Med., INIS Atomind., Ind.Med. (1957-), Nutr.Abstr.
—BLDSC (3553.290000), CASDDS, CISTI, GNLM, ingenta. **CCC.**
Published by: W.B. Saunders Co. (Subsidiary of: Harcourt Publishers Ltd.), 11830 Westline Industrial Dr, St Louis, MO 63146. TEL 800-325-4177, http://www.wbsaunders.com. **Subscr. to:** Periodicals Fulfillment, W B Saunders Co, 6277 Sea Harbor Dr, 4th Fl, Orlando, FL 32891-4800.

DENTAL COMPUTER NEWSLETTER. see *MEDICAL SCIENCES—Computer Applications*

M

617.6 IND ISSN 0970-4167
DENTAL DIALOGUE. Text in English. 1974. q. USD 5.
Indexed: Dent.Ind.
—GNLM.
Address: Government Dental College & Hospital, Nagpur, Maharashtra 440 003, India. Ed. Dr. V K Hazarey. Circ: 1,500.

617.6 330 ESP ISSN 1135-4534
DENTAL ECONOMICS; revista de la gestion de la clinica dental. Text in Spanish. 1995. bi-m. USD 125. **Document type:** *Academic/Scholarly.*
Related titles: Online - full text ed.: (from Northern Light Technology, Inc.).
Published by: Ediciones Doyma S.A., Traversa de Gracia, 17-21, Barcelona 08021, Spain. TEL 34-93-200-0711, FAX 34-93-209-1136. Ed. J Geli I Burgues. adv.: page ESP 195,000. Circ: 3,000.

617.6 USA ISSN 0011-8583
RK1
DENTAL ECONOMICS. Text in English. 1911. m. USD 82 domestic; USD 105 foreign; USD 9 newsstand/cover (effective 2001). adv. illus. index. back issues avail.; reprints avail. **Document type:** *Trade.* **Description:** Helps dentists combine their clinical skills and product knowledge with sound management decisions. Includes articles on marketing, financial and investment information.
Formerly: Oral Hygiene
Related titles: Online - full text ed.: (from ProQuest Information & Learning, Northern Light Technology, Inc., Factiva); Supplement: Dental Graduate.
Indexed: Account.Ind. (1987-), Dent.Abstr., Dent.Ind.
—BLDSC (3553.321000), GNLM, ingenta. **CCC.**
Published by: PennWell Publishing Co., Dental Economics Division, PO Box 3408, Tulsa, OK 74101. joeb@pennwell.com, http://www.dentaleconomics.com, http://www.pennwell.com. Ed., R&P Dr. Joe Blaes TEL 314-434-6808. Pub. Lyle Hoyt. Adv. contact Margaret Pagel. B&W page USD 6,797, color page USD 8,387. Circ: 100,000 (controlled).

617.6 CAN ISSN 0070-3656
DENTAL GUIDE (DON MILLS). Text in English. 1965. a. CND 15 domestic; USD 15 foreign (effective 1999). adv.
Published by: Southam Magazine Group, 1450 Don Mills Rd, Don Mills, ON M3B 2X7, Canada. TEL 416-445-6641, FAX 416-442-2261. Circ: 13,663.

DENTAL GUIDE (SCARBOROUGH); the CE planner for the dental profession. see *MEETINGS AND CONGRESSES*

617.6 GBR ISSN 0011-8605
DENTAL HEALTH. Text in English. 1962. bi-m. GBP 50 domestic; GBP 59 foreign (effective 2000). adv. bk.rev. charts, illus. index. reprint service avail. from PQC. *Refereed.* **Document type:** *Academic/Scholarly, Abstract/Index.*
Related titles: Microform ed.: (from PQC).
Indexed: Biol.Abstr., Dent.Ind., NRN.
—BLDSC (3553.325000), GNLM.
Published by: British Dental Hygienists' Association, 21 Cross Common Rd, Dinas Powis, S Glam CF64 4TP, United Kingdom. TEL 44-1222-514822, FAX 44-1222-514822, lewismao@cardiff.ac.uk. Ed., R&P Heather Lewis. Adv. contact Freda Rimini. B&W page GBP 307; trim 298 x 210. Circ: 2,500 (controlled).

617.6 GBR ISSN 0958-6687
DENTAL HISTORIAN. Text in English. s-a. GBP 12. **Document type:** *Academic/Scholarly.*
—GNLM.
Published by: Lindsay Society for the History of Dentistry, c/o Christine Hillam, University of Liverpool,, Department of Clinical Dental Sciences,, Pembroke Pl, Liverpool, Merseyside L3 5PS, United Kingdom.

M

617.6 USA ISSN 0070-3664
DENTAL IMAGES. Text in English. 1961. 3/yr. free per issue. adv. **Document type:** *Academic/Scholarly.* **Description:** For alumni and friends. Covers the school, the university, and the alumni.
Indexed: Dent.Ind.
Published by: Marquette University, School of Dentistry, 604 N 16th St, Milwaukee, WI 53233. TEL 414-288-7738. Ed. Dr. Robert B Morris. Adv. contact Carol Trecek. Circ: 8,400.

617.6 USA ISSN 1062-0346
DENTAL IMPLANTOLOGY UPDATE. Text in English. 1990. m. USD 497 domestic; USD 527 foreign; USD 83 newsstand/cover (effective 2001). **Document type:** *Newsletter.* **Description:** Presents practical information for both general dentists and specialists on materials, procedures and techniques.
Incorporates (1992-1994?): G P (General Practitioner) (1063-3324); Which was formed by the merger of (1989-1991): Endodontics for G Ps (1050-8767); (in 1991): Periodontics for G Ps (1057-445X); which was formerly (1989-1991): Soft Tissue Care for G Ps (1050-8783); (1988-1991): Cosmetic Dentistry for G Ps (1042-1092); which superseded: Dental Practice Success (1053-153X); which was previously (until 1990): Dental Update on Practice Management (1043-4178); (until 1989): Dental Management Update (1042-167X); (until 1988): Procom Update (1043-4178)
Indexed: Ref.Zh.
—BLDSC (3553.332200), GNLM.
Published by: American Health Consultants (Subsidiary of: Medical Economics Co., Inc.), 3525 Piedmont Rd, N E, 6 Piedmont Center, Ste 400, Atlanta, GA 30305. TEL 404-262-5476, 800-688-2421, FAX 404-262-7837, 800-284-3291, custserv@ahcpub.com, http://www.ahcpub.com. Circ: 1,140.

617.6 USA ISSN 0146-9738
DENTAL LAB PRODUCTS. Text in English. 1976. bi-m. USD 35 domestic; USD 41 foreign (effective 2000). adv. bk.rev. illus, tr.lit. **Document type:** *Trade.* **Description:** Provides news, new products and step-by-step procedures for dental laboratory owners and managers.
Related titles: Microform ed.: (from PQC).
Published by: MEDEC Dental Communications (Subsidiary of: Medical Economics Co., Inc.), 2 Northfield Plaza, Ste 300, Northfield, IL 60093-1219. TEL 847-441-3700, 800-451-7838. Ed. D Kaplan. Circ: 20,983.

617.6 DEU ISSN 0011-8656
DAS DENTAL-LABOR; internationales Fachblatt fuer die gesamte Zahntechnik und ihre Randgebiete. Text in German. 1953. m. DEM 166.25; EUR 85 domestic; DEM 197.54, EUR 101 foreign; DEM 16.62, EUR 8.50 newsstand/cover domestic; DEM 19.56, EUR 10 newsstand/cover foreign (effective 2001). adv. bk.rev. charts, illus, pat, stat. index. **Document type:** *Trade.*
Indexed: Curr.Tit.Dent., Dent.Ind.
—CISTI, GNLM.
Published by: Verlag Neuer Merkur GmbH, Anton-Ditt-Bogen 23, Munich 80939, Germany. TEL 49-89-318905-0, FAX 49-89-31890538, info@vnm-gmbh.de, info@vnmonline.de, http://www.vnmonline.de. Ed. Dr. Joerg Lingenberg. Circ: 19,000.

617.6 DNK ISSN 0070-3672
DENTAL LABORATORIE BLADET. Text in Danish. 1949. 4/yr. DKK 150. adv. bk.rev.
Published by: (Association of Dental Laboratories in Denmark/Danske Dental Laboratorier), D L B -Bladforlag A-S, Rentemestervej 64, Copenhagen Nv 2400, Denmark. TEL 31-10-76-83, FAX 38-33-16-07. Eds. Alf Rasmussen, Vibeke Fialla. Circ: 500.

617.6 GBR ISSN 0957-5138
DENTAL LABORATORY. Text in English. 1975. m. GBP 20 registered dental technicians; GBP 28 domestic; GBP 60 foreign; GBP 2.50 newsstand/cover (effective 2000). adv. bk.rev. Supplement avail. **Document type:** *Trade.* **Description:** Directed at dental laboratory owners. Covers all aspects of dental technology, including product features and articles aimed at technicians.
Published by: Dental Laboratories Association Ltd., N Sherwood St, Nottingham NG1 4EE, United Kingdom. TEL 44-115-948-2400, FAX 44-115-948-2777. Ed. William Courtney. R&P, Adv. contact Christian Dunn. page GBP 400. Circ: 3,000.

617.6 USA
DENTAL LABORATORY CONFERENCE. NEWS & VIEWS✶. Text in English. 1976. q. membership. adv. back issues avail.
Published by: Dental Laboratory Conference, Packman Gitman Market, Box 3427, Maple Glen, PA 19002-8427. FAX 215-546-9595. Ed. Robert C Gitman. Circ: 700.

617.6 DEU ISSN 0176-7291
DENTAL-MAGAZIN. Text in German. 1983. q. adv. **Document type:** *Journal, Trade.*
Published by: Deutscher Aerzte-Verlag GmbH, Dieselstr 2, Cologne 50859, Germany. TEL 49-2234-7011233, FAX 49-2234-7011515, info@dental-magazin.de, verlag@aerzteblatt.de, http://www.aerzteblatt.de. Ed. Dr. Kerstin Graupner. Circ: 53,000 (paid and controlled).

617.6 USA ISSN 0109-5641
CODEN: DEMAEP
DENTAL MATERIALS. Text in English. 1985. bi-m. EUR 210 in Europe to individuals; JPY 27,900 in Japan to individuals; USD 235 elsewhere to individuals; EUR 304 in Europe to institutions; JPY 40,300 in Japan to institutions; USD 235 elsewhere to institutions (effective 2002). adv. bk.rev. abstr. index. back issues avail. *Refereed.* **Document type:** *Academic/Scholarly.* **Description:** Devoted to the materials used in dentistry; covers all aspects of dental materials science, such as laboratory, clinical, and biocompatibility testing of materials and their components, as well as instruments and equipment; interactions of dental materials, testing methods, and protocols.
Related titles: Microfilm ed.: (from PQC); Online - full text ed.: (from ingenta, Swets Blackwell, ScienceDirect, Institute for Scientific Information).
Indexed: Alloys Ind., Curr.Cont. (coverage dropped), Curr.Tit.Dent., Dent.Abstr., Eng.Mat.Abstr., Inpharma, METADEX, Mat.Sci.Cit.Ind., Met.Abstr., Met.Abstr.Ind., Nonfer.Met.Alert, PCC Alert, Reac., Sci.Cit.Ind. (coverage dropped), Steels Alert, World Alum.Abstr.
—BLDSC (3553.365800), CASDDS, CISTI, GNLM, IDS, ingenta.
Published by: Academy of Dental Materials, 3302 Gaston Ave, Dallas, TX 75246. TEL 214-828-8378, FAX 214-874-4503, http://www.elsevier.com/locate/dental. Ed. D Watts. Adv. contact Dr. Victoria A Marker. B&W page USD 350, color page USD 1,650. Circ: 780 (paid).

617.6 PHL ISSN 0011-8699
DENTAL MIRROR✶; journal of Philippine dentistry. Text in English. 1965 (vol.2). s-a. adv.
Published by: Philippine Medical - Dental Publications, c/o Philippine Medical Association, PMA Bldg, North Ave, Quezon City, Philippines. Ed. P V Norona.

617.6 JPN ISSN 0011-8702
DENTAL OUTLOOK/SHIKAI TENBO. Text in Japanese. 1921. m. JPY 1,300 per issue. adv. bk.rev. abstr, charts, illus. s-a. index.
Indexed: Dent.Ind., INIS Atomind.
—BLDSC (3553.370000), CISTI, GNLM.
Published by: Ishiyaku Publishers Inc., 7-10 Honkomagome 1-chome, Bunkyo-ku, Tokyo 113-0021, Japan. Ed. Hiroshi Miura. Circ: 24,500.

617.6 GBR ISSN 0011-8710
DENTAL PRACTICE; the journal of modern techniques, equipment and materials. Text in English. 1970 (vol.2). m. GBP 30; GBP 40 elsewhere (effective 2002). adv. bk.rev. abstr, charts, illus. 5 cols./p. reprint service avail. from PQC. **Document type:** *Trade.* **Description:** Entertaining and informative reading for dentists, including up-to-date articles on products and news.
Incorporating: Dental News
Related titles: Microform ed.: (from PQC).
Indexed: Curr.Tit.Dent., Dent.Ind.
—BLDSC (3553.372300), GNLM.
Published by: A.E. Morgan Publications Ltd., Stanley House, 9 West St, Epsom, Surrey KT18 7RL, United Kingdom. TEL 44-1372-741411, FAX 44-1372-744493. Ed. Mary Newing. Pub. Terence Morgan. Adv. contact Frank Archer. color page GBP 1,530; 215 x 300. Circ: 15,000.

338.436176 USA ISSN 1078-1250
DENTAL PRACTICE & FINANCE. Text in English. 1993. bi-m. USD 55 in United States; USD 75 foreign (effective 2000). **Document type:** *Trade.* **Description:** Publishes information designed to help dentists better manage their technology, practices and personal finances in a rapidly changing business environment.
Published by: MEDEC Dental Communications (Subsidiary of: Medical Economics Co., Inc.), 2 Northfield Plaza, Ste 300, Northfield, IL 60093-1219. TEL 847-441-3700, 800-451-7838.

617.6 658 CAN ISSN 0827-1305
DENTAL PRACTICE MANAGEMENT. Text in English. 1985. q. CND 20.95 domestic; USD 25.95 in United States; USD 41.95 elsewhere (effective 1999). back issues avail. **Description:** Provides business management information to dentists, hygienists, dental assistants and office managers. Covers topics from investment planning to life-style issues.
Indexed: CBCA Bus. (1996-), Dent.Abstr.
—BLDSC (3553.372700), GNLM, ingenta.
Published by: Southam Magazine Group, 1450 Don Mills Rd, Don Mills, ON M3B 2X7, Canada. TEL 416-442-2193, FAX 416-442-2214. Pub. Melissa Summerfield. Circ: 16,100.

617.6 DEU
DENTAL PRAXIS. Text in German. 1983. bi-m. DEM 179.94, EUR 92; DEM 205.36, EUR 105 foreign; DEM 34.23, EUR 17.50 newsstand/cover; DEM 39.12, EUR 20 newsstand/cover foreign (effective 2001). adv. bk.rev. **Document type:** *Magazine, Trade.*
Former titles (until 2000): Phillip Journal (0945-1412); Philip Journal fuer Restaurative Zahnmedizin (0174-5980)
—BLDSC (3553.378500), GNLM.
Published by: Verlag Neuer Merkur GmbH, Anton-Ditt-Bogen 23, Munich 80939, Germany. TEL 49-89-318905-0, FAX 49-89-31890553, info@vnm-gmbh.de, info@vnmonline.de, http://www.vnmonline.de. Pub. Burkhard Bierschenck. Circ: 5,200.

617.6 USA ISSN 0011-8737 CODEN: DPREE3
DENTAL PRODUCTS REPORT; trends in dentistry. Text in English. 1967. m. (11/yr.). USD 120 domestic; USD 135 foreign (effective 2000). adv. bk.rev. illus, tr.lit. **Document type:** *Trade.* **Description:** Focuses on the latest innovations in products, literature, techniques, continuing education opportunities and services of interest to practicing dentists.
Formerly: Dental Products Annual Report (0070-3702)
Related titles: Microform ed.: (from PQC).
Published by: Medical Economics Co., Inc., MEDEC Dental Communications, 5 Paragon Dr, Montvale, NJ 07645-1742. Ed. Jeanne K Matson. Circ: 147,801 (controlled).

617.6 HKG ISSN 1016-5037
DENTAL REVIEW; continuing clinical education journal for practising dentists in Asia. (Regional editions avail. for Hong Kong, Indonesia, Malaysia, Philippines, Thailand, Singapore) Text in English. 1989. bi-m. HKD 54. adv. index. back issues avail. *Refereed.* **Document type:** *Trade.* **Description:** Contains abstracts and reviews of articles in dentistry published for continuing education of dentists in Asia.
Published by: MediMedia Asia (Subsidiary of: MediMedia Pacific Ltd.), 2102 Tung Sun Commercial Centre, 194-200 Lockhart Rd, Wanchai, Hong Kong, Hong Kong. TEL 852-2559-5888, 852-2511-0765, FAX 852-2559-6910, 852-2507-3817, http://www.medimedia.com.hk/. Ed. H Edward Lyon. Adv. contact Mary Ng. color page HKD 496; trim 276 x 206. Circ: 12,200.

617.6 PHL
DENTAL SERVICE QUARTERLY. Text in English. 4/yr. adv.
Published by: Philippines Dental Society, Armed Forces, 23 Zamboanga St, Diliman, Quezon City Mm 1128, Philippines. Circ: 1,200.

617.6 USA
DENTAL SOCIETY OF WESTERN PENNSYLVANIA. BULLETIN. Text in English. 1900. bi-m. USD 36. adv. bk.rev. charts, illus. **Document type:** *Bulletin.*
Formerly: Odontological Bulletin (0029-8433)
Indexed: Dent.Ind.
Published by: Dental Society of Western Pennsylvania, 900 Cedar Ave, Pittsburgh, PA 15212. TEL 412-321-5810, FAX 412-321-7719. Ed., Pub. Dr. Joel A Casar. Circ: 1,600.

617.6 GBR ISSN 0011-8796
DENTAL TECHNICIAN. Text in English. 1948. m. GBP 17 in United Kingdom; GBP 20 elsewhere (effective 2002); subscr. includes Dental Technician Yearbook & Directory. adv. bk.rev. illus. 20 p./no. 6 cols./p. **Document type:** *Directory, Trade.* **Description:** Lists suppliers and contact persons for dental technicians.
Indexed: Br.Ceram.Abstr., Curr.Tit.Dent., Dent.Ind.
—GNLM.
Published by: A.E. Morgan Publications Ltd., Stanley House, 9 West St, Epsom, Surrey KT18 7RL, United Kingdom. TEL 44-1372-741411, FAX 44-1372-744493. Ed. D Ritchie. Pub. Terence Morgan. Adv. contact Frank Archer. B&W page GBP 530; 214 x 250. Circ: 3,500.

617.6025 GBR
DENTAL TECHNICIAN DIRECTORY OF DENTAL LABORATORIES AND SERVICES. Text in English. 1979. a., latest vol.30. GBP 9.50 (effective 2001). adv. 220 p./no. 2 cols./p. **Document type:** *Directory, Trade.*
Formerly: Dental Technician Yearbook & Directory
Published by: A.E. Morgan Publications Ltd., Stanley House, 9 West St, Epsom, Surrey KT18 7RL, United Kingdom. TEL 44-1372-741411, FAX 44-1372-744493. Ed. D Ritchie. Pub. Terence Morgan. Adv. contact Frank Archer. B&W page GBP 350; 125 x 155.

617.6 DNK ISSN 1600-4469 CODEN: EDTRED
DENTAL TRAUMATOLOGY. Text and summaries in English. 1985. bi-m. USD 331 in the Americas to institutions print & online eds. combined; GBP 230 elsewhere to institutions print & online eds. combined (effective 2002). adv. bk.rev. illus. back issues avail. *Refereed.* **Document type:** *Journal, Academic/Scholarly.*
Formerly: Endodontics & Dental Traumatology (0109-2502)
Related titles: ♦ Online - full text ed.: Dental Traumatology Online.
Indexed: ASCA, Biol.Abstr., Chem.Abstr., Chem.Indus.Notes, Chem.Titles, Curr.Cont., Curr.Tit.Dent., Dent.Abstr., Inpharma, Reac., Rev.Med.& Vet.Mycol.
—BLDSC (3553.512500), CASDDS, CISTI, GNLM, IDS, ingenta. **CCC.**
Published by: (International Association for Dental Traumatology), Blackwell Munksgaard, Noerre Soegade 35, PO Box 2148, Copenhagen K 1016, Denmark. TEL 45-77-33-33-33, FAX 45-77-33-33-77, customerservice@munksgaard.dk, http://www.munksgaard.dk. Ed. Leif Tronstad. Circ: 900.

617.6 DNK
DENTAL TRAUMATOLOGY ONLINE. Text in English. bi-m. DKK 2,070 (effective 2001). **Document type:** *Academic/Scholarly.*
Media: Online - full text (from EBSCO Publishing, ingenta, Munksgaard & Blackwell Science's Synergy, Swets Blackwell, Institute for Scientific Information). **Related titles:** ♦ Print ed.: Dental Traumatology. ISSN 1600-4469.
Published by: Blackwell Munksgaard, Noerre Soegade 35, PO Box 2148, Copenhagen K 1016, Denmark. TEL 45-77-33-33-33, FAX 45-77-33-33-77, fsub@mail.munksgaard.dk, http://www.ingenta.com/journals/browse/mksg/edt, http://www.munksgaard.dk.

617.3 GBR ISSN 0305-5000
DENTAL UPDATE. Text in English. 1973. 10/yr. GBP 65 in United Kingdom; GBP 78 rest of Europe; GBP 80 rest of world; GBP 29 to students (effective 2000). adv. bk.rev. cum.index. *Refereed.* **Document type:** *Academic/Scholarly.* **Description:** Provides dentists with in-depth clinical information on orthodontics, preventative, restorative and conservative dentistry.
Related titles: ♦ English ed.: Dental Update (South African Edition). ISSN 1011-5986.
Indexed: Curr.Adv.Ecol.Sci., Curr.Tit.Dent., Dent.Ind.
—BLDSC (3553.515000), CISTI, GNLM.
Published by: George Warman Publications Ltd., Unit 2, Riverview Business Park, Walnut Tree Close, Guildford, Surrey GU1 4QT, United Kingdom. TEL 44-1483-304944, FAX 44-1483-303191. Ed. Angela Stroud. Adv. contact Erica Kilburn. Circ: 7,500.

617.6 ZAF ISSN 1011-5986
DENTAL UPDATE (SOUTH AFRICAN EDITION); the journal for the general dental practitioner. Text in English. 1987. m. ZAR 102.60; ZAR 160 foreign (effective 1997). adv. back issues avail. **Document type:** *Trade, Academic/Scholarly.* **Description:** Clinical journal for the continuing education of dentists.
Related titles: ♦ English ed.: Dental Update. ISSN 0305-5000.
Published by: George Warman Publications (Pty.) Ltd., PO Box 704, Cape Town 8000, South Africa. TEL 27-21-24-5320, FAX 27-21-26-1332. Ed. A Rademeyer. Circ: 2,679.

617.6 USA
THE DENTAL ZONE NEWSLETTER. Text in English. m. **Document type:** *Newsletter.* **Description:** Provides easy to read and understand information for better oral health and a brighter smile.
Media: Online - full text.
Published by: Dental Zone Newsletter, 3900 Walnut St, PO Box H71, Philadelphia, PA 19104. TEL 215-417-3215, FAX 215-893-4376, chapz@mindspring.com, htpp://www.saveyoursmile.com/newsletter/dznewsletterrequest.html. Ed. Chuck Peters.

617.6 CAN ISSN 0822-1596
DENTALETTER. Text in English. 11/yr. CND 119. **Document type:** *Newsletter.* **Description:** Consists of a professional source letter for the practicing dentist.
Published by: M P L Communications Inc., 133 Richmond St W, Ste 700, Toronto, ON M5H 3M8, Canada. TEL 416-869-1177, FAX 416-869-0456.

617.6 CHE
DENTALHYGIENE. Text in French, German. 1976. bi-m. CHF 85 (effective 2001). adv. bk.rev. *Refereed.* **Document type:** *Journal, Trade.*
Formerly: Dentalhygienikerin
Published by: Swiss Dental Hygienists' Association, Oberstadt 8, Sempach Stadt 6204, Switzerland. TEL 41-41-4627065, FAX 41-41-4627061. Ed. Vreni Steinegger. Adv. contact Vreni Koch. Circ: 1,623.

617.6 GBR ISSN 0266-3414
DENTIST. Text in English. m. GBP 29. back issues avail. **—CCC.**
Published by: Reed Business Publishing Group, Carew Division (Subsidiary of: Reed International PLC), Quadrant House, The Quadrant, Brighton Rd, Sutton, Surrey SM2 5AS, United Kingdom. TEL 081-661-3500. Ed. Jennifer C Dyer.

617.643 ITA
DENTISTA MODERNO. Text in Italian. m. (except July & Aug.). ITL 100,000. adv.
Published by: U T E T SpA, Corso Raffaello 28, Turin 10125, Italy. TEL 39-2-29003555, FAX 39-2-6599049. Ed. Paolo Pegoraro. Adv. contact Corrado Trevisani. B&W page ITL 2,640,000, color page ITL 3,795,000; trim 250 x 185. Circ: 22,600.

617.6 JPN ISSN 0070-3737
DENTISTRY IN JAPAN. Text in English. 1964. a. membership. **Document type:** *Academic/Scholarly.*
Formerly (until 1968): Japanese Dental Journal
—BLDSC (3553.545000), GNLM.
Published by: Japanese Dental Association/Nihon Shika Ishikai, 4-1-20 Kudan-Kita, Chiyoda-ku, Tokyo 102-0073, Japan. TEL 81-3-3262-9214, FAX 81-3-3262-9885. Ed. Dr. Isao Ishikawa. Pub. Dr. Yoshikage Higashi. Circ: 2,400 (controlled).

617.6 USA
DENTISTRY IN SOUTH DAKOTA. Text in English. 1962. q. USD 20 to non-members (effective 1999). adv. **Document type:** *Newsletter.*
Formerly (until 1995): South Dakota Dental Association. Newsletter (0038-3287)
Published by: South Dakota Dental Association, 330 S Poplar Ave, Box 1194, Pierre, SD 57501-1194. TEL 605-224-9133, FAX 605-224-9168. Ed., Pub., R&P Paul Knecht. Adv. contact Bobbi Martin. page USD 500. Circ: 530 (controlled).

617.6 GBR ISSN 1359-7647
DENTISTRY ON-LINE. Text in English. m. free per issue. bk.rev., software rev., video rev., Website rev. *Refereed.* **Document type:** *Journal, Academic/Scholarly.* **Description:** Dedicated to dental surgeons, dentists, dental assistants and hygienists.
Media: Online - full text.
Published by: Priory Lodge Education Ltd., 2 Cornflower Way, Moreton, Wirral CH46 1SV, United Kingdom. TEL 44-151-606-1796, FAX 44-151-606-1812, solutions@priory.com, http://www.priory.com/dent.htm. Ed. Dr. R. Glenning. Circ: 40,000 (controlled).

617.6 USA ISSN 8750-2186
DENTISTRY TODAY. Text in English. 1982. 11/yr. USD 65 domestic; USD 95 in Canada; USD 120 elsewhere (effective 2000). tr.lit. reprints avail. *Refereed.* **Document type:** *Magazine, Trade.*
—BLDSC (3553.546500), GNLM.
Published by: Dentistry Today, Inc., Greenbrook Corporate Center, 100 Passaic Ave FIR.2, Fairfield, NJ 07004. TEL 201-783-3190, FAX 201-783-6835, dent2day@aol.com. Ed. Ted Fetner. Pub. Paul Radcliffe. R&P Michele Herrmann. Adv. contact James Radcliffe. Circ: 147,000 (controlled).

DENTISTS' COMPUTER NEWS. see *MEDICAL SCIENCES—Computer Applications*

617.6 USA
DENTIST'S PATIENT NEWSLETTER. Text in English. 1983. q. USD 645 per quarter for 1000 copies (effective 2001). index. 4 p./no. 3 cols./p. **Document type:** *Newsletter, Consumer.* **Description:** Provides dental health information for dentists to use to market their practice.
Published by: Newsletters Ink, PO Box 2019, Lancaster, PA 17608-2019. TEL 717-393-1000, 800-379-5585, FAX 717-393-4702, http://www.newslettersink.com. Ed. Ann Mead Ash. Pub. Gregory A Gilson.

M

617.6 USA ISSN 0011-9601
DETROIT DENTAL BULLETIN* . Text in English. 1939. m. (8/yr.). USD 25 to non-members. adv. bk.rev. abstr. **Document type:** *Bulletin, Trade.*
Indexed: Dent.Ind.
—BLDSC (3561.500000).
Published by: Detroit District Dental Society, 460 Fisher Bldg, Detroit, MI 48202. TEL 313-871-3500, FAX 313-871-3503. Ed. Edward H Hirisch. Circ: 1,400.

617.6 DEU ISSN 0012-1029
CODEN: DZZEA7
DEUTSCHE ZAHNAERZTLICHE ZEITSCHRIFT. Text in German; Summaries in English. 1946. m. DEM 368 domestic; DEM 384 foreign (effective 2001). adv. bk.rev. abstr, charts, illus. **Document type:** *Journal, Trade.*
Indexed: Biol.Abstr., Chem.Abstr., Chem.Indus.Notes, Chem.Titles, Curr.Cont. (coverage dropped), Curr.Tit.Dent., Dent.Ind., INIS Atomind., Ind.Med. (coverage dropped).
—BLDSC (3575.694000), CASDDS, CISTI, GNLM, Infotrieve. **CCC.**
Published by: (Deutsche Gesellschaft fuer Zahn-, Mund- und Kieferheilkunde), Carl Hanser Verlag, Kolbergerstr 22, Munich 81679, Germany. TEL 49-89-99830-0, FAX 49-89-984809, info@hanser.de, http://www.zahnheilkunde.de/dzz/set.htm, http://www.hanser.de. Circ: 5,300.

DEUTSCHER KONGRESS KALENDER ZAHNMEDIZINER. see *MEETINGS AND CONGRESSES*

617.6 DEU ISSN 0344-2926
DEUTSCHER ZAHNAERZTEKALENDER. Text in German. 1941. a. DEM 74 (effective 2001). adv. **Document type:** *Journal, Trade.*
Related titles: Online - full text ed.
—GNLM.
Published by: Carl Hanser Verlag, Kolbergerstr 22, Munich 81679, Germany. TEL 49-89-99830-0, FAX 49-89-984809, info@zahnheilkunde.de, http://www.zahnheilkunde.de/dzk/. Ed. Dr. Werner Ketterl. Circ: 6,000.

617.5 MEX
DICCIONARIO DE ESPECIALIDADES ODONTOLOGICAS. Text in Spanish. 1984. a.
Published by: Ediciones P L M S.A. de C.V., San BERNADINO 17, Col del Valle, Mexico City, DF 03100, Mexico. TEL 687-1311, FAX 536-5027, TELEX 01772912 EPLM ME. Ed. Patricia Calderon. Circ: 5,000.

617.6 USA
DISTRIBUTION OF DENTISTS IN THE U S. Text in English. triennial. USD 100 to non-members; USD 25 to members. **Document type:** *Monographic series.*
Published by: American Dental Association, Survey Center, 211 E Chicago Ave, Chicago, IL 60611. TEL 312-440-2500, FAX 312-440-2790.

617.6 USA
DISTRICT OF COLUMBIA DENTAL SOCIETY. NEWSLETTER. Text in English. 1915. 10/yr. membership. adv. **Document type:** *Newsletter.* **Description:** Contains news of particular interest to District of Columbia and surrounding metropolitan area practitioners, such as Society activities, legislative and political developments, community activities, as well as news of general interest.
Published by: District of Columbia Dental Society, 502 C St, N E, Washington, DC 20002-5810. TEL 202-547-7613, FAX 202-546-1482, info@dcdental.org, http://www.dcdental.org. Ed., R&P, Adv. contact Danielle A Dobiesz. Circ: 850.

617.643 ITA
DOCTOR OS. Text in Italian. 1990. 9/yr. ITL 75,000. adv. bk.rev.
Published by: Ariesdue s.r.l., Via P A Galletti, 4, Carimate, CO 22060, Italy. TEL 39-31-792135, FAX 39-31-790743, ariesdue@tin.it. Ed. Sergio Porro. Circ: 17,500.

617.634 ITA
DOSSIER DEL DENTISTA MODERNO. Text in Italian. irreg. (7-8/yr.). adv.
Published by: U T E T SpA, Corso Raffaello 28, Turin 10125, Italy. TEL 39-2-29003555, FAX 39-2-6599049. Ed. Paolo Pegoraro. Adv. contact Corrado Trevisan. B&W page ITL 2,640,000, color page ITL 3,795,000; trim 250 x 185. Circ: 22,470.

617.6 USA ISSN 0012-8759
EASTERN DENTAL SOCIETY BULLETIN✶. Text in English. 1968 (vol.11). m. membership. bk.rev. illus.
Published by: Eastern Dental Society, c/o Tim Wong, D D S, 85 Fourth Ave, New York, NY 10003.

617.6 EGY ISSN 0070-9484
EGYPTIAN DENTAL JOURNAL. Text in English; Summaries in Arabic. 1955. q., latest vol.47, 2001. EGP 60 domestic; USD 150 foreign (effective 2002).
Indexed: Biol.Abstr., Dent.Ind.
Published by: Egyptian Dental Association, 84A Mathaf El-Manial Street, El-Manial, Cairo 11451, Egypt. TEL 20-2-3658568, FAX 20-2-5319143, eda@internetegypt.com, malatif@soficom.com.eg. Ed. Dr. M El Sadeek.

617.6 GRC
ELLINIKI ODONTIATRIKI OMOSPONDIA. ENEMEROTIKO DELTIO/HELLENIC DENTAL ASSOCIATION. JOURNAL. Text in Greek. bi-m. free per issue to qualified personnel. **Document type:** *Academic/Scholarly.*
Published by: Hellenic Dental Association, 38 Themistokleous St, Athens 106 78, Greece. TEL 30-1-3803-816, FAX 30-1-3834-385. Ed. Dimitrios Damoulis.

617.6 FRA ISSN 1283-0860
ENCYCLOPEDIE MEDICO-CHIRURGICALE. ODONTOLOGIE. Cover title: Traite d'Ontologie. Text in French. 1939. 6 base vols. plus q. updates. bibl, charts, illus. **Document type:** *Academic/Scholarly.* **Description:** Provides a comprehensive and up-to-date reference for dental professionals.
Former titles (until 1997): Encyclopedie Medico-Chirurgicale. Odontologie et Stomatologie. Tome 2 (1258-9802); (until 1981): Encyclopedie Medico-Chirurgicale. Stomatologie. Tome 2 (0246-1048); Which superseded in part (1939-1949): Encyclopedie Medico-Chirurgicale. Stomatologie (0246-0386)
Published by: Elsevier Paris, Editions Scientifiques et Medicales (Subsidiary of: Reed Elsevier plc. group), 23 rue Linois, Paris 75015, France. TEL 33-1-44589110, FAX 33-1-45589425, redaction-emc@elsevier.fr, redacion-emc@elsevier.fr, http://www.elsevier.fr, http://www.elsevier.com.

617.6 FRA ISSN 1283-0852
ENCYCLOPEDIE MEDICO-CHIRURGICALE. STOMATOLOGIE. Text in French. 1939. 7 base vols. plus q. updates. bibl, charts, illus. *Refereed.* **Document type:** *Academic/Scholarly.* **Description:** Offers a comprehensive and up-to-date reference for medical specialists who diagnose and treat diseases of the mouth.
Former titles (until 1997): Encyclopedie Medico-Chirurgicale. Odontologie et Stomatologie. Tome 1 (1154-2934); (until 1987): Encyclopedie Medico-Chirurgicale. Stomatologie. Tome 1 (0246-103X); Which superseded in part (1939-1949): Encyclopedie Medico-Chirurgicale. Stomatologie (0246-0386)
Published by: Elsevier Paris, Editions Scientifiques et Medicales (Subsidiary of: Reed Elsevier plc. group), 23 rue Linois, Paris 75015, France. TEL 33-1-45589110, FAX 33-1-45589425, redaction-emc@elsevier.fr, redacion-emc@elsevier.fr, http://www.elsevier.fr, http://www.elsevier.com.

617.6 FRA ISSN 1168-5476
ENDO✶; revue Francaise d'endodontie. Text in French. 4/yr. adv.
Formerly (until 1992): Revue Francaise d'Endodontie (0294-1813)
—GNLM.
Address: 58 rue de la Procession, Suresnes 92150, France. TEL 40-99-90-67, FAX 45-06-04-74. Ed. Jean Marie Laurichesse. Adv. contact Chantal Daly. Circ: 3,000.

617.6 ESP ISSN 1130-9903
ENDODONCIA. Text in Spanish; Summaries in English. 1982. q. ESP 3,600, USD 26. adv. bk.rev. index. back issues avail. **Document type:** *Academic/Scholarly.*
Formerly: Revista Espanola de Endodoncia (0212-4688)
—GNLM.
Published by: (Asociacion Espanola de Endodoncia), Ediciones Ergon S.A., Pza. Josep Pallach 10, 1o, Barcelona 08035, Spain. TEL 34-93-428-5500, FAX 34-93-428-5660. **Subscr. to:** Ergon, Antonio Lopez Aguado, 1, Madrid 28029, Spain.

617.6 GBR ISSN 1465-9417
ENDODONTIC PRACTICE. Text in English. 1998. q. GBP 87 to individuals; GBP 150 to institutions (effective 2000). **Description:** Promotes excellence in endodontics to dental practitioners with a variety of articles by leading dentists and endodontists covering the full range of clinical and management topics.
—BLDSC (3743.113000).
Published by: Finlayson Media Communications, Ltd, 524 Watford Way, Mill Hill, London NW7 4SY, United Kingdom. TEL 44-20-8906-4003, FAX 44-20-8906-8808, endo@fmc.co.uk.

617.6 USA
ENDODONTICS NEWSLETTER. Text in English. q. **Document type:** *Newsletter.* **Description:** Each issue contains summaries of research findings in endodontics. Aims to enable non-specialists to keep current with significant developments in the field of endodontics.
Related titles: Diskette ed.
Published by: W P I Communications Inc., 55 Morris Ave, Springfield, NJ 07081. TEL 973-467-8700, 800-323-4995, FAX 973-467-0368, http://www.wpicomm.com. Ed. Ken Berry. Pub. Steven H Klinghoffer.

617.6 DEU ISSN 0940-9505
ENDODONTIE; Zeitschrift fuer die Praxis. Text in German. 1992. 4/yr. EUR 108 domestic; EUR 114 foreign; EUR 66 domestic to students; EUR 72 foreign to students (effective 2002). adv. **Document type:** *Magazine, Trade.*
—GNLM.
Published by: Quintessenz Verlags GmbH, Ifenpfad 2-4, Berlin 12107, Germany. TEL 49-30-76180646, FAX 49-30-76180680, central@quintessenz.de, http://www.quintessenz.de. Adv. contact Gudrun Matthes.

617.6 USA ISSN 1045-9812
ESTHETIC DENTISTRY UPDATE✶; endorsed by the American Academy of Cosmetic Dentistry. Text in English. 1990. bi-m. USD 125; USD 152 foreign (effective 1996). adv. illus. *Refereed.* **Document type:** *Academic/Scholarly.* **Description:** Provides information on restorative dentistry to practitioners seeking to expand their practices.
—GNLM.
Published by: Health Care Advancements Inc., c/o Dr Lenin, 10 New Plant Ct, Owings, MD 21117-3514. Ed. Dr. Roger P Levin. Adv. contact Steve Gray. B&W page USD 580, color page USD 1,380. Circ: 1,390.

617.7 DNK ISSN 1396-5883
EUROPEAN JOURNAL OF DENTAL EDUCATION. Text in English. 1997. q. USD 241 in the Americas to institutions print & online eds. combines; GBP 168 elsewhere to institutions print & online eds. combined (2002). **Document type:** *Academic/Scholarly.*
Related titles: ♦ Online - full text ed.: European Journal of Dental Education Online.
—BLDSC (3829.728255), CISTI.
Published by: (Association for Dental Education in Europe), Blackwell Munksgaard, Noerre Soegade 35, PO Box 2148, Copenhagen K 1016, Denmark. TEL 45-77-33-33-33, FAX 45-77-33-33-77, customerservice@munksgaard.dk, http://www.munksgaard.dk. Ed. John Scott.

617.7 DNK
EUROPEAN JOURNAL OF DENTAL EDUCATION ONLINE. Text in English. q. DKK 864 to individuals; DKK 1,674 to institutions (effective 2001). **Document type:** *Academic/Scholarly.*
Media: Online - full text (from EBSCO Publishing, ingenta, Swets Blackwell). **Related titles:** ♦ Print ed.: European Journal of Dental Education. ISSN 1396-5883.
Published by: Blackwell Munksgaard, Noerre Soegade 35, PO Box 2148, Copenhagen K 1016, Denmark. TEL 45-77-33-33-33, FAX 45-77-33-33-77, fsub@mail.munksgaard.dk, http://www.ingenta.com/journals/browse/mksg/eje, http://www.munksgaard.dk.

617.6 DNK ISSN 0909-8836
CODEN: SJDRAN
EUROPEAN JOURNAL OF ORAL SCIENCES. Text and summaries in English. 1893. bi-m. USD 300 in the Americas to institutions print & online eds. combined; GBP 208 elsewhere to institutions print & online eds. combined (effective 2002). adv. illus. index. reprint service avail. from SWZ,ISI. *Refereed.* **Document type:** *Academic/Scholarly.*
Former titles: Scandinavian Journal of Dental Research (0029-845X); (until 1970): Odontologisk Tidskrift (0472-514X)
Related titles: Microform ed.: (from SWZ); ♦ Online - full text ed.: European Journal of Oral Sciences Online; ♦ Supplement: European Journal of Oral Sciences. Supplement (CD-ROM Edition). ISSN 1398-3393; ♦ European Journal of Oral Sciences. Supplement (Print Edition). ISSN 1397-7555.
Indexed: ASCA, Biol.Abstr., Chem.Abstr., Chem.Indus.Notes, Chem.Titles, Curr.Adv.Ecol.Sci., Curr.Cont., Curr.Tit.Dent., Dent.Abstr., Dent.Ind., Environ.Sci.Poll.Mgmt., Excerp.Med., INIS Atomind., Ind.Med. (1995-), Ind.Sci.Rev., Inpharma, Med.& Surg.Dermat., NRN, Nutr.Abstr., Pollut.Abstr., Reac., Risk Abstr., Saf.Sci.Abstr., Sci.Cit.Ind., Sugar Ind.Abstr.
—BLDSC (3829.733250), CASDDS, CISTI, GNLM, IDS, Infotrieve, ingenta, KNAW. **CCC.**

M

Published by: (Nordiska Odontologiska Foreningen), Blackwell Munksgaard, Noerre Soegade 35, PO Box 2148, Copenhagen K 1016, Denmark. TEL 45-77-33-33-33, FAX 45-77-33-33-77, fsub@munksgaard.dk, http://www.munksgaard.dk. Ed. Anders Linde. Circ: 2,000.

617.6 DNK
EUROPEAN JOURNAL OF ORAL SCIENCES ONLINE. Text in English. bi-m. DKK 1,953 (effective 2001). **Document type:** *Academic/Scholarly.*
Media: Online - full text (from Swets Blackwell, Institute for Scientific Information). **Related titles:** Microform ed.: (from SWZ); ♦ Print ed.: European Journal of Oral Sciences. ISSN 0909-8836.
Published by: Blackwell Munksgaard, Noerre Soegade 35, PO Box 2148, Copenhagen K 1016, Denmark. TEL 45-77-33-33-33, FAX 45-77-33-33-77, fsub@mail.munksgaard.dk, http://www.ingenta.com/journals/browse/mksg/eos, http://www.munksgaard.dk.

617.6 DNK ISSN 1398-3393
EUROPEAN JOURNAL OF ORAL SCIENCES. SUPPLEMENT (CD-ROM EDITION). Text in English. 1998. irreg.
Media: CD-ROM. **Related titles:** ♦ Supplement to: European Journal of Oral Sciences. ISSN 0909-8836.
Published by: Blackwell Munksgaard, Noerre Soegade 35, PO Box 2148, Copenhagen K 1016, Denmark. TEL 45-77-33-33-33. Ed. Edward Valauskas.

617.6 DNK ISSN 1397-7555
EUROPEAN JOURNAL OF ORAL SCIENCES. SUPPLEMENT (PRINT EDITION). Text in English. 1998. irreg.
Related titles: ♦ Supplement to: European Journal of Oral Sciences. ISSN 0909-8836.
Published by: Blackwell Munksgaard, Noerre Soegade 35, PO Box 2148, Copenhagen K 1016, Denmark. FAX 45-77-33-33-77. Ed. Edward Valauskas.

617.6 GBR ISSN 0141-5387
EUROPEAN JOURNAL OF ORTHODONTICS. Text in English. 1979. bi-m. GBP 160, USD 265 to individuals; GBP 195, USD 330 to institutions (effective Feb. 2002). adv. bk.rev. back issues avail. *Refereed.* **Document type:** *Journal, Academic/Scholarly.* **Description:** Presents research or clinical papers of interest to all orthodontists.
Related titles: Online - full content ed.: ISSN 1460-2210. GBP 175, USD 295 to institutions Online only (effective Feb. 2002) (from EBSCO Publishing, O C L C Online Computer Library Center, Inc., ingenta, Swets Blackwell); Online - full text ed.: (from Institute for Scientific Information, RoweCom Information Quest).
Indexed: ASCA, Biol.Abstr., Curr.Cont., Dent.Ind., Excerp.Med., Ind.Med. (1979-), Ind.Sci.Rev., Inpharma, Reac., Ref.Zh., Sci.Cit.Ind.
—BLDSC (3829.733300), CISTI, GNLM, IDS, ingenta. **CCC.**
Published by: (European Association of Orthodontics), Oxford University Press, Academic Division, Great Clarendon St, Oxford OX2 6DP, United Kingdom. TEL 44-1865-267907, FAX 44-1865-267835, jnl.info@oup.co.uk, http://www.ejo.oupjournals.org, http://www.oup.co.uk/journals. Ed. Fraser McDonald. Pub. Mandy Sketch. R&P Fionna Willis. adv.: page GBP 410, page USD 740. Circ: 3,350. **U.S. subscr. to:** Oxford University Press, Journals, 2001 Evans Rd, Cary, NC 27513. TEL 800-852-7323, FAX 919-677-1714, jnlorders@oup-usa.org; **Subscr. to:** Journals Marketing, Great Clarendon St, Oxford OX2 6DP, United Kingdom.

617.6 GBR ISSN 0965-7452
EUROPEAN JOURNAL OF PROSTHODONTICS AND RESTORATIVE DENTISTRY. Abbreviated title: E J P R D. Text in English. 1962. q. GBP 42 in Europe to non-members; GBP 47 elsewhere to non-members; GBP 34 in Europe to members; GBP 38 elsewhere to members; GBP 73.50 in Europe to institutions; GBP 79 elsewhere to institutions (effective 1999). adv. bk.rev. **Document type:** *Academic/Scholarly.* **Description:** Covers all aspects of prosthodontics and restorative dentistry.
Former titles (until 1992): Restorative Dentistry; Anglo-Continental Dental Society. Journal (0003-3324)
—BLDSC (3829.737550), GNLM.
Published by: (F D I World Dental Federation), F D I World Dental Press Ltd., 7 Carlisle St, London W1V 5RG, United Kingdom. TEL 44-2079-357852, FAX 44-2074-860183. Ed. Paul S Wright. Circ: 1,000.

616.645 DEU
EUROPEAN WORKSHOP ON PERIODONTOLOGY. PROCEEDINGS. Text mainly in English. 1993. irreg., latest vol.3, 1999. membership. back issues avail. **Document type:** *Proceedings, Academic/Scholarly.* **Description:** Publishes research on gum diseases and conditions presented at the European Workshop on Periodontology.
—BLDSC (6843.843730).
Published by: Quintessenz Verlags GmbH, Ifenpfad 2-4, Berlin 12107, Germany. TEL 49-30-76180646, 49-30-74006-0, FAX 49-30-76180680, TELEX 183815-QUINT-D, http://www.molar.unibe.ch/perio/ittingen, http://www.quintessenz.de. **Co-sponsors:** European Federation of Periodontology; European Federation of Osseointegration; Swiss Society of Periodontology/Schweizerische Gesellschaft fuer Parodontologie.

617.6 GBR ISSN 1462-0049
EVIDENCE - BASED DENTISTRY. Text in English. 1998. q. GBP 30 in Europe to individuals for print ed; GBP 30, USD 48 rest of world to individuals for print ed.; GBP 75 in Europe to institutions for print ed.; GBP 80, USD 128 rest of world to institutions for print ed.; GBP 33 in Europe to individuals for print and online eds.; GBP 33, USD 53 rest of world to individuals for print and online eds.; GBP 83 in Europe to institutions for print and online eds.; GBP 88, USD 141 rest of world to institutions for print and online eds. (effective 2001); Free to members of British Dental Association.
Related titles: Online - full text ed.: GBP 30 to individuals; USD 48, GBP 75, USD 120 to institutions (effective 2001) (from ingenta, Swets Blackwell, RoweCom Information Quest).
Published by: (British Dental Association), Nature Publishing Group Specialist Journals (Subsidiary of: Holtzbrink Publishers), Houndmills, Basingstoke, Hants RG21 6XS, United Kingdom. TEL 44-1256-329242, FAX 44-1256-328339, subscriptions@nature.com, http://www.stockton-press.co.uk/ebd/, http://www.nature.com. **Affiliate:** Nature Publishing Group Specialist Journals.

617.6 NLD ISSN 0928-4109
EXKIES; vaktijdschrift voor tandartsen en tandtechnici. Text in Dutch. 1981. 8/yr. NLG 135. **Document type:** *Trade.*
Published by: Van Zuiden Communications B.V., Postbus 2122, Alphen aan den Rijn 2400 CC, Netherlands. TEL 31-1720-76191, FAX 31-1720-71882. Ed. L J van Zuiden. Circ: 6,000.

617.6 USA ISSN 0894-7929
EXPLORER (FALLS CHURCH). Text in English. 1974. m. USD 15 domestic; USD 20 foreign (effective 2000).
Published by: National Association of Dental Assistants, 900 S Washington St, Ste G13, Falls Church, VA 22046. TEL 703-237-8616. Ed. S Young. Adv. contact Ruth Ludeman. Circ: 4,000.

617.6 USA
EXPLORER (LAKE WORTH). Text in English. 1972. s-a. membership. adv. tr.lit. *Refereed.* **Document type:** *Newsletter.*
Indexed: Biol.Abstr., Biol.Dig., GeoRef.
Published by: Atlantic Coast District Dental Association, 5700 Lake Worth Rd, Ste 208 3, Lake Worth, FL 33463. TEL 561-968-7714, FAX 561-968-4834, acdda@aol.com. Ed., R&P, Adv. contact Catherine Sanson. Circ: 1,260.

617.6 GBR
F D I WORLD. Text in English. 1952. bi-m. GBP 32 in Europe to non-members; GBP 37 elsewhere to non-members (effective 1999). adv. illus. **Document type:** *Newsletter.* **Description:** Includes clinical articles, dental news from around the world, news of F.D.I. activities, and the trade industry; also contains features and congress news.
Former titles (until 1992): F D I Dental World (0965-9986); F D I News; F D I Newsletter (0014-5777)
Related titles: French ed.; German ed.; Spanish ed.
—GNLM.
Published by: (Federation Dentaire Internationale), F D I World Dental Press Ltd., 7 Carlisle St, London W1V 5RG, United Kingdom. TEL 44-2079-357852, FAX 44-2074-860183. Ed. Peter Swiss. Circ: 30,000.

617.6 USA
FACETS (SAN DIEGO). Text in English. 1930. m. USD 20. adv. **Document type:** *Newsletter.* **Description:** Provides in-house information to the membership.
Former titles: San Diego County Dental Society. News; San Diego County Dental Society. Bulletin (0036-4010)
Indexed: Dent.Ind.
Published by: San Diego County Dental Society, 1275 W Morena Blvd, Ste B, San Diego, CA 92110-3837. TEL 619-275-0244, FAX 619-275-0646. Ed. Clayton S Fuller. R&P, Adv. contact Shirlee Smith. Circ: 1,500.

617.6 BRA
FACULDADE DE ODONTOLOGIA DE BAURU. REVISTA. Text in Portuguese; Abstracts in English, Portuguese. 1993. q. BRL 15 (effective 1994). bibl.
Published by: Universidade de Sao Paulo, Faculdade de Odontologia de Bauru, AL DR O P BRISOLLA, 9-75, Centro, Caixa Postal 73, Bauru, SP 17001-970, Brazil. TEL 55-142-234133, FAX 55-142-230415, TELEX 142314 FOBU.

617.6 BRA ISSN 0104-7582
FACULDADE DE ODONTOLOGIA DE LINS. REVISTA. Text in Portuguese; Summaries in English, Portuguese. 1988. s-a. BRL 20 domestic; BRL 40 foreign (effective 1999). adv. bibl, charts, illus. **Document type:** *Academic/Scholarly.*
Indexed: Bibliogr.Bras.Odontol., Cal.Tiss.Abstr., Tox.Abstr. (coverage dropped).
Published by: Unidade Universitaria de Lins - U.N.I.M.E.P., Faculdade de Odontologia, Rua Tenente Florencio Pupo Netto no. 300, Jardim Americano, Lins, SP 16400-000, Brazil. TEL 55-145-225088, FAX 55-145-224611, editora@unimep.br, http://www.unimep.br/~editora. Ed. Casimiro Cabrera Peralta. Circ: 1,000 (paid).

617.6 BRA ISSN 0048-3419
FACULDADE DE ODONTOLOGIA DE PERNAMBUCO. REVISTA. Text in Portuguese; Summaries in English, Portuguese. 1968. s-a. free per issue. illus. index. **Document type:** *Newspaper.*
Indexed: Dent.Ind.
Published by: Faculdade de Odontologia de Pernambuco, Biblioteca, Av General Niwton Cavalcante, 1650, Primavera, Camaragibe, PE 54753-220, Brazil. TEL 55-81-4581088. Ed., R&P Jose Thadeu Pinheiro.

617.6 BRA ISSN 0566-1854
FACULDADE DE ODONTOLOGIA DE PORTO ALEGRE. REVISTA. Text in Portuguese; Summaries in English. 1958. s-a. per issue exchange basis only. adv. **Document type:** *Academic/Scholarly.* **Description:** Covers orthodontics, dental occlusion, pathology, preventive dentistry and dental care.
Formerly: Universidade Federal do Rio Grande do Sul. Faculdade de Odontologia. Revista (0477-6763)
Indexed: Bibliogr.Bras.Odontol., Dent.Ind.
Published by: Universidade Federal do Rio Grande do Sul, Faculdade de Odontologia, Rua Ramiro Barcelos, 2492, PO Box 1118, Porto Alegre, RGS 90035-003, Brazil. TEL 55-512-3165011, FAX 55-512-3165023. Ed. Pantelis Varvaki Rados. Circ: 3,500.

617.6 BRA
FACULDADE DE ODONTOLOGIA. REVISTA. Text in Portuguese. 1997. s-a. free per issue. **Document type:** *Academic/Scholarly.*
Published by: Universidade Federal de Goias, Faculdade de Odontologia, Av. Universitaria s-n, Setor Universitario, Goiania, Goias 74605-020, Brazil. TEL 55-62-261-2518, FAX 55-62-261-2518, cai@reitoria.ufg.br, http://www.ufg.br.

617.6 COL ISSN 0046-354X
FEDERACION ODONTOLOGICA COLOMBIANA. REVISTA. Text in Spanish. 1950. 4/yr. adv. illus.
Indexed: Dent.Ind., Ind.Med. (coverage dropped).
—BLDSC (7815.800000), GNLM.
Published by: Federacion Odontologica Colombiana, Calle 71, 11-10, Of 1101, Apartado Aereo 52925, Bogota, CUND, Colombia. Ed. Edmundo Alberto Noguera.

617.6 USA
FIFTH DISTRICT DENTAL SOCIETY, FRESNO, CALIFORNIA. BULLETIN. Text in English. 1953. bi-m. membership. adv. *Refereed.* **Document type:** *Newsletter.*
Former titles: Thirtieth District Dental Society, Fresno, California. Bulletin.; Thirteenth District Dental Society. Bulletin; Fifth District Dental Society. Bulletin (0071-9544)
Published by: Fresno-Madera Dental Society, 371 E Bullard Ave, Ste 120, Fresno, CA 93710-5217. TEL 559-438-7284, FAX 559-438-7287, fmds@pacdell.net. Ed. Dr. Treva Lee. R&P, Adv. contact Valjean Xaiz. Circ: 600.

FINLAND. LAAKINTOHALLITUS. LAAKARIT - LAKARE/FINLAND. MEDICINALSTYRELSEN. LAEKARE. see *MEDICAL SCIENCES*

M

614 USA ISSN 0092-3664
TD467
FLUORIDATION CENSUS. Text in English. 1954. quinquennial. free (effective 2001). **Document type:** *Government.*
Published by: National Center for Disease Prevention, Division of Oral Health, Program Services Branch, 4770 Buford Hwy NE, MS F-10, Atlanta, GA 30341-3717. TEL 770-488-6056, FAX 770-488-6080, ccdinfo@cdc.gov, http://www.cdc.gov/nohss.

FLUORIDE; journal of the international society for fluoride research. see *MEDICAL SCIENCES—Abstracting, Bibliographies, Statistics*

617.6 USA
FOCUS M D A. Text in English. 1934. every 6 wks. USD 12 to non-members; USD 5 to members (effective 1999). adv. bk.rev. illus. reprint service avail. from PQC. **Document type:** *Trade.*
Former titles: Missouri Dental Journal (0887-4646); (until 1985): Missouri Dental Association. Journal (0273-3463); (until I980): M D A Journal (0199-6584); (until 1979): Missouri Dental Association. Journal (0026-6523); (until 1961): Missouri State Dental Association. Journal (1041-1178)
Related titles: Microform ed.: (from PQC).
Indexed: Dent.Abstr., Dent.Ind., Med.Care Rev.
—BLDSC (3964.219250), GNLM.
Published by: Missouri Dental Association, 230 W McCarty St, Box 1707, Jefferson City, MO 65102. TEL 573-634-3436, FAX 573-635-0764, modental@sockits.net. Ed. Dr. Elizabeth Ward. Adv. contact Cristin Clark. B&W page USD 340; trim 9.5 x 7.25. Circ: 2,700.

617.6 USA ISSN 1042-2528
FOCUS ON OHIO DENTISTRY. Text in English. 1926. m. USD 60 to non-members; USD 15 to members (effective 2000). adv. **Document type:** *Newsletter.* **Description:** Includes information on legislation, regulations, nutrition, practice management, and new products related to dentistry.
—BLDSC (3964.232730).
Published by: Ohio Dental Association, 1370 Dublin Rd, Columbus, OH 43215-1098. TEL 614-486-2700, FAX 614-486-0381, dentist2oda.org, http://www.oda.org. Ed. Dr. Robert Buchholz. R&P Stacy Wendt. Adv. contact Amy Szmania. Circ: 5,500.

617.6 USA ISSN 0071-9285
LJ105.P75
FRATER OF PSI OMEGA. Text in English. 1901. 3/yr. membership. **Document type:** *Newsletter.*
Published by: Psi Omega Fraternity, 1040 Savannah Hwy, Charleston, SC 29407. Circ: 8,500.

617.6 DEU ISSN 0340-1766
DER FREIE ZAHNARZT. Text in German. 1958. m. DEM 4 (effective 1997 & 1998). bk.rev. **Document type:** *Trade.*
Formerly: Monatschrift Deutscher Zahnaerzte (0047-7842)
Indexed: Curr.Tit.Dent., Dent.Ind.
—CISTI, GNLM.
Published by: (Freier Verband Deutscher Zahnaerzte e.V.), Kern und Birner GmbH und Co., Werrastr 4, Frankfurt Am Main 60486, Germany. TEL 49-69-970807-0, FAX 49-69-9708076. Ed. Peter Kind. adv.: B&W page DEM 5,700, color page DEM 9,150; trim 253 x 185. Circ: 51,000.

617.643 CHE ISSN 1420-2433
CODEN: FROPBK
FRONTIERS OF ORAL BIOLOGY. Text in English. 1974. irreg., latest vol.11. CHF 180 in Europe; DEM 190 in Germany; USD 155 in United States (2001). reprint service avail. from ISI. *Refereed.* **Document type:** *Monographic series, Academic/Scholarly.* **Description:** Contains information on vital topics in the theoretical and technical development of dental and oral medicine.
Formerly: Frontiers of Oral Physiology (0301-536X)
Related titles: Online - full text ed.: (from Institute for Scientific Information).
Indexed: Biol.Abstr., Chem.Abstr., Chem.Indus.Notes, Chem.Titles, Curr.Cont. (coverage dropped), Ind.Med. (coverage dropped).
—BLDSC (4042.044000), CASDDS, CISTI, Infotrieve. **CCC.**
Published by: S. Karger AG, Allschwilerstr 10, PO Box, Basel 4009, Switzerland. TEL 41-61-306-1111, FAX 41-61-306-1234, karger@karger.ch, http://www.karger.com/bookseries/FORBI. Ed. R W A Linden.

617.6 USA ISSN 8756-3150
FUNCTIONAL ORTHODONTIST; a journal of functional jaw orthopedics. Text in English. 1984. q. USD 89 domestic; USD 99 foreign (effective 2000).
—BLDSC (4055.630000), GNLM, ingenta.
Address: c/o The AAFO, 106 S Kent St, Winchester, VA 22601. TEL 540-662-2200. Ed. Dr. Craig C Stoner.

617.6 GBR
THE G D P; the voice of general practice. Text in English. 1959. m. (10/yr.). GBP 60; GBP 6 newsstand/cover (effective 2000). adv. bk.rev., video rev. tr.lit. back issues avail. *Refereed.* **Document type:** *Academic/Scholarly.* **Description:** Covers political issues and negotiations with government.
Former titles (until 1998): General Dental Practitioner (0954-4186); (until 1988): Probe (0032-9185)
Indexed: Can.Mus.Per.Ind. (1990-1993), Dent.Ind.
—GNLM.
Published by: General Dental Practitioners Association, Victoria House, Victoria Rd, Barnsley, Yorks S70 2BB, United Kingdom. TEL 44-1303-252082, FAX 44-1303-240882, GDPJournal@hotmail.com. Ed., R&P Dr. Joe Sullivan. Adv. contact Freda Rimini. B&W page GBP 200, color page GBP 360. Circ: 2,500 (controlled).

617.6 USA
G M D A JOURNAL. Text in English. 1934. q. USD 30; USD 40 foreign. adv. charts, illus. **Document type:** *Bulletin.*
Former titles (until 1995): G M D A Bulletin (0884-6898); Greater Milwaukee Dental Bulletin (0017-3754)
Indexed: Dent.Ind.
—CISTI, GNLM.
Published by: Greater Milwaukee Dental Association, 111 E Wisconsin Ave, Ste 1300, Milwaukee, WI 53202-4807. TEL 414-276-9911. Ed. Dr. Anthony Ziebert. Adv. contact Nanci Dabareiner. Circ: 1,000.

617.6 ESP
GACETA DENTAL. Text in Spanish. m.
Published by: Pues S.L., Canillas, 2 (local, Madrid 28002, Spain. TEL 34-91-563-4907, FAX 34-91-564-3216. Ed. Jose Ma Herran. Circ: 17,000.

617.6 RUS
GAZETA DLA STOMATOLOGOV, ZUBNYCH TECHNIKOV... I NE TOLKO. Text in Russian.
Related titles: Online - full text ed.
Published by: OOO Neodent, ul. Fabrichnaya 5, Krasnodar 350018, Russian Federation. TEL 7-8612-398668, neodent@mail.kubtelecom.ru, http://www.stom.ru/kuban/. Ed. D. Orfanidi.

617.6 GBR ISSN 0072-0674
GENERAL DENTAL COUNCIL. DENTISTS REGISTER. Text in English. 1878. a. GBP 15.50 domestic; GBP 18.50 overseas. back issues avail. **Document type:** *Directory.*
Published by: General Dental Council, 37 Wimpole St, London W1M 8DQ, United Kingdom. TEL 44-20-7887-3800, FAX 44-20-7224-3294. Ed. Chris Collins.

617.6 GBR ISSN 0072-0682
GENERAL DENTAL COUNCIL. MINUTES OF THE PROCEEDINGS. Text in English. 1956. a. GBP 10. **Document type:** *Proceedings.*
Published by: General Dental Council, 37 Wimpole St, London W1M 8DQ, United Kingdom. TEL 44-20-7887-3800, FAX 44-20-7224-3294.

617.6 USA ISSN 0363-6771
GENERAL DENTISTRY. Text in English. 1952. bi-m. USD 30 domestic to individuals; USD 35 in Canada to individuals; USD 50 elsewhere to individuals; USD 48 domestic to institutions; USD 53 in Canada to institutions; USD 68 elsewhere to institutions (effective 2001). adv. bk.rev. illus. index. back issues avail. *Refereed.* **Document type:** *Academic/Scholarly.* **Description:** Features clinical data, techniques, self-instruction program for the general dentist.
Former titles: Academy of General Dentistry. Journal (0001-4265); Academy of General Dentistry. Bulletin (0098-3810)
Related titles: Microform ed.: (from PQC).
Indexed: Biol.Abstr., CINAHL, Dent.Abstr., Dent.Ind., Energy Res.Abstr., INIS Atomind.
—BLDSC (4103.430000), GNLM, ingenta. **CCC.**
Published by: Academy of General Dentistry, 211 E Chicago Ave, Ste 900, Chicago, IL 60611-1999. TEL 312-440-4300, 888-243-3368, FAX 312-440-4261, AGDJournal@agd.org, http://www.agd.org. Ed. Dr. Roger D Winland. R&P Jo-Ellyn Posselt TEL 312-440-4307. Adv. contact Todd Goldman. B&W page USD 3,075, color page USD 4,200. Circ: 65,000.
Subscr. to: Allen Press Inc.

617.6 USA
RK58.5
GETTING THROUGH DENTAL SCHOOL; A S D A's guide for dental students. Text in English. a. USD 20 domestic; USD 35 foreign (effective 2001). adv. **Document type:** *Directory.* **Description:** Reference guide for dental students. Contains information on applying to dental schools, financial aid, ASDA membership benefits, post doctoral opportunities.
Formerly: A S D A Handbook (0277-3619)
Published by: American Student Dental Association, 211 E Chicago Ave, Ste. 1160, Chicago, IL 60611-2616. TEL 312-440-2795, FAX 312-440-2820, asda@asdanet.org, editors@asdanet.org. Pub. Cynthia L Kennedy. R&P Lauren Waggoner. Adv. contact Stephanie Cesna TEL 312-440-2845. Circ: 18,000.

617.6 ITA ISSN 0393-067X
GIORNALE DELL'ODONTOIATRA/DENTAL FLASH. Text in Italian. 1984. 18/yr. ITL 27,000 (effective 1999).
Published by: Masson S.p.A., Divisione Periodici, Via F.lli Bressan 2, Milan, MI 20126, Italy. TEL 39-2-270741, FAX 39-2-27074210. adv.: B&W page ITL 3,420,000, color page ITL 4,570,000; trim 265 x 193. Circ: 19,000.

617.643 ITA ISSN 1122-1038
GIORNALE DI STOMATOLOGIA E DI ORTOGNATODONZIA. Text in Italian. 1982. q. USD 50. adv. bk.rev.
—GNLM.
Published by: Poliambulatorio Odontoiatrico Riunito S.r.l., Pza Castello, 9, Oderzo, TV 31046, Italy. Ed. Dr Lorenzo Favero. Circ: 5,000.

617.643 ITA
GIOVANE ODONTOIATRA. Cover title: G O - Giovane Odontoiatra. Text in Italian. 1984. 4/yr. ITL 39,000 (effective 1999). **Document type:** *Academic/Scholarly.*
Formerly: Bollettino Nazionale A I S O (1120-8686)
Published by: (Associazione Italiana Studenti in Odontoiatria), Masson S.p.A., Divisione Periodici, Via F.lli Bressan 2, Milan, MI 20126, Italy. TEL 39-2-270741, FAX 39-2-2707210. adv.: color page ITL 1,680,000; trim 265 x 193. Circ: 2,200.

617.6 USA ISSN 1062-0265
GREATER HOUSTON DENTAL SOCIETY. JOURNAL. Text in English. 1993 (vol.64, no.6). 9/yr. USD 50; USD 60 foreign (effective 1999). adv. *Refereed.* **Document type:** *Academic/Scholarly.*
—BLDSC (4757.639000).
Published by: Greater Houston Dental Society, One Greenway Plaza, Ste 110, Houston, TX 77046. TEL 713-961-4337, FAX 713-961-3617, ghds@flash.net, http://www.ghds.com. Ed. Dr. Janet Harrison. R&P, Adv. contact Charlotte Bolls. Circ: 1,700.

616.7 BEL ISSN 0303-7479
CODEN: BGEODI
GROUPEMENT INTERNATIONAL POUR LA RECHERCHE EN STOMATOLOGIE ET ODONTOLOGIE. BULLETIN. Text in French. 1957. q. EUR 95 in Europe to individuals; EUR 105 elsewhere to individuals; EUR 105 in Europe to institutions; EUR 115 elsewhere to institutions (effective 2000). adv. **Document type:** *Bulletin.*
Indexed: Curr.Adv.Ecol.Sci., Excerp.Med., Ind.Med. (coverage dropped).
—GNLM.
Published by: Groupement International pour la Recherche Stomatologie et Odontologie/International Group for Research in Stomatology and Odontology, Faculte de Medecine ULB Erasme, Rte de Lennik 808-621, Brussels 1070, Belgium. Ed. L Fonzi. Adv. contact G Anastasi.

617.6 USA
THE GUIDE TO IMPLANT RESEARCH. Text in English. irreg. **Document type:** *Magazine, Academic/Scholarly.* **Description:** Dedicated to international and university-based implant research.
Published by: Montage Media Corp., 1000 Wyckoff Ave, Mahwah, NJ 07430. TEL 201-891-3200, FAX 201-891-2626, info@montagemedia.com, http://www.montagemedia.com/ir.html.

617.6 TUR ISSN 0250-5207
HACETTEPE DIS HEKIMLIGI FAKULTESI DERGISI/HACETTEPE FACULTY OF DENTISTRY JOURNAL. Text in Turkish; Summaries in English, French, German. 1977. q. USD 60 to individuals; USD 100 foreign to individuals; USD 150 to institutions. *Refereed.* **Document type:** *Academic/Scholarly.* **Description:** Keeps dentists informed on research being done in the field of dentistry and related areas.

M

Published by: Hacettepe Universitesi, Dis Hekimligi Fakultesi/Hacettepe University, Faculty of Dentistry, Yayin Kurulu Sekreterligi, Sihhiye - Ankara 06100, Turkey. TEL 90-312-3116461, FAX 90-312-3091138. Ed. Ayhan Enacar. Circ: 1,200.

617.6 USA
HARTFORD DENTAL SOCIETY NEWSLETTER. Text in English. 1897. m. membership. **Document type:** *Newsletter, Trade.* **Description:** Announces upcoming meetings and programs, lists new members, course offerings, provides comment and editorial.
Published by: Hartford Dental Society, 230 Scarborough St, Hartford, CT 06105. TEL 860-523-8657, FAX 860-236-8401. Ed. Dr. Janel Johnson. R&P Joyce Cote. Circ: 600 (controlled).

617.6 USA ISSN 1062-029X
HARVARD DENTAL BULLETIN. Text in English. 1940. s-a. free per issue. illus. **Document type:** *Bulletin.* **Description:** Provides information on teaching, research and clinical activities of the school. Presents articles on students, faculty and alumni.
Former titles (until 1990): Harvard Dental Alumni Bulletin (0046-6891); Harvard Dental Record
Indexed: Ind.Med. (coverage dropped).
—BLDSC (4265.886100).
Published by: Harvard School of Dental Medicine, 188 Longwood Ave, Boston, MA 02115. TEL 617-432-1533, FAX 617-432-4266. Ed., R&P Patricia A Flint TEL 617-432-1534. Circ: 2,500 (controlled). **Co-sponsor:** Harvard Dental Alumni Association.

617.6 USA ISSN 0073-1021
HAWAII DENTAL ASSOCIATION. TRANSACTIONS. Text in English. a. **Document type:** *Academic/Scholarly.*
Published by: Hawaii Dental Association, 1345 S Beretania St, 301, Honolulu, HI 96814-1821. TEL 808-536-2135, FAX 808-536-2137. Ed. Dr. George Wessberg. Adv. contact Sherry Goya.

617.6 USA ISSN 0891-9933
HAWAII DENTAL JOURNAL. Text in English. 1967. m. USD 25 domestic; USD 30 foreign (effective 2000). adv. illus. **Document type:** *Academic/Scholarly.*
Formerly: Hawaii State Dental Association. Journal (0017-8616)
Indexed: Dent.Abstr., Dent.Ind.
—GNLM.
Published by: Hawaii Dental Association, 1345 S Beretania St, 301, Honolulu, HI 96814-1821. TEL 808-536-2135, FAX 808-536-2137, hda@lava.net. Ed. Dr. Wynn Okuda. Circ: 950 (controlled).

617.3 USA ISSN 0073-1404
HAYES DIRECTORY OF DENTAL SUPPLY HOUSES*. Text in English. 1935. a. USD 80. **Document type:** *Directory.*
Published by: Edward N. Hayes, Ed. & Pub., 4229 Birch St, Box 3436, Mission Viejo, CA 92690-1436. TEL 714-756-9063, FAX 714-756-0921.

HEALTHSTATE. see *MEDICAL SCIENCES*

617.6 GRC ISSN 1011-4181
HELLENIC STOMATOLOGICAL REVIEW. Text in Greek; Summaries in English. 1957. q. GRD 4,000, USD 30. adv. bk.rev. bibl, charts, illus. index. **Document type:** *Academic/Scholarly.*
Former titles: Hellenic Stomatological Annals; Acta Stomatologica Hellenica
—GNLM.
Published by: Hellenic Dental Association, 38 Themistocleous St, Athens 106 78, Greece. TEL 30-1-3803-816, FAX 30-1-3834-385. Circ: 7,000.

617.6 JPN ISSN 0046-7472
CODEN: HUDJAN
HIROSHIMA UNIVERSITY DENTAL SOCIETY. JOURNAL/HIROSHIMA DAIGAKU SHIGAKU ZASSHI. Text in English, Japanese. 1969. s-a. USD 12. adv. illus. reprint service avail. from PQC.
Related titles: Microform ed.: (from PQC).
Indexed: Chem.Abstr., Chem.Indus.Notes, Chem.Titles, Dent.Ind., INIS Atomind.
—BLDSC (4758.330000), CASDDS, GNLM, KNAW.
Published by: Hiroshima Daigaku Shigakkai/Hiroshima University Dental Society, Daigaku, 2-3 Kasumi 1-chome, Minami-ku, Hiroshima-shi 734-0037, Japan. Ed. Nobuo Nagasaka.

617.6 AUS
▼ **HISTOLOGY**; Royal Australasian College of Dental Surgeons. Lecture notes in histology. Text in English. 1999. irreg. AUD 36 newsstand/cover (effective 2001). 70 p./no. **Document type:** *Academic/Scholarly.* **Description:** Contains lecture notes in the basic sicence subject of oral histology.
Published by: Royal Australasian College of Dental Surgeons, 64 Castlereagh St, Sydney, NSW 2000, Australia. TEL 61-2-9232-3800, FAX 61-2-9221-8108, registrar@racds.org, http://www.racds.org. Circ: 132 (controlled).

617.6 CHN ISSN 1000-1182
RC815
HUAXI KOUQIANG YIXUE ZAZHI/WEST CHINA JOURNAL OF STOMATOLOGY. Text in Chinese; Summaries in English. 1983. q. CNY 7.20.
Indexed: Ind.Med. (1983-).
—GNLM.
Published by: Huaxi Yike Daxue/West China University of Medical Sciences, 17 Renmin Nanlu 3 Duan, Chengdu, Sichuan 610041, China. FAX 028-583252. Ed. Wang Hanzhang. **Co-sponsor:** Sichuan Branch of the Chinese Medical Association.

617.6 USA
I A O STRAIGHT TALK*. Text in English. 1968. m. USD 15; USD 20 foreign (effective 1998). back issues avail. **Document type:** *Newsletter.* **Description:** Contains news and concerns of association members.
Formerly: Bandelette
Published by: International Association for Orthodontics, 735 N. Water St., Ste. 617, Milwaykee, WI 53202-4104. TEL 708-445-0320, FAX 708-445-0321. Ed., R&P Detlef B Moore. Circ: 2,100 (controlled).

617.6 USA
I C D GLOBE*. Variant title: I C D Key. Text in English. 1970 (vol.2). a. membership.
Formerly: I C D Letterette (0018-8875)
Published by: International College of Dentists, PO Box 62258, Phoenix, AZ 85082-2258. TEL 602-248-9445. Circ: 6,000.

617.6 USA ISSN 1084-8282
RK1
ILLINOIS DENTAL NEWS. Text in English. 1905. m., latest vol.70, 2001. USD 45 to non-members; USD 75 foreign to non-members (effective 2001). adv. illus. 16 p./no. 4 cols./p. reprints avail. **Document type:** *Magazine, Trade.* **Description:** Contains news of interest, editorials, and official business of ISDS including legislative affairs and policies affecting the dental profession in Illinois.
Formerly (until 1995): Illinois Dental Journal (0019-1973)
Related titles: Microfiche ed.; Microfilm ed.: (from PQC).
Indexed: Chem.Abstr., Dent.Abstr., Dent.Ind.
—GNLM.
Published by: Illinois State Dental Society, 1010 S Second St, Springfield, IL 62705. TEL 217-525-1406, FAX 217-525-8872, http://www.isds.org. Ed. Dr. D Milton Salzer. R&P Lee Ann Beanne. Adv. contact Jennifer Walker. page USD 980; trim 14 x 10. Circ: 6,300 (controlled).

617.6 FRA ISSN 1254-2431
IMPLANT. Text in French. 1992. q. FRF 1,100 domestic; FRF 1,150 foreign (effective 2000). adv. bk.rev. back issues avail. **Document type:** *Academic/Scholarly.* **Description:** Provides a continuous update on current scientific, theoretical, experimental and clinical knowledge in the field of implantology.
Formerly (until 1994): Cahiers de Prothese. Implant (1286-9066)
Published by: Editions C D P, 1 ave. Edouard Belin, Rueil-Malmaison 92856, France. TEL 33-1-34633341, FAX 33-1-34633388. Ed. Xavier Assemat Tessandier. Pub. Stephane Tschanz. Adv. contact Sybille Barbera. B&W page FRF 5,900, color page FRF 10,100; 270 x 210. Circ: 2,500.

617.6 USA ISSN 1056-6163
IMPLANT DENTISTRY. Text in English. 1992. q. USD 182 domestic to individuals; USD 216 foreign to individuals; USD 225 domestic to institutions; USD 258 foreign to institutions; USD 62 newsstand/cover (effective 2002). adv. bk.rev. *Refereed.* **Document type:** *Academic/Scholarly.* **Description:** Scientific, clinical, educational and research articles on oral implantology and related dental and medical topics.
Former titles (until 1992): International Journal of Oral Implantology (1048-1842); Implantologist (0190-2024)
Related titles: Microfilm ed.: (from WWS).
Indexed: Dent.Abstr.
—BLDSC (4371.436300), CISTI, GNLM, ingenta.
Published by: (International Congress of Oral Implantologists), Williams & Wilkins (Subsidiary of: Waverly International), 351 W Camden St, Baltimore, MD 21201-2436. TEL 410-528-4068, 800-222-3790, FAX 410-528-4452, mricks@wwilkins.com, http://www.wwilkins.com, http://www.Lww.com. Ed. Dr. Sheldon Winkler. Adv. contact Melanie Ricks. B&W page USD 750; trim 10.88 x 8.13. Circ: 4,878; 4,782 (paid).

617.6 USA ISSN 1059-3489
IMPLANT SOCIETY; dedicated to the highest quality dentistry. Text in English. 1990. bi-m. USD 125. **Document type:** *Academic/Scholarly.*
—GNLM.
Published by: Implant Society, Inc., PO Box 1264, Westborough, MA 01581. TEL 617-621-7170, FAX 508-366-3637. Pub. Richard Ciambrone.

617.7 DEU ISSN 0943-9692
IMPLANTOLOGIE. Text in German. q. EUR 108 domestic; EUR 114 foreign; EUR 66 domestic to students; EUR 72 foreign to students (effective 2002). **Document type:** *Magazine, Academic/Scholarly.*
—GNLM.
Published by: Quintessenz Verlags GmbH, Ifenpfad 2-4, Berlin 12107, Germany. TEL 49-30-76180646, FAX 49-30-76180680, central@quintessenz.de, http://www.quintessenz.de.

617.6 615.842 IND ISSN 0972-1363
INDIAN ACADEMY OF ORAL MEDICINE AND RADIOLOGY. JOURNAL. Text in English. 4/yr. INR 400, USD 40 (effective 2000). adv. reprints avail. *Refereed.* **Description:** Aims at promoting research and academic activities concerning the speciality of Oral Medicine & Radiology.
Published by: The Indian Academy of Oral Medicine and Radiology, c/o P.K. Dayal, EIC, Associate Dean, College of Dental Surgery, Mangalore, Karnataka 575 001, India. TEL 91-824-423452, 91-824-442539, FAX 91-824-428183, dayalpk@hotmail.com. Ed., Pub. P K Dayal. adv.: page INR 1,500. Circ: 1,000.

617.6 IND ISSN 0019-4611
CODEN: IDAJA2
INDIAN DENTAL ASSOCIATION. JOURNAL. Text in English. 1925. m. INR 300, USD 70. bk.rev. abstr, charts, illus. index.
Former titles (until 1966): All India Dental Association. Journal (0377-0516); (until 1947): Indian Dental Journal (0971-1147)
Indexed: Dent.Abstr., Dent.Ind., INIS Atomind.
—CASDDS, CISTI, GNLM.
Published by: Indian Dental Association, 532, 10th Main, 5th Block, Jayanagar, Bangalore, Karnataka 560 041, India. TEL 91-253-78443, FAX 91-253-77234. Ed. K G Ghorpade. adv.: B&W page INR 2,500, color page INR 5,000. Circ: 3,000.

617.6 IND ISSN 0970-9290
INDIAN JOURNAL OF DENTAL RESEARCH. Text in English. 1989. q. INR 400 domestic; USD 40 foreign (effective 2000). adv. bk.rev. index. back issues avail. *Refereed.* **Document type:** *Academic/Scholarly.* **Description:** Aims to promote research activities in dental field.
Media: Fax. **Related titles:** Fax ed.
Indexed: Dent.Ind.
—BLDSC (4411.100000), GNLM.
Published by: Indian Society for Dental Research, College of Dental Surgery, Mangalore, Karnataka 575 001, India. TEL 91-824-423452, FAX 91-824-428183, dayalpk@hotmail.com. Ed. P K Dayal. Pub., Adv. contact P.K. Dayal. page INR 1,500; trim 220 x 160. Circ: 1,000.

617.6 IND ISSN 0970-4388
INDIAN SOCIETY OF PEDODONTICS AND PREVENTIVE DENTISTRY. JOURNAL. Text in English. 1983. q. INR 225 to individuals; INR 600 to institutions; USD 26 foreign.
—BLDSC (4768.900000), GNLM.
Published by: Indian Society of Pedodontics and Preventive Dentistry, c/o H.S. Chawka, Ed., Dept. of Dentistry, P.G.I.M.E.R., Chandigarh, Haryana 160 012, India. Ed. H S Chawla.

M

617.6 USA ISSN 0019-6568 CODEN: IDNJBY
INDIANA DENTAL ASSOCIATION. JOURNAL. Text in English. 1921. q. USD 25; USD 40 foreign (effective 1999). adv. bk.rev. charts. back issues avail. *Refereed.* **Document type:** *Trade.* **Description:** It provides a forum for dentists in practice. Articles in each issue address topics identified by members of the Indiana Dental Association and it also includes IDA membership news and benefits information.
Indexed: Dent.Abstr., Dent.Ind.
—BLDSC (4769.070000), GNLM.
Published by: Indiana Dental Association, 401 W Michigan St, Suite 1000, Indianapolis, IN 46202-3233. TEL 317-634-2610, FAX 317-634-2612, orders@allenpress.com, http://www.allenpress.com. Ed. Dr. H William Gilmore. R&P Jennifer Hawke. Adv. contact Jody Cleary. Circ: 3,000. **Subscr. to:** Allen Press Inc., PO Box 1897, Lawrence, KS 66044-8897.

617.6 USA
INDIANAPOLIS DISTRICT DENTAL SOCIETY. NEWSLETTER✶ . Text in English. 1957 (vol.11). q. USD 35. adv. bk.rev. **Document type:** *Newsletter.*
Formerly: Indianapolis District Dental Society. Journal (0073-7135)
Published by: Indianapolis District Dental Society, 8780 Purdue Rd, Ste 8, Indianapolis, IN 46268-1173. TEL 317-923-8421, FAX 317-923-8575. Ed. Dr. Desiree Dimond. Adv. contact Sara M Snyder. Circ: 860.

INDICE DE LA LITERATURA DENTAL EN CASTELLANO. see *MEDICAL SCIENCES—Abstracting, Bibliographies, Statistics*

617.6 ITA
INFODENT INTERNATIONAL. Text in Italian. 198?. q. USD 34, EUR 30. adv. **Document type:** *Trade.*
Formerly (until 1994): Infodent
Published by: B & C s.r.l., Via Str Teverina Km, 3600, Viterbo, VT 01100, Italy. TEL 39-07-61393218, FAX 39-07-61393222. Ed. Tina Persson. adv.: color page ITL 3,500,000; trim 280 x 210. Circ: 13,000.

617.6 FRA ISSN 0020-0018
INFORMATION DENTAIRE; hebdomadaire independant. Text in French. 1918. 44/yr. FRF 930 (effective 2000). adv. bk.rev. abstr. illus. reprint service avail. from ISI.
Indexed: Biol.Abstr., Chem.Abstr., Curr.Tit.Dent., Dent.Ind., Dok.Arbeitsmed.
—BLDSC (4493.530000), CISTI, GNLM.
Address: 40 av. Bugeaud, Paris Cedex 16 75784, France. TEL 33-1-56265000, FAX 33-1-56265001, http://www.information-dentaire.com. Eds. Marylene Scagni, Sophie Bour. Pub. Marylene Scagni. Adv. contact Florence Gouaux. Circ: 20,000.

617.43 DEU ISSN 0020-0336
INFORMATIONEN AUS ORTHODONTIE UND KIEFERORTHOPAEDIE. Text in German. 1968. q. EUR 212.80 domestic to institutions; EUR 215.90 in Europe to institutions; EUR 219.80 elsewhere to institutions; EUR 55 newsstand/cover (effective 2002). adv. bk.rev. illus. **Document type:** *Journal, Academic/Scholarly.*
Related titles: Online - full text ed.: ISSN 1439-4200.
Indexed: Dent.Ind.
—GNLM.
Published by: Georg Thieme Verlag, Ruedigerstr 14, Stuttgart 70469, Germany. TEL 49-711-8931-0, FAX 49-711-8931258, iok@medizinverlage.de, kunden.service@thieme.de, http://www.thieme.de/iok. adv.: B&W page DEM 1,900; trim 210 x 275. Circ: 2,400.

617.6 618.97 USA ISSN 0887-6304
INTERFACE (CHICAGO, 1984). Text in English. 1984. q. USD 25. adv. **Document type:** *Newsletter.*
Published by: American Society for Geriatric Dentistry, 211 E Chicago Ave, Chicago, IL 60611. TEL 312-440-2660. Ed. Gretchen Gibson. R&P John S Rutkovskas. Adv. contact John S Rutkavskas. Circ: 600.

617.632 GBR ISSN 1466-2094
INTERNATIONAL ACADEMY OF PERIODONTOLOGY. JOURNAL. Text in English. q. adv.
—BLDSC (4802.067700).
Published by: FDI World Dental Press Ltd., IAP Secretariat, 7 Carlisle St, London W1V 5RG, United Kingdom. TEL 44-207-9357852, FAX 44-207-4860183, iap@fdi.org.uk. Ed. Dr. Mark Patters.

INTERNATIONAL ASSOCIATION FOR DENTAL RESEARCH. ABSTRACTS OF THE GENERAL MEETING. see *MEDICAL SCIENCES—Abstracting, Bibliographies, Statistics*

617.6 GBR ISSN 0257-2796
INTERNATIONAL COLLEGE OF DENTISTS. EUROPEAN SECTION. NEWSLETTER. Text in English. 1956. a. membership. bk.rev. **Document type:** *Newsletter.*
Published by: (International College of Dentists), F D I World Dental Press Ltd., 7 Carlisle St, London W1V 5RG, United Kingdom. TEL 44-2079-357852, FAX 44-2074-860183. Ed. Dr. M Seward. Circ: 600.

617.6 USA
INTERNATIONAL COLLEGE OF DENTISTS. KEY; journal of events. Text in English. a. **Description:** Publishes report of past meetings, promotions, future meetings, biography of leaders, reports from districts.
Published by: International College of Dentists, 51 Monroe St, Ste 1501, Rockville, MD 20850-2408. TEL 301-251-8861, FAX 301-738-9143. Ed. Robert L Smith. Circ: 4,800.

617.6 USA ISSN 1057-5235
INTERNATIONAL COMMUNICATOR✶ . Text in English. 1976. 2/yr. membership. **Document type:** *Newsletter, Directory.* **Description:** Informs membership of news, actions of the Board of Regents, and meetings.
Published by: Academy of Dentistry International, PO Box 307, Hicksville, OH 43526-0307. TEL 202-364-8349, FAX 202-364-8349, adintl@mindspring.com, http://www.adint.org. Eds. Dr. Henry J Sazima, Robert L Ramus. R&P Dr. Henry J Sazima. Circ: 2,500 (controlled).

617.6 GBR ISSN 0020-6539 CODEN: IDJOAS
INTERNATIONAL DENTAL JOURNAL. Text in English. 1951. bi-m. GBP 63 in Europe to non-members; GBP 68 rest of world to non-members; GBP 40 in Europe to members; GBP 100 in Europe to institutional members; GBP 105 rest of world to institutional members (effective 1999). adv. bk.rev. illus, abstr. index. reprint service avail. from PQC. **Document type:** *Academic/Scholarly.* **Description:** Peer reviewed papers/research on clinical dentistry of international interest and significance.
Related titles: Microfilm ed.: (from PQC); Online - full text ed.: (from Institute for Scientific Information).
Indexed: Biol.Abstr., Chem.Abstr., Curr.Adv.Ecol.Sci., Curr.Cont., Curr.Tit.Dent., Dent.Ind., Dok.Arbeitsmed., Environ.Sci.Poll.Mgmt., Ind.Med. (1950-), Ind.Sci.Rev., NRN, Nutr.Abstr., Pollut.Abstr., Saf.Sci.Abstr., Sci.Cit.Ind. (coverage dropped).
—BLDSC (4539.520000), CASDDS, CISTI, GNLM, ingenta.
Published by: F D I World Dental Press Ltd., 7 Carlisle St, London W1V 5RG, United Kingdom. TEL 44-2079-357852, FAX 44-2074-860183. Ed. Dr. Margaret Seward. Circ: 3,000.

617.6 GBR ISSN 0143-2885 CODEN: IENJEA
INTERNATIONAL ENDODONTIC JOURNAL. Text in English. 1981 (vol.14). 8/yr., latest vol.35, 2002. GBP 208 in Europe to individuals; USD 330 in North America to individuals; GBP 229 elsewhere to individuals; GBP 449 in Europe to institutions; USD 712 in North America to institutions; GBP 494 elsewhere to institutions (effective 2002). adv. bibl, illus. index. back issues avail. *Refereed.* **Document type:** *Journal, Academic/Scholarly.* **Description:** Contains research into the diseases of the dental pulp and periapical tissues, and their treatment.
Formerly (until 1980): British Endodontic Society Journal (0007-0653)
Related titles: ♦ Online - full text ed.: International Endodontic Journal Online. ISSN 1365-2591.
Indexed: ASCA, Curr.Cont., Curr.Tit.Dent., Dent.Ind., Inpharma, Reac., Rev.Med.& Vet.Mycol., SSCI (coverage dropped).
—BLDSC (4539.975000), CISTI, GNLM, IDS, ingenta. CCC.
Published by: (British Endodontic Society), Blackwell Science Ltd., PO Box 88, Oxford OX2 0NE, United Kingdom. TEL 44-1865-206180, 44-1865-206002, FAX 44-1865-206219, jnl.orders@blacksci.co.uk, http://www.blackwell-science.com/~cgilib/jnlpage.asp?Journal=iej&File=iej, http://www.blackwellpublishing.com. Ed. P Dummer. Pub. Elaine Stott. R&P Sophie Savage. Adv. contact Jenny Applin. Circ: 2,300. **Co-sponsors:** Dutch Society for Endodontology; European Society of Endodontology; Portuguese Society of Endodontology; Irish Endodonic Society.

617.6 GBR ISSN 1365-2591
▼ **INTERNATIONAL ENDODONTIC JOURNAL ONLINE.** Text in English. 1999. 8/yr. GBP 188 in Europe to individuals; USD 297 in North America to individuals; GBP 188 elsewhere to individuals; GBP 405 in Europe to institutions; USD 641 in North America to institutions; GBP 405 elsewhere to institutions (effective 2002). *Refereed.* **Document type:** *Academic/Scholarly.*
Media: Online - full text (from EBSCO Publishing, O C L C Online Computer Library Center, Inc., RoweCom Information Quest, ingenta, Munksgaard & Blackwell Science's Synergy, Swets Blackwell, Institute for Scientific Information). **Related titles:** ♦ Print ed.: International Endodontic Journal. ISSN 0143-2885.
Published by: Blackwell Science Ltd., Osney Mead, Oxford OX2 0EL, United Kingdom. TEL 44-1685-206206, FAX 44-1685-721205, website@blacksci.com, journals.cs@blacksci.co.uk, http://www.blackwell-science.com/~cgilib/jnlpage.bin?Journal=iej&File=iej&Page=aims.

617.6 617 USA ISSN 0742-1931 CODEN: IAOSEE
INTERNATIONAL JOURNAL OF ADULT ORTHODONTICS AND ORTHOGNATHIC SURGERY. Text in English. 1986. q. USD 116, GBP 83, EUR 132 to individuals; USD 166, GBP 119, EUR 188 to institutions; USD 76, GBP 54, EUR 86 to students (effective 2002). adv. charts, illus. index. back issues avail. *Refereed.* **Document type:** *Magazine, Trade.* **Description:** Conveys advances in orthodontics and orthognathic surgery care of interest to general practitioners, orthodontists, oral surgeons and periodontists.
Related titles: Online - full text ed.
Indexed: Curr.Tit.Dent., Dent.Abstr.
—BLDSC (4541.571000), CISTI, GNLM, Infotrieve, ingenta. CCC.
Published by: Quintessence Publishing Co., Inc., 551 Kimberly Dr, Carol Stream, IL 60188-1881. TEL 630-682-3223, FAX 630-682-3288, quintpub@aol.com, http://www.quintpub.com. Eds. Dr. Raymond White, Dr. Robert Vanarsdall. Pub. H W Haase. R&P Kathy Monteleone. Adv. contact William G Hartman. Circ: 3,200.

617.607 DEU ISSN 1463-4201
INTERNATIONAL JOURNAL OF COMPUTERIZED DENTISTRY; computer application in clinical treatment. Text in English. 1998. 4/yr. EUR 88, USD 78, GBP 70; EUR 46, USD 40, GBP 43 to students (effective 2002). **Document type:** *Journal, Academic/Scholarly.*
—BLDSC (4542.175300).
Published by: Quintessenz Verlags GmbH, Ifenpfad 2-4, Berlin 12107, Germany. TEL 49-30-74006-0, FAX 49-30-7415080, central@quintessenz.de, http://www.quintessenz.de.

617.6 USA
INTERNATIONAL JOURNAL OF DENTAL SYMPOSIA. Text in English. 1993. irreg. **Document type:** *Magazine, Trade.* **Description:** Showcases the exceptional dental techniques presented during leading conferences and symposia by national and international professionals.
Published by: Montage Media Corp., 1000 Wyckoff Ave, Mahwah, NJ 07430. TEL 201-891-3200, FAX 201-891-2626, info@montagemedia.com, http://www.montagemedia.com/jds.html.

617.6 USA ISSN 0882-2786 CODEN: IJOIED
INTERNATIONAL JOURNAL OF ORAL & MAXILLOFACIAL IMPLANTS. Text in English. 1986. bi-m. USD 176, GBP 126, EUR 198 to individuals; USD 250, GBP 179, EUR 282 to institutions; USD 115, GBP 81, EUR 130 to students (effective 2002). adv. charts, illus. index. back issues avail. *Refereed.* **Document type:** *Magazine, Trade.* **Description:** Tracks developments in reconstructive dentistry and implantology by compiling research, technology, clinical applications, symposia proceedings and review treatises.
Related titles: Online - full text ed.: (from Institute for Scientific Information).
Indexed: Curr.Cont., Dent.Abstr., Excerp.Med., INIS Atomind., Ind.Med. (1986-), Inpharma, Reac., Sci.Cit.Ind.
—BLDSC (4542.429600), CISTI, GNLM, IDS, ingenta. CCC.
Published by: (Academy of Osseointegration), Quintessence Publishing Co., Inc., 551 Kimberly Dr, Carol Stream, IL 60188-1881. TEL 630-682-3223, FAX 630-682-3288, quintpub@aol.com, http://www.quintpub.com. Ed. Dr. William Laney. Pub. H W Haase. Adv. contact William G Hartman. Circ: 6,800.

M

617.6 GBR ISSN 0901-5027 CODEN: IJOSE9
INTERNATIONAL JOURNAL OF ORAL & MAXILLOFACIAL SURGERY. Text in English. 1972. bi-m. GBP 278 to individuals (effective 2002). adv. bk.rev. charts, illus. reprint service avail. from SWZ,ISI. *Refereed.* **Document type:** *Academic/Scholarly.* **Description:** Covers work in oral and maxillofacial surgery and supporting specialies, including interactions with neighboring surgical specialties.
Formerly: International Journal of Oral Surgery (0300-9785)
Related titles: Online - full text ed.: (from Ovid Technologies, Inc., EBSCO Publishing, O C L C Online Computer Library Center, Inc., RoweCom Information Quest, Munksgaard & Blackwell Science's Synergy, Swets Blackwell, IDEAL Online Library, Institute for Scientific Information).
Indexed: ASCA, Biol.Abstr., C.I.J.E. (coverage dropped), Chem.Abstr., Curr.Cont., Curr.Tit.Dent., Dent.Abstr., Dent.Ind., Excerp.Med., INIS Atomind., Ind.Med. (1986-), Ind.Sci.Rev., Ind.Vet., Inpharma, Nutr.Abstr., Reac., Rev.Appl.Entomol., Sci.Cit.Ind.
—BLDSC (4542.429800), CASDDS, CISTI, EMDOCS, GNLM, IDS, ingenta, KNAW. **CCC.**
Published by: (International Association of Oral and Maxillofacial Surgeons DNK), Churchill Livingstone (Subsidiary of: Harcourt Publishers Ltd.), Robert Stevenson House, 1-3 Baxter's Pl, Leith Walk, Edinburgh, Midlothian EH1 3AF, United Kingdom. TEL 44-131-556-2424, FAX 44-131-489-1177, cservice@harcourt.com. Circ: 3,200. **Subscr. to:** Harcourt Publishers Ltd., Foots Cray High St, Sidcup, Kent DA14 5HP, United Kingdom. TEL 44-20-8308-5700, FAX 44-20-8309-0807.

617.6 GBR ISSN 0960-7439 CODEN: IJPDE3
INTERNATIONAL JOURNAL OF PAEDIATRIC DENTISTRY. Text in English. 1971. q., latest vol.12, 2002. GBP 359 in Europe; USD 569 in North America; GBP 395 elsewhere (effective 2002). adv. bk.rev. abstr, illus. index. back issues avail. *Refereed.* **Document type:** *Academic/Scholarly.*
Incorporates (in 1991): International Association of Dentistry for Children. Journal (0309-6858); Former titles: Journal of Paediatric Dentistry (0267-2073); British Paedodontic Society. Proceedings (0308-4922)
Related titles: Microform ed.: (from PQC); ♦ Online - full text ed.: International Journal of Paediatric Dentistry Online. ISSN 1365-263X.
—GNLM, Infotrieve. **CCC.**
Published by: (British Society of Paediatric Dentistry), Blackwell Science Ltd., PO Box 88, Oxford OX2 0NE, United Kingdom. TEL 44-1865-206180, 44-1865-206002, FAX 44-1865-206219, jnl.orders@blacksci.co.uk, http://www.blackwell-science.com/~cgilib/jnlpage.asp?Journal=ijpd&File=ijpd, http://www.blackwellpublishing.com. Pub. Elaine Stott. R&P Sophie Savage. Adv. contact Jenny Applin. Circ: 1,470. **Co-sponsor:** International Association of Paediatric Dentistry.

617.6 GBR ISSN 1365-263X
INTERNATIONAL JOURNAL OF PAEDIATRIC DENTISTRY ONLINE. Text in English. 1998. bi-m. GBP 324 in Europe; USD 513 in North America; GBP 324 elsewhere (effective 2002). *Refereed.* **Document type:** *Academic/Scholarly.*
Media: Online - full text (from EBSCO Publishing, Munksgaard & Blackwell Science's Synergy, Swets Blackwell, RoweCom Information Quest). **Related titles:** Microform ed.: (from PQC); ♦ Print ed.: International Journal of Paediatric Dentistry. ISSN 0960-7439.
Published by: Blackwell Science Ltd., Osney Mead, Oxford OX2 0EL, United Kingdom. TEL 44-1685-206206, FAX 44-1685-721205, website@blacksci.com, journals.cs@blacksci.co.uk, http://www.blackwell-science.com.

617.6 USA ISSN 0198-7569
INTERNATIONAL JOURNAL OF PERIODONTICS & RESTORATIVE DENTISTRY. Text in English. 1981. bi-m. USD 225, GBP 160, EUR 254 to individuals; USD 326, GBP 233, EUR 366 to institutions; USD 178, GBP 127, EUR 200 to students (effective 2002). adv. charts, illus. index. back issues avail. *Refereed.* **Document type:** *Magazine, Academic/Scholarly.* **Description:** Provides clinically oriented coverage of the relationship between a healthy periodontium and precise restorations.
Related titles: Online - full text ed.: (from Institute for Scientific Information); ♦ German ed.: Internationales Journal fuer Paradontologie und Restaurative Zahnheilkund. ISSN 0721-0051; Japanese ed.; Italian ed.: Revista Internazionale di Parodontologia & Odontoiatria Ricostruttiva. ISSN 0721-006X; Spanish ed.: Revista Internacional de Periodoncia y Odontologia Restauradora. ISSN 0275-2867.
Indexed: ASCA, Curr.Cont., Curr.Tit.Dent., Dent.Abstr., Sci.Cit.Ind.
—BLDSC (4542.452400), GNLM, IDS, ingenta. **CCC.**
Published by: Quintessence Publishing Co., Inc., 551 Kimberly Dr, Carol Stream, IL 60188-1881. TEL 630-682-3223, FAX 630-682-3288, quintpub@aol.com, http://www.quintpub.com. Ed. Dr. Myron Nevins. Pub. H W Haase. Adv. contact William G Hartman. Circ: 5,800.

617.6 USA ISSN 0893-2174 CODEN: IJLPEJ
INTERNATIONAL JOURNAL OF PROSTHODONTICS. Text in English. 1988. bi-m. USD 158, GBP 113, EUR 178 to individuals; USD 228, GBP 163, EUR 258 to institutions; USD 108, GBP 77 to students (effective 2002). adv. charts, illus. index. back issues avail. *Refereed.* **Document type:** *Magazine, Academic/Scholarly.* **Description:** Provides prosthodontists throughout the world with research articles on prosthodontics and interrelated disciplines.
Related titles: Online - full text ed.: (from Institute for Scientific Information).
Indexed: Curr.Cont., Dent.Abstr., Inpharma, Reac.
—BLDSC (4542.488000), GNLM, IDS, Infotrieve. **CCC.**
Published by: (International College of Prosthodontists), Quintessence Publishing Co., Inc., 551 Kimberly Dr, Carol Stream, IL 60188-1881. TEL 630-682-3223, FAX 630-682-3288, quintpub@aol.com. Ed. Dr. Gunnar E Carlson. Pub. H W Haase. Adv. contact William G Hartman. Circ: 3,100.

617.6 DEU ISSN 0721-0051
INTERNATIONALES JOURNAL FUER PARADONTOLOGIE UND RESTAURATIVE ZAHNHEILKUND. Text in German. 1981. bi-m. EUR 165 domestic; EUR 180 foreign; EUR 98 domestic to students; EUR 115 foreign to students (effective 2002). **Document type:** *Magazine, Academic/Scholarly.*
Related titles: ♦ English ed.: International Journal of Periodontics & Restorative Dentistry. ISSN 0198-7569; Italian ed.: Revista Internazionale di Parodontologia & Odontoiatria Ricostruttiva. ISSN 0721-006X; Spanish ed.: Revista Internacional de Periodoncia y Odontologia Restauradora. ISSN 0275-2867.
Indexed: Curr.Tit.Dent., Inpharma, Reac.
Published by: Quintessenz Verlags GmbH, Ifenpfad 2-4, Berlin 12107, Germany. TEL 49-30-76180646, FAX 49-30-76180680, central@quintessenz.de, http://www.quintessenz.de.

617.6 USA ISSN 0021-0498
IOWA DENTAL JOURNAL. Text in English. 1929 (vol.15). 4/yr. USD 30; USD 35 foreign. adv. bk.rev. charts, illus, stat. **Document type:** *Trade.*
Indexed: Curr.Tit.Dent., Dent.Abstr., Dent.Ind.
—CISTI, GNLM.
Published by: (Iowa Dental Association), Sutherland Printing, 505 5th Ave, Ste 333, Des Moines, IA 50309-2379. TEL 515-282-7250, FAX 515-282-7256. Ed., R&P Dr. Francis Keith. Adv. contact Barbara Blough. Circ: 2,250.

ISHI SHIKAISHI YAKUZAISHI CHOSA/SURVEY ON PHYSICIANS, DENTISTS AND PHARMACEUTISTS. see *MEDICAL SCIENCES*

617.6 JPN ISSN 0385-1311
IWATE MEDICAL UNIVERSITY. DENTAL JOURNAL/IWATE IKA DAIGAKU SHIGAKU ZASSHI. Text in Japanese; Summaries in English. 1976. 3/yr. JPY 4,000, USD 32. back issues avail. **Document type:** *Academic/Scholarly.*
Indexed: INIS Atomind.
Published by: Iwate Medical University, Dental Society, c/o Iwate Ika Daigaku Shigakubu, 3-27 Chuodori 1-chome, Morioka, Iwate-ken 020-0021, Japan. TEL 81-196-51-5111, FAX 81-196-52-4131. Ed. Dr. Yohichiro Nozaka. Pub. Takashi A Suzuki. Circ: 900.

617.7 ITA ISSN 0393-800X
J D; rivista d'informazione dentale. (Junior Dental) Text in Italian. 1986. q. free in Italy. adv. bk.rev. illus. index. 24 p./no. **Document type:** *Newspaper.*
Published by: Imadent s.n.c., Via Locana, 14-A, Turin, TO 10143, Italy. TEL 39-011-7492333, FAX 39-011-747718, imadent@nevib.it, imadent_snc@libero.it. Ed. Federico Manassero. adv.: B&W page ITL 1,650,000; 195 x 265. Circ: 20,000.

617.6 CAN ISSN 0845-9320
J D Q: JOURNAL DENTAIRE DU QUEBEC. Text in English, French. 1963. 10/yr. CND 69.88; CND 80 foreign (effective 1999). adv. bk.rev. charts, illus. cum.index: 1963-1966. **Document type:** *Academic/Scholarly.*
Formerly (until 1987): Journal Dentaire du Quebec (0021-7999)
Indexed: Dent.Ind., Pt.de Rep. (1988-).
—BLDSC (4968.400000), CISTI, GNLM.
Published by: Ordre des Dentistes du Quebec, 625 Rene Levesque Ouest 15th Fl, Montreal, PQ H3B 1R2, Canada. TEL 514-875-8511, FAX 514-393-9248, journal@odq.qc.ca, http://www.odq.qc.ca. Ed., R&P Denis Forest. Adv. contact Johanne Erdelyon. Circ: 5,100.

617.6 JAM
JAMAICA DENTAL ASSOCIATION. NEWSLETTER. Text in English. irreg. **Document type:** *Newsletter.*
Published by: Jamaica Dental Association, PO Box 19, Kingston 5, Jamaica.

617.6 IRN
JAME'E DANDANPEZESHKI IRAN. NAMAH-I/IRANIAN DENTAL ASSOCIATION. BULLETIN. Text in Persian, Modern. m.
Published by: (Iranian Dental Association), Hamid Adeli-Najafi, Ed. & Pub., No. 94, W. Piroozi Str., Nasr Place, P O Box 14155-3695, Tehran, Iran. TEL 98-21-639591, FAX 98-21-639592.

617.6 JPN ISSN 0021-5163 CODEN: NGGZAK
JAPANESE JOURNAL OF ORAL AND MAXILLOFACIAL SURGERY. Key Title: Nippon Koku Geka Gakkai Zasshi. Text mainly in Japanese. 1954. bi-m. adv. charts, illus. index.
Formerly: Japanese Journal of Oral Surgery (0454-1693)
Related titles: Diskette ed.: USD 49.95 per issue (effective 2000).
Indexed: Chem.Abstr., Chem.Indus.Notes, Chem.Titles, Dent.Ind., INIS Atomind.
—BLDSC (4656.785000), CISTI. **CCC.**
Published by: Japanese Society of Oral and Maxillofacial Surgeons/Nippon Koku Geka Gakkai, 1-15-2-502 Nakaza-To, Kita-ku, Tokyo 114-0015, Japan. Circ: 2,500 (controlled).

617.6 FRA ISSN 1256-6128
JOURNAL DE PARODONTOLOGIE ET D'IMPLANTOLOGIE ORALE. Abbreviated title: J P I O. Text in English, French. 1982. q. FRF 950 to individuals; FRF 410 to students; FRF 300 newsstand/cover. adv. **Document type:** *Academic/Scholarly.* **Description:** For specialists and general practitioners interested in the connective tissues of the teeth and their influence on odontology and general health.
Formerly (until 1994): Journal de Parodontologie (0750-1838)
—BLDSC (5029.260000), GNLM.
Published by: (Societe Francaise de Parodontologie), Editions C D P, 1 av. Edward Belin, Rueil Malmaison 92856, France. TEL 33-1-34633333, FAX 33-1-34633388. Adv. contact Sybille Barbera. Circ: 3,500.

617.6 BEL ISSN 1370-2602
LE JOURNAL DU DENTISTE. Text in French. 1990. s-m. EUR 49 (effective 2001). 8 p./no. 5 cols./p. **Document type:** *Newspaper.*
Related titles: Diskette ed.
Published by: Medical Integrated Communication, Rue du Duc 94, Brussels 1150, Belgium. TEL 32-2-7706847, FAX 32-2-7792171, micbel@skynet.be. Ed. Beatrice Couteaux. Circ: 8,000.

617.6 USA ISSN 1461-5185
▼ **THE JOURNAL OF ADHESIVE DENTISTRY.** Text in English. 1999. 4/yr. USD 68, GBP 63, EUR 78; USD 35, GBP 39, EUR 40 to students (effective 2002). **Document type:** *Journal, Academic/Scholarly.*
—BLDSC (4918.937000).
Published by: Quintessence Publishing Co., Inc., 551 Kimberly Dr, Carol Stream, IL 60188-1881. TEL 630-682-3223, FAX 630-682-3288, quintpub@aol.com, http://www.quintpub.com. Eds. Dr. Jean-Francois Roulet, Dr. Michel Degrange.

617.3 USA ISSN 0895-8831
THE JOURNAL OF CLINICAL DENTISTRY; the international journal of applied dental research. Text in English. 1988. q. USD 70; USD 100 foreign (effective 1999). *Refereed.* **Document type:** *Academic/Scholarly.* **Description:** Dedicated to the rapid dissemination of significant laboratory and clinical dental product research and reviews.
Indexed: Curr.Cont. (coverage dropped), Excerp.Med., Inpharma, Reac.
—BLDSC (4958.389000), GNLM.
Published by: Professional Audience Communications, Inc., PO Box 243, Yardley, PA 19067. TEL 215-493-7400, FAX 215-493-9804, dntlpblshr@jclindent.com, http://jclindent.com. Ed. Dr. Robert Emling. Pub. Stephen Siegel.

617.643 USA ISSN 0022-3875
JOURNAL OF CLINICAL ORTHODONTICS. Text in English. 1967. m. USD 147 domestic to individuals; USD 195 foreign to individuals; USD 205 domestic to institutions; USD 245 foreign to institutions (effective 2000 - 2001). adv. bk.rev. index. back issues avail. *Refereed.* **Document type:** *Academic/Scholarly.*
Indexed: Curr.Tit.Dent., Dent.Abstr., Dent.Ind.
—BLDSC (4958.630000), CISTI, GNLM, ingenta.
Published by: J C O Inc., 1828 Pearl St, Boulder, CO 80302. FAX 303-443-9356. Ed. David Vogels. Adv. contact Lynn Bollinger. Circ: 11,000.

617.6 618.92 USA ISSN 1053-4628
RK55.C5 CODEN: JCPDEX
JOURNAL OF CLINICAL PEDIATRIC DENTISTRY. Text in English. 1977. q. USD 129 domestic to individuals; USD 149 foreign to individuals; USD 139 domestic to institutions; USD 159 foreign to institutions (effective 2000). bk.rev. index. reprint service avail. from PQC. *Refereed.* **Document type:** *Academic/Scholarly.*
Formerly: Journal of Pedodontics (0145-5508)
Related titles: Microform ed.: (from PQC).
Indexed: Behav.Med.Abstr., Biol.Abstr., Chem.Abstr., Dent.Abstr., Dent.Ind., Excerp.Med.
—BLDSC (4958.665000), CASDDS, CISTI, GNLM, ingenta.
Address: Tufts University, School of Dental Medicine, Dept of Pediatric Dentistry, 1 Kneeland St, Boston, MA 02111. TEL 617-636-6902, FAX 205-995-1588, jcpd@world.std.com, http://www.pediatricdentistry.com. Ed., R&P Dr. George E White. Circ: 2,600. **Subscr. to:** PO Box 830259, Birmingham, AL 35283-0259.

617.6 DNK ISSN 0303-6979
CODEN: JCPEDZ
JOURNAL OF CLINICAL PERIODONTOLOGY. Text in English; Summaries in German, French. 1974. m. USD 370 in the Americas to institutions print & online eds. combined; GBP 257 elsewhere to institutions print and online eds combined (effective 2002). adv. illus. reprint service avail. from SWZ,ISI. *Refereed.* **Document type:** *Journal, Academic/Scholarly.*
Related titles: Microform ed.: (from SWZ); Online - full text ed.: DKK 2,412 (2001) (from Ovid Technologies, Inc., EBSCO Publishing, ingenta, Munksgaard & Blackwell Science's Synergy, Swets Blackwell, Institute for Scientific Information).
Indexed: ASCA, Biol.Abstr., Chem.Abstr., Chem.Indus.Notes, Curr.Cont., Curr.Tit.Dent., Dent.Abstr., Dent.Ind., Environ.Sci.Poll.Mgmt., Excerp.Med., Ind.Med. (1974-), Ind.Sci.Rev., Inpharma, Pharm.&Out.News, Pollut.Abstr., Reac., Rev.Arom.& Med.Plants, Risk Abstr., Saf.Sci.Abstr., Sci.Cit.Ind.
—BLDSC (4958.672000), CASDDS, CISTI, EMDOCS, GNLM, IDS, ingenta, KNAW. **CCC.**
Published by: (European Federation of Periodontology), Blackwell Munksgaard, Noerre Soegade 35, PO Box 2148, Copenhagen K 1016, Denmark. TEL 45-77-33-33-33, FAX 45-77-33-33-77, customerservice@munksgaard.dk, http://www.munksgaard.dk/journals/periodontology, http://www.munksgaard.dk. Ed. Jan Lindhe. Circ: 11,000.

JOURNAL OF CRANIO-MAXILLOFACIAL TRAUMA. see *MEDICAL SCIENCES—Surgery*

JOURNAL OF DENTAL EDUCATION. see *EDUCATION—Higher Education*

617.6 USA ISSN 1043-254X
RK1
JOURNAL OF DENTAL HYGIENE. Text in English. 1927. 9/yr. USD 35 (effective 2000). adv. bk.rev. abstr, bibl, charts, illus, stat. index. reprint service avail. from PQC. *Refereed.* **Document type:** *Academic/Scholarly.* **Description:** Scientific journal with articles pertaining to dental hygiene practice, education, and research.
Former titles (until Oct. 1988): Dental Hygiene (0091-3979); American Dental Hygienists Association. Journal (0002-8185)
Related titles: Microform ed.: (from PQC); Online - full text ed.: (from Northern Light Technology, Inc., Gale Group).
Indexed: AgeLine, Biol.Abstr., CINAHL, Curr.Tit.Dent., Dent.Abstr., Dent.Ind., INIS Atomind.
—BLDSC (4968.470000), GNLM, Infotrieve, ingenta. **CCC.**
Published by: American Dental Hygienists' Association, 444 N Michigan Ave, Ste 3400, Chicago, IL 60611. TEL 312-440-8900, 800-243-2342, FAX 312-440-8929, adha@ix.netcom.org, http://www.adha.org. Ed. Mary Alice Gaston. Pub. Banta Greenfield. Adv. contact Wesley Blaszczynski. Circ: 30,000.

617.6 JPN ISSN 0285-0508
JOURNAL OF DENTAL HYGIENE. Text in Japanese. 1981. m. JPY 850 per issue. adv. bk.rev. charts, illus.
Related titles: Online - full text ed.: (from Northern Light Technology, Inc.).
Published by: Ishiyaku Publishers Inc., 7-10 Honkomagome 1-chome, Bunkyo-ku, Tokyo 113-0021, Japan. Ed. Hiroshi Miura. Circ: 15,000.

617.6 USA ISSN 0022-0345
RK1 CODEN: JDREAF
JOURNAL OF DENTAL RESEARCH. Text in English. 1919. m. USD 350 domestic; USD 360 foreign; USD 70 to members (effective 2001). adv. charts, illus, stat. index. back issues avail.; reprint service avail. from PQC. *Refereed.* **Document type:** *Academic/Scholarly.* **Description:** Publishes original research on the oral cavity, its contiguous parts and its effect on the total human organism in health and disease.
Related titles: Microform ed.: (from PQC,PMC); Online - full text ed.: (from Northern Light Technology, Inc., ProQuest Information & Learning, Institute for Scientific Information); ♦ Special ed.: International Association for Dental Research. Abstracts of the General Meeting. ISSN 0534-669X; ♦ Supplement: Advances in Dental Research. ISSN 0895-9374.
Indexed: ASCA, Abstr.Anthropol., Alloys Ind., Biol.Abstr., Cal.Tiss.Abstr., Chem.Abstr., Chem.Indus.Notes, Chem.Titles, Curr.Cont., Curr.Tit.Dent., Dairy Sci.Abstr., Dent.Abstr., Dent.Ind., Eng.Mat.Abstr., Environ.Sci.Poll.Mgmt., Excerp.Med., GeoRef, INIS Atomind., Ind.Med. (1919-), Ind.Sci.Rev., Inpharma, Mass Spectr.Bull., Mat.Sci.Cit.Ind. (coverage dropped), Met.Abstr., Met.Abstr.Ind., NRN, Neurosci.Cit.Ind., Nonfer.Met.Alert, Nutr.Abstr., PCC Alert, Pollut.Abstr., Reac., Rev.Med.& Vet.Mycol., Risk Abstr., SSCI (coverage dropped), Saf.Sci.Abstr., Sci.Cit.Ind., Steels Alert, Tox.Abstr. (coverage dropped), World Alum.Abstr.
—BLDSC (4968.500000), ADONIS, CASDDS, CISTI, GNLM, IDS, ingenta, KNAW, Linda Hall. **CCC.**
Published by: (International and American Associations for Dental Research), American Association for Dental Research, 1619 Duke St, Alexandria, VA 22314-3406. TEL 703-548-0066, FAX 703-548-1883, research@iadr.com, http://www.dentalresearch.org, http://www.iadr.com. Ed. Dr. Mark C Herzberg. adv.: B&W page USD 945, color page USD 1,690; trim 10 x 7. Circ: 7,237.

617.6 USA ISSN 1088-3118
RK1.N28
JOURNAL OF DENTAL TECHNOLOGY. Text in English. 1954. 10/yr. USD 40 domestic; USD 50 foreign (effective 2000). adv. bk.rev. illus. **Document type:** *Trade.* **Description:** Published for dental technicians and laboratory owners. Covers technical issues, association activities and business management, as well as industry news and new products.
Former titles: Trends & Techniques in the Contemporary Dental Laboratory (0746-8962); N A D L Journal (0360-5361); N A C D L Journal (0027-5735)
Indexed: Dent.Ind.
—GNLM.
Published by: National Association of Dental Laboratories, 8201 Greensboro Dr., Ste. 300, Mclean, VA 22102-3810. Ed. Cathy Jones. Circ: 17,000.

617.6 GBR ISSN 0300-5712
CODEN: JDENAB
THE JOURNAL OF DENTISTRY. Text in English. 1972. 8/yr. EUR 698 in Europe to institutions; JPY 92,600 in Japan to institutions; USD 780 elsewhere to institutions (effective 2002). bk.rev. illus. index. back issues avail.; reprint service avail. from PQC. *Refereed.* **Document type:** *Academic/Scholarly.* **Description:** Reports on all issues relating to research, innovations and the practice of restorative dentistry, including dental materials science.
Incorporates: Quarterly Dental Review (0033-5479); Dental Practitioner and Dental Record (0011-8729)
Related titles: Microform ed.: (from PQC); Online - full text ed.: (from ingenta, ScienceDirect, Swets Blackwell, Institute for Scientific Information).
Indexed: ASCA, Chem.Abstr., Chem.Indus.Notes, Chem.Titles, Curr.Cont., Curr.Tit.Dent., Dent.Abstr., Dent.Ind., Ind.Med. (1972-), Ind.Sci.Rev., Inpharma, Mat.Sci.Cit.Ind. (coverage dropped), NRN, Nutr.Abstr., Pharm.&Out.News, Reac., Sci.Cit.Ind., Sugar Ind.Abstr.
—BLDSC (4968.670000), CASDDS, CISTI, GNLM, IDS, ingenta. **CCC.**
Published by: Pergamon (Subsidiary of: Elsevier Science), The Boulevard, Langford Ln, East Park, Kidlington, Oxford OXB 1GB, United Kingdom. FAX 44-1865-843010, http://www.elsevier.nl/locate/jdent. Eds. Miss Jeniifer M Middleton, Neil Meredith. **Subscr. in Australasia and the Far East to:** Elsevier Science (Singapore) Pte Ltd, No.1 Temasek Ave, 17-01 Millenia Tower, Singapore 039192, Singapore. TEL 65-434-3727, FAX 65-337-2230; **Subscr. in the Americas to:** Elsevier Science, PO Box 945, New York, NY 10159-0945. TEL 212-633-3730, FAX 212-633-3680, usinfo-f@elsevier.com; **Subscr. to:** Elsevier Science BV, PO Box 211, Amsterdam 1000 AE, Netherlands. TEL 31-20-485-3757, nlinfo-f@elsevier.nl, http://www.elsevier.nl.

617.64 618.92 USA ISSN 0022-0353
CODEN: JDCHAH
JOURNAL OF DENTISTRY FOR CHILDREN. Text in English. 1933. bi-m. USD 140 domestic to institutions; USD 175 foreign to institutions (effective 2001). adv. bk.rev. abstr, charts, illus, stat. index. reprint service avail. from PSC,PQC. *Refereed.* **Document type:** *Journal, Academic/Scholarly.* **Description:** Covers field of pediatric and general dentistry.
Related titles: Microform ed.: (from PQC,WWS); Online - full text ed.: (from Institute for Scientific Information).
Indexed: ASCA, Behav.Med.Abstr., Biol.Abstr., CINAHL, Chem.Abstr., Chic.Per.Ind., Curr.Cont., Curr.Tit.Dent., Dairy Sci.Abstr., Dent.Abstr., Dent.Ind., Ind.Med. (1968-), Ind.Sci.Rev., Inpharma, NRN, Nutr.Abstr., Reac., SSCI (coverage dropped), Sci.Cit.Ind., Trop.Dis.Bull.
—BLDSC (1739.600000), CISTI, GNLM, IDS, ingenta.
Published by: American Society of Dentistry for Children, 211 E Chicago Ave, Ste 710, Chicago, IL 60611. TEL 312-943-1244, FAX 312-943-5341, asdckids@aol.com, http://cudental.creighton.edu/asdc. Ed. Dr. George W Teuscher. Adv. contact Anthony Jannetti. Circ: 3,783 (controlled and free).

617.6 USA ISSN 0099-2399
RK351
THE JOURNAL OF ENDODONTICS. Text in English. 1975. m. USD 130 domestic to individuals; USD 188 foreign to institutions; USD 203 domestic to individuals; USD 261 foreign to institutions; USD 24 newsstand/cover (effective 2002). adv. abstr, illus. index. 2 cols./p. back issues avail.; reprints avail. *Refereed.* **Document type:** *Academic/Scholarly.* **Description:** Explores methods of pulp conservation, root canal instrumentation and endodontic treatment.
Related titles: Microfilm ed.: (from PMC,WWS); Online - full text ed.: (from Ovid Technologies, Inc., Institute for Scientific Information).
Indexed: ASCA, Biol.Abstr., Curr.Cont., Curr.Tit.Dent., Dent.Abstr., Dent.Ind., Excerp.Med., INIS Atomind., Inpharma, Reac., SSCI (coverage dropped), Sci.Cit.Ind.
—BLDSC (4978.200000), CISTI, GNLM, IDS, ingenta.
Published by: (American Association of Endodontics), Lippincott Williams & Wilkins (Baltimore) (Subsidiary of: Wolters Kluwer N.V.), 351 W Camden St, Baltimore, MD 21201-2436. TEL 410-528-4192, FAX 410-361-8034, mricks@wwilkins.com, http://www.wwilkins.com. Ed. Dr. Henry Van Hassel. Pub. Marjory Spraycar. Adv. contact Sherry Reed. B&W page USD 1,220, color page USD 3,220; trim 10.88 x 8.13. Circ: 6,800 (paid).

617.6 CAN
JOURNAL OF ESTHETIC AND RESTORATIVE DENTISTRY. Text in English. 1988. bi-m. USD 179 in US & Canada to individuals; USD 229 elsewhere to individuals; USD 279 in US & Canada to institutions; USD 309 elsewhere to institutions (effective 2001). adv. back issues avail. *Refereed.* **Document type:** *Journal, Academic/Scholarly.* **Description:** Provides information relative to the fields of esthetic dentistry.
Formerly (until 2001): Journal of Esthetic Dentistry (1040-1466)
Related titles: CD-ROM ed.; Online - full text ed.: (from Northern Light Technology, Inc., ProQuest Information & Learning).
Indexed: e-psyche.
—GNLM, Infotrieve. **CCC.**

Published by: B.C. Decker Inc., 20 Hughson St S, LCD 1, P O Box 620, Hamilton, ON L8N 3K7, Canada. TEL 905-522-7017, 800-568-7281, FAX 905-522-7839, info@bcdecker.com, http://www.bcdecker.com. Ed. Harald Heymann. Pub. David LeGallais. R&P Paula Presutti. Adv. contact Bob Sutherland. Circ: 25,000. **Co-sponsors:** American Academy of Esthetic Dentistry; Japan Academy of Esthetic Dentistry; International Federation of Esthetic Dentistry.

617.6 ESP
JOURNAL OF ESTHETIC DENTISTRY (EDICION ESPANOLA)✶ . Text in Spanish. 1991. q. adv. bk.rev. index. back issues avail.
Published by: (Rhone-Poulenc Rorer), Ediciones Ergon S.A., Pza. Josep Pallach 10, 1o, Barcelona 08035, Spain. TEL 2010911, FAX 2015911. **Subscr. to:** Cempro, Plaza Conde Valle Suchil 20, Madrid 28015, Spain.

617.6 USA ISSN 1532-3382
▼ **THE JOURNAL OF EVIDENCE-BASED DENTAL PRACTICE.** Text in English. 2001 (Jun.). q. USD 59 domestic to individuals; USD 73 foreign to individuals; USD 89 domestic to institutions; USD 103 foreign to institutions; USD 29 domestic to students; USD 43 foreign to students; USD 26 per issue (effective 2001). adv. reprints avail. *Refereed.* **Document type:** *Journal, Academic/Scholarly.* **Description:** Contains original articles and reviews of articles on the results and outcomes of clinical procedures and treatment.
Related titles: Online - full text ed.: forthcoming 2001.
Published by: Mosby, Inc. (Subsidiary of: Elsevier Science), 11830 Westline Industrial Dr, St Louis, MO 63146-3318. TEL 314-872-8370, 800-432-4177, FAX 314-432-1380, http://www.mosby.com/ebdp. Ed. Michael G Newman. Pub. Cynthia Baudendistel. Adv. contact Carol Kilzer TEL 314-453-4307. B&W page USD 895, color page USD 1,820; trim 10.88 x 8.13. Circ: 6,000.

617.643 USA ISSN 1048-1990
JOURNAL OF GENERAL ORTHODONTICS✶ . Text in English. 1990. q. USD 40; USD 60 foreign (effective 1998). adv. bk.rev. **Document type:** *Trade.* **Description:** Contains scientific and clinical articles on orthodontic techniques.
—BLDSC (4988.300000), GNLM.
Published by: International Association for Orthodontics, 735 N. Water St., Ste. 617, Milwaykee, WI 53202-4104. TEL 708-445-0320, FAX 708-445-0321. Ed. Yosh Jefferson. R&P Joanna Carey. Circ: 3,800 (controlled).

617.6 DEU ISSN 0891-8171
THE JOURNAL OF GNATHOLOGY. Text in English. 1981. a. DEM 50, USD 28; DEM 32, USD 18 to students (effective 2000). adv. **Document type:** *Magazine, Academic/Scholarly.*
—GNLM.
Published by: (International Academy of Gnathology), Quintessenz Verlags GmbH, Ifenpfad 2-4, Berlin 12107, Germany. TEL 49-30-76180646, FAX 49-30-76180680, central@quinline.com, central@quintessenz.de, http://www.quinline.com, http://www.quintessenz.de. Ed. Dr. Axel Bauer. Adv. contact Marlies Kauffeldt. B&W page DEM 1,980; trim 210 x 280.

617.6 CAN ISSN 1464-3294
▼ **JOURNAL OF LINGUAL ORTHODONTICS.** Text in English. 1999. q. USD 120 domestic; USD 139 foreign (effective 2001). adv. 24 p./no. back issues avail.; reprints avail. *Refereed.* **Document type:** *Journal, Academic/Scholarly.* **Description:** Designed to provide a dedicated scientific organ for those committed pioneers, teachers and practitioners who, seeing the potential for treating greater numbers of patients, particularly adults, using a discreet appliance, persevered in difficult conditions to improve the technique.
—BLDSC (5010.474700).
Published by: B.C. Decker Inc, Decker Europe Ltd., 20 Hughson St, S, 10th Fl, PO Box 620, LCD 1, Hamilton, ON L8N 3K7, Canada. TEL 905-522-7017, 800-568-7281, FAX 905-522-7839, info@bcdecker.com, http://www.bcdecker.com/. Ed. Didier Fillion. Pub. Vivienne Oakes. R&P Paula Presutti TEL 905-522-7017. **Affiliate:** Decker Europe Ltd.

617.6 GBR ISSN 1366-4697
RD130
THE JOURNAL OF MAXILLOFACIAL PROSTHETICS AND TECHNOLOGY. Text in English. 1997. a. GBP 24; GBP 29 foreign (effective 2000). adv. **Document type:** *Academic/Scholarly.*
—BLDSC (5015.405000).
Published by: (Institute of Maxillofacial Prosthetists and Technologists), Matrix Marketing, 30 New Brighton, Cottingley, Bingley BD16 1UR, United Kingdom. TEL 44-1274-584730, FAX 44-1274-584730, matrixm@btinternet.com. Ed. Ian Collins. Adv. contact Frank Johnson.

JOURNAL OF MEDICAL AND DENTAL SCIENCES. see *MEDICAL SCIENCES*

617.6 USA ISSN 0278-2391
RK1 CODEN: JOMSDA
JOURNAL OF ORAL AND MAXILLOFACIAL SURGERY. Text in English. 1943. m. USD 145 domestic to individuals Full text online included; USD 230 foreign to individuals Full text online included; USD 195 domestic to institutions Full text online included; USD 274 foreign to institutions Full text online included; USD 106 domestic to students Full text online included; USD 148 foreign to students Full text online included; USD 23 per issue (effective 2001). adv. bk.rev. abstr, bibl, charts, illus. index. reprint service avail. from PQC. *Refereed.* **Document type:** *Journal, Academic/Scholarly.* **Description:** Serves oral and maxillofacial surgeons and other health care professionals interested in the field with scientific reports, case studies, news articles, and editorials.
Former titles (until 1982): Journal of Oral Surgery (0022-3255); Journal of Oral Surgery, Anesthesia and Hospital Dental Service (0095-9618)
Related titles: Diskette ed.: USD 49.95 per issue (effective 2000); Microform ed.: (from PQC); Online - full text ed.: (from IDEAL Online Library, Institute for Scientific Information).
Indexed: AIM, ASCA, Abstr.Hyg., Biol.Abstr., Cal.Tiss.Abstr., Chem.Abstr., Curr.Cont., Curr.Tit.Dent., Dent.Abstr., Dent.Ind., Environ.Sci.Poll.Mgmt., Excerp.Med., Helminthol.Abstr., INIS Atomind., Ind.Med. (1982-), Ind.Sci.Rev., Inpharma, Neurosci.Cit.Ind., Pollut.Abstr., Reac., Rev.Med.& Vet.Mycol., Risk Abstr., Saf.Sci.Abstr., Sci.Cit.Ind., Tox.Abstr. (coverage dropped).
—BLDSC (5026.385000), CISTI, EMDOCS, GNLM, IDS, ingenta, KNAW. **CCC.**
Published by: (American Association of Oral and Maxillofacial Surgeons), W.B. Saunders Co. (Subsidiary of: Harcourt Publishers Ltd.), 11830 Westline Industrial Dr, St Louis, MO 63146. TEL 800-325-4177, http://www.joms.org, http://www.wbsaunders.com. Ed. Dr. Daniel M Laskin. adv.: B&W page USD 1,680, color page USD 2,755; trim 7 x 10. Circ: 9,894 (paid). **Subscr. to:** Periodicals Fulfillment, W B Saunders Co, 6277 Sea Harbor Dr, 4th Fl, Orlando, FL 32891-4800.

617.6 USA ISSN 0160-6972
JOURNAL OF ORAL IMPLANTOLOGY; the official journal of the American Academy of Implant Dentistry. Text in English. 1975. q. USD 145 domestic to institutions; USD 165 foreign to institutions (effective 2001). adv. bk.rev. abstr, illus, stat. back issues avail. *Refereed.* **Document type:** *Academic/Scholarly.* **Description:** Brings information of interest on all areas of implant dentistry to scientists, clinicians, laboratory owners, technicians, manufacturers, and educators.
Formerly (until 1977): Oral Implantology (0048-2064); Which incorporates: American Academy of Implant Dentistry. Newsletter
Related titles: Microform ed.: (from PQC).
Indexed: Dent.Ind.
—BLDSC (5026.410000), CISTI, GNLM, ingenta, KNAW. **CCC.**
Published by: (American Academy of Implant Dentistry), Allen Press, Inc., Division Alliance Communications Group, PO Box 1897, Lawrence, KS 66044. TEL 785-843-1235, FAX 785-843-1274, orim@allenpress.com, orim@allenpress.com, http://www.aaid-implant.org. Ed. A Norman Cranin. Pub. Angela Pfeifer. R&P Ethel Burke. adv.: B&W page USD 710, color page USD 780; trim 11 x 8.25. Circ: 2,565 (paid).

617.6 USA
▼ **JOURNAL OF ORAL LASER APPLICATIONS.** Text in English. forthcoming 2002 (Apr.). q. USD 98, GBP 69, EUR 118; USD 50, GBP 36, EUR 60 to students (effective 2002). **Document type:** *Magazine, Academic/Scholarly, Trade.* **Description:** Presents overviews of established indications and applications in all fields of dentistry, as well as reports of ongoing scientific developments in laser technology that will impact dental practice in the future.
Published by: (European Society for Oral Laser Applications AUT), Quintessence Publishing Co., Inc., 551 Kimberly Dr, Carol Stream, IL 60188-1881. TEL 630-682-3223, FAX 630-682-3288, quintpub@aol.com, http://www.quintpub.com. Eds. Dr. Andreas Moritz, Dr. Lynn Powell.

617.6 DNK ISSN 0904-2512
CODEN: JPMEEA
JOURNAL OF ORAL PATHOLOGY & MEDICINE. Text in English. 1972. 10/yr. USD 462 in the Americas to institutions print & online eds. combined; GBP 321 elsewhere to institutions print & online eds. combined (effective 2002). adv. bk.rev. charts, illus, bibl. reprint service avail. from SWZ,ISI. *Refereed.* **Document type:** *Academic/Scholarly.*
Formerly: Journal of Oral Pathology (0300-9777)
Related titles: Microform ed.: (from SWZ); Online - full text ed.: DKK 3,132 (effective 2001) (from Ovid Technologies, Inc., EBSCO Publishing, ingenta, Swets Blackwell, Institute for Scientific Information).
Indexed: ASCA, Biol.Abstr., Cal.Tiss.Abstr. (coverage dropped), Chem.Abstr., Chem.Indus.Notes, Chem.Titles, Curr.Adv.Ecol.Sci., Curr.Cont., Curr.Tit.Dent., Dent.Abstr., Dent.Ind., Excerp.Med., INIS Atomind., Ind.Med. (1989-), Ind.Sci.Rev., Inpharma, Int.Abstr.Biol.Sci., Med.& Surg.Dermat., Nutr.Abstr., Pharm.&Out.News, Reac., Rev.Med.& Vet.Mycol., Rev.Plant Path., Sci.Cit.Ind., Tox.Abstr. (coverage dropped), Virol.Abstr. (coverage dropped).
—BLDSC (5026.435000), CASDDS, CISTI, EMDOCS, GNLM, IDS, ingenta, KNAW. **CCC.**
Published by: (International Association of Oral Pathologists), Blackwell Munksgaard, Noerre Soegade 35, PO Box 2148, Copenhagen K 1016, Denmark. TEL 45-77-33-33-33, FAX 45-77-33-33-77, customerservice@munksgaard.dk, http://www.munksgaard.dk. Ed. Eric Dabelsteen. Circ: 900. **Co-sponsors:** American Academy of Oral and Maxillofacial Pathology; International Association of Oral Pathology; British Society for Oral Pathology; British Society for Oral Medicine.

617.6 GBR ISSN 0305-182X
CODEN: JORHBY
JOURNAL OF ORAL REHABILITATION; clinical dental science and materials. Text in English. 1974. m., latest vol.29, 2002. GBP 129 in Europe to individuals; USD 205 in North America to individuals; GBP 142 elsewhere to individuals; GBP 829 in Europe to institutions; USD 1,314 in North America to institutions; GBP 912 elsewhere to institutions (effective 2002). adv. bk.rev. bibl, illus. index. back issues avail.; reprint service avail. from ISI. *Refereed.* **Document type:** *Journal, Academic/Scholarly.* **Description:** Devoted to original comment and research in subjects relevant to the practice and development or oral rehabilitation.
Related titles: Microform ed.: (from PQC); ♦ Online - full text ed.: Journal of Oral Rehabilitation Online. ISSN 1365-2842.
Indexed: AMED, ASCA, Behav.Med.Abstr., Chem.Abstr., Chem.Indus.Notes, Chem.Titles, Curr.Cont., Curr.Tit.Dent., Dent.Abstr., Dent.Ind., Excerp.Med., Ind.Med. (1974-), Ind.Sci.Rev., Inpharma, Mat.Sci.Cit.Ind. (coverage dropped), Reac., Rev.Med.& Vet.Mycol., Sci.Cit.Ind.
—BLDSC (5026.440000), CASDDS, GNLM, IDS, ingenta. **CCC.**
Published by: Blackwell Science Ltd., PO Box 88, Oxford OX2 0NE, United Kingdom. TEL 44-1865-206180, 44-1865-206002, FAX 44-1865-206219, jnl.orders@blacksci.co.uk, http://www.blackwell-science.com/products/journals/jor.htm, http://www.blackwellpublishing.com. Ed. A S T Franks. Pub. Elaine Stott. R&P Sophie Savage. Adv. contact Jenny Applin. Circ: 430.

617.6 GBR ISSN 1365-2842
▼ **JOURNAL OF ORAL REHABILITATION ONLINE.** Text in English. 1999. m. GBP 117 in Europe to individuals; USD 185 in North America to individuals; GBP 117 elsewhere to individuals; GBP 747 in Europe to institutions; USD 1,183 in North America to institutions; GBP 747 elsewhere to institutions (effective 2002). *Refereed.* **Document type:** *Academic/Scholarly.*
Media: Online - full text (from EBSCO Publishing, Munksgaard & Blackwell Science's Synergy, Swets Blackwell, Institute for Scientific Information, RoweCom Information Quest). **Related titles:** Microform ed.: (from PQC); ♦ Print ed.: Journal of Oral Rehabilitation. ISSN 0305-182X.
Published by: Blackwell Science Ltd., Osney Mead, Oxford OX2 0EL, United Kingdom. TEL 44-1685-206206, FAX 44-1685-721205, journals.cs@blacksci.co.uk, http://www.blackwell-science.com.

617.6 JPN ISSN 1343-4934
CODEN: JORSF3
JOURNAL OF ORAL SCIENCE. Text in English. 1958. q. JPY 5,000 (effective 2001). bk.rev. abstr, charts, illus. index. 60 p./no. *Refereed.* **Document type:** *Journal, Academic/Scholarly.* **Description:** Contains academic research papers and case reports.

M

Formerly (until vol.39, no.4): Nihon University. School of Dentistry. Journal (Nihon Daigaku Shigakubu Obun Zasshi) (0029-0432)
Related titles: Online - full text ed.
Indexed: Biol.Abstr., Chem.Abstr., Chem.Indus.Notes, Chem.Titles, Curr.Tit.Dent., Dent.Ind., INIS Atomind., Ind.Med. (1998-), Med.Abstr.
—BLDSC (5026.445000), CASDDS, CISTI, GNLM, ingenta.
Published by: Nihon University, School of Dentistry/Nihon Daigaku Shigakubu, 1-8-13 Kanda-Surugadai, Chiyoda-ku, Tokyo 101-8310, Japan. TEL 81-3-3219-8060, FAX 81-3-3219-8324, institute@nc.dent.nihon-u.ac.jp, http://www.dent.nihon-u.ac.jp/publ/journal/e-jou00.html. Ed. Minoru Takagi. Circ: 1,000 (controlled).

617.6 USA ISSN 1064-6655
CODEN: JOROEO
JOURNAL OF OROFACIAL PAIN. Text in English. 1987. q. USD 106, GBP 76, EUR 120 to individuals; USD 152, GBP 109, EUR 172 to institutions; USD 68, GBP 49, EUR 78 to students (effective 2002). adv. charts, illus. index. back issues avail. *Refereed.* **Document type:** *Magazine, Academic/Scholarly.* **Description:** Reports research, clinical material and treatment therapies on facial pain, headaches, occlusion, physiology and physical therapy.
Formerly (until 1993): Journal of Craniomandibular Disorders (0890-2739)
Related titles: Online - full text ed.: (from Institute for Scientific Information).
Indexed: Curr.Cont., Dent.Abstr., Sci.Cit.Ind.
—BLDSC (5027.530000), CISTI, GNLM, IDS, ingenta. **CCC.**
Published by: (American Academy of Orofacial Pain), Quintessence Publishing Co., Inc., 551 Kimberly Dr, Carol Stream, IL 60188-1881. TEL 630-682-3223, FAX 630-682-3288, quintpub@aol.com, http://www.quintpub.com. Ed. Dr. Barry J Sessle. Pub. H W Haase. Adv. contact William G Hartman. Circ: 3,000. **Co-sponsor:** European Academy of Craniomandibular Disorders.

617.643 GBR ISSN 1465-3125
THE JOURNAL OF ORTHODONTICS. Text in English. 1974. q. GBP 140, USD 230 includes print & online (effective Mar. 2002). adv. bk.rev. index. back issues avail. *Refereed.* **Document type:** *Journal, Academic/Scholarly.* **Description:** Contains original articles, reviews, critical commentaries, editorials, and correspondence on features of orthodontic practice, teaching and research.
Formerly (until 2000): British Journal of Orthodontics (0301-228X)
Related titles: Microform ed.: (from PQC); Online - full text ed.: ISSN 1460-2164. GBP 125, USD 205 to institutions Online only (effective Mar. 2002) (from HighWire Pr., EBSCO Publishing, O C L C Online Computer Library Center, Inc., RoweCom Information Quest, ingenta, Swets Blackwell).
Indexed: Curr.Adv.Ecol.Sci., Curr.Tit.Dent., Dent.Abstr., Dent.Ind., Ind.Med. (2000-), Ref.Zh.
—CISTI, GNLM, ingenta. **CCC.**
Published by: (British Society of the Study of Orthodontics), Oxford University Press, Academic Division, Great Clarendon St, Oxford OX2 6DP, United Kingdom. TEL 44-1865-267907, FAX 44-1865-267835, jnl.info@oup.co.uk, http://ortho.oupjournals.org/, http://www.oup.co.uk/journals. Ed. M L Jones. Pub. Mandy Sketch. R&P Fionna Willis. Adv. contact Helen Pearson TEL 44-1235-201904. Circ: 2,700. **US subscr. to:** Oxford University Press, Journals, 2001 Evans Rd, Cary, NC 27513. TEL 800-852-7323, FAX 919-677-1714, jnlorders@oup-usa.org.

617.632 DNK ISSN 0022-3484
RK361.A1 CODEN: JPDRAY
JOURNAL OF PERIODONTAL RESEARCH. Text in English. 1966. 6/yr. USD 357 in the Americas to institutions print & online eds. combined; GBP 248 elsewhere to institutions print & online eds. combined (effective 2002). adv. bibl, charts, illus. reprint service avail. from SWZ,ISI. *Refereed.* **Document type:** *Academic/Scholarly.*
Related titles: Microform ed.: (from SWZ); Online - full text ed.: DKK 2,232 (effective 2001) (from Ovid Technologies, Inc., EBSCO Publishing, ingenta, Swets Blackwell, Institute for Scientific Information).
Indexed: ASCA, Biol.Abstr., Chem.Abstr., Chem.Indus.Notes, Chem.Titles, Curr.Adv.Ecol.Sci., Curr.Cont., Curr.Tit.Dent., Dairy Sci.Abstr., Dent.Abstr., Dent.Ind., Excerp.Med., INIS Atomind., Ind.Med. (1966-), Ind.Sci.Rev., Inpharma, Reac., SSCI (coverage dropped), Sci.Cit.Ind.
—BLDSC (5030.600000), CASDDS, CISTI, GNLM, IDS, ingenta, KNAW. **CCC.**
Published by: Blackwell Munksgaard, Noerre Soegade 35, PO Box 2148, Copenhagen K 1016, Denmark. TEL 45-77-33-33-33, FAX 45-77-33-33-77, customerservice@munksgaard.dk, http://www.munksgaard.dk. Ed. Roy C Page. Circ: 1,000.

617.632 USA ISSN 0022-3492
RK1.A512 CODEN: JOPRAJ
JOURNAL OF PERIODONTOLOGY. Text in English. 1930. m. USD 130 in US & Canada to individuals; USD 160 elsewhere to individuals; USD 230 in US & Canada to institutions; USD 275 elsewhere to institutions (effective 2001). adv. abstr, bibl, illus. index. back issues avail.; reprint service avail. from PQC. *Refereed.* **Document type:** *Academic/Scholarly.* **Description:** Contains papers of clinical and scientific interest to periodontists and other members of the dental community.
Formerly: Journal of Periodontology - Periodontics
Related titles: CD-ROM ed.; Microform ed.: (from PQC,PMC); Online - full text ed.: (from Institute for Scientific Information).
Indexed: AIDS Abstr., ASCA, Biol.Abstr., Biol.Dig., Chem.Abstr., Chem.Indus.Notes, Chem.Titles, Curr.Adv.Ecol.Sci., Curr.Cont., Curr.Tit.Dent., Dent.Abstr., Dent.Ind., Excerp.Med., INIS Atomind., Ind.Med. (1970-), Ind.Sci.Rev., Inpharma, Mat.Sci.Cit.Ind. (coverage dropped), Microbiol.Abstr., Nutr.Abstr., Pharm.&Out.News, Reac., Sci.Cit.Ind.
—BLDSC (5030.700000), CASDDS, CISTI, GNLM, IDS, ingenta, KNAW. **CCC.**
Published by: American Academy of Periodontology, 737 N Michigan, Ste 800, Chicago, IL 60611. TEL 312-573-3220, 312-787-5518, FAX 312-573-3225, 312-787-3670, lee@perio.org, orders@perio.org, http://www.perio.org. Ed. Robert Genco. R&P Rita Shafer. Adv. contact Katie Goss. Circ: 9,000.

617.6 USA ISSN 1072-7965
THE JOURNAL OF PRACTICAL HYGIENE. Variant title: J P H. Text in English. 1991. bi-m. USD 58 domestic to individuals; USD 95 foreign to individuals (effective 2001). adv. back issues avail.; reprints avail. *Refereed.* **Document type:** *Academic/Scholarly.* **Description:** Clinical publication disseminating information on practical applications of soft tissue management and oral hygiene, as well as applications in restorative and implant treatments.
Published by: Montage Media Corp., 1000 Wyckoff Ave, Mahwah, NJ 07430. TEL 201-891-3200, FAX 201-891-2626, jph@montagemedia.com, info@mantagemedia.com, http://www.montagemedia.com/jph.html. Ed. Miriam Rinn. Pub., R&P Stephen E Sweeney. Adv. contact Jim King. B&W page USD 5,232, color page USD 6,932; trim 10.88 x 8.13. Circ: 60,400 (controlled).

617.69 USA ISSN 0022-3913
RK1 CODEN: JPDEAT
THE JOURNAL OF PROSTHETIC DENTISTRY. Text in English. 1951. m. USD 145 domestic to individuals; USD 179 foreign to individuals; USD 299 domestic to institutions; USD 333 foreign to institutions; USD 75 domestic to students; USD 109 foreign to students; USD 28 newsstand/cover (effective 2001). adv. bk.rev. charts, illus. s-a. index. back issues avail.; reprint service avail. from PQC. *Refereed.* **Document type:** *Journal, Academic/Scholarly.* **Description:** New techniques, evaluation of dental materials, and patient psychology relevant to practitioners of prosthetic dentistry.
Related titles: Microfilm ed.: (from PQC); Online - full text ed.: (from EBSCO Publishing, IDEAL Online Library, Institute for Scientific Information, RoweCom Information Quest).
Indexed: ASCA, AgeLine, Alloys Ind., Biol.Abstr., Br.Ceram.Abstr., CINAHL, Ceram.Abstr., Chem.Abstr., Chem.Indus.Notes, Chem.Titles, Curr.Adv.Ecol.Sci., Curr.Cont., Curr.Tit.Dent., Dent.Abstr., Dent.Ind., Eng.Mat.Abstr., Environ.Sci.Poll.Mgmt., INIS Atomind., Ind.Med. (1951-), Ind.Sci.Rev., Inpharma, METADEX, Met.Abstr., Met.Abstr.Ind., Nonfer.Met.Alert, PCC Alert, Pollut.Abstr., Reac., Risk Abstr., Saf.Sci.Abstr., Sci.Cit.Ind., Steels Alert, World Alum.Abstr.
—BLDSC (5042.900000), CASDDS, CISTI, GNLM, IDS, ingenta. **CCC.**
Published by: (Academy of Prosthodontics), Mosby, Inc. (Subsidiary of: Elsevier Science), 11830 Westline Industrial Dr, St Louis, MO 63146-3318. TEL 314-872-8370, 800-325-4177, FAX 314-432-1380, http://www.mosby.com/periodicals. Ed. Dr. Glen P McGivney. Pub. Cynthia Baudendistel. Adv. contact Grace Williams TEL 314-453-4689. B&W page USD 1,485, color page USD 2,660; trim 10.88 x 8.13. Circ: 8,311. **Co-sponsors:** American Prosthodontic Society; Pacific Coast Society of Prosthodontists.

617.6 USA ISSN 1059-941X
JOURNAL OF PROSTHODONTICS. Text in English. 1992. q. USD 125 domestic to individuals; USD 151 foreign to individuals; USD 175 domestic to institutions; USD 199 foreign to institutions; USD 91 domestic to students; USD 140 foreign to students; USD 50 newsstand/cover (effective 2001). adv. *Refereed.* **Document type:** *Academic/Scholarly.* **Description:** Contains original articles, reviews of new techniques and instrumentation, and instructive case reports.
Related titles: Online - full text ed.: (from IDEAL Online Library).
—BLDSC (5042.920000), CISTI, GNLM, Infotrieve. **CCC.**
Published by: (American College of Prosthodontists), W.B. Saunders Co. (Subsidiary of: Harcourt Publishers Ltd.), 11830 Westline Industrial Dr, St Louis, MO 63146. TEL 800-325-4177, http://www.wbsaunders.com. Ed. Dr. Patrick M Lloyd. adv.: B&W page USD 1,065, color page USD 2,165; trim 10 x 7. Circ: 3,072. **Subscr. to:** Periodicals Fulfillment, W B Saunders Co, 6277 Sea Harbor Dr, 4th Fl, Orlando, FL 32891-4800.

617.6 614.8 USA ISSN 0022-4006
RK52 CODEN: JPHDAC
JOURNAL OF PUBLIC HEALTH DENTISTRY. Text in English. 1941. q. USD 100 (effective 2000). adv. bk.rev. bibl, charts, illus, stat. reprint service avail. from PQC. *Refereed.* **Document type:** *Academic/Scholarly.* **Description:** Contains news about dentistry practices.
Former titles: Public Health Dentistry; American Association of Public Health Dentists. Bulletin
Related titles: Microform ed.: (from PQC); Online - full text ed.: (from Institute for Scientific Information).
Indexed: ASCA, Abstr.Health Care Manage.Stud., AgeLine, Biol.Abstr., Curr.Cont., Curr.Tit.Dent., Dent.Abstr., Dent.Ind., Excerp.Med., Ind.Med. (1965-), Ind.Sci.Rev., Inpharma, NRN, Reac., SSCI (coverage dropped), Sci.Cit.Ind.
—BLDSC (5043.550000), CISTI, GNLM, IDS, ingenta.
Published by: American Association of Public Health Dentistry, 3760 S W, Lyle Ct, Portland, OR 97221. TEL 503-242-0712, FAX 503-242-0721, natoff@aol.com. Ed. R Gary Rozier. Adv. contact J Toothaker. Circ: 1,200.

617.6 USA ISSN 0743-491X
JOURNAL OF THE AMERICAN ASSOCIATION OF FORENSIC DENTISTS. Text in English. 1978. q. USD 5 (effective 1999). adv. **Description:** News journal on the subjects of forensic dentistry, forensic odontology, dental identification, dental anthropology, law enforcement and pathology.
Published by: Andent, Inc., 1000 North Ave, Waukegan, IL 60085. TEL 847-223-5077, eneiburger@cs.com, http://www.andent.net. Ed., Pub. E J Neiburger. adv.: B&W page USD 125; trim 8 x 11. Circ: 3,000 (paid).

617.6 USA ISSN 1089-6287
JOURNAL OF THE HISTORY OF DENTISTRY. Text in English. 1952. 3/yr., latest vol.50, 2002. USD 60 domestic; USD 65 foreign (effective 2001). adv. bk.rev. bibl, illus. cum.index every 5 yrs. 48 p./no. back issues avail.; reprint service avail. from PQC. *Refereed.* **Document type:** *Journal, Academic/Scholarly.* **Description:** Covers all areas relating to dental history.
Formerly (until Mar. 1996): Bulletin of the History of Dentistry (0007-5132)
Related titles: Microfilm ed.: (from PQC).
Indexed: Curr.Tit.Dent., Dent.Abstr., Dent.Ind., INIS Atomind., Ind.Med. (coverage dropped).
—GNLM, ingenta.
Published by: American Academy of the History of Dentistry, c/o Aletha Kowitz, 100 S Vail Ave, Arlington, IL 60005-1866. TEL 847-670-7561. Ed. H T Loevy. R&P, Adv. contact Aletha Kowitz TEL 312-996-1991. Circ: 800 (paid).

JOURNAL OF THE MEDICAL AND DENTAL DEFENCE UNIONS. see *MEDICAL SCIENCES*

617.6 JPN ISSN 0385-1443
CODEN: BKDCD5
KANAGAWA DENTAL COLLEGE. BULLETIN. Text in English. 1973. s-a. free per issue. **Document type:** *Bulletin.*
Indexed: Chem.Abstr., Chem.Indus.Notes, Chem.Titles.
—BLDSC (2597.959000), CASDDS, GNLM.
Published by: Kanagawa Dental College Society/Kanagawa Shika Daigaku Gakkai, 82 Inaoka-cho, Yokosuka-shi, Kanagawa-ken 238-0003, Japan. TEL 0468-25-1500, FAX 0468-23-9415. Ed. Akiya Yamanaka. Circ: 1,000.

617.6 JPN ISSN 0454-8302
CODEN: KSHGDM
KANAGAWA SHIGAKU/KANAGAWA ODONTOLOGICAL SOCIETY. JOURNAL. Text in Japanese. 1967. q. JPY 1,500.

M

Indexed: Chem.Abstr., Chem.Indus.Notes, Chem.Titles, INIS Atomind.
—BLDSC (4810.229000), CASDDS, GNLM.
Published by: Kanagawa Dental College Society/Kanagawa Shika Daigaku Gakkai, 82 Inaoka-cho, Yokosuka-shi, Kanagawa-ken 238-0003, Japan. TEL 0468-25-1500, FAX 0468-23-9415. Ed. Tsugio Iwamoto. Circ: 3,000.

617.6 USA ISSN 0888-7063
KANSAS DENTAL ASSOCIATION. JOURNAL. Text in English. 1973 (vol.57). q. USD 35 (effective 1998). adv. illus.
Formerly (until July 1981): Kansas State Dental Association. Journal (0022-8796)
Indexed: Dent.Abstr., Dent.Ind., Med.Care Rev.
—CISTI, GNLM.
Published by: Kansas Dental Association, 5200 S W Huntoon St, Topeka, KS 66604-2365. FAX 785-272-2301, kda@cjnetworks.com. Ed. Dr. Eugene McGill. Circ: 1,200.

617.6 USA ISSN 0744-396X
KENTUCKY DENTAL ASSOCIATION. JOURNAL*. Text in English. 1949. bi-m. USD 20. adv. bk.rev. illus.
Indexed: Dent.Abstr., Dent.Ind.
—GNLM.
Published by: Kentucky Dental Association, 1725 Hillcrest Dr, Madisonville, KY 42431. Ed. Joe W Jones Jr. Circ: 1,900.

617.6 USA
KERN COUNTY DENTAL SOCIETY OCCLUSAL REGISTER. Text in English. 1967. bi-m. free per issue. adv. charts, illus, stat.
Formerly: Kern County Dental Society Newsletter (0023-0634)
Published by: Kern County Dental Society, 1701 Westwind Dr, Ste 209, Bakersfield, CA 93301. TEL 805-327-2666, FAX 805-327-1229. Ed. Dr. Karen Yoon. Circ: 180.

617.6 DEU
KIEFERORTHOPAEDIE; die Zeitschrift fuer die Praxis. Text in German. 1987. q. EUR 108 domestic to individuals; EUR 114 foreign to individuals; EUR 66 domestic to students; EUR 72 foreign to students (effective 2002). back issues avail. **Document type:** *Magazine, Academic/Scholarly.* **Description:** Further education for dentists and orthodontists.
Formerly: Praktische Kieferorthopaedie (0931-6965)
—GNLM.
Published by: Quintessenz Verlags GmbH, Ifenpfad 2-4, Berlin 12107, Germany. TEL 49-30-76180646, FAX 49-30-76180680, central@quintessenz.de, http://www.quintessenz.de. Eds. Dieter Drescher, Rainer Reginald Miethke. Circ: 3,000.

617.6 RUS
KLINICHESKAYA IMPLANTOLOGIYA I STOMATOLOGIYA; mezhdunarodnyi nauchno-prakticheskii zhurnal. Text in Russian. 1997. q.
Related titles: Online - full text ed.
Published by: OOO Nordmed, Ul. Tverskaya 12/15, Sankt-Peterburg 193124, Russian Federation. TEL 7-812-2754197, FAX 7-812-1100206, dantist@stom.ru, http://www.stom.ru/implant, http://www.stom.ru/dentist. Ed. K. Vuraki. Circ: 1,000.

617.6 RUS
KLINICHESKAYA STOMATOLOGIYA. Text in Russian; Contents page in English, Russian. q. USD 36 domestic; USD 75 foreign (effective 2002). adv. *Refereed.*
Indexed: Ref.Zh.
Published by: (Stomatologicheskaya Assotsiatsia Rossii/Association of Stomatology of Russia), TBI, Ostozhenka 6, Moscow 119034, Russian Federation. stoma@glasnet.ru, http://www.stoma.ru. adv.: page USD 2,000. Circ: 5,000 (paid and controlled). **US dist. addr.:** East View Publications, 3020 Harbor Ln N, Minneapolis, MN 55447. TEL 612-550-0961.

617.6 SWE ISSN 0281-7020
KLINIK OCH TERAPI FOER TANDLAEKARE. Text in Swedish. 1970-1976; resumed 1980-1987; resumed 1991. s-a.
Formerly (until 1982): Astranytt
Published by: Astra Laekemedel AB, Soedertaelje 15185, Sweden.

617.6 JPN ISSN 0023-2831
CODEN: KEGZA7
KOKU EISEI GAKKAI ZASSHI* /JAPANESE JOURNAL OF ORAL HYGIENE. Text in Japanese. 1952. q. adv. index.
Indexed: Biol.Abstr., Chem.Abstr., Dent.Ind.
—BLDSC (4968.460000), GNLM.
Published by: Tokyo Medical and Dental University, Faculty of Dentistry, 1-5-45 Yushima, Bunkyo-ku, Tokyo 113-8549, Japan. Ed. Masao Onisi.

617.6 KOR ISSN 0023-3927
KOREA RESEARCH SOCIETY FOR DENTAL MATERIALS. JOURNAL*. Text in Korean; Abstracts and contents page in English. 1966. q. free per issue. adv. abstr, bibl, charts, illus.
Published by: Seoul National University, College of Dentistry, San 56-1 Sinlim-dong, Kwanak-ku, Seoul 151742, Korea, S.. Ed. Dr. Yang Shok Yoo.

617.6 RUS
KVINTESSENTSIYA; mezhdunarodnyi stomotalogicheskii zhurnal. Text in Russian. 1991. 6/yr.
Address: c/o Yu E Shirokov, Ed, A-ya, Moscow 125190, Russian Federation. TEL 203-99-88.

617.6 USA ISSN 1058-7845
LAB MANAGEMENT TODAY. Text in English. 1984. 10/yr. USD 17; USD 18.50 in Canada; USD 45 foreign; USD 5 newsstand/cover (effective 2000); free to qualified personnel. adv. tr.lit. reprints avail. *Refereed.* **Document type:** *Trade.* **Description:** Provides management and marketing strategies for dental laboratory decision makers.
Formerly: Dental Lab Management Today (8750-9539)
—GNLM.
Published by: L M T Communications, Inc., 731 Main St, Ste. A2, Monroe, CT 06468. TEL 203-459-2888, FAX 203-459-2889, info@lmtcommunications.com, http://www.lmtcommunications.com. Ed., R&P Kelly Fessel Carr. Pub. Judy Fishman. Adv. contact James Pouilliard. B&W page USD 2,840, color page USD 4,240; trim 14.5 x 10.88. Circ: 17,500.

617.6 USA ISSN 1091-5184
LABORATORY DIGEST. Text in English. 1995. q. **Document type:** *Magazine, Academic/Scholarly, Trade.* **Description:** Provides current information on new trends, innovative techniques, and state-of-the-art laboratory technology and fabrication procedures.
Published by: Montage Media Corp., 1000 Wyckoff Ave, Mahwah, NJ 07430. TEL 201-891-3200, FAX 201-891-2626, info@montagemedia.com, http://www.montagemedia.com/lab.html.

617.6 HKG ISSN 1022-7970
LATIN AMERICAN DENTAL NEWS. Text in English, Spanish. 1994. q. **Document type:** *Trade.*
Published by: MediMedia Asia (Subsidiary of: MediMedia Pacific Ltd.), 2102 Tung Sun Commercial Centre, 194-200 Lockhart Rd, Wanchai, Hong Kong, Hong Kong. TEL 852-2511-0765, FAX 852-2507-3817, http://www.medimedia.com.hk/.

617.6 USA ISSN 0023-9062
LAVENDER BAND. Text in English. 1961. bi-m. USD 20 to non-members (effective 1998). adv. **Document type:** *Newsletter.*
Published by: Iowa Dental Hygienists' Association, 1231 21st St, Rock Island, IL 61201. TEL 309-788-8858, FAX 309-788-8858. Ed., R&P, Adv. contact Linda Rowe. Circ: 575.

617.6 USA ISSN 0024-6786
LOUISIANA DENTAL ASSOCIATION. JOURNAL. Text in English. 1966 (vol.23). q. USD 15. adv. illus.
Indexed: Dent.Abstr., Dent.Ind.
Published by: Louisiana Dental Association, 8510 Line Ave, Shreveport, LA 71106. FAX 318-869-3111. Ed. Dr. Gary L Roberts. Circ: 1,650.

617.6 SWE ISSN 0076-3438
LUND UNIVERSITY. SCHOOL OF DENTISTRY. FACULTY OF ODONTOLOGY. ANNUAL PUBLICATIONS. Text in English. 1958. a. free per issue. bk.rev. **Document type:** *Academic/Scholarly.*
Published by: Lund University, Faculty of Odontology, School of Dentistry, Malmo 21421, Sweden. FAX 46-40-92-53-59. Ed. Krister Nilner. Circ: 750.

617.6 USA ISSN 0738-4556
M D S NEWS*. Text in English. 1964. 6/yr. USD 20. back issues avail.
Published by: Massachusetts Dental Society, 2 Willow St No 200, Southborough, MA 01745-1027. TEL 508-651-7511, FAX 508-653-7115. Ed. Margaret Quinlan. Circ: 4,250.

617.6 IDN ISSN 0024-9548
MADJALAH PERSATUAN DOKTER GIGI INDONESIA*. Summaries in English. 1951. 4/yr. USD 10.
Published by: Indonesian Dental Association, Jalan Prapatan 14, Jakarta, Indonesia. Ed. Geri Pandjaitan. Circ: 1,000.

617.6 POL ISSN 1230-0888
MAGAZYN STOMATOLOGICZNY. Text in Polish. 1991. m. USD 99 (effective 1998). adv. bk.rev. abstr, bibl, charts, illus. index. back issues avail. **Document type:** *Academic/Scholarly.* **Description:** Covers all dental fields and related branches.
Published by: Wydawnictwo Medyczne Sanmedica Sp. z o.o., Ul Nowy Zjazd 1, Warsaw 00301, Poland. TEL 48-22-8262287, FAX 48-22-8263182. Ed. Wanda Rytlowa. Adv. contact Jolanta Paterczyk. B&W page USD 800, color page USD 1,000. Circ: 4,500.

617.6 IRN
MAJDA. Text in Persian, Modern; Summaries in English. 1964. 3/yr. membership.
Formerly: Iranian Dental Association. Journal - Jame'e-Ye Dandanpezeshkan-e Iran. Majalleh
Published by: (Iranian Dental Association), Hamid Adeli-Najafi, Ed. & Pub., No. 94, W. Piroozi Str., Nasr Place, P O Box 14155-3695, Tehran, Iran. TEL 98-21-639591, FAX 98-21-639592.

617.6 658 USA ISSN 1083-3641
MANAGED DENTAL CARE. Text in English. 1995. m. USD 277 domestic; USD 287 in Canada; USD 301 elsewhere (effective 2000). charts, mkt. back issues avail. **Document type:** *Newsletter.* **Description:** Provides business intelligence on dental regulatory developments, quality of care concerns, Medicaid and Medicare issues and new contracts.
—CCC.
Published by: Business Information Services, Inc, 12811 North Point Ln, Laurel, MD 20708. TEL 301-604-4001, FAX 301-604-5126, businfosvc@aol.com. Ed. Sheila Moldover. Pub. James H Gutman. R&P Seth Sprecher.

617.6 TUR ISSN 1018-5992
MARMARA UNIVERSITY. FACULTY OF DENTISTRY. JOURNAL. Key Title: Journal of Marmara University Dental Faculty. Text in English. 1990. a. USD 15 (effective 1997 & 1998). back issues avail. *Refereed.* **Document type:** *Academic/Scholarly.*
—GNLM.
Published by: Marmara University, Faculty of Dentistry, Buyukciftlik Sok. No. 6, Nisantasi - Istanbul 80200, Turkey. TEL 90-212-2483127, FAX 90-212-2465247. Ed. Dr. Nesrin Emekli. Pub. Dr. Nesrin Emelki. Circ: 1,200 (controlled).

617.6 USA ISSN 0025-4355
MARYLAND STATE DENTAL ASSOCIATION. JOURNAL. Text in English. 1958. q. USD 40 to non-members; USD 5 to members; USD 12 newsstand/cover. adv. bk.rev. charts, illus, stat. index. *Refereed.* **Document type:** *Academic/Scholarly.*
Indexed: Dent.Abstr., Dent.Ind., INIS Atomind.
—CISTI, GNLM.
Published by: Maryland State Dental Association, 6450 Dobbin Rd, Columbia Business Center, Columbia, MD 21045-4744. TEL 410-964-2880, FAX 410-964-0583. Ed., R&P Harold Goodman. Adv. contact Rosemaria Richardson. Circ: 2,800.

617.6 USA ISSN 0025-4800
MASSACHUSETTS DENTAL SOCIETY. JOURNAL*. Text in English. 1951. q. USD 12 domestic; USD 23.40 in Canada; USD 35.40 elsewhere. adv. bk.rev. illus, abstr. **Document type:** *Academic/Scholarly.*
Indexed: Dent.Abstr., Dent.Ind.
—BLDSC (4821.600000), CISTI, GNLM.
Published by: Massachusetts Dental Society, 2 Willow St No 200, Southborough, MA 01745-1027. TEL 508-651-7511, FAX 508-653-7115, madental@massdental.org. Ed. Dr. Norman Becker. R&P Catherine Peterson. Circ: 4,166.

MATSUMOTO SHIGAKU/MATSUMOTO DENTAL UNIVERSITY SOCIETY. JOURNAL. see *BIOLOGY*

MEDICAL AND DENTAL ASSOCIATION OF BOTSWANA. JOURNAL. see *MEDICAL SCIENCES*

MEDICAL MALPRACTICE: HANDLING DENTAL CASES. see *LAW—Civil Law*

617.6 HRV ISSN 0025-7966
MEDICINAR; glasnk studentica i studenata Medicinskog Fakulteta Sveucilista u Zagrebu. Text in Croatian, English. 1946. 2/yr., latest vol.42. USD 28. adv. bk.rev. abstr, bibl, charts, illus, stat. index. **Document type:** *Journal.*

M

Published by: Sveuciliste u Zagrebu, Medicinski Fakultet, Salata 3-b, Zagreb 10000, Croatia. TEL 385-1-4566720, medicinar@mef.hr, http://www.mef.hr. Ed. Dinka Pavicic. Circ: 3,500.

617.6 BGR ISSN 1310-8999
MEDITSINSKI PREGLED. SUVREMENNA STOMATOLOGIA. Text in Bulgarian; Summaries in Bulgarian, English. 1997. bi-m., latest vol.32, 2001. BGL 21 domestic; BGL 35 foreign (effective 2001 - 2002). adv. abstr, bibl, illus. 52 p./no. **Document type:** *Journal.* **Description:** Covers general, pediatric, therapeutic, prosthetic, and surgical dentistry; maxillofacial surgery; and orthodontics.
Indexed: Ref.Zh.
Published by: Meditsinski Universitet - Sofia, Tsentur za Informatsiia po Meditsina/Medical University - Sofia, Medical Information Center, 1Sv Georgi Sofiiski ul 1, Sofia 1431, Bulgaria. TEL 359-2-9522342, FAX 359-2-9522393, mutafov@sun.medun.acad.bg, http://www.medun.acad.bg. Ed. B Indzhov. R&P, Adv. contact Dr. Christo Mutafov. B&W page USD 50, color page USD 200; 12 x 18. Circ: 300. **Dist. by:** Sofia Books, Ul Silivria 16, Sofia 1404, Bulgaria. TEL 359-2-9586257, sofiabooks@hotmail.com, http://www.sofiabooks.hit.bg. **Co-sponsor:** ORMED Ltd.

617.6 DEU ISSN 0940-2500
MEDIZIN DENTAL MAGAZIN; der Wegbegleiter vom Studienanfaenger zum Praxisgruender. Key Title: Med.-dent.-Magazin. Text in German. 1987. bi-m. DEM 24 (effective 2000). adv. bk.rev. **Document type:** *Magazine, Trade.*
Published by: H.P. Kuechenmeister Hochschulverlag, Daldorferstr 15, Rickling 24635, Germany. TEL 49-4328-722477, FAX 49-4328-722478. Ed. Hans Peter Kuechenmeister. Circ: 13,000.

617.6 JPN ISSN 0916-0701
CODEN: JSDKD3
MEIKAI DAIGAKU SHIGAKU ZASSHI/MEIKAI UNIVERSITY DENTAL JOURNAL/MEIKAI UNIVERSITY SCHOOL OF DENTISTRY. JOURNAL. Text mainly in Japanese; Text occasionally in English. 1972. 2/yr. *Refereed.* **Document type:** *Academic/Scholarly.* **Description:** Covers dental and medical science.
Formerly: Josai Shika Daigaku Kiyo (0301-2662)
Indexed: Chem.Abstr., Chem.Titles, INIS Atomind.
—BLDSC (5536.394000), CASDDS, CISTI, GNLM.
Published by: Meikai University, School of Dentistry, 1-1 Keyakidai, Sakado-shi, Saitama-ken 350-0248, Japan. TEL 81-492-79-2770, FAX 81-492-87-4712, ueha@dent.meikai.ac.jp, http://www.dent.meikai.ac.jp, http://www.dental.meikai.ac.jp. Ed. Takao Ueha. Circ: 1,000.

617.6 USA ISSN 0026-2102
MICHIGAN DENTAL ASSOCIATION. JOURNAL. Text in English. 1919. 9/yr., latest vol.83. USD 70 to non-members; USD 15 to libraries; USD 5 to students (effective 2001). adv. bk.rev. illus. back issues avail. **Document type:** *Journal, Trade.* **Description:** Seeks to publish news and feature articles useful to the average practitioner.
Former titles (until 1968): Michigan State Dental Association. Journal (0098-7107); (until 1951): Michigan State Dental Society. Journal
Indexed: Abstr.Health Care Manage.Stud., Biol.Abstr., Dent.Abstr., Dent.Ind., INIS Atomind.
—BLDSC (4825.600000), CISTI, GNLM.
Published by: Michigan Dental Association, 230 N Washington Sq, Ste 208, Lansing, MI 48933. TEL 517-372-9070, FAX 517-372-0008, mdadtp@smilemichigan.com, http://www.smilemichigan.com, http://www.michigandental.org. Ed. Dr. Michael G Mailhofer. Adv. contacts David Foe TEL 517-346-9421, Jackie Lovaas TEL 517-346-9419. B&W page USD 565, color page USD 1,265. Circ: 6,300 (paid).

617.6 USA ISSN 0047-7095
MICHIGAN DENTAL HYGIENIST ASSOCIATION. BULLETIN. Text in English. 1973. 3/yr. USD 20 domestic; USD 25 foreign (effective 2000). adv. bk.rev. illus. **Document type:** *Trade.*
Indexed: Dent.Ind.
Published by: Michigan Dental Hygienists Association, 600 S Capitol Ave, Lansing, MI 48933-2308. TEL 517-484-1352, FAX 517-484-8174. Ed., Pub., Adv. contact Chris Farrell. R&P Becky Forest. Circ: 1,400.

610 579 AUS
▼ **MICROBIOLOGY**; Royal Australasian College of Dental Surgeons. Lecture notes in microbiology. Text in English. 1999. a. AUD 36 newsstand/cover (effective 2001 & 2002). **Document type:** *Academic/Scholarly.*
Published by: Royal Australasian College of Dental Surgeons, 64 Castlereagh St, Sydney, NSW 2000, Australia. TEL 61-2-9232-3800, FAX 61-2-9221-8108, registrar@racds.org, http://www.racds.org. Ed. Laurance Walsh.

617.6 USA ISSN 0026-3478
MIDWESTERN DENTIST. Text in English. 1925. m. (except June, July, Aug.). USD 18 (effective 1999); only to qualified personnel in the U.S.. adv. bk.rev. **Document type:** *Newsletter.*
Former titles (until 1959): Kansas City District Dental Society. Journal; (until 1947): Kansas City Dental Society Bulletin; (until 1932): Kansas City Dental Society. Monthly Bulletin
—GNLM.
Published by: Greater Kansas City Dental Society, 5907 Raytown Trafficway, Kansas City, MO 64133. TEL 816-737-5353. Ed. Dr. Robert Nelson. Adv. contact Pamela Ratliff. Circ: 800 (controlled).

617.6 ITA ISSN 0394-168X
MINERVA ORTOGNATODONTICA; rivista trimestrale di ortognatodonzia, gnatologia, odontoiatria preventiva. Text in Italian. q. USD 105 to individuals; USD 155 to institutions (effective 1999). adv. *Refereed.* **Document type:** *Academic/Scholarly.* **Description:** Covers orthognathodontics, gnathology, and preventive dentistry.
Formerly: Minerva Odontoiatrica
—GNLM.
Published by: Edizioni Minerva Medica, Corso Bramante, 83-85, Turin, TO 10126, Italy. TEL 39-11-678282, FAX 39-11-674502. Ed. P Bracco. Pub. Alberto Oliaro. Adv. contact F Filippo. B&W page USD 1,200, color page USD 2,000; trim 270 x 190. Circ: 2,000 (paid).

617.6 ITA ISSN 0026-4970
MINERVA STOMATOLOGICA. Text in Italian; Summaries in English, Italian. 1952. m. (10/yr.). USD 130 to individuals; USD 165 to institutions (effective 2000 - 2001). adv. bk.rev. abstr, bibl, charts, illus. index. *Refereed.* **Document type:** *Academic/Scholarly.* **Description:** Covers odontostomatology and maxillofacial surgery.
Related titles: Microform ed.: (from PQC).
Indexed: Abstr.Hyg., Biol.Abstr., Chem.Abstr., Dent.Ind., Excerp.Med., Ind.Med. (1952-), Nutr.Abstr., Rev.Med.& Vet.Mycol.
—BLDSC (5794.600000), CISTI, KNAW.
Published by: (Societa Italiana di Odontostomatologia e Chirurgia Maxillo-Facciale), Edizioni Minerva Medica, Corso Bramante, 83-85, Turin, TO 10126, Italy. TEL 39-11-678282, FAX 39-11-674502. Ed. R Modica. Pub. Alberto Oliaro. Adv. contact F Filippo. B&W page USD 1,200, color page USD 2,000; trim 270 x 190. Circ: 4,000 (paid).

617.6 LKA
MIRROR AND PROBE✱. Text in English; Summaries in Singhalese, Tamil. 1963. a. adv. charts, illus, stat.
Published by: Dental Students' Association, University of Sri Lanka, University Park, Peradeniya, Sri Lanka. Circ: (controlled).

617.6 USA
MOMENTUM (ROCHESTER). Text in English. 1974. q.
Published by: Eastman Dental Center, 625 Elmwood Ave, Rochester, NY 14620. TEL 716-275-5064, FAX 716-244-8772. Ed. Teresa A O'Loughlin. Circ: 1,800.

617.6 BEL
MONDE DENTAIRE/TANDARTSEN WERELD. Text in French, Dutch. 1982. bi-m. BEF 1,000. adv. illus. index. back issues avail. **Document type:** *Magazine, Trade.*
Related titles: Dutch ed.: Tandartsen Wereld.
Published by: C.E.P. s.r.l., Av de Tervuren 298, Brussels 1150, Belgium. TEL 32-2-7623458, FAX 32-2-7716351, cep@cep.be, http://www.cep.be. Ed. Emmanuel M G Steinbach. adv.: B&W page XEU 1,545, color page XEU 2,111; 184 x 254. Circ: 9,200.

617.6 ITA ISSN 0391-2000
CODEN: MOORDG
MONDO ORTODONTICO. Text in Italian. 1975. 6/yr. ITL 159,000 (effective 1999). **Document type:** *Academic/Scholarly.*
Indexed: Biol.Abstr., Dent.Ind., Excerp.Med.
—BLDSC (5908.235000), GNLM.
Published by: Masson S.p.A., Divisione Periodici, Via F.lli Bressan 2, Milan, MI 20126, Italy. TEL 39-2-270741, FAX 39-2-27074210. adv.: B&W page ITL 1,510,000, color page ITL 2,160,000; trim 265 x 193. Circ: 4,000.

617.6 CHE ISSN 0077-0892
CODEN: MGUSCU
MONOGRAPHS IN ORAL SCIENCE. Text in English. 1972. irreg., latest vol.18. CHF 180 in Europe; DEM 215 in Germany; USD 145 in United States (2001). reprint service avail. from ISI. *Refereed.* **Document type:** *Monographic series, Academic/Scholarly.* **Description:** Summaries of important topics in oral biology.
Related titles: Online - full text ed.: (from Institute for Scientific Information).
Indexed: Biol.Abstr., Chem.Abstr., Curr.Cont. (coverage dropped), Ind.Med. (1971-).
—BLDSC (5915.830000), CISTI, GNLM, KNAW. **CCC.**
Published by: S. Karger AG, Allschwilerstr 10, PO Box, Basel 4009, Switzerland. TEL 41-61-306-1111, FAX 41-61-306-1234, karger@karger.ch, http://www.karger.com/bookseries/MOORS. Ed. G M Whitford.

617.6 USA ISSN 0027-0156
MONTGOMERY - BUCKS DENTAL SOCIETY. BULLETIN. Text in English. 1955. 7/yr. membership. adv. bk.rev. bibl. **Document type:** *Bulletin.*
Indexed: Dent.Ind.
Published by: Montgomery - Bucks County Dental Society, 85 Old Eagle School Rd, Wayne, PA 19087. TEL 610-995-0109, FAX 610-995-0107. Ed. Dr. Bruce R Terry. Adv. contact Dr. Bruce Terry. Circ: 800.

617.6 USA
CODEN: DENTEJ
MOUTH (YEAR). Text in English. 1981. q. USD 16 domestic; USD 24 foreign (effective 2001). adv. 30 p./no. reprints avail. **Document type:** *Academic/Scholarly, Trade.* **Description:** For dental students and young dental professionals. Discusses issues, trends and new developments in dentistry.
Formerly: Dentistry (Year) (0277-3635)
Indexed: INIS Atomind.
—GNLM, ingenta.
Published by: American Student Dental Association, 211 E Chicago Ave, Ste. 1160, Chicago, IL 60611-2616. TEL 312-440-2795, editors@asdanet.org, asda@asdanet.org, http://www.asdanet.org. Pub. Cynthia L Kennedy. R&P Lauren Waggoner. Adv. contact Stephanie Cesna TEL 312-440-2845. B&W page USD 950; trim 10.88 x 8.25. Circ: 16,000.

617.6 USA
MOUTHPIECE (CHICAGO). Text in English. 1983. q. USD 56 to non-members; USD 40 to members. illus. **Document type:** *Trade.*
Indexed: Sports Per.Ind.
Published by: American Dental Association, 211 E Chicago Ave, Chicago, IL 60611. TEL 312-440-2602, FAX 312-440-2790. Ed. Alanna Gordon.

617.6 USA
MOUTHPIECE (REDWOOD CITY). Text in English. 1965. m. USD 15. adv. **Document type:** *Newsletter.* **Description:** General information for dentists with emphasis on local impact.
Formerly: San Mateo County Dental Society. Bulletin (0080-598X)
Published by: San Mateo County Dental Society, 240 Twin Dolphin Dr, Ste A, Redwood City, CA 94065-1403. TEL 650-637-1121. Ed., R&P Adrian Vogt TEL 650-342-5801. Adv. contact David E Moore. Circ: 525.

617.6 NOR ISSN 0047-8377
MUNNPLEIEN✱. Text in Norwegian. 1916. 4/yr. NOK 300. adv. bk.rev.
Indexed: Dent.Ind.
Published by: Norsk Tannvern/Oral Health of Norway, Postboks 9341, Groenland, Oslo 0188, Norway. TEL 47-22-44-28-66, FAX 47-22-56-36-93. Ed. Gerd M Brandt. Circ: 5,000.

617.6 USA ISSN 1524-4938
N D A JOURNAL. Text in English. q. USD 20 domestic; USD 30 foreign; USD 6 newsstand/cover (effective 1999). adv. back issues avail. *Refereed.* **Document type:** *Academic/Scholarly.* **Description:** Addresses issues of particular interest to African-American oral health providers and the communities they serve.
Published by: (National Dental Association), Heritage Information Publishers, 1101 Pennsylvania Ave, N W, Ste 820, Washington, DC 20004. TEL 202-347-3820, FAX 202-347-4096. Ed. Dr. Georgetta Manning Cox. R&P Lee Wellman TEL 202-588-1697. Circ: 24,000.
Subscr. to: Lee Wellman, National Dental Association, 3517 16th St, N W, Washington, DC 20010. TEL 202-588-1697, FAX 202-588-1244.

617.6 USA ISSN 0027-6545
N H D S NEWSLETTER. Text in English. 1939. bi-m. membership. adv. bk.rev. illus, stat. **Document type:** *Newsletter.*
Indexed: Dent.Abstr.
Published by: New Hampshire Dental Society, PO Box 2229, Concord, NH 03301-1772. Ed. Dr. Richard P Berryman. R&P H. Dougherty. Circ: 600.

617.6 USA
NASSAU COUNTY DENTAL SOCIETY. NEWSLETTER. Text in English. 1949. 6/yr. USD 15 per issue. adv. bk.rev. *Refereed.* **Document type:** *Bulletin, Academic/Scholarly.*
Former titles (until 1994): Nassau Dental News; (until 1984): Nassau County Dental Society. Bulletin; (until 1981): Tenth District Dental Society of the State of New York. Bulletin (0070-3729)
Published by: Nassau County Dental Society Headquarters, 377 Oak St, 205, Garden City, NY 11530-6543. TEL 516-764-9620, FAX 516-227-1114. Ed. Dr. Steven Kerpen. R&P Dr. William F Boyd. Adv. contact Irene Cruz. Circ: 2,000 (controlled).

617.6 USA
NATIONAL ASSOCIATION OF DENTAL LABORATORIES. MEMBERSHIP MEMO✶ . Text in English. q. membership. **Document type:** *Newsletter.*
Published by: National Association of Dental Laboratories, 8201 Greensboro Dr., Ste. 300, Mclean, VA 22102-3810.

614.5996 617.6 USA ISSN 0027-9269
NATIONAL FLUORIDATION NEWS✶ . Text in English. 1955. q. USD 10. bk.rev. illus. **Document type:** *Newspaper.* **Description:** Reports on research into the toxicity of fluoride, news on accidents, election outcomes and general information on the issue.
Published by: Shirley Graves, Ed. & Pub., 57 Bahama Reef, Novato, CA 94949-5357. TEL 415-453-0158. Circ: 5,000.

NATIONAL MEDICAL AND DENTAL ASSOCIATION. BULLETIN. see *MEDICAL SCIENCES*

617.6 NLD ISSN 0028-2111
NEDERLANDS TANDARTSENBLAD. Text in Dutch. 1942. fortn. NLG 260 in Europe; NLG 312 rest of world; (outside Europe fl.312). bk.rev. index. **Document type:** *Trade.*
—CISTI.
Published by: Nederlandse Maatschappij tot Bevordering der Tandheelkunde, Postbus 2000, Nieuwegein 3430 CA, Netherlands. TEL 31-30-6076251, FAX 31-30-6076301, nt@nmt.nl. Ed. J H Schotte. R&P J A van der Horst. adv.: B&W page NLG 2,005, color page NLG 2,665; trim 297 x 210. Circ: 8,600 (paid).

617.6 NLD ISSN 1384-3966
NEDERLANDS TIJDSCHRIFT VOOR MONDHYGIENE. Text in Dutch. 1977. bi-m. adv. **Document type:** *Trade.* **Description:** Offers dental hygienists practical information.
Formerly (Until 1996): N V M Tijdschrift (0169-0892)
Published by: Wegener Tijdschriften Groep BV (Subsidiary of: Wegener Arcade NV), Wildenborch 5, Postbus 1860, Diemen 1112 CD, Netherlands. TEL 31-20-660-3300, FAX 31-20-660-3303, info@wtg.wegener.nl, http://www.wegener.nl. Adv. contact Peter Buitendijk. B&W page NLG 1,890, color page NLG 4,480. Circ: 2,000.

617.6 NLD ISSN 0028-2200 CODEN: NTTAAX
NEDERLANDS TIJDSCHRIFT VOOR TANDHEELKUNDE. Text in Dutch. 1894. m. NLG 166.40; BEF 3,250 in Belgium; NLG 192 elsewhere (effective 1999); free to qualified personnel. adv. bk.rev. illus, tr.lit. index. **Document type:** *Trade.* **Description:** Reports on the newest patient-care methods and techniques, developments in oral hygiene, and economic and practice-management issues.
Related titles: Online - full text ed.
Indexed: Biol.Abstr., Dent.Ind.
—CISTI, GNLM, KNAW.
Published by: Wegener Tijdschriften Groep BV (Subsidiary of: Wegener Arcade NV), Wildenborch 5, Postbus 1860, Diemen 1112 CD, Netherlands. TEL 31-20-660-3300, FAX 31-20-660-3303, info@wtg.wegener.nl; ntvtred@wxs.nl, http://www.wegener.nl; http://www.ntvt.nl. Ed. Dr. A M Kuijpers Jagtman. Pub. Mark Hoogeveen. Adv. contact Peter Buitendijk. B&W page NLG 2,330, color page NLG 5,115. Circ: 5,500 (controlled).

617.6 USA ISSN 0093-7347
NEW JERSEY DENTAL ASSOCIATION. JOURNAL. Text in English. 1912. q. USD 50 to non-members; USD 20 to members (effective 2000). adv. bk.rev. bibl, charts, illus, stat. back issues avail. **Document type:** *Academic/Scholarly.*
Indexed: Dent.Abstr., Dent.Ind., INIS Atomind.
—BLDSC (4832.200000), GNLM.
Published by: New Jersey Dental Association, 1 Dental Plaza, Box 6020, North Brunswick, NJ 08902-6020. TEL 732-821-9400, FAX 732-821-1082, http://www.njda.org. Ed. Dr. Harvey S Nisselson. Pub. Arthur Meisel. R&P, Adv. contact Lynn M Foley. Circ: 5,000 (paid).

617.6 USA ISSN 0028-7571
THE NEW YORK STATE DENTAL JOURNAL. Text in English. 1933. 10/yr. USD 54 domestic to non-members; USD 89 foreign (effective 2001); Free to members. adv. bk.rev. bibl, illus, stat. index. back issues avail.; reprint service avail. from PQC. *Refereed.* **Document type:** *Journal, Trade.* **Description:** Features scientific articles covering research reports, case studies, and experiences with new techniques. Includes general and technical information of interest to dental practitioners.
Related titles: Microform ed.: (from PQC); Online - full text ed.: (from Northern Light Technology, Inc., ProQuest Information & Learning).
Indexed: AgeLine, Biol.Abstr., Chem.Abstr., Curr.Tit.Dent., Dent.Abstr., Dent.Ind., Dok.Arbeitsmed., Excerp.Med., INIS Atomind., Ind.Med. (1947-), Med.Care Rev.
—BLDSC (6089.730000), CISTI, GNLM.
Published by: New York State Dental Association, 121 State St, Fourth Fl, Albany, NY 12207. TEL 518-465-0044, FAX 518-427-0461, http://www.nysdental.org. Ed. Sheridan B Albert. Adv. contact Christine Noon TEL 518-465-0044 ext 271. Circ: 13,950 (paid).

617.6 NZL ISSN 0028-8047 CODEN: NZDJAM
NEW ZEALAND DENTAL JOURNAL. Text in English. 1905. q. NZD 80; NZD 105 foreign. adv. bk.rev. abstr, charts, illus. index. *Refereed.* **Document type:** *Academic/Scholarly.* **Description:** Presents scientific and clinical articles related to dentistry and the dental sciences; correspondence and news about dentistry; personal items and obituaries.
Indexed: Biol.Abstr., Dent.Abstr., Dent.Ind., Excerp.Med., INIS Atomind., Ind.Med. (1905-), Ind.N.Z.Per., NRN.
—BLDSC (6089.970000), CISTI, GNLM, ingenta. **CCC.**
Published by: New Zealand Dental Association, PO Box 647, Dunedin, New Zealand. TEL 64-3-4797040, FAX 64-03-4790673. Ed. R H Brown. R&P R.H. Brown. Adv. contact Maureen McCort. Circ: 1,660; 1,600 (controlled).

617.632 NZL ISSN 0111-1485
NEW ZEALAND SOCIETY OF PERIODONTOLOGY. JOURNAL. Text in English. 1956. s-a. NZD 80 (effective 2000). adv. bk.rev. stat. *Refereed.* **Document type:** *Academic/Scholarly.*
Formerly: New Zealand Society of Periodontology. Bulletin (0028-8705)
Indexed: Curr.Tit.Dent., Dent.Ind.
—BLDSC (4833.070000), GNLM, Infotrieve. **CCC.**
Published by: New Zealand Society of Periodontology, PO Box 647, Dunedin, New Zealand. TEL 64-3-4797-108, FAX 64-3-4790-673, angela.pack@stonebow.otago.ac.nz. Ed. Angela R C Pack. R&P, Adv. contact Angela R.C. Pack. Circ: 600.

617.6 USA
NEWS AND VIEWS (BETHESDA). Text in English. 1972. q. membership. back issues avail. **Document type:** *Newsletter.* **Description:** Covers the activities and projects of the College and its 41 sections.
Published by: American College of Dentists, 839 J Quince Orchard Blvd, Bethesda, MD 20878-1614. TEL 301-977-3223, 888-223-1920, FAX 301-977-3330, robyn@acdentists.org. Ed. David Chambers. R&P Robyn Hulvey.

617.6 JPN ISSN 0385-0102
NICHIDAI SHIGAKU/NIHON UNIVERSITY DENTAL JOURNAL. Text in Japanese; Summaries in English. 1921. bi-m. JPY 5,000 (effective 2001). *Refereed.*
Indexed: INIS Atomind.
Published by: Nihon Daigaku Shigakukai, c/o Mayumi Nomura Secy., Nihon University School of Dentistry, 1-8-13 Kanda-Surugadai, Chiyoda-ku, Tokyo 101-8310, Japan. FAX 81-3-3219-8310. Ed. Yoshihiko Moriya. Circ: 2,170.

617.6 JPN ISSN 0029-0297 CODEN: NKOGAV
NIHON KOKUKA GAKKAI ZASSHI/JAPANESE STOMATOLOGICAL SOCIETY. JOURNAL. Text in Japanese. 1952. q. JPY 5,200, USD 3.50.
Indexed: Chem.Abstr., INIS Atomind., Ind.Med. (coverage dropped).
—BLDSC (4809.550000), CASDDS, CISTI, GNLM, Infotrieve. **CCC.**
Published by: Nihon Kokuka Gakkai/Japanese Stomatological Society, Department of Oral Surgery School of Medicine, University of, 7-3-1 Hongo, Bunkyo-ku, Tokyo 113-0033, Japan. Circ: 1,900.

617.6 JPN ISSN 0047-1763 CODEN: NISIA9
NIHON SHIKA ISHIKAI ZASSHI/JAPAN DENTAL ASSOCIATION. JOURNAL. Text in Japanese. 1948. m. JPY 4,896 (effective 2001). adv. illus. index. reprint service avail. from PQC. **Document type:** *Academic/Scholarly.*
Related titles: Microform ed.: (from PQC).
Indexed: Dent.Ind., INIS Atomind., Ind.Med. (coverage dropped).
—CASDDS, CISTI, GNLM.
Published by: Japanese Dental Association/Nihon Shika Ishikai, 4-1-20 Kudan-Kita, Chiyoda-ku, Tokyo 102-0073, Japan. TEL 81-3-3262-9213, FAX 81-3-3262-9885. Circ: 63,000.

NIHON SHIKA MASUI GAKKAI ZASSHI/JAPANESE DENTAL SOCIETY OF ANESTHESIOLOGY. JOURNAL. see *MEDICAL SCIENCES—Anaesthesiology*

617.6 JPN ISSN 0385-0110 CODEN: NSKADI
NIHON SHISHUBYO GAKKAI KAISHI/JAPANESE ASSOCIATION OF PERIODONTOLOGY. JOURNAL. Text in Japanese. 1968. q. JPY 9,000, USD 100 (effective 2000). adv. bk.rev. *Refereed.* **Document type:** *Academic/Scholarly.* **Description:** Publishes articles relevant to science and practice of the periodontal disease and related fields.
Indexed: Chem.Abstr., Dent.Ind., Eng.Ind.
—CASDDS, CISTI, GNLM.
Published by: Nihon Shishubyo Gakkai, Koku Hoken Kyokai, 44-9 Komagome 1-chome, Toshima-ku, Tokyo 170-0003, Japan. TEL 81-52-3-3947-8891, FAX 81-52-3-3947-8341. Ed. Satoru Yamada. R&P Isao Ishikawa. Adv. contact Koku Hoken Kyokai. Circ: 4,300.

617.6 JPN ISSN 0385-0145 CODEN: NKOKDC
NIHON UNIVERSITY. JOURNAL OF ORAL SCIENCE/NICHIDAI KOKU KAGAKU. Text in Japanese. 1975. q. per issue exchange basis. index. *Refereed.* **Document type:** *Academic/Scholarly.*
Indexed: INIS Atomind.
—BLDSC (6113.150000), CASDDS, GNLM.
Published by: Nihon University, School of Dentistry at Matsudo, 870-1 Sakaecho-Nishi -2, Matsudo-shi, Chiba-ken 271-0061, Japan. TEL 81-47-368-6111, FAX 81-47-364-6295, msr@mascat.nihon-u.ac.jp, http://www.mascat.nihon-u.ac.jp/. Ed. Yukishige Kozawa. Circ: 900.

617.6 JPN ISSN 0549-5245
NIPPON DENTAL UNIVERSITY. ANNUAL PUBLICATIONS. Text in English. 1964. a. per issue exchange basis. **Document type:** *Academic/Scholarly.*
Formerly: Society of Nippon Dental College. Annual Publications
Indexed: INIS Atomind.
—**CCC.**
Published by: Society of the Nippon Dental University/Nippon Shika Daigaku Shigakukai, 9-20 Fujimi 1-chome, Chiyoda-ku, Tokyo 102-0071, Japan. FAX 81-3-3264-8745. Ed. Arika Hasegawa. Circ: 2,000.

617.6 NOR ISSN 0029-2303
DEN NORSKE TANNLEGEFORENINGS TIDENDE/NORWEGIAN DENTAL JOURNAL. Text in Norwegian; Summaries in English. 1890. 17/yr. NOK 1,075 domestic; USD 135 foreign (effective 2000). adv. bk.rev. charts, illus, stat, tr.lit. index. *Refereed.* **Document type:** *Journal, Academic/Scholarly.* **Description:** Contains scientific articles, health, politics, etc.
Former titles (until 1946): Norges Tannlaegeforbunds Tidsskrift (0801-4477); (until 1941): Norske Tannlaegeforenings Tidsskrift (0801-4469)
Related titles: Online - full text ed.
Indexed: Dent.Abstr., Dent.Ind., INIS Atomind., Ind.Med. (coverage dropped).
—CISTI, GNLM, Infotrieve. **CCC.**

M

Published by: Norske Tannlegeforening/Norwegian Dental Association, Postboks 3063, Elisenberg, Oslo 0207, Norway. TEL 47-22-54-74-00, FAX 47-22-55-11-09, tannlegeforeningen@tannlegeforeningen.no, http://www.tannlegeforeningen.no. Ed. Gudrun Sangnes. Adv. contact Nina Smedstad. B&W page NOK 6,700, color page NOK 13,500; trim 188 x 250. Circ: 5,300 (controlled).

617.6 USA
NORTH CAROLINA DENTAL REVIEW. Text in English. 1983. s-a. USD 10 (effective 2000). adv. **Document type:** *Newsletter, Academic/Scholarly.* **Description:** Supports the school's missions of dental education, patient care, research and service.
Published by: University of North Carolina, School of Dentistry, Brauer Hall, Rm 410, CB 7450, Chapel Hill, NC 27599-7450. TEL 919-966-2730, FAX 919-966-0482, Sharon_Grayden@dentistry.unc.edu. Ed., R&P Sharon K Grayden. Circ: 6,200 (controlled).
Co-sponsor: U N C Dental Alumni Association.

617.6 USA ISSN 0029-2915
RK1
NORTHWEST DENTISTRY. Text in English. 1930. bi-m. USD 20 to non-members. adv. **Document type:** *Trade.*
Indexed: Dent.Ind., INIS Atomind.
—BLDSC (6151.710000), CISTI, GNLM, ingenta.
Published by: Minnesota Dental Association, 2236, Marshall, MN 55104. TEL 612-646-7457, FAX 612-646-8246. Ed. Alan Quam. R&P Claudia Kanter. Adv. contact Patty Lien. Circ: 3,100. **Co-sponsor:** North Dakota Dental Association.

617.6 CAN
NOVA SCOTIA DENTIST. Text in English. 1985. bi-m. membership. adv. **Document type:** *Newsletter.*
Formerly (until 1985): Nova Scotia Dental Association. Newsletter
Published by: Nova Scotia Dental Association, 5991 Spring Garden Rd, Ste 604, Halifax, NS B3H 1Y6, Canada. TEL 902-420-0088, FAX 902-423-6537. Ed. D V Pamenter. Adv. contact Steve Jennex. Circ: 1,000 (controlled).

617.6 USA
O D A NEWSLETTER. Text in English. 1987 (vol.17). q. USD 20 to non-members; USD 15 to members; (includes subscr. to Journal of the Oregon Dental Association). **Document type:** *Newsletter.*
Published by: Oregon Dental Association, 17898 S W McEwan Rd, Portland, OR 97224. Ed. Dr. James P Fratzke.

617.6 FRA ISSN 0251-172X
ODONTO-STOMATOLOGIE TROPICALE/TROPICAL DENTAL JOURNAL. Text in English, French. 1972. q. EUR 56.41 domestic; EUR 38.11 in Africa; EUR 67.08 elsewhere (effective 2001). adv. bk.rev. charts. index. back issues avail.; reprint service avail. from IRC. **Description:** Addresses numerous oral health problems in various tropical countries and efforts to treat them.
Formerly (until 1978): Secretariat de Sante Dentaire de l'Afrique. Revue
Indexed: Biol.Abstr., So.Pac.Per.Ind.
—BLDSC (9055.800000), GNLM.
Published by: (Secretariat de Sante Dentaire de l'Afrique), Edition Communication (N G - Com), 2799 avenue J.F. Kennedy, Six Fours les Plages 83140, France. TEL 33-04-94109999, FAX 33-04-94061703, TELEX IN UB2 572 237 F, info@santetropicale.com, http://www.santetropicale.com. Ed., Pub. Nicolas Gabella. Circ: 2,500. **Co-sponsor:** Commonwealth Foundation.

617.6 DNK ISSN 0105-0141
ODONTOLOGI. Text in Danish, Norwegian, Swedish. 1976. a. price varies. illus. **Document type:** *Academic/Scholarly.*
Published by: Blackwell Munksgaard, Book Division, Noerre Soegade 35, PO Box 2148, Copenhagen K 1016, Denmark. FAX 45-77-33-33-77. Ed. Hanne Terp.

617.6 URY ISSN 0029-8425
ODONTOLOGIA URUGUAYA. Text in Spanish. 1965 (vol.21). s-a. membership. adv. bk.rev. bibl, charts, illus, stat.
—CISTI.
Published by: Asociacion Odontologica Uruguaya, Durazno, 937-39, Montevideo 11109, Uruguay. TEL 901572. Circ: 3,000.

617.6 FIN ISSN 0078-3358
ODONTOLOGISKA SAMFUNDET I FINLAND. AARSBOK. Text in Finnish. 1946. a. FIM 50. adv. bk.rev. **Document type:** *Proceedings.*
Indexed: Biol.Abstr.
Published by: Odontologiska Samfundets i Finland, Bergmansg 11 D 11, Helsinki 00140, Finland. Ed. Marianne Lenander Lumikari. Adv. contact Harriet Bergman. Circ: 500.

617.6 PAN ISSN 0472-5158
ODONTOLOGO. Text in Spanish; Abstracts in English. 1975. s-a. USD 10 (effective 1997). adv. *Refereed.* **Document type:** *Trade.*
Published by: Asociacion Odontologica Panamena/Panamanian Dental Association, Apdo 6777, Zona 5, Panama City, Panama. TEL 507-269-1603, FAX 507-269-3749. Ed., Adv. contact Miriam Enith Bullen Cabrera. Circ: 1,000 (controlled).

617.6 ITA
ODONTOSTOMATOLOGIA. Text in Italian. 1974. m. ITL 150,000; ITL 300,000 foreign (effective 1998). adv. bk.rev.
Formerly: Odontostomatologia e Implantoprotesi (0391-3783)
Indexed: Dent.Ind.
—GNLM.
Published by: Stammer S.p.A., Via della Liberazione, 1, Peschiera Borromeo, MI 20068, Italy. TEL 30-2-55302606, FAX 39-2-5530-2700, stammer@micronet.it, http://stammer.it. Circ: 20,000.

617.6 GRC ISSN 0029-8506
ODONTOSTOMATOLOGICAL PROGRESS. Text in Greek; Summaries in English. 1947. bi-m. USD 60. adv. bk.rev. charts, illus. **Document type:** *Academic/Scholarly.*
—GNLM.
Published by: Society of Odontostomatological Research, 70 Mikras Asias St, Athens 115 27, Greece. TEL 30-11-301-7780671. Ed. John A Vrotsos. Pub. N Spyropulos. Circ: 3,000.

617.6 AUT ISSN 0029-9596
OESTERREICHISCHE ZAHNAERZTE - ZEITUNG. Text in German. 1950. m. adv. bk.rev. charts, stat. **Document type:** *Newsletter.*
Incorporates (1949-1989): Oesterreichische Dentistenzeitschrift (0029-9006)
—CISTI, GNLM.
Published by: Bundesfachgruppe fuer Zahn-, Mund- und Kieferheilkunde, Weihburgstrasse 1012, Vienna, W 1010, Austria. Circ: 4,900.

617.6 AUT
DAS OESTERREICHISCHE ZAHNTECHNIKER HANDWERK. Text in German. 1955. bi-m. adv. tr.lit. **Document type:** *Trade.*
Former titles: Oesterreichische Zahntechniker; Oesterreichische Zahnprothetik; Oesterreichische Zahntechnikerhandwerk
Published by: (Bundesinnung der Zahntechniker), Oesterreichischer Wirtschaftsverlag GmbH, Nikolsdorfer Gasse 7-11, Vienna, W 1051, Austria. TEL 43-1-54664, FAX 43-1-54664360, office@oewv.at, http://www.oewv.at. Ed. Wolfgang Biedermann. Adv. contact Karl Weidschacher. B&W page ATS 16,100, color page ATS 26,100; trim 252 x 172. Circ: 4,200.

617.6 USA ISSN 0164-9442
OKLAHOMA DENTAL ASSOCIATION JOURNAL. Text in English. 1973 (vol.64). q. USD 12; USD 18 foreign. adv. illus. *Refereed.* **Document type:** *Academic/Scholarly.*
Former titles: Your Oklahoma Dental Association. Journal (0149-2594); Oklahoma State Dental Association. Journal (0030-1868)
Indexed: Dent.Abstr., Dent.Ind.
—GNLM.
Published by: Oklahoma Dental Association, c/o Suzie J Weir, 629 W I 44 Service Rd, Oklahoma City, OK 73118-6098. TEL 405-848-8873, FAX 405-848-8875, odamail@okdental.org, http://www.okdentassoc.org. Ed. Manville Duncanson D D S. R&P Suzie J Weir. Adv. contact Suzie Weir. Circ: 1,500.

617.6 CAN ISSN 0300-5275
ONTARIO DENTIST. Text in English. 1925. m. CND 70. adv. bk.rev. bibl, illus.
Formerly: Ontario Dental Association. Journal (0030-2864)
Indexed: Dent.Abstr., Dent.Ind.
—BLDSC (6261.890000), CISTI, GNLM, Infotrieve. **CCC.**
Published by: Ontario Dental Association, 4 New St, Toronto, ON M5R 1P6, Canada. TEL 416-922-3900, FAX 416-922-9005. Ed. Dr. James Shosenberg. Pub. Peter James. Adv. contact Doug Lawson. Circ: 6,500.

617.6 USA ISSN 0361-7734
RK501
OPERATIVE DENTISTRY. Variant title: Journal of Operative Dentistry. Text in English. 1976. bi-m., latest vol.26, 2001. USD 70 domestic to individuals; USD 80 foreign to individuals; USD 80 domestic to institutions; USD 90 foreign to institutions (effective 2001). bk.rev. illus. back issues avail. *Refereed.* **Document type:** *Journal, Academic/Scholarly.* **Description:** Covers conservation and restoration of teeth; the scientific foundation of operative dental therapy; dental materials; dental education; and the social, political, and economic aspects of dental practice.
Supersedes: American Academy of Gold Foil Operators. Journal (0002-7146)
Related titles: Microfilm ed.: (from PQC); Online - full text ed.: (from Institute for Scientific Information); ♦ Supplement: Operative Dentistry. Supplement. ISSN 0163-3473.
Indexed: ASCA, Curr.Cont., Curr.Tit.Dent., Dent.Abstr., Dent.Ind., Inpharma, Mat.Sci.Cit.Ind. (coverage dropped), Reac., Sci.Cit.Ind.
—BLDSC (6269.375000), CISTI, GNLM, IDS, ingenta.
Address: c/o Indiana University School of Dentistry, 1121 W. Michigan St., Rm. S411, Indiana, Indianapolis, IA 46202-5186. TEL 317-278-4800, FAX 317-278-4900, editor@jopdent.org, mcochran@iupui.edu, http://www.jopdent.org. Ed., R&P Michael A Cochran.
Subscr. to: Allen Press Inc., PO Box 1897, Lawrence, KS 66044-8897. **Co-sponsor:** American Academy of Gold Foil Operators.

617.6 USA ISSN 0163-3473
OPERATIVE DENTISTRY. SUPPLEMENT. Text in English. 1977. latest vol.6. back issues avail.; reprints avail. **Document type:** *Journal, Academic/Scholarly.*
Related titles: ♦ Supplement to: Operative Dentistry. ISSN 0361-7734.
Published by: Operative Dentistry, c/o Indiana University School of Dentistry, 1121 W. Michigan St., Rm. S411, Indiana, Indianapolis, IA 46202-5186. TEL 317-278-4800, FAX 317-278-4900. R&P Michael A Cochran.

OPPORTUNITIES FOR MINORITY STUDENTS IN THE U.S. DENTAL SCHOOLS. see *EDUCATION—Higher Education*

617.6 USA
ORACLE (FAIRFIELD). Text in English. 1964. m. USD 2 (effective 2000). adv. **Description:** Contains organization news.
Formerly: Napa-Solano Dental Society. District Six. Newsletter (0027-7800)
Published by: Napa-Solano Dental Society, 1023 Empire St, Fairfield, CA 94533-5706. Ed. Dr. Mark Bowen. Circ: 195.

ORAL AND MAXILLOFACIAL SURGERY CLINICS OF NORTH AMERICA. see *MEDICAL SCIENCES—Surgery*

617.6 DNK ISSN 1354-523X
CODEN: ORDIFD
ORAL DISEASES. Text in English. 1995. q. USD 462 in the Americas to institutions print & online combined; GBP 321 elsewhere to institutions print & online combined (effective 2002). adv. back issues avail. **Document type:** *Journal, Academic/Scholarly.* **Description:** Covers all research related to oral diseases, including the basic sciences, well designed and controlled clinical research and analytical epidemiology.
Related titles: Online - full text ed.: (from EBSCO Publishing, O C L C Online Computer Library Center, Inc., RoweCom Information Quest, ingenta, Swets Blackwell, Institute for Scientific Information).
Indexed: CINAHL, Curr.Cont., Int.Abstr.Biol.Sci.
—BLDSC (6277.470000), CISTI, EMDOCS, GNLM, Infotrieve. **CCC.**
Published by: Munksgaard (Subsidiary of: Blackwell Science Ltd.), 35 Norre Sogade, PO Box 2148, Copenhagen K 1016, Denmark. TEL 45-7733-3333, FAX 45-7733-3377, nbc@munksgaard.dk, http://www.munksgaard.dk/. Eds. Crispian Scully, Newell Johnson.

617.6 CAN ISSN 0030-4204
ORAL HEALTH; a clinical journal devoted to the advancement of the dental profession. Text in English. 1911. m. CND 52.95 domestic; USD 59.95 in United States; USD 89.95 elsewhere (effective 2000). adv. bk.rev. illus. **Document type:** *Trade.* **Description:** Consists of clinical articles from the world's dental literature.
Related titles: Microfiche ed.: (from MML); Microform ed.: (from MML).

M

Indexed: CBCA Bus. (1996-), CBCA Ref., Chem.Abstr., Dent.Abstr., Dent.Ind., NRN.
—BLDSC (6277.500000), CISTI, GNLM. **CCC.**
Published by: Southam Magazine Group, 1450 Don Mills Rd, Don Mills, ON M3B 2X7, Canada. TEL 416-442-2046, FAX 416-442-2214. Pub. Melissa Summerfield. Adv. contact Ursula Krieger. Circ: 17,132.

617.6 615.842 JPN ISSN 0911-6028
ORAL RADIOLOGY. Text in English. 1985. 2/yr. (in one vol.). JPY 5,000 (effective 1999). adv. **Document type:** *Academic/Scholarly.*
Related titles: ♦ Japanese ed.: Shika Hoshasen. ISSN 0389-9705.
Indexed: CINAHL, INIS Atomind.
—BLDSC (6277.595000), EMDOCS, GNLM.
Published by: Nihon Shika Hoshasen Gakkai/Japanese Society for Oral and Maxillofacial Radiology, c/o Hitotsubashi Printing Co Ltd., Gakkai Business Center, 3-12-15 Kami-Osaki, Shinagawa-ku, Tokyo 141-0021, Japan. Ed. Kanji Kishi. R&P Hajime Fuchinata. Adv. contact Hajime Fuchihata.

617.6 USA ISSN 1079-2104
RD1
ORAL SURGERY, ORAL MEDICINE, ORAL PATHOLOGY, ORAL RADIOLOGY, AND ENDODONTICS. Text in English. 1948. m. USD 141 domestic to individuals; USD 170 foreign to individuals; USD 307 domestic to institutions; USD 336 foreign to institutions; USD 69 domestic to students; USD 98 foreign to students; USD 29 newsstand/cover (effective 2001). adv. bk.rev. abstr, illus. s-a. index. reprint service avail. from PQC. *Refereed.* **Document type:** *Journal, Academic/Scholarly, Trade.* **Description:** Provides comprehensive coverage of the field including identification of abnormalities and use of specialized diagnostic techniques.
Formerly: Oral Surgery, Oral Medicine, Oral Pathology (0030-4220)
Related titles: Microfilm ed.: (from PQC); Online - full text ed.: (from Ovid Technologies, Inc., EBSCO Publishing, IDEAL Online Library, Institute for Scientific Information, RoweCom Information Quest).
Indexed: ASCA, Abstr.Anthropol., Apic.Abstr., CINAHL, Chem.Abstr., Curr.Adv.Cancer Res., Curr.Adv.Ecol.Sci., Curr.Cont., Curr.Tit.Dent., Dent.Abstr., Dent.Ind., Environ.Sci.Poll.Mgmt., Excerp.Med., Helminthol.Abstr., INIS Atomind., Ind.Med. (1995-), Ind.Sci.Rev., Inpharma, Med.& Surg.Dermat., NRN, Neurosci.Cit.Ind., Nutr.Abstr., Pharm.&Out.News, Pollut.Abstr., Reac., Rev.Med.& Vet.Mycol., Rev.Plant Path., Risk Abstr., SSCI (coverage dropped), Saf.Sci.Abstr., Sci.Cit.Ind.
—BLDSC (6277.800500), CASDDS, CISTI, GNLM, IDS, ingenta, KNAW. **CCC.**
Published by: (American Academy of Oral and Maxillofacial Radiology), Mosby, Inc. (Subsidiary of: Elsevier Science), 11830 Westline Industrial Dr, St Louis, MO 63146-3318. TEL 314-872-8370, 800-325-4177, FAX 314-432-1380, http://www.mosby.com/periodicals. Ed. Dr. Larry J Peterson. Pub. Cynthia Baudendistel. Adv. contact Carol Kilzer TEL 314-453-4307. B&W page USD 1,230, color page USD 2,265; trim 10.88 x 8.13. Circ: 5,999 (paid and controlled). **Co-sponsors:** American Academy of Oral Medicine; American Academy of Oral and Maxillofacial Pathology; Organization of Teachers of Oral Diagnosis.

617.6 DEU ISSN 0724-4991
ORALPROPHYLAXE. Text in German. 1984. q. DEM 87 domestic; DEM 90 foreign (effective 2001). adv. bk.rev. *Refereed.* **Document type:** *Journal, Trade.* **Description:** Contains current information and research concerning dental and mouth hygiene. Covers flouride, oral hygiene, nutrition, professional prevention of oral diseases, and childrens' dental care.
—BLDSC (6277.808000), Infotrieve. **CCC.**
Published by: (Verein fuer Zahnhygiene e.V.), Carl Hanser Verlag, Kolbergerstr 22, Munich 81679, Germany. TEL 49-89-99830603, FAX 49-89-99830623, hanser@compuserve.com, info@hanser.de, http://www.zahnheilkunde.de, http://www.hanser.de. Adv. contact Rolf Hoerr. Circ: 5,000.

617.6 FRA ISSN 0755-2378
ORDRE NATIONAL DES CHIRURGIENS- DENTISTES. CONSEIL NATIONAL. BULLETIN OFFICIEL. Text in French. 1976. q. FRF 190 to members. charts, illus. **Document type:** *Bulletin.*
Published by: Ordre National des Chirurgiens- Dentistes, Conseil National, 22 rue Emile Menier, Paris 75116, France. TEL 33-1-45534005. Ed. M Andre Robert.

617.6 USA
OREGON DENTAL ASSOCIATION. DENTAL OFFICE SAFETY & HEALTH MANUAL. Text in English. a. membership. **Description:** Provides information for dentist and dental office staff concerning potential occupational hazards and compliance with Oregon OSHA rules and regulations.
Published by: Oregon Dental Association, 17898 S W McEwan Rd, Portland, OR 97224. TEL 503-620-3230.

617.6 USA
OREGON DENTAL ASSOCIATION. JOURNAL. Text in English. 1930. q. USD 20 to non-members; USD 15 to members; includes ODA newsletter. adv. bk.rev. charts, illus. **Document type:** *Trade.* **Description:** Covers the current news in the science of dentistry.
Formerly: Oregon State Dental Journal
Indexed: Dent.Abstr., Dent.Ind.
Published by: Oregon Dental Association, 17898 S W McEwan Rd, Portland, OR 97224. TEL 503-620-3230. Ed. Dr. Marion S Ratliff. Circ: 2,000.

617.643 USA ISSN 1097-797X
ORTHODONTIC PRODUCTS. Text in English. 199?. 8/yr. USD 16 (effective 2000). adv. **Document type:** *Magazine, Trade.* **Description:** Offers the latest clinical and practical information for the orthodontist.
Published by: Novicom, Inc. (Subsidiary of: Medical World Communications), 4676 Admiralty Way, Ste 202, Marina Del Rey, CA 90292-6603. TEL 310-642-4400, FAX 310-641-1511, http://www.novicom.com. Ed. Christina Chang. Adv. contacts Jacques Montague, Lisa Chose. B&W page USD 1,512, color page USD 2,212; trim 8.125 x 10.825. Circ: 12,000 (paid and controlled).

617.643 USA ISSN 0895-5034
ORTHODONTIC REVIEW*. Text in English. 1987. q. USD 93.
Published by: University of Missouri at Kansas City, School of Dentistry, 650 E 25th St, Kansas City, MO 64108. TEL 816-235-2100. Ed. Dr. Katherine Kula.

617.643 JPN ISSN 1344-0241
ORTHODONTIC WAVES. Variant title: Japanese Orthodontic Society. Journal. Text in Japanese; Summaries in English. 1932. bi-m. JPY 9,000 (effective 2000). adv. *Refereed.* **Document type:** *Academic/Scholarly.*
Formerly (until 1998): Nihon Kyosei Shika Gakkai Zasshi (0021-454X)
Indexed: Dent.Ind.
—BLDSC (6296.109500), CISTI, GNLM.
Published by: Japanese Orthodontic Society/Nihon Kyosei Shika Gakkai, c/o Oral health Association of Japan, 1-43-9 Komagome, Toshima-ku, Tokyo 170-0003, Japan. TEL 81-3-3947-8891, FAX 81-3-3947-8341. Ed., R&P Kenji Takada. Pub. Kooji Hanada. Adv. contact Shoji Iinuma. Circ: 5,400.

617.6 FRA ISSN 0078-6608
ORTHODONTIE FRANCAISE. Text in French. 1921. a. FRF 1,600 (effective 1999). adv. back issues avail. **Document type:** *Academic/Scholarly.*
Indexed: Ind.Med. (1921-).
—CISTI, GNLM.
Published by: Societe d'Information et de Diffusion, Librarie International, 9 rue Christine, Paris 75006, France. TEL 33-1-43293101, FAX 33-1-43293262, flancou@mail.easynet.fr, http://www.sdid.org/, http://www.editionsid.com/. Ed. Charles Bolender. Pub., R&P, Adv. contact Fatima Lancou.

617.6 ARG ISSN 0030-5936
ORTODONCIA. Text in Spanish; Summaries in English, French, German, Spanish. 1937. s-a. USD 56. bk.rev. abstr, bibl, charts, illus, stat. index.
Indexed: Biol.Abstr., Dent.Ind.
—CISTI, GNLM.
Published by: Sociedad Argentina de Ortodoncia, Montevideo, 971, Capital Federal, Buenos Aires 1019, Argentina. TEL 54-114-8115569, FAX 54-114-8155804. Ed. Dr. Marcos M Rose. adv.: page USD 400. Circ: 1,500.

617.6 ESP
ORTODONCIA CLINICA. Text in Spanish. 1998. 3/yr. ESP 4,300, USD 115 (effective 1999). **Document type:** *Trade.*
Published by: Editorial Dips Rocas, Muntaner, 393 pral. 4, Barcelona 08021, Spain. TEL 34-93-2001389, FAX 34-93-2021958, edipsro@intercom.es. Ed. Eduardo Padros Serrat. Circ: 2,000 (paid).

617.643 ESP ISSN 0210-1637
ORTODONCIA ESPANOLA; revista de clinica e investigacion en ortodoncia. Text in Spanish. 1955. q. ESP 9,180 to individuals; ESP 13,700 to institutions; ESP 7,350 to students (effective 2001). adv. back issues avail.; reprints avail. *Refereed.* **Document type:** *Academic/Scholarly.* **Description:** Publishes original clinical research for orthodontists and informs them of noteworthy congresses and symposia. Provides a forum for ideas and opinion.
Related titles: Online - full text ed.: 1996.
Published by: (Sociedad Espanol de Ortodoncia), Ediciones Doyma S.A., Traversa de Gracia, 17-21, Barcelona 08021, Spain. TEL 34-93-200-0711, ro@doyma.es, doyma@doyma.es, http://www.doyma.es/ro. Ed. Joaquin Travesi Gomez. R&P Monica Barnes. Adv. contact Jose Antonio Hernandez. B&W page ESP 122,000, color page ESP 152,000; 280 x 210. Circ: 1,500 (paid).

617.6 BRA ISSN 0030-5944
ORTODONTIA*. Text in Portuguese; Summaries in English. 1968. 3/yr. per issue exchange basis. adv. bk.rev. bibl, charts, illus. index. **Description:** Presents results of research in orthodontics.
Related titles: Microform ed.: 1968.
Indexed: Dent.Ind.
—GNLM.
Published by: Sociedade Paulista de Ortodontia, Rua do Livramento, 243, Vl Mariana, Sao Paulo, SP 04008-030, Brazil. Ed. Dr Julio W Vigorito. Circ: 5,000.

617.6 JPN ISSN 0473-4629
CODEN: ODSZA2
OSAKA DAIGAKU SHIGAKU ZASSHI/OSAKA UNIVERSITY DENTAL SOCIETY. JOURNAL. Text in Japanese. 1956. s-a. JPY 3,000. adv. **Description:** Contains mini-reviews, original articles, and case reports on dental science.
Indexed: Dent.Ind., Excerp.Med., INIS Atomind.
—BLDSC (4839.370000), CISTI, GNLM.
Published by: Osaka Daigaku Shigakkai/Osaka University Dental Society, 1-8 Yamada-Oka, Suita-shi, Osaka-fu 565-0871, Japan. TEL 06-876-5711, FAX 06-876-7931. Ed. Yoshio Shigenaga. Circ: 1,700.

617.6 JPN ISSN 0475-2058
CODEN: JODUA2
OSAKA DENTAL UNIVERSITY. JOURNAL. Text and summaries in English. 1967. s-a. per issue exchange basis. abstr, charts, illus, stat, tr.lit. index. back issues avail. **Document type:** *Academic/Scholarly.*
Indexed: Biol.Abstr., Chem.Abstr., Chem.Indus.Notes, Chem.Titles, Curr.Tit.Dent., Dent.Ind., Excerp.Med., Ind.Med. (coverage dropped), Oral Res.Abstr.
—BLDSC (4838.500000), CASDDS, CISTI, GNLM, ingenta.
Published by: Osaka Odontological Society/Osaka Shika Gakkai, 8-1 Kuzuha-Hanazono-cho, Hirakata-shi, Osaka-fu 573-1121, Japan. FAX 81-720-643164. Ed. Tatsuo Kawamoto.

617.6 USA ISSN 1091-5168
OSSTIUM. Text in English. 1994. q. **Document type:** *Magazine, Trade.* **Description:** Provides information about important clinical applications and breakthroughs in implantology.
Related titles: Spanish ed.: ISSN 1091-5176. 1994; Italian ed.: ISSN 1092-5686. 1994; German ed.: ISSN 1092-5678. 1994; French ed.: ISSN 1092-5694. 1994.
Published by: (Steri-Oss), Montage Media Corp., 1000 Wyckoff Ave, Mahwah, NJ 07430. TEL 201-891-3200, FAX 201-891-2626, info@montagemedia.com, http://www.montagemedia.com/oss.html.

617.6 PAK ISSN 0030-9710
CODEN: PKDRAV
PAKISTAN DENTAL REVIEW. Text in English. 1951. q. USD 30. adv. bk.rev. bibl, charts, illus, stat. index.
Indexed: Biol.Abstr., Dent.Ind.
—CISTI.
Address: Shahrah e Quaid e Azam 26, Lahore 54000, Pakistan. Ed. S Eckbelle. Circ: 5,000.

617.6 ITA
PARODONTOLOGIA E STOMATOLOGIA NUOVA. Text in Italian; Summaries in English, French, German. 1965 (vol.9). q. ITL 50,000. adv. bk.rev. charts, illus. index.
Formerly: Stomatologica (0039-1727)
Indexed: Chem.Abstr., INIS Atomind.
Published by: Istituto Clinico di Odontostomatologia, Viale Benedetto 15, Genoa, GE, Italy. Eds. F Torrielli, I Jonata.

M

617.6 DEU ISSN 0937-1532
PARODONTOLOGIE. Text in German. 1990. q. EUR 108 domestic; EUR 114 foreign; EUR 66 domestic to students; EUR 72 foreign to students (effective 2002). **Document type:** *Magazine, Academic/Scholarly.*
Indexed: Curr.Tit.Dent.
—GNLM.
Published by: Quintessenz Verlags GmbH, Ifenpfad 2-4, Berlin 12107, Germany. TEL 49-30-76180646, FAX 49-30-76180680, central@quintessenz.de, http://www.quintessenz.de.

617.6 USA
PASSAIC COUNTY DENTAL SOCIETY NEWSLETTER✱ . Text in English. 1979. m. (Oct.-May). USD 60 (effective 2000). adv. **Document type:** *Bulletin.*
Formerly (until 1981): Passaic County Dental Society. Bulletin (0079-0125)
Indexed: Dent.Ind.
Published by: Passaic County Dental Society, 205 US Hwy 46 #205, Totowa, NJ 075121838. Ed. Dr. Barry Raphael. Pub., R&P, Adv. contact Rhoda Wachsstock. Circ: 300.

617.6 AUS
▼ **PATHOLOGY**; Royal Australasian College of Dental Surgeons. Lecture notes in pathology. Text in English. 1999. irreg. AUD 36 newsstand/cover (effective 2001). 70 p./no. **Document type:** *Academic/Scholarly.* **Description:** Covers lecture notes in the basic science subject of pathology.
Published by: Royal Australasian College of Dental Surgeons, 64 Castlereagh St, Sydney, NSW 2000, Australia. TEL 61-2-9232-3800, FAX 61-2-9221-8108, registrar@racds.org, http://www.racds.org. Circ: 129 (controlled).

617.6 618.92 JPN ISSN 0917-2394
PEDIATRIC DENTAL JOURNAL. Variant title: International Journal of Japanese Society of Pediatric Dentistry. Text in English. 1991. a. USD 10. **Description:** Promotes research, practice and education specifically related to pediatric dentistry.
—BLDSC (6417.575000), GNLM.
Published by: Japanese Society of Pediatric Dentistry, Oral Health Association, 1-44-2 Komagome, Toshima-ku, Tokyo 170-0003, Japan. Ed. Mizuho Nishino.

617.6 USA ISSN 0164-1263
CODEN: PEDEDL
PEDIATRIC DENTISTRY. Text in English. 1979. bi-m. (7/yr.). USD 120 domestic to individuals; USD 175 foreign to individuals; USD 175 domestic to institutions; USD 210 foreign to institutions (effective 2000). adv. bk.rev. *Refereed.* **Document type:** *Trade.* **Description:** Promotes the practice, education, and research of pediatric dentistry.
Indexed: Behav.Med.Abstr., Biol.Abstr., Biol.Dig., Curr.Tit.Dent., Dent.Abstr., Dent.Ind., INIS Atomind., Ind.Med. (1979-).
—BLDSC (6417.580000), CISTI, GNLM.
Published by: American Academy of Pediatric Dentistry, 211 E Chicago Ave, Ste 700, Chicago, IL 60611-2616. TEL 312-337-2169, FAX 312-337-6329, http://aapd.org. Ed. Dr. Paul S Casamassimo. R&P Sara Pullan Geimer. Adv. contact Margitta Winkler. B&W page USD 380; trim 10.88 x 8.25. Circ: 4,210 (paid).

617.6 618.92 USA ISSN 1046-2791
PEDIATRIC DENTISTRY TODAY. Text in English. bi-m. USD 20 to members; USD 30 foreign to members. adv. back issues avail.; reprints avail. **Document type:** *Newsletter.*
Published by: American Academy of Pediatric Dentistry, 211 E Chicago Ave, Ste 700, Chicago, IL 60611-2616. TEL 312-337-2169, FAX 312-337-6329, http:/aapd.org, http://aapd.org. Ed. Amy Fox. R&P Sara Pullan Geimer. Adv. contact Margitta Winkler. B&W page USD 228; trim 11 x 8.5. Circ: 3,100.

617.6 USA ISSN 0031-4331
PENN DENTAL JOURNAL. Text in English. 1897. s-a. USD 40. adv. bk.rev. charts, illus. index. **Document type:** *Academic/Scholarly.* **Description:** A progressive, clinical journal of dentistry, containing articles by faculty and students.
Related titles: Microform ed.: (from PQC).
Indexed: Dent.Ind.
—GNLM.
Published by: University of Pennsylvania, School of Dental Medicine, 4001 Spruce St, Philadelphia, PA 19104. TEL 215-898-8951, FAX 215-898-5243. Ed., Pub., R&P, Adv. contact Tobe Amsterdam. Circ: 7,500.

617.6 USA ISSN 0031-4439
RK1
PENNSYLVANIA DENTAL JOURNAL. Text in English. 1933. bi-m. USD 36 domestic; USD 60 foreign (effective 2000). adv. index. reprint service avail. from PQC. *Refereed.* **Document type:** *Trade.* **Description:** Covers topics of interest to members of the dental professions: dentistry techniques, breakthroughs, governmental regulations, and other items.
Related titles: Microfilm ed.: (from PQC).
Indexed: Dent.Abstr., Dent.Ind., INIS Atomind., Med.Care Rev.
—BLDSC (6421.705000), CISTI, GNLM.
Published by: Pennsylvania Dental Association, PO Box 3341, Harrisburg, PA 17105. TEL 717-234-5941, FAX 717-232-7169, rap@padental.org, http:// www.padental.org. Eds. Dr. Judith McFadden, Dr. Richard Galeone. R&P, Adv. contact Rob Pugliese. B&W page USD 565, color page USD 1,315; trim 11 x 8.5. Circ: 7,000.

617.6 USA
PENNSYLVANIA SOCIETY OF DENTISTRY FOR CHILDREN NEWSLETTER. Text in English. 1968. q. bk.rev. **Document type:** *Newsletter.*
Published by: Pennsylvania Society of Dentistry for Children, c/o Dr W F Hrin, Ed, 227 Franklin St, Ste 220, Johnstown, PA 15901. Circ: 1,100.

617.6 ESP
PERIODONCIA. Text in Spanish; Summaries in English. 1991. 4/yr. ESP 6,000, USD 9,000. adv. bk.rev. abstr. index. back issues avail.
Published by: (Sociedad Espanola de Periodoncia), Ediciones Ergon S.A., Pza. Josep Pallach 10, 1o, Barcelona 08035, Spain. TEL 91-3142715, FAX 91-3235745, seponet@infomed.es, http:// www.infomed.es/seponet. R&P Monica Guinea. Circ: 10,000. **Subscr. to:** Ergon, Antonio Lopez Aguado, 1, Madrid 28029, Spain.

617.6 AUS ISSN 0726-5247
PERIODONTOLOGY. Text in English. 1967. s-a. AUD 40 domestic; AUD 50 foreign (effective 2001). adv. bk.rev. back issues avail. *Refereed.* **Document type:** *Magazine, Academic/Scholarly.* **Description:** Publishes clinical papers, original research, review articles, case reports and items of general interest in the field of periodontology.
Formerly (until 1980): A S P Newsletter
Published by: Australian Society of Periodontology, Dept. of Periodontics, United Dental Hopsital of Sydney, 2 chalmers St, Surry Hills, NSW 2010, Australia. TEL 61-2-92933274, FAX 61-7-92933488, gumnut@udh3.udh, gumnut@udh3.udh.cs.nsw.gov.au, http://www.cs.nsw.gov.au. Ed., R&P B A Taylor. adv.: B&W page AUD 500, color page AUD 1,000; trim 210 x 295. Circ: 400 (paid).

617.632 DNK ISSN 0906-6713
PERIODONTOLOGY 2000. Text in English. 1993. 3/yr. USD 288 in the Americas to institutions print & online eds. combined; GBP 200 elsewhere to institutions print & online eds. combined (effective 2002). adv. illus. reprints avail. *Refereed.* **Document type:** *Academic/Scholarly.*
Related titles: ♦ Online - full text ed.: Periodontology 2000 Online.
Indexed: ASCA, Curr.Cont., Inpharma, Reac., Rev.Med.& Vet.Mycol., Sci.Cit.Ind.
—BLDSC (6426.452300), CISTI, GNLM, IDS, Infotrieve. CCC.
Published by: Blackwell Munksgaard, Noerre Soegade 35, PO Box 2148, Copenhagen K 1016, Denmark. TEL 45-77-33-33-33, FAX 45-77-33-33-77, customerservice@munksgaard.dk, http:// www.munksgaard.dk. Ed. Joergen Slots. Circ: 3,000.

617.632 DNK
PERIODONTOLOGY 2000 ONLINE. Text in English. 3/yr. DKK 990 to individuals; DKK 1,890 to institutions (effective 2001). *Refereed.* **Document type:** *Academic/Scholarly.*
Media: Online - full text (from EBSCO Publishing, ingenta, Munksgaard & Blackwell Science's Synergy, Swets Blackwell, Institute for Scientific Information). **Related titles:** ♦ Print ed.: Periodontology 2000. ISSN 0906-6713.
Published by: Blackwell Munksgaard, Noerre Soegade 35, PO Box 2148, Copenhagen K 1016, Denmark. TEL 45-77-33-33-33, FAX 45-77-33-33-77, fsub@mail.munksgaard.dk, http://www.ingenta.com/ journals/browse/mksg/pe2, http://www.munksgaard.dk.

617.6 BRA ISSN 1517-7491
CODEN: ROUPES
PESQUISA ODONTOLOGICA BRASILEIRA. Text and summaries in English, Portuguese. 1987. q. USD 40 domestic; USD 60 foreign (effective 2000). adv. bk.rev. abstr, bibl, charts, illus, stat. reprint service avail. from PQC. **Document type:** *Academic/Scholarly.*
Formerly (until 2000): Universidade de Sao Paulo. Revista de Odontologia (0103-0663); Formed by the merger of (1968-1986): Estomatologia e Cultura (0014-1364); (1964-1986): Faculdade de Odontologia de Ribeirao Preto. Revista (0102-129X); Which was formerly (until 1983): Faculdade de Farmacia e Odontologia de Ribeirao Preto. Revista (0006-9418); (until 1970): Faculdade de Farmacia e Odontologia de Ribeirao Preto. Boletim (0080-2913); (1963-1986): Universidade de Sao Paulo. Faculdade de Odontologia. Revista (0581-6866); Which superseded in part (1939-1962): Universidade de Sao Paulo. Faculdade de Farmacia. Anais (0365-2181)
Related titles: Online - full text ed.: (from SciELO).
Indexed: Biol.Abstr., Cal.Tiss.Abstr. (coverage dropped), Chem.Abstr., Dent.Ind., INIS Atomind.
—BLDSC (6428.243870), CASDDS, GNLM.
Published by: Universidade de Sao Paulo, Faculdade de Odontologia, Servico de Documentacao Odontologica, Seccao de Documentacao Odontologica, Centro, Caixa Postal 8216, Sao Paulo, SP 01065970, Brazil. TEL 55-11-8187861, FAX 55-11-8187413, rousp@siso.fo.usp.br, http://www.scielo.br/. Ed., R&P Esther Goldenberg Birman. Circ: 2,000.

617.6 USA ISSN 0031-7268
PHILADELPHIA COUNTY DENTAL SOCIETY. BULLETIN. Text in English. 1936. bi-m. membership. adv. illus. **Document type:** *Bulletin.*
Indexed: Dent.Ind., Med.Care Rev.
—GNLM.
Published by: Philadelphia County Dental Society, 225 E Washington Sq, Philadelphia, PA 19106. TEL 215-925-6050, FAX 215-925-6998. Ed. Dr. James H Dyen. Circ: 2,500.

617.6 PHL ISSN 0031-7497
PHILIPPINE DENTAL ASSOCIATION. JOURNAL. Text in English. 1908. q. PHP 200 to non-members; USD 25 foreign. adv. bk.rev. bibl, illus. index. back issues avail. **Document type:** *Academic/Scholarly.*
Related titles: CD-ROM ed.
Indexed: Dent.Ind., ExtraMED.
—GNLM.
Published by: Philippines Dental Association, Ayala Ave corner Kamagong St, Makati, Quezon City, Philippines. TEL 818-6144, FAX 816-3034. Ed. Dr. Francisco M Herbosa. Adv. contact Leo G Espina. Circ: 5,000.

610 571 AUS
▼ **PHYSIOLOGY**; Royal Australasian College of Dental Surgeons. Lecture notes in physiology. Text in English. 2000. a. AUD 36 newsstand/cover (effective 2001). **Document type:** *Academic/Scholarly.* **Description:** Covers lecture notes in the basic science of physiology.
Published by: Royal Australasian College of Dental Surgeons, 64 Castlereagh St, Sydney, NSW 2000, Australia. TEL 61-2-9232-3800, FAX 61-2-9221-8108, registrar@racds.org, http://www.racds.org. Ed. Timothy Miles. Circ: 100 (controlled).

617.6 BRA ISSN 0102-9460
RK1
PONTIFICIA UNIVERSIDADE CATOLICA DO RIO GRANDE DO SUL. REVISTA ODONTOCIENCIA. Key Title: Revista Odonto Ciencia. Text in Portuguese. 1986. 2/yr. BRL 10, USD 20.
Published by: (Pontificia Universidade Catolica do Rio Grande do Sul), Editora da P U C R S, c/o Antoninho M. Naime, Partenon, Caixa Postal 12001, Porto Alegre, RGS 90651-970, Brazil. Circ: 1,000.

617.6 GBR ISSN 0959-6666
POSTGRADUATE DENTIST: MIDDLE EAST✱ . Text in English. 1990. q. GBP 20 in Europe; GBP 30 elsewhere. adv. bk.rev. charts, illus. back issues avail. **Document type:** *Academic/Scholarly.* **Description:** Contains specially commissioned postgraduate-level review articles on all aspects of clinical dentistry for practicing dentists in the Middle East.
Published by: George Warman Publications Ltd., Unit 2, Riverview Business Park, Walnut Tree Close, Guildford, Surrey GU1 4QT, United Kingdom. TEL 44-1483-304944, FAX 44-1483-303191. Ed. David Croser. Circ: 6,150.

617.6 MEX ISSN 0185-5905
PRACTICA ODONTOLOGICA. Text in Spanish. 1979. m.
—BLDSC (6593.809000), GNLM.

M

Published by: Mundo Medico S.A., Ejercito Nacional 381, Mexico City, DF 11520, Mexico. TEL 525-545-17-98, FAX 525-203-64-18. Ed. Maria Beatriz Elizalde Vergara.

617.632 USA ISSN 1042-2722
PRACTICAL PERIODONTICS AND AESTHETIC DENTISTRY. Variant title: P P A D. Text in English. 1988. 9/yr. USD 98 domestic; USD 168 foreign (effective 2000). adv. back issues avail. *Refereed.* **Document type:** *Academic/Scholarly.* **Description:** Presents practical applications of soft tissue management and all aspects of restorative and aesthetic dentistry.
Related titles: ♦ Supplement: Signature (Mahwah). ISSN 1091-5222.
—GNLM.
Published by: Montage Media Corp., 1000 Wyckoff Ave, Mahwah, NJ 07430. TEL 201-891-3200, FAX 201-891-2626, editorial@montagemedia.com, http://www.montagemedia.com. Ed. Bernard Touati. Pub., R&P Stephen E Sweeney. Adv. contact Jim King. B&W page USD 5,721, color page USD 7,421; trim 10.88 x 8.13. Circ: 86,400.

617.69 JPN ISSN 0018-6341
PRACTICE IN PROSTHODONTICS/HOTETSU RINSHO. Text in Japanese. 1968. bi-m. JPY 1,300 per issue. adv. bk.rev. index.
Indexed: Dent.Ind.
Published by: Ishiyaku Publishers Inc., 7-10 Honkomagome 1-chome, Bunkyo-ku, Tokyo 113-0021, Japan. Ed. Hiroshi Miura. Circ: 16,200.

617.6 362.1 SWE ISSN 1103-1727
PRAKTIKAN. Text in Swedish. 1986. 9/yr.
Published by: Praktikertjaenst AB, Stockholm 10355, Sweden. TEL 46-8-789-40-00, FAX 46-8-789-45-42, malin.bergh@hq.ptj.se, http://www.ptj.se. Ed., Pub. Malin Bergh. adv.: B&W page SEK 8,500; trim 267 x 167. Circ: 12,000.

617.6 ITA ISSN 0393-9960
PREVENZIONE & ASSISTENZA DENTALE. Text in Italian. 1975. 6/yr. ITL 64,000 (effective 1999). **Document type:** *Academic/Scholarly.*
Formerly (until 1985): Prevenzione Stomatologica (0390-1033)
—BLDSC (6612.795300), GNLM.
Published by: Masson S.p.A., Divisione Periodici, Via F.lli Bressan 2, Milan, MI 20126, Italy. TEL 39-2-270741, FAX 39-2-27074210. Ed. Carlo Guastamacchia. adv.: B&W page ITL 1,520,000, color page ITL 2,160,000; trim 265 x 193. Circ: 4,000.

617.6 USA ISSN 1079-0187
PREVIEW (COLLINSVILLE). Text in English. 1991. s-a. free per issue. adv. **Document type:** *Trade.* **Description:** Covers practice set-up and management, dental equipment and material selection, office design, practice purchase, associateship, and advanced dental education.
Published by: Stehman Publications, 300 W Main St, Collinsville, IL 62234. TEL 618-345-7559. Ed., Pub. James J Stehman. adv.: B&W page USD 1,260, color page USD 1,660. Circ: (controlled).

617.6 GBR ISSN 1355-7610
PRIMARY DENTAL CARE; journal of the Faculty of General Dental Practitioners (UK). Text in English. 1994. q. GBP 170 domestic; GBP 184 foreign (effective 2001). adv. abstr, bibl, charts, illus, stat. Annual article index. back issues avail. *Refereed.* **Document type:** *Journal, Academic/Scholarly.* **Description:** Contains peer-reviewed articles by general dental practitioners on scientific dental topics.
Related titles: Online - full content ed.
—BLDSC (6612.908570).
Published by: (Royal College of Surgeons of England), Faculty of Dental Practitioners (Subsidiary of: Royal College of Surgeons of England), 35-43 Lincoln's Inn Fields, London WC2A 3PE, United Kingdom. TEL 44-20-7869-6759, FAX 44-20-7869-6765, lrsmith@rcseng.ac.uk, lsmith@rcseng.ac.uk, http://www.rcseng.ac.uk/fgdp. Ed. Edward Renson. R&P, Adv. contact Lee Smith. color page GBP 500; trim 188 x 270. Circ: 3,050 (controlled); 40 (paid); 50 (free).

617.6 AUS ISSN 0079-5631
PROBE. Text in English. 1949. a. AUD 15. adv. bk.rev. **Document type:** *Newsletter.*
Published by: Adelaide University Dental Students Society (AUDSS), School of Dentistry, Undergraduate Mailbox, 5th Fl. Dental Hospital, Frome Rd., Adelaide, SA 5000, Australia. TEL 618-223-9211, FAX 61-8-232-4061. Eds. K Tabalotny, M Bilski. Circ: 220 (paid).

617.6 KAZ
PROBLEMY STOMATOOGII; ezhekvartal'nyi nauchno-prakticheskii zhurnal. Text in Russian. 1998. q. **Document type:** *Journal, Academic/Scholarly.*
Related titles: Online - full text ed.
Published by: Stomatologiya, Ul. Bagenbai Batyra 149, Almata 480012, Kazakstan. TEL 3272-695149, FAX 3272-692492, http://www.stom.ru/trouble/. Ed. T. Supiev.

617.6 DEU ISSN 0932-4488
PRODENT✱ ; Zahntechnik-Gesundheit-Soziales-Arbeit. Text in German. 1988. q. adv. bk.rev. back issues avail.
Published by: Deutscher Zahntechniker Verband e.V., Neustaedter Str 21, Bielefeld 33602, Germany. TEL 49-521-179674. Ed. Dr. Ulrich Weisemann. Circ: 3,500.

617.643 DNK ISSN 1399-7513
▼ **PROGRESS IN ORTHODONTICS.** Text in English. 2000. a. USD 58 in the Americas to institutions print & online eds. combined; GBP 41 elsewhere to institutions print & online eds. combined (effective 2002). *Refereed.* **Document type:** *Journal, Academic/Scholarly.*
Related titles: ♦ Online - full text ed.: Progress in Orthodontics Online.
—BLDSC (6872.230000).
Published by: Blackwell Munksgaard, Noerre Soegade 35, PO Box 2148, Copenhagen K 1016, Denmark. TEL 45-77-33-33-33, FAX 45-77-33-33-77, customerservice@munksgaard.dk, http://www.munksgaard.dk.

617.643 DNK
▼ **PROGRESS IN ORTHODONTICS ONLINE.** Text in English. 2000. a. DKK 405 (effective 2001). **Document type:** *Academic/Scholarly.*
Media: Online - full text (from Swets Blackwell). **Related titles:** ♦ Print ed.: Progress in Orthodontics. ISSN 1399-7513.
Published by: Blackwell Munksgaard, Noerre Soegade 35, PO Box 2148, Copenhagen K 1016, Denmark. TEL 45-77-33-33-33, FAX 45-77-33-33-77, fsub@mail.munksgaard.dk, http://www.munksgaard.dk.

617.6 USA ISSN 0033-1236
RK1
PROOFS; the magazine of dental sales. Text in English. 1918. 5/yr. USD 35 domestic; USD 37.95 in Canada & Mexico; USD 82.95 elsewhere; USD 5 newsstand/cover (effective 2001). adv. illus. **Document type:** *Trade.* **Description:** Directed to dental sales and marketing sales personnel and staff, and to key executives and marketing personnel of dental manufacturing firms.
Published by: PennWell Publishing Co., Dental Economics Division, PO Box 3408, Tulsa, OK 74101. TEL 918-835-3161, 847-559-7501, FAX 918-831-9804, julieh@pennwell.com, http://www.pennwell.com. Ed. Mary Elizabeth Good. Pub., R&P Lyle Hoyt. Adv. contact Margaret Pagel. Circ: 4,000.

617.6 USA ISSN 1060-1341
Q D T. (Quintessence of Dental Technology) Text in English. 1976. a. USD 60 (effective 1999). adv. illus. index. **Document type:** *Academic/Scholarly.*
Former titles: Q D T Yearbook (0896-6532); (until 1987): Quintessence of Dental Technology (0362-0913)
Related titles: German ed.; Italian ed.; Japanese ed.
Indexed: Dent.Abstr., Dent.Ind.
—GNLM, Infotrieve. **CCC.**
Published by: Quintessence Publishing Co., Inc., 551 Kimberly Dr, Carol Stream, IL 60188-1881. TEL 630-682-3223, FAX 630-682-3288. Ed. John Sorensen. Pub. H W Haase. Adv. contact William G Hartman.

617.6 USA
QUEENS COUNTY DENTAL SOCIETY. BULLETIN. Text in English. 1962. bi-m. USD 30. adv. bk.rev. illus. **Document type:** *Bulletin.* **Description:** Covers news of the society and the dental profession.
Formerly: Eleventh District Dental Society. Bulletin (0013-6166)
Indexed: Dent.Ind.
Published by: Queens County Dental Society, 86 90 188th St, Jamaica, NY 11423. TEL 718-454-8344, FAX 718-454-8818. Ed., R&P Alan N Queen. Circ: 1,500.

617.6 ESP ISSN 0214-0985
QUINTESSENCE (EDICION ESPANOLA); publicacion internacional de odontologia. Text in Spanish. 1988. m. (10/yr.). USD 188. adv. **Document type:** *Academic/Scholarly.* **Description:** Contains scientific and technical information from clinical centers in Europe and North America. Covers hygiene and prophylaxis, implantology, periodontics, pediatric dentistry, maxofacial surgery and prothesis.
Published by: Ediciones Doyma S.A., Traversa de Gracia, 17-21, Barcelona 08021, Spain. TEL 34-93-200-0711, FAX 34-93-209-1136. Ed. S Campi Schoeller. Adv. contact Marte Vidal. color page ESP 292,000; trim 210 x 280. Circ: 6,700.

617.6 USA ISSN 0033-6572
QUINTESSENCE INTERNATIONAL. Text in English. 1970. m. USD 98, GBP 91, EUR 118; USD 50, GBP 43, EUR 46 to students (effective 2002). adv. *Refereed.* **Document type:** *Magazine, Academic/Scholarly, Trade.* **Description:** Targets general practitioners. Covers all areas of dentistry, including oral surgery, preventive and pediatric dentistry, practice administration, and clinical communication.
Incorporates: Dental Digest (0011-8567)
Related titles: Online - full text ed.: (from Institute for Scientific Information).
Indexed: Curr.Cont., Curr.Tit.Dent., Dent.Abstr., Dent.Ind.
—BLDSC (7218.120000), CISTI, GNLM, IDS. **CCC.**
Published by: Quintessence Publishing Co., Inc., 551 Kimberly Dr, Carol Stream, IL 60188-1881. TEL 630-682-3223, FAX 630-682-3288, quintpub@aol.com. Ed. Dr. William Wathen. Pub. H W Haase. Adv. contact William G Hartman. Circ: 19,800.

617.6 ESP ISSN 1130-5339
QUINTESSENCE TECNICA (EDICION ESPANOLA); publicacion internacional de protesis dental. Text in Spanish. 1990. m. (10/yr). USD 113. adv. **Document type:** *Academic/Scholarly.* **Description:** Covers dental prosthesis. Contains photographs and schematics of new techniques to facilitate their immediate practical application.
Related titles: ♦ Translation of: Quintessenz der Zahntechnik. ISSN 0340-4641.
Published by: Ediciones Doyma S.A., Traversa de Gracia, 17-21, Barcelona 08021, Spain. TEL 34-93-200-0711, FAX 34-93-209-1136. Ed. G Sierra Del Hoyo. Adv. contact Marte Vidal. page ESP 170,000; trim 210 x 150. Circ: 4,500.

617.6 DEU ISSN 0033-6580
DIE QUINTESSENZ (BERLIN); die Monatszeitschrift fuer den praktizierenden Zahnarzt. Text in German. 1950. m. EUR 128 domestic; EUR 134 foreign; EUR 76 domestic to students; EUR 82 foreign to students (effective 2002). **Document type:** *Magazine, Academic/Scholarly.*
Indexed: Curr.Tit.Dent., Dok.Arbeitsmed.
—CISTI, GNLM.
Published by: Quintessenz Verlags GmbH, Ifenpfad 2-4, Berlin 12107, Germany. TEL 49-30-76180646, FAX 49-30-76180680, central@quintessenz.de, http://www.quintessenz.de.

617.6 DEU ISSN 0340-4641
QUINTESSENZ DER ZAHNTECHNIK. Text in German. 1975. m. EUR 108 domestic; EUR 112 foreign; EUR 78 domestic to students; EUR 84 foreign to students (effective 2002). **Document type:** *Magazine, Academic/Scholarly.*
Related titles: ♦ Spanish Translation: Quintessence Tecnica (Edicion Espanola). ISSN 1130-5339.
Indexed: Curr.Tit.Dent., Dok.Arbeitsmed.
—BLDSC (7218.160000), GNLM.
Published by: Quintessenz Verlags GmbH, Ifenpfad 2-4, Berlin 12107, Germany. TEL 49-30-76180646, FAX 49-30-76180680, central@quintessenz.de, http://www.quintessenz.de.

617.6 DEU
QUINTESSENZ TEAM - JOURNAL; die Zeitschrift fuer die zahnaerztliche Praxis. Text in German. 1971. 11/yr. EUR 72 domestic; EUR 76 foreign (effective 2002). adv. **Document type:** *Magazine, Academic/Scholarly.*
Formerly (until 1998): Quintessenz Journal (0033-6599)
Indexed: Dent.Ind., Dok.Arbeitsmed., So.Pac.Per.Ind.
—BLDSC, CISTI, GNLM.
Published by: Quintessenz Verlags GmbH, Ifenpfad 2-4, Berlin 12107, Germany. TEL 49-30-76180646, FAX 49-30-76180680, TELEX 183815-QUINT-D, central@quintessenz.de, http://www.quintessenz.de. Eds. Ilona Kronfeld, Susanne Fath. Adv. contact Marlies Kauffeldt.

617.6 USA ISSN 0279-7720
R D H; the national magazine for dental hygiene professionals. (Registered Dental Hygienist) Text in English. 1981. m. USD 50 domestic; USD 65 in Canada & Mexico; USD 82 elsewhere; USD 6 newsstand/cover (effective 2001). adv. **Document type:** *Trade.*
—BLDSC (7300.251200), GNLM, Infotrieve. **CCC.**

M

Published by: PennWell Publishing Co., Dental Economics Division, PO Box 3408, Tulsa, OK 74101. TEL 918-835-3161, 847-559-7501, FAX 918-832-9295, http://www.pennwell.com. Ed., R&P Mark Hartley. Pub. Lyle Hoyt. Adv. contact Margaret Pagel. Circ: 66,835.

617.643 FRA ISSN 0997-3397
R F P D ACTUALITES. (Revue Francaise des Prothesistes Dentaires) Text in French. 10/yr. FRF 70 (effective 1997). adv.
Formerly (until 1987): Revue Francaise des Prothesistes Dentaires (0242-1828)
—GNLM.
Published by: Promo U.N., 80 rue de la Roquette, Paris 75011, France. TEL 33-1-49294619, FAX 33-1-49294626. Ed. Robert Frederic Dumont. Pub. Maurice Dauvois. Adv. contact Carla Pelmard. B&W page FRF 2,800, color page FRF 8,900; 270 x 210. Circ: 6,000.

617.6 ITA ISSN 0048-6787
RASSEGNA ODONTOTECNICA. Text in Italian. 1954. bi-m. ITL 120,000; ITL 240,000 foreign. **Document type:** *Corporate.*
Indexed: Dent.Ind.
Published by: Sindacato Nazionale Odontotecnici, Via Termopili, 12, Milan, MI 20127, Italy. Ed. Francesco Palladini.

617.6 ITA ISSN 0033-9911
RASSEGNA TRIMESTRALE DI ODONTOIATRIA. Text in Italian; Summaries in English, French, German. 1920. q. ITL 5,000. adv. charts, illus. index.
Indexed: Biol.Abstr., INIS Atomind., Ind.Med. (coverage dropped).
—CISTI, GNLM.
Published by: Istituto Stomatologico Italiano, Via della Pace 21, Milan, MI 20122, Italy. Ed. Oscar Hoffer.

617.6 FRA ISSN 0999-5021
REALITES CLINIQUES; revue europeenne d'odontologie. Text in French. 1990. q. FRF 950 (effective 2000). adv. **Document type:** *Academic/Scholarly.*
—BLDSC (7303.287500), GNLM.
Published by: Societe Editrice de la Revue Realites Cliniques, 4o av. Bugeaud, Paris 75116, France. TEL 33-1-56265000, FAX 33-1-56265001, info@information-dentaire.fr, http://www.information-dentaire.com. Ed. Jean Jacques Lasfargues. Pub. Marylene Scagni. Adv. contact Florence Gouaux.

617.6 USA ISSN 1041-8199
REALITY (HOUSTON). Text in English. 1986. a. USD 141.55 domestic to individuals; USD 164.10 in Canada to individuals; USD 164.10 in Mexico to individuals; USD 194.10 elsewhere to individuals; USD 208.05 domestic to institutions; USD 242.10 in Canada & Mexico to institutions; USD 272.10 elsewhere to institutions (effective 2002).
Related titles: ♦ Supplement: Reality Now. ISSN 1041-8253.
Published by: (Esthetic Dentistry Research Group), Reality Publishing Co., 11757 Katy Freeway, Ste 210, Houston, TX 77079-1717. TEL 281-588-9101, 800-544-4999, FAX 281-493-1558, sales@realityesthetics.com.

617.6 USA ISSN 1041-8253
REALITY NOW. Text in English. 1989. 11/yr. USD 159 domestic to individuals; USD 197 in Canada & Mexico to individuals; USD 227 elsewhere to individuals; USD 217 domestic to institutions; USD 257 in Canada & Mexico to institutions; USD 286 elsewhere to institutions (effective 2000).
Related titles: ♦ Supplement to: Reality (Houston). ISSN 1041-8199.
Published by: (Esthetic Dentistry Research Group), Reality Publishing Co., 11757 Katy Freeway, Ste 210, Houston, TX 77079-1717. TEL 281-558-9101, 800-544-4999, FAX 281-493-1558, realnow@ix.netcom.com. Ed., Pub. Michael B Miller.

617.6 ZAF
RECOMMENDED SCALES OF BENEFITS. DENTAL PRACTITIONERS. Text in English. 1994. a.
Published by: Representative Association of Medical Schemes, PO Box 2324, Parklands, Johannesburg 2121, South Africa.

617.6 BRA ISSN 0034-7272
REVISTA BRASILEIRA DE ODONTOLOGIA. Text in Portuguese; Summaries in English, Portuguese. 1942. bi-m. BRL 2,000, USD 15. adv. bk.rev. abstr. back issues avail.
Indexed: Biol.Abstr.
—CISTI, GNLM.
Published by: Associacao Brasileira de Odontologia, Secao do Rio de Janeiro, Rua Barao de Sertorio, 75, R Comprido, Rio De Janeiro, RJ 20261-050, Brazil. TEL 021-293-5322, FAX 021-293-3893. Ed. Francisco Nader. Circ: 15,000.

617.6 CUB ISSN 0034-7507
CODEN: RCUEA9
REVISTA CUBANA DE ESTOMATOLOGIA. Text in Spanish; Summaries in English, French, Spanish. 1965. 3/yr. USD 38 in the Americas; USD 46 in Europe; USD 54 elsewhere. bibl, abstr, charts, illus. index.
Indexed: Biol.Abstr., Dent.Ind., Ind.Med. (coverage dropped).
—CASDDS, CISTI.
Published by: (Cuba. Ministerio de Salud Publica, Centro Nacional de Informacion de Ciencias Medicas), Editorial de Ciencias Medicas, O'Reilly No. 4, Habana, Cuba. TEL 809-62-8091. Ed. Grisell Concepcion. Circ: 2,500.
Co-sponsor: Sociedad Cubana de Estomatologia.

617.643 CUB ISSN 0864-3784
REVISTA CUBANA DE ORTODONCIA. Text in Spanish; Summaries in English, Spanish. 1985. s-a. USD 36 in the Americas; USD 44 in Europe; USD 52 elsewhere. **Document type:** *Government.* **Description:** Covers the field of orthodontics and related specialties.
Published by: (Cuba. Ministerio de Salud Publica, Centro Nacional de Informacion de Ciencias Medicas), Editorial de Ciencias Medicas, O'Reilly No. 4, Habana, Cuba. TEL 809-62-8091. Ed. Fidel Araujo. Circ: 1,000.
Co-sponsor: Sociedad Cubana de Ortodoncia.

617.6 BRA ISSN 1415-5419
REVISTA DENTAL PRESS DE ORTODONTIA E ORTOPEDIA FACIAL. Text in Portuguese. 1996. bi-m. BRL 189 domestic; USD 290 foreign (effective 2001). adv. abstr. charts. Index. *Refereed.* **Document type:** *Academic/Scholarly.* **Description:** Presents the results of scientific research, original articles, translated articles, congress announcements, new products.
Formerly (until 1997): Revista Dental Press de Ortodontia e Ortopedia Maxilar (1413-4446)
Related titles: Diskette ed.: Abstracts Dental Press de Ortodontia e Ortopedia Facial.
Published by: Dental Press Editora Ltda., Av Euclides da Cunha, 1718, Maringa, Zona, PR 87015-180, Brazil. FAX 55-44-2622425, biblioteca@dentalpress.com.br, http://www.dentalpress.com.br. Ed. Laurindo Z Furquim. Circ: 2,000.

REVISTA ESPANOLA DE CIRUGIA ORAL Y MAXILOFACIAL. see *MEDICAL SCIENCES—Surgery*

617.6 ESP ISSN 0210-0576
REVISTA ESPANOLA DE ORTODONCIA. Text in Spanish. 1971. q. ESP 5,000, USD 90 (effective 1999). adv. bk.rev. abstr, bibl. back issues avail. *Refereed.*
Indexed: Dent.Abstr., Ind.Med.Esp.
Published by: Publicaciones Permanyer, Mallorca, 310, Barcelona 08037, Spain. TEL 34-93-207-5920, FAX 34-93-457-6642, permanyer@bcn.servicom.es. Ed., R&P Arturo Costa. Circ: 1,000.

617.6 ESP ISSN 1133-1615
REVISTA ESPANOLA ODONTOESTOMATOLOGICA DE IMPLANTES. Text in Spanish. 1993. q. ESP 6,500, USD 115 (effective 1999). adv. **Document type:** *Trade.*
Published by: Editorial Dips Rocas, Muntaner, 393 pral. 4, Barcelona 08021, Spain. TEL 39-3-2001389, FAX 39-3-2021958, edipsro@intercom.es. Ed. Dr. Esteban Padulles. R&P Alvaro Treviso. Adv. contact Alvaro Trevino. color page ESP 105,000. Circ: 2,000.

617.6 BRA ISSN 0034-9542
REVISTA GAUCHA DE ODONTOLOGIA. Text in Portuguese; Summaries in English. 1953. q. USD 21. adv. bk.rev. abstr, bibl, illus. index.
Indexed: Dent.Ind.
Address: Estrada da Ponta Grossa 5311, Porto Alegre, RGS 9000, Brazil. Ed. Ricardo Cauduro Neto. Circ: 22,680.

617.6 COL ISSN 0120-2855
REVISTA ODONTOLOGIA. Text in Spanish. 1963. 3/yr. adv. bibl, illus.
Formerly: Odontologia (0029-8409)
Published by: Universidad Nacional de Colombia, Facultad de Odontologia, Ciudad Universitaria, Bogota, CUND, Colombia. Ed. Oscar Monroy Vega. Circ: 2,000.

617.6 BRA ISSN 0100-705X
REVISTA PAULISTA DE ODONTOLOGIA. Text in Portuguese. 1979. bi-m. USD 50 (effective 2001). adv. back issues avail.; reprints avail.
Published by: Sindicato dos Odontologistas do Estado de Sao Paulo, Rua Humaita, 349-1a, sobreloja, B Vista, Sao Paulo, SP 01321-010, Brazil. TEL 55-11-31077567, FAX 55-11-31069364, soesp@soesp.com.br, http://www.soesp.com.br. Ed. Henrique Motilinsky. Pub. Jairo Correa. R&P, Adv. contact Ernesto Leme F. B&W page USD 1,440, color page USD 1,720; trim 280 x 210. Circ: 20,000.

617.6 PRT ISSN 0035-0397
REVISTA PORTUGUESA DE ESTOMATOLOGIA E CIRURGIA MAXILO-FACIAL. Text in Portuguese; Summaries in English, French. 1944. q. PTE 5,000 (effective 1998). adv. bk.rev. abstr, bibl, charts, illus, stat. index. *Refereed.* **Document type:** *Academic/Scholarly.*
Indexed: Biol.Abstr., Dent.Ind., Ind.Med. (coverage dropped).
—CISTI, GNLM.
Published by: Sociedade Portuguesa de Estomatologia e Medicina Dentaria, Rua Professor Fernando da Fonseca No 10A, Escritorio 7, Lisbon 1600-618, Portugal. TEL 351-21-7520056, FAX 351-21-7520057. Ed. Dr. Carlos Portugal. Adv. contact Luis Lopes. Circ: 1,800.

617.6 FRA ISSN 0300-9815
REVUE D'ODONTO-STOMATOLOGIE. Text in French; Summaries in English. 1954. bi-m. FRF 920 (effective 2000). adv. bk.rev. bibl, charts, illus, tr.lit. index, cum.index: 1954-1961. **Document type:** *Newspaper.*
Formerly: Revue Francaise d'Odonto-Stomatologie (0035-3043)
Indexed: Chem.Abstr., Curr.Tit.Dent., Dent.Ind., Ind.Med. (coverage dropped).
—BLDSC (7938.710000), CISTI, GNLM, Infotrieve. **CCC.**
Published by: Societe Odontologique de Paris, 239 rue du Faubourg Saint-Martin, Paris 75010, France. TEL 33-1-42092913, FAX 33-1-42092908, secretariat@sop.asso.fr, http://www.sop.assoc.fr. Ed. Dr. Gerard Mandel. Adv. contact Louis Verchere.

617.6 FRA ISSN 0035-2470
REVUE D'ODONTO-STOMATOLOGIE DU MIDI DE LA FRANCE. Text in French; Summaries in English. 1937. 4/yr. USD 45. adv. bk.rev. abstr, bibl, charts.
Indexed: Dent.Ind.
—CISTI, GNLM.
Published by: Faculte de Medecine, 3 T place de la Victoire, Bordeaux Cedex 33076, France. Ed. P Benoit. Circ: 2,000.

617.6 FRA ISSN 0337-9736
REVUE D'ORTHOPEDIE DENTO-FACIALE. Text in French, English. 1967. q. FRF 1,010 domestic; FRF 1,102 foreign (effective 2000). adv. bk.rev. back issues avail. **Document type:** *Journal, Academic/Scholarly.*
Indexed: Dent.Ind.
—BLDSC (7940.070000), GNLM.
Published by: (Association de la Revue d'Orthopedie Dento-Faciale), Societe d'Information et de Diffusion, Librarie International, 9 rue Christine, Paris 75006, France. TEL 33-1-43293101, FAX 33-1-43293262, flancou@mail.easynet.fr, http://www.editionsid.com/. Ed. Charles Bolender. Pub., R&P, Adv. contact Fatima Lancou. B&W page FRF 3,900, color page FRF 8,780; trim. Circ: 2,200.

617.6 FRA ISSN 0035-4147
REVUE STOMATO-ODONTOLOGIQUE DU NORD DE LA FRANCE✶ . Text in French. 1970 (vol.25). q. FRF 25. adv. illus. index.
Indexed: Biol.Abstr.
—CISTI, GNLM.
Address: Place de Verdun, Lille 59, France.

617.6 DEU ISSN 0035-4503
RHEINISCHES ZAHNAERZTEBLATT. Text in German. m. **Document type:** *Newsletter, Trade.*
—GNLM.
Published by: Vereinigte Verlagsanstalten GmbH, Hoeherweg 278, Duesseldorf 40231, Germany. TEL 49-211-7357589, FAX 49-211-7357507, am@vva.de, http://www.vva.de. Circ: 9,000 (controlled).

617.6 USA
CODEN: RIDJEJ
RHODE ISLAND DENTAL ASSOCIATION. JOURNAL. Text in English. 1968. q. USD 20 (effective 2000). adv. bk.rev. illus. **Document type:** *Newsletter, Trade.*
Formerly (until 1975): Rhode Island State Dental Society. Journal (0035-4643)
Indexed: Dent.Ind.

M

Published by: Rhode Island Dental Association, 200 Centerville Pl, Warwick, RI 02886. TEL 401-732-6833. Ed., Adv. contact Dr. Jan Feldman. R&P Valerie G Donnelly. Circ: 700.

617.6 USA
RHODE ISLAND DENTAL ASSOCIATION. NEWSLETTER. Text in English. 1972. s-a. membership only.
Published by: Rhode Island Dental Association, 200 Centerville Pl, Warwick, RI 02886. TEL 401-732-6833. R&P Valerie G Donnelly. Circ: 600.

617.6 ITA ISSN 0391-5611
RIVISTA ITALIANA DEGLI ODONTOTECNICI - DENTAL PRESS. Text in Italian. 1964. 9/yr. ITL 92,000 (effective 1999). bk.rev. **Document type:** *Academic/Scholarly.*
Former titles (until 1983): Dental Press (0391-5883); (until 1965): Rivista Italiana degli Odontotecnici
Indexed: Dent.Ind.
Published by: Masson S.p.A., Divisione Periodici, Via F.lli Bressan 2, Milan, MI 20126, Italy. TEL 39-2-270741, FAX 39-2-27074210. adv.: B&W page ITL 1,580,000, color page ITL 2,110,000; trim 280 x 210. Circ: 7,000.

617.6 ITA ISSN 1120-7558
RIVISTA ITALIANA DI CHIRURGIA MAXILLO-FACCIALE. Text in Italian; Summaries in English, Italian. 1990. 3/yr. ITL 90,000 (effective 2000). adv. abstr, bibl, charts, illus. back issues avail. **Document type:** *Academic/Scholarly.*
Published by: (Societa Italiana di Chirurgia Maxillo-Facciale), Edizioni Calderini, Via Emilia Levante 31, Bologna, BO 40139, Italy. TEL 39-51-62267, FAX 39-51-490200, stampa@calolerini.agriline.it. Ed. Danio Romagnoli. Adv. contact F Metri. B&W page ITL 787,500, color page ITL 1,837,500.

617.6 ITA ISSN 0035-6905
RIVISTA ITALIANA DI STOMATOLOGIA*. Text in Italian. 1931. m. ITL 65,000. bk.rev.
Indexed: Dent.Ind.
—CISTI, GNLM.
Published by: (Associazione Medici Dentisti Italiani), Attualita Dentale S.r.l., Via Ludovico Da Viadana, 9, Milan, MI 20122, Italy. Circ: 15,000.

617.6 GBR
ROLLS OF DENTAL AUXILIARIES. Text in English. a. GBP 8. back issues avail.
Formerly: Rolls of Ancilliary Dental Workers
Published by: General Dental Council, 37 Wimpole St, London W1M 8DQ, United Kingdom. TEL 44-20-7887-3800, FAX 44-20-7224-3294.

617.6 RUS
ROSSIISKII STOMATOLOGICHESKII ZHURNAL. Text in Russian; Summaries in English. 1997. q. RUR 45; USD 125 foreign. adv. abstr, bibl, illus. back issues avail.
Formerly: Problemy Neirostomatologii i Stomatologii (1560-9553)
Related titles: Fax ed.
Published by: Izdatel'stvo Meditsina, Petroverigskii per 6-8, Moscow 101000, Russian Federation. TEL 7-095-9248785, FAX 7-095-9286003. Ed. M.N. Puzin. Pub. A M Stochik. R&P M N Puzin. Adv. contact O A Fadeeva TEL 7-095-923-51-40. Circ: 400. **Dist by:** Mezhdunarodnaya Kniga, B Yakimanka 39, Moscow 117049, Russian Federation. TEL 7-095-2384967, FAX 7-095-2384634; **US dist. addr.:** East View Publications, 3020 Harbor Ln N, Minneapolis, MN 55447. TEL 612-550-0961.

617.6 AUS ISSN 0158-1570
ROYAL AUSTRALASIAN COLLEGE OF DENTAL SURGEONS. ANNALS. Text in English. 1967. irreg., latest vol.15, 2000. AUD 42 newsstand/cover (effective 2001). 394 p./no. **Document type:** *Proceedings.* **Description:** Contains papers and abstracts from the Convocation and associated oral and maxillofacial surgery and periodontics meeting.
Former titles: Royal Australian College of Dental Surgeons. Annals (0312-7923); Australian College of Dental Surgeons. Annals. (0004-8895)
—BLDSC (1031.492000), GNLM.
Published by: Royal Australasian College of Dental Surgeons, 64 Castlereagh St, Sydney, NSW 2000, Australia. TEL 61-2-9232-3800, FAX 61-2-9221-8108, registrar@racds.org, http://www.racds.org. Ed., R&P John K Harcourt, O A M TEL 61-2-9232-3800. Adv. contact Neil J Peppitt. Circ: 1,800.

617.6 GBR ISSN 0049-1160
S A A D DIGEST. Text in English. 1970. q. GBP 30 (effective 2002). adv. bk.rev. illus. **Document type:** *Academic/Scholarly.*
Indexed: Curr.Adv.Ecol.Sci.
—BLDSC (8055.110000), GNLM.
Published by: Society for the Advancement of Anaesthesia in Dentistry, 53 Wimpole St, London W1M 7DP, United Kingdom. TEL 44-20-7935-0476. Ed. Andrea Wraith. Circ: 1,500.

617.6 USA
SAN ANTONIO DISTRICT DENTAL SOCIETY NEWSLETTER*. Text in English. 1946. m. USD 40. adv. illus.
Supersedes (in 1970): San Antonio District Dental Society. Journal (0036-3979)
Indexed: Dent.Ind.
Published by: San Antonio District Dental Society, 3355 Cherry Ridge St Ste 214, San Antonio, TX 78230-4818. TEL 512-732-1264. Ed. Dr. Dave C Bensh. Circ: 1,100.

617.6 CHE ISSN 0256-2855 CODEN: SMOZEP
SCHWEIZERISCHE MONATSSCHRIFT FUER ZAHNMEDIZIN/REVUE MENSUELLE SUISSE D'ODONTO-STOMATOLOGIE/RIVISTA MENSILE SVIZZERA DI ODONTOLOGIA E STOMATOLOGIA. Text in English, French, German, Italian. 1891. m. CHF 250. adv. bk.rev. abstr, bibl, charts, illus. index. **Document type:** *Academic/Scholarly.*
Formerly (until 1984): Schweizerische Monatsschrift fuer Zahnheilkunde (0036-7702); Incorporates: Helvetica Odontologica Acta (0018-0211); Helvetica Odontologica Acta. Supplementum (0073-1803)
Indexed: Biol.Abstr., Chem.Abstr., Curr.Adv.Ecol.Sci., Curr.Tit.Dent., Dent.Ind., Excerp.Med., Ind.Med. (coverage dropped).
—BLDSC (8112.360000), CASDDS, CISTI, GNLM.
Published by: Schweizerische Zahnaerztegesellschaft, Postfach, Bern, 8 3000, Switzerland. TEL 41-31-3120377, FAX 41-31-3113534. Circ: 5,300.

617.6 USA ISSN 0037-0452
SEATTLE - KING COUNTY DENTAL SOCIETY. JOURNAL. Text in English. 1962. m. (Aug.-May). USD 16. bk.rev.
Formerly: Seattle District Dental Society. Journal
Indexed: Dent.Ind.
Published by: (Seattle-King County Dental Society), Journal and Bulletin Agency, PO Box 10249, Bainbridge Island, WA 98110. TEL 206-682-7813. adv.: B&W page USD 140; trim 7.5 x 4.75. Circ: 1,500.

SELECTED READINGS IN ORAL AND MAXILLOFACIAL SURGERY. see *MEDICAL SCIENCES—Surgery*

617.643 USA ISSN 1073-8746
SEMINARS IN ORTHODONTICS. Text in English. 1995. q. USD 125 domestic to individuals; USD 156 foreign to individuals; USD 154 domestic to institutions; USD 186 foreign to institutions; USD 72 domestic to students; USD 94 foreign to students; USD 47 newsstand/cover (effective 2001). adv. bibl, illus. index. **Document type:** *Academic/Scholarly.* **Description:** Provides authoritative, up-to-date coverage of innovative techniques, new instruments and other products, and new uses for existing material.
—BLDSC (8239.456690), CISTI.
Published by: W.B. Saunders Co. (Subsidiary of: Harcourt Publishers Ltd.), 11830 Westline Industrial Dr, St Louis, MO 63146. TEL 800-325-4177, wbsaunders.co, http://www.wbsaunders.com. Ed. Dr. P Lionel Sadowsky. adv.: B&W page USD 645, color page USD 1,570; trim 10 x 7. Circ: 2,209. **Subscr. to:** Periodicals Fulfillment, W B Saunders Co, 6277 Sea Harbor Dr, 4th Fl, Orlando, FL 32891-4800. FAX 800-574-6418.

617.6 IRN
SHAHEED BEHESHTI UNIVERSITY. FACULTY OF DENTISTRY. JOURNAL. Text in Persian, Modern; Abstracts in English. 1968. q., latest 2000, Mar. adv. **Document type:** *Academic/Scholarly.*
Formerly (until 1983): National University of Iran. Dental School. Journal (0011-8745)
Published by: Shaheed Beheshti University, Faculty of Dentistry, Shahid Chamran Ave., Tehran 19834, Iran. TEL 98-21-2255537, 98-21-2255958, TELEX 215464, bujdent@hotmail.com. Ed., Adv. contact Dr. Ghassem Ansari.

617.6 JPN ISSN 0029-8484 CODEN: SHIGAZ
SHIGAKU/ODONTOLOGY. Text in Japanese; Summaries in English. 1941. bi-m. JPY 6,000 (effective 1999). charts, illus. **Document type:** *Academic/Scholarly.*
Indexed: Biol.Abstr., Chem.Abstr., Chem.Titles, Dent.Ind., Hist.Abstr. (until 1992, dropped), INIS Atomind.
—BLDSC (6235.230000), CASDDS, CISTI, GNLM, Infotrieve. **CCC.**
Published by: Society of the Nippon Dental University/Nippon Shika Daigaku Shigakukai, 9-20 Fujimi 1-chome, Chiyoda-ku, Tokyo 102-0071, Japan. FAX 81-3-3264-8745. Ed. Motoo Niwa. Circ: 2,650.

617.6 JPN ISSN 0037-3710 CODEN: SHGKA3
SHIKA GAKUHO/TOKYO DENTAL COLLEGE SOCIETY JOURNAL. Text in English, Japanese. 1895. m. JPY 5,000, USD 8.60. adv. bk.rev. abstr, bibl, charts, illus, stat, tr.lit. index.
Indexed: Biol.Abstr., Chem.Abstr., Chem.Indus.Notes, Chem.Titles, Dent.Ind., Excerp.Med., INIS Atomind.
—BLDSC (4908.920000), CASDDS, CISTI, GNLM.
Published by: Tokyo Shika Daigaku Gakkai/Tokyo Dental College Society, Tokyo Dental College, 2-2 Masago 1-chome, Chiba 260, Japan. Ed. Dr. Tetsuya Kanatake. Circ: 4,600. **Order from:** Import and Export Department, P.O. Box 5050, Tokyo International, Tokyo 100-31, Japan; Maruzen Co., 2-3-10 Nihonbashi, Chuo-ku, Tokyo 103-0027, Japan.

617.6 JPN ISSN 0389-1895 CODEN: SHGKD6
SHIKA GIKO/JOURNAL OF DENTAL TECHNICS. Text in Japanese. 1973. m. JPY 1,200 per issue. adv. bk.rev. charts, illus. Supplement avail.
Indexed: Chem.Abstr., Chem.Titles.
—CASDDS.
Published by: Ishiyaku Publishers Inc., 7-10 Honkomagome 1-chome, Bunkyo-ku, Tokyo 113-0021, Japan. Ed. Hiroshi Miura. Circ: 20,000.

617.6 615.84 JPN ISSN 0389-9705
SHIKA HOSHASEN. Text in Japanese. 1960. q. JPY 10,000; includes English edition. adv. **Document type:** *Academic/Scholarly.*
Related titles: ♦ English ed.: Oral Radiology. ISSN 0911-6028.
Indexed: INIS Atomind.
—BLDSC (3553.430000).
Published by: Nihon Shika Hoshasen Gakkai/Japanese Society for Oral and Maxillofacial Radiology, c/o Hitotsubashi Printing Co Ltd., Gakkai Business Center, 3-12-15 Kami-Osaki, Shinagawa-ku, Tokyo 141-0021, Japan. Ed. Tomohiro Okano. R&P Hajime Fuchihata. Adv. contact Hajime Fuchinata.

617.6 JPN ISSN 0030-6150 CODEN: SIGAAE
SHIKA IGAKU/ODONTOLOGICAL MEDICINE. Variant title: Osaka Odontological Society. Journal. Text in Japanese; Summaries in English. 1930. q. adv. charts, illus. **Document type:** *Academic/Scholarly.* **Description:** Contains numerous studies in dental research, including new technologies and treatments.
Indexed: Biol.Abstr., Chem.Abstr., Chem.Indus.Notes, Chem.Titles, INIS Atomind.
—BLDSC (4839.300000), CASDDS, GNLM, Infotrieve. **CCC.**
Published by: Osaka Odontological Society/Osaka Shika Gakkai, 8-1 Kuzuha-Hanazono-cho, Hirakata-shi, Osaka-fu 573-1121, Japan. FAX 83-720-643164. Ed. Tatsuo Kawamoto.

617 USA ISSN 1091-5222
SIGNATURE (MAHWAH). Text in English. 1996. irreg. **Document type:** *Trade.*
Related titles: ♦ Supplement to: Practical Periodontics and Aesthetic Dentistry. ISSN 1042-2722.
—BLDSC (8276.135000).
Published by: Montage Media Corp., 1000 Wyckoff Ave, Mahwah, NJ 07430. TEL 201-891-3200, FAX 201-891-2626, editorial@montagemedia.com, http://www.montagemedia.com.

SOUTH AFRICA. STATISTICS SOUTH AFRICA. CENSUS OF MEDICAL, DENTAL AND OTHER HEALTH SERVICES - DENTISTS. see *MEDICAL SCIENCES—Abstracting, Bibliographies, Statistics*

617.6 ZAF ISSN 1029-4864 CODEN: DASJAG
SOUTH AFRICAN DENTAL JOURNAL. Text and summaries in Afrikaans, English. 1945. m., latest vol.56. ZAR 1,300 (effective 2001). adv. bk.rev., music rev. charts, illus, abstr. index. 56 p./no. back issues avail. *Refereed.* **Document type:** *Journal, Academic/Scholarly.* **Description:** Original scientific research articles of interest to association members.
Formerly: Dental Association of South Africa. Journal (0011-8516)
Indexed: Biol.Abstr., Dent.Abstr., Dent.Ind., INIS Atomind., I.P.A., Ind.S.A.Per., Ref.Zh.
—CASDDS, CISTI, GNLM.

M

Published by: African Medical Association, Health & Medical Publication Group, Private Bag 1, Houghton, Johannesburg 2041, South Africa. TEL 27-11-4845288, 27-11-5306520, FAX 27-11-6425718, 27-11-5314126. Ed., R&P, Adv. contact Dr. Adrian W R Rademeyer TEL 27-11-671-2233. Circ: 3,750.

617.6 USA ISSN 0038-3945
SOUTHERN CALIFORNIA DENTAL LABORATORY ASSOCIATION. BULLETIN✱. Text in English. 1944. bi-m. USD 5. adv. illus.
Formerly (until 1969): Southern California State Dental Laboratory Association Bulletin (0091-3308)
Published by: Southern California Dental Laboratory Association, 195 S C St, Ste 250, Tustin, CA 92680-3666. TEL 213-661-2188. Ed. James C Powell. Circ: 2,000.

617.6 USA ISSN 0275-1879
RK55.H28
SPECIAL CARE IN DENTISTRY; managing special patients, settings, and situations. Text in English. 1981. bi-m. USD 60 domestic to individuals; USD 90 foreign to individuals; USD 102 domestic to corporations; USD 132 foreign to corporations (effective 1999). adv. back issues avail. *Refereed.* **Document type:** *Academic/Scholarly.* **Description:** Provides oral health care professionals with information to enhance their ability to address special patient needs.
Formed by merger of (1974-1981): Journal of Dentistry for the Handicapped (0163-8629); (1967-1981): Journal of Hospital Dental Practice (0022-1600); (1966-1981): American Society for Geriatric Dentistry. Journal (0003-1054)
Related titles: Microform ed.: (from PQC).
Indexed: AgeLine, CINAHL, Curr.Tit.Dent., Dent.Abstr., Dent.Ind., INIS Atomind.
—BLDSC (8365.680000), GNLM, ingenta.
Published by: Federation of Special Care Organizations in Dentistry, 211 East Chicago Ave, Chicago, IL 60611. TEL 312-440-2661, http://www.iadr.com. Ed. Dr. Ronald Ettinger. R&P John S Rutkavskas TEL 312-440-2660. Circ: 2,500. **Co-sponsors:** Academy of Dentistry for Persons with Disabilities; American Association of Hospital Dentists; American Society for Geriatric Dentistry.

617.643 LKA ISSN 1391-0728
SRI LANKA DENTAL JOURNAL. Text in English. 1970. s-a. LKR 100; USD 5 foreign. adv. charts, illus, stat. back issues avail. *Refereed.* **Document type:** *Academic/Scholarly.*
Published by: Sri Lanka Dental Association, Office of the SLDA, Professional Centre, No.275-75 Bauddhaloka Mawatha, Colombo 7, Sri Lanka. TEL 94-1-595147, FAX 94-1-595147, slda@sri.lanka.net. adv.: B&W page USD 45. Circ: 300.

617.6 NLD ISSN 0922-310X
STANDBY; vaktijdschrift voor tandartsassistenten. Text in Dutch. 1988. bi-m. NLG 63.20 (effective 1999). adv. bk.rev. *Refereed.* **Document type:** *Trade.* **Description:** Offers dental assistants and hygienists practical tips and information.
Published by: Wegener Tijdschriften Groep BV (Subsidiary of: Wegener Arcade NV), Wildenborch 5, Postbus 1860, Diemen 1112 CD, Netherlands. TEL 31-20-660-3300, FAX 31-20-660-3303, info@wtg.wegener.nl, http://www.wegener.nl. Adv. contact Peter Buitendijk. B&W page NLG 1,990, color page NLG 4,490. Circ: 3,000.

617.6 PRT ISSN 0870-4287
STOMA; cadernos de estomatologia, cirurgia maxilo-facial e medicina dentaria. Text in Portuguese. 1986. q. PTE 10,000 in the European Union; PTE 10,250 elsewhere. adv. **Description:** Publishes scientific works on dentistry, maxillo traumatology, dental surgery and dental forensic sciences. Includes information on new products and services, meetings and congresses.
—BLDSC (8465.863000).
Published by: Edicoes Vade-mecum Lda., Calcada do Tijolo, 45, Lisbon 1200, Portugal. TEL 351-1-3420518, FAX 351-1-3420682. Ed. Dr. Pedro Graca Castel Branco. Adv. contact Joaquim Azevedo. Circ: 3,000.

617.6 ITA ISSN 1120-9402
STOMATOLOGIA MEDITERRANEA; rivista trimestrale di odontoiatria e chirurgia maxillo-facciale. Text in Italian; Summaries in English. 1981. q. ITL 70,000, USD 80. adv. bk.rev. bibl, charts, illus, stat.
—GNLM.
Address: Via Emerico Amari, 32, Palermo, PA 90139, Italy. TEL 091-32-82-69. Ed. Giuseppe Messina. Circ: 1,500.

617.6 BGR ISSN 0204-6415
STOMATOLOGICHEN PREGLED. Text in Bulgarian. 1970. q. BGL 4,000 domestic; USD 30 foreign (effective 2000). adv. abstr. index. back issues avail. **Document type:** *Academic/Scholarly.* **Description:** Presents original articles and abstracts of foreign publications on prevention, diagnosis and treatment of stomatological conditions, new materials and techniques in dental practice.
Published by: Meditsinski Universitet - Sofia, Tsentur za Informatsiia po Meditsina/Medical University - Sofia, Medical Information Center, 1 Sv Georgi Sofiiski ul, Sofia 1431, Bulgaria. TEL 359-2-9522342, FAX 359-2-9522393, mutafov@sun.medun.acad.bg, http://www.medun.acad.bg. Ed. N Polichronov. adv.: B&W page USD 50, color page USD 150; trim 160 x 110.

617.6 AUT ISSN 0946-3151
STOMATOLOGIE. Text in German; Summaries in English. 1903. 8/yr. EUR 156; EUR 23 newsstand/cover (effective 2002). adv. bk.rev. bibl, illus, abstr. index. back issues avail. *Refereed.* **Document type:** *Journal, Academic/Scholarly.* **Description:** Publishes original papers, survey articles, and case reports on dentistry and oral surgery.
Former titles: Zeitschrift fuer Stomatologie (0175-7784); Oesterreichische Zeitschrift fuer Stomatologie (0029-9642)
Related titles: Microform ed.; Online - full text ed.: (from Springer LINK); Supplement: Zeitschrift fuer Stomatologie. Supplementem. ISSN 0178-4595.
Indexed: Biol.Abstr., Curr.Cont. (coverage dropped), Curr.Tit.Dent., Dent.Ind.
—CISTI, GNLM, Infotrieve. **CCC.**
Published by: Springer-Verlag Wien (Subsidiary of: BertelsmannSpringer), Sachsenplatz 4-6, PO Box 89, Vienna, W 1201, Austria. TEL 43-1-3302415-0, FAX 43-1-330242665, journals@springer.at, http://www.springer.at/stomatologie. Eds. M Matejka, R Fischer. R&P Angela Foessl TEL 43-1-3302415517. Adv. contact Michael Katzenberger TEL 43-1-3302415220. B&W page XEU 1,470, color page XEU 1,911; 180 x 260. Circ: 3,500. **Subscr. in N. America to:** Springer-Verlag, Journals. TEL 212-460-1500, FAX 212-473-6272, orders@springer-ny.com, http://www.springer-ny.com.

617.6 BGR ISSN 0491-0982
CODEN: STMYAN
STOMATOLOGIJA. Text in Bulgarian; Summaries in English, Russian. 1951. bi-m. BGL 16.
Indexed: Abstr.Bulg.Sci.Med.Lit., INIS Atomind.
—CASDDS, CISTI, GNLM.
Published by: (Bulgaria. Ministerstvo na Narodnoto Zdrave), Izdatelstvo Meditsina i Fizkultura, 11 Pl Slaveikov, Sofia 1080, Bulgaria. Ed. E Atanassova. Circ: 2,581. **Distr. by:** Hemus, 6 Rouski blvd, Sofia 1000, Bulgaria. **Co-sponsor:** Nauchno Druzhestvo po Stomatologija.

617.6 RUS ISSN 0039-1735
CODEN: STOAAT
STOMATOLOGIYA/STOMATOLOGY. Text in Russian. 1922. bi-m. RUR 288 for 6 mos. to individuals; RUR 720 for 6 mos. to institutions (effective 2002). adv. bk.rev. index. **Description:** Reports on theoretical and practical problems of therapeutic, operative and orthopedic stomatology, stomatology of childhood, the etiology, pathogenesis, prophylaxis and treatment of diseases of the teeth, oral cavity and the maxillofacial region.
Indexed: Biol.Abstr., Chem.Abstr., Chem.Indus.Notes, Chem.Titles, Dent.Ind., Excerp.Med., INIS Atomind., Ind.Med. (1937-), Nutr.Abstr., Ref.Zh., Rev.Med.& Vet.Mycol., Sugar Ind.Abstr.
—BLDSC (0169.500000), CASDDS, CISTI, East View, GNLM, Infotrieve. **CCC.**
Published by: (A-O Stomatologiya), Media Sfera, Dmitrovskoe shosse 46, korp 2, etazh 4, P.O. Box 54, Moscow 127238, Russian Federation. TEL 7-095-4824329, FAX 7-095-4824312, mediashp@mediasphera.ru. Ed. O M Bezrukov. Adv. contact Valery Nemtsov. **Dist. by:** Mezhdunarodnaya Kniga, B Yakimanka 39, Moscow 117049, Russian Federation. TEL 7-095-2384967, FAX 7-095-2384634; **US dist. addr.:** East View Publications, 3020 Harbor Ln N, Minneapolis, MN 55447. TEL 612-550-0961. **Co-sponsor:** Ministerstvo Zdravookhraneniya.

617.6 RUS
STOMATOLOGIYA ROSSII/RUSSIAN STOMATOLOGY. Text in Russian. 1997. a. RUR 200 (effective 2002). **Document type:** *Directory.*
Published by: Chelovek, Malyi Pr. V.O., # 26, office 2, Sankt-Peterburg 199004, Russian Federation. TEL 7-812-3252564, http://www.stom.ru/stom2000/english.shtml. Ed. Anatoliy Dudarev.

617.6 YUG ISSN 0039-1743
CODEN: SGLSAB
STOMATOLOSKI GLASNIK SRBIJE✱. Text in Serbian; Summaries in English, French, German. 1954. bi-m. USD 25. adv. bk.rev. charts, illus. **Document type:** *Academic/Scholarly.*
Indexed: Dent.Ind.
—BLDSC (8465.920000), CASDDS, GNLM.
Published by: Srpsko Lekarsko Drustvo/Serbian Medical Association, Vase Stajica 9, Novi Sad 21000, Yugoslavia. TEL 381-11-3246539, kentera@eunet.yu. Ed. Vladimir Slavkovic. Circ: 2,000.

617.6 USA
SUFFOLK DENTISTRY; bulletin of the Suffolk County Dental Society. Variant title: Suffolk Dental Bulletin. Text in English. 1970 (vol.16). bi-m. USD 12. adv. bk.rev. **Document type:** *Bulletin.*
Formerly: Suffolk County Dental Society. Bulletin (0039-4688)
Published by: Suffolk County Dental Society, 1727 Veterans Hwy, Islandia, NY 11749-1520. TEL 631-232-1400, FAX 631-232-1402, exec@sc-ds.org, http://www.sc-ds.org. Adv. contact Dr. Jane S Meslin. Circ: 1,100.

617.6 USA
SURGICAL UPDATE. Text in English. 1985. 3/yr. back issues avail. *Refereed.* **Document type:** *Newsletter.* **Description:** Provides information on oral and maxillofacial surgery for general dentists.
Published by: American Association of Oral and Maxillofacial Surgeons, 9700 W. Bryn Mawr Ave., Rosemont, IL 60018. TEL 708-678-6200, FAX 708-678-6286. Circ: 150,000 (controlled).

617.6 USA
SURVEY OF DENTAL PRACTICE. Text in English. a. USD 200 to non-members; USD 75 to members. **Document type:** *Trade.*
Indexed: SRI.
Published by: American Dental Association, Survey Center, 211 E Chicago Ave, Chicago, IL 60611. TEL 312-440-2500, FAX 312-440-2790.

617.6 SWE ISSN 0348-0011
SVENSK SJUKHUSTANDLAEKARTIDNING. Text in Swedish. 1976. q. SEK 140 (effective 1998). adv. bk.rev. **Document type:** *Academic/Scholarly.*
Published by: Svensk Sjukhustandlaekarfoerening, Sjukhustandvaarden KKK, Uppsala 75185, Sweden. TEL 47-31-374842, FAX 47-18-1764-50. Ed. Christina Engqvist.

617.6 SWE ISSN 0347-9994
CODEN: SDJOD5
SWEDISH DENTAL JOURNAL. Text in English. 1908. bi-m. SEK 700; SEK 800 foreign (effective 1999). adv. bk.rev. charts, illus. index, cum.index: 1908-1953. *Refereed.* **Document type:** *Academic/Scholarly.*
Formed by the merger of: Odontologisk Revy (0029-8441); Svensk Tandlaekare-Tidskrift (0039-6745)
Related titles: Online - full text ed.: (from Institute for Scientific Information); ♦ Supplement: Swedish Dental Journal. Supplement. ISSN 0348-6672.
Indexed: ASCA, Biol.Abstr., Chem.Abstr., Curr.Adv.Ecol.Sci., Curr.Cont., Curr.Tit.Dent., Dent.Abstr., Dent.Ind., Excerp.Med., INIS Atomind., Ind.Med. (1977-), Inpharma, NRN, Reac., Sci.Cit.Ind.
—BLDSC (8573.865000), CASDDS, CISTI, GNLM, IDS, ingenta.
Published by: Sveriges Tandlaekarfoerbund/Swedish Dental Association, Box 1217, Stockholm 11182, Sweden. TEL 46-8-666-15-00. Ed., R&P Goeran Koch TEL 46-36-324604. Adv. contact Elisabeth Hedman. Circ: 12,000.

617.6 SWE ISSN 0348-6672
SWEDISH DENTAL JOURNAL. SUPPLEMENT. Text in English. 1977. irreg.
Related titles: ♦ Supplement to: Swedish Dental Journal. ISSN 0347-9994.
Indexed: Ind.Med. (1977-).
—BLDSC (8573.865100).
Published by: Sveriges Tandlaekarfoerbund/Swedish Dental Association, Box 1217, Stockholm 11182, Sweden. TEL 46-8-666-15-00, FAX 46-8-666-15-95.

M

617.6 CHE ISSN 0251-1657
SWISS DENT; Schweizerische Zeitschrift fuer orale Praeventiv- und Kurativmedizin. Text in German. 1980. 10/yr. CHF 180 domestic; CHF 200 in Europe; CHF 340 elsewhere; CHF 20 newsstand/cover (effective 2001). adv. back issues avail. *Refereed.* **Document type:** *Journal, Trade.* **Description:** Publishes interviews with dental professors and companies as well as selected papers and reports.
—GNLM.
Published by: Verlag Dr. Felix Wuest AG, Kuesnachterstr 36, Postfach 161, Zumikon 8126, Switzerland. TEL 41-1-919-80-60, FAX 41-1-919-80-69. Ed., Pub., Adv. contact Dr. Felix Wuest. B&W page CHF 2,150, color page CHF 3,590; trim 185 x 265. Circ: 3,200 (paid and controlled).

617.6 BEL
TANDARTSENKRANT. Text in Dutch. 1990. s-m. EUR 49 (effective 2001). 8 p./no. 5 cols./p. **Document type:** *Newspaper.*
Related titles: Diskette ed.
Published by: Medical Integrated Communication, Rue du Duc 94, Brussels 1150, Belgium. TEL 32-2-7706847, FAX 32-2-7792171, micbel@skynet.be. Ed. Beatrice Couteaux. Circ: 8,000 (paid).

617.6 NLD ISSN 0167-1685
TANDARTSPRAKTIJK; onafhankelijk vaktijdschrift voor tandartsen. Text in Dutch. 1979. 10/yr. NLG 103.20; BEF 1,920 in Belgium; NLG 164 in Europe. adv. **Document type:** *Trade.* **Description:** Offers dentists practical information on a light scientific foundation.
Published by: Wegener Tijdschriften Groep BV (Subsidiary of: Wegener Arcade NV), Wildenborch 5, Postbus 1860, Diemen 1112 CD, Netherlands. TEL 31-20-660-3300, FAX 31-20-660-3303, info@wtg.wegener.nl, http://www.wegener.nl. Ed. J G Advokaat. Adv. contact Peter Buitendijk. B&W page NLG 2,260, color page NLG 5,045. Circ: 6,100 (paid).

617.6 SWE ISSN 1102-6146
TANDHYGIENIST TIDNINGEN. Text in Swedish. 1977. bi-m. SEK 276 (effective 2000). **Document type:** *Newspaper, Trade.*
Formerly (until 1991): Tandhygienistbladet (0349-9456)
Published by: Sveriges Tandhygienistfoerening (SRAT), Magnus Ladulaasgata 8, Fack 38401, Stockholm 10064, Sweden. Ed. Margaretha Malmquist. Adv. contact Lillemor Norfenhammar.

617.6 DNK ISSN 0039-9353
TANDLAEGEBLADET/DANISH DENTAL JOURNAL. Text in Danish. 1897. 18/yr. DKK 1,150 in Europe; DKK 1,925 elsewhere. adv. bk.rev. index.
Indexed: Dent.Ind., Ind.Med. (coverage dropped).
—BLDSC (8601.700000), CISTI, GNLM.
Published by: Dansk Tandlaegeforening/Danish Dental Association, Amaliegade 17, PO Box 143, Copenhagen K 1004, Denmark. TEL 45-33-15-77-11, FAX 45-33-13-10-03. Eds. Chr Nissen, Ib Paul Sewerin. Circ: 7,269.

617.6 DNK ISSN 0901-9898
TANDLAEGERNES NYE TIDSSKRIFT. Variant title: T N T. Text in Danish. 1976. m. membership. adv. bk.rev. illus. **Document type:** *Trade.*
Former titles (until 1986): D B - D Bat (0109-3592); (until 1980): D Bat (0109-4475)
Published by: Tandlaegernes Nye Landsforening - T N L, Kompagnistraede 14 D, Copenhagen K 1208, Denmark. TEL 45-33-14-00-65, FAX 45-33-14-03-24. Ed. Peter Simonsen. Adv. contact Dorthe Medjhede. Circ: 1,500.

617.6 SWE ISSN 0039-6982
TANDLAEKARTIDNINGEN. Text in Swedish. 1909. 15/yr. SEK 1,480 (effective 2001). adv. bk.rev. illus, stat. index. **Document type:** *Magazine, Trade.*
Formerly (until 1971): Sveriges Tandlaekarfoerbunds Tidning
Indexed: Dent.Ind.
—GNLM.
Published by: Sveriges Tandlaekarfoerbund/Swedish Dental Association, Box 1217, Stockholm 11182, Sweden. TEL 46-8-666-15-00, FAX 46-8-666-15-95, redaktionen.tlt@tandlakarforbundet.se, http://www.tandlakarforbundet.se/swe/tidning/. Ed., Pub. Christina Moerk. Adv. contact Christer Johansson. B&W page SEK 17,900, color page SEK 24,700; trim 174 x 245. Circ: 11,300.

617.6 331.8 DNK ISSN 0900-257X
TANDPLEJEREN. Text in Danish. 1976. m. DKK 255 (effective 1999). adv. **Document type:** *Trade.*
Published by: Dansk Tandplejerforening, Sundhedsorganisationernes Hus, Noerre Voldgade 90, Copenhagen K 1358, Denmark. TEL 45-33-13-82-11, FAX 45-33-93-82-14. Ed. Eva Lis Pedersen. Circ: 1,500.

617.6 SWE ISSN 0346-2617
TANDSKOETERSKETIDNINGEN. Text in Swedish. 1946. q. SEK 100 (effective 1990).
Formerly (until vol.3, 1974): Svenska Tandskoeterskefoerbundets Tidskrift
Published by: Svenska Tandskoeterskefoerbundet, Fack 30102, Stockholm 10425, Sweden.

617.6 NLD ISSN 0929-2934
TANDTECHNISCH MAGAZINE; onafhankelijk magazine voor tandartsen en tandtechnici. Text in Dutch. 1993. bi-m. NLG 106, USD 125. bk.rev. stat. back issues avail. **Document type:** *Trade.* **Description:** Publishes articles of interest to dentists and dental technicians.
Published by: Stichting Public Affairs, Postbus 658, Zeist 3700 AR, Netherlands. TEL 31-30-691-5754, FAX 31-30-691-7045. Ed. N J C Eikmans. adv.: B&W page NLG 2,215, color page NLG 5,165; trim 297 x 210. Circ: 10,000.

617.6 SWE ISSN 0039-9361
TANDTEKNIKERN* . Text in Swedish. 1932. m. SEK 700 (effective 1998). adv. **Document type:** *Trade.*
—GNLM.
Published by: Tandteknikerfoerbundet, c/o Svenges Tandlakarforbund, Fack 5843, Stockholm 10248, Sweden. TEL 46-8-703-23-98, FAX 46-8-752-60-36. Ed. Kerstin Orsen. adv.: B&W page SEK 5,100. Circ: 1,800.

617.6 DEU
TEAMWORK; interdisziplinaeres Journal fuer prothetische Zahnheilkunde. Text in German. 1998. q. DEM 160; DEM 195 foreign (effective 2000). **Document type:** *Trade.*
Published by: Teamwork Medien GmbH, Jakob Strobl Str 11, Fuchstal 86925, Germany. TEL 49-8243-96920, FAX 49-8243-969222, ct.verlag@t-online.de. Ed. Ralf Suckert. Circ: 12,000 (paid).

617.6 USA ISSN 0040-3385
CODEN: JTDAAB
TENNESSEE DENTAL ASSOCIATION. JOURNAL. Text in English. 1919. q. USD 15; USD 17.50 in Canada; USD 20 elsewhere. adv. bk.rev. illus. index. back issues avail. **Document type:** *Academic/Scholarly, Trade.*
Formerly: Tennessee State Dental Association. Journal
Indexed: Dent.Abstr., Dent.Ind., INIS Atomind.
—BLDSC (4907.100000), CISTI, GNLM.
Published by: Tennessee Dental Association, 2104 Sunset Pl, Box 120188, Nashville, TN 37212. TEL 615-383-8962. Ed., R&P Dr. Stephen Brooks. Adv. contact Sharon Melvin. Circ: 2,100.

617.6 USA
TENTH TIMES* . Text in English. 1962. m. USD 15. adv.
Formerly: Austin Dental News (0004-8267)
Published by: Texas Dental Association, Tenth District Dental Society, 3305 Northland, 515, Austin, TX 78731. TEL 512-452-9296. Ed. Dr. Mark Sweeney. Circ: 450 (controlled).

617.6 USA
TEXAS DENTAL ASSISTANTS ASSOCIATION. BULLETIN. Text in English. 195?. 3/yr. USD 10. adv. illus. **Document type:** *Bulletin.* **Description:** Information for association members.
Former titles: Texas Dental Assistants Association. Newsletter; Texas Dental Assistants Association. Bulletin (0049-3503)
Indexed: Dent.Ind.
Published by: Texas Dental Assistants Association, 4948 Colonial Park Dr., Haltom City, TX 76117-1009. TEL 817-281-3949. Ed. Dennise Jennings. Circ: 500.

617.6 USA ISSN 0040-4284
TEXAS DENTAL JOURNAL. Text in English. 1883. m., latest vol.119, 2002. USD 82.50 to non-members; USD 49.50 to members (effective 1999). adv. bk.rev., Website rev. charts, illus, stat, abstr, bibl, tr.lit. 100 p./no. 3 cols./p. back issues avail. *Refereed.* **Document type:** *Journal, Trade.* **Description:** Professional journal, (Dental).
Indexed: Dent.Abstr., Dent.Ind.
—BLDSC (8798.690000), CISTI, GNLM.
Published by: Texas Dental Association, S IH-35', Austin, TX 78704. TEL 512-443-3675, FAX 512-443-3031, tda@tda.org, http://www.tda.org. R&P, Adv. contact Paul Schlesinger. Circ: 7,600.

617.6 DEU ISSN 0939-5687
THUERINGER ZAHNAERZTEBLATT. Text in German. 1991. m. DEM 88 domestic; DEM 102 foreign (effective 2000). bk.rev. *Refereed.* **Document type:** *Newspaper, Trade.*
—GNLM.
Published by: Landeszahnaerztekammer Thueringen, Barbarossahof 16, Erfurt 99092, Germany. TEL 49-361-7432-0, FAX 49-361-7432150, webmaster@lzaekthue.de, http://www.landeszahnaerztekammer-thueringen.de. Ed. Gottfried Wolf.

617.6 USA ISSN 1048-5317
TODAY'S F D A. (Florida Dental Association) Text in English. 1989. m. USD 42.80 (effective 2001). adv. bk.rev. charts, illus, abstr. 32 p./no. back issues avail. *Refereed.* **Document type:** *Magazine, Trade.* **Description:** Contains news, features, commentary, and scientific information for the Florida dentist.
Incorporates (in 1989): Dental Team; Formed by the merger of (19??-1989): Dental Times Dispatch (0886-5094); (1938-1989): Florida Dental Journal (0015-3990); Which was formerly (until 1967): Florida State Dental Society. Journal (0360-1676); F D A Dispatch; F D A Intaglio
Related titles: Online - full text ed.
Indexed: Dent.Ind.
—CISTI, GNLM.
Published by: Florida Dental Association, 1111 E Tennessee St, Tallahassee, FL 32308-6914. TEL 850-681-3629, FAX 850-561-0504, fda@floridadental.org, http://www.floridadental.org. Ed. Dr. Edward F Gonsky Jr. R&P Karen Thurston Chavez TEL 850-681-3629 ext 115. Adv. contact Janie Brannon TEL 850-681-3629 ext 116. Circ: 7,000 (paid and controlled).

617.6 JPN ISSN 0040-8891
CODEN: BTDCAV
TOKYO DENTAL COLLEGE. BULLETIN/TOKYO SHIKA DAIGAKU OBUN KIYO. Text in English. 1960. q. JPY 6,000 (effective 2001). charts, illus. back issues avail. *Refereed.* **Document type:** *Bulletin, Academic/Scholarly.*
Related titles: Microfiche ed.
Indexed: Biol.Abstr., Chem.Abstr., Chem.Indus.Notes, Chem.Titles, Curr.Adv.Ecol.Sci., Curr.Tit.Dent., Dent.Abstr., Dent.Ind., INIS Atomind.
—BLDSC (2780.300000), CASDDS, GNLM, ingenta, KNAW. **CCC.**
Published by: Tokyo Shika Daigaku/Tokyo Dental College, 1-2-2 Masago, Mihama-ku, Chiba-shi 261-0011, Japan. TEL 81-43-270-3985, FAX 81-43-270-3986. Ed., R&P Tatsuya Ishikawa. Circ: 700.

TOKYO IKA SHIKA DAIGAKU SEITAI ZAIRYO KOGAKU KENKYUJO HOKOKU/TOKYO MEDICAL AND DENTAL UNIVERSITY. INSTITUTE OF BIOMATERIALS AND BIOENGINEERING. REPORTS. see *MEDICAL SCIENCES*

617.6 COL ISSN 0121-246X
UNIVERSIDAD DE ANTIOQUIA. FACULTAD DE ODONTOLOGIA. REVISTA. Text in Spanish. 1984. s-a. COP 13,000 domestic; USD 20 foreign (effective 2000).
Published by: Universidad de Antioquia, Facultad de Odontologia, Apartado Postal 1226, Medellin, Colombia. TEL 57-4-510-5740, FAX 57-4-263-1230.

617.643 ARG ISSN 1515-372X
UNIVERSIDAD DE BUENOS AIRES. FACULTAD DE ODONTOLOGIA. MUSEO Y CENTRO DE ESTUDIOS HISTORICOS. REVISTA. Key Title: Revista del Museo y Centro de Estudios Historicos de la Facultad de Odontologia de Buenos Aires. Text in Spanish. 1986. s-a. **Document type:** *Academic/Scholarly.*
Formerly (until 1992): Universidad de Buenos Aires. Facultad de Odontologia. Museo. Revista (0327-2745)
Published by: Universidad de Buenos Aires, Facultad de Odontologia de Buenos Aires, Museo y Centro de Estudios Historicos, Marcelo T. De Alvear, 2142, Capital Federal, Buenos Aires 1122, Argentina. TEL 54-114-9641271, FAX 54-114-45083958, postmast@legal.odon.uba.ar, http://www.odon.uba.ar. Ed. Orestes Walter Siutti. Pub. Esteban Garcia.

617.6 URY ISSN 0083-4785
UNIVERSIDAD DE LA REPUBLICA. FACULTAD DE ODONTOLOGIA. ANALES. Text in Spanish. 1955. irreg. per issue exchange basis. Supplement avail.
Indexed: Biol.Abstr., Dent.Ind.
Published by: Universidad de la Republica, Facultad de Odontologia, Gl. Las Heras, 1925, Montevideo 11609, Uruguay.

M

617.6 VEN
UNIVERSIDAD DE LOS ANDES. FACULTAD DE ODONTOLOGIA. REVISTA✱. Text in Spanish. 1958. s-a. per issue exchange basis. illus.
Formerly: Revista Odontologica de Merida (0035-0273)
Published by: Universidad de Los Andes, Facultad de Odontologia, Via los Chorras de Milla, Merida, Tchira 5101, Venezuela.

617.6 BRA ISSN 0101-1774
CODEN: ROUNDL
UNIVERSIDADE ESTADUAL PAULISTA. REVISTA DE ODONTOLOGIA. Key Title: Revista de Odontologia da Unesp. Text in Portuguese; Summaries in English, Portuguese. 1979. a., latest vol.28, 1999. USD 30 (effective 2001); or exchange basis. bibl, charts, illus, stat, abstr. back issues avail. *Refereed.* **Document type:** *Journal, Academic/Scholarly.* **Description:** Publishes original articles in the study and research of odontology.
Formed by the merger of (1972-1979): Universidade Estadual Paulista. Faculdade de Odontologia de Aracatuba. Revista (0300-1350); Which was formerly: Revista F O A (0300-2837); (1967-1979): Faculdade de Odontologia de Araraquara. Revista (0101-1820); Which was formerly (until 1977): Faculdade de Farmacia e Odontologia de Araraquara. Revista (0014-6684); (1972-1977): Faculdade de Odontologia de Sao Jose dos Campos. Revista (0301-1119)
Indexed: Bibliogr.Bras.Odontol., Biol.Abstr., Cal.Tiss.Abstr., Environ.Sci.Poll.Mgmt., INIS Atomind., Risk Abstr., Saf.Sci.Abstr., Tox.Abstr. (coverage dropped).
—BLDSC (7869.080000), CASDDS, CISTI, GNLM, KNAW.
Published by: Universidade Estadual Paulista, Ave. VICENTE FERREIRA, 1278, Centro, Caixa Postal 71, Marilia, SP 17515-901, Brazil. TEL 55-144-222504, FAX 55-144-222504, cgb@marilia.unesp.br. Ed. Yasmin Robe Carvalho. Circ: 1,000 (controlled).

617.6 BRA ISSN 1516-0939
CODEN: ACECDB
UNIVERSIDADE FEDERAL DE MINAS GERAIS. FACULDADE DE ODONTOLOGIA. ARQUIVOS EM ODONTOLOGIA. Text in Portuguese; Summaries in English. 1964. s-a. BRL 20 newsstand/cover. bibl, charts, illus.
Former titles (until 1997): Arquivos do Centro de Estudos do Curso de Odontologia (0102-5902); (until 1974): Universidade Federal de Minas Gerais. Faculdade de Odontologia. Arquivos do Centro de Estudos (0365-1142)
Indexed: Biol.Abstr., Chem.Abstr., Dent.Ind., Oral Res.Abstr.
—BLDSC (1695.715000), CISTI.
Published by: Universidade Federal de Minas Gerais, Faculdade de Odontologia, Rua Conde de Linhares, 141, C Jardim, Belo Horizonte, MG 30000, Brazil. Ed. Mario Lucio Jardim Parreira.

617.6 BRA ISSN 0083-3908
UNIVERSIDADE FEDERAL DE PERNAMBUCO. FACULDADE DE ODONTOLOGIA. ANAIS. Text in Portuguese; Summaries in English. 1960. a.
Formerly (until vol.5): Universidade do Recife. Faculdade de Odontologia. Anais
Published by: Universidade Federal de Pernambuco, Faculdade de Odontologia, Recife, Pernambuco, Brazil.

617.6 BRA ISSN 0041-8919
UNIVERSIDADE FEDERAL DO RIO DE JANEIRO. FACULDADE DE ODONTOLOGIA. ANAIS✱. Text in Portuguese; Summaries in English. 1947. a. illus, stat.
Indexed: Biol.Abstr.
—CISTI.
Published by: Universidade Federal do Rio de Janeiro, Faculdade de Odontologia, Ilha da Cidade Universitaria, Rio De Janeiro, RJ, Brazil. Circ: (controlled).

378.1 617.6 GBR
UNIVERSITY COLLEGE LONDON. EASTMAN ACADEMY. NEWSLETTER. Text in English. m. **Document type:** *Newsletter, Academic/Scholarly.*
Related titles: Online - full content ed.
Published by: University College London, Eastman Dental Institute, 256 Gray's Inn Road, London WC1X 8LD, United Kingdom. TEL 44-20-79151038, http://www.eastman.ucl.ac.uk/academy/.

UNIVERSITY OF ILLINOIS AT CHICAGO. COLLEGE OF DENTISTRY. ALUMNI REPORT. see *COLLEGE AND ALUMNI*

617.6 USA ISSN 0076-843X
UNIVERSITY OF MICHIGAN. SCHOOL OF DENTISTRY. ALUMNI BULLETIN. Text in English. 1937. a.
Indexed: Dent.Ind.
Published by: University of Michigan, School of Dentistry, Ann Arbor, MI 48104. TEL 313-764-1817. Ed. Charles C Kelsey. Circ: 6,000.

617.6 USA ISSN 1524-2706
VERBATIM; the new word in dentistry. Text in English. 1998. 3/yr. **Document type:** *Magazine, Trade.* **Description:** Provides a forum for dental professionals to disseminate the latest innovative technologies, procedures, and restorative products in the industry.
Related titles: Online - full text ed.
Published by: Montage Media Corp., 1000 Wyckoff Ave, Mahwah, NJ 07430. TEL 201-891-3200, FAX 201-891-2626, info@montagemedia.com, http://www.montagemedia.com/verbatim.html.

617.6 RUS
VESTNIK STAR. Text in Russian. q.
Related titles: Online - full content ed.
Published by: (Stomatologicheskaya Assotsiatsia Rossii/Association of Stomatology of Russia), A-O Stomatologiya, Novyi Arbat 34, # 203, Moscow 121099, Russian Federation. http://www.e-stomatology.ru/periodika/veststar/vstar.html.

617.6 USA ISSN 0049-6472
VIRGINIA DENTAL JOURNAL. Text in English. 1924. q. USD 12 to non-members. adv. bk.rev. illus.
Supersedes: Virginia Dental Association. Bulletin
Indexed: Dent.Ind., INIS Atomind., Ind.Med. (coverage dropped).
—BLDSC (9238.400000), GNLM.
Published by: Virginia Dental Association, c/o Leslie S Webb, Jr, D D S Ed, Box 6906, Richmond, VA 23230. TEL 804-358-4927, FAX 804-353-7342. Adv. contact Tanya Moore. Circ: 2,900.

617.643 ITA ISSN 1128-6547
VIRTUAL JOURNAL OF ORTHODONTICS (ONLINE). Text in Italian, English, Spanish. q. free. adv. bk.rev., software rev., Website rev. abstr, bibl, mkt, stat. 50 p./no. back issues avail. *Refereed.* **Document type:** *Journal, Academic/Scholarly.* **Description:** Publishes research, reviews, and news in the field of clinical orthodontics.
Formerly (until 1996): Virtual Journal of Clinical Orthodontics (Print)
Media: Online - full content. **Related titles:** English ed.; Spanish ed.
Published by: Virtual Journal of Orthodontics, Via Giovanni Boccaccio, 89, Florence, FI 50133, Italy. TEL 39-055-5048054, FAX 39-055-5057015, staff@vjco.it, http://vjco.it/. Ed., R&P Dr. Gabriele Floria. Adv. contact Dr. Yasemin Yaleinkaya.

617.6 USA ISSN 1046-9338
CODEN: WDJOEG
W D A JOURNAL. Text in English. 1973 (vol.49). m. USD 45 domestic to Libraries and dental agencies; USD 85 foreign; USD 75 to non-members (effective 2001). adv. charts, illus. **Document type:** *Journal, Academic/Scholarly.*
Former titles (until 1988): Wisconsin Dental Association. Journal (0887-9699); Wisconsin State Dental Society. Journal (0043-6674)
Indexed: Dent.Abstr., Dent.Ind., Med.Care Rev.
Published by: Wisconsin Dental Association, 111 E Wisconsin Ave, Ste 1300, Milwaukee, WI 53202. TEL 414-276-4520, FAX 414-276-8431. Ed. Dr. Dennis W Engel. R&P, Adv. contact Heather Breed. Circ: 3,100 (controlled).

617.6 USA
W S D A MEMBERSHIP DIRECTORY & RESOURCE GUIDE. Text in English. 1934. a. included with W S D A News subscr.. adv. **Document type:** *Directory, Trade.*
Formerly (until 1993): Washington State Dental Journal. Membership Roster (0083-7431)
Indexed: Dent.Ind.
—GNLM.
Published by: Washington State Dental Association, 2033 Sixth Ave, 333, Seattle, WA 98121-2514. TEL 206-448-1914. Ed. Dr. Richard J Mielke. R&P Jean M Cerar. Adv. contact Tim Conklin. Circ: 3,900.

617.6 USA ISSN 1064-0835
W S D A NEWS. Text in English. 1960. m. (11/yr.). USD 43.28; USD 75.44 foreign; includes W S D A Membership Directory & Resource Guide. adv. illus. **Document type:** *Newsletter.* **Description:** Contains brief articles of interest to members.
—GNLM.
Published by: Washington State Dental Association, 2033 Sixth Ave, 333, Seattle, WA 98121-2514. TEL 206-448-1914. Ed. Dr. Richard J Mielke. R&P Jean Cerar. Adv. contact Tim Conklin. Circ: 3,900.

617.6 JPN ISSN 0386-1449
WAY. Text in Japanese. 1975. q.
Published by: Kawamura Dental Clinic, Matsuzakaya, 2-chome, Kyobashi, Higashi-ku, Osaka-shi, Japan.

617.6 USA ISSN 0043-3225
WEST VIRGINIA DENTAL JOURNAL✱. Text in English. 1966 (vol.40). q. USD 10. adv. bk.rev. illus.
Indexed: Dent.Abstr., Dent.Ind., Med.Care Rev.
—GNLM.
Published by: West Virginia Dental Association, 2003 Quarrier St, Charleston, WV 25311-2212. TEL 304-925-7201. Ed. R D Smith. Circ: 1,100.

WESTERN SOCIETY OF PERIODONTOLOGY. JOURNAL. PERIODONTAL ABSTRACTS. see *MEDICAL SCIENCES—Abstracting, Bibliographies, Statistics*

617.6 USA
WESTVIEWS. Text in English. 1972. bi-m. USD 20. adv. **Document type:** *Newsletter.*
Formerly: Western Los Angeles Dental Society. Newsletter
Published by: Western Dental Society, 14722 Hawthorne Blvd #B, Lawndale, CA 90260. TEL 310-641-5561, FAX 310-641-3258, wlads@pacbell.net. Ed. Arta Farahmand. Adv. contact Katherine Orlin TEL 310-349-2199. Circ: 910.

617.6 USA ISSN 1062-8746
WIRELINE (DALLAS). Variant title: Wire Line (Dallas). Text in English. 1978. q. adv. back issues avail. **Document type:** *Trade.* **Description:** Provides information relating to changes within the organization, as well as dental and orthodontic information.
Formerly (until 1992): American Orthodontic Society. Newsletter
Published by: American Orthodontic Society, 11884 Greenville Ave, 112, Dallas, TX 75243-3537. TEL 972-234-4000, FAX 972-234-4290. Ed. Tom Chapman. Circ: 15,000 (controlled).

617.6 USA
WORD OF MOUTH (SAN FRANCISCO). Text in English. 1975. q. free to program purchasers and brokers. adv. *Refereed.* **Document type:** *Newsletter.* **Description:** Provides news and dental health tips for California dental program purchasers and brokers.
Address: c/o Delta Dental Plan of CA, Box 7736, San Francisco, CA 94120. TEL 415-972-8300. Ed. Jeannine Rucker. Circ: 9,000 (controlled).

617.6 USA ISSN 1534-2530
▼ **WORLD DENTISTRY.** Text in English. 2001. m. USD 48 for Print or CD-ROM Edition (effective 2001). adv. **Document type:** *Academic/Scholarly.* **Description:** Contains feature articles on the latest dental procedures, clinical techniques, patient care and related topics; also includes reviews of journal articles and oral medicine.
Related titles: CD-ROM ed.; Online - full content ed.
Published by: World Dentistry, Inc., 808 Newtown Rd, Berwyn, PA 19312. TEL 610-725-9994, 888-725-9994, FAX 610-993-8636, info@worlddent.com, http://www.worlddent.com/, http://www.worlddent.com/about/contact_us.xml. Pub. H Frank McCranie. Adv. contact Joseph E McCabe.

617.6 USA
▼ **WORLD JOURNAL OF ORTHODONTICS.** Text in English. 2000. q. USD 128, GBP 91, EUR 148 to individuals for 6 nos.; USD 228, GBP 163, EUR 260 to institutions for 6 nos.; USD 80, GBP 57, EUR 92 to students for 6 nos. (effective 2002). **Document type:** *Journal, Academic/Scholarly.* **Description:** Provides evidence-based, clinically relevant information to orthodontic clinicians.
Related titles: Online - full text ed.: 2000.
Published by: Quintessence Publishing Co., Inc., 551 Kimberly Dr, Carol Stream, IL 60188-1881. TEL 630-682-3223, FAX 630-682-3288, quintpub@aol.com, http://www.quintpub.com. Ed. Dr. T M Graber.

THE WORLD MARKET FOR ORAL HYGIENE. see *BEAUTY CULTURE*

617.6 USA ISSN 0049-8262
XI PSI PHI QUARTERLY✱. Text in English. 1906. q. USD 6. bk.rev. illus.
Indexed: Dent.Ind.
Published by: Xi Psi Phi Fraternity, c/o Dr Leighton A Wier, Ed, 104 Magnolia Ave, San Antonio, TX 78212. TEL 512-733-1961. Circ: 3,000.

M

617.643 CHN ISSN 1005-2593
YATI YASUI YAZHOUBINGXUE ZAZHI/CHINESE JOURNAL OF CONSERVATIVE DENTISTRY. Text in Chinese; Summaries in Chinese, English. 1991. bi-m. CNY 36 (effective 1999). adv. bk.rev. stat. back issues avail. *Refereed.* **Document type:** *Academic/Scholarly.*
Description: Covers conservative dentistry and the improvements in clinical and basic research in the field of conservative dentistry.
Published by: Fourth Military Medical University, School of Stomatology, 1 Kang Fu Rd, Xian, Shaanxi 710032, China. TEL 86-29-3376082, FAX 86-29-3224432, kqybk@fmmu.edu.cn. Ed. Junnan Shi. Circ: 7,000.

617.6058 USA ISSN 0084-3717
RK16
THE YEAR BOOK OF DENTISTRY. Text in English. 1936. a. USD 85 domestic; USD 91 foreign (effective 2001). illus. **Document type:** *Academic/Scholarly, Abstract/Index.* **Description:** Presents abstracts of pertinent literature with commentary by leading experts in the field.
Related titles: CD-ROM ed.
Indexed: Curr.Adv.Ecol.Sci.
—CISTI, GNLM.
Published by: Mosby, Inc., Continuity Division (Subsidiary of: Harcourt Health Sciences), 11830 Westline Industrial Dr, St Louis, MO 63146-3313. TEL 314-872-8370, 800-325-4177, FAX 314-432-1380, http://www.mosby.com/periodicals. Ed. Dr. Kenneth Zakariasen.

617.6 JPN ISSN 0914-9554
YOKOHAMA GAKU GANMEN KOKU GEKA GAKKAISHI/YOKOHAMA JOURNAL OF ORAL AND MAXILLOFACIAL SURGERY. Text in Japanese; Summaries in English. 1988. s-a.
Published by: Yokohama Gaku Ganmen Koku Geka Gakkai/Yokohama Society of Oral and Maxillofacial Surgery, Yokohama Shiritsu Daigaku Igakubu Koku Gekagaku Koza, 3-46 Urafune-cho, Minami-ku, Yokohama-shi, Kanagawa-ken 232-0024, Japan.

617.6 DEU ISSN 1432-2390
Z M K. (Zahnheilkunde, Management und Kultur) Text in German. 1985. 10/yr. DEM 120 (effective 1999). **Document type:** *Academic/Scholarly.*
Formerly (until 1990): Z M K Heute (0930-0139)
—GNLM.
Published by: Spitta Verlag GmbH und Co. KG, Ammonitenstr 1, Balingen 72336, Germany. TEL 49-7433-952-0, FAX 49-7433-952185.

617.6 DEU ISSN 0949-6092
Z T; Magazin fuer innovative Zahntechnik. (Zahntechnik) Text in German. 1996. bi-m. DEM 48 (effective 1999). **Document type:** *Academic/Scholarly.*
Published by: Spitta Verlag GmbH und Co. KG, Ammonitenstr 1, Balingen 72336, Germany. TEL 49-7433-952-0, FAX 49-7433-952185.

617.6 DEU ISSN 0044-166X
Z W R; das Deutsche Zahnaerzteblatt. (Zahnaerztliche Welt Rundschau) Text in German. 1891. 10/yr. EUR 184.80 domestic to institutions; EUR 205.40 in Europe to institutions; EUR 212.80 elsewhere to institutions; EUR 78 to students; EUR 18 newsstand/cover (effective 2002). bk.rev. illus. index. **Document type:** *Journal, Trade.* **Description:** Professional journal for dentists, dental technicians and their support staff.
Incorporates (1968-1986): Zahnarzt (0044-1678); (1948-1971): Stoma (0039-1697); Formerly (until 1970): Z W R - Zahnaerztliche Welt, Zahnaerztliche Rundschau (0301-1607)
Indexed: Biol.Abstr., Chem.Abstr., Curr.Tit.Dent., Dent.Ind., Ind.Med. (coverage dropped).
—CISTI, GNLM. **CCC.**
Published by: Georg Thieme Verlag, Ruedigerstr 14, Stuttgart 70469, Germany. TEL 49-711-8931-0, FAX 49-711-8931258, kunden.service@thieme.de, http://www.thieme.de. Circ: 20,000.

617.6 DEU ISSN 0933-1786
ZAHN MAGAZIN. Text in German. 1987. q. **Document type:** *Bulletin.*
Published by: (Kassenzahnaerztliche Vereinigung Berlin), Quintessenz Verlags GmbH, Ifenpfad 2-4, Berlin 12107, Germany. TEL 49-30-74006-0, FAX 49-30-7415080, central@quinline.com, central@quintessenz.de, http://www.quinline.com, http://www.quintessenz.de. Pub. Horst Wolfgang Haase. adv.: B&W page DEM 4,200; trim 175 x 276. Circ: 48,000 (controlled).

617.6 DEU ISSN 0724-0376
ZAHNAERZTE WIRTSCHAFTSDIENST. Text in German. 1982. m. EUR 180 in Germany; EUR 180 foreign (effective 2002). **Document type:** *Journal, Trade.*
Published by: (Institut fuer Wirtschaftspublizistik), Vogel Verlag und Druck GmbH & Co. KG, Max-Planck-Str 7-9, Wuerzburg 97064, Germany. TEL 49-931-45353-0, FAX 49-931-4535399, http://www.vogel-medien.de. **Subscr. to:** DataM-Services GmbH, Fichtestr 9, Wuerzburg 97074, Germany. TEL 49-931-417001, FAX 49-931-4170499, swestenberger@datam-services.de, http://www.datam-services.de.

617.6 DEU ISSN 0340-3017
ZAHNAERZTEBLATT BADEN-WUERTTEMBERG. Text in German. 1972. m. DEM 174, EUR 88.96 (effective 2000). **Document type:** *Magazine, Trade.*
Indexed: Dent.Ind.
—GNLM.
Published by: (Landeszahnaerztekammer Baden-Wuerttemberg), Deutscher Aerzte-Verlag GmbH, Dieselstr 2, Cologne 50859, Germany. TEL 49-2234-7011-0, FAX 49-2234-7011515, http://www.aerzteverlag.de. Eds. J Glueck, Johannes Clausen. Circ: 10,800.

617.6 DEU ISSN 0938-8486
ZAHNAERZTEBLATT SACHSEN. Text in German. 1989. m. DEM 87.50 (effective 2000). adv. **Document type:** *Journal, Academic/Scholarly.*
Published by: (Landeszahnaerztekammer Sachsen), Satztechnik Meissen GmbH, Am Sand 1 c, Nieschuetz 01665, Germany. TEL 49-3525-7186-0, FAX 49-3525-718610, satztechnik.meissen@t-online.de, http://www.satztechnik-meissen.de. Circ: 4,800.

617.6 DEU ISSN 0341-8995
ZAHNAERZTLICHE MITTEILUNGEN. Text in German. 1910. s-m. DEM 300, EUR 153.39; DEM 95 to students (effective 2000). adv. bk.rev. charts, illus, stat, tr.lit. index. **Document type:** *Journal, Trade.*
Indexed: Curr.Tit.Dent., Dent.Ind., INIS Atomind., Ind.Med. (coverage dropped).
—CISTI.
Published by: (Bundesverband der Deutschen Zahnaerzte e.V.), Deutscher Aerzte-Verlag GmbH, Dieselstr 2, Cologne 50859, Germany. TEL 49-2234-7011-0, FAX 49-2234-7011515, zm@aerzteverlag.de, http://www.zm-online.de, http://www.aerzteverlag.de. Circ: 78,900.

617.6 DEU ISSN 0934-9634
DIE ZAHNARZTHELFERIN. Text in German. 1987. m. DEM 70.80 (effective 2000). **Document type:** *Magazine, Trade.*
—GNLM.
Published by: Friedrich Kiehl Verlag GmbH, Pfaustr 13, Ludwigshafen 67063, Germany. TEL 49-621-63502-0, FAX 49-621-6350222. Ed. Lothar Kurz. Circ: 8,500 (paid).

617.6 DEU ISSN 1435-2508
ZAHNRAT; die Patientenzeitung der Zahnaerzte Brandenburgs, Sachsens, Mecklenburg-Vorpommerns, Sachsen-Anhalts und Thueringen. Text in German. 1995. q. **Document type:** *Newspaper, Consumer, Trade.*
Published by: (Landeszahnaerztekammer Brandenburg), Satztechnik Meissen GmbH, Am Sand 1 c, Nieschuetz 01665, Germany. TEL 49-3525-718600, FAX 49-3525-718610, satztechnik.meissen@t-online.de, http://www.satztechnik-meissen.de. Circ: 55,000 (controlled). **Co-sponsors:** Landeszahnaerztekammer Sachsen; Zahnaerztekammer Mecklenburg-Vorpommern; Zahnaerztekammer Sachsen-Anhalt; Landeszahnaerztekammer Thueringen.

617.6 DEU
ZEITSCHRIFT FUER ZAHNAERZTLICHE IMPLANTOLOGIE. Text in German; Summaries in English. 1984. q. DEM 297 domestic; DEM 302 foreign (effective 2001). adv. bk.rev. charts, illus. reprint service avail. from SCH. **Document type:** *Journal, Trade.*
Formerly: Fortschritte der Zahnaertzliche Implantologie (0177-3348)
Indexed: Curr.Tit.Dent.
—GNLM, Infotrieve. **CCC.**
Published by: (Deutsche Gesellschaft fuer Zahn-, Mund- und Kieferheilkunde), Carl Hanser Verlag, Kolbergerstr 22, Munich 81679, Germany. TEL 49-89-99830-0, FAX 49-89-984809, info@hanser.de, http://www.zahnheilkunde.de/imp/set.htm, http://www.hanser.de. Circ: 1,700.

ZHONGGUO YIXUE WENZHAI (KOUQIANG YIXUE)/CHINA MEDICAL ABSTRACTS (STOMATOLOGY). see *MEDICAL SCIENCES—Abstracting, Bibliographies, Statistics*

617.6 SVN ISSN 0044-4928
CODEN: ZOVEAG
ZOBOZDRAVSTVENI VESTNIK. Text in Slovenian; Summaries in English, German. 1946. bi-m. SIT 100, USD 20.85. adv. bk.rev. illus. index.
Indexed: Chem.Abstr., Dent.Ind.
—BLDSC (9514.950000), CASDDS, CISTI, GNLM.
Published by: Drustvo Zobozdrastvenih Delavcev Slovenije, Hrvatski trg 6, Ljubljana, Slovenia. Ed. Rajko Sedej. Circ: 1,500.

MEDICAL SCIENCES—Dermatology And Venereology

616.5 616.95 NOR ISSN 0001-5555
CODEN: ADVEA4
ACTA DERMATO-VENEREOLOGICA. Text and summaries in English. 1920. 6/yr. GBP 103, USD 170 to individuals; GBP 173, USD 285 to institutions (effective 2002). adv. illus. index. *Refereed.* **Document type:** *Academic/Scholarly.* **Description:** Focuses on clinical and experimental research in the field of dermatology and venereology.
Related titles: Online - full text ed.: (from EBSCO Publishing, O C L C Online Computer Library Center, Inc., RoweCom Information Quest, CatchWord Ltd., ingenta, Swets Blackwell, Institute for Scientific Information); ♦ Supplement: Acta Dermato-Venereologica. Supplementum. ISSN 0365-8341.
Indexed: ASCA, Abstr.Hyg., Agri.& Environ.Biotech.Abstr. (coverage dropped), Biol.Abstr., C.I.S. Abstr., Chem.Abstr., Curr.Adv.Cancer Res., Curr.Adv.Ecol.Sci., Curr.Cont., Dairy Sci.Abstr., Dent.Ind., Derwent Biotech.Abstr., Dok.Arbeitsmed., Excerp.Med., Helminthol.Abstr., INIS Atomind., Ind.Med. (1920-), Ind.Sci.Rev., Inpharma, Int.Abstr.Biol.Sci., Int.Nurs.Ind., Jrnl.Watch Derm., Kidney, Med.& Surg.Dermat., Nutr.Abstr., Pharm.&Out.News, Protozool.Abstr., Reac., Rev.Appl.Entomol., Rev.Med.& Vet.Mycol., Rev.Plant Path., Sci.Cit.Ind., THA, Trop.Dis.Bull., Weed Abstr.
—BLDSC (0612.320000), ADONIS, CASDDS, CISTI, EMDOCS, GNLM, IDS, ingenta, KNAW. **CCC.**
Published by: Taylor & Francis AS (Subsidiary of: Taylor & Francis Group), Cort Adelersgt. 17, Solli, PO Box 2562, Oslo 0202, Norway. TEL 47-22-12-98-80, FAX 47-22-12-98-90, journals@tandf.no, http://www.tandf.co.uk/tfas. Ed. Anders Vahlquist. Circ: 1,100.

616.5 NOR ISSN 0365-8341
CODEN: AVSUAR
ACTA DERMATO-VENEREOLOGICA. SUPPLEMENTUM. Text in Norwegian. 1929. irreg. **Document type:** *Monographic series, Academic/Scholarly.*
Related titles: Online - full text ed.: (from Swets Blackwell); ♦ Supplement to: Acta Dermato-Venereologica. ISSN 0001-5555.
Indexed: Curr.Cont. (coverage dropped), Environ.Sci.Poll.Mgmt., Ind.Med. (1929-), Int.Abstr.Biol.Sci., Pollut.Abstr., Rev.Appl.Entomol., Risk Abstr., Saf.Sci.Abstr.
—BLDSC (0612.322000), ADONIS, CASDDS, CISTI, EMDOCS, ingenta, KNAW. **CCC.**
Published by: Scandinavian University Press (Subsidiary of: Taylor & Francis Ltd.), Postboks 2959, Toeyen, Oslo 0608, Norway. FAX 47-22-57-53-53, journals@scup.no, http://www.scup.no/dermato.

616.5 SVN ISSN 1318-4458
CODEN: ADIGAD
ACTA DERMATOVENEROLOGICA ALPINA, PANNONICA ET ADRIATICA. Text in Slovenian. 1974. q. DEM 105 (effective 1999). adv. bk.rev. *Refereed.* **Document type:** *Academic/Scholarly.*
Formerly (until 1992): Acta Dermatovenerologica Iugoslavica (0302-4466)
Indexed: Biol.Abstr., Excerp.Med. (1994-).
—BLDSC (0612.328000), CASDDS, CISTI, EMDOCS, GNLM, KNAW.
Published by: Slovene Medical Society, Dermatological Section, Dermatoloska Klinika, Zaloska 2, Ljubljana 1525, Slovenia. TEL 386-61-312559. Ed., R&P Aleksej Kansky. Adv. contact Aloisia Miklic. B&W page DEM 500, color page DEM 1,000. Circ: 440. **Subscr. to:** DZS d.d. Import - Export, Slovenska 55, Ljubljana 1000, Slovenia. TEL 386-61-1332316, FAX 386-61-310737.

616.5 HRV ISSN 1330-027X
ACTA DERMATOVENEROLOGICA CROATICA. Text in Croatian. 1993. q. DEM 100. adv. bk.rev. *Refereed.* **Document type:** *Academic/Scholarly, Abstract/Index.*

M

Indexed: Excerp.Med. (1994-).
—BLDSC (0612.323000), EMDOCS.
Published by: Sveuciliste u Zagrebu, Dermatologski Odjel/Croatian Dermatological Society, Dept of Dermatology & Venerology, Zagreb University Hospital Center, Salata 4, Zagreb 10000, Croatia. Ed. Dr. Vladimir Cajkovac. Adv. contact Branka Marinovic. **Co-sponsor:** Hravatska Akademija Medicinskih Znanosti/Croatian Academy of Medical Sciences.

616.5 ESP ISSN 0001-7310
ACTAS DERMO-SIFILIOGRAFICAS. Text in Spanish. 1989. m. (10/yr.). ESP 17,300 to individuals; ESP 24,000 to institutions; ESP 13,890 to students (effective 2001). adv. bk.rev. illus. index. back issues avail.; reprints avail. *Refereed.* **Document type:** *Journal, Academic/Scholarly.*
Related titles: Online - full text ed.: 1996.
Indexed: Chem.Abstr., Dent.Ind., Excerp.Med., Ind.Med. (coverage dropped), Ind.Med.Esp., Med.& Surg.Dermat., Ref.Zh., Rev.Med.& Vet.Mycol., Rev.Plant Path.
—BLDSC (0612.330000), CINDOC, CISTI, EMDOCS, GNLM, Infotrieve, KNAW. **CCC.**
Published by: (Asociacion Espanola de Dermatologia, Sifiliografia y Venerologia), Ediciones Doyma S.A., Traversa de Gracia, 17-21, Barcelona 08021, Spain. TEL 34-93-200-0711, doyma@doyma.es, http://www.doyma.es/. Ed. Luis Requena Caballero. Pub. Evaristo Sanchez Yus. R&P Monica Barnes. Adv. contact Jose Antonio Hernandez. B&W page ESP 122,000, color page ESP 152,000; 280 x 210. Circ: 1,500.

616.5 ESP ISSN 0210-279X
ACTUALIDAD DERMATOLOGICA. Text in Spanish. 1962. m. (11/yr.).
Address: Corsega, 83, 6o 2a, Barcelona 08029, Spain. TEL 34-93-439-2541.

616.5 USA ISSN 0882-0880
CODEN: ADDEEK
ADVANCES IN DERMATOLOGY. Text in English. 1986. a. USD 95 domestic; USD 101 foreign (effective 2001). illus. **Document type:** *Academic/Scholarly.*
Description: Presents a collection of fully referenced articles from experts in dermatology.
Indexed: INIS Atomind., Ind.Med. (1986-).
—BLDSC (0704.242300), CISTI, GNLM, ingenta, KNAW.
Published by: Mosby, Inc. (Subsidiary of: Elsevier Science), 11830 Westline Industrial Dr, St Louis, MO 63146-3313. TEL 314-872-8370, 800-325-4177, FAX 314-432-1380, http://www.mosby.com/periodicals. Ed. Dr. William D James.

616.5 USA ISSN 1527-7941
ADVANCES IN SKIN AND WOUND CARE; the journal for wound prevention and healing. Text in English. 1988. bi-m. USD 49 domestic to individuals; USD 54 in Canada to individuals; USD 79 elsewhere to individuals; USD 139 domestic to institutions; USD 144 in Canada to institutions; USD 183.50 elsewhere to institutions (effective 2001); USD 9 newsstand/cover (effective 2002). adv. tr.lit. reprints avail. *Refereed.* **Document type:** *Academic/Scholarly.* **Description:** Publishes original research, clinical reviews and short reports on all aspects of wound management.
Former titles (until 2000): Advances in Wound Care (1076-2191); (until 1994): Decubitus: The Journal of Skin Ulcers (0898-1655)
Related titles: Online - full text ed.: (from Gale Group).
Indexed: CINAHL, Int.Nurs.Ind., Med.& Surg.Dermat.
—BLDSC (0711.389000), GNLM, Infotrieve. **CCC.**
Published by: Springhouse Corporation (Subsidiary of: Lippincott Williams & Wilkins (Philadelphia)), 1111 Bethlehem Tpk, Springhouse, PA 19477. TEL 215-646-8700, 800-950-0879, FAX 215-643-4153, http://www.woundcarenet.com/advances.htm. Ed. Susan Doan Johnson. Circ: 20,000. **Subscr. to:** Advances in Wound Care, 434 W Downer Pl, Aurora, IL 60506. TEL 800-950-0879, FAX 708-892-7466.

646.72 DEU ISSN 1436-2635
CODEN: TWDEEM
AERZTLICHE PRAXIS. DERMATOLOGIE. Short title: Ae P Dermatologie. Text in German. 1971. m. DEM 89 domestic; DEM 112 foreign; DEM 44.50 domestic to students; DEM 56 foreign to students (effective 2001). adv. **Document type:** *Journal, Trade.*
Former titles (until 1998): T und E Dermatologie (1435-7747); T W Dermatologie (0939-0448); Aerztliche Kosmetologie (0340-5702); Kosmetologie
Indexed: Chem.Abstr., Excerp.Med. (until 1988, 1994-), Ref.Zh.
—BLDSC (1567.767000), CASDDS, CISTI, EMDOCS, GNLM, Infotrieve, KNAW. **CCC.**
Published by: Reed Elsevier Deutschland GmbH (Subsidiary of: Reed Elsevier group), Gabrielenstr 9, Munich 80636, Germany. TEL 49-89-89817-0, FAX 49-89-89817400, http://aep.r-e.de. Ed. Hans Juergen Kuntze. Pub. Wolfram Haase. Adv. contact Marina Vasilj. Circ: 5,000.

AIDS INFORMATION EXCHANGE. (Acquired Immune Deficiency Syndrome) see *MEDICAL SCIENCES—Communicable Diseases*

616.5 DEU ISSN 0340-2541
AKTUELLE DERMATOLOGIE; Angiologie - Allergologie - Umweltmedizin - Photodermatologie - Mykologie - Infektiologie. Text in German. 1975. m. EUR 194.40 domestic to institutions; EUR 206.80 in Europe to institutions; EUR 219.80 elsewhere to institutions; EUR 19 newsstand/cover (effective 2002). adv. index. back issues avail.; reprint service avail. from PQC. *Refereed.* **Document type:** *Journal, Academic/Scholarly.*
Related titles: Online - full text ed.: ISSN 1438-938X.
Indexed: Biol.Abstr., Excerp.Med.
—BLDSC (0785.729700), CISTI, EMDOCS, GNLM, Infotrieve, KNAW. **CCC.**
Published by: (Deutsche Gesellschaft fuer Lichtforschung), Georg Thieme Verlag, Ruedigerstr 14, Stuttgart 70469, Germany. TEL 49-711-8931-0, FAX 49-711-8931298, kunden.service@thieme.de, http://www.thieme.de/derma/index.html. R&P Peter Eich. adv.: page DEM 3,300; 175 x 250. Circ: 4,600.

616.5 USA ISSN 0278-9000
RL43
AMERICAN ACADEMY OF DERMATOLOGY. DIRECTORY. Text in English. irreg. **Document type:** *Directory.*
Formerly: American Academy of Dermatology. Roster: Bylaws, Officers, Committees (0162-0037)
Published by: American Academy of Dermatology, 930 N Meacham Rd, Schaumburg, IL 60173-4965. TEL 847-330-0230, FAX 847-330-0050.

616.5 USA ISSN 0190-9622
RL1 CODEN: JAADDB
AMERICAN ACADEMY OF DERMATOLOGY. JOURNAL. Text in English. 1979. m. USD 191 domestic to individuals; USD 231 foreign to individuals; USD 366 domestic to institutions; USD 411 foreign to institutions; USD 96 domestic to students; USD 136 foreign to students; USD 35 newsstand/cover (effective 2001). adv. bk.rev. s-a. index. Supplement avail.; back issues avail.; reprint service avail. from PQC. *Refereed.* **Document type:** *Journal, Academic/Scholarly.*
Description: Provides a clinical perspective on manifestations of skin disease.
Related titles: Microfilm ed.: (from PQC); Online - full text ed.: (from Ovid Technologies, Inc., EBSCO Publishing, IDEAL Online Library, Institute for Scientific Information, RoweCom Information Quest).
Indexed: AIDS Abstr., ASCA, Abstr.Hyg., Biol.Abstr., Curr.Adv.Cancer Res., Curr.Cont., Dok.Arbeitsmed., Excerp.Med., Helminthol.Abstr., Hort.Abstr., INIS Atomind., I.P.A., Ind.Med. (1979-), Ind.Sci.Rev., Inpharma, Int.Abstr.Biol.Sci., Int.Nurs.Ind., Jrnl.Watch Derm., Kidney, Lab.Haz.Bull., Med.& Surg.Dermat., NRN, Nutr.Abstr., Pharm.&Out.News, Protozool.Abstr., Reac., Rev.Appl.Entomol., Rev.Med.& Vet.Mycol., SSCI (coverage dropped), Sci.Cit.Ind., Small Anim.Abstr., THA, Trop.Dis.Bull.
—BLDSC (4683.703000), CISTI, GNLM, IDS, ingenta, KNAW. **CCC.**
Published by: (American Academy of Dermatology), Mosby, Inc. (Subsidiary of: Elsevier Science), 11830 Westline Industrial Dr, St Louis, MO 63146-3318. TEL 314-872-8370, 800-325-4177, FAX 314-432-1380, http://www.eblue.org, http://www.mosby.com/periodicals. Ed. Dr. Jeffrey D Bernhard. Adv. contact Tracey Schriefer TEL 314-453-4304. B&W page USD 1,930, color page USD 3,280; trim 10.88 x 8.13. Circ: 18,541.

616.5 USA ISSN 1175-0561
▼ **AMERICAN JOURNAL OF CLINICAL DERMATOLOGY.** Text in English. 2000. bi-m. USD 150 to individuals Print or Online ed.; USD 180 to individuals Print and Online combined eds.; USD 385 to institutions Print or Online ed.; USD 462 to institutions Print and Online combined eds. (effective 2001). abstr. back issues avail. *Refereed.* **Document type:** *Journal, Academic/Scholarly.* **Description:** Forum for discussing, evaluating and disseminating the latest information about dermatology and appearance medicine. Provides indepdendent review articles covering important issues in the management of dermatological conditions.
Related titles: Online - full text ed.: (from Ovid Technologies, Inc., ingenta, Swets Blackwell, RoweCom Information Quest).
—BLDSC (0822.790000), ADONIS.
Published by: Adis International Limited, Mairangi Bay, Private Bag 65901, Auckland 1010, New Zealand. http://www.adis.com. Ed. Rosie Stather.

616.5 USA ISSN 1046-199X
CODEN: AJCDFL
AMERICAN JOURNAL OF CONTACT DERMATITIS. Text in English. 1990. q. USD 173 domestic to individuals; USD 223 foreign to individuals; USD 244 domestic to institutions; USD 288 foreign to institutions; USD 107 domestic to students; USD 151 foreign to students; USD 73 newsstand/cover (effective 2001). adv. bk.rev. abstr. back issues avail. *Refereed.* **Document type:** *Academic/Scholarly.* **Description:** Provides clinically focused articles on diagnosing and treating dermatologic conditions caused by irritants and allergic reactions.
Related titles: Online - full text ed.: (from IDEAL Online Library).
Indexed: Excerp.Med. (1995-), Ind.Med. (1990-), Med.& Surg.Dermat.
—BLDSC (0824.150000), EMDOCS, GNLM, Infotrieve, ingenta, KNAW. **CCC.**
Published by: (American Contact Dermatitis Society), W.B. Saunders Co. (Subsidiary of: Harcourt Publishers Ltd.), 11830 Westline Industrial Dr, St Louis, MO 63146. TEL 800-325-4177, http://www.wbsaunders.com. Ed. Dr. Ponciano D Cruz Jr. adv.: B&W page USD 850, color page USD 1,950; trim 10 x 7. Circ: 828. **Subscr. to:** Periodicals Fulfillment, W B Saunders Co, 6277 Sea Harbor Dr, 4th Fl, Orlando, FL 32891-4800.

AMERICAN JOURNAL OF DERMATOPATHOLOGY. see *MEDICAL SCIENCES*

616.5 BRA ISSN 0365-0596
CODEN: ABDEB3
ANAIS BRASILEIROS DE DERMATOLOGIA. Text in Portuguese; Summaries in English, Portuguese. 1925. bi-m. USD 90 (effective 2000). adv. bk.rev. abstr, bibl, charts, illus, stat. index, cum.index. back issues avail. *Refereed.* **Document type:** *Academic/Scholarly.*
Description: Contains original research papers, review articles and case reports in dermatology.
Related titles: Microform ed.: (from PQC).
Indexed: Abstr.Hyg., Biol.Abstr., Chem.Abstr., Curr.Cont. (coverage dropped), Dairy Sci.Abstr., Excerp.Med., Helminthol.Abstr., INIS Atomind., Ind.Med. (coverage dropped), Nutr.Abstr., Protozool.Abstr., Rev.Appl.Entomol., Rev.Med.& Vet.Mycol., Tox.Abstr., Trop.Dis.Bull., Virol.Abstr., Weed Abstr.
—CISTI, EMDOCS, GNLM, KNAW.
Published by: Sociedade Brasileira de Dermatologia, Av Rio Branco, 39/Andar 18, Centro, Rio De Janeiro, RJ 20090-003, Brazil. TEL 55-21-2631377, FAX 55-21-2536747, anais@sbd.org.br, http://www.sbd.org.br. Ed. Leninha Nascimento. R&P Carla Noroes. Adv. contact Paulo Borges. Circ: 4,200.

616.5 616.951 FRA ISSN 0151-9638
CODEN: ADVED7
ANNALES DE DERMATOLOGIE ET DE VENEREOLOGIE. Text in French; Summaries in English. 1869. 11/yr. FRF 1,458; FRF 1,751 foreign (effective 2000). adv. bk.rev. illus, abstr. index. reprint service avail. from ISI. *Refereed.* **Document type:** *Academic/Scholarly.*
Description: Publishes original work from numerous schools of dermatology. Provides both clinical and therapeutic points of view.
Former titles: Annales de Dermatologie et de Syphiligraphie; Societe Francaise de Dermatologie et de Syphiligraphie. Bulletin (0003-3979)
Related titles: Microform ed.: (from PQC); Online - full text ed.: (from Institute for Scientific Information, RoweCom Information Quest).
Indexed: ASCA, Abstr.Hyg., Biol.Abstr., C.I.S. Abstr., CSNB, Chem.Abstr., Curr.Adv.Ecol.Sci., Curr.Cont., Dent.Ind., Excerp.Med., Helminthol.Abstr., Ind.Med. (1977-), Ind.Sci.Rev., Ind.Vet., Inpharma, Int.Nurs.Ind., Lab.Haz.Bull., Med.& Surg.Dermat., Nutr.Abstr., Pharm.&Out.News, Protozool.Abstr., Reac., Rev.Appl.Entomol., Rev.Med.& Vet.Mycol., Rev.Plant Path., Sci.Cit.Ind. (coverage dropped).
—BLDSC (0971.600000), CISTI, EMDOCS, GNLM, IDS, Infotrieve, KNAW. **CCC.**
Published by: (Societe Francaise de Dermatologie et de l'Association des Dermatologistes Francophones), Masson - Periodiques, 120 bd. St. Germain, Paris 75006, France. TEL 33-1-40466200, FAX 33-1-40466201. Ed. E Grosshans. Circ: 3,900. **Subscr. to:** Societe de Periodiques Specialises, BP 22, Vineuil Cedex 41354, France. TEL 33-2-54504612, FAX 33-2-54504611.

616.5 ITA ISSN 1592-6826
ANNALI ITALIANI DI DERMATOLOGIA ALLERGOLOGICA CLINICA E SPERIMENTALE. Text in English, Italian. 1945. q. USD 89 (effective 2000). adv. bk.rev. 64 p./no. **Document type:** *Journal, Academic/Scholarly.*
Former titles: Annali Italiani di Dermatologia Clinica e Sperimentale (0365-169X); (until 1961): Annali Italiani di Dermatologia e Sifilologia (0003-4703)
Indexed: Biol.Abstr., Chem.Abstr., Excerp.Med., Ind.Med. (coverage dropped), Ref.Zh.
—BLDSC (1014.325000), GNLM.
Published by: Il Pensiero Scientifico Editore s.r.l., Via Bradano, 3-C, Rome, RM 00199, Italy. TEL 39-06-862821, FAX 39-06-86282250, pensiero@pensiero.it, http://www.pensiero.it. Ed. Stefano Simonetti. Pub. Luca De Fiore. R&P Andrea De Fiore. Adv. contact Luciano De Fiore. Circ: 400 (controlled).

616.5 DEU ISSN 0340-3696
CODEN: ADREDL
ARCHIVES OF DERMATOLOGICAL RESEARCH. Text in English. 1869. m. EUR 2,211.10 domestic; EUR 1,110.70 in Germany; EUR 109 foreign (effective 2002). adv. bibl, charts, illus. index. back issues avail.; reprint service avail. from ISI. *Refereed.* **Document type:** *Journal, Academic/Scholarly.* **Description:** Publishes original contributions in the field of experimental dermatology, including biochemistry, morphology and immunology of the skin.
Former titles: Archiv fuer Dermatologische Forschung (0003-9187); Archiv fuer Klinische und Experimentelle Dermatologie
Related titles: Microfilm ed.: (from PQC); Online - full text ed.: ISSN 1432-069X (from EBSCO Publishing, RoweCom Information Quest, Swets Blackwell, Springer LINK, Institute for Scientific Information); ♦ Supplement: Archives of Dermatological Research. Supplement. ISSN 0944-1948.
Indexed: ASCA, Agri.& Environ.Biotech.Abstr. (coverage dropped), Biol.Abstr., Chem.Abstr., Chem.Indus.Notes, Chem.Titles, Curr.Adv.Ecol.Sci., Curr.Cont., Dairy Sci.Abstr., Derwent Biotech.Abstr., Excerp.Med., Helminthol.Abstr., INIS Atomind., Ind.Med. (1978-), Ind.Sci.Rev., Inpharma, Med.& Surg.Dermat., NRN, Nutr.Abstr., Ornam.Hort., Pharm.&Out.News, Protozool.Abstr., Reac., Rev.Appl.Entomol., Rev.Med.& Vet.Mycol., Rev.Plant Path., Risk Abstr., Sci.Cit.Ind.
—BLDSC (1634.130000), ADONIS, CASDDS, CISTI, EMDOCS, GNLM, IDS, ingenta, KNAW. **CCC.**
Published by: Springer-Verlag (Subsidiary of: BertelsmannSpringer), Tiergartenstr 17, Heidelberg 69121, Germany. TEL 49-6221-345-0, FAX 49-6221-345229, subscriptions@springer.de, http://link.springer.de/link/service/journals/00403/index.htm, http://www.springer.de. Ed. E Christophers. **Subscr. in N. America to:** Springer-Verlag New York Inc., PO Box 2485, Secaucus, NJ 07096-2485. TEL 212-460-1500, FAX 212-473-6272.

616.5 DEU ISSN 0944-1948
ARCHIVES OF DERMATOLOGICAL RESEARCH. SUPPLEMENT. Text in English. irreg. **Document type:** *Monographic series, Academic/Scholarly.*
Related titles: ♦ Supplement to: Archives of Dermatological Research. ISSN 0340-3696.
—ADONIS.
Published by: Springer-Verlag (Subsidiary of: BertelsmannSpringer), Tiergartenstr 17, Heidelberg 69121, Germany. TEL 49-6221-345-0, FAX 49-6221-345229, subscriptions@springer.de, http://www.springer.de.

616.5 USA ISSN 0003-987X
RL1 CODEN: ARDEAC
ARCHIVES OF DERMATOLOGY. Text in English. 1882. m. USD 350 in North America to institutions; USD 450 to institutions Central & S. America; GBP 295 elsewhere to institutions (effective 2001). adv. bk.rev. abstr, charts, illus. index. back issues avail.; reprints avail. *Refereed.* **Document type:** *Academic/Scholarly.* **Description:** Enhances the understanding of skin and its diseases by publishing original articles.
Related titles: CD-ROM ed.: (from Ovid Technologies, Inc.); Microform ed.: (from PQC); Online - full text ed.: (from The Dialog Corporation, Gale Group, Ovid Technologies, Inc., EBSCO Publishing, Institute for Scientific Information); ♦ Spanish Translation: Archives of Dermatology (Edicion Espanola). ISSN 1130-1910.
Indexed: AIM, ASCA, Abstr.Hyg., Abstr.Inter.Med., Agri.& Environ.Biotech.Abstr. (coverage dropped), Biol.Abstr., C.I.S. Abstr., Chem.Abstr., Chem.Indus.Notes, Chem.Titles, Curr.Adv.Cancer Res., Curr.Adv.Ecol.Sci., Curr.Adv.Gen.& Molec.Biol., Curr.Cont., Dairy Sci.Abstr., Dent.Ind., Derwent Biotech.Abstr., Dok.Arbeitsmed., Environ.Sci.Poll.Mgmt., Excerp.Med., Helminthol.Abstr., INIS Atomind., I.P.A., Ind.Med. (1960-), Ind.Sci.Rev., Inpharma, Int.Abstr.Biol.Sci., Jrnl.Watch Derm., Med.& Surg.Dermat., NRN, Nutr.Abstr., Pharm.&Out.News, Pollut.Abstr., Protozool.Abstr., Reac., Rev.Appl.Entomol., Rev.Med.& Vet.Mycol., Risk Abstr., SSCI (coverage dropped), Saf.Sci.Abstr., Sci.Cit.Ind., THA, Trop.Dis.Bull., Weed Abstr.
—BLDSC (1634.150000), CASDDS, CISTI, GNLM, IDS, ingenta, KNAW. **CCC.**
Published by: American Medical Association, 515 N State St, P O Box 10946, Chicago, IL 60610-0946. http://www.ama-assn.org/public/journals/derm/dermhome.htm, http://www.archdermatol.com. Ed. Dr. Kenneth A Arndt. R&P Ada Jimenez Walker. Adv. contact Philip B Altamore. Circ: 14,500.

616.5 ESP ISSN 1130-1910
ARCHIVES OF DERMATOLOGY (EDICION ESPANOLA). Text in Spanish. bi-m. USD 101. adv. **Document type:** *Academic/Scholarly.* **Description:** Contains translations of articles on investigative dermatology from the US edition.
Related titles: ♦ Translation of: Archives of Dermatology. ISSN 0003-987X.
Indexed: Sci.Cit.Ind. (coverage dropped).
Published by: (American Medical Association USA), Ediciones Doyma S.A., Traversa de Gracia, 17-21, Barcelona 08021, Spain. TEL 34-93-200-0711, FAX 34-93-209-1136. Ed. J M Mascaro Ballester. Adv. contact Olga Gomez. B&W page ESP 227,000; trim 280 x 210. Circ: 2,000.

616.5 ARG ISSN 0066-6750
ARCHIVOS ARGENTINOS DE DERMATOLOGIA. Text in Spanish; Abstracts in English. 1951. bi-m., latest vol.51. USD 140 (effective 2000). adv. bk.rev. 48 p./no. back issues avail. *Refereed.* **Document type:** *Journal, Academic/Scholarly.*
Indexed: Excerp.Med., Ind.Med. (coverage dropped).
—CISTI, GNLM.
Address: Parana, 731 2o A, Capital Federal, Buenos Aires 1017, Argentina. TEL 54-114-3732458, FAX 54-114-3732458. Ed. Dr. Adrian M Pierini. Adv. contact Dagoberto E Pierini. Circ: 1,600 (controlled).

616.5 AUS ISSN 0004-8380
CODEN: AJDEBP
AUSTRALASIAN JOURNAL OF DERMATOLOGY. Text in English. 1951. q. AUD 165 domestic to individuals; AUD 150 in New Zealand to individuals; USD 125 elsewhere to individuals; AUD 314 domestic to institutions; AUD 285 in New Zealand to institutions; USD 275 elsewhere to institutions; AUD 182 domestic to individuals paper & online eds. combined; AUD 165 in New Zealand to individuals paper & onlined eds. combined; USD 138 elsewhere to individuals paper & online eds. combined; AUD 346 domestic to institutions paper & online eds. combined; AUD 314 in New Zealand to institutions paper & online eds. combined; USD 303 elsewhere to institutions paper & online eds. combined (effective 2001). adv. bk.rev. back issues avail. *Refereed.* **Document type:** *Academic/Scholarly.* **Description:** Presents research and review articles on recent advances in therapeutics and pharmacology dealing with normal and pathological skin conditions.
Formerly (until 1960): Australian Journal of Dermatology
Related titles: Online - full text ed.: ISSN 1440-0960. AUD 149 domestic to individuals; AUD 135 in New Zealand to individuals; USD 113 elsewhere to individuals; AUD 283 domestic to institutions; AUD 257 in New Zealand to institutions; USD 248 elsewhere to institutions (effective 2001) (from EBSCO Publishing, O C L C Online Computer Library Center, Inc., RoweCom Information Quest, ingenta, Munksgaard & Blackwell Science's Synergy, Swets Blackwell).
Indexed: Abstr.Hyg., Biol.Abstr., Chem.Abstr., Curr.Cont. (coverage dropped), Dent.Ind., Environ.Sci.Poll.Mgmt., Excerp.Med., INIS Atomind., Ind.Med. (1967-), Inpharma, Med.& Surg.Dermat., NRN, Nutr.Abstr., Pharm.&Out.News, Pollut.Abstr., Reac., Rev.Appl.Entomol., Rev.Med.& Vet.Mycol., Rev.Plant Path., Risk Abstr., Saf.Sci.Abstr., Trop.Dis.Bull., Weed Abstr.
—BLDSC (1794.900000), ADONIS, CASDDS, CISTI, GNLM, ingenta, KNAW. **CCC.**
Published by: (Australasian College of Dermatologists), Blackwell Science Asia Pty Ltd, PO Box 378, Carlton South, VIC 3053, Australia. TEL 61-3-9347-0300, FAX 61-3-9347-5001, info@blacksci-asia.com.au, http://www.blacksci.co.uk. Ed. D Dyall-Smith. Adv. contact Kathryn O'Brien. B&W page AUD 920, color page AUD 1,870; trim 210 x 275. Circ: 800. **Co-sponsor:** New Zealand Dermatological Society, NZ.

616.5 GBR
B A D NEWS. Variant title: British Association of Dermatologists. Newsletter. Text in English. 1997. q. **Document type:** *Newsletter.*
Published by: (British Association of Dermatologists), Hayward Medical Communications Ltd., Covent Garden, Seven Dials Warehouse, 44 Earlham St, London WC2H 9LA, United Kingdom. TEL 44-20-7240-4493, FAX 44-20-7240-4479, admin@hayward.co.uk, http://www.hayward.co.uk. Ed. D Black. Circ: 900. **Subscr. to:** Rosemary House, Lanwades Park, Kentford, Near, Newmarket, Suffolk CB8 7PW, United Kingdom. TEL 44-1638-751515, FAX 44-1638-751517.

616.5 BGD
BANGLADESH JOURNAL OF DERMATOLOGY, VENEREOLOGY AND LEPROLOGY. Text in Bengali. s-a. **Document type:** *Academic/Scholarly.*
Indexed: Excerp.Med. (1995-).
Published by: Bangladesh Dermatological Society, Dept. of Dermatology and Venereology, University of Dhaka, Dhaka 1000, Bangladesh. TEL 2-500658.

616.5 GBR ISSN 0007-0963
CODEN: BJDEAZ
BRITISH JOURNAL OF DERMATOLOGY. Text in English. 1886. m., latest vol.146, 2002. GBP 127 in Europe to individuals; USD 201 in North America to individuals; GBP 139 elsewhere to individuals; GBP 560 in Europe to institutions; USD 888 in North America to institutions; GBP 616 elsewhere to institutions (effective 2002). adv. bk.rev. abstr, bibl, illus. index. back issues avail.; reprint service avail. from ISI. *Refereed.* **Document type:** *Academic/Scholarly.* **Description:** Publishes papers on all aspects of the biology and pathology of the skin.
Related titles: Microform ed.: (from PQC); Online - full text ed.: ISSN 1365-2133. 1997. GBP 115 in Europe to individuals; USD 181 in North America to individuals; GBP 115 elsewhere to individuals; GBP 504 in Europe to institutions; USD 800 in North America to institutions; GBP 504 elsewhere to institutions (effective 2002) (from Ovid Technologies, Inc., EBSCO Publishing, O C L C Online Computer Library Center, Inc., RoweCom Information Quest, ingenta, Munksgaard & Blackwell Science's Synergy, Swets Blackwell, Institute for Scientific Information); ♦ Supplement: British Journal of Dermatology. Supplement. ISSN 0366-077X.
Indexed: AIDS Abstr., ASCA, Abstr.Hyg., Abstr.Inter.Med., Agri.& Environ.Biotech.Abstr. (coverage dropped), Biol.Abstr., C.I.S. Abstr., Chem.Abstr., Chem.Indus.Notes, Chem.Titles, Curr.Adv.Cancer Res., Curr.Adv.Gen.& Molec.Biol., Curr.Cont., Dairy Sci.Abstr., Dent.Ind., Derwent Biotech.Abstr., Environ.Sci.Poll.Mgmt., Excerp.Med., Forest Prod.Abstr., Helminthol.Abstr., INIS Atomind., I.P.A., Ind.Med. (1951-), Ind.Sci.Rev., Ind.Vet., Inpharma, Int.Abstr.Biol.Sci., Jrnl.Watch Derm., Lab.Haz.Bull., Med.& Surg.Dermat., NRN, Nutr.Abstr., Pharm.&Out.News, Pig News & Info., Pollut.Abstr., Protozool.Abstr., Reac., Rev.Appl.Entomol., Rev.Arom.& Med.Plants, Rev.Med.& Vet.Mycol., Rev.Plant Path., Risk Abstr., Saf.Sci.Abstr., Sci.Cit.Ind., Triticale Abstr., Trop.Dis.Bull.
—BLDSC (2307.400000), ADONIS, CASDDS, CISTI, EMDOCS, GNLM, IDS, ingenta, KNAW. **CCC.**
Published by: (British Association of Dermatologists), Blackwell Science Ltd., PO Box 88, Oxford OX2 0NE, United Kingdom. TEL 44-1865-206180, 44-1865-206002, FAX 44-1865-206219, jnl.orders@blacksci.co.uk, http://www.blackwell-science.com/products/journals/bjd.htm, http://www.blackwellpublishing.com. Eds. N H Cox, S M Breathnach. Pub. Allen Stevens. R&P Sophie Savage. Adv. contact Jenny Applin. Circ: 2,895.

615.5 GBR
BRITISH JOURNAL OF DERMATOLOGY NURSING. Abbreviated title: B J D N. Text in English. 1997. q. bk.rev. **Document type:** *Academic/Scholarly.*
—BLDSC (2307.430000).
Published by: Hayward Medical Communications Ltd., Covent Garden, Seven Dials Warehouse, 44 Earlham St, London WC2H 9LA, United Kingdom. TEL 44-20-7240-4493, FAX 44-20-7240-4479, admin@hayward.co.uk, http://www.hayward.co.uk, http://www.ejpc.co.uk. Ed. Julie Van Onselen. Circ: 600. **Subscr. to:** Rosemary House, Lanwades Park, Kentford, Near, Newmarket, Suffolk CB8 7PW, United Kingdom. TEL 4-1638-751515, FAX 44-1638-751517.

M

616.5 GBR ISSN 0366-077X
CODEN: BJDSA9

BRITISH JOURNAL OF DERMATOLOGY. SUPPLEMENT. Text in English. 1969. irreg. adv. **Document type:** *Academic/Scholarly.*

Related titles: Microform ed.: (from PQC); Online - full text ed.: (from Ovid Technologies, Inc., Swets Blackwell); ♦ Supplement to: British Journal of Dermatology. ISSN 0007-0963.

Indexed: ASCA, Biol.Abstr., Chem.Abstr., Curr.Cont. (coverage dropped), Excerp.Med., Helminthol.Abstr., I.P.A., Ind.Med. (coverage dropped), Int.Abstr.Biol.Sci., Nutr.Abstr., Rev.Plant Path., Sci.Cit.Ind. (coverage dropped).

—BLDSC (2307.405000), ADONIS, CASDDS, CISTI, EMDOCS, Infotrieve, KNAW. **CCC.**

Published by: (British Association of Dermatologists), Blackwell Science Ltd., Osney Mead, Oxford OX2 0EL, United Kingdom. TEL 44-1865-206206, FAX 44-1865-721205, journals.cs@blacksci.co.uk, http://www.blackwell-science.com. Pub. Allen Stevens. R&P Sophie Savage. Adv. contact Jenny Applin.

▼ **BURNS SOURCEBOOK.** see *MEDICAL SCIENCES—Orthopedics And Traumatology*

616.5 GBR ISSN 1367-0123

C M E BULLETIN DERMATOLOGY. (Continuing Medical Education) Text in English. 1997. 3/yr. (1 volume per annum). GBP 45 domestic to individuals; GBP 60 foreign to individuals; GBP 60 domestic to institutions; GBP 90 foreign to institutions (effective 2001). adv. Website rev. abstr. 24 p./no. 2 cols./p. reprints avail. **Document type:** *Journal, Academic/Scholarly.*

—BLDSC (3287.223020).

Published by: Rila Publications Ltd., 73 Newman St, London W1A 4PG, United Kingdom. TEL 44-20-7631-1299, FAX 44-20-7580-7166, admin@rila.co.uk, http://www.rila.co.uk. Ed. Saleem Goolamali. Pub., Adv. contact G Da'Cambra. Circ: 600 (paid).

616.521 CAN ISSN 0833-1464

CELIAC NEWS. Text in English. 1986. q. CND 25, USD 30 (effective 2000). adv. bk.rev. back issues avail. **Document type:** *Newsletter.* **Description:** Provides information on celiac disease and dermatitis herpetiformis for the purposes of education and updating.

Published by: Canadian Celiac Association, 190 Britannia Rd E, Unit 11, Mississauga, ON L4Z 1W6, Canada. TEL 905-507-6208, FAX 905-507-4673. Ed., R&P Judi Farrell. Adv. contact Donna Mason. Circ: 3,500.

616.5 CZE ISSN 0009-0514
CODEN: CEDEAB

CESKO-SLOVENSKA DERMATOLOGIE. Text in Czech, Slovak; Summaries in Czech, English. 1925. 6/yr. EUR 126, USD 168 (effective 2001). adv. bk.rev. *Refereed.*

Indexed: Biol.Abstr., C.I.S. Abstr., Chem.Abstr., Curr.Adv.Ecol.Sci., Excerp.Med., INIS Atomind., Ind.Med. (coverage dropped).

—BLDSC (3120.550000), CASDDS, CISTI, EMDOCS, GNLM, Infotrieve. **CCC.**

Published by: (Ceska Lekarska Spolecnost J.E. Purkyne/Czech Medical Association), Nakladatelske Stredisko C L S J.E. Purkyne, Sokolska 31, Prague 12026, Czech Republic. TEL 42-2-24911420, FAX 42-2-24911420, nts@iol.cz, http://www.clsjep.cz, http://www.medical.cz. Ed. F Vosmik. adv.: color page CZK 44,000, B&W page CZK 31,000; 250 x 170. Circ: 2,100. **Dist. by:** Abont s.r.o., Chlumova 17, Prague, 3 130 00, Czech Republic; **Dist. in Western Countries by:** Kubon & Sagner, Hesstr 39-41, Munich 80798, Germany. **Co-sponsor:** Ceska Dermato-Venerologicka Spolecnost.

616.5 ITA ISSN 0011-1759

CHRONICA DERMATOLOGICA. Text in Italian; Summaries in English, Italian. 1946. bi-m. ITL 150,000; ITL 300,000 foreign. adv. bk.rev. abstr, bibl, charts, illus, stat. index. *Refereed.* **Document type:** *Academic/Scholarly.*

Formerly: I D I Cronache

Indexed: Excerp.Med.

—CISTI, EMDOCS, GNLM, KNAW.

Published by: Istituto Dermopatico dell'Immacolata, Via Dei Monti Di Creta, 104, Rome, RM 00167, Italy. FAX 39-6-66464437. Ed. Rino Cavalieri. R&P Gesaldo Scriva TEL 39-6-66464610. Circ: 7,000 (controlled).

616.5 GBR ISSN 0307-6938
CODEN: CEDEDE

CLINICAL AND EXPERIMENTAL DERMATOLOGY. Text in English. 1976. 8/yr., latest vol.27, 2002. GBP 99 in Europe to individuals; USD 157 in North America to individuals; GBP 109 elsewhere to individuals; GBP 549 in Europe to institutions; USD 870 in North America to institutions; GBP 604 elsewhere to institutions (effective 2002). adv. back issues avail.; reprint service avail. from ISI. *Refereed.* **Document type:** *Academic/Scholarly.* **Description:** Aims to publish a variety of review articles, original papers, concise reports and correspondence concerned with clinical and experimental aspects of dematology.

Formerly (until 1976): St. John's Hospital Dermatological Society. Transactions (0036-2891)

Related titles: Microform ed.: (from PQC); Online - full text ed.: ISSN 1365-2230. 1997. GBP 90 in Europe to individuals; USD 142 in North America to individuals; GBP 90 elsewhere to individuals; GBP 495 in Europe to institutions; USD 783 in North America to institutions; GBP 495 elsewhere to institutions (effective 2002) (from Ovid Technologies, Inc., EBSCO Publishing, O C L C Online Computer Library Center, Inc., RoweCom Information Quest, ingenta, Munksgaard & Blackwell Science's Synergy, Swets Blackwell, Institute for Scientific Information); ♦ Supplement: Clinical and Experimental Dermatology. Supplement. ISSN 0966-3487.

Indexed: AIDS Abstr., ASCA, Agri.& Environ.Biotech.Abstr. (coverage dropped), Chem.Abstr., Curr.Adv.Ecol.Sci., Curr.Cont., Dent.Ind., Derwent Biotech.Abstr., Dok.Arbeitsmed., Excerp.Med., Helminthol.Abstr., INIS Atomind., Ind.Med. (1976-), Ind.Sci.Rev., Ind.Vet., Inpharma, Int.Abstr.Biol.Sci., Jrnl.Watch Derm., Med.& Surg.Dermat., NRN, Nutr.Abstr., Pharm.&Out.News, Protozool.Abstr., Reac., Rev.Med.& Vet.Mycol., Rev.Plant Path., Sci.Cit.Ind., Small Anim.Abstr., Trop.Dis.Bull.

—BLDSC (3286.250000), ADONIS, CASDDS, CISTI, EMDOCS, GNLM, IDS, ingenta, KNAW. **CCC.**

Published by: Blackwell Science Ltd., PO Box 88, Oxford OX2 0NE, United Kingdom. TEL 44-1865-206180, 44-1865-206002, FAX 44-1865-206219, jnl.orders@blacksci.co.uk, http://www.blackwell-science.com/products/journals/ced.htm, http://www.blackwellpublishing.com. Ed. J Barker. Pub. Allen Stevens. R&P Sophie Savage. Adv. contact Jenny Applin. Circ: 805.

616.5 GBR ISSN 0966-3487

CLINICAL AND EXPERIMENTAL DERMATOLOGY. SUPPLEMENT. Text in English. irreg. adv. **Document type:** *Academic/Scholarly.*

Related titles: ♦ Supplement to: Clinical and Experimental Dermatology. ISSN 0307-6938.

Indexed: Excerp.Med. (1993-).

—ADONIS.

Published by: Blackwell Science Ltd., Osney Mead, Oxford OX2 0EL, United Kingdom. TEL 44-1865-206206, FAX 44-1865-721205, journals.cs@blacksci.co.uk, http://www.blackwell-science.com. Pub. Allen Stevens. R&P Sophie Savage. Adv. contact Jenny Applin.

616.5 JPN ISSN 0018-1404

CLINICAL DERMATOLOGY/HIFUKA NO RINSHO. Text in Japanese. 1959. m. JPY 1,950 per issue. bk.rev. illus. index.

Indexed: INIS Atomind.

—BLDSC (7971.620000), CISTI.

Published by: Kanehara & Co. Ltd., 2-31-14 Yushima, Bunkyo-ku, Tokyo 113-0034, Japan. Ed. Dr. Kenichi Ueno. Circ: 4,500.

616.5 USA ISSN 0738-081X
RL1

CLINICS IN DERMATOLOGY. Text in English. 1983. bi-m. EUR 175 in Europe to individuals; JPY 23,200 in Japan to individuals; USD 197 elsewhere to individuals; EUR 458 in Europe to institutions; JPY 60,800 in Japan to institutions; USD 511 elsewhere to institutions (effective 2002). illus. index. back issues avail. *Refereed.* **Document type:** *Academic/Scholarly.* **Description:** Provides information on the treatment and care of skin disorders.

Related titles: Microform ed.: (from PQC); Online - full text ed.: (from ingenta, Swets Blackwell, ScienceDirect, Institute for Scientific Information).

Indexed: ASCA, Abstr.Hyg., Curr.Cont., Excerp.Med., Ind.Med. (1983-), Inpharma, Int.Abstr.Biol.Sci., Nutr.Abstr., Pharm.&Out.News, Protozool.Abstr., Reac., Rev.Appl.Entomol., Rev.Med.& Vet.Mycol., SSCI (coverage dropped), Trop.Dis.Bull.

—BLDSC (3286.548000), CISTI, EMDOCS, GNLM, IDS, Infotrieve, ingenta, KNAW. **CCC.**

Published by: Elsevier Science, 655 Ave of the Americas, New York, NY 10010. TEL 212-633-3686, FAX 212-633-3820, usinfo-f@elsevier.com, http://www.elsevier.com/locate/clindermatol. Ed. Dr. Lawrence Charles Parish. Adv. contact Georgia Nikolaros. Circ: 1,500. **Subscr. in Australasia and the Far East to:** Elsevier Science (Singapore) Pte Ltd. TEL 65-434-3727, FAX 65-337-2230; **Subscr. in Japan to:** Elsevier Science Inc - Japan Regional Office. TEL 81-3-5561-5033, FAX 81-3-5561-5047; **Subscr. outside the Americas to:** Elsevier Science BV. TEL 31-20-485-3757, FAX 31-20-485-3432.

COMMON SENSE ABOUT AIDS. see *MEDICAL SCIENCES—Communicable Diseases*

616.5 DNK ISSN 0105-1873
CODEN: CODEDG

CONTACT DERMATITIS; environmental and occupational dermatitis. Text in English. 1975. m. USD 420 in the Americas to institutions print & online eds. combined; GBP 292 elsewhere to institutions print & online eds. combined (effective 2002). bk.rev. illus. reprint service avail. from SWZ,ISI. *Refereed.* **Document type:** *Academic/Scholarly.*

Related titles: Microform ed.: (from SWZ); Online - full text ed.: ISSN 1600-0536. GBP 263 (2002) (from Ovid Technologies, Inc., EBSCO Publishing, O C L C Online Computer Library Center, Inc., ingenta, Munksgaard & Blackwell Science's Synergy, Swets Blackwell, Institute for Scientific Information); ♦ Supplement: Contact Dermatitis. Supplement. ISSN 1396-6669.

Indexed: ASCA, Abstr.Hyg., Arts & Hum.Cit.Ind. (coverage dropped), Biol.Abstr., C.I.S. Abstr., CSNB, Chem.Abstr., Chem.Indus.Notes, Chem.Titles, Curr.Adv.Ecol.Sci., Curr.Cont., Dairy Sci.Abstr., Dent.Ind., Dok.Arbeitsmed., Environ.Sci.Poll.Mgmt., Excerp.Med., Forest Prod.Abstr., Helminthol.Abstr., Hort.Abstr., INIS Atomind., Ind.Hyg.Dig., Ind.Med. (1975-), Ind.Sci.Rev., Ind.Vet., Inpharma, Int.Abstr.Biol.Sci., Jrnl.Watch Derm., Lab.Haz.Bull., Mass Spectr.Bull., Med.& Surg.Dermat., Nutr.Abstr., Ornam.Hort., Pharm.&Out.News, Pollut.Abstr., Reac., Rev.Appl.Entomol., Rev.Arom.& Med.Plants, Rev.Med.& Vet.Mycol., Rev.Plant Path., Risk Abstr., Saf.Sci.Abstr., Sci.Cit.Ind., Sugar Ind.Abstr., THA, Triticale Abstr., Trop.Dis.Bull., Weed Abstr.

—BLDSC (3424.960000), ADONIS, CASDDS, CISTI, EMDOCS, GNLM, IDS, ingenta, KNAW. **CCC.**

Published by: (European Society of Contact Dermatitis), Blackwell Munksgaard, Noerre Soegade 35, PO Box 2148, Copenhagen K 1016, Denmark. TEL 45-77-33-33-33, FAX 45-77-33-33-77, customerservice@munksgaard.dk, http://www.munksgaard.dk/contactdermatitis. Ed. Dr. Richard Rycroft. Adv. contact Eric Rozario TEL 45-77-33-33-01. Circ: 1,600.

616.5 DNK ISSN 1396-6669

CONTACT DERMATITIS. SUPPLEMENT. Text in English. irreg. **Document type:** *Monographic series, Academic/Scholarly.*

Related titles: ♦ Supplement to: Contact Dermatitis. ISSN 0105-1873.

—ADONIS.

Published by: Blackwell Munksgaard, Noerre Soegade 35, PO Box 2148, Copenhagen K 1016, Denmark. TEL 45-77-33-33-33, FAX 45-77-33-33-77, customerservice@munksgaard.dk, http://www.munksgaard.dk.

CORE JOURNALS IN DERMATOLOGY. see *MEDICAL SCIENCES—Abstracting, Bibliographies, Statistics*

616.5 USA ISSN 1041-3766

COSMETIC DERMATOLOGY. Text in English. m. USD 160 in United States to institutions; USD 107 out of North America to institutions. adv. **Document type:** *Trade.* **Description:** Presents news and clinical information focusing on the cosmetic aspects of dermatology. Includes coverage of clinical meetings and industry events as well as news from Washington, DC, legal information and new products.

Indexed: I.P.A., Med.& Surg.Dermat.

—BLDSC (3477.174690), GNLM, Infotrieve. **CCC.**

Published by: Quadrant HealthCom, 26 Main St, Ste A, Chatham, NJ 07928-2402. Ed. Suzanne Ludlum. Pub. Linda Fox. Adv. contact Denise Andrade. Circ: 13,403 (controlled).

COSMETIC SURGERY TIMES; a magazine for the innovative cosmetic surgery practice. see *MEDICAL SCIENCES—Surgery*

CURRENT MEDICAL LITERATURE. DERMATOLOGY. see *MEDICAL SCIENCES—Abstracting, Bibliographies, Statistics*

M

616.5 GBR ISSN 1068-381X
CURRENT OPINION IN DERMATOLOGY. Text in English. 1993. a. GBP 154.95, USD 239.95. **Document type:** *Academic/Scholarly.*
Related titles: CD-ROM ed.; Online - full text ed.; Supplement: Slide Atlas of Current Dermatology. ISSN 1076-7770. 1994.
Indexed: Biotech.& Bioeng.Abstr. (coverage dropped), Cal.Tiss.Abstr., Chemorec.Abstr., Environ.Sci.Poll.Mgmt., Microbiol.Abstr., Neurosci.Abstr. (coverage dropped), Pollut.Abstr., Saf.Sci.Abstr.
Published by: Rapid Science Publishers, 2-6 Boundary Row, London SE1 8HN, United Kingdom. TEL 44-207-865-0198, FAX 44-207-410-6600, rapid@rapidcom.co.uk; info@hugo.curbio.com, http://BioMedNet.com/cgi-bin/members1/titles.pl. Eds. M V Dahl, P J Lynch.

616.5 CHE ISSN 0070-2064
CODEN: APDEBX
CURRENT PROBLEMS IN DERMATOLOGY. Text in English. 1959. irreg., latest vol.30. CHF 220 in Europe; DEM 265 in Germany; USD 180 in United States (effective 2001). reprint service avail. from ISI. *Refereed.* **Document type:** *Monographic series, Academic/Scholarly.* **Description:** Contains reports from the most active areas of dermatology and skin research.
Indexed: ASCA, Biol.Abstr., Chem.Abstr., Curr.Cont. (coverage dropped), Dent.Ind., Ind.Med. (1968-).
—BLDSC (3501.370000), CASDDS, CISTI, GNLM, ingenta, KNAW. **CCC.**
Published by: S. Karger AG, Allschwilerstr 10, PO Box, Basel 4009, Switzerland. TEL 41-61-306-1111, FAX 41-61-306-1234, karger@karger.ch, http://www.karger.com/bookseries/CUPDE. Ed. G Burg.

616.5 USA ISSN 1040-0486
CURRENT PROBLEMS IN DERMATOLOGY. Text in English. 1989. bi-m. USD 96 domestic to individuals; USD 105 foreign to individuals; USD 155 domestic to institutions; USD 164 foreign to institutions; USD 51 domestic to students; USD 60 foreign to students; USD 28 (effective 2001). **Document type:** *Trade.* **Description:** Covers current concerns of the dermatologist in everyday practice.
Related titles: Online - full text ed.: (from Institute for Scientific Information).
Indexed: Curr.Cont., Excerp.Med. (1996-), Sci.Cit.Ind.
—EMDOCS, GNLM, IDS, Infotrieve. **CCC.**
Published by: Mosby, Inc. (Subsidiary of: Elsevier Science), 11830 Westline Industrial Dr, St Louis, MO 63146-3318. TEL 314-872-8370, 800-325-4177, FAX 314-432-1380, customerservice@mosby.com, http://www.mosby.com/cpderm, http://www.mosby.com/periodicals. Ed. Jeffrey P Callen. Circ: 2,402.

616.5 USA ISSN 0011-4162
RL1 CODEN: CUTIB
CUTIS; cutaneous medicine for the practitioner. Text in English. 1965. m. USD 170 in the Americas to institutions; USD 255 elsewhere to institutions (effective 2000). adv. bk.rev. charts, illus. reprint service avail. from PQC. *Refereed.* **Document type:** *Academic/Scholarly, Trade.* **Description:** Provides practical information on skin diseases and allergies, with clinical observations and discussions of therapeutic techniques.
Related titles: Microform ed.: (from PQC); Online - full text ed.: (from Northern Light Technology, Inc., ProQuest Information & Learning, Institute for Scientific Information).
Indexed: ASCA, Abstr.Inter.Med., Curr.Cont., Dent.Ind., Excerp.Med., Forest.Abstr., Helminthol.Abstr., INIS Atomind., Ind.Med. (1965-), Ind.Sci.Rev., Ind.Vet., Inpharma, Med.& Surg.Dermat., NRN, Nutr.Abstr., Pharm.&Out.News, Protozool.Abstr., Reac., Rev.Appl.Entomol., Rev.Med.& Vet.Mycol., SSCI (coverage dropped), Sci.Cit.Ind., Weed Abstr.
—BLDSC (3506.150000), CISTI, EMDOCS, GNLM, IDS, ingenta, KNAW. **CCC.**
Published by: Quadrant HealthCom, 26 Main St, Ste A, Chatham, NJ 07928-2402. TEL 973-701-8900, FAX 973-701-8892. Ed. Christine McCrary-Sisk. Pub. Sharon Finch. Adv. contact Denise Andrade. Circ: 49,300.

616.95 ROM
DERMATO-VENEROLOGIE. Text in Romanian. 1956. 3/yr.
Formerly: Revista de Medicina Interna, Neurologie, Psihiatrie, Neuro-Chirurgie, Dermato-Venerologie. Series Dermato-Venerologie.; Supersedes: Dermato-Venerologie (0011-9024)
—GNLM.
Published by: Asociatia Medicala Romana, Societatea Romana de Dermatologie, Str. Progresului 8, Bucharest 70754, Romania. Ed. Dr. Stefan Antonescu.

616.5 MEX ISSN 0185-4038
DERMATOLOGIA; revista mexicana. Text in Spanish; Summaries in English, Spanish. 1952. bi-m. MXP 300, USD 55 (effective 1996 & 1997). bk.rev. cum.index: 1952-1981. *Refereed.* **Document type:** *Academic/Scholarly.* **Description:** Contains original articles, revision articles, clinical cases, and notices.
Indexed: Biol.Abstr., Excerp.Med., Trop.Dis.Bull.
Published by: (Sociedad Mexicana de Dermatologia), Obsidiana Editores S.A., CZDA DE TLALPAN 2365, Col Ciudad Jardin, Mexico City, DF 04370, Mexico. TEL 52-5-689-9133. Eds. Dr. Clemente Moreno Collado, Dr. Roberto Arenas. Pub. Jorge Godoy-Gutierrez. Circ: 2,400. **Dist. by:** Distribuidora Editorial de Mexico SA de CV, P.O. Box 76-026, Mexico City, DF 04201, Mexico. TEL 52-5-544-7953, FAX 52-5-689-6545. **Co-sponsor:** Academia Mexicana de Dermatologia.

616.5 ITA ISSN 0392-1395
DERMATOLOGIA CLINICA. Text in Italian; Summaries in English. 1981. q. ITL 80,000, USD 70 (effective 2001). adv.
Indexed: Excerp.Med., Ref.Zh.
—BLDSC (3555.110000), CISTI, EMDOCS, GNLM, KNAW. **CCC.**
Published by: C I C Edizioni Internazionali s.r.l., Corso Trieste 42, Rome, RM 00198, Italy. TEL 39-06-8412673, FAX 39-06-8412688, info@gruppocic.it, 1160199510. Ed. O A Carlesimo. Pub. A Salvati. adv.: B&W page ITL 2,400,000, color page ITL 3,300,000; trim 210 x 280.

616.5 616.95 BGR ISSN 0417-0792
CODEN: DVENA3
DERMATOLOGIA I VENEROLOGIA. Text in Bulgarian; Summaries in Russian, English. 1962. q. BGL 15, USD 5.
Indexed: Abstr.Bulg.Sci.Med.Lit., Biol.Abstr., C.I.S. Abstr., Chem.Abstr., Excerp.Med. (until 1993).
—CASDDS, CISTI, GNLM.
Published by: (Bulgaria. Ministerstvo na Narodnoto Zdrave), Izdatelstvo Meditsina i Fizkultura, 11 Pl Slaveikov, Sofia 1080, Bulgaria. Ed. N Z Catkov. Circ: 988. **Dist by:** Hemus, 6 Rouski blvd, Sofia 1000, Bulgaria. **Co-sponsor:** Nauchno Druzhestvo po Dermatologia.

616.5 ESP ISSN 1130-605X
DERMATOLOGIA & COSMETICA. Text in Spanish. 1990. q. ESP 8,600, USD 85 to individuals; USD 10,200 to institutions; USD 6,800 to students. adv. back issues avail.; reprints avail. *Refereed.* **Document type:** *Academic/Scholarly.*
Related titles: Online - full text ed.
—CISTI.
Published by: (Grupo Espanol de Dermatologia Cosmetica), Editorial Garsi S.A. (Subsidiary of: Grupo Masson), Juan Bravo, 46, Madrid 28006, Spain. TEL 34-91-402-1212, FAX 34-91-402-0954, garsi@mad.servicom.es, http://www.masson.es. Ed. M E de las Heras Alonso. Pub. M Asin Llorca. adv.: B&W page ESP 120,000, color page ESP 150,000; 280 x 210.

616.5 USA ISSN 0733-8635
RL1 CODEN: DRMCDJ
DERMATOLOGIC CLINICS. Text in English. 1983. q. USD 174 domestic to individuals; USD 199 in Canada to individuals; USD 224 elsewhere to individuals; USD 228 domestic to institutions; USD 278 foreign to institutions; USD 70 per issue (effective 2001). *Refereed.* **Document type:** *Journal, Academic/Scholarly.* **Description:** Each issue covers a single topic of skin disease or therapy in detail.
Related titles: Microform ed.: (from PQC); Online - full text ed.: (from Institute for Scientific Information).
Indexed: ASCA, CINAHL, Chem.Abstr., Chem.Indus.Notes, Chem.Titles, Curr.Cont., Excerp.Med., INIS Atomind., Ind.Med. (1983-), Inpharma, Int.Nurs.Ind., Ornam.Hort., Pharm.&Out.News, Protozool.Abstr., Reac., Rev.Appl.Entomol., Rev.Med.& Vet.Mycol.
—BLDSC (3555.138000), CASDDS, CISTI, EMDOCS, GNLM, IDS, ingenta, KNAW. **CCC.**
Published by: W.B. Saunders Co. (Subsidiary of: Harcourt Publishers Ltd.), 11830 Westline Industrial Dr, St Louis, MO 63146. TEL 800-325-4177, http://www.wbsaunders.com. Ed. Bruce H Thiers. **Subscr. to:** Periodicals Fulfillment, W B Saunders Co, 6277 Sea Harbor Dr, 4th Fl, Orlando, FL 32891-4800.

DERMATOLOGIC SURGERY. see *MEDICAL SCIENCES—Surgery*

DERMATOLOGIC SURGERY ONLINE. see *MEDICAL SCIENCES—Surgery*

616.5 USA ISSN 1396-0296
DERMATOLOGIC THERAPY. Text in English. 1996. 4/yr. USD 100 domestic to individuals; USD 115 in Canada & Mexico to individuals; USD 125 elsewhere to individuals; USD 295 domestic to institutions; USD 310 in Canada & Mexico to institutions; USD 320 elsewhere to institutions; USD 110 to individuals print & online eds. combined; USD 324.50 to institutions print & online eds. combined (effective 2001). adv. illus. **Document type:** *Journal, Academic/Scholarly.*
Announced as: Dermatologic Therapy 2000
Related titles: Online - full text ed.: ISSN 1529-8019. USD 90 to individuals; USD 266 to institutions (effective 2001) (from Ovid Technologies, Inc., O C L C Online Computer Library Center, Inc., ingenta, Munksgaard & Blackwell Science's Synergy, Swets Blackwell).
—BLDSC (3555.143000), Infotrieve. **CCC.**
Published by: Blackwell Science Inc., Commerce Pl, 350 Main St, Malden, MA 02148-5018. TEL 781-388-8250, 800-759-6102, FAX 781-388-8255, journals@blacksci.com, http://www.blackwell-science.com.

616.5 DEU ISSN 1438-776X
CODEN: DBUMDB
DERMATOLOGIE IN BERUF UND UMWELT/ OCCUPATIONAL AND ENVIRONMENTAL DERMATOLOGY. Text in English, German; Summaries in English, German. 1952. bi-m. DEM 78.23, EUR 40 domestic; DEM 88.01, EUR 45 foreign; DEM 89.97, EUR 46 domestic print & online eds. combined; DEM 101.70, EUR 52 foreign print & online eds. combined (effective 2001). adv. bk.rev. abstr, bibl, charts, illus. index. back issues avail.; reprint service avail. from IRC,ISI. *Refereed.* **Document type:** *Journal, Trade, Academic/Scholarly.* **Description:** Provides information on all questions pertaining to the relationship between skin and the environment.
Former titles (until 2000): Dermatosen in Beruf und Umwelt (0343-2432); (until 1978): Berufs-Dermatosen (0005-9498)
Related titles: Online - full text ed.
Indexed: ASCA, Abstr.Hyg., Biol.Abstr., C.I.S. Abstr., Chem.Abstr., Chem.Indus.Notes, Chem.Titles, Curr.Cont. (coverage dropped), Excerp.Med., INIS Atomind., Ind.Med. (coverage dropped), Int.Abstr.Biol.Sci., Lab.Haz.Bull., Protozool.Abstr., SSCI (coverage dropped), Trop.Dis.Bull.
—BLDSC (3555.185000), CASDDS, CISTI, EMDOCS, GNLM, IDS, Infotrieve, KNAW. **CCC.**
Published by: Editio Cantor Verlag, Postfach 1255, Aulendorf 88322, Germany. TEL 49-7525-940135, FAX 49-7525-940180, info@ecv.de, http://www.ecv.de/dermhome.htm. Ed. Hans Joachim Schwanitz. Adv. contact Holger Leupoldt. Circ: 6,850.

616.5 FRA ISSN 0982-8567
DERMATOLOGIE PRATIQUE. Text in French. 1986. m. (10/yr.). EUR 39 domestic to individuals; EUR 53 foreign to individuals; EUR 27 domestic to libraries; EUR 42 foreign to libraries (effective 2002). **Document type:** *Newspaper.*
Published by: L E N Medical, 15 rue des Sablons, Paris 75116, France. TEL 33-1-47553131, FAX 33-1-47553132, lenmed@club-internet.fr, http://www.webmedguide.com. Ed. Dr. C P Morel.

616.5 ITA
IL DERMATOLOGO. Text in Italian. 1979. 10/yr. ITL 40,000, USD 30 (effective 2001). adv. bk.rev.
Formerly: Il Dermatologo Ospedaliero (0391-8912)
Published by: C I C Edizioni Internazionali s.r.l., Corso Trieste 42, Rome, RM 00198, Italy. TEL 39-06-8412673, FAX 39-06-8412688, info@gruppocic.it, 1160199510. Ed. A Salvati. adv.: B&W page ITL 4,000,000, color page ITL 5,100,000; trim 300 x 420.

616.5 CHE ISSN 1018-8665
CODEN: DERAEG
DERMATOLOGY; international journal for clinical and investigative dermatology. Text in English. 1893. 8/yr. (in 2 vols.). CHF 1,368 in Europe to institutions; CHF 1,391.20 overseas to institutions; EUR 976.40 in Europe to institutions; USD 1,064 overseas to institutions (effective 2002). adv. bk.rev. bibl, illus. index. back issues avail. *Refereed.* **Document type:** *Journal, Academic/Scholarly.* **Description:** Provides a worldwide survey of clinical and investigative dermatology.
Formerly: Dermatologica (0011-9075)
Related titles: Microform ed.: (from PQC,PMC); Online - full text ed.: ISSN 1421-9832. CHF 116, EUR 84, USD 90 to institutions with print edition (effective 2002) (from EBSCO Publishing, O C L C Online Computer Library Center, Inc., RoweCom Information Quest, Swets Blackwell, Institute for Scientific Information).

M

Indexed: Abstr.Hyg., Agri.& Environ.Biotech.Abstr. (coverage dropped), Biol.Abstr., C.I.S. Abstr., Chem.Abstr., Curr.Adv.Ecol.Sci., Curr.Cont., Dent.Ind., Derwent Biotech.Abstr., Excerp.Med., Helminthol.Abstr., INIS Atomind., Ind.Med. (1992-), Ind.Sci.Rev., Med.& Surg.Dermat., NRN, Nutr.Abstr., Protozool.Abstr., Rev.Appl.Entomol., Rev.Arom.& Med.Plants, Rev.Med.& Vet.Mycol., Rev.Plant Path., Rural Recreat.Tour.Abstr., SSCI (coverage dropped), Sci.Cit.Ind., Trop.Dis.Bull.
—BLDSC (3555.213000), CASDDS, CISTI, EMDOCS, GNLM, IDS, ingenta, KNAW. **CCC.**
Published by: S. Karger AG, Allschwilerstr 10, PO Box, Basel 4009, Switzerland. TEL 41-61-306-1111, FAX 41-61-306-1234, karger@karger.ch, http://www.online.karger.com/journals/drm, http://www.karger.com. Ed. J H Saurat. adv.: page USD 1,205. Circ: 2,350. **Co-sponsor:** Belgian Society for Dermatology and Syphiligraphy, Schweizerische Gesellschaft fuer Dermatologie und Venerologie.

616.5 CHE ISSN 1422-9196
▼ **DERMATOLOGY AND PSYCHOSOMATICS/ DERMATOLOGIE UND PSYCHOSOMATIK.** Text in English, German. 2000. 4/yr. CHF 171, EUR 116 in Europe to institutions; CHF 182.60, USD 137 overseas to institutions (effective 2002). **Document type:** *Journal, Academic/Scholarly.* **Description:** Provides a forum for the rapid transfer of new findings in basic and therapy research into clinic and practice as well as a platform for the exchange between clinical dermatology and psychosomatic-psychiatric research.
Related titles: Online - full text ed.: ISSN 1424-0564. CHF 58, EUR 42, USD 45 to institutions with print edition (effective 2002) (from EBSCO Publishing, O C L C Online Computer Library Center, Inc., RoweCom Information Quest, Swets Blackwell).
—BLDSC (3555.225000).
Published by: S. Karger AG, Allschwilerstr 10, PO Box, Basel 4009, Switzerland. TEL 41-61-306-1111, FAX 41-61-306-1234, karger@karger.ch, http://www.online.karger.com/journals/dps, http://www.karger.com.

616.5 GBR ISSN 0262-5504
DERMATOLOGY IN PRACTICE. Text in English. 1982-1990; resumed 1994. bi-m. bk.rev. illus. **Document type:** *Academic/Scholarly.*
—BLDSC (3555.232980).
Published by: Hayward Medical Communications Ltd., Covent Garden, Seven Dials Warehouse, 44 Earlham St, London WC2H 9LA, United Kingdom. TEL 44-20-7240-4493, FAX 44-20-7240-4479, admin@hayward.co.uk, http://www.hayward.co.uk. Ed. Dr. John Sovin. Circ: 19,000. **Subscr. to:** Rosemary House, Lanwades Park, Kentford, Near, Newmarket, Suffolk CB8 7PW, United Kingdom. TEL 44-1638-751515, FAX 44-1638-751517.

616.5 USA
▼ **DERMATOLOGY INSIGHTS.** Text in English. 2000. s-a. adv. **Description:** Covers a wide range of dermatologic conditions for patients. Also includes tips for keeping skin, hair and nails healthy.
Published by: American Academy of Dermatology, 930 N Meacham Rd, Schaumburg, IL 60173-4965. TEL 847-330-0230, FAX 847-330-8907, http://www.aad.org/2001_DermatologyInsights.pdf. Ed. Dean Monti. Pub. Anne Allodi. Adv. contact Tim McCormack TEL 913-469-1110. B&W page USD 5,950, color page USD 7,900; trim 8.125 x 10.875.

616.5 USA ISSN 1060-3441
DERMATOLOGY NURSING. Text in English. 1989. bi-m. USD 24 in United States to individuals; USD 47 elsewhere to individuals; USD 45 in United States to institutions; USD 60 elsewhere to institutions; USD 8 newsstand/cover (effective 2001). adv. back issues avail. *Refereed.* **Document type:** *Journal, Academic/Scholarly.* **Description:** Strives to develop and foster the highest standards of dermatology and wound nursing care through education and research.
Related titles: CD-ROM ed.: (from Ovid Technologies, Inc.); Online - full text ed.: (from Ovid Technologies, Inc., Northern Light Technology, Inc., Gale Group).
Indexed: Brit.Nur.Ind., CINAHL, Int.Nurs.Ind.
—BLDSC (3555.232600), CISTI, GNLM, Infotrieve, ingenta. **CCC.**
Published by: (Dermatology Nurses' Association), Jannetti Publications, Inc., East Holly Ave, Box 56, Pitman, NJ 08071-0056. TEL 856-256-2300, FAX 856-589-7463, DNJRNL@.ajj.com, http://www.ajj.com/services/pblshng/dnj/default.htm, http://www.cinahl.com/jrnls/DERN/dern.htm, http://www.ajj.com/services/pblshng/jrnls.htm. Ed. Marcia Hill. Adv. contact Michael Cunningham. Circ: 6,000 (paid).

616.9 USA ISSN 1051-8258
DERMATOLOGY (STAMFORD). Text in English. 1990. biennial. **Document type:** *Monographic series.*
Published by: Appleton & Lange, Journal Division (Subsidiary of: Simon & Schuster Company), 11 W 19th St, New York, CT 10011-4209. TEL 203-406-4500, FAX 203-406-4600.

616.5 USA ISSN 0196-6197
CODEN: DETIEG
DERMATOLOGY TIMES. Text in English. 1979. m., latest vol.22. USD 95 United States & Possessions; USD 140 in Canada & Mexico; USD 185 elsewhere; USD 10 newsstand/cover United States & Possessions (effective 2001). adv. tr.lit. back issues avail. *Refereed.* **Document type:** *Trade.* **Description:** Industry news and developments, and meeting announcements for office- and hospital-based dermatology professionals.
Related titles: Microform ed.: (from PQC); Online - full text ed.: (from The Dialog Corporation, Gale Group, Northern Light Technology, Inc., ProQuest Information & Learning).
—BLDSC (3555.233600). **CCC.**
Published by: Advanstar Communications Inc., Healthcare Group, 7500 Old Oak Blvd, Cleveland, OH 44130-3369. TEL 440-243-8100, FAX 440-891-2735, dermtines@advanstar.com, http://www.advanstar.com, http://www.modernmedicine.com/derm. Ed. Tom Skernivitz. Pub. Claudia Shayne-Ferguson. adv.: B&W page USD 2,335, color page USD 3,745; trim 10.75 x 14.5. Circ: 9,372. **Subscr. to:** 131 W First St, Duluth, MN 55802. TEL 888-527-7008.

616.5 DEU ISSN 0340-8078
DER DEUTSCHE DERMATOLOGE. Text in German. 1952. m. EUR 136.30 domestic; EUR 140.30 foreign; EUR 105.46 domestic to students; EUR 109.46 foreign to students; EUR 18.69 newsstand/cover (effective 2002). adv. reprint service avail. from PQC. **Document type:** *Journal, Academic/Scholarly.*
Formerly (until 1977): Dermatologen-Mitteilungsblatt (0340-806X)
—BLDSC (3564.420000), GNLM. **CCC.**
Published by: Urban und Vogel Medien und Medizin Verlagsgesellschaft mbH (Subsidiary of: BertelsmannSpringer), Neumarkter Str 43, Munich 81673, Germany. TEL 49-89-43721411, FAX 49-89-43721410, verlag@urban-vogel.de, http://www.urban-vogel.de. Ed. R Blumenthal. R&P Friederik Klein. Adv. contact Christiane Loichinger. Circ: 5,000. **Subscr. to:** Springer Auslieferungs Gesellschaft, Postfach 105160, Heidelberg 69041, Germany. TEL 49-6221-345244, FAX 49-6221-345244.

616.5 616.95 USA
DIALOGUES IN DERMATOLOGY; the audiojournal of dermatology. Text in English. 1977. m., latest vol.48. USD 300 to non-members; USD 150 to members (effective 2001). bibl, illus. cum.index: 1977-present. back issues avail. **Document type:** *Academic/Scholarly.* **Description:** Features interviews with experts on recent advances in the field of dermatology.
Media: Audio cassette/tape.
Published by: American Academy of Dermatology, 930 N Meacham Rd, Schaumburg, IL 60173-4965. TEL 847-330-0230, FAX 847-330-0050, mktg@aad.org. Ed. Dr. Warren Heymann. R&P Thomas Pearson. Adv. contact Jennie McGuire. Circ: 2,500.

616.5 GBR
DIRECTORY OF TRAINING POSTS IN DERMATOLOGY. Text in English. a. GBP 10 (effective 2001). **Document type:** *Directory.*
Published by: (British Association of Dermatologists), Hawker Publications Ltd., Culvert House, Culvert Rd, London SW11 5AP, United Kingdom. TEL 44-20-7720-2108, FAX 44-20-7498-3023, hawker@hawkerpubs.demon.co.uk, http://www.careinfo.org/.

616.5 646.7 USA
ELECTROLYSIS WORLD✱. Text in English. 1982. q. membership. back issues avail.
Published by: American Electrolysis Association, 7332 E Camelback Rd, No D, Scottsdale, AZ 85251. TEL 602-945-4245. Ed. Gail J Walker. Circ: 1,700.

616.5 FRA ISSN 0246-0319
ENCYCLOPEDIE MEDICO-CHIRURGICALE. DERMATOLOGIE. Cover title: Traite de Dermatologie. Variant title: Encyclopedie Medico-Chirurgicale, Instantanes Medicaux. Dermatologie. Receuil Periodique de l'Encyclopedie Medico-Chirurgicale. Dermatologie. Text in French. 1936. 3 base vols. plus q. updates. bibl, charts, illus. *Refereed.* **Document type:** *Academic/Scholarly.* **Description:** Offers dermatologists a comprehensive and up-to-date reference to diagnose and treat various skin conditions.
Published by: Elsevier Paris, Editions Scientifiques et Medicales (Subsidiary of: Reed Elsevier plc. group), 23 rue Linois, Paris 75015, France. TEL 33-1-45589110, FAX 33-1-45589425, redaction-emc@elsevier.fr, redacion-emc@elsevier.fr, http://www.elsevier.fr, http://www.elsevier.com.

616.5 616.9 GBR ISSN 0926-9959
CODEN: JEAVEQ
EUROPEAN ACADEMY OF DERMATOLOGY AND VENEREOLOGY. JOURNAL. Short title: J E A D V(Journal of the European Academy of Dermatology and Venereology). Text in English. 1992. bi-m., latest vol.16, 2002. GBP 110 in Europe to individuals; USD 121 in North America to individuals; GBP 175 elsewhere to individuals; GBP 452 in Europe to institutions; USD 718 in North America to institutions; GBP 498 elsewhere to institutions (effective 2002). back issues avail. *Refereed.* **Document type:** *Academic/Scholarly.* **Description:** Publishes articles of general and practical interest in the field of dermatology and venereology on clinical and basic science topics, as well as research with practical implications.
Related titles: Microform ed.: (from PQC); Online - full text ed.: ISSN 1468-3083. GBP 99 in Europe to individuals; USD 158 in North America to individuals; GBP 99 elsewhere to individuals; GBP 407 in Europe to institutions; USD 647 in North America to institutions; GBP 407 elsewhere to institutions (effective 2002) (from EBSCO Publishing, O C L C Online Computer Library Center, Inc., ingenta, ScienceDirect, Munksgaard & Blackwell Science's Synergy, Swets Blackwell, Institute for Scientific Information); ♦ Supplement to: European Academy of Dermatology and Venereology. Journal. Supplement. ISSN 0929-0168.
Indexed: Curr.Cont., Excerp.Med. (1992-), Ind.Med. (1992-), Inpharma, Med.& Surg.Dermat., Pharm.&Out.News, Protozool.Abstr., Reac., Rev.Appl.Entomol., Rev.Med.& Vet.Mycol.
—BLDSC (4741.624000), CISTI, EMDOCS, GNLM, IDS, Infotrieve, KNAW. **CCC.**
Published by: (European Academy of Dermatology and Venereology BEL), Blackwell Science Ltd., PO Box 88, Oxford OX2 0NE, United Kingdom. TEL 44-1865-206180, 44-1865-206002, FAX 44-1865-206219, jnl.orders@blacksci.co.uk, http://www.blackwell-science.com/~cgilib/jnlpage.asp?Journal=jdv&File=jdv, http://www.blackwellpublishing.com. Eds. D Freedman, T Lotti. Pub. Allen Stevens. R&P Sophie Savage. Adv. contact Jenny Applin. Circ: 1,800.

616.5 616.9 NLD ISSN 0929-0168
EUROPEAN ACADEMY OF DERMATOLOGY AND VENEREOLOGY. JOURNAL. SUPPLEMENT. Key Title: JEADV. Journal of the European Academy of Dermatology and Venereology. Supplement. Text in English. 1992. irreg., latest vol.12. abstr, illus. *Refereed.* **Document type:** *Monographic series, Proceedings, Academic/Scholarly.*
Related titles: ♦ Supplement: European Academy of Dermatology and Venereology. Journal. ISSN 0926-9959.
—KNAW.
Published by: (European Academy of Dermatology and Venereology BEL), Elsevier Science BV, PO Box 211, Amsterdam 1000 AE, Netherlands. TEL 31-20-485-3757, TELEX 18582 ESPA NL, http://www.elsevier.nl.

616.5 FRA ISSN 1167-1122
CODEN: EJDEE4
EUROPEAN JOURNAL OF DERMATOLOGY. Text in English. 1991. 8/yr. FRF 1,350 domestic to individuals; FRF 224 in Europe to individuals; USD 250 elsewhere to individuals; FRF 2,100 domestic to institutions; EUR 338 in Europe to institutions; USD 360 elsewhere to institutions; FRF 600 domestic to students; EUR 123 in Europe to students; USD 135 elsewhere to students; FRF 270 newsstand/cover (effective 2001). *Refereed.* **Document type:** *Academic/Scholarly.* **Description:** Provides up-to-date information and works in all fields of dermatology and skin biology.
Related titles: Online - full text ed.: FRF 1,350 to individuals; FRF 2,100 to institutions; FRF 600 to students (effective 2001) (from Institute for Scientific Information).

M

Indexed: ASCA, Chem.Abstr., Chem.Indus.Notes, Chem.Titles, Curr.Cont., Excerp.Med. (1993-), I.P.A., Ind.Med. (1991-), Inpharma, Int.Nurs.Ind., Lab.Haz.Bull., Nutr.Abstr., Pharm.&Out.News, Protozool.Abstr., Reac., Rev.Appl.Entomol., Rev.Arom.& Med.Plants, Rev.Med.& Vet.Mycol., Sci.Cit.Ind., Trop.Dis.Bull.
—BLDSC (3668.416000), ADONIS, CASDDS, CISTI, EMDOCS, GNLM, IDS, KNAW.
Published by: John Libbey Eurotext, 127 av. de la Republique, Montrouge 92120, France. TEL 33-01-46730660, FAX 33-01-40840999, marketing@jle.com, http://www.john-libbey-eurotext.fr/. Ed. Jean Thivolet. **Subscr. to:** A T E I, 3 av. Pierre Keraudren, Romainville 92230, France. TEL 33-1-48408686, FAX 33-1-48400731, atei@club-internet.fr.

616.5 618.92 ITA ISSN 1122-7788
EUROPEAN JOURNAL OF PEDIATRIC DERMATOLOGY (EDIZIONE ITALIANA). Key Title: P D. European Journal of Pediatric Dermatology (Ed. Italiana). Text in Italian. 1982. q. ITL 85,000 domestic; ITL 125,000 foreign (effective 2000). Index. 64 p./no. back issues avail. **Document type:** *Academic/Scholarly.*
Supersedes (in 1991): Bollettino di Dermatologia Pediatrica (1122-5793)
Related titles: Online - full text ed.; ♦ Italian ed.: European Journal of Pediatric Dermatology (English Edition). ISSN 1122-7672.
Published by: Dermatologia Pediatrica Association, Via Bitritto, 131, Bari, BA 70124, Italy. FAX 39-80-5478927. Ed. Ernesto Bonifazi.

616.5 ITA ISSN 1122-7672
CODEN: EPDDE
EUROPEAN JOURNAL OF PEDIATRIC DERMATOLOGY (ENGLISH EDITION). Key Title: P D. European Journal of Pediatric Dermatology (English Ed.). Text in Italian. 1982. q. ITL 75,000 domestic; ITL 125,000 foreign (effective 2000). **Document type:** *Academic/Scholarly.*
Supersedes (in 1991): Pediatric Dermatology News (1122-8644)
Related titles: ♦ Italian ed.: European Journal of Pediatric Dermatology (Edizione Italiana). ISSN 1122-7788.
Indexed: Excerp.Med. (1994-).
—BLDSC (3829.733440), GNLM, KNAW.
Published by: Dermatologia Pediatrica Association, Via Bitritto, 131, Bari, BA 70124, Italy. FAX 39-80-5478927. Ed. Ernesto Bonifazi.

EXCERPTA MEDICA. SECTION 13: DERMATOLOGY AND VENEREOLOGY. see *MEDICAL SCIENCES—Abstracting, Bibliographies, Statistics*

616.5 CHE ISSN 1424-4616
▼ **EXOGENOUS DERMATOLOGY**; physical - chemical - biological. Text in English. forthcoming 2002. bi-m. CHF 798, EUR 570.80 in Europe to institutions; CHF 815.40, USD 623 elsewhere to institutions (effective 2002). **Document type:** *Journal, Academic/Scholarly.*
Related titles: Online - full text ed.: ISSN 1424-4624. forthcoming 2002. CHF 58, EUR 42, USD 45 to institutions (effective 2002).
Published by: S. Karger AG, Allschwilerstr 10, PO Box, Basel 4009, Switzerland. TEL 41-61-3061111, FAX 41-61-3061234, karger@karger.ch, http://www.online.karger.com/journals/EXD, http://www.karger.com.

616.5 616.95 DNK ISSN 0906-6705
CODEN: EXDEEY
EXPERIMENTAL DERMATOLOGY. Text in English. 1992. bi-m. USD 300 in the Americas to institutions print & online eds. combined; GBP 208 elsewhere to institutions print & online eds. cimbined (effective 2002). adv. illus. reprints avail. *Refereed.* **Document type:** *Academic/Scholarly.*
Related titles: ♦ Online - full text ed.: Experimental Dermatology Online. ISSN 1600-0625.
Indexed: Chem.Abstr., Chem.Indus.Notes, Chem.Titles, Curr.Cont., Excerp.Med. (1993-), INIS Atomind., Ind.Med. (1992-), Inpharma, Int.Abstr.Biol.Sci., Pharm.&Out.News, Reac., Sci.Cit.Ind.
—BLDSC (3839.070000), CASDDS, CISTI, EMDOCS, GNLM, IDS, Infotrieve, KNAW. **CCC.**
Published by: Blackwell Munksgaard, Noerre Soegade 35, PO Box 2148, Copenhagen K 1016, Denmark. TEL 45-77-33-33-33, FAX 45-77-33-33-77, fsub@munksgard.dk, http://www.munksgard.dk/experimentaldermatology, http://www.munksgaard.dk. Eds. Angela Christiano, T A Luger. Adv. contact Eric Rozario TEL 45-77-33-33-01.

616.5 DNK ISSN 1600-0625
EXPERIMENTAL DERMATOLOGY ONLINE. Text in English. bi-m. GBP 187 (effective 2002). **Document type:** *Academic/Scholarly.*
Media: Online - full text (from EBSCO Publishing, ingenta, Munksgaard & Blackwell Science's Synergy, Swets Blackwell, Institute for Scientific Information). **Related titles:** ♦ Print ed.: Experimental Dermatology. ISSN 0906-6705.
Published by: Blackwell Munksgaard, Noerre Soegade 35, PO Box 2148, Copenhagen K 1016, Denmark. TEL 45-77-33-33-33, FAX 45-77-33-33-77, fsub@mail.munksgaard.dk, http://www.munksgaard.dk.

EXTRACTA DERMATOLOGICA; weltweit Auserlesen. see *MEDICAL SCIENCES—Abstracting, Bibliographies, Statistics*

616.5 616.95 USA ISSN 0071-7932
FORTSCHRITTE DER PRAKTISCHEN DERMATOLOGIE UND VENEROLOGIE. Text in English. 1952. irreg., latest vol.14, 1995. price varies. reprint service avail. from ISI. **Document type:** *Monographic series.*
—GNLM, KNAW.
Published by: Springer-Verlag, Journals (Subsidiary of: BertelsmannSpringer), 175 Fifth Ave, New York, NY 10010. TEL 212-460-1500, FAX 212-473-6272.

616.5 616.951 ITA ISSN 0392-0488
CODEN: GIDVDZ
GIORNALE ITALIANO DI DERMATOLOGIA E VENEREOLOGIA. Text in Italian; Summaries in English, Italian. 1866. bi-m. USD 125 to individuals; USD 165 to institutions (effective 2000 - 2001). adv. abstr, bibl, charts, illus. index. **Document type:** *Academic/Scholarly.* **Description:** Covers dermatological and venereological biology, histology, clinical medicine and therapy.
Supersedes (in 1979): Giornale Italiano di Dermatologia. Minerva Dermatologica (0300-1318); Which was formed by the 1969 merger of: Giornale Italiano di Dermatologia (0376-0901); Minerva Dermatologica (0026-4741); Which was formerly (until 1950): Dermosifilografo (0366-886X); Cosmetologia
Related titles: Microform ed.
Indexed: Abstr.Hyg., C.I.S. Abstr., Chem.Abstr., Dent.Ind., Excerp.Med., Ind.Med. (coverage dropped), Med.& Surg.Dermat., Nutr.Abstr., Protozool.Abstr., Ref.Zh., Rev.Appl.Entomol., Rev.Arom.& Med.Plants, Rev.Med.& Vet.Mycol., Soils & Fert., Trop.Dis.Bull.
—BLDSC (4178.214000), CASDDS, CISTI, GNLM, KNAW.
Published by: (Societa Italiana di Dermatologia e Venereologia), Edizioni Minerva Medica, Corso Bramante, 83-85, Turin, TO 10126, Italy. TEL 39-11-678282, FAX 39-11-674502. Ed. M Pippione. Pub. Alberto Oliaro. Adv. contact F Filippo. B&W page USD 1,400, color page USD 2,300; trim 280 x 215. Circ: 3,000 (paid).

GLOSSARIUM DERMATOLOGIA. see *PHARMACY AND PHARMACOLOGY*

616.5 CHN ISSN 1001-3504
GUOWAI YIXUE (PIFUBINGXUE FENCE)/FOREIGN MEDICAL SCIENCES (DERMATOSES). Text in Chinese. 1979. bi-m. USD 22.20; USD 3.70 newsstand/cover (effective 2001). **Document type:** *Academic/Scholarly.*
Published by: China International Book Trading Corp/Zhongguo Guoji Tushu Maoyi Zonggongsi cibtc@mail.cibtc.com.cn, http://www.cibtc.com.cn. **Dist. by:** 35, Chegongzhuang Xilu, Haidian District, Beijing 100044, China.

616.5 616.95 DEU ISSN 0017-8470
CODEN: HAUTAW
DER HAUTARZT; Zeitschrift fuer Dermatologie, Allergologie, Venerologie und verwandte Gebiete. Text in German. 1950. m. EUR 361.76 domestic; EUR 333.16 in Germany; EUR 31.80 newsstand/cover foreign (effective 2002). adv. bk.rev. illus. index. back issues avail.; reprint service avail. from ISI. *Refereed.* **Document type:** *Journal, Academic/Scholarly.* **Description:** Covers all aspects of dermatology and related sciences.
Related titles: Microform ed.: (from PQC); Online - full text ed.: Elektronische Ausgabe. ISSN 1432-1173 (from EBSCO Publishing, RoweCom Information Quest, Swets Blackwell, Springer LINK, Institute for Scientific Information); ♦ Supplement: Der Hautarzt. Supplementum. ISSN 0172-9713.
Indexed: ASCA, Abstr.Hyg., Agri.& Environ.Biotech.Abstr. (coverage dropped), Biol.Abstr., Chem.Abstr., Curr.Adv.Cancer Res., Curr.Cont., Dent.Ind., Derwent Biotech.Abstr., Dok.Arbeitsmed., Excerp.Med., INIS Atomind., Ind.Med. (1950-), Ind.Sci.Rev., Ind.Vet., Inpharma, Int.Nurs.Ind., Med.& Surg.Dermat., Nutr.Abstr., Pharm.&Out.News, Pig News & Info., Protozool.Abstr., Reac., Rev.Appl.Entomol., Rev.Med.& Vet.Mycol., SSCI (coverage dropped), Sci.Cit.Ind.
—BLDSC (4273.760000), CASDDS, CISTI, GNLM, IDS, Infotrieve, KNAW. **CCC.**
Published by: Springer-Verlag (Subsidiary of: BertelsmannSpringer), Tiergartenstr 17, Heidelberg 69121, Germany. TEL 49-6221-345-0, FAX 49-6221-345229, subscriptions@springer.de, http://link.springer.de/link/service/journals/00105/index.htm, http://www.springer.de. Ed. D Petzoldt. **Subscr. in N. America to:** Springer-Verlag New York Inc., PO Box 2485, Secaucus, NJ 07096-2485. TEL 212-460-1500, FAX 212-473-6272.

616.5 DEU ISSN 0172-9713
DER HAUTARZT. SUPPLEMENTUM. Text in German. 1976. irreg.
Related titles: ♦ Supplement to: Der Hautarzt. ISSN 0017-8470.
Published by: Springer-Verlag (Subsidiary of: BertelsmannSpringer), Haber Str 7, Heidelberg 69126, Germany. TEL 49-30-8207448. Ed. Dr. Beate Fruhstorfer.

616.5 DEU ISSN 0933-7385
HAUTFREUND. Text in German. 1986. bi-m. DEM 66 (effective 2000). adv. bk.rev. back issues avail. **Document type:** *Journal, Academic/Scholarly.*
Published by: (Deutscher Neurodermitiker Bund e.V.), Schwennessen Verlag, Postfach 202313, Hamburg 20216, Germany. TEL 49-40-510619, FAX 49-40-5110605, info@hautfreund.de, http://www.hautfreund.de. Ed., Pub., Adv. contact Thomas Schwennesen. Circ: 10,000 (paid and controlled).

616.5 DEU ISSN 0938-0221
HAUTNAH DERMATOLOGIE. Text in German. 1985. bi-m. EUR 70.68 domestic; EUR 81.68 foreign; EUR 55.73 domestic to students; EUR 66.73 foreign to students; EUR 15.89 newsstand/cover (effective 2002). adv. bk.rev. **Document type:** *Journal, Academic/Scholarly.*
Supersedes in part: Hautnah (0930-7109)
—GNLM.
Published by: Urban und Vogel Medien und Medizin Verlagsgesellschaft mbH (Subsidiary of: BertelsmannSpringer), Neumarkter Str 43, Munich 81673, Germany. TEL 49-89-43721411, FAX 49-89-43721410, verlag@urban-vogel.de, http://www.urban-vogel.de. Ed., R&P Friederik Klein. Adv. contact Christiane Loichinger. Circ: 7,500. **Subscr. to:** Springer Auslieferungs Gesellschaft, Postfach 105160, Heidelberg 69041, Germany. TEL 49-6221-345244, FAX 49-6221-345244.

616.5 JPN
HIFU SHIKKAN SAISHIN NO CHIRYO. Text in Japanese. 1987. biennial. JPY 7,000 per issue.
Published by: Nankodo Co. Ltd., 42-6 Hongo 3-chome, Bunkyo-ku, Tokyo 113-0033, Japan. FAX 03-3811-7230.

616.5 AUS ISSN 1028-9623
HONG KONG DERMATOLOGY & VENEREOLOGY BULLETIN. Text in English. 1992. q. AUD 377 domestic; AUD 343 in New Zealand; USD 209 elsewhere; AUD 415 domestic print & online eds.; AUD 378 in New Zealand print & online eds.; USD 230 elsewhere print & online eds. (effective 2001). adv. **Document type:** *Journal, Academic/Scholarly.* **Description:** Provides a forum for the discussion of problems related to dermatology and venereology.
Related titles: Online - full text ed.: AUD 340 domestic; AUD 309 in New Zealand; USD 189 elsewhere (effective 2001).
Published by: (Hong Kong Society of Dermatology & Venereology HKG), Blackwell Science Asia Pty Ltd, PO Box 378, Carlton South, VIC 3053, Australia. TEL 61-3-9347-0300, FAX 61-3-9347-5001, info@blacksci-asia.com.au, http://www.blacksci.co.uk/australi. Ed. Dr. Chong Lai-yin.

616.5 USA
ICHTHYOSIS FOCUS* . Text in English. 1981. q. USD 35 to membership (effective 1999). adv. bk.rev. back issues avail. *Refereed.* **Document type:** *Consumer.* **Description:** Provides information on support services, treatments and research for a group of rare genetic skin disorders collectively called ichthyosis.
Indexed: Aquacult.Abstr.
Published by: Foundation for Ichthyosis and Related Skin Types, Inc., 650 N Cannon Ave Ste 17, Lansdale, PA 19446-1874. TEL 610-789-3995, 800-545-3286, ichthyosis@aol.com, http://www.libertynet.org/~ichthyos. Ed., R&P, Adv. contact Elena Levitan. Circ: 3,000.

M

616.5 IND ISSN 0019-5154
CODEN: IJDEAA

INDIAN JOURNAL OF DERMATOLOGY. Abbreviated title: I J D. Text in English. 1955. q. INR 240 domestic; USD 50 foreign; INR 75 newsstand/cover domestic; USD 15 newsstand/cover foreign (effective 2001). adv. bk.rev. charts, illus, abstr, stat. Index. back issues avail.; reprints avail. *Refereed.* **Document type:** *Journal, Academic/Scholarly.* **Description:** Publishes information relating to skin, it's ailments and the different modes of therapeutics. This journal is circulated among Dermatologists, Medical Professionals and Institutions.
Related titles: Online - full text ed.
Indexed: Biol.Abstr., Curr.Adv.Ecol.Sci., Excerp.Med., Ind.Med. (coverage dropped), Nutr.Abstr., Rev.Appl.Entomol.
—BLDSC (4411.500000), CISTI, GNLM.
Published by: Indian Association of Dermatologists, Venereologists and Leprologists, W B State Branch, I M A House, 53 Creek Row, Kolkata, West Bengal 700 014, India. TEL 91-33-2349536, FAX 91-33-2366437, iadvlwb@vsnl.net, http://www.e-ijd.org. Ed. Sujit R Sengupta. Pub., Adv. contact Dr. Koushik Lahiri. B&W page INR 7,500, color page INR 20,000, online banner INR 25,000; trim 180 x 235. Circ: 1,000 (paid); 50 (controlled).

616.5 616.951 IND ISSN 0378-6323
CODEN: IJDLDY

INDIAN JOURNAL OF DERMATOLOGY, VENEREOLOGY AND LEPROLOGY. Text in English. 1935. bi-m. INR 500, USD 100 (effective 1996). adv. bk.rev. charts, illus, stat. index. reprint service avail. from PQC. **Document type:** *Academic/Scholarly.*
Supersedes (in 1976): Indian Journal of Dermatology and Venereology (0019-5162)
Related titles: CD-ROM ed.; Microform ed.: (from PQC).
Indexed: Biol.Abstr., Chem.Abstr., Excerp.Med., ExtraMED, Indian Sci.Abstr., Rev.Plant Path.
—BLDSC (4411.610000), CISTI, EMDOCS, GNLM, ingenta, KNAW.
Published by: Indian Association of Dermatologists Venereologists and Leprologists, c/o Dr. Gurmohan Singh, Ed., New D-7, Banaras Hindu University, Varanasi, Uttar Pradesh 221 005, India. TEL 91-542-310845. Adv. contact S S Pandey. Circ: 2,000.

616.5 617.520592 USA ISSN 1530-8200

▼ **INTERNATIONAL JOURNAL OF COSMETIC SURGERY AND AESTHETIC DERMATOLOGY.** Text in English. 1999. q. USD 381 domestic; USD 458 foreign; USD 457 domestic to institutions print and online eds.; USD 534 foreign to institutions print and online eds.; USD 172 domestic to individuals print eds.; USD 248 foreign to individuals print eds.; USD 215 domestic to individuals print and online eds.; USD 283 foreign to individuals print and online eds. (effective 2002). back issues avail.; reprints avail. *Refereed.* **Document type:** *Journal, Academic/Scholarly.* **Description:** Devoted to dermatology for aesthetic or cosmetic purposes.
Formerly: Journal of Aesthetic Dermatology and Cosmetic Dermatologic Surgery (1096-6226)
Related titles: Online - full content ed.: USD 381 to institutions; USD 179 to individuals (effective 2002) (from Swets Blackwell); Online - full text ed.: (from CatchWord Ltd., RoweCom Information Quest).
—BLDSC (4542.178600). **CCC.**
Published by: Mary Ann Liebert, Inc. Publishers, 2 Madison Ave, Larchmont, NY 10538. TEL 914—834-3100, FAX 914-834-1388, info@liebertpub.com, http://www.liebertpub.com/cos. Ed. Dr. Howard Sobel.

616.5 GBR ISSN 0011-9059
RL1 CODEN: IJDEBB

INTERNATIONAL JOURNAL OF DERMATOLOGY. Text in English. 1962. m., latest vol.41, 2002. GBP 115 in Europe to individuals; USD 166 in North America to individuals; GBP 115 elsewhere to individuals; GBP 298 in Europe to institutions; USD 430 in North America to institutions; GBP 298 elsewhere to institutions (effective 2002); GBP 294.80 in Europe to institutions print & online eds.; GBP 117.70 in Europe to individuals print & online eds.; USD 454.30 in North America to institutions print & online eds.; USD 181.50 in North America to individuals print & online eds.; GBP 294.80 elsewhere to institutions print & online eds.; GBP 117.70 elsewhere to individuals print & online eds. (effective 2001). adv. illus. index. *Refereed.* **Document type:** *Academic/Scholarly.*
Formerly: Dermatologia Internationalis
Related titles: Microform ed.: (from PQC); Online - full text ed.: ISSN 1365-4632. GBP 104 in Europe to individuals; USD 150 in North America to individuals; GBP 104 elsewhere to individuals; GBP 269 in Europe to institutions; USD 387 in North America to institutions; GBP 269 elsewhere to institutions (effective 2002) (from Ovid Technologies, Inc., EBSCO Publishing, O C L C Online Computer Library Center, Inc., RoweCom Information Quest, ingenta, Munksgaard & Blackwell Science's Synergy, Swets Blackwell, Institute for Scientific Information).
Indexed: ASCA, Abstr.Hyg., Biol.Abstr., Chem.Abstr., Curr.Adv.Ecol.Sci., Curr.Cont., Dairy Sci.Abstr., Dent.Ind., Dok.Arbeitsmed., Excerp.Med., Helminthol.Abstr., INIS Atomind., Ind.Med. (1970-), Ind.Sci.Rev., Ind.Vet., Inpharma, Int.Nurs.Ind., Jrnl.Watch Derm., Med.& Surg.Dermat., NRN, Pharm.&Out.News, Protozool.Abstr., Reac., Rev.Appl.Entomol., Rev.Med.& Vet.Mycol., SSCI (coverage dropped), Sci.Cit.Ind., Trop.Dis.Bull.
—BLDSC (4542.185000), CASDDS, CISTI, GNLM, IDS, ingenta, KNAW. **CCC.**
Published by: (International Society of Dermatology: Tropical, Geographic, and Ecologic), Blackwell Science Ltd., PO Box 88, Oxford OX2 0NE, United Kingdom. TEL 44-1865-206180, 44-1865-206002, FAX 44-1865-206219, jnl.orders@blacksci.co.uk, http://www.blackwell-science.com/~cgilib/jnlpage.asp?Journal=ijd&File=ijd, http://www.blackwellpublishing.com. Ed. Dr. Lawrence C Parish. Pub. Allen Stevens. R&P Sophie Savage. Adv. contact Jenny Applin. Circ: 2,730.

616.5 JPN ISSN 0021-4973

JAPANESE JOURNAL OF CLINICAL DERMATOLOGY/ RINSHO HIFUKA. Text in Japanese. 1946. m. JPY 30,330, USD 233.
Indexed: INIS Atomind.
—BLDSC (4651.373000), CISTI, GNLM.
Published by: Igaku-Shoin Ltd., 5-24-3 Hongo, Bunkyo-ku, Tokyo 113-0033, Japan. TEL 81-3-3817-5716, FAX 81-3-3815-4145. Ed. Takeji Nishikawa. Circ: 4,000.

616.5 JPN ISSN 0021-499X
CODEN: NHKZAD

JAPANESE JOURNAL OF DERMATOLOGY: SERIES A. Key Title: Nihon Hifuka Gakkai Zasshi. Text in Japanese. 1901. m. JPY 7,000. bk.rev. charts, illus. index. **Document type:** *Academic/Scholarly.*
Former titles (until 1957): Hifuka Seibyoka Zasshi (0368-3524); (until 1942): Hifuka Hinyokika Zasshi (0368-2846)
Indexed: Biol.Abstr., Chem.Abstr., Dent.Ind., INIS Atomind., Ind.Med. (coverage dropped), Rev.Med.& Vet.Mycol.
—BLDSC (4651.550000), CASDDS, CISTI, GNLM.
Published by: Japanese Dermatological Association/Nihon Hifuka Gakkai, Taisei Bldg, 14-10 Hongo 3-chome, Bunkyo-ku, Tokyo 113-0033, Japan. Ed. M Takenouchi.

616.5 DEU ISSN 1432-511X

JATROS DERMA. Text in German. 1987. 12/yr. DEM 140 (effective 1998). back issues avail. **Document type:** *Academic/Scholarly.* **Description:** Seminar papers including summaries of articles, interviews and congress reports on dermatology.
Formerly: Jatros Dermatologie (0932-8661)
—GNLM.
Published by: Hoffmann und Hoffmann GmbH, August-Schanz-Str 8-II, Frankfurt A.m. 60433, Germany. TEL 49-69-54800015, FAX 49-69-54800080, TELEX 412952-PMI-D, huhgmbh@aol.com. Ed. Peter Hoffmann. Circ: 3,000.

616.5 ITA ISSN 0392-8543
CODEN: JACOEL

JOURNAL OF APPLIED COSMETOLOGY; quarterly review of cosmetic dermatology. Text in Italian. 1983. q. ITL 180,000 domestic; USD 100 foreign (effective 2000). adv. bk.rev.
Indexed: Chem.Abstr., Chem.Indus.Notes, Chem.Titles, Eng.Ind., Excerp.Med.
—BLDSC (4942.380000), CASDDS, Ei, EMDOCS, GNLM, KNAW, Linda Hall.
Published by: (International Society of Cosmetic Dermatology), International Ediemme, Via Innocenzo XI, 41, Rome, RM 00165, Italy. TEL 39-6-9286261, FAX 39-6-9281523, mavi@colosseum.it. Ed. Pierfrancesco Morganti. R&P, Adv. contact Maria Luisa Numbiata. Circ: 5,000.

616.5 615.8 GBR ISSN 1462-883X

▼ **JOURNAL OF CUTANEOUS LASER THERAPY.** Text in English. 1999. q. GBP 78, USD 125 to individuals; GBP 185, USD 300 to institutions (effective 2002). index. *Refereed.* **Document type:** *Academic/Scholarly.* **Description:** Covers new lasers and new applications in the use of laser therapy for cosmetic dermatology and plastic surgery.
Related titles: Online - full content ed.: ISSN 1471-1761; Online - full text ed.: (from CatchWord Ltd.).
Indexed: Jrnl.Watch Derm.
—BLDSC (4965.957700), CatchWord.
Published by: Martin Dunitz Ltd. (Subsidiary of: Taylor & Francis Group), 7-9 Pratt St, London NW1 0AE, United Kingdom. TEL 44-20-7482-2202, FAX 44-20-7482-7088, info@dunitz.co.uk, http://www.dunitz.co.uk. Eds. Gary Lask, Nicholas Lowe. Circ: 1,400 (paid).

616.5 617 CAN ISSN 1203-4754
CODEN: JCMSFU

JOURNAL OF CUTANEOUS MEDICINE AND SURGERY. Text in English. 1997. bi-m. USD 218.90 domestic; USD 212.60 in Germany; USD 37.10 newsstand/cover foreign (effective 2002). back issues avail. **Document type:** *Journal, Academic/Scholarly.* **Description:** Examines major advances in clinical and academic dermatology, design measurement and analysis, gene therapy and other related issues.
Incorporates (1994-2001): Medical & Surgical Dermatology (0944-5196)
Related titles: Online - full text ed.: ISSN 1615-7109 (from ProQuest Information & Learning, Swets Blackwell, Springer LINK, RoweCom Information Quest).
Indexed: Ind.Med. (1996-).
—BLDSC (4965.959000), GNLM, Infotrieve. **CCC.**
Published by: Springer-Verlag, Journals (Subsidiary of: BertelsmannSpringer), 175 Fifth Ave, New York, NY 10010. TEL 212-460-1575, FAX 212-473-6292, info@bcdecker.com, journals@springer-ny.com, http://www.bcdecker.com, http://www.springer-ny.com. Ed. Daniel N Sauder. Circ: 2,286 (paid).

616.5 DNK ISSN 0303-6987
CODEN: JCUPBN

JOURNAL OF CUTANEOUS PATHOLOGY. Text and summaries in English. 1974. 10/yr. USD 420 Sat. in the Americas to institutions print & online eds. combined; GBP 292 elsewhere to institutions print & online eds. combined (effective 2002). adv. bibl, charts, illus. reprint service avail. from ISI. *Refereed.* **Document type:** *Academic/Scholarly.*
Related titles: Online - full text ed.: ISSN 1600-0560. GBP 263 (2002) (from Ovid Technologies, Inc., EBSCO Publishing, ingenta, Munksgaard & Blackwell Science's Synergy, Swets Blackwell, Institute for Scientific Information).
Indexed: ASCA, Abstr.Hyg., Biol.Abstr., Chem.Abstr., Curr.Adv.Biochem., Curr.Cont., Dent.Ind., Excerp.Med., Helminthol.Abstr., INIS Atomind., Immun.Abstr., Ind.Med. (1974-), Ind.Sci.Rev., Inpharma, Jrnl.Watch Derm., Med.& Surg.Dermat., Neurosci.Cit.Ind., Nutr.Abstr., Protozool.Abstr., Reac., Rev.Appl.Entomol., Rev.Med.& Vet.Mycol., Rev.Plant Path., Sci.Cit.Ind., Trop.Dis.Bull.
—BLDSC (4965.960000), ADONIS, CISTI, EMDOCS, GNLM, IDS, ingenta, KNAW. **CCC.**
Published by: (American Society for Dermatopathology USA), Blackwell Munksgaard, Noerre Soegade 35, PO Box 2148, Copenhagen K 1016, Denmark. TEL 45-77-33-33-33, FAX 45-77-33-33-77, fsub@munksgaard.dk, http://journals.munksgaard.dk/cutaneouspathology, http://www.munksgaard.dk. Ed. Bruce R Smoller. Adv. contact Eric Rozario TEL 45-77-33-33-01. Circ: 1,800.

616.5 IRL ISSN 0923-1811
CODEN: JDSCEI

JOURNAL OF DERMATOLOGICAL SCIENCE. Text in English. 1990. 9/yr. EUR 889 in Europe to institutions; JPY 118,200 in Japan to institutions; USD 995 elsewhere to institutions (effective 2002). adv. bk.rev. back issues avail. *Refereed.* **Document type:** *Academic/Scholarly.* **Description:** Publishes manuscripts covering the entire scope of dermatology, from molecular studies to clinical investigations.
Related titles: Online - full text ed.: (from ingenta, ScienceDirect, Swets Blackwell, Institute for Scientific Information).
Indexed: ASCA, Biol.Abstr., Chem.Abstr., Chem.Indus.Notes, Chem.Titles, Curr.Cont., Excerp.Med., Ind.Med. (1990-), Inpharma, Int.Abstr.Biol.Sci., Med.& Surg.Dermat., Pharm.&Out.News, Reac., Rev.Appl.Entomol., Rev.Med.& Vet.Mycol., Sci.Cit.Ind.
—BLDSC (4968.766500), CASDDS, CISTI, EMDOCS, GNLM, IDS, Infotrieve, KNAW. **CCC.**

Published by: (Japanese Society for Investigative Dermatology JPN), Elsevier Science Ireland Ltd, Elsevier House, Brookvale Plaza, E. Park, Shannon, Co. Clare, Ireland. TEL 353-61-471944, FAX 353-61-472144, http://www.elsevier.nl/locate/jdermsci. Ed. Hideoki Ogawa. R&P Annette Moloney. Circ: 1,500. **Subscr. in Australasia and the Far East to:** Elsevier Science (Singapore) Pte Ltd, No.1 Temasek Ave, 17-01 Millenia Tower, Singapore 039192, Singapore. TEL 65-434-3727, FAX 65-337-2230; **Subscr. in the Americas to:** Elsevier Science, PO Box 945, New York, NY 10159-0945. TEL 212-633-3730, FAX 212-633-3680; **Subscr. to:** Elsevier Science BV, PO Box 211, Amsterdam 1000 AE, Netherlands. TEL 31-20-485-3757.

616.5 GBR ISSN 0954-6634
CODEN: JDTREY
JOURNAL OF DERMATOLOGICAL TREATMENT. Text in English. 1989. q. GBP 83, USD 130 to individuals; GBP 190, USD 305 to institutions (effective 2002). adv. bk.rev. illus. index. back issues avail. *Refereed.* **Document type:** *Academic/Scholarly.* **Description:** Examines all aspects of the diagnosis and treatment of skin conditions and disorders.
Related titles: Online - full content ed.: ISSN 1471-1753; Online - full text ed.: (from CatchWord Ltd., Institute for Scientific Information).
Indexed: ASCA, Chem.Abstr., Curr.Cont., Excerp.Med., Ind.Sci.Rev., Inpharma, Med.& Surg.Dermat., Microbiol.Abstr., Pharm.&Out.News, Reac., Rev.Arom.& Med.Plants, Rev.Med.& Vet.Mycol., Sci.Cit.Ind.
—BLDSC (4968.767000), CASDDS, CISTI, EMDOCS, GNLM, Infotrieve, KNAW. **CCC.**
Published by: Martin Dunitz Ltd. (Subsidiary of: Taylor & Francis Group), 7-9 Pratt St, London NW1 0AE, United Kingdom. TEL 44-20-7482-2202, FAX 44-20-7482-7088, info@dunitz.co.uk, http://www.dunitz.co.uk. Eds. Christopher E M Griffiths, Jean Paul Ortonne. Circ: 2,500 (paid).

616.5 JPN ISSN 0385-2407
CODEN: JDMYAG
JOURNAL OF DERMATOLOGY. Text in English. 1974. m. bk.rev. charts, illus. index. **Document type:** *Academic/Scholarly.*
Supersedes (1963-1972): Japanese Journal of Dermatology: Series B (0368-282X)
Indexed: Biol.Abstr., Chem.Abstr., Chem.Indus.Notes, Chem.Titles, Dent.Ind., Excerp.Med., INIS Atomind., Ind.Med. (1974-), Med.& Surg.Dermat., NRN, Rev.Appl.Entomol., Rev.Med.& Vet.Mycol., THA.
—BLDSC (4968.770000), CASDDS, CISTI, EMDOCS, GNLM, KNAW.
Published by: Japanese Dermatological Association/Nihon Hifuka Gakkai, Taisei Bldg, 14-10 Hongo 3-chome, Bunkyo-ku, Tokyo 113-0033, Japan. TEL 81-3-3811-5099. Ed. Shinji Shimada.

616.5 USA ISSN 0022-202X
RL1 CODEN: JIDEAE
THE JOURNAL OF INVESTIGATIVE DERMATOLOGY; an international journal for research in cutaneous biology. Text in English. 1938. m. USD 390 domestic to individuals; USD 420 in Canada & Mexico to individuals; USD 465 elsewhere to individuals; USD 535 domestic to institutions; USD 565 in Canada & Mexico to institutions; USD 610 elsewhere to institutions; USD 429 to individuals print & online eds. combined; USD 588.50 to institutions print & online eds. combined (effective 2001). adv. bk.rev. bibl, illus, abstr. index. back issues avail.; reprints avail. *Refereed.* **Document type:** *Academic/Scholarly.* **Description:** Presents original papers and reviews pertinent to the normal and abnormal function of the skin.
Related titles: Microform ed.: (from WWS); Online - full text ed.: ISSN 1523-1747. USD 351 to individuals; USD 482 to institutions (effective 2001) (from Ovid Technologies, Inc., HighWire Pr., EBSCO Publishing, O C L C Online Computer Library Center, Inc., RoweCom Information Quest, ingenta, Munksgaard & Blackwell Science's Synergy, Swets Blackwell, Institute for Scientific Information).
Indexed: ASCA, Abstr.Hyg., AgBiotech, Agri.& Environ.Biotech.Abstr. (coverage dropped), Anim.Breed.Abstr., Biol.Abstr., C.I.S. Abstr., Chem.Abstr., Chem.Titles, Curr.Adv.Biochem., Curr.Adv.Cancer Res., Curr.Adv.Cell & Devel.Biol., Curr.Adv.Ecol.Sci., Curr.Adv.Gen.& Molec.Biol., Curr.Cont., Dent.Ind., Derwent Biotech.Abstr., Excerp.Med., Forest Prod.Abstr., INIS Atomind., I.P.A., Ind.Med. (1938-), Ind.Sci.Rev., Ind.Vet., Inpharma, Int.Abstr.Biol.Sci., Jrnl.Watch Derm., Med.& Surg.Dermat., Neurosci.Cit.Ind., Nutr.Abstr., Pharm.&Out.News, Pig News & Info., Poult.Abstr., Reac., Rev.Appl.Entomol., Rev.Arom.& Med.Plants, Rev.Med.& Vet.Mycol., Sci.Cit.Ind., Small Anim.Abstr., Vet.Bull., Weed Abstr.
—BLDSC (5008.000000), ADONIS, CASDDS, CISTI, GNLM, IDS, ingenta, KNAW. **CCC.**
Published by: (Society of Investigative Dermatology, Inc.), Blackwell Science Inc., Commerce Pl, 350 Main St, Malden, MA 02148-5018. TEL 781-388-8250, 800-759-6102, FAX 781-388-8255, journals@blacksci.com, http://www.jidonline.org/, http://www.blackwell-science.com. Ed. Dr. David Norris. R&P Tracey Davies. Adv. contact Jenny Applin. Circ: 4,800. **Co-sponsor:** European Society for Dermatological Research.

616.5 USA ISSN 1087-0024
THE JOURNAL OF INVESTIGATIVE DERMATOLOGY SYMPOSIUM PROCEEDINGS. Text in English. 1996. s-a. **Document type:** *Proceedings, Academic/Scholarly.*
Related titles: Online - full text ed.: (from Institute for Scientific Information).
Indexed: Ind.Med.
—ADONIS.
Published by: (Society For Investigative Dermatology, European Society for Dermatological Research), Blackwell Science Inc., Commerce Pl, 350 Main St, Malden, MA 02148-5018. http://www.blackwell-science.com.

616.5 PAK ISSN 1560-9014
CODEN: JPADFG
JOURNAL OF PAKISTAN ASSOCIATION OF DERMATOLOGISTS. Text in English. 1997. q. GBP 80 in United Kingdom; USD 120 elsewhere (effective 2001). adv. charts, stat, illus. back issues avail. *Refereed.* **Document type:** *Journal, Academic/Scholarly.* **Description:** Contains editorial, news and views, case reports, and information on continuing medical education involving dermatology.
Published by: Pakistan Association of Dermatologists, 17-B Khyabanijanbaz Phase 5, Defence Housing Authority, Karachi, Pakistan. TEL 92-5854535, FAX 92-5846248, http://www.who.sci.eg/library/index.htm. Ed., Pub. Yasmeena Khan.

616.5 GBR ISSN 0965-206X
JOURNAL OF TISSUE VIABILITY. Text in English. 1981. q. GBP 20 in the European Union; GBP 25 elsewhere (effective 2000). adv. bk.rev. back issues avail. *Refereed.* **Document type:** *Academic/Scholarly.*
Formerly (until 1991): Care - Science and Practice (0268-0009)
Indexed: AMED, Brit.Nur.Ind., Int.Nurs.Ind.
—BLDSC (5069.540000), CISTI, GNLM. **CCC.**
Published by: Tissue Viability Society, Glanville Centre Association, Salisbury District Hospital, Salisbury, Wilts SP2 8BJ, United Kingdom. TEL 44-1722-429057, FAX 44-1722-425263, tvs@dial.pipex.com, http://www.tvs.org.uk. Ed. K S Gebhardt. R&P, Adv. contact D Roberts. page GBP 300.

JOURNAL OF TOXICOLOGY. CUTANEOUS AND OCULAR TOXICOLOGY. see *PHARMACY AND PHARMACOLOGY*

016.6165 USA ISSN 1521-3595
JOURNAL WATCH DERMATOLOGY. Key Title: Journal Watch for Dermatology. Text in English. 1993 (Mar.). m. USD 98. 8 p./no. **Document type:** *Newsletter.* **Description:** Presents concise summaries of important research appearing in the dermatology literature.
Published by: Massachusetts Medical Society, P O Box 9085, Waltham, MA 02254-9085. http://mms.org.

616.5 ITA
LEXICON VEVY EUROPE SKIN CARE INSTANT REPORTS. Text in Italian. 1984. q. free per issue to qualified personnel. bk.rev. **Document type:** *Trade.* **Description:** Contains international information on dermo-pharmaceutics, cosmetics and toiletries.
Formerly (until 1989): Lexicon Vevy Skin Care Instant Reports
—BLDSC (5185.14780).
Published by: Vevy Europe S.p.A., Casella Postale 81570, Genoa, GE 16131, Italy. TEL 39-10-5221515, FAX 39-10-5221530, TELEX 281257 VEVY I. Ed. Dr. Giorgio Rialdi. Circ: 12,900 (controlled). **Co-sponsor:** Skin Applied Sciences Associates.

616.5 CHN ISSN 1000-4963
CODEN: LPZAEH
LINCHUANG PIFUKE ZAZHI/JOURNAL OF CLINICAL DERMATOLOGY. Text in Chinese; Abstracts in English. 1972. m. (bi-m. until 2001, vol. 30). CNY 115.20, USD 60 (effective 2002). adv. bk.rev. **Document type:** *Journal, Academic/Scholarly.* **Description:** Contains original papers on clinical and laboratory studies, therapies, case reports and reviews.
Related titles: CD-ROM ed.
Indexed: ExtraMED, Poult.Abstr., Rev.Appl.Entomol., Rev.Arom.& Med.Plants, Rev.Med.& Vet.Mycol., Trop.Dis.Bull.
Published by: First Affiliated Hospital of Nanjing Medical University, 300 Guangzhou Lu, Nanjing 210029, China. TEL 86-25-372-9951, FAX 86-25-651-6459, jcdch@jlonline.com. Ed., R&P Zhao Bian. Adv. contact Xu Zu Jian. Circ: 20,000.

LOOSE CONNECTIONS. see *SOCIAL SERVICES AND WELFARE*

616.5 ESP ISSN 0210-5187
MEDICINA CUTANEA IBERO-LATINO-AMERICANA. Text in Spanish. 1973. bi-m. USD 119 (effective 1999). adv. bk.rev. **Document type:** *Academic/Scholarly.*
Formed by the merger of: Medicina Cutanea (0025-7788); Dermatologia Ibero Latino-Americano (0011-9040)
Indexed: Biol.Abstr., Dent.Ind., Excerp.Med., Ind.Med. (coverage dropped), Ind.Vet., Med.& Surg.Dermat., Protozool.Abstr., Rev.Appl.Entomol., Rev.Arom.& Med.Plants, Rev.Med.& Vet.Mycol., Trop.Dis.Bull., Vet.Bull.
—BLDSC (5532.790000), CISTI, GNLM, KNAW.
Published by: (Colegio Ibero-Latino-Americano de Dermatologia ARG), Editorial Dips Rocas, Muntaner, 393 pral. 4, Barcelona 08021, Spain. TEL 39-3-2001389, FAX 34-3-2021958, edipsro@intercom.es. Ed. Mario Lecha. Circ: 2,000.

616.5 616.99 USA
MELANOMA LETTER. Text in English. q. USD 25. **Document type:** *Bulletin, Newsletter.* **Description:** Features articles by prominent medical authorities to inform health care professionals of the latest advances in melanoma research and treatment.
Published by: Skin Cancer Foundation, 245 Fifth Ave, Ste 2402, New York, NY 10016. TEL 212-725-5176, FAX 212-725-5751. Ed. Joyce Weisbach Ayoub.

616.5 ESP ISSN 0214-4735
CODEN: MONDE4
MONOGRAFIAS DE DERMATOLOGIA. Text in Spanish. 6/yr. ESP 10,500 to individuals; ESP 12,360 domestic to institutions; ESP 18,500 foreign to institutions (effective 2000). adv. **Document type:** *Monographic series.*
Indexed: Excerp.Med.
—BLDSC (5912.655500), KNAW.
Published by: Grupo Aula Medica S.A., C.I. Venecia 2 Alfa III, Isabel Colbrand, 10-12, Madrid 28050, Spain. TEL 34-1-3588657, FAX 34-1-3589067. Eds. J A Ruiz, Francisco Camacho. Adv. contact J.A. Ruiz.

616.5 616.4 646.7 USA ISSN 0894-1769
NATIONAL ALOPECIA AREATA FOUNDATION NEWSLETTER. Text in English. 1981. bi-m. USD 35. adv. back issues avail. **Document type:** *Newsletter.*
Published by: National Alopecia Areata Foundation, 710 C St, Ste 11, San Rafael, CA 94901. TEL 415-456-4644, FAX 415-456-4274, naaf@compuserve.com, http://www.alopeciaareata.com. Ed. Rose Kozar. Circ: 7,000.

616.5 USA ISSN 8756-2243
RL321
NATIONAL PSORIASIS FOUNDATION. ANNUAL REPORT. Text in English. a. donation. adv. **Document type:** *Corporate.* **Description:** Provides a summary of the foundation's major activities, programs, and research involvement, in addition to financial statements.
Published by: National Psoriasis Foundation, 6600 S W 92nd Ave, Ste 300, Portland, OR 97223. TEL 503-244-7404, FAX 503-245-0626, getinfo@npfusa.org, http://www.psorias.org. Ed., R&P Sheri Decker. Adv. contact Matt Merenda. Circ: 39,000.

616.5 USA ISSN 1040-0060
NATIONAL PSORIASIS FOUNDATION. BULLETIN. Text in English. 1968. bi-m. donation. adv. **Document type:** *Bulletin.* **Description:** Provides information on psoriasis treatments and includes news of the Foundation's research and activities.
Published by: National Psoriasis Foundation, 6600 S W 92nd Ave, Ste 300, Portland, OR 97223. TEL 503-244-7404, FAX 503-245-0626, getinfo@npfusa.org, http://www.psorias.org. R&P Sheri Decker. Adv. contact Norah Barward. Circ: 39,000.

M

616.5 616.95 NLD ISSN 0925-8604
NEDERLANDS TIJDSCHRIFT VOOR DERMATOLOGIE EN VENEREOLOGIE. Text in Dutch; Summaries in Dutch, English. 1991. 10/yr. NLG 199; NLG 318 foreign (effective 1999). adv. abstr. **Document type:** *Academic/Scholarly.* **Description:** Covers dermatology, dermato-surgery, allergies, and scholarships; also includes original articles and a congress calendar.
Incorporates (1985-1989): Psoriasis News (0920-4520)
—KNAW.
Published by: (Nederlandse Vereniging voor Dermatologie en Venereologie), Elsevier Gezondheidszorg B.V., Tijdstroom (Subsidiary of: Reed Elsevier plc Group), Planetenbaan 1, Maarssen 3600 AK, Netherlands. TEL 31-346-577577, FAX 31-346-554287, http://www.tijdstroom.nl. Ed. M J Korstanje. Pub. C Stauenuiter. Adv. contact Johnan Ysebrands. Circ: 1,425. **Subscr. to:** Elsevier Den Haag, Postbus 16500, The Hague 2500 BM, Netherlands. TEL 31-70-381-9900, FAX 31-70-333-8399.

NETWORK (DURHAM). see *BIRTH CONTROL*

616.5 JPN ISSN 0386-9784
CODEN: NNHIAN
NISHINIHON JOURNAL OF DERMATOLOGY/NISHINIHON HIFUKA. Text in Japanese; Summaries in English. 1933. bi-m. JPY 8,000. adv. bk.rev. bibl, charts, illus. **Document type:** *Academic/Scholarly.*
Supersedes in part: Dermatology and Urology - Hifu to Hinyo (0011-9091)
Indexed: Biol.Abstr., Chem.Abstr., Excerp.Med., INIS Atomind., Ind.Med. (coverage dropped).
—BLDSC (6113.603000), CISTI, EMDOCS, GNLM, KNAW.
Published by: Kyushu University, Faculty of Medicine, Department of Dermatology, 3-1-1 Maidashi, Higashi-ku, Fukuoka-shi 812-0054, Japan. TEL 81-92-641-1151, FAX 81-92-651-0165. Ed. Yoshiaki Hori. Circ: 3,500.

616 FRA ISSN 0752-5370
CODEN: NODEE
NOUVELLES DERMATOLOGIQUES. Text in French. 1982. 10/yr. FRF 450 domestic to individuals; FRF 530 foreign to individuals; FRF 340 to students.
Indexed: Excerp.Med. (1994-).
—BLDSC (6176.762000), EMDOCS, GNLM, Infotrieve, KNAW. **CCC.**
Published by: Initiatives Sante, 26 av. de l'Europe, BP 60, Velizy Villacoublay Cedex 78141, France. TEL 33-1-34633333, FAX 33-1-34653985.

616.5 SWE ISSN 0345-9616
P S O - AKTUELLT. Text in Swedish. 1963. q. bk.rev.
Published by: Svenska Psoriasisfoerbundet, Rokerigatan 19, Johanneshov 12162, Sweden. TEL 46-8-600-36-36, FAX 46-8-600-22-84, pso@pso.se, http://www.pso.se. Ed. Maria G Darin. Pub. Lars Ettarp. adv.: B&W page SEK 7,900, color page SEK 7,900; trim 270 x 190. Circ: 19,800.

PAEDIATRIE HAUTNAH. see *MEDICAL SCIENCES—Pediatrics*

616.5 618.92 USA ISSN 0736-8046
PEDIATRIC DERMATOLOGY. Text in English. 1983. bi-m. USD 230 domestic to individuals; USD 245 in Canada & Mexico to individuals; USD 260 elsewhere to individuals; USD 430 domestic to institutions; USD 445 in Canada & Mexico to institutions; USD 460 elsewhere to institutions; USD 253 domestic to individuals print & online eds. combined; USD 269.50 in Canada & Mexico to individuals print & online eds. combined; USD 286 elsewhere to individuals print & online eds. combined; USD 473 domestic to institutions print & online eds. combined; USD 489.50 in Canada & Mexico to institutions print & online eds. combined; USD 506 elsewhere to institutions print & online eds. combined (effective 2001). adv. bk.rev. reprints avail. *Refereed.* **Document type:** *Academic/Scholarly.* **Description:** Answers the need for new ideas and strategies for today's pediatrician or dematologist.
Related titles: Online - full text ed.: ISSN 1525-1470. USD 207 to individuals; USD 387 to institutions (effective 2001) (from Ovid Technologies, Inc., EBSCO Publishing, O C L C Online Computer Library Center, Inc., RoweCom Information Quest, ingenta, Munksgaard & Blackwell Science's Synergy, Swets Blackwell, Institute for Scientific Information).
Indexed: ASCA, Curr.Cont., INIS Atomind., Ind.Med. (1983-), Inpharma, Int.Abstr.Biol.Sci., Jrnl.Watch Derm., Med.& Surg.Dermat., Nutr.Abstr., Pharm.&Out.News, Protozool.Abstr., Reac., Rev.Appl.Entomol., Rev.Med.& Vet.Mycol., Trop.Dis.Bull.
—BLDSC (6417.582000), CISTI, EMDOCS, GNLM, IDS, ingenta, KNAW. **CCC.**
Published by: (Society for Pediatric Dermatology), Blackwell Science Inc., Commerce Pl, 350 Main St, Malden, MA 02148-5018. TEL 781-388-8250, 800-759-6102, FAX 781-388-8255, journals@blacksci.com, http://www.blackwell-science.com. Ed. Dr. N Esterly. R&P Heather Beal. Adv. contact Tom Palmisano. Circ: 1,300. **Co-sponsor:** International Society of Pediatric Dermatology.

616.5 CHE ISSN 1011-291X
CODEN: PHSKEY
PHARMACOLOGY AND THE SKIN. Text in English. 1987. irreg., latest vol.5. price varies. *Refereed.* **Document type:** *Monographic series, Academic/Scholarly.* **Description:** Spotlights topics at the center of interest in skin pharmacology.
Indexed: Chem.Abstr., Chem.Titles.
—BLDSC (6447.061500), CASDDS, EMDOCS, Infotrieve. **CCC.**
Published by: S. Karger AG, Allschwilerstr 10, PO Box, Basel 4009, Switzerland. TEL 41-61-306-1111, FAX 41-61-306-1234, karger@karger.ch, http://www.karger.com/bookseries/PSKIN. Eds. B Shroot, H Schaefer.

616.5 DNK ISSN 0905-4383
CODEN: PPPHEW
PHOTODERMATOLOGY, PHOTOIMMUNOLOGY & PHOTOMEDICINE. Text and summaries in English. 1984. bi-m. USD 264 in the Americas to institutions print & online eds. combined; GBP 183 elsewhere to institutions print & online eds. combined (effective 2002). adv. illus. *Refereed.* **Document type:** *Academic/Scholarly.*
Formerly: Photodermatology (0108-9684)
Related titles: ♦ Online - full text ed.: Photodermatology, Photoimmunology & Photomedicine Online. ISSN 1600-0781.
Indexed: ASCA, Chem.Abstr., Chem.Indus.Notes, Chem.Titles, Curr.Adv.Ecol.Sci., Curr.Cont., Excerp.Med., INIS Atomind., Ind.Med. (1990-), Inpharma, Int.Abstr.Biol.Sci., Jrnl.Watch Derm., Pharm.&Out.News, Reac., Rev.Arom.& Med.Plants, Sci.Cit.Ind. (coverage dropped).
—BLDSC (6465.991500), CASDDS, CISTI, EMDOCS, GNLM, IDS, Infotrieve, ingenta, KNAW. **CCC.**
Published by: Blackwell Munksgaard, Noerre Soegade 35, PO Box 2148, Copenhagen K 1016, Denmark. TEL 45-77-33-33-33, FAX 45-77-33-33-77, fsub@munksgaard.dk, http://www.munksgaard.dk.photodermatology. Ed. Henry Lim. Adv. contact Eric Rozario TEL 45-77-33-33-01. Circ: 800.

616.5 DNK ISSN 1600-0781
PHOTODERMATOLOGY, PHOTOIMMUNOLOGY & PHOTOMEDICINE ONLINE. Text in English. bi-m. GBP 165 (effective 2002). *Refereed.* **Document type:** *Academic/Scholarly.*
Media: Online - full text (from EBSCO Publishing, ingenta, Swets Blackwell, Institute for Scientific Information). **Related titles:** ♦ Print ed.: Photodermatology, Photoimmunology & Photomedicine. ISSN 0905-4383.
Published by: Blackwell Munksgaard, Noerre Soegade 35, PO Box 2148, Copenhagen K 1016, Denmark. TEL 45-77-33-33-33, FAX 45-77-33-33-77, fsub@mail.munksgaard.dk, http://www.munksgaard.dk.

616.5 ESP ISSN 0213-9251
PIEL. Text in Spanish. 1986. m. (10/yr..). USD 116. adv. reprint service avail. from PQC. **Document type:** *Academic/Scholarly.* **Description:** Offers articles for the continuing education of physicians concerned with dermatology.
Indexed: Ind.Med.Esp.
Published by: Ediciones Doyma S.A., Traversa de Gracia, 17-21, Barcelona 08021, Spain. TEL 34-93-200-0711, FAX 34-93-209-1136. Ed. Carlos Ferrandiz Foraster. Adv. contact Anna Pahissa. color page ESP 292,000; trim 280 x 210. Circ: 3,500.

616.5 USA ISSN 0033-0639
PROGRESS IN DERMATOLOGY. Text in English. 1966. q. membership only. adv. **Document type:** *Academic/Scholarly.*
Published by: Dermatology Foundation, 1560 Sherman Ave, Ste 302, Evanston, IL 60201-4802. Ed. Dr. Thomas Lawley. Circ: 3,000 (controlled).

616.5 POL ISSN 0033-2526
CODEN: PRDEA7
PRZEGLAD DERMATOLOGICZNY. Text in Polish; Summaries in English. 1959. bi-m. USD 1,500. bk.rev. abstr, charts, illus. index. **Document type:** *Academic/Scholarly.* **Description:** Addresses skin problems and sexually transmitted diseases.
Indexed: Biol.Abstr., Chem.Abstr., Dent.Ind., Dok.Arbeitsmed., Excerp.Med., INIS Atomind., Ind.Med. (coverage dropped), Rev.Med.& Vet.Mycol.
—BLDSC (6939.700000), CASDDS, CISTI, GNLM, KNAW.
Published by: (Polskie Towarzystwo Dermatologiczne), Wydawnictwo Medyczne Sanmedica Sp. z o.o., Ul Nowy Zjazd 1, Warsaw 00301, Poland. TEL 48-22-6215180, FAX 48-22-6215180. Ed. Ewa Dabrowska. adv.: B&W page USD 600, color page USD 750. **Dist. by:** Ars Polona, Krakowskie Przedmiescie 7, Warsaw, Poland.

616.5 DEU ISSN 0931-1521
PSO MAGAZIN. Text in German. 1973. 6/yr. membership. adv. Website rev. charts, illus. *Refereed.* **Document type:** *Magazine, Academic/Scholarly.*
Formerly: Psoriasis Magazin
Published by: Deutscher Psoriasis Bund e.V., Oberaltenallee 20A, Hamburg 22081, Germany. TEL 49-40-2233990, FAX 49-40-22339922, dpb.hamburg@t-online.de, http://www.psoriasis-bund.de. Ed. Peter Dlugi.

616.5 AUS
PSORI NEWSLETTER. Text in English. 1979. bi-m. AUD 25 to members. back issues avail. **Document type:** *Newsletter.* **Description:** Articles by dermatologists directed to the general public.
Formerly (until 1986): Skin and Psoriasis Newsletter (1030-7257)
Published by: Psoriasis Association of Victoria Inc., PO Box 1151, Glen Waverley, VIC 3150, Australia. TEL 61-3-95304454, FAX 61-3-95633489. Ed. Helen McNair. Circ: 500.

616.5 USA
PSORIASIS NEWSLETTER. Text in English. 1980. s-a. free per issue. **Document type:** *Newsletter.* **Description:** Reports research advances in the field of dermatology relevant to psoriasis. Directed to the general public.
Published by: Psoriasis Research Institute, 600 Town and Country Village, Palo Alto, CA 94301-2326. TEL 415-326-1848, FAX 415-326-1262. Ed. Dr. Warren Gibson. Circ: 14,000.

616.5 615 USA
PSORIASIS RESOURCE. Text in English. 1989. 3/yr. membership. adv. **Document type:** *Newsletter, Catalog.* **Description:** Provides consumer related articles about over-the-counter and prescription products for psoriasis and ways to cope with psoriasis.
Formerly (until 199?): Pharmacy News (1089-3512)
Published by: National Psoriasis Foundation, 6600 S W 92nd Ave, Ste 300, Portland, OR 97223. TEL 503-244-7404, FAX 503-245-0626, getinfo@npfusa.org, http://www.psoriasis.org. Ed. Sheri Decker. Adv. contact Norah Barnard.

616.5 ITA ISSN 0033-9490
CODEN: RDSIAI
RASSEGNA DI DERMATOLOGIA E SIFILOGRAFIA. Text in Italian. 1948. s-a. ITL 50,000; ITL 100,000 foreign (effective 1998). **Document type:** *Academic/Scholarly.*
Indexed: Excerp.Med. (1994-).
—CISTI, EMDOCS, GNLM.
Published by: Casa Editrice Maccari, Via Palermo, 44, Parma, PR 43100, Italy. TEL 39-521-771268. Circ: 1,200.

616.5 GBR ISSN 0309-2747
RECENT ADVANCES IN DERMATOLOGY. Text in English. 1938. irreg., latest vol.9. **Document type:** *Monographic series, Academic/Scholarly.*
—GNLM, KNAW. **CCC.**
Published by: Churchill Livingstone (Subsidiary of: Harcourt Publishers Ltd.), Robert Stevenson House, 1-3 Baxter's Pl, Leith Walk, Edinburgh, Midlothian EH1 3AF, United Kingdom. TEL 44-131-556-2424, FAX 44-131-459-1177, http://www.churchillmed.com. **US subscr. to:** Churchill Livingstone, 650 Ave of the Americas, New York, NY 10011. TEL 212-206-5000.

616.951 GBR ISSN 0143-6805
RECENT ADVANCES IN SEXUALLY TRANSMITTED DISEASES. Text in English. 1975. irreg., latest vol.4. **Document type:** *Monographic series, Academic/Scholarly.*
—KNAW.
Published by: Churchill Livingstone (Subsidiary of: Harcourt Publishers Ltd.), Robert Stevenson House, 1-3 Baxter's Pl, Leith Walk, Edinburgh, Midlothian EH1 3AF, United Kingdom. TEL 44-131-556-2424, FAX 44-131-459-1177, http://www.churchillmed.com. **US subscr. to:** Churchill Livingstone, 650 Ave of the Americas, New York, NY 10011. TEL 212-206-5000.

REFERATOVY VYBER Z DERMATOVENEROLOGIE/ ABSTRACTS OF DERMATOLOGY AND VENEROLOGY. see *MEDICAL SCIENCES—Abstracting, Bibliographies, Statistics*

616.506 619.9 GBR ISSN 1367-5559
RETINOIDS AND LIPID-SOLUBLE VITAMINS IN CLINICAL PRACTICE. Text in English. 1984. q. GBP 35; GBP 60 foreign. adv. bk.rev. bibl, tr.lit. back issues avail. *Refereed.* **Document type:** *Academic/Scholarly.* **Description:** Contains articles and reviews on the use of retinoids and other lipid-soluble vitamins in dermatology and oncology.
Formerly (until 1997): Retinoids Today and Tomorrow (0953-7368)
Published by: Mediscript Ltd., 1 Mountview Ct, 310 Friern Barnet Ln, London N20 0LD, United Kingdom. TEL 44-20-8446-8898, FAX 44-20-8446-9194, 101607.3205@compuserve.com. Ed., R&P, Adv. contact Linda Lazarus. Pub. Fatima Patel. Circ: 7,000 (paid).

616.95 ESP ISSN 1132-032X
REVISTA IBERO-AMERICANA E T S. (Enfermedades de Transmision Sexual) Text in Spanish; Abstracts in Spanish, English. 1987. bi-m. ESP 8,000; USD 200 foreign (effective 2000). adv. abstr, bibl, illus, stat. *Refereed.* **Document type:** *Academic/Scholarly.*
Published by: Aran Ediciones S.A., Castello, 128 1o, Madrid 28006, Spain. TEL 34-91-782-0030, FAX 34-91-561-5787, edita@grupoaran.com, http://www.grupoaran.com. Pub. Jose Jimenez. R&P Maria Dolores Linares TEL 34-1-7820035. Circ: 2,000.

616.5 ESP ISSN 1138-9427
REVISTA INTERNACIONAL DE DERMATOLOGIA Y DERMOCOSMETICA CLINICA. Text in Spanish. 1993. bi-m. **Document type:** *Academic/Scholarly.* **Description:** Covers various aspects in dermatology and plastic surgery.
Formerly (until 1998): Dermocosmetica Clinica (1132-9513)
Published by: Saned S.A., Capitan Haya, 60, Madrid 28020, Spain. TEL 34-91-749-9506, FAX 34-91-749-9507, saned@meditex.es. Ed. Dr. J Vilata Corell. adv.: page ESP 240,000.

616.9 JPN
S T D: JAPANESE JOURNAL OF THE SEXUALLY TRANSMITTED DISEASES. Text in Japanese. 1921. q. JPY 2,000. adv. stat. **Document type:** *Academic/Scholarly.*
Formerly (until vol.64, 1983): V D: Japanese Journal of Venereal Diseases
Published by: Japanese Association for the Prevention of Venereal Diseases/Nihon Seibyo Yobo Kyokai, 3-14-10 Hongo, Bunkyo-ku, Tokyo 113-0033, Japan. FAX 03-3814-4117. Ed. Tadao Niijima. Circ: 880.

616.5 ITA ISSN 1121-1881
SEMINARI IN DERMATOLOGIA. Text in Italian. 1992. q. adv. 96 p./no. **Document type:** *Journal, Academic/Scholarly.*
Related titles: ♦ English ed.: Seminars in Cutaneous Medicine & Surgery. ISSN 1085-5629.
Indexed: Rev.Med.& Vet.Mycol., Weed Abstr.
Published by: Il Pensiero Scientifico Editore s.r.l., Via Bradano, 3-C, Rome, RM 00199, Italy. TEL 39-06-862821, FAX 39-06-86282250. Pub. Luca De Fiore. Adv. contact Luciano De Fiore. Circ: 5,000.

616.5 USA ISSN 1085-5629
CODEN: SDERDN
SEMINARS IN CUTANEOUS MEDICINE & SURGERY. Text in English. 1982. q. USD 135 domestic to individuals; USD 194 foreign to individuals; USD 197 domestic to institutions; USD 245 foreign to institutions; USD 94 domestic to students; USD 116 foreign to students; USD 62 newsstand/cover (effective 2001). adv. bibl, charts, illus, stat. index. back issues avail. *Refereed.* **Document type:** *Academic/Scholarly.* **Description:** Each issue focuses on a single aspect of the field from several angles as it applies to daily practice.
Formerly (until 1996): Seminars in Dermatology (0278-145X)
Related titles: Microform ed.: (from PQC); Online - full text ed.: (from Institute for Scientific Information); ♦ Italian ed.: Seminari in Dermatologia. ISSN 1121-1881.
Indexed: ASCA, Curr.Cont., Ind.Med. (1996-), Inpharma, Med.& Surg.Dermat., Pharm.&Out.News, Reac.
—BLDSC (8239.448600), CISTI, EMDOCS, GNLM, IDS, Infotrieve, ingenta. **CCC.**
Published by: W.B. Saunders Co. (Subsidiary of: Harcourt Publishers Ltd.), 11830 Westline Industrial Dr, St Louis, MO 63146. TEL 800-325-4177, http://www.wbsaunders.com. adv.: B&W page USD 900, color page USD 1,975; trim 10 x 7. Circ: 1,081. **Subscr. to:** Periodicals Fulfillment, W B Saunders Co, 6277 Sea Harbor Dr, 4th Fl, Orlando, FL 32891-4800.

SEXUAL HEALTH EXCHANGE. see *MEDICAL SCIENCES—Communicable Diseases*

616.951 USA ISSN 0148-5717
RC201.A1 CODEN: STRDDM
SEXUALLY TRANSMITTED DISEASES. Text in English. 1974. m., latest vol.28. USD 235 domestic to individuals; USD 253 foreign to individuals; USD 391 domestic to institutions; USD 415 foreign to institutions; USD 32 newsstand/cover (effective 2002); Print & Online eds. combined. adv. illus. index. *Refereed.* **Document type:** *Academic/Scholarly.* **Description:** Covers all of the human sexually transmitted diseases through original, peer-reviewed articles and special reports from the NIH, the CDC and the ASTDA.
Formerly: American Venereal Disease Association. Journal (0095-148X)
Related titles: Online - full text ed.: USD 508.30 domestic academic site license; USD 532.30 foreign academic site license; USD 566.95 domestic corporate site license; USD 590.95 foreign corporate site license (2002) (from Ovid Technologies, Inc., Gale Group, Factiva, Institute for Scientific Information).
Indexed: AIDS Abstr., CINAHL, Chem.Abstr., Curr.Adv.Ecol.Sci., Curr.Cont., Dent.Ind., Derwent Biotech.Abstr., Excerp.Med. (1993-), Helminthol.Abstr., INIS Atomind., Ind.Med. (1977-), Ind.Sci.Rev., Inpharma, Int.Nurs.Ind., Jrnl.Watch Inf.Dis., Med.& Surg.Dermat., Pharm.&Out.News, Reac., SSCI (coverage dropped), Sci.Cit.Ind.
—BLDSC (8254.486500), CISTI, GNLM, IDS, ingenta, KNAW.
Published by: (American Venereal Disease Association), Lippincott Williams & Wilkins (Philadelphia) (Subsidiary of: Wolters Kluwer N.V.), 530 Walnut St, Philadelphia, PA 19106-3621. TEL 215-521-8300, FAX 215-521-8902, http://www.stdjournal.com, http://www.lww.com. Ed. Julius Schachter. Pub. Shelley Johnson. R&P Margaret Becker. Adv. contact Ray Thibodeau. B&W page USD 645, color page USD 1,605; trim 11 x 8.13. Circ: 1,401. **Subscr. to:** PO Box 1600, Hagerstown, MD 21740-1600. TEL 800-777-2295, FAX 301-824-7390.

616.951 GBR ISSN 1368-4973
RC201.A1 CODEN: STINF9
SEXUALLY TRANSMITTED INFECTIONS; the journal of sexual health and HIV. Text in English. 1925. bi-m. GBP 97, USD 155 combined subscription to individuals includes print & online eds.; GBP 205, USD 324 to institutions for print only (effective 2002). adv. bk.rev. abstr, charts, illus. index. Supplement avail. *Refereed.* **Document type:** *Academic/Scholarly.* **Description:** Presents an international forum for experts in the clinical, microbiological, immunological, behavioral, epidemiological, social, and historical aspects of sexually transmitted diseases.
Former titles (until 1998): Genitourinary Medicine (0266-4348); (until 1984): British Journal of Venereal Diseases (0007-134X); Incorporated: International Union Against the Venereal Diseases and the Treponematoses. Proceedings of Assemblies (0074-9230)
Related titles: CD-ROM ed.: (from Ovid Technologies, Inc.); Microform ed.: (from PQC); Online - full text ed.: S T I Online. ISSN 1472-3263. 2000. GBP 65, USD 99 to individuals (effective 2002); Institutions please contact publisher for online rates. (from ProQuest Information & Learning, Ovid Technologies, Inc., HighWire Pr., EBSCO Publishing, O C L C Online Computer Library Center, Inc., RoweCom Information Quest, ingenta, Swets Blackwell, SilverPlatter Information, Inc., Institute for Scientific Information).
Indexed: AIDS Abstr., ASCA, Abstr.Hyg., Addic.Abstr., Agri.& Environ.Biotech.Abstr. (coverage dropped), Biol.Abstr., Chem.Abstr., Curr.Adv.Ecol.Sci., Curr.Cont., Dent.Ind., Derwent Biotech.Abstr., Excerp.Med., Helminthol.Abstr., Ind.Med. (1998-), Ind.Sci.Rev., Inpharma, Int.Abstr.Biol.Sci., Int.Nurs.Ind., Med.& Surg.Dermat., Pharm.&Out.News, Protozool.Abstr., Reac., Ref.Zh., Rev.Med.& Vet.Mycol., Rev.Plant Path., SSCI (coverage dropped), Sci.Cit.Ind., Trop.Dis.Bull.
—BLDSC (8254.488700), ADONIS, CASDDS, CISTI, EMDOCS, GNLM, IDS, Infotrieve, ingenta, KNAW. **CCC.**
Published by: B M J Publishing Group, B M A House, Tavistock Sq, London WC1H 9JR, United Kingdom. TEL 44-20-7387-4499, FAX 44-20-7383-6400, info.norththames@bma.org.uk, http://www.sextransinf.com, http://www.bma.org.uk. Ed. Mohsen Shahmanesh. Pub. Alex Williamson. R&P Carol Torselli TEL 44-20-7383-6674. Adv. contact Euan Currer TEL 44-20-7383-6181.

SKIN & AGING; the journal of geriatric dermatology. see *GERONTOLOGY AND GERIATRICS*

616.5 USA ISSN 0037-6337
CODEN: SKANB4
SKIN & ALLERGY NEWS. Text in English. 1970. m. USD 70. adv. bk.rev. **Document type:** *Newspaper.*
Related titles: Microform ed.: (from PQC).
—BLDSC (8295.910000), GNLM, Infotrieve. **CCC.**
Published by: International Medical News Group, 12230 Wilkins Ave, Rockville, MD 20852. TEL 301-816-8700. Ed. Catherine Nellist. Circ: 17,500.

SKIN CANCER FOUNDATION JOURNAL. see *MEDICAL SCIENCES—Oncology*

616.5 USA ISSN 0898-6525
SKIN INC.; business and science for skin care professionals. Text in English. 1988. bi-m. USD 49 domestic; USD 57 in Canada; USD 75 elsewhere; USD 10 newsstand/cover in US & Canada; USD 16 newsstand/cover elsewhere (effective 2001). adv. bk.rev. index. back issues avail. **Document type:** *Magazine, Trade.* **Description:** For the aesthetician and skin care professional. Includes treatments, physiology and business articles.
Published by: Allured Publishing, P O Box 506, Mt. Morris, IL 61054-0506. TEL 815-734-1147, 800-469-7445, FAX 815-734-5880, skininc@allured.com, allured@allured.com, http://www.skininc.com, http://www.allured.com. Ed. Marian Raney. Circ: 15,000.

SKIN PHARMACOLOGY AND APPLIED SKIN PHYSIOLOGY. see *PHARMACY AND PHARMACOLOGY*

616.5 JPN ISSN 0018-1390
CODEN: HIFUAG
SKIN RESEARCH* /HIFU. Text in Japanese; Summaries in English. 1959. bi-m. adv. index. **Document type:** *Academic/Scholarly.*
Indexed: Biol.Abstr., Chem.Abstr., INIS Atomind.
—BLDSC (8295.940000), CASDDS, CISTI, GNLM.
Published by: (Osaka Dermatological Association/Nihon Hifukagakkai Osaka Chihokai), Osaka University Press, c/o Osaka Daigaku Jimukyoku, 1-1 Yamada-Oka, Suita-shi, Osaka-fu 565-0871, Japan. Ed. Dr. Minoru Yasuhara. Circ: 1,050.

616.5 DNK ISSN 0909-752X
CODEN: SRTEFN
SKIN RESEARCH AND TECHNOLOGY. Text in English. 1995. q. USD 276 in the Americas to institutions print & online eds. combined; GBP 192 elsewhere to institutions print & online eds. combined (effective 2002). adv. illus. *Refereed.* **Document type:** *Academic/Scholarly.*
Related titles: Online - full text ed.: ISSN 1600-0846. GBP 173 (2001) (from Ovid Technologies, Inc., EBSCO Publishing, O C L C Online Computer Library Center, Inc., ingenta, Swets Blackwell, Institute for Scientific Information).
Indexed: Curr.Cont., INIS Atomind., Int.Abstr.Biol.Sci., Sci.Cit.Ind.
—BLDSC (8295.948000), CISTI, EMDOCS, GNLM, Infotrieve, KNAW. **CCC.**
Published by: Blackwell Munksgaard, Noerre Soegade 35, PO Box 2148, Copenhagen K 1016, Denmark. TEL 45-77-33-33-33, FAX 45-77-33-33-77, fsub@munksgaard.dk, http://www.munksgaard.dk/srt. Ed. Jorgen Serup. Adv. contact Eric Rozario TEL 45-77-33-33-01. Circ: 700.

615.778 CAN ISSN 1201-5989
SKIN THERAPY LETTER. Text in English. 1950. bi-m. CND 85 domestic to individuals; CND 155 domestic to institutions; USD 60 in United States to individuals; USD 110 in United States to institutions; USD 80 out of North America to individuals; USD 130 out of North America to institutions (effective 2000). illus. back issues avail. **Document type:** *Newsletter.* **Description:** Provide information from authoritative sources concerning the treatment of patients, including material on new and existing drugs, that is practical and balanced and has immediate clinical relevance to both clinical practitioners and hospital-based dermatologists.
Media: Online - full text.
Indexed: Ind.Med. (1995-).

M

—BLDSC (8295.949000).
Published by: International Skin Therapy Newsletter, Inc., 835 W Tenth Ave, Vancouver, BC V5Z 4E8, Canada. TEL 604-874-6112, FAX 604-873-9919, smaddin@vanhosp.bc.ca, http://www.derm.ubc.ca. Ed. Dr. Stuart Maddin.

616.5 ZAF ISSN 1015-8782
SOUTHERN AFRICAN JOURNAL OF EPIDEMIOLOGY AND INFECTION. Text in English. 1982. q. ZAR 70; ZAR 180 foreign (effective 1997). adv. bk.rev. charts, illus. back issues avail. *Refereed.* **Document type:** *Academic/Scholarly.* **Description:** Contains articles on infectious diseases, sexually transmitted diseases and epidemiology.
Incorporates: Southern African Journal of Sexually Transmitted Diseases
Indexed: Ind.S.A.Per., Ind.Vet., Nutr.Abstr., Protozool.Abstr., Rev.Med.& Vet.Mycol., Rural Devel.Abstr., Trop.Dis.Bull.
Address: PO Box 1038, Johannesburg 2000, South Africa. TEL 27-11-4899021, FAX 27-11-4899022. Ed. H J Koornhoff. R&P Priscilla May. Adv. contact Louise Blake. Circ: 1,800. **Co-sponsors:** Epidemiological Society of Southern Africa; Infections Diseases Society of Southern Africa; Sexually Transmitted Diseases Society of Southern Africa; South African Institute for Medical Research.

616.5 ITA ISSN 1121-1946
CODEN: GSDOE
GLI SPECIALIZZATI OGGI - DERMATOLOGIA. Text in Italian. 1986. q. ITL 25,000. adv. bk.rev.
Formerly (until 1992): Dermatologia Oggi (0394-2503)
Indexed: Excerp.Med.
—EMDOCS, GNLM.
Published by: E S I Stampa Medica s.r.l., Largo Volontari Del Sangue, 10, Casella Postale 42, San Donato, MI 20133, Italy. TEL 39-2-5274241, FAX 39-2-55600670. Ed. Diego Onestinghel. Adv. contact Ornella Galbiati. B&W page ITL 5,200,000, color page ITL 6,800,000; trim 242 x 162. Circ: 8,700.

616.5 USA
SUN & SKIN NEWS. Text in English. q. USD 25. **Document type:** *Newsletter.* **Description:** Alerts the general public on sun protection, skin health, and skin cancer prevention and treatment.
Published by: Skin Cancer Foundation, 245 Fifth Ave, Ste 2402, New York, NY 10016. TEL 212-725-5176, FAX 212-725-5751. Ed. Joyce Weisbach Ayoub.

616.5 AUS ISSN 1440-6357
▼ **THERAPEUTIC GUIDELINES. DERMATOLOGY.** Text in English. 1999. irreg., latest version 1 (every 3-4 yrs.). AUD 31.90 newsstand/cover (effective 2001). **Document type:** *Academic/Scholarly.*
Related titles: CD-ROM ed.
Published by: Therapeutic Guidelines Ltd., Chelsea House, Level 2, 55 Flemington Rd, North Melbourne, VIC 3051, Australia. TEL 61-3-9329-1566, FAX 61-3-9326-5632, sales@tg.com.au, http://www.tg.com.au. Ed., R&P Mary Hemming. Circ: 18,000.

TOILETRIES, FRAGRANCES AND SKIN CARE: THE ROSE SHEET. see *BEAUTY CULTURE—Perfumes And Cosmetics*

616.5 TUR
CODEN: DHFAE
TURKDERM. Text in Turkish. 1967. q. adv. **Document type:** *Academic/Scholarly.*
Formerly: Deri Hastaliklari ve Frengi Arsivi / Turkish Archives of Dermatology and Syphilology (1019-214X)
Indexed: Excerp.Med.
—EMDOCS, GNLM, KNAW.
Published by: Deri ve Zuhrevi Hastaliklar Dernegi/Istanbul Association of Dermatology and Venereology, Istanbul Universitesi, Tip Fakultesi, Dermatoloji Anabilim Dali, Cerrahpasa - Istanbul 34303, Turkey. TEL 90-212-5313899, FAX 90-212-2345139. Ed. Nahide Onsun.

616.5 TUR ISSN 1300-4301
TURKISH JOURNAL OF DERMATOPATHOLOGY/ DERMATOPATOLOJI DERGESI. Text in English, Turkish. 1991. q. USD 10 to membership; USD 100 foreign to membership. adv. bk.rev. *Refereed.* **Document type:** *Academic/Scholarly.* **Description:** Publishes clinical, pathological and laboratory studies, case reports, reviews and other items of significance to the dermatologic and pathologic community.
Related titles: Online - full text ed.
Indexed: Excerp.Med. (1994-).
—BLDSC (3555.238100).
Published by: Turkish Society of Dermatopathology/ Dermatopatoloji Dernegi, Yenisehir, Mithatpasa Cad 16-11, Ankara 06420, Turkey. TEL 90-312-4300221, FAX 90-312-4300221, cmcelebi@rorqual.cc.metu.edu.tr, http://www.ato.org.tr/konuk/tdp. Ed. Dr. Cengizhan Erdem. R&P, Adv. contact Celalettin R Celebi TEL 90-312-433-1717. Circ: 1,000 (paid).

616.95 AUS ISSN 1032-1012
CODEN: VNERE
VENEREOLOGY; the interdisciplinary international journal of sexual health. Text in English. 1988. q. AUD 110 domestic to individuals; AUD 121 to individuals in New Zealand & Asia; AUD 138 elsewhere to individuals; AUD 165 domestic to institutions; AUD 187 to institutions in New Zealand & Asia; AUD 209 elsewhere to institutions (effective 2001). adv. bk.rev., video rev. charts, illus. cum.index. back issues avail. *Refereed.* **Document type:** *Magazine, Academic/Scholarly.* **Description:** Provides information to those in clinical practice and public health as well as those working in social sciences.
Related titles: Online - full text ed.: (from Institute for Scientific Information).
Indexed: AIDS Abstr., ASCA, ASSIA, Abstr.Hyg., CINAHL, Curr.Cont., Excerp.Med. (1994-), Fam.Ind., Helminthol.Abstr., Lang.& Lang.Behav.Abstr., SOPODA, SSCI, Soc.Serv.Abstr., Sociol.Abstr.
—BLDSC (9154.425400), EMDOCS, GNLM, IDS, ingenta, KNAW.
Published by: Venereology Publishing Inc., National Centre in HIV Social Research, University of New South Wales, Sydney, NSW 2052, Australia. TEL 61-2-9385-6404, FAX 61-2-9385-6455, venereology@unsw.edu.au, http://www.venereology.com. Eds. Basil Donovan, Juliet Richters. Pub. Juliet Richters. R&P Jo Healy-North. adv.: B&W page AUD 880, color page AUD 1,760; trim 297 x 210. Circ: 600 (paid); 100 (controlled).

616.5 616.951 RUS ISSN 0042-4609
CODEN: VDVEAV
VESTNIK DERMATOLOGII I VENEROLOGII/ANNALS OF DERMATOLOGY AND VENEREOLOGY. Text in Russian; Summaries in English. 1924. bi-m. RUR 216 for 6 mos. to individuals; RUR 540 for 6 mos. to institutions (effective 2002). adv. bk.rev. bibl, illus. **Description:** Deals with experimental and clinical dermatology and venereology, control of skin and venereal diseases.
Indexed: Abstr.Hyg., Biol.Abstr., Chem.Abstr., Chem.Indus.Notes, Curr.Cont. (coverage dropped), Dent.Ind., Dok.Arbeitsmed., Excerp.Med., Helminthol.Abstr., INIS Atomind., Ind.Med. (coverage dropped), Protozool.Abstr., Ref.Zh., Sci.Cit.Ind. (coverage dropped), Trop.Dis.Bull.
—CASDDS, CISTI, East View, GNLM, IDS, Infotrieve, KNAW. **CCC.**
Published by: (Nauchnoe Obshchestvo Dermatologov i Venerologov), Media Sfera, Dmitrovskoe shosse 46, korp 2, etazh 4, P.O. Box 54, Moscow 127238, Russian Federation. TEL 7-095-4824329, FAX 7-095-4824312, mediashp@mediasphera.ru. Ed. V A Samsonov. Adv. contact Valery Nemtsov. **Dist. by:** Mezhdunarodnaya Kniga, B Yakimanka 39, Moscow 117049, Russian Federation. TEL 7-095-2384967, FAX 7-095-2384634; **US dist. addr.:** East View Publications, 3020 Harbor Ln N, Minneapolis, MN 55447. TEL 612-550-0961.

VETERINARY DERMATOLOGY; an international journal. see *VETERINARY SCIENCE*

▼ **VETERINARY DERMATOLOGY ONLINE.** see *VETERINARY SCIENCE*

THE WORLD MARKET FOR SKIN CARE AND SUN CARE. see *BEAUTY CULTURE*

WOUND CARE. see *MEDICAL SCIENCES—Communicable Diseases*

616.5 USA
WOUND CARE SOURCEBOOK. Text in English. 1997. a. USD 269; USD 229 foreign (effective 1999). **Document type:** *Trade.*
Published by: American Health Consultants (Subsidiary of: Medical Economics Co., Inc.), 3525 Piedmont Rd, N E, 6 Piedmont Center, Ste 400, Atlanta, GA 30305. TEL 404-262-5476, custserv@ahcpub.com, http://www.ahcpub.com.

▼ **THE YEAR BOOK OF DERMATOLOGY AND DERMATOLOGIC SURGERY.** see *MEDICAL SCIENCES—Abstracting, Bibliographies, Statistics*

616.5 DEU
CODEN: DMONBP
ZEITSCHRIFT FUER DERMATOLOGIE*. Text in German. 1892. bi-m. DEM 99; DEM 105 foreign (effective 1999). adv. bk.rev. bibl, charts, illus, stat. index. **Document type:** *Academic/Scholarly.*
Former titles: Zeitschrift fuer Dermatologie und deren Grenzgebiete (0946-4115); (until 1994): Dermatologische Monatsschrift (0011-9083); Dermatologische Wochenschrift
Indexed: Biol.Abstr., C.I.S. Abstr., Chem.Abstr., Curr.Adv.Ecol.Sci., Dent.Ind., Excerp.Med., Hort.Abstr., INIS Atomind., Ind.Med. (coverage dropped), Rev.Plant Path.
—CASDDS, CISTI, GNLM, Infotrieve, KNAW. **CCC.**
Published by: Johann Ambrosius Barth Verlag in Medizinverlage Heidelberg GmbH & Co. KG, Ruedigerstr 14, Stuttgart 70469, Germany. TEL 49-6221-489281, FAX 49-711-8931422, http://www.thieme.de.

616.5 DEU ISSN 0301-0481
CODEN: ZHKRAJ
ZEITSCHRIFT FUER HAUTKRANKHEITEN H & G. Text in German. 1946. m. DEM 711.92 in Europe to institutions; DEM 375.52 in Europe to individuals; DEM 786.24 elsewhere to institutions; DEM 449.84 elsewhere to individuals; DEM 783.11 in Europe to institutions print & online eds. combined; DEM 413.07 in Europe to individuals print & online eds. combined; DEM 864.86 elsewhere to institutions print & online eds. combined; DEM 494.82 elsewhere to individuals print & online eds. combined (effective 2001). adv. bk.rev. charts, illus, tr.lit. index. *Refereed.* **Document type:** *Journal, Academic/Scholarly.* **Description:** Covers all aspects of clinical dermatology.
Formerly: Zeitschrift fuer Haut- und Geschlechtskrankheiten (0044-2844)
Related titles: ♦ Online - full text ed.: Zeitschrift fuer Hautkrankheiten H & G Online. ISSN 1439-0353.
Indexed: A.D.& D., Agri.& Environ.Biotech.Abstr. (coverage dropped), Biol.Abstr., Curr.Cont. (coverage dropped), Dent.Ind., Derwent Biotech.Abstr., Excerp.Med., Helminthol.Abstr., INIS Atomind., Ind.Med. (coverage dropped), Inpharma, Reac., Ref.Zh., Rev.Med.& Vet.Mycol., Rev.Plant Path.
—BLDSC (9464.322000), CASDDS, CISTI, EMDOCS, GNLM, KNAW. **CCC.**
Published by: (Berliner Dermatologische Gesellschaft), Blackwell Wissenschafts Verlag GmbH, Kurfuerstendamm 57, Berlin 10707, Germany. TEL 49-30-32790624, FAX 49-30-32790610, abo@blackwis.de, http://www.blackwell.de. Eds. Dr. H F Merk, Dr. T Krieg. Adv. contact Jutta Weber-Pianka. Circ: 4,000.

616.5 DEU ISSN 1439-0353
ZEITSCHRIFT FUER HAUTKRANKHEITEN H & G ONLINE. Text in German. m. DEM 338 to individuals; DEM 641 to institutions (effective 2001). *Refereed.* **Document type:** *Academic/Scholarly.*
Media: Online - full text. **Related titles:** ♦ Print ed.: Zeitschrift fuer Hautkrankheiten H & G. ISSN 0301-0481.
Published by: Blackwell Wissenschafts Verlag GmbH, Kurfuerstendamm 57, Berlin 10707, Germany. TEL 49-30-32790624, FAX 49-30-32790610, abo@blackwis.de, http://www.blackwell.de/hg.htm.

ZHONGGUO SHAOSHANG CHUANGSHANG ZAZHI/CHINESE JOURNAL OF BURNS, WOUNDS & SURFACE ULCERS. see *MEDICAL SCIENCES—Orthopedics And Traumatology*

616.5 CHN ISSN 0412-4030
ZHONGHUA PIFUKE ZAZHI/CHINESE JOURNAL OF DERMATOLOGY. Text in Chinese. 1953. bi-m. USD 104.40 foreign; CNY 60 domestic; USD 17.40 newsstand/cover foreign; CNY 10 newsstand/cover domestic (effective 2001). **Document type:** *Academic/Scholarly.*
Published by: Zhonghua Yixue Kexueyuan, Pifu Yanjiusuo, Taipingmen-wai, 14, Jiangwangmiao Jie, Nanjing 210042, China. TEL 86-25-5420299, ZPBJB@public.ptt.js.cn. Ed. Wen-yan Xu. **Dist. by:** China International Book Trading Corp, 35, Chegongzhuang Xilu, Haidian District, Beijing 100044, China. TEL 86-1-68413849, FAX 86-1-68412048, cibtc@mail.cibtc.com.cn, http://www.cibtc.com.cn.

617.11 CHN
ZHONGHUA SHAOSHANG ZAZHI/CHINESE JOURNAL OF BURNS. Text in Chinese. bi-m. USD 31.20; USD 5.20 newsstand/cover (effective 2001). **Document type:** *Academic/Scholarly.*

Published by: Zhonghua Yixuehui Zazhishe, 42 Dongsi Xidajie, Beijing 100710, China. **Dist. by:** China International Book Trading Corp, 35, Chegongzhuang Xilu, Haidian District, Beijing 100044, China. TEL 86-1-68413849, FAX 86-1-68412048, cibtc@mail.cibtc.com.cn, http://www.cibtc.com.cn.

MEDICAL SCIENCES—Endocrinology

616.462 DEU ISSN 0940-5429 CODEN: ACDAEZ
ACTA DIABETOLOGICA; an international journal devoted to the study of clinical and experimental diabetes and metabolism. Text in English. 1964. q. EUR 322.70 domestic; EUR 318.80 in Germany; EUR 91.80 newsstand/cover foreign (effective 2002). bk.rev. abstr, bibl, illus. index. *Refereed.* **Document type:** *Academic/Scholarly.*
Formerly (until 1991): Acta Diabetologica Latina (0001-5563)
Related titles: Microfiche ed.: (from PQC); Online - full text ed.: (from EBSCO Publishing, RoweCom Information Quest, Swets Blackwell, Springer LINK, Institute for Scientific Information).
Indexed: ASCA, Biol.Abstr., Chem.Abstr., Chem.Indus.Notes, Chem.Titles, Curr.Adv.Ecol.Sci., Curr.Cont., Diab.Cont., Excerp.Med., Ind.Med. (1991-), Ind.Sci.Rev., Inpharma, Int.Abstr.Biol.Sci., Nutr.Abstr., Pharm.&Out.News, Reac., Sci.Cit.Ind., Sugar Ind.Abstr.
—BLDSC (0612.399900), CASDDS, CISTI, EMDOCS, GNLM, IDS, Infotrieve, KNAW. **CCC.**
Published by: Springer-Verlag (Subsidiary of: BertelsmannSpringer), Haber Str 7, Heidelberg 69126, Germany. FAX 49-30-82787448, subscriptions@springer.de, http://link.springer.de/link/service/journals/00592/index.htm. Ed. G Pozza. Circ: 5,000. **Subscr. in N. America to:** Springer-Verlag New York Inc., PO Box 2485, Secaucus, NJ 07096-2485. TEL 212-460-1500, FAX 212-473-6272.

616.4 ARG ISSN 0065-1192
ACTA ENDOCRINOLOGICA PANAMERICANA* . Text in Spanish. 1970. irreg. **Document type:** *Proceedings.*
Indexed: INIS Atomind.
Published by: Panamerican Federation of Endocrine Societies, c/o Dr. Noe Altschuler, 25 De Mayo, 648, Vicente Lopez, Buenos Aires 1638, Argentina.

616.4 618.2 610.73 ITA ISSN 0001-6004 CODEN: AMAXBK
ACTA MEDICA AUXOLOGICA. Text in English, Italian. 1969. 3/yr. ITL 87,000, USD 90 (effective 2000). adv. bk.rev. abstr, bibl, illus. index. back issues avail. *Refereed.* **Document type:** *Journal, Academic/Scholarly.*
Indexed: Biol.Abstr., Curr.Adv.Ecol.Sci., Curr.Cont. (coverage dropped), Excerp.Med., Ind.Med. (coverage dropped), Nutr.Abstr., Psychol.Abstr., Ref.Zh.
—BLDSC (0633.200000), GNLM.
Published by: Istituto Auxologico Italiano, Via Lodovico Ariosto, 13, Milan, MI 20145, Italy. TEL 39-2-58216896, FAX 39-2-58216901, info@masson.it, http://www.masson.it. Ed. Francesco Morabito. Circ: 3,000. **Subscr. to:** Masson S.p.A., Divisione Periodici, Via F.lli Bressan 2, Milan, MI 20126, Italy.

616.4 USA
RC620.A1 CODEN: AMTDAK
ADVANCES IN METABOLISM. Text in English. 1964. irreg., latest vol.13, 1987. reprint service avail. from ISI. *Refereed.*
Formerly (until vol.11): Advances in Metabolic Disorders (0065-2903); Which supersedes: Advances in Metabolic Disorders. Supplements (0587-4394)
Indexed: Biol.Abstr., Curr.Adv.Ecol.Sci.
—CASDDS, CISTI, GNLM, Infotrieve, Linda Hall. **CCC.**
Published by: Academic Press, Inc., Journal Division (Subsidiary of: Harcourt Brace & Company), 525 B St, Ste 1900, San Diego, CA 92101-4495. TEL 619-231-0926, FAX 619-699-6715. **Subscr. to:** Order Dept., 6277 Sea Harbor Dr, 4th Fl, Orlando, FL 32887. TEL 800-321-5068.

616.4 GBR ISSN 1362-9670 CODEN: ARENFF
ADVANCES IN REPRODUCTIVE ENDOCRINOLOGY. Text in English. 1989. irreg., latest vol.8. adv. **Document type:** *Monographic series.*
Indexed: Chem.Abstr., Chem.Indus.Notes, Chem.Titles.
—CASDDS.
Published by: Parthenon Publishing Group (Subsidiary of: C R C Press (New York)), Casterton Hall, Casterton, Carnforth, Lancs LA6 2LA, United Kingdom. TEL 44-1524-272084, FAX 44-1524-271587, mail@parthpub.com, http://www.parthpub.com/. R&P Jean Wright. Adv. contact Julia Tissington.

616.46 362.1 AUS ISSN 0706-1870
ALERT (ADELAIDE). Text in English. 1980. q. AUD 27 to members. adv. bk.rev. *Refereed.* **Document type:** *Consumer.* **Description:** Contains articles and general items related to diabetes management and the products and services offered by Diabetes Australia to make the task of diabetes management easier.
Published by: Diabetic Association of South Australia, Unit 4, 159 Burbridge Rd., Hilton, SA 5033, Australia. TEL 61-8-8234-1977, FAX 61-8-8234-2013. Ed. Jennifer Barber. Adv. contact Cheryl Bawden. Circ: 14,200 (paid).

AMERICAN JOURNAL OF KIDNEY DISEASES. see *MEDICAL SCIENCES—Urology And Nephrology*

AMERICAN JOURNAL OF PHYSIOLOGY: ENDOCRINOLOGY AND METABOLISM. see *BIOLOGY—Physiology*

616.4 FRA ISSN 0003-4266 CODEN: ANENAG
ANNALES D'ENDOCRINOLOGIE. Text and summaries in English, French. 1939. bi-m. FRF 1,308; FRF 1,584 foreign (effective 2000). adv. bk.rev. illus. index. reprint service avail. from ISI. *Refereed.* **Document type:** *Academic/Scholarly.* **Description:** Publishes reports of meetings of Belgian and French societies, original articles, biological and clinical notes and commentaries.
Related titles: Microform ed.: (from PQC); Online - full text ed.: (from Institute for Scientific Information, RoweCom Information Quest).
Indexed: ASCA, Anim.Breed.Abstr., Biol.Abstr., Chem.Abstr., Chem.Indus.Notes, Chem.Titles, Curr.Adv.Ecol.Sci., Curr.Cont., Dairy Sci.Abstr., Excerp.Med., INIS Atomind., Ind.Med. (1939-), Ind.Sci.Rev., Inpharma, Int.Abstr.Biol.Sci., Nutr.Abstr., Pharm.&Out.News, Reac., Sci.Cit.Ind.
—BLDSC (0972.000000), CASDDS, CISTI, EMDOCS, GNLM, IDS, Infotrieve, KNAW. **CCC.**
Published by: (Societe Francaise d'Endocrinologie), Masson - Periodiques, 120 bd. St. Germain, Paris 75006, France. TEL 33-1-40466200, FAX 33-1-40466201. Ed. P J Leclere. Circ: 1,500. **Subscr. to:** Societe de Periodiques Specialises, BP 22, Vineuil Cedex 41354, France. TEL 33-2-54504612, FAX 33-2-54504611.

616.4 JPN
ANNUAL REVIEW NAIBUNPI TAISHA/ANNUAL REVIEW. ENDOCRINE AND METABOLISM. Text in Japanese. a. JPY 9,975 (effective 1998). adv. **Document type:** *Academic/Scholarly.*
Published by: Chugai Igakusha, 62 Yarai-cho, Shinjuku-ku, Tokyo 162-0805, Japan. R&P M Takahashi. Adv. contact M. Takahashi.

APOTHEKEN-MAGAZIN FUER SENIOREN & DIABETIKER. see *PHYSICAL FITNESS AND HYGIENE*

616.4 BRA ISSN 0004-2730 CODEN: ABENAY
ARQUIVOS BRASILEIROS DE ENDOCRINOLOGIA E METABOLOGIA. Text in English, French, Portuguese, Spanish. 1951-1973; resumed 1978. q. free per issue. bk.rev. bibl, charts, illus. index.
Indexed: Biol.Abstr., Chem.Abstr., Excerp.Med., INIS Atomind., Ind.Med. (coverage dropped), Nutr.Abstr.
—CASDDS, GNLM.
Published by: Universidade de Sao Paulo, Faculdade de Filosofia, Letras e Ciencias Humanas, Av Dr Arnaldo, 455, Pacaembu, Caixa Postal 8100, Sao Paulo, SP 01246-000, Brazil. Ed. Antonio Roberto Chacra.

573.4 USA ISSN 1522-4120
ARTHROPOD ENDOCRINOLOGY NEWS. Text in English. 1998. m. USD 190; USD 220 foreign (effective 1999). **Document type:** *Academic/Scholarly.* **Description:** Designed to keep readers abreast of the latest development in the field of endocrinology.
Related titles: Online - full text ed.
Published by: Scientific Reference Resources, PO Box 73674, Davis, CA 95616. aen@sciref.org, http://www.sciref.org/aen/arthendo.htm. Ed. Michael L Grieneisen.

ATRIAL NATRIURETIC FACTORS. see *MEDICAL SCIENCES—Abstracting, Bibliographies, Statistics*

AUSTRALIA. BUREAU OF STATISTICS. NATIONAL HEALTH SURVEY: DIABETES, AUSTRALIA. see *MEDICAL SCIENCES—Abstracting, Bibliographies, Statistics*

616.4 GBR ISSN 1521-690X CODEN: BBPMFY
BAILLIERE'S BEST PRACTICE & RESEARCH IN CLINICAL ENDOCRINOLOGY AND METABOLISM. Text in English. 1987. q. GBP 111 to individuals; GBP 187 to institutions (effective 2002). *Refereed.* **Document type:** *Academic/Scholarly.*
Formerly: Bailliere's Clinical Endocrinology and Metabolism (0950-351X)
Related titles: Online - full text ed.: (from EBSCO Publishing, O C L C Online Computer Library Center, Inc., Swets Blackwell, IDEAL Online Library, Institute for Scientific Information, RoweCom Information Quest).
Indexed: ASCA, Curr.Cont., Diab.Cont., Excerp.Med., Ind.Med. (1999-), Ind.Sci.Rev., Inpharma, Pharm.&Out.News, Reac., Ref.Zh., SSCI (coverage dropped), Sci.Cit.Ind., Soyabean Abstr.
—BLDSC (3286.279200), CISTI, EMDOCS, GNLM, IDS, ingenta, KNAW. **CCC.**
Published by: Bailliere Tindall (Subsidiary of: Harcourt Publishers Ltd.), 24-28 Oval Rd, London NW1 7DX, United Kingdom. TEL 44-20-7424-4200, FAX 44-20-7424-4515, cservice@harcourt.com, http://www.harcourt-international.com/journals/beem/. **Subscr to:** Harcourt Publishers Ltd., Foots Cray High St, Sidcup, Kent DA14 5HP, United Kingdom. TEL 44-20-8308-5700, FAX 44-20-8309-0807.

616.462 GBR ISSN 0005-4216
BALANCE. Text in English. 1935. bi-m. GBP 2 newsstand/cover (effective 2000). adv. bk.rev. illus. **Document type:** *Magazine, Consumer.* **Description:** For people with diabetes and their families: medical and dietary information and research news.
Published by: Diabetes UK, 10 Queen Anne St, London W1G 9LH, United Kingdom. TEL 44-207-323-1531, FAX 44-207-636-5762, balance@diabetes.org.uk, http://www.diabetes.org.uk. Ed. Lesley Hallett. Pub. John Isitt. adv.: B&W page GBP 2,430, color page GBP 3,500; trim 210 x 297. Circ: 208,000. **Dist. by:** Seymour, 86 Newman St, London W1P 3EX, United Kingdom. TEL 44-20-7396-8000, FAX 44-20-7396-8002.

BARIATRICIAN. see *MEDICAL SCIENCES—Internal Medicine*

616.4 USA ISSN 0891-2068
RC648.A1
BASIC & CLINICAL ENDOCRINOLOGY. Text in English. 1981. irreg., latest vol.9, 1987. adv. *Refereed.*
Indexed: Chem.Abstr., Chem.Indus.Notes, Chem.Titles.
—CCC.
Published by: Marcel Dekker, Inc., Attn: Eridania Perrez, 270 Madison Ave, New York, NY 10016-0602. TEL 212-696-9000, 800-228-1160, FAX 212-685-4540, marketing@dekker.com, http://www.dekker.com. Pub. Russell Dekker. R&P Julia Mulligan. Adv. contact Eridania Perez.

▼ **BEST RECIPES DIABETIC COOKING.** see *FOOD AND FOOD INDUSTRIES*

BONE. see *MEDICAL SCIENCES—Orthopedics And Traumatology*

616.462 GBR ISSN 1474-6514
▼ **THE BRITISH JOURNAL OF DIABETES AND VASCULAR DISEASE.** Text in English. 2001 (Aug.). q. GBP 75 in United Kingdom to individuals; GBP 95 in Europe to individuals; GBP 100 elsewhere to individuals; GBP 150 in United Kingdom to institutions; GBP 175 in Europe to institutions; GBP 200 elsewhere to institutions (effective 2002).
Published by: MediNews (Diabetes) Ltd. (Subsidiary of: J R A A S Ltd), Edgbaston House, 3 Duchess Pl, Birmingham B16 8NH, United Kingdom. TEL 44-121-454-4114, FAX 44-121-454-1190, ngibbs@sherbornegibbs@co.uk.

616.4 617.3 USA ISSN 0171-967X
QP88 CODEN: CTINDZ
CALCIFIED TISSUE INTERNATIONAL. Text in English. 1967. m. (in 2 vols., 6 nos./vol.). USD 974 domestic for Print & Online Eds.; USD 1,982.30 in Germany for Print & Online Eds.; USD 96.40 newsstand/cover foreign (effective 2002). adv. back issues avail.; reprints avail. *Refereed.* **Document type:** *Academic/Scholarly.* **Description:** Serves as a forum to explore biochemical, biophysical, and clinical aspects of bone structure, function, and metabolism.
Formerly: Calcified Tissue Research (0008-0594)
Related titles: Microform ed.: (from PQC); Online - full text ed.: ISSN 1432-0827 (from EBSCO Publishing, RoweCom Information Quest, Swets Blackwell, Springer LINK, Institute for Scientific Information).

M

Indexed: ASCA, Abstr.Anthropol., Aqua.Sci.& Fish.Abstr., Biol.Abstr., Cal.Tiss.Abstr., Chem.Abstr., Chem.Indus.Notes, Chem.Titles, Curr.Adv.Cell & Devel.Biol., Curr.Adv.Ecol.Sci., Curr.Cont., Curr.Tit.Dent., Dairy Sci.Abstr., Dent.Ind., Environ.Sci.Poll.Mgmt., Excerp.Med., GeoRef, INIS Atomind., Ind.Med. (1979-), Ind.Sci.Rev., Ind.Vet., Inpharma, Int.Aerosp.Abstr., NRN, Nutr.Abstr., Pharm.&Out.News, Pig News & Info., Poult.Abstr., Reac., Risk Abstr., SSCI (coverage dropped), Sci.Cit.Ind., Tox.Abstr. (coverage dropped), Vet.Bull.
—BLDSC (2952.840000), CASDDS, CISTI, EMDOCS, GNLM, IDS, ingenta, KNAW, Linda Hall. **CCC.**
Published by: Springer-Verlag, Journals (Subsidiary of: BertelsmannSpringer), 175 Fifth Ave, New York, NY 10010. TEL 212-460-1500, FAX 212-473-6272, orders@springer-ny.com, http://www.springer-ny.com. Eds. A. Ralston, K. Hruska, R. Civitelli. R&P Ian Gross. Adv. contact Jay Feinman. **N. American subscr. to:** Journal Fulfillment Services, PO Box 2485, Secaucus, NJ 07096-2485. TEL 800-777-4643, FAX 201-348-4505.

616.462 CAN
CANADIAN JOURNAL OF DIABETES CARE. Text in English; Summaries in English, French. q. CND 35. adv. bk.rev. *Refereed.* **Document type:** *Academic/Scholarly.*
Formerly: Beta Release (0710-0248)
Indexed: CINAHL.
—CISTI. **CCC.**
Published by: Canadian Diabetes Association, 15 Toronto St, Ste 800, Toronto, ON M5C 2E3, Canada. TEL 416-363-3373, FAX 416-363-7465, info@diabetes.ca, http://www.diabetes.ca; http://www.medscape.com. Ed. George Fantus. R&P Jeanne McKane. Adv. contact Tom Cowell. Circ: 4,500 (controlled).

CHRONOBIOLOGIA. see *BIOLOGY*

616.4 615.533 JPN ISSN 0917-5857
CODEN: CLCCEJ
CLINICAL CALCIUM. Text in Japanese. 1991. m. JPY 31,500 (effective 2000). adv. **Document type:** *Academic/Scholarly.*
Indexed: Chem.Abstr., Chem.Indus.Notes, Chem.Titles.
—BLDSC (3286.264400), CASDDS.
Published by: Iyaku Journal-sha/Medicine & Drug Journal Co., Ltd., 2-8 Hirano-Machi 3-chome, Chuo-ku, Osaka-shi 541-0046, Japan. TEL 81-6-6202-7280, FAX 81-6-6202-5295, iyakujor@skyblue.ocn.ne.jp, http://www.so-net.ne.jp/medipro/iyaku. R&P, Adv. contact Kiriko Numata.

616.46 USA ISSN 0891-8929
CODEN: CLDIE8
CLINICAL DIABETES. Text in English. 1983. q. USD 50 to individuals in United States & Mexico; USD 53.50 in Canada to individuals; USD 61 elsewhere to individuals; USD 100 to institutions in United States & Mexico; USD 107 in Canada to institutions; USD 85 elsewhere to institutions (effective 2001). adv. back issues avail. *Refereed.* **Description:** Provides physicians and clinicians with information on advances and state of the art care for people with diabetes. Includes issues in practice, medical-legal issues, recent research and patient education materials.
Related titles: Online - full text ed.: (from Gale Group, Ovid Technologies, Inc., Northern Light Technology, Inc., EBSCO Publishing, ProQuest Information & Learning, Factiva).
Indexed: Diab.Cont.
—BLDSC (3286.272700), CISTI, GNLM, Infotrieve. **CCC.**
Published by: American Diabetes Association, 1701 N. Beauregard St., Alexandria, VA 22311-1717. TEL 800-232-3472, FAX 703-549-6995, 703-683-2890, http://diabetes.diabetesjournals.org/, http://www.diabetes.org. Circ: 50,000 (paid and controlled).

616.4 GBR ISSN 0300-0664
CODEN: CLECAP
CLINICAL ENDOCRINOLOGY. Text in English. 1972. m., latest vol.56, 2002. GBP 628 in Europe; USD 996 in North America; GBP 691 elsewhere (effective 2002). adv. bk.rev. index. back issues avail.; reprint service avail. from ISI. *Refereed.* **Document type:** *Academic/Scholarly.* **Description:** Publishes papers and reviews which focus on the practical aspects of clinical endocrinology, such as protocols for investigation of endocrine disorders, imaging in endocrinology and the clinical application of molecular endocrinology.
Related titles: Microform ed.: (from PQC); Online - full text ed.: ISSN 1365-2265. 1997. GBP 566 in Europe; USD 897 in North America; GBP 566 elsewhere (effective 2002) (from Ovid Technologies, Inc., EBSCO Publishing, O C L C Online Computer Library Center, Inc., RoweCom Information Quest, ingenta, Munksgaard & Blackwell Science's Synergy, Swets Blackwell, Institute for Scientific Information).
Indexed: ASCA, Abstr.Inter.Med., Agri.& Environ.Biotech.Abstr. (coverage dropped), Biol.Abstr., Chem.Abstr., Chem.Indus.Notes, Chem.Titles, Curr.Adv.Ecol.Sci., Curr.Adv.Gen.& Molec.Biol., Curr.Cont., Dairy Sci.Abstr., Derwent Biotech.Abstr., Diab.Cont., Excerp.Med., INIS Atomind., Ind.Med. (1972-), Ind.Sci.Rev., Inpharma, Int.Abstr.Biol.Sci., Nutr.Abstr., Pharm.&Out.News, Reac., Ref.Zh., Sci.Cit.Ind., THA.
—BLDSC (3286.278000), ADONIS, CASDDS, CISTI, EMDOCS, GNLM, IDS, ingenta, KNAW. **CCC.**
Published by: Blackwell Science Ltd., PO Box 88, Oxford OX2 0NE, United Kingdom. TEL 44-1865-206180, 44-1865-206002, FAX 44-1865-206219, jnl.orders@blacksci.co.uk, http://www.blackwell-science.com/products/journals/cend.htm, http://www.blackwellpublishing.com. Ed. S Franks. Pub. Allen Stevens. R&P Sophie Savage. Adv. contact Jenny Applin. Circ: 1,810.

616.4 616.15 DEU ISSN 1433-6510
CODEN: KLLAEA
CLINICAL LABORATORY; journal for clinical laboratories and laboratories related to blood transfusion. Text and summaries in English. 1955. 6/yr. DEM 139.50 domestic; DEM 150 foreign (effective 2000). bk.rev. bibl, charts, illus. cum.index. back issues avail. *Refereed.* **Document type:** *Journal, Academic/Scholarly.* **Description:** Publication for physicians concerning the latest research and findings in medical laboratories. Covers all fields of medicine and includes announcements of events and list of suppliers.
Former titles (until 1995): Klinisches Labor (0941-2131); Aerztliche Laboratorium (0001-9526)
Indexed: Biol.Abstr., Chem.Abstr., Chem.Indus.Notes, Chem.Titles, Curr.Adv.Ecol.Sci., Curr.Cont. (coverage dropped), Excerp.Med., INIS Atomind., Ind.Med. (1997-), Int.Abstr.Biol.Sci., Mass Spectr.Bull., Ref.Zh.
—BLDSC (3286.295600), CASDDS, CISTI, EMDOCS, GNLM, IDS, Infotrieve, KNAW. **CCC.**
Published by: Clinical Laboratory Publications, Im Breitspiel 15, Heidelberg 69126, Germany. TEL 49-6221-3432115, FAX 49-6221-300291, clin.lab.publications@t-online.de, http://www.clin-lab-publications.de. Ed., R&P Heinrich Schmidt-Gayk. Adv. contact Ellen Buck TEL 49-6221-3432133. Circ: 3,000; 2,000 (paid).

CLINICAL PEDIATRIC ENDOCRINOLOGY. see *MEDICAL SCIENCES—Pediatrics*

616.462 USA
CLINICAL PRACTICE RECOMMENDATIONS. Text in English. a. USD 13.60 to individuals; free with subscr. to Diabetes Care.
Related titles: ♦ Supplement to: Diabetes Care. ISSN 0149-5992.
Published by: American Diabetes Association, 1701 N. Beauregard St., Alexandria, VA 22311-1717. TEL 703-549-1500, FAX 703-836-7439.

616.4 USA ISSN 1050-3374
CLINICAL SURVEYS IN ENDOCRINOLOGY. Text in English. 1987. irreg., latest vol.2, 1988. price varies. back issues avail. *Refereed.* **Document type:** *Monographic series.*
Published by: Kluwer Academic - Plenum Publishers (Subsidiary of: Wolters Kluwer N.V.), 233 Spring St, New York, NY 10013-1578. TEL 212-620-8000, 800-221-9369, FAX 212-463-0742, info@plenum.com, http://www.plenum.com. Ed. C R Kannan.

616.4 USA ISSN 0160-242X
COMPREHENSIVE ENDOCRINOLOGY. Text in English. 1978. irreg. reprint service avail. from PQC. *Refereed.* **Document type:** *Monographic series.*
—KNAW.
Published by: Lippincott Williams & Wilkins (Philadelphia) (Subsidiary of: Wolters Kluwer N.V.), 530 Walnut St, Philadelphia, PA 19106-3621. TEL 301-223-2300, 800-638-3030, FAX 301-223-2400.

616.4 USA ISSN 0196-8653
QP187.A1 CODEN: CNEND7
CONTEMPORARY ENDOCRINOLOGY. Text in English. 1976; N.S. 1996. irreg., latest vol.21, 1999. price varies. illus. back issues avail. *Refereed.* **Document type:** *Monographic series, Academic/Scholarly.* **Description:** Provides a forum whereby endocrinologists and other medical professionals (physicians and researchers) review the latest research, treatment protocols, and drug regimens for patients suffering from metabolic and other endocrine disorders.
Formerly (until 1979): Year in Endocrinology (0146-4078)
Indexed: Chem.Abstr.
—CASDDS, CISTI, GNLM. **CCC.**
Published by: Humana Press Inc., 999 Riverview Dr, Ste 208, Totowa, NJ 07512. TEL 973-256-1699, FAX 973-256-8341, humana@humanapr.com, http://humanapress.com. Ed. P Michael Conn. R&P Richard Hruska.

616.4 USA ISSN 0193-340X
RC627.5 CODEN: CONMDM
CONTEMPORARY METABOLISM; analytical reviews of basic & clinical progress. Text in English. 1976. irreg., latest vol.2, 1982. *Refereed.* **Document type:** *Monographic series.*
Formerly: Year in Metabolism (0147-4189)
—CASDDS, CISTI, GNLM.
Published by: Kluwer Academic - Plenum Publishers (Subsidiary of: Wolters Kluwer N.V.), 233 Spring St, New York, NY 10013-1578. TEL 212-620-8000, 800-221-9369, FAX 212-463-0742, info@plenum.com, http://www.plenum.com. Ed. Norbert Freinkel.

616.4 DEU ISSN 0933-002X
CORTISON SPIEGEL. Text in German. 1988. q. back issues avail. **Document type:** *Academic/Scholarly.*
Published by: P M I Verlag AG, August-Schanz-Str 8, Frankfurt Am Main 60433, Germany. TEL 49-69-548000-0, FAX 49-69-548000-77, pmiverlag@aol.com. Ed. E Merck. Circ: 60,000.

612.4 GBR ISSN 0964-8720
QP1
CURRENT ADVANCES IN ENDOCRINOLOGY & METABOLISM. Text in English. 1984. m. EUR 120 in Europe to qualified personnel; JPY 16,275 in Japan to qualified personnel; USD 135 elsewhere to qualified personnel; EUR 1,184 in Europe to institutions; JPY 156,991 in Japan to institutions; USD 1,325 elsewhere to institutions (effective 2002). adv. **Document type:** *Abstract/Index.* **Description:** Provides current awareness service in the fields of endocrinology and metabolic studies. Gives listings of titles of these papers published throughout the world classified into 149 main areas and provides a comprehensive listing of review articles.
Formerly (until 1992): Current Advances in Physiology (0741-1693)
Related titles: Diskette ed.; Microfilm ed.: (from PQC); Online - full text ed.
Indexed: Curr.Cont. (coverage dropped).
—BLDSC (3494.063700), GNLM, Infotrieve. **CCC.**
Published by: Elsevier Science BV, PO Box 211, Amsterdam 1000 AE, Netherlands. TEL 31-20-485-2911, FAX 31-20-485-2457, http://www.elsevier.com/locate/caendo, http://www.elsevier.nl. **Subscr. in Australasia and the Far East to:** Elsevier Science (Singapore) Pte Ltd, No.1 Temasek Ave, 17-01 Millenia Tower, Singapore 039192, Singapore. TEL 65-434-3727, FAX 65-337-2230; **Subscr. in Japan to:** Elsevier Science Inc - Japan Regional Office, 9-15 Higashi-Azabu 1-chome, Minato-ku, Tokyo 106-0044, Japan. TEL 81-3-5561-5033; **Subscr. in the Americas to:** Elsevier Science, PO Box 945, New York, NY 10159-0945. TEL 212-633-3730, FAX 212-633-3680, usinfo-f@elsevier.com.

616.4 JPN ISSN 0912-2249
CURRENT CONCEPTS IN MAGNESIUM METABOLISM/MAGUNESHUMU TAISHA KONNICHI NO KANAEKATA. Text in Japanese. 1985. q.
Published by: Standard McIntyre/Sutandado Makkintaiya, 3-7 Irifune 2-chome, Chuo-ku, Tokyo 104-0042, Japan.

CURRENT MEDICAL LITERATURE. DIABETES. see *MEDICAL SCIENCES—Abstracting, Bibliographies, Statistics*

M

616.4 USA ISSN 1068-3097
CODEN: CENDES
CURRENT OPINION IN ENDOCRINOLOGY & DIABETES. Text in English. 1994. bi-m. USD 230 domestic to individuals for print & online eds.; USD 230 foreign to individuals for print & online eds.; USD 83 newsstand/cover; USD 539 per issue domestic to institutions; USD 539 per issue foreign to institutions (effective 2002). adv. **Document type:** *Academic/Scholarly.*
Related titles: Online - full text ed.: USD 700.70 domestic academic site license; USD 700.70 foreign academic site license; USD 781.55 domestic corporate site license; USD 781.55 foreign corporate site license (effective 2002) (from Ovid Technologies, Inc., EBSCO Publishing, Swets Blackwell).
Indexed: Biotech.& Bioeng.Abstr. (coverage dropped), CINAHL, Cal.Tiss.Abstr., Chem.Abstr., Chem.Indus.Notes, Chem.Titles, Chemorec.Abstr., Genet.Abstr. (coverage dropped), Neurosci.Abstr. (coverage dropped), Nuc.Acids Abstr.
—BLDSC (3500.774200), ADONIS, CASDDS, GNLM.
Published by: Lippincott Williams & Wilkins (Philadelphia) (Subsidiary of: Wolters Kluwer N.V.), 530 Walnut St, Philadelphia, PA 19106-3621. FAX 215-521-8902, 215-521-8902, http://www.Lww.com. Ed. Lewis E Braverman. Pub. Maria McMichael. R&P Tobias Weschler. Adv. contact Kelly Adamitis. **Subscr. to:** PO Box 1600, Hagerstown, MD 21740-1600.

CURRENT TOPICS IN NEUROENDOCRINOLOGY. see *MEDICAL SCIENCES—Psychiatry And Neurology*

616.462 NLD ISSN 0166-7629
DIABC. Text in Dutch. 1970. 11/yr. NLG 7.50. **Document type:** *Bulletin.*
Published by: Diabetes Vereniging Nederland, Postbus 933, Amersfoort 3800 AX, Netherlands. TEL 31-33-4630566, FAX 31-33-4630930. Ed. Gaby de Reus. R&P Mrs. P Kaatee-Bieler. Circ: 49,000.

616.46 ITA ISSN 0394-901X
IL DIABETE. Text in Italian. 1989. q. EUR 51.65 domestic; USD 80 foreign (effective 2002).
Related titles: Online - full text ed.: EUR 25.82 (effective 2002).
Published by: (Italian Society of Diabetology), Editrice Kurtis s.r.l., Via Luigi Zoja, 30, Milan, MI 20153, Italy. TEL 39-02-48202740, FAX 39-02-4820-1219, info@kurtis.it, http://www.kurtis.it. Ed. Riccardo Vigneri.

616.462 DNK ISSN 0901-3652
DIABETES. Text in Danish. 1941. bi-m. DKK 110. **Document type:** *Academic/Scholarly.*
Former titles (until 1985): Tidsskrift for Sukkersyge (0900-3215); (until 1948): Landsforeningen for Sukkersyge (0909-6949)
Related titles: Online - full text ed.: (from Northern Light Technology, Inc.).
Published by: Diabetesforeningen/Danish Diabetes Association, Filosofgangen 24, Odense C 5000, Denmark. TEL 45-66-12-90-06, FAX 45-66-13-58-83. Ed. Flemming Kjaersgaard Johansen. adv.: B&W page DKK 8,710, color page DKK 16,648. Circ: 40,000.

616.462 SWE ISSN 0419-0459
DIABETES. Text in Swedish. 1948. bi-m. SEK 190. adv. 40 p./no. 3 cols./p. **Document type:** *Magazine, Consumer.*
Related titles: Online - full text ed.: (from Northern Light Technology, Inc.).
Published by: Svenska Diabetesfoerbundet, Fack 1107, Sundbyberg 17222, Sweden. TEL 46-8-564-821-00, FAX 46-8-564-821-39, info@diabetes.se, http://www.diabetes.se. Eds. Ann Sofie Lindberg, Ulla Emstroem. Pub. Anders Ericson. adv.: B&W page SEK 14,400, color page SEK 21,500; trim 195 x 270. Circ: 33,900.

616.462 FIN ISSN 0046-0192
DIABETES. Text in Finnish; Section in Swedish. 1949. 10/yr. FIM 150 to non-members; FIM 40 to members (effective 2000). adv. illus. *Refereed.* **Document type:** *Journal, Academic/Scholarly.* **Description:** Covers diabetes care and health care, research, psychological and social aspects of diabetes, for persons with diabetes and health professionals.
Related titles: Online - full text ed.: (from Northern Light Technology, Inc.).
Indexed: Abstr.Inter.Med., Curr.Adv.Biochem., Curr.Cont. (coverage dropped), NRN.
Published by: Finnish Diabetes Association, Kirjoniementie 15, Tampere 33680, Finland. TEL 358-3-28-60-111, FAX 358-3-3600-462, lehdet@diabetes.fi, http://www.diabetes.fi. Ed. Tarja Sampo Makinen. Circ: 53,271 (controlled).

616.462 USA ISSN 0012-1797
RC660.A1 CODEN: DIAEAZ
DIABETES. Text in English. 1952. m. USD 280 to individuals in USA & Mexico; USD 299 in Canada to individuals; USD 260 elsewhere to individuals; USD 560 to institutions in USA & Mexico; USD 599 in Canada to institutions; USD 380 elsewhere to institutions (effective 2001). adv. abstr, charts, illus. index. back issues avail.; reprint service avail. from PQC. *Refereed.* **Document type:** *Journal, Academic/Scholarly.* **Description:** Diabetes explores the physiology and pathophysiology of diabetes. It offers information on the pathogenesis of diabetes and its complications, normal and pathological pancreatic islet function and intermediary metabolism, and mechanisms of drug and hormone action.
Related titles: CD-ROM ed.: (from Ovid Technologies, Inc.); Microform ed.: (from PQC,PMC); Online - full text ed.: (from Gale Group, Ovid Technologies, Inc., Northern Light Technology, Inc., EBSCO Publishing, ProQuest Information & Learning, Factiva, Institute for Scientific Information); ♦ Supplement: Diabetes-Related Literature Index by Authors and Key Words in the Title. ISSN 0070-4652.
Indexed: AIM, Abstr.Hyg., Abstr.Inter.Med., Agri.& Environ.Biotech.Abstr. (coverage dropped), Biol.Abstr., CINAHL, Chem.Abstr., Chem.Indus.Notes, Chem.Titles, Curr.Adv.Biochem., Curr.Adv.Cancer Res., Curr.Adv.Cell & Devel.Biol., Curr.Adv.Ecol.Sci., Curr.Adv.Gen.& Molec.Biol., Curr.Cont., Curr.Ind.Stat., Dairy Sci.Abstr., Derwent Biotech.Abstr., Diab.Cont., Excerp.Med., INIS Atomind., Ind.Med. (1952-), Ind.Sci.Rev., Inpharma, Int.Abstr.Biol.Sci., Kidney, Nutr.Abstr., Pharm.&Out.News, Reac., Ref.Zh., SSCI (coverage dropped), Sci.Cit.Ind., So.Pac.Per.Ind., Sugar Ind.Abstr., THA, Trop.Dis.Bull.
—BLDSC (3579.600000), CASDDS, CISTI, GNLM, IDS, ingenta, KNAW. **CCC.**
Published by: American Diabetes Association, 1701 N. Beauregard St., Alexandria, VA 22311-1717. TEL 703-549-1500, 800-232-3472, FAX 703-549-6995, orders@allenpress.com, http://diabetes.diabetesjournals.org/, http://www.diabetes.org. Ed. Dr. Gordon C. Weir. Pub. Peter Banks. Adv. contact Kimberly Kelemen. B&W page USD 1,775, color page USD 3,539. Circ: 9,000 (paid). **Subscr. to:** Allen Press Inc., PO Box 1897, Lawrence, KS 66044-8897. http://www.allenpress.com. **Dist. by:** PO Box 0028, Washionton, DC 20073-0028.

616.462 FRA ISSN 1262-3636
CODEN: DIMEDU
DIABETES & METABOLISM. Text in English, French. 1975. bi-m. FRF 1,208; FRF 1,510 foreign (effective 2000). adv. illus. index. reprint service avail. from ISI. **Document type:** *Academic/Scholarly.* **Description:** Presents original clinical and laboratory work of high quality.
Former titles (until 1995): Diabete et Metabolisme (0338-1684); (until 1975): Diabete (0012-1770)
Related titles: Microform ed.: (from PQC); Online - full text ed.: (from Institute for Scientific Information, RoweCom Information Quest).
Indexed: ASCA, Apic.Abstr., Biol.Abstr., Chem.Abstr., Curr.Adv.Ecol.Sci., Curr.Cont., Diab.Cont., Excerp.Med., Ind.Med. (1996-), Ind.Sci.Rev., Inpharma, Int.Abstr.Biol.Sci., Int.Nurs.Ind., Nutr.Abstr., Pharm.&Out.News, Reac., Risk Abstr., SSCI (coverage dropped), Sci.Cit.Ind., THA.
—CASDDS, CISTI, EMDOCS, GNLM, IDS, ingenta, KNAW.
Published by: (Association de Langue Francaise pour l'Etude du Diabete et des Maladies Metaboliques), Masson - Periodiques, 120 bd. St. Germain, Paris 75006, France. TEL 33-1-40466200, FAX 33-1-40466201. Ed. P Sai. Circ: 1,500.

616.462 GBR ISSN 1466-8955
▼ **DIABETES AND PRIMARY CARE.** Text in English. 1999. q. GBP 30 in United Kingdom to individuals; GBP 48 foreign to individuals; GBP 50 in United Kingdom to institutions; GBP 66 foreign to institutions (effective (No. 2001). back issues avail. *Refereed.* **Document type:** *Trade.* **Description:** For health professionals of all disciplines working in diabetes care in primary care in the community. Covers clinical practiced, organization of care and current controversial topics.
—BLDSC (3579.600515).
Published by: S B Communications Group, 15 Mandeville Courtyard, 142 Battersea Park Rd, London SW11 4NB, United Kingdom. TEL 44-20-7627-1510, FAX 44-20-7627-1570, sbcomm@dial.pipex.com, info@sbcommunicationsgroup.com, http://www.sbcomm.dial.pipex.com, http://www.sbcommunicationsgroup.com. Ed. Eugene Hughes.

616.4 NLD ISSN 0168-9282
RC660.A1 CODEN: DIANEW
DIABETES ANNUAL. Text in Dutch. 1985. a., latest vol.10, 1996. USD 237.25 (effective 1996). *Refereed.* **Document type:** *Monographic series.* **Description:** Publishes reviews in basic science and clinical practice.
—BLDSC (3579.600520), CASDDS, CISTI, GNLM, ingenta, KNAW. **CCC.**
Published by: Elsevier Science BV, Regional Sales Office, PO Box 211, Amsterdam 1000 AE, Netherlands. nlinfo-f@elsevier.nl; usinfo-f@elsevier.com; info@elsevier.co.jp; asiainfo@elsevier.com.sg, http://www.elsevier.nl/. **Subscr. in Australasia and the Far East to:** Elsevier Science (Singapore) Pte Ltd, No.1 Temasek Ave, 17-01 Millenia Tower, Singapore 039192, Singapore. TEL 65-434-3727, FAX 65-337-2230; **Subscr. in Japan to:** Elsevier Science Inc - Japan Regional Office, 9-15 Higashi-Azabu 1-chome, Minato-ku, Tokyo 106-0044, Japan. TEL 81-3-5561-5033, FAX 81-3-5561-5047; **Subscr. in the Americas to:** Elsevier Science, PO Box 945, New York, NY 10159-0945. TEL 212-633-3730, FAX 212-633-3680, http://www.elsevier.com.

616.462 USA ISSN 0149-5992
RC660.A1 CODEN: DICAD2
DIABETES CARE. Text in English. 1978. m. USD 280 to individuals in USA & Mexico; USD 299.60 in Canada to individuals; USD 260 elsewhere to individuals; USD 560 to institutions in USA & Mexico; USD 599.20 in Canada to institutions; USD 380 elsewhere to institutions (effective 2001). adv. charts, illus, stat. index. back issues avail.; reprint service avail. from PQC. *Refereed.* **Document type:** *Journal, Academic/Scholarly.* **Description:** Contains articles dealing with research, etiology. and treatment of diabetes.
Related titles: CD-ROM ed.: (from Ovid Technologies, Inc.); Microform ed.: (from PQC); Online - full text ed.: (from Ovid Technologies, Inc., Northern Light Technology, Inc., EBSCO Publishing, ProQuest Information & Learning, Gale Group, Institute for Scientific Information); ♦ Supplement: Clinical Practice Recommendations; ♦ Diabetes Care. Supplement. ISSN 1064-9131.
Indexed: ASCA, Abstr.Inter.Med., Agricola, Behav.Med.Abstr., Bibl.Agri., CINAHL, Chem.Abstr., Chic.Per.Ind., Curr.Cont., Dairy Sci.Abstr., Diab.Cont., Excerp.Med., INIS Atomind., Ind.Med. (1978-), Ind.Sci.Rev., Inpharma, Int.Nurs.Ind., Jrnl.Watch Wom.Hlth., Kidney, NRN, Neurosci.Cit.Ind., Nutr.Abstr., Pharm.&Out.News, Reac., Ref.Zh., Rev.Med.& Vet.Mycol., SSCI (coverage dropped), Sci.Cit.Ind., Sugar Ind.Abstr., THA.
—BLDSC (3579.600600), CASDDS, CISTI, GNLM, IDS, ingenta, KNAW. **CCC.**
Published by: American Diabetes Association, 1701 N. Beauregard St., Alexandria, VA 22311-1717. TEL 703-549-1500, 1-800-342-2383, FAX 703-549-6995, customerservice@diabetes.org, http://diabetes.diabetesjournals.org/, http://www.diabetes.org. Ed. Dr. Charles M Clark Jr. Pub. Peter Banks. Adv. contact Kimberly Kelemen. B&W page USD 2,084, color page USD 4,012. Circ: 13,500 (paid). **Subscr. to:** Allen Press Inc., PO Box 1897, Lawrence, KS 66044-8897. TEL 785-843-1235, FAX 785-843-1274, http://www.allenpress.com/catalog/pdfs/diabetes_care.pdf. **Dist. by:** PO Box 0028, Washionton, DC 20073-0028. FAX 703-549-6995.

616.462 USA ISSN 1064-9131
DIABETES CARE. SUPPLEMENT. Text in English. irreg.
Related titles: ♦ Supplement to: Diabetes Care. ISSN 0149-5992.
Published by: American Diabetes Association, 1701 N. Beauregard St., Alexandria, VA 22311-1717. TEL 703-549-1500, FAX 703-683-2890.

616.4 USA
DIABETES COUNTDOWN✱ . Text in English. 1982. q. USD 25. adv. **Document type:** *Consumer.* **Description:** Offers the latest information in diabetes research and treatment, as the foundation strives for a cure.
Published by: Juvenile Diabetes Foundation International, 120 Wall St, New York, NY 10005-3904. TEL 212-889-7575, FAX 212-532-8791. Ed. Julie Mettenburg. Circ: 240,042.

616.462 CAN ISSN 0703-5764
DIABETES DIALOGUE. Text in English. 1954. q. CND 20 to members. adv. bk.rev. illus. *Refereed.* **Document type:** *Consumer.* **Description:** Geared to readers with either Type 1 (insulin dependent) and Type 2 (non-insulin dependent) diabetes. Covers topics such as exercise, nutrition, food choices, foot care, health care, medical updates, research, life-style management, travel, book reviews, advice columns, skin care, products and policy statements.

M

Formerly (until vol.24, 1977): C D A Newsletter (0007-8018)
Related titles: Audio cassette/tape ed.
Published by: Canadian Diabetes Association, 15 Toronto St, Ste 800, Toronto, ON M5C 2E3, Canada. TEL 416-363-3373, FAX 416-363-7465, info@diabetes.ca, http://www.diabetes.ca. Ed. Dr. Amir Hanna. R&P Bill Clarke. Adv. contact Tom Cowell. Circ: 60,000.

616.462 USA
DIABETES: DISEASE STATE MANAGEMENT RESOURCE. Text in English. 1996. a., latest vol.3, 1999. USD 295 domestic; USD 325 foreign (effective 2001). **Document type:** *Trade.*
Published by: American Health Consultants (Subsidiary of: Medical Economics Co., Inc.), 3525 Piedmont Rd, N E, 6 Piedmont Center, Ste 400, Atlanta, GA 30305. TEL 404-262-5476, 404-262-7436, 800-688-2421, FAX 404-262-7837, 800-284-3291, custserv@ahcpub.com, http://www.ahcpub.com.

DIABETES EDUCATION REIMBURSEMENTS & POLICY REPORT. see *LAW*

616.46 USA ISSN 0145-7217
RC660.A1 CODEN: DIEDEM
THE DIABETES EDUCATOR. Text in English. 1975. bi-m. USD 55 domestic; USD 62 in Canada; USD 75 elsewhere (effective 2001). adv. bk.rev. back issues avail. *Refereed.* **Document type:** *Journal, Academic/Scholarly, Consumer.*
Related titles: Online - full text ed.: (from Institute for Scientific Information).
Indexed: ASCA, Agricola, Behav.Med.Abstr., Bibl.Agri., CINAHL, Curr.Cont., Diab.Cont., Ind.Med. (coverage dropped), Inpharma, Int.Nurs.Ind., NRN, Pharm.&Out.News, Reac., Ref.Zh.
—BLDSC (3579.600650), GNLM, ingenta.
Published by: Stenson Bauer Communications, Inc, 100 W Monroe St, 400, Chicago, IL 60603-1901. TEL 312-424-2426, FAX 312-424-2427. Ed. James A Fain. R&P Mary Beach TEL 312-654-1710. Adv. contact Traci K Treinen. Circ: 12,000.

616.462 USA ISSN 0095-8301
RC660.A1
DIABETES FORECAST; the healthy living magazine for 50 years. Text in English. 1948. m. USD 28 domestic to membership; USD 46 in Canada to membership; USD 39 in Mexico to membership; USD 59 elsewhere to membership; USD 4 newsstand/cover to membership; USD 5.99 newsstand/cover in Canada to membership (effective 2000 - 2001). adv. charts, illus. back issues avail.; reprints avail. **Document type:** *Magazine, Consumer.* **Description:** Covers diabetes, nutrition, and health research findings.
Formerly: A.D.A. Forecast (0001-0847)
Related titles: Diskette ed.; Online - full text ed.: (from Gale Group, Northern Light Technology, Inc., ProQuest Information & Learning, Factiva).
Indexed: Agricola, CHNI, CINAHL, Hlth.Ind., Ref.Zh.
—BLDSC (3579.600670), CISTI, GNLM, Infotrieve, ingenta. **CCC.**
Published by: American Diabetes Association, 1701 N. Beauregard St., Alexandria, VA 22311-1717. TEL 703-549-1500, 800-232-3472, FAX 703-549-6995, TELEX 901132, akeegan@diabetes.org, http://www.diabetes.org/diabetesforecast. Ed. Andrew Keegan. Pub. Peter Banks. Adv. contact Kimberly Kelemen. Circ: 400,000.

616.462 JPN ISSN 0915-6593
CODEN: DIFREZ
DIABETES FRONTIER. Text in Japanese. 1990. 6/yr. JPY 2,400 (effective 1998). **Document type:** *Academic/Scholarly.*
—BLDSC (3579.600680).
Published by: Medikaru Rebyusha/Medical Review Co., Ltd., 7-3 Hirano-Machi 1-chome, Chuo-ku, Osaka-shi 541-0046, Japan. TEL 81-6-223-1556, FAX 81-6-223-1414, medrev@osk2.3web.ne.jp. Ed. Mitsuaki Matsuoka.

616.462 USA
DIABETES HEALTH MONITOR. Text in English. bi-m. **Document type:** *Newsletter.* **Description:** Seeks to educate patients about diabetes.
Published by: Data Centrum Communications, Inc., 21 W 38th St, 4th fl, New York, NY 10018. TEL 212-997-9800, FAX 212-997-0078. Eds. Karen Seigal, Anny Queyroy. Pub. Eric Jensen.

616.46 GBR ISSN 1468-6570
DIABETES INTERNATIONAL. Text in English. 3/yr. GBP 32.50, USD 52 (effective 2002).
Published by: F S G MediMedia Ltd., Vine House, The Barn, Fair Green, Reach, Cambridge CB5 0JD, United Kingdom. TEL 44-1638-743633, FAX 44-1638-743998, info@fsg.co.uk.

616 USA ISSN 1523-1003
DIABETES INTERVIEW. Text in English. 1991. m. adv. **Description:** Shows diabetes patients how to stay upbeat and sensibly deal with their condition.
Formerly (until 199?): Scott King's Diabetes Interview (1058-6598)
Address: 3715 Balboa St, San Francisco, CA 94121. TEL 415-387-4002, 800-234-1218, FAX 415-387-3604, webmgr@diabetesinterview.com, http://www.diabetesinterview.com.

616.462 FIN ISSN 1455-7827
DIABETES JA LAAKARI. Text in Finnish. 1972. 6/yr. FIM 70 (effective 2000). adv. **Document type:** *Journal, Academic/Scholarly.* **Description:** Information concerning diabetes for physicians and other health professionals.
Formerly (until 1988): Laakarililte (0787-4758)
Published by: Finnish Diabetes Association, Kirjoniementie 15, Tampere 33680, Finland. TEL 358-3-28-60-111, FAX 358-3-3600-462, mervi.pohjalainen@diabetes.fi. Ed. Mervi Pohjalainen. Circ: 15,000 (paid).

616.462 DEU ISSN 0341-8812
CODEN: DIJODB
DIABETES - JOURNAL. Text in German. 1951. m. DEM 67.20 (effective 1999). adv. bk.rev. charts, illus. **Document type:** *Academic/Scholarly.*
Formerly: Diabetiker (0012-1851)
Indexed: Chem.Abstr.
—CASDDS, GNLM. **CCC.**
Published by: (Deutscher Diabetikerbund e.V.), Verlag Kirchheim und Co. GmbH, Kaiserstr 41, Mainz 55116, Germany. TEL 49-6131-96070-0, FAX 49-6131-9607070, kirchheim@aol.com. Ed. Dr. Eberhard Standl. Circ: 52,000.

DIABETES MELLITUS. see *MEDICAL SCIENCES—Abstracting, Bibliographies, Statistics*

616.4 GBR ISSN 1520-7552
CODEN: DMRREG
DIABETES - METABOLISM RESEARCH AND REVIEWS. Text in English. 1985. bi-m. USD 430 in United States; USD 430 in Canada & Mexico; USD 430 elsewhere; USD 452 combined subscription in United States for print and online eds.; USD 452 combined subscription in Canada & Mexico for print and online eds.; USD 452 combined subscription elsewhere for print and online eds. (effective 2002). adv. back issues avail.; reprint service avail. from SWZ. *Refereed.* **Document type:** *Academic/Scholarly.* **Description:** Covers clinical and basic scientific advances in endocrinology, insulin secretion, resistance, ketone metabolism, obesity and lipid metabolism, pathogenesis and cellular action of insulin.
Formerly (until 1999): Diabetes - Metabolism Reviews (0742-4221)
Related titles: Microform ed.: (from PQC); Online - full text ed.: ISSN 1520-7560. USD 430 in United States; USD 430 in Canada & Mexico; USD 430 elsewhere (effective 2002) (from EBSCO Publishing, Wiley InterScience, Institute for Scientific Information).
Indexed: ASCA, Chem.Indus.Notes, Chem.Titles, Curr.Cont., Diab.Cont., Excerp.Med., INIS Atomind., Ind.Med. (1999-), Inpharma, Int.Abstr.Biol.Sci., NRN, Nutr.Abstr., Reac., Sci.Cit.Ind., THA.
—BLDSC (3579.601870), CASDDS, CISTI, EMDOCS, GNLM, IDS, ingenta. **CCC.**
Published by: Wiley Europe Ltd., Baffins Ln, Chichester, W Sussex PO19 1UD, United Kingdom. TEL 44-1243-779777, FAX 44-1243-775878, customer@wiley.co.uk, http://www.wiley.co.uk. adv.: B&W page GBP 750, color page GBP 1,650; trim 210 x 297. Circ: 700. **Subscr. in the Americas to:** John Wiley & Sons, Inc., Journals, 605 Third Ave, New York, NY 10158. TEL 212-850-6021, 212-850-6645, subinfo@jwiley.com.

616.462 ITA ISSN 0394-3402
CODEN: DNMEEW
DIABETES, NUTRITION & METABOLISM, CLINICAL AND EXPERIMENTAL. Text in English. 1988. bi-m. EUR 77.47 domestic; USD 100 (effective 2002). *Refereed.* **Description:** Publishes original papers on diabetes, nutrition and metabolism research.
Related titles: Online - full text ed.: EUR 38.73 (effective 2002) (from Institute for Scientific Information).
Indexed: ASCA, Curr.Cont., Diab.Cont., Ind.Med. (1988-), Ind.Sci.Rev., Inpharma, Nutr.Abstr., Pharm.&Out.News, Reac., Sci.Cit.Ind., Soils & Fert., Triticale Abstr.
—BLDSC (3579.601950), CASDDS, CISTI, EMDOCS, GNLM, IDS, KNAW.
Published by: Editrice Kurtis s.r.l., Via Luigi Zoja, 30, Milan, MI 20153, Italy. TEL 39-02-48202740, FAX 39-02-4820-1219, info@kurtis.it, http://www.kurtis.it. Ed. P Brunetti.

616.4 GBR ISSN 1462-8902
CODEN: DOMEF6
▼ **DIABETES, OBESITY AND METABOLISM.** Text in English. 1999. bi-m., latest vol.4, 2002. GBP 57 in Europe to individuals; USD 103 in North America to individuals; GBP 63 elsewhere to individuals; GBP 250 in Europe to institutions; USD 396 in North America to institutions; GBP 275 elsewhere to institutions (effective 2002). adv. **Document type:** *Academic/Scholarly.* **Description:** Aims to provide a forum for publication of clinical and experimental pharmacology studies related to diabetes, obesity and metabolism.
Related titles: ♦ Online - full text ed.: Diabetes, Obesity and Metabolism Online. ISSN 1463-1326.
Indexed: Curr.Cont., Ind.Med., Nutr.Abstr.
—BLDSC (3579.601970). **CCC.**
Published by: Blackwell Science Ltd., PO Box 88, Oxford OX2 0NE, United Kingdom. TEL 44-1865-206180, 44-1865-206002, FAX 44-1865-206219, jnl.orders@blacksci.co.uk, http://www.blackwell-science.com/~cgilib/jnlpage.asp?Journal=dom&File=dom, http://www.blackwellpublishing.com. Eds. A Garber, R Donnelly. Pub. Allen Stevens. R&P Sophie Savage. Adv. contact Jenny Applin. Circ: 1,000.

616.4 GBR ISSN 1463-1326
DIABETES, OBESITY AND METABOLISM ONLINE. Text in English. bi-m. GBP 52 in Europe to individuals; USD 93 in North America to individuals; GBP 52 elsewhere to individuals; GBP 225 in Europe to institutions; USD 357 in North America to institutions; GBP 225 elsewhere to institutions (effective 2002). **Document type:** *Academic/Scholarly.*
Media: Online - full text (from EBSCO Publishing, O C L C Online Computer Library Center, Inc., RoweCom Information Quest, ingenta, Munksgaard & Blackwell Science's Synergy, Swets Blackwell, Institute for Scientific Information). **Related titles:** ♦ Print ed.: Diabetes, Obesity and Metabolism. ISSN 1462-8902.
Published by: Blackwell Science Ltd., Osney Mead, Oxford OX2 0EL, United Kingdom. TEL 44-1685-206206, FAX 44-1685-721205, website@blacksci.com, journals.cs@blacksci.co.uk, http://www.blackwell-science.com.

616.46 NOR ISSN 1502-1424
DIABETES (OSLO). Text in Norwegian. 1950. bi-m. NOK 290 (effective 2001). adv. bk.rev. **Document type:** *Bulletin.*
Formerly (until 2000): Diabetikeren (0419-0505)
Published by: Norges Diabetesforbund/Norwegian Diabetic Association, Postboks 6442, Etterstad, Oslo 0605, Norway. TEL 47-23-05-18-00, FAX 47-33-05-18-01, diabetes@dianet.no. Ed. Erik Lie. Adv. contact Kari Aasen TEL 47-23-05-18-12. Circ: 30,082.

616.46 USA
DIABETES PATH FINDER. Text in English. 1978. q. USD 12. bk.rev.
Formerly (until 1994): W A News
Published by: American Diabetes Association, Washington Affiliate, Inc., 557 Roy St, Lower Lever, Seattle, WA 98109. TEL 206-282-4616, 800-628-8808, FAX 206-282-4729. Ed. Clair Sagiv. Circ: 15,000 (controlled).

616.4 IRL ISSN 0168-8227
CODEN: DRCPE9
DIABETES RESEARCH AND CLINICAL PRACTICE. Text in English. m. EUR 1,459 in Europe to individuals; JPY 18,800 in Japan to individuals; USD 157 elsewhere to individuals; EUR 1,459 in Europe to institutions; JPY 193,600 in Japan to institutions; USD 1,632 elsewhere to institutions (effective 2002). abstr. back issues avail. *Refereed.* **Document type:** *Academic/Scholarly.* **Description:** Covers diabetes research, experimental biology, molecular biology and immunology, clinical practice, epidemiology and diabetes education.
Related titles: Online - full text ed.: (from ingenta, Swets Blackwell, ScienceDirect, Institute for Scientific Information).
Indexed: ASCA, Chem.Abstr., Chem.Indus.Notes, Chem.Titles, Curr.Cont., Diab.Cont., Excerp.Med., Ind.Med. (1985-), Ind.Sci.Rev., Inpharma, Int.Abstr.Biol.Sci., NRN, Nutr.Abstr., Pharm.&Out.News, Reac., SSCI (coverage dropped), Sci.Cit.Ind., Soyabean Abstr., THA, Trop.Dis.Bull.
—BLDSC (3579.603700), CASDDS, CISTI, GNLM, IDS, Infotrieve, ingenta, KNAW. **CCC.**

M

Published by: (International Diabetes Federation/ Federation Internationale du Diabete BEL), Elsevier Science Ireland Ltd, Elsevier House, Brookvale Plaza, E. Park, Shannon, Co. Clare, Ireland. TEL 353-61-471944, FAX 353-61-472144, http://www.elsevier.com/inca/publications/store/5/0/5/9/4/9/. Ed. S Baba. R&P Annette Moloney. **Subscr. in Australasia and the Far East to:** Elsevier Science (Singapore) Pte Ltd, No.1 Temasek Ave, 17-01 Millenia Tower, Singapore 039192, Singapore. TEL 65-434-3727, FAX 65-337-2230; **Subscr. in the Americas to:** Elsevier Science, PO Box 945, New York, NY 10159-0945. TEL 212-633-3730, FAX 212-633-3680, usinfo-f@elsevier.com; **Subscr. to:** Elsevier Science BV, PO Box 211, Amsterdam 1000 AE, Netherlands. TEL 31-20-485-3757, FAX 31-20-485-3432.

616.462 USA

▼ **DIABETES RESEARCH AND WELLNESS DIRECT.** Text in English. 2001. q. **Description:** Serves as a health resource for diabetics and their families.

Published by: Diabetes Research and Wellness Foundation, 189 Bradley Pl, Palm Beach, FL 33480. TEL 561-802-3600, FAX 561-802-3860, http://www.diabeteswellness.org/magazinepage.asp. Ed. Charlotte Green. Pub. Mike Gretschel. Adv. contact Carol Archebelle.

616.46 GBR ISSN 0265-5985 CODEN: DIREEM

DIABETES RESEARCH: CLINICAL & EXPERIMENTAL. Text in English. 1984. bi-m. GBP 395 domestic; GBP 495 in the European Union; GBP 975 in Asia. adv. bk.rev. **Document type:** *Academic/Scholarly.*

Indexed: Curr.Adv.Cell & Devel.Biol., Curr.Adv.Ecol.Sci., Curr.Cont. (coverage dropped), Excerp.Med.

—BLDSC (3579.603600), CASDDS, CISTI, EMDOCS, GNLM, ingenta, KNAW. **CCC.**

Published by: Teviot Scientific Publications Ltd., 82 Great King St, Edinburgh EH3 6QU, United Kingdom. TEL 44-131-226-5435, FAX 44-131-220-8209. Ed. W James Irvine.

616.4 USA ISSN 1066-9442 RC660.A1 CODEN: DBRVEO

DIABETES REVIEWS. Text in English. ceased; resumed 1993. q. USD 95 to individuals; USD 150 to institutions. *Refereed.* **Document type:** *Academic/Scholarly.*

Related titles: Online - full text ed.: (from EBSCO Publishing).

Indexed: Curr.Cont., Diab.Cont., Excerp.Med. (1994-), Sci.Cit.Ind.

—CISTI, GNLM, IDS, Infotrieve, KNAW. **CCC.**

Published by: American Diabetes Association, 1701 N. Beauregard St., Alexandria, VA 22311-1717. TEL 703-549-1500, FAX 703-683-2890. Ed. Dr. Ralph A Defronzo.

616.46 613.7 USA ISSN 0741-6253 CODEN: DSMAEL

DIABETES SELF-MANAGEMENT. Text in English. 1983. bi-m. USD 18; USD 4 newsstand/cover (effective 2001). adv. charts, illus. back issues avail.; reprints avail. *Refereed.* **Document type:** *Magazine, Consumer, Trade.* **Description:** Provides practical and instructive "how-to" information for people with diabetes.

Indexed: CHNI, CINAHL.

—BLDSC (3579.603900).

Published by: R.A. Rapaport Publishing, Inc., 150 W 22nd St, New York, NY 10011. TEL 212-989-0200, FAX 212-989-4786, staff@diabetes-self-mgmt.com, http://www.diabetes-self-mgmt.com. Ed., R&P James Hazlett. Pub. Richard A Rapaport. Adv. contact Kathy Jones. B&W page USD 10,500. Circ: 470,000 (paid). **Subscr. to:** PO Box 52890, Boulder, CO 80322-2890.

616.46 USA

DIABETES SOURCEBOOK. Text in English. 1994. irreg., latest vol.2, 1999. USD 78 per vol. (effective 2001). charts, illus, stat. master index. **Document type:** *Consumer.* **Description:** Provides laypersons with basic information on all forms of diabetes and related disorders. Offers advice on treatment options and finding help.

Published by: Omnigraphics, Inc., 615 Griswold St, Detroit, MI 48226. TEL 313-961-1340, 800-234-1340, FAX 313-961-1383, 800-875-1340, info@omnigraphics.com, http://www.omnigraphics.com. Ed. Karen Bellenir. Pub. Frederick G Ruffner Jr.

616.4 USA ISSN 1040-9165 RC660.A1

DIABETES SPECTRUM; from research to practice. Text in English. 1988. q. USD 70 to individuals in United States & Mexico; USD 74.50 in Canada to individuals; USD 71 elsewhere to individuals; USD 140 to institutions in United States & Mexico; USD 149.80 in Canada to institutions; USD 101 elsewhere to institutions (effective 2001). adv. illus. *Refereed.* **Document type:** *Journal, Academic/Scholarly.* **Description:** Explores diabetes care topics in-depth and practical applications of current research findings.

Related titles: Online - full text ed.: (from Northern Light Technology, Inc., ProQuest Information & Learning, Gale Group, EBSCO Publishing, Factiva).

Indexed: CINAHL, Inpharma, Pharm.&Out.News, Reac.

—BLDSC (3579.603950), Infotrieve. **CCC.**

Published by: American Diabetes Association, 1701 N. Beauregard St., Alexandria, VA 22311-1717. TEL 703-549-1500, 800-232-3472, FAX 703-549-6995, http://diabetes.diabetesjournals.org/. Ed. Belinda P. Childs. Pub. Peter Banks. Adv. contact Kimberly Kelemen. Circ: 10,500.

616.462 USA ISSN 1520-9156 CODEN: DTTHFH

▼ **DIABETES TECHNOLOGY & THERAPEUTICS.** Text in English. 1999. bi-m. USD 179 domestic to individuals; USD 229 foreign to individuals; USD 215 domestic to individuals print and online eds. combined; USD 265 foreign to individuals print and online eds. combined; USD 309 domestic to institutions print and online eds. combined; USD 368 foreign to institutions print and online eds. combined (effective 2002). charts, illus. back issues avail.; reprints avail. *Refereed.* **Document type:** *Journal, Academic/Scholarly.* **Description:** Reports on innovative invasive and noninvasive technologies for diagnosing and treating all forms of diabetes.

Related titles: Online - full text ed.: USD 179 to individuals; USD 309 to institutions (effective 2002) (from CatchWord Ltd., EBSCO Publishing, O C L C Online Computer Library Center, Inc., RoweCom Information Quest, Swets Blackwell).

—BLDSC (3579.603960), CatchWord.

Published by: Mary Ann Liebert, Inc. Publishers, 2 Madison Ave, Larchmont, NY 10538. TEL 914-834-3100, FAX 914-834-1388, info@liebertpub.com, http://www.liebertpub.com/dia. Ed. David C Klonoff. Adv. contact Carl Maury.

616.462 GBR ISSN 1464-5009

DIABETES TODAY. Text in English. 1998. bi-m. GBP 18 domestic to individuals; GBP 30 foreign to individuals; GBP 30 domestic to institutions; GBP 50 foreign to institutions (effective 2000). **Document type:** *Journal.*

—BLDSC (3579603965).

Published by: Media Publishing Company, Media House, 41 Crayford Way, Dartford, Kent DA1 4JY, United Kingdom. TEL 44-1322-558029, FAX 44-1322-558524, medipub@aol.com.

616.4 DEU ISSN 0942-0037

DIABETES UND STOFFWECHSEL. Text in German; Summaries in English, German. 1992. bi-m. DEM 162; DEM 84 to students. adv. bk.rev. index. back issues avail. **Document type:** *Academic/Scholarly.*

Indexed: Excerp.Med. (1995-).

—BLDSC (3579.604100), GNLM, Infotrieve. **CCC.**

Published by: (Deutscher Diabetes-Gesellschaft), Verlag Kirchheim und Co. GmbH, Kaiserstr 41, Mainz 55116, Germany. TEL 49-6131-96070-0, FAX 49-6131-9607070, kirchheim@aol.com. Eds. B Willms, E Standl. Adv. contact Andreas Goerner. Circ: 13,000 (controlled).

616.462 USA

DIABETES UPDATE. Text in English. 1955. q. USD 10 domestic to non-members; USD 20 foreign to non-members. adv. bk.rev. **Description:** News, information, and announcements pertaining to the members and activities of the Greater Boston Diabetes Society with medical and nutritional information on inhibiting and controlling the disorder and information about diet and exercise to help prevent or delay the onset of diabetes.

Former titles (until 1985): Diabetes Dialogue; Diabetes Newsletter (0012-1827)

Published by: Greater Boston Diabetes Society Inc., 1330 Beacon St, Ste 345, Brookline, MA 02146. TEL 617-731-2972. Ed. Thelma Gruenbaum. Circ: 4,000.

616.462 BEL ISSN 1437-4064 CODEN: IDFBD6

DIABETES VOICE; bulletin of the International Diabetes Federation. Text in English, French, Spanish. 1954. q. (plus 2/yr special issues). USD 40 to non-members includes online ed; USD 30 to institutions includes online ed (effective 2000). adv. bk.rev., Website rev. 44 p./no. back issues avail. **Document type:** *Bulletin, Academic/Scholarly.* **Description:** Covers diabetes, health economics, and relevant developments in endocrinology and medicine.

Former titles (until 1999): I D F Bulletin (0306-4980); (until 1974): International Diabetes Foundation. News Bulletin (0534-9753)

Related titles: Online - full content ed.: 2000. USD 30 to non-members; USD 20 to institutions (effective 2000); French ed.: Voix du Diabete. ISSN 1437-6547; Spanish ed.: Voz de Diabetes. ISSN 1437-6555.

Indexed: Diab.Cont.

—BLDSC (3579.604250), GNLM.

Published by: International Diabetes Federation/Federation Internationale du Diabete, Rue Defacqz 1, Brussels 1000, Belgium. TEL 32-2-538-5511, FAX 32-2-538-5514, http://www.idf.org, http://www.diabetesvoice.com. Ed. Leena Etu-Seppala. R&P Delice Gan. Adv. contact Kristina Hawthorne TEL 49-6131-9607031. Circ: 6,000. **Co-publisher:** Verlag Kirchheim und Co. GmbH.

616.46 USA

THE DIABETESCARE GUIDE. Text in English. 1991. 3/yr. USD 6. adv. back issues avail. **Description:** Reference guide distributed to newly diagnosed adults. Covers the practical aspects of controlling and managing diabetes.

Published by: Bounty/SCA Worldwide, 550 W Washington, 1000, Chicago, IL 60661. TEL 312-799-7000, FAX 312-799-7100. adv.: B&W page USD 12,225, color page USD 14,450; trim 7.5 x 5.25. Circ: 200,000.

616.462 DEU ISSN 1435-3644

DIABETESPROFI; Forum fuer professionelle Diabetiker-Versorgung. Text in German. 1992. bi-m. DEM 42 (effective 1999). **Document type:** *Academic/Scholarly.*

Former titles: Schulungsprofi Diabetes (1433-903X); (until 1997): Diabetes Journal Schulungsprofi (0946-9877)

Published by: (Deutscher Diabetiker-Bund), Verlag Kirchheim und Co. GmbH, Kaiserstr 41, Mainz 55116, Germany. TEL 49-6131-96070-0, FAX 49-6131-9607070, kirchheim@aol.com. Ed. Dr. Eberhard Standl. **Co-sponsors:** Deutsche Diabetes-Gesellschaft; Deutsche Diabetes-Union.

616.462 IND ISSN 0970-4035 CODEN: JDAIBB

DIABETIC ASSOCIATION OF INDIA. JOURNAL. EDUCATION SECTION. Text in English. 1960. q. **Document type:** *Academic/Scholarly.*

Supersedes in part (in 1988): Diabetic Association of India. Journal (0304-4513); Which was formerly (until 1974): Madhumeh (0024-9424)

Indexed: Excerp.Med. (until 19??).

—CASDDS, CISTI, GNLM.

Published by: Diabetic Association of India, S.L. Raheja Hospital, Raheja Rugnalaya Marg Mahim, Mumbai, Maharashtra 400 016, India.

616.462 IND ISSN 0970-4027 CODEN: JDAIB

DIABETIC ASSOCIATION OF INDIA. JOURNAL. SCIENTIFIC SECTION. Text in English. 1960. q. adv. bk.rev. illus. **Document type:** *Academic/Scholarly.*

Supersedes in part (in 1988): Diabetic Association of India. Journal (0304-4513); Which was formerly (until 1974): Madhumeh (0024-9424)

Indexed: Biol.Abstr., Excerp.Med.

—BLDSC (4734.542000), CASDDS, CISTI, EMDOCS, GNLM.

Published by: Diabetic Association of India, S.L. Raheja Hospital, Raheja Rugnalaya Marg Mahim, Mumbai, Maharashtra 400 016, India. Circ: 3,000.

641.563 USA

▼ **DIABETIC COOKING.** Text in English. 1999. bi-m. USD 14.95 (effective 2001); USD 3.50 newsstand/cover (effective 1999). adv. **Document type:** *Consumer.* **Description:** Contains recipes specifically designed for people with diabetes; also includes cooking tips, baking ideas, menus suggestions, and seasons ideas.

Published by: Publications International Ltd., 7373 N Cicero Ave, Lincolnwood, IL 60646. TEL 847-676-3470, 800-777-5582, FAX 847-676-3671, mbowen@pubint.com, http://www.diabeticcooking.com/. Pub. Louis Weber. Adv. contact Patrick Bachler. color page USD 16,000; trim 7.75 x 4.88. Circ: 250,000.

M

616.46 617.585 GBR ISSN 1462-2041
THE DIABETIC FOOT. Text in English. 1998. q. GBP 30 domestic to individuals; GBP 48 foreign to individuals; GBP 50 domestic to institutions; GBP 66 foreign to institutions (effective 2001). adv. *Refereed.*
Description: For health care professionals involved in the care of the diabetic foot. Contains an editorial and 5-6 key articles per issue. Sections include education, prevention, treatment, case reports, wound care, imaging, vascular intervention, and foot pressure interest group, plus a digest round-up of recent research articles.
Indexed: CINAHL, Rev.Appl.Entomol.
—BLDSC (3579.604500).
Published by: S B Communications Group, 15 Mandeville Courtyard, 142 Battersea Park Rd, London SW11 4NB, United Kingdom. TEL 44-20-7627-1510, FAX 44-20-7627-1570, sbcomm@dial.pipex.com, info@sbcommunicationsgroup.com, http://www.sbcomm.dial.pipex.com, http://www.sbcommunicationsgroup.com. Ed. Alistair McInnes. Pub., Adv. contact Simon Breed. R&P Sophie Perks.

616.46 616.3 610.73 GBR ISSN 0742-3071 CODEN: DIMEEV
DIABETIC MEDICINE. Text in English. 1984. m., latest vol.19, 2002. GBP 115 in Europe to individuals; USD 257 in North America to individuals; GBP 178 elsewhere to individuals; GBP 472 in Europe to institutions; USD 749 in North America to institutions; GBP 520 elsewhere to institutions (effective 2002). adv. bk.rev. back issues avail.; reprint service avail. from SWZ. *Refereed.* **Document type:** *Academic/Scholarly.*
Description: Designed as an information exchange on all aspects of diabetes mellitus and aims to interest everyone helping diabetic patients whether through fundamental research or better health care.
Related titles: Microform ed.: (from PQC); ♦ Online - full text ed.: Diabetic Medicine Online. ISSN 1464-5491.
Indexed: ASCA, Behav.Med.Abstr., Brit.Nur.Ind., CINAHL, Curr.Adv.Ecol.Sci., Curr.Cont., Diab.Cont., Environ.Sci.Poll.Mgmt., Excerp.Med., Ind.Med. (1984-), Inpharma, Int.Abstr.Biol.Sci., NRN, Neurosci.Cit.Ind., Nutr.Abstr., Pharm.&Out.News, Reac., Rev.Med.& Vet.Mycol., Risk Abstr., SSCI (coverage dropped), Sugar Ind.Abstr., THA, Triticale Abstr.
—BLDSC (3579.606000), ADONIS, CISTI, EMDOCS, GNLM, IDS, ingenta, KNAW. **CCC.**
Published by: (British Diabetic Association), Blackwell Science Ltd., PO Box 88, Oxford OX2 0NE, United Kingdom. TEL 44-1865-206180, 44-1865-206002, FAX 44-1865-206219, jnl.orders@blacksci.co.uk, http://www.blackwell-science.com/~cgilib/jnlpage.asp?Journal=dme&File=dme, http://www.blackwellpublishing.com. Ed. Simon Heller. Pub. Allen Stevens. R&P Sophie Savage. Adv. contact Jenny Applin. Circ: 2,033.

616.46 GBR ISSN 1464-5491
DIABETIC MEDICINE ONLINE. Text in English. m. GBP 104 in Europe to individuals; USD 232 in North America to individuals; GBP 104 elsewhere to individuals; GBP 425 in Europe to institutions; USD 675 in North America to institutions; GBP 425 elsewhere to institutions (effective 2002). *Refereed.* **Document type:** *Academic/Scholarly.*
Media: Online - full text (from EBSCO Publishing, Munksgaard & Blackwell Science's Synergy, O C L C Online Computer Library Center, Inc., RoweCom Information Quest, ingenta, Swets Blackwell, Institute for Scientific Information). **Related titles:** Microform ed.: (from PQC); ♦ Print ed.: Diabetic Medicine. ISSN 0742-3071.
Published by: Blackwell Science Ltd., Osney Mead, Oxford OX2 0EL, United Kingdom. TEL 44-1685-206206, FAX 44-1685-721205, website@blacksci.com, journals.cs@blacksci.co.uk, http://www.blackwell-science.com/~cgilib/jnlpage.bin?Journal=dme&File=dme&Page=aims.

616.46 USA
DIABETIC READER; we read to know we're not alone. Text in English. 1981. s-a. USD 5. adv. bk.rev.
Document type: *Newsletter, Consumer.* **Description:** Offers support, advice, and practical information to persons with diabetes and family members.
Formerly (until 1991): Health-O-Gram
Media: Online - full text.
Published by: Online Diabetes, 5623 Matilija Ave, Van Nuys, CA 91401. TEL 818-780-1308, 800-735-7726, FAX 818-786-7359, prana2@aol.com, http://www.diabeteswebsite.com. Ed. June Bierman. Pubs. Barbara Toohey, June Biermann. R&P, Adv. contact Barbara Toohey. Circ: 45,000 (paid).

616.462 DEU ISSN 0172-2166
DIABETIKER RATGEBER. Text in German. 1978. m. adv. **Document type:** *Consumer.*
Published by: Wort und Bild Verlag Konradshoehe GmbH, Konradshoehe, Baierbrunn 82065, Germany. TEL 49-89-74433-0, FAX 49-89-74433150, http://www.wortundbild.de. Adv. contact Wolfgang Smeilus.

616.462 DEU ISSN 0012-186X
RC660.A1 CODEN: DBTGAJ
DIABETOLOGIA; clinical and experimental diabetes and metabolism. Text in English. 1965. m. EUR 895.90 domestic; EUR 876.70 in Germany; EUR 85 newsstand/cover foreign (effective 2002). adv. bibl, charts, illus, tr.lit. back issues avail.; reprint service avail. from ISI. *Refereed.* **Document type:** *Journal, Academic/Scholarly.* **Description:** Reports of clinical and experimental work on all aspects of diabetes research and related medicine, metabolic diseases, and physiology.
Related titles: Microform ed.: (from PQC); Online - full text ed.: ISSN 1432-0428 (from EBSCO Publishing, RoweCom Information Quest, Swets Blackwell, Springer LINK, Institute for Scientific Information).
Indexed: ASCA, Agri.& Environ.Biotech.Abstr. (coverage dropped), Behav.Med.Abstr., Biol.Abstr., Chem.Abstr., Chem.Indus.Notes, Chem.Titles, Curr.Adv.Cell & Devel.Biol., Curr.Adv.Ecol.Sci., Curr.Adv.Gen.& Molec.Biol., Curr.Cont., Derwent Biotech.Abstr., Diab.Cont., Excerp.Med., INIS Atomind., Ind.Med. (1965-), Ind.Sci.Rev., Inpharma, Int.Abstr.Biol.Sci., NRN, Neurosci.Cit.Ind., Nutr.Abstr., Pharm.&Out.News, Reac., Ref.Zh., SSCI (coverage dropped), Sci.Cit.Ind., Small Anim.Abstr., THA.
—BLDSC (3579.615000), ADONIS, CASDDS, CISTI, GNLM, IDS, ingenta, KNAW. **CCC.**
Published by: (European Association for the Study of Diabetes), Springer-Verlag (Subsidiary of: BertelsmannSpringer), Tiergartenstr 17, Heidelberg 69121, Germany. TEL 49-6221-345-0, FAX 49-6221-345229, subscriptions@springer.de, http://link.springer.de/link/service/journals/00125/index.htm, http://www.springer.de. Ed. W Waldhaeusl. **Subscr. in N. America to:** Springer-Verlag New York Inc., PO Box 2485, Secaucus, NJ 07096-2485. TEL 212-460-1500, FAX 213-473-6272.

616.46 619 HRV ISSN 0351-0042 CODEN: DBCRB2
DIABETOLOGIA CROATICA. Text and summaries in English. 1972. q. USD 45 (effective 2000). adv. bk.rev. *Refereed.* **Document type:** *Academic/Scholarly.*
Incorporates: Bulletin - Delivery of Health Care for Diabetics Worldwide (0353-3395); Which was formerly (1980-1988): Bulletin - Delivery of Health Care for Diabetics in Developing Countries (0352-4442)
Related titles: Online - full text ed.; ♦ Supplement: Diabetologia Croatica. Supplement. ISSN 0351-1995.
Indexed: Biol.Abstr., Chem.Abstr., Excerp.Med.
—CASDDS, CISTI, EMDOCS, GNLM.
Published by: Vuk Vrhovac Institute for Diabetes Endocrinology and Metabolic Diseases, Dugi dol 4-a, Zagreb 10000, Croatia. TEL 385-1-2332222, FAX 385-1-2331515, mail@idb.hr, http://www.indija.idb.hr. Ed., R&P Zeljko Metelko TEL 385-1-2331480. Adv. contact Bozica Mandic. Circ: 750.

616.46 HRV ISSN 0351-1995
DIABETOLOGIA CROATICA. SUPPLEMENT. Text in English. 1977. a.
Related titles: ♦ Supplement to: Diabetologia Croatica. ISSN 0351-0042.
Published by: Vuk Vrhovac Institute for Diabetes Endocrinology and Metabolic Diseases, Dugi dol 4-a, Zagreb 10000, Croatia. TEL 385-1-2332222, FAX 385-1-2331515, mail@idb.hr.

616.4 DEU ISSN 0171-8045
DIABETOLOGIE INFORMATIONEN. Text in German. q. DEM 56; DEM 59 foreign (effective 2000). **Document type:** *Bulletin, Consumer.*
Indexed: Ref.Zh.
—GNLM.
Published by: (Deutsche Diabetes Gesellschaft), Hansisches Verlagskontor, Mengstr 16, Luebeck 23552, Germany. TEL 49-451-7031-01, FAX 49-451-7031281.

616.462 SWE ISSN 1401-2618
DIABETOLOGNYTT. Text in Swedish. 1995. q. SEK 200 (effective 2001). **Document type:** *Journal, Academic/Scholarly.* **Description:** Covers all aspects of research and studies involving diabetes and diabetics.
Published by: Svensk Foerening foer Diabetologi, Diabetescentrum, Sahlgrenska Sjukhuset, Goeteborg 41345, Sweden. TEL 46-31-3421000, FAX 46-31-270087, http://www.diabetolognytt.nu. Ed., Adv. contact Stig Attvall.

DOMESTIC ANIMAL ENDOCRINOLOGY. see *VETERINARY SCIENCE*

616.462 UKR
DYABETIK. Text in Russian, Ukrainian. m. USD 115 in United States.
Published by: Telepresskorporatsiya, Ul Pushkinskaya 33, Kiev, Ukraine. TEL 380-294-7200. **US dist. addr.:** East View Publications, 3020 Harbor Ln N, Minneapolis, MN 55447. TEL 612-550-0961.

616.462 RUS
DYABETOGRAFIYA. Text in Russian. q. USD 99.95 in United States.
Published by: Farmatsevticheskaya Gruppa Serv'e, Chasovaya ul 20, Moscow 125315, Russian Federation. **US dist. addr.:** East View Publications, 3020 Harbor Ln N, Minneapolis, MN 55447. TEL 612-550-0961.

▼ **E D NEWS.** see *MEDICAL SCIENCES—Urology And Nephrology*

616.4 EGY ISSN 0070-9506
EGYPTIAN SOCIETY OF ENDOCRINOLOGY AND METABOLISM. JOURNAL✱. Text in English. 1955-1968; resumed 1971. irreg.
Published by: Egyptian Society of Endocrinology and Metabolism, 42 Sharia Kasr el-Aini, Cairo, Egypt.

616.4 613.2 FRA ISSN 1155-1941
ENCYCLOPEDIE MEDICO-CHIRURGICALE. ENDOCRINOLOGIE - NUTRITION. Cover title: Traite d'Endocrinologie - Nutrition. Variant title: Encyclopedie Medico-Chirurgicale. Endocrinologie - Nutrition. Text in French. 1936. 4 base vols. plus q. updates. bibl, charts, illus. *Refereed.* **Document type:** *Academic/Scholarly.*
Description: Offers endocrinologists, internists, and nutritionists a comprehensive, up-to-date reference for diagnosing and treating related conditions and disorders.
Former titles (until 1990): Encyclopedie Medico-Chirurgicale. Glandes Endocrines, Maladies de la Nutrition, Pathologie Generale (0246-0548); (until 1967): Encyclopedie Medico-Chirurgicale. Glandes Endocrines, Maladies de la Nutrition (0246-1056)
Published by: Elsevier Paris, Editions Scientifiques et Medicales (Subsidiary of: Reed Elsevier plc. group), 23 rue Linois, Paris 75015, France. TEL 33-1-45589110, FAX 33-1-45589425, redacion-emc@elsevier.fr, http://www.elsevier.fr, http://www.elsevier.com.

612.4 USA ISSN 1355-008X CODEN: EOCRE5
ENDOCRINE. Text in English. 1993. bi-m. USD 540 domestic; USD 550 foreign (effective 2000). adv. **Document type:** *Journal, Academic/Scholarly.*
Description: Publishes full-length articles devoted to the molecular, cellular, biochemical, and physiological aspects of endocrinology, including clinical papers on significant endocrine phenomena that are appropriately controlled, as well as methodological papers of special interest to endocrine investigators.
Formerly (until 1994): Endocrine Journal (0969-711X)
Related titles: Online - full text ed.: (from Institute for Scientific Information).
Indexed: ASCA, Chem.Abstr., Chem.Indus.Notes, Chem.Titles, Curr.Cont., Excerp.Med. (1995-), Ind.Med. (1994-), Ind.Sci.Rev., Inpharma, Int.Abstr.Biol.Sci., Pharm.&Out.News, Reac., Sci.Cit.Ind.
—BLDSC (3740.440000), ADONIS, CASDDS, CISTI, GNLM, IDS, Infotrieve, ingenta, KNAW. **CCC.**
Published by: Humana Press Inc., 999 Riverview Dr, Ste 208, Totowa, NJ 07512. TEL 973-256-1699, FAX 973-256-8341, humana@humanapr.com, http://humanapress.com. Ed. P Michael Conn. R&P Richard Hruska. Adv. contact Thomas B Lanigan Jr.

616.4 618.92 CHE ISSN 1421-7082
ENDOCRINE DEVELOPMENT. Text in English. 1998. irreg., latest vol.4. CHF 190 in Europe; DEM 230 in Germany; USD 190 in United States (2001). **Document type:** *Monographic series, Academic/Scholarly.* **Description:** Series of specialist publications devoted to specific areas of fetal, neonatal, pediatric and adolescent endocrinology.
—BLDSC (3740.451000).
Published by: S. Karger AG, Allschwilerstr 10, PO Box, Basel 4009, Switzerland. TEL 41-61-306-1111, FAX 41-61-306-1234, karger@karger.ch, http://www.karger.com/bookseries/ENDEV. Ed. M O Savage.

M

616.4 JPN ISSN 0918-8959
CODEN: ECJPAE
ENDOCRINE JOURNAL. Text in English. 1954. bi-m. JPY 12,000, USD 70 to individuals; USD 100 to institutions (effective 2001). bk.rev. abstr, charts, illus. index. 135 p./no. back issues avail. *Refereed.* **Document type:** *Journal, Academic/Scholarly.* **Description:** Publishes papers which contribute either experimentally, theoretically or clinically to knowledge in the field of endocrinology.
Formerly (until Feb. 1993): Endocrinologia Japonica (0013-7219)
Related titles: Online - full text ed.: (from Institute for Scientific Information).
Indexed: ASCA, Anim.Breed.Abstr., Aqua.Sci.& Fish.Abstr., Biol.Abstr., Cal.Tiss.Abstr. (coverage dropped), Chem.Abstr., Chem.Indus.Notes, Chem.Titles, Curr.Adv.Ecol.Sci., Curr.Cont., Curr.Ref.Fish Res., Dairy Sci.Abstr., Dent.Ind., Excerp.Med., INIS Atomind., Ind.Med. (1993-), Ind.Sci.Rev., Ind.Vet., Int.Abstr.Biol.Sci., Neurosci.Cit.Ind., Nutr.Abstr., Sci.Cit.Ind., THA, Tox.Abstr. (coverage dropped), Vet.Bull.
—BLDSC (3740.453000), CASDDS, CISTI, EMDOCS, GNLM, IDS, ingenta, KNAW, Linda Hall.
Published by: Japan Endocrine Society/Nihon Naibunpi Gakkai, Kinki Invention Center, 14 Yosida Kawahara-cho, Sakyo-ku, Kyoto 606-8305, Japan. TEL 81-75-752-2955, FAX 81-75-752-2963, endo-soc-japan@ml.infoweb.ne.jp, http://square.umin.ac.jp/endocrine, http://square.umin.ac.jp/endocrine/. Ed. Hajime Nawata. Circ: 6,000.

616.4 USA ISSN 1046-3976
RC648.A1 CODEN: ENPAFD
ENDOCRINE PATHOLOGY. Text in English. 1989. q. USD 385 domestic; USD 405 foreign (effective 2000). adv. bk.rev. abstr, bibl, charts, illus. index. *Refereed.* **Document type:** *Journal, Academic/Scholarly.* **Description:** Focuses on the diagnostic aspects of endocrine pathology and developments in the diagnostic applications of molecular biology and immunohistochemistry to endocrine pathology.
Related titles: Online - full text ed.: (from Institute for Scientific Information).
Indexed: ASCA, Chem.Abstr., Chem.Indus.Notes, Chem.Titles, Curr.Cont., Ind.Sci.Rev., Inpharma, Pharm.&Out.News, Reac., Sci.Cit.Ind.
—BLDSC (3740.460000), ADONIS, CASDDS, CISTI, GNLM, IDS, Infotrieve, KNAW. **CCC.**
Published by: (Endocrine Pathology Society), Humana Press Inc., 999 Riverview Dr, Ste 208, Totowa, NJ 07512. TEL 973-256-1699, FAX 973-256-8341, humana@humanapr.com, http://humanapress.com. Ed. Dr. Ricardo V Lloyd. R&P Richard Hruska. Adv. contact Thomas B Lanigan Jr. **Dist. in Japan by:** Maruzen Co., Ltd., International Division, Export Dept, P.O. Box 5050, Tokyo International 100-3191, Japan. TEL 81-3-3275-8591.

616.4 SVK ISSN 1210-0668
CODEN: EREGE3
ENDOCRINE REGULATIONS. Text and summaries in English. 1967. q. USD 100 (effective 2001 - 2002). bk.rev. charts, illus, stat. index. **Description:** Publishes original works that deal with the contemporary problems of experimental endocrinology of morphologic, physiologic, biochemical, pathophysiological or pharmacologic character.
Formerly (until 1991): Endocrinologia Experimentalis (0013-7200)
Indexed: Anim.Behav.Abstr., Aqua.Sci.& Fish.Abstr., Biol.Abstr., Chem.Abstr., Chem.Indus.Notes, Chem.Titles, Curr.Adv.Ecol.Sci., Curr.Cont. (coverage dropped), Dairy Sci.Abstr., Environ.Sci.Poll.Mgmt., Excerp.Med., INIS Atomind., Ind.Med. (1991-), Ind.Sci.Rev., Ind.Vet., Microbiol.Abstr., Nutr.Abstr., Pig News & Info., Sci.Cit.Ind. (coverage dropped), Vet.Bull.
—BLDSC (3740.467000), CASDDS, CISTI, GNLM, KNAW.
Published by: (Slovenska Akademia Vied/Slovak Academy of Sciences), Slovak Academic Press Ltd., Nam Slobody 6, PO Box 57, Bratislava 81005, Slovakia. TEL 42-12-54772800, http://www.savba.sk/logos/journals/ap/ap.html. Ed. Richard Kvetnansky. Circ: 800.

616.4 GBR ISSN 1351-0088
CODEN: ERCAE9
ENDOCRINE - RELATED CANCER. Text in English. q. GBP 190 in Europe; USD 350 in the Americas; GBP 210 elsewhere (effective 2002). charts, illus. back issues avail.; reprints avail. *Refereed.* **Document type:** *Journal, Academic/Scholarly.* **Description:** Provides an international forum for the presentation of all types of basic, clinical, and experimental investigations and observations which concern endocrine-related cancers.
Formerly (until 1993): Reviews on Endocrine - Related Cancer (0260-0897)
Related titles: Online - full text ed.: 1998 (from EBSCO Publishing, Swets Blackwell, Institute for Scientific Information).
Indexed: ASCA, Chem.Abstr., Chem.Indus.Notes, Chem.Titles, Curr.Cont., Excerp.Med., Ind.Med. (1994-), Ind.Sci.Rev., Inpharma, Int.Abstr.Biol.Sci., Pharm.&Out.News, Reac., Ref.Zh., Sci.Cit.Ind.
—BLDSC (3740.467500), CASDDS, CISTI, EMDOCS, GNLM, IDS, Infotrieve, KNAW. **CCC.**
Published by: Society for Endocrinology, 17-18 The Courtyard, Woodlands, Bradley Stoke, Bristol BS32 4NQ, United Kingdom. TEL 44-1454-642220, FAX 44-1454-642222, sales@portlandpress.co.uk, editorial@endocrinology.org, http://www.endocrinology.org. Ed. M Lippman. R&P Lyn Cole. Adv. contact Ailsa Bailey. **Subscr.in N. America to:** Allen Press Inc., PO Box 1897, Lawrence, KS 66044-8897. **Dist. by:** Portland Press Ltd., Commerce Way, Colchester, Essex CO2 8HP, United Kingdom. TEL 44-1206-796351, FAX 44-1206-799331.; **Dist. in Japan by:** Kinokuniya Co. Ltd., Journal Department, Chitose, P.O. Box 55, Tokyo 156, Japan.

616.4 USA ISSN 0743-5800
QP187.A1 CODEN: ENRSE8
ENDOCRINE RESEARCH. Text in English. 1965. q. USD 110 to individuals print & online eds.; USD 950 to institutions print only (effective 2002). adv. *Refereed.* **Document type:** *Journal, Academic/Scholarly.* **Description:** Coverage spans the entire field, providing the latest laboratory findings and developments in all areas of active investigation. Presents proceedings of conferences on endocrinology in addition to basic and applied research papers, technical comments, brief review articles, short reports, and laboratory protocols.
Formerly: Endocrine Research Communications (0093-6391); Supersedes: Endocrinological Communications
Related titles: Microform ed.: (from RPI); Online - full content ed.; Online - full text ed.: (from Institute for Scientific Information).
Indexed: ASCA, Anim.Breed.Abstr., BBCI, Biol.Abstr., Chem.Abstr., Chem.Indus.Notes, Chem.Titles, Curr.Adv.Ecol.Sci., Curr.Cont., Dairy Sci.Abstr., Excerp.Med., INIS Atomind., Ind.Med. (1984-), Ind.Sci.Rev., Inpharma, Int.Abstr.Biol.Sci., Nutr.Abstr., Pharm.&Out.News, Pig News & Info., Reac., Ref.Zh., Sci.Cit.Ind.
—BLDSC (3740.469000), CASDDS, CISTI, EMDOCS, GNLM, IDS, ingenta, KNAW. **CCC.**
Published by: Marcel Dekker Inc., 270 Madison Ave, New York, NY 10016. TEL 212-696-9000, 800-228-1160, FAX 212-685-4540, journals@dekker.com, custserv@dekker.com, http://www.dekker.com/servlet/product/productid/ERC. Ed. Alexander C Brownie. R&P Julia Mulligan. Adv. contact Anne Mullins. B&W page USD 800. Circ: 350. **Dist. addr. in Europe, Far East, Middle East & Africa:** Marcel Dekker AG, Hutgasse 4, PO Box 812, Basel 4001, Switzerland. TEL 41-61-261-8482, FAX 41-61-261-8896, intlcustserv@dekker.com.

616.4 USA ISSN 0163-769X
QP187.A1 CODEN: ERVIDP
ENDOCRINE REVIEWS. Text in English. 1980. bi-m. USD 168 domestic to individuals; USD 218 domestic to individuals Print & Online eds.; USD 204 foreign to individuals; USD 254 foreign to individuals Print & Online eds.; USD 278 domestic to institutions; USD 361 domestic to institutions Print & Online eds.; USD 318 foreign to institutions; USD 401 foreign to institutions Print & Online eds. (effective 2001). adv. back issues avail. *Refereed.* **Document type:** *Academic/Scholarly.* **Description:** Review articles explore clinical and experimental endocrinology topics.
Related titles: Microform ed.: (from WWS); Online - full text ed.: (from Ovid Technologies, Inc., HighWire Pr., EBSCO Publishing, Institute for Scientific Information).
Indexed: ASCA, Anim.Behav.Abstr., Anim.Breed.Abstr., Aqua.Sci.& Fish.Abstr., Chem.Abstr., Chem.Indus.Notes, Chem.Titles, Curr.Adv.Ecol.Sci., Curr.Cont., Diab.Cont., Excerp.Med., INIS Atomind., Ind.Med. (1980-), Ind.Sci.Rev., Inpharma, Int.Abstr.Biol.Sci., Neurosci.Abstr., Pharm.&Out.News, Pig News & Info., Poult.Abstr., Reac., Ref.Zh., SSCI (coverage dropped), Sci.Cit.Ind., THA.
—BLDSC (3740.480000), ADONIS, CASDDS, CISTI, GNLM, IDS, ingenta, KNAW. **CCC.**
Published by: Endocrine Society, 4350 East West Hwy, Ste 500, Bethesda, MD 20814-4410. TEL 301-941-0230, FAX 301-941-0259, endoreviews@endo-society.org; orders@allenpress.com, http://www.endosociety.org; http://www.allenpress.com. Ed. Marc G Caron. R&P Catherine Ang. Circ: 4,800. **Subscr. to:** Allen Press Inc., PO Box 1897, Lawrence, KS 66044-8897.

616.4 AUS ISSN 0312-4738
CODEN: ESAUAS
ENDOCRINE SOCIETY OF AUSTRALIA. PROCEEDINGS. Text in English. 1958. a. AUD 45 domestic; USD 55 foreign (effective 2000). adv. back issues avail. *Refereed.* **Document type:** *Proceedings.* **Description:** Covers endocrinology research in Australia.
Indexed: Biol.Abstr., Excerp.Med.
—BLDSC (6695.900000), CASDDS.
Published by: Endocrine Society of Australia, c/o Ivone Johnson, ESA Secretariat, 145 Macquarie St, Sydney, NSW 5405, Australia. TEL 61-8-83035342, FAX 61-8-83033356, c.coulter@physiol.adelaide.edu.au, esa@racp.edu.au, http://www.mmcc.monash.edu.au/endocrine/endoc.htm. Ed., R&P, Adv. contact Dr. Catherine Coulter. B&W page AUD 800, color page AUD 1,100; trim 170 x 245. Circ: 1,000.

616.4 ESP ISSN 0211-2299
CODEN: ENDCDP
ENDOCRINOLOGIA. Text in Spanish; Summaries in English. 1953. m. (10/yr.). USD 113 to non-members. adv. reprint service avail. from PQC. **Document type:** *Academic/Scholarly.* **Description:** Publishes clinical and experimental research in endocrinology.
Indexed: Chem.Abstr., Chem.Indus.Notes, Chem.Titles, Excerp.Med., Ind.Med.Esp.
—CASDDS, CISTI, GNLM, Infotrieve, KNAW. **CCC.**
Published by: (Sociedad Espanola de Endocrinologia), Ediciones Doyma S.A., Traversa de Gracia, 17-21, Barcelona 08021, Spain. TEL 34-93-200-0711, FAX 34-93-209-1136. Ed. R Gomis Barbera. Adv. contact Marte Vidal. color page ESP 238,000; trim 180 x 210. Circ: 2,000.

616.4 SVN ISSN 0351-1677
ENDOCRINOLOGIA IUGOSLAVICA. Text in Serbo-Croatian; Summaries in English. 1977. s-a. SIT 1,800, USD 20. adv. bk.rev. **Description:** Research reports on clinical endocrinology and diabetology for internists, endocrinologists, gynecologists and pediatricians.
Published by: (Raziskovalna Skupnost Slovenija), Tiskarna Tone Tomsic, Gregorciceua 25-a, Ljubljana 61000, Slovenia. Ed. Andreja Kocijancic. Circ: 400. **Subscr. to:** Nusa Bambic, Dispanzer za Diabetike, UKC Njegoseva 4, Ljubljana 61000, Slovenia.

616.4 USA ISSN 1051-2144
CODEN: EDOCEB
THE ENDOCRINOLOGIST. Text in English. 1991. bi-m. USD 155 domestic to individuals; USD 190 foreign to individuals; USD 294 domestic to institutions; USD 338 foreign to institutions; USD 51 newsstand/cover (effective 2002). adv. *Refereed.* **Document type:** *Academic/Scholarly.* **Description:** Directed exclusively to clinicians interested in practical applications of new discoveries in endocrinology, diabetes, and metabolism.
Related titles: Microfilm ed.: (from WWS); Online - full text ed.: USD 382.20 domestic academic site license; USD 426.20 foreign academic site license; USD 426.30 domestic corporate site license; USD 470.30 foreign corporate site license (2002) (from Ovid Technologies, Inc., Institute for Scientific Information).
Indexed: ASCA, Curr.Cont., Excerp.Med. (1993-), Ind.Sci.Rev., Inpharma, Pharm.&Out.News, Reac., Sci.Cit.Ind.
—BLDSC (3741.750000), EMDOCS, GNLM, IDS, KNAW.
Published by: Williams & Wilkins (Subsidiary of: Waverly International), 351 W Camden St, Baltimore, MD 21201-2436. TEL 410-528-4068, 800-222-3790, FAX 410-528-4452, custserv@wwilkins.com, http://www.wwilkins.com, http://www.Lww.com. Ed. Dr. Lynn Loriaux. Adv. contact Sharlene Isaacson. B&W page USD 785; trim 10.88 x 8.13. Circ: 3,555; 3,360 (paid).

616.4 USA ISSN 0013-7227
QP187 CODEN: ENDOAO
ENDOCRINOLOGY. Text in English. 1917. m. USD 60, USD 20 domestic to individuals; USD 140 domestic to institutions; USD 40 elsewhere to institutions (effective 2002). adv. bibl, charts, illus. index. back issues avail.; reprints avail. *Refereed.* **Document type:** *Academic/Scholarly.* **Description:** Covers all aspects of research on endocrine glands and their hormones.
Related titles: Microform ed.: (from PMC); Online - full text ed.: (from Ovid Technologies, Inc., HighWire Pr., EBSCO Publishing, Institute for Scientific Information).

M

Indexed: AIM, ASCA, AgBiotech, Agri.& Environ.Biotech.Abstr. (coverage dropped), Anim.Breed.Abstr., Aqua.Sci.& Fish.Abstr., Biol.Abstr., Cal.Tiss.Abstr., Chem.Abstr., Chem.Indus.Notes, Chem.Titles, Curr.Adv.Biochem., Curr.Adv.Cancer Res., Curr.Adv.Cell & Devel.Biol., Curr.Adv.Ecol.Sci., Curr.Adv.Gen.& Molec.Biol., Curr.Cont., Curr.Ref.Fish Res., Dairy Sci.Abstr., Dent.Ind., Derwent Biotech.Abstr., Diab.Cont., Environ.Sci.Poll.Mgmt., Excerp.Med., Hum.Gen.Abstr., INIS Atomind., Ind.Med. (1917-), Ind.Sci.Rev., Ind.Vet., Inpharma, Int.Abstr.Biol.Sci., Mass Spectr.Bull., Neurosci.Cit.Ind., Nuc.Acids Abstr., Nutr.Abstr., Pharm.&Out.News, Pig News & Info., Poult.Abstr., Reac., Ref.Zh., Rev.Appl.Entomol., Rev.Arom.& Med.Plants, Rev.Med.& Vet.Mycol., Sci.Cit.Ind., Small Anim.Abstr., Soils & Fert., Soyabean Abstr., Sport Fish.Abstr., THA, Tox.Abstr. (coverage dropped), Trop.Dis.Bull., Vet.Bull., Wild.Rev., Zoo.Rec.
—BLDSC (3742.000000), ADONIS, CASDDS, CISTI, GNLM, IDS, ingenta, KNAW, Linda Hall. **CCC.**
Published by: Endocrine Society, 4350 East West Hwy, Ste 500, Bethesda, MD 20814-4410. TEL 301-941-0230, FAX 301-941-0259, endocrinology@endo-society.org; orders@allenpress.com, http://www.endo-society.org; http://www.allenpress.com, http://www.endosociety.org; http://www.allenpress.com. Ed. Kenneth Korach. R&P Catherine Ang. Circ: 5,800. **Subscr. to:** Allen Press Inc., PO Box 1897, Lawrence, KS 66044-8897.

616.4 USA ISSN 0889-8529
RC648.A1 CODEN: ECNAER
ENDOCRINOLOGY AND METABOLISM CLINICS OF NORTH AMERICA. Text in English. 1972. q. USD 157 domestic to individuals; USD 175 in Canada to individuals; USD 204 elsewhere to individuals; USD 205 domestic to institutions; USD 245 foreign to institutions; USD 62 per issue (effective 2001). *Refereed.* **Document type:** *Journal, Academic/Scholarly.* **Description:** Delivers practical advice from experts in specialty covered as well as the information on new developments and controversies.
Formerly: Clinics in Endocrinology and Metabolism (0300-595X)
Related titles: Online - full text ed.: (from Institute for Scientific Information).
Indexed: ASCA, Biol.Abstr., CINAHL, Chem.Abstr., Chem.Indus.Notes, Chem.Titles, Curr.Adv.Ecol.Sci., Curr.Cont., Dent.Ind., Excerp.Med., INIS Atomind., Ind.Med. (1987-), Ind.Sci.Rev., Inpharma, Neurosci.Cit.Ind., Nutr.Abstr., Pharm.&Out.News, Reac., SSCI (coverage dropped), Sci.Cit.Ind.
—BLDSC (3743.052000), CASDDS, CISTI, EMDOCS, GNLM, IDS, ingenta, KNAW. **CCC.**
Published by: W.B. Saunders Co. (Subsidiary of: Harcourt Publishers Ltd.), 11830 Westline Industrial Dr, St Louis, MO 63146. TEL 800-325-4177, http://www.wbsaunders.com. **Subscr. to:** Periodicals Fulfillment, W B Saunders Co, 6277 Sea Harbor Dr, 4th Fl, Orlando, FL 32891-4800.

616.4 DEU ISSN 0721-667X
ENDOKRINOLOGIE - INFORMATIONEN. Text in German; Summaries in English. 1977. 4/yr. **Document type:** *Journal, Academic/Scholarly.*
—GNLM.
Published by: (Deutsche Gesellschaft fuer Endokrinologie), Georg Thieme Verlag, Ruedigerstr 14, Stuttgart 70469, Germany. TEL 49-711-8931-0, FAX 49-711-8931298, kunden.service@thieme.de, http://www.thieme.de. Circ: 1,600.

616.4 UKR
ENDOKRINOLOHIYA. Text in Ukrainian, Russian. 1996. s-a. USD 125 in the Americas (effective 2000).
Published by: Akademiya Medychnykh Nauk Ukrainy, Institut Endokrinologii i Obmena Veshchestv, Ul Vyshgorodskaya 69, Kiev, Ukraine. TEL 430-36-94, FAX 430-37-18. **Dist. by:** East View Publications, 3020 Harbor Ln N, Minneapolis, MN 55447. TEL 763-550-0961, FAX 763-559-2931.

616.4 POL ISSN 0423-104X
CODEN: EDPKA2
ENDOKRYNOLOGIA POLSKA. Text in Polish; Summaries in English, Russian. 1951. bi-m. USD 30. adv. bk.rev. bibl, charts, illus. index. **Description:** Papers on practical and theoretical aspects of Polish research on endocrinology.
Indexed: Anim.Breed.Abstr., Biol.Abstr., Chem.Abstr., Dent.Ind., Excerp.Med. (until 1993), INIS Atomind., Ind.Med. (coverage dropped).
—BLDSC (3743.300000), CASDDS, CISTI, GNLM.
Published by: Polskie Towarzystwo Endokrynologiczne/ Polish Endocrinological Association, Pl Starynkiewicza 3, Warsaw 02015, Poland. Ed. Zbigniew Szybinski. **Dist. by:** Ars Polona, Krakowskie Przedmiescie 7, Warsaw, Poland.

612.4 USA ISSN 1534-7621
ENDOTRENDS. Text in English. 1994. q. abstr. **Document type:** *Newsletter.* **Description:** Publishes articles describing new research developments in endocrinology, patient case studies, grant information, career counseling tips, a medical meetings calendar, and other clinical and practical information for endocrine fellows.
Related titles: Online - full text ed.: ISSN 1534-763X (from IDEAL Online Library).
Published by: (Endocrine Fellows Foundation), Academic Press, Inc., Journal Division (Subsidiary of: Harcourt Brace & Company), 525 B St, Ste 1900, San Diego, CA 92101-4495. TEL 619-231-6616.

616.4 GBR ISSN 0804-4643
QP187.A1 CODEN: EJOEEP
EUROPEAN JOURNAL OF ENDOCRINOLOGY. Text in English. 1948. m. GBP 410, USD 655 (effective 2002). adv. abstr, charts, illus. index. 2 cols./p. back issues avail.; reprints avail. *Refereed.* **Document type:** *Journal, Academic/Scholarly.* **Description:** Publishes original scientific papers and critical reviews within clinical and experimental endocrinology.
Formerly (until 1994): Acta Endocrinologica (0001-5598)
Related titles: Online - full text ed.: (from EBSCO Publishing, Swets Blackwell, Institute for Scientific Information); ♦ Supplement: European Journal of Endocrinology. Supplement. ISSN 0804-4635.
Indexed: ASCA, Abstr.Inter.Med., AgBiotech, Agri.& Environ.Biotech.Abstr. (coverage dropped), Anim.Breed.Abstr., Aqua.Sci.& Fish.Abstr., Aquacult.Abstr., Behav.Med.Abstr., Biol.Abstr., C.I.S. Abstr., Chem.Abstr., Chem.Indus.Notes, Chem.Titles, Curr.Adv.Cancer Res., Curr.Adv.Cell & Devel.Biol., Curr.Adv.Ecol.Sci., Curr.Adv.Gen.& Molec.Biol., Curr.Cont., Dairy Sci.Abstr., Dent.Ind., Derwent Biotech.Abstr., Diab.Cont., Environ.Sci.Poll.Mgmt., Excerp.Med., INIS Atomind., Ind.Med. (1994-), Ind.Sci.Rev., Ind.Vet., Inpharma, Int.Abstr.Biol.Sci., Mass Spectr.Bull., Neurosci.Cit.Ind., Nutr.Abstr., Pharm.&Out.News, Pig News & Info., Reac., Rev.Arom.& Med.Plants, SSCI (coverage dropped), Sci.Cit.Ind., Small Anim.Abstr., Sport Fish.Abstr., Trop.Dis.Bull., Vet.Bull., Wild.Rev., Zoo.Rec.
—BLDSC (3829.728700), CASDDS, CISTI, EMDOCS, GNLM, IDS, ingenta, KNAW. **CCC.**
Published by: (European Federation of Endocrine Societies), BioScientifica Ltd., 16 The Courtyard, Woodlands, Bradley Stoke, Bristol BS32 4NQ, United Kingdom. TEL 44-1454-642240, FAX 44-1454-642222, info@eje.org, sales@portlandpress.co.uk, http://www.eje.org. Ed. Paolo Beck-Peccoz. R&P Lyn Cole. Adv. contact Lara Thompson. B&W page GBP 450, color page GBP 995; bleed 221 x 286. Circ: 1,200. **Subscr. in US to:** Allen Press Inc., PO Box 1897, Lawrence, KS 66044-8897. TEL 785-843-1235, FAX 785-843-1274; **Subscr. to:** Portland Press Ltd., Customer Service, Commerce Way, Colchester, Essex CO2 8HP, United Kingdom.

616.4 GBR ISSN 0804-4635
QP1 CODEN: EJESE
EUROPEAN JOURNAL OF ENDOCRINOLOGY. SUPPLEMENT. Text in English. 1948. irreg., latest 1998. GBP 410, USD 655 (effective 2002). abstr, illus, charts. back issues avail.; reprints avail. **Document type:** *Journal, Academic/Scholarly.*
Formerly (until 1994): Acta Endocrinologica. Supplementum (0300-9750)
Related titles: ♦ Supplement to: European Journal of Endocrinology. ISSN 0804-4643.
Indexed: Biol.Abstr., Chem.Abstr., Curr.Adv.Ecol.Sci., Curr.Cont. (coverage dropped), Dairy Sci.Abstr., Excerp.Med. (1993-), INIS Atomind., Ind.Med. (coverage dropped), Int.Abstr.Biol.Sci., Nutr.Abstr.
—BLDSC (3829.728710), CASDDS, CISTI, ingenta, KNAW. **CCC.**
Published by: (European Federation of Endocrine Societies), BioScientifica Ltd., 16 The Courtyard, Woodlands, Bradley Stoke, Bristol BS32 4NQ, United Kingdom. TEL 44-1454-642240, FAX 44-1454-642222, info@eje.org, http://www.eje.org; http://www.bioscientifica.com. Ed. Paolo Beck-Peccoz. R&P Lyn Cole. Adv. contact Lara Thompson. **Subscr. to:** Portland Press Ltd., Commerce Way, PO Box 32, Colchester CO2 8HP, United Kingdom.

EXCERPTA MEDICA. SECTION 3: ENDOCRINOLOGY. see *MEDICAL SCIENCES—Abstracting, Bibliographies, Statistics*

616.4 DEU ISSN 0947-7349
QP187.A1 CODEN: ECEDFQ
EXPERIMENTAL AND CLINICAL ENDOCRINOLOGY AND DIABETES. Text in English. 1928. 8/yr. EUR 268.40 domestic to institutions; EUR 278.80 in Europe to institutions; EUR 282.80 elsewhere to institutions; EUR 36 newsstand/cover (effective 2002). adv. abstr, bibl, charts, illus. index. 65 p./no. *Refereed.* **Document type:** *Journal, Academic/Scholarly.* **Description:** Covers the entire field of endocrinology from molecular biology to the clinic.
Former titles: Experimental and Clinical Endocrinology (0232-7384); Endokrinologie (0013-7251)
Related titles: Online - full text ed.: ISSN 1439-3646 (from Institute for Scientific Information); ♦ Supplement: Experimental and Clinical Endocrinology & Diabetes. Supplement. ISSN 0948-146X.
Indexed: ASCA, Agri.& Environ.Biotech.Abstr. (coverage dropped), Anim.Breed.Abstr., Biol.Abstr., Chem.Abstr., Chem.Indus.Notes, Chem.Titles, Curr.Adv.Cancer Res., Curr.Cont., Dairy Sci.Abstr., Dent.Ind., Derwent Biotech.Abstr., Dok.Arbeitsmed., Excerp.Med., INIS Atomind., Ind.Med. (1995-), Ind.Sci.Rev., Ind.Vet., Inpharma, Int.Abstr.Biol.Sci., Neurosci.Cit.Ind., Nutr.Abstr., Pharm.&Out.News, Pig News & Info., Protozool.Abstr., Reac., Rev.Med.& Vet.Mycol., Sci.Cit.Ind., Vet.Bull.
—BLDSC (3838.630100), CASDDS, CISTI, EMDOCS, GNLM, IDS, Infotrieve, ingenta, KNAW. **CCC.**
Published by: (Deutsche Gesellschaft fuer Endokrinologie), Johann Ambrosius Barth Verlag in Medizinverlage Heidelberg GmbH & Co. KG, Ruedigerstr 14, Stuttgart 70469, Germany. TEL 49-711-8931-0, FAX 49-711-8931422, eced@medizinverlage.de, kunden.service@thieme.de, http://www.eced.org, http://www.thieme.de. Eds. H Schatz, M Wehling. Adv. contact Irmgard Mayer TEL 49-711-8931469. B&W page DEM 1,900; trim 210 x 280. Circ: 2,500.

616.4 DEU ISSN 0948-146X
EXPERIMENTAL AND CLINICAL ENDOCRINOLOGY & DIABETES. SUPPLEMENT. Text in English. 1995. irreg.
Related titles: ♦ Supplement to: Experimental and Clinical Endocrinology and Diabetes. ISSN 0947-7349.
Published by: Johann Ambrosius Barth Verlag in Medizinverlage Heidelberg GmbH & Co. KG, Ruedigerstr 14, Stuttgart 70469, Germany. TEL 49-6221-489251, FAX 49-711-8931422. Ed. S Hofmann von Kap-herr.

616.4 CHE ISSN 0251-5342
CODEN: FDIADJ
FRONTIERS IN DIABETES. Text in English. irreg., latest vol.15. CHF 200 in Europe; DEM 240 in Germany; CHF 160 in United States (effective 2001). reprint service avail. from ISI. *Refereed.* **Document type:** *Journal, Academic/Scholarly.* **Description:** Provides a reference tool for workers who need convenient, well-ordered access to the latest information.
Related titles: Online - full text ed.
Indexed: Biol.Abstr., Chem.Abstr., Chem.Indus.Notes, Chem.Titles, Mass Spectr.Bull.
—BLDSC (4042.003000), CASDDS, CISTI, Infotrieve, KNAW. **CCC.**
Published by: S. Karger AG, Allschwilerstr 10, PO Box, Basel 4009, Switzerland. TEL 41-61-306-1111, FAX 41-61-306-1234, karger@karger.ch, http://www.karger.com/bookseries/FDIAB. Ed. F Belfiore.

616.4 GBR ISSN 0959-6623
RC660.A1
FRONTIERS IN DIABETES RESEARCH. Text in English. 1984. biennial. **Document type:** *Academic/Scholarly.*
Formerly (until 1988): Lessons from Animal Diabetes (0953-4318)
—BLDSC (5184.611000).
Published by: Smith-Gordon and Co. Ltd., 13 Shalcomb St, London SW10 0HZ, United Kingdom. TEL 44-171-351-7042, FAX 44-171-351-1250. Ed. Eldred Smith Gordon. **Dist. in US by:** Books International, PO Box 605, Herndon, VA 20172. TEL 703-435-7064, 703-689-0660.

616.4 616.8 USA ISSN 0091-3022
QP187.A1 CODEN: FNEDA7
FRONTIERS IN NEUROENDOCRINOLOGY. Text in English. 1962. q. USD 330 in US & Canada to institutions; USD 360 elsewhere to institutions (effective 2001). reprint service avail. from PQC. *Refereed.* **Document type:** *Academic/Scholarly.* **Description:** Contains review coverage of major clinical issues.
Related titles: Online - full text ed.: (from EBSCO Publishing, O C L C Online Computer Library Center, Inc., RoweCom Information Quest, ingenta, Swets Blackwell, IDEAL Online Library, Institute for Scientific Information).

M

Indexed: ASCA, Biol.Abstr., Chem.Abstr., Chem.Indus.Notes, Chem.Titles, Curr.Cont., Excerp.Med., Ind.Med. (1969-), Ind.Sci.Rev., Inpharma, Neurosci.Cit.Ind., Pharm.&Out.News, Reac., Sci.Cit.Ind. —BLDSC (4042.040000), ADONIS, CASDDS, CISTI, IDS, ingenta. **CCC.**
Published by: Academic Press, Inc., Journal Division (Subsidiary of: Harcourt Brace & Company), 528 B St, Ste 1900, San Diego, CA 92101-4495. TEL 619-230-1840, FAX 619-699-6800, TELEX 181726, apsubs@acad.com, http://www.academicpress.com/fine. Eds. Luciano Martini, William F Ganong.

616.4 CHE ISSN 0301-3073 CODEN: FHRSA7
FRONTIERS OF HORMONE RESEARCH. Text in English. 1972. irreg., latest vol.30. CHF 180 in Europe; DEM 215 in Germany; USD 145 in United States (effective 2001). reprint service avail. from ISI. *Refereed.* **Document type:** *Journal, Academic/Scholarly.* **Description:** Information on how findings from hormone research can be used in clinical medicine.
Formerly: Monographs in Hormone Research (0077-0868)
Related titles: Online - full text ed.: (from Institute for Scientific Information).
Indexed: ASCA, Biol.Abstr., Chem.Abstr., Chem.Indus.Notes, Chem.Titles, Curr.Cont. (coverage dropped), Ind.Med. (1972-), Ind.Sci.Rev., Ind.Vet., Sci.Cit.Ind., Small Anim.Abstr., Vet.Bull. —BLDSC (4042.025000), GNLM, Infotrieve, ingenta, KNAW. **CCC.**
Published by: S. Karger AG, Allschwilerstr 10, PO Box, Basel 4009, Switzerland. TEL 41-61-306-1111, FAX 41-61-306-1234, karger@karger.ch, http://www.karger.com/bookseries/FHORE. Ed. A Grossman.

616.4 USA ISSN 0016-6480 QP187 CODEN: GCENA5
GENERAL AND COMPARATIVE ENDOCRINOLOGY; an international journal. Text in English. 1961. m. USD 1,799 in US & Canada to institutions; USD 2,000 elsewhere to institutions (effective 2001). adv. bk.rev. bibl, charts, illus. index. back issues avail. *Refereed.* **Document type:** *Academic/Scholarly.* **Description:** Devoted to basic endocrinological research; emphasizes fundamental research; features occasional brief reviews that deal with a particular field or problem.
Related titles: Online - full text ed.: (from EBSCO Publishing, O C L C Online Computer Library Center, Inc., RoweCom Information Quest, ingenta, Swets Blackwell, IDEAL Online Library, Institute for Scientific Information).
Indexed: ASCA, AgBiotech, Agri.Eng.Abstr., Agricola, Anim.Behav.Abstr., Anim.Breed.Abstr., Aqua.Sci.& Fish.Abstr., Bibl.Agri., Biol.Abstr., Cal.Tiss.Abstr., Chem.Abstr., Chem.Indus.Notes, Chem.Titles, Curr.Adv.Cell & Devel.Biol., Curr.Adv.Ecol.Sci., Curr.Cont., Dairy Sci.Abstr., Entomol.Abstr., Environ.Sci.Poll.Mgmt., Excerp.Med., Helminthol.Abstr., INIS Atomind., Ind.Med. (1961-), Ind.Sci.Rev., Ind.Vet., Inpharma, Int.Abstr.Biol.Sci., Neurosci.Abstr. (coverage dropped), Neurosci.Cit.Ind., Nutr.Abstr., Pig News & Info., Pollut.Abstr., Poult.Abstr., Reac., Rev.Appl.Entomol., Sci.Cit.Ind., Sport Fish.Abstr., Vet.Bull., Wild.Rev., Zoo.Rec. —BLDSC (4097.400000), ADONIS, CASDDS, CISTI, GNLM, IDS, ingenta, Linda Hall. **CCC.**
Published by: Academic Press, Inc., Journal Division (Subsidiary of: Harcourt Brace & Company), 525 B St, Ste 1900, San Diego, CA 92101-4495. TEL 619-230-1840, FAX 619-699-6800, apsubs@acad.com, http://www.academicpress.com/gce. Eds. Frank L Moore, Ian W Henderson.

616.46 ITA CODEN: GIDIDU
GIORNALE ITALIANO DI DIABETOLOGIA E METABOLISMO. Text in Italian; Summaries in English, Italian, Spanish. 1981. q. ITL 60,000, USD 52. adv. bk.rev. abstr, charts, illus, stat. index. **Document type:** *Academic/Scholarly.* **Description:** Features original articles, reviews and edited letters on topics of physiopathology, clinics, and the therapy of diabetic illnesses. Includes columns on domestic and international cultural, social and sanitary-political activities for the diabetic.
Formerly (until 2000): Giornale Italiano di Diabetologia (0391-7525)
Indexed: Chem.Abstr., Chem.Indus.Notes, Chem.Titles, Excerp.Med., Inpharma, Reac. —BLDSC (4178.214350), CASDDS, EMDOCS, GNLM, KNAW.
Published by: Boehringer Mannheim Italia S.p.A., Viale G.B. Stucchi, 110, Milan, MI 20052, Italy. TEL 39-247-4068, FAX 39-247-4084, karin-berger@bmg.boehringer-manheim.com. Ed. Gianmichele Molinatti. Circ: 2,300.

GROWTH FACTORS & CYTOKINES - CLINICAL. see *MEDICAL SCIENCES—Abstracting, Bibliographies, Statistics*

GROWTH FACTORS & CYTOKINES - RESEARCH. see *MEDICAL SCIENCES—Abstracting, Bibliographies, Statistics*

616.4 GBR ISSN 1096-6374 CODEN: GHIRF9
GROWTH HORMONE AND I G F RESEARCH. Text in English. 1991. bi-m. GBP 101 to individuals; GBP 258 to institutions (effective 2002). adv. *Refereed.* **Document type:** *Academic/Scholarly.* **Description:** Provides a forum for research on the regulation of growth in humans, animals, tissues and cells. Publishes articles on all aspects of growth-promoting and growth-inhibiting hormones and factors.
Formed by the merger of: Growth Regulation (0956-523X); Endocrinology and Metabolism (1074-939X); Which was formerly (until 1995): Clinical and Experimental Metabolism
Related titles: Online - full text ed.: (from EBSCO Publishing, RoweCom Information Quest, Swets Blackwell, IDEAL Online Library, Institute for Scientific Information).
Indexed: ASCA, BBCI, Biol.Abstr., Chem.Abstr., Chem.Indus.Notes, Chem.Titles, Curr.Cont., Excerp.Med. (1993-), Ind.Med. (1998-), Ind.Sci.Rev., Inpharma, Int.Abstr.Biol.Sci., Pharm.&Out.News, Reac., Ref.Zh., Sci.Cit.Ind. —BLDSC (4223.033700), CASDDS, EMDOCS, GNLM, IDS, Infotrieve, KNAW. **CCC.**
Published by: (Growth Hormone Research Society), Churchill Livingstone (Subsidiary of: Harcourt Publishers Ltd.), Robert Stevenson House, 1-3 Baxter's Pl, Leith Walk, Edinburgh, Midlothian EH1 3AF, United Kingdom. TEL 44-131-556-2424, FAX 44-131-535-1704, cservice@harcourt.com, http://www.harcourt-international.com/journals/ghir. Eds. D Le Roith, P H Sondsen. Adv. contact David Dunnachie. **Subscr. to:** Harcourt Publishers Ltd., Foots Cray High St, Sidcup, Kent DA14 5HP, United Kingdom. TEL 44-20-8308-5700, FAX 44-20-8309-0807. **Co-sponsor:** International I G F Research Society.

612.4008042 GBR ISSN 0951-3590
GYNECOLOGICAL ENDOCRINOLOGY. Text in English. 1987. bi-m. GBP 85, USD 145 to individuals; GBP 155, USD 255 to institutions (effective 2000). adv. back issues avail. *Refereed.* **Document type:** *Academic/Scholarly.*
Related titles: Online - full text ed.: ISSN 1473-0766 (from CatchWord Ltd., Institute for Scientific Information).
Indexed: ASCA, Curr.Cont., Excerp.Med., Ind.Med. (1987-), Inpharma, Int.Abstr.Biol.Sci., Pharm.&Out.News, Reac. —BLDSC (4233.720000), ADONIS, CISTI, EMDOCS, GNLM, IDS, Infotrieve, ingenta, KNAW. **CCC.**
Published by: (International Society of Gynecological Endocrinology), Parthenon Publishing Group (Subsidiary of: C R C Press (New York)), Casterton Hall, Casterton, Carnforth, Lancs LA6 2LA, United Kingdom. TEL 44-1524-272084, FAX 44-1524-271587, mail@parthpub.com, http://www.parthpub.com/gynend/home.html. Ed., R&P Jean Wright. Adv. contact Julia Tissington. Circ: 1,200 (paid).

616.4 USA
HOMEOSTASIS QUARTERLY* . Text in English. 1971. q. USD 5. bk.rev.
Published by: Hypoglycemia Foundation, Inc., Adrenal Metabolic Research Society, 32 Sunrise Ter, Clifton Park, NY 12065-2327. Ed. Marilyn Hamilton Light. Circ: 5,000.

616.4 DEU ISSN 0018-5043 QP801.H7 CODEN: HMMRA2
HORMONE AND METABOLIC RESEARCH. Text in English. 1969. 12/yr. EUR 372.40 domestic to institutions; EUR 375.80 in Europe to institutions; EUR 382.80 elsewhere to institutions; EUR 38 newsstand/cover (effective 2002). adv. bibl, charts, illus, stat. index. reprint service avail. from PQC. *Refereed.* **Document type:** *Journal, Academic/Scholarly.*
Related titles: Microform ed.: (from PQC); Online - full text ed.: ISSN 1439-4286 (from Institute for Scientific Information); ♦ Supplement: Hormone and Metabolic Research. Supplement. ISSN 0170-5903.
Indexed: ASCA, Agri.& Environ.Biotech.Abstr. (coverage dropped), Anim.Breed.Abstr., Apic.Abstr., BBCI, Biol.Abstr., Chem.Abstr., Chem.Indus.Notes, Chem.Titles, Curr.Adv.Biochem., Curr.Adv.Cell & Devel.Biol., Curr.Adv.Ecol.Sci., Curr.Cont., Dairy Sci.Abstr., Dent.Ind., Derwent Biotech.Abstr., Diab.Cont., Excerp.Med., INIS Atomind., Ind.Med. (1969-), Ind.Sci.Rev., Ind.Vet., Inpharma, Int.Abstr.Biol.Sci., Nutr.Abstr., Pharm.&Out.News, Pig News & Info., Poult.Abstr., Reac., Risk Abstr., Sci.Cit.Ind., Sugar Ind.Abstr., THA, Vet.Bull. —BLDSC (4327.300000), ADONIS, CASDDS, CISTI, GNLM, IDS, ingenta, KNAW, Linda Hall. **CCC.**
Published by: Georg Thieme Verlag, Ruedigerstr 14, Stuttgart 70469, Germany. TEL 49-711-8931-0, FAX 49-711-8931298, hmr@thieme.de, kunden.service@thieme.de, leser.service@thieme.de, http://www.thieme.de/hmr, http://www.thieme-connect.de. Ed. W A Scherbaum. R&P Michael Wachinger. Circ: 1,100.

616.4 DEU ISSN 0170-5903 CODEN: HMRSAU
HORMONE AND METABOLIC RESEARCH. SUPPLEMENT. Text in German. irreg. back issues avail. **Document type:** *Monographic series, Academic/Scholarly.*
Related titles: Online - full text ed.; ♦ Supplement to: Hormone and Metabolic Research. ISSN 0018-5043.
Indexed: Chem.Abstr., Chem.Indus.Notes, Chem.Titles, Curr.Cont. (coverage dropped), Excerp.Med. (1994-), Ind.Med. (coverage dropped), Int.Abstr.Biol.Sci., Neurosci.Cit.Ind. —CASDDS, CISTI, KNAW. **CCC.**
Published by: Georg Thieme Verlag, Ruedigerstr 14, Stuttgart 70469, Germany. TEL 49-711-8931-0, FAX 49-711-8931298, hmr@thieme.de, kunden.service@thieme.de, leser.service@thieme.de, http://www.thieme.de/hmr, http://www.thieme-connect.de. Ed. W A Scherbaum. R&P Michael Wachinger.

HORMONE FRONTIER IN GYNECOLOGY. see *MEDICAL SCIENCES—Obstetrics And Gynecology*

616.4 CHE ISSN 0301-0163 QP187.A1 CODEN: HRMRA3
HORMONE RESEARCH; international journal of experimental and clinical endocrinology. Text in English. 1970. m. (2 vols.). CHF 1,508, EUR 1,077.60 in Europe to institutions; CHF 1,542.80, USD 1,176 elsewhere to institutions (effective 2002). adv. bk.rev. bibl, charts, stat. back issues avail. *Refereed.* **Document type:** *Journal, Academic/Scholarly.* **Description:** Facilitates the interchange of ideas by placing findings at all levels and from all branches side by side in a single source. Provides a background of experimental data on the pathology, cytology, histology, biochemistry, pharmacology and regulation of hormones.
Incorporates: Hormones (0018-5051); Steroids and Lipids Research (0300-0621); Which was formerly: Steroidologica (0049-2221)
Related titles: Microform ed.; Online - full text ed.: ISSN 1423-0046. CHF 116 with print edition; EUR 84, USD 90 to institutions with print edition (effective 2002) (from EBSCO Publishing, O C L C Online Computer Library Center, Inc., RoweCom Information Quest, Swets Blackwell, Institute for Scientific Information).
Indexed: ASCA, Agri.& Environ.Biotech.Abstr. (coverage dropped), Anim.Breed.Abstr., Aqua.Sci.& Fish.Abstr., Biol.Abstr., Cal.Tiss.Abstr. (coverage dropped), Chem.Abstr., Chem.Indus.Notes, Chem.Titles, Curr.Adv.Ecol.Sci., Curr.Cont., Dairy Sci.Abstr., Dent.Ind., Derwent Biotech.Abstr., Diab.Cont., Excerp.Med., INIS Atomind., Ind.Med. (1973-), Ind.Sci.Rev., Inpharma, Int.Nurs.Ind., Neurosci.Abstr. (coverage dropped), Neurosci.Cit.Ind., Nutr.Abstr., Pharm.&Out.News, Pig News & Info., Reac., SSCI (coverage dropped), Sci.Cit.Ind., Tox.Abstr. (coverage dropped). —BLDSC (4327.400000), CASDDS, CISTI, EMDOCS, GNLM, IDS, Infotrieve, ingenta, KNAW. **CCC.**
Published by: S. Karger AG, Allschwilerstr 10, PO Box, Basel 4009, Switzerland. TEL 41-61-306-1111, FAX 41-61-306-1234, karger@karger.ch, http://www.online.karger.com/journals/hed, http://www.karger.com. Ed. M B Ranke. adv.: page USD 1,195. Circ: 1,000.

616.4 156 USA ISSN 0018-506X QP187.A1 CODEN: HOBEAO
HORMONES AND BEHAVIOR. Text in English. 1969. 8/yr. USD 660 in US & Canada to institutions; USD 699 elsewhere to institutions (effective 2001). adv. back issues avail. *Refereed.* **Document type:** *Academic/Scholarly.* **Description:** Publishes original articles concerned with behavioral systems that are known to be hormonally influenced.

M

Related titles: Online - full text ed.: (from EBSCO Publishing, O C L C Online Computer Library Center, Inc., RoweCom Information Quest, ingenta, Swets Blackwell, IDEAL Online Library, Institute for Scientific Information).

Indexed: ASCA, Abstr.Anthropol., Anim.Behav.Abstr., Anim.Breed.Abstr., Aqua.Sci.& Fish.Abstr., Biol.Abstr., Chem.Abstr., Chem.Indus.Notes, Chem.Titles, Chemorec.Abstr., Curr.Adv.Ecol.Sci., Curr.Cont., Dairy Sci.Abstr., Environ.Sci.Poll.Mgmt., Excerp.Med., Ind.Med. (1969-), Ind.Sci.Rev., Inpharma, Mid.East: Abstr.& Ind., Neurosci.Abstr. (coverage dropped), Neurosci.Cit.Ind., Nutr.Abstr., Poult.Abstr., PsycInfo, Psychol.Abstr. (1971-), Reac., Risk Abstr., SSCI (coverage dropped), Saf.Sci.Abstr., Sci.Cit.Ind., Zoo.Rec., e-psyche.

—BLDSC (4328.050000), ADONIS, CASDDS, CISTI, GNLM, IDS, ingenta. **CCC.**

Published by: Academic Press, Inc., Journal Division (Subsidiary of: Harcourt Brace & Company), 525 B St, Ste 1900, San Diego, CA 92101-4495. TEL 619-230-1840, FAX 619-699-6800, apsubs@acad.com, http://www.apnet.com/www/journal/hb.htm; http://www.idealibrary.com/. Ed. Michael Baum.

616.4 JPN ISSN 0045-7167 CODEN: HORIAE

HORUMON TO RINSHO/CLINICAL ENDOCRINOLOGY. Text in Japanese. 1953. m. JPY 2,000 per issue.

Indexed: Chem.Abstr., Chem.Indus.Notes, Chem.Titles, INIS Atomind., Jap.Per.Ind.

—BLDSC (3286.279000), CASDDS, CISTI, GNLM.

Published by: Igaku no Sekaisha, 12-4 Kudan-Kita 1-chome, Chiyoda-ku, Tokyo 102-0073, Japan.

HUMAN FERTILITY. see *MEDICAL SCIENCES—Obstetrics And Gynecology*

HUMAN REPRODUCTION. see *MEDICAL SCIENCES—Obstetrics And Gynecology*

616.33 570 JPN ISSN 0289-2057

I-BUNPI KENKYUKAISHI/JAPANESE SOCIETY OF GASTRIC SECRETION RESEARCH. PROCEEDINGS. Variant title: I-bunpi Kenkyukai Kiroku. Text in Japanese. 1971. a. JPY 3,000 (effective 2000). adv. back issues avail. **Document type:** *Proceedings.*

Published by: Japanese Society of Gastric Secretion Research/I-bunpi Kenkyukai, c/o Tokyo Jikaijai Ika Daigaku Dai-2 Geka, 25-8 Nishi-Shinbashi 3-chome, Minato-ku, Tokyo 105-0000, Japan. TEL 81-3-3433-1111, FAX 86-3-3578-9075. Ed., R&P, Adv. contact Teruaki Aoki. Circ: 1,000.

616.3 USA ISSN 0169-4197 CODEN: IJPNEX

INTERNATIONAL JOURNAL OF PANCREATOLOGY. Text in English. 1986. bi-m. USD 465 domestic; USD 530 foreign (effective 2000). adv. bk.rev. abstr, bibl, charts, illus. index. back issues avail. *Refereed.* **Document type:** *Journal, Academic/Scholarly.* **Description:** Multidisciplinary forum for original clinical research on the exocrine and endocrine pancreas.

Related titles: Online - full text ed.: (from Institute for Scientific Information).

Indexed: ASCA, Biol.Abstr., Chem.Abstr., Chem.Indus.Notes, Chem.Titles, Curr.Cont., Excerp.Med., INIS Atomind., Ind.Med. (1986-), Ind.Sci.Rev., Inpharma, Jrnl.Watch Gastr., Pharm.&Out.News, Reac., Sci.Cit.Ind.

—BLDSC (4542.441000), ADONIS, CASDDS, CISTI, GNLM, IDS, ingenta, KNAW. **CCC.**

Published by: (International Association of Pancreatology), Humana Press Inc., 999 Riverview Dr, Ste 208, Totowa, NJ 07512. TEL 973-256-1699, FAX 973-256-8341, humana@humanapr.com, http://humanapress.com. Eds. Dr. C.W. Imrie, Dr. Manfred Singer. R&P Richard Hruska. Adv. contact Thomas B Lanigan Jr. **Dist. in Japan by:** Maruzen Co., Ltd., International Division, Export Dept, P.O. Box 5050, Tokyo International 100-3191, Japan. TEL 81-3-3275-8591.

616.4 DEU ISSN 0943-1675 CODEN: IJTYEI

INTERNATIONAL JOURNAL OF THYMOLOGY. Text in English. 1993. 2/yr. DEM 50. bk.rev. *Refereed.* **Document type:** *Academic/Scholarly.*

Indexed: Aqua.Sci.& Fish.Abstr., Chem.Abstr., Chem.Indus.Notes, Chem.Titles, Excerp.Med. (1995-), Ind.Vet., Vet.Bull.

—BLDSC (4542.695300), CASDDS, GNLM.

Published by: Thymus Medizinischer Fachbuchverlag, Rudolf Huch Str 14, Bad Harzburg 38667, Germany. TEL 49-5322-960532, FAX 49-5322-3017, drspiggelk@aol.com.de. Ed. Dr. Milan Jevremovic.

IRON METABOLISM. see *BIOLOGY—Abstracting, Bibliographies, Statistics*

616.15 USA ISSN 0895-7762

IRONIC BLOOD; information on iron overload. Text in English. 1981. bi-m. free per issue. back issues avail. **Document type:** *Newsletter, Academic/Scholarly, Consumer.* **Description:** Contains the latest information about hemochromatosis and other iron overload diseases for doctors, patients, and the public.

Published by: Iron Overload Diseases Association, Inc., International Clearinghouse, 433 Westwind Dr, N, Palm Beach, FL 33408. TEL 561-840-8512, FAX 561-842-9881, iod@ironoverload.org, http://www.ironoverload.org. Ed. Roberta Crawford. Circ: 8,000.

616.462 JPN ISSN 0021-437X CODEN: TONYA4

JAPAN DIABETES SOCIETY. JOURNAL/TONYOBYO. Text in Japanese; Summaries in English. 1958. m. JPY 20,280, USD 65. adv. charts. index. **Document type:** *Academic/Scholarly.*

Formerly: Japan Diabetic Society. Journal

Indexed: Biol.Abstr., Chem.Abstr., Diab.Cont., Excerp.Med., INIS Atomind., Ref.Zh.

—BLDSC (4804.840000), CASDDS, CISTI, GNLM.

Published by: Japan Diabetes Society/Nihon Tonyobyo Gakkai, Sky Bldg Rm 403, 3-38-11 Hongo, Bunkyo-ku, Tokyo 113-0033, Japan. TEL 81-3-3815-4364, FAX 81-3-3815-7985. Ed. Dr. K Yamashita. Circ: 4,800.

616.4 570 JPN ISSN 0913-9036 CODEN: PJSEEU

JAPAN SOCIETY FOR COMPARATIVE ENDOCRINOLOGY. PROCEEDINGS. Text in English. 1986. a. JPY 3,000. back issues avail. **Document type:** *Proceedings.*

Indexed: Zoo.Rec.

—BLDSC (6742.312000).

Published by: Japan Society for Comparative Endocrinology/Nihon Hikaku Naibunpi Gakkai, c/o Zoology Institute, Faculty of Science University of, 3-1 Hongo 7-chome, Bunkyo-ku, Tokyo 113-0033, Japan. TEL 03-3812-2111, FAX 81-3-3816-1965. Ed. Yuichi Sasayama. Circ: 600.

616.462 USA

JOSLIN MAGAZINE. Text in English. 1985. 4/yr. USD 25 (effective 2000). illus. back issues avail. **Description:** Covers articles on patient care and research on diabetes and its complications.

Former titles: Joslin Diabetes Center Newsletter; Joslin Diabetes Foundation. Newsletter (0021-7611)

Published by: Joslin Diabetes Center, Inc., One Joslin Pl, Boston, MA 02215. TEL 617-732-2415, FAX 617-732-2562, http://www.joslin.org. Ed., Pub., R&P Julie F Rafferty. Circ: 30,000.

616.4 CHE

JOURNAL DES DIABETIQUES. Text in French. 1962. 5/yr. CHF 30. adv. bk.rev. **Document type:** *Academic/Scholarly.*

Address: 2 Rue du Moulin, Moutier 2740, Switzerland. TEL 032-935908, FAX 032-936234. Ed. J J Grimm. Circ: 7,000.

JOURNAL FUER MINERALSTOFFWECHSEL; Zeitschrift fuer Physiologie, Pathophysiologie und Klinik des Mineralstoffwechsels. see *BIOLOGY—Biochemistry*

616.4 JPN ISSN 0914-8779 CODEN: JBMME4

JOURNAL OF BONE AND MINERAL METABOLISM. Text in English. 1988. bi-m. (in 1 vol., 6 nos./vol.). JPY 22,000 domestic; USD 229 in North America; DEM 438 elsewhere; DEM 213, EUR 108.91 in Germany for Print & Online Eds.; DEM 215.40, EUR 110.14 elsewhere for Print & Online Eds. (effective 2001). **Document type:** *Academic/Scholarly.* **Description:** Serves as the official publication of the Society.

Related titles: Online - full text ed.: ISSN 1435-5604 (from EBSCO Publishing, RoweCom Information Quest, Swets Blackwell, Springer LINK, Institute for Scientific Information); ♦ Japanese ed.: Nihon Kotsu Taisha Gakkai Zasshi. ISSN 0910-0067.

Indexed: BBCI, Cal.Tiss.Abstr., Chem.Abstr., Chem.Indus.Notes, Chem.Titles, Ind.Med. (1988-).

—BLDSC (4954.255500), CASDDS, CISTI, GNLM, IDS, Infotrieve. **CCC.**

Published by: (Nihon Kotsu Taisha Gakkai/Japan Society for Bone and Metabolism Research), Springer-Verlag Tokyo, Eastern Book Service, Inc. (Subsidiary of: BertelsmannSpringer), 3-13 Hongo 3-chome, Bunkyo-ku, Tokyo 113-0033, Japan. TEL 81-3-5395-6366, FAX 81-3-5395-6876, orders@svt-ebs.co.jp, http://link.springer-ny.com/link/service/journals/00774/index.htm, http://www.springer.ny.com, http://link.springer.de. Ed. Fujio Suzuki. **Subscr. in N. America to:** Springer-Verlag New York Inc., PO Box 2485, Secaucus, NJ 07096-2485. TEL 800-777-4643, 212-460-1526, FAX 201-348-4505, orders@springer-ny.com; **Subscr. outside N. America & Japan to:** Springer-Verlag, c/o Gabriele Kubitza, Haberstrasse 7, Heidelberg 69126, Germany. FAX 49-30-82787448, 49-6221-345229, subscriptions@springer.de, http://link.springer-ny.com; **Subscr. to:** Eastern Book Service, Inc., 3-13 Hongo 3-chome, Bunkyo-ku, Tokyo 113-8480, Japan.

616.4 USA ISSN 0021-972X CODEN: JCEMAZ

JOURNAL OF CLINICAL ENDOCRINOLOGY AND METABOLISM. Text in English. 1941. m. USD 259 domestic to individuals; USD 337 domestic to individuals Print & Online eds.; USD 344 foreign to individuals (effective 2001); USD 422 foreign to individuals Print & Online eds.; USD 443 domestic to institutions; USD 576 domestic to institutions Print & Online eds.; USD 516 foreign to institutions; USD 649 foreign to institutions Print & Online eds. (effective 1999). adv. charts, illus. back issues avail.; reprints avail. *Refereed.* **Document type:** *Academic/Scholarly.* **Description:** Information on the clinical applications of endocrine research.

Related titles: Microform ed.: (from PMC); Online - full text ed.: (from Ovid Technologies, Inc., HighWire Pr., EBSCO Publishing, Institute for Scientific Information).

Indexed: AIM, ASCA, Agri.& Environ.Biotech.Abstr. (coverage dropped), Behav.Med.Abstr., Biol.Abstr., Cal.Tiss.Abstr. (coverage dropped), Chem.Abstr., Chem.Indus.Notes, Chem.Titles, Curr.Adv.Biochem., Curr.Adv.Cancer Res., Curr.Adv.Cell & Devel.Biol., Curr.Adv.Gen.& Molec.Biol., Curr.Cont., Dairy Sci.Abstr., Dent.Ind., Derwent Biotech.Abstr., Diab.Cont., Diar.Dis.Res., Excerp.Med., Food Sci.& Tech.Abstr., Forest Prod.Abstr., Helminthol.Abstr., INIS Atomind., Ind.Med. (1952-), Ind.Sci.Rev., Inpharma, Int.Abstr.Biol.Sci., Int.Nurs.Ind., Jrnl.Watch, Jrnl.Watch Wom.Hlth., Kidney, Med.& Surg.Dermat., Neurosci.Cit.Ind., Nutr.Abstr., Pharm.&Out.News, Protozool.Abstr., Reac., Risk Abstr., SSCI (coverage dropped), Sci.Cit.Ind., Soyabean Abstr., Sport Fish.Abstr., THA, Tox.Abstr. (coverage dropped), Trop.Dis.Bull., Wild.Rev.

—BLDSC (4958.400000), ADONIS, CASDDS, CISTI, GNLM, IDS, ingenta, KNAW. **CCC.**

Published by: Endocrine Society, 4350 East West Hwy, Ste 500, Bethesda, MD 20814-4410. TEL 301-941-0230, FAX 301-941-0259, jcem@endo-society.org; orders@allenpress.com, http://www.endo-society.org; http://www.allenpress.com, http://www.endosociety.org; http://www.allenpress.com. R&P Catherine Ang. Circ: 9,400. **Subscr. to:** Allen Press Inc., PO Box 1897, Lawrence, KS 66044-8897.

616.4 USA ISSN 1056-8727 CODEN: JDICE2

JOURNAL OF DIABETES AND ITS COMPLICATIONS. Text in English. 1987. bi-m. EUR 199 in Europe to individuals; JPY 26,400 in Japan to individuals; USD 223 elsewhere to individuals; EUR 422 in Europe to institutions; JPY 56,000 in Japan to institutions; USD 472 elsewhere to institutions (effective 2002). back issues avail.; reprints avail. *Refereed.* **Document type:** *Academic/Scholarly.* **Description:** Publishes original contributions developed from clinical investigation, as well as brief review articles.

Formerly (until 1992): Journal of Diabetic Complications (0891-6632)

Related titles: Microform ed.: (from PQC); Online - full text ed.: (from ingenta, ScienceDirect, Swets Blackwell, Institute for Scientific Information).

Indexed: ASCA, Curr.Cont., Diab.Cont., Excerp.Med., INIS Atomind., Ind.Med. (1992-), Inpharma, Int.Abstr.Biol.Sci., NRN, Pharm.&Out.News, Reac., THA.

—BLDSC (4969.407000), CISTI, EMDOCS, GNLM, IDS, Infotrieve, KNAW. **CCC.**

M

Published by: Elsevier Science, PO Box 945, New York, NY 10159-0945. TEL 212-989-5800, FAX 212-633-3990, usinfo-f@elsevier.com, http://www.elsevier.com/locate/jdiacomp. Eds. C E Mogensen, Dr. Philip Raskin. **Subscr. in Australasia and the Far East to:** Elsevier Science (Singapore) Pte Ltd, No.1 Temasek Ave, 17-01 Millenia Tower, Singapore 039192, Singapore. TEL 65-434-3727, FAX 65-337-2230; **Subscr. in Japan to:** Elsevier Science Inc - Japan Regional Office, 9-15 Higashi-Azabu 1-chome, Minato-ku, Tokyo 106-0044, Japan. TEL 81-3-5561-5033; **Subscr. outside the Americas to:** Elsevier Science BV, PO Box 211, Amsterdam 1000 AE, Netherlands. TEL 31-20-485-3757, nlinfo-f@elsevier.nl.

JOURNAL OF DIABETES NURSING; the journal for professionals working in the field of diabetes nursing. see *MEDICAL SCIENCES—Nurses And Nursing*

616.4 599.9 ISR ISSN 1565-012X CODEN: JEGEF6

▼ **JOURNAL OF ENDOCRINE GENETICS.** Text in English. 1999. q., latest vol.3. USD 260 (effective 2002). adv. **Document type:** *Academic/Scholarly.*
—BLDSC (4977.880000).
Published by: Freund Publishing House, Ltd., P O Box 35010, Tel Aviv 61350, Israel. TEL 972-3-562-8540, FAX 972-3-562-8540, h_freund@netvision.net.il, http://www.angelfire.com/il/freund. Ed. C Stratakis. adv.: B&W page USD 1,000, color page USD 2,000.

616.4 ITA ISSN 0391-4097 CODEN: JEIND7

JOURNAL OF ENDOCRINOLOGICAL INVESTIGATION. Text in English. 1978. 11/yr. EUR 100.71 domestic; USD 140 foreign (effective 2002). charts, illus, stat. *Refereed.* **Document type:** *Academic/Scholarly.* **Description:** Publishes original studies on clinical and experimental research in endocrinology and related fields.
Related titles: Online - full text ed.: EUR 50.35 (effective 2002) (from Institute for Scientific Information); ♦ Supplement: Journal of Endocrinological Investigation. Supplement. ISSN 1121-1369.
Indexed: ASCA, Chem.Abstr., Chem.Indus.Notes, Chem.Titles, Curr.Adv.Biochem., Curr.Adv.Cell & Devel.Biol., Curr.Cont., Dairy Sci.Abstr., Excerp.Med., Ind.Med. (1978-), Ind.Sci.Rev., Inpharma, Med.& Surg.Dermat., Neurosci.Cit.Ind., Nutr.Abstr., Pharm.&Out.News, Reac., Sci.Cit.Ind., THA.
—BLDSC (4977.900000), CASDDS, CISTI, EMDOCS, GNLM, IDS, ingenta, KNAW.
Published by: (Societa Italiana di Endocrinologia/Italian Society of Endocrinology), Editrice Kurtis s.r.l., Via Luigi Zoja, 30, Milan, MI 20153, Italy. TEL 39-02-48202740, FAX 39-02-4820-1219, info@kurtis.it, http://www.kurtis.it. Ed. Aldo Pinchera.

616.4 GBR ISSN 0022-0795
QP187.A1 CODEN: JOENAK

JOURNAL OF ENDOCRINOLOGY. Text in English. 1939. m. GBP 473 in Europe; USD 795 North & South America; GBP 492 elsewhere (effective 2002). adv. charts, illus. index, cum.index: vols.1-20, 21-40. 2 cols./p. Supplement avail.; back issues avail.; reprints avail. *Refereed.* **Document type:** *Journal, Academic/Scholarly.* **Description:** Covers all aspects of the nature and functions of the endocrine system in animals and man. Contains research papers, reviews, rapid communications, and commentaries.
Related titles: Online - full text ed.: 1997 (from EBSCO Publishing, Swets Blackwell, Institute for Scientific Information).
Indexed: ASCA, AgBiotech, Agri.& Environ.Biotech.Abstr. (coverage dropped), Anal.Abstr., Anim.Behav.Abstr. (coverage dropped), Anim.Breed.Abstr., Aqua.Sci.& Fish.Abstr., Behav.Med.Abstr., Biol.Abstr., Chem.Abstr., Chem.Indus.Notes, Chem.Titles, Curr.Adv.Biochem., Curr.Adv.Cell & Devel.Biol., Curr.Adv.Gen.& Molec.Biol., Curr.Cont., Curr.Ref.Fish Res., Dairy Sci.Abstr., Dent.Ind., Derwent Biotech.Abstr., Diab.Cont., Excerp.Med., INIS Atomind., Ind.Med. (1939-), Ind.Sci.Rev., Ind.Vet., Inpharma, Int.Abstr.Biol.Sci., Kidney, Mass Spectr.Bull., NRN, Neurosci.Abstr. (coverage dropped), Neurosci.Cit.Ind., Nutr.Abstr., Pharm.&Out.News, Pig News & Info., Poult.Abstr., Reac., Ref.Zh., Rev.Arom.& Med.Plants, SSCI (coverage dropped), Sci.Cit.Ind., Sport Fish.Abstr., THA, Vet.Bull., Wild.Rev., Zoo.Rec.
—BLDSC (4978.000000), CASDDS, CISTI, GNLM, IDS, ingenta, KNAW, Linda Hall. **CCC.**
Published by: Society for Endocrinology, 17-18 The Courtyard, Woodlands, Bradley Stoke, Bristol BS32 4NQ, United Kingdom. TEL 44-1454-642220, FAX 44-1454-642222, editorial@endocrinology.org, orders@allenpress.com, sales@portlandpress.co.uk, http://www.endocrinology.org. Ed. S G Hillier. R&P Lyn Cole. Adv. contact Ailsa Bailey. Circ: 1,500. **Subscr. to:** Allen Press Inc., PO Box 1897, Lawrence, KS 66044-8897. TEL 785-843-1235, FAX 875-843-1274. **Dist. by:** Portland Press Ltd., Commerce Way, Colchester, Essex CO2 8HP, United Kingdom. TEL 44-1206-796351, FAX 44-1206-799331.; **Dist. in Japan by:** Kinokuniya Co. Ltd., Journal Department, Chitose, P.O. Box 55, Tokyo 156, Japan.

JOURNAL OF ENDOCRINOLOGY & REPRODUCTION. see *BIOLOGY*

616.4 GBR ISSN 0968-0519
QP632.E4 CODEN: JENREB

JOURNAL OF ENDOTOXIN RESEARCH. Text in English. 1994. bi-m. GBP 116 to individuals; USD 184 in United States to individuals; GBP 318 to institutions; USD 478 in United States to institutions (effective 2002). bk.rev. back issues avail. *Refereed.* **Document type:** *Academic/Scholarly.* **Description:** Covers developments in endotoxin research.
Related titles: Online - full text ed.: (from Institute for Scientific Information).
Indexed: ASCA, Aqua.Sci.& Fish.Abstr., BBCI, Chem.Abstr., Chem.Indus.Notes, Chem.Titles, Curr.Cont., Environ.Sci.Poll.Mgmt., Excerp.Med. (1995-), Ind.Med., Inpharma, Int.Abstr.Biol.Sci., Microbiol.Abstr., Pollut.Abstr., Reac., Tox.Abstr.
—BLDSC (4978.205000), CASDDS, CISTI, GNLM, IDS, Infotrieve, KNAW. **CCC.**
Published by: Maney Publishing, Hudson Rd, Leeds, W Yorks LS9 7DL, United Kingdom. TEL 44-113-249-7481, FAX 44-113-248-6983, maney@maney.co.uk, http://www.maney.co.uk. Ed. Jack Levin.

616.4 ZAF

JOURNAL OF METABOLISM, DIABETES AND ENDOCRINOLOGY IN SOUTH AFRICA. Text in English. 3/yr. USD 15 foreign (effective 2000). back issues avail. *Refereed.* **Document type:** *Journal, Academic/Scholarly.* **Description:** Discusses clinical and experimental topics in endocrinology, including issues metabolism and diabetic disorders.
Published by: South African Medical Association, Health and Medical Publishing Group, 14 Central Sq, Pinelands 7430, South Africa. TEL 27-21-531-3081, FAX 27-21-531-4126, annp@smedical.org, publishing@samedical.org, http://www.samedical.org. R&P Peter Roberts. **Subscr. to:** PO Box 74789, Lynnwood Ridge, Pretoria 0040, South Africa. TEL 27-12-481-2010, FAX 27-12-481-2061, ann@samedical.org. **Dist. by:** Private Bag X1, Pinelands 7430, South Africa. TEL 27-21-531-3081, FAX 27-21-531-4126.

616.4 GBR ISSN 0952-5041
QP187.3.M64 CODEN: JMLEEI

JOURNAL OF MOLECULAR ENDOCRINOLOGY. Text in English. 1988. bi-m. GBP 270 domestic; USD 477 in the Americas; GBP 288 elsewhere (effective 2002); includes online ed.. adv. charts, illus. index. back issues avail.; reprints avail. *Refereed.* **Document type:** *Journal, Academic/Scholarly.* **Description:** Publishes research and review papers on molecular and cellular aspects of endocrine and related systems.
Related titles: Online - full text ed.: 1997 (from EBSCO Publishing, Swets Blackwell, Institute for Scientific Information).
Indexed: ASCA, AgBiotech, Anim.Breed.Abstr., BBCI, Chem.Abstr., Chem.Indus.Notes, Chem.Titles, Curr.Cont., Diab.Cont., Excerp.Med., Ind.Med. (1988-), Ind.Sci.Rev., Inpharma, Int.Abstr.Biol.Sci., Pharm.&Out.News, Reac., Ref.Zh., Sci.Cit.Ind., Zoo.Rec.
—BLDSC (5020.709000), CASDDS, CISTI, EMDOCS, GNLM, IDS, ingenta, KNAW. **CCC.**
Published by: Society for Endocrinology, 17-18 The Courtyard, Woodlands, Bradley Stoke, Bristol BS32 4NQ, United Kingdom. TEL 44-1454-642220, FAX 44-1454-642222, info@endocrinology.org; orders@allenpress.com, editorial@endocrinology.org, sales@portlandpress.co.uk, http:// www.endocrinology.org; http://www.allenpress.com. Ed. J I Mason. R&P Lyn Cole. Adv. contact Lara Thompson. Circ: 550. **Subscr. to:** Allen Press Inc., PO Box 1897, Lawrence, KS 66044-8897; Portland Press Ltd., Customer Service, Commerce Way, Colchester, Essex CO2 8HP, United Kingdom. **Dist. in Japan by:** Kinokuniya Co. Ltd., Journal Department, Chitose, P.O. Box 55, Tokyo 156, Japan.

JOURNAL OF NEUROENDOCRINOLOGY. see *MEDICAL SCIENCES—Psychiatry And Neurology*

JOURNAL OF NEUROENDOCRINOLOGY ONLINE. see *MEDICAL SCIENCES—Psychiatry And Neurology*

616.4 618.92 ISR ISSN 0334-018X CODEN: JPENEV

JOURNAL OF PEDIATRIC ENDOCRINOLOGY & METABOLISM. Variant title: Journal of Pediatric Endocrinology. Text in English. 1985. 9/yr., latest vol.15 (plus supplements). USD 460 (effective 2002). adv. bk.rev. back issues avail. *Refereed.* **Document type:** *Academic/Scholarly.*
Related titles: Online - full text ed.: (from Institute for Scientific Information).
Indexed: ASCA, Curr.Adv.Ecol.Sci., Curr.Cont., Excerp.Med., Ind.Med. (1993-, dropped), Ind.Sci.Rev., Inpharma, Kidney, Reac., Sci.Cit.Ind.
—BLDSC (5030.174000), CASDDS, CISTI, EMDOCS, GNLM, ingenta, KNAW.
Published by: Freund Publishing House, Ltd., P O Box 35010, Tel Aviv 61350, Israel. TEL 972-3-562-8540, FAX 972-3-652-8538, h_freund@netvision.net.il, http://www.angelfire.com/il/freund. Ed. Z Laron. Circ: 1,000.

616.4 JPN ISSN 0289-4947 CODEN: PRCTEH

JOURNAL OF PRACTICAL DIABETES; practice. Text in Japanese. 1984. q. JPY 800 per issue. adv. bk.rev. charts, illus.
Published by: Ishiyaku Publishers Inc., 7-10 Honkomagome 1-chome, Bunkyo-ku, Tokyo 113-0021, Japan. Ed. Hiroshi Miura. Circ: 10,000.

▼ **JOURNAL OF THE PANCREAS.** see *MEDICAL SCIENCES—Gastroenterology*

616.4 FRA ISSN 0075-4439 CODEN: JDBHAC

JOURNEES ANNUELLES DE DIABETOLOGIE DE L'HOTEL DIEU. Text in French. 1961. a. price varies.
Indexed: Biol.Abstr., Chem.Abstr., Chem.Titles, Dent.Ind., Ind.Med. (1961-).
—BLDSC (5072.940000), CASDDS, CISTI, GNLM, Infotrieve, KNAW. **CCC.**
Published by: (Hotel-Dieu, Clinique Medico-Sociale du Diabete et des Maladies Metaboliques), Flammarion Medecine Sciences, 4 rue Casimir Delavigne, Paris 75006, France. Ed. Dr. Rathery. **U.S. subscr. addr.:** S.F.P.A., c/o Mr Benech, 14 E 60th St, New York, NY 10022.

616.4 RUS

KLINICHESKAYA ENDOKRINOLOGIYA. Text in Russian. 1997. m. USD 195 in United States.
Published by: Vserossiiskii Institut Nauchnoi i Tekhnicheskoi Informatsii (VINITI), Usievicha ul 20-a, Moscow 125315, Russian Federation. TEL 7-095-1526441, FAX 7-095-943-0060. **US dist. addr.:** East View Publications, 3020 Harbor Ln N, Minneapolis, MN 55447. TEL 612-550-0961.

L M S ALERT. DIABETES. (Literature Monitoring and Evaluation Service) see *MEDICAL SCIENCES—Abstracting, Bibliographies, Statistics*

616.4 FRA

LA LETTRE DU SENOLOGUE. Text in French. 1998. q. FRF 300 domestic to individuals; FRF 420, USD 76 foreign to individuals; FRF 380 domestic to institutions; FRF 500, USD 91 foreign to institutions; FRF 190 domestic to students; USD 56 foreign to students (effective 2000). *Refereed.* **Document type:** *Academic/Scholarly.*
Published by: Edimark S.A., 62-64 rue Jean Jaures, Puteaux 92800, France. TEL 33-1-414-58000, FAX 33-1-41458025, contact@edimark.fr, http://www.edimark.fr. Ed. Dr. Anne Lesur. Pub. Claudie Damour-Terrasson.

616.4 IND ISSN 0971-5053 CODEN: LSAEE

LIFE SCIENCE ADVANCES: EXPERIMENTAL & CLINICAL ENDOCRINOLOGY. Key Title: Experimental & Clinical Endocrinology - Life Science Advances. Text in English. 1982. 4/yr. **Document type:** *Academic/Scholarly.*
Indexed: Excerp.Med. (1994-).
—GNLM.
Published by: Council of Scientific Research Integration, T.C. 28-408 (3), Vilayal Gardens, Kaithamukku, Thiruvananthapuram, Kerala 695 024, India. TEL 91-471-77305.

M

616.4 DEU ISSN 1433-5255
CODEN: LFPRFH

LYMPHOLOGIE IN FORSCHUNG UND PRAXIS. Text in German. s-a. DEM 116; DEM 50 to students. adv. **Document type:** *Academic/Scholarly.*
—BLDSC (5311.295000), GNLM.
Published by: (Deutscher Gesellschaft fuer Lymphologie), Kagerer Kommunikation, Koblenzer Str 18, Bonn 53173, Germany. TEL 49-228-95696-0, FAX 49-228-9569640. Ed. Dr. H Weissleder. Adv. contact Bettina Thiemeyer.

616.4 USA ISSN 0024-7766
RC646 CODEN: LYMPBN

LYMPHOLOGY. Text in English. 1968. q. USD 75 (effective 2000). adv. abstr, charts, illus, stat. index. reprint service avail. from PQC. *Refereed.* **Document type:** *Proceedings, Newsletter, Academic/Scholarly.*
Related titles: Online - full text ed.: (from Institute for Scientific Information).
Indexed: ASCA, Biol.Abstr., Chem.Abstr., Curr.Adv.Cancer Res., Curr.Adv.Ecol.Sci., Curr.Cont., Dairy Sci.Abstr., Dent.Ind., Excerp.Med., Helminthol.Abstr., INIS Atomind., Ind.Med. (1968-), Ind.Sci.Rev., Inpharma, Int.Abstr.Biol.Sci., Reac., Sci.Cit.Ind., Vet.Bull.
—BLDSC (5311.300000), CASDDS, CISTI, GNLM, IDS, KNAW. **CCC.**
Published by: International Society of Lymphology, c/o Dr Charles L Witte, Ed, Dept of Surgery Trauma, Arizona Health Sciences Center, Box 245063, Tucson, AZ 85724-5063. TEL 520-626-6118, FAX 520-626-0822, lymph@u.arizona.edu. R&P Dr. Charles L Witte. Circ: 1,100.

616.4 JPN ISSN 0913-4867
CODEN: MAGUEO

MAGUNESHUMU✶ /MAGNESIUM. Variant title: Japanese Society for Magnesium Research. Journal. Text in English, Japanese; Summaries in English. 1982. s-a.
Indexed: Chem.Abstr., Chem.Indus.Notes, Chem.Titles.
—BLDSC (4809.464000), CASDDS.
Published by: Nihon Maguneshumu Kenkyukai/Japanese Society for Magnesium Research, 4 Yoshidakawara-chyo, Sakyou-ku, Kyoto 606-8315, Japan.

616.4 FRA ISSN 1295-9359

▼ **MEDECINE THERAPEUTIQUE - ENDOCRINOLOGIE.** Abbreviated title: M T E. Text in French. 1999. bi-m. FRF 670 domestic to individuals; EUR 114 in Europe to individuals; FRF 790 elsewhere to individuals; FRF 1,120 domestic to institutions; EUR 183 in Europe to institutions; FRF 1,240 elsewhere to institutions; FRF 420 domestic to students; EUR 76 in Europe to students; FRF 540 elsewhere to students (effective 2001).
Related titles: Online - full text ed.: FRF 670 to individuals; FRF 1,120 to institutions; FRF 420 to students.
Published by: John Libbey Eurotext, 127 av. de la Republique, Montrouge 92120, France. TEL 33-01-46730660, FAX 33-01-40840999, marketing@jle.com, http://www.john-libbey-eurotext.fr/. Eds. Christian Boitard, Pierre Bougneres. **Subscr. to:** A T E I. atei@club-internet.fr.

616.4 BGR ISSN 0324-1475

MEDITSINSKI PREGLED. ENDOKRINNI ZABOLIAVANIIA. Text in Bulgarian. 1972. q., latest vol.30, 2001. BGL 14 domestic; USD 48 foreign (effective 2002). adv. abstr, bibl, illus. 48 p./no. back issues avail. *Refereed.* **Document type:** *Journal, Academic/Scholarly, Abstract/Index, Bibliography.* **Description:** Presents original articles and abstracts of foreign publications in the field of endocrinology.
Published by: Meditsinski Universitet - Sofia, Tsentur za Informatsiia po Meditsina/Medical University - Sofia, Medical Information Center, 1 Sv Georgi Sofiiski ul, Sofia 1431, Bulgaria. TEL 359-2-9522342, FAX 359-2-9522393, mutafov@sun.medun.acad.bg, http://www.medun.acad.bg. Ed. Dr. D Koev. R&P, Adv. contact Dr. Christo Mutafov. B&W page USD 50, color page USD 150; 12 x 18. Circ: 250. **Dist. by:** Sofia Books, Ul Silivria 16, Sofia 1404, Bulgaria. TEL 359-2-9586257, sofiabooks@hotmail.com, http://www.sofiabooks.hit.bg.

MENOPAUSE. see *MEDICAL SCIENCES—Obstetrics And Gynecology*

MENOPAUSE NEWS. see *WOMEN'S HEALTH*

616.4 574.133 USA ISSN 0026-0495
RB147 CODEN: METAAJ

METABOLISM: CLINICAL AND EXPERIMENTAL. Text in English. 1952. m. USD 269 domestic to individuals; USD 411 foreign to individuals; USD 388 domestic to institutions; USD 494 foreign to institutions; USD 203 domestic to students; USD 249 foreign to students; USD 42 newsstand/cover (effective 2001). adv. abstr, bibl, charts, illus. index. *Refereed.* **Document type:** *Journal, Academic/Scholarly.* **Description:** Reports on research into the metabolic aspects of nutrition, endocrines, genetics, dystrophies, diabetes, and gout.
Related titles: Online - full text ed.: (from IDEAL Online Library, Institute for Scientific Information).
Indexed: ASCA, Abstr.Hyg., Agri.& Environ.Biotech.Abstr. (coverage dropped), Anim.Breed.Abstr., BBCI, Bibl.Agri., Biol.Abstr., Chem.Abstr., Chem.Indus.Notes, Chem.Titles, Curr.Adv.Biochem., Curr.Adv.Cell & Devel.Biol., Curr.Adv.Ecol.Sci., Curr.Cont., Dairy Sci.Abstr., Derwent Biotech.Abstr., Diab.Cont., Excerp.Med., Food Sci.& Tech.Abstr., Helminthol.Abstr., INIS Atomind., Ind.Med. (1952-), Ind.Sci.Rev., Ind.Vet., Inpharma, Int.Abstr.Biol.Sci., Maize Abstr., Mass Spectr.Bull., NRN, Neurosci.Cit.Ind., Nutr.Abstr., Pharm.&Out.News, Protozool.Abstr., Reac., Rev.Appl.Entomol., SSCI (coverage dropped), Sci.Cit.Ind., Soyabean Abstr., Sugar Ind.Abstr., THA, Trop.Dis.Bull.
—BLDSC (5683.300000), CASDDS, CISTI, GNLM, IDS, ingenta, KNAW. **CCC.**
Published by: W.B. Saunders Co. (Subsidiary of: Harcourt Publishers Ltd.), 11830 Westline Industrial Dr, St Louis, MO 63146. TEL 800-325-4177, http://www.wbsaunders.com. Ed. Dr. James B Field. adv.: B&W page USD 890, color page USD 1,940; trim 10 x 7. Circ: 1,909. **Subscr. to:** Periodicals Fulfillment, W B Saunders Co, 6277 Sea Harbor Dr, 4th Fl, Orlando, FL 32891-4800.

616.4 FRA

METABOLISMES - HORMONES - NUTRITION. Text in French. bi-m. FRF 300, EUR 45.73 domestic to individuals; FRF 420, USD 76 foreign to individuals; FRF 380, EUR 57.93 domestic to institutions; FRF 500, USD 91 foreign to institutions (effective 2000). adv. *Refereed.* **Document type:** *Academic/Scholarly.*
Published by: Medica-Press International, 62-64 rue Jean-Jaures, Puteaux 92800, France. TEL 33-1-41458000, FAX 33-1-41458025, contact@edimark.fr, http://www.edimark.fr. Ed. J M Kuhn. Pub. Claudie Damour Terrasson.

616.4 ITA ISSN 0391-1977
CODEN: MNREDJ

MINERVA ENDOCRINOLOGICA; rivista trimestrale di fisiopatologia e clinica delle ghiandole endocrine. Text in Italian. 1976. q. USD 105 to individuals; USD 155 to institutions (effective 2000 - 2001). adv. *Refereed.* **Document type:** *Academic/Scholarly.*
Indexed: Chem.Abstr., Ind.Med. (1976-), Inpharma, Reac.
—BLDSC (5794.153000), CASDDS, CISTI, GNLM.
Published by: Edizioni Minerva Medica, Corso Bramante, 83-85, Turin, TO 10126, Italy. TEL 39-11-678282, FAX 39-11-674502. Ed. G H Molinatti. Pub. Alberto Oliaro. Adv. contact F Filippo. B&W page USD 1,200, color page USD 2,000; trim 270 x 190. Circ: 1,900 (paid).

616.46 ITA

MODUS. Text in Italian. 1982. 3/yr. free per issue to qualified personnel. **Description:** For diabetics, their families, doctors and medical students.
Formerly: Diabete Oggi e Domani
Published by: Boehringer Mannheim Italia, Via G B Stucchi, 110, Monza, MI 20052, Italy. TEL 39-2474271, FAX 39-2474290. Ed. Rodolfo Colarizi. adv.: B&W page ITL 2,800,000, color page ITL 5,500,000; trim 248 x 188. Circ: 130,000.

616.4 IRL ISSN 0303-7207
QP187.A1 CODEN: MCEND6

MOLECULAR AND CELLULAR ENDOCRINOLOGY. Text in English. 1974. 26/yr. EUR 3,489 in Europe to institutions; JPY 463,400 in Japan to institutions; USD 3,904 elsewhere to institutions (effective 2002). abstr. back issues avail. *Refereed.* **Document type:** *Academic/Scholarly.* **Description:** Integrates all aspects related to the biochemical effects, synthesis and secretions of ectracellular signals and to the understanding of cellular regulatory mechanisms.
Related titles: Microform ed.: (from PQC); Online - full text ed.: (from ingenta, ScienceDirect, Swets Blackwell, Institute for Scientific Information).
Indexed: ASCA, AgBiotech, Anim.Breed.Abstr., Aqua.Sci.& Fish.Abstr., BBCI, Biol.Abstr., Chem.Abstr., Chem.Indus.Notes, Chem.Titles, Curr.Adv.Biochem., Curr.Adv.Cell & Devel.Biol., Curr.Adv.Ecol.Sci., Curr.Adv.Gen.& Molec.Biol., Curr.Cont., Dairy Sci.Abstr., Environ.Sci.Poll.Mgmt., Excerp.Med., INIS Atomind., Ind.Med. (1974-), Ind.Sci.Rev., Inpharma, Int.Abstr.Biol.Sci., Neurosci.Cit.Ind., Nuc.Acids Abstr., Nutr.Abstr., Pig News & Info., Pollut.Abstr., Poult.Abstr., Reac., Rev.Appl.Entomol., Rev.Med.& Vet.Mycol., SSCI (coverage dropped), Sci.Cit.Ind., Sport Fish.Abstr.
—BLDSC (5900.760000), CASDDS, CISTI, EMDOCS, GNLM, IDS, ingenta, KNAW. **CCC.**
Published by: Elsevier Science Ireland Ltd, Elsevier House, Brookvale Plaza, E. Park, Shannon, Co. Clare, Ireland. TEL 353-61-471944, FAX 353-61-472144, http://www.elsevier.com/locate/mce. Ed. B A Cooke. R&P Annette Moloney. **Subscr. in Australasia and the Far East to:** Elsevier Science (Singapore) Pte Ltd, No.1 Temasek Ave, 17-01 Millenia Tower, Singapore 039192, Singapore. TEL 65-434-3727, FAX 65-337-2230; **Subscr. in the Americas to:** Elsevier Science, PO Box 945, New York, NY 10159-0945. TEL 212-633-3730, FAX 212-633-3680; **Subscr. to:** Elsevier Science BV, PO Box 211, Amsterdam 1000 AE, Netherlands. TEL 31-20-485-3757, nlinfo-f@elsevier.nl.

616.4 USA ISSN 0888-8809
QP187.3.M64 CODEN: MOENEN

MOLECULAR ENDOCRINOLOGY. Text in English. m. USD 251 domestic to individuals; USD 326 domestic to individuals Print & Online eds.; USD 329 foreign to individuals; USD 404 foreign to individuals Print & Online eds.; USD 416 domestic to institutions; USD 541 domestic to institutions Print & Online eds.; USD 490 foreign to institutions; USD 615 foreign to institutions Print & Online eds. (effective 2001). adv. back issues avail. *Refereed.* **Document type:** *Academic/Scholarly.* **Description:** Forum for molecular and cellular biologists investigating the molecular mechanisms of cellular regulatory processes.
Related titles: Microfilm ed.: (from WWS); Online - full text ed.: (from Ovid Technologies, Inc., HighWire Pr., EBSCO Publishing, Institute for Scientific Information).
Indexed: ASCA, AgBiotech, Anim.Breed.Abstr., Aqua.Sci.& Fish.Abstr., BBCI, Chem.Abstr., Chem.Indus.Notes, Chem.Titles, Curr.Adv.Biochem., Curr.Adv.Cancer Res., Curr.Adv.Cell & Devel.Biol., Curr.Adv.Gen.& Molec.Biol., Curr.Cont., Dairy Sci.Abstr., Genet.Abstr., Hum.Gen.Abstr., INIS Atomind., Ind.Med. (1987-), Ind.Sci.Rev., Inpharma, Int.Abstr.Biol.Sci., Neurosci.Abstr. (coverage dropped), Neurosci.Cit.Ind., Nuc.Acids Abstr., Nutr.Abstr., Pharm.&Out.News, Poult.Abstr., Reac., Sci.Cit.Ind., Sport Fish.Abstr., Wild.Rev.
—BLDSC (5900.817390), ADONIS, CASDDS, CISTI, EMDOCS, GNLM, IDS, ingenta, KNAW. **CCC.**
Published by: Endocrine Society, 4350 East West Hwy, Ste 500, Bethesda, MD 20814-4410. TEL 301-941-0230, FAX 301-941-0259, molendo@endo-society.org; orders@allenpress.com, http://www.endo-society.org; http://www.allenpress.com, http://www.endosociety.org; http://www.allenpress.com. Ed. John H Wilson. R&P Catherine Ang. Circ: 1,900. **Subscr. to:** Allen Press Inc., PO Box 1897, Lawrence, KS 66044-8897.

616.4 JPN ISSN 0918-6557
CODEN: MOLMEL

MOLECULAR MEDICINE. Text in Japanese. 1964. m. JPY 2,550 per issue. adv. bk.rev. **Document type:** *Academic/Scholarly.*
Formerly (until vol.30, no.1, 1993): Taisha - Metabolism and Diseases (0372-1566)
Indexed: Chem.Abstr., Helminthol.Abstr., INIS Atomind., Inpharma, Jap.Per.Ind., Pharm.&Out.News, Protozool.Abstr., Reac.
—BLDSC (5900.817950), CASDDS, CISTI, GNLM.
Published by: Nakayama Shoten, 25-14 Hakusan 1-chome, Bunkyo-ku, Tokyo 113-0001, Japan. TEL 81-3-3813-1103, FAX 81-3-3814-6336, koume@nakayamashoten.co.jp. Ed. Makiko Umehara. Adv. contact Takeshi Fukadas.

616.4 USA ISSN 0077-1015
CODEN: MOENBK

MONOGRAPHS ON ENDOCRINOLOGY. Text in English. 1967. irreg., latest vol.30, 1988. price varies. reprint service avail. from ISI. **Document type:** *Monographic series.*
Indexed: Biol.Abstr., Chem.Abstr., Ind.Med. (coverage dropped).
—CASDDS, CISTI, GNLM, KNAW.
Published by: Springer-Verlag, Journals (Subsidiary of: BertelsmannSpringer), 175 Fifth Ave, New York, NY 10010. TEL 212-460-1500, FAX 212-473-6272.

M

616.4 617 JPN ISSN 0914-9953
NAIBUNPI GEKA/ENDOCRINE SURGERY. Text in English, Japanese; Summaries in English. 1984. q. JPY 15,100 (effective 2001). bk.rev. back issues avail. *Refereed.* **Document type:** *Journal, Academic/Scholarly.*
Indexed: INIS Atomind.
Published by: Intermerc Co. Ltd., 39-15-105 Eifuku 1-chome, Suginami-ku, Tokyo 168-0064, Japan. TEL 81-3-5376-2820, FAX 81-3-5376-5790.

NATIONAL ALOPECIA AREATA FOUNDATION NEWSLETTER. see *MEDICAL SCIENCES—Dermatology And Venereology*

NEUROENDOCRINE PERSPECTIVES. see *MEDICAL SCIENCES—Psychiatry And Neurology*

616.4 616.8 CHE ISSN 0028-3835
QP187.A1 CODEN: NUNDAJ
NEUROENDOCRINOLOGY; international journal for basic and clinical studies on neuroendocrine relationships. Text in English. 1965. m. (2 vols./yr.). CHF 2,662, EUR 1,901.60 in Europe to institutions; CHF 2,696.80, USD 2,064 elsewhere to institutions (effective 2002). adv. illus. back issues avail. *Refereed.* **Document type:** *Journal, Academic/Scholarly.* **Description:** Publishes papers reporting original research in basic and clinical neuroendocrinology. Explores the complex interactions between neuronal networks and endrocrine glands.
Related titles: Microform ed.; Online - full text ed.: ISSN 1423-0194. CHF 116, EUR 84, USD 90 to institutions with print edition (effective 2002) (from Northern Light Technology, Inc., EBSCO Publishing, O C L C Online Computer Library Center, Inc., RoweCom Information Quest, ProQuest Information & Learning, Swets Blackwell, Institute for Scientific Information).
Indexed: ASCA, AgBiotech, Agri.& Environ.Biotech.Abstr. (coverage dropped), Anim.Breed.Abstr., Aqua.Sci.& Fish.Abstr., Biol.Abstr., Biotech.& Bioeng.Abstr., Cal.Tiss.Abstr., Chem.Abstr., Chem.Indus.Notes, Chem.Titles, Chemorec.Abstr., Curr.Adv.Cell & Devel.Biol., Curr.Adv.Ecol.Sci., Curr.Adv.Gen.& Molec.Biol., Curr.Cont., Dairy Sci.Abstr., Derwent Biotech.Abstr., Excerp.Med., Ind.Med. (1965-), Ind.Sci.Rev., Ind.Vet., Inpharma, Int.Abstr.Biol.Sci., Int.Aerosp.Abstr., Neurosci.Abstr., Neurosci.Cit.Ind., Nutr.Abstr., Pharm.&Out.News, Poult.Abstr., Protozool.Abstr., Reac., Sci.Cit.Ind., Sport Fish.Abstr., THA, Vet.Bull., Wild.Rev., Zoo.Rec., e-psyche.
—BLDSC (6081.370000), CASDDS, CISTI, GNLM, IDS, ingenta, KNAW. **CCC.**
Published by: (International Society of Neuroendocrinology), S. Karger AG, Allschwilerstr 10, PO Box, Basel 4009, Switzerland. TEL 41-61-306-1111, FAX 41-61-306-1234, karger@karger.ch, http://www.online.karger.com/journals/nen, http://www.karger.com. Ed. C Kordon. adv.: page USD 1,195. Circ: 1,650.

NIHON DAEKISEN GAKKAISHI/JAPAN SALIVARY GLAND SOCIETY. JOURNAL. see *BIOLOGY—Physiology*

616.4 JPN ISSN 0913-9044
NIHON HIKAKU NAIBUNPI GAKKAI NYUSU/JAPAN SOCIETY FOR COMPARATIVE ENDOCRINOLOGY. NEWSLETTER. Text in Japanese. 1975. q. JPY 1,000 (effective 2000). adv. bk.rev. *Refereed.* **Document type:** *Newsletter.*
Published by: Nihon Hikaku Naibunpi Gakkai/Japan Society for Comparative Endocrinology, Ocean Research Institute, University of, 1-15-1 Minami-Dai, Nakano-ku, Tokyo 164-0014, Japan. TEL 81-52-789-4073, FAX 81-52-789-4072, keimaeda@nuagr1.agr.nagoya-u.ac.jp, http://wwwsoc.nacsis.ac.jp/j5ce3/index.html. Ed. Kei Ichiro Maeda. R&P, Adv. contact Yoshio Takei TEL 81-3-5351-6467. Circ: 600.

616.4 JPN ISSN 0910-0067
CODEN: NKTZEF
NIHON KOTSU TAISHA GAKKAI ZASSHI. Text in Japanese. 1984. 3/yr. JPY 9,000 domestic; USD 100 foreign (effective 2000). *Refereed.* **Document type:** *Academic/Scholarly.* **Description:** Provides an international forum for researchers and clinicians to present and discuss relevant issues in bone and mineral research.
Related titles: ♦ English ed.: Journal of Bone and Mineral Metabolism. ISSN 0914-8779.
Indexed: INIS Atomind.
—CASDDS, CISTI.
Published by: Nihon Kotsu Taisha Gakkai/Japan Society for Bone and Metabolism Research, TS Bldg, 43-9, Komagome 1-chome, Toshima-ku, Tokyo 170-0003, Japan. TEL 81-3-5395-6366, FAX 81-3-5395-6876. Ed. Hidehiro Ozawa. Circ: 2,500.

616.4 JPN ISSN 0029-0661
CODEN: NNGZAZ
NIHON NAIBUNPI GAKKAI ZASSHI/FOLIA ENDOCRINOLOGICA JAPONICA. Text in Japanese; Summaries in English. 1925. m. JPY 700 per issue. adv. bk.rev.
Indexed: Anim.Breed.Abstr., Biol.Abstr., Dent.Ind., Excerp.Med., INIS Atomind., Ind.Med. (coverage dropped), Pig News & Info.
—CASDDS, CISTI, GNLM.
Published by: Nihon Naibunpi Gakkai/Japan Endocrine Society, Kinki Chiho Hatsumei Center, 14, Yoshida Kawara-machi, Sakyo-ku, Kyoto-shi 606, Japan.

616.4 JPN ISSN 0912-2532
NO CHO HORUMON GAKKAI NYUSU/NEWS OF THE BRAIN-GUT HORMONE RESEARCH. Text in Japanese. 1986. q.
Published by: No Cho Horumon Gakkai/Society of Brain-Gut Hormone Research, Niigata Daigaku Igakubu Dai 3 Kaibogaku Kyoshitsu, 757, Ichibancho, Asahimachi Dori, Niigata-shi, Niigata-ken 951, Japan.

616.4 FRA ISSN 0985-0562
CODEN: NCMEEV
NUTRITION CLINIQUE ET METABOLISME. Text in French. 1987. q. FRF 925 domestic to institutions; EUR 151 in Europe to institutions; USD 196 in the Americas to institutions; FRF 1,141 elsewhere to institutions (effective 2002). back issues avail. *Refereed.* **Document type:** *Academic/Scholarly.* **Description:** Brings together clinicians, biologists, pharmacologists, gastroenterologists, dieticians, endocrinologists and anesthesiologists in a forum for clinical and theoretical articles on nutrition and metabolism.
Related titles: Online - full text ed.
Indexed: Chem.Abstr., Chem.Indus.Notes, Chem.Titles, Food Sci.& Tech.Abstr., Nutr.Abstr.
—BLDSC (6188.133000), CASDDS, EMDOCS, GNLM, Infotrieve. **CCC.**
Published by: (Societe Francophone de Nutrition Enterale et Parenterale), Elsevier Paris, Editions Scientifiques et Medicales (Subsidiary of: Reed Elsevier plc. group), 23 rue Linois, Paris 75015, France. TEL 33-1-45589110, FAX 33-1-45589419, medecine@elsevier.fr; academic@elsevier-fr.com, http://www.elsevier.com/locate/nupar. Eds. J F Zazzo, J F de Brandt.

616.4 USA ISSN 0885-3177
CODEN: PANCE4
PANCREAS. Text in English. 1986. 8/yr., latest vol.23. USD 610 domestic to individuals Print & Online eds. combined; USD 719 foreign to individuals Print & Online eds. combined; USD 1,147 domestic to institutions Print & Online eds. combined; USD 1,147 per issue foreign to institutions Print & Online eds. combined; USD 128 newsstand/cover Print & Online eds. combined (effective 2002). adv. bk.rev. charts, illus. index. back issues avail.; reprint service avail. from PQC. *Refereed.* **Document type:** *Academic/Scholarly.* **Description:** Publishes both basic and clinical work on the exocrine and endocrine pancreas, their interrelationship, and consequences in disease states.
Related titles: Online - full text ed.: USD 1,491.10 domestic academic site license; USD 1,491.10 foreign academic site license; USD 1,663.15 domestic corporate site license; USD 1,663.15 foreign corporate site license (2002) (from Ovid Technologies, Inc., Institute for Scientific Information).
Indexed: ASCA, Curr.Adv.Biochem., Curr.Adv.Cell & Devel.Biol., Curr.Cont., Excerp.Med., INIS Atomind., Ind.Med. (1986-), Ind.Sci.Rev., Inpharma, Int.Abstr.Biol.Sci., Jrnl.Watch Gastr., Nutr.Abstr., Pharm.&Out.News, Reac., Sci.Cit.Ind., THA.
—BLDSC (6357.351500), CASDDS, CISTI, EMDOCS, GNLM, IDS, ingenta, KNAW.
Published by: Lippincott Williams & Wilkins (Philadelphia) (Subsidiary of: Wolters Kluwer N.V.), 530 Walnut St, Philadelphia, PA 19106-3621. TEL 215-521-8300, FAX 215-521-8902, http://www.pancreasjournal.com, http://www.lww.com. Ed. Dr. Vay Liang W Go. Pub. Jim Merritt. R&P Alice McElhinney. Adv. contact Ray Thibodeau. B&W page USD 775, color page USD 1,905. Circ: 863 (paid). **Subscr. to:** PO Box 1600, Hagerstown, MD 21740-1600. TEL 800-777-2295, FAX 301-824-7390.

PANCREATIC AND SALIVARY SECRETION. see *BIOLOGY—Abstracting, Bibliographies, Statistics*

612.34 CHE ISSN 1424-3903
▼ **PANCREATOLOGY.** Text in English. 2001. 6/yr. CHF 467.80 in Europe to individuals; USD 366.30 in United States to individuals; CHF 481.70 elsewhere to individuals; CHF 914, EUR 652.80 in Europe to institutions; USD 711, CHF 931.40 elsewhere to institutions (effective 2002). adv. *Refereed.* **Document type:** *Journal, Academic/Scholarly.* **Description:** Covers research and treatment of the endocrine and exocrine pancreas.
Related titles: Online - full text ed.: ISSN 1424-3911. CHF 39, USD 30 to individuals Only in addition to the print subscription. (effective 2001); CHF 58, EUR 42, USD 45 to institutions Only in addition to the print subscription. (effective 2002) (from Swets Blackwell).
—BLDSC (6357.352500).
Published by: (European Pancreatic Club GBR, International Association of Pancreatology USA), S. Karger AG, Allschwilerstr 10, PO Box, Basel 4009, Switzerland. TEL 41-61-3061111, FAX 41-61-3061234, karger@karger.ch, http://www.pancreatology.com, http://www.karger.ch. Eds. C W Imrie, M V Singer. adv.: B&W page CHF 1,475, B&W page USD 1,185, color page CHF 2,975, color page USD 2,235. **Subscr. to:** S Karger Publishers Inc.

▼ **PEDIATRIC DIABETES.** see *MEDICAL SCIENCES—Pediatrics*

▼ **PEDIATRIC DIABETES ONLINE.** see *MEDICAL SCIENCES—Pediatrics*

PINEAL GLAND: ITS MOLECULAR SIGNALS. see *BIOLOGY*

616.4 NLD ISSN 1386-341X
CODEN: PITUF9
PITUITARY. Text in English. 1998. q. EUR 330 to institutions for print or online ed.; EUR 394.80 to institutions print & online eds.combined (effective 2002). *Refereed.* **Description:** Covers basic and clinical aspects of the pituitary gland. It is designed to publish original, high quality research in both basic and pituitary function as well as clinical pituitary disease.
Related titles: Online - full text ed.: (from EBSCO Publishing, O C L C Online Computer Library Center, Inc., RoweCom Information Quest, Swets Blackwell, Kluwer Online).
Indexed: Dairy Sci.Abstr., Ind.Med., Neurosci.Abstr.
—BLDSC (6506.050000). **CCC.**
Published by: Kluwer Academic Publishers Group (Subsidiary of: Wolters Kluwer N.V.), Spuiboulevard 50, PO Box 17, Dordrecht 3300 AA, Netherlands. FAX 31-78-639-2254, services@wkap.nl, http://www.wkap.nl. Ed. Shlomo Melmed. **Dist. by:** Journals Department, PO Box 322, Dordrecht 3300 AH, Netherlands. TEL 781-871-6600, FAX 31-78-654-6474.

616.462 CAN ISSN 0384-7810
PLEIN SOLEIL. Text in English. 1958. q. CND 20 (effective 1999). adv. bk.rev. *Refereed.* **Document type:** *Consumer.*
Formerly: Survivre (0562-7087)
Related titles: Audio cassette/tape ed.
Indexed: Pt.de Rep. (1979-).
Published by: Association Diabete Quebec Inc., 5635 rue Sherbrooke E, Montreal, PQ H1N 1A2, Canada. TEL 514-259-3422, FAX 514-259-9286, adq@cam.org, http://www.diabete.qc.ca. Ed. Aline Toupin. R&P, Adv. contact Louise Bouchard TEL 574-259-3422. Circ: 17,000.

616.5 GBR ISSN 1357-8170
CODEN: PDINFY
PRACTICAL DIABETES INTERNATIONAL; the international journal for diabetes care teams worldwide. Text in English. 1984. 9/yr. USD 85 in Europe; USD 125 elsewhere; USD 90 combined subscription in Europe for print and online eds.; USD 132 combined subscription elsewhere for print and online eds. (effective 2002). adv. back issues avail. **Document type:** *Academic/Scholarly.* **Description:** Delivers important educational service to all health professionals involved in diabetes care.
Formerly (until vol.12, 1995): Practical Diabetes (0266-447X)
Related titles: Online - full text ed.: ISSN 1528-252X. USD 85 in Europe; USD 125 elsewhere (effective 2002) (from Wiley InterScience).
Indexed: CINAHL, Diab.Cont.
—BLDSC (6593.980157), CISTI, EMDOCS, GNLM, ingenta, KNAW.

Published by: Wiley Europe Ltd., Baffins Ln, Chichester, W Sussex PO19 1UD, United Kingdom. TEL 44-1243-779777, FAX 44-1243-843232, customer@wiley.co.uk, http://www.wiley.co.uk. Ed. Kenneth Shaw. R&P Roslyn Elson. Adv. contact James Wroe. Circ: 17,500. **Subscr. in the Americas to:** John Wiley & Sons, Inc., Journals, 605 Third Ave, New York, NY 10158. TEL 212-850-6645, FAX 212-850-6021, uscs-wis@wiley.com; **Subscr. to:** John Wiley & Sons Ltd., Baffins Ln, Chichester, Sussex PO19 IUD, United Kingdom. cs-journals@wiley.co.uk.

616.4 USA ISSN 0730-3491
PRACTICAL DIABETOLOGY. Text in English. 1982. q. USD 48 (effective 2000). adv. back issues avail. *Refereed.* **Document type:** *Trade, Consumer.*
Description: Practical diabetes information for the busy physician and pharmacist.
—BLDSC (6593.980300), GNLM.
Published by: R.A. Rapaport Publishing, Inc., 150 W 22nd St, New York, NY 10011. TEL 212-989-0200, FAX 212-989-4786, staff@diabetes-selg-mgmt.com, http://www.diabetes-self-mgmt.com. Ed., R&P James Hazlett. Pub. Richard A Rapaport. Adv. contact Kathy Jones. B&W page USD 5,100. Circ: 52,000 (controlled).

616.4 612.405 RUS ISSN 0375-9660
CODEN: PROEAS
PROBLEMY ENDOKRINOLOGII/PROBLEMS OF ENDOCRINOLOGY. Text in Russian; Summaries in English. 1955. bi-m. USD 150 foreign (effective 2000). adv. bk.rev., Website rev. **Document type:** *Journal.*
Description: Covers the most pressing problems of modern endocrinology, such as chemical structure, biosynthesis and metabolism of hormones, the metabolism of their action at cellular and molecular levels, as well as the pathogenesis and clinical picture of endocrine diseases and new methods of their diagnosis and treatment.
Formerly: Problemy Endokrinologii i Gormonoterapii (0032-9509)
Indexed: Agri.& Environ.Biotech.Abstr. (coverage dropped), Biol.Abstr., Chem.Abstr., Chem.Indus.Notes, Chem.Titles, Derwent Biotech.Abstr., Excerp.Med., Ind.Med. (coverage dropped), Int.Aerosp.Abstr., Nutr.Abstr., Ref.Zh.
—BLDSC (0133.980000), CASDDS, CISTI, East View, EMDOCS, GNLM. **CCC.**
Published by: Izdatel'stvo Meditsina, Petroverigskii per 6-8, Moscow 101000, Russian Federation. TEL 7-095-9248785, 7-095-928-86-48, FAX 7-095-9211355, 7-095-9286003, meditsina@iname.com, http://www.medit.ru. Ed. Yu P Fedotov. Pub. A M Stochik. R&P T Kravchenko. Adv. contact O A Fadeeva TEL 7-095-923-51-40. Circ: 2,000. **Dist. by:** Mezhdunarodnaya Kniga, B Yakimanka 39, Moscow 117049, Russian Federation. TEL 7-095-2384967, FAX 7-095-2384634; **US dist. addr.:** East View Publications, 3020 Harbor Ln N, Minneapolis, MN 55447. TEL 612-550-0961.

616.4 USA ISSN 0890-7048
CODEN: PERTEZ
PROGRESS IN ENDOCRINE RESEARCH AND THERAPY. Text in English. 1984. irreg. price varies. reprint service avail. from PQC. *Refereed.* **Document type:** *Proceedings.*
Indexed: Chem.Abstr., Chem.Titles.
—CASDDS, CISTI.
Published by: Lippincott Williams & Wilkins (Philadelphia) (Subsidiary of: Wolters Kluwer N.V.), 530 Walnut St, Philadelphia, PA 19106-3621. TEL 215-521-8300, FAX 215-521-8902, custserv@lww.com, http://www.lww.com/. **Subscr. to:** PO Box 1600, Hagerstown, MD 21740-1600. TEL 310-223-2300, 800-638-3030, FAX 310-223-2400, CustomerService@LWW.com.

▼ **PROGRESS IN OSTEOPOROSIS.** see *MEDICAL SCIENCES*

PROLACTIN. see *MEDICAL SCIENCES—Abstracting, Bibliographies, Statistics*

616.4 USA ISSN 1098-8823
QP801.P68 CODEN: PRGLBA
PROSTAGLANDINS AND OTHER LIPID MEDIATORS. Text in English. 1997. 12/yr. EUR 286 in Europe to individuals; JPY 37,800 in Japan to individuals; USD 319 elsewhere to individuals; EUR 1,190 in Europe to institutions; JPY 157,800 in Japan to institutions; USD 1,331 elsewhere to institutions (effective 2002). back issues avail. *Refereed.* **Document type:** *Academic/Scholarly.* **Description:** Covers all areas of prostaglandin research, including chemistry, endocrinology, immunology, and oncology.
Formed by the merger of (1972-1997): Prostaglandins (0090-6980); (1994-1997): Journal of Lipid Mediators and Cell Signaling (0929-7855); Which was formerly (1989-1994): Journal of Lipid Mediators (0921-8319)
Related titles: Microform ed.: (from PQC,PMC); Online - full text ed.: (from ingenta, ScienceDirect, Swets Blackwell, Institute for Scientific Information).
Indexed: ASCA, Agri.& Environ.Biotech.Abstr. (coverage dropped), Agricola, Anal.Abstr., Anim.Breed.Abstr., Biol.Abstr., Chem.Abstr., Chem.Indus.Notes, Chem.Titles, Curr.Adv.Biochem., Curr.Adv.Cancer Res., Curr.Adv.Cell & Devel.Biol., Curr.Adv.Ecol.Sci., Curr.Chem.React., Curr.Cont. (coverage dropped), Dairy Sci.Abstr., Dent.Ind., Derwent Biotech.Abstr., Excerp.Med., Helminthol.Abstr., INIS Atomind., Ind.Chem., Ind.Med. (1998-), Ind.Sci.Rev., Ind.Vet., Inpharma, Int.Abstr.Biol.Sci., Mass Spectr.Bull., NPU, Nutr.Abstr., Pharm.&Out.News, Pig News & Info., RCI, Reac., Sci.Cit.Ind. (coverage dropped), Telegen, Vet.Bull.
—BLDSC, ADONIS, CASDDS, CISTI, GNLM, IDS, Infotrieve, ingenta. **CCC.**
Published by: Elsevier Science, 655 Ave of the Americas, New York, NY 10010. TEL 212-989-5800, FAX 212-633-3990, usinfo-f@elsevier.com, http://www.elsevier.nl/locate/prostaglandins. Ed. Peter W Ramwell. **Subscr. in Australasia and the Far East to:** Elsevier Science (Singapore) Pte Ltd, No.1 Temasek Ave, 17-01 Millenia Tower, Singapore 039192, Singapore. TEL 65-434-3727, FAX 65-337-2230; **Subscr. in Japan to:** Elsevier Science Inc - Japan Regional Office, 9-15 Higashi-Azabu 1-chome, Minato-ku, Tokyo 106-0044, Japan. TEL 81-3-5561-5033; **Subscr. outside the Americas to:** Elsevier Science BV, PO Box 211, Amsterdam 1000 AE, Netherlands. TEL 31-20-485-3757.

PROSTAGLANDINS - BIOLOGY. see *MEDICAL SCIENCES—Abstracting, Bibliographies, Statistics*

616.4 GBR ISSN 0952-3278
CODEN: PLEAEU
PROSTAGLANDINS, LEUKOTRIENES AND ESSENTIAL FATTY ACIDS. Text in English. 1978. m. GBP 1,684 to institutions (effective 2002). adv. back issues avail. *Refereed.* **Document type:** *Journal, Academic/Scholarly.* **Description:** Covers all aspects of the roles of lipids in cellular, organ and whole organism function, and places a particular emphasis on human studies.
Former titles (until 1988): Prostaglandins, Leukotrienes and Medicine (0262-1746); Prostaglandins and Medicine (0161-4630)
Related titles: Microform ed.: (from PQC); Online - full text ed.: (from EBSCO Publishing, RoweCom Information Quest, Swets Blackwell, IDEAL Online Library, Institute for Scientific Information).
Indexed: ASCA, Anim.Breed.Abstr., Aqua.Sci.& Fish.Abstr., BBCI, Chem.Abstr., Chem.Titles, Curr.Adv.Ecol.Sci., Curr.Cont., Dairy Sci.Abstr., Derwent Biotech.Abstr., Excerp.Med., INIS Atomind., Ind.Med. (1988-), Ind.Sci.Rev., Inpharma, Int.Abstr.Biol.Sci., Neurosci.Cit.Ind., Nutr.Abstr., Pharm.&Out.News, Poult.Abstr., Protozool.Abstr., Reac., Ref.Zh., Rev.Appl.Entomol., Rev.Arom.& Med.Plants, Rev.Med.& Vet.Mycol., SSCI (coverage dropped), Sci.Cit.Ind., THA.
—BLDSC (6935.190900), ADONIS, CASDDS, CISTI, EMDOCS, GNLM, IDS, ingenta, KNAW. **CCC.**
Published by: Churchill Livingstone (Subsidiary of: Harcourt Publishers Ltd.), Robert Stevenson House, 1-3 Baxter's Pl, Leith Walk, Edinburgh, Midlothian EH1 3AF, United Kingdom. TEL 44-131-556-2424, FAX 44-131-459-1177, cservice@harcourt.com, http://www.harcourt-international.com/journals/plef. Ed. Dr. David F Horrobin. Pub. Gillian Griffith. R&P Catherine John TEL 212-424-4200. Adv. contact David Dunnachie. Circ: 450. **Subscr. to:** Harcourt Publishers Ltd., Foots Cray High St, Sidcup, Kent DA14 5HP, United Kingdom. TEL 44-20-8308-5700, FAX 44-20-8309-0807.

PSYCHONEUROENDOCRINOLOGY. see *MEDICAL SCIENCES—Psychiatry And Neurology*

616.462 GBR ISSN 0264-7397
CODEN: RADIES
RECENT ADVANCES IN DIABETES. Text in English. 1984. irreg. **Document type:** *Monographic series, Academic/Scholarly.*
—CASDDS.
Published by: Churchill Livingstone (Subsidiary of: Harcourt Publishers Ltd.), Robert Stevenson House, 1-3 Baxter's Pl, Leith Walk, Edinburgh, Midlothian EH1 3AF, United Kingdom. TEL 44-131-556-2424, FAX 44-131-459-1177, http://www.churchillmed.com. **US subscr. to:** Churchill Livingstone, 650 Ave of the Americas, New York, NY 10011. TEL 212-206-5000.

616.4 GBR ISSN 0140-9123
RC648.A1 CODEN: RAEMDA
RECENT ADVANCES IN ENDOCRINOLOGY AND METABOLISM. Text in English. 1978. irreg. **Document type:** *Monographic series, Academic/Scholarly.*
—CASDDS, CISTI, GNLM.
Published by: Churchill Livingstone (Subsidiary of: Harcourt Publishers Ltd.), Robert Stevenson House, 1-3 Baxter's Pl, Leith Walk, Edinburgh, Midlothian EH1 3AF, United Kingdom. TEL 44-131-556-2424, FAX 44-131-459-1177, http://www.churchilmed.com.

616.4 574.192 USA ISSN 0079-9963
QP187 CODEN: RPHRA6
RECENT PROGRESS IN HORMONE RESEARCH. PROCEEDINGS OF THE LAURENTIAN HORMONE CONFERENCE. Text in English. 1947. irreg., latest vol.50, 1995. index, cum.index: vols.1-10 (1947-1954). reprint service avail. from ISI. *Refereed.* **Document type:** *Proceedings.*
Related titles: Online - full text ed.: (from Institute for Scientific Information).
Indexed: ASCA, Anim.Breed.Abstr., Biol.Abstr., Chem.Abstr., Chem.Indus.Notes, Chem.Titles, Dairy Sci.Abstr., Excerp.Med., Ind.Med. (1947-), Ind.Sci.Rev., Ind.Vet., Nutr.Abstr., Sci.Cit.Ind., Vet.Bull.
—BLDSC (7305.000000), CASDDS, CISTI, GNLM, ingenta, Linda Hall. **CCC.**
Published by: Academic Press, Inc., Journal Division (Subsidiary of: Harcourt Brace & Company), 525 B St, Ste 1900, San Diego, CA 92101-4495. TEL 619-231-0926, FAX 619-699-6715. Ed. Roy O Greep. **Subscr. to:** Order Dept., 6277 Sea Harbor Dr, 4th Fl, Orlando, FL 32887. TEL 800-321-5068.

RENIN, ANGIOTENSIN & KININS. see *BIOLOGY—Abstracting, Bibliographies, Statistics*

616.4 USA ISSN 1389-9155
▼ **REVIEWS IN ENDOCRINE & METABOLIC DISORDERS.** Text in English. 2000. q. USD 322, EUR 322 to institutions for print or online ed.; USD 386.40, EUR 386.40 to institutions print & online eds.combined (effective 2002). **Document type:** *Academic/Scholarly.*
Description: Informs the students, clinicians and researchers involved in the broad area of endocrinology and metabolism of all the latest exciting advancements that are essential to their research or clinical practice.
Related titles: Online - full text ed.: (from EBSCO Publishing, O C L C Online Computer Library Center, Inc., RoweCom Information Quest, Swets Blackwell, Kluwer Online).
—BLDSC (7790.369000).
Published by: Kluwer Academic Publishers Boston, 101 Philip Dr, Assinippi Park, Norwell, MA 02061. TEL 781-871-6600, FAX 781-871-9045, services@wkap.nl, http://www.wkap.nl/journalhome.htm/1389-9155. Ed. Derek Leroith. R&P Rose Luongo TEL 781-871-6311. **Subscr. outside the Americas to:** Kluwer Academic Publishers Group, Journals Department, PO Box 322, Dordrecht 3300 AH, Netherlands. TEL 31-78-639-2392, FAX 31-78-654-6474; **Subscr. to:** Kluwer Academic - Plenum Publishers, 233 Spring St, New York, NY 10013-1578. TEL 212-620-8468, FAX 212-807-1047.

616.4 CUB ISSN 0864-4462
REVISTA CUBANA DE ENDOCRINOLOGIA. Text in Spanish; Summaries in English, Spanish. 1990. 3/yr. USD 34 in North America; USD 42 in Europe; USD 50 elsewhere. **Description:** Covers the fields of endocrinology, metabolic illnesses and related specialties.
Published by: (Cuba. Ministerio de Salud Publica, Centro Nacional de Informacion de Ciencias Medicas), Editorial de Ciencias Medicas, O'Reilly No. 4, Habana, Cuba. TEL 809-62-8091. Ed. Milagros de los Reyes. Circ: 1,000. **Co-sponsors:** Instituto Nacional de Endocrinologia y Enfermedades Metabolicas; Sociedad Cubana de Endocrinologia.

616.4 FRA ISSN 0048-8062
CODEN: RECNAS
REVUE FRANCAISE D'ENDOCRINOLOGIE CLINIQUE, NUTRITION ET METABOLISME✶ . Text in French; Abstracts occasionally in English. 1960. bi-m. illus.
Indexed: Biol.Abstr., C.I.S. Abstr., Chem.Abstr., Chem.Indus.Notes, Chem.Titles, Excerp.Med., Ind.Med. (coverage dropped), Rev.Appl.Entomol.
—BLDSC (7903.800000), CASDDS, CISTI, EMDOCS, GNLM, Infotrieve, KNAW. **CCC.**
Published by: Editions de Medecine Pratique, 132 av. du General Leclerc, Paris 75014, France. TEL 33-1-47910910.

M

616.4 JPN ISSN 0910-4186
CODEN: RINPEJ
RINPAGAKU/JAPANESE JOURNAL OF LYMPHOLOGY. Text in English, Japanese; Summaries in English. 1978. 2/yr. JPY 6,000.
Indexed: Chem.Abstr., Chem.Titles, INIS Atomind.
—CASDDS.
Published by: Nihon Rinpa Gakkai/Japanese Society of Lymphology, Ika Daigaku Dai 1 Kaibogaku Kyoshitsu, 1-1 Shinjuku 6-chome, Shinjuku-ku, Tokyo 160-0022, Japan.

616.4 ROM ISSN 1221-356X
CODEN: RJENE9
ROMANIAN JOURNAL OF ENDOCRINOLOGY/REVUE ROUMAINE D'ENDOCRINOLOGIE. Text in English, French, German, Russian, Spanish. 1964. q. adv. bk.rev. abstr, bibl, illus. index. **Document type:** *Academic/Scholarly.* **Description:** Presents original papers (studies and researches in experimental and clinical endocrinology), short articles on unusual cases and techniques, editorials and endocrinological news.
Former titles (until 1992): Endocrinologie (1220-4722); (until 1988): Revue Roumaine de Medecine. Endocrinologie (0253-1801); Supersedes in part (in 1975); Revue Romaine de Medicine (0303-822X); Which was formed by the 1974 merger of: Revue Roumaine de Medecine Interne (0484-8632); Revue Roumaine d'Endocrinologie (0035-4015); Revue Roumaine de Neurologie et de Psychiatrie (0301-7303)
Indexed: Biol.Abstr., Chem.Abstr., Chem.Titles, Curr.Adv.Ecol.Sci., Curr.Cont. (coverage dropped), Excerp.Med. (until 1993), Ind.Med. (coverage dropped).
—BLDSC, CASDDS, CISTI, GNLM.
Published by: (Academia de Stiinte Medicale), Editura Academiei Romane, Calea 13 Septembrie 13, Bucharest 76117, Romania. Ed. Marcela Pitis. Circ: 1,050. **Dist. by:** Rodipet S.A.. TEL 401-618-5103, FAX 401-222-6407.

616.462 ZAF
S A DIABETIESE TYDSKRIF/S A DIABETIC JOURNAL. Text in Afrikaans, English. 1992. q. illus.
Published by: Dia Kure, Posbus 1908, Bloemfontein 9300, South Africa.

616.4 USA ISSN 1526-8004
RC963.A1
SEMINARS IN REPRODUCTIVE MEDICINE. Text in English. q. EUR 182 to individuals; EUR 363 to institutions; EUR 84 newsstand/cover (effective 2002). adv. abstr, bibl, illus. **Document type:** *Journal, Academic/Scholarly.* **Description:** Provides in-depth coverage of important advances in the understanding of normal and disordered human reproduction, as well as new diagnostic and interventional techniques destined to become standard procedures in the future.
Former titles: Seminars in Reproductive Endocrinology (0734-8630); Reproductive Endocrinology
Related titles: Online - full text ed.: ISSN 1526-4564 (from RoweCom Information Quest, Institute for Scientific Information).
Indexed: Curr.Adv.Cell & Devel.Biol., Curr.Adv.Ecol.Sci., Curr.Adv.Gen.& Molec.Biol., Curr.Cont., Ind.Med. (2000-), Inpharma, Int.Abstr.Biol.Sci., Pharm.&Out.News, Reac.
—BLDSC, CISTI, EMDOCS, GNLM, IDS, Infotrieve, ingenta, KNAW. **CCC.**
Published by: Thieme Medical Publishers, 333 Seventh Ave, New York, NY 10001. TEL 212-760-0888, 800-782-3488, FAX 212-947-1112, http://www.thieme.com. Ed. Dr. Leon Speroff. Adv. contact Jean Azzato. Circ: 1,900. **Orders in Europe to:** Thieme International, Postfach 3001120, Stuttgart 70451, Germany. TEL 49-711-8931-0.

SEMINARS IN RESPIRATORY INFECTIONS. see *MEDICAL SCIENCES—Respiratory Diseases*

616.4 COL ISSN 0120-1182
SOCIEDAD COLOMBIANA DE ENDOCRINOLOGIA. REVISTA. Text in Spanish; Summaries in English, Spanish. 1958. s-a. USD 6. adv. index.
Indexed: Biol.Abstr.
Published by: Sociedad Colombiana de Endocrinologia, Apartado Aereo 29714, Bogota, DE, Colombia. Ed. Dr. Alfredo F Jacome. Circ: 2,000.

616.44 USA
STICKING OUT OUR NECKS - THE THYROID DISEASE NEWS REPORT; we're patients....NOT lab values!. Text in English. bi-m. USD 25 domestic; USD 35 foreign (effective 2000). adv. bk.rev., software rev. stat. back issues avail. **Document type:** *Newsletter.* **Description:** Features the latest conventional & alternative thyroid-related news and therapies from around the world.
Formerly: Thyroid Newsletter Online
Related titles: E-mail ed.: 1997. free per issue; Online - full text ed.
Published by: Shomon, PO Box 0385, Palm Harbor, FL 34682. FAX 425-977-1175, 888-810-9471, mshomon@pop.dn.net, news@thyroid-info.com, http://www.thyroid-info.com. Adv. contact Mary Shomon. Circ: 1,000.

616.4 USA
▼ **SUCCESSFUL LIVING WITH DIABETES.** Text in English. 2000. bi-m. USD 21; USD 3.99 newsstand/cover (effective 2001). **Document type:** *Consumer.*
Published by: Oxmoor House, 2100 Lakeshore Dr, Birmingham, AL 35209. TEL 205-877-6000. Ed. Nancy Fitzpatrick Wyatt. Pub. Bruce Akin.

616.4 SAU ISSN 1319-7266
AS-SUKKARYOUN; diabetic education. Text in Arabic. 1998. bi-m. SAR 45 (effective 1999); USD 12. charts, illus, stat. back issues avail. *Refereed.* **Document type:** *Monographic series, Academic/Scholarly.* **Description:** Caters to diabetics and those concerned with their care. Highlights diabetes, the concept of preventative medicine, detection, treatment research, and future developments of the disease.
Published by: Makkah Advertising, P O Box 4288, Jeddah 21491, Saudi Arabia. TEL 966-2651-4148, FAX 966-2653-0693, info@makkahadv.com. Ed. Dr. Zohair J Gazzaz. Pub. Mohammed Salahuddin. adv.: color page SAR 5,000; trim 150 x 210. Circ: 10,000.

616.46 USA
TEAMWORK (NEW YORK). Text in English. 1995. 3/yr. illus. **Document type:** *Newsletter.* **Description:** Provides information that will enable people with diabetes to live better. Informs about activities and events at the Joslin Center.
Published by: Joslin Center for Diabetes, St Luke s Roosevelt Hospital Center, 425 W 59th St, New York, NY 10019. TEL 212-523-8353, FAX 212-523-2617. Ed. Sandra Salisbury. Circ: 15,000.

616.4 AUS ISSN 1327-9505
THERAPEUTIC GUIDELINES. ENDOCRINOLOGY. Text in English. 1998. irreg., latest version 2 (every 3-4 yrs.). AUD 31.90 newsstand/cover (effective 2001). **Document type:** *Academic/Scholarly.* **Description:** Offers recommendations for drug therapy to treat or manage endocrinologic diseases and conditions and, where applicable, alternative approaches to overall patient management.
Formerly: Endocrinology Guidelines
Related titles: CD-ROM ed.
Published by: Therapeutic Guidelines Ltd., Chelsea House, Level 2, 55 Flemington Rd, North Melbourne, VIC 3051, Australia. TEL 61-3-9329-1566, FAX 61-3-9326-5632, sales@tg.com.au, http://www.tg.com.au. Ed., R&P Mary Hemming. Circ: 18,000.

616.44 USA ISSN 1050-7256
CODEN: THYRER
THYROID. Text in English. 1991. m. USD 179 domestic to individuals; USD 259 foreign to individuals; USD 215 domestic to individuals print and online eds. combined; USD 295 foreign to individuals print and online eds. combined; USD 398 domestic to institutions; USD 498 foreign to institutions; USD 478 domestic to institutions print and online eds. combined; USD 578 foreign to institutions print and online eds. combined (effective 2002). back issues avail.; reprints avail. *Refereed.* **Document type:** *Journal, Academic/Scholarly.* **Description:** Covers all aspects of thyroid medicine, from the molecular biology of the cell to clinical management of thyroid disorders.
Related titles: Online - full content ed.: USD 179 to individuals; USD 398 to institutions (effective 2002); Online - full text ed.: (from CatchWord Ltd., Institute for Scientific Information, RoweCom Information Quest).
Indexed: ASCA, Curr.Cont., Excerp.Med. (1992-), Ind.Med. (1990-), Ind.Sci.Rev., Inpharma, Nutr.Abstr., Pharm.&Out.News, Reac., Rev.Med.& Vet.Mycol., Sci.Cit.Ind.
—BLDSC (8820.383300), CISTI, EMDOCS, GNLM, IDS, Infotrieve, ingenta, KNAW. **CCC.**
Published by: (American Thyroid Association), Mary Ann Liebert, Inc. Publishers, 2 Madison Ave, Larchmont, NY 10538. TEL 914—834-3100, FAX 914-834-1388, terry.davies@mssm.edu, info@liebertpub.com, http://www.liebertpub.com/thy. Ed. Dr. Terry F Davies.

THYROID HORMONES. see *MEDICAL SCIENCES—Abstracting, Bibliographies, Statistics*

616.44 ITA ISSN 1121-7596
THYROIDOLOGY: CLINICAL AND EXPERIMENTAL. Text in Italian. 1989. 3/yr. ITL 50,000, USD 40 to individuals; ITL 60,000, USD 50 to institutions. **Document type:** *Academic/Scholarly.*
—BLDSC (8820.384500), GNLM, KNAW.
Published by: Pacini Editore, Via Alessandro Gherardesca, 1, Ospedaletto, PI 56121, Italy. TEL 39-050-313011, FAX 39-050-3130300, pacini@cibernet.it, http://www.cibernet.it/pacini, http://www.pacinieditore.it. Ed. A Carpi.

616.462 USA ISSN 1042-2838
TODAY IN MEDICINE. DIABETOLOGY AND ENDOCRINOLOGY. Text in English. 198?. bi-m.
Published by: Data Centrum Communications, Inc., 21 W 38th St, 4th fl, New York, NY 10018.

616.46 GBR ISSN 1043-2760
RC648.A1 CODEN: TENME4
TRENDS IN ENDOCRINOLOGY AND METABOLISM. Text in English. 1989. 10/yr. GBP 81 in Europe to individuals; EUR 102 to individuals; JPY 12,400 in Japan to individuals; USD 111 elsewhere to individuals; EUR 797 in Europe to institutions; JPY 110,600 in Japan to institutions; USD 891 elsewhere to institutions; GBP 42 in Europe to students; JPY 9,000 in Japan to students; USD 70 elsewhere to students; USD 1,146 to institutions Print & online eds. combined; EUR 127 to qualified personnel; JPY 15,500 in Japan to qualified personnel; USD 139 elsewhere to qualified personnel (effective 2002). adv. bk.rev. back issues avail.; reprints avail. *Refereed.* **Document type:** *Academic/Scholarly.* **Description:** Keeps researchers and clinicians informed of advances across the field of endocrinology, with emphasis on research.
Related titles: Microform ed.: (from PQC); Online - full text ed.: (from ingenta, Swets Blackwell, Institute for Scientific Information, ScienceDirect).
Indexed: ASCA, Biol.Abstr., Chem.Abstr., Chem.Titles, Curr.Cont., Excerp.Med., Ind.Med., Ind.Sci.Rev., Inpharma, Int.Abstr.Biol.Sci., Pharm.&Out.News, Reac., Sci.Cit.Ind.
—BLDSC (9049.590500), CASDDS, CISTI, EMDOCS, GNLM, IDS, ingenta, KNAW. **CCC.**
Published by: Elsevier Science Ltd., Elsevier Trends Journals, 68 Hills Rd, Cambridge CB2 1LA, United Kingdom. TEL 44-1223-315961, FAX 44-1223-464430, TEM@elsevier.co.uk, http://www.elsevier.com/locate/issn/10432760. Ed. N S Halmi. Adv. contact Thelma Reid. **Subscr. in Australasia and the Far East to:** Elsevier Science (Singapore) Pte Ltd, No. 1 Temasek Ave, 17-01 Millenia Tower, Singapore 039192, Singapore. TEL 65-434-3727; **Subscr. in the Americas to:** Elsevier Science, PO Box 945, New York, NY 10159-0945. TEL 212-633-3730, FAX 212-633-3680, http://www.elsevier.com; **Subscr. to:** Elsevier Current Trends Subscriptions, PO Box 331, Haywards Heath, W Sussex RH16 3FG, United Kingdom. TEL 44-1444-475650, FAX 44-1444-445423.

616.462 USA
UNA VIDA SALUDABLE CON DIABETES. Text in Spanish. bi-m. USD 6.95; USD 1.95 newsstand/cover (effective 2001). adv. **Description:** Contains information on diabetes for patients, focusing on recent developments in treatment.
Published by: Data Centrum Communications, Inc., 21 W 38th St, 4th fl, New York, NY 10018. TEL 212-997-9800, FAX 212-997-0078. Eds. Karen Seigal, Anny Queyroy. Pub. Eric Jensen.

VOICE OF THE DIABETIC; a support and information network. see *HANDICAPPED—Visually Impaired*

616.4058 USA ISSN 0084-3741
RC648
THE YEAR BOOK OF ENDOCRINOLOGY. Text in English. 1934. a. USD 91 domestic; USD 97 foreign (effective 2001). **Document type:** *Abstract/Index, Academic/Scholarly.* **Description:** Presents abstracts of pertinent literature with commentary by leading experts in the field.
Supersedes in part: Year Book of Endocrinology, Metabolism and Nutrition (0196-836X); Which superseded in part (in 1946): Year Book of Neurology, Psychiatry and Endocrinology (0887-3941)
Related titles: CD-ROM ed.
Indexed: Anim.Breed.Abstr., Curr.Adv.Ecol.Sci.
—CISTI, GNLM.
Published by: Mosby, Inc., Continuity Division (Subsidiary of: Harcourt Health Sciences), 11830 Westline Industrial Dr, St Louis, MO 63146-3313. TEL 314-872-8370, 800-325-4177, FAX 314-432-1380, http://www.mosby.com/periodicals. Ed. Dr. John D Bagdade.

616.46 CHN
ZHONGGUO TANGNIAOBING ZAZHI/CHINESE DIABETES MAGAZINE. Text in English. 1993. q. 68 p./no. **Document type:** *Academic/Scholarly.*
Description: Reports on new technology and medicine in diagnosing and treating diabetes.
Published by: (Zhonggua Yixuehui, Tangniaobing Xuehui), Zhongguo Tangniaobing Zazhishe, Jia-7 Dongdan Santiao, Beijing 100005, China. TEL 86-10-5223466. Ed. Chi Zhisheng. **Dist. overseas by:** China International Book Trading Corp, 35 Chegongzhuang Xilu, Haidian District, Beijing 100044, China.

616.4 CHN ISSN 1000-6699
CODEN: ZNDZEK
ZHONGHUA NEIFENMI DAIXIE ZAZHI/CHINESE JOURNAL OF ENDOCRINOLOGY AND METABOLISM. Text in Chinese; Summaries in Chinese, English. 1985. bi-m. CNY 47.40 domestic; USD 31.20 foreign; CNY 7.90 newsstand/cover per academic year domestic; USD 5.20 newsstand/cover foreign (effective 2001). adv. back issues avail. **Document type:** *Academic/Scholarly.*
Related titles: CD-ROM ed.; Online - full content ed.: (from WanFang Data Corp.).
Indexed: Chem.Abstr., ExtraMED.
—CASDDS.
Published by: Shanghai-shi Neifenmi Yanjiusuo/Shanghai Institute of Endocrinology, 197, Ruijin 2 Lu, Shanghai 200025, China. TEL 86-21-8431-5587, FAX 86-21-6431-5587, cjeme@online.sh.cn, http://www.chinainfo.gov.cn/periodical. Ed. Yifan Shi. R&P, Adv. contact Ming-Dao Chen. Circ: 10,000. **Dist. by:** China International Book Trading Corp, 35, Chegongzhuang Xilu, Haidian District, Beijing 100044, China. TEL 86-1-68413849, FAX 86-1-68412048, cibtc@mail.cibtc.com.cn, http://www.cibtc.com.cn.
Co-sponsor: Chinese Medical Association - Zhonghua Yixue Hui.

616.4 CHN ISSN 1001-7097
ZHONGHUA SHENZANGBING ZAZHI/CHINESE JOURNAL OF NEPHROLOGY. Text in Chinese. 1985. bi-m. USD 25.20; USD 4.20 newsstand/cover (effective 2001). **Document type:** *Academic/Scholarly.*
Published by: Zhonghua Yixuehui Zazhishe, 42 Dongsi Xidajie, Beijing 100710, China. **Dist. by:** China International Book Trading Corp, 35, Chegongzhuang Xilu, Haidian District, Beijing 100044, China. TEL 86-1-68413849, FAX 86-1-68412048, cibtc@mail.cibtc.com.cn, http://www.cibtc.com.cn.

616.4 CHN ISSN 1007-5232
ZHONGHUA XIAOHUA NEIJING ZAZHI/CHINESE JOURNAL OF DIGESTIVE ENDOSCOPY. Text in Chinese. 1984. bi-m. USD 24.60; USD 4.10 newsstand/cover (effective 2001). **Document type:** *Academic/Scholarly.*
Formerly: Neijing (1004-9827)
Published by: China International Book Trading Corp/Zhongguo Guoji Tushu Maoyi Zonggongsi cibtc@mail.cibtc.com.cn, http://www.cibtc.com.cn. **Dist. by:** 35, Chegongzhuang Xilu, Haidian District, Beijing 100044, China.

MEDICAL SCIENCES—Experimental Medicine, Laboratory Technique

616 USA
A A B BULLETIN. Text in English. 1965. bi-m. membership. **Document type:** *Bulletin.*
Published by: American Association of Bioanalysts, 917 Locust St., Ste. 1100, St. Louis, MO 63101-1419. TEL 314-241-1445, FAX 314-241-1449. Ed. Mark S Birenbaum. Circ: 4,500 (controlled).

A A M I NEWS. see *INSTRUMENTS*

616 USA
A C I L NEWSLETTER. Text in English. m. **Document type:** *Newsletter.*
Published by: American Council of Independent Laboratories, 1629 K St, N W, Washington, DC 20006. TEL 202-887-5872, FAX 202-887-0021. Ed. Joseph F O'Neil.

619 USA
A C S DIGEST. Text in English. 1984. q. USD 35; includes The Immortalist. adv. bk.rev. **Document type:** *Newsletter.* **Description:** Reports on cryonics, cryobiology, and life extension; articles speculating on future medicine, and life; how current discoveries may change lifestyles.
Former titles: American Cryonics; A C S Notebook; A C S Journal
Published by: American Cryonics Society, PO Box 1509, Cupertino, CA 95015-0761. TEL 415-254-2001, FAX 415-967-4444. Ed. Shane Mohler. Pub., Adv. contact Jim Yount. R&P Edgar Swank. Circ: 500.

616 USA ISSN 0732-8753
RB155.6
A C T INTERNATIONAL CYTOGENETICS LABORATORY DIRECTORY. Text in English. a. USD 60. **Document type:** *Directory.*
Published by: Association of Cytogenetic Technologists, c/o A C T Association Manager, Box 15945-288, Lenexa, KS 66285. TEL 913-541-9077, FAX 913-541-0156. Ed. Turid Knutsen. Circ: 1,700.

A I CH E EQUIPMENT TESTING PROCEDURES SERIES. see *ENGINEERING—Chemical Engineering*

616.15 AUS
A I M S SELF ASSESSMENT PROGRAMMES SERIES. Text in English. 1988. s-a. AUD 25 (effective 2000). adv. back issues avail.
Formerly: A I M L S Self Assessment Programmes Series (1031-7074)
Published by: Australian Institute of Medical Scientists, PO Box 1911, Milton, QLD 4064, Australia. TEL 61-7-3876-2988, FAX 61-7-3876-2999. Adv. contact William Stewart. Circ: 400.

616 IND
A M T CHRONICLE. Text in English. q.
Published by: Association of Medical Technologists, 55 Harish Mukherjee, Kolkata, West Bengal 700 025, India.

A S A I O JOURNAL. see *MEDICAL SCIENCES*

619 USA ISSN 1073-466X
A S C L S TODAY. Text in English. 1965. 11/yr. **Document type:** *Newsletter.*
Former titles (until 1993): A S M T Today (0895-3597); A S M T News (0001-2564)
Published by: American Society for Clinical Laboratory Science, 7910 Woodmont Ave, Ste 530, Bethesda, MD 20814-3015. TEL 301-657-2768, FAX 301-657-2909. Ed. Mary Jean Rutherford. R&P Elissa Passiment. Circ: 20,000.

619 616 BGR ISSN 0324-1750
CODEN: AMBUCH
ACTA MEDICA BULGARICA. Abbreviated title: A M B. Text and summaries in English. 1974. s-a., latest vol.27, 2001. BGL 12 domestic; USD 28 foreign (effective 2001 - 2002). adv. abstr, bibl, illus. index. 60 p./no. back issues avail. *Refereed.* **Document type:** *Journal, Academic/Scholarly, Abstract/Index, Bibliography.*
Description: Publishes original articles by Bulgarian authors covering experimental and clinical developments in all fields of medicine.
Indexed: Abstr.Bulg.Sci.Med.Lit., INIS Atomind., Ref.Zh.
—CASDDS, CISTI, KNAW.
Published by: Meditsinski Universitet - Sofia, Tsentur za Informatsiia po Meditsina/Medical University - Sofia, Medical Information Center, 1 Sv Georgi Sofiiski ul, Sofia 1431, Bulgaria. TEL 359-2-9522342, FAX 359-2-9522393, mutafov@sun.medun.acad.bg, http://www.medun.acad.bg. Ed. D Djerov. R&P, Adv. contact Dr. Christo Mutafov. B&W page USD 50, color page USD 200; 12 x 18. Circ: 300.

ACTA MYOLOGICA; myopathies and cardiomyopathies. see *MEDICAL SCIENCES—Cardiovascular Diseases*

ACTA TOXICOLOGICA ET THERAPEUTICA; international journal of toxicology, pharmacology and therapy. see *ENVIRONMENTAL STUDIES—Toxicology And Environmental Safety*

619 651 USA ISSN 1096-6269
ADVANCE FOR ADMINISTRATORS OF THE LABORATORY. Text in English. 1992. m. *Refereed.* **Document type:** *Trade.*
Published by: Merion Publications, Inc., 2900 Horizon Dr, PO Box 61556, King Of Prussia, PA 19406. TEL 610-278-1400, 800-355-5627, FAX 610-278-1421, advance@merion.com, http://www.advanceweb.com. Ed. Lynn Nace. Pub. Ann Kielinski. adv.: B&W page USD 2,437, color page USD 3,237; trim 10.88 x 8.38. Circ: 29,400.

619 USA ISSN 1088-5676
ADVANCE FOR MEDICAL LABORATORY PROFESSIONALS. Text in English. 1989-199?; N.S.. bi-w. Free to qualified subscribers.. adv. illus. reprints avail. *Refereed.* **Document type:** *Magazine, Trade.*
Formerly (until 199?): Advance for Medical Technologists (1044-2898)
Related titles: Online - full content ed.
—ingenta.
Published by: Merion Publications, Inc., 2900 Horizon Dr, PO Box 61556, King Of Prussia, PA 19406. TEL 610-278-1400, 800-355-5627, FAX 610-278-1421, 610-278-1425, lbrzezicki@merion.com, advance@merion.com, http://www.advanceformlp.com/, http://www.advanceweb.com. Ed. Bette Mooney. Pub. Ann Kielinski. adv.: B&W page USD 3,500, color page USD 3,800; trim 10.88 x 8.38. Circ: 61,800.

619 POL ISSN 1230-025X
ADVANCES IN CLINICAL AND EXPERIMENTAL MEDICINE/POSTEPY MEDYCYNY KLINICZNEJ I DOSWIADCZALNEJ. Text and summaries in English, Polish. 1992. q. EUR 40 to individuals; EUR 80 to institutions (effective 2001). adv. *Refereed.*
Description: Publishes original and clinical studies, review articles, and case reports on various aspects of medicine.
—BLDSC (0703.864000).
Published by: Akademia Medyczna we Wroclawiu/Wroclaw University of Medicine, Wybrzeze L Pasteura 2, Wroclaw 50367, Poland. TEL 48-71-3285154, FAX 48-71-3285154, http://www.am.wroc.pl/advances/advances.html. Ed. Antonina Harlozinska-Szmyrka. Adv. contact Urszula Madrzak. page PLZ 3,000, page XEU 750;.

619 USA
ALBERT HOFMANN'S STRANGE MISTAKE. Text in English. 1993. a. **Document type:** *Bulletin.*
Description: Techno-oral histories of non-ordinary reality and psychotropic experience.
Media: Online - full text.
Address: Box 1852, Brown University, Providence, RI 02912. bobby@rabyd.com, http://www.rabyd.com/lsd. Ed. Bobby Rabyd.

619 016 GBR ISSN 0261-1929
QH301 CODEN: AALADQ
ALTERNATIVES TO LABORATORY ANIMALS. Abbreviated title: A T L A. Text in English. 1973. bi-m. USD 190 in United States to individuals; GBP 95 elsewhere to individuals (effective 2002); Subscription is free in Argentina, Brazil, Bulgaria, Chile, China, Colombia, Costa Rica, Croatia, Czech Republic, Cuba, the former East Germany, Egypt, India, Iran, Iraq, Mexico, Nigeria, Paraguay, Peru, Poland, Romania, Slovakia, the former Soviet Republic, Thailand, Turkey, Uraguay,Yugoslavia, Zimbabwe and others. Please contact publisher.. adv. bk.rev. bibl, illus. Index. back issues avail.; reprints avail. *Refereed.* **Document type:** *Academic/Scholarly.* **Description:** Covers all aspects of the development, validation, introduction and implementation of alternatives to the use of laboratory animals in biomedical research and toxicity testing.
Formerly (until 1983): A T L A Abstracts (0306-2465)
Related titles: Online - full text ed.: (from Institute for Scientific Information); Supplement: Animal Experimentation. Improvements and Alternatives.
Indexed: ASCA, Abstr.Hyg., AgBiotech, Agri.Eng.Abstr., Agricola, Anim.Breed.Abstr., Bibl.Agri., Bio-Contr.News & Info., Biol.Abstr., Curr.Adv.Ecol.Sci., Curr.Cont., Dairy Sci.Abstr., Focus on: Vet.Sci.& Med., Ind.Med., Ind.Vet., Inpharma, Nutr.Abstr., Poult.Abstr., Reac., Ref.Zh., Rev.Appl.Entomol., SSCI (coverage dropped), Sci.Cit.Ind., Soils & Fert., Vet.Bull., Weed Abstr.
—BLDSC (1765.890900), CASDDS, GNLM, IDS. **CCC.**
Published by: Fund for the Replacement of Animals in Medical Experiments, Russell & Burch House, 96-98 N. Sherwood St, Nottingham NG1 4EE, United Kingdom. TEL 44-115-958-4740, FAX 44-115-950-3570, atla@frame.org.uk, http://www.frame.org.uk. Ed. Michael Balls. Adv. contact Richard McGowan. Circ: 850.

619 179 DEU ISSN 0946-7785
ALTEX. Text in German. 1984. q. DEM 98 to individuals; DEM 195 to institutions; DEM 30 to students (effective 2000). **Document type:** *Journal, Academic/Scholarly.*
Formerly (until 1994): Alternativen zu Tierexperimenten (1018-4562)
Related titles: Online - full text ed.: (from Institute for Scientific Information).
Indexed: Curr.Cont., Ind.Med., Inpharma, Pharm.&Out.News, Reac.
—GNLM, IDS.
Published by: (Mitteleuropaeischen Gesellschaft fuer Alternativen zu Tierversuchen), Spektrum Akademischer Verlag GmbH, Vangerowstr 20, Heidelberg 69115, Germany. TEL 49-6221-912645, FAX 49-6221-912638, service@mediapoly.com, http://www.spektrum-verlag.com.

AMERICAN BIOTECHNOLOGY LABORATORY. see *BIOLOGY—Biotechnology*

619 USA ISSN 8750-9490
CODEN: ACPREA
AMERICAN CLINICAL LABORATORY. Text in English. 1982. 10/yr. USD 237; USD 280 foreign. adv. bk.rev. charts, illus, stat, tr.lit. **Document type:** *Trade.*
Formerly: American Clinical Products Review
Indexed: Chem.Abstr., Chem.Indus.Notes, Chem.Titles, Mass Spectr.Bull.
—BLDSC (0812.590500), CASDDS, GNLM, Linda Hall.
Published by: International Scientific Communications, Inc., 30 Controls Dr, Box 870, Shelton, CT 06484-0870. TEL 203-926-9300, FAX 203-926-9310, iscpubs@iscpubs.com, http://www.iscpubs.com. Ed. Brian Howard. Pub. William Wham. R&P Gina Lascola. Adv. contact Thomas G Thomas. B&W page USD 3,995, color page USD 5,305. Circ: 62,050 (controlled).

619 USA
AMERICAN COLLEGE OF LABORATORY ANIMAL MEDICINE SERIES. Text in English. 1974. irreg. back issues avail. *Refereed.* **Document type:** *Monographic series.*
Published by: Academic Press, Inc., Journal Division (Subsidiary of: Harcourt Brace & Company), 525 B St, Ste 1900, San Diego, CA 92101-4495. TEL 619-231-6616, FAX 619-699-6715. **Subscr. to:** Order Dept., 6277 Sea Harbor Dr, 4th Fl, Orlando, FL 32887. TEL 800-321-5068.

AMERICAN JOURNAL OF EMERGENCY MEDICINE. see *MEDICAL SCIENCES—Orthopedics And Traumatology*

AMERICAN POLYGRAPH ASSOCIATION NEWSLETTER. see *CRIMINOLOGY AND LAW ENFORCEMENT*

616 NLD ISSN 0166-7688
ANALYSE. Text in Dutch. 1946. 10/yr. NLG 200 to non-members; NLG 140 to members. adv. bk.rev. illus. index. *Refereed.* **Document type:** *Newsletter.*
Formerly: Tijdschrift voor Medische Analisten
Related titles: Online - full text ed.
Indexed: INIS Atomind.
—KNAW.
Published by: Nederlandse Vereniging van BioMedische Laboratoriummedewerkers/Dutch Association of Bio-Medical Laboratory Technologists, Wilhelminapark 52, Utrecht 3581 NM, Netherlands. TEL 31-30-252-2881, FAX 31-30-254-1814. Ed. Dr. M A Kusters Van Someren. Circ: 3,500 (controlled). **Co-sponsor:** International Association of Medical Technologists.

619 JPN ISSN 0910-0911
ANIMARUZU NYUSU/ANIMALS NEWS. Text in Japanese. 1978. a.
—CCC.
Published by: Niigata Daigaku, Igakubu/Niigata University, School of Medicine, Fuzoku Dobutsu Jikken Shisetsu, 757, Asahimachi Dori Ichibancho, Niigata-shi, Niigata-ken 951, Japan.

616 JPN ISSN 0915-3667
ANITEKKUSU/LABORATORY ANIMAL TECHNOLOGY AND SCIENCE. Text in Japanese. 1989. bi-m. JPY 1,100 per issue.
Published by: Kenseisha Inc., 6-4 Kakigaracho-Nihonbashi 1-chome, Chuo-ku, Tokyo 103-0000, Japan.

ANLEITUNG FUER DIE CHEMISCHE LABORATORIUMSPRAXIS - CHEMICAL LABORATORY PRACTICE. see *CHEMISTRY*

616 CAN ISSN 0709-8502
CODEN: ABCQD2
ANNALES DE BIOCHIMIE CLINIQUE DU QUEBEC. Text in French. 1980. q. free per issue. adv. bk.rev. abstr. index. back issues avail. *Refereed.* **Document type:** *Bulletin, Academic/Scholarly.* **Description:** Studies clinical biochemistry.
Indexed: Biol.Abstr., Chem.Abstr., Chem.Indus.Notes, Chem.Titles, Curr.Adv.Ecol.Sci.
—BLDSC (0967.590000), CASDDS, CISTI.
Published by: (Societe Quebecoise de Biochimie Clinique), Marc Letellier, Ed. & Pub., c/o Marc Letellier, Ed, Dept de Biochimie Clinique, C H U S, Sherbrooke, PQ J1H 5N4, Canada. TEL 819-563-5555, FAX 819-820-6425. Ed. Mar Letellier. R&P Marc Letellier. Circ: 900.

616 USA ISSN 0091-7370
RB37.A1 CODEN: ACLSCP
ANNALS OF CLINICAL AND LABORATORY SCIENCE. Text in English. 1971. bi-m. USD 85 to individuals; USD 120 foreign to individuals; USD 120 to institutions; USD 130 foreign to institutions. adv. bk.rev. abstr, charts, illus. index. *Refereed.* **Document type:** *Academic/Scholarly.*
Related titles: Online - full text ed.: (from Institute for Scientific Information).
Indexed: ASCA, Biol.Abstr., Chem.Abstr., Chem.Indus.Notes, Chem.Titles, Curr.Adv.Cancer Res., Curr.Adv.Ecol.Sci., Curr.Cont., Dent.Ind., Dok.Arbeitsmed., Excerp.Med., INIS Atomind., Ind.Med. (1973-), Ind.Sci.Rev., Inpharma, Int.Abstr.Biol.Sci., Nutr.Abstr., Pharm.&Out.News, Reac., Sci.Cit.Ind., THA.
—BLDSC (1040.228000), CASDDS, CISTI, EMDOCS, GNLM, IDS, ingenta, KNAW. **CCC.**
Published by: (Association of Clinical Scientists), Institute for Clinical Science, 1833 Delancey Pl, Philadelphia, PA 19103. TEL 215-829-7068, FAX 215-829-3094, 104657.346@compuserve.com. Ed. Dr. F William Sunderman. Circ: 2,000.

616 GBR ISSN 0785-3890
CODEN: ANMDEU
ANNALS OF MEDICINE. Text in English. 1969. 8/yr. GBP 64, USD 105 to individuals; GBP 288, USD 475 to institutions (effective 2002). bk.rev. charts, illus. index. back issues avail. *Refereed.* **Document type:** *Academic/Scholarly.* **Description:** Publishes a wide range of papers which bridge the gap between basic science and clinical medicine.
Formed by the merger of (1969-1989): Annals of Clinical Research (0003-4762); Which was formed by the merger of: Annales Paediatriae Fenniae (0570-1732); Annales Medininae Internae Fenniae (0365-4362); (1974-1989): Medical Biology (0302-2137); Which superseded: Annales Medicinae Experimentalis et Biologiae Fenniae (0003-4479)
Related titles: Microform ed.: (from PQC); Online - full text ed.: (from Ovid Technologies, Inc., EBSCO Publishing, Swets Blackwell, Institute for Scientific Information, CatchWord Ltd.).
Indexed: ASCA, Abstr.Hyg., Biol.Abstr., Chem.Abstr., Chem.Indus.Notes, Chem.Titles, Child Devel.Abstr., Compumath, Curr.Adv.Ecol.Sci., Curr.Cont., Dairy Sci.Abstr., Derwent Biotech.Abstr., Diar.Dis.Res., Environ.Sci.Poll.Mgmt., Excerp.Med., Helminthol.Abstr., INIS Atomind., Ind.Med. (1989-), Ind.Sci.Rev., Inpharma, Int.Abstr.Biol.Sci., Med.& Surg.Dermat., NRN, Neurosci.Abstr. (coverage dropped), Nutr.Abstr., Pharm.&Out.News, Pollut.Abstr., PsycInfo, Psychol.Abstr. (1989-), Reac., Ref.Zh., Risk Abstr., SSCI (coverage dropped), Saf.Sci.Abstr., Sci.Cit.Ind., Trop.Dis.Bull., e-psyche.
—BLDSC (1043.131000), ADONIS, CASDDS, CISTI, EMDOCS, GNLM, IDS, ingenta, KNAW. **CCC.**
Published by: (Finnish Medical Society Duodecim), Royal Society of Medicine Press Ltd, 1 Wimpole St, London W1M 8AE, United Kingdom. TEL 44-207-290-2929, rsmjournals@roysocmed.ac.uk, http://www.roysocmed.ac.uk. Ed. Dr. P T Kovanen. Circ: 995.

ANTHROZOOS; a multidisciplinary journal on the interactions of people and animals. see *BIOLOGY—Zoology*

APPLIED NURSING RESEARCH. see *MEDICAL SCIENCES—Nurses And Nursing*

APPLIED RADIATION AND ISOTOPES. see *PHYSICS—Nuclear Physics*

ARCHIVES OF PATHOLOGY & LABORATORY MEDICINE. see *MEDICAL SCIENCES*

ARQUIVOS DE CIRURGIA CLINICA E EXPERIMENTAL. see *MEDICAL SCIENCES—Surgery*

610.28 660 USA ISSN 1073-1199
R856.A1 CODEN: ABSBE4
ARTIFICIAL CELLS, BLOOD SUBSTITUTES, AND IMMOBILIZATION BIOTECHNOLOGY. Text in English. 1973. bi-m. USD 145 to individuals print & online eds.; USD 1,395 to institutions print only (effective 2002). adv. illus. *Refereed.* **Document type:** *Academic/Scholarly.* **Description:** Covers artificial cells, blood substitutes, and immobilization biotechnology from an interdisciplinary perspective.
Former titles (until 1993): Biomaterials, Artificial Cells and Immobilization Biotechnology (1055-7172); (until 1991): Biomaterials, Artificial Cells and Artificial Organs; (until 1987): Biomaterials, Medical Devices, and Artificial Organs (0890-5533)
Related titles: Microform ed.: (from RPI); Online - full text ed.: (from Institute for Scientific Information, RoweCom Information Quest).
Indexed: ASCA, Alloys Ind. (1978-), Bioeng.Abstr., Biol.Abstr., Biotech.& Bioeng.Abstr., Chem.Abstr., Chem.Indus.Notes, Chem.Titles, Curr.Cont. (coverage dropped), Dent.Ind., Eng.Ind., Eng.Mat.Abstr., Excerp.Med., INIS Atomind., INSPEC (1975-), Ind.Med. (1994-), Ind.Sci.Rev., Inpharma, Mat.Sci.Cit.Ind., Met.Abstr. (1978-), Met.Abstr.Ind. (1978-), Nonfer.Met.Alert (1978-), PCC Alert (1978-), Pharm.&Out.News, Reac., Ref.Zh., Sci.Cit.Ind., Steels Alert (1978-), World Alum.Abstr.
—BLDSC (1735.022500), AskIEEE, CASDDS, CISTI, Ei, EMDOCS, GNLM, IDS, ingenta, KNAW. **CCC.**
Published by: Marcel Dekker Inc., 270 Madison Ave, New York, NY 10016. TEL 212-696-9000, 800-228-1160, FAX 212-685-4540, http://www.dekker.com/servlet/product/productid/BIO. Ed. T M S Chang. R&P Julia Mulligan. Adv. contact Anne Mullins. B&W page USD 800. Circ: 325.

619 USA ISSN 0160-564X
RD130 CODEN: ARORD7
ARTIFICIAL ORGANS. Text in English. 1977. m. USD 515 domestic to individuals; USD 535 in Canada & Mexico to individuals; USD 555 overseas to individuals; USD 810 domestic to institutions; USD 830 in Canada & Mexico to institutions; USD 850 overseas to institutions; USD 566.50 to individuals print & online eds. combined; USD 891 to institutions print & online eds. combined (effective 2001). adv. bk.rev. charts, illus. index. back issues avail.; reprints avail. *Refereed.* **Document type:** *Academic/Scholarly.* **Description:** Multidisciplinary journal publishing reports on the design, performance and evaluation of biomaterials and devices used in artificial organs for the medical, scientific and engineering communities; includes relevant coverage of biomechanics, bioelectronics, hemodynamics, and plasmapheresis.
Related titles: Online - full text ed.: ISSN 1525-1594. USD 464 to individuals; USD 729 to institutions (effective 2001) (from Ovid Technologies, Inc., EBSCO Publishing, O C L C Online Computer Library Center, Inc., RoweCom Information Quest, ingenta, Munksgaard & Blackwell Science's Synergy, Swets Blackwell, Institute for Scientific Information).
Indexed: ASCA, Biol.Abstr., Chem.Abstr., Chem.Indus.Notes, Chem.Titles, Curr.Cont., Dent.Ind., Environ.Sci.Poll.Mgmt., Excerp.Med., INIS Atomind., Ind.Med. (1977-), Ind.Sci.Rev., Inpharma, Mat.Sci.Cit.Ind., Pharm.&Out.News, Pollut.Abstr., Reac., Rev.Med.& Vet.Mycol., Risk Abstr., SSCI (coverage dropped), Saf.Sci.Abstr., Sci.Cit.Ind.
—BLDSC (1735.052000), ADONIS, CASDDS, CISTI, EMDOCS, GNLM, IDS, ingenta. **CCC.**
Published by: (International Society for Artificial Organs), Blackwell Science Inc., Commerce Pl, 350 Main St, Malden, MA 02148-5018. TEL 781-388-8250, 800-759-6102, FAX 781-388-8255, journals@blacksci.com, http://www.blackwell-science.com. Ed. Dr. Yukihiko Nose. R&P Tracey Davies. Adv. contact Jenny Applin. Circ: 1,400.

619 530 AUS ISSN 0158-9938
CODEN: AUPMDI
AUSTRALASIAN PHYSICAL & ENGINEERING SCIENCES IN MEDICINE. Text in English. 1977. q. AUD 55 domestic to individuals; AUD 60 foreign to individuals; AUD 99 domestic to libraries; AUD 100 foreign to libraries (effective 2001). adv. bk.rev. index. 70 p./no. back issues avail. *Refereed.* **Document type:** *Academic/Scholarly.* **Description:** Covers applications of the physical sciences and engineering on medicine and biology; papers, reviews, technical reports and letters.
Formerly: Australasian Physical Sciences in Medicine
Related titles: Online - full text ed.: 1977.
Indexed: Bioeng.Abstr., Biotech.& Bioeng.Abstr., Chem.Abstr., Comput.& Info.Sys., Electron.& Communic.Abstr.J., Eng.Ind., Excerp.Med., INIS Atomind., INSPEC (May 1979-), ISMEC, Ind.Med. (1980-).
—BLDSC (1796.030000), AskIEEE, CASDDS, CISTI, Ei, GNLM, ingenta, KNAW, Linda Hall.
Published by: Australasian College of Physical Scientists and Engineers in Medicine, Dept. of Medical Physics, Royal Adelaide Hospital, Adelaide, SA, ACT 5000, Australia. TEL 61-8-8222-5536, FAX 61-8-8222-5937, szavgoro@mail.rah.sa.gov.au, http://www.sci.qut.edu.au/phys/apesm. Ed., R&P Dr. Sergei F Zavgorodni TEL 61-8-8222-5539. Adv. contact Ms. C Robinson. Circ: 450. **Co-sponsor:** College of Biomedical Engineers, Institution of Engineers, Australia.

AUSTRALIAN JOURNAL OF MEDICAL SCIENCE. see *MEDICAL SCIENCES*

B B A - GENE STRUCTURE AND EXPRESSION. see *BIOLOGY—Genetics*

619 LVA ISSN 1407-0944
BALTIC JOURNAL OF LABORATORY ANIMAL SCIENCE. Text in English, Russian. 1991. q. USD 90 in Europe; USD 100 elsewhere (effective 2000). adv. bk.rev. abstr, bibl, charts, illus. index. back issues avail. *Refereed.* **Document type:** *Academic/Scholarly.* **Description:** Publishes original scientific articles, reviews on all problems of laboratory animal science and technology, educational articles and practical recommendations.
Formerly (until 1996): Laboratornye Zhyvotnye (0869-0219)
Indexed: AgBiotech, Anim.Breed.Abstr., Ind.Vet., Poult.Abstr., Ref.Zh., Rev.Med.& Vet.Mycol., Vet.Bull., Zoo.Rec.
—BLDSC (1861.316620), Linda Hall.
Published by: Public Joint Stock Company Grindeks, Krustpils iela 53, Riga 1057, Latvia. TEL 371-7104547, FAX 371-7138683, bjlanim@grindeks.lv, http://www.vip.latnet.lv/journalLAS/. Ed. Elena Porunkevich. R&P Guna Jacobson TEL 371-7139461. Adv. contact Ludmila Vandish. page USD 150; trim 240 x 170. Circ: 200.

BIOLOGICAL RESEARCH. see *BIOLOGY*

619 GBR ISSN 0269-3879
CODEN: BICHE2
BIOMEDICAL CHROMATOGRAPHY. Text in English. 1986. 8/yr. USD 1,695 in United States; USD 1,695 in Canada & Mexico; USD 1,695 elsewhere; USD 1,780 combined subscription in United States for print and online eds.; USD 1,780 combined subscription in Canada & Mexico for print and online eds.; USD 1,780 combined subscription elsewhere for print and online eds. (effective 2002). adv. reprint service avail. from SWZ. *Refereed.* **Document type:** *Academic/Scholarly.* **Description:** Devoted to the publication of original papers on the applications of chromatography and allied techniques in the biological and medical sciences.
Related titles: Microform ed.: (from PQC); Online - full text ed.: ISSN 1099-0801. 1997. USD 1,695 in United States; USD 1,695 in Canada & Mexico; USD 1,695 elsewhere (effective 2002) (from EBSCO Publishing, Wiley InterScience, Institute for Scientific Information).
Indexed: ASCA, Anal.Abstr., BBCI, Chem.Abstr., Chem.Cit.Ind., Chem.Indus.Notes, Chem.Titles, Chromat.Abstr., Curr.Cont., Dairy Sci.Abstr., Eng.Ind., Excerp.Med., Ind.Med. (1986-), Ind.Sci.Rev., Inpharma, Int.Abstr.Biol.Sci., Mass Spectr.Bull., Nutr.Abstr., RCI, Reac., Sci.Cit.Ind.
—BLDSC (2087.758000), CASDDS, CISTI, Ei, EMDOCS, GNLM, IDS, Infotrieve, ingenta. **CCC.**
Published by: Wiley Europe Ltd., Baffins Ln, Chichester, W Sussex PO19 1UD, United Kingdom. TEL 44-1243-779777, FAX 44-1243-775878, customer@wiley.co.uk, http://www.interscience.wiley.com/jpages/0269-3879/, http://www.wiley.co.uk. adv.: B&W page GBP 650, color page GBP 1,550; trim 210 x 297. Circ: 300. **Subscr. in the Americas to:** John Wiley & Sons, Inc., Journals, 605 Third Ave, New York, NY 10158. TEL 212-850-6021, 212-850-6645, subinfo@jwiley.com.

BIOMEDICAL INFORMATICS. JOURNAL. see *MEDICAL SCIENCES*

BIOMEDICAL PRODUCTS. see *MEDICAL SCIENCES*

616 GBR ISSN 1352-7673
BIOMEDICAL SCIENTIST. Text in English. 1951. m. GBP 60; GBP 75 foreign (effective 1999). adv. bk.rev. **Document type:** *Trade.* **Description:** Provides news and management ideas for biomedical laboratory scientists.
Former titles (until 1994): I M L S Gazette (0267-2928); Institute of Medical Laboratory Science. Gazette (0307-5656); Institute of Medical Laboratory Technology. Gazette (0020-2959)
Related titles: ♦ Supplement: Pathology in Practice. ISSN 1465-9131.
Indexed: CINAHL.
—BLDSC (2087.880150).
Published by: (Institute of Biomedical Science), Step Publishing Ltd., Lower Green Rd, Rusthall, Turnbridge Wells TN4 8TT, United Kingdom. TEL 44-1892-518877, mail@stepex.co.uk, http://www.stepex.co.uk. Ed. Roy Owen. Adv. contact Gill Ansell. Circ: 14,000.

619 USA
BIONICS✱. Text in English. 1988. q. USD 20. adv. film rev. charts, illus, pat, tr.lit. cum.index: 1989-1990. **Description:** Reports on bionics, bio-sensors, artificial organs, cybernetics, industrial and governmental research, investment news.
Related titles: Microfilm ed.: 1988.
Published by: Bionics Industry Association, c/o Ben Campbell, Ed, 917 S Park St, Owosso, MI 48867-4422. TEL 517-485-7800. Circ: 4,000.

BIOPSY INTERPRETATION SERIES. see *MEDICAL SCIENCES*

BIOTECH SOFTWARE AND INTERNET REPORT; the computer software journal for scientists. see *BIOLOGY—Biotechnology*

619 USA
BLOOD & MARROW TRANSPLANT NEWSLETTER. Text in English. 1990. q. free per issue. adv. **Document type:** *Newsletter.* **Description:** Aimed at bone marrow, stem cell, and cord blood transplant patients and survivors.
Formerly (until Aug. 1996): Bone and Marrow Transplant Newsletter
Related titles: Online - full text ed.
Address: 2900 Skokie Valley Road, Highland, IL 60035. TEL 847-433-3313, FAX 847-433-4599, help@bmtnews.org, http://www.BMTNews.org. Ed. Susan Stewart. R&P, Adv. contact Carol Fradkin.

619 GBR ISSN 0268-3369
CODEN: BMTRE9
BONE MARROW TRANSPLANTATION. Text in English. 1986. 24/yr. GBP 207 in Europe to individuals for print or online ed.; USD 405 elsewhere to individuals for print or online ed.; GBP 297 combined subscription in Europe to individuals print & online eds.; USD 446 combined subscription elsewhere to individuals print & online eds.; GBP 660 in Europe to institutions for print or online ed.; USD 990 elsewhere to institutions for print or online ed.; GBP 726 combined subscription in Europe to institutions print & online ed.; USD 1,089 combined subscription elsewhere to institutions print & online ed. (effective 2002). adv. bk.rev. abstr, illus, charts. index. back issues avail.; reprints avail. *Refereed.* **Document type:** *Journal, Academic/Scholarly.* **Description:** Clinical results of bone marrow transplantation in man and experimental results with animals.
Related titles: Online - full text ed.: 1997 (from Northern Light Technology, Inc., EBSCO Publishing, O C L C Online Computer Library Center, Inc., RoweCom Information Quest, ingenta, Swets Blackwell, Institute for Scientific Information); ♦ Supplement: Bone Marrow Transplantation. Supplement. ISSN 0951-3078.
Indexed: AIDS & Cancer Res., ASCA, Abstr.Hyg., Curr.Adv.Cancer Res., Curr.Adv.Cell & Devel.Biol., Curr.Adv.Ecol.Sci., Curr.Adv.Gen.& Molec.Biol., Curr.Cont., Environ.Sci.Poll.Mgmt., Excerp.Med., Helminthol.Abstr., Immun.Abstr., Ind.Med. (1986-), Ind.Sci.Rev., Inpharma, Int.Abstr.Biol.Sci., Med.& Surg.Dermat., Microbiol.Abstr., Pharm.&Out.News, Protozool.Abstr., Reac., Ref.Zh., Rev.Med.& Vet.Mycol., SSCI (coverage dropped), Sci.Cit.Ind., Trop.Dis.Bull.
—BLDSC (2247.358000), CISTI, EMDOCS, GNLM, IDS, ingenta, KNAW. **CCC.**
Published by: (European Group for Blood and Marrow Transplantation), Nature Publishing Group Specialist Journals (Subsidiary of: Holtzbrink Publishers), Houndmills, Basingstoke, Hants RG21 6XS, United Kingdom. TEL 44-1256-329242, FAX 44-1256-328339, subscriptions@nature.com, http://www.nature.com/bmt. Ed. John M Golman. Pub. Sue Deeley. R&P Trace Noel. Adv. contact Robert Sloan TEL 44-20-8882-7199.

619 GBR ISSN 0951-3078
BONE MARROW TRANSPLANTATION. SUPPLEMENT. Text in English. 1986. 24/yr. GBP 207 in Europe to individuals for print or online ed.; USD 405 elsewhere to individuals for print or online ed.; GBP 297 combined subscription in Europe to individuals print & online; USD 446 combined subscription elsewhere to individuals print & online; GBP 660 in Europe to institutions for print or online ed.; USD 990 elsewhere to institutions for print or online ed.; GBP 726 combined subscription in Europe to institutions print & online; USD 1,089 combined subscription elsewhere to institutions print & online (effective 2002). abstr, illus. back issues avail.; reprints avail. **Document type:** *Academic/Scholarly.*
Related titles: Online - full content ed.; ♦ Supplement to: Bone Marrow Transplantation. ISSN 0268-3369.
—KNAW.
Published by: (European Group for Blood and Marrow Transplantation), Nature Publishing Group Specialist Journals (Subsidiary of: Holtzbrink Publishers), Houndmills, Basingstoke, Hants RG21 6XS, United Kingdom. TEL 44-1256-329242, FAX 44-1256-328339, subscriptions@nature.com, http://www.nature.com/bmt. Ed. John M Goldman TEL 44-20-8383-3233. Pub. Sue Deeley. R&P Trace Noel. Adv. contact Robert Sloan TEL 44-20-8882-7199.

BRAIN PATHOLOGY. see *MEDICAL SCIENCES—Psychiatry And Neurology*

616 GBR ISSN 0967-4845
CODEN: BJMSEO
BRITISH JOURNAL OF BIOMEDICAL SCIENCE. Text in English. 1951. q. GBP 110; USD 208 foreign. adv. bk.rev. abstr, bibl, charts, illus. index. *Refereed.* **Document type:** *Academic/Scholarly.*
Former titles: Medical Laboratory Sciences (0308-3616); Medical Laboratory Technology (0022-2607); Journal of Medical Laboratory Technology
Related titles: Online - full text ed.: (from Northern Light Technology, Inc., ProQuest Information & Learning, Institute for Scientific Information).
Indexed: ASCA, Abstr.Hyg., AgBiotech, Biol.Abstr., CINAHL, Chem.Abstr., Chem.Indus.Notes, Chem.Titles, Curr.Adv.Cancer Res., Curr.Adv.Ecol.Sci., Curr.Cont., Dairy Sci.Abstr., Diar.Dis.Res., Environ.Sci.Poll.Mgmt., Excerp.Med., INIS Atomind., Ind.Med. (1993-), Ind.Sci.Rev., Ind.Vet., Inpharma, Int.Abstr.Biol.Sci., Med.& Surg.Dermat., Microbiol.Abstr., NRN, Nutr.Abstr., Pharm.&Out.News, Poult.Abstr., Protozool.Abstr., Reac., Ref.Zh., Rev.Arom.& Med.Plants, Rev.Med.& Vet.Mycol., Rev.Plant Path., SSCI (coverage dropped), Sci.Cit.Ind., Telegen, Trop.Dis.Bull., Vet.Bull.
—BLDSC (2306.730000), ADONIS, CASDDS, CISTI, EMDOCS, GNLM, IDS, ingenta, KNAW. **CCC.**
Published by: (Institute of Biomedical Science), Royal Society of Medicine Press Ltd, 1 Wimpole St, London W1M 8AE, United Kingdom. FAX 44-207-290-2929. R&P Caroline McLaughlin. Circ: 15,000.

C I T PLUS. (Chemie Ingenieur Technik) see *ENGINEERING—Chemical Engineering*

542 681.2 USA ISSN 0093-8076
RB36.2
C L R. (Clinical Laboratory Reference) Text in English. 1974. a. USD 32 domestic; USD 38 foreign; USD 32 newsstand/cover (effective 2001). adv. reprints avail. **Document type:** *Trade.* **Description:** Includes product information on diagnostic reagents, test systems, instruments, and equipment for the medical laboratory.
Published by: Medical Economics Co., Inc., 5 Paragon Dr, Montvale, NJ 07645-1742. TEL 201-358-7200. Circ: 59,000 (controlled).

C M B E S - S C G B NEWSLETTER. see *MEDICAL SCIENCES*

619 CAN ISSN 0045-4354
CANADIAN ASSOCIATION FOR LABORATORY ANIMAL SCIENCE NEWSLETTER. Text and summaries in English, French. 1968. bi-m. membership. adv. bk.rev. bibl, charts, illus. **Document type:** *Newsletter.*
Published by: Canadian Association for Laboratory Animal Science (CALAS), c/o Dr Donald G McKay, Biosciences Animal Service, University of Alberta, Edmonton, AB T6G 2E9, Canada. Ed. M Buckley. Circ: 1,000 (controlled).

CANADIAN JOURNAL OF CARDIOLOGY. see *MEDICAL SCIENCES—Cardiovascular Diseases*

616 CAN ISSN 1207-5833
CODEN: CJMTAY
CANADIAN JOURNAL OF MEDICAL LABORATORY SCIENCE. Text in English. 1938. bi-m. CND 21.40 domestic; CND 24 in United States; CND 35 foreign (effective 2000). adv. bk.rev. bibl, charts, illus, tr.lit. index. **Document type:** *Journal, Trade.* **Description:** Explores medical laboratory technology, management and education.
Formerly: Canadian Journal of Medical Technology (0008-4158)
Related titles: French ed.: ISSN 1207-5825. 1985.
Indexed: Biol.Abstr., CINAHL, Chem.Abstr., Curr.Adv.Ecol.Sci., Curr.Cont. (coverage dropped), GeoRef, Helminthol.Abstr., INIS Atomind., Ind.Med. (coverage dropped), Nutr.Abstr., Ref.Zh., Rev.Med.& Vet.Mycol., Sci.Cit.Ind. (coverage dropped).
—BLDSC (3032.200000), CASDDS, CISTI, GNLM, ingenta. **CCC.**
Published by: Canadian Society for Medical Laboratory Science/Societe Canadienne de Science de Laboratoire Medical, LCD 1, P O Box 2830, Hamilton, ON L8N 3N8, Canada. TEL 905-528-8642, FAX 905-528-4968, cjmls@csmls.org. Ed., Pub., R&P, Adv. contact Alison Toupitch. Circ: 13,805.

CELL DEATH AND DIFFERENTIATION. see *BIOLOGY—Cytology And Histology*

CHEMIE-INGENIEUR-TECHNIK; Verfahrenstechnik, Technische Chemie, Apparatewaren, Biotechnologie. see *ENGINEERING—Chemical Engineering*

▼ **CLINICAL AND EXPERIMENTAL MEDICINE.** see *MEDICAL SCIENCES*

619 616 USA ISSN 0009-9147
RB1 CODEN: CLCHAU
CLINICAL CHEMISTRY; international journal of laboratory medicine and molecular diagnostics. Text in English. 1955. m. USD 171 domestic to individuals; USD 217 in Canada & Mexico to individuals; USD 264 elsewhere to individuals; USD 561 domestic to institutions; USD 607 in Canada & Mexico to institutions; USD 653 elsewhere to institutions (effective 2000); includes print & online eds.. adv. bk.rev. abstr, bibl, charts, illus. index, cum.index. back issues avail.; reprints avail. *Refereed.* **Document type:** *Academic/Scholarly.* **Description:** Covers analytical and molecular diagnostic techniques, instrumentation, statistical analysis of data, clinical investigations in which clinical chemistry has played a major role, and a variety of in vivo and in vitro studies of human disease.
Related titles: Microfiche ed.; Microfilm ed.; Online - full text ed.: (from HighWire Pr., EBSCO Publishing, Institute for Scientific Information).
Indexed: ASCA, Anal.Abstr., BBCI, Biodet.Abstr., Biol.Abstr., C.I.S. Abstr., Chem.Abstr., Chem.Cit.Ind., Chem.Indus.Notes, Chem.Titles, Chromat.Abstr., Compumath, Curr.Adv.Cancer Res., Curr.Adv.Ecol.Sci., Curr.Cont., Dairy Sci.Abstr., Dent.Ind., Derwent Biotech.Abstr., Diar.Dis.Res., Excerp.Med., INIS Atomind., Ind.Med. (1955-), Ind.Sci.Rev., Ind.Vet., Inpharma, Int.Abstr.Biol.Sci., Mass Spectr.Bull., Neurosci.Cit.Ind., Nutr.Abstr., Pharm.&Out.News, Reac., Ref.Zh., Rev.Appl.Entomol., Rev.Med.& Vet.Mycol., SSCI (coverage dropped), Sci.Cit.Ind., So.Pac.Per.Ind., Soyabean Abstr., THA, Vet.Bull.
—BLDSC (3286.268000), ADONIS, CASDDS, CISTI, EMDOCS, GNLM, IDS, ingenta, KNAW, Linda Hall. **CCC.**
Published by: American Association for Clinical Chemistry, Inc., 2101 L St N W, Ste 202, Washington, DC 20037-1526. TEL 800-892-1400, FAX 202-887-5093, clinchem@aacc.org, http://www.clinchem.org. Ed. David E Bruns. Pub., R&P Mac Fancher TEL 202-857-0717. Circ: 15,000.

616 USA ISSN 0197-8454
CODEN: CLLEE2
CLINICAL LAB LETTER. Text in English. 1980. 22/yr., latest vol.22 (m. in Jan. & Aug.). USD 349 domestic to individuals; USD 389 foreign to individuals; USD 440 domestic to institutions; USD 499 foreign to institutions; USD 23 newsstand/cover (effective 2002). bk.rev. tr.lit. index. back issues avail. **Document type:** *Newsletter.* **Description:** Published for clinical lab personnel. Covers latest diagnostic technology, safety hazards, recalls, legislation, standards, products, legal issues and education.
Related titles: Online - full text ed.: USD 572 domestic academic site license; USD 631 foreign academic site license; USD 638 domestic corporate site license; USD 697 foreign corporate site license (2002) (from ProQuest Information & Learning).
Indexed: P.N.I.
Published by: Lippincott Williams & Wilkins (Philadelphia) (Subsidiary of: Wolters Kluwer N.V.), 530 Walnut St, Philadelphia, PA 19106-3621. TEL 215-521-8300, FAX 215-521-8902, http://www.lww.com. Ed. Linda G Huang. **Subscr. to:** PO Box 1600, Hagerstown, MD 21740-1600. TEL 800-777-2295, FAX 301-824-7390.

616 USA ISSN 0192-1282
CLINICAL LAB PRODUCTS. Text in English. 1972. m. USD 60; USD 6 newsstand/cover; free to qualified personnel (effective 2001). adv. back issues avail.; reprints avail. **Document type:** *Magazine, Trade.* **Description:** News items concerning instruments, diagnostics and supplies used in clinical laboratory. Provides a news digest, product development, lab economics, and disease management.
Related titles: Online - full text ed.
Published by: Medical World Communications, Allied Healthcare Group, 295 Promenade St, Ste 2, Providence, RI 02908-5720. TEL 401-455-0555, FAX 401-455-1555, sandersen@mwc.com, info@healthtechnet.com, http://www.clpmag.com, http://www.healthtechnet.com. Ed. Coleen Curran. Pub. Scott Andersen. Circ: 51,500 (controlled).

542 USA
CLINICAL LAB PRODUCTS BUYERS GUIDE. Text in English. 1975. a. adv. **Document type:** *Catalog, Trade.*
Formerly: Clinical Lab Products Annual Guide
Published by: Medical World Communications, Allied Healthcare Group, 295 Promenade St, Ste 2, Providence, RI 02908-5720. TEL 401-455-0555, FAX 401-455-1555, info@healthtechnet.com, http://www.clpmag.com, http://www.healthtechnet.com. Circ: 48,000.

619 BEL
CLINICAL LABORATORY INTERNATIONAL. Text in English. 1977. 8/yr. USD 90 in Europe; USD 95 in South America; free to qualified personnel. adv. bk.rev. **Document type:** *Magazine, Trade.* **Description:** Reports on new clinical laboratory instrumentation, reagents, and test kits for use in medical and blood bank laboratories.
Indexed: CSNB, Lab.Haz.Bull.
—BLDSC (3286.295850).
Published by: Elsevier Business Information - Belgium (Subsidiary of: Reed Elsevier plc), Rue des Palais 100, Brussels B-1030, Belgium. TEL 32-2-240-2611, FAX 32-2-242-7111, pepco@pepco.be, http://www.pepco.be, http://www.ebi.be. Ed. Joanna Winstone. Pub., R&P Dr. Bernard Leger. Adv. contact Astrid Wydouw. B&W page USD 7,430; 7.875 x 10.4375. Circ: 27,010 (controlled).

616 USA
CLINICAL LABORATORY METHODS AND TECHNIQUES. Text in English. 1991. q.?. USD 125 to individuals; USD 159 to institutions. *Refereed.* **Document type:** *Academic/Scholarly.*
Published by: Field & Wood, Medical Periodicals, Inc., PO Box 975, Blue Bell, PA 19422. TEL 610-828-4010, FAX 610-482-0226. Ed. Dr. Sun.

681 USA
CLINICAL LABORATORY PRODUCT COMPARISON SYSTEM. Variant title: Healthcare Product Comparison System: Clinical Laboratory Edition. Text in English. m. USD 1,027.40 domestic; USD 1,075.40 in Canada; USD 1,145 elsewhere (effective 2002). *Refereed.* **Description:** Covers laboratory instrumentation, such as amino acid and blood chemistry analyzers, to labware washers and centrifuges.
Related titles: CD-ROM ed.
Published by: (Emergency Care Research Institute), E C R I, 5200 Butler Pike, Plymouth, PA 19462. TEL 610-825-6000, FAX 610-834-1275, info@ecri.org, http://www.ecri.org. Ed. Nanette Bross.

616 USA ISSN 0894-959X
CLINICAL LABORATORY SCIENCE. Text in English. 1984. bi-m. USD 40 to individuals; USD 60 to institutions; USD 80 foreign (effective 2001). adv. bk.rev. back issues avail. **Document type:** *Academic/Scholarly.* **Description:** Written for all clinical laboratory professionals, including senior management, mid-level supervisors, and staff technologists and technicians. Editorial is based on the common body of knowledge that unites all clinical laboratory scientists, and articles cover all subspecialties of medical technology.
Formerly (until 1988): Journal of Medical Technology (0741-5397); Which was formed by the 1984 merger of part of: American Medical Technologists. Journal (0002-9963); Which was formerly (until 1966): American Medical Technologists. Official Journal (0092-6485); (1940-1959): American Medical Technologists. Journal (0360-0645); and (1977-1984): American Journal of Medical Technology (0148-8759); Which was formerly: Medical Technology (0146-8596); (1936-1977): American Journal of Medical Technology (0002-9335)
Related titles: Microform ed.: (from PQC); Online - full text ed.: (from Northern Light Technology, Inc., ProQuest Information & Learning).
Indexed: CINAHL, Ind.Vet., Rev.Med.& Vet.Mycol.
—BLDSC (3286.295880), CISTI, EMDOCS, GNLM, ingenta.
Published by: American Society for Clinical Laboratory Science, 7910 Woodmont Ave, Ste 530, Bethesda, MD 20814-3015. TEL 301-657-2768, FAX 301-657-2909, ascls@ascls.org, http://www.ascls.org/. Ed. Marian Schwaubauer. R&P Elissa Passiment. Adv. contact Larry Lothridge. Circ: 22,000.

616 658 USA ISSN 1527-3954
CLINICAL LEADERSHIP & MANAGEMENT REVIEW. Text in English. 1985. bi-m. USD 124 domestic to individuals; USD 184 foreign to individuals; USD 170 domestic to institutions; USD 230 foreign to institutions; USD 37 newsstand/cover (effective 2002). adv. *Refereed.* **Document type:** *Journal, Academic/Scholarly.* **Description:** Geared toward the clinical laboratory professional. Includes general management, federal regulations, and general health care issues.
Formerly: Clinical Laboratory Management Review (0888-7950)
Related titles: Microform ed.: (from WWS); Online - full text ed.: (from Institute for Scientific Information).
Indexed: CINAHL, Ind.Med. (coverage dropped), Int.Nurs.Ind.
—BLDSC (3286.295870), EMDOCS, GNLM, IDS.
Published by: (Clinical Laboratory Management Association), Williams & Wilkins (Subsidiary of: Waverly International), 351 W Camden St, Baltimore, MD 21201-2436. TEL 410-528-4068, 800-222-3790, FAX 410-528-4452, cbrooks@wwilkins.com, http://www.wwilkins.com, http://www.Lww.com. Ed. David Wilkinson. R&P Patricia Bergbauer. Adv. contact Carol Brooks. B&W page USD 1,015; trim 10.88 x 8.13. Circ: 8,870 (paid).

CLINICAL RESEARCH RESOURCES DIRECTORY. see *MEDICAL SCIENCES—Abstracting, Bibliographies, Statistics*

619 USA ISSN 0272-2712
RB37.A1 CODEN: CLMED6
CLINICS IN LABORATORY MEDICINE. Text in English. 1981. q. USD 131 domestic to individuals; USD 152 in Canada to individuals; USD 178 elsewhere to individuals; USD 179 domestic to institutions; USD 219 foreign to institutions; USD 55 per issue (effective 2001). *Refereed.* **Document type:** *Journal, Academic/Scholarly.* **Description:** Delivers practical advice from experts in specialty covered as well as information on new developments in a variety of specialties with a fresh perspective on problems and controversies.
Related titles: Microform ed.: (from PQC); Online - full text ed.: (from Institute for Scientific Information).
Indexed: ASCA, CINAHL, Curr.Adv.Ecol.Sci., Curr.Cont., Dok.Arbeitsmed., Excerp.Med., Ind.Med. (1981-), Inpharma, Pharm.&Out.News, Reac., SSCI (coverage dropped).
—BLDSC (3286.575000), CISTI, EMDOCS, GNLM, IDS, ingenta, KNAW. **CCC.**
Published by: W.B. Saunders Co. (Subsidiary of: Harcourt Publishers Ltd.), 11830 Westline Industrial Dr, St Louis, MO 63146. TEL 800-325-4177, http://www.wbsaunders.com. **Subscr. to:** Periodicals Fulfillment, W B Saunders Co, 6277 Sea Harbor Dr, 4th Fl, Orlando, FL 32891-4800.

COMPARATIVE MEDICINE (MEMPHIS). see *BIOLOGY—Zoology*

COMPARATIVE MEDICINE RESEARCH RESOURCES. see *MEDICAL SCIENCES—Abstracting, Bibliographies, Statistics*

616 USA ISSN 1060-0558
CONTEMPORARY TOPICS IN LABORATORY ANIMAL SCIENCE. Text in English. 1961. 6/yr. USD 150 domestic; USD 165 in Canada & Mexico (effective 2001). adv. back issues avail. *Refereed.* **Document type:** *Academic/Scholarly.* **Description:** Contains clinical, technical, managerial, and philosophical articles.
Formerly (until Dec. 1991): A A L A S Bulletin (1056-1471)
Media: Duplicated (not offset). **Related titles:** Online - full text ed.: (from Institute for Scientific Information).
Indexed: ASCA, Agricola, Anim.Breed.Abstr., Aqua.Sci.& Fish.Abstr., Curr.Cont., Focus on: Vet.Sci.& Med., Ind.Med., Ind.Vet., Nutr.Abstr., Pig News & Info., Rev.Appl.Entomol., Rev.Med.& Vet.Mycol., Vet.Bull.
—BLDSC (0537.309200), IDS.
Published by: American Association for Laboratory Animal Science, 9190 Crestwyn Hills Drive, Memphis, TN 38125. TEL 901-754-8620, FAX 901-753-0046, info@aalas.org, http://www.aalas.org. R&P Chris Lyons. Circ: 3,000.

619 USA ISSN 0197-2456
R850.A1 CODEN: CCLTDH
CONTROLLED CLINICAL TRIALS; design, methods, and analysis. Text in English. 1979. 6/yr. EUR 255 in Europe to individuals; JPY 33,800 in Japan to individuals; USD 255 elsewhere to individuals; EUR 519 in Europe to institutions; JPY 68,900 in Japan to institutions; USD 581 elsewhere to institutions (effective 2002). Supplement avail.; back issues avail. *Refereed.* **Document type:** *Academic/Scholarly.* **Description:** Provides current information on the design, methods, and operational aspects of controlled clinical trials and follow-up studies.
Related titles: Microform ed.: (from PQC); Online - full text ed.: (from ingenta, Swets Blackwell, ScienceDirect, Institute for Scientific Information).
Indexed: ASCA, Abstr.Hyg., Agri.& Environ.Biotech.Abstr. (coverage dropped), Behav.Med.Abstr., Biol.Abstr., Biostat., Curr.Adv.Ecol.Sci., Curr.Cont., Curr.Ind.Stat., Derwent Biotech.Abstr., Diar.Dis.Res., Environ.Sci.Poll.Mgmt., Excerp.Med., I.P.A., Ind.Med. (1980-), Ind.Sci.Rev., Inpharma, Int.Abstr.Biol.Sci., Int.Nurs.Ind., Nutr.Abstr., Oper.Res.Manage.Sci., Pharm.&Out.News, Pollut.Abstr., Qual.Contr.Appl.Stat., Reac., Risk Abstr., Saf.Sci.Abstr., Sci.Cit.Ind., THA.
—BLDSC (3463.060000), ADONIS, CASDDS, CISTI, EMDOCS, GNLM, IDS, ingenta, KNAW. **CCC.**

M

Published by: (Society for Clinical Trials), Elsevier Science, 655 Ave of the Americas, New York, NY 10010. TEL 212-989-5800, FAX 212-633-3990, usinfo-f@elsevier.com, http://www.elsevier.com/locate/conclintrial. Ed. Janet Wittes. **Subscr. in Australasia and the Far East to:** Elsevier Science (Singapore) Pte Ltd, No.1 Temasek Ave, 17-01 Millenia Tower, Singapore 039192, Singapore. TEL 65-434-3727, FAX 65-337-2230; **Subscr. in Japan to:** Elsevier Science Inc - Japan Regional Office, 9-15 Higashi-Azabu 1-chome, Minato-ku, Tokyo 106-0044, Japan. TEL 81-3-5561-5033; **Subscr. outside the Americas to:** Elsevier Science BV, PO Box 211, Amsterdam 1000 AE, Netherlands. TEL 31-20-485-3757.

619 USA ISSN 1054-4305
RA624
CRYONICS. Text in English. 1981. q. USD 15; USD 20 in Canada & Mexico; USD 25 elsewhere. adv. bk.rev. **Document type:** *Academic/Scholarly.* **Description:** Covers the new medical and legal developments of the cryonics movement.
Published by: Alcor Life Extension Foundation, 7895 E Acoma Dr, Ste 110, Scottsdale, AZ 85260-6916. TEL 602-922-9013, FAX 602-922-9027, info@alcor.org, http://www.webcom.com/~alcor. Ed., Adv. contact Ralph Whelan. R&P Stephen W Bridge. Circ: 925 (paid).

619 USA ISSN 0892-5798
CURRENT COMMENTS; the newsletter of discovery and innovation. Text in English. 1986. 10/yr. USD 145. **Description:** Emerging research and innovation in life sciences.
Indexed: ABC.
Published by: Chocorua Group, PO Box 193, Woodstock, CT 06281. TEL 203-928-3692. Ed. Thompson E Upham.

619 AUT ISSN 1563-311X
▼ **CURRENT OPINION IN CLINICAL EXPERIMENTAL RESEARCH.** Text in English. 1999. q. USD 75 domestic; USD 115 foreign; USD 35 newsstand/cover (effective 2001). adv. back issues avail. *Refereed.* **Document type:** *Journal, Academic/Scholarly.* **Description:** Provides comprehensive coverage of current clinical and experimental research from a multidisciplinary vierw.
Related titles: Online - full text ed.: ISSN 1606-0180.
Published by: V I C E R Publishing, PO Box 14, Vienna A-1097, Austria. TEL 43-676-9568085, FAX 43-676-9568086, vicer@vicer.org, http://www.vicer.org/clinexpres1.html. Ed., R&P Roland Hofbauer. adv.: B&W page USD 1,700, color page USD 2,200. Circ: 1,000 (paid and controlled).

D.L.A.N.Y. NEWSLETTER. see *MEDICAL SCIENCES—Dentistry*

DECHEMA MONOGRAPHIEN. see *CHEMISTRY—Analytical Chemistry*

DEVICES & DIAGNOSTICS LETTER. see *INSTRUMENTS*

DIABETOLOGIA CROATICA. see *MEDICAL SCIENCES—Endocrinology*

DIABETOLOGIA CROATICA. SUPPLEMENT. see *MEDICAL SCIENCES—Endocrinology*

616 CHE ISSN 1070-3608
CODEN: DTENER
DIAGNOSTIC AND THERAPEUTIC ENDOSCOPY. Text in English. 1994. 4/yr. EUR 294 to institutions; EUR 465 to corporations; USD 106 to individuals (effective 2001). back issues avail. *Refereed.* **Document type:** *Journal, Academic/Scholarly.* **Description:** Reports on preclinical and clinical research on all applications of endoscopy.
Related titles: CD-ROM ed.; Online - full text ed.: (from EBSCO Publishing, RoweCom Information Quest).
Indexed: Excerp.Med. (1995-).
—GNLM, KNAW.
Published by: Gordon and Breach - Harwood Academic (Subsidiary of: Taylor & Francis Group), PO Box 531, Lausanne 1000, Switzerland. TEL 41-21-6411280, FAX 41-21-6411281, info@gbhap.com, http://www.gbhap.com/Diagnostic_Therapeutic_Endoscopy/. Ed. Harubuni Kato. **Subscr. addr. in US:** International Publishers Direct, PO Box 32160, Newark, NJ 07102. FAX 215-750-6343.

DIAGNOSTYKA LABORATORYJNA. see *MEDICAL SCIENCES*

619 USA
DIRECTORY OF FEDERAL LABORATORY TECHNOLOGIES AND RESOURCES. Text in English. biennial. USD 600 in North America; USD 900 elsewhere (effective 1999). **Document type:** *Directory.* **Description:** Includes detailed summaries of over 1,100 resources and descriptions of over 90 technical information centers.
Published by: U.S. National Technical Information Service, 5285 Port Royal Rd, Springfield, VA 22161. TEL 703-605-6060, FAX 703-650-6880. Ed. Ed Lehmann.

616 FRA ISSN 0183-0856
▼ **DROIT & DISPOSITIFS MEDICAUX ACTUALITES.** Text in French. 1999. 11/yr. EUR 406.28 (effective 2001). **Document type:** *Journal, Trade.* **Description:** Contains comprehensive technical, economic and regulatory information on medical devices.
Published by: Droit & Pharmacie, 12 rue de Lorraine, Levallois-Perret Cedex 92309, France. TEL 33-1-55-46-91-00, FAX 33-1-55-46-91-01, info@droit-et-pharmacie.fr, http://www.droit-et-pharmacie.fr.

619 USA
DRUG AND DEVICE PRODUCT APPROVAL LIST. Text in English. m. USD 150 in North America; USD 300 elsewhere. **Document type:** *Government.* **Description:** Lists the most recent new drug approvals, new animal and drug devices, and licenses issued for biological products.
Published by: U.S. Food and Drug Administration, Office of Public Affairs, 5600 Fishers Ln, Rockville, MD 20857. TEL 301-443-3220. **Orders to:** National Technical Information Service, Government Research Center. FAX 703-321-8547.

DRUG TARGETING. see *PHARMACY AND PHARMACOLOGY—Abstracting, Bibliographies, Statistics*

619 EGY ISSN 1012-5558
CODEN: EJBEDR
EGYPTIAN JOURNAL OF BIOMEDICAL ENGINEERING. Text in English; Summaries in Arabic, English. 1980. a. USD 42 (effective 2000). charts, illus. reprint service avail. from IRC. **Document type:** *Academic/Scholarly.*
Indexed: INSPEC (1982-1992, dropped), Ind.Vet.
—CISTI.
Published by: (Egyptian Society of Biomedical Engineering, Research Department), National Information and Documentation Centre (NIDOC), Tahrir St., Dokki, Awqaf P.O., Cairo, Egypt. TEL 20-2-3371696. Ed. M I El Gouhary. Circ: 1,000.

619 JPN ISSN 0915-5422
EIJU SOGO BYOIN KIYO/EIJU GENERAL HOSPITAL. JOURNAL. Text in Japanese. 1989. a.
Published by: Raifu Ekusutenshon Kenkyujo/Research Institute for Life Extension, 11-7 Motoasakusa 2-chome, Taito-ku, Tokyo 111-0041, Japan.

EKSPERIMENTAL'NAYA ONKOLOGIYA/EXPERIMENTAL ONCOLOGY; nauchno-tekhnicheskii zhurnal. see *MEDICAL SCIENCES—Oncology*

ELECTRON MICROSCOPY IN BIOLOGY AND MEDICINE. see *BIOLOGY—Microscopy*

619 340 USA ISSN 1070-2504
ENVIRONMENTAL LABORATORY WASHINGTON REPORT. Text in English. 1990. bi-w. USD 349 (effective 1999). index. back issues avail. **Document type:** *Newsletter.* **Description:** Reports on regulations of environmental testing written exclusively for lab managers, directors and quality assurance professionals. Covers federal regulations as well as consumers and insurance groups.
Formerly: Laboratory Regulation News (1048-0706)
Related titles: Online - full text ed.: (from LexisNexis).
—CCC.
Published by: L R P Publications, 747 Dresher Rd, Box 980, Horsham, PA 19044. TEL 215-784-0941, 800-341-7874, FAX 215-784-9014, custserve@lrp.com, http://www.lrp.com. Ed. Carrie Trutwin.

619 179 AUT ISSN 0948-5155
ERSATZ- UND ERGAENZUNGSMETHODEN ZU TIERVERSUCHEN. Text in German. 1993. irreg. price varies. **Document type:** *Monographic series, Academic/Scholarly.*
Published by: Springer-Verlag Wien (Subsidiary of: BertelsmannSpringer), Sachsenplatz 4-6, PO Box 89, Vienna, W 1201, Austria. TEL 43-1-3302415-0, FAX 43-1-330242665, books@springer.at, http://www.springer.at. Eds. H A Tritthart, H Schoeffl, H Spielmann. R&P Angela Foessl TEL 43-1-3302415517. **Dist. in N. America by:** Springer-Verlag, Journals. books@springer.at.

619 USA ISSN 0888-7128
EUROPEAN CLINICAL LABORATORY. Text in English. 1982. 7/yr. USD 162; USD 147 foreign. bk.rev. charts, illus, stat, tr.lit. **Document type:** *Trade.*
Formerly: International Clinical Products Review
Related titles: Special ed.: European Clinical Laboratory. Buyers' Guide.
Indexed: ABC, Anal.Abstr., Lab.Haz.Bull.
—BLDSC (3829.606800), GNLM.
Published by: International Scientific Communications, Inc., 30 Controls Dr, Box 870, Shelton, CT 06484-0870. TEL 203-926-9300, FAX 203-926-9310, iscpubs@iscpubs.com, http://www.iscpubs.com. Ed. Brian Howard. Pub. William Wham. adv.: B&W page USD 5,085, color page USD 6,455. Circ: 32,801 (controlled). **U.K. subscr. to:** I.S.C. House, Progress Business Centre, Whittle Parkway, 5 Whittle Pkwy, Slough, Berks SL1 6DQ, United Kingdom. TEL 44-1628-669199, 44-1628-668881.

616 ITA ISSN 1122-8652
CODEN: EJLAEW
EUROPEAN JOURNAL OF LABORATORY MEDICINE. Text in English. 1987. 6/yr. USD 100 (effective 1997). **Document type:** *Academic/Scholarly.*
Formerly (until 1993): Progressi in Medicina di Laboratorio (1120-995X)
Indexed: Chem.Abstr., Chem.Indus.Notes, Chem.Titles, Excerp.Med. (1994-), Int.Abstr.Biol.Sci.
—BLDSC (3829.730950), CASDDS, GNLM.
Published by: T H Editing, Via Cristoforo Colombo, 63, Turin, TO 10129, Italy. TEL 39-11-500497.

EXCERPTA MEDICA. SECTION 29: CLINICAL AND EXPERIMENTAL BIOCHEMISTRY. see *BIOLOGY—Abstracting, Bibliographies, Statistics*

619 JPN ISSN 1341-1357
CODEN: JIDOAA
EXPERIMENTAL ANIMALS. Text in English, Japanese; Summaries in English. 1952. q. JPY 3,000 newsstand/cover (effective 2000). adv. bk.rev. charts, illus. cum.index. *Refereed.* **Document type:** *Academic/Scholarly.*
Formerly (until 1995): Jikken Dobutsu (0007-5124)
Related titles: Online - full text ed.: (from Institute for Scientific Information).
Indexed: ASCA, AgBiotech, Anim.Breed.Abstr., Biol.Abstr., Chem.Abstr., Chem.Indus.Notes, Chem.Titles, Curr.Adv.Ecol.Sci., Curr.Cont., Dairy Sci.Abstr., Dent.Ind., Excerp.Med., Focus on: Vet.Sci.& Med., Helminthol.Abstr., Ind.Med. (1995-), Ind.Vet., Nutr.Abstr., Pig News & Info., Poult.Abstr., Rev.Arom.& Med.Plants, Rev.Med.& Vet.Mycol., Small Anim.Abstr., Vet.Bull., Zoo.Rec.
—BLDSC (3838.730000), CASDDS, CISTI, GNLM, IDS, Infotrieve, KNAW, Linda Hall. **CCC.**
Published by: Japanese Association for Laboratory Animal Science/Nihon Jikken Dobutsu Gakkai, Akamon Royal Heights, Rm 1103, 5-29-12 Hongo, Bunkyo-ku, Tokyo 113-0033, Japan. TEL 81-3-3814-8276, FAX 81-3-3814-3990, http://www.jalas.or.jp/. Ed. Yasuhiro Yoshikawa. Circ: 2,300.

EXPERIMENTAL BIOLOGY AND MEDICINE (MAYWOOD). see *BIOLOGY*

619 572 USA
EXPERIMENTAL BIOLOGY AND MEDICINE (TOTOWA). Text in English. 1980. irreg., latest vol.28, 1997. price varies. illus. back issues avail. *Refereed.* **Document type:** *Monographic series, Academic/Scholarly.* **Description:** Publishes research on the ways new pharmacologic compounds affect the human biochemical makeup.
Published by: Humana Press Inc., 999 Riverview Dr, Ste 208, Totowa, NJ 07512. TEL 973-256-1699, FAX 973-256-8341, humana@humanapr.com, http://humanapress.com. R&P Richard Hruska.

619 DEU ISSN 0936-0506
FIBRINOLYSE. Text in German. q. DEM 48 in Europe; USD 40 elsewhere (effective 2001). **Document type:** *Journal, Academic/Scholarly.*

M

Published by: Schattauer GmbH, Hoelderlinstr 3, Stuttgart 70174, Germany. TEL 49-711-22987-0, FAX 49-711-2298750, info@schattauer.de, http://www.schattauer.com. R&P Annika Schmidt TEL 49-711-2298713. **Subscr. to:** CSJ, Postfach 140220, Munich 80452, Germany. TEL 49-89-20959129, schattauer@csj.de.

619 GBR ISSN 1369-0191 CODEN: FBRIE7
FIBRINOLYSIS & PROTEOLYSIS. Text in English. 1987. bi-m. GBP 380 to institutions; USD 585 in North America (effective 2001). adv. *Refereed.* **Document type:** *Academic/Scholarly.* **Description:** Covers molecular biology of fibrinolysis and clinical trials of thrombolytic agents.
Former titles (until 1997): Fibrinolysis (0268-9499); Journal of Fibrinolysis
Related titles: Online - full text ed.: (from EBSCO Publishing, O C L C Online Computer Library Center, Inc., Swets Blackwell, IDEAL Online Library, Institute for Scientific Information).
Indexed: ASCA, Curr.Cont., Ind.Sci.Rev., Inpharma, Int.Abstr.Biol.Sci., Pharm.&Out.News, Reac., Ref.Zh., Sci.Cit.Ind.
—BLDSC (3918.119000), ADONIS, CASDDS, CISTI, EMDOCS, GNLM, IDS, Infotrieve, KNAW. **CCC.**
Published by: (International Society for Fibrinolysis and Thrombosis), Churchill Livingstone (Subsidiary of: Harcourt Publishers Ltd.), Robert Stevenson House, 1-3 Baxter's Pl, Leith Walk, Edinburgh, Midlothian EH1 3AF, United Kingdom. TEL 44-131-556-2424, FAX 44-131-459-1177, cservice@harcourt.com, http://www.harcourt-international.com/journals/fipr. Eds. D C Rijken, J H Verheijen. Adv. contact David Dunnachie. Circ: 650. **Subscr. to:** Harcourt Publishers Ltd., Foots Cray High St, Sidcup, Kent DA14 5HP, United Kingdom. TEL 44-20-8308-5700, FAX 44-20-8309-0807.

619 PRT ISSN 0374-7638 CODEN: FAUCAR
FOLIA ANATOMICA UNIVERSITATIS CONIMBRICENSIS. Text in English, French, Portuguese. 1926. a. free per issue or exchange basis. bibl, illus. index.
Indexed: Biol.Abstr.
Published by: Imprensa de Coimbra Ltd., Largo de S. Salvador, Coimbra 3000, Portugal. Ed. A Simoes de Carvalho.

619 ITA ISSN 1121-8142 CODEN: FTCME
FORUM: TRENDS IN EXPERIMENTAL AND CLINICAL MEDICINE. Key Title: Forum (Genova). Text in English. 1991. q. ITL 180,000 domestic; USD 180 foreign (effective 2000). adv. bibl, charts, illus. back issues avail.; reprints avail. *Refereed.* **Document type:** *Journal, Academic/Scholarly.* **Description:** Reviews scientific articles for medical staff and researchers.
Related titles: Online - full text ed.
Indexed: Excerp.Med. (1993-), Ind.Med. (1991-).
—BLDSC (4024.117000), EMDOCS, GNLM, KNAW.
Published by: Scuola Internazionale di Oncologia e Medicina Sperimentale, Piazza Della Vittoria, 15-1, Genoa, GE 16121, Italy. TEL 39-10-5458612, FAX 39-10-5450056, forum@accmed.net, journal@accmed.net, http://www.accmed.net. Ed. Luigi Frati. R&P Remy Adatia TEL 39-10-5458621. adv.: B&W page ITL 2,355, color page ITL 3,090; trim 204 x 275. Circ: 3,000.

FUJIAN ZHONGYI YAO/FUJIAN JOURNAL OF TRADITIONAL CHINESE MEDICINE. see *ALTERNATIVE MEDICINE*

616 DEU ISSN 0016-3538 CODEN: GITEAR
G I T; Fachzeitschrift fuer das Laboratorium. Summaries in English, German. 1957. m. DEM 176 (effective 1999). adv. bk.rev. charts, illus, pat, tr.lit. index. **Document type:** *Trade.*
Indexed: Anal.Abstr., CEABA, Chem.Abstr., Dok.Arbeitsmed., Excerp.Med., INIS Atomind., Mass Spectr.Bull., Sugar Ind.Abstr.
—CASDDS, CISTI, Infotrieve, Linda Hall. **CCC.**
Published by: G I T Verlag GmbH, Roesslerstr 90, Darmstadt 64293, Germany. TEL 49-6151-8090-0, FAX 49-6151-8090144, gitverlaggmbh@gitverlag.com, http://www.gitverlag.com. Ed. Ernst Giebeler. Adv. contact Hubert Schulz TEL 49-6151-8090116. B&W page DEM 9,230, color page DEM 12,545; trim 260 x 185. Circ: 25,000.

G I T LABORATORY JOURNAL. see *MEDICAL SCIENCES*

619 616.9 USA
GAY MEN'S HEALTH CRISIS. Text in English. 1989. a. USD 30. **Document type:** *Newsletter.* **Description:** Devoted to providing reliable information on experimental therapies for people living with AIDS and HIV infections.
Related titles: Online - full text ed.
Published by: (Gay Men's Health Crisis), G M H C, Inc., 129 W 20th St, 2nd Fl, New York, NY 10011-0022. TEL 212-367-1000, FAX 212-337-3656, http://www.thebody.com/gmhc/gmhcix.html. Circ: 30,000.

616 USA
GUIDE FOR THE CARE AND USE OF LABORATORY ANIMALS. Text in English. 1963. irreg. free per issue. **Document type:** *Government.* **Description:** Contains guidelines to assist institutions in appropriately caring for and using laboratory research animals.
Formerly (until 1985): Guide for Laboratory Animal Facilities and Care (0072-8098)
Published by: (National Research Council), National Academy of Sciences, 2101 Constitution Ave, Washington, DC 20418. **Subscr. to:** National Academy Press, 2101 Constitution Ave, N W, Washington, DC 20418. TEL 202-334-3313, FAX 202-334-2451.

610 GUY
GUYANA ASSOCIATION OF MEDICAL TECHNOLOGISTS. NEWSLETTER. Text in English. s-a.
Published by: Guyana Association of Medical Technologists, c/o Central Medical Laboratory, Public Hospital, Middle St., Georgetown, Guyana.

619 USA ISSN 0887-3712
H L B NEWSLETTER; reporting on heart, lung and blood disease research policy development. Text in English. 1985. 24/yr. USD 325; USD 375 foreign (effective 2000). bk.rev. charts. back issues avail. **Document type:** *Newsletter.* **Description:** Researches policy development in heart, lungs and blood.
Related titles: E-mail ed.; Fax ed.
Published by: British Trading Company, 860 N DeWitt Pl, no 1704, Chicago, IL 60611. TEL 312-932-0166, FAX 312-640-0339, adonatan02@m8.sprynet.com. Ed., Pub. Natan Polster. R&P Gerlinde Kubitz.

HAYASTANI BZHSHKAGITUTYUN/ARMENIAN MEDICAL JOURNAL/MEDITSINSKAYA NAUKA ARMENII. see *MEDICAL SCIENCES*

HOOFDLIJNEN. see *MEDICAL SCIENCES—Psychiatry And Neurology*

381.45681761 SGP ISSN 0218-9542
HOSPITAL PRODUCTS ASIA. Text in English. 1996. bi-m. USD 210. **Document type:** *Trade.* **Description:** Offers news and product coverage for hospital and healthcare administrators and professionals in the Asia-Pacific region.
Published by: First Asia Publishing Pte. Ltd., 6 New Industrial Rd 02-02-04, Singapore 536199, Singapore. TEL 65-858-0040, FAX 65-858-1141, jovankahuer@firstasia.com.sg.

616 DNK ISSN 0900-3630
HOSPITALSLABORANTEN* . Text in Danish. fortn. adv.
Formerly (until 1984): Nyt for Hospitalslaboranter (0029-683X)
Published by: Landssammenslutningen af Hospitalslaboranter/Danish Association of Medical Laboratory Technologists, Noerre Voldgade 90, Copenhagen K 1358, Denmark. Circ: 4,500.

619 USA ISSN 0885-0615
R853.H8
HUMAN RESEARCH REPORT; protecting researchers and research subjects. Text in English. 1986. m. USD 264 domestic; USD 285 in Canada & Mexico; USD 264 elsewhere (effective 2002). 16 p./no. back issues avail. **Document type:** *Newsletter.* **Description:** Contains notices and explanations of research regulations, ethics, laws, lawsuits and case studies of government investigation of biomedical and behavioral research institutions.
Published by: Deem Corporation, PO Box 44069, Omaha, NE 68144-0069. TEL 402-895-5748, 800-786-5748, FAX 402-895-2306, dennis@humansubjects.com, den@deemcorp.com, http://www.humansubjects.com, http://www.deemcorp.com. Ed., R&P Dennis M Maloney.

I E E E BIOMEDICAL ENGINEERING DAYS. see *BIOLOGY—Biotechnology*

I L A R JOURNAL. see *BIOLOGY—Zoology*

619 USA ISSN 0193-7758
I R B: A REVIEW OF HUMAN SUBJECTS RESEARCH. (Institutional Review Board) Text in English. 1979. bi-m. USD 48 to individuals; USD 70 to libraries; USD 320 to institutions (effective 2000). bk.rev. bibl. back issues avail. **Document type:** *Journal, Academic/Scholarly.*
Indexed: Ind.Per.Art.Relat.Law, PsycInfo, Psychol.Abstr. (1984-), e-psyche.
—BLDSC (4567.631000), ingenta.
Published by: Hastings Center, Rte 9D, Garrison, NY 10524. TEL 914-424-4040, FAX 914-424-4545. Ed. Robert J Levine. R&P Bette Crigger. Circ: 5,000.

619 USA ISSN 1079-7823
THE IMMORTALIST. Text in English. 1970. m. USD 25 domestic; USD 50 foreign; USD 2.50 newsstand/cover domestic (effective 2000). bk.rev. **Document type:** *Newsletter.* **Description:** Contains news, information, conjecture, and opinion related to cryonics and life extension.
Formerly: Outlook
Published by: Immortalist Society, 24355 Sorrentino Ct, Clinton, MI 48035. TEL 810-791-5961, FAX 810-791-5961, cryonics@cryonics.org; cryonics@jps.net, http://www.cryonics.org; http://www.jps.net/cryonics. Ed., R&P John Bull. Circ: 420. **Co-sponsor:** American Cryonics Society.

619 GRC ISSN 0258-851X CODEN: IVIVE4
IN VIVO; international journal of in vivo research. Text in English. 1987. bi-m. USD 395 to individuals; USD 630 to institutions; USD 105 per issue (effective 2002). index. back issues avail. *Refereed.* **Document type:** *Journal, Academic/Scholarly.* **Description:** Takes a multidisciplinary approach to the study of biomedical research involving experimental systems. Covers oncology, chemotherapy, pharmacology, immunology, radiology, toxicology, genetics, cytology, endocrinology biotechnology, comparative pathology, and nutrition.
Related titles: Online - full text ed.: (from Institute for Scientific Information).
Indexed: ASCA, BBCI, Biol.Abstr., Biol.Dig., Chem.Abstr., Chem.Indus.Notes, Chem.Titles, Excerp.Med., Ind.Med. (1987-), Inpharma, Int.Abstr.Biol.Sci., Neurosci.Abstr. (coverage dropped), Pharm.&Out.News, Reac.
—BLDSC (4372.507000), CASDDS, CISTI, EMDOCS, GNLM, IDS, Infotrieve, KNAW. **CCC.**
Published by: International Institute of Anticancer Research, Kapandritiou Kalamou Rd, km 1, PO Box 22, Kapandriti, Attiki 190 14, Greece. TEL 30-295-52945, FAX 30-295-53389, journals@iiar-anticancer.org, http://www.iiar-anticancer.org. R&P John G Delinassios. Circ: 520.

570 FRA ISSN 0989-8735
INFORMATION DU TECHNICIEN BIOLOGISTE* . Text in French. 4/yr. FRF 318; FRF 428 foreign. **Document type:** *Academic/Scholarly.*
Published by: Doin Editeurs, 26 av. de l'Europe, B.P. 60, Velizy Cedex 78141, France. TEL 1-45481210, FAX 1-45444331.

INSTITUTION OF CHEMISTS (INDIA). JOURNAL. see *CHEMISTRY*

INSTITUTION OF CHEMISTS (INDIA). PROCEEDINGS. see *CHEMISTRY*

INSTRUMENTATION SCIENCE & TECHNOLOGY. see *CHEMISTRY—Analytical Chemistry*

INTERNATIONAL BIOTECHNOLOGY LABORATORY. see *BIOLOGY—Biotechnology*

INTERNATIONAL JOURNAL OF ARTIFICIAL ORGANS. see *MEDICAL SCIENCES*

INTERNATIONAL JOURNAL OF COSMETIC SCIENCE. see *BEAUTY CULTURE—Perfumes And Cosmetics*

619 GBR ISSN 0266-4623
R855
INTERNATIONAL JOURNAL OF TECHNOLOGY ASSESSMENT IN HEALTH CARE. Text in English. 1985. q. GBP 124 to individuals; USD 218 to institutions (effective 2002). adv. bk.rev. back issues avail.; reprint service avail. from SWZ. *Refereed.* **Document type:** *Academic/Scholarly.* **Description:** Forum for professionals interested in the assessment of medical technology, its consequences for patients and its impact on society.
Related titles: Microform ed.: (from PQC); Online - full text ed.: (from Swets Blackwell, Institute for Scientific Information).

M

Indexed: ASCA, Abstr.Health Care Manage.Stud., AgeLine, Curr.Cont., EEA, Environ.Sci.Poll.Mgmt., Excerp.Med., Human Resour.Abstr., Ind.Med. (1985-), Inpharma, Int.Nurs.Ind., Lang.& Lang.Behav.Abstr., Pharm.&Out.News, Pollut.Abstr., Reac., Risk Abstr., SOPODA, Saf.Sci.Abstr., Sci.Cit.Ind., Sociol.Abstr.
—BLDSC (4542.693300), CISTI, EMDOCS, GNLM, IDS, ingenta, KNAW. **CCC.**
Published by: Cambridge University Press, Edinburgh Bldg, Shaftesbury Rd, Cambridge CB2 2RU, United Kingdom. FAX 44-1223-315052, information@cup.cam.ac.uk, information@cambridge.org, http://www.cup.cam.ac.uk, http://www.uk.cambridge.org/journals/pmu. Eds. Egon Jonsson, Stanley J Reiser. R&P Linda Nicol. Adv. contact Rebecca Symons.

616 542 GBR ISSN 0143-5140
INTERNATIONAL LABMATE. Text in English. 1976. 7/yr. GBP 65, USD 105 (effective 2000). adv. stat, tr.lit. back issues avail. **Document type:** *Trade.* **Description:** Presents the latest in laboratory equipment and chemicals.
Indexed: Anal.Abstr., CEABA, INIS Atomind., Ref.Zh., World Surf.Coat.
—BLDSC (4542.702850).
Published by: International Labmate Ltd., 12 Alban Park, Hatfield Rd, St Albans, Herts AL4 0JJ, United Kingdom. TEL 44-1727-855574, FAX 44-1727-841694. Ed. Michael H Pattison. Adv. contact Russell Purvis. Circ: 41,935.

J E O L NEWS: ANALYTICAL INSTRUMENTATION. see *INSTRUMENTS*

J E O L NEWS: ELECTRON OPTICS INSTRUMENTATION. see *INSTRUMENTS*

619 JPN ISSN 0021-4965
JAPANESE JOURNAL OF CLINICAL AND EXPERIMENTAL MEDICINE/RINSHO TO KENKYU. Text in English, Japanese. 1924. m. JPY 11,760, USD 40. **Description:** Covers clinical and experimental medicine.
Indexed: Biol.Abstr., INIS Atomind.
—GNLM.
Published by: Daido Gakkan Shuppan-bu, Kyushu University Medical School, 3576 Hakozaki, Higashi-ku, Fukuoka-shi 812-0053, Japan.

619 JPN ISSN 0910-7967
CODEN: JICHBJ
JIKKEN CHIRYO/EXPERIMENT & THERAPY. Text in Japanese. 1921. q. JPY 5,100. **Document type:** *Academic/Scholarly.*
—CASDDS.
Published by: Takeda Yakuhin Kogyo K.K./Takeda Chemical Industries, Ltd., 4-1-1 Dosho-Machi, Chuo-ku, Osaka-shi 541-0045, Japan.

JOURNAL OF APPLIED ANIMAL WELFARE SCIENCE. see *ANIMAL WELFARE*

619 USA ISSN 1526-9914
▼ **JOURNAL OF APPLIED CLINICAL MEDICAL PHYSICS.** Text in English. 2000. free. **Description:** Publishes papers that will help clinical medical physicists perform their responsibilities more effectively and efficiently, and for the increased benefit of the patient.
Indexed: C.P.I., INSPEC.
Published by: (American College of Medical Physics), American Institute of Physics, 2 Huntington Quadrangle, Suite 1NO1, Melville, NY 11747-4502. FAX 516-576-2374, subs@aip.org, http://www.acmp.org/acm, http://www.aip.org.

610 619 JPN ISSN 1434-7229
CODEN: JAORFN
JOURNAL OF ARTIFICIAL ORGANS. Text in English. 1998. q. (in 1 vol., 2 nos./vol.). JPY 18,000 domestic; USD 209 in North America; DEM 356 elsewhere; DEM 213, EUR 108.91 in Germany for Print & Online Eds.; DEM 215.40, EUR 110.14 elsewhere for Print & Online Eds. (effective 2001). **Document type:** *Academic/Scholarly.*
Related titles: Online - full text ed.: (from EBSCO Publishing, Springer LINK).
—BLDSC (4947.211920), CASDDS, CISTI, GNLM.
Published by: Springer-Verlag Tokyo, Eastern Book Service, Inc. (Subsidiary of: BertelsmannSpringer), 3-13 Hongo 3-chome, Bunkyo-ku, Tokyo 113-0033, Japan. TEL 81-3-38120331, FAX 81-3-3812-0719, order@svt-ebs.co.jp, http://link.springer-ny.com/link/service/journals/10047/index.htm. Ed. Hikaru Matsuda,. **Subscr. in N. America to:** Springer-Verlag New York Inc., PO Box 2485, Secaucus, NJ 07096-2485. TEL 800-777-4643, 212-460-1526, FAX 201-348-4505, orders@springer-ny.com; **Subscr. outside N. America & Japan to:** Springer-Verlag, c/o Gabriele Kubitza, Haberstrasse 7, Heidelberg 69126, Germany. TEL 49-6221-345242, FAX 49-30-82787448, 49-6221-345229, subscriptions@springer.de, http://link.springer.de, http://link.springer-ny.com; **Subscr. to:** Eastern Book Service, Inc., 3-13 Hongo 3-chome, Bunkyo-ku, Tokyo 113-8480, Japan. TEL 81-3-3818-0861, FAX 81-3-3818-0864, orders@svt-ebs.co.jp.

▼ **JOURNAL OF CANNABIS THERAPEUTICS;** studies in endogenous, herbal, and synthetic cannabinoids. see *ALTERNATIVE MEDICINE*

619 USA ISSN 0887-8013
CODEN: JCANEM
JOURNAL OF CLINICAL LABORATORY ANALYSIS. Text in English. 1987. bi-m. USD 1,125 in United States; USD 1,185 in Canada & Mexico; USD 1,236 elsewhere; USD 1,182 combined subscription in United States for print and online eds.; USD 1,242 combined subscription in Canada & Mexico for print and online eds.; USD 1,293 combined subscription elsewhere for print and online eds. (effective 2002). adv. back issues avail. *Refereed.* **Document type:** *Academic/Scholarly.* **Description:** Includes articles about immunochemistry, toxicology, hematology, immunopathology, microbiology, genetic testing, immunohematology, and clinical chemistry.
Related titles: Microform ed.: (from PQC); Online - full text ed.: ISSN 1098-2825. 1996. USD 1,125 in United States; USD 1,125 in Canada & Mexico; USD 1,125 elsewhere (effective 2002) (from EBSCO Publishing, Wiley InterScience, Institute for Scientific Information).
Indexed: ASCA, Anal.Abstr., Biol.Abstr., Chem.Abstr., Chem.Indus.Notes, Chem.Titles, Curr.Cont., Dairy Sci.Abstr., Environ.Sci.Poll.Mgmt., Food Sci.& Tech.Abstr., INIS Atomind., Ind.Med. (1987-), Ind.Sci.Rev., Inpharma, Nutr.Abstr., Pharm.&Out.News, Pollut.Abstr., Protozool.Abstr., Reac., Rev.Med.& Vet.Mycol., Risk Abstr., Saf.Sci.Abstr., Sci.Cit.Ind., THA.
—BLDSC (4958.520000), CASDDS, CISTI, EMDOCS, GNLM, IDS, ingenta, KNAW. **CCC.**
Published by: John Wiley & Sons, Inc., Journals (Subsidiary of: Wiley InterScience), 605 Third Ave, New York, NY 10158. TEL 212-850-6645, FAX 212-850-6021, subinfo@wiley.com, uscs-wis@wiley.com, http://www.wiley.com. adv.: B&W page GBP 640, color page GBP 1,515; trim 210 x 279. Circ: 550. **Subscr. outside the Americas to:** John Wiley & Sons Ltd., Baffins Ln, Chichester, Sussex PO19 IUD, United Kingdom. TEL 44-1243-779777, FAX 44-1243-843232, cs-journals@wiley.co.uk, http://www.wiley.co.uk.

619 DEU ISSN 0939-8600
CODEN: JEXSEU
JOURNAL OF EXPERIMENTAL ANIMAL SCIENCE. Text in English. 1961. irreg. (4 nos./vol.). EUR 198, GBP 161 (effective 2002). adv. bk.rev. abstr, bibl, charts, illus. index, cum.index. reprint service avail. from ISI. *Refereed.* **Document type:** *Journal, Academic/Scholarly.*
Formerly (until 1991): Zeitschrift fuer Versuchstierkunde (0044-3697)
Related titles: Online - full text ed.: (from Institute for Scientific Information).
Indexed: ASCA, AgBiotech, Agri.& Environ.Biotech.Abstr. (coverage dropped), Anim.Breed.Abstr., Bibl.Agri., Biol.Abstr., Chem.Abstr., Chem.Indus.Notes, Chem.Titles, Curr.Adv.Cancer Res., Curr.Adv.Ecol.Sci., Curr.Adv.Gen.& Molec.Biol., Curr.Cont., Dairy Sci.Abstr., Dent.Ind., Excerp.Med., Focus on: Vet.Sci.& Med., Helminthol.Abstr., INIS Atomind., Ind.Med. (coverage dropped), Ind.Vet., Inpharma, Int.Abstr.Biol.Sci., Nutr.Abstr., Pig News & Info., Protozool.Abstr., Reac., Sci.Cit.Ind. (coverage dropped), Vet.Bull.
—BLDSC (4979.850000), CASDDS, CISTI, EMDOCS, GNLM, IDS, Infotrieve, Linda Hall. **CCC.**
Published by: Urban & Fischer Verlag, Loebdergraben 14A, Jena 07743, Germany. TEL 49-3641-626444, FAX 49-3641-626500, info@urbanfischer.de, http://www.urbanfischer.de/journals. Ed. H J Hedrich. Adv. contact Sabine Schroeter. page DEM 750; trim 200 x 135. Circ: 350.

610 USA ISSN 0022-1007
R11 CODEN: JEMEAV
THE JOURNAL OF EXPERIMENTAL MEDICINE. Text in English. 1896. bi-m. (in 2 vols., 12 nos./vol.), latest vol.194. USD 615 in US & Canada to institutions print ed.; USD 775 elsewhere to institutions print ed.; USD 490 to institutions online ed.; USD 1,105 in US & Canada to institutions print and online ed.; USD 1,265 elsewhere to institutions print and online ed. (effective 2001). adv. charts, illus. 146 p./no. back issues avail.; reprint service avail. from PQC,ISI. *Refereed.* **Document type:** *Journal, Academic/Scholarly.* **Description:** Provides significant research in immunology and experimental medicine.
Related titles: Microform ed.: (from PQC); Online - full text ed.: (from HighWire Pr., EBSCO Publishing, RoweCom Information Quest, Institute for Scientific Information).
Indexed: AIDS & Cancer Res., AIDS Abstr., Abstr.Hyg., AgBiotech, Agri.& Environ.Biotech.Abstr. (coverage dropped), Anim.Breed.Abstr., Aqua.Sci.& Fish.Abstr., Biol.Abstr., Chem.Abstr., Chem.Indus.Notes, Chem.Titles, Curr.Adv.Cancer Res., Curr.Adv.Cell & Devel.Biol., Curr.Adv.Gen.& Molec.Biol., Curr.Cont., Dairy Sci.Abstr., Derwent Biotech.Abstr., Diar.Dis.Res., Excerp.Med., Genet.Abstr., Helminthol.Abstr., Hum.Gen.Abstr., INIS Atomind., Immun.Abstr., Ind.Med. (1896-), Ind.Sci.Rev., Ind.Vet., Inpharma, Int.Abstr.Biol.Sci., Med.& Surg.Dermat., Microbiol.Abstr., Neurosci.Abstr., Neurosci.Cit.Ind., Nuc.Acids Abstr., Nutr.Abstr., Pharm.&Out.News, Poult.Abstr., Protozool.Abstr., Reac., Ref.Zh., Rev.Appl.Entomol., Rev.Med.& Vet.Mycol., Sci.Cit.Ind., Trop.Dis.Bull., Vet.Bull., Virol.Abstr. (coverage dropped).
—BLDSC (4982.000000), CASDDS, CISTI, GNLM, IDS, ingenta, KNAW. **CCC.**
Published by: Rockefeller University Press, 1114 First Ave, New York, NY 10021. TEL 212-327-8522, FAX 212-327-8513, jem@rockefeller.edu, rupress@rockefeller.edu, http://www.jem.org, http://www.rockefeller.edu/rupress. Ed. Philip L. Bernstein. R&P Laura Smith TEL 212-327-8025. Adv. contact Lorna Peterson TEL 212-327-8880. Circ: 2,730.

JOURNAL OF EXPERIMENTAL ZOOLOGY. see *BIOLOGY—Zoology*

JOURNAL OF EXPERIMENTAL ZOOLOGY. SUPPLEMENT. see *BIOLOGY—Zoology*

610 USA ISSN 0022-2143
R13 CODEN: JLCMAK
THE JOURNAL OF LABORATORY AND CLINICAL MEDICINE. Text in English. 1915. m. USD 160 domestic to individuals; USD 196 foreign to individuals; USD 365 domestic to institutions; USD 399 foreign to institutions; USD 80 domestic to students; USD 105 foreign to students; USD 34 newsstand/cover (effective 2001). adv. abstr, bibl, charts, illus. s-a. index. reprint service avail. from PQC. *Refereed.* **Document type:** *Proceedings, Academic/Scholarly.* **Description:** Information on clinical investigation and research with advanced information on hematology, nephrology, organ transplantation, cardiology and immunology.
Related titles: Microfilm ed.: (from PQC,PMC); Online - full text ed.: (from Ovid Technologies, Inc., IDEAL Online Library, Institute for Scientific Information, RoweCom Information Quest).
Indexed: AIM, ASCA, Abstr.Hyg., Agri.& Environ.Biotech.Abstr. (coverage dropped), BBCI, Biol.Abstr., CINAHL, Chem.Abstr., Chem.Titles, Curr.Adv.Biochem., Curr.Adv.Cancer Res., Curr.Adv.Ecol.Sci., Curr.Cont., Dairy Sci.Abstr., Derwent Biotech.Abstr., Diar.Dis.Res., Excerp.Med., Helminthol.Abstr., INIS Atomind., Ind.Med. (1915-), Ind.Sci.Rev., Ind.Vet., Inpharma, Int.Abstr.Biol.Sci., Kidney, Med.& Surg.Dermat., Nutr.Abstr., Pharm.&Out.News, Reac., Rev.Med.& Vet.Mycol., Rev.Plant Path., SSCI (coverage dropped), Sci.Cit.Ind., THA, Telegen, Trop.Dis.Bull., Vet.Bull.
—BLDSC (5010.000000), ADONIS, CASDDS, CISTI, GNLM, IDS, Infotrieve, ingenta, KNAW. **CCC.**
Published by: (Central Society for Clinical Research), Mosby, Inc. (Subsidiary of: Elsevier Science), 11830 Westline Industrial Dr, St Louis, MO 63146-3318. TEL 314-872-8370, 800-325-4177, FAX 314-432-1380, http://www.mosby.com/lab, http://www.mosby.com/periodicals. Ed. Dr. Dale Hammerschmidt. adv.: B&W page USD 795, color page USD 1,645; trim 10.88 x 8.25. Circ: 2,923.

610 JPN ISSN 1343-1420
CODEN: JMIVFL
JOURNAL OF MEDICAL INVESTIGATION. Text in English, Multiple languages. 1954. s-a. per issue exchange basis. adv. charts, illus. back issues avail.; reprints avail. *Refereed.* **Document type:** *Journal, Academic/Scholarly.*

M

Formerly (until 1997, vol.44): Tokushima Journal of Experimental Medicine (0040-8875)
Indexed: Abstr.Hyg., Biol.Abstr., Chem.Abstr., Curr.Adv.Ecol.Sci., Excerp.Med., INIS Atomind., Ind.Med. (1997-), Nutr.Abstr., Trop.Dis.Bull.
—BLDSC (5017.072800), CASDDS, CISTI, GNLM, ingenta, KNAW.
Published by: Tokushima Daigaku, Igakubu/Tokushima University, School of Medicine, 18-15 Kuramoto-cho 3-chome, Tokushima-shi 770-8503, Japan. TEL 81-88-633-7104, FAX 81-88-633-7115, ssone@clin.med.tokushima-u.ac.jp, jmi@basic.med.tokushima-u.ac.jp. R&P, Adv. contact Kazuko Miyamoto.

619 611.01816 USA ISSN 0896-548X
CODEN: JTEMEM
THE JOURNAL OF TRACE ELEMENTS IN EXPERIMENTAL MEDICINE. Text in English. 1988. q. USD 645 in United States; USD 685 in Canada & Mexico; USD 719 elsewhere; USD 678 combined subscription in United States for print and online eds.; USD 718 combined subscription in Canada & Mexico for print and online eds.; USD 752 combined subscription elsewhere for print and online eds. (effective 2002). adv. back issues avail. *Refereed.* **Document type:** *Academic/Scholarly.* **Description:** Focuses on the role of trace elements in human health and disease. Provides special attention to their clinical, nutritional, biochemical, immunological, and toxicological aspects.
Related titles: Microform ed.: (from PQC); Online - full text ed.: ISSN 1520-670X. 1996. USD 645 in United States; USD 645 in Canada & Mexico; USD 645 elsewhere (effective 2002) (from EBSCO Publishing, Wiley InterScience, Institute for Scientific Information).
Indexed: ASCA, Anim.Breed.Abstr., BBCI, Chem.Abstr., Chem.Indus.Notes, Chem.Titles, Curr.Cont., Dairy Sci.Abstr., Environ.Sci.Poll.Mgmt., Excerp.Med., Ind.Vet., Inpharma, NRN, Nutr.Abstr., Pharm.&Out.News, Pig News & Info., Reac., Ref.Zh., Saf.Sci.Abstr.
—BLDSC (5069.744300), CASDDS, CISTI, EMDOCS, GNLM, IDS, Infotrieve, KNAW. **CCC.**
Published by: (International Society for Trace Element Research in Humans), John Wiley & Sons, Inc., Journals (Subsidiary of: Wiley InterScience), 605 Third Ave, New York, NY 10158. TEL 212-850-6645, FAX 212-850-6021, subinfo@wiley.com, uscs-wis@wiley.com, http://www.wiley.com. Ed. Ananda S Prasad. adv.: B&W page GBP 640, color page GBP 1,515; trim 174 x 254. Circ: 350. **Subscr. outside the Americas to:** John Wiley & Sons Ltd., Baffins Ln, Chichester, Sussex PO19 IUD, United Kingdom. TEL 44-1243-779777, FAX 44-1243-843232, cs-journals@wiley.co.uk.

619 JPN ISSN 0301-2611
CODEN: KTGIDU
KENSA TO GIJUTSU/MODERN MEDICAL LABORATORY. Text in Japanese. 1973. m. JPY 16,100, USD 170.
Indexed: Chem.Titles, Mass Spectr.Bull.
—CASDDS, CISTI.
Published by: Igaku-Shoin Ltd., 5-24-3 Hongo, Bunkyo-ku, Tokyo 113-0033, Japan. TEL 81-3-3817-5713, FAX 81-3-3815-7802, kensa@nna.so-net.or.jp. Circ: 9,000.

616 RUS ISSN 0869-2084
RB1 CODEN: KLDIES
KLINICHESKAYA LABORATORNAYA DIAGNOSTIKA/ CLINICAL AND LABORATORY DIAGNOSIS. Text in Russian; Summaries in English. 1955. m. USD 170 foreign (effective 2000). adv. bk.rev., Website rev. bibl. **Document type:** *Journal.* **Description:** Covers clinical laboratory diagnosis - hematology, cytology, coagulation, biochemistry, immunology.
Formerly: Laboratornoe Delo (0023-6748)
Indexed: Anal.Abstr., Biol.Abstr., Chem.Abstr., Chem.Titles, Dent.Ind., INIS Atomind., Ind.Med. (1992-), Nutr.Abstr., Ref.Zh.
—BLDSC (0089.238000), CASDDS, CISTI, East View, GNLM, Infotrieve. **CCC.**
Published by: Izdatel'stvo Meditsina, Petroverigskii per 6-8, Moscow 101000, Russian Federation. TEL 7-095-9248785, 7-095-928-86-48, FAX 7-095-9211355, 7-095-9286003, meditsina@iname.com, http://www.medit.ru. Ed. V V Men'shikov. Pub. A M Stochik. R&P L Shankina. Adv. contact O A Fadeeva TEL 7-095-923-51-40. Circ: 3,300. **Dist. by:** Mezhdunarodnaya Kniga, B Yakimanka 39, Moscow 117049, Russian Federation. TEL 7-095-2384967, FAX 7-095-2384634; **US dist. addr.:** East View Publications, 3020 Harbor Ln N, Minneapolis, MN 55447. TEL 612-550-0961.

619 ZAF ISSN 1013-1205
L M S; new developments in laboratory equipment. (Laboratory Marketing Spectrum) Text in English. 1982. bi-m. adv. bk.rev. index. back issues avail. **Document type:** *Trade.* **Description:** Provides product data on laboratory equipment and materials.
Published by: George Warman Publications (Pty.) Ltd., PO Box 704, Cape Town 8000, South Africa. TEL 27-21-24-5320, FAX 27-21-26-1332. Ed. Wendy Borland. Circ: 5,500 (controlled).

542 ZAF
L M S - LABORATORY EQUIPMENT BUYERS GUIDE. (Laboratory Marketing Spectrum) Text in English. 1989. a. ZAR 110. **Document type:** *Directory.* **Description:** Guide for buyers of laboratory equipment.
Published by: George Warman Publications (Pty.) Ltd., PO Box 704, Cape Town 8000, South Africa. TEL 27-21-24-5320, FAX 27-21-26-1332. Ed. Abdul Rawoot.

619 USA ISSN 0093-7355
LAB ANIMAL. Text in English. 1972. 11/yr. USD 135 domestic in US & Canada; USD 145 elsewhere (effective 2001). adv. bk.rev. charts, illus, tr.lit. back issues avail.; reprints avail. *Refereed.* **Document type:** *Journal.* **Description:** Provides users of laboratory animals with review articles on the following subjects; new animal models, breeds or breeding practices, and in vitro or computer alternatives to animal use; lab animal care and nutrition; diagnostic activities; toxicology, genetics and ambryology as they relate to the animal research field.
Related titles: Online - full text ed.: (from Institute for Scientific Information).
Indexed: ASCA, Agricola, Focus on: Vet.Sci.& Med.
—BLDSC (5137.700000), CISTI, IDS. **CCC.**
Published by: Nature Publishing Co. (Subsidiary of: Macmillan Magazines, Ltd.), 345 Park Ave S, 10th Fl, New York, NY 10012-2467. TEL 212-726-9200, labanimal@natureny.com, http://www.labanimal.com. Ed. Julia Schuloff. Pub. James Skowrenski. Adv. contact Shelia Killeen. Circ: 10,000 (controlled). **Subscr. to:** Lab Animal Subscription Fulfillment, PO Box 1710, Riverton, NJ 08077-7310.

542 DEU ISSN 0343-9100
LAB-COMPACT SERVICE; Produkte fuer das Labor. Text in German. 1971. 4/yr. free per issue to qualified personnel. adv. illus, tr.lit. **Document type:** *Trade.* **Description:** Consists of requests-for-information postcards.
Published by: G I T Verlag GmbH, Roesslerstr 90, Darmstadt 64293, Germany. TEL 49-6151-8090-0, FAX 49-6151-809044, gitverlaggmbh@gitverlag.com, http://www.gitverlag.com. Ed. Joerg Peter Matthes. Adv. contact Hubert Schulz TEL 49-6151-8090116. Circ: 14,000.

619 USA
LAB HOTLINE. Text in English. 1965. m. free per issue. charts, stat. **Document type:** *Academic/Scholarly.*
Published by: University of Iowa, University Hygienic Laboratory, Oakdale Campus, Iowa City, IA 52242. TEL 319-335-4500, FAX 319-335-4555. Ed. Tex Heald. Circ: 1,000.

619 BEL
LAB PLUS INTERNATIONAL. Text in English. 1987. 6/yr. BEF 3,000 in Europe; USD 90 in Africa; USD 95 in the Americas; free to qualified personnel (effective 1999). adv. bk.rev. illus. **Document type:** *Magazine, Trade.* **Description:** Reports on new instruments and technologies available in Europe and Asia for use in industrial and analytical laboratories.
Former title: Lab Products International (0775-602X)
Published by: Elsevier Business Information - Belgium (Subsidiary of: Reed Elsevier plc), Rue des Palais 100, Brussels B-1030, Belgium. TEL 32-2-240-2611, FAX 32-2-242-7111, lpi@ebi.be, http://www.ebi.be. Ed. Joanna Winstone. Pub., R&P Dr. Bernard Leger. Adv. contact Astrid Wydouw. B&W page USD 11,000; 20 x 26.5. Circ: 40,011 (controlled).

616 542 GBR ISSN 1463-080X
LAB SOUTH AMERICA. Text in English. 1998. 3/yr. GBP 45 (effective 2000). adv. **Document type:** *Trade.* **Description:** Presents the latest in laboratory equipment and chemicals.
Published by: International Labmate Ltd., 12 Alban Park, Hatfield Rd, St Albans, Herts AL4 0JJ, United Kingdom. TEL 44-1727-855574, FAX 44-1727-841694.

616 USA ISSN 1068-1760
LABMEDICA INTERNATIONAL. Text in English; Summaries in French, German, Italian, Spanish. 1982. 6/yr. USD 80 to non-members. adv. bk.rev. index. *Refereed.* **Document type:** *Trade.* **Description:** Covers the latest developments in laboratory technology, including: microbiology, clinical chemistry, hematology and immunology.
Former titles (until 1990): LabMedica (1054-0970); (until 1984): Medilab
—GNLM.
Published by: Globetech Publishing, 8 Cannon Rd, Wilton, CT 06897. TEL 203-762-3432, FAX 203-762-8640. Ed. Jill Quigley Roberge. Pub. Marc Gueron. Adv. contact Chrys Emery. Circ: 26,000 (controlled).

542 DEU ISSN 0344-5208
LABO; Magazin fuer Labortechnik. Text in German. 1970. 12/yr. free per issue. adv. bk.rev. **Document type:** *Trade.*
Indexed: CEABA.
Published by: Verlag Hoppenstedt GmbH, Havelstr 9, Darmstadt 64295, Germany. TEL 49-6151-380326, FAX 49-6151-380341. Ed. Rainer Jupe. Circ: 25,000 (controlled).

658.5 DEU
LABOR 2000. Text in German. 1976. s-a. DEM 22. adv. **Document type:** *Bulletin.*
Formerly: Labor Praxis in der Medizin (0171-4279)
Related titles: ♦ Supplement to: LaborPraxis. ISSN 0344-1733.
Indexed: Chem.Abstr., Excerp.Med., INIS Atomind., Sugar Ind.Abstr.
—CISTI, GNLM. **CCC.**
Published by: Vogel Verlag und Druck GmbH & Co. KG, Max-Planck-Str 7-9, Wuerzburg 97064, Germany. TEL 49-931-4182518, FAX 49-931-4182750. Adv. contact Ludwig Springauf. Circ: 14,000 (controlled).

616 CHE
LABOR AND MEDIZIN. Text in German. 1973. 11/yr. CHF 80. adv. bk.rev. **Document type:** *Academic/Scholarly.*
Published by: Swiss Association of Medical Laboratory Technologists, Chemin de Carles, Corcelles Ne 2035, Switzerland. TEL 41-38-318838, FAX 41-38-305766. Ed., R&P Jacqueline Merlotti. Circ: 2,900.

616 CHE
LABOR FLASH. Text in German. 9/yr. adv. **Document type:** *Trade.*
Published by: Kretz AG, Postfach, Feldmeilen 8706, Switzerland. TEL 41-1-9237656, FAX 41-1-9237657, kretz_ag@bluewin.ch. Ed. H Zullinger. Adv. contact Esther Kretz. B&W page CHF 2,410, color page CHF 3,470; trim 265 x 185. Circ: 6,400.

616 DEU ISSN 0931-7570
LABOR JAHRBUCH. Text in German. 1983. a. adv. **Document type:** *Directory.*
—GNLM.
Published by: G I T Verlag GmbH, Roesslerstr 90, Darmstadt 64293, Germany. TEL 49-6151-8090-0, FAX 49-6151-8090183, gitverlaggmbh@gitverlag.com, http://www.gitverlag.com. Adv. contact Christa Trumpfheller.

616 SWE ISSN 0345-696X
LABORATORIET. Variant title: Tidskriften Laboratoriet. Text in Swedish. 1953. 6/yr. SEK 275 (effective 1999). adv. bk.rev. **Document type:** *Bulletin.*
Published by: (Biomedicinska Analytiker), Institutet foer Biomedicinsk Laboratorivetenskap, Adolf Fredriks Kyrkogata 11, Stockholm 11137, Sweden. TEL 46-8-24-01-31, FAX 46-8-24-01-24, http://www.lbt-inst.se. Ed. Bodil Persson. Adv. contact Barbro Soederberg. B&W page SEK 7,600, color page SEK 14,600; trim 269 x 180. Circ: 9,900 (controlled).

616 NLD ISSN 0924-4433
LABORATORIUM PRAKTIJK. Text in Dutch. 1979. 10/yr. NLG 164; NLG 275 foreign (effective 1998). adv. **Document type:** *Trade.* **Description:** Covers developments, new methods and techniques of interest to laboratory staff and management.
Former titles (until 1992): Lab - A B C (0168-7417); (until 1983): Para Medica (0927-0582)
Published by: Ten Hagen & Stam b.v. (Subsidiary of: Wolters Kluwer N.V.), Regulusweg 11, The Hague 2516 AC, Netherlands. Ed. H Buskes. Adv. contact Herman Voois. B&W page NLG 3,400, color page NLG 5,700; trim 210 x 297. Circ: 3,940 (paid).

M

616.07 DEU ISSN 0342-3026
CODEN: LABOD3

LABORATORIUMS MEDIZIN. Text and summaries in English, German. 1976. 12/yr. DEM 469.13 in Europe; DEM 566.92 elsewhere; DEM 516.04 in Europe print & online eds. combined; DEM 623.61 elsewhere print & online eds. combined (effective 2001). adv. charts, illus. *Refereed.* **Document type:** *Journal, Academic/Scholarly.* **Description:** Covers chemical and microbiological analysis of body fluids, evaluation of diagnostic tools, and quality assurance of medical therapies.
Related titles: ♦ Online - full text ed.: Laboratoriums Medizin Online. ISSN 1439-0477.
Indexed: Chem.Abstr., Chem.Indus.Notes, Chem.Titles, Int.Abstr.Biol.Sci., Ref.Zh.
—BLDSC (5137.974000), CASDDS, CISTI, EMDOCS, GNLM, Infotrieve, KNAW. **CCC.**
Published by: (Deutschen Gesellschaft fuer Laboratoriumsmedizin e.V.), Blackwell Wissenschafts Verlag GmbH, Kurfuerstendamm 57, Berlin 10707, Germany. TEL 49-30-32790624, FAX 49-30-32790610, abo@blackwis.de, http://www.blackwell.de. Ed. Dr. Arnold von Eckardstein. Adv. contact Jutta Weber-Pianka. B&W page DEM 3,500, color page DEM 6,200; trim 178 x 250. Circ: 7,000.

616.07 DEU ISSN 1439-0477

LABORATORIUMS MEDIZIN ONLINE. Text in German. m. DEM 423 (effective 2001). **Document type:** *Academic/Scholarly.*
Media: Online - full text. **Related titles:** ♦ Print ed.: Laboratoriums Medizin. ISSN 0342-3026.
Published by: Blackwell Wissenschafts Verlag GmbH, Kurfuerstendamm 57, Berlin 10707, Germany. TEL 49-30-32790624, FAX 49-30-32790610, abo@blackwis.de, http://www.blackwell.de/labmed.htm.

616 GBR ISSN 0458-5933
CODEN: LAHBA

LABORATORY ANIMAL HANDBOOKS. Text in English. 1968. irreg. **Document type:** *Monographic series.*
Formerly (until 1969): Laboratory Animal Symposia (0374-8855)
Indexed: Biol.Abstr., Excerp.Med.
—BLDSC (5138.530000), CISTI.
Published by: Laboratory Animals Ltd., c/o Royal Society of Medicine Press Ltd., 1 Wimpole St, London W1M 8AE, United Kingdom. TEL 44-20-7290-2900, FAX 44-20-7290-2929.

LABORATORY ANIMALS. see *BIOLOGY—Zoology*

619 GBR ISSN 0309-7382

LABORATORY ANIMALS. BUYERS GUIDE. Text in English. 1977. irreg. **Document type:** *Directory.*
Published by: Laboratory Animals Ltd., c/o Royal Society of Medicine Press Ltd., 1 Wimpole St, London W1M 8AE, United Kingdom. TEL 44-20-7290-2900, FAX 44-20-7290-2929.

619 CAN ISSN 0381-6729

LABORATORY BUYERS GUIDE. Text in English. a. CND 70 domestic; USD 70 foreign (effective 1999). adv. **Document type:** *Trade.* **Description:** Lists suppliers of laboratory equipment and chemicals, major manufacturers along with their Canadian sales agents. Includes alphabetical listing of allied products and an advertisers index.
Published by: Southam Magazine Group, 1450 Don Mills Rd, Don Mills, ON M3B 2X7, Canada. TEL 416-445-6641, FAX 416-442-2213. Ed., R&P Rita Tate. Adv. contact Anita Havas.

542 USA ISSN 0023-6810

LABORATORY EQUIPMENT. Text in English. 1966. 12/yr. (plus annual directory). USD 65.95 domestic; USD 68.95 in Canada & Mexico; USD 85.95 elsewhere; USD 8 newsstand/cover domestic; USD 10 newsstand/cover foreign (effective 2001). adv. illus. **Document type:** *Trade.* **Description:** Reaches managers, supervisors and research directors with buying responsibility in laboratories located in industry, government and universities.
Related titles: Microform ed.: (from PQC); Online - full text ed.: (from Gale Group).
Indexed: Curr.Pack.Abstr., Graph.Arts Lit.Abstr., World Text.Abstr.
—Infotrieve, Linda Hall. **CCC.**
Published by: Cahners Business Information, New Product Information Unit (Subsidiary of: Reed Elsevier plc), 301 Gibraltar Dr, P O Box 650, Morris Plains, NJ 07950-0650. TEL 973-292-5100 ext.381, FAX 973-539-3476, http://www.laboratoryequipment.com. Ed. Helen Robinson TEL 973-292-5100 x260. Pub. Timothy J Canny. adv.: page USD 11,920; trim 10.5 x 15. Circ: 120,018.

619 AUS

LABORATORY INFORMATION BULLETIN. Text in English. a. free. **Document type:** *Government.* **Description:** Reports significant work undertaken by the laboratories of the TGA. It is a source of information relevant to the work of the laboratories in monitoring the quality, safety and efficacy of therapeutic goods.
Media: Online - full content.
Published by: Therapeutic Goods Administration, PO Box 100, Woden, ACT 2606, Australia. TEL 61-2-6232-8610, 61-2-6232-8444, FAX 61-2-6232-8222, tga-information-officer@health.gov.au, http://www.health.gov.au/tga/docs/html/lib/libindex.htm, http://www.anzfa.gov.au/.

616 USA ISSN 0023-6837
RB1 CODEN: LAINAW

LABORATORY INVESTIGATION; a journal of experimental methods and pathology. Text in English. 1952. m. USD 209 domestic to individuals for print & online eds.; USD 281 foreign to individuals for print & online eds.; USD 523 domestic to institutions for print & online eds.; USD 595 foreign to institutions for print & online eds.; USD 50 newsstand/cover (effective 2002). adv. abstr, bibl, charts, illus. *Refereed.* **Document type:** *Academic/Scholarly.* **Description:** Experimental, anatomical and comparative pathology, cytologic and histologic methods, tissue culturing for pathologists and laboratory technicians.
Related titles: E-mail ed.; Microfilm ed.: (from WWS); Online - full text ed.: ISSN 1530-0307. USD 679.90 domestic academic site license; USD 751.90 foreign academic site license; USD 758.35 domestic corporate site license; USD 830.45 foreign corporate site license (effective 2002) (from Ovid Technologies, Inc., HighWire Pr., Institute for Scientific Information).
Indexed: ASCA, Aqua.Sci.& Fish.Abstr., Biol.Abstr., Chem.Abstr., Chem.Indus.Notes, Chem.Titles, Curr.Adv.Cancer Res., Curr.Adv.Cell & Devel.Biol., Curr.Adv.Ecol.Sci., Curr.Adv.Gen.& Molec.Biol., Curr.Cont., Dairy Sci.Abstr., Dent.Ind., Diar.Dis.Res., Excerp.Med., Helminthol.Abstr., INIS Atomind., Ind.Med. (1952-), Ind.Sci.Rev., Ind.Vet., Inpharma, Int.Abstr.Biol.Sci., Neurosci.Cit.Ind., Nutr.Abstr., Pharm.&Out.News, Pig News & Info., Protozool.Abstr., Reac., Rev.Appl.Entomol., Rev.Med.& Vet.Mycol., Sci.Cit.Ind., Small Anim.Abstr., Sport Fish.Abstr., THA, Vet.Bull., Wild.Rev.
—BLDSC (5140.000000), CASDDS, CISTI, GNLM, IDS, ingenta, KNAW, Linda Hall.
Published by: (United States and Canadian Academy of Pathology), Williams & Wilkins (Subsidiary of: Waverly International), 351 W Camden St, Baltimore, MD 21201-2436. TEL 410-528-4068, 800-222-3790, FAX 410-528-4452, sisaacson@wwilkins.com, http://labinvest.uscapjournals.org/, http://www.Lww.com. Eds. Dr. Jon S Morrow, Dr. Jordan S Pober. Adv. contact Sharlene Isaacson. B&W page USD 865; trim 10.88 x 8.13. Circ: 2,718; 2,627 (paid).

616.07 USA ISSN 0007-5027
RB37.A1 CODEN: LBMEBX

LABORATORY MEDICINE. Text in English. 1965. m. USD 55 domestic to individuals; USD 70 foreign to individuals; USD 60 domestic to institutions; USD 75 foreign to institutions (effective 2000). adv. bk.rev. charts, illus, stat, tr.lit. back issues avail.; reprints avail. *Refereed.* **Document type:** *Bulletin, Academic/Scholarly.* **Description:** Devoted to the continuing education of laboratory professionals. Presents original scientific articles from laboratory professionals containing both theoretical and practical information on the most recent ideas and the latest research.
Formerly (until 1970): Bulletin of Pathology; Incorporates: Technical Improvement Service Bulletin
Related titles: Microform ed.: (from PQC); Online - full text ed.: (from Institute for Scientific Information).
Indexed: ASCA, CINAHL, C.I.S. Abstr., Chem.Abstr., Curr.Adv.Cell & Devel.Biol., Curr.Adv.Ecol.Sci., Curr.Adv.Gen.& Molec.Biol., Curr.Cont., Excerp.Med., Helminthol.Abstr., Inpharma, Int.Abstr.Biol.Sci., Nutr.Abstr., Pharm.&Out.News, Protozool.Abstr., Reac., Rev.Med.& Vet.Mycol., SSCI (coverage dropped), Trop.Dis.Bull.
—BLDSC (5140.400000), CASDDS, CISTI, GNLM, IDS, ingenta, KNAW.
Published by: American Society of Clinical Pathologists, 2100 W Harrison St, Chicago, IL 60612. TEL 312-738-1336, 800-633-4931, FAX 312-738-0101, http://www.ascp.org. Ed. Paul Philipsher. Pub. Joshua Weikersheimer. R&P Robert Behr. Adv. contact Joe Dingee. Circ: 160,567. **Subscr. in Japan to:** Igaku-Shoin, 1-28-36 Hongo, Bunkyo-ku, Tokyo 113-0033, Japan.

619 GBR ISSN 0266-7169
CODEN: LANEEY

LABORATORY NEWS. Text in English. 1971. fortn. GBP 125. adv. bk.rev. **Description:** Provides news of experimental medicine and laboratory technique.
Indexed: ABC, Anal.Abstr., Br.Tech.Ind., CEABA, Curr.Biotech.Abstr., INIS Atomind.
—BLDSC (5140.570000), CISTI.
Published by: Quantum Publishing Ltd., Quantum House, 19 Scarbrook Rd, Croydon, Surrey CR9 1LX, United Kingdom. TEL 44-20-8565-4290, FAX 44-20-8565-4302. Ed. Alex Crawford. Circ: 16,000.

616 542 GBR ISSN 0023-6853
Q183 CODEN: LABPA3

LABORATORY PRACTICE; research techniques and equipment. Text in English; Summaries in French, German. 1952. m. GBP 39, USD 170. adv. bk.rev. abstr, charts, illus. index, cum.index.
Indexed: Abstr.Hyg., Alloys Ind., Anal.Abstr., Biol.Abstr., Br.Ceram.Abstr., Br.Tech.Ind., Chem.Abstr., Curr.Adv.Ecol.Sci., Dairy Sci.Abstr., Excerp.Med., Field Crop Abstr., Fluidex, Food Sci.& Tech.Abstr., Herb.Abstr., Hort.Abstr., IBR, INIS Atomind., INSPEC (pre-1969-Dec.1988, dropped), Ind.Vet., Lab.Haz.Bull., Mass Spectr.Bull., Met.Abstr., Met.Abstr.Ind., Nonfer.Met.Alert, PCC Alert, RAPRA, Soils & Fert., Steels Alert, Trop.Dis.Bull., Vet.Bull., W.R.C.Inf., World Surf.Coat.
—CASDDS, CISTI, GNLM, ingenta, Linda Hall.
Published by: United Trade Press Ltd., UTP House, 33-35 Bowling Green Ln, London EC1R 0DA, United Kingdom. TEL 01-837 1212. Ed. Richard Davies. Circ: 15,669.

616 CAN ISSN 0047-3855

LABORATORY PRODUCT NEWS. Text in English. 1971. 7/yr. CND 30.95 domestic; USD 57.95 in United States; USD 93.95 elsewhere (effective 1999). adv. **Document type:** *Trade.* **Description:** Provides concise product data for buyers, specifiers and users of laboratory equipment. Industrial, hospital, university, private and government users are informed about the latest equipment suitable for their particular branch of science.
Indexed: CBCA Bus. (1996-).
Published by: Southam Magazine Group, 1450 Don Mills Rd, Don Mills, ON M3B 2X7, Canada. TEL 416-445-6641, FAX 416-442-2213. Ed. Rita Tate. Circ: 20,000 (controlled).

619 USA ISSN 0272-3778

LABORATORY REGULATION MANUAL. Text in English. 1976. q. USD 719; USD 863 foreign. **Description:** Covers existing or proposed state and federal laws and regulations affecting the operation of clinical laboratories.
Published by: Aspen Publishers, Inc., 200 Orchard Ridge Dr, Ste 200, Gaithersburg, MD 20878. TEL 800-638-8437, FAX 301-417-7550. Eds. H Robert Halper, Hope S Foster.

LABORATORY TECHNIQUES IN BIOCHEMISTRY AND MOLECULAR BIOLOGY. see *BIOLOGY—Biochemistry*

LABORATORY YELLOW PAGES. see *BUSINESS AND ECONOMICS—Trade And Industrial Directories*

619 DEU ISSN 0170-2572

LABORMEDIZIN. Text in German. 1978. bi-m. DEM 98 (effective 1999). adv. **Document type:** *Academic/Scholarly.*
Indexed: INIS Atomind.
Published by: G I T Verlag GmbH, Roesslerstr 90, Darmstadt 64293, Germany. TEL 49-6151-8090-0, FAX 49-6151-809044, gitverlaggmbh@gitverlag.com, http://www.gitverlag.com. Ed. Ernst Giebeler. Adv. contact Walter Depner. B&W page DEM 6,235, color page DEM 8,995; trim 260 x 185. Circ: 11,000.

619 DEU ISSN 0344-1733
CODEN: LAPRDE

LABORPRAXIS. Text in German. 1976. m. EUR 105 domestic; EUR 123.40 foreign (effective 2002). adv. bk.rev. **Document type:** *Journal, Trade.*
Related titles: ♦ Supplement: Labor 2000.
Indexed: Anal.Abstr., CEABA, Chem.Abstr., Chem.Indus.Notes, Chem.Titles, INIS Atomind., Mass Spectr.Bull., Ref.Zh.
—BLDSC (5141.942000), CASDDS, GNLM, Infotrieve. **CCC.**

M

Published by: Vogel Verlag und Druck GmbH & Co. KG, Max-Planck-Str 7-9, Wuerzburg 97064, Germany. TEL 49-931-4182518, FAX 49-931-4182750, laborpraxis@vogel-medien.de, http://www.laborpraxis.de, http://www.vogel-medien.de. Ed. Dieter Kneucker. Adv. contact Ludwig Springauf. B&W page DEM 8,360, color page DEM 10,780; trim 190 x 270. Circ: 24,969 (controlled). **Subscr. to:** DataM-Services GmbH, Fichtestr 9, Wuerzburg 97074, Germany. TEL 49-931-417001, FAX 49-931-4170499, swestenberger@datam-services.de, http://www.datam-services.de. **Dist. in US by:** Vogel Europublishing Inc., 632 Sunflower Ct., San Ramos, CA 94583. TEL 510-648-1170.

542 CHE
LABORSCOPE; Messtechnik - Regelung und Steuerung - Datentechnik. Text in German. 1974. 8/yr. CHF 35; CHF 66 foreign (effective 1996). adv. bk.rev. illus. **Document type:** *Trade.*
Published by: Verlag Laupper AG, Emil-Frey-Str 70, Muenchenstein 4142, Switzerland. TEL 41-61-3321616, FAX 41-61-3321600. Circ: 6,250.

616 USA ISSN 0580-7247
RB36 CODEN: MLOBAC
M L O. (Medical Laboratory Observer) Text in English. 1969. m. USD 70 domestic; USD 80 foreign; USD 12 newsstand/cover (effective 2001). adv. charts, illus, stat. index. back issues avail. **Description:** Contains information to improving the business management and leadership skills of laboratory directors, managers and other providers of clinical laboratory services.
Related titles: Microform ed.: (from PQC); Online - full text ed.: (from Gale Group, ProQuest Information & Learning, Factiva).
Indexed: Bus.Ind., CINAHL, Int.Nurs.Ind., Tr.& Indus.Ind.
—BLDSC (5529.387000), GNLM, ingenta. **CCC.**
Published by: Medical Economics Co., Inc., 5 Paragon Dr, Montvale, NJ 07645-1742. TEL 201-358-7200. Ed. Darlene Berger. Circ: 59,000.

M T A - FACHZEITSCHRIFT DER TECHNISCHE ASSISTENTEN DER MEDIZIN; Monatszeitschrift fuer MTA's, Labormediziner, Fachleute Radio-Diagnostik, Lehrer und Studenten. (Medizinisch-Technische Assistenten) see *MEDICAL SCIENCES*

M T A - REPETITORIUM. (Medizinisch- Technische Assistenten) see *MEDICAL SCIENCES*

MEDICAL AND RADIOLOGICAL DEVICES GUIDANCE MANUAL. see *PUBLIC HEALTH AND SAFETY*

619 681 USA
MEDICAL DEVICE APPROVAL LETTER WITH G M P - DESIGN CONTROLS REVIEWS. Text in English. ceased; resumed 1992. m. USD 599 (effective 2000). bk.rev. back issues avail. **Document type:** *Newsletter.*
Formerly: Medical Device Approval Letter (1060-8338)
Related titles: Online - full text ed.: (from Gale Group, Factiva).
—CCC.
Published by: Washington Information Source, 6506 Old Stage Rd, Ste 100, Rockville, MD 20852-4326. TEL 301-770-5553. Ed., Pub., R&P Ken Reid.

MEDICAL DEVICE ESTABLISHMENT REGISTRATION MASTER FILE. see *PUBLIC HEALTH AND SAFETY*

MEDICAL DEVICE PROBLEMS REPORT FROM THE D E N: REPORTS FROM MEDICAL DEVICE USERS. (Device Experience Network) see *PUBLIC HEALTH AND SAFETY*

MEDICAL DEVICE REPORTING FROM THE D E N: REPORTS FROM MEDICAL DEVICE MANUFACTURERS. (Device Experience Network) see *PUBLIC HEALTH AND SAFETY*

MEDICAL EQUIPMENT AND SUPPLY GUIDE. see *MEDICAL SCIENCES*

610 GBR ISSN 0140-3028
CODEN: MLWODQ
MEDICAL LABORATORY WORLD. Text in English. 1977. m. (10/yr.). GBP 62; GBP 78 in Europe; USD 216 in US & Canada; GBP 115 elsewhere (effective 1999). **Document type:** *Trade.*
Indexed: ABC, Br.Tech.Ind., CBNB (1994-), Chem.Abstr.
—BLDSC (5529.420000), CASDDS, CISTI.
Published by: Wilmington Publishing Ltd., Wilmington House, Church Hill, Wilmington, Dartford, Kent DA2 7EF, United Kingdom. TEL 44-1322-277788, FAX 44-1322-276474, wbp@wilmington.co.uk. Ed. Dominic Mason. Circ: 8,072.

681 DEU ISSN 1615-1615
CODEN: LASMEF
MEDICAL LASER APPLICATION; international journal for laser treatment and research. Text in English. 1985. q. EUR 230 (effective 2002). **Document type:** *Journal, Academic/Scholarly.* **Description:** Publishes articles and papers from all fields of technical and scientific research and clinical applications of lasers in medicine for therapy and diagnostics.
Formerly (until 2001): Lasermedizin (0938-765X)
—BLDSC (5529.430000), CISTI, GNLM.
Published by: Urban & Fischer Verlag, Loebdergraben 14a, Jena 07743, Germany. TEL 49-3641-626444, FAX 49-3641-626500, journals@urbanfischer.de, http://www.urbanfischer.de/journals. R&P Martin Huber TEL 49-3641-626430. **Subscr. to:** Nature Publishing Group, Brunel Rd, Basingstoke RG21 6XS, United Kingdom. TEL 44-1256-302629, FAX 44-1256-463570, j.stephens@macmillan.com.

619 ITA ISSN 0393-7623
LA MEDICINA DI LABORATORIO. Text in Italian. 1985. q. USD 180 (effective 1999). **Document type:** *Academic/Scholarly.*
Published by: Piccin Nuova Libraria, Via Altinate, 107, Padua, PD 35121, Italy. TEL 39-49-655566, FAX 39-49-8750693, TELEX 432074 PICCIN I. Circ: 3,000.

▼ **MICROSPHERES, MICROCAPSULES & LIPOSOMES.** see *PHARMACY AND PHARMACOLOGY*

MICROSURGERY. see *MEDICAL SCIENCES—Surgery*

619 540 GBR ISSN 0890-8508
RB43.7
MOLECULAR AND CELLULAR PROBES; the location, diagnosis, and monitoring of disease by nucleic acid techniques. Text in English. 1987. bi-m. GBP 215 to institutions (effective 2001). adv. index. back issues avail.; reprint service avail. from SWZ. *Refereed.* **Document type:** *Academic/Scholarly.* **Description:** Examines location, diagnosis, and monitoring of both infectious and inherited diseases.
Related titles: Online - full text ed.: (from EBSCO Publishing, O C L C Online Computer Library Center, Inc., RoweCom Information Quest, ingenta, Swets Blackwell, IDEAL Online Library, Institute for Scientific Information).
Indexed: ASCA, AgBiotech, Anim.Breed.Abstr., Biotech.Cit.Ind., Chem.Abstr., Chem.Indus.Notes, Chem.Titles, Curr.Cont., Derwent Biotech.Abstr., Excerp.Med. (1993-), Food Sci.& Tech.Abstr., Helminthol.Abstr., Ind.Med. (1987-), Ind.Vet., Inpharma, Protozool.Abstr., Reac., Rev.Appl.Entomol., Rev.Med.& Vet.Mycol., Sci.Cit.Ind.
—BLDSC (5900.761000), ADONIS, CASDDS, CISTI, EMDOCS, GNLM, IDS, ingenta, KNAW. **CCC.**
Published by: Academic Press (Subsidiary of: Harcourt Publishers Ltd.), 24 Oval Rd, London NW1 7DX, United Kingdom. TEL 44-20-7267-4466, FAX 44-20-7482-2293, apsubs@acad.com, http://www.academicpress.com/mcp; http://www.europe.idealibrary.com/. Ed. D J H Brock J L Waner. R&P Catherine John. Adv. contact Nik Screen. **Subscr. to:** Harcourt Publishers Ltd., Foots Cray High St, Sidcup, Kent DA14 5HP, United Kingdom. TEL 44-20-8300-3322, FAX 44-20-8309-0807.

619 GBR ISSN 1366-8714
RB113 CODEN: MOPAF6
MOLECULAR PATHOLOGY. Text in English. 1995. bi-m. GBP 108, USD 173 combined subscription to individuals includes print & online eds. (effective 2002). adv. bk.rev. abstr, charts, illus. index. Supplement avail.; reprint service avail. from PQC. *Refereed.* **Document type:** *Journal, Academic/Scholarly.* **Description:** Includes original articles of molecular studies on human material relating to pathogenesis and disease processes.
Formerly (until 1996): Clinical Molecular Pathology (1355-2910)
Related titles: Microfilm ed.: (from PQC); Online - full text ed.: M P Online. 2000. GBP 50, USD 75 (effective 2002) (from Ovid Technologies, Inc., EBSCO Publishing, O C L C Online Computer Library Center, Inc., RoweCom Information Quest, ingenta, HighWire Pr., Swets Blackwell, Institute for Scientific Information); ♦ Supplement to: Journal of Clinical Pathology. ISSN 0021-9746.
Indexed: Chem.Abstr., Chem.Indus.Notes, Chem.Titles, Curr.Cont., Derwent Biotech.Abstr., Excerp.Med. (1996-), Ind.Med. (1997-), Inpharma, Protozool.Abstr., Reac., Rev.Appl.Entomol., Rev.Med.& Vet.Mycol., Sci.Cit.Ind.
—BLDSC (5900.817994), ADONIS, CASDDS, CISTI, GNLM, IDS, Infotrieve, ingenta, KNAW. **CCC.**

Published by: B M J Publishing Group, B M A House, Tavistock Sq, London WC1H 9JR, United Kingdom. TEL 44-20-7387-4499, FAX 44-20-7383-6400, info.norththames@bma.org.uk, http://mp.bmjjournals.com/, http://www.bma.org.uk. Eds. David Burnett, John Crocker. Adv. contact Euan Currer TEL 44-20-7383-6181. **U.S. subscr. to:** PO Box 590A, Kennebunkport, ME 04046. TEL 800-236-6265, FAX 800-232-9265.

MONOCLONAL ANTIBODIES. see *BIOLOGY—Abstracting, Bibliographies, Statistics*

619 USA ISSN 0177-7475
MONOGRAPHS ON PATHOLOGY OF LABORATORY ANIMALS. Text in English. 1983. irreg., latest 1995. price varies. **Document type:** *Monographic series.*
Published by: (International Life Sciences Institute), Springer-Verlag, Journals (Subsidiary of: BertelsmannSpringer), 175 Fifth Ave, New York, NY 10010. TEL 212-460-1500, FAX 212-473-6272. Ed. T C Jones.

619 NLD
NEDERLANDSE VERENIGING VOOR KLINISCHE CHEMIE. ALMANAK. Text in Dutch. a. membership. adv.
Published by: Nederlandse Vereniging voor Klinische Chemie, Vredenburg 134, 2nd Fl., Utrecht 3511 BG, Netherlands. TEL 31-30-232-8623, FAX 31-30-231-1178. Ed. F van der Graaf. R&P S Bendien. Adv. contact Mrs. S. Bendien. B&W page NLG 1,095, color page NLG 2,190. Circ: 650.

NIHON JIKKEN DOBUTSU GIJUTSUSHA KYOKAI HOKKAIDO SHIBU KAISHI/JAPANESE ASSOCIATION FOR EXPERIMENTAL ANIMAL TECHNOLOGISTS. HOKKAIDO BRANCH. JOURNAL. see *BIOLOGY—Zoology*

616 USA ISSN 0048-069X
NORTH DAKOTA SOCIETY OF MEDICAL TECHNOLOGISTS. NEWSLETTER. Text in English. 1972 (vol.24). q. USD 6 to non-members. adv. bk.rev., film rev. bibl, charts, illus. **Document type:** *Newsletter.*
Indexed: Ind.Med. (coverage dropped).
Published by: (North Dakota Society for Medical Technology), University of North Dakota, Department of Pathology, Grand Forks, ND 58201. TEL 701-777-2563, FAX 701-772-9636. Eds. Eileen Nelson, Linda Larson. Circ: 400.

619 681 ITA
▼ **NUOVE TECNOLOGIE IN MEDICINA, INFORMATICA, TELEMATICA APPLICAZIONI.** Text in Italian. 1999. q. ITL 90,000 (effective 2000). **Document type:** *Academic/Scholarly.*
Formerly: Nuove Tecnologie in Medicina, Informatica, Telematica
Published by: Sirse S.r.l., Via Confu 51, Brescia, BS 25124, Italy. TEL 39-03-0221522, info@sirse.com, http://www.sirse.com. Ed. R Cataneo.

NURSE RESEARCHER. see *MEDICAL SCIENCES—Nurses And Nursing*

542 CAN ISSN 1200-751X
O S M T ADVOCATE. Text in English. 1985. 4/yr. CND 100; free per issue to members. adv. bk.rev. *Refereed.* **Document type:** *Newsletter, Abstract/Index, Academic/Scholarly.* **Description:** Deals with the developments in medical technology and the latest OSMT news and views.
Formerly: O S M T Update (0832-5332)
Published by: Ontario Society of Medical Technologists, 234 Eglinton Ave E, Ste 402, Toronto, ON M4P 1K5, Canada. TEL 416-485-6768, 800-461-6768, FAX 416-485-7660, bmcarthur@osmt.org, http://www.osmt.org. Ed. Blanca McArthur. adv.: B&W page CND 600, color page CND 1,300; trim 11 x 8.5. Circ: 3,500 (controlled).

ONKOLOGIYA. see *MEDICAL SCIENCES—Oncology*

616 USA ISSN 1521-7418
PATHOLOGY AND LABORATORY MEDICINE. Text in English. 1996. irreg., latest vol.3, 1998. price varies. illus. back issues avail. *Refereed.* **Document type:** *Monographic series, Academic/Scholarly.* **Description:** Discusses techniques and materials in diagnosing and monitoring medical conditions.
Published by: Humana Press Inc., 999 Riverview Dr, Ste 208, Totowa, NJ 07512. TEL 973-256-1699, FAX 973-256-8341, humana@humanapr.com, http://humanapress.com. R&P Richard Hruska.

M

PERITONEAL DIALYSIS INTERNATIONAL. see *MEDICAL SCIENCES*

619.05 USA ISSN 1053-8984
QL55
PERSPECTIVES ON MEDICAL RESEARCH. Text in English. 1989. irreg. USD 10 per issue to non-members (effective 2001). bk.rev. back issues avail. *Refereed.* **Document type:** *Monographic series.* **Description:** Critically evaluates various research methods to assess their scientific validity and clinical utility.
Formerly (until 1990): Perspectives on Animal Research (1045-0424)
—GNLM.
Published by: Medical Research Modernization Committee, PO Box 201791, Cleveland, OH 44120. TEL 216-283-6702, FAX 216-283-6702, stkaufman@mindspring.com, stkaufman@pol.net, http://www.mrmcmed.org. Eds. Dr. Murry J Cohen, Dr. Stephen R Kaufman. Circ: 1,200 (controlled).

▼ **POINT OF CARE**; the journal of near-patient testing and technology. see *MEDICAL SCIENCES*

619 GBR ISSN 0966-4068
CODEN: POPPEF
PORTLAND PRESS PROCEEDINGS. Text in English. 1992. irreg., latest vol.16, 1999. back issues avail. *Refereed.* **Document type:** *Proceedings.*
Indexed: Chem.Abstr., Chem.Indus.Notes, Chem.Titles.
—BLDSC (6555.657000), CASDDS, CISTI, Infotrieve. **CCC.**
Published by: Portland Press Ltd., 59 Portland Pl, London W1N 3AJ, United Kingdom. TEL 44-20-7580-5530, FAX 44-20-7323-1136, sales@portland-service.com, http://www.portlandpress.com/bst/default.htm. R&P Adam Marshall. **Subscr. to:** Commerce Way, Colchester, Essex CO2 8HP, United Kingdom. TEL 44-1206-796351, FAX 44-1206-799331.

PROCESS CONTROL; vakblad voor procesbesturing en analysetechniek. see *COMPUTERS—Automation*

PROEFDIERVRIJ. see *ANIMAL WELFARE*

619 DNK ISSN 0105-9173
REGISTER OVER AUTORISEREDE LABORATORIER* /REGISTER OF AUTHORIZED LABORATORIES. Text in Danish. 1978. a. free per issue. illus.
Formerly: Autorisationsregister
Published by: (Denmark. Teknologistyrelsen), Dansk Teknologisk Instituts Forlag, Teknologiparken, Aarhus C 8000, Denmark. Circ: 3,000.

REPRODUKTIONSMEDIZIN. see *MEDICAL SCIENCES—Obstetrics And Gynecology*

619 616 FRA ISSN 0296-5321
REVUE DES LABORATOIRES D'ESSAIS. Text in French. 1978. q.
Formerly (until 1984): Association pour le Developpement des Sciences et Techniques de l'Environnement. Revue (0249-6658)
Indexed: GeoRef, INIS Atomind.
Published by: A.S.T.E., 8 rue Roquepine, Paris 75008, France. TEL 42-66-58-29, FAX 42-66-12-06. Ed. Jean Delatte. Circ: 3,000.

619 JPN ISSN 0485-1420
CODEN: RNKNAT
RINSHO KENSA/JOURNAL OF MEDICAL TECHNOLOGY. Text in Japanese. 1957. m. JPY 21,500, USD 219.
Indexed: Chem.Abstr., Chem.Indus.Notes, Chem.Titles, INIS Atomind.
—BLDSC (5017.090000), CASDDS, CISTI.
Published by: Igaku-Shoin Ltd., 5-24-3 Hongo, Bunkyo-ku, Tokyo 113-0033, Japan. TEL 81-3-3817-5712, FAX 81-3-3815-7802, rinkensa@nna.so-net.or.jp. Circ: 10,000.

619 ITA ISSN 0394-1671
RIVISTA DI MUSICOTERAPIA. Text in Italian. s-a. USD 40.
Published by: Edizioni Minerva Medica, Corso Bramante, 83-85, Turin, TO 10126, Italy. TEL 39-11-678282, FAX 39-11-674502.

S E R B OFFICIAL REPORTER. (State Employment Relations Board) see *LAW*

616 FRA ISSN 0339-722X
CODEN: STALDT
S T A L. (Sciences et Techniques de l'Animal de Laboratoire) Text in English, French. 1976. q. FRF 350. adv. bk.rev. *Refereed.*
Formerly: Association des Techniciens d'Animaux de Laboratoire. Bulletin Trimestriel (0339-7238)
Indexed: ASCA, Anim.Breed.Abstr., Biol.Abstr., Curr.Adv.Ecol.Sci., Curr.Cont., Dairy Sci.Abstr., Focus on: Vet.Sci.& Med., Helminthol.Abstr., Ind.Vet., Int.Aerosp.Abstr., Met.Abstr., Ref.Zh., SSCI (coverage dropped), Vet.Bull.
—BLDSC (8430.123000), Linda Hall.
Published by: Societe Francaise d'Experimentation Animale (SFEA), Centre d'Experimentation Animale et de Recherches Chirurgicales, 6 rue du General Sarrail, Creteil 94000, France. TEL 31-47-02-00. Ed. J Duteil. Circ: 1,000. **Subscr. to:** C. Bugiani, Laboratoire Roussel-Uclaf, 102 route de Noisy, Romainville 93230, France. TEL 1-48-91-51-90.

616 NOR ISSN 0036-5513
RB1 CODEN: SJCLAY
SCANDINAVIAN JOURNAL OF CLINICAL & LABORATORY INVESTIGATION. Text in English. 1949. 8/yr. GBP 230, USD 380 to institutions (effective 2002). adv. bibl, charts, illus. index. back issues avail.; reprint service avail. from ISI. *Refereed.* **Document type:** *Academic/Scholarly.*
Related titles: Microform ed.: (from PQC); Online - full text ed.: (from EBSCO Publishing, O C L C Online Computer Library Center, Inc., RoweCom Information Quest, CatchWord Ltd., ingenta, Swets Blackwell, Institute for Scientific Information); ♦ Supplement: Scandinavian Journal of Clinical and Laboratory Investigation. Supplement. ISSN 0085-591X.
Indexed: ASCA, Abstr.Hyg., Agri.& Environ.Biotech.Abstr. (coverage dropped), BBCI, Biol.Abstr., C.I.S. Abstr., Cal.Tiss.Abstr., Chem.Abstr., Chem.Titles, Chemorec.Abstr., Curr.Adv.Cancer Res., Curr.Adv.Ecol.Sci., Curr.Cont., Dairy Sci.Abstr., Derwent Biotech.Abstr., Environ.Sci.Poll.Mgmt., Excerp.Med., Helminthol.Abstr., INIS Atomind., Ind.Med. (1949-), Ind.Sci.Rev., Ind.Vet., Inpharma, Int.Abstr.Biol.Sci., Mass Spectr.Bull., Nutr.Abstr., Pharm.&Out.News, Pig News & Info., Reac., SSCI (coverage dropped), Sci.Cit.Ind., THA, Trop.Dis.Bull., Vet.Bull.
—BLDSC (8087.500000), ADONIS, CASDDS, CISTI, GNLM, IDS, ingenta, KNAW. **CCC.**
Published by: (Scandinavian Society for Clinical Chemistry), Taylor & Francis AS (Subsidiary of: Taylor & Francis Group), Cort Adelersgt. 17, Solli, PO Box 2562, Oslo 0202, Norway. TEL 47-22-12-98-80, FAX 47-22-12-98-90, journals@tandf.no, http://www.tandf.co.uk/tfas. Ed. Tor-Arne Hagre. Circ: 1,200.

616 NOR ISSN 0085-591X
CODEN: SJCLAY
SCANDINAVIAN JOURNAL OF CLINICAL AND LABORATORY INVESTIGATION. SUPPLEMENT. Text in English. 1951. irreg. adv. back issues avail.; reprint service avail. from ISI. **Document type:** *Academic/Scholarly.*
Related titles: Microform ed.: (from PQC); Online - full text ed.: (from Swets Blackwell); ♦ Supplement to: Scandinavian Journal of Clinical & Laboratory Investigation. ISSN 0036-5513.
Indexed: Biol.Abstr., Chem.Abstr., Chem.Indus.Notes, Chem.Titles, Curr.Adv.Biochem., Curr.Adv.Cell & Devel.Biol., Curr.Adv.Ecol.Sci., Curr.Cont. (coverage dropped), Excerp.Med., Ind.Med. (1951-), Int.Abstr.Biol.Sci., Nutr.Abstr.
—BLDSC (8087.505000), ADONIS, CASDDS, CISTI, ingenta, KNAW. **CCC.**
Published by: (Scandinavian Society for Clinical Chemistry and Clinical Physiology), Scandinavian University Press (Subsidiary of: Taylor & Francis Ltd.), Postboks 2959, Toeyen, Oslo 0608, Norway. FAX 47-22-57-53-53, journals@scup.no, http://www.scup.no/sjcli. Ed. O Stokke. Circ: 1,200.

616 DNK ISSN 0901-3393
SCANDINAVIAN JOURNAL OF LABORATORY ANIMAL SCIENCE. Text in English. 1974. q. SEK 250 (effective 2001). *Refereed.* **Document type:** *Journal, Academic/Scholarly.* **Description:** Covers all aspects of laboratory animal science from an international perspective.
Formerly (until 1985): Scand L A S Nyt (0901-3792)
Related titles: Online - full text ed.: (from Institute for Scientific Information).
Indexed: Focus on: Vet.Sci.& Med., Ind.Vet., Rev.Med.& Vet.Mycol.
—BLDSC (8087.517200).
Published by: R R Consult, Skomagerkrogen 14, Roskilde 4000, Denmark. TEL 45-46-35-31-68, rrcons@get2net.dk, http://biomedicum.ut.ee/sjlas. Ed. Jann Hau.

SCANNING MICROSCOPY; an international journal of scanning electron microscopy, related techniques, and applications. see *BIOLOGY—Microscopy*

616 CHE ISSN 0253-5211
CODEN: SSLADA
SCHWEIZERISCHE LABORATORIUMS ZEITSCHRIFT. Text in French, German, Italian. 1943. 10/yr. CHF 90 domestic; CHF 120 foreign (effective 2001). adv. bk.rev. **Document type:** *Journal, Academic/Scholarly.*
Indexed: Chem.Abstr., Chem.Titles.
—BLDSC (8117.855000), CASDDS.
Published by: Schweizerischer Laborpersonal Verband, Postfach, Basel 4002, Switzerland. TEL 41-61-3242759. Ed. Christian Beerli. Adv. contact Ursula Schmidt TEL 41-31-3006383. B&W page CHF 1,385, color page CHF 2,585; trim 185 x 270. Circ: 2,500.

619 USA ISSN 1087-3309
R11 CODEN: SCMEFJ
SCIENCE & MEDICINE. Text in English. 1994. bi-m. USD 59 domestic; USD 75 foreign; USD 9.95 newsstand/cover (effective 2000). adv. illus. reprints avail. **Document type:** *Journal, Academic/Scholarly.* **Description:** Provides medical scientists with an opportunity to interpret their biomedical research to a wide audience.
Formerly (until 1996): Scientific American Science and Medicine (1068-6746)
Indexed: Aqua.Sci.& Fish.Abstr., Biol.Dig., Chem.Abstr., Chem.Titles, Environ.Sci.Poll.Mgmt., Inpharma, Pharm.&Out.News, Pollut.Abstr., Reac.
—BLDSC (8134.175100), CASDDS, GNLM, Infotrieve, KNAW. **CCC.**
Address: PO Box 313, Narberth, PA 19072. TEL 800-888-0028, FAX 215-545-5056. Ed., Pub., R&P Albert E Meier. Adv. contact R K Bussy.

SCRIPTA SCIENTIFICA MEDICA. see *MEDICAL SCIENCES—Oncology*

619 ITA ISSN 0390-8283
SOCIETA MEDICO CHIRURGICA DI PAVIA. BOLLETTINO. Text in Italian; Summaries in English, Italian. 1886. q. bibl. Index.
—GNLM.
Published by: Societa Medico Chirurgica di Pavia, Palazzo Universita, Strada Nuova, 65, Pavia, PV 27100, Italy. TEL 39-322-422932. Ed. Vittorio Malamavi. Circ: 300.
Co-sponsor: Universita di Pavia, Facolta Medica.

SOUTHERN CALIFORNIA DENTAL LABORATORY ASSOCIATION. BULLETIN. see *MEDICAL SCIENCES—Dentistry*

570 FRA ISSN 0766-5725
CODEN: TEBIEY
TECHNIQUE ET BIOLOGIE; revue de documentation scientifique et d'information professionnelle. Text in French. 1975. bi-m. FRF 300; FRF 400 foreign (effective 1998). adv. charts, illus.
Formerly: Technicien Biologiste (0337-9965)
Indexed: C.I.S. Abstr., Chem.Abstr.
—CASDDS. **CCC.**
Published by: Editions Scientifiques et Medicales Elsevier, 141 rue de Javel, Paris Cedex 15 75747, France. TEL 33-1-45589022, FAX 33-1-45589421. Ed. Colette Gallula.

TECHNIQUES OF CHEMISTRY. see *CHEMISTRY*

616 ESP ISSN 0371-5728
CODEN: TCLBAB
TECNICAS DE LABORATORIO. Text in Spanish. 1969. 10/yr. ESP 9,900, USD 110 (effective 1999). adv. bk.rev. bibl, charts, illus. **Document type:** *Trade.*
Indexed: Chem.Abstr., Chem.Indus.Notes, Chem.Titles, Food Sci.& Tech.Abstr., GeoRef, Ind.Med.Esp., Ind.SST, Ref.Zh.
—BLDSC (8762.710000), CASDDS, CINDOC. **CCC.**
Published by: Publica S.A., Ecuador, 75, entlo., Barcelona 08029, Spain. TEL 34-93-3215046, FAX 34-93-4391027, publica@publica.es. Ed. Carlos Romagosa. Circ: 3,000.

610 JPN ISSN 0040-8727
CODEN: TJEMAO
TOHOKU JOURNAL OF EXPERIMENTAL MEDICINE. Text in English. 1920. m. (3 vols./yr.). USD 410 (effective 2000). abstr, bibl, charts, illus. reprint service avail. from PQC. *Refereed.* **Document type:** *Academic/Scholarly.*
Related titles: Microform ed.: (from PQC,PMC); Online - full text ed.: (from Institute for Scientific Information).

M

Indexed: ASCA, Abstr.Hyg., AgBiotech, Anim.Breed.Abstr., Biol.Abstr., C.I.S. Abstr., Chem.Abstr., Chem.Indus.Notes, Chem.Titles, Curr.Adv.Ecol.Sci., Curr.Cont., Dairy Sci.Abstr., Dent.Ind., Excerp.Med., Helminthol.Abstr., INIS Atomind., Ind.Med. (1920-), Ind.Sci.Rev., Ind.Vet., Inpharma, Mass Spectr.Bull., Neurosci.Cit.Ind., Nutr.Abstr., Pharm.&Out.News, Reac., Rev.Appl.Entomol., Rev.Med.& Vet.Mycol., Risk Abstr., Sci.Cit.Ind., Trop.Dis.Bull.
—BLDSC (8861.000000), CASDDS, CISTI, GNLM, IDS, ingenta, KNAW. **CCC.**
Published by: Tohoku University Medical Press, 2-1 Seiryo-cho, Aoba-ku, Sendai-shi, Miyagi-ken 980-8575, Japan. TEL 81-22-717-8184, FAX 81-22-717-8185, http://www.journal.med.tohoku.ac.jp/, http://journal.med.tohoku.ac.jp/. Ed. Hiroshi Satoh. Circ: 800.

TRANSPLANTATION PROCEEDINGS. see *MEDICAL SCIENCES—Surgery*

U.S. NATIONAL INSTITUTES OF HEALTH. NATIONAL CENTER FOR RESEARCH RESOURCES. SCIENTIFIC HIGHLIGHTS. see *MEDICAL SCIENCES—Abstracting, Bibliographies, Statistics*

616 USA
VANTAGE POINT. Text in English. 1979. s-m. USD 37 to non-members; USD 21 to members (effective 1999). adv. **Document type:** *Newsletter.* **Description:** To keep association members updated on general healthcare management issues.
Former titles (until Dec. 1996): Management Briefs (1048-5007); (until 1989): Clinical Laboratory Management Newsletter
Indexed: Excerp.Med.
Published by: Clinical Laboratory Management Association, 989 Old Eagle School Rd, Ste 815, Wayne, PA 19087-1704. TEL 610-995-9580, FAX 610-995-9568, http://www.clma.org. Ed., R&P Beth Barrow. Adv. contact Jason Pointe. Circ: 9,000 (controlled).

YAOWU SHIPIN FENXI/JOURNAL OF FOOD AND DRUG ANALYSIS. see *FOOD AND FOOD INDUSTRIES*

619 CHN ISSN 0253-973X
ZHONGHUA YIXUE JIANYAN ZAZHI/CHINESE JOURNAL OF MEDICAL LABORATORY TECHNOLOGY. Text in Chinese. 1978. q. USD 25.20; USD 4.20 newsstand/cover (effective 2001). **Document type:** *Academic/Scholarly.*
Related titles: Online - full content ed.: (from WanFang Data Corp.).
Published by: Zhonghua Yixuehui Zazhishe, 42 Dongsi Xidajie, Beijing 100710, China. **Dist. by:** China International Book Trading Corp, 35, Chegongzhuang Xilu, Haidian District, Beijing 100044, China. TEL 86-1-68413849, FAX 86-1-68412048, cibtc@mail.cibtc.com.cn, http://www.cibtc.com.cn.

MEDICAL SCIENCES—Forensic Sciences

614.19 USA ISSN 0739-7666
RA1001.A35
ACADEMY NEWS (COLORADO SPRINGS). Text in English. 1955. bi-m. USD 15 to non-members (effective 2000). adv. illus. back issues avail. **Document type:** *Newsletter.* **Description:** Informs membership of professional issues, upcoming forensic meetings and conferences, job opportunities, section news and Forensic Science Foundation activities.
Published by: American Academy of Forensic Sciences, PO Box 669, Colorado Springs, CO 80901. TEL 719-636-1100, FAX 719-636-1993, kreynolds@aafs.org, http://www.aafs.org. Ed., R&P, Adv. contact Kathy Reynolds. Pub. Anne Warren. B&W page USD 400; trim 10 x 7.5. Circ: 5,400.

ACCIDENT RECONSTRUCTION JOURNAL. see *LAW*

ACTA CRIMINOLOGIAE ET MEDICINAE LEGALIS JAPONICA/HANZAIGAKU ZASSHI. see *CRIMINOLOGY AND LAW ENFORCEMENT*

340.6 CHE
ACTA MEDICINAE LEGALIS. Text in English, French. 1948. a. **Document type:** *Proceedings, Academic/Scholarly.*
Formerly: Acta Medicinae Legalis et Socialis (0065-1397)
Indexed: Biol.Abstr., Chem.Abstr., Ind.Med. (coverage dropped).
—GNLM.
Published by: International Academy of Legal Medicine, c/o Institut fuer Rechtsmedizin, Universitaet Zuerich, Winterthurerstr 190/52, Zurich 8057, Switzerland. TEL 41-1-6355611, FAX 41-1-6356815, baer@irm.unizh.ch, http://www.irm.unizh.ch/ialm. Circ: 450.

614.19 TUR ISSN 1018-5275
CODEN: ATDEE
ADLI TIP DERGISI. Text in Turkish. 1985. 3/yr.
Indexed: Chem.Abstr., Chem.Indus.Notes, Chem.Titles, Excerp.Med. (1994-).
—BLDSC (0681.746000), CASDDS, EMDOCS, GNLM.
Published by: (Malawi. Ministry of Justice MWI), Council of Forensic Medicine of Turkey, Cerrahpasa Medical Faculty, Istanbul 34303, Turkey. TEL 5880873.

614.19 USA ISSN 0195-7910
RA1001
AMERICAN JOURNAL OF FORENSIC MEDICINE AND PATHOLOGY. Text in English. 1980. q. USD 245 domestic to individuals for print & online eds.; USD 311 foreign to individuals for print & online eds; USD 409 domestic to institutions for print & online eds; USD 488 foreign to institutions for print & online eds; USD 111 newsstand/cover (effective 2002). adv. bk.rev. charts, illus, stat. index. back issues avail.; reprint service avail. from PQC. *Refereed.* **Document type:** *Academic/Scholarly.* **Description:** Features original articles on new examination and documentation procedures, case reports, new devices, and medico-legal aspects.
Related titles: Microform ed.; Online - full text ed.: USD 531.70 domestic academic site license; USD 610.70 foreign academic site license; USD 593.05 domestic corporate site license; USD 672.05 foreign corporate site license (effective 2001) (from Ovid Technologies, Inc., Institute for Scientific Information).
Indexed: ASCA, Abstr.Anthropol., C.L.I., Crim.Just.Abstr., Curr.Cont., Dent.Ind., Excerp.Med., INIS Atomind., Ind.Med. (1980-), Inpharma, Int.Nurs.Ind., Leg.Per. (coverage dropped), Reac., Rev.Appl.Entomol., SSCI (coverage dropped).
—BLDSC (0824.630000), CISTI, EMDOCS, GNLM, IDS, ingenta, KNAW.
Published by: (National Association of Medical Examiners), Lippincott Williams & Wilkins (Philadelphia) (Subsidiary of: Wolters Kluwer N.V.), 530 Walnut St, Philadelphia, PA 19106-3621. TEL 215-521-8300, FAX 215-521-8902, http://www.Lww.com. Ed. Dr. Vincent J M Dimaio. Pub. Jim Merritt. R&P Margaret Becker. Adv. contact Ray Thibodeau. B&W page USD 875, color page USD 1,950. Circ: 1,806 (paid). **Subscr. to:** PO Box 1600, Hagerstown, MD 21740-1600. TEL 800-777-2295, FAX 301-824-7390.

616.8 340 USA ISSN 0163-1942
RA1151 CODEN: AFPSFZ
AMERICAN JOURNAL OF FORENSIC PSYCHIATRY. Text in English. 1978. q., latest vol.23, 2002. USD 75 in US & Canada; USD 100 elsewhere (effective 2002). bk.rev. 90 p./no. 1 cols./p. back issues avail.; reprint service avail. from WSH. *Refereed.* **Document type:** *Journal, Academic/Scholarly.* **Description:** For psychiatrists used as expert witnesses in civil and criminal court cases.
Related titles: Microfiche ed.: (from WSH); Microfilm ed.: (from WSH,PMC); Microform ed.: (from WSH).
Indexed: Abstr.Bk.Rev.Curr.Leg.Per., Psychol.Abstr. (1983-), e-psyche.
—BLDSC (0824.640000), EMDOCS, GNLM, KNAW.
Published by: American College of Forensic Psychology, PO Box 5870, Balboa Island, CA 92662. TEL 949-673-7773, FAX 949-673-7710, psychlaw@sover.net, http://www.forensicpsychiatry.cc, http://www.forensicpsychonline.com. Ed., Pub. Edward Miller. Circ: 1,000.

614.19 DEU ISSN 0570-5886
ARBEITSMETHODEN DER MEDIZINISCHEN UND NATURWISSENSCHAFTLICHEN KRIMINALISTIK. Text in German. 1962. irreg., latest vol.24, 2000. price varies. **Document type:** *Monographic series, Academic/Scholarly.*
Published by: Schmidt-Roemhild Verlag, Mengstr 16, Luebeck 23552, Germany. TEL 49-451-7031-01, FAX 49-451-7031253, msr-luebeck@t-online.de, http://www.schmidt-roemhild.de. Eds. Dr. B Brinkmann, Dr. Steffen Berg.

ARCHIVUM IMMUNOLOGIAE ET THERAPIAE EXPERIMENTALIS. see *MEDICAL SCIENCES*

614.19 364 POL ISSN 0324-8267
CODEN: AMSKA2
ARCHIWUM MEDYCYNY SADOWEJ I KRIMINOLOGII. Text in Polish. 1950. q. PLZ 40; USD 100 foreign. bk.rev. *Refereed.* **Document type:** *Monographic series, Academic/Scholarly.* **Description:** Covers forensic medicine and criminology.
Formerly (until 1966): Archiwum Medycyny Sadowej, Psychiatrii Sadowej i Kryminalistyki (0402-9178)
—CASDDS.
Published by: Polskie Towarzystwo Medycyny Sadowej i Kryminologii, Ul Grzegorzecka 16, Krakow 31531, Poland. TEL 48-12-211113, http://www.cyf~kr.edu.pl/acdemic/cmuj/medsad/med-sad.html. Ed., R&P Erazm Baran.

614.19 AUS ISSN 0045-0618
K1 CODEN: AJFSB9
AUSTRALIAN JOURNAL OF FORENSIC SCIENCES. Text in English. 1968. 2/yr. AUD 60 domestic; AUD 60 foreign (effective 2002). adv. bk.rev. cum.index: 1968-1998 in vol.30. back issues avail. *Refereed.* **Document type:** *Journal, Academic/Scholarly.* **Description:** Interdisciplinary forum on law, medicine and science.
Related titles: Online - full text ed.: (from Gale Group).
Indexed: Aus.P.A.I.S., C.L.I., Chem.Abstr., Excerp.Med., INIS Atomind., L.R.I. (Mar.1980-).
—BLDSC (1808.100000), CASDDS, EMDOCS, GNLM, ingenta.
Published by: Australian Academy of Forensic Sciences, c/o John Rowe Publishing Consultant, 359 Clovelly Rd, Clovelly, NSW 2031, Australia. TEL 61-2-96655909, FAX 61-2-96645909, jcprowe@ozemail.com.au, http://www.forensicacademy.org. Ed. David Bell. R&P, Adv. contact John Rowe. Circ: 400.

340.6 AUT ISSN 0067-5016
RA1001 CODEN: BEGMA5
BEITRAEGE ZUR GERICHTLICHEN MEDIZIN. Text in German. 1911. a. price varies. cum.index (vols. 1-20 in vol. 20; vols. 21-30 in vol. 31). back issues avail. **Document type:** *Journal, Academic/Scholarly.*
Indexed: Chem.Abstr., Chem.Indus.Notes, Chem.Titles, Dent.Ind., Excerp.Med., Ind.Med. (coverage dropped).
—CASDDS, CISTI, GNLM.
Published by: Franz Deuticke Verlag GmbH, Hegelgasse 21, Vienna, W 1015, Austria. TEL 43-1-5121544258, FAX 43-1-5121544289, info@deuticke.at, http://www.deuticke.at. Ed. W Holczobek. Circ: 250.

360 614.19 GBR ISSN 1463-6646
▼ **THE BRITISH JOURNAL OF FORENSIC PRACTICE.** Text in English. 1999. q. GBP 39 to individuals; GBP 79 to institutions. bk.rev. back issues avail. *Refereed.* **Document type:** *Bulletin, Academic/Scholarly.* **Description:** Aims at managers and practitioners responsible for delivering, commissioning, planning, and running services for people in forensic settings across all client groups.
—BLDSC (2308.330000).
Published by: (Forensic Psychiatric Nurses Association), Pavilian Publishing Ltd., 8 St George's Pl, Brighton, E Essex BN1 4GB, United Kingdom. TEL 44-1273-623222, FAX 44-1273-625526, pavpub@pavilian.co.uk, http://www.pavpub.com. Ed. Graham Towl.

614.1 ESP ISSN 1575-6793
▼ **CIENCIA FORENSE**; revista aragonesa de medicina legal. Text in Spanish. 1999. a. ESP 2,000, EUR 12.02 (effective 2001).
Published by: Institucion "Fernando el Catolico", Plaza Espana, 2, Zaragoza 50004, Spain. TEL 34-976-288878, FAX 34-976-288869, ifc@dpz.es, http://www.dpz.es/ifc/default.html.

340.6 USA ISSN 0009-7446
KF3821.A59
CITATION; current legal developments relating to medicine and allied professions. Text in English. 1958. s-m. USD 130; (Canadian $150; elsewhere $160) (effective 1998). index. **Document type:** *Newsletter.*
Indexed: I.P.A.
Published by: (Health Law Division, American Medical Association), Citation Publishing Corp., PO Box 3538 RFD, Long Grove, IL 60047. TEL 847-438-2020, FAX 847-438-2299. Ed. Sheri Thomsen. Pub. Dean E Snyder. Circ: 1,000.

614.1 USA
COMPOSITE ART MANUAL. Text in English. irreg. USD 15 (effective 2002). **Document type:** *Journal, Academic/Scholarly.*

Published by: International Association for Identification, c/o Joseph Polski, 2535 Pilot Knob Rd, Ste 117, Mendota Heights, MN 55120-1120. TEL 651-681-8566, FAX 651-681-8443, iaisecty@theiai.org, http://www.theiai.org/.

614.1 USA
COURTROOM MEDICINE SERIES: DEATH. Text in English. 1966. irreg. (in 3 vols.). USD 680 (effective 1999).
Published by: Matthew Bender & Co., Inc. (Subsidiary of: Lexis Law Publishing), 2 Park Ave, New York, NY 10016. TEL 212-448-2000, international@bender.com, http://www.bender.com. Eds. Irwin Hauts, Marshall Houts.

CRIMINALIST'S SOURCE BOOK. see *CRIMINOLOGY AND LAW ENFORCEMENT—Abstracting, Bibliographies, Statistics*

EXCERPTA MEDICA. SECTION 49: FORENSIC SCIENCE ABSTRACTS. see *MEDICAL SCIENCES—Abstracting, Bibliographies, Statistics*

THE EXPERT AND THE LAW. see *LAW*

FINGERPRINT WORLD. see *CRIMINOLOGY AND LAW ENFORCEMENT*

614.19 DEU ISSN 0724-844X
FORENSIA; interdisziplinaere Jahrbuch fuer Psychiatrie, Psychologie, Kriminologie und Recht. Text in German. 1983 (vol.4). a. reprint service avail. from ISI. **Document type:** *Monographic series.*
Related titles: Microform ed.: (from PQC).
Indexed: Excerp.Med., IBR.
—GNLM, Infotrieve. **CCC.**
Published by: (Gesellschaft Oesterreichischer Nervenaerzte und Psychiater), Springer-Verlag (Subsidiary of: BertelsmannSpringer), Haber Str 7, Heidelberg 69126, Germany. FAX 49-30-82787448, subscriptions@springer.de, http://www.springer.de, http://link.springer-ny.com. Ed. G Harrer.

347.066 USA
FORENSIC ACCIDENT INVESTIGATION: MOTOR VEHICLES. Text in English. base vol. plus a. updates. USD 95. Supplement avail. **Description:** Explains the physical laws underlying motor vehicle accident reconstruction and the way to present physical evidence most effectively.
Published by: Lexis Law Publishing (Subsidiary of: Reed Elsevier plc), PO Box 7587, Charlottesville, VA 22906-7587. TEL 804-972-7600, 800-562-1197, FAX 804-972-7666, llp.customer.support@lexis-nexis.com, http://www.lexislawpublishing.com. Eds. Arthur C Damask, Thomas L Bohan.

FORENSIC DRUG ABUSE ADVISOR; a monthly digest of information on the forensic aspects of drug abuse. see *DRUG ABUSE AND ALCOHOLISM*

614.19 USA ISSN 1084-5569
FORENSIC EXAMINER. Text in English. 1993. bi-m. USD 100 domestic; USD 125 foreign (effective 2000). adv. bk.rev. back issues avail. *Refereed.* **Document type:** *Trade.* **Description:** Includes scientific articles, case studies, and new research in the areas of forensic examination.
Published by: American College of Forensic Examiners, 2750 E Sunshine, Springfield, MO 65804. TEL 417-881-3818, 800-423-9737, FAX 417-881-4702, editor@acfe.com; orders@allenpress.com, http://www.acfe.com; http://www.allenpress.com. Ed., Adv. contact Daphne Greenlee. Pub. Robert O'Block. Circ: 13,000. **Subscr. to:** Allen Press Inc., PO Box 1897, Lawrence, KS 66044-8897.

614.1 USA
▼ **FORENSIC MEDICINE SOURCEBOOK.** Text in English. 1999 (May). irreg., latest vol.1. USD 78 per issue (effective 2001). charts. master index. **Description:** Contains basic information for the Layperson about forensic medicine, including crime scene investigation, evidence collection and analysis, expert testimony, accident reconstruction, autopsies, ballistics, craniofacial identification, fingerprinting, DNA profiling, handwriting analysis, and establishing paternity, along with statistical data, a glossary, and listings of sources for further help and information.
Published by: Omnigraphics, Inc., 615 Griswold St, Detroit, MI 48226. TEL 313-961-1340, 800-234-1340, 800-234-1340, FAX 313-961-1383, info@omnigraphics.com, http://www.omnigraphics.com. Ed. Annemarie S Muth.

614.1 USA
▼ **FORENSIC NURSE.** Text in English. 2001. m. USD 19.95 (effective 2002). adv. **Document type:** *Magazine, Trade.* **Description:** Reports on important trend and news on the topic of frensic science, provideing a forum for the exchange of ideas, insights and information pertinent to professionals in all forensic nursing specialties: Clinical, psychiatric, corrections and legal.
Published by: Virgo Publishing, Inc., 3300 N Central Ave, Ste 2500, Phoenix, AZ 85012. TEL 480-990-1101, FAX 480-990-0819, kpyrek@vpico.com, virgopub@vpico.com, http://www.forensicnursemag.com, http://www.vpico.com. Ed. Kelly M Pyrek. adv.: B&W page USD 2,025, color page USD 3,325; trim 8.125 x 10.875. Circ: 8,000 (paid and controlled).

614.19 USA
▼ **FORENSIC SCIENCE AND MEDICINE.** Text in English. 2000. irreg. price varies. illus. back issues avail. *Refereed.* **Document type:** *Monographic series, Academic/Scholarly.* **Description:** Focuses on topics of vital interest to a wide range of forensic specialists, including those in forensic sciences, toxicology, pathology, medicine, and law and police administration.
Published by: Humana Press Inc., 999 Riverview Dr, Ste 208, Totowa, NJ 07512. TEL 973-256-1699, FAX 973-256-8341, humana@humanapr.com, http://humanapress.com. Ed. Steven Karch. R&P Wendy A Warren.

363.2 IRL ISSN 0379-0738
RA1001 CODEN: FSINDR
FORENSIC SCIENCE INTERNATIONAL; an international journal dedicated to the applications of science to the administration of justice. Text in English. 1972. 24/yr. NLG 3,675, EUR 1,667.64 in Europe to institutions; JPY 230,900 in Japan to institutions; USD 1,865 elsewhere to institutions; NLG 3,872, EUR 1,757.04 in Europe to institutions combined with Legal Medicine; JPY 243,800 in Japan to institutions combined with Legal Medicine; USD 1,965 elsewhere to institutions combined with Legal Medicine (effective 2001). charts, illus. back issues avail.; reprint service avail. from WSH. *Refereed.* **Document type:** *Academic/Scholarly.* **Description:** Publishes original contributions in the many different scientific disciplines pertaining to the forensic sciences.
Former titles (until vol.13, no.1, 1979): Forensic Science (0300-9432); Journal of Forensic Medicine (0022-1171)
Related titles: Microform ed.: (from PQC); Online - full text ed.: (from ingenta, Gale Group, Swets Blackwell, ScienceDirect, Institute for Scientific Information).
Indexed: ASCA, Abstr.Anthropol., Abstr.Crim.& Pen., Anal.Abstr., Biol.Abstr., C.L.I., Cal.Tiss.Abstr., Chem.Abstr., Chem.Indus.Notes, Chem.Titles, Crim.Just.Abstr., Curr.Cont., Dent.Ind., Environ.Sci.Poll.Mgmt., Excerp.Med., GeoRef, HRIS, Hlth.Ind., Ind.Med. (1978-), Ind.Sci.Rev., Inpharma, L.R.I. (Jan.1980-), Leg.Per. (coverage dropped), Mass Spectr.Bull., Nutr.Abstr., Pollut.Abstr., Reac., Rev.Appl.Entomol., Rev.Med.& Vet.Mycol., Risk Abstr., Russ.Acad.Sci.Bibl., SSCI (coverage dropped), Saf.Sci.Abstr., Sci.Cit.Ind., Tox.Abstr., Weed Abstr.
—BLDSC (3987.764000), CASDDS, CISTI, EMDOCS, GNLM, IDS, Infotrieve, ingenta. **CCC.**
Published by: Elsevier Science Ireland Ltd, Elsevier House, Brookvale Plaza, E. Park, Shannon, Co. Clare, Ireland. TEL 353-61-471944, FAX 353-61-472144, http://www.elsevier.com/locate/forsciint. Ed. B Knight. R&P Annette Moloney. **Subscr. in Australasia and the Far East to:** Elsevier Science (Singapore) Pte Ltd, No.1 Temasek Ave, 17-01 Millenia Tower, Singapore 039192, Singapore. TEL 65-434-3727, FAX 65-337-2230; **Subscr. in the Americas to:** Elsevier Science, PO Box 945, New York, NY 10159-0945. TEL 212-633-3730, FAX 212-633-3680, usinfo-f@elsevier.com; **Subscr. to:** Elsevier Science BV, PO Box 211, Amsterdam 1000 AE, Netherlands. TEL 31-20-485-3757.

614.19 USA ISSN 0930-1461
HV8073 CODEN: FSPRE7
FORENSIC SCIENCE PROGRESS. Text in English. 1986. irreg., latest vol.6, 1991. price varies. reprints avail. **Document type:** *Academic/Scholarly.*
Indexed: Chem.Abstr., Chem.Indus.Notes, Chem.Titles.
—CASDDS, Linda Hall.
Published by: Springer-Verlag, Journals (Subsidiary of: BertelsmannSpringer), 175 Fifth Ave, New York, NY 10010. TEL 212-460-1550, FAX 212-473-6272.

614.19 USA
FORENSIC SCIENCES. Text in English. 1981. irreg. (in 5 vols.). USD 680 (effective 1999).
Published by: Matthew Bender & Co., Inc. (Subsidiary of: Lexis Law Publishing), 2 Park Ave, New York, NY 10016. TEL 212-448-2000, international@bender.com, http://www.bender.com. Ed. Cyril Wacht.

FORENSIC SERVICES DIRECTORY; national register of experts, engineers, scientific advisors, medical specialists, technical consultants and sources of specialized knowledge. see *LAW*

340.6 CAN ISSN 0226-8841
KE3646.A13
HEALTH LAW IN CANADA. Text in English. 1980. q. CND 200 (effective 2001). **Document type:** *Trade.* **Description:** Covers all major aspects of Canadian health law.
Related titles: Online - full text ed.: (from Gale Group).
Indexed: C.L.I., Hlth.Ind., Ind.Can.L.P.L., L.R.I. (Jan.1981-).
—BLDSC (4275.016174), CISTI, ingenta. **CCC.**
Published by: Butterworths Canada Ltd., Part of the Reed Elsevier group, 75 Clegg Rd, Markham, ON L6G 1A1, Canada. TEL 905-479-2665, FAX 905-479-2826, http://www.lexisnexis.ca/healthlawincanada.htm. Ed. Gilbert Sharpe.

614.19 JPN ISSN 0289-0755
HOIGAKU NO JISSAI TO KENKYU/RESEARCH AND PRACTICE IN FORENSIC MEDICINE. Text in English, Japanese; Summaries in English. 1954. a. JPY 4,000 to individuals; JPY 5,000 to institutions. back issues avail. **Document type:** *Academic/Scholarly.*
—BLDSC (7715.695000). **CCC.**
Published by: Tohoku Daigaku, Igakubu Hoigaku Danwakai/Tohoku University, School of Medicine, Department of Forensic Medicine, Sendai-shi, Miyagi-ken 980, Japan. TEL 81-22-717-8110, FAX 81-22-717-8112, sagisaka@forensic.med.tohoku.ac.jp. Ed. Kaoru Sagisaka. Circ: 1,000.

340.6 USA
INFORM QUARTERLY NEWSLETTER. Text in English. 1969. q. USD 25. bibl.
Formerly: Inform - Letter (0019-9702)
Indexed: Excerp.Med.
Published by: International Reference Organization in Forensic Medicine & Sciences, PO Box 8282, Wichita, KS 67208. TEL 316-685-7612. Circ: 1,500.

INFORMATION EXCHANGE. see *MEDICAL SCIENCES—Pediatrics*

614.19 345 364 COL ISSN 0120-0097
RA1001 CODEN: RINCDD
INSTITUTO NACIONAL DE MEDICINA LEGAL DE COLOMBIA. REVISTA. Text in Spanish. 1975. a. COP 9,500 (effective 2001). bk.rev. *Refereed.* **Document type:** *Magazine, Academic/Scholarly.* **Description:** Contains scientific and technical information on legal medicine, forensic sciences, criminology, medical liability, violence, and other related topics for forensic experts, lawyers, law enforcement and judicial authorities.
Indexed: Excerp.Med.
—CASDDS.
Published by: Instituto Nacional de Medicina Legal y Ciencias Forenses, Division de Normalizacion y Certificacion Forense, Calle 7A No. 12-61, Bogota, CUND, Colombia. TEL 57-1-2339883, FAX 57-1-2338534, im12@gaitana.interred.net.co, http://www.medicinalegui.gov.co. Ed. Ricardo Mora Izquierdo. Pub., R&P Ana Maria Berenguer. Circ: 2,000.

340.6 BEL ISSN 0074-1248
INTERNATIONAL ACADEMY OF LEGAL MEDICINE AND SOCIAL MEDICINE. CONGRESS REPORTS. Text in English. triennial, latest 1994, 16th, Strasbourg. **Document type:** *Proceedings.*
Published by: University of Turku, c/o Professor Pekka Saukko, Dept of Forensic Medicine, Turku 20520, Finland. TEL 32-87-229821.

614.19 BEL ISSN 1016-829X
INTERNATIONAL ACADEMY OF LEGAL MEDICINE AND SOCIAL MEDICINE. NEWSLETTER. Text in English. 3/yr. free per issue. bk.rev. **Document type:** *Newsletter.*
Published by: University of Turku, c/o Professor Pekka Saukko, Dept of Forensic Medicine, Turku 20520, Finland. TEL 32-87-229821.

614.19 DEU ISSN 0937-9827
RA1001 CODEN: IJLMEA
INTERNATIONAL JOURNAL OF LEGAL MEDICINE. Text in English. 1922. bi-m. EUR 846.20 domestic; EUR 860.40 in Germany; EUR 170 newsstand/cover foreign (effective 2002). adv. illus. index. back issues avail.; reprint service avail. from ISI. *Refereed.* **Document type:** *Journal, Academic/Scholarly.* **Description:** Provides research articles in the areas of forensic pathology, clinical forensic pathology, forensic hemogenetics and stain identification, forensic toxicology, and traffic medicine.

M

Former titles (until 1992): Zeitschrift fuer Rechtsmedizin - Journal of Legal Medicine (0044-3433); Deutsche Zeitschrift fuer die Gesamte Gerichtliche Medizin
Related titles: Microform ed.: (from PQC); Online - full text ed.: ISSN 1437-1596 (from EBSCO Publishing, RoweCom Information Quest, Swets Blackwell, Springer LINK, Institute for Scientific Information).
Indexed: ASCA, Biol.Abstr., C.L.I., Chem.Abstr., Curr.Cont., Excerp.Med., Ind.Med. (1990-), Ind.Sci.Rev., Inpharma, L.R.I., Leg.Per. (coverage dropped), Pharm.&Out.News, Reac., Rev.Appl.Entomol., SSCI (coverage dropped), Sci.Cit.Ind., Weed Abstr.
—BLDSC (4542.315500), CASDDS, CISTI, EMDOCS, GNLM, IDS, Infotrieve, KNAW. **CCC.**
Published by: (International Academy of Legal Medicine), Springer-Verlag (Subsidiary of: BertelsmannSpringer), Haber Str 7, Heidelberg 69126, Germany. subscriptions@springer.de, http://link.springer.de/link/service/journals/00414/index.htm. Ed. B Brinkmann. **Subscr. in N. America to:** Springer-Verlag New York Inc., PO Box 2485, Secaucus, NJ 07096-2485. TEL 212-460-1500, FAX 212-473-6272.

INTERNATIONAL SYMPOSIUM ON FINGERPRINT DETECTION AND IDENTIFICATION. PROCEEDINGS. see *CRIMINOLOGY AND LAW ENFORCEMENT*

614.1 USA ISSN 1528-8250
▼ **THE INTERNET JOURNAL OF LAW, HEALTHCARE AND ETHICS.** Text in English. 2000. s-a. free. adv. bk.rev. back issues avail. *Refereed.* **Document type:** *Academic/Scholarly.* **Description:** Contains information from the field of medical legal issues and ethics in healthcare. Original articles, reviews, case reports, streaming slid shows, streaming videos, letters to the editor, press releases, meeting information.
Media: Online - full content.
Published by: Internet Scientific Publications, L.L.C., 23 Rippling Creek Dr, Sugar Land, TX 77479. TEL 281-240-1533, FAX 281-240-1533, http://www.ispub.com/journals/ijlhe.htm. Ed. Lee Parmlee. R&P, Adv. contact Hope Morrow TEL 832-754-0335.

614.1 JPN ISSN 0915-9606
CODEN: HOCHE8
JAPANESE JOURNAL OF FORENSIC TOXICOLOGY/HO CHUDOKU. Text in English, Japanese. 1983. 3/yr. JPY 5,000. adv. **Document type:** *Proceedings, Academic/Scholarly.*
Indexed: Chem.Abstr., Chem.Indus.Notes, Chem.Titles, Excerp.Med. (1993-), Int.Abstr.Biol.Sci., Mass Spectr.Bull.
—BLDSC (4651.955000), CASDDS, EMDOCS, GNLM, KNAW.
Published by: (Hamamatsu University School of Medicine, Department of Legal Medicine), Japanese Association of Forensic Toxicology (JAFT Bureau)/Nihon Ho Chudoku Gakkai, Hokuriku University, Faculty of Pharmaceutical Sciences, Department of Hygienic Chemistry, Kanagawa-machi, Kanazawa 920-1181, Japan. TEL 81-76-229-1165, FAX 81-76-229-2781, houigaku@akiha.hama_med.ac.jp. Ed. Osamu Suzuki. Circ: 500.

614.19 JPN ISSN 0047-1887
CODEN: NHOZAX
JAPANESE JOURNAL OF LEGAL MEDICINE/NIPPON HOIGAKU ZASSHI. Abstracts and contents page in English. 1944. bi-m. USD 49.50. illus. Supplement avail.
Indexed: Chem.Abstr., Chem.Indus.Notes, Chem.Titles, Dent.Ind., Excerp.Med., INIS Atomind., Ind.Med. (1944-), Mass Spectr.Bull.
—BLDSC (4655.850000), CASDDS, CISTI, GNLM, KNAW.
Published by: Medico-Legal Society of Japan/Nihon Hoi Gakkai, Faculty of Medicine, University of, 7-3-1 Hongo, Bunkyo-ku, Tokyo 113-0033, Japan. **Subscr. to:** Japan Publications Trading Co. Ltd., Tokyo International, PO Box 5030, Tokyo 100-31, Japan.

614.19 364 GBR ISSN 1353-1131
CODEN: JCFMEA
JOURNAL OF CLINICAL FORENSIC MEDICINE. Text in English. 1972. q. GBP 104 to individuals; GBP 211 to institutions (effective 2002). adv. bk.rev. **Document type:** *Academic/Scholarly.* **Description:** Provides a forum for the rapid publication of topical articles on the clinical aspects of forensic medical work.
Formerly (until 1994): Police Surgeon (0308-0242)
Related titles: Online - full text ed.: (from Swets Blackwell, IDEAL Online Library).
Indexed: Cal.Tiss.Abstr., Environ.Sci.Poll.Mgmt., IBZ, Pollut.Abstr., Risk Abstr., Saf.Sci.Abstr.
—BLDSC (4958.460000), CISTI, EMDOCS, GNLM, Infotrieve, KNAW. **CCC.**
Published by: (Association of Police Surgeons), Churchill Livingstone (Subsidiary of: Harcourt Publishers Ltd.), Robert Stevenson House, 1-3 Baxter's Pl, Leith Walk, Edinburgh, Midlothian EH1 3AF, United Kingdom. TEL 44-131-556-2424, FAX 44-131-459-1177, cservice@harcourt.com, http://www.harcourt-international.com/journals/jcfm. Ed. Jason Payne James. Adv. contact David Dunnachie. **Subscr. to:** Harcourt Publishers Ltd., Foots Cray High St, Sidcup, Kent DA14 5HP, United Kingdom. TEL 44-20-8308-5700, FAX 44-20-8309-0807.

JOURNAL OF EVIDENCE PHOTOGRAPHY. see *PHOTOGRAPHY*

614.19 USA ISSN 0895-173X
HV8073 CODEN: JFIDFK
JOURNAL OF FORENSIC IDENTIFICATION. Text in English. 1960. bi-m. USD 90 in North America to membership to individuals; USD 110 in North America to membership to institutions & libraries; USD 130 elsewhere (effective 2002). Index. 115 p./no. *Refereed.* **Document type:** *Journal, Academic/Scholarly.* **Description:** Devoted to the publication of information about forensic identification in its various disciplines, including document examination, imprint evidence, polygraph examination, crime scene investigation, forensic reconstruction, blood stain pattern identification, and other pertinent subjects.
Formerly (until 1987): Identification News (0019-1450)
Related titles: Online - full text ed.: (from Northern Light Technology, Inc., ProQuest Information & Learning).
Indexed: CJPI, Excerp.Med. (1996-).
—BLDSC (4984.588000), EMDOCS.
Published by: International Association for Identification, c/o Joseph Polski, 2535 Pilot Knob Rd, Ste 117, Mendota Heights, MN 55120-1120. TEL 651-681-8566, FAX 651-681-8443, iaisecty@theiai.org, http://www.theiai.org/. Ed. Alan McRoberts. Circ: 3,800 (paid).

614.19 CHN ISSN 1004-5619
JOURNAL OF FORENSIC MEDICINE/FAYIXUE ZAZHI. Text in Chinese; Summaries in English. 1985. q. USD 55 (effective 2001). adv. bk.rev. 64 p./no. reprint service avail. from WSH. *Refereed.* **Document type:** *Journal, Academic/Scholarly.* **Description:** Publishes original contributions in the fields of forensic pathology, histochemistry, serology, toxicology, odontology, psychiatry and anthropology.
Indexed: Ind.Med. (1985-).
—BLDSC (4984.591000).
Published by: Ministry of Justice, Institute of Forensic Sciences, 1347 West Guangfu Rd, Shanghai 200063, China. TEL 86-21-2440148, FAX 86-21-2442691, fyxzz@online.sh.cn. Ed. Yu-Chang Gong. adv.: B&W page USD 300, color page USD 600. Circ: 5,000 (paid).

JOURNAL OF FORENSIC PSYCHIATRY. see *MEDICAL SCIENCES—Psychiatry And Neurology*

340.6 614.19 USA ISSN 0022-1198
RA1001 CODEN: JFSCAS
JOURNAL OF FORENSIC SCIENCES. Text in English. 1956. bi-m. USD 249 in North America; USD 274 elsewhere (effective 2001). adv. bk.rev. charts, illus. index. reprint service avail. from PQC,WSH. *Refereed.* **Document type:** *Academic/Scholarly.*
Supersedes: What's New in Forensic Sciences (0511-8662)
Related titles: Microform ed.: (from PQC); Online - full text ed.: (from ProQuest Information & Learning, Institute for Scientific Information).
Indexed: ASCA, Abstr.Anthropol., Abstr.Bk.Rev.Curr.Leg.Per., Abstr.Bull.Inst.Pap.Chem., Abstr.Crim.& Pen., Anal.Abstr., Art & Archaeol.Tech.Abstr., Biol.Abstr., CJPI, C.L.I., Chem.Abstr., Chem.Cit.Ind., Chem.Indus.Notes, Chem.Titles, Compumath, Crim.Just.Abstr., Curr.Cont., Dent.Ind., Excerp.Med., HRIS, Hlth.Ind., INIS Atomind., Ind.Med. (1956-), Ind.Sci.Rev., Inpharma, L.R.I. (Jan.1980-Nov.1995), Lab.Haz.Bull., Leg.Per. (coverage dropped), Mass Spectr.Bull., Pharm.&Out.News, Protozool.Abstr., PsycInfo, Psychol.Abstr. (1989-), Reac., Rev.Appl.Entomol., Rev.Med.& Vet.Mycol., Russ.Acad.Sci.Bibl., SSCI (coverage dropped), Sci.Cit.Ind., Soils & Fert., THA, W.R.C.Inf., Wild.Rev., Zoo.Rec., e-psyche.
—BLDSC (4984.600000), CASDDS, CISTI, GNLM, IDS, ingenta, KNAW, Linda Hall. **CCC.**
Published by: American Academy of Forensic Sciences, PO Box 669, Colorado Springs, CO 80901. TEL 719-636-1100, FAX 719-636-1993, http://www.aafs.org. Ed. R E Gaensslen. Circ: 4,200. **Subscr. to:** American Society for Testing and Materials. http://www.astm.org.

610 USA ISSN 1081-5589
R11 CODEN: JINVFI
JOURNAL OF INVESTIGATIVE MEDICINE. Text in English. 1953. bi-m. USD 204 domestic to individuals; USD 256 foreign to individuals; USD 237 domestic to institutions; USD 274 foreign to institutions (2002). adv. abstr, illus. index. *Refereed.* **Description:** Publishes original articles and reviews of broad interest to academic physicians and scientists.
Formerly (until Dec. 1994): Clinical Research (0009-9279)
Related titles: Microform ed.: (from PQC); Online - full text ed.: (from Northern Light Technology, Inc., ProQuest Information & Learning, Institute for Scientific Information).
Indexed: ASCA, Agri.& Environ.Biotech.Abstr. (coverage dropped), Biol.Abstr., Chem.Abstr., Curr.Adv.Ecol.Sci., Curr.Cont., Derwent Biotech.Abstr., Diar.Dis.Res., Excerp.Med., Helminthol.Abstr., Ind.Med. (1994-), Ind.Sci.Rev., Inpharma, Med.& Surg.Dermat., NRN, Neurosci.Cit.Ind., Nutr.Abstr., Pharm.&Out.News, Reac., Risk Abstr., SSCI (coverage dropped), Sci.Cit.Ind., THA, Telegen.
—BLDSC (5008.010000), CISTI, GNLM, IDS, ingenta, KNAW.
Published by: (American Federation for Clinical Research), Slack, Inc., 6900 Grove Rd, Thorofare, NJ 08086-9447. TEL 856-848-1000, 800-257-8290, FAX 856-853-5991, http://www.slackinc.com. Eds. Dr. Barbara Hempstead, Dr. Jonathan Weissler. Circ: 11,675.

347.006 USA ISSN 1533-2608
▼ **JOURNAL OF THREAT ASSESSMENT.** Text in English. 2001. q. USD 60 domestic to individuals; USD 81 in Canada to individuals; USD 87 elsewhere to individuals; USD 95 domestic to institutions; USD 128 in Canada to institutions; USD 138 elsewhere to institutions; USD 125 domestic to libraries; USD 169 in Canada to libraries; USD 181 elsewhere to libraries (effective Aug. 2001). adv. **Document type:** *Journal, Academic/Scholarly.* **Description:** Offers information on the assessment and management of threats in relation to forensic psychology.
Published by: Haworth Press, Inc., 10 Alice St, Binghamton, NY 13904-1580. TEL 607-722-5857, 800-429-6784, FAX 607-722-6362, 800-895-0582, http://www.haworthpress.com/journals/journallist.asp. Ed. Joseph T McCann. Pub. William Cohen. adv.: B&W page USD 315, color page USD 550; trim 6 x 8.5.

614 340 ITA ISSN 0394-8218
CODEN: JUMEE
JURA MEDICA; rivista di medicina legale. Text in Italian. 1988. 3/yr. ITL 120,000; ITL 150,000 foreign (effective 1997). bk.rev. **Document type:** *Academic/Scholarly.* **Description:** Presents updates of legal guidelines in the medical field.
Indexed: Excerp.Med. (1995-).
—BLDSC (5075.552400).
Published by: Edizioni Colosseum, Viale Delle Milizie, 52, Rome, RM 00192, Italy. TEL 39-6-3722050, FAX 39-6-3721238. Ed. Giancarlo Umani Ronchi.

614.19 JPN ISSN 0285-7960
HV6005 CODEN: KKHKA9
KAGAKU KEISATSU KENKYUJO HOKOKU HOKAGAKU HEN/NATIONAL RESEARCH INSTITUTE OF POLICE SCIENCE. REPORT. RESEARCH OF FORENSIC SCIENCE. Text in Japanese; Summaries in English. 1948. s-a. **Document type:** *Academic/Scholarly.*
Formerly: National Research Institute of Police Science. Report (0451-1980)
Indexed: Crim.Just.Abstr., INIS Atomind., Psychol.Abstr.
—BLDSC (7570.222600).
Published by: Kagaku Keisatsu Kenkyujo/National Research Institute of Police Science, 6 Sanban-cho, Chiyoda-ku, Tokyo 102-0075, Japan. TEL 81-3-3261-9986, FAX 81-3-3221-1245. Ed. Taizo Nagano. Circ: 1,000.

616 CHE ISSN 1019-4231
LABOLIFE. Text in English, French, German, Italian. 1992. 6/yr. CHF 30; CHF 50 foreign (effective 1999). adv. bk.rev. **Document type:** *Academic/Scholarly.* **Description:** Covers laboratory medicine, including clinical chemistry, hematology, microbiology, immunology and endocrinology.
Indexed: Ref.Zh.
—GNLM, KNAW.
Published by: Labolife Verlagsgemeinschaft, Postfach 415, Rotkreuz 6343, Switzerland. TEL 41-41-7904860, FAX 41-41-7905323, verlag@labolife.ch. Ed. Peter Hagemann. Pub. Rolf Rueegg. R&P Prisca Rueegg. Adv. contact Prisca Rueegg. Circ: 4,000.

LEBENSMITTELCHEMIE; Zeitschrift des Lebensmittelchemischen Gesellschaft. see *FOOD AND FOOD INDUSTRIES*

M

LEGAL AND CRIMINOLOGICAL PSYCHOLOGY. see *PSYCHOLOGY*

614.190971 USA ISSN 0703-1211
LEGAL MEDICAL QUARTERLY. Text in English. 1977. bi-m. USD 135 (effective 2001). adv. back issues avail.; reprint service avail. from WSH. **Document type:** *Academic/Scholarly.* **Description:** Publishes articles of concern to attorneys, judges, doctors, psychiatrists, mental health care professionals and veterinarians.
Indexed: CINAHL, C.L.I., I.P.A., Ind.Can.L.P.L., L.R.I. (Jan.1980-Jan.1986), Leg.Per. (coverage dropped).
Published by: Jonah Publications, 554 Pleasant St, New Bedford, MA 02740-6236. TEL 508-994-5515, FAX 508-994-1119, editor@jonahlaw.com, http://www.jonahlaw.com. Ed., Pub., Adv. contact David A Silverman.

614.1 NLD ISSN 1344-6223
▼ **LEGAL MEDICINE.** Text in English. 1999. q. EUR 191 in Europe to institutions; JPY 25,300 in Japan to institutions; USD 213 elsewhere to institutions (effective 2002). **Description:** Provides an international forum for publication of original articles, reviews and correspondence on subjects that cover practical and theoretical areas of interest relating to the wide range of legal medicine.
Related titles: Online - full text ed.: (from ScienceDirect).
Indexed: Tox.Abstr.
—BLDSC (5181.329970).
Published by: (Japanese Society of Legal Medicine JPN), Elsevier Science BV, Sara Burgerhartstraat 25, Amsterdam 1055 KV, Netherlands. TEL 31-20-485-2911, FAX 31-20-485-2457, nlinfo-f@elsevier.nl, http://www.elsevier.com/locate/legalmed, http://www.elsevier.nl. Eds. A Takatsu, H Takizawa.

614 363.2 FRA ISSN 1246-7391
CODEN: MEDRFT
MEDECINE ET DROIT; information ethique et juridique du pracicien. Text in French. 1993. bi-m. EUR 117 in Europe to institutions; USD 144 elsewhere to institutions (effective 2002). reprints avail. *Refereed.* **Document type:** *Academic/Scholarly.* **Description:** Examines issues in bioethics, philosophical ethics, and professional duties and responsibilities common to professionals in both medicine and the law.
Related titles: Microform ed.: (from PQC); Online - full text ed.: (from ingenta, ScienceDirect, Swets Blackwell).
—EMDOCS.
Published by: Elsevier Paris, Editions Scientifiques et Medicales (Subsidiary of: Reed Elsevier plc. group), 23 rue Linois, Paris 75015, France. TEL 33-1-71724500, FAX 33-1-71724664, m&d@elsevier.fr, http://www.elsevier.com/locate/meddro. Eds. F Lesaulnier, P Biclet.

340.6 614.19 IND ISSN 0047-6536
MEDICAL NEWS, MEDICINE AND LAW. Text in English. 1970. m. INR 15, USD 7.50. bk.rev.
Related titles: Microfilm ed.: (from PQC).
Published by: Joshi Hospital, 778 Shivajinagar, Pune, Maharashtra 411 004, India. Ed. Dr. L B Joshi. Circ: 2,500.

MEDICINE AND LAW; an international journal. see *LAW*

614.19 GBR ISSN 0025-8024
K13 CODEN: MDSLA6
MEDICINE, SCIENCE AND THE LAW. Text in English. 1960. q. GBP 64 domestic; GBP 75 overseas (effective 1999). adv. bk.rev. reprint service avail. from WSH. *Refereed.* **Document type:** *Academic/Scholarly.* **Description:** Publishes original contributions on topics in the forensic sciences and medicolegal issues.
Related titles: Online - full text ed.: (from Institute for Scientific Information).
Indexed: ASCA, Abstr.Crim.& Pen., Adol.Ment.Hlth.Abstr., AgeLine, Anal.Abstr., Biol.Abstr., C.I.S. Abstr., C.L.I., Chem.Abstr., Crim.Just.Abstr., Curr.Adv.Ecol.Sci., Curr.Cont., Dent.Ind., Euro.LJI, Excerp.Med., Fam.Ind., HRIS, Hlth.Ind., Ind.Med. (1960-), Ind.Sci.Rev., Inpharma, LJI, L.R.I. (Jan.1980-Oct.1995), Leg.Per. (coverage dropped), Nutr.Abstr., P C I, Pharm.&Out.News, Reac., Risk Abstr., SSCI, Sci.Cit.Ind., Weed Abstr.
—BLDSC (5534.100000), CASDDS, CISTI, GNLM, ingenta, KNAW. **CCC.**
Published by: (British Academy of Forensic Science), Chiltern Publishing, 34 Aylesbury End, Beaconsfield, Bucks HP9 1LW, United Kingdom. TEL 44-1494-678914, FAX 44-1494-678914, chipub@globalnet.co.uk. Ed. Hazel Powell. Circ: 1,600.

614.19 IRL ISSN 1393-1792
K13
MEDICO-LEGAL JOURNAL OF IRELAND. Text in English. 1995. 2/yr. IEP 95, EUR 120.61 in the European Union; IEP 120 rest of world (effective 2000). back issues avail. **Document type:** *Academic/Scholarly, Trade.* **Description:** Aims to inform concerned professionals of current scientific and clinical research in forensic medicine, and of current legal and ethical issues related to patient care and the health services.
—BLDSC (5534.201500).
Published by: Round Hall Sweet & Maxwell, 4 Upper Ormond Quay, Dublin 7, Ireland. TEL 353-1-8730101, FAX 353-1-8720078. Ed. Denis Cusack.

340.6 LKA
MEDICO-LEGAL SOCIETY OF SRI LANKA. PROCEEDINGS. Text in English. irreg. **Document type:** *Proceedings.*
Published by: Medico-Legal Society of Sri Lanka, 111 Francis Rd., Colombo 10, Sri Lanka.

614.19 DEU ISSN 0723-8886
KK6206.A13
MEDIZINRECHT. Variant title: MedR. Text in German. 1983. m. EUR 518; EUR 51.80 newsstand/cover (effective 2002). adv. *Refereed.* **Document type:** *Journal, Academic/Scholarly.* **Description:** Covers legal issues for physicians and judges.
Formerly: Med R-Medizinrecht
Related titles: Online - full text ed.: ISSN 1433-8629 (from EBSCO Publishing, RoweCom Information Quest, Swets Blackwell, Springer LINK).
Indexed: INIS Atomind.
—GNLM, Infotrieve. **CCC.**
Published by: (Deutsche Gesellschaft fuer Medizinrecht), Springer-Verlag (Subsidiary of: BertelsmannSpringer), Tiergartenstr 17, Heidelberg 69121, Germany. TEL 49-6221-345-0, FAX 49-6221-345229, subscriptions@springer.de, http://link.springer.de/link/service/journals/00350/index.htm, http://www.springer.de. Eds. A Laufs, H.-J Rieger. adv.: B&W page DEM 1,740, color page DEM 3,480; trim 186 x 260. **Subscr. in N. America to:** Springer-Verlag New York Inc., PO Box 2485, Secaucus, NJ 07096-2485. TEL 212-460-1500, FAX 212-473-6272. **Co-publisher:** Verlag C.H. Beck.

340.6 ITA ISSN 0026-4849
HV6004
MINERVA MEDICOLEGALE; archivio di antropologia criminale. Text in Italian; Summaries in English, Italian. 1880. q. USD 105 to individuals; USD 155 to institutions (effective 2000 - 2001). adv. bk.rev. bibl, charts, illus. index. **Document type:** *Academic/Scholarly.* **Description:** Covers forensic medicine, criminal anthropology and insurance medicine.
Related titles: Microform ed.: (from PQC).
Indexed: C.I.S. Abstr., Chem.Abstr., Excerp.Med., Ind.Med. (coverage dropped).
—CISTI, GNLM.
Published by: Edizioni Minerva Medica, Corso Bramante, 83-85, Turin, TO 10126, Italy. TEL 39-11-678282, FAX 39-11-674502. Ed. P L Baima Bollone. Pub. Alberto Oliaro. Adv. contact F Filippo. B&W page USD 1,200, color page USD 2,000; trim 270 x 190. Circ: 2,000 (paid).

614.19 NLD ISSN 0927-2216
MODUS✶ ; tijdschrift voor recherche en forensische wetenschappen. Text in Dutch. 1992. 6/yr. NLG 149 (effective 2001). adv. illus. **Document type:** *Trade.* **Description:** Covers current issues, technical developments and other topics relating to forensic sciences.
Incorporates (1982-1992): Nederlands Forensisch Tijdschrift (0920-363X)
—KNAW.
Published by: Uitgeverijten Brink Meppel BV/Elsevier Business Information, The Hague (Subsidiary of: Reed Elsevier plc), Postbus 16500, The Hague 2500 BK, Netherlands. TEL 31-70-4415000, FAX 31-70-4415900. adv.: B&W page NLG 1,115, color page NLG 2,735; trim 297 x 210. **Co-sponsors:** Rechercheschool; Divisie Centrale Recherche Informatie; Gerechtelijk Laboratorium; Forensisch Medisch Genootschap; Stichting Landelijk Kontakt van Technische Recherche-en Forensische Wetenschappen; Ministerie van Justitie.

NATIONAL LAW ENFORCEMENT AND CORRECTIONS TECHNOLOGY NEWS SUMMARY. see *CRIMINOLOGY AND LAW ENFORCEMENT*

344.73 614.19 USA ISSN 1052-309X
K14
NATIONAL MEDICAL-LEGAL JOURNAL. Text in English. 1990. q. USD 60 to individuals; USD 75 foreign to individuals. adv. software rev., video rev. bibl, charts, illus. back issues avail. **Document type:** *Newsletter.* **Description:** Written for legal nurse consultants and dedicated to innovative career opportunities and defensive legal strategies.
Indexed: CINAHL.
—BLDSC (6027.095000).
Published by: Medical - Legal Consulting Institute, Inc., 2476 Bolsover St, Ste 632, Houston, TX 77005. TEL 713-942-2200, 800-880-0944, FAX 713-942-8075, mail@legalnurse.com, http://www.legalnurse.com. Ed. Vickie L Milazzo. R&P Thomas M Ziemba. Adv. contact Karen M Jones. Circ: 1,300.

RECHT & PSYCHIATRIE. see *PSYCHOLOGY*

610 DEU ISSN 0937-9819
RECHTSMEDIZIN. Text in German. 1991. bi-m. EUR 284.63 domestic; EUR 281.03 in Germany; EUR 54.20 newsstand/cover foreign (effective 2002). *Refereed.* **Document type:** *Journal, Academic/Scholarly.*
Related titles: Online - full text ed.: ISSN 1434-5196 (from EBSCO Publishing, RoweCom Information Quest, Swets Blackwell, Springer LINK).
—GNLM, Infotrieve. **CCC.**
Published by: (Deutschen Gesellschaft fuer Rechtsmedizin), Springer-Verlag (Subsidiary of: BertelsmannSpringer), Tiergartenstr 17, Heidelberg 69121, Germany. TEL 49-6221-345-0, FAX 49-6221-345229, subscriptions@springer.de, http://link.springer.de/link/service/journals/00194/index.htm, http://www.springer.de. Ed. M Staak. **Subscr. in N. America to:** Springer-Verlag New York Inc., PO Box 2485, Secaucus, NJ 07096-2485. TEL 212-460-1500, FAX 212-473-6272.

REGULATORY TOXICOLOGY AND PHARMACOLOGY. see *ENVIRONMENTAL STUDIES—Toxicology And Environmental Safety*

344.041 ROM ISSN 1221-8618
CODEN: RMLGB
REVISTA DE MEDICINA LEGALA/ROMANIAN JOURNAL OF LEGAL MEDICINE. Text in English, Romanian; Summaries in English. 1993. q. USD 70 in Europe to individuals; USD 100 elsewhere to individuals; USD 110 in Europe to institutions; USD 120 elsewhere to institutions (effective 2000). adv. bk.rev. charts, illus, stat. back issues avail. *Refereed.* **Document type:** *Academic/Scholarly.* **Description:** Covers forensic pathology, clinical forensic medicine, medical malpractice, drug trafficing, thanatochemistry, forensic toxicology, paternity, forensic psychiatry, forensic odontology, law and ethics.
Related titles: CD-ROM ed.
Indexed: Excerp.Med. (1995-).
—BLDSC (8019.632500).
Published by: (Societatea de Medicina Legala din Romania/Romanian Legal Medicine Society), Bucura Mond Prod Com S R L, Str. Ral Ipatescu 10 G, Sector 2, Bucharest 70317, Romania. TEL 40-1-6430329, 40-1-6343880, FAX 40-1-3124180, 40-1-3210260, bucura@ul.ici.ro, bucura@dial.rocknet.ro. Ed., R&P Vladimir Belis TEL 40-1-3325035. Adv. contact Dan Demengiu. B&W page USD 250, color page USD 1,000. Circ: 800 (paid); 200 (controlled).

614.19 URY
REVISTA DE TECNICA FORENSE. Text in Spanish. irreg., latest vol.6. USD 25 (effective 1999). **Document type:** *Academic/Scholarly, Trade.*
Published by: (Instituto de Tecnica Forense), Fundacion de Cultura Universitaria, Veinticinco de Mayo, 568, Casilla de Correos 1155, Montevideo 11003, Uruguay. TEL 598-2-9161152, FAX 598-2-9152549, fcuventa@multi.com.uy, http://www.fcu.com.uy.

340.6 ESP ISSN 0377-4732
CODEN: REMLE8
REVISTA ESPANOLA DE MEDICINA LEGAL. Text in Spanish; Summaries in English, Portuguese, Spanish. 1974. q. ESP 7,500 to individuals; ESP 10,000 to institutions (effective 1999). bk.rev. **Document type:** *Academic/Scholarly.* **Description:** Offers advice to professionals in Ibero-American legal medicine and forensic sciences.
Indexed: Abstr.Crim.& Pen., Ind.Med.Esp.
—CINDOC, GNLM.
Published by: Asociacion Nacional de Medicos Forenses/National Association of Forensic Doctors, Esc. D 1o Dcha., Goya, 99, Madrid 28009, Spain. anmf@arrakis.es, http://www.arrakis.es/~anmf. Ed. Dr. Carmen Baladia. Circ: 1,000.

614.19 FRA
REVUE FRANCAISE DU DOMMAGE CORPOREL✱. Text in French. 1975. q. FRF 360. bibl, charts, illus, stat. index.
Published by: (Federation Francaise des Associations de Medecins-Conseils de Societes d'Assurances), Editions J.B. Bailliere, 46 rue la Boetie -Elysees, Paris Cedex 8 75379, France. TEL 33-1-49536900. Ed. C Rousseau.

RIDGE DETAIL IN NATURE. see *CRIMINOLOGY AND LAW ENFORCEMENT*

614.19 ITA ISSN 1124-3376
RIVISTA ITALIANA DI MEDICINA LEGALE; dottrina, casistica, ricerca sperimentale, giurisprudenza e legislazione. Text in Italian. 1979. bi-m. EUR 103.29 in the European Union; EUR 154.94 elsewhere (effective 2001). adv. bk.rev. index. back issues avail. **Description:** Concerns the problematic legal and legislative issues surrounding the medical field.
Indexed: Excerp.Med., IBZ.
Published by: Casa Editrice Dott. A. Giuffre, Via Busto Arsizio, 40, Milan, MI 20151, Italy. FAX 39-2-38009582, giuffre@giuffre.it, http://www.giuffre.it. Ed. Francesco Introna. Circ: 2,200.

340.6 614.19 GBR ISSN 1355-0306
HV6001 CODEN: SJUSFE
SCIENCE AND JUSTICE. Text in English. 1960. q. GBP 100, USD 230; GBP 25, USD 57.50 newsstand/cover (effective 2001). adv. bk.rev. charts, illus. index. *Refereed.* **Document type:** *Journal, Academic/Scholarly.* **Description:** Seeks to advance the study, application and standing of forensic science and to facilitate cooperation among persons interested in forensic science throughout the world.
Formerly: Forensic Science Society. Journal (0015-7368)
Related titles: Online - full text ed.: (from Gale Group, Institute for Scientific Information).
Indexed: ASCA, Abstr.Crim.& Pen., Biol.Abstr., C.L.I., Chem.Abstr., Chem.Indus.Notes, Chem.Titles, Crim.Just.Abstr., Curr.Adv.Ecol.Sci., Curr.Adv.Gen.& Molec.Biol., Curr.Cont., Excerp.Med., Hlth.Ind., INIS Atomind., Ind.Med. (1995-), Ind.Sci.Rev., Ind.Vet., Inpharma, L.R.I. (Jan.1980-Oct.1994, Mar.1995-), Mass Spectr.Bull., Reac., Ref.Zh., Russ.Acad.Sci.Bibl., SSCI (coverage dropped), Sci.Cit.Ind., Vet.Bull.
—BLDSC (8134.129500), CASDDS, CISTI, GNLM, IDS, Infotrieve, ingenta, Linda Hall. **CCC.**
Published by: Forensic Science Society, 18a Mount Parade, Harrogate, Yorks HG1 1BX, United Kingdom. TEL 44-1423-506068, FAX 44-1423-566391, journal@forensic-science-society.org.uk, http://www.forensic-science-society.org.uk/. Ed. B Caddy. Adv. contact Jane Cross. Circ: 2,600.

347.06 USA
SCIENTIFIC EVIDENCE. Text in English. 1993 (2nd ed.). 2 base vols. plus a. updates. USD 175. **Description:** Explains the latest forensic techniques and scientific concepts used in collecting and evaluating evidence.
Published by: Lexis Law Publishing (Subsidiary of: Reed Elsevier plc), PO Box 7587, Charlottesville, VA 22906-7587. TEL 804-972-7600, 800-562-1197, FAX 804-972-7666, llp.customer.support@lexis-nexis.com, http://www.lexislawpublishing.com. Eds. Edward J Imwinkelried, Paul C Giannelli.

614.19 345 USA ISSN 1043-4224
KF9214
SCIENTIFIC SLEUTHING REVIEW; a quarterly of forensic science in law enforcement. Text in English. 1976. q., latest vol.25. USD 30 domestic; USD 35 foreign (effective 2001). adv. bk.rev. 20 p./no. back issues avail. **Document type:** *Newsletter, Academic/Scholarly.* **Description:** Covers applications of forensic sciences in both criminal and civil cases.
Former titles: Scientific Sleuthing Newsletter (0749-1395); Science in Criminal Law Newsletter; Scientific Sleuthing Newsletter
Published by: Scientific Sleuthing, Inc., c/o James E Starrs, Pub, George Washington University, Law School, Washington, DC 20052. TEL 202-994-6770, FAX 202-994-9446, jstarrs@main.nic.gwu.edu. Ed. Barbara Murillo. Pub., R&P, Adv. contact James E Starrs. page USD 600; 8 x 10. Circ: 800 (paid).

614.19 ITA
SOCIETA LOMBARDA DI MEDICINA LEGALE E DELLE ASSICURAZIONI. ARCHIVIO. Text in Italian. 1965. q. ITL 15,000.
Published by: (Societa Lombarda di Medicina Legale e delle Assicurazioni), Universita degli Studi di Milano, Istituto di Medicina Legale, Via Luigi Mangiagalli, 37, Milan, MI 20133, Italy. Ed. A Fornari.

610 RUS ISSN 0039-4521
CODEN: SMEZA5
SUDEBNO-MEDITSINSKAYA EKSPERTIZA/MEDICO-LEGAL EXPERT TESTIMONY. Text in Russian; Summaries in English. 1958. q. USD 150 foreign (effective 2000). adv. bk.rev. abstr, charts, illus. **Document type:** *Journal, Academic/Scholarly.* **Description:** Concerned with the theory and practice of forensic medicine. Examines the problems of thanatology, traumatology, toxicology, serology, forensic obstetrics, stomatology, psychiatry, chemistry, history of forensic medicine and certain problems of criminology and legal laws as they relate to forensic medicine.
Indexed: Biol.Abstr., Chem.Abstr., Chem.Indus.Notes, Chem.Titles, Dent.Ind., Excerp.Med., INIS Atomind., Ind.Med. (1958-), Ref.Zh., Russ.Acad.Sci.Bibl.
—BLDSC (0174.500000), CASDDS, CISTI, East View, GNLM.
Published by: Izdatel'stvo Meditsina, Petroverigskii per 6-8, Moscow 101000, Russian Federation. TEL 7-095-9248785, FAX 7-095-9211355, 7-095-9286003, meditsina, http://www.medit.ru. Ed. V V Tomilin. Pub. A M Stochik. R&P A Nikolaeva. Adv. contact O A Fadeeva TEL 7-095-923-51-40. Circ: 1,000. **Dist. by:** Mezhdunarodnaya Kniga, B Yakimanka 39, Moscow 117049, Russian Federation. TEL 7-095-2384967, FAX 7-095-2384634.

SYNOPSIS (COLUMBIA). see *MEDICAL SCIENCES—Pediatrics*

355 USA ISSN 1055-0305
RA1121 CODEN: WBREFD
WOUND BALLISTICS REVIEW. Text in English. 1991. s-a. USD 40 for 2 yrs. domestic; USD 48 for 2 yrs. in Canada & Mexico; USD 58 for 2 yrs. elsewhere (effective 1999 & 2000). bk.rev. abstr, charts, illus. back issues avail. *Refereed.* **Document type:** *Academic/Scholarly.* **Description:** Looks at the effects of projectiles on tissue, medical treatment of ballistic trauma, law enforcement equipment and procedures. Also studies projectile design, testing and evaluation.
Published by: International Wound Ballistics Association, PO Box 701, El Segundo, CA 90245. TEL 310-640-6065, http://www.iwba.com. Ed. Dr. Martin Fackler. R&P Robyn Townsend. Circ: 800 (paid).

614.19 ITA ISSN 0044-1570
CODEN: ZACCAL
ZACCHIA; archivio di medicina legale, sociale e criminologica. Text and summaries in English, Italian, French, German, Spanish. 1921. q. ITL 20,000, USD 40. adv. bk.rev. abstr, bibl, charts, illus, stat. index.
Indexed: Biol.Abstr., Chem.Abstr., Excerp.Med., Ind.Med. (coverage dropped).
—BLDSC (9425.200000), CASDDS, CISTI, GNLM.
Published by: (Universita degli Studi di Roma, Istituto di Medicina Legale), Societa Editrice Universo, Via Giovanni Battista Morgagni, 1, Rome, RM 00161, Italy. Ed. Cesare Gerin. Circ: 900.

614.1 CHN ISSN 1001-5728
ZHONGGUO FAYIXUE ZAZHI/CHINESE JOURNAL OF FORENSIC SCIENCES. Text in Chinese. 1986. q. CNY 2.55 per issue. adv. bk.rev. **Document type:** *Academic/Scholarly.*
Published by: Zhongguo Fayi Xuehui/Forensic Medicine Association of China, No 17 Muxidi Nanli, Beijing 100038, China. TEL 01-3264488. Ed. Wu Jiayi. Circ: 3,000.

MEDICAL SCIENCES—Gastroenterology

616.33 USA
A G A NEWS. Text in English. m. **Document type:** *Newsletter.*
Media: Online - full text.
Published by: American Gastroenterological Association, 7910 Woodmont Ave 7th Fl, Bethesda, MD 20814. TEL 301-654-2055, FAX 301-652-3890, mgoslin@gastro.org, http://www.gastro.org/news/.

616.3 616.07 USA ISSN 0942-8925
CODEN: ABIMEL
ABDOMINAL IMAGING. Text in English. 1976. bi-m. (in 1 vol., 6 nos./vol.). USD 493.30 domestic for Print & Online Eds.; USD 466.60 in Germany for Print & Online Eds.; USD 87.90 newsstand/cover domestic (effective 2002). adv. reprints avail. *Refereed.* **Document type:** *Academic/Scholarly.* **Description:** Brings together previously disparate information of value to radiologists, internists, and surgeons involved in diagnostic imaging of the alimentary tract and the genitourinary system.
Formerly: Gastrointestinal Radiology (0364-2356); Incorporates (in 1993): Urologic Radiology (0171-1091)
Related titles: Microform ed.: (from PQC); Online - full text ed.: ISSN 1432-0509 (from EBSCO Publishing, RoweCom Information Quest, Swets Blackwell, Springer LINK, Institute for Scientific Information).
Indexed: ASCA, Curr.Cont., Excerp.Med., Helminthol.Abstr., INIS Atomind., Ind.Imag.Lit., Ind.Med. (1993-), Ind.Sci.Rev., Inpharma, Jrnl.Watch Gastr., Reac., Rev.Med.& Vet.Mycol., Sci.Cit.Ind., Trop.Dis.Bull.
—BLDSC (0537.809800), CISTI, EMDOCS, GNLM, IDS, ingenta, KNAW. **CCC.**
Published by: Springer-Verlag, Journals (Subsidiary of: BertelsmannSpringer), 175 Fifth Ave, New York, NY 10010. TEL 212-460-1500, FAX 212-473-6272, orders@springer-ny.com; link@springer.de, http://www.springer-ny.com. Ed. Morton A Meyers. R&P Ian Gross. Adv. contact Jay Feinman. **N. America subscr. to:** Journal Fulfillment Services, PO Box 2485, Secaucus, NJ 07096-2485. TEL 800-777-4643, FAX 201-348-4505.

616.4 616.3 FRA ISSN 0240-642X
CODEN: AENDD5
ACTA ENDOSCOPICA. Text in English, French. 1970. 5/yr. (plus 2 special issues). EUR 178; EUR 42 newsstand/cover (effective 2002). adv. bk.rev. **Document type:** *Academic/Scholarly.*
Indexed: Excerp.Med.
—BLDSC (0614.620000), CISTI, EMDOCS, GNLM, Infotrieve, KNAW. **CCC.**
Published by: Endoscopica, 127 rue Saint Dizier, Nancy 54000, France. TEL 33-3-83374438, FAX 33-3-83353453. Ed. Dr. Fernand Vicari. Adv. contact Lydie Devred. Circ: 4,500. **Co-sponsors:** Societe Medicale d'Imagerie, Enseignement et Recherche; Interamerican Society for Digestive Endoscopy.

616.3 POL ISSN 0867-4140
CODEN: AEPOEF
ACTA ENDOSCOPICA POLONA. Text in Polish. 1991. q. PLZ 25 (effective 2000). adv. *Refereed.* **Document type:** *Academic/Scholarly.*
Indexed: Excerp.Med. (1993-).
—BLDSC (0614.625000), EMDOCS, GNLM.
Published by: Krakowskie Stowarzyszenie im. Ludwika Rydygiera, Ul Kopernika 40, Krakow 31501, Poland. TEL 48-12-4213583, FAX 48-12-4213583. Ed. Tadeusz Popiela. Circ: 800.

616.3 BEL ISSN 0001-5644
CODEN: AGEBAX
ACTA GASTRO-ENTEROLOGICA BELGICA. Text mainly in French; Text occasionally in English, German. 1933. q. EUR 54.55 domestic; EUR 64.45 foreign; EUR 14.85 per issue domestic; EUR 17.35 per issue foreign (effective 2002). adv. bk.rev. abstr, bibl, charts, illus. index. Supplement avail. *Refereed.* **Document type:** *Journal, Academic/Scholarly.*
Related titles: Online - full text ed.: (from Institute for Scientific Information).
Indexed: ASCA, Biol.Abstr., Chem.Abstr., Curr.Adv.Cancer Res., Curr.Cont., Excerp.Med., Helminthol.Abstr., Ind.Med. (1946-), Inpharma, Nutr.Abstr., Pharm.&Out.News, Reac.
—BLDSC (0616.700000), CASDDS, CISTI, EMDOCS, GNLM, IDS, KNAW.
Published by: (Association des Societes Scientifiques Medicales Belges/Vereiniging van de Belgische Wetenschappelijke Genootschappen), Acta Medica Belgica, Av Circulaire 138A, Brussels 1180, Belgium. TEL 32-2-374-5158, FAX 32-2-3749628, amb@skynet.be, http://www.ulb.ac.be/medecine/loce/amb.htm. Circ: 1,000.

616.3 ARG ISSN 0300-9033
CODEN: AGLTBL
ACTA GASTROENTEROLOGICA LATINOAMERICANA. Text in Spanish. 1969. 5/yr. USD 100 (effective 1998). adv. bk.rev. *Refereed.* **Document type:** *Academic/Scholarly.* **Description:** Contains original research in clinical or basic gastroenterology.
Related titles: CD-ROM ed.
Indexed: Biol.Abstr., Chem.Abstr., Excerp.Med., Ind.Med. (1969-).
—BLDSC (0616.730000), CASDDS, CISTI, GNLM, KNAW.
Address: Planta Baja B, Juncal, 2134, Capital Federal, Buenos Aires 1125, Argentina. TEL 54-114-8250050, FAX 54-114-8222139. Eds. Mauricio Schraier, Pablo Mazure. Circ: 3,500 (controlled).

616.3 GBR ISSN 0269-2813
CODEN: APTHEN
ALIMENTARY PHARMACOLOGY AND THERAPEUTICS. Text in English. 1987. m., latest vol.16, 2002. GBP 111 in Europe to individuals; USD 176 in North America to individuals; GBP 122 elsewhere to individuals; GBP 617 in Europe to institutions; USD 977 in North America to institutions; GBP 678 elsewhere to institutions (effective 2002). adv. bk.rev. illus. index. back issues avail. *Refereed.* **Document type:** *Academic/Scholarly.*
Related titles: Microform ed.: (from PQC); Online - full text ed.: ISSN 1365-2036. GBP 100 in Europe to individuals; USD 159 in North America to individuals; GBP 100 elsewhere to individuals; GBP 556 in Europe to institutions; USD 880 in North America to institutions; GBP 556 elsewhere to institutions (effective 2002) (from Ovid Technologies, Inc., EBSCO Publishing, O C L C Online Computer Library Center, Inc., RoweCom Information Quest, ingenta, Munksgaard & Blackwell Science's Synergy, Swets Blackwell, Institute for Scientific Information); ♦ Supplement: Alimentary Pharmacology and Therapeutics. Supplement. ISSN 0953-0673.
Indexed: ASCA, Chem.Abstr., Chem.Indus.Notes, Chem.Titles, Curr.Cont., Derwent Biotech.Abstr., Excerp.Med., Ind.Med. (1987-), Ind.Sci.Rev., Inpharma, Jrnl.Watch Gastr., Nutr.Abstr., Pharm.&Out.News, Protozool.Abstr., Reac., Sci.Cit.Ind., Sugar Ind.Abstr., Trop.Dis.Bull.
—BLDSC (0787.886000), ADONIS, CASDDS, CISTI, EMDOCS, GNLM, IDS, ingenta, KNAW. **CCC.**
Published by: Blackwell Science Ltd., PO Box 88, Oxford OX2 0NE, United Kingdom. TEL 44-1865-206180, 44-1865-206002, FAX 44-1865-206219, jnl.orders@blacksci.co.uk, http://www.blackwell-science.com/~cgilib/jnlpage.asp?Journal=apt&File=apt, http://www.blackwellpublishing.com. Eds. R E Pounder, W L Peterson. Pub. Allen Stevens. R&P Sophie Savage. Adv. contact Jenny Applin. Circ: 1,920.

616.3 GBR ISSN 0953-0673
ALIMENTARY PHARMACOLOGY AND THERAPEUTICS. SUPPLEMENT. Text in English. 1987. irreg. adv. **Document type:** *Academic/Scholarly.*
Related titles: Online - full text ed.: (from Ovid Technologies, Inc.); ♦ Supplement to: Alimentary Pharmacology and Therapeutics. ISSN 0269-2813.
Indexed: Curr.Cont. (coverage dropped).
—ADONIS, EMDOCS, Infotrieve, KNAW. **CCC.**
Published by: Blackwell Science Ltd., Osney Mead, Oxford OX2 0EL, United Kingdom. TEL 44-1865-206206, FAX 44-1865-721205, journals.cs@blacksci.co.uk, http://www.blackwell-science.com. Pub. Allen Stevens. R&P Sophie Savage. Adv. contact Jenny Applin.

617.5 USA ISSN 0065-7204
AMERICAN ASSOCIATION OF GENITO-URINARY SURGEONS. TRANSACTIONS. Text in English. a.
Related titles: Microform ed.: (from PQC).
Indexed: Ind.Med. (coverage dropped).
—CISTI, GNLM.
Published by: American Association of Genito-Urinary Surgeons, 22 W Greene St, Baltimore, MD 21201.

616.3 NLD ISSN 0002-9270
RC799 CODEN: AJGAAR
AMERICAN JOURNAL OF GASTROENTEROLOGY. Text in Dutch. 1934. m. EUR 358 in Europe to individuals; JPY 47,600 in Japan to individuals; USD 401 elsewhere to individuals; EUR 405 in Europe to institutions; JPY 53,800 in Japan to institutions; USD 373 in United States to institutions; USD 454 elsewhere to institutions; USD 247 in United States to qualified personnel Nurses; USD 89 in United States to qualified personnel Residents (effective 2002). adv. bk.rev. abstr, bibl, illus, stat. index. *Refereed.* **Document type:** *Academic/Scholarly.* **Description:** Contains articles and reviews of current topics for gastroenterologists and internists.
Related titles: Microfilm ed.: (from WWS); Microform ed.; Online - full text ed.: (from Institute for Scientific Information).
Indexed: AIDS Abstr., ASCA, Abstr.Hyg., Agri.& Environ.Biotech.Abstr. (coverage dropped), Behav.Med.Abstr., Biol.Abstr., Chem.Abstr., Chem.Indus.Notes, Chem.Titles, Curr.Adv.Cancer Res., Curr.Adv.Ecol.Sci., Curr.Cont., Dairy Sci.Abstr., Dent.Ind., Derwent Biotech.Abstr., Diar.Dis.Res., Environ.Sci.Poll.Mgmt., Excerp.Med., Helminthol.Abstr., INIS Atomind., Ind.Med. (1954-), Ind.Sci.Rev., Ind.Vet., Inpharma, Int.Abstr.Biol.Sci., Int.Nurs.Ind., Jrnl.Watch Gastr., Maize Abstr., Microbiol.Abstr., NRN, Neurosci.Cit.Ind., Nutr.Abstr., Pharm.&Out.News, Pollut.Abstr., Protozool.Abstr., Reac., Rev.Appl.Entomol., Rev.Arom.& Med.Plants, Rev.Med.& Vet.Mycol., Rev.Plant Path., Risk Abstr., SSCI (coverage dropped), Saf.Sci.Abstr., Sci.Cit.Ind., Sugar Ind.Abstr., THA, Triticale Abstr., Trop.Dis.Bull., Weed Abstr.
—BLDSC (0824.650000), CASDDS, CISTI, EMDOCS, GNLM, IDS, ingenta, KNAW. **CCC.**
Published by: (American College of Gastroenterology, Inc. USA), Elsevier Science BV, PO Box 211, Amsterdam 1000 AE, Netherlands. TEL 31-20-485-3911, FAX 31-20-485-2457, nlinfo-f@elsevier.nl, http://www.elsevier.com/locate/amjgastroenterol. Ed. Dr. E M M Quigley. Circ: 9,884. **Subscr. in Australasia and the Far East to:** Elsevier Science (Singapore) Pte Ltd, No.1 Temasek Ave, 17-01 Millenia Tower, Singapore 039192, Singapore. TEL 65-434-3727, FAX 65-337-2230; **Subscr. in Japan to:** Elsevier Science Inc - Japan Regional Office, 9-15 Higashi-Azabu 1-chome, Minato-ku, Tokyo 106-0044, Japan. TEL 81-3-5561-5033, FAX 81-3-5561-5047; **Subscr. in the Americas to:** Elsevier Science, PO Box 945, New York, NY 10159-0945. TEL 212-633-3730, FAX 212-633-3680.

AMERICAN JOURNAL OF PHYSIOLOGY: GASTROINTESTINAL AND LIVER PHYSIOLOGY. see *BIOLOGY—Physiology*

616.3 FRA ISSN 0066-2070
CODEN: AGHPBN
ANNALES DE GASTROENTEROLOGIE ET D'HEPATOLOGIE. Text in French. 1963. 5/yr. FRF 1,150 domestic to individuals; FRF 1,600 foreign to individuals; FRF 575 domestic to students; FRF 800 foreign to students. adv. bk.rev. *Refereed.* **Document type:** *Academic/Scholarly.*
Incorporates: Actualites Hepato-Gastro-Enterologiques de l'Hotel Dieu
Indexed: ASCA, Biol.Abstr., Curr.Cont. (coverage dropped), Excerp.Med., Helminthol.Abstr., INIS Atomind., Inpharma, Pharm.&Out.News, Protozool.Abstr., Reac., Rev.Med.& Vet.Mycol.
—CISTI, EMDOCS, GNLM, IDS, Infotrieve, KNAW. **CCC.**
Published by: Expansion Scientifique Francaise, 31 bd. de la Tour Maubourg, Paris Cedex 7 75343, France. TEL 33-1-40626400, FAX 33-1-45556920. Eds. J Cosnes, Y Ngo. Circ: 3,500.

616.3 GRC ISSN 1108-7471
ANNALS OF GASTROENTEROLOGY. Text in English. 1988. q. GRD 8,000 to individuals; GRD 10,000 to institutions; GRD 5,000 to students; USD 60 foreign (effective 2001). adv. bk.rev. *Refereed.* **Document type:** *Academic/Scholarly.*
Formerly (until 2000): Ellenike Gastroenterologia / Hellenic Journal of Gastroenterology (1012-0424)
Related titles: CD-ROM ed.
Indexed: Excerp.Med. (1994-).
—BLDSC (1040.660000), CISTI, EMDOCS, GNLM.
Published by: (Hellenike Gastroenterologike Etaireia/Hellenic Society of Gastroenterology), Beta Medical Publishers Ltd., 3 Adrianiou St, Athens 115 25, Greece. hsg@hol.gr. Ed., Pub. J K Triantafillidis. Circ: 1,500 (paid).

ANNUAL OF GASTROINTESTINAL ENDOSCOPY. see *MEDICAL SCIENCES—Abstracting, Bibliographies, Statistics*

616.3 ARG ISSN 0004-0517
ARCHIVOS ARGENTINOS ENFERMEDADES DEL APARATO DIGESTIVO. Text in Spanish. 1971 (vol.46). bi-m. USD 25. adv. bk.rev.
—CISTI.
Published by: Sociedad Argentina de Gastroenterologia, Jeronimo Salguero, 88 A, Capital Federal, Buenos Aires 1177, Argentina. TEL 54-114-9830863, FAX 54-114-9814936. Ed. Dr. Leonardo Pinchuck. Circ: 1,350.

ARCHIVOS DE ODONTOESTOMATOLOGIA. see *MEDICAL SCIENCES—Dentistry*

616.3 ITA ISSN 1120-8651
ARGOMENTI DI GASTROENTEROLOGIA CLINICA. Text in Italian. 1988. 6/yr. ITL 28,000 (effective 1999).
Indexed: Excerp.Med., Inpharma, Reac.
—BLDSC (1664.344950), EMDOCS, GNLM, KNAW.
Published by: Masson S.p.A., Divisione Periodici, Via F.lli Bressan 2, Milan, MI 20126, Italy. TEL 39-2-270741, FAX 39-2-27074210. Ed. Gabriele Bianchi Porro. adv.: B&W page ITL 4,600,000, color page ITL 6,600,000; trim 265 x 195. Circ: 6,000.

617.43 BRA ISSN 0102-6720
ARQUIVOS BRASILEIROS DE CIRURGIA DIGESTIVA. Abbreviated title: A B C D. Text in English; Summaries in Portuguese. 1985. q. adv. bk.rev. cum.index. back issues avail. *Refereed.* **Document type:** *Academic/Scholarly.*
Related titles: Online - full text ed.
Indexed: Helminthol.Abstr.
—CISTI, GNLM.
Published by: Lemos Editorial & Graficos Ltda., Rua Rui Barbosa, 70, B Vista, Sao Paulo, SP 01326-010, Brazil. TEL 55-11-251-4300, FAX 55-11-251-4300, lemospl@netpoint.com.br, http://www.lemos.com.br. Ed. Dr. Bruno Zilberstein. Adv. contact Paulo Lemos. Circ: 3,000 (controlled).

616.3 BRA ISSN 0004-2803
CODEN: ARQGAF
ARQUIVOS DE GASTROENTEROLOGIA. Text in English, French, Portuguese, Spanish; Summaries in English, Portuguese. 1964. q. BRL 50, USD 50 (effective 1997). adv. bk.rev. charts, illus. index. reprint service avail. from IRC,PQC. *Refereed.* **Description:** Publishes original papers, review articles, and case reports concerning all aspects of the digestive tract, including the liver.
Related titles: Microfilm ed.: (from PQC).
Indexed: Abstr.Hyg., Biol.Abstr., Chem.Abstr., Dairy Sci.Abstr., Diar.Dis.Res., Excerp.Med., Ind.Med. (1964-), Nutr.Abstr., Protozool.Abstr., Rev.Appl.Entomol., Rice Abstr., Soyabean Abstr., Triticale Abstr., Trop.Dis.Bull.
—BLDSC (1695.430000), CASDDS, CISTI, EMDOCS, GNLM, KNAW.
Published by: Instituto Brasileiro de Estudos e Pesquisas de Gastroenterologia/Brazilian Institute for Studies and Research in Gastroenterology, Rua Dr Seng, 320, B Vista, Sao Paulo, SP 01331-020, Brazil. TEL 55-11-2882119, FAX 55-11-2892768. Ed. Nelson Henrique Michelsohn. Circ: 5,000 (controlled). **Co-sponsor:** Brazilian Society of Digestive Motility.

616.3 USA ISSN 0892-9386
AUDIO-DIGEST GASTROENTEROLOGY. Text in English. 1987. m. USD 84 (effective 2000). *Refereed.*
Media: Audio cassette/tape.
Published by: Audio-Digest Foundation (Subsidiary of: California Medical Association), 1577 E Chevy Chase Dr, Glendale, CA 91206. TEL 213-245-8505, 800-423-2308, FAX 818-240-7379, 800-845-4375. Ed. Claron L Oakley. Circ: (controlled).

616.3 GBR ISSN 1521-6918
CODEN: BBPGFG
BAILLIERE'S BEST PRACTICE & RESEARCH IN CLINICAL GASTROENTEROLOGY. Text in English. 1987. bi-m. GBP 172 to individuals; GBP 228 to institutions (effective 2002). *Refereed.* **Document type:** *Journal, Academic/Scholarly.* **Description:** Provides a comprehensive review of current clinical practice and thinking within the specialty of gastroenterology.
Formerly (until 1999): Bailliere's Clinical Gastroenterology (0950-3528); Which superseded in part (in 1987): Clinics in Gastroenterology (0300-5089)
Related titles: Online - full text ed.: (from EBSCO Publishing, O C L C Online Computer Library Center, Inc., Swets Blackwell, IDEAL Online Library, Institute for Scientific Information, RoweCom Information Quest).
Indexed: ASCA, Abstr.Hyg., Curr.Cont., Ind.Med. (1999-), Ind.Sci.Rev., Inpharma, Pharm.&Out.News, Reac., Ref.Zh., Rev.Med.& Vet.Mycol., Sci.Cit.Ind., Trop.Dis.Bull.
—CISTI, EMDOCS, GNLM, IDS, Infotrieve, ingenta, KNAW. **CCC.**
Published by: Bailliere Tindall (Subsidiary of: Harcourt Publishers Ltd.), 24-28 Oval Rd, London NW1 7DX, United Kingdom. TEL 44-20-7424-4200, FAX 44-20-7424-4515, cservice@harcourt.com, http://www.harcourt-international.com/journals/bega/. Ed. G N Tytgat. **Subscr to:** Harcourt Publishers Ltd., Foots Cray High St, Sidcup, Kent DA14 5HP, United Kingdom. TEL 44-20-8308-5700, FAX 44-20-8309-0807.

616.3 USA
C C F A COMMUNIQUE. (Crohn's and Colitis Foundation of America, Inc.) Text in English. q. membership. **Document type:** *Newsletter.*
Published by: Crohn's and Colitis Foundation of America, Inc., Philadelphia - Delaware Valley Chapter, Philadelphia, PA 19053-7711. TEL 215-396-9100, FAX 215-396-1170, ccfasilly@aol.com. Ed. Barbara Berman.

616.3 CAN ISSN 0835-7900
CANADIAN JOURNAL OF GASTROENTEROLOGY. Text in English. 1987. 9/yr. CND 230 domestic to institutions; CND 285 foreign to institutions (effective 2000). adv. bk.rev. *Refereed.* **Document type:** *Academic/Scholarly.* **Description:** Original papers, case reports and reviews pertaining to gastroenterology and hepatology.
Related titles: Online - full text ed.: (from Institute for Scientific Information).
Indexed: ASCA, Curr.Cont., Excerp.Med., Ind.Med. (1987-), Inpharma, NRN, Nutr.Abstr., Pharm.&Out.News, Reac.
—BLDSC (3031.550000), CISTI, EMDOCS, GNLM, IDS, Infotrieve, ingenta, KNAW. **CCC.**

M

Published by: Pulsus Group Inc., 2902 S Sheridan Way, Oakville, ON L6J 7L6, Canada. TEL 905-829-4770, FAX 905-829-4799, pulsus@pulsus.com, http://www.pulsus.com. Eds. A B R Thomson, Dr. C N Williams. Circ: 15,500 (controlled).

616.3 CZE ISSN 1210-7824 CODEN: CSGAEE
CESKA A SLOVENSKA GASTROENTEROLOGIE/CZECH AND SLOVAK GASTROENTEROLOGY. Text in Czech, Slovak; Summaries in Czech, English. 1947. 6/yr. EUR 84, USD 108 (effective 2001). adv. bk.rev. abstr, charts, illus. index. *Refereed.* **Document type:** *Academic/Scholarly.* **Description:** Publishes original papers on the digestive system including liver, gastronintestinal endoscopy, gastroenterosurgery, clinical nutrition and allied disorders, as well as articles serving postgraduate education of gastroenterologists in practice.
Formerly (until Aug. 1994): Cesko-Slovenska Gastroenterologie a Vyziva (0009-0565)
Indexed: Biol.Abstr., C.I.S. Abstr., Chem.Abstr., Chem.Indus.Notes, Chem.Titles, Curr.Adv.Ecol.Sci., Excerp.Med., Food Sci.& Tech.Abstr., INIS Atomind., Ind.Med. (coverage dropped), Nutr.Abstr.
—BLDSC, CASDDS, CISTI, EMDOCS, GNLM. **CCC.**
Published by: (Ceska Lekarska Spolecnost J.E. Purkyne/Czech Medical Association), Nakladatelske Stredisko C L S J.E. Purkyne, Sokolska 31, Prague 12026, Czech Republic. TEL 42-2-24911420, FAX 42-2-24911420, nts@iol.cz, http://www.clsjep.cz, http://www.medical.cz. Ed. Milan Kment. adv.: B&W page CZK 27,500, color page CZK 39,800; 244 x 167. Circ: 900. **Dist in Western countries by:** Kubon & Sagner, Hesstr 39-41, Munich 80798, Germany**; Dist. by:** Abont s.r.o., Chlumova 17, Prague, 3 130 00, Czech Republic.

616.3 AUS ISSN 1443-9611
▼ **CHINESE JOURNAL OF DIGESTIVE DISEASES.** Text in English. 2000. q. AUD 209 domestic; AUD 190 in New Zealand; USD 198 elsewhere; AUD 230 domestic print & online eds.; AUD 209 in New Zealand print & online eds.; USD 218 elsewhere print & online eds. (effective 2001). adv. **Document type:** *Journal, Academic/Scholarly.*
Related titles: ♦ Online - full text ed.: Chinese Journal of Digestive Diseases Online. ISSN 1443-9573.
Published by: Blackwell Science Asia Pty Ltd, PO Box 378, Carlton South, VIC 3053, Australia. TEL 61-3-9347-0300, FAX 61-3-9347-5001, info@blacksci-asia.com.au, http://www.blacksci.co.uk/australi. Ed. Xiao Shudong.

616.3 AUS ISSN 1443-9573
▼ **CHINESE JOURNAL OF DIGESTIVE DISEASES ONLINE.** Text in English. 2000. q. AUD 188 domestic; AUD 171 in New Zealand; USD 179 elsewhere (effective 2001). **Document type:** *Academic/Scholarly.*
Media: Online - full text (from ingenta, Munksgaard & Blackwell Science's Synergy, Swets Blackwell, RoweCom Information Quest). **Related titles:** ♦ Print ed.: Chinese Journal of Digestive Diseases. ISSN 1443-9611.
Published by: Blackwell Science Asia Pty Ltd, PO Box 378, Carlton South, VIC 3053, Australia. TEL 61-3-9347-0300, FAX 61-3-9347-3016, info@blacksci-asia.com.au, http://www.blacksci.co.uk/australi.

616.3 ITA ISSN 0009-4765
CHIRURGIA GASTROENTEROLOGICA; rassegna trimestrale di chirurgia dell'apparato digerente e degli organi addominali. Text in Italian; Summaries in English, Italian. 1967. q. ITL 90,000, USD 80 (effective 1995). adv. bk.rev.
Indexed: Excerp.Med.
—CISTI, GNLM.
Published by: Giovanni Battista Grassi, C.P. 4236, Rome Appio, RM 00100, Italy. FAX 06-70454246.

616.3 CHE ISSN 0177-9990
CHIRURGISCHE GASTROENTEROLOGIE; Interdisziplinaer. Text in English, German. 1985. 4/yr. CHF 226 in Europe to institutions; CHF 237.60 overseas to institutions; EUR 155 in Europe to institutions; USD 179 overseas to institutions (effective 2002). *Refereed.* **Document type:** *Journal, Academic/Scholarly.*
Related titles: Microform ed.: (from PQC); Online - full text ed.: ISSN 1421-9808. CHF 58, EUR 42 to institutions with print edition (effective 2002); USD 45 to institutions with print edition (effective 2001) (from EBSCO Publishing, O C L C Online Computer Library Center, Inc., RoweCom Information Quest, Swets Blackwell, Institute for Scientific Information).
Indexed: ASCA, Excerp.Med. (1995-).
—BLDSC (3181.470700), EMDOCS, GNLM, IDS, Infotrieve, KNAW. **CCC.**
Published by: S. Karger AG, Allschwilerstr 10, PO Box, Basel 4009, Switzerland. TEL 41-61-306-1111, FAX 41-61-306-1234, karger@karger.ch, http://www.online.karger.com/journals/cga, http://www.karger.com. Ed. R Bittner.

663 USA
▼ **CLINICAL GASTROENTEROLOGY.** Text in English. 2001. irreg. price varies. illus. back issues avail. *Refereed.* **Document type:** *Monographic series, Academic/Scholarly.* **Description:** Covers all aspects of gastroenterology, including related diseases and general medicine.
Published by: Humana Press Inc., 999 Riverview Dr, Ste 208, Totowa, NJ 07512. TEL 973-256-1699, FAX 973-256-8341, humana@humanapr.com, http://humanapress.com. Ed. George Wu. R&P Wendy A Warren.

CLINICAL NUTRITION. see *NUTRITION AND DIETETICS*

616.33 USA ISSN 1098-8351
▼ **CLINICAL PERSPECTIVES IN GASTROENTEROLOGY.** Text in English. 1999. bi-m. USD 69 domestic to individuals; USD 99 foreign to individuals; USD 149 domestic to institutions; USD 185 foreign to institutions; USD 57 domestic to students; USD 76 foreign to students; USD 31 per issue (effective 2001). **Document type:** *Journal, Academic/Scholarly.* **Description:** Features timely, relevant articles, columns and stories on managed care, patient care and digestive disease prevention, diagnosis and management.
—BLDSC (3286.326350).
Published by: (American Gastroenterological Association), W.B. Saunders Co. (Subsidiary of: Harcourt Publishers Ltd.), Curtis Center, Independence Sq W, Philadelphia, PA 19106-3399. TEL 215-238-2800, FAX 215-238-6490, http://www.wbsaunders.com. Ed. Martin D Gelfand.

CLINICS IN COLON & RECTAL SURGERY. see *MEDICAL SCIENCES—Surgery*

616.362 USA ISSN 1089-3261
CLINICS IN LIVER DISEASE. Text in English. q. USD 139 domestic to individuals; USD 158 in Canada to individuals; USD 174 elsewhere to individuals; USD 173 domestic to institutions; USD 200 foreign to institutions; USD 51 per issue (effective 2001). **Description:** Covers each month a single issue in liver disease. Year 2000 issues to focus on the progress of hepatology over the course of the last century, the pathophysiology of liver disease, advances in liver transplantation, as well as pediatric hepatology of liver disease.
Indexed: Ind.Med. (1997-).
—BLDSC (3286.576000).
Published by: W.B. Saunders Co. (Subsidiary of: Harcourt Publishers Ltd.), 11830 Westline Industrial Dr, St Louis, MO 63146. TEL 800-325-4177, wbspcs@harcourtbrace.com, http://www.wbsaunders.com.

COLON AND RECTAL SURGERY OUTLOOK. see *MEDICAL SCIENCES—Abstracting, Bibliographies, Statistics*

616.3 DEU ISSN 0174-2442
COLOPROCTOLOGY. Text in German. 1979. bi-m. EUR 167.94 domestic; EUR 174.94 foreign; EUR 95.98 domestic to students; EUR 102.98 foreign to students; EUR 31.78 newsstand/cover (effective 2002). adv. bk.rev. index. back issues avail. *Refereed.* **Document type:** *Journal, Academic/Scholarly.* **Description:** Covers case reports and techniques in proctology. Includes new product information, calendar of events and reviews of journal articles.
Formerly: Proktologie (0174-240X)
Related titles: Online - full text ed.: ISSN 1615-6730 (from RoweCom Information Quest, Swets Blackwell, Springer LINK).
—GNLM.
Published by: (Berufsverband der Coloproktologen Deutschland), Urban und Vogel Medien und Medizin Verlagsgesellschaft mbH (Subsidiary of: BertelsmannSpringer), Neumarkter Str 43, Munich 81673, Germany. TEL 49-89-43721411, FAX 49-89-43721410, verlag@urban-vogel.de, http://www.urban-vogel.de. Ed. T Hager. Pub., R&P Oliver Renn. Adv. contact Sibylle Schurr TEL 49-89-43721353. Circ: 4,000. **Co-sponsor:** Deutsche Gesellschaft fuer Koloproktologie.

616.3 GBR ISSN 1462-8910 CODEN: CODIFU
▼ **COLORECTAL DISEASE.** Text in English. 1999. bi-m., latest vol.4, 2002. GBP 85 in Europe to individuals; USD 144 in North America to individuals; GBP 93 elsewhere to individuals; GBP 201 in Europe to institutions; USD 319 in North America to institutions; GBP 221 elsewhere to institutions (effective 2002). adv. *Refereed.* **Document type:** *Academic/Scholarly.* **Description:** Publishes original research in any discipline relating to colorectal pathology.
Related titles: ♦ Online - full text ed.: Colorectal Disease Online. ISSN 1463-1318.
—BLDSC (3322.110000). **CCC.**
Published by: (Association of Coloproctology of Great Britain and Ireland DEU), Blackwell Science Ltd., PO Box 88, Oxford OX2 0NE, United Kingdom. TEL 44-1865-206180, 44-1865-206002, FAX 44-1865-206219, jnl.orders@blacksci.co.uk, http://www.blackwell-science.com/~cgilib/jnlpage.asp?Journal=cdi&File=cdi, http://www.blackwellpublishing.com. Ed. R J Nicholls. Pub. Allen Stevens. R&P Sophie Savage. Adv. contact Jenny Applin. Circ: 1,000.

616.3 GBR ISSN 1463-1318
COLORECTAL DISEASE ONLINE. Text in English. bi-m. GBP 77 in Europe to individuals; USD 130 in North America to individuals; GBP 77 elsewhere to individuals; GBP 181 in Europe to institutions; USD 288 in North America to institutions; GBP 181 elsewhere to institutions (effective 2002). *Refereed.* **Document type:** *Academic/Scholarly.*
Media: Online - full text (from EBSCO Publishing, O C L C Online Computer Library Center, Inc., RoweCom Information Quest, ingenta, Munksgaard & Blackwell Science's Synergy, Swets Blackwell). **Related titles:** ♦ Print ed.: Colorectal Disease. ISSN 1462-8910.
Published by: Blackwell Science Ltd., Osney Mead, Oxford OX2 0EL, United Kingdom. TEL 44-1685-206206, FAX 44-1685-721205, website@blacksci.com, journals.cs@blacksci.co.uk, http://www.blackwell-science.com/~cgilib/jnlpage.bin?Journal=cdi&File=cdi&Page=aims.

CORE JOURNALS IN GASTROENTEROLOGY. see *MEDICAL SCIENCES—Abstracting, Bibliographies, Statistics*

616.3 HRV ISSN 0353-9296 CODEN: CJGHE6
CROATIAN JOURNAL OF GASTROENTEROLOGY AND HEPATOLOGY. Text in Croatian. 1992. q.
Indexed: Excerp.Med. (1993-).
—BLDSC (3487.498100), EMDOCS, GNLM, KNAW.
Published by: Medicinska Naklada Co., Vlaska 69, Zagreb 41000, Croatia. TEL 41-447255.

616.3 USA ISSN 0198-8085
RC799 CODEN: CUGADR
CURRENT GASTROENTEROLOGY* . Text in English. 1980. a. USD 79.95 domestic; USD 88 foreign (effective 2000). illus. **Document type:** *Academic/Scholarly.* **Description:** Surveys developments in gastroenterology and provides synopses of the past 12 months of medical literature.
—CASDDS, GNLM.
Published by: Mosby, Inc. (Subsidiary of: Elsevier Science), 11830 Westline Industrial Dr, St Louis, MO 63146-3313. TEL 314-872-8370, 800-325-4177, FAX 314-432-1380, http://www.mosby.com/periodicals. Ed. Dr. Gary Gitnick.

616.33 USA ISSN 1522-8037
CURRENT GASTROENTEROLOGY REPORTS. Text in English. 6/yr. USD 163.95, GBP 120 to individuals; USD 327.95 to institutions; USD 80, GBP 60 to students (effective 2002); Subscr. includes print & onlines eds..
Related titles: Online - full content ed.: USD 85, GBP 65 (effective 2002).
Indexed: Ind.Med.
—BLDSC (3496.940000).
Published by: Current Science Inc., 400 Market St, Ste 700, Philadelphia, PA 19106. TEL 800-427-1796, FAX 215-574-2225, info@current-reports.com, http://www.current-reports.com/cr_jrnl_home.cfm?JournalID=GR, http://www.current-science.com/, http://www.current-science-group.com/. Ed. Joel E Richter. **Affiliate:** Current Science Ltd.

M

616.3 USA ISSN 0198-8093
RC845 CODEN: CUHEDA

CURRENT HEPATOLOGY. Text in English. 1980. a. USD 79.95 domestic; USD 88 foreign (effective 2000). **Document type:** *Academic/Scholarly.* **Description:** Surveys developments in hepatology and provides synopses of the past 12 months of medical literature.
—CASDDS, CISTI, GNLM, KNAW.
Published by: Mosby, Inc. (Subsidiary of: Elsevier Science), 11830 Westline Industrial Dr, St Louis, MO 63146-3313. TEL 314-872-8370, 800-432-4177, FAX 314-432-1380, http://www.mosby.com/periodicals. Ed. Dr. Gary L Gitnick.

CURRENT MEDICAL LITERATURE. COLORECTAL CANCER. see *MEDICAL SCIENCES—Abstracting, Bibliographies, Statistics*

CURRENT MEDICAL LITERATURE. GASTROENTEROLOGY. see *MEDICAL SCIENCES—Abstracting, Bibliographies, Statistics*

616.3 USA ISSN 0267-1379
CODEN: COGAEK

CURRENT OPINION IN GASTROENTEROLOGY. Text in English. 1985. bi-m. USD 249 domestic to individuals for print & online eds.; USD 249 foreign to individuals for print & online eds.; USD 585 per issue domestic to institutions; USD 585 per issue foreign to institutions; USD 91 newsstand/cover (effective 2002). adv. bibl, illus. *Refereed.* **Document type:** *Academic/Scholarly.* **Description:** Directed toward clinicians, surgeons and endoscopists. Presents review articles followed by annotated bibliographies of references consulted. A bibliography of the current world literature published during the previous year.
Related titles: CD-ROM ed.; Online - full text ed.: USD 760.50 domestic academic site license; USD 760.50 foreign academic site license; USD 848.25 domestic corporate site license; USD 848.25 foreign corporate site license (effective 2002) (from Ovid Technologies, Inc., EBSCO Publishing, Swets Blackwell, Institute for Scientific Information); ◆ Supplement: The Year In Helicobacter Pylori. ISSN 1358-7269.
Indexed: ASCA, Abstr.Hyg., CINAHL, Chem.Abstr., Chem.Indus.Notes, Chem.Titles, Curr.Adv.Cancer Res., Curr.Cont., Dairy Sci.Abstr., Diar.Dis.Res., Excerp.Med., Helminthol.Abstr., Inpharma, Int.Abstr.Biol.Sci., Nutr.Abstr., Pharm.&Out.News, Pig News & Info., Protozool.Abstr., Reac.
—BLDSC (3500.775000), ADONIS, CASDDS, CISTI, EMDOCS, GNLM, IDS, ingenta, KNAW.
Published by: Lippincott Williams & Wilkins (Philadelphia) (Subsidiary of: Wolters Kluwer N.V.), 530 Walnut St, Philadelphia, PA 19106-3621. FAX 215-521-8902, 215-521-8902, http://www.Lww.com. Ed. Tadataka Yamada. Pub. Maria McMichael. R&P Tobias Weschler. Adv. contact Kelly Adamitis. Circ: 4,222. **Subscr. to:** PO Box 1600, Hagerstown, MD 21740-1600.

616.33 USA ISSN 1092-8472

CURRENT TREATMENT OPTIONS IN GASTROENTEROLOGY. Text in English. 6/yr. USD 163.95 to individuals; USD 80 to students (effective 2002); Subscr. includes both print & online eds.. **Document type:** *Journal, Academic/Scholarly.*
Related titles: Online - full content ed.: USD 75 (effective 2002).
Published by: Current Science Inc., 400 Market St, Ste 700, Philadelphia, PA 19106. TEL 800-427-1796, FAX 215-574-2225, info@phl.cursci.com, http://www.treatment-options.com/cto_jrnl_home.cfm?JournalID=GA. Ed. Mark Feldman. **Affiliate:** Current Science Ltd.

616.3 NLD ISSN 0167-935X

DEVELOPMENTS IN GASTROENTEROLOGY. Text in English. 1981. irreg., latest vol.13, 1991. price varies. *Refereed.* **Document type:** *Monographic series.*
—BLDSC (3579.071870), CISTI, KNAW.
Published by: Kluwer Academic Publishers Group (Subsidiary of: Wolters Kluwer N.V.), Spuiboulevard 50, PO Box 17, Dordrecht 3300 AA, Netherlands. FAX 31-78-639-2254, services@wkap.nl, http://www.wkap.nl. **Dist. by:** Journals Department, PO Box 322, Dordrecht 3300 AH, Netherlands. FAX 31-78-654-6474.

DIABETIC MEDICINE. see *MEDICAL SCIENCES—Endocrinology*

DIABETIC MEDICINE ONLINE. see *MEDICAL SCIENCES—Endocrinology*

616.3 CHE ISSN 0012-2823
QP141.A1 CODEN: DIGEBW

DIGESTION; international journal of gastroenterology. Text in English. 1968. 8/yr. CHF 1,420 in Europe to institutions; CHF 1,443.20 overseas to institutions; EUR 1,014.40 in Europe to institutions; USD 1,104 overseas to institutions (effective 2002). adv. bibl, illus. back issues avail. *Refereed.* **Document type:** *Journal, Academic/Scholarly.* **Description:** Publishes research reports on diseases and pathophysiology of the gastrointestinal tract, liver and pancreas and on gastrointestinal endocrinology.
Formerly: Gastroenterologia
Related titles: Microform ed.; Online - full text ed.: ISSN 1421-9867. CHF 116, EUR 84, USD 90 to institutions with print edition (effective 2002) (from Northern Light Technology, Inc., EBSCO Publishing, O C L C Online Computer Library Center, Inc., RoweCom Information Quest, ProQuest Information & Learning, Swets Blackwell, Institute for Scientific Information).
Indexed: ASCA, Abstr.Hyg., Biol.Abstr., Chem.Abstr., Chem.Indus.Notes, Chem.Titles, Curr.Adv.Ecol.Sci., Curr.Cont., Dairy Sci.Abstr., Dent.Ind., Excerp.Med., Helminthol.Abstr., Ind.Med. (1968-), Ind.Sci.Rev., Inpharma, Int.Abstr.Biol.Sci., Jrnl.Watch Gastr., NRN, Nutr.Abstr., Pharm.&Out.News, Protozool.Abstr., Reac., Rev.Arom.& Med.Plants, Sci.Cit.Ind., Sugar Ind.Abstr.
—BLDSC (3588.345000), CASDDS, CISTI, GNLM, IDS, ingenta, KNAW. **CCC.**
Published by: S. Karger AG, Allschwilerstr 10, PO Box, Basel 4009, Switzerland. TEL 41-61-306-1111, FAX 41-61-306-1234, karger@karger.ch, http://www.online.karger.com/journals/dig, http://www.karger.com. Ed. R Arnold. adv.: page USD 1,185. Circ: 1,250.

616.3 ITA ISSN 1590-8658
CODEN: ITJGDH

DIGESTIVE AND LIVER DISEASE. Text in English; Summaries in English, Italian. 1969. m. (9/yr.). USD 180 to individuals; USD 260 to institutions. adv. bk.rev. index, cum.index. reprints avail. *Refereed.* **Document type:** *Academic/Scholarly.* **Description:** Publishes original articles concerning basic and clinical research, case reports, editorials, articles discussing hypotheses and interpretations, and the proceedings of the national congresses on gastroenterology and hepatology.
Former titles (until 2000): Italian Journal of Gastroenterology and Hepatology (1125-8055); (until 1997): Italian Journal of Gastroenterology (0392-0623); (until 1978): Rendiconti di Gastroenterologia (0300-0877); (until 1971): Rendiconti Romani di Gastro-Enterologia (0300-0524); (until 1970): Rendiconti delle Romane di Gastro-Enterology
Related titles: Microform ed.: (from PQC); Online - full text ed.: (from Institute for Scientific Information).
Indexed: ASCA, Chem.Abstr., Chem.Indus.Notes, Chem.Titles, Curr.Cont., Diar.Dis.Res., Excerp.Med., Ind.Med. (coverage dropped), Ind.Sci.Rev., Inpharma, Nutr.Abstr., Pharm.&Out.News, Reac., Rev.Med.& Vet.Mycol., Sci.Cit.Ind.
—BLDSC (4588.340410), CASDDS, CISTI, EMDOCS, GNLM, IDS, KNAW.
Published by: (Italian Society of Gastroenterology), Pacini Editore, Via Alessandro Gherardesca, 1, Ospedaletto, PI 56121, Italy. TEL 39-06-5411000, FAX 39-06-86211026. Ed. Romano Carratu. Adv. contact Isabella Leonardo. B&W page USD 1,400, color page USD 2,150; trim 235 x 179. Circ: 3,000. **Co-sponsor:** Italian Association for the Study of the Liver.

616.3 CHE ISSN 0257-2753
CODEN: DIDIEW

DIGESTIVE DISEASES; clinical reviews. Text in English. 1983. 4/yr. CHF 1,012 in Europe to institutions; CHF 1,023.60 overseas to institutions; EUR 723.20 in Europe to institutions; USD 784 overseas to institutions (effective 2002). adv. illus. index. back issues avail. *Refereed.* **Document type:** *Journal, Academic/Scholarly.* **Description:** Covers both clinical and basic science topics in gastrointestinal function and disorders, including medicine, liver disease, surgery, nutrition, pathology and the basic sciences.
Formerly: Survey of Digestive Diseases (0253-4398)
Related titles: Online - full text ed.: ISSN 1421-9875. CHF 58, EUR 42, USD 45 to institutions with print edition (effective 2002) (from EBSCO Publishing, O C L C Online Computer Library Center, Inc., RoweCom Information Quest, Swets Blackwell, Institute for Scientific Information).
Indexed: ASCA, Chem.Abstr., Curr.Cont., Ind.Med. (1986-), Inpharma, NRN, Pharm.&Out.News, Reac., SSCI (coverage dropped).
—BLDSC (3588.346000), CASDDS, CISTI, GNLM, IDS, Infotrieve, KNAW. **CCC.**
Published by: S. Karger AG, Allschwilerstr 10, PO Box, Basel 4009, Switzerland. TEL 41-61-306-1111, FAX 41-61-306-1234, karger@karger.ch, http://www.online.karger.com/journals/ddi. Ed. S R Achem. adv.: page USD 1,185. Circ: 800.

616.3 USA

▼ **DIGESTIVE DISEASES & DISORDERS SOURCEBOOK.** Text in English. 1999. irreg., latest 1999. USD 48 per issue (effective 2001). charts. Index. **Document type:** *Consumer.* **Description:** Basic consumer health information about common disorders of the upper and lower digestive tract. It also includes information about medications and recommendations for maintaining a healthy digestive tract. A glossary of important terms and a directory of digestive diseases organizations are also provided.
Published by: Omnigraphics, Inc., 615 Griswold St, Detroit, MI 48226. TEL 313-961-1340, 800-234-1340, FAX 313-961-1383, 800-875-1340, info@omnigraphics.com, jjts@sprynet.com, http://www.omnigraphics.com/cgi-bin/loadpage.cgi?user_id=1567&file=0-7808-0327-2.html. Ed. Karen Bellenir.

616.3 USA ISSN 0163-2116
RC799 CODEN: DDSCDJ

DIGESTIVE DISEASES AND SCIENCES. Text in English. 1934. m. USD 899, EUR 898 to institutions for print or online ed.; USD 1,078.80, EUR 1,077.60 to institutions for print & online eds.combined (effective 2002). adv. bk.rev. illus. back issues avail. *Refereed.* **Document type:** *Journal, Academic/Scholarly.* **Description:** Disseminates articles on basic research and clinical practice in gastroenterology and related fields.
Formerly (until vol.24, no.1, 1979): American Journal of Digestive Diseases (0002-9211)
Related titles: Microfilm ed.: (from PQC); Online - full text ed.: (from CatchWord Ltd., Ovid Technologies, Inc., EBSCO Publishing, O C L C Online Computer Library Center, Inc., RoweCom Information Quest, Swets Blackwell, Kluwer Online, Institute for Scientific Information).
Indexed: AIM, ASCA, Abstr.Hyg., Abstr.Inter.Med., Behav.Med.Abstr., Biol.Abstr., Chem.Abstr., Chem.Indus.Notes, Chem.Titles, Chic.Per.Ind., Curr.Adv.Cancer Res., Curr.Adv.Ecol.Sci., Curr.Adv.Gen.& Molec.Biol., Curr.Cont., Dairy Sci.Abstr., Dent.Ind., Derwent Biotech.Abstr., Diar.Dis.Res., Excerp.Med., Fababean Abstr., Helminthol.Abstr., INIS Atomind., Ind.Med. (1979-), Ind.Sci.Rev., Ind.Vet., Inpharma, Int.Abstr.Biol.Sci., Int.Nurs.Ind., Jrnl.Watch Gastr., Maize Abstr., NRN, Neurosci.Cit.Ind., Nutr.Abstr., Pharm.&Out.News, Pig News & Info., Protozool.Abstr., Reac., Ref.Zh., Rev.Appl.Entomol., Rev.Med.& Vet.Mycol., SSCI (coverage dropped), Sci.Cit.Ind., Small Anim.Abstr., Sugar Ind.Abstr., THA, Triticale Abstr., Trop.Dis.Bull., Vet.Bull.
—BLDSC (3588.346100), ADONIS, CASDDS, CatchWord, CISTI, GNLM, IDS, ingenta, KNAW. **CCC.**
Published by: Kluwer Academic - Plenum Publishers (Subsidiary of: Wolters Kluwer N.V.), 233 Spring St, New York, NY 10013-1578. TEL 212-620-8000, 800-221-9369, FAX 212-463-0742, services@wkap.nl, info@plenum.com, http://www.wkap.nl/journalhome.htm/0163-2116. Ed. Richard L Wechsler. R&P Rose Luongo TEL 781-871-6311. **Subscr. outside the Americas to:** Kluwer Academic Publishers Group, Journals Department, PO Box 322, Dordrecht 3300 AH, Netherlands. TEL 31-78-639-2392, FAX 31-78-654-6474.

616.3 AUS ISSN 0915-5635

DIGESTIVE ENDOSCOPY. Text in English. 1989. q. AUD 207 domestic to individuals; AUD 189 in New Zealand to individuals; USD 115 elsewhere to individuals; AUD 739 domestic to institutions; AUD 672 in New Zealand to institutions; JPY 49,220 in Japan to institutions; USD 410 elsewhere to institutions; AUD 228 domestic to individuals paper & online eds. combined; AUD 208 in New Zealand to individuals paper & online eds. combined; USD 127 elsewhere to individuals paper & online eds. combined; AUD 813 domestic to institutions paper & online eds. combined; AUD 740 in New Zealand to institutions paper & online eds. combined; JPY 54,142 in Japan to institutions paper & online eds. combined; USD 451 elsewhere to institutions paper & online eds. combined (effective 2001). adv. bk.rev. abstr. *Refereed.* **Document type:** *Journal, Academic/Scholarly.* **Description:** Covers the study and investigation relating to the various endoscopic techniques used in diagnosis and treatment of digestive disease.
Related titles: ◆ Online - full text ed.: Digestive Endoscopy Online. ISSN 1443-1661.
Indexed: INIS Atomind.
—BLDSC (3588.346200), EMDOCS, GNLM, KNAW.

M

Published by: (Japan Gastroenterological Endoscopy Society JPN), Blackwell Science Asia Pty Ltd, PO Box 378, Carlton South, VIC 3053, Australia. TEL 61-3-9347-0300, FAX 61-3-9347-5001, info@blacksci-asia.com.au, http://www.blacksci.co.uk/australi. Ed. Hirohumi Niwa. Circ: 1,000.

616.3 AUS ISSN 1443-1661
DIGESTIVE ENDOSCOPY ONLINE. Text in English. q. AUD 187 domestic to individuals; AUD 171 in New Zealand to individuals; USD 104 elsewhere to individuals; AUD 666 domestic to institutions; AUD 606 in New Zealand to institutions; JPY 44,298 in Japan to institutions; USD 369 elsewhere to institutions (effective 2001). **Document type:** *Academic/Scholarly.*
Media: Online - full text (from EBSCO Publishing, O C L C Online Computer Library Center, Inc., ingenta, Munksgaard & Blackwell Science's Synergy, Swets Blackwell). **Related titles:** ♦ Print ed.: Digestive Endoscopy. ISSN 0915-5635.
Published by: (Japan Gastroenterological Endoscopy Society JPN), Blackwell Science Asia Pty Ltd, PO Box 378, Carlton South, VIC 3053, Australia. TEL 61-3-9347-0300, FAX 61-3-9347-3016, website@blacksci.com, info@blacksci-asia.com.au, http://www.blackwell-science.com/~cgilib/jnlpage.bin?Journal=den&File=den&Page=aims, http://www.blacksci.co.uk/australi.

616.33 USA
DIGESTIVE HEALTH & NUTRITION. Text in English. bi-m. USD 12.95 domestic; USD 22 foreign (effective 2001). back issues avail. **Description:** Provides up-to-date tips and treatment information for sufferers of digestive disorders.
Related titles: Online - full text ed.
Published by: American Gastroenterological Association, 7910 Woodmont Ave 7th Fl, Bethesda, MD 20814. TEL 301-654-2055, FAX 301-652-3890, mgoslin@gastro.org, http://www.gastro.org/.

DIGESTIVE SURGERY. see *MEDICAL SCIENCES—Surgery*

616.3 FRA ISSN 1155-1968
ENCYCLOPEDIE MEDICO-CHIRURGICALE. GASTRO-ENTEROLOGIE. Cover title: Traite de Gastro-Enterologie. Variant title: Encyclopedie Medico-Chirurgicale, Instantanes Medicaux. Gastro-Enterologie. Text in French. 1936. 4 base vols. plus q. updates. bibl, charts, illus. *Refereed.* **Document type:** *Academic/Scholarly.* **Description:** Provides gastroenterologists with a comprehensive, up-to-date reference for diagnosing and treating various conditions and disorders.
Formerly (until 1991): Encyclopedie Medico-Chirurgicale. Estomac - Intestin (0246-0327)
Published by: Elsevier Paris, Editions Scientifiques et Medicales (Subsidiary of: Reed Elsevier plc. group), 23 rue Linois, Paris 75015, France. TEL 33-1-44589110, FAX 33-1-45589425, redaction-emc@elsevier.fr, redacion-emc@elsevier.fr, http://www.elsevier.fr, http://www.elsevier.com.

616.3 FRA ISSN 1155-1976
ENCYCLOPEDIE MEDICO-CHIRURGICALE. HEPATOLOGIE. Cover title: Traite d'Hepatologie. Variant title: Enclyclopedie Medico-Chirurgicale, Instantanes Medicaux. Hepatologie. Text in French. 1935. 3 base vols. plus q. updates. bibl, charts, illus. *Refereed.* **Document type:** *Academic/Scholarly.* **Description:** Offers hepatologists a comprehensive, up-to-date reference for diagnosing and treating disorders and conditions of the liver.
Former titles (until 1991): Encyclopedie Medico-Chirurgicale. Foie - Pancreas (0246-053X); (until 1960): Encyclopedie Medico-Chirurgicale. Foie (0246-0688)
Published by: Elsevier Paris, Editions Scientifiques et Medicales (Subsidiary of: Reed Elsevier plc. group), 23 rue Linois, Paris 75015, France. TEL 33-1-45589110, FAX 33-1-44589425, redaction-emc@elsevier.fr, redacion-emc@elsevier.fr, http://www.elsevier.fr, http://www.elsevier.com.

ENCYCLOPEDIE MEDICO-CHIRURGICALE. TECHNIQUES CHIRURGICALES. APPAREIL DIGESTIF; la reference du chirurgien - actualisee en permanence. see *MEDICAL SCIENCES—Surgery*

ENCYCLOPEDIE MEDICO-CHIRURGICALE. TECNICHE CHIRURGICHE. CHIRURGIA ADDOMINALE. see *MEDICAL SCIENCES—Surgery*

ENCYCLOPEDIE MEDICO-CHIRURGICALE. TRAITE DE RADIODIAGNOSTIC: APPAREIL DIGESTIF. see *MEDICAL SCIENCES—Radiology And Nuclear Medicine*

616.3 DEU ISSN 0177-4077
ENDOPRAXIS. Text in German. 1987. q. EUR 28.60 domestic to institutions; EUR 30.80 in Europe to institutions; EUR 36.20 elsewhere to institutions; EUR 8 newsstand/cover (effective 2002). **Document type:** *Journal, Academic/Scholarly.*
Published by: Georg Thieme Verlag, Ruedigerstr 14, Stuttgart 70469, Germany. TEL 49-711-8931-0, FAX 49-711-8931298, kunden.service@thieme.de, http://www.thieme.de. R&P Peter Eich. Adv. contact Manfred Marggraf.

616.3 DEU ISSN 0013-726X
CODEN: ENDCAM
ENDOSCOPY. Text in English. 1969. 12/yr. EUR 230.40 domestic to individuals; EUR 230.80 in Europe to individuals; EUR 246.80 elsewhere to individuals; EUR 428.40 domestic to institutions; EUR 428.80 in Europe to institutions; EUR 444.80 elsewhere to institutions (effective 2002). adv. bk.rev. abstr, bibl, charts, illus, stat. index. reprint service avail. from PQC. *Refereed.* **Document type:** *Journal, Academic/Scholarly.*
Related titles: Microform ed.: (from PQC); Online - full text ed.: ISSN 1438-8812; (from Institute for Scientific Information).
Indexed: ASCA, Biol.Abstr., Curr.Cont., Dent.Ind., Excerp.Med., Helminthol.Abstr., INIS Atomind., Ind.Med. (1969-), Ind.Sci.Rev., Inpharma, Jrnl.Watch Gastr., Nutr.Abstr., Pharm.&Out.News, Reac., Ref.Zh., Rev.Med.& Vet.Mycol., Sci.Cit.Ind., Trop.Dis.Bull.
—BLDSC (3743.600000), CISTI, GNLM, IDS, ingenta, KNAW. **CCC.**
Published by: Georg Thieme Verlag, Ruedigerstr 14, Stuttgart 70469, Germany. TEL 49-711-8931-0, FAX 49-711-8931298, endoscopy@thieme.de, leser.service@thieme.de, http://www.thieme.de/endoscopy/index.html. Ed. M Classen. R&P Michael Wachinger. Circ: 9,000 (paid and controlled).

616.3 DEU ISSN 0933-811X
CODEN: ENDHE7
ENDOSKOPIE HEUTE; forum bildgebender verfahren. Text in German. 1988. q. EUR 94.80 domestic to institutions; EUR 98.40 in Europe to institutions; EUR 102.80 elsewhere to institutions; EUR 27 newsstand/cover to institutions (effective 2002). **Document type:** *Journal, Academic/Scholarly.*
Related titles: Online - full text ed.: ISSN 1439-2577.
—BLDSC (3743.630000), CISTI, EMDOCS, GNLM.
Published by: Demeter Verlag GmbH und Co. KG, Ruedigerstr 14, Stuttgart 70469, Germany. TEL 49-711-8931-0, FAX 49-711-8931322, custserv@thieme.de, http://www.demeter-verlag.de. Eds. J F Riemann, Dr. R Ottenjann. Circ: 2,500.

616.362 ITA
CODEN: EPATA4
EPATOLOGIA E MALATTIE DEL RICAMBIO. Text in Italian. 1955. 3/yr. ITL 48,000; ITL 96,000 foreign.
Formerly (until 1984): Epatologia (0013-9475)
Indexed: Biol.Abstr., Chem.Abstr., Excerp.Med.
—CASDDS, CISTI, GNLM.
Published by: Societa Editrice Universo, Via Giovanni Battista Morgagni, 1, Rome, RM 00161, Italy.

616.3 USA ISSN 0954-691X
CODEN: EJGHES
EUROPEAN JOURNAL OF GASTROENTEROLOGY AND HEPATOLOGY. Text in English. 1989. m. USD 347 domestic to individuals for print & online eds.; USD 347 foreign to individuals unknown; USD 782 per issue domestic to institutions; USD 782 per issue foreign to institutions; USD 58 newsstand/cover (effective 2002). adv. bibl, illus. index. *Refereed.* **Document type:** *Academic/Scholarly.* **Description:** Directed toward practicing gastroenterologists, hepatologists and researchers. Presents review articles followed by annotated bibliographies of references consulted. Includes a bibliography of the current world literature published during the previous year.
Related titles: CD-ROM ed.; Diskette ed.; Online - full text ed.: USD 1,016.60 domestic academic site license; USD 1,016.60 foreign academic site license; USD 1,133.90 domestic corporate site license; USD 1,133.90 foreign corporate site license (effective 2002) (from Ovid Technologies, Inc., EBSCO Publishing, Institute for Scientific Information); Hungarian ed.; ♦ Supplement: European Journal of Gastroenterology and Hepatology. Supplement. ISSN 0969-9163.
Indexed: ASCA, Abstr.Hyg., CINAHL, Curr.Cont., Diar.Dis.Res., Excerp.Med., Helminthol.Abstr., Ind.Med. (1989-), Inpharma, Int.Abstr.Biol.Sci., Jrnl.Watch Gastr., Nutr.Abstr., Pharm.&Out.News, Reac., Rev.Med.& Vet.Mycol., SSCI (coverage dropped), Soyabean Abstr., Trop.Dis.Bull.
—BLDSC (3829.729400), ADONIS, CISTI, EMDOCS, GNLM, IDS, KNAW.
Published by: Lippincott Williams & Wilkins (Philadelphia) (Subsidiary of: Wolters Kluwer N.V.), 530 Walnut St, Philadelphia, PA 19106-3621. TEL 215-521-8300, FAX 215-521-8902, http://www.Lww.com. Ed. J J Misiewicz. Adv. contact Anthony Gresford. Circ: 2,347. **Subscr. to:** PO Box 1600, Hagerstown, MD 21740-1600. TEL 800-777-2295, FAX 301-824-7390.

616.3 USA ISSN 0969-9163
CODEN: EJGSF
EUROPEAN JOURNAL OF GASTROENTEROLOGY AND HEPATOLOGY. SUPPLEMENT. Text in English. irreg. **Document type:** *Academic/Scholarly.*
Related titles: ♦ Supplement to: European Journal of Gastroenterology and Hepatology. ISSN 0954-691X.
Indexed: Excerp.Med. (1996-), Int.Abstr.Biol.Sci.
—ADONIS, KNAW.
Published by: Lippincott Williams & Wilkins (Philadelphia) (Subsidiary of: Wolters Kluwer N.V.), 530 Walnut St, Philadelphia, PA 19106-3621. TEL 215-521-8300, FAX 215-521-8902, http://www.lww.com. **Subscr. to:** PO Box 1600, Hagerstown, MD 21740-1600. TEL 800-777-2295, FAX 301-824-7390.

663 USA ISSN 1527-8557
▼ **EVIDENCE - BASED GASTROENTEROLOGY.** Text in English. 2000. q. USD 99 to individuals; USD 135 to institutions (effective 2002). *Refereed.* **Document type:** *Journal, Academic/Scholarly.* **Description:** Contains research and reports on new procedures and advances in gastroenterology.
Related titles: Online - full text ed.: USD 175.50 academic site license; USD 195.75 corporate site license (effective 2002).
Published by: Lippincott Williams & Wilkins (Philadelphia) (Subsidiary of: Wolters Kluwer N.V.), 530 Walnut St, Philadelphia, PA 19106-3621. TEL 215-521-8300, FAX 215-521-8902, custserv@lww.com, http://www.evidence-basedgastro.com, http://www.lww.com/. Eds. Dr. Glenn M. Eisen, Dr. John F. Johanson. **Subscr. to:** PO Box 1600, Hagerstown, MD 21740-1600. TEL 800-638-3030, FAX 310-223-2400.

EXCERPTA MEDICA. SECTION 48: GASTROENTEROLOGY. see *MEDICAL SCIENCES—Abstracting, Bibliographies, Statistics*

▼ **FOODBORNE PATHOGENS AND DISEASE.** see *MEDICAL SCIENCES—Communicable Diseases*

616.3 USA ISSN 0897-6759
FOUNDATION FOCUS. Text in English. 1977. 3/yr. USD 25 to members (effective 1999). adv. bk.rev. back issues avail. **Document type:** *Newsletter.* **Description:** Features stories about coping with Crohn's disease (ileitis) and ulcerative colitis; articles on CCFA-sponsored research and education programs; medical news and profiles of individuals.
Published by: Crohn's & Colitis Foundation of America, Inc., 386 Park Ave S, New York, NY 10016-7374. TEL 212-685-3440, 800-932-2423, FAX 212-779-4098, info@ccfa.org. R&P Rosemary Bimculli. Circ: 65,000.

616.3 CHE ISSN 0302-0665
CODEN: FGREDT
FRONTIERS OF GASTROINTESTINAL RESEARCH. Text in English. 1960. irreg., latest vol.24. CHF 280 per issue in Europe; DEM 330 per issue in Germany; USD 240 per issue in United States (effective 2001). reprint service avail. from ISI. *Refereed.* **Document type:** *Monographic series, Academic/Scholarly.*
Formerly (until 1975): Bibliotheca Gastroenterologica (0067-7949)
Related titles: Online - full text ed.: (from Institute for Scientific Information).
Indexed: ASCA, Biol.Abstr., Chem.Abstr., Chem.Indus.Notes, Chem.Titles, Curr.Cont. (coverage dropped), Ind.Med. (coverage dropped).
—BLDSC (4042.022000), CASDDS, CISTI, GNLM, Infotrieve, ingenta, KNAW. **CCC.**
Published by: S. Karger AG, Allschwilerstr 10, PO Box, Basel 4009, Switzerland. TEL 41-61-306-1111, FAX 41-61-306-1234, karger@karger.ch, http://www.karger.com/bookseries/FGARE. Eds. C Scarpignato, I M Modlin, P Rozen.

M

616.3 BRA ISSN 0101-7772
G E D. (Gastroenterologia e Endoscopia Digestiva) Text in Portuguese; Summaries in English, Portuguese. 1982. bi-m. BRL 72. abstr, bibl, illus.
Published by: (Sociedade Brasileira de Endoscopia Digestiva), Redprint Editora Ltda., Rua Domingos de Morais 2777, 15o cjs 151 e 154, Sao Paulo, SP 04035-001, Brazil. TEL 55-11-5724813, FAX 55-11-5711719.

616.3 VEN ISSN 0016-3503
G E N. Text in Spanish; Summaries in English, Spanish. 1946. q. VEB 4,000, USD 70. adv. bk.rev. abstr, bibl, charts, illus. **Document type:** *Academic/Scholarly.*
Indexed: Abstr.Hyg., Biol.Abstr., Excerp.Med., Helminthol.Abstr., Ind.Med. (coverage dropped), Trop.Dis.Bull.
—BLDSC (4096.385000), CISTI, GNLM.
Published by: Sociedad Venezolana de Gastroenterologia/Venezuelan Society of Gastroenterology, Torre del Colegio Piso 2, Ave. Jose Maria Vargas, Santa Fe Norte, Caracas, DF 1080, Venezuela. TEL 58-2-9765520, FAX 58-2-9799380. Ed. Dr. Mercedes Alvarado. Circ: 1,200.

G I CANCER; an international journal on gastrointestinal oncology. (Gastrointestinal) see *MEDICAL SCIENCES—Oncology*

G I G NEWSLETTER. see *NUTRITION AND DIETETICS*

▼ **GASTRIC CANCER.** see *MEDICAL SCIENCES—Oncology*

616.3 FRA ISSN 0399-8320
CODEN: GCBIDC
GASTRO-ENTEROLOGIE CLINIQUE ET BIOLOGIQUE. Text in French; Summaries in English. 1907. 10/yr. FRF 1,432; FRF 1,724 foreign (effective 2000). adv. bk.rev. illus. index. reprint service avail. from ISI. *Refereed.* **Document type:** *Academic/Scholarly.* **Description:** Publishes original work, clinical radiological laboratory and pathological documents related to gastroenterology, laboratory or experimental research on the digestive tract and related glands.
Former titles: Archives Francaises des Maladies de l'Appareil Digestif (0003-9772); Biologie et Gastro-Enterologie (0006-3258); Archives Francaises des Maladies de l'Appareil Digestif et des Maladies de la Nutrition
Related titles: Online - full text ed.: (from Institute for Scientific Information, RoweCom Information Quest).
Indexed: Biol.Abstr., Chem.Abstr., Chem.Indus.Notes, Chem.Titles, Curr.Adv.Biochem., Curr.Adv.Cancer Res., Curr.Adv.Ecol.Sci., Curr.Adv.Gen.& Molec.Biol., Curr.Cont., Dairy Sci.Abstr., Dent.Ind., Excerp.Med., Helminthol.Abstr., INIS Atomind., Ind.Med. (1977-), Inpharma, Nutr.Abstr., Pharm.&Out.News, Protozool.Abstr., Reac., Risk Abstr., Sci.Cit.Ind.
—BLDSC (4088.973000), CASDDS, CISTI, EMDOCS, GNLM, IDS, KNAW. **CCC.**
Published by: (Societe Nationale Francaise de Gastro-Enterologie), Masson - Periodiques, 120 bd. St. Germain, Paris 75006, France. TEL 33-1-40466200, FAX 33-1-40466201. Ed. Dr. Robaszkiewicz. Circ: 4,500. **Subscr. to:** Societe de Periodiques Specialises, BP 22, Vineuil Cedex 41354, France. TEL 33-2-54504612, FAX 33-1-54504611.

616.3 FRA ISSN 0995-7278
GASTRO-ENTEROLOGIE PRATIQUE. Text in French. 1989. m. (10/yr.). FRF 39 domestic to individuals; FRF 53 foreign to individuals; FRF 27 domestic to libraries; FRF 42 foreign to libraries (effective 2002). **Document type:** *Newspaper.*
Published by: L E N Medical, 15 rue des Sablons, Paris 75116, France. TEL 33-1-47553131, FAX 33-1-47553132, lenmed@club-internet.fr, http://www.webmedguide.com. Ed. Dr. Philippe Levy.

616.3 FRA ISSN 0016-5077
GASTRO-ENTEROLOGIE QUOTIDIENNE. Text in French. 1967. 3/yr. free per issue. adv. illus, tr.mk.
Published by: Laboratoires Beaufour, 18 place Doguereau, Dreux 28100, France. Ed. P Bernades. Circ: 30,000.

616.3 ITA ISSN 1120-3757
GASTROENTEROLOGIA CLINICA. Text in Italian. 1972. q., latest vol.30, 2001. USD 107 (effective 2000). adv. 48 p./no. **Document type:** *Academic/Scholarly.*
Related titles: ♦ Translation of: Gastroenterology Clinics of North America. ISSN 0889-8553.
Published by: Il Pensiero Scientifico Editore s.r.l., Via Bradano, 3-C, Rome, RM 00199, Italy. TEL 39-06-862821, FAX 39-06-86282250, pensiero@pensiero.it, http://www.pensiero.it. Pub. Luca De Fiore. R&P Andrea De Fiore. Adv. contact Luciano De Fiore. Circ: 350.

616.3 ESP ISSN 0210-5705
CODEN: GHEPDF
GASTROENTEROLOGIA Y HEPATOLOGIA. Text in Spanish; Summaries in English. 1978. m. (10/yr.). USD 116; free to qualified personnel. adv. reprint service avail. from PQC. **Document type:** *Academic/Scholarly.* **Description:** Covers gastroenterology, hepatology and pathology of the digestive tract, liver, pancreas and biliary paths.
Indexed: Excerp.Med., Ind.Med. (1978-), Ind.Med.Esp.
—EMDOCS, GNLM, Infotrieve, KNAW. **CCC.**
Published by: Ediciones Doyma S.A., Traversa de Gracia, 17-21, Barcelona 08021, Spain. TEL 34-93-200-0711, FAX 34-93-209-1136. Ed. Dr. J Rodes Teixidor. Adv. contact Eulalia Valls. color page ESP 259,000; trim 280 x 210. Circ: 2,500.

616.3 JPN ISSN 0387-1207
GASTROENTEROLOGICAL ENDOSCOPY. Text in Japanese. 1958. m. JPY 12,000, USD 120 to members (effective 2001). adv. charts, illus, abstr. 10 p./no. back issues avail. *Refereed.* **Document type:** *Academic/Scholarly.* **Description:** Serves as a medium for presenting original articles that offer significant contributions to knowledge in the broad field of endoscopy; also includes case reports, informal editorial opinions, abstracts, and news items that maybe of interest to endoscopists.
Indexed: Excerp.Med., INIS Atomind.
—BLDSC (4088.965000), EMDOCS, GNLM, KNAW. **CCC.**
Published by: Nihon Shokaki Naishikyo Gakkai/Japan Gastroenterological Endoscopy Society, Taimei Bldg, 3-22, Kanda Ogawa-machi, Chiyoda-ku, Tokyo 101-0052, Japan. TEL 81-3-3291-4111, FAX 81-3-3291-5568, info@jges.or.jp, http://www.jges.net. Ed. Takashi Nakamura. adv.: page JPY 78,000; 182 x 256. Circ: 27,500.

616.35 FRA ISSN 0989-263X
GASTROENTEROLOGIE. Variant title: Actualites Medicales Internationales. Gastroenterologie. Text in French. 1987. m. FRF 460, EUR 70.12 domestic to individuals; FRF 580, USD 105 foreign to individuals; FRF 580, EUR 88.42 domestic to institutions; FRF 700, USD 127 foreign to institutions; FRF 290 domestic to students; USD 75 foreign to students (effective 2000). adv. Supplement avail. *Refereed.* **Document type:** *Academic/Scholarly.* **Description:** Covers clinical and applied research in the field.
Published by: Medica-Press International, 62-64 rue Jean-Jaures, Puteaux 92800, France. TEL 33-1-41458000, FAX 33-1-41458025, contact@edimark.fr, http://www.edimark.fr. Ed. T Vallot. Pub. Claudie Damour Terrasson. Adv. contact Chantal Zuili.

616.3 USA ISSN 1065-2477
CODEN: GASTFG
THE GASTROENTEROLOGIST. Text in English. 1993. q. USD 114 domestic to individuals; USD 150 foreign to individuals; USD 201 domestic to institutions; USD 242 foreign to institutions; USD 61 newsstand/cover. adv. **Document type:** *Trade.* **Description:** Covers the latest in diagnosis and treatment in gastroenterology and nutrition through review articles. Other sections include New Techniques, Therapeutic Recommendations, and Grand Rounds.
Indexed: Excerp.Med. (1995-), Ind.Med. (1994-, dropped).
—GNLM.
Published by: Little, Brown & Co, 34 Beacon St, Boston, MA 02108. TEL 617-859-5500. adv.: B&W page USD 740, color page USD 1,710; trim 8.25 x 11. Circ: 984.

616.3 ITA ISSN 0391-8939
IL GASTROENTEROLOGO. Text in Italian; Summaries in Italian, English. 1979. 10/yr. ITL 40,000, USD 30 (effective 2001). adv.
Published by: C I C Edizioni Internazionali s.r.l., Corso Trieste 42, Rome, RM 00198, Italy. TEL 39-06-8412673, FAX 39-06-8412688, info@gruppocic.it, 1160199510. Pub. A Salvati. adv.: B&W page XEU 1,626.8, color page XEU 2,065.83; 210 x 290.

616.3 USA ISSN 0016-5085
RC799 CODEN: GASTAB
GASTROENTEROLOGY; a journal devoted to the clinical and basic studies of the digestive tract and liver. Text in English. 1943. 13/yr. USD 299 domestic to individuals Full text online included; USD 465 foreign to individuals Full text online included; USD 493 domestic to institutions Full text online included; USD 617 foreign to institutions Full text online included; USD 112 domestic to students Full text online included; USD 266 foreign to students Full text online included; USD 48 newsstand/cover (effective 2001). adv. bk.rev. abstr, charts, illus. cum.index. Supplement avail.; reprint service avail. from PQC. *Refereed.* **Document type:** *Journal, Academic/Scholarly.* **Description:** Provides clinical coverage of all areas of the digestive tract, including the liver.
Related titles: Microform ed.: (from PQC,WWS); Online - full text ed.: ISSN 1528-0012 (from HighWire Pr., EBSCO Publishing, IDEAL Online Library, Institute for Scientific Information).
Indexed: AIM, ASCA, Abstr.Hyg., Abstr.Inter.Med., Agri.& Environ.Biotech.Abstr. (coverage dropped), Behav.Med.Abstr., Biol.Abstr., C.I.S. Abstr., Chem.Abstr., Chem.Indus.Notes, Chem.Titles, Curr.Adv.Biochem., Curr.Adv.Cancer Res., Curr.Adv.Cell & Devel.Biol., Curr.Adv.Ecol.Sci., Curr.Cont., Dairy Sci.Abstr., Dent.Ind., Derwent Biotech.Abstr., Diar.Dis.Res., Excerp.Med., Food Sci.& Tech.Abstr., Helminthol.Abstr., INIS Atomind., Ind.Med. (1943-), Ind.Sci.Rev., Ind.Vet., Inpharma, Int.Abstr.Biol.Sci., Int.Nurs.Ind., Jrnl.Watch, Jrnl.Watch Gastr., Jrnl.Watch Inf.Dis., Kidney, Med.& Surg.Dermat., NRN, Neurosci.Cit.Ind., Nutr.Abstr., Pharm.&Out.News, Pig News & Info., Protozool.Abstr., Reac., Rev.Arom.& Med.Plants, Rev.Med.& Vet.Mycol., Rice Abstr., Risk Abstr., SSCI (coverage dropped), Sci.Cit.Ind., Small Anim.Abstr., Soyabean Abstr., THA, Trop.Dis.Bull., Vet.Bull.
—BLDSC (4089.000000), CASDDS, CISTI, GNLM, IDS, ingenta, KNAW. **CCC.**
Published by: (American Gastroenterological Association), W.B. Saunders Co. (Subsidiary of: Harcourt Publishers Ltd.), Curtis Center, Independence Sq W, Philadelphia, PA 19106-3399. TEL 215-238-7800, FAX 215-238-6445, http://www.gastrojournal.org/, http://www.wbsaunders.com. Ed. Dr. David Brenner. adv.: B&W page USD 1,990, color page USD 3,890; trim 10 x 7. Circ: 16,608. **Subscr. to:** Periodicals Fulfillment, W B Saunders Co, 6277 Sea Harbor Dr, 4th Fl, Orlando, FL 32891-4800. TEL 800-654-2542, FAX 800-874-6418.

616.35 USA ISSN 0883-8348
RC864.A1
GASTROENTEROLOGY AND ENDOSCOPY NEWS. Text in English. 1978. m. USD 60; USD 75 foreign (effective 1999). adv. bk.rev. bibl, illus. index. *Refereed.* **Document type:** *Academic/Scholarly.*
Former titles (until 1985): American Journal of Proctology, Gastroenterology and Colon and Rectal Surgery (0162-6566); (until 1977): American Journal of Proctology (0002-9521)
Related titles: Microform ed.: (from PQC); Online - full text ed.
Indexed: Biol.Abstr., Curr.Cont. (coverage dropped), Excerp.Med., INIS Atomind., Ind.Med. (coverage dropped).
—GNLM, IDS.
Published by: McMahon Group, 545 W 45th St, 8th Fl, New York, NY 10036. TEL 212-957-5300, FAX 212-957-7230. Ed. Kirell Lakhman. Circ: 8,000.

616.3 USA ISSN 0889-8553
RC799 CODEN: GCNAEF
GASTROENTEROLOGY CLINICS OF NORTH AMERICA. Text in English. 1972. q. USD 158 domestic to individuals; USD 172 in Canada to individuals; USD 203 elsewhere to individuals; USD 207 domestic to institutions; USD 249 foreign to institutions; USD 63 per issue (effective 2001). *Refereed.* **Document type:** *Journal, Academic/Scholarly.* **Description:** Delivers practical advice from experts in specialty covered, gives information on new developments in a variety of specialties, plus a fresh perspective on problems and controversies.
Supersedes in part (in 1987): Clinics in Gastroenterology (0300-5089)
Related titles: Online - full text ed.: (from Institute for Scientific Information); ♦ Italian Translation: Gastroenterologia Clinica. ISSN 1120-3757.
Indexed: ASCA, Biol.Abstr., CINAHL, Chem.Abstr., Curr.Adv.Ecol.Sci., Curr.Cont., Dent.Ind., Diar.Dis.Res., Excerp.Med., Helminthol.Abstr., INIS Atomind., Ind.Med. (1987-), Ind.Sci.Rev., Inpharma, Nutr.Abstr., Pharm.&Out.News, Reac., SSCI (coverage dropped), Sci.Cit.Ind.
—BLDSC (4089.031500), CASDDS, CISTI, EMDOCS, GNLM, IDS, ingenta, KNAW. **CCC.**

Published by: W.B. Saunders Co. (Subsidiary of: Harcourt Publishers Ltd.), 11830 Westline Industrial Dr, St Louis, MO 63146. TEL 800-325-4177, http://www.wbsaunders.com. **Subscr. to:** Periodicals Fulfillment, W B Saunders Co, 6277 Sea Harbor Dr, 4th Fl, Orlando, FL 32891-4800.

616.3 ITA ISSN 0950-5911
CODEN: GASIEG
GASTROENTEROLOGY INTERNATIONAL (INTERNATIONAL EDITION). Text in English. 1988. q. USD 160 to individuals; USD 190 to institutions. adv. back issues avail.; reprints avail. **Document type:** *Academic/Scholarly.* **Description:** Publishes reports from international working teams, composed of leading clinicians and appointed by the editors, on controversial clinical topics. Provides information on the activities of the major international gastroenterological organizations.
Indexed: Int.Abstr.Biol.Sci.
—BLDSC (4089.032000), CISTI, EMDOCS, GNLM, KNAW.
Published by: International University Press, Via Monte Delle Gioie, 22, Rome, RM 00199, Italy. TEL 39-6-86211027, FAX 39-6-86211026, univpres@tin.it. Ed. Juan Malagelada. Pub., R&P Giulio Bertolaccini TEL 39-6-862110278. Adv. contact Isabella Leonardo. B&W page USD 1,200, color page USD 2,150; trim 235 x 179. Circ: 3,000.

616.3 USA ISSN 1042-895X
RC804.E6 CODEN: GANUER
GASTROENTEROLOGY NURSING. Text in English. 1977. bi-m. USD 99 domestic to individuals; USD 149 foreign to individuals; USD 169 domestic to institutions; USD 199 foreign to institutions; USD 34 newsstand/cover (effective 2002). adv. bk.rev. back issues avail. **Document type:** *Academic/Scholarly.* **Description:** Describes new procedures, techniques and equipment for gastroenterology nurses and associates.
Formerly: S G A Journal (0149-6212)
Related titles: Microfilm ed.: (from WWS); Online - full text ed.: (from Ovid Technologies, Inc.).
Indexed: CINAHL, INIS Atomind., Int.Nurs.Ind.
—BLDSC (4089.032300), CISTI, GNLM, KNAW.
Published by: (Society of Gastroenterology Nurses and Associates), Williams & Wilkins (Subsidiary of: Waverly International), 351 W Camden St, Baltimore, MD 21201-2436. TEL 410-528-4068, 800-222-3790, FAX 410-528-4452, gpessagno@wwilkins.com, http://www.wwilkins.com, http://www.Lww.com. Ed. Belinda E Puetz. Adv. contact Greg Pessagno. B&W page USD 1,010; 10.88 x 8.13. Circ: 7,146; 6,780 (paid).

616.3 USA
GASTROENTEROLOGY NURSING BUYER'S GUIDE. Text in English. a. free per issue to qualified personnel. adv. **Description:** Comprehensive directory of manufacturers and service providers in the gastroenterology marketplace.
Published by: Williams & Wilkins (Subsidiary of: Waverly International), 351 W Camden St, Baltimore, MD 21201-2436. TEL 410-528-4068, 800-222-3790, FAX 410-528-4452, gpessagno@wwilkins.com, http://www.wilkins.com. Ed., Adv. contact Greg Pessagno.

616.3 GBR ISSN 0969-0131
GASTROENTEROLOGY TODAY. Text in English. 1991. q. GBP 18 domestic to individuals; GBP 30 foreign to individuals; GBP 30 domestic to institutions; GBP 50 foreign to institutions (effective 2000). **Document type:** *Trade.*
Published by: Media Publishing Company, Media House, 41 Crayford Way, Dartford, Kent DA1 4JY, United Kingdom. TEL 44-1322-558029, FAX 44-1322-558524, medipub@aol.com. Ed. M Goldman.

616.3 USA ISSN 0016-5107
RC804.E6 CODEN: GAENBQ
GASTROINTESTINAL ENDOSCOPY. Text in English. 1954. m. USD 171 domestic to individuals; USD 224 foreign to individuals; USD 239 domestic to institutions; USD 299 foreign to institutions; USD 94 domestic to students; USD 147 foreign to students; USD 25 newsstand/cover domestic (effective 2001). adv. bk.rev. abstr. index. back issues avail.; reprints avail. *Refereed.* **Document type:** *Journal, Academic/Scholarly.* **Description:** Contains current papers in endoscopy for gastroenterologists and general surgeons.
Formerly: Bulletin of Gastrointestinal Endoscopy
Related titles: Microfilm ed.: (from WWS); Online - full text ed.: (from EBSCO Publishing, IDEAL Online Library, Institute for Scientific Information, RoweCom Information Quest).
Indexed: AMED, ASCA, Abstr.Hyg., Biol.Abstr., CINAHL, Curr.Adv.Cancer Res., Curr.Cont., Excerp.Med., Helminthol.Abstr., INIS Atomind., Ind.Med. (1965-), Ind.Sci.Rev., Inpharma, Int.Nurs.Ind., Jrnl.Watch Gastr., Nutr.Abstr., Pharm.&Out.News, Protozool.Abstr., Reac., Rev.Med.& Vet.Mycol., Sci.Cit.Ind., Sugar Ind.Abstr., Trop.Dis.Bull.
—BLDSC (4089.050000), CISTI, GNLM, IDS, ingenta, KNAW. **CCC.**
Published by: (American Society for Gastrointestinal Endoscopy), Mosby, Inc. (Subsidiary of: Elsevier Science), 11830 Westline Industrial Dr, St Louis, MO 63146-3318. TEL 314-453-4307, 800-325-4177, FAX 314-872-9164, customerservice@mosby.com, http://www.mosby.com/gie, http://www.mosby.com/periodicals. Ed. Dr. Michael V Sivak Jr. Pub. Terrie Duhadway. Adv. contact Gina Burkert TEL 314-453-4306. B&W page USD 1,080, color page USD 2,430; trim 10.88 x 8.13. Circ: 10,228.

616.3 USA ISSN 1052-5157
CODEN: GECNED
GASTROINTESTINAL ENDOSCOPY CLINICS OF NORTH AMERICA. Text in English. 1991. q. USD 158 domestic to individuals; USD 172 in Canada to individuals; USD 188 elsewhere to individuals; USD 195 domestic to institutions; USD 242 foreign to institutions; USD 61 per issue (effective 2001). **Document type:** *Academic/Scholarly.* **Description:** Each issue focuses on the treatment or diagnosis of a condition or disease of the digestive tract.
Related titles: Microform ed.: (from PQC).
Indexed: CINAHL, Excerp.Med. (1993-), Ind.Med. (1991-).
—BLDSC (4089.052000), EMDOCS, GNLM, KNAW.
Published by: W.B. Saunders Co. (Subsidiary of: Harcourt Publishers Ltd.), 11830 Westline Industrial Dr, St Louis, MO 63146. TEL 800-325-4177, http://www.wbsaunders.com. Ed. Dr. Charles J Lightdale. **Subscr. to:** Periodicals Fulfillment, W B Saunders Co, 6277 Sea Harbor Dr, 4th Fl, Orlando, FL 32891-4800.

GASTROINTESTINAL HORMONES AND GASTRIC SECRETION. see *MEDICAL SCIENCES—Abstracting, Bibliographies, Statistics*

616.3 ESP ISSN 0211-058X
GASTRUM PATOLOGIA DEL APARATO DIGESTIVO. Text in Spanish. 1977. 4/yr. ESP 6,000 (effective 2001). adv. **Document type:** *Monographic series.*
Address: Antonio Lopez Aguado, 4, Madrid 28029, Spain. TEL 1-314-43-38, FAX 1-314-44-99, editorial@jarpyo.es, http://jarpyo.es/. Ed. Dr. Jose Mora Sainz. Circ: 2,838.

616.3 ITA
GIORNALE DI GASTROENTEROLOGY. Text in Italian. 1990. q. USD 80 to individuals; USD 120 to institutions. adv. back issues avail.; reprints avail. **Document type:** *Academic/Scholarly.* **Description:** Devoted to education and international cooperation in the field of digestive disease.
Formerly: Gastroenterology International (Italian Edition) (1120-4818)
Published by: International University Press, Via Monte Delle Gioie, 22, Rome, RM 00199, Italy. TEL 39-6-86211027, FAX 39-6-86211026, univpres@tin.it. Ed. Renzo Caprilli. Pub., R&P Giulio Bertolaccini TEL 39-6-862110278. Adv. contact Isabella Leonardo. B&W page USD 3,500, color page USD 7,800; trim 28 x 21. Circ: 10,000.

616.3 ITA ISSN 0394-0225
GIORNALE ITALIANO DI ENDOSCOPIA DIGESTIVA. Text in Italian; Summaries in English. 1978. 4/yr. ITL 88,000 (effective 1999). reprint service avail. from PQC. **Document type:** *Academic/Scholarly.*
Formerly (until 1980): Giornale di Gastroenterologia ed Endoscopia (0394-0489)
Indexed: Excerp.Med.
—EMDOCS, GNLM.
Published by: (Societa Italiana di Endoscopia Digestiva), Masson S.p.A., Divisione Periodici, Via F.lli Bressan 2, Milan, MI 20126, Italy. TEL 39-2-270741, FAX 39-2-27074210. Ed. Renzo Cestari. adv.: B&W page ITL 2,100,000, color page ITL 2,900,000; trim 280 x 210. Circ: 2,000.

616.3 GBR ISSN 0017-5749
CODEN: GUTTAK
GUT; an international journal of gastroenterology & hepatology. Text in English. 1960. m. GBP 129, USD 205 combined subscription to individuals includes print & online eds.; GBP 309 to institutions for print ed. only.; USD 476 to institutions for print ed. only (effective 2002). adv. bk.rev. charts, illus. index. reprint service avail. from PQC. *Refereed.* **Document type:** *Journal, Academic/Scholarly.* **Description:** Covers all diseases of the alimentary tract, liver, biliary tree, and pancreas.
Related titles: CD-ROM ed.: (from Ovid Technologies, Inc.); Microform ed.: (from PQC); Online - full text ed.: Gut Online. ISSN 1468-3288. GBP 85, USD 125 to individuals for online ed. (effective 2001); Institutions please contact publisher for online only rates. (from HighWire Pr., Ovid Technologies, Inc., Northern Light Technology, Inc., EBSCO Publishing, RoweCom Information Quest, ProQuest Information & Learning, ingenta, Swets Blackwell, SilverPlatter Information, Inc., Institute for Scientific Information).
Indexed: AIM, Agri.& Environ.Biotech.Abstr. (coverage dropped), Behav.Med.Abstr., Biol.Abstr., Chem.Abstr., Chem.Indus.Notes, Chem.Titles, Curr.Adv.Ecol.Sci., Curr.Cont., Dairy Sci.Abstr., Dent.Ind., Derwent Biotech.Abstr., Diar.Dis.Res., Excerp.Med., Helminthol.Abstr., INIS Atomind., I.P.A., Ind.Med. (1960-), Ind.Sci.Rev., Ind.Vet., Inpharma, Int.Abstr.Biol.Sci., Int.Nurs.Ind., Jrnl.Watch Gastr., NRN, Nutr.Abstr., Pharm.&Out.News, Protozool.Abstr., Reac., Rev.Arom.& Med.Plants, SSCI (coverage dropped), Sci.Cit.Ind., Triticale Abstr., Trop.Dis.Bull., Vet.Bull.
—BLDSC (4232.400000), ADONIS, CASDDS, CISTI, GNLM, IDS, ingenta, KNAW. **CCC.**
Published by: (British Society of Gastroenterology), B M J Publishing Group, B M A House, Tavistock Sq, London WC1H 9JR, United Kingdom. TEL 44-20-7387-4499, FAX 44-20-7383-6400, info.norththames@bma.org.uk, http://www.gutjnl.com, http://www.bma.org.uk. Ed. M Farthing. Pub. Alex Williamson. R&P Carol Torselli TEL 44-20-7383-6674. Adv. contact Euan Currer TEL 44-20-7383-6181.

616.36 GBR ISSN 1365-182X
H P B. Variant title: Hepato Pancreato Biliary. Text in English. 1997. q. GBP 90, USD 150 to individuals; GBP 165, USD 270 to institutions (effective 2002). **Document type:** *Journal, Academic/Scholarly.* **Description:** Contains original research, reviews, HPB images, editorials, case reports and reader correspondence connected with the various scientific and clinical interests involved in hepatic, pancreatic and biliary disease, along with the latest news from the IHPBA.
Related titles: Online - full content ed.; Online - full text ed.: (from CatchWord Ltd.).
Published by: (International Hepato Pancreato Biliary Association JPN), Isis Medical Media Ltd. (Subsidiary of: Martin Dunitz Ltd.), The Livery House, 7-9 Pratt St, London NW1 0AE, United Kingdom. TEL 44-20-7482-2202, FAX 44-20-7267-0159, info@dunitz.co.uk, http://www.dunitz.co.uk/. Ed. Robin Williamson.

HELICOBACTER. see *BIOLOGY—Microbiology*

616.362 USA
HEPATITIS SOURCEBOOK. Text in English. 1997. a. USD 269; USD 229 foreign (effective 1999). **Document type:** *Trade.*
Published by: American Health Consultants (Subsidiary of: Medical Economics Co., Inc.), 3525 Piedmont Rd, N E, 6 Piedmont Center, Ste 400, Atlanta, GA 30305. TEL 404-262-5476, custserv@ahcpub.com, http://www.ahcpub.com.

616.3 FRA ISSN 1253-7020
CODEN: HEGAF6
HEPATO - GASTRO. Text in French. 1994. bi-m. FRF 670 domestic to individuals; EUR 114 in Europe to individuals; FRF 790 elsewhere to individuals; FRF 1,120 domestic to institutions; EUR 183 in Europe to institutions; FRF 1,240 elsewhere to institutions; FRF 390 domestic to students; EUR 72 in Europe to students; FRF 520 elsewhere to students (effective 2001). **Document type:** *Trade.* **Description:** Used as a training and updating tool in digestive pathology. Includes bibliographical synopses, mini-reviews and annotated clinical cases.
Related titles: CD-ROM ed.: FRF 590 domestic; FRF 620 foreign (effective 2001); Online - full text ed.: FRF 670 to individuals; FRF 1,120 to institutions; FRF 390 to students (effective 2001).
Indexed: Excerp.Med. (1996-), Inpharma, Reac.
—BLDSC (4295.833000), GNLM, KNAW.

Published by: John Libbey Eurotext, 127 av. de la Republique, Montrouge 92120, France. TEL 33-01-46730660, FAX 33-01-40840999, marketing@jle.com, http://www.john-libbey-eurotext.fr/. Eds. Jean Paul Galmiche, Jean Pierre Benhamou. Circ: 1,000. **Subscr. to:** A T E I, 3 av. Pierre Keraútret, Romainville 92230, France. TEL 33-1-48408686, atei@club-internet.fr.

616.3 GRC ISSN 0172-6390
CODEN: HEGAD4

HEPATO-GASTROENTEROLOGY. Text in English; Summaries in English, German. 1954. bi-m. EUR 332 to institutions; EUR 58 newsstand/cover (effective 2002). adv. bk.rev. abstr, bibl, charts, illus, stat. index. back issues avail.; reprint service avail. from PQC. *Refereed.* **Document type:** *Journal, Academic/Scholarly.*

Former titles: Acta Hepato-Gastroenterologica (0300-970X); Acta Hepato- Splenologica (0001-5822)

Related titles: Microform ed.: (from PQC); Online - full text ed.: (from Institute for Scientific Information).

Indexed: ASCA, Biol.Abstr., Chem.Abstr., Curr.Adv.Ecol.Sci., Curr.Cont., Dent.Ind., Excerp.Med., Helminthol.Abstr., INIS Atomind., Ind.Med. (1980-), Ind.Sci.Rev., Inpharma, Int.Abstr.Biol.Sci., Int.Nurs.Ind., Jrnl.Watch Gastr., Mass Spectr.Bull., Nutr.Abstr., Pharm.&Out.News, Reac., Rev.Med.& Vet.Mycol., Sci.Cit.Ind.

—BLDSC (4295.835000), ADONIS, CASDDS, CISTI, GNLM, ingenta, KNAW. **CCC.**

Address: PO Box 17160, Athens 100 24, Greece. TEL 30-1-3623333, FAX 30-1-7245988. Ed. N J Lygidakis. Circ: 2,700.

616.362 USA ISSN 0270-9139
RC845 CODEN: HPTLD9

HEPATOLOGY. Text in English. 1981. m. USD 422 domestic to individuals print & online eds. combined; USD 500 foreign to individuals print & online eds. combined; USD 685 domestic to institutions print & online eds. combined; USD 768 foreign to institutions print & online eds. combined; USD 122 domestic to students print & online eds. combined; USD 195 foreign to students print & online eds. combined; USD 65 per issue domestic (effective 2001). adv. bk.rev. back issues avail. *Refereed.* **Document type:** *Journal, Academic/Scholarly.* **Description:** Examines hepatitis, gallstone formation, drug injury, liver physiology and disease. For gastroenterologists and internists.

Related titles: Microform ed.: (from WWS); Online - full text ed.: (from HighWire Pr., EBSCO Publishing, IDEAL Online Library, Institute for Scientific Information).

Indexed: ASCA, Addic.Abstr., Chem.Abstr., Chem.Indus.Notes, Chem.Titles, Curr.Adv.Cancer Res., Curr.Adv.Ecol.Sci., Curr.Cont., Excerp.Med., INIS Atomind., Ind.Med. (1981-), Ind.Sci.Rev., Ind.Vet., Inpharma, Int.Abstr.Biol.Sci., Jrnl.Watch Gastr., Kidney, Neurosci.Cit.Ind., Nutr.Abstr., Pharm.&Out.News, Pig News & Info., Poult.Abstr., Protozool.Abstr., Reac., Rev.Med.& Vet.Mycol., Risk Abstr., SSCI (coverage dropped), Sci.Cit.Ind., Sugar Ind.Abstr., Vet.Bull.

—BLDSC (4295.836000), CASDDS, CISTI, EMDOCS, GNLM, IDS, ingenta, KNAW. **CCC.**

Published by: (American Association for the Study of Liver Diseases), W.B. Saunders Co. (Subsidiary of: Harcourt Publishers Ltd.), Curtis Center, 3rd Fl, Independence Sq W, Philadelphia, PA 19106-3399. TEL 215-238-7800, FAX 215-238-6445, http://www.hepatology.org/. Ed. Dr. Andres Blei. adv.: B&W page USD 860; trim 10 x 7. Circ: 5,718. **Subscr. to:** Periodicals Fulfillment, W B Saunders Co, 6277 Sea Harbor Dr, 4th Fl, Orlando, FL 32891-4800.

616.362 IRL ISSN 1386-6346
CODEN: HPRSFM

HEPATOLOGY RESEARCH; an international journal for the rapid dissemination of original short communications in hepatology. Text in English. 1993. 9/yr. EUR 813 in Europe to institutions; JPY 107,800 in Japan to institutions; USD 910 elsewhere to institutions (effective 2002). back issues avail. *Refereed.* **Document type:** *Academic/Scholarly.* **Description:** Publishes reports of basic and clinical research in the field of hepatology, and reviews on selected aspects of hepatology undergoing rapid change.

Formerly (until 1997, vol.7): International Hepatology Communications (0928-4346); Which was previously announced as: Hepatology Letters

Related titles: Microform ed.: (from PQC); Online - full text ed.: (from ingenta, Swets Blackwell, ScienceDirect, Institute for Scientific Information).

Indexed: ASCA, Curr.Cont., Excerp.Med. (1994-), Inpharma, Pharm.&Out.News, Reac.

—BLDSC (4295.845000), CISTI, EMDOCS, GNLM, IDS, Infotrieve, KNAW. **CCC.**

Published by: Elsevier Science Ireland Ltd, Elsevier House, Brookvale Plaza, E. Park, Shannon, Co. Clare, Ireland. TEL 353-61-471944, FAX 353-61-472144, http://www.elsevier.com/locate/ihepcom. Eds. T W Okita, T Tsujii. **Subscr. in Australasia and the Far East to:** Elsevier Science (Singapore) Pte Ltd, No.1 Temasek Ave, 17-01 Millenia Tower, Singapore 039192, Singapore. TEL 65-434-3727, FAX 65-337-2230; **Subscr. in the Americas to:** Elsevier Science, PO Box 945, New York, NY 10159-0945. TEL 212-633-3730, FAX 212-633-3680; **Subscr. to:** Elsevier Science BV, PO Box 211, Amsterdam 1000 AE, Netherlands. TEL 31-20-485-3757.

I E H REPORT ON FACTORS AFFECTING THE ABSORPTION OF TOXIC METALS FROM THE DIET. see *ENVIRONMENTAL STUDIES—Toxicology And Environmental Safety*

616.3 JPN ISSN 0536-2180

I TO CHO/STOMACH AND INTESTINE. Text in Japanese; Summaries in English. 1966. m. JPY 29,600, USD 292.70.

Related titles: Online - full text ed.: (from JICST).

Indexed: INIS Atomind.

—BLDSC (8465.870000), CISTI, EMDOCS, GNLM.

Published by: Igaku-Shoin Ltd., 5-24-3 Hongo, Bunkyo-ku, Tokyo 113-0033, Japan. TEL 81-3-3817-5714, FAX 81-3-3815-7802, itocyo@nna.so.net.or.jp. Circ: 15,000.

616.3 GBR ISSN 1352-8513
CODEN: ICRGF8

ILLUSTRATED CASE REPORTS IN GASTROENTEROLOGY. Text in English. 1994. q. USD 145 to individuals; USD 265 to institutions. adv. illus. reprints avail. *Refereed.* **Document type:** *Academic/Scholarly.* **Description:** Covers all research and clinical aspects of gastroenterology.

Related titles: Online - full text ed.: (from Swets Blackwell).

Published by: Chapman & Hall, Journals Department (Subsidiary of: International Thomson Publishing Group), Chapman & Hall, 2-6 Boundary Row, London SE1 8HN, United Kingdom. TEL 44-20-7865-0066, FAX 44-20-7522-9323, jhelp@chall.co.uk, http://www.chaphall.com/chaphall/journals.html. Ed. K R F Schiller. **Subscr. to:** International Thompson Publishing Services Ltd.

616.3 IND ISSN 0970-0935

INDIAN JOURNAL OF COLO-PROCTOLOGY. Text in English. 1986. s-a. INR 500, USD 100 (effective 2000). adv. bk.rev. index. *Refereed.* **Document type:** *Academic/Scholarly.* **Description:** Contains original papers, research articles, and case reports in the field of colo-proctology.

Published by: Association of Colon and Rectal Surgeons of India, Tata Memorial Hospital, Parel, Mumbai, Maharashtra 400 012, India. TEL 91-22-4137316, jaganath@bom3.vsnl.net.in. Ed. Dr. P Jagannath. Circ: 500.

616.3 IND ISSN 0254-8860
CODEN: IJOGD

INDIAN JOURNAL OF GASTROENTEROLOGY. Text in English. 1982. q. INR 350 domestic; USD 75 foreign (effective 2000). adv. bk.rev. abstr, bibl. back issues avail. *Refereed.* **Document type:** *Proceedings, Academic/Scholarly.*

Related titles: Online - full text ed.; ♦ Supplement: Indian Society of Gastroenterology. Proceedings of the Annual Conference.

Indexed: Abstr.Hyg., Diar.Dis.Res., Excerp.Med., Helminthol.Abstr., Ind.Med. (1982-), Ind.Vet., Nutr.Abstr., Protozool.Abstr., Rev.Arom.& Med.Plants, Trop.Dis.Bull.

—BLDSC (4412.760000), CISTI, EMDOCS, GNLM, Infotrieve, KNAW. **CCC.**

Published by: Indian Society of Gastroenterology, 23 Bombay Mutual Terrace, 534 Sandhurst Bridge, Mumbai, Maharashtra 400 007, India. TEL 91-22-3613344, FAX 91-22-4143435, editor@indianjgastro.com, http://www.indianjgastro.com. Ed. Philip Abraham. Circ: 1,200.

616.3 IND

INDIAN SOCIETY OF GASTROENTEROLOGY. PROCEEDINGS OF THE ANNUAL CONFERENCE. Text in English. 1962. a. USD 25 (effective 2000). adv. bk.rev. **Document type:** *Academic/Scholarly.*

Related titles: ♦ Supplement to: Indian Journal of Gastroenterology. ISSN 0254-8860.

Indexed: Excerp.Med., Ind.Med. (coverage dropped).

Published by: Indian Society of Gastroenterology, 23 Bombay Mutual Terrace, 534 Sandhurst Bridge, Mumbai, Maharashtra 400 007, India. TEL 91-22-3613344, FAX 91-22-4143435, editor@indianjgastro.com, http://www.indianjgastro.com. Ed., R&P Philip Abraham. Circ: 1,800.

616.3 USA ISSN 1078-0998

INFLAMMATORY BOWEL DISEASES. Text in English. 1976. q. USD 183 domestic to individuals; USD 183 foreign to individuals; USD 228 domestic to institutions; USD 228 foreign to institutions (effective 2002); USD 47 newsstand/cover. adv. bk.rev. abstr, bibl. back issues avail. *Refereed.* **Document type:** *Academic/Scholarly.* **Description:** Articles on basic research and clinical studies related to Crohn's disease and ulcerative colitis, also known as inflammatory bowel disease.

Former titles (until 1995): Progress in Inflammatory Bowel Disease; (until 1990): I B D News

Related titles: Microfiche ed.: (from PQC); Online - full text ed.: (from Institute for Scientific Information).

Indexed: Curr.Cont., Ind.Med. (1995-), Inpharma, Int.Nurs.Ind., Jrnl.Watch Gastr., Nutr.Abstr., Pharm.&Out.News, Reac.

—BLDSC (4478.845400), GNLM, IDS.

Published by: (Crohn's & Colitis Foundation of America, Inc.), Lippincott Williams & Wilkins (Philadelphia) (Subsidiary of: Wolters Kluwer N.V.), 530 Walnut St, Philadelphia, PA 19106-3621. TEL 215-521-8300, FAX 215-521-8902, http://www.lww.com. Eds. Dr. Richard P MacDermott, Dr. Robert Burakoff. Pub. Shelley Johnson. R&P Margaret Becker. Adv. contact Ray Thibodeau. B&W page USD 940, color page USD 2,010. Circ: 3,688 (paid). **In Japan subscr. to:** Igaku-Shoin, 1-28-36 Hongo, Bunkyo-ku, Tokyo 113-0033, Japan; **Subscr. to:** PO Box 1600, Hagerstown, MD 21740-1600. TEL 800-777-2295, FAX 301-824-7390.

616.3 USA ISSN 1047-5028
CODEN: IDITE8

INFLAMMATORY DISEASE AND THERAPY. Text in English. 1989. irreg., latest vol.12, 1993. price varies. adv. **Document type:** *Monographic series.*

Indexed: Chem.Abstr., Chem.Indus.Notes, Chem.Titles.

—CASDDS, Infotrieve, KNAW. **CCC.**

Published by: Marcel Dekker, Inc., Attn: Eridania Perrez, 270 Madison Ave, New York, NY 10016-0602. TEL 212-696-9000, 800-228-1160, FAX 212-685-4540, marketing@dekker.com, http://www.dekker.com. Pub. Russell Dekker. R&P Julia Mulligan. Adv. contact Eridania Perez.

616.3 GBR ISSN 1363-4534

INTERNATIONAL JOURNAL OF GASTROENTEROLOGY. Text in English. 1990. q. adv. bk.rev. **Document type:** *Academic/Scholarly.*

Formerly (until 1996): Gastroenterology in Practice (0966-6311); Supersedes in part (in 1991): Gastroenterology and Rheumatology in Practice (0959-3314); Which was formed by the merger of (1983-1990): Gastroenterology in Practice (0264-7478); (1981-1990): Rheumatology in Practice (0262-5512)

—BLDSC (4542.262500).

Published by: Hayward Medical Communications Ltd., 44 Earlham St, Covent Garden, London WC2H 7LA, United Kingdom. TEL 44-20-7240-4493, FAX 44-20-7240-4479, admin@hayward.co.uk, http://www.hayward.co.uk. Ed. Dr. Val Heatley. Circ: 27,000. **Subscr. to:** Rosemary House, Lanwades Park, Kentford, Near, Newmarket, Suffolk CB8 7PW, United Kingdom. TEL 44-1638-751515, FAX 44-1638-751517.

INTERNATIONAL JOURNAL OF PANCREATOLOGY. see *MEDICAL SCIENCES—Endocrinology*

616.3 CAN ISSN 1188-4525

INTERNATIONAL SEMINARS IN PAEDIATRIC GASTROENTEROLOGY AND NUTRITION. Text in English. 1990. q. USD 65 in US & Canada to individuals; USD 90 elsewhere to individuals; USD 95 in US & Canada to institutions; USD 125 elsewhere to institutions. back issues avail. **Document type:** *Newsletter, Academic/Scholarly.* **Description:** Offers a review of current investigation and clinical practice in the nutritional management of children.

Formerly (until 1992): Seminars in Paediatric Gastroenterology and Nutrition (1188-0244)

Related titles: Online - full text ed.: (from ProQuest Information & Learning).

—Infotrieve, KNAW. **CCC.**

Published by: B.C. Decker Inc., 20 Hughson St S, LCD 1, P O Box 620, Hamilton, ON L8N 3K7, Canada. TEL 905-522-7017, 800-568-7281, FAX 905-522-7839, info@bcdecker.com, http://www.bcdecker.com. Ed. W Allan Walker.

M

616.3 USA

▼ **THE INTERNET JOURNAL OF GASTROENTEROLOGY.** Text in English. 2000. s-a. free per issue. adv. bk.rev. back issues avail. *Refereed.* **Document type:** *Academic/Scholarly.* **Description:** Provides information from the field of gastroenterology and digestive diseases; contains original articles, reviews, case reports, streaming slide shows, streaming videos, letters to the editor, press releases, and meeting information.
Media: Online - full content.
Published by: Internet Scientific Publications, L.L.C., 23 Rippling Creek Dr, Sugar Land, TX 77479. TEL 281-240-1533, FAX 281-240-1533, http://www.ispub.com/. Ed. Sandeep Lahoti. R&P, Adv. contact Hope Morrow TEL 832-754-0335.

INTESTINAL FUNCTION. see *MEDICAL SCIENCES—Abstracting, Bibliographies, Statistics*

616.3 USA ISSN 0192-0790
RC799

JOURNAL OF CLINICAL GASTROENTEROLOGY. Text in English. 1979. 10/yr. USD 229 domestic to individuals; USD 307 foreign to individuals; USD 490 domestic to institutions; USD 499 foreign to institutions; USD 46 newsstand/cover (effective 2002). adv. bk.rev. charts, illus, stat. index. back issues avail.; reprint service avail. from PQC. *Refereed.* **Document type:** *Academic/Scholarly.* **Description:** Focuses on essential advances in the field of digestive diseases that relate directly to clinical practice and patient care problems.
Related titles: Online - full text ed.: USD 637 domestic academic site license; USD 646 foreign academic site license; USD 710.50 domestic corporate site license; USD 719.50 foreign corporate site license (2002) (from Ovid Technologies, Inc., Swets Blackwell, Institute for Scientific Information).
Indexed: ASCA, Curr.Adv.Cancer Res., Curr.Cont., Dairy Sci.Abstr., Excerp.Med., Helminthol.Abstr., INIS Atomind., Ind.Med. (1979-), Ind.Sci.Rev., Inpharma, Int.Abstr.Biol.Sci., Int.Nurs.Ind., Jrnl.Watch Gastr., NRN, Neurosci.Cit.Ind., Nutr.Abstr., Pharm.&Out.News, Protozool.Abstr., Reac., Rev.Med.& Vet.Mycol., SSCI (coverage dropped), Sci.Cit.Ind., THA, Trop.Dis.Bull.
—BLDSC (4958.470000), CISTI, GNLM, IDS, ingenta, KNAW.
Published by: Lippincott Williams & Wilkins (Philadelphia) (Subsidiary of: Wolters Kluwer N.V.), 530 Walnut St, Philadelphia, PA 19106-3621. TEL 215-521-8300, FAX 215-521-8902, http://www.Lww.com. Ed. Dr. Martin H Floch. Pub. Shelley Johnson. R&P Margaret Becker. Adv. contact Ray Thibodeau. B&W page USD 895, color page USD 1,990. Circ: 2,531 (paid). **Subscr. to:** PO Box 1600, Hagerstown, MD 21740-1600. TEL 800-777-2295, FAX 301-824-7390.

616.37 NLD

▼ **JOURNAL OF CYSTIC FIBROSIS.** Text in English. 2002. q. EUR 204 in Europe to institutions; JPY 27,100 in Japan to institutions; USD 228 elsewhere to institutions (effective 2002). *Refereed.* **Description:** Devoted to promoting the research and treatment of cystic fibrosis.
Published by: Elsevier Science, 211, Amsterdam 1000 AE, Netherlands. http://www.elsevier.com/locate/jcf. **Co-publisher:** European Cystic Fibrosis Society.

616.3 JPN ISSN 0944-1174
CODEN: JOGAET

JOURNAL OF GASTROENTEROLOGY. Text in English. 1966. m. (in 1 vol., 12 nos./vol.). JPY 40,000 domestic; USD 370 in North America; DEM 698 elsewhere; DEM 788, EUR 402.09 in Germany for Print & Online Eds.; DEM 802.40, EUR 410.26 elsewhere for Print & Online Eds. (effective 2001). adv. abstr. back issues avail. *Refereed.* **Document type:** *Academic/Scholarly.* **Description:** Publishes original papers, case reports, reports of multi-center trials, and review articles on all aspects of the field of gastroenterology.
Formerly (until 1993): Gastroenterologia Japonica (0435-1339)
Related titles: Online - full text ed.: ISSN 1435-5922 (from EBSCO Publishing, RoweCom Information Quest, Swets Blackwell, Springer LINK, Institute for Scientific Information).
Indexed: ASCA, Biol.Abstr., CINAHL, Chem.Abstr., Chem.Indus.Notes, Chem.Titles, Curr.Cont., Excerp.Med., INIS Atomind., Ind.Med. (1994-), Inpharma, Nutr.Abstr., Pharm.&Out.News, Reac., Rev.Med.& Vet.Mycol., SSCI (coverage dropped).
—BLDSC (4987.610000), CASDDS, CISTI, EMDOCS, GNLM, IDS, KNAW.
Published by: (Japanese Society of Gastroenterology/ Nihon Gan Chiryo Gakkai), Springer-Verlag Tokyo, Eastern Book Service, Inc. (Subsidiary of: BertelsmannSpringer), 3-13 Hongo 3-chome, Bunkyo-ku, Tokyo 113-0033, Japan. TEL 81-3-3812-0617, FAX 81-3-3812-4699, orders@svt-ebs.co.jp; helpdesk@link.springer.de, http://link.springer-ny.com/link/service/journals/00535/index.htm, http://link.springer.de. Ed. Tsutomu Chiba. Circ: 4,500. **Subscr. in N. America to:** Springer-Verlag New York Inc., PO Box 2485, Secaucus, NJ 07096-2485. TEL 800-777-4643, 201-348-4033, 212-460-1526, FAX 201-348-4505, orders@springer-ny.com; **Subscr. to:** Eastern Book Service, Inc., 3-13 Hongo 3-chome, Bunkyo-ku, Tokyo 113-8480, Japan. TEL 81-3-3818-0861, FAX 81-3-3818-0864, orders@svt-ebs.co.jp; Springer-Verlag, c/o Gabriele Kubitza, Haberstrasse 7, Heidelberg 69126, Germany. TEL 49-6221-345242, FAX 49-6221-345229, subscriptions@springer.de.

616.3 AUS ISSN 0815-9319
CODEN: JGHEEO

JOURNAL OF GASTROENTEROLOGY AND HEPATOLOGY. Text in English. 1986. m. AUD 1,293 domestic to institutions; AUD 1,175 in New Zealand to institutions; USD 699 elsewhere to institutions; AUD 1,423 domestic to institutions paper & online eds. combined; AUD 1,293 in New Zealand to institutions paper & onlined eds. combined; USD 769 elsewhere to institutions paper & online eds. combined (effective 2001). adv. illus. index. back issues avail.; reprint service avail. from PQC. *Refereed.* **Document type:** *Academic/Scholarly.* **Description:** Covers original contributions concerned with clinical practice and research in the fields of gastroenterology and hepatology.
Related titles: Microform ed.: (from PQC); Online - full text ed.: ISSN 1440-1746. AUD 1,164 domestic to institutions; AUD 1,058 in New Zealand to institutions; USD 630 elsewhere to institutions (effective 2001) (from Ovid Technologies, Inc., EBSCO Publishing, O C L C Online Computer Library Center, Inc., RoweCom Information Quest, ingenta, Munksgaard & Blackwell Science's Synergy, Swets Blackwell, Institute for Scientific Information).
Indexed: ASCA, Abstr.Hyg., Chem.Abstr., Chem.Indus.Notes, Chem.Titles, Curr.Adv.Cancer Res., Curr.Cont., Excerp.Med., Helminthol.Abstr., Ind.Med. (1986-), Ind.Sci.Rev., Inpharma, Int.Abstr.Biol.Sci., Nutr.Abstr., Pharm.&Out.News, Protozool.Abstr., Reac., Rev.Arom.& Med.Plants, Rev.Med.& Vet.Mycol., Sci.Cit.Ind., Sugar Ind.Abstr., Triticale Abstr., Trop.Dis.Bull.
—BLDSC (4987.615000), ADONIS, CASDDS, CISTI, EMDOCS, GNLM, IDS, Infotrieve, ingenta, KNAW. **CCC.**
Published by: (Asian Pacific Association for the Study of the Liver), Blackwell Science Asia Pty Ltd, PO Box 378, Carlton South, VIC 3053, Australia. TEL 61-3-9347-0300, FAX 61-3-9347-5001, info@blacksci-asia.com.au, http://www.blacksci.co.uk. Eds. K Okuda, S K Lam. Adv. contact Kathryn O'Brien. B&W page AUD 1,375, color page AUD 2,585; trim 210 x 275. Circ: 3,000. **Co-sponsor:** Asian Pacific Association for Gastroenterology.

JOURNAL OF HEALTH POPULATION AND NUTRITION. see *MEDICAL SCIENCES—Abstracting, Bibliographies, Statistics*

616.3 NLD ISSN 0168-8278
CODEN: JOHEEC

JOURNAL OF HEPATOLOGY. Text and summaries in English. 1985. m. (in 2 vols., 6 nos./vol.). USD 289 elsewhere to individuals; JPY 24,868 in Japan to individuals; EUR 275 in Europe to individuals; USD 783 elsewhere to institutions; JPY 66,868 in Japan to institutions; EUR 746 in Europe to institutions (effective 2002). adv. bk.rev. illus. index. back issues avail.; reprint service avail. from SWZ,ISI. *Refereed.* **Document type:** *Academic/Scholarly.* **Description:** Publishes original papers and reviews concerned with practice and research in the field of hepatology.
Related titles: Online - full text ed.: DKK 1,710 to individuals; DKK 4,860 to institutions (effective 2001) (from EBSCO Publishing, ingenta, ScienceDirect, Swets Blackwell, Institute for Scientific Information); ♦ Supplement: Journal of Hepatology. Supplement. ISSN 0169-5185.
Indexed: ASCA, Addic.Abstr., Chem.Abstr., Chem.Indus.Notes, Chem.Titles, Curr.Adv.Cell & Devel.Biol., Curr.Adv.Ecol.Sci., Curr.Cont., Excerp.Med., Helminthol.Abstr., INIS Atomind., Ind.Med. (1985-), Inpharma, Int.Abstr.Biol.Sci., Int.Nurs.Ind., Nutr.Abstr., Pharm.&Out.News, Reac., Rev.Med.& Vet.Mycol., Sci.Cit.Ind.
—BLDSC (4997.700000), ADONIS, CASDDS, CISTI, GNLM, IDS, Infotrieve, ingenta, KNAW. **CCC.**
Published by: (European Association for the Study of the Liver DNK), Elsevier Science BV, Life Sciences Department, Molenwerf 1, Amsterdam 1014 AG, Netherlands. http://www.jhep-elsevier.com. Ed. Juan Rodes TEL 34-93-453-64-97. Circ: 2,000.

616.3 NLD ISSN 0169-5185

JOURNAL OF HEPATOLOGY. SUPPLEMENT. Text in English. 1985. irreg.
Related titles: ♦ Supplement to: Journal of Hepatology. ISSN 0168-8278.
Indexed: Int.Abstr.Biol.Sci.
—ADONIS.
Published by: Elsevier Science BV, Life Sciences Department, Molenwerf 1, Amsterdam 1014 AG, Netherlands.

JOURNAL OF PEDIATRIC GASTROENTEROLOGY AND NUTRITION. see *NUTRITION AND DIETETICS*

JOURNAL OF PEPTIDE SCIENCE. see *CHEMISTRY—Organic Chemistry*

616.3 ITA ISSN 1590-8577

▼ **JOURNAL OF THE PANCREAS.** Abbreviated title: J O P. Text in English. 2000. bi-m., latest vol.2. free. abstr, illus. back issues avail. *Refereed.* **Document type:** *Academic/Scholarly.* **Description:** Focuses on the entire spectrum of the pancreatic gland aspects: normal function, etiology, epidemiology, prevention, genetics, pathophysiology, diagnosis, surgical and medical management of pancreatic diseases including cancer, inflammatory diseases, diabetes mellitus, cystic fibrosis and other congenital disorders. JOP also publishes: case reports, state-of-the-art reviews, book reviews, hypotheses and letters to the Editors. Comments on controversial issues and reviews of articles are also considered.
Media: Online - full content.
Published by: E S Burioni Ricerche Bibliografiche, Corso Firenze 41/2, Genova 16136, Italy. TEL 39-010-2722178, FAX 39-010-2722913, info@burioni.it, http://www.joplink.net. Eds. Generoso Uomo, Raffaele Pezzilli.

616.3 GBR ISSN 1352-0504
CODEN: JVHEER

JOURNAL OF VIRAL HEPATITIS. Text in English. 1994. bi-m., latest vol.9, 2002. GBP 79 in Europe to individuals; USD 133 in North America to individuals; GBP 86 elsewhere to individuals; GBP 372 in Europe to institutions; USD 591 in North America to institutions; GBP 410 elsewhere to institutions (effective 2002). adv. reprints avail. *Refereed.* **Document type:** *Academic/Scholarly.* **Description:** Publishes reviews, original research, and short rapid communications in the area of viral hepatitis.
Related titles: Microform ed.: (from PQC); Online - full text ed.: ISSN 1365-2893. 1999. GBP 72 in Europe to individuals; USD 120 in North America to individuals; GBP 72 elsewhere to individuals; GBP 335 in Europe to institutions; USD 532 in North America to institutions; GBP 335 elsewhere to institutions (effective 2002) (from Ovid Technologies, Inc., EBSCO Publishing, O C L C Online Computer Library Center, Inc., RoweCom Information Quest, ingenta, Munksgaard & Blackwell Science's Synergy, Swets Blackwell, Institute for Scientific Information).
Indexed: AIDS & Cancer Res., ASCA, Curr.Cont., Environ.Sci.Poll.Mgmt., Ind.Med. (1994-), Inpharma, Pharm.&Out.News, Pollut.Abstr., Reac., Risk Abstr., Saf.Sci.Abstr., Sci.Cit.Ind., Virol.Abstr.
—BLDSC (5072.485500), ADONIS, CISTI, GNLM, IDS, Infotrieve, KNAW. **CCC.**
Published by: Blackwell Science Ltd., PO Box 88, Oxford OX2 0NE, United Kingdom. TEL 44-1865-206180, 44-1865-206002, FAX 44-1865-206219, jnl.orders@blacksci.co.uk, http://www.blackwell-science.com/~cgilib/jnlpage.asp?Journal=jvh&File=jvh, http://www.blackwellpublishing.com. Eds. G D Foster, H C Thomas. Pub. Elizabeth Whelan. R&P Sophie Savage. Adv. contact Jenny Applin. Circ: 385.

▼ **JOURNAL WATCH GASTROENTEROLOGY.** see *MEDICAL SCIENCES—Abstracting, Bibliographies, Statistics*

616.362 JPN ISSN 0451-4203
CODEN: KNZOA

KANZO/ACTA HEPATOLOGICA JAPONICA. Text in Japanese; Summaries in English, Japanese. 1960. m. **Document type:** *Academic/Scholarly.*
Indexed: Chem.Abstr., Chem.Indus.Notes, Chem.Titles, Excerp.Med., INIS Atomind.
—CASDDS, CISTI, EMDOCS, GNLM, KNAW.

M

Published by: Nihon Kanzo Gakkai/Japanese Society of Hepatology, 28-10 Hongo 3-chome, Bunkyo-ku, Tokyo 113-0033, Japan. TEL 03-3812-1567.

616.3 DEU ISSN 0940-9092
KONTINENZ; Zeitschrift fuer Funktionsstoerungen von Blase und Darm. Text in German. 1992. bi-m. DEM 104. **Document type:** *Academic/Scholarly.*
—GNLM.
Published by: Hippokrates Verlag GmbH, Postfach 300504, Stuttgart 70445, Germany. TEL 0711-8931-0, FAX 0711-8931453. Ed. W Jost.

L M S ALERT. PEPTIC ULCER DISEASE. (Literature Monitoring and Evaluation Service) see *MEDICAL SCIENCES—Abstracting, Bibliographies, Statistics*

616.3 DEU ISSN 0300-8622
CODEN: LBMDAT
LEBER MAGEN DARM; zeitschrift fuer angewandte gastroenterologie und stoffwechsel. Text in German. 1971. 6/yr. DEM 129; DEM 138 in Europe. adv. bk.rev. *Refereed.* **Document type:** *Academic/Scholarly.*
Incorporates: Innere Medizin (0303-4305)
Related titles: Online - full text ed.: (from Institute for Scientific Information).
Indexed: ASCA, Curr.Cont. (coverage dropped), Excerp.Med., Helminthol.Abstr., INIS Atomind., Ind.Med. (coverage dropped), Ind.Sci.Rev., Inpharma, Nutr.Abstr., Pharm.&Out.News, Reac.
—CASDDS, CISTI, EMDOCS, GNLM, IDS, Infotrieve, KNAW. **CCC.**
Published by: Richard Pflaum Verlag GmbH und Co. KG, Lazarettstr 4, Munich 80636, West Germany. TEL 49-89-12607-0, FAX 49-89-12607202. Ed. P Fruehmorgen. Adv. contact I Brandl. Circ: 14,000.

616.3 FRA ISSN 1286-580X
LA LETTRE DE L'HEPATO-GASTROENTEROLOGUE. Text in French. 1998. bi-m. FRF 300 domestic to individuals; FRF 420, USD 76 foreign to individuals; FRF 380 domestic to institutions; FRF 500, USD 91 foreign to institutions; FRF 190 domestic to students; FRF 310, USD 56 foreign to students (effective 2000). *Refereed.* **Document type:** *Academic/Scholarly.*
Published by: Edimark S.A., 62-64 rue Jean Jaures, Puteaux 92800, France. TEL 33-1-414-58000, FAX 33-1-41458025, contact@edimark.fr, http://www.edimark.fr. Ed. M A Bigard.

LIFELINELETTER. see *NUTRITION AND DIETETICS*

616.3 DNK ISSN 0106-9543
CODEN: LIVEDR
LIVER; an international journal. Text in English. 1981. bi-m. USD 324 in the Americas to institutions print & online eds. combined; GBP 225 elsewhere to institutions print & online eds. combined (effective 2002). adv. bk.rev. illus, stat. index. reprint service avail. from ISI. *Refereed.* **Document type:** *Academic/Scholarly.*
Related titles: Online - full text ed.: ISSN 1600-0676. GBP 202 (effective 2002) (from Ovid Technologies, Inc., EBSCO Publishing, O C L C Online Computer Library Center, Inc., ingenta, Munksgaard & Blackwell Science's Synergy, Swets Blackwell, Institute for Scientific Information).
Indexed: ASCA, Biol.Abstr., Curr.Adv.Biochem., Curr.Adv.Cell & Devel.Biol., Curr.Cont., Excerp.Med., Helminthol.Abstr., INIS Atomind., Ind.Med. (1981-), Inpharma, Int.Abstr.Biol.Sci., Nutr.Abstr., Pharm.&Out.News, Reac., Rev.Med.& Vet.Mycol., Sci.Cit.Ind.
—BLDSC (5280.400000), CASDDS, CISTI, GNLM, IDS, ingenta, KNAW. **CCC.**
Published by: Blackwell Munksgaard, Noerre Soegade 35, PO Box 2148, Copenhagen K 1016, Denmark. FAX 45-77-33-33-77, fsub@munksgaard.dk, http://journals.munksgaard.dk/liver, http://www.munksgaard.dk. Ed. Alaistair Burt. Adv. contact Eric Rozario TEL 45-77-33-33-01. Circ: 800.

616.02 USA
▼ **LIVER DISORDERS SOURCEBOOK.** Text in English. 1999. irreg., latest 1999. USD 78 per issue (effective 2001). charts. Index. **Document type:** *Consumer.* **Description:** Contains basic consumer health information about the liver, how it works, and how to keep it healthy.
Published by: Omnigraphics, Inc., 615 Griswold St, Detroit, MI 48226. TEL 313-961-1340, 800-234-1340, FAX 313-961-1383, 800-875-1340, info@omnigraphics.com, jjts@sprynet.com, http://www.omnigraphics.com/cgi-bin/loadpage.cgi?user_id=20756&file=0-7808-0383-3.html. Ed. Joyce Brennfleck Shannon.

617 616.362 USA ISSN 1527-6465
CODEN: LTSUF3
LIVER TRANSPLANTATION. Text in English. 1995. m. USD 283 domestic to individuals Full text online included; USD 351 foreign to individuals Full text online included; USD 428 domestic to institutions Full text online included; USD 494 foreign to institutions Full text online included; USD 112 domestic to students Full text online included; USD 128 foreign to students Full text online included; USD 42 newsstand/cover (effective 2001). adv. back issues avail. *Refereed.* **Document type:** *Academic/Scholarly.* **Description:** Discusses surgical techniques, clinical investigations, and drug research in the subspecialties of liver transplantation and surgery.
Formerly (until 2000): Liver Transplantation and Surgery (1074-3022)
Related titles: Online - full text ed.: ISSN 1527-6473 (from HighWire Pr., EBSCO Publishing, IDEAL Online Library, Institute for Scientific Information).
Indexed: Curr.Cont., Ind.Med. (2000-), Inpharma, Int.Nurs.Ind., Pharm.&Out.News, Reac., Sci.Cit.Ind.
—BLDSC (5280.522000), EMDOCS, GNLM, IDS.
Published by: (American Association for the Study of Liver Diseases), W.B. Saunders Co. (Subsidiary of: Harcourt Publishers Ltd.), 11830 Westline Industrial Dr, St Louis, MO 63146. TEL 800-325-4177, http://www.ltsjournal.org, http://www.wbsaunders.com. Eds. Dr. Russell H. Wiesner, Dr. Ruud A. Krom. adv.: B&W page USD 720, color page USD 1,795. Circ: 1,429. **Subscr. to:** Journals Fulfillment, W B Saunders Co, 6277 Sea Harbor Dr, 4th Fl, Orlando, FL 32891-4800. TEL 800-654-2452, FAX 800-874-6418. **Co-sponsor:** International Liver Transplantation Society.

616.02 USA
LIVER UPDATE. Text in English. 1988. irreg. (2-4/yr.). USD 40. **Document type:** *Newsletter.*
Published by: American Liver Foundation, 1425 Pompton Ave, Cedar Grove, NJ 07009-1043. TEL 973-256-2550, 800-232-0179, info@liverfoundation.org, http://www.liverfoundation.org. Ed. Dr. Anna Mae Diehl. Circ: 70,000 (controlled).

616.3 BGR ISSN 1311-5030
MEDITSINSKI PREGLED. GASTROENTEROLOGIIA. Text in Bulgarian; Summaries in Bulgarian, English. 1970. q., latest vol.32, 2001. BGL 14 domestic; USD 30 foreign (effective 2001 - 2002). adv. bk.rev. abstr, bibl. index. back issues avail. *Refereed.* **Document type:** *Journal, Academic/Scholarly, Abstract/Index, Bibliography.* **Description:** Presents original articles and abstracts of foreign publications in the field of gastroenterology, including methods and techniques of diagnosis, drug therapy, risk factors.
Former titles: Gastroenterologiia; Gastroenterologichni Zaboliavaniia (0324-1513)
Published by: Meditsinski Universitet - Sofia, Tsentur za Informatsiia po Meditsina/Medical University - Sofia, Medical Information Center, 1 Sv Georgi Sofiiski ul, Sofia 1431, Bulgaria. TEL 359-2-9522342, FAX 359-2-9522393, mutafov@sun.medun.acad.bg, http://www.medun.acad.bg. Ed. S Stoinov. R&P, Adv. contact Dr. Christo Mutafov. B&W page USD 50, color page USD 150; 12 x 18. Circ: 300. **Dist. by:** Sofia Books, Ul Silivria 16, Sofia 1404, Bulgaria. TEL 359-2-9586257, sofiabooks@hotmail.com, http://www.sofiabooks.hit.bg.

616.3 ITA ISSN 1121-421X
RC799 CODEN: MDGADI
MINERVA GASTROENTEROLOGICA E DIETOLOGICA; rivista trimestrale di gastroenterologia e nutrizione clinica. Text in Italian; Summaries in English, Italian. 1960. q. USD 105 to individuals; USD 155 to institutions (effective 2000 - 2001). adv. bk.rev. bibl, charts, illus. index. *Refereed.* **Document type:** *Academic/Scholarly.*
Formerly (until 1990): Minerva Dietologica e Gastroenterologica (0391-1993); Which was formed by the merger of: Minerva Dietologica (0026-475X); Minerva Gastroenterologica (0026-4776)
Related titles: Microform ed.: (from PQC).
Indexed: Abstr.Hyg., Biol.Abstr., Chem.Abstr., Dent.Ind., Excerp.Med., Helminthol.Abstr., Ind.Med. (coverage dropped), Nutr.Abstr., Protozool.Abstr., Rice Abstr.
—BLDSC (5794.178000), CASDDS, CISTI, GNLM, KNAW.
Published by: Edizioni Minerva Medica, Corso Bramante, 83-85, Turin, TO 10126, Italy. TEL 39-11-678282, FAX 39-11-674502. Ed. M Rizzetto. Pub. A Oliaro. Adv. contact F Filippo. B&W page USD 1,200, color page USD 2,000; trim 270 x 190. Circ: 3,000 (paid).

616.3 GBR ISSN 0969-935X
N A C C NEWS. Text in English. 1980. 2/yr. GBP 12 to membership for the first year and then GBP 10 per year thereafter. (effective 2001). adv. bk.rev. **Document type:** *Newsletter.* **Description:** The National Association for Colitis and Crohn's Disease (NACC) is a registered charity providing support and information for patients and families living with these conditions.
Formerly (until 1990): N A C C Newsletter (0144-6967)
Published by: National Association for Colitis and Crohn's Disease, 4 Beaumont House, 4 Beaumont Works, 4 Sutton Rd, St Albans, Herts AL1 5HH, United Kingdom. TEL 44-1727-844296, FAX 44-1727-862550, nacc@nacc.org.uk, http://www.nacc.org.uk. Ed. Sarah Masters. Circ: 31,000.

616.3 GBR ISSN 1350-1925
CODEN: NMOTEK
NEUROGASTROENTEROLOGY AND MOTILITY. Text in English. 1989. bi-m., latest vol.14, 2002. GBP 132 in Europe to individuals; USD 209 in North America to individuals; GBP 145 elsewhere to individuals; GBP 409 in Europe to institutions; USD 633 in North America to institutions; GBP 439 elsewhere to institutions (effective 2002). adv. bk.rev. abstr, bibl, illus. index. back issues avail. *Refereed.* **Document type:** *Academic/Scholarly.* **Description:** Contains papers on all basic and clinical aspects of gastrointestinal motility and its control by myogenic, neural and chemical mechanisms.
Formerly (until 1994): Journal of Gastrointestinal Motility (1043-4518)
Related titles: Microform ed.: (from PQC); ♦ Online - full text ed.: Neurogastroenterology and Motility Online. ISSN 1365-2982.
Indexed: ASCA, Curr.Cont., Ind.Med. (1994-), Ind.Sci.Rev., Inpharma, Int.Abstr.Biol.Sci., Neurosci.Cit.Ind., Nutr.Abstr., Pharm.&Out.News, Protozool.Abstr., Reac., Sci.Cit.Ind.
—BLDSC (6081.371450), ADONIS, EMDOCS, GNLM, IDS, Infotrieve, ingenta, KNAW. **CCC.**
Published by: (European Society of Neurogastroenterology and Motility), Blackwell Science Ltd., PO Box 88, Oxford OX2 0NE, United Kingdom. TEL 44-1865-206180, 44-1865-206002, FAX 44-1865-206219, jnl.orders@blacksci.co.uk, http://www.blackwell-science.com/~cgilib/jnlpage.asp?Journal=ngem&File=ngem, http://www.blackwellpublishing.com. Eds. D Grundy, D Wingate. Pub. Allen Stevens. R&P Sophie Savage. Adv. contact Jenny Applin. Circ: 850.

616.3 GBR ISSN 1365-2982
▼ **NEUROGASTROENTEROLOGY AND MOTILITY ONLINE.** Text in English. 1999. bi-m. GBP 119 in Europe to individuals; USD 189 in North America to individuals; GBP 119 elsewhere to individuals; GBP 369 in Europe to institutions; USD 570 in North America to institutions; GBP 369 elsewhere to institutions (effective 2002). *Refereed.* **Document type:** *Academic/Scholarly.*
Media: Online - full text (from EBSCO Publishing, ingenta, Munksgaard & Blackwell Science's Synergy, Swets Blackwell, Institute for Scientific Information, RoweCom Information Quest). **Related titles:** Microform ed.: (from PQC); ♦ Print ed.: Neurogastroenterology and Motility. ISSN 1350-1925.
Published by: Blackwell Science Ltd., Osney Mead, Oxford OX2 0EL, United Kingdom. TEL 44-1685-206206, FAX 44-1685-721205, website@blacksci.com, journals.cs@blacksci.co.uk, http://www.blackwell-science.com/~cgilib/jnlpage.bin?Journal=ngem&File=ngem&Page=aims.

616.3 NLD
NEW CLINICAL APPLICATIONS. GASTROENTEROLOGY. Text in English. irreg. price varies. *Refereed.* **Document type:** *Monographic series.*
Published by: Kluwer Academic Publishers Group (Subsidiary of: Wolters Kluwer N.V.), Spuiboulevard 50, PO Box 17, Dordrecht 3300 AA, Netherlands. FAX 31-78-639-2254, services@wkap.nl, http://www.wkap.nl. **Dist. by:** Journals Department, PO Box 322, Dordrecht 3300 AH, Netherlands. FAX 31-78-654-6474.

NIHON KIKAN SHOKUDOKA GAKKAI KAIHO/JAPAN BRONCHO-ESOPHAGOLOGICAL SOCIETY. JOURNAL. see *MEDICAL SCIENCES—Respiratory Diseases*

616.3 JPN ISSN 0386-9768
NIHON SHOKAKI GEKA GAKKAI ZASSHI/JAPANESE JOURNAL OF GASTROENTEROLOGICAL SURGERY. Text in Japanese; Summaries in English, Japanese. 1969. m. JPY 1,000 per issue.
Indexed: INIS Atomind.

M

Published by: Nihon Shokaki Geka Gakkai/Japanese Society of Gastroenterological Surgery, 2-4 Kudan-Minami 2-chome, Chiyoda-ku, Tokyo 102-0074, Japan.

616.3 JPN ISSN 0912-0505
CODEN: EFDDE7
NIHON SHOKAKI NAISHIKYO GAKKAI KOSHIN'ETSU CHIHOKAI ZASSHI/ENDOSCOPIC FORUM FOR DIGESTIVE DISEASE. Text in Japanese; Summaries in English. 1986. s-a. JPY 10,400 (effective 2001). adv. bk.rev. **Document type:** *Journal, Academic/Scholarly.*
Indexed: Excerp.Med. (1993-).
—BLDSC (3743.560000), EMDOCS, GNLM.
Published by: Japanese Journal of Cancer and Chemotherapy Publishers Inc., Risshu Bldg, 2-2-3 Nihonbashi, Chuo-ku, Tokyo 103-0027, Japan. TEL 81-3-3278-0052, FAX 81-3-3281-0435. Ed., Pub. Masayuki A Fujino. Adv. contact Hachiro Sato.

616.3 JPN ISSN 0047-1801
CODEN: NDKGAU
NIPPON DAICHO KOMONBYO GAKKAI ZASSHI/JAPAN SOCIETY OF COLO-PROCTOLOGY. JOURNAL. Text in Japanese. 1940. 10/yr. **Document type:** *Academic/Scholarly.*
Indexed: Excerp.Med., INIS Atomind.
—BLDSC (4807.030000), CISTI, GNLM, KNAW.
Published by: Nippon Daicho Komonbyo Gakkai/Japan Society of Colo-Proctology, 11-1 Omori-Nishi 6-chome, Ota-ku, Tokyo 143-0015, Japan. TEL 03-3762-4151.

PANCREAS. see *MEDICAL SCIENCES—Endocrinology*

616.3 USA ISSN 0277-4208
CODEN: PRGAEE
PRACTICAL GASTROENTEROLOGY; for the busy gastroenterologist. Text in English. 1977. 12/yr. USD 125 domestic; USD 180 foreign (effective 2000). adv. bk.rev. abstr, bibl, charts, illus, tr.lit. index. back issues avail.; reprint service avail. from PQC,ISI. *Refereed.* **Document type:** *Trade.* **Description:** For the gastroenterologist on the diagnosis, therapy and management of digestive disorders. Includes articles on topics that the practitioner encounters in daily practice.
Former titles: Primary Care Physician's Guide to Practical Gastroenterology (0163-7894); Physician's Guide to Practical Gastroenterology (0149-9912)
Related titles: Microfilm ed.: (from PQC); Online - full text ed.
Indexed: AgeLine, Curr.Cont. (coverage dropped), Excerp.Med.
—BLDSC (6594.062000), CISTI, EMDOCS, GNLM, Infotrieve, KNAW. **CCC.**
Published by: Shugar Publishing, 99-B Main St, Westhampton Beach, NY 11978-2311. TEL 631-288-4404, FAX 631-288-4435, shugarpub@aol.com, http://www.practicalgastro.com. Ed. Dorine Kitay. Pub., R&P, Adv. contact Vivian Mahl. B&W page USD 2,560. Circ: 19,000 (controlled).

616.02 USA
PROGRESS (CEDAR GROVE). Text in English. irreg. (approx. 4/yr.). membership. **Document type:** *Newsletter.* **Description:** Reports on A.L.F. research, education and prevention, and lobbying efforts.
Published by: American Liver Foundation, 1425 Pompton Ave, Cedar Grove, NJ 07009-1043. TEL 973-256-2550, 800-465-4837, info@liverfoundation.org, http://www.liverfoundation.org. Ed. Julie Lehane.

PROTEASE INHIBITOR REFERENCE. see *BIOLOGY—Biochemistry*

616.3 GBR ISSN 0141-5581
RC799 CODEN: RAGADI
RECENT ADVANCES IN GASTROENTEROLOGY. Text in English. 1965. irreg. **Document type:** *Monographic series, Academic/Scholarly.*
—CASDDS, CISTI, GNLM, Infotrieve. **CCC.**
Published by: Churchill Livingstone (Subsidiary of: Harcourt Publishers Ltd.), Robert Stevenson House, 1-3 Baxter's Pl, Leith Walk, Edinburgh, Midlothian EH1 3AF, United Kingdom. TEL 44-131-556-2424, FAX 44-131-459-1177, http://www.churchillmed.com.

616.362 GBR ISSN 0264-7532
RECENT ADVANCES IN HEPATOLOGY. Text in English. 1983. irreg. **Document type:** *Monographic series, Academic/Scholarly.*
Published by: Churchill Livingstone (Subsidiary of: Harcourt Publishers Ltd.), Robert Stevenson House, 1-3 Baxter's Pl, Leith Walk, Edinburgh, Midlothian EH1 3AF, United Kingdom. TEL 44-131-556-2424, FAX 44-131-459-1177, http://www.churchillmed.com. **US subscr. to:** Churchill Livingstone, 650 Ave of the Americas, New York, NY 10011. TEL 212-206-5000.

REFERATIVNYI ZHURNAL. ENDOSKOPIYA. see *MEDICAL SCIENCES—Abstracting, Bibliographies, Statistics*

RENAL PHYSIOLOGY. see *BIOLOGY—Abstracting, Bibliographies, Statistics*

616.3 ESP ISSN 1138-6010
REVISIONES EN GASTROENTEROLOGIA. Text in Spanish; Abstracts in Spanish, English. 1997. bi-m. ESP 8,000; USD 300 foreign (effective 2000). adv. abstr, bibl, illus, stat. back issues avail. *Refereed.* **Document type:** *Academic/Scholarly.*
Related titles: CD-ROM ed.
Published by: Aran Ediciones S.A., Castello, 128 1o, Madrid 28006, Spain. TEL 34-91-782-0030, FAX 34-91-561-5787, edita@grupoaran.com, http://www.grupoaran.com. Ed. J.M. Herrerias Gutierrez. Pub. Jose Jimenez. R&P Maria Dolores Linares TEL 34-1-7820035. Circ: 5,000.

616.3 MEX ISSN 0375-0906
CODEN: RGMXA
REVISTA DE GASTROENTEROLOGIA DE MEXICO. Text in Spanish; Summaries in English. 1935. q. MXP 300, USD 80 (effective 1996 & 1997). *Refereed.* **Document type:** *Academic/Scholarly.* **Description:** Contains original articles, research reports, review articles, clinical cases, and notices related to gastroenterology.
Related titles: CD-ROM ed.
Indexed: Ind.Med. (1935-).
—BLDSC (7856.520000), GNLM.
Published by: (Asociacion Mexicana de Gastroenterologia), Obsidiana Editores S.A., CZDA DE TLALPAN 2365, Col Ciudad Jardin, Mexico City, DF 04370, Mexico. TEL 52-5-689-9133. Eds. Dr. Eduardo Marin-Lopez, Dr. Lorenzo de la Garza-Villasenor. Pub. Jorge Godoy-Gutierrez. Circ: 2,400. **Dist. by:** Distribuidora Editorial de Mexico SA de CV, P.O. Box 76-026, Mexico City, DF 04201, Mexico. TEL 52-5-544-7953, FAX 52-5-689-6545.

616.3 PER ISSN 1022-5129
REVISTA DE GASTROENTEROLOGIA DEL PERU. Text in Spanish. 1981. 3/yr. USD 25; USD 50 foreign. adv. Supplement avail. *Refereed.* **Document type:** *Trade.* **Description:** Contains gastroenterology articles, reviews and case reports.
Indexed: INIS Atomind.
—BLDSC (7856.550000).
Published by: Sociedad de Gastroenterologia del Peru, Juan de Aliaga 204, Magdalena del Mar, Lima 17, Peru. TEL 51-1-2640157, FAX 51-1-2641400, abussalleu@upch.edu.pe. Ed. Dr. Herman Vildosola G.

616.3 ESP
REVISTA ESPANOLA DE ECOGRAFIA DIGESTIVA. Text in Spanish. q. ESP 7,000; USD 200 foreign. adv. illus, stat, bibl. back issues avail. *Refereed.* **Document type:** *Academic/Scholarly.*
Published by: Aran Ediciones S.A., Castello, 128 1o, Madrid 28006, Spain. TEL 34-91-782-0030, FAX 34-91-561-5787, edita@grupoaran.com, http://www.grupoaran.com. Ed. L. Martin Herrera. Pub. Jose Jimenez. R&P Maria Dolores Linares TEL 34-1-7820035. Circ: 3,000.

616.3 ESP ISSN 1130-0108
CODEN: REDIE
REVISTA ESPANOLA DE ENFERMEDADES DIGESTIVAS. Text in Spanish; Summaries in English, Spanish. 1918. m. ESP 13,700 to individuals; ESP 16,500 to institutions; ESP 10,900 to students. adv. bk.rev. abstr, bibl, charts, illus, stat. back issues avail.; reprint service avail. from PQC. *Refereed.* **Document type:** *Academic/Scholarly.*
Former titles (until 1989): Revista Espanola de las Enfermedades del Aparato Digestivo (0034-9437); (until 1967): Revista Espanola de las Enfermedades del Aparato Digestivo y de la Nutricion (0370-4343); (until 1934): Archivos Espanoles de las Enfermedades del Aparato Digestivo y de la Nutrition (0210-1556)
Related titles: Microform ed.: (from PQC); Online - full text ed.: (from Institute for Scientific Information); Supplement: Revista Espanola de Enfermedades Digestivas. Suplemento. ISSN 1130-4588. 1990.
Indexed: Biol.Abstr., CINAHL, Chem.Abstr., Chem.Titles, Curr.Cont., Excerp.Med., Helminthol.Abstr., Ind.Med. (1990-), Ind.Med.Esp., Inpharma, Nutr.Abstr., Protozool.Abstr., Reac., Ref.Zh., Tox.Abstr., Virol.Abstr.
—BLDSC (7853.970000), CASDDS, CINDOC, CISTI, GNLM, IDS, Infotrieve, KNAW. **CCC.**
Published by: (Sociedad Espanola de Patologia Digestiva), Aran Ediciones S.A., Castello, 128 1o, Madrid 28006, Spain. TEL 34-91-782-0030, FAX 34-91-561-5787, edita@grupoaran.com, http://www.grupoaran.com. adv.: B&W page ESP 145,000, color page ESP 177,000; 280 x 210. Circ: 3,500.

616.3 FRA ISSN 0035-2888
REVUE FRANCAISE DE GASTRO ENTEROLOGIE. Text in French. 6/yr. FRF 480 domestic to individuals; EUR 106.71, FRF 700 foreign to individuals; FRF 335 to students (effective 2001).
Indexed: Excerp.Med., Inpharma, Reac.
—BLDSC (7904.140000), CISTI, GNLM, KNAW.
Published by: Galliena Promotion, 62 rue Amelot, Paris 75011, France. TEL 33-1-53360180, FAX 33-1-53360164.

616.3 ITA ISSN 0035-6255
RIVISTA DI GASTROENTEROLOGIA. Text in Italian; Summaries in English. 1949. s-a. ITL 50,000; ITL 100,000 foreign (effective 1998). adv. bk.rev. **Document type:** *Academic/Scholarly.*
Indexed: Chem.Abstr., Excerp.Med.
—CISTI, GNLM.
Published by: Casa Editrice Maccari, Via Palermo, 44, Parma, PR 43100, Italy. TEL 39-521-771268. Circ: 1,200.

616.3 SAU ISSN 1319-3767
THE SAUDI JOURNAL OF GASTROENTEROLOGY. Text in English. 1994. 3/yr. *Refereed.* **Document type:** *Journal, Academic/Scholarly.* **Description:** Publishes clinical and experimental research in diseases and conditions of the digestive tract.
Published by: Saudi Gastroenterology Association, c/o Dallah Hospital, Riyadh 11652, Saudi Arabia. TEL 966-1-454-5277 ext 2152, FAX 966-1-454-5253.

616.3 SWE ISSN 0036-5521
CODEN: SJGRA4
SCANDINAVIAN JOURNAL OF GASTROENTEROLOGY. Text in English. 1966. m. GBP 175, USD 289 to individuals; GBP 412, USD 680 to institutions (effective 2002). adv. bk.rev. charts, illus. index. *Refereed.* **Document type:** *Journal, Academic/Scholarly.* **Description:** Membership journal for the gastroenterologic societies of Denmark, Finland, Iceland, Norway and Sweden.
Related titles: Microform ed.: (from PQC); Online - full text ed.: (from EBSCO Publishing, O C L C Online Computer Library Center, Inc., RoweCom Information Quest, CatchWord Ltd., ingenta, Swets Blackwell, Institute for Scientific Information); Chinese ed.; Spanish ed.; ♦ Supplement: Scandinavian Journal of Gastroenterology. Supplement. ISSN 0085-5928.
Indexed: Abstr.Hyg., Agri.& Environ.Biotech.Abstr. (coverage dropped), Biol.Abstr., Chem.Abstr., Chem.Indus.Notes, Chem.Titles, Curr.Adv.Cancer Res., Curr.Adv.Ecol.Sci., Curr.Adv.Gen.& Molec.Biol., Curr.Cont., Dairy Sci.Abstr., Dent.Ind., Derwent Biotech.Abstr., Diar.Dis.Res., Excerp.Med., Helminthol.Abstr., INIS Atomind., Ind.Med. (1966-), Ind.Sci.Rev., Ind.Vet., Inpharma, Int.Abstr.Biol.Sci., Jrnl.Watch Gastr., NRN, Nutr.Abstr., Pharm.&Out.News, Pig News & Info., Protozool.Abstr., Reac., Ref.Zh., Rev.Appl.Entomol., Rev.Med.& Vet.Mycol., Sci.Cit.Ind., Soyabean Abstr., Sugar Ind.Abstr., Trop.Dis.Bull., Vet.Bull.
—BLDSC (8087.507000), ADONIS, CASDDS, CISTI, GNLM, IDS, ingenta, KNAW. **CCC.**
Published by: Taylor & Francis AS (Subsidiary of: Taylor & Francis Group), Cort Adelersgt. 17, Solli, PO Box 2562, Oslo 0202, Norway. TEL 47-22-12-98-80, FAX 47-22-12-98-90, journals@tandf.no, http://www.tandf.co.uk/tfas. Ed. E Schumpf. adv.: B&W page SEK 8,500, color page SEK 16,500; trim 190 x 260.

616.3 SWE ISSN 0085-5928
CODEN: SJGSB8
SCANDINAVIAN JOURNAL OF GASTROENTEROLOGY. SUPPLEMENT. Text in English. 1968. irreg. back issues avail.; reprint service avail. from ISI.
Related titles: Microform ed.: (from PQC); Online - full text ed.: (from Swets Blackwell); ♦ Supplement to: Scandinavian Journal of Gastroenterology. ISSN 0036-5521.

M

Indexed: Biol.Abstr., Cal.Tiss.Abstr., Chem.Abstr., Chem.Titles, Chemorec.Abstr., Curr.Adv.Ecol.Sci., Dairy Sci.Abstr., Dent.Ind., Excerp.Med., Ind.Med. (1968-), Neurosci.Abstr. (coverage dropped), Nutr.Abstr., Ref.Zh., THA.
—BLDSC (8087.508000), ADONIS, CASDDS, CISTI, ingenta, KNAW. **CCC.**
Published by: Taylor & Francis AB (Subsidiary of: Taylor & Francis Group), Hollaendargatan 20, PO Box 3255, Stockholm 11160, Sweden. TEL 46-8-4408040, FAX 46-8-4408050, journals@se.tandf.no, http://www.tandf.co.uk/journals/tfas.html.

SEMINARS IN COLON AND RECTAL SURGERY. see *MEDICAL SCIENCES—Surgery*

616.3 USA ISSN 1049-5118 CODEN: SGDIED
SEMINARS IN GASTROINTESTINAL DISEASE. Text in English. 1990. q. USD 150 domestic to individuals; USD 211 foreign to individuals; USD 205 domestic to institutions; USD 256 foreign to institutions; USD 94 domestic to students; USD 127 foreign to students; USD 65 newsstand/cover (effective 2001). **Document type:** *Academic/Scholarly.* **Description:** Serves specialists caring for patients suffering disorders of the digestive tract and liver by focusing on a single topic in each issue on treatment options, complications, and alternative approaches.
Indexed: Excerp.Med. (1993-), Ind.Med. (1990-), Protozool.Abstr.
—BLDSC (8239.449600), CISTI, EMDOCS, GNLM, Infotrieve, KNAW. **CCC.**
Published by: W.B. Saunders Co. (Subsidiary of: Harcourt Publishers Ltd.), 11830 Westline Industrial Dr, St Louis, MO 63146. TEL 800-325-4177, http://www.wbsaunders.com. Ed. Marvin H Sleisenger. **Subscr. to:** Periodicals Fulfillment, W B Saunders Co, 6277 Sea Harbor Dr, 4th Fl, Orlando, FL 32891-4800.

616.3 USA ISSN 0272-8087 CODEN: SLDIEE
SEMINARS IN LIVER DISEASES. Text in English. 1981. q. EUR 186 to individuals; EUR 369 to institutions; EUR 86 newsstand/cover (effective 2002). adv. abstr. reprint service avail. from PQC. *Refereed.* **Document type:** *Journal, Academic/Scholarly.* **Description:** Offers guidelines for diagnosing and treating hepatic diseases.
Related titles: Microform ed.: (from PQC); Online - full text ed.: ISSN 1098-8971 (from Ovid Technologies, Inc., EBSCO Publishing, O C L C Online Computer Library Center, Inc., RoweCom Information Quest, Institute for Scientific Information).
Indexed: ASCA, Abstr.Hyg., Biol.Abstr., Curr.Adv.Gen.& Molec.Biol., Curr.Cont., Excerp.Med., Ind.Med. (1981-), Ind.Sci.Rev., Inpharma, Pharm.&Out.News, Reac., Rev.Med.& Vet.Mycol., Sci.Cit.Ind.
—BLDSC (8239.454000), CASDDS, CISTI, EMDOCS, GNLM, IDS, ingenta, KNAW. **CCC.**
Published by: Thieme Medical Publishers, 333 Seventh Ave, New York, NY 10001. TEL 212-760-0888, 800-782-3488, FAX 212-947-1112, http://www.thieme.com. Ed. Dr. Paul D Berk. Circ: 2,800. **Orders in Europe to:** Thieme International, Postfach 3001120, Stuttgart 70451, Germany. TEL 49-711-8931-0, 49-711-8931-298.

616.3 CHN CODEN: WJGAF2
SHIJIE HUAREN XIAOHUA ZAZHI/WORLD CHINESE JOURNAL OF DIGESTOLOGY. Text in Chinese; Summaries in English. 1995. m. USD 139.20; USD 11.60 newsstand/cover (effective 2001). adv. bk.rev. abstr, bibl, illus, mkt, stat. back issues avail. **Document type:** *Academic/Scholarly, Abstract/Index.* **Description:** Covers all aspects of gastroenterology, including hepatology, oncology, and radiology, in basic and clinical medicine. Publishes mainly original research articles and clinical trials, case reports, reviews, comments, and news.
Former titles (until 1998): Huaren Hiaohua Zazhi - Chinese Digestology Journal; (until 1997): Xin Xiaohuabingxueazhi - China National Journal of New Gastroenterology
Related titles: Diskette ed.; E-mail ed.; Fax ed.
Indexed: Ref.Zh.
—BLDSC, CASDDS.
Published by: (Shijie Xiaohuaxue Wang/World Digestology Network), W J G Press, 381 Shuangta Xijie, Taiyuan, Shanxi 030001, China. TEL 86-1-6589-1901, FAX 86-1-6589-1893, wcjd@public.bta.net.cn, http://www.wd.org.cn. Ed. Bo Rong Pan. Pub. Ma Lian Sheng. R&P Lian-Sheng Ma. Adv. contact Lian Sheng Ma. Circ: 9,000. **Subscr. to:** PO Box 2345, Beijing 100023, China. **Dist. overseas by:** China International Book Trading Corp, 35, Chegongzhuang Xilu, Haidian District, Beijing 100044, China. TEL 86-1-68413849, FAX 86-1-68412048, cibtc@mail.cibtc.com.cn, http://www.cibtc.com.cn.

616.3 JPN ISSN 0387-2645
SHOKAKI GEKA/GASTROENTEROLOGICAL SURGERY. Text in Japanese; Contents page in English. 1978. m. JPY 1,900 per issue.
Indexed: INIS Atomind.
—BLDSC (4088.966000).
Published by: Herusu Publishing Co. Inc., 2-3 Nakano 2-chome, Nakano-ku, Tokyo 164-0001, Japan. Eds. Aki Ishibashi, Keizo Shogenji.

616.3 JPN ISSN 0915-3217
SHOKAKI NAISHIKYO/ENDOSCOPIA DIGESTIVA. Text in Japanese; Summaries in English. 1989. m. JPY 37,000; JPY 2,800 newsstand/cover (effective 1999).
—BLDSC (3743.550000).
Published by: Tokyo Igakusha Ltd., 35-4 Hongo 3-chome, Bunkyo-ku, Tokyo 113-0033, Japan. TEL 03-3814-8541, FAX 81-3-3811-4119.

616.3 JPN ISSN 0389-9403
SHOKAKI NAISHIKYO NO SHINPO/PROGRESS OF DIGESTIVE ENDOSCOPY. Text in Japanese; Summaries in English. 1972. s-a. JPY 10,300. charts, illus. back issues avail.
—BLDSC (6868.155000).
Published by: Kyowa Kikaku Tsushin, 2-20 Shinbashi, Minato-ku, Tokyo 105-0004, Japan. TEL 03-3575-0181. Circ: 2,000.

616.3 GBR
SLIDE ATLAS OF GASTROINTESTINAL ENDOSCOPY (YEAR). Text in English. bi-m. USD 195. **Document type:** *Academic/Scholarly.* **Description:** Provides authoritative presentations of new techniques, procedures, clinical applications, material and equipment in over 115 slides.
Related titles: ♦ Supplement to: Annual of Gastrointestinal Endoscopy. ISSN 0952-6293.
Published by: Rapid Science Publishers, 2-6 Boundary Row, London SE1 8HN, United Kingdom. TEL 44-207-865-0198, FAX 44-207-410-6600, rapid@rapidcom.co.uk.

616.3 ESP ISSN 0301-1143
SOCIEDAD VALENCIANA DE PATOLOGIA DIGESTIVA. REVISTA. Text in Spanish. 1982. q. ESP 7,600 to individuals; ESP 10,860 to institutions; ESP 6,080 to students (effective 2001). adv. back issues avail.; reprints avail. *Refereed.* **Document type:** *Journal, Academic/Scholarly.*
Related titles: Online - full text ed.: 1996.
Published by: Ediciones Doyma S.A., Traversa de Gracia, 17-21, Barcelona 08021, Spain. TEL 34-93-200-0711, supd@doyma.es, doyma@doyma.es, http://www.doyma.es/supd. Ed. M Bixquert Jimenez. R&P Monica Barnes. Adv. contact Jose Antonio Hernandez. B&W page ESP 122,000, color page ESP 152,000; 280 x 210.

616.3 ITA
GLI SPECIALIZZATI. GASTROENTEROLOGIA. Text in Italian. 1990. q. ITL 25,000. adv. bk.rev.
Formerly: Gastroenterologia Oggi (1120-3641)
Published by: E S I Stampa Medica s.r.l., Largo Volontari Del Sangue, 10, Casella Postale 42, San Donato, MI 20133, Italy. TEL 39-2-5274241, FAX 39-2-55600670, TELEX 324-894. Ed. Diego Onestinghel. Adv. contact Ornella Galbiati. B&W page ITL 5,200,000, color page ITL 6,800,000; trim 235 x 171. Circ: 5,900.

SULLY'S LIVING WITHOUT; a lifestyle guide for people with food and chemical sensitivity. see *LIFESTYLE*

SURGICAL LAPAROSCOPY, ENDOSCOPY AND PERCUTANEOUS TECHNIQUES. see *MEDICAL SCIENCES—Surgery*

616.3 ITA ISSN 1128-045X
TECHNIQUES IN COLOPROCTOLOGY ONLINE. Text in English. 3/yr. *Refereed.* **Document type:** *Journal, Academic/Scholarly.*
Media: Online - full text (from EBSCO Publishing, RoweCom Information Quest, Swets Blackwell, Springer LINK). **Related titles:** ♦ Print ed.: Techniques in Coloproctology. ISSN 1123-6337.
Published by: Springer-Verlag Italia Srl (Subsidiary of: BertelsmannSpringer), Via Podgora, 4, Milan, MI 20122, Italy. TEL 39-2-55194656, FAX 39-2-55193360, springer@springer.it, http://link.springer.de.

616.3 ITA ISSN 1123-6337
TECHNIQUES IN COLORPROCTOLOGY. Variant title: U C P News. Text in English. 1995. 3/yr. USD 196.75; USD 77.30 newsstand/cover (effective 2001). **Document type:** *Journal, Academic/Scholarly, Trade.*
Related titles: ♦ Online - full text ed.: Techniques in Coloproctology Online. ISSN 1128-045X.
—BLDSC (8743.875000).
Published by: (Italian Association of Coloproctology Units, U C P Club), Springer-Verlag Italia Srl (Subsidiary of: BertelsmannSpringer), Via Podgora, 4, Milan, MI 20122, Italy. TEL 39-2-55194656, FAX 39-2-55193360, springer@springer.it, http://link.springer.de. Ed. Mario Pescatori.

663 USA ISSN 1096-2883
▼ **TECHNIQUES IN GASTROINTESTINAL ENDOSCOPY.** Text in English. 1999. q. USD 116 domestic to individuals; USD 144 foreign to individuals; USD 180 domestic to institutions; USD 209 foreign to institutions; USD 69 domestic to students; USD 86 foreign to students; USD 53 newsstand/cover (effective 2001). illus. *Refereed.* **Document type:** *Journal, Academic/Scholarly.* **Description:** Reports that illustrate diagnosis, rationale for and against a procedure, actual technique, management, and prevention of complications.
—BLDSC (8745.055000).
Published by: W.B. Saunders Co. (Subsidiary of: Harcourt Publishers Ltd.), Curtis Center, Independence Sq W, Philadelphia, PA 19106-3399. TEL 215-238-2800, FAX 215-238-6490, http://www.wbsaunders.com.

616.3 AUS
THERAPEUTIC GUIDELINES. GASTROINTESTINAL. Text in English. 1994. irreg., latest version 2 (every 3-4 yrs.). AUD 31.90 newsstand/cover (effective 2001). **Document type:** *Academic/Scholarly.* **Description:** Gives concrete recommendations for rational therapy of gastrointestinal disease and where necessary justifies the choice of therapy.
Formerly: Gastrointestinal Drug Guidelines
Related titles: CD-ROM ed.
Published by: Therapeutic Guidelines Ltd., Chelsea House, Level 2, 55 Flemington Rd, North Melbourne, VIC 3051, Australia. TEL 61-3-9329-1566, FAX 61-3-9326-5632, sales@tg.com.au, http://www.tg.com.au. Ed., R&P Mary Hemming. Circ: 20,000.

616.3 DEU ISSN 0303-6294
TIPS FUER DIE GASTROENTEROLOGISCHE PRAXIS*. Text in German. 1974. s-a. **Document type:** *Academic/Scholarly.*
—GNLM.
Published by: (Gesellschaft fuer Gastroenterologie in Bayern e.V.), Demeter Verlag GmbH und Co. KG, Ammonitenstr 1, Balingen 72336, Germany. Circ: 2,500.

616.3 USA ISSN 1048-6771
TODAY IN MEDICINE. GASTROENTEROLOGY. Text in English. 1990. bi-m.
Published by: Data Centrum Communications, Inc., 21 W 38th St, 4th fl, New York, NY 10018.

616.3 USA
TOPICS IN GASTROENTEROLOGY. Text in English. 1979. irreg., latest 1992. price varies. *Refereed.* **Document type:** *Monographic series.*
Indexed: Biol.Abstr.
Published by: Kluwer Academic - Plenum Publishers (Subsidiary of: Wolters Kluwer N.V.), 233 Spring St, New York, NY 10013-1578. TEL 212-620-8000, FAX 212-463-0742, books@plenum.com. Ed. Howard M Spiro.

616.33 TUR ISSN 1300-4948 CODEN: TJGAF
TURKISH JOURNAL OF GASTROENTEROLOGY/TURK GASTROENTEROLOJI DERGISI. Text in English, Turkish. 1990. q. *Refereed.* **Document type:** *Academic/Scholarly.*
Formerly (until 1995): Gastroenteroloji (1300-2856)
Indexed: Abstr.Hyg., Excerp.Med. (1996-), Protozool.Abstr., Trop.Dis.Bull.
—BLDSC (9072.468760), EMDOCS, GNLM.

M

Published by: Turkish Society of Gastroenterology, Bayindir Sokak 17-7, Kizilay - Ankara 06420, Turkey. TEL 90-312-4354373.

616.3 AUS ISSN 0819-4610
WORLD COUNCIL OF ENTEROSTOMAL THERAPISTS JOURNAL*. Text in English. 1986. q. USD 48. adv. bk.rev. back issues avail. **Description:** Specializes in the care of patients who have had their bowel or bladder removed and are given an alternative method of elimination. Covers draining wounds and fistulae.
Indexed: CINAHL.
Published by: (World Council of Enterostomal Therapists), Ink Press International, PO Box 846, Ashfield, NSW 1800, Australia. Ed. Pat Blackley. Circ: 6,000.

616.3 CHN ISSN 1007-9327
WORLD JOURNAL OF GASTROENTEROLOGY. Text in English. 1995 (Oct). bi-m. USD 145.20; USD 24.20 newsstand/cover (effective 2001). **Document type:** *Academic/Scholarly.*
Formerly: China National Journal of New Gastroenterology
Related titles: Online - full content ed.: (from WanFang Data Corp.); Online - full text ed.: (from Institute for Scientific Information).
Indexed: Ref.Zh.
—BLDSC (9356.073300).
Published by: (Chinese Association of the Integrated Traditional Chinese and Western Medicine), W J G Press, 381 Shuangta Xijie, Taiyuan, Shanxi 030001, China. TEL 86-1-6589-1893, FAX 86-1-6589-1893. Ed. Bo Rong Pan. Adv. contact Lian Sheng Ma. **Dist. by:** China International Book Trading Corp, 35, Chegongzhuang Xilu, Haidian District, Beijing 100044, China. TEL 86-1-68413849, FAX 86-1-68412048, cibtc@mail.cibtc.com.cn, http://www.cibtc.com.cn.

616.3 USA ISSN 0739-5930
RC799
THE YEAR BOOK OF GASTROENTEROLOGY. Text in English. a. USD 87 domestic; USD 93 foreign (effective 2001). illus. **Document type:** *Academic/Scholarly, Abstract/Index.* **Description:** Presents abstracts of pertinent literature with commentary by leading experts in the field.
Formerly: Year Book of Digestive Diseases (0739-5930)
Related titles: CD-ROM ed.
—GNLM.
Published by: Mosby, Inc., Continuity Division (Subsidiary of: Harcourt Health Sciences), 11830 Westline Industrial Dr, St Louis, MO 63146-3313. TEL 314-872-8370, 800-325-4177, FAX 314-432-1380, http://www.mosby.com/periodicals. Ed. Dr. Gary Lichtenstein.

616.3 GBR ISSN 1358-7269
THE YEAR IN HELICOBACTER PYLORI. Text in English. 1994. a.
Related titles: ♦ Supplement to: Current Opinion in Gastroenterology. ISSN 0267-1379.
—ADONIS.
Published by: (European Helicobacter Pylori Study Group), Lippincott Williams & Wilkins (Philadelphia) (Subsidiary of: Wolters Kluwer N.V.), 227 E Washington Sq, Philadelphia, PA 19106-3780. Eds. Francis Megraud, Peter Malfertheiner, Pierre Michetti.

616 DEU ISSN 0044-2771
CODEN: ZGASAX
ZEITSCHRIFT FUER GASTROENTEROLOGIE. Text in German. 1963. m. EUR 196.80 domestic to institutions; EUR 215.80 in Europe to institutions; EUR 219.80 elsewhere to institutions; EUR 20.50 newsstand/cover (effective 2002). adv. bk.rev. abstr, charts, illus, stat, tr.lit. *Refereed.* **Document type:** *Journal, Academic/Scholarly.*
Related titles: Online - full text ed.: ISSN 1439-7803 (from Institute for Scientific Information).
Indexed: ASCA, Biol.Abstr., Chem.Abstr., Chem.Indus.Notes, Chem.Titles, Curr.Cont., Excerp.Med., Helminthol.Abstr., INIS Atomind., Ind.Med. (1963-), Ind.Sci.Rev., Inpharma, Int.Nurs.Ind., Nutr.Abstr., Protozool.Abstr., Reac., Rev.Med.& Vet.Mycol., Sci.Cit.Ind.
—BLDSC (9462.350000), CASDDS, CISTI, GNLM, IDS, Infotrieve, KNAW. **CCC.**
Published by: (Deutsche Gesellschaft fuer Verdauungs- und Stoffwechselkrankheiten), Demeter Verlag GmbH und Co. KG, Ammonitenstr 1, Balingen 72336, Germany. Ed. Dr. F W Caspary. Circ: 2,000. **Co-sponsors:** Deutsche Gesellschaft fuer Gastroenterologische Endoskopie; Oesterreichische Gesellschaft fuer Gastroenterologie.

616.3 CHN ISSN 1000-1174
ZHONGGUO GANGCHANGBING ZAZHI/CHINESE JOURNAL OF COLO-PROCTOLOGY. Text in Chinese; Abstracts in Chinese, English. 1981. m. USD 10. adv. *Refereed.* **Document type:** *Academic/Scholarly.* **Description:** Covers the latest achievements in scientific research on the prevention, diagnosis and treatment of anorectal diseases in China.
Published by: Zhongguo Gangchangbing Zazhi Bianjibu, No 42 Wenhua Xilu, Jinan, Shandong 250011, China. TEL 86-531-2963276. Ed. Huang Naijian. Adv. contact Li Wenfu. Circ: 15,000 (paid).

616.3 CHN
ZHONGGUO ZHONGXIYI JIEHE ZAZHI (GASTRO-SPLEEN)/CHINESE JOURNAL OF INTEGRATED TRADITIONAL AND WESTERN MEDICINE (GASTRO-SPLEEN). Text in Chinese. bi-m. USD 16.80; USD 2.80 newsstand/cover (effective 2001). **Document type:** *Academic/Scholarly.*
Published by: China International Book Trading Corp/Zhongguo Guoji Tushu Maoyi Zonggongsi cibtc@mail.cibtc.com.cn, http://www.cibtc.com.cn. **Dist. by:** 35, Chegongzhuang Xilu, Haidian District, Beijing 100044, China.

617.6 CHN ISSN 1002-0098
ZHONGHUA KOUQIANG YIXUE ZAZHI/CHINESE JOURNAL OF STOMATOLOGY. Text in Chinese. 1953-1959; resumed 1987. bi-m. CNY 67.20 domestic; CNY 11.20 newsstand/cover domestic; USD 35.40 foreign; USD 5.90 newsstand/cover foreign (effective 2000). **Document type:** *Academic/Scholarly.*
Formerly (1953-1959): Chung-Hua K'ou Ch'iang K'o Tsa Chih (0412-4014)
Related titles: Online - full content ed.
Indexed: Ind.Med. (1987-).
Published by: Zhonghua Yixuehui Zazhishe, 42 Dongsi Xidajie, Beijing 100710, China. TEL 86-1-65251918, cmakq@public.sti.ac.cn. **Dist. by:** China International Book Trading Corp, 35, Chegongzhuang Xilu, Haidian District, Beijing 100044, China. TEL 86-1-68413849, FAX 86-1-68412048, cibtc@mail.cibtc.com.cn, http://www.cibtc.com.cn.

616.3 TWN ISSN 1013-7696
CODEN: CMHCE
ZHONGHUA MINGUO XIAOHUA XIYI XUEHUI ZAZHI/GASTROENTEROLOGICAL SOCIETY OF TAIWAN. JOURNAL. Text in Chinese. 1982. q. **Document type:** *Trade.*
Indexed: Excerp.Med.
—EMDOCS.
Published by: Zhonghua Minguo Xiaohua Xiyi Xuehui/Gastroenterological Society of the Republic of China, Taita Jing-fu Alumni Bldg, 2nd Fl, 7 Chung-San South Rd, Taipei, Taiwan. TEL 02-3119062, FAX 02-3114182. Ed. Shiann Pan. Pub. Teh Hong Wang.

616.3 CHN ISSN 0254-1432
ZHONGHUA XIAOHUA ZAZHI/CHINESE JOURNAL OF DIGESTION. Text in Chinese; Abstracts in Chinese, English. bi-m. CNY 45 domestic; USD 23.40 foreign; CNY 7.50 newsstand/cover domestic; USD 3.90 newsstand/cover foreign (effective 2001). reprints avail.
Related titles: CD-ROM ed.; Online - full content ed.: (from WanFang Data Corp.).
Indexed: ExtraMED.
Published by: Zhonghua Yixuehui (Shanghai Fenhui)/Chinese Medical Association (Shanghai Branch), 1623 Beijing Xilu, Shanghai 200040, China. TEL 86-21-62531885, FAX 86-21-62550842, cma-sb@online.sh.cn. Ed. Shu-Dong Xiao. Circ: 13,000. **Dist. by:** China International Book Trading Corp, 35, Chegongzhuang Xilu, Haidian District, Beijing 100044, China. TEL 86-1-68413849, FAX 86-1-68412048, cibtc@mail.cibtc.com.cn, http://www.cibtc.com.cn.

MEDICAL SCIENCES—Hematology

613.7 616.15 USA ISSN 1092-0412
A B C NEWSLETTER. Text in English. 1978. w. USD 264 in North America; USD 288 elsewhere (effective 2000). adv. bk.rev. index. back issues avail. **Document type:** *Newsletter.* **Description:** Current events and trends in community blood services and transfusion medicine.
Formerly: C C B C Newsletter (1083-3811)
Related titles: E-mail ed.: USD 216 (effective 2000).
Published by: America's Blood Centers, 725 15th St, N W, Ste 700, Washington, DC 20005-2109. TEL 202-393-5725, 888-872-5663, FAX 202-393-1282, abc@americasblood.org, http://www.americasblood.org. Ed. Jane M Starkey. Circ: 580 (paid).

616.15 CHE ISSN 0001-5792
CODEN: ACHAAH
ACTA HAEMATOLOGICA. Text in English. 1948. 8/yr. (2 vols. per yr.). CHF 1,336, EUR 954.40 in Europe to institutions; CHF 1,359.20, USD 1,038 overseas to institutions (effective 2002). adv. bk.rev. abstr, illus. index. back issues avail. *Refereed.* **Document type:** *Journal, Academic/Scholarly.* **Description:** Features balanced, wide-ranging coverage of current hematology research.
Related titles: Online - full text ed.: ISSN 1421-9662. CHF 116, EUR 84, USD 90 with print edition (effective 2002) (from EBSCO Publishing, O C L C Online Computer Library Center, Inc., RoweCom Information Quest, Swets Blackwell, Institute for Scientific Information).
Indexed: ASCA, Biol.Abstr., Chem.Abstr., Chem.Indus.Notes, Chem.Titles, Curr.Adv.Cancer Res., Curr.Adv.Ecol.Sci., Curr.Cont., Excerp.Med., INIS Atomind., Ind.Med. (1948-), Ind.Sci.Rev., Ind.Vet., Inpharma, Nutr.Abstr., Pharm.&Out.News, Protozool.Abstr., Reac., Sci.Cit.Ind., So.Pac.Per.Ind., Telegen, Vet.Bull.
—BLDSC (0623.000000), CASDDS, CISTI, EMDOCS, GNLM, IDS, ingenta, KNAW. **CCC.**
Published by: S. Karger AG, Allschwilerstr 10, PO Box, Basel 4009, Switzerland. TEL 41-61-306-1111, FAX 41-61-306-1234, karger@karger.ch, http://www.online.karger.com/journals/aha. Ed. I Ben Bassat. adv.: page USD 1,185. Circ: 1,600.

616.15 POL ISSN 0001-5814
CODEN: AHPLBO
ACTA HAEMATOLOGICA POLONICA. Text and summaries in Polish, English. 1970. 4/yr. PLZ 55 domestic; USD 60 foreign (effective 2000). adv. bk.rev. index. *Refereed.* **Document type:** *Monographic series, Academic/Scholarly.* **Description:** Features case reports on hematology, transfusion and immunology.
Media: Duplicated (not offset). **Related titles:** Cards ed.
Indexed: Biol.Abstr., Chem.Abstr., Excerp.Med., INIS Atomind., Ind.Med. (coverage dropped), Ref.Zh.
—BLDSC (0623.200000), CASDDS, CISTI, EMDOCS, GNLM, KNAW.
Published by: Polskie Towarzystwo Hematologow i Transfuzjologow/Polish Society of Hematology and Transfusiology, c/o Klinika Hematologii Akademii Medycznej, Ul Pabianicka 62, Lodz 93513, Poland. TEL 48-42-6846890, FAX 48-42-6846890, korycka@psk2.am.lodz.pl. Ed. Tadeusz Robak. Adv. contact Anna Korycka. B&W page PLZ 1,500, B&W page USD 30, color page PLZ 2,500, color page USD 50. Circ: 1,150. **Co-sponsor:** Instytut Hematologii i Transfuzjologii.

616.15 CHE ISSN 1074-3944
ADVANCES IN BLOOD DISORDERS. Text in English. 1995. irreg., latest vol.3. price varies. **Document type:** *Monographic series.*
—CISTI.
Published by: Gordon and Breach - Harwood Academic (Subsidiary of: Taylor & Francis Group), PO Box 531, Lausanne 1000, Switzerland. **Subscr. addr. in US:** International Publishers Direct, PO Box 32160, Newark, NJ 07102. FAX 215-750-6343.

616.1 USA ISSN 0361-8609
QP91 CODEN: AJHEDD
AMERICAN JOURNAL OF HEMATOLOGY. Text in English. 1976. m. USD 2,595 in United States; USD 2,715 in Canada & Mexico; USD 2,817 elsewhere; USD 2,725 combined subscription in United States for print and online eds.; USD 2,845 combined subscription in Canada & Mexico for print and online eds.; USD 2,947 combined subscription elsewhere for print and online eds. (effective 2002). adv. bibl, illus. back issues avail.; reprint service avail. from ISI. *Refereed.* **Document type:** *Academic/Scholarly.* **Description:** Provides broad coverage of both human and animal hematologic topics and publishes original contributions from investigators and clinicians in hematology, as well as related areas such as immunology, blood banking, genetics, chemotherapy, and cell biology.
Related titles: Microform ed.: (from PQC); Online - full text ed.: ISSN 1096-8652. USD 2,595 in United States; USD 2,595 in Canada & Mexico; USD 2,595 elsewhere (effective 2002) (from EBSCO Publishing, Wiley InterScience, Institute for Scientific Information).
Indexed: ASCA, Abstr.Hyg., Abstr.Inter.Med., Biol.Abstr., Chem.Abstr., Chem.Indus.Notes, Chem.Titles, Curr.Adv.Ecol.Sci., Curr.Adv.Gen.& Molec.Biol., Curr.Cont., Dent.Ind., Environ.Sci.Poll.Mgmt., Excerp.Med., Helminthol.Abstr., INIS Atomind., Ind.Med. (1976-), Ind.Sci.Rev., Inpharma, Int.Abstr.Biol.Sci., Nutr.Abstr., Pharm.&Out.News, Pollut.Abstr., Protozool.Abstr., Reac., Ref.Zh., Rev.Med.& Vet.Mycol., Risk Abstr., SSCI (coverage dropped), Saf.Sci.Abstr., Sci.Cit.Ind., Trop.Dis.Bull.

M

—BLDSC (0824.800000), CASDDS, CISTI, EMDOCS, GNLM, IDS, ingenta, KNAW. **CCC.**
Published by: John Wiley & Sons, Inc., Journals (Subsidiary of: Wiley InterScience), 605 Third Ave, New York, NY 10158. TEL 212-850-6645, FAX 212-850-6021, subinfo@jwiley.com, uscs-wis@wiley.com, http://www.wiley.com. Ed. Ananda S Prasad. adv.: B&W page GBP 640, color page GBP 1,515; trim 210 x 279. Circ: 1,350. **Subscr. outside the Americas to:** John Wiley & Sons Ltd., Baffins Ln, Chichester, Sussex PO19 IUD, United Kingdom. TEL 44-1243-779777, FAX 44-1243-843232, cs-journals@wiley.co.uk, http://www.wiley.co.uk.

AMERICAN JOURNAL OF KIDNEY DISEASES. see *MEDICAL SCIENCES—Urology And Nephrology*

616.15 DEU ISSN 0939-5555
CODEN: ANHEE8
ANNALS OF HEMATOLOGY. Text in English. 1950. m. EUR 1,058.20 domestic; EUR 1,050.70 in Germany; EUR 103 newsstand/cover foreign (effective 2002). adv. bk.rev. abstr, bibl, charts, illus. index. reprint service avail. from ISI. *Refereed.* **Document type:** *Journal, Academic/Scholarly.* **Description:** Covers the entire spectrum of clinical and experimental hematology, hemostasiology, immunohematology and blood transfusion, including the diagnosis and treatment of hematopoietic and lymphatic neoplasis and of bone marrow transplantation.
Formerly (until 1991): Blut (0006-5242)
Related titles: Microform ed.: (from PQC); Online - full text ed.: ISSN 1432-0584 (from EBSCO Publishing, RoweCom Information Quest, Swets Blackwell, Springer LINK, Institute for Scientific Information); ♦ Supplement: Haematologie und Bluttransfusion. ISSN 0440-0607.
Indexed: ASCA, Biol.Abstr., Chem.Abstr., Chem.Indus.Notes, Chem.Titles, Curr.Adv.Cancer Res., Curr.Adv.Ecol.Sci., Curr.Cont., Excerp.Med., Helminthol.Abstr., INIS Atomind., Ind.Med. (1991-), Ind.Sci.Rev., Ind.Vet., Inpharma, Kidney, Nutr.Abstr., Pharm.&Out.News, Protozool.Abstr., Reac., Rev.Med.& Vet.Mycol., Sci.Cit.Ind., Vet.Bull.
—BLDSC (1040.855000), CASDDS, CISTI, EMDOCS, GNLM, IDS, ingenta, KNAW. **CCC.**
Published by: (Gesellschaft fuer Thrombose und Haemostaseforschung), Springer-Verlag (Subsidiary of: BertelsmannSpringer), Tiergartenstr 17, Heidelberg 69121, Germany. TEL 49-6221-345-0, FAX 49-6221-345229, subscriptions@springer.de, http://link.springer.de/link/service/journals/00277/index.htm, http://www.springer.de. Ed. G Brittinger. **Subscr. in N. America to:** Springer-Verlag New York Inc., PO Box 2485, Secaucus, NJ 07096-2485. TEL 212-460-1500. **Co-sponsors:** Deutsche Gesellschaft fuer Haematologie und Onkologie; Deutsche Gesellschaft fuer Transfusionsmedizin und Immunhaematologie.

616.15 JPN
ANNUAL REVIEW KETSUEKI/ANNUAL REVIEW. BLOOD. Text in Japanese. 1988. a. JPY 8,925 (effective 1998). adv. **Document type:** *Academic/Scholarly.*
Published by: Chugai Igakusha, 62 Yarai-cho, Shinjuku-ku, Tokyo 162-0805, Japan. R&P M Takahashi. Adv. contact M. Takahashi.

616.15 USA
APLASTIC ANEMIA & M D S INTERNATIONAL FOUNDATION. NEWSLETTER. Text in English. 1987. q. free. back issues avail. **Document type:** *Newsletter.*
Formerly: Aplastic Anemia Foundation of America. Newsletter
Published by: Aplastic Anemia & M D S International Foundation, Inc., PO Box 613, Annapolis, MD 21404-0613. TEL 410-867-0242, 800-747-2820, FAX 410-867-0240, aamdsoffice@aol.com, http://www.aamds.org. Ed., R&P Marilyn Baker. Circ: 15,000.

616.5 GBR ISSN 1521-6926
BAILLIERE'S BEST PRACTICE & RESEARCH IN CLINICAL HAEMATOLOGY. Text in English. 1987. q. GBP 112 to individuals; GBP 174 to institutions (effective 2002). *Refereed.* **Document type:** *Journal, Academic/Scholarly.* **Description:** Provides a comprehensive review of current clinical practice and thinking within the specialty of haematology.
Formerly: Bailliere's Clinical Haematology (0950-3536)
Related titles: Online - full text ed.: (from EBSCO Publishing, O C L C Online Computer Library Center, Inc., Swets Blackwell, IDEAL Online Library, Institute for Scientific Information, RoweCom Information Quest).
Indexed: ASCA, Curr.Cont., Ind.Med. (1999-), Ind.Sci.Rev., Inpharma, Pharm.&Out.News, Reac., Ref.Zh., Sci.Cit.Ind.
—BLDSC (3286.289100), CISTI, EMDOCS, GNLM, IDS, Infotrieve, ingenta, KNAW. **CCC.**
Published by: Bailliere Tindall (Subsidiary of: Harcourt Publishers Ltd.), 24-28 Oval Rd, London NW1 7DX, United Kingdom. TEL 44-20-7424-4200, FAX 44-20-7424-4515, cservice@harcourt.com, http://www.harcourt-international.com/journals/beha/. **Subscr to:** Harcourt Publishers Ltd., Foots Cray High St, Sidcup, Kent DA14 5HP, United Kingdom. TEL 44-20-8308-5700, FAX 44-20-8309-0807.

362.19699419 CHN ISSN 1006-6934
BAIXUEBING/JOURNAL OF LEUKEMIA. Text in Chinese. bi-m. back issues avail. **Document type:** *Academic/Scholarly.*
Formerly: Shanxi Baixuebing (1004-3683)
Related titles: Online - full content ed.: (from WanFang Data Corp.).
Published by: Shanxi-sheng Zhongliu Yanjiusuo, Zigong Xinjie 3 Hao, Taiyuan, Shanxi 030013, China. TEL 86-351-4425911. Ed. Yu Luan Wang.

616.15 YUG ISSN 0354-4494
BILTEN ZA TRANSFUZIOLOGIJU. Text in Serbian; Summaries in English. 1954. s-a. YUN 100 domestic; USD 10 foreign (effective 1999). adv. bk.rev. back issues avail. **Document type:** *Academic/Scholarly.* **Description:** Covers current topics, original and professional papers in the transfusion medicine and hematology fields.
Former titles (until 1994): Bilten za Hematologiju i Transfuziologiju (0354-1142); (until 1991): Bilten za Hematologiju i Transfuziju (0350-2023); (until 1973): Bilten za Transfuzije (0523-6150)
Related titles: Diskette ed.; Fax ed.
Indexed: Ind.Med. (coverage dropped).
—GNLM.
Published by: Zavod za Transfuziju Krvi Srbije/National Blood Transfusion Institute, Svetog Save 39, Belgrade 11000, Yugoslavia. TEL 381-11-4318861, FAX 381-11-458328, simzor@evnet.yu. Ed. Baklaja Radmila. Pub. Vukman Gligorovic. R&P, Adv. contact Antuljeskov Gordana TEL 381-1-431886. B&W page USD 50. Circ: 300. **Co-sponsor:** Ministry of Science and Technology.

616.15 USA ISSN 1083-8791
CODEN: BBMTF6
BIOLOGY OF BLOOD AND MARROW TRANSPLANTATION. Text in English. 1995. bi-m. USD 225 to individuals; USD 250 to institutions; USD 250 foreign to individuals; USD 275 foreign to institutions. adv. **Document type:** *Academic/Scholarly.* **Description:** Describes blood and marrow transplantation processes for the medical profession.
Related titles: Online - full text ed.: (from Institute for Scientific Information).
Indexed: Curr.Cont., Ind.Med. (1995-), Sci.Cit.Ind.
—BLDSC (2087.013000), CASDDS.
Published by: (American Society for Blood and Marrow Transplantation), Carden Jennings Publishing, 1224 W Main St, Ste 200, Charlottesville, VA 22903-2858. TEL 804-979-4913, FAX 804-979-4025. Ed. Dr. Richard J O'Reilly. Adv. contact David Ern. color page USD 1,565.

616.15 DEU ISSN 0934-0734
BIOMEDICAL PROGRESS; clinical trends in coagulation and fibrinolysis. Text in English. 1988. q. USD 32 (effective 2001). *Refereed.* **Document type:** *Journal, Academic/Scholarly.*
—GNLM.
Published by: Die Medizinische Verlagsgesellschaft Umwelt & Medizin mbH, Scharderhohlweg 35, Koenigstein 61462, Germany. TEL 49-69-638204, FAX 49-69-637109. Ed. Dr. Eberhard Mammen. Circ: 14,000 (paid).

616.15 USA ISSN 0006-4971
RB145 CODEN: BLOOAW
BLOOD. Text in English. 1945. 24/yr. USD 532 domestic to individuals; USD 747 foreign to individuals; USD 748 domestic to institutions; USD 897 foreign to institutions; USD 244 domestic to students; USD 667 foreign to students; USD 38 newsstand/cover domestic (effective 2000). adv. bk.rev. abstr, bibl, charts, illus. index. *Refereed.* **Document type:** *Academic/Scholarly.* **Description:** Publishes original articles relating to all phases of hematology.
Formerly: Blood: The Journal of Hematology
Related titles: Online - full text ed.: (from HighWire Pr., EBSCO Publishing, Institute for Scientific Information).
Indexed: AIDS Abstr., AIM, ASCA, Abstr.Hyg., Abstr.Inter.Med., AgBiotech, Agri.& Environ.Biotech.Abstr. (coverage dropped), Anim.Breed.Abstr., Biol.Abstr., Chem.Abstr., Chem.Indus.Notes, Chem.Titles, Curr.Adv.Cancer Res., Curr.Adv.Ecol.Sci., Curr.Cont., Dairy Sci.Abstr., Dent.Ind., Derwent Biotech.Abstr., Excerp.Med., Helminthol.Abstr., INIS Atomind., Ind.Med. (1946-), Ind.Sci.Rev., Ind.Vet., Inpharma, Int.Abstr.Biol.Sci., Neurosci.Cit.Ind., Nutr.Abstr., Pharm.&Out.News, Protozool.Abstr., Reac., Ref.Zh., Rev.Arom.& Med.Plants, Rev.Med.& Vet.Mycol., Risk Abstr., SSCI (coverage dropped), Sci.Cit.Ind., Small Anim.Abstr., Telegen, Trop.Dis.Bull., Vet.Bull.
—BLDSC (2112.000000), CASDDS, CISTI, EMDOCS, GNLM, IDS, ingenta, KNAW, Linda Hall. **CCC.**
Published by: American Society of Hematology, 1900 M St, NW, Ste 200, Washington, DC 20036. TEL 202-776-0544, 202-776-0548, 202-776-0550, FAX 202-776-0545, 202-776-0549, 202-776-0551, ash@hematology.org, editorial@hematology.org, publishing@hematology.org, http://www.bloodjournal.org/. Ed. Kenneth Kaushansky. adv.: B&W page USD 1,840, color page USD 3,290; trim 10 x 7. Circ: 13,835. **Subscr. to:** Periodicals Fulfillment, W B Saunders Co, 6277 Sea Harbor Dr, 4th Fl, Orlando, FL 32891-4800. TEL 800-654-2452, FAX 800-874-6418. **Dist. by:** W.B. Saunders Co.. http://www.wbsaunders.com.

BLOOD CELL BIOCHEMISTRY. see *BIOLOGY—Biochemistry*

616.1 USA ISSN 1079-9796
CODEN: BCMDFX
BLOOD CELLS, MOLECULES, AND DISEASES. Text in English. 1975. 6/yr. USD 499 in US & Canada to institutions; USD 518 elsewhere to institutions (effective 2001). reprints avail. *Refereed.* **Document type:** *Academic/Scholarly.* **Description:** Aimed at researchers involved in physiology, ultrastructure, immunology, and biophysics of blood cells.
Formerly (until 1995): Blood Cells (0340-4684)
Related titles: Microform ed.: (from PQC); Online - full text ed.: (from EBSCO Publishing, O C L C Online Computer Library Center, Inc., RoweCom Information Quest, ProQuest Information & Learning, ingenta, Swets Blackwell, IDEAL Online Library, Institute for Scientific Information).
Indexed: ASCA, Anim.Breed.Abstr., Chem.Abstr., Chem.Indus.Notes, Chem.Titles, Curr.Adv.Cell & Devel.Biol., Curr.Adv.Ecol.Sci., Curr.Adv.Gen.& Molec.Biol., Curr.Cont., Excerp.Med., INIS Atomind., Ind.Med. (1995-), Ind.Sci.Rev., Inpharma, Pharm.&Out.News, Reac., Sci.Cit.Ind.
—BLDSC (2112.300000), ADONIS, CASDDS, CISTI, EMDOCS, GNLM, IDS, ingenta, KNAW. **CCC.**
Published by: (Blood Cells Foundation), Academic Press, Inc., Journal Division (Subsidiary of: Harcourt Brace & Company), 525 B St, Ste 1900, San Diego, CA 92101-4495. TEL 619-230-1840, FAX 619-699-6800, apsubs@acad.com, http://www.academicpress.com/bcmd. Ed. Dr. Ernest Beutler.

616.15 USA ISSN 0957-5235
CODEN: BLFIE7
BLOOD COAGULATION AND FIBRINOLYSIS; international journal in haemostasis and thrombosis. Text in English. 1990. 8/yr. USD 297 domestic to individuals; USD 297 foreign to individuals; USD 1,202 per issue domestic to institutions; USD 1,202 per issue foreign to institutions; USD 132 newsstand/cover (effective 2002). adv. bk.rev. *Refereed.* **Document type:** *Academic/Scholarly.* **Description:** Features review and original research articles on all clinical, laboratory and experimental aspects of haemostasis and thrombosis.
Related titles: Online - full text ed.: USD 1,562.60 domestic academic site license; USD 1,562.60 foreign academic site license; USD 1,742.90 domestic corporate site license; USD 1,742.90 foreign corporate site license (2002) (from Ovid Technologies, Inc., EBSCO Publishing, Institute for Scientific Information).
Indexed: ASCA, Chem.Abstr., Chem.Indus.Notes, Chem.Titles, Curr.Cont., Excerp.Med. (1993-), Ind.Med. (1990-), Ind.Sci.Rev., Inpharma, Int.Abstr.Biol.Sci., Pharm.&Out.News, Reac., Sci.Cit.Ind.
—BLDSC (2112.650000), ADONIS, CASDDS, CISTI, EMDOCS, GNLM, IDS, ingenta, KNAW.
Published by: Lippincott Williams & Wilkins (Philadelphia) (Subsidiary of: Wolters Kluwer N.V.), 530 Walnut St, Philadelphia, PA 19106-3621. TEL 215-521-8300, FAX 215-521-8902, http://www.lww.com/productdetailresults/1,2265,0957-5235,00.html?PromoCD=W1P567ZZ, http://www.Lww.com. Eds. E G D Tuddentram, Dr. R Marlar. Adv. contact Gemma Heiser. **Subscr. to:** PO Box 1600, Hagerstown, MD 21740-1600. TEL 800-777-2295, FAX 301-824-7390.

BLOOD COAGULATION FACTORS; current awareness service for researchers in life sciences. see *MEDICAL SCIENCES—Abstracting, Bibliographies, Statistics*

BLOOD PRESSURE MONITORING. see *MEDICAL SCIENCES—Cardiovascular Diseases*

616.15 CHE ISSN 0253-5068 CODEN: BLPUDO
BLOOD PURIFICATION. Text and summaries in English. 1983. q. CHF 870, EUR 621.80 in Europe to institutions; CHF 887.40, USD 677 overseas to institutions (effective 2002). adv. illus. index. back issues avail. *Refereed.* **Document type:** *Journal, Academic/Scholarly.* **Description:** Includes practical information on hemodialysis, hemofiltration, peritoneal dialysis and plasma filtration.
Related titles: Microform ed.: (from PQC); Online - full text ed.: ISSN 1421-9735. CHF 58, EUR 42, USD 45 to institutions with print edition (effective 2002) (from EBSCO Publishing, O C L C Online Computer Library Center, Inc., RoweCom Information Quest, Swets Blackwell, Institute for Scientific Information).
Indexed: ASCA, Chem.Abstr., Chem.Indus.Notes, Chem.Titles, Curr.Cont., Excerp.Med., Ind.Med. (1983-), Inpharma, Pharm.&Out.News, Reac.
—BLDSC (2113.037000), CASDDS, CISTI, EMDOCS, GNLM, IDS, ingenta, KNAW. **CCC.**
Published by: S. Karger AG, Allschwilerstr 10, PO Box, Basel 4009, Switzerland. TEL 41-61-306-1111, FAX 41-61-306-1234, karger@karger.ch, http://www.online.karger.com/journals/bpu, http://www.karger.com. Eds. K M Leunissen, L W Henderson. adv.: page USD 1,195. Circ: 950.

616.15 GBR ISSN 0268-960X CODEN: BLOREB
BLOOD REVIEWS. Text in English. 1987. q. GBP 139 to individuals; GBP 233 to institutions (effective 2002). adv. *Refereed.* **Document type:** *Journal, Academic/Scholarly.* **Description:** Covers all aspects of hematology - current ideas in clinical and laboratory practice.
Related titles: Online - full text ed.: (from EBSCO Publishing, O C L C Online Computer Library Center, Inc., Swets Blackwell, IDEAL Online Library, Institute for Scientific Information).
Indexed: ASCA, Curr.Cont., Ind.Med. (1987-), Ind.Sci.Rev., Inpharma, Int.Abstr.Biol.Sci., Pharm.&Out.News, Reac., Ref.Zh., Sci.Cit.Ind.
—BLDSC (2113.038000), CISTI, EMDOCS, GNLM, IDS, ingenta, KNAW. **CCC.**
Published by: Churchill Livingstone (Subsidiary of: Harcourt Publishers Ltd.), Robert Stevenson House, 1-3 Baxter's Pl, Leith Walk, Edinburgh, Midlothian EH1 3AF, United Kingdom. TEL 44-131-556-2424, FAX 44-131-459-1177, cservice@harcourt.com, http://www.harcourt-international.com/journals/blre. Eds. Ian Franklin, Jacob Rowe. Pub. Gillian Griffith. R&P Catherine John TEL 212-424-4200. Adv. contact David Dunnachie. Circ: 990. **Subscr. to:** Harcourt Publishers Ltd., Foots Cray High St, Sidcup, Kent DA14 5HP, United Kingdom. TEL 44-20-8308-5700, FAX 44-20-8309-0807.

616.15 IND ISSN 0006-5005
BLOOD THERAPY JOURNAL INTERNATIONAL; committed to the cause of eradication of blood diseases & cancer. Text in English, Hindi; Summaries in English. 1965. bi-m. INR 120, USD 50. adv. bk.rev. abstr, bibl, charts, illus. *Refereed.*
Supersedes (in 1980): Blood Therapy Journal
—CISTI.
Published by: Institute of Haematology, 11 6 B Pusa Rd., New Delhi 110 005, India. TEL 91-11-2246228, FAX 91-11-2247189. Ed. Dr. V B Lal. R&P A M Bande. Adv. contact A.M. Bande. Circ: 3,000.

616.6 USA ISSN 1065-6073
BLOOD WEEKLY. Text in English. 1993. w. (43/yr.). USD 1,549 in North America; USD 1,649 elsewhere. **Document type:** *Newsletter.* **Description:** Concentrates on blood-related news and research worldwide, with original reporting, reviews of periodicals and journal articles and calendars of forthcoming professional meetings. Covers blood products and substitutes, blood-related diseases, including AIDS, tissue transplants and blood-borne pathogens.
Related titles: Microform ed.: (from PQC); Online - full text ed.: (from CompuServe, Inc., Data-Star, The Dialog Corporation, Dow Jones Interactive, Gale Group, NewsNet, Northern Light Technology, Inc., Factiva).
Indexed: Bus.& Indus. (Jan.1995-).
—Infotrieve. **CCC.**
Published by: Charles W. Henderson, Ed. & Pub., PO Box 5528, Atlanta, GA 31107-0528. TEL 770-507-7777, FAX 770-507-7788, info@hendersonnet.atl.ga.us, http://www.newsfile.com.

616.15 GBR ISSN 0007-1048 CODEN: BJHEAL
BRITISH JOURNAL OF HAEMATOLOGY. Text in English. 1955. 16/yr., latest vol.116, 2002. GBP 114 in Europe to individuals; USD 190 in North America to individuals; GBP 129 elsewhere to individuals; GBP 622 in Europe to institutions; USD 982 in North America to institutions; GBP 682 elsewhere to institutions (effective 2002). adv. bk.rev. bibl, charts, illus. index. back issues avail.; reprint service avail. from ISI. *Refereed.* **Document type:** *Academic/Scholarly.* **Description:** Publishes original research papers in clinical, laboratory and experimental haematology.
Related titles: CD-ROM ed.: (from Ovid Technologies, Inc.); Microform ed.: (from PQC); Online - full text ed.: ISSN 1365-2141. 1997. GBP 103 in Europe to individuals; USD 171 in North America to individuals; GBP 103 elsewhere to individuals; GBP 560 in Europe to institutions; USD 884 in North America to institutions; GBP 560 elsewhere to institutions (effective 2002) (from Ovid Technologies, Inc., EBSCO Publishing, O C L C Online Computer Library Center, Inc., RoweCom Information Quest, ingenta, Munksgaard & Blackwell Science's Synergy, Swets Blackwell, Institute for Scientific Information); ♦ Supplement: British Journal of Haematology. Supplement. ISSN 0963-1860.
Indexed: ASCA, Abstr.Hyg., Biol.Abstr., Chem.Abstr., Chem.Indus.Notes, Chem.Titles, Curr.Adv.Biochem., Curr.Adv.Cancer Res., Curr.Adv.Cell & Devel.Biol., Curr.Adv.Ecol.Sci., Curr.Adv.Gen.& Molec.Biol., Curr.Cont., Dairy Sci.Abstr., Dent.Ind., Derwent Biotech.Abstr., Excerp.Med., Helminthol.Abstr., INIS Atomind., Ind.Med. (1955-), Ind.Sci.Rev., Ind.Vet., Inpharma, Int.Abstr.Biol.Sci., Int.Nurs.Ind., Mass Spectr.Bull., Nutr.Abstr., Pharm.&Out.News, Protozool.Abstr., Reac., Ref.Zh., Rev.Med.& Vet.Mycol., Sci.Cit.Ind., Telegen, Trop.Dis.Bull., Vet.Bull.
—BLDSC (2309.000000), ADONIS, CASDDS, CISTI, EMDOCS, GNLM, IDS, ingenta, KNAW. **CCC.**
Published by: Blackwell Science Ltd., PO Box 88, Oxford OX2 0NE, United Kingdom. TEL 44-1865-206180, 44-1865-206002, FAX 44-1865-206219, jnl.orders@blacksci.co.uk, http://www.blackwell-science.com/products/journals/bjh.htm, http://www.blackwellpublishing.com. Ed. M Greaves. Pub. Allen Stevens. R&P Sophie Savage. Adv. contact Jenny Applin. Circ: 3,430. **Co-sponsors:** British Society for Haematology; European Haematology Association.

616.15 GBR ISSN 0963-1860
BRITISH JOURNAL OF HAEMATOLOGY. SUPPLEMENT. Text in English. irreg. adv. **Document type:** *Academic/Scholarly.*
Related titles: Online - full text ed.: (from Ovid Technologies, Inc.); ♦ Supplement to: British Journal of Haematology. ISSN 0007-1048.
Indexed: Excerp.Med.
—ADONIS, EMDOCS, KNAW.
Published by: Blackwell Science Ltd., Osney Mead, Oxford OX2 0EL, United Kingdom. TEL 44-1865-206206, FAX 44-1865-721205, journals.cs@blacksci.co.uk, http://www.blackwell-science.com. Pub. Allen Stevens. R&P Sophie Savage. Adv. contact Jenny Applin.

616.15 USA ISSN 0895-1934 CODEN: BMPSEQ
BRUNNER - MAZEL PSYCHOSOCIAL STRESS SERIES*. Text in English. 1978. irreg., latest vol.23. **Document type:** *Monographic series.*
Indexed: e-psyche.
Published by: Brunner - Routledge (Subsidiary of: Taylor & Francis Group), 325 Chestnut St, Ste 800, Philadelphia, PA 19106. TEL 215-269-0400, FAX 215-269-0363, postmaster@bmpub.com.

CALCIFIED TISSUE INTERNATIONAL. see *MEDICAL SCIENCES—Endocrinology*

616.15 CAN ISSN 0840-5360
CANADIAN RED CROSS SOCIETY. BLOOD SERVICES. ANNUAL REPORT. Text in English, French. 1946. a. free per issue.
Formerly (until 1986): Canadian Red Cross Blood Transfusion Service. Annual Report (0708-7047)
Related titles: French ed.: Societe Canadienne de la Croix-Rouge. Services Transfusionnels. Rapport Annuel. ISSN 0840-6103.
Published by: Canadian Red Cross Society, National Headquarters, 5700 Cancross Court, Mississauga, ON L5R 3E9, Canada. TEL 416-890-1000. Circ: 6,000.

CANCER DRUG DISCOVERY AND DEVELOPMENT. see *MEDICAL SCIENCES—Oncology*

CEREBROVASCULAR DISEASES. see *MEDICAL SCIENCES—Psychiatry And Neurology*

616.15 USA ISSN 1076-0296 CODEN: CATHF9
CLINICAL AND APPLIED THROMBOSIS - HEMOSTASIS. Text in English. 1995. q. USD 208 to individuals; USD 258 to institutions; USD 64 newsstand/cover (effective 2001). adv. back issues avail. *Refereed.* **Document type:** *Academic/Scholarly.* **Description:** Publishes the latest results of new clinical trials and studies, discussions of new pharmacologic methodologies, and new management strategies.
Related titles: Microform ed.: (from PQC); Online - full text ed.: (from Institute for Scientific Information).
Indexed: ASCA, Curr.Cont., Helminthol.Abstr., Ind.Med. (1995-), Inpharma, Pharm.&Out.News, Reac.
—BLDSC (3286.247800), CASDDS, CISTI, GNLM, IDS, KNAW.
Published by: (Academy of Clinical and Applied Thrombosis - Hemostasis), Lippincott Williams & Wilkins (Philadelphia) (Subsidiary of: Wolters Kluwer N.V.), 530 Walnut St, Philadelphia, PA 19106-3621. TEL 301-223-2300, 800-638-3030, FAX 301-223-2400, http://www.thrombosis-hemostasis.com, http://www.Lww.com. Ed. Rodger L Bick. adv.: B&W page USD 620, color page USD 1,555. Circ: 684. **Subscr. to:** PO Box 1600, Hagerstown, MD 21740-1600.

616.15 GBR ISSN 0141-9854 CODEN: CLHAD3
CLINICAL AND LABORATORY HAEMATOLOGY. Text in English. 1979. bi-m., latest vol.24, 2002. GBP 348 in Europe to institutions; USD 552 in North America to institutions; GBP 383 elsewhere to institutions (effective 2002). adv. bk.rev. abstr, bibl, charts, illus. index. back issues avail.; reprint service avail. from ISI. *Refereed.* **Document type:** *Academic/Scholarly.* **Description:** Aims to be a forum for the communication of new developments, research topics and the practice of clinical and laboratory haematology.
Related titles: Microform ed.: (from PQC); Online - full text ed.: ISSN 1365-2257. GBP 314 in Europe; USD 497 in North America; GBP 314 elsewhere (effective 2002) (from Ovid Technologies, Inc., EBSCO Publishing, O C L C Online Computer Library Center, Inc., RoweCom Information Quest, ingenta, Munksgaard & Blackwell Science's Synergy, Swets Blackwell, Institute for Scientific Information); ♦ Partial English Translation: Clinical and Laboratory Haematology. Supplement. ISSN 0960-3964.
Indexed: ASCA, Curr.Adv.Ecol.Sci., Curr.Cont., Excerp.Med., Ind.Med. (1979-), Ind.Sci.Rev., Inpharma, Pharm.&Out.News, Reac., Rev.Med.& Vet.Mycol., Sci.Cit.Ind.
—BLDSC (3286.253200), ADONIS, CASDDS, CISTI, EMDOCS, GNLM, IDS, ingenta. **CCC.**
Published by: Blackwell Science Ltd., PO Box 88, Oxford OX2 0NE, United Kingdom. TEL 44-1865-206180, 44-1865-206002, FAX 44-1865-206219, jnl.orders@blacksci.co.uk, http://www.blackwell-science.com/products/journals/clh.htm, http://www.blackwellpublishing.com. Ed. I Cavill. Pub. Elizabeth Whelan. R&P Sophie Savage. Adv. contact Jenny Applin. Circ: 720.

616.15 GBR ISSN 0960-3964
CLINICAL AND LABORATORY HAEMATOLOGY. SUPPLEMENT. Text in English. 1990. s-a.
Related titles: ♦ Partial translation of: Clinical and Laboratory Haematology. ISSN 0141-9854.
—ADONIS.
Published by: Blackwell Science Ltd., Osney Mead, Oxford OX2 0EL, United Kingdom. TEL 44-1685-206206, FAX 44-1685-721205, journals.cs@blacksci.co.uk, http://www.blackwell-science.com.

616.15 NLD ISSN 1386-0291 CODEN: CHMIFQ
CLINICAL HEMORHEOLOGY AND MICROCIRCULATION; an international journal on blood flow, vessel wall, interstitium: transport and interactions. Text in English. 1981. 8/yr. (in 2 vols.). EUR 620, USD 584 to institutions (effective 2002). adv. *Refereed.* **Document type:** *Journal, Academic/Scholarly.* **Description:** Topics covered include pathogenesis, symptomatology, and diagnostic, prophylactic and therapeutic methods.
Formerly (until 1997): Clinical Hemorheology (0271-5198)
Related titles: Microfilm ed.: (from PQC); Online - full text ed.: (from EBSCO Publishing, O C L C Online Computer Library Center, Inc., ingenta, Swets Blackwell, Institute for Scientific Information, RoweCom Information Quest).

M

Indexed: ASCA, Chem.Abstr., Curr.Adv.Ecol.Sci., Curr.Cont., Excerp.Med., Helminthol.Abstr., Ind.Med. (1997-), Inpharma, Int.Abstr.Biol.Sci., Nutr.Abstr., Pharm.&Out.News, Reac., Sci.Cit.Ind.
—BLDSC (3286.290050), ADONIS, CASDDS, CISTI, EMDOCS, GNLM, IDS, Infotrieve, ingenta, KNAW. **CCC.**
Published by: I O S Press, Nieuwe Hemweg 6B, Amsterdam 1013 BG, Netherlands. TEL 31-20-688-3355, FAX 31-20-620-3419, prof_witte@yahoo.de, market@iospress.nl, http://www.iospress.nl. Eds. Jean Francois Stoltz, Siegfried Witte. **Subscr. to:** Globe Publication Pvt. Ltd., C-62 Inderpuri, New Delhi 100 012, India. TEL 91-11-579-3211, 91-11-579-3212, FAX 91-11-579-8876, custserve@globepub.com, http://www.globepub.com; Kinokuniya Company Ltd, Shinjuku 3-chome, Shinjuku-ku, Tokyo 160-0022, Japan. FAX 81-3-3439-1094, journal@kinokuniya.co.jp, http://www.kinokuniya.co.jp; I O S Press, Inc, 5795-G Burke Centre Pkwy, Burke, VA 22015. TEL 703-323-5554, FAX 703-323-3668, iosbooks@iospress.com.

CLINICAL LABORATORY; journal for clinical laboratories and laboratories related to blood transfusion. see *MEDICAL SCIENCES—Endocrinology*

616.15 ITA ISSN 0393-487X
CLOT AND HEMATOLOGIC MALIGNANCIES; journal of blood coagulation, hemostasis, thrombosis, hemorheology, and malignant hemopathies. Text in Italian. 1981. bi-m. adv. bk.rev. index. **Document type:** *Academic/Scholarly.*
Formerly (until 1984): Clot
—CISTI, GNLM.
Address: Via le Unita d'Italia, 743, Talsano, TA 74029, Italy. Ed. Teodoro Ripa. Circ: 2,500.

616.15 GBR ISSN 0938-7714
QP91 CODEN: CHAIEX
COMPARATIVE HAEMATOLOGY INTERNATIONAL. Text in English. 1991. q. USD 406; USD 120.40 newsstand/cover (effective 2001). back issues avail. *Refereed.* **Document type:** *Academic/Scholarly.* **Description:** Publishes papers encompassing the entire spectrum of comparative haematology, including immunological, toxicological and cellular aspects, data from human, veterinary and zoological studies, as well as experimental and diagnostic studies.
Related titles: Online - full text ed.: ISSN 1433-2973 (from EBSCO Publishing, RoweCom Information Quest, Swets Blackwell, Springer LINK, Institute for Scientific Information).
Indexed: ASCA, Chem.Abstr., Chem.Indus.Notes, Chem.Titles, Curr.Cont., Excerp.Med. (1993-), Ind.Sci.Rev., Inpharma, Pharm.&Out.News, Reac., Sci.Cit.Ind., Zoo.Rec.
—BLDSC (3363.782200), CASDDS, CISTI, EMDOCS, GNLM, IDS, Infotrieve, KNAW. **CCC.**
Published by: Springer-Verlag London Ltd. (Subsidiary of: BertelsmannSpringer), Sweetapple House, Catteshall Rd, Godalming, Surrey GU7 3DJ, United Kingdom. TEL 44-1483-418800, FAX 44-1483-415144, link@springer-ny.com, http://link.springer.de/link/service/journals/00580/. Eds. Geoff Brown, Nemi C Jain, Paul Sibbons. **U.S. subscr. to:** Springer-Verlag New York Inc., PO Box 2485, Secaucus, NJ 07096-2485.

616.15 USA
RB145
CONTEMPORARY HEMATOLOGY. Text in English. 1977-1984; resumed 1997. irreg., latest 1999. *Refereed.* **Document type:** *Monographic series, Academic/Scholarly.*
Former titles: Contemporary Hematology - Oncology (0197-3649); (until 1980): Year in Hematology (0160-7014)
Indexed: Biol.Abstr.
—CASDDS, CISTI, GNLM.
Published by: Humana Press Inc., 999 Riverview Dr, Ste 208, Totowa, NJ 07512. TEL 973-256-1699, FAX 973-256-8341, humana@humanapr.com, http://humanapress.com. R&P Richard Hruska.

CRITICAL REVIEWS IN ONCOLOGY - HEMATOLOGY. see *MEDICAL SCIENCES—Oncology*

▼ **CURRENT CLINICAL ONCOLOGY.** see *MEDICAL SCIENCES—Oncology*

616.15 USA ISSN 1065-6251
RC633.A1 CODEN: COHEF4
CURRENT OPINION IN HEMATOLOGY. Text in English. 1994. bi-m. USD 273 domestic to individuals for print & online eds.; USD 273 foreign to individuals for print & online eds.; USD 665 per issue domestic to institutions; USD 665 per issue to institutions; USD 103 newsstand/cover (effective 2002). adv. **Document type:** *Academic/Scholarly.*
Related titles: Online - full text ed.: USD 864.50 domestic academic site license; USD 864.50 foreign academic site license; USD 964.25 domestic corporate site license; USD 964.25 foreign corporate site license (effective 2002) (from Ovid Technologies, Inc., EBSCO Publishing, Swets Blackwell, Institute for Scientific Information).
Indexed: Curr.Cont., Excerp.Med. (1996-), Ind.Med. (1993-), Inpharma, Pharm.&Out.News, Reac.
—BLDSC (3500.775200), ADONIS, CISTI, EMDOCS, GNLM, KNAW.
Published by: Lippincott Williams & Wilkins (Philadelphia) (Subsidiary of: Wolters Kluwer N.V.), 530 Walnut St, Philadelphia, PA 19106-3621. FAX 215-521-8902, 215-521-8902, http://www.Lww.com. Ed. Thomas P Stossel. Pub. Maria McMichael. R&P Tobias Weschler. Adv. contact Kelly Adamitis. Circ: 707. **Subscr. to:** PO Box 1600, Hagerstown, MD 21740-1600.

CURRENT REVIEW OF CEREBROVASCULAR DISEASE. see *MEDICAL SCIENCES—Psychiatry And Neurology*

616.1 CHE ISSN 0258-0330
CODEN: CSHTE8
CURRENT STUDIES IN HEMATOLOGY AND BLOOD TRANSFUSION. Text in English. 1955. irreg., latest vol.62. CHF 230 in Europe; DEM 280 in Germany; USD 185 in United States (effective 2001). reprint service avail. from ISI. *Refereed.* **Document type:** *Journal, Academic/Scholarly.* **Description:** Presents current data in areas of hematology and transfusion medicine where problems are far from solved.
Formerly: Bibliotheca Haematologica
Related titles: Online - full text ed.: (from Institute for Scientific Information).
Indexed: Biol.Abstr., Chem.Abstr., Chem.Indus.Notes, Chem.Titles, Curr.Cont. (coverage dropped), Excerp.Med., Ind.Med. (1986-).
—BLDSC (3504.041000), CASDDS, CISTI, EMDOCS, GNLM, Infotrieve, ingenta, KNAW. **CCC.**
Published by: (European Society of Hematology), S. Karger AG, Allschwilerstr 10, PO Box, Basel 4009, Switzerland. TEL 41-61-306-1111, FAX 41-61-306-1234, karger@karger.ch, http://www.karger.com/bookseries/CSHBT.

616.15 616.99 USA ISSN 0899-6857
RC633.A1
CURRENT THERAPY IN HEMATOLOGY - ONCOLOGY. Text in English. 1984. irreg. **Document type:** *Monographic series, Academic/Scholarly.*
—CISTI, Infotrieve. **CCC.**
Published by: Mosby, Inc. (Subsidiary of: Elsevier Science), 11830 Westline Industrial Dr, St Louis, MO 63146-3318. TEL 314-872-8370, 800-325-4177, FAX 314-432-1380, http://www.mosby.com/periodicals.

616.15 GBR ISSN 1368-4736
RM282.C95 CODEN: CCMTFO
CYTOKINES, CELLULAR & MOLECULAR THERAPY. Text in English. 1995. q. GBP 72, USD 115 to individuals; GBP 185, USD 295 to institutions (effective 2002). adv. bk.rev. index. back issues avail. *Refereed.* **Document type:** *Academic/Scholarly.* **Description:** Includes research and clinical application of new therapies using cytokines, stem cells, growth factors, interferons and other cellular and molecular products, particularly in oncology, hematology and immunology.
Formerly (until 1997): Cytokines and Molecular Therapy (1355-6568)
Related titles: Online - full content ed.: ISSN 1466-0830; Online - full text ed.: (from CatchWord Ltd., Institute for Scientific Information).
Indexed: AIDS & Cancer Res., ASCA, Biotech.Cit.Ind., Chem.Abstr., Chem.Indus.Notes, Chem.Titles, Curr.Cont., Excerp.Med. (1996-), Genet.Abstr. (coverage dropped), Immun.Abstr., Ind.Med. (1997-), Inpharma, Int.Abstr.Biol.Sci., Med.& Pharm.Biotech.Abstr., Pharm.&Out.News, Reac., Sci.Cit.Ind. (coverage dropped).
—BLDSC (3506.788000), CASDDS, CatchWord, CISTI, EMDOCS, GNLM, KNAW.
Published by: Martin Dunitz Ltd. (Subsidiary of: Taylor & Francis Group), 7-9 Pratt St, London NW1 0AE, United Kingdom. TEL 44-20-7482-2202, FAX 44-20-7482-7088, info@dunitz.co.uk, http://www.dunitz.co.uk. Ed. Dr. David W Golde. R&P, Adv. contact Ian Mellor. Circ: 2,000 (paid).

615.505 GBR ISSN 1465-3249
▼ **CYTOTHERAPY.** Text in English. 1999. bi-m. GBP 175, USD 285 to individuals; GBP 325, USD 520 to institutions (effective 2002). *Refereed.* **Document type:** *Academic/Scholarly.*
Related titles: Online - full text ed.: (from CatchWord Ltd., Institute for Scientific Information).
Indexed: Biotech.Cit.Ind., Curr.Cont.
—BLDSC (3506.883500).
Published by: (International Society for Hematotherapy and Graft Engineering), Isis Medical Media Ltd. (Subsidiary of: Martin Dunitz Ltd.), The Livery House, 7-9 Pratt St, London NW1 0AE, United Kingdom. TEL 44-20-7482-2202, FAX 44-20-7267-0159, info@dunitz.co.uk, http://www.dunitz.co.uk/. Eds. John Barrett, Nancy H Collins.

616.15 DEU ISSN 0931-5551
DEUTSCHE GESELLSCHAFT FUER ANGIOLOGIE. MITTEILUNGEN. Text in German. q. EUR 44.80 domestic to institutions; EUR 48.80 in Europe to institutions; EUR 52.80 elsewhere to institutions; EUR 13 newsstand/cover (effective 2002). **Document type:** *Journal, Academic/Scholarly.*
—GNLM.
Published by: (Deutsche Gesellschaft fuer Angiologie), Demeter Verlag GmbH und Co. KG, Ammonitenstr 1, Balingen 72336, Germany. TEL 49-711-8931-0, FAX 49-711-8931322, custserv@thieme.de, http://www.demeter-verlag.de. Circ: 1,000.

616.15 NLD ISSN 0167-9201
CODEN: DHIMDR
DEVELOPMENTS IN HEMATOLOGY AND IMMUNOLOGY. Text in English. 1980. irreg., latest vol.28, 1993. price varies. *Refereed.* **Document type:** *Monographic series, Proceedings.*
Formerly (until 1982): Developments in Hematology (0167-448X)
Indexed: Chem.Abstr., Chem.Indus.Notes, Chem.Titles.
—BLDSC (3579.075400), CASDDS, CISTI, KNAW. **CCC.**
Published by: Kluwer Academic Publishers Group (Subsidiary of: Wolters Kluwer N.V.), Spuiboulevard 50, PO Box 17, Dordrecht 3300 AA, Netherlands. FAX 31-78-639-2254, services@wkap.nl, http://www.wkap.nl. **Dist. by:** Journals Department, PO Box 322, Dordrecht 3300 AH, Netherlands. FAX 31-78-654-6474.

ERYTHROCYTES. see *MEDICAL SCIENCES—Abstracting, Bibliographies, Statistics*

616.15 GBR ISSN 0956-6309
CODEN: ERYTE
ERYTHROPOIESIS; new dimensions in the treatment of anaemia. Text in English. 1989. q. abstr. *Refereed.* **Document type:** *Academic/Scholarly.* **Description:** Discusses recent research into the production of red blood cells and developments in the treatment of anemia.
Indexed: Excerp.Med. (1995-).
—BLDSC (3810.885000), GNLM.
Published by: (Janssen-Cilag), Adis International Ltd., Chowley Oak Ln, Tattenhall, Chester, Ches CH3 9GA, United Kingdom. TEL 44-1829-771155, FAX 44-1829-770330, Christine.Gardner@adis-europe.co.uk. Ed. Dr. Helen L Ross. Pub. Mr. M Nelson. Circ: 8,500 (controlled).

616.15 DNK ISSN 0902-4441
CODEN: EJHAEC
EUROPEAN JOURNAL OF HAEMATOLOGY. Text in English. 1964. m. USD 506 in the Americas to institutions print & online eds. combined; GBP 352 elsewhere to institutions print & online eds. combined (effective 2002). adv. bk.rev. bibl, charts, illus. reprint service avail. from ISI. *Refereed.* **Document type:** *Academic/Scholarly.*
Formerly: Scandinavian Journal of Haematology (0036-553X)
Related titles: Online - full text ed.: ISSN 1600-0609. GBP 317 (effective 2002) (from Ovid Technologies, Inc., EBSCO Publishing, ingenta, Munksgaard & Blackwell Science's Synergy, Swets Blackwell, Institute for Scientific Information).
Indexed: ASCA, Biol.Abstr., Chem.Abstr., Chem.Indus.Notes, Chem.Titles, Curr.Adv.Ecol.Sci., Curr.Cont., Dairy Sci.Abstr., Dent.Ind., Excerp.Med., Helminthol.Abstr., INIS Atomind., Ind.Med. (1987-), Ind.Sci.Rev., Inpharma, Int.Abstr.Biol.Sci., Nutr.Abstr., Pharm.&Out.News, Protozool.Abstr., Reac., Rev.Med.& Vet.Mycol., Sci.Cit.Ind.
—BLDSC (3829.729700), ADONIS, CASDDS, CISTI, EMDOCS, GNLM, IDS, ingenta, KNAW, Linda Hall. **CCC.**

M

Published by: Blackwell Munksgaard, Noerre Soegade 35, PO Box 2148, Copenhagen K 1016, Denmark. TEL 45-77-33-33-33, FAX 45-77-33-33-77, fsub@munksgaard.dk, http://journals.munksgaard.dk/ejh, http://www.munksgaard.dk. Adv. contact Eric Rozario TEL 45-77-33-33-01. Circ: 1,200.

616.15 DNK ISSN 0902-4506 CODEN: EJHSEW
EUROPEAN JOURNAL OF HAEMATOLOGY. SUPPLEMENTUM. Text in English. 1964. irreg. free with subscription to European Journal of Haematology. adv. reprint service avail. from ISI. *Refereed.* **Document type:** *Academic/Scholarly.*
Formerly: Scandinavian Journal of Haematology. Supplementum (0080-6722)
Related titles: Online - full text ed.: (from Ovid Technologies, Inc.).
Indexed: Biol.Abstr., Chem.Abstr., Chem.Indus.Notes, Chem.Titles, Curr.Cont. (coverage dropped), Excerp.Med., INIS Atomind., Ind.Med. (1987-), Int.Abstr.Biol.Sci., Nutr.Abstr.
—BLDSC (3829.729800), ADONIS, CASDDS, CISTI, EMDOCS, KNAW, Linda Hall. **CCC.**
Published by: Blackwell Munksgaard, Noerre Soegade 35, PO Box 2148, Copenhagen K 1016, Denmark. TEL 45-77-33-33-33, FAX 45-77-33-33-77, customerservice@munksgaard.dk, http://www.munksgaard.dk/ejh. Ed. Niels Borregaard. Adv. contact Eric Rozario TEL 45-77-33-33-01.

EXCERPTA MEDICA. SECTION 25: HEMATOLOGY. see *MEDICAL SCIENCES—Abstracting, Bibliographies, Statistics*

616.15 USA ISSN 0301-472X CODEN: EXHMA6
EXPERIMENTAL HEMATOLOGY. Text in English. 1973. m. EUR 236 in Europe to individuals; JPY 31,300 in Japan to individuals; USD 264 elsewhere to individuals; EUR 488 in Europe to institutions; JPY 64,800 in Japan to institutions; USD 546 elsewhere to institutions (effective 2002). adv. reprint service avail. from ISI. *Refereed.* **Document type:** *Academic/Scholarly.* **Description:** Covers all aspects of experimental hematology including hematopoiesis, cytokine biology, radiobiology, experimental clinical stem cell transplantations, cellular immunotherapy, and gene therapy.
Related titles: Online - full text ed.: (from ingenta, Swets Blackwell, ScienceDirect, Institute for Scientific Information); ♦ Supplement: Experimental Hematology. Supplement. ISSN 0256-9280.
Indexed: ASCA, Biol.Abstr., Chem.Abstr., Chem.Indus.Notes, Chem.Titles, Curr.Adv.Cell & Devel.Biol., Curr.Adv.Ecol.Sci., Curr.Cont., Dent.Ind., Excerp.Med., INIS Atomind., Ind.Med. (1973-), Ind.Sci.Rev., Inpharma, Pharm.&Out.News, Reac., Sci.Cit.Ind.
—BLDSC (3839.360000), CASDDS, CISTI, EMDOCS, GNLM, IDS, ingenta, KNAW. **CCC.**
Published by: (International Society for Experimental Hematology), Elsevier Science, 655 Ave of the Americas, New York, NY 10010. TEL 212-989-5800, FAX 212-633-3990, usinfo-f@elsevier.com, http://www.elsevier.com/locate/exphem. Eds. M Hoffman, V Johnston. Circ: 1,700 (paid). **Subscr. in Australasia and the Far East to:** Elsevier Science (Singapore) Pte Ltd, No.1 Temasek Ave, 17-01 Millenia Tower, Singapore 039192, Singapore. TEL 65-434-3727, FAX 65-337-2230; **Subscr. in Japan to:** Elsevier Science Inc - Japan Regional Office, 9-15 Higashi-Azabu 1-chome, Minato-ku, Tokyo 106-0044, Japan. TEL 81-3-5561-5033; **Subscr. outside the Americas to:** Elsevier Science BV, PO Box 211, Amsterdam 1000 AE, Netherlands. TEL 31-20-485-3757.

616.15 USA ISSN 0256-9280
EXPERIMENTAL HEMATOLOGY. SUPPLEMENT. Text in English. 1976.
Related titles: ♦ Supplement to: Experimental Hematology. ISSN 0301-472X.
Published by: Elsevier Science, 655 Ave of the Americas, New York, NY 10010. TEL 212-989-5800, FAX 212-633-3990.

FEDERAZIONE DELLE SOCIETA MEDICO-SCIENTIFICHE ITALIANE. CONGRESSI (YEAR). see *MEDICAL SCIENCES*

616.15 RUS ISSN 0234-5730 CODEN: GETRE8
GEMATOLOGIYA I TRANSFUSIOLOGIYA/HEMATOLOGY AND TRANSFUSIOLOGY. Text in Russian; Summaries in English. 1956. bi-m. USD 129 foreign (effective 2000). adv. Website rev. *Refereed.* **Document type:** *Journal, Academic/Scholarly.* **Description:** Publishes original theoretical and clinical investigations, reviews and clinical notes concerning different problems of hematology and blood transfusion.
Formerly (until 1983): Problemy Gematologii i Perelivaniya Krovi (0552-2080)
Related titles: Online - full text ed.: (from Institute for Scientific Information).
Indexed: ASCA, Biol.Abstr., Chem.Abstr., Chem.Indus.Notes, Chem.Titles, Curr.Cont., Excerp.Med., INIS Atomind., Ind.Med. (coverage dropped), Inpharma, Nutr.Abstr., Pharm.&Out.News, Reac., Ref.Zh.
—BLDSC (0047.072000), CASDDS, CISTI, East View, EMDOCS, GNLM, IDS, KNAW. **CCC.**
Published by: Izdatel'stvo Meditsina, Petroverigskii per 6-8, Moscow 101000, Russian Federation. TEL 7-095-9248785, 7-095-928-86-48, FAX 7-095-9211355, 7-095-9286003, http://www.medit.ru. Ed. A I Vorebyeb. Pub. A M Stochik. R&P L Kosmodemyanskaya. Adv. contact O A Fadeeva TEL 7-095-923-51-40. Circ: 1,100. **Dist. by:** Mezhdunarodnaya Kniga, B Yakimanka 39, Moscow 117049, Russian Federation. TEL 7-095-2384967, FAX 7-095-2384634; **US dist. addr.:** East View Publications, 3020 Harbor Ln N, Minneapolis, MN 55447. TEL 612-550-0961.

616.15 CHN ISSN 1001-1013
GUOWAI YIXUE (SHUXUE YU XUEYEXUE FENCE)/FOREIGN MEDICAL SCIENCES (BLOOD TRANSFUSION AND HEMATOLOGY). Text in Chinese. 1979. bi-m. USD 15; USD 2.50 newsstand/cover (effective 2001).
Published by: Chinese Academy of Medical Sciences, Blood Transfusion Research Institute, San Xiang, Xiaojiacun, Renmin Beilu, Chengdu, Sichuan 610081, China. **Dist. by:** China International Book Trading Corp. cibtc@mail.cibtc.com.cn, http://www.cibtc.com.cn.

H L B NEWSLETTER; reporting on heart, lung and blood disease research policy development. see *MEDICAL SCIENCES—Experimental Medicine, Laboratory Technique*

616.15 GRC ISSN 1108-2682
HAEMA. Text in English. 1998. q. free (effective 2001).
Related titles: Online - full text ed.
Published by: Haema Jornal, Epsilon, 20 Potamianou St., Athens 11528, Greece. TEL 30-1-7487587, FAX 30-1-7487588, http://www.mednet.gr/eae/haema/top.htm. Ed. John Meletis.

616.15 NLD ISSN 0017-6559 CODEN: HAEMBY
HAEMATOLOGIA; international quarterly of haematology. Text in English. 1967. q. EUR 299, USD 346 includes online ed. (effective 2002). adv. bk.rev. back issues avail. *Refereed.* **Document type:** *Journal, Academic/Scholarly.* **Description:** Publishes original papers, preliminary reports and reviews of basic and clinical research in hematology and related fields, including immunology, blood transfusion, transplantation and oncology.
Related titles: Online - full content ed.: 2000 (from EBSCO Publishing, Swets Blackwell); Online - full text ed.: (from CatchWord Ltd., Institute for Scientific Information).
Indexed: ASCA, Biol.Abstr., Chem.Abstr., Chem.Indus.Notes, Chem.Titles, Curr.Adv.Ecol.Sci., Curr.Adv.Gen.& Molec.Biol., Curr.Cont., Excerp.Med., INIS Atomind., Ind.Med. (1967-), Ind.Sci.Rev., Inpharma, Pharm.&Out.News, Protozool.Abstr., Reac., Sci.Cit.Ind. (coverage dropped), Trop.Dis.Bull.
—BLDSC (4237.800000), CASDDS, CISTI, GNLM, ingenta, KNAW.
Published by: (Magyar Tudomanyos Akademia HUN), V S P (Subsidiary of: Brill Academic Publishers), PO Box 346, Zeist 3700 AH, Netherlands. TEL 31-30-692-5790, FAX 31-30-693-2081, vsppub@compuserve.com, http://www.vsppub.com/journals/jn-Hae.html. Ed. Susan R Hollan.

616.1 ITA ISSN 0390-6078 CODEN: HAEMAX
HAEMATOLOGICA. Text and summaries in English. 1914. m. ITL 220,000 (effective 1998). adv. bk.rev. abstr, bibl, charts, illus. index. back issues avail.; reprint service avail. from ISI. *Refereed.* **Document type:** *Academic/Scholarly.*
Related titles: Online - full text ed.: (from Institute for Scientific Information).
Indexed: ASCA, Aqua.Sci.& Fish.Abstr., Biol.Abstr., Chem.Abstr., Chem.Indus.Notes, Chem.Titles, Curr.Adv.Cell & Devel.Biol., Curr.Adv.Ecol.Sci., Curr.Adv.Gen.& Molec.Biol., Curr.Cont., Environ.Sci.Poll.Mgmt., Excerp.Med., INIS Atomind., Ind.Med. (1920-), Ind.Sci.Rev., Inpharma, Int.Nurs.Ind., Pharm.&Out.News, Plant Breed.Abstr., Pollut.Abstr., Protozool.Abstr., Reac., Rev.Med.& Vet.Mycol., Risk Abstr., Saf.Sci.Abstr., Sci.Cit.Ind.
—BLDSC (4238.000000), CASDDS, CISTI, EMDOCS, GNLM, IDS, KNAW.
Published by: Ferrata Storti Foundation, Strada Nuova, 134, Pavia, PV 27100, Italy. http://www.haematologica.it/, http://www.ferratastorti.org. Ed. Edoardo Ascari. Adv. contact Luciano Defiore. Circ: 2,000.

616.15 ESP ISSN 1138-0381
HAEMATOLOGICA; journal of Hematology. Text in English, Spanish. 1997. m. **Document type:** *Academic/Scholarly.* **Description:** Publishes research into all areas of hematology.
Published by: Ediciones Doyma S.A., Traversa de Gracia, 17-21, Barcelona 08021, Spain. TEL 34-93-200-0711, FAX 34-93-209-1136, comercial@doymanet.es, http://www.doyma.es, http://www.doymanet.es/. Ed. Maite Vidal. adv.: color page ESP 259,000; trim 280 x 210. Circ: 2,000.

616.15 USA ISSN 0440-0607 CODEN: HABLAF
HAEMATOLOGIE UND BLUTTRANSFUSION. Text in English, German. 1962. irreg., latest 1995, Oct. price varies. reprint service avail. from ISI. **Document type:** *Academic/Scholarly.*
Formerly: Haematology and Blood Transfusion (0171-7111)
Related titles: Microform ed.: (from PQC); ♦ Supplement to: Annals of Hematology. ISSN 0939-5555.
Indexed: Chem.Abstr., Chem.Indus.Notes, Chem.Titles, Excerp.Med. (1996-).
—CASDDS, CISTI, GNLM, KNAW. **CCC.**
Published by: Springer-Verlag, Journals (Subsidiary of: BertelsmannSpringer), 175 Fifth Ave, New York, NY 10010. TEL 212-460-1500, FAX 212-473-6272. Eds. G Ruhenstroth Bauer, W Stich.

616.1572 GBR ISSN 1351-8216
HAEMOPHILIA. Text in English. 1994. bi-m., latest vol.8, 2002. GBP 118 in Europe to individuals; USD 189 in North America to individuals; GBP 131 elsewhere to individuals; GBP 311 in Europe to institutions; USD 497 in North America to institutions; GBP 345 elsewhere to institutions (effective 2002). adv. back issues avail. *Refereed.* **Document type:** *Academic/Scholarly.* **Description:** Provides a forum regarding the comprehensive care of hemophilia.
Related titles: ♦ Online - full text ed.: Haemophilia Online. ISSN 1365-2516; ♦ Supplement: Haemophilia. Supplement. ISSN 1355-0691.
Indexed: ASCA, Curr.Cont., Excerp.Med. (1996-), Ind.Med. (1995-), Inpharma, Pharm.&Out.News, Protozool.Abstr., Reac., Rev.Med.& Vet.Mycol.
—BLDSC (4238.086500), CISTI, GNLM, IDS, Infotrieve, KNAW. **CCC.**
Published by: (World Federation of Haemophilia), Blackwell Science Ltd., PO Box 88, Oxford OX2 0NE, United Kingdom. TEL 44-1865-206180, 44-1865-206002, FAX 44-1865-206219, jnl.orders@blacksci.co.uk, http://www.blackwell-science.com/~cgilib/jnlpage.asp?Journal=haem&File=haem, http://www.blackwellpublishing.com. Eds. Christine A Lee, Craig Kessler. Pub. Allen Stevens. R&P Sophie Savage. Adv. contact Jenny Applin. Circ: 975.

616.15 AUS
HAEMOPHILIA FOUNDATION, VICTORIA. NEWSLETTER. Text in English. 1955. q. AUD 20 (effective 2000). bk.rev. back issues avail. **Document type:** *Newsletter.* **Description:** Information for people with haemophilia and related bleeding disorders on their families and careers.
Formerly: Haemophilia Society of Victoria. Newsletter
Published by: Haemophilia Foundation Victoria, Ste. 5, Ground Fl., 860 Nepean Hwy, Moorabbin, VIC 3189, Australia. TEL 61-3-95557595, FAX 61-3-95557375, hfvic@vicnet.net.au, http://www.vicnet.net.au/~haemvic. Ed., R&P Natalie Lonsdale. Circ: 480.

616.1572 GBR ISSN 1365-2516
HAEMOPHILIA ONLINE. Text in English. 1998. bi-m. GBP 107 in Europe to individuals; USD 171 in North America to individuals; GBP 107 elsewhere to individuals; GBP 280 in Europe to institutions; USD 448 in North America to institutions; GBP 280 elsewhere to institutions (effective 2002). *Refereed.* **Document type:** *Academic/Scholarly.*

Media: Online - full text (from EBSCO Publishing, O C L C Online Computer Library Center, Inc., RoweCom Information Quest, ingenta, Munksgaard & Blackwell Science's Synergy, Swets Blackwell, Institute for Scientific Information). **Related titles:** ♦ Print ed.: Haemophilia. ISSN 1351-8216.
Published by: Blackwell Science Ltd., Osney Mead, Oxford OX2 0EL, United Kingdom. TEL 44-1685-206206, FAX 44-1685-721205, website@blacksci.com, journals.cs@blacksci.co.uk, http://www.blackwell-science.com/~cgilib/jnlpage.bin?Journal=haem&File=haem&Page=aims.

615.1572 GBR ISSN 1355-0691
HAEMOPHILIA. SUPPLEMENT. Text in English. 1994. irreg. adv. back issues avail. **Document type:** *Academic/Scholarly.*
Related titles: Online - full text ed.: (from RoweCom Information Quest); ♦ Supplement to: Haemophilia. ISSN 1351-8216.
—EMDOCS, KNAW.
Published by: (World Federation of Haemophilia), Blackwell Science Ltd., Osney Mead, Oxford OX2 0EL, United Kingdom. TEL 44-1865-206206, FAX 44-1865-721205, journals.cs@blacksci.co.uk, http://www.blackwell-science.com. Pub. Allen Stevens. R&P Sophie Savage. Adv. contact Jenny Applin.

616.15 DEU ISSN 0720-9355
CODEN: HAEMD2
HAEMOSTASEOLOGIE; Diagnostik, Therapie und Grundlagenforschung von Haemorrhagien und Thromboembolien. Text in German. 1981. q. DEM 210 to individuals; DEM 260 to institutions; DEM 100 to students (effective 2001). adv. *Refereed.* **Document type:** *Journal, Academic/Scholarly.*
Indexed: Chem.Abstr., Chem.Indus.Notes, Chem.Titles, Excerp.Med.
—CASDDS, CISTI, EMDOCS, GNLM, Infotrieve, KNAW. **CCC.**
Published by: Schattauer GmbH, Hoelderlinstr 3, Stuttgart 70174, Germany. TEL 49-711-22987-0, FAX 49-711-2298750, info@schattauer.de, http://www.schattauer.com. Pub. Dieter Bergemann. R&P Annika Schmidt TEL 49-711-2298713. Adv. contact Hans-Georg Schwarz. B&W page XEU 1,685.22, color page XEU 2,650.03; 183 x 227. Circ: 3,800. **Subscr. to:** CSJ, Postfach 140220, Munich 80452, Germany. TEL 49-89-20959129, schattauer@csj.de.

616.15 USA ISSN 1088-7008
HEM AWARE. Text in English. 1996. bi-m. free per issue to members. adv. illus. **Document type:** *Consumer.* **Description:** Offers treatment news about bleeding disorders, highlights new programs and new resources in the field of hemophiliac research.
Published by: National Hemophilia Foundation, 116 W 32nd St, 11th Fl, New York, NY 10001. TEL 212-328-3700, 800-42-HANDI, FAX 212-328-3799, info@hemophilia.org, http://www.hemophilia.org. Ed. Blake Zeff. Pub., R&P Jodie Landes Corngold. Adv. contact Jacqueline Cortez.

616.15 616.07 ESP ISSN 1138-6029
HEMATOLOGIA, CITOQUINAS, INMUNOTERAPIA Y TERAPIA CELULAR. Text in Spanish; Abstracts in Spanish, English. bi-m. ESP 10,000; USD 350 foreign (effective 2000). adv. abstr, bibl, illus, stat. back issues avail. *Refereed.* **Document type:** *Academic/Scholarly.*
Related titles: CD-ROM ed.
Published by: Aran Ediciones S.A., Castello, 128 1o, Madrid 28006, Spain. TEL 34-91-782-0030, FAX 34-91-561-5787, edita@grupoaran.com, http://www.grupoaran.com. Ed. J. Garcia Conde. Pub. Jose Jimenez. R&P Maria Dolores Linares TEL 34-1-7820035. Circ: 3,000.

616.15 GBR ISSN 0278-0232
CODEN: HAONDL
HEMATOLOGICAL ONCOLOGY. Text in English. 1983. q. USD 915 in United States; USD 915 in Canada & Mexico; USD 915 elsewhere; USD 961 combined subscription in United States for print and online eds.; USD 961 combined subscription in Canada & Mexico for print and online eds.; USD 961 combined subscription elsewhere for print and online eds. (effective 2002). adv. bk.rev. charts, illus. index. back issues avail.; reprint service avail. from SWZ,PQC. *Refereed.* **Document type:** *Academic/Scholarly.* **Description:** Presents a variety of clinical and scientific specialties concerned with neoplastic disease of the hemopoietic system, and any neoplastic or related process that may directly or indirectly involve the hemopoietic system.
Related titles: Microform ed.: (from PQC); Online - full text ed.: ISSN 1099-1069. USD 915 in United States; USD 915 in Canada & Mexico; USD 915 elsewhere (effective 2002) (from EBSCO Publishing, Wiley InterScience, Institute for Scientific Information).
Indexed: ASCA, Cal.Tiss.Abstr., Chem.Abstr., Curr.Adv.Ecol.Sci., Curr.Adv.Gen.& Molec.Biol., Curr.Cont., Excerp.Med., INIS Atomind., Ind.Med. (1983-), Inpharma, Int.Abstr.Biol.Sci., Pharm.&Out.News, Reac., SSCI (coverage dropped), Sci.Cit.Ind., Telegen.
—BLDSC (4291.550000), CASDDS, CISTI, EMDOCS, GNLM, IDS, ingenta, KNAW. **CCC.**
Published by: Wiley Europe Ltd., Baffins Ln, Chichester, W Sussex PO19 1UD, United Kingdom. TEL 44-1243-779777, FAX 44-1243-775878, customer@wiley.co.uk, http://www.wiley.co.uk. adv.: B&W page GBP 650, color page GBP 1,550; trim 200 x 260. Circ: 400. **Subscr. to:** John Wiley & Sons, Inc., Journals, 605 Third Ave, New York, NY 10158. TEL 201-850-6021, 212-850-6645, subinfo@jwiley.com.

616.1 FRA ISSN 1264-7527
HEMATOLOGIE. Text in French. 1995. bi-m. FRF 670 domestic to individuals; EUR 114 in Europe to individuals; FRF 790 elsewhere to individuals; FRF 1,120 domestic to institutions; EUR 183 in Europe to institutions; FRF 1,240 elsewhere to institutions; FRF 190 newsstand/cover (effective 2001). *Refereed.* **Document type:** *Academic/Scholarly.*
Related titles: CD-ROM ed.: FRF 590 domestic; FRF 620 foreign (effective 2001); Online - full text ed.: FRF 670 to individuals; FRF 1,120 to institutions (effective 2001).
Indexed: Excerp.Med. (1996-), Inpharma, Reac.
—BLDSC (4291.552000), KNAW.
Published by: John Libbey Eurotext, 127 av. de la Republique, Montrouge 92120, France. TEL 33-01-46730660, FAX 33-01-40840999, marketing@jle.com, http://www.john-libbey-eurotext.fr/. Ed. Francois Sigaux. **Subscr. to:** A T E I, 3 av. Pierre Kerautret, Romainville 92230, France. TEL 33-1-48408686, FAX 33-1-48400731, atei@club-internet.fr.

616.15 GBR ISSN 1024-5332
CODEN: HMATFL
HEMATOLOGY. Text in French. 1985. 6/yr. GBP 72, USD 87, EUR 96 to individuals; GBP 295, USD 382, EUR 392 to institutions; GBP 481, USD 625, EUR 641 to corporations (effective 2002). *Refereed.* **Document type:** *Journal, Academic/Scholarly.*
Supersedes (with vol.9): Hematology Reviews and Communications (0882-8083)
Related titles: CD-ROM ed.; Microform ed.; Online - full text ed.: ISSN 1607-8454 (from RoweCom Information Quest).
Indexed: ASCA, Environ.Sci.Poll.Mgmt., Excerp.Med., Pollut.Abstr., Risk Abstr., Saf.Sci.Abstr.
—BLDSC (4291.565000), CISTI, EMDOCS, GNLM, Infotrieve, KNAW. **CCC.**
Published by: The Gordon & Breach Publishing Group, Harwood Academic Publishers, Ste K101 Tower Bridge Business Complex, 100 Clements Rd, London SE16 4DG, United Kingdom. TEL 44-20-7740-1382, FAX 44-20-7252-3510, http://www.gbhap.com/Hematology/. Ed. A C Newland. **Subscr. addr. in US:** International Publishers Direct, PO Box 32160, Newark, NJ 07102. FAX 215-750-6343.

616.15 FRA ISSN 1269-3286
RC633.A1 CODEN: HCTHFA
HEMATOLOGY AND CELL THERAPY. Text in English; Summaries in English, French. 1958. bi-m. FRF 2,400 (effective 2000). adv. bk.rev. illus. index. reprint service avail. from ISI. *Refereed.* **Document type:** *Academic/Scholarly.* **Description:** Provides editorials, original articles, and congress reports on the clinical, genetic, and experimental aspects of hematology. For physiologists, pathologists, oncologists, and physicians.
Formerly (until 1997): Nouvelle Revue Francaise d'Hematologie - Journal of Experimental and Clinical Hematology (0029-4810)
Related titles: Microform ed.: (from PQC); Online - full text ed.: ISSN 1279-8509 (from EBSCO Publishing, RoweCom Information Quest, Swets Blackwell, Springer LINK).
Indexed: ASCA, Biol.Abstr., Chem.Abstr., Chem.Indus.Notes, Chem.Titles, Curr.Adv.Cancer Res., Curr.Adv.Ecol.Sci., Curr.Cont. (coverage dropped), Dent.Ind., Excerp.Med., INIS Atomind., Ind.Med. (1996-), Ind.Sci.Rev., Inpharma, Nutr.Abstr., Pharm.&Out.News, Reac., Ref.Zh., Rev.Med.& Vet.Mycol., Sci.Cit.Ind.
—BLDSC (4291.593000), CASDDS, CISTI, GNLM, IDS. **CCC.**
Published by: (French Society of Bone Marrow Transplantation), Springer-Verlag France (Subsidiary of: BertelsmannSpringer), 1 rue Paul Cezanne, Paris 75008, France. TEL 33-1-53933644, FAX 33-1-53933683, access@link.springer.de; york@springer-paris.fr, http://link.springer.de/link/service/journals/00590/index.htm. adv.: B&W page FRF 5,200, color page FRF 11,500; trim 210 x 275. **Subscr. in N. America to:** Springer-Verlag New York Inc., PO Box 2485, Secaucus, NJ 07096-2485. TEL 201-348-4403, FAX 212-473-6272.

616.15 USA
HEMATOLOGY SERIES. Text in English. irreg., latest vol.16, 1993. adv. *Refereed.* **Document type:** *Monographic series.*
Published by: Marcel Dekker, Inc., Attn: Eridania Perrez, 270 Madison Ave, New York, NY 10016-0602. TEL 212-696-9000, 800-228-1160, FAX 212-658-4540, marketing@dekker.com, http://www.dekker.com. Ed. Kenneth M Brinkhous. R&P Julia Mulligan. Adv. contact Eridania Perez.

616.15 USA ISSN 0363-0269
RC641.7.H35 CODEN: HEMOD8
HEMOGLOBIN; international journal for hemoglobin research. Text in English. 1977. q. USD 115 to individuals for print and online eds.; USD 1,095 to institutions print only (effective 2002). adv. *Refereed.* **Document type:** *Academic/Scholarly.* **Description:** Emphasizes several topic areas concerning normal, modified, and abnormal human hemoglobins.
Related titles: Microform ed.: (from RPI); Online - full text ed.: (from Institute for Scientific Information, RoweCom Information Quest).
Indexed: ASCA, BBCI, Chem.Abstr., Chem.Indus.Notes, Chem.Titles, Curr.Adv.Ecol.Sci., Curr.Cont., Excerp.Med., Ind.Med. (1976-), Ind.Sci.Rev., Inpharma, Int.Abstr.Biol.Sci., Pharm.&Out.News, Reac., Ref.Zh., SSCI (coverage dropped), Sci.Cit.Ind., THA.
—BLDSC (4295.040000), CASDDS, CISTI, EMDOCS, GNLM, IDS, ingenta, KNAW. **CCC.**
Published by: Marcel Dekker Inc., 270 Madison Ave, New York, NY 10016. TEL 212-696-9000, 800-228-1160, FAX 212-685-4540, http://www.dekker.com/servlet/product/productid/HEM. Ed. Henri Wajcman. R&P Julia Mulligan. Adv. contact Anne Mullins. B&W page USD 800. Circ: 325.

616.15 CAN ISSN 0046-7251
HEMOPHILIA TODAY* . Text in English. 1964. q. free per issue.
Related titles: French ed.: 1964.
Published by: Canadian Hemophilia Society, 625 President Kennedy, Ste 1210, Montreal, PQ H3A 1K2, Canada. TEL 514-848-0503, FAX 514-848-9661. Ed. Barry Issac. Circ: 6,000.

▼ **I E H REPORT ON U K BLOOD LEAD SURVEYS.** see *ENVIRONMENTAL STUDIES—Toxicology And Environmental Safety*

616.15 BRA ISSN 0103-3263
CODEN: RIECF4
INSTITUTO ESTADUAL DE HEMATOLOGIA ARTHUR DE SIQUEIRA CAVALCANTI. REVISTA. Text in Portuguese; Summaries in English. 1971. s-a. per issue exchange basis. bk.rev. bibl, charts. reprint service avail. from IRC.
Formerly (until vol.4, no.2, 1976): Instituto Estadual de Hematologia Arthur de Siqueira Cavalcanti. Boletim (0046-9963)
Indexed: Excerp.Med., INIS Atomind.
Published by: Instituto Estadual de Hematologia Arthur de Siqueira Cavalcanti, Biblioteca, Rua Frei Caneca, 08, Rio de Janiero, RJ 20211, Brazil. TEL 021-242-6080, FAX 021-252-3739. Ed. Jose Moreira Pereira. Circ: 1,000.

INTERNATIONAL ANGIOLOGY. see *MEDICAL SCIENCES—Cardiovascular Diseases*

612.1 USA ISSN 0074-3682
INTERNATIONAL CONGRESS OF HEMATOLOGY. PROCEEDINGS. (Proceedings Published in host country) Text in English. 1958. biennial, latest 1992, 24th, London. **Document type:** *Newsletter, Proceedings.*
Published by: International Society of Hematology, c/o Dr. Guillermo Ruiz-Arguelles, Blvd. Dizz Ordaz 808, Puebla 71530, Mexico. Circ: 2,000 (controlled).

M

616.15 JPN ISSN 0925-5710
CODEN: IJHEEY
INTERNATIONAL JOURNAL OF HEMATOLOGY. Text in English. 1938. 10/yr. (8/yr before 2002). JPY 150 to individuals print & online eds.; JPY 225 to institutions print & online eds. (effective 2002). adv. bk.rev. *Refereed.* **Document type:** *Journal, Academic/Scholarly.* **Description:** Publishes original papers and reviews of international origin in basic and clinical hematology.
Formerly (until 1991): Acta Haematologica Japonica (0001-5806)
Related titles: Microform ed.: (from PQC); Online - full text ed.: 2001. USD 80 to individuals; USD 175 to institutions (effective 2002) (from ingenta, Institute for Scientific Information).
Indexed: ASCA, Aqua.Sci.& Fish.Abstr., Biol.Abstr., Chem.Abstr., Chem.Indus.Notes, Chem.Titles, Curr.Adv.Biochem., Curr.Adv.Cancer Res., Curr.Adv.Cell & Devel.Biol., Curr.Adv.Ecol.Sci., Curr.Cont., Dent.Ind., Environ.Sci.Poll.Mgmt., Excerp.Med., INIS Atomind., Ind.Med. (1991-), Inpharma, Int.Abstr.Biol.Sci., Nutr.Abstr., Pharm.&Out.News, Reac., SSCI (coverage dropped), Sport Fish.Abstr.
—BLDSC (4542.280400), CASDDS, CISTI, EMDOCS, GNLM, IDS, Infotrieve, KNAW. **CCC.**
Published by: Japanese Society of Hematology, Kinki Chihou Hatsumei Center, 14 Kawaramachi Yoshida, Sakyo-ku, Kyoto 606-8305, Japan. TEL 81-75-751-8982, FAX 81-75-752-0761, ijh-ind@umin.ac.jp. Eds. E Yoshida, Yataro Yoshida. Circ: 5,000. **Dist. in the US by:** Carden Jennings Publishing, 1224 W Main St, Ste 200, Charlottesville, VA 22903-2858. TEL 804-817-2000, FAX 804-817-2020, ijh@cjp.com, http://www.cjp.com/.

INTERNATIONAL JOURNAL OF PEDIATRIC HEMATOLOGY - ONCOLOGY. see *MEDICAL SCIENCES—Oncology*

616.5 612.1 FRA ISSN 0074-8528
INTERNATIONAL SOCIETY OF BLOOD TRANSFUSION. PROCEEDINGS OF THE CONGRESS. Text in Multiple languages. biennial, latest 1992, 22nd, Sao Paolo. **Document type:** *Proceedings.*
Indexed: Biol.Abstr.
Published by: Societe Internationale de Transfusion Sanguine/International Society of Blood Transfusion, c/o C N T S, B.P. 100, Les Ulis Cedex 91943, France. TEL 69-07-20-40, FAX 69-07-41-85, TELEX 603218. Circ: (controlled).

IRON METABOLISM. see *BIOLOGY—Abstracting, Bibliographies, Statistics*

IRONIC BLOOD; information on iron overload. see *MEDICAL SCIENCES—Endocrinology*

616.15 CAN ISSN 0715-8602
JOURNAL: NEWS OF THE BLOOD PROGRAMME IN CANADA. Text in English, French. 1983. q. free per issue.
Published by: Canadian Red Cross Society, National Headquarters, 5700 Cancross Court, Mississauga, ON L5R 3E9, Canada. TEL 416-890-1000. Circ: 4,000.

616.15 USA ISSN 0733-2459
CODEN: JCAPES
JOURNAL OF CLINICAL APHERESIS. Text in English. 1982. q. USD 715 in United States; USD 755 in Canada & Mexico; USD 789 elsewhere; USD 751 combined subscription in United States for print and online eds.; USD 791 combined subscription in Canada & Mexico for print and online eds.; USD 825 combined subscription elsewhere for print and online eds. (effective 2002). adv. back issues avail. *Refereed.* **Document type:** *Journal, Academic/Scholarly.* **Description:** Examines research articles on all topics relating to apheresis: plasmapheresis, lymphoplasmapheresis, and ctyapheresis, including experimental and technical developments.
Related titles: Microform ed.: (from PQC); Online - full text ed.: ISSN 1098-1101. 1996. USD 715 in United States; USD 715 in Canada & Mexico; USD 715 elsewhere (effective 2002) (from EBSCO Publishing, Wiley InterScience, Institute for Scientific Information).
Indexed: ASCA, Curr.Cont., Excerp.Med., Ind.Med. (1982-), Ind.Sci.Rev., Inpharma, Int.Nurs.Ind., Pharm.&Out.News, Reac., Sci.Cit.Ind.
—BLDSC (4958.381500), CISTI, EMDOCS, GNLM, IDS, ingenta, KNAW. **CCC.**
Published by: (American Society for Apheresis), John Wiley & Sons, Inc., Journals (Subsidiary of: Wiley InterScience), 605 Third Ave, New York, NY 10158. TEL 212-850-6645, FAX 212-850-6021, subinfo@wiley.com, uscs-wis@wiley.com, http://www.interscience.wiley.com/jpages/0733-2459/, http://www.wiley.com. Ed. Alvaro A Pineda. adv.: B&W page GBP 640, color page GBP 1,515; trim 210 x 279. Circ: 1,300. **Subscr. outside the Americas to:** John Wiley & Sons Ltd., Baffins Ln, Chichester, Sussex PO19 IUD, United Kingdom. TEL 44-1243-779777, FAX 44-1243-843232, cs-journals@wiley.co.uk, http://www.wiley.co.uk.

616.15 USA ISSN 1525-8165
CODEN: JOEMEL
JOURNAL OF HEMATOTHERAPY & STEM CELL RESEARCH. Text in English. 1993. bi-m. USD 119 domestic to individuals; USD 209 foreign to individuals; USD 143 domestic to individuals print and online eds. combined; USD 233 foreign to individuals print and online eds. combined; USD 320 domestic to institutions; USD 438 foreign to institutions; USD 384 domestic to institutions print and online eds. combined; USD 502 foreign to institutions print and online eds. combined (effective 2002). back issues avail.; reprints avail. *Refereed.* **Document type:** *Journal, Academic/Scholarly.* **Description:** Focuses on a specific area of clinical research that ranges over several disciplines; that of ex vivo manipulation of hematopoietic cells for in vivo therapy.
Formerly (until 2000): Journal of Hematotherapy (1061-6128)
Related titles: Online - full text ed.: USD 119 to individuals; USD 320 to institutions (effective 2002) (from CatchWord Ltd., EBSCO Publishing, O C L C Online Computer Library Center, Inc., RoweCom Information Quest, Swets Blackwell, Institute for Scientific Information).
Indexed: Curr.Cont., Derwent Biotech.Abstr., Excerp.Med. (1993-), Ind.Med. (1999-), Inpharma, Int.Abstr.Biol.Sci., Reac., Sci.Cit.Ind.
—BLDSC (4997.605000), CASDDS, CatchWord, EMDOCS, GNLM, IDS, Infotrieve, KNAW. **CCC.**
Published by: Mary Ann Liebert, Inc. Publishers, 2 Madison Ave, Larchmont, NY 10538. TEL 914—834-3100, FAX 914-834-1388, info@liebertpub.com, http://www.liebertpub.com/jht. Ed. Denis English.

JOURNAL OF PEDIATRIC HEMATOLOGY - ONCOLOGY. see *MEDICAL SCIENCES—Oncology*

616 JPN
KENKETSU JIGYO NO GENKYO/BLOOD DONATION IN NARA PREFECTURE. Text in Japanese. a.
Published by: Naraken Hoken Kankyobu/Nara Prefectural Government, Public Health and Environment Affairs Department, Noborioji-cho, Nara-shi 630-8213, Japan.

616.15 JPN ISSN 0913-9532
KESSEI HANNO NO AYUMI/STUDY REPORT OF SERUM REACTION. Text in Japanese. 1972. irreg. **Document type:** *Academic/Scholarly.*
Published by: Nihon Toketsu Kanso Kenkyujo/Japan Lyophilization Laboratory, 2-6 Kohinata 4-chome, Bunkyo-ku, Tokyo 112-0006, Japan. TEL 03-5800-5310, FAX 03-5800-5352, TELEX 2322357 BCGLAB J. Ed. Kuniyoshi Kikuchi.

616.15 JPN ISSN 1344-6940
KETSUEKI FRONTIER/PRACTICAL HEMATOLOGY. Text in Japanese. 1991. m. JPY 27,720 (effective 2000). adv. **Document type:** *Academic/Scholarly.*
Formerly: Nichijo Shinryo to Ketsueki (0917-5776)
—BLDSC (4291.602000).
Published by: Iyaku Journal-sha/Medicine & Drug Journal Co., Ltd., 2-8 Hirano-Machi 3-chome, Chuo-ku, Osaka-shi 541-0046, Japan. TEL 81-6-6202-7280, FAX 81-6-6202-5295, iyakujor@skyblue.ocn.ne.jp, http://www.so-net.ne.jp/medipro/iyaku. R&P, Adv. contact Kiriko Numata.

616.15 JPN
KETSUEKI JIGYO/BLOOD PROGRAMME. Text in Japanese. q. JPY 1,000 per issue.
Published by: Nihon Ketsueki Jigyo Gakkai/Society for Japanese Blood Programme, Nihon Sekijujisha Ketsueki Jigyobu, 1-3 Shiba-Daimon 1-chome, Minato-ku, Tokyo 105-0000, Japan.

616.15 JPN
KETSUEKIGAKU SEMINA/SEMINAR IN HEMATOLOGY. Text in Japanese. 1983. a. membership.
Indexed: Chem.Abstr., Chem.Titles.
Published by: Osaka Shiritsu Daigaku, Byoin Ketsueki Kenkyukai, Shiritsu Daigaku Igakubu Fuzoku Byoin, 4-54 Asahi-Machi 1-chome, Abeno-ku, Osaka-shi 545-0051, Japan.

616.15 BGR ISSN 0861-7880
KLINICHNA I TRANSFUZIONNA HEMATOLOGIIA. Text in Bulgarian; Summaries in Bulgarian, English. 1965. q., latest vol.36, 2000. BGL 10 domestic (effective 2001); USD 64 foreign (effective 2002). adv. bk.rev. abstr, bibl. index. 48 p./no. back issues avail. *Refereed.* **Document type:** *Journal, Academic/Scholarly, Abstract/Index, Bibliography.* **Description:** Presents original articles of Bulgarian medical researchers and practitioners and abstracts of foreign publications in the field of hematology and blood transfusion.
Indexed: Abstr.Bulg.Sci.Med.Lit.
Published by: Meditsinski Universitet - Sofia, Tsentur za Informatsiia po Meditsina/Medical University - Sofia, Medical Information Center, 1 Sv Georgi Sofiiski ul, Sofia 1431, Bulgaria. TEL 359-2-9522342, FAX 359-2-9522393, mutafov@sun.medun.acad.bg, http://www.medun.acad.bg. Ed. Dr. Georgi Balacenko. R&P, Adv. contact Dr. Christo Mutafov. B&W page USD 50, color page USD 200; 12 x 18. Circ: 250. **Dist. by:** Sofia Books, Ul Silivria 16, Sofia 1404, Bulgaria. TEL 359-2-9586257, sofiabooks@hotmail.com, http://www.sofiabooks.hit.bg.

616.15 USA ISSN 1080-2924
LABORATORY HEMATOLOGY. Text in English. 1995. q. USD 125; USD 155 foreign. **Description:** Publishes high-quality reports of original research, reviews, editorials and letters to the editor in all fields of laboratory hematology.
—BLDSC (5139.880000), CISTI, GNLM, Infotrieve. **CCC.**
Published by: (International Society for Laboratory Hematology), Kluge Carden Jennings Publishing Co. Ltd., Blake Center, Ste 200, 1224 W Main St, Charlottesville, VA 22903. TEL 804-979-9413, FAX 804-295-0612, wendy_passerell@kcj.ccmail.compuserve). Ed. Dr. Kenneth A Ault.

LEUCOCYTES. see *MEDICAL SCIENCES—Abstracting, Bibliographies, Statistics*

616.15 GBR ISSN 0887-6924
CODEN: LEUKED
LEUKEMIA; normal and malignant hemopoiesis. Text in English. 1987. m. GBP 260, USD 408 worldwide to individuals; GBP 695 in Europe to institutions; GBP 715, USD 1,123 elsewhere to institutions; GBP 286, USD 449 worldwide to individuals Print & Online eds.; GBP 765 in Europe to institutions Print & Online eds.; GBP 787, USD 1,235 elsewhere to institutions Print & Online eds. (effective 2000). adv. inde. back issues avail. *Refereed.* **Document type:** *Academic/Scholarly.* **Description:** Articles on leukemia, germane diseases and normal hemopoiesis by specialists.
Related titles: Online - full text ed.: (from EBSCO Publishing, O C L C Online Computer Library Center, Inc., RoweCom Information Quest, ingenta, Swets Blackwell, Institute for Scientific Information).
Indexed: ASCA, Aqua.Sci.& Fish.Abstr., Curr.Adv.Cell & Devel.Biol., Curr.Adv.Gen.& Molec.Biol., Curr.Cont., Excerp.Med., Genet.Abstr., Hum.Gen.Abstr., INIS Atomind., Immun.Abstr., Ind.Med. (1987-), Inpharma, Int.Abstr.Biol.Sci., Nuc.Acids Abstr., Oncog.G.F.Abstr., Reac., Rev.Med.& Vet.Mycol., Sci.Cit.Ind., Telegen.
—BLDSC (5185.249000), CASDDS, CISTI, EMDOCS, GNLM, IDS, ingenta, KNAW. **CCC.**
Published by: (Sven-Adge Killmann Leukemia Foundation), Nature Publishing Group Specialist Journals (Subsidiary of: Holtzbrink Publishers), Houndmills, Basingstoke, Hants RG21 6XS, United Kingdom. TEL 44-1256-329242, FAX 44-1256-328339, k.hinton@stockton-press.co.uk, subscriptions@nature.com, http://www.stockton-press.co.uk/leu/, http://www.nature.com. Ed. Nicole Muller Berat Killman. Pub. Harry Holt. R&P Pat Blower. Adv. contact Robert Sloan TEL 44-20-8882-7199. B&W page GBP 595, color page GBP 1,150; trim 210 x 280.
Co-sponsor: Leukemia Research Fund.

616.15 CHE ISSN 1042-8194
CODEN: LELYEA
LEUKEMIA AND LYMPHOMA. Text in English. 12/yr. (in 4 vols., 6 nos./vol.). GBP 368, USD 540, EUR 492 to individuals; GBP 1,848, USD 2,420, EUR 2,460 to institutions; GBP 3,091, USD 3,965, EUR 4,116 to corporations (effective 2002). *Refereed.* **Document type:** *Journal, Academic/Scholarly.* **Description:** Offers clinical-pathologic correlation and brings together clinical and laboratory data on lymphomas, leukemias, and allied disorders, including myeloma and myelodysplastic syndromes.

M

Related titles: CD-ROM ed.; Microform ed.; Online - full text ed.: (from EBSCO Publishing, Institute for Scientific Information, RoweCom Information Quest).
Indexed: AIDS & Cancer Res., AIDS Abstr., ASCA, Curr.Cont., Excerp.Med., Immun.Abstr., Ind.Med. (1989-), Inpharma, Int.Abstr.Biol.Sci., Oncog.G.F.Abstr., Protozool.Abstr., Reac.
—BLDSC (5185.251500), EMDOCS, GNLM, ingenta, KNAW. **CCC.**
Published by: Gordon and Breach - Harwood Academic (Subsidiary of: Taylor & Francis Group), PO Box 531, Lausanne 1000, Switzerland. TEL 41-21-6411280, FAX 41-21-6411281, info@gbhap.com, http://www.gbhap.com/Leukemia_Lymphoma/. Ed. Aaron Polliak. **Subscr. addr. in US:** International Publishers Direct, PO Box 32160, Newark, NJ 07102. FAX 215-750-6343.

616 GBR ISSN 0145-2126
CODEN: LEREDD
LEUKEMIA RESEARCH. Text in English. 1977. m. EUR 249 in Europe to individuals; JPY 33,000 in Japan to individuals; USD 278 elsewhere to individuals; EUR 1,761 in Europe to institutions; JPY 233,800 in Japan to institutions; USD 1,969 elsewhere to institutions (effective 2002). adv. bk.rev. abstr, bibl, charts, illus. index. back issues avail. *Refereed.* **Document type:** *Academic/Scholarly.* **Description:** Integrates basic research in leukemia with recent reports of clinical applications.
Related titles: Microfilm ed.: (from PQC); Online - full text ed.: (from ingenta, ScienceDirect, Swets Blackwell, Institute for Scientific Information).
Indexed: AIDS & Cancer Res., ASCA, Abstr.Hyg., Biol.Abstr., Chem.Abstr., Chem.Indus.Notes, Chem.Titles, Curr.Adv.Ecol.Sci., Curr.Cont., Excerp.Med., INIS Atomind., Immun.Abstr., Ind.Med. (1977-), Ind.Sci.Rev., Inpharma, Oncog.G.F.Abstr., Pharm.&Out.News, Reac., Ref.Zh., Rev.Med.& Vet.Mycol., Risk Abstr., Sci.Cit.Ind., Telegen, Trop.Dis.Bull., Vet.Bull.
—BLDSC (5185.270000), CASDDS, CISTI, GNLM, IDS, ingenta, KNAW. **CCC.**
Published by: Pergamon (Subsidiary of: Elsevier Science), The Boulevard, Langford Ln, East Park, Kidlington, Oxford OXB 1GB, United Kingdom. FAX 44-1865-843010, http://www.elsevier.nl/locate/leukres. Eds. Peter Reizenstein, Terry Hamblin. Circ: 1,100. **Subscr. in Australasia and the Far East to:** Elsevier Science (Singapore) Pte Ltd, No.1 Temasek Ave, 17-01 Millenia Tower, Singapore 039192, Singapore. TEL 65-434-3727, FAX 65-337-2230; **Subscr. in the Americas to:** Elsevier Science, PO Box 945, New York, NY 10159-0945. TEL 212-633-3730, FAX 212-633-3680, usinfo-f@elsevier.com; **Subscr. to:** Elsevier Science BV, PO Box 211, Amsterdam 1000 AE, Netherlands. TEL 31-20-485-3757.

616.15 USA ISSN 0740-9451
QP106.6 CODEN: MELYEL
MICROCIRCULATION, ENDOTHELIUM AND LYMPHATICS✱ . Text in English. 1984. bi-m. USD 230; USD 288 foreign. adv. abstr, illus. index. back issues avail. *Refereed.* **Document type:** *Academic/Scholarly.*
Related titles: Microform ed.: 1984 (from PQC).
Indexed: Chem.Abstr., Chem.Titles, Curr.Cont. (coverage dropped), INIS Atomind.
—CASDDS, CISTI, GNLM. **CCC.**
Published by: B M A Publications, 31 Willows Rd, PO Box 562, Ayer, MA 01432-0562. TEL 212-270-2194.

NOU TO JONKAN/BRAIN AND CIRCULATION. see *MEDICAL SCIENCES—Psychiatry And Neurology*

THE ONCOLOGIST. see *MEDICAL SCIENCES—Oncology*

615.15 GBR ISSN 1362-6795
OPINION: SPECIALIST REVIEWS OF KEY PAPERS IN HAEMATOLOGY. Abbreviated title: Opinion: Haematology. Text in English. 1996. 3/yr. bk.rev. **Document type:** *Academic/Scholarly.*
Published by: Hayward Medical Communications Ltd., Covent Garden, Seven Dials Warehouse, 44 Earlham St, London WC2H 9LA, United Kingdom. TEL 44-20-7240-4493, FAX 44-20-7240-4479, admin@hayward.co.uk, http://www.hayward.co.uk. Ed. Dr. J Wainscoat. Circ: 2,000. **Subscr. to:** Rosemary House, Lanwades Park, Kentford, Near, Newmarket, Suffolk CB8 7PW, United Kingdom. TEL 44-1638-751515, FAX 44-1638-751517.

616.15 CHE ISSN 1424-8832
CODEN: HMTSB7
PATHOPHYSIOLOGY OF HAEMOSTASIS AND THROMBOSIS; international journal on haemostasis and thrombosis research. Text in English. 1968. bi-m. CHF 914, EUR 652.80 in Europe to institutions; CHF 931.40, USD 711 elsewhere to institutions (effective 2002). adv. bk.rev. back issues avail. *Refereed.* **Document type:** *Journal, Academic/Scholarly.* **Description:** Reports the latest findings on the pathology, physiology and biochemistry of hemorrhagic disease and thrombosis. In addition to in-depth studies of such topics as blood coagulation factors and fibrinolysis.
Former titles: Haemostasis (0301-0147); (until 1972): Coagulation (0009-9902)
Related titles: Microform ed.; Online - full text ed.: ISSN 1424-8840. CHF 58, EUR 42, USD 45 with print edition (effective 2002) (from EBSCO Publishing, O C L C Online Computer Library Center, Inc., RoweCom Information Quest, Swets Blackwell, Institute for Scientific Information).
Indexed: ASCA, Biol.Abstr., Chem.Abstr., Chem.Indus.Notes, Chem.Titles, Curr.Adv.Biochem., Curr.Adv.Cancer Res., Curr.Adv.Cell & Devel.Biol., Curr.Adv.Ecol.Sci., Curr.Cont., Excerp.Med., Helminthol.Abstr., Ind.Med. (1972-), Ind.Sci.Rev., Inpharma, Kidney, Pharm.&Out.News, Reac., Sci.Cit.Ind.
—BLDSC (4238.090000), CASDDS, CISTI, EMDOCS, GNLM, IDS, ingenta, KNAW. **CCC.**
Published by: S. Karger AG, Allschwilerstr 10, PO Box, Basel 4009, Switzerland. TEL 41-61-306-1111, FAX 41-61-306-1234, karger@karger.ch, http://www.karger.com/journals/hae/hae_jh.htm. Ed. H C Hemker. adv.: page USD 1,185. Circ: 1,150.

PEDIATRIC HEMATOLOGY & ONCOLOGY. see *MEDICAL SCIENCES—Pediatrics*

PEDIATRIC HEMATOLOGY - ONCOLOGY SERIES. see *MEDICAL SCIENCES—Oncology*

PERFUSION; Kreislauferkrankungen in Klinik und Praxis. see *MEDICAL SCIENCES—Cardiovascular Diseases*

615.15 ITA
POLICLINICO DI MILANO. NOTIZIE BREVI. Text in Italian. 1982. bi-m. free per issue. bibl, illus, stat. back issues avail. **Document type:** *Newsletter, Bibliography.* **Description:** Provides information on their transfusion service's activities, transplantation data in the Nord Italia Transplant Organization, and general medical information for blood donors.
Related titles: Fax ed.
Published by: Ospedale Maggiore Policlinico, Centro Transf., Via Francesco Sforza, 35, Milan, MI 20122, Italy. TEL 39-02-59901338, FAX 39-02-5458129, ctit@polic.cilea.it. Ed. Dr. Girolamo Sirchia. R&P Giusi Baldocchi TEL 39-02-55034002. Circ: 30,000.

PROGRESS IN CARDIOVASCULAR DISEASES. see *MEDICAL SCIENCES—Cardiovascular Diseases*

616.15 GBR ISSN 1357-2520
PROGRESS IN GROWTH FACTORS. Text in English. 1995. q. GBP 40; GBP 68 foreign. adv. bk.rev. bibl, tr.lit. back issues avail. *Refereed.* **Document type:** *Academic/Scholarly.* **Description:** Contains reviews of current literature on haematopoietic growth factors, both pre-clinical and clinical.
Published by: Mediscript Ltd., 1 Mountview Ct, 310 Friern Barnet Ln, London N20 0LD, United Kingdom. TEL 44-20-8446-8898, FAX 44-20-8446-9194, 101607.3205@compuserve.com. Ed., R&P, Adv. contact Linda Lazarus. Pub. Fatima Patel. Circ: 7,000 (paid).

616.15 GBR ISSN 0143-6740
CODEN: RADVDW
RECENT ADVANCES IN BLOOD COAGULATION. Text in English. 1969. irreg., latest vol.6. **Document type:** *Monographic series, Academic/Scholarly.*
—BLDSC (7303.800500), CASDDS, CISTI, GNLM, Infotrieve, KNAW. **CCC.**
Published by: Churchill Livingstone (Subsidiary of: Harcourt Publishers Ltd.), Robert Stevenson House, 1-3 Baxter's Pl, Leith Walk, Edinburgh, Midlothian EH1 3AF, United Kingdom. TEL 44-131-556-2424, FAX 44-131-459-1177, http://www.churchillmed.com. **Subscr. to:** Harcourt Publishers Ltd., Foots Cray High St, Sidcup, Kent DA14 5HP, United Kingdom. TEL 44-20-8308-5700, FAX 44-20-8309-0807.

616.15 GBR ISSN 0143-697X
CODEN: RAHADN
RECENT ADVANCES IN HAEMATOLOGY. Text in English. 1971. irreg., latest vol.7. **Document type:** *Monographic series, Academic/Scholarly.*
—BLDSC (7303.842000), CASDDS, GNLM, KNAW.
Published by: Churchill Livingstone (Subsidiary of: Harcourt Publishers Ltd.), Robert Stevenson House, 1-3 Baxter's Pl, Leith Walk, Edinburgh, Midlothian EH1 3AF, United Kingdom. TEL 44-131-556-2424, FAX 44-131-459-1177, http://www.churchillmed.com. **US subscr. to:** Churchill Livingstone, 650 Ave of the Americas, New York, NY 10011. TEL 212-206-5000.

REFERATIVNYI ZHURNAL. GEMATOLOGIYA. see *MEDICAL SCIENCES—Abstracting, Bibliographies, Statistics*

616.15 GBR ISSN 1127-0020
REVIEWS IN CLINICAL AND EXPERIMENTAL HEMATOLOGY. Text in English. 1997. q., latest vol.6, 2002. GBP 54 in Europe to individuals; USD 98 in North America to individuals; GBP 59 elsewhere to individuals; GBP 215 in Europe to institutions; USD 342 in North America to institutions; GBP 237 elsewhere to institutions (effective 2002). back issues avail. *Refereed.* **Document type:** *Academic/Scholarly.* **Description:** Includes current topics in haematology which specifically highlights the role of the laboratory and its different aspects and applications: diagnosis, prognosis, treatment, follow-up, etc.
Related titles: Online - full text ed.: ISSN 1468-0734. GBP 49 in Europe to individuals; USD 89 in North America to individuals; GBP 49 elsewhere to individuals; GBP 194 in Europe to institutions; USD 308 in North America to institutions; GBP 194 elsewhere to institutions (effective 2002) (from EBSCO Publishing, O C L C Online Computer Library Center, Inc., ingenta, Munksgaard & Blackwell Science's Synergy, Swets Blackwell).
—BLDSC (7788.978500).
Published by: (Accademia Nazionale di Medicina ITA), Blackwell Science Ltd., Osney Mead, Oxford OX2 0EL, United Kingdom. TEL 44-1865-206206, FAX 44-1865-721205, journals.cs@blacksci.co.uk, http://www.blackwell-science.com. Ed. R Foa. Pub. Allen Stevens. R&P Sophie Savage. Adv. contact Jenny Applin. Circ: 1,200.

616.15 CUB ISSN 0864-0289
REVISTA CUBANA DE HEMATOLOGIA, INMUNOLOGIA Y HEMATERAPIA. Text in Spanish; Summaries in English, Spanish. s-a. USD 34 in the Americas; USD 42 in Europe; USD 50 elsewhere. adv. charts, illus, stat. index. **Description:** Covers immunology, hematologic and hematopoietic system diseases, AIDS research and the application of hemotherapy techniques.
Published by: (Cuba. Ministerio de Salud Publica, Centro Nacional de Informacion de Ciencias Medicas), Editorial de Ciencias Medicas, O'Reilly No. 4, Habana, Cuba. TEL 809-62-8091. Ed. Ivette Cabrera. Circ: 1,200.
Co-sponsors: sociedad Cubana de Hematologia; Instituto Nacional Hematologia e Inmunologia.

REVISTA IBEROAMERICANA DE TROMBOSIS Y HEMOSTASIA. see *MEDICAL SCIENCES—Cardiovascular Diseases*

REVISTA IBEROAMERICANA DE TROMBOSIS Y HEMOSTASIA. SUPLEMENTO. see *MEDICAL SCIENCES—Cardiovascular Diseases*

616.15 FRA ISSN 0999-7385
CODEN: STVAEY
SANG THROMBOSE VAISSEAUX. Abbreviated title: S T V. Text in French. 10/yr. FRF 630 domestic to individuals; EUR 114 in Europe to individuals; FRF 800 elsewhere to individuals; FRF 1,120 domestic to institutions; EUR 189 in Europe to institutions; FRF 1,290 elsewhere to institutions; FRF 430 domestic to students; EUR 84 in Europe to students; FRF 600 elsewhere to students; FRF 120 newsstand/cover (effective 2001). **Document type:** *Academic/Scholarly.* **Description:** Studies fundamental and practical aspects of blood and vascular problems.
Related titles: Online - full text ed.: FRF 630 to individuals; FRF 1,120 to institutions; FRF 430 to students (effective 2001).
Indexed: Inpharma, Reac., Ref.Zh.
—BLDSC (8073.160000), EMDOCS, GNLM, KNAW.
Published by: John Libbey Eurotext, 127 av. de la Republique, Montrouge 92120, France. TEL 33-01-46730660, FAX 33-01-40840999, marketing@jle.com, http://www.john-libbey-eurotext.fr/. Ed. Gerard Tobelem. **Subscr. to:** A T E I, 3 av. Pierre Keraütret, Romainville 92230, France. TEL 33-1-48408686, FAX 33-1-48400731, atei@club-internet.fr.

616.1 ESP ISSN 0036-4355
RC633.A1 CODEN: SNGRAW
SANGRE; trabajos de hematologia y hemoterapia. Text mainly in Spanish; Summaries in English, Spanish. 1956. bi-m. ESP 5,300, USD 70. adv. bk.rev. index. back issues avail.
Indexed: Biol.Abstr., Chem.Abstr., Curr.Adv.Gen.& Molec.Biol., Curr.Cont. (coverage dropped), Dent.Ind., Excerp.Med., Ind.Med. (coverage dropped), Ind.Med.Esp., Inpharma, Nutr.Abstr., Reac., Ref.Zh.
—CASDDS, CINDOC, CISTI, GNLM, IDS, Infotrieve, KNAW. **CCC.**
Published by: Revista Sangre S.A., General Sueiro, 35 pral.dcha, PO Box 687, Zaragoza 50008, Spain. TEL 76-222638, FAX 76-222638. Ed. M Giralt. Circ: 2,200.

▼ **SEMINARS IN CEREBROVASCULAR DISEASES AND STROKE.** see *MEDICAL SCIENCES—Psychiatry And Neurology*

616.15 USA ISSN 0037-1963
RC633.A1 CODEN: SEHEA3
SEMINARS IN HEMATOLOGY. Text in English. 1964. q. USD 143 domestic to individuals; USD 217 foreign to individuals; USD 207 domestic to institutions; USD 263 foreign to institutions; USD 80 domestic to students; USD 130 foreign to students; USD 66 newsstand/cover (effective 2001). adv. bibl, charts, illus. index. *Refereed.* **Document type:** *Journal, Academic/Scholarly.* **Description:** Publishes original articles of current importance in clinical hematology and related fields.
Related titles: Microform ed.: (from SWZ); Online - full text ed.: (from Institute for Scientific Information).
Indexed: Biol.Abstr., Chem.Abstr., Chem.Titles, Curr.Adv.Cancer Res., Curr.Adv.Ecol.Sci., Curr.Cont., Excerp.Med., INIS Atomind., Ind.Med. (1964-), Ind.Sci.Rev., Inpharma, Int.Abstr.Biol.Sci., Nutr.Abstr., Pharm.&Out.News, Reac., Sci.Cit.Ind.
—BLDSC (8239.450000), CASDDS, CISTI, GNLM, IDS, ingenta, KNAW. **CCC.**
Published by: W.B. Saunders Co. (Subsidiary of: Harcourt Publishers Ltd.), 11830 Westline Industrial Dr, St Louis, MO 63146. TEL 800-325-4177, http://www.wbsaunders.com. Eds. Dr. Neal S. Young, Dr. Photis Beris. adv.: B&W page USD 1,235, color page USD 2,485; trim 10 x 7. Circ: 4,680. **Subscr. to:** Periodicals Fulfillment, W B Saunders Co, 6277 Sea Harbor Dr, 4th Fl, Orlando, FL 32891-4800.

616.15 USA ISSN 0094-6176
CODEN: STHMBV
SEMINARS IN THROMBOSIS AND HEMOSTASIS. Text in English. bi-m. EUR 222 to individuals; EUR 455 to institutions; EUR 70 newsstand/cover (effective 2002). adv. reprint service avail. from PQC. *Refereed.* **Document type:** *Monographic series, Academic/Scholarly.* **Description:** Covers a specific advance in clinical and laboratory diagnosis and therapeutic intervention in this specialty.
Related titles: Microform ed.: (from PQC); Online - full text ed.: ISSN 1098-9064 (from Ovid Technologies, Inc., EBSCO Publishing, O C L C Online Computer Library Center, Inc., RoweCom Information Quest, Institute for Scientific Information).
Indexed: ASCA, Biol.Abstr., Chem.Abstr., Curr.Adv.Ecol.Sci., Curr.Cont., Excerp.Med., INIS Atomind., Ind.Med. (1974-), Ind.Sci.Rev., Inpharma, Pharm.&Out.News, Reac., SSCI (coverage dropped), Sci.Cit.Ind.
—BLDSC (8239.480000), ADONIS, CASDDS, CISTI, GNLM, IDS, ingenta, KNAW. **CCC.**
Published by: Thieme Medical Publishers, 333 Seventh Ave, New York, NY 10001. TEL 212-760-0888, 800-782-3488, FAX 212-947-1112, http://www.thieme.com. Ed. Dr. Eberhard F Mammen. Circ: 2,493. **Orders in Europe to:** Thieme International, Postfach 3001120, Stuttgart 70451, Germany. TEL 49-711-8931-0.

LA STILLA; organo di stampa dell'A.V.I.S. provinciale di Montova. see *SOCIAL SERVICES AND WELFARE*

TETSU TAISHA KENKYUKAI PUROGURAMU SHOROKUSHU/CONFERENCE ON CURRENT TOPICS FOR IRON METABOLISM. PROGRAM AND ABSTRACTS. see *BIOLOGY—Biochemistry*

616.15 FRA
TRAITE D'HEMATOLOGIE. Cover title: Traite d'Hematologie. Variant title: Encyclopedie Medico-Chirurgicale, Instantanes Medicaux. Hematologie. Text in French. 1937. 3 base vols. plus q. updates. bibl, charts, illus. *Refereed.* **Document type:** *Academic/Scholarly.* **Description:** Provides a comprehensive, up-to-date reference for diagnosing conditions in hematology.
Former titles: Encyclopedie Medico-Chirurgicale. Hematologie (1155-1984); (until 1990): Encyclopedie Medico-Chirurgicale, Instantanes Medicaux. Sang, Organes Hematopoietiques (0246-0556); (until 1959): Encyclopedie Medico-Chirurgicale. Sang, Organes Hematopoietiques, Systeme Vegetatif (0246-0696); (until 1951): Encyclopedie Medico-Chirurgicale. Sang, Systeme Vegetatif (0246-070X)
Published by: Elsevier Paris, Editions Scientifiques et Medicales (Subsidiary of: Reed Elsevier plc. group), 3 rue Linois, Paris Cedex 15 75015, France. TEL 33-45589110, FAX 33-1-45589425, redaction-emc@elsevier.fr, redacion-emc@elsevier.fr, http://www.elsevier.fr, http://www.elsevier.com.

616.15 GBR ISSN 1473-0502
CODEN: TRASEE
TRANSFUSION AND APHERESIS SCIENCE. Text in English. 6/yr. EUR 256 in Europe to individuals; JPY 34,000 in Japan to individuals; USD 286 elsewhere to individuals; EUR 808 in Europe to institutions; JPY 107,400 in Japan to institutions; USD 904 elsewhere to institutions (effective 2002). back issues avail. *Refereed.* **Document type:** *Academic/Scholarly.* **Description:** Presents scientific and clinical studies in the areas of immunohematology, transfusion practice and apheresis.
Former titles: Transfusion Science (0955-3886); (until 1989): Plasma Therapy and Transfusion Technology (0278-6222); (until 1981): Plasma Therapy (0196-4267); Incorporates: Apheresis Bulletin
Related titles: Microfilm ed.: (from PQC); Online - full text ed.: (from ingenta, Swets Blackwell, Institute for Scientific Information, ScienceDirect).
Indexed: ASCA, Curr.Cont., Excerp.Med., Inpharma, Int.Abstr.Biol.Sci., Pharm.&Out.News, Reac.
—BLDSC (9020.704500), CISTI, EMDOCS, GNLM, IDS, Infotrieve, ingenta, KNAW. **CCC.**
Published by: (European Society for Haemapheresis), Pergamon (Subsidiary of: Elsevier Science), The Boulevard, Langford Ln, East Park, Kidlington, Oxford OXB 1GB, United Kingdom. FAX 44-1865-843010, http://www.elsevier.com/locate/transci. Eds. Dr. Gail Rock, T J Hamblin. Circ: 2,000. **Subscr. in Australasia and the Far East to:** Elsevier Science (Singapore) Pte Ltd, No.1 Temasek Ave, 17-01 Millenia Tower, Singapore 039192, Singapore. TEL 65-434-3727, FAX 65-337-2230; **Subscr. in the Americas to:** Elsevier Science, PO Box 945, New York, NY 10159-0945. TEL 212-633-3730, FAX 212-633-3680, usinfo-f@elsevier.com; **Subscr. to:** Elsevier Science BV, PO Box 211, Amsterdam 1000 AE, Netherlands. TEL 31-20-485-3757.

616.1 FRA ISSN 1246-7820
CODEN: RFTID6
TRANSFUSION CLINIQUE ET BIOLOGIQUE. Text mainly in French; Text occasionally in English; Abstracts in English, French. 1958. bi-m. FRF 1,478 domestic to institutions; EUR 234 in Europe to institutions; USD 294 in the Americas to institutions; FRF 1,660, EUR 253.07 elsewhere to institutions (effective 2002). bk.rev. index. reprint service avail. from PQC. *Refereed.* **Document type:** *Academic/Scholarly.* **Description:** Bridges the gap between fundamental research and everyday applications in blood transfusion.
Former titles (until 1994): Revue Francaise de Transfusion et d'Hemobiologie (1140-4639); (until 1989): Revue Francaise de Transfusion et Immuno-Hematologie (0338-4535); (until 1975): Revue Francaise de Transfusion (0035-2977); Transfusion
Related titles: Microform ed.: (from PQC); Online - full text ed.: (from ingenta, Institute for Scientific Information, ScienceDirect).
Indexed: ASCA, Biol.Abstr., Chem.Abstr., Curr.Cont., Dent.Ind., Excerp.Med., Ind.Med. (1994-), Ind.Sci.Rev., Ind.Vet., Inpharma, Int.Nurs.Ind., Pharm.&Out.News, Protozool.Abstr., Reac., Rev.Med.& Vet.Mycol., Sci.Cit.Ind., Vet.Bull.
—BLDSC (9020.705000), CASDDS, CISTI, GNLM, IDS, Infotrieve, KNAW. **CCC.**
Published by: (Societe Francaise de Transfusion Sanguine), Elsevier Paris, Editions Scientifiques et Medicales (Subsidiary of: Reed Elsevier plc. group), 23 rue Linois, Paris 75015, France. TEL 33-1-45589110, FAX 33-1-45589419, tcb@elsevier.fr; academic@elsevier-fr.com, http://www.elsevier.nl/inca/publications/store/6/0/1/0/2/0/. Eds. H Klinkmann, U E Nydegger. Circ: 1,000.

616.15 GBR ISSN 0958-7578
CODEN: TRMDET
TRANSFUSION MEDICINE. Text in English. 1991. bi-m., latest vol.12, 2002. GBP 80 in Europe to individuals; USD 127 in North America to individuals; GBP 88 elsewhere to individuals; GBP 252 in Europe to institutions; USD 399 in North America to institutions; GBP 277 elsewhere to institutions (effective 2002). adv. bk.rev. illus. index. *Refereed.* **Document type:** *Academic/Scholarly.* **Description:** Reflects the interest of clinicians, scientists and other professionals working in the broad field of blood transfusion medicine.
Related titles: Microform ed.: (from PQC); Online - full text ed.: ISSN 1365-3148. 1999. GBP 72 in Europe to individuals; USD 115 in North America to individuals; GBP 72 elsewhere to individuals; GBP 227 in Europe to institutions; USD 360 in North America to institutions; GBP 227 elsewhere to institutions (effective 2002) (from Ovid Technologies, Inc., EBSCO Publishing, O C L C Online Computer Library Center, Inc., RoweCom Information Quest, ingenta, Munksgaard & Blackwell Science's Synergy, Swets Blackwell, Institute for Scientific Information).
Indexed: ASCA, Curr.Cont., Ind.Med. (1991-), Ind.Sci.Rev., Inpharma, Int.Abstr.Biol.Sci., Int.Nurs.Ind., Pharm.&Out.News, Reac., Sci.Cit.Ind.
—BLDSC (9020.706000), CISTI, EMDOCS, IDS, Infotrieve, KNAW. **CCC.**
Published by: (British Blood Transfusion Society), Blackwell Science Ltd., Osney Mead, Oxford OX2 0EL, United Kingdom. TEL 44-1865-206206, FAX 44-1865-721205, journals.cs@blacksci.co.uk, http://www.blackwell-science.com. Ed. D J Anstee. Pub. Allen Stevens. R&P Sophie Savage. Adv. contact Jenny Applin. Circ: 1,665.

616.15 USA ISSN 0887-7963
CODEN: TMEREU
TRANSFUSION MEDICINE REVIEWS. Text in English. 1987 (Apr.). q. USD 117 domestic to individuals; USD 185 foreign to individuals; USD 173 domestic to institutions; USD 225 foreign to institutions; USD 87 domestic to students; USD 111 foreign to students; USD 57 newsstand/cover (effective 2001). adv. abstr, bibl, charts, illus. index. *Refereed.* **Document type:** *Academic/Scholarly.* **Description:** Provides a forum for important clinical and research topics in the field.
Related titles: Online - full text ed.: (from Institute for Scientific Information).
Indexed: ASCA, CINAHL, Curr.Cont., Excerp.Med. (1993-), Ind.Med. (1987-), Ind.Sci.Rev., Inpharma, Protozool.Abstr., Reac., Sci.Cit.Ind.
—BLDSC (9020.707000), CISTI, EMDOCS, GNLM, IDS, ingenta, KNAW. **CCC.**
Published by: W.B. Saunders Co. (Subsidiary of: Harcourt Publishers Ltd.), 11830 Westline Industrial Dr, St Louis, MO 63146. TEL 800-325-4177, http://www.wbsaunders.com. Ed. Dr. Morris A Blajchman. adv.: B&W page USD 765, color page USD 1,790; trim 10 x 7. Circ: 1,367. **Subscr. to:** Periodicals Fulfillment, W B Saunders Co, 6277 Sea Harbor Dr, 4th Fl, Orlando, FL 32891-4800.

616.15 FRA ISSN 1015-3276
TRANSFUSION TODAY. Text in English. 1989. q. membership. adv. bk.rev. **Description:** Articles on blood transfusion and related topics.
Related titles: French ed.: ISSN 1015-3284; Spanish ed.: ISSN 1015-3292.
—BLDSC (9020.711000).
Published by: Societe Internationale de Transfusion Sanguine/International Society of Blood Transfusion, c/o C N T S, B.P. 100, Les Ulis Cedex 91943, France. TEL 69-07-20-40, FAX 69-07-41-85. Ed. Bahman Habibi. Circ: 7,000.

616.15 ITA ISSN 0041-1787
CODEN: TRSABD
LA TRASFUSIONE DEL SANGUE. Text mainly in Italian, English; Summaries in Italian, English. 1956. bi-m. ITL 200,000 domestic to individuals; ITL 300,000 foreign to individuals; ITL 250,000 domestic to institutions (effective 2000). adv. bk.rev. abstr, bibl, charts, illus. index. **Document type:** *Academic/Scholarly.*
Indexed: Biol.Abstr., Excerp.Med.
—CASDDS, GNLM.
Published by: (Societa Italiana di Medicina Trasfusionale e Immunoematologia), S I M T I Editore, Viale Beatrice D'Este, 5, Milan, MI 20122, Italy. TEL 39-2-58316515, FAX 39-2-58316353. Ed. Dr. Giorgio Reali. Adv. contact Gianalfredo Sciorelli. Circ: 700.

616.15 CHN
ZHONGGUO SHIYAN XIEYEXUE ZAZHI/JOURNAL OF EXPERIMENTAL HEMATOLOGY. Text in Chinese. q. USD 20.80; USD 5.20 newsstand/cover (effective 2000). **Document type:** *Academic/Scholarly.*

Published by: China International Book Trading Corp/Zhongguo Guoji Tushu Maoyi Zonggongsi cibtc@mail.cibtc.com.cn, http://www.cibtc.com.cn. **Dist. by:** 35, Chegongzhuang Xilu, Haidian District, Beijing 100044, China.

616.15 CHN ISSN 0253-2727
CODEN: CHTCD7

ZHONGHUA XUEYEXUE ZAZHI/CHINESE JOURNAL OF HEMATOLOGY. Text in Chinese; Abstracts in Chinese, English. 1980. m. CNY 96 domestic; USD 50.40 foreign; CNY 8 newsstand/cover domestic; USD 4.20 newsstand/cover foreign (effective 2001). adv. **Document type:** *Academic/Scholarly.* **Description:** Covers the latest development on hematology in China. Contains original articles, case reports and laboratory techniques.
Related titles: CD-ROM ed.; Online - full content ed.: (from WanFang Data Corp.).
Indexed: Chem.Abstr., ExtraMED, Ind.Med. (1980-).
—CASDDS.
Published by: Zhongguo Yixue Kexueyuan, Xueye Yanjiusuo/Chinese Academy of Medical Sciences, Institute of Hematology, 288 Nanjing Lu, Tianjin 300020, China. TEL 86-22-2730-4167, FAX 86-22-2730-4167, cnblood@shell.tjvan.net.cn. Ed. Jiazeng Li. R&P Zhifang Zhang. Adv. contact Rurui Wang. B&W page USD 1,400, color page USD 3,000. Circ: 10,000. **Subscr. to:** China International Book Trading Corp, 35, Chegongzhuang Xilu, Haidian District, Beijing 100044, China. TEL 86-1-68413849, FAX 86-1-68412048, cibtc@mail.cibtc.com.cn, http://www.cibtc.com.cn.

MEDICAL SCIENCES—Hypnosis

154.7 616.891 USA ISSN 0002-9157
RC490 CODEN: AJHNA3

AMERICAN JOURNAL OF CLINICAL HYPNOSIS. Text in English. 1958. q. USD 62.50 to individuals; USD 125 to institutions (effective 2001). adv. bk.rev. illus. abstr. index, cum.index. 88 p./no. 1 cols./p. back issues avail.; reprint service avail. from PQC,PSC,SCH. *Refereed.* **Document type:** *Journal, Academic/Scholarly.* **Description:** Provides peer reviewed research and case reports on clinical hypnosis.
Related titles: Microform ed.: 1958 (from PQC); Online - full text ed.: (from Institute for Scientific Information).
Indexed: AMED, Adol.Ment.Hlth.Abstr., AgeLine, Arts & Hum.Cit.Ind. (coverage dropped), Behav.Med.Abstr., Bibl.Ind., Biol.Abstr., Curr.Cont., Excerp.Med., Ind.Med. (1958-), Mid.East: Abstr.& Ind., PsycInfo, Psychol.Abstr. (1966-), SSCI, e-psyche.
—BLDSC (0822.800000), EMDOCS, GNLM, IDS, ingenta, KNAW.
Published by: American Society of Clinical Hypnosis, 130 East Elm Court, Ste 201, Roselle, IL 60172-2000. TEL 630-980-4740, FAX 630-351-8490, info@asch.net, http://www.asch.net/journal.htm. Ed. Thurman Mott. Adv. contact Melanie Datz. page USD 400; 5.5 x 8.5. Circ: 3,000.

ANESTEZIOLOGIIA I INTENSIVNO LECHENIE. see *MEDICAL SCIENCES—Anaesthesiology*

▼ **ARCHIVES OF PSYCHIATRY AND PSYCHOTHERAPY.** see *MEDICAL SCIENCES—Psychiatry And Neurology*

616.891 AUS ISSN 0156-0417
CODEN: AJCHDV

AUSTRALIAN JOURNAL OF CLINICAL AND EXPERIMENTAL HYPNOSIS. Text in English. 1977. s-a. AUD 40 to individuals; AUD 45 foreign to individuals; AUD 50 to institutions; AUD 55 foreign to institutions (effective 2000). adv. bk.rev. back issues avail. **Document type:** *Academic/Scholarly.*
Former titles: Australian Society of Hypnosis. Journal; Australian Society of Clinical and Experimental Hypnosis. Journal
Indexed: Excerp.Med., Ind.Med. (coverage dropped), PsycInfo, Psychol.Abstr. (1978-), Sci.Cit.Ind. (coverage dropped), e-psyche.
—BLDSC (1806.200000), CISTI, GNLM, ingenta, KNAW.
Published by: Australian Society of Hypnosis, PO Box 592, Heidelberg, VIC 3084, Australia. TEL 61-3-92431274, FAX 61-3-92431158. Ed., Adv. contact Barry J Evans. Circ: 1,100.

616.891 AUS ISSN 0810-0713

AUSTRALIAN JOURNAL OF CLINICAL HYPNOTHERAPY AND HYPNOSIS. Text in English. 1980. s-a. AUD 25 to individuals; AUD 32 to institutions (effective 2000). bk.rev. back issues avail. **Document type:** *Academic/Scholarly.* **Description:** Publishes original clinical, research, review, theoretical, historical and related reports dealing with the professional application of hypnosis and hypnotherapy.
Related titles: Microform ed.: (from PQC); Online - full text ed.: (from ProQuest Information & Learning).
Indexed: AMED, Excerp.Med., PsycInfo, Psychol.Abstr. (1980-), e-psyche.
—BLDSC (1806.353000), CISTI, EMDOCS, GNLM.
Published by: (Australian Society of Clinical Hypnotherapists), Australian Academic Press Pty. Ltd., 32 Jeays St, Bowen Hills, QLD 4006, Australia. TEL 61-7-32571176, FAX 61-7-32525908, australianacademicpress@compuserve.com, http://www.australianacademicpress.com.au. Ed. Zoltan A Kelemen.

COMPREHENSIVE PSYCHIATRY. see *MEDICAL SCIENCES—Psychiatry And Neurology*

616.89 GBR ISSN 0960-5290
CODEN: COHYET

CONTEMPORARY HYPNOSIS. Text in English. 1983. q. USD 99 in North America to individuals; GBP 55 rest of world to individuals; USD 199 in North America to institutions; GBP 110 rest of world to institutions (effective 2001). adv. bk.rev. index. back issues avail. *Refereed.* **Document type:** *Academic/Scholarly.* **Description:** Covers all aspects of theory, research and practice of hypnosis.
Formerly: British Journal of Experimental and Clinical Hypnosis (0265-1033)
Related titles: Online - full text ed.: (from ProQuest Information & Learning).
Indexed: AMED, ASSIA, Behav.Med.Abstr., CINAHL, PsycInfo, Psychol.Abstr. (1982-), e-psyche.
—BLDSC (3425.182900), ADONIS, CISTI, EMDOCS, GNLM.
Published by: (British Society of Experimental and Clinical Hypnosis), Whurr Publishers Ltd., 19b Compton Terr, London N1 2UN, United Kingdom. TEL 44-20-7359-5979, FAX 44-20-7226-5290, info@whurr.co.uk, http://www.whurr.co.uk. Ed. David Oakley. Adv. contact Maggy Park. page GBP 200. Circ: 450. **Subscr. in N. America to:** Whurr Publishers Ltd., PO Box 1897, Lawrence, KS 66044-8897. TEL 913-843-1221, FAX 913-843-1274, am&m@allenpress.com. **Subscr. to:** Turpin Distribution Services Ltd., Blackhorse Rd, Letchworth, Herts SG6 1HN, United Kingdom. TEL 44-1462-488900, FAX 44-1462-483011, custservturpin@turpinltd.com.

616.891 DEU ISSN 0933-1093

EXPERIMENTELLE UND KLINISCHE HYPNOSE. Text in German; Summaries in English, German. 1983. s-a. DEM 28 (effective 2000). adv. bk.rev. abstr, bibl. back issues avail. **Document type:** *Journal, Academic/Scholarly.* **Description:** Concerns clinical and therapeutic applications of hypnosis. Affiliated with the German Association of Hypnosis and aimed at an audience of psychologists and therapeutic workers in the public health sector.
Indexed: PsycInfo, Psychol.Abstr. (1987-), e-psyche.
—GNLM.
Published by: (Deutsche Gesellschaft fuer Hypnose), D G V T - Verlag, Hechinger Str 203, Tuebingen 72072, Germany. TEL 49-7071-792850, FAX 49-7071-792851. Ed., R&P Detlef W Timp. adv.: B&W page DEM 600; trim 115 x 185. Circ: 1,100.

616.891 370.15 USA ISSN 0882-8652

HYPNOTHERAPY TODAY. Text in English. 1980. q. membership. bk.rev. tr.lit. **Document type:** *Newsletter, Directory, Trade, Academic/Scholarly.* **Description:** Studies the therapeutic uses of hypnosis for the body, mind and spiritual needs.
Related titles: E-mail ed.; Online - full text ed.
Indexed: e-psyche.
Published by: American Association of Professional Hypnotherapists, 4149 El Camino Way No A, Palo Alto, CA 94306-4036. TEL 650-323-3224, http://www.aaph.org. Ed. Mary Horngren. Pub. Josie Hadley. Circ: 1,000.

154.7 616.891 USA ISSN 0020-7144
RC490 CODEN: IJEHAO

INTERNATIONAL JOURNAL OF CLINICAL AND EXPERIMENTAL HYPNOSIS. Text in English; Summaries in French, German, Spanish. 1953. q. USD 80 to individuals; USD 320 to institutions; USD 25 newsstand/cover to individuals; USD 80 newsstand/cover to institutions (effective 2002). adv. bk.rev. illus. cum.index. back issues avail.; reprint service avail. from PQC. *Refereed.* **Document type:** *Academic/Scholarly.* **Description:** Publishes research papers dealing with hypnosis in psychology, psychiatry, the medical and dental specialties, and related studies.
Formerly (until 1958): Journal of Clinical and Experimental Hypnosis (0095-988X)
Related titles: Microfilm ed.: (from PQC); Online - full text ed.: (from Institute for Scientific Information).
Indexed: AMED, ASCA, Adol.Ment.Hlth.Abstr., Behav.Med.Abstr., Biol.Abstr., Curr.Cont., Excerp.Med., Ind.Med. (1959-), Ind.Sci.Rev., Mid.East: Abstr.& Ind., PsycInfo, Psychol.Abstr. (1959-), Ref.Zh., SSCI, Sci.Cit.Ind. (coverage dropped), Soc.Work Res.& Abstr., Viol.& Abuse Abstr., e-psyche.
—BLDSC (4542.170000), CISTI, GNLM, ingenta, KNAW.
Published by: (Society for Clinical and Experimental Hypnosis), Sage Publications, Inc., 2455 Teller Rd, Thousand Oaks, CA 91320. TEL 805-499-0721, info@sagepub.com, http://www.sagepub.com. Eds. Mia Consalvo, Michael Nash. R&P Tanya Udin. Adv. contact DeAnna Vega Hammersley. Circ: 2,500. **Overseas subscr. to:** Sage Publications Ltd., 6 Bonhill St, London EC2A 4PU, United Kingdom; Sage Publications India Pvt. Ltd., P O Box 4215, New Delhi 110 048, India.

615.8 USA

JOURNAL OF HYPNOTHERAPY AND HYPNOANALYSIS✱. Text in English. 1994. q. USD 42.50 domestic to individuals; USD 86.50 foreign to individuals; USD 70 domestic to institutions; USD 104 foreign to institutions. **Document type:** *Academic/Scholarly.*
Published by: Institute for Research on Hypnotherapy and Hypnoanalysis, 1991 Broadway, Ste 18 B, New York, NY 10023. TEL 212-533-4042. Ed. Milton V Kline. **Co-sponsor:** International Society for Medical and Psychological Hypnosis.

KWARTAALSCHRIFT VOOR DIRECTIEVE THERAPIE EN HYPNOSE. see *PSYCHOLOGY*

614.8512 154.7 USA ISSN 0894-5098
RC490

MEDICAL HYPNOANALYSIS JOURNAL✱. Text in English. 1980. q. USD 40 (effective 2000). film rev. tr.lit. cum.index. back issues avail. **Document type:** *Academic/Scholarly, Trade.* **Description:** Presents information about medical hypnoanalysis that clinicians can use immediately. Technique, as well as hypnotic scripts, are clearly written and include mind, body and spirit orientation.
Indexed: AMED, Psychol.Abstr. (1986-), e-psyche.
—BLDSC (5527.525000), CISTI, GNLM.
Published by: (American Academy of Medical Hypnoanalysts), A A M H, 5628 Murray Rd, Ste 4, Memphis, TN 38119-3876. TEL 888-454-9766, 800-344-9766, FAX 413-589-7560. Ed. Roxanne Lewis. Circ: 334 (paid).

616.8 USA

NATIONAL REGISTER OF PROFESSIONAL HYPNOTHERAPISTS✱. Text in English. 1983. a. membership. **Document type:** *Directory.* **Description:** Lists hypnotherapy practitioners state-by-state and in 20 foreign countries.
Indexed: e-psyche.
Published by: American Association of Professional Hypnotherapists, 4149 El Camino Way No A, Palo Alto, CA 94306-4036. TEL 650-323-3224. Circ: 2,000.

616.891 USA

NEW YORK SOCIETY OF ETHICAL HYPNOSIS. NEWSLETTER✱. Text in English. 4/yr. USD 10. **Document type:** *Newsletter.*
Published by: New York Society of Ethical Hypnosis, c/o Carol Styron Gore, Ed, Box 818, Skyland, NC 28776-0818.

PSYCHOTERAPIA. see *MEDICAL SCIENCES—Psychiatry And Neurology*

154.7 616.891 USA ISSN 0583-8975

S C E H NEWSLETTER. Text in English. 1955. q. USD 10; USD 13 foreign. bk.rev. **Document type:** *Newsletter.*
Published by: Society for Clinical and Experimental Hypnosis, 2201 Haeder Rd 1, Pullman, WA 99163-8619. TEL 509-332-7555, FAX 509-332-5907, peeblemj@menninger.edu, sceh@pullman.com. Ed. Mary Jo Peebles Kleiger TEL 785-554-3088. Circ: 1,200.

SEMINARS IN ANESTHESIA, PERIOPERATIVE MEDICINE AND PAIN. see *MEDICAL SCIENCES—Anaesthesiology*

MEDICAL SCIENCES—Internal Medicine

see also MEDICAL SCIENCES—Cardiovascular Diseases; MEDICAL SCIENCES—Communicable Diseases; MEDICAL SCIENCES—Endocrinology; MEDICAL SCIENCES—Gastroenterology; MEDICAL SCIENCES—Hematology; MEDICAL

M

SCIENCES—Oncology; MEDICAL SCIENCES—Respiratory Diseases; MEDICAL SCIENCES—Rheumatology; MEDICAL SCIENCES—Urology And Nephrology

A C P JOURNAL CLUB. see *MEDICAL SCIENCES—Abstracting, Bibliographies, Statistics*

616 BRA
ACADEMIA NACIONAL DE MEDICINA. ANAIS. Text in Portuguese; Summaries in English, Portuguese. 1841. q. BRL 29, USD 72. adv. charts, bibl, illus. back issues avail. **Document type:** *Academic/Scholarly.* **Description:** Presents studies in clinical medicine.
Former titles: Academia Nacional de Medicina. Boletim (0001-3838); (until 1918): Academia Nacional de Medicina. Revista
Indexed: Biol.Abstr., Chem.Abstr., Helminthol.Abstr. —CISTI, GNLM.
Published by: Academia Nacional de Medicina, Av General Justo, 365 7o, Centro, Caixa Postal 459, Rio De Janeiro, RJ 20021-130, Brazil. TEL 55-21-2621732, FAX 55-21-2408673. Ed. Ruben David Azulay. Adv. contact Maria Luiza C Doneda. Circ: 3,000.

616 USA ISSN 0065-2822
RC46 CODEN: AIMNAL
ADVANCES IN INTERNAL MEDICINE. Text in English. 1954. a. USD 89 domestic; USD 95 foreign (effective 2001). reprint service avail. from PQC. **Document type:** *Academic/Scholarly.* **Description:** Presents a collection of original fully referenced clinical reviews from the experts in the field.
Related titles: Microfilm ed.: (from PQC); Online - full text ed.: (from Institute for Scientific Information).
Indexed: ASCA, Biol.Abstr., Chem.Abstr., Curr.Adv.Ecol.Sci., Curr.Adv.Gen.& Molec.Biol., Dent.Ind., Diar.Dis.Res., INIS Atomind., Ind.Med. (1942-), Ind.Sci.Rev., Sci.Cit.Ind.
—BLDSC (0709.250000), CASDDS, CISTI, GNLM, ingenta, KNAW.
Published by: Mosby, Inc. (Subsidiary of: Elsevier Science) TEL 314-872-8370, 800-325-4177, FAX 314-432-1380, http://www.mosby.com/periodicals. Ed. Robert W Schrier.

616 USA
AMERICAN SOCIETY OF BARIATRIC PHYSICIANS. NEWS. Short title: News from A S B P. Text in English. 1986. bi-m. **Document type:** *Newsletter.*
Published by: American Society of Bariatric Physicians, 5453 East Evans Place, Denver, CO 80222-5234. TEL 303-770-2526, bariatric@asbp.org, http://www.asbp.org. Ed. Lola M Fehr. R&P, Adv. contact Diane Hawken.

616.02 ESP ISSN 0212-7199
ANALES DE MEDICINA INTERNA. Text in Spanish; Abstracts in Spanish, English. 1983. m. ESP 10,000; USD 200 foreign (effective 2000). adv. abstr, bibl, illus, stat. back issues avail. *Refereed.* **Document type:** *Academic/Scholarly.*
Related titles: ♦ Special ed.: Anales de Medicina Interna. Seminarios.
Indexed: Ind.Med. (1984-), Int.Nurs.Ind., Virol.Abstr.
—BLDSC (0890.018000), CISTI, EMDOCS, GNLM, Infotrieve, KNAW. **CCC.**
Published by: (Sociedad Espanola de Medicina Interna), Aran Ediciones S.A., Castello, 128 1o, Madrid 28006, Spain. TEL 34-91-782-0030, FAX 34-91-561-5787, edita@grupoaran.com, http://www.grupoaran.com. Ed. Dr. J Portugal Alvarez. Pub. Jose Jimenez. R&P Maria Dolores Linares TEL 34-1-7820035. Circ: 5,000.

616 ESP
ANALES DE MEDICINA INTERNA. SEMINARIOS. Text in Spanish; Abstracts in Spanish, English. q. ESP 2,000; USD 200 foreign (effective 2000). adv. abstr, bibl, illus, stat. back issues avail. *Refereed.* **Document type:** *Academic/Scholarly.*
Related titles: ♦ Special ed. of: Anales de Medicina Interna. ISSN 0212-7199.
Published by: Aran Ediciones S.A., Castello, 128 1o, Madrid 28006, Spain. TEL 34-91-782-0030, FAX 34-91-561-5787, edita@grupoaran.com, http://www.grupoaran.com. Ed. Dr. J Portugal Alvarez. Pub. Jose Jimenez. R&P Maria Dolores Linares TEL 34-1-7820035. Circ: 5,000.

616.026 FRA ISSN 0003-410X
CODEN: AMDIBO
ANNALES DE MEDECINE INTERNE. Text in French. 1848. 8/yr. FRF 1,678; FRF 1,890 foreign (effective 2000). adv. index. reprint service avail. from ISI. *Refereed.* **Document type:** *Academic/Scholarly.* **Description:** Covers equipment, techniques, and economic surveys relating to medical bioengineering.
Supersedes: Societe Medicale des Hopitaux de Paris. Bulletins et Memoires
Related titles: Microform ed.: (from PQC); Online - full text ed.: (from Institute for Scientific Information, RoweCom Information Quest).
Indexed: ASCA, Biol.Abstr., C.I.S. Abstr., Chem.Abstr., Chem.Indus.Notes, Chem.Titles, Curr.Cont., Dent.Ind., Environ.Sci.Poll.Mgmt., Excerp.Med., Helminthol.Abstr., INIS Atomind., Ind.Med. (1969-), Ind.Sci.Rev., Inpharma, Neurosci.Cit.Ind., Pharm.&Out.News, Pollut.Abstr., Protozool.Abstr., Reac., Rev.Appl.Entomol., Rev.Med.& Vet.Mycol., Rev.Plant Path., Risk Abstr., SSCI (coverage dropped), Saf.Sci.Abstr., Sci.Cit.Ind.
—BLDSC (0981.800000), CASDDS, CISTI, EMDOCS, GNLM, IDS, Infotrieve, KNAW. **CCC.**
Published by: (Societe Medicale des Hopitaux de Paris (SMHP)), Masson - Periodiques, 120 bd. St. Germain, Paris 75006, France. TEL 33-1-40466200, FAX 33-1-40466201. Ed. P Guillevin. Circ: 1,500. **Subscr. to:** Societe de Periodiques Specialises, BP 22, Vineuil Cedex 41354, France. TEL 33-2-54504612, FAX 33-2-54504611.

616.02 ITA ISSN 0393-9340
CODEN: AIMIEA
ANNALI ITALIANI DI MEDICINA INTERNA. Text in Italian. 1986. q. USD 90. adv. bk.rev. **Document type:** *Proceedings, Academic/Scholarly.*
Indexed: Ind.Med. (1986-).
—BLDSC (1014.460000), CISTI, EMDOCS, GNLM, KNAW.
Published by: C E P I - Centro Editoriale Pubblicitario Italiano s.r.l., Via Nicolo' Tartaglia, 3, Rome, RM 00197, Italy. TEL 39-6-8082101, FAX 39-6-8072458. Ed. Alberico Borghetti. Adv. contact Enzo Buongiorno.

616.026 USA ISSN 0003-4819
R11 CODEN: AIMEAS
ANNALS OF INTERNAL MEDICINE. Text in English. 1922. s-m. USD 131 domestic to individuals; USD 153 in Canada to individuals; USD 222 elsewhere to individuals; USD 177 domestic to institutions; USD 199 in Canada to institutions; USD 275 elsewhere to institutions (effective 2000). adv. bk.rev. charts, illus. index, cum.index. back issues avail. *Refereed.* **Document type:** *Academic/Scholarly.* **Description:** Contains reports of original clinical research, reviews, and commentaries.
Related titles: CD-ROM ed.: (from Ovid Technologies, Inc.); Microform ed.: (from PQC,PMC); Online - full text ed.: (from Ovid Technologies, Inc., EBSCO Publishing, Gale Group, Institute for Scientific Information).
Indexed: AIDS Abstr., AIM, AMED, ASCA, Abstr.Anthropol., Abstr.Health Care Manage.Stud., Abstr.Hyg., Abstr.Inter.Med., Addic.Abstr., AgeLine, Agri.& Environ.Biotech.Abstr. (coverage dropped), Behav.Med.Abstr., Biol.Abstr., CINAHL, C.I.S. Abstr., Chem.Abstr., Chem.Indus.Notes, Chem.Titles, Curr.Adv.Cancer Res., Curr.Adv.Ecol.Sci., Curr.Cont., Curr.Ind.Stat., Dairy Sci.Abstr., Dent.Ind., Derwent Biotech.Abstr., Diab.Cont., Diar.Dis.Res., Dok.Arbeitsmed., Environ.Sci.Poll.Mgmt., Excerp.Med., FAMLI, Helminthol.Abstr., Hosp.Lit.Ind., INIS Atomind., I.P.A., Ind.Med. (1927-), Ind.Sci.Rev., Ind.Vet., Inpharma, Int.Nurs.Ind., Jrnl.Watch, Jrnl.Watch Card., Jrnl.Watch Derm., Jrnl.Watch Emer.Med., Jrnl.Watch Gastr., Jrnl.Watch Inf.Dis., Jrnl.Watch Neuro., Jrnl.Watch Psych., Jrnl.Watch Wom.Hlth., Kidney, L.R.I., Med.& Surg.Dermat., Med.Care Rev., NRN, Neurosci.Cit.Ind., Nutr.Abstr., Pharm.&Out.News, Pollut.Abstr., Protozool.Abstr., Reac., Rev.Appl.Entomol., Rev.Med.& Vet.Mycol., Rev.Plant Path., Risk Abstr., Rural Devel.Abstr., Rural Recreat.Tour.Abstr., SSCI (coverage dropped), Saf.Sci.Abstr., Sci.Cit.Ind., Sugar Ind.Abstr., THA, Trop.Dis.Bull., Virol.Abstr. (coverage dropped).
—BLDSC (1041.200000), CASDDS, CISTI, EMDOCS, GNLM, IDS, ingenta, KNAW. **CCC.**
Published by: American College of Physicians/Co-sponsor: American Society of Internal Medicine, 190 N. Independence Mall W, Philadelphia, PA 19106-1572. TEL 215-351-2600, FAX 215-351-2799, custserv@mail.acponline.org, http://www.annalsonline.org. Ed. Dr. Frank Davidoff. R&P Joshua Roberts TEL 215-351-2630. Adv. contact Ron Taylor. B&W page USD 5,390. Circ: 97,000. **Subscr. to:** Allen Press Inc., PO Box 1897, Lawrence, KS 66044-8897.

616 USA ISSN 0003-9926
R11 CODEN: AIMDAP
ARCHIVES OF INTERNAL MEDICINE. Text in English. 1908. 22/yr. USD 325 in North America to institutions; USD 425 to institutions Central & S. America; GBP 275 elsewhere to institutions (effective 2001). adv. charts, illus. index. back issues avail. *Refereed.* **Document type:** *Academic/Scholarly.* **Description:** Publishes clinically relevant science in internal medicine and the subspecialties.
Related titles: CD-ROM ed.: (from Ovid Technologies, Inc.); Microform ed.: (from PQC,PMC); Online - full text ed.: (from The Dialog Corporation, Gale Group, Ovid Technologies, Inc., EBSCO Publishing, Institute for Scientific Information).
Indexed: AIDS Abstr., AIM, AMED, ASCA, Abstr.Health Care Manage.Stud., Abstr.Hyg., Abstr.Inter.Med., AgeLine, Agri.& Environ.Biotech.Abstr. (coverage dropped), Biol.Abstr., Biol.Dig., CINAHL, C.I.S. Abstr., Chem.Abstr., Chem.Indus.Notes, Chem.Titles, Crim.Just.Abstr., Curr.Adv.Cancer Res., Curr.Adv.Ecol.Sci., Curr.Cont., Curr.Ind.Stat., Curr.Lit.Fam.Plan., Dairy Sci.Abstr., Dent.Ind., Derwent Biotech.Abstr., Diab.Cont., Diar.Dis.Res., Dok.Arbeitsmed., Environ.Sci.Poll.Mgmt., Excerp.Med., Gen.Sci.Ind. (Jul.1997-), Helminthol.Abstr., Hosp.Lit.Ind., INIS Atomind., I.P.A., Ind.Med. (1960-), Ind.Sci.Rev., Ind.Vet., Inpharma, Int.Abstr.Biol.Sci., Int.Nurs.Ind., Jrnl.Watch, Jrnl.Watch Card., Jrnl.Watch Gastr., Jrnl.Watch Inf.Dis., Jrnl.Watch Neuro., Jrnl.Watch Wom.Hlth., Kidney, Med.& Surg.Dermat., NRN, Neurosci.Cit.Ind., Nutr.Abstr., Pharm.&Out.News, Poult.Abstr., Protozool.Abstr., Reac., Rev.Appl.Entomol., Rev.Arom.& Med.Plants, Rev.Med.& Vet.Mycol., Rev.Plant Path., Risk Abstr., SSCI (coverage dropped), Sci.Cit.Ind., Soyabean Abstr., THA, Trop.Dis.Bull., Vet.Bull., Virol.Abstr. (coverage dropped).
—BLDSC (1634.850000), CASDDS, CISTI, EMDOCS, GNLM, IDS, ingenta, KNAW. **CCC.**
Published by: American Medical Association, 515 N State St, P O Box 10946, Chicago, IL 60610-0946. ama-subs@ama-assn.org, http://www.archinternmed.com. Ed. James E Dalen. R&P Ada Jimenez Walker. Adv. contact Phillip B Altamore. B&W page USD 4,270, color page USD 6,050. Circ: 999,000. **Subscr. outside the Americas to:** JAMA, Readers Services, PO Box 299, London WC1H 9TD, United Kingdom.

616 ITA ISSN 0004-010X
CODEN: AMITAD
ARCHIVIO DI MEDICINA INTERNA. Text in Italian. 1949. bi-m. ITL 80,000; ITL 160,000 foreign (effective 1998). **Document type:** *Academic/Scholarly.*
Indexed: Excerp.Med.
—BLDSC (1647.650000), CISTI, EMDOCS, GNLM.
Published by: Casa Editrice Maccari, Via Palermo, 44, Parma, PR 43100, Italy. TEL 39-521-771268. Circ: 1,000.

616 BRA ISSN 0365-0723
CODEN: ABMEAD
ARQUIVOS BRASILEIROS DE MEDICINA. Text in Portuguese; Summaries in English, Portuguese. 1911. bi-m. BRL 54 domestic; USD 72 foreign (effective 2000). adv. bk.rev. index, cum.index. back issues avail. **Document type:** *Academic/Scholarly.* **Description:** Presents studies in internal medicine.
Indexed: Biol.Abstr., Excerp.Med., INIS Atomind., Ind.Med. (coverage dropped), Ref.Zh.
—BLDSC (1695.220000), EMDOCS, GNLM, KNAW.
Published by: (Universidade Federal Fluminense, Faculdade de Medicina), ECN - Editora Cientifica Nacional Ltda., Rua da Gloria, 366 Andar 3, Gloria, Rio De Janeiro, RJ 20241-180, Brazil. TEL 55-21-2213235, FAX 55-21-2213235, ecn@rj.sol.com.br. Ed. Antonio Alves de Couto. R&P, Adv. contact Maria Luiza Carvalho. Circ: 10,000.

610 BRA ISSN 0571-1320
ARS CURANDI. CLINICA MEDICA. Text in Portuguese. 1968. m. BRL 120, USD 145.20 (effective 2000). adv. back issues avail. *Refereed.* **Document type:** *Academic/Scholarly.* **Description:** Publishes a variety of research and clinical articles in general-practice medicine.
Indexed: INIS Atomind.
Published by: Elea Ciencia Editorial Ltda., Rua Haddock Lobo, 86 Andar 6, Estacio, Rio De Janeiro, RJ 20260-132, Brazil. TEL 55-21-293-2112, FAX 55-21-293-7818, elea@openlink.com.br. Ed. Luiz Augusto Rodrigues. Adv. contact Alexandre Augusto Rodrigues.

616 ITA ISSN 1123-1378
ARTERIOSCLEROSI NEWS. Text in Italian. 1994. 3/yr. adv. **Document type:** *Newsletter.*
Published by: (Societa Italiana per lo Studio dell'Arteriosclerosi), C I C Edizioni Internazionali s.r.l., Corso Trieste 42, Rome, RM 00198, Italy. TEL 39-06-8412673, FAX 39-06-8412688, info@gruppocic.it, 1160199510. Ed. G Ricci. adv.: B&W page ITL 3,100,000, color page ITL 3,900,000; trim 210 x 290.

▼ **ATKINS: A PASSION FOR HEALTHY LIVING.** see *NUTRITION AND DIETETICS*

M

616 016 USA ISSN 0271-1303
AUDIO-DIGEST INTERNAL MEDICINE. Text in English. 1954. s-m. USD 168 (effective 2000). index. *Refereed.*
Media: Audio cassette/tape.
Published by: Audio-Digest Foundation (Subsidiary of: California Medical Association), 1577 E Chevy Chase Dr, Glendale, CA 91206. TEL 213-245-8505, 800-423-2308, FAX 818-240-7379, 800-845-4375. Ed. Claron L Oakley. Circ: (controlled).

616 USA ISSN 1099-4521
BARIATRICIAN. Variant title: American Journal of Bariatric Medicine. Text in English. 1988. q. USD 48 domestic; USD 72 foreign (effective 2001). adv. illus, stat, tr.lit. reprints avail. *Refereed.* **Document type:** *Journal, Trade, Academic/Scholarly.* **Description:** Deals with various aspects of the medical treatment of overweight, obesity and associated conditions, and with administrative aspects of operating a bariatrics practice.
Published by: American Society of Bariatric Physicians, 5453 East Evans Place, Denver, CO 80222-5234. TEL 303-770-2526, FAX 303-779-4834, bariatric@asbp.org, http://www.asbp.org. Ed. Lola M Fehr. R&P, Adv. contact Diane Hawken. B&W page USD 800, color page USD 1,400; trim 11 x 8.5. Circ: 50 (paid); 1,100 (controlled).

616 GBR ISSN 0956-3075
CODEN: CICAEQ
CLINICAL INTENSIVE CARE; international journal of critical care medicine. Text in English. 1989. bi-m. GBP 76 in the European Union to individuals; USD 122 in North Africa to individuals; GBP 88 rest of world to individuals; GBP 157 in the European Union to institutions; USD 251 in North America to institutions; GBP 178 rest of world to institutions; GBP 30 per issue in the European Union price applies to current subscr, year; USD 48 per issue in North America price applies to current subscr, year; GBP 30 per issue rest of world price applies to current subscr, year (effective 2001); Online access free with print subscr.. adv. bk.rev. abstr, illus. index. 64 p./no. back issues avail.; reprints avail. *Refereed.* **Document type:** *Journal, Academic/Scholarly.* **Description:** Aims for rapid publication of original research, case reports and state-of-the-art reviews in all areas of critical care.
Related titles: Online - full content ed.: 2000 (issues from 1995 onwards available). free; Online free with print (from EBSCO Publishing); Online - full text ed.: (from CatchWord Ltd., RoweCom Information Quest).
Indexed: Excerp.Med.
—BLDSC (3286.293910), CatchWord, CISTI, EMDOCS, GNLM, KNAW.
Published by: BIOS Scientific Publishers Ltd., 9 Newtec Pl, Magdalen Rd, Oxford, Berks OX4 1RE, United Kingdom. TEL 44-1865-726286, FAX 44-1865-200386, cic@bios.co.uk, mansell@bios.co.uk, http://www.bios.co.uk/journals/cic/intensivej.htm. Ed. Dr. E D Bennett. Pub. Lisa Mansell. R&P Andrea Bosher. Adv. contact Amanda Whiting. Circ: 185 (paid). **Dist. by:** Turpin Distribution Services Ltd., Blackhorse Rd, Letchworth, Herts SG6 1HN, United Kingdom. TEL 44-1462-488900, FAX 44-1462-483011.

CLINICS ATLAS OF OFFICE PROCEDURES. see *MEDICAL SCIENCES*

616 JPN ISSN 1342-4904
CODEN: CTKEFK
COMPLICATION/TONYOBYO TO KEKKAN. Text in Japanese. 1996. 2/yr. JPY 2,400 per issue (effective 1998). **Document type:** *Academic/Scholarly.*
—CASDDS.
Published by: Medikaru Rebyusha/Medical Review Co., Ltd., 7-3 Hirano-Machi 1-chome, Chuo-ku, Osaka-shi 541-0046, Japan. TEL 81-6-223-1556, FAX 81-6-223-1414, medrev@osk2.3web.ne.jp.

616 USA ISSN 1042-9646
CONTEMPORARY INTERNAL MEDICINE✱ . Text in English. 1989. m. USD 94 domestic to individuals; USD 116 in Canada to individuals; USD 171 elsewhere to individuals; USD 165 domestic to institutions; USD 193 in Canada to institutions; USD 219 elsewhere to institutions. adv. *Refereed.* **Document type:** *Trade, Academic/Scholarly.* **Description:** Provides clinically practical and authoritative information in areas of high interest to internists and specialist physicians.
—Infotrieve. **CCC.**
Published by: Appleton & Lange, Journal Division (Subsidiary of: Simon & Schuster Company), 11 W 19th St, New York, CT 10011-4209. TEL 203-406-4500, FAX 203-406-4603. Ed. Harriet Lebowitz. Circ: 75,000 (controlled). **Subscr. to:** PO Box 89, Congers, NY 10920-0086.

616 GBR ISSN 0968-6053
CODEN: CDPAFN
CURRENT DIAGNOSTIC PATHOLOGY. Text in English. 1994. bi-m. GBP 135 to individuals; GBP 271 to institutions (effective 2002). adv. bk.rev. **Document type:** *Academic/Scholarly.* **Description:** Publishes reviews in histopathology and cytology for the diagnostic pathollist.
Related titles: Online - full text ed.: (from EBSCO Publishing, O C L C Online Computer Library Center, Inc., Swets Blackwell, IDEAL Online Library).
—BLDSC (3496.315000), GNLM.
Published by: Churchill Livingstone (Subsidiary of: Harcourt Publishers Ltd.), Robert Stevenson House, 1-3 Baxter's Pl, Leith Walk, Edinburgh, Midlothian EH1 3AF, United Kingdom. TEL 44-131-556-2424, FAX 44-131-459-1177, cservice@harcourt.com, http://www.harcourt-international.com/journals/cdip. Ed. Simon Harrington. R&P Catherine John TEL 212-424-4200. Adv. contact David Dunnachie. **Subscr. to:** Harcourt Publishers Ltd., Foots Cray High St, Sidcup, Kent DA14 5HP, United Kingdom. TEL 44-20-8308-5700, FAX 44-20-8309-0807.

616 NLD ISSN 0272-1465
CURRENT HISTOPATHOLOGY. Text in English. irreg., latest vol.23, 1993. price varies. *Refereed.* **Document type:** *Monographic series.*
—CISTI.
Published by: Kluwer Academic Publishers Group (Subsidiary of: Wolters Kluwer N.V.), Spuiboulevard 50, PO Box 17, Dordrecht 3300 AA, Netherlands. FAX 31-78-639-2254, services@wkap.nl, http://www.wkap.nl. **Dist. by:** Journals Department, PO Box 322, Dordrecht 3300 AH, Netherlands. FAX 31-78-654-6474.

616.026 BRA ISSN 1413-9979
DIAGNOSTICO & TRATAMENTO. Text in English; Summaries in Portuguese. 1996. bi-m. adv. bk.rev. back issues avail. *Refereed.* **Document type:** *Academic/Scholarly.*
Related titles: Online - full text ed.
Published by: (Associacao Paulista de Medicina), Lemos Editorial & Graficos Ltda., Rua Rui Barbosa, 70, B Vista, Sao Paulo, SP 01326-010, Brazil. TEL 55-11-251-4300, FAX 55-11-251-4300, lemospl@netpoint.com.br, http://www.lemos.com.br. Ed. Dr. Alvaro Nagib Atallah. Adv. contact Paulo Lemos. Circ: 50,000 (controlled).

616 FRA ISSN 1283-0836
ENCYCLOPEDIE MEDICO-CHIRURGICALE. TRATADO DE PRAXIS MEDICA. Key Title: Praxis Medica (Tomos I a VII). Cover title: Tratado de Praxis Medica. Text in Spanish. 1998. 7 base vols. plus q. updates. bibl, charts, illus. *Refereed.* **Document type:** *Academic/Scholarly.* **Description:** Offers Spanish-speaking general practitioners a comprehensive, up-to-date reference for diagnosing and treating all types of ailments, disorders, and conditions.
Published by: Elsevier Paris, Editions Scientifiques et Medicales (Subsidiary of: Reed Elsevier plc. group), 23 rue Linois, Paris 75015, France. TEL 33-1-45589110, FAX 33-1-45589425, mgarcia@elsevier-fr.com, http://www.elsevier.fr, http://www.elsevier.com.

616 USA ISSN 0953-6205
CODEN: EJIMEJ
EUROPEAN JOURNAL OF INTERNAL MEDICINE. Text in English; Summaries in French. 1990. bi-m. EUR 223 in Europe to institutions; JPY 28,100 in Japan to institutions; USD 249 elsewhere to institutions (effective 2002). *Refereed.* **Document type:** *Academic/Scholarly.* **Description:** Covers all aspects of internal medicine.
Related titles: Online - full text ed.: (from ingenta, Swets Blackwell, ScienceDirect).
Indexed: Excerp.Med.
—BLDSC (3829.730700), EMDOCS, GNLM, KNAW.
Published by: Elsevier Science, PO Box 945, New York, NY 10159-0945. TEL 212-989-5800, FAX 212-633-3990, usinfo-f@elsevier.com, http://www.elsevier.com/locate/ejim. Ed. U Carcassi. Circ: 1,200. **Subscr. outside the Americas to:** Elsevier Science BV, PO Box 211, Amsterdam 1000 AE, Netherlands. TEL 31-20-485-3757.

616 GBR
EUROPEAN JOURNAL OF PALLIATIVE CARE. Text in English. 1994. bi-m. GBP 48 in Europe; USD 75 in United States; GBP 72 elsewhere. **Document type:** *Academic/Scholarly.* **Description:** Covers the many clinical and social aspects of palliative care.
Related titles: French ed.
Indexed: Brit.Nur.Ind., CINAHL.
—BLDSC (3829.733390).
Published by: (European Association for Palliative Care), Hayward Medical Communications Ltd., Covent Garden, Seven Dials Warehouse, 44 Earlham St, London WC2H 9LA, United Kingdom. TEL 44-20-7240-4493, FAX 44-20-7240-4479, admin@hayward.co.uk, http://www.ejpc.co.uk, http://www.hayward.co.uk. Ed. Dr. Andrew Hoy. Circ: 2,000. **Subscr. to:** Rosemary House, Lanwades Park, Kentford, Near, Newmarket, Suffolk CB8 7PW, United Kingdom. TEL 44-1638-751515, FAX 44-1638-751517.

EXCERPTA MEDICA. SECTION 6: INTERNAL MEDICINE. see *MEDICAL SCIENCES—Abstracting, Bibliographies, Statistics*

616.042 GBR ISSN 1462-3994
EXPERT REVIEWS IN MOLECULAR MEDICINE. Text in English. 1997. irreg. (electronic journal constantly updated). free. bk.rev. back issues avail. **Description:** Comprises an expanding collection of review articles in the area of molecular medicine.
Media: Online - full text.
Published by: (University of Cambridge, School of Clinical Medicine, Clinical and Biomedical Computing Unit), Cambridge University Press, Edinburgh Bldg, Shaftesbury Rd, Cambridge CB2 2RU, United Kingdom. FAX 44-1223-315052, information@cup.cam.ac.uk, information@cambridge.org, http://www.cup.cam.ac.uk/, http://www.uk.cambridge.org/journals/pmu. Eds. Louise Walsh, Rebecca Jones, Rosemary Boddington.

616 DEU ISSN 0931-1130
FORTSCHRITTE IN DER HOCHDRUCKFORSCHUNG. Text in German. 1986. irreg., latest vol.5, 1992. **Document type:** *Academic/Scholarly.*
—CISTI.
Published by: W. Zuckschwerdt Verlag GmbH, Industriestr 1, Germering 82110, Germany. TEL 49-89-894349-0, FAX 49-89-89434950. Ed. J Rosenthal.

616 CHN
GUOWAI YIXUE (NEIKEXUE FENCE)/FOREIGN MEDICAL SCIENCES (INTERNAL MEDICINE). Text in Chinese. m.
Published by: Zhongshan Yike Daxue/Sun Yat-sen Medical University, 74 Zhongshan Erlu, Guangzhou, Guangdong 510089, China. TEL 778223. Ed. Liang Sudi.

616 USA
I M ADVANTAGE. Text in English. m. membership only. **Document type:** *Newsletter.* **Description:** Covers the socioeconomics of internal medicine practice.
Formerly: Internist's Intercom (0164-6419)
Published by: American Society of Internal Medicine, 2011 Pennsylvania Ave, N W, Ste 800, Washington, DC 20006-1834. TEL 202-835-2746, FAX 202-835-0441, blauter@asim.org. Ed. Barbara Lauter. R&P Stacy Rosenberg. Circ: 20,000.

616.1 IND ISSN 0377-9343
THE INDIAN JOURNAL OF CHEST DISEASES AND ALLIED SCIENCES. Text in English. 1959. q. INR 500 domestic; USD 75 foreign (effective 2001). adv. bk.rev. abstr, illus. 60 p./no. 2 cols./p. *Refereed.* **Document type:** *Academic/Scholarly.* **Description:** Contains original research in cardiopulmonary medicine, including radiology. Provides case studies.
Formerly (until vol.18, Jan. 1976): Indian Journal of Chest Diseases
Related titles: CD-ROM ed.
Indexed: Biol.Abstr., Chem.Abstr., Curr.Cont. (coverage dropped), Dent.Ind., Dok.Arbeitsmed., Excerp.Med. (until 19??), ExtraMED, Helminthol.Abstr., Ind.Med. (1976-).
—BLDSC (4410.710000), CISTI, GNLM, ingenta. **CCC.**
Published by: University of Delhi, Vallabhbhai Patel Chest Institute, New Delhi 110 007, India. TEL 91-11-7667102, FAX 91-11-7667420, vpci@delnet.ren.nic.in, http://www.vpci.org. Ed., Pub. V K Vijayan. adv.: color page INR 3,750, page INR 2,500; 24 x 17. Circ: 1,000. **Co-sponsor:** National College of Chest Physicians.

616 USA ISSN 1056-9286
R11 CODEN: IMEIEI
INTERNAL MEDICINE. Variant title: I M. Text in English. 1980. m. USD 75 domestic; USD 99 foreign (effective 2000). **Document type:** *Trade.* **Description:** Presents current approach to diagnostic and management problems of particular interest to internists, with emphasis on cardiovascular and pulmonary medicine, gastroenterology, infectious disease, rheumatology, oncology, nephrology and allergy.
Formerly (until 1990): Internal Medicine for the Specialist (0273-6608)
Related titles: Microform ed.: (from PQC); Online - full text ed.: (from Gale Group).

M

Indexed: Excerp.Med., Inpharma, Neurosci.Cit.Ind., Pharm.&Out.News, Reac.
—EMDOCS, GNLM, Infotrieve, KNAW. **CCC.**
Published by: Medical Economics Co., Inc., 5 Paragon Dr, Montvale, NJ 07645-1742. Ed. Martin Di Carlantonio. Circ: 81,000.

616 USA ISSN 0195-315X
INTERNAL MEDICINE ALERT. Text in English. 1979. s-m. USD 199 domestic; USD 229 foreign; USD 17 newsstand/cover (effective 2001). index. reprints avail. **Document type:** *Newsletter.*
Incorporates (1985-1991): Diagnostic Testing Alert (8756-7474)
Related titles: Audio cassette/tape ed.; Online - full text ed.: (from Northern Light Technology, Inc., Gale Group).
Published by: American Health Consultants (Subsidiary of: Medical Economics Co., Inc.), 3525 Piedmont Rd, N E, 6 Piedmont Center, Ste 400, Atlanta, GA 30305. TEL 404-262-5476, 404-262-7436, 800-688-2421, FAX 404-262-7837, 800-284-3291, custserv@ahcpub.com, http://www.ahcpub.com. Circ: 6,345.

616 ITA
INTERNAL MEDICINE; CLINICAL AND LABORATORY. Text in Italian. 1993. 3/yr. ITL 50,000, USD 50 to individuals; ITL 60,000, USD 60 to institutions.
Published by: Pacini Editore, Via Alessandro Gherardesca, 1, Ospedaletto, PI 56121, Italy. TEL 39-050-313011, FAX 39-050-3130300, pacini@cibernet.it, http://www.cibernet.it/pacini, http://www.pacinieditore.it. Eds. A Capri, A Sagripanti.

616 AUS ISSN 1444-0903
INTERNAL MEDICINE JOURNAL. Text in English. 1971. bi-m. AUD 154 domestic to individuals; AUD 140 in New Zealand to individuals; USD 150 elsewhere to individuals; AUD 374 domestic to institutions; AUD 340 in New Zealand to institutions; USD 450 elsewhere to institutions; AUD 170 domestic to individuals print & online eds.; AUD 154 in New Zealand to individuals print & online eds.; USD 165 elsewhere to individuals print & online eds.; AUD 412 domestic to institutions print & online eds.; AUD 374 in New Zealand to institutions print & online eds.; USD 495 elsewhere to institutions print & online eds. (effective 2001). **Document type:** *Journal, Academic/Scholarly.*
Former titles (until Jan.2001): Australian and New Zealand Journal of Medicine (0004-8291); (until 1971): Australasian Annals of Medicine (0571-9283); (until 1952): Australasian College of Physicians. Proceedings
Related titles: ♦ Online - full text ed.: Internal Medicine Journal Online.
Indexed: Abstr.Hyg., Curr.Cont., Nutr.Abstr., Trop.Dis.Bull.
—BLDSC (1796.888000), ADONIS.
Published by: Blackwell Science Asia Pty Ltd, PO Box 378, Carlton South, VIC 3053, Australia. TEL 61-3-9347-0300, FAX 61-3-9347-5001, info@blacksci-asia.com.au, http://www.blacksci.co.uk/australi. Ed. Edward Byrne.

616 AUS
INTERNAL MEDICINE JOURNAL ONLINE. Text in English. bi-m. AUD 139 domestic to individuals; AUD 126 in New Zealand to individuals; USD 135 elsewhere to individuals; AUD 337 domestic to institutions; AUD 306 in New Zealand to institutions; USD 405 elsewhere to institutions (effective 2001). **Document type:** *Academic/Scholarly.*
Media: Online - full text (from Swets Blackwell, Institute for Scientific Information, RoweCom Information Quest). **Related titles:** ♦ Print ed.: Internal Medicine Journal. ISSN 1444-0903.
Published by: Blackwell Science Asia Pty Ltd, PO Box 378, Carlton South, VIC 3053, Australia. TEL 61-3-9347-0300, FAX 61-3-9347-3016, info@blacksci-asia.com.au, http://www.blacksci.co.uk/australi.

616 USA ISSN 1097-8690
INTERNAL MEDICINE NEWS. Text in English. 1968. bi-m. USD 96 (effective 2000). adv. bk.rev. **Document type:** *Newspaper.* **Description:** Covers internal medicine and associated specialties.
Former titles (until 1994): Internal Medicine News and Cardiology News (0274-5542); (until 1980): Internal Medicine News (0099-152X); (until 1975): Internal Medicine News and Diagnosis News (0099-1538); (until 1971): Internal Medicine and Diagnosis News (0012-1908); (until 1968): Diagnosis News
Related titles: Microform ed.: (from PQC).
—Infotrieve. **CCC.**
Published by: International Medical News Group, 12230 Wilkins Ave, Rockville, MD 20852. TEL 301-816-8700, FAX 301-816-8738. Ed. Mary Jo Dales. adv.: B&W page USD 8,675, color page USD 10,590. Circ: 99,995.

616 JPN ISSN 0918-2918
CODEN: IEDIEP
INTERNAL MEDICINE (TOKYO, 1992). Text and summaries in English. 1962. m. JPY 20,000 to non-members; JPY 3,000 to members; USD 270 foreign (effective 2000). abstr, charts, illus. back issues avail. *Refereed.* **Document type:** *Academic/Scholarly.*
Formerly (until 1992): Japanese Journal of Medicine (0021-5120)
Related titles: Online - full text ed.: (from Institute for Scientific Information).
Indexed: Abstr.Hyg., Biol.Abstr., Chem.Abstr., Chem.Indus.Notes, Chem.Titles, Curr.Cont., Excerp.Med., Helminthol.Abstr., INIS Atomind., Ind.Med. (1992-), Nutr.Abstr., Protozool.Abstr., Rev.Med.& Vet.Mycol., Trop.Dis.Bull.
—BLDSC (4534.880000), CASDDS, CISTI, EMDOCS, GNLM, IDS, Infotrieve, KNAW. **CCC.**
Published by: Japanese Society of Internal Medicine/Nihon Naika Gakkai, Hongo Daiichi Bldg 8F, 34-3, 3-chome, Hongo, Bunkyo-ku, Tokyo 113-8433, Japan. TEL 81-3-3813-5991, FAX 81-3-3818-1556, naika@mb.infoweb.or.jp, naika@mb.infoweb.ne.jp, http://www.niaka.or.jp, http://www.naika.or.jp. Ed. Hidehiko Saito. Pub. Satoshi Kimura. Circ: 6,500 (paid). **Dist. overseas by:** Japan Publications Trading Co. Ltd., Tokyo International, PO Box 5030, Tokyo 100-31, Japan. TEL 81-3-3292-3753; **Dist. to non-members by:** Nankodo Co. Ltd., 42-6 Hongo 3-chome, Bunkyo-ku, Tokyo 113-0033, Japan. TEL 03-3811-7239, FAX 81-3-3811-7230.

616 USA
INTERNAL MEDICINE WORLD REPORT. Text in English. 12/yr. USD 170 (effective 2000). adv. **Document type:** *Newspaper, Trade.* **Description:** Provides internists and subspecialists with comprehensive resource for the most significant and current news in worldwide health care.
Published by: Medical World Business Press, Inc. (Subsidiary of: Medical World Communications), 241 Forsgate Dr, Jamesburg, NJ 08831. TEL 732-656-1140, FAX 732-656-1142. Ed. Karen Rosenberg. Pub. Lisa M Greene. Adv. contact Mary Jo Fencel. Circ: 102,424 (controlled).

616 USA
▼ **THE INTERNET JOURNAL OF FAMILY PRACTICE.** Text in English. 2000. s-a. free per issue. adv. bk.rev. back issues avail. *Refereed.* **Document type:** *Academic/Scholarly.* **Description:** Provides information from the field of family practice medicine; contains original articles, reviews, case reports, streaming slide shows, streaming videos, letters to the editor, press releases, and meeting information.
Media: Online - full content.
Published by: Internet Scientific Publications, L.L.C., 23 Rippling Creek Dr, Sugar Land, TX 77479. TEL 281-240-1533, FAX 281-240-1533, http://www.ispub.com/. R&P, Adv. contact Oliver Wenker TEL 832-754-0335.

616 USA
▼ **THE INTERNET JOURNAL OF INTERNAL MEDICINE.** Text in English. 2000. s-a. free per issue. bk.rev. back issues avail. *Refereed.* **Document type:** *Academic/Scholarly.* **Description:** Provides information from the field of general and internal medicine; contains original articles, reviews, case reports, streaming slide shows, streaming videos, letters to the editor, press releases and meeting information.
Media: Online - full content.
Published by: Internet Scientific Publications, L.L.C., 23 Rippling Creek Dr, Sugar Land, TX 77479. TEL 281-240-1533, FAX 281-240-1533, http://www.ispub.com/. R&P, Adv. contact Hope Morrow TEL 832-754-0335.

616 DEU ISSN 0020-9554
CODEN: INTEAG
DER INTERNIST. Text in German. 1960. m. EUR 319.62 domestic; EUR 305.82 in Germany; EUR 29 newsstand/cover foreign (effective 2002). adv. bk.rev. charts, illus. index, cum.index. back issues avail.; reprint service avail. from ISI. *Refereed.* **Document type:** *Journal, Academic/Scholarly.* **Description:** Contains research articles and papers of interest to internists and general practitioners.
Related titles: Microform ed.: (from PQC); Online - full text ed.: ISSN 1432-1289 (from EBSCO Publishing, RoweCom Information Quest, Swets Blackwell, Springer LINK, Institute for Scientific Information).
Indexed: ASCA, Agri.& Environ.Biotech.Abstr. (coverage dropped), Biol.Abstr., Curr.Cont., Derwent Biotech.Abstr., Excerp.Med., INIS Atomind., Ind.Med. (1960-), Ind.Sci.Rev., Inpharma, Int.Nurs.Ind., Nutr.Abstr., Pharm.&Out.News, Reac., Sci.Cit.Ind.
—BLDSC (4557.200000), ADONIS, CASDDS, CISTI, GNLM, IDS, Infotrieve, KNAW. **CCC.**
Published by: (Berufsverband Deutscher Internisten), Springer-Verlag (Subsidiary of: BertelsmannSpringer), Tiergartenstr 17, Heidelberg 69121, Germany. TEL 49-6221-345-0, FAX 49-6221-345229, subscriptions@springer.de, http://link.springer.de/link/service/journals/00108/index.htm, http://www.springer.de. Eds. M Classen, V Diehl. **Subscr. in N. America to:** Springer-Verlag New York Inc., PO Box 2485, Secaucus, NJ 07096-2485. TEL 212-460-1500, FAX 212-473-6272. **Co-sponsor:** Deutsche Gesellschaft fuer Innere Medizin.

616 ITA ISSN 1121-9017
CODEN: IRNIE
L'INTERNISTA; giornale di medicina interna. Text and summaries in English, Italian. 1993. 3/yr. ITL 60,000; USD 60 foreign. adv. bk.rev. index. *Refereed.* **Document type:** *Academic/Scholarly.* **Description:** Provides editorials, reviews, original clinical works and case reports, news, scientific notes, and letters to the editor.
Indexed: Excerp.Med. (1994-).
—BLDSC (4557.208000), EMDOCS, GNLM.
Published by: (Ospedale Niguarda - Ca Grande), P C A Publishing, Via Clerici 12, Brusuglio Di Corman, MI 20032, Italy. TEL 39-02-6630-0802, FAX 39-02-6151239, p.c.a@galactica.it. R&P Lorna Simpson. Adv. contact Liliana Succio. color page ITL 5,000,000. Circ: 2,000.

616 DEU ISSN 0020-9570
CODEN: INPXAJ
INTERNISTISCHE PRAXIS; taegliche Praxis der gesamten Inneren Medizin. Text in German. 1961. 4/yr. EUR 162; EUR 45 newsstand/cover (effective 2002). bk.rev. abstr, bibl, charts, illus. index, cum.index every 5 yrs. reprint service avail. from PQC. **Document type:** *Journal, Academic/Scholarly.* **Description:** Practical information of interest to specialists in internal medicine. Features the latest research in the field. Includes questions and answers.
Related titles: Microfilm ed.: (from PQC).
Indexed: AMED, Biol.Abstr., Excerp.Med., Ind.Med. (coverage dropped).
—BLDSC (4557.220000), CISTI, GNLM, Infotrieve. **CCC.**
Published by: Hans Marseille Vertrieb Medizinischer Zeitschriften, Buerkleinstr 12, Munich 80538, Germany. TEL 49-89-227988, FAX 49-89-2904643, marseille-verlag@t-online.de, http://www.marseille-verlag.com. Eds. H Feiereis, R Saller. Circ: 4,800.

616.02 DEU ISSN 0344-4201
DIE INTERNISTISCHE WELT. Text in German. 1978. 6/yr. DEM 110; DEM 60 to students (effective 2001). *Refereed.* **Document type:** *Journal, Academic/Scholarly.*
Indexed: Excerp.Med., INIS Atomind.
—BLDSC (4557.220200), GNLM, Infotrieve, KNAW. **CCC.**
Published by: Schattauer GmbH, Hoelderlinstr 3, Stuttgart 70174, Germany. TEL 49-711-2298714, FAX 49-711-2298775, info@schattauer.de, http://www.schattauer.com. Ed. G Oehler. Pub. Dieter Bergemann. R&P Hannelore Hensen.

616 JPN ISSN 0021-5384
CODEN: NNGAAS
JAPANESE SOCIETY OF INTERNAL MEDICINE. JOURNAL/NIHON NAIKA GAKKAI ZASSHI. Text in Japanese. 1913. m. JPY 9,000 to non-members. adv. charts, illus. index, cum.index. **Document type:** *Academic/Scholarly.* **Description:** Covers internal medicine.
Related titles: Online - full text ed.: (from Institute for Scientific Information).
Indexed: Biol.Abstr., Curr.Cont. (coverage dropped), Dent.Ind., Ind.Med. (1913-), Int.Nurs.Ind.
—CASDDS, CISTI, GNLM, IDS, Infotrieve, KNAW. **CCC.**
Published by: Japanese Society of Internal Medicine/Nihon Naika Gakkai, Hongo Daiichi Bldg 8F, 34-3, 3-chome, Hongo, Bunkyo-ku, Tokyo 113-8433, Japan. TEL 81-3-3813-5991, FAX 81-3-3818-1556, naika@mb.infoweb.ne.jp, http://www.naika.or.jp. Ed. Hidehiko Saito. Circ: 77,000.

M

616 USA ISSN 0884-8734
R11 CODEN: JGIMEJ
JOURNAL OF GENERAL INTERNAL MEDICINE. Short title: J G I M. Text in English. m. USD 125 domestic to individuals; USD 135 in Canada & Mexico to individuals; USD 150 elsewhere to individuals; USD 195 domestic to institutions; USD 205 in Canada & Mexico to institutions; USD 220 elsewhere to institutions; USD 137.50 to individuals print & online eds. combined; USD 214.50 to institutions print & online eds. combined (effective 2001). adv. reprints avail. *Refereed.* **Document type:** *Academic/Scholarly.* **Description:** Focuses on the training and practice of the general internist.
Related titles: Online - full text ed.: ISSN 1525-1497. USD 113 to individuals; USD 176 to institutions (effective 2001) (from Ovid Technologies, Inc., EBSCO Publishing, O C L C Online Computer Library Center, Inc., RoweCom Information Quest, ingenta, Munksgaard & Blackwell Science's Synergy, Swets Blackwell, Institute for Scientific Information); ♦ Supplement: S G I M Forum.
Indexed: ASCA, Behav.Med.Abstr., Curr.Cont., Excerp.Med., INIS Atomind., Ind.Med. (1986-), Inpharma, Int.Nurs.Ind., Jrnl.Watch Wom.Hlth., NRN, Pharm.&Out.News, Reac., Rev.Med.& Vet.Mycol., SSCI (coverage dropped), THA.
—BLDSC (4987.827000), ADONIS, CISTI, EMDOCS, GNLM, IDS, ingenta, KNAW. **CCC.**
Published by: (Society for General Internal Medicine, American College of Physicians/Co-sponsor: American Society of Internal Medicine), Blackwell Science Inc., Commerce Pl, 350 Main St, Malden, MA 02148-5018. TEL 781-388-8250, 800-759-6102, FAX 781-388-8255, journals@blacksci.com, http://www.blackwell-science.com. Ed. Sankey V Williams. R&P Tracey Davies. Adv. contact Jenny Applin. Circ: 3,000.

616 615.89 USA ISSN 1522-8940
▼ **JOURNAL OF HERBAL PHARMACOTHERAPY;** innovations in clinical & applied evidence-based herbal medicinals. Text in English. 2001 (Spring). q. USD 50 domestic to individuals; USD 68 in Canada to individuals; USD 73 elsewhere to individuals; USD 75 domestic to institutions; USD 101 in Canada to institutions; USD 109 elsewhere to institutions; USD 125 domestic to libraries; USD 169 in Canada to libraries; USD 181 elsewhere to libraries (effective Aug. 2001). adv. *Refereed.* **Document type:** *Journal, Academic/Scholarly.* **Description:** Offers peer-reviewed, scientifically based articles and original research. Also assists in understanding and prescribing herbal medications.
Indexed: AMED.
—BLDSC (4997.760000), Haworth.
Published by: Haworth Press, Inc., 10 Alice St, Binghamton, NY 13904-1580. TEL 607-722-5857, 800-429-6784, FAX 607-722-6362, 800-895-0582, getinfo@haworthpressinc.com, http://www.haworthpress.com/journals/journallist.asp. Ed. Lucinda G Miller. Pub. William Cohen. R&P Ruth Ann Heath. Adv. contact Jackie Blakeslee TEL 607-722-5857 ext 346. B&W page USD 315, color page USD 550; trim 6 x 8.5.

610 GBR ISSN 0954-6820
CODEN: JINMEO
JOURNAL OF INTERNAL MEDICINE. Text in English. 1869. m., latest vol.251, 2002. GBP 78 in Europe to individuals; USD 119 in North America to individuals; GBP 78 elsewhere to individuals; GBP 369 in Europe to institutions; USD 532 in North America to institutions; GBP 369 elsewhere to institutions (effective 2002); GBP 376.20 in Europe to institutions print & online eds.; GBP 82.50 in Europe to individuals print & online eds.; USD 579.70 in North America to institutions print & online eds.; USD 130.90 in North America to individuals print & online eds.; GBP 376.20 elsewhere to institutions print & online eds.; GBP 82.50 elsewhere to individuals print & online eds. (effective 2001). adv. abstr, bibl, charts, illus. index. cum.index: vols.52-140. back issues avail. *Refereed.* **Document type:** *Academic/Scholarly.*
Formerly (until 1989): Acta Medica Scandinavica (0001-6101)
Related titles: Microform ed.: (from PQC); Online - full text ed.: ISSN 1365-2796. GBP 71 in Europe to individuals; USD 108 in North America to individuals; GBP 71 elsewhere to individuals; GBP 333 in Europe to institutions; USD 479 in North America to institutions; GBP 333 elsewhere to institutions (effective 2002) (from Ovid Technologies, Inc., EBSCO Publishing, O C L C Online Computer Library Center, Inc., RoweCom Information Quest, ingenta, Munksgaard & Blackwell Science's Synergy, Swets Blackwell, Institute for Scientific Information); ♦ Supplement: Journal of Internal Medicine. Supplement. ISSN 0955-7873.
Indexed: ASCA, Abstr.Inter.Med., Agri.& Environ.Biotech.Abstr. (coverage dropped), Biol.Abstr., C.I.S. Abstr., Chem.Abstr., Chem.Titles, Curr.Adv.Ecol.Sci., Curr.Cont., Dairy Sci.Abstr., Dent.Ind., Derwent Biotech.Abstr., Diar.Dis.Res., Energy Ind., Energy Info.Abstr., Excerp.Med., Helminthol.Abstr., INIS Atomind., Ind.Med. (1989-), Ind.Sci.Rev., Inpharma, Int.Abstr.Biol.Sci., Kidney, Med.& Surg.Dermat., NRN, Neurosci.Cit.Ind., Nutr.Abstr., Pharm.&Out.News, Protozool.Abstr., Reac., Rev.Arom.& Med.Plants, Rev.Med.& Vet.Mycol., Risk Abstr., SSCI (coverage dropped), Sci.Cit.Ind., THA.
—BLDSC (5007.548700), ADONIS, CASDDS, CISTI, EMDOCS, GNLM, IDS, ingenta, KNAW. **CCC.**
Published by: Blackwell Science Ltd., PO Box 88, Oxford OX2 0NE, United Kingdom. TEL 44-1865-206180, 44-1865-206002, FAX 44-1865-206219, jnl.orders@blacksci.co.uk, http://www.blackwell-science.com/~cgilib/jnlpage.asp?Journal=jint&File=jint, http://www.blackwellpublishing.com. Ed. Goran Holm. Pub. Allen Stevens. R&P Sophie Savage. Adv. contact Jenny Applin. Circ: 1,735.

616 GBR ISSN 0955-7873
CODEN: JIMSE3
JOURNAL OF INTERNAL MEDICINE. SUPPLEMENT. Text in English. 1989. q. adv. **Document type:** *Academic/Scholarly.*
Related titles: Online - full text ed.: (from Ovid Technologies, Inc.); ♦ Supplement to: Journal of Internal Medicine. ISSN 0954-6820.
Indexed: Chem.Abstr., Chem.Indus.Notes, Chem.Titles, Excerp.Med., Ind.Med. (1989-), Int.Abstr.Biol.Sci.
—ADONIS, CASDDS, CISTI, EMDOCS, KNAW. **CCC.**
Published by: Blackwell Science Ltd., Osney Mead, Oxford OX2 0EL, United Kingdom. TEL 44-1865-206206, FAX 44-1865-721205, journals.cs@blacksci.co.uk, http://www.blackwell-science.com. Pub. Allen Stevens. R&P Sophie Savage. Adv. contact Jenny Applin.

612.67 USA ISSN 1279-7707
QP86
JOURNAL OF NUTRITION, HEALTH AND AGING. Text in English. 1997. 3/yr. USD 80 in United States to individuals; USD 135 for 2 yrs. in United States to individuals; USD 95 foreign to individuals; USD 160 for 2 yrs. foreign to individuals; USD 120 in United States to institutions; USD 210 for 2 yrs. in United States to institutions; USD 140 foreign to institutional members; USD 245 for 2 yrs. foreign to institutions (effective 2000). **Document type:** *Academic/Scholarly.* **Description:** Features studies about nutrition's effect on the elderly, includes reports on research funding, international conferences and literature abstracts of interest to professionals in gerontology, geridrics, medicine, community health, public health, biology, social medicine, epidemiology and biostatistics.
Indexed: AgeLine, Ind.Med. (1997-), Nutr.Abstr.
—BLDSC (5024.716000).
Published by: Serdi Publishers, 320 rue Saint-Honore, Paris 75001, France. TEL 33-561-75-79-12, FAX 33-561-75-11-28, springer@springer.pub.com, http://www.springerpub.com. **Dist. in US by:** Springer Publishing Company, 536 Broadway, New York, NY 10012. TEL 212-941-7842, http://www.springerpub.com.

616 JPN ISSN 0913-2384
CODEN: KRRYEI
KAGAKU RYOHO NO RYOIKI/ANTIBIOTICS AND CHEMOTHERAPY. Text in Japanese. 1985. m. JPY 32,865 (effective 2000). **Document type:** *Academic/Scholarly.*
Indexed: Chem.Abstr., Chem.Indus.Notes, Chem.Titles.
—CASDDS, GNLM.
Published by: (Kagaku Ryoho Kenkyukai/Committee of Chemotherapy), Iyaku Journal-sha/Medicine & Drug Journal Co., Ltd., 2-8 Hirano-Machi 3-chome, Chuo-ku, Osaka-shi 541-0046, Japan. TEL 81-6-6202-7280, FAX 81-6-6202-5295, iyakujor@skyblue.ocn.ne.jp, http://www.so-net.ne.jp/medipro/iyaku.

616 KOR ISSN 0494-4712
R97.7.K6 CODEN: TNHCA3
KOREAN JOURNAL OF INTERNAL MEDICINE/DAIHAN NAIGWA HAGHOI JABJI. Text in Korean. 1958. m. **Document type:** *Academic/Scholarly.*
Indexed: Excerp.Med. (1993-), INIS Atomind., Ind.Med. (1986-).
—BLDSC (5113.561000), CASDDS, CISTI, EMDOCS, GNLM.
Published by: Korean Association of Internal Medicine/Daihan Naigwa Haghoi, Korean Medical Association Bldg., PO Box 2062, Seoul 140031, Korea, S..

L M S ALERT. HYPERLIPIDAEMIA. (Literature Monitoring and Evaluation Service) see *MEDICAL SCIENCES—Abstracting, Bibliographies, Statistics*

616 JPN ISSN 0025-7699
CODEN: MDCHBH
MEDICINA; journal of internal medicine. Text in Japanese. 1964. m. JPY 30,950. adv. charts, illus. index.
Indexed: Chem.Abstr., Chem.Indus.Notes, Chem.Titles, INIS Atomind.
—BLDSC (5532.400000), CASDDS, CISTI.
Published by: Igaku-Shoin Ltd., 5-24-3 Hongo, Bunkyo-ku, Tokyo 113-0033, Japan. TEL 81-3-3817-5717. Circ: 19,000.

616 MEX ISSN 0186-4866
MEDICINA INTERNA. Text in Spanish; Summaries in English, Spanish. 1985. q. MXP 210, USD 40 (effective 1996 & 1997). *Refereed.* **Document type:** *Academic/Scholarly.* **Description:** Contains original articles, research reports, review articles, clinical cases and notices related to internal medicine.
Published by: (Asociacion de Medicina Interna de Mexico), Obsidiana Editores S.A., CZDA DE TLALPAN 2365, Col Ciudad Jardin, Mexico City, DF 04370, Mexico. TEL 52-5-689-9133. Eds. Dr. Manuel Ramiro Hernandez, Dr. Oscar Saita Kamino. Pub. Jorge Godoy-Gutierrez. Circ: 3,000. **Dist. by:** Distribuidora Editorial de Mexico SA de CV, P.O. Box 76-026, Mexico City, DF 04201, Mexico. TEL 52-5-544-7953, FAX 52-5-689-6545.

616.026 ROM ISSN 1220-5818
MEDICINA INTERNA. Text in Romanian; Summaries in English, French, German, Russian. 1905. q. USD 20. adv. bk.rev. abstr, bibl, charts, illus.
Former titles (until 1991): Revista de Medicina Interna, Neurologie, Psihiatrie, Neuro-Chirurgie, Dermato-Venerologie. Series Medicina Interna (1220-0905); (until 1974): Medicina Interna (0025-7869); (until 1954): Revista Stiintelor Medicale (1013-414X)
Indexed: Biol.Abstr., Chem.Abstr., Dent.Ind., INIS Atomind., Ind.Med. (1991-).
—CISTI, GNLM.
Published by: Societatea de Medicina Interna, Str. Progresului 8, Bucharest 70754, Romania. **Subscr. to:** ILEXIM, Str. 13 Decembrie 3, PO Box 136-137, Bucharest 70116, Romania.

616.042 USA
METHODS IN MOLECULAR MEDICINE. Text in English. 1996. irreg. price varies. adv. **Document type:** *Monographic series, Academic/Scholarly.* **Description:** Contains protocols essential to the study of the molecular basis of disease processes.
Related titles: Online - full text ed.
—BLDSC (5748.202250).
Published by: Humana Press Inc., 999 Riverview Dr, Ste 208, Totowa, NJ 07512. TEL 973-256-1699, FAX 973-256-8341, humana@humanapr.com, http://humanapress.com. R&P Richard Hrsuka. Adv. contact Thomas B Lanigan Jr.

616 ITA ISSN 0026-4806
R61 CODEN: MIMEAO
MINERVA MEDICA; rivista mensile di medicina interna. Text in Italian; Summaries in English, Italian. 1909. m. (in 10 vols.). USD 125 to individuals; USD 165 to institutions (effective 2000 - 2001). adv. bibl, illus. *Refereed.* **Document type:** *Academic/Scholarly.*
Supersedes (1963-1969): Minerva Medica Siciliana (0026-4822); Which was formerly (1869-1963): Gazzetta Medica Siciliana (0540-1585)
Related titles: Microform ed.: (from PQC); ♦ Supplement: Istituzione Italiana di Cardio-Chirurgia. Giornale. ISSN 0391-1969.
Indexed: Agri.& Environ.Biotech.Abstr. (coverage dropped), Biol.Abstr., C.I.S. Abstr., Chem.Abstr., Curr.Adv.Cancer Res., Curr.Adv.Ecol.Sci., Curr.Cont. (coverage dropped), Dent.Ind., Derwent Biotech.Abstr., Dok.Arbeitsmed., Excerp.Med., Helminthol.Abstr., INIS Atomind., Ind.Med. (1909-), Inpharma, Nutr.Abstr., Reac., Ref.Zh., Rev.Med.& Vet.Mycol.
—CASDDS, CISTI, GNLM, KNAW.
Published by: Edizioni Minerva Medica, Corso Bramante, 83-85, Turin, TO 10126, Italy. TEL 39-11-678282, FAX 39-11-674502. Ed. M L Benzo. Pub. Alberto Oliaro. Adv. contact F Filippo. B&W page USD 1,200, color page USD 2,000; trim 270 x 190. Circ: 5,000 (paid).

616 JPN ISSN 0022-1961
NAIKA/INTERNAL MEDICINE (TOKYO, 1958). Text in Japanese. 1958. m. JPY 47,000. adv. charts, illus. s-a. index. **Description:** Covers internal medicine.
Indexed: Aqua.Sci.& Fish.Abstr., Aquacult.Abstr., Biol.Abstr., Curr.Adv.Cancer Res., Environ.Sci.Poll.Mgmt., INIS Atomind., So.Pac.Per.Ind.
—BLDSC (4534.890000), CISTI, GNLM.

Published by: Nankodo Co. Ltd., 42-6 Hongo 3-chome, Bunkyo-ku, Tokyo 113-0033, Japan. FAX 03-3811-7230. Ed. Kiyoshi Kurokawa. Circ: 13,000.

616 TWN ISSN 1016-7390
R97.7.C5
NEIKE XUEZHI* /JOURNAL OF INTERNAL MEDICINE R O C. Text in Chinese. 1990. q.
Published by: Zhonghua Minguo Neike Yixuehui/Society of Internal Medicine of Taiwan, Zhong Xiao Xi Lu, Sec.1, no.50, 22nd Fl, Rm 26, Taipei, Taiwan. TEL 886-2-23758068, FAX 886-2-23758072, intmed@tpts1.seed.net.tw, http://www.sim.org.tw/.

616 NLD ISSN 0300-2977
CODEN: NLJMAV
NETHERLANDS JOURNAL OF MEDICINE. Text in English. 1958. m. NLG 1,401, EUR 635.75 in Europe to institutions; JPY 8,800 in Japan to institutions; USD 711 elsewhere to institutions (effective 2001). adv. bk.rev. bibl, charts, illus. back issues avail. *Refereed.* **Document type:** *Academic/Scholarly.* **Description:** Publishes original articles and reviews in all relevant fields of internal medicine.
Formerly (until 1973): Folia Medica Neerlandica (0015-5624)
Related titles: Microform ed.: (from PQC); Online - full text ed.: (from ingenta, ScienceDirect, Swets Blackwell, Institute for Scientific Information).
Indexed: ASCA, Abstr.Hyg., Biol.Abstr., Chem.Abstr., Chem.Indus.Notes, Chem.Titles, Curr.Adv.Biochem., Curr.Cont., Derwent Biotech.Abstr., Excerp.Med., Helminthol.Abstr., INIS Atomind., Ind.Med. (1973-), Ind.Sci.Rev., Inpharma, Int.Abstr.Biol.Sci., Int.Nurs.Ind., NRN, Nutr.Abstr., Pharm.&Out.News, Reac., Rev.Appl.Entomol., Rev.Med.& Vet.Mycol., Sci.Cit.Ind., Sugar Ind.Abstr.
—BLDSC (6077.003000), CASDDS, CISTI, EMDOCS, GNLM, IDS, Infotrieve, KNAW. **CCC.**
Published by: (Nederlandse Internisten Vereniging), Elsevier Science BV, PO Box 211, Amsterdam 1000 AE, Netherlands. TEL 31-20-485-3757, FAX 31-20-485-3432, TELEX 18582 ESPA NL, nlinfo-f@elsevier.nl; usinfo-f@elsevier.com; forinfo-kyf04035@niftyserve.or.jp, http://www.elsevier.com/locate/nljmed. Circ: 1,600. **Subscr. in Australasia and the Far East to:** Elsevier Science (Singapore) Pte Ltd, No.1 Temasek Ave, 17-01 Millenia Tower, Singapore 039192, Singapore. TEL 65-434-3727, FAX 65-337-2230, asiainfo@elsevier.com.sg; **Subscr. in Japan to:** Elsevier Science Inc - Japan Regional Office, 9-15 Higashi-Azabu 1-chome, Minato-ku, Tokyo 106-0044, Japan. TEL 81-3-5561-5033, FAX 81-3-5561-5047, info@elsevier.co.jp; **Subscr. in the Americas to:** Elsevier Science, PO Box 945, New York, NY 10159-0945. TEL 212-633-3730, 888-437-4636, FAX 212-633-3680, usinfo-f@elsevier.com, http://www.elsevier.com. **Dist. by:** Elsevier Science (Brazil).

NIHON SHOKAKI NAISHIKYO GAKKAI KOSHIN'ETSU CHIHOKAI ZASSHI/ENDOSCOPIC FORUM FOR DIGESTIVE DISEASE. see *MEDICAL SCIENCES—Gastroenterology*

THE ORIGINAL INTERNIST; Official publication of the AIMA (American Integrative Medical Association). see *MEDICAL SCIENCES—Chiropractic, Homeopathy, Osteopathy*

616 ITA ISSN 1127-4867
▼ **OSPEDALI SAN CAMILLO E FORLANINI. ANNALI.** Text in Italian; Summaries in English. 1999. q. ITL 180,000, USD 107 (effective 2000). **Document type:** *Academic/Scholarly.*
Published by: (Azienda Ospedaliera San Camillo - Forlanini), Il Pensiero Scientifico Editore s.r.l., Via Bradano, 3-C, Rome, RM 00199, Italy. TEL 39-06-862821, FAX 39-06-86282250, pensiero@pensiero.it, http://www.pensiero.it. Ed. Franco Salvati. Pub. Francesco De Fiore. Circ: 2,000.

616 PHL ISSN 0556-0071
PHILIPPINE JOURNAL OF INTERNAL MEDICINE. Text in English. 1963. bi-m. **Document type:** *Academic/Scholarly.*
Related titles: CD-ROM ed.
Indexed: Excerp.Med., ExtraMED, INIS Atomind.
—EMDOCS, GNLM.
Published by: Philippine College of Physicians, Facilities Central Bldg, 548 Shaw Blvd, Mandaluyong Mm, Philippines. TEL 2-780233.

616.026 POL ISSN 0032-3772
CODEN: PAMWAL
POLSKIE ARCHIWUM MEDYCYNY WEWNETRZNEJ/ POLISH ARCHIVES OF INTERNAL MEDICINE. Text in English, Polish; Summaries in English. 1923. m. PLZ 120 domestic to non-members; USD 30 foreign to non-members; PLZ 96 domestic to members; USD 24 foreign to members; PLZ 216 domestic to institutions; USD 54 foreign to institutions (effective 2000). adv. bk.rev. charts, illus. index. back issues avail. *Refereed.* **Document type:** *Academic/Scholarly.* **Description:** Covers internal medicine.
Indexed: Biol.Abstr., Chem.Abstr., Dent.Ind., Excerp.Med. (until 1993, 1995-), INIS Atomind., Ind.Med. (1923-).
—BLDSC (6546.500000), CASDDS, CISTI, GNLM.
Published by: Towarzystwo Internistow Polskich/Polish Society of Internal Medicine, c/o Szpital Praski, III Oddzial Wewnetrzny, Pl Weteranow 4, Warsaw 03701, Poland. TEL 48-22-6190897, FAX 48-22-6189666. Ed. Artur Czyzyk. R&P Janusz Bolanowski TEL 48-71-3285487. Adv. contact Jozef Malolepszy TEL 48-71-3700102. Circ: 4,100 (paid and controlled).

616 FRA ISSN 0248-8663
CODEN: RMEIDE
LA REVUE DE MEDECINE INTERNE. Text in French; Summaries in English, French. 1962; N.S. 1980. m. EUR 267 in Europe to individuals; USD 334 elsewhere to individuals; EUR 312 in Europe to institutions; USD 392 elsewhere to institutions (effective 2002). adv. bk.rev. illus. index. *Refereed.* **Document type:** *Academic/Scholarly.* **Description:** Covers internal medicine.
Formerly (until 1980): Coeur et Medecine Interne (0010-0234)
Related titles: Microform ed.: N.S. (from PQC); Online - full text ed.: (from ingenta, Swets Blackwell, Institute for Scientific Information).
Indexed: ASCA, Abstr.Hyg., Biol.Abstr., C.I.S. Abstr., Chem.Abstr., Curr.Adv.Ecol.Sci., Curr.Cont., Excerp.Med., Ind.Med. (1980-), Ind.Vet., Inpharma, Int.Abstr.Biol.Sci., Int.Nurs.Ind., Nutr.Abstr., Pharm.&Out.News, Protozool.Abstr., Reac., Rev.Appl.Entomol., Rev.Med.& Vet.Mycol., SSCI (coverage dropped), Sugar Ind.Abstr., Trop.Dis.Bull.
—BLDSC (7930.940000), CISTI, EMDOCS, GNLM, IDS, Infotrieve, KNAW. **CCC.**
Published by: (Societe Nationale Francaise de Medecine Interne), Elsevier Paris, Editions Scientifiques et Medicales (Subsidiary of: Reed Elsevier plc. group), 23 rue Linois, Paris 75015, France. TEL 33-1-71724500, FAX 33-1-71724664, http://www.elsevier.com/locate/revmed. Eds. B Devulder, C Canuel. **Subscr. to:** Elsevier Science.

616.026 ROM ISSN 1220-4749
CODEN: RRINEH
ROMANIAN JOURNAL OF INTERNAL MEDICINE/REVUE ROUMAINE DE MEDECINE INTERNE. Text in English, French, German, Russian. 1964. 4/yr. bk.rev. charts, illus. index. reprint service avail. from PQC. **Document type:** *Academic/Scholarly.* **Description:** Contains reviews, articles, results of experimental studies and new book information.
Formerly (until 1990): Revue Roumaine de Medecine. Serie Medecine Interne (0377-1202); Which supersedes in part (in 1975): Revue Roumaine de Medecine (0303-822X); Which was formed by the 1974 merger of: Revue Roumaine de Neurologie et de Psychiatrie (0301-7303); Which was formerly (1964-1974): Revue Roumaine de Neurologie (0035-3981); Revue Roumaine d'Endocrinologie (0035-4015); Revue Roumaine de Medecine Interne (0035-3973); Which was formerly (1964-1974): Revue de Sciences Medicales (0484-8632)
Related titles: Microform ed.: (from PQC).
Indexed: Biol.Abstr., Chem.Abstr., Curr.Cont. (coverage dropped), Environ.Sci.Poll.Mgmt., Excerp.Med., Helminthol.Abstr., Ind.Med. (1991-), Nutr.Abstr., Pollut.Abstr., PsycInfo, Risk Abstr.
—BLDSC (8019.632000), CASDDS, CISTI, GNLM, KNAW.
Published by: (Academia de Stiinte Medicale), Editura Academiei Romane, Calea 13 Septembrie 13, Bucharest 76117, Romania. Ed. S Purice. Circ: 1,500. **Dist. by:** Rodipet S.A.. TEL 401-618-5103, FAX 401-222-6407.

616 USA
S G I M FORUM. Text in English. m. **Description:** Seeks to provide a forum for information and opinions of interest to SGIM members and to general internists and those engaged in the study, teaching or operation of general internal medicine.
Related titles: Online - full text ed.: (from Ovid Technologies, Inc.); ♦ Supplement to: Journal of General Internal Medicine. ISSN 0884-8734.

Published by: Society of General Internal Medicine, 2011 Pennsylvania Ave, N W, Ste 800, Washington, DC 20006-1813. TEL 202-393-1662, 800-822-3060, erhodes@gwuvm.gwu.edu. Ed. Harry Selker.

616 USA ISSN 1048-6755
TODAY IN MEDICINE. INTERNAL MEDICINE REPORT. Text in English. 1990. m.
Published by: Data Centrum Communications, Inc., 21 W 38th St, 4th fl, New York, NY 10018.

616 ITA ISSN 1125-0747
UNIVERSITA DI FERRARA. ANNALI. SEZIONE 12: MEDICINA INTERNA. Text in Italian. 1953. a.
Published by: (Universita di Ferrara), Casa Editrice Leo S. Olschki, Viuzzo Del Pozzetto, Florence, FI 50126, Italy. TEL 39-55-6530684, FAX 39-55-6530214.

616 BGR ISSN 0506-2772
CODEN: VTBLAU
VUTRESHNI BOLESTI. Text in Bulgarian; Summaries in English, Russian. 1969. q., latest vol.33, 2001. BGL 20,000 domestic; USD 50 foreign; BGL 2,500 newsstand/cover (effective 2001 - 2002). adv. abstr, bibl, illus. index. 56 p./no. back issues avail. *Refereed.* **Document type:** *Abstract/Index, Academic/Scholarly, Bibliography.* **Description:** Includes articles, reports, and reviews on internal medicine.
Indexed: Abstr.Bulg.Sci.Med.Lit., INIS Atomind., Ind.Med. (1962-).
—CASDDS, CISTI, GNLM.
Published by: (Bulgaria. Ministerstvo na Narodnoto Zdrave), Meditsinski Universitet - Sofia, Tsentur za Informatsiia po Meditsina/Medical University - Sofia, Medical Information Center, 1Sv Georgi Sofiiski ul 1, Sofia 1431, Bulgaria. TEL 359-2-5222342, FAX 359-2-9522393, mutafov@sun.medun.acad.bg, http://www.medun.acad.bg. Ed. Dr. Ch Nachev. Adv. contact Dr. Christo Mutafov. B&W page USD 50, color page USD 150; 18 x 27. Circ: 500. **Co-sponsor:** Nauchno Druzhestvo po V'treshni Bolesti.

617 CHN
ZHONGGUO GANDAN WAIKE ZAZHI/CHINESE JOURNAL OF HEPATOBILIARY SURGERY. Text in Chinese. bi-m. USD 22.80, USD 3.80 (effective 2001). **Document type:** *Academic/Scholarly.*
Published by: China International Book Trading Corp/Zhongguo Guoji Tushu Maoyi Zonggongsi cibtc@mail.cibtc.com.cn, http://www.cibtc.com.cn. **Dist. by:** 35, Chegongzhuang Xilu, Haidian District, Beijing 100044, China.

616 CHN ISSN 1005-2194
ZHONGGUO SHIYONG NEIKE ZAZHI/CHINESE JOURNAL OF PRACTICAL INTERNAL MEDICINE. Text in Chinese; Abstracts in English. 1981. m. CNY 48, USD 60 (effective 1997 & 1998). adv. *Refereed.* **Document type:** *Academic/Scholarly.* **Description:** Features new developments and methods of practical diagnosis, treatment and prevention of internal diseases.
Formerly: Shiyong Neike Zazhi - Journal of Practical Internal Medicine (1001-084X)
Published by: Zhongguo Shiyong Yixue Zazhishe/Chinese Journals' Society of Practical Medicine, 44-1, Jixian St, Heping-qu, Shenyang, Liaoning 110005, China. TEL 86-24-3395218, FAX 86-24-3391212. Eds. Qingli Wang, Runjiang Yu. R&P Qingli Wang. Adv. contact Jianguo Li. page USD 2,000. Circ: 80,000.

ZHONGGUO YIXUE WENZHAI (NEIKE XUE). see *MEDICAL SCIENCES—Abstracting, Bibliographies, Statistics*

616.362 CHN ISSN 1007-3418
ZHONGHUA GANZANGBING ZAZHI/CHINESE JOURNAL OF HEPATOLOGY. Text in Chinese. 1996. bi-m. USD 27; USD 4.50 newsstand/cover (effective 2001). **Document type:** *Academic/Scholarly.*
Indexed: Ind.Med.
—BLDSC (3180.350500).
Published by: Zhonghua Yixuehui Zazhishe, 42 Dongsi Xidajie, Beijing 100710, China. **Dist. by:** China International Book Trading Corp, 35, Chegongzhuang Xilu, Haidian District, Beijing 100044, China. TEL 86-1-68413849, FAX 86-1-68412048, cibtc@mail.cibtc.com.cn, http://www.cibtc.com.cn.

616.02 CHN
ZHONGHUA NEIKE ZAZHI/CHINESE JOURNAL OF INTERNAL MEDICINE. Text in Chinese. m. USD 55.20; USD 4.60 newsstand/cover (effective 2001). **Document type:** *Journal, Academic/Scholarly.*
Related titles: CD-ROM ed.

Indexed: Chem.Abstr., ExtraMED, Ind.Med. (coverage dropped).
—BLDSC (3180.360000).
Published by: China International Book Trading Corp/Zhongguo Guoji Tushu Maoyi Zonggongsi cibtc@mail.cibtc.com.cn, http://www.cibtc.com.cn. **Dist. by:** 35, Chegongzhuang Xilu, Haidian District, Beijing 100044, China.

MEDICAL SCIENCES—Nurses And Nursing

see also GERONTOLOGY AND GERIATRICS; HEALTH FACILITIES AND ADMINISTRATION

610.73 USA ISSN 0094-6354
CODEN: ANJOEE
A A N A JOURNAL. Text in English. 1933. bi-m. USD 30 (effective 2001). adv. bk.rev. back issues avail. *Refereed.* **Document type:** *Academic/Scholarly.* **Description:** Publishes original manuscripts that foster understanding of the science of anesthesia delivery and investigate issues, ideas and innovations that advance the practice of nurse anesthesia.
Formerly: American Association of Nurse Anesthetists. Journal (0002-7448)
Related titles: Microform ed.: (from MIM,PMC,PQC).
Indexed: CINAHL, Excerp.Med., Hosp.Lit.Ind., INIS Atomind., Int.Nurs.Ind.
—BLDSC (0537.340000), EMDOCS, GNLM, ingenta, KNAW, Linda Hall.
Published by: (American Association of Nurse Anesthetists), A A N A Publishing, Inc., 222 S Prospect Ave, Park Ridge, IL 60068. TEL 847-692-7137, FAX 847-692-6968, publications@aana.com, http://www.aana.com. Ed. Chuck Biddle. R&P Sally Aquino. Adv. contact Wayne McCourt. B&W page USD 2,910, color page USD 4,760. Circ: 21,151 (controlled).

610.73 USA
A A N N SYNAPSE. Text in English. bi-m. membership only. **Document type:** *Newsletter.*
Indexed: CINAHL.
Published by: American Association of Neuroscience Nurses, 4700 W Lake Ave, Glenview, IL 60025-1468. TEL 847-375-4733, 888-557-2266, FAX 847-375-6333, bsimmons@amctec.com, http://www.AANN.org. R&P Barbara Simmons. Circ: 4,000.

610.73 USA ISSN 1046-7041
A B N F JOURNAL. Text in English. 1990. bi-m. USD 90 domestic to individuals; USD 210 foreign to individuals; USD 185 domestic to institutions; USD 250 foreign to institutions (effective 2001). adv. bk.rev. *Refereed.* **Document type:** *Academic/Scholarly.*
Related titles: Online - full text ed.: (from ProQuest Information & Learning).
Indexed: CINAHL, Int.Nurs.Ind.
—BLDSC (0549.610000), ingenta. **CCC.**
Published by: (Association of Black Nursing Faculty in Higher Education, Inc.), Tucker Publications, Inc., PO Box 580, Lisle, IL 60532. TEL 630-969-3809, FAX 630-969-3895, callen@tuckerpub.com, http://www.tuckerpub.com. Ed., Pub. Dr. Sallie Tucker-Allen. R&P Clay Allen. Adv. contact S Monique Allen. Circ: 450 (paid).

613.7 615.53 USA
A F H H A INSIDER. Text in English. 1984. m. free per issue to members. adv. bk.rev. back issues avail. **Document type:** *Newsletter.* **Description:** Explores home health care industry issues.
Published by: American Federation of Home Health Agencies, 1320 Fenwick Ln, Ste 100, Silver Spring, MD 20910. TEL 301-588-1454, FAX 301-588-4732. Ed. Ann Howard. Circ: 500.

610.73 USA
A J N GUIDE; to nursing career opportunities. Text in English. 1982. a. USD 10 (effective 2000). adv. *Refereed.* **Document type:** *Directory.*
Related titles: Microform ed.
Published by: Lippincott Williams & Wilkins, 345 Hudson St, 16th Fl, New York, NY 10014-4502. TEL 212-886-1200, FAX 212-886-1215, orders@lww.com, http://www.lww.com, http://www.Lww.com. Ed. Diana J Mason. Pub. Donna Hilton. R&P Hop Welscher. Adv. contact Steve Kurlander. Circ: 150,000 (paid).

610.73 COL ISSN 0120-1832
A N E C. Text in Spanish. 1966. irreg. COP 15,000; COP 5,000 per issue (effective 2000 - 2001). adv. bk.rev. illus.
Formerly: Asociacion Nacional de Enfermeras de Colombia. A N E C. Revista
Indexed: Int.Nurs.Ind.
Published by: Asociacion Nacional de Enfermeras de Colombia, Apartado Aereo 059871, Bogota, DE, Colombia. TEL 57-1-2683535, FAX 57-1-2683535, anecnal@andinet.lat.net. Eds. Beatriz Carballo, Esperanza Morales. Circ: 1,500,811.

610.73 PHL ISSN 0065-0676
A N P H I PAPERS. Text in English. 1966. a. PHP 30, USD 10. bk.rev. **Document type:** *Academic/Scholarly.*
Related titles: Microfilm ed.: (from PQC).
Indexed: CINAHL, Int.Nurs.Ind.
Published by: Academy of Nursing of the Philippines, College of Nursing, University of the, Padre Faura, Manila, Philippines. TEL 58-49-39. Ed. Cecilia M Laurente. Circ: 400.

610.73 USA
RD99.A1 CODEN: AOJOEL
A O R N JOURNAL. Text in English. 1963. m. USD 80 domestic to non-members; USD 90 foreign to non-members; USD 28 to members; USD 87 to libraries (effective 2001). adv. bk.rev. abstr, bibl, charts, illus, stat. index, cum.index. *Refereed.* **Document type:** *Journal, Trade.* **Description:** Contains clinical information, research articles, and perioperative nursing standards of practice.
Supersedes: O R Nursing
Related titles: CD-ROM ed.: (from Ovid Technologies, Inc.); Microfilm ed.: (from PQC); Online - full text ed.: (from Ovid Technologies, Inc., ProQuest Information & Learning, Gale Group).
Indexed: AMED, Abstr.Health Care Manage.Stud., Brit.Nur.Ind., CINAHL, Hosp.Lit.Ind., INIS Atomind., I.P.A., Ind.Med. (1963-), Int.Nurs.Ind., Nurs.Abstr.
—BLDSC (1567.727000), CISTI, GNLM, ingenta, KNAW. **CCC.**
Published by: Association of periOperative Registered Nurses, Inc., 2170 S Parker Rd, Ste 300, Denver, CO 80231-5711. TEL 303-755-6300, 800-755-2676, FAX 303-750-3441, http://www.aorn.org. Ed. Brenda Gregory Dawes. Adv. contact Janet Mongeon. Circ: 50,389.

610.73 CAN
A R N N L ACCESS. Text in English. 1981. q. USD 10 (effective 2000). adv. **Document type:** *Newsletter.* **Description:** Deals with issues affecting nurses in the province. It is sent to all practicing nurses in the province.
Former titles: A R N N Access (1182-8897); (until 1990): A R N N News News News (0822-7160); (until 1981): News! News! News! (0319-7611)
Published by: Association of Registered Nurses of Newfoundland and Labrador, 55 Military Rd, P O Box 6116, St. John's, NF A1C 5X8, Canada. TEL 709-753-6040, FAX 709-753-4940, cfitzgerald@nf.aibn.com, http://www.arnn.nf.ca. Ed. Jeanette Andrews. Adv. contact Christine Fitzgerald. B&W page USD 425, color page USD 450. Circ: 6,300.

610.73 USA
A R N NETWORK. Text in English. 1976. 6/yr. adv. **Document type:** *Newsletter.* **Description:** Focuses on association news, upcoming educational events, committee functions, and new items of interest to those in the field of nursing and the specialty of rehabilitation nursing.
Formerly: A R N News (1075-5764)
Published by: Association of Rehabilitation Nurses, 4700 W Lake Ave, Glenview, IL 60025-1485. TEL 847-375-4710, FAX 847-375-4777. Circ: 11,000.

A W H O N N LIFELINES; promoting the health of women and newborns. see *WOMEN'S HEALTH*

610.73 618 USA ISSN 1066-2944
A W H O N N NEWSLETTER✱. Text in English. 1974. 10/yr. USD 35; to individuals (foreign $45); institutions $69 (effective 1996). adv. index. back issues avail. **Document type:** *Newsletter.* **Description:** For nurses and others interested in women's health nursing issues.
Formerly (until 1993): N A A C O G Newsletter (0889-0579)
Published by: Association of Women's Health, Obstetric, and Neonatal Nurses, 2000 L St NW, Ste 740, Washington, DC 20036-4907. TEL 202-622-1600. Ed., R&P, Adv. contact Angela Fowler. Circ: 22,000.

610.73 USA
THE ACADEMIC NURSE. Text in English. 1906. 2/yr. free per issue. **Document type:** *Academic/Scholarly.*
Formerly: Alumnae Magazine (0069-634X)
Indexed: CINAHL.
—BLDSC (0570.513970).
Published by: Columbia University, School of Nursing, 617 W 168th St, New York, NY 10032. TEL 212-305-3254, FAX 212-305-6020, capsona@columbia.edu. Ed. Mary Mundinger. Circ: 2,700.

610.73 GBR ISSN 0965-2302
ACCIDENT AND EMERGENCY NURSING. Text in English. 1993. q. GBP 42 to individuals; GBP 163 to institutions (effective 2002). adv. bk.rev. 64 p./no. 2 cols./p. back issues avail.; reprints avail. *Refereed.* **Document type:** *Journal, Academic/Scholarly.* **Description:** Covers various topics in emergency-care nursing.
Related titles: Online - full text ed.: (from Swets Blackwell, IDEAL Online Library).
Indexed: ASSIA, Brit.Nur.Ind., CINAHL, Fam.Ind., Int.Nurs.Ind.
—BLDSC (0573.137000), CISTI, GNLM, Infotrieve. **CCC.**
Published by: Churchill Livingstone (Subsidiary of: Harcourt Publishers Ltd.), Robert Stevenson House, 1-3 Baxter's Pl, Leith Walk, Edinburgh, Midlothian EH1 3AF, United Kingdom. TEL 44-131-556-2424, FAX 44-131-558-1278, journals@harcourt.com, http://www.harcourt-international.com/journals/aaen/. Ed. Bob Wright. R&P Sharon Boyle TEL 44-131-524-1747. Adv. contact Deborah Watkins TEL 44-207-424-4280. Circ: 725. **Subscr. in the Us:** Harcourt Health Sciences, Journals Subscription Department, PO Box 156, Avenel, NJ 07001. TEL 877-839-7126; **Subscr. to:** Harcourt Publishers Ltd., Foots Cray High St, Sidcup, Kent DA14 5HP, United Kingdom. TEL 44-20-8308-5700, FAX 44-20-8309-0807.

ACTA MEDICA AUXOLOGICA. see *MEDICAL SCIENCES—Endocrinology*

610.73 USA ISSN 1096-6293
ADVANCE FOR NURSE PRACTITIONERS. Text in English. 1993. m. *Refereed.*
Indexed: Int.Nurs.Ind.
Published by: Merion Publications, Inc., 2900 Horizon Dr., PO Box 61556, King of Prussia, PA 19406. TEL 610-278-1400, 800-355-5627, FAX 610-278-1421, advance@merion.com, http://www.advanceweb.com. Ed. Michelle Pronsati.

610.73 USA
ADVANCE FOR NURSES. Text in English. bi-w. Free to qualified subscribers.. adv. **Document type:** *Magazine, Trade.* **Description:** Covers clinical and management issues for nurses of all specialties.
Related titles: Online - full content ed.
Published by: Merion Publications, Inc., 2900 Horizon Dr, PO Box 61556, King Of Prussia, PA 19406. TEL 800-355-5627, FAX 610-278-1421, 610-278-1425, gguterl@merion.com, http://www.advancefornurses.com/ , http://www.advanceweb.com. adv.: B&W page USD 6,275, color page USD 8,835.

610.7361 USA
ADVANCE FOR PROVIDERS OF POST-ACUTE CARE. Text in English. m. Free to qualified subscribers. adv. **Document type:** *Magazine, Trade.* **Description:** Covers both business and clinical information for providers of long-term care, home care and subacute care.
Related titles: Online - full content ed.
Published by: Merion Publications, Inc., 2900 Horizon Dr, PO Box 61556, King Of Prussia, PA 19406. TEL 800-355-5627, FAX 610-278-1421, 610-278-1425, cadkins@merion.com, http://www.advanceforpac.com/, http://www.advanceweb.com.

ADVANCES IN GERONTOLOGICAL NURSING. see *GERONTOLOGY AND GERIATRICS*

610.73 USA ISSN 0161-9268
RT1
ADVANCES IN NURSING SCIENCE. Text in English. 1978. q. USD 132 to individuals; USD 40 newsstand/cover (effective 2002). adv. index. back issues avail. *Refereed.* **Document type:** *Academic/Scholarly.*
Related titles: CD-ROM ed.: (from Ovid Technologies, Inc.); Online - full text ed.: (from Ovid Technologies, Inc., ProQuest Information & Learning, Gale Group, Institute for Scientific Information).
Indexed: ASCA, AgeLine, Arts & Hum.Cit.Ind. (coverage dropped), Behav.Med.Abstr., Brit.Nur.Ind., CINAHL, Compumath, Curr.Cont., Fam.Ind., IMFL, Ind.Med. (1978-), Int.Nurs.Ind., Nurs.Abstr., PsycInfo, Psychol.Abstr. (1984-), SSCI, e-psyche.
—BLDSC (0709.508000), CISTI, GNLM, IDS, ingenta, KNAW. **CCC.**
Published by: Aspen Publishers, Inc., 200 Orchard Ridge Dr, Ste 200, Gaithersburg, MD 20878. TEL 301-417-7500, 800-638-8437, FAX 301-695-7931, customer.service@aspenpubl.com, http:// www.aspenpub.com. Ed. Dr. Peggy L Chinn. Adv. contact Frances S Ray. Circ: 3,277 (paid). **Dist. by:** Aspen Publishers Inc., Distribution Center, 7201 McKinney Circle, Frederick, MD 21701. TEL 301-698-7100, FAX 301-417-7550.

610.73 FRA ISSN 1166-3413
L'AIDE SOIGNANTE. Text in French. 10/yr. EUR 60 in Europe to individuals; USD 69 elsewhere to individuals; EUR 60 in Europe to institutions; USD 69 elsewhere to institutions (effective 2002). **Document type:** *Academic/Scholarly.*
Formerly (until 1992): L' Ami de la Petite Camargue Alsacienne (0987-8947)
Related titles: Online - full text ed.
Published by: Elsevier Paris, Editions Scientifiques et Medicales (Subsidiary of: Reed Elsevier plc. group), 23 rue Linois, Paris 75015, France. http://www.elsevier.com/locate/soign. Circ: 20,000.

610.73 USA ISSN 0002-4317
ALABAMA NURSE. Text in English. q. Free to qualified subscribers. adv. 24 p./no. **Document type:** *Newsletter, Trade.* **Description:** Covers issues and employment opportunities of interest to licensed nursing professionals.
Published by: (Alabama State Nurses' Association), Arthur L. Davis Publishing Agency, Inc., 517 Washington St, P O Box 216, Cedar Falls, IA 50613. TEL 319-277-2414, 800-626-4081, FAX 319-277-4055, sales@aldpub.com, http://www.aldpub.com/. Ed. Mark Miller. R&P Karen Pakkala. Adv. contact Jim Larson. Circ: 57,000 (free).

610.73 USA ISSN 0002-4546
ALASKA NURSE. Text in English. 1951. q. USD 15 domestic to non-members; USD 20 foreign to non-members (effective 2000). adv. bk.rev. illus.
Indexed: CINAHL, Int.Nurs.Ind.
—GNLM.
Published by: Alaska Nurses Association, 237 E Third Ave, 3, Anchorage, AK 99501. TEL 907-274-0827, FAX 907-272-0292, aknurse@ptialaska.net. Ed. Kathy North. R&P, Adv. contact Wanda Katinscky. Circ: 650 (paid).

610.73 CAN ISSN 1481-9988
ALBERTA R N. (Registered Nurses) Text in English. 1948. 6/yr. CND 35; CND 40 foreign (effective 1999). adv. bk.rev. illus, stat. **Document type:** *Trade.* **Description:** Provides information on current trends and issues in nursing in Alberta. Lists educational and career opportunities and a calendar of events.
Formerly (until 1998): A A R N Newsletter (0001-0197)
Indexed: CINAHL, Int.Nurs.Ind.
—BLDSC (0786.588700), GNLM, Infotrieve, KNAW. **CCC.**
Published by: Alberta Association of Registered Nurses, 11620 168 St, Edmonton, AB T5M 4A6, Canada. TEL 780-451-0043, FAX 780-452-3276, http://www.nurses.ab.ca. Ed. Michaleen Elabdi. Adv. contact Jan Henry. B&W page CND 1,300, color page CND 1,750; trim 10 x 7.75. Circ: 24,000 (controlled).

610.73 DEU ISSN 0002-6573
ALTENHEIM; Zeitschrift fuer das Altenhilfe Management. Text in German. 1962. m. EUR 90 domestic; EUR 92 foreign (effective 2002). adv. bk.rev. charts, illus, stat. index. **Document type:** *Magazine, Trade.*
Indexed: Dok.Arbeitsmed.
—GNLM, Infotrieve. **CCC.**
Published by: Vincentz Verlag, Schiffgraben 43, Hannover 30175, Germany. TEL 49-511-9910000, FAX 49-511-9910099, info@vincentz.de, http://www.vincentz.de. Ed. Reinhard Hein. Circ: 8,297. **Subscr. to:** Postfach 6247, Hannover 30062, Germany.

610.73 DEU ISSN 0341-0455
ALTENPFLEGE; Fachmagazin fuer ambulante und stationaere Altenpflege. Text in German. 1976. m. EUR 50 domestic; EUR 60 foreign (effective 2002). adv. bk.rev. charts, illus, stat. index. **Document type:** *Journal, Trade.*
—GNLM, Infotrieve. **CCC.**
Published by: Vincentz Verlag, Schiffgraben 43, Hannover 30175, Germany. TEL 49-511-9910000, FAX 49-511-9910099, info@vincentz.de, http://www.vincentz.de. Ed. Holger Jenrich. Circ: 30,126.

610.73 USA ISSN 1041-2972
RT82.8 CODEN: JANPEB
AMERICAN ACADEMY OF NURSE PRACTITIONERS. JOURNAL. Text in English. 1988. m. USD 32 domestic to individuals; USD 57 in Canada to individuals; USD 102 elsewhere to individuals; USD 58 domestic to institutions; USD 83 in Canada to institutions; USD 128 elsewhere to institutions. *Refereed.* **Document type:** *Academic/Scholarly.* **Description:** Captures what's happening in clinical practice, management, education, research and legislation.
Related titles: Online - full text ed.: (from ProQuest Information & Learning).
Indexed: CINAHL, Fam.Ind., INIS Atomind., Int.Nurs.Ind.
—BLDSC (4683.731500), CISTI, GNLM, ingenta.
Published by: (American Academy of Nurse Practitioners), Slack, Inc., 6900 Grove Rd, Thorofare, NJ 08086-9447. TEL 856-848-1000, 800-257-8290, FAX 856-853-5991, http://www.slackinc.com. Ed. Donna Nativio Jan Towers.

610.73 USA ISSN 0891-0162
RC966
AMERICAN ASSOCIATION OF OCCUPATIONAL HEALTH NURSES JOURNAL. Abbreviated title: A A O H N Journal. Text in English. 1953. m. USD 56 to individuals; USD 81 in Canada to individuals; USD 96 elsewhere to individuals; USD 75 to institutions; USD 100 in Canada to institutions; USD 115 elsewhere to institutions. adv. bk.rev. charts, illus. index. *Refereed.* **Document type:** *Academic/Scholarly.* **Description:** Offers original articles of professional interest to the occupational health nurse.
Former titles: Occupational Health Nursing (0029-7933); (until 1968): American Association of Industrial Nurses Journal (0098-6097)
Related titles: Microfilm ed.; Online - full text ed.: (from ProQuest Information & Learning).
Indexed: CINAHL, C.I.S. Abstr., CSNB, Excerp.Med., Ind.Hyg.Dig., Int.Nurs.Ind., Noise Pollut.Publ.Abstr., Nurs.Abstr.
—BLDSC (0537.501300), CISTI, EMDOCS, GNLM, ingenta, KNAW.
Published by: (American Association of Occupational Health Nurses, Inc.), Slack, Inc., 6900 Grove Rd, Thorofare, NJ 08086-9447. TEL 856-848-1000, 800-257-8290, FAX 856-853-5991, http://www.slackinc.com/. Circ: 14,000.

610.73 616 USA ISSN 1062-3264
AMERICAN JOURNAL OF CRITICAL CARE. Text in English. 1992. bi-m. USD 48 domestic to individuals; USD 66 foreign to individuals; USD 116 domestic to institutions; USD 150 foreign to institutions. *Refereed.* **Document type:** *Academic/Scholarly.* **Description:** Communicates important advances in clinical science and research in critical care.
Related titles: CD-ROM ed.: (from SilverPlatter Information, Inc.); Online - full text ed.: (from Northern Light Technology, Inc., ProQuest Information & Learning).
Indexed: CINAHL, Environ.Sci.Poll.Mgmt., Ind.Med. (1992-), Int.Nurs.Ind., Pollut.Abstr., Risk Abstr., Saf.Sci.Abstr.
—BLDSC (0824.210000), CISTI, GNLM, KNAW. **CCC.**
Published by: American Association of Critical Care Nurses, 101 Columbia, Aliso Viejo, CA 92656. TEL 949-362-2000, FAX 949-362-2020, ajcc@aol.com. Eds. Dr. Christopher Dryan Brown, Kathleen Dracup. Pub. Bonnie Horrigan. R&P Beth Wos TEL 800-899-1712. Circ: 74,000. **Subscr. to:** PO Box 626, Holmes, PA 19043.

610.73 USA ISSN 0002-936X
RT1
AMERICAN JOURNAL OF NURSING. Text in English. 1900. m. USD 29.95 domestic to individuals; USD 44.95 in Canada to individuals; USD 49.95 elsewhere to individuals; USD 79.95 domestic to institutions; USD 94.95 foreign to institutions; USD 9 newsstand/cover (effective 2001). adv. bk.rev. bibl, charts, illus, tr.lit. index, cum.index: 1961-65, 1966-70, 1971-75. back issues avail.; reprint service avail. from PQC. *Refereed.* **Document type:** *Trade.* **Description:** Provides comprehensive and in-depth information to help nurses stay current in their profession. Content includes practical, hands-on clinical articles on essential topics, vital information on drugs, trends in nursing and legal advice.
Related titles: CD-ROM ed.: (from Ovid Technologies, Inc.); Microform ed.: (from PMC,PQC); Online - full text ed.: (from Ovid Technologies, Inc., Gale Group, Factiva, Institute for Scientific Information).
Indexed: AIM, AMED, ASCA, ASSIA, Abstr.Health Care Manage.Stud., Abstr.Soc.Geront., Acad.Ind., Adol.Ment.Hlth.Abstr., AgeLine, Brit.Nur.Ind., CINAHL, Chem.Abstr., Curr.Cont., Curr.Lit.Fam.Plan., Dent.Ind., Dok.Arbeitsmed., Environ.Sci.Poll.Mgmt., Except.Child Educ.Abstr., Fam.Ind., Gen.Sci.Ind. (Mar.1984-), Hlth.Ind., Hosp.Lit.Ind., IMFL, INIS Atomind., I.P.A., Ind.Med. (1900-), Ind.Sci.Rev., Int.Nurs.Ind., Med.Care Rev., NRN, Neurosci.Cit.Ind., Nurs.Abstr., Nutr.Abstr., P.A.I.S., Pollut.Abstr., Psychol.Abstr., Risk Abstr., SSCI, Saf.Sci.Abstr., Sci.Cit.Ind. (coverage dropped), Soc.Sci.Ind. (coverage dropped), Soc.Work Res.& Abstr., Stud.Wom.Abstr., Tr.& Indus.Ind.
—BLDSC (0828.500000), CISTI, GNLM, IDS, ingenta, KNAW, Linda Hall.
Published by: (American Nurses Association), Lippincott Williams & Wilkins, 345 Hudson St, 16th Fl, New York, NY 10014-4502. TEL 303-604-1464, 800-677-3361, FAX 215-627-4856, ajn@lww.com, http://www.nursingcenter.com, http://www.Lww.com. Ed. Diana J Mason. R&P Tobiaj Weclsler. Adv. contact Steven Curlander. B&W page USD 2,995, color page USD 4,295. Circ: 347,781. **Subscr. to:** Centrobe Agents Department, PO Box 8035, Boulder, CO 80306-8035.

610.73 USA ISSN 0098-1486
THE AMERICAN NURSE. Text in English. 1969. 6/yr. USD 20 (effective 2000). adv. reprint service avail. from PQC. **Document type:** *Newspaper.* **Description:** Covers trends and issues affecting staff nurses.
Formerly (until 1974): A N A in Action (0587-3053)
Related titles: Microform ed.: (from PQC); Online - full text ed.: (from Northern Light Technology, Inc., ProQuest Information & Learning).
Indexed: CINAHL, Hosp.Lit.Ind., Int.Nurs.Ind., Nurs.Abstr.
—GNLM, KNAW.
Published by: American Nurses Association, 600 Maryland Ave S W, Ste 100 W, Washington, DC 20024-2571. TEL 202-651-7000, FAX 202-651-7005, http://www.nursingworld.org. Ed. Connie Helmlinger. R&P Sheila Lindsay. Adv. contact Betty Whitaker. Circ: 185,000.

610.73 616.89 USA ISSN 1078-3903
AMERICAN PSYCHIATRIC NURSES ASSOCIATION. JOURNAL. Text in English. 1995. bi-m. USD 59 domestic to individuals; USD 77 foreign to individuals; USD 110 domestic to institutions; USD 129 foreign to institutions; USD 30 domestic to students; USD 46 foreign to students; USD 22 newsstand/cover (effective 2001). adv. index. Supplement avail.; back issues avail.; reprints avail. *Refereed.* **Document type:** *Journal, Academic/Scholarly.* **Description:** Covers a blend of clinical and research topics, practice challenges, and changes occurring in this ever-changing field.
Related titles: Online - full text ed.: (from IDEAL Online Library, RoweCom Information Quest).
Indexed: CINAHL, Nurs.Abstr., PsycInfo, e-psyche.
—BLDSC (4692.068000), Infotrieve. **CCC.**
Published by: (American Psychiatric Nurses Association), Mosby, Inc. (Subsidiary of: Elsevier Science), 11830 Westline Industrial Dr, St Louis, MO 63146-3318. TEL 314-872-8370, 800-325-4177, FAX 314-872-9164, http://www.mosby.com/periodicals. Eds. Grayce M Sills, Nikki S Polis. Pub. Pat Nornhold. Adv. contact Gina Burkert TEL 314-453-4306. B&W page USD 875, color page USD 1,840; trim 10.88 x 8.25. Circ: 4,949.

610.73 USA ISSN 0739-6686
RT81.5
ANNUAL REVIEW OF NURSING RESEARCH. Text in English. 1983. a., latest vol.17, 1999. USD 46; USD 51 foreign (effective 1999). back issues avail. **Document type:** *Academic/Scholarly.* **Description:** Focuses on Complementary Health and Pain Management.
Indexed: CINAHL, Ind.Med. (1983-), Int.Nurs.Ind.
—BLDSC (1524.200000), CISTI, GNLM, ingenta, KNAW.
Published by: Springer Publishing Company, 536 Broadway, New York, NY 10012. TEL 212-431-4370, FAX 212-941-7842, springer@springerpub.com, htp://www.springerpub.com, http://www.springerpub.com. Ed. Joyce J Fitzpatrick. Circ: 1,500.

610.73 616 USA ISSN 0897-1897
CODEN: ANUREA
APPLIED NURSING RESEARCH. Text in English. 1988. q. USD 70 domestic to individuals; USD 156 foreign to individuals; USD 143 domestic to institutions; USD 216 foreign to institutions; USD 53 domestic to students; USD 99 foreign to students; USD 55 newsstand/cover (effective 2001). adv. *Refereed.* **Document type:** *Academic/Scholarly.* **Description:** Devoted to advancing nursing as a research-based profession and bridging the gap between research and practice in nursing.
Related titles: Online - full text ed.: (from IDEAL Online Library, Institute for Scientific Information).
Indexed: ASCA, AgeLine, CINAHL, Curr.Cont., Fam.Ind., Ind.Med. (1988-), Int.Nurs.Ind., SSCI.
—BLDSC (1576.236000), GNLM, IDS, ingenta. **CCC.**
Published by: W.B. Saunders Co. (Subsidiary of: Harcourt Publishers Ltd.), 11830 Westline Industrial Dr, St Louis, MO 63146. TEL 800-325-4177, http://www.wbsaunders.com. Ed. Joyce J Fitzpatrick. Adv. contact Steve Gray. B&W page USD 615, color page USD 1,540; trim 10 x 7. Circ: 1,625. **Subscr. to:** Periodicals Fulfillment, W B Saunders Co, 6277 Sea Harbor Dr, 4th Fl, Orlando, FL 32891-4800.

M

610.73 616.8 USA ISSN 0883-9417
ARCHIVES OF PSYCHIATRIC NURSING. Text in English. 1987. bi-m. USD 70 domestic to individuals; USD 125 foreign to individuals; USD 118 domestic to institutions; USD 161 foreign to institutions; USD 50 domestic to students; USD 75 foreign to students; USD 27 newsstand/cover domestic (effective 2001). adv. bk.rev. abstr, bibl, charts, illus. index. *Refereed.* **Document type:** *Journal, Academic/Scholarly.* **Description:** Approaches the field from the broadest possible perspective through articles and case reports relating to theories, practices, and research applications.
Related titles: Online - full text ed.: (from IDEAL Online Library, Institute for Scientific Information).
Indexed: ASCA, AgeLine, Brit.Nur.Ind., CINAHL, Chic.Per.Ind., Curr.Cont., Fam.Ind., Ind.Med. (1987-), Int.Nurs.Ind., Nurs.Abstr., PsycInfo, Psychol.Abstr. (1988-), SSCI, e-psyche.
—BLDSC (1640.410000), CISTI, GNLM, IDS, ingenta. **CCC.**
Published by: (Society for Education and Research in Psychiatric-Mental Health Nursing), W.B. Saunders Co. (Subsidiary of: Harcourt Publishers Ltd.), 11830 Westline Industrial Dr, St Louis, MO 63146. TEL 800-325-4177, http://www.wbsaunders.com. Ed. Judith B Krauss. Adv. contact Steve Gray. B&W page USD 820, color page USD 1,765; trim 10 x 7. Circ: 2,537. **Subscr. to:** Periodicals Fulfillment, W B Saunders Co, 6277 Sea Harbor Dr, 4th Fl, Orlando, FL 32891-4800.

610.73 USA ISSN 0004-1599
ARIZONA NURSE. Text in English. 1947. 6/yr. USD 30. adv. bk.rev. illus. reprint service avail. from PQC. **Document type:** *Newsletter.*
Related titles: Microfilm ed.: (from PQC); Online - full text ed.: (from Northern Light Technology, Inc., ProQuest Information & Learning).
Indexed: CINAHL, Int.Nurs.Ind.
—GNLM.
Published by: Arizona Nurses Association, 1850 E Southern Ave, Ste 1, Tempe, AZ 85282. FAX 602-839-4780. Ed. Ela Joy Lehrman. R&P Lyndall Eddy. Adv. contact Jennifer McAfee. Circ: 2,000.

610.73 USA
ARIZONA STATE BOARD OF NURSING. NEWSLETTER. Text in English. q. Free to qualified subscribers. 28 p./no. **Document type:** *Newsletter, Trade.* **Description:** Covers issues and employment opportunities of interest to licensed nursing professionals.
Published by: (Arizona State Board of Nursing), Arthur L. Davis Publishing Agency, Inc., 517 Washington St, P O Box 216, Cedar Falls, IA 50613. TEL 319-277-2414, 800-626-4081, FAX 319-277-4055, sales@aldpub.com, http://www.aldpub.com/. Ed. Mark Miller. R&P Joey Ridenour. Adv. contact Jim Larson. Circ: 85,000 (free).

610.73 DEU ISSN 0931-5853
DIE ARZTHELFERIN. Text in German. 1963. m. DEM 70.80 (effective 2000). adv. bk.rev. index. **Document type:** *Magazine, Trade.*
Incorporates (in 1989): Helferin des Arztes (0017-9949)
—CCC.
Published by: Friedrich Kiehl Verlag GmbH, Pfaustr 13, Ludwigshafen 67063, Germany. TEL 49-621-63502-0, FAX 49-621-6350222. Ed. Lothar Kurz. Adv. contact Joern Mueller Grote. Circ: 13,500.

610.73 ITA ISSN 1592-5986
ASSISTENZA INFERMIERISTICA E RICERCA. Text in Italian. q. ITL 80,000, EUR 62, USD 67 to individuals; ITL 100,000 to institutions and libraries (effective 2000). adv. 64 p./no. **Document type:** *Journal, Academic/Scholarly.*
Formerly (until 1999): Rivista dell'Infermiere (1120-3803)
Indexed: CINAHL, Int.Nurs.Ind.
—BLDSC (1746.661970), GNLM.
Published by: Il Pensiero Scientifico Editore s.r.l., Via Bradano, 3-C, Rome, RM 00199, Italy. TEL 39-06-862821, FAX 39-06-86282250, pensiero@pensiero.it, http://www.pensiero.it. Ed. Paola Di Giulio. Pub. Luca De Fiore. R&P Andrea De Fiore. Adv. contact Luciano De Fiore. Circ: 1,000.

ASSOCIATION OF MEDICAL WOMEN IN INDIA. JOURNAL. see *WOMEN'S HEALTH*

ASSOCIATION OF NURSES IN AIDS CARE. JOURNAL. see *MEDICAL SCIENCES—Communicable Diseases*

AUSTRALASIAN JOURNAL OF EMERGENCY CARE. see *MEDICAL SCIENCES—Orthopedics And Traumatology*

610.73 618.92 AUS ISSN 1036-5060
AUSTRALIA PAEDIATRIC NURSE JOURNAL. Abbreviated title: A P N J. Text in English. 1988-1993; resumed 1994. 3/yr. **Description:** Provides a means for the publication of articles in the field of healthcare for infants, children, and their families. Promotes the sharing of information among networks of nurses and other health care providers to improve the quality of care.
Formerly (until 1991): Queensland Paediatric Nurses Association Journal (1035-2600)
Published by: Queensland Paediatric Nurses Association, c/o Education Centre, Royal Children's Hospital, Herston Rd., Herston, QLD 4029, Australia.

AUSTRALIAN AND NEW ZEALAND JOURNAL OF MENTAL HEALTH NURSING. see *MEDICAL SCIENCES—Psychiatry And Neurology*

610.73 AUS ISSN 1036-7314
AUSTRALIAN CRITICAL CARE✶. Text in English. 1988. q. AUD 70. adv. bk.rev. abstr. back issues avail. *Refereed.* **Document type:** *Academic/Scholarly.* **Description:** For critical care nurses, universities, hospital libraries, agencies.
Indexed: CINAHL, Int.Nurs.Ind.
—BLDSC (1798.264300), GNLM.
Published by: Cambridge Media, 17 Northwood St, West Leederville, W.A. 6007, Australia. TEL 61-8-9382-3911, FAX 61-8-9382-3187, info@cambridgemedia.com.au, http://www.cambridgemedia.com.au. Ed. Dr. Gavin Leslie. adv.: page AUD 600; trim 296 x 210. Circ: 2,600.

610.73 AUS ISSN 0813-0531
AUSTRALIAN JOURNAL OF ADVANCED NURSING. Text in English. 1983. q. AUD 85 domestic to non-members; AUD 75 domestic to members; AUD 175 domestic to libraries; AUD 95 foreign to individuals; AUD 195 foreign to institutions (effective 2001). adv. 48 p./no. back issues avail. *Refereed.* **Document type:** *Journal, Academic/Scholarly.* **Description:** Covers nursing research and allied philosophical study.
Indexed: Brit.Nur.Ind., CINAHL, Int.Nurs.Ind.
—BLDSC (1801.830000), CISTI, GNLM, ingenta, KNAW. **CCC.**
Published by: Australian Nursing Federation, Level 2, 21 Victoria St, Melbourne, VIC 3000, Australia. TEL 61-3-96395211, FAX 61-3-96520567, http://www.anf.org.au. Ed., R&P Heather Byrne TEL 61-3-9652-0507. Pub. Jill Iliffe. Adv. contact Barry Telfer TEL 61-3-9563-6602. Circ: 1,300.

AUSTRALIAN JOURNAL OF RURAL HEALTH. see *PUBLIC HEALTH AND SAFETY*

610.73 AUS
AUSTRALIAN NURSING COUNCIL. ANNUAL REPORT. Text in English. 1993. a. free per issue. back issues avail. **Document type:** *Newsletter.* **Description:** Includes the purposes and objects of the council, program structure and goals, organizational structure, professional activities, staff and financial statements.
Published by: Australian Nursing Council Inc., PO Box 873, Dickson, ACT 2602, Australia. TEL 61-2-62577960, FAX 61-2-62577955. Ed. Jan Duke. Circ: 300.

610.73 AUS ISSN 1321-117X
AUSTRALIAN NURSING COUNCIL NEWSLETTER. Text in English. 1993. 3/yr. free per issue. adv. **Document type:** *Newsletter.* **Description:** Contains news on current activities of the organization and other issues on nursing nationally and internationally.
Published by: Australian Nursing Council Inc., PO Box 873, Dickson, ACT 2602, Australia. TEL 61-2-62577960, FAX 61-2-62577955. Circ: 750.

610.73 AUS ISSN 1320-3185
RT15
AUSTRALIAN NURSING JOURNAL. Text in English. 1962. 11/yr. AUD 50 to non-members; AUD 25 to members; AUD 70 domestic to institutions; AUD 85 foreign to institutions (effective 2001). adv. bk.rev. reprint service avail. from PQC. **Document type:** *Academic/Scholarly.* **Description:** Multi-purpose professional and trade union nursing journal.
Formerly: Australian Nurses' Journal (0045-0758)
Related titles: Microfiche ed.: (from PQC); Online - full text ed.: (from Northern Light Technology, Inc., ProQuest Information & Learning).
Indexed: AMED, Brit.Nur.Ind., CINAHL, INIS Atomind., Int.Nurs.Ind., NRN, WMB.
—BLDSC (1815.830000), CISTI, GNLM, Infotrieve, ingenta, KNAW. **CCC.**
Published by: Australian Nursing Federation, Level 2, 21 Victoria St, Melbourne, VIC 3000, Australia. TEL 61-3-96395211, FAX 61-3-96520567, anj2@anf.org.au, http://www.anf.org.au. Ed., R&P Heather Byrne TEL 61-3-9652-0507. Adv. contact Barry Telfer TEL 61-3-9563-6602. Circ: 56,000.

610.73 DEU ISSN 1434-9574
B A L K INFO. Text in German. 1990. bi-m. USD 92; USD 17 newsstand/cover (effective 2001). **Document type:** *Bulletin, Trade.*
Published by: (Bundesarbeitsgemeinschaft Leitender Krankenpflegepersonen e.V.), Springer-Verlag (Subsidiary of: BertelsmannSpringer), Haber Str 7, Heidelberg 69126, Germany. FAX 49-30-82787448, subscriptions@springer.de, http://link.springer.de/link/service/journals/15003/index.htm.

610.73 GBR
BAILLIERE'S NURSES' DICTIONARY. Text in English. 1912. irreg., latest 2000, no.23/e. GBP 6.95 (effective 2000). back issues avail. **Document type:** *Academic/Scholarly.*
Published by: Bailliere Tindall (Subsidiary of: Harcourt Publishers Ltd.), 24-28 Oval Rd, London NW1 7DX, United Kingdom. TEL 44-20-7485-4752, FAX 44—20-7267-4466, http://www..hbuk.co.uk.

BALANCE (ALEXANDRIA). see *GERONTOLOGY AND GERIATRICS*

610.73 BRB ISSN 0572-6042
BARBADOS NURSING JOURNAL. Text in English. a. membership.
Published by: Barbados Registered Nurses Association, Gibson House, Spry Street, Bridgetown, Barbados.

BARNBLADET; tidskrift foer Sveriges barnsjukskoeterskor. see *MEDICAL SCIENCES—Pediatrics*

610.73 NOR
BASIS. Text in Norwegian. 1967. 12/yr. NOK 600. adv. bk.rev. **Document type:** *Trade.*
Formerly: Hjelpepleiren (0332-7841)
—CCC.
Published by: Norsk Hjelpepleierforbund, Nordsk Helse - og Sosialforbund, Oslo 0611, Norway. FAX 645602. Ed. Solveig Steien. Adv. contact Lillian Lindberg. Circ: 59,459 (controlled).

610.73 USA ISSN 1071-2984
BEGINNINGS (FLAGSTAFF); the official newslettr of the American holistic nurses' association. Text in English. 1981. m. (10/yr.). USD 25 domestic; USD 30 in Canada; USD 35 elsewhere (effective 2000). adv. bk.rev. tr.lit. **Document type:** *Newsletter.* **Description:** Promotes the education of nurses and the public in the concepts and practice of health of the whole person.
Indexed: CINAHL, Int.Nurs.Ind.
—BLDSC (1876.607000).
Published by: American Holistic Nurses' Association, PO Box 2130, Flagstaff, AZ 86003. TEL 520-526-2196, 800-278-AHNA, FAX 520-526-2752, ahna-flag@flaglink.com, http://www.ahna.org. Ed. Marie Fasano Ramos. R&P, Adv. contact Michael French TEL 800-278-2462. B&W page USD 570; trim 10 x 7.5. Circ: 3,500 (paid).

610.73 USA ISSN 1099-8004
▼ **BIOLOGICAL RESEARCH FOR NURSING.** Text in English. 1999. q. USD 410 domestic; USD 426 elsewhere (effective 2002). 88 p./no. back issues avail.; reprints avail. *Refereed.* **Document type:** *Journal, Academic/Scholarly, Trade.* **Description:** Provides nurses with a forum for dialogue concerning substantive, theoretical, and methodological research related to normal and abnormal function.
Formerly (until 1999): Biological Nursing Research
Related titles: Online - full text ed.: (from EBSCO Publishing, O C L C Online Computer Library Center, Inc., RoweCom Information Quest, ingenta, Swets Blackwell).
Indexed: Human Resour.Abstr., Ind.Med.
—BLDSC (2077.679000).
Published by: Sage Publications, Inc., Sage Science Press, 2455 Teller Rd, Thousand Oaks, CA 91320. TEL 805-499-0721, FAX 805-499-0871, info@sagepub.com, http://www.sagesciencepress.com. Eds. Christine E Kasper, Pat Perry. R&P Peter Marino. Adv. contact Robert Vrooman. Circ: 200 (paid). **Overseas subscr. to:** Sage Publications Ltd., 6 Bonhill St, London EC2A 4PU, United Kingdom. TEL 44-20-7374-0645, 44-20-7374-8741.

M

BIRTH; issues in perinatal care. see *MEDICAL SCIENCES—Obstetrics And Gynecology*

BLAETTER AUS DEM HENRIETTENSTIFT. see *HEALTH FACILITIES AND ADMINISTRATION*

BREATHLINE. see *MEDICAL SCIENCES—Anaesthesiology*

610.73 GBR ISSN 1462-4753
BRITISH JOURNAL OF COMMUNITY NURSING. Text in English. 1996. m. GBP 54 to individuals; GBP 60 to institutions; GBP 94 to libraries.
Formerly (until 1997): British Journal of Community Health Nursing (1362-4407)
Indexed: Brit.Nur.Ind.
—BLDSC (2307.280000).
Published by: Mark Allen Publishing Ltd., Croxted Mews, 286-288a Croxted Rd, London SE24 9BY, United Kingdom. TEL 44-20-8671-7521, FAX 44-20-8671-1722, http://www.MarAllenGroup.com/bjcn.htm. Ed. Georgina Stevens.

▼ **BRITISH JOURNAL OF HOMECARE.** see *SOCIAL SERVICES AND WELFARE*

610.73 GBR ISSN 0966-0461
RT1
BRITISH JOURNAL OF NURSING. Text in English. 1979. fortn. GBP 78 to individuals; GBP 170 foreign to individuals; GBP 160 to institutions; GBP 230 foreign to institutions (effective 1999). adv. **Document type:** *Academic/Scholarly, Trade.*
Formerly: Nursing (0142-0372)
Related titles: Online - full text ed.: (from Northern Light Technology, Inc., ProQuest Information & Learning).
Indexed: AMED, ASSIA, Addic.Abstr., Brit.Nur.Ind., CINAHL, Curr.Adv.Ecol.Sci., Diab.Cont., Fam.Ind., Int.Nurs.Ind., Nurs.Abstr., Tr.& Indus.Ind.
—BLDSC (2311.980100), CISTI, GNLM, Infotrieve. **CCC.**
Published by: Mark Allen Publishing Ltd., Croxted Mews, 286-288a Croxted Rd, London SE24 9BY, United Kingdom. TEL 44-208-671-7521, FAX 44-208-671-1722, http://www.markallengroup.com/bjn.htm. Ed. George Castledine. Pub. Mark Allen. Adv. contact Edward Rusling. **Dist. by:** Comag, Tavistock Works, Tavistock Rd, W Drayton, Middx UB7 7QX, United Kingdom. TEL 44-1895-444055, FAX 44-1895-433602.

610.73 GBR
BRITISH JOURNAL OF PERIOPERATIVE NURSING. Text in English. 1965. m. GBP 35 domestic; GBP 45 foreign (effective 2000). adv. bk.rev. back issues avail. *Refereed.* **Document type:** *Academic/Scholarly.* **Description:** News and research articles on the professional, technological, administrative, and procedural aspects of providing care and services to patients in the operating room, with announcements of the educational activities and membership of the association.
Former titles (until 2000): British Journal of Theatre Nursing (1353-0224); (until 1991): N A T News (0027-6049)
Related titles: Online - full text ed.: (from Northern Light Technology, Inc., ProQuest Information & Learning).
Indexed: Brit.Nur.Ind., CINAHL, Int.Nurs.Ind.
—BLDSC (2314.630000), CISTI, GNLM, ingenta, KNAW.
Published by: National Association of Theatre Nurses, Daisy Ayris House, 6 Grove Park Ct, Harrogate, Yorks HG1 4DP, United Kingdom. TEL 44-1423-508079, FAX 44-1423-531613, http://www.natn.org.uk. Ed. Paul Wicker. Adv. contact John Matthews. Circ: 8,000 (controlled).

BRITISH NURSING INDEX; index of journal articles of interest to nurses, midwives and community staff. see *MEDICAL SCIENCES—Abstracting, Bibliographies, Statistics*

610.73 616.6 CAN
C A N N T JOURNAL. Text in English, French. q. CND 30. adv. **Document type:** *Trade.*
Indexed: CINAHL, Int.Nurs.Ind.
Published by: (Canadian Association of Nephrology Nurses and Technologists), Pappin Communications, The Victoria Centre, 84 Isabella St, Pembroke, ON K8A 5S5, Canada. TEL 613-735-0952, FAX 613-735-7983. Eds. Colleen Turpin, Gillian Brunier. R&P Debbie Maure TEL 905-436-0145. Adv. contact C B Pappin.

610.73 BEL ISSN 0926-3209
C I C I A M S NOUVELLES (MULTILINGUAL EDITION). Text in English, French, German, Spanish. 1975. 3/yr. BEF 1,200, USD 40. adv. bk.rev. bibl, illus.
Formed by the 1975 merger of: C I C I A M S Nouvelles (French Edition) (0773-0594); (1965-1975): C I C I A M S News (English Edition) (0007-8417)
—GNLM.
Published by: International Catholic Committee of Nurses and Medico Social Assistants/C I C I A M S - Comite International Catholique des Infirmieres et des Assistantes Medico-Sociales, Sq Vergote 43, Brussels 1030, Belgium. TEL 32-2-7321050, FAX 32-2-7348460. Ed. Mrs. Du Verlunde. Circ: 700.

610.73 CAN
C I N A. Text in English. 1975. a. adv. **Document type:** *Trade.*
Indexed: CINAHL.
—BLDSC (3198.496830).
Published by: (Canadian Intravenous Nurses Association), Pappin Communications, The Victoria Centre, 84 Isabella St, Pembroke, ON K8A 5S5, Canada. TEL 613-735-0952, FAX 613-735-7983. Ed. Elaine Walker. R&P Pam Smith TEL 416-292-0687. Adv. contact C B Pappin.

C I N PLUS. (Computers in Nursing) see *MEDICAL SCIENCES—Computer Applications*

C N N T NEWSLETTER. see *MEDICAL SCIENCES—Urology And Nephrology*

610.73 USA
C N S: THE JOURNAL FOR ADVANCED NURSING PRACTICE. Text in English. 1987. bi-m. USD 87 domestic to individuals; USD 127 foreign to individuals; USD 157 domestic to institutions; USD 197 foreign to institutions (effective 2002). adv. *Refereed.* **Document type:** *Journal, Academic/Scholarly.* **Description:** Information for the clinician, consultant, executive, peer, and patient educator.
Formerly: Clinical Nurse Specialist (0887-6274)
Related titles: Microfilm ed.: (from WWS); Online - full text ed.: USD 204.10 domestic academic site license; USD 227.65 domestic corporate site license; USD 244.10 foreign academic site license; USD 267.65 foreign corporate site license (effective 2002) (from Ovid Technologies, Inc.).
Indexed: CINAHL, Int.Nurs.Ind., Nurs.Abstr.
—BLDSC (3286.314100), GNLM, ingenta.
Published by: Lippincott Williams & Wilkins (Philadelphia) (Subsidiary of: Wolters Kluwer N.V.), 530 Walnut St, Philadelphia, PA 19106-3621. TEL 215-521-8300, FAX 215-521-8902, custserv@lww.com, http://www.lww.com/. Ed. Pauline C. Beecroft. Circ: 3,600. **Subscr. to:** PO Box 1600, Hagerstown, MD 21740-1600. TEL 800-638-3030, FAX 310-223-2400.

610.73 USA ISSN 0008-1310
CALIFORNIA NURSE. Text in English. 1904. 10/yr. USD 40 (effective 2001). adv. bk.rev. back issues avail.; reprint service avail. from PQC,ISI. **Document type:** *Bulletin.* **Description:** Provides news of the California Nurses Association's activities reports on developments of concern to all RNs in the state. Also carries general coverage and commentory on matters of nursing practice, community health and healthcare policy.
Formerly: C N A Bulletin
Related titles: Microfilm ed.: 1904 (from PQC); Online - full text ed.
Indexed: CINAHL, Cal.Per.Ind. (1978-), Int.Nurs.Ind.
—BLDSC (3015.085000), GNLM.
Published by: California Nurses' Association, 2000 Franklin St 300, Oakland, CA 94612-0000. TEL 510-273-2200, FAX 510-663-2761, http://www.calnurse.org/cna/calnurseapror. Ed. Carl Bloice. Adv. contact Felicia Mello TEL 510-273-2251. page USD 1,300; 8.75 x 10. Circ: 30,200 (controlled and free).

610.73 USA
CALIFORNIA SCHOOL NURSE✱ . Text in English. 3/yr.
Published by: Health Information Publications, Inc., 200 Valley Rd Ste 405, Mount Arlington, NJ 07856-1320. TEL 973-267-8938, FAX 973-267-8926. Ed. Barbara Bradstock. Circ: 1,888.

610.73 CAN ISSN 0843-6096
CANADIAN JOURNAL OF CARDIOVASCULAR NURSING. Text in English, French. 1973. q. CND 28 to individuals; CND 42 to institutions; CND 20 to students. adv. bk.rev. *Refereed.* **Description:** Concerned with health care issues related to cardiovascular diseases.
Supersedes (in Apr. 1989): Canadian Bulletin of Cardiovascular Nursing (0831-4462)
Indexed: CINAHL, Int.Nurs.Ind.
—BLDSC (3030.600000), CISTI, GNLM, Infotrieve. **CCC.**
Published by: Canadian Council of Cardiovascular Nurses, 222 Queen St, Ste 1402, Ottawa, ON K1P 5V9, Canada. TEL 613-569-4361, FAX 613-569-3278, http://www.cardiovascularnurse.com. Ed. Ellen Rukholm. Circ: 1,200.

610.73 CAN
CANADIAN JOURNAL OF NURSING LEADERSHIP. Text in English. 1988. q. CND 28. *Refereed.* **Document type:** *Trade.* **Description:** For Canadian nurse administrators, managers and educators.
Supersedes (in 1999): Canadian Journal of Nursing Administration (0838-2948)
Indexed: CINAHL, Int.Nurs.Ind., Nurs.Abstr.
—BLDSC (3033.370000), GNLM, Infotrieve. **CCC.**
Published by: Health Media Inc., 14453 29A Ave, White Rock, BC V4A 9K8, Canada. TEL 604-535-7933.

610.73 CAN ISSN 0844-5621
CODEN: CJNRE3
THE CANADIAN JOURNAL OF NURSING RESEARCH/REVUE CANADIENNE DE RECHERCHE EN SCIENCES INFIRMIERES. Text in English, French. 1969. q. CND 80.25 to individuals; CND 91 foreign to individuals; CND 171.20 to institutions; CND 176 foreign to institutions; CND 48.15 to students; CND 61 foreign to students. adv. *Refereed.* **Document type:** *Academic/Scholarly.* **Description:** Provides a forum for research and articles relevant to nursing and health. Covers clinical research, methodological issues, education research, and theory.
Formerly: Nursing Papers - Perspectives en Nursing (0318-1006)
Indexed: Abstr.Health Care Manage.Stud., Brit.Nur.Ind., CBCA Ref., CINAHL, Fam.Ind., Hosp.Abstr., Int.Nurs.Ind., Lang.& Lang.Behav.Abstr., Nurs.Abstr., Pt.de Rep. (1988-), SOPODA, Sociol.Abstr.
—BLDSC (3033.400000), CISTI, GNLM, ingenta, KNAW. **CCC.**
Published by: McGill University, School of Nursing, 3506 University St, Montreal, PQ H3A 2A7, Canada. TEL 514-398-6172, FAX 514-398-8455, jtoti@po-box.mcgill.ca, http://www.nursing.mcgill.ca. Ed. Laurie Gottlieb. R&P, Adv. contact Joanne Toti. B&W page CND 294.25.

610.73 CAN
CANADIAN NURSE/L'INFIRMIERE CANADIENNE. Text in English. 1905. 10/yr. CND 36 domestic; USD 50 in United States; CND 60 elsewhere. adv. bk.rev., film rev. bibl, charts, illus, stat, tr.lit. index. reprint service avail. from PQC.
Formed by the merger of: Infirmiere Canadienne (0019-9605); Canadian Nurse (0008-4581)
Related titles: Microfilm ed.: (from PQC,PMC).
Indexed: AMED, AgeLine, Brit.Nur.Ind., CBCA Ref., CINAHL, Can.B.P.I., Can.Per.Ind. (Jan.1988-), Hosp.Abstr., INIS Atomind., Int.Nurs.Ind., Nurs.Abstr., Pt.de Rep. (1979-).
—BLDSC (4478.830000), CISTI, GNLM, ingenta, Linda Hall. **CCC.**
Published by: Canadian Nurses Association/Association des Infirmieres et Infirmiers du Canada, 50 Drway, Ottawa, ON K2P 1E2, Canada. TEL 613-237-2133, FAX 613-237-3520, pubss@cna-nurses.ca. Ed. Judith Haines. Circ: 112,000.

610.73 CAN
CANADIAN NURSING MANAGEMENT. Text in English. 1987. 10/yr. CND 109. **Document type:** *Newsletter.*
Published by: M P L Communications Inc., 133 Richmond St W, Ste 700, Toronto, ON M5H 3M8, Canada. TEL 416-869-1177, FAX 416-869-0456. Ed. John Hobel. Circ: 800.

610.73 616.99 CAN ISSN 1181-912X
CANADIAN ONCOLOGY NURSING JOURNAL/REVUE CANADIENNE DE NURSING ONCOLOGIQUE. Text and summaries in English, French. 1991. 4/yr. CND 44.94 to individuals; CND 64.20 to institutions; CND 75 foreign. adv. *Refereed.* **Document type:** *Trade.* **Description:** Covers clinical oncology nursing practice, education and research. Also serves as newsletter and networking vehicle for nurses.
Indexed: CINAHL, Int.Nurs.Ind.
—BLDSC (3043.176000), Infotrieve. **CCC.**
Published by: (Canadian Association of Nurses in Oncology), Pappin Communications, The Victoria Centre, 84 Isabella St, Pembroke, ON K8A 5S5, Canada. TEL 613-735-0952, FAX 613-735-7983. Ed. Beverley Page. adv.: B&W page CND 950, color page CND 1,550; trim 11 x 8.5. Circ: 1,100. **Subscr. to:** CANO, 111 Peter St., Ste 219, Toronto, ON M5V 2H1, Canada.

610.73 CAN ISSN 0712-6778
CANADIAN OPERATING ROOM NURSING JOURNAL. Text in English. 1983. 4/yr. CND 18, USD 20.
Indexed: CINAHL, Int.Nurs.Ind.
—BLDSC (3043.177000), GNLM, Infotrieve. **CCC.**

M

Published by: (Operating Room Nurses Association of Canada), Health Media Inc., 14453 29A Ave, White Rock, BC V4A 9K8, Canada. TEL 604-535-7933. Ed. Agnes Forster. Circ: 4,020.

610.73 616.99 USA ISSN 0162-220X
RC266
CANCER NURSING; an international journal for cancer care. Text in English. 1978. bi-m. USD 75 domestic to individuals; USD 105 foreign to individuals; USD 169 domestic to institutions; USD 195 foreign to institutions; USD 31 newsstand/cover (effective 2002). adv. bk.rev. charts, illus, stat, tr.lit. back issues avail.; reprint service avail. from PQC. *Refereed.* **Document type:** *Academic/Scholarly.* **Description:** Covers problems arising in the care of cancer patients.
Related titles: CD-ROM ed.: (from Ovid Technologies, Inc.); Microform ed.; Online - full text ed.: USD 219.70 domestic academic site license; USD 245.70 foreign academic site license; USD 245.05 domestic corporate site license; USD 271.05 foreign corporate site license (effective 2002) (from Ovid Technologies, Inc., Institute for Scientific Information).
Indexed: AMED, ASCA, AgeLine, Brit.Nur.Ind., CINAHL, Curr.Cont., Dent.Ind., Fam.Ind., INIS Atomind., Ind.Med. (1978-), Int.Nurs.Ind., Nurs.Abstr., SSCI, THA.
—BLDSC (3046.491000), CISTI, EMDOCS, GNLM, IDS, ingenta, KNAW.
Published by: Lippincott Williams & Wilkins (Philadelphia) (Subsidiary of: Wolters Kluwer N.V.), 530 Walnut St, Philadelphia, PA 19106-3621. TEL 301-223-2300, 800-638-3030, FAX 301-223-2400, http:// www.nursingcenter.com, http://www.Lww.com. Ed. Carol Reed Ash. Circ: 7,300. **Subscr. to:** PO Box 1600, Hagerstown, MD 21740-1600.

610.736 616.994 GBR
CANCER NURSING PRACTICE. Text in English. 10/yr. GBP 67.50 in Europe to institutions and libraries; GBP 84.38 elsewhere to institutions and libraries (effective 2002). **Document type:** *Journal, Academic/Scholarly.*
Published by: R C N Publishing Co. (Subsidiary of: B M J Publishing Group), R C N Direct, Copse Walk, Cardiff Gate Business Park, Cardiff CF23 8XG, United Kingdom. TEL 44-29-2054-6450, FAX 44-29-2054-6401, directjournalsteam@rcn.org.uk, http://www.rcn.org.uk/.

610.73 USA
CAPITAL NURSING. Text in English. 1984. q. adv. index. back issues avail. **Description:** Covers news and activities of the Association.
Published by: District of Columbia Nurses Association, 5100 Wisconsin Ave, N W, Ste 306, Washington, DC 20016. TEL 202-244-2705, FAX 202-362-8285. Ed. Evelyn Sommers. Adv. contact Nancy Kofie. page USD 1,000. Circ: 15,000 (controlled).

610.73 CAN ISSN 0843-9966
CARE CONNECTION. Text in English. 1985. q. CND 23.50; CND 29 foreign. adv. bk.rev. illus, tr.lit. back issues avail. **Document type:** *Newsletter.* **Description:** Contains educational articles and health care issue updates.
Former tites: Bedside Specialist (0835-6203); Green Band
Indexed: CINAHL.
Published by: Registered Practical Nurses Association of Ontario (RPNAO), 5025 Orbitor Dr, Ste 200, Bldg 4, Mississauga, ON L4W 4Y5, Canada. TEL 905-602-4664, FAX 905-602-4666, rpnao@istar.ca, http://www.cdn-domain.com/rpnao. Ed., R&P Barbara Thornber. Adv. contact Bonnie Krakenberg. B&W page CND 450; trim 11 x 8.5. Circ: 5,500.

610.73 USA ISSN 1521-0987
▼ **CARE MANAGEMENT JOURNALS**; journal of case management and the journal of long term home health care. Text in English. 1999. q. USD 56 domestic to individuals; USD 65 foreign to individuals; USD 123 domestic to institutions; USD 141 foreign to institutions (effective 2001). adv. bk.rev., software rev., video rev. 80 p./no. back issues avail.; reprints avail. *Refereed.* **Document type:** *Journal, Academic/Scholarly.* **Description:** Comprehensive resource for professional care givers, nurses, nursing home administrators and case managers.
Formed by the merger of (1992-1998): Journal of Case Management (1061-3706); (1994-1998): Journal of Long Term Home Health Care (1072-4281); Which was formerly (1982-1994): Pride Institute Journal of Long Term Home Health Care (0743-5088)
Indexed: Abstr.Soc.Geront., AgeLine, CINAHL, Hospit.Ind., Ind.Med. (1999-), Int.Nurs.Ind., Lang.& Lang.Behav.Abstr., Psychol.Abstr. (1986-), SOPODA, Soc.Serv.Abstr., Soc.Work Res.& Abstr.
—BLDSC (3051.572000), GNLM, Infotrieve, ingenta, KNAW. **CCC.**
Published by: (St. Vincent's Hospital, Pride Institute), Springer Publishing Company, 536 Broadway, New York, NY 10012. TEL 212-431-4370, FAX 212-941-7842, springer@springerpub.com, http://www.springerpub.com. R&P Dorothy Kouwenberg. Adv. contact Bob Friel. B&W page USD 300.

610.73 VIR
CARIBBEAN CHRONICLE* . Text in English. bi-m.
Published by: Caribbean Nurses Organization, P O Box 583, Christiansted, VI 00820.

610.73 USA
CARIBBEAN NURSES ORGANIZATION. NEWSLETTER* . Text in English. q.
Published by: Caribbean Nurses Organization, P O Box 583, Christiansted, VI 00820.

610.73 CAN
CARING. Text in English. 1945. bi-m. membership. adv. **Document type:** *Newsletter, Bulletin.*
Formerly (until 1990): Nurses News
Published by: Manitoba Association of Licensed Practical Nurses, 200 1601 Regent Ave W, Winnipeg, MB R2C 3B3, Canada. TEL 204-663-1212, FAX 204-663-1207. Ed., R&P, Adv. contact Verna Holgate.

658 610 USA ISSN 0738-467X
RA645.35 CODEN: CARGET
CARING (WASHINGTON). Text in English. 1982. m. USD 45 (effective 2000). adv. bk.rev. charts, stat, illus. index. back issues avail.; reprints avail. **Description:** Contains articles, special sections and departments covering national and international aspects of the home care field.
Supersedes: Home Health Review (0193-2683)
Indexed: Abstr.Health Care Manage.Stud., Abstr.Soc.Geront., AgeLine, CINAHL, Hosp.Lit.Ind., I.P.A., Int.Nurs.Ind.
—BLDSC (3053.222000), GNLM, ingenta.
Published by: National Association for Home Care, 228 Seventh St, S E, Washington, DC 20003-4306. TEL 202-547-5277, FAX 202-547-7518, http://www.nahc.org. Ed. Margaret J Cushman. Pub. Val Halamandaris. R&P Patty Esseusee. Adv. contact Cathrine Wolden. Circ: 5,927.

613 DEU ISSN 0948-003X
CARITAS UND PFLEGE. Text in German. q. DEM 30. adv.
Former titles (until 1993): Caritas-Gemeinschaft. Publication; Caritasschwester
—GNLM.
Published by: Caritas-Gemeinschaft fuer Pflege- und Sozialberufe e.V., Maria-Theresia-Str 10, Freiburg Im Breisgau 79102, Germany. TEL 49-761-70861-0, FAX 49-761-7086116. Ed. Renate Heinzmann. Circ: 4,500.

610.73 USA ISSN 0069-2778
CHART* . Text in English. 1904. 12/yr. USD 30 to institutions (effective 1999). adv. **Document type:** *Newsletter.* **Description:** Covers health care and professional issues of importance to all nurses.
Related titles: Microfilm ed.: (from PQC); Online - full text ed.: (from ProQuest Information & Learning).
Indexed: CBCA Ref., CINAHL, Can.Per.Ind. (Sep.1986-), Int.Nurs.Ind.
—BLDSC (3129.960000), GNLM.
Published by: Illinois Nurses Association, 105 W Adams St #2101, Chicago, IL 60603-4109. TEL 312-360-2300, FAX 312-360-9380. Ed. Pamela Towne. Circ: 8,000.

610.73 USA ISSN 0199-2066
CHICAGO NURSE. Text in English. 1946. q. USD 15 (effective 1998). adv. bk.rev. **Document type:** *Newspaper.*
Former titles (until 1979): Chicago District; First (0015-2749)
Published by: Chicago Nurses' Association, 203 N Wabash, Ste 1507, Chicago, IL 60601-2415. TEL 312-263-2708, FAX 312-263-2737. Ed., R&P, Adv. contact Renata Hornick. page USD 300. Circ: 1,400.

610.73 CHL ISSN 0717-2079
CIENCIA Y ENFERMERIA. Text in Spanish. 1995. s-a. CLP 20 domestic; USD 60 foreign (effective 2001). **Document type:** *Academic/Scholarly.* **Description:** Includes news and in-depth articles on nursing and general well being.
Published by: Universidad de Concepcion, Departamento de Enfermeria, Casilla 160-C, Concepcion, Chile. TEL 56-41-204948, FAX 56-41-228353, smendoza@udec.cl.

610.73 GBR ISSN 1361-9004
CLINICAL EFFECTIVENESS IN NURSING. Text in English. 1997. q., latest vol.5. GBP 42 to individuals; GBP 179 to institutions (effective 2002). bk.rev. abstr. 64 p./no. 2 cols./p. back issues avail.; reprints avail. *Refereed.* **Document type:** *Journal, Academic/Scholarly.* **Description:** Aims to address the effects of interventions on patient well-being by publishing work from nursing, midwifery, health visiting and allied disciplines directly relevant to the clinical work of nursing.
Related titles: Online - full text ed.: (from Swets Blackwell, IDEAL Online Library).
Indexed: Brit.Nur.Ind., CINAHL.
—BLDSC (3286.273950).
Published by: Churchill Livingstone (Subsidiary of: Harcourt Publishers Ltd.), Robert Stevenson House, 1-3 Baxter's Pl, Leith Walk, Edinburgh, Midlothian EH1 3AF, United Kingdom. TEL 44-131-556-2424, FAX 44-131-558-1278, journals@harcourt.com, http://www.harcourt-international.com/journals/cein. Eds. Rob Newell, Ruth Hughes. R&P Sharon Boyle TEL 44-131-524-1747. Circ: 500 (paid). **Subscr. in the US:** Harcourt Health Sciences, Journals Subscription Department, PO Box 156, Avenel, NJ 07001. TEL 877-839-7126; **Subscr. to:** Harcourt Publishers Ltd., Journal Sales & Marketing Dept., 32 Jamestown Rd, London NW1 7BY, United Kingdom. TEL 44-20-8308-5700.

610.73 USA ISSN 1085-2360
RT82.8
CLINICAL EXCELLENCE FOR NURSE PRACTITIONERS. Text in English. 1997. bi-m. USD 57 domestic to individuals; USD 100 foreign to individuals; USD 149 domestic to institutions; USD 197 foreign to institutions; USD 33 per issue (effective 2001). **Document type:** *Academic/Scholarly.* **Description:** Publishes articles addressing clinical advances, issues and problems, and outcomes research that serve the continuing education and professional development needs of nurse practitioners.
Indexed: Brit.Nur.Ind., CINAHL, Int.Nurs.Ind.
—BLDSC (3286.285050). **CCC.**
Published by: Churchill Livingstone (Subsidiary of: Harcourt Health Sciences), The Curtis Center, Independence Square West, Philadelphia, PA 19106-3399. http://www.churchillmed.com. Ed. Joellen W Hawkins.

610.73 616.99 USA ISSN 1092-1095
RC266
CLINICAL JOURNAL OF ONCOLOGY NURSING. Text in English. 1997. bi-m. USD 95 domestic; USD 110 foreign; USD 170 domestic for print & online eds.; USD 185 foreign for print & online eds. (effective 2001). adv. 56 p./no. 3 cols./p. back issues avail.; reprints avail. *Refereed.* **Document type:** *Journal, Academic/Scholarly.* **Description:** Provides practical information for direct care of patients and their families across the cancer continuum.
Related titles: Online - full text ed.
Indexed: CINAHL, Int.Nurs.Ind.
—BLDSC (3286.294100), CISTI.
Published by: Oncology Nursing Society, 501 Holiday Dr, Pittsburgh, PA 15220-2749. TEL 412-921-7373, FAX 412-921-6565, http://www.ons.org. Ed. Lisa Scholmeister. Pub. Leonard Mafria. R&P Jeanette M Kent TEL 412-921-7373 ext. 246. Adv. contact Jack Edelman TEL 856-256-2313. Circ: 27,964.

610.73 USA ISSN 1089-1145
THE CLINICAL LETTER FOR NURSE PRACTITIONERS. Text in English. 1997. bi-m., latest vol.5. USD 47 domestic to individuals; USD 76 foreign to individuals; USD 79 domestic to institutions; USD 107 foreign to institutions; USD 19 newsstand/cover (effective 2001). **Document type:** *Newsletter.* **Description:** Provides clinically applicable information relevant to patient practice.
—BLDSC (3286.296500).
Published by: Williams & Wilkins, Newsletters (Subsidiary of: Waverly International), 351 W Camden St, Baltimore, MD 21201-2436. TEL 410-528-8555, FAX 410-528-8596, custserv@wwilkins.com, http://www.wwilkins.com.

610.73 USA ISSN 1054-7738
RT81.5 CODEN: CNREFD
CLINICAL NURSING RESEARCH. Text in English. 1992. q. USD 65 to individuals; USD 260 to institutions; USD 25 newsstand/cover to individuals; USD 70 newsstand/cover to institutions (effective 2002). adv. back issues avail.; reprints avail. *Refereed.* **Document type:** *Academic/Scholarly.* **Description:** Provides an international forum for scholarly research focusing on clinical nursing practice, including the clinical application of research findings.

Related titles: Online - full text ed.: (from EBSCO Publishing, O C L C Online Computer Library Center, Inc., RoweCom Information Quest, ProQuest Information & Learning, Gale Group, ingenta, Swets Blackwell, Factiva).
Indexed: AMED, ASSIA, CINAHL, Fam.Ind., Int.Nurs.Ind., Lang.& Lang.Behav.Abstr., PsycInfo, SOPODA, Sage Fam.Stud.Abstr., Sociol.Abstr., Viol.& Abuse Abstr., e-psyche.
—BLDSC (3286.314150), CISTI, GNLM, Infotrieve, ingenta. **CCC.**
Published by: (University of Alberta CAN), Sage Publications, Inc., 2455 Teller Rd, Thousand Oaks, CA 91320. TEL 805-499-0721, FAX 805-499-0871, info@sagepub.com, http://www.sagepub.com. Eds. Marilynn J Wood, Patricia Hayes. Adv. contact DeAnna Vega Hammersley. Circ: 1,250. **Overseas subscr. to:** Sage Publications Ltd., 6 Bonhill St, London EC2A 4PU, United Kingdom. TEL 44-20-7374-0645, FAX 44-20-7374-8741; Sage Publications India Pvt. Ltd., 4215, New Delhi 110 048, India. TEL 91-11-641-9884, FAX 91-11-647-2426.

610.73 ESP
COLECCION LIBROS DE ENFERMERIA. Text in Spanish. 1975. irreg. price varies. **Document type:** *Monographic series.*
Published by: (Universidad de Navarra, Escuela de Enfermeras), Ediciones Universidad de Navarra, S.A. (EUNSA), Pza. Los Sauces, 1-2, Baranain, (Navarra) 31010, Spain. TEL 34-648-256850, FAX 34-648-256854, eunsaedi@abc.ibernet.com, http://www.unav.es.

610.73 ZAF
COLIMPEX PAEDIATRIC EXECUPAD. Text in Afrikaans, English. a. free per issue to qualified personnel. adv.
Published by: Colimpex Africa (Pty) Ltd., PO Box 5838, Johannesburg 2000, South Africa.

610.73 AUS ISSN 1322-7696
RT1
COLLEGIAN. Text in English. 1994. q. AUD 110 domestic to non-members individuals; AUD 130 foreign to non-members individuals; AUD 220 domestic to institutions; AUD 230 foreign to institutions (effective 2001). adv. 44 p./no. back issues avail. *Refereed.* **Document type:** *Journal, Academic/Scholarly, Consumer.* **Description:** Seeks to educate, inform and stimulate the nursing profession with articles broad in scope. Discusses topical issues, focusing on practice and professional and policy issues. Aimed primarily at nurse practicioners and educators.
Indexed: CINAHL.
—BLDSC (3311.326300).
Published by: Royal College of Nursing Australia, 1 Napier Close, Deakin, ACT 2600, Australia. TEL 61-2-6282-5633, FAX 61-2-6282-3565, canberra@rcna.org.au, http://www.rcna.org.au. Ed., R&P Glenn Gardner. Adv. contact Dominique Hanlon TEL 61-3-9392-1191. B&W page AUD 1,300, color page AUD 1,695; trim 210 x 297.

610.73 USA ISSN 0010-1680
COLORADO NURSE. Text in English. 1973 (vol.73). q. Free to qualified subscribers. adv. 28 p./no. back issues avail. **Document type:** *Newsletter, Trade.* **Description:** Covers issues and employment opportunities of interest to licensed nursing professionals.
Indexed: CINAHL, Int.Nurs.Ind.
—GNLM.
Published by: (Colorado Nurses Association), Arthur L. Davis Publishing Agency, Inc., 517 Washington St, P O Box 216, Cedar Falls, IA 50613. TEL 319-277-2414, 800-626-4081, FAX 319-277-4055, sales@aldpub.com, http://www.aldpub.com/. Ed. Mark Miller. R&P Linda Metzner. Adv. contact Jim Larson. Circ: 54,000 (free).

COMMUNITY NURSE. see *MEDICAL SCIENCES*

610.73 GBR
RT97
COMMUNITY PRACTITIONER. Text in English. 1927. m. GBP 78.50 domestic; GBP 82 foreign (effective 2001). adv. bk.rev., film rev. illus. index. reprint service avail. from PQC. *Refereed.* **Document type:** *Academic/Scholarly.*
Formerly (until 1998): Health Visitor (0017-9140)
Related titles: Microfilm ed.: (from PQC).
Indexed: ASSIA, Abstr.Hyg., Brit.Nur.Ind., CINAHL, Curr.Adv.Ecol.Sci., Dent.Ind., Fam.Ind., Int.Nurs.Ind., Mult.Ed.Abstr., Sp.Ed.Needs Abstr., Trop.Dis.Bull.
—BLDSC (3363.648420), GNLM, KNAW.
Published by: (Community Practitioners' and Health Visitors' Association), T G Scott, Pl, Strand, 1 Lancaster Rd, London W11 1QL, United Kingdom. TEL 44-171-240-2032, FAX 44-171-379-7155. Ed. N Robin. Adv. contact Gillian Notton. Circ: 18,000.

610.73 616.8 GBR
COMMUNITY PSYCHIATRIC NURSING. Text in English. irreg., latest vol.3, 1995. price varies. **Document type:** *Monographic series.*
Indexed: e-psyche.
Published by: Chapman & Hall Ltd. (Subsidiary of: International Thomson Publishing Group), Journals Department, Chapman & Hall, 2-6 Boundary Row, London SE1 8HN, United Kingdom. TEL 44-20-7865-0066, FAX 44-20-7522-9623. **Dist. in N. America by:** Singular Publishing Group, 4284 41st St, San Diego, CA 92105.

362 051 USA ISSN 1070-0323
COMPLEAT NURSE*. Text in English. 1991. m. USD 12 (effective 1999). adv. bk.rev. **Document type:** *Newsletter.* **Description:** Publishes news, features, poetry and other materials of interest to nurses and their patients.
Published by: Jim Rankin, Ed. & Pub., PO Box 597, Roseville, CA 95678-0597. TEL 415-292-7371, FAX 415-292-7314. R&P J Rankin. Adv. contact J. Rankin. Circ: 750.

610.73 618.202 GBR ISSN 1353-6117
COMPLEMENTARY THERAPIES IN NURSING & MIDWIFERY. Text in English. 1995. q. GBP 44 to individuals; GBP 174 to institutions (effective 2002). adv. bk.rev. 56 p./no. 2 cols./p. back issues avail.; reprints avail. *Refereed.* **Document type:** *Journal, Academic/Scholarly.* **Description:** Publishes articles on all aspects of individual therapies and includes original research in nursing practice.
Related titles: Online - full text ed.: (from Swets Blackwell, IDEAL Online Library).
Indexed: AMED, ASSIA, Brit.Nur.Ind., CINAHL, Int.Nurs.Ind.
—BLDSC (3364.203780), GNLM, Infotrieve. **CCC.**
Published by: Churchill Livingstone (Subsidiary of: Harcourt Publishers Ltd.), Robert Stevenson House, 1-3 Baxter's Pl, Leith Walk, Edinburgh, Midlothian EH1 3AF, United Kingdom. TEL 44-131-556-2424, FAX 44-131-558-1278, journals@harcourt.com, http://www.harcourt-international.com/journals/ctnm. Eds. Claire Ancell, Denise Rankin-Box. R&P Sharon Boyle TEL 44-131-524-1747. Adv. contact Deborah Watkins TEL 44-207-424-4280. Circ: 700 (paid). **Subscr. in the US to:** Harcourt Health Sciences, Journals Subscription Department, PO Box 156, Avenel, NJ 07001. TEL 877-839-7126; **Subscr. to:** Harcourt Publishers Ltd., Journal Sales & Marketing Dept., 32 Jamestown Rd, London NW1 7BY, United Kingdom. TEL 44-20-8308-5700.

COMPUTERS IN NURSING. see *MEDICAL SCIENCES—Computer Applications*

610.73 CAN
CONCERN. Text in English. 1968. 6/yr. adv.
Published by: ProWest Publications, 208, 438 Victoria Ave E, Regina, SK S4N 0N7, Canada. TEL 306-352-3400, FAX 306-525-0960. Circ: 9,700.

610.73 USA ISSN 0278-4092
CONNECTICUT NURSING NEWS. Text in English. 1921. q. Free to qualified subscribers. adv. 24 p./no. back issues avail.; reprint service avail. from PQC. **Document type:** *Newspaper, Trade.* **Description:** Covers issues and employment opportunities of interest to licensed nursing professionals.
Formerly: Nursing News (Meriden) (0029-652X)
Related titles: Microform ed.: (from PQC); Online - full text ed.: (from ProQuest Information & Learning).
Indexed: CINAHL, Int.Nurs.Ind.
—GNLM.
Published by: (Connecticut Nurses Association), Arthur L. Davis Publishing Agency, Inc., 517 Washington St, P O Box 216, Cedar Falls, IA 50613. TEL 319-277-2414, 800-626-4081, FAX 319-277-4055, sales@aldpub.com, http://www.aldpub.com/. Ed. Mark Miller. R&P Polly Barey. Adv. contact Jim Larson. Circ: 48,000 (free).

610.730994 AUS ISSN 1037-6178
CONTEMPORARY NURSE; a journal for the Australian nursing profession. Text in English. 1992. q. AUD 75 domestic to individuals; USD 65 in North America to individuals; AUD 105 elsewhere to individuals; AUD 175 domestic to institutions; USD 140, AUD 225 in North America to institutions; AUD 50 domestic to students (effective 2000). adv. bk.rev. back issues avail. *Refereed.* **Document type:** *Academic/Scholarly.*
Indexed: CINAHL, Int.Nurs.Ind.
—BLDSC (3425.195500), ingenta.
Published by: John Libbey & Company Pty. Ltd., Level 10, 15-17 Young St, Sydney, NSW 2000, Australia. TEL 61-2-9251-4099, FAX 61-2-9251-4428, churchill@pp.com.au, jlsydney@mpx.com.au, http://www.churchillmed.com. **US subscr. to:** Churchill Livingstone, PO Box 3217, Secaucus, NJ 07096-3217. TEL 800-553-5426.

610.736 616.1 GBR ISSN 1362-3265
CORONARY HEALTH CARE. Text in English. 1997. q. USD 71 in North America to individuals; USD 259 in North America to institutions; GBP 46 to individuals; GBP 168 to institutions (effective 2001). adv. bk.rev. abstr. 64 p./no. 2 cols./p. back issues avail.; reprints avail. *Refereed.* **Document type:** *Journal, Academic/Scholarly.* **Description:** Promotes clinical practice based on evidence gathered from sound scientific research; disseminates the concepts of primary and secondary prevention of coronary heart disease; and provides a forum for healthcare professionals engaged in the day-to-day management and rehabilitation of patients with coronary heart disease.
Related titles: Online - full text ed.: (from EBSCO Publishing, O C L C Online Computer Library Center, Inc., Swets Blackwell, IDEAL Online Library).
Indexed: Brit.Nur.Ind.
—BLDSC (3472.049500).
Published by: Churchill Livingstone (Subsidiary of: Harcourt Publishers Ltd.), Robert Stevenson House, 1-3 Baxter's Pl, Leith Walk, Edinburgh, Midlothian EH1 3AF, United Kingdom. TEL 44-131-556-2424, FAX 44-131-558-1278, journals@harcourt.com, http://www.harcourt-international.com/journals/chec. Eds. Ann Taylor, Grace Lindsay. R&P Sharon Boyle TEL 44-131-524-1747. Adv. contact Deborah Watkins TEL 44-207-424-4280. Circ: 500 (paid). **Subscr. in the US to:** Harcourt Health Sciences, Journals Subscription Department, PO Box 156, Avenel, NJ 07001. TEL 877-839-7126; **Subscr. to:** Harcourt Publishers Ltd., Journal Sales & Marketing Dept., 32 Jamestown Rd, London NW1 7BY, United Kingdom. TEL 44-20-8308-5700, http://www.harcourthealth.com/.

610.73 USA ISSN 1078-4535
CREATIVE NURSING; a journal of values, issues, experience & collaboration. Text in English. 1982. 4/yr. USD 35; USD 42 foreign (effective 1999). adv. bk.rev. back issues avail. *Refereed.* **Document type:** *Trade.* **Description:** Features interviews with nursing leaders, cutting edge information and analysis from a national and international perspective.
Formerly (until Sep. 1994): Primarily Nursing (0739-4446)
Indexed: CINAHL, Int.Nurs.Ind.
—BLDSC (3487.240500), GNLM.
Published by: Creative Nursing Management, Inc., 1701 E. 79th St., Ste. 1, Bloomington, MN 55425-1151. TEL 612-339-7766, 800-728-7766, FAX 612-339-2065, chcm@chcm.com, http://www.chcm.com. Ed. Lisa Legge. Pub. Marie Manthey. R&P, Adv. contact Beth Beaty TEL 612-854-9015. page USD 650; trim 9.63 x 7.75. Circ: 1,000 (paid).

610.73 USA ISSN 0279-5442
RT120.I5 CODEN: CCNUEV
CRITICAL CARE NURSE. Text in English. 1980. bi-m. USD 39 domestic to individuals; USD 120 domestic to institutions; USD 8 newsstand/cover (effective 2001). adv. back issues avail.; reprint service avail. from PQC. *Refereed.* **Document type:** *Academic/Scholarly.* **Description:** Provides current information and perspectives on a wide range of topics in critical care nursing.
Related titles: Online - full text ed.: (from Northern Light Technology, Inc., ProQuest Information & Learning).
Indexed: CINAHL, Fam.Ind., INIS Atomind., Int.Nurs.Ind., Nurs.Abstr.
—BLDSC (3487.451100), GNLM, ingenta, KNAW. **CCC.**
Published by: American Association of Critical Care Nurses, 101 Columbia, Aliso Viejo, CA 92656. TEL 714-362-2000, FAX 949-362-2020, critnurse@aol.com, http://www.critical-care-nurse.org/, http://www.aacn.org. Ed. Grif Alspach. Pub. Bonnie Harrigan. R&P Beth Wos TEL 800-899-1712. adv.: B&W page USD 5,235, color page USD 6,855. Circ: 78,000 (paid). **Subscr. to:** PO Box 611, Holmes, PA 19043.

M

610.7 USA ISSN 0899-5885
RT120.I5
CRITICAL CARE NURSING CLINICS OF NORTH AMERICA. Text in English. 1989. q. USD 83 domestic to individuals; USD 117 foreign to individuals; USD 121 domestic to institutions; USD 149 foreign to institutions; USD 83 domestic to students; USD 38 per issue (effective 2001). index. back issues avail. **Document type:** *Academic/Scholarly.* **Description:** Delivers practical advice from experts in specialty covered with a fresh perspective on problems and controversies.
Related titles: Microform ed.: (from PQC).
Indexed: CINAHL, Int.Nurs.Ind.
—BLDSC (3487.451150), GNLM, ingenta.
Published by: W.B. Saunders Co. (Subsidiary of: Harcourt Publishers Ltd.), 11830 Westline Industrial Dr, St Louis, MO 63146. TEL 800-325-4177, http://www.wbsaunders.com. Ed. Suzanne S Prevost. **Subscr. to:** Periodicals Fulfillment, 6277 Sea Harbor Dr, 4th Fl, Orlando, FL 32891-4800. TEL 800-654-2452, FAX 800-874-6418.

610 USA ISSN 0887-9303
CODEN: CCNQEJ
CRITICAL CARE NURSING QUARTERLY. Text in English. 1978. q. USD 132 to individuals; USD 40 newsstand/cover (effective 2002). reprint service avail. from PQC. **Document type:** *Journal, Academic/Scholarly.* **Description:** Presents current, proven, hands-on procedures for improving clinical practice.
Formerly: Critical Care Quarterly (0160-2551)
Related titles: Microform ed.: (from PQC); Online - full text ed.: (from Ovid Technologies, Inc., ProQuest Information & Learning, Gale Group).
Indexed: Biol.Abstr., CINAHL, Excerp.Med., Fam.Ind., IMFL, Int.Nurs.Ind., Nurs.Abstr., Psychol.Abstr.
—BLDSC (3487.451200), CISTI, EMDOCS, GNLM, ingenta, KNAW. **CCC.**
Published by: Aspen Publishers, Inc., 200 Orchard Ridge Dr, Ste 200, Gaithersburg, MD 20878. TEL 301-417-7500, FAX 301-417-7550, customer.service@aspenpubl.com, http://www.aspenpub.com. Ed. Janet M Barber. Pub. Jack Bruggeman. Circ: 4,429 (paid). **Dist. by:** Aspen Publishers Inc., Distribution Center, 7201 McKinney Circle, Frederick, MD 21701. TEL 301-698-7100, FAX 301-417-7550.

610.73 618.202 ZAF ISSN 0379-8577
CURATIONIS; accredited research journal of the Democratic Nursing Organisation of South Africa. Text in Afrikaans, English. 1977. q., latest vol.24. ZAR 120, USD 50 (effective 2001). adv. bk.rev. charts, illus. 88 p./no. back issues avail. *Refereed.* **Document type:** *Journal, Academic/Scholarly.* **Description:** Publishes accredited research articles.
Indexed: CINAHL, Ind.S.A.Per., Int.Nurs.Ind.
—BLDSC (3493.458000), GNLM.
Published by: Democratic Nursing Organisation of South Africa, PO Box 1280, Pretoria 0001, South Africa. TEL 27-12-3432315, FAX 27-12-3445750, info@denosa.org.za, http://www.denosa.org.za. Eds. Bhungani ka Mzolo, Nelouise Geyer. Adv. contact Bhungani ka Mzolo. Circ: 600 (paid).

CURRENT REVIEWS FOR PERIANESTHESIA NURSES. see *MEDICAL SCIENCES—Anaesthesiology*

DAGENS MEDICIN. see *MEDICAL SCIENCES*

610.73 USA
DELAWARE NURSES' ASSOCIATION REPORTER. Text in English. 1968. q. USD 20 (effective 2001). adv. bk.rev. 24 p./no. back issues avail. **Document type:** *Newsletter, Trade.* **Description:** Covers issues and employment opportunities of interest to licensed nursing professionals.
Supersedes: Delaware Nurse (0070-3281)
Indexed: CINAHL.
Published by: (Delaware Nurses Association), Arthur L. Davis Publishing Agency, Inc., 517 Washington St, P O Box 216, Cedar Falls, IA 50613. TEL 319-277-2414, 800-626-4081, FAX 319-277-4055, sales@aldpub.com, http://www.aldpub.com/. Ed. Mark Miller. R&P Ruth Bashford. Adv. contact Jim Larson. B&W page USD 150; trim 7.25 x 9.5. Circ: 15,000 (free).

DELMAR'S DRUG GUIDE FOR NURSES. see *PHARMACY AND PHARMACOLOGY*

610.73698 USA ISSN 1091-4587
DEVELOPMENT IN SUPPORTIVE CANCER CARE✱. Text in English. 1996. q. free per issue. **Document type:** *Trade.* **Description:** Provides clinically relevant, state-of-the-art information to nurses in various settings who care for and interact with patients facing cancer.
Indexed: CINAHL.
Published by: Meniscus Educational Institute (Subsidiary of: Meniscus Ltd.), 18 Elizabeth St, West Conshohocken, PA 19428-2935. TEL 610-660-8080, FAX 610-660-9583, email@meniscus.com, http://www.meniscus.com. Ed. Susan B Baird. Pub. Lois Trench Hines.

DIABETIC MEDICINE. see *MEDICAL SCIENCES—Endocrinology*

DIABETIC MEDICINE ONLINE. see *MEDICAL SCIENCES—Endocrinology*

DIALAESEN; tidningen foer personal inom nyursyukvaard. see *MEDICAL SCIENCES—Urology And Nephrology*

610.73 USA ISSN 0730-4625
DIMENSIONS OF CRITICAL CARE NURSING. Abbreviated title: D C C N. Text in English. 1982. bi-m. USD 55 domestic to individuals; USD 65 in Canada to individuals; USD 73 elsewhere to individuals; USD 86 domestic to institutions; USD 96 in Canada to institutions; USD 104 elsewhere to institutions; USD 17 newsstand/cover (effective 2001). adv. illus. index. back issues avail. *Refereed.* **Description:** Focuses on research, educational, leadership and practice issues for experienced critical care nurses.
Related titles: Online - full text ed.: (from ProQuest Information & Learning).
Indexed: CINAHL, Fam.Ind., Int.Nurs.Ind., Nurs.Abstr.
—BLDSC (3588.471200), GNLM, ingenta. **CCC.**
Published by: Springhouse Corporation (Subsidiary of: Lippincott Williams & Wilkins (Philadelphia)), 1111 Bethlehem Tpk., Springhouse, PA 19477-0908. TEL 215-646-8700, 800-783-4903, FAX 215-646-4399, http://www.springnet.com/criticalcare/dccn99.htm, http://www.springnet.com; http://www.cinahl.com/jrnls/index.htm. Ed. Jan Corwin Enger. Circ: 3,000. **Subscr. to:** 30 Broad St, PO Box 3000, Denville, NJ 07834.

610.73 GBR
DIRECTORY OF COMMUNITY NURSING. Text in English. 1980. a. GBP 24.95 (effective 2002). adv. **Document type:** *Trade.*
Published by: P M H Publications Ltd., PO Box 100, Chichester, W Sussex PO18 8HD, United Kingdom. TEL 44-1243-576444, FAX 44-1243-576456, admin@pmh.uk.com, http://www.pmh.uk.com. Ed. Pat Scowen. Pub. Linda Edmondson.

DIRECTORY OF FUNDING SOURCES. see *EDUCATION—Higher Education*

610.73025 AUS ISSN 0812-5856
DIRECTORY OF HIGHER EDUCATION NURSING COURSES. Text in English. 1984. a. AUD 14.95 to non-members; AUD 12.95 to members. adv. back issues avail. **Document type:** *Directory.* **Description:** Provides alphabetical listing of pre- and post-registration nursing courses in Australia.
Published by: Royal College of Nursing Australia, 1 Napier Close, Deakin, ACT 2600, Australia. TEL 61-2-6282-5633, FAX 61-2-6282-3565. Adv. contact Joanne Ramadge.

610.73 USA ISSN 1062-8835
DIRECTORY OF NURSE-MIDWIFERY PRACTICES (YEAR). Text in English. a. membership. adv. **Document type:** *Directory.* **Description:** Lists nurse-midwifery practices.
Formerly: Registry of Nurse-Midwifery Services and Practices
Published by: American College of Nurse-Midwives, 818 Connecticut Ave, Ste 900, Washington, DC 20005. TEL 202-728-9860, FAX 202-728-9897. Ed. John Boggess. Circ: 6,000.

610.73 CAN
THE DOGWOOD NEWS. Text in English. 1957. q. free per issue to members. **Description:** Includes information for the association general membership, as well as, pertinent articles relating to Licensed Practical Nurses practicing in the health care field, provincially and nationally.
Published by: Licenced Practical Nurses Association of British Columbia, 3302 McIver Rd, Westbank, BC V4T 1G2, Canada. TEL 604-768-2482. Ed. Barry E Phillips.

610.73 DMA
DOMINICA NURSES ASSOCIATION. NEWSLETTER. Text in English. q. membership. **Document type:** *Newsletter.*
Published by: Dominica Nurses Association, Roseau, Dominica.

DRUGS AND DEVICE RECALL BULLETIN. see *PHARMACY AND PHARMACOLOGY*

610.736 USA
E D NURSING. (Emergency Department) Text in English. 1997. m. USD 299 domestic; USD 329 foreign; USD 48 newsstand/cover (effective 2001). **Description:** Provides emergency department nurses with solutions for difficult procedures, uncooperative patients, and other tough clinical situations they face on a daily basis.
Published by: American Health Consultants (Subsidiary of: Medical Economics Co., Inc.), 3525 Piedmont Rd, N E, 6 Piedmont Center, Ste 400, Atlanta, GA 30305. TEL 404-262-5476, 404-262-7436, 800-688-2421, FAX 404-262-7837, 800-284-3291, custserv@ahcpub.com, http://www.ahcpub.com.

E D T N A - E R C A JOURNAL. see *MEDICAL SCIENCES—Urology And Nephrology*

610.73 618 GBR
E N B NEWS. Text in English. 1991. q. free per issue. adv. **Document type:** *Newsletter.* **Description:** Contains information about the decisions, activities, policy statements and publications of the board.
Formerly (until 1990): Feedback
Related titles: CD-ROM ed.: E N B Link CD-ROM; Online - full text ed.
Published by: English National Board for Nursing, Midwifery, and Health Visiting, Victory House, 170 Tottenham Ct Rd, London W1P 0HA, United Kingdom. TEL 44-171-388-3131, FAX 44-171-383-4031, enb.link@easynet.co.uk, http://www.eng.org.uk. Ed. Jill Rogers. Circ: 19,000 (controlled).

610.73 GBR ISSN 1354-5752
EMERGENCY NURSE. Text in English. 1994. 10/yr. GBP 80 in Europe to institutions; GBP 96 elsewhere to institutions (effective 2002). adv. **Document type:** *Trade.*
Related titles: Online - full text ed.: (from Northern Light Technology, Inc.).
Indexed: Brit.Nur.Ind., CINAHL, Int.Nurs.Ind.
—BLDSC (3733.192900).
Published by: (R C N Accident & Emergency Nursing Association), R C N Publishing Co. (Subsidiary of: B M J Publishing Group), R C N Direct, Copse Walk, Cardiff Gate Business Park, Cardiff CF23 8XG, United Kingdom. TEL 44-29-2054-6450, FAX 44-29-2054-6401, directjournalsteam@rcn.org.uk, http://www.rcn.org.uk/. Ed. Brian Dolan. Adv. contact Phil Whomes. Circ: 3,106.

610 340 USA ISSN 0098-1516
KF2915.N8
EMERGENCY NURSE LEGAL BULLETIN. Abbreviated title: E N L B. Text in English. 1975. q. USD 20. **Document type:** *Newsletter, Bulletin.*
Indexed: CINAHL, Int.Nurs.Ind.
—BLDSC (3733.193000).
Published by: Med-Law Publishers, Inc., PO Box 293, Westville, NJ 08093. TEL 609-848-3817, FAX 609-848-1431. Ed. Dr. James E George.

610.73 BRA
ENFERMAGEM; o jornal brasileiro de enfermagem. Text in Portuguese. 1977. bi-m. USD 50. adv.
Published by: (Associacao Brasileira de Enfermagem), Cidade - Editora Cientifica Ltda., Rua Mexico, 90-Andar 2, Centro, Rio De Janeiro, RJ 20031-141, Brazil. TEL 021-240-4578. Ed. Fernando Moyses. Circ: 31,000.

610.73 MEX
ENFERMERAS. Text in Spanish. 1953. 3/yr. MXP 75 (effective 1999 & 2000). adv. charts, illus, stat. back issues avail. **Document type:** *Newsletter, Trade.* **Description:** Covers nursing research, practice and news on events of interest to nurses. Presents scientific and technical advances in the Mexican nursing field.
Former titles: Colegio Nacional de Enfermeras. Revista (0045-7329); Asociacion Mexicana de Enfermeras. Revista
Indexed: Int.Nurs.Ind.
Published by: Colegio Nacional de Enfermeras, OBRERO MUNDIAL 229, Col Del Valle, Mexic City, DF 03100, Mexico. TEL 525-5436637, FAX 525-6694031, conalenf@df1.telmex.net.mx. Ed. Ezequiel Canela. Pub., Adv. contact Bertha Delgado. R&P Josefina Reyes Gonzalez. B&W page USD 300, color page USD 400. Circ: 1,300 (paid); 700 (controlled).

610.73 ESP ISSN 0211-9005
ENFERMERIA CIENTIFICA. Text in Spanish. 12/yr.
Address: Francisca Armada, 38, Madrid 28047, Spain. TEL 1-255-68-09, FAX 1-46-48-613. Ed. Jesus Sanchez Martos.

M

610.73 ESP ISSN 1130-8621
ENFERMERIA CLINICA. Text in Spanish. 1990. bi-m. USD 75. adv. **Document type:** *Academic/Scholarly.* **Description:** Studies clinical nursing to promote a solution to the health problems of individuals, families and communities. Contributes to the theoretical and practical development of the profession in Spain.
Indexed: CINAHL.
—BLDSC (3747.900700).
Published by: Ediciones Doyma S.A., Traversa de Gracia, 17-21, Barcelona 08021, Spain. TEL 34-93-200-0711, FAX 34-93-209-1136. Ed. P Vilagrasa. Adv. contact Anna Pahissa. page ESP 225,000; trim 280 x 210. Circ: 4,500.

610.73 ESP ISSN 1130-2399
ENFERMERIA INTENSIVA. Text in Spanish. 1990. q. ESP 7,000 to individuals; ESP 10,300 to institutions; ESP 5,600 to students (effective 2001). adv. bk.rev. index. back issues avail.; reprints avail. *Refereed.* **Document type:** *Journal, Academic/Scholarly.*
Related titles: Online - full text ed.
Indexed: Ind.Med.Esp., Int.Nurs.Ind.
—BLDSC (3747.900800), Infotrieve. **CCC.**
Published by: (Sociedad Espanola de Enfermeria Intensiva y Unidades Coronarias), Ediciones Doyma S.A., Traversa de Gracia, 17-21, Barcelona 08021, Spain. TEL 34-93-200-0711, ei@doyma.es, doyma@doyma.es, http://www.doyma.es/ei. Ed. Maria del Carmen Asiain Erro. R&P Monica Barnes. Adv. contact Jose Antonio Hernandez. B&W page ESP 117,000, color page ESP 139,000; 280 x 210.

610.73 ESP ISSN 1576-5520
ENFERMERIA ONCOLOGICA. Variant title: Revista de Enfermeria Oncologica. Text in Spanish; Abstracts in English, Spanish. 1986. q. ESP 3,750 to membership (effective 2001). abstr. back issues avail.
Related titles: E-mail ed.
Published by: Sociedad Espanola de Enfermeria Oncologica, Apdo Postal 46-351, Madrid, Spain. info@seeo.org, http://www.seeo.org. Ed. Pilar O'Kelly.

610.73 GBR
EUROFORUM. Text in English. q. **Document type:** *Bulletin.*
Indexed: CINAHL.
—BLDSC (3829.268430).
Published by: Royal College of Nursing, 20 Cavendish Sq, London W1M 0AB, United Kingdom. TEL 44-171-409-3333, FAX 44-171-355-1379. Ed. Susan Williams.

610.73 616.9 GBR ISSN 1462-3889
EUROPEAN JOURNAL OF ONCOLOGY NURSING. Text in English. 1997. q. GBP 44 to individuals; GBP 170 to institutions (effective 2002). adv. bk.rev. abstr. bibl. 72 p./no. 2 cols./p. back issues avail.; reprints avail. *Refereed.* **Document type:** *Journal, Academic/Scholarly.* **Description:** Discusses clinical and experimental trends and techniques in nursing for cancer-care patients.
Formerly: Journal of Cancer Nursing
Related titles: Online - full text ed.: (from EBSCO Publishing, O C L C Online Computer Library Center, Inc., Swets Blackwell, IDEAL Online Library).
Indexed: Brit.Nur.Ind., CINAHL.
—BLDSC (3829.733100).
Published by: (European Oncology Nursing Society BEL), Churchill Livingstone (Subsidiary of: Harcourt Publishers Ltd.), Robert Stevenson House, 1-3 Baxter's Pl, Leith Walk, Edinburgh, Midlothian EH1 3AF, United Kingdom. TEL 44-131-556-2424, FAX 44-131-558-1278, ejon@harcourt.com, journals@harcourt.com, http://www.harcourt-international.com/journals/ejon. Ed. Alison Richardson. R&P Sharon Boyle TEL 44-131-524-1747. Adv. contact Deborah Watkins TEL 44-207-424-4280. Circ: 750 (paid). **Subscr. in the US to:** Harcourt Health Sciences, Journals Subscription Department, PO Box 156, Avenel, NJ 07001. TEL 877-839-7126; **Subscr. to:** Harcourt Publishers Ltd., Journal Sales & Marketing Dept., 32 Jamestown Rd, London NW1 7BY, United Kingdom. TEL 44-20-8308-5700.

610.73 GBR ISSN 1367-6539
EVIDENCE - BASED NURSING. Text in English. 1997. q. GBP 47 combined subscription in Europe to individuals includes print & online eds.; USD 118 combined subscription elsewhere to individuals includes print & online eds.; GBP 99 in Europe to institutions for print only; USD 178 elsewhere to institutions for print only (effective 2002). **Document type:** *Academic/Scholarly.* **Description:** Helps nurses base their clinical decisions on the best current clinical evidence.
Related titles: E-mail ed.; Online - full text ed.: ISSN 1468-9618. 1998. GBP 30, USD 50 to individuals (effective 2002) (from O C L C Online Computer Library Center, Inc., HighWire Pr.).
Indexed: Brit.Nur.Ind., CINAHL.
Published by: B M J Publishing Group, R C N Publishing Co. nso@nursing-standard.co.uk, subscriptions@bmjgroup.com, http://wbn.bmjjournals.com/. Circ: 6,150. **Co-publisher:** R C N Publishing Co.

610.73 BEL ISSN 0774-935X
F.N.I.B. - INFO. Text in French. 1921. bi-m. BEF 1,500 (effective 1998 & 1999). adv. illus.
Former titles (until 1987): Flash-informations (0771-8187); (until 1983): F.N.I.B. - N.V.B.V. (0301-0813); (until 1971): Infirmiere (0019-9591)
—CISTI, GNLM.
Published by: Federation Nationale Neutre des Infirmieres de Belgique, Rue de la Source 18, Brussels 1060, Belgium. TEL 32-75-365153, FAX 32-75-365153. Ed. Yves Mengal. **Subscr. to:** c/o Dominique Rombaux, Rue Warmonceau 32, Charleroi 6000, Belgium. TEL 32-71-433453, FAX 32-71-251498.

610.73 USA ISSN 0172-5238
FACHSCHWESTER - FACHPFLEGER. Text in English. 1975. irreg., latest 1990. price varies. reprint service avail. from ISI. **Document type:** *Monographic series.*
—GNLM.
Published by: Springer-Verlag, Journals (Subsidiary of: BertelsmannSpringer), 175 Fifth Ave, New York, NY 10010. TEL 212-460-1500, FAX 212-473-6272.

610.73 615.82 ESP ISSN 0211-5638
FISIOTERAPIA. Text in Spanish; Summaries in English. 1979. q. ESP 10,300 to individuals; USD 14,750 to institutions; USD 8,240 to students (effective 2001). bk.rev. index. back issues avail.; reprints avail. *Refereed.* **Document type:** *Journal, Academic/Scholarly.*
Related titles: Online - full text ed.: 1996.
Published by: (Sociedad Espanola de Fisioterapia), Ediciones Doyma S.A., Traversa de Gracia, 17-21, Barcelona 08021, Spain. TEL 34-93-200-0711, ft@doyma.es, doyma@doyma.es, http://www.doyma.es/ft. Ed. Santos Sastre Fernandez. R&P Monica Barnes. Adv. contact Jose Antonio Hernandez.

610.73 USA ISSN 0015-4199
FLORIDA NURSE. Text in English. 1952. q. Free to qualified subscribers. adv. bk.rev. illus. 36 p./no. back issues avail.; reprint service avail. from PQC. **Document type:** *Newsletter, Trade.* **Description:** Covers issues and employment opportunities of interest to licensed nursing professionals.
Related titles: Online - full text ed.: (from Northern Light Technology, Inc., ProQuest Information & Learning).
Indexed: AMED, CINAHL, Int.Nurs.Ind.
—BLDSC (3956.080000), GNLM.
Published by: (Florida Nurses Association), Arthur L. Davis Publishing Agency, Inc., 517 Washington St, P O Box 216, Cedar Falls, IA 50613. Ed. Mark Miller. R&P Paula Massey. Adv. contact Jim Larson. Circ: 185,000 (free).

610.73 USA
FLORIDA NURSING NEWS*. (In 2 editions: South Florida and Gulf-Central) Text in English. 1981. fortn. USD 9.95. adv.
Published by: Nursing News, Inc., 127 Signal Ridge Dr, Dawsonville, GA 30534-8244. Ed. Steven Ricci. Circ: 55,000.

610.73 SWE ISSN 0283-913X
FOERETAGSSKOETERSKAN. Text in Swedish. 1957. q. SEK 250 (effective 2000). adv. **Document type:** *Newsletter, Trade.*
Supersedes: Industriskoeterskan
Published by: Riksfoereningen foer Foeretagsskoeterskor, c/o Birgitta Langlet Soederholm, Loevdalsvaegen 5A, Saltsjoe-Boo 13241, Sweden. Ed., Pub., R&P Birgitta Langlet Soederholm TEL 46-8-7158530.

610.73 USA ISSN 0016-2116
FRONTIER NURSING SERVICE QUARTERLY BULLETIN. Text in English. 1925. q. USD 6 to individuals; USD 10 to institutions (effective 2000). adv. illus. back issues avail. **Document type:** *Newsletter.* **Description:** Provides an overview of the Frontier Nursing Service of Eastern Kentucky.
Related titles: Microform ed.: (from PQC).
Indexed: CINAHL, Int.Nurs.Ind.
—BLDSC (4041.200000), GNLM.
Published by: Frontier Nursing Service, Inc., 132 FNS Dr, Wendover, KY 41775. TEL 606-672-2317, FAX 606-672-3022. Ed., R&P Barb Gibson. Circ: 8,000.

610.73 USA ISSN 0016-8335
GEORGIA NURSING. Text in English. 1945. q. Free to qualified subscribers. adv. 36 p./no. back issues avail. **Document type:** *Newsletter, Trade.* **Description:** Covers issues and employment opportunities of interest to licensed nursing professionals.
Related titles: Online - full text ed.: (from Northern Light Technology, Inc., ProQuest Information & Learning).
Indexed: CINAHL, Int.Nurs.Ind.
—BLDSC (4158.457000), GNLM.
Published by: (Georgia Nurses Association), Arthur L. Davis Publishing Agency, Inc., 517 Washington St, P O Box 216, Cedar Falls, IA 50613. TEL 319-277-2414, 800-626-4081, FAX 319-277-4055, sales@aldpub.com, http://www.aldpub.com/. Ed. Mark Miller. R&P Deborah Hackman. Adv. contact Jim Larson. Circ: 86,000 (free).

GERIATRIC NURSING. see *GERONTOLOGY AND GERIATRICS*

GEROKOMOS. see *GERONTOLOGY AND GERIATRICS*

610.73 BEL ISSN 0778-4457
GEST HOME; la revue des gestionnaires et du personnel soignant des maisons de repos, centres hopitaliers, c.p.a.s., centre de sante et de soins. Text in Dutch, French. 1986. q. BEF 450. adv. bk.rev. **Description:** Intended to serve those involved and working in the health care profession, nursing homes, rehabilitation centers, and hospitals.
Published by: Socorema s.c.r.l., Rue du Merlo 28, Brussels 1180, Belgium. TEL 02-376-62-28, FAX 02-376-12-80. Ed. J Laffineur Brouhon. Circ: 5,000.

GUIDE TO SUCCESSFUL GRANT APPLICATIONS. see *EDUCATION—Higher Education*

610.73 CHN ISSN 1001-1099
GUOWAI YIXUE (HULIXUE FENCE)/FOREIGN MEDICAL SCIENCES (NURSING). Text in Chinese. 1980. m. USD 20.40; USD 1.70 newsstand/cover (effective 2001). **Document type:** *Academic/Scholarly.*
Published by: China International Book Trading Corp/Zhongguo Guoji Tushu Maoyi Zonggongsi cibtc@mail.cibtc.com.cn, http://www.cibtc.com.cn. **Dist. by:** 35, Chegongzhuang Xilu, Haidian District, Beijing 100044, China.

610.73 CAN
HAND IN HAND. Text in English. 3/yr. membership. **Document type:** *Newspaper.*
Formerly: S N A A Newsletter
Published by: Saskatchewan Association of Licensed Practical Nurses, 2310 Smith, Regina, SK S4P 2P6, Canada. TEL 306-525-1436, FAX 306-347-7784. Ed., R&P, Adv. contact Ede Leeson. Circ: 2,600.

THE HEALTH CARE MANAGER. see *HEALTH FACILITIES AND ADMINISTRATION*

HEALTH CAREER POST. see *HEALTH FACILITIES AND ADMINISTRATION*

610.73 USA ISSN 0199-8552
HEALTHWIRE. Text in English. 1980. bi-m. membership. adv. **Document type:** *Newsletter.* **Description:** Describes membership and local union activities, provides readers with national union news and an update on activities organized at the national level. Covers topics of interest to healthcare professionals and provides information on professional development workshops, conferences and publications.
Indexed: Genet.Abstr. (coverage dropped).
Published by: (American Federation of Teachers), Federation of Nurses and Health Professionals (Subsidiary of: American Federation of Teachers), 555 New Jersey Ave, N W, Washington, DC 20001. TEL 202-879-4430, afteditor@aol.com, http://www.aft.org. Ed., R&P Pricilla Nemeth TEL 202-393-5661. Adv. contact Sharon Wright. Circ: 63,000 (paid).

HELEN K. MUSSALLEM LIBRARY SELECTED ACQUISITIONS. see *MEDICAL SCIENCES—Abstracting, Bibliographies, Statistics*

HELEN K. MUSSALLEM. PERIODICAL HOLDINGS LIST. see *MEDICAL SCIENCES—Abstracting, Bibliographies, Statistics*

M

610.73 616 FIN ISSN 0786-5686
HOITOTIEDE/NURSING SCIENCE; journal of Nurshing Science. Text in Finnish. 1989. bi-m. FIM 200 in Scandinavia; FIM 300 elsewhere (effective 2001). adv. *Refereed.* **Document type:** *Journal, Academic/Scholarly, Trade.* **Description:** Reports about the results of nursing research, actual events in nursing research and provides a discussion forum for nurse researches.
Indexed: CINAHL, Int.Nurs.Ind.
—BLDSC (4322.216500).
Published by: (Department of Nursing Science), Finnish Association of Caring Sciences, PL 1627, Kuopio 70211, Finland. TEL 358-17-162610, FAX 358-17-162632, arja.isola@uku.fi. Ed. Arja Isola. R&P Pirjo Laitinin-Junkkari TEL 358-17-162-628. Adv. contact Jaino Viitaniemi TEL 358-3-3141-7826. B&W page FIM 2,000.

610.73 JPN ISSN 0018-3369
HOKENFU NO KEKKAKU TENBO/REVIEW OF TUBERCULOSIS FOR PUBLIC HEALTH NURSE. Text in Japanese. 1963. s-a. JPY 1,700 (effective 2001). adv. bk.rev. charts, illus, stat. 100 p./no. **Document type:** *Academic/Scholarly.*
Published by: Japan Anti-Tuberculosis Association/Kekkaku Yobokai, 1-3-12 Misaki-cho, Chiyoda-ku, Tokyo 101-0061, Japan. TEL 81-3-3292-0211, FAX 81-3-3292-9208, jata@jatahq.org, http://www.jatahq.org. Pub. Toru Mori. Circ: 1,700.

610.73 JPN ISSN 0047-1844
HOKENFU ZASSHI/JAPANESE JOURNAL FOR PUBLIC HEALTH NURSE. Text in Japanese. 1951. m. JPY 16,200, USD 93.
—BLDSC (4658.420000), GNLM.
Published by: Igaku-Shoin Ltd., 5-24-3 Hongo, Bunkyo-ku, Tokyo 113-0033, Japan. TEL 81-3-3817-5774, FAX 81-3-3815-4145, ysekiyama@nna.so.net.or.jp. Circ: 8,500.

610.73 USA ISSN 0887-9311
HOLISTIC NURSING PRACTICE. Text in English. 1979. q. USD 132 to individuals; USD 40 newsstand/cover (effective 2002). **Document type:** *Journal, Academic/Scholarly.* **Description:** Provides nurse clinicians and educators with information on holistic approaches to nursing practice in clinical settings.
Formerly (until 1985): Topics in Clinical Nursing (0164-0534)
Related titles: Online - full text ed.: (from Ovid Technologies, Inc., ProQuest Information & Learning, Gale Group).
Indexed: AMED, CINAHL, Fam.Ind., IMFL, Int.Nurs.Ind., Nurs.Abstr.
—BLDSC (4322.302600), CISTI, GNLM, ingenta. **CCC.**
Published by: Aspen Publishers, Inc., 200 Orchard Ridge Dr, Ste 200, Gaithersburg, MD 20878. TEL 301-417-7500, 800-638-8437, FAX 301-695-7931, customer.service@aspenpubl.com, http://www.aspenpub.com. Pub. Jack Bruggeman. Circ: 3,000 (paid). **Dist. by:** Aspen Publishers Inc., Distribution Center, 7201 McKinney Circle, Frederick, MD 21701. TEL 301-698-7100, FAX 301-417-7550.

610.73 GBR ISSN 1364-3029
HOME AND COMMUNITY HEALTHCARE. Text in English. a. GBP 55. **Document type:** *Trade.*
Published by: Sterling Publications Ltd. (Subsidiary of: Sterling Publishing Group Plc.), Brunel House, 55-57 North Wharf Rd, London W2 1LA, United Kingdom. FAX 44-20-7724-2089, http://www.sterlingpublications.com. R&P Sandy Tucker. Circ: 10,000 (controlled).

610.73 USA
HOME CARE AND HOSPICE UPDATE. Text in English. 1994. m. **Description:** Provides timely and useful information to clinician and managers practicing or managing in home care and hospice.
Formerly (until 1999): Home Care Nurse News (1077-2251)
—BLDSC (4326.000450).
Address: Box 629, Boca Grande, FL 33921-0629. FAX 941-697-2901, 800-993-6397, news@marrelli.com.

610.736 362.14 USA ISSN 1087-0385
HOME CARE EDUCATION MANAGEMENT. Text in English. 1996. m. USD 299; USD 306 foreign (effective 1999). back issues avail. **Document type:** *Newsletter.* **Description:** Discusses trends and tips for educating home-care professionals.
Indexed: CINAHL.
Published by: American Health Consultants (Subsidiary of: Medical Economics Co., Inc.), 3525 Piedmont Rd, N E, 6 Piedmont Center, Ste 400, Atlanta, GA 30305. TEL 404-262-5476, custserv@ahcpub.com, http://www.ahcpub.com. Ed. Melinda G Young. Pub. Donald R Johnston.

610.73 USA ISSN 1084-628X
HOME CARE PROVIDER. Text in English. 1996. bi-m. USD 34 domestic to individuals; USD 51 foreign to individuals; USD 106 domestic to institutions; USD 123 foreign to institutions; USD 25 domestic to students; USD 42 foreign to students; USD 21 newsstand/cover (effective 2001). adv. Supplement avail.; reprints avail. **Document type:** *Journal, Trade.* **Description:** Contains how-to articles addressing clinical issues, patient education, practice management tips, pharmacology information, research findings, legal and reimbursement issues for home care providers.
Related titles: Online - full text ed.: (from EBSCO Publishing, IDEAL Online Library, RoweCom Information Quest).
Indexed: CINAHL, Int.Nurs.Ind.
—BLDSC (4326.000900), GNLM, Infotrieve. **CCC.**
Published by: (Joint Commission on Accreditation of Healthcare Organizations (JCAHO)), Mosby, Inc. (Subsidiary of: Elsevier Science), 11830 Westline Industrial Dr, St Louis, MO 63146-3318. TEL 314-872-8370, 800-325-4177, FAX 314-432-1380, journals.service@mosby.com, http://www.mosby.com/homecare, http://www.mosby.com/periodicals. Ed. Tina M Marelli. Pub. Nathania Sawyer. Adv. contact Gina Burkert TEL 314-453-4306. B&W page USD 210, color page USD 1,010; trim 10.88 x 8.13. Circ: 1,375. **Co-sponsor:** National Association for Medical Equipment Services (NAMEA).

610.736 362.14 USA ISSN 1087-0407
HOME CARE QUALITY MANAGEMENT. Text in English. 1995. m. USD 319 domestic; USD 349 foreign; USD 53 newsstand/cover (effective 2001). **Document type:** *Newsletter.* **Description:** Discusses the monitoring of quality in administering home care.
Indexed: CINAHL.
—BLDSC (4326.175452).
Published by: American Health Consultants (Subsidiary of: Medical Economics Co., Inc.), 3525 Piedmont Rd, N E, 6 Piedmont Center, Ste 400, Atlanta, GA 30305. TEL 404-262-5476, 404-262-7436, 800-688-2421, FAX 404-262-7837, 800-284-3291, custserv@ahcpub.com, http://www.ahcpub.com.

610.736 USA ISSN 1099-5323
HOME HEALTH CARE CONSULTANT; journal of alternative site medicine and management. Text in English. m. USD 95 domestic; USD 145 foreign; USD 9.50 newsstand/cover domestic; USD 11.50 newsstand/cover foreign (effective 2000). **Document type:** *Magazine, Academic/Scholarly.* **Description:** Provides a forum for disseminating important and unique perspectives on the care of home bound patients and their caregivers.
Indexed: CINAHL.
—BLDSC (4326.053750).
Published by: MultiMedia Healthcare Inc., Office Center of Princeton Meadows, Bldg 300, Plainsboro, NJ 08536. TEL 609-275-7355, FAX 609-275-7369, info@mmhc.com, http://www.mmhc.com/hhcc. Ed. Barbara Weinfeld.

362.16 USA ISSN 1075-2188
HOME HEALTH FOCUS. Text in English. 1994. m. USD 33 domestic to individuals; USD 51 foreign to individuals; USD 81 domestic to institutions; USD 99 foreign to institutions (effective 2000). **Document type:** *Newsletter.* **Description:** Designed for the home health professional with practical clinical articles, regulation and documentation updates, advice and counsel from colleagues, patient education tools and more.
Indexed: CINAHL.
—Infotrieve. **CCC.**
Published by: Mosby, Inc. (Subsidiary of: Elsevier Science), 11830 Westline Industrial Dr, St Louis, MO 63146-3318. TEL 314-453-4351, FAX 314-431-1158, journals.service@mosby.com, http;//wwwLww.com. Ed. Karen S Martin.

362.14 330 USA ISSN 0882-2700
HOMECARE. Text in English. 1978. m. USD 65 in United States; USD 75 in Canada; USD 150 elsewhere (effective 1999). adv. **Description:** Provides comprehensive coverage of the home health care industry, including trends, issues, acquisitions, products and legislation.
Formerly (until 1984): Homecare Rental - Sales
Related titles: Online - full text ed.
—CCC.
Published by: Primedia Business Magazines & Media, Inc. (Subsidiary of: Primedia Inc.), 23815 Stuart Ranch Rd, Box 8987, Malibu, CA 90265-8987. TEL 310-317-4522, FAX 310-317-9644, http://www.homecaremag.com. Ed. Susanne Hopkins. Pub., Adv. contact Sally Matteson. R&P Greg Vargas TEL 800-543-4116. Circ: 16,000. **Subscr. to:** Homecare, P.O. Box 16837, N. Hollywood, CA 91615-6837.

362.14 USA
HOMECARE MONDAY. Text in English. 1997. w. USD 297 domestic; USD 319 in Canada; USD 339 elsewhere. adv. **Document type:** *Newsletter.* **Description:** Provides the latest industry and financial news, including legislation, products, and trends.
Media: Fax. **Related titles:** Fax ed.
Published by: Primedia Business Magazines & Media, Inc. (Subsidiary of: Primedia Inc.), 23815 Stuart Ranch Rd, Box 8987, Malibu, CA 90265-8987. TEL 310-317-4522, FAX 310-317-9644, inquiries@primediabusiness.com, http://www.primediabusiness.com. Ed. Kimberly Schworm. Pub., Adv. contact Sally Matteson. R&P Greg Vargas TEL 800-543-4116. **Subscr. to:** PO Box 12914, Overland Park, KS 66282-2914. TEL 800-441-0294, FAX 913-967-1903.

610.73 USA ISSN 1045-1242
HOMECARE NEWS. Text in English. q. USD 20 (effective 2000). **Document type:** *Newspaper.*
Published by: National Association for Home Care, 228 Seventh St, S E, Washington, DC 20003-4306. TEL 202-547-7424, FAX 202-547-3540. Ed., R&P Janet Neigh. Pub. Val Halamandaris. Adv. contact Cathrine Wolden. Circ: 28,000.

610.73 AUS ISSN 0073-3253
HONG KONG NURSING JOURNAL/HSIANG KANG HU LI TSA CHIH. Key Title: Xianggang Huli Zazhi. Text in Chinese, English. 1965. q. AUD 436 domestic; AUD 397 in New Zealand; USD 242 elsewhere; AUD 480 domestic print & online eds. combined; AUD 437 in New Zealand print & online eds. combined; USD 267 elsewhere print & online eds. combined (effective 2001). adv. bk.rev. *Refereed.* **Document type:** *Journal, Academic/Scholarly.* **Description:** Contains articles on all issues relating to nursing.
Related titles: ♦ Online - full text ed.: Hong ong Nursing Journal Online.
Indexed: CINAHL, HongKongiana.
—BLDSC (4326.402000), CISTI. **CCC.**
Published by: (Hong Kong Nurses Association HKG), Blackwell Science Asia Pty Ltd, PO Box 378, Carlton South, VIC 3053, Australia. TEL 61-3-9347-0300, FAX 61-3-9347-5001, info@blacksci-asia.com.au, http://www.medicine.org.hk/conhk/hknj/home.htm, http://www.blacksci.co.uk/australi. Ed. Filomena Lai Wan Chow. Circ: 4,500.

610.73 AUS
HONG ONG NURSING JOURNAL ONLINE. Text in Chinese, English. q. AUD 393 domestic; AUD 358 in New Zealand; USD 382 elsewhere (effective 2001). *Refereed.* **Document type:** *Academic/Scholarly.*
Media: Online - full text. **Related titles:** ♦ Print ed.: Hong Kong Nursing Journal. ISSN 0073-3253.
Published by: (Hong Kong Nurses Association HKG), Blackwell Science Asia Pty Ltd, PO Box 378, Carlton South, VIC 3053, Australia. TEL 61-3-9347-0300, FAX 61-3-9347-3016, info@blacksci-asia.com.au, http://www.medicine.org.hk/conhk/hknj/home.htm, http://www.blacksci.co.uk/australi.

HOSPICE BULLETIN. see *HEALTH FACILITIES AND ADMINISTRATION*

HOSPITAL & HEALTHCARE NEWS. see *HEALTH FACILITIES AND ADMINISTRATION*

HOSPITAL PHARMACY DIRECTOR'S MONTHLY MANAGEMENT SERIES. see *PHARMACY AND PHARMACOLOGY*

610.73 NLD ISSN 1013-1779
I C H S INFORMATION BULLETIN. Text in Dutch. irreg. (approx. 3-4/yr.). **Document type:** *Bulletin.*
Published by: International Council of Homehelp Services, c/o R Kalfsbeek, Exec Sec, Postbus 100, Bunnik 3980 CC, Netherlands. TEL 31-3405-96211, FAX 31-3405-63994.

M

610.736 GRC ISSN 1108-7366
I C U S AND NURSING WEB JOURNAL. Variant title: I C U s and Nursing Web Journal(ICU NURS WEB J). Text in English, Greek. q. free (effective 2001). adv. *Refereed.* **Document type:** *Academic/Scholarly.* **Description:** Dedicated to the dissemination of knowledge generated in the critical care and emergency nursing practice setting.
Media: Online - full text.
Address: 121 Tzavella St, Nikea, Piraeus 18450, Greece. nursing@nursing.gr, editor@nursing.gr, http://www.nursing.gr/. Pub., Adv. contact Ioannis Caldfissudis.

610.73 USA
I N S NEWSLINE. Text in English. 1973. bi-m. membership. adv. bk.rev. stat. **Document type:** *Newsletter.* **Description:** Offers timely coverage on clinical issues, product developments, IV drug safety, legislative and entrepreneurial topics affecting IV nurse specialists, and opportunities for continuing education and professional advancement.
Former titles: I N S Update; N I T A Update
Published by: Intravenous Nurses Society, 10 Fawcett St, Cambridge, MA 02138-1110. TEL 617-441-3008, FAX 617-441-3009. Ed. Danielle R Patrella. R&P Sarah Kill Kelly TEL 800-694-0298. Adv. contact Danielle R Petrella. Circ: 8,000.

610.73 USA
I S N A BULLETIN. (Indiana State Nursing Association) Text in English. q. Free to qualified subscribers. adv. back issues avail. **Document type:** *Newsletter, Trade.* **Description:** Covers issues and employment opportunities of interest to licensed nursing professionals.
Published by: (Indiana State Nurses Association), Arthur L. Davis Publishing Agency, Inc., 517 Washington St, P O Box 216, Cedar Falls, IA 50613. TEL 319-277-2414, 800-626-4081, FAX 319-277-4055, sales@aldpub.com, http://www.aldpub.com/. Ed. Mark Miller. R&P Ernest Klein. Adv. contact Jim Larson. Circ: 98,000 (free).

610.73 USA ISSN 0019-3062
IMPRINT (NEW YORK). Text in English. 1968. 5/yr. USD 15. adv. illus. index. reprints avail. **Description:** Provides organization news.
Formerly: N S N A Newsletter
Indexed: BHA, CINAHL, Int.Nurs.Ind.
—BLDSC (4371.486500), ingenta, KNAW.
Published by: National Student Nurses' Association, 555 W 57 St, New York, NY 10019. TEL 212-581-2211, http://www.nsna.org/pubs/index_imprint.html. Ed. Caroline Jaffe. Circ: 34,000.

INDUSTRIAL HEALTH FOUNDATION. NURSING SERIES. BULLETINS. see *OCCUPATIONAL HEALTH AND SAFETY*

INFECTION CONTROL AND WOUNDCARE YEARBOOK. see *MEDICAL SCIENCES—Communicable Diseases*

610.73 CAN ISSN 0822-8558
L'INFIRMIERE AUXILIAIRE. Text in French. 1928. 4/yr. CND 20; CND 25 foreign (effective 2000). adv. bk.rev. charts, illus. index. **Document type:** *Bulletin.*
Former titles: Auxiliaire (0703-9484); Revue des Infirmieres et Infirmiers Auxiliaires du Quebec; Cahiers du Nursing (0316-411X)
—GNLM.
Published by: Ordre des Infirmieres et Infirmiers Auxiliaires du Quebec, 531 Sherbrooke E, Montreal, PQ H2L 1K2, Canada. TEL 514-282-9511, FAX 514-282-0631. Ed., R&P Francine Saucier TEL 514-282-8511. Adv. contact Sylvie Lariviere. Circ: 23,000.

610.73 CAN ISSN 1195-2695
INFIRMIERE DU QUEBEC. Text in French. 1976. bi-m. CND 25 to individuals; CND 36 in United States to individuals; CND 46 elsewhere to individuals; CND 36 to institutions; CND 47 in United States to institutions; CND 57 elsewhere to institutions (effective 1999). adv. bk.rev. illus. *Refereed.* **Document type:** *Newsletter.*
Former titles (until Sep. 1993): Nursing Quebec (0381-6419); (until 1980): Order of Nurses of Quebec. News and Notes (0319-2636)
Indexed: Can.Per.Ind. (Oct.1993-), Int.Nurs.Ind., Pt.de Rep. (1982-).
—GNLM, KNAW.
Published by: Ordre des Infirmieres et Infirmiers du Quebec/Ordre of Nurses of Quebec, 4200 Dorchester Blvd W, Montreal, PQ H3Z 1V4, Canada. TEL 514-935-2501, FAX 514-935-2055, inf@oiiq.org, http://www.oiiq.org. Ed. Diane Iezzi. R&P Marlene Lavoie. Adv. contact Ghislaine Brunet. B&W page CND 1,865, color page CND 3,235; trim 10.88 x 8.13. Circ: 61,803 (controlled).

610.73 FRA
INFIRMIERE LIBERALE. Text in French. 6/yr. FRF 420 to individuals; FRF 490 to institutions; FRF 260 to students; FRF 56 newsstand/cover.
Published by: Initiatives Sante, 26 av. de l'Europe, BP 60, Velizy Villacoublay Cedex 78141, France. TEL 33-1-34633333, FAX 33-1-34653985. Circ: 55,000.

610.73 CAN ISSN 0846-524X
INFO NURSING. Text in English, French. 1967. 4/yr. CND 25 domestic; USD 30 foreign (effective 2000). adv. bk.rev. illus. **Document type:** *Newsletter.*
Former titles (until 1989): Info - Nurses Association of New Brunswick (0842-3210); (until 1984): Info - New Brunswick Association of Registered Nurses (0382-5574); (until 1975): N B A R N News (0382-5566)
Indexed: CINAHL.
—BLDSC (4478.876830), Infotrieve. **CCC.**
Published by: Nurses Association of New Brunswick/Association des Infirmieres et Infirmiers du Nouveau-Brunswick, 165 Regent St, Fredericton, NB E3B 7B4, Canada. TEL 506-458-8731, FAX 506-459-2838. Ed., Adv. contact George Bergeron. Circ: 8,900.

610.73 BEL
INFO-NURSING. Text in English. 1929. 8/yr. BEF 2,000 domestic; BEF 2,500 foreign (effective 2000). adv. **Document type:** *Bulletin, Trade.*
Published by: Association Nationale Catholique du Nursing, Av Hippocrate 91, Brussels 1200, Belgium. TEL 32-2-7625618, FAX 32-2-7725219. Ed., Pub., R&P, Adv. contact Hans Sabine TEL 32-21762-5618.

INFORMATIONSDIENST KRANKENHAUSWESEN/ HEALTH CARE INFORMATION SERVICE. see *HEALTH FACILITIES AND ADMINISTRATION*

INSIGHT (ST. LOUIS). see *MEDICAL SCIENCES—Ophthalmology And Optometry*

610.73 GBR ISSN 0964-3397
INTENSIVE AND CRITICAL CARE NURSING. Text in English. 1985. bi-m. GBP 50 to individuals; GBP 208 to institutions (effective 2002). adv. bk.rev. abstr. 64 p./no. 2 cols./p. back issues avail.; reprints avail. *Refereed.* **Document type:** *Journal, Academic/Scholarly.* **Description:** International and interdisciplinary forum for specialist nurses.
Formerly (until Mar. 1992): Intensive Care Nursing (0266-612X)
Related titles: Online - full text ed.: (from Swets Blackwell, IDEAL Online Library).
Indexed: ASSIA, Brit.Nur.Ind., CINAHL, Fam.Ind., Int.Nurs.Ind.
—BLDSC (4531.836000), CISTI, GNLM, ingenta. **CCC.**
Published by: Churchill Livingstone (Subsidiary of: Harcourt Publishers Ltd.), Robert Stevenson House, 1-3 Baxter's Pl, Leith Walk, Edinburgh, Midlothian EH1 3AF, United Kingdom. TEL 44-131-556-2424, FAX 44-131-558-1278, iccn@harcourt.com, journals@harcourt.com, ejon@harcourt.com, http://www.harcourt-international.com/journals/iccn. Ed. Carol Ball. R&P Sharon Boyle TEL 44-131-524-1747. Adv. contact Deborah Watkins TEL 44-207-424-4280. Circ: 4,000. **Subscr. in the US to:** Harcourt Health Sciences, Journals Subscription Department, PO Box 156, Avenel, NJ 07001. TEL 877-839-7126; **Subscr. to:** Harcourt Publishers Ltd., Journal Sales & Marketing Dept., 32 Jamestown Rd, London NW1 7BY, United Kingdom. TEL 44-20-8308-5700.

610.73 FRA ISSN 0242-3960
INTERBLOC; la revue des infirmiers et infirmieres de salles d'operations. Text in French. 4/yr. FRF 350; FRF 406 foreign (effective 2000). **Document type:** *Academic/Scholarly.* **Description:** Topics covered include hygiene, surgical technique and technology, and legal and professional aspects.
Formerly: Journal of Operating Theatre Male and Female Nurses
—BLDSC (4531.850200). **CCC.**
Published by: (Association des Enseignants des Ecoles d'Infirmieres de Bloc Operatoire), Masson - Periodiques, 120 bd. St. Germain, Paris 75006, France. TEL 33-1-40466200, FAX 33-1-40466201. Ed. A Blanchart. Circ: 2,500. **Subscr. to:** Societe de Periodiques Specialises, BP 22, Vineuil Cedex 41354, France. TEL 33-2-54504612, FAX 33-2-54504611.

610.73 NLD ISSN 0074-4360
INTERNATIONAL COUNCIL OF HOMEHELP SERVICES. REPORTS OF CONGRESS. Text in Dutch. 1959. quadrennial, latest 1989, 8th, Noordwijkerhout, NE. **Document type:** *Proceedings.*
Published by: International Council of Homehelp Services, c/o R Kalfsbeek, Exec Sec, Postbus 100, Bunnik 3980 CC, Netherlands. TEL 31-3405-96211, FAX 31-3405-63994.

610.73 GBR ISSN 1360-1105
INTERNATIONAL HISTORY OF NURSING JOURNAL. Text in English. 1983. s-a. GBP 60 in Europe; GBP 76 elsewhere (effective 2002). bk.rev. back issues avail. **Document type:** *Bulletin.*
Former titles (until 1995): History of Nursing Journal (0960-2348); History of Nursing Bulletin (0265-3834)
Indexed: Brit.Nur.Ind., CINAHL.
—BLDSC (4540.724150), GNLM.
Published by: (Royal College of Nursing), R C N Publishing Co. (Subsidiary of: B M J Publishing Group), R C N Direct, Copse Walk, Cardiff Gate Business Park, Cardiff CF23 8XG, United Kingdom. TEL 44-29-2054-6450, FAX 44-29-2054-6401, directjournalsteam@rcn.org.uk, http://www.rcn.org.uk/. Ed. Steven Black. Circ: 450.

610.73 USA ISSN 1091-5710
RT86
INTERNATIONAL JOURNAL FOR HUMAN CARING. Text in English. 1997. 3/yr. USD 75 domestic to individuals; USD 85 in Canada to individuals; USD 91 elsewhere to individuals; USD 125 domestic to institutions; USD 135 in Canada to institutions; USD 141 elsewhere to institutions (effective 2000). back issues avail. *Refereed.* **Document type:** *Academic/Scholarly.* **Description:** It serves as a scholarly forum for nurses to advance knowledge of care and caring within the discipline of nursing.
Indexed: CINAHL.
—BLDSC (4542.286000).
Published by: International Association for Human Caring, 1770 E Lancaster Ave, Ste 1B, Paoli, PA 19301. TEL 503-646-8974, FAX 503-646-8974, orders@allnenpress.com, http://www.allenpress.com. Ed. Kathleen Valentine. **Subscr. to:** Allen Press Inc., PO Box 1897, Lawrence, KS 66044-8897. **Dist. by:** TEL 610-640-5755, FAX 610-640-3863.

610.73 AUS ISSN 1322-7114
INTERNATIONAL JOURNAL OF NURSING PRACTICE. Text in English. 1995. bi-m. AUD 160 domestic to individuals; AUD 145 in New Zealand to individuals; USD 145 elsewhere to individuals; AUD 501 domestic to institutions; AUD 455 in New Zealand to institutions; USD 455 elsewhere to institutions; AUD 176 domestic to individuals paper & online eds. combined; AUD 160 in New Zealand to individuals paper & online eds. combined; USD 160 elsewhere to individuals paper & online eds. combined; AUD 552 domestic to institutions paper & online eds. combined; AUD 501 in New Zealand to institutions paper & online eds. combined; USD 501 elsewhere to institutions paper & online eds. combined (effective 2001). adv. back issues avail. *Refereed.* **Document type:** *Academic/Scholarly.* **Description:** Explores and promotes nursing as both a profession and an academic discipline.
Related titles: Online - full text ed.: ISSN 1440-172X. AUD 144 domestic to individuals (effective 2001); AUD 131 in New Zealand to individuals; USD 131 elsewhere to individuals; AUD 451 domestic to institutions; AUD 410 in New Zealand to institutions; USD 410 elsewhere to institutions (effective 1999) (from Ovid Technologies, Inc., EBSCO Publishing, O C L C Online Computer Library Center, Inc., RoweCom Information Quest, ingenta, Munksgaard & Blackwell Science's Synergy, Swets Blackwell).
Indexed: ASSIA, Brit.Nur.Ind., CINAHL, Environ.Sci.Poll.Mgmt., Int.Nurs.Ind., Pollut.Abstr., Risk Abstr., Saf.Sci.Abstr.
—BLDSC (4542.406800), GNLM, Infotrieve, ingenta. **CCC.**
Published by: Blackwell Science Asia Pty Ltd, PO Box 378, Carlton South, VIC 3053, Australia. TEL 61-3-9347-0300, FAX 61-3-9347-5001, info@blacksci-asia.com.au; apearson@medicinen.adelaide.edu.au, http://www.blacksci.co.uk. Ed. Alan Pearson. Adv. contact Kathryn O'Brien. B&W page AUD 935, color page AUD 1,950; trim 210 x 275.

M

610.730 GBR ISSN 0020-7489
RT1
INTERNATIONAL JOURNAL OF NURSING STUDIES. Text in English. 1965. bi-m. EUR 106 in Europe to individuals; JPY 14,100 in Japan to individuals; USD 119 elsewhere to individuals; EUR 727 in Europe to institutions; JPY 91,640 in Japan to institutions; USD 814 elsewhere to institutions (effective 2002). adv. bk.rev. charts, illus. index. back issues avail.; reprint service avail. from PQC. *Refereed.* **Document type:** *Academic/Scholarly.* **Description:** Publishes material of interest to an international readership of nurses, midwives and others interested in nursing and caring sciences.
Related titles: Microfilm ed.: (from PQC); Online - full text ed.: (from ingenta, Swets Blackwell, ScienceDirect, Institute for Scientific Information).
Indexed: ASCA, ASSIA, Abstr.Health Care Manage.Stud., AgeLine, Brit.Nur.Ind., CINAHL, Curr.Cont., ERA, Educ.Tech.Abstr., Fam.Ind., Hosp.Abstr., Ind.Med. (1963-), Int.Nurs.Ind., PsycInfo, Psychol.Abstr. (1982-), SSCI, Stud.Wom.Abstr., Tech.Educ.Abstr., e-psyche.
—BLDSC (4542.407000), CISTI, GNLM, IDS, ingenta, KNAW. **CCC.**
Published by: Pergamon (Subsidiary of: Elsevier Science), The Boulevard, Langford Ln, East Park, Kidlington, Oxford OX8 1GB, United Kingdom. FAX 44-1865-843010, http://www.elsevier.com/locate/ijnurstu. Eds. J Alexander, Jenifer Wilson-Barnett. Circ: 1,150. **Subscr. in Australasia and the Far East to:** Elsevier Science (Singapore) Pte Ltd, No.1 Temasek Ave, 17-01 Millenia Tower, Singapore 039192, Singapore. TEL 65-434-3727, FAX 65-337-2230; **Subscr. in the Americas to:** Elsevier Science, PO Box 945, New York, NY 10159-0945. TEL 212-633-3730, FAX 212-633-3680, usinfo-f@elsevier.com; **Subscr. to:** Elsevier Science BV, PO Box 211, Amsterdam 1000 AE, Netherlands. TEL 31-20-485-3757.

610.73 GBR ISSN 1357-6321
INTERNATIONAL JOURNAL OF PALLIATIVE NURSING. Text in English. 1995. bi-m. back issues avail. **Document type:** *Academic/Scholarly.* **Description:** Specialist journal on palliative care for nurses with an international focus.
Indexed: AMED, Brit.Nur.Ind., CINAHL.
—BLDSC (4542.440900).
Published by: Mark Allen Publishing Ltd., Croxted Mews, 286-288a Croxted Rd, London SE24 9BY, United Kingdom. TEL 44-20-8671-7521, FAX 44-20-8671-4454, editorial@markallengroup.com. Ed. Gwen Clarke. Pub. Mark Allen. R&P Roger Allen. adv.: B&W page GBP 990, color page GBP 1,390; trim 215 x 292. Circ: 2,500 (paid). **Subscr. to:** Jesses Farm, Dinton, Salisbury, Wilts SP3 5HN, United Kingdom. TEL 44-1722-716997.

THE INTERNATIONAL JOURNAL OF PSYCHIATRIC NURSING RESEARCH. see *MEDICAL SCIENCES—Psychiatry And Neurology*

610.73 617.1 USA ISSN 1075-4210
INTERNATIONAL JOURNAL OF TRAUMA NURSING. Text in English. 1995. q. USD 39 domestic to individuals; USD 63 foreign to individuals; USD 90 domestic to institutions; USD 114 foreign to institutions; USD 25 domestic to students; USD 49 foreign to students; USD 29 per issue domestic (effective 2001). adv. *Refereed.* **Document type:** *Academic/Scholarly.* **Description:** Written especially for the nursing professionals working in trauma care, from scene of injury through rehabilitation. Original articles focus on topics of key interest to readers and are clinically relevant to trauma nurses.
Related titles: Online - full text ed.: (from EBSCO Publishing, IDEAL Online Library, RoweCom Information Quest).
Indexed: CINAHL, Int.Nurs.Ind.
—BLDSC (4542.696050). **CCC.**
Published by: (Trauma Nursing Coalition), Mosby, Inc. (Subsidiary of: Elsevier Science), 11830 Westline Industrial Dr, St Louis, MO 63146-3318. TEL 314-872-8370, 800-325-4177, FAX 314-432-1380, http://www.mosby.com/ijtn, http://www.mosby.com/periodicals. Ed. Judith Stoner Halpern. Adv. contact Gina Burkert TEL 314-453-4306. B&W page USD 545, color page USD 1,495; trim 10.88 x 8.25. Circ: 1,118. **Co-sponsors:** American Association of Nurse Anesthetists; Emergency Nurses Association; Air and Surface Transport Nurses Association; American Association of Critical Care Nurses; Association of Rehabilitation Nurses; Association of periOperative Registered Nurses, Inc.

610.73 GBR ISSN 0020-8132
RT1
INTERNATIONAL NURSING REVIEW. Text in English. 1926. q., latest vol.49, 2002. GBP 38 in Europe to individuals; USD 61 in North America to individuals; GBP 42 elsewhere to individuals; GBP 59 in Europe to institutions; USD 94 in North America to institutions; GBP 65 elsewhere to institutions (effective 2002). adv. bk.rev. illus. index. reprint service avail. from PQC. *Refereed.* **Document type:** *Academic/Scholarly.* **Description:** Examines the current concerns and issues of modern day nursing and health care from an international perspective.
Related titles: Microform ed.: (from PQC); ◆ Online - full text ed.: International Nursing Review Online. ISSN 1466-7657.
Indexed: ASSIA, Abstr.Health Care Manage.Stud., CINAHL, Fam.Ind., Ind.Med. (1954-), Int.Nurs.Ind.
—BLDSC (4544.500000), CISTI, GNLM, ingenta.
Published by: (International Council of Nurses CHE), Blackwell Science Ltd., PO Box 88, Oxford OX2 0NE, United Kingdom. TEL 44-1865-206180, 44-1865-206002, FAX 44-1865-206219, icn@uni2a.unige.ch, jnl.orders@blacksci.co.uk, http://www.blackwell-science.com/~cgilib/jnlpage.asp?Journal=inr&File=inr, http://www.blackwellpublishing.com. Pub. Griselda Campbell. Circ: 3,500.

610.73 GBR ISSN 1466-7657
INTERNATIONAL NURSING REVIEW ONLINE. Text in English. q. GBP 35 in Europe to individuals; USD 55 in North America to individuals; GBP 35 elsewhere to individuals; GBP 54 in Europe to institutions; USD 85 in North America to institutions; GBP 54 elsewhere to institutions (effective 2002). *Refereed.* **Document type:** *Academic/Scholarly.*
Media: Online - full text (from EBSCO Publishing, Munksgaard & Blackwell Science's Synergy, O C L C Online Computer Library Center, Inc., RoweCom Information Quest, ingenta, Swets Blackwell). **Related titles:** Microform ed.: (from PQC); ◆ Print ed.: International Nursing Review. ISSN 0020-8132.
Published by: Blackwell Science Ltd., Osney Mead, Oxford OX2 0EL, United Kingdom. TEL 44-1685-206206, FAX 44-1685-721205, website@blacksci.com, journals.cs@blacksci.co.uk, http://www.blackwell-science.com.

610.73 USA ISSN 1081-7700
THE INTERNATIONAL OREM SOCIETY NEWSLETTER. Text in English. 1994. s-a. USD 5 to non-members (effective 2000).
—BLDSC (6107.451400).
Published by: International Orem Society for Nursing Science and Scholarship, S428 School of Nursing, University of Missouri, Columbia, MO 65211. FAX 573-884-4544.

610.73 USA ISSN 1523-6064
THE INTERNET JOURNAL OF ADVANCED NURSING PRACTICE. Text in English. 1997. s-a. free per issue. bk.rev. back issues avail. *Refereed.* **Document type:** *Academic/Scholarly.* **Description:** Contains information from the field of nursing. Original articles, reviews, case reports, streaming slide shows, streaming videos, letters to the editor, press releases, meeting information.
Media: Online - full text.
Published by: Internet Scientific Publications, L.L.C., 23 Rippling Creek Dr, Sugar Land, TX 77479. TEL 281-240-1533, FAX 281-240-1533, sruppert@ispub.com, http://www.ispub.com/journals/ijanp.htm. Pub., R&P, Adv. contact Hope Morrow TEL 832-754-0335.

610.73 GBR
INTERNURSE. Text in English. m. adv. *Refereed.*
Media: Online - full text.
Published by: Mark Allen Group.com Ltd, Croxted Mews, 288 Croxted Rd, London SE24 9BY, United Kingdom. TEL 44-20-8671-7521, http://www.internurse.com/. Ed. Paul Mangan.

610.73 COL ISSN 0120-5307
INVESTIGACION Y EDUCACION EN ENFERMERIA. Text in Spanish; Summaries in English, Spanish. 1983. s-a. COP 12,000 domestic; USD 25 foreign (effective 2000). adv. bk.rev. bibl. **Document type:** *Academic/Scholarly.* **Description:** Publishes works from Latin American institutions that are of importance to health and social science workers.
—GNLM. **CCC.**
Published by: Universidad de Antioquia, Facultad de Enfermeria, Carrera 53 no. 62-65, Apartado Aereo 1226, Medellin, ANT, Colombia. TEL 57-4-510-6335, FAX 57-4-211-0058, rieenf@caribe.udea.edu.co, meruiz@catios.udea.edu.co, http://caribe.udea.edu.co. Ed. Luz Elena Ospina Llano. Adv. contact Luz Angela Ramirez. page USD 300. Circ: 1,000 (controlled).

610.73 USA
IOWA BOARD OF NURSING. NEWSLETTER. Text in English. q. Free to qualified subscribers. 32 p./no. back issues avail. **Document type:** *Newsletter, Trade.* **Description:** Covers issues and employment opportunities of interest to licensed nursing professionals.
Published by: (Iowa Board of Nursing), Arthur L. Davis Publishing Agency, Inc., 517 Washington St, P O Box 216, Cedar Falls, IA 50613. TEL 319-277-2414, 800-626-4081, FAX 319-277-4055, sales@aldpub.com, http://www.aldpub.com/. Ed. Mark Miller. R&P Lorinda Inman. Adv. contact Jim Larson. Circ: 46,000 (free).

610.73 IRL ISSN 0790-7257
IRISH NURSING FORUM & HEALTH SERVICES. Text in English. 6/yr.
Address: 127 Lower Baggot St., Dublin 2, Ireland. TEL 789318, FAX 767072. Ed. Eivlin Roden.

610.73 USA ISSN 0146-0862
UNC CODEN: ICNUDS
ISSUES IN COMPREHENSIVE PEDIATRIC NURSING. Text in English. 1976. q. GBP 43, USD 71 to individuals; GBP 112, USD 184 to institutions (effective 2002). adv. bk.rev. bibl, charts, illus. index. back issues avail.; reprint service avail. from PQC. *Refereed.* **Document type:** *Academic/Scholarly.* **Description:** Publishes articles pertinent to the critical aspects of pediatric nursing.
Related titles: Online - full text ed.: ISSN 1521-043X (from CatchWord Ltd., EBSCO Publishing, O C L C Online Computer Library Center, Inc., RoweCom Information Quest, Swets Blackwell).
Indexed: CINAHL, Fam.Ind., INIS Atomind., Int.Nurs.Ind., J.of Abstr.Int.Educ., Lang.& Lang.Behav.Abstr., PsycInfo, Psychol.Abstr. (1981-), SOPODA, Sage Fam.Stud.Abstr., Sociol.Abstr., e-psyche.
—BLDSC (4584.160000), CatchWord, GNLM, ingenta, KNAW. **CCC.**
Published by: Taylor & Francis Ltd. (Subsidiary of: Taylor & Francis Group), 325 Chestnut St, Suite 800, Philadelphia, PA 19016. TEL 215-625-8900, FAX 215-625-2940, info@taylorandfrancis.com, http://www.taylorandfrancis.com/. Ed. Jane Bliss-Holtz. Circ: 1,200. **Subscr. addr. in Europe:** Taylor & Francis Group, Journals Customer Service, Rankine Rd, Basingstoke, Hants RG24 8PR, United Kingdom. TEL 44-1256-813000, FAX 44-1256-479438, enquiry@tanf.co.uk, http://www.tandf.co.uk/journals.

616.8 USA ISSN 0161-2840
Discard CODEN: IHNUDT
ISSUES IN MENTAL HEALTH NURSING. Text in English. 1978. 8/yr. GBP 68, USD 113 to individuals; GBP 215, USD 354 to institutions (effective 2002). adv. bk.rev., film rev. bibl, charts, illus. index. back issues avail.; reprint service avail. from PQC. *Refereed.* **Document type:** *Academic/Scholarly.* **Description:** Presents practical information about psychosocial and mental health issues in nursing.
Related titles: Online - full text ed.: ISSN 1096-4673 (from CatchWord Ltd., EBSCO Publishing, O C L C Online Computer Library Center, Inc., RoweCom Information Quest, Swets Blackwell).
Indexed: CINAHL, Fam.Ind., Int.Nurs.Ind., J.of Abstr.Int.Educ., Lang.& Lang.Behav.Abstr., Nurs.Abstr., Peace Res.Abstr., PsycInfo, Psychol.Abstr. (1981-), SOPODA, Sage Fam.Stud.Abstr., Sociol.Abstr., Viol.& Abuse Abstr., e-psyche.
—BLDSC (4584.305000), CatchWord, GNLM, ingenta. **CCC.**
Published by: Taylor & Francis Ltd. (Subsidiary of: Taylor & Francis Group), 325 Chestnut St, Suite 800, Philadelphia, PA 19016. TEL 215-625-8900, FAX 215-625-2940, info@taylorandfrancis.com, http://www.taylorandfrancis.com/. Ed. Sandra P Thomas. Circ: 600. **Subscr. addr. in Europe:** Taylor & Francis Group, Journals Customer Service, Rankine Rd, Basingstoke, Hants RG24 8PR, United Kingdom. TEL 44-1256-813000, FAX 44-1256-479438, enquiry@tanf.co.uk, http://www.tandf.co.uk/journals.

610.73 JPN ISSN 0912-3741
J N SUPESHARU/JAPANESE JOURNAL OF NURSING SPECIAL. Text in Japanese. 1986. irreg. JPY 2,200, USD 12 per issue.

M

Published by: Igaku-Shoin Ltd., 5-24-3 Hongo, Bunkyo-ku, Tokyo 113-0033, Japan. TEL 81-3-3817-5771, FAX 81-3-3815-4145, nishii@nna.so-net.or.jp. Circ: 30,000.

616.98023 USA ISSN 1070-4329
J M N R. (Journal of Military Nursing & Research) Text in English. 1993. q. USD 29.95 to individuals; USD 49.95 to institutions; USD 9 newsstand/cover. adv. bk.rev., software rev., video rev. illus. *Refereed.* **Document type:** *Trade.* **Description:** Covers nursing and medical research for military, veteran administration and US Public Health Service professionals.
Indexed: CINAHL, Ind.Med. (coverage dropped).
Published by: E.J. Gossett Publishing, Inc, 7145 S Maplewood Ave, Chicago, IL 60629-2045. TEL 312-476-5978, 800-779-JMNR, FAX 312-476-3259, evalyng@aol.com. Ed., Pub. Evalyn J Gossett. Circ: 2,000.

618 USA ISSN 0884-2175
RG951 CODEN: JOGNEY
J O G N N. (Journal of Obstetric, Gynecologic, and Neonatal Nursing) Text in English. 1972. bi-m. USD 64 in United States to individuals; USD 147 foreign to individuals; USD 348 in United States to institutions; USD 396 foreign to institutions; USD 20 newsstand/cover in United States to individuals; USD 90 newsstand/cover in United States to institutions (effective 2001). adv. bk.rev. illus. 120 p./no. back issues avail.; reprints avail. *Refereed.* **Document type:** *Journal, Academic/Scholarly.*
Former titles: J O G N Nursing (0090-0311); Nurses Association of the American College of Obstetricians and Gynecologists. Bulletin News (0044-7641); Nurses Association of A.C.O.G. Bulletin (0095-2982)
Related titles: CD-ROM ed.: (from Ovid Technologies, Inc.); Microform ed.: (from PQC); Online - full text ed.: (from ingenta, Swets Blackwell, RoweCom Information Quest).
Indexed: Brit.Nur.Ind., CINAHL, Chic.Per.Ind., Fam.Ind., INIS Atomind., Ind.Med. (1985-), Int.Nurs.Ind., Nurs.Abstr.
—BLDSC (4670.352000), CISTI, GNLM, ingenta.
Published by: (Association of Women's Health, Obstetric, and Neonatal Nurses), Sage Publications, Inc., Sage Science Press, 2455 Teller Rd, Thousand Oaks, CA 91320. TEL 805-499-0721, FAX 805-499-0871, info@sagepub.com, http://www.sagesciencepress.com/. Ed. Karen B Haller. R&P Peter Marino. Adv. contact David Baker TEL 410-638-6831. B&W page USD 2,494, color page USD 4,399; bleed 8.375 x 11.125. Circ: 24,042.

610.73 JAM ISSN 0021-4140
JAMAICAN NURSE. Text in English. 1961. 3/yr. USD 25 (effective 1998). adv. bk.rev. charts, illus. cum.index. **Document type:** *Academic/Scholarly.*
Indexed: CINAHL, Int.Nurs.Ind.
—CISTI, GNLM.
Published by: Nurses Association of Jamaica, Mary Seacole Annex, 4 Trevennion Park Rd, PO Box 277, Kingston 5, Jamaica. TEL 876-929-5213. Ed. Cyringa Marshall Burnett. Circ: 2,500.

610.73 JPN ISSN 0389-8326
JAPANESE JOURNAL OF NURSING. Text in Japanese. 1981. m. JPY 9,600.
Indexed: Dent.Ind.
—BLDSC (4656.700000).
Published by: Gakken Co. Ltd., 40-5 Kami-Ikedai 4-chome, Ota-ku, Tokyo 145-0064, Japan. Ed. Hisashi Nakamura.

610.73 371.42 JPN ISSN 0911-0844
JAPANESE NURSING ASSOCIATION RESEARCH REPORT. Text in Japanese; Summaries in English. 1975. irreg. JPY 1,500. **Document type:** *Academic/Scholarly.* **Description:** Reports on status of nursing personnel.
Published by: Japanese Nursing Association, 8-2 Jingu-Mae 5-chome, Shibuya-ku, Tokyo 150-0001, Japan. http://www.nurse.or.jp. Ed. Kiyoko Iwashita.

610.73 USA ISSN 0002-6700
JOHNS HOPKINS HOSPITAL SCHOOL OF NURSING. ALUMNI MAGAZINE*. Text in English. 1971 (vol.70). q. USD 6. adv. illus.
Indexed: CINAHL.
Published by: Johns Hopkins Hospital School of Nursing, c/o Allie Saularn, 515 N Washington, Baltimore, MD 21205. Ed. Mary Kuntz.

JORDMORBLADET. see *MEDICAL SCIENCES—Obstetrics And Gynecology*

JOSANPU ZASSHI/JAPANESE JOURNAL FOR MIDWIVES. see *MEDICAL SCIENCES—Obstetrics And Gynecology*

658 USA ISSN 1098-7886
RT76
JOURNAL FOR NURSES IN STAFF DEVELOPMENT. Text in English. 1985. bi-m. USD 77 domestic to individuals; USD 137 foreign to individuals; USD 237 domestic to institutions; USD 287 foreign to institutions; USD 47 newsstand/cover (effective 2002). illus. index. **Document type:** *Journal, Academic/Scholarly.*
Formerly (until 1998): Journal of Nursing Staff Development (0882-0627)
Related titles: CD-ROM ed.: (from Ovid Technologies, Inc.); Microform ed.: (from PQC); Online - full text ed.: USD 308.10 domestic academic site license; USD 358.10 foreign academic site license; USD 343.65 domestic corporate site license; USD 393.65 foreign corporate site license (2002) (from Ovid Technologies, Inc.).
Indexed: CINAHL, Int.Nurs.Ind.
—BLDSC (5023.660000), GNLM, IDS, ingenta.
Published by: Lippincott Williams & Wilkins (Philadelphia) (Subsidiary of: Wolters Kluwer N.V.), 530 Walnut St, Philadelphia, PA 19106-3621. TEL 301-223-2300, 800-638-3030, FAX 301-223-2400, http://www.Lww.com. Ed. Belinda Puetz. Pub. Lisa Marshall. Adv. contact Tyra London. Circ: 4,361. **Subscr. to:** PO Box 1600, Hagerstown, MD 21740-1600.

JOURNAL MIDWIFERY AND WOMEN'S HEALTH. see *MEDICAL SCIENCES—Obstetrics And Gynecology*

610.73 362.29 USA ISSN 1088-4602
CODEN: ADNUFH
JOURNAL OF ADDICTIONS NURSING. Text in English. 1989. q. USD 89 domestic to individuals; USD 179 foreign to individuals; USD 259 domestic to institutions; USD 376 foreign to institutions (effective 2002). reprints avail. *Refereed.* **Document type:** *Journal, Academic/Scholarly.* **Description:** Recognizes the major role of nurses in identifying and intervening with drug and alcohol abuse. Provides current information on serious health problems, as well as specialties of addictions nursing.
Former titles (until 1996): Addictions Nursing (1073-886X); (until 1994): Addictions Nursing Network (0899-9112)
Indexed: CINAHL, Fam.Ind., THA.
—BLDSC (4918.934030), Infotrieve. **CCC.**
Published by: Mary Ann Liebert, Inc. Publishers, 2 Madison Ave, Larchmont, NY 10538. TEL 914—834-3100, FAX 914-834-1388, info@liebertpub.com, www.liebertpub.com/jan, http://www.liebertpub.com. Ed. Christine Vourakis.

610.73 GBR ISSN 0309-2402
RT1
JOURNAL OF ADVANCED NURSING. Text in English. 1976. 24/yr., latest vol.37, 2002. GBP 119 in Europe to individuals; USD 107 in North America to individuals; GBP 131 elsewhere to individuals; GBP 695 in Europe to institutions; USD 1,102 in North America to institutions; GBP 765 elsewhere to institutions (effective 2002). adv. bk.rev. bibl, illus. index. back issues avail.; reprint service avail. from ISI. *Refereed.* **Document type:** *Academic/Scholarly.*
Related titles: CD-ROM ed.: (from Ovid Technologies, Inc.); Microform ed.: (from PQC); Online - full text ed.: ISSN 1365-2648. GBP 108 in Europe to individuals; USD 97 in North America to individuals; GBP 108 elsewhere to individuals; GBP 626 in Europe to institutions; USD 992 in North America to institutions; GBP 626 elsewhere to institutions (effective 2002) (from Ovid Technologies, Inc., EBSCO Publishing, O C L C Online Computer Library Center, Inc., RoweCom Information Quest, ingenta, Munksgaard & Blackwell Science's Synergy, Swets Blackwell, Institute for Scientific Information).
Indexed: AMED, ASCA, ASSIA, Abstr.Health Care Manage.Stud., AgeLine, Arts & Hum.Cit.Ind. (coverage dropped), Behav.Med.Abstr., Brit.Nur.Ind., CINAHL, Curr.Cont., Diab.Cont., ERA, Excerp.Med., Fam.Ind., Ind.Med. (1976-), Int.Nurs.Ind., Mult.Ed.Abstr., Res.High.Educ.Abstr., Risk Abstr., SSCI, Stud.Wom.Abstr., Tech.Educ.Abstr.
—BLDSC (4918.947000), CISTI, GNLM, IDS, ingenta, KNAW. **CCC.**
Published by: Blackwell Science Ltd., PO Box 88, Oxford OX2 0NE, United Kingdom. TEL 44-1865-206180, 44-1865-206002, FAX 44-1865-206219, jnl.orders@blacksci.co.uk, http://www.blackwell-science.com/jan/, http://www.blackwellpublishing.com. Eds. J Robinson, J P Smith. Pub. Elaine Stott. R&P Sophie Savage. Adv. contact Jenny Applin. Circ: 2,205.

JOURNAL OF CARDIOVASCULAR NURSING. see *MEDICAL SCIENCES—Cardiovascular Diseases*

616.89 155.4 USA ISSN 1073-6077
RJ499.A1
JOURNAL OF CHILD AND ADOLESCENT PSYCHIATRIC NURSING. Abbreviated title: J C A P N. Text in English. 1987-1991; resumed 1994. q. USD 54 domestic to individuals; USD 61 elsewhere to individuals; USD 36 domestic to students; USD 79 domestic to institutions; USD 91 elsewhere to institutions; USD 26 newsstand/cover domestic; USD 30 newsstand/cover elsewhere (effective 2002). adv. bk.rev. back issues avail.; reprints avail. *Refereed.* **Document type:** *Academic/Scholarly.* **Description:** Provides a professional forum for nurses involved in promoting the mental health of children and adolescents and caring for emotionally disturbed youth and their families.
Formerly: Journal of Child and Adolescent Psychiatric and Mental Health Nursing (0897-9685)
Related titles: Online - full text ed.: (from ProQuest Information & Learning, Gale Group).
Indexed: CINAHL, Fam.Ind., Int.Nurs.Ind.
—BLDSC (4957.423500), GNLM, ingenta.
Published by: (Association of Child & Adolescent Psychiatric Nurses), Nursecom, Inc., 1211 Locust St, Philadelphia, PA 19107. TEL 215-545-7222, 800-242-6757, FAX 215-545-1807, customer.service@nursecominc.com, http://www.cinahl.com/jrnls/JCAP/jcap.htm, http://www.nursecominc.com. Ed. Elizabeth Poster. Pub. Margo C Neal. R&P Timothy Bower. Adv. contact Alison L Graham. B&W page USD 875, color page USD 1,425. Circ: 1,700.

610.73 USA ISSN 0743-2550
JOURNAL OF CHRISTIAN NURSING. Text in English. 1984. q. USD 22.95 domestic; USD 25.45 foreign (effective 2001). adv. bk.rev., film rev., video rev. abstr. cum.index. back issues avail. **Document type:** *Trade.* **Description:** Offers biblically based articles to help nurses and students meet patients' spiritual needs and ethical dilemmas and helps them grow spiritually.
Related titles: Microform ed.: (from PQC); Online - full text ed.
Indexed: CINAHL, Chr.Per.Ind., Fam.Ind., Int.Nurs.Ind., Nurs.Abstr., Ref.Zh.
—BLDSC (4958.275000), GNLM, Infotrieve, ingenta. **CCC.**
Published by: InterVarsity Christian Fellowship, Nurses Christian Fellowship, 430 E Plaza Dr, Westmont, IL 60559. TEL 630-734-4030, FAX 630-734-4200, jcn@ivpress.com, http://www.ncf-jcn.org. Ed. Judith Allen Shelly. R&P Melodee Yohe. Adv. contact Elaine Johns TEL 608-274-4823. Circ: 10,000. **Subscr. to:** PO Box 7895, Madison, WI 53707-7895.

610.73 GBR ISSN 0962-1067
RT41 CODEN: JCCNEW
JOURNAL OF CLINICAL NURSING. Text in English. 1992. bi-m., latest vol.11, 2002. GBP 99 in Europe to individuals; USD 157 in North America to individuals; GBP 109 elsewhere to individuals; GBP 399 in Europe to institutions; USD 633 in North America to institutions; GBP 439 elsewhere to institutions (effective 2002). adv. bk.rev. bibl. index. back issues avail. *Refereed.* **Document type:** *Academic/Scholarly.* **Description:** Seeks to enhance nurses practice, focusing directly on the theory and practice of nursing and highlighting matters of concern to practicing nurses.
Related titles: CD-ROM ed.: (from Ovid Technologies, Inc.); Microform ed.: (from PQC); Online - full text ed.: ISSN 1365-2702. GBP 90 in Europe to individuals; USD 142 in North America to individuals; GBP 90 elsewhere to individuals; GBP 360 in Europe to institutions; USD 570 in North America to institutions; GBP 360 elsewhere to institutions (effective 2002) (from Ovid Technologies, Inc., EBSCO Publishing, O C L C Online Computer Library Center, Inc., RoweCom Information Quest, ingenta, Munksgaard & Blackwell Science's Synergy, Swets Blackwell, Institute for Scientific Information).
Indexed: ASCA, ASSIA, AgeLine, Brit.Nur.Ind., CINAHL, Curr.Cont., Diab.Cont., Fam.Ind., Int.Nurs.Ind., SSCI.
—BLDSC (4958.595000), GNLM, IDS, Infotrieve. **CCC.**
Published by: Blackwell Science Ltd., PO Box 88, Oxford OX2 0NE, United Kingdom. TEL 44-1865-206180, 44-1865-206002, FAX 44-1865-206219, jnl.orders@blacksci.co.uk, http://www.blackwell-science.com/~cgilib/jnlpage.asp?Journal=jcn&File=jcn, http://www.blackwellpublishing.com. Ed. Christine Webb. Pub. Elaine Stott. R&P Sophie Savage. Adv. contact Jenny Applin. Circ: 610.

M

610.73 USA ISSN 0737-0016
JOURNAL OF COMMUNITY HEALTH NURSING. Text in English. 1984. q. USD 35 in US & Canada to individuals; USD 65 elsewhere to individuals; USD 335 in US & Canada to institutions; USD 365 elsewhere to institutions (effective 2002). adv. bk.rev. abstr, charts, illus. *Refereed.* **Document type:** *Journal, Academic/Scholarly.* **Description:** Focuses on health care issues relevant to all aspects of community practice - schools, homes, visiting nursing services, clinics, hospices, education, and public health administration.
Related titles: Online - full text ed.: ISSN 1532-7655. USD 31.50 to individuals; USD 301.50 to institutions (effective 2002) (from CatchWord Ltd., EBSCO Publishing, O C L C Online Computer Library Center, Inc., RoweCom Information Quest, Swets Blackwell).
Indexed: ASSIA, CINAHL, Environ.Sci.Poll.Mgmt., Excerp.Med., Ind.Med. (1984-), Int.Nurs.Ind., PsycInfo, Risk Abstr., Saf.Sci.Abstr., THA, e-psyche.
—BLDSC (4961.722000), CatchWord, CISTI, EMDOCS, GNLM, ingenta, KNAW. **CCC.**
Published by: Lawrence Erlbaum Associates, Inc., 10 Industrial Ave, Mahwah, NJ 07430-2262. TEL 201-760-3735, 800-926-6579, FAX 201-236-0072, journals@erlbaum.com, http://www.erlbaum.com/ Journals/journals/JCHN/jchn.htm. Eds. Alice Schroeder, Arlene O'Brien. adv.: page USD 525; trim 6 x 9.

610.73 GBR
JOURNAL OF COMMUNITY NURSING. Text in English. 1977. m. GBP 40; GBP 75 foreign. adv. bk.rev. *Refereed.* **Document type:** *Trade.*
Former titles: Journal of District Nursing (0263-4465); Journal of Community Nursing (0140-0908)
Indexed: Brit.Nur.Ind.
—BLDSC (4961.730000).
Published by: P T M Publishers Ltd., 282 High St, Sutton, Surrey SM1 1PQ, United Kingdom. TEL 44-20-8642-0162, FAX 44-20-8643-2275, 44-20-8643-2275, mail@ptmpublishers.com. Ed. Fiona Meehan. Pub., Adv. contact Stephen Mell TEL 44-20-8642-0162. R&P Linda King. Circ: 25,000.

610.73 USA ISSN 0022-0124
RT90
JOURNAL OF CONTINUING EDUCATION IN NURSING. Text in English. 1970. bi-m. USD 54 domestic to individuals; USD 69 in Canada to individuals; USD 89 elsewhere to individuals; USD 80 domestic to institutions; USD 95 in Canada to institutions; USD 115 elsewhere to institutions. adv. bk.rev. reprint service avail. from PQC,SCH,PSC. *Refereed.* **Document type:** *Academic/Scholarly.* **Description:** Provides articles on continuing nursing education.
Related titles: Microform ed.: (from PQC); Online - full text ed.: (from Northern Light Technology, Inc., H. W. Wilson, ProQuest Information & Learning).
Indexed: AMED, AgeLine, Brit.Nur.Ind., C.I.J.E. (coverage dropped), CINAHL, Cont.Pg.Educ., ERA, Educ.Ind. (Nov.1983-), Educ.Tech.Abstr., Fam.Ind., Int.Nurs.Ind., Nurs.Abstr., Tech.Educ.Abstr.
—BLDSC (4965.246000), CISTI, GNLM, ingenta, KNAW. **CCC.**
Published by: Slack, Inc., 6900 Grove Rd, Thorofare, NJ 08086-9447. TEL 856-848-1000, 800-257-8290, FAX 856-853-5991, http://www.slackinc.com. Ed. Patricia S Yoder Wise. Circ: 3,800.

306 USA ISSN 1071-5568
JOURNAL OF CULTURAL DIVERSITY; an interdisciplinary journal. Text in English. 1994. q. USD 60 domestic to individuals; USD 100 elsewhere to individuals; USD 100 domestic to institutions; USD 200 foreign to institutions (effective 2001). adv. bk.rev., software rev., video rev. abstr, charts, illus. index. *Refereed.* **Document type:** *Academic/Scholarly.* **Description:** Documents the distinct nature and needs of the multicultural person, family and community with original research and manuscripts, materials and reviews.
Related titles: Online - full text ed.: (from Northern Light Technology, Inc., ProQuest Information & Learning).
Indexed: CINAHL, Fam.Ind., Int.Nurs.Ind.
—BLDSC (4965.842000), GNLM, Infotrieve, ingenta. **CCC.**
Published by: Tucker Publications, Inc., PO Box 580, Lisle, IL 60532. TEL 630-969-3809, FAX 630-969-3895, callen@tuckerpub.com, http://www.tuckerpub.com. Eds. Dr. Joseph Hoff, Dr. Kay Edwards. R&P, Adv. contact Clay Allen.

610.736 616.462 GBR ISSN 1368-1109
JOURNAL OF DIABETES NURSING; the journal for professionals working in the field of diabetes nursing. Text in English. 1997. bi-m. GBP 38 domestic to individuals; GBP 62 foreign to individuals; GBP 58 domestic to institutions; GBP 78 foreign to institutions (effective 2001). *Refereed.* **Document type:** *Trade.* **Description:** Covers clinical, professional issues, education, research, and primary and secondary care interface, along with diabetes nursing. Allows for commentary and debate.
Indexed: Brit.Nur.Ind., CINAHL.
—BLDSC (4969.408000).
Published by: S B Communications Group, 15 Mandeville Courtyard, 142 Battersea Park Rd, London SW11 4NB, United Kingdom. TEL 44-20-7627-1510, FAX 44-20-7627-1570, sbcomm@dial.pipex.com, info@sbcommunicationsgroup.com, http:// www.sbcomm.dial.pipex.com, http:// www.sbcommunicationsgroup.com. Ed. Maggie Watkinson. Pub. Simon Breed. R&P Sophie Perks.

610.73 USA ISSN 0099-1767
RT120.E4
JOURNAL OF EMERGENCY NURSING. Key Title: JEN, Journal of Emergency Nursing. Variant title: J E N. Text in English. 1975. bi-m. USD 62 domestic to individuals; USD 80 foreign to individuals; USD 205 domestic to institutions; USD 225 foreign to institutions; USD 33 domestic to students; USD 51 foreign to students; USD 38 (effective 2001). adv. bk.rev. illus. index. Supplement avail.; reprint service avail. from PQC. **Document type:** *Journal, Academic/Scholarly.* **Description:** Information on emergency care with articles written and reviewed by emergency nurses.
Related titles: CD-ROM ed.: (from Ovid Technologies, Inc.); Microfilm ed.: (from PQC); Online - full text ed.: ISSN 1527-2966 (from Ovid Technologies, Inc., EBSCO Publishing, IDEAL Online Library, RoweCom Information Quest).
Indexed: AgeLine, Brit.Nur.Ind., CINAHL, Int.Nurs.Ind., Nurs.Abstr.
—BLDSC (4977.300000), CISTI, GNLM, ingenta, KNAW. **CCC.**
Published by: (Emergency Nurses Association), Mosby, Inc. (Subsidiary of: Elsevier Science), 11830 Westline Industrial Dr, St Louis, MO 63146-3318. TEL 314-872-8370, 800-325-4177, FAX 314-432-1380, http://www.mosby.com/jen, http://www.mosby.com/ periodicals. Ed. Gail Pisarcik Lenehan. Pub. Pat Nornhold. Adv. contact Tracey Schriefer TEL 314-453-4304. B&W page USD 1,790, color page USD 3,040; trim 10.88 x 8.13. Circ: 27,240.

610.73 USA ISSN 1074-8407
RT120.F34 CODEN: JFNUFS
JOURNAL OF FAMILY NURSING. Text in English. 1995. q. USD 65 to individuals; USD 395 to institutions; USD 25 newsstand/cover to individuals; USD 100 newsstand/cover to institutions (effective 2002). adv. bk.rev. back issues avail.; reprints avail. *Refereed.* **Document type:** *Academic/Scholarly.* **Description:** Publishes empirical and theoretical analyses and scholarly work on nursing research, education, and policy issues pertaining to family health and illness.
Related titles: Online - full content ed.: (from EBSCO Publishing, O C L C Online Computer Library Center, Inc., ProQuest Information & Learning, ingenta, Swets Blackwell); Online - full text ed.: (from RoweCom Information Quest).
Indexed: ASSIA, CINAHL, Fam.Ind., Lang.& Lang.Behav.Abstr., SOPODA, Sociol.Abstr.
—BLDSC (4983.720000), CISTI, Infotrieve, ingenta. **CCC.**
Published by: (Faculty of Nursing CAN, University of Calgary CAN), Sage Publications, Inc., 2455 Teller Rd, Thousand Oaks, CA 91320. TEL 805-499-0721, FAX 805-499-0871, info@sagepub.com, http:// www.sagepub.com. Ed. Janice M Bell. Pub. Sara Miller McCune. R&P Tanya Udin. Adv. contact DeAnna Vega Hammersley. **Subscr. to:** Sage Publications Ltd., 6 Bonhill St, London EC2A 4PU, United Kingdom; Sage Publications India Pvt. Ltd., 4215, New Delhi 110 048, India.

JOURNAL OF GERONTOLOGICAL NURSING; for nursing care of older adults. see *GERONTOLOGY AND GERIATRICS*

610.73 USA ISSN 0898-0101
RT42 CODEN: JHNUF8
JOURNAL OF HOLISTIC NURSING. Text in English. 1983. q. USD 60 to individuals; USD 225 to institutions; USD 25 newsstand/cover to individuals; USD 60 newsstand/cover to institutions (effective 2002). adv. index. back issues avail.; reprints avail. **Document type:** *Academic/Scholarly.* **Description:** Offers a holistic nursing foundation for practitioners and educators through shared research and clinical experience; publishes original work and disseminates the ideals of holistic nursing to the health care community.
Related titles: Online - full text ed.: (from ProQuest Information & Learning, ingenta).
Indexed: AMED, CINAHL, Fam.Ind., Int.Nurs.Ind., Lang.& Lang.Behav.Abstr., SOPODA, Sociol.Abstr., Viol.& Abuse Abstr.
—BLDSC (5002.710000), GNLM, Infotrieve, ingenta. **CCC.**
Published by: (American Holistic Nurses' Association), Sage Publications, Inc., 2455 Teller Rd, Thousand Oaks, CA 91320. TEL 805-499-0721, FAX 805-499-0871, info@sagepub.com, http:// www.sagepub.com. Ed. Lynn Rew. Pub. Sara Miller McCune. R&P Tanya Udin. Adv. contact DeAnna Vega Hammersley. Circ: 3,600. **Overseas subscr. to:** Sage Publications Ltd., 6 Bonhill St, London EC2A 4PU, United Kingdom. TEL 44-20-7374-0645, FAX 44-20-7374-8741, subscription@sagepub.co.uk, http://www.sagepub.co.uk; Sage Publications India Pvt. Ltd., 4215, New Delhi 110 048, India. TEL 91-11-641-9884, FAX 91-11-647-2426.

610.73 USA ISSN 1522-2179
▼ **JOURNAL OF HOSPICE AND PALLIATIVE NURSING.** Text in English. 1999. q. USD 45 domestic to individuals; USD 50 foreign to individuals; USD 90 domestic to institutions; USD 100 foreign to institutions (effective 2002). reprints avail. *Refereed.* **Document type:** *Academic/Scholarly.* **Description:** Focuses on clinical articles of interest to nurses caring for patients enrolled in hospice programs and nurses providing palliative care in a variety of settings. Relevant research is included along with a pharmacy corner, case studies, use of technology in the field and clinical practice tips.
—BLDSC (4668.393500).
Published by: Nursecom, Inc., 1211 Locust St, Philadelphia, PA 19107. TEL 215-545-7222, FAX 215-545-8107, rosemary@earthlink.net, http://www.nursecominc.com. Ed. Rose Mary Carroll Johnson. Pub. Margo C Neal.

658 USA ISSN 1533-1458
JOURNAL OF INFUSION NURSING. Text in English. 1978. bi-m. USD 97 domestic to individuals; USD 137 foreign to individuals; USD 197 domestic to institutions; USD 237 foreign to institutions (effective 2002). adv. abstr, bibl, charts, illus. index. back issues avail. *Refereed.* **Document type:** *Journal, Academic/Scholarly, Trade.* **Description:** News of Society activities and clinical developments affecting intravenous therapy practice.
Former titles: Journal of Intravenous Nursing (0896-5846); (until 1988): N I T A (0160-3930)
Related titles: CD-ROM ed.: (from Ovid Technologies, Inc.); Microform ed.: (from PQC); Online - full text ed.: (from Ovid Technologies, Inc.).
Indexed: AgeLine, CINAHL, Excerp.Med., I.P.A., Int.Nurs.Ind., Nurs.Abstr.
—BLDSC (5007.698000), EMDOCS, GNLM, ingenta, KNAW.
Published by: (Intravenous Nurses Society), Lippincott Williams & Wilkins (Philadelphia) (Subsidiary of: Wolters Kluwer N.V.), 530 Walnut St, Philadelphia, PA 19106-3621. TEL 215-521-8300, FAX 215-521-8902, custserv@lww.com, http://www.nursingcenter.com, http://www.lww.com/. Ed. Mary Alexander. adv.: B&W page USD 1,770; 10 x 7. Circ: 10,107. **Subscr. to:** PO Box 1600, Hagerstown, MD 21740-1600. TEL 800-638-3030, FAX 310-223-2400.

610.73 USA ISSN 0194-1658
JOURNAL OF INTRAVENOUS THERAPY. Text in English. 1976. bi-m. USD 24 domestic; USD 32 in Canada; USD 35 elsewhere (effective 2001). adv. bk.rev. **Document type:** *Journal, Academic/Scholarly, Trade.*
Indexed: I.P.A.
Published by: (I.V. Therapy Association of the USA), Medical Education Consultants, PO Box 67159, Los Angeles, CA 90067. TEL 310-475-5339, FAX 310-475-5339. Ed., Pub. William J Kurdi. R&P Kurt J Kurdi. Adv. contact Kevin J Kurdi. Circ: 1,000.

JOURNAL OF LEARNING DISABILITIES. see *EDUCATION—Special Education And Rehabilitation*

M

610.73 340 USA ISSN 1080-3297
THE JOURNAL OF LEGAL NURSE CONSULTING. Text in English. 1990. q. USD 115 (effective 1999). adv. bk.rev. back issues avail. **Document type:** *Newsletter.* **Description:** Provides a forum for continuing education, facilities and exchange of information; establishes a communication network for its members; it also functions as a resource to other professional organizations of similar interest.
Formerly (until vol.6, 1995): American Association of Legal Nurse Consultants Network (1065-3449)
Indexed: CINAHL.
—BLDSC (5010.271500).
Published by: American Association of Legal Nurse Consultants, 4700 W Lake Ave, Glenview, IL 60025-1485. TEL 847-375-4713, FAX 847-375-4777. Ed. S Fandray. Adv. contact Pat Delaney. Circ: 1,800 (paid).

610.73 USA ISSN 1526-8233
JOURNAL OF MULTICULTURAL NURSING AND HEALTH. Text in English. 1994. 3/yr. USD 55 to individuals; USD 80 to institutions (effective 2000). adv. *Refereed.* **Document type:** *Academic/Scholarly.* **Description:** Addresses issues of multiculturalism in nursing education and health.
Formerly (until 1994): Journal of Multicultural Nursing (1076-0210)
Indexed: CINAHL, Ind.Med. (coverage dropped), Nurs.Abstr., Sage Race Rel.Abstr.
—BLDSC (5021.058300).
Published by: (Center for the Study of Multiculturalism and Health), Riley Publications, Inc., Chautauqua Institution, PO Box 889, Chautauqua, NY 14722. TEL 716-357-2479, FAX 716-357-2479. Ed., R&P Essie A Riley Eddins. Adv. contact Berkley Eddins.

612.652 GBR ISSN 1355-1841
THE JOURNAL OF NEONATAL NURSING. Abbreviated title: J N N. Text in English. 1994. bi-m. GBP 38 domestic to individuals; GBP 47 in Europe to individuals; GBP 52 elsewhere to individuals; GBP 60 domestic to institutions; GBP 70 in Europe to institutions; GBP 75 elsewhere to institutions; GBP 9 newsstand/cover (effective 2000). adv. bk.rev. abstr, charts, illus. *Refereed.* **Document type:** *Journal, Academic/Scholarly.* **Description:** Aimed at nurses, midwives and all other professionals concerned with the care of preterm infants and small, vulnerable term infants and their families.
Related titles: Online - full text ed.: GBP 40 foreign to individuals; GBP 60 foreign to institutions (effective 2000).
Indexed: Brit.Nur.Ind., CINAHL.
—BLDSC (5021.399200).
Published by: Stansted News Ltd., 134 South St, Bishop's Stortford, Herts CM23 3BQ, United Kingdom. TEL 44-1279-714510, FAX 44-1279-714519, jnn@bizjet.com, http://ww.bizjet.com/jnn/. Ed. Barbara Weller. Pub., R&P Christine Bishop. Adv. contact Barry Dawkins. B&W page GBP 830, color page GBP 1,260; trim 210 x 297. Circ: 3,750 (paid); 500 (controlled).

610.73 USA ISSN 0888-0395
RC350.5 CODEN: JNNUEF
JOURNAL OF NEUROSCIENCE NURSING. Text in English. 1969. bi-m. USD 110 domestic to individuals; USD 135 domestic to libraries; USD 135 foreign to individuals; USD 160 foreign to libraries (effective 2000). adv. bk.rev. illus. reprint service avail. from PQC. *Refereed.* **Document type:** *Newsletter, Trade.* **Description:** Contains original articles on advances in neurosurgical and neurological techniques as they affect nursing procedures and commentary on the role of the neuroscience nurse in the health care team.
Formerly (until 1986): Journal of Neurosurgical Nursing (0047-2603)
Related titles: Microform ed.: (from PQC); Online - full text ed.: (from Northern Light Technology, Inc., ProQuest Information & Learning, Gale Group).
Indexed: CINAHL, Fam.Ind., Hosp.Lit.Ind., INIS Atomind., Ind.Med. (1986-), Int.Nurs.Ind., Nurs.Abstr.
—BLDSC (5022.085000), GNLM, ingenta. **CCC.**
Published by: American Association of Neuroscience Nurses, 4700 W Lake Ave, Glenview, IL 60025-1468. TEL 847-375-4733, 888-557-2266, FAX 847-375-6333, bsimmons@amctec.com, http://www.AANN.org. Ed. Christina Stewart Amidi. R&P, Adv. contact Barbara Simmons. Circ: 5,300.

610.73 TWN ISSN 0047-262X
JOURNAL OF NURSING/HU LI TSA CHIH. Text in Chinese. 1954. bi-m. USD 70 (effective 2001). adv. bk.rev. illus. cum.index: 1954-1997. back issues avail. *Refereed.* **Document type:** *Academic/Scholarly.*
Indexed: CINAHL, Int.Nurs.Ind.
—BLDSC (5023.690000), CISTI.
Published by: Taiwan Nurses Association, 4F, 281 Sec 4, Hsin-Yi Rd, Taipei 106, Taiwan. TEL 886-2-2755-2291, FAX 886-2-2701-9817, tnaj@twna.org.tw, twna@twna.org.tw, http://www.twna.org.tw. Ed. Ming Rung Lee. Adv. contact Ming-Rung Lee. B&W page USD 250, color page USD 720; trim 210 x 150. Circ: 28,300.

610.73 USA ISSN 0002-0443
RT89 CODEN: JNUAA
JOURNAL OF NURSING ADMINISTRATION. Abbreviated title: J O N A. Text in English. 1971. 11/yr. USD 95 domestic to individuals; USD 167 foreign to individuals; USD 295 domestic to institutions; USD 375 foreign to institutions; USD 34 newsstand/cover (effective 2002). adv. illus. index. reprints avail. *Refereed.* **Document type:** *Academic/Scholarly.*
Related titles: CD-ROM ed.: (from Ovid Technologies, Inc.); Microform ed.: (from PQC); Online - full text ed.: USD 383.50 domestic academic site license; USD 463.50 foreign academic site license; USD 427.75 domestic corporate site license; USD 507.75 foreign corporate site license (2002) (from Ovid Technologies, Inc., Institute for Scientific Information).
Indexed: AIM, ASCA, Abstr.Health Care Manage.Stud., AgeLine, C.I.J.E. (coverage dropped), CINAHL, Curr.Cont., Hosp.Lit.Ind., INIS Atomind., Ind.Med. (1971-), Int.Nurs.Ind., Nurs.Abstr., SSCI.
—BLDSC (5023.700000), CISTI, GNLM, IDS, ingenta, KNAW.
Published by: Lippincott Williams & Wilkins (Philadelphia) (Subsidiary of: Wolters Kluwer N.V.), 530 Walnut St, Philadelphia, PA 19106-3621. TEL 301-223-2300, 800-638-3030, FAX 301-223-2400, http://www.lww.com. Ed. Suzanne P Smith. Circ: 11,397. **Subscr. to:** PO Box 1600, Hagerstown, MD 21740-1600.

610.73 USA ISSN 1057-3631
RT85.5
JOURNAL OF NURSING CARE QUALITY. Text in English. 1986. q. USD 149 to individuals; USD 45 newsstand/cover (effective 2002). back issues avail. *Refereed.* **Document type:** *Journal.* **Description:** Nursing QA programs, especially in the application of QA principles and concepts in the practice setting.
Formerly (until 1991): Journal of Nursing Quality Assurance (0889-4647)
Related titles: Microfiche ed.; Online - full text ed.: (from Ovid Technologies, Inc., ProQuest Information & Learning, Gale Group, Institute for Scientific Information).
Indexed: AgeLine, CINAHL, Curr.Cont., Environ.Sci.Poll.Mgmt., Fam.Ind., Ind.Med. (1991-), Int.Nurs.Ind., Nurs.Abstr., SSCI.
—BLDSC (5023.770000), GNLM, IDS, ingenta. **CCC.**
Published by: Aspen Publishers, Inc., 200 Orchard Ridge Dr, Ste 200, Gaithersburg, MD 20878. TEL 800-638-8437, FAX 301-417-7550, customer.service@aspenpubl.com, http://www.nursingcenter.com, http://www.aspenpub.com. Ed. Martha Sasser. Pub. Jack Bruggeman. Circ: 4,300 (paid). **Dist. by:** Aspen Publishers Inc., Distribution Center, 7201 McKinney Circle, Frederick, MD 21701. TEL 301-698-7100, FAX 301-417-7550.

610.73 USA ISSN 0022-3158
JOURNAL OF NURSING EDUCATION. Text in English. 1962. 9/yr. USD 68 to individuals; USD 84 to institutions. adv. illus. index. reprint service avail. from PQC,SCH,PSC. **Document type:** *Academic/Scholarly.* **Description:** Provides a forum for original articles and new ideas for nursing educators in various types and levels of nursing programs.
Formerly (until 1983): J N E: Journal of Nursing Education (0148-4834)
Related titles: Microform ed.: (from PQC); Online - full text ed.: (from Northern Light Technology, Inc., H. W. Wilson, ProQuest Information & Learning, Institute for Scientific Information).
Indexed: ASCA, AgeLine, Brit.Nur.Ind., CINAHL, Cont.Pg.Educ., Curr.Cont., ERA, Educ.Ind. (May 1983-), Educ.Tech.Abstr., Hosp.Lit.Ind., Ind.Med. (1962-), Ind.Sci.Rev., Int.Nurs.Ind., Mult.Ed.Abstr., Nurs.Abstr., SSCI, Tech.Educ.Abstr.
—BLDSC (5023.800000), CISTI, GNLM, IDS, Infotrieve, ingenta. **CCC.**
Published by: Slack, Inc., 6900 Grove Rd, Thorofare, NJ 08086-9447. TEL 856-848-1000, 800-257-8290, FAX 856-853-5991, http://www.slackinc.com. Ed. Christine Tanner. Adv. contact Kelly Wark. B&W page USD 815, color page USD 2,025. Circ: 4,800 (paid).

610.73 340 USA ISSN 1073-7472
K10
JOURNAL OF NURSING LAW. Text in English. 1993. q. USD 75 domestic to individuals; USD 95 foreign to individuals; USD 145 domestic to institutions; USD 165 foreign to institutions. abstr. back issues avail. *Refereed.* **Document type:** *Academic/Scholarly, Trade.*
Related titles: Microform ed.
Indexed: CINAHL.
—BLDSC (5023.828000).
Published by: P E S I Health Care LLC., 200 Spring St, Eau Claire, WI 54703. TEL 715-933-5288, mconner@pesi.com. Ed. Diane K Kjervik. Pub. Mike Conner. R&P Shelly Kistner. Circ: 1,000.

610.73 658 GBR ISSN 0966-0429
CODEN: JNMNEN
JOURNAL OF NURSING MANAGEMENT. Text in English. 1993. bi-m., latest vol.10, 2002. GBP 59 in Europe to individuals; USD 94 in North America to individuals; GBP 65 elsewhere to individuals; GBP 219 in Europe to institutions; USD 348 in North America to institutions; GBP 241 elsewhere to institutions (effective 2002). adv. bk.rev. bibl, illus. index. back issues avail. *Refereed.* **Document type:** *Academic/Scholarly.* **Description:** Disseminates scholarly papers on all aspects of nursing management, that is, management practice, education, and research.
Related titles: Microform ed.: (from PQC); Online - full text ed.: ISSN 1365-2834. GBP 54 in Europe to individuals; USD 85 in North America to individuals; GBP 54 elsewhere to individuals; GBP 198 in Europe to institutions; USD 314 in North America to institutions; GBP 198 elsewhere to institutions (effective 2002) (from Ovid Technologies, Inc., EBSCO Publishing, O C L C Online Computer Library Center, Inc., RoweCom Information Quest, ingenta, Munksgaard & Blackwell Science's Synergy, Swets Blackwell).
Indexed: ASSIA, Brit.Nur.Ind., CINAHL, Int.Nurs.Ind.
—BLDSC (5023.830000), GNLM, Infotrieve. **CCC.**
Published by: Blackwell Science Ltd., PO Box 88, Oxford OX2 0NE, United Kingdom. TEL 44-1865-206180, 44-1865-206002, FAX 44-1865-206219, jnl.orders@blacksci.co.uk, http://www.blackwell-science.com/products/journals/jnm.htm, http://www.blackwellpublishing.com. Ed. A M Palmer. Pub. Elaine Stott. R&P Sophie Savage. Adv. contact Jenny Applin. Circ: 520.

610.73 USA ISSN 1061-3749
RT81.5
JOURNAL OF NURSING MEASUREMENT. Text in English. 1993. 3/yr. USD 38 in United States to individual members; USD 66 for 2 yrs. in United States to individual members; USD 45 foreign to individual members; USD 77 for 2 yrs. foreign to individual members; USD 78 in United States to institutions; USD 133 for 2 yrs. in United States to institutions; USD 90 foreign to institutions; USD 153 for 2 yrs. foreign to institutions (effective 2000). adv. bk.rev. abstr, charts, stat. 100 p./no. back issues avail.; reprints avail. *Refereed.* **Document type:** *Journal, Academic/Scholarly.* **Description:** Provides a forum for disseminating information on instruments, tools, approaches, and procedures developed or used to measure variables in nursing, spanning practice, education, and research.
Indexed: AgeLine, CINAHL, Fam.Ind., Ind.Med. (1993-), Int.Nurs.Ind., PsycInfo, SOPODA, Sociol.Abstr., e-psyche.
—BLDSC (5023.832000), CISTI, GNLM, Infotrieve, ingenta. **CCC.**
Published by: Springer Publishing Company, 526 Broadway, New York, NY 10012-3955. TEL 212-431-4370, FAX 212-941-7842, springer@springerpub.com, http://www.springerjournals.com/. Eds. Ada Sue Hinshaw, Ora L Strickland. Pub. Ursula Springer. R&P Dorothy Kouwenberg. Adv. contact Bob Friel. B&W page USD 300; 6 x 9. Circ: 300 (paid); 50 (controlled).

610.73 TWN
JOURNAL OF NURSING RESEARCH. (special double issue vol.9, no.3 (Jun. 2001) text in Chinese & English) Text in English. 1993. q. (Bi-m. until Jun., 2001). USD 69 (effective until 2001); USD 48 (effective until 2002). bk.rev. cum.index: 1993-1997. back issues avail. *Refereed.* **Document type:** *Academic/Scholarly.*
Formerly: Nursing Research (1022-6265)
Indexed: Addic.Abstr., CINAHL.
—BLDSC (6187.111000).
Published by: Taiwan Nurses Association, 4F, 281 Sec 4, Hsin-Yi Rd, Taipei 106, Taiwan. TEL 886-2-2755-2291, FAX 886-2-2701-9817, twna@twna.org.tw, http://www.twna.org.tw. Eds. Min Rung Lee, Ming Rung Lee. Adv. contact Ming-Rung Lee. Circ: 6,500.

610.73 USA ISSN 1527-6546
RT1 CODEN: IMNSEP
JOURNAL OF NURSING SCHOLARSHIP. Text in English. 1967. q. USD 39 to individuals; USD 63 to institutions (effective 2001). adv. back issues avail. *Refereed.* **Document type:** *Academic/Scholarly.* **Description:** Presents cutting-edge thinking from top writers and researchers in nursing.
Former titles (until 2000): Image: Journal of Nursing Scholarship (0743-5150); Image (0363-2792)
Related titles: CD-ROM ed.: (from Ovid Technologies, Inc.); Microfiche ed.; Online - full text ed.: (from Gale Group, Institute for Scientific Information).
Indexed: AgeLine, Brit.Nur.Ind., CINAHL, Curr.Cont., Ind.Med. (2000-), Int.Nurs.Ind., Nurs.Abstr., PsycInfo, Psychol.Abstr. (1983-), SSCI, e-psyche.
—BLDSC (5023.850000), GNLM, ingenta.
Published by: Sigma Theta Tau International Honor Society of Nursing, 550 W North St, Indianapolis, IN 46202. TEL 317-634-8171, FAX 317-634-8188, http://nursingsociety.org/publications/main.html. Ed. Dr. Sue Hegyvary. R&P Melody Jones. Adv. contact Rachael McLaughlin. B&W page USD 2,895. Circ: 125,000 (paid and controlled).

610.73 USA ISSN 0744-7132
RE88
JOURNAL OF OPHTHALMIC NURSING & TECHNOLOGY. Text in English. 1982. bi-m. USD 42 domestic to individuals; USD 57 in Canada to individuals; USD 72 elsewhere to individuals; USD 60 domestic to institutions; USD 75 in Canada to institutions; USD 90 elsewhere to institutions. adv. **Document type:** *Trade, Academic/Scholarly.* **Description:** Forum for original articles that explore topics of interest to ophthalmic nurses and technicians.
Related titles: Online - full text ed.: (from ProQuest Information & Learning).
Indexed: CINAHL, Int.Nurs.Ind., Nurs.Abstr.
—BLDSC (5026.344000), GNLM, Infotrieve, ingenta. **CCC.**
Published by: Slack, Inc., 6900 Grove Rd, Thorofare, NJ 08086-9447. TEL 856-848-1000, 800-257-8290, FAX 856-853-5991, http://www.slackinc.com. Ed. Heather Boyd Monk. Circ: 3,000.

610.73 617 GBR ISSN 1361-3111
JOURNAL OF ORTHOPAEDIC NURSING. Text in English. 1997. q. GBP 45 to individuals; GBP 163 to institutions (effective 2002). adv. bk.rev. abstr. 64 p./no. 2 cols./p. back issues avail.; reprints avail. *Refereed.* **Document type:** *Journal, Academic/Scholarly.* **Description:** Aims to move health professionals forward to improve their patients' outcomes, at home and in the hospital.
Related titles: Online - full text ed.: (from Swets Blackwell, IDEAL Online Library).
Indexed: Brit.Nur.Ind.
—BLDSC (5027.663000).
Published by: Churchill Livingstone (Subsidiary of: Harcourt Publishers Ltd.), Robert Stevenson House, 1-3 Baxter's Pl, Leith Walk, Edinburgh, Midlothian EH1 3AF, United Kingdom. TEL 44-131-556-2424, FAX 44-131-558-1278, journals@harcourt.com, http://www.harcourt-international.com/journals/joon. Eds. Claire Ancell, Peter Davis. R&P Sharon Boyle TEL 44-131-524-1747. Adv. contact Deborah Watkins TEL 44-207-424-4280. Circ: 1,200 (paid). **Subscr. in the US to:** Harcourt Health Sciences, Journals Subscription Department, PO Box 156, Avenel, NJ 07001. TEL 877-839-7126; **Subscr. to:** Harcourt Publishers Ltd., Journal Sales & Marketing Dept., 32 Jamestown Rd, London NW1 7BY, United Kingdom. TEL 44-20-8308-5700.

610.73 USA ISSN 0882-5963
CODEN: JLPNEO
JOURNAL OF PEDIATRIC NURSING; nursing care of children and families. Text in English. 1986. bi-m. USD 81 domestic to individuals; USD 154 foreign to individuals; USD 136 domestic to institutions; USD 200 foreign to institutions; USD 41 domestic to students; USD 92 foreign to students; USD 34 newsstand/cover (effective 2001). adv. bk.rev. bibl, charts, illus. index. *Refereed.* **Document type:** *Journal, Academic/Scholarly.* **Description:** Taking a family-centered approach, presents comprehensive discussions of topics of interest to pediatric and maternal nurses from several points of view.
Related titles: Online - full text ed.: (from IDEAL Online Library).
Indexed: CINAHL, Fam.Ind., Ind.Med. (1986-), Int.Nurs.Ind., THA.
—BLDSC (5030.190000), CISTI, GNLM, ingenta. **CCC.**
Published by: W.B. Saunders Co. (Subsidiary of: Harcourt Publishers Ltd.), 11830 Westline Industrial Dr, St Louis, MO 63146. TEL 800-325-4177, http://www.wbsaunders.com. Ed. Cecily Lynn Betz. adv.: B&W page USD 785, color page USD 910; trim 10 x 7. Circ: 2,579. **Subscr. to:** Periodicals Fulfillment, W B Saunders Co, 6277 Sea Harbor Dr, 4th Fl, Orlando, FL 32891-4800.

JOURNAL OF PEDIATRIC ONCOLOGY NURSING. see *MEDICAL SCIENCES—Oncology*

610.73 617.96 USA
JOURNAL OF PERIANESTHESIA NURSING. Text in English. 1986. bi-m. USD 89 domestic to individuals Full text online included; USD 179 foreign to individuals Full text online included; USD 158 domestic to institutions Full text online included; USD 220 foreign to institutions Full text online included; USD 56 domestic to students Full text online included; USD 107 foreign to students Full text online included; USD 37 per issue (effective 2001). adv. bibl, charts, illus. cum.index. *Refereed.* **Document type:** *Journal, Academic/Scholarly.* **Description:** Aimed primarily at nurses engaged in the practice of postsurgical nursing and the management of patients in postanesthesia care units; covers standards of care, educational resources, pharmacology, and legal and ethical issues.
Formerly (until 1996): Journal of Post Anasthesia Nursing (1089-9472)
Related titles: Online - full text ed.: (from IDEAL Online Library).
Indexed: Brit.Nur.Ind., CINAHL, Int.Nurs.Ind.
—BLDSC (5030.546000), Infotrieve. **CCC.**
Published by: (American Society of PeriAnesthesia Nurses), W.B. Saunders Co. (Subsidiary of: Harcourt Publishers Ltd.), 11830 Westline Industrial Dr, St Louis, MO 63146. TEL 800-325-4177, http://www.jopan.org, http://www.wbsaunders.com. Eds. Jan Odom, Vallire Hooper. adv.: B&W page USD 895, color page USD 1,995; trim 10 x 7. Circ: 12,674. **Subscr. to:** Periodicals Fulfillment, W B Saunders Co, 6277 Sea Harbor Dr, 4th Fl, Orlando, FL 32891-4800. TEL 800-654-2452, FAX 800-874-6418.

610.73 618.2 USA ISSN 0893-2190
CODEN: JPNNE8
JOURNAL OF PERINATAL AND NEONATAL NURSING. Text in English. 1987. q. USD 132 to individuals; USD 40 newsstand/cover (effective 2002). *Refereed.* **Document type:** *Journal, Trade.* **Description:** Covers topics in critical care, obstetrics, neonatal intensive care, intervention outcomes, home care, professional development, and state-of-the-art technological advances.
Related titles: Online - full text ed.: (from Ovid Technologies, Inc., ProQuest Information & Learning, Gale Group, Institute for Scientific Information).
Indexed: ASCA, CINAHL, Curr.Cont., Fam.Ind., IMFL, Int.Nurs.Ind., Nurs.Abstr., SSCI.
—BLDSC (5030.548000), CISTI, GNLM, IDS, ingenta. **CCC.**
Published by: Aspen Publishers, Inc., 200 Orchard Ridge Dr, Ste 200, Gaithersburg, MD 20878. TEL 301-417-7500, 800-638-8437, FAX 301-695-7931, customer.service@aspenpubl.com, http://www.aspenpub.com. Eds. Diane J Angelini, Susan Blackburn. **Dist. by:** Aspen Publishers Inc., Distribution Center, 7201 McKinney Circle, Frederick, MD 21701. TEL 301-698-7100, FAX 301-417-7550.

610.73 USA ISSN 0022-3867
JOURNAL OF PRACTICAL NURSING. Text in English. 1951. q. USD 15; USD 25 foreign (effective 1994). adv. bk.rev. abstr, bibl, charts, illus, stat. index, cum.index. reprint service avail. from PQC. *Refereed.* **Document type:** *Trade.*
Related titles: Microform ed.: (from PQC).
Indexed: AgeLine, CINAHL, Dent.Ind., Hosp.Lit.Ind., INIS Atomind., Int.Nurs.Ind., Rehabil.Lit.
—BLDSC (5041.600000), CISTI, GNLM, ingenta, KNAW.
Published by: National Association for Practical Nurse Education and Service, Inc., 1400 Spring St, Ste 330, Silver Spring, MD 20910. TEL 301-588-2491, FAX 301-588-2839. Ed., R&P, Adv. contact Helen Larsen. B&W page USD 695, color page USD 1,345; trim 9.88 x 7. Circ: 13,000.

JOURNAL OF PRACTICE TEACHING IN HEALTH & SOCIAL WORK. see *SOCIAL SERVICES AND WELFARE*

610.73 USA ISSN 8755-7223
RT1 CODEN: JPNUET
JOURNAL OF PROFESSIONAL NURSING. Text in English. 1985. bi-m. USD 103 domestic to individuals Full text online included; USD 208 foreign to individuals Full text online included; USD 199 domestic to institutions Full text online included; USD 245 foreign to institutions Full text online included; USD 71 domestic to students Full text online included; USD 129 foreign to students Full text online included; USD 41 per issue (effective 2001). adv. bk.rev. back issues avail. *Refereed.* **Document type:** *Academic/Scholarly.* **Description:** Addresses the practice, research, and policy roles of nurses through general articles, research articles, reviews, and editorials.
Related titles: Online - full text ed.: (from IDEAL Online Library, Institute for Scientific Information).
Indexed: AMED, ASCA, AgeLine, C.I.J.E., CINAHL, Curr.Cont., INIS Atomind., Ind.Med. (1985-), Int.Nurs.Ind., Nurs.Abstr., SSCI.
—BLDSC (5042.697000), CISTI, GNLM, IDS, ingenta. **CCC.**
Published by: (American Association of Colleges of Nursing), W.B. Saunders Co. (Subsidiary of: Harcourt Publishers Ltd.), 11830 Westline Industrial Dr, St Louis, MO 63146. TEL 800-325-4177, http://www.professionalnursing.org, http://www.wbsaunders.com. Ed. Eleanor J Sullivan. Adv. contact Steve Gray. B&W page USD 720, color page USD 1,670; trim 10 x 7. Circ: 2,396. **Subscr. to:** Periodicals Fulfillment, W B Saunders Co, 6277 Sea Harbor Dr, 4th Fl, Orlando, FL 32891-4800.

610.736 USA ISSN 0279-3695
RC440
JOURNAL OF PSYCHOSOCIAL NURSING AND MENTAL HEALTH SERVICES. Text in English. 1962. m. USD 48 to individuals; USD 68 in Canada to individuals; USD 88 elsewhere to individuals; USD 58 to institutions; USD 78 in Canada to institutions; USD 98 elsewhere to institutions (effective 1999). adv. bk.rev. charts, illus. index. reprint service avail. from PQC. *Refereed.* **Document type:** *Academic/Scholarly.* **Description:** Provides up-to-date practical information for today's psychosocial nurse.
Former titles: Journal of Psychiatric Nursing and Mental Health Services (0360-5973); Journal of Psychiatric Nursing (0022-3948)
Related titles: Microform ed.: (from PQC); Online - full text ed.: (from ProQuest Information & Learning, Institute for Scientific Information).
Indexed: Adol.Ment.Hlth.Abstr., AgeLine, Brit.Nur.Ind., CINAHL, Chic.Per.Ind., Fam.Ind., Ind.Med. (1981-), Int.Nurs.Ind., Mid.East: Abstr.& Ind., Nurs.Abstr., Psychol.Abstr.
—BLDSC (5043.475000), CISTI, GNLM, IDS, Infotrieve, ingenta. **CCC.**
Published by: Slack, Inc., 6900 Grove Rd, Thorofare, NJ 08086-9447. TEL 856-848-1000, 800-257-8290, FAX 856-853-5991, fdestefano@slackinc.com, http://www.slackinc.com/allied/jpn/jpnhome.htm. Ed. Shirley Smoyak. Circ: 12,800.

610.73 371.7 USA ISSN 1059-8405
JOURNAL OF SCHOOL NURSING. Text in English. 1970; N.S. 1985. bi-m. USD 95 domestic to institutions; USD 120 foreign to institutions (effective 2002). adv. 64 p./no. back issues avail. *Refereed.* **Document type:** *Journal, Academic/Scholarly.* **Description:** Professional journal for school nurses. Contains articles on the practice of school nursing, pertinent research projects, and legal issues which will affect school nurses.
Formerly (until vol.7, no.3, 1991): School Nurse (0048-945X)
Indexed: CINAHL, Int.Nurs.Ind.
—BLDSC (5052.665000), GNLM, Infotrieve. **CCC.**
Published by: (National Association of School Nurses, Inc.), Alliance Communications Group (Subsidiary of: Allen Press Inc.), PO Box 7065, Lawrence, KS 66044-8897. TEL 785-843-1235, 800-627-0629, FAX 480-843-1274, nasn@allenpress.com, http://www.nasn.org. Ed. Janice Denehy. Pub., R&P Beth Pine TEL 785-843-1235 ext 237. adv.: B&W page USD 1,635, color page USD 2,530; bleed 11.25 x 8.75. Circ: 9,500 (paid). **Subscr. to:** Allen Press Inc.. http://www.allenpress.com.

JOURNAL OF SUBSTANCE USE; for nursing, health and social care. see *DRUG ABUSE AND ALCOHOLISM*

610.73 USA ISSN 1086-4431
JOURNAL OF THEORY CONSTRUCTION AND TESTING. Text in English. 1997. s-a. USD 45, USD 60 to individuals; USD 75, USD 160 to institutions (effective 2001). *Refereed.* **Document type:** *Academic/Scholarly.* **Description:** Committed to the advancement and development of the scientific base of nursing as a practice discipline.

M

Related titles: Online - full text ed.: (from ProQuest Information & Learning).
Indexed: CINAHL.
—BLDSC (5069.075890).
Published by: Tucker Publications, Inc., PO Box 580, Lisle, IL 60532. TEL 630-969-3809, FAX 630-969-3895, callen@tuckerpub.com, http://www.tuckerpub.com. Ed. Dr. Margaret T Beard. R&P Clay Tucker.

610.73 USA ISSN 1043-6596
RT86.54
JOURNAL OF TRANSCULTURAL NURSING. Text in English. 1989. q. USD 75 to individuals; USD 160 to institutions; USD 25 newsstand/cover to individuals; USD 50 newsstand/cover to institutions (effective 2002). adv. bk.rev. back issues avail. *Refereed.* **Document type:** *Academic/Scholarly.* **Description:** Serves as an international forum for researchers who desire to share their ideas culturally congruent health care delivery.
Related titles: Online - full content ed.: (from EBSCO Publishing, O C L C Online Computer Library Center, Inc., ingenta, Swets Blackwell); Online - full text ed.: (from RoweCom Information Quest).
Indexed: Brit.Nur.Ind., CINAHL, Fam.Ind., Human Resour.Abstr., Int.Nurs.Ind.
—BLDSC (5069.795000), GNLM, ingenta. **CCC.**
Published by: (Transcultural Nursing Society), Sage Publications, Inc., 2455 Teller Rd, Thousand Oaks, CA 91320. TEL 805-499-0721, FAX 805-499-0871, info@sagepub.com, http://www.sagepub.com. Ed. Marilyn Marty Douglas. Pub. Sara Miller McCune. R&P Tanya Udin. Adv. contact DeAnna Vega Hammersley.

610.73 USA ISSN 1078-7496
JOURNAL OF TRAUMA NURSING. Text in English. 1994. q. USD 110 domestic to institutions; USD 140 foreign to institutions (effective 2002). adv. bk.rev., software rev., video rev. abstr. back issues avail. *Refereed.* **Document type:** *Journal, Academic/Scholarly.*
Formerly: S T N's Journal of Trauma Nursing (1076-4747)
Related titles: Online - full text ed.: (from Northern Light Technology, Inc., ProQuest Information & Learning, Gale Group).
Indexed: CINAHL, Int.Nurs.Ind.
—BLDSC (5070.515000), CISTI, GNLM.
Published by: Society of Trauma Nurses, 2743 S Veterans Pkwy, PMB 193, Springfield, IL 62704-6536. TEL 217-787-3281, FAX 217-787-3285, stnexecdir@aol.com, STNexecdir@aol.com, http://www.cinahl.com/jrnls/intro.htm/, http://www.traumamursesoc.org/. Ed. B Anderson. adv.: B&W page USD 700, color page USD 1,100. Circ: 800 (paid); 700 (controlled).

610.736 616.1 USA ISSN 1062-0303
JOURNAL OF VASCULAR NURSING. Text in English. 1982. q. USD 60 domestic to individuals; USD 73 foreign to individuals; USD 99 domestic to institutions; USD 112 foreign to institutions; USD 33 domestic to students; USD 46 foreign to students; USD 29 newsstand/cover (effective 2001). adv. *Refereed.* **Document type:** *Journal, Academic/Scholarly.* **Description:** Provides coverage of state-of-the-art nursing techniques in the care of vascular patients, valuable insights on surgical implications, and product information.
Related titles: Online - full text ed.: (from IDEAL Online Library, RoweCom Information Quest).
Indexed: CINAHL, Int.Nurs.Ind.
—BLDSC (5072.268500), CISTI, GNLM, Infotrieve. **CCC.**
Published by: (Society for Vascular Nursing, Inc.), Mosby, Inc. (Subsidiary of: Elsevier Science), 11830 Westline Industrial Dr, St Louis, MO 63146-3318. TEL 314-872-8370, 800-325-4177, FAX 314-432-1380, http://www.mosby.com/vascnurs, http://www.mosby.com/periodicals. Eds. Janice D Nunnelee, Victora A Fahey. Adv. contact Tracey Schriefer TEL 314-453-4304. B&W page USD 910, color page USD 1,860; trim 10.88 x 8.25. Circ: 1,546.

610.73 NZL ISSN 1173-2032
KAI TIAKI: NURSING NEW ZEALAND. Text in English. 1993; N.S. 1995. m. NZD 100 domestic; AUD 100 in Australasia; USD 100 elsewhere (effective 2001). adv. bk.rev. charts, illus, stat. 48 p./no. back issues avail. *Refereed.* **Document type:** *Academic/Scholarly, Trade.* **Description:** Contains information on professional issues and issues concerning nurses' pay and conditions. Includes clinical and research articles, news and events and reports from staff around the country.
Formerly (until Feb. 1995): Nursing New Zealand (1172-1979); Formed by the merger of (1909-1993): New Zealand Nursing Journal (0028-8535); (1982-1993): N Z N U News (0111-865X); Which was formed by the merger of (1979-1982): N.Z. Nurses News (0111-297X); New Zealand Nurses Union News
Indexed: CINAHL, Fam.Ind., Ind.N.Z.Per., Int.Nurs.Ind.
—BLDSC (5081.173000), CISTI, GNLM, ingenta, KNAW. **CCC.**
Published by: New Zealand Nurses' Organisation, PO Box 2128, Wellington, New Zealand. TEL 64-4-385-0847, FAX 64-4-382-9993, teresao@nzno.org.nz, http://www.nzno.org.nz. Eds. Anne Manchester, Teresa O'Connor TEL 64-3-548-0018. R&P Teresa O'Connor TEL 64-3-548-0018. Adv. contact Evelyn Nelson TEL 64-4-384-4952. B&W page NZD 1,500, color page NZD 2,100; trim 210 x 285. Circ: 27,000 (controlled).

610.73 SWE
KANALEN. Variant title: Vaardfoerbundet Kanalen. Text in Swedish. 11/yr. **Document type:** *Magazine, Trade.*
Published by: Vaardfoerbundet, Box 3207, Stockholm 10364, Sweden. TEL 46-8-14-77-00, FAX 46-8-411-19-93, http://www.vardforbundet.se.

610.73 JPN ISSN 0022-8362
KANGO/NURSING. Text in Japanese. 1949. m. JPY 900 per issue. adv. bk.rev., film rev., play rev. abstr, bibl, charts, illus, stat. index, cum.index. **Document type:** *Trade.*
Indexed: Int.Nurs.Ind.
—BLDSC (5085.356000), CISTI, GNLM.
Published by: Japanese Nursing Association, 8-11 Jingu-Mae 5-chome, Shibuya-ku, Tokyo 150-0001, Japan. http://www.nurse.or.jp. Ed. Shinya Sato. Circ: 50,000.

610.73 JPN ISSN 0385-5988
KANGO GAKUSEI/NURSE STUDENT. Text in Japanese. 1951. m. JPY 12,300. Supplement avail.; back issues avail. **Document type:** *Academic/Scholarly.* **Description:** Learning guide and drills for student nurses.
Published by: Medical Friend Co. Ltd./Mejikaru Furendo Sha, 2-4 Kudan-Kita 3-chome, Chiyoda-ku, Tokyo 102-0073, Japan. FAX 81-3-3261-6602. Circ: 30,000.

610.7 JPN ISSN 0449-752X
KANGO GIJUTSU/JAPANESE JOURNAL OF NURSING ARTS. Text in Japanese. 1950. m. JPY 17,600, USD 133. bk.rev. Supplement avail.; back issues avail. **Document type:** *Academic/Scholarly.* **Description:** Case studies in clinical nursing.
Indexed: Dent.Ind., Int.Nurs.Ind.
—BLDSC (4656.740500), GNLM.
Published by: Medical Friend Co. Ltd./Mejikaru Furendo Sha, 2-4 Kudan-Kita 3-chome, Chiyoda-ku, Tokyo 102-0073, Japan. FAX 81-3-3261-6602. Circ: 100,000.

610.73 JPN ISSN 0022-8370
KANGO KENKYU/JAPANESE JOURNAL OF NURSING RESEARCH. Text in Japanese. 1968. q. JPY 9,600.
Indexed: Int.Nurs.Ind.
—BLDSC (4656.745000), CISTI, GNLM, Linda Hall.
Published by: Igaku-Shoin Ltd., 5-24-3 Hongo, Bunkyo-ku, Tokyo 113-0033, Japan. TEL 81-3-3817-5775, FAX 81-3-3815-4145, ykawada@nna.so-net.or.jp. Circ: 8,000.

610.73 JPN ISSN 0047-1895
KANGO KYOIKU/JAPANESE JOURNAL OF NURSING EDUCATION. Text in Japanese. 1960. m. JPY 16,900. illus.
Indexed: Int.Nurs.Ind.
—GNLM.
Published by: Igaku-Shoin Ltd., 5-24-3 Hongo, Bunkyo-ku, Tokyo 113-0033, Japan. TEL 81-3-3817-5776, FAX 81-3-3815-4145, ykawada@nna.so-net.or.jp. Circ: 10,000.

610.73 JPN ISSN 0385-549X
KANGO TENBO/JAPANESE JOURNAL OF NURSING SCIENCE. Text in Japanese. 1976. m. JPY 18,000. index. Supplement avail.; back issues avail. **Document type:** *Academic/Scholarly.* **Description:** Covers the administrative issues of nursing and contains various discussions on nursing education.
Indexed: Int.Nurs.Ind., Intl.Bibl.Soc.Sci.
—CISTI, GNLM.
Published by: Medical Friend Co. Ltd./Mejikaru Furendo Sha, 2-4 Kudan-Kita 3-chome, Chiyoda-ku, Tokyo 102-0073, Japan. FAX 81-3-3261-6602. Circ: 30,000.

610.73 JPN ISSN 0387-351X
KANGOGAKU ZASSHI/NURSING MAGAZINE. Text in Japanese. 1946. m. JPY 12,000.
Published by: Igaku-Shoin Ltd., 5-24-3 Hongo, Bunkyo-ku, Tokyo 113-0033, Japan. TEL 81-3-3817-5772, FAX 81-3-3815-4145, ysekiyama@nna.so-net.or.jp, ysekiyama@nna.so.net.or.jp. Circ: 50,000.

610.73 USA ISSN 0022-8710
KANSAS NURSE*. Text in English. 1973 (vol.48). 10/yr. USD 30 domestic to non-members; USD 45 foreign to non-members (effective 1999). adv. bk.rev. illus. reprint service avail. from PQC. **Document type:** *Trade.*
Related titles: Microform ed.: (from PQC); Online - full text ed.: (from Northern Light Technology, Inc., ProQuest Information & Learning).
Indexed: CINAHL, Int.Nurs.Ind.
—BLDSC (5085.648000), GNLM.
Published by: Kansas State Nurses Association, 1208 S W Tyler St, Topeka, KS 66612-1735. TEL 785-233-8638, FAX 785-233-5222, troberts@echo.sound.net, http://www.nursingworld.org/sna/ks. Ed., R&P Shellanne Flyntz. Adv. contact Margaret Krog. Circ: 2,360.

610.73 USA
KANSAS STATE BOARD OF NURSING. NEWSLETTER. Text in English. q. Free to qualified subscribers. 32 p./no. **Document type:** *Newsletter, Trade.* **Description:** Covers issues and employment opportunities of interest to licensed nursing professionals.
Published by: (Kansas State Board of Nursing), Arthur L. Davis Publishing Agency, Inc., 517 Washington St, P O Box 216, Cedar Falls, IA 50613. TEL 319-277-2414, 800-626-4081, FAX 319-277-4055, sales@aldpub.com, http://www.aldpub.com/. Ed. Mark Miller. R&P Mary Blubaugh. Adv. contact Jim Larson. Circ: 41,000 (free).

610.73 USA ISSN 0742-8367
KENTUCKY NURSE. Text in English. 1952. q. USD 18 domestic; USD 26 foreign; free to membership (effective 2001). adv. bk.rev. 32 p./no. back issues avail. **Document type:** *Newsletter, Trade.* **Description:** Covers issues and employment opportunities of interest to licensed nursing professionals.
Formerly: Kentucky Nurse Association Newsletter (0023-0316)
Related titles: Microform ed.: (from PQC).
Indexed: CINAHL.
—BLDSC (5089.653500).
Published by: (Kentucky Nurses Association), Arthur L. Davis Publishing Agency, Inc., 517 Washington St, P O Box 216, Cedar Falls, IA 50613. TEL 319-277-2414, 800-626-4081, FAX 319-277-4055, kentucky.nurses@prodigy.net, sales@aldpub.com, http://www.kentucky-nurses.org, http://www.aldpub.com/. Ed. Mark Miller. R&P Anne Powell. Adv. contact Jim Larson. Circ: 61,000 (free).

610.73 KEN ISSN 0301-0333
KENYA NURSING JOURNAL. Text in English. 1972. s-a. KES 7.50, USD 1 per issue. adv. bk.rev. back issues avail.
Indexed: Int.Nurs.Ind.
Published by: National Nurses Association of Kenya, PO Box 49422, Nairobi, Kenya. Ed. J B Khachina. Circ: 2,750.

610.73 GBR
KEY NOTE MARKET REPORT: NURSING CARE. Variant title: Nursing Care. Text in English. irreg. GBP 265 (effective 1999). **Document type:** *Trade.*
Published by: Key Note Ltd., Field House, 72 Oldfield Rd, Hampton, Mddx TW12 2HQ, United Kingdom. TEL 44-20-8481-8750, FAX 44-20-8783-0049, http://www.keynote.co.uk.

610.73 618.92 DEU ISSN 0723-2276
KINDERKRANKENSCHWESTER. Text in German. 1982. m. DEM 62 domestic; DEM 80 foreign (effective 2001). adv. bk.rev. back issues avail. **Document type:** *Journal, Trade.*
Indexed: Int.Nurs.Ind.
—BLDSC (5095.637000), GNLM.
Published by: Schmidt-Roemhild Verlag, Mengstr 16, Luebeck 23552, Germany. TEL 49-451-7031-01, FAX 49-451-7031253, msr-luebeck@t-online.de, http://www.schmidt-roemhild.de. Circ: 17,000.

610.73 DNK ISSN 0902-2767
KLINISK SYGEPLEJE. Text in Danish. 1987. bi-m. DKK 350 (effective 2001). index. back issues avail. **Document type:** *Academic/Scholarly.*
Published by: Blackwell Munksgaard, Noerre Soegade 35, PO Box 2148, Copenhagen K 1016, Denmark. FAX 45-77-33-33-77, fsub@mail.munksgaard.dk, http://www.munksgaard.dk. Ed. Kirsten Eeg. Circ: 3,500.

610.73 KOR ISSN 0047-3618
RT1
KOREAN NURSE/TAEHAN KANHO. Text in Korean. 1961. bi-m. USD 1.49. adv. bk.rev. illus.
Related titles: CD-ROM ed.
Indexed: ExtraMED, Int.Nurs.Ind.

M

—CISTI.
Published by: Korean Nurses' Association, 88-7 Sanglim-Dong, Choong Ku, Seoul, Korea, S.. Ed. San Cho Chun.

KRANKENDIENST; Zeitschrift fuer kath. Krankenhaeuser, Sozialstationen und Pflegeberufe. see *HEALTH FACILITIES AND ADMINISTRATION*

610.73 DEU ISSN 0174-108X
KRANKENPFLEGE JOURNAL; Krankenhaus Magazin. Text in German. 1963. m. DEM 36.40. adv. illus.
Formerly: Schwestern Revue (0048-9549)
Indexed: Int.Nurs.Ind.
—BLDSC (5118.146600), CISTI, GNLM, Infotrieve, KNAW. **CCC.**
Published by: Die Schwestern Revue GmbH, Am Schwarzenberg 28, Wuerzburg 97078, Germany. Ed. Knut Wenzel Backe.

610.73 JPN ISSN 0388-5585
KURINIKARU SUTADI/CLINICAL STUDY. Text in Japanese. 1980. m. JPY 15,000. Supplement avail.; back issues avail. **Document type:** *Academic/Scholarly.* **Description:** Case studies in nursing process and miscellanies for student nurses.
Indexed: Int.Nurs.Ind.
Published by: Medical Friend Co. Ltd./Mejikaru Furendo Sha, 2-4 Kudan-Kita 3-chome, Chiyoda-ku, Tokyo 102-0073, Japan. TEL 81-3-3261-6602. Ed. Yoshihiro Ogura. Circ: 60,000.

610.73 CAN
L P N ASSOCIATION OF BRITISH COLUMBIA NEWSLETTER. Text in English. 1957. q. free per issue to members. **Document type:** *Bulletin, Newsletter.*
Published by: Licensed Practical Nurses of British Columbia, 3302 McIvor Rd, Westbank, BC V4T 1G2, Canada. TEL 604-768-2482. Ed. Barry Philips.

610.7 AUS ISSN 0047-3936
LAMP. Text in English. 1943. m. AUD 55 domestic to non-members; AUD 27.50 domestic to members; AUD 85 foreign (effective 2001). adv. bk.rev. **Document type:** *Journal, Trade.* **Description:** Features industrial and professional news and development of interest to nurses.
Related titles: Microfiche ed.
Indexed: CINAHL, HRIS, Int.Nurs.Ind.
—BLDSC (5145.050000), GNLM, ingenta, KNAW.
Published by: New South Wales Nurses Association, 43 Australia St, Camperdown, NSW 2050, Australia. TEL 61-2-550-3244, FAX 61-2-550-3667. Pub. Julie Venamore. Adv. contact Patricia Purcell TEL 61-2-8595-2139. page AUD 1,707; trim 200 x 275. Circ: 39,500. **Subscr. to:** PO Box 40, Camperdown, NSW 2050, Australia. TEL 61-2-8595-2153, FAX 61-2-9565-2891.

610.7365 AUT ISSN 1024-6908
LAZARUS; Oesterreichs Zeitschrift fuer Kranken- und Altenpflege. Text in German. 1986. m. ATS 550 (effective 2001). adv. bk.rev. **Document type:** *Journal, Trade.*
Published by: Verein Lazarus Press, Doppel 29, Kirchstetten, N 3062, Austria. TEL 43-2743-8797, FAX 43-2743-8797, lazarus@netway.at, http://www.austrocare.org. Ed., R&P, Adv. contact Erich Hofer. B&W page ATS 22,000, color page ATS 30,000; trim 251 x 191. Circ: 24,000.

610.73 340 USA ISSN 8756-0054
LEGISLATIVE NETWORK FOR NURSES; policy and politics for the nursing profession. Text in English. 1984. bi-w. USD 287 in US & Canada (effective 2001). **Document type:** *Newsletter.* **Description:** Covers regulations and how they affect the nursing profession - salaries, training, recruiting, and unionizing.
Related titles: E-mail ed.; Online - full text ed.
—CCC.
Published by: Business Publishers, Inc., 8737 Colesville Rd, 11th Fl, Silver Spring, MD 20910-3928. TEL 301-587-6300, 800-274-6737, FAX 301-589-8493, bpinews@bpinews.com, http://www.bpinews.com. Ed. Sarah Spencer. Pub. Leonard A Eiserer.

610.73 GBR ISSN 1354-1412
LIBRARIES FOR NURSING BULLETIN. Text in English. 1981. q. GBP 10; GBP 30 foreign. adv. bk.rev. **Document type:** *Bulletin.* **Description:** Includes news, articles, reviews, and reports relevant to the provision of library services to nurses and the nursing profession.
Formerly (until 1993): N I S G Newsletter (0263-4945)
—BLDSC (5186.094000).
Published by: Library Association Health Libraries Group, Libraries for Nursing, St George's Hospital, London SW17 0RE, United Kingdom. TEL 44-181-725-5466, FAX 44-181-767-4696, lbrymw@ford.anglia.ac.uk. Eds. Maurice Wakeham, Paul Moorbath. Adv. contact Sue David. page GBP 50. Circ: 150 (paid).

LINK (WOODLAND HILLS). see *MEDICAL SCIENCES—Psychiatry And Neurology*

610.73 USA ISSN 1529-7764
LIPPINCOTT'S CASE MANAGEMENT; managing the process of patient care. Text in English. 1996. bi-m. USD 55 domestic to individuals; USD 85 foreign to individuals; USD 115 domestic to institutions; USD 139 foreign to institutions; USD 21 newsstand/cover (effective 2002). adv. **Document type:** *Journal, Academic/Scholarly.*
Formerly (until 2000): Nursing Case Management (1084-3647)
Related titles: CD-ROM ed.: (from Ovid Technologies, Inc.); Online - full text ed.: USD 149.50 domestic academic site license; USD 173.50 foreign academic site license; USD 166.75 domestic corporate site license; USD 190.75 foreign corporate site license (2002) (from Ovid Technologies, Inc.).
Indexed: CINAHL, Int.Nurs.Ind.
—BLDSC (5221.874800).
Published by: Lippincott Williams & Wilkins (Philadelphia) (Subsidiary of: Wolters Kluwer N.V.), 530 Walnut St, Philadelphia, PA 19106-3621. TEL 301-223-2300, 800-638-3030, FAX 301-223-2400, nursingcm@aol.com, http://www.lww.com. Ed. Diane Williams. Pub. Sandra Kasko. Adv. contact Ted D'Elia TEL 212-886-1386.

LIPPINCOTT'S NURSING DRUG GUIDE. see *PHARMACY AND PHARMACOLOGY*

LIST OF CANADIAN NURSING-RELATED PERIODICALS. see *MEDICAL SCIENCES—Abstracting, Bibliographies, Statistics*

LONG TERM CARE. see *GERONTOLOGY AND GERIATRICS*

610.73 USA
LOUISIANA. STATE BOARD OF NURSING. REPORT (CALENDAR YEAR). Text in English. 1973. a. USD 30. **Document type:** *Government.*
Formerly (until 1976): Louisiana. State Board of Nurse Examiners. Report (0095-5884)
Published by: State Board of Nursing, 3510 N. Causeway, Ste. 501, Metrarie, LA 70002. TEL 504-838-5332, FAX 504-838-5349, isbn@isbn.state.la.us, http://www.lsbn.state.la.us. Ed. Barbara L Morvant. R&P Barbara Morvant. Circ: 150.

610.73 USA ISSN 0361-929X
RG951 CODEN: MCNNEI
M C N: AMERICAN JOURNAL OF MATERNAL CHILD NURSING. Text in English. 1976. bi-m., latest vol.26. USD 35 domestic to individuals; USD 67 elsewhere to individuals; USD 87 domestic to institutions; USD 107 elsewhere to institutions; USD 18 newsstand/cover (effective 2002). adv. bk.rev. bibl, charts, illus. index. reprint service avail. from PQC. *Refereed.* **Document type:** *Trade.*
Related titles: CD-ROM ed.: (from Ovid Technologies, Inc.); Microform ed.: (from PQC); Online - full text ed.: USD 113.10 domestic academic site license; USD 133.10 foreign academic site license; USD 126.15 domestic corporate site license; USD 146.15 foreign corporate site license (2002) (from Ovid Technologies, Inc.).
Indexed: AgeLine, Brit.Nur.Ind., CINAHL, Fam.Ind., IMFL, Ind.Med. (1976-), Int.Nurs.Ind., Nurs.Abstr.
—BLDSC (5413.499800), GNLM, ingenta, KNAW.
Published by: Lippincott Williams & Wilkins (Philadelphia) (Subsidiary of: Wolters Kluwer N.V.), 530 Walnut St, Philadelphia, PA 19106-3621. TEL 301-223-2300, 800-638-3030, FAX 301-223-2400, http://www.nursingcenter.com, http://www.lww.com. Ed. Margaret Comerford Freda. Circ: 22,000.

610.73 362 NLD ISSN 0165-2923
M G Z. (Maatschappelijke Gezondheidszorg) Text in Dutch. 1973. m. adv. bk.rev. illus. index. **Document type:** *Trade.* **Description:** For professionals in home care and preventive health care, including district nurses, midwives, dieticians, doctors, and home nursing services.
Formed by the merger of (1910-1972): Gezondheidszorg (0016-9528); Katholieke Gezondheidszorg (0022-9369); Oranje - Groene Kruis
Published by: Elsevier Bedrijfsinformatie BV, Misset (Subsidiary of: Reed Elsevier plc), Postbus 4, Doetinchem 7000 BA, Netherlands. TEL 31-314-349371, FAX 31-314-363638, info@ebi.nl, http://www.ebi.nl. Adv. contact Cor van Nek. B&W page NLG 2,178, color page NLG 4,768; trim 297 x 210. Circ: 5,900.

610.73 GBR
MACMILLAN NURSE. Text in English. 1995. 3/yr.
Published by: Hayward Medical Communications Ltd., Covent Garden, Seven Dials Warehouse, 44 Earlham St, London WC2H 9LA, United Kingdom. TEL 44-20-7240-4493, FAX 44-20-7240-4479, admin@hayward.co.uk, http://www.hayward.co.uk. Circ: 2,000. **Subscr. to:** Rosemary House, Lanwades Park, Kentford, Near, Newmarket, Suffolk CB8 7PW, United Kingdom. TEL 44-1638-751515, FAX 44-1638-751517.

610.73 618 POL ISSN 1425-6789
MAGAZYN PIELEGNIARKI I POLOZNEJ. Text in Polish. 1995. m. USD 45 (effective 1998). adv. illus. reprints avail. **Document type:** *Academic/Scholarly.* **Description:** Covers all fields of nursing and midwifery.
Published by: (Naczelna Rada Pielegniarek i Poloznych), Wydawnictwo Medyczne Sanmedica Sp. z o.o., Ul Nowy Zjazd 1, Warsaw 00301, Poland. TEL 48-22-8262287, FAX 48-22-8263182. Ed. Barbara Dworak Bator. Adv. contact Jolanta Paterczyk. color page USD 850. Circ: 12,000.

610.73 USA
THE MAINE NURSE. Text in English. q. Free to qulified subscribers. 20 p./no. **Document type:** *Newsletter, Trade.* **Description:** Covers issues and employment opportunities of interest to licensed nursing professionals.
Published by: (Maine State Nurses Association), Arthur L. Davis Publishing Agency, Inc., 517 Washington St, P O Box 216, Cedar Falls, IA 50613. TEL 319-277-2414, 800-626-4081, FAX 319-277-4055, sales@aldpub.com, http://www.aldpub.com/. Ed. Mark Miller. R&P Tammy McLaughlin. Adv. contact Jim Larson. Circ: 18,000 (free).

610.73 USA ISSN 0047-6080
MARYLAND NURSE. Text in English. 1970. 4/yr. Free to qualified subscribers. adv. 32 p./no. back issues avail. **Document type:** *Newsletter, Trade.* **Description:** Covers issues and employment opportunities of interest to licensed nursing professionals.
Supersedes: Maryland Nurses News
Related titles: Microfilm ed.: (from PQC).
Indexed: CINAHL, Int.Nurs.Ind.
—BLDSC (5383.518000), GNLM.
Published by: (Maryland Nurses Association), Arthur L. Davis Publishing Agency, Inc., 517 Washington St, P O Box 216, Cedar Falls, IA 50613. TEL 319-277-2414, 800-626-4081, FAX 319-277-4055, sales@aldpub.com, http://www.aldpub.com/. Ed. Mark Miller. R&P Kathryn V Hall. Adv. contact Jim Larson. Circ: 59,000.

610.73 USA ISSN 0163-0784
MASSACHUSETTS NURSE. Text in English. 1932. q. Free to qualified subscribers. adv. 36 p./no. back issues avail. **Document type:** *Newsletter, Trade.* **Description:** Covers issues and employment opportunities of interest to licensed nursing professionals.
Formerly (until vol. 44, 1975): Massachusetts Nurses Association. Bulletin (0025-4843)
Indexed: CINAHL, Int.Nurs.Ind.
—GNLM.
Published by: (Massachusetts Nurses Association), Arthur L. Davis Publishing Agency, Inc., 517 Washington St, P O Box 216, Cedar Falls, IA 50613. TEL 319-277-2414, 800-626-4081, FAX 319-277-4055, sales@aldpub.com, http://www.aldpub.com/. Ed. Mark Miller. R&P David Schildmeier. Adv. contact Jim Larson. Circ: 107,000 (free).

610.73 RUS ISSN 0869-7760
CODEN: MESEAQ
MEDITSINSKAYA POMOSHCH/MEDICAL CARE. Text in Russian; Summaries in English. 1942. bi-m. USD 87 foreign (effective 2000). adv. bk.rev., Website rev. index. **Document type:** *Journal, Academic/Scholarly.* **Description:** Publishes articles on the care of patients, medical technique, medical advances, and sanitary education.
Formerly (until 1993): Meditsinskaya Sestra (0025-8342)
Indexed: Biol.Abstr., Chem.Abstr., Dent.Ind., INIS Atomind., Ind.Sci.Rev., Int.Nurs.Ind., Ref.Zh.
—CISTI, East View, GNLM, Infotrieve. **CCC.**

Published by: Izdatel'stvo Meditsina, Petroverigskii per 6-8, Moscow 101000, Russian Federation. TEL 7-095-9248785, 7-095-928-86-48, FAX 7-095-9211355, 7-095-9286003, meditsina@iname.com, http://www.medit.ru. Ed. Kh A Musalatov. Pub. A M Stochik. R&P L Vecherkina. Adv. contact O A Fadeeva TEL 7-095-923-51-40. Circ: 12,000. **Dist. by:** Mezhdunarodnaya Kniga, B Yakimanka 39, Moscow 117049, Russian Federation. TEL 7-095-2384967, FAX 7-095-2384634; **US dist. addr.:** East View Publications, 3020 Harbor Ln N, Minneapolis, MN 55447. TEL 612-550-0961.

610.73 BGR ISSN 1310-7496
MEDITSINSKI PREGLED. SESTRINSKO DELO. Text in Bulgarian; Summaries in Bulgarian, English. 1969. q., latest vol.33, 2001. BGL 14 domestic; USD 35 foreign (effective 2001 - 2002). adv. bk.rev. 48 p./no. back issues avail. *Refereed.* **Document type:** *Journal, Academic/Scholarly, Abstract/Index, Bibliography.* **Description:** Presents original articles and abstracts of foreign publications in the fields of nursing care, education, nursing services, nurse-patient relations, hospital nursing staff.
Formerly: Za Srednite Meditsinski Kadri (0324-1726)
Indexed: Ref.Zh.
Published by: Meditsinski Universitet - Sofia, Tsentur za Informatsiia po Meditsina/Medical University - Sofia, Medical Information Center, 1 Sv Georgi Sofiiski ul, Sofia 1431, Bulgaria. TEL 359-2-9522342, FAX 359-2-9522393, mutafov@sun.medun.acad.bg, http://www.medun.acad.bg. Ed. Dr. K Iurukova. R&P, Adv. contact Dr. Christo Mutafov. B&W page USD 50, color page USD 150; trim 160 x 110. Circ: 300. **Dist. by:** Sofia Books, Ul Silivria 16, Sofia 1404, Bulgaria. TEL 359-2-9586257, sofiabooks@hotmail.com, http://www.sofiabooks.hit.bg.

MEDSURG NURSING. see *MEDICAL SCIENCES—Surgery*

MENTAL HEALTH NURSING JOURNAL. see *MEDICAL SCIENCES—Psychiatry And Neurology*

MENTAL HEALTH PRACTICE. see *MEDICAL SCIENCES—Psychiatry And Neurology*

610.73 USA ISSN 0026-2366
MICHIGAN NURSE. Text in English. 1924. 11/yr., latest vol.74, no.5. USD 33 domestic; USD 50 foreign (effective 2001). adv. illus. index. back issues avail. **Document type:** *Trade.* **Description:** Publishes information of interest to nurses, including topics related to the profession, announcements of continuing education opportunities, and convention reports. Reports on Michigan Nurses Association programs, elections, and committee activities.
Related titles: Microform ed.: (from PQC).
Indexed: CINAHL, Int.Nurs.Ind., Mich.Mag.Ind.
—BLDSC (5755.540000), GNLM, Linda Hall.
Published by: Michigan Nurses Association, 2310 Jolly Oak Rd, Okemos, MI 48864-4599. TEL 517-349-5640, FAX 517-349-5818, minurses@minurses.org, http://www.minurses.org. Ed., R&P Ann Kettering Sincox. Adv. contacts Ann Kettering Sincox, Lisa Gottlieb-Kinnaird. Circ: 10,000.

MIDWIFERY. see *MEDICAL SCIENCES—Obstetrics And Gynecology*

610.736 GBR ISSN 0961-1479
MIDWIFERY MATTERS. Text in English. 1978. q. GBP 25 in United Kingdom; GBP 30 overseas (effective 2000). adv. bk.rev. **Document type:** *Trade, Consumer.* **Description:** Disseminates ideas, skills and information with colleagues and clients. Helps midwives develop their role as advocates for women's active participation in maternity care.
Former titles (until 1990): Association of Radical Midwives Magazine (0951-5488); (until 1986): Association of Radical Midwives. Newsletter (0142-4610)
Indexed: Brit.Nur.Ind., CINAHL, Gend.Watch.
—BLDSC (5761.449232).
Published by: Association of Radical Midwives, 62 Greetby Hill, Ormskirk, Lancs L39 2DT, United Kingdom. TEL 44-1695-572776, arm@radmid.demon.co.uk, http://www.radmid.demon.co.uk. Ed. Margaret Jowitt. Adv. contact Ishbel Kargar. Circ: 1,200.

610.73 ARE
MINBAR AL-TAMRID/NURSING FORUM. Text in Arabic, English. 1987. 5/yr. free per issue. **Description:** Scientific articles in the field of nursing, and news of interest to the nursing profession.
Published by: Ministry of Health, School of Nursing/Wizarat al-Sihhah, Madrasat al-Tamrid, PO Box 3798, Abu Dhabi, United Arab Emirates. TEL 668591, FAX 665472, TELEX 22678 MEDAD EM. Ed. Nabil Kronfol. Circ: 1,000 (controlled).

610.73 USA ISSN 0026-5586
MINNESOTA NURSING ACCENT. Variant title: M N A Accent. Text in English. 1927. 10/yr. USD 25 domestic to non-members; USD 45 foreign to non-members (effective 2001). adv. bk.rev. illus. **Document type:** *Trade.*
Indexed: CINAHL, Int.Nurs.Ind.
—BLDSC (5810.290000), GNLM.
Published by: Minnesota Nurses Association, 1295 Bandana Blvd., Ste. 140, St. Paul, MN 55108. FAX 612-646-4807, http://www.mnnurses.org. Ed., R&P, Adv. contact Jan Rabbers TEL 612-646-4807 ext 161. Pub. Marilyn Cunningham. Circ: 14,000.

MINORITY NURSE. see *OCCUPATIONS AND CAREERS*

610.73 910.03 USA ISSN 1071-9946
MINORITY NURSE NEWSLETTER. Text in English. 1994. q. USD 50 domestic to individuals; USD 75 foreign to individuals; USD 100 domestic to institutions; USD 125 foreign to institutions (effective 2001). **Document type:** *Newsletter.* **Description:** Looks at timely issues affecting minority patients, families, communities, nurses, students and faculty members.
Related titles: Online - full text ed.: (from Northern Light Technology, Inc., ProQuest Information & Learning).
Indexed: CINAHL, Int.Nurs.Ind.
Published by: Tucker Publications, Inc., PO Box 580, Lisle, IL 60532. TEL 630-969-3809, FAX 630-969-3895, callen@tuckerpub.com, http://www.tuckerpub.com. Eds. Mary Anderson, Mary Branch. R&P Clay Allen.

610.73 USA ISSN 0026-6388
MISSISSIPPI R N. (Registered Nurse) Text in English. 1939. bi-m. USD 18 domestic; USD 25 foreign (effective 2000). adv. bk.rev. illus. **Document type:** *Trade.*
Indexed: CINAHL, Int.Nurs.Ind.
—GNLM.
Published by: Mississippi Nurses' Association, 31 Woodgreen Pl, Madison, MS 39110-9531. TEL 601-898-0670, FAX 601-898-0190, mna@netdoor.com. Ed. Betty Dickson. Adv. contact Clay Cazier. Circ: 2,000.

610.73 USA
MISSOURI STATE BOARD OF NURSING. NEWSLETTER. Text in English. q. Free to qualified subscribers. 24 p./no. **Document type:** *Newsletter, Trade.* **Description:** Covers issues and employment opportunities of interest to licensed nursing professionals.
Published by: (Missouri State Board of Nursing), Arthur L. Davis Publishing Agency, Inc., 517 Washington St, P O Box 216, Cedar Falls, IA 50613. TEL 319-277-2414, 800-626-4081, FAX 319-277-4055, sales@aldpub.com, http://www.aldpub.com/. Ed. Mark Miller. R&P Calvina Thomas. Adv. contact Jim Larson. Circ: 102,000 (free).

612.652 USA ISSN 1080-3807
N A N N CENTRAL LINES✱. Text in English. 199?. q. USD 65 in US & Canada to membership; USD 101 elsewhere to membership (effective 2000). **Document type:** *Newsletter, Trade.* **Description:** Announces news and events of interest to nurses working with neonatal patients.
Published by: National Association of Neonatal Nurses, 4700 West Lake Ave, Glenview, IL 60025-1468. TEL 847-299-6266, 847-299-NANN, 800-451-3795, FAX 847-297-6768, info@nann.org, http://www.nann.org.

610.73 USA ISSN 1047-4757
N A S N NEWSLETTER✱. Text in English. 1986. 5/yr. membership. **Document type:** *Newsletter.* **Description:** Covers news, issues, conferences and resources of interest to school nurses.
Published by: (National Association of School Nurses, Inc.), Health Information Publications, Inc., 200 Valley Rd Ste 405, Mount Arlington, NJ 07856-1320. TEL 973-267-8938, FAX 973-267-8926. Ed. Debbie Iiardi. adv.: B&W page USD 1,075, color page USD 1,925; bleed 11.25 x 8.5. Circ: 9,000 (paid). **Subscr. to:** PO Box 1300, Scarborough, ME 04070-1300.

610.736 362.1 GBR
N B S GAZETTE. Text in English. 1997. irreg. **Document type:** *Bulletin.*
—BLDSC (6067.748500).
Published by: National Board for Nursing, Midwifery and Health Visiting for Scotland, 22 Queen St, Edinburgh, Midlothian EH2 1NT, United Kingdom. TEL 44-131-226-7371, FAX 44-131-225-9970.

610.73 GBR ISSN 1361-4096
N T RESEARCH. (Nursing Times) Text in English. 1995. bi-m. GBP 39 domestic to individuals; GBP 52.50 in Europe to individuals; GBP 131 domestic to institutions; GBP 136.50 in Europe to institutions (effective 2000). **Document type:** *Trade.* **Description:** Aims to make formal, well-tested expertise in nursing research accessible to practitioners.
Indexed: Brit.Nur.Ind., CINAHL.
—BLDSC (6180.592200).
Published by: Emap Healthcare Ltd. (Subsidiary of: Emap Business Communications Ltd.), Greater London House, Hampstead Rd, London NW1 7EJ, United Kingdom. TEL 44-20-7874-0502, FAX 44-20-7874-0505, ntresearch@healthcare.emap.co.uk. Ed. Veronica Bishop. Pub. John Barnes. **Subscr. to:** Emap Readerlink Ltd., Audit House, 260 Field End Rd, Ruislip, Mddx HA4 9LT, United Kingdom. TEL 44-181-956-3000.

612.652 USA
NATIONAL ASSOCIATION OF NEONATAL NURSES. POSITION STATEMENT✱. Text in English. irreg. USD 15 per issue to members; USD 25 per issue to non-members (effective 2000). back issues avail. **Document type:** *Monographic series.* **Description:** Discusses important issues in neonatal and pediatric nursing.
Published by: National Association of Neonatal Nurses, 4700 West Lake Ave, Glenview, IL 60025-1468. TEL 847-299-6266, 847-299-NANN, 800-451-3795, FAX 847-297-6768, info@nann.org, http://www.nann.org/resource/publctns/pstmts.

610.73 GBR ISSN 0956-9715
NATIONAL BOARD FOR NURSING, MIDWIFERY AND HEALTH VISITING FOR NORTHERN IRELAND. CONSOLIDATED ACCOUNTS (YEAR). Text in English. 1984. a. **Document type:** *Government.*
Formerly (until 1987): National Board for Nursing, Midwifery and Health Visiting for Northern Ireland. Accounts (0956-9707)
Published by: National Board for Nursing, Midwifery and Health Visiting for Northern Ireland, c/o H.M.S.O. Publications Centre, PO Box 276, London SW8 5DT, United Kingdom. TEL 44-171-873-9090, FAX 44-171-873-8200.

610.73 USA ISSN 0028-1921
NEBRASKA NURSE. Text in English. 1947. q. Free to qualified subscribers. adv. 36 p./no. back issues avail. **Document type:** *Newsletter, Trade.* **Description:** Covers issues and employment opportunities of interest to licensed nursing professionals.
Indexed: CINAHL, Int.Nurs.Ind.
—GNLM.
Published by: (Nebraska Nurses' Association), Arthur L. Davis Publishing Agency, Inc., 517 Washington St, P O Box 216, Cedar Falls, IA 50613. TEL 319-277-2414, 800-626-4081, FAX 319-277-4055, sales@aldpub.com, http://www.aldpub.com/. Ed. Mark Miller. R&P Chuck Stepanek. Adv. contact Jim Larson. Circ: 26,000 (free).

610.73 USA ISSN 0730-0832
CODEN: NEONEE
NEONATAL NETWORK; the journal of neonatal nursing. Variant title: Journal of Neonatal Nursing. Text in English. 1982. 8/yr., latest vol.20, 2001. USD 44 domestic to individuals; USD 48 in Canada to individuals; USD 80 elsewhere to individuals; USD 56 domestic to institutions; USD 60 in Canada to institutions; USD 80 elsewhere to institutions (effective 2001). adv. bk.rev. illus. index. back issues avail. *Refereed.* **Document type:** *Journal, Academic/Scholarly.*
Indexed: Brit.Nur.Ind., CINAHL, Fam.Ind., Ind.Med. (coverage dropped), Int.Nurs.Ind.
—GNLM, ingenta, KNAW.
Published by: (National Association of Neonatal Nurses), Neonatal Network, 1410 Neotomas Ave, Ste 107, Santa Rosa, CA 95405-7533. TEL 707-569-1415, FAX 707-569-0786, editorial@neonatalnetwork.com, http://www.neonatalnetwork.com. Ed. Charles Rait. R&P Judyann Silbo. Adv. contact A J Janetti. Circ: 9,800.

610.7362 AUS ISSN 1441-6638
NEONATAL, PAEDIATRIC AND CHILD HEALTH NURSING*. Abbreviated title: N P C H N. Text in English. 1986. q. AUD 60 domestic to individuals; AUD 80 foreign to individuals; AUD 75 domestic to institutions; AUD 100 foreign to institutions (effective 2000). adv. bk.rev. illus. *Refereed.* **Document type:** *Journal, Academic/Scholarly.* **Description:** Presents a broad range of content in the specialties of neonatal, pediatric, and child health nursing, including original research, discussion papers, and case studies.
Formerly (until 1998): Paediatric Nursing Review (1038-5029)
Indexed: CINAHL.
—BLDSC (6075.624200).
Published by: (Australian Confederation of Paediatric and Child Health Nurses, N S W Branch), Ink Press International, PO Box 846, Ashfield, NSW 1800, Australia. npchn@hotmail.com. Ed., R&P Fiona Ferguson. Adv. contact Sandra Ashby. Circ: 500.
Co-sponsors: Australian Neonatal Nurses Association; New Zealand Association of Neonatal Nurses/Nga Tapuhi Whare Kohanga o Aotearoa.

610.73 616.1 USA ISSN 1526-744X
RC902.A1
NEPHROLOGY NURSING JOURNAL. Text in English. 1974. bi-m. USD 30 domestic to individuals; USD 45 foreign to individuals; USD 42 domestic to institutions; USD 57 foreign to institutions (effective 2000). adv. bk.rev. *Refereed.* **Document type:** *Academic/Scholarly.*
Former titles (until 2000): A N N A Journal (8750-0779); (until 1984): A A N N T Journal (0744-1479); (until 1980): American Association of Nephrology Nurses and Technicians (0360-7615)
Related titles: Online - full text ed.: (from Gale Group).
Indexed: CINAHL, Ind.Med. (coverage dropped), Int.Nurs.Ind., Nurs.Abstr.
—BLDSC (6075.686500), GNLM, ingenta, KNAW. **CCC.**
Published by: (American Nephrology Nurses' Association), Jannetti Publications, Inc., East Holly Ave, Box 56, Pitman, NJ 08071-0056. TEL 856-256-2300, FAX 856-589-7463, anna@ajj.com. Ed. Sally Downs McCulloch. Circ: 5,743.

610.73 USA ISSN 0273-4117
NEVADA R N FORMATION. Key Title: Nevada RNformation. Variant title: Nevada Registered Nurse Information. Text in English. 1931. q. Free to qualified subscribers. adv. 36 p./no. back issues avail.
Document type: *Newsletter, Trade.* **Description:** Reports information on topics of concern to registered nurses in Nevada, as well as association business.
Indexed: CINAHL, Int.Nurs.Ind.
Published by: (Nevada Nurses Association), Arthur L. Davis Publishing Agency, Inc., 517 Washington St, P O Box 216, Cedar Falls, IA 50613. TEL 319-277-2414, 800-626-4081, FAX 319-277-4055, sales@aldpub.com, http://www.nvnurses.org/, http://www.aldpub.com/. Ed. Mark Miller. R&P Richard Schlegel. Adv. contact Jim Larson. Circ: 17,000 (free).

610.73 USA ISSN 0196-4895
NEW JERSEY NURSE. Text in English. 1970 (vol.26). 10/yr. USD 22 (effective 2000). adv. bk.rev. **Document type:** *Newsletter.* **Description:** News and information of interest to association members.
Formerly: N J S N A Newsletter (0028-5870)
Indexed: CINAHL, Int.Nurs.Ind.
—BLDSC (6084.312000).
Published by: New Jersey State Nurses' Association, 1479 Pennington Rd, Trenton, NJ 08618-2661. TEL 609-883-5335, FAX 609-883-5343. Ed. Andrea Aughenbaugh. R&P Sandra Kerr. Adv. contact Julia Schneider. Circ: 6,000.

610.73 USA
NEW YORK STATE ASSOCIATION OF SCHOOL NURSES COMMUNICATOR*. Text in English. s-a. membership. **Document type:** *Newsletter.*
Published by: (New York State Association of School Nurses), Health Information Publications, Inc., 200 Valley Rd Ste 405, Mount Arlington, NJ 07856-1320. TEL 973-267-8938, FAX 973-267-8926. Ed. Ruth Papagni. adv.: B&W page USD 500. Circ: 800 (paid).

610.73 USA ISSN 0028-7644
CODEN: JNYNA
NEW YORK STATE NURSES ASSOCIATION. JOURNAL. Text in English. 1970. biennial, latest vol.32, no.1. USD 30 domestic; USD 35 in Canada; USD 40 in Mexico (effective 2001). bk.rev. abstr, bibl, charts, illus, stat. back issues avail. *Refereed.* **Document type:** *Academic/Scholarly.* **Description:** Publishes research reports and scholarly articles on nurses and nursing.
Formerly: New York State Nurse
Related titles: Microform ed.: (from PQC).
Indexed: CINAHL, Int.Nurs.Ind., Soc.Work Res.& Abstr.
—BLDSC (4832.940000), GNLM.
Published by: New York State Nurses Association, 11 Cornell Rd, Latham, NY 12110-1403. TEL 518-782-9400, FAX 518-782-9533, info@nysna.org., http://www.nysna.org. Ed., R&P Anne Schott. Circ: 35,000.

610.73 USA ISSN 0028-7652
NEW YORK STATE NURSES ASSOCIATION. REPORT. Text in English. 1969. 10/yr., latest vol.32, no.7. USD 30 domestic; USD 44.56 in Canada; USD 42.88 in Mexico; USD 58 elsewhere (effective 2000). adv. charts, illus, stat. back issues avail. **Document type:** *Newsletter.* **Description:** Covers news of interest to nurses, and reports activities of the Association.
Incorporates (in 1978): N Y S N A Legislative Bulletin
Published by: New York State Nurses Association, 11 Cornell Rd, Latham, NY 12110-1403. TEL 518-782-9400, FAX 518-782-9533, info@nysna.org, http://www.nysna.org. Ed. Anne Schott. Adv. contact Nancy Webber. Circ: 35,000.

610.73 NZL ISSN 0110-7968
NEW ZEALAND NURSING FORUM. Text in English. 1973-199?; resumed 1995. q. NZD 45. adv. bk.rev. abstr, bibl, charts, illus, stat. **Document type:** *Academic/Scholarly.* **Description:** Original papers, abstracts and reviews on nursing.
Formerly (until 1978): Nursing Forum (0110-0890)
Indexed: CINAHL, Int.Nurs.Ind.
—Infotrieve. **CCC.**
Published by: Nurses Society of New Zealand., P.O. Box 3195, Auckland, 1, New Zealand. TEL 64-9-8178412, FAX 64-9-817-6833. Ed. David Wills. Circ: 12,500.

610.73 AUS ISSN 1175-2904
▼ **NEW ZEALAND NURSING REVIEW.** Text in English. 2000. m. NZD 48 domestic; NZD 98 foreign (effective 2001).
Published by: A P N Educational Media Pty. Ltd., ERCNA, PO Box 6097, North Sydney, NSW 2060, Australia. TEL 61-2-9936-8666, FAX 61-2-9954-0565.

610.7362 USA ISSN 1527-3369
▼ **NEWBORN AND INFANT NURSING REVIEWS.** Text in English. 2001. q. USD 69 domestic to individuals; USD 93 foreign to individuals; USD 96 domestic to institutions; USD 120 foreign to institutions; USD 49 domestic to students; USD 93 foreign to students (effective 2001). adv. *Refereed.* **Document type:** *Journal, Academic/Scholarly.* **Description:** Contains articles and information on neonatal nursing subjects of interest to clinicians, educators and researchers.
Published by: W.B. Saunders Co. (Subsidiary of: Harcourt Publishers Ltd.), 11830 Westline Industrial Dr, St Louis, MO 63146. TEL 800-325-4177, http://www.wbsaunders.com. Ed. Carole Ann Kenner.

NIEUWSBRIEF ZORGVISIE. see *HEALTH FACILITIES AND ADMINISTRATION*

610.73 NGA ISSN 0331-4448
NIGERIAN NURSE. Text in English. 1973. bi-m. USD 13.50 (effective 2000). bibl, illus. **Document type:** *Journal, Academic/Scholarly.*
Indexed: CINAHL.
Published by: (National Association of Nigeria Nurses and Midwives), Literamed Publications Nigeria Ltd, PMB 21068, Ikeja, Oregun Village, Lagos, Nigeria. TEL 234-64-962512, FAX 234-64-961037. Ed. Anu Adegoroye. Pub. O M Lawal Solarin. Circ: 10,000.

610.73 USA ISSN 0894-5780
NIGHTINGALE. Text in English. 1973. m. USD 15 (effective 2000). stat, tr.lit. back issues avail.
Related titles: Microform ed.: (from PQC).
Published by: National Association of Physician Nurses, 900 S Washington St, Ste G 13, Falls Church, VA 22046. TEL 703-237-8616. Ed. Terri Hughes Lazzell.

610.73 JPN ISSN 0917-513X
NIHON KANGO GAKKAISHI/JOURNAL OF JAPANESE NURSING RESEARCH. Text in Japanese. 1991. s-a. **Document type:** *Journal, Academic/Scholarly.* **Description:** Publishes selected papers presented at the JNA department research conferences.
Indexed: Int.Nurs.Ind.
—BLDSC (5009.250000).
Published by: J N A Publishing Company, Japanese Nursing Association, Nursing Education and Research Center, 1-2-3 Umezono, Kiyose-shi, Tokyo 204-0024, Japan. TEL 81-3-3499-7335, FAX 81-3-3499-5943, http://www.nurse.or.jp/. Ed. Kayoko Matsumoto. Adv. contact Toshiaki Okuno.

610.73 CHE ISSN 1422-4178
NOVA. Text in French, German, Italian. 11/yr. CHF 92 (effective 2001). adv. **Document type:** *Magazine, Trade.*
Published by: Schweizer Berufs- und Fachverband der Geriatrie-, Rehabilitations- und Langzeitpflege, Obergrundstr 44, Luzern 6003, Switzerland. TEL 41-41-2407822, FAX 41-41-2407820, info@sbgrl.ch, http://www.sbgrl.ch. Circ: 6,000.

610.73 HUN ISSN 0864-7003
NOVER; az apolas elmelete es gyakorlata. Text in Hungarian; Abstracts in English. 1988. bi-m. HUF 750; USD 60 foreign. adv. bk.rev. index. **Document type:** *Academic/Scholarly.* **Description:** Directed at the continuing education of nurses, nursing theory and practice.
Indexed: CINAHL.
—BLDSC (6180.365000).
Published by: Orszagos Orvostudomanyi Informacios Intezet es Konyvtar/National Institute for Medical Information and Library of Medicine, Szentkiralyi utca 21, PO Box 278, Budapest 1444, Hungary. TEL 36-1-384133, FAX 36-1-266-9710, konyvtar@nt-ph.medinfo.hu. Pub. Dr. Alexander Fedinecz. R&P Katalin Vittay TEL 36-1-1176352. Adv. contact Ilona Borbas. B&W page HUF 30,000, color page HUF 45,000. Circ: 3,500. **Co-sponsor:** Egeszsegugyi Szakkepzo es Tovabbkepzo Intezet.

610.73 ESP ISSN 0210-8275
NUEVA ENFERMERIA. Text in Spanish. m. free per issue to qualified personnel. adv. bk.rev. **Document type:** *Bulletin.*
Formerly (until 1979): A T S Boletin Cultural e Informativo (0210-8186); Which was formed by the merger of (1928-1977): Boletin Oficial de los Practicantes de Medicina y Cirugia (0210-833X); Boletin de las Enfermeras Espanoles y A T S de Espana (0304-9213); Which was formerly (1963-1968): Caridad, Ciencia y Arte (0069-0546)
Indexed: Int.Nurs.Ind.
Published by: Consejo Nacional de Ayudantes Tecnicos Sanitarios y Diplomados en Enfermeria, Buen Suceso, 6 2o, Madrid 28008, Spain. TEL 1-541-60-73. Ed. Luis A Jurjo Alonso.

610.73 AUS ISSN 1440-1541
NURITINGA; an electronic journal of nursing. Text in English. 1998. m. bk.rev. back issues avail. *Refereed.*
Media: Online - full text. **Related titles:** E-mail ed.
Published by: University of Tasmania, School of Nursing, GPO Box 252-52, Hobart, TAS 7001, Australia. TEL 61-3-6324-3318, http://www.healthsci.utas.edu.au/nursing/nuritinga/. Ed. Sheryl Brennan.

610.73 CAN ISSN 0382-8476
NURSCENE. Text in English. 1967. 4/yr. CND 30; CND 40 foreign. bk.rev. **Document type:** *Trade.* **Description:** Includes articles on healthcare, profiles of nurses, updates on education, seminars, meetings and forums dealing with the provision and administration of healthcare in Manitoba and elsewhere.
Formerly: Marnews
Published by: Manitoba Association of Registered Nurses, 647 Broadway, Winnipeg, MB R3C 0X2, Canada. TEL 204-774-3477, 800-665-2027, FAX 204-775-6052, marn@marn.mb.ca. Ed., R&P Linda Neyedly. adv.: B&W page CND 825. Circ: 12,000 (controlled).

NURSE AIDE - V I P; published especially for those very important people who care for the elderly. see *GERONTOLOGY AND GERIATRICS*

NURSE AUTHOR AND EDITOR; a newsletter for nurse authors, editors, and editorial board members. see *JOURNALISM*

610.73 USA
NURSE - BEAT; a cardiac nursing electronic journal. Text in English. bi-m. **Document type:** *Trade.* **Description:** Dedicated to the use of health care professionals who exercise their own professional judgment in assessing and treating individual patients.
Media: Online - full text.
Address: TEL 610-967-6161, nurse-beat@drafx.com, http://badman.drafx.com/nurse-beat. Ed. Deborah W Kumar.

M

610.73 GBR ISSN 1471-5953
▼ **NURSE EDUCATION IN PRACTICE.** Text in English. 2001 (Mar). q. GBP 90 combined subscription to individuals for Nurse Education Today & Nurse Education in Practice; GBP 410 combined subscription to institutions for Nurse Education Today & Nurse Education in Practice (effective 2002). adv. bk.rev. abstr. 48 p./no. 2 cols./p. back issues avail.; reprints avail. *Refereed.* **Document type:** *Journal, Academic/Scholarly.* **Description:** Features articles on using research evidence in teaching and learning, developing practice through education, and collaborative education development.
Related titles: Online - full text ed.: (from Swets Blackwell, IDEAL Online Library).
Indexed: Brit.Nur.Ind.
—BLDSC (6187.028370).
Published by: Churchill Livingstone (Subsidiary of: Harcourt Publishers Ltd.), Robert Stevenson House, 1-3 Baxter's Pl, Leith Walk, Edinburgh, Midlothian EH1 3AF, United Kingdom. TEL 44-131-556-2424, FAX 44-131-558-1278, journals@harcourt.com, http://www.harcourt-international.com/journals/nepr. Eds. Claire Ancell, Karen Holland. R&P Sharon Boyle TEL 44-131-524-1747. Adv. contact Deborah Watkins TEL 44-207-424-4280. Circ: 850 (paid). **Subscr. in the US to:** Harcourt Health Sciences, Journals Subscription Department, PO Box 156, Avenel, NJ 07001. TEL 877-839-7126; **Subscr. to:** Harcourt Publishers Ltd., Journal Sales & Marketing Dept., 32 Jamestown Rd, London NW1 7BY, United Kingdom. TEL 44-20-8308-5700.

610.73 GBR ISSN 0260-6917
NURSE EDUCATION TODAY. Text in English. 1981. 12/yr. GBP 90, GBP 410 combined subscription to individuals for Nurse Education Today & Nurse Education in Practice (effective 2002). adv. bk.rev. illus, abstr. 88 p./no. 2 cols./p. back issues avail.; reprints avail. *Refereed.* **Document type:** *Journal, Academic/Scholarly.* **Description:** Publishes information and articles on aspects of nurse education in all parts of the world and covers a broad range of disciplines.
Related titles: Microform ed.: (from PQC); Online - full text ed.: (from EBSCO Publishing, O C L C Online Computer Library Center, Inc., ingenta, Swets Blackwell, IDEAL Online Library, Institute for Scientific Information).
Indexed: ASCA, ASSIA, AgeLine, Arts & Hum.Cit.Ind. (coverage dropped), Brit.Nur.Ind., C.I.J.E., CINAHL, Cont.Pg.Educ., Curr.Cont., ERA, Educ.Tech.Abstr., Hosp.Abstr., IBZ, Int.Nurs.Ind., Mult.Ed.Abstr., SSCI, Sociol.Educ.Abstr., Stud.Wom.Abstr., Tech.Educ.Abstr.
—BLDSC (6187.028400), GNLM, IDS, Infotrieve. **CCC.**
Published by: Churchill Livingstone (Subsidiary of: Harcourt Publishers Ltd.), Robert Stevenson House, 1-3 Baxter's Pl, Leith Walk, Edinburgh, Midlothian EH1 3AF, United Kingdom. TEL 44-131-556-2424, FAX 44-131-558-1278, journals@harcourt.com, http://www.harcourt-international.com/journals/nedt. Eds. Claire Ancell, Peter Birchenall. R&P Sharon Boyle TEL 44-131-524-1747. Adv. contact Deborah Watkins TEL 44-207-424-4280. Circ: 990. **Subscr. addr. in the US to:** Harcourt Health Sciences, Journals Subscription Department, PO Box 156, Avenel, NJ 07001. TEL 877-839-7126; **Subscr. to:** Harcourt Publishers Ltd., Journal Sales & Marketing Dept., 32 Jamestown Rd, London NW1 7BY, United Kingdom. TEL 44-20-8308-5700.

610.73 USA ISSN 0363-3624
RT71 CODEN: NUEDEC
NURSE EDUCATOR. Text in English. 1976. bi-m., latest vol.26. USD 77 domestic to individuals; USD 137 foreign to individuals; USD 187 domestic to institutions; USD 237 foreign to institutions; USD 39 newsstand/cover (effective 2002). adv. bk.rev. index. **Document type:** *Academic/Scholarly.*
Related titles: CD-ROM ed.: (from Ovid Technologies, Inc.); Microform ed.: (from PQC); Online - full text ed.: USD 243.10 domestic academic site license; USD 293.10 foreign academic site license; USD 271.15 domestic corporate site license; USD 321.15 foreign corporate site license (2002) (from Ovid Technologies, Inc.).
Indexed: C.I.J.E. (coverage dropped), CINAHL, Educ.Ind. (Jul.1992-), Int.Nurs.Ind., Nurs.Abstr.
—BLDSC (6187.028500), GNLM, ingenta.
Published by: Lippincott Williams & Wilkins (Philadelphia) (Subsidiary of: Wolters Kluwer N.V.), 530 Walnut St, Philadelphia, PA 19106-3621. TEL 301-223-2300, 800-638-3030, FAX 301-223-2400, http://www.nursingcenter.com, http://www.lww.com. Ed. Suzanne P Smith. Circ: 3,416.

610.73 USA ISSN 0361-1817
RT1 CODEN: NRPRDJ
THE NURSE PRACTITIONER; the American journal of primary health care. Text in English. 1975. m. USD 50 domestic to individuals; USD 67 in Canada to individuals; AUD 125 in Australia to individuals; USD 73 elsewhere to individuals; USD 90 domestic to institutions; USD 105 in Canada to institutions; USD 112 elsewhere to institutions; USD 10 newsstand/cover (effective 2001). adv. charts, illus, stat. index. reprint service avail. from PQC. *Refereed.* **Document type:** *Trade.* **Description:** Provides practical clinical and professional information for nurse practitioners.
Related titles: Microform ed.: (from PQC); Online - full text ed.: (from Northern Light Technology, Inc., ProQuest Information & Learning, Gale Group).
Indexed: AgeLine, Brit.Nur.Ind., CINAHL, Curr.Lit.Fam.Plan., FAMLI, Hosp.Lit.Ind., INIS Atomind., I.P.A., Ind.Med. (1975-), Int.Nurs.Ind., Nurs.Abstr.
—BLDSC (6187.028700), CISTI, GNLM, ingenta, KNAW. **CCC.**
Published by: Springhouse Corporation (Subsidiary of: Lippincott Williams & Wilkins (Philadelphia)), 1111 Bethlehem Tpk, Springhouse, PA 19477. TEL 215-646-8700, 800-490-6580, FAX 215-646-4399, http://www.springnet.com/np/nursepract.htm. Ed. Linda J Pearson. Circ: 24,653. **Subscr. to:** Nurse Practitioner, 307 Southgate Ct, Brentwood, TN 37027. TEL 800-490-6580, FAX 615-377-0525.

610.73 USA ISSN 1045-5485
NURSE PRACTITIONER FORUM. Text in English. 1990. q. USD 62 domestic to individuals; USD 121 foreign to individuals; USD 99 domestic to institutions; USD 140 foreign to institutions; USD 49 domestic to students; USD 121 foreign to students; USD 36 newsstand/cover (effective 2000). adv. *Refereed.* **Document type:** *Academic/Scholarly.* **Description:** Each issue covers a single clinical topic, emphasizing diagnostic and therapeutic measures performed by the nurse practitioner.
Related titles: Online - full text ed.: (from Institute for Scientific Information).
Indexed: ASCA, AgeLine, Brit.Nur.Ind., CINAHL, Curr.Cont., Fam.Ind., Int.Nurs.Ind., SSCI.
—BLDSC (6187.028720), GNLM, IDS, Infotrieve, ingenta. **CCC.**
Published by: W.B. Saunders Co. (Subsidiary of: Harcourt Publishers Ltd.), Curtis Center, Independence Sq W, Philadelphia, PA 19106-3399. http://www.wbsaunders.com. Ed. Charon A Pierson. Adv. contact Steve Gray. B&W page USD 695, color page USD 1,645; trim 10 x 7. Circ: 1,100. **Subscr. to:** Periodicals Fulfillment, W B Saunders Co, 6277 Sea Harbor Dr, 4th Fl, Orlando, FL 32891-4800.

NURSE PRACTITIONERS' PRESCRIBING REFERENCE. see *PHARMACY AND PHARMACOLOGY*

610.73 616 GBR ISSN 1351-5578
NURSE RESEARCHER. Text in English. 1993. q. GBP 60 in Europe to institutions; GBP 76 elsewhere to institutions (effective 2002). back issues avail. *Refereed.* **Document type:** *Academic/Scholarly.* **Description:** Contains authoritative papers on the appropriate application and relevance of research methods to nursing.
Related titles: CD-ROM ed.: (from Ovid Technologies, Inc.); Online - full text ed.: (from Ovid Technologies, Inc., Northern Light Technology, Inc., ProQuest Information & Learning).
Indexed: Brit.Nur.Ind., CINAHL.
—BLDSC (6187.028730), GNLM, Infotrieve. **CCC.**
Published by: R C N Publishing Co. (Subsidiary of: B M J Publishing Group), R C N Direct, Copse Walk, Cardiff Gate Business Park, Cardiff CF23 8XG, United Kingdom. TEL 44-29-2054-6450, FAX 44-29-2054-6401, directjournalsteam@rcn.org.uk, http://www.rcn.org.uk/. Ed. Stephen Black.

610.73 340 USA ISSN 0196-6790
KFC615.A15
THE NURSE, THE PATIENT AND THE LAW✶ ; the journal of nursing law & risk management. Text in English. 1977-1983; resumed 1984. m. USD 250. index. *Refereed.* **Description:** Discusses nursing negligence cases from a risk management perspective; keeps readers current on new standards of care, new methods to reduce or eliminate risks and new laws affecting patient care and nursing practice.
Indexed: CINAHL.
Published by: Cox Publications, 1908 Colton Blvd, Billings, MT 59102-2316. TEL 406-256-2248, FAX 406-256-7550. Ed. Meridith B Cox. Circ: 1,046.

610.73 USA
NURSE-ZINE. Variant title: Nursing Electronic Newsletter. Text in English. 1997. m. adv. back issues avail. **Document type:** *Newsletter.*
Media: Online - full text.
Published by: Worldwide Nurse TEL 612-816-8773, nurse-zine@wwnurse.com, http://www.wwnurse.com/Nurse-zine/. Ed. Brian Short. Circ: 21,000.

610.73 USA
NURSELINX. Text in English. d. adv. **Document type:** *Newsletter.* **Description:** Includes current nursing news and medical information for nurses and healthcare professionals.
Media: Online - full text. **Related titles:** E-mail ed.
Published by: MDLinx.com Inc, 316 F St NE Ste 200, Washington, DC 20002. TEL 202-543-6544, FAX 202-543-6674, info@mdlinx.com, http://www.nurselinx.com. Ed. Dave Rothenberg.

610.73 615 USA ISSN 0191-2291
NURSES' DRUG ALERT. Text in English. 1976. m., latest vol.25, 2001. USD 25.95; USD 34 in Canada; USD 39 elsewhere (effective 2001). index. back issues avail. **Document type:** *Newsletter.*
Indexed: CINAHL, Nurs.Abstr.
—BLDSC (6187.034000).
Published by: M.J. Powers & Co. Publishers, 65 Madison Ave Ste 220, Morristown, NJ 07960-6088. TEL 973-898-1200, FAX 973-898-1201, psych@alertpubs.com, http://www.alertpubs.com. Ed. Trish Elliott. Pub. Michael Powers. R&P Jenny Marie DeJesus.

610.73 615.53 USA
NURSES IN TRANSITION✶ . Text in English. 4/yr. USD 5.
Address: c/o Marta Johnson, 38921 Prindle Rd, Mokelumne Hill, CA 95245-9547. Ed. Claudia Deyton.

610.73 USA ISSN 1063-2859
NURSEWEEK. Text in English. 1989. bi-w. USD 24.95 in state California; USD 45 domestic; USD 75 foreign (effective 2001); Free to qualified subscribers.. adv. **Document type:** *Magazine, Trade.* **Description:** Reports on news and issues about nursing.
Related titles: Online - full content ed.; ♦ Regional ed.: NurseWeek South Central Edition; NurseWeek Mountain West Edition; NurseWeek Midwest Edition; NurseWeek Great Lakes Edition.
Indexed: CINAHL.
—BLDSC (6187.036000).
Published by: Nurseweek Publishing, Inc., 1156 Aster Ave, Ste C, Sunnyvale, CA 94086-6801. TEL 408-249-5877, 800-859-2091, FAX 408-249-3756, nursewked@aol.com, http://www.nurseweek.com. Eds. Mary Elizabeth Hopkins, Tim Graham. Pub. Ray Riordan. Circ: 1,225,000 (controlled).

610.73 USA
NURSEWEEK SOUTH CENTRAL EDITION. Text in English. 1994. bi-w. USD 40. adv. back issues avail. **Document type:** *Magazine, Trade.* **Description:** Includes healthcare news and information with a nursing and allied health angle.
Formerly: HealthWeek; Formed by the 1996 merger of: Nurseweek (Dallas); Allied Healthweek
Related titles: Online - full text ed.; ♦ Regional ed.: NurseWeek. ISSN 1063-2859; NurseWeek Mountain West Edition; NurseWeek Midwest Edition; NurseWeek Great Lakes Edition.
Indexed: CINAHL, Environ.Abstr.
Published by: Nurseweek Publishing, Inc., 1156 Aster Ave, Ste C, Sunnyvale, CA 94086-6801. TEL 408-249-5877, 800-859-2091, FAX 408-249-3756, editor@nurseweek.com, nursewked@aol.com, http://www.nurseweek.com. Ed. Barbara Bronson Gray. Pubs. Dennis Riordan, Ray Riordan. Circ: 100,000 (controlled).

610.73 PRT ISSN 0871-6196
NURSING. Variant title: Revista Tecnica de Enfermagem. Text in Portuguese. 1988. m. (11/yr.). PTE 6,080. **Document type:** *Trade.*
Related titles: Online - full text ed.: (from Northern Light Technology, Inc.).
Address: Rua D. Estefania 32-1o, Lisbon 1000, Portugal. TEL 351-1-791-2500, TELEX 64198 FERBEN P, http://www.fbento.pt/FB. Circ: 15,000.

610.73 USA ISSN 0363-9568
RT89

NURSING ADMINISTRATION QUARTERLY. Text in English. 1976. q. USD 149 to individuals; USD 45 newsstand/cover (effective 2002). adv. bk.rev. illus. reprint service avail. from PQC. *Refereed.* **Document type:** *Journal, Trade.* **Description:** Focuses on a selected aspect of nursing administration that offers new opportunities for patient-care and institutional leadership in today's fast-evolving health care setting.

Related titles: Microform ed.: (from PQC); Online - full text ed.: (from Ovid Technologies, Inc., ProQuest Information & Learning, Gale Group).

Indexed: Abstr.Health Care Manage.Stud., AgeLine, CINAHL, Int.Nurs.Ind., Nurs.Abstr.

—BLDSC (6187.038400), CISTI, GNLM. **CCC.**

Published by: Aspen Publishers, Inc., 200 Orchard Ridge Dr, Ste 200, Gaithersburg, MD 20878. TEL 301-417-7500, 800-638-8437, FAX 301-695-7931, customer.service@aspenpubl.com, http://www.aspenpub.com. **Dist. by:** Aspen Publishers Inc., Distribution Center, 7201 McKinney Circle, Frederick, MD 21701. TEL 301-698-7100, FAX 301-417-7550.

610.73 USA ISSN 1094-2831
RT1

NURSING AND HEALTH CARE PERSPECTIVES. Text in English. 1952. bi-m. USD 40 domestic to individuals; USD 50 foreign to individuals; USD 65 domestic to institutions; USD 75 foreign to institutions (effective 2000). adv. bk.rev. illus. reprint service avail. from PQC. *Refereed.* **Document type:** *Journal, Academic/Scholarly.* **Description:** Features news and articles on interdisciplinary, community-based health care delivery, education amd research, as well as social and economic issues that affect health care and higher education.

Former titles: N and H C Perspectives on Community (1081-8731); (until 1995): Nursing and Health Care (0276-5284); Supersedes (1952-1980): N L N News (0027-6804)

Related titles: CD-ROM ed.: (from Ovid Technologies, Inc.); Microfiche ed.: 1952 (from CIS); Microform ed.: 1952 (from PQC); Online - full text ed.: 1952 (from Ovid Technologies, Inc., Gale Group, Institute for Scientific Information).

Indexed: AMED, AgeLine, C.I.J.E., CINAHL, Curr.Cont., Int.Nurs.Ind., Med.Care Rev., Nurs.Abstr., SRI, SSCI.

—BLDSC (6187.038810), GNLM, IDS, ingenta. **CCC.**

Published by: National League for Nursing, 61 Broadway, New York, NY 10006-2701. TEL 212-363-5555, 800-669-1656, FAX 212-812-0393, nlnweb@nln.org, http://www.nln.org. Ed., R&P Leslie Block. Circ: 9,000 (paid).

610.73 USA ISSN 1533-208X

▼ **NURSING & HEALTH POLICY REVIEW.** Text in English. 2001. 3/yr. USD 44 domestic to individuals; USD 52 foreign to individuals; USD 98 domestic to institutions; USD 106 foreign to institutions (effective 2001).

Published by: Springer Publishing Company, 536 Broadway, New York, NY 10012. TEL 212-431-4370, FAX 212-941-4370, springer@springerpub.com, http://www.springerjournals.com/.

610.73 AUS ISSN 1033-6303

▼ **NURSING AND HEALTH SCIENCE EDUCATION.** Text in English. 2000. s-a. USD 60 to individuals; USD 120 to institutions (effective 2000). adv. bk.rev. index. *Refereed.* **Document type:** *Academic/Scholarly.* **Description:** Provides nursing practitioners, nursing educators, hospital administrators and health science educators with current and innovative theory and practice in various major areas of nursing and health science education.

Published by: James Nicholas Publishers, PO Box 244, Albert Park, VIC 3206, Australia. TEL 61-3-9696-5545, FAX 61-3-9699-2040, reazajda@jamesnicholaspublishers.com.au, http://www.jamesnicholaspublishers.com.au. Ed. Joseph Zajda. Pub. Rea Zajda. R&P Mary Berchmans. Adv. contact Dorothy Murphy.

610.736 AUS ISSN 1441-0745

▼ **NURSING AND HEALTH SCIENCES.** Text in English. 1999. q. AUD 198 domestic to individuals; AUD 180 in New Zealand to individuals; JPY 13,100 in Japan to individuals; USD 110 elsewhere to individuals; AUD 577 domestic to institutions; AUD 525 in New Zealand to institutions; JPY 38,500 in Japan to institutions; USD 320 elsewhere to institutions; AUD 218 domestic to individuals paper & online eds. combined; AUD 198 in New Zealand to individuals paper & online eds. combined; JPY 14,410 in Japan to individuals paper & online eds. combined; USD 121 elsewhere to individuals paper & online eds. combined; AUD 635 domestic to institutions paper & online eds. combined; AUD 578 in New Zealand to institutions paper & online eds. combined; JPY 42,350 in Japan to institutions paper & online eds. combined; USD 352 elsewhere to institutions paper & online eds. combined (effective 2001). adv. back issues avail.; reprints avail. *Refereed.* **Document type:** *Academic/Scholarly.* **Description:** Publishes research in all areas of nursing and related fields.

Related titles: Online - full text ed.: ISSN 1442-2018. AUD 179 domestic to individuals; AUD 162 in New Zealand to individuals; JPY 11,790 in Japan to individuals; USD 99 elsewhere to individuals; AUD 520 domestic to institutions; AUD 473 in New Zealand to institutions; JPY 34,650 in Japan to institutions; USD 288 elsewhere to institutions (effective 2001) (from EBSCO Publishing, O C L C Online Computer Library Center, Inc., RoweCom Information Quest, ingenta, Munksgaard & Blackwell Science's Synergy, Swets Blackwell).

—BLDSC (6187.038820). **CCC.**

Published by: (Japanese Urological Association/Shadan Hojin, Nihon Hinyokika Gakkai JPN, Yamaguchi University, School of Allied Health Sciences JPN), Blackwell Science Asia Pty Ltd, PO Box 378, Carlton South, VIC 3053, Australia. TEL 61-3-9347-0300, FAX 61-3-9347-5001, info@blacksci.co.uk; nhs@po.cc.yamaguchi-u.ac.jp, http://www.blacksci.co.uk. Eds. Masato Tsukahara, Patricia R Underwood. Pub. Heisuke Hironaka. R&P Chris Hum. Adv. contact Kathryn O'Brien.

610.73 362.1 USA

NURSING & POLICY FORUM. Text in English. 1995. bi-m. adv. **Description:** Addresses the professional nurse's need for communication about policy issues, education, and relevant research findings. Aims to challenge, mobilize and empower nurses who share an interest in public policy, and to showcase nursing's unique contributions to the field of public health.

Published by: NEX - Wolfe Publishing, PO Box 48, Eden, MD 21822. TEL 410-749-3200, 800-520-6685. Ed. Carole P Jennings. Pub. Walter W Moore. Adv. contact Alexis B O'Leary.

610.73 GBR ISSN 1465-9301

NURSING & RESIDENTIAL CARE. Text in English. m. GBP 60 domestic to individuals; GBP 160 foreign to individuals; GBP 150 domestic to institutions; GBP 220 foreign to institutions; GBP 46 domestic to students (effective 2000). **Description:** Serves care workers, nurses, and managers working in health and social care.

—BLDSC (6187.038840).

Published by: Mark Allen Publishing Ltd., Croxted Mews, 286A-288 Croxted Road, London SE24 9BY, United Kingdom. TEL 44-20-8671-7521, FAX 44-20-8671-4454. Ed. Nicola Lloyd. Pub. Mark Allen.

610.73 USA

NURSING ARCHIVES NEWS. Text in English. 1981. a. bk.rev. back issues avail. **Document type:** *Newsletter.* **Description:** Information for the Nursing Archives Associates membership and others about the activities of the Nursing Archives.

Published by: Boston University, Mugar Memorial Library, Department of Special Collections, Nursing Archives, Charles River Campus, 771 Commonwealth Ave, Boston, MA 02215. TEL 617-353-3696, FAX 617-353-2838. Ed. Sean Noel. Circ: 300.

610.73 CAN ISSN 1185-3638

NURSING B C. Text in English. 1968. 5/yr. CND 55 to non-members (effective 2000). adv. bk.rev. illus. reprint service avail. from PQC. **Document type:** *Trade.* **Description:** Official publication of the Registered Nurses Association of British Columbia; reports on significant issues affecting nurses' ability to practice safely and competently.

Formerly: R N A B C News (0048-7104)

Related titles: Microform ed.: (from PQC); Online - full text ed.: (from ProQuest Information & Learning).

Indexed: CINAHL, Int.Nurs.Ind.

—BLDSC (6187.038950), GNLM, Infotrieve. **CCC.**

Published by: Registered Nurses Association of British Columbia, 2855 Arbutus St, Vancouver, BC V6J 3Y8, Canada. TEL 604-736-7331, FAX 604-738-2272, nursingbc@rnabc.bc.ca. Ed., R&P Bruce Wells. Adv. contact Gord Smart. Circ: 35,000 (controlled).

610.73 USA ISSN 0029-6465
RT1 CODEN: NCNAAK

NURSING CLINICS OF NORTH AMERICA. Text in English. 1966. q. USD 91 domestic to individuals; USD 119 in Canada to individuals; USD 139 elsewhere to individuals; USD 138 domestic to institutions; USD 174 foreign to institutions; USD 44 per issue to non-members (effective 2001). index. reprint service avail. from PQC,ISI. *Refereed.* **Document type:** *Journal, Trade.* **Description:** Aimed at students and graduate nurses.

Related titles: Microform ed.: (from PQC); Online - full text ed.: (from Institute for Scientific Information).

Indexed: AIM, AMED, ASCA, Abstr.Health Care Manage.Stud., AgeLine, Brit.Nur.Ind., CINAHL, Chem.Abstr., Curr.Cont., Excerp.Med., Fam.Ind., Hosp.Lit.Ind., INIS Atomind., Ind.Med. (1966-), Int.Nurs.Ind., Nurs.Abstr., SSCI.

—BLDSC (6187.040000), CISTI, GNLM, IDS, ingenta, KNAW. **CCC.**

Published by: W.B. Saunders Co. (Subsidiary of: Harcourt Publishers Ltd.), 11830 Westline Industrial Dr, St Louis, MO 63146. TEL 800-325-4177, http://www.wbsaunders.com. **Subscr. to:** Periodicals Fulfillment, W B Saunders Co, 6277 Sea Harbor Dr, 4th Fl, Orlando, FL 32891-4800.

610.73 USA ISSN 1046-7459
RT48.6

NURSING DIAGNOSIS; the journal of nursing language & classification. Text in English. 1974. q. USD 54 domestic to individuals; USD 70 elsewhere to individuals; USD 36 domestic to students; USD 81 domestic to institutions; USD 97 elsewhere to institutions; USD 23 newsstand/cover domestic; USD 28 newsstand/cover elsewhere (effective 2002). adv. back issues avail.; reprints avail. *Refereed.* **Document type:** *Academic/Scholarly.* **Description:** Promotes the development, refinement, and utilization of nursing language and classification.

Formerly (until 1990): Nursing Diagnosis Newsletter (0890-7188)

Related titles: Microform ed.: (from PQC); Online - full text ed.: (from Northern Light Technology, Inc., ProQuest Information & Learning, Gale Group).

Indexed: CINAHL, Int.Nurs.Ind.

—BLDSC (6187.043000), CISTI, GNLM, ingenta.

Published by: (North American Nursing Diagnosis Association), Nursecom, Inc., 1211 Locust St, Philadelphia, PA 19107. TEL 215-545-7222, 800-242-6757, FAX 215-545-8107, customer.service@nursecominc.com, http://www.nursecominc.com; http://www.cinahl.com/jrnls/index.htm. Ed. Jolene M Simon. Pub. Margo C Neal. R&P, Adv. contact Timothy Bower.

610.73 USA ISSN 0746-1739

NURSING ECONOMICS; the journal for health care leaders. Text in English. 1983. bi-m. USD 45 domestic to individuals; USD 60 foreign to individuals; USD 60 domestic to institutions; USD 75 foreign to institutions (effective 2000). illus. Index. back issues avail.; reprints avail. *Refereed.* **Document type:** *Academic/Scholarly.*

Related titles: Online - full text ed.: (from Northern Light Technology, Inc., ProQuest Information & Learning, Gale Group, Institute for Scientific Information).

Indexed: ASCA, AgeLine, CINAHL, Curr.Cont., Fam.Ind., Int.Nurs.Ind., Nurs.Abstr., SSCI.

—BLDSC (6187.046800), CISTI, GNLM, IDS, ingenta. **CCC.**

Published by: Jannetti Publications, Inc., East Holly Ave, Box 56, Pitman, NJ 08071-0056. TEL 856-256-2300, FAX 856-589-7463, nejrnl@ajj.com, NEJRNL@ajj.com, http://www.cinahl.com/jrnls/NECO/neco.htm.

610.73 GBR ISSN 0969-7330
NURSING ETHICS; an international journal for health care professionals. Text in English. 1994. bi-m. GBP 56 in Europe to individuals; USD 102 in North America to individuals; GBP 64 rest of world to individuals; GBP 193 in Europe to institutions; USD 341 in North America to institutions; GBP 208 rest of world to institutions; GBP 49 in Europe to members International Nursing Ethics Network (INEN); USD 91 in North America to members International Nursing Ethics Network (INEN); GBP 53 rest of world to members International Nursing Ethics Network (INEN); GBP 104 in developing nations; GBP 55 newsstand/cover in Europe; USD 91 newsstand/cover in North America; GBP 59 newsstand/cover rest of world (effective 2002). adv. back issues avail.; reprints avail. *Refereed.* **Document type:** *Journal, Academic/Scholarly.* **Description:** Examines ethical issues as an integral part of nursing practice, education and research.
Related titles: Online - full text ed.: (from EBSCO Publishing, O C L C Online Computer Library Center, Inc., RoweCom Information Quest, ingenta, Swets Blackwell, Institute for Scientific Information).
Indexed: ASCA, ASSIA, AgeLine, Brit.Nur.Ind., CINAHL, Curr.Cont., Fam.Ind., Int.Nurs.Ind., SSCI.
—BLDSC (6187.046970), GNLM, IDS, Infotrieve, ingenta. **CCC.**
Published by: Arnold Publishers (Subsidiary of: Hodder Headline plc.), 338 Euston Rd, London NW1 3BH, United Kingdom. TEL 44-20-7873-6337, FAX 44-20-7873-6325, arnoldjournals@hodder.co.uk, http://www.arnoldpublishers.com/journals/journtitles.htm, http://www.palliativemedjournal.com. Ed. Verena Tschudin. Adv. contact Mary Attree. **Subscr. to:** Turpin Distribution Services Ltd., Blackhorse Rd, Letchworth, Herts SG6 1HN, United Kingdom. TEL 44-1462-488900, FAX 44-1462-483011.

610.73 USA ISSN 0029-6473
RT1 CODEN: NUFOA
NURSING FORUM; an independent voice for nursing. Text in English. 1961. q. USD 54 domestic to individuals; USD 68 elsewhere to individuals; USD 36 domestic to students; USD 65 domestic to institutions; USD 81 elsewhere to institutions; USD 21 newsstand/cover domestic; USD 24 newsstand/cover elsewhere (effective 2002). adv. bk.rev. charts, illus. index. back issues avail.; reprint service avail. from PQC. *Refereed.* **Document type:** *Academic/Scholarly.* **Description:** Presents innovative ideas and emerging issues in nursing.
Related titles: Microfilm ed.: (from PQC); Online - full text ed.: (from Northern Light Technology, Inc., ProQuest Information & Learning, Gale Group).
Indexed: AgeLine, Brit.Nur.Ind., CINAHL, Excerp.Med., Hosp.Lit.Ind., Ind.Med. (coverage dropped), Int.Nurs.Ind.
—BLDSC (6187.050000), CISTI, GNLM, ingenta.
Published by: Nursecom, Inc., 1211 Locust St, Philadelphia, PA 19107. TEL 215-545-7222, 800-242-6757, FAX 215-545-8107, http://www.nursecominc.com; http://www.cinahl.com/jrnls/NFOR/nfor.htm. Ed. Lynda Juall Carpenito. Pub. Margo C Neal. R&P Alison L Graham. Adv. contact Timothy Bower. B&W page USD 700, color page USD 1,100; trim 10.88 x 8.25. Circ: 2,050.

610.73 USA ISSN 1062-8061
RT31
NURSING HISTORY REVIEW. Text in English. 1993. a. USD 36 in United States to individuals; USD 66 for 2 yrs. in United States to individuals; USD 43 foreign to individuals; USD 77 for 2 yrs. foreign to individuals; USD 68 in United States to institutions; USD 120 for 2 yrs. in United States to institutions; USD 80 foreign to institutions; USD 140 for 2 yrs. foreign to institutions (effective 2000). adv. bk.rev. **Document type:** *Academic/Scholarly.* **Description:** Traces new and developing work in the fields of nursing and health care history. Includes coverage of national and international activities in health care history.
Related titles: Online - full text ed.: (from Institute for Scientific Information).
Indexed: ASCA, Amer.Hist.& Life, Arts & Hum.Cit.Ind. (coverage dropped), CINAHL, Curr.Cont., Hist.Abstr. (1993-), Ind.Med. (1993-), Int.Nurs.Ind., SSCI.
—BLDSC (6187.051000), GNLM, IDS. **CCC.**
Published by: (American Association for the History of Nursing), Springer Publishing Company, 526 Broadway, New York, NY 10012-3955. TEL 212-431-4370, FAX 212-941-7842, springer@springerpub.com, http://www.springerpub.com. Ed. Joan E Lynaugh. Adv. contact Rafael Ortiz. B&W page USD 300.

610.73 GBR
NURSING HOME BUSINESS. Text in English. 1997. m. GBP 50 domestic; GBP 100 foreign; GBP 2.50 newsstand/cover. adv. bk.rev. tr.lit. back issues avail. **Document type:** *Trade.* **Description:** Covers nursing home training, finances, medical information, health, and safety management for proprietors and managers.
Published by: Park View Publishing Ltd., Park View House, 19 The Ave, Eastbourne, E Sussex BN21 3YD, United Kingdom. TEL 44-1323-411601, FAX 44-1323-411654, editorial@nhb.argonet.co.uk. Ed. Stephanie Richman. Pub. B T Collins. R&P B.T. Collins. adv.: B&W page GBP 700, color page GBP 995; trim 188 x 265. Circ: 7,500 (paid).

649.8 USA ISSN 1061-4753
RA997.A1
NURSING HOMES; long term care management. Text in English. 1950. m. USD 95 domestic; USD 100 in Canada & Mexico; USD 110 elsewhere. adv. illus. stat. back issues avail.; reprints avail. **Description:** For professionals in planning, directing, organizing and delivering quality long-term care in the proprietary nursing home field.
Former titles: Nursing Homes and Senior Citizen Care (0896-6915); (until 1986): Nursing Homes (0029-649X)
Related titles: Microform ed.: (from PQC); Online - full text ed.: (from The Dialog Corporation, Gale Group, ProQuest Information & Learning, Northern Light Technology, Inc., Factiva).
Indexed: ABI Inform. (Jan.1991-), Account.Ind. (1974-), AgeLine, B.P.I. (Nov.1986-Sep.1991), Bus.Ind., CINAHL, Hosp.Lit.Ind., I.P.A., Int.Nurs.Ind., L.R.I., Rehabil.Lit., Tr.& Indus.Ind.
—BLDSC (6187.060000), GNLM, Infotrieve, ingenta. **CCC.**
Published by: Medquest Communications, LLC, 629 Euclid Ave, Ste 1200, Cleveland, OH 44114-3003. TEL 216-522-9700, FAX 216-522-9707. Ed. Richard L Peck. Pub. Mark Goodman III. Circ: 45,000.

610.73 GBR ISSN 1362-1017
NURSING IN CRITICAL CARE. Text in English. 1996. bi-m. GBP 40 domestic to individuals; GBP 50 in Europe to individuals; GBP 60 elsewhere to individuals; GBP 120 domestic to institutions; GBP 150 in Europe to institutions; GBP 180 elsewhere to institutions. adv. **Description:** Focuses on topics of particular interest to specialist nurses working in accident and emergency, coronary care, renal care, and adult, pediatric and neonatal intensive care.
Indexed: Brit.Nur.Ind., CINAHL, Int.Nurs.Ind.
—BLDSC (6187.042200).
Published by: (British Association of Critical Care Nurses), Greycoat Publishing, 1 Harley St, London W1N 1DA, United Kingdom. TEL 44-20-7637-1828. Eds. Julie Pearce, Kim Manley. R&P Guy Wallis. Adv. contact Ashley Wallis. B&W page GBP 780, color page GBP 1,155; trim 210 x 297. Circ: 2,400 (paid); 1,100 (controlled).

610.73 CAN ISSN 1492-2878
NURSING IN FOCUS. Text in English. 1961. 3/yr. CND 30 to non-members (effective 2000). adv. bk.rev. *Refereed.* **Document type:** *Journal, Trade.*
Former titles (until 2000): Nurse to Nurse (0849-3383); (until 1990): R N A N S Bulletin (0319-4604)
Indexed: CINAHL.
—BLDSC (6187.047700).
Published by: Registered Nurses Association of Nova Scotia, Ste 600, Barrington Tower, Scotia Square, 1849 Barrington St, Halifax, NS B3J 2A8, Canada. TEL 902-471-9744, FAX 902-471-9510, info@rnans.ns.ca, http://www.rnans.ns.ca. Ed. Marie Dauphinee Booth. Adv. contact Colleen Burke. Circ: 10,000.

610.73 GBR ISSN 1320-7881
NURSING INQUIRY. Text in English. 1994. q., latest vol.9, 2002. GBP 89 in Europe to individuals; USD 140 in North America to individuals; GBP 79 elsewhere to individuals; GBP 197 in Europe to institutions; USD 342 in North America to institutions; GBP 169 elsewhere to institutions (effective 2002). adv. bk.rev. illus. back issues avail. *Refereed.* **Document type:** *Academic/Scholarly.* **Description:** Discusses the practical, methodological, ethical, and philosophical issues in nursing from a variety of perspectives.
Related titles: Online - full text ed.: ISSN 1440-1800. GBP 81 in Europe to individuals; USD 126 in North America to individuals; GBP 81 elsewhere to individuals; GBP 178 in Europe to institutions; USD 308 in North America to institutions; GBP 178 elsewhere to institutions (effective 2002) (from EBSCO Publishing, O C L C Online Computer Library Center, Inc., RoweCom Information Quest, ingenta, Munksgaard & Blackwell Science's Synergy, Swets Blackwell).
Indexed: ASSIA, Brit.Nur.Ind., CINAHL, Fam.Ind., Int.Nurs.Ind., PsycInfo, e-psyche.
—BLDSC (6187.072000), Infotrieve. **CCC.**
Published by: (University of Melbourne, School of Postgraduate Nursing AUS), Blackwell Science Ltd., PO Box 88, Oxford OX2 0NE, United Kingdom. TEL 44-1865-206180, 44-1865-206002, FAX 44-1865-206219, jnl.orders@blacksci.co.uk, http://www.blackwell-science.com/~cgilib/jnlpage.asp?Journal=xninq&File=xninq, http://www.blackwellpublishing.com. Eds. Judith Parker, Nelson Sioban. Pub. Elaine Stott. R&P Sophie Savage. Adv. contact Jenny Applin. Circ: 195.

610.73 LKA
NURSING JOURNAL. Text in English. a.
Indexed: CINAHL.
Published by: Sri Lanka Nurses Association, Post Basic School of Nursing, Regent St., Colombo 10, Sri Lanka.

610.73 IND ISSN 0029-6503
RT13
NURSING JOURNAL OF INDIA. Text in English, Hindi. 1910. m. INR 250, USD 50 (effective 1999). adv. bk.rev. charts, illus. index. reprint service avail. from PQC. *Refereed.* **Document type:** *Academic/Scholarly.* **Description:** For members of the Trained Nurses' Association of India. Keeps them informed of the latest developments in the field of Nursing and allied subjects.
Related titles: Microfilm ed.: (from PQC).
Indexed: CINAHL, Int.Nurs.Ind.
—BLDSC (6187.080000), GNLM.
Published by: Trained Nurses Association of India, L-17 Green Park, New Delhi 110 016, India. TEL 91-11-6566665, FAX 91-11-6858306. Ed. Jaiwanti P Dhaulta. Circ: 60,000.

610.73 344.01 USA
NURSING LAW'S REGAN REPORT. Text in English. 1960. m. USD 52 domestic; USD 64 foreign (effective 2000). stat. reprints avail. **Description:** Reports the latest appellate court decisions on nursing law in a case and comment format.
Formerly: Regan Report on Nursing Law (0034-3196)
Related titles: Microform ed.: (from PQC); Online - full text ed.: (from Northern Light Technology, Inc., Gale Group).
Indexed: CINAHL, Int.Nurs.Ind.
—BLDSC (6187.091200), GNLM. **CCC.**
Published by: Medica Press Inc., 10 Dorrance St, Ste 500, Providence, RI 02903-2018. TEL 401-521-9226. Ed., R&P, Adv. contact A David Tammelleo. Circ: 10,000.

610.73 USA ISSN 1076-1632
CODEN: NLFOFM
NURSING LEADERSHIP FORUM. Text in English. 1995. 4/school-academic yr., latest vol.5, no.3, 2001, Spring. USD 52 domestic to individuals; USD 61 foreign to individuals; USD 112 domestic to institutions; USD 128 foreign to institutions (effective 2001). bk.rev., software rev., video rev., Website rev. abstr, bibl, charts, illus. 40 p./no. back issues avail.; reprints avail. *Refereed.* **Document type:** *Journal, Academic/Scholarly, Abstract/Index, Bibliography.* **Description:** Aimed at nurses in management positions in practice, education, research, administration, or politics.
Indexed: CINAHL, Int.Nurs.Ind., Lang.& Lang.Behav.Abstr., SOPODA, Sociol.Abstr.
—BLDSC (6187.091550), Infotrieve. **CCC.**
Published by: Springer Publishing Company, 536 Broadway, New York, NY 10012. TEL 212-431-4370, FAX 212-941-7842, springer@springerpub.com, http://www.springerjournals.com/nlf/home.htm, http://www.springerpub.com. Ed. Harriet R Feldman. Pub. Ursula Springer. R&P Dorothy Kouwenberg. Circ: 350 (paid).

610.73 USA ISSN 0744-6314
RT89
NURSING MANAGEMENT. Text in English. 1970. m. USD 38 domestic to individuals; USD 45 per issue in Canada to individuals; AUD 80 in Australia to individuals; USD 58 elsewhere to individuals; USD 60 domestic to institutions; USD 70 in Canada to institutions; USD 85 elsewhere to institutions; USD 9 newsstand/cover (effective 2001). adv. bk.rev. illus. index. back issues avail.; reprint service avail. from PQC. *Refereed.* **Description:** Addresses aspects of nursing management and related medical, legal, economic, personnel and ethical issues. Emphasizes new skills requiredin today's health care arena.
Formerly (until 1981): Supervisor Nurse (0039-5870)
Related titles: Microform ed.: (from PQC); Online - full text ed.: (from Northern Light Technology, Inc., ProQuest Information & Learning, Gale Group, Factiva).
Indexed: ABI Inform. (Dec.1987-), AMED, AgeLine, Brit.Nur.Ind., CINAHL, Hosp.Lit.Ind., Int.Nurs.Ind., Nurs.Abstr.
—BLDSC (6187.094000), CISTI, GNLM, ingenta, KNAW. **CCC.**

M

Published by: Springhouse Corporation (Subsidiary of: Lippincott Williams & Wilkins (Philadelphia)), 1111 Bethlehem Tpk, Springhouse, PA 19477. TEL 215-646-8700, FAX 215-646-4399, http://www.springnet.com/nm/nurseman.htm. Ed. Theresa M Steltzer. Circ: 98,789 (controlled). **Subscr. to:** Nursing Management, 434 W Downer Pl, Aurora, IL 60506. TEL 800-950-0879, FAX 708-892-7466.

610.73 GBR ISSN 1354-5760
NURSING MANAGEMENT. Text in English. 1979. 10/yr. GBP 80 in Europe to institutions; GBP 102.65 elsewhere to institutions (effective 2002). *Refereed.* **Document type:** *Trade.* **Description:** For senior clinical nurses and administrative nurse managers.
Former titles (until 1994): Senior Nurse (0265-9999); (until 1984): Nursing Focus (0144-4069)
Related titles: CD-ROM ed.: (from Ovid Technologies, Inc.); Microform ed.: (from PQC); Online - full text ed.: (from Ovid Technologies, Inc., Northern Light Technology, Inc., ProQuest Information & Learning).
Indexed: ASSIA, Brit.Nur.Ind., CINAHL, Curr.Cont. (coverage dropped).
—BLDSC (6187.093500), GNLM.
Published by: (Royal College of Nursing), R C N Publishing Co. (Subsidiary of: B M J Publishing Group), R C N Direct, Copse Walk, Cardiff Gate Business Park, Cardiff CF23 8XG, United Kingdom. TEL 44-29-2054-6450, FAX 44-29-2054-6401, directjournalsteam@rcn.org.uk, http://www.rcn.org.uk/. Ed. Tom Keighley. Circ: 2,300.

610.73 USA ISSN 0029-6538
NURSING NEWS (CONCORD). Text in English. 1949. q. Free to qualified subscribers. adv. 28 p./no. back issues avail. **Document type:** *Newsletter, Trade.* **Description:** Covers issues and employment opportunities of interest to licensed nursing professionals.
Indexed: CINAHL, Int.Nurs.Ind.
—BLDSC (6187.104000).
Published by: (New Hampshire Nurses' Association), Arthur L. Davis Publishing Agency, Inc., 517 Washington St, P O Box 216, Cedar Falls, IA 50613. TEL 319-277-2414, 800-626-4081, FAX 319-277-4055, sales@aldpub.com, http://nhnurses.myassociation.com/home.jsp, http://www.aldpub.com/. Ed. Mark Miller. R&P Robert Best. Adv. contact Jim Larson. Circ: 19,000 (free).

610.73 USA ISSN 0029-6546
NURSING NEWS (FLORAL PARK). Text in English. 1944. q. USD 25 to non-members (effective 2000). adv. bk.rev. illus. *Refereed.* **Document type:** *Newsletter, Trade.* **Description:** Provides updates on current affairs in the nursing profession and healthcare in general. Aims for the education and motivation of people in the nursing profession.
Published by: Nurses Association of the Counties of Long Island, 99 Tulip Ave, 404, Floral Park, NY 11001-1959. TEL 516-352-0717, FAX 516-352-4993, nacli@worldnet.att.net. Ed., Adv. contact Anne J Quashen. Circ: 3,500.

610.73 USA
NURSING OPPORTUNITIES. Text in English. 1970. a. USD 9.95 domestic; USD 15 foreign (effective 2000). adv. bk.rev. **Document type:** *Trade.* **Description:** Features comprehensive profiles of hundreds of hospitals emphasizing specific employment opportunities for nurses, and related information.
Related titles: Microform ed.: (from PQC); ♦ Supplement to: R N. ISSN 0033-7021.
Published by: (R N Magazine), Medical Economics Co., Inc., 5 Paragon Dr, Montvale, NJ 07645-1742. Circ: 130,000.

610.73 USA ISSN 0029-6554
RT1
NURSING OUTLOOK. Text in English. 1953. bi-m. USD 49 domestic to individuals; USD 73 foreign to individuals; USD 91 domestic to institutions; USD 115 foreign to institutions; USD 30 domestic to students; USD 54 foreign to students; USD 20 newsstand/cover (effective 2001). adv. bk.rev. charts, illus, tr.lit. index. reprint service avail. from PQC. *Refereed.* **Document type:** *Journal, Academic/Scholarly.*
Related titles: Microform ed.: (from PQC); Online - full text ed.: (from EBSCO Publishing, IDEAL Online Library, Institute for Scientific Information, RoweCom Information Quest).
Indexed: AIM, ASCA, ASSIA, Abstr.Health Care Manage.Stud., AgeLine, Brit.Nur.Ind., C.I.J.E., CINAHL, C.I.S. Abstr., Curr.Cont., Curr.Lit.Fam.Plan., Except.Child Educ.Abstr., I.P.A., Ind.Med. (1953-), Int.Nurs.Ind., Med.Care Rev., Nurs.Abstr., Psychol.Abstr., Rehabil.Lit., SSCI, Soc.Sci.Ind. (coverage dropped), Soc.Work Res.& Abstr.
—BLDSC (6187.108000), CISTI, GNLM, IDS, ingenta, KNAW, Linda Hall. **CCC.**
Published by: (American Academy of Nursing), Mosby, Inc. (Subsidiary of: Elsevier Science), 11830 Westline Industrial Dr, St Louis, MO 63146-3318. TEL 314-872-8370, 800-325-4177, FAX 314-432-1380, http://www.mosby.com/nursoutlook, http://www.mosby.com/periodicals. Ed. Carole A Anderson. Pub. Todd Hummel. Adv. contact Gina Burkert TEL 314-453-4306. B&W page USD 1,180, color page USD 2,280; trim 10.88 x 8.13. Circ: 5,852. **Subscr. to:** Journal Subscription Service, 11830 Westline Industrial Dr., St. Louis, MO 63146. TEL 800-325-4177.

610.73 100 GBR ISSN 1466-7681
▼ **NURSING PHILOSOPHY**; an international journal for healthcare professionals. Text in English. 2000. 2/yr., latest vol.3, 2002. GBP 45 in Europe to individuals; USD 72 in North America to individuals; GBP 49.50 elsewhere to individuals; GBP 146 in Europe to institutions; USD 232 in North America to institutions; GBP 161 elsewhere to institutions (effective 2002). adv. **Document type:** *Journal.* **Description:** Provides a forum for discussion of philosophical issues in nursing.
Related titles: Online - full text ed.: Nursing Philosophy Online. ISSN 1466-769X. 2000. GBP 41 in Europe to individuals; USD 65 in North America to individuals; GBP 41 elsewhere to individuals; GBP 132 in Europe to institutions; USD 209 in North America to institutions; GBP 132 elsewhere to institutions (effective 2002) (from EBSCO Publishing, ingenta, Munksgaard & Blackwell Science's Synergy, Swets Blackwell, RoweCom Information Quest).
Indexed: Brit.Nur.Ind.
—BLDSC (6187.109020).
Published by: Blackwell Science Ltd., PO Box 88, Oxford OX2 0NE, United Kingdom. TEL 44-1865-206180, 44-1865-206002, FAX 44-1865-206219, jnl.orders@blacksci.co.uk, http://www.blackwell-science.com/nup, http://www.blackwellpublishing.com. Eds. J Liaschenko, S Edwards. Pub. Elaine Stott. R&P Sophie Savage. Adv. contact Jenny Applin. B&W page GBP 400, color page GBP 1,000. Circ: 500.

610.73 NZL ISSN 0112-7438
NURSING PRAXIS IN NEW ZEALAND. Text in English. 1985. 3/yr. NZD 90. bk.rev. back issues avail. *Refereed.* **Document type:** *Academic/Scholarly.* **Description:** Presents articles of interest to the international nursing community. Focuses on publishing New Zealand nurses writing about issues relevant to New Zealand nursing.
Indexed: CINAHL, Ind.N.Z.Per., Int.Nurs.Ind.
—BLDSC (6187.109210), GNLM.
Published by: Nursing Praxis in N.Z., P.O. Box 1984, Palmerston North, New Zealand. TEL 6-3555002, FAX 6-35550003. Ed. Tina Smith. Circ: 750.

610.73 378 USA
NURSING PROGRESS. Text in English. 1988. 3/yr. adv. back issues avail.
Published by: Oregon Health Sciences University, School of Nursing Alumni Association, 1121 S W Salmon St, Ste 200, Portland, OR 97205. TEL 503-228-8337, FAX 503-228-9588, schwartt@ohsu.edu. Ed., Adv. contact Todd Schwartz. page USD 650; trim 11 x 8.5. Circ: 8,000.

610.73 USA ISSN 0029-6562
RT1 CODEN: NURNA
NURSING RESEARCH. Text in English. 1952. bi-m., latest vol.50. USD 67 domestic to individuals; USD 97 foreign to individuals; USD 167 domestic to institutions; USD 197 foreign to institutions; USD 33 (effective 2002). adv. bk.rev. abstr, charts, stat. index. cum.index: 1952-1963. reprint service avail. from PQC. *Refereed.*
Related titles: CD-ROM ed.: (from Ovid Technologies, Inc.); Microform ed.: (from PQC); Online - full text ed.: (from Ovid Technologies, Inc., Institute for Scientific Information).
Indexed: AIM, AMED, ASCA, ASSIA, Abstr.Health Care Manage.Stud., AgeLine, Behav.Med.Abstr., Brit.Nur.Ind., CINAHL, Child Devel.Abstr., Curr.Cont., Curr.Ind.Stat., Dent.Ind., ERA, Excerp.Med., Fam.Ind., Hosp.Lit.Ind., IMFL, INIS Atomind., I.P.A., Ind.Med. (1952-), Ind.Sci.Rev., Int.Nurs.Ind., MEDSOC, Med.Care Rev., Ment.Retard.Abstr., Mid.East: Abstr.& Ind., Mult.Ed.Abstr., Nurs.Abstr., PsycInfo, Psychol.Abstr. (1952-), Risk Abstr., SSCI, Sci.Cit.Ind. (coverage dropped), Soc.Work Res.& Abstr., Sp.Ed.Needs Abstr., Stud.Wom.Abstr., e-psyche.
—BLDSC (6187.110000), CISTI, GNLM, ingenta, KNAW, Linda Hall.
Published by: Lippincott Williams & Wilkins (Philadelphia) (Subsidiary of: Wolters Kluwer N.V.), 530 Walnut St, Philadelphia, PA 19106-3621. TEL 301-223-2300, 800-638-3030, FAX 301-223-2400, http://www.lww.com. Ed. Molly C Dougherty. Circ: 13,000.

610.73 AUS
NURSING REVIEW. Text in English. m. AUD 36 to non-members; AUD 40 to institutions. adv. **Document type:** *Newspaper.* **Description:** Deals with practice, research, education, policy and more.
Indexed: Brit.Nur.Ind., CINAHL.
Published by: (Royal College of Nursing, Australia), A P N Educational Media Pty. Ltd., ERCNA, PO Box 6097, North Sydney, NSW 2060, Australia. TEL 61-2-9936-8666, FAX 61-2-9954-0565. Ed., R&P, Adv. contact Joanne Ramadge TEL 61-2-6283-3404. **Co-sponsor:** Australian Provincial Newspapers.

610.73 USA ISSN 0894-3184
NURSING SCIENCE QUARTERLY; theory, research and practice. Text in English. 1988. q. USD 75 to individuals; USD 195 to institutions; USD 25 newsstand/cover to individuals; USD 50 newsstand/cover to institutions (effective 2002). adv. bk.rev. abstr, bibl, charts, illus, stat. index. back issues avail. *Refereed.* **Document type:** *Academic/Scholarly.* **Description:** Covers key aspects of nursing science, such as theoretical dilemmas, research issues, and practice applications.
Related titles: Microfilm ed.: (from WWS); Online - full text ed.: (from EBSCO Publishing, O C L C Online Computer Library Center, Inc., RoweCom Information Quest, ProQuest Information & Learning, ingenta, Swets Blackwell, Institute for Scientific Information).
Indexed: ASCA, AgeLine, CINAHL, Curr.Cont., Fam.Ind., Human Resour.Abstr., Int.Nurs.Ind., Nurs.Abstr., SSCI.
—BLDSC (6187.116340), CISTI, GNLM, ingenta.
Published by: Sage Publications, Inc., 2455 Teller Rd, Thousand Oaks, CA 91320. TEL 805-499-0721, FAX 805-499-0871, info@sagepub.com, http://www.sagepub.com. Ed. Rosemarie Rizzo Parse. Pub. Sara Miller McCune. R&P Tanya Udin. Adv. contact DeAnna Vega Hammersley.

610.73 USA
NURSING SPECTRUM - FLORIDA EDITION. Text in English. 1991. bi-w. adv. **Document type:** *Trade.* **Description:** Designed for people interested in registered nursing as a career.
Related titles: Online - full text ed.
Indexed: CINAHL.
Published by: Nursing Spectrum, Inc., 1001 W Cypress Creed Rd, Ste 300, Fort Lauderdale, FL 33309. TEL 954-776-1455, FAX 954-776-1456, pclass@nursingspectrum.com, http://www.nursingspectrum.com. Ed. Phyllis Class. Pub. Patti Roger. Circ: 53,928.

610.73 USA
NURSING SPECTRUM - GREATER PHILADELPHIA - TRI-STATE EDITION. Text in English. 1992. bi-w. **Document type:** *Trade.*
Published by: Nursing Spectrum, Inc., 2002 Renaissance Blvd, Ste 250, King of Prussia, PA 19406. TEL 610-292-8000, FAX 610-292-0179, rhess@nursingspectrum.com, http://www.nursingspectrum.com. Ed. Cheryl Barrett. Circ: 59,553.

610.73 USA
NURSING SPECTRUM - NEW ENGLAND EDITION. Text in English. 1997. bi-w. **Document type:** *Trade.*
Published by: Nursing Spectrum, Inc., 1050 Waltham St, Ste 510, Waltham, MA 02421. TEL 781-863-2300, FAX 781-863-6277, jborgatti@nursingspectrum.com, http://www.nursingspectrum.com. Ed. Joan Borgatti. Circ: 114,555.

610.73 USA
NURSING SPECTRUM - WASHINGTON DC - BALTIMORE EDITION. Text in English. 1990. bi-w. **Document type:** *Trade.*
Published by: Nursing Spectrum, Inc., 803 W Broad St, Ste 500, Falls Church, VA 22046. TEL 703-237-6515, FAX 703-237-6299, lesposito@nursingspectrum.com, http://www.nursingspectrum.com. Ed. Cynthia L Saver. Circ: 55,000.

610.73 GBR ISSN 0029-6570
CODEN: NSTAEU
NURSING STANDARD. Text in English. 1968. 50/yr. GBP 86.50 in Europe to institutions; GBP 173 elsewhere to institutions (effective 2002). adv. bk.rev. illus. reprint service avail. from IRC. **Document type:** *Academic/Scholarly.*
Incorporated: Lampada (0266-8769); Tradimus (0269-0977)
Related titles: CD-ROM ed.: (from Ovid Technologies, Inc.); Online - full text ed.: (from Ovid Technologies, Inc., Northern Light Technology, Inc.).
Indexed: AMED, Brit.Nur.Ind., CINAHL, Fam.Ind., INIS Atomind., Int.Nurs.Ind.

M

—BLDSC (6187.116700), CISTI, GNLM.
Published by: (Royal College of Nursing), R C N Publishing Co. (Subsidiary of: B M J Publishing Group), R C N Direct, Copse Walk, Cardiff Gate Business Park, Cardiff CF23 8XG, United Kingdom. TEL 44-29-2054-6450, FAX 44-29-2054-6401, nso@nursing-standard.co.uk, directjournalsteam@rcn.org.uk, http://www.nursing-standard.co.uk, http://www.rcn.org.uk/. Ed. Norah Casey. Adv. contact Phil Whomes. Circ: 70,000.

610.73 IND
NURSING TECHNOLOGY. Text in English. 1991. bi-m. INR 640, USD 45 (effective 2000). adv. abstr, bibl. index.
Published by: K.K. Roy (Private) Ltd., 55 Gariahat Rd., P O Box 10210, Kolkata, West Bengal 700 019, India. Ed. K K Roy. R&P M Misra TEL 91-33-475-4872. Circ: 2,240.

610.73 GBR ISSN 0954-7762
NURSING TIMES; the independent voice of nursing. Text in English. 1905. w. GBP 67 domestic; GBP 190 in Europe; GBP 1.10 newsstand/cover (effective 2000). adv. bk.rev. illus. index. reprint service avail. from PQC. **Document type:** *Trade.* **Description:** Aims to inform, inspire and entertain as it campaigns for a better deal for patients and for the nurses, midwives and health visitors who care for them.
Formerly (until 1987): Nursing Times, Nursing Mirror (0269-7289); Which was formed by the 1985 merger of: Nursing Times (0029-6589); Nursing Mirror (0029-6511); Which incorporates (in 1978): Nursing Mirror and Midwives Journal (0143-2524); Which was formerly: Queen's Nursing Journal (0301-0821); District Nursing (0012-4044)
Related titles: Microfilm ed.: (from BHP); Microform ed.: (from PQC); Online - full text ed.: (from Gale Group).
Indexed: AMED, ASSIA, Abstr.Health Care Manage.Stud., Addic.Abstr., AgeLine, Brit.Nur.Ind., CINAHL, C.I.S. Abstr., Curr.Adv.Ecol.Sci., Dent.Ind., Fam.Ind., Hosp.Abstr., Hosp.Lit.Ind., INIS Atomind., Ind.Med. (coverage dropped), Int.Nurs.Ind., Sp.Ed.Needs Abstr.
—BLDSC (6187.120000), CISTI, GNLM, ingenta, KNAW, Linda Hall. **CCC.**
Published by: Emap Healthcare Ltd. (Subsidiary of: Emap Business Communications Ltd.), Greater London House, Hampstead Rd, London NW1 7EJ, United Kingdom. TEL 44-20-7874-0200, FAX 44-20-7874-0201, nt@healthcare.emap.co.uk, http://www.emap.com. Ed. Tricia Reid. Pub. John Barnes. Adv. contact Heather Simmons. Circ: 63,500. **Subscr. to:** Emap Readerlink Ltd., Audit House, 260 Field End Rd, Ruislip, Mddx HA4 9LT, United Kingdom. TEL 44-181-956-3522, FAX 44-181-956-3175. **Dist. by:** Seymour, 86 Newman St, London W1P 3EX, United Kingdom. TEL 44-20-7396-8000, FAX 44-207-396-8002.

610.73 618.202 ZAF
NURSING UPDATE. Text in English. 1935. m. ZAR 300, USD 80 (effective 2001). adv. bk.rev. illus. 66 p./no. back issues avail. *Refereed.* **Document type:** *Magazine, Academic/Scholarly.* **Description:** Nursing magazine including news and educational articles.
Formerly: Nursing News (1018-9238); Supersedes in 1978: South African Nursing Journal (0038-2507)
Indexed: CINAHL.
—GNLM, KNAW.
Published by: Democratic Nursing Organisation of South Africa, PO Box 1280, Pretoria 0001, South Africa. TEL 27-12-3432315, FAX 27-12-3440750, denosahq@cis.co.za, info@denosa.org.za, http://www.denosa.org.za. Eds., R&Ps, Adv. contacts Bhungani ka Mzolo, Darryl Egnal. B&W page ZAR 3,864, color page ZAR 5,620; bleed 273 x 210. Circ: 92,000 (paid).

610.73 NLD ISSN 1381-5911
NURSING (YEAR). Text in Dutch. 1994. m. NLG 132.50. adv. illus. **Document type:** *Trade.* **Description:** Offers nurses in all areas of medical care practical professional and clinical advice.
Incorporates (in 1944-1996): Verpleegkundigen en Gemeenschapszorg
Published by: Elsevier Gezondheidszorg B.V., Tijdstroom (Subsidiary of: Reed Elsevier plc Group), Planetenbaan 1, Maarssen 3600 AK, Netherlands. TEL 31-346-577577, FAX 31-346-554287, http://www.tijdstroom.nl. Adv. contact Cor Vannek. Circ: 50,000. **Subscr. to:** Elsevier Den Haag, Postbus 16500, The Hague 2500 BM, Netherlands. TEL 31-70-381-9900, FAX 31-70-333-8399.

610.73 USA ISSN 0360-4039
RT1
NURSING (YEAR); the voice and vision of nursing. Text in English. 1971. m. USD 42 domestic to individuals; USD 47 in Canada to individuals; AUD 54 in Australia to individuals; USD 51 elsewhere to individuals; USD 66 domestic to institutions; USD 83 in Canada to institutions; USD 94 elsewhere to institutions; USD 5 newsstand/cover (effective 2001). adv. bibl, charts, illus. index. back issues avail.; reprints avail. *Refereed.* **Document type:** *Trade.* **Description:** Addresses the practical needs of nurses who are direct caregivers, focusing on clinical, legal, ethical, career and professional issues. Includes special sections for hospital, critical care and home health nurses.
Related titles: Diskette ed.; Magnetic Tape ed.; Microform ed.: (from PQC); Online - full text ed.: (from ProQuest Information & Learning, Gale Group, Factiva).
Indexed: AMED, AgeLine, CINAHL, Curr.Lit.Fam.Plan., Gen.Sci.Ind. (Jan.1999-Dec.1999), Hosp.Lit.Ind., INIS Atomind., I.P.A., Ind.Med. (coverage dropped), Int.Nurs.Ind., Nurs.Abstr., Tr.& Indus.Ind.
—BLDSC (6187.037500), CISTI, GNLM, ingenta, KNAW, Linda Hall. **CCC.**
Published by: Springhouse Corporation (Subsidiary of: Lippincott Williams & Wilkins (Philadelphia)), 1111 Bethlehem Tpk, Springhouse, PA 19477. TEL 215-646-8700, 800-346-7844, FAX 215-646-4399, http://www.springnet.com/pn/nurse98.htm. Ed. Jane Benner. Pub. Summer Mering. adv.: B&W page USD 15,590, color page USD 18,585. Circ: 300,424 (paid).

610.73 ITA
NURSING (YEAR). Text in Italian. q.
Published by: Systems Comunicazioni, Via Olanda, 6, Gaggiano, MI 20083, Italy. TEL 02-90811814, FAX 02-90841682. adv.: B&W page ITL 1,300,000, color page ITL 2,000,000; trim 240 x 180. Circ: 5,000.

610.73025 USA ISSN 0192-2394
RT82
NURSING (YEAR) CAREER DIRECTORY. Text in English. 1979. a. free per issue. adv. charts, illus, tr.lit. **Document type:** *Directory.* **Description:** Directed to Registered Nurses and nursing graduate students seeking employment in American hospitals.
—CCC.
Published by: Springhouse Corporation (Subsidiary of: Lippincott Williams & Wilkins (Philadelphia)), 1111 Bethlehem Tpk., Springhouse, PA 19477-0908. TEL 215-646-8700, 800-346-7844, FAX 215-646-4399. Circ: 100,000 (controlled).

610.73 USA ISSN 0273-320X
RM301.12
NURSING (YEAR) DRUG HANDBOOK. Text in English. a. USD 34.95 (effective 1998). **Document type:** *Trade.*
Published by: Springhouse Corporation (Subsidiary of: Lippincott Williams & Wilkins (Philadelphia)), 1111 Bethlehem Tpk., Springhouse, PA 19477-0908. TEL 215-646-8700, 800-346-7844, FAX 215-646-4508. Pub. Donna Carpenter.

610.73 ESP ISSN 0212-5382
NURSING (YEAR) (EDICION ESPANOLA). Text in Spanish. 1983. m. (10/yr..). USD 95. adv. reprint service avail. from PQC. **Document type:** *Academic/Scholarly.* **Description:** Covers nursing within and outside of the hospital environment. Serves the continuing education needs of nurses on a scientific and technical level.
Published by: Ediciones Doyma S.A., Traversa de Gracia, 17-21, Barcelona 08021, Spain. TEL 34-93-200-0711, FAX 34-93-209-1136. Ed. Margarita Peya. Adv. contact Julio Esteva. color page ESP 421,000; trim 273 x 200. Circ: 25,000.

610.73 USA
NURSING2000. Text in English. 1971. m. **Document type:** *Trade.*
Published by: Springhouse Corporation (Subsidiary of: Lippincott Williams & Wilkins (Philadelphia)), 1111 Bethlehem Tpk, Springhouse, PA 19477. TEL 215-646-8700, FAX 215-653-0826, nursing@springnet.com, http://www.springnet.com. Ed. Jane Benner. Circ: 300,000. **Subscr. to:** 30 Broad St, PO Box 3000, Denville, NJ 07834.

610.73 USA
NURSINGMATTERS: WISCONSIN EDITION; envisioning a future for nursing. Text in English. 1997 (vol.8, no.12). m. USD 15. adv. **Description:** Focuses on supporting and fostering the growth of professional nursing.
Indexed: CINAHL.
Published by: Madison Newspapers, Inc., PO Box 8056, Madison, WI 53708. TEL 414-637-6937. Ed. Margo O'Brien Hokanson. Adv. contact Cynthia T Wheeler.

O N S NEWS. see *MEDICAL SCIENCES—Oncology*

613.62 610.73 CAN ISSN 0828-542X
O O H N A JOURNAL. Text in English. 1980. 3/yr. CND 25 (effective 1999). adv. bk.rev. bibl, charts, illus, stat. *Refereed.* **Document type:** *Academic/Scholarly.*
Published by: Ontario Occupational Health Nurses Association, Ste 605, 302 The East Mall, Etobicoke, ON M9B 6C7, Canada. TEL 416-239-6462, FAX 416-239-5462, journal@oohna.on.ca. Ed., Adv. contact Frances MacCusworth. R&P Brian Verrall. Circ: 1,200 (paid).

O R L - HEAD AND NECK NURSING. see *MEDICAL SCIENCES—Otorhinolaryngology*

610.73 FRA ISSN 1163-4634
OBJECTIF SOINS* ; la revue professionnelle du nouveau science de soins infirmieres. Text in French. 1992. 10/yr. FRF 490 to individuals; FRF 590 to institutions; FRF 58 newsstand/cover. adv. **Document type:** *Trade.*
Published by: Editions Lamarre-Poinat, Initatives Sante, 26 av. de l'Europe, Velizy-Villacoublay 78140, France. Ed. Christian Moreau. Pub. Thierry Verret. Adv. contact Pascale Bernanose.

610.73 SVN ISSN 1318-2951
CODEN: OZNEF5
OBZORNIK ZDRAVSTVENE NEGE. Text in Slovenian; Summaries in English, Slovenian. 1966. q. SIT 300. adv. bk.rev. index. back issues avail. *Refereed.* **Document type:** *Academic/Scholarly.*
Formerly (until vol.27, 1993): Zdravstveni Obzornik (0350-9516)
Indexed: Vet.Bull.
Published by: Zveza Drustev Medicinskih Sester Slovenije/Nurses Association of Slovenia, Vidovdanska 9, Ljubljana 1000, Slovenia. TEL 386-1-2316055, zveza.med.sester@siol.net. Ed. Vera Grbec. Circ: 5,000.

610.73 GBR ISSN 0029-7917
OCCUPATIONAL HEALTH; a journal for the occupational health team. Text in English. 1949. m. GBP 75 domestic; GBP 93, USD 140 elsewhere (effective 2000). adv. bk.rev. illus. index. *Refereed.* **Document type:** *Academic/Scholarly.* **Description:** Provides expert advice on how to develop and implement workable health and safety policies for your organization.
Related titles: Microform ed.: (from PQC).
Indexed: ASSIA, Alloys Ind., Brit.Nur.Ind., CINAHL, C.I.S. Abstr., CSNB, Curr.Adv.Ecol.Sci., Excerp.Med., INIS Atomind., Int.Nurs.Ind., Lab.Haz.Bull., Met.Abstr., Met.Abstr.Ind., Nonfer.Met.Alert, PCC Alert, Steels Alert.
—BLDSC (6228.849000), CISTI, GNLM, Infotrieve, KNAW. **CCC.**
Published by: Reed Business Information (Subsidiary of: Reed Elsevier plc), Quadrant House, The Quadrant, Brighton Rd, Sutton, Surrey SM2 5AS, United Kingdom. TEL 44-20-8652-3946, FAX 44-208-652-8977, rbp.subscriptions@rbi.co.uk, http://www.reedbusiness.com. Ed. Catriona Marchant. Pub. Susan Downey. Adv. contact Peter Collis TEL 44-20-8652-4668. **Subscr. to:** Quadrant Subscription Services, PO Box 302, Haywards Heath, W Sussex RH16 3YY, United Kingdom. TEL 44-1444-445566, FAX 44-1444-445447.

610.73 AUT ISSN 0303-4461
OESTERREICHISCHE KRANKENPFLEGEZEITSCHRIFT. Text in German. 1948. 10/yr. ATS 480; ATS 560 foreign (effective 2000). adv. bk.rev. abstr, illus. **Document type:** *Newsletter.*
Indexed: Int.Nurs.Ind.
—CISTI, GNLM, KNAW.
Published by: Oesterreichischer Krankenpflegeverband, Mollgasse 3 a, Vienna, W 1180, Austria. TEL 43-1-4782710. Ed. Harald Verworner. Adv. contact Ernst Stempfel. B&W page ATS 18,700, color page ATS 32,700; trim 260 x 180. Circ: 12,500.

610.73 AUT
OESTERREICHISCHER KRANKENPFLEGEVERBAND. FORTBILDUNGSPROGRAMM. Text in German. 1969. a. free. adv. **Document type:** *Academic/Scholarly.*
Published by: Oesterreichischer Krankenpflegeverband, Mollgasse 3 a, Vienna, W 1180, Austria. TEL 43-1-4782710. Ed. Harald Verworwer. Adv. contact Ernst Stempfel. Circ: 15,000.

610.73 USA ISSN 0893-6595
OFFICE NURSE. Text in English. 1988. 10/yr. USD 25.97 domestic; USD 31.97 in Canada & Mexico; USD 37.97 elsewhere (effective 2000).
Related titles: Online - full text ed.: (from Gale Group).
Indexed: CINAHL.

—Infotrieve. **CCC.**
Published by: (American Association of Office Nurses), Medical Economics Co., Inc., 5 Paragon Dr, Montvale, NJ 07645-1742. customerservice@medec.com, http://www.medec.com. Ed. Marianne Dekker Mattera.

OFFICIEL DE LA SAGE-FEMME. see *MEDICAL SCIENCES—Obstetrics And Gynecology*

610.73 USA ISSN 0030-0993
OHIO NURSES REVIEW. Text in English. 1926. m. USD 30; USD 35 foreign (effective 1997). index. *Refereed.* **Document type:** *Trade.*
Indexed: CINAHL, Int.Nurs.Ind.
—BLDSC (6247.150000).
Published by: Ohio Nurses Association, 4000 E Main St, Columbus, OH 43213-2983. TEL 614-237-5414, FAX 614-237-6074. Ed. Carol A Jenkins. adv.: B&W page USD 580; 10 x 7. Circ: 10,000 (controlled).

OMVAARDAREN. see *SOCIAL SERVICES AND WELFARE*

610.736 616.992 NLD ISSN 1386-1263
ONCOLOGY NURSES TODAY. Text in English. 1996. q. illus. back issues avail. *Refereed.* **Document type:** *Newsletter, Academic/Scholarly, Trade.* **Description:** Provides a forum for cancer nurses throughout Europe to communicate with each other, exchange ideas, and provide information about the state of cancer nursing in various European countries.
Related titles: Danish ed.: Oncology Nurses i Dag. ISSN 1386-1344; Dutch ed.: Oncology Nurses Vandaag. ISSN 1386-1271; French ed.: Oncology Nurses Aujourd'hui. ISSN 1386-1298; Ed.: Oncology Nurses Heute. ISSN 1386-128X; Italian ed.: Oncology Nurses Oggi. ISSN 1386-131X; Portuguese ed.: Oncology Nurses Hoje. ISSN 1386-1328; Spanish ed.: Oncology Nurses Hoy. ISSN 1386-1301.
—BLDSC (6256.977500).
Published by: (European Oncology Nursing Society BEL), Excerpta Medica Medical Communications BV (Subsidiary of: Reed Elsevier plc), Rooseveltweg 15, Almere-Stad 1314 SJ, Netherlands. TEL 31-36-538-5600, FAX 31-36-538-5650, http://www.excerptamedica.com.

610.73 616.99 USA ISSN 0190-535X
ONCOLOGY NURSING FORUM. Text in English. 1974. 10/yr. USD 115 domestic; USD 130 foreign; USD 170 Print & online eds. (effective 2001). adv. bk.rev., video rev., Website rev. index. 170 p./no. 3 cols./p. back issues avail. *Refereed.* **Document type:** *Journal, Academic/Scholarly.* **Description:** Publishes articles related to developments in oncology nursing practice, technology, and research. Focuses on promoting a positive image of professional specialized nursing.
Related titles: Microfilm ed.: (from PQC); Online - full text ed.: USD 150 (effective 2001).
Indexed: AMED, Brit.Nur.Ind., CINAHL, Chic.Per.Ind., Fam.Ind., INIS Atomind., Ind.Med. (1977-), Int.Nurs.Ind., Nurs.Abstr.
—BLDSC (6256.980000), CISTI, GNLM, ingenta, KNAW.
Published by: Oncology Nursing Society, 501 Holiday Dr, Pittsburgh, PA 15220-2749. TEL 412-921-7373, FAX 412-921-6565, publishing@ons.org, http://www.ons.org; http://www.allenpress.com. Ed. Rose Mary Carroll Johnson Rn. Pub. Leonard Mafrica. R&P Jeanette M Kent TEL 412-921-7373 ext. 246. Adv. contact Jack Edelman TEL 856-256-2313. Circ: 28,169.

016.616 USA ISSN 1521-219X
ONLINE JOURNAL OF CLINICAL INNOVATIONS. Text in English. 1998. q. USD 40 to individuals; USD 100 to institutions. bk.rev. back issues avail. **Document type:** *Academic/Scholarly, Bibliography.*
Media: Online - full text.
Indexed: CINAHL.
Published by: Cinahl Information Systems, 1509 Wilson Terrace, Glendale, CA 91206. TEL 818-409-8005, 800-959-7167, FAX 818-546-5633, http://www.cinahl.com/jrnls/OJCI/clinical.htm. Eds. Dana Rutledge, Nancy E Donaldson.

610.73 USA ISSN 1091-3734
ONLINE JOURNAL OF ISSUES IN NURSING. Text in English. 1996. q. free. back issues avail. *Refereed.* **Document type:** *Academic/Scholarly.* **Description:** Provides a forum for discussion of pertinent issues in nursing. It provides different viewson topics that affect nursing research, education and practice. The interactive format encourages dialogue with raders, resulting i a comprehensive discussion of topics.
Media: Online - full text.
Indexed: CINAHL, Ind.Med.
Published by: (Kent State University), American Nurses Association, 600 Maryland Ave S W, Ste 100 W, Washington, DC 20024-2571. TEL 202-651-7000, 800-274-4262, FAX 202-651-7005, http://www.nursingworld.org/ojin/. Ed. Harrcet Coeling.

610.73 USA ISSN 1072-7639
ONLINE JOURNAL OF KNOWLEDGE SYNTHESIS FOR NURSING. Text in English. 1993. irreg. (updated approx. bi-w.). USD 60 to individuals; USD 250 to institutions (effective 2000). adv. abstr, bibl, charts, stat. back issues avail. *Refereed.* **Document type:** *Academic/Scholarly.* **Description:** Provides critical reviews of research literature of interest to clinical nurses, academicians and researchers.
Media: Online - full text (from EBSCO Publishing, Institute for Scientific Information).
Indexed: ASCA, CINAHL, Curr.Cont. (1994-), SSCI (1994-).
—IDS.
Published by: Sigma Theta Tau International Honor Society of Nursing, 550 W North St, Indianapolis, IN 46202. TEL 317-634-8171, FAX 317-634-8188. Ed. Dr. Kathleen Stevens. Pub. Nancy Dickenseon-Hazard. R&P Lorraine R Swedberg. Adv. contact Rachael McLaughlin.

610.73 GBR ISSN 1368-1249
OPHTHALMIC NURSING; international journal of ophthalmic nursing. Text in English. 1997. q. GBP 16 domestic to individuals; GBP 25 in the European Union to individuals; GBP 45 elsewhere to individuals; GBP 50 domestic to institutions; GBP 60 in the European Union to institutions; GBP 75 elsewhere to institutions (effective 2000). adv. back issues avail. *Refereed.* **Document type:** *Academic/Scholarly, Trade.* **Description:** Contains research papers, clinical articles, news features, letters page, noticeboard of events, and book review page.
Indexed: Brit.Nur.Ind.
—BLDSC (6271.080000).
Published by: T M & D Press Ltd., United House, 41 North Rd, London N7 9DP, United Kingdom. TEL 44-20-7700-3479, FAX 44-20-7700-2049, tmd.press@btinternet.com. Ed. Heather Waterman. Pub. Kevin Kibble. R&P Penny Stephens. Adv. contact Mike Brearley. B&W page GBP 795, color page GBP 1,020; trim 210 x 297. Circ: 3,500 (paid).

610.73 617 GBR ISSN 0961-1258
OPPORTUNITIES FOR THEATRE STAFF & OTHER SPECIALISTS. Text in English. 1980. fortn. adv. bk.rev. **Document type:** *Newsletter.*
Published by: Newton Mann Ltd., Stretton Rd, Tansley, Matlock, Derbys DE4 5GE, United Kingdom. TEL 44-1629-583941, FAX 44-1629-580479, admin@opps.co.uk, http://www.opps.co.uk. Ed. Mark Moore. Pub. Charles Mann. Adv. contact John Eaton TEL 0207-878-2317. Circ: 7,000 (controlled).

610.73 USA ISSN 0030-4751
RT1
OREGON NURSE. Text in English. 1932. 4/yr. USD 25; USD 35 foreign (effective 1999). adv. bk.rev. illus. *Refereed.* **Document type:** *Newsletter.* **Description:** Provides articles about nursing issues, health care trends, collective bargaining for nurses; legislative health care issues.
Related titles: Online - full text ed.
Indexed: CINAHL, Int.Nurs.Ind.
—BLDSC (6281.600000).
Published by: Oregon Nurses Association, 9600 S W Oak St, Ste 550, Portland, OR 97223-6599. TEL 503-293-0011, FAX 503-293-0013, ona@oregonrn.org, http://www.oregonrn.org. Ed., R&P Sandy Marron. Adv. contact Debra Feammelli. B&W page USD 735; trim 11 x 17. Circ: 6,000. **Subscr. to:** ONA, 9600 SW Oak St, Ste 550, Portland, OR 97223.

610.73 617.3 USA ISSN 0744-6020
ORTHOPAEDIC NURSING JOURNAL. Text in English. 1981. bi-m. USD 28 domestic to individuals; USD 43 foreign to individuals; USD 40 domestic to institutions; USD 55 foreign to institutions (effective 2000). adv. bk.rev. *Refereed.* **Document type:** *Academic/Scholarly.*
Related titles: Online - full text ed.: (from ProQuest Information & Learning, Gale Group).
Indexed: AgeLine, Brit.Nur.Ind., CINAHL, Nurs.Abstr.
—BLDSC (6296.125300), GNLM, ingenta. **CCC.**
Published by: (National Association of Orthopaedic Nurses), Jannetti Publications, Inc., East Holly Ave, Box 56, Pitman, NJ 08071-0056. TEL 856-256-2300, FAX 856-589-7463. Ed. Ann Maher. Circ: 10,000.

ORTHOSCOPE. see *MEDICAL SCIENCES—Orthopedics And Traumatology*

610.73068 USA ISSN 1535-2765
RT85.5
OUTCOMES MANAGEMENT. Text in English. 1998. q., latest vol.5. USD 57 domestic to individuals; USD 77 foreign to individuals; USD 117 domestic to institutions; USD 147 foreign to institutions (effective 2002). adv. illus. index. *Refereed.* **Document type:** *Journal, Academic/Scholarly, Trade.*
Formerly: Outcomes Management for Nursing Practice (1093-1783)
Related titles: CD-ROM ed.: (from Ovid Technologies, Inc.); Online - full text ed.: USD 152.10 domestic academic site license; USD 169.65 domestic corporate site license; USD 182.10 foreign academic site license; USD 199.65 foreign corporate site license (effective 2002) (from Ovid Technologies, Inc.).
Indexed: CINAHL, Int.Nurs.Ind.
—BLDSC (6314.409575), Infotrieve.
Published by: Lippincott Williams & Wilkins (Philadelphia) (Subsidiary of: Wolters Kluwer N.V.), 530 Walnut St, Philadelphia, PA 19106-3621. TEL 301-223-2300, 800-638-3030, FAX 301-223-2400, http://www.nursingcenter.com, http://www.lww.com. Ed. Marilyn H Oermann.

610.7362 GBR ISSN 0962-9513
PAEDIATRIC NURSING. Text in English. 1988. 10/yr. GBP 80 in Europe to institutions; GBP 96 elsewhere to institutions (effective 2002). adv. *Refereed.* **Document type:** *Trade.*
Indexed: Brit.Nur.Ind., CINAHL, Int.Nurs.Ind.
—BLDSC (6333.399760).
Published by: (Royal College of Nursing), R C N Publishing Co. (Subsidiary of: B M J Publishing Group), R C N Direct, Copse Walk, Cardiff Gate Business Park, Cardiff CF23 8XG, United Kingdom. TEL 44-29-2054-6450, FAX 44-29-2054-6401, directjournalsteam@rcn.org.uk, http://www.rcn.org.uk/. Ed. Anne Casey. Adv. contact Phil Whomes. Circ: 9,100.

▼ **PAIN MANAGEMENT NURSING.** see *MEDICAL SCIENCES—Anaesthesiology*

610.73 PAK ISSN 0078-8376
PAKISTAN NURSING AND HEALTH REVIEW. Text in English. 1951. q.
Indexed: Int.Nurs.Ind.
Published by: Pakistan Nurses Federation, c/o College of Nursing, Jinnah Postgraduate Medical Centre, Karachi, 35, Pakistan. Ed. Mushtaq Ahmad. Circ: 2,000.

PALLIATIVE CARE TODAY; the journal for today's palliative care team. see *MEDICAL SCIENCES—Oncology*

610.73 USA
PATIENT CARE FOR THE NURSE PRACTITIONER. Text in English. m. USD 55; USD 10 newsstand/cover (effective 2001).
Media: Online - full content.
—BLDSC (6412.862500).
Published by: Medical Economics Company, Five Paragon Dr, Montvale, NJ 07645-1742. TEL 201-358-7200, http://www.patientcarenp.com/.

610.73 USA
PATIENT CARE MANAGEMENT. Text in English. 1985. m. USD 245 to individuals; USD 25 newsstand/cover (effective 2002). **Document type:** *Newsletter.* **Description:** Covers strategies; financial techniques; new ventures; human resources; and legislative, legal, and labor issues, all presented from the perspective of the nurse executive.
Former titles: Aspen's Nurse Executive Network; (until 1993): Aspen's Advisor for Nurse Executives (0883-9743)
Related titles: Online - full text ed.: (from ProQuest Information & Learning).
Indexed: CINAHL, Int.Nurs.Ind.
—BLDSC (1745.932000), GNLM, Infotrieve. **CCC.**
Published by: Aspen Publishers, Inc., 200 Orchard Ridge Dr, Ste 200, Gaithersburg, MD 20878. TEL 301-417-7500, 800-638-8437, FAX 301-695-7931, customer.service@aspenpubl.com, http://www.aspenpub.com. **Dist. by:** Aspen Publishers Inc., Distribution Center, 7201 McKinney Circle, Frederick, MD 21701. TEL 301-698-7100, FAX 301-417-7550.

616.8 USA
PATIENT CARE STAFFING REPORT. Text in English. m. USD 128 for 6 mos. (effective 2001). **Document type:** *Trade.* **Description:** Covers in-depth case studies, news, analysis, practical tools and tips.
Related titles: Online - full content ed.

Published by: C O R Health, LLC, PO Box 50507, Santa Barbara, CA 93150. TEL 805-564-2177, FAX 805-564-2146, info@corhealth.com, http://www.corhealth.com. Ed. Marilyn Lang. Pub. Dean H. Anderson.

610.73 AUS ISSN 1031-3443
PATRICIA CHOMLEY ORATIONS; nursing and human service. Text in English. a. AUD 5 to non-members; AUD 4.50 to members. back issues avail. **Document type:** *Trade.* **Description:** Publishes historical speeches on nursing.
Published by: Royal College of Nursing Australia, 1 Napier Close, Deakin, ACT 2600, Australia. TEL 61-2-6282-5633, FAX 61-2-6282-3565. R&P, Adv. contact Lisa Howdin.

610.73 USA ISSN 0886-9006
PEDIATRIC NURSE PRACTITIONER. Text in English. bi-m. **Document type:** *Newsletter.*
Published by: National Association of Pediatric Nurse Associates and Practitioners, 1101 Kings Hwy N, 206, Cherry Hill, NJ 08034. TEL 609-667-1773, FAX 609-667-7187. Ed. Timothy W Gordon. R&P Joe Casey. Circ: 4,000.

610.73 USA ISSN 0097-9805
RJ245 CODEN: PENUEI
PEDIATRIC NURSING. Text in English. 1975. bi-m. USD 30 domestic to individuals; USD 45 foreign to individuals; USD 42 domestic to institutions; USD 57 foreign to institutions (effective 2000). adv. bk.rev. illus. back issues avail.; reprint service avail. from PQC. *Refereed.* **Document type:** *Academic/Scholarly.*
Related titles: Microfilm ed.: (from PQC); Online - full text ed.: (from Northern Light Technology, Inc., ProQuest Information & Learning, Gale Group).
Indexed: CINAHL, Dent.Ind., Fam.Ind., INIS Atomind., Int.Nurs.Ind., Nurs.Abstr.
—BLDSC (6417.605300), CISTI, GNLM, ingenta, KNAW. **CCC.**
Published by: Jannetti Publications, Inc., East Holly Ave, Box 56, Pitman, NJ 08071-0056. TEL 856-256-2300, FAX 856-589-7463, PNJRNL@ajj.com, http://www.cinahl.com/jrnls/PEDN/pedn.htm. Ed. Veronica Feeg. Circ: 12,000.

610.73 USA ISSN 0031-4617
THE PENNSYLVANIA NURSE. Text in English. 1946. 6/yr., latest vol.56. USD 15. adv. bk.rev. illus. back issues avail. *Refereed.* **Document type:** *Magazine.* **Description:** Keeps Pennsylvania nurses informed of events affecting nursing, with timely reporting of professional, practice, economic, legislative, legal, ethical and education issues.
Indexed: CINAHL, Int.Nurs.Ind.
—BLDSC (6421.747000), GNLM.
Published by: Pennsylvania State Nurses Association, Editorial Board, PO Box 68525, Harrisburg, PA 17106-8525. TEL 717-657-1222, FAX 717-657-3796, communications@psna.org, http://www.psna.org. Ed. Lori Anne Artz. adv.: B&W page USD 449; trim 15 x 11.5. Circ: 3,000.

610.73 617 USA ISSN 1089-9480
PERIANESTHESIA AND AMBULATORY SURGERY NURSING UPDATE. Text in English. 1993. bi-m. USD 81 domestic to individuals; USD 147 foreign to individuals; USD 142 domestic to institutions; USD 168 foreign to institutions; USD 81 domestic to students; USD 147 foreign to students; USD 29 newsstand/cover (effective 2001). **Document type:** *Newsletter, Abstract/Index.* **Description:** Informs post-anesthesia nurses, nurse anesthetists, and nurses in ambulatory surgery about developments in their field. Also summarizes current literature.
Formerly (until 1992): Post Anesthesia and Ambulatory Surgery Nursing Update (1066-8977)
—Infotrieve. **CCC.**
Published by: (American Society of PeriAnesthesia Nurses), W.B. Saunders Co. (Subsidiary of: Harcourt Publishers Ltd.), 11830 Westline Industrial Dr, St Louis, MO 63146. TEL 800-325-4177, http://www.wbsaunders.com. Ed. Nancy Burden. **Subscr. to:** Periodicals Fulfillment, W B Saunders Co, 6277 Sea Harbor Dr, 4th Fl, Orlando, FL 32891-4800.

610.73 617 USA
PERIOPERATIVE SERVICES MANAGEMENT RESOURCE. Text in English. 1997. a. USD 269; USD 229 foreign (effective 1999). **Document type:** *Trade.*
Published by: American Health Consultants (Subsidiary of: Medical Economics Co., Inc.), 3525 Piedmont Rd, N E, 6 Piedmont Center, Ste 400, Atlanta, GA 30305. TEL 404-262-5476, custserv@ahcpub.com, http://www.ahcpub.com.

610.73 USA ISSN 0894-1076
RT3
PERSPECTIVES IN NURSING*. Text in English. 1985. triennial. **Document type:** *Monographic series.*
Published by: National League for Nursing, 61 Broadway, New York, NY 10006-2701. TEL 800-669-1656.

610.736 USA ISSN 0031-5990
RC475 CODEN: PEPYA
PERSPECTIVES IN PSYCHIATRIC CARE. Text in English. 1963. q. USD 54 domestic to individuals; USD 68 elsewhere to individuals; USD 34 domestic to students; USD 65 domestic to institutions; USD 81 elsewhere to institutions; USD 21 newsstand/cover domestic; USD 24 newsstand/cover elsewhere (effective 2002). adv. bk.rev. index. back issues avail.; reprint service avail. from PQC,PSC,SCH. *Refereed.* **Document type:** *Academic/Scholarly.* **Description:** Focuses on research, clinical practice, trends and innovations in psychiatric and mental-health nursing.
Related titles: Microfilm ed.: (from PQC); Online - full text ed.: (from Northern Light Technology, Inc., ProQuest Information & Learning, Gale Group, Institute for Scientific Information).
Indexed: ASCA, AgeLine, CINAHL, Curr.Cont., Excerp.Med., Fam.Ind., Hosp.Lit.Ind., Ind.Med. (coverage dropped), Int.Nurs.Ind., Nurs.Abstr., PsycInfo, Psychol.Abstr. (1972-), SSCI, e-psyche.
—BLDSC (6428.160000), GNLM, IDS, ingenta, KNAW.
Published by: Nursecom, Inc., 1211 Locust St, Philadelphia, PA 19107. TEL 215-545-7222, 800-242-6757, FAX 215-545-8107, customer.service@nursecominc.com, http://www.nursecominc.com; http://www.cinahl.com/jrnls/PPCJ/ppcj.htm. Ed. Mary Paquette. Pub. Margo C Neal. R&P, Adv. contact Timothy Bower. B&W page USD 700, color page USD 1,100; trim 10.88 x 8.13. Circ: 2,580.

PERSPECTIVES (TORONTO). see *GERONTOLOGY AND GERIATRICS*

610.73025 USA ISSN 1073-7820
RT79
PETERSON'S GUIDE TO NURSING PROGRAMS. Variant title: Guide to Nursing Programs. Text in English. 1994. irreg. **Document type:** *Directory.*
Published by: (American Association of Colleges of Nursing), Peterson's Magazine Group, 202 Carnegie Center, PO Box 2123, Princeton, NJ 08543-2123. TEL 609-243-9111, FAX 609-243-9150.

610.73 CHE ISSN 1012-5302
PFLEGE; die wissenschaftliche Zeitschrift fuer Pflegeberufe. Text in German. 1988. bi-m. CHF 104 domestic; CHF 117 foreign (effective 2001). adv. 64 p./no. **Document type:** *Journal, Academic/Scholarly.*
Indexed: CINAHL, Int.Nurs.Ind.
—BLDSC (6440.710000), GNLM.
Published by: Hans Huber AG, Laengassstr 76, Bern, 9 3000, Switzerland. TEL 41-31-3004500, FAX 41-31-3004591, zeitschriften@hanshuber.com, http://www.hanshuber.com. Adv. contact Rene Waelchli. color page CHF 2,314; trim 167 x 263. Circ: 3,300.

610.73 DEU ISSN 0944-8918
PFLEGE AKTUELL. Text in German. 1946. m. DEM 75. adv. bk.rev. illus. index. **Document type:** *Trade.*
Formerly (until 1993): Krankenpflege (0002-1008)
Indexed: Dok.Arbeitsmed., Int.Nurs.Ind.
—BLDSC (6440.711000), CISTI, GNLM, KNAW.
Published by: Deutscher Berufsverband fuer Pflegeberufe, Hauptstr 392, Eschborn 65760, Germany. TEL 49-6173-63016, FAX 49-6173-640913. Ed. Eva Maria Krampe. Circ: 26,000.

610.73 DEU ISSN 1433-1985
DER PFLEGEBRIEF (EMAIL EDITION); das Online-Magazin fuer die Pflege. Text in German. 1995. m. back issues avail. **Document type:** *Trade.*
Media: E-mail. **Related titles:** Fax ed.: Der Pflegebrief (Fax Edition). ISSN 1433-1993; ♦ Online - full content ed.: Der Pflegebrief (Online Edition). ISSN 1433-2795.
Published by: Pflegebrief, Germany. bruehe@uke.uni-hamburg.de; pflegebrief@iname.com, http://www.pflegenet.com/. Ed. Roland Bruehe.

610.73 DEU ISSN 1433-2795
DER PFLEGEBRIEF (ONLINE EDITION); das Online-Magazin fuer die Pflege. Text in German. 1995. m. free per issue. abstr. illus. back issues avail. **Document type:** *Newsletter, Academic/Scholarly.* **Description:** Contains topics on nursing care.
Media: Online - full content. **Related titles:** ♦ E-mail ed.: Der Pflegebrief (Email Edition). ISSN 1433-1985; Fax ed.: Der Pflegebrief (Fax Edition). ISSN 1433-1993.
Published by: Pflegebrief, Geschwister-Scholl-Str 106, Hamburg 20251, Germany. TEL 49-410-5660421, FAX 49-410-5660423, bruehe@uke.uni-hamburg.de, http://www.pflegenet.com/ezine/. Ed., Pub., R&P Roland Bruehe. Circ: 1,300.

▼ **PFLEGEMAGAZIN**; Zeitschrift fuer den gesamten Pflegebereich. see *PUBLIC HEALTH AND SAFETY*

610.73 DEU ISSN 0945-1129
PFLEGEZEITSCHRIFT. Text in German. 1948. m. EUR 48, CHF 94; EUR 29.10, CHF 56.90 to students; EUR 8.20, CHF 16 newsstand/cover (effective 2002). bk.rev. **Document type:** *Journal, Academic/Scholarly.*
Former titles: Deutsche Krankenpflege-Zeitschrift (0012-074X); Deutsche Schwesternzeitung
Indexed: Dok.Arbeitsmed., Int.Nurs.Ind.
—BLDSC (6440.715000), CISTI, GNLM, Infotrieve. **CCC.**
Published by: W. Kohlhammer GmbH, Hessbruehlstr 69, Stuttgart 70565, Germany. TEL 49-711-7863-1, FAX 49-711-7863263, info@kohlhammer-katalog.de, http://www.kohlhammer.de. Circ: 20,000.

PHARMACY HEALTH-LINE. see *PHARMACY AND PHARMACOLOGY*

610.73 PHL ISSN 0048-3818
PHILIPPINE JOURNAL OF NURSING. Text in English. 1953. q. PHP 100 domestic; USD 35 foreign (effective 2001). adv. bk.rev. illus, abstr. 56 p./no. *Refereed.* **Document type:** *Academic/Scholarly.*
Formerly: Filipino Nurse
Indexed: CINAHL, Ind.Phil.Per., Int.Nurs.Ind.
—BLDSC (6455.629000), GNLM.
Published by: Philippine Nurses Association, 1663 F Tirena Benitez St, Malate, Manila 1004, Philippines. TEL 63-2-536-1888, FAX 63-2-525-1596, pna@the.net.ph. Eds. Shirley V Pena, Victoria L Vidal. Adv. contacts Lily Ann Baldago, Mrs. Rosie S de Leon. Circ: 13,000.

PHYSICIAN ASSISTANTS' PRESCRIBING REFERENCE. see *PHARMACY AND PHARMACOLOGY*

610.73 POL ISSN 0860-8466
PIELEGNIARSTWO POLSKIE. Text and summaries in English, Polish. 1989. irreg. price varies.
Published by: (Poland. Ministerstwo Zdrowia i Opieki Spolecznej/Ministry of Health and Social Welfare), Wydawnictwo Naukowe P W Nowe, Ul Miodowa 10, Warsaw 00251, Poland. TEL 48-22-6954321, FAX 48-22-6954288. Ed. Laura Wolowicka. **Dist. by:** Redakcja Pielegniarsto Polskie, c/o Akademia Medyczna, Wydzial Pielegniarski, ul Dabrowskiego 79, Poznan 60529, Poland.

610.73 617.95 USA ISSN 0741-5206
CODEN: PSNUEE
PLASTIC SURGICAL NURSING. Text in English. q. USD 30 domestic to individuals; USD 40 foreign to individuals; USD 40 domestic to institutions; USD 50 foreign to institutions (effective 2000). **Document type:** *Academic/Scholarly.*
Related titles: Online - full text ed.: (from Northern Light Technology, Inc., ProQuest Information & Learning, Gale Group).
Indexed: Brit.Nur.Ind., CINAHL, Int.Nurs.Ind., Nurs.Abstr.
—BLDSC (6528.938100), GNLM, Infotrieve. **CCC.**
Published by: (American Society of Plastic and Reconstructive Surgical Nurses), Jannetti Publications, Inc., East Holly Ave, Box 56, Pitman, NJ 08071-0056. TEL 856-256-2300, FAX 856-689-7463, ASPRSN@ajj.com.

610.73 USA ISSN 1527-1544
POLICY, POLITICS & NURSING PRACTICE. Text in English. q. USD 60 to individuals; USD 250 to institutions; USD 25 newsstand/cover to individuals; USD 70 newsstand/cover to institutions (effective 2002). back issues avail. *Refereed.* **Description:** Serves as a forum for examining policies, political activities and health services research that affect nursing practice across all venues of care delivery. Topics including legislation affecting nursing practice and health care, case studies involving policy and political action, interviews with government and other policy makers and health professionals, international health policy issues, related conferences and media reviews.
Related titles: Online - full text ed.: (from EBSCO Publishing, O C L C Online Computer Library Center, Inc., RoweCom Information Quest, ingenta, Swets Blackwell).
—BLDSC (6543.327388).
Published by: Sage Publications, Inc., 2455 Teller Rd, Thousand Oaks, CA 91320. TEL 805-499-9821, FAX 805-499-0721, http://www.sagepub.com. Ed. Carole Pe Jennings.

610.7365 USA ISSN 1090-3909
POST ACUTE CARE STRATEGY REPORT; the newsletter for integrating post acute services. Text in English. 1996. m. USD 297 (effective 2000). charts, stat. back issues avail. *Refereed.* **Document type:** *Newsletter.* **Description:** Provides strategic advice and case studies to hospital and nursing home administrators, nursing staff and company recruiters on how to integrate post acute services such as rehab, home health, skilled nursing into a network. Contains regulatory and medical reimbursement news.
Published by: Harling Communications, Inc., 18 2 E Dundee Rd, Ste 200, Barrington, IL 60010. TEL 847-304-1011, 800-894-8786, FAX 847-304-1035, postacute@aol.com. Eds. Harriet Gill, Matthew Hay. Pub., R&P Mark Harling TEL 516-379-7097.

610.73 GBR ISSN 0953-6612
PRACTICE NURSE. Text in English. 1988. fortn. GBP 51 domestic; GBP 92, USD 138 elsewhere (effective 2000). adv. index. **Document type:** *Trade.* **Description:** Covers news, clinical features, self-assessment tests and research.
Indexed: Brit.Nur.Ind., CINAHL.
—BLDSC (6597.170000), Infotrieve. **CCC.**
Published by: Reed Business Information (Subsidiary of: Reed Elsevier plc), Quadrant House, The Quadrant, Brighton Rd, Sutton, Surrey SM2 5AS, United Kingdom. TEL 44-208-652-3500, FAX 44-208-652-8977, rbp.subscriptions@rbi.co.uk, http://www.reedbusiness.com. Ed. Carolyn Scott. Circ: 6,500. **Subscr. to:** Quadrant Subscription Services, PO Box 302, Haywards Heath, W Sussex RH16 3YY, United Kingdom. TEL 44-1444-445566, FAX 44-1444-445447.

610.73 GBR ISSN 0964-9271
PRACTICE NURSING. Text in English. 1990. fortn. GBP 44; GBP 90 foreign. **Document type:** *Academic/Scholarly.*
Indexed: Brit.Nur.Ind.
—BLDSC (6597.175000).
Published by: Mark Allen Publishing Ltd., Croxted Mews, 286-288a Croxted Rd, London SE24 9BY, United Kingdom. TEL 44-208-671-7521, FAX 44-208-671-1722. Ed. Elizabeth Gledhill. Pub. Mark Allen.

PRACTISING MIDWIFE; the voice of clinical midwifery. see *MEDICAL SCIENCES—Obstetrics And Gynecology*

610.73 USA ISSN 0032-6666
PRAIRIE ROSE. Text in English. 1931. q. USD 10 (effective 2001). adv. bk.rev. 32 p./no. back issues avail. **Document type:** *Newsletter, Trade.* **Description:** Covers issues and employment opportunities of interest to licensed nursing professionals.
Indexed: CINAHL, Int.Nurs.Ind.
Published by: (North Dakota Nurses Association), Arthur L. Davis Publishing Agency, Inc., 517 Washington St, P O Box 216, Cedar Falls, IA 50613. TEL 319-277-2414, 800-626-4081, FAX 319-277-4055, sales@aldpub.com, http://www.aldpub.com/. Ed., R&P Mark Miller. Adv. contact Jim Larson. Circ: 12,000.

PRAXIS NAH. see *MEDICAL SCIENCES—Surgery*

610.73 CAN ISSN 1197-2297
PRE & POST NATAL NEWS. Text in English. 1987. 3/yr. adv. **Document type:** *Newsletter.* **Description:** Covers the latest medical and social research affecting pregnancy, birth and infant care.
Formerly: Canadian Childbirth Educator (0835-586X)
Published by: (Today's Parent Group), Professional Publishing Associates, 269 Richmond St W, Toronto, ON M5V 1X1, Canada. TEL 416-596-8680, FAX 416-596-1991. Ed. Jennifer Elliott. Circ: 7,000 (controlled).

610.73 AUT ISSN 0949-7323
PROCARE; das Fortbildungsmagazin fuer Pflegeberufe. Text in German. 1996. m. EUR 81 domestic; EUR 75.40 in Germany; EUR 6 newsstand/cover foreign (effective 2002). adv. **Document type:** *Journal, Trade.* **Description:** Contains articles of interest to health care aides.
Related titles: Online - full text ed.: (from Springer LINK).
Published by: Springer-Verlag Wien (Subsidiary of: BertelsmannSpringer), Sachsenplatz 4-6, PO Box 89, Vienna, W 1201, Austria. TEL 43-1-3302415-0, FAX 43-1-330242665, journals@springer.at, http://www.springer.at/procare. Eds. R Hoehl, V Kienast. R&P Angela Foessl TEL 43-1-3302415517. Adv. contact Michael Katzenberger TEL 43-1-3302415220. B&W page XEU 1,925, color page XEU 2,503; 180 x 260. **Subscr. in N. America to:** Springer-Verlag, Journals. TEL 212-460-1500, FAX 212-473-6272, orders@springer-ny.com, http://www.springer-ny.com.

PROFESSION SAGE-FEMME. see *MEDICAL SCIENCES—Obstetrics And Gynecology*

614 GBR ISSN 0964-4156
PROFESSIONAL CARE OF MOTHER & CHILD; journal of family healthcare. Text in English. 1965. bi-m. GBP 20 to individuals; GBP 36 to institutions; GBP 9 to students; GBP 38 in Europe; GBP 45 rest of world (effective 2002). adv. bk.rev. index. **Document type:** *Academic/Scholarly.*
Former titles: Midwife, Health and Community Nurse (0306-9699); Midwife and Health Visitor (0026-3516)
Indexed: ASSIA, Brit.Nur.Ind., CINAHL, Dent.Ind., Fam.Ind., Int.Nurs.Ind.
—BLDSC (6857.395000), GNLM, ingenta.
Published by: P M H Publications Ltd., PO Box 100, Chichester, W Sussex PO18 8HD, United Kingdom. TEL 44-1243-576444, FAX 44-1243-576456, admin@pmh.uk.com, http://www.pmh.uk.com. Ed. Pat Scowen. Pub. Linda Edmondson. Adv. contact Andrea Turner. Circ: 5,330.

610.73 AUS ISSN 1325-7706
PROFESSIONAL DEVELOPMENT SERIES. Text in English. 1995. q. AUD 35 to non-members; AUD 27 to members. adv. **Document type:** *Trade.* **Description:** Publishes several perspectives on a topic of immediate concern for the nursing profession and other health disciplines.
Published by: Royal College of Nursing Australia, 1 Napier Close, Deakin, ACT 2600, Australia. TEL 61-2-6282-5633, FAX 61-2-6282-3565. Adv. contact Joanne Ramadge.

610.73 USA ISSN 0033-0140
R728.8
PROFESSIONAL MEDICAL ASSISTANT. Cover title: P M A. Text in English. 1956. bi-m. USD 30. adv. bk.rev. illus. index. **Document type:** *Trade.* **Description:** Educational articles of interest to medical assistants in the office, hospital, clinic or school setting.
Formerly: A A M A Bulletin
Related titles: Microform ed.: (from PQC); Online - full text ed.: (from ProQuest Information & Learning).
Indexed: CINAHL.
—BLDSC (6541.079200), ingenta.
Published by: American Association of Medical Assistants, Inc., 20 N Wacker Dr, Ste 1575, Chicago, IL 60606-2903. TEL 312-899-1500, 800-228-2262, FAX 312-899-1259. Ed. Donald A Balasa. R&P Jean Lynch. Adv. contact Eileen Ford. B&W page USD 940; trim 10.88 x 8.25. Circ: 16,000.

610.73 GBR ISSN 0266-8130
RT1
PROFESSIONAL NURSE; the leading update for clinical nurses. Text in English. 1985. m. GBP 36 domestic to individuals; GBP 45 in Europe to individuals; GBP 75 elsewhere to individuals; GBP 72 domestic to institutions; GBP 78 in Europe to institutions; GBP 96 elsewhere to institutions; GBP 3.50 newsstand/cover (effective 2000). adv. bk.rev. index. back issues avail. **Document type:** *Academic/Scholarly, Trade.* **Description:** Primarily clinical magazine with the aim of keeping nurses up to date on practice issues and improving their effectiveness.
Indexed: AMED, Brit.Nur.Ind., CINAHL.
—BLDSC (6860.300000), CISTI, GNLM, Infotrieve. **CCC.**
Published by: Emap Healthcare Ltd. (Subsidiary of: Emap Business Communications Ltd.), Greater London House, Hampstead Rd, London NW1 7EJ, United Kingdom. TEL 44-20-7874-0200, FAX 44-20-7874-0201, http://www.emap.com. Ed. Carolyn Scott. Pub. Rosemarie Finley. Adv. contact Gillian Johnson. Circ: 29,493 (paid). **Subscr. to:** Emap Readerlink Ltd., Audit House, 260 Field End Rd, Ruislip, Mddx HA4 9LT, United Kingdom. TEL 44-181-956-3170. **Dist. by:** Seymour Ltd., 86 Newman St, London W1P 3LD, United Kingdom.

610.73 USA ISSN 0734-1431
PROGRAM PLANS: NURSING BASIC SERIES. Text in English. 1979. m. USD 89 in North America; USD 98 elsewhere (effective 2000). bk.rev. bibl, charts, illus, stat. index. 6 p./no. back issues avail. **Document type:** *Journal, Trade.* **Description:** Offers training programs for non-professional staff in health service organizations.
Indexed: CINAHL.
—**CCC.**
Published by: (Educational Planning Services Corp.), E P S C O, 923 Rte 6A, Yarmouth, MA 02675. TEL 508-375-0155, FAX 508-375-0156, reterrill@capecod.net, http://www.educationalplanning.com. Ed. Jessica D Terrill. R&P Robert Terrill. Circ: 3,000 (paid).

PROGRESS IN CARDIOVASCULAR NURSING. see *MEDICAL SCIENCES—Cardiovascular Diseases*

610.73 USA ISSN 0737-1209
PUBLIC HEALTH NURSING. Text in English. bi-m. USD 90 domestic to individuals; USD 105 in Canada & Mexico to individuals; USD 120 elsewhere to individuals; USD 245 domestic to institutions; USD 260 in Canada & Mexico to institutions; USD 275 elsewhere to institutions; USD 99 domestic to individuals print & online eds. combined; USD 115.50 in Canada & Mexico to individuals print & online eds. combined; USD 132 elsewhere to individuals print & online eds. combined; USD 269.50 domestic to institutions print & online eds. combined; USD 286 in Canada & Mexico to institutions print & online eds. combined; USD 302.50 elsewhere to institutions print & online eds. combined (effective 2001). adv. back issues avail. *Refereed.* **Document type:** *Trade, Academic/Scholarly.* **Description:** Publishes theoretical and practical discussions, reviews, and clinical reports in the field of public-health nursing.
Related titles: Online - full text ed.: ISSN 1525-1446. USD 81 to individuals; USD 221 to institutions (effective 2001) (from Ovid Technologies, Inc., EBSCO Publishing, O C L C Online Computer Library Center, Inc., RoweCom Information Quest, ingenta, Munksgaard & Blackwell Science's Synergy, Swets Blackwell, Institute for Scientific Information).
Indexed: ASCA, AgeLine, CINAHL, Curr.Cont., Fam.Ind., Ind.Med. (1984-), Int.Nurs.Ind., Nurs.Abstr., PsycInfo, Psychol.Abstr. (1993-), SSCI, THA, e-psyche.
—GNLM, IDS, ingenta, KNAW. **CCC.**
Published by: Blackwell Science Inc., Commerce Pl., 350 Main St., Malden, MA 02148-5018. TEL 781-388-8250, 800-759-6102, FAX 781-388-8255, http://www.blacksci.co.uk. Eds. Katherine J Young Graham, Sherry Shamansky. R&P Tracey Davies. Adv. contact Jenny Applin.

610.73 USA
THE PULSE (CEDAR FALLS). Text in English. q. Free to qualified subscribers. 20 p./no. **Document type:** *Newsletter, Trade.* **Description:** Covers issues and employment opportunities of interest to licensed nursing professionals.
Published by: (Montana Nurses' Association), Arthur L. Davis Publishing Agency, Inc., 517 Washington St, P O Box 216, Cedar Falls, IA 50613. TEL 319-277-2414, 800-626-4081, FAX 319-277-4055, sales@aldpub.com, http://www.aldpub.com/. Circ: 13,000 (free).

QUALITY OF LIFE; a nursing challenge. see *MEDICAL SCIENCES*

610.73 USA ISSN 0196-3805
QUICKENING. Text in English. bi-m. membership only. **Document type:** *Newsletter.*
Published by: American College of Nurse-Midwives, 818 Connecticut Ave, Ste 900, Washington, DC 20005. TEL 202-728-9860, FAX 202-728-9897. Ed. Gina Harps. Circ: 5,000.

610.73 GBR
R C N INSTITUTE. REPORT. Text in English. irreg. **Document type:** *Monographic series, Academic/Scholarly.* **Description:** Examines topics in professional nurse training.
Published by: (R C N Institute), Royal College of Nursing, School Nurse's Forum, 20 Cavendish Sq, London W1M 0AB, United Kingdom. http://www.rcn.org.uk/instit.

610.73 GBR
R C N NATIONAL HEALTH MANIFESTO. ANNUAL REPORT. (Royal College of Nursing) Text in English. 1973. a. free per issue. bibl. **Document type:** *Corporate.*
Formerly (until 1996): Study of Nursing Care: Research Project Series (0302-1440)
Published by: Royal College of Nursing, 20 Cavendish Sq, London W1M 0AB, United Kingdom. TEL 44-171-409-3333, FAX 44-171-355-1379.

610.73 USA ISSN 0033-7021
RT1
R N. (Registered Nurse) Text in English. 1937. m. USD 35 domestic; USD 50 foreign; USD 10 newsstand/cover (effective 2001). adv. illus. index. back issues avail.; reprints avail. *Refereed.* **Document type:** *Trade.* **Description:** Articles of interest to registered nurses, particularly those in the hospital environment.
Related titles: CD-ROM ed.: (from Ovid Technologies, Inc.); Microform ed.: (from RPI,PQC); Online - full text ed.: R N Web (from Gale Group, Ovid Technologies, Inc., H. W. Wilson, ProQuest Information & Learning, Factiva); ♦ Supplement: Nursing Opportunities.

M

Indexed: AMED, Acad.Ind., AgeLine, Brit.Nur.Ind., Bus.Ind., CINAHL, Curr.Cont. (coverage dropped), Curr.Lit.Fam.Plan., Gen.Sci.Ind. (Mar.1984-), Hlth.Ind., Hosp.Lit.Ind., INIS Atomind., I.P.A., Int.Nurs.Ind., L.R.I., Nurs.Abstr., Tr.& Indus.Ind.
—BLDSC (7993.980000), GNLM, ingenta, KNAW, Linda Hall. **CCC.**
Published by: Medical Economics Co., Inc., 5 Paragon Dr, Montvale, NJ 07645-1742. http://rn.pdr.net/rn/. Ed. Marianne Dekker Mattera. adv.: B&W page USD 10,360, color page USD 13,735. Circ: 250,000. **Subscr. to:** Medical Economics Co, Inc, P D R, PO Box 162, Montvale, NJ 07645-1742. TEL 800-232-7379, FAX 201-722-2680.

610.73 USA ISSN 0192-298X
R.N. IDAHO. Text in English. 1942. q. USD 25 to non-members. adv. **Document type:** *Newsletter.*
Former titles: Gem State R N Newsletter; Gem State R N (0072-0569); Idaho State Bulletin
Published by: Idaho Nurses Association, 200 N Fourth St, Ste 20, Boise, ID 83702-6001. TEL 208-345-0500, FAX 208-385-0166, idanurse@rmci.net. Ed. Myrl Wheeler. Circ: 600.

RECENT ADVANCES IN OPHTHALMOLOGY/YANKE XIN JINZHAN. see *MEDICAL SCIENCES—Ophthalmology And Optometry*

610.73 USA
RECRUITMENT, RETENTION & RESTRUCTURING REPORT; strategies for recruiters, managers, R&R committees, & human resource directors. Text in English. 1988. bi-m. USD 128 (effective 1998). adv. bk.rev. abstr, bibl, charts. back issues avail. **Document type:** *Newsletter.* **Description:** Offers strategies for nursing recruitment, retention, restructuring, and improving nurse satisfaction.
Formerly (until 1994): Recruitment and Retention Report (1044-0666)
Related titles: Online - full text ed.
Indexed: CINAHL.
—CCC.
Published by: Springhouse Corporation (Subsidiary of: Lippincott Williams & Wilkins (Philadelphia)), 1111 Bethlehem Tpk., Springhouse, PA 19477-0908. TEL 215-646-8700, cinahl@cinahl.com, http://www.cinahl.com/jrnls/RRRR/rrrr.htm. Ed. Suzanne Hall Johnson.

REFLECTIONS ON NURSING LEADERSHIP. see *CLUBS*

610.73 CAN ISSN 1484-0863
REGISTERED NURSE. Short title: R N. Text in English. 6/yr. CND 36 domestic; CND 42 foreign (effective 1999). adv. **Document type:** *Magazine.* **Description:** Acts as a forum between the association and its members, discussing ethical, legal, moral, professional and economic issues within the profession.
Former titles (until 1996): Registered Nurse Journal (1203-9659); Registered Nurse (0840-8831)
Indexed: CINAHL.
—BLDSC (7344.160000). **CCC.**
Published by: Registered Nurses Association of Ontario, 438 University Ave, Ste 1600, Toronto, ON M5G 2K8, Canada. TEL 416-599-1925, 800-268-7199, FAX 416-599-1926, info@rnao.org, http://www.rnao.org. Ed., R&P Lesley Frey. Pub. Sine MacKinnon. Adv. contact Kimberley Kearsey. B&W page CND 1,215, color page CND 2,015; trim 10.75 x 8.13. Circ: 16,000.

610.73 CAN
REGISTERED PSYCHIATRIC NURSES' ASSOCIATION OF SASKATCHEWAN. R P NEWS. Text in English. q. CND 10. adv. **Document type:** *Newsletter.*
Formerly: Saskatchewan Psychiatric Nurses' Association. Newsletter
Published by: Registered Psychiatric Nurses Association of Saskatchewan, 2055 Lorne St, Regina, SK S4P 2M4, Canada. TEL 306-586-4617, FAX 306-586-6000. Ed., R&P, Adv. contact Marion Rieger. Circ: 1,400.

610.73 615.82 USA ISSN 0278-4807
RT120.R4
REHABILITATION NURSING. Text in English. 1975. bi-m. USD 75 to individuals; USD 125 to institutions; USD 125 in Canada; USD 135 elsewhere (effective 2001). adv. bk.rev. charts, illus. index. back issues avail.; reprint service avail. from PQC. **Document type:** *Academic/Scholarly.*
Formerly (until 1981): A R N Journal (0362-3505)
Related titles: Microform ed.: (from PQC); Online - full text ed.: (from Northern Light Technology, Inc., ProQuest Information & Learning).
Indexed: AMED, Brit.Nur.Ind., CINAHL, Fam.Ind., Int.Nurs.Ind., Nurs.Abstr.
—BLDSC (7350.285000), GNLM, Infotrieve, ingenta, KNAW. **CCC.**
Published by: Association of Rehabilitation Nurses, 4700 W Lake Ave, Glenview, IL 60025-1485. TEL 847-375-4710, FAX 847-375-4777. Ed. Susan Dean-Baar. Circ: 13,000.

610.73 USA ISSN 0160-6891
RT81.5
RESEARCH IN NURSING & HEALTH. Text in English. 1978. bi-m. USD 760 in United States; USD 820 in Canada & Mexico; USD 871 elsewhere; USD 798 combined subscription in United States for print and online eds.; USD 858 combined subscription in Canada & Mexico for print and online eds.; USD 909 combined subscription elsewhere for print and online eds. (effective 2002). adv. back issues avail.; reprint service avail. from PQC. *Refereed.* **Document type:** *Academic/Scholarly.* **Description:** Covers nursing practice, education and administration.
Related titles: Microform ed.: (from PQC); Online - full text ed.: ISSN 1098-240X. 1996. USD 760 in United States; USD 760 in Canada & Mexico; USD 760 elsewhere (effective 2002) (from EBSCO Publishing, Wiley InterScience, Institute for Scientific Information).
Indexed: ASCA, AgeLine, Behav.Med.Abstr., CINAHL, Curr.Cont., Fam.Ind., Ind.Med. (1978-), Int.Nurs.Ind., Lang.& Lang.Behav.Abstr., Nurs.Abstr., PsycInfo, Psychol.Abstr. (1980-), SOPODA, SSCI, Sage Race Rel.Abstr., Sociol.Abstr., THA, e-psyche.
—BLDSC (7750.150000), CISTI, GNLM, IDS, ingenta, KNAW. **CCC.**
Published by: John Wiley & Sons, Inc., Journals (Subsidiary of: Wiley InterScience), 605 Third Ave, New York, NY 10158. TEL 212-850-6645, FAX 212-850-6021, subinfo@wiley.com, uscs-wis@wiley.com, http://www.wiley.com. Ed. Marilyn T Oberst. adv.: B&W page GBP 640, color page GBP 1,515; trim 172 x 254. Circ: 1,900. **Subscr. outside the Americas to:** John Wiley & Sons Ltd., Baffins Ln, Chichester, Sussex PO19 IUD, United Kingdom. TEL 44-1243-779777, FAX 44-1243-843232, cs-journals@wiley.co.uk.

610.73 GBR
RESOURCES FOR NURSING RESEARCH. Text in English. irreg., latest vol.2, 1994. USD 75 (effective 2000). **Document type:** *Directory.*
Published by: (Library Association), Library Association Publishing Ltd., 7 Ridgmount St, London WC1E 7AE, United Kingdom. TEL 44-20-7255-0500, FAX 44-20-7255-0501, lapublishing@lahq.org.uk, info@la-hq.org.uk, http://www.la-hq.org.uk/. **Dist. by:** Bernan Associates, 4611 F Assembly Dr, Lanham, MD 20706. TEL 800-274-4447, FAX 800-865-3450.

610.73 USA ISSN 1040-3957
RESPONSE (LEBANON)∗ . Text in English. 1988. m. USD 19.95. adv. bk.rev. charts, illus, pat. back issues avail. **Description:** Potpourri of clinical data, personal insights and humor. For all nurses: active, retired, students, or those with advanced degrees.
Address: c/o D J Russell, Pub, 1002 Smith Ave, Lebanon, PA 17042-7144. Ed. Terrilynn M Quillen. Circ: 600.

610.73 USA ISSN 0898-5316
REVIEW OF RESEARCH IN NURSING EDUCATION∗ . Text in English. 1986. irreg., latest vol.6. **Document type:** *Monographic series, Academic/Scholarly.*
Published by: National League for Nursing, 61 Broadway, New York, NY 10006-2701. TEL 800-669-1656.

610.73 BRA ISSN 0034-7167
REVISTA BRASILEIRA DE ENFERMAGEM. Text in Portuguese; Abstracts in English. 1932. q. BRL 67 domestic; USD 77 foreign (effective 1999). bk.rev. abstr, bibl, charts, illus, stat. back issues avail. *Refereed.* **Document type:** *Academic/Scholarly.* **Description:** Provides nurses and health professionals with information from different knowledge areas of nursing, aimed at scientific, technical and cultural development.
Formerly (until 1954): Anais de Enfermagen (0100-6843)
Related titles: Online - full text ed.
Indexed: Int.Nurs.Ind.
—GNLM.
Published by: Associacao Brasileira de Enfermagem, Av. L2 Norte Q. 603, Modulo B, Brasilia, DF, Brazil. TEL 55-61-2260653, FAX 55-61-2254473, reben@persocom.com.br, http://www.persocom.com.br/aben. Ed. Maria Therezinha Nobrega da Silva. Circ: 2,400.

610.73 CUB ISSN 0864-0319
RT7.C9
REVISTA CUBANA DE ENFERMERIA. Text in Spanish; Summaries in English, French, Spanish. 1985. 3/yr. USD 30 in the Americas; USD 38 in Europe; USD 46 elsewhere. bibl, charts, illus. index.
Indexed: Int.Nurs.Ind.
—BLDSC (7852.104000), GNLM.
Published by: (Cuba. Ministerio de Salud Publica, Centro Nacional de Informacion de Ciencias Medicas), Editorial de Ciencias Medicas, O'Reilly No. 4, Habana, Cuba. TEL 809-62-8091. Ed. Fredesvinda Blanco. Circ: 2,500. **Co-sponsor:** Sociedad Cubana de Enfermeria.

610.73 BRA ISSN 0102-6933
REVISTA GAUCHA DE ENFERMAGEM. Text in Burmese. 1976. s-a. BRL 20 domestic; USD 45 foreign; BRL 15 newsstand/cover (effective 2001). abstr, bibl. cum.index: 1976-1986, 1987-1990, 1991-1995. back issues avail. *Refereed.* **Document type:** *Academic/Scholarly, Consumer, Internal.* **Description:** Presents articles, research, and monographs done by nurses throughout Brazil.
Indexed: Ind.Med. (coverage dropped), Int.Nurs.Ind.
Published by: Universidade Federal do Rio Grande do Sul, Escola de Enfermagem, Rua Sao Manoel, 963, Campus da Saude, Porto Alegre, RGS 90620-110, Brazil. TEL 55-51-3165242, FAX 55-51-3321601, revista@enf.ufrgs.br, http://www.ufrgs.br/eenf/revist.htm. Ed. Anne Marie Weissheimer. Pub. Ida H de Freitas Xavier. Circ: 300 (paid).

610.73 BRA ISSN 0104-1169
REVISTA LATINO-AMERICANA DE ENFERMAGEM. Text in English, Portuguese, Spanish. 1993. bi-m. abstr. *Refereed.* **Document type:** *Journal, Academic/Scholarly.* **Description:** Covers issues about all areas of nursing: practice, education, research, policies, etc..
Indexed: CINAHL.
—BLDSC (7863.410000).
Published by: University of Sao Paulo, Ribeirao Preto College of Nursing, Escola de Enfermagem de Ribeirao Preto, Av. Bandeirantes, 3900, Ribeirao Preto, Sao Paulo 14040-902, Brazil. TEL 55-16-3023451, FAX 55-16-6333271, http://www.eerp.usp.br/rlannf. Ed. Dr. Maria Helena Palucci-Marziale.

658 ESP ISSN 0210-5020
REVISTA ROL DE ENFERMERIA. Text in Spanish. 1978. 12/yr. ESP 9,500, USD 67 (effective 2001). adv. *Refereed.* **Document type:** *Newsletter.* **Description:** Updates, developments, and research in nursing in hospitals, first aid, teaching, public health, health administration and management.
Indexed: CINAHL.
—BLDSC (7870.510000), GNLM, Infotrieve. **CCC.**
Published by: Ediciones Rol S.A., San Elias, 29, Barcelona 08006, Spain. TEL 34-93-2008033, FAX 34-93-2002762, redaccion@e.zol.es, zol@e.zol.es, http://www.e.zol.es/. Ed. Julia Martinez Saavedra. Adv. contact Jose Garcia Rey. page ESP 217,000, page XEU 1,370.31. Circ: 25,000.

610.73 URY ISSN 0797-6194
REVISTA URUGUAYA DE ENFERMERIA. Text in Spanish. 1989. 3/yr., latest 2000. UYP 220 domestic; UYP 170 domestic to students; UYP 90 newsstand/cover domestic (effective 2001). charts, illus. back issues avail. **Document type:** *Journal, Academic/Scholarly.* **Description:** Its objective is to spread scientific and technical information on advances in the field of health, especially nursing. It also aims at building theories, revise methodologies and procedures and investigate unexplored issues.
Published by: (Universidad de la Republica, Instituto Nacional de Enfermeria, Universidad de la Republica, Colegio de Enfermeras del Uruguay), Ediciones Sciencias Biologicas Pub. Pablo Anzalone.

610.73 USA ISSN 1059-0927
RT1
REVOLUTION; the journal for RNs and patient advocacy. Text in English. 1991. bi-m. USD 30 in United States to individuals; USD 35 in Canada to individuals; USD 100 to institutions; USD 7 newsstand/cover (effective 2001). adv. 32 p./no. 3 cols./p. back issues avail. *Refereed.* **Document type:** *Journal, Magazine, Trade.* **Description:** Covers major issues that face nurses and patients, such as short staffing, unethical medical practice, fighting against corporate power which has taken over the healthcare industry.
Indexed: CINAHL.
—CISTI.

M

Published by: Center For Caregiver and Patient Advocacy, 2000 Franklin St, Ste 400, Oakland, CA 94612. TEL 510-273-2290, FAX 510-663-0629, http://www.revolutionmag.com/. adv.: page USD 2,600. Circ: 2,500 (paid).

610.73 FRA ISSN 1293-8505
REVUE DE L'INFIRMIERE. Text in French. 1951. 10/yr. EUR 71 in Europe to individuals; EUR 100 in Europe to institutions; USD 121 rest of world to institutions (effective 2002). adv. bk.rev. charts, illus. index. back issues avail. *Refereed.* **Document type:** *Journal, Academic/Scholarly.* **Description:** Offers practical, up-to-date information on all aspects of nursing.
Formerly (until 1971): Revue de l'Infirmiere et de l'Assistante Sociale (0397-7900)
Related titles: Online - full text ed.
Indexed: AMED, Dent.Ind., Int.Nurs.Ind., Pt.de Rep. (1979-).
—BLDSC (7924.170000), CISTI, GNLM, Infotrieve. **CCC.**
Published by: Elsevier Paris, Editions Scientifiques et Medicales (Subsidiary of: Reed Elsevier plc. group), 23 rue Linois, Paris 75015, France. TEL 33-1-45589110, FAX 33-1-45589419, e.durant@elsevier.fr, academic@elsevier-fr, http://www.elsevier.com/locate/revinf, http://www.elsevier.fr. Eds. Elisabeth Durant TEL 33-1-45-58-98-74, Lise Kipman TEL 33-1-45-58-98-78. Circ: 60,000.

610.736 USA ISSN 1050-9089
ROGERIAN NURSING SCIENCE NEWS. Text in English. 1988. q. USD 24. bk.rev. 10 p./no. 2 cols./p. *Refereed.* **Document type:** *Newsletter.* **Description:** Presents articles relating to the studies of Martha Rogers.
Indexed: CINAHL.
—BLDSC (8019.172400).
Published by: Society of Rogerian Scholars, PO Box 1195, Canal Street Sta, New York, NY 10013-0867. TEL 804-828-0836, wcowling@hsc.vcu.edu. Ed. W Richard Cowling. Circ: 250.

610.73 CAN ISSN 1180-3983
SANTE QUEBEC. Text in French, English. 1990. q. CND 20; CND 0.25 foreign (effective 1999). adv. bk.rev. back issues avail. **Document type:** *Bulletin.* **Description:** Contains information for nursing assistants.
Published by: Ordre des Infirmieres et Infirmiers Auxiliaires du Quebec, 531 Sherbrooke E, Montreal, PQ H2L 1K2, Canada. TEL 514-282-9511, FAX 514-282-0631, service.communications@oiiaq.org. R&P Francine Saucier TEL 514-282-8511. Adv. contact Francine Soucier. B&W page CND 1,000, color page CND 1,300; 10.5 x 8.

610.73 PHL ISSN 0048-9123
SANTO TOMAS NURSING JOURNAL; devoted to the collegiate programmes of nursing in the Philippines. Text in English. 1962-1976; resumed 1978. s-a. USD 8. adv. bk.rev. illus.
Indexed: CINAHL, Int.Nurs.Ind.
—CISTI.
Published by: (University of Santo Tomas), University Of Santo Tomas, College of Nursing (Subsidiary of: University of Santo Tomas), Espana St., Sampaloc, Manila, Philippines. Ed. Conchita Torres-Maceda. Circ: 2,000.

610.73 CAN ISSN 0836-7310
SASKATCHEWAN CONCE R N. Text in English. 1948. bi-m. CND 20; USD 30 foreign (effective 1999). adv. bk.rev. **Document type:** *Academic/Scholarly.* **Description:** Information about the association's activities in nursing education.
Formerly (until 1987): Saskatchewan Registered Nurses' Association. Bulletin (0319-8499)
Related titles: Online - full text ed.: (from ProQuest Information & Learning).
—BLDSC (3399.430105).
Published by: Saskatchewan Registered Nurses' Association, 2066 Retallack St, Regina, SK S4T 7X5, Canada. TEL 306-359-4245, FAX 306-525-0849, http://www.srna.org. Ed. Joy Johnson. Adv. contact Linda Laxdal. Circ: 10,000.

SCANDINAVIAN JOURNAL OF PRIMARY HEALTH CARE. see *MEDICAL SCIENCES*

SCANDINAVIAN JOURNAL OF PRIMARY HEALTH CARE. SUPPLEMENT. see *MEDICAL SCIENCES*

610.73 USA ISSN 0889-7182 CODEN: SINPFV
SCHOLARLY INQUIRY FOR NURSING PRACTICE; an international journal. Text in English. 1986. 4/yr., latest vol.15, no.1, 2001, Spring. USD 56 domestic to individuals; USD 65 foreign to individuals; USD 123 domestic to institutions; USD 141 foreign to institutions (effective 2001). adv. 80 p./no. back issues avail.; reprints avail. *Refereed.* **Document type:** *Journal, Academic/Scholarly.* **Description:** Publishes original manuscripts concerned with the development and testing of theory relevant to nursing practice to facilitate the integration of theory, research and practice.
Indexed: Behav.Med.Abstr., CINAHL, Fam.Ind., Ind.Med. (1987-), Int.Nurs.Ind., PsycInfo, Psychol.Abstr. (1987-), SOPODA, Sociol.Abstr., e-psyche.
—BLDSC (8092.540300), CISTI, GNLM, ingenta. **CCC.**
Published by: Springer Publishing Company, 536 Broadway, New York, NY 10012. TEL 212-431-4370, FAX 212-941-7842, springer@springerpub.com, http://www.springerjournals.com/sinp/home.htm, http://www.springerpub.com. Pub. Ursula Springer. R&P Dorothy Kouwenberg. Adv. contact Bob Friel. B&W page USD 300; 4.5 x 7.5. Circ: 580 (paid).

610.73 USA ISSN 1048-3896
SCHOOL HEALTH ALERT. Text in English. 1984. m. (10/yr.). USD 34 domestic; USD 49 foreign (effective 2000). adv. bk.rev. *Refereed.* **Document type:** *Newsletter.* **Description:** Addresses the needs of school nurses, health educators, and special education teachers and administrators to remain current with professional, and clinical matters.
Address: PO Box 150127, Nashville, TN 37215-0127. TEL 615-370-7899, FAX 615-370-9993, publisher@schoolnurse.com, http://www.schoolnurse.com. Eds. Dr. Jan Ozias, Richard M. Adams. Pub. Robert Andrews. Circ: 9,000 (paid).

610.73 USA ISSN 1080-7543
SCHOOL NURSE NEWS* ; current issues affecting school nurses. Text in English. 1994 (vol.11). 5/yr. adv. illus. **Document type:** *Trade.* **Description:** Reports on current medical and professional developments of interest to school nurses.
Indexed: CINAHL.
—CCC.
Published by: Health Information Publications, Inc., 200 Valley Rd Ste 405, Mount Arlington, NJ 07856-1320. TEL 973-267-8938, FAX 973-267-8926. Ed. Linda Dychkowski. Pub. Michael Franklin. Adv. contact Rhonda Guthoff. B&W page USD 1,190, color page USD 395; trim 14.25 x 11.13. Circ: 10,000 (paid).

610.73 CHE ISSN 1422-4526
SCHWEIZER HEBAMME. Text in French, German. 1903. m. CHF 89; CHF 110 foreign (effective 1999). adv. bk.rev. *Refereed.* **Document type:** *Newsletter.*
Published by: Schweizer Hebammenverband, Flurstr 26, Bern, 22 3000, Switzerland. TEL 41-31-3313520, FAX 41-31-3313520, sh.redakmichel@bluewin.ch. Ed. Gerlinde Michel. R&P G Michel TEL 41-31-331-35-20. Adv. contact Kunzler Bachmann St Gallen. Circ: 2,900.

610.73 DEU ISSN 0340-5303
DIE SCHWESTER - DER PFLEGER. Text in German. 1962. m. DEM 73.20, EUR 37.43 domestic; DEM 85.80, EUR 43.87 foreign; DEM 12, EUR 6.14 newsstand/cover (effective 2001). adv. bk.rev. **Document type:** *Journal, Academic/Scholarly.*
Indexed: Dok.Arbeitsmed., Ref.Zh.
—GNLM.
Published by: Bibliomed - Medizinische Verlagsgesellschaft mbH, Postfach 1150, Melsungen 34201, Germany. TEL 49-5661-7344-0, FAX 49-5661-8360, info@bibliomed.de, http://www.bibliomed.de. Circ: 42,000.

610.73 USA ISSN 1066-3851
RT89
SEMINARS FOR NURSE MANAGERS. Text in English. 1993. q. USD 81 domestic to individuals; USD 130 foreign to individuals; USD 117 domestic to institutions; USD 169 foreign to institutions; USD 49 domestic to students; USD 78 foreign to students; USD 43 newsstand/cover (effective 2001). adv. back issues avail. **Document type:** *Academic/Scholarly.* **Description:** Provides detailed reviews of the challenges nurse managers face; each issue covers a single topic in detail through clinical review articles and regular columns.
Indexed: CINAHL, Int.Nurs.Ind.
—BLDSC (8239.456050), GNLM, Infotrieve. **CCC.**
Published by: W.B. Saunders Co. (Subsidiary of: Harcourt Publishers Ltd.), 11830 Westline Industrial Dr, St Louis, MO 63146. TEL 800-325-4177, http://www.wbsaunders.com. Ed. Roxane B Spitzer. Adv. contact Steve Gray. B&W page USD 660, color page USD 1,610; 10 x 7. Circ: 1,386. **Subscr. to:** Periodicals Fulfillment, W B Saunders Co, 6277 Sea Harbor Dr, 4th Fl, Orlando, FL 32891-4800.

610.736 616.992 USA ISSN 0749-2081
SEMINARS IN ONCOLOGY NURSING. Text in English. 1985. q. USD 85 domestic to individuals; USD 151 foreign to individuals; USD 154 domestic to institutions; USD 204 foreign to institutions; USD 77 domestic to students; USD 91 foreign to students; USD 52 newsstand/cover (effective 2001). adv. bibl, charts, illus. index. **Document type:** *Journal, Academic/Scholarly.* **Description:** Each issue focuses on a single theme on cancer-patient nursing.
Indexed: AMED, CINAHL, INIS Atomind., Ind.Med. (1985-), Int.Nurs.Ind., Nurs.Abstr.
—BLDSC (8239.456600), CISTI, GNLM, ingenta, KNAW. **CCC.**
Published by: W.B. Saunders Co. (Subsidiary of: Harcourt Publishers Ltd.), 11830 Westline Industrial Dr, St Louis, MO 63146. TEL 800-325-4177, http://www.wbsaunders.com. Ed. Connie H Yarbro. adv.: B&W page USD 885, color page USD 2,060; trim 10 x 7. Circ: 2,062. **Subscr. to:** Periodicals Fulfillment, W B Saunders Co, 6277 Sea Harbor Dr, 4th Fl, Orlando, FL 32891-4800.

610.73 617 USA ISSN 1056-8670
SEMINARS IN PERIOPERATIVE NURSING. Text in English. 1992. q. USD 84 domestic to individuals; USD 141 foreign to individuals; USD 122 domestic to institutions; USD 173 foreign to institutions; USD 62 domestic to students; USD 85 foreign to students; USD 44 newsstand/cover (effective 2001). adv. **Document type:** *Academic/Scholarly.* **Description:** Reviews a clinical topic of operating-room nursing in each issue.
Indexed: CINAHL, Int.Nurs.Ind.
—BLDSC (8239.456900), CISTI, GNLM, Infotrieve. **CCC.**
Published by: W.B. Saunders Co. (Subsidiary of: Harcourt Publishers Ltd.), 11830 Westline Industrial Dr, St Louis, MO 63146. TEL 800-325-4177, http://www.wbsaunders.com. Ed. Nancy Girard. Adv. contact Cindy Gray. B&W page USD 745, color page USD 1,695; trim 9.5 x 6. Circ: 764. **Subscr. to:** Periodicals Fulfillment, W B Saunders Co, 6277 Sea Harbor Dr, 4th Fl, Orlando, FL 32891-4800.

610.73 CAN ISSN 1192-5299
SERVO. Text in English, French. 1967. 2/yr. CND 5. adv. back issues avail. **Document type:** *Newsletter, Bulletin.* **Description:** For hospital auxiliary volunteers.
Published by: Association of Hospital Auxiliaries of the Province of Quebec, 505 Maisonneuve W, Ste 400, Montreal, PQ H3A 3C2, Canada. TEL 514-282-4264, FAX 514-282-4289. Adv. contact Andree Quinn. Circ: 300.

610.73 CZE ISSN 1210-0404
SESTRA. Text in Czech. 1951. 10/yr. illus. Supplement avail. **Document type:** *Journal, Academic/Scholarly.*
Formerly (until 1991): Zdravotnicka Pracovnice (0049-8572)
Indexed: Int.Nurs.Ind.
—CISTI.
Published by: (Ceska Lekarska Spolecnost J.E. Purkyne/Czech Medical Association), Strategie Praha s.r.o., Drtinova 8, Prague, 5 150 00, Czech Republic. TEL 420-2-57323578, FAX 420-2-57018362, strategie.praha@istrategie.cz, http://www.istrategie.cz.

610.73 SGP
SINGAPORE NURSING JOURNAL. Text in English. 1972. q. SGD 40 (effective 2001). adv. **Document type:** *Trade.* **Description:** Contains president's message, from the editor's desk, clinical focus, research education, words of wisdom, occasional papers, local and international news and reports.
Former titles (until 1998): Professional Nurse (0218-0995); (until 1987): Nursing Journal of Singapore - Berita Jururawat (0067-5814); S T N A Newsletter
Indexed: CINAHL, Diab.Cont., Int.Nurs.Ind.
—BLDSC.
Published by: Singapore Nurses' Association, 77 Maude Rd, Singapore 208353, Singapore. TEL 65-3920770, FAX 65-3927877, sna@pacific.net.sg, http://www.sna.org.sg. Ed., R&P Tan Wee King. Circ: 4,000.

610.73 SWE
▼ **SKANDINAVIEN DIREKT.** Text in Swedish. 1999. 13/yr. free to qualified personnel; SEK 35 newsstand/cover. adv. **Document type:** *Magazine, Trade.*

M

Published by: Florence Kompetensutveckling AB, Box 3348, Stockholm 10367, Sweden. TEL 46-8-10-66-00, FAX 46-8-10-25-04, info@skandinaviendirekt.se, http://www.skandinaviendirekt.se, http://www.florence.se. Ed. Anna-Karin Andersson. Adv. contact Magnus Sjoeberg. page SEK 39,000; trim 250 x 370. Circ: 12,000 (controlled).

610.73 SWE ISSN 0284-284X
SKOLHAELSAN. Text in Swedish. 1993. q. SEK 150; SEK 50 newsstand/cover (effective 2000 & 2001). **Document type:** *Trade.*
Published by: (Riksfoereningen foer Skolskoeterskor), Via Media, Fack 640, Landskrona 26125, Sweden. TEL 46-418-10780, FAX 46-418-12394, viamedia@nornemark.com, http://www.nornemark.com/viamedia. Ed. Kaerstin Loeoef. Circ: 2,300 (paid).

610.736 SWE ISSN 1402-1048
SMAERTA. Text in Swedish. 1996. q. SEK 250; SEK 70 newsstand/cover (effective 2000 & 2001). **Document type:** *Trade.*
Published by: (Riksfoereningen mot Smaerta), Via Media, Fack 640, Landskrona 26125, Sweden. TEL 46-418-10780, FAX 46-418-12394, viamedia@nornemark.com, http://www.nornemark.com/viamedia. Ed. Leena Sundberg. Circ: 2,500 (paid).

610.73 USA ISSN 1088-145X
RJ245 CODEN: MCNJA2
SOCIETY OF PEDIATRIC NURSES. JOURNAL. Variant title: J S P N. Text in English. 1972. q. USD 54 domestic to individuals; USD 68 elsewhere to individuals; USD 36 domestic to students; USD 59 domestic to institutions; USD 75 elsewhere to institutions; USD 21 newsstand/cover domestic; USD 24 newsstand/cover elsewhere (effective 2002). adv. bk.rev. back issues avail.; reprint service avail. from PQC,WSH. *Refereed.* **Document type:** *Academic/Scholarly.* **Description:** Publishes articles on the professional care of mothers and children for the expert nurse practitioner.
Formerly (until 1996): Maternal - Child Nursing Journal (0090-0702)
Related titles: Microform ed.: (from PQC); Online - full text ed.: (from ProQuest Information & Learning, Gale Group).
Indexed: CINAHL, Excerp.Med., Ind.Med. (1996-), Int.Nurs.Ind., Nurs.Abstr., PsycInfo, Psychol.Abstr. (1972-), e-psyche.
—BLDSC (4894.690000), CISTI, GNLM, ingenta.
Published by: (Society of Pediatric Nurses), Nursecom, Inc., 1211 Locust St, Philadelphia, PA 19107. TEL 215-545-7222, 800-242-6757, FAX 215-545-8107, 73764.123@compuserve.com, customer.service@nursecominc.com, http://www.cinahl.com/jrnls/JSPN/jspn.htm, http://www.nursecominc.com. Ed. Rose Foster. Pub. Margo C Neal. Adv. contact Alison L Graham. B&W page USD 925, color page USD 1,475. Circ: 2,500.

610.73 JPN ISSN 0038-0660
SOGO KANGO; comprehensive nursing quarterly. Text in Japanese. 1966. q. JPY 4,000. adv. bk.rev. **Document type:** *Academic/Scholarly.*
Indexed: Int.Nurs.Ind.
Published by: Gendaisha Publishing Co. Ltd., 514 Waseda, Tsurumaki-cho, Shinjuku-ku, Tokyo 162, Japan. TEL 81-3-3202-5061. Ed., Adv. contact Yoshio Takeuchi. Pub., R&P Yoshihiko Kominami. Circ: 12,000.

610.73 FRA ISSN 0038-0814
SOINS; la revue de reference infirmiere. Text in French. 1956. 10/yr. FRF 396 to individuals; FRF 507 foreign to individuals; FRF 690 to institutions; FRF 863 foreign to institutions (effective 2000). adv. bk.rev. **Document type:** *Academic/Scholarly.* **Description:** Covers management, communication, health, psychology, education as they relate to nursing and nurses.
Indexed: AMED, Int.Nurs.Ind., Pt.de Rep. (1979-).
—BLDSC (8327.117000), CISTI, GNLM, KNAW.
Published by: Masson - Periodiques, 120 bd. St. Germain, Paris 75006, France. TEL 33-1-40466280, FAX 33-1-40466221. Ed. Bernard Goddet. adv.: B&W page FRF 16,900, color page FRF 29,300; trim 210 x 297. Circ: 30,000. **Subscr. to:** Societe de Periodiques Specialises, BP 22, Vineuil Cedex 41354, France. TEL 33-2-54504612, FAX 33-2-54504611.

910.73 617 FRA ISSN 0249-6429
SOINS - CHIRURGIE. Text in French. 1981. 6/yr. FRF 281 to individuals; FRF 490 to institutions; FRF 245 to students. adv. **Document type:** *Academic/Scholarly.*
—GNLM.
Published by: Masson - Periodiques, 120 bd. St. Germain, Paris 75006, France. TEL 33-1-40466255, FAX 33-1-40466201. Eds. Bernard Goddet, Chantal Toucheboeuf. Circ: 5,000. **Subscr. to:** Societe de Periodiques Specialises, BP 22, Vineuil Cedex 41354, France. TEL 33-2-54504612, FAX 33-2-54504611.

610.73 FRA ISSN 1163-4723
SOINS - ENCADREMENT, FORMATION. Text in French. 1992. 4/yr. FRF 456 domestic to individuals; FRF 524 foreign to individuals; FRF 550 domestic to institutions; FRF 633 foreign to institutions. adv. bk.rev. **Document type:** *Academic/Scholarly.* **Description:** Looks at the initial and continuing education of nurses.
Formerly: Soins - Formation, Pedagogie, Encadrement
Published by: Masson - Periodiques, 120 bd. St. Germain, Paris 75006, France. TEL 33-1-40466200, FAX 33-1-40466201. Ed., R&P Chantal Toucheboeuf. Adv. contact Nathalie Gerard. B&W page FRF 11,300, color page FRF 20,200; trim 210 x 297. Circ: 5,000. **Subscr. to:** Societe de Periodiques Specialises, BP 22, Vineuil Cedex 41354, France. TEL 33-2-54504612, FAX 33-2-54504611.

610.736 FRA ISSN 1268-6034
SOINS GERONTOLOGIE. Text in French. 1996. 5/yr. FRF 350 domestic to individuals; FRF 525 foreign to individuals; FRF 550 domestic to institutions; FRF 638 foreign to institutions (effective 2000). adv.
Indexed: Int.Nurs.Ind.
—BLDSC (8327.117270).
Published by: Masson - Periodiques, 120 bd. St. Germain, Paris 75006, France. TEL 33-1-40466200, FAX 33-1-40466201. Ed. Bernard Goddet. adv.: B&W page FRF 11,300, color page FRF 20,200; trim 210 x 297. **Subscr. to:** Societe de Periodiques Specialises, BP 22, Vineuil Cedex 41354, France. TEL 33-2-54504612, FAX 33-2-54504611.

610.73 FRA ISSN 1259-4792
SOINS - PEDIATRIE, PUERICULTURE. Text in French. 1980. 6/yr. FRF 350 domestic to individuals (effective 2000); FRF 560 foreign to individuals; FRF 550 domestic to institutions; FRF 770 foreign to institutions. adv. **Document type:** *Academic/Scholarly.* **Description:** Each issue covers a clinical case.
Former titles (until 1995): Soins - Gynecologie, Obstetrique, Puericulture, Pediatrie (0766-1193); (until 1981): Soins - Gynecologie, Obstetrique, Puericulture (0151-6655)
Indexed: Int.Nurs.Ind.
—BLDSC (8327.117550), GNLM.
Published by: Masson - Periodiques, 120 bd. St. Germain, Paris 75006, France. TEL 33-1-40466200, FAX 33-1-40466201. Ed. Bernard Goddet. adv.: B&W page FRF 11,300, color page FRF 20,200; trim 210 x 270. Circ: 5,000. **Subscr. to:** Societe de Periodiques Specialises, BP 22, Vineuil Cedex 41354, France. TEL 33-2-54504612, FAX 33-2-54504611.

610.73 616.8 FRA ISSN 0241-6972
SOINS - PSYCHIATRIE. Text in French. 1980. 6/yr. FRF 350 domestic to individuals (effective 2000); FRF 466 foreign to individuals; FRF 550 domestic to institutions; FRF 713 foreign to institutions. adv. **Document type:** *Academic/Scholarly.* **Description:** Specializes in the training of psychiatric nurses.
Indexed: e-psyche.
—BLDSC (8327.117600), GNLM.
Published by: Masson - Periodiques, 120 bd. St. Germain, Paris 75006, France. TEL 33-1-40466200, FAX 33-1-40466201. Eds. Bernard Goddet, Chantal Toucheboeuf. adv.: B&W page FRF 11,300, color page FRF 20,200; trim 210 x 297. Circ: 5,000. **Subscr. to:** Societe de Periodiques Specialises, BP 22, Vineuil Cedex 41354, France. TEL 33-2-54504612, FAX 33-2-54504611.

610.73 USA ISSN 1046-7394
SOUTH CAROLINA NURSE. Text in English. 1979. q. Free to qualified subscribers. 32 p./no. back issues avail. **Document type:** *Newsletter, Trade.* **Description:** Covers issues and employment opportunities of interest to licensed nursing professionals.
Formerly (until 1985): S C N A Newsletter (0199-3399)
—BLDSC (8350.139000).
Published by: (South Carolina Nurses Association), Arthur L. Davis Publishing Agency, Inc., 517 Washington St, P O Box 216, Cedar Falls, IA 50613. TEL 319-277-2414, 800-626-4081, FAX 319-277-4055, sales@aldpub.com, http://www.aldpub.com/. Ed. Mark Miller. R&P Judith Thompson. Adv. contact Jim Larson. Circ: 48,000 (free).

610.73 USA
SPRINGER SERIES ON ADVANCED PRACTICE NURSING. Text in English. 1993. irreg., latest 2001. price varies. back issues avail. **Document type:** *Monographic series.*
Published by: Springer Publishing Company, 536 Broadway, New York, NY 10012. TEL 212-431-1370, FAX 212-941-7842, springer@springerpub.com, http://www.springerpub.com. Ed. Terry T Fulmer. R&P Dorothy Kouwenberg.

SPRINGER SERIES ON GERIATRIC NURSING. see *GERONTOLOGY AND GERIATRICS*

610.73 USA ISSN 0272-1473
SPRINGER SERIES ON THE TEACHING OF NURSING. Text in English. 1977. irreg., latest vol.20, 1998. price varies. back issues avail. **Document type:** *Monographic series.* **Description:** Deals with various aspects of professional training in nursing.
Published by: Springer Publishing Company, 536 Broadway, New York, NY 10012. TEL 212-431-4370, FAX 212-941-7842, springer@springerpub.com, http://www.springerpub.com. Ed. Patricia Moccia. R&P Dorothy Kouwenberg.

610.73 USA
STANFORD NURSE. Text in English. 197?. s-a. free per issue to qualified personnel. illus. *Refereed.* **Document type:** *Academic/Scholarly, Trade.* **Description:** Discusses ways in which nurses can and have enhanced their profession and their own fulfillment.
Indexed: CINAHL.
—BLDSC.
Published by: Stanford Health Services, Division of Patient Care Services, Center for Education and Professional Development, 300 Pasteur Dr., Ste. NOB, Stanford, CA 94305. Ed. Candice Speers. Pub. Sharon Flynn Hollander.

610.73 USA ISSN 0038-9986
STAT (MADISON). Text in English. 1941. m. USD 45 to members (effective 2000). illus. **Document type:** *Newsletter, Bulletin.*
Indexed: CINAHL, Int.Nurs.Ind.
Published by: Wisconsin Nurses Association, 6117 Monona Dr, Madison, WI 53716-3932. FAX 608-221-2788. Ed., R&P, Adv. contact Susan Carter TEL 608-221-0383. Circ: 2,700.

610.73025 USA ISSN 0081-4423
RT74
STATE-APPROVED SCHOOLS OF NURSING - L.P.N. - L.V.N.* . Text in English. 1959. a. USD 27.95.
Formerly (until 1967): State-Approved Schools of Practical and Vocational Nursing (0095-6570)
Related titles: Microfiche ed.: 1959 (from CIS).
Indexed: SRI.
Published by: National League for Nursing, 61 Broadway, New York, NY 10006-2701. TEL 800-669-1656.

610.73025 USA ISSN 0081-4431
STATE-APPROVED SCHOOLS OF NURSING - R.N.* . Text in English. a. USD 27.95.
Related titles: Microfiche ed.: (from CIS).
Indexed: SRI.
Published by: National League for Nursing, 61 Broadway, New York, NY 10006-2701. TEL 800-669-1656.

SUGGESTED LIST OF PERIODICALS FOR NURSES FOR THE CANADIAN HEALTH SCIENCE LIBRARY. see *MEDICAL SCIENCES—Abstracting, Bibliographies, Statistics*

610.73 DNK ISSN 0106-8350
SYGEPLEJERSKEN. Text in Danish. 1901. w. DKK 860 domestic (effective 2001); USD 168 foreign (effective 2000); DKK 18.25 per issue (effective 2001). adv. bk.rev. illus. **Document type:** *Academic/Scholarly.*
Former titles (until 1972): Tidsskrift for Sygeplejersker (0049-3856); (until 1950): Tidsskrift for Sygepleje (0909-4032)
Indexed: Dent.Ind., Ind.Med. (coverage dropped), Int.Nurs.Ind.
—BLDSC (8579.400000), CISTI.
Published by: Dansk Sygeplejeraad/Danish Nurses' Organization, Vimmelskaftet 38, PO Box 1084, Copenhagen K 1008, Denmark. TEL 45-33-15-15-55, FAX 45-33-93-47-82, redaktionen@dsr.dk, http://www.dsr.dk/sygeplejersken. Ed., R&P Peter Skeel Hjorth TEL 45-33-15-15-55. Circ: 72,969.

610.73 NLD ISSN 1380-3425
T V Z: TIJDSCHRIFT VOOR VERPLEEGKUNDIGEN. Text in Dutch. 1890. s-m. (23/yr.). NLG 182.75. adv. bk.rev. charts, illus. index. **Document type:** *Academic/Scholarly, Trade.* **Description:** Reports on issues of concern to nurses and other nursing professionals.
Former titles (until 1994): Tijdschrift voor Ziekenverpleging (0303-6456); (until 1914): Maandblad voor Ziekenverpleging (0926-342X)
Indexed: C.I.S. Abstr., Dent.Ind., Int.Nurs.Ind.
—CISTI, GNLM, KNAW.
Published by: (Stichting Publikaties voor Verpleegkundigen en Verzorgenden), Elsevier Gezondheidszorg B.V., Tijdstroom (Subsidiary of: Reed Elsevier plc Group), Planetenbaan 1, Maarssen 3600 AK, Netherlands. TEL 31-346-577577, FAX 31-346-554287, http://www.tijdstroom.nl. Circ: 18,000. **Subscr. to:** Elsevier Den Haag, Postbus 16500, The Hague 2500 BM, Netherlands. TEL 31-70-381-9900, FAX 31-70-333-8399.

610.73 USA ISSN 0039-9620
TAR HEEL NURSE. Text in English. 1939. bi-m. USD 25 to non-members (effective 2001); USD 50 foreign; free to members. adv. charts, illus. reprint service avail. from PQC. **Document type:** *Newsletter.*
Related titles: Microform ed.: (from PQC).
Indexed: CINAHL, Int.Nurs.Ind.
Published by: North Carolina Nurses Association, PO Box 12025, Raleigh, NC 27605. TEL 919-821-4250, FAX 919-829-5807, http://www.ncnurses.org. Ed., R&P Sindy Barker. Adv. contact Beth Holder. Circ: 3,500.

610.73 FIN ISSN 0358-4038
TEHY. Text in Finnish, Swedish. 1925. s-m. FIM 550 (effective 1998). adv. bk.rev., film rev. bibl, charts, illus.
Former titles (until 1981): Laboratoriohoitaja; Lastenhoitajalehti (0355-5089); Sairaanhoitaja - Sjukskoterskan (0036-3278); Sairaanhoitajalehti
—CISTI.
Published by: Union of Health and Social Care Services, TEHY/Terveyden- ja Sosiaalhihuoltoalan Ammatijarjesto Tehy ry., PL 10, Tehy 0060, Finland. TEL 358-9-1551, FAX 358-9-148-3038, TELEX 122505. Ed., R&P Sinikka Kivela. Adv. contact Tuire Sillanpaa. Circ: 110,000.

610.73 USA
TELEPHONE NURSING TELEZINE. Short title: T N T. Text in English. 1996. m. **Description:** For nurses, physicians and other health professionals involved in the specialty of telephone triage or telephone nursing.
Media: Online - full text.
Indexed: CINAHL.
Address: 4012 W Fig St, Tampa, FL 33609. webster@cyberspy.com, http://ally.ios.com/~webster/telezine.html. Ed. Kathi Webster.

610.73 USA ISSN 1055-3134
TENNESSEE NURSE. Text in English. 1934. bi-m. USD 20 (effective 2000 - 2001). adv. bk.rev. illus. *Refereed.* **Document type:** *Trade.*
Formerly (until 1990): Tennessee Nurses Association. Bulletin (0040-3342)
Related titles: Microform ed.: (from PQC).
Indexed: CINAHL, Int.Nurs.Ind.
—BLDSC (8790.733500), GNLM.
Published by: Tennessee Nurses Association, 545 Mainstream Dr, Ste 405, Nashville, TN 37228-1296. TEL 615-254-0350, FAX 615-254-0303. Ed., R&P, Adv. contact Heather Wicks. Circ: 5,000.

610.73 USA ISSN 0095-036X
TEXAS NURSING. Text in English. 1925. m. USD 30. adv. bk.rev. back issues avail. **Document type:** *Trade.*
Related titles: Microform ed.
Indexed: CINAHL, Int.Nurs.Ind.
—BLDSC (8799.560000), GNLM.
Published by: Texas Nurses Association, 7600 Burnet Rd, 440, Austin, TX 78757-1241. TEL 512-452-0645, FAX 512-452-0648, http://www.texasnurses.org. Ed. John Levis Brown. Circ: 6,000.

610.73 DNK ISSN 0900-3002
TIDSKRIFT FOR SYGEPLEJEFORSKNING. Text in Danish. 1985. 3/yr. DKK 200 (effective 2001). adv. bk.rev. **Document type:** *Academic/Scholarly.*
Published by: Dansk Selskab for Sygeplejeforskning/ Danish Nursing Research Society, PO Box 37, Klampenborg 2930, Denmark. Ed. Lise Hounsgaard TEL 45-89-42-48-47. Circ: 1,000.

610.7306 332.88 NOR ISSN 0806-7511
TIDSKRIFTET SYKEPLEIEN. Text in Norwegian. 1912. 21/yr. NOK 645; NOK 45 newsstand/cover (effective 1999). adv. bk.rev. **Document type:** *Trade.*
Formed by the merger of (1990-1995): Sykepleien. Journal (0802-9776); (1992-1995): Sykepleien Fag (0804-1342); Which was formerly (until 1990): Sykepleien Fagtidskriftet (0802-9768); Sykepleien (0039-7628)
Indexed: Dent.Ind., Int.Nurs.Ind.
—CISTI, Infotrieve. **CCC.**
Published by: Norsk Sykepleierforbund/Norwegian Nurses Association, Postboks 2633, St Hanshaugen, Oslo 0131, Norway. TEL 47-22-04-33-04, FAX 47-22-38-35-36. Ed. Morten E Mathiesen. Adv. contact Maud P Kaino. B&W page NOK 19,900, color page NOK 21,200; trim 185 x 260. Circ: 55,009 (controlled).

610.73 NLD ISSN 0921-5832
HET TIJDSCHRIFT VOOR VERZORGENDEN. Text in Dutch. 1968. m. (11/yr.). NLG 116. adv. bk.rev. tr.lit. index. **Document type:** *Trade.* **Description:** Offers clinical and professional advice to nurses and caregivers for ailing persons in every sector.
Former titles (until 1988): B K Z (0169-7765); (until 1983): Tijdschrift voor Bejaarden-, Kraam- en Ziekenverzorging (0049-3880)
Indexed: Int.Nurs.Ind.
—CISTI.
Published by: Elsevier Gezondheidszorg B.V., Tijdstroom (Subsidiary of: Reed Elsevier plc Group), Planetenbaan 1, Maarssen 3600 AK, Netherlands. TEL 31-346-577577, FAX 31-346-554287, http://www.tijdstroom.nl. **Subscr. to:** Elsevier Den Haag, Postbus 16500, The Hague 2500 BM, Netherlands. TEL 31-70-381-9900, FAX 31-70-333-8399.

610.73 ISL ISSN 1022-2278
TIMARIT HJUKRUNARFRAEDINGA. Text in Icelandic. 1925. 5/yr. USD 50 to members (effective 2001). adv. bk.rev. illus. *Refereed.* **Document type:** *Newsletter, Academic/Scholarly, Trade.* **Description:** Publishes a wide variety of articles and news relevant to nursing as a profession and trade.
Former titles (until 1993): Hjukrun (0250-4731); (until 1978): Timarit Hjukrunarfelags Islands (0046-7634); (until 1959): Hjukrunarkvennabladid (0258-3798)
Indexed: Int.Nurs.Ind.
Published by: Felag islenskra hjukrunarfraedinga/Icelandic Nurses' Association, Sudurlandsbraut 22, Reykjavik 108, Iceland. TEL 354-568-7575, FAX 354-568-0727, hjukrun@hjukrun.is, http://www.hjukrun.is. Ed., R&P Valgerdur Katrin Jonsdottir. Circ: 3,500.

610.73 USA ISSN 1087-1667
TODAY'S SURGICAL NURSE. Text in English. 1979. bi-m. USD 38 to individuals; USD 58 in Canada to individuals; USD 78 elsewhere to individuals; USD 48 to institutions; USD 68 in Canada to institutions; USD 88 elsewhere to institutions. adv. bk.rev. back issues avail. **Document type:** *Trade.* **Description:** Provides up-to-the-minute information for the practicing operating room nurse.
Formerly (until 1996): Today's O R Nurse (0194-5181)
Related titles: Online - full text ed.: (from Northern Light Technology, Inc., ProQuest Information & Learning).
Indexed: CINAHL, Dent.Ind., Int.Nurs.Ind., Nurs.Abstr.
—GNLM, Infotrieve, ingenta. **CCC.**
Published by: Slack, Inc., 6900 Grove Rd, Thorofare, NJ 08086-9447. TEL 856-848-1000, 800-257-8290, FAX 856-853-5991, http://www.slackinc.com. Ed. Rose Marie McWilliams. Circ: 8,000.

610.73 617 AUS
TRANSPLANT NURSES JOURNAL✶. Text in English. 1992. 3/yr. AUD 40 to individuals; AUD 60 foreign to individuals. **Document type:** *Trade.*
Indexed: CINAHL.
Published by: Transplant Nurses' Association, c/o Health Services Union of Australia, 88 Mount Alexander Rd., Flemington, VIC, VIC 4066, Australia. TEL 61-7-3253-8748, FAX 61-7-3253-1382. Ed. Cecilia Boyd.

U.S. HEALTH CARE FINANCING ADMINISTRATION. MEDICARE SKILLED NURSING FACILITY MANUAL. see *INSURANCE*

610.73 BRA ISSN 0080-6234
UNIVERSIDADE DE SAO PAULO. ESCOLA DE ENFERMAGEM. REVISTA. Text in Portuguese. 1967. 4/yr. USD 100 (effective 2000). adv. index, cum.index. **Document type:** *Academic/Scholarly.*
Indexed: Ind.Med. (coverage dropped), Int.Nurs.Ind.
—BLDSC (7805.530000).
Published by: Universidade de Sao Paulo, Escola de Enfermagem, Av Dr Eneas Carvalho de Aguiar, 419, C Cesar, Sao Paulo, SP 05403-000, Brazil. TEL 55-11-30667524, FAX 55-11-30667524. Ed. Paulina Kurcgant. Pub., R&P Regina Toshie Takahashi. Adv. contact Alaide Moura de Oliveira. Circ: 1,000 (controlled).

610.73 GBR
UNIVERSITY OF SHEFFIELD. SCHOOL OF NURSING AND MIDWIFERY. RESEARCH REPORT. Text in English. 1996. irreg. **Document type:** *Monographic series, Academic/Scholarly.*
—BLDSC.
Published by: School of Nursing and Midwifery, 8 Brunswick Centre, Sheffield, S Yorks S10 2FN, United Kingdom. Ed. University Of Sheffield.

610.73 AUS ISSN 1442-617X
UNIVERSITY OF TECHNOLOGY, SYDNEY. FACULTY OF NURSING, MIDWIFERY AND HEALTH HANDBOOK. Text in English. 1990. a. AUD 11 domestic; AUD 13 foreign (effective 2000). **Document type:** *Catalog, Academic/Scholarly.* **Description:** Contains details about the faculty, schools, staff, courses, and other information pertaining to nursing students.
Formerly (until 1999): University of Technology, Sydney. Faculty of Nursing Handbook (1036-0700)
Published by: University of Technology, Sydney, City Campus, PO Box 123, Broadway, NSW 2007, Australia. TEL 61-2-9514-2000, FAX 61-2-9514-1551, publications@uts.eou.au, http://www.uts.eou.au/div/publications, http://www.uts.edu.au/div/publications. Circ: 3,000.

UROLOGIC NURSING. see *MEDICAL SCIENCES—Urology And Nephrology*

610.73 USA
UTAH NURSE. Text in English. 1975. q. free to members (effective 2001). adv. 24 p./no. back issues avail. **Document type:** *Newsletter, Trade.* **Description:** Covers issues and employment opportunities of interest to licensed nursing professionals.
Former titles: Pro Re Nata (1044-4025); (until 1987): One on One (0270-6628); U N A Communique; Utah Nurse
Indexed: CINAHL.
Published by: (Utah Nurses Association), Arthur L. Davis Publishing Agency, Inc., 517 Washington St, P O Box 216, Cedar Falls, IA 50613. TEL 319-277-2414, 800-626-4081, FAX 319-277-4055, http://www.utahnurses.com. Eds. Carol Roberts, Karen Dewey. R&P Karen Dewey. Circ: 22,000 (free).

610.73 VIR ISSN 0049-6464
V I N A QUARTERLY✶. Text in English. 1964. q. illus.
Indexed: Int.Nurs.Ind.
Published by: Virgin Islands Nurses Association, PO Box 2866, Charlotte Amalie, St. Thomas, Virgin Isl., US.

610.73 USA
V N A B NEWSLETTER. (Visiting Nurse Association of Brooklyn) Text in English. 1970. s-a. free per issue. charts, illus. **Document type:** *Newsletter.* **Description:** Covers news and services of the Visiting Nurse Association of Brooklyn.
Former titles: V N A Newsletter; In Step with the Visiting Nurse Association of Brooklyn (0046-8770)
Published by: Visiting Nurse Association of Brooklyn, 111 Livingston St, Brooklyn, NY 11201. TEL 718-923-7100, FAX 718-636-7572, http://www.vnabklyn.org. Ed. Jane Gould. R&P Glynis McBean TEL 718-230-6921. Circ: 5,000.

610.73 CAN
V O N CANADA ANNUAL REPORT (YEAR). Text in English. a. adv. **Document type:** *Corporate.*
Published by: Victorian Order of Nurses for Canada, 5 Blackburn Ave, Ottawa, ON K1N 8A2, Canada. TEL 613-233-5694, comm@von.ca, http://www.von.ca. Ed. Richard Marritt. R&P, Adv. contact Marie Belanger.

610.73 CAN ISSN 0846-135X
V O N CANADA REPORT. Text in English. q. **Document type:** *Newsletter.* **Description:** Reports on VON's commitment to innovative community based nursing and other health care and support services.
Published by: Victorian Order of Nurses for Canada, 5 Blackburn Ave, Ottawa, ON K1N 8A2, Canada. TEL 613-233-5694, comm@von.ca, http://www.von.ca. Ed. Richard Marritt. R&P Marie Belanger.

M

610.73 NOR ISSN 0107-4083
VAARD I NORDEN; sykepleievitenskap, omvaardnadsforskning og utvikling. Text in Danish, English, Norwegian, Swedish; Abstracts in English. 1981. q. NOK 280; NOK 125 to students (effective 2001). bk.rev. charts, illus. back issues avail. *Refereed.* **Document type:** *Journal, Abstract/Index, Academic/Scholarly.* **Description:** Focuses on development and research in nursing in the Nordic countries.
Related titles: CD-ROM ed.; E-mail ed.; Fax ed.; Online - full text ed.
Indexed: ASSIA.
—BLDSC (9146.090000).
Published by: Sykepleiernes Samarbeid i Norden/Northern Nurses Federation, Postboks 456, Sentrum, Oslo N-0104, Norway. TEL 47-22-04-33-04, FAX 47-22-41-48-68, marithelgerud@nosf.no. Ed. Martha Quivey. Circ: 1,500.

610.73 SWE ISSN 0347-0911
VAARDFACKET. Text in Swedish. 1934. 11/yr. SEK 590; SEK 53 newsstand/cover (effective 2001). adv. bk.rev. charts, illus, stat. index. **Document type:** *Magazine, Trade.*
Formerly (until 1978): Tidskrift foer Sveriges Sjukskoeterskor (0037-6027)
—CISTI, GNLM.
Published by: Vaardfoerbundet, Box 3207, Stockholm 10364, Sweden. TEL 46-8-14-77-00, FAX 46-8-411-19-93, http://www.vardforbundet.se/vf2/vf.htm. Ed., Pub., R&P Irene Wanland. Adv. contact Barbro Dahlqvist. B&W page SEK 22,740, color page SEK 30,930; trim 185 x 266. Circ: 113,800 (paid).

610.73 USA ISSN 1529-4609
VERMONT NURSE CONNECTION. Text in English. 199?. q. Free to qualified subscribers. adv. 20 p./no. **Document type:** *Newsletter, Trade.* **Description:** Covers issues and employment opportunities of interest to licensed nursing professionals.
Published by: (Vermont State Nurses' Association), Arthur L. Davis Publishing Agency, Inc., 517 Washington St, P O Box 216, Cedar Falls, IA 50613. TEL 319-277-2414, 800-626-4081, FAX 319-277-4055, sales@aldpub.com, http://www.aldpub.com/. Ed. Mark Miller. R&P Fran Keeler. Adv. contact Jim Larson. Circ: 10,000 (free).

610.73 USA ISSN 0191-1880
VERMONT REGISTERED NURSE. Text in English. 1934. q. USD 18. adv. **Document type:** *Newsletter.* **Description:** Contains association news and feature articles for members.
Indexed: CINAHL, Int.Nurs.Ind.
Published by: Vermont State Nurses' Association, 1 Main St, 26, Winooski, VT 05404-2230. TEL 802-655-7123, FAX 802-655-7187. Ed. Bonnie Stiles. R&P, Adv. contact Lynne Dapice. page USD 165. Circ: 500.

610.73 NLD ISSN 0920-3273
VERPLEEGKUNDE; Nederlandse-Vlaams tijdschrift voor verpleegkundigen. Text in Dutch, Flemish. 1986. q. NLG 79.25 domestic to individuals; NLG 148.75 foreign to individuals; NLG 152 to institutions. adv. bk.rev. **Document type:** *Academic/Scholarly.* **Description:** Covers case studies, research and items of interest to nursing leaders and teachers.
—GNLM.
Published by: Elsevier Gezondheidszorg B.V., Tijdstroom (Subsidiary of: Reed Elsevier plc Group), Planetenbaan 1, Maarssen 3600 AK, Netherlands. TEL 31-346-577577, FAX 31-346-554287, http://www.tijdstroom.nl. Ed. C L M Wiebnga. Circ: 2,500. **Subscr. to:** Elsevier Den Haag, Postbus 16500, The Hague 2500 BM, Netherlands. TEL 31-70-381-9900, FAX 31-70-333-8399.

610.73 USA ISSN 1084-4740
VIRGINIA NURSES TODAY. Text in English. 1976. q. Free to qualified subscribers. adv. bk.rev. 28 p./no. back issues avail. **Document type:** *Newsletter, Trade.* **Description:** Covers issues and employment opportunities of interest to licensed nursing professionals.
Former titles (until 1992): Virginia Nurse (0270-7780); Virginia Nurse Quarterly (0042-6695)
Indexed: CINAHL, Int.Nurs.Ind.
Published by: (Virginia Nurses Association), Arthur L. Davis Publishing Agency, Inc., 517 Washington St, P O Box 216, Cedar Falls, IA 50613. TEL 319-277-2414, 800-626-4081, FAX 319-277-4055, sales@aldpub.com, http://www.aldpub.com/. Ed. Mark Miller. R&P Jan Johnson. Adv. contact Jim Larson. Circ: 83,000 (free).

VITAL SIGNS PHARMACY SERVICES NEWSLETTER. see *PHARMACY AND PHARMACOLOGY*

610.73 USA ISSN 0734-5666
WASHINGTON NURSE✱. Text in English. 1929. q. USD 20 domestic; USD 26 in Canada & Mexico; USD 39 elsewhere (effective 1999). adv. bk.rev. back issues avail. **Document type:** *Trade.* **Description:** Provides information about professional, educational, ethical, legal, economic, and legislative issues affecting the practice of nursing.
Supersedes (in 1977): W S N A Mini Journal
Indexed: CINAHL, Int.Nurs.Ind.
—BLDSC (9263.210000).
Published by: Washington State Nurses Association, 575 Andover Park W #101, Seattle, WA 981188-3348. TEL 206-443-9762, FAX 206-728-2074, dshepard@wsna.org. Ed., R&P, Adv. contact Denise Shepard. page USD 499; 9 x 6.5. Circ: 7,000 (paid).

610.73 USA ISSN 1074-8091
WEST VIRGINIA NURSE. Text in English. 1927. q. Free to qualified subscribers. adv. 20 p./no. back issues avail. **Document type:** *Newsletter, Trade.* **Description:** Covers issues and employment opportunities of interest to licensed nursing professionals.
Formerly: Weather Vane (0043-1664)
Indexed: CINAHL, Int.Nurs.Ind.
Published by: (West Virginia Nurses Association), Arthur L. Davis Publishing Agency, Inc., 517 Washington St, P O Box 216, Cedar Falls, IA 50613. TEL 319-277-2414, 800-626-4081, FAX 319-277-4055, sales@aldpub.com, http://www.aldpub.com/. Ed. Mark Miller. R&P Cher Montgomery. Adv. contact Jim Larson. Circ: 31,000 (free).

610.73 USA ISSN 0193-9459
WESTERN JOURNAL OF NURSING RESEARCH; an international forum for communicating nursing research. Text in English. 1979. 8/yr. USD 100 to individuals; USD 510 to institutions; USD 20 newsstand/cover to individuals; USD 75 newsstand/cover to institutions (effective 2002). adv. bk.rev., film rev. abstr, bibl, charts, illus, stat. cum.index. back issues avail.; reprints avail. *Refereed.* **Document type:** *Academic/Scholarly.* **Description:** Provides a forum for scholarly debate and for research and theoretical papers. Clinical studies have commentaries and rebuttals.
Related titles: Online - full text ed.: (from EBSCO Publishing, O C L C Online Computer Library Center, Inc., RoweCom Information Quest, ProQuest Information & Learning, Gale Group, ingenta, Swets Blackwell, Institute for Scientific Information).
Indexed: ASCA, ASSIA, AgeLine, Behav.Med.Abstr., CINAHL, Chic.Per.Ind., Curr.Cont., Fam.Ind., Human Resour.Abstr., Ind.Med. (1979-), Int.Nurs.Ind., PsycInfo, Psychol.Abstr. (1991-), SSCI, Sage Fam.Stud.Abstr., THA, Viol.& Abuse Abstr., e-psyche.
—BLDSC (9300.835000), GNLM, IDS, ingenta, KNAW. **CCC.**
Published by: Sage Publications, Inc., 2455 Teller Rd, Thousand Oaks, CA 91320. TEL 805-499-0721, FAX 805-499-0871, info@sagepub.com, http://www.sagepub.com. Ed. Pamela J Brink. Pub. Sara Miller McCune. R&P Tanya Udin. Adv. contact DeAnna Vega Hammersley. Circ: 2,000. **Overseas subscr. to:** Sage Publications Ltd., 6 Bonhill St, London EC2A 4PU, United Kingdom; Sage Publications India Pvt. Ltd., 4215, New Delhi 110 048, India.

610.73 920 USA
WHO'S WHO IN AMERICAN NURSING. Text in English. 1984. irreg., latest 1995. USD 149.95. **Document type:** *Directory.* **Description:** Lists biographies of over 22,000 leading American primary care nurses, nursing administrators, educators, researchers, and other specialists. These individuals are indexed by city and state within their specialties.
Formed by the 1991 merger of: Who's Who in American Nursing. Administrators, Educators, and Other Nursing Professionals (1062-2411); Who's Who in American Nursing. Primary Care Nurses in Clinical Settings (1062-242X); Which was formerly (until 1989): Who's Who in American Nursing (0740-7912)
Related titles: CD-ROM ed.: (from Bowker Electronic Publishing); Magnetic Tape ed.
Published by: Marquis Who's Who (Subsidiary of: Reed Elsevier plc Group), 121 Chanlon Rd, New Providence, NJ 07964. TEL 908-464-6800, FAX 908-665-6688, info@reedref.com, http://www.reedref.com. **Subscr. to:** Order Dept., PO Box 31, New Providence, NJ 07974-9903. TEL 800-521-8110.

610.73 USA
WYOMING NURSE. Text in English. 1926. q. Free to qualified subscribers. adv. 24 p./no. **Document type:** *Newsletter, Trade.* **Description:** Covers issues and employment opportunities of interest to licensed nursing professionals.
Formerly: Wyoming Nurses Newsletter (0084-3164)
Indexed: CINAHL.
Published by: (Wyoming Nurses Association), Arthur L. Davis Publishing Agency, Inc., 517 Washington St, P O Box 216, Cedar Falls, IA 50613. TEL 319-277-2414, 800-626-4081, FAX 319-277-4055, sales@aldpub.com, http://www.aldpub.com/. Ed. Mark Miller. R&P Beverly J McDermott. Adv. contact Jim Larson. Circ: 6,000 (free).

610.73 ZMB
ZAMBIA NURSE✱. Text in English. 1965. 3/yr. ZMK 5. adv. bk.rev.
Indexed: CINAHL, Int.Nurs.Ind.
Published by: (Zambia Nurses Association), Mission Press, PO Box 71581, Ndola, Zambia. Eds. N Booth, P S Chibuye. Circ: 1,000.

610.73 CHN ISSN 0254-1769
ZHONGHUA HULI ZAZHI/CHINESE JOURNAL OF NURSING. Text in Chinese. m. CNY 5 newsstand/cover domestic; USD 39.60 foreign; USD 3.30 newsstand/cover foreign (effective 2001). **Document type:** *Academic/Scholarly.*
Related titles: Online - full content ed.: (from WanFang Data Corp.).
—BLDSC (3180.439000).
Published by: Zhonghua Huli Xuehui, 42, Dong 4-Xi Dajie, Beijing 100710, China. TEL 86-1-64013293. **Dist. by:** China International Book Trading Corp, 35, Chegongzhuang Xilu, Haidian District, Beijing 100044, China. TEL 86-1-68413849, FAX 86-1-68412048, cibtc@mail.cibtc.com.cn, http://www.cibtc.com.cn.

ZORGVISIE. see *HEALTH FACILITIES AND ADMINISTRATION*

MEDICAL SCIENCES—Obstetrics And Gynecology

see also WOMEN'S HEALTH

618.202 AUS ISSN 1031-170X
A C M I JOURNAL. (Australian College of Midwives Incorporated) Text in English. 1988. q. AUD 60 domestic; AUD 75 foreign (effective 2001). adv. bk.rev., video rev. stat, tr.lit. back issues avail. *Refereed.* **Document type:** *Academic/Scholarly.*
—BLDSC (1798.183000), GNLM.
Published by: Australian College of Midwives Inc., 1st Fl., 3 Bowen Cresent, Melbourne, VIC 3000, Australia. TEL 61-3-9804-5071, FAX 61-3-9866-1370, austmid@ozemail.com.au. Ed. Pauline Glover. R&P, Adv. contact Alanna Street. B&W page AUD 500, color page AUD 1,000. Circ: 3,000.

A C O G CLINICAL REVIEW. see *MEDICAL SCIENCES—Abstracting, Bibliographies, Statistics*

A I U M REPORTER. see *MEDICAL SCIENCES—Radiology And Nuclear Medicine*

A W H O N N NEWSLETTER. see *MEDICAL SCIENCES—Nurses And Nursing*

ACTA CHIRURGICA MEDITERRANEA. see *MEDICAL SCIENCES—Surgery*

618 ESP ISSN 0001-5776
CODEN: ACGLA
ACTA GINECOLOGICA. Text in Spanish; Summaries in English. 1958. 10/yr. ESP 9,000 domestic; USD 100 foreign (effective 2001). adv. bk.rev. illus. index. **Document type:** *Academic/Scholarly.*
Related titles: Translation of: Journal of Gynaecology & Obstetrics.
Indexed: Biol.Abstr., Chem.Abstr., Excerp.Med., Helminthol.Abstr., Ind.Med. (coverage dropped), Ind.Med.Esp.
—BLDSC (0622.600000), CISTI, EMDOCS, GNLM, Infotrieve, KNAW. **CCC.**
Published by: Editores Medicos S.A., Gabriela Mistral, 2, Madrid 28035, Spain. TEL 34-91-3768140, FAX 34-91-3739907. Circ: 2,000.

ACTA MEDICA AUXOLOGICA. see *MEDICAL SCIENCES—Endocrinology*

618 ESP
ACTA OBSTETRICA ET GYNECOLOGICA. Text in Spanish. 1988. bi-m. **Document type:** *Academic/Scholarly.* **Description:** Publishes clinical and research articles in obstetrics and gynecology.
Formerly: Acta Obstetrica et Gynecologica Scandinavica (Edicion Espanola) (0214-0977)
Indexed: Ind.Vet., Inpharma, Int.Nurs.Ind., Reac., THA.

M

Published by: Saned S.A., Capitan Haya, 60, Madrid 28020, Spain. TEL 34-91-749-9507, FAX 34-91-749-9507, saned@meditex.es. Ed. M Escudero. adv.: page ESP 200,000. Circ: 3,000.

618 DNK ISSN 0001-6349 CODEN: AOGSAE
ACTA OBSTETRICA ET GYNECOLOGICA SCANDINAVICA. Text in English. 1921. 12/yr. USD 444 in the Americas to institutions print & online eds. combined; GBP 308 elsewhere to institutions print & online eds. combined (effective 2002). adv. bk.rev. bibl, charts, illus. cum.index: 1922-1952; 1953-1962. back issues avail. *Refereed.* **Document type:** *Academic/Scholarly.*
Formerly (until 1925): Acta Gynecologica Scandinavica
Related titles: Microfiche ed.; Online - full text ed.: ISSN 1600-0412. GBP 270 (effective 2002) (from Ovid Technologies, Inc., ingenta, Munksgaard & Blackwell Science's Synergy, Swets Blackwell, Institute for Scientific Information).
Indexed: ASCA, Abstr.Hyg., Agri.& Environ.Biotech.Abstr. (coverage dropped), Biol.Abstr., Chem.Abstr., Curr.Adv.Ecol.Sci., Curr.Cont., Curr.Lit.Fam.Plan., Dairy Sci.Abstr., Derwent Biotech.Abstr., Excerp.Med., INIS Atomind., Ind.Med. (1926-), Ind.Sci.Rev., Inpharma, NRN, Nutr.Abstr., Pharm.&Out.News, Protozool.Abstr., Reac., Rev.Med.& Vet.Mycol., Risk Abstr., Rural Devel.Abstr., SSCI (coverage dropped), Sci.Cit.Ind., Sugar Ind.Abstr., Trop.Dis.Bull.
—BLDSC (0641.600000), ADONIS, CASDDS, CISTI, EMDOCS, GNLM, IDS, ingenta, KNAW. **CCC.**
Published by: (Federation of Scandinavian Societies of Obstetrics and Gynecology), Blackwell Munksgaard, Noerre Soegade 35, PO Box 2148, Copenhagen K 1016, Denmark. FAX 45-77-33-33-77, customerservice@munksgaard.dk, http://www.munksgaard.dk/actaobstetgynecol. Ed. Per-Olof Janson. Adv. contact Eric Rozario TEL 45-77-33-33-01. Circ: 4,600.

618 DNK ISSN 0300-8835 CODEN: AGSSAI
ACTA OBSTETRICA ET GYNECOLOGICA SCANDINAVICA. SUPPLEMENT. Text in English. irreg. free to subscribers of Acta Obstetrica et Gynecologica Scandinavica. **Document type:** *Academic/Scholarly.*
Related titles: Online - full text ed.: ISSN 1600-5457 (from Ovid Technologies, Inc.).
Indexed: Arts & Hum.Cit.Ind. (coverage dropped), Biol.Abstr., Chem.Abstr., Curr.Adv.Ecol.Sci., Dairy Sci.Abstr., Excerp.Med., Helminthol.Abstr., INIS Atomind., Ind.Med. (1926-), Ind.Sci.Rev., Nutr.Abstr.
—BLDSC (0641.605000), ADONIS, CASDDS, CISTI, EMDOCS, KNAW. **CCC.**
Published by: (Association of Scandinavian Societies of Obstetric and Gynecology Publishers), Blackwell Munksgaard, Noerre Soegade 35, PO Box 2148, Copenhagen K 1016, Denmark. TEL 45-77-33-33-33, FAX 45-77-33-33-77, customerservice@munksgaard.dk, http://www.munksgaard.dk/actaobstetgynecol. Ed. Per-Olof Janson. Adv. contact Eric Rozario TEL 45-77-33-33-01.

618 TUR ISSN 0252-9696 CODEN: ARTUD7
ACTA REPRODUCTIVA TURCICA. Text and summaries in English. 1979-19??; resumed 1992. q. TRL 110,000 (effective 1993). adv. abstr, charts, illus. *Refereed.* **Document type:** *Academic/Scholarly.* **Description:** Publishes original research studies in obstetrics and gynecology, reproductive biology, public health, and related fields, including endocrinology, pediatrics, surgery and population studies.
Indexed: Bibl.Repro., Biol.Abstr.
—CISTI.
Published by: Hacettepe University, Department of Gynecology and Obstetrics, Ankara, Turkey. Ed. Dr. Husnu A Kisnisci. Circ: 1,000. **Co-sponsor:** Hacettepe University, Department of Public Health.

618.3 USA ISSN 0731-1400 CODEN: APMDD9
ADVANCES IN PERINATAL MEDICINE. Text in English. 1981. irreg., latest vol.5. **Document type:** *Monographic series, Academic/Scholarly.*
—CASDDS, GNLM.
Published by: Kluwer Academic - Plenum Publishers (Subsidiary of: Wolters Kluwer N.V.), 233 Spring St, New York, NY 10013-1578. TEL 212-620-8000, 800-221-9369, FAX 212-463-0742, info@plenum.com, http://www.plenum.com.

618 616.6 NLD
ADVANCES IN REPRODUCTIVE HEALTH CARE. Text in English. irreg., latest vol.6, 1984. price varies. back issues avail. *Refereed.* **Document type:** *Monographic series.*
Published by: Kluwer Academic Publishers Group (Subsidiary of: Wolters Kluwer N.V.), Spuiboulevard 50, PO Box 17, Dordrecht 3300 AA, Netherlands. FAX 31-78-639-2254, services@wkap.nl, http://www.wkap.nl. **Dist. by:** Journals Department, PO Box 322, Dordrecht 3300 AH, Netherlands. FAX 31-78-654-6474.

618 DEU ISSN 1436-2627 CODEN: TWGYE
AERZTLICHE PRAXIS. GYNAEKOLOGIE. Short title: Ae P Gynaekologie. Text in German. 1988. 12/yr. DEM 98; DEM 126 foreign (effective 1998). adv. **Document type:** *Trade.*
Former titles (until 1998): T und E Gynaekologie (1435-7739); (until 1997): T W Gynaekologie (0935-3208)
Indexed: Excerp.Med.
—BLDSC (1738.516000), EMDOCS, GNLM. **CCC.**
Published by: Reed Elsevier Deutschland GmbH (Subsidiary of: Reed Elsevier group), Gabrielenstr 9, Munich 80636, Germany. TEL 49-89-89817-0, FAX 49-89-89817400, http://aep.r-e.de. Ed. Annette Leinberger. Pub. Wolfram Haase. Adv. contact Marina Vasilj.

618.2 DEU ISSN 0935-0810
AERZTLICHER RATGEBER FUER WERDENDE UND JUNGE MUETTER; die Schwangerschaft, Geburt und Babyzeit. Text in German. 1964. 3/yr. free per issue. adv. **Document type:** *Consumer.* **Description:** Supplies useful information to expectant mothers as well as single mothers and fathers.
Published by: (Deutsches Gruenes Kreuz e.V.), Wort und Bild Verlag Konradshoehe GmbH, Konradshoehe, Baierbrunn 82065, Germany. TEL 49-89-74433-0, FAX 49-89-74433155. Ed. Dorothee Walzel. R&P Harald Pohl TEL 49-89-74433164. Adv. contact Christine Waeninger. Circ: 240,000 (controlled).

618 JPN ISSN 0917-0162
AICHI BOSEI EISEI GAKKAISHI/AICHI JOURNAL OF MATERNAL HEALTH. Text in Japanese. 1985. a. JPY 2,000. adv. bk.rev., film rev., software rev. bibl, illus. **Document type:** *Bulletin.*
Published by: Aichi Bosei Eisei Gakkai/Aichi Society of Maternal Health, Nagoya Daigaku Iryo Gijutsu Tanki Daigaku, 1-20 Taiko-Minami 1-chome, Higashi-ku, Nagoya-shi, Aichi-ken 461-0000, Japan. TEL 052-723-1111, FAX 052-723-0290. Ed. Miyoko Ogiso. Circ: 300.

618 JPN
AKITA SANFUJINKA IHO/AKITA JOURNAL OF OBSTETRICIANS AND GYNECOLOGISTS. Text in Japanese. 1976. bi-m. free per issue. **Document type:** *Bulletin.*
Published by: Nihon Sanka Fujinka Gakkai, Akita Chiho Bukai/Japan Society of Obstetrics and Gynecology, Akita Branch, Akita-ken Ishi Kaikan, 6-6 Senshu-kubota-cho, Akita-shi 010-0000, Japan. TEL 81-188-33-7401, FAX 81-188-32-1356. Ed. Toshiya Ohkura. Circ: 100.

618 RUS ISSN 0300-9092
AKUSHERSTVO I GINEKOLOGIYA/OBSTETRICS AND GYNECOLOGY. Text in Russian; Summaries in English. 1922. bi-m. USD 105 foreign (effective 2000). adv. bk.rev., Website rev. illus. index. **Document type:** *Journal, Academic/Scholarly.* **Description:** Publishes original and survey papers dealing with modern scientific achievements in the field of obstetrics and gynecology. Covers physiology and pathology of the fetus and the newborn, scientific and practical problems of diagnosis, treatment of complications in pregnancy, labor and gynecologic diseases.
Indexed: Abstr.Bulg.Sci.Med.Lit., Biol.Abstr., Chem.Abstr., Chem.Indus.Notes, Chem.Titles, Dairy Sci.Abstr., Excerp.Med., INIS Atomind., Ind.Med. (1962-), Ind.Sci.Rev., Nutr.Abstr., Ref.Zh.
—CISTI, East View, EMDOCS, GNLM, Infotrieve. **CCC.**
Published by: Izdatel'stvo Meditsina, Petroverigskii per 6-8, Moscow 101000, Russian Federation. TEL 7-095-9248785, 7-095-928-86-48, FAX 7-095-9211355, meditisina@iname.com, http://www.medit.ru. Ed. A P Kiryushchenkov. Pub. A M Stochik. R&P N Biyatova. Adv. contact O A Fadeeva TEL 7-095-923-51-40. Circ: 6,000. **Dist. by:** Mezhdunarodnaya Kniga, B Yakimanka 39, Moscow 117049, Russian Federation. TEL 7-095-2384967, FAX 7-095-2384634; **US dist. addr.:** East View Publications, 3020 Harbor Ln N, Minneapolis, MN 55447. TEL 612-550-0961.

AMERICAN ASSOCIATION OF GENITO-URINARY SURGEONS. TRANSACTIONS. see *MEDICAL SCIENCES—Gastroenterology*

618 USA ISSN 1074-3804 CODEN: JAALF3
AMERICAN ASSOCIATION OF GYNECOLOGIC LAPAROSCOPISTS. JOURNAL. Text in English. 1993. q. USD 115 to non-members; USD 145 to institutions. adv. bk.rev. *Refereed.* **Document type:** *Academic/Scholarly.* **Description:** Articles to educate, inform, and update ob-gyn doctors, residents, fellows, and operating room personnel.
Related titles: Online - full text ed.: (from Institute for Scientific Information).
Indexed: ASCA, Curr.Cont., Excerp.Med. (1995-), Ind.Med. (1993-), Inpharma, Reac.
—BLDSC (4683.830000), CISTI, EMDOCS, GNLM, IDS, KNAW.
Published by: American Association of Gynecologic Laparoscopists, 13021 E Florence Ave, Santa Fe Springs, CA 90670-4505. TEL 562-946-8774, 800-554-2245, FAX 562-946-9204, journal@aagl.com, http://www.aagl.com. Ed. Robert B Hunt. R&P Clifford K Chu. Adv. contact James T Brady.

618 USA ISSN 0002-9378
RG1 CODEN: AJOGAH
AMERICAN JOURNAL OF OBSTETRICS AND GYNECOLOGY. Text in English. 1920. m. USD 174 domestic to individuals; USD 215 foreign to individuals; USD 370 domestic to institutions; USD 411 foreign to institutions; USD 83 domestic to students; USD 124 foreign to students; USD 35 newsstand/cover domestic (effective 2001). adv. illus. s-a. index. reprint service avail. from PQC. *Refereed.* **Document type:** *Journal, Academic/Scholarly.* **Description:** Devoted to obstetrics, gynecology, fetuses, the placenta and the newborn.
Related titles: CD-ROM ed.: (from Ovid Technologies, Inc.); Microform ed.: (from PQC,PMC); Online - full text ed.: (from Ovid Technologies, Inc., EBSCO Publishing, Gale Group, IDEAL Online Library, Institute for Scientific Information, RoweCom Information Quest).
Indexed: AIM, ASCA, Abstr.Anthropol., Abstr.Hyg., Agri.& Environ.Biotech.Abstr. (coverage dropped), Anim.Breed.Abstr., Behav.Med.Abstr., Bibl.Dev.Med.& Child Neur., Biol.Abstr., Biol.Dig., Brit.Nur.Ind., C.C.I.Ob.Gyn., CINAHL, Chem.Abstr., Chem.Indus.Notes, Chem.Titles, Curr.Adv.Biochem., Curr.Adv.Cancer Res., Curr.Adv.Cell & Devel.Biol., Curr.Adv.Ecol.Sci., Curr.Adv.Gen.& Molec.Biol., Curr.Cont., Curr.Lit.Fam.Plan., Dairy Sci.Abstr., Derwent Biotech.Abstr., Diab.Cont., Dok.Arbeitsmed., Excerp.Med., FAMLI, Fam.Ind., INIS Atomind., I.P.A., Ind.Med. (1920-), Ind.Sci.Rev., Ind.Vet., Inpharma, Int.Abstr.Biol.Sci., Int.Nurs.Ind., Jrnl.Watch Wom.Hlth., Kidney, Med.& Surg.Dermat., NRN, Neurosci.Cit.Ind., Nutr.Abstr., Pharm.&Out.News, Protozool.Abstr., Reac., Rel.Ind.One, Rel.Ind.Two, Rev.Med.& Vet.Mycol., Rev.Plant Path., Risk Abstr., SSCI (coverage dropped), Sage Fam.Stud.Abstr., Sci.Cit.Ind., THA, Trop.Dis.Bull., Vet.Bull.
—BLDSC (0828.700000), ADONIS, CASDDS, CISTI, EMDOCS, GNLM, IDS, ingenta, KNAW. **CCC.**
Published by: (American Gynecological and Obstetrical Society), Mosby, Inc. (Subsidiary of: Elsevier Science), 11830 Westline Industrial Dr, St Louis, MO 63146-3318. TEL 314-872-8370, 800-325-4177, FAX 314-432-1380, http://www.mosby.com/ajog, http://www.mosby.com/periodicals. Eds. E J Quilligan, Dr. Frederick P Zuspan. Pub. Cheryl A Smart. Adv. contact Gale Schlogl TEL 314-453-4337. B&W page USD 1,650, color page USD 2,925; trim 10.88 x 8.13. Circ: 13,804 (paid and free). **Co-sponsor:** American Board of Obstetrics and Gynecology, Society of Gynecologic Surgeons, Society of Perinatal Obstetricians.

618.3 USA ISSN 0735-1631
RG600
AMERICAN JOURNAL OF PERINATOLOGY. Text in English. 1983. 8/yr. EUR 185 to individuals; EUR 410 to institutions; EUR 51 newsstand/cover (effective 2002). adv. bk.rev. reprints avail. *Refereed.* **Document type:** *Journal, Academic/Scholarly.* **Description:** Examines all aspects of perinatal and critical-care management, including maternal risk factors, antenatal diagnosis and intervention, abnormalities and complications of pregnancy, labor and delivery, and congenital and acquired diseases and disorders in newborns.
Related titles: Online - full text ed.: ISSN 1098-8785 (from Ovid Technologies, Inc., EBSCO Publishing, O C L C Online Computer Library Center, Inc., RoweCom Information Quest, Institute for Scientific Information).
Indexed: ASCA, Bibl.Dev.Med.& Child Neur., CINAHL, Curr.Cont., Excerp.Med., INIS Atomind., Ind.Med. (1983-), Inpharma, Int.Nurs.Ind., Pharm.&Out.News, Protozool.Abstr., Reac., SSCI (coverage dropped), Sci.Cit.Ind. (coverage dropped).

M

—BLDSC (0829.900000), CISTI, EMDOCS, GNLM, IDS, ingenta, KNAW. **CCC.**

Published by: Thieme Medical Publishers, 333 Seventh Ave, New York, NY 10001. TEL 212-760-0888, 800-782-3488, FAX 212-947-1112, http://www.thieme.com. Adv. contact Jean Azzato. Circ: 1,600. **Orders in Europe to:** Thieme International, Postfach 301120, Stuttgart 70451, Germany. TEL 49-711-8931-0, 49-711-8931-298.

AMERICAN JOURNAL OF REPRODUCTIVE IMMUNOLOGY. see *MEDICAL SCIENCES—Allergology And Immunology*

AMERICAN JOURNAL OF REPRODUCTIVE IMMUNOLOGY ONLINE. see *MEDICAL SCIENCES—Allergology And Immunology*

ANNALES CHIRURGIAE ET GYNAECOLOGIAE. see *MEDICAL SCIENCES—Surgery*

618 ITA ISSN 0300-0087
CODEN: AOGMAU

ANNALI DI OSTETRICIA GINECOLOGIA MEDICINA PERINATALE. Summaries in English, Italian. 1879. bi-m. ITL 70,000; ITL 100,000 foreign. adv. bibl, charts, illus. index.

Formerly (until 1971): Annali di Ostetricia e Ginecologia (0003-4657)

Indexed: Biol.Abstr., Chem.Abstr., Excerp.Med., Ind.Med. (coverage dropped).

—BLDSC (1016.190000), CASDDS, CISTI, GNLM.

Published by: (Universita degli Studi di Milano, Clinica Ostetrica e Ginecologica), Istituti Clinici di Perfezionamento, Via Francesco Daverio, 6, Milan, MI 20122, Italy. Ed. G B Candiani.

618 JPN ISSN 0913-8307

AOMORIKEN RINSHO SANFUJINKA IKAISHI/AOMORI SOCIETY OF OBSTETRICIANS AND GYNECOLOGISTS. JOURNAL. Text in English, Japanese; Summaries in English. 1986. s-a.

Published by: Aomoriken Rinsho Sanfujinka Ikai, Hirosaki Daigaku Igakubu Sanfujinka Kyoshitsu, 5 Zaifu-cho, Hirosaki-shi, Aomori-ken 036-8216, Japan.

618.92 GBR ISSN 1359-2998

ARCHIVES OF DISEASE IN CHILDHOOD. FETAL AND NEONATAL EDITION. Text in English. 1988. bi-m. GBP 85 combined subscription to individuals includes print & online eds.; USD 136 combined subscription to individuals includes print & online eds (effective 2002). adv. bk.rev. abstr, charts, illus. index. reprint service avail. from PQC. *Refereed.* **Document type:** *Journal, Academic/Scholarly.* **Description:** Focuses on research in neonatology, genetics, fetal medicine, neurodevelopmental medicine, fetal physiology, and perinatal epidemiology.

Related titles: Microfilm ed.: (from PQC); Online - full text ed.: e A D C - F & N. ISSN 1468-2052. 1997. GBP 50, USD 75 to individuals (effective 2002) (from Ovid Technologies, Inc., EBSCO Publishing, O C L C Online Computer Library Center, Inc., RoweCom Information Quest, ingenta, Swets Blackwell); ♦ Supplement to: Archives of Disease in Childhood. ISSN 0003-9888.

Indexed: Abstr.Hyg., Dairy Sci.Abstr., Ind.Med. (1988-), Int.Nurs.Ind., Nutr.Abstr., Rev.Arom.& Med.Plants, Rural Devel.Abstr., THA, Trop.Dis.Bull.

—ADONIS.

Published by: B M J Publishing Group, B M A House, Tavistock Sq, London WC1H 9JR, United Kingdom. TEL 44-20-7387-4499, FAX 44-20-7383-6400, info.norththames@bma.org.uk, http://www.archdischild.com/, http://www.bma.org.uk. Ed. H Marcovitch. Adv. contact Euan Currer TEL 44-20-7383-6181.

618.1 DEU ISSN 0932-0067
CODEN: AGOBEJ

ARCHIVES OF GYNECOLOGY AND OBSTETRICS. Text in English. 1870. 4/yr. EUR 469.40 domestic; EUR 466.90 in Germany; EUR 138 newsstand/cover foreign (effective 2002). adv. bibl, charts, illus. index. back issues avail.; reprint service avail. from ISI. *Refereed.* **Document type:** *Journal, Academic/Scholarly.* **Description:** Informs about the latest advances in gynecology and allied fields.

Former titles: Archives of Gynecology (0170-9925); Archiv fuer Gynaekologie (0003-9128)

Related titles: Microfiche ed.: (from BHP); Microform ed.: (from PQC); Online - full text ed.: ISSN 1432-0711 (from EBSCO Publishing, RoweCom Information Quest, Swets Blackwell, Springer LINK, Institute for Scientific Information).

Indexed: ASCA, Anim.Breed.Abstr., Biol.Abstr., Chem.Abstr., Chem.Indus.Notes, Chem.Titles, Curr.Adv.Cancer Res., Curr.Adv.Cell & Devel.Biol., Curr.Adv.Ecol.Sci., Curr.Cont. (coverage dropped), Dairy Sci.Abstr., Excerp.Med., INIS Atomind., Ind.Med. (1987-), Ind.Sci.Rev., Inpharma, NRN, Nutr.Abstr., Pharm.&Out.News, Reac., SSCI (coverage dropped), Sci.Cit.Ind.

—BLDSC (1634.404000), CASDDS, CISTI, EMDOCS, GNLM, IDS, Infotrieve, ingenta, KNAW. **CCC.**

Published by: (Deutschen Gesellschaft fuer Gynaekologie und Geburtshilfe), Springer-Verlag (Subsidiary of: BertelsmannSpringer), Tiergartenstr 17, Heidelberg 69121, Germany. TEL 49-6221-345-0, FAX 49-6221-345229, subscriptions@springer.de, http://link.springer.de/link/service/journals/00404/index.htm, http://www.springer.de. **Subscr. in N. America to:** Springer-Verlag New York Inc., PO Box 2485, Secaucus, NJ 07096-2485. TEL 212-460-1500, FAX 212-473-6272.

618 ITA ISSN 0004-0126
CODEN: AOGNAX

ARCHIVIO DI OSTETRICIA E GINECOLOGIA. Text in Italian. 1975 (vol.80). q. ITL 60,000; USD 90 foreign (effective 1999). **Document type:** *Academic/Scholarly.*

Indexed: Biol.Abstr., Chem.Abstr., Excerp.Med., Ind.Med. (coverage dropped).

—CASDDS, CISTI, GNLM.

Published by: (Universita di Napoli, Clinica Ostetrica e Ginecologica), Giannini Editore, Via Cisterna dell'Olio, Naples, NA 80134, Italy. TEL 39-81-5513928. Ed. Enzo Martella.

ASIAN AND PACIFIC WOMEN'S RESOURCE AND ACTION SERIES. see *WOMEN'S INTERESTS*

618.2 FRA

ASSOCIATION DES SAGES-FEMMES DE LA MATERNITE DE NANCY. BULLETIN. Text in French. 1946. q. FRF 75. adv.

Published by: Association des Sages-Femmes de l'Ecole d'Accouchement de la Maternite de Nancy, rue du Docteur-Heydendreich, Nancy 54000, France. Ed. Mme Poutas. Circ: 1,400.

618 ITA ISSN 0004-7317

ATTUALITA DI OSTETRICIA E GINECOLOGIA. Text in Italian; Summaries in English, French, German, Italian. 1955. bi-m. ITL 20,000.

Indexed: Biol.Abstr.

—CISTI, GNLM.

Published by: (Universita degli Studi di Padova, Facolta di Medicina e Chirurgia), Societa Editrice Universo, Via Giovanni Battista Morgagni, 1, Rome, RM 00161, Italy. Ed. Giuseppe Vecchietti.

618 USA ISSN 0271-129X

AUDIO-DIGEST OBSTETRICS - GYNECOLOGY. Text in English. 1954. s-m. USD 168 (effective 2000). *Refereed.*

Media: Audio cassette/tape.

—ingenta.

Published by: Audio-Digest Foundation (Subsidiary of: California Medical Association), 1577 E Chevy Chase Dr, Glendale, CA 91206. TEL 213-245-8505, 800-423-2308, FAX 818-240-7379, 800-845-4375. Ed. Claron L Oakley. Circ: (controlled).

618 AUS ISSN 0004-8666
CODEN: AZOGBS

AUSTRALIAN AND NEW ZEALAND JOURNAL OF OBSTETRICS AND GYNECOLOGY. Text in English. 1961. q. AUD 75 to Australia, Papua New Guinea, New Zealand; AUD 85 elsewhere (effective 2000). adv. bk.rev. charts, illus. index. back issues avail. *Refereed.* **Document type:** *Academic/Scholarly.* **Description:** Covers clinical obstetrics and gynaecology and related research.

Related titles: Online - full text ed.: (from Institute for Scientific Information).

Indexed: ASCA, Bibl.Dev.Med.& Child Neur., Biol.Abstr., Curr.Adv.Ecol.Sci., Curr.Cont., Excerp.Med., Fam.Ind., Helminthol.Abstr., INIS Atomind., Ind.Med. (1961-), Inpharma, NRN, Nutr.Abstr., Pharm.&Out.News, Reac., SSCI (coverage dropped), So.Pac.Per.Ind., THA.

—BLDSC (1796.890000), CASDDS, CISTI, GNLM, IDS, ingenta, KNAW.

Published by: Royal Australian & New Zealand College of Obstetricians & Gynecologists, 254-260 Albert St, East Melbourne, VIC 3002, Australia. TEL 61-3-94171699, FAX 61-3-94190672, 61-3-9415-9306, racog@racog.edu.au, ranzcog@ranzcog.edu.au, http://medrwh.unimelb.edu.au/anzjog/anzjog-index.htm. Ed., R&P Shaun A Brennecke. Adv. contact Bill Minnis. Circ: 5,300 (paid and controlled).

618 GBR ISSN 1521-6934
CODEN: BPRGFM

BAILLIERE'S BEST PRACTICE & RESEARCH IN CLINICAL OBSTETRICS AND GYNAECOLOGY. Text in English. 1974. bi-m. GBP 134 to individuals; GBP 230 to institutions (effective 2002). *Refereed.* **Document type:** *Academic/Scholarly.*

Formerly (until 1999): Bailliere's Clinical Obstetrics and Gynaecology (0950-3552); Which superseded in part (in 1987): Clinics in Obstetrics and Gynaecology (0306-3356)

Related titles: Online - full text ed.: (from EBSCO Publishing, O C L C Online Computer Library Center, Inc., Swets Blackwell, IDEAL Online Library, Institute for Scientific Information, RoweCom Information Quest).

Indexed: ASCA, Curr.Cont., Ind.Med. (1999-), Ind.Sci.Rev., Inpharma, Reac., Ref.Zh., SSCI (coverage dropped), Sci.Cit.Ind.

—BLDSC (1942.327832), EMDOCS, GNLM, IDS, ingenta, KNAW. **CCC.**

Published by: Bailliere Tindall (Subsidiary of: Harcourt Publishers Ltd.), 24-28 Oval Rd, London NW1 7DX, United Kingdom. TEL 44-20-7424-4200, FAX 44-20-7424-4515, cjournals@harcourt.com, http://www.harcourt-international.com/journals/beog/. **Subscr. to:** Harcourt Publishers Ltd., Foots Cray High St, Sidcup, Kent DA14 5HP, United Kingdom. TEL 44-20-8308-5700, FAX 44-20-8309-0807.

618.2 GBR

BAILLIERE'S MIDWIVES' DICTIONARY. Text in English. 1951. irreg., latest vol.8, 1992. GBP 5.95 (effective 1996). back issues avail. **Document type:** *Academic/Scholarly.*

Published by: Bailliere Tindall (Subsidiary of: Harcourt Publishers Ltd.), 24-28 Oval Rd, London NW1 7DX, United Kingdom. TEL 44-20-7485-4752, FAX 44—20-7267-4466, http://www.hbuk.co.uk. **Orders in N. America to:** W.B. Saunders Co., Journal Subscription Fulfillment, 6277 Sea Harbor Dr, 4th Fl, Orlando, FL 32887-4800. TEL 800-874-6418; **Orders to:** Harcourt Publishers Ltd., Foots Cray High St, Sidcup, Kent DA14 5HP, United Kingdom. TEL 44-20-8300-3322, FAX 44-20-8309-0807.

BELIZE FAMILY HEALTH SURVEY. see *MEDICAL SCIENCES—Abstracting, Bibliographies, Statistics*

571.86 612.64 CHE ISSN 0006-3126
RJ251 CODEN: BNEOBV

BIOLOGY OF THE NEONATE; foetal and neonatal research. Text in English. 1959. m. (2 vols./yr.). CHF 1,534, EUR 1,096.40 in Europe to institutions; CHF 1,557.20, USD 1,192 overseas to institutions (effective 2002). adv. bibl, charts, illus. back issues avail. *Refereed.* **Document type:** *Journal, Academic/Scholarly.* **Description:** Original papers present laboratory findings from both human and animal studies covering the physiological and biochemical events taking place during the period leading up to and immediately following birth, whether fullterm or premature.

Incorporates (in 1995): Developmental Pharmacology and Therapeutics (0379-8305); Formerly: Biologia Neonatorum

Related titles: Microform ed.: (from PQC); Online - full text ed.: ISSN 1421-9727. CHF 116, EUR 84, USD 90 to institutions with print edition (effective 2002) (from EBSCO Publishing, O C L C Online Computer Library Center, Inc., RoweCom Information Quest, Swets Blackwell, Institute for Scientific Information).

Indexed: ASCA, Abstr.Hyg., Anim.Breed.Abstr., Bibl.Dev.Med.& Child Neur., Biol.Abstr., Chem.Abstr., Chem.Indus.Notes, Chem.Titles, Curr.Adv.Ecol.Sci., Curr.Cont., Dairy Sci.Abstr., Derwent Biotech.Abstr., Environ.Sci.Poll.Mgmt., Excerp.Med., Fam.Ind., Ind.Med. (1970-), Ind.Sci.Rev., Ind.Vet., Inpharma, Int.Abstr.Biol.Sci., Neurosci.Cit.Ind., Nutr.Abstr., Pharm.&Out.News, Pig News & Info., Pollut.Abstr., Poult.Abstr., Protozool.Abstr., Reac., Risk Abstr., SSCI (coverage dropped), Saf.Sci.Abstr., Sci.Cit.Ind., Vet.Bull.

—BLDSC (2087.100000), CASDDS, CISTI, EMDOCS, GNLM, IDS, ingenta, KNAW. **CCC.**

Published by: S. Karger AG, Allschwilerstr 10, PO Box, Basel 4009, Switzerland. TEL 41-61-306-1111, FAX 41-61-306-1234, karger@karger.ch, http://www.online.karger.com/journals/bon, http://www.karger.com. Ed. J P Relier. adv.: page USD 1,185. Circ: 1,150.

301.4 618 USA ISSN 0730-7659
RG651
BIRTH; issues in perinatal care. Text in English. 1973. q. USD 60 domestic to individuals; USD 70 in Canada & Mexico to individuals; USD 90 overseas to individuals; USD 195 domestic to institutions; USD 210 in Canada & Mexico to institutions; USD 225 overseas to institutions; USD 66 to individuals print & online eds. combined; USD 214.50 to institutions print & online eds. combined (effective 2001). adv. bk.rev. illus. Index. back issues avail.; reprint service avail. from PQC,ISI. *Refereed.* **Document type:** *Academic/Scholarly.* **Description:** Covers education and technology regarding childbirth for childbirth educators, midwives and physicians.
Formerly (until 1981): Birth and the Family Journal (0098-860X)
Related titles: Microform ed.: (from PQC); Online - full text ed.: ISSN 1523-536X. USD 54 to individuals; USD 176 to institutions (effective 2001) (from Ovid Technologies, Inc., EBSCO Publishing, O C L C Online Computer Library Center, Inc., RoweCom Information Quest, ingenta, Munksgaard & Blackwell Science's Synergy, Swets Blackwell, Institute for Scientific Information).
Indexed: ASSIA, Brit.Nur.Ind., CINAHL, Curr.Cont., Dairy Sci.Abstr., Dok.Arbeitsmed., Ind.Med. (1982-), Int.Nurs.Ind., NRN, Nutr.Abstr., Psychol.Abstr., SSCI.
—BLDSC (2094.081000), ADONIS, GNLM, IDS, Infotrieve, ingenta, KNAW. **CCC.**
Published by: Blackwell Science Inc., Commerce Pl, 350 Main St, Malden, MA 02148-5018. TEL 781-388-8250, 800-759-6102, FAX 781-388-8255, journals@blacksci.com, http://www.blackwell-science.com. Ed. Diony Young. R&P Tracey Davies. Adv. contact Jenny Applin. Circ: 3,500.

618 AUS ISSN 1032-9625
BIRTH. Text in English. 1989. a. AUD 7.95; AUD 9.50 foreign (effective 1999). adv. bk.rev. **Document type:** *Consumer.* **Description:** Offers important information for expectant mothers.
Published by: Magazine House Pty. Ltd., PO Box 1067, Crows Nest, NSW 1585, Australia. TEL 61-2-94382399, FAX 61-2-94363014. Ed. Carol Fallows. Pub., R&P Martin Fallows. Adv. contact Paola Forlano. Circ: 40,000.

618 USA ISSN 0890-3255
BIRTH GAZETTE. Text in English. 1977; N.S. 1985. q. USD 35 to individuals; USD 40 in Canada & Mexico to individuals; USD 42 elsewhere to individuals; USD 50 to institutions (effective 2000). adv. bk.rev. illus, stat. reprint service avail. from PQC. **Document type:** *Consumer.* **Description:** Covers midwifery, childbirth issues, and access to maternity care.
Formerly (until vol.11, no.4, 1985): Practicing Midwife (0733-8317)
Related titles: Microform ed.: N.S. (from PQC).
Indexed: CINAHL, Gend.Watch, Int.Nurs.Ind.
—GNLM.
Published by: Second Foundation, 42 The Farm, Summertown, TN 38483. TEL 615-964-2519, brthgzt@usit.net. Ed., Pub. Ina May Gaskin. Adv. contact Kim Trainor. B&W page USD 650, color page USD 1,200. Circ: 3,000.

BIRTH PSYCHOLOGY BULLETIN. see *PSYCHOLOGY*

618.202 USA ISSN 1075-4733
THE BIRTHKIT. Key Title: Birthkit (Eugene, Or.). Text in English. 1994. q. USD 25; USD 28 in Canada & Mexico; USD 30 elsewhere. adv. bk.rev. illus, tr.lit. back issues avail. **Document type:** *Newsletter.* **Description:** Carries news, articles reviews and information for midwives, doulas, birth educators and other birth practitioners.
Related titles: Online - full text ed.: (from LexisNexis).
Indexed: CWI, Gend.Watch.
Published by: Midwifery Today Association, PO Box 2672, Eugene, OR 97402. TEL 541-344-7438, 800-743-0974, FAX 541-344-1422, midwifery@aol.com, http://www.midwiferytoday.com/. Ed., Pub., R&P Jan Tritten. Adv. contact Heather Maurer. Circ: 500.

618 IRL
THE BOUNTY PREGNANCY GUIDE. Text in English. 1991. a. adv. **Document type:** *Journal, Consumer.*
Published by: Bounty Services (Ireland) Ltd., Bromhill Rd, Unit 66, Tallaght, Dublin 24, Ireland. TEL 353-1-4596066, FAX 353-1-4596082.

618 GBR
THE BOUNTY PREGNANCY GUIDE. Text in English. 1982. a. adv. **Document type:** *Journal, Consumer.*
Published by: Bounty Publications Ltd., 3 Theobald Ct, Theobald St, Borehamwood, Herts WD6 4RN, United Kingdom. TEL 44-181-207-4040, FAX 44-181-207-6966, http://www.bounty.com.

618.1 GBR ISSN 0960-9776
CODEN: BREAEK
THE BREAST. Text in English. 1992. bi-m. GBP 150 to individuals; GBP 390 to institutions (effective 2002). adv. abstr, bibl. *Refereed.* **Document type:** *Journal, Academic/Scholarly.* **Description:** Covers the physiology of the normal breast and the etiology, biology, investigation, medical and surgical treatment and management of benign and malignant breast diseases.
Related titles: Online - full text ed.: (from EBSCO Publishing, O C L C Online Computer Library Center, Inc., Swets Blackwell, IDEAL Online Library, Institute for Scientific Information).
Indexed: Curr.Cont., Excerp.Med. (1993-), Inpharma, Int.Abstr.Biol.Sci., Pharm.&Out.News, Reac.
—BLDSC (2277.492700), EMDOCS, GNLM, IDS, Infotrieve, KNAW. **CCC.**
Published by: Churchill Livingstone (Subsidiary of: Harcourt Publishers Ltd.), Robert Stevenson House, 1-3 Baxter's Pl, Leith Walk, Edinburgh, Midlothian EH1 3AF, United Kingdom. TEL 44-131-459-1177, FAX 44-131-535-1704, cservice@harcourt.com, http://www.harcourt-international.com/journals/brst. Ed. J Michael Dixon. Pub. Gillian Griffith. R&P Catherine John TEL 212-424-4200. Adv. contact David Dunnachie. Circ: 955. **Subscr. to:** Harcourt Publishers Ltd., Foots Cray High St, Sidcup, Kent DA14 5HP, United Kingdom. TEL 44-20-8308-5700, FAX 44-20-8309-0807.

BREAST CANCER; evolution of concepts. see *MEDICAL SCIENCES—Oncology*

618.1 616.99 613.082 NLD ISSN 0888-6008
RC280.B8 CODEN: BRDIE5
BREAST DISEASE; an international journal. Text in English. 1987. a. EUR 234, USD 212 to institutions (effective 2002). back issues avail. *Refereed.* **Document type:** *Journal, Academic/Scholarly.* **Description:** Provides information on all aspects of human breast disease - benign and malignant - to help improve the health care and management of patients.
Related titles: Online - full text ed.: (from EBSCO Publishing, ingenta, Swets Blackwell, RoweCom Information Quest).
Indexed: Excerp.Med., Int.Abstr.Biol.Sci., NRN.
—BLDSC (2277.494070), CASDDS, CISTI, EMDOCS, GNLM, Infotrieve, KNAW. **CCC.**
Published by: I O S Press, Nieuwe Hemweg 6B, Amsterdam 1013 BG, Netherlands. TEL 31-20-688-3355, FAX 31-20-620-3419, liue@nih.gov, market@iospress.nl, http://www.iospress.nl. Ed. Dr. Edison T Liu TEL 301-496-3251. **Subscr. to:** I O S Press, Inc, 5795-G Burke Centre Pkwy, Burke, VA 22015. TEL 703-323-5554, FAX 703-323-3668, iosbooks@iospress.com; Kinokuniya Company Ltd, Shinjuku 3-chome, Shinjuku-ku, Tokyo 160-0022, Japan; Globe Publication Pvt. Ltd., C-62 Inderpuri, New Delhi 100 012, India. TEL 91-11-579-3211, 91-11-579-3212, FAX 91-11-579-8876, custserve@globepub.com, http://www.globepub.com.

016.61819 USA ISSN 1043-321X
BREAST DISEASES. Text in English. 1990. q. USD 99 domestic to individuals; USD 118 foreign to individuals; USD 161 domestic to institutions; USD 182 foreign to institutions; USD 59 domestic to students; USD 77 foreign to students; USD 46 newsstand/cover (effective 2001). reprint service avail. from PQC. **Document type:** *Yearbook.* **Description:** Provides an interdisciplinary perspective on advances in prevention, diagnosis, and management of breast diseases. Each issue includes more than 40 abstracts selected from 700 different journals worldwide.
Related titles: Microfilm ed.: (from PQC).
—Infotrieve. **CCC.**
Published by: Mosby, Inc. (Subsidiary of: Elsevier Science), 11830 Westline Industrial Dr, St Louis, MO 63146-3318. TEL 314-872-8370, FAX 314-432-1380, periodical.service@mosby.com, http://www.mosby.com/periodicals.

618.19 USA ISSN 1075-122X
CODEN: BRJOFK
THE BREAST JOURNAL. Text in English. 1995. bi-m. USD 115 domestic to individuals; USD 125 in Canada & Mexico to individuals; USD 145 elsewhere to individuals; USD 220 domestic to institutions; USD 230 in Canada & Mexico to institutions; USD 250 elsewhere to institutions; USD 126.50 to individuals print & online eds. combined; USD 242 to institutions print & online eds. combined (effective 2001). adv. back issues avail.; reprints avail. *Refereed.* **Document type:** *Academic/Scholarly.*
Related titles: ♦ Online - full text ed.: The Breast Journal Online. ISSN 1524-4741.
Indexed: CINAHL.
—BLDSC (2277.494100), GNLM, Infotrieve, KNAW. **CCC.**
Published by: (University of Florida, Health Science Center, Jacksonville), Blackwell Science Inc., Commerce Pl, 350 Main St, Malden, MA 02148-5018. TEL 781-388-8250, 800-759-6102, FAX 781-388-8255, journals@blacksci.com, http://www.blackwell-science.com. R&P Tracey Davies. Adv. contact Jenny Applin.

618.19 USA ISSN 1524-4741
THE BREAST JOURNAL ONLINE. Text in English. bi-m. USD 104 to individuals; USD 198 to institutions (effective 2001). **Document type:** *Academic/Scholarly.*
Media: Online - full text (from EBSCO Publishing, O C L C Online Computer Library Center, Inc., RoweCom Information Quest, ingenta, Munksgaard & Blackwell Science's Synergy, Swets Blackwell). **Related titles:** ♦ Print ed.: The Breast Journal. ISSN 1075-122X.
Published by: Blackwell Science Inc., Commerce Pl, 350 Main St, Malden, MA 02148-5018. TEL 781-388-8250, 800-759-6102, FAX 781-388-8255, website@blacksci.com, journals@blacksci.com, http://www.blackwell-science.com.

BREAST NEWS. see *MEDICAL SCIENCES—Oncology*

618.3 USA ISSN 0897-6112
BRIGGS UPDATE: DRUGS IN PREGNANCY AND LACTATION. Key Title: Drugs in Pregnancy and Lactation. Text in English. 1983. q., latest vol.14. USD 63 domestic to individuals; USD 74 foreign to individuals; USD 109 domestic to institutions; USD 26 newsstand/cover; USD 109 per issue foreign to institutions (effective 2002). **Document type:** *Newsletter.* **Description:** Publishes news on prescription and nonprescription drugs.
Published by: Lippincott Williams & Wilkins (Philadelphia) (Subsidiary of: Wolters Kluwer N.V.), 530 Walnut St, Philadelphia, PA 19106-3621. TEL 215-521-8300, FAX 215-521-8902, http://www.lww.com. Eds. Gerald G Briggs, Dr. Roger K Freeman. **Subscr. to:** PO Box 1600, Hagerstown, MD 21740-1600. TEL 800-777-2295, FAX 301-824-7390.

618 GBR ISSN 0969-4900
BRITISH JOURNAL OF MIDWIFERY. Text in English. 1993. m. GBP 50.40; GBP 4.99 newsstand/cover (effective 1999). adv. **Document type:** *Academic/Scholarly, Consumer.*
Indexed: Brit.Nur.Ind., CINAHL.
—BLDSC (2311.885000).
Published by: Mark Allen Publishing Ltd., Croxted Mews, 286-288a Croxted Rd, London SE24 9BY, United Kingdom. TEL 44-208-671-7521, FAX 44-208-671-4454, http://www.markallengroup.com/bjm.htm. Ed. Christine Henderson. Pub. Mark Allen. Adv. contact Ian White.

618 GBR ISSN 0306-5456
CODEN: BJOGAS
BRITISH JOURNAL OF OBSTETRICS & GYNAECOLOGY. Text in English. 1902. m. EUR 283 in Europe to institutions; JPY 42,490 in Japan to institutions; USD 363 elsewhere to institutions (effective 2002). adv. bk.rev. abstr, bibl, charts, illus. index. back issues avail. *Refereed.* **Document type:** *Academic/Scholarly.*
Formerly: Journal of Obstetrics and Gynaecology of the British Commonwealth (0022-3204)
Related titles: Online - full text ed.: (from EBSCO Publishing, RoweCom Information Quest, ScienceDirect, Institute for Scientific Information); ♦ Supplement: British Journal of Obstetrics & Gynaecology. Supplement. ISSN 0140-7686.

Indexed: AIM, ASCA, Agri.& Environ.Biotech.Abstr. (coverage dropped), Arts & Hum.Cit.Ind. (coverage dropped), Bibl.Dev.Med.& Child Neur., Biol.Abstr., Brit.Nur.Ind., CINAHL, Chem.Abstr., Chem.Indus.Notes, Chem.Titles, Curr.Adv.Cancer Res., Curr.Adv.Ecol.Sci., Curr.Cont., Curr.Lit.Fam.Plan., Dairy Sci.Abstr., Dent.Ind., Derwent Biotech.Abstr., Diab.Cont., Excerp.Med., Fam.Ind., Helminthol.Abstr., INIS Atomind., Ind.Med. (coverage dropped), Ind.Sci.Rev., Ind.Vet., Inpharma, Int.Nurs.Ind., Jrnl.Watch Wom.Hlth., Kidney, Med.& Surg.Dermat., NRN, Neurosci.Cit.Ind., Nutr.Abstr., Pharm.&Out.News, Protozool.Abstr., Reac., Ref.Zh., Risk Abstr., SSCI (coverage dropped), Sci.Cit.Ind., THA, Vet.Bull.
—BLDSC (2312.300000), ADONIS, CASDDS, CISTI, EMDOCS, GNLM, IDS, KNAW. **CCC.**
Published by: (Royal College of Obstetricians and Gynaecologists), Blackwell Science Ltd., Osney Mead, Oxford OX2 0EL, United Kingdom. TEL 44-1865-206206, FAX 44-1865-721205, journals.cs@blacksci.co.uk, http://www.elsevier.com/locate/bjog, http://www.blackwell-science.com. Ed. J M Grant. Pub. Allen Stevens. R&P Sophie Savage. Adv. contact Jenny Applin. Circ: 6,400.

618 016 GBR ISSN 0140-7686
BRITISH JOURNAL OF OBSTETRICS & GYNAECOLOGY. SUPPLEMENT. Text in English. 1977. irreg. adv. **Document type:** *Academic/Scholarly.*
Related titles: ♦ Supplement to: British Journal of Obstetrics & Gynaecology. ISSN 0306-5456.
Indexed: Curr.Cont. (coverage dropped).
—BLDSC (2312.310000), ADONIS, CISTI, EMDOCS, ingenta, KNAW. **CCC.**
Published by: (Royal College of Obstetricians and Gynaecologists), Blackwell Science Ltd., Osney Mead, Oxford OX2 0EL, United Kingdom. TEL 44-1865-206206, FAX 44-1865-721205, journals.cs@blacksci.co.uk, http://www.blackwell-science.com. Pub. Allen Stevens. R&P Sarah Pollard. Adv. contact Jenny Applin.

618.2 617.96 JPN ISSN 0387-2653
BUNBEN TO MASUI/JOURNAL OF OBSTETRICS AND ANESTHESIA. Text in Japanese; Summaries in English. 1961. irreg.
Published by: (Bunben to Masui Kenkyukai), Kokuseido Publishing Co. Ltd., 23-5-202 Hongo 3-chome, Bunkyo-ku, Tokyo 113-0033, Japan. TEL 81-3-3811-0995, FAX 81-3-3813-1866.

CARING NOTES; a professional newsletter by S H A R E. see *PSYCHOLOGY*

618 CZE ISSN 1210-7832
CESKA GYNEKOLOGIE/CZECH GYNAECOLOGY. Text in Czech, Slovak; Summaries in English, Russian. 1936. 6/yr. EUR 108, USD 138 (effective 2001). adv. bk.rev. *Refereed.* **Document type:** *Academic/Scholarly.* **Description:** Publishes original papers from clinical practice, as well as information on the activities of professional societies.
Formerly (until 1993): Ceskoslovenska Gynekologie (0374-6852)
Indexed: Biol.Abstr., Excerp.Med., INIS Atomind., Ind.Med. (1994-).
—CISTI, EMDOCS, GNLM, Infotrieve. **CCC.**
Published by: (Ceska Lekarska Spolecnost J.E. Purkyne/Czech Medical Association), Nakladatelske Stredisko C L S J.E. Purkyne, Sokolska 31, Prague 12026, Czech Republic. TEL 42-2-24911420, FAX 42-2-24911420, nts@iol.cz, http://www.clsjep.cz, http://www.medical.cz. Ed. Jaroslav Zivny. adv.: B&W page CZK 27,300, color page CZK 39,700; 244 x 167. Circ: 2,400. **Dist. by:** Abont s.r.o., Chlumova 17, Prague, 3 130 00, Czech Republic; **Dist. in Western countries by:** Kubon & Sagner, Hesstr 39-41, Munich 80798, Germany. **Co-sponsor:** Ceska Spolecnost Gynekologicka a Porodnicka.

618 LKA
CEYLON COLLEGE OF OBSTETRICIANS AND GYNAECOLOGISTS. JOURNAL. Text in English. q. LKR 25.
Published by: Ceylon College of Obstetricians and Gynaecologists, C.M.A. House, 6 Wijerama Mawatha, Colombo 7, Sri Lanka.

618.45 USA
CHILDBIRTH WITHOUT PAIN EDUCATION ASSOCIATION. MEMO. Text in English. 1960. bi-m. membership. adv. bk.rev. tr.mk. **Document type:** *Newsletter.*
Formerly: Childbirth Without Pain Education Association. Newsletter (0009-4048)
Media: Duplicated (not offset).
Published by: Childbirth Without Pain Education Association, 20134 Snowden, Detroit, MI 48235. TEL 313-341-3816. Ed. Flora Hommel. Circ: 3,000.

618 USA
CHILDBIRTH (YEAR); your guide to the last trimester. Text in English. 1984. s-a. Dist. with The American Baby Basket for Expectant Parents through participating childbirth educators only. adv. illus. **Document type:** *Consumer.* **Description:** Answers the questions of couples approaching the birth of their child. The magazine's four sections include: your pregnant body, getting ready for baby, labor and birth, and baby's early weeks.
Indexed: CINAHL.
Published by: Primedia Consumer Media & Magazine Group, 249 W 17th St, New York, NY 10011-5300. TEL 212-462-3500, FAX 212-367-8333, http://www.americanbaby.com, http://www.primedia.com/. Ed. Judith Nolte. Pub. Bob Davidowitz. Adv. contact Jeff Christian. B&W page USD 92,700, color page USD 128,800; trim 10.5 x 7.88. Circ: 2,300,000 (controlled).

618.1 ESP ISSN 1137-2273
CIENCIA GINECOLOGIKA. Text in Spanish. 1996. bi-m., latest vol.4, 2000. ESP 6,000 domestic; USD 65 in Europe; USD 70 elsewhere (effective 2001). adv. charts. *Refereed.* **Document type:** *Academic/Scholarly.* **Description:** Offers OB-GYNs original clinical and research articles as well as reviews on all aspects of gynecological medicine.
—BLDSC (3196.322000), CINDOC.
Published by: (Sociedad de Obstetricia y Ginecologia de la Comunidad Valenciana), Alpe Editores S.A., Pedro Rico, 27, Madrid 28029, Spain. TEL 34-91-733-8811, FAX 34-91-315-9652, alpeeditores@sistelcom.com. Eds. Eduardo Vilar Checa, Juan Jose Vidal Pelaez. Pub. Angeles Alvarez Sanchez. Adv. contact Ana Jurado. Circ: 5,000 (controlled).

CLIMACTERIC. see *WOMEN'S HEALTH*

618 ESP ISSN 0210-573X
CODEN: CIGODJ
CLINICA E INVESTIGACION EN GINECOLOGIA Y OBSTETRICIA. Text in Spanish; Summaries in English. 1974. m. (10/yr.). USD 113. adv. reprint service avail. from PQC. **Document type:** *Academic/Scholarly.* **Description:** Covers the early detection of gynecological diseases and conditions, the improvement of family planning methods, the treatment of sterility and infertility, and the mother-child relationship during pregnancy.
Indexed: Excerp.Med., Ind.Med.Esp., Ref.Zh.
—BLDSC (3286.202000), CISTI, EMDOCS, GNLM, KNAW. **CCC.**
Published by: Ediciones Doyma S.A., Traversa de Gracia, 17-21, Barcelona 08021, Spain. TEL 34-93-200-0711, FAX 34-93-209-1136. Ed. J Esteban Altirriba. Adv. contact Olga Gomez. color page ESP 238,000; trim 280 x 210. Circ: 2,500.

618 CAN ISSN 0390-6663
CODEN: CEOGA4
CLINICAL AND EXPERIMENTAL OBSTETRICS AND GYNECOLOGY. Text and summaries in English. 1974. q. USD 150 to individuals; USD 250 to institutions (effective 1999). adv. back issues avail. *Refereed.* **Document type:** *Academic/Scholarly.*
Indexed: Biol.Abstr., Chem.Abstr., Excerp.Med., Ind.Med. (1974-).
—BLDSC (3286.251900), CASDDS, CISTI, EMDOCS, GNLM, Infotrieve, KNAW. **CCC.**
Published by: S O G Canada, Inc., 4900 Cote St Luc, Apt 212, Montreal, PQ H3W 2H3, Canada. TEL 514-489-3242, FAX 514-485-4513. Ed. Antonio Onnis. Adv. contact Moriuz Morsoui.

618 USA ISSN 0009-9201
RG101 CODEN: COGYAK
CLINICAL OBSTETRICS AND GYNECOLOGY. Text in English. 1958. q. USD 189 domestic to individuals for print & online eds.; USD 245 foreign to individuals for print & online eds.; USD 396 domestic to institutions for print & online eds.; USD 471 foreign to institutions for print & online eds.; USD 107 newsstand/cover (effective 2002). adv. *Refereed.* **Document type:** *Academic/Scholarly.*
Related titles: Microform ed.: (from PQC); Online - full text ed.: USD 514.80 domestic academic site license; USD 589.80 foreign academic site license; USD 574.20 domestic corporate site license; USD 649.20 foreign corporate site license (effective 2002) (from Ovid Technologies, Inc., Institute for Scientific Information).
Indexed: Bibl.Dev.Med.& Child Neur., Biol.Abstr., C.C.I.Ob.Gyn., Chem.Abstr., Curr.Adv.Cancer Res., Curr.Adv.Ecol.Sci., Curr.Cont., Dok.Arbeitsmed., Excerp.Med., Hosp.Lit.Ind., INIS Atomind., Ind.Med. (1958-), Ind.Sci.Rev., Inpharma, Pharm.&Out.News, Protozool.Abstr., Reac., SSCI (coverage dropped), Sci.Cit.Ind.
—BLDSC (3286.316000), CASDDS, CISTI, EMDOCS, GNLM, IDS, ingenta, KNAW.
Published by: Lippincott Williams & Wilkins (Philadelphia) (Subsidiary of: Wolters Kluwer N.V.), 530 Walnut St, Philadelphia, PA 19106-3621. TEL 215-521-8300, FAX 215-521-8902, http://www.Lww.com. Eds. Dr. James R Scott, Dr. Roy M Pitkin. Pub. Kathleen Gaffney. R&P Alice McElhinney. Adv. contact Ray Thibodeau. Circ: 7,273. **Subscr. to:** PO Box 1600, Hagerstown, MD 21740-1600. TEL 800-777-2295, FAX 301-824-7390.

618 USA ISSN 0178-0328
CLINICAL PERSPECTIVES IN OBSTETRICS AND GYNECOLOGY. Text in English. 1983. irreg., latest 1995. price varies. **Document type:** *Monographic series.*
Published by: Springer-Verlag, Journals (Subsidiary of: BertelsmannSpringer), 175 Fifth Ave, New York, NY 10010. TEL 212-460-1500, FAX 212-473-6272.

618 USA ISSN 1043-3198
RG1 CODEN: CPGYEV
CLINICAL PRACTICE OF GYNECOLOGY. Text in English. 1991. 3/yr. *Refereed.* **Document type:** *Academic/Scholarly.* **Description:** Covers all aspects of gynecology from diagnosis to treatment.
—CISTI, GNLM. **CCC.**
Published by: Elsevier Science, PO Box 945, New York, NY 10159-0945. TEL 212-989-5800, FAX 212-633-3990, usinfo-f@elsevier.com, http://www.wlsevier.nl/, http://www.elsevier.com. Ed. Michael S Baggish. **Subscr. in Australasia and the Far East to:** Elsevier Science (Singapore) Pte Ltd, No.1 Temasek Ave, 17-01 Millenia Tower, Singapore 039192, Singapore. TEL 65-434-3727, FAX 65-337-2230; **Subscr. in Japan to:** Elsevier Science Inc - Japan Regional Office, 9-15 Higashi-Azabu 1-chome, Minato-ku, Tokyo 106-0044, Japan. TEL 81-3-5561-5033, FAX 81-3-5561-5047; **Subscr. outside the Americas to:** Elsevier Science BV, PO Box 211, Amsterdam 1000 AE, Netherlands. TEL 31-20-485-3757, FAX 31-20-485-3432, nlinfo-f@elsevier.nl.

618 USA ISSN 0095-5108
CODEN: CLPEDL
CLINICS IN PERINATOLOGY. Text in English. 1974. q. USD 129 domestic to individuals; USD 152 in Canada to individuals; USD 178 elsewhere to individuals; USD 175 domestic to institutions; USD 220 foreign to institutions; USD 56 per issue (effective 2001). reprint service avail. from PQC,ISI. *Refereed.* **Document type:** *Journal, Academic/Scholarly.* **Description:** Delivers practical advice from experts in specialty covered as well as information on new developments in a variety of specialties with a fresh perspective on problems and controversies.
Related titles: Online - full text ed.: (from Institute for Scientific Information); ♦ Spanish Translation: Clinicas de Perinatologia de Norteamerica.
Indexed: ASCA, Bibl.Dev.Med.& Child Neur., Biol.Abstr., CINAHL, Chem.Abstr., Chem.Indus.Notes, Chem.Titles, Curr.Adv.Ecol.Sci., Curr.Cont., Dairy Sci.Abstr., Dent.Ind., Excerp.Med., Helminthol.Abstr., INIS Atomind., Ind.Med. (1974-), Ind.Sci.Rev., Inpharma, Neurosci.Cit.Ind., Nutr.Abstr., Pharm.&Out.News, Reac., SSCI (coverage dropped), Sci.Cit.Ind.
—BLDSC (3286.585000), CASDDS, CISTI, EMDOCS, GNLM, IDS, ingenta, KNAW. **CCC.**
Published by: W.B. Saunders Co. (Subsidiary of: Harcourt Publishers Ltd.), 11830 Westline Industrial Dr, St Louis, MO 63146. TEL 800-325-4177, http://www.wbsaunders.com. **Subscr. to:** Periodicals Fulfillment, W B Saunders Co, 6277 Sea Harbor Dr, 4th Fl, Orlando, FL 32891-4800.

CLIO; die Zeitschrift fuer Frauengesundheit. see *WOMEN'S HEALTH*

618 649 USA ISSN 0829-8564
THE COMPLEAT MOTHER; the magazine of pregnancy, birth and breastfeeding. Text in English. 1985. q. adv. bk.rev. illus. Index. reprints avail. **Document type:** *Consumer.*
Published by: Compleat Mother, 720 Fourth Ave, N W, Box 209, Minot, ND 58702. TEL 701-852-2822, http://www.CompleatMother.com. Ed. Jody McLaughlin. adv.: B&W page USD 350. Circ: 20,000.

M

COMPLEMENTARY THERAPIES IN NURSING & MIDWIFERY. see *MEDICAL SCIENCES—Nurses And Nursing*

618 USA ISSN 0090-3159
RG1
CONTEMPORARY OB-GYN. Text in English. 1973. m. (plus 1 special issue). USD 99 domestic; USD 127 foreign; USD 10 newsstand/cover (effective 2001). adv. charts, illus, stat. index. *Refereed.* **Description:** Sets the standards for women's health. Includes practical advice by leading authorities in the ob-gyn field emphasizing clinical problems.
Related titles: Microfilm ed.: (from PQC); Online - full text ed.: (from Gale Group, Institute for Scientific Information).
Indexed: Curr.Cont. (coverage dropped), Curr.Lit.Fam.Plan.
—BLDSC (3425.196000), GNLM, IDS, ingenta, KNAW. **CCC.**
Published by: Medical Economics Co., Inc., 5 Paragon Dr, Montvale, NJ 07645-1742. TEL 201-358-7500, http://www.contobgyn.com. Ed. Judy Orvas. Circ: 39,255.

618 CAN ISSN 1194-7519
CONTEMPORARY OB-GYN. Text in English. 1993. 6/yr. CND 38; CND 54 foreign. adv.
Indexed: CINAHL, Fam.Ind.
Published by: Thomson Healthcare Communications, 1120 Birchmount Rd, Ste 200, Scarborough, ON M1K 5G4, Canada. TEL 416-750-8900, FAX 416-751-8126. Ed. Vil Meere. Adv. contact Alexandra Hamilton. B&W page CND 1,695, color page CND 2,790; trim 10.88 x 8.13. Circ: 10,832.

618.1 GBR ISSN 0953-9182
CODEN: CROGEV
CONTEMPORARY REVIEWS IN OBSTETRICS AND GYNAECOLOGY. Text in English. 1989. q. GBP 58, USD 95 to individuals; GBP 120, USD 195 to institutions (effective 2000). adv. bk.rev. back issues avail. *Refereed.* **Document type:** *Academic/Scholarly.* **Description:** Aims to provide an up-to-date source on the latest trends and developments in obstetrics and gynecology.
Indexed: Excerp.Med.
—BLDSC (3425.300100), EMDOCS, GNLM, Infotrieve, KNAW. **CCC.**
Published by: Parthenon Publishing Group (Subsidiary of: C R C Press (New York)), Casterton Hall, Casterton, Carnforth, Lancs LA6 2LA, United Kingdom. TEL 44-1524-272084, FAX 44-1524-271587, mail@parthpub.com, http://www.parthpub.com/. Ed., R&P Jean Wright. Adv. contact Julia Tissington.

CONTRACEPTION. see *BIRTH CONTROL*

618.1 618.2 CHE ISSN 0304-4246
CODEN: CGOBD6
CONTRIBUTIONS TO GYNECOLOGY AND OBSTETRICS. Text in English. 1950. irreg., latest vol.20. price varies. back issues avail.; reprint service avail. from ISI. *Refereed.* **Document type:** *Monographic series, Academic/Scholarly.*
Formerly: Advances in Obstetrics and Gynaecology (0065-2997)
Related titles: Online - full text ed.: (from Institute for Scientific Information).
Indexed: ASCA, Biol.Abstr., Chem.Abstr., Chem.Indus.Notes, Chem.Titles, Curr.Adv.Ecol.Sci., Curr.Cont. (coverage dropped), Excerp.Med., Ind.Med. (1976-).
—BLDSC (3458.610000), CASDDS, CISTI, GNLM, Infotrieve, ingenta, KNAW. **CCC.**
Published by: S. Karger AG, Allschwilerstr 10, PO Box, Basel 4009, Switzerland. TEL 41-61-306-1111, FAX 41-61-306-1234, karger@karger.ch, http://www.karger.com/bookseries/COGYO. Ed. O R Koechli.

618 ECU
CUADERNOS DE SALUD DE LA MUJER. Text in Spanish. 1990. q. USD 10. bk.rev. bibl, illus.
Published by: Centro de Estudios y Asesoria en Salud, Dpto. 602, Calle ROCA, 549, Quito, Ecuador. TEL 593-2-466714, FAX 593-2-566714. Ed. Dr. Jose Yepez.
Co-sponsor: Panamerican Health Organization.

CURATIONIS; accredited research journal of the Democratic Nursing Organisation of South Africa. see *MEDICAL SCIENCES—Nurses And Nursing*

CURRENT MEDICAL LITERATURE. GYNAECOLOGY AND OBSTETRICS. see *MEDICAL SCIENCES—Abstracting, Bibliographies, Statistics*

618 GBR ISSN 0957-5847
CURRENT OBSTETRICS AND GYNAECOLOGY. Text in English. 1991. bi-m. GBP 93 to individuals; GBP 265 to institutions (effective 2002). adv. **Document type:** *Academic/Scholarly.* **Description:** Provides reviews on themes of current interest and educational values for both practicing clinicians and training grade staff; includes self-evaluation sections for the examination candidate.
Related titles: Online - full text ed.: (from EBSCO Publishing, O C L C Online Computer Library Center, Inc., Swets Blackwell, IDEAL Online Library).
Indexed: Excerp.Med. (1995-), Ref.Zh.
—BLDSC (3500.715000), GNLM, Infotrieve, KNAW. **CCC.**
Published by: Churchill Livingstone (Subsidiary of: Harcourt Publishers Ltd.), Robert Stevenson House, 1-3 Baxter's Pl, Leith Walk, Edinburgh, Midlothian EH1 3AF, United Kingdom. TEL 44-131-556-2424, FAX 44-131-459-1177, cservice@harcourt.com, http://www.harcourt-international.com/journals/cuog/. Ed. E M Symonds. Pub. Gillian Griffith. R&P Catherine John TEL 212-424-4200. Adv. contact David Dunnachie. Circ: 890. **Subscr. to:** Harcourt Publishers Ltd., Foots Cray High St, Sidcup, Kent DA14 5HP, United Kingdom. TEL 44-20-8308-5700, FAX 44-20-8309-0807.

618 ITA
CURRENT OBSTETRICS AND GYNAECOLOGY - EDIZIONE ITALIANA. Text in Italian. 1992. q.
Published by: Gruppo Editoriale Faenza Editrice s.p.a., Via Pier de Crescenzi, 44, Faenza, RA 48018, Italy. TEL 39-0546-663488, FAX 39-0546-660440, info@faenza.com. adv.: B&W page ITL 4,230,000, color page ITL 5,690,000.

618 USA ISSN 1040-872X
RG1 CODEN: COOGEA
CURRENT OPINION IN OBSTETRICS & GYNECOLOGY. Text in English. 1989. bi-m. USD 249 domestic to individuals for print & online eds.; USD 249 foreign to individuals for print & online eds.; USD 611 per issue domestic to institutions; USD 611 per issue foreign to institutions (effective 2002). adv. bibl, illus. index. back issues avail. *Refereed.* **Document type:** *Academic/Scholarly.* **Description:** Directed toward researchers and practicing obstetricians and gynecologists. Presents review articles followed by annotated bibliographies of references consulted. A bibliography of the current world literature published during the previous year is available.
Related titles: CD-ROM ed.; Diskette ed.; Online - full text ed.: USD 794.30 domestic academic site license; USD 794.30 foreign academic site license; USD 885.95 domestic corporate site license; USD 885.95 foreign corporate site license (effective 2002) (from Ovid Technologies, Inc., EBSCO Publishing, Swets Blackwell, Institute for Scientific Information).
Indexed: ASCA, CINAHL, Curr.Cont., Excerp.Med., INIS Atomind., Ind.Med. (1989-), Inpharma, Int.Abstr.Biol.Sci., Pharm.&Out.News, Reac., SSCI (coverage dropped).
—BLDSC (3500.776200), ADONIS, CISTI, EMDOCS, GNLM, IDS, KNAW.
Published by: Lippincott Williams & Wilkins (Philadelphia) (Subsidiary of: Wolters Kluwer N.V.), 530 Walnut St, Philadelphia, PA 19106-3621. FAX 215-521-8902, 215-521-8902, http://www.Lww.com. Eds. Dr. Alan H Decherney, Stuart Campbell. Adv. contact Gemma Heiser. color page GBP 1,145. Circ: 3,381. **Subscr. to:** PO Box 1600, Hagerstown, MD 21740-1600.

618 USA ISSN 8756-0410
CODEN: CPOIEN
CURRENT PROBLEMS IN OBSTETRICS, GYNECOLOGY AND FERTILITY. Text in English. 1978. bi-m. USD 89 domestic to individuals; USD 99 foreign to individuals; USD 149 domestic to institutions; USD 159 foreign to institutions; USD 49 domestic to students; USD 58 foreign to students; USD 27 per issue domestic (effective 2001). illus. cum.index. reprint service avail. from PQC. **Description:** Provides clinical monographic reviews in obstetrics, gynecology and fertility.
Formerly: Current Problems in Obstetrics and Gynecology (0147-1988)
Related titles: Microform ed.: (from PQC).
Indexed: ASCA, Curr.Cont. (coverage dropped), Excerp.Med., Ind.Med. (coverage dropped).
—BLDSC (3501.387200), CASDDS, EMDOCS, GNLM, IDS, ingenta, KNAW. **CCC.**
Published by: Mosby, Inc. (Subsidiary of: Elsevier Science), 11830 Westline Industrial Dr, St Louis, MO 63146-3318. TEL 314-872-8370, 800-325-4177, FAX 314-432-1380, customerservice@mosby.com, http://www.mosby.com/periodicals. Ed. Sarah L Berga. Circ: 1,220.

618 DEU ISSN 0012-026X
DEUTSCHE HEBAMMEN-ZEITSCHRIFT; Fachblatt fuer Hebammern und Entbildungspfleger. Text in German. 1886. m. DEM 63. adv. bk.rev. charts, illus, stat. index.
—GNLM, Infotrieve. **CCC.**
Published by: (Bund Deutscher Hebammen), Elwin Staude Verlag GmbH, Fuchsrain 18A, Hannover 30657, Germany. Ed. Dr. H W Vasterling. Circ: 9,200.

DISABILITY, PREGNANCY & PARENTHOOD INTERNATIONAL; a forum for disabled parents and professionals to exchange information and experience. see *HANDICAPPED*

E N B NEWS. see *MEDICAL SCIENCES—Nurses And Nursing*

618.2 IRL ISSN 0378-3782
RG600 CODEN: EHDEDN
EARLY HUMAN DEVELOPMENT; an international journal concerned with the continuity of fetal and post natal life. Text in English. 1977. 10/yr. EUR 107 in Europe to individuals; JPY 14,000 in Japan to individuals; USD 120 elsewhere to individuals; EUR 1,112 in Europe to institutions; JPY 147,500 in Japan to institutions; USD 1,244 elsewhere to institutions (effective 2002). adv. bk.rev. back issues avail. *Refereed.* **Document type:** *Academic/Scholarly.* **Description:** Publishes original research papers with particular emphasis on the continuum between fetal life and the perinatal period; aspects of postnatal growth influenced by early events; and the safeguarding of the quality of human survival.
Incorporates (1992-1996): Screening (0925-6164); Which was previously announced as: International Journal of Neonatal and Later Screening
Related titles: Microform ed.: (from PQC); Online - full text ed.: (from ingenta, Swets Blackwell, ScienceDirect, Institute for Scientific Information).
Indexed: Abstr.Hyg., Bibl.Dev.Med.& Child Neur., Biol.Abstr., CINAHL, Chem.Abstr., Chem.Indus.Notes, Chem.Titles, Curr.Adv.Cell & Devel.Biol., Curr.Adv.Ecol.Sci., Curr.Cont., Dairy Sci.Abstr., Excerp.Med., Fam.Ind., Ind.Med. (1977-), Ind.Sci.Rev., Inpharma, Int.Abstr.Biol.Sci., Int.Nurs.Ind., NRN, Neurosci.Cit.Ind., Nutr.Abstr., Pharm.&Out.News, Protozool.Abstr., PsycInfo, Psychol.Abstr. (1979-), Reac., Ref.Zh., SSCI (coverage dropped), Sci.Cit.Ind., THA, Trop.Dis.Bull., e-psyche.
—BLDSC (3642.983000), CASDDS, CISTI, EMDOCS, GNLM, IDS, Infotrieve, ingenta, KNAW. **CCC.**
Published by: Elsevier Science Ireland Ltd, Elsevier House, Brookvale Plaza, E. Park, Shannon, Co. Clare, Ireland. TEL 353-61-471944, FAX 353-61-472144, http://www.elsevier.com/inca/publications/store/5/0/5/9/5/6/. Ed. David R Harvey. R&P Annette Moloney. **Subscr. in Australasia and the Far East to:** Elsevier Science (Singapore) Pte Ltd, No.1 Temasek Ave, 17-01 Millenia Tower, Singapore 039192, Singapore. TEL 65-434-3727, FAX 65-337-2230**; Subscr. in the Americas to:** Elsevier Science, PO Box 945, New York, NY 10159-0945. TEL 212-633-3730, FAX 212-633-3680**; Subscr. to:** Elsevier Science BV, PO Box 211, Amsterdam 1000 AE, Netherlands. TEL 31-20-485-3757.

618 ITA ISSN 1123-8399
ECO NEWS. Text in Italian. 1995. q. adv. **Document type:** *Newsletter.*
Published by: (Societa Italiana di Ecografia Ostetrico-Ginecologica e Metodologie Biofisiche Correlate), C I C Edizioni Internazionali s.r.l., Corso Trieste 42, Rome, RM 00198, Italy. TEL 39-06-8412673, FAX 39-06-8412688, info@gruppocic.it, 1160199510. Ed. G Mommi. adv.: B&W page ITL 3,100,000, color page ITL 3,900,000; trim 210 x 290.

618 GBR
EMMA'S DIARY. Text in English. 1992. 2/yr. free per issue. adv. **Document type:** *Magazine, Consumer.* **Description:** Designed to provide pregnant mothers with an up-to-date guide to pregnancy.
Published by: (Royal College of General Practitioners), Lifecycle Marketing Ltd., 1-3 Malvern Rd, Maidenhead, Berkshire SL6 7QY, United Kingdom. TEL 44-1628-771232, FAX 44-1628-770705.

618 FRA ISSN 1283-081X
ENCYCLOPEDIE MEDICO-CHIRURGICALE. GINECOLOGIA - OBSTETRICIA. Cover title: Tratado de Ginecologia - Obstetricia. Text in Spanish. 1998. 5 base vols. plus q. updates. bibl, charts, illus. **Document type:** *Academic/Scholarly.* **Description:** Provides a comprehensive, up-to-date reference for topics in gynecology and obstetrics.
Related titles: ♦ Italian ed.: Encyclopedie Medico-Chirurgicale. Ginecologia - Ostetricia. ISSN 1293-2639.

Published by: Elsevier Paris, Editions Scientifiques et Medicales (Subsidiary of: Reed Elsevier plc. group), 23 rue Linois, Paris 75015, France. TEL 33-1-45589110, FAX 33-1-45589425, redaction-emc@elsevier.fr, redacion-emc@elsevier.fr, http://www.elsevier.fr, http://www.elsevier.com. Ed. Caroline Chaine.

618 FRA ISSN 1293-2639
ENCYCLOPEDIE MEDICO-CHIRURGICALE. GINECOLOGIA - OSTETRICIA; la collana della donna, dalla prevenzione alla condotta terapeutica. Cover title: Trattato di Ginecologia - Ostetricia. Text in Italian. 1998. 5 base vols. plus q. updates. bibl, charts, illus. **Document type:** *Academic/Scholarly.* **Description:** Provides up-to-date reference topics in gynecology and obstetrics.
Related titles: ♦ Spanish ed.: Encyclopedie Medico-Chirurgicale. Ginecologia - Obstetricia. ISSN 1283-081X.
Published by: Elsevier Paris, Editions Scientifiques et Medicales (Subsidiary of: Reed Elsevier plc. group), 23 rue Linois, Paris 75015, France. TEL 33-1-45589110, FAX 33-1-45589425, redaction-emc@elsevier.fr, redacion-emc@elsevier.fr, http://www.elsevier.fr, http://www.elsevier.com. Ed. Caroline Chaine.

618 FRA ISSN 0246-1064
ENCYCLOPEDIE MEDICO-CHIRURGICALE. GYNECOLOGIE. Cover title: Traite de Gynecologie. Variant title: Encyclopedie Medico-Chirurgicale, Instantanes Medicaux. Gynecologie. Receuil Periodique de l'Encyclopedie Medico-Chirurgicale. Gynecologie. Text in French. 1930. 4 base vols. plus q. updates. bibl, charts, illus. *Refereed.* **Document type:** *Academic/Scholarly.* **Description:** Offers gynecologists and obstetricians a comprehensive, up-to-date reference for diagnosing and treating gynecologic conditions and disorders.
Formerly: Encyclopedie Medico-Chirurgicale. Gynecologie - Mamelle (0246-067X)
Published by: Elsevier Paris, Editions Scientifiques et Medicales (Subsidiary of: Reed Elsevier plc. group), 23 rue Linois, Paris 75015, France. TEL 33-1-45589110, FAX 33-1-45589425, redaction-emc@elsevier.fr, redacion-emc@elsevier.fr, http://www.elsevier.fr, http://www.elsevier.com.

618.2 FRA ISSN 0246-0335
ENCYCLOPEDIE MEDICO-CHIRURGICALE. OBSTETRIQUE. Cover title: Traite d'Obstetrique. Variant title: Enclyclopedie Medico-Chirurgicale, Instantanes Medicaux. Obstetrique. Text in French. 4 base vols. plus q. updates. bibl, charts, illus. *Refereed.* **Document type:** *Academic/Scholarly.* **Description:** Provides a comprehensive, up-to-date reference for diagnosing and treating obstetric conditions and disorders.
Published by: Elsevier Paris, Editions Scientifiques et Medicales (Subsidiary of: Reed Elsevier plc. group), 23 rue Linois, Paris 75015, France. TEL 33-1-45589110, FAX 33-1-45589425, redaction-emc@elsevier.fr, redacion-emc@elsevier.fr, http://www.elsevier.fr, http://www.elsevier.com.

ENCYCLOPEDIE MEDICO-CHIRURGICALE. TRAITE DE RADIODIAGNOSTIC: UROLOGIE - GYNECOLOGIE. see *MEDICAL SCIENCES—Radiology And Nuclear Medicine*

ENCYCLOPEDIE MEDICO-CHIRURGICALE. TRAITE DE TECHNIQUES CHIRURGICALES. GYNECOLOGIE. see *MEDICAL SCIENCES—Surgery*

EUROPEAN JOURNAL OF CONTRACEPTION AND REPRODUCTIVE HEALTH CARE. see *BIRTH CONTROL*

EUROPEAN JOURNAL OF GYNECOLOGICAL ONCOLOGY. see *MEDICAL SCIENCES—Oncology*

618 IRL ISSN 0301-2115
CODEN: EOGRAL
EUROPEAN JOURNAL OF OBSTETRICS & GYNECOLOGY AND REPRODUCTIVE BIOLOGY. Text in English. 1971. m. EUR 2,046 in Europe to institutions; JPY 271,800 in Japan to institutions; USD 2,289 elsewhere to institutions (effective 2002). adv. bk.rev. bibl, charts. back issues avail. *Refereed.* **Document type:** *Academic/Scholarly.* **Description:** Serves both the clinical practitioner and researcher by publishing studies, case reports and reviews of developments, as well as basic biochemical, physiological, embryological and genetic research related to human reproduction.
Formerly: European Journal of Obstetrics and Gynecology (0028-2243)
Related titles: Microform ed.: (from PQC); Online - full text ed.: (from ingenta, Swets Blackwell, ScienceDirect, Institute for Scientific Information); ♦ Supplement: European Journal of Obstetrics, Gynaecology and Reproductive Biology. Supplement. ISSN 0921-8750.
Indexed: ASCA, Biol.Abstr., Chem.Abstr., Chem.Indus.Notes, Chem.Titles, Curr.Adv.Cancer Res., Curr.Adv.Ecol.Sci., Curr.Cont., Dairy Sci.Abstr., Dent.Ind., Excerp.Med., Ind.Med. (1973-), Ind.Sci.Rev., Inpharma, Int.Abstr.Biol.Sci., Int.Nurs.Ind., NRN, Nutr.Abstr., Pharm.&Out.News, Protozool.Abstr., Reac., Rev.Med.& Vet.Mycol., SSCI (coverage dropped), Sci.Cit.Ind., Sugar Ind.Abstr.
—BLDSC (3829.733000), CASDDS, CISTI, GNLM, IDS, Infotrieve, ingenta, KNAW. **CCC.**
Published by: (European Association of Gynaecologists and Obstetricians), Elsevier Science Ireland Ltd, Elsevier House, Brookvale Plaza, E. Park, Shannon, Co. Clare, Ireland. TEL 353-61-471944, FAX 353-61-472144, http://www.elsevier.com/locate/ejogrb. Ed. Dr. T K A B Eskes. R&P Annette Moloney. **Subscr. in Australasia and the Far East to:** Elsevier Science (Singapore) Pte Ltd, No.1 Temasek Ave, 17-01 Millenia Tower, Singapore 039192, Singapore. TEL 65-434-3727, FAX 65-337-2230; **Subscr. in the Americas to:** Elsevier Science, PO Box 945, New York, NY 10159-0945. TEL 212-633-3730, FAX 212-633-3680, usinfo-f@elsevier.com; **Subscr. to:** Elsevier Science BV, PO Box 211, Amsterdam 1000 AE, Netherlands. TEL 31-20-485-3757.

618 IRL ISSN 0921-8750
EUROPEAN JOURNAL OF OBSTETRICS, GYNAECOLOGY AND REPRODUCTIVE BIOLOGY. SUPPLEMENT. Text in English. 1988. irreg.
Related titles: ♦ Supplement to: European Journal of Obstetrics & Gynecology and Reproductive Biology. ISSN 0301-2115.
Published by: Elsevier Science Ireland Ltd, Elsevier House, Brookvale Plaza, E. Park, Shannon, Co. Clare, Ireland. TEL 353-61-471944, FAX 353-61-472144.

618 GBR ISSN 1361-259X
EVIDENCE - BASED OBSTETRICS & GYNAECOLOGY. Text in English. 1997. q. GBP 45 to individuals; GBP 185 to institutions (effective 2002). adv. *Refereed.* **Document type:** *Journal, Academic/Scholarly.* **Description:** Helps clinicians to combine the best external evidence from systematic research with individual clinical expertise to make effective decisions about patient treatment and care through abstracts and commentaries on key articles from current literature.
Related titles: Online - full text ed.: (from EBSCO Publishing, O C L C Online Computer Library Center, Inc., Swets Blackwell, IDEAL Online Library).
Published by: Churchill Livingstone (Subsidiary of: Harcourt Publishers Ltd.), Robert Stevenson House, 1-3 Baxter's Pl, Leith Walk, Edinburgh, Midlothian EH1 3AF, United Kingdom. TEL 44-131-556-2424, FAX 44-131-459-1177, cservice@harcourt.com, http://www.harcourt-international.com/journals/ebog. Ed. Dr. Salim Daya. Adv. contact David Dunnachie. **Subscr. to:** Harcourt Publishers Ltd., Foots Cray High St, Sidcup, Kent DA14 5HP, United Kingdom. TEL 44-20-8308-5700, FAX 44-20-8309-0807.

EXCERPTA MEDICA. SECTION 10: OBSTETRICS AND GYNECOLOGY. see *MEDICAL SCIENCES—Abstracting, Bibliographies, Statistics*

EXCERPTA MEDICA. SECTION 21: DEVELOPMENTAL BIOLOGY AND TERATOLOGY. see *BIOLOGY—Abstracting, Bibliographies, Statistics*

618 GBR
EXPECTING OUR BABY. Text in English. 1994. m. GBP 2.20 newsstand/cover (effective 2000). adv. **Document type:** *Magazine, Consumer.* **Description:** Presents informative information and advice for expectant parents.
Published by: Southbank Publishing Company Ltd., King's Reach Tower, Stamford St, London SE1 9LS, United Kingdom. TEL 44-171-261-6860, FAX 44-171-261-5260.

F P A B HIGHLIGHTS. see *BIRTH CONTROL*

618 USA
▼ **FAMILY BUILDING.** Text in English. 2001. q. **Description:** Covers infertility issues from medical options, treatments, psychological issues, adoption, and other related topics.
Published by: RESOLVE: The National Infertility Association, 1310 Broadway, Somerville, MA 02144 . TEL 617-623-0744, FAX 617-623-0252, resolveinc@aol.com, http://www.resolve.org/.

FAMILY MEDICINE; medical advances in practice. see *MEDICAL SCIENCES—Pediatrics*

FAMILY PLANNING ASSOCIATION OF FIJI. NEWS. see *BIRTH CONTROL*

301.426 USA ISSN 0014-7354
HQ763 CODEN: FPGPA
FAMILY PLANNING PERSPECTIVES. Text in English. 1969. bi-m. USD 42 to individuals; USD 52 domestic to institutions; USD 62 foreign to institutions (effective 2001). adv. bk.rev. charts, illus. index. 50 p./no. 3 cols./p. back issues avail.; reprint service avail. from PQC,PSC,SCH. *Refereed.* **Document type:** *Academic/Scholarly.* **Description:** Focuses on the country's most pressing reproductive health issues, providing key findings from the institute's research and work of other distinguished social scientists.
Related titles: Microfilm ed.: (from PQC,CIS); Online - full text ed.: (from ProQuest Information & Learning, JSTOR (Web-based Journal Archive), Northern Light Technology, Inc., Gale Group, LexisNexis, Factiva, Institute for Scientific Information).
Indexed: ASCA, Abstr.Anthropol., Adol.Ment.Hlth.Abstr., Bibl.Agri., Biol.Abstr., Biol.Dig., CINAHL, CWI, Curr.Cont., Curr.Lit.Fam.Plan., Environ.Abstr., Excerp.Med., Fam.Ind., Human Resour.Abstr., IMFL, Ind.Med. (1969-), Int.Nurs.Ind., Jrnl.Watch Wom.Hlth., Lang.& Lang.Behav.Abstr., Mid.East: Abstr.& Ind., Mult.Ed.Abstr., P.A.I.S., Popul.Ind., Psychol.Abstr., Risk Abstr., Russ.Acad.Sci.Bibl., SOPODA, SRI, SSCI, Sage Fam.Stud.Abstr., Soc.Work Res.& Abstr., Sociol.Abstr., Stud.Wom.Abstr.
—BLDSC (3865.572000), CIS, GNLM, IDS, ingenta, KNAW.
Published by: Alan Guttmacher Institute, 120 Wall St, New York, NY 10005. TEL 212-248-1111, FAX 212-248-1951, llebran@AGI-USA.org, http://www.AGI-USA.org. Ed. Michael Klitsch. R&P Kaylynn Chiarello. Adv. contact Jennifer Nadeau. Circ: 5,000 (paid and free).

618.2 649 USA
FAMILY WAYS; education resources for pregnancy to parenthood. Text in English. m. **Description:** Provides mothers and mothers-to-be advice on feeding baby and other parenthood issues.
Published by: 30 West Advertising (Subsidiary of: Wyeth-Ayerst), 130 Radnor, Chester, PA 19087. TEL 610-902-2800, 800-234-WAYS.

618 JPN ISSN 0915-6852
FEMALE PATIENT* . Text in Japanese. 1988. 2/yr. **Document type:** *Academic/Scholarly.*
Published by: (Nihon Scherin KK), OCC Japan KK, KIT Building, 2-8-16 Yuten-Ji, Meguro-ku, Tokyo 153-0052, Japan. TEL 81-3-5721-0411, FAX 81-3-5721-0445. Pub. Dan Feldman.

618.1 USA ISSN 0888-2401
CODEN: FPPME5
FEMALE PATIENT: PRACTICAL OB-GYN MEDICINE; total health care for women. Text in English. 1976. m. USD 93 in the Americas to institutions; USD 140 elsewhere to institutions (effective 2000). adv. illus. reprint service avail. from PQC. *Refereed.* **Document type:** *Trade.*
Supersedes in part (in 1981): Female Patient (0364-1198)
Related titles: Microform ed.: (from PQC); Online - full text ed.: (from Northern Light Technology, Inc., ProQuest Information & Learning).
Indexed: Curr.Lit.Fam.Plan., FAMLI, Inpharma, Pharm.&Out.News, Reac.
—BLDSC (3905.168000), CISTI, EMDOCS, GNLM, Infotrieve, KNAW. **CCC.**
Published by: Quadrant HealthCom, 26 Main St, Ste A, Chatham, NJ 07928-2402. TEL 973-701-8900, FAX 973-701-8892. Ed. Caroline Tredway. Pub. Kathy McShea. Adv. contact Denise Andrade. Circ: 36,000.

618.178 USA ISSN 0015-0282
RC889 CODEN: FESTAS
FERTILITY AND STERILITY. Text in English. 1949. m. NLG 523, EUR 237.33 in Europe to individuals; JPY 32,900 in Japan to individuals; USD 266 elsewhere to individuals; NLG 771, EUR 349.86 in Europe to institutions; JPY 48,400 in Japan to institutions; USD 391 elsewhere to institutions (effective 2001). adv. bk.rev. bibl, charts, illus. index, cum.index: vols.1-50. back issues avail. *Refereed.* **Document type:** *Journal, Academic/Scholarly.* **Description:** Includes ethical guidelines governing the new reproductive technologies; protocols for management and standards and guidelines for practice as determined by the ASRM Practice Committee.
Related titles: CD-ROM ed.: (from Ovid Technologies, Inc.); Online - full text ed.: (from Ovid Technologies, Inc., ingenta, Swets Blackwell, ScienceDirect, Institute for Scientific Information).

M

Indexed: ASCA, Abstr.Anthropol., Anim.Breed.Abstr., Biol.Abstr., C.C.I.Ob.Gyn., Chem.Abstr., Curr.Adv.Cancer Res., Curr.Adv.Cell & Devel.Biol., Curr.Adv.Ecol.Sci., Curr.Cont., Curr.Lit.Fam.Plan., Dairy Sci.Abstr., Dent.Ind., Derwent Biotech.Abstr., Excerp.Med., Fam.Ind., Helminthol.Abstr., INIS Atomind., I.P.A., Ind.Med. (1950-), Ind.Sci.Rev., Ind.Vet., Inpharma, Jrnl.Watch Wom.Hlth., Med.& Surg.Dermat., Nutr.Abstr., Pharm.&Out.News, Reac., Risk Abstr., SSCI (coverage dropped), Sci.Cit.Ind., THA, Vet.Bull.
—BLDSC (3909.750000), CASDDS, CISTI, GNLM, IDS, ingenta, KNAW. **CCC.**
Published by: (American Society for Reproductive Medicine), Elsevier Science, Box 945, New York, NY 10159-0945. TEL 212-989-5800, FAX 212-633-3990, adechern@obgyn.medsch.ucla.edu, usinfo-f@elsevier.com, http://www.elsevier.com/locate/fertnstert. Ed. Dr. Roger D Kempers. R&P Joyce Zeitz. Adv. contact Jackson Gaeta. B&W page USD 1,194. Circ: 14,000. **Subscr. in Australasia and the Far East to:** Elsevier Science (Singapore) Pte Ltd, No.1 Temasek Ave, 17-01 Millenia Tower, Singapore 039192, Singapore. TEL 65-434-3727, FAX 65-337-2230; **Subscr. in Japan to:** Elsevier Science Inc - Japan Regional Office, 9-15 Higashi-Azabu 1-chome, Minato-ku, Tokyo 106-0044, Japan. TEL 81-3-5561-5033; **Subscr. outside the Americas to:** Elsevier Science BV, PO Box 211, Amsterdam 1000 AE, Netherlands. TEL 31-20-485-3757. **Co-sponsor:** Pacific Coast Fertility Society, Canadian Fertility Society.

618 USA ISSN 1086-1068
FERTILITY WEEKLY. Text in English. w. (48/yr.). USD 695 domestic; USD 895 out of North America (effective 2000). **Document type:** *Newsletter.* **Description:** Covers research, discoveries, news and conferences on fertility and human reproductive science, including such areas as infertility, assisted reproductive techniques, sterility, reproductive law, andrology, and more.
Related titles: Online - full text ed.
Address: PO Box 43054, Atlanta, GA 30336. FAX 205-991-1198, kkey@atl.mindspring.com, http://www.newsfile.com/lf.htm. Ed., Pub., R&P Keith K Key TEL 770-889-6970. Adv. contact Mike Chrisptopher.

618 GBR ISSN 0965-5395
CODEN: FMMREI
FETAL AND MATERNAL MEDICINE REVIEW. Text in English. 1989. q. GBP 106 to individuals; USD 200 to institutions (effective 2002). adv. back issues avail. *Refereed.* **Document type:** *Academic/Scholarly.* **Description:** Aims to bring together all multidisciplinary interests and approaches appropriate to the advancement of knowledge and clinical practice in obstetrics.
Formerly (until 1993): Fetal Medicine Review (0953-8267)
Related titles: Online - full text ed.: (from EBSCO Publishing, O C L C Online Computer Library Center, Inc., RoweCom Information Quest, Swets Blackwell).
Indexed: Excerp.Med. (1993-), Int.Abstr.Biol.Sci.
—BLDSC (3910.846000), EMDOCS, GNLM, Infotrieve, KNAW. **CCC.**
Published by: Cambridge University Press, Edinburgh Bldg, Shaftesbury Rd, Cambridge CB2 2RU, United Kingdom. FAX 44-1223-315052, TELEX 851817556, information@cup.cam.ac.uk, information@cambridge.org, http://www.cup.cam.ac.uk, http://www.uk.cambridge.org/journals/pmu. Eds. Stephen Robson, William Dunlop. R&P Linda Nicol. Adv. contact Rebecca Symons.

618 CHE ISSN 1015-3837
CODEN: FDTHES
FETAL DIAGNOSIS AND THERAPY; clinical advances and basic research. Text in English. 1986. bi-m. CHF 809 in Europe to institutions; CHF 826.40 elsewhere to institutions; EUR 577.80 in Europe to institutions; USD 631 elsewhere to institutions (effective 2002). adv. back issues avail. *Refereed.* **Document type:** *Journal, Academic/Scholarly.* **Description:** Focuses on the fetus as a patient. Provides a wide range of biomedical specialists with a unique single source of reports aimed at ameliorating and/or preventing congenital abnormalities.
Formerly: Fetal Therapy (0257-2788)
Related titles: Microform ed.: (from PQC); Online - full text ed.: ISSN 1421-9964. CHF 58, EUR 42 to institutions with print edition (effective 2002); USD 45 to institutions with print edition (effective 2001) (from EBSCO Publishing, O C L C Online Computer Library Center, Inc., RoweCom Information Quest, Swets Blackwell, Institute for Scientific Information).
Indexed: ASCA, Curr.Cont., Excerp.Med., Ind.Med. (1990-), Inpharma, Pharm.&Out.News, Reac., SSCI (coverage dropped).
—BLDSC (3910.848000), CISTI, EMDOCS, GNLM, IDS, ingenta, KNAW. **CCC.**
Published by: (International Fetal Medicine and Surgery Society), S. Karger AG, Allschwilerstr 10, PO Box, Basel 4009, Switzerland. TEL 41-61-306-1111, FAX 41-61-306-1234, karger@karger.ch, http://www.online.karger.com/journals/fdt, http://www.karger.com. Ed. W Holzgreve. adv.: page USD 1,185. Circ: 800. **U.S. and Canada subscr. to:** S. Karger Publishers Inc.

FIRST YEAR OF LIFE; a guide to your baby's growth and development month by month. see *CHILDREN AND YOUTH—About*

618 613.7 USA ISSN 1079-3615
FIT PREGNANCY. Variant title: Shape Presents Fit Pregnancy. Text in English. 1995. bi-m. USD 9.97 domestic; USD 17.97 foreign; USD 3.95 newsstand/cover domestic; GBP 2.95 newsstand/cover in United Kingdom; CND 4.95 newsstand/cover in Canada (effective 2001). adv. **Document type:** *Magazine, Consumer.* **Description:** Contains all the necessary information and advice about having babies and taking care of babies.
Related titles: Online - full text ed.: (from America Online, Inc.); ♦ Spanish ed.: Fit Pregnancy en Espanol.
Published by: Weider Publications, 21100 Erwin St, Woodland Hills, CA 91367. TEL 818-884-6800, FAX 818-716-5626, http://www.fitpregnancy.com. Ed. Peg Moline. Pub. Kevin Walsh. **Dist. in UK by:** Comag, Tavistock Works, Tavistock Rd, W Drayton, Middx UB7 7QX, United Kingdom. TEL 44-1895-433600, FAX 44-189-543-3606.

618 613.7 USA
▼ **FIT PREGNANCY EN ESPANOL.** Text in Spanish. 2000. bi-m. USD 4.95 newsstand/cover (effective 2001). adv. **Document type:** *Magazine, Consumer.*
Related titles: ♦ English ed.: Fit Pregnancy. ISSN 1079-3615.
Published by: Weider Publications, 21100 Erwin St, Woodland Hills, CA 91367. TEL 818-884-6800, FAX 818-716-5626. Pub. Kevin Walsh. Circ: 250,000.

▼ **FIT PREGNANCY STYLE.** see *LIFESTYLE*

618.2 649 SWE ISSN 1400-268X
FOEDSEL & FOERAELDRASKAP. Text in Swedish. 1981. q. SEK 200 domestic; SEK 330 in Europe; SEK 360 elsewhere. adv. bk.rev. **Document type:** *Newsletter, Consumer.*
Formerly (until 1994): Foeda Hemma (0282-4272)
Published by: Foereningen Foeda Hemma, c/o Sjoegren, Naadhammar 357, Molnbo 15021, Sweden. TEL 46-158231-58, FAX 46-8-550-131-33, bo.diane@gnesta.mail.telia.com, http://www.antronet.se/fodhem/. Eds. Helena Lindgren, Karin Salomonsson. Pub. Anna Whitaker. R&P Diane Sjoegren. Adv. contact Monica Winiger. Circ: 3,600.

618 ESP ISSN 1137-2990
FOLIA CLINICA EN OBSTETRICIA Y GINECOLOGIA. Text in Spanish. 1996. 6/yr. ESP 6,000 domestic; EUR 36.15 in Europe; USD 40 in United States (effective 2001).
Published by: Ediciones Mayo S.A., Muntaner, 374-376 4o, Barcelona 08006, Spain. TEL 34-93-2090255, FAX 34-93-2020643, foliagin@edicionesmayo.es, foliagin@edicionesmayo.es, http://www.edicionesmayo.es. Ed. Dr. Luis Cabero Roura.

618.1 DEU ISSN 0016-0237
DER FRAUENARZT✶. Text in German. 1951. 9/yr. DEM 198. adv. bk.rev. bibl, illus. **Document type:** *Academic/Scholarly.*
—GNLM.
Published by: (Berufsverband der Frauenaerzte e.V.), Demeter Verlag GmbH und Co. KG, Ammonitenstr 1, Balingen 72336, Germany. Circ: 5,300.

618 DEU ISSN 0016-5751
CODEN: GEFRA2
GEBURTSHILFE UND FRAUENHEILKUNDE. Text in German; Summaries in English, German. 1940. m. EUR 248.80 domestic to institutions; EUR 270.60 in Europe to institutions; EUR 291.80 elsewhere to institutions; EUR 24 newsstand/cover (effective 2002). adv. bk.rev. abstr, bibl, stat. index. reprint service avail. from PQC. *Refereed.* **Document type:** *Journal, Academic/Scholarly.*
Related titles: Online - full text ed.: ISSN 1438-8804 (from Institute for Scientific Information).
Indexed: ASCA, Agri.& Environ.Biotech.Abstr. (coverage dropped), Biol.Abstr., Chem.Abstr., Chem.Indus.Notes, Chem.Titles, Curr.Adv.Cancer Res., Curr.Cont., Derwent Biotech.Abstr., Excerp.Med., INIS Atomind., Ind.Med. (coverage dropped), Ind.Sci.Rev., Inpharma, Pharm.&Out.News, Reac., Rev.Med.& Vet.Mycol., SSCI (coverage dropped), Sci.Cit.Ind.
—BLDSC (4095.650000), CASDDS, CISTI, GNLM, IDS, KNAW. **CCC.**
Published by: (Deutsche Gesellschaft fuer Gynokologie und Geburtshilfe), Georg Thieme Verlag, Ruedigerstr 14, Stuttgart 70469, Germany. TEL 49-711-8931-0, FAX 49-711-8931298, gebfra@thieme.de, leser.service@thieme.de, http://www.thieme.de/gebfra. Eds. J Baltzer, M Breckwoldt. R&P Alessandra Kreibaum. Circ: 6,400.

618 USA ISSN 0744-0596
GENESIS (WASHINGTON). Text in English. 1966. q. USD 95 to members. adv. bk.rev. **Document type:** *Newsletter.*
Former titles: A.S.P.O. Genesis; (until 1978): Conceptions; A.S.P.O. Newsletter
Indexed: Gend.Watch.
Published by: Lamaze International, Inc., 1200 19th St, N W, Washington, DC 20036. TEL 202-857-1128, FAX 202-223-4579, Chris_Murphy@dcsba.com, http://www.lamaze-childbirth.com. Ed. Roberta Scaer. Adv. contact Karen Thompson. Circ: 4,000.

618.1 ESP ISSN 0211-6901
GINE DIPS. Text mainly in Spanish; Summaries in English, Spanish. 1970. 5/yr. ESP 6,300, USD 115 (effective 1999). adv. abstr, bibl, charts, illus, stat. **Document type:** *Trade.*
Indexed: Excerp.Med. (1995-), Ind.Med.Esp., Ref.Zh.
Published by: (Facultad de Medicina de Barcelona, Departamento de Ostetricia y Ginecologia), Editorial Dips Rocas, Muntaner, 393 pral. 4, Barcelona 08021, Spain. TEL 39-3-2001389, FAX 39-3-2021958, edipsro@intercom.es. Ed. Lorenzo Belaguero. R&P Alvaro Trevino. Adv. contact Carlos Martin. color page ESP 105,000. Circ: 5,000.

618 ITA
CODEN: GICLDY
GINECOLOGIA CLINICA E ONCOLOGICA. Text in Italian; Summaries in English. 1980. q. ITL 80,000, USD 90 domestic; ITL 150,000 foreign (effective 1999). adv. back issues avail. *Refereed.* **Document type:** *Academic/Scholarly.*
Formerly (until 1995): Ginecologia Clinica (0392-2944)
Indexed: Biol.Abstr.
—CISTI, GNLM.
Published by: Tipografia Editrice La Garangola, Via Montona, 6, Padua, PD 35137, Italy. TEL 39-49-8750550, FAX 39-49-8751743. Ed. Antonio Onnis. Adv. contact G Callegaro.

618 ITA ISSN 0393-5337
GINECOLOGIA DELL'INFANZIA E DELL'ADOLESCENZA. Text in Italian; Summaries in English. 1985-1992 (Jan.); resumed 2001. q. ITL 50,000, USD 50. adv. **Document type:** *Directory.*
Published by: (Societa Italiana di Ginecologia dell'Infanzia e dell'Adolescenza), C I C Edizioni Internazionali s.r.l., Corso Trieste 42, Rome, RM 00198, Italy. TEL 06-8412673, FAX 06-8443365, info@gruppocic.it, http://www.gruppocic.it. Ed. V Bruni. Pub. A Salvati.

618 MEX ISSN 0300-9041
CODEN: GOMEAY
GINECOLOGIA Y OBSTETRICIA DE MEXICO. Text in Spanish. 1946. m. USD 135. **Document type:** *Academic/Scholarly.*
Related titles: CD-ROM ed.
Indexed: Artemisa, Excerp.Med., INIS Atomind., Ind.Med. (1946-).
—BLDSC (4176.400000), CASDDS, EMDOCS, GNLM, KNAW.
Published by: Asociacion Mexicana de Ginecologia y Obstetricia, Ave. AMSTERDAM 214-PH2, Col Hipodromo, Mexico City, DF 06100, Mexico. TEL 5645463, FAX 2641745. Ed. Dr. Jose Ahved Ahved.

618.1 ITA ISSN 0391-8920
GINECORAMA. Text in Italian. 1979. 10/yr. ITL 40,000, USD 30 (effective 2001). adv.
Published by: C I C Edizioni Internazionali s.r.l., Corso Trieste 42, Rome, RM 00198, Italy. TEL 39-06-8412673, FAX 39-06-8412688, info@gruppocic.it, 1160199510. Ed. A Salvati. adv.: B&W page XEU 2,065.83, color page XEU 2,633.93; 300 x 420.

M

618.1 POL ISSN 0017-0011
CODEN: GIPOA3
GINEKOLOGIA POLSKA✱. Text in Polish; Summaries in English, Russian. 1922. m. USD 180. adv. bk.rev. abstr, bibl, charts, illus. index; cum.index.
Indexed: Biol.Abstr., Chem.Abstr., Curr.Adv.Ecol.Sci., Dok.Arbeitsmed., Excerp.Med., INIS Atomind., Ind.Med. (1922-).
—BLDSC (4176.500000), CASDDS, CISTI, GNLM.
Published by: Polskie Towarzystwo Ginekologiczne/Polish Society of Gynaecology, Ul Czerniakowska 231, Warsaw 01416, Poland. Ed. Z Slomko. Circ: 2,600. **Subscr. to:** RSW Prasa-Ksiazka-Ruch, Centrala Kolportazu Prasy i Wydawnictw, ul Towarowa 28, Warsaw 00958, Poland.

618 ITA ISSN 0391-9013
GIORNALE ITALIANO DI OSTETRICIA E GINECOLOGIA. Text in Italian; Summaries in English. 1979. m. ITL 130,000, USD 100 (effective 2001). adv.
Indexed: Excerp.Med., Ref.Zh.
—BLDSC (4178.237000), CISTI, EMDOCS, GNLM, Infotrieve, KNAW. **CCC.**
Published by: C I C Edizioni Internazionali s.r.l., Corso Trieste 42, Rome, RM 00198, Italy. TEL 39-06-8412673, FAX 39-06-8412688, info@gruppocic.it, 1160199510. Pub. A Salvati. adv.: B&W page XEU 1,239.5, color page XEU 1,704.31; 210 x 280. **Co-sponsors:** Gruppo di Ricerca ed Applicazioni Tecnologiche in Ostetricia e Ginecologia; Gruppo Operativo per la Ricerca Clinica in Ostetricia e Ginecologia.

618.2 618.1 BRA ISSN 1414-3534
GO ATUAL. Text in Portuguese. 1992. 10/yr. USD 450 (effective 2000 - 2001). abstr, bibl. Index.
Published by: Editora de Publicacoes Cientificas Ltda., Rua Major Suckow, 30, Rocha, Rio De Janeiro, RJ 20911-160, Brazil. TEL 55-21-2013722, 55-21-5010057, FAX 55-21-2613749. Eds. Paulo Belfort, J M Melo. R&P, Adv. contact Ana Paula. Circ: 14,500.

GREAT BRITAIN. GOVERNMENT STATISTICAL SERVICE. ABORTION STATISTICS. see *BIRTH CONTROL—Abstracting, Bibliographies, Statistics*

305.42 CAN ISSN 0823-9266
GREAT EXPECTATIONS. Text in English. 1972. 3/yr. CND 12, USD 18 (effective 2000). adv. bk.rev. back issues avail. **Document type:** *Consumer.* **Description:** Focus on pregnancy, birth, postpartum care, breastfeeding and parenting the newborn.
Published by: (Today's Parent Group), Professional Publishing Associates, 269 Richmond St W, Toronto, ON M5V 1X1, Canada. TEL 416-596-8680, FAX 416-596-1991. Ed. Holly Bennett. adv.: B&W page CND 13,120, color page CND 16,400. Circ: 200,000 (controlled).

618.4 ESP ISSN 1138-8412
GUIA DE EMBARAZO Y PARTO. Text in Spanish. 1996. s-a. free per issue to qualified personnel. adv. **Description:** Presents information on childbirth for pregnant women.
Formerly (until 1998): Enhorabuena Futura Mama (1136-3320)
Published by: Sfera Editores S.L., Pol. Mas Blau Ed. Muntadas, planta baja Esc. B, SOLSONES, 2, El Prat De Llobregat, Barcelona 08820, Spain. TEL 34-93-370-8585, FAX 34-93-370-5060, sfera@intercom.es. Ed. Juan Turu. adv.: page ESP 110,000; 205 x 270. Circ: 104,076.

618 USA
GUIDELINES FOR PERINATAL CARE. Text in English. 1983. irreg., latest vol.4, 1997. USD 60 (effective 2001). **Document type:** *Monographic series.* **Description:** Guidelines for care of pregnant women, fetuses, and neonates including discussion of preconceptional and antenatal screening, adoption, perinatal infections, and fetal monitoring.
Published by: American Academy of Pediatrics, 141 Northwest Point Blvd, Box 927, Elk Grove Village, IL 60009-0927. TEL 847-228-5005, 800-433-9016, FAX 847-228-1281, http://www.aap.org. **Co-sponsor:** American College of Obstetricians and Gynecologists.

618 CHN
GUOWAI YIXUE (FUCHAN KEXUE FENCE)/FOREIGN MEDICAL SCIENCES (GYNECOLOGY & OBSTETRICS). Text in Chinese. q.
Published by: Tianjin Yixue Keji Qingbao Yanjiusuo/Tianjin Medical Science and Technology Information Institute, 131 Chengdu Dao, Heping-qu, Tianjin 300050, China. TEL 302570. Ed. Yu Aifeng.

618 FRA ISSN 0240-172X
GYN OBS - LA MEDECINE ET LA FEMME. Text in French. 1979. 18/yr. EUR 99 in Europe to institutions; USD 116 elsewhere to institutions (effective 2002). illus. back issues avail. *Refereed.* **Document type:** *Journal, Academic/Scholarly, Trade.* **Description:** Provides obestetricians and gynecologists with updated information and commentary on women's medicine.
Indexed: Ref.Zh.
Published by: Elsevier Paris, Editions Scientifiques et Medicales (Subsidiary of: Reed Elsevier plc. group), 23 rue Linois, Paris 75015, France. TEL 33-1-45589110, FAX 33-1-45589419, gynobs@elsevier.fr, academic@elsevier-fr, http://www.elsevier.fr. Ed. Christian Rayr. Pub. Jean Cohen. Circ: 10,000.

618 HRV ISSN 1330-0091
CODEN: GYPREQ
GYNAECOLOGIA ET PERINATOLOGIA; journal for gynaecology, perinatology, reproductive medicine, and ultrasonic diagnostics. Text in Croatian, English; Summaries in English. 1960. q., latest vol.10, 2001. USD 30. adv. bk.rev. bibl, charts, illus. index. 60 p./no. back issues avail.; reprints avail. *Refereed.* **Document type:** *Journal, Academic/Scholarly.*
Former titles (until 1992): Jugoslavenska Ginekologija i Perinatologija (0352-5562); (until 1985): Jugoslavenska Ginekologija i Opstetricija (0017-002X); Ginekologija i Opstetricija
Indexed: Biol.Abstr., Dent.Ind., Excerp.Med., Ind.Med. (coverage dropped).
—CISTI, EMDOCS, GNLM.
Published by: Hrvatsko Drustvo Ginekologa i Opstetricara/Croatian Society of Gynecology & Obstetrics, Petrova 13, Zagreb 10000, Croatia. TEL 385-1-4604616, FAX 385-1-4633512. Eds. Dr. Ante Drazancic, Dr. Asim Kurjak, Dr. Zdravko Pavlic. Circ: 1,350.

618 GBR ISSN 0962-1091
CODEN: GYNEEB
GYNAECOLOGICAL ENDOSCOPY. Text in English. 1992. bi-m., latest vol.11, 2002. GBP 107 in Europe to individuals; USD 173 in North America to individuals; GBP 117 elsewhere to individuals; GBP 322 in Europe to institutions; USD 507 in North America to institutions; GBP 352 elsewhere to institutions (effective 2002). adv. bk.rev. abstr, bibl, illus. index. back issues avail. *Refereed.* **Document type:** *Academic/Scholarly.* **Description:** Contains reviews articles, research papers, short communications and letters on development of endoscopic techniques in gynecological practice.
Related titles: Microform ed.: (from PQC); Online - full text ed.: ISSN 1365-2508. GBP 97 in Europe to individuals; USD 156 in North America to individuals; GBP 97 elsewhere to individuals; GBP 290 in Europe to institutions; USD 457 in North America to institutions; GBP 290 elsewhere to institutions (effective 2002) (from Ovid Technologies, Inc., EBSCO Publishing, O C L C Online Computer Library Center, Inc., RoweCom Information Quest, ingenta, Munksgaard & Blackwell Science's Synergy, Swets Blackwell, Institute for Scientific Information); ♦ Supplement: Gynaecological Endoscopy. Supplement. ISSN 1354-5167.
Indexed: Curr.Cont., Excerp.Med. (1993-), Inpharma, Pharm.&Out.News, Reac.
—BLDSC (4233.510000), ADONIS, EMDOCS, GNLM, IDS, Infotrieve, KNAW. **CCC.**
Published by: (British Society for Gynaecological Endoscopy), Blackwell Science Ltd., PO Box 88, Oxford OX2 0NE, United Kingdom. TEL 44-1865-206180, 44-1865-206002, FAX 44-1865-206219, jnl.orders@blacksci.co.uk, http://www.blackwell-science.com/~cgilib/jnlpage.asp?Journal=gendo&File=gendo, http://www.blackwellpublishing.com. Ed. R Garry. Pub. Allen Stevens. R&P Sophie Savage. Adv. contact Jenny Applin. Circ: 1,525.

618 GBR ISSN 1354-5167
GYNAECOLOGICAL ENDOSCOPY. SUPPLEMENT. Text in English. irreg.
Related titles: ♦ Supplement to: Gynaecological Endoscopy. ISSN 0962-1091.
—ADONIS.
Published by: Blackwell Science Ltd., Osney Mead, Oxford OX2 0EL, United Kingdom. TEL 44-1865-206206, FAX 44-1865-721205, journals.cs@blacksci.co.uk, http://www.blackwell-science.com/.

618.1 NLD ISSN 1384-5454
GYNAECOLOGY FORUM. Text in English. 1996. q. USD 125 to individuals; USD 150 to institutions (effective 2000). **Document type:** *Academic/Scholarly.*
—BLDSC (4233.515000), KNAW.
Published by: Medical Forum International, PO Box 655, Zeist 3700 AR, Netherlands. FAX 31-30-6930162, correspondence@medforum.nl, http://www.medforum.nl/. Ed. Stephen R Killick. Pub. K Polack.

618.1 DEU ISSN 0017-5994
CODEN: GYNKAP
DER GYNAEKOLOGE. Text in German. 1968. m. EUR 296.54 domestic; EUR 267.74 foreign; EUR 25.20 newsstand/cover (effective 2002). adv. back issues avail.; reprint service avail. from ISI. *Refereed.* **Document type:** *Journal, Academic/Scholarly.* **Description:** Covers all aspects of gynecology and women's health.
Related titles: Microform ed.: (from PQC); Online - full text ed.: ISSN 1433-0393 (from EBSCO Publishing, RoweCom Information Quest, Swets Blackwell, Springer LINK, Institute for Scientific Information).
Indexed: ASCA, Biol.Abstr., Curr.Adv.Ecol.Sci., Curr.Cont., Excerp.Med., INIS Atomind., Ind.Med. (coverage dropped), Pharm.&Out.News.
—BLDSC (4233.550000), CISTI, GNLM, IDS, Infotrieve, KNAW. **CCC.**
Published by: Springer-Verlag (Subsidiary of: BertelsmannSpringer), Tiergartenstr 17, Heidelberg 69121, Germany. TEL 49-6221-345-0, FAX 49-6221-345229, subscriptions@springer.de, http://link.springer.de/service/journals/00129/index.htm, http://www.springer.de. Eds. H G Bender, L Beck. **Subscr. in N. America to:** Springer-Verlag New York Inc., PO Box 2485, Secaucus, NJ 07096-2485. TEL 212-460-1500, FAX 212-473-6272.

618.1 CHE ISSN 1420-6811
GYNAEKOLOGIE FUER HAUSAERZTE. Text in German. 1996. q. CHF 36; CHF 46 in Europe; CHF 62 elsewhere (effective 2000). adv. **Document type:** *Magazine, Academic/Scholarly, Trade.*
Related titles: ♦ Supplement to: Ars Medici. ISSN 0004-2897.
—GNLM.
Published by: Rosenfluh Publikationen, Rosenbergstr 115, Neuhausen 8212, Switzerland. TEL 41-52-6727822, FAX 41-52-6727823. Ed. Dr. Barbel Hirrle. **Subscr. to:** EDP Services, Ebenaustr, Horw 6048, Switzerland. TEL 41-41-3491760, FAX 41-41-3491718.

618 DEU ISSN 1439-3557
GYNAEKOLOGIE UND GEBURTSHILFE. Text in German. 1996. bi-m. EUR 70.68 domestic; EUR 81.68 foreign; EUR 55.73 domestic to students; EUR 66.73 foreign to students; EUR 15.89 newsstand/cover (effective 2002). adv. **Document type:** *Journal, Academic/Scholarly.*
Formerly (until 1998): Hautnah Gynaekologie und Geburtshilfe (1431-5688)
Published by: Urban und Vogel Medien und Medizin Verlagsgesellschaft mbH (Subsidiary of: BertelsmannSpringer), Neumarkter Str 43, Munich 81673, Germany. TEL 49-89-43721411, FAX 49-89-43721410, verlag@urban-vogel.de, http://www.urban-vogel.de. Ed. Dr. B Kleine-Gunk. R&P Friederik Klein. Adv. contact Christiane Loichinger. Circ: 13,000 (paid). **Subscr. to:** Springer Auslieferungs Gesellschaft, Postfach 105160, Heidelberg 69041, Germany. TEL 49-6221-345244, FAX 49-6221-345244.

618.1 CHE ISSN 1018-8843
CODEN: GGRUEL
GYNAEKOLOGISCH - GEBURTSHILFLICHE RUNDSCHAU. Text in English, French, German. 1964. q. CHF 643, EUR 459.20 in Europe to institutions; CHF 654.60, USD 500 elsewhere to institutions (effective 2002). adv. illus. Supplement avail.; back issues avail.; reprint service avail. from ISI. *Refereed.* **Document type:** *Journal, Academic/Scholarly.* **Description:** Publishes selected original articles and practice-oriented studies on particular themes in the fields of obstetrics and gynecology.
Formerly: Gynaekologische Rundschau (0017-6001)
Related titles: Online - full text ed.: ISSN 1423-0011. CHF 58, EUR 42, USD 45 to institutions with print edition (effective 2002) (from EBSCO Publishing, O C L C Online Computer Library Center, Inc., RoweCom Information Quest, Swets Blackwell).
Indexed: ASCA, Biol.Abstr., Curr.Cont., Ind.Med. (1992-), Inpharma, Pharm.&Out.News, Reac., Rev.Appl.Entomol.
—BLDSC (4233.565000), CISTI, GNLM, IDS, Infotrieve, KNAW. **CCC.**
Published by: (Oesterreichische Gesellschaft fuer Gynaekologie und Geburtshilfe), S. Karger AG, Allschwilerstr 10, PO Box, Basel 4009, Switzerland. TEL 41-61-306-1111, FAX 41-61-306-1234, karger@karger.ch, http://www.online.karger.com/journals/ggr, http://www.karger.com. adv.: page USD 1,195. Circ: 1,500.

M

618 DEU ISSN 0341-8677
GYNAEKOLOGISCHE PRAXIS. Text in German. 4/yr. EUR 162; EUR 45 newsstand/cover (effective 2002). **Document type:** *Journal, Academic/Scholarly.*
—BLDSC (4233.570000), GNLM. **CCC.**
Published by: Hans Marseille Vertrieb Medizinischer Zeitschriften, Buerkleinstr 12, Munich 80538, Germany. TEL 49-89-227988, FAX 49-89-2904643, marseille-verlag@t-online.de, http://www.marseille-verlag.com. Ed. W Siebert.

618 DEU ISSN 0179-9185
GYNE. Text in German. 1980. m. DEM 60; DEM 5.50 newsstand/cover (effective 2000). adv. index. back issues avail. **Document type:** *Magazine, Academic/Scholarly.*
Related titles: ♦ Supplement: Horme. ISSN 0935-2880; ♦ Korasion. ISSN 0932-0601; ♦ Ikon. ISSN 0941-911X.
—BLDSC (4233.630000), GNLM.
Published by: H U F Verlag, Lindenhof 47, Muehlheim 45481, Germany. TEL 49-208-480027, FAX 49-208-485899. Circ: 10,450.

618 CHE ISSN 0378-7346
CODEN: GOBIDS
GYNECOLOGIC AND OBSTETRIC INVESTIGATION. Text in English. 1895. 8/yr. (in 2 vols.). CHF 1,534, EUR 1,096.40 in Europe to institutions; CHF 1,557.20, USD 1,192 elsewhere to institutions (effective 2002). adv. bibl, illus. index. back issues avail. *Refereed.* **Document type:** *Journal, Academic/Scholarly.* **Description:** Covers the most active and promising areas of current research in gynecology and obstetrics. Original papers report selected experimental and clinical investigations in all fields related to gynecology, obstetrics and reproduction.
Former titles: Gynecologic Investigation (0017-5986); Gynaecologia
Related titles: Microform ed.; Online - full text ed.: ISSN 1423-002X. CHF 116, EUR 84, USD 90 to institutions with print edition (effective 2002) (from EBSCO Publishing, O C L C Online Computer Library Center, Inc., RoweCom Information Quest, Swets Blackwell, Institute for Scientific Information).
Indexed: ASCA, Anim.Breed.Abstr., Biol.Abstr., Chem.Abstr., Chem.Indus.Notes, Chem.Titles, Curr.Adv.Ecol.Sci., Curr.Cont., Dairy Sci.Abstr., Excerp.Med., Ind.Med. (1978-), Ind.Sci.Rev., Inpharma, NRN, Pharm.&Out.News, Reac., Rev.Appl.Entomol., Rev.Med.& Vet.Mycol., Sci.Cit.Ind., THA.
—BLDSC (4233.650000), CASDDS, CISTI, EMDOCS, GNLM, IDS, ingenta, KNAW. **CCC.**
Published by: S. Karger AG, Allschwilerstr 10, PO Box, Basel 4009, Switzerland. TEL 41-61-306-1111, FAX 41-61-306-1234, karger@karger.ch, http://www.online.karger.com/journals/goi, http://www.karger.com. Ed. G Zador. adv.: page USD 1,195. Circ: 950.

618.1 USA ISSN 0090-8258
RC280.G5 CODEN: GYNOA3
GYNECOLOGIC ONCOLOGY; an international journal. Text in English. 1972. m. USD 1,755 in US & Canada to institutions; USD 1,999 elsewhere to institutions (effective 2001). adv. index. back issues avail. *Refereed.* **Document type:** *Academic/Scholarly.* **Description:** Serves as an archive devoted to the publication of clinical and investigative articles that concern tumors of the female reproductive tract.
Related titles: Online - full text ed.: (from EBSCO Publishing, O C L C Online Computer Library Center, Inc., RoweCom Information Quest, ingenta, Swets Blackwell, IDEAL Online Library, Institute for Scientific Information).
Indexed: ASCA, Apic.Abstr., Biol.Abstr., Chem.Abstr., Chem.Indus.Notes, Chem.Titles, Curr.Adv.Ecol.Sci., Curr.Cont., Excerp.Med., INIS Atomind., Ind.Med. (1972-), Ind.Sci.Rev., Inpharma, Int.Abstr.Biol.Sci., NRN, Pharm.&Out.News, Reac., Sci.Cit.Ind., THA.
—BLDSC (4233.710000), ADONIS, CASDDS, CISTI, GNLM, IDS, ingenta, KNAW. **CCC.**
Published by: Academic Press, Inc., Journal Division (Subsidiary of: Harcourt Brace & Company), 525 B St, Ste 1900, San Diego, CA 92101-4495. TEL 619-230-1840, FAX 619-699-6800, apsubs@acad.com, http://www.academicpress.com/gyn. Ed. David Gershenson.

618 617 USA
GYNECOLOGIC SURGERY SOCIETY. MEMBERSHIP NEWSLETTER. Text in English. 1993. s-a. USD 95 to members (effective 1995). bk.rev. back issues avail. **Document type:** *Newsletter.* **Description:** Reports and analyzes developments in surgical procedures, complications, instruments and other trends of interest.
Formerly: Gynecologic Laser and Advanced Technology Society. Membership Newsletter
Published by: (Gynecologic Surgery Society), Mary Ann Liebert, Inc. Publishers, 2 Madison Ave, Larchmont, NY 10538. Circ: 1,000.

GYNECOLOGICAL ENDOCRINOLOGY. see *MEDICAL SCIENCES—Endocrinology*

618 FRA ISSN 1167-2420
GYNECOLOGIE INTERNATIONALE; recherche et clinique en gynecologie obstetrique. Text in French. 1992. m. (10/yr). FRF 300 domestic to individuals; FRF 450 foreign to individuals; FRF 210 domestic to libraries; FRF 360 foreign to libraries (effective 2001). adv. *Refereed.* **Document type:** *Academic/Scholarly.*
Published by: L E N Medical, 15 rue des Sablons, Paris 75116, France. TEL 33-1-47553131, FAX 33-1-47553132. Ed. Dr. Louis Elgozi. Adv. contact Emmanuelle Guiard Schmid. Circ: 8,000.

618 301.426 FRA ISSN 1297-9589
GYNECOLOGIE OBSTETRIQUE ET FERTILITE. Text in French. 1973. m. USD 273 in United States to institutions; EUR 224 in Europe to institutions (effective 2002). adv. bk.rev. **Description:** Explores various planned parenthood issues.
Former titles (until 2000): Contraception - Fertilite - Sexualite (1165-1083); (until 1992): Fertilite, Contraception, Sexualite (1164-7418); (until 1992): Contraception Fertilite Sexualite (1157-8181); (until 1991): Fertilite Contraception Sexualite (0980-3904); (until 1986): Contraception Fertilite Sexualite (0301-861X)
Related titles: Online - full text ed.: (from ingenta, Institute for Scientific Information).
Indexed: ASCA, Biol.Abstr., Curr.Adv.Cancer Res., Curr.Adv.Cell & Devel.Biol., Curr.Cont. (coverage dropped), Excerp.Med., Ind.Med. (2000-), Inpharma, Pharm.&Out.News, Reac., SSCI (coverage dropped).
—BLDSC (4233.765000), CISTI, EMDOCS, GNLM, IDS, Infotrieve, KNAW. **CCC.**
Published by: Elsevier Paris, Editions Scientifiques et Medicales (Subsidiary of: Reed Elsevier plc. group), 23 rue Linois, Paris 75015, France. TEL 33-1-45589110, FAX 33-1-45589419. Circ: 5,000.

618 FRA ISSN 0988-6990
GYNECOLOGIE - OBSTETRIQUE PRATIQUE. Text in French. 1988. m. (10/yr.). EUR 39 domestic to individuals; EUR 53 foreign to individuals; EUR 27 domestic to libraries; EUR 42 foreign to libraries (effective 2002).
Published by: L E N Medical, 15 rue des Sablons, Paris 75116, France. TEL 33-1-47553131, FAX 33-1-47553132, lenmed@club-internet.fr, http://www.webmedguide.com. Ed. Dr. D Zarca. Circ: 7,800.

618.1 FRA ISSN 1250-3347
CODEN: GRGYE
GYNECOLOGIE - REVUE DU GYNECOLOGUE. Text in French; Summaries in English. 1950. 8/yr. FRF 750; FRF 927 foreign (effective 1996). adv. bk.rev. abstr, bibl, charts, illus, stat. index. reprint service avail. from ISI. **Document type:** *Academic/Scholarly.* **Description:** Publishes original papers, general reviews, and round tables.
Formed by the 1993 merger of: Revue du Gynecologue Obstetricien (1141-5886); Gynecologie (0301-2204); Which was formerly: Gynecologie Pratique (0017-6028)
Indexed: Biol.Abstr., Excerp.Med., Ind.Med. (coverage dropped).
—CISTI, EMDOCS, GNLM, Infotrieve. **CCC.**
Published by: (Societe Francaise de Gynecologie), Masson - Periodiques, 120 bd. St. Germain, Paris 75006, France. TEL 33-1-40466200, FAX 33-1-40466201. Ed. Hoang Mgnoc Minh. Circ: 6,000. **Co-sponsor:** Federation Internationale de Gynecologie et du Partheriologie.

618.1 301.5 USA ISSN 0892-628X
H E R S NEWSLETTER. Text in English. 1982. q. USD 20 (effective 2001). bk.rev. abstr, stat. cum.index. back issues avail. **Document type:** *Newsletter, Proceedings, Consumer.* **Description:** Presents medical and scientific reviews discussing alternatives and consequences of hysterectomies.
Published by: (Hysterectomy Educational Resources & Services), H E R S Foundation, 422 Bryn Mawr Ave, Bala Cynwyd, PA 19004. TEL 610-667-7757, FAX 610-667-8096, hersfdn@aol.com, http://www.hersfoundation.com/. Ed. Joanne West. R&P Nora W Coffey. Circ: 15,000.

618 ZAF ISSN 1023-4802
HAPPY, HEALTHY AND PREGNANT; for mums & dads to be. Text in English. 1994. s-a. ZAR 4.96. adv. illus. **Document type:** *Consumer.*
Published by: Grape Publishing, PO Box 467, Dunnottar 1590, South Africa.

HAVING A BABY. see *CHILDREN AND YOUTH—About*

HEALTH CARE FOR WOMEN INTERNATIONAL. see *WOMEN'S HEALTH*

HEALTH LAW LITIGATION REPORTER; the monthly national journal of record reporting general medical malpractice, obstetrical and gynecological litigation. see *LAW—Civil Law*

618.202 DEU ISSN 0932-8122
DIE HEBAMME; Fortbildungszeitschrift fuer Hebammen und Entbildungspfleger. Text in German. 1988. q. EUR 54.40 domestic to institutions; EUR 60.90 in Europe to institutions; EUR 63.80 elsewhere to institutions; EUR 15.90 newsstand/cover (effective 2002). adv. reprint service avail. from IRC. **Document type:** *Journal, Academic/Scholarly.*
—GNLM.
Published by: Ferdinand Enke Verlag, Ruedigerstr 14, Stuttgart 70469, Germany. TEL 49-711-25520-0, FAX 49-711-2552030, http://www.thieme.de. Eds. G Martius, J W Dudenhausen. R&P, Adv. contact Babette Kehrenberg.

618 JPN ISSN 0367-6277
HOKKAIDO SANKA FUJINKA GAKKAI KAISHI/HOKKAIDO OBSTETRICAL AND GYNECOLOGICAL SOCIETY. JOURNAL. Text in Japanese. 1950. a. JPY 8,000. **Document type:** *Academic/Scholarly.*
Published by: Nihon Sanfujinka Gakkai, Hokkaido Chiho Bukai/Japan Society of Obstetrics and Gynecology, Hokkaido Branch, c/o Hokkaido Daigaku Igakubu Sanfujinka Kyoshitsu, Nishi 7-chome, Kita 15-jo, Kita-ku, Sapporo-shi, Hokkaido 060, Japan. TEL 011-716-1161, FAX 011-707-5767. Ed. Hiroshi Satoh. Circ: 650.

618 DEU ISSN 0935-2880
HORME. Text in German. 1988. 3/yr. **Document type:** *Journal, Academic/Scholarly.*
Related titles: ♦ Supplement to: Gyne. ISSN 0179-9185.
—GNLM.
Published by: H U F Verlag, Lindenhof 47, Muehlheim 45481, Germany. TEL 49-208-480027, FAX 49-208-485899.

618 616.4 JPN ISSN 1340-220X
CODEN: HFGYFH
HORMONE FRONTIER IN GYNECOLOGY. Text in Japanese. 1994. 4/yr. JPY 2,400 per issue (effective 1998).
Indexed: Chem.Abstr., Chem.Indus.Notes, Chem.Titles.
—CASDDS.
Published by: Medikaru Rebyusha/Medical Review Co., Ltd., 7-3 Hirano-Machi 1-chome, Chuo-ku, Osaka-shi 541-0046, Japan. TEL 81-6-223-1667, FAX 81-6-223-1338, meview@osk3.3web.ne.jp.

618 GBR
HUMAN CONCERN NEWSPAPER. Text in English. 1968. q. membership. adv. bk.rev. stat. **Document type:** *Newspaper.*
Formerly: Society for the Protection of Unborn Children. Bulletin
Published by: Society for the Protection of Unborn Children, Phyllis Bowman House, 5 St Matthew St, London SW1P 2JT, United Kingdom. TEL 44-171-222-5845, FAX 44-171-222-0630, sysop@spuc.org.uk. Ed. Phyllis Bowman. Circ: 65,000.

618 GBR ISSN 1464-7273
HUMAN FERTILITY. Text in English. 1996. q. GBP 160 to libraries (effective 2001). adv. 72 p./no. 2 cols./p. back issues avail. *Refereed.* **Document type:** *Journal, Academic/Scholarly.* **Description:** Publishes research into all aspects of human fertility and reproduction.
Formerly (until 1998): British Fertility Society. Journal (1363-9579)
—BLDSC (4336.086000). **CCC.**
Published by: (British Fertility Society), Journals of Reproduction & Fertility Ltd, 22 Newmarket Rd, Cambridge CB5 8DT, United Kingdom. TEL 44-1223-351809, FAX 44-1223-359754, jrf@journals-of-reproduction.org.uk, http://www.journals-of-reproduction.org.uk. Ed. Henry Leese. adv.: page GBP 405; trim 170 x 240.

M

618 616.4 GBR ISSN 0268-1161
CODEN: HUREEE
HUMAN REPRODUCTION. Text in English. 1986. m. GBP 290, USD 495 to individuals; GBP 630, USD 1,165 to institutions (effective 2002). adv. illus. index. back issues avail.; reprint service avail. from SWZ. *Refereed.* **Document type:** *Journal, Academic/Scholarly.* **Description:** For scientists and clinicians working in international human reproduction research and practice.
Related titles: Online - full text ed.: ISSN 1460-2350. GBP 565, USD 1,050 to institutions Online only (effective 2002) (from HighWire Pr., EBSCO Publishing, O C L C Online Computer Library Center, Inc., RoweCom Information Quest, ingenta, Swets Blackwell, Institute for Scientific Information).
Indexed: ASCA, Anim.Breed.Abstr., Biol.Abstr., Chem.Abstr., Chem.Indus.Notes, Chem.Titles, Curr.Adv.Ecol.Sci., Curr.Cont., Dairy Sci.Abstr., Excerp.Med., Fam.Ind., Ind.Med. (1986-), Ind.Sci.Rev., Inpharma, Neurosci.Cit.Ind., Nutr.Abstr., Pharm.&Out.News, Reac., SSCI (coverage dropped), Sci.Cit.Ind., THA.
—BLDSC (4336.431000), CASDDS, CISTI, EMDOCS, GNLM, IDS, ingenta, KNAW. **CCC.**
Published by: (European Society of Human Reproduction and Embryology BEL), Oxford University Press, Academic Division, Great Clarendon St, Oxford OX2 6DP, United Kingdom. TEL 44-1865-267907, FAX 44-1865-267835, jnl.info@oup.co.uk, http://www.oup.co.uk/humrep/, http://www.oup.co.uk/journals. Eds. H K Beard, D H Barlow. Pub. J Boullin. R&P Fionna Willis. adv.: page GBP 450, page USD 800. Circ: 3,600. **Subscr. in the Americas to:** Oxford University Press, Journals, 2001 Evans Rd, Cary, NC 27513. TEL 800-852-7323, FAX 919-677-1714, jnlorders@oup-usa.org; **Subscr. to:** Journals Marketing, Great Clarendon St, Oxford OX2 6DP, United Kingdom.

HYPERTENSION IN PREGNANCY. see *MEDICAL SCIENCES—Cardiovascular Diseases*

618 DEU ISSN 0941-911X
IKON. Text in German. 1991. s-a. **Document type:** *Magazine, Academic/Scholarly.*
Related titles: ♦ Supplement to: Gyne. ISSN 0179-9185.
Published by: H U F Verlag, Lindenhof 47, Muehlheim 45481, Germany. TEL 49-208-480027, FAX 49-208-485899.

IN VERWACHTING. see *CHILDREN AND YOUTH—About*

618 USA ISSN 1064-7449
CODEN: IDOGEX
INFECTIOUS DISEASES IN OBSTETRICS AND GYNECOLOGY. Text in English. 1993. bi-m. GBP 50 domestic to individuals; USD 75 in United States to individuals; GBP 125 domestic to institutions; USD 195 in United States to institutions (effective 2000). adv. back issues avail. *Refereed.* **Document type:** *Academic/Scholarly.* **Description:** Publishes original papers focusing on the study or treatment of infectious disease in the obstetric patient or the female reproductive organs. Provides detailed coverage of such areas as viral, microbial, and bacterial infections; sexually transmitted disease and HIV; ante-partum infections, opportunistic infection in chemotherapy patients; and new developments in antibiotics and other therapeutic measures.
Related titles: Microform ed.: (from PQC); Online - full text ed.: ISSN 1098-0997. 1996 (from EBSCO Publishing, CatchWord Ltd., Wiley InterScience).
Indexed: Abstr.Hyg., Dairy Sci.Abstr., Environ.Sci.Poll.Mgmt., Helminthol.Abstr., Ind.Med. (1993-), Microbiol.Abstr., Pollut.Abstr., Protozool.Abstr., Ref.Zh., Rev.Appl.Entomol., Rev.Med.& Vet.Mycol., Risk Abstr., Saf.Sci.Abstr., Trop.Dis.Bull., Virol.Abstr. (coverage dropped).
—BLDSC (4478.729100), GNLM, Infotrieve, KNAW. **CCC.**
Published by: Parthenon Publishing Group (Subsidiary of: C R C Press (New York)), Casterton Hall, Casterton, Carnforth, Lancs LA6 2LA, United Kingdom. TEL 44-1524-272084, FAX 44-1524-271587, mail@parthpub.com, http://www.parthpub.com/. adv.: B&W page GBP 640, color page GBP 1,515; trim 210 x 279. Circ: 550.

618 USA ISSN 0160-7626
RC889 CODEN: INFEDH
INFERTILITY* ; an interdisciplinary journal devoted to the rapid communication of clinical aspects of human infertility. Text in English. 1978. q. USD 65 to individuals; USD 147 to institutions. adv. charts, illus. index. back issues avail.; reprint service avail. from PQC. *Refereed.* **Document type:** *Academic/Scholarly.* **Description:** Examines female infertility, andrology, endocrinology, genetics, extra-corporeal fertilization and other aspects of human fertility.
Related titles: Online - full text ed.: 1978.
Indexed: Biol.Abstr., Chem.Abstr., Curr.Adv.Ecol.Sci., Curr.Cont. (coverage dropped), Excerp.Med., I.P.A.
—CASDDS, CISTI, GNLM, ingenta. **CCC.**
Address: c/o Dr Louis A Mucelli, Ed, 131 E 65th St, New York, NY 10021-7006. TEL 212-684-4242, FAX 212-684-4290.

618 USA ISSN 1047-9422
RG133.5 CODEN: IRMCF8
INFERTILITY AND REPRODUCTIVE MEDICINE CLINICS OF NORTH AMERICA. Text in English. 1990. q. USD 132 domestic to individuals; USD 174 in Canada to individuals; USD 185 elsewhere to individuals; USD 199 domestic to institutions; USD 252 foreign to institutions; USD 129 domestic to students; USD 64 per issue (effective 2001). index. back issues avail. **Document type:** *Academic/Scholarly.* **Description:** Each issue approaches a specific topic in the field.
Related titles: Microform ed.: (from PQC).
Indexed: CINAHL, Excerp.Med. (1995-).
—BLDSC (4478.791000), GNLM, KNAW.
Published by: W.B. Saunders Co. (Subsidiary of: Harcourt Publishers Ltd.), 11830 Westline Industrial Dr, St Louis, MO 63146. TEL 800-325-4177, http://www.wbsaunders.com. Eds. Alan H Decherney, Michael P Diamond. **Subscr. to:** Periodicals Fulfillment, W B Saunders Co, 6277 Sea Harbor Dr, 4th Fl, Orlando, FL 32891-4800.

618.202 GBR
INTERNATIONAL CONFEDERATION OF MIDWIVES. ANNUAL REPORT. Text in English. 1993. a. **Description:** Includes summary of the Confederation's membership, activities,and finance over three years.
Formerly: International Confederation of Midwives. Triennial Report
Published by: International Confederation of Midwives/Confederation Internationale des Sages-femmes, Eisenhowerlaan 138, The Hague 2517, United Kingdom. TEL 44-181-995-1332, FAX 44-181-995-1332.

610.73 GBR ISSN 0074-2880
INTERNATIONAL CONFEDERATION OF MIDWIVES. CONGRESS REPORTS. Text in English. triennial, latest 1996, 24th, Oslo. GBP 25 (effective 1998). **Document type:** *Proceedings, Abstract/Index.* **Description:** Lists over 200 papers given at the Triennial Congress.
Published by: International Confederation of Midwives/Confederation Internationale des Sages-femmes, Eisenhowerlaan 138, The Hague 2517, United Kingdom. TEL 44-181-995-1332, FAX 44-181-995-1332.

618 GBR
INTERNATIONAL CONFEDERATION OF MIDWIVES. POSITION STATEMENTS. Text in English. 1990. 3/yr. GBP 0.50 per issue (effective 1998). **Document type:** *Monographic series.* **Description:** Includes statements agreed by the Confederation on professional, clinical, ethical, and statutory issues relating to midwifery.
Published by: International Confederation of Midwives/Confederation Internationale des Sages-femmes, Eisenhowerlaan 138, The Hague 2517, United Kingdom. TEL 44-181-995-1332, FAX 44-181-995-1332.

301.426 USA ISSN 0190-3187
HQ763
INTERNATIONAL FAMILY PLANNING PERSPECTIVES. Text in English. 1975. q. USD 36 to individuals; USD 46 domestic to institutions; USD 56 foreign to institutions (effective 2001). adv. charts, illus, stat. reprint service avail. from PQC. *Refereed.* **Document type:** *Academic/Scholarly.* **Description:** Highlights population research and program achievements of prime interest to those concerned with the growing family planning challenges faced by developing countries.
Former titles (until vol.4, no.4, 1978): International Family Planning Perspectives and Digest (0162-2749); (until vol.3, no.4, 1977): International Family Planning Digest
Related titles: Microfilm ed.: (from PQC); Online - full text ed.: (from JSTOR (Web-based Journal Archive), Northern Light Technology, Inc., ProQuest Information & Learning, LexisNexis, Institute for Scientific Information); ♦ Spanish ed.: Perspectivas Internacionales en Planificacion Familiar. ISSN 0190-3195; ♦ French ed.: Perspectives Internationales sur le Planning Familial.
Indexed: ASCA, Abstr.Hyg., Abstr.Rural Dev.Trop., Bibl.Asian Stud. (1988-1991), Biol.Dig., CWI, Curr.Cont., Curr.Cont.M.E., Curr.Lit.Fam.Plan., Ekist.Ind., Excerp.Med., Fam.Ind., Lang.& Lang.Behav.Abstr., Mult.Ed.Abstr., P.A.I.S., Popul.Ind., Ref.Zh., Rural Devel.Abstr., SOPODA, SRI, SSCI, Soc.Serv.Abstr., Sociol.Abstr., Stud.Wom.Abstr., Trop.Dis.Bull.
—BLDSC (4540.150000), GNLM, IDS, ingenta, KNAW.
Published by: Alan Guttmacher Institute, 120 Wall St, New York, NY 10005. TEL 212-248-1111, FAX 212-248-1951, llebran@AGI-USA.org, http://www.AGI-USA.org. Ed. Patricia Donovan. R&P Kaylynn Chiarello. Adv. contact Mark Hildebrand. Circ: 20,000.

618 USA ISSN 0887-8625
INTERNATIONAL JOURNAL OF CHILDBIRTH EDUCATION. Text in English. 1961. q. USD 25. adv. bk.rev. bibl. *Refereed.* **Document type:** *Consumer.* **Description:** Covers maternity and infant care.
Formerly (until 1986): I C E A News (0445-0485)
Related titles: Online - full text ed.: (from Northern Light Technology, Inc., ProQuest Information & Learning).
Indexed: CINAHL, Curr.Lit.Fam.Plan., Fam.Ind., Gend.Watch.
—BLDSC (4542.165400).
Published by: International Childbirth Education Association, PO Box 20048, Minneapolis, MN 55420-0048. TEL 612-854-8660, FAX 612-854-8772. Ed. Trudy Keller. Adv. contact Doris Olson. Circ: 12,000.

618 616.99 USA ISSN 1048-891X
CODEN: IJGCEN
INTERNATIONAL JOURNAL OF GYNECOLOGICAL CANCER. Text in English. 1991. bi-m. USD 335 domestic to individuals; USD 350 in Canada & Mexico to individuals; USD 375 elsewhere to individuals; USD 465 domestic to institutions; USD 480 in Canada & Mexico to institutions; USD 505 elsewhere to institutions; USD 368.50, USD 511.50 to institutions print & online eds. combined (effective 2001). adv. reprints avail. *Refereed.* **Document type:** *Academic/Scholarly.* **Description:** Covers topics in gynecology, oncology, radiation therapy and pathology from an interdisciplinary perspective.
Related titles: Online - full text ed.: ISSN 1525-1438. USD 302 to individuals; USD 419 to institutions (effective 2001) (from Ovid Technologies, Inc., EBSCO Publishing, O C L C Online Computer Library Center, Inc., RoweCom Information Quest, ingenta, Munksgaard & Blackwell Science's Synergy, Swets Blackwell, Institute for Scientific Information).
Indexed: ASCA, Curr.Cont., Excerp.Med. (1993-), Ind.Sci.Rev., Inpharma, Int.Abstr.Biol.Sci., Pharm.&Out.News, Reac., Sci.Cit.Ind., Trop.Dis.Bull.
—BLDSC (4542.273500), EMDOCS, GNLM, IDS, Infotrieve, KNAW. **CCC.**
Published by: (International Gynecological Cancer Society), Blackwell Science Inc., Commerce Pl, 350 Main St, Malden, MA 02148-5018. TEL 781-388-8250, 800-759-6102, FAX 781-388-8255, journals@blacksci.com, http://www.blackwell-science.com. Ed. Harold Fox. R&P Tracey Davies. Adv. contact Jenny Applin.

618.1 USA ISSN 0277-1691
INTERNATIONAL JOURNAL OF GYNECOLOGICAL PATHOLOGY. Text in English. 1982. q. USD 288 domestic to individuals; USD 355 foreign to individuals; USD 430 domestic to institutions; USD 497 foreign to institutions; USD 114 newsstand/cover (effective 2002). adv. index. reprint service avail. from PQC. *Refereed.* **Document type:** *Academic/Scholarly.* **Description:** Reports on advances in the understanding and management of gynecological disease.
Related titles: Online - full text ed.: USD 559 domestic academic site license; USD 626 foreign academic site license; USD 623.50 domestic corporate site license; USD 690.50 foreign corporate site license (effective 2002) (from Ovid Technologies, Inc., Institute for Scientific Information).
Indexed: ASCA, Curr.Adv.Cancer Res., Curr.Cont., Excerp.Med., INIS Atomind., Ind.Med. (1982-), Ind.Sci.Rev., Inpharma, Int.Abstr.Biol.Sci., Pharm.&Out.News, Reac., Sci.Cit.Ind.
—BLDSC (4542.274000), CISTI, EMDOCS, GNLM, IDS, ingenta, KNAW.
Published by: (International Society of Gynecological Pathologists), Lippincott Williams & Wilkins (Philadelphia) (Subsidiary of: Wolters Kluwer N.V.), 530 Walnut St, Philadelphia, PA 19106-3621. TEL 215-521-8300, http://www.Lww.com. Ed. Dr. Philip B Clement. Pub. Shelley Johnsony. R&P Margaret Becker. Adv. contact Ray Thibodeau. B&W page USD 710, color page USD 1,790. Circ: 1,176 (paid). **Subscr. to:** PO Box 1600, Hagerstown, MD 21740-1600. TEL 800-777-2295, FAX 301-824-7390.

618 IRL ISSN 0020-7292
RG1 CODEN: IJGOAL
INTERNATIONAL JOURNAL OF GYNECOLOGY AND OBSTETRICS. Text in English. 1963. m. EUR 177 in Europe to individuals; JPY 23,600 in Japan to individuals; USD 199 elsewhere to individuals; EUR 1,269 in Europe to institutions; JPY 168,400 in Japan to institutions; USD 1,420 elsewhere to institutions (effective 2002). adv. bibl, illus. index. back issues avail. *Refereed.* **Document type:** *Journal, Academic/Scholarly.* **Description:** Publishes articles on all aspects of basic and clinical research in the fields of obstetrics and gynecology and related subjects, with emphasis on matters of worldwide interest.
Supersedes: International Federation of Gynaecology and Obstetrics. Journal (0020-6695)
Related titles: Microform ed.: (from PQC); Online - full text ed.: (from ingenta, Swets Blackwell, ScienceDirect, Institute for Scientific Information).
Indexed: ASCA, Abstr.Hyg., Arts & Hum.Cit.Ind. (coverage dropped), Biol.Abstr., Chem.Abstr., Chem.Indus.Notes, Chem.Titles, Curr.Adv.Ecol.Sci., Curr.Cont., Curr.Lit.Fam.Plan., Dairy Sci.Abstr., Dent.Ind., Excerp.Med., INIS Atomind., Ind.Med. (1969-), Ind.Sci.Rev., Inpharma, Int.Abstr.Biol.Sci., Int.Nurs.Ind., NRN, Nutr.Abstr., Pharm.&Out.News, Protozool.Abstr., Reac., Rev.Appl.Entomol., Rev.Med.& Vet.Mycol., Rural Devel.Abstr., SSCI (coverage dropped), Sci.Cit.Ind., THA, Trop.Dis.Bull.
—BLDSC (4542.273000), CASDDS, CISTI, GNLM, IDS, ingenta, KNAW. **CCC.**
Published by: (International Federation of Gynaecology and Obstetrics NGA), Elsevier Science Ireland Ltd, Elsevier House, Brookvale Plaza, E. Park, Shannon, Co. Clare, Ireland. TEL 353-61-709600, FAX 353-61-709100, http://www.elsevier.com/locate/ijgo. Ed. J J Sciarra. R&P Annette Moloney. Circ: 4,000. **Subscr. in Australasia and the Far East to:** Elsevier Science (Singapore) Pte Ltd, No.1 Temasek Ave, 17-01 Millenia Tower, Singapore 039192, Singapore. TEL 65-434-3727, FAX 65-337-2230; **Subscr. in the Americas to:** Elsevier Science, PO Box 945, New York, NY 10159-0945. TEL 212-633-3730, 888-437-4636, FAX 212-633-3680, usinfo-f@elsevier.com, http://www.elsevier.com; **Subscr. to:** Elsevier Science Inc - Japan Regional Office, 9-15 Higashi-Azabu 1-chome, Minato-ku, Tokyo 106-0044, Japan. TEL 81-3-5561-5033, FAX 81-3-5561-5047. **Subscr. to:** Elsevier Science BV, PO Box 211, Amsterdam 1000 AE, Netherlands. TEL 31-20-485-3757, FAX 31-20-485-3432.; **Dist. by:** Elsevier Science (Brazil).

618 GBR ISSN 0959-289X
CODEN: IOANER
INTERNATIONAL JOURNAL OF OBSTETRIC ANESTHESIA. Text in English. q. GBP 127 to individuals; GBP 230 to institutions (effective 2002). adv. *Refereed.* **Document type:** *Academic/Scholarly.* **Description:** Presents research papers on obstetric anaesthesia, analgesia and related topics.
Related titles: Online - full text ed.: (from IDEAL Online Library, Institute for Scientific Information).
Indexed: Curr.Cont., Excerp.Med. (1993-), Inpharma, Pharm.&Out.News, Reac., Ref.Zh.
—BLDSC (4542.410500), EMDOCS, GNLM, IDS, Infotrieve, KNAW. **CCC.**
Published by: Churchill Livingstone (Subsidiary of: Harcourt Publishers Ltd.), Robert Stevenson House, 1-3 Baxter's Pl, Leith Walk, Edinburgh, Midlothian EH1 3AF, United Kingdom. TEL 44-131-556-2424, FAX 44-131-459-1177, cservice@harcourt.com, http://www.harcourt-international.com/journals/ijoa. Eds. D A Rocke, S C Hughes. Pub. Gillian Griffith. R&P Catherine John TEL 212-424-4200. Adv. contact David Dunnachie. Circ: 625. **Subscr. to:** Harcourt Publishers Ltd., Foots Cray High St, Sidcup, Kent DA14 5HP, United Kingdom. TEL 44-20-8308-5700, FAX 44-20-8309-0807.

618 DEU ISSN 0943-5417
INTERNATIONAL JOURNAL OF PRENATAL AND PERINATAL PSYCHOLOGY AND MEDICINE. Text in English, German. 1989. 4/yr. DEM 120 to individuals; DEM 160 to institutions (effective 2001 & 2002). adv. bk.rev. **Document type:** *Journal, Academic/Scholarly.*
Formerly (until 1993): International Journal of Prenatal and Perinatal Studies (0954-8629)
—BLDSC (4542.481800), GNLM.
Published by: Mattes Verlag GmbH, Postfach 103866, Heidelberg 69028, Germany. TEL 49-6221-459321, FAX 49-6221-459322, journals@mattes.de. Eds. L Janus, P Fedor Freybergh. Pub. Kurt Mattes.

618 GBR
INTERNATIONAL MIDWIFERY. Text in English. 6/yr. NLG 85, EUR 40 (effective 1998). **Document type:** *Newsletter.* **Description:** News and listings of events and publications both from member associations and relating to midwifery worldwide.
Former titles (until 1998): International Midwifery Matters (1025-1669); (until 1994): International Confederation of Midwives. Newsletter
Indexed: Brit.Nur.Ind., CINAHL.
Published by: International Confederation of Midwives/Confederation Internationale des Sages-femmes, Eisenhowerlaan 138, The Hague 2517, United Kingdom. TEL 44-181-995-1332, FAX 44-181-995-1332, intimidwives@compuserve.com, 100702.2405@compuserve.com. Ed. Elizabeth Duff.

618 616.6 GBR ISSN 0937-3462
CODEN: IUJOEF
INTERNATIONAL UROGYNECOLOGY JOURNAL. Text in English. 1990. bi-m. EUR 373.30 domestic; EUR 357.10 in Germany; EUR 68.80 newsstand/cover foreign (effective 2002). back issues avail. *Refereed.* **Document type:** *Academic/Scholarly.* **Description:** Emphasizes a clinical approach to urogynecological topics of interest to urologists, gynecologists, nurses and basic scientists.
Related titles: Microform ed.: (from PQC); Online - full text ed.: ISSN 1433-3023. 1999 (from EBSCO Publishing, RoweCom Information Quest, Swets Blackwell, Springer LINK, Institute for Scientific Information).
Indexed: Curr.Cont., Excerp.Med. (1993-), Ind.Med. (coverage dropped).
—BLDSC (4551.567800), EMDOCS, GNLM, Infotrieve, KNAW. **CCC.**
Published by: Springer-Verlag London Ltd. (Subsidiary of: BertelsmannSpringer), Sweetapple House, Catteshall Rd, Godalming, Surrey GU7 3DJ, United Kingdom. TEL 44-1483-418800, FAX 44-1483-415144. Ed. Ó C Ortiz. **U.S. subscr. to:** Springer-Verlag New York Inc., PO Box 2485, Secaucus, NJ 07096-2485.

618 USA
▼ **THE INTERNET JOURNAL OF GYNECOLOGY AND OBSTETRICS.** Text in English. 2000. s-a. free per issue. adv. bk.rev. back issues avail. *Refereed.* **Document type:** *Academic/Scholarly.* **Description:** Provides information from the field of gynecology and obstetrics; contains original articles, reviews, case reports, streaming slide shows, streaming videos, letters to the editor, press releases and meeting information.
Media: Online - full content.
Published by: Internet Scientific Publications, L.L.C., 23 Rippling Creek Dr, Sugar Land, TX 77479. TEL 281-240-1533, FAX 281-240-1533, http://www.ispub.com/. R&P, Adv. contact Hope Morrow TEL 832-754-0335.

618 ITA ISSN 1121-8339
ITALIAN JOURNAL OF GYNAECOLOGY & OBSTETRICS. Text in Italian. 1989. q.
—BLDSC (4588.340430), EMDOCS, GNLM, KNAW.
Published by: Societa Italiana di Ginecologia e Ostetricia, Via dei Soldati 25, Rome, RM 00186, Italy.

618 360 JPN
J A O G NEWS. Text in Japanese. 1949. m. JPY 10,000. adv. bk.rev. *Refereed.* **Document type:** *Newsletter.*
Former titles (until May 1995): Nihon Bosei Hogo Sanfujinka Ikai; (until Mar. 1994): Nichibo Iho (0288-8270)
Published by: Japan Association of Obstetricians & Gynecologists/Japan Association for Maternal Welfare, 1-2 Ichigaya-Sadohara-cho, Shinjuku-ku, Tokyo 162-0842, Japan. TEL 81-3-3269-4739, FAX 81-3-3269-4730, jimu@jaog.or.jp, http://www.jaog.or.jp. Ed., Pub. Shoichi Sakamoto. Circ: 14,800.

J O G N N. (Journal of Obstetric, Gynecologic, and Neonatal Nursing) see *MEDICAL SCIENCES—Nurses And Nursing*

618 DEU ISSN 0941-5246
JAHRBUCH DER GYNAEKOLOGIE UND GEBURTSHILFE. Text in German; Summaries in English, German. 1991. a. DEM 126.40. back issues avail. **Document type:** *Academic/Scholarly.*
—GNLM.
Published by: Biermann Verlag GmbH, Nideggenerstr 18, Zuelpich 53909, Germany. TEL 49-2252-9410-0, FAX 49-2252-941015. Ed. W Schmidt.

618.202 JAM
JAMAICA MIDWIVES ASSOCIATION. NEWSLETTER. Text in English. bi-m. membership.
Published by: Jamaica Midwives Association, c/o Victoria Jubilee Hospital, Kingston, Jamaica.

618 DEU ISSN 1432-5128
JATROS GYN. Text in German. 1985. 12/yr. DEM 140 (effective 1998). back issues avail. **Document type:** *Academic/Scholarly.* **Description:** Seminar papers including summaries of original articles, interviews and congress reports.
Formerly: Jatros Gynaekologie (0177-9109)
—GNLM.
Published by: Hoffmann und Hoffmann GmbH, August-Schanz-Str 8-II, Frankfurt A.m. 60433, Germany. TEL 49-69-54800015, FAX 49-69-54800080, huhgmbh@aol.com. Ed. Peter Hoffman. Circ: 8,500.

618 TUR ISSN 1016-5126
CODEN: JODEE
JINEKOLOJI VE OBSTETRIK DERGISI/JOURNAL OF GYNECOLOGY AND OBSTETRICS. Text in Turkish; Summaries in English. 1987. q. USD 60 (effective 2001). adv. **Document type:** *Journal, Academic/Scholarly.*
Indexed: Excerp.Med. (1994-).
—BLDSC (4669.029380), EMDOCS.
Published by: Logos Yayincilik Ticaret A.S., Yildiz Posta Cad., Sinan Apt. No. 36 D 66-67, Gayrettepe, Istanbul 80280, Turkey. TEL 90-212-2880541, FAX 90-212-3116185, info@logos.com.tr, http://logos.com.tr. Ed. Dr. Turgay Atasu. Adv. contact Sukran Oznalga.

618.2 SWE
JORDEMODERN/MIDWIFE; Svenska Barnmorskefoerbundet tids tidskrift. Text in Swedish. 1888. m. SEK 300 (effective 2001). adv. bk.rev. illus. 48 p./no. **Document type:** *Newspaper, Journal, Academic/Scholarly, Internal.*
Indexed: Int.Nurs.Ind.
—BLDSC (4673.940000), GNLM.
Published by: Svenska Barnmorskefoerbundet/Swedish Association of Midwives, Ostermalmsgatan 19, Stockholm 11426, Sweden. TEL 46-8-10-70-88, FAX 46-8-24-49-46, barnmorskeforbundet@swemidwife.a.se, http://www.barnmorskefoerbundet.a.se. Ed. Ann Nordfell. Pub. Ingera Radesrnd. Adv. contact Karsn Westwnd. Circ: 7,300.

618.2 610.73 NOR ISSN 0805-0562
JORDMORBLADET. Text in Norwegian. 1994. 10/yr. bk.rev. **Document type:** *Trade.* **Description:** Contains professional articles on obstetrics, midwifery, pregnancy and childbirth.
Indexed: Int.Nurs.Ind.
Published by: Norsk Sykepleierforbund/Norwegian Nurses Association, Postboks 2633, St Hanshaugen, Oslo 0131, Norway. TEL 47-22-04-33-04, FAX 47-22-38-35-36. Circ: 1,900.

618.1 BRA ISSN 0368-1416
CODEN: JBGCA8
JORNAL BRASILEIRO DE GINECOLOGIA. Text and summaries in English, Portuguese. 1935. m. USD 200. adv. bk.rev. bibl, charts, illus.
Indexed: Biol.Abstr., Excerp.Med., INIS Atomind., Ind.Med. (coverage dropped).
—BLDSC (4674.637000), CISTI, EMDOCS, GNLM.
Published by: (Universidade Federal do Rio de Janeiro, Centro de Estudos da Maternidade), Cidade - Editora Cientifica Ltda., Rua Mexico, 90-Andar 2, Centro, Rio De Janeiro, RJ 20031-141, Brazil. Ed. Fernando Moyses. R&P Jose Soly Torres. Adv. contact Sergio Hardy. Circ: 9,000.

618.202 JPN ISSN 0389-9063
JOSANPU/JAPANESE MIDWIFE. Text in Japanese. 1947. 4/yr. JPY 6,300 per issue. **Document type:** *Trade.*
Published by: Nihon Josanpukai Shuppanbu/Japan Midwives Association, 8-21 Fujimi 1-chome, Chiyoda-ku, Tokyo 102-0071, Japan. TEL 813-3262-9923, FAX 813-3262-8933. Ed. Shigeko Horiuchi.

618.202 610.73 JPN ISSN 0047-1836
JOSANPU ZASSHI/JAPANESE JOURNAL FOR MIDWIVES. Text in Japanese. 1952. m. JPY 14,400. adv. illus.
Indexed: Int.Nurs.Ind., Ref.Zh.
—BLDSC (4656.510000), GNLM.
Published by: Igaku-Shoin Ltd., 5-24-3 Hongo, Bunkyo-ku, Tokyo 113-0033, Japan. TEL 81-3-3817-5773, FAX 81-3-3825-4145, ysekiyama@nna.so.net.or.jp. Circ: 12,000.

618 FRA ISSN 0368-2315
CODEN: JGOBAC
JOURNAL DE GYNECOLOGIE OBSTETRIQUE ET BIOLOGIE DE LA REPRODUCTION. Text in French; Summaries in English, French. 1920. 8/yr. FRF 1,135; FRF 1,363 foreign (effective 2000). adv. bk.rev. abstr, illus. index. reprint service avail. from ISI. **Document type:** *Academic/Scholarly.* **Description:** Focuses on the entire field of medical and surgical gynecology as well as obstetrics and perinatal medicine.
Formerly: Gynecologie et Obstetrique et Federation des Societes de Gynecologie et d'Obstetrique. Bulletin (0017-601X)
Related titles: Microform ed.: (from PQC); Online - full text ed.: (from RoweCom Information Quest).
Indexed: Biol.Abstr., Chem.Abstr., Excerp.Med., Ind.Med. (1972-), Int.Nurs.Ind., Nutr.Abstr.
—BLDSC (4996.600000), CASDDS, CISTI, EMDOCS, GNLM, Infotrieve, KNAW. **CCC.**
Published by: (Federation des Gynecologues et Obstetriciens de Langue Francaise. College National des Gynecologues et Obstetriciens), Masson - Periodiques, 120 bd. St. Germain, Paris 75006, France. TEL 33-1-40466200, FAX 33-1-40466201. Ed. G Magnin. Circ: 5,000. **Subscr. to:** Societe de Periodiques Specialises, BP 22, Vineuil Cedex 41354, France. TEL 33-2-54504612, FAX 33-2-54504611.

618 FRA ISSN 1241-4727
JOURNAL D'OBSTETRIQUE ET DE GYNECOLOGIE. Key Title: Jobgyn. Text in French. 1993. bi-m. FRF 485 domestic to doctors; USD 100 foreign to doctors; FRF 980 domestic to institutions; USD 195 foreign to institutions; FRF 350 domestic to students; USD 68 foreign to students.
Published by: Sedip Medical, 75 Cours Albert Thomas, Lyon Cedex 3 69447, France. TEL 72-35-23-72, FAX 72-35-23-75.

612.6 AUT ISSN 1019-066X
JOURNAL FUER FERTILITAET UND REPRODUKTION; Zeitschrift fuer In-Vitro-Fertilisation, assistierte Reproduktion und Kontrazeption. Text in German. 1991. q. ATS 400; ATS 120 newsstand/cover (effective 2001). adv. bk.rev. abstr, bibl. back issues avail. *Refereed.* **Document type:** *Journal, Academic/Scholarly.* **Description:** Contains research into all aspects of in-vitro fertilization and other forms of artificial reproduction.
—BLDSC (4984.035000).
Published by: Krause & Pachernegg GmbH, Mozartgasse 10, Gablitz 3003, Austria. TEL 43-2231-61258-0, FAX 43-2231-6125810, k_u_p@eunet.at, http://members.eunet.at/k_u_p/fert.htm, http://members.eunet.at/k_u_p/verlag.htm. Ed. Dr. Franz Fischl.

618.173 AUT ISSN 1023-0904
JOURNAL FUER MENOPAUSE; Zeitschrift fuer diagnostische, therapeutische und prophylaktische Aspekte im Klimakterium. Text in German. 1994. q. ATS 400 (effective 2001). abstr, bibl. back issues avail. *Refereed.* **Document type:** *Journal, Academic/Scholarly.* **Description:** Contains research into all aspects of menopause.
—BLDSC (5017.643000).
Published by: Krause & Pachernegg GmbH, Mozartgasse 10, Gablitz 3003, Austria. TEL 43-2231-61258-0, FAX 43-2231-6125810, k_u_p@eunet.at, http://members.eunet.at/k_u_p/meno.htm, http://members.eunet.at/k_u_p/verlag.htm. Ed. Dr. Franz Fischl.

JOURNAL FUER UROLOGIE UND UROGYNAEKOLOGIE; Zeitschrift fuer Urologie und Urogynaekologie in Klinik und Praxis. see *MEDICAL SCIENCES—Urology And Nephrology*

610.73 618 USA ISSN 1526-9523
CODEN: JNUMEQ
JOURNAL MIDWIFERY AND WOMEN'S HEALTH. Text in English. 1955. bi-m. EUR 99 in Europe to individuals; JPY 13,200 in Japan to individuals; USD 112 elsewhere to individuals; EUR 237 in Europe to institutions; JPY 31,500 in Japan to institutions; USD 265 elsewhere to institutions; EUR 64 in Europe student price; JPY 8,500 in Japan student price; USD 72 elsewhere student price (effective 2002). adv. bk.rev. bibl, charts, illus. cum.index. back issues avail.; reprints avail. *Refereed.* **Document type:** *Journal, Academic/Scholarly.* **Description:** Includes the presentation of current knowledge in the fields of nurse-midwifery, parent-child health, obstetric, well-woman gynecology, family planning and neonatology.
Former titles (1973-1999): Journal of Nurse - Midwifery (0091-2182); American College of Nurse - Midwives. Bulletin (0002-8002); (until 1969): American College of Nurse - Midwifery. Bulletin (0098-3721)
Related titles: Microform ed.: (from PQC); Online - full text ed.: (from ingenta, ScienceDirect, Swets Blackwell, Institute for Scientific Information).
Indexed: ASCA, ASSIA, AgeLine, CINAHL, Curr.Cont., Excerp.Med., Fam.Ind., Ind.Med. (2000-), Int.Nurs.Ind., Jrnl.Watch Wom.Hlth., Nurs.Abstr., SSCI.
—BLDSC (5019.935000), GNLM, IDS, Infotrieve, ingenta, KNAW. **CCC.**
Published by: (American College of Nurse-Midwives), Elsevier Science, Box 945, New York, NY 10159-0945. TEL 212-989-5800, FAX 212-633-3990, info@acnm.org, usinfo-f@elsevier.com, http://www.elsevier.com/locate/jmwh. Eds. L L Paine, Mary Ann Shah. **Subscr. in Australasia and the Far East to:** Elsevier Science (Singapore) Pte Ltd, No.1 Temasek Ave, 17-01 Millenia Tower, Singapore 039192, Singapore. TEL 65-434-3727, FAX 65-337-2230**; Subscr. in Japan to:** Elsevier Science Inc - Japan Regional Office, 9-15 Higashi-Azabu 1-chome, Minato-ku, Tokyo 106-0044, Japan. TEL 81-3-5561-5033**; Subscr. outside the Americas to:** Elsevier Science BV, PO Box 211, Amsterdam 1000 AE, Netherlands. TEL 31-20-485-3757.

618 USA ISSN 1058-0468
RG135 CODEN: JARGE4
JOURNAL OF ASSISTED REPRODUCTION AND GENETICS. Text in English. 1984. m. USD 899, EUR 897 to institutions for print or online ed.; USD 152, EUR 152 to individuals for print or online ed.; USD 1,078.80, EUR 1,076.40 to institutions for print & online eds.combined (effective 2002). adv. back issues avail. *Refereed.* **Document type:** *Journal, Academic/Scholarly.* **Description:** Covers research in the reproductive sciences, including assisted reproduction technologies, genetics of early gestation, relevant contributions from laboratory sciences affecting diagnosis and treatment of infertility, preimplantation genetics, and controversies in assisted reproduction.
Formerly (until 1992): Journal of in Vitro Fertilization and Embryo Transfer (0740-7769)
Related titles: Microfilm ed.: (from PQC); Online - full text ed.: (from Ovid Technologies, Inc., EBSCO Publishing, O C L C Online Computer Library Center, Inc., RoweCom Information Quest, Swets Blackwell, Kluwer Online, Institute for Scientific Information).
Indexed: ASCA, AgBiotech, Anim.Breed.Abstr., Curr.Cont., Excerp.Med., INIS Atomind., Ind.Med. (1992-), Inpharma, Pharm.&Out.News, Reac., Rel.Ind.One, Rel.Ind.Two.
—BLDSC (4947.286000), CISTI, EMDOCS, GNLM, IDS, Infotrieve, ingenta, KNAW. **CCC.**
Published by: (International Working Group on Preimplanation Genetics), Kluwer Academic - Plenum Publishers (Subsidiary of: Wolters Kluwer N.V.), 233 Spring St, New York, NY 10013-1578. TEL 212-620-8000, 800-221-9369, FAX 212-463-0742, info@plenum.com, http://www.wkap.nl; http://www.wkap.nl/journalhome.htm/1058-0468. Ed. Norbert Gleicher. R&P Rose Luongo TEL 781-871-6311. **Subscr. outside the Americas to:** Kluwer Academic Publishers Group, Journals Department, PO Box 322, Dordrecht 3300 AH, Netherlands. TEL 31-78-639-2392, FAX 31-78-654-6474.

JOURNAL OF DIAGNOSTIC MEDICAL SONOGRAPHY. see *MEDICAL SCIENCES—Radiology And Nuclear Medicine*

618 JPN ISSN 0914-6776
JOURNAL OF FERTILIZATION AND IMPLANTATION. Key Title: Nihon Jusei Chakusho Gakkai Zasshi. Text in English, Japanese. 1984. a. JPY 6,000. **Document type:** *Academic/Scholarly.*
Published by: Japan Society of Fertilization and Implantation/Nihon Jusei Chakusho Gakkai, c/o Convex Inc., Ichijoji Bldg, 2-3-22 Azabudai, Minato-ku, Tokyo 106-0041, Japan. TEL 81-3-3589-3460, FAX 81-3-3589-3974, convex@po.iijnet.or.jp. Ed. Masahiko Hiroi. Circ: 1,400.

618.1059 USA ISSN 1042-4067
CODEN: JGYSEF
JOURNAL OF GYNECOLOGIC SURGERY. Text in English. 1984. q. USD 149 domestic to individuals; USD 268 foreign to individuals; USD 179 domestic to individuals print and online eds. combined; USD 298 foreign to individuals print and online eds. combine; USD 417 domestic to institutions; USD 532 foreign to institutions; USD 500 domestic to institutions print and online eds. combined; USD 615 foreign to institutions print and online eds. combined (effective 2002). adv. bk.rev. abstr. back issues avail.; reprints avail. *Refereed.* **Document type:** *Journal, Academic/Scholarly.* **Description:** Deals with all aspects of operative and office gynecology, including colposcopy, endoscopy (hysteroscopy and laparoscopy), laser and conventional surgery, female urology, microsurgery, and in vitro fertilization.
Formerly (until 1989): Colposcopy and Gynecologic Laser Surgery (0741-6113)
Related titles: Online - full content ed.: USD 417 to institutions; USD 149 to individuals (effective 2002); Online - full text ed.: (from CatchWord Ltd., Institute for Scientific Information, RoweCom Information Quest).
Indexed: ASCA, Curr.Adv.Cancer Res., Curr.Cont. (coverage dropped), Excerp.Med., Inpharma, Pharm.&Out.News, Reac., Sci.Cit.Ind. (coverage dropped).
—BLDSC (4996.595000), CISTI, EMDOCS, GNLM, IDS, Infotrieve, KNAW. **CCC.**
Published by: (Gynecologic Laser Society), Mary Ann Liebert, Inc. Publishers, 2 Madison Ave, Larchmont, NY 10538. TEL 914—834-3100, FAX 914-834-1388, info@liebertpub.com, http://www.liebertpub.com/gyn. Ed. Michael S Baggish. **Co-sponsors:** Gynecologic Surgery Society; International Society for Gynecologic Endoscopy: British Society for Cervical Pathology.

618.1 USA ISSN 1069-2673
JOURNAL OF GYNECOLOGIC TECHNIQUES. Text in English. 1995. q. USD 111 domestic to individuals; USD 149 foreign to individuals; USD 176 domestic to institutions; USD 229 foreign to institutions; USD 58 domestic to students; USD 92 foreign to students; USD 58 per issue (effective 2000). *Refereed.* **Document type:** *Academic/Scholarly.* **Description:** Features original and review articles on techniques and methods, particularly those that are innovative, and general advances in diagnostic, operative, and other therapeutic techniques related to the specialty of gynecology.
—CISTI, GNLM, Infotrieve, KNAW. **CCC.**
Published by: Saunders Company (Subsidiary of: Pearson Professional), 15 E 26th St, Fl 15, New York, NY 10010-1505. TEL 212-238-7800, FAX 212-727-7808, http://www.wbsaunders.com. Ed. Jonathan Berek. Pub. Jane Grochowski. **Subscr. in the UK to:** Pearson Professional Ltd., Journals Subscription Department, Fourth Ave., PO Box 77, Harlow, Essex CM19 5AA, United Kingdom. TEL 44-1279-623924, FAX 44-1279-639609.

618.71 USA ISSN 0890-3344
CODEN: JHLAE5
JOURNAL OF HUMAN LACTATION. Text in English. 1984. q. USD 340 domestic; USD 356 foreign (effective 2002). adv. bk.rev., film rev., video rev. bibl, illus. index. 96 p./no. back issues avail.; reprints avail. *Refereed.* **Document type:** *Journal, Academic/Scholarly.* **Description:** Publishes scientific articles and commentaries on human lactation and breastfeeding, and discussions of clinical case reports relevant to practicing lactation consultants.
Related titles: Online - full text ed.: (from EBSCO Publishing, O C L C Online Computer Library Center, Inc., ingenta, Swets Blackwell, RoweCom Information Quest).
Indexed: CINAHL, Fam.Ind., IMFL, Int.Nurs.Ind.
—BLDSC (5003.417000), GNLM, ingenta, KNAW.
Published by: (International Lactation Consultant Association), Sage Publications, Inc., Sage Science Press, 2455 Teller Rd, Thousand Oaks, CA 91320. TEL 805-499-0721, FAX 805-499-0871, info@sagepub.com, http://www.sagesciencepress.com/. Ed. M Jane Heinig. Pub. Susan Hanscom. R&P Peter Marino. Adv. contact Robert Vrooman. B&W page USD 635, color page USD 1,895; bleed 8.375 x 11.125. Circ: 2,000.

618 616.6 USA ISSN 1089-2591
JOURNAL OF LOWER GENITAL TRACT DISEASE. Text in English. 1997. q. USD 105 domestic to individuals; USD 115 in Canada & Mexico to individuals; USD 135 elsewhere to individuals; USD 170 domestic to institutions; USD 180 in Canada & Mexico to institutions; USD 200 elsewhere to institutions; USD 115.50 to individuals print & online eds. combined; USD 187 to institutions print & online eds. combined (effective 2001). adv. reprints avail. *Refereed.* **Document type:** *Journal, Academic/Scholarly.* **Description:** Acts as a source for the latest science in the field of diagnosis, etiology and therapy of pathologic conditions of the cervix, vagina and vulva.
Related titles: ♦ Online - full text ed.: Journal of Lower Genital Tract Disease Online. ISSN 1526-0976.
—BLDSC (5010.590000), Infotrieve. **CCC.**
Published by: (American Society for Colposcopy and Cervical Pathology), Blackwell Science Inc., Commerce Pl, 350 Main St, Malden, MA 02148-5018. TEL 781-388-8250, journals@blacksci.com, http://www.blackwell-science.com. Ed. Leo V Twiggs. R&P Tracey Davies. Adv. contact Jenny Applin. **Co-sponsor:** International Federation of Cervical Pathology and Coloscopy.

618 USA ISSN 1526-0976
JOURNAL OF LOWER GENITAL TRACT DISEASE ONLINE. Text in English. q. USD 95 to individuals; USD 153 to institutions (effective 2001). **Document type:** *Academic/Scholarly.*
Media: Online - full text (from EBSCO Publishing, O C L C Online Computer Library Center, Inc., RoweCom Information Quest, ingenta, Munksgaard & Blackwell Science's Synergy, Swets Blackwell). **Related titles:** ♦ Print ed.: Journal of Lower Genital Tract Disease. ISSN 1089-2591.
Published by: Blackwell Science Inc., Commerce Pl, 350 Main St, Malden, MA 02148-5018. TEL 781-388-8250, 800-759-6102, FAX 781-388-8255, website@blacksci.com, journals@blacksci.com, http://www.blackwell-science.com.

THE JOURNAL OF NEONATAL NURSING. see *MEDICAL SCIENCES—Nurses And Nursing*

618 GBR ISSN 0144-3615
CODEN: JOGYDW
JOURNAL OF OBSTETRICS AND GYNAECOLOGY. Text in English. 1980. bi-m. GBP 70, USD 131 to individuals; GBP 234, USD 409 to institutions (effective 2002). adv. bk.rev. index. *Refereed.* **Document type:** *Academic/Scholarly.*
Related titles: Online - full text ed.: ISSN 1364-6893 (from CatchWord Ltd., EBSCO Publishing, O C L C Online Computer Library Center, Inc., RoweCom Information Quest, ProQuest Information & Learning, Swets Blackwell).
Indexed: Chem.Abstr., Curr.Adv.Cancer Res., Curr.Adv.Ecol.Sci., Curr.Cont. (coverage dropped), Excerp.Med., Nutr.Abstr., Protozool.Abstr.
—BLDSC (5025.400000), ADONIS, CASDDS, CatchWord, CISTI, GNLM, ingenta, KNAW. **CCC.**
Published by: (Institute of Obstetrics and Gynaecology Trust), Carfax Publishing Limited (Subsidiary of: Taylor & Francis Group), PO Box 25, Abingdon, Oxon OX14 3UE, United Kingdom. TEL 44-1235-401000, FAX 44-1235-401550, enquiries@carfax.co.uk, enquiry@tandf.co.uk, http://www.carfax.co.uk. Ed. D F Hawkins. Circ: 500.

618 JPN ISSN 1341-8076
CODEN: AOJGDU
JOURNAL OF OBSTETRICS AND GYNAECOLOGY. Text in English. 1970. 6/yr. JPY 12,000 domestic; JPY 15,000 foreign (effective 2000); free per issue to qualified personnel. abstr. *Refereed.* **Document type:** *Academic/Scholarly.* **Description:** Contains open announcement, clinical investigations, fundamental investigations, abstracts, and congress lists.
Formerly: Asia - Oceania Journal of Obstetrics and Gynaecology (0389-2328)
Related titles: CD-ROM ed.
Indexed: Chem.Abstr., Excerp.Med. (1993-), ExtraMED, INIS Atomind., Ind.Med. (1996-), Int.Nurs.Ind.
—BLDSC (5026.055000), CASDDS, CISTI, EMDOCS, GNLM.
Published by: (Juntendo University, School of Medicine, Department of Obstetrics and Gynaecology), University of Tokyo Press Production Center, 2-4-16 Yayoi, Bunkyo-ku, Tokyo 113-0032, Japan. Circ: 4,000 (paid and controlled).

618 IND ISSN 0022-3190
CODEN: JOBYA4
JOURNAL OF OBSTETRICS AND GYNAECOLOGY OF INDIA. Text in English. 1950. bi-m. INR 600, USD 35. adv. bk.rev. charts, illus, stat. reprint service avail. from IRC. *Refereed.* **Document type:** *Academic/Scholarly.*
Related titles: CD-ROM ed.
Indexed: Biol.Abstr., Chem.Abstr., Chem.Indus.Notes, Chem.Titles, ExtraMED.
—CASDDS, CISTI, GNLM.
Published by: Federation of Obstetric & Gynaecological Societies of India, Cama & Albelass Hospital, New Bldg., 6th Fl., Mahapalika Marg, Mumbai, Maharashtra 400 007, India. TEL 2642308, FAX 2676405. Ed. Dr. R D Pandit. Circ: 13,500.

618 618.92 HKG ISSN 1012-8875
JOURNAL OF PAEDIATRICS, OBSTETRICS AND GYNAECOLOGY (HONG KONG EDITION). Text and summaries in English. 1975. bi-m. USD 42 domestic; USD 48 foreign (effective 1999). adv. illus. *Refereed.* **Description:** Reviews papers in the field of pediatrics and in obstetrics and gynecology.
Formerly: Mother and Child
Related titles: ♦ Regional ed.: Journal of Paediatrics, Obstetrics and Gynaecology (Taiwan Edition). ISSN 1015-4337; ♦ Journal of Paediatrics, Obstetrics and Gynaecology (Thailand Edition). ISSN 1015-4345.
Indexed: Abstr.Hyg.
—BLDSC (5027.780000), GNLM.
Published by: Medimedia, 8-F Pacific Plaza, 410 Des Voeux Rd W, Hong Kong, Hong Kong. TEL 852-2559-5888, FAX 852-2559-6910, mmp@medimedia.com.hk, http://www.medimedia.com.hk/. Ed. Sarah Aguoniby. Pub. Edgar Richards. Circ: 17,100 (controlled).

618 618.92 HKG ISSN 1015-4337
JOURNAL OF PAEDIATRICS, OBSTETRICS AND GYNAECOLOGY (TAIWAN EDITION). Text and summaries in English. 1974. bi-m. **Document type:** *Academic/Scholarly, Trade.*
Related titles: ♦ Regional ed.: Journal of Paediatrics, Obstetrics and Gynaecology (Hong Kong Edition). ISSN 1012-8875; ♦ Journal of Paediatrics, Obstetrics and Gynaecology (Thailand Edition). ISSN 1015-4345.
Published by: Medimedia, 8-F Pacific Plaza, 410 Des Voeux Rd W, Hong Kong, Hong Kong. TEL 852-2559-5888, FAX 852-2559-6910, mmp@medimedia.com.hk, http://www.medimedia.com.hk/.

618 618.92 HKG ISSN 1015-4345
JOURNAL OF PAEDIATRICS, OBSTETRICS AND GYNAECOLOGY (THAILAND EDITION). Text and summaries in English. 1974. bi-m. **Document type:** *Academic/Scholarly, Trade.*
Related titles: ♦ Regional ed.: Journal of Paediatrics, Obstetrics and Gynaecology (Hong Kong Edition). ISSN 1012-8875; ♦ Journal of Paediatrics, Obstetrics and Gynaecology (Taiwan Edition). ISSN 1015-4337.
Published by: Medimedia, 8-F Pacific Plaza, 410 Des Voeux Rd W, Hong Kong, Hong Kong. TEL 852-2559-5888, FAX 852-2559-6910, mmp@medimedia.com.hk, http://www.medimedia.com.hk/.

JOURNAL OF PEDIATRIC AND ADOLESCENT GYNECOLOGY. see *MEDICAL SCIENCES—Pediatrics*

JOURNAL OF PEDIATRIC SURGERY. see *MEDICAL SCIENCES—Surgery*

JOURNAL OF PERINATAL AND NEONATAL NURSING. see *MEDICAL SCIENCES—Nurses And Nursing*

618 USA ISSN 1058-1243
JOURNAL OF PERINATAL EDUCATION. Text in English. 1992. q. USD 55 to individuals; USD 150 to institutions (effective 2000). **Document type:** *Academic/Scholarly.* **Description:** Covers breastfeeding, labor, birth, maternal child health, clinical issues and more.
Indexed: CINAHL, Gend.Watch.
—BLDSC (5030.549000), Infotrieve, ingenta. **CCC.**
Published by: (Lamaze International, Inc.), Jones & Bartlett, 1200 19th St, N W, Ste 300, Washington, DC 20036. TEL 202-857-1128, FAX 202-223-4579. Ed., R&P Shanon Humenick. Adv. contact Sandra Hagan. Circ: 4,000.

618 DEU ISSN 0300-5577
CODEN: JPEMAO
JOURNAL OF PERINATAL MEDICINE. Text in German. 1973. 6/yr. EUR 205.65 domestic to individuals; EUR 209.75 foreign to individuals; EUR 335.65 domestic to institutions; EUR 339.75 foreign to institutions; EUR 308 online ed. only; EUR 64 newsstand/cover (effective 2002). adv. *Refereed.* **Document type:** *Journal, Academic/Scholarly.* **Description:** Covers the whole field of perinatal medicine and neonatalogy.
Related titles: Online - full text ed.: (from EBSCO Publishing, O C L C Online Computer Library Center, Inc., Swets Blackwell, Institute for Scientific Information).
Indexed: ASCA, Bibl.Dev.Med.& Child Neur., Biol.Abstr., Chem.Abstr., Chem.Titles, Curr.Adv.Biochem., Curr.Adv.Ecol.Sci., Curr.Cont., Dairy Sci.Abstr., Environ.Sci.Poll.Mgmt., Excerp.Med., Fam.Ind., INIS Atomind., Ind.Med. (1973-), Ind.Sci.Rev., Inpharma, Nutr.Abstr., Pharm.&Out.News, Pollut.Abstr., Reac., Risk Abstr., SSCI (coverage dropped), Saf.Sci.Abstr., Sci.Cit.Ind., THA.
—BLDSC (5030.550000), CASDDS, CISTI, EMDOCS, GNLM, IDS, ingenta, KNAW. **CCC.**
Published by: Walter de Gruyter und Co., Genthiner Str 13, Berlin 10785, Germany. TEL 49-30-26005-0, FAX 49-30-26005-251, wdg-info@degruyter.de, http://www.degruyter.de. Ed. Joachim Dudenhausen. adv.: page DEM 1,000; trim 170 x 240. Circ: 700 (paid and controlled).

618.3 GBR ISSN 0743-8346
CODEN: JOPEEI
JOURNAL OF PERINATOLOGY. Text in English. 1981. 8/yr. EUR 73 in Europe to individuals for print or online ed.; EUR 73 elsewhere to individuals for print or online ed; GBP 73 combined subscription in Europe to individuals print & online; USD 110 combined subscription rest of world to individuals print & online; EUR 147 in Europe to institutions for print only; USD 198 elsewhere to institutions for print or online ed.; GBP 147 combined subscription in Europe to institutions print & online; EUR 132 combined subscription rest of world to institutions print & online (effective 2002). adv. bk.rev. charts, illus, stat. index. back issues avail.; reprints avail. *Refereed.* **Document type:** *Journal, Academic/Scholarly.* **Description:** Contains original clinical articles, commentaries, current concepts, case reports, editorials, and letters on all aspects of perinatal medicine from pregnancy through neonatal period.
Related titles: Microform ed.: (from PQC); Online - full text ed.: GBP 120 in Europe to institutions (effective 2002) (from EBSCO Publishing, O C L C Online Computer Library Center, Inc., RoweCom Information Quest, ingenta, Swets Blackwell).
Indexed: C.C.I.P., CINAHL, Fam.Ind., Ind.Med. (1984-), Int.Abstr.Biol.Sci., Sage Race Rel.Abstr.
—BLDSC (5030.570000), CISTI, GNLM, ingenta, KNAW.
Published by: (National Perinatal Association), Nature Publishing Group Specialist Journals (Subsidiary of: Holtzbrink Publishers), Houndmills, Basingstoke, Hants RG21 6XS, United Kingdom. TEL 44-1256-329242, FAX 44-1256-328339, subscriptions@nature.com, http://www.nature.com/jp. Ed. Edward Lawson. Pub. Julia Schulhof. R&P Trace Noel. Circ: 3,529. **Co-sponsor:** California Perinatal Association.

618.2 613.9 USA ISSN 1097-8003
RG635 CODEN: PPPJE4
JOURNAL OF PRENATAL & PERINATAL PSYCHOLOGY & HEALTH. Text in English. 1986. q. USD 50 domestic to individuals; USD 60 in Canada & Mexico to individuals; USD 65 elsewhere to individuals; USD 200 for 18 mos. domestic to institutions; USD 220 for 18 mos. elsewhere to institutions (effective 2001). adv. back issues avail.; reprint service avail. from PQC. *Refereed.* **Document type:** *Academic/Scholarly.* **Description:** Explores the psychological dimensions of human reproduction and pregnancy and the mental and emotional development of the unborn and newborn child.
Formerly (until vol.11, no.4, 1997): Pre- and Perinatal Psychology Journal (0883-3095)
Indexed: IMFL, PsycInfo, Psychol.Abstr. (1986-), e-psyche.
—BLDSC (5042.162000), GNLM, Infotrieve, ingenta. **CCC.**
Published by: (Pre- and Peri-Natal Psychology Association of North America), Kluwer Academic - Human Sciences Press (Subsidiary of: Wolters Kluwer N.V.), 233 Spring St, New York, NY 10013-1578. TEL 212-620-8000, 707-857-4041, FAX 212-463-0742, 707-857-4042, apppah@aol.com, http://www.birthdaypsychology.com. Ed. Ruth Carter.

618 GBR ISSN 0167-482X CODEN: JPOGD
JOURNAL OF PSYCHOSOMATIC OBSTETRICS AND GYNECOLOGY. Text in English. 1982. q. GBP 85, USD 145 to individuals; GBP 170, USD 275 to institutions (effective 2000). adv. bk.rev. charts, illus. back issues avail. *Refereed.* **Document type:** *Academic/Scholarly.*
Related titles: Online - full text ed.: (from Institute for Scientific Information).
Indexed: ASCA, AgeLine, Curr.Cont., Dok.Arbeitsmed., Excerp.Med., Fam.Ind., Ind.Med. (1982-), Inpharma, Nutr.Abstr., Pharm.&Out.News, Psychol.Abstr., Reac., SSCI, Sci.Cit.Ind. (coverage dropped), e-psyche.
—BLDSC (5043.479000), ADONIS, CISTI, GNLM, IDS, Infotrieve, ingenta, KNAW. **CCC.**
Published by: (International Society of Psychosomatic Obstetrics and Gynecology), Parthenon Publishing Group (Subsidiary of: C R C Press (New York)), Casterton Hall, Casterton, Carnforth, Lancs LA6 2LA, United Kingdom. TEL 44-1524-272084, FAX 44-1524-271587, mail@parthpub.com, http://www.parthpub.com/pog/home.html. Ed., R&P Jean Wright. Adv. contact Julia Tissington. Circ: 1,000 (paid).

JOURNAL OF REPRODUCTIVE IMMUNOLOGY. see *MEDICAL SCIENCES—Allergology And Immunology*

618.05 USA ISSN 0024-7758 RG1 CODEN: JRPMAP
JOURNAL OF REPRODUCTIVE MEDICINE; for the obstetrician and gynecologist. Text in English. 1968. m. USD 135 domestic to individuals; USD 160 foreign to individuals; USD 210 domestic to institutions; USD 235 foreign to institutions (effective 2000). adv. bk.rev. illus. index. back issues avail.; reprint service avail. from ISI. *Refereed.* **Document type:** *Academic/Scholarly.* **Description:** Peer-reviewed original and clinical articles, case reports, and letters to the editor.
Continues: Lying-in (0096-7033)
Related titles: Microform ed.: (from PQC,PMC); Online - full text ed.: (from Institute for Scientific Information).
Indexed: ASCA, Abstr.Hyg., Anim.Breed.Abstr., Arts & Hum.Cit.Ind. (coverage dropped), Biol.Abstr., C.C.I.Ob.Gyn., CINAHL, Chem.Abstr., Chem.Indus.Notes, Chem.Titles, Curr.Adv.Ecol.Sci., Curr.Cont., Curr.Lit.Fam.Plan., Excerp.Med., Fam.Ind., INIS Atomind., Ind.Med. (1969-), Ind.Sci.Rev., Inpharma, Int.Nurs.Ind., Med.& Surg.Dermat., NRN, Nutr.Abstr., Pharm.&Out.News, Protozool.Abstr., Reac., Ref.Zh., Rev.Med.& Vet.Mycol., SSCI (coverage dropped), Sci.Cit.Ind., THA.
—BLDSC (5049.700000), CASDDS, CISTI, GNLM, IDS, ingenta, KNAW. **CCC.**
Published by: Science Printers and Publishers, Inc., 8342 Olive Blvd., St. Louis, MO 63132. TEL 314-991-4440, FAX 314-991-4654, editor@aqch.com. Ed. Dr. George L Wied. R&P Donna Kessel. Adv. contact Al Heidler. Circ: 31,758.

618 JPN ISSN 0916-2747
KAGAKU RYOHO KENKYUJO KIYO/INSTITUTE OF CHEMOTHERAPY. BULLETIN. Text in English, Japanese. 1989. a.
Published by: Kagaku Ryoho Kenkyujo, 1-14 Kono-Dai 6-chome, Ichikawa-shi, Chiba-ken 272-0827, Japan.

618 DEU ISSN 0932-0601
KORASION. Text in German. 1986. q. **Document type:** *Magazine, Academic/Scholarly.*
Related titles: ♦ Supplement to: Gyne. ISSN 0179-9185.
—GNLM.
Published by: H U F Verlag, Lindenhof 47, Muehlheim 45481, Germany. TEL 49-208-480027, FAX 49-208-485899.

618.202 JPN ISSN 0917-3641
KYOTO DAIGAKU JOSANPU DOSOKAISHI/MIDWIVES ASSOCIATION OF KYOTO UNIVERSITY. ANNALS. Text in Japanese. a.
Published by: Kyoto Daigaku Josanpu Dosokai, Kyoto Daigaku Igakubu, Fanfujinkagaku Kyoshitsu, Shogoin Kawaramachi, Sakyo-ku, Kyoto-shi, Kyoto 606, Japan.

618.45 USA
LAMAZE PARA PADRES* . Text in Spanish. 1994. a. free per issue to qualified personnel. adv. **Document type:** *Consumer.* **Description:** Offers information to Spanish-speaking expectant couples on prenatal and postpartum care through Lamaze classes.
Published by: (American Society for Psychoprophylaxis in Obstetrics, Inc.), Lamaze Publishing Co., 9 Old Kings Hwy S, Darien, CT 06820-4505. TEL 203-656-3600. Ed. Susan Strecker Richard. adv.: page USD 48,075. Circ: 575,028 (controlled).

618 USA
LAMAZE PARENTS' MAGAZINE. Text in English. 1983. a. free per issue to qualified personnel. adv. **Document type:** *Consumer.* **Description:** Offers prenatal and postpartum information to expectant couples who are preparing for birth through Lamaze classes.
Published by: (Lamaze International, Inc.), Lamaze Publishing Co., 9 Old Kings Hwy S, Darien, CT 06820-4505. TEL 203-656-3600, FAX 203-656-2221. Ed. Patricia Duarte. adv.: page USD 135,300. Circ: 2,417,489 (controlled).

618.45 USA
LAMAZEBABY. Text in English. 1993. s-a. free per issue to qualified personnel. adv. **Document type:** *Consumer.* **Description:** Addressed to new parents on baby's first year.
Published by: (Lamaze International, Inc.), Lamaze Publishing Co., 9 Old Kings Hwy S, Darien, CT 06820-4505. TEL 203-834-2711, FAX 203-761-8696. Ed. Patricia Duarte. adv.: page USD 158,750. Circ: 3,023,076 (controlled).

618.1 FRA ISSN 0759-1594
LA LETTRE DU GYNECOLOGUE. Text in French. 1984. m. FRF 460 domestic to individuals; FRF 580, USD 105 foreign to individuals; FRF 580 domestic to institutions; FRF 700, USD 127 foreign to institutions; FRF 290 domestic to students; USD 75 foreign to students (effective 2000). Supplement avail. *Refereed.* **Document type:** *Academic/Scholarly.*
Published by: Edimark S.A., 62-64 rue Jean Jaures, Puteaux 92800, France. TEL 33-1-414-58000, FAX 33-1-41458025, contact@edimark.fr, http://www.edimark.fr. Ed. P Madelenat. Pub. Claudie Damour-Terrasson.

THE LOCAL BABY DIRECTORY: BRISTOL & BATH. see *CHILDREN AND YOUTH—About*

▼ **THE LOCAL BABY DIRECTORY: HERTS & MIDDLESEX;** an a-z of everything for pregnant women, babies and children. see *CHILDREN AND YOUTH—About*

THE LOCAL BABY DIRECTORY: OXFORDSHIRE, BERKS & BUCKS; an a-z of everything for pregnant women, babies and children. see *CHILDREN AND YOUTH—About*

THE LOCAL BABY DIRECTORY: SOUTH WALES; an a-z of everything for pregnant women, babies and children. see *CHILDREN AND YOUTH—About*

THE LOCAL BABY DIRECTORY: SURREY; an a-z everything for pregnant women, babies and children. see *CHILDREN AND YOUTH—About*

THE LOCAL BABY DIRECTORY: SUSSEX & HAMPSHIRE; an a-z of everything for pregnant women, babies and children. see *CHILDREN AND YOUTH—About*

THE LONDON BABY DIRECTORY; an a-z of everything for pregnant women, babies and children. see *CHILDREN AND YOUTH—About*

618 ITA
LUCINA. Text in Italian. 1934. m. free per issue. adv. **Document type:** *Bulletin.*
Published by: Federazione Nazionale dei Collegi delle Ostetriche, Piazza Tarquinia, 5-D, Rome, RM 00183, Italy. TEL 39-6-7000943. Ed. Berta Comitini. Circ: 20,000.

618.202 GBR ISSN 0961-5555
M I D I R S MIDWIFERY DIGEST. Text in English. 1986. q. GBP 39 domestic to individuals; GBP 45 in Europe to individuals; GBP 50 elsewhere to individuals; GBP 80 domestic to institutions; GBP 86 in Europe to institutions; GBP 90 elsewhere to institutions (effective 2000). adv. back issues avail. **Document type:** *Academic/Scholarly.* **Description:** Enables midwives and other childbirth professionals to keep up to date with the latest research and information in the field.
Formerly (until 1991): M I D I R S Information Pack (0955-8683)
Indexed: Brit.Nur.Ind., CINAHL.
—BLDSC (5761.413886).
Published by: Midwives Information and Resource Service, 9 Elmdale Rd, Tyndalls Park, Clifton, Bristol, Glos BS8 1SL, United Kingdom. TEL 44-117-925-1791, FAX 44-117-925-1792, digest@midirs.org, http://www.midirs.org. Ed. Julie Frohlich. R&P Val Dickens. Adv. contact Sue Penn.

618 USA
M I D S NEWSLETTER. (Miscarriage, Infant Death, and Stillbirth) Text in English. 1983. 4/yr. USD 30 (effective 2000). **Document type:** *Newsletter.* **Description:** Newsletter of announcements for families suffering miscarriages, infant deaths, and stillbirths.
Indexed: e-psyche.
Published by: M I D S Inc., 16 Crescent Dr, Parsippany, NJ 07054. mids@nac.net.

M O M MAGAZINE. see *WOMEN'S HEALTH*

MAGAZYN PIELEGNIARKI I POLOZNEJ. see *MEDICAL SCIENCES—Nurses And Nursing*

610 HUN ISSN 0025-021X CODEN: MNLAA8
MAGYAR NOORVOSOK LAPJA. Text in Hungarian; Summaries in English. 1937. bi-m. HUF 3,000 domestic; HUF 5,000 foreign (effective 2000). bibl, charts, illus.
Indexed: Chem.Abstr., Chem.Titles, Excerp.Med., INIS Atomind., Ind.Med. (coverage dropped).
—BLDSC (5345.010000), CASDDS, CISTI.
Published by: Magyar Noorvos Tarsasag, Szabolcs utca 35, PO Box 112, Budapest 1135, Hungary. TEL 36-1-3506502, FAX 36-1-3506502. Ed. Dr. Jozsef Doszpod. **Subscr. to:** Kultura, PO Box 149, Budapest 1389, Hungary.

613.9 MYS ISSN 0127-3213
MALAYSIAN JOURNAL OF REPRODUCTIVE HEALTH. Text in English. 1983. a. USD 25. **Document type:** *Government.* **Description:** Discusses various aspects of reproductive health.
Published by: National Population and Family Development Board, Jalan Raja Laut, PO Box 10416, Kuala Lumpur 50712, Malaysia. TEL 2937555. Ed. Dr. Mohd Ismail Thambi. Circ: 618.

MAMM; women, cancer and community. see *WOMEN'S HEALTH*

MAMMARY GLAND. see *BIOLOGY—Abstracting, Bibliographies, Statistics*

618.1 USA
THE MANAGEMENT OF THE MENOPAUSE: ANNUAL REVIEW. Text in English. 1998. a. GBP 38, USD 55 per issue (effective 2000).
—BLDSC (5359.043800).
Published by: Parthenon Publishing Group (Subsidiary of: C R C Press (New York)), One Blue Hill Plaza, PO Box 1564, Pearl River, NY 10965. TEL 914-735-9363, FAX 914-735-1385. Ed. John Studd.

618 USA ISSN 1091-5680
MANAGING MENOPAUSE. Text in English. s-a. adv.
Published by: American College of Obstetricians and Gynecologists, 409 12th St, S W, Washington, DC 20024. TEL 202-484-3321, FAX 202-479-6826.

618.1 ESP ISSN 1138-8196
MASSON NEWSLETTER DE GINECOLOGIA. Text in Spanish. 1998. 3/yr. **Document type:** *Newsletter.*
—BLDSC (5388.749600).
Published by: Editorial Garsi, S.A., Grupo Masson, AV. Diagonal, 427bis-429, Barcelona 08036, Spain. TEL 34-932418800, 34-932418800, masson@masson.es.

618 USA ISSN 1092-7875 RJ102 CODEN: MCHJFB
MATERNAL AND CHILD HEALTH JOURNAL. Text in English. 1997. q. EUR 219 to institutions for print or online ed.; EUR 262.80 to institutions print & online eds.combined (effective 2002). *Refereed.* **Document type:** *Academic/Scholarly.* **Description:** Investigates all areas of the maternal and child health field, including MCH epidemiology, demography, and health status assessment; innovative MCH initiatives; carrying out MCH programs; MCH policy analysis and advocacy;and MCH professional development.
Related titles: Online - full text ed.: (from EBSCO Publishing, O C L C Online Computer Library Center, Inc., Swets Blackwell, Kluwer Online, RoweCom Information Quest).
Indexed: CINAHL, Ind.Med. (1997-).
—BLDSC (5399.272500), ingenta. **CCC.**

M

Published by: (Association of Maternal and Child Health Programs), Kluwer Academic - Plenum Publishers (Subsidiary of: Wolters Kluwer N.V.), 233 Spring St, New York, NY 10013-1578. TEL 212-620-8000, 800-221-9369, FAX 212-463-0742, info@plenum.com; kluwer@wkap.com; services@wkap.nl; kotelchuck@unc.edu, http://www.plenum.com. Ed. Milton Kotelchuck. **Co-sponsors:** Association of Teachers of Maternal and Child Health; CityMatCH; American Public Health Association, Maternal and Child Health Section.

612.665 IRL ISSN 0378-5122 CODEN: MATUDK

MATURITAS; international journal for the study of the climacteric. Text in English. 1978. 9/yr. EUR 156 in Europe to individuals; JPY 20,700 in Japan to individuals; USD 173 elsewhere to individuals; EUR 833 in Europe to institutions; JPY 110,700 in Japan to institutions; USD 932 elsewhere to institutions (effective 2002). bk.rev. reprint service avail. from SWZ. *Refereed.* **Document type:** *Academic/Scholarly.* **Description:** For gynecologists, endocrinologists, geriatricians, andrologists, sociologists, psychologists. Publishes original research on the physiological, psychological and sociological changes in function related to the climacteric in both men and women.
Incorporates (1994-1998): European Menopause Journal (1381-2858)
Related titles: Microform ed.: (from PQC); Online - full text ed.: (from ingenta, ScienceDirect, Swets Blackwell, Institute for Scientific Information).
Indexed: ASCA, Biol.Abstr., Chem.Abstr., Chem.Indus.Notes, Chem.Titles, Curr.Adv.Ecol.Sci., Curr.Cont., Excerp.Med., Ind.Med. (1978-), Ind.Sci.Rev., Inpharma, Int.Abstr.Biol.Sci., Nutr.Abstr., Pharm.&Out.News, Protozool.Abstr., PsycInfo, Psychol.Abstr. (1993-), Reac., SSCI (coverage dropped), Sci.Cit.Ind., e-psyche.
—BLDSC (5413.265000), ADONIS, CASDDS, CISTI, EMDOCS, GNLM, IDS, ingenta, KNAW. **CCC.**
Published by: (International Menopause Society), Elsevier Science Ireland Ltd, Elsevier House, Brookvale Plaza, E. Park, Shannon, Co. Clare, Ireland. TEL 353-61-709600, FAX 353-61-709100, http://www.elsevier.nl/locate/maturitas. Eds. H Kopera, W H Utian. R&P Annette Moloney. **Subscr. in Australasia and the Far East to:** Elsevier Science (Singapore) Pte Ltd, No.1 Temasek Ave, 17-01 Millenia Tower, Singapore 039192, Singapore. TEL 65-434-3727, FAX 65-337-2230, asiainfo@elsevier.com.sg; **Subscr. in the Americas to:** Elsevier Science, PO Box 945, New York, NY 10159-0945. TEL 212-633-3730, 888-437-4636, FAX 212-633-3680, usinfo-f@elsevier.com, http://www.elsevier.com; **Subscr. to:** Elsevier Science BV, PO Box 211, Amsterdam 1000 AE, Netherlands. TEL 31-20-485-3757, FAX 31-20-485-3432, nlinfo-f@elsevier.nl; **Subscr. to:** Elsevier Science Inc - Japan Regional Office, 9-15 Higashi-Azabu 1-chome, Minato-ku, Tokyo 106-0044, Japan. TEL 81-3-5561-5033, FAX 81-3-5561-5047, info@elsevier.co.jp. **Dist. by:** Elsevier Science (Brazil).

MEALEY'S LITIGATION REPORT: DRUGS AND MEDICAL DEVICES. see *LAW—Corporate Law*

MEDICAL MALPRACTICE: HANDLING OBSTETRIC AND NEONATAL CASES. see *LAW—Civil Law*

618 613 BGR ISSN 0204-0956 CODEN: AKGIBP

MEDITSINSKI PREGLED. AKUSHERSTVO I GINEKOLOGIIA. Text in Bulgarian; Summaries in Bulgarian, English. 1970. q., latest vol.32, 2001. BGL 14 domestic; USD 48 foreign (effective 2001 - 2002). adv. bk.rev. abstr, bibl. index. 48 p./no. back issues avail. *Refereed.* **Document type:** *Journal, Academic/Scholarly, Abstract/Index, Bibliography.* **Description:** Publishes original articles and abstracts of foreign publications on gynecologic diseases and obstetrics - pregnancy complications, risk factors, neonatal diseases and abnormalities.
Indexed: Abstr.Bulg.Sci.Med.Lit., Excerp.Med., INIS Atomind., Ind.Med. (coverage dropped).
—BLDSC (0006.300000), CASDDS, CISTI, EMDOCS.
Published by: Meditsinski Universitet - Sofia, Tsentur za Informatsiia po Meditsina/Medical University - Sofia, Medical Information Center, 1 Sv Georgi Sofiiski ul, Sofia 1431, Bulgaria. TEL 359-2-9522342, FAX 359-2-9522393, mutafov@sun.medun.acad.bg, http://www.medun.acad.bg. Ed. Dr. B Marinov. R&P, Adv. contact Dr. Christo Mutafov. B&W page USD 50, color page USD 150; trim 160 x 110. Circ: 350.

618 POL

MEDYCYNA PRAKTYCZNA. GINEKOLOGIA I POLOZNICTWO. Text in Polish. bi-m. PLZ 120 (effective 2000).
Published by: Medycyna Praktyczna, Ul Skawinska 8, Krakow 31066, Poland. TEL 48-12-4305520, FAX 48-12-4305536, listy@mp.pl, http://mp.pl/czasop.htm. Ed. Andrzej Bacz.

618.175 ITA ISSN 1123-699X

MENOPAUSA NEWS. Text in Italian. 1995. q. adv. **Document type:** *Newsletter.*
Published by: (Societa Italiana della Menopausa), C I C Edizioni Internazionali s.r.l., Corso Trieste 42, Rome, RM 00198, Italy. TEL 39-06-8412673, FAX 39-06-8412688, info@gruppocic.it, 1160199510. Ed. G B Serra. adv.: B&W page ITL 3,100,000, color page ITL 3,900,000; trim 210 x 290.

618 USA ISSN 1072-3714
RG186 CODEN: MENOF2

MENOPAUSE. Text in English. 1994. bi-m., latest vol.8. USD 177 domestic to individuals; USD 208 foreign to individuals; USD 287 domestic to institutions; USD 316 foreign to institutions; USD 50 newsstand/cover (effective 2002). adv. charts, illus. back issues avail. *Refereed.* **Document type:** *Academic/Scholarly.* **Description:** Forum for new research and scholarly material relating to all aspects of the human female menopause, from physiological, pathological, sociocultural and medical perspectives.
Related titles: Microform ed.: (from PQC); Online - full text ed.: USD 373.10 domestic academic site license; USD 402.10 foreign academic site license; USD 416.15 domestic corporate site license; USD 445.15 foreign corporate site license (2002) (from Ovid Technologies, Inc., Institute for Scientific Information).
Indexed: ASCA, Curr.Cont., Ind.Med. (1994-), Ind.Sci.Rev., Inpharma, Jrnl.Watch Wom.Hlth., Nutr.Abstr., Pharm.&Out.News, Reac., Sci.Cit.Ind., Soyabean Abstr.
—BLDSC (5678.457030), IDS, KNAW.
Published by: (North American Menopause Society), Lippincott Williams & Wilkins (Philadelphia) (Subsidiary of: Wolters Kluwer N.V.), 530 Walnut St, Philadelphia, PA 19106-3621. TEL 215-521-8300, FAX 215-521-8902, http://www.lww.com. Eds. Isaac Schiff, Wulf H Utian. Pub. Marcia Serepy. R&P Margaret Becker. Adv. contact Ray Thibodeau. B&W page USD 805, color page USD 1,810. Circ: 2,806. **Subscr. to:** PO Box 1600, Hagerstown, MD 21740-1600. TEL 800-777-2295, FAX 301-824-7390.

618.2 EGY ISSN 1110-5690

MIDDLE EAST FERTILITY SOCIETY. JOURNAL. Text in English. 1996. 3/yr. USD 25 to individuals; USD 35 to institutions (effective 2000). adv. bk.rev. abstr, charts, illus. back issues avail. *Refereed.* **Document type:** *Journal, Academic/Scholarly.*
—BLDSC (5761.374250).
Published by: Middle East Fertility Society, 10 Geziret El Arab St., Mohandessin, Cairo 12411, Egypt. TEL 202-749-8488, FAX 20-2-338-3049, ghar@link.net, www.mefsjournal.com. Ed. Dr. Mohamed A Aboulghar. adv.: color page USD 1,480; 25.5 x 17.8. Circ: 1,500 (paid); 500 (controlled).

MIDLIFE WOMEN'S HEALTH SOURCEBOOK. see *WOMEN'S HEALTH*

618 GBR ISSN 0266-6138

MIDWIFERY. Text in English. 1984. q. GBP 58 to individuals; GBP 176 to institutions (effective 2002). adv. bk.rev. abstr. back issues avail.; reprints avail. *Refereed.* **Document type:** *Journal, Academic/Scholarly.* **Description:** Provides an international and interdisciplinary forum for the discussion of advances, controversies and current research. Actively promotes continuing education through publication of reviews and updates on all aspects of midwifery.
Related titles: Online - full text ed.: (from EBSCO Publishing, O C L C Online Computer Library Center, Inc., Swets Blackwell, IDEAL Online Library, Institute for Scientific Information).
Indexed: ASCA, ASSIA, Brit.Nur.Ind., CINAHL, Curr.Adv.Ecol.Sci., Curr.Cont., Fam.Ind., Int.Nurs.Ind., SSCI.
—BLDSC (5761.449220), CISTI, GNLM, IDS, Infotrieve, ingenta, KNAW. **CCC.**
Published by: Churchill Livingstone (Subsidiary of: Harcourt Publishers Ltd.), Robert Stevenson House, 1-3 Baxter's Pl, Leith Walk, Edinburgh, Midlothian EH1 3AF, United Kingdom. TEL 44-131-556-2424, FAX 44-131-558-1278, journals@harcourt.com, http://www.harcourt-international.com/journals/midw. Eds. Ann Thomson, Barbara McAviney. R&P Sharon Boyle TEL 44-131-524-1747. Adv. contact Deborah Watkins TEL 44-207-424-4280. Circ: 1,100. **Subscr. addr. in the US:** Harcourt Health Sciences, Journals Subscription Department, PO Box 156, Avenel, NJ 07001. TEL 877-839-7126; **Subscr. to:** Harcourt Publishers Ltd., Journal Sales & Marketing Dept., 32 Jamestown Rd, London NW1 7BY, United Kingdom. TEL 44-20-8308-5700.

MIDWIFERY MATTERS. see *MEDICAL SCIENCES—Nurses And Nursing*

618.202 USA

MIDWIFERY TODAY WITH INTERNATIONAL MIDWIFE. Text in English. 1987. q., latest vol.59, 2001. USD 50 domestic; USD 60 in Canada & Mexico; USD 75 elsewhere; USD 12.50 newsstand/cover (effective 2000). adv. bk.rev., video rev. bibl, illus, tr.lit. Index. 72 p./no. back issues avail.; reprints avail. **Document type:** *Magazine, Trade.* **Description:** Directs professionals and non-professionals alike; balances technical articles with personal accounts and photography to present a wide range of options and perspectives on current birth care issues.
Former titles (until 199?): Midwifery Today and Childbirth Education with International Midwife (1522-2888); Formed by the merger of (1987-1996): Midwifery Today (0891-7701); (1995-1996): International Midwife (1080-9023)
Related titles: Online - full text ed.: (from LexisNexis).
Indexed: CINAHL, CWI, Fam.Ind., Fem.Per. (1993-), Gend.Watch, Int.Nurs.Ind.
—BLDSC (5761.449240), GNLM.
Address: PO Box 2672, Eugene, OR 97402. TEL 541-344-7438, 800-743-0974, FAX 541-344-1422, editorial@midwiferytoday.com, http://www.midwiferytoday.com/magazine. Eds. Alice Evans, Jan Tritten. R&P Jan Tritten. adv.: B&W page USD 150; trim 10 x 7.5. Circ: 2,500.

618 JPN

MIEKEN SANFUJINKA IHO/MIE SOCIETY OF OBSTETRICIANS AND GYNECOLOGISTS. ANNUAL BULLETIN. Text in Japanese. 1982. a. **Document type:** *Bulletin.*
Published by: Mieken Sanfujinka Ikai, c/o Mr Mizuno, 97-52 Otani-cho, Tsu-shi, Mie-ken 514-0007, Japan.

618 ITA ISSN 0026-4784

MINERVA GINECOLOGICA. Text in Italian; Summaries in English, Italian. 1949. m. (10/yr.). USD 125 to individuals; USD 165 to institutions (effective 2000 - 2001). adv. bk.rev. bibl, charts, illus. index. *Refereed.* **Document type:** *Academic/Scholarly.*
Incorporates: Folia Gynaecologica; Ginecologia; Aggiornamenti di Ostetricia e Ginecologia (0002-0931)
Related titles: Microform ed.: (from PQC).
Indexed: Biol.Abstr., Chem.Abstr., Excerp.Med., Helminthol.Abstr., Ind.Med. (1949-), Ref.Zh., Zoo.Rec.
—BLDSC (5794.185000), CISTI, GNLM, KNAW.
Published by: Edizioni Minerva Medica, Corso Bramante, 83-85, Turin, TO 10126, Italy. TEL 39-11-678282, FAX 39-11-674502. Ed., Pub. Alberto Oliaro. Adv. contact F Filippo. B&W page USD 1,400, color page USD 2,300; trim 270 x 190. Circ: 4,000 (paid).

612.6 571.8 GBR ISSN 1360-9947 CODEN: MHREFD

MOLECULAR HUMAN REPRODUCTION. Text in English. 1995. m. GBP 145, USD 245 to individuals; GBP 455, USD 840 to institutions (effective 2002). adv. 108 p./no. back issues avail. *Refereed.* **Document type:** *Journal, Academic/Scholarly.* **Description:** Fields covered include the molecular control of development and senescence, paracrines in embryonic growth and reproductive organs, genetic factors in reproduction and development, cell proliferations and apoptosis, and transport systems within cells and across membranes.
Related titles: Online - full text ed.: ISSN 1460-2407. GBP 410, USD 755 in United Kingdom to institutions Online only (effective 2002) (from HighWire Pr., EBSCO Publishing, O C L C Online Computer Library Center, Inc., RoweCom Information Quest, ingenta, Swets Blackwell, Institute for Scientific Information).
Indexed: Chem.Abstr., Chem.Indus.Notes, Chem.Titles, Curr.Cont., Ind.Med. (1995-), Inpharma, Pharm.&Out.News, Reac., Sci.Cit.Ind.
—BLDSC (5900.817650), CASDDS, CISTI, GNLM, IDS, Infotrieve, KNAW. **CCC.**

M

Published by: Oxford University Press, Academic Division, Great Clarendon St, Oxford OX2 6DP, United Kingdom. TEL 44-1865-267907, FAX 44-1865-267835, jnl.orders@oup.co.uk, jnl.info@oup.co.uk, http://www.oup.co.uk/molehr/, http://www.oup.co.uk/journals. Ed. R Ivell. Pub. J Boullin. R&P Fionna Willis. adv.: page GBP 315, page USD 595. Circ: 1,000. **Subscr. in the Americas to:** Oxford University Press, Journals, 2001 Evans Rd, Cary, NC 27513. TEL 800-852-7323, FAX 919-677-1714, jnlorders@oup-usa.org.

618.2 AUS
MOTHER & BABY. Text in English. bi-m. AUD 4.50 newsstand/cover (effective 2000). adv. **Document type:** *Consumer.* **Description:** Discusses pregnancy, babycare and children's development up to 4 years of age.
Published by: Bounty Services Pty. Ltd. (Subsidiary of: Emap International), 187 Thomas St., Level 6, Haymarket, NSW 2000, Australia. TEL 61-2-9581-9555. Ed. Margaret Rafferty. R&P Wisal Masri. Adv. contacts Dempster Clare, Sarah Fleischer. page AUD 8,635. Circ: 99,631. **Subscr. to:** PO Box 1014, Haymarket, NSW 1240, Australia. FAX 61-2-9581-9556.

MOTHERING; the magazine of natural family living. see *WOMEN'S HEALTH*

N A B C O BREAST CANCER RESOURCE LIST. see *MEDICAL SCIENCES—Oncology*

N A B C O NEWS. see *MEDICAL SCIENCES—Oncology*

N A N N CENTRAL LINES. see *MEDICAL SCIENCES—Nurses And Nursing*

N H S CERVICAL SCREENING PROGRAMME (YEAR). (National Health Service) see *WOMEN'S HEALTH*

618.1 JPN
NAGANOKEN SANKA FUJINKA IKAIHO/ GYNECOLOGICAL SOCIETY OF NAGANO. BULLETIN. Text in Japanese. 1962. s-a. free per issue. **Document type:** *Bulletin.*
Published by: Naganoken Sanka Fujinka Ikai, Shinshu Daigaku Igakubu Sanfujinka Kyoshitsu, 1-1 Asahi 3-chome, Matsumoto-shi, Nagano-ken 390-0802, Japan. Ed. Hiroo Linumd.

NATIONAL ASSOCIATION OF NEONATAL NURSES. POSITION STATEMENT. see *MEDICAL SCIENCES—Nurses And Nursing*

618.2 USA
NATIONAL PERINATAL ASSOCIATION. BULLETIN. Text in English. 1980. q. USD 15 to non-members. adv. bk.rev. **Document type:** *Newsletter.* **Description:** Information for association members.
Published by: National Perinatal Association, 3500 E Fletcher Ave, Ste 209, Tampa, FL 33613-4712. TEL 813-971-1008, FAX 813-971-9306. Ed. Julie A Leachman. Circ: 1,500.

618 NLD ISSN 0921-4011
NEDERLANDS TIJDSCHRIFT VOOR OBSTETRIE & GYNAECOLOGIE. Text in Dutch. 1980. 5/yr. NLG 265; to foreign members. bk.rev. abstr, charts, illus. reprint service avail. from PQC. **Document type:** *Academic/Scholarly, Trade.* **Description:** Informs association members about developments in the field of obstetrics and gynecology.
Incorporates (in 1987): Ob-Gyn Digest (English Edition) (0198-9197); Which was formed by the merger of (1976-1980): Medilex Digest Ob-Gyn (0921-402X); (1977-1980): Journal of Continuing Education in Obstetrics and Gynecology (0148-5164); Which superseded (1959-1977): Ob-Gyn Digest (0029-7429); And incorporated: Ob-Gyn Abstracts
Related titles: Microform ed.: (from PQC).
Published by: (Nederlandse Verengiging voor Obstetrie en Gynaecologie), Elsevier Gezondheidszorg B.V., Tijdstroom (Subsidiary of: Reed Elsevier plc Group), Planetenbaan 1, Maarssen 3600 AK, Netherlands. TEL 31-346-577577, FAX 31-346-554287, http://www.tijdstroom.nl. **Subscr. to:** Elsevier Den Haag, Postbus 16500, The Hague 2500 BM, Netherlands. TEL 31-70-381-9900, FAX 31-70-333-8399.

618 618.92 USA ISSN 1062-2454
NEONATAL INTENSIVE CARE; the journal of perinatology - neonatology. Text in English. 1988. bi-m. USD 80; USD 110 foreign (effective 1999). adv. *Refereed.* **Description:** Covers diagnostic techniques, case studies and research findings in perinatology and neonatology.
Indexed: CINAHL.
—CISTI.
Published by: Goldstein and Associates, 1150 Yale St, Ste 12, Santa Monica, CA 90403-4738. TEL 310-828-1309. Ed. Les Plesko. Pub. Steve Goldstein.

NEONATAL NETWORK; the journal of neonatal nursing. see *MEDICAL SCIENCES—Nurses And Nursing*

NETWORK (DURHAM). see *BIRTH CONTROL*

618 NLD
NEW CLINICAL APPLICATIONS. GYNAECOLOGY. Text in English. irreg. price varies. **Document type:** *Monographic series.*
Published by: Kluwer Academic Publishers Group (Subsidiary of: Wolters Kluwer N.V.), Spuiboulevard 50, PO Box 17, Dordrecht 3300 AA, Netherlands. FAX 31-78-639-2254, services@wkap.nl, http://www.wkap.nl. **Dist. by:** Journals Department, PO Box 322, Dordrecht 3300 AH, Netherlands. FAX 31-78-654-6474.

618 GBR
NEW DIGEST. Text in English. 1993. q. GBP 6 (effective 2000). **Document type:** *Consumer.*
Formerly: New Generation Digest (1350-2735)
—BLDSC (6083.150000).
Published by: National Childbirth Trust, Alexandra House, Oldham Terr, Acton, London W3 6NH, United Kingdom. TEL 44-20-8992-8637, 44-20-8992-2616, FAX 44-20-8466-5307. Ed. Amanda Saunders.

618 GBR ISSN 0263-5429
NEW GENERATION. Text in English. 1982. q. GBP 6 (effective 2000). bk.rev. **Document type:** *Consumer.*
Indexed: Hist.Abstr. (1969-1974, dropped).
—BLDSC (6084.210900).
Published by: National Childbirth Trust, Alexandra House, Oldham Terr, Acton, London W3 6NH, United Kingdom. TEL 44-20-8992-8637, FAX 44-20-8992-5929. Ed. Gerry Gulliver. Circ: 43,000.

NEW MOTHER. see *CHILDREN AND YOUTH—About*

618 613.9 AUS ISSN 1030-3987
NEW PARENT. Text in English. 1968. q. AUD 20. adv. bk.rev. **Description:** Provides information to general public about birthing and parenting options and practices.
Published by: Parents Centers Australia, 71 Grand Ave., Westmead, NSW 2150, Australia. TEL 02-633 5899. Ed. Beth Mitchell. Circ: 2,000.

363.46 310 NZL
NEW ZEALAND. STATISTICS NEW ZEALAND. ABORTION STATISTICS (YEAR). Text in English. a. **Document type:** *Government.*
Published by: Statistics New Zealand/Te Tari Tatau, PO Box 2922, Wellington, New Zealand. TEL 64-4-495-4600, FAX 64-4-473-2626, info@stats.govt.nz, http://www.stats.govt.nz.

618.1 JPN
NIHON FUJINKA BYORI KORUPOSUKOPI GAKKAI ZASSHI/JAPAN SOCIETY OF GYNECOLOGIC PATHOLOGY AND COLPOSCOPY. JOURNAL. Text in Japanese; Summaries in English, Japanese. 1982. s-a.
Published by: Nihon Fujinka Byori Koruposukopi Gakkai, Keio Gijuku Daigaku Igakubu Sanfujinkagaku Kyoshitsu, 35 Shinano-Machi, Shinjuku-ku, Tokyo 160-0016, Japan.

618.202 JPN ISSN 0917-6357
NIHON JOSAN GAKKAISHI/JAPAN ACADEMY OF MIDWIFERY. JOURNAL. Text in Japanese; Summaries in English, Japanese. 1987. s-a.
Published by: Nihon Josan Gakkai, Josanpu Kaikan, 8-21 Fujimi 1-chome, Chiyoda-ku, Tokyo 102-0071, Japan.

618 616.9 JPN ISSN 0918-4031
NIHON SANFUJINKA KANSENSHO KENKYUKAI GAKUJUTSU KOENKAI KIROKUSHU/CONFERENCE ON OBSTETRICAL AND GYNECOLOGICAL INFECTION. PROCEEDINGS. Text in Japanese; Summaries in English, Japanese. 1983. a. **Document type:** *Proceedings, Academic/Scholarly.*
Published by: Nihon Sanfujinka Kansensho Kenkyukai/Japan Association of Obstetrical and Gynecological Infection, Koto Byoin Sanfujinka, 8-5 Ojima 6-chome, Koto-ku, Tokyo 136-0072, Japan.

618 JPN ISSN 0916-8796
NIHON SANFUJINKA SHINSEIJI KETSUEKI GAKKAISHI/JAPANESE JOURNAL OF OBSTETRICAL, GYNECOLOGICAL AND NEONATAL HEMATOLOGY. Text in English, Japanese. 1977. q. JPY 8,000. adv. bk.rev. *Refereed.* **Document type:** *Academic/Scholarly.* **Description:** Contains papers with laboratory or clinical orientation, case reports and revew articles.
Published by: Japanese Society of Obstetrical Gynecological and Neonatal Hematology, Hamamatsu University School of Medicine, Department of Obstetrics and Gynecology, 3600 Handa-cho, Hamamatsu-shi, Shizuoka-ken 431-3124, Japan. TEL 81-53-435-2309, FAX 81-53-435-2308, terao@hama-med.ac.jp. Ed. Terao Toshihiko. Adv. contact Maeda Makoto. Circ: 1,500.

618 JPN ISSN 0546-1790
NIHON SANKA FUJINKA GAKKAI CHUGOKU SHIKOKU GODO CHIHO BUKAI ZASSHI/JAPAN SOCIETY OF OBSTETRICS AND GYNECOLOGY. CHUGOKU AND SHIKOKU DISTRICTS JOURNAL. Text in Japanese. 1951. s-a.
Indexed: INIS Atomind.
Published by: Nihon Sanka Fujinka Gakkai, Chuoku Shikoku Godo Chiho Bukai, c/o Okayama Daigaku Igakubu Sanfujinkagaku Kyoshitsu, 5-1 Shikata-cho 2-chome, Okayama-shi 700-0914, Japan.

618 JPN ISSN 0910-2485
NIHON SANKA FUJINKA GAKKAI KANAGAWA CHIHO BUKAI KAISHI/JAPAN SOCIETY OF OBSTETRICS AND GYNECOLOGY. KANAGAWA DISTRICT JOURNAL. Text in Japanese. 1964. s-a.
Published by: Nihon Sanka Fujinka Gakkai, Kanagawa Chiho Bukai, Kanagawaken Ishi Kaikan, 4-104 Hanasaki-cho, Nishi-ku, Yokohama-shi, Kanagawa-ken 220-0022, Japan.

618 JPN ISSN 1341-5050
NIHON SANKA FUJINKA GAKKAI KUMAMOTO CHIHO BUKAI ZASSHI/JAPAN SOCIETY OF OBSTETRICS AND GYNECOLOGY. KUMAMOTO DISTRICT JOURNAL. Text in Japanese. 1949. a. JPY 13,000 for 5 years. adv. **Document type:** *Academic/Scholarly.*
Published by: Nihon Sanka Fujinka Gakkai, Kumamoto Chiho Bukai, c/o Kumamoto Daigaku Igakubu Sanfujinka Kyoshitsu, 1-1 Honjo 1-chome, Kumamoto-shi 860-0811, Japan. Ed. H Okamura.

618 JPN ISSN 0913-2368
NIHON SANKA FUJINKA GAKKAI KYUSHU RENGO CHIHO BUKAI ZASSHI/JAPAN SOCIETY OF OBSTETRICS AND GYNECOLOGY. KYUSHU DISTRICT JOURNAL. Text in Japanese. a.
Published by: Nihon Sanka Fujinka Gakkai, Kyushu Rengo Chiho Bukai/Japan Society of Obstetrics and Gynecology, Kurume Daigaku Igakubu Sanfujinkagaku Kyoshitsu, 67 Asahi-Machi, Kurume-shi, Fukuoka-ken 830-0011, Japan.

618 JPN ISSN 0285-3485
NIHON SANKA FUJINKA GAKKAI NIIGATA CHIHO BUKAI KAISSHI/JAPAN SOCIETY OF OBSTETRICS AND GYNECOLOGY. NIIGATA DISTRICTS JOURNAL. Text in Japanese. 1972. q. membership.
Published by: Nihon Sanka Fujinka Gakkai, Niigata Chiho Bukai, c/o Niigata Daigaku Igakubu Sanfujinka Kyoshitsu, 1-757, Asahi-machi Dori, Niigata-shi, Niigata-ken 951, Japan.

618 JPN ISSN 0911-6281
NIHON SANKA FUJINKA GAKKAI SAITAMA CHIHO BUKAI KAISHI/JAPAN SOCIETY OF OBSTETRICS AND GYNECOLOGY. SAITAMA DISTRICT JOURNAL. Text in Japanese. 1971. s-a. JPY 2,500 per issue.
Published by: Nihon Sanka Fujinka Gakkai, Saitama Chiho Bukai, Saitama Kenmin Kenko Senta, 5-1 Naka-cho 3-chome, Urawa-shi, Saitama-ken 336-0007, Japan.

618 JPN ISSN 0300-9165
CODEN: NISFAY
NIHON SANKA FUJINKA GAKKAI ZASSHI/ACTA OBSTETRICA ET GYNAECOLOGICA JAPONICA. Text in English, Japanese. 1949. m. JPY 1,100. adv. bibl, charts. index.
Incorporates (in 1969): Acta Obstetrica et Gynaecologica Japonica (0001-6330); Which was formerly (1954-1968): Japanese Obstetrical and Gynecological Society. Journal (0388-0486)
Indexed: Anim.Breed.Abstr., Biol.Abstr., Chem.Abstr., Excerp.Med., INIS Atomind., Ind.Med. (coverage dropped).
—BLDSC (0641.571000), CASDDS, CISTI, EMDOCS, GNLM, KNAW.

Published by: Nihon Sanka Fujinka Gakkai/Japan Society of Obstetrics and Gynecology, Hoken Kaikan Bekkan, 1-1 Ichigaya-Sadohara-cho, Shinjuku-ku, Tokyo 162-0842, Japan. Circ: 2,500.

618 JPN
NIHON SANKA FUJINKA NAISHIKYO GAKKAI ZASSHI/JAPANESE JOURNAL OF GYNECOLOGIC AND OBSTETRIC ENDOSCOPY. Text in Japanese. 1985. irreg.
Published by: Nihon Sanka Fujinka Naishinkyo Gakkai/Japan Endoscopy Society of Obstetrics and Gynecology, c/o Mr Iwata, Kawasaki Byoin Sanfujinka, 12-1, Shinkawa Dori, Kawasaki-ku, Kawasaki-shi, Kanagawa-ken 210, Japan.

618 JPN
NISSANFUKAI TOHOKU RENGO CHIHO BUKAIHO/TOHOKU JOURNAL OF OBSTETRICS AND GYNECOLOGY. Text in Japanese. a.
Published by: Nihon Sanka Fujinka Gakkai, Tohoku Rengo Chiho Bukai/Japan Society of Obstetrics and Gynecology, Tohoku Branch, Tohoku Daigaku Igakubu Sankafujinka Kyoshitsu, 1-1 Seiryo-cho, Aoba-ku, Sendai-shi, Miyagi-ken 980-0872, Japan.

NURSING UPDATE. see *MEDICAL SCIENCES—Nurses And Nursing*

NYUSEN HINYU KENKYUKAI KOEN YOSHISHU/ SOCIETY FOR MAMMARY GLANDS AND LACTATION RESEARCH. ABSTRACTS OF THE MEETING. see *MEDICAL SCIENCES—Abstracting, Bibliographies, Statistics*

618 658 USA ISSN 1044-307X
O B G MANAGEMENT. (Obstetrics and Gynecology) Text in English. 1989. m. USD 97 (effective 2000). adv.
Description: Provides information on how to make patient care decisions that take into account clinical and nonclinical factors, such as reimbursement, government regulation, technology, ethics and patient relations.
—BLDSC (6196.954000). **CCC.**
Published by: Dowden Health Media, Inc, 110 Summit Ave, Montvale, NJ 07645. TEL 201-391-9100, FAX 201-391-2778. Ed. Jeffrey Phelan. Circ: 34,500 (controlled).

618 USA
O B - G Y N SPECIAL EDITION. Text in English. a. USD 30 domestic; USD 35 foreign (effective 2001); Free to qualified subscribers. adv. **Document type:** *Trade.*
Description: Publishes a compendium of educational reviews that explore the full range of women's health issues.
Published by: McMahon Group, 545 W 45th St, 8th Fl, New York, NY 10036. TEL 212-957-5300, FAX 212-957-7230, stilyou@mcmahonmed.com, http://www.mcmahonmed.com/se/indexse.htm. Ed. Sara Tilyou. adv.: B&W page USD 4,200, color page USD 1,200.

618 USA ISSN 0743-8354
RG1
OB-GYN CLINICAL ALERT. Text in English. 1982. m. USD 199 domestic; USD 229 foreign; USD 33 newsstand/cover (effective 2001). index. reprints avail. **Document type:** *Newsletter.*
Related titles: Audio cassette/tape ed.
Published by: American Health Consultants (Subsidiary of: Medical Economics Co., Inc.), 3525 Piedmont Rd, N E, 6 Piedmont Center, Ste 400, Atlanta, GA 30305. TEL 404-262-5476, 404-262-7436, 800-688-2421, FAX 404-262-7837, 800-284-3291, custserv@ahcpub.com, http://www.ahcpub.com. Circ: 2,810.

618 CAN
OB-GYN INTERACTIONS: PROGRAMS IN CLINICAL DECISION MAKING. Text in English. 1988. bi-m. USD 365 to individuals; USD 215 to residents (effective 2000). abstr. **Description:** Focuses on a challenging clinical topic in OB-GYN and combines case studies, animated color graphics, management options and references.
Formerly: A C O G Interactions: Programs in Clinical Decision Making
Media: Diskette.
Published by: B.C. Decker, LCD 1, P O Box 620, Hamilton, ON L8N 3K7, Canada. TEL 905-522-7017, 800-568-7281, FAX 905-522-7839, info@bcdecker.com, http://www.bcdecker.com. Ed. Dr. Alan H Decherney.

OB-GYN MALPRACTICE PREVENTION. see *LAW*

618 USA ISSN 0029-7437
RG1
OB-GYN NEWS. Text in English. 1966. s-m. USD 96. adv. bk.rev. **Document type:** *Newspaper.*
Related titles: Microform ed.: (from PQC); Online - full text ed.: (from Gale Group).
Indexed: Curr.Lit.Fam.Plan.
—**CCC.**
Published by: International Medical News Group, 12230 Wilkins Ave, Rockville, MD 20852. TEL 301-816-8700. Ed. Kathleen Scarbeck. Circ: 31,000 (controlled).

OB-GYN PRACTICE ADVISOR. see *HEALTH FACILITIES AND ADMINISTRATION*

OBSTETRIC ANESTHESIA DIGEST. see *MEDICAL SCIENCES—Anaesthesiology*

618 ROM ISSN 1220-5532
OBSTETRICA SI GINECOLOGIE. Text in Romanian; Summaries in English, French, German, Russian. 1920. 4/yr. USD 20. adv. bk.rev. bibl, charts, illus.
Former titles (until 1990): Revista de Pediatrie, Obstetrica si Ginecologie. Obstetrica di Ginecologie (1220-0913); (until 1975): Obstetrica si Ginecologie (0029-781X); (until 1953): Revista de Obstetrica - Ginecologie (1220-5524); (until 1946): Revista de Obstetrica - Ginecologie, Puericultura (1220-5540)
Indexed: Biol.Abstr., Chem.Abstr., Dent.Ind.
—CISTI, GNLM.
Published by: Romanian Medical Association, Str. Ionel Perlea Nr.10, Bucharest 70754, Romania. **Subscr. to:** ILEXIM, Str. 13 Decembrie 3, PO Box 136-137, Bucharest 70116, Romania.

618 USA ISSN 0029-7828
RG1 CODEN: OGSUA8
OBSTETRICAL & GYNECOLOGICAL SURVEY. Text in English. 1946. m., latest vol.56. USD 165 domestic to individuals Print & Online eds. combined; USD 214 foreign to individuals Print & Online eds. combined; USD 331 domestic to institutions Print & Online eds. combined; USD 331 foreign to institutions Print & Online eds. combined; USD 28 newsstand/cover (effective 2002). adv. bk.rev. abstr, bibl, charts, illus. **Document type:** *Academic/Scholarly, Abstract/Index.* **Description:** Reviews articles and in-depth condensations of important obstetrical and gynecological articles from nearly 100 US and international journals.
Related titles: CD-ROM ed.: (from Ovid Technologies, Inc.); Microfilm ed.: (from WWS); Online - full text ed.: USD 430.30 domestic academic site license; USD 430.30 foreign academic site license; USD 479.95 domestic corporate site license; USD 479.95 foreign corporate site license (effective 2002) (from Ovid Technologies, Inc., Swets Blackwell, Institute for Scientific Information).
Indexed: Biol.Abstr., C.C.I.Ob.Gyn., Chem.Abstr., Curr.Adv.Cancer Res., Curr.Adv.Ecol.Sci., Curr.Cont., Curr.Lit.Fam.Plan., Excerp.Med., INIS Atomind., Ind.Med. (1946-), Int.Nurs.Ind., Med.& Surg.Dermat., NRN.
—BLDSC (6208.172000), CASDDS, CISTI, GNLM, IDS, ingenta, KNAW.
Published by: Williams & Wilkins (Subsidiary of: Waverly International), 351 W Camden St, Baltimore, MD 21201-2436. TEL 410-528-4068, 800-222-3790, FAX 410-528-4452, Kmalamphy@wwilkins.com, http://www.obgynsurvey.com, http://www.wwilkins.com. Ed. Dr. Howard Jones III. Adv. contact Kathleen Malamphy. Circ: 9,900.

618 ESP ISSN 1130-7919
OBSTETRICIA Y GINECOLOGIA ESPANOLA. Text in Spanish. 1991. bi-m.
—GNLM.
Published by: Obstetricia y Ginecologia Espanola S.L., C MAESTRO LOPE, 59, Burjassot, Valencia 46100, Spain. TEL 363-82-02, FAX 363-85-52. Ed. F Bonilla Musoles.

618.2 GBR ISSN 1467-2561
▼ **THE OBSTETRICIAN & GYNAECOLOGIST.** Text in English. 1999. q. GBP 25 to individuals; GBP 50 to institutions (effective 2002).
—BLDSC (6208.178000).
Published by: P M H Publications Ltd., PO Box 100, Chichester, W Sussex PO18 8HD, United Kingdom. TEL 44-1243-576444, FAX 44-1243-576456, admin@pmh.uk.com, http://www.pmh.uk.com. Ed. Shaughn O'Brien. Adv. contact Sarah Monger.

618 ZAF ISSN 1029-1962
OBSTETRICS & GYNAECOLOGY FORUM. Text in English. 1990. q., latest vol.11, no.2, 2001. free per issue domestic; USD 60 foreign (effective 2001). adv. back issues avail. *Refereed.* **Document type:** *Journal, Trade.* **Description:** Targets gynecologists and general practitioners with an interest in gynecology.
Related titles: Online - full text ed.
Published by: In House Publications, PO Box 412748, Craighall, Johannesburg 2024, South Africa. TEL 27-11-4429759, FAX 27-11-8807898, inhouse@iafrica.com, http://www.inhousepub.co.za. Ed. B G Lindeque. Pub., R&P A. Thomas. Adv. contact A Thomas. B&W page USD 887, color page USD 1,200; 210 x 297.

618 USA ISSN 0029-7844
RG1 CODEN: OBGNAS
OBSTETRICS AND GYNECOLOGY. Text in English. 1952. m. EUR 310 in Europe to individuals; JPY 39,800 in Japan to individuals; USD 222 elsewhere to individuals; EUR 429 in Europe to institutions; JPY 57,000 in Japan to institutions; USD 479 elsewhere to institutions; EUR 91 in Europe to Residents; JPY 12,000, USD 101 in Japan to Residents (effective 2002). adv. bk.rev. bibl, charts, illus. s-a. index. back issues avail.; reprint service avail. from PQC. *Refereed.* **Document type:** *Academic/Scholarly.* **Description:** Provides information on current developments in obstetrics, gynecology, and women's total health care.
Related titles: Microform ed.: (from PQC,WWS); Online - full text ed.: (from ingenta, ScienceDirect, Swets Blackwell, Institute for Scientific Information).
Indexed: AIDS Abstr., AIM, ASCA, Agri.& Environ.Biotech.Abstr. (coverage dropped), Behav.Med.Abstr., Bibl.Dev.Med.& Child Neur., Biol.Abstr., C.C.I.Ob.Gyn., CINAHL, Chem.Abstr., Chem.Indus.Notes, Chem.Titles, Curr.Adv.Cancer Res., Curr.Adv.Ecol.Sci., Curr.Adv.Gen.& Molec.Biol., Curr.Cont., Curr.Lit.Fam.Plan., Dairy Sci.Abstr., Dent.Ind., Derwent Biotech.Abstr., Diab.Cont., Excerp.Med., Helminthol.Abstr., INIS Atomind., I.P.A., Ind.Med. (1953-), Ind.Sci.Rev., Inpharma, Int.Abstr.Biol.Sci., Int.Nurs.Ind., Jrnl.Watch, Jrnl.Watch Wom.Hlth., Kidney, Med.& Surg.Dermat., NRN, Neurosci.Cit.Ind., Nutr.Abstr., Pharm.&Out.News, Reac., Rev.Appl.Entomol., Rev.Med.& Vet.Mycol., Risk Abstr., SSCI (coverage dropped), Sci.Cit.Ind., Soyabean Abstr.
—BLDSC (6208.200000), ADONIS, CASDDS, CISTI, GNLM, IDS, ingenta, KNAW. **CCC.**
Published by: (American College of Obstetricians and Gynecologists), Elsevier Science, PO Box 945, New York, NY 10159-0945. TEL 212-989-5800, FAX 212-633-3990, usinfo-f@elsevier.com, http://www.elsevier.com/locate/obstgyn. Ed. Dr. Roy M Pitkin. **Subscr. in Australasia and the Far East to:** Elsevier Science (Singapore) Pte Ltd, No.1 Temasek Ave, 17-01 Millenia Tower, Singapore 039192, Singapore. TEL 65-434-3727, FAX 65-337-2230; **Subscr. in Japan to:** Elsevier Science Inc - Japan Regional Office, 9-15 Higashi-Azabu 1-chome, Minato-ku, Tokyo 106-0044, Japan. TEL 81-3-5561-5033; **Subscr. outside the Americas to:** Elsevier Science BV, PO Box 211, Amsterdam 1000 AE, Netherlands. TEL 31-20-485-3757.

618 USA ISSN 0889-8545
CODEN: OGCAE8
OBSTETRICS AND GYNECOLOGY CLINICS OF NORTH AMERICA. Text in English. 1974. q. USD 145 domestic to individuals; USD 175 in Canada to individuals; USD 199 foreign to individuals; USD 212 domestic to institutions; USD 256 foreign to institutions; USD 65 per issue (effective 2001). *Refereed.* **Document type:** *Journal, Academic/Scholarly.* **Description:** Each issue addresses a single topic in obstetric and gynecological care.
Supersedes in part (in 1987): Clinics in Obstetrics and Gynaecology (0306-3356)
Related titles: Online - full text ed.: (from Institute for Scientific Information); ♦ Spanish Translation: Clinicas Obstetricas y Ginecologicas de Norteamerica. ISSN 0009-9333.
Indexed: ASCA, Bibl.Dev.Med.& Child Neur., Biol.Abstr., CINAHL, Curr.Adv.Ecol.Sci., Curr.Cont., Curr.Lit.Fam.Plan., Dok.Arbeitsmed., Excerp.Med., Ind.Med. (1987-), Ind.Sci.Rev., Inpharma, Int.Nurs.Ind., Pharm.&Out.News, Reac., SSCI (coverage dropped), Sci.Cit.Ind.
—BLDSC (6208.206300), CISTI, EMDOCS, GNLM, IDS, ingenta, KNAW. **CCC.**
Published by: W.B. Saunders Co. (Subsidiary of: Harcourt Publishers Ltd.), 11830 Westline Industrial Dr, St Louis, MO 63146. TEL 800-325-4177, http://www.wbsaunders.com. **Subscr. to:** Periodicals Fulfillment, W B Saunders Co, 6277 Sea Harbor Dr, 4th Fl, Orlando, FL 32891-4800.

618 FRA ISSN 0223-4211
OFFICIEL DE LA SAGE-FEMME* . Text in French. 1953. 10/yr. FRF 330 (effective 1999). adv. **Document type:** *Newsletter.*
Published by: Organisation Nationale des Syndicats de Sages Femmes (ONSSF), 7 rue Rougemont, Paris 75009, France. TEL 33-1-48245020, FAX 33-1-45231961. Adv. contact Francine Dauphin. Circ: 3,500.

618.178019 USA
▼ **ON FERTILE GROUND.** Text in English. 1999. m. free per issue. back issues avail. **Document type:** *Newsletter.* **Description:** Focuses on developing coping skills for managing infertility.
Media: Online - full text.
Published by: Fertility Coach, 2004 Cliff Valley Way, Atlanta, GA 30329. TEL 404-728-0728, FAX 404-845-9988, http://www.fertilitycoach.com/. Ed. Linda Tillman.

618 JPN
ONCHIKAI KAIHO/NEWS OF ONCHIKAI. Text in Japanese. a.
Published by: Onchikai, Kyoto Daigaku Igakubu, Fuzoku Byoin Sanfujinkagaku Kyoshitsu, 54, Kawara-cho Shogoin, Sakyo-ku, Kyoto-shi, Kyoto 606, Japan.

618 ITA
ONCO GYN NEWS. Text in Italian. 1995. 3/yr. adv. **Document type:** *Newsletter.*
Published by: (Societa Italiana di Oncologia Ginecologia), C I C Edizioni Internazionali s.r.l., Corso Trieste 42, Rome, RM 00198, Italy. TEL 39-06-8412673, FAX 39-06-8412688, info@gruppocic.it, 1160199510. Eds. G Atlante, G De Palo. adv.: B&W page XEU 1,601.02, color page XEU 2,014.18; 210 x 290.

ONCOLOGY & CHEMOTHERAPY. see *MEDICAL SCIENCES—Oncology*

618 USA
ONLINE BIRTH CENTER NEWS. Text in English. 1996. w. free per issue. adv. **Document type:** *Consumer.* **Description:** Issues are sent out every Tuesday. Focuses on pregnancy, birth, breastfeeding and early child care as well as other items that might be of interest.
Media: Online - full text.
Published by: Midwifery Today Association, PO Box 2672, Eugene, OR 97402. TEL 541-344-7438, FAX 541-344-1422, djz@efn.org, http://www.efn.org/~djz/birth/obcnews.html. Pub. Donna Dolezal Zelzer. R&P Jan Tritten. Adv. contact Heather Maurer.

OPERATIVE TECHNIQUES IN GYNECOLOGIC SURGERY. see *MEDICAL SCIENCES—Surgery*

618 JPN
OSAKA SOCIETY OF OBSTETRICIANS AND GYNECOLOGISTS. JOURNAL. Text in Japanese. 1977. biennial.
Published by: Osaka Society of Obstetricians and Gynecologists/Osaka Sanfujinka Ikai, 8-25 Karakiyo-cho, Tennoji-ku, Osaka-shi 543-0018, Japan.

PAEDIATRIA CROATICA; the journal for the. see *MEDICAL SCIENCES—Pediatrics*

PAIS E FILHOS; revista mensal da familia moderna. see *CHILDREN AND YOUTH—About*

649 USA ISSN 1091-0387
PARENTING'S HEALTHY PREGNANCY. Text in English. 1990. a. (in 2 printings). USD 2.95 newsstand/cover; USD 3.50 newsstand/cover in Canada (effective 2001). adv. illus. **Document type:** *Magazine, Consumer.* **Description:** Guide to a healthy pregnancy, labor and delivery, and taking care of a newborn.
Formerly (until 1996): Baby on the Way: Basics (1173-0269)
Published by: (American College of Obstetricians and Gynecologists (ACOG)), Time Publishing Ventures (Subsidiary of: Time - Warner Inc.), 1325 Ave of the Americas, 27th Fl, New York, NY 10019. TEL 212-522-8989, FAX 212-522-8159. Ed. Susan Kane. Pub. Risa Crandell. adv.: B&W page USD 59,130, color page USD 73,910. Circ: 2,400,000.

618 USA ISSN 0014-472X
PARENTS EXPECTING. Text in English. 1967. q. free to qualified persons. adv. bk.rev. illus. reprint service avail. from PQC. **Document type:** *Consumer.* **Description:** Presents various health and beauty topics to expectant moms and dads.
Related titles: Microform ed.: (from PQC).
Published by: Gruner + Jahr U.S.A. Publishing (Subsidiary of: Gruner und Jahr AG & Co.), 375 Lexington Ave, New York, NY 10017-5514. TEL 212-499-2000, FAX 212-499-2097, http://www.parents.com. Ed. Sally Lee. Pub. Beth Ann Burzon. adv.: B&W page USD 46,950, color page USD 62,600; trim 7.875 x 10.5. Circ: 5,200,000.

618 USA
PARENTS PREGNANCY. Text in English. s-a. adv.
Published by: Gruner + Jahr U.S.A. Publishing (Subsidiary of: Gruner und Jahr AG & Co.), 375 Lexington Ave, New York, NY 10017-5514. TEL 212-499-2119, FAX 212-499-2097, http://www.gjusa.com/parentsbaby.cfm, http://www.gjusa.com. Ed. Sally Lee. Pub. Mary Jo Romeo. Circ: 1,000,000.

PEDIATRIYA, AKUSHERSTVO TA GINEKOLOGIYA. see *MEDICAL SCIENCES—Pediatrics*

618 JPN ISSN 0910-8718
PERINATAL CARE. Text in Japanese. 1982. m. JPY 1,631 per issue.
Published by: Medika Shuppan/Medicus Publishing Inc., 18-24 Hiroshiba-cho, Suita-shi, Osaka-fu 564-0052, Japan. TEL 81-6-385-6911, FAX 81-6-385-6721. Ed. Takahiki Matsui.

618.3 USA ISSN 0893-6293
PERINATAL PRACTICE. Text in English. 1984. irreg., latest vol.7. **Document type:** *Monographic series.*
Published by: John Wiley & Sons, Inc., Journals (Subsidiary of: Wiley InterScience), 605 Third Ave, New York, NY 10158. **Subscr. outside the Americas to:** John Wiley & Sons Ltd., Baffins Ln, Chichester, Sussex PO19 IUD, United Kingdom. FAX 44-1243-776128.

618 JPN ISSN 0910-3570
PERINATOLOGY SYMPOSIUM. Text in Japanese. 1984. a. JPY 6,000 (effective 1999). **Document type:** *Proceedings.* **Description:** Contains the annual proceedings of the Society.
Published by: (Japan Society of Perinatology/Nihon Shusanki Gakkai), Medical View Co. Ltd./Mejikaru Byusha, 2-30 Ichigaya-Honmura-cho, Shinjuku-ku, Tokyo 162-0845, Japan. Circ: 5,000 (controlled).

613.9 USA ISSN 0190-3195
PERSPECTIVAS INTERNACIONALES EN PLANIFICACION FAMILIAR. Text in Spanish. a. USD 10 (effective 2001). adv. bk.rev. **Description:** Focuses on the population concerns of Latin America.
Related titles: ♦ English ed.: International Family Planning Perspectives. ISSN 0190-3187; ♦ French ed.: Perspectives Internationales sur le Planning Familial.
Indexed: Hisp.Amer.Per.Ind. (1994).
Published by: Alan Guttmacher Institute, 120 Wall St, New York, NY 10005. TEL 212-248-1111, FAX 212-248-1951, llebran@AGI-USA.org, http://www.AGI-USA.org. Ed. Patricia Donovan. R&P Kaylynn Chiarello. Adv. contact Mark Hildebrand.

301.426 USA
PERSPECTIVES INTERNATIONALES SUR LE PLANNING FAMILIAL. Text in French. a. USD 10 (effective 2001). adv. bk.rev. **Description:** Focuses on the population concerns of francophone Africa.
Related titles: ♦ English ed.: International Family Planning Perspectives. ISSN 0190-3187; ♦ Spanish ed.: Perspectivas Internacionales en Planificacion Familiar. ISSN 0190-3195.
Published by: Alan Guttmacher Institute, 120 Wall St, New York, NY 10005. TEL 212-248-1111, FAX 212-248-1951, llebran@AGI-USA.org, http://www.AGI-USA.org. Ed. Patricia Donovan. R&P Kaylynn Chiarello. Adv. contact Mark Hildebrand.

618 GBR ISSN 1461-3123
PRACTISING MIDWIFE; the voice of clinical midwifery. Text in English. 1991. m. GBP 35; GBP 64 foreign. adv. bk.rev. back issues avail. *Refereed.* **Document type:** *Academic/Scholarly.*
Formerly (until Dec. 1997): Modern Midwife
Indexed: Brit.Nur.Ind., CINAHL, Fam.Ind.
—BLDSC (6597.820000), GNLM.
Published by: Hochland & Hochland Ltd., 174A Ashley Rd, Hale, Altrincham, Ches WA15 95F, United Kingdom. TEL 44-161-929-0190, FAX 44-161-929-1818, practimid@hochland.demon.co.uk. Ed. Jilly Rosser. Pub. Henry Hochland. R&P Jane Bowler. Adv. contact M Henwood. B&W page GBP 600, color page GBP 900; trim 2100 x 297. Circ: 5,000. **Subscr. to:** Proact Marketing, The Foot & Bowden Bldg, 19th Crescent, Plymouth, Devon PL1 3AD, United Kingdom. TEL 44-1752-675175, FAX 44-1752-675176.

618 USA
▼ **PREGNANCY.** Text in English. 2000. bi-m. USD 19.99; USD 5.99 newsstand/cover (effective 2001). adv. **Document type:** *Consumer.*
Published by: Highbury House Communications, Inc., 1925 Vaughn Rd Ste 235, Kennesaw, GA 30411. TEL 770-422-3225, feedback@ePregnancy.com, http://www.ePregnancy.com. Pub. Paul Jackson.

618 AUS ISSN 1035-5448
PREGNANCY. Text in English. 1986. q. AUD 4.95; AUD 9.50 foreign (effective 1999). adv. bk.rev. **Document type:** *Consumer.* **Description:** Covers birth process, moods of pregnancy, exercizes, beauty, breastfeeding, and choosing a birth place.
Formerly: Pregnancy, Birth and the Next 6 Months (0817-2420)
Published by: Magazine House Pty. Ltd., PO Box 1067, Crows Nest, NSW 1585, Australia. TEL 61-2-94382399, FAX 61-2-94363014. Ed. Carol Fallows. Pub., R&P Martin Fallows. Adv. contact Paola Forlano. B&W page AUD 3,600, color page AUD 4,900. Circ: 45,000.

618 GBR ISSN 1368-6194
PREGNANCY. Text in English. 1997. m. GBP 2.50 newsstand/cover. **Document type:** *Consumer.*
Published by: W V Publications and Exhibitions Ltd., 57-59 Rochester Pl, London NW1 9JG, United Kingdom. TEL 44-20-7485-0011, FAX 44-20-7482-6269, wvmags@computer.com. **Dist. by:** Comag, Tavistock Works, Tavistock Rd, W Drayton, Middx UB7 7QX, United Kingdom. TEL 44-1895-433600, FAX 44-1895-433602.

618.2 AUS
PREGNANCY & BIRTH. Text in English. bi-m. AUD 5.95 newsstand/cover (effective 2000). adv. **Document type:** *Consumer.* **Description:** Guides the expectant mother through the nine months of her pregnancy, informing and reassuring her about he changes she's facing; offers facts on their changing bodies and lifestyles, gives insight into what they can expect from birth to their baby and includes suggestion on how to cope during the exciting, early days of motherhood.
Published by: Bounty Services Pty. Ltd. (Subsidiary of: Emap International), 187 Thomas St., Level 6, Haymarket, NSW 2000, Australia. TEL 61-2-9581-9555. Ed. Margaret Rafferty. R&P Wisal Masri. Adv. contacts Dempster Clare, Sarah Fleischer. page AUD 3,350. Circ: 21,500 (paid).

618.2 AUS ISSN 1328-5661
THE PREGNANCY BOOK. Text in English. 1986. a. free per issue. adv. illus. **Document type:** *Consumer.* **Description:** Provides a complete guide to pregnancy, approved and distributed by hospitals.
Published by: Bounty Services Pty. Ltd. (Subsidiary of: Emap International), 187 Thomas St., Level 6, Haymarket, NSW 2000, Australia. TEL 61-2-9581-9555. Ed. Margaret Rafferty. Pub. Mandy Key. R&P Wisal Masri. Adv. contacts Dempster Clare, Sarah Fleischer. page AUD 12,930; trim 148 x 210. Circ: 205,000.

618 GBR ISSN 1359-8635
CODEN: PNMEFT
PRENATAL AND NEONATAL MEDICINE. Text in English. 1996. bi-m. GBP 85, USD 145 to individuals; GBP 155, USD 250 to institutions. adv. *Refereed.* **Document type:** *Academic/Scholarly.*
Related titles: Online - full text ed.: ISSN 1473-0774 (from CatchWord Ltd., Institute for Scientific Information).
Indexed: Curr.Cont., Inpharma, Pharm.&Out.News, Reac.
—BLDSC (6607.644900), ADONIS, CASDDS, GNLM, IDS, Infotrieve. **CCC.**
Published by: Parthenon Publishing Group (Subsidiary of: C R C Press (New York)), Casterton Hall, Casterton, Carnforth, Lancs LA6 2LA, United Kingdom. TEL 44-1524-272084, FAX 44-1524-271587, mail@parthpub.com, http://www.parthpub.com/pan/home.html. Ed., R&P Jean Wright. Adv. contact Julia Tissington.

M

618 GBR ISSN 0197-3851
CODEN: PRDIDM

PRENATAL DIAGNOSIS. Text in English. 1981. 13/yr. USD 1,645 in United States; USD 1,645 in Canada & Mexico; USD 1,645 elsewhere; USD 1,728 combined subscription in United States for print and online eds.; USD 1,728 combined subscription in Canada & Mexico for print and online eds.; USD 1,728 combined subscription elsewhere for print and online eds. (effective 2002). adv. back issues avail.; reprint service avail. from SWZ,PQC,ISI. *Refereed.* **Document type:** *Academic/Scholarly.* **Description:** Communicates the results of original research in a variety of clinical and scientific specialties concerned with human in utero diagnosis of fetal abnormality resulting from genetic and environmental factors.
Related titles: Microform ed.: (from PQC); Online - full text ed.: ISSN 1097-0223. 1996. USD 1,645 in United States; USD 1,645 in Canada & Mexico; USD 1,645 elsewhere (effective 2002) (from EBSCO Publishing, Wiley InterScience, Institute for Scientific Information).
Indexed: ASCA, Aqua.Sci.& Fish.Abstr., Bibl.Dev.Med.& Child Neur., Biol.Abstr., Biotech.Cit.Ind., Cal.Tiss.Abstr., Chem.Abstr., Chem.Indus.Notes, Chem.Titles, Curr.Adv.Ecol.Sci., Curr.Adv.Gen.& Molec.Biol., Curr.Cont., Dent.Ind., Environ.Sci.Poll.Mgmt., Excerp.Med., Fam.Ind., Genet.Abstr., Hum.Gen.Abstr., Ind.Med. (1981-), Ind.Sci.Rev., Inpharma, Int.Abstr.Biol.Sci., Int.Nurs.Ind., Med.& Surg.Dermat., Neurosci.Cit.Ind., Pharm.&Out.News, Pollut.Abstr., Reac., Ref.Zh., Risk Abstr., SSCI (coverage dropped), Saf.Sci.Abstr., Sci.Cit.Ind.
—BLDSC (6607.646000), CASDDS, CISTI, GNLM, IDS, ingenta, KNAW. **CCC.**
Published by: Wiley Europe Ltd., Baffins Ln, Chichester, W Sussex PO19 1UD, United Kingdom. TEL 44-1243-779777, FAX 44-1243-843232, customer@wiley.co.uk, http://www.wiley.co.uk. Ed. M A Ferguson Smith. Pub. Sally Betteridge. R&P Diane Southern TEL 44-1243-770347. adv.: B&W page GBP 750, color page GBP 1,650; trim 210 x 297. Circ: 1,500. **Subscr. in the Americas to:** John Wiley & Sons, Inc., Journals, 605 Third Ave, New York, NY 10158. TEL 212-850-6645, FAX 212-850-6021, uscs-wis@wiley.com; **Subscr. to:** John Wiley & Sons Ltd., Baffins Ln, Chichester, Sussex PO19 IUD, United Kingdom. cs-journals@wiley.co.uk.

PRESCRIBING REFERENCE FOR OBSTETRICIANS AND GYNECOLOGISTS. see *PHARMACY AND PHARMACOLOGY*

618 USA ISSN 1068-607X
CODEN: PUOGEP

PRIMARY CARE UPDATE FOR OB - GYNS. Text in English. 1994. bi-m. EUR 82 in Europe to individuals; JPY 10,900 in Japan to individuals; USD 93 elsewhere to individuals; EUR 165 in Europe to institutions; JPY 21,900 in Japan to institutions; USD 184 elsewhere to institutions (effective 2002). *Refereed.* **Document type:** *Academic/Scholarly.* **Description:** Serves as a current resource on primary and preventive health care for women, focusing on practical clinical information pertaining to the diagnosis, treatment and management of non-Ob/gyn disorders in women.
Related titles: Microform ed.: (from PQC); Online - full text ed.: (from ingenta, Swets Blackwell, ScienceDirect).
Indexed: Abstr.Hyg., Dairy Sci.Abstr., Environ.Sci.Poll.Mgmt., Excerp.Med. (1995-), Nutr.Abstr., Protozool.Abstr., Saf.Sci.Abstr., Stud.Wom.Abstr.
—BLDSC (6612.908450), CISTI, GNLM, Infotrieve, KNAW. **CCC.**
Published by: (American College of Obstetricians and Gynecologists), Elsevier Science, PO Box 945, New York, NY 10159-0945. TEL 212-989-5800, FAX 212-633-3990, usinfo-f@elsevier.com, http://www.elsevier.com/locate/primcareob. Ed. Dr. V L Seltzer. **Subscr. in Australasia and the Far East to:** Elsevier Science (Singapore) Pte Ltd, No.1 Temasek Ave, 17-01 Millenia Tower, Singapore 039192, Singapore. TEL 65-434-3727, FAX 65-337-2230; **Subscr. in Japan to:** Elsevier Science Inc - Japan Regional Office, 9-15 Higashi-Azabu 1-chome, Minato-ku, Tokyo 106-0044, Japan. TEL 81-3-5561-5033; **Subscr. outside the Americas to:** Elsevier Science BV, PO Box 211, Amsterdam 1000 AE, Netherlands. TEL 31-20-485-3757.

618 USA

PRINCIPLES AND TECHNIQUES IN GYNECOLOGIC SURGERY SERIES. Text in English. 1992. irreg. price varies. **Document type:** *Monographic series.*
Published by: Lippincott Williams & Wilkins (Philadelphia) (Subsidiary of: Wolters Kluwer N.V.), 530 Walnut St, Philadelphia, PA 19106-3621. TEL 301-223-2300, 800-638-3030, FAX 301-223-2400, http://www.lww.com.

618.202 FRA ISSN 1251-9839

PROFESSION SAGE-FEMME. Text in French. 1994. m. FRF 360 domestic; FRF 420 foreign (effective 2000). adv. bk.rev. bibl, stat. back issues avail. **Document type:** *Academic/Scholarly.* **Description:** Features articles about obstetrics and midwifery. Informs readers about the profession as well as new technologies.
Published by: Paganelle, 94-96 bd. Magenta, Paris 75010, France. TEL 33-140346473, FAX 33-140345938. Pub. Jean Pascal Fix. adv.: B&W page FRF 7,400, color page FRF 9,600; trim 210 x 297.

PROFESSIONAL CARE OF MOTHER & CHILD; journal of family healthcare. see *MEDICAL SCIENCES—Nurses And Nursing*

618 ITA ISSN 1122-0961

PROGESSI CLINICI: GINECOLOGIA E OSTETRICIA. Text in Italian. 1992. q. ITL 160,000, USD 180 (effective 1998).
Published by: Piccin Editore, Via Altinate, 107, Padua, PD 35121, Italy. TEL 39-049-655566, FAX 39-049-8750693.

618 ESP ISSN 0304-5013

PROGRESOS DE OBSTETRICIA Y GINECOLOGIA. Text in Spanish; Summaries in English. 1958. 10/yr. ESP 21,100 to individuals; ESP 29,000 to institutions (effective 2001). bk.rev. index. back issues avail.; reprints avail. *Refereed.* **Document type:** *Journal, Academic/Scholarly.*
Related titles: Online - full text ed.: 1996.
Indexed: Excerp.Med., Ind.Med.Esp.
—BLDSC (6864.939800), CINDOC, EMDOCS, GNLM, KNAW.
Published by: (Sociedad Espanola de Ginecologia e Obstetricia), Ediciones Doyma S.A., Traversa de Gracia, 17-21, Barcelona 08021, Spain. TEL 34-93-200-0711, pog@doyma.es, doyma@doyma.es, http://www.doyma.es/pog. Eds. Jesus Gonzales Merlo, Santiago Dexeus. R&P Monica Barnes. Adv. contact Jose Antonio Hernandez. Circ: 3,000.

618 ESP ISSN 1130-0523

PROGRESOS EN DIAGNOSTICO PRENATAL/ PROGRESS IN PRENATAL DIAGNOSIS. Text in Spanish; Summaries in English. 1989. 10/yr. ESP 13,400 to individuals; ESP 15,800 to institutions; ESP 10,600 to students (effective 2001). bk.rev. index. back issues avail.; reprints avail. *Refereed.* **Document type:** *Journal, Academic/Scholarly.*
Related titles: Online - full text ed.: 1996.
Published by: (Asociacion Espanola de Diagnostico Prenatal), Ediciones Doyma S.A., Traversa de Gracia, 17-21, Barcelona 08021, Spain. TEL 34-93-200-0711, pdp@doyma.es, doyma@doyma.es, http://www.doyma.es/pdp. Ed. J M Carrera. R&P Monica Barnes. Adv. contact Jose Antonio Hernandez. Circ: 2,000.

618 ITA ISSN 0033-491X

QUADERNI DI CLINICA OSTETRICA E GINECOLOGICA. Text in Italian; Summaries in English. 1946. bi-m. ITL 80,000; ITL 160,000 foreign (effective 1998). **Document type:** *Academic/Scholarly.*
Indexed: Chem.Abstr., Excerp.Med., Ind.Med. (coverage dropped).
—CISTI, GNLM.
Published by: Casa Editrice Maccari, Via Palermo, 44, Parma, PR 43100, Italy. TEL 39-521-771268. Eds. Eugenio Maurizio, Giuseppe Dellepiane. Circ: 1,000.

618.202 GBR

R C M MIDWIVES JOURNAL. Text in English. 1888. m. GBP 75 domestic; GBP 100 in Europe; GBP 106 elsewhere (effective 2001). adv. bk.rev. index. reprint service avail. from PQC. *Refereed.* **Document type:** *Trade.* **Description:** Presents articles, features and news relevant to midwives, obstetricians and others interested in the health and care of mothers and infants.
Former titles (until 1998): Midwives (1355-8404); (until 1995): Midwives Chronicle (0026-3524)
Related titles: Microform ed.: (from PQC).
Indexed: ASSIA, Brit.Nur.Ind., CINAHL, Curr.Adv.Ecol.Sci., Int.Nurs.Ind.
—BLDSC, CISTI, GNLM, KNAW.
Published by: (Royal College of Midwives), T G Scott & Son Ltd., Brettenham House, Savoy St, Strand, London WC2E 7HR, United Kingdom. TEL 44-20-7240-2032, FAX 44-20-7379-7155, midwives@dial.pipex.com. Ed. Matthew Pulzer. Adv. contact Gillian Norton. Circ: 35,000. **Subscr. to:** TG Scott Subscriber Services, 6 Bourne Enterprise Centre, Bourne Industrial Estate, Wrotham Rd, Borough Green, Sevenoaks, Kent TN15 8DG, United Kingdom. TEL 44-1732-884023, FAX 44-1732-884034.

618 GBR ISSN 0143-6848
RG1

RECENT ADVANCES IN OBSTETRICS AND GYNAECOLOGY. Text in English. 1926. irreg., latest vol.18. **Document type:** *Monographic series, Academic/Scholarly.*
—BLDSC (7303.865000), CISTI, GNLM, KNAW.
Published by: Churchill Livingstone (Subsidiary of: Harcourt Publishers Ltd.), Robert Stevenson House, 1-3 Baxter's Pl, Leith Walk, Edinburgh, Midlothian EH1 3AF, United Kingdom. TEL 44-131-556-2424, FAX 44-131-459-1177, http://www.churchillmed.com. **US subscr. to:** Churchill Livingstone, 650 Ave of the Americas, New York, NY 10011. TEL 212-206-5000.

618 FRA ISSN 1244-8168
CODEN: RGOBE2

REFERENCES EN GYNECOLOGIE OBSTETRIQUE. Text in English, French. 1993. 6/yr. EUR 192 domestic to individuals; EUR 48 newsstand/cover foreign to institutions (effective 2002). adv. *Refereed.* **Document type:** *Academic/Scholarly.* **Description:** Contains articles on techniques for diagnosing and treating various gynecological and obstetrical conditions and diseases.
Indexed: Excerp.Med. (1994-).
—BLDSC (7332.020000), CISTI, GNLM.
Published by: (Editions Mellet), Springer-Verlag France (Subsidiary of: BertelsmannSpringer), 1 rue Paul Cezanne, Paris 75008, France. TEL 33-1-53933644, FAX 33-1-53933683, access@link.springer.de; york@springer-paris.fr, http://link.springer.de/link/service/journals/00590/index.htm. Ed. P Bouchard. adv.: B&W page FRF 19,500, color page FRF 25,800; trim 220 x 285. **Subscr. in N. America to:** Springer-Verlag New York Inc., PO Box 2485, Secaucus, NJ 07096-2485.

612.6 GBR ISSN 0962-2799
QP251 CODEN: RMERE8

REPRODUCTIVE MEDICINE REVIEW. Text in English. 1992. 3/yr. GBP 90 to individuals; USD 198 to institutions (effective 2002). adv. bk.rev. **Document type:** *Academic/Scholarly.* **Description:** Addresses topics of interest to obstetricians involved in reproductive medicine, reproductive endocrinologists, clinicians in fertility and in-vitro fertilization clinics, and scientific staff in all these areas.
Related titles: Online - full text ed.: (from EBSCO Publishing, O C L C Online Computer Library Center, Inc., RoweCom Information Quest, Swets Blackwell).
Indexed: Excerp.Med. (1994-).
—BLDSC (7713.706200), EMDOCS, GNLM, Infotrieve. **CCC.**
Published by: Cambridge University Press, Edinburgh Bldg, Shaftesbury Rd, Cambridge CB2 2RU, United Kingdom. FAX 44-1223-315052, information@cup.cam.ac.uk, information@cambridge.org, http://www.cup.cam.ac.uk, http://www.uk.cambridge.org/journals/pmu. Ed. Iain T. Cameron. R&P Linda Nicol. Adv. contact Rebecca Symons.

618 CAN ISSN 1528-4840
RG133.5 CODEN: AEPEEJ

REPRODUCTIVE TECHNOLOGIES. Text in English. 1991. bi-m. USD 220 in US & Canada to individuals; USD 245 elsewhere to individuals; USD 279 in US & Canada to institutions; USD 305 elsewhere to institutions. back issues avail. *Refereed.* **Document type:** *Journal, Academic/Scholarly.* **Description:** Publishes reviews covering advances in reproductive medicine directed to obstetricians, gynecologists, urologists, endocrinologists and biologists.
Formerly (until 2000): Assisted Reproduction (1051-2446)
Related titles: CD-ROM ed.
Indexed: Excerp.Med. (1993-), Rel.Ind.One, Rel.Ind.Two.
—BLDSC (7713.706400), EMDOCS, GNLM.
Published by: B.C. Decker, LCD 1, P O Box 620, Hamilton, ON L8N 3K7, Canada. TEL 905-522-7017, 800-568-7281, FAX 905-522-7839, info@bcdecker.com, http://www.bcdecker.com. Ed. Dr. Alan H Decherney. Adv. contact John Birkby. Circ: 400.

618 619 DEU ISSN 1434-6931
CODEN: FSIKEJ

REPRODUKTIONSMEDIZIN. Text in German. 1985. 6/yr. EUR 340.70 domestic; EUR 337.10 in Germany; EUR 65.40 newsstand/cover foreign (effective 2002). back issues avail.; reprint service avail. from ISI. *Refereed.* **Document type:** *Journal, Academic/Scholarly.* **Description:** Covers all aspects of reproductive medicine and procedures.
Formerly (until 1998): Fertilitaet, Sterilitaet, In-Vitro-Fertilisation, Sexualitaet, Kontrazeption (0179-1796)

Related titles: Microform ed.: (from PQC); Online - full text ed.: ISSN 1434-808X (from EBSCO Publishing, RoweCom Information Quest, Swets Blackwell, Springer LINK).
Indexed: Agri.& Environ.Biotech.Abstr. (coverage dropped). —CASDDS, GNLM, Infotrieve, KNAW. **CCC.**
Published by: Springer-Verlag (Subsidiary of: BertelsmannSpringer), Tiergartenstr 17, Heidelberg 69121, Germany. TEL 49-6221-345-0, FAX 49-6221-345229, subscriptions@springer.de, http://link.springer.de/link/service/journals/00444/index.htm, http://www.springer.de. Eds. E Nieschlag, W Holzgreve. **Subscr. in N. America to:** Springer-Verlag New York Inc., PO Box 2485, Secaucus, NJ 07096-2485. TEL 212-460-1500, FAX 212-473-6272.

618 USA
RESOLVE NATIONAL NEWSLETTER. Text in English. q. free with membership. **Document type:** *Newsletter, Consumer.* **Description:** Covers all aspects of infertility with topics such as: medical information, adoption advise, advocacy, expert answers to reader questions.
Published by: RESOLVE: The National Infertility Association, 1310 Broadway, Somerville, MA 02144 . TEL 617-623-0744, FAX 617-623-0252, resolveinc@aol.com, http://www.resolve.org/newslett.htm.

618.3 USA ISSN 0362-5699
RG600 CODEN: PPMED7
REVIEWS IN PERINATAL MEDICINE. Text in English. 1976. a. reprint service avail. from PQC. *Refereed.* **Document type:** *Monographic series.*
Indexed: Biol.Abstr.
—CASDDS, CISTI, GNLM.
Published by: Lippincott Williams & Wilkins (Philadelphia) (Subsidiary of: Wolters Kluwer N.V.), 530 Walnut St, Philadelphia, PA 19106-3621. TEL 301-223-2300, 800-638-3030, FAX 301-223-2400, http://www.lww.com.

618 ESP
▼ **REVISIONES EN GINECOLOGIA Y OBSTETRICIA.** Text in Spanish; Abstracts in Spanish, English. 1999. q. ESP 6,000; USD 200 foreign (effective 2000). adv. abstr, bibl, illus, stat. back issues avail. *Refereed.* **Document type:** *Academic/Scholarly.*
Published by: Aran Ediciones S.A., Castello, 128 1o, Madrid 28006, Spain. TEL 34-91-782-0030, FAX 34-91-561-5787, edita@grupoaran.com, http://www.grupoaran.com. Ed. A. Cano. Pub. Jose Jimenez. R&P Maria Dolores Linares TEL 34-1-7820035. Circ: 5,000.

REVISTA BRASILEIRA DE MASTOLOGIA. see *MEDICAL SCIENCES—Oncology*

618 CHL ISSN 0048-766X
REVISTA CHILENA DE OBSTETRICIA Y GINECOLOGIA. Text in Spanish. 1935. bi-m. illus. 80 p./no. **Document type:** *Journal, Abstract/Index, Bibliography.*
Supersedes (in 1961): Sociedad Chilena de Obstetricia y Ginecologia. Boletin (0366-3140)
Related titles: E-mail ed.; Fax ed.
Indexed: Chem.Abstr., Excerp.Med., Ind.Med. (coverage dropped).
—BLDSC (7848.930000), CISTI, GNLM, KNAW.
Published by: Sociedad Chilena de Obstetricia y Ginecologia, Roman Diaz, 205, Of 205, Providencia, Santiago, Chile. TEL 562-235-0133, FAX 562-235-1294, sochog@entel-chile.net. Ed. Mario Herrera.

618 COL ISSN 0034-7434
REVISTA COLOMBIANA DE OBSTETRICIA Y GINECOLOGIA* . Text in Spanish. 1950. bi-m. COP 2,000, USD 50. adv. bk.rev. bibl, charts, illus. index.
Indexed: Biol.Abstr., Excerp.Med., Ind.Med. (coverage dropped).
—BLDSC (7851.405000), CISTI, GNLM.
Published by: (Sociedad Colombiana de Obstetricia y Ginecologia), Federacion Medica Colombiana, Calle 72, No 6-44, Piso 11, Bogota, Colombia. Eds. Enrique Archila, Jose Gabriel Acuna. Circ: 2,000. **Co-sponsor:** Federacion Colombiana de Sociedades de Obstetricia y Ginecologia.

618 CUB ISSN 0138-600X
REVISTA CUBANA DE OBSTETRICIA Y GINECOLOGIA. Text in Spanish; Summaries in English, Spanish. 1975. 3/yr. USD 36 in the Americas; USD 44 in Europe; USD 52 elsewhere. bibl, charts, illus. index.
Published by: (Cuba. Ministerio de Salud Publica, Centro Nacional de Informacion de Ciencias Medicas), Editorial de Ciencias Medicas, O'Reilly No. 4, Habana, Cuba. TEL 809-62-8091. Ed. Fredesvinda Blanco. Circ: 1,500. **Co-sponsor:** Sociedad Cubana de Obstetricia y Ginecologia.

618 VEN ISSN 0048-7732
REVISTA DE OBSTETRICIA Y GINECOLOGIA DE VENEZUELA. Text in Spanish. 1941. q. USD 50. adv. bk.rev. **Document type:** *Academic/Scholarly.*
Indexed: Biol.Abstr., Chem.Abstr., Excerp.Med., Ind.Med. (coverage dropped).
—CISTI, GNLM.
Published by: Sociedad de Obstetricia y Ginecologia de Venezuela, Biblioteca, Ave. San Martin, Apdo 20081, Caracas, DF 1020-A, Venezuela. TEL 58-2-4515955, FAX 58-2-4510895. Ed. Jacqueline Saulni de Jorges. Circ: 2,000.

618 ESP ISSN 0214-1582
REVISTA DE SENOLOGIA Y PATOLOGIA MAMARIA. Text in Spanish. q. ESP 11,900 to individuals; ESP 17,000 to institutions; ESP 9,520 to students (effective 2001). adv. back issues avail.; reprints avail. *Refereed.* **Document type:** *Journal, Academic/Scholarly.*
Related titles: Online - full text ed.: 1996.
Indexed: Ind.Med.Esp.
Published by: (Sociedad Espanola de Senologia y Patologia Mamaria), Ediciones Doyma S.A., Traversa de Gracia, 17-21, Barcelona 08021, Spain. TEL 34-93-200-0711, rspm@doyma.es, doyma@doyma.es, http://www.doyma.es/rspm. Ed. Miguel Prats Esteve. R&P Monica Barnes. Adv. contact Jose Antonio Hernandez. B&W page ESP 122,000, color page ESP 152,000; 280 x 210. Circ: 1,000.

618 ESP ISSN 0034-9445
CODEN: REOGAX
REVISTA ESPANOLA DE OBSTETRICIA Y GINECOLOGIA. Text in Spanish; Summaries in English, Spanish. 1944. bi-m. ESP 6,000. adv. bk.rev. bibl, charts, illus.
Indexed: Biol.Abstr., Chem.Abstr., Dairy Sci.Abstr., Ind.Med. (coverage dropped), Ind.Med.Esp.
—CASDDS, CISTI, GNLM, Infotrieve. **CCC.**
Published by: (Asociacion de Obstetricia y Ginecologia), Editorial Facta, Menendez y Pelayo, 5-7, Valencia 46010, Spain. Ed. Dr. F Gomar Sancho. Circ: 3,500.

618 FRA ISSN 0035-290X
CODEN: RFGOAO
REVUE FRANCAISE DE GYNECOLOGIE ET D'OBSTETRIQUE. Text in French; Summaries in English, French, German. 1906. 6/yr. FRF 1,100 domestic to individuals; FRF 1,390 foreign to individuals; FRF 550 domestic to students; FRF 695 foreign to students (effective 1999). adv. bk.rev. abstr, charts, illus, stat, tr.lit. reprint service avail. from PQC.
Related titles: Microform ed.: (from PQC).
Indexed: Biol.Abstr., Chem.Abstr., Curr.Cont. (coverage dropped), Excerp.Med., Ind.Med. (coverage dropped), Ref.Zh., Rev.Plant Path.
—CASDDS, CISTI, GNLM, KNAW. **CCC.**
Published by: Expansion Scientifique Francaise, 31 bd. de la Tour Maubourg, Paris Cedex 7 75343, France. TEL 33-1-40626400, FAX 33-1-45556920. Eds. J Seneze, Y Malinas. Circ: 5,000.

618 JPN ISSN 0386-9865
CODEN: RFUSA4
RINSHO FUJINKA SANKA/CLINICAL GYNECOLOGY AND OBSTETRICS. Text in Japanese. 1946. m. JPY 2,400 per issue.
Indexed: Biol.Abstr., Chem.Abstr., Chem.Titles, INIS Atomind.
—BLDSC (3286.289000), CASDDS, CISTI.
Published by: Igaku-Shoin Ltd., 5-24-3 Hongo, Bunkyo-ku, Tokyo 113-0033, Japan. TEL 81-3-3817-5709. Circ: 3,000.

618 ITA
RISVEGLIO OSTETRICO. Text in Italian. 1922. m. ITL 8,000. adv.
Published by: Editoriale Emme 3, Corso Venezia, 24, Milan, MI 20121, Italy. TEL 2-66-91-97. Circ: 20,000.

618.1 RUS
ROSSIISKAYA ASSOTSIATSAYA AKUSHEROV-GINEKOLOGOV. VESTNIK. Text in Russian. q. USD 99.95 in United States.
Indexed: Ref.Zh., Russ.Acad.Sci.Bibl.
—BLDSC (0032.754500).
Published by: (Rossiiskii Assotsyatsii Akusherov-Ginekologov), Passport International Ltd., Ul Pokrovka 22-a, Moscow 101000, Russian Federation. TEL 7-095-9231610, FAX 7-095-9231720. **US dist. addr.:** East View Publications, 3020 Harbor Ln N, Minneapolis, MN 55447. TEL 612-550-0961.

618 RUS
CODEN: VOMDAQ
ROSSIISKII VESTNIK PERINATOLOGII I PEDIATRII. Text in Russian. 1956. bi-m. RUR 216 for 6 mos. to individuals; RUR 450 for 6 mos. to institutions (effective 2002). adv. bk.rev. bibl. index. **Document type:** *Trade.* **Description:** For pediatricians, obstetricians and gynecologists, working in different fields of maternal and child health at maternity and pediatric health centers, hospitals, nurseries and kindergarten, schools, rural medical centers.
Former titles: Materinstvo i Detstvo (0869-2114); (until 1992): Voprosy Okhrany Materinstva i Detstva (0042-8825)
Indexed: Bibl.Dev.Med.& Child Neur., Biol.Abstr., Chem.Abstr., Excerp.Med., Ind.Med. (coverage dropped), Nutr.Abstr., Ref.Zh., Russ.Acad.Sci.Bibl., World Bibl.Soc.Sec.
—BLDSC (0154.059180), CASDDS, CISTI, GNLM, Infotrieve, KNAW. **CCC.**
Published by: Media Sfera, Dmitrovskoe shosse 46, korp 2, etazh 4, P.O. Box 54, Moscow 127238, Russian Federation. TEL 7-095-4824329, FAX 7-095-4824312, mediashp@mediasphera.ru. Ed. Yu. E Vel'tishchev. Adv. contact Valery Nemtsov. **Dist. by:** Mezhdunarodnaya Kniga, B Yakimanka 39, Moscow 117049, Russian Federation. TEL 7-095-2384967, FAX 7-095-2384634; **US dist. addr.:** East View Publications, 3020 Harbor Ln N, Minneapolis, MN 55447. TEL 612-550-0961.

618 GBR
▼ **ROYAL COLLEGE OF OBSTETRICIANS AND GYNAECOLOGISTS. AUDIT.** Text in English. 2001.
Published by: (Royal College of Obstetricians and Gynaecologists), Royal College of Obstetricians and Gynaecologists Press, 27 Sussex Place, Regent's Park, London NW1 4RG, United Kingdom.

618 GBR
ROYAL FREE AND UNIVERSITY COLLEGE MEDICAL SCHOOL. DEPARTMENT OF OBSTETRICS & GYNAECOLOGY. NEWSLETTER. Text in English. m. **Document type:** *Newsletter, Academic/Scholarly.*
Published by: Royal Free and University College Medical School. Department of Obstetrics & Gynaecology (Subsidiary of: University College London), 86-96 Chenies Mews, London WC1E 6HX, United Kingdom. TEL 44-20-76796056, FAX 44-20-73837429, http://www.ucl.ac.uk/obstetrics-gynaecology/Newsletter/Archive/newsletter_archive.htm.

618 JPN ISSN 0912-2966
SAITAMA-KEN SANFUJINKA IKAIHO/SAITAMA SOCIETY OF OBSTETRICIANS AND GYNECOLOGISTS. Text in Japanese. 1970. a.
Published by: Saitamaken Sanfujinka Ikai, Saitamaken Ishikai, 5-1 Naka-cho 3-chome, Urawa-shi, Saitama-ken 336-0007, Japan.

618 JPN ISSN 0558-471X
CODEN: RKAKDK
SANFUJINKA CHIRYO/OBSTETRICAL AND GYNECOLOGICAL THERAPY. Text in Japanese. 1960. m. USD 354 (effective 2000). **Document type:** *Academic/Scholarly.*
Indexed: INIS Atomind.
—BLDSC (6208.173000), CASDDS, CISTI.
Published by: Nagai Shoten Co. Ltd., 21-15 Fukushima 8-chome, Fukushima-ku, Osaka-shi 553-0003, Japan. Ed. T Nagai.

618 617 JPN
SANFUJINKA MAIKURO SAJARI GAKKAI ZASSHI/JAPANESE JOURNAL OF GYNECOLOGICAL MICROSURGERY. Text in Japanese. a.
Published by: Sanfujinka Maikuro Sajari Gakkai/Japan Society for Gynecological Microsurgery, Tokai Daigaku Igakubu Sanfujinka Kyoshitsu, 143 Shimoka-Suya, Isehara-shi, Kanagawa-ken 259-1143, Japan.

618 JPN ISSN 0558-4728
SANFUJINKA NO JISSAI/OBSTETRICAL AND GYNECOLOGICAL PRACTICE. Text in Japanese. 1952. m. JPY 2,000 per issue.
Indexed: INIS Atomind.
—CISTI, GNLM.
Published by: Kanehara Shuppan Ltd., 2-31-14 Yushima, Bunkyo-ku, Tokyo 113-0034, Japan.

618 JPN ISSN 0386-9873
CODEN: SASEAU
SANFUJINKA NO SEKAI/WORLD OF OBSTETRICS AND GYNECOLOGY. Text in Japanese. 1949. m. JPY 1,900 per issue.
Indexed: Chem.Abstr., Chem.Indus.Notes, Chem.Titles, INIS Atomind.

M

—BLDSC (9356.900000), CASDDS.
Published by: Igaku no Sekaisha, 12-4 Kudan-Kita 1-chome, Chiyoda-ku, Tokyo 102-0073, Japan.

618 617 JPN ISSN 0915-8375
SANFUJINKA SHUJUTSU/GYNECOLOGIC AND OBSTETRIC SURGERY. Text in Japanese. 1990. a. JPY 7,000 (effective 1999). **Document type:** *Proceedings.* **Description:** Contains annual proceedings of the Society.
Indexed: Curr.Cont. (coverage dropped).
Published by: (Japan Society of Gynecological and Obstetrical Surgery), Medical View Co. Ltd./Mejikaru Byusha, 2-30 Ichigaya-Honmura-cho, Shinjuku-ku, Tokyo 162-0845, Japan. Circ: 4,000 (controlled).

618 616.99 USA ISSN 1092-4450
CODEN: SBDSF9
SEMINARS IN BREAST DISEASE; diagnostic imaging, medical oncology, pathology, radiation oncology, surgery. Text in English. 1998. q. USD 131 domestic to individuals; USD 174 foreign to individuals; USD 193 domestic to institutions; USD 237 foreign to institutions; USD 76 domestic to students; USD 104 foreign to students; USD 60 newsstand/cover (effective 2001). **Document type:** *Journal, Academic/Scholarly.* **Description:** Each issue contains a comprehensive, current overview of a single problem in breast disease.
—BLDSC (8239.448320).
Published by: W.B. Saunders Co. (Subsidiary of: Harcourt Publishers Ltd.), 11830 Westline Industrial Dr, St Louis, MO 63146. TEL 800-325-4177, wbspcs@harcourtbrace.com, http://www.wbsaunders.com. Ed. Dr. Stephen Feig.

SEMINARS IN LAPAROSCOPIC SURGERY. see *MEDICAL SCIENCES—Surgery*

618.92 GBR ISSN 1084-2756
CODEN: SNEOFI
SEMINARS IN NEONATOLOGY. Text in English. 1996. bi-m. GBP 73 to individuals; GBP 183 to institutions (effective 2002). adv. **Document type:** *Academic/Scholarly.* **Description:** Each issue offers current, clinical information on a single topic in the care and treatment of the neonate.
Related titles: Online - full text ed.: (from EBSCO Publishing, O C L C Online Computer Library Center, Inc., Swets Blackwell, IDEAL Online Library).
Indexed: Ind.Med. (1996-).
—BLDSC (8239.455100), GNLM, Infotrieve, KNAW. **CCC.**
Published by: W.B. Saunders Co. (Subsidiary of: Harcourt Publishers Ltd.), 24-28 Oval Rd, London NW1 7DX, United Kingdom. TEL 44-20-7424-4200, FAX 44-20-7424-4515, cservice@harcourt.com, http://www.harcourt-international.com/journals/siny. Ed. S W Ryan. Adv. contact Nik Screen. **Subscr. to:** Harcourt Publishers Ltd., Foots Cray High St, Sidcup, Kent DA14 5HP, United Kingdom. TEL 44-20-8308-5700, FAX 44-20-8309-0807.

SEMINARS IN PERINATOLOGY. see *MEDICAL SCIENCES—Pediatrics*

SHARING (ST. CHARLES); the official newsletter of S H A R E. see *PSYCHOLOGY*

618 JPN ISSN 0386-9881
CODEN: SHUIAX
SHUSANKI IGAKU/PERINATAL MEDICINE. Text in Japanese. 1971. m. JPY 37,300 per issue; JPY 2,400 newsstand/cover (effective 1999). **Document type:** *Academic/Scholarly.*
—CASDDS.
Published by: Tokyo Igakusha Ltd., 35-4 Hongo 3-chome, Bunkyo-ku, Tokyo 113-0033, Japan. TEL 81-3-3811-4119, FAX 81-3-3811-6135.

618 SGP ISSN 0129-3273
CODEN: SJOGDE
SINGAPORE JOURNAL OF OBSTETRICS & GYNAECOLOGY. Text in English. 1967 (vol.6). 3/yr. USD 25 to individuals; USD 6 to students (effective 2000). adv. bk.rev. charts, illus. reprint service avail. from ISI. **Document type:** *Academic/Scholarly.* **Description:** Original and review articles on all aspects of obstetrics and gynaecology.
Formerly: Kandang Kerbau Hospital Bulletin (0022-8346)
Related titles: CD-ROM ed.
Indexed: ASCA, Biol.Abstr., Chem.Abstr., Curr.Cont. (coverage dropped), ExtraMED.
—BLDSC (8285.463800), CASDDS, CISTI, GNLM, KNAW.
Published by: Obstetrical and Gynaecological Society of Singapore, c/o National University Hospital, Dept. of O & G, Lower Kent Ridge Rd, Singapore 0511, Singapore. ogss@pacific.net.sg. Ed. Dr. Loganath K Annamalai. Circ: 1,000.

618.2 FRA
SOCIETE FRANCAISE DE PSYCHO-PROPHYLAXIE OBSTETRICALE. BULLETIN OFFICIEL. Text in French. 1959. q. FRF 350. adv. bk.rev. **Document type:** *Bulletin.*
Formerly: Societe Internationale de Psycho-Prophylaxie Obstetricale. Bulletin Officiel (0037-9468)
Published by: Societe Internationale de Psycho-Prophylaxie Obstetricale, 31 rue Saint Guillaume, Paris 75007, France. Ed. Daniel Lipszyc.

618 BEL ISSN 0037-9522
SOCIETE ROYALE BELGE DE GYNECOLOGIE ET D'OBSTETRIQUE. BULLETIN* . Text in French. 1966 (vol.36). bi-m. adv.
Indexed: Biol.Abstr.
—GNLM.
Published by: Societe Royale Belge de Gynecologie et d'Obstetrique, Av Moliere 309, Brussels, Belgium.

618 USA ISSN 1071-5576
CODEN: JSGIED
SOCIETY FOR GYNECOLOGIC INVESTIGATION. JOURNAL. Text in English. 1994. bi-m. EUR 160 in Europe to individuals; JPY 21,300 in Japan to individuals; USD 180 elsewhere to individuals; EUR 303 in Europe to institutions; JPY 40,200 in Japan to institutions; USD 339 elsewhere to institutions; EUR 111 in Europe to institutions residents price; JPY 14,700 in Japan to institutions residents price; USD 123 elsewhere to institutions residents price (effective 2002). adv. back issues avail. *Refereed.* **Document type:** *Academic/Scholarly.* **Description:** Publishes timely and important scientific papers on all aspects of reproductive biology, including the disciplines of perinatology, obstetrics, gynecology, infertility and other related fields.
Related titles: Microform ed.: (from PQC); Online - full text ed.: (from ingenta, ScienceDirect, Swets Blackwell, Institute for Scientific Information).
Indexed: ASCA, AgBiotech, Anim.Breed.Abstr., Chem.Abstr., Chem.Indus.Notes, Chem.Titles, Curr.Cont., Dairy Sci.Abstr., Excerp.Med. (1995-), Ind.Med. (1994-), Inpharma, Int.Abstr.Biol.Sci., Pharm.&Out.News, Reac., Sci.Cit.Ind.
—BLDSC (4888.100000), CASDDS, CISTI, GNLM, IDS, Infotrieve, KNAW. **CCC.**
Published by: (Society for Gynecologic Investigation), Elsevier Science, PO Box 945, New York, NY 10159-0945. TEL 212-989-5800, FAX 212-633-3990, usinfo-f@elsevier.com, http://www.elsevier.com/locate/jsgi. Eds. G Mills, Dr. R A Lobo. **Subscr. in Australasia and the Far East to:** Elsevier Science (Singapore) Pte Ltd, No.1 Temasek Ave, 17-01 Millenia Tower, Singapore 039192, Singapore. FAX 65-337-2230; **Subscr. in Japan to:** Elsevier Science Inc - Japan Regional Office, 9-15 Higashi-Azabu 1-chome, Minato-ku, Tokyo 106-0044, Japan. TEL 81-3-5561-5033; **Subscr. outside the Americas to:** Elsevier Science BV, PO Box 211, Amsterdam 1000 AE, Netherlands. TEL 31-20-485-3757.

618 ZAF ISSN 0038-2329
CODEN: SAJOA
SOUTH AFRICAN JOURNAL OF OBSTETRICS AND GYNAECOLOGY. Text in English. 3/yr. USD 15 foreign (effective 2000). adv. illus. back issues avail. *Refereed.* **Document type:** *Journal, Academic/Scholarly.* **Description:** Discusses clinical and experimental topics in obstetrics and gynecology.
Related titles: ♦ Supplement to: S A M J South African Medical Journal. ISSN 0256-9574.
Indexed: Environ.Sci.Poll.Mgmt., Ind.S.A.Per., Pollut.Abstr., Risk Abstr., Saf.Sci.Abstr., Trop.Dis.Bull.
—BLDSC (8339.300000).
Published by: South African Medical Association, Health and Medical Publishing Group, 14 Central Sq, Pinelands 7430, South Africa. TEL 27-21-531-3081, FAX 27-21-531-4126, annp@samedical.org, publishing@samedical.org, http://www.samedical.org. R&P Peter Roberts. **Subscr. to:** PO Box 74789, Lynnwood Ridge, Pretoria 0040, South Africa. TEL 27-12-481-2010, FAX 27-12-481-2061, ann@samedical.org. **Dist. by:** Private Bag X1, Pinelands 7430, South Africa. TEL 27-21-531-3081, FAX 27-21-531-4126.

SOUTH EAST THAMES PERINATAL MONITORING GROUP. PROVISIONAL STATISTICS. see *STATISTICS*

618.202 USA ISSN 1083-5008
SPECIAL DELIVERY. Text in English. 1977. q. USD 20; USD 25 foreign (effective 1999). adv. bk.rev. illus. back issues avail.; reprints avail. **Document type:** *Newsletter.* **Description:** Discusses midwifery, alternatives in birth, parenting, early childhood education, women's health.
Related titles: Online - full text ed.: (from Gale Group, Northern Light Technology, Inc.).
Indexed: Gend.Watch, Hlth.Ind.
Published by: Association of Labor Assistants & Childbirth Educators, PO Box 382724, Cambridge, MA 02238. TEL 617-441-2500, FAX 617-441-3167, http://www.alace.org. Ed. Annmarie Kalmar. Pub., R&P, Adv. contact Jessica Porter. Circ: 2,000 (paid).

618.1 ITA
GLI SPECIALIZZATI. GINECOLOGIA. Text in Italian. 1990. q. ITL 25,000. adv. bk.rev.
Formerly: Ginecologia Oggi (1120-365X)
Published by: E S I Stampa Medica s.r.l., Largo Volontari Del Sangue, 10, Casella Postale 42, San Donato, MI 20133, Italy. TEL 39-2-5274241, FAX 39-2-55600670. Ed. Diego Onestinghel. Adv. contact Ornella Galbiati. B&W page ITL 5,200,000, color page ITL 6,800,000; trim 235 x 171. Circ: 8,870.

612.6 AUT ISSN 1011-8772
SPECULUM; Geburtshilfe - Frauen-Heilkunde - Strahlen-Heilkunde Forschung - Konsequenzen. Text in German. 1983. q. adv. abstr, bibl. back issues avail. **Document type:** *Journal, Academic/Scholarly.*
Published by: Krause & Pachernegg GmbH, Mozartgasse 10, Gablitz 3003, Austria. TEL 43-2231-61258-0, FAX 43-2231-6125810, k_u_p@eunet.at, http://members.eunet.at/k_u_p/spec.htm, http://members.eunet.at/k_u_p/verlag.htm. Ed. Dr. Kinga Chalubinski.

618 346.01 USA ISSN 1046-6703
KF3771.Z95
STATE REPRODUCTIVE HEALTH MONITOR; legislative proposals and actions. Text in English. q. USD 80 to individuals; USD 96 domestic to institutions; USD 100 foreign to institutions (effective 2001). adv. **Description:** Compiles state legislation dealing with reproductive health.
Related titles: Online - full text ed.: (from Northern Light Technology, Inc.).
Indexed: CWI.
—ingenta.
Published by: Alan Guttmacher Institute, 120 Wall St, New York, NY 10005. TEL 212-248-1111, FAX 212-248-1951, llebran@AGI-USA.org, http://www.AGI-USA.org. R&P Lori Gertein. Adv. contact Mark Hildebrand.

SURGICAL LAPAROSCOPY, ENDOSCOPY AND PERCUTANEOUS TECHNIQUES. see *MEDICAL SCIENCES—Surgery*

618 TWN ISSN 1028-4559
TAIWANESE JOURNAL OF OBSTETRICS AND GYNECOLOGY. Text and summaries in Chinese, English. 1962. q. TWD 1,500; USD 65 foreign (effective 1999). adv. reprint service avail. from PQC. **Document type:** *Academic/Scholarly, Trade.*
Formerly (until vol.36, no.1, 1997): Journal of Obstetrics and Gynecology of the Republic of China
Related titles: Microform ed.: (from PQC).
Published by: Taiwan Association of Obstetrics and Gynecology, No1 Chang-Te St, Taipei, Taiwan. TEL 886-2-25684819, FAX 886-2-25684820, http://med.mc.ntu.edu.tw/~obsgyn/assoc/. Ed. Tsang Ming Ko. Pub. Min Shyan Tsai. Adv. contact Tsung Hsien Su. Circ: 2,400.

618.202 DNK ISSN 0106-1836
TIDSSKRIFT FOR JORDEMOEDRE. Text in Danish. m. DKK 350; DKK 30 newsstand/cover (effective 1998). **Document type:** *Bulletin, Academic/Scholarly.* **Description:** Seeks to spread knowledge about professional and trade-political matters for the awareness of the profession of midwifery and its developments.
Published by: Almindelige Danske Jordemoderforening/ Danish Association of Midwives, Noerre Voldgade 90, Copenhagen K 1358, Denmark. TEL 45-32-51-66-66, FAX 45-32-51-08-66. Ed. Anne Marie Kjeldset. adv.: B&W page DKK 5,090, color page DKK 9,815; trim 186 x 236. Circ: 2,000.

618 NLD ISSN 0921-7304
CODEN: TIFEE
TIJDSCHRIFT VOOR FERTILITEITSONDERZOEK. Text in Dutch. 1987. q. free to qualified personnel. adv. *Refereed.* **Document type:** *Academic/Scholarly.* **Description:** Contains research information for gynecologists and fertility consultants in the Netherlands, Belgium, and Luxembourg.
Indexed: Excerp.Med. (1994-).
—BLDSC (8841.130000), EMDOCS.

Published by: (Organon), Excerpta Medica Medical Communications BV (Subsidiary of: Reed Elsevier plc), Rooseveltweg 15, Almere-Stad 1314 SJ, Netherlands. TEL 31-36-538-5600, FAX 31-36-538-5650, http://www.excerptamedica.com. Ed. Dr. A T Alberda. Circ: 2,225 (controlled).

618 USA ISSN 1053-7651
TODAY IN MEDICINE. OBSTETRICS & GYNECOLOGY. Text in English. 198?. bi-m.
Former titles (until 199?): Today in Medicine. Ob-Gyn Report (1049-5479); (until 198?): Today in Medicine. Ob-Gyn Disorders (1042-2854)
Published by: Data Centrum Communications, Inc., 21 W 38th St, 4th fl, New York, NY 10018.

618 JPN ISSN 0915-7204
TOKAI SANKA FUJINKA GAKKAI ZASSHI/TOKAI JOURNAL OF OBSTETRICS AND GYNECOLOGY. Text in English, Japanese. 1981. a.
Published by: Tokai Sanka Fujinka Gakkai/Tokai Society of Obstetrics and Gynecology, Nogoya Daigaku Iryo Gijutsu Tanki Daigakubu, 1-20, Daiko Minami 1-chome, Higashi-ku, Nagoya-shi, Aichi-ken 461, Japan.

618.1 ESP ISSN 0040-8867
TOKO-GINECOLOGIA PRACTICA. Text in Spanish. 1936. m. (10/yr.). ESP 7,200 to individuals; ESP 8,900 to institutions; ESP 5,800 to students. adv. bk.rev. charts, stat. back issues avail. *Refereed.* **Document type:** *Academic/Scholarly.*
Related titles: Online - full text ed.: 1996.
Indexed: Biol.Abstr., Excerp.Med., Ind.Med.Esp., Nutr.Abstr., Ref.Zh.
—BLDSC (8862.885000), CISTI, GNLM.
Published by: Ediciones Doyma S.A., Traversa de Gracia, 17-21, Barcelona 08021, Spain. TEL 34-93-200-0711, tp@doyma.es, doyma@doyma.es, http://www.doyma.es/tp. Ed. J Cruz Hermida. R&P Monica Barnes. Adv. contact Jose Antonio Hernandez. B&W page ESP 122,000, color page ESP 152,000; 280 x 210. Circ: 3,000.

618 ZAF ISSN 1023-4047
TOPICS IN OBSTETRICS AND GYNAECOLOGY. Text in English. 1994. a. illus. **Document type:** *Academic/Scholarly.*
Published by: Julmar Communications, PO Box 1474, Highlands North, Johannesburg 2037, South Africa. Ed. Julian Bassin.

618 USA ISSN 0891-9925
CODEN: TRREEN
TROPHOBLAST RESEARCH. Text in English. 1984. irreg., latest vol.4, 1990. price varies. back issues avail. *Refereed.* **Document type:** *Monographic series, Proceedings.*
Indexed: Chem.Abstr. (1984-), Chem.Indus.Notes, Chem.Titles.
—BLDSC (9051.930000), CASDDS, CISTI, Infotrieve. **CCC.**
Published by: Kluwer Academic - Plenum Publishers (Subsidiary of: Wolters Kluwer N.V.), 233 Spring St, New York, NY 10013-1578. TEL 212-620-8000, 800-221-9369, FAX 212-463-0742, info@plenum.com, http://www.plenum.com. Eds. Henry A Thiede, Richard K Miller.

618 NGA ISSN 0189-5117
TROPICAL JOURNAL OF OBSTETRICS AND GYNAECOLOGY. Text in English. 1981. q. USD 60. **Document type:** *Journal, Academic/Scholarly.*
Published by: (International Federation of Gynaecology and Obstetrics), Fourth Dimension Publishing Co. Ltd., House 16, Fifth Ave., PMB 01164, New Haven, Enugu State, Nigeria. TEL 234-42-459969, FAX 234-42-453739. Circ: 1,000. **Co-sponsor:** Society of Gynaecology and Obstetrics of Nigeria.

618 616.07 GBR ISSN 0960-7692
CODEN: UOGYFJ
ULTRASOUND IN OBSTETRICS & GYNECOLOGY. Text in English. 1991. 13/yr., latest vol.19, 2002. GBP 270 in Europe to individuals; USD 442 in North America to individuals; GBP 297 elsewhere to individuals; GBP 441 in Europe to institutions; USD 699 in North America to institutions; GBP 485 elsewhere to institutions (effective 2002). adv. bk.rev. *Refereed.* **Document type:** *Academic/Scholarly.* **Description:** Publishes clinical research in the field.
Related titles: Online - full text ed.: ISSN 1469-0705. GBP 243 in Europe to individuals; USD 398 in North America to individuals; GBP 243 elsewhere to individuals; GBP 397 in Europe to institutions; USD 630 in North America to institutions; GBP 397 elsewhere to institutions (effective 2002) (from EBSCO Publishing, O C L C Online Computer Library Center, Inc., ingenta, Munksgaard & Blackwell Science's Synergy, Swets Blackwell, Institute for Scientific Information, RoweCom Information Quest).
Indexed: ASCA, Curr.Cont., Excerp.Med., Ind.Med. (1991-), Inpharma, Pharm.&Out.News, Reac., SSCI (coverage dropped), Sci.Cit.Ind.
—BLDSC (9082.815300), ADONIS, CISTI, GNLM, IDS, Infotrieve, KNAW. **CCC.**
Published by: (International Society of Ultrasound in Obstetrics and Gynecology), Blackwell Science Ltd., Osney Mead, Oxford OX2 0EL, United Kingdom. TEL 44-1865-206206, FAX 44-1865-721205, journals.cs@blacksci.co.uk, http://www.blackwell-science.com. Ed. S Campbell. Pub. Allen Stevens. R&P Sophie Savage. Adv. contact Jenny Applin. Circ: 2,500.

618 GBR ISSN 1472-2240
▼ **THE ULTRASOUND REVIEW OF OBSTETRICS AND GYNECOLOGY**; the international journal of continuing education and current awareness. Text in English. 2001. q.
Published by: Parthenon Publishing Group (Subsidiary of: C R C Press (New York)), Casterton Hall, Casterton, Carnforth, Lancs LA6 2LA, United Kingdom. TEL 44-1524-272084, FAX 44-1524-271587, mail@parthpub.com, http://www.parthpub.com/. Eds. A. Kurjak, F. Chervenak.

618.1 ZAF ISSN 0254-184X
UNIVERSITY OF CAPE TOWN. DEPARTMENT OF OBSTETRICS AND GYNAECOLOGY. ANNUAL REPORT. Text in English. 1952. a. free per issue. **Document type:** *Corporate.* **Description:** Lists personnel, research in progress, publications and programs available in the department.
Formerly: University of Cape Town. Department of Gynaecology. Annual Report (0069-0228)
Published by: University of Cape Town, Department of Obstetrics and Gynaecology, Medical School, Anzio Rd, Observatory, Cape Town 7925, South Africa. TEL 27-21-4066114, FAX 27-21-4486921. Ed. Herman A van Coeverden de Groot. Circ: 100. **Co-sponsor:** Cape Provincial Administration.

618 616.6 ITA ISSN 1121-3086
CODEN: UIJOFU
UROGYNAECOLOGIA INTERNATIONAL JOURNAL. Text in English. 1987. 3/yr. ITL 100,000, USD 65. adv. bk.rev. abstr, bibl, illus, stat. back issues avail. *Refereed.* **Document type:** *Journal, Academic/Scholarly.* **Description:** Deals with urogynaecology, especially physiology of female lower urinary tract, urinary incontinence, urogenital fistula, pelvic surgery, pharmacological treatment and medical rehabilitation of incontinence.
Indexed: Excerp.Med. (1995-).
—BLDSC (9124.397000).
Address: Via Di Ponte Salario, 290, Rome, RM 00199, Italy. TEL 39-06-8080114, FAX 39-06-8549024, urogyn@tin.it. Ed., Pub. Dr. Maurizio Bologna. Adv. contact Antonella Rizzo. Circ: 3,500.

VIDEO JOURNAL OF COLOR FLOW IMAGING. see *MEDICAL SCIENCES—Radiology And Nuclear Medicine*

WOMEN'S HEALTH ADVISOR. see *WOMEN'S HEALTH*

WOMEN'S HEALTH ISSUES. see *WOMEN'S HEALTH*

WOMEN'S HEALTH SOURCE BOOK. see *WOMEN'S HEALTH*

618.1 USA ISSN 1082-1899
WOMEN'S IMAGING; the journal of breast imaging. Text in English. 1994. bi-m. USD 42 to individuals; USD 80 to institutions (effective 2000). adv. bk.rev. *Refereed.* **Document type:** *Academic/Scholarly.*
Formerly: Mammography Today (1071-8001)
Published by: Durantech Publishing Co., 3870 La Sierra Ave, Ste 392, Riverside, CA 92505. TEL 818-413-0826. Pub., Adv. contact Rod Durant. R&P S John Curtis.

618.2 USA ISSN 8756-5005
RG631
THE YEAR BOOK OF NEONATAL AND PERINATAL MEDICINE. Text in English. 1987. a. USD 95 domestic; USD 101 foreign (effective 2001). illus. reprints avail. **Document type:** *Abstract/Index, Academic/Scholarly.* **Description:** Presents abstracts of pertinent literature with commentary by leading experts in the field.
Formerly (until 1989): Year Book of Perinatal - Neonatal Medicine (8756-5005)
Related titles: CD-ROM ed.
—GNLM, Infotrieve. **CCC.**
Published by: Mosby, Inc., Continuity Division (Subsidiary of: Harcourt Health Sciences), 11830 Westline Industrial Dr, St Louis, MO 63146-3313. TEL 314-872-8370, 800-325-4177, FAX 314-432-1380, http://www.mosby.com/periodicals. Ed. Dr. Avroy Fanaroff.

618.1 618.082 USA ISSN 1090-798X
RG26
THE YEAR BOOK OF OBSTETRICS, GYNECOLOGY, AND WOMEN'S HEALTH. Text in English. 1901. a. USD 93 domestic; USD 99 foreign (effective 2001). illus. **Document type:** *Academic/Scholarly, Abstract/Index.* **Description:** Presents abstracts of pertinent literature with commentary by leading experts in the field.
Formerly: Year Book of Obstetrics and Gynecology (0084-3911)
Related titles: CD-ROM ed.
Indexed: Curr.Adv.Ecol.Sci.
—BLDSC (9414.652500), CISTI, GNLM.
Published by: Mosby, Inc., Continuity Division (Subsidiary of: Harcourt Health Sciences), 11830 Westline Industrial Dr, St Louis, MO 63146-3313. TEL 314-872-8370, 800-325-4177, FAX 314-432-1380, http://www.mosby.com/periodicals. Ed. Dr. Daniel R Mishell Jr.

618 GBR ISSN 1465-9255
RG1
YEARBOOK OF OBSTETRICS AND GYNAECOLOGY. Text in English. 1993. a. GBP 46.67 (effective 2001). subject. back issues avail. **Document type:** *Yearbook, Academic/Scholarly.*
Formerly (until 1996): Royal College of Obstetricians and Gynaecologists. Yearbook (1351-4148)
—BLDSC (9414.648000), GNLM.
Published by: (Royal College of Obstetricians and Gynaecologists), R C O G Press, 27 Sussex Pl, Regent's Park, London NW1 4RG, United Kingdom. TEL 44-152-427-2084, FAX 44-152-427-1587. Eds. David Stwdec, Delan Keaue, Karl Olah. Pub., R&P Jane Moody TEL 44-20-7772-6300.

618 DEU ISSN 0948-2393
RG1 CODEN: ZGNEFR
ZEITSCHRIFT FUER GEBURTSHILFE UND NEONATOLOGIE. Text in German; Summaries in English, German. 1876. bi-m. EUR 248.20 domestic to institutions; EUR 251.80 in Europe to institutions; EUR 261.60 elsewhere to institutions; EUR 132 to students; EUR 52 newsstand/cover (effective 2002). adv. bk.rev. charts, illus. index per vol. reprint service avail. from IRC. *Refereed.* **Document type:** *Journal, Academic/Scholarly.*
Former titles: Zeitschrift fuer Geburtshilfe und Perinatologie (0300-967X); Zeitschrift fuer Geburtshilfe und Gynaekologie (0044-278X)
Related titles: Microfiche ed.: 1876 (from BHP); Online - full text ed.: ISSN 1439-1651; (from Institute for Scientific Information); ♦ Supplement: Buecherei des Frauenarztes. ISSN 0068-337X.
Indexed: ASCA, Bibl.Dev.Med.& Child Neur., Biol.Abstr., Chem.Abstr., Curr.Cont., Dairy Sci.Abstr., Dent.Ind., Excerp.Med., INIS Atomind., Ind.Med. (1995-), Inpharma, Nutr.Abstr., Protozool.Abstr., Reac., Sci.Cit.Ind. (coverage dropped).
—BLDSC (9462.452000), ADONIS, CASDDS, CISTI, EMDOCS, GNLM, IDS, Infotrieve, KNAW. **CCC.**
Published by: Georg Thieme Verlag, Ruedigerstr 14, Stuttgart 70469, Germany. TEL 49-711-8931-0, FAX 49-711-8931298, zgn@thieme.de, leser.service@thieme.de, http://www.thieme.de/zgn/index.html.

618.1 DEU ISSN 0044-4197
CODEN: ZEGYAX
ZENTRALBLATT FUER GYNAEKOLOGIE. Text in German; Summaries in English. 1877. m. EUR 239.80 domestic to institutions; EUR 250.80 in Europe to institutions; EUR 255.30 elsewhere to institutions; EUR 106 to students; EUR 23 newsstand/cover (effective 2002). adv. bk.rev. charts, illus. index. 75 p./no. *Refereed.* **Document type:** *Journal, Academic/Scholarly.* **Description:** Covers all areas of gynecology and obstetrics.

M

Related titles: Microfiche ed.: (from BHP); Online - full text ed.: ISSN 1438-9762; (from Institute for Scientific Information).
Indexed: Biol.Abstr., Chem.Abstr., Chem.Indus.Notes, Chem.Titles, Curr.Adv.Cancer Res., Curr.Adv.Ecol.Sci., Curr.Cont. (coverage dropped), Dent.Ind., Excerp.Med., INIS Atomind., Ind.Med. (1903-), Nutr.Abstr., Ref.Zh.
—BLDSC (9508.400000), CASDDS, CISTI, GNLM, IDS, KNAW. **CCC.**
Published by: Johann Ambrosius Barth Verlag in Medizinverlage Heidelberg GmbH & Co. KG, Ruedigerstr 14, Stuttgart 70469, Germany. TEL 49-711-8931-0, FAX 49-711-8931422, zblgyn@medizinverlage.de, kunden.service@thieme.de, http://www.thieme.de/zblgyn. Adv. contact Irmgard Mayer TEL 49-711-8931469. B&W page DEM 2,000; trim. Circ: 2,000.

618 CHN
ZHONGGUO FUYOU BAOJIAN/CHINESE WOMEN AND CHILDREN'S HEALTH. Text in Chinese. bi-m.
Published by: Jilin Sheng Weisheng Ting/Jilin Provincial Bureau of Health, Fu 2, Dong Minzhu Dajie, Changchun, Jilin 130061, China. TEL 825027. Ed. He Jiesheng.

618 CHN ISSN 1005-2216
ZHONGGUO SHIYONG FUKE YU CHANKE ZAZHI/CHINESE JOURNAL OF PRACTICAL GYNECOLOGY AND OBSTETRICS. Text in Chinese; Abstracts in English. 1985. bi-m. CNY 24, USD 30 (effective 1997). adv. *Refereed.* **Document type:** *Academic/Scholarly.* **Description:** Features new developments and methods of practical diagnosis, treatment, and prevention of gynecological and obstetrical diseases.
Formerly: Shiyong Fuke yu Chanke Zazhi - Journal of Practical Gynecology and Obstetrics (1001-0858)
Published by: Zhongguo Shiyong Yixue Zazhishe/Chinese Journals' Society of Practical Medicine, 44-1, Jixian St, Heping-qu, Shenyang, Liaoning 110005, China. TEL 86-24-3394474, FAX 86-24-3391212. Eds. Dezhi Wang, Qingli Wang. R&P Qingli Wang. Adv. contact Jianguo Li. page USD 1,500. Circ: 55,000.

ZHONGGUO YIXUE WENZHAI (JIHUA SHENGYU, FUCHAN KEXUE)/CHINA MEDICAL ABSTRACTS (BIRTH CONTROL AND GYNECOLOGY). see *MEDICAL SCIENCES—Abstracting, Bibliographies, Statistics*

ZHONGGUO YOUSHENG YOUYU/JOURNAL OF IMPROVING BIRTH OUTCOME AND CHILD DEVELOPMENT OF CHINA. see *BIRTH CONTROL*

618 CHN ISSN 0529-567X
ZHONGHUA FUCHANKE ZAZHI/CHINESE JOURNAL OF OBSTETRICS AND GYNECOLOGY. Text in Chinese. q. CNY 99.60 domestic; USD 52.80 foreign; CNY 8.30 newsstand/cover domestic; USD 4.40 newsstand/cover foreign (effective 2001). **Document type:** *Academic/Scholarly.*
Related titles: CD-ROM ed.; Online - full content ed.: (from WanFang Data Corp.).
Indexed: Chem.Abstr., ExtraMED, Ind.Med. (1953-).
—BLDSC (3180.440000).
Published by: Zhonghua Yixuehui Zazhishe, 42 Dongsi Xidajie, Beijing 100710, China. TEL 86-1-65273375, cmafc@public.sti.ac.cn. Ed. Zeyi Cao. **Dist. by:** China International Book Trading Corp, 35 Chegongzhuang Xilu, Haidian District, Beijing 100044, China. TEL 86-1-68413849, FAX 86-1-68412048, cibtc@mail.cibtc.com.cn, http://www.cibtc.com.cn.

ZHONGHUA NEIFENMI DAIXIE ZAZHI/CHINESE JOURNAL OF ENDOCRINOLOGY AND METABOLISM. see *MEDICAL SCIENCES—Endocrinology*

MEDICAL SCIENCES—Oncology

see also MEDICAL SCIENCES—Radiology And Nuclear Medicine

616.99 DEU CODEN: ADRCEG
A D C NEWS. Text in German. 1994. irreg. bk.rev. *Refereed.* **Document type:** *Journal, Academic/Scholarly.* **Description:** Publishes information regarding new therapeutic approaches for treating infection and malignant disease.
Formerly (until 2001): Antiinfective Drugs and Chemotherapy (0946-4832); Which incorporates: Journal on Chemotherapy of Infectious Diseases and Malignancies (0724-9004)
Indexed: Chem.Abstr., Chem.Indus.Notes, Chem.Titles.
—BLDSC (1547.534480), CASDDS, EMDOCS, GNLM, Infotrieve, KNAW. **CCC.**
Published by: (European Society for Biomodulation and Chemotherapy), Futuramed Publishers GmbH, Postfach 830358, Munich 81703, Germany. TEL 49-89-674047, FAX 49-89-6701434, futuramed@algora.de, http://www.futuramed.de.

616.9 ESP ISSN 1133-3871
A E C C. Text in Spanish. 1993. q. free per issue. **Description:** Cover cancer issues and notices about association activities.
Published by: Asociacion Espanola Contra el Cancer, Amador de los Rios, 5, Madrid 28010, Spain. TEL 34-1-3194138, FAX 34-1-3190966. Ed. Lolina Perez Caballero. Circ: 20,000.

616.99 USA
A F I P ATLAS OF TUMOR PATHOLOGY. Text in English. 1949; N.S. 1990. irreg., latest vol.22, 1998, July. price varies. back issues avail. **Document type:** *Monographic series, Government, Academic/Scholarly.* **Description:** Reports on research in the treatment and management of various tumors.
Published by: (Armed Forces Institute of Pathology), American Registry of Pathology, 14th St & Alaska Ave, N W, Washington, DC 20306-6000. TEL 301-319-0093, FAX 301-319-0630, jonstone@afip.asd.mil, http://www.afip.org.

A L R A NEWSLETTER. see *BIRTH CONTROL*

616.99 340 USA
A V A ADVISOR*. Text in English. 1980. q. USD 25; membership; reduced rate for asbestos victims. adv. back issues avail. **Document type:** *Newsletter.* **Description:** Coverage of medical, legal, and social aspects of asbestos, including worker safety, scientific data, medical treatments, laws governing uses and exposure, legislative developments, and legal remedies.
Published by: Asbestos Victims of America, PO Box 66594, Scotts Valley, CA 95067-6594. TEL 408-438-5864. Ed. H R Maurer. Circ: 18,000.

ACOUSTIC NEUROMA ASSOCIATION NOTES. see *MEDICAL SCIENCES—Otorhinolaryngology*

616.994 PER ISSN 1013-5545
ACTA CANCEROLOGICA. Text in Spanish; Summaries in English. 1960; N.S. 1987. s-a. PEN 240, USD 15. adv. bibl, charts, illus. **Description:** Covers the study and research of cancer.
Indexed: Biol.Abstr., INIS Atomind.
Published by: Peruvian Society of Cancerology, Ave. Angamos Este, 2520, Surquillo, Lima 34, Peru. Ed. Dr. Juvenal Sanchez. Circ: 500.

616.99 NOR ISSN 0284-186X CODEN: ACTOEL
ACTA ONCOLOGICA. Text in English. 1921. 8/yr. GBP 137, USD 226, GBP 275 to individuals; USD 453 to institutions (effective 2002). adv. bk.rev. bibl, illus. index, cum.index. *Refereed.* **Document type:** *Academic/Scholarly.* **Description:** Focuses on all fields of clinical cancer research including cancer nursing and psychological and social aspects of cancer.
Former titles (until 1986): Acta Radiologica. Oncology (0349-652X); (until 1979): Acta Radiologica. Oncology, Radiation, Physics, Biology (0348-5196); (until 1977): Acta Radiologica. Therapy, Physics, Biology (0567-8064); Which superseded in part (in 1962): Acta Radiologica (0001-6926)
Related titles: Online - full text ed.: (from EBSCO Publishing, O C L C Online Computer Library Center, Inc., RoweCom Information Quest, CatchWord Ltd., ingenta, Swets Blackwell, Institute for Scientific Information); ♦ Supplement: Acta Oncologica. Supplement. ISSN 1100-1704.
Indexed: ASCA, Agri.& Environ.Biotech.Abstr. (coverage dropped), Bioeng.Abstr., Biol.Abstr., Biotech.& Bioeng.Abstr., Chem.Abstr., Curr.Adv.Cell & Devel.Biol., Curr.Adv.Ecol.Sci., Curr.Cont., Dent.Ind., Derwent Biotech.Abstr., Excerp.Med., INIS Atomind., INSPEC (Jun.1973-1993, dropped), Ind.Imag.Lit., Ind.Med. (1987-), Ind.Sci.Rev., Inpharma, Int.Abstr.Biol.Sci., Med.& Surg.Dermat., Pharm.&Out.News, Reac., SSCI (coverage dropped), Sci.Cit.Ind.
—BLDSC (0641.705000), ADONIS, AskIEEE, CASDDS, CISTI, Ei, EMDOCS, GNLM, IDS, Infotrieve, ingenta, KNAW. **CCC.**
Published by: (Acta Radiologica), Taylor & Francis AS (Subsidiary of: Taylor & Francis Group), Cort Adelersgt. 17, Solli, PO Box 2562, Oslo 0202, Norway. TEL 47-22-12-98-80, FAX 47-22-12-98-90, journals@tandf.no, http://www.tandf.co.uk/tfas. Ed. Bengt Glimelius. Circ: 1,400.

616.99 NOR ISSN 1100-1704 CODEN: AOSPEZ
ACTA ONCOLOGICA. SUPPLEMENT. Text in Norwegian. irreg. **Document type:** *Academic/Scholarly.*
Related titles: ♦ Supplement to: Acta Oncologica. ISSN 0284-186X.
Indexed: Excerp.Med. (1993-), INIS Atomind.
—ADONIS, EMDOCS, Infotrieve, KNAW. **CCC.**
Published by: Scandinavian University Press (Subsidiary of: Taylor & Francis Ltd.), Postboks 2959, Toeyen, Oslo 0608, Norway. FAX 47-22-57-53-53, journals@scup.no, http://www.scup.no/oncol.

616.994 USA ISSN 0065-230X
RC267 CODEN: ACRSAJ
ADVANCES IN CANCER RESEARCH. Text in English. 1953. irreg., latest vol.74, 1998. reprint service avail. from ISI. *Refereed.* **Document type:** *Monographic series.*
Related titles: Online - full text ed.: (from Institute for Scientific Information).
Indexed: AIDS & Cancer Res., ASCA, Agri.& Environ.Biotech.Abstr. (coverage dropped), Biol.Abstr., Chem.Abstr., Chem.Indus.Notes, Chem.Titles, Dent.Ind., Derwent Biotech.Abstr., Excerp.Med., INIS Atomind., Ind.Med. (1953-), Ind.Sci.Rev., Ind.Vet., Oncog.G.F.Abstr., Sci.Cit.Ind., Sport Fish.Abstr., Telegen, Vet.Bull.
—BLDSC (0701.000000), CASDDS, CISTI, EMDOCS, GNLM, ingenta, KNAW, Linda Hall. **CCC.**
Published by: Academic Press, Inc., Journal Division (Subsidiary of: Harcourt Brace & Company), 525 B St, Ste 1900, San Diego, CA 92101-4495. TEL 619-231-0926, FAX 619-699-6715. Eds. George Klein, Sidney Weinhouse. **Subscr. to:** Order Dept., 6277 Sea Harbor Dr, 4th Fl, Orlando, FL 32887. TEL 800-321-5068.

616.99 USA
ADVANCES IN ONCOBIOLOGY. Text in English. 1996. irreg. USD 128.50. **Document type:** *Monographic series, Academic/Scholarly.*
—BLDSC (0709.535600).
Published by: J A I Press Inc., 100 Prospect St, Box 811, Stamford, CT 06904-0811. TEL 203-323-9606, FAX 203-357-8446.

616.99 USA
ADVANCES IN ONCOLOGY. Text in English. 1985. q. **Document type:** *Academic/Scholarly.*
Published by: (Bristol-Myers Squibb, Oncology - Immunology Division), Cliggott Publishing Co. (Subsidiary of: S C P Communications, Inc.), 55 Holly Hill Ln, Box 4010, Greenwich, CT 06831. TEL 203-661-0600, http://medserv.com/onco/journals/aio/. Ed. Jenevieve Blair Polin. Pub. Warren Gordon.

616.99 USA ISSN 0735-0104 CODEN: AVONDN
ADVANCES IN VIRAL ONCOLOGY. Text in English. 1982. irreg. price varies. reprint service avail. from PQC. *Refereed.* **Document type:** *Monographic series.*
—CASDDS, CISTI, KNAW.
Published by: Lippincott Williams & Wilkins (Philadelphia) (Subsidiary of: Wolters Kluwer N.V.), 530 Walnut St, Philadelphia, PA 19106-3621. TEL 301-223-2300, 800-638-3030, FAX 301-223-2400.

616.99 JPN ISSN 0916-068X
AICHI CANCER CENTER RESEARCH INSTITUTE. SCIENTIFIC REPORT. Text in English. 1968. biennial. free per issue. **Document type:** *Government.* **Description:** Covers the scientific research activities conducted by the institute.
Formerly: Aichi Cancer Center Research Institute. Annual Report (0374-5295)
—GNLM.
Published by: Aichi Cancer Center Research Institute, Kanoko-Den, Chikusa-ku, Nagoya-shi, Aichi-ken 464-0021, Japan. TEL 052-762-6111, FAX 052-763-5233. Ed. Akio Matsukaga. Circ: 1,000.

AIDS & CANCER RESEARCH. see *MEDICAL SCIENCES—Abstracting, Bibliographies, Statistics*

616.99 CHN ISSN 1000-467X
AIZHENG/CHINESE JOURNAL OF CANCER. Text in Chinese; Abstracts in English. 1982. m. CNY 108 domestic; USD 60 foreign; CNY 9 newsstand/cover domestic; USD 5 newsstand/cover foreign (effective 2000).
Related titles: Online - full content ed.: (from WanFang Data Corp.).

M

Published by: Zhongshan Yike Daxue, Zhongliuzhi Zhongxin, Dongfeng Dong Lu 651 Hao, Guangzhou, Guangdong 510060, China. TEL 86-20-87777136, FAX 86-20-87777136, cjcgz@gzsums.edu.cn. Ed. Yixin Ceng. **Co-sponsor:** Shijie Weisheng Zuzhi Yanzheng Yanjiu Hezuo Zhongxin.

616.99 DEU ISSN 0174-2744
CODEN: AKONFG
AKTUELLE ONKOLOGIE. Text in German. 1981. irreg., latest vol.104, 1999. **Document type:** *Academic/Scholarly.*
—BLDSC (0785.778000), CASDDS, CISTI, Infotrieve. **CCC.**
Published by: W. Zuckschwerdt Verlag GmbH, Industriestr 1, Germering 82110, Germany. TEL 49-89-894349-0, FAX 49-89-89434950.

616.99 USA ISSN 0197-016X
RC261.A1
AMERICAN ASSOCIATION FOR CANCER RESEARCH. PROCEEDINGS OF THE ANNUAL MEETING. Text in English. 1953. a. USD 45 domestic; USD 51 foreign (effective 2000). adv. *Refereed.* **Document type:** *Proceedings.* **Description:** Publishes papers on original research presented at the annual meeting.
Former titles (until 1974): Annual Meeting of the American Association for Cancer Research. Proceedings (0197-0151); (until 1971): American Association for Cancer Research. Proceedings (0569-2261)
Related titles: Online - full text ed.: (from Institute for Scientific Information).
Indexed: Derwent Biotech.Abstr., INIS Atomind.
—BLDSC (6841.204900), CINDOC, CISTI, GNLM, KNAW.
Published by: American Association for Cancer Research, Public Ledger Bldg, 150 S Independence Mall W, Ste 826, Philadelphia, PA 19106. TEL 215-440-9300, FAX 215-440-9354, http://www.aacr.org. R&P Margaret Foti. Adv. contact Morgan Robinson.

616.99 USA ISSN 1044-4580
AMERICAN INSTITUTE FOR CANCER RESEARCH NEWSLETTER. Text in English. 1983. q. free per issue. adv. charts, illus. back issues avail. **Document type:** *Newsletter.* **Description:** Covers diet, nutrition, and dietary guidelines for reducing cancer risk.
Indexed: CHNI, Ref.Zh.
Published by: American Institute for Cancer Research (AICR), 1759 R St, N W, Washington, DC 20009. TEL 202-328-7744, FAX 202-328-7226, aicrweb@aicr.org, http://www.aicr.org. Ed. Catherine McPherson. R&P, Adv. contact Susan Simolunas. Circ: 1,500,000 (controlled).

616.99 USA ISSN 0277-3732
CODEN: AJCODI
AMERICAN JOURNAL OF CLINICAL ONCOLOGY; cancer clinical trials. Text in English. 1978. bi-m. USD 276 domestic to individuals for print & online eds.; USD 336 foreign to individuals for print & online eds.; USD 444 domestic to institutions for print & online eds.; USD 518 foreign to institutions for print & online eds.; USD 80 newsstand/cover (effective 2002). adv. bk.rev. charts, illus. index. back issues avail.; reprint service avail. from PQC. *Refereed.* **Document type:** *Academic/Scholarly.* **Description:** Presents pathologic, surgical, and clinical data related to all aspects of metastatic and neoplastic diseases and localized tumors.
Formerly: Cancer Clinical Trials (0190-1206)
Related titles: Microform ed.; Online - full text ed.: USD 577.20 domestic academic site license; USD 651.20 foreign academic site license; USD 643.80 domestic corporate site license; USD 717.80 foreign corporate site license (2002) (from Ovid Technologies, Inc., Institute for Scientific Information).
Indexed: ASCA, Agri.& Environ.Biotech.Abstr. (coverage dropped), Biol.Abstr., Chem.Abstr., Curr.Cont., Curr.Ind.Stat., Dent.Ind., Derwent Biotech.Abstr., Excerp.Med., INIS Atomind., Ind.Med. (1982-), Ind.Sci.Rev., Inpharma, Int.Abstr.Biol.Sci., Med.& Surg.Dermat., NRN, Pharm.&Out.News, Reac., SSCI (coverage dropped), Sci.Cit.Ind., THA, Telegen.
—BLDSC (0823.500000), CASDDS, CISTI, EMDOCS, GNLM, IDS, ingenta, KNAW.
Published by: Lippincott Williams & Wilkins (Philadelphia) (Subsidiary of: Wolters Kluwer N.V.), 530 Walnut St, Philadelphia, PA 19106-3621. TEL 215-521-8300, FAX 215-521-8902, http://www.Lww.com. Ed. Dr. Luther W Brady. Pub. Christine Rullo. R&P Margaret Becker. Adv. contact Ray Thibodeau. B&W page USD 885, color page USD 1,970. Circ: 1,780. **Subscr. to:** PO Box 1600, Hagerstown, MD 21740-1600. TEL 800-777-2295, FAX 301-824-7390.

616.994 NLD
ANALOGUES IN CANCER AND HUMAN REPRODUCTION. Text in English. irreg. price varies. **Document type:** *Monographic series.*
Published by: Kluwer Academic Publishers Group (Subsidiary of: Wolters Kluwer N.V.), Spuiboulevard 50, PO Box 17, Dordrecht 3300 AA, Netherlands. FAX 31-78-639-2254, services@wkap.nl, http://www.wkap.nl. **Dist. by:** Journals Department, PO Box 322, Dordrecht 3300 AH, Netherlands. FAX 31-78-654-6474.

616.99 GBR ISSN 0969-6970
CODEN: AGIOFT
ANGIOGENESIS. Text in English. 1997. q. USD 525, EUR 525 to institutions for print or online ed.; USD 631.20, EUR 630 to institutions for print & online eds. combined (effective 2002). adv. *Refereed.* **Document type:** *Academic/Scholarly.* **Description:** Encourages active research toward the development of practical therapies aimed at angiogenic diseases.
Incorporates (1998-1999): Angiogenesis Research (1386-2049)
Related titles: Online - full text ed.: (from EBSCO Publishing, O C L C Online Computer Library Center, Inc., RoweCom Information Quest, Swets Blackwell, Kluwer Online).
Indexed: Biotech.& Bioeng.Abstr., Ind.Med. (1997-), Med.& Pharm.Biotech.Abstr.
—BLDSC (0902.630000), CASDDS, Infotrieve. **CCC.**
Published by: Kluwer Academic & Lippencott-Raven (Subsidiary of: Wolters Kluwer N.V.), 2-6 Boundary Row, London SE1 8HN, United Kingdom. TEL 44-171-865-0198, FAX 44-171-928-0726, services@wkap.nl, http://angiogenesis.rapidscience.com, http://www.Lww.com. Ed. Tai Ping Fan. R&P Annemeike Dolfing. Adv. contact Gemma Heiser. **Dist. by:** I T P S Ltd., Cheriton House, North Way, Walworth Industrial Estate, Andover, Hants SP10 5BE, United Kingdom. TEL 44-1264-342773, FAX 44-1264-342807.

616.99 GBR ISSN 0923-7534
CODEN: ANONE2
ANNALS OF ONCOLOGY. Text in English. 1990. m. GBP 665, USD 1,090 to individuals; GBP 665, USD 1,090 to institutions (effective 2002). bk.rev. 150 p./no. back issues avail.; reprint service avail. from SWZ. *Refereed.* **Document type:** *Journal, Academic/Scholarly.* **Description:** Publishes research in medical oncology, surgery, radiotherapy, pediatric oncology, basic research, and the comprehensive management of patients with malignant diseases.
Related titles: Microform ed.: (from PQC); Online - full text ed.: (from Ovid Technologies, Inc., EBSCO Publishing, O C L C Online Computer Library Center, Inc., RoweCom Information Quest, Swets Blackwell, Kluwer Online, Institute for Scientific Information).
Indexed: AIDS Abstr., ASCA, Abstr.Hyg., Curr.Cont., Excerp.Med., Helminthol.Abstr., Ind.Med. (1990-), Ind.Sci.Rev., Inpharma, Int.Abstr.Biol.Sci., Int.Nurs.Ind., NRN, Nutr.Abstr., Pharm.&Out.News, Reac., Rev.Appl.Entomol., Rev.Arom.& Med.Plants, Rev.Plant Path., SSCI (coverage dropped), Sci.Cit.Ind., Trop.Dis.Bull., Weed Abstr.
—BLDSC (1043.320000), CISTI, EMDOCS, GNLM, IDS, KNAW. **CCC.**
Published by: (European Society for Medical Oncology NLD), Oxford University Press, Academic Division, Great Clarendon St, Oxford OX2 6DP, United Kingdom. TEL 44-1865-267907, FAX 44-1865-267835, jnl.info@oup.co.uk, http://www3.oup.co.uk/annonc/, http://www.oup.co.uk/journals. Ed. David Kerr. Pub. Mandy Sketch. R&P Fionna Willis. Adv. contact Helen Pearson TEL 44-1235-201904. Circ: 3,850. **Subscr. to:** Journals Marketing, Great Clarendon St, Oxford OX2 6DP, United Kingdom.

ANNALS OF SURGICAL ONCOLOGY. see *MEDICAL SCIENCES—Surgery*

616.99 SWE ISSN 0348-8799
ANNUAL REPORT ON THE RESULTS OF TREATMENT IN GYNECOLOGICAL CANCER. Text in Swedish. 1937. triennial. USD 45. adv. charts. **Document type:** *Monographic series.*
Former titles (until 1977): Annual Report on the Results of Treatment in Carcinoma of the Uterus, Vagina and Ovary (0346-7503); (until 1973): Annual Report on the Results of Treatment in Carcinoma of the Uterus and Vagina
Indexed: Excerp.Med.
—GNLM.
Published by: Annual Report, Radiumhemmet, Stockholm 17176, Sweden. TEL 08-328752. Ed. Dr. Folke Pettersson. Circ: 2,000.

616.994 GBR ISSN 0266-9536
CODEN: ACDDEA
ANTI-CANCER DRUG DESIGN. Text in English. 1985. 6/yr. GBP 385, USD 610 to institutions (effective Feb. 2001). adv. index, cum.index. 88 p./no. back issues avail. *Refereed.* **Document type:** *Academic/Scholarly.* **Description:** Forum for original research in medicinal chemistry, cell and molecular biology, biophysics, molecular virology, and molecular pharmacology.
Related titles: Microfilm ed.; Online - full text ed.: ISSN 1460-2148. GBP 333, USD 504 (effective 2000) (from HighWire Pr., EBSCO Publishing, O C L C Online Computer Library Center, Inc., RoweCom Information Quest, ingenta, Swets Blackwell, Institute for Scientific Information).
Indexed: ASCA, BBCI, Chem.Abstr., Chem.Cit.Ind., Chem.Indus.Notes, Chem.Titles, Curr.Cont., Derwent Biotech.Abstr., Excerp.Med., Ind.Med. (1985-), Ind.Sci.Rev., Inpharma, Pharm.&Out.News, Reac., Sci.Cit.Ind., Telegen.
—BLDSC (1547.287000), CASDDS, CISTI, EMDOCS, GNLM, IDS, ingenta, KNAW. **CCC.**
Published by: (Cancer Research Campaign), Oxford University Press, Academic Division, Great Clarendon St, Oxford OX2 6DP, United Kingdom. TEL 44-1865-267907, FAX 44-1865-267835, jnl.info@oup.co.uk, http://www3.oup.co.uk/antcan/, http://www.oup.co.uk/journals. Ed. Stephen Neidle. Pub. J Boullin. R&P Fionna Willis. Circ: 300. **Subscr. in the Americas to:** Oxford University Press, Journals, 2001 Evans Rd, Cary, NC 27513. TEL 800-852-7323, FAX 919-677-1714, jnlorders@oup-usa.org.

616.99 USA ISSN 0959-4973
CODEN: ANTDEV
ANTI-CANCER DRUGS; international journal on anti-cancer agents. Text in English. 1990. 10/yr. USD 330 domestic to individuals; USD 330 foreign to individuals; USD 1,404 newsstand/cover domestic to institutions; USD 1,404 newsstand/cover foreign to institutions; USD 142 newsstand/cover (effective 2002). adv. bk.rev. reprints avail. *Refereed.* **Document type:** *Academic/Scholarly.* **Description:** Aims to stimulate and report both clinical and experimental results of research on toxic and non-toxic anti-cancer agents.
Related titles: CD-ROM ed.; Online - full text ed.: USD 1,825 domestic academic site license; USD 1,825 foreign academic site license; USD 2,035.80 domestic corporate site license; USD 2,035.80 foreign corporate site license (effective 2002) (from Ovid Technologies, Inc., EBSCO Publishing, Institute for Scientific Information).
Indexed: ASCA, Biotech.& Bioeng.Abstr., Chem.Abstr., Chem.Indus.Notes, Chem.Titles, Curr.Cont., Environ.Sci.Poll.Mgmt., Excerp.Med. (1993-), Ind.Med. (1990-), Ind.Sci.Rev., Inpharma, Int.Abstr.Biol.Sci., Int.Nurs.Ind., Med.& Pharm.Biotech.Abstr., Pharm.&Out.News, Reac., Rev.Arom.& Med.Plants, Sci.Cit.Ind., Tox.Abstr.
—BLDSC (1547.287300), ADONIS, CASDDS, CISTI, EMDOCS, GNLM, IDS, KNAW.
Published by: Lippincott Williams & Wilkins (Philadelphia) (Subsidiary of: Wolters Kluwer N.V.), 530 Walnut St, Philadelphia, PA 19106-3621. TEL 215-521-8300, FAX 215-521-8902, http://www.anti-cancerdrugs.com, http://www.Lww.com. Ed. Dr. Mels Sluyser. Adv. contact Gemma Heiser. Circ: 127. **Subscr. to:** PO Box 1600, Hagerstown, MD 21740-1600. TEL 800-777-2295, FAX 301-824-7390.

616.99 GRC ISSN 0250-7005
CODEN: ANTRD4
ANTICANCER RESEARCH; international journal of cancer research and treatment. Text and summaries in English. 1981. bi-m. USD 540 in Europe to individuals; USD 590 elsewhere to individuals; USD 1,130 in Europe to institutions; USD 1,200 elsewhere to institutions; USD 205 per issue (effective 2002). adv. bk.rev. index. back issues avail. *Refereed.* **Document type:** *Journal, Academic/Scholarly.* **Description:** Contains high-quality works on all aspects of experimental and clinical cancer research.
Related titles: Online - full text ed.: (from Institute for Scientific Information).

M

Indexed: AIDS & Cancer Res., AIDS Abstr., ASCA, Biol.Abstr., Biol.Dig., Biotech.& Bioeng.Abstr., Chem.Abstr., Chem.Cit.Ind., Chem.Indus.Notes, Chem.Titles, Curr.Adv.Biochem., Curr.Adv.Cell & Devel.Biol., Curr.Adv.Ecol.Sci., Curr.Adv.Gen.& Molec.Biol., Curr.Cont., Curr.Tit.Dent., Dairy Sci.Abstr., Environ.Sci.Poll.Mgmt., Excerp.Med., Genet.Abstr. (coverage dropped), Ind.Med. (1981-), Ind.Sci.Rev., Ind.Vet., Inpharma, Int.Abstr.Biol.Sci., Med.& Pharm.Biotech.Abstr., NRN, Neurosci.Cit.Ind., Nutr.Abstr., Oncog.G.F.Abstr., Pharm.&Out.News, Pollut.Abstr., Protozool.Abstr., Reac., Ref.Zh., Rev.Arom.& Med.Plants, Rev.Med.& Vet.Mycol., Rice Abstr., Risk Abstr., Saf.Sci.Abstr., Sci.Cit.Ind., THA, Telegen, Triticale Abstr., Trop.Dis.Bull., Vet.Bull., Weed Abstr.
—BLDSC (1547.290000), CASDDS, CISTI, EMDOCS, GNLM, IDS, ingenta, KNAW. **CCC.**
Published by: International Institute of Anticancer Research, Kapandritiou Kalamou Rd, km 1, PO Box 22, Kapandriti, Attiki 190 14, Greece. TEL 30-295-52945, FAX 30-295-53389, journals@iiar-anticancer.org, http://www.iiar-anticancer.org. Ed., Pub., R&P, Adv. contact John G Delinassios. Circ: 1,400.

ANTIMICROBIAL AGENTS AND CHEMOTHERAPY. see *BIOLOGY—Microbiology*

616.99 YUG ISSN 0354-7310
ARCHIVE OF ONCOLOGY. Text in English. 1993. q. YUN 480 domestic to individuals; YUN 1,000 domestic to institutions (effective 2001). adv. bk.rev. *Refereed.* **Document type:** *Journal, Academic/Scholarly.* **Description:** Original articles, actual problems, review articles, case reports, brief communications (short reports), letters to the editor, news, books received, book reviews, congress reports, calendar of medical and scientific meetings, ONCONET, editorials.
Formerly: Onkoloski Arhiv (0354-2351)
Related titles: Online - full content ed.; ♦ Supplement: Archive of Oncology. Supplement. ISSN 0354-8139.
—BLDSC (1638.438000).
Published by: Institut za Onkologiju/Institute of Oncology, Institutski put 4, Sremska Kamenica 21204, Yugoslavia. TEL 381-21-611061, FAX 381-21-613741, archive@onko.onk.ns.ac.yu, http://www.onk.ns.ac.yu. Ed. Vladimir V Baltic. R&P, Adv. contact Ljiljana Zegarac. Circ: 300.

616.99 YUG ISSN 0354-8139
ARCHIVE OF ONCOLOGY. SUPPLEMENT. Text in English. 1995. a. YUN 1,000 domestic to individuals; YUN 2,000 domestic to institutions; USD 60 foreign to individuals; USD 90 foreign to institutions (effective 2001). adv. back issues avail. *Refereed.* **Document type:** *Academic/Scholarly.* **Description:** Presents abstracts, sometimes combined with original articles, as well as actual cases, problems, review articles, and short reports.
Related titles: ♦ Supplement to: Archive of Oncology. ISSN 0354-7310.
Published by: Institut za Onkologiju/Institute of Oncology, Institutski put 4, Sremska Kamenica 21204, Yugoslavia. TEL 381-21-611061, FAX 381-21-613741, onkons@eunet.yu, baltic@uns.ns.ac.yu, http://www.onk.ns.ac.yu. Ed. Vladimir V Baltic. R&P, Adv. contact Ljiljana Zegarac. Circ: 200.

616.994 ITA ISSN 0004-0266
ARCHIVIO ITALIANO DI PATOLOGIA E CLINICA DEI TUMORI. Text in English, Italian. 1971 (vol.14). q. ITL 6,000. charts, illus.
Indexed: Biol.Abstr., Chem.Abstr., Ind.Med. (coverage dropped).
—CISTI, GNLM.
Published by: Universita degli Studi di Milano, Istituto di Farmacologia, Via Luigi Vanvitelli, 32, Milan, MI 20129, Italy.

616.9 ESP
ASOCIACION ESPANOLA CONTRA EL CANCER. MEMORIA. Text in Spanish. 1958. a. free per issue. charts, stat.
Former titles: Asociacion Espanola Contra el Cancer. Memoria Tecnico-Administrativa; Asociacion Espanola Contra el Cancer. Memoria de la Asamblea General (0066-8540)
Published by: Asociacion Espanola Contra el Cancer, Amador de los Rios, 5, Madrid 28010, Spain. TEL 34-1-3194138, FAX 34-1-3190966.

616.99 GBR ISSN 1350-9667
AUDIO JOURNAL OF ONCOLOGY. Text in English. 1995. q. GBP 69 in the European Union to individuals; GBP 130 in the European Union to institutions. adv. reprints avail. *Refereed.* **Document type:** *Academic/Scholarly.* **Description:** Covers research in cancer.
Media: Audio cassette/tape.
Published by: Chapman & Hall, Journals Department (Subsidiary of: International Thomson Publishing Group), Chapman & Hall, 2-6 Boundary Row, London SE1 8HN, United Kingdom. TEL 44-20-7865-0066, FAX 44-20-7522-9623, jhelp@chall.co.uk. **Subscr. to:** International Thompson Publishing Services Ltd.

616.99021 AUS
AUSTRALIA. BUREAU OF STATISTICS. CANCER IN AUSTRALIA. Text in English. 1996. a. AUD 23.50 (effective 2001). **Document type:** *Government.*
Published by: Australian Bureau of Statistics, PO Box 10, Belconnen, ACT 2616, Australia. TEL 61-2-6252-5249, FAX 61-2-6252-6778, http://www.abs.gov.au.

AUSTRALIA. BUREAU OF STATISTICS. NATIONAL HEALTH SURVEY: CANCER SCREENING, AUSTRALIA. see *MEDICAL SCIENCES—Abstracting, Bibliographies, Statistics*

616.994 NLD ISSN 0304-419X
QD1 CODEN: BBACE
B B A - REVIEWS ON CANCER. Text in Dutch. 1977 (vol.605). q. EUR 695 in Europe to institutions; JPY 92,200 in Japan to institutions; USD 777 elsewhere to institutions (effective 2002). reprint service avail. from ISI. *Refereed.* **Document type:** *Academic/Scholarly.* **Description:** Presents critical reviews on new developments in cancer investigation at the biochemical level.
Related titles: Microform ed.: (from PQC); Online - full text ed.: (from EBSCO Publishing, ingenta, Swets Blackwell, ScienceDirect, Institute for Scientific Information).
Indexed: ASCA, BBCI, Curr.Adv.Ecol.Sci., Curr.Cont., Derwent Biotech.Abstr., Excerp.Med., Ind.Vet., Inpharma, Int.Abstr.Biol.Sci., Reac., Ref.Zh., Sci.Cit.Ind.
—ADONIS, CISTI, EMDOCS, IDS. **CCC.**
Published by: Elsevier Science BV, PO Box 211, Amsterdam 1000 AE, Netherlands. TEL 31-20-485-2911, FAX 31-20-485-2457, nlinfo-f@elsevier.nl, http://www.elsevier.com/locate/bbaroco. Ed. N P Jones. **Subscr. in Australasia and the Far East to:** Elsevier Science (Singapore) Pte Ltd, No.1 Temasek Ave, 17-01 Millenia Tower, Singapore 039192, Singapore. TEL 65-434-3727, FAX 65-337-2230; **Subscr. in Japan to:** Elsevier Science Inc - Japan Regional Office, 9-15 Higashi-Azabu 1-chome, Minato-ku, Tokyo 106-0044, Japan. TEL 81-3-5561-5033, FAX 81-3-5561-5047; **Subscr. in the Americas to:** Elsevier Science, PO Box 945, New York, NY 10159-0945. TEL 212-633-3730, FAX 212-633-3680, usinfo-f@elsevier.com.

616.992 GRC ISSN 1107-0625
BALKAN UNION OF ONCOLOGY. JOURNAL. Variant title: The Journal of B U On. Text in English. 1996. q. USD 60 to individuals; USD 100 to institutions; USD 20 newsstand/cover (effective 2001); Free for members.
—BLDSC (4707.645500).
Published by: (Balkan Union of Oncology), Zerbinis Medical Publications, 42 Antifilou St., Athens 15771, Greece.

616.99 ISR
BAMAH (GIVATAYIM); journal for health professionals in the field of cancer. Text in Hebrew. 1983. irreg. free per issue.
Published by: Israel Cancer Association, Revivim 7, P O Box 437, Giv'atayim 51304, Israel. TEL 972-3-5721616, FAX 972-3-5719578, debby@cancer.org.il, http://www.cancer.org.il. Ed. Miri Ziv. Circ: 10,000.

616.99 USA ISSN 1073-0028
CODEN: BCLOEQ
BASIC AND CLINICAL ONCOLOGY. Text in English. 1993. irreg., latest vol.18. adv. **Document type:** *Monographic series.*
Indexed: Chem.Abstr., Chem.Indus.Notes, Chem.Titles.
—BLDSC (1863.914100), CASDDS, CISTI, Infotrieve. **CCC.**
Published by: Marcel Dekker, Inc., Attn: Eridania Perrez, 270 Madison Ave, New York, NY 10016-0602. TEL 212-696-9000, 800-228-1160, FAX 212-685-4540, marketing@dekker.com, http://www.dekker.com. Pub. Russell Dekker. R&P Julia Mulligan. Adv. contact Eridania Perez.

616.99449 AUS
THE BEACON. Text in English. 1998. q. **Document type:** *Newsletter, Consumer.* **Description:** Meets the needs of those affected by breast cancer through communication, shared information and experiences, and education.
Published by: Breast Cancer Network Australia, PO Box 4082, Auburn South, VIC 3122, Australia. TEL 61-3-9805-2500, FAX 61-3-9805-2599, beacon@bcna.org.au, http://www.bcna.org.au. Ed. Lyn Swinburne. Circ: 5,500 (controlled).

616.994 JPN ISSN 1433-7398
CODEN: BTPAFM
BRAIN TUMOR PATHOLOGY. Text in English. 1983. s-a. (in 1 vol., 2 nos./vol.). EUR 118.20 foreign; EUR 116.40 in Germany; EUR 64.80 newsstand/cover foreign (effective 2002). **Document type:** *Academic/Scholarly.* **Description:** Documents the latest research and topical debate in all clinical and experimental fields related to brain tumors.
Related titles: Online - full text ed.: (from RoweCom Information Quest, Springer LINK).
Indexed: Ind.Med. (1997-), e-psyche.
—BLDSC (2268.221500), CASDDS.
Published by: Springer-Verlag Tokyo, Eastern Book Service, Inc. (Subsidiary of: BertelsmannSpringer), 3-13 Hongo 3-chome, Bunkyo-ku, Tokyo 113-0033, Japan. TEL 81-3-38180861, FAX 81-3-38180864, orders@svt-ebs.co.jp, http://link.springer-ny.com/link/service/journals/10014/index.htm. Ed. Kintomo Takakura. **Subscr. in US to:** Springer-Verlag New York Inc., PO Box 2485, Secaucus, NJ 07096-2485. TEL 800-777-4643, 212-460-1526, FAX 201-348-4505, orders@springer-ny.com; **Subscr. to:** Springer-Verlag, c/o Gabriele Kubitza, Haberstrasse 7, Heidelberg 69126, Germany. TEL 49-6221-345242, FAX 49-6221-345229, subscriptions@springer.de, http://link.springer.de, http://link.springer-ny.com. **Dist. by:** Eastern Book Service, Inc.. TEL 81-3-3818-0861, FAX 81-3-3818-0864, orders@svt-ebs.co.jp.

616.99249 USA ISSN 1074-6900
BREAST CANCER; evolution of concepts. Text in English. 1996. q. USD 145 to individuals; USD 225 to institutions. *Refereed.* **Document type:** *Academic/Scholarly.*
Related titles: Online - full text ed.: (from Northern Light Technology, Inc.).
—GNLM, KNAW.
Published by: Field & Wood, Medical Periodicals, Inc., PO Box 975, Blue Bell, PA 19422. TEL 610-828-4010, FAX 215-482-0226. Ed. Dr. Gruhn.

616.99449 USA
BREAST CANCER: DISEASE STATE MANAGEMENT RESEARCH. Text in English. 1997. a., latest vol.1, 1997. USD 295 domestic; USD 325 foreign (effective 2001). **Document type:** *Trade.*
Published by: American Health Consultants (Subsidiary of: Medical Economics Co., Inc.), 3525 Piedmont Rd, N E, 6 Piedmont Center, Ste 400, Atlanta, GA 30305. TEL 404-262-5476, 404-262-7436, 800-688-2421, FAX 404-262-7837, 800-284-3291, custserv@ahcpub.com, http://www.ahcpub.com.

616.99449 USA
BREAST CANCER NEWSLETTER. Text in English. d. **Document type:** *Newsletter.* **Description:** Devoted to breaking news about the prevention, screening and treatment of breast cancer.
Media: E-mail.
Address: webfeats@breastcancer.net. Ed. Steven Craig Sicles.

616.9949059 GBR ISSN 1465-5411
▼ **BREAST CANCER RESEARCH.** Text in English. 1999. 6/yr. GBP 200 in United Kingdom; USD 300 elsewhere (effective 2001). illus. back issues avail. **Document type:** *Journal, Academic/Scholarly.* **Description:** Aims to ensure that researchers and clinicians have easy access to the latest research and analysis, particularly in the areas of genetics, biochemistry and cell biology.
Related titles: Online - full content ed.: ISSN 1465-542X. 1999; Online - full text ed.: (from Institute for Scientific Information).
Indexed: Genet.Abstr. (coverage dropped).
—BLDSC (2277.493900).
Published by: Current Science Ltd, Middlesex House, 34-42 Cleveland St, London W1P 6LB, United Kingdom. TEL 44-20-7323-0323, FAX 44-20-7580-1938, info@breast-cancer-research.com, http://www.biomedcentral.com/1465-5411/, http://www.currentsciencegroup.com. Ed. Bruce AJ Ponder.

616.99249 USA ISSN 0167-6806
CODEN: BCTRD6

BREAST CANCER RESEARCH AND TREATMENT. Text in English. 1981. 18/yr. USD 735, EUR 734 to individuals for print or online ed.; USD 1,553, EUR 1,551 to institutions for print or online ed.; USD 1,863.60, EUR 1,861.20 to institutions for print & online eds. combined (effective 2002). adv. bk.rev. back issues avail.; reprint service avail. from SWZ. *Refereed.* **Document type:** *Journal, Academic/Scholarly.* **Description:** Seeks to develop a new focus and new perspectives for all those concerned with breast cancer.

Related titles: Microform ed.: (from PQC); Online - full text ed.: (from Ovid Technologies, Inc., EBSCO Publishing, O C L C Online Computer Library Center, Inc., RoweCom Information Quest, Swets Blackwell, Kluwer Online, Institute for Scientific Information).

Indexed: ASCA, Biol.Abstr., Chem.Abstr., Chem.Indus.Notes, Chem.Titles, Compumath, Curr.Adv.Cancer Res., Curr.Adv.Ecol.Sci., Curr.Cont., Dairy Sci.Abstr., Excerp.Med., INIS Atomind., Ind.Med. (1981-), Ind.Sci.Rev., Ind.Vet., Inpharma, Int.Abstr.Biol.Sci., NRN, Nutr.Abstr., Pharm.&Out.News, Reac., Sci.Cit.Ind., Vet.Bull.

—BLDSC (2277.494000), ADONIS, CASDDS, CISTI, EMDOCS, GNLM, IDS, ingenta, KNAW. **CCC.**

Published by: Kluwer Academic Publishers Boston, 101 Philip Dr, Assinippi Park, Norwell, MA 02061. TEL 781-871-6600, FAX 781-871-9045, services@wkap.nl, http://www.wkap.nl/journalhome.htm/0167-6806. Eds. Robert B Dickson, Marc E Lippman. R&P Rose Luongo TEL 781-871-6311. **Subscr. outside N America to:** Kluwer Academic Publishers Group, Journals Department, PO Box 322, Dordrecht 3300 AH, Netherlands. TEL 31-78-639-2392, FAX 31-78-654-6474; **Subscr. to:** Kluwer Academic - Plenum Publishers, 233 Spring St, New York, NY 10013-1578. TEL 212-620-8468, FAX 212-807-1047.

BREAST DISEASE; an international journal. see *MEDICAL SCIENCES—Obstetrics And Gynecology*

616.99249 AUS ISSN 1324-7077

BREAST NEWS. Text in English. 1995. q. free in Australia. **Document type:** *Newsletter.* **Description:** Covers current research and issues in breast cancer management and control.

Related titles: Online - full text ed.

Published by: N H M R C National Breast Cancer Centre, PO Box 572, Kings Cross, NSW 2011, Australia. TEL 61-2-9334-1700, FAX 61-2-9326-9329, directorate@nbcc.org.au, http://www.nbcc.org.au/pages/info/resource/nbccpubs/brnews/contents.htm. Ed. Debra Lee. Circ: 6,500.

616.99 USA
CODEN: BCSYDM

BRISTOL-MYERS - SQUIBB CANCER SYMPOSIA. Text in English. 1979. irreg. price varies. reprint service avail. from ISI. **Document type:** *Proceedings.*

Formerly (until 1990): Bristol-Meyers Cancer Symposia. Proceedings (0197-8756)

Indexed: Chem.Abstr., Chem.Indus.Notes, Chem.Titles.

—CASDDS, CISTI, KNAW.

Published by: Lippincott Williams & Wilkins (Philadelphia) (Subsidiary of: Wolters Kluwer N.V.), 530 Walnut St, Philadelphia, PA 19106-3621. TEL 301-223-2300, 800-638-3030, FAX 301-223-2400.

616.992 CAN ISSN 1185-1031

BRITISH COLUMBIA CANCER RESEARCH CENTRE. ANNUAL REPORT. Text in English. 1950. a. free per issue. **Document type:** *Corporate.*

Former titles (until 1990): British Columbia. Cancer Control Agency. Annual Report (0849-4703); British Columbia. Cancer Foundation. Annual Report (0068-1423)

Published by: British Columbia Cancer Agency, 600 W Tenth Ave, Vancouver, BC V5Z 4E6, Canada. TEL 604-877-6000, FAX 604-877-6146. Circ: 6,000.
Co-sponsor: British Columbia Cancer Foundation.

616.994 GBR ISSN 0007-0920
CODEN: BJCAAI

BRITISH JOURNAL OF CANCER. Text in English. 1947. s-m. USD 323 in North America to individuals; USD 1,386 in North America to institutions; GBP 210 to individuals; GBP 900 to institutions (effective 2001). adv. bk.rev. illus. index. reprint service avail. from PQC. *Refereed.* **Document type:** *Journal, Academic/Scholarly.* **Description:** Clinical and experimental aspects of cancer research.

Related titles: Microform ed.: (from PQC,PMC); Online - full text ed.: (from EBSCO Publishing, Swets Blackwell, IDEAL Online Library, Institute for Scientific Information).

Indexed: AIDS & Cancer Res., ASCA, Abstr.Hyg., Agri.& Environ.Biotech.Abstr. (coverage dropped), Anim.Breed.Abstr., Biol.Abstr., C.I.S. Abstr., Chem.Abstr., Chem.Indus.Notes, Chem.Titles, Curr.Adv.Biochem., Curr.Adv.Cell & Devel.Biol., Curr.Adv.Ecol.Sci., Curr.Adv.Gen.& Molec.Biol., Curr.Cont., Curr.Ind.Stat., Dairy Sci.Abstr., Dent.Ind., Derwent Biotech.Abstr., Dok.Arbeitsmed., Environ.Sci.Poll.Mgmt., Excerp.Med., Herb.Abstr., INIS Atomind., Ind.Med. (1947-), Ind.Sci.Rev., Ind.Vet., Inpharma, Int.Abstr.Biol.Sci., Int.Nurs.Ind., Med.& Surg.Dermat., NRN, Neurosci.Cit.Ind., Nutr.Abstr., Oncog.G.F.Abstr., Pharm.&Out.News, Pollut.Abstr., Reac., Rev.Arom.& Med.Plants, Rev.Med.& Vet.Mycol., Rev.Plant Path., Risk Abstr., SSCI (coverage dropped), Saf.Sci.Abstr., Sci.Cit.Ind., Small Anim.Abstr., Soyabean Abstr., Sugar Ind.Abstr., THA, Trop.Dis.Bull., Vet.Bull., Weed Abstr.

—BLDSC (2307.000000), ADONIS, CASDDS, CINDOC, CISTI, GNLM, IDS, ingenta, KNAW. **CCC.**

Published by: (Cancer Research Campaign), Churchill Livingstone (Subsidiary of: Harcourt Publishers Ltd.), Robert Stevenson House, 1-3 Baxter's Pl, Leith Walk, Edinburgh, Midlothian EH1 3AF, United Kingdom. TEL 44-131-556-2424, FAX 44-131-459-1177, cservice@harcourt.com, http://www.harcourt-international.com/journals/bjoc. Ed. Robin Weiss. Pub. Gillian Griffith. R&P Catherine John TEL 212-424-4200. Adv. contact David Dunnachie. Circ: 2,000. **Subscr. to:** Harcourt Publishers Ltd., Foots Cray High St, Sidcup, Kent DA14 5HP, United Kingdom. TEL 44-20-8308-5700, FAX 44-20-8309-0807.

616.994 FRA ISSN 0007-4551
CODEN: BUCABS

BULLETIN DU CANCER. Text and summaries in English, French. 1908. m. FRF 1,600 domestic; EUR 262 in Europe; FRF 1,780 elsewhere (effective 2001). adv. bk.rev. illus. index. reprint service avail. from ISI. *Refereed.* **Document type:** *Academic/Scholarly.* **Description:** Publishes original articles on clinical oncology, basic cancer research and related fields. Includes review articles, editorials, brief notes, letters to the editor.

Formerly: Association Francaise pour l'Etude du Cancer. Bulletin (0004-5497)

Related titles: Microform ed.: (from PQC); Online - full text ed.: FRF 1,600 (effective 2001) (from Institute for Scientific Information).

Indexed: ASCA, Biol.Abstr., Chem.Abstr., Curr.Adv.Cancer Res., Curr.Adv.Ecol.Sci., Curr.Cont., Dent.Ind., Derwent Biotech.Abstr., Excerp.Med., INIS Atomind., Ind.Med. (1966-), Ind.Sci.Rev., Ind.Vet., Inpharma, Nutr.Abstr., Pharm.&Out.News, Reac., SSCI (coverage dropped), Sci.Cit.Ind., Vet.Bull.

—BLDSC (2837.970000), ADONIS, CASDDS, CISTI, EMDOCS, GNLM, IDS, Infotrieve, KNAW. **CCC.**

Published by: (Societe Francaise du Cancer), John Libbey Eurotext, 127 av. de la Republique, Montrouge 92120, France. TEL 33-01-46730660, FAX 33-01-40840999, marketing@jle.com, http://www.john-libbey-eurotext.fr/. Eds. Paul Cappelaere, Philippe Jeanteur. Circ: 3,500. **Subscr. to:** A T E I, 3 av. Pierre Kerautret, Romainville 92230, France. TEL 33-1-48408686, FAX 33-1-48400731, atei@club-internet.fr.

616.994 USA ISSN 0007-9235
CODEN: CAMCAM

C A - A CANCER JOURNAL FOR CLINICIANS; a cancer journal for clinicians. Key Title: Ca. Text in English. 1950. bi-m. USD 4 domestic to individuals; USD 93 foreign to individuals; USD 48 domestic to institutions; USD 135 foreign to institutions (effective 2002); USD 22 newsstand/cover (effective 2002). adv. bibl, charts, illus. index, cum.index: 1971-80. reprint service avail. from PQC. *Refereed.* **Document type:** *Academic/Scholarly.* **Description:** Covers all aspects of cancer management for clinicians in primary care, oncology and related specialties.

Related titles: Microform ed.: (from PQC); Online - full text ed.: (from Gale Group, EBSCO Publishing, Factiva, Institute for Scientific Information).

Indexed: AIM, Biol.Abstr., CINAHL, Curr.Cont., Environ.Sci.Poll.Mgmt., Excerp.Med., INIS Atomind., Ind.Med. (1950-), Inpharma, Med.& Surg.Dermat., Pharm.&Out.News, Reac., Ref.Zh., Risk Abstr., Sci.Cit.Ind.

—BLDSC (2943.180000), CISTI, EMDOCS, GNLM, IDS, ingenta, KNAW.

Published by: (American Cancer Society, Inc.), Lippincott Williams & Wilkins, PO Box 1600, Hagerstown, MD 21740-1600. TEL 800-638-3030, orders@lww.com, http://www.ca-journal.org/, http://www.Lww.com. Ed. Margie Miller. Pub. Vicky Thaw. Adv. contact Ray Thibodeau. Circ: 150,000 (controlled).

C A SELECTS. NUTRITIONAL ASPECTS OF CANCER. see *MEDICAL SCIENCES—Abstracting, Bibliographies, Statistics*

C A SELECTS PLUS. ANTITUMOR AGENTS. see *MEDICAL SCIENCES—Abstracting, Bibliographies, Statistics*

616.992 GBR ISSN 1367-9031

C M E BULLETIN ONCOLOGY. (Continuing Medical Education) Variant title: Continuing Medical Education Bulletin. Oncology. Text in English. 1997. 3/yr. (1 volume per annum). GBP 45 domestic to individuals; GBP 60 foreign to individuals; GBP 60 domestic to institutions; GBP 90 foreign to institutions (effective 2000). adv. bk.rev., Website rev. abstr. 24 p./no. 2 cols./p. *Refereed.* **Document type:** *Journal.* **Description:** Provides information, reviews and research relating to oncology.

—BLDSC (3287.223035).

Published by: Rila Publications Ltd., 73 Newman St, London W1A 4PG, United Kingdom. TEL 44-20-7631-1299, FAX 44-20-7580-7166, admin@rila.co.uk, subscriptions@rila.co.uk, http://www.rila.co.uk. Ed. Peter Barrett-Lee. Pub., Adv. contact G Da'Cambra. Circ: 700 (paid).

C R C FACTSHEETS. (Cancer Research Campaign) see *MEDICAL SCIENCES—Abstracting, Bibliographies, Statistics*

CANADIAN ONCOLOGY NURSING JOURNAL/REVUE CANADIENNE DE NURSING ONCOLOGIQUE. see *MEDICAL SCIENCES—Nurses And Nursing*

616.994 USA ISSN 0008-543X
RC261 CODEN: CANCAR

CANCER. Text in English. 1948. 30/yr. USD 437 in United States to institutions; USD 577 in Canada & Mexico to institutions; USD 655 elsewhere to institutions (effective 2001). adv. illus. index. *Refereed.* **Document type:** *Academic/Scholarly.* **Description:** Provides an international, interdisciplinary forum for the exchnage of information among all specialists concerned with cancer prevention, early detection, diagnosis, cure, and rehabilitation.

Related titles: CD-ROM ed.: Cancer on Disk. ISSN 1045-7410; Microform ed.: (from PQC); Online - full text ed.: ISSN 1097-0142. 1998 (from EBSCO Publishing, Gale Group, Wiley InterScience, Institute for Scientific Information); Supplement: Cancer Cytopathology.

Indexed: AIDS Abstr., AIM, Abstr.Hyg., AgeLine, Agri.& Environ.Biotech.Abstr. (coverage dropped), Anim.Breed.Abstr., Behav.Med.Abstr., Biol.Abstr., Biol.Dig., CINAHL, Chem.Abstr., Curr.Adv.Cancer Res., Curr.Adv.Ecol.Sci., Curr.Adv.Gen.& Molec.Biol., Curr.Cont., Dairy Sci.Abstr., Dent.Ind., Derwent Biotech.Abstr., Dok.Arbeitsmed., Environ.Sci.Poll.Mgmt., Excerp.Med., Helminthol.Abstr., Hosp.Lit.Ind., INIS Atomind., Ind.Med. (1948-), Ind.Sci.Rev., Ind.Vet., Inpharma, Int.Abstr.Biol.Sci., Int.Nurs.Ind., Kidney, Mass Spectr.Bull., Med.& Surg.Dermat., NRN, Neurosci.Cit.Ind., Nutr.Abstr., Oncog.G.F.Abstr., Pharm.&Out.News, Reac., Rev.Med.& Vet.Mycol., Risk Abstr., SSCI (coverage dropped), Sci.Cit.Ind., Small Anim.Abstr., Telegen, Trop.Dis.Bull., Vet.Bull.

—BLDSC (3046.477300), CASDDS, CISTI, EMDOCS, GNLM, IDS, ingenta, KNAW. **CCC.**

Published by: (American Cancer Society, Inc.), John Wiley & Sons, Inc., Journals (Subsidiary of: Wiley InterScience), 605 Third Ave, New York, NY 10158. TEL 212-850-6645, FAX 212-850-6021, madarden@wiley.com, uscs-wis@wiley.com, http://www.wiley.co.uk, http://www.wiley.com. Ed. Dr. Robert V P Hutter. adv.: B&W page GBP 2,270, color page GBP 3,570; trim 10.88 x 8.5. Circ: 10,116. **Subscr. outside the Americas to:** John Wiley & Sons Ltd., Baffins Ln, Chichester, Sussex PO19 IUD, United Kingdom. TEL 44-1243-779777, FAX 44-1243-843232, cs-journals@wiley.co.uk, http://www.wiley.co.uk.

616.99 USA ISSN 0167-7659
CODEN: CMRED4

CANCER AND METASTASIS REVIEWS. Text in English. 1981. q. USD 263, EUR 262 to individuals for print or online ed.; USD 397, EUR 396 to institutions for print or online ed.; USD 476.40, EUR 475.20 to institutions for print & online eds. combined (effective 2002). adv. bk.rev. back issues avail.; reprint service avail. from SWZ,PQC. *Refereed.* **Document type:** *Journal, Academic/Scholarly.* **Description:** Reviews some of the more important and interesting recent developments in the biology and treatment of malignant disease, as well as to highlight new and promising directions, be theytechnological or conceptual.

Formerly: Cancer Metastasis

Related titles: Microform ed.: (from PQC); Online - full text ed.: (from EBSCO Publishing, O C L C Online Computer Library Center, Inc., RoweCom Information Quest, Swets Blackwell, Kluwer Online, Institute for Scientific Information).
Indexed: ASCA, CBCA Ref., Chem.Abstr., Chem.Indus.Notes, Chem.Titles, Curr.Adv.Ecol.Sci., Curr.Adv.Gen.& Molec.Biol., Curr.Cont., Excerp.Med., INIS Atomind., Ind.Med. (coverage dropped), Ind.Sci.Rev., Inpharma, Int.Abstr.Biol.Sci., Pharm.&Out.News, Reac., Sci.Cit.Ind.
—BLDSC (3046.455700), ADONIS, CASDDS, CISTI, EMDOCS, GNLM, IDS, ingenta, KNAW. **CCC.**
Published by: Kluwer Academic Publishers Boston, 101 Philip Dr, Assinippi Park, Norwell, MA 02061. TEL 781-871-6600, FAX 781-871-9045, services@wkap.nl, http://www.wkap.nl/journalhome.htm/0167-7659. Eds. Ian Hart, Philip Frost, Robert S Kerbel. Pub. Melissa Ramondetta. R&P Rose Luongo TEL 781-871-6311. **Subscr. outside N America to:** Kluwer Academic Publishers Group, Journals Department, PO Box 322, Dordrecht 3300 AH, Netherlands. TEL 31-78-639-2392, FAX 31-78-654-6474; **Subscr. to:** Kluwer Academic - Plenum Publishers, 233 Spring St, New York, NY 10013-1578. TEL 212-620-8468, FAX 212-807-1047.

616.994 CHE ISSN 0305-7232
RC261.A1 CODEN: CABCD4
CANCER BIOCHEMISTRY BIOPHYSICS. Text in English. 1975. q. EUR 900, USD 1,001 to institutions; EUR 1,400, USD 1,580 to corporations; USD 336 to individuals (effective 2001). adv. *Refereed.* **Document type:** *Journal, Academic/Scholarly.*
Related titles: Microform ed.
Indexed: ASCA, Agri.& Environ.Biotech.Abstr. (coverage dropped), Biol.Abstr., Chem.Abstr., Curr.Adv.Ecol.Sci., Curr.Cont. (coverage dropped), Dairy Sci.Abstr., Derwent Biotech.Abstr., Excerp.Med., Helminthol.Abstr., Ind.Med. (1974-), Ind.Sci.Rev., Int.Abstr.Biol.Sci., Sci.Cit.Ind. (coverage dropped).
—BLDSC (3046.456000), CISTI, EMDOCS, GNLM, Infotrieve, KNAW. **CCC.**
Published by: Gordon and Breach - Harwood Academic (Subsidiary of: Taylor & Francis Group), PO Box 531, Lausanne 1000, Switzerland. TEL 41-21-6411280, FAX 41-21-6411281, info@gbhap.com, http:// www.gbhap.com. Ed. Harry Darrow Brown. **Subscr. addr. in US:** International Publishers Direct, PO Box 32160, Newark, NJ 07102. FAX 215-750-6343.

616.994 NLD
CANCER BIOLOGY AND MEDICINE. Text in English. irreg., latest vol.3, 1992. price varies. **Document type:** *Monographic series.*
Published by: Kluwer Academic Publishers Group (Subsidiary of: Wolters Kluwer N.V.), Spuiboulevard 50, PO Box 17, Dordrecht 3300 AA, Netherlands. FAX 31-78-639-2254, services@wkap.nl, http://www.wkap.nl. **Dist. by:** Journals Department, PO Box 322, Dordrecht 3300 AH, Netherlands. FAX 31-78-654-6474.

616.99 USA ISSN 1084-9785
RC271.C5 CODEN: CBRAFJ
CANCER BIOTHERAPY & RADIOPHARMACEUTICALS. Text in English. 1983. bi-m. USD 218 domestic to individuals; USD 319 foreign to individuals; USD 262 domestic to individuals print and online eds. combined; USD 362 foreign to individuals print and online eds. combined; USD 447 domestic to institutions; USD 555 foreign to institutions; USD 536 domestic to institutions print and online eds. combined; USD 645 foreign to institutions print and online eds. combined (effective 2002). adv. back issues avail.; reprints avail. *Refereed.* **Document type:** *Journal, Academic/Scholarly.* **Description:** Reports on research and advances in cancer therapy, including more selective delivery of drugs, biologicals, radiopharmaceuticals, and advances in delivery instrumentation and technology.
Incorporates (in 1996): Antibody, Immunoconjugates, and Radiopharmaceuticals (0892-7049); Former titles (until 1996): Cancer Biotherapy (1062-8401); (until 1991): Selective Cancer Therapeutics (1043-0733); (until 1989): Cancer Drug Delivery (0732-9482)
Related titles: Online - full content ed.: USD 218 to individuals; USD 447 to institutions (effective 2002) (from EBSCO Publishing, Swets Blackwell); Online - full text ed.: (from CatchWord Ltd., Institute for Scientific Information, RoweCom Information Quest).
Indexed: ASCA, Biotech.& Bioeng.Abstr., Chem.Abstr., Chem.Indus.Notes, Chem.Titles, Curr.Adv.Ecol.Sci., Curr.Cont., Derwent Biotech.Abstr., Environ.Sci.Poll.Mgmt., Excerp.Med., INIS Atomind., Ind.Med. (1996-), Ind.Sci.Rev., Inpharma, Med.& Pharm.Biotech.Abstr., Nutr.Abstr., Pharm.&Out.News, Pollut.Abstr., Reac., Risk Abstr., Saf.Sci.Abstr., Sci.Cit.Ind., Telegen.
—BLDSC (3046.457600), CASDDS, CISTI, EMDOCS, GNLM, IDS, Infotrieve, ingenta, KNAW. **CCC.**
Published by: Mary Ann Liebert, Inc. Publishers, 2 Madison Ave, Larchmont, NY 10538. TEL 914—834-3100, FAX 914-834-1388, info@liebertpub.com, http://www.liebertpub.com/cbr. Ed. Robert K Oldham.

616.99 USA ISSN 1090-7491
CANCER CASE PRESENTATIONS: THE TUMOR BOARD. Text in English. 1997. bi-m. USD 111 domestic to individuals; USD 126 foreign to individuals; USD 143 domestic to institutions; USD 166 foreign to institutions (effective 2001); USD 28 newsstand/cover. adv. **Document type:** *Academic/Scholarly.*
Published by: Lippincott Williams & Wilkins (Philadelphia) (Subsidiary of: Wolters Kluwer N.V.), 530 Walnut St, Philadelphia, PA 19106-3621. TEL 215-521-8300, FAX 215-521-8902, http://www.Lww.com. Eds. Dr. Glenn D Steele Jr., Dr. Monica Morrow. adv.: B&W page USD 500, color page USD 1,390. **Subscr. to:** PO Box 1600, Hagerstown, MD 21740-1600. TEL 800-777-2295, FAX 301-824-7390.

616.99 NLD ISSN 0957-5243
CODEN: CCCNEN
CANCER CAUSES & CONTROL; an international journal of studies of cancer in human populations. Text in Dutch. 1990. bi-m. EUR 1,290, USD 1,291 to institutions for print or online ed.; EUR 1,548, USD 1,549.20 to institutions for print & online eds. combined (effective 2002). adv. *Refereed.* **Document type:** *Journal, Academic/Scholarly.* **Description:** Reports and stimulates new avenues of investigation into the causes, control and subsequent prevention of cancer.
Related titles: CD-ROM ed.; Online - full text ed.: (from EBSCO Publishing, O C L C Online Computer Library Center, Inc., RoweCom Information Quest, Swets Blackwell, Kluwer Online, Institute for Scientific Information).
Indexed: AESIS, ASCA, Curr.Cont., Dairy Sci.Abstr., Environ.Sci.Poll.Mgmt., Excerp.Med. (1993-), Ind.Med. (1990-), Ind.Sci.Rev., Inpharma, Int.Abstr.Biol.Sci., NRN, Nutr.Abstr., Pharm.&Out.News, Pollut.Abstr., Reac., Risk Abstr., Saf.Sci.Abstr., Sci.Cit.Ind., Soyabean Abstr., THA, Tox.Abstr.
—BLDSC (3046.464150), ADONIS, CISTI, EMDOCS, GNLM, IDS, ingenta, KNAW. **CCC.**
Published by: Kluwer Academic Publishers Group (Subsidiary of: Wolters Kluwer N.V.), Spuiboulevard 50, PO Box 17, Dordrecht 3300 AA, Netherlands. TEL 31-78-639-2392, FAX 31-78-654-2254, services@wkap.nl, http://www.wkap.nl/journalhome.htm/ 0957-5243. Ed. Graham A Colditz. Adv. contact Gemma Heiser. **Subscr. in N America to:** Kluwer Academic - Plenum Publishers, 233 Spring St, New York, NY 10013-1578. TEL 212-620-8468, FAX 212-807-1047; **Subscr. to:** Journals Department, PO Box 322, Dordrecht 3300 AH, Netherlands. TEL 31-78-639-2392, FAX 31-78-654-6474.

616.99 NLD ISSN 0921-4410
CODEN: CCBAED
CANCER CHEMOTHERAPY AND BIOLOGICAL RESPONSE MODIFIERS. Text in Dutch. 1979. a., latest vol.16, 1996. back issues avail. *Refereed.* **Document type:** *Monographic series.* **Description:** Reviews recent major developments in pharmacology of anti-cancer agents, biologicals, and clinical management of the cancer patient.
Former titles (until vol.9, 1987): Cancer Chemotherapy Annual; (until vol.2, 1980): Cancer Chemotherapy (0167-7853)
Indexed: Chem.Abstr., Chem.Indus.Notes, Chem.Titles, Ind.Med. (1987-).
—BLDSC (3046.466000), CASDDS, CISTI, GNLM, ingenta, KNAW. **CCC.**
Published by: Elsevier Science BV, Regional Sales Office, PO Box 211, Amsterdam 1000 AE, Netherlands. TEL 31-20-485-2911, nlinfo-f@elsevier.nl; usinfo-f@elsevier.com; info@elsevier.co.jp; asiainfo@elsevier.com.sg, http://www.elsevier.nl/. **Subscr. in Australasia and the Far East to:** Elsevier Science (Singapore) Pte Ltd, No.1 Temasek Ave, 17-01 Millenia Tower, Singapore 039192, Singapore. TEL 65-434-3727, FAX 65-337-2230; **Subscr. in Japan to:** Elsevier Science Inc - Japan Regional Office, 9-15 Higashi-Azabu 1-chome, Minato-ku, Tokyo 106-0044, Japan. TEL 81-3-5561-5033, FAX 81-3-5561-5047; **Subscr. in the Americas to:** Elsevier Science, PO Box 945, New York, NY 10159-0945. TEL 212-633-3730, FAX 212-633-3680, http://www.elsevier.com.

616.99 DEU ISSN 0344-5704
CODEN: CCPHDZ
CANCER CHEMOTHERAPY AND PHARMACOLOGY. Text in English. 1978. m. EUR 2,171 domestic; EUR 2,160.70 in Germany; EUR 214 newsstand/cover foreign (effective 2002). adv. index. reprint service avail. from ISI. *Refereed.* **Document type:** *Journal, Academic/Scholarly.* **Description:** Addresses a wide range of pharmacologic and oncologic concerns on both the experimental and clinical levels.
Related titles: Microform ed.: (from PQC); Online - full text ed.: ISSN 1432-0843 (from EBSCO Publishing, RoweCom Information Quest, Swets Blackwell, Springer LINK, Institute for Scientific Information); ♦ Supplement: Cancer Chemotherapy and Pharmacology. Supplement. ISSN 0943-9404.
Indexed: ASCA, Agri.& Environ.Biotech.Abstr. (coverage dropped), Chem.Abstr., Chem.Indus.Notes, Chem.Titles, Curr.Adv.Cancer Res., Curr.Adv.Ecol.Sci., Curr.Cont., Dent.Ind., Derwent Biotech.Abstr., Excerp.Med., INIS Atomind., Ind.Med. (1978-), Ind.Sci.Rev., Ind.Vet., Inpharma, Int.Abstr.Biol.Sci., Neurosci.Cit.Ind., Pharm.&Out.News, Reac., Sci.Cit.Ind.
—BLDSC (3046.467000), ADONIS, CASDDS, CISTI, EMDOCS, GNLM, IDS, ingenta, KNAW. **CCC.**
Published by: Springer-Verlag (Subsidiary of: BertelsmannSpringer), Tiergartenstr 17, Heidelberg 69121, Germany. TEL 49-6221-345-0, FAX 49-6221-345229, subscriptions@springer.de, http://link.springer.de/link/service/journals/00280/ index.htm, http://www.springer.de. **Subscr. in N. America to:** Springer-Verlag New York Inc., PO Box 2485, Secaucus, NJ 07096-2485. TEL 212-460-1500, FAX 212-473-6272.

616.99 DEU ISSN 0943-9404
CODEN: CCHSE
CANCER CHEMOTHERAPY AND PHARMACOLOGY. SUPPLEMENT. Text in German. irreg. **Document type:** *Academic/Scholarly.*
Related titles: ♦ Supplement to: Cancer Chemotherapy and Pharmacology. ISSN 0344-5704.
Indexed: Excerp.Med. (1995-), Int.Abstr.Biol.Sci.
—ADONIS, EMDOCS, Infotrieve, KNAW. **CCC.**
Published by: Springer-Verlag (Subsidiary of: BertelsmannSpringer), Haber Str 7, Heidelberg 69126, Germany. FAX 49-30-82787448, subscriptions@springer.de.

616.99 USA ISSN 1073-2748
CODEN: CACOFD
CANCER CONTROL; journal of the Moffitt Cancer Centeer. Text in English. 1994. bi-m. USD 60 domestic to individuals; USD 75 foreign to individuals; USD 120 domestic to institutions; USD 135 foreign to institutions (effective 2000). adv. *Refereed.* **Document type:** *Academic/Scholarly.* **Description:** Each issue contains a series of articles that present original research and review a specific theme.
Related titles: Online - full text ed.
Indexed: Environ.Sci.Poll.Mgmt., Excerp.Med. (1995-), Ind.Med. (1994-), Inpharma, Pharm.&Out.News, Pollut.Abstr., Reac., Saf.Sci.Abstr.
—BLDSC (3046.472100), GNLM.
Published by: Moffitt Cancer Center, 12902 Magnolia Dr, Tampa, FL 33612. TEL 813-632-1349, FAX 813-632-1380, ccjournal@moffitt.usf.edu, http://www.moffitt.usf.edu/pubs/ccj/. Ed. John Horton. R&P Jean Joy TEL 813-632-1348. Adv. contact Tony Dibiase Jr. Circ: 25,000 (controlled).

616 USA ISSN 0191-3794
CANCER CONTROL JOURNAL. Text in English. 1973. irreg. membership. bk.rev. back issues avail.
Published by: Cancer Control Society, Cancer Book House, 2043 N Berendo, Los Angeles, CA 90027. TEL 323-663-7801. Circ: 10,000.

616.994 USA ISSN 0361-090X
RC268 CODEN: CDPRD4
CANCER DETECTION AND PREVENTION. Text in English. 1976. bi-m. USD 210 domestic to individuals; USD 220 in Canada & Mexico to individuals; USD 260 elsewhere to individuals; USD 650 domestic to institutions; USD 660 in Canada & Mexico to institutions; USD 700 elsewhere to institutions (effective 2000). adv. reprint service avail. from ISI. *Refereed.* **Document type:** *Academic/Scholarly.* **Description:** Publishes current scientific data on cancer epidemiology, biomarkers, and the identification and management of patients at risk for cancer development.
Related titles: Microfilm ed.; Online - full text ed.: ISSN 1525-1500 (from Ovid Technologies, Inc., EBSCO Publishing, O C L C Online Computer Library Center, Inc., RoweCom Information Quest, ingenta, Swets Blackwell, Institute for Scientific Information).

M

Indexed: ASCA, Abstr.Hyg., Biol.Abstr., Chem.Abstr., Chem.Indus.Notes, Chem.Titles, Curr.Cont., Dent.Ind., Dok.Arbeitsmed., Environ.Sci.Poll.Mgmt., Excerp.Med., INIS Atomind., Ind.Med. (1976-), Inpharma, Int.Abstr.Biol.Sci., Nutr.Abstr., Pharm.&Out.News, Pollut.Abstr., Reac., Risk Abstr., SSCI (coverage dropped), Saf.Sci.Abstr., THA, Trop.Dis.Bull.
—BLDSC (3046.477500), CASDDS, CISTI, GNLM, IDS, ingenta, KNAW. **CCC.**
Published by: (International Society of Preventive Oncology), Blackwell Science Inc., Commerce Pl, Malden, MA 02148-5018. TEL 781-388-8250, 800-759-6102, FAX 781-388-8255, journals@blacksci.com, http://www.blackwell-science.com. R&P Tracey Davies. Adv. contact Jenny Applin.

616.99 616.15 USA
CANCER DRUG DISCOVERY AND DEVELOPMENT. Text in English. 1996. irreg., latest vol.6, 1999. price varies. illus. *Refereed.* **Document type:** *Monographic series, Academic/Scholarly.* **Description:** Provides pharmacologists and oncologists with reviews of the latest research in the development of new pharmacological agents, or approaches to the treatment and cure of cancer.
Published by: Humana Press Inc., 999 Riverview Dr, Ste 208, Totowa, NJ 07512. TEL 973-256-1699, FAX 973-256-8341, humana@humanapr.com, http://humanapress.com. Ed. Beverly A Teicher. R&P Richard Hruska.

616.99 GBR ISSN 1369-7129
CANCER DRUG NEWS (C D N). Text in English. 1997. m. GBP 395 (effective 2000). **Document type:** *Newsletter, Trade.*
Related titles: CD-ROM ed.: ISSN 1461-7617.
Published by: Espicom Business Intelligence, Lincoln House, City Fields Business Park, City Fields Way, Tangmere, Chichester, W Sussex PO20 6FS, United Kingdom. TEL 44-1243-533322, FAX 44-1243-533418, general@espicom.com, http://www.espicom.com. Ed. Kay Griffin. R&P Nigel Chivers.

616.994 USA ISSN 1053-9611
CANCER ECONOMICS. Text in English. 1987.
Related titles: ♦ Supplement to: Cancer Letter. ISSN 0096-3917.
Published by: Cancer Letter Inc., PO Box 9905, Washington, DC 20016. TEL 202-362-1809, FAX 202-362-1681.

CANCER EPIDEMIOLOGY. see *MEDICAL SCIENCES—Abstracting, Bibliographies, Statistics*

616.99 USA ISSN 1055-9965
RC268.48 CODEN: CEBPE4
CANCER EPIDEMIOLOGY, BIOMARKERS & PREVENTION. Text in English. 1991. m. USD 140 domestic to individuals; USD 180 foreign to individuals; USD 365 domestic to institutions; USD 405 foreign to institutions (effective 2000). adv. *Refereed.* **Document type:** *Academic/Scholarly.* **Description:** Contains research on the causes and prevention of cancer in humans.
Related titles: Online - full text ed.: (from HighWire Pr., Institute for Scientific Information).
Indexed: ASCA, Abstr.Hyg., Chem.Abstr., Chem.Indus.Notes, Chem.Titles, Curr.Cont., Dairy Sci.Abstr., Excerp.Med. (1993-), Helminthol.Abstr., Ind.Med. (1991-), Ind.Sci.Rev., Ind.Vet., Inpharma, Int.Abstr.Biol.Sci., NRN, Nutr.Abstr., Pharm.&Out.News, Reac., Rev.Appl.Entomol., Rev.Med.& Vet.Mycol., SSCI (coverage dropped), Sci.Cit.Ind., Soyabean Abstr., Sugar Ind.Abstr., THA, Triticale Abstr., Trop.Dis.Bull., Vet.Bull.
—BLDSC (3046.477930), CASDDS, CISTI, EMDOCS, GNLM, ingenta, KNAW.
Published by: American Association for Cancer Research, Public Ledger Bldg, 150 S Independence Mall W, Ste 826, Philadelphia, PA 19106. TEL 215-440-9300, FAX 215-440-9354, http://www.aacr.org. Ed. Frederick P Li. R&P Margaret Foti. Adv. contact Morgan Robinson. Circ: 1,540. **Subscr. to:** Subscription Office, P O Box 11806, Birmingham, AL 35202. TEL 205-995-1567, FAX 205-995-1588.

616.994 USA ISSN 0069-0147
RC261
CANCER FACTS AND FIGURES. Text in English. 1951. a. free per issue. **Description:** Provides the latest estimates of cancer incidence and morality.
Indexed: SRI.
—BLDSC (3046.478000), GNLM.
Published by: American Cancer Society, Inc., 1599 Clifton Rd, N E, Atlanta, GA 30329. TEL 404-329-5735, 800-ACS-2345, FAX 404-329-5787, http://www.cancer.org. Ed. Joann Schellenbach. Circ: 300,000 (controlled).

616.99 AUS ISSN 0311-306X
CANCER FORUM. Text in English. 1974. 3/yr. free per issue. bk.rev. abstr. back issues avail. *Refereed.* **Document type:** *Journal, Academic/Scholarly.* **Description:** Publishes original articles concerning medical, scientific, political, social, educational or administrative aspects of cancer.
Related titles: Online - full content ed.
Indexed: Biol.Abstr., Excerp.Med. (1993-), INIS Atomind.
—BLDSC (3046.478200), CISTI, EMDOCS, GNLM, ingenta, KNAW.
Published by: Cancer Council Australia, GPO Box 4708, Sydney, NSW 2000, Australia. TEL 61-2-93809022, FAX 61-2-93809033, thecancercouncil@cancer.org.au, http://www.cancer.org.au/pubforum.htm. Eds. Bernard Stewart, Lawrence A Wright, Les White, Robyn Ward. Circ: 4,000.

616.992 DEU
▼ **CANCER FUTURES.** Text in English. forthcoming 2002. a. EUR 46 (effective 2002). **Document type:** *Magazine, Academic/Scholarly.* **Description:** Focuses on oncology news, reports and issues concerning new diagnostic techniques, treatment strategies and the follow-up methodology for malignancies.
Related titles: Online - full text ed.: forthcoming.
Published by: Springer-Verlag (Subsidiary of: BertelsmannSpringer), Haber Str 7, Heidelberg 69126, Germany. TEL 49-30-82787-0, FAX 49-30-82787301, service@springer.de, http://www.springer.de. Ed. Maurice Schneider.

616.994 USA ISSN 0929-1903
CODEN: CGTHEG
CANCER GENE THERAPY. Text in English. 1994. m. EUR 207 in Europe to individuals; USD 330 rest of world to individuals; EUR 587 in Europe to institutions; USD 880 rest of world to institutions (effective 2002). adv. abstr, bibl, charts, illus, stat. back issues avail. *Refereed.* **Document type:** *Academic/Scholarly.* **Description:** Publishes original research, clinical reviews, literature reviews, patents listings, and all clinical protocols relating to gene transfer and therapy of cancer.
Related titles: Online - full text ed.: (from EBSCO Publishing, O C L C Online Computer Library Center, Inc., RoweCom Information Quest, ingenta, Swets Blackwell, Institute for Scientific Information).
Indexed: ASCA, Biotech.& Bioeng.Abstr., Biotech.Cit.Ind., Chem.Abstr., Chem.Indus.Notes, Chem.Titles, Curr.Cont., Derwent Biotech.Abstr., Ind.Med. (1994-), Ind.Sci.Rev., Inpharma, Med.& Pharm.Biotech.Abstr., Oncog.G.F.Abstr., Pharm.&Out.News, Reac., Sci.Cit.Ind.
—BLDSC (3046.478350), CASDDS, GNLM, IDS, Infotrieve, KNAW. **CCC.**
Published by: Nature Publishing Group Specialist Journals (Subsidiary of: Macmillan Publishers Ltd.), 345 Park Ave S, New York, NY 10010-1707. TEL 212-726-9264, FAX 212-696-0052, d.ramsay@natureny.com, http://www.nature.com/cgt, http://www.nature.com/het. Ed. Robert E Sobol. Pub. Chris Rawlins. R&P Chris J Rawlins.

616.99 USA ISSN 0165-4608
RC268.4 CODEN: CGCYDF
CANCER GENETICS & CYTOGENETICS. Text in English. 1979. 16/yr. EUR 2,475 in Europe to institutions; JPY 328,800 in Japan to institutions; USD 2,768 elsewhere to institutions (effective 2002). back issues avail.; reprint service avail. from SWZ. *Refereed.* **Document type:** *Academic/Scholarly.* **Description:** Covers the cellular and molecular aspects of cancer research.
Related titles: Microform ed.: (from PQC); Online - full text ed.: (from ingenta, Swets Blackwell, ScienceDirect, Institute for Scientific Information).
Indexed: ASCA, Biol.Abstr., Biotech.Cit.Ind., Chem.Abstr., Curr.Adv.Cancer Res., Curr.Adv.Ecol.Sci., Curr.Adv.Gen.& Molec.Biol., Curr.Cont., Dent.Ind., Dok.Arbeitsmed., Excerp.Med., Genet.Abstr., Hum.Gen.Abstr., INIS Atomind., Ind.Med. (1979-), Ind.Sci.Rev., Inpharma, Int.Abstr.Biol.Sci., Neurosci.Cit.Ind., Nuc.Acids Abstr., Pharm.&Out.News, Reac., Ref.Zh., Sci.Cit.Ind., THA.
—BLDSC (3046.478400), CASDDS, CISTI, EMDOCS, GNLM, IDS, ingenta, KNAW. **CCC.**
Published by: Elsevier Science, 655 Ave of the Americas, New York, NY 10010. TEL 212-989-5800, FAX 212-633-3990, usinfo-f@elsevier.com, http://www.elsevier.nl/locate/cancergene, http://www.elsevier.com. Ed. Avery A Sandberg. **Subscr. in Australasia and the Far East to:** Elsevier Science (Singapore) Pte Ltd, No.1 Temasek Ave, 17-01 Millenia Tower, Singapore 039192, Singapore. TEL 65-434-3727, FAX 65-337-2230; **Subscr. in Japan to:** Elsevier Science Inc - Japan Regional Office, 9-15 Higashi-Azabu 1-chome, Minato-ku, Tokyo 106-0044, Japan. TEL 81-3-5561-5033, FAX 81-3-5561-5047; **Subscr. outside the Americas to:** Elsevier Science BV, PO Box 211, Amsterdam 1000 AE, Netherlands. TEL 31-20-485-3757, FAX 31-20-485-3432, http://www.elsevier.nl.

616.9 NLD
CANCER GROWTH AND PROGRESSION. Text in English. irreg. price varies. **Document type:** *Monographic series.*
Published by: Kluwer Academic Publishers Group (Subsidiary of: Wolters Kluwer N.V.), Spuiboulevard 50, PO Box 17, Dordrecht 3300 AA, Netherlands. FAX 31-78-639-2254, services@wkap.nl, http://www.wkap.nl. **Dist. by:** Journals Department, PO Box 322, Dordrecht 3300 AH, Netherlands. FAX 31-78-654-6474.

615 619 DEU ISSN 0340-7004
CODEN: CIIMDN
CANCER IMMUNOLOGY, IMMUNOTHERAPY; other biological response modifications. Text in English. 1976. m. EUR 1,628 domestic; EUR 2,160.70 in Germany; EUR 160 newsstand/cover foreign (effective 2002). adv. reprint service avail. from ISI. *Refereed.* **Document type:** *Journal, Academic/Scholarly.* **Description:** Presents the latest research results and clinical findings in oncology and immunology, including the latest developments in understanding tumor-host interactions.
Related titles: Microfiche ed.: (from PQC); Online - full text ed.: ISSN 1432-0851 (from EBSCO Publishing, RoweCom Information Quest, Swets Blackwell, Springer LINK, Institute for Scientific Information).
Indexed: ASCA, Biotech.& Bioeng.Abstr., Chem.Abstr., Chem.Indus.Notes, Chem.Titles, Curr.Adv.Cancer Res., Curr.Adv.Ecol.Sci., Curr.Cont., Derwent Biotech.Abstr., Excerp.Med., Helminthol.Abstr., INIS Atomind., Immun.Abstr., Ind.Med. (1982-), Ind.Sci.Rev., Inpharma, Int.Abstr.Biol.Sci., Med.& Pharm.Biotech.Abstr., Pharm.&Out.News, Reac., Rev.Arom.& Med.Plants, Sci.Cit.Ind., Telegen.
—BLDSC (3046.478600), ADONIS, CASDDS, CISTI, EMDOCS, GNLM, IDS, ingenta, KNAW. **CCC.**
Published by: Springer-Verlag (Subsidiary of: BertelsmannSpringer), Tiergartenstr 17, Heidelberg 69121, Germany. TEL 49-6221-345-0, FAX 49-6221-345229, subscriptions@springer.de, http://link.springer.de/link/service/journals/00262/index.htm, http://www.springer.de. Eds. E Mihich, R W Baldwin. **Subscr. in N. America to:** Springer-Verlag New York Inc., PO Box 2485, Secaucus, NJ 07096-2485. TEL 212-460-1500, FAX 212-473-6272.

616.99 CAN
CANCER IN FOCUS. Text in English. 1984. q. free per issue. stat. back issues avail. *Refereed.* **Document type:** *Newsletter.* **Description:** Summarizes current research into all aspects of cancer: causation, detection, prevention, treatment, epidemiology, survival.
Formerly (until 1997): Cancer Research News
Published by: Canadian Cancer Society, B.C. and Yukon Division, 565 W 10th Ave, Vancouver, BC V5Z 4J4, Canada. TEL 604-872-4400, FAX 604-879-4533, brichards@bc.cancer.ca, cmspinder@bc.cancer.ca, http://www.bc.cancer.ca. Ed., R&P Bernadette Richards. Circ: 4,800.

616.9 PRI ISSN 0896-9035
RC279.P8
CANCER IN PUERTO RICO. Text in English, Spanish. 1950. a. free per issue. adv. bk.rev.
Indexed: Excerp.Med.
Published by: (Puerto Rico. Department of Health USA, Puerto Rico. Cancer Control Program USA, Puerto Rico. NCI-BIO Branch USA), Cancer Registry of Puerto Rico, Department of Health, P.O. Box 9342, Santurce, PR 00657. TEL 787-764-7453. Ed. Dr. Isidro Martinez. Circ: 1,000.

CANCER INCIDENCE AND MORTALITY MICHIGAN. see *PUBLIC HEALTH AND SAFETY—Abstracting, Bibliographies, Statistics*

CANCER INCIDENCE IN SWEDEN. see *MEDICAL SCIENCES—Abstracting, Bibliographies, Statistics*

M

616.99 USA ISSN 0735-7907
RC261.A1 CODEN: CINVD7

CANCER INVESTIGATION. Text in English. 1983. 8/yr. USD 175 to individuals print & online eds.; USD 1,275 to institutions print only (effective 2002). adv. bk.rev. charts, illus. index. *Refereed.* **Document type:** *Academic/Scholarly.* **Description:** Informs about the current stateof progress in the cancer field with the broad background of reliable information necessary for effective decision making.

Related titles: Microform ed.: (from RPI); Online - full content ed.; Online - full text ed.: (from Institute for Scientific Information, RoweCom Information Quest).

Indexed: AIDS & Cancer Res., ASCA, Arts & Hum.Cit.Ind. (coverage dropped), Biol.Abstr., Biol.Dig., Chem.Abstr., Chem.Indus.Notes, Chem.Titles, Curr.Adv.Ecol.Sci., Curr.Cont., Dok.Arbeitsmed., Environ.Abstr., Environ.Sci.Poll.Mgmt., Excerp.Med., INIS Atomind., Ind.Med. (1983-), Ind.Sci.Rev., Inpharma, Int.Nurs.Ind., NRN, Oncog.G.F.Abstr., Pharm.&Out.News, Pollut.Abstr., Reac., Ref.Zh., Rev.Med.& Vet.Mycol., Risk Abstr., SSCI (coverage dropped), Saf.Sci.Abstr., Sci.Cit.Ind., THA, Telegen.

—BLDSC (3046.479500), CASDDS, CISTI, EMDOCS, GNLM, IDS, ingenta, KNAW. **CCC.**

Published by: (Inter-American Society for Chemotherapy, Cancer Section), Marcel Dekker Inc., 270 Madison Ave, New York, NY 10016. TEL 212-696-9000, 800-228-1160, FAX 212-685-4540, http://www.dekker.com/servlet/product/productid/CNV. Ed. Dr. Yashar Hirshaut. R&P Julia Mulligan. Adv. contact James T Brady Jr. B&W page USD 1,620. Circ: 23,500 (paid and free). **Co-sponsor:** Chemotherapy Foundation.

616.99 USA ISSN 1081-4442
RC261.A1 CODEN: CJSAFC

THE CANCER JOURNAL FROM SCIENTIFIC AMERICAN (ENGLISH EDITION). Abbreviated title: T C J F S A. Text in English. 1995. bi-m. USD 129 domestic to individuals; USD 139 in Canada to individuals; USD 144 elsewhere to individuals; USD 179 domestic to institutions; USD 189 in Canada to institutions; USD 194 elsewhere to institutions. adv. charts, illus. back issues avail. *Refereed.* **Document type:** *Academic/Scholarly.* **Description:** Presents an integrated view of modern oncology across all disciplines, and reports noteworthy research at the interface between laboratory and clinic.

Related titles: Online - full text ed.: ISSN 1464-0678 (from EBSCO Publishing, ProQuest Information & Learning); Spanish ed.: The Cancer Journal from Scientific American (Spanish Edition). ISSN 1405-5643.

Indexed: AIDS & Cancer Res., ASCA, CINAHL, Curr.Cont., Environ.Sci.Poll.Mgmt., Excerp.Med., Ind.Med. (coverage dropped), Ind.Sci.Rev., Inpharma, Oncog.G.F.Abstr., Pharm.&Out.News, Pollut.Abstr., Reac., Risk Abstr., SSCI (coverage dropped), Saf.Sci.Abstr., Sci.Cit.Ind.

—BLDSC (3046.479850), CISTI, GNLM, IDS, Infotrieve, KNAW. **CCC.**

Published by: (American Radium Society), Scientific American, Inc., 415 Madison Ave, New York, NY 10017-1111. TEL 212-754-0550, 800-545-0554, FAX 212-980-3062, samedinfo@sciam.com, http://www.samonline.com. Eds. Samuel Hellman, Steven A, Vincent T. DeVita II. Pub. John J Hanley. R&P Maya Harty TEL 212-451-8861. Adv. contact Steve Kavalgan. B&W page USD 1,496, color page USD 2,761; trim 10.75 x 8.13. Circ: 2,737 (paid); 3,513 (controlled).

616.994 USA ISSN 0096-3917

CANCER LETTER. Text in English. 1974. 48/yr. USD 275 (effective 2000). bk.rev. **Document type:** *Newsletter.* **Description:** Covers funding policy and research news about the National Cancer Program.

Related titles: ♦ Supplement: Cancer Economics. ISSN 1053-9611.

Indexed: Curr.Adv.Biochem., Curr.Adv.Cancer Res., Curr.Adv.Cell & Devel.Biol., Food Sci.& Tech.Abstr.

Published by: Cancer Letter Inc., PO Box 9905, Washington, DC 20016. TEL 202-362-1809, FAX 202-362-1681. Ed. Kirsten B Goldberg. R&P Kirsten Boyd Goldberg.

616.994 IRL ISSN 0304-3835
RC261.A1 CODEN: CALEDQ

CANCER LETTERS; an international journal providing a forum for original and pertinent contributions in cancer research. Text in English. 1975. 28/yr. EUR 3,804 in Europe to institutions; JPY 505,400 in Japan to institutions; USD 4,255 elsewhere to institutions (effective 2002). adv. charts, illus, abstr. index. back issues avail.; reprint service avail. from SWZ. *Refereed.* **Document type:** *Academic/Scholarly.* **Description:** Covers all areas of cancer research, including: molecular biology of cancer, oncogenes, carcinogenesis, hormones and cancer, viral oncology, chemotherapy, epidemiology, biology of cancer and metastasis.

Related titles: Microform ed.: (from PQC); Online - full text ed.: (from ingenta, Swets Blackwell, ScienceDirect, Institute for Scientific Information).

Indexed: AIDS & Cancer Res., ASCA, Biol.Abstr., Chem.Abstr., Chem.Indus.Notes, Chem.Titles, Curr.Adv.Biochem., Curr.Adv.Ecol.Sci., Curr.Cont., Dairy Sci.Abstr., Dent.Ind., Environ.Sci.Poll.Mgmt., Excerp.Med., INIS Atomind., Ind.Med. (1975-), Ind.Sci.Rev., Ind.Vet., Inpharma, Int.Abstr.Biol.Sci., Maize Abstr., Med.& Surg.Dermat., NRN, Nuc.Acids Abstr., Nutr.Abstr., Oncog.G.F.Abstr., Pharm.&Out.News, Reac., Rev.Appl.Entomol., Rev.Arom.& Med.Plants, Rev.Med.& Vet.Mycol., Risk Abstr., Sci.Cit.Ind., Small Anim.Abstr., THA, Telegen, Vet.Bull., Weed Abstr.

—BLDSC (3046.485000), ADONIS, CASDDS, CISTI, EMDOCS, GNLM, IDS, ingenta, KNAW. **CCC.**

Published by: Elsevier Science Ireland Ltd, Elsevier House, Brookvale Plaza, E. Park, Shannon, Co. Clare, Ireland. TEL 353-61-471944, FAX 353-61-472144, http://www.elsevier.com/locate/canlet. Eds. F Beland, R J Muschel. R&P Annette Moloney. **Subscr. in Australasia and the Far East to:** Elsevier Science (Singapore) Pte Ltd, No.1 Temasek Ave, 17-01 Millenia Tower, Singapore 039192, Singapore. TEL 65-434-3727, FAX 65-337-2230; **Subscr. in the Americas to:** Elsevier Science, PO Box 945, New York, NY 10159-0945. TEL 212-633-3730, FAX 212-633-3680; **Subscr. to:** Elsevier Science BV, PO Box 211, Amsterdam 1000 AE, Netherlands. TEL 31-20-485-3757.

616.99 EGY

CANCER MOLECULAR BIOLOGY; international journal of cancer molecular biology research. Cover title: C M B. Text in English. 1994. 6/yr. USD 120 in the Middle East to individuals; USD 200 elsewhere to individuals; USD 180 in the Middle East to institutions; USD 220 elsewhere to institutions. adv. index. *Refereed.* **Document type:** *Academic/Scholarly.* **Description:** Publishes full papers and short communications that cover all aspects of cancer molecular biology research.

Indexed: AIDS & Cancer Res., Chem.Abstr., Chem.Indus.Notes, Chem.Titles, Environ.Sci.Poll.Mgmt., Excerp.Med. (1995-), Int.Abstr.Biol.Sci., Oncog.G.F.Abstr., Pollut.Abstr., Risk Abstr., Saf.Sci.Abstr.

—BLDSC (3046.487500).

Published by: Ain Shams Medical Faculty, Oncology Diagnostic Unit, Abbassia, Cairo, Egypt. TEL 20-2-2858940, FAX 20-2-2859928. Ed. A Khalifa.

CANCER NURSING; an international journal for cancer care. see *MEDICAL SCIENCES—Nurses And Nursing*

CANCER NURSING PRACTICE. see *MEDICAL SCIENCES—Nurses And Nursing*

616.99 617.96 USA ISSN 1013-3097

CANCER PAIN RELEASE; publication of the World Health Organization Collaborating Center for Policy & Communications in Cancer Care. Text in English. 1988. q. USD 12 domestic; USD 17 foreign (effective 2000). bk.rev. abstr, bibl, maps, stat. back issues avail. **Document type:** *Newsletter, Bulletin, Academic/Scholarly, Abstract/Index.* **Description:** Covers information on the improvement of cancer pain control and palliative and supportive care. Aims to keep a worldwide and mutidisciplinary audience in the health professions and government abreast of relevant information and developments in clinical medicine, education and policy.

Related titles: Online - full text ed.; French ed.; Spanish ed.

Published by: World Health Organization, Collaborating Center for Policy & Communications in Cancer Care, 1900 University Ave, Madison, WI 53705. TEL 608-263-0727, FAX 608-263-0259, http://www.medsch.wisc.edu/WHOcancerpain. Ed., R&P Dr. Sophie M Colleau. Circ: 90,000.

616.99 NLD ISSN 0920-7848

CANCER PHARMACOLOGY ANNUAL. Text in Dutch. 1983. a. **Document type:** *Monographic series.*
—CISTI, GNLM.

Published by: Elsevier Science BV, PO Box 211, Amsterdam 1000 AE, Netherlands. TEL 31-20-485-2911, FAX 31-20-485-2457, nlinfo-f@elsevier.nl; usinfo-f@elsevier.com; forinfo-kyf04035@niftyserve.or.jp, http://www.elsevier.nl/. **Subscr. in Australasia and the Far East to:** Elsevier Science (Singapore) Pte Ltd, No.1 Temasek Ave, 17-01 Millenia Tower, Singapore 039192, Singapore. TEL 65-434-3727, FAX 65-337-2230; **Subscr. in Japan to:** Elsevier Science Inc - Japan Regional Office, 9-15 Higashi-Azabu 1-chome, Minato-ku, Tokyo 106-0044, Japan. TEL 81-3-5561-5033, FAX 81-3-5561-5047; **Subscr. in the Americas to:** Elsevier Science, PO Box 945, New York, NY 10159-0945. TEL 212-633-3730, FAX 212-633-3680, usinfo-f@elsevier.com, http://www.elsevier.com.

616.99 USA ISSN 1065-4704
CODEN: CAPRFJ

CANCER PRACTICE. Text in English. 1993. bi-m. USD 49.50 domestic to individuals; USD 64.50 in Canada & Mexico to individuals; USD 74.50 elsewhere to individuals; USD 175 domestic to institutions; USD 190 in Canada & Mexico to institutions; USD 200 elsewhere to institutions; USD 45 to individuals print & online eds. combined; USD 158 to institutions print & online eds. combined (effective 2001). reprints avail. *Refereed.* **Document type:** *Journal, Academic/Scholarly.*

Related titles: Microform ed.: (from PQC); ♦ Online - full text ed.: Cancer Practice Online. ISSN 1523-5394.

Indexed: AgeLine, CINAHL, Curr.Cont., Excerp.Med. (1995-), Fam.Ind., Int.Nurs.Ind., SSCI.

—BLDSC (3046.492906), GNLM, IDS, Infotrieve, KNAW. **CCC.**

Published by: Blackwell Science Inc., Commerce Pl, 350 Main St, Malden, MA 02148-5018. TEL 781-388-8250, FAX 781-388-8255, journals@blacksci.com, http://www.blackwell-science.com. Ed. Genevieve V Foley. R&P Tracey Davies. Adv. contact Jenny Applin. Circ: 10,333.

616.99 USA ISSN 1523-5394

CANCER PRACTICE ONLINE. Text in English. bi-m. USD 45 to individuals; USD 158 to institutions (effective 2001). **Document type:** *Academic/Scholarly.*

Media: Online - full text (from EBSCO Publishing, ingenta, Munksgaard & Blackwell Science's Synergy, Swets Blackwell, Institute for Scientific Information, RoweCom Information Quest). **Related titles:** Microform ed.: (from PQC); ♦ Print ed.: Cancer Practice. ISSN 1065-4704.

Published by: Blackwell Science Inc., Commerce Pl, 350 Main St, Malden, MA 02148-5018. TEL 781-388-8250, 888-661-5800, FAX 781-388-8255, journals@blacksci.com, http://www.blackwell-science.com.

616.99 615.84 FRA ISSN 1278-3218
CODEN: BCRAEE

CANCER - RADIOTHERAPIE. Text in French; Summaries in English, French. 1990. bi-m. EUR 181 in Europe to individuals; USD 224 elsewhere to individuals; EUR 215 in Europe to institutions; USD 268 elsewhere to institutions (effective 2002). back issues avail. *Refereed.* **Document type:** *Academic/Scholarly.* **Description:** Provides a forum within the field of oncology for the dissemination of knowledge in all areas relating to therapeutic radiation oncology: technology, radiophysics, radiobiology and clinical radiotherapy.

Former titles (until 1997): Bulletin du Cancer - Radiotherapie (0924-4212); Which superseded in part (in 1990): Bulletin du Cancer (0007-4551)

Related titles: Microform ed.: (from PQC); Online - full text ed.: (from ingenta, ScienceDirect, Institute for Scientific Information).

Indexed: Biol.Abstr., Curr.Cont. (coverage dropped), Excerp.Med., INIS Atomind., Ind.Med. (1997-), Sci.Cit.Ind. (coverage dropped).

—BLDSC (3046.494000), ADONIS, CISTI, EMDOCS, GNLM, IDS, Infotrieve. **CCC.**

Published by: (Societe Francaise de Radiotherapie Oncologique), Elsevier Paris, Editions Scientifiques et Medicales (Subsidiary of: Reed Elsevier plc. group), 23 rue Linois, Paris 75015, France. TEL 33-1-45589110, FAX 33-1-45589419, cancer-radio@elsevier.fr; academic@elsevier-fr.com, http://www.elsevier.com/locate/canrad. Ed. J J Mazeron. Circ: 3,500. **Dist. by:** Centre des Tumeurs, Hopital de la Pitie-Salpetriere, 47-83, Bd. de l'Hopital, Paris Cedex 13 75651, France. TEL 33-1-42178171, 33-1-42178250.

616.994 USA ISSN 0008-5472
RC261 CODEN: CNREA8
CANCER RESEARCH. Text in English. 1941. s-m. USD 555 domestic to individuals; USD 645 foreign to individuals; USD 1,030 domestic to institutions; USD 1,155 foreign to institutions (effective 2000); includes Clinical Cancer Research. adv. abstr, bibl, charts, illus. index. *Refereed.* **Document type:** *Academic/Scholarly.* **Description:** Contains original basic, clinical, and translational research into all areas of cancer investigation.
Related titles: Microfilm ed.: (from PMC); Online - full text ed.: (from HighWire Pr., Institute for Scientific Information).
Indexed: ABC, AIDS & Cancer Res., AIDS Abstr., ASCA, Abstr.Hyg., Agri.& Environ.Biotech.Abstr. (coverage dropped), Anim.Breed.Abstr., BBCI, Biol.Abstr., Cal.Tiss.Abstr. (coverage dropped), Chem.Abstr., Chem.Cit.Ind., Chem.Indus.Notes, Chem.Titles, Curr.Adv.Biochem., Curr.Adv.Cancer Res., Curr.Adv.Cell & Devel.Biol., Curr.Adv.Ecol.Sci., Curr.Adv.Gen.& Molec.Biol., Curr.Biotech.Abstr., Curr.Cont., Curr.Ind.Stat., Dairy Sci.Abstr., Dent.Ind., Derwent Biotech.Abstr., Dok.Arbeitsmed., Environ.Sci.Poll.Mgmt., Excerp.Med., Food Sci.& Tech.Abstr., Genet.Abstr., Helminthol.Abstr., Hum.Gen.Abstr., INIS Atomind., I.P.A., Immun.Abstr. (coverage dropped), Ind.Med. (1941-), Ind.Sci.Rev., Ind.Vet., Inpharma, Int.Abstr.Biol.Sci., Int.Nurs.Ind., Lab.Haz.Bull., Maize Abstr., Mass Spectr.Bull., Med.& Pharm.Biotech.Abstr., Med.& Surg.Dermat., NRN, Neurosci.Abstr. (coverage dropped), Neurosci.Cit.Ind., Nuc.Acids Abstr., Nutr.Abstr., Oncog.G.F.Abstr., Pharm.&Out.News, Pig News & Info., Poult.Abstr., Reac., Ref.Zh., Rev.Appl.Entomol., Rev.Arom.& Med.Plants, Rev.Med.& Vet.Mycol., Rev.Plant Path., Risk Abstr., SSCI (coverage dropped), Saf.Sci.Abstr., Sci.Cit.Ind., Small Anim.Abstr., Soyabean Abstr., Sport Fish.Abstr., THA, Telegen, Tox.Abstr. (coverage dropped), Trop.Dis.Bull., Vet.Bull.
—BLDSC (3046.500000), CASDDS, CINDOC, CISTI, EMDOCS, GNLM, IDS, ingenta, KNAW, Linda Hall. **CCC.**
Published by: American Association for Cancer Research, Public Ledger Bldg, 150 S Independence Mall W, Ste 826, Philadelphia, PA 19106. TEL 215-440-9300, FAX 215-440-9354, http://www.aacr.org. Ed. Carlo M Croce. R&P Margaret Foti. Adv. contact Morgan Robinson. Circ: 8,550. **Subscr. to:** Subscr. to, P O Box 11806, Birmingham, AL 35202. TEL 205-995-1567, FAX 205-995-1588.

616.994 GBR
RC261
CANCER RESEARCH CAMPAIGN. SCIENTIFIC YEARBOOK. Text in English. 1924. a. GBP 5. adv. illus. **Document type:** *Academic/Scholarly.* **Description:** Provides reviews of contemporary topics in cancer research and details the scope and availability of Campaign funding and a full listing of all current CRC research projects and programmes.
Former titles: Cancer Research Campaign. Annual Report (0365-9623); (until 1971): British Empire Cancer Campaign For Research (0268-5612)
—CISTI, GNLM, KNAW.
Published by: Cancer Research Campaign, Information Unit, 10 Cambridge Terr, Regent's Park, London NW1 4JL, United Kingdom. TEL 44-171-224-1333, FAX 44-171-486-8317, http://www.crc.org.uk. Ed., R&P Dr. Lesley Walker.

616.99 USA ISSN 0892-0001
CODEN: CREMEX
CANCER RESEARCH MONOGRAPHS. Text in English. 1983. irreg., latest vol.5. **Document type:** *Monographic series.*
—CASDDS, CISTI.
Published by: Greenwood Press, Inc. (Subsidiary of: Greenwood Publishing Group Inc.), 88 Post Rd W, Box 5007, Westport, CT 06881. TEL 203-226-3571, FAX 203-226-1502.

616.99 CHE ISSN 1064-0525
RC261.A1 CODEN: CRTCEA
CANCER RESEARCH, THERAPY AND CONTROL. Text in English. 1989. 4/yr. EUR 535 to institutions; EUR 856 to corporations; USD 130 to individuals (effective 2001). **Document type:** *Journal, Academic/Scholarly.*
Formerly (until 1992): Cancer Therapy and Control (0896-5080)
Related titles: Microform ed.
Indexed: AMED, ASCA, Curr.Cont. (coverage dropped), Excerp.Med. (1995-), Ind.Sci.Rev., Inpharma, Int.Abstr.Biol.Sci., Reac., Sci.Cit.Ind. (coverage dropped).
—BLDSC (3046.506000), CISTI, EMDOCS, GNLM, Infotrieve, KNAW. **CCC.**
Published by: Gordon and Breach - Harwood Academic (Subsidiary of: Taylor & Francis Group), PO Box 531, Lausanne 1000, Switzerland. TEL 41-21-6411280, FAX 41-21-6411281, info@gbhap.com, http://www.gbhap.com. Ed. Samuel Gross. **Subscr. addr. in US:** International Publishers Direct, PO Box 32160, Newark, NJ 07102. FAX 215-750-6343.

616.99 USA
CANCER REVIEW* . Text in English. 1980. 3/yr. illus.
Formerly: Quest (Dallas)
Published by: (Cancer Center at Wadley), Wadley Institutes of Molecular Medicine, 9000 Harry Hines Blvd, PO Box 35988, Dallas, TX 75235. TEL 214-351-8111. Ed. Christine Donovan. Circ: 50,000.

616.99 USA
CANCER SOURCEBOOK. Text in English. 1990. irreg., latest vol.3, 1999. USD 78 per vol. (effective 2001). illus, stat. master index. **Document type:** *Consumer.* **Description:** Offers basic information about the most common forms of cancer and their stages. Includes facts on primary and secondary neoplasms of all kinds, along with treatment options and advice on coping.
Former titles (until 1999): New Cancer Sourcebook; (until 1996): Cancer Sourcebook
Published by: Omnigraphics, Inc., 615 Griswold St, Detroit, MI 48226. TEL 313-961-1340, 800-234-1340, FAX 313-961-1383, 800-875-1340, info@omnigraphics.com, http://www.omnigraphics.com. Ed. Edward J Prucha. Pub. Frederick G Ruffner Jr.

616.99 613.082 USA
CANCER SOURCEBOOK FOR WOMEN. Text in English. 1996. irreg., latest vol.2, 2002. USD 78 per vol. (effective 2001). charts, illus. master index. **Document type:** *Consumer.* **Description:** Offers laypersons information on forms of cancer specific to women: breast cancer, cervical cancer, ovarian cancer, cancer of the uterus and uterine sarcoma, and cancer of the vulva, along with advice on coping and seeking treatment.
Published by: Omnigraphics, Inc., 615 Griswold St, Detroit, MI 48226. TEL 313-961-1340, 800-234-1340, FAX 313-961-1383, 800-875-1340, info@omnigraphics.com, http://www.omnigraphics.com. Ed. Edward J Prucha. Pub. Frederick G Ruffner Jr.

616.99 USA ISSN 0261-2429
CODEN: CASUD7
CANCER SURVEYS; advances and prospects in clinical, epidemiological, and laboratory oncology. Text in English. 1982. irreg. *Refereed.* **Document type:** *Monographic series, Academic/Scholarly.* **Description:** Provides comprehensive coverage of current and future developments in well-defined areas in oncology. Each issues deals with a specific topic and has guest editors with an expert knowledge of the subject.
Related titles: Microform ed.: (from PQC).
Indexed: AIDS & Cancer Res., ASCA, Abstr.Hyg., Chem.Abstr., Chem.Indus.Notes, Chem.Titles, Curr.Adv.Ecol.Sci., Curr.Cont. (coverage dropped), Excerp.Med., Ind.Med. (1982-), Ind.Sci.Rev., Ind.Vet., Inpharma, Int.Abstr.Biol.Sci., Med.& Surg.Dermat., Oncog.G.F.Abstr., Pharm.&Out.News, Poult.Abstr., Reac., Sci.Cit.Ind. (coverage dropped), Small Anim.Abstr., Telegen, Vet.Bull.
—CASDDS, CISTI, EMDOCS, GNLM, IDS, ingenta, KNAW. **CCC.**
Published by: Cold Spring Harbor Laboratory Press, Publications Department, 10 Skyline Dr, Plainview, NY 11803. TEL 800-843-4388, FAX 516-349-1946, cshpress@cshl.org, http://www.cshl.org. Ed. John Tooze. **Subscr. to:** Fulfillment Center.

616.99 NZL ISSN 1174-5916
▼ **CANCER TODAY.** Text in English. 1999. m. USD 95 to individuals; USD 545 to institutions (effective 2001). back issues avail. **Description:** Rapid alerts service on all aspects of drug therapy and disease management of cancer.
Indexed: Inpharma, Pharm.&Out.News, Reac.
Published by: Adis International Limited, Mairangi Bay, Private Bag 65901, Auckland 1010, New Zealand. TEL 64-9-477-0700, FAX 64-9-477-0766, http://www.adis.com. **Americas subscr. to:** Adis International Inc., Attn: Subscription Dept, 860 Town Center Dr, Langhorne, PA 19047. TEL 877-872-2347.

616.99 GBR ISSN 0265-1319
CANCER TOPICS; regular news and reviews of cancer therapy. Text in English. 1972. 3/yr. free in United Kingdom; GBP 15 foreign. adv. bk.rev. abstr. back issues avail. *Refereed.* **Document type:** *Academic/Scholarly.* **Description:** Covers all aspects of cancer research and therapy.
Incorporates (1981-199?): Cancer Topics Abstracts
Indexed: INIS Atomind.
—BLDSC (3046.623000).
Published by: (Wyeth Laboratories USA), Eurocommunica Publications, Caxton House, 51 Barnham Rd, Barnham, W Sussex PO22 OER, United Kingdom. TEL 44-1234-555041, FAX 44-1234-555043. Ed. Rod Robinson. Circ: 13,000.

616.99 NLD ISSN 0927-3042
CODEN: CTRREP
CANCER TREATMENT AND RESEARCH. Text in English. 1981. irreg., latest vol.68, 1993. price varies. back issues avail. *Refereed.* **Document type:** *Monographic series.*
Indexed: Chem.Abstr., Chem.Indus.Notes, Chem.Titles, Ind.Med. (1981-).
—BLDSC (3046.625000), CASDDS, CISTI, GNLM, Infotrieve, KNAW. **CCC.**
Published by: Kluwer Academic Publishers Group (Subsidiary of: Wolters Kluwer N.V.), Spuiboulevard 50, PO Box 17, Dordrecht 3300 AA, Netherlands. FAX 31-78-639-2254, services@wkap.nl, http://www.wkap.nl. **Dist. by:** Journals Department, PO Box 322, Dordrecht 3300 AH, Netherlands. FAX 31-78-654-6474.

616.994 GBR ISSN 0305-7372
CODEN: CTREDJ
CANCER TREATMENT REVIEWS. Text in English. 1974. bi-m. GBP 86 to individuals; GBP 233 to institutions (effective 2002). adv. illus. index. back issues avail.; reprint service avail. from SWZ. *Refereed.* **Document type:** *Journal, Academic/Scholarly.* **Description:** Devoted to important advances in the field of cancer treatment for oncologists and physicians.
Related titles: Online - full text ed.: (from EBSCO Publishing, RoweCom Information Quest, Swets Blackwell, IDEAL Online Library, Institute for Scientific Information).
Indexed: ASCA, Biol.Abstr., Chem.Abstr., Chem.Indus.Notes, Chem.Titles, Curr.Cont., Dent.Ind., Environ.Sci.Poll.Mgmt., Excerp.Med., INIS Atomind., Ind.Med. (1974-), Ind.Sci.Rev., Inpharma, Int.Nurs.Ind., Pharm.&Out.News, Pollut.Abstr., Reac., Ref.Zh., Risk Abstr., SSCI (coverage dropped), Saf.Sci.Abstr., Sci.Cit.Ind., Tox.Abstr.
—BLDSC (3046.630000), CASDDS, CISTI, EMDOCS, GNLM, IDS, ingenta, KNAW. **CCC.**
Published by: W.B. Saunders Co. Ltd. (Subsidiary of: Harcourt Publishers Ltd.), 24-28 Oval Rd, London NW1 7DX, United Kingdom. TEL 44-20-7424-4200, FAX 44-20-7424-4515, cservice.harcourt.com, http://www.harcourt-international.com/journals/ctrv. Eds. R Coleman, R Rubens. **Subscr. to:** Harcourt Publishers Ltd., Foots Cray High St, Sidcup, Kent DA14 5HP, United Kingdom. TEL 44-20-8308-5700, FAX 44-20-8309-0807.

616.99 USA ISSN 1059-3802
CANCER WATCH; the monthly news and educational magazine of cancer research. Text in English. 1992. m. USD 50 domestic to individuals; USD 60 in Canada & Mexico to individuals; USD 70 elsewhere to individuals; USD 70 domestic to institutions; USD 80 in Canada & Mexico to institutions; USD 90 elsewhere to institutions (effective 2000). adv. **Document type:** *Newsletter.*
Indexed: Inpharma, Pharm.&Out.News, Reac.
Published by: Adenine Press, 2066 Central Ave, Schenectady, NY 12304. TEL 518-456-0784, FAX 518-452-4955, stone@adeninepress.com, http://www.adeninepress.com. Ed., Adv. contact M H Sarma. R&P Shawn Stone.

616.99 USA
CANCER WEEKLY PLUS. Text in English. 1988. w. (43/yr.). USD 1,895 in North America; USD 2,095 elsewhere. **Document type:** *Newsletter.*
Former titles: Cancer Researcher Weekly (1071-7226); (until 1993): Cancerweekly (1071-7218); (until 1991): N C I Cancer Weekly (0896-7385)
Related titles: Microform ed.: (from PQC); Online - full text ed.: (from CompuServe, Inc., Data-Star, Dow Jones Interactive, Gale Group, The Dialog Corporation, NewsNet).
Indexed: Bus.& Indus. (Aug.1996-), CWI.
—**CCC.**
Published by: Charles W. Henderson, Ed. & Pub., PO Box 5528, Atlanta, GA 31107-0528. TEL 770-507-7777, FAX 770-507-7788, TELEX 78-2661, cwhender@newsfile.com; info@hendersonnet.atl.ga.us, http://www.newsfile.com.

616.9 CAN
CANCERCARE MANITOBA REPORT. Text in English. 1957. a. free per issue. **Document type:** *Corporate.*
Formerly: Manitoba Cancer Treatment and Research Foundation. Report (0076-3802)

Published by: Manitoba Cancer Treatment and Research Foundation, 100 Olivia St, Winnipeg, MB R3E 0V9, Canada. TEL 204-787-2241, FAX 204-787-1184. Ed. Julia De Fehr. R&P Brent Schacter. Circ: 1,000.

616.99 FRA ISSN 1140-9916
CANCEROLOGIE AUJOURD'HUI. Text in French. 1991. bi-m. FRF 200; FRF 400 foreign (effective 2000). adv. **Document type:** *Academic/Scholarly.*
Related titles: Online - full text ed.
Address: 7 rue Jacquemont, Paris 75017, France. TEL 33-1-53069494, FAX 33-1-53069400, http://www.medkiosk.org. Pub. Arnaud Dupin. Adv. contact Laurence Delorne. Circ: 3,000.

616.994 ITA ISSN 0008-5480
CANCRO. Summaries in English. 1970 (vol.23). bi-m. ITL 4,000. adv. bk.rev. charts, illus.
Indexed: Biol.Abstr., Chem.Abstr., Dent.Ind., INIS Atomind., Ind.Med. (coverage dropped).
—CISTI, GNLM.
Published by: Istituto di Oncologia, Via Cavour 31, Turin, TO 10123, Italy.

618.92 616.99 USA
CANDLELIGHTERS CHILDHOOD CANCER FOUNDATION QUARTERLY NEWSLETTER. Text in English. q. USD 25 to institutions (effective 1999). bk.rev. **Document type:** *Newsletter.* **Description:** Provides information and support for families of children and teens with cancer; for interested health or education professionals as well.
Formerly: Candlelighters Foundation Quarterly Newsletter
Indexed: Rehabil.Lit.
Published by: Candlelighters Childhood Cancer Foundation, 3910 Warner St, Kensington, MD 20895-3931. TEL 301-657-8401, 800-366-2223. Circ: 40,000.

616.99 649 USA
CANDLELIGHTERS CHILDHOOD CANCER FOUNDATION YOUTH NEWSLETTER. Text in English. 1979. q. USD 25 (effective 1999); to health professionals and institutions. **Document type:** *Newsletter.* **Description:** Contains information and creative expressions by and for young people with cancer and their siblings.
Formerly: Candlelighters Foundation Youth Newsletter
Published by: Candlelighters Childhood Cancer Foundation, 3910 Warner St, Kensington, MD 20895-3931. TEL 301-657-8401, 800-366-2223. Circ: 17,000.

616 GBR ISSN 0143-3334
RC268.5 CODEN: CRNGDP
CARCINOGENESIS. Text in English. 1980. m. GBP 250, USD 385 to individuals; GBP 625, USD 1,020 to institutions (effective 2002). adv. illus. index. back issues avail.; reprint service avail. from SWZ. *Refereed.* **Document type:** *Journal, Academic/Scholarly.* **Description:** Multi-disciplinary research journal in the areas of viral, physical and chemical carcinogenesis and mutagenesis.
Related titles: Online - full text ed.: ISSN 1460-2180. GBP 562, USD 918 to institutions Online only (effective 2002) (from HighWire Pr., Northern Light Technology, Inc., EBSCO Publishing, O C L C Online Computer Library Center, Inc., RoweCom Information Quest, ingenta, Swets Blackwell, Institute for Scientific Information).
Indexed: AIDS & Cancer Res., Abstr.Hyg., Anim.Breed.Abstr., BBCI, Biotech.& Bioeng.Abstr., Chem.Cit.Ind., Curr.Adv.Cancer Res., Curr.Adv.Cell & Devel.Biol., Curr.Adv.Ecol.Sci., Curr.Adv.Gen.& Molec.Biol., Curr.Cont., Dairy Sci.Abstr., Derwent Biotech.Abstr., Environ.Sci.Poll.Mgmt., Excerp.Med., Food Sci.& Tech.Abstr., Genet.Abstr., Hum.Gen.Abstr., INIS Atomind., Ind.Med. (1980-), Inpharma, Int.Abstr.Biol.Sci., NRN, Nuc.Acids Abstr., Nutr.Abstr., Oncog.G.F.Abstr., Pharm.&Out.News, Reac., Rev.Arom.& Med.Plants, Rev.Med.& Vet.Mycol., Rice Abstr., Sci.Cit.Ind., Soyabean Abstr., Sugar Ind.Abstr., THA, Tox.Abstr., Triticale Abstr., Trop.Dis.Bull., Weed Abstr.
—BLDSC (3051.007000), CASDDS, CISTI, EMDOCS, GNLM, IDS, ingenta, KNAW. **CCC.**
Published by: Oxford University Press, Academic Division, Great Clarendon St, Oxford OX2 6DP, United Kingdom. TEL 44-1865-267907, FAX 44-1865-267835, jnl.info@oup.co.uk, http://www.oup.co.uk/carcin/, http://www.oup.co.uk/journals. Eds. A Balmain, Curtis C Harris, R Brown. Pub. Mandy Sketch. adv.: page GBP 270, page USD 485. Circ: 1,050. **Subscr. in the Americas to:** Oxford University Press, Journals, 2001 Evans Rd, Cary, NC 27513. TEL 800-852-7323, FAX 919-677-1714, jnlorders@oup-usa.org; **Subscr. to:** Journals Marketing, Great Clarendon St, Oxford OX2 6DP, United Kingdom.

616 USA ISSN 0147-4006
RC268.5 CODEN: CCSUDL
CARCINOGENESIS; a comprehensive survey. Text in English. 1976. irreg. price varies. reprint service avail. from PQC. *Refereed.* **Document type:** *Monographic series.*
Related titles: Online - full text ed.: (from Northern Light Technology, Inc.).
Indexed: Biol.Abstr., Chem.Abstr., Chem.Cit.Ind., Chem.Indus.Notes, Chem.Titles, Dairy Sci.Abstr., Dent.Ind., Dok.Arbeitsmed., INIS Atomind., Ind.Med. (1976-), Ind.Sci.Rev., Rev.Med.& Vet.Mycol., Rev.Plant Path., Risk Abstr., Sci.Cit.Ind. (coverage dropped).
—CASDDS, CISTI, KNAW.
Published by: Lippincott Williams & Wilkins (Philadelphia) (Subsidiary of: Wolters Kluwer N.V.), 530 Walnut St, Philadelphia, PA 19106-3621. TEL 301-223-2300, 800-638-3030, FAX 301-223-2400.

616.99 JPN ISSN 0918-1989
CARCINOLOGICAL SOCIETY OF JAPAN. CANCER. Text in Japanese. 1972. a.
Formerly (until 1991): Nihon Kokakurui Gakkai Nyusu - Carcinological Society of Japan. News
Published by: Nihon Kokakurui Gakkai/Carcinological Society of Japan, University of Fisheries, Dept of Aquatic Bioscience, 4-5-7 Ko-Unan, Minato-ku, Tokyo 108-0075, Japan. TEL 81-3-5463-0535, FAX 81-3-5463-0684.

616.99 USA ISSN 1044-9523
RC261.A1 CODEN: CGDIE7
CELL GROWTH & DIFFERENTIATION. Text in English. 1990. m. USD 140 domestic to individuals; USD 180 foreign to individuals; USD 385 domestic to institutions; USD 425 foreign to institutions (effective 1999). adv. *Refereed.* **Document type:** *Journal, Academic/Scholarly.* **Description:** Publishes original research in all areas of the molecular biology of cancer.
Related titles: Online - full text ed.: (from HighWire Pr., Institute for Scientific Information).
Indexed: ASCA, BBCI, Biol.Abstr., Chem.Abstr., Chem.Indus.Notes, Chem.Titles, Curr.Cont., Excerp.Med. (1993-), INIS Atomind., Ind.Med. (1990-), Ind.Sci.Rev., Inpharma, Int.Abstr.Biol.Sci., Pharm.&Out.News, Reac., Sci.Cit.Ind., THA.
—BLDSC (3097.790000), CASDDS, CISTI, EMDOCS, GNLM, ingenta, KNAW.
Published by: American Association for Cancer Research, Public Ledger Bldg, 150 S Independence Mall W, Ste 826, Philadelphia, PA 19106. TEL 215-440-9300, FAX 215-440-9354, http://www.aacr.org. Ed. Joseph R Nevins. R&P Margaret Foti. Adv. contact Morgan Robinson. Circ: 1,830. **Subscr. to:** Cell Growth & Differentiation, Subscription Office, Box 11806, Birmingham, AL 35202. TEL 205-995-1567, FAX 205-995-1588.

616.99 USA
CENTER NEWS. Text in English. 1975. bi-m. donation. **Document type:** *Newsletter.* **Description:** Lay language coverage of treatment advances, basic and clinical research, and other programs and activities at Memorial Sloan-Kettering Cancer Center.
Published by: Memorial Sloan-Kettering Cancer Center, Department of Public Affairs, 1275 York Ave, New York, NY 10021. TEL 212-639-3573, FAX 212-639-3576, http://www.mskcc.org. Ed. Debbie Rosenberg Bush. Circ: 250,000 (controlled).

616.99 USA
THE CHALLENGE (BANNING). Text in English. 1978. q. USD 20; USD 35 foreign (effective 1999). bk.rev. back issues avail. *Refereed.* **Document type:** *Academic/Scholarly.* **Description:** Covers cancer immunology and biological modifiers.
Published by: Cancer Federation, Inc., PO Box 1298, Banning, CA 92220-0009. TEL 909-849-4325, FAX 909-849-0156, cancerfed@msn.com, http://www.cancerfed.com. Ed. John Steinbacher. Circ: 2,000.

616.99 DEU ISSN 0940-6735
CODEN: CHJOFT
CHEMOTHERAPIE JOURNAL. Text in German. 1992. bi-m. EUR 101.52 domestic; EUR 105.60 foreign; EUR 22 newsstand/cover (effective 2002). *Refereed.* **Document type:** *Journal, Academic/Scholarly.*
Indexed: Chem.Abstr., Chem.Indus.Notes, Chem.Titles, Excerp.Med. (1996-).
—BLDSC (3172.303000), CASDDS, EMDOCS, GNLM, Infotrieve, KNAW. **CCC.**
Published by: (Paul-Ehrlich-Gesellschaft fuer Chemotherapie e.V.), Wissenschaftliche Verlagsgesellschaft mbH, Postfach 101061, Stuttgart 70009, Germany. TEL 49-711-2582-0, FAX 49-711-2582-290, sheinz@wissenschaftliche-verlagsgesellschaft.de, http://www.wissenschaftliche-verlagsgesellschaft.de. Eds. B Wiedemann, G Hoeffken.

616.99 CHN ISSN 1000-9604
CODEN: CJCRFH
CHINESE JOURNAL OF CANCER RESEARCH/ ZHONGGUO AIZHENG YANJIU. Text in English. 1989. q. CNY 40 domestic; USD 120 foreign (effective 2000). back issues avail. *Refereed.* **Document type:** *Academic/Scholarly.* **Description:** Contains research papers, clinical observations and traditional Chinese medicine in the field of cancer research.
Related titles: CD-ROM ed.; Online - full content ed.: (from WanFang Data Corp.).
Indexed: Ref.Zh.
—BLDSC (3180.297700), CASDDS, CISTI, GNLM.
Published by: (Beijing Institute for Cancer Research), China Anti-Cancer Association, Da-Hong-Luo-Chang St, Western District, Beijing 100034, China. TEL 86-10-66124844, FAX 86-22-23374477, chjcacnr@public3.bta.net.cn; qingbaoy@public2.east.net.cn. Ed. Qibo Ling. Circ: 300 (controlled).

616 USA
CHOICE (CHULA VISTA). Text in English. 1975. 3/yr. USD 16 (effective 1999). adv. bk.rev. illus, stat. back issues avail. **Document type:** *Newsletter, Consumer.* **Description:** Devoted to news about medicine, medical politics, and "alternative" therapies.
Indexed: Bk.Rev.Dig. (coverage dropped), Lib.Lit. (coverage dropped).
Published by: Committee for Freedom of Choice in Medicine, Inc., c/o American Biologics, 1180 Walnut St, Chula Vista, CA 91911. TEL 619-429-8200, FAX 619-429-8004, cfcm@americanbiologics.com, http://www.americanbiologics.com. Ed., R&P Carole Bradford. adv.: B&W page USD 400. Circ: 8,000.

616.992 USA ISSN 1086-4601
CLASSIC PAPER AND CURRENT COMMENTS; highlights of cancer research. Text in English. 1996. q. USD 111 domestic to individuals; USD 127 foreign to individuals; USD 142 domestic to institutions; USD 158 foreign to institutions (effective 2002). *Refereed.* **Document type:** *Journal, Academic/Scholarly.* **Description:** Compiles some of the most important papers on the diagnosis and management of particular disease states previously published in the Journal of Clinical Oncology.
Published by: Lippincott Williams & Wilkins (Philadelphia) (Subsidiary of: Wolters Kluwer N.V.), 530 Walnut St, Philadelphia, PA 19106-3621. TEL 215-521-8300, FAX 215-521-8902, custserv@lww.com, http://www.lww.com/. Ed. Dr. George Canellos. **Subscr. to:** PO Box 1600, Hagerstown, MD 21740-1600. TEL 800-638-3030, FAX 310-223-2400.

616.99 NLD ISSN 0262-0898
CODEN: CEXMD2
CLINICAL AND EXPERIMENTAL METASTASIS. Text in Dutch. 1982. 8/yr. USD 1,271 in the Americas to institutions for print or online ed.; EUR 1,269 elsewhere to institutions for print or online ed.; USD 1,525.50 in the Americas to institutions for print & online eds; EUR 1,522.80 elsewhere to institutions for print & online eds (effective 2002). adv. bk.rev. index. *Refereed.* **Document type:** *Journal, Academic/Scholarly.* **Description:** Focuses on the crucial process of dissemination and metastasis formation.
Related titles: CD-ROM ed.; Online - full text ed.: (from EBSCO Publishing, O C L C Online Computer Library Center, Inc., RoweCom Information Quest, Swets Blackwell, Kluwer Online, Institute for Scientific Information).
Indexed: AIDS & Cancer Res., ASCA, Chem.Abstr., Chem.Indus.Notes, Chem.Titles, Curr.Adv.Ecol.Sci., Curr.Cont., Excerp.Med., Ind.Med. (1983-), Ind.Sci.Rev., Inpharma, Int.Abstr.Biol.Sci., Oncog.G.F.Abstr., Pharm.&Out.News, Reac., Sci.Cit.Ind.
—BLDSC (3286.251400), ADONIS, CASDDS, CISTI, EMDOCS, GNLM, IDS, ingenta, KNAW. **CCC.**

M

Published by: Kluwer Academic Publishers Group (Subsidiary of: Wolters Kluwer N.V.), Spuiboulevard 50, PO Box 17, Dordrecht 3300 AA, Netherlands. TEL 31-78-639-2392, FAX 31-78-654-2254, services@wkap.nl, http://www.wkap.nl/journalhome.htm/0262-0898. Eds. Garth L Nicolson, Suzanne A Eccles, Tatsuro Irimura. Adv. contact Gemma Heiser. **Subscr. in the Americas to:** Kluwer Academic - Plenum Publishers, 233 Spring St, New York, NY 10013-1578. TEL 212-620-8468, FAX 212-807-1047

616.99 USA ISSN 0164-985X
CLINICAL CANCER LETTER. Text in English. 1978. m. USD 89 (effective 2000). **Document type:** *Newsletter.* **Description:** Covers new clinical developments, clinical trials, and research on cancer.
—BLDSC (3286.264500).
Published by: Cancer Letter Inc., PO Box 9905, Washington, DC 20016. TEL 202-362-1809, FAX 202-362-1681. Ed. Kirsten B Goldberg.

616.99 USA ISSN 1078-0432
RC267 CODEN: CCREF4
CLINICAL CANCER RESEARCH. Text in English. 1995. m. USD 155 domestic to individuals; USD 195 foreign to individuals; USD 1,030 domestic to institutions; USD 1,155 foreign to institutions (effective 2000); includes Cancer Research. adv. *Refereed.* **Document type:** *Academic/Scholarly.* **Description:** Cutting edge clinical and transnational cancer research that has implications for patient care.
Related titles: Online - full text ed.: (from HighWire Pr., Institute for Scientific Information).
Indexed: ASCA, Abstr.Hyg., Chem.Abstr., Chem.Indus.Notes, Chem.Titles, Curr.Cont., Dairy Sci.Abstr., Derwent Biotech.Abstr., Excerp.Med. (1996-), Helminthol.Abstr., Ind.Med. (1995-), Ind.Vet., Inpharma, Int.Abstr.Biol.Sci., NRN, Nutr.Abstr., Pharm.&Out.News, Reac., Rev.Arom.& Med.Plants, Sci.Cit.Ind., Soyabean Abstr., Vet.Bull.
—BLDSC (3286.264750), CASDDS, CINDOC, CISTI, EMDOCS, GNLM, ingenta, KNAW.
Published by: American Association for Cancer Research, Public Ledger Bldg, 150 S Independence Mall W, Ste 826, Philadelphia, PA 19106. TEL 215-440-9300, FAX 215-440-9354, http://www.aacr.org. Ed. Dr. John Mendelsohn. R&P Margaret Foti. Adv. contact Morgan Robinson. Circ: 4,552. **Subscr. to:** Subscription Office, P O Box 11806, Birmingham, AL 35202. TEL 205-995-1567, FAX 205-995-1588.

CLINICAL JOURNAL OF ONCOLOGY NURSING. see *MEDICAL SCIENCES—Nurses And Nursing*

616.994 GBR ISSN 0936-6555
CODEN: CLIOEH
CLINICAL ONCOLOGY. (To be published by W.B. Saunders from February 2002 (44-20-8300-3322) Subscr. prices: GBP 78.00 (to individuals), GBP 295.00 (to institutions) (effective 2002)) Text in English. 1989. bi-m. back issues avail. **Document type:** *Academic/Scholarly.* **Description:** International, multidisciplinary research covering all aspects of the clinical management of cancer patients.
Related titles: Online - full text ed.: ISSN 1433-2981 (from EBSCO Publishing, RoweCom Information Quest, Swets Blackwell, Springer LINK, Institute for Scientific Information).
Indexed: Curr.Cont., Excerp.Med. (1993-), INIS Atomind., Ind.Med. (1989-), Int.Nurs.Ind.
—BLDSC (3286.317000), CISTI, EMDOCS, GNLM, Infotrieve, KNAW. **CCC.**
Published by: (Royal College of Radiologists), Springer-Verlag London Ltd. (Subsidiary of: BertelsmannSpringer), Sweetapple House, Catteshall Rd, Godalming, Surrey GU7 3DJ, United Kingdom. TEL 44-1483-418800, FAX 44-1483-415144. Ed. T J Priestman. **U.S. subscr. to:** Springer-Verlag New York Inc., PO Box 2485, Secaucus, NJ 07096-2485.

616.99 USA ISSN 0886-7186
CLINICAL ONCOLOGY ALERT. Text in English. 1986. m. USD 219 domestic; USD 249 foreign; USD 37 newsstand/cover (effective 2001). index. reprints avail. *Refereed.* **Document type:** *Newsletter.*
Related titles: Audio cassette/tape ed.; Online - full text ed.: (from Gale Group).
Published by: American Health Consultants (Subsidiary of: Medical Economics Co., Inc.), 3525 Piedmont Rd, N E, 6 Piedmont Center, Ste 400, Atlanta, GA 30305. TEL 404-262-5476, custserv@ahcpub.com, http://www.ahcpub.com. Circ: 2,225.

CLINICAL RADIOLOGY. see *MEDICAL SCIENCES—Radiology And Nuclear Medicine*

616.992 USA
CLINICAL TRIALS NEWS. Text in English. w. bk.rev. back issues avail. **Document type:** *Newsletter.* **Description:** Features special reports and clinical briefs dealing with all aspects of cancer.
Media: Online - full text.
Published by: University of Pennsylvania, Cancer Center Clinical Trials Group, 1223 Penn Tower, 3400 Spruce St, Philadelphia, PA 19104. FAX 215-349-8299, http://www.oncolink.upenn.edu/upcc/clin_trials/spr94/. Ed. Maggie Hampshire.

616.992 AUS ISSN 1328-9454
CLINICAL UPDATE. Text in English. 1998. s-a. free per issue to qualified personnel. **Description:** Provides surgeons, medical and radiation oncologists with information about recent breast cancer research with immediate signifance to clinical practice.
Related titles: Online - full text ed.
Published by: (N H M R C National Breast Cancer Center), Kings Cross, N.S.W. 1340, Kings Cross, NSW 2011, Australia. TEL 61-2-9634-1700, FAX 61-2-9326-9329, directorate@nbcc.org.au, http://www.nbcc.org.au/pages/info/resource/nbccpubs/clinicup/contents.htm. Ed. Karen Luxford. Circ: 1,200.

616.99 USA ISSN 0743-5061
COMMUNITY CANCER PROGRAMS IN THE UNITED STATES. Text in English. 1980. a. USD 150 (effective 2001). back issues avail. **Document type:** *Directory.* **Description:** Summaries of close to 600 cancer programs in the U.S. Includes medical contacts, a cancer program narrative description, and cancer program data.
Published by: Association of Community Cancer Centers, 11600 Nebel St, Ste 201, Rockville, MD 20852. TEL 301-984-9496, FAX 301-770-1949. Ed. Lee E Mortenson. R&P Donald Jewler.

616.992 USA
CONRAD NOTES. Text in English. irreg. **Document type:** *Newsletter.* **Description:** Provides information to healthcare professionals, patients, information specialists and marketing executives. Presents succinct analyses of key presentations on therapy and clinical research on pain, colorectal cancer and other types of cancer.
Media: Online - full text.
Published by: Ultitech, Inc., Foot of Broad St, Stratford, CT 06497. TEL 203-375-7300, FAX 203-375-6699, comcowic@meds.com, http://www.meds.com/conradnotes.html. Ed. William J Comcowich.

616.99 USA
CONTEMPORARY CANCER RESEARCH. Text in English. 1998. irreg., latest vol.4, 1999. price varies. illus. *Refereed.* **Document type:** *Monographic series, Academic/Scholarly.* **Description:** Provides state-of-the-art scientific and medical reviews on the subject of cutting-edge cancer research. Intended for all those conducting both basic and clinical cancer research.
Indexed: Biotech.& Bioeng.Abstr., Hum.Gen.Abstr., Nuc.Acids Abstr.
Published by: Humana Press Inc., 999 Riverview Dr, Ste 208, Totowa, NJ 07512. TEL 973-256-1699, FAX 973-256-8341, humana@humanapr.com, http://humanapress.com. Ed. Jac A Nickoloff. R&P Richard Hruska.

616.99 CHE ISSN 0250-3220
CODEN: COONEV
CONTRIBUTIONS TO ONCOLOGY/BEITRAEGE ZUR ONKOLOGIE. Text in English, German. 1979. irreg., latest vol.55. CHF 120 in Europe; DEM 145 in Germany; USD 105 in United States (effective 2001). index. *Refereed.* **Document type:** *Monographic series, Academic/Scholarly.*
Indexed: Biol.Abstr., Chem.Abstr., Chem.Indus.Notes, Chem.Titles, Curr.Cont. (coverage dropped).
—BLDSC (1887.090000), CASDDS, CISTI, GNLM, KNAW. **CCC.**
Published by: S. Karger AG, Allschwilerstr 10, PO Box, Basel 4009, Switzerland. TEL 41-61-306-1111, FAX 41-61-306-1234, karger@karger.ch, http://www.karger.com/bookseries/COONC. Eds. W Queisser, W Scheithauer.

616.994 USA
RC261.A1
COPING WITH CANCER. Text in English. 1986. bi-m. USD 19 domestic; USD 25 foreign (effective 2001). adv. bk.rev. illus. back issues avail.; reprints avail. *Refereed.* **Document type:** *Magazine, Consumer.* **Description:** Targets those affected by cancer. Empowers readers by providing the knowledge they need to cope with the many issues in their daily lives. Aims to inspire patients and survivors to assume greater responsibility for, and participation in, the many aspects of their disease.
Formerly: Coping (1043-8637)
Published by: Media America, PO Box 682268, Franklin, TN 37068-2268. TEL 615-790-2400, FAX 615-794-0179, copingmag@aol.com. Ed. Kay Thomas. Pub. Michael D Holt. R&P Marsha Moore TEL 615-790-2400 ext 27. Adv. contact Paula K Chadwell. Circ: 80,000 (paid and controlled).

COURTROOM MEDICINE SERIES: CANCER. see *LAW*

616.99 USA ISSN 0893-9675
CODEN: CRONEI
CRITICAL REVIEWS IN ONCOGENESIS. Text in English. 1989. q. USD 99.95 to individuals; USD 312 to institutions (effective 2000). adv. *Refereed.* **Document type:** *Academic/Scholarly.* **Description:** Offers a selection of reviews on topics of current interest in the field of basic oncology.
Related titles: Online - full text ed.: (from Institute for Scientific Information).
Indexed: AIDS & Cancer Res., ASCA, Chem.Abstr., Chem.Indus.Notes, Chem.Titles, Curr.Cont. (coverage dropped), Excerp.Med. (1995-), INIS Atomind., Ind.Med. (1989-), Ind.Sci.Rev., Inpharma, Int.Abstr.Biol.Sci., Oncog.G.F.Abstr., Pharm.&Out.News, Reac., Sci.Cit.Ind. (coverage dropped).
—BLDSC (3487.478900), CASDDS, CISTI, EMDOCS, GNLM, IDS, Infotrieve, ingenta, KNAW. **CCC.**
Published by: Begell House Inc., 79 Madison Ave, Ste 1205, New York, NY 10016-7892. TEL 212-725-1999, FAX 212-213-8368, begellhouse@worldnet.att.nct, orders@begellhouse.com. Pub. William Begell. R&P, Adv. contact Jung K Ra.

616.99 616.15 IRL ISSN 1040-8428
RC254.A1 CODEN: CCRHEC
CRITICAL REVIEWS IN ONCOLOGY - HEMATOLOGY. Text in English. 1981. m. EUR 191 in Europe to individuals; JPY 25,200 in Japan to individuals; USD 214 elsewhere to individuals; EUR 1,364 in Europe to institutions; JPY 181,200 in Japan to institutions; USD 1,526 elsewhere to institutions (effective 2002). back issues avail. *Refereed.* **Document type:** *Academic/Scholarly.* **Description:** Publishes scholarly, critical reviews in the fields of oncology and hematology.
Formerly: C R C Critical Reviews in Oncology - Hematology (0737-9587)
Related titles: Online - full text ed.: (from ingenta, Swets Blackwell, ScienceDirect, Institute for Scientific Information).
Indexed: ASCA, Curr.Cont., Excerp.Med., INIS Atomind., Ind.Med. (1983-), Ind.Sci.Rev., Inpharma, Int.Abstr.Biol.Sci., Pharm.&Out.News, Reac., Sci.Cit.Ind., Telegen.
—BLDSC (3487.479000), CISTI, EMDOCS, GNLM, IDS. **CCC.**
Published by: Elsevier Science Ireland Ltd, Elsevier House, Brookvale Plaza, E. Park, Shannon, Co. Clare, Ireland. TEL 353-61-471944, FAX 353-61-472144, http://www.elsevier.com/inca/publications/store/5/2/2/3/4/5/. Eds. A Surbone, M S Aapro, Stephen Davis. R&P Annette Moloney. **Subscr. in Australasia and the Far East to:** Elsevier Science (Singapore) Pte Ltd, No.1 Temasek Ave, 17-01 Millenia Tower, Singapore 039192, Singapore. TEL 65-434-3727, FAX 65-337-2230; **Subscr. in the Americas to:** Elsevier Science, PO Box 945, New York, NY 10159-0945. TEL 212-633-3730, FAX 212-633-3680; **Subscr. to:** Elsevier Science BV, PO Box 211, Amsterdam 1000 AE, Netherlands. TEL 31-20-485-3757.

CURRENT ADVANCES IN CANCER RESEARCH. see *MEDICAL SCIENCES—Abstracting, Bibliographies, Statistics*

616.994 NLD ISSN 1568-0096
▼ **CURRENT CANCER DRUG TARGETS.** Text in English. 2001. q.
Published by: Bentham Science Publishers, P.O. Box 1673, Hilversum BR 1200, Netherlands. FAX 31-35-6980150.

616.99 DEU ISSN 0940-0745
CURRENT CANCER RESEARCH. Text in German. 1986. irreg. DEM 35 (effective 2000). **Document type:** *Academic/Scholarly, Corporate.*
Published by: Deutsches Krebsforschungszentrum, Im Neuenheimer Feld 280, Heidelberg 69120, Germany. TEL 49-6221-422854, FAX 49-6221-422995.

616.99 USA ISSN 1074-2816
CURRENT CANCER THERAPEUTICS. Text in English. 1994. a. **Document type:** *Trade, Academic/Scholarly.*
Published by: Current Medicine, 400 Market St, Ste 700, Philadelphia, PA 19106. TEL 800-427-1796, FAX 215-574-2225. Ed. Lori J Bainbridge.

616.99 616.15 USA
▼ **CURRENT CLINICAL ONCOLOGY.** Text in English. 1999. irreg. price varies. illus. *Refereed.* **Document type:** *Monographic series, Academic/Scholarly.*
Description: Covers the latest therapies and treatment regimens for physicians treating patients with cancer.
Published by: Humana Press Inc., 999 Riverview Dr, Ste 208, Totowa, NJ 07512. TEL 973-256-1699, FAX 973-256-8341, humana@humanapr.com, http://humanapress.com. Ed. Maurie Markman. R&P Richard Hruska.

CURRENT MEDICAL LITERATURE. BREAST CANCER. see *MEDICAL SCIENCES—Abstracting, Bibliographies, Statistics*

CURRENT MEDICAL LITERATURE. COLORECTAL CANCER. see *MEDICAL SCIENCES—Abstracting, Bibliographies, Statistics*

CURRENT MEDICAL LITERATURE. LEUKAEMIA AND LYMPHOMA. see *MEDICAL SCIENCES—Abstracting, Bibliographies, Statistics*

616.992 USA ISSN 1523-3790
CURRENT ONCOLOGY REPORTS. Text in English. 2/yr. USD 163.95, GBP 120 to individuals; USD 327.95 to institutions; USD 85, GBP 60 to students (effective 2002); Subscr. includes both print & online eds..
Related titles: Online - full content ed.: USD 85, GBP 65 (effective 2002).
Indexed: Ind.Med.
Published by: Current Science Inc., 400 Market St, Ste 700, Philadelphia, PA 19106. TEL 800-427-1796, FAX 215-574-2225, info@current-reports.com, http://www.current-reports.com/cr_jrnl_home.cfm?JournalID=OR, http://www.current-science.com/, http://www.current-science-group.com/. Ed. Maurie Markman. **Affiliate:** Current Science Ltd.

616.99 CAN ISSN 1198-0052
CODEN: CUONF6
CURRENT ONCOLOGY (TORONTO)✶. Text in English. 1994. q. adv. *Refereed.* **Document type:** *Academic/Scholarly.*
—GNLM, Infotrieve. **CCC.**
Published by: Multimed, Inc., 66 Martin St, Milton, ON L9T R2R, Canada. TEL 416-650-0610, FAX 416-650-0639. Ed. M McLean. Adv. contact Harriet Cooper.

616.99 USA ISSN 1040-8746
RC254.A1 CODEN: CUOOE8
CURRENT OPINION IN ONCOLOGY. Text in English. 1989. bi-m. USD 273 domestic to individuals for print & online eds.; USD 273 foreign to individuals for print & online eds.; USD 665 per issue domestic to institutions; USD 665 per issue foreign to institutions; USD 103 newsstand/cover (effective 2002). adv. bibl, illus. **Document type:** *Academic/Scholarly.* **Description:** Directed toward researchers and practicing oncologists. Presents review articles followed by annotated bibliographies of references consulted. A bibliography of the current world literature published during the previous year is available.
Related titles: Online - full text ed.: USD 864.50 domestic academic site license; USD 864.50 foreign academic site license; USD 964.25 domestic corporate site license; USD 964.25 foreign corporate site license (effective 2002) (from Ovid Technologies, Inc., EBSCO Publishing, Swets Blackwell, Institute for Scientific Information).
Indexed: CINAHL, Chem.Abstr., Chem.Indus.Notes, Chem.Titles, Curr.Cont., Excerp.Med., INIS Atomind., Ind.Med. (1989-), Inpharma, Pharm.&Out.News, Reac., Sci.Cit.Ind.
—BLDSC (3500.776400), ADONIS, CASDDS, CISTI, EMDOCS, GNLM, ingenta, KNAW.
Published by: Lippincott Williams & Wilkins (Philadelphia) (Subsidiary of: Wolters Kluwer N.V.), 530 Walnut St, Philadelphia, PA 19106-3621. FAX 215-521-8902, 215-521-8902, http://www.Lww.com. Ed. Martin D Abeloff. Pub. Maria McMichael. R&P Tobias Weschler. Adv. contact Kelly Adamitis. Circ: 1,183. **Subscr. to:** PO Box 1600, Hagerstown, MD 21740-1600.

616.99 USA ISSN 0147-0272
RC261.A1 CODEN: CPRCDJ
CURRENT PROBLEMS IN CANCER. Short title: C P Ca. Text in English. 1977. bi-m. USD 96 domestic to individuals; USD 108 foreign to individuals; USD 145 domestic to institutions; USD 162 foreign to institutions; USD 51 domestic to students; USD 60 foreign to students; USD 28 per issue domestic (effective 2001). index. reprint service avail. from PQC. *Refereed.*
Description: A fully referenced monographic journal with information from recognized experts on practical clinical care.
Related titles: Microform ed.: (from PQC); Online - full text ed.: (from Institute for Scientific Information).
Indexed: ASCA, Biol.Abstr., Curr.Cont., Dent.Ind., Dok.Arbeitsmed., INIS Atomind., Ind.Med. (1976-), Ind.Sci.Rev., Inpharma, Pharm.&Out.News, Reac., Sci.Cit.Ind.
—BLDSC (3501.345000), CISTI, GNLM, IDS, ingenta, KNAW. **CCC.**
Published by: Mosby, Inc. (Subsidiary of: Elsevier Science), 11830 Westline Industrial Dr, St Louis, MO 63146-3318. TEL 314-872-8370, 800-325-4177, FAX 314-432-1380, periodical.service@mosby.com, http://www.mosby.com/cpcancer, http://www.mosby.com/periodicals. Ed. Stephen D Williams. Circ: 1,407.

616.99 USA ISSN 0266-9927
CURRENT PROBLEMS IN TUMOUR PATHOLOGY✶. Text in English. 1985. irreg., latest vol.6. **Document type:** *Monographic series.*
—KNAW.
Published by: Churchill Livingstone (Subsidiary of: Harcourt Health Sciences), 15 E 26th St, Fl 15, New York, NY 10010-1505. TEL 212-206-5040, FAX 212-727-7808, http://www.churchillmed.com.

CURRENT THERAPY IN HEMATOLOGY - ONCOLOGY. see *MEDICAL SCIENCES—Hematology*

CYTOKINES, CELLULAR & MOLECULAR THERAPY. see *MEDICAL SCIENCES—Hematology*

362.1 USA ISSN 0095-6775
RC267
DAMON RUNYON - WALTER WINCHELL CANCER RESEARCH FUND. ANNUAL REPORT✶. Key Title: Annual Report, Damon Runyon - Walter Winchell Cancer Research Fund. Text in English. 1973. a. free per issue.
Formerly (until 1973): Damon Runyon Memorial Fund for Cancer Research. Annual Report (0416-6639)
Published by: Damon Runyon Walter Winchell Cancer Research Fund, 675 Third Ave, New York, NY 10017-5704. Circ: 1,000.

DERMATOLOGIC SURGERY. see *MEDICAL SCIENCES—Surgery*

DERMATOLOGIC SURGERY ONLINE. see *MEDICAL SCIENCES—Surgery*

616.99 DEU ISSN 0932-7479
DEUTSCHE KREBSGESELLSCHAFT. MITTEILUNGEN✶. Text in German. 1986. q. DEM 60. **Document type:** *Newsletter.*
Published by: Deutsche Krebsgesellschaft, Paul-Ehrlich-Str 41, Frankfurt Am Main 60596, Germany. Circ: 2,400.

616.99 DEU ISSN 1617-5891
CODEN: DZONEH
DEUTSCHE ZEITSCHRIFT FUER ONKOLOGIE/GERMAN JOURNAL OF ONCOLOGY. Text in German; Summaries in English. q. EUR 59.40 domestic to institutions; EUR 63.40 in Europe to institutions; EUR 69.80 elsewhere to institutions; EUR 15.90 newsstand/cover to institutions (effective 2002). adv. back issues avail. **Document type:** *Journal, Academic/Scholarly.*
Former titles (until 2001): Zeitschrift fuer Onkologie (1432-2919); (until 1996): Deutsche Zeitschrift fuer Onkologie (0931-0037); (until 1987): Krebsgeschehen (0340-5672)
Related titles: Online - full text ed.: ISSN 1439-0930.
Indexed: Excerp.Med., Ref.Zh.
—EMDOCS, GNLM, Infotrieve. **CCC.**
Published by: (Deutsche Gesellschaft fuer Onkologie e.V.), Karl F. Haug Verlag, Fritz-Frey-Str 21, Heidelberg 69121, Germany. TEL 49-6221-489445, FAX 49-6221-489584, http://www.haug-verlag.de. Circ: 5,000.

616.99 DEU ISSN 0932-6235
DEUTSCHES KREBSFORSCHUNGSZENTRUM. RESEARCH REPORT. Text in German. 1986. biennial. free per issue. **Document type:** *Academic/Scholarly.*
Published by: Deutsches Krebsforschungszentrum, Im Neuenheimer Feld 280, Heidelberg 69120, Germany. TEL 49-6221-423666, FAX 49-6221-423668.

616.9 DEU ISSN 0070-4229
DEUTSCHES KREBSFORSCHUNGSZENTRUM. VEROEFFENTLICHUNGEN. Text in German. 1965. a. **Document type:** *Academic/Scholarly.*
Published by: Deutsches Krebsforschungszentrum, Im Neuenheimer Feld 280, Heidelberg 69120, Germany. TEL 49-6221-422854, FAX 49-6221-422995, TELEX 461562-DKFZ-D. Circ: 1,000.

DEVELOPMENT IN SUPPORTIVE CANCER CARE. see *MEDICAL SCIENCES—Nurses And Nursing*

619.99 NLD ISSN 0167-4927
CODEN: DEOND5
DEVELOPMENTS IN ONCOLOGY. Text in Dutch. 1980. irreg., latest vol.74, 1994. price varies. *Refereed.* **Document type:** *Monographic series.*
Indexed: Chem.Abstr., Chem.Indus.Notes, Chem.Titles.
—BLDSC (3579.085470), CASDDS, CISTI. **CCC.**
Published by: Kluwer Academic Publishers Group (Subsidiary of: Wolters Kluwer N.V.), Spuiboulevard 50, PO Box 17, Dordrecht 3300 AA, Netherlands. FAX 31-78-639-2254, services@wkap.nl, http://www.wkap.nl. **Dist. by:** Journals Department, PO Box 322, Dordrecht 3300 AH, Netherlands. FAX 31-78-654-6474.

616.99 NLD ISSN 0278-0240
CODEN: DMARD3
DISEASE MARKERS. Text in English. 1982. q. EUR 516, USD 473 to institutions (effective 2002). adv. bk.rev. charts, illus. index. reprint service avail. from SWZ. *Refereed.* **Document type:** *Academic/Scholarly.*
Description: Addresses original research findings and reviews on the subject of the identification of markers associated with the disease process, whether they are an integral part of the pathological lesion.
Related titles: Online - full text ed.: (from EBSCO Publishing, O C L C Online Computer Library Center, Inc., Swets Blackwell, Institute for Scientific Information, RoweCom Information Quest).
Indexed: ASCA, AgBiotech, Biotech.Cit.Ind., Chem.Abstr., Chem.Indus.Notes, Chem.Titles, Curr.Adv.Ecol.Sci., Curr.Adv.Gen.& Molec.Biol., Curr.Cont., Environ.Sci.Poll.Mgmt., Excerp.Med., Ind.Med. (1983-), Inpharma, Int.Abstr.Biol.Sci., Microbiol.Abstr., Nutr.Abstr., Pharm.&Out.News, Pollut.Abstr., Reac., Rev.Appl.Entomol., SSCI (coverage dropped), Saf.Sci.Abstr., Sci.Cit.Ind., Telegen.
—BLDSC (3598.090000), ADONIS, CASDDS, CISTI, EMDOCS, GNLM, IDS, ingenta. **CCC.**
Published by: I O S Press, Nieuwe Hemweg 6B, Amsterdam 1013 BG, Netherlands. TEL 31-20-688-3355, FAX 31-20-620-3419, market@iospress.nl, http://www.iospress.nl. Ed. Suhdir Srivastava. Circ: 171. **Subscr. to:** I O S Press, Inc, 5795-G Burke Centre Pkwy, Burke, VA 22015. TEL 703-323-5554, FAX 703-323-3668, iosbooks@iospress.com; Globe Publication Pvt. Ltd., C-62 Inderpuri, New Delhi 100 012, India. TEL 91-11-579-3211, 91-11-579-3212, FAX 91-11-579-8876, custserve@globepub.com, http://www.globepub.com; Kinokuniya Company Ltd, Shinjuku 3-chome, Shinjuku-ku, Tokyo 160-0022, Japan. FAX 81-3-3439-1094, journal@kinokuniya.co.jp, http://www.kinokuniya.co.jp.

616.99 NLD ISSN 0927-328X
E C C NEWSLETTER. Text in English. 1992. q. NLG 75, USD 66. bk.rev. back issues avail.
Published by: (European Cancer Centre), Van Zuiden Communications B.V., Postbus 2122, Alphen aan den Rijn 2400 CC, Netherlands. TEL 31-172-476191, FAX 31-172-471882, 101617.2211@compuserve.com. Ed. P A Voute. adv.: color page NLG 4,000; trim 297 x 210.

616.99 DEU ISSN 0933-128X
EINBLICK. Text in German. 1987. 4/yr. free per issue. **Document type:** *Academic/Scholarly.*
—GNLM.
Published by: Deutsches Krebsforschungszentrum, Im Neuenheimer Feld 280, Heidelberg 69120, Germany. TEL 49-6221-422854, FAX 49-6221-422995.

M

616.99 619 UKR ISSN 0204-3564 CODEN: EKSODD

EKSPERIMENTAL'NAYA ONKOLOGIYA/EXPERIMENTAL ONCOLOGY; nauchno-tekhnicheskii zhurnal. Text in Russian, English, Ukrainian; Summaries in English, Russian. 1979. q. USD 95 (effective 2001). bk.rev. *Refereed.* **Document type:** *Journal, Academic/Scholarly.*

Related titles: Online - full text ed.: (from Institute for Scientific Information).

Indexed: ASCA, Biol.Abstr., Chem.Abstr., Curr.Adv.Ecol.Sci., Curr.Cont., Djerelo, Excerp.Med., INIS Atomind., Ind.Med. (coverage dropped), Ind.Sci.Rev., Inpharma, Pharm.&Out.News, Reac., Sci.Cit.Ind.

—CASDDS, CISTI, East View, EMDOCS, GNLM, IDS, Infotrieve, KNAW, Linda Hall. **CCC.**

Published by: (Natsional'na Akademiya Nauk Ukrainy, Institut Eksperymental'noi Patologii Onkologii i Radiobiologii im. R.E. Kavets'kogo), Morion LLC, Vladimirskaya ul 42, Kiev 01034, Ukraine. exponcol@onconet.kiev.ua, http://www.onconet.kiev.ua. Ed. V F Chekhun. Circ: 300. **Dist. by:** Mezhdunarodnaya Kniga, B Yakimanka 39, Moscow 117049, Russian Federation. TEL 7-095-2384967, FAX 7-095-2384634; **US dist. addr.:** East View Publications, 3020 Harbor Ln N, Minneapolis, MN 55447. TEL 612-550-0961.

616.994 FRA

▼ **ELECTRONIC JOURNAL OF ONCOLOGY.** Text in English. 1999. q. back issues avail. *Refereed.* **Description:** Publishes original articles in the fields of oncology and hematology.

Media: Online - full text.

Published by: Federation Nationale des Centres de Lutte contre le Cancer, 101 rue de Tolbiac, Paris Cedex 13 75654, France. TEL 33-1-44230404, FAX 33-1-45846682, ejo@univ-lyon1.fr, http://ejo.univ-lyon1.fr. Eds. Charles Dumontet, Jean Yves Blay.

ENFERMERIA ONCOLOGICA. see *MEDICAL SCIENCES—Nurses And Nursing*

ETESIA STATISTIKE. EREVNA TOU KARKINOU/ANNUAL STATISTICAL SURVEY OF CANCER. see *MEDICAL SCIENCES—Abstracting, Bibliographies, Statistics*

616.99 FRA ISSN 1253-0727

EUROCANCER (YEAR). Text in English. 1958. a.

Supersedes in part (in 1995): Pathologie et Biologie (0369-8114); Which was formerly (until 1959): Archives de Biologie Medicale, Anales de la Recherche Medicale (0150-7265); Which was formed by the 1958 merger of: Annales de la Recherche Medicale (0997-4415); Societe Francaise de Biologie Medicale. Archives (0997-4423)

—BLDSC (3829.247755).

Published by: John Libbey Eurotext, 127 av. de la Republique, Montrouge 92120, France. TEL 33-01-46730660, FAX 1-40-84-09-99, http://www.john-libbey-eurotext.fr. Eds. Michel Boiron, Michel Marty.

616.994 GBR
RC261.A1 CODEN: EJCAEL

EUROPEAN JOURNAL OF CANCER. Text in English. 1965. 18/yr. EUR 85 in Europe to individuals; JPY 11,200 in Japan to individuals; USD 95 elsewhere to individuals; EUR 1,968 in Europe to institutions; EUR 261,300 in Japan to institutions; USD 2,200 elsewhere to institutions (effective 2002). adv. bk.rev. charts, illus. index. back issues avail. *Refereed.* **Document type:** *Academic/Scholarly.* **Description:** Provides an integrated forum for publication of clinical and laboratory research in all specializations of oncology.

Formerly: European Journal of Cancer. Part A: General Topics; Which superseded in part (in 1992): European Journal of Cancer (0959-8049); Which was formerly (until 1990): European Journal of Cancer and Clinical Oncology (0277-5379); (until 1981): European Journal of Cancer (0014-2964)

Related titles: Microfilm ed.: (from PQC); Online - full text ed.: (from ingenta, Swets Blackwell, ScienceDirect, Institute for Scientific Information).

Indexed: AIDS & Cancer Res., AIDS Abstr., ASCA, Abstr.Health Care Manage.Stud., Abstr.Hyg., Agri.& Environ.Biotech.Abstr. (coverage dropped), Biol.Abstr., Chem.Abstr., Chem.Indus.Notes, Chem.Titles, Curr.Adv.Biochem., Curr.Adv.Cancer Res., Curr.Adv.Cell & Devel.Biol., Curr.Adv.Ecol.Sci., Curr.Adv.Gen.& Molec.Biol., Curr.Cont. (coverage dropped), Dairy Sci.Abstr., Dent.Ind., Derwent Biotech.Abstr., Dok.Arbeitsmed., Excerp.Med., INIS Atomind., Ind.Med. (coverage dropped), Ind.Sci.Rev., Ind.Vet., Inpharma, Int.Abstr.Biol.Sci., Med.& Surg.Dermat., NRN, Neurosci.Cit.Ind., Nutr.Abstr., Oncog.G.F.Abstr. (coverage dropped), Pharm.&Out.News, Reac., Rev.Arom.& Med.Plants, Rev.Med.& Vet.Mycol., Risk Abstr., SSCI (coverage dropped), Saf.Sci.Abstr., Sci.Cit.Ind. (coverage dropped), THA, Vet.Bull.

—BLDSC (3829.725100), ADONIS, CASDDS, CISTI, EMDOCS, GNLM, IDS, ingenta, KNAW. **CCC.**

Published by: (Federation of European Cancer Societies), Pergamon (Subsidiary of: Elsevier Science), The Boulevard, Langford Ln, East Park, Kidlington, Oxford OXB 1GB, United Kingdom. FAX 44-1865-843010, dpurves@ejcancer.demon.co.uk, http://www.elsevier.com/locate/ejca. Ed. J Smyth. Adv. contact Rachel Gresle Farthing. Circ: 3,500. **Subscr. in Australasia and the Far East to:** Elsevier Science (Singapore) Pte Ltd, No.1 Temasek Ave, 17-01 Millenia Tower, Singapore 039192, Singapore. TEL 65-434-3727, FAX 65-337-2230; **Subscr. in the Americas to:** Elsevier Science, PO Box 945, New York, NY 10159-0945. TEL 212-633-3730, FAX 212-633-3680; **Subscr. to:** Elsevier Science BV, PO Box 211, Amsterdam 1000 AE, Netherlands. TEL 31-20-485-3757. **Co-sponsors:** European Organization for Research on Treatment of Cancer; European School of Oncology; European Association for Cancer Research.

616.99 GBR ISSN 0961-5423 CODEN: EUCAEU

EUROPEAN JOURNAL OF CANCER CARE. Text in English. 1992. q., latest vol.11, 2002. GBP 75 in Europe to individuals; USD 120 in North America to individuals; GBP 83 elsewhere to individuals; GBP 251 in Europe to institutions; USD 399 in North America to institutions; GBP 277 elsewhere to institutions (effective 2002). adv. bk.rev. bibl, illus. index. *Refereed.* **Document type:** *Journal, Academic/Scholarly.* **Description:** Provides a medium for communicating comprehensive, multiprofessional cancer care across Europe and beyond.

Related titles: Microform ed.: (from PQC); ♦ Online - full text ed.: European Journal of Cancer Care Online. ISSN 1365-2354.

Indexed: AMED, ASSIA, Brit.Nur.Ind., CINAHL, Curr.Cont., Inpharma, Int.Nurs.Ind., Nutr.Abstr., Pharm.&Out.News, Reac.

—BLDSC (3829.725350), CISTI, Infotrieve, KNAW. **CCC.**

Published by: Blackwell Science Ltd., PO Box 88, Oxford OX2 0NE, United Kingdom. TEL 44-1865-206180, 44-1865-206002, FAX 44-1865-206219, jnl.orders@blacksci.co.uk, http://www.blackwell-science.com/products/journals/ejcc.htm, http://www.blackwellpublishing.com. Ed. Pat Webb. Pub. Elaine Stott. R&P Sohpie Savage. Adv. contact Jenny Applin. Circ: 430.

616.99 GBR ISSN 1365-2354

▼ **EUROPEAN JOURNAL OF CANCER CARE ONLINE.** Text in English. 1999. q. GBP 68 in Europe to individuals; USD 108 in North America to individuals; GBP 68 elsewhere to individuals; GBP 226 in Europe to institutions; USD 360 in North America to institutions; GBP 226 elsewhere to institutions (effective 2002). *Refereed.* **Document type:** *Academic/Scholarly.*

Media: Online - full text (from EBSCO Publishing, Munksgaard & Blackwell Science's Synergy, O C L C Online Computer Library Center, Inc., RoweCom Information Quest, ingenta, Swets Blackwell, Institute for Scientific Information). **Related titles:** Microform ed.: (from PQC); ♦ Print ed.: European Journal of Cancer Care. ISSN 0961-5423.

Published by: Blackwell Science Ltd., Osney Mead, Oxford OX2 0EL, United Kingdom. TEL 44-1685-206206, FAX 44-1685-721205, website@blacksci.com, journals.cs@blacksci.co.uk, http://www.blackwell-science.com.

616.99 USA ISSN 0959-8278 CODEN: EJUPEK

EUROPEAN JOURNAL OF CANCER PREVENTION. Text in English. 1992. bi-m. USD 216 domestic to individuals; USD 216 foreign to individuals; USD 838 per issue domestic to institutions; USD 838 per issue foreign to institutions; USD 127 newsstand/cover (effective 2002). adv. reprints avail. *Refereed.* **Document type:** *Academic/Scholarly.* **Description:** Aims to promote an increased awareness of all aspects of cancer prevention and to stimulate new ideas and innovations.

Related titles: CD-ROM ed.; Online - full text ed.: USD 1,089.40 domestic academic site license; USD 1,089.40 foreign academic site license; USD 1,215.10 domestic corporate site license; USD 1,215.10 foreign corporate site license (effective 2002) (from Ovid Technologies, Inc., EBSCO Publishing, Institute for Scientific Information).

Indexed: ASCA, Abstr.Hyg., Curr.Cont., Dairy Sci.Abstr., Excerp.Med. (1994-), Ind.Med. (1991-), Inpharma, Int.Abstr.Biol.Sci., Nutr.Abstr., Pharm.&Out.News, Postharvest, Poult.Abstr., Reac., Rev.Arom.& Med.Plants, Sugar Ind.Abstr., THA, Trop.Dis.Bull.

—BLDSC (3829.725400), ADONIS, CISTI, EMDOCS, GNLM, IDS, KNAW.

Published by: (European Cancer Prevention Organisation), Lippincott Williams & Wilkins (Philadelphia) (Subsidiary of: Wolters Kluwer N.V.), 530 Walnut St, Philadelphia, PA 19106-3621. TEL 215-521-8300, FAX 215-521-8902, http://www.Lww.com. Eds. Dr. A Giacosa, Michael J Hill. Adv. contact Gemma Heiser. Circ: 203. **Subscr. to:** PO Box 1600, Hagerstown, MD 21740-1600. TEL 800-777-2295, FAX 301-824-7390.

616.99 618.1 CAN ISSN 0392-2936 CODEN: EJGODE

EUROPEAN JOURNAL OF GYNECOLOGICAL ONCOLOGY. Text and summaries in English. 1980. bi-m., latest vol.23. USD 260 to individuals; USD 360 to institutions; USD 95 per issue to institutions (effective 2002). adv. bk.rev. back issues avail. *Refereed.* **Document type:** *Academic/Scholarly.*

Related titles: Online - full text ed.: (from Institute for Scientific Information).

Indexed: Biol.Abstr., Curr.Cont., Excerp.Med., Ind.Med. (1980-), Inpharma, NRN, Pharm.&Out.News, Reac., Rev.Med.& Vet.Mycol.

—BLDSC (3829.729600), CISTI, EMDOCS, GNLM, IDS, ingenta, KNAW. **CCC.**

Published by: (European Society of Gynecological Oncology), S O G Canada, Inc., 4900 Cote St Luc, Apt 212, Montreal, PQ H3W 2H3, Canada. TEL 514-489-3242, 39-49-8758644, FAX 514-485-4513. Ed. Antonio Onnis. Adv. contact Moriuz Morsoui. Circ: 600.

EUROPEAN JOURNAL OF ONCOLOGY NURSING. see *MEDICAL SCIENCES—Nurses And Nursing*

616.994 GBR ISSN 0748-7983

EUROPEAN JOURNAL OF SURGICAL ONCOLOGY. Text in English. 1975. 8/yr. GBP 155 to individuals; GBP 298 to institutions (effective 2002). adv. illus. index. reprint service avail. from SWZ. *Refereed.* **Document type:** *Academic/Scholarly.* **Description:** Presents original articles and state-of-the-art reviews of immediate interest to surgical oncologists.

Formerly: Clinical Oncology (0305-7399)

Related titles: Online - full text ed.: (from EBSCO Publishing, RoweCom Information Quest, Swets Blackwell, IDEAL Online Library, Institute for Scientific Information).

Indexed: AMED, Biol.Abstr., Curr.Adv.Cancer Res., Curr.Adv.Ecol.Sci., Curr.Adv.Gen.& Molec.Biol., Curr.Cont., Excerp.Med., INIS Atomind., Ind.Med. (1985-), Inpharma, Int.Nurs.Ind., Nutr.Abstr., Pharm.&Out.News, Reac.

—BLDSC (3829.745500), CISTI, EMDOCS, GNLM, IDS, Infotrieve, ingenta, KNAW. **CCC.**

Published by: (British Association of Surgical Oncology), W.B. Saunders Co. Ltd. (Subsidiary of: Harcourt Publishers Ltd.), 24-28 Oval Rd, London NW1 7DX, United Kingdom. TEL 44-20-7424-4200, FAX 44-20-7424-4515, cservice@harcourt.com, http://www.harcourt-international.com/journals/ejso. Ed. Irving Taylor. **Subscr. to:** Harcourt Publishers Ltd., Foots Cray High St, Sidcup, Kent DA14 5HP, United Kingdom. TEL 44-20-8308-5700, FAX 44-20-8309-0807. **Co-sponsor:** European Society of Surgical Oncology.

616 USA ISSN 0146-0447 CODEN: MSECDH

EUROPEAN ORGANIZATION FOR RESEARCH ON TREATMENT OF CANCER. MONOGRAPH SERIES. Short title: E O R T C Monograph Series. Text in English. 1975. irreg. price varies. reprint service avail. from PQC. *Refereed.* **Document type:** *Monographic series.*

M

Indexed: Biol.Abstr., Curr.Cont. (coverage dropped). —CASDDS, CISTI, KNAW.
Published by: (European Organization for Research on Treatment of Cancer), Lippincott Williams & Wilkins (Philadelphia) (Subsidiary of: Wolters Kluwer N.V.), 530 Walnut St, Philadelphia, PA 19106-3621. TEL 301-223-2300, 800-638-3030, FAX 301-223-2400.

616.99 DEU
EUROPEAN SCHOOL OF ONCOLOGY. MONOGRAPHS. Text in German. irreg. **Document type:** *Monographic series.* **Description:** Publishes new cancer research.
Published by: (European School of Oncology), Springer-Verlag (Subsidiary of: BertelsmannSpringer), Haber Str 7, Heidelberg 69126, Germany. FAX 49-30-82787448, subscriptions@springer.de, http://www.springer.de, http://link.springer-ny.com. Ed. U Veronesi.

EUROPEAN UROLOGY. see *MEDICAL SCIENCES—Urology And Nephrology*

616.89 GBR ISSN 1363-4054
▼ **EVIDENCE - BASED ONCOLOGY.** Text in English. 2000 (Mar.). q. GBP 70 to individuals; GBP 185 to institutions (effective 2002). *Refereed.* **Document type:** *Journal, Academic/Scholarly.* **Description:** External evidence from systematic research combined with individual clinical expertise assists clinicians in making effective decisions about patient treatment and care.
Related titles: Online - full text ed.: (from EBSCO Publishing, O C L C Online Computer Library Center, Inc., Swets Blackwell, IDEAL Online Library).
Published by: Churchill Livingstone (Subsidiary of: Harcourt Publishers Ltd.), Robert Stevenson House, 1-3 Baxter's Pl, Leith Walk, Edinburgh, Midlothian EH1 3AF, United Kingdom. TEL 44-131-556-2424, FAX 44-131-489-1177, cservice@harcourt.com, http://www.harcourt-international.com/journals/ebon. Eds. Benjamin Djulbegovic, Dr. Gary Lyman. **Subscr. to:** Harcourt Publishers Ltd., Foots Cray High St, Sidcup, Kent DA14 5HP, United Kingdom. TEL 44-20-8308-5700, FAX 44-20-8309-0807.

EXCERPTA MEDICA. SECTION 16: CANCER. see *MEDICAL SCIENCES—Abstracting, Bibliographies, Statistics*

▼ **EXPERT REVIEW OF ANTICANCER THERAPY**; an essential contribution to decision making in cancer care. see *PHARMACY AND PHARMACOLOGY*

616.2 599.935 NLD ISSN 1389-9600
▼ **FAMILIAL CANCER.** Text in English. 2000. q. EUR 264, USD 264 to institutions for print & online eds.combined (effective 2002). reprints avail. *Refereed.* **Document type:** *Journal, Academic/Scholarly.* **Description:** Publishes research into the hereditary aspects of cancer, with material of interest to the clinician, geneticist, and counselor.
Related titles: Online - full text ed.: (from O C L C Online Computer Library Center, Inc., RoweCom Information Quest, Swets Blackwell, Kluwer Online).
—BLDSC (3865.553881).
Published by: Kluwer Academic Publishers Group (Subsidiary of: Wolters Kluwer N.V.), Spuiboulevard 50, PO Box 17, Dordrecht 3300 AA, Netherlands. TEL 31-78-639-2392, FAX 31-78-654-2254, services@wkap.nl, http://www.wkap.nl/journalhome.htm/1389-9600. Eds. Fred H Menko, Hans Vasen, Henry Lynch. Pub. Carolijn van den Reydt. **Subscr. in the Americas to:** Kluwer Academic - Plenum Publishers, 233 Spring St, New York, NY 10013-1578. TEL 212-620-8468, FAX 212-807-1047; **Subscr. to:** Journals Department, PO Box 322, Dordrecht 3300 AH, Netherlands. TEL 31-78-639-2392, FAX 31-78-654-6474.

616.99 DEU
FOCUS ON CANCER. Text in English. 1995. irreg., latest vol.3, 1996. **Document type:** *Monographic series.* **Description:** Provides overviews of general aspects of cancer for oncologists as well as for involved professionals who are not specialists.
Published by: Springer-Verlag (Subsidiary of: BertelsmannSpringer), Haber Str 7, Heidelberg 69126, Germany. FAX 49-30-82787448, orders@springer.de, http://www.springer.de, http://link.springer-ny.com. Ed. D Malkin.

616.99 DEU ISSN 1435-7402
FOCUS ONKOLOGIE. Text in German. 1998. 8/yr. EUR 80.29 domestic; EUR 87.29 foreign; EUR 46.64 domestic to students; EUR 53.64 foreign to students; EUR 15.89 newsstand/cover (effective 2002). adv. **Document type:** *Journal, Academic/Scholarly.*
Published by: Urban und Vogel Medien und Medizin Verlagsgesellschaft mbH (Subsidiary of: BertelsmannSpringer), Neumarkter Str 43, Munich 81673, Germany. TEL 49-89-43721411, FAX 49-89-43721410, verlag@urban-vogel.de, http://www.urban-vogel.de. Ed. Martin Roos. R&P Friederik Klein. Adv. contact Sibylle Schurr TEL 49-89-43721353. Circ: 12,000 (paid). **Subscr. to:** Springer Auslieferungs Gesellschaft, Postfach 105160, Heidelberg 69041, Germany. TEL 49-6221-345244, FAX 49-6221-345244.

616.994 ITA ISSN 0392-047X
FOLIA ONCOLOGICA. Text in English, Italian; Summaries in English. 1978. q. ITL 50,000, USD 50 (effective 1994). bk.rev. **Document type:** *Academic/Scholarly.*
Indexed: Excerp.Med.
—EMDOCS, GNLM.
Published by: (Istituto Scientifico Oncologico), Ciemme, Via Curzio dei Mille, 2, Bari, BA 70122, Italy. TEL 39-80-5555480, FAX 39-80-5555119. Ed. Luigi Marinaccio. Circ: 600. **Subscr. to:** I.S.O., Via Giovanni Amendola, 209, Bari, BA 70126, Italy.

616.99 362.1 FRA ISSN 0180-9792
FONDAMENTAL✱. Text in French. 1978. q. FRF 40; FRF 10 newsstand/cover (effective 1997). adv. bk.rev. **Description:** Informs on cancer research and prevention.
Published by: Association pour la Recherche sur le Cancer (ARC), 16 av. Paul Vaillant Couturier, Villejuif Cedex 94800, France. TEL 33-1-45595959, FAX 33-1-47260475. Ed. Thierry Hercend. Adv. contact Michel Lucas.

FRONTIERS OF RADIATION THERAPY AND ONCOLOGY. see *MEDICAL SCIENCES—Radiology And Nuclear Medicine*

616.99 616.3 CHE ISSN 1064-9700 CODEN: GICAE2
G I CANCER; an international journal on gastrointestinal oncology. (Gastrointestinal) Text in English. 1993. 4/yr. GBP 80, USD 118 to individuals; GBP 234, USD 350 to institutions (effective 2002). **Document type:** *Academic/Scholarly.* **Description:** Features multidisciplinary clinical and laboratory data on gastrointestinal oncology for all physicians, urgeons, pure scientists, epidemiologists, pathologists, oncologists, radiologists and radiotherapists.
Related titles: CD-ROM ed.; Microform ed.; Online - full text ed.: (from RoweCom Information Quest).
Indexed: Curr.Cont. (coverage dropped), Excerp.Med. (1996-), Inpharma, Pharm.&Out.News, Reac., Sci.Cit.Ind. (coverage dropped).
—BLDSC (4169.100000), CISTI, GNLM, Infotrieve, KNAW. **CCC.**
Published by: Gordon and Breach - Harwood Academic (Subsidiary of: Taylor & Francis Group), PO Box 531, Lausanne 1000, Switzerland. http://www.gbhap.com/GI_Cancer/. Ed. John W L Fielding. **Subscr. addr. in US:** International Publishers Direct, PO Box 32160, Newark, NJ 07102. FAX 215-750-6343.

616.994 JPN
GAN KANGO/JAPANESE JOURNAL OF CANCER CARE. Text in Japanese. 3/yr. JPY 10,000. **Document type:** *Academic/Scholarly.*
Published by: Nankodo Co. Ltd., 42-6 Hongo 3-chome, Bunkyo-ku, Tokyo 113-0033, Japan. FAX 03-3811-7230.

616.99 JPN
GAN KANJA TO TAISHO RYOHO/SYMPTOM CONTROL IN CANCER PATIENTS. Text in Japanese. 1989. a. JPY 2,400 (effective 1998).
Published by: Medikaru Rebyusha/Medical Review Co., Ltd., 7-3 Hirano-Machi 1-chome, Chuo-ku, Osaka-shi 541-0046, Japan. TEL 81-6-223-1667, FAX 81-6-223-1338, mreview@osk3.3web.ne.jp.

616.9 JPN ISSN 0385-0684 CODEN: GTKRDX
GAN TO KAGAKU RYOHO/JAPANESE JOURNAL OF CANCER AND CHEMOTHERAPY. Text in Japanese; Summaries in English. 1974. m. JPY 39,840 (effective 2001). adv. bk.rev. Supplement avail. *Refereed.* **Document type:** *Journal, Academic/Scholarly.*
Indexed: Chem.Abstr., Chem.Indus.Notes, Chem.Titles, Excerp.Med., INIS Atomind., Ind.Med. (1974-), Inpharma, Int.Nurs.Ind., Reac.
—BLDSC (4651.230000), CASDDS, CISTI, EMDOCS, GNLM, KNAW.
Published by: Japanese Journal of Cancer and Chemotherapy Publishers Inc., Risshu Bldg, 2-2-3 Nihonbashi, Chuo-ku, Tokyo 103-0027, Japan. TEL 81-3-3278-0052, FAX 81-3-3281-0435. Ed., Pub. Tetsuo Taguchi. Adv. contact Hachiro Sato. Circ: 6,000 (paid).

616.9 CHE ISSN 0072-0151 CODEN: GMCRDC
GANN MONOGRAPHS ON CANCER RESEARCH. Text in English. 1966. irreg., latest vol.49. CHF 280 per issue. bk.rev. *Refereed.* **Document type:** *Monographic series, Academic/Scholarly.* **Description:** Includes collected contributions on current topics in cancer problems and allied fields.
Indexed: Biol.Abstr., Chem.Abstr., Chem.Indus.Notes, Chem.Titles, Excerp.Med., INIS Atomind.
—BLDSC (4069.310500), CASDDS, CISTI, GNLM, KNAW.
Published by: (Japanese Cancer Association JPN), S. Karger AG, Allschwilerstr 10, PO Box, Basel 4009, Switzerland. TEL 41-61-306-1111, FAX 41-61-306-1234, karger@karger.ch, http://www.karger.com/bookseries/GAMOC. Circ: 2,000.

616.99 663 JPN ISSN 1436-3291
▼ **GASTRIC CANCER.** Text in English. 1999. q. (in 1 vol., 4 nos./vol.). EUR 220.40 domestic; EUR 216.80 in Germany for print & online eds.; EUR 60 newsstand/cover foreign for print & online eds. (effective 2002). **Document type:** *Academic/Scholarly.* **Description:** Devoted exclusively to studies of stomach neoplasms.
Related titles: Online - full content ed.: ISSN 1436-3305 (from EBSCO Publishing, Swets Blackwell); Online - full text ed.: (from Springer LINK, RoweCom Information Quest).
Published by: (Japanese Gastric Cancer Association), Springer-Verlag Tokyo, Eastern Book Service, Inc. (Subsidiary of: BertelsmannSpringer), 3-13 Hongo 3-chome, Bunkyo-ku, Tokyo 113-0033, Japan. TEL 81-3-3812-0617, orders@svt-ebs.co.jp, http://link.springer-ny.com/link/service/journals/10120/index.htm, http://link.springer.de. Eds. J R Siewert, O Kobori. **Subscr. in N. America to:** Springer-Verlag New York Inc., PO Box 2485, Secaucus, NJ 07096-2485. TEL 800-777-4643, 212-460-1500, 212-460-1526, FAX 201-348-4505, 212-473-6272, orders@springer-ny.com; **Subscr. to:** Springer-Verlag, c/o Gabriele Kubitza, Haberstrasse 7, Heidelberg 69126, Germany. TEL 49-6221-345242, FAX 49-6221-345229, subscriptions@springer.de, http://link.springer-ny.com. **Dist. by:** Eastern Book Service, Inc.. TEL 81-3-3818-0861, FAX 81-3-3818-0864, orders@svt-ebs.co.jp.

GENES, CHROMOSOMES & CANCER. see *BIOLOGY—Genetics*

616.99 ITA ISSN 0392-128X
GIORNALE ITALIANO DI ONCOLOGIA. Text in Italian; Summaries in English. 1981. q. ITL 80,000, USD 70 (effective 2001).
Indexed: Excerp.Med., Ref.Zh.
—BLDSC (4178.236000), CISTI, EMDOCS, GNLM, Infotrieve, KNAW. **CCC.**
Published by: C I C Edizioni Internazionali s.r.l., Corso Trieste 42, Rome, RM 00198, Italy. TEL 39-06-8412673, FAX 39-06-8412688, info@gruppocic.it, 1160199510. Pub. A Salvati.

616.99 150 ITA ISSN 1128-5516
▼ **GIORNALE ITALIANO DI PSICO-ONCOLOGIA.** Text in Italian; Summaries in Italian, English. 1999. s-a., latest vol.3, 2001. ITL 70,000, EUR 68 (effective 2000). adv. bk.rev. abstr. illus. 64 p./no. back issues avail.; reprints avail. *Refereed.* **Document type:** *Journal, Academic/Scholarly.* **Description:** Publishes original articles, case reports, editorials in the field of psycho-oncology. For oncologists and psychologists.
Published by: (Societa Italiana di Psico-Oncologica), Il Pensiero Scientifico Editore s.r.l., Via Bradano, 3-C, Rome, RM 00199, Italy. TEL 39-06-862821, FAX 39-06-86282250, pensiero@pensiero.it, http://www.pensiero.it. Eds. Gabriella Morasso, Luigi Grassi. Pub. Francesco De Fiore. Adv. contact Luciano De Fiore. B&W page XEU 955, color page XEU 1,291; 21 x 28. Circ: 1,200.

GLOSSARIUM ONCOLOGIA. see *PHARMACY AND PHARMACOLOGY*

GREAT BRITAIN. GOVERNMENT STATISTICAL SERVICE. CANCER STATISTICS REGISTRATIONS. ENGLAND AND WALES. see *MEDICAL SCIENCES—Abstracting, Bibliographies, Statistics*

616.99 USA
HEALTH VICTORY BULLETIN. Text in English. 1975. m. USD 20 (effective 1998). adv. bk.rev. index. back issues avail. **Document type:** *Bulletin, Newsletter.* **Description:** Covers current developments in cancer, health and nutrition with emphasis on practical information for the patient.
Formerly (until 1982): Cancer Victory Bulletin

M

Published by: Arlin J. Brown Information Center, Inc., PO Box 251, Fort Belvoir, VA 22060. TEL 540-752-9511, FAX 540-752-4324. Ed., Pub., R&P, Adv. contact Arlin J Brown. Circ: 300.

HELICOBACTER. see *BIOLOGY—Microbiology*

616.99 USA ISSN 0889-8588
RB145 CODEN: HCNAEQ
HEMATOLOGY - ONCOLOGY CLINICS OF NORTH AMERICA. Text in English. 1987. bi-m. USD 175 domestic to individuals; USD 199 in Canada to individuals; USD 225 elsewhere to individuals; USD 227 domestic to institutions; USD 277 foreign to institutions; USD 47 per issue foreign (effective 2001). *Refereed.* **Document type:** *Journal, Academic/Scholarly.* **Description:** Addresses a single topic in the management of patients with cancer and systemic disease.
Formed by the merger of (1982-1987): Clinics in Oncology (0261-9873); (1972-1987): Clinics in Haematology (0308-2261)
Related titles: Microform ed.: (from PQC); Online - full text ed.: (from Institute for Scientific Information).
Indexed: Biol.Abstr., CINAHL, Chem.Abstr., Curr.Adv.Ecol.Sci., Curr.Cont., Excerp.Med., Helminthol.Abstr., INIS Atomind., Ind.Med. (1987-), Ind.Sci.Rev., Inpharma, Nutr.Abstr., Pharm.&Out.News, Reac., Sci.Cit.Ind.
—BLDSC (4291.610000), CASDDS, CISTI, EMDOCS, GNLM, IDS, Infotrieve, ingenta, KNAW. **CCC.**
Published by: W.B. Saunders Co. (Subsidiary of: Harcourt Publishers Ltd.), 11830 Westline Industrial Dr, St Louis, MO 63146. TEL 800-325-4177, http://www.wbsaunders.com. **Subscr. to:** Periodicals Fulfillment, W B Saunders Co, 6277 Sea Harbor Dr, 4th Fl, Orlando, FL 32891-4800.

616.994 GBR ISSN 0309-0167
CODEN: HISTDD
HISTOPATHOLOGY. Text in English. 1977. m., latest vol.40, 2002. GBP 150 in Europe to individuals; USD 220 in North America to individuals; GBP 150 elsewhere to individuals; GBP 487 in Europe to institutions; USD 772 in North America to institutions; GBP 536 elsewhere to institutions (effective 2002). adv. bk.rev. illus. index. back issues avail.; reprint service avail. from ISI. *Refereed.* **Document type:** *Academic/Scholarly.* **Description:** Publishes original histopathological material with clinical application in the study of human disease. Designed to be of practical importance to diagnostic histopathologists and to investigate workers in clinicopathological fields of study.
Related titles: Online - full text ed.: ISSN 1365-2559. GBP 135 in Europe to individuals; USD 198 in North America to individuals; GBP 135 elsewhere to individuals; GBP 439 in Europe to institutions; USD 695 in North America to institutions; GBP 439 elsewhere to institutions (effective 2002) (from Ovid Technologies, Inc., EBSCO Publishing, O C L C Online Computer Library Center, Inc., RoweCom Information Quest, ingenta, Munksgaard & Blackwell Science's Synergy, Swets Blackwell, Institute for Scientific Information).
Indexed: ASCA, BBCI, Biol.Abstr., Curr.Adv.Cancer Res., Curr.Adv.Ecol.Sci., Curr.Cont., Dent.Ind., Dok.Arbeitsmed., Excerp.Med., Helminthol.Abstr., Ind.Med. (1977-), Ind.Sci.Rev., Inpharma, Int.Abstr.Biol.Sci., Neurosci.Cit.Ind., Pharm.&Out.News, Protozool.Abstr., Reac., Rev.Med.& Vet.Mycol., Sci.Cit.Ind., Vet.Bull.
—BLDSC (4316.027000), ADONIS, CISTI, EMDOCS, GNLM, IDS, ingenta, KNAW. **CCC.**
Published by: (International Academy of Pathology. British Division), Blackwell Science Ltd., PO Box 88, Oxford OX2 0NE, United Kingdom. TEL 44-1865-206180, 44-1865-206002, FAX 44-1865-206219, jnl.orders@blacksci.co.uk, http://www.blackwell-science.com/~cgilib/jnlpage.asp?Journal=histo&File=histo, http://www.blackwellpublishing.com. Ed. J C E Underwood. Pub. Elizabeth Whelan. R&P Sophie Savage. Adv. contact Jenny Applin. Circ: 2,850.

HORIZONS (LIVINGSTON). see *PHYSICAL FITNESS AND HYGIENE*

HUMAN ANTIBODIES. see *MEDICAL SCIENCES—Allergology And Immunology*

616.99 NLD ISSN 1389-2142
▼ **HUMAN CELL CULTURE.** Text in English. 1999. irreg. bk.rev. back issues avail. **Document type:** *Academic/Scholarly.*
—BLDSC (4336.034000).
Published by: Kluwer Law International (Subsidiary of: Wolters Kluwer N.V.), Laan van Meerdervoort 70, PO Box 85889, The Hague 2508 CN, Netherlands.

616.9 JPN ISSN 0913-8927
HYOGO KENRITSU SEIJINBYO SENTA KIYO/HYOGO MEDICAL CENTER FOR ADULTS. BULLETIN. Text in Japanese; Summaries in English, Japanese. 1962. a. **Document type:** *Bulletin.*
Former titles (until 1984): Hyogo Kenritsu Byoin Gan Senta Kiyo - Hyogo Cancer Hospital. Bulletin (0387-0944); (until 1973): Hyogoken Gan Senta Nenpo (0441-537X)
Indexed: INIS Atomind.
—CCC.
Published by: Hyogo Kenritsu Seijinbyo Senta, 13-17 Kita-Oji-cho, Akashi-shi, Hyogo-ken 673-0021, Japan.

616.994 GBR
I A QUARTERLY JOURNAL. Text in English. 1956. q. GBP 12. adv. pat, stat.
Published by: Ileostomy and Internal Pouch Support Group, Amblehurst House, PO Box 23, Mansfield, Notts NG18 4TT, United Kingdom. TEL 01623-28099. Ed. David Eades. Circ: 11,400.

616.99 FRA ISSN 0250-8613
I A R C BIENNIAL REPORT. Text in English. 1987. biennial. USD 13.
Formerly: I A R C Annual Report
Related titles: Microfiche ed.: (from CIS); French ed.: ISSN 1017-3412.
Indexed: IIS.
—GNLM.
Published by: (International Agency for Research on Cancer), I A R C, 150 Cours Albert Thomas, Lyon Cedex 8 69372, France. TEL 33-4-72-738485, FAX 33-4-72-738302, http://www.iarc.fr/. Circ: 3,000.

616.99 FRA ISSN 1027-5622
I A R C HANDBOOKS OF CANCER PREVENTION. (International Agency for Research on Cancer) Text in English. 1997. irreg., latest vol.4, 1999.
Published by: World Health Organization, International Agency for Research on Cancer, 150 Cours Albert Thomas, Lyon F-69372, France.

616.994 FRA ISSN 1017-1606
RC268.6 CODEN: IARMB8
I A R C MONOGRAPHS ON THE EVALUATION OF CARCINOGENIC RISKS TO HUMANS. Text in English. 1972. 3/yr. price varies. **Description:** Monographs comprise sections on physical and chemical data, technical products, use, occurrence and analysis, carcinogenicity in animals, other biological data, human epidemiological results and evaluations.
Former titles: I A R C Monographs on the Evaluation of the Carcinogenic Risk of Chemicals to Humans (0250-9555); (until 1978): I A R C Monographs on the Evaluation of Carcinogenic Risk of Chemicals to Man (0301-3944)
Indexed: Abstr.Hyg., Anal.Abstr., Biol.Abstr., Curr.Cont. (coverage dropped), Food Sci.& Tech.Abstr., Ind.Med. (1988-), Int.Abstr.Biol.Sci., NRN, Trop.Dis.Bull.
—BLDSC (4359.536700), CASDDS, CISTI, EMDOCS, GNLM, KNAW. **CCC.**
Published by: (International Agency for Research on Cancer), I A R C, 150 Cours Albert Thomas, Lyon Cedex 8 69372, France. TEL 33-4-72-738485, FAX 33-4-72-738302, TELEX 380023, press@iarc.fr, http://www.iarc.fr/. **Subscr. addr.:** I A R C Press or World Health Organization, Distribution and Sales Services, Geneva, 27 1211, Switzerland.

616.994 FRA ISSN 0300-5038
CODEN: IARCCD
I A R C SCIENTIFIC PUBLICATIONS. Text in French. 1971. irreg., latest vol.151. price varies. bk.rev. **Document type:** *Monographic series, Academic/Scholarly.* **Description:** Reviews issues concerning the epidemiology of cancer and the study of potential carcinogens in the human environment.
Indexed: Abstr.Hyg., Anal.Abstr., Biol.Abstr., Chem.Abstr., Curr.Cont. (coverage dropped), Dent.Ind., Dok.Arbeitsmed., Excerp.Med., Food Sci.& Tech.Abstr., Ind.Med. (1979-), Trop.Dis.Bull.
—BLDSC (4359.537000), CASDDS, CISTI, GNLM, KNAW. **CCC.**
Published by: (International Agency for Research on Cancer), I A R C, 150 Cours Albert Thomas, Lyon Cedex 8 69372, France. TEL 33-4-72-738485, FAX 33-4-72-738302, press@iarc.fr, http://www.iarc.fr/. **U.S. subscr. to:** I A R C Press Oxford University Press, 200 Madison Ave, New York, NY 10016.

616.99 FRA ISSN 1012-7348
I A R C TECHNICAL REPORTS. Text mainly in French; Text occasionally in English, Spanish. 1988. irreg., latest vol.36, 2000. price varies. **Document type:** *Monographic series.*
Published by: (International Agency for Research on Cancer), I A R C, 150 Cours Albert Thomas, Lyon Cedex 8 69372, France. TEL 33-4-72-738485, FAX 33-4-72-738302, press@iarc.fr, http://www.iarc.fr/.

616.99 362.1 DEU ISSN 0724-8016
ILCO-PRAXIS. Text in German. 1974. q. EUR 30 to membership. adv. bk.rev. **Document type:** *Newsletter.*
Formerly (until 1982): Deutsche Ilco-Praxis (0724-8024)
Published by: Deutsche Ilco, Landshuter Str 30, Freising 85356, Germany. FAX 49-8161-9343, deutsche.ilco@t-online.de, info@ilco.de, http://www.ilco.de. Ed. Helga Englert. Circ: 12,000.

616.994 GBR ISSN 0306-4905
IMPERIAL CANCER RESEARCH FUND. SCIENTIFIC REPORT. Text in English. 1973. a. free per issue to qualified personnel. **Document type:** *Academic/Scholarly.*
Related titles: Online - full text ed.
—BLDSC (8197.900000).
Published by: Imperial Cancer Research Fund, Lincoln's Inn Fields, Imperial Cancer Research Fund, London WC2A 3PX, United Kingdom. TEL 44-20-7269-3206, FAX 44-20-7269-3084, lib_info@icrf.icnet.uk, http://www.icnet.uk. Ed., R&P Angela Aldam TEL 44-20-7269-3371. Circ: 1,700 (controlled).

616.99 USA ISSN 1522-7510
▼ **IN TOUCH (MELVILLE)**; cancer prevention and treatment: the good health guide. Text in English. 1999. bi-m. USD 19.50 domestic; USD 25.50 in Canada; USD 34.50 elsewhere (effective 2001). adv. **Description:** Helps to improve the dialogue between cancer experts and the public.
Published by: P R R, Inc., 48 S Service Rd, Melville, NY 11747-2335. TEL 631-777-3800, 877-246-8682, FAX 631-777-8700, intouch@cancernetwork.com, http://www.intouchlive.com, http://www.cancernetwork.com. Eds. Randi Londer Gould, Dr. Steve Rosen. R&P Lisa Klepacki TEL 631-777-3800 ext 366. Adv. contact Jeannine Coronna. Circ: 80,000 (paid and controlled).

616.9 SVN ISSN 0079-9580
INCIDENCA RAKA V SLOVENIJI/CANCER INCIDENCE IN SLOVENIA. Text in English, Slovenian. 1957. a. free per issue. index. **Document type:** *Yearbook, Academic/Scholarly.*
Formerly: Rak v Sloveniji. Tabele
Published by: Onkoloski Institut/Institute of Oncology, Zaloska 2, Ljubljana 1000, Slovenia. TEL 386-1-4324113, vpompe@onko-i.si, http://www.onko-i.si. Ed. Gregor Sersia. Circ: 750.

616.994 IND ISSN 0019-509X
CODEN: IJCAAR
INDIAN JOURNAL OF CANCER. Text in English. 1963. q. (in 38 vols.). INR 240, USD 55 (effective 2001). adv. bk.rev. charts, illus, stat. 60 p./no. 2 cols./p. back issues avail.; reprint service avail. from IRC,PQC. *Refereed.* **Document type:** *Journal, Academic/Scholarly.* **Description:** Contains researches in the field of cancer.
Related titles: CD-ROM ed.; Microfilm ed.: (from PQC).
Indexed: Biol.Abstr., Chem.Abstr., Dent.Ind., Excerp.Med. (until 199?), ExtraMED, INIS Atomind., Ind.Med. (1963-), Vet.Bull.
—BLDSC (4410.550000), CASDDS, CISTI, GNLM, ingenta, KNAW, Linda Hall.
Published by: Indian Cancer Society, 74 Jerbai Wadia Rd., Parel, Mumbai, Maharashtra 400 012, India. TEL 91-22-4125238, FAX 91-22-4122351, bcrics@vsnl.com. Eds. Dr. Anita Borges, Dr. D J Jussawalla. adv.: B&W page INR 900, color page INR 1,200; 20 x 14.5. Circ: 1,500. **Co-sponsor:** Indian Association of Oncology.

616.994 DEU ISSN 1435-2486
INFO ONKOLOGIE. Text in German. 1998. bi-m. EUR 104.33 domestic; EUR 117.33 foreign; EUR 85.64 domestic to students; EUR 98.64 foreign to students; EUR 20.56 newsstand/cover (effective 2002). **Document type:** *Journal, Academic/Scholarly.*
Related titles: CD-ROM ed.
Published by: (Deutscher Krebsgesellschaft e.V., Arbeitsgemeinschaft Internistische Onkologie), Urban und Vogel Medien und Medizin Verlagsgesellschaft mbH (Subsidiary of: BertelsmannSpringer), Neumarkter Str 43, Munich 81673, Germany. TEL 49-89-43721411, FAX 49-89-43721410, verlag@urban-vogel.de, http://www.urban-vogel.de.

661.994 USA ISSN 1082-1341
INNOVATIONS IN BREAST CANCER CARE✶. Text in English. 1995. q.
Indexed: CINAHL.

M

Published by: Meniscus Educational Institute (Subsidiary of: Meniscus Ltd.), 18 Elizabeth St, West Conshohocken, PA 19428-2935. TEL 610-660-8080, FAX 610-660-9583, email@meniscus.com, http://www.meniscus.com. Ed. Susan B Baird.

616.994 MEX ISSN 0076-7131
INSTITUTO NACIONAL DE CANCEROLOGIA. REVISTA. Text in Spanish; Summaries in English. 1954. 4/yr. MXP 100 to individuals; MXP 120 domestic to institutions; USD 60 foreign to institutions. adv. charts, illus, stat. *Refereed.* **Document type:** *Academic/Scholarly.* **Description:** Provides original papers and clinal case work on cancer.
Related titles: CD-ROM ed.
Indexed: Excerp.Med., Ind.Med. (coverage dropped).
—BLDSC (7819.920000).
Published by: Instituto Nacional de Cancerologia, Ave. San FERNANDO 22, Centro Tlalpan, Mexico City, DF 14000, Mexico. TEL 52-5-6551437, FAX 52-5-5733627, mohar@cenids.ssa.gob.mx. Ed. Dr. Alejandro Mohar-Betancourt. R&P Alejandro Mohar Betancourt. Adv. contact Alicia Garfias Flores. Circ: 1,500 (paid). **Co-sponsors:** Sociedad Mexicana de Estudios Oncologicos; Union Internacional Contral el Cancer en Latinoamerica; Federacion Latinoamericana de Sociedades Contra el Cancer.

616.994 USA ISSN 0020-7136
RC261 CODEN: IJCNAW
INTERNATIONAL JOURNAL OF CANCER/JOURNAL INTERNATIONAL DU CANCER. Variant title: Predictive Oncology. Text in English, French. 1966. 30/yr. USD 2,495 worldwide to institutions (effective 2001). adv. bk.rev. charts, illus, abstr. s-a. index. back issues avail.; reprint service avail. from SWZ. *Refereed.* **Document type:** *Journal, Academic/Scholarly.* **Description:** Examines all topics relevant to experimental and clinical cancer research, with an emphasis on fundamental studies that have relevance to the understanding of human cancer.
Incorporates (1993-2000): Radiation Oncology Investigation (1065-7541)
Related titles: Microform ed.: (from PQC); Online - full text ed.: ISSN 1097-0215. 1996 (from EBSCO Publishing, Wiley InterScience, Institute for Scientific Information); ♦ Supplement: International Journal of Cancer. Supplement. ISSN 0898-6924.
Indexed: AIDS & Cancer Res., AIDS Abstr., ASCA, Abstr.Hyg., Agri.& Environ.Biotech.Abstr. (coverage dropped), Biol.Abstr., Biotech.& Bioeng.Abstr., C.I.S. Abstr., Chem.Abstr., Chem.Indus.Notes, Chem.Titles, Curr.Adv.Cell & Devel.Biol., Curr.Adv.Ecol.Sci., Curr.Adv.Gen.& Molec.Biol., Curr.Cont., Dairy Sci.Abstr., Dent.Ind., Derwent Biotech.Abstr., Dok.Arbeitsmed., Environ.Sci.Poll.Mgmt., Excerp.Med., Helminthol.Abstr., INIS Atomind., Ind.Med. (1966-), Ind.Sci.Rev., Ind.Vet., Inpharma, Int.Abstr.Biol.Sci., Int.Nurs.Ind., Med.& Pharm.Biotech.Abstr., Med.& Surg.Dermat., NRN, Neurosci.Cit.Ind., Nuc.Acids Abstr., Nutr.Abstr., Oncog.G.F.Abstr., Pharm.&Out.News, Pollut.Abstr., Poult.Abstr., Reac., Ref.Zh., Rev.Arom.& Med.Plants, Rev.Med.& Vet.Mycol., Risk Abstr., SSCI (coverage dropped), Saf.Sci.Abstr., Sci.Cit.Ind., Small Anim.Abstr., THA, Telegen, Trop.Dis.Bull., Vet.Bull., Virol.Abstr. (coverage dropped).
—BLDSC (4542.156000), CASDDS, CISTI, GNLM, IDS, ingenta, KNAW, Linda Hall. **CCC.**
Published by: (International Union Against Cancer), John Wiley & Sons, Inc., Journals (Subsidiary of: Wiley InterScience), 605 Third Ave, New York, NY 10158. TEL 212-850-6645, FAX 212-850-6021, subinfo@wiley.com, uscs-wis@wiley.com, http://journals.wiley.com/0020-7136/, http://www.wiley.com. Ed. N Odartchenko. adv.: B&W page GBP 640, color page GBP 1,515; trim 210 x 279. Circ: 1,350. **Subscr. outside the Americas to:** John Wiley & Sons Ltd., Baffins Ln, Chichester, Sussex PO19 IUD, United Kingdom. TEL 44-1243-779777, FAX 44-1243-843232, cs-journals@wiley.co.uk, http://www.wiley.co.uk.

616.994 USA ISSN 0898-6924
INTERNATIONAL JOURNAL OF CANCER. SUPPLEMENT. Text in English. 1987. irreg.
Related titles: ♦ Supplement to: International Journal of Cancer. ISSN 0020-7136.
Indexed: Ind.Med. (1987-).
—BLDSC (4542.156100).
Published by: John Wiley & Sons, Inc., Journals (Subsidiary of: Wiley InterScience), 605 Third Ave, New York, NY 10158. TEL 212-570-6645, 212-850-6645, FAX 212-850-6021, uscs-wis@wiley.com, http://www.wiley.com.

616.994 JPN ISSN 1341-9625
CODEN: IJCOF6
INTERNATIONAL JOURNAL OF CLINICAL ONCOLOGY. Text in English, Japanese. 1996. bi-m. (in 1 vol., 6 nos./vol.). EUR 215.40 domestic; EUR 211.80 in Germany for Print & Online Eds.; EUR 39 newsstand/cover foreign for Print & Online Eds. (effective 2002). adv. bk.rev. abstr, bibl, charts, illus. **Document type:** *Academic/Scholarly.*
Formerly (until 1996): Japan Society for Cancer Therapy. Journal (0021-4671)
Related titles: ♦ Online - full text ed.: International Journal of Clinical Oncology Online. ISSN 1437-7772.
Indexed: Biol.Abstr., Chem.Abstr., Chem.Titles, Dent.Ind., Excerp.Med., INIS Atomind., Ind.Med. (coverage dropped), Inpharma, Pharm.&Out.News, Reac.
—BLDSC (4542.170500), CASDDS, CISTI, GNLM, KNAW.
Published by: (Japan Society of Clinical Oncology/Nihon Gan Chiryo Gakkai), Springer-Verlag Tokyo, Eastern Book Service, Inc. (Subsidiary of: BertelsmannSpringer), 3-13 Hongo 3-chome, Bunkyo-ku, Tokyo 113-0033, Japan. TEL 81-3-3812-0617, FAX 81-3-3812-4699, orders@svt-ebs.co.jp, http://link.springer-ny.com/link/service/journals/10147/. Ed. Yoshio Yamaoka. **Subscr. in N. America to:** Springer-Verlag New York Inc., PO Box 2485, Secaucus, NJ 07096-2485. TEL 800-777-4643, 212-460-1526, FAX 201-348-4505, orders@springer-ny.com; **Subscr. outside N. America & Japan to:** Springer-Verlag, c/o Gabriele Kubitza, Haberstrasse 7, Heidelberg 69126, Germany. TEL 49-6221-345242, FAX 49-6221-345229, subscriptions@springer.de, http://link.springer.de, http://link.springer-ny.com; **Subscr. to:** Eastern Book Service, Inc., 3-13 Hongo 3-chome, Bunkyo-ku, Tokyo 113-8480, Japan.

616.994 JPN ISSN 1437-7772
INTERNATIONAL JOURNAL OF CLINICAL ONCOLOGY ONLINE. Text in English. bi-m. **Document type:** *Journal, Academic/Scholarly.*
Media: Online - full text (from EBSCO Publishing, RoweCom Information Quest, Swets Blackwell, Springer LINK). **Related titles:** ♦ Print ed.: International Journal of Clinical Oncology. ISSN 1341-9625.
Published by: Springer-Verlag Tokyo, Eastern Book Service, Inc. (Subsidiary of: BertelsmannSpringer), 3-13 Hongo 3-chome, Bunkyo-ku, Tokyo 113-0033, Japan. TEL 81-3-38120331, FAX 81-3-3812-0719, orders@svt-ebs.co.jp, http://link.springer.de, http://www.springer.de. **Subscr. in N. America to:** Springer-Verlag New York Inc., PO Box 2485, Secaucus, NJ 07096-2485. TEL 800-777-4643, FAX 201-348-4505; **Subscr. to:** Eastern Book Service, Inc., 3-13 Hongo 3-chome, Bunkyo-ku, Tokyo 113-8480, Japan. TEL 81-3-3818-0861, FAX 81-3-3818-0864, orders@svt-ebs.co.jp.

INTERNATIONAL JOURNAL OF GYNECOLOGICAL CANCER. see *MEDICAL SCIENCES—Obstetrics And Gynecology*

616.99 GBR ISSN 0265-6736
CODEN: IJHYEQ
INTERNATIONAL JOURNAL OF HYPERTHERMIA. Text in English. bi-m. GBP 597, USD 986 to institutions (effective 2002). adv. *Refereed.* **Document type:** *Academic/Scholarly.* **Description:** Provides a forum for the publication of research and clinical papers on hyperthermia, which fall largely into the three main categories: clinical studies, biological studies and techniques of heat delivery and temperature measurement.
Related titles: Online - full text ed.: ISSN 1464-5157 (from CatchWord Ltd., EBSCO Publishing, O C L C Online Computer Library Center, Inc., RoweCom Information Quest, Swets Blackwell, Institute for Scientific Information).
Indexed: ASCA, Chem.Abstr., Chem.Indus.Notes, Chem.Titles, Curr.Adv.Cancer Res., Curr.Adv.Cell & Devel.Biol., Curr.Adv.Ecol.Sci., Curr.Cont., Excerp.Med., INSPEC (Jan.1986-), Ind.Med. (1985-), Ind.Sci.Rev., Inpharma, Int.Abstr.Biol.Sci., Pharm.&Out.News, Reac., Sci.Cit.Ind.
—BLDSC (4542.297000), AskIEEE, CASDDS, CatchWord, CISTI, EMDOCS, GNLM, IDS, ingenta, KNAW. **CCC.**
Published by: (North American Hyperthermia Group), Taylor & Francis Group, Taylor & Francis Ltd., 11 New Fetter Ln, London EC4P 4EE, United Kingdom. TEL 44-20-7583-9855, FAX 44-20-7842-2298, info@tandf.co.uk, http://www.tandf.co.uk. Eds. Jens Overgaard, Mark Dewhirst, Y Tanaka. **Subscr. in N. America to:** Taylor & Francis Ltd., 325 Chestnut St, Suite 800, Philadelphia, PA 19016. TEL 800-354-1420, FAX 215-625-8914, info@taylorandfrancis.com, http://www.taylorandfrancis.com/.

616.98 574 ITA ISSN 1128-935X
QH301 CODEN: MBENDX
INTERNATIONAL JOURNAL OF MEDICINE, BIOLOGY AND THE ENVIRONMENT. Text in English. 1971. s-a. USD 110 to individuals; USD 50 to members (effective 2000). adv. charts, illus. index. *Refereed.* **Document type:** *Journal, Academic/Scholarly.* **Description:** Disseminates information of relevance to histo-cytological, molecular and clinical pathology, oncology, radio-photo-biology, pharmacology, nutrition and health.
Formerly: Medecine, Biologie, Environnement (0302-0800)
Indexed: Chem.Abstr., Chem.Indus.Notes, Chem.Titles, Excerp.Med.
—BLDSC (4542.351100), CASDDS, EMDOCS.
Published by: (International Society for Nutrition and Cancer (I S N A C) USA, European Institute of Ecology and Cancer), Medicine Biologie Environnement I N E C, c/o Lega Italiana Lotta Contro i Tumori, Piazza Botta, 10, Pavia, PV 27100, Italy. TEL 39-0382-506333, FAX 39-0382-303673, 39-0382-303673, http://w3.unipv.it/mbe/mbe.htm. Ed., R&P, Adv. contact Leonida Santamaria. Circ: 3,000 (paid and controlled).

616.99 GRC ISSN 1019-6439
CODEN: IJONES
INTERNATIONAL JOURNAL OF ONCOLOGY; an international journal devoted to oncology research and cancer treatment. Text in Greek. 1992. m. USD 350 in Europe to individuals (effective 2002); USD 390 elsewhere to individuals; USD 720 in Europe to institutions; USD 770 elsewhere to institutions (effective 2002). adv. bk.rev. charts, illus. *Refereed.* **Document type:** *Journal, Academic/Scholarly.* **Description:** Publishes original high-quality articles and reports in experimental and clinical cancer research.
Related titles: Online - full text ed.: (from Institute for Scientific Information).
Indexed: AIDS & Cancer Res., ASCA, Aqua.Sci.& Fish.Abstr., Cal.Tiss.Abstr., Chem.Abstr., Chem.Indus.Notes, Chem.Titles, Curr.Cont., Environ.Sci.Poll.Mgmt., Excerp.Med. (1993-), Ind.Med. (1992-), Ind.Sci.Rev., Inpharma, Int.Abstr.Biol.Sci., Neurosci.Cit.Ind., Oncog.G.F.Abstr., Pharm.&Out.News, Reac., Rev.Arom.& Med.Plants, Saf.Sci.Abstr., Sci.Cit.Ind., Virol.Abstr. (coverage dropped), Weed Abstr.
—BLDSC (4542.424600), CASDDS, CISTI, EMDOCS, GNLM, IDS, Infotrieve, KNAW. **CCC.**
Published by: Demetrios A. Spandidos Ed. & Pub., PO Box 18179, Athens 116 10, Greece. TEL 30-1-722-7809, FAX 30-1-752-3866, spandido@hol.gr. Circ: 700.

INTERNATIONAL JOURNAL OF PANCREATOLOGY. see *MEDICAL SCIENCES—Endocrinology*

618.92 CHE ISSN 1070-2903
INTERNATIONAL JOURNAL OF PEDIATRIC HEMATOLOGY - ONCOLOGY. Text in English. 1994. 6/yr. EUR 514 to institutions; EUR 803 to corporations (effective 2000). back issues avail. *Refereed.* **Document type:** *Academic/Scholarly.* **Description:** Provides a global forum for publication of papers on laboratory and clinical investigations encompassed by pediatric hematology and oncology. Promotes cross-fertilization of ideas among clinicians and scientists in pediatric hematology/oncology and related fields and facilitates productive interchanges of information among clinical investigators worldwide.
Related titles: CD-ROM ed.; Online - full text ed.: (from EBSCO Publishing, RoweCom Information Quest).
Indexed: ASCA, Curr.Cont. (coverage dropped), Excerp.Med. (1996-), Inpharma, Int.Abstr.Biol.Sci., Reac., Rev.Med.& Vet.Mycol.
—BLDSC (4542.449900), GNLM, Infotrieve. **CCC.**
Published by: Gordon and Breach - Harwood Academic (Subsidiary of: Taylor & Francis Group), PO Box 531, Lausanne 1000, Switzerland. http://www.gbhap.com/Pediatric_Hematology-Oncology/; http://biomednet.com/library/387. Ed. Erlinda Maria Gordon. **Subscr. addr. in US:** International Publishers Direct, PO Box 32160, Newark, NJ 07102. FAX 215-750-6343.

616.99 571.4 GBR ISSN 0955-3002
QH652 CODEN: IJRBE7
INTERNATIONAL JOURNAL OF RADIATION BIOLOGY. Text and summaries in English, French, German. 1959. m. GBP 493, USD 815 to individuals; GBP 1,170, USD 1,930 to institutions (effective 2002). adv. charts, illus. index. *Refereed.* **Document type:** *Academic/Scholarly.* **Description:** Contains original research and review papers on the effects of ionization, ultraviolet and visible radiation, accelerated particles, microwaves, ultrasound and heat and related modalities.
Formerly (until 1988): International Journal of Radiation Biology and Related Studies in Physics, Chemistry and Medicine (0020-7616)

Related titles: Microform ed.; Online - full text ed.: ISSN 1362-3095. 1996 (from CatchWord Ltd., EBSCO Publishing, O C L C Online Computer Library Center, Inc., RoweCom Information Quest, Swets Blackwell, Institute for Scientific Information).
Indexed: ASCA, BBCI, Biol.Abstr., Chem.Abstr., Chem.Cit.Ind., Chem.Indus.Notes, Chem.Titles, Crop Physiol.Abstr., Curr.Adv.Biochem., Curr.Adv.Cancer Res., Curr.Adv.Cell & Devel.Biol., Curr.Adv.Gen.& Molec.Biol., Curr.Cont., Curr.Ind.Stat., Dairy Sci.Abstr., Eng.Ind., Environ.Sci.Poll.Mgmt., Excerp.Med., Field Crop Abstr., Food Sci.& Tech.Abstr., Helminthol.Abstr., Herb.Abstr., Hort.Abstr., INIS Atomind., INSPEC (1971-), Ind.Med. (1988-), Ind.Sci.Rev., Ind.Vet., Inpharma, Int.Abstr.Biol.Sci., Nutr.Abstr., Pollut.Abstr., Poult.Abstr., Reac., Ref.Zh., Saf.Sci.Abstr., Sci.Cit.Ind., Seed Abstr., THA, Tox.Abstr., Vet.Bull.
—BLDSC (4542.517900), ADONIS, AskIEEE, CASDDS, CatchWord, CISTI, Ei, EMDOCS, GNLM, IDS, ingenta, Linda Hall. **CCC.**
Published by: Taylor & Francis Group, Taylor & Francis Ltd., 11 New Fetter Ln, London EC4P 4EE, United Kingdom. TEL 44-20-7583-9855, FAX 44-20-7842-2298, info@tandf.co.uk, http://www.tandf.co.uk. Ed. G Gordon Steel. **Subscr. in N. America to:** Taylor & Francis Ltd., 325 Chestnut St, Suite 800, Philadelphia, PA 19016. TEL 800-354-1420, FAX 215-625-8914, info@taylorandfrancis.com, http://www.taylorandfrancis.com/.

INTERNATIONAL JOURNAL OF SURGICAL PATHOLOGY. see *MEDICAL SCIENCES—Surgery*

616.992 ITA ISSN 1125-632X
INTERNATIONAL TRENDS IN ONCOLOGY. Text in Multiple languages. 1997. q. ITL 25,000, USD 15 (effective 2001). adv.
Published by: C I C Edizioni Internazionali s.r.l., Corso Trieste 42, Rome, RM 00198, Italy. TEL 39-06-8412673, FAX 39-06-8412688, info@gruppocic.it, 1160199510. Ed. A Salvati. adv.: B&W page XEU 2,065.83, color page XEU 2,633.93; 275 x 375.

616.994 CHE ISSN 0074-9206
INTERNATIONAL UNION AGAINST CANCER. PROCEEDINGS OF CONGRESS. Text in Multiple languages. quadrennial, latest 1994, 16th, New Delhi. **Document type:** *Proceedings.*
Published by: International Union Against Cancer, 3 rue de Conseil General, Geneva 1205, Switzerland. TEL 41-22-8091811, FAX 41-22-8091810, info@uicc.ch, http://www.uicc.ch.

616.992 USA
▼ **THE INTERNET JOURNAL OF ONCOLOGY.** Text in English. 2000. a. free per issue. adv. bk.rev. back issues avail. *Refereed.* **Document type:** *Academic/Scholarly.* **Description:** Provides information from the field of oncology, cancer prevention and cancer treatment; contains original articles, reviews, case reports, streaming slide shows, streaming videos, letters to the editor, press releases, and meeting information.
Media: Online - full content.
Published by: Internet Scientific Publications, L.L.C., 23 Rippling Creek Dr, Sugar Land, TX 77479. TEL 281-240-1533, FAX 281-240-1533, http://www.ispub.com/. Ed. Claire Verschraegen. R&P Hope Morrow TEL 832-754-0335.

▼ **THE INTERNET JOURNAL OF PAIN, SYMPTOM CONTROL AND PALLIATIVE CARE.** see *MEDICAL SCIENCES—Anaesthesiology*

INTERSCIENCE CONFERENCE ON ANTIMICROBIAL AGENTS AND CHEMOTHERAPY. PROGRAM AND ABSTRACTS. see *BIOLOGY—Microbiology*

616.99 RUS ISSN 0202-7127
RC280.B6
ITOGI NAUKI I TEKHNIKI. ONKOLOGIYA. Text in Russian. irreg., latest vol.18, 1989.
—GNLM, Linda Hall.
Published by: Vserossiiskii Institut Nauchnoi i Tekhnicheskoi Informatsii (VINITI), Usievicha ul 20-a, Moscow 125315, Russian Federation. TEL 7-095-1526441, FAX 7-095-943-0060. **Dist. by:** Mezhdunarodnaya Kniga, B Yakimanka 39, Moscow 117049, Russian Federation. TEL 7-095-2384967, FAX 7-095-2384634; **US dist. addr.:** East View Publications, 3020 Harbor Ln N, Minneapolis, MN 55447. TEL 612-550-0961.

616.99 158 AUT ISSN 0949-0213
JAHRBUCH DER PSYCHOONKOLOGIE. Text in German. 1993. irreg. price varies. **Document type:** *Monographic series, Academic/Scholarly.*
Published by: (Oesterreichische Gesellschaft fuer Psychoonkologie), Springer-Verlag Wien (Subsidiary of: BertelsmannSpringer), Sachsenplatz 4-6, PO Box 89, Vienna, W 1201, Austria. TEL 43-1-3302415-0, FAX 43-1-330242665, books@springer.at, http://www.springer.at. R&P Angela Foessl TEL 43-1-3302415517. **Dist. in N. America by:** Springer-Verlag, Journals. TEL 212-460-1500, FAX 212-473-6272, orders@springer-ny.com, books@springer.at, http://www.springer-ny.com.

616.994 JPN ISSN 0021-4949
CODEN: GANRAE
JAPANESE JOURNAL OF CANCER CLINICS/GAN NO RINSHO. Text in Japanese; Summaries in English. 1954. m. JPY 34,820. adv. bk.rev. abstr, charts, illus. index.
Indexed: Chem.Abstr., Dent.Ind., INIS Atomind., Ind.Med. (coverage dropped), Inpharma, Reac., Telegen.
—BLDSC (4651.250000), CASDDS, CISTI, GNLM.
Published by: Shinohara Publishers Inc., Yaguchi Bldg, 11-7 Hongo 2-chome, Bunkyo-ku, Tokyo 113-0033, Japan. TEL 03-3816-5311, FAX 03-3816-5314. Ed. Yoshikuni Shinohara. Circ: 3,800.

616.994 GBR ISSN 0910-5050
CODEN: JJCREP
JAPANESE JOURNAL OF CANCER RESEARCH. Text and summaries in English. 1907. m. GBP 125, USD 200 to individuals; GBP 425, USD 680 to institutions (effective 2002). adv. illus. index, cum.index. back issues avail.; reprint service avail. from ISI. *Refereed.* **Document type:** *Journal, Academic/Scholarly.* **Description:** Provides an overview of state-of-the-art cancer research in Japan.
Formerly (until 1985): Gann (0016-450X)
Related titles: Microform ed.: (from PQC,PMC); Online - full text ed.: (from ingenta, Institute for Scientific Information).
Indexed: AIDS & Cancer Res., ASCA, Biol.Abstr., Chem.Abstr., Chem.Indus.Notes, Chem.Titles, Curr.Adv.Biochem., Curr.Adv.Cancer Res., Curr.Adv.Cell & Devel.Biol., Curr.Adv.Ecol.Sci., Curr.Adv.Gen.& Molec.Biol., Curr.Cont., Dairy Sci.Abstr., Environ.Sci.Poll.Mgmt., Excerp.Med., INIS Atomind., Ind.Med. (1985-), Ind.Sci.Rev., Ind.Vet., Inpharma, Int.Abstr.Biol.Sci., NRN, Nutr.Abstr., Oncog.G.F.Abstr., Pharm.&Out.News, Pollut.Abstr., Reac., Ref.Zh., Rev.Med.& Vet.Mycol., Risk Abstr., SSCI (coverage dropped), Saf.Sci.Abstr., Sci.Cit.Ind., THA.
—BLDSC (4651.270000), CASDDS, CISTI, EMDOCS, GNLM, IDS, ingenta, KNAW. **CCC.**
Published by: (Japanese Cancer Association JPN), Oxford University Press, Academic Division, Great Clarendon St, Oxford OX2 6DP, United Kingdom. TEL 44-1865-267907, FAX 44-1865-267835, jjcr@bcasj.or.jp, jnl.info@oup.co.uk, http://www3.oup.co.uk/jjcanr/, http://www.oup.co.uk/journals. Ed. Masaaki Terada. Circ: 17,500. **Subscr. addr. in the Americas:** Oxford University Press, Journals, 2001 Evans Rd, Cary, NC 27513. TEL 919-677-0977, 800-852-7323, FAX 919-677-1714, jnlorders@oup-usa.org; **Subscr. to:** Journals Marketing, Great Clarendon St, Oxford OX2 6DP, United Kingdom.

616.994 GBR ISSN 0368-2811
CODEN: JJCOAC
JAPANESE JOURNAL OF CLINICAL ONCOLOGY. Text in English. 1971. m. GBP 70, USD 100 to individuals; GBP 105, USD 170 to institutions (effective 2002). bibl, charts, illus. back issues avail.; reprint service avail. from ISI. *Refereed.* **Document type:** *Journal, Academic/Scholarly.* **Description:** Publishes original high-quality articles and reviews on all aspects of clinical oncology; also epidemiology notes, clinical trial notes, interesting case reports with merits for clical oncologists, as well as data of basic research with relevance to clinical oncology are welcomed.
Related titles: CD-ROM ed.; Online - full text ed.: ISSN 1465-3621. GBP 94, USD 153 to institutions Online only (effective 2002) (from JICST, EBSCO Publishing, O C L C Online Computer Library Center, Inc., RoweCom Information Quest, ingenta, Swets Blackwell, Institute for Scientific Information).
Indexed: ASCA, Chem.Abstr., Curr.Cont., Dent.Ind., Excerp.Med., INIS Atomind., Ind.Med. (1971-), Inpharma, NRN, Oncog.G.F.Abstr., Pharm.&Out.News, Reac., Rev.Med.& Vet.Mycol., SSCI (coverage dropped), THA.
—BLDSC (4651.378000), CISTI, GNLM, IDS, ingenta, KNAW.
Published by: Oxford University Press, Academic Division, Great Clarendon St, Oxford OX2 6DP, United Kingdom. TEL 44-1865-267907, FAX 44-1865-267835, jnl.info@oup.co.uk, http://jjco.oupjournals.org/, http://www.oup.co.uk/journals. Ed. Dr. Kaoru Abe. R&P Masako Noda. Circ: 1,100. **US Subscr. addr.:** Oxford University Press, Journals, 2001 Evans Rd, Cary, NC 27513. TEL 800-852-7323, FAX 919-677-1714; **Subscr. to:** Journals Marketing, Great Clarendon St, Oxford OX2 6DP, United Kingdom.

616.9 USA ISSN 1094-4540
CODEN: JOBRFM
JOURNAL OF BRACHYTHERAPY INTERNATIONAL. Variant title: Brachytherapy International. Journal of Brachytherapy. Text in English. 1985. q. USD 70 domestic to individuals; USD 80 in Europe to individuals; USD 85 elsewhere to individuals; USD 150 domestic to institutions; USD 160 in Europe to institutions; USD 170 elsewhere to institutions (effective 2000). adv. bk.rev. illus, stat. back issues avail. *Refereed.* **Document type:** *Proceedings, Academic/Scholarly.* **Description:** Publishes original articles, reviews of selected subjects, and information on the techniques and clinical applications of interstitial irradiation, endovascular brachytherapy, systemic brachytherapy, and hyperthermia in the management of cancer, cardiac and other patients, including laboratory and experimental research relevant to clinical practice.
Formerly (until 1997): Endocurietherapy - Hyperthermia Oncology (8756-1689)
Indexed: Excerp.Med. (1995-).
—BLDSC (4954.280000), GNLM.
Published by: Endocurietherapy Research Foundation, Dept. of Radiation Oncology, Long Beach Memorial Medical Center, 2801 Atlantic Ave, Long Beach, CA 90806. TEL 562-933-2929, FAX 562-490-3738, ksheikh@memorialcare.org. Ed. A M Nisar Syed. Pub., R&P, Adv. contact Khalid M Sheikh. B&W page USD 700; trim 11 x 8.25. Circ: 1,000.

616.99 USA ISSN 0885-8195
RC266.5
JOURNAL OF CANCER EDUCATION. Text in English. 1986. q., latest vol.16, 2001. USD 104 domestic to individuals; USD 116 foreign to individuals; USD 174 domestic to institutions; USD 186 foreign to institutions; USD 30 newsstand/cover (effective 2001). adv. index. back issues avail. *Refereed.* **Document type:** *Journal, Academic/Scholarly.* **Description:** Addresses varied aspects of cancer education for physicians, dentists, nurses, students, social workers and other allied health professionals. Articles include reports of original results of educational research and discussions of current problems and techniques in cancer education.
Related titles: Microform ed.: (from PQC); Online - full text ed.: (from Institute for Scientific Information).
Indexed: CINAHL, Cont.Pg.Educ., Curr.Cont., ERA, Educ.Tech.Abstr., Excerp.Med., Ind.Med. (1986-), Int.Nurs.Ind., NRN, THA, Tech.Educ.Abstr.
—BLDSC (4954.843000), EMDOCS, GNLM, Infotrieve, ingenta. **CCC.**
Published by: (American Association for Cancer Education), Hanley & Belfus, Inc., 210 S 13th St, Philadelphia, PA 19107. TEL 215-546-7293, FAX 215-790-9330. Ed. Richard F Bakemeier. Adv. contact Diane R Sherel. B&W page USD 590;. Circ: 1,000.
Co-sponsor: European Association for Cancer Education.

616.994 DEU ISSN 0171-5216
CODEN: JCROD7
JOURNAL OF CANCER RESEARCH AND CLINICAL ONCOLOGY. Text in English. 1903. m. EUR 1,800.70 domestic; EUR 1,811.10 foreign; EUR 178 newsstand/cover foreign (effective 2002). adv. back issues avail.; reprint service avail. from ISI. *Refereed.* **Document type:** *Journal, Academic/Scholarly.* **Description:** Contains up-to-date articles within the fields of experimental and clinical oncology.
Formerly: Zeitschrift fuer Krebsforschung und Klinische Onkologie (0084-5353)
Related titles: Microform ed.: (from PQC); Online - full text ed.: ISSN 1432-1335 (from EBSCO Publishing, RoweCom Information Quest, Swets Blackwell, Springer LINK, Institute for Scientific Information); ♦ Supplement: Journal of Cancer Research and Clinical Oncology. Supplement. ISSN 0943-9382.

M

Indexed: ASCA, Agri.& Environ.Biotech.Abstr. (coverage dropped), Biol.Abstr., C.I.S. Abstr., Chem.Abstr., Chem.Indus.Notes, Chem.Titles, Curr.Adv.Cancer Res., Curr.Cont., Dairy Sci.Abstr., Derwent Biotech.Abstr., Environ.Sci.Poll.Mgmt., Excerp.Med., INIS Atomind., Ind.Med. (1979-), Ind.Sci.Rev., Ind.Vet., Inpharma, Int.Abstr.Biol.Sci., Med.& Surg.Dermat., NRN, Nutr.Abstr., Pharm.&Out.News, Pollut.Abstr., Protozool.Abstr., Reac., Rev.Med.& Vet.Mycol., Risk Abstr., SSCI (coverage dropped), Saf.Sci.Abstr., Sci.Cit.Ind., Vet.Bull.
—BLDSC (4954.851000), ADONIS, CASDDS, CISTI, GNLM, IDS, ingenta, KNAW. **CCC.**
Published by: (Deutsche Krebsgesellschaft), Springer-Verlag (Subsidiary of: BertelsmannSpringer), Tiergartenstr 17, Heidelberg 69121, Germany. TEL 49-6221-345-0, FAX 49-6221-345229, subscriptions@springer.de, http://link.springer.de/link/service/journals/00432/index.htm, http://www.springer.de. Ed. K Hoeffken. **Subscr. in N. America to:** Springer-Verlag New York Inc., PO Box 2485, Secaucus, NJ 07096-2485. TEL 212-460-1500, FAX 212-473-6272.

616.994 DEU ISSN 0943-9382
CODEN: JCCSE
JOURNAL OF CANCER RESEARCH AND CLINICAL ONCOLOGY. SUPPLEMENT. Text in English. irreg. **Document type:** *Academic/Scholarly.*
Related titles: ♦ Supplement to: Journal of Cancer Research and Clinical Oncology. ISSN 0171-5216.
Indexed: Excerp.Med. (1995-), Int.Abstr.Biol.Sci.
—ADONIS, KNAW.
Published by: (Deutsche Krebsgesellschaft), Springer-Verlag (Subsidiary of: BertelsmannSpringer), Haber Str 7, Heidelberg 69126, Germany. TEL 49-30-8207-0, FAX 49-30-8214091, orders@springer.de. **Subscr. in N. America to:** Springer-Verlag New York Inc., New York, NY 07096-2491. TEL 201-348-4505, 201-348-4033.

616.99 615.8 616.2 ITA ISSN 1120-009X
CODEN: JCHEEU
JOURNAL OF CHEMOTHERAPY. Text in English. 1978. bi-m., latest vol.13, 2001. EUR 150 domestic; USD 200 foreign (effective 2001). adv. abstr. index. back issues avail. *Refereed.* **Document type:** *Journal, Academic/Scholarly.* **Description:** Publishes original articles on experimental and clinical studies in antimicrobial and oncologic chemotherapy.
Former titles (until 1989): Chemioterapia (0392-906X); Which was formed by the 1982 merger of: Chemoterapia Antimicrobica (0391-9862); Chemoterapia Oncologica (0392-0968)
Related titles: CD-ROM ed.; Online - full text ed.: (from Institute for Scientific Information).
Indexed: ASCA, Chem.Abstr., Chem.Indus.Notes, Chem.Titles, Curr.Cont., Excerp.Med., Ind.Med. (1989-), Inpharma, Pharm.&Out.News, Protozool.Abstr., Reac., Ref.Zh., Rev.Med.& Vet.Mycol.
—BLDSC (4957.390000), ADONIS, CASDDS, CISTI, EMDOCS, GNLM, IDS, Infotrieve, ingenta, KNAW. **CCC.**
Published by: (Italian Society of Immunopharmacology), E I F T srl, Via Venti Settembre, 102, Florence, FI 50129, Italy. TEL 39-055-486147, FAX 39-055-474426, info@jchemother.it, http://www.jchemother.it. Eds. Piero Periti, Teresita Mazzei. Pub. Piero Periti. R&P, Adv. contact Mary Forrest. Circ: 700.

616.992 USA ISSN 0732-183X
RC254.A1 CODEN: JCONDN
JOURNAL OF CLINICAL ONCOLOGY. Text in English. 1983. 24/yr. USD 319 domestic to individuals for print & online eds.; USD 450 foreign to individuals for print & online eds.; USD 446 domestic to institutions for print & online eds.; USD 577 foreign to institutions for print & online eds.; USD 24 newsstand/cover (effective 2002). adv. abstr, bibl, charts, illus. index. back issues avail. *Refereed.* **Document type:** *Academic/Scholarly.* **Description:** Contains articles from around the world discussing the diagnosis, management, treatment, and prevention of cancer.
Related titles: Online - full text ed.: 1983. USD 579.80 domestic academic site license; USD 710.80 foreign academic site license; USD 646.70 domestic corporate site license; USD 777.70 foreign corporate site license (effective 2002) (from EBSCO Publishing, Institute for Scientific Information).
Indexed: ASCA, Abstr.Health Care Manage.Stud., CINAHL, Chem.Abstr., Chem.Indus.Notes, Chem.Titles, Chic.Per.Ind., Curr.Cont., Dent.Ind., Derwent Biotech.Abstr., Excerp.Med., INIS Atomind., I.P.A., Ind.Med. (1983-), Ind.Sci.Rev., Inpharma, Int.Abstr.Biol.Sci., Jrnl.Watch, Kidney, Med.& Surg.Dermat., NRN, Neurosci.Cit.Ind., Pharm.&Out.News, Reac., Rev.Med.& Vet.Mycol., SSCI (coverage dropped), Sci.Cit.Ind., Soyabean Abstr., THA.
—BLDSC (4958.615000), CASDDS, CISTI, EMDOCS, GNLM, IDS, ingenta, KNAW. **CCC.**
Published by: (American Society of Clinical Oncology), Lippincott Williams & Wilkins (Philadelphia) (Subsidiary of: Wolters Kluwer N.V.), 530 Walnut St, Philadelphia, PA 19106-3621. TEL 301-223-2300, 800-638-3030, FAX 301-223-2400, jco-fb@highwire.stanford.edu, http://www.jco.org/, http://www.lww.com. adv.: B&W page USD 1,715, color page USD 3,215; 10 x 7. Circ: 17,658. **Subscr. to:** Periodicals Fulfillment.

JOURNAL OF ENVIRONMENTAL SCIENCE AND HEALTH. PART C: ENVIRONMENTAL CARCINOGENESIS & ECOTOXICOLOGY REVIEWS. see *ENVIRONMENTAL STUDIES—Toxicology And Environmental Safety*

616.99 ITA ISSN 0392-9078
CODEN: JECRDN
JOURNAL OF EXPERIMENTAL AND CLINICAL CANCER RESEARCH. Text in English. 1982. q. ITL 100,000, USD 100 (effective 1994). *Refereed.* **Document type:** *Academic/Scholarly.* **Description:** Publishes original contributions dealing with basic and applied research in the field of experimental and clinical oncology.
Related titles: Online - full text ed.: (from Institute for Scientific Information).
Indexed: ASCA, Abstr.Hyg., Chem.Abstr., Chem.Indus.Notes, Chem.Titles, Curr.Cont., INIS Atomind., Ind.Med. (1982-), Inpharma, NRN, Nutr.Abstr., Pharm.&Out.News, Reac., Ref.Zh., Rev.Arom.& Med.Plants, Rev.Med.& Vet.Mycol.
—BLDSC (4979.740000), CASDDS, CISTI, EMDOCS, GNLM, IDS, KNAW.
Published by: Regina Elena Institute for Cancer Research, Via Delle Messi D'Oro, 156, Rome, RM 00158, Italy. TEL 39-6-4985536, FAX 39-6-4180473. Ed. Dr. Ercole Sega.

THE JOURNAL OF EXPERIMENTAL MEDICINE. see *MEDICAL SCIENCES—Experimental Medicine, Laboratory Technique*

616.99 USA ISSN 1359-4117
CODEN: JETOFX
JOURNAL OF EXPERIMENTAL THERAPEUTICS AND ONCOLOGY. Text in English. 1996. bi-m. USD 150 domestic to individuals; USD 170 in Canada & Mexico to individuals; USD 200 elsewhere to individuals; USD 495 domestic to institutions; USD 515 in Canada & Mexico to institutions; USD 545 elsewhere to institutions; USD 165 to individuals print & online eds. combined; USD 544.50 to institutions print & online eds. combined (effective 2001). adv. *Refereed.* **Document type:** *Journal, Academic/Scholarly.* **Description:** Designed to communicate, encourage, and support the work of those dedicating their time and effort to cancer treatments.
Related titles: ♦ Online - full text ed.: Journal of Experimental Therapeutics and Oncology Online.
Indexed: Chem.Abstr., Chem.Indus.Notes, Chem.Titles.
—CASDDS, CISTI, GNLM, Infotrieve. **CCC.**
Published by: (Anticancer Therapeutics and Oncology Society GBR), Blackwell Science Inc., Commerce Pl, 350 Main St, Malden, MA 02148-5018. TEL 781-388-8250, 888-661-5800, FAX 781-388-8255, journals@blacksci.com, http://www.blackwell-science.com. Ed. Dominic Fan.

616.99 USA
▼ **JOURNAL OF EXPERIMENTAL THERAPEUTICS AND ONCOLOGY ONLINE.** Text in English. 2000. bi-m. USD 135 to individuals; USD 446 to institutions (effective 2001). **Document type:** *Academic/Scholarly.*
Media: Online - full text (from Swets Blackwell). **Related titles:** ♦ Print ed.: Journal of Experimental Therapeutics and Oncology. ISSN 1359-4117.
Published by: Blackwell Science Inc., Commerce Pl, 350 Main St, Malden, MA 02148-5018. TEL 781-388-8250, 888-661-5800, FAX 781-388-8255, journals@blacksci.com, http://www.blackwell-science.com.

616.99 USA ISSN 0167-594X
CODEN: JNODD2
JOURNAL OF NEURO-ONCOLOGY. Text in English. 1983. 15/yr. USD 1,400, EUR 1,397 to institutions for print or online ed.; USD 1,680, EUR 1,676.40 to institutions for print & online eds.combined (effective 2002). adv. bk.rev. back issues avail.; reprint service avail. from SWZ,PQC. *Refereed.* **Document type:** *Journal, Academic/Scholarly.* **Description:** Encompasses basic, applied and clinical investigations in all research areas as they relate to cancer and the central nervous system.
Related titles: Microform ed.: (from PQC); Online - full text ed.: (from Ovid Technologies, Inc., EBSCO Publishing, O C L C Online Computer Library Center, Inc., RoweCom Information Quest, Swets Blackwell, Kluwer Online, Institute for Scientific Information).
Indexed: ASCA, Chem.Abstr., Curr.Adv.Biochem., Curr.Adv.Cell & Devel.Biol., Curr.Cont., Excerp.Med., Ind.Med. (1983-), Ind.Sci.Rev., Inpharma, Int.Abstr.Biol.Sci., Neurosci.Cit.Ind., Reac., Rev.Med.& Vet.Mycol., Sci.Cit.Ind.
—BLDSC (5021.650000), CASDDS, CISTI, GNLM, IDS, ingenta, KNAW. **CCC.**
Published by: Kluwer Academic Publishers Boston, 101 Philip Dr, Assinippi Park, Norwell, MA 02061. TEL 781-871-6600, FAX 781-871-9045, services@wkap.nl, http://www.wkap.nl/journalhome.htm/0167-594X. Ed. Joseph M Piepmeier. R&P Rose Luongo TEL 781-871-6311. **Subscr. outside the Americas to:** Kluwer Academic Publishers Group, Journals Department, PO Box 322, Dordrecht 3300 AH, Netherlands. TEL 31-78-639-2392, FAX 31-78-654-6474; **Subscr. to:** Kluwer Academic - Plenum Publishers, 233 Spring St, New York, NY 10013-1578. TEL 212-620-8468, FAX 212-807-1047.

616.99 USA ISSN 1061-9364
JOURNAL OF ONCOLOGY MANAGEMENT✱. Text in English. 1992. bi-m. USD 45; USD 54 in Canada; USD 60 elsewhere. adv. **Description:** Disseminates information and ideas among professionals involved in day-to-day management and administrative duties in hospital, university and freestanding cancer programs.
—BLDSC (5026.314550).
Published by: Knolls Publishing Group, Inc., 105 Raider Blvd, Belle Mead, NJ 08502-1510. TEL 201-285-0855, FAX 201-285-1472. Ed. Nancy Salerno Davis. Adv. contact Stuart G Mann. Circ: 11,564.

JOURNAL OF ONCOLOGY PHARMACY PRACTICE. see *PHARMACY AND PHARMACOLOGY*

618.92 616.99 USA ISSN 1077-4114
RJ411 CODEN: JPHOFG
JOURNAL OF PEDIATRIC HEMATOLOGY - ONCOLOGY. Text in English. 1979. 9/yr. USD 280 domestic to individuals; USD 336 foreign to individuals; USD 455 domestic to institutions; USD 528 foreign to institutions (effective 2002). adv. bk.rev. abstr, bibl, charts, illus, stat, tr.lit. index. back issues avail.; reprint service avail. from PQC. *Refereed.* **Document type:** *Journal, Academic/Scholarly.* **Description:** Reports on advances in the diagnosis and treatment of cancer and blood diseases in children.
Formerly (until 1995): American Journal of Pediatric Hematology - Oncology (0192-8562)
Related titles: Microform ed.; Online - full text ed.: USD 591.50 domestic academic site license; USD 659.75 domestic corporate site license; USD 664.50 foreign academic site license; USD 732.75 foreign corporate site license (effective 2002) (from Ovid Technologies, Inc., Institute for Scientific Information).
Indexed: ASCA, Curr.Cont., Dent.Ind., Excerp.Med., INIS Atomind., Ind.Med. (1995-), Ind.Sci.Rev., Inpharma, Int.Abstr.Biol.Sci., Int.Nurs.Ind., Pharm.&Out.News, Reac., Rev.Med.& Vet.Mycol., Sci.Cit.Ind.
—BLDSC (5030.183000), CASDDS, CISTI, EMDOCS, GNLM, IDS, ingenta, KNAW.
Published by: (American Society of Pediatric Hematology, Oncology), Lippincott Williams & Wilkins (Philadelphia) (Subsidiary of: Wolters Kluwer N.V.), 530 Walnut St, Philadelphia, PA 19106-3621. TEL 215-521-8300, FAX 215-521-8902, http://www.lrpub.com. Ed. Dr. Robert J Arceci. Pub. Robert Emenecker. R&P Margaret Becker. Adv. contact Ray Thibodeau. B&W page USD 1,055, color page USD 2,150. Circ: 1,800. **Subscr. to:** PO Box 1600, Hagerstown, MD 21740-1600. TEL 800-777-2295, FAX 301-824-7390.

616.99 610.73 USA ISSN 1043-4542
CODEN: JONUEM
JOURNAL OF PEDIATRIC ONCOLOGY NURSING. Text in English. 1984. bi-m. USD 89 domestic to individuals; USD 145 foreign to individuals; USD 175 domestic to institutions; USD 211 foreign to institutions; USD 53 domestic to students; USD 87 foreign to students; USD 36 newsstand/cover (effective 2001). adv. bk.rev. bibl. *Refereed.* **Document type:** *Journal, Academic/Scholarly.* **Description:** Stimulates and disseminates research in the treatment of young cancer patients with emphasis on holistic, family-centered care.
Related titles: Online - full text ed.: (from IDEAL Online Library).
Indexed: AMED, CINAHL, Fam.Ind., Ind.Med. (1989-), Int.Nurs.Ind.
—BLDSC (5030.195000), GNLM, Infotrieve, ingenta. **CCC.**

M

Published by: (Association of Pediatric Oncology Nurses), W.B. Saunders Co. (Subsidiary of: Harcourt Publishers Ltd.), 11830 Westline Industrial Dr, St Louis, MO 63146. TEL 800-325-4177, http://www.wbsaunders.com. Ed. Nancy E Kline. adv.: B&W page USD 865, color page USD 2,065; trim 10 x 7. Circ: 2,660. **Subscr. to:** Journal Subscription Fulfillment, 6277 Sea Harbor Dr, 4th Fl, Orlando, FL 32887-4800. TEL 800-654-2452, FAX 800-874-6418.

616.9 USA ISSN 0734-7332
RC261.A1
JOURNAL OF PSYCHOSOCIAL ONCOLOGY; the official journal of the association of oncology social work. Text in English. 1983. q. USD 75 to individuals; USD 101 in Canada to individuals; USD 109 elsewhere to individuals; USD 240 to institutions; USD 324 in Canada to institutions; USD 348 elsewhere to institutions; USD 420 to libraries; USD 567 in Canada to libraries; USD 609 elsewhere to libraries (effective Aug. 2001). adv. bk.rev. back issues avail.; reprint service avail. from HAW. *Refereed.* **Document type:** *Journal, Academic/Scholarly.* **Description:** Publishes for health professionals responsible for psychosocial needs of cancer patients and their families.
Related titles: Microfiche ed.: (from PQC); Microform ed.; Online - full text ed.: (from Institute for Scientific Information).
Indexed: AMED, ASCA, Abstr.Soc.Geront., Behav.Med.Abstr., CINAHL, Curr.Cont., Environ.Sci.Poll.Mgmt., Excerp.Med., Fam.Ind., IMFL, Lang.& Lang.Behav.Abstr., Past.Care & Couns.Abstr., PsycInfo, Psychol.Abstr. (1983-), Ref.Zh., Rehabil.Lit., SOPODA, SSCI, Saf.Sci.Abstr., Soc.Serv.Abstr., Soc.Work Res.& Abstr., Sociol.Abstr., Sp.Ed.Needs Abstr., e-psyche.
—BLDSC (5043.476000), EMDOCS, GNLM, Haworth, IDS, ingenta, KNAW.
Published by: Haworth Press, Inc., 10 Alice St, Binghamton, NY 13904-1580. TEL 607-722-5857, 800-429-6784, FAX 607-722-6362, 800-895-0582, getinfo@haworthpressinc.com, http://www.haworthpress.com/journals/journallist.asp. Eds. Grace H Christ, James R Zabora. Pub. William Cohen. R&P Ruthann Heath TEL 607-723-5857 ext 316. Adv. contact Jackie Blakeslee TEL 607-722-5857 ext 346. B&W page USD 315, color page USD 550; trim 6 x 8.5. Circ: 2,400.

JOURNAL OF SURGICAL ONCOLOGY. see *MEDICAL SCIENCES—Surgery*

JOURNAL OF TOXICOLOGY AND ENVIRONMENTAL HEALTH. PART A. see *ENVIRONMENTAL STUDIES—Toxicology And Environmental Safety*

JOURNAL OF TOXICOLOGY AND ENVIRONMENTAL HEALTH. PART B: CRITICAL REVIEWS. see *ENVIRONMENTAL STUDIES—Toxicology And Environmental Safety*

616.99 USA ISSN 0886-3849
CODEN: JTMOEY
JOURNAL OF TUMOR MARKER ONCOLOGY. Text in English. 1986. q. USD 120; USD 160 foreign. *Refereed.* **Description:** Covers tumor markers and their applications in the diagnosis and treatment of malignant neoplasms. Includes new markers for clinical application, and basic research on their physiological behavior and role in malignant neoplasms.
Related titles: Online - full text ed.: (from Institute for Scientific Information).
Indexed: ASCA, Biotech.Cit.Ind., Curr.Cont., Excerp.Med., Inpharma, Pharm.&Out.News, Reac., Sci.Cit.Ind.
—BLDSC (5071.250000), CASDDS, CISTI, GNLM, IDS.
Published by: International Academy of Tumor Marker Oncology, Schwarzspanierstr. 15, Vienna 1090, Austria.

KOSANKINBYO KENKYUSHO ZASSHI. see *MEDICAL SCIENCES—Communicable Diseases*

616.99 DEU ISSN 0177-0853
RC267
KREBSFORSCHUNG HEUTE. Text in German. 1978. biennial. DEM 35 (effective 2000). **Document type:** *Academic/Scholarly, Corporate.*
—GNLM.
Published by: Deutsches Krebsforschungszentrum, Im Neuenheimer Feld 280, Heidelberg 69120, Germany. TEL 49-6221-422854, FAX 49-6221-422995.

616.99 DEU
KREBSNACHSORGE UND REHABILITATION. Text in German. 1989. irreg., latest vol.5, 1995. **Document type:** *Academic/Scholarly.*
Published by: W. Zuckschwerdt Verlag GmbH, Industriestr 1, Germering 82110, Germany. TEL 49-89-894349-0, FAX 49-89-89434950. Ed. H G Delbrueck.

L M S ALERT. CANCER CHEMOTHERAPY. (Literature Monitoring and Evaluation Service) see *MEDICAL SCIENCES—Abstracting, Bibliographies, Statistics*

616.992 GBR ISSN 1470-2045
▼ **THE LANCET ONCOLOGY.** Text in English. 2000. m. USD 330 in United States to institutions print with multiple access; GBP 205 elsewhere to institutions print with multiple access (effective 2002).
Related titles: Online - full text ed.: (from ScienceDirect).
—BLDSC (5146.090000).
Published by: The Lancet Publishing Group (Subsidiary of: Reed Elsevier plc), 84 Theobald's Rd, London WC1X 8RR, United Kingdom. TEL 44-20-7436-4981, 44-20-7611-4102, FAX 44-20-7611-4479, lanceteditorial@elsevier.co.uk, custserv@lancet.com, http://www.elsevier.com/locate, http://www.thelancet.com. Eds. E Hutchinson, S Silver.

616.99 FRA ISSN 1165-113X
LA LETTRE DU CANCEROLOGUE. Text in French. 1992. bi-m. FRF 300 domestic to individuals; FRF 420, USD 76 foreign to individuals; FRF 380 domestic to institutions; FRF 500, USD 91 foreign to institutions; FRF 190 domestic to students; USD 56 foreign to students (effective 2000). Supplement avail. *Refereed.* **Document type:** *Academic/Scholarly.*
Published by: Edimark S.A., 62-64 rue Jean Jaures, Puteaux 92800, France. TEL 33-1-414-58000, FAX 33-1-41458025, contact@edimark.fr, http://www.edimark.fr. Ed. J F Morere. Pub. Claudie Damour-Terrasson.

LEUKEMIA; normal and malignant hemopoiesis. see *MEDICAL SCIENCES—Hematology*

LEUKEMIA AND LYMPHOMA. see *MEDICAL SCIENCES—Hematology*

LEUKEMIA RESEARCH. see *MEDICAL SCIENCES—Hematology*

616.99 USA
LEUKEMIA SOCIETY OF AMERICA. NEWSLINE. Text in English. 1983. q. free per issue. bk.rev. illus. back issues avail.; reprints avail. **Document type:** *Newsletter.* **Description:** Informs patients, volunteers, grantees, and the public about the society's programs and advances in research.
Formerly: Leukemia Society of America. Society News
Published by: Leukemia Society of America, Inc., 600 Third Ave, 4th Fl, New York, NY 10016. TEL 212-573-8484, FAX 212-856-9686, http://www.leukemia.org. Ed., R&P Julie Farin TEL 212-450-8861. Circ: 86,000 (controlled).

616 HRV ISSN 0300-8142
CODEN: LBOCB3
LIBRI ONCOLOGICI; Croatian journal of oncology. Text in English; Summaries in Croatian. 1972. 3/yr. HRK 80; USD 30 foreign (effective 1999). adv. back issues avail. *Refereed.* **Document type:** *Academic/Scholarly.* **Description:** Examines primary and secondary prevention of malignant diseases, early diagnosis, screening, advances in treatments, terminal care, and basic research work in Molecular Biology, Genetics, Biochemistry & Immunology.
Indexed: Chem.Abstr., Excerp.Med.
—BLDSC (5207.350000), CASDDS, EMDOCS, GNLM.
Published by: University Hospital for Tumors, Ilica 197, Zagreb 10000, Croatia. TEL 385-1-3783555, FAX 385-1-3775536. Ed. Marco Turic. Adv. contact Morana Simat. Circ: 300.

616.99 IND ISSN 0971-5134
LIFE SCIENCE ADVANCES: ONCOLOGY. Key Title: Oncology - Life Science Advances. Text in English. 1983. 4/yr. **Document type:** *Academic/Scholarly.*
Indexed: Excerp.Med. (1995-).
Published by: Council of Scientific Research Integration, T.C. 28-408 (3), Vilayal Gardens, Kaithamukku, Thiruvananthapuram, Kerala 695 024, India. TEL 91-471-77305.

616.99 USA
LIVE WELL WITH CANCER. Text in English. 1982. s-a. USD 15 (effective 2000). **Document type:** *Newsletter.* **Description:** Covers current activities related to cancer in the Western Pennsylvania region.
Formerly (until 1988): Cancer Challenge
Published by: Cancer Caring Center, 4117 Liberty Ave, Pittsburgh, PA 15224-1424. TEL 412-622-1212, FAX 412-622-1216, cancercr@sgi.net, http://trfn.clpgh.org/cancercaring. Ed. Rebecca Whitlinger. Circ: 10,000.

LIVEWELL. see *PHYSICAL FITNESS AND HYGIENE*

616.994 USA
LIVINGRIGHT. Text in English. 1970. 3/yr. free per issue. adv. bk.rev. **Document type:** *Consumer.* **Description:** Health promotion and lifestyle information for the mature audience. Not cancer specific.
Formerly (until 1990): Florida Cancer News (0015-3931)
Published by: American Cancer Society, Inc., Florida Division, 3709 W Jetton Ave, Tampa, FL 33629. TEL 813-253-0541, FAX 813-254-5857. Ed. Sheila Buchert. Adv. contact Sheila H Buchert. Circ: 350,000 (controlled).

616.99 USA ISSN 0737-142X
LUDWIG SYMPOSIA. Text in English. 1981. irreg. **Document type:** *Monographic series.*
Published by: (Ludwig Institute for Cancer Research), Academic Press, Inc., Journal Division (Subsidiary of: Harcourt Brace & Company), 525 B St, Ste 1900, San Diego, CA 92101-4495. TEL 619-230-1840, FAX 619-699-6800, http://www.apnet.com.

616.99 IRL ISSN 0169-5002
LUNG CANCER. Text in English. 1986. m. EUR 1,616 in Europe to individuals; JPY 189,212 in Japan to individuals; USD 1,808 elsewhere to individuals (effective 2002). back issues avail.; reprints avail. *Refereed.* **Document type:** *Academic/Scholarly.* **Description:** Reports new findings and advances in therapy, etiology and related aspects.
Related titles: Online - full text ed.: (from ingenta, ScienceDirect, Swets Blackwell, Institute for Scientific Information).
Indexed: ASCA, Curr.Cont., Excerp.Med., Ind.Med. (1985-), Inpharma, Int.Abstr.Biol.Sci., Pharm.&Out.News, Reac., Rev.Med.& Vet.Mycol., Sci.Cit.Ind., Trop.Dis.Bull.
—BLDSC (5307.245000), CISTI, GNLM, IDS, Infotrieve, KNAW. **CCC.**
Published by: (International Association for the Study of Lung Cancer), Elsevier Science Ireland Ltd, Elsevier House, Brookvale Plaza, E. Park, Shannon, Co. Clare, Ireland. TEL 353-61-471944, FAX 353-61-472144, http://www.elsevier.com/locate/lungcan. Ed. H H Hansen. R&P Annette Moloney. **Subscr. in Australasia and the Far East to:** Elsevier Science (Singapore) Pte Ltd, No.1 Temasek Ave, 17-01 Millenia Tower, Singapore 039192, Singapore. TEL 65-434-3727, FAX 65-337-2230; **Subscr. in the Americas to:** Elsevier Science, PO Box 945, New York, NY 10159-0945. TEL 212-633-3730, FAX 212-633-3680, usinfo-f@elsevier.com; **Subscr. to:** Elsevier Science BV, PO Box 211, Amsterdam 1000 AE, Netherlands. TEL 31-20-485-3757.

616.99 AUT ISSN 1609-7041
▼ **MALIGNANT HYPERTHERMIA.** Text in English. 2000. q. USD 75 domestic; USD 115 foreign; USD 35 newsstand/cover (effective 2001). adv. back issues avail. *Refereed.* **Document type:** *Journal, Academic/Scholarly.* **Description:** Publishes articles, case reports, reviews, and letters on improving communications in understanding malignant hyperthermia reactions.
Related titles: Online - full text ed.
Published by: V I C E R Publishing, PO Box 14, Vienna A-1097, Austria. TEL 43-676-9568085, FAX 43-676-9568086, vicer@vicer.org, http://www.vicer.org. Ed., R&P Roland Hofbauer. adv.: B&W page USD 1,700, color page USD 2,200. Circ: 1,000 (paid and controlled).

MAMM; women, cancer and community. see *WOMEN'S HEALTH*

616.99 USA ISSN 1522-6395
▼ **MANAGED CARE & CANCER**; the journal of cancer economics & policy. Text in English. 1999. bi-m. USD 50; USD 56 in Canada; USD 62 foreign; USD 45 nurses; USD 40 to students; USD 10 newsstand/cover (effective 1999). adv. *Refereed.* **Document type:** *Magazine, Academic/Scholarly.* **Description:** Presents articles and commentary on the latest diagnostic approaches, treatments and study outcomes involving all aspects of oncology.
Published by: P R R, Inc., 48 S Service Rd, Melville, NY 11747-2335. TEL 516-777-3800, FAX 631-777-8700, intouch@cancernetwork.com, http://www.cancernetwork.com. Ed. Dr. Joseph Bailes. Pub. Jennifer Tashner.

616.99 USA ISSN 1046-638X
MANUAL OF ONCOLOGIC THERAPEUTICS. Text in English. 1990. irreg. **Document type:** *Monographic series.*
Published by: Lippincott Williams & Wilkins (Philadelphia) (Subsidiary of: Wolters Kluwer N.V.), 530 Walnut St, Philadelphia, PA 19106-3621. TEL 301-223-2300, 800-638-3030, FAX 301-223-2400, http://www.lww.com.

616.99 NOR ISSN 1400-7347
MEDDELANDE FRAAN S O F. (Svensk Onkologisk Foerening) Text in Swedish. 1995. 8/yr. USD 25 elsewhere to institutions (effective 2002). **Document type:** *Academic/Scholarly.*
Published by: (Svensk Onkologisk Foerening), Taylor & Francis AS (Subsidiary of: Taylor & Francis Group), Cort Adelersgt. 17, Solli, PO Box 2562, Oslo 0202, Norway. TEL 47-22-12-98-80, FAX 47-22-12-98-90, journals@tandf.no, http://www.tandf.co.uk.tfas. Ed. Jan-Erik Froedin.

616.994 618.92 USA ISSN 0098-1532
RC261.A1 CODEN: MPONDB
MEDICAL AND PEDIATRIC ONCOLOGY. Text in English. 1975. m. USD 1,965 in United States; USD 2,085 in Canada & Mexico; USD 2,187 elsewhere; USD 2,064 combined subscription in United States for print and online eds.; USD 2,184 combined subscription in Canada & Mexico for print and online eds.; USD 2,286 combined subscription elsewhere for print and online eds. (effective 2002). adv. charts, illus. index. back issues avail.; reprint service avail. from ISI. *Refereed.* **Document type:** *Academic/Scholarly.* **Description:** Provides broad coverage of advances in clinical oncology in children and adults; presents original articles on the diagnosis and treatment of malignant cancerous diseases.
Related titles: Microform ed.: (from PQC); Online - full text ed.: ISSN 1096-911X. 1996. USD 1,965 in United States; USD 1,965 in Canada & Mexico; USD 1,965 elsewhere (effective 2002) (from EBSCO Publishing, Wiley InterScience, Institute for Scientific Information); ♦ Supplement: Medical and Pediatric Oncology. Supplement. ISSN 0740-8226.
Indexed: ASCA, Biol.Abstr., Curr.Adv.Ecol.Sci., Curr.Cont., Curr.Ind.Stat., Dent.Ind., Excerp.Med., INIS Atomind., Ind.Med. (1975-), Ind.Sci.Rev., Inpharma, Int.Abstr.Biol.Sci., Int.Nurs.Ind., Neurosci.Cit.Ind., Nutr.Abstr., Pharm.&Out.News, Reac., Ref.Zh., Rev.Med.& Vet.Mycol., Sci.Cit.Ind., THA, Trop.Dis.Bull.
—BLDSC (5525.980000), CASDDS, CISTI, GNLM, IDS, ingenta, KNAW. **CCC.**
Published by: (International Society of Pediatric Oncology), John Wiley & Sons, Inc., Journals (Subsidiary of: Wiley InterScience), 605 Third Ave, New York, NY 10158. TEL 212-850-6645, FAX 212-850-6021, subinfo@wiley.com, uscs-wis@wiley.com, http://www.wiley.com. Ed. Giulio J D'Angio. adv.: B&W page USD 640, color page USD 1,515; trim 210 x 279. Circ: 1,650. **Subscr. outside the Americas to:** John Wiley & Sons Ltd., Baffins Ln, Chichester, Sussex PO19 IUD, United Kingdom. TEL 44-1243-779777, FAX 44-1243-843232, cs-journals@wiley.co.uk.

616.994 USA ISSN 0740-8226
MEDICAL AND PEDIATRIC ONCOLOGY. SUPPLEMENT. Text in English. 1982. irreg. price varies. back issues avail. *Refereed.* **Document type:** *Academic/Scholarly.*
Related titles: Microform ed.: (from PQC); ♦ Supplement to: Medical and Pediatric Oncology. ISSN 0098-1532.
Indexed: Curr.Cont. (coverage dropped), Ind.Med. (1982-).
—KNAW.
Published by: (International Society of Pediatric Oncology), John Wiley & Sons, Inc., Journals (Subsidiary of: Wiley InterScience), 605 Third Ave, New York, NY 10158. SUBINFO@JWILEY.COM. **Subscr. outside the Americas to:** John Wiley & Sons Ltd., Baffins Ln, Chichester, Sussex PO19 IUD, United Kingdom. TEL 44-243-779777, 44-243-776128.

M

616.99 USA ISSN 1357-0560
CODEN: MOTPE2
MEDICAL ONCOLOGY; a leading journal in clinical oncology. Text in English. 1984. q. USD 365 to institutions for print ed.; USD 400 combined subscription to individuals for print & online eds. (effective 2001). adv. back issues avail.; reprints avail. *Refereed.* **Document type:** *Journal, Academic/Scholarly.* **Description:** Studies the chemistry, biochemistry, biology, epidemiology, pathology, virology, and genetics of malignant tumors, along with clinical aspects of cancer.
Formerly (until 1994): Medical Oncology and Tumor Pharmacotherapy (0736-0118)
Related titles: Microform ed.: (from PQC); Online - full text ed.: USD 365 (effective 2001) (from EBSCO Publishing, O C L C Online Computer Library Center, Inc., RoweCom Information Quest, ProQuest Information & Learning, ingenta, Swets Blackwell, Institute for Scientific Information).
Indexed: ASCA, Aqua.Sci.& Fish.Abstr., Curr.Adv.Cancer Res., Curr.Adv.Ecol.Sci., Curr.Cont., Derwent Biotech.Abstr., Environ.Sci.Poll.Mgmt., Excerp.Med., Ind.Med. (1994-), Inpharma, Int.Abstr.Biol.Sci., Pharm.&Out.News, Reac.
—ADONIS, CASDDS, CISTI, EMDOCS, GNLM, IDS, Infotrieve, ingenta. **CCC.**
Published by: Humana Press Inc., 999 Riverview Dr, Ste 208, Totowa, NJ 07512. TEL 973-256-1699, FAX 973-256-8341, jumana@humanapr.com, http://www.humanapress.com/JournalDetail.pasp?journal=14, http;//humanapress.com. Eds. Anders Osterborg, Peter H Wiernik.

016.61699 BGR ISSN 1311-4573
MEDITSINSKI PREGLED. KLINICHNA ONKOLOGIIA. Text in Bulgarian. 1994. q., latest vol.8, 2001. BGL 14 domestic; USD 30 foreign (effective 2001 - 2002). adv. abstr, bibl, illus. back issues avail. *Refereed.* **Document type:** *Journal, Academic/Scholarly, Abstract/Index, Bibliography.* **Description:** Publishes original articles and abstracts of foreign publications on diagnosis and treatment of oncologic diseases.
Formerly: Onkologichen Pregled (1310-1714)
Indexed: INIS Atomind.
—BLDSC (5099.284797), GNLM.
Published by: Meditsinski Universitet - Sofia, Tsentur za Informatsiia po Meditsina/Medical University - Sofia, Medical Information Center, 1 Sv Georgi Sofiiski ul, Sofia 1431, Bulgaria. TEL 359-2-9522342, FAX 359-2-9522393, mutafov@sun.medun.acad.bg, http://www.medun.acad.bg. Ed. Dr. D Todorov. R&P, Adv. contact Dr. Christo Mutafov. B&W page USD 50, color page USD 150; 12 x 18. Circ: 200. **Dist. by:** Sofia Books, Ul Silivria 16, Sofia 1404, Bulgaria. TEL 359-2-9586257, sofiabooks@hotmail.com, http://www.sofiabooks.hit.bg.

MEDITSINSKI PREGLED. RADIATSIIA I MEDITSINA. see *MEDICAL SCIENCES—Radiology And Nuclear Medicine*

616.99 USA
MEDSCAPE ONCOLOGY. Text in English. 1997. w. **Description:** Provides clinicians with information on the broad range of issues affecting the care of patients presenting with cancer and its complications.
Media: Online - full text.
Published by: Medscape, Inc., 134 W 29th St, New York, NY 10001-5399. TEL 212-760-3193, FAX 212-760-3140, http://www.medscape.com.

MELANOMA LETTER. see *MEDICAL SCIENCES—Dermatology And Venereology*

616.99 GBR ISSN 0960-8931
CODEN: MREEEH
MELANOMA RESEARCH. Text in English. 1990. bi-m., latest vol.11. USD 299 domestic to individuals; USD 299 foreign to individuals; USD 899 domestic to institutions; USD 899 per issue foreign to institutions; USD 139 newsstand/cover (effective 2002). adv. reprints avail. *Refereed.* **Document type:** *Academic/Scholarly.* **Description:** Provides an international forum for the rapid dissemination of research on melanoma both at basic and clinical levels.
Related titles: CD-ROM ed.: USD 1,168.70 domestic academic site license; USD 1,168.70 foreign academic site license; USD 1,303.55 domestic corporate site license; USD 1,303.55 foreign corporate site license (effective 2002); Online - full text ed.: (from Ovid Technologies, Inc., EBSCO Publishing, Institute for Scientific Information).
Indexed: ASCA, Chem.Abstr., Chem.Titles, Curr.Cont., Excerp.Med. (1992-), Ind.Med. (1991-), Inpharma, Int.Abstr.Biol.Sci., Med.& Surg.Dermat., Pharm.&Out.News, Reac., Sci.Cit.Ind.
—BLDSC (5536.813450), ADONIS, CASDDS, CISTI, EMDOCS, GNLM, IDS, ingenta, KNAW.
Published by: Lippincott Williams & Wilkins (Philadelphia) (Subsidiary of: Wolters Kluwer N.V.), 530 Walnut St, Philadelphia, PA 19106-3621. TEL 215-238-4200, FAX 215-238-4478, http://www.melanomaresearch.com, http://www.lww.com. R&P Annemeike Dolfing. Adv. contact Gemma Heiser. Circ: 200.

616.99 USA
MEMORIAL SLOAN-KETTERING CANCER CENTER. ANNUAL REPORT. Text in English. a. free per issue. charts, illus. **Document type:** *Corporate.* **Description:** Reviews research in the detection, prevention, and treatment of cancer conducted at Memorial Sloan-Kettering Cancer Center.
Published by: Memorial Sloan-Kettering Cancer Center, Department of Public Affairs, 1275 York Ave, New York, NY 10021. TEL 212-639-3573, FAX 212-639-3576, http://www.mskcc.org.

616.99 USA ISSN 1060-233X
MESSAGE LINE. Text in English. 1974. 3/yr. free per issue. 24 p./no. 4 cols./p. back issues avail. **Document type:** *Newsletter, Consumer.* **Description:** Updates on research advances in the treatment of brain tumors.
Related titles: E-mail ed.
Published by: American Brain Tumor Association, 2720 River Rd, Ste 146, Des Plaines, IL 60018-4110. TEL 847-827-9910, 800-886-2282, FAX 847-827-9918. Circ: 40,000.

616.992 GBR
MITOMYCIN-C KYOWA UPDATE. Text in English. 3/yr. **Document type:** *Academic/Scholarly.* **Description:** Provides information on recent clinical applications of mitomycin-C in relation to cancer.
Published by: Leeds Medical Information, University of Leeds, Leeds, W Yorks LS2 9JT, United Kingdom. TEL 44-113-233-5550, FAX 44-113-233-5568, lmi@leeds.ac.uk, http://www.leeds.ac.uk/lmi/bespoke/mmc.html, http://www.leeds.ac.uk/lmi/intro.html. **Co-sponsor:** Kyowa Hakko U.K. Ltd.

616.992 USA
MOLECULAR CANCER THERAPEUTICS. Text in English.
Media: Online - full text (from HighWire Pr.).
Published by: American Association for Cancer Research, Public Ledger Bldg, 150 S Independence Mall W, Ste 826, Philadelphia, PA 19106. TEL 215-440-9300, FAX 215-440-9354, http://www.aacr.org.

616.994071 USA ISSN 0899-1987
CODEN: MOCAE8
MOLECULAR CARCINOGENESIS. Text in English. 12/yr. (in 3 vols., 4 nos./vol.). USD 1,635 in United States; USD 1,755 in Canada & Mexico; USD 1,857 elsewhere; USD 1,717 combined subscription in United States for print and online eds.; USD 1,837 combined subscription in Canada & Mexico for print and online eds.; USD 1,837 combined subscription elsewhere for print and online eds. (effective 2002). adv. bk.rev. back issues avail. *Refereed.* **Document type:** *Academic/Scholarly.* **Description:** Devoted to the study of the molecular aspects of mechanisms involved in chemical, physical and viral (biological) carcinogenesis.
Related titles: Microform ed.: (from PQC); Online - full text ed.: ISSN 1098-2744. 1996. USD 1,635 in United States; USD 1,635 in Canada & Mexico; USD 1,635 elsewhere (effective 2002) (from EBSCO Publishing, Wiley InterScience, Institute for Scientific Information).
Indexed: AIDS & Cancer Res., ASCA, BBCI, Biotech.& Bioeng.Abstr., Biotech.Cit.Ind., Chem.Abstr., Chem.Indus.Notes, Chem.Titles, Curr.Cont., Environ.Sci.Poll.Mgmt., Focus on: Mol.Med., Genet.Abstr., Hum.Gen.Abstr., INIS Atomind., Ind.Med. (1988-), Ind.Sci.Rev., Inpharma, Int.Abstr.Biol.Sci., Nuc.Acids Abstr., Nutr.Abstr., Oncog.G.F.Abstr., Pharm.&Out.News, Pollut.Abstr., Reac., Ref.Zh., Rev.Med.& Vet.Mycol., Saf.Sci.Abstr., Sci.Cit.Ind., THA, Tox.Abstr.
—BLDSC (5900.802000), CASDDS, CISTI, EMDOCS, GNLM, IDS, ingenta, KNAW. **CCC.**
Published by: (University of Texas), John Wiley & Sons, Inc., Journals (Subsidiary of: Wiley InterScience), 605 Third Ave, New York, NY 10158. TEL 212-850-6645, FAX 212-850-6021, subinfo@wiley.com, uscs-wis@wiley.com, http://www.wiley.com. Eds. J Carl Barrett, Thomas Slaga. adv.: B&W page GBP 640, color page GBP 1,515; trim 210 x 279. Circ: 600. **Subscr. outside the Americas to:** John Wiley & Sons Ltd., Baffins Ln, Chichester, Sussex PO19 IUD, United Kingdom. TEL 44-1243-779777, FAX 44-1243-843232, cs-journals@wiley.co.uk.

572.8 USA ISSN 1525-0016
MOLECULAR THERAPY. Text in English. m. USD 299 in US & Canada; USD 305 elsewhere (effective 2001). back issues avail.; reprints avail. **Document type:** *Academic/Scholarly.* **Description:** Publishes scientific meritorious papers in the areas of gene transfer, gene regulation, gene discovery, cell therapy, experimental models, correction of genetic and acquired diseases, clinical trials and significant methodological advances. It also publish timely reviews, scientific correspondence and commentaries.

Related titles: Online - full text ed.: (from EBSCO Publishing, O C L C Online Computer Library Center, Inc., ingenta, Swets Blackwell, IDEAL Online Library, Institute for Scientific Information).
Indexed: Biotech.Cit.Ind., Curr.Cont., Ind.Med.
—BLDSC (5900.856500).
Published by: Academic Press, Inc., Journal Division (Subsidiary of: Harcourt Brace & Company), 525 B St, Ste 1900, San Diego, CA 92101-4495. TEL 800-543-9534, apsubs@acad.com, http://www.apnet.com/moltherapy. Ed. Dr. Inder Verma.

616.994 USA ISSN 1526-5803
N A B C O BREAST CANCER RESOURCE LIST. Text in English. a. USD 50 to members (effective 2000). **Document type:** *Directory.* **Description:** Compiles books, brochures, hotlines, and video resources useful to breast cancer patients and professionals.
Published by: National Alliance of Breast Cancer Organizations, 9 E 37th St, 10th Fl, New York, NY 10016-2822. TEL 212-889-0606, FAX 212-689-1213, nabcoinfo@aol.com, http://www.nabco.org.

616.99 USA
N A B C O NEWS. Text in English. 1987. q. USD 50 to members (effective 2000). bk.rev. index. back issues avail. **Document type:** *Newsletter.* **Description:** Contains updates on breast cancer research, treatment, policy programs, and detection.
Related titles: Online - full text ed.
Published by: National Alliance of Breast Cancer Organizations, 9 E 37th St, 10th Fl, New York, NY 10016-2822. TEL 212-889-0606, FAX 212-689-1213, nabcoinfo@aol.com, http://www.nabco.org. Ed. Ruth Spear. Circ: 7,000.

616.99 USA ISSN 0270-7950
RC267
N C I FACT BOOK. Text in English. a. **Document type:** *Government.*
Formerly: National Cancer Institute Fact Book
Published by: National Cancer Institute, Financial Management Branch, 9000 Rockville Pike, Bethesda, MD 20892.

616.994 USA ISSN 0027-8874
CODEN: JNCIEQ
NATIONAL CANCER INSTITUTE. JOURNAL. Abbreviated title: J N C I. Text in English. 1940. s-m. GBP 180 in Europe to individuals Print and online; USD 190 in North America to individuals Print and online; USD 260 rest of world to individuals Print and online; GBP 825, USD 1,235 to institutions For large institutions, print and online; GBP 615, USD 935 to institutions For medium institutions, print and online; GBP 275, USD 415 to institutions For small institutions, print and online (effective 2002). adv. bk.rev. bibl, charts, illus. index. back issues avail.; reprint service avail. from CIS. *Refereed.* **Document type:** *Journal, Academic/Scholarly.* **Description:** Contains original reports, articles, reviews, editorials, and commentaries on new findings in clinical and laboratory cancer research.
Incorporates (in 1987): Cancer Treatment Reports (0361-5960); Which was formed by the 1976 merger of: Cancer Chemotherapy Reports. Part 1 (0069-0112); Cancer Chemotherapy Reports. Part 2 (0069-0120); Cancer Chemotherapy Reports. Part 3 (0069-0139)
Related titles: Microfiche ed.: (from CIS); Microform ed.: (from PQC,PMC); Online - full text ed.: ISSN 1460-2105 (from HighWire Pr., LexisNexis, EBSCO Publishing, O C L C Online Computer Library Center, Inc., RoweCom Information Quest, ProQuest Information & Learning, ingenta, Gale Group, Swets Blackwell, Institute for Scientific Information); ♦ Supplement: National Cancer Institute. Journal. Monographs. ISSN 1052-6773.
Indexed: AIDS & Cancer Res., ASCA, Abstr.Hyg., Agri.& Environ.Biotech.Abstr. (coverage dropped), Amer.Stat.Ind. (1985-), Behav.Med.Abstr., Biol.Abstr., CINAHL, C.I.S. Abstr., Chem.Abstr., Chem.Indus.Notes, Chem.Titles, Chic.Per.Ind., Curr.Adv.Biochem., Curr.Adv.Cancer Res., Curr.Adv.Ecol.Sci., Curr.Adv.Gen.& Molec.Biol., Curr.Cont., Curr.Ind.Stat., Dairy Sci.Abstr., Dent.Ind., Derwent Biotech.Abstr., Dok.Arbeitsmed., Environ.Sci.Poll.Mgmt., Excerp.Med., Food Sci.& Tech.Abstr., INIS Atomind., I.P.A., Ind.Med. (1940-), Ind.U.S.Gov.Per., Ind.Vet., Inpharma, Int.Abstr.Biol.Sci., Int.Nurs.Ind., Med.& Surg.Dermat., NRN, Nutr.Abstr., Oncog.G.F.Abstr., Pharm.&Out.News, Pollut.Abstr., Poult.Abstr., Reac., Rev.Med.& Vet.Mycol., Risk Abstr., SRI, Saf.Sci.Abstr., Sage Race Rel.Abstr., Sci.Cit.Ind., Sport Fish.Abstr., THA, Telegen, Triticale Abstr., Trop.Dis.Bull., Vet.Bull.
—BLDSC (4830.000000), CASDDS, CINDOC, CISTI, EMDOCS, GNLM, IDS, ingenta, KNAW. **CCC.**
Published by: (U.S. National Cancer Institute), Oxford University Press, Academic Division, Great Clarendon St, Oxford OX2 6DP, United Kingdom. TEL 44-1865-267907, FAX 44-1865-267835, jnlorders@oup-usa.org, jnl.info@oup.co.uk, http://jnci.oupjournals.org/, http://www.oup.co.uk/journals. Eds. Gordon J McVie, Richard E Manrow, Barnett S Kramer. Pubs. J Boullin, J Fox. R&P Fionna Willis. Adv. contact Helen Pearson TEL 44-1235-201904. B&W page USD 1,300, B&W page GBP 720. Circ: 10,000. **Subscr. outside the Americas to:** Journals Marketing, Great Clarendon St, Oxford OX2 6DP, United Kingdom.

616.994 USA ISSN 1052-6773
RC261.A2 CODEN: JNCME4
NATIONAL CANCER INSTITUTE. JOURNAL. MONOGRAPHS. Key Title: Journal of the National Cancer Institute. Monographs. Text in English. 1986. irreg., latest vol.24, 1998. USD 25 (effective 2000). *Refereed.* **Document type:** *Monographic series.* **Description:** Provides in-depth examinations of critical issues in cancer research, treatment, prevention, and control.
Former titles (until 1990): N C I Monographs (0893-2751); Which was formed by the 1986 merger of: Cancer Treament Sympoia (0742-1761); National Cancer Institute. Monographs (0083-1921)
Media: Microfiche. **Related titles:** Online - full text ed.: (from HighWire Pr.); ♦ Supplement to: National Cancer Institute. Journal. ISSN 0027-8874.
Indexed: AgeLine, Biol.Abstr., Chic.Per.Ind., Excerp.Med. (until 1993), INIS Atomind., Ind.Med. (1990-), Inpharma, Nutr.Abstr., Pharm.&Out.News, Reac., SSCI (coverage dropped).
—BLDSC (5914.670000), CASDDS, CINDOC, CISTI, GNLM, Infotrieve, KNAW. **CCC.**
Published by: (U.S. National Cancer Institute), Oxford University Press, Journals, 2001 Evans Rd, Cary, NC 27513. FAX 919-677-1714, jnl.info@oup.co.uk, http://jnci.oupjournals.org. Ed. Barnett S Kramer. R&P Fionna Willis. **Subscr. outside U.S. to:** Oxford University Press, Great Clarendon St, Oxford OX2 6DP, United Kingdom. TEL 44-1865-267907, jnl.info@oup.co.uk.

616.9 CAN ISSN 0077-3689
NATIONAL CANCER INSTITUTE OF CANADA. ANNUAL REPORT. Text in English. 1947. a. free per issue.
Published by: National Cancer Institute of Canada, 10 Alcorn Ave, Ste 200, Toronto, ON M4V 3B1, Canada. TEL 416-961-7223, FAX 416-961-4189. Ed. Dr. M Wosnick. Circ: 1,000.

616.99 ESP ISSN 0212-9787
NEOPLASIA; oncologia multidisciplinaria. Text in Spanish. 1984. bi-m. USD 99. adv. **Document type:** *Academic/Scholarly.* **Description:** For oncologists, epidemiologists, pathologists, surgeons, internists and specialists interested in oncology and neoplasia.
Indexed: Excerp.Med. (1993-).
—EMDOCS, GNLM. **CCC.**
Published by: Ediciones Doyma S.A., Traversa de Gracia, 17-21, Barcelona 08021, Spain. TEL 34-93-200-0711, FAX 34-93-209-1136. Ed. J Estape Rodriguez. Adv. contact Olga Gomez. page ESP 195,000; trim 280 x 210. Circ: 2,000.

616.99 USA ISSN 1522-8002
CODEN: NEOPFL
▼ **NEOPLASIA.** Text in English. 1999. bi-m. USD 129 in Europe to individuals; USD 194 rest of world to individuals; EUR 259 in Europe to institutions; USD 389 rest of world to institutions (effective 2002). adv. abstr, bibl, charts, illus, stat. back issues avail. *Refereed.* **Document type:** *Academic/Scholarly.* **Description:** Publishes laboratory and clinical studies describing new molecular and genetic findings relating to the neoplastic phenotype.
Related titles: Online - full text ed.: (from EBSCO Publishing, O C L C Online Computer Library Center, Inc., RoweCom Information Quest, ingenta, Swets Blackwell, Institute for Scientific Information).
Indexed: Biotech.& Bioeng.Abstr., Curr.Cont., Ind.Med., Oncog.G.F.Abstr.
—BLDSC (6075.628100).
Published by: Nature Publishing Group Specialist Journals (Subsidiary of: Macmillan Publishers Ltd.), 345 Park Ave S, New York, NY 10010-1707. TEL 212-726-9264, FAX 212-696-0052, d.ramsay@natureny.com, http://www.nature.com/neo, http://www.neoplasia.org. Ed. Brian D Ross. Pub. Chris Rawlins.

616.994 SVK ISSN 0028-2685
CODEN: NEOLA4
NEOPLASMA. Text in English. 1954. bi-m., latest vol.48. USD 295 (effective 2001). bk.rev. charts, illus. index. 80 p./no. reprints avail. *Refereed.* **Document type:** *Journal, Academic/Scholarly.* **Description:** Publishes original works of Czechoslovak and foreign authors in the fields of experimental and clinical oncology. Covers the biochemistry of tumors, the biology and genetics of oncology, and significant causistry. Includes statistics of oncology.
Related titles: Online - full text ed.: (from Institute for Scientific Information).
Indexed: ASCA, Aqua.Sci.& Fish.Abstr., Biol.Abstr., C.I.S. Abstr., Chem.Abstr., Chem.Indus.Notes, Chem.Titles, Curr.Adv.Cancer Res., Curr.Adv.Gen.& Molec.Biol., Curr.Cont., Dent.Ind., Excerp.Med., INIS Atomind., Ind.Med. (1957-), Ind.Sci.Rev., Ind.Vet., Inpharma, NRN, Nutr.Abstr., Pharm.&Out.News, Reac., Ref.Zh., Risk Abstr., Sci.Cit.Ind., Vet.Bull.
—BLDSC (6075.630000), CASDDS, CISTI, GNLM, IDS, ingenta, KNAW.
Published by: (Cancer Research Institute), Veda Publishing House of the Slovak Academy of Sciences FAX 421-2-59127250, http://www.elis.sk. Ed. Viliam Ujhazy. **Dist. by:** Mezhdunarodnaya Kniga, B Yakimanka 39, Moscow 117049, Russian Federation. TEL 7-095-2384967, FAX 7-095-2384634.

616.99383 USA
NEURO-FIBROMA-TOSIS NEWS. Text in English. q. USD 35 (effective 1999). **Document type:** *Newsletter.*
Formerly: Neuro-Fibroma-Tosis
Published by: National Neurofibromatosis Foundation, Inc., 95 Pine St, Fl 16, New York, NY 10005-1611. TEL 212-344-6633, FAX 212-747-0004, nnff@nf.org, http://www.nf.org. R&P Francine Morris. Circ: 35,000.

616.994 USA ISSN 1522-8517
▼ **NEURO-ONCOLOGY.** Text in English. 1999. q.
Related titles: Online - full text ed.: (from Institute for Scientific Information).
Indexed: Curr.Cont., Ind.Med.
—BLDSC (6081.288000).
Published by: Carden Jennings Publishing, 1224 W Main St, Ste 200, Charlottesville, VA 22903-2858. TEL 804-979-4913, FAX 804-979-4025. Ed. Darell D Bigner.

616 USA
NORTHWESTERN UNIVERSITY. ROBERT H. LURIE COMPREHENSIVE CANCER CENTER. JOURNAL. Text in English. 1977. s-a. free per issue. bk.rev. charts, illus. index. *Refereed.* **Document type:** *Academic/Scholarly.* **Description:** Covers topics of interest to members of the center; faculty and staff of Northwestern University; and oncologists, nurses, clinicians and officials of cancer centers and programs throughout the U.S.
Former titles (until vol.2, no.2., 1991): Northwestern University Cancer Center. Journal (1049-6025); Supersedes (1977-1987): Cancer Focus (0147-1155)
Published by: Northwestern University, Robert H. Lurie Comprehensive Cancer Center, Office of Public Affairs and Communications, Olson Pavilion 8250, 303 E Chicago Ave, Chicago, IL 60611. TEL 312-908-6346, FAX 312-908-1372. Ed., R&P Dr. Steven T Rosen TEL 312-908-5250. Circ: 2,000.

616.994 POL ISSN 0029-540X
CODEN: NOWOAL
NOWOTWORY. Text in Polish; Summaries in English. 1923. bi-m. USD 80 (effective 1999). adv. bk.rev. index. reprints avail. *Refereed.* **Document type:** *Academic/Scholarly.* **Description:** Highlights oncology, radio-chemotherapy and surgery, cancer biology, epidemiology and control.
Indexed: Biol.Abstr., Chem.Abstr., Chem.Indus.Notes, Chem.Titles, Dent.Ind., Excerp.Med., INIS Atomind., Ind.Med. (coverage dropped).
—BLDSC (6180.479000), CASDDS, CISTI, GNLM.
Published by: Maria Curie-Sklodowska Memorial Cancer Center and Institute of Oncology, Ul Roentgena 5, Warsaw 02781, Poland. TEL 48-22-6445024, FAX 48-22-6439380, redakcja@coi.waw.pl. Ed. Edward Towpik. Adv. contact Danuta Sadowska Osmycka. Circ: 1,200. **Co-sponsor:** Polskie Towarzystwo Onkologiczne.

NUTRITION AND CANCER; an international journal. see *NUTRITION AND DIETETICS*

616.99 618.082 JPN ISSN 0911-2251
NYUGAN NO RINSHO/JAPANESE JOURNAL OF BREAST CANCER. Text in English; Summaries in Japanese. 1986. q. JPY 2,200 per issue.
Indexed: INIS Atomind.

M

Published by: Shinohara Publishers Inc., Yaguchi Bldg, 11-7 Hongo 2-chome, Bunkyo-ku, Tokyo 113-0033, Japan.

616.9 610.73 USA ISSN 0890-5215
O N S NEWS. Text in English. 1986. m. USD 10 (effective 2001). 16 p./no. 3 cols./p. back issues avail. **Document type:** *Newsletter.* **Description:** News and information of interest to Oncology Nursing Society members and other oncology nursing professionals.
Indexed: CINAHL, Int.Nurs.Ind.
—BLDSC (6261.570000).
Published by: Oncology Nursing Society, 501 Holiday Dr, Pittsburgh, PA 15220-2749. TEL 412-921-7373, FAX 412-921-2131, publishing@ons.org, http://www.ons.org. Ed. Debra Wujcik Rn. Pub. Leonard Mafrica. R&P Jeanette M Kent TEL 412-921-7373 ext. 246. Adv. contact Jack Edelman TEL 856-256-2313. Circ: 25,665.

ONCO GYN NEWS. see *MEDICAL SCIENCES—Obstetrics And Gynecology*

616.994 GBR ISSN 0950-9232
CODEN: ONCNES
ONCOGENE. Text in English. 1987. w. GBP 576 in Europe to individuals for print or online; USD 922 elsewhere to individuals for print or online; GBP 633 combined subscription in Europe to individuals print & online; USD 1,013 combined subscription elsewhere to individuals print & online; GBP 2,100 in Europe to individuals for print or online; USD 3,520 elsewhere to institutions for print only; GBP 2,310 combined subscription in Europe to institutions print & online; USD 3,872 combined subscription elsewhere to institutions print & online (effective 2001). adv. bk.rev. charts, illus, stat. index. back issues avail.; reprints avail. *Refereed.* **Document type:** *Journal, Academic/Scholarly.* **Description:** Studies all aspects of oncogene research and relationships to cancer.
Related titles: Microfilm ed.: (from PQC); Online - full text ed.: USD 3,360 to institutions outside of Europe (effective 2001) (from EBSCO Publishing, O C L C Online Computer Library Center, Inc., RoweCom Information Quest, ingenta, Swets Blackwell, Institute for Scientific Information).
Indexed: AIDS & Cancer Res., AIDS Abstr., ASCA, Anim.Breed.Abstr., BBCI, Biotech.& Bioeng.Abstr., Biotech.Cit.Ind., Cal.Tiss.Abstr. (coverage dropped), Chem.Abstr., Chem.Titles, Curr.Cont., Excerp.Med., Focus on: Mol.Med., Genet.Abstr., Hum.Gen.Abstr., Ind.Med. (1987-), Ind.Vet., Inpharma, Int.Abstr.Biol.Sci., Neurosci.Abstr., Neurosci.Cit.Ind., Nuc.Acids Abstr., Oncog.G.F.Abstr., Pharm.&Out.News, Reac., Rev.Med.& Vet.Mycol., Sci.Cit.Ind., Small Anim.Abstr., Sport Fish.Abstr., THA, Telegen, Tox.Abstr. (coverage dropped), Vet.Bull., Virol.Abstr.
—BLDSC (6256.782000), ADONIS, CASDDS, CISTI, EMDOCS, GNLM, IDS, ingenta, KNAW. **CCC.**
Published by: Nature Publishing Group Specialist Journals (Subsidiary of: Holtzbrink Publishers), Houndmills, Basingstoke, Hants RG21 6XS, United Kingdom. TEL 44-1256-329242, FAX 44-1256-328339, subscriptions@nature.com, http://www.nature.com/onc. Eds. E Reddy, J Jenkins. Pub. Sue Deeley. R&P Trace Noel. Adv. contact Robert Sloan TEL 44-20-8882-7199.

ONCOGENES. see *MEDICAL SCIENCES—Abstracting, Bibliographies, Statistics*

616.99 ESP ISSN 0378-4835
CODEN: NCLGDV
ONCOLOGIA. Text in Spanish. 1976. m. ESP 10,500 domestic; USD 105 in Europe; USD 132 elsewhere (effective 2001). adv. charts, illus, bibl. *Refereed.* **Document type:** *Academic/Scholarly.* **Description:** Presents original articles, reviews, case studies, and clinical notes in the treatment of all types of cancer.
Indexed: Biol.Abstr., Chem.Abstr., Excerp.Med., INIS Atomind., Ind.Med.Esp.
—BLDSC (6256.790000), CASDDS, CINDOC, CISTI, EMDOCS, GNLM, Infotrieve, KNAW. **CCC.**
Published by: (Federacion de Sociedades Espanolas de Oncologia), Alpe Editores S.A., Pedro Rico, 27, Madrid 28029, Spain. TEL 34-91-733-8811, FAX 34-91-315-9652, oncologia@sistelcom.com. Eds. Dr. Alejandro de la Torre, Dr. Jesus Vicente, Dr. Ysmael Alvarez. Pub. Esther Martinez Cuesta. Adv. contact Ana Jurado. color page ESP 180,000; 280 x 210. Circ: 4,500 (controlled).

616.99 ECU ISSN 1390-0110
ONCOLOGIA. Text in Spanish. 1993. q. ECS 100,000 domestic to doctors; USD 80 foreign to doctors; ECS 150,000 domestic to institutions; USD 100 foreign to institutions (effective 1999). adv. *Refereed.* **Description:** Publishes original research and study cases on oncology.
Indexed: AMED, Excerp.Med., INIS Atomind.
Published by: Sociedad de Lucha contra el Cancer, Ave. PEDRO J MENENDEZ GILBERT, Apdo 5255 O 3626, Guayaquil, Guayas, Ecuador. TEL 593-4-281744, FAX 593-4-287151, revista@solca.med.ed and oncologia@solsa.med.ec. Ed. Jaime Sanchez Sabando. R&P Juan Tanca Campozano TEL 593-4-288-088 ext. 128-208. Adv. contact Amado Freire Torres.

616.99 FRA ISSN 1292-3818
CODEN: CIOCEO
ONCOLOGIE. Text in French. 1992. 8/yr. EUR 154 domestic; EUR 27 newsstand/cover foreign (effective 2002). adv. reprints avail. *Refereed.* **Document type:** *Journal, Academic/Scholarly.* **Description:** Gives information on recent advances in cancer therapy to clinicians and all related personnel.
Formerly (until 1999): Cahiers d'Oncologie (0941-3804)
Related titles: Microform ed.
Indexed: Excerp.Med. (1995-).
—BLDSC (6256.887500), EMDOCS, GNLM, Infotrieve, KNAW. **CCC.**
Published by: Springer-Verlag France (Subsidiary of: BertelsmannSpringer), 1 rue Paul Cezanne, Paris 75008, France. TEL 33-1-53933644, FAX 33-1-53933683, access@link.sprintm; york@springer-paris.fr, http://link.springer.de/link/service/journals/00590/index.htm. adv.: B&W page FRF 12,200, color page FRF 21,700; trim 210 x 275.

616.99 616.15 USA ISSN 1083-7159
CODEN: OCOLF6
THE ONCOLOGIST. Text in English. 1996. bi-m. USD 155 domestic to individuals; USD 175 in Canada to individuals; USD 190 foreign to individuals; USD 225 domestic to institutions; USD 245 in Canada to institutions; USD 260 foreign to institutions (effective 2002). adv. bk.rev. abstr. 100 p./no. 2 cols./p. back issues avail.; reprints avail. *Refereed.* **Document type:** *Journal, Academic/Scholarly.* **Description:** Designed for the practicing oncologist and hematologist. Reports on the multimodality diagnosis and treatment of the cancer patient.
Related titles: Online - full text ed.: (from HighWire Pr., EBSCO Publishing); Spanish ed.
Indexed: Ind.Med. (1996-), Int.Nurs.Ind.
—BLDSC (6256.890000), CASDDS, GNLM, Infotrieve, KNAW. **CCC.**
Published by: AlphaMed Press, Inc., One Prestige Pl, Ste 290, Miamisburg, OH 45342-3758. TEL 937-291-2355, FAX 937-291-4229, theoncologist@alphamedpress.com, alphamedpress@alphamedpress.com; subscribers@alphamedpress.com, http://www.theoncologist.com. Ed. Bruce A Chabner. R&P Tim Sparling. Adv. contact Ann Murphy. B&W page USD 1,500, color page USD 1,625. Circ: 17,000.
The Oncologist is devoted to medical and practice issues for surgical, radiation, and medical oncologists and is designed for busy practitioners entrusted with the care of cancer patients. The journal's articles are meant to impact the practice of oncology and facilitate significant communications of new medical treatments and technologies. This bimonthly, international peer-reviewed journal publishes original papers, reviews, and commentaries addressing the multimodality diagnosis, treatment, and quality of life of the cancer patient.
Publisher provided annotation.

616.99 DEU
ONCOLOGY. Text in English. 1992. irreg., latest vol.3, 1995. **Document type:** *Proceedings.*
Indexed: Ind.Sci.Rev.
Published by: Sympomed Medical Publishers, Hohenbrunner Weg 150, Taufkirchen 82024, Germany. TEL 49-89-6124411, FAX 49-89-6123770. Pub. Siegfried Bezold.

616.99 USA ISSN 0890-9091
RC254.A1 CODEN: OCLGE9
ONCOLOGY. Text in English. 1987. 12/yr. USD 99 domestic; USD 105 in Canada; USD 121 elsewhere (effective 2000). adv. bk.rev. cum.index. *Refereed.* **Description:** Publishes articles reviewing recent trends in the clinical practice of oncology, original research or results of trials having clinical relevance.
Related titles: Online - full text ed.: (from Institute for Scientific Information); Supplement: A Supplement to Oncology.
Indexed: AMED, Curr.Cont., Excerp.Med., INIS Atomind., Ind.Med. (1987-), Ind.Sci.Rev., Inpharma, Int.Nurs.Ind., Pharm.&Out.News, Reac.
—BLDSC (6256.930000), CISTI, EMDOCS, GNLM, IDS, KNAW. **CCC.**
Published by: P R R, Inc., 48 S Service Rd, Melville, NY 11747-2335. TEL 631-777-3800, FAX 631-777-8700, info.prr@scp.com, http://www.cancernetwork.com. Ed. Dr. Robert F Wittes. Pub. Robert C Canale. adv.: B&W page USD 2,040, color page USD 3,290; trim 10.75 x 7.88. Circ: 26,265 (controlled).

616.994 CHE ISSN 0030-2414
RC261 CODEN: ONCOBS
ONCOLOGY; international journal of cancer research and treatment. Text in English. 1948. 8/yr. (in 2 vols.). CHF 1,594, EUR 1,138.40 in Europe to institutions; CHF 1,617.20, USD 1,238 elsewhere to institutions (effective 2002). adv. bk.rev. abstr, bibl, charts, illus. index. back issues avail. *Refereed.* **Document type:** *Journal, Academic/Scholarly.* **Description:** Works to accelerate the adaptation of experimental results to the clinic.
Supersedes: Oncologia
Related titles: Microform ed.; Online - full content ed.: ISSN 1423-0232. CHF 116, EUR 84, USD 90 to institutions with print edition (effective 2002) (from EBSCO Publishing, O C L C Online Computer Library Center, Inc., Swets Blackwell); Online - full text ed.: (from Institute for Scientific Information, RoweCom Information Quest).
Indexed: Biol.Abstr., Chem.Abstr., Chem.Indus.Notes, Chem.Titles, Curr.Adv.Ecol.Sci., Curr.Cont., Dairy Sci.Abstr., Dent.Ind., Excerp.Med., Ind.Med. (1967-), Ind.Sci.Rev., Ind.Vet., Med.& Surg.Dermat., NRN, Nutr.Abstr., Sci.Cit.Ind., Telegen, Vet.Bull.
—BLDSC (6256.900000), CASDDS, CISTI, GNLM, IDS, ingenta, KNAW. **CCC.**
Published by: S. Karger AG, Allschwilerstr 10, PO Box, Basel 4009, Switzerland. TEL 41-61-306-1111, FAX 41-61-306-1234, karger@karger.ch, http://www.online.karger.com/journals/ocl, http://www.karger.com. Ed. P P Carbone. adv.: page USD 1,185. Circ: 1,500.

616.99 618 JPN ISSN 0913-9834
ONCOLOGY & CHEMOTHERAPY. Text in Japanese. 1985. q. JPY 1,500 per issue (effective 2000).
Formerly (until 1986): Research Society on Oncology and Chemotherapy in Gynecology (0912-1013)
—BLDSC (6256.965000).
Published by: Japanese Association for Oncology and Chemotherapy, Topuki Yoshida-Bldg 301, 4-1-31 kudan-Kita, Chiyoda-ku, Tokyo 102-0073, Japan.

616.99 USA ISSN 1046-3356
ONCOLOGY ISSUES. Text in English. 1986. bi-m. USD 20 to individuals; USD 40 to corporations (effective 2001). adv. back issues avail. **Document type:** *Trade.* **Description:** Provides economic, health policy and planning information to United States cancer programs.
Related titles: Online - full text ed.
—BLDSC (6256.972000).
Published by: Association of Community Cancer Centers, 11600 Nebel St, Ste 201, Rockville, MD 20852. TEL 301-984-9496, FAX 301-770-1949, http://www.medscape.com/ACCC/OncIssues/public/journal.OncIssues.html. Ed., R&P Donald Jewler. Adv. contact Mal Milburn TEL 301-984-9496. Circ: 17,000.

616.99 USA
▼ **ONCOLOGY NET GUIDE;** internet guide to cancer sites. Text in English. 2000. q. **Document type:** *Journal, Trade.* **Description:** Reviews, describes and compiles online resources for oncologists.
Related titles: ♦ E-mail ed.: Oncology net guide eNewsletter; ♦ Online - full content ed.: Oncology net guide Online.

M

Published by: Intellisphere (Subsidiary of: MultiMedia Healthcare Inc.), Office Center at Princeton Meadows, Ste 400, Plainsboro, NJ 08536. TEL 609-275-3800, FAX 609-275-6076, info@mdnetguide.com, http://www.oncologynetguide.com. Ed. Mary Jardem.

616.99 USA
▼ **ONCOLOGY NET GUIDE ENEWSLETTER.** Text in English. 2000. bi-m. **Document type:** *Trade.* **Description:** Provides information on headlines, upcoming events, and special promotions related to oncology.
Media: E-mail. **Related titles:** ♦ Online - full content ed.: Oncology net guide Online; ♦ Print ed.: Oncology net guide.
Published by: Intellisphere (Subsidiary of: MultiMedia Healthcare Inc.), Office Center at Princeton Meadows, Ste 400, Plainsboro, NJ 08536. TEL 609-275-3800, FAX 609-275-6076, info@mdnetguide.com, http://www.oncologynetguide.com. Ed. Mary Jardem.

616.99 USA
▼ **ONCOLOGY NET GUIDE ONLINE**; internet guide to cancer sites. Text in English. 2000. d. **Document type:** *Trade.* **Description:** Provides a health care global network for oncology clinicians and researchers by compiling useful and pertinent websites.
Media: Online - full content. **Related titles:** ♦ E-mail ed.: Oncology net guide eNewsletter; ♦ Print ed.: Oncology net guide.
Published by: Intellisphere (Subsidiary of: MultiMedia Healthcare Inc.), Office Center at Princeton Meadows, Ste 400, Plainsboro, NJ 08536. TEL 609-275-3800, FAX 609-275-6076, info@mdnetguide.com, http://www.oncologynetguide.com. Ed. Mary Jardem.

616.99 USA ISSN 1065-2957
ONCOLOGY NEWS INTERNATIONAL. Text in English. 1992. 12/yr. USD 97 domestic; USD 103 in Canada; USD 122 elsewhere; USD 82 to students; USD 16 newsstand/cover (effective 2001). adv. **Document type:** *Newspaper, Academic/Scholarly.* **Description:** Publishes timely reports on news and developments from around the world in all areas of interest to the cancer specialist.
Related titles: ♦ Supplement: A Supplement to Oncology News International.
—**CCC.**
Published by: P R R, Inc., 48 S Service Rd, Melville, NY 11747-2335. TEL 631-777-3800, FAX 631-777-8700. Ed. Dr. Martin Abeloff. Pub. Joseph Schuldner. adv.: B&W page USD 3,090, color page USD 4,380; trim 14.75 x 10.88. Circ: 907 (paid); 26,722 (controlled).

ONCOLOGY NURSES TODAY. see *MEDICAL SCIENCES—Nurses And Nursing*

ONCOLOGY NURSING FORUM. see *MEDICAL SCIENCES—Nurses And Nursing*

616.99 GRC ISSN 1021-335X
CODEN: OCRPEW
ONCOLOGY REPORTS; an international journal devoted to fundamental and applied research in oncology. Text in Greek. 1994. bi-m. USD 190 in Europe to individuals; USD 210 elsewhere to individuals; USD 450 in Europe to institutions; USD 500 elsewhere to institutions (effective 2002). adv. bk.rev. index. *Refereed.* **Document type:** *Journal, Academic/Scholarly.* **Description:** Covers the spectrum of cancer research; aimed at a multidisciplinary readership.
Related titles: Online - full text ed.: (from Institute for Scientific Information).
Indexed: ASCA, Aqua.Sci.& Fish.Abstr., Chem.Abstr., Chem.Titles, Curr.Cont., Dairy Sci.Abstr., Environ.Sci.Poll.Mgmt., Excerp.Med. (1995-), Helminthol.Abstr., Ind.Med. (1994-), Inpharma, Int.Abstr.Biol.Sci., Nutr.Abstr., Pharm.&Out.News, Pollut.Abstr., Reac., Rev.Med.& Vet.Mycol., Sci.Cit.Ind.
—BLDSC (6256.983350), CASDDS, GNLM, IDS, Infotrieve, KNAW. **CCC.**
Published by: Demetrios A. Spandidos Ed. & Pub., PO Box 18179, Athens 116 10, Greece. TEL 30-1-722-7809, FAX 30-1-752-3866, spandido@hol.gr.

616.99 USA ISSN 0965-0407
RC261.A1 CODEN: ONREE8
ONCOLOGY RESEARCH. Text in English. 1989. m. USD 825 domestic; USD 875 foreign (effective 2001). adv. back issues avail. *Refereed.* **Document type:** *Academic/Scholarly.* **Description:** Rapid dissemination journal for full research papers and short communications contributing to the understanding of cancer in areas of molecular biology, cell biology, biochemistry, biophysics, genetics, virology, endocrinology and immunology.
Formerly (until 1992): Cancer Communications (0955-3541)
Related titles: Microfilm ed.: (from PQC); Online - full text ed.: (from Institute for Scientific Information).
Indexed: ASCA, Chem.Abstr., Chem.Indus.Notes, Chem.Titles, Curr.Cont., Excerp.Med., Genet.Abstr. (coverage dropped), INIS Atomind., Ind.Med. (1992-), Ind.Sci.Rev., Inpharma, Pharm.&Out.News, Reac., Sci.Cit.Ind.
—BLDSC (6256.983400), CASDDS, CISTI, EMDOCS, GNLM, IDS, KNAW. **CCC.**
Published by: Cognizant Communication Corporation, 3 Hartsdale Rd, Elmsford, NY 10523-3701. TEL 914-592-7720, FAX 914-592-8981, cogcomm@aol.com, http://www.cognizantcommunication.com. Eds. Alan C Sartorelli, Takashi Tsurno. Pub., R&P Robert N Miranda. Adv. contact Lori Miranda.

616.99 GBR ISSN 0265-7945
ONCOLOGY REVIEW. Text in English. 1984. irreg. **Document type:** *Monographic series, Academic/Scholarly.* **Description:** Contains highlights from major international cancer conferences.
Indexed: Ref.Zh.
—BLDSC (6256.983500).
Published by: Gardiner - Caldwell Communications Ltd., Victoria Mill, Windmill St, Macclesfield, Ches SK11 7HQ, United Kingdom. TEL 44-1625-664000, FAX 44-1625-610260, louise_garrod@gardiner-caldwell.com. Circ: 100.

616.992 USA
ONCOLOGY SPECIAL EDITION. Text in English. a. **Document type:** *Trade.* **Description:** Publishes a collection of relevant clinical reviews devoted exclusively to exploring the latest drug information in succinct educational summaries.
Published by: McMahon Group, 545 W 45th St, 8th Fl, New York, NY 10036. TEL 212-957-5300, FAX 212-957-7230, cdeluca@mcmahonmed.com, http://www.mcmahonmed.com/se/indexse.htm.

616.99 USA ISSN 0276-2234
ONCOLOGY TIMES; the independent newspaper for cancer specialists. Text in English. 1979. m., latest vol.23. USD 165 domestic to individuals; USD 214 foreign to individuals; USD 331 domestic to institutions; USD 331 foreign to institutions; USD 21 newsstand/cover (effective 2002). adv. bk.rev. index. back issues avail. *Refereed.* **Document type:** *Newspaper.* **Description:** Covers all aspects of the diagnosis, treatment, and care of the cancer patient.
Indexed: Biol.Dig.
Published by: Lippincott Williams & Wilkins, 345 Hudson St, 16th Fl, New York, NY 10014-4502. TEL 212-840-7760, FAX 212-840-7813, oncologytimes@compuserve.com, http://www.oncology-times.com, http://www.lrpub.com. Ed. Serena Stockwell. Pub. Nhora Cortes Comerer. R&P Kyle Booth. Adv. contact Ray Thibodeau. B&W page USD 3,340, color page USD 4,740. Circ: 38,513.

616.99 DEU ISSN 0947-8965
DER ONKOLOGE. Text in German. 1995. m. EUR 219.77 domestic; EUR 192.97 in Germany; EUR 17.80 newsstand/cover foreign (effective 2002). adv. back issues avail. *Refereed.* **Document type:** *Journal, Academic/Scholarly.*
Related titles: Online - full text ed.: ISSN 1433-0415 (from EBSCO Publishing, RoweCom Information Quest, Swets Blackwell, Springer LINK).
—BLDSC (6260.580000), EMDOCS, GNLM, KNAW. **CCC.**
Published by: Springer-Verlag (Subsidiary of: BertelsmannSpringer), Tiergartenstr 17, Heidelberg 69121, Germany. TEL 49-6221-345-0, FAX 49-6221-345229, subscriptions@springer.de, http://link.springer.de/link/service/journals/00761/index.htm, http://www.springer.de. Ed. M Bamberg. **Subscr. in N. America to:** Springer-Verlag New York Inc., PO Box 2485, Secaucus, NJ 07096-2485. TEL 212-460-1500, FAX 212-473-6272.

616.99 RUS
ONKOLOGICHESKII NAUCHNYI TSENTR. VESTNIK. Text in Russian. q. USD 129.95 in United States.
Published by: Onkologicheskii Nauchnyi Tsentr, Kashirskoe shosse 24, Moscow 115478, Russian Federation. TEL 7-095-3241891. **US dist. addr.:** East View Publications, 3020 Harbor Ln N, Minneapolis, MN 55447. TEL 612-550-0961.

616 CHE ISSN 0378-584X
CODEN: ONKOD2
ONKOLOGIE; international journal for cancer research and treatment. Text in English, German. bi-m. CHF 229 in Europe to institutions; CHF 246.40 elsewhere to institutions; EUR 150 in Europe to institutions; USD 184 elsewhere to institutions (effective 2002). adv. illus. index. back issues avail. *Refereed.* **Document type:** *Journal, Academic/Scholarly.*
Formerly: Oesterreichische Zeitschrift fuer Onkologie
Related titles: Microform ed.: (from PQC); Online - full text ed.: ISSN 1423-0240. CHF 58 in Europe with print edition; CHF 58 overseas with print edition; DEM 78 in Germany with print edition; USD 45 in United States with print edition (effective 2001) (from EBSCO Publishing, O C L C Online Computer Library Center, Inc., RoweCom Information Quest, Swets Blackwell, Institute for Scientific Information).
Indexed: ASCA, Biol.Abstr., Curr.Adv.Cancer Res., Curr.Adv.Ecol.Sci., Curr.Cont., Dent.Ind., Excerp.Med., Ind.Med. (coverage dropped), Ind.Sci.Rev., Inpharma, Pharm.&Out.News, Reac., Ref.Zh., Rev.Med.& Vet.Mycol., SSCI (coverage dropped), Sci.Cit.Ind.
—CASDDS, CISTI, EMDOCS, GNLM, IDS, Infotrieve, KNAW. **CCC.**
Published by: (Deutsche und Oesterreichische Gesellschaft fuer Haematologie und Onkologie), S. Karger AG, Allschwilerstr 10, PO Box, Basel 4009, Switzerland. TEL 41-61-306-1111, FAX 41-61-306-1234, karger@karger.ch, http://www.online.karger.com/journals/onk, http://www.karger.com. Eds. W Queisser, W Scheithauer. Circ: 11,000. **Co-sponsor:** Oesterreichische Krebsgesellschaft-Krebsliga.

616.99 AUT ISSN 1436-1280
▼ **ONKOLOGIE HEUTE.** Text in German. 1999. irreg. price varies. **Document type:** *Monographic series, Academic/Scholarly.*
Published by: Springer-Verlag Wien (Subsidiary of: BertelsmannSpringer), Sachsenplatz 4-6, PO Box 89, Vienna, W 1201, Austria. TEL 43-1-3302415-0, FAX 43-1-330242665, books@springer.at, http://www.springer.at. Eds. C Zielinski, R Jakesz. R&P Angela Foessl TEL 43-1-3302415517. **Dist. in N. America by:** Springer-Verlag, Journals. books@springer.at, http://www.springer-ny.com.

616.99 AUT
ONKOLOGIE IN DER PRAXIS. Text in German. 4/yr. **Document type:** *Journal, Trade, Academic/Scholarly.* **Description:** Covers all aspects of cancer detection, treatment and research.
Published by: Aerzte Woche Zeitungsverlagsgesellschaft mbH (Subsidiary of: BertelsmannSpringer), Wiesingerstr 1, Vienna 1010, Austria. TEL 43-1-5131047, FAX 43-1-5134783, aerzte@aerztewoche.at, http://www.aerztewoche.at. Ed. Dr. Monika Steinmassl-Wirrer.

616 BGR ISSN 0369-7649
CODEN: ONKLAO
ONKOLOGIJA. Text in Bulgarian; Summaries in English, Russian. 1964. q. BGL 10, USD 6.
Indexed: Abstr.Bulg.Sci.Med.Lit., Excerp.Med., INIS Atomind.
—CASDDS, CISTI, GNLM.
Published by: (Bulgaria. Ministerstvo na Narodnoto Zdrave), Izdatelstvo Meditsina i Fizkultura, 11 Pl Slaveikov, Sofia 1080, Bulgaria. Ed. T Tchernozemski. Circ: 713. **Dist. by:** Hemus, 6 Rouski blvd, Sofia 1000, Bulgaria. **Co-sponsor:** Nauchno Druzhestvo op Onkologija.

616.9 619 UKR ISSN 1562-1774
ONKOLOGIYA. Text in Russian, Ukrainian; Abstracts in English; Summaries in English. q.
Published by: (Natsional'na Akademiya Nauk Ukrainy, Institut Eksperymental'noi Patologii Onkologii i Radiobiologii im. R.E. Kavets'kogo), Morion LLC, a/c A-82, Kiev 01001, Ukraine. TEL 380-44-2386860, exponcol@onconet.kiev.ua.

616.99 GBR ISSN 1362-6817
OPINION: SPECIALIST REVIEWS OF KEY PAPERS IN ONCOLOGY. Abbreviated title: Opinion: Oncology. Text in English. 1996. 3/yr. bk.rev. **Document type:** *Academic/Scholarly.*
Published by: Hayward Medical Communications Ltd., 44 Earlham St, Covent Garden, London WC2H 7LA, United Kingdom. TEL 44-20-7240-4493, FAX 44-20-7240-4479, admin@hayward.co.uk, http://www.hayward.co.uk. Ed. J Carmichael. Circ: 1,500. **Subscr. to:** Rosemary House, Lanwades Park, Kentford, Near, Newmarket, Suffolk CB8 7PW, United Kingdom. TEL 44-1638-751515, FAX 44-1638-751517.

616.99 GBR ISSN 1368-8375
RC280.M6 CODEN: EJCCER
ORAL ONCOLOGY. Text in English. 1965. 8/yr. EUR 97 in Europe to individuals; JPY 12,900 in Japan to individuals; USD 109 elsewhere to individuals; EUR 717 in Europe to institutions; JPY 95,200 in Japan to institutions; USD 802 elsewhere to institutions (effective 2002). *Refereed.* **Document type:** *Academic/Scholarly.* **Description:** Discusses issues relating to aetiopathogenesis, epidemiology, prevention and management of oral cancer.
Formerly (until 1997): European Journal of Cancer. Part B: Oral Oncology (0964-1955); Which superseded in part (in 1992): European Journal of Cancer (0959-8049); Which was formerly (until 1990): European Journal of Cancer and Clinical Oncology (0277-5379); (until 1981): European Journal of Cancer (0014-2964)
Related titles: Microfilm ed.: (from PQC); Online - full text ed.: (from ingenta, Swets Blackwell, ScienceDirect, Institute for Scientific Information).
Indexed: AIDS & Cancer Res., ASCA, Abstr.Hyg., Chem.Abstr., Chem.Indus.Notes, Chem.Titles, Curr.Cont., Derwent Biotech.Abstr., Environ.Sci.Poll.Mgmt., Excerp.Med. (1993-), INIS Atomind., Ind.Med. (1997-), Ind.Sci.Rev., Inpharma, Int.Abstr.Biol.Sci., Nutr.Abstr., Oncog.G.F.Abstr., Pharm.&Out.News, Reac., Sci.Cit.Ind., THA, Trop.Dis.Bull.
—BLDSC (6277.592000), ADONIS, CASDDS, CISTI, EMDOCS, IDS, Infotrieve, ingenta, KNAW. **CCC.**
Published by: Pergamon (Subsidiary of: Elsevier Science), The Boulevard, Langford Ln, East Park, Kidlington, Oxford OXB 1GB, United Kingdom. FAX 44-1865-843010, http://www.elsevier.com/locate/oraloncology. Ed. Crispian Scully. **Subscr. in Australasia and the Far East to:** Elsevier Science (Singapore) Pte Ltd, No.1 Temasek Ave, 17-01 Millenia Tower, Singapore 039192, Singapore. TEL 65-434-3727, FAX 65-337-2230; **Subscr. in the Americas to:** Elsevier Science, PO Box 945, New York, NY 10159-0945. TEL 212-633-3730, FAX 212-633-3680, usinfo-f@elsevier.com; **Subscr. to:** Elsevier Science BV, PO Box 211, Amsterdam 1000 AE, Netherlands. TEL 31-20-485-3757.

616 JPN
OSAKA UNIVERSITY. INSTITUTE FOR CANCER RESEARCH. ANNUAL REPORT✱ . Text in English. irreg. per issue exchange basis.
Published by: (Osaka Daigaku, Igakubu Fuzoku Gankenku Shisetsu), Osaka University Press, c/o Osaka Daigaku Jimukyoku, 1-1 Yamada-Oka, Suita-shi, Osaka-fu 565-0871, Japan.

616.9 USA
P P O UPDATE. (Principles and Practices of Oncology) Text in English. 1987. m. USD 99 (effective 2000). **Document type:** *Academic/Scholarly.* **Description:** Provides updated information for the textbook Principles and Practices of Oncology.
Published by: Lippincott Williams & Wilkins (Philadelphia) (Subsidiary of: Wolters Kluwer N.V.), 530 Walnut St, Philadelphia, PA 19106-3621. TEL 301-223-2300, 800-638-3030, FAX 301-223-2400, http://www.lww.com. Circ: 25,000 (controlled).

THE PAIN CLINIC. see *MEDICAL SCIENCES—Anaesthesiology*

▼ **THE PAIN CLINIC: A MULTIDISCIPLINARY APPROACH TO ACUTE AND CHRONIC PAIN MANAGEMENT.** see *MEDICAL SCIENCES—Orthopedics And Traumatology*

THE PAIN CLINIC (PROCEEDINGS). see *MEDICAL SCIENCES—Anaesthesiology*

616.99 610.73 362.1 GBR ISSN 0969-7853
PALLIATIVE CARE TODAY; the journal for today's palliative care team. Text in English. 1992. q. free per issue to qualified personnel. bk.rev. *Refereed.* **Document type:** *Academic/Scholarly, Trade.* **Description:** Discusses various topics in treating and offering comfort to persons with terminal illnesses.
Indexed: AMED.
—BLDSC (6345.562058).
Published by: (N A P P in Palliative Care), C C T Healthcare Communications Ltd., C C T Healthcare Communications Ltd, 50-52 Union St, London SE1 1TD, United Kingdom. TEL 0171-407-9731, FAX 0171-407-7083. Eds. Ilora Finlay, Dr. John Ellershaw. Pub. Cath Hawkings. Circ: 8,000 (controlled).

616.994 GBR ISSN 1219-4956
CODEN: POREFR
PATHOLOGY AND ONCOLOGY RESEARCH. Text in English. 1995. q. GBP 52 to individuals; USD 84 in United States to individuals; GBP 96 to institutions (effective 2000). adv. **Document type:** *Academic/Scholarly.* **Description:** Provides an international forum for the communication of reviews, original research and critical and topical reports in pathology and oncology covering basic research and clinicopathological developments.
Related titles: Online - full text ed.: (from EBSCO Publishing, RoweCom Information Quest, Swets Blackwell, IDEAL Online Library).
Indexed: Environ.Sci.Poll.Mgmt., Ind.Med. (1995-), Int.Nurs.Ind., Oncog.G.F.Abstr. (coverage dropped), Ref.Zh., Risk Abstr., Saf.Sci.Abstr.
—CASDDS, GNLM.
Published by: (Aranyi Lajos Foundation), W.B. Saunders Co. Ltd. (Subsidiary of: Harcourt Publishers Ltd.), 24-28 Oval Rd, London NW1 7DX, United Kingdom. TEL 44-20-7424-4200, FAX 44-20-7424-4515, http://www.harcourt-international.com/journals/paor, http://www.wbsaunders.com. Eds. Jozsef Timar, Laszlo Kopper. **Subscr. addr. in US:** Harcourt Health Sciences; **Subscr. to:** Harcourt Publishers Ltd., Foots Cray High St, Sidcup, Kent DA14 5HP, United Kingdom. TEL 44-20-8308-5700, FAX 44-20-8309-0807.

616.992 USA
▼ **PEDIATRIC CANCER SOURCEBOOK.** Text in English. 1999. irreg., latest 1999. USD 78 per issue (effective 2001). charts. Index. **Document type:** *Consumer.* **Description:** Basic consumer health information about cancers in infants, children, and adolescents.
Published by: Omnigraphics, Inc., 615 Griswold St, Detroit, MI 48226. TEL 313-961-1340, 800-234-1340, FAX 313-961-1383, 800-875-1340, info@omnigraphics.com, http://www.omnigraphics.com. Ed. Edward J Prucha.

PEDIATRIC HEMATOLOGY & ONCOLOGY. see *MEDICAL SCIENCES—Pediatrics*

618.92 616 USA ISSN 1054-2086
PEDIATRIC HEMATOLOGY - ONCOLOGY SERIES. Text in English. 1988. irreg., latest 1990. price varies. reprint service avail. from PQC. *Refereed.* **Document type:** *Monographic series.*
Published by: Lippincott Williams & Wilkins (Philadelphia) (Subsidiary of: Wolters Kluwer N.V.), 530 Walnut St, Philadelphia, PA 19106-3621. TEL 215-521-8300, FAX 215-521-8902, custserv@lww.com, http://www.lww.com/. **Subscr. to:** Lippincott Williams & Wilkins (Baltimore), 12107 Insurance Way, Hagerstown, MD 21740. TEL 301-714-2300, FAX 301-714-2398, 800-638-3030.

PEDIATRIC PATHOLOGY & MOLECULAR MEDICINE. see *MEDICAL SCIENCES—Pediatrics*

616.994 ITA ISSN 0069-8520
CODEN: PPQCDL
PERUGIA QUADRENNIAL INTERNATIONAL CONFERENCES ON CANCER. PROCEEDINGS. Text in Italian. 1957. quadrennial. price varies. index. **Document type:** *Proceedings.*
—CASDDS.
Published by: Universita degli Studi di Perugia, Division of Cancer Research, P.O. Box 327, P O Box 327, Monteluce, PG 06100, Italy. Ed. Lucio Severi.

616.994 PHL ISSN 0031-7608
PHILIPPINE JOURNAL OF CANCER✱ . Text in English. 1970 (vol.12). q. PHP 10. charts, illus, stat. index.
Indexed: Chem.Abstr., Ind.Med. (coverage dropped).
Published by: Philippine Cancer Society, 310 San Rafael, Manila, Philippines. Ed. Dr. C P Manahan. Circ: 1,000.

618.92 616.99 USA
PHOENIX (BETHESDA). Text in English. 1993. 2/yr. USD 25 to institutions. **Document type:** *Newsletter.* **Description:** Newsletter for adult survivors of childhood cancer.
Published by: Candlelighters Childhood Cancer Foundation, 3910 Warner St, Kensington, MD 20895-3931. TEL 301-657-8401, 800-366-2223. Circ: 1,300.

616.99 USA ISSN 0743-8176
RC261.A1
PRIMARY CARE & CANCER. Text in English. 1981. 10/yr. USD 90 domestic; USD 96 in Canada & Mexico; USD 105 elsewhere (effective 2000). adv. charts, illus, stat. reprint service avail. from PQC. **Description:** Reports on the latest developments in cancer prevention, early detection, diagnosis, and follow-up.
Formerly (until 1984): Your Patient and Cancer (0272-6955)
Related titles: Microform ed.: (from PQC); Online - full text ed.
Indexed: Ref.Zh.
—BLDSC (6612.908100), CISTI, GNLM, Infotrieve. **CCC.**
Published by: P R R, Inc., 48 S Service Rd, Melville, NY 11747-2335. TEL 631-777-3800, FAX 631-777-8700, info.prr@scp.com. Ed. Dr. Robert F Wittes. Pub. John J Coronna. adv.: B&W page USD 4,800, color page USD 6,050; trim 14.75 x 10.88. Circ: 70,440 (controlled).

616.994 CAN ISSN 0033-0604
PROGRESS AGAINST CANCER. Text in English. 1948. 3/yr. free per issue. illus. **Document type:** *Consumer.*
Related titles: French ed.: Progres Contre le Cancer.
Published by: Canadian Cancer Society, 10 Alcorn Ave, Ste 200, Toronto, ON M4V 3B1, Canada. TEL 416-961-7223. Ed. Kerstin Ring. Circ: 8,000.

616 USA ISSN 0145-3726
CODEN: PCRTDK
PROGRESS IN CANCER RESEARCH AND THERAPY. Text in English. 1976. irreg. price varies. reprint service avail. from PQC. *Refereed.* **Document type:** *Proceedings.*
Indexed: Biol.Abstr., Chem.Abstr., Dairy Sci.Abstr., Hort.Abstr., Nutr.Abstr.
—CASDDS, CISTI, KNAW.
Published by: Lippincott Williams & Wilkins (Philadelphia) (Subsidiary of: Wolters Kluwer N.V.), 530 Walnut St, Philadelphia, PA 19106-3621. TEL 301-223-2300, 800-638-3030, FAX 301-223-2400, http://www.lww.com.

616.994 CHE ISSN 0079-6263
RC254 CODEN: PEXTAR
PROGRESS IN EXPERIMENTAL TUMOR RESEARCH. Text in English. 1960. irreg., latest vol.37. price varies. back issues avail.; reprint service avail. from ISI. *Refereed.* **Document type:** *Monographic series, Academic/Scholarly.* **Description:** Overviews of experimental work in key areas of tumor research.
Related titles: Online - full text ed.: (from Institute for Scientific Information).
Indexed: ASCA, Biol.Abstr., Chem.Abstr., Chem.Titles, Curr.Cont. (coverage dropped), INIS Atomind., Ind.Med. (1960-), Ind.Sci.Rev., Rev.Med.& Vet.Mycol., Sci.Cit.Ind.
—CASDDS, CISTI, GNLM, ingenta, KNAW. **CCC.**
Published by: S. Karger AG, Allschwilerstr 10, PO Box, Basel 4009, Switzerland. TEL 41-61-306-1111, FAX 41-61-306-1234, karger@karger.ch, http://www.karger.com/bookseries/PRETR. Ed. J R Bertino.

571.86 USA ISSN 0884-6790
CODEN: PLBIE5
PROGRESS IN LEUKOCYTE BIOLOGY. Text in English. 1985. irreg. **Document type:** *Monographic series.*
Indexed: Chem.Abstr., Chem.Indus.Notes, Chem.Titles.
—CASDDS, CISTI, KNAW.
Published by: John Wiley & Sons, Inc., Journals (Subsidiary of: Wiley InterScience), 605 Third Ave, New York, NY 10158. **Subscr. outside of the Americas to:** John Wiley & Sons Ltd., Baffins Ln, Chichester, Sussex PO19 IUD, United Kingdom. FAX 44-1243-776128.

616.99 GBR ISSN 0969-9260
PROGRESS IN PALLIATIVE CARE. Text in English. 1993. bi-m. USD 118 in United States to individuals; GBP 67 in the European Union to individuals; USD 274 in United States to institutions; GBP 164 in the European Union to institutions (effective 2002). back issues avail. **Document type:** *Academic/Scholarly.* **Description:** Locates and reports the scholarly literature on all aspects of the management of the problems of end-stage disease, and issues pertinent to living with chronic or progressive disease.
Indexed: AMED.
—BLDSC (6872.285000).
Published by: Maney Publishing, Hudson Rd, Leeds, W Yorks LS9 7DL, United Kingdom. TEL 44-113-249-7481, FAX 44-113-248-6983, maney@maney.co.uk, http://www.maney.co.uk. Ed. Ian Maddocks.

616.99 NLD ISSN 0924-1914
PROSTAGLANDINS, LEUKOTRIENES AND CANCER. Text in English. 1985. irreg. price varies. *Refereed.* **Document type:** *Monographic series.*
Indexed: Curr.Cont. (coverage dropped).
—CISTI, KNAW.
Published by: Kluwer Academic Publishers Group (Subsidiary of: Wolters Kluwer N.V.), Spuiboulevard 50, PO Box 17, Dordrecht 3300 AA, Netherlands. FAX 31-78-639-2254, services@wkap.nl, http://www.wkap.nl. **Dist. by:** Journals Department, PO Box 322, Dordrecht 3300 AH, Netherlands. FAX 31-78-654-6474.

M

THE PROSTATE. see *MEDICAL SCIENCES*

616.65 GBR
PROSTATE CANCER. Text in English. 1997. bi-m. **Document type:** *Academic/Scholarly.*
Published by: Macmillan Magazines Ltd, Porters South, 4 Crinan Street, London N1 9XW, United Kingdom. TEL 44-171-843-4962, FAX 44-171-843-4998. **Subscr. to:** Brunel Rd., Houndmills, ., Basingstoke, Hants RG21 2BR, United Kingdom. TEL 44-1256-29242, 44-1256-612358; **Subscr. to:** 345 Park Ave S, New York, NY 10010-1707.

616.65 GBR ISSN 1365-7852
CODEN: PCPDFW
PROSTATE CANCER AND PROSTATIC DISEASES. Text in English. 1997. bi-m. GBP 223 in Europe to individuals print or online ed.; USD 173 in United States to individuals print or online ed.; GBP 225 elsewhere to individuals print or online ed.; GBP 127 combined subscription in Europe to individuals print & online; USD 191 combined subscription elsewhere to individuals print & online; GBP 225 in Europe to institutions print or online ed.; USD 338 elsewhere to institutions print or online ed.; GBP 248 combined subscription in Europe to institutions print & online; USD 372 combined subscription elsewhere to institutions print & online (effective 2002). adv. bk.rev. charts, illus, stat. index. back issues avail.; reprints avail. *Refereed.* **Document type:** *Journal, Academic/Scholarly.* **Description:** Focuses on all aspects of prostate cancer and prostatic diseases, and covers both clinical and basic research.
Related titles: Online - full text ed.: (from EBSCO Publishing, O C L C Online Computer Library Center, Inc., RoweCom Information Quest, ingenta, Swets Blackwell, Institute for Scientific Information).
Indexed: Curr.Cont., Inpharma, Pharm.&Out.News, Reac.
—BLDSC (6935.194500), CASDDS, CISTI, IDS, Infotrieve. **CCC.**
Published by: Nature Publishing Group Specialist Journals (Subsidiary of: Holtzbrink Publishers), Houndmills, Basingstoke, Hants RG21 6XS, United Kingdom. TEL 44-1256-329242, FAX 44-1256-328339, subscriptions@nature.com, http://www.nature.com/pcan. Eds. Judd W Moul, Michael K Brawer, Roger S Kirby. Pub. Sue Deeley. R&P Trace Noel. Adv. contact Robert Sloan TEL 44-20-8882-7199. B&W page GBP 595, color page GBP 1,150; trim 210 x 280.

▼ **THE PROSTATE JOURNAL.** see *MEDICAL SCIENCES*

THE PROSTATE JOURNAL ONLINE. see *MEDICAL SCIENCES*

616.99 GBR ISSN 1057-9249
RC261.A1 CODEN: POJCEE
PSYCHO-ONCOLOGY; journal of the psychological, social and behavioral dimensions of cancer. Text in English. 1992. 8/yr. USD 710 in United States; USD 710 in Canada & Mexico; USD 710 elsewhere; USD 746 combined subscription in United States for print and online eds.; USD 746 combined subscription in Canada & Mexico for print and online eds.; USD 746 combined subscription elsewhere for print and online eds. (effective 2002). adv. back issues avail.; reprint service avail. from SWZ. *Refereed.* **Document type:** *Academic/Scholarly.* **Description:** Covers the the psychological, social, behavioral, and ethical aspects of cancer.
Related titles: Microform ed.: (from PQC); Online - full text ed.: ISSN 1099-1611. 1996. USD 710 in United States; USD 710 in Canada & Mexico; USD 710 elsewhere (effective 2002) (from EBSCO Publishing, Wiley InterScience, Institute for Scientific Information).
Indexed: ASSIA, AgeLine, Brit.Nur.Ind., CINAHL, Curr.Cont., Excerp.Med. (1994-), Fam.Ind., Ind.Med. (1992-), Int.Nurs.Ind., PsycInfo, Ref.Zh., SSCI, e-psyche.
—BLDSC (6946.543200), GNLM, IDS, Infotrieve, KNAW. **CCC.**
Published by: Wiley Europe Ltd., Baffins Ln, Chichester, W Sussex PO19 1UD, United Kingdom. TEL 44-1243-779777, FAX 44-1243-843232, customer@wiley.co.uk, http://www.wiley.co.uk. Eds. Jimmie C Holland, Maggie Watson. Pub. Richard Edelstein. R&P Diane Southern TEL 44-1243-770347. adv.: B&W page GBP 750, color page GBP 1,650; trim 200 x 260. Circ: 1,100. **Subscr. in the Americas to:** John Wiley & Sons, Inc., Journals, 605 Third Ave, New York, NY 10158. TEL 212-850-6645, FAX 212-850-6021, uscs-wis@wiley.com; **Subscr. to:** John Wiley & Sons Ltd., Baffins Ln, Chichester, Sussex PO19 IUD, United Kingdom. cs-journals@wiley.co.uk.

PUBLIC HEALTH REVIEWS; an international quarterly. see *PUBLIC HEALTH AND SAFETY*

616.99 ITA ISSN 1122-0260
QUADERNI DI CURE PALLIATIVE. Text in Italian. 1993. 4/yr. ITL 95,000 (effective 1999). **Document type:** *Academic/Scholarly.*
Published by: Masson S.p.A., Divisione Periodici, Via F.lli Bressan 2, Milan, MI 20126, Italy. TEL 39-2-270741, FAX 39-2-27074210. Ed. F Martino. adv.: B&W page ITL 2,950,000, color page ITL 4,200,000. Circ: 3,000.

RADIATION MEDICINE; medical imaging and radiation oncology. see *MEDICAL SCIENCES—Radiology And Nuclear Medicine*

RADIATION THERAPIST. see *MEDICAL SCIENCES—Radiology And Nuclear Medicine*

RADIOTHERAPY AND ONCOLOGY. see *MEDICAL SCIENCES—Radiology And Nuclear Medicine*

616.99 GBR ISSN 0261-7013
RECENT ADVANCES IN CLINICAL ONCOLOGY. Text in English. 1982. irreg. **Document type:** *Monographic series, Academic/Scholarly.*
Published by: Churchill Livingstone (Subsidiary of: Harcourt Publishers Ltd.), Robert Stevenson House, 1-3 Baxter's Pl, Leith Walk, Edinburgh, Midlothian EH1 3AF, United Kingdom. TEL 44-131-556-2424, FAX 44-131-459-1177, http://www.churchillmed.com. **US subscr. to:** Churchill Livingstone, 650 Ave of the Americas, New York, NY 10011. TEL 212-206-5000.

RECENT ADVANCES IN OPHTHALMOLOGY/YANKE XIN JINZHAN. see *MEDICAL SCIENCES—Ophthalmology And Optometry*

616.994 USA ISSN 0080-0015
RC261 CODEN: RRCRBU
RECENT RESULTS IN CANCER RESEARCH/ FORTSCHRITTE DER KREBSFORSCHUNG. Text in English; Text occasionally in French, German. 1965. irreg., latest vol.136, 1994. price varies. reprint service avail. from ISI. **Document type:** *Academic/Scholarly.*
Related titles: Online - full text ed.: (from Institute for Scientific Information).
Indexed: Biol.Abstr., Chem.Abstr., Dent.Ind., Excerp.Med., INIS Atomind., Ind.Med. (1965-), THA.
—BLDSC (7305.090000), CASDDS, CISTI, GNLM, IDS, ingenta, KNAW, Linda Hall. **CCC.**
Published by: Springer-Verlag, Journals (Subsidiary of: BertelsmannSpringer), 175 Fifth Ave, New York, NY 10010. TEL 212-460-1500, FAX 212-473-6272. Ed. P Rentchnick.

REFERATIVNYI ZHURNAL. ONKOLOGIYA. see *MEDICAL SCIENCES—Abstracting, Bibliographies, Statistics*

REFERATIVNYI ZHURNAL. ONKOLOGIYA: EKSPERIMENTALNAYA. see *MEDICAL SCIENCES—Abstracting, Bibliographies, Statistics*

REFERATIVNYI ZHURNAL. ONKOLOGIYA: TERAPIYA OPUKHOLEI. see *MEDICAL SCIENCES—Abstracting, Bibliographies, Statistics*

RETINOIDS AND LIPID-SOLUBLE VITAMINS IN CLINICAL PRACTICE. see *MEDICAL SCIENCES—Dermatology And Venereology*

616.99 ESP ISSN 0213-8573
REVISIONES EN CANCER. Text in Spanish; Abstracts in Spanish, English. 1987. bi-m. ESP 7,000; USD 200 foreign (effective 2000). adv. abstr, bibl, illus, stat. back issues avail. *Refereed.* **Document type:** *Academic/Scholarly.*
—BLDSC (7800.572000), GNLM.
Published by: Aran Ediciones S.A., Castello, 128 1o, Madrid 28006, Spain. TEL 34-91-782-0030, FAX 34-91-561-5787, edita@grupoaran.com, http://www.grupoaran.com. Ed. Dr. E. Diaz-Rubio. Pub. Jose Jimenez. R&P Maria Dolores Linares TEL 34-1-7820035. Circ: 3,000.

616.994 BRA ISSN 0034-7116
CODEN: RVBCA7
REVISTA BRASILEIRA DE CANCEROLOGIA. Text in Portuguese; Summaries in English, Portuguese. 1947. bi-m. free to qualified personnel; exchange requested. adv. bibl, charts, illus. **Document type:** *Academic/Scholarly.*
Indexed: Chem.Abstr., Excerp.Med., INIS Atomind., Ind.Med. (coverage dropped).
—CASDDS, GNLM.
Address: Pro-Onco/INCa-MS,, Av Venezuela, 134, bl. A 9o andar, Rio De Janeiro, RJ 20081-310, Brazil. TEL 55-21-2638565, FAX 55-21-2638297, atalecio@venus.rdc.puc-rio.br. Ed. Luiz Eduardo Atalecio. Adv. contact Marcos Morais. Circ: 3,000.

616.99 618.1 BRA ISSN 0104-8058
REVISTA BRASILEIRA DE MASTOLOGIA. Text in Portuguese. 1990. q. adv. bk.rev. back issues avail. **Document type:** *Academic/Scholarly.*
Related titles: Online - full text ed.
Published by: Lemos Editorial & Graficos Ltda., Rua Rui Barbosa, 70, B Vista, Sao Paulo, SP 01326-010, Brazil. TEL 55-11-251-4300, FAX 55-11-251-4300, lemospl@netpoint.com.br, http://www.lemos.com.br. Ed. Dr. Alfredo Carlos S D Barros. Adv. contact Paulo Lemos. Circ: 3,000 (controlled).

616.99 CUB ISSN 0864-0297
REVISTA CUBANA DE ONCOLOGIA. Text in Spanish; Summaries in English, Spanish. 1985. 3/yr. USD 36 in the Americas; USD 44 in Europe; USD 52 elsewhere. bibl, charts, illus. index.
Indexed: Excerp.Med. (until 1993), INIS Atomind., Ind.Hyg.Dig.
Published by: (Cuba. Ministerio de Salud Publica, Centro Nacional de Informacion de Ciencias Medicas), Editorial de Ciencias Medicas, O'Reilly No. 4, Habana, Cuba. TEL 809-62-8091. Ed. Frances Saiz. Circ: 1,000. **Co-sponsors:** Sociedad Cubana de Oncologia; Instituto Nacional de Oncologia y Radiobiologia de Cuba.

616.992 USA
ROSEWELLNESS. Text in English. 3/yr. **Document type:** *Magazine, Consumer.*
Published by: Roswell Park Cancer Institute, Elm and Carlton St, Buffalo, NY 14263. TEL 716-845-2300, http://www.roswellpark.org/document_16.html.

616.99 RUS
ROSSIISKII ONKOLOGICHESKII ZHURNAL/RUSSIAN ANEOLOGICAL JOURNAL. Text in Russian; Summaries in English. 1996. bi-m. USD 155 foreign (effective 2000). adv. bk.rev. **Document type:** *Academic/Scholarly.* **Description:** Publishes papers on all aspects of cancer research, ranging from basic investigations to the results of experimental and clinical studies, new trends in the treatment of cancer and cancer control.
Indexed: Ref.Zh.
—BLDSC (0154.059257).
Published by: Izdatel'stvo Meditsina, Petroverigskii per 6-8, Moscow 101000, Russian Federation. TEL 7-095-9456497, 7-095-928-86-48, FAX 7-095-9211355, meditsina@iname.com, http://www.medit.ru. Ed. V I Chissov. Pub. A M Stochik. R&P I Sokolova. Adv. contact O A Fadeeva TEL 7-095-923-51-40. **Dist. by:** Mezhdunarodnaya Kniga, B Yakimanka 39, Moscow 117049, Russian Federation. TEL 7-095-2384967, FAX 7-095-2384634.

616.994 JPN ISSN 0022-2119
CODEN: SKBZAA
SAIBOKAKU BYORIGAKU ZASSHI/JOURNAL OF KARYOPATHOLOGY; tumor and tumor virus. Text in Japanese; Summaries in English. 1953. irreg. USD 2. adv. reprint service avail. from ISI.
Indexed: Biol.Abstr., Ind.Med. (coverage dropped).
—CASDDS.
Published by: (Okayama Daigaku, Igakubu/Okayama University, School of Medicine), Department of Pathology (Subsidiary of: Okayama Daigaku, Igakubu/Okayama University, School of Medicine), 2-5-1 Shikata-cho, Okayama 700, Japan. Ed. Y Hamazaki.

616.99 ITA ISSN 1124-0490
SARCOIDOSIS VASCULITIS AND DIFFUSE LUNG DISEASES. Text in English. 1984. s-a. ITL 68,500; USD 67 foreign. adv. bk.rev. index. Supplement avail. *Refereed.* **Document type:** *Academic/Scholarly.* **Description:** Publishes editorials, original clinical works and case reports, news, scientific notes, and letters to the editor.
Formerly (until 1995): Sarcoidosis (0393-1447)
Related titles: Online - full text ed.: (from Institute for Scientific Information).
Indexed: ASCA, Curr.Cont., Excerp.Med., Ind.Med. (1996-), Ind.Sci.Rev., Inpharma, Reac., SSCI (coverage dropped), Sci.Cit.Ind.
—BLDSC (8076.025300), CISTI, EMDOCS, GNLM, IDS, KNAW.

Published by: (World Association of Sarcoidosis and Other Granulomatous Disorders), P C A Publishing, Via Clerici 12, Brusuglio Di Corman, MI 20032, Italy. TEL 39-02-6630-0802, FAX 39-02-6151239, p.c.a@galactica.it. Ed. D G James. Pub. Gianfranco Boldrini. R&P Lorna Simpson. Adv. contact Liliana Succio. color page ITL 5,000,000. Circ: 1,000.

616.99 GBR ISSN 1357-714X CODEN: SARCFO

SARCOMA. Text in English. 1997. q. GBP 65, USD 106 to individuals; GBP 215, USD 354 to institutions (effective 2002). *Refereed.* **Document type:** *Academic/Scholarly.* **Description:** Publishes papers covering all aspects of connective tissue oncology research. Covers molecular biology and pathology and the clinical sciences of epidemiology, surgery, radiotherapy and chemotherapy.
Related titles: Online - full text ed.: ISSN 1369-1643 (from CatchWord Ltd., EBSCO Publishing, O C L C Online Computer Library Center, Inc., RoweCom Information Quest, Swets Blackwell).
—BLDSC (8076.026000), ADONIS, CASDDS, CatchWord, CISTI, Infotrieve. **CCC.**
Published by: Carfax Publishing Limited (Subsidiary of: Taylor & Francis Group), PO Box 25, Abingdon, Oxon OX14 3UE, United Kingdom. TEL 44-1235-401000, FAX 44-1235-401550, enquiries@carfax.co.uk, enquiry@tandf.co.uk, http://www.carfax.co.uk. Ed. Martin Robinson.

616.99 BGR ISSN 0582-3250 CODEN: SSCMBX

SCRIPTA SCIENTIFICA MEDICA* . Text in English; Summaries in Russian. 1962. a. BGL 10. Supplement avail.; back issues avail.
Indexed: Abstr.Bulg.Sci.Med.Lit., Abstr.Hyg., BSL Biol., Biol.Abstr., Chem.Abstr., Chem.Titles, Trop.Dis.Bull.
—CASDDS, GNLM, KNAW.
Published by: Higher Medical Institute, V Aprilov 15-A, Plovdiv 4000, Bulgaria. Ed. G Marinov. **Subscr. to:** Martinus Nijhoff, PO Box 269, The Hague 2501 AX, Netherlands. TEL 31-79-684400.

SEMINARS IN BREAST DISEASE; diagnostic imaging, medical oncology, pathology, radiation oncology, surgery. see *MEDICAL SCIENCES—Obstetrics And Gynecology*

SEMINARS IN CANCER BIOLOGY. see *BIOLOGY—Physiology*

616.994 USA ISSN 0093-7754
RC261 CODEN: SOLGAV

SEMINARS IN ONCOLOGY. Text in English. 1974 (Mar.). bi-m. USD 181 domestic to individuals; USD 278 foreign to individuals; USD 272 domestic to institutions; USD 334 foreign to institutions; USD 97 domestic to students; USD 167 foreign to students; USD 56 newsstand/cover (effective 2001). adv. bibl, charts, illus. index. *Refereed.* **Document type:** *Journal, Academic/Scholarly.* **Description:** Reviews recent developments in cancer applicable to clinical oncology for general physicians.
Related titles: Online - full text ed.: (from Institute for Scientific Information).
Indexed: ASCA, Biol.Abstr., CINAHL, C.I.S. Abstr., Chem.Abstr., Chem.Indus.Notes, Chem.Titles, Curr.Adv.Cell & Devel.Biol., Curr.Adv.Ecol.Sci., Curr.Adv.Gen.& Molec.Biol., Curr.Cont., Dent.Ind., Excerp.Med., INIS Atomind., Ind.Med. (1974-), Ind.Sci.Rev., Inpharma, NRN, Pharm.&Out.News, Reac., SSCI (coverage dropped), Sci.Cit.Ind.
—BLDSC (8239.456500), CASDDS, CISTI, GNLM, IDS, ingenta, KNAW. **CCC.**
Published by: W.B. Saunders Co. (Subsidiary of: Harcourt Publishers Ltd.), 11830 Westline Industrial Dr, St Louis, MO 63146. TEL 800-325-4177, http:// www.wbsaunders.com. Eds. Dr. John W Yarbro, Dr. Michael J Mastrangelo. adv.: B&W page USD 1,245, color page USD 2,495. Circ: 10,723. **Subscr. to:** Periodicals Fulfillment, W B Saunders Co, 6277 Sea Harbor Dr, 4th Fl, Orlando, FL 32891-4800.

SEMINARS IN ONCOLOGY NURSING. see *MEDICAL SCIENCES—Nurses And Nursing*

616.99 616.07 USA ISSN 1053-4296 CODEN: SRONEO

SEMINARS IN RADIATION ONCOLOGY. Text in English. 1991 (Oct.). q. USD 139 domestic to individuals; USD 182 foreign to individuals; USD 182 domestic to institutions; USD 231 foreign to institutions; USD 70 domestic to students; USD 109 foreign to students; USD 58 newsstand/cover (effective 2001). adv. *Refereed.* **Document type:** *Academic/Scholarly.* **Description:** Discusses the use of radiation in cancer treatment from both clinical and scientific perspectives.
Related titles: Online - full text ed.: (from EBSCO Publishing, Institute for Scientific Information).
Indexed: CINAHL, Curr.Cont., Excerp.Med. (1993-), Ind.Med. (1991-), Inpharma, Int.Nurs.Ind., Pharm.&Out.News, Reac., Sci.Cit.Ind.
—BLDSC (8239.457300), EMDOCS, GNLM, IDS, Infotrieve, KNAW. **CCC.**
Published by: W.B. Saunders Co. (Subsidiary of: Harcourt Publishers Ltd.), 11830 Westline Industrial Dr, St Louis, MO 63146. TEL 800-325-4177, http:// www.wbsaunders.com. Ed. Dr. Joel E Tepper. adv.: B&W page USD 780, color page USD 1,930; trim 10 x 7. Circ: 2,644. **Subscr. to:** Periodicals Fulfillment, W B Saunders Co, 6277 Sea Harbor Dr, 4th Fl, Orlando, FL 32891-4800.

616.99 USA ISSN 8756-0437
RD651 CODEN: SSONEV

SEMINARS IN SURGICAL ONCOLOGY. Text in English. 1978. 8/yr. (in 2 vols., 4 nos./vol.). USD 1,175 in United States; USD 1,255 in Canada & Mexico; USD 1,323 elsewhere; USD 1,234 combined subscription in United States for print and online eds.; USD 1,314 combined subscription in Canada & Mexico for print and online eds.; USD 1,382 combined subscription elsewhere for print and online eds. (effective 2002). adv. back issues avail. *Refereed.* **Document type:** *Academic/Scholarly.* **Description:** Offers invited review articles about topics in the field of surgical oncology. Each issue focuses on a particular disease entity or therapeutic approach.
Formerly (until 1985): International Advances in Surgical Oncology (0190-1575)
Related titles: Microform ed.: (from PQC); Online - full text ed.: ISSN 1098-2388. 1996. USD 1,175 in United States; USD 1,175 in Canada & Mexico; USD 1,175 elsewhere (effective 2002) (from EBSCO Publishing, Wiley InterScience, Institute for Scientific Information).
Indexed: ASCA, Curr.Cont., Excerp.Med., INIS Atomind., Ind.Med. (1985-), Inpharma, Pharm.&Out.News, Reac.
—BLDSC (8239.470000), CASDDS, CISTI, EMDOCS, GNLM, IDS, ingenta, KNAW. **CCC.**
Published by: John Wiley & Sons, Inc., Journals (Subsidiary of: Wiley InterScience), 605 Third Ave, New York, NY 10158. TEL 212-850-6645, FAX 212-850-6021, subinfo@wiley.com, uscs-wis@wiley.com, http://www.wiley.com. Ed. Gerald P Murphy. adv.: B&W page GBP 640, color page GBP 1,515; trim 210 x 279. **Subscr. outside the Americas to:** John Wiley & Sons Ltd., Baffins Ln, Chichester, Sussex PO19 IUD, United Kingdom. TEL 44-1243-779777, FAX 44-1243-843232, cs-journals@wiley.co.uk.

616.99 USA ISSN 1081-0943

SEMINARS IN UROLOGIC ONCOLOGY. Text in English. 1983. q. USD 119 domestic to individuals; USD 167 foreign to individuals; USD 169 domestic to institutions; USD 208 foreign to institutions; USD 59 domestic to students; USD 99 foreign to students; USD 53 newsstand/cover (effective 2001). adv. bibl, charts, illus. index. **Document type:** *Journal, Academic/Scholarly.* **Description:** Each issue covers a specific area, which experts discuss in detail from their clinical experience.
Formerly (until 1995): Seminars in Urology (0730-9147)
Indexed: CINAHL, Ind.Med. (1995-), NRN.
—BLDSC (8239.485508), EMDOCS, GNLM, ingenta, KNAW. **CCC.**
Published by: W.B. Saunders Co. (Subsidiary of: Harcourt Publishers Ltd.), 11830 Westline Industrial Dr, St Louis, MO 63146. TEL 800-325-4177, http:// www.wbsaunders.com. Ed. Dr. James Montie. adv.: B&W page USD 875, color page USD 2,050; trim 10 x 7. Circ: 1,515. **Subscr. to:** Periodicals Fulfillment, W B Saunders Co, 6277 Sea Harbor Dr, 4th Fl, Orlando, FL 32891-4800.

616.99 CHN ISSN 1001-1692

SHIYONG ZHONGLIU ZAZHI/JOURNAL OF PRACTICAL ONCOLOGY. Text in Chinese. q. CNY 4.40. *Refereed.*
Published by: Zhejiang Yike Daxue/Zhejiang Medical University, Population Research Institute, 353 Yan'an Lu, Hangzhou, Zhejiang 310006, China. TEL 86-571-7217265, FAX 86-571-7217044. Ed. Zheng Shu. **Dist. outside China by:** China International Book Trading Corp, 35 Chegongzhuang Xilu, Haidian District, Beijing 100044, China.

616.99 CHN ISSN 1002-3070

SHIYONG ZHONGLIUXUE ZAZHI/JOURNAL OF APPLIED ONCOLOGY. Text in Chinese. 1987. q. CNY 4.80. **Document type:** *Academic/Scholarly.*
Published by: Heilongjiang Zhongliu Fangzhi Bangongshi/Heilongjiang Cancer Prevention and Treatment Office, Haping Lu, Harbin, Heilongjiang 150040, China. TEL 65003. Ed. Ding Li. Circ: 4,000.

616.99 DEU ISSN 0721-6831

SIGNAL; Leben mit Krebs. Text in German. 4/yr. EUR 25.20 domestic to institutions; EUR 29.20 in Europe to institutions; EUR 34.60 elsewhere to institutions; EUR 5.40 newsstand/cover (effective 2002). **Document type:** *Journal, Academic/Scholarly.*
Related titles: Online - full text ed.: (from Northern Light Technology, Inc.).
Indexed: Abstr.Engl.Stud.
—GNLM, Infotrieve. **CCC.**
Published by: Karl F. Haug Verlag, Fritz-Frey-Str 21, Heidelberg 69121, Germany. TEL 49-6221-489445, FAX 49-6221-489584, http://www.haug-verlag.de. Ed. Arndt Kroedel. Adv. contact Guenter Fecke.

616 USA ISSN 0898-6665

SKIN CANCER FOUNDATION JOURNAL. Text in English. a. **Document type:** *Academic/Scholarly.* **Description:** Compiles short articles to strengthen public awareness of the importance of prevention and early detection of skin cancer.
Related titles: Special ed.: Fourth World Congress of Cancers of the Skin.
Published by: Skin Cancer Foundation, 245 Fifth Ave, Ste 2402, New York, NY 10016. TEL 212-725-5176, FAX 212-725-5751. Ed. Lucy Kaveler.

616.992 ITA ISSN 1123-7112

SOCIETA ITALIANA DI CHIRURGIA ONCOLOGICA. NEWS. Key Title: S I C O News. Text in Italian. 1995. s-a. adv. **Document type:** *Newsletter.*
Published by: (Societa Italiana di Chirurgia Oncologica), C I C Edizioni Internazionali s.r.l., Corso Trieste 42, Rome, RM 00198, Italy. TEL 39-06-8412673, FAX 39-06-8412688, info@gruppocic.it, 1160199510. Ed. F Badellino. adv.: B&W page XEU 1,601.02, color page XEU 2,014.18; 210 x 290.

616.99 FRA ISSN 0753-7417 CODEN: BFCPE5

SOCIETE FRANCAISE DE CANCEROLOGIE PRIVEE. BULLETIN. Text in French. 1982. 4/yr. FRF 850. adv. **Document type:** *Bulletin.*
Indexed: Curr.Cont. (coverage dropped), Excerp.Med. (1993-).
—EMDOCS, KNAW.
Published by: Societe Francaise de Cancerologie Privee, 25 rue Henry Dunant, Thiais 94320, France. TEL 1-46-87-20-57. Ed. Dr. H Lauche.

616.99 USA

A SUPPLEMENT TO ONCOLOGY NEWS INTERNATIONAL. Text in English. irreg. **Document type:** *Monographic series, Academic/Scholarly.*
Related titles: ♦ Supplement to: Oncology News International. ISSN 1065-2957.
Published by: P R R, Inc., 48 S Service Rd, Melville, NY 11747-2335. TEL 516-424-8900, FAX 516-424-8503. Ed. Dr. Martin Abeloff.

616.99 DEU ISSN 0941-4355 CODEN: SCCAEO

SUPPORTIVE CARE IN CANCER. Text in English. 1992. bi-m. DEM 516.60 domestic; DEM 524.40 foreign (effective 2001). *Refereed.* **Document type:** *Journal, Academic/Scholarly.* **Description:** Provides the most recent scientific and social information on all aspects of supportive care for cancer patients.
Related titles: Microform ed.: (from PQC); Online - full text ed.: ISSN 1433-7339 (from EBSCO Publishing, RoweCom Information Quest, Swets Blackwell, Springer LINK, Institute for Scientific Information).
Indexed: AMED, ASCA, Abstr.Hyg., Curr.Cont., Ind.Med. (1993-), Ind.Sci.Rev., Inpharma, Int.Nurs.Ind., Pharm.&Out.News, Reac., Rev.Med.& Vet.Mycol., SSCI (coverage dropped), Sci.Cit.Ind.
—BLDSC (8547.638620), CISTI, GNLM, IDS, Infotrieve, KNAW. **CCC.**
Published by: (Multinational Association of Supportive Care in Cancer), Springer-Verlag (Subsidiary of: BertelsmannSpringer), Tiergartenstr 17, Heidelberg 69121, Germany. TEL 49-6221-345-0, FAX 49-6221-345229, subscriptions@springer.de, http://link.springer.de/link/service/journals/00520/ index.htm, http://www.springer.de. Ed. H.-J Senn. **Subscr. in N. America to:** Springer-Verlag New York Inc., PO Box 2485, Secaucus, NJ 07096-2485. TEL 212-460-1500, FAX 212-473-6272.

616.99 GBR ISSN 0960-7404 CODEN: SUOCEC
SURGICAL ONCOLOGY. Text in English. 1992. q. EUR 96 in Europe to individuals; JPY 12,700 in Japan to individuals; USD 107 elsewhere to individuals; EUR 440 in Europe to institutions; JPY 58,500 in Japan to institutions; USD 492 elsewhere to institutions (effective 2002). adv. bk.rev. illus. index. reprints avail. *Refereed.* **Document type:** *Academic/Scholarly.* **Description:** Publishes review articles that contribute to the advancement of knowledge in surgical oncology and related fields.
Related titles: Microform ed.: (from PQC); Online - full text ed.: (from EBSCO Publishing, ingenta, Swets Blackwell, Institute for Scientific Information, ScienceDirect).
Indexed: ASCA, Curr.Cont., Excerp.Med. (1993-), Ind.Med. (1992-), Inpharma, Int.Abstr.Biol.Sci., Pharm.&Out.News, Reac.
—BLDSC (8548.242000), ADONIS, CISTI, EMDOCS, GNLM, IDS, Infotrieve, KNAW. **CCC.**
Published by: Elsevier Science, The Boulevard, Langford Ln, Kidlington, Oxon OX5 1GB, United Kingdom. TEL 44-1865-843000, FAX 44-1865-843010, usinfo-f@elsevier.com, http://www.elsevier.nl/locate/issn/09607404, http://www.elsevier.com. Circ: 180.

616.992 BEL
SURGICAL ONCOLOGY/ONCOLOGISCHE HEELKUNDE. Text in Dutch, English. 1995. irreg. price varies. **Document type:** *Academic/Scholarly.*
Published by: Leuven University Press, Blijde Inkomststraat 5, Leuven 3000, Belgium. TEL 32-16-325345, FAX 32-16-325352, university.press@upers.kuleuven.ac.be, http://www.lup.be.

616.99 617 USA ISSN 1055-3207
SURGICAL ONCOLOGY CLINICS OF NORTH AMERICA. Text in English. 1992. q. USD 137 domestic to individuals; USD 156 in Canada to individuals; USD 185 elsewhere to individuals; USD 179 domestic to institutions; USD 218 foreign to institutions; USD 55 per issue (effective 2001). adv. index. back issues avail. **Document type:** *Academic/Scholarly.* **Description:** Discusses diagnostic techniques, surgical procedures, and radiation therapy for the treatment of cancer patients.
Related titles: Microform ed.: (from PQC).
Indexed: CINAHL, Ind.Med. (1992-), Int.Nurs.Ind.
—BLDSC (8548.242100), CISTI, EMDOCS, GNLM, KNAW.
Published by: W.B. Saunders Co. (Subsidiary of: Harcourt Publishers Ltd.), 11830 Westline Industrial Dr, St Louis, MO 63146. TEL 800-325-4177, http://www.wbsaunders.com. Ed. Dr. Blake Cady. **Subscr. to:** Periodicals Fulfillment, W B Saunders Co, 6277 Sea Harbor Dr, 4th Fl, Orlando, FL 32891-4800.

▼ **SURGICAL THEATRE EQUIPMENT AND TECHNNOLOGY (S T E T).** see *MEDICAL SCIENCES—Surgery*

616.994 FIN ISSN 0356-3081
SYOPA/CANCER. Text in Finnish, Swedish. 1969. 6/yr. FIM 170 to non-members (effective 2001). adv. bk.rev. 32 p./no. 3 cols./p. **Document type:** *Magazine, Consumer.* **Description:** Contains articles and information about the latest discoveries in cancer treatment, information on rehabilitation, personal stories and other material of interest to cancer patients and their families.
Former titles: Syovantorjunta - Kampen Mot Kraefta - Against Cancer; Terveystyo (0049-2787)
Related titles: Online - full text ed.
Indexed: Risk Abstr.
Published by: Suomen Syopayhdistys/Cancer Society of Finland, Liisankatu 21 B, Helsinki 00170, Finland. TEL 358-9-135331, FAX 358-9-1351093, satu.lipponen@cancer.fi, http://www.cancer.fi. Eds. Satu Lipponen, Seppo Pyrhoenen. Circ: 134,000.

616.994 NLD ISSN 0166-3925
TIJDSCHRIFT KANKER. Text in Dutch. 1977. 6/yr. NLG 72; NLG 45 to students (effective 2001). adv. bk.rev. **Document type:** *Journal, Academic/Scholarly.*
Formerly: K.W.F. Nieuws (0022-7447)
—KNAW.
Published by: (Nederlandse Vereniging tot Steun aan het Koningin Wilhelmina Fonds voor de Kankerbestrijding), K B U Uitgevers B.V., Postbus 24, Oisterwyk 5060 AA, Netherlands. TEL 31-13-5216665, FAX 31-13-5235255, kbu@vandenboogaardgroep.nl, http://www.vandenboogaardgroep.nl. Circ: 3,000.

TOXIC EXPOSURE ADVISORY NEWSLETTER. see *ENVIRONMENTAL STUDIES—Toxicology And Environmental Safety*

616.992 CHE ISSN 1010-4283 CODEN: OBIMD4
TUMOR BIOLOGY; from basic science to clinical application. Text in English. 1980. bi-m. CHF 980, EUR 699.80 in Europe to institutions; CHF 997.40, USD 762 elsewhere to institutions (effective 2002). adv. back issues avail. *Refereed.* **Document type:** *Journal, Academic/Scholarly.* **Description:** Focuses on the basic biology of tumor markers, the crucial indicators of the onset of cancer. Reflects new approaches analyzing the structural and functional properties, differentiation status and lineage derivation of individual cells in normal and neoplastic populations.
Former titles: Oncodevelopmental Biology and Medicine (0167-1618); Tumour Biology (0289-5447)
Related titles: Online - full text ed.: ISSN 1423-0380. CHF 58, EUR 42, USD 45 to institutions with print edition (effective 2002) (from EBSCO Publishing, O C L C Online Computer Library Center, Inc., RoweCom Information Quest, Swets Blackwell, Institute for Scientific Information).
Indexed: AIDS & Cancer Res., ASCA, Curr.Adv.Biochem., Curr.Adv.Cancer Res., Curr.Adv.Cell & Devel.Biol., Curr.Cont., INIS Atomind., Ind.Med. (1984-), Ind.Sci.Rev., Inpharma, Oncog.G.F.Abstr., Pharm.&Out.News, Reac., Sci.Cit.Ind.
—BLDSC (9070.645500), CASDDS, CISTI, EMDOCS, GNLM, IDS, ingenta, KNAW. **CCC.**
Published by: (International Society for Oncodevelopmental Biology and Medicine), S. Karger AG, Allschwilerstr 10, PO Box, Basel 4009, Switzerland. TEL 41-61-306-1111, FAX 41-61-306-1234, karger@karger.ch, http://www.online.karger.com/journals/tbi, http://www.karger.com. Ed. T Stigbrand. adv.: page USD 1,195.

616.99 USA
TUMOR DIAGNOSIS. Text in English. 1996. q. USD 67 to individuals; USD 95 to institutions. *Refereed.* **Document type:** *Academic/Scholarly.* **Description:** Devoted to the problems involved in the diagnosis of a tumor. Places special emphasis on the utilization of modern techniques of molecular biology.
Published by: Field & Wood, Medical Periodicals, Inc., PO Box 975, Blue Bell, PA 19422. TEL 610-828-4010, FAX 215-482-0226. Eds. Dr. Irma Russo, Dr. Jose Russo.

616.994 JPN ISSN 0041-4093 CODEN: TUREA6
TUMOR RESEARCH: EXPERIMENTAL AND CLINICAL/GAN KENKYU, JIKKEN TO RINSHO. Text in English. 1966. a. per issue exchange basis. abstr, bibl, charts, illus, stat. *Refereed.* **Document type:** *Academic/Scholarly.*
Related titles: Microfilm ed.: (from PQC).
Indexed: Biol.Abstr., Chem.Abstr., Curr.Adv.Ecol.Sci., Excerp.Med., INIS Atomind., Ref.Zh.
—BLDSC (9070.650000), CASDDS, CISTI, GNLM, KNAW.
Published by: Sapporo Ika Daigaku/Sapporo Medical University, Fuzoku Gan Kenkyujo, Nishi-17-chome, Minami-1-jo, Chuo-ku, Sapporo-shi, Hokkaido 060-8556, Japan. TEL 81-11-611-2111, FAX 81-11-615-3099. Ed. Yohichi Mochizuki. Circ: 550.

616.99 DEU ISSN 0722-219X
TUMORDIAGNOSTIK & THERAPIE. Text in German; Summaries in English, German. bi-m. EUR 165.80 domestic to institutions; EUR 171.80 in Europe to institutions; EUR 181.60 elsewhere to institutions; EUR 32 newsstand/cover (effective 2002). *Refereed.* **Document type:** *Journal, Academic/Scholarly.*
Related titles: Online - full text ed.: ISSN 1439-1279.
Indexed: ASCA, Curr.Cont. (coverage dropped), INIS Atomind., Ind.Sci.Rev., Inpharma, Pharm.&Out.News, Reac., Sci.Cit.Ind. (coverage dropped).
—BLDSC (9070.675000), CISTI, EMDOCS, GNLM, IDS, Infotrieve, KNAW. **CCC.**
Published by: Georg Thieme Verlag, Ruedigerstr 14, Stuttgart 70469, Germany. TEL 49-711-8931-0, FAX 49-711-8931133, tumor@thieme.de, leser.service@thieme.de, http://www.thieme.de/tumor, http://www.thieme-connect.de. Eds. J Schuette, S Seeber. R&P Michael Wachinger. Circ: 6,000.

616.994 ITA ISSN 0300-8916 CODEN: TUMOAB
TUMORI; a journal of experimental and clinical oncology. Text in English; Abstracts in English. 1911. bi-m., latest vol.87. USD 150 (effective 2000). adv. bk.rev. bibl, illus. index, cum.index. 96 p./no. back issues avail.; reprints avail. *Refereed.* **Document type:** *Journal, Academic/Scholarly.*
Related titles: Online - full text ed.: (from Institute for Scientific Information).
Indexed: ASCA, Biol.Abstr., Chem.Abstr., Chem.Indus.Notes, Chem.Titles, Curr.Adv.Biochem., Curr.Adv.Cancer Res., Curr.Adv.Ecol.Sci., Curr.Adv.Gen.& Molec.Biol., Curr.Cont., Dent.Ind., Excerp.Med., INIS Atomind., Ind.Med. (1911-), Ind.Sci.Rev., Ind.Vet., Inpharma, Int.Abstr.Biol.Sci., Nutr.Abstr., Pharm.&Out.News, Reac., Risk Abstr., Sci.Cit.Ind., Vet.Bull.
—BLDSC (9070.700000), CASDDS, CISTI, EMDOCS, GNLM, IDS, KNAW.
Published by: (Istituto Nazionale per lo Studio e la Cura dei Tumori), Il Pensiero Scientifico Editore s.r.l., Via Bradano, 3-C, Rome, RM 00199, Italy. TEL 39-06-862821, FAX 39-06-86282250, tumori@istitutotumori.mi.it, http://www.cilea.it/tumori. Eds. Franco Zunino, Natale Cascinelli. Adv. contact Luciano De Fiore. B&W page XEU 1,032, color page XEU 1,653; 21 x 28. Circ: 3,700.

616.99 GBR ISSN 0955-5102
TUMOUR MARKER UPDATE. Text in English. 1989. bi-m. GBP 66 domestic to individuals; USD 132 in United States to individuals; GBP 83 elsewhere to individuals; GBP 90 domestic to institutions; USD 190 in United States to institutions; GBP 112 elsewhere to institutions. **Document type:** *Abstract/Index, Academic/Scholarly.* **Description:** Locates and reports the scientific literature on circulating, genetic and immunohistochemical tumor markers from more than 1,000 international biomedical titles.
Published by: Leeds Medical Information, University of Leeds, Leeds, W Yorks LS2 9JT, United Kingdom. lmi@leeds.ac.uk, http://www.leeds.ac.uk/lmi/intro.html. Circ: 400. **Subscr. to:** Royal Society of Medicine Press Ltd, PO Box 9002, London W1A 0ZA, United Kingdom. TEL 44-20-7290-2927.

616.99 TUR ISSN 1019-3103
TURKISH JOURNAL OF CANCER. Text in English. 1967. 4/yr. USD 100 (effective 2001). adv. bk.rev. back issues avail. *Refereed.* **Document type:** *Academic/Scholarly.* **Description:** Contains scientific research articles, reviews, editorials, and letters to the editor in the fields of basic and clinical oncology.
Formerly (until 1992): Kanser (0377-9750)
Related titles: Online - full text ed.
—BLDSC (9072.468000).
Published by: Turkish Association for Cancer Research and Control/Turk Kanser Arastirma ve Savas Kurumu, Atac Sokak No. 21, 06420 Yenisehir, Ankara, Turkey. TEL 90-312-4312950, FAX 90-312-4313958, http://www.turkcancer.org.tr. Ed. Dr. Dincer Firat. Circ: 1,000 (paid).

U I C C INTERNATIONAL CALENDAR OF MEETINGS ON CANCER. see *MEETINGS AND CONGRESSES*

616.99 CHE
U I C C INTERNATIONAL DIRECTORY OF CANCER INSTITUTES AND ORGANIZATIONS. Text in English. 1976. quadrennial, latest vol.6, 1994. CHF 100. **Document type:** *Directory.*
Formerly: International Directory of Specialized Cancer Research and Treatment Establishments
Published by: Union Internationale Contre le Cancer/International Union Against Cancer, 3 rue de Conseil General, Geneva 1205, Switzerland. TEL 41-22-8091811, FAX 41-22-8091810, info@uicc.org, http://www.uicc.org.

616.992 USA
RC268.6
U.S. NATIONAL TOXICOLOGY PROGRAM. REPORT ON CARCINOGENS. Text in English. 1980. a. USD 68; USD 73 foreign (effective 1998). *Refereed.* **Document type:** *Government.*
Formerly: U.S. National Toxicology Program. Annual Report on Carcinogens (0272-2836)
Related titles: Online - full text ed.
Published by: U.S. National Toxicology Program, PO Box 12233, Research Triangle Park, NC 27709. TEL 919-541-3841, FAX 919-541-0763, ehis@niehs.nih.gov, http://ehis.niehs.nih.gov. Ed. C W Jameson.

616.992 USA ISSN 0191-3123
RB25 CODEN: ULPAD3
ULTRASTRUCTURAL PATHOLOGY. Text in English. 1980. bi-m. GBP 306, USD 505 to individuals; GBP 645, USD 1,064 to institutions (effective 2002). adv. bk.rev. abstr, bibl, illus, stat. index. back issues avail.; reprint service avail. from PQC. *Refereed.* **Document type:** *Academic/Scholarly.* **Description:** Covers electron microscopy, immunohistochemistry, the study and diagnosis of human diseases, EM and oncology, theory, and possible applications.

M

Related titles: Microform ed.: (from PQC); Online - full text ed.: ISSN 1521-0758 (from CatchWord Ltd., EBSCO Publishing, O C L C Online Computer Library Center, Inc., RoweCom Information Quest, Swets Blackwell, Institute for Scientific Information).
Indexed: ASCA, Biol.Abstr., Chem.Abstr., Curr.Adv.Ecol.Sci., Curr.Cont., Dent.Ind., Excerp.Med., Helminthol.Abstr., INIS Atomind., Ind.Med. (1980-), Ind.Sci.Rev., Inpharma, Int.Abstr.Biol.Sci., Med.& Surg.Dermat., Neurosci.Cit.Ind., Protozool.Abstr., Reac., Rev.Med.& Vet.Mycol., Sci.Cit.Ind.
—BLDSC (9082.816000), ADONIS, CASDDS, CatchWord, CISTI, GNLM, IDS, ingenta, KNAW. **CCC.**
Published by: Taylor & Francis Ltd. (Subsidiary of: Taylor & Francis Group), 325 Chestnut St, Suite 800, Philadelphia, PA 19016. TEL 215-625-8900, FAX 215-625-2940, info@taylorandfrancis.com, http://www.taylorandfrancis.com/. Eds. Victor E Gould, Jan Vincents Johannessen. Circ: 750. **Subscr. addr. in Europe:** Taylor & Francis Group, Journals Customer Service, Rankine Rd, Basingstoke, Hants RG24 8PR, United Kingdom. TEL 44-1256-813000, FAX 44-1256-479438, enquiry@tanf.co.uk, http://www.tandf.co.uk/journals.

616.9 USA
UNIVERSITY OF TEXAS. M.D. ANDERSON CANCER CENTER. RESEARCH REPORT. Text in English. 1955. a. free per issue. charts, illus, pat. **Document type:** *Academic/Scholarly.* **Description:** Compendium of research accomplishments at the center.
Formerly (until 1977): M.D. Anderson Hospital and Tumor Institute. Research Report (0066-1635)
Related titles: Online - full text ed.
Published by: University of Texas, M.D. Anderson Cancer Center, Scientific Publications, 1515 Holcombe, PO Box 234, Houston, TX 77030. TEL 713-792-3175, FAX 713-794-1370, jrichard@mdanderson.org, http://www.mdanderson.org/~resrep. Ed. Jude Richard. Pub. John Mendelsohn. R&P Walter Pagel TEL 713-792-3305. Circ: 5,500.

616.9 USA ISSN 1078-1439
CODEN: URONEC
UROLOGIC ONCOLOGY. Text in English. 1995. 6/yr. EUR 146 in Europe to individuals; JPY 19,300 in Japan to individuals; USD 163 elsewhere to individuals; EUR 246 in Europe to institutions; JPY 32,700 in Japan to institutions; USD 275 elsewhere to institutions (effective 2002). back issues avail. *Refereed.* **Document type:** *Academic/Scholarly.* **Description:** Covers all aspects of cancers of the genitourinary system.
Related titles: Online - full text ed.: (from ingenta, Swets Blackwell, Institute for Scientific Information, ScienceDirect).
Indexed: Curr.Cont., Int.Abstr.Biol.Sci.
—BLDSC (9124.627000), CASDDS, EMDOCS, GNLM, KNAW. **CCC.**
Published by: Elsevier Science, PO Box 945, New York, NY 10159-0945. TEL 212-989-5800, FAX 212-633-3990, usinfo-f@elsevier.com, http://www.elsevier.nl/locate/issn/10781439. Eds. Dr. George R Prout Jr., L J Schwartz, M J Droller. **Subscr. in Australasia and the Far East to:** Elsevier Science (Singapore) Pte Ltd, No.1 Temasek Ave, 17-01 Millenia Tower, Singapore 039192, Singapore. TEL 65-434-3727, FAX 65-337-2230; **Subscr. in Japan to:** Elsevier Science Inc - Japan Regional Office, 9-15 Higashi-Azabu 1-chome, Minato-ku, Tokyo 106-0044, Japan. TEL 81-3-5561-5033; **Subscr. outside the Americas to:** Elsevier Science BV, PO Box 211, Amsterdam 1000 AE, Netherlands. TEL 31-20-485-3757.

616.99 616.6 CHE ISSN 1561-0950
UROONCOLOGY. Text in English. q. GBP 59, USD 90, EUR 99 to individuals; GBP 130, USD 200, EUR 213 to institutions; GBP 189, USD 290, EUR 312 to corporations (effective 2002).
Published by: Gordon and Breach - Harwood Academic (Subsidiary of: Taylor & Francis Group), PO Box 531, Lausanne 1000, Switzerland. TEL 41-21-6411280, FAX 41-21-6411281, info@gbhap.com, http://www.gbhap.com/UroOncology/. Ed. Leslie E F Moffat. **Dist. by:** International Publishers Direct.

616.994 FRA ISSN 0249-0358
VIVRE. Text in French. 1923. q. FRF 25; FRF 10 newsstand/cover (effective 2000). bk.rev. bibl, charts, illus, stat. **Document type:** *Magazine, Consumer.* **Description:** Information on cancer research, prevention, and treatments.
Formerly: Lutte Contre le Cancer (0024-7642)
Indexed: Biol.Abstr., Ind.Med. (coverage dropped), Ref.Zh.
—BLDSC (9244.470000).
Published by: Ligue Nationale Francaise Contre le Cancer, 1 av. Stephen Pichon, Paris 75013, France. TEL 33-1-44068080, http://www.ligue-cancer.net. Eds. Anne Leclerc, Michel Miegnier. Circ: 120,000.

616.994 RUS ISSN 0507-3758
CODEN: VOONAW
VOPROSY ONKOLOGII/PROBLEMS IN ONCOLOGY. Text in Russian; Summaries in Russian, English. 1955. bi-m. RUR 60; USD 10 foreign (effective 1999). adv. bk.rev. abstr, bibl, charts, illus, stat. Index. back issues avail. *Refereed.* **Document type:** *Academic/Scholarly.* **Description:** Discusses problems of experimental and clinical oncology (origin, development, course, diagnosis and methods of treating neoplasms), the problems of the organization of oncological aid to the population, prevention and treatment of malignant tumors and precancerous conditions.
Related titles: Diskette ed.; E-mail ed.; Fax ed.; Online - full text ed.
Indexed: Agri.& Environ.Biotech.Abstr. (coverage dropped), Biol.Abstr., Chem.Abstr., Chem.Indus.Notes, Chem.Titles, Curr.Cont. (coverage dropped), Dent.Ind., Derwent Biotech.Abstr., Dok.Arbeitsmed., Excerp.Med., INIS Atomind., Ind.Med. (1955-), Ind.Vet., Nutr.Abstr., Ref.Zh., Sci.Cit.Ind. (coverage dropped), Vet.Bull.
—CASDDS, CISTI, EMDOCS, GNLM, Infotrieve. **CCC.**
Published by: Vsesoyuznoe Nauchnoe Obshchestvo Onkologov, B Zelenina 43-a, St Petersburg 197110, Russian Federation. TEL 7-812-235-3009, FAX 7-812-235-0986, aesculap@amil.wplus.net, http://www.awsculap.ru. Ed. Sergei V Kanayev. Pub. Catherine Tkalenko. R&P, Adv. contact Alexei Belkin TEL 7-812-235-1719. B&W page USD 600, color page USD 2,000; trim 205 x 210. Circ: 1,000. **Subscr. to:** Mezhdunarodnaya Kniga, B Yakimanka 39, Moscow 117049, Russian Federation. **US dist. addr.:** East View Publications, 3020 Harbor Ln N, Minneapolis, MN 55447. TEL 612-550-0961.

616.99 DEU ISSN 0931-8364
WISSENSCHAFTLICHER ERGEBNISBERICHT. Text in German. 1982. biennial. free. **Document type:** *Academic/Scholarly.*
Published by: Deutsches Krebsforschungszentrum, Im Neuenheimer Feld 280, Heidelberg 69120, Germany. TEL 49-6221-423666, FAX 49-6221-423668.

616.994071 616.043 616.042 CHN
YANBIAN - JIBIAN - TUBIAN/CARCINOGENSIS, TERATOGENSIS AND MUTAGENESIS. Text in Chinese. q. USD 13.60; USD 3.40 newsstand/cover (effective 2001). **Document type:** *Academic/Scholarly.*
Published by: China International Book Trading Corp/Zhongguo Guoji Tushu Maoyi Zonggongsi cibtc@mail.cibtc.com.cn, http://www.cibtc.com.cn. **Dist. by:** 35, Chegongzhuang Xilu, Haidian District, Beijing 100044, China.

616.994 USA ISSN 1040-1741
RC261 CODEN: YEONEX
THE YEAR BOOK OF ONCOLOGY. Text in English. 1957. a. USD 96 domestic; USD 102 foreign (effective 2001). illus. **Document type:** *Abstract/Index, Academic/Scholarly.* **Description:** Presents abstracts of pertinent literature with commentary by leading experts in the field.
Formerly (until 1958): Year Book of Cancer (0084-3679)
Related titles: CD-ROM ed.
—CISTI, GNLM.
Published by: Mosby, Inc., Continuity Division (Subsidiary of: Harcourt Health Sciences), 11830 Westline Industrial Dr, St Louis, MO 63146-3313. TEL 314-872-8370, 800-325-4177, FAX 314-432-1380, http://www.mosby.com/periodicals. Ed. Dr. Patrick Loehrer.

616.99 CHN ISSN 1000-8179
CODEN: ZZLIEP
ZHONGGUO ZHONGLIU LINCHUANG/CHINESE JOURNAL OF CLINICAL ONCOLOGY. Text in Chinese; Abstracts in English. 1984. m. USD 22.20; CNY 8, USD 4.70 newsstand/cover (effective 2001). adv. **Document type:** *Academic/Scholarly.* **Description:** Publishes original articles pertaining to the clinical disciplines of oncology and the related laboratory studies.
Related titles: CD-ROM ed.
Indexed: Excerp.Med., ExtraMED.
—CASDDS, EMDOCS, GNLM.
Published by: Tianjin Zhongliu Yanjiusuo, Zhongguo Kang-Ai Xiehui/Tianjin Cancer Institute, China Anti-Cancer Association, Huan-hu-xi Lu Tiyuanbei, Hexi-qu, Tianjin 300060, China. cjco@pulic.tpt.tj.cn. Ed. Tian-Ze Zhang. Pub. Lian Zhong Zhao. Adv. contact Hong Xin Yang. color page CNY 6,000. Circ: 10,000. **Dist. overseas by:** China International Book Trading Corp, 35, Chegongzhuang Xilu, Haidian District, Beijing 100044, China. TEL 86-1-68413849, FAX 86-1-68412048, cibtc@mail.cibtc.com.cn, http://www.cibtc.com.cn.

ZHONGHUA SHENJING WAIKE ZAZHI/CHINESE JOURNAL OF NEUROSURGERY. see *MEDICAL SCIENCES—Psychiatry And Neurology*

616.99 CHN ISSN 0253-3766
CODEN: CCLCDY
ZHONGHUA ZHONGLIU ZAZHI/CHINESE JOURNAL OF ONCOLOGY. Text in Chinese. bi-m. USD 11.50 foreign; CNY 11.50 newsstand/cover domestic; USD 6.30 newsstand/cover per academic year foreign (effective 2001). **Document type:** *Academic/Scholarly.*
Related titles: CD-ROM ed.; Online - full content ed.: (from WanFang Data Corp.).
Indexed: Biol.Abstr., Chem.Abstr., Excerp.Med., ExtraMED, Ind.Med. (1979-), Maize Abstr., Rev.Med.& Vet.Mycol.
—BLDSC (3180.460000), CASDDS, CISTI, EMDOCS, GNLM.
Published by: Zhongguo Kexue Yixue Kexueyuan, Zhaoyang-qu, Panjiayuan #17, Beijing 100021, China. TEL 86-1-67762118, cmazhl@public.sti.ac.cn. **Dist. by:** China International Book Trading Corp, 35, Chegongzhuang Xilu, Haidian District, Beijing 100044, China. TEL 86-1-68413849, FAX 86-1-68412048, cibtc@mail.cibtc.com.cn, http://www.cibtc.com.cn. **Co-publisher:** Zhonggo Xiehe Yike Daxue, Zhongliu Yiyuan.

616.992 CHN ISSN 1000-8578
ZHONGLIU FANGZHI YANJIU/CANCER RESEARCH ON PREVENTION AND TREATMENT. Text in Chinese. 1973. q. CNY 36 domestic; USD 22.20 foreign; CNY 6 newsstand/cover domestic; USD 3.70 newsstand/cover foreign (effective 2001). **Document type:** *Academic/Scholarly.*
Related titles: Online - full content ed.: (from WanFang Data Corp.).
Published by: Zhongguo Kangyan Xiehui, 16, Zhuodaoquan Nan Lu, Wuchang 430079, China. TEL 86-27-87393126, http://www.tumorh.gzsums.edu.cn. Ed. Minghe Zhang. **Dist. by:** China International Book Trading Corp, 35, Chegongzhuang Xilu, Haidian District, Beijing 100044, China. TEL 86-1-68413849, FAX 86-1-68412048, cibtc@mail.cibtc.com.cn, http://www.cibtc.com.cn.

MEDICAL SCIENCES—Ophthalmology And Optometry

617.7 USA ISSN 0192-1304
20 - 20. Text in English. 1974. m. USD 165, CND 265 (effective 2000); free per issue to qualified personnel. adv. illus.
Published by: Jobson Publishing LLC, 100 Ave of Americas, New York, NY 10013-1678. TEL 212-274-7000, 800-747-1652, FAX 212-431-0500, http://www.jobson.com. Circ: 495,000.

617.7 USA ISSN 1353-3290
20-20 EUROPE. Text in English. m.
Published by: Jobson Publishing LLC, 100 Ave of Americas, New York, NY 10013-1678. TEL 212-274-7000, 800-747-1652, FAX 212-431-0500, http://www.jobson.com.

617.7 HRV ISSN 0001-6403
CODEN: AOPIBU
ACTA OPHTHALMOLOGICA IUGOSLAVICA. Text in Serbo-Croatian; Summaries in English, French, German. 1963. s-a. adv. bk.rev. abstr. index.
Indexed: Biol.Abstr., C.I.S. Abstr.
Published by: Zbor Lijecnika Hrvatske, Oftalmoloska Sekcija, Subiceva 12, Zagreb 41000, Croatia. Ed. Dr. Kresimir Cupak. Circ: 1,200.

617.7 DNK ISSN 1395-3907
RE1 CODEN: AOSCFV
ACTA OPHTHALMOLOGICA SCANDINAVICA. Text in English. 1923. bi-m. USD 192 in the Americas to institutions print & online eds. combined; GBP 133 elsewhere to institutions print & online eds. combined (effective 2002). adv. bibl, charts, illus. index, cum.index: vols.1-25. *Refereed.* **Document type:** *Academic/Scholarly.*
Formerly (until 1995): Acta Ophthalmologica (0001-639X)

Related titles: ♦ Online - full text ed.: Acta Ophthamologica Scandinavica Online. ISSN 1600-5465; ♦ Supplement: Acta Ophthalmologica Scandinavica. Supplementum. ISSN 1395-3931.
Indexed: ASCA, Biol.Abstr., Chem.Abstr., Chem.Indus.Notes, Chem.Titles, Curr.Adv.Cancer Res., Curr.Adv.Ecol.Sci., Curr.Cont., Dok.Arbeitsmed., Environ.Sci.Poll.Mgmt., Excerp.Med., Helminthol.Abstr., INIS Atomind., Ind.Med. (1995-), Ind.Sci.Rev., Inpharma, Int.Nurs.Ind., Neurosci.Cit.Ind., Pharm.&Out.News, Pollut.Abstr., Protozool.Abstr., Psychol.Abstr., Reac., Rev.Appl.Entomol., Rev.Med.& Vet.Mycol., Risk Abstr., SSCI (coverage dropped), Saf.Sci.Abstr., Sci.Cit.Ind., Trop.Dis.Bull.
—BLDSC (0641.753000), CASDDS, CISTI, EMDOCS, GNLM, IDS, ingenta, KNAW. **CCC.**
Published by: Blackwell Munksgaard, Noerre Soegade 35, PO Box 2148, Copenhagen K 1016, Denmark. TEL 45-77-33-33-33, FAX 45-77-33-33-77, fsub@mail.munksgaard.dk, http://www.munksgaard.dk/actaopthalmologica. Ed. Anders Heijl. Adv. contact Eric Rozario TEL 45-77-33-33-01. Circ: 2,500.

617.7 DNK ISSN 1395-3931
RE1 CODEN: AOSSFB
ACTA OPHTHALMOLOGICA SCANDINAVICA. SUPPLEMENTUM. Text in English. 1932. irreg. free to subscribers to Acta Ophthalmologica. adv. **Document type:** *Academic/Scholarly.*
Formerly (until 1995): Acta Ophthalmologica. Supplementum (0065-1451)
Related titles: ♦ Supplement to: Acta Ophthalmologica Scandinavica. ISSN 1395-3907.
Indexed: Biol.Abstr., Curr.Cont. (coverage dropped), Dent.Ind., Dok.Arbeitsmed., Excerp.Med. (1996-), INIS Atomind., Ind.Med. (1995-).
—BLDSC (0641.754000), CASDDS, CISTI, EMDOCS, ingenta, KNAW. **CCC.**
Published by: Scriptor Publisher ApS, Soevangsvej 1-5, Hvidovre 2650, Denmark. TEL 45-36-77-41-13, FAX 45-35-77-41-15. Ed. Gunnar Lennerstrand. R&P Vibeke Allen.

617.7 DNK ISSN 1600-5465
ACTA OPHTHAMOLOGICA SCANDINAVICA ONLINE. Text in English. bi-m. GBP 120 (effective 2002). **Document type:** *Academic/Scholarly.*
Media: Online - full text (from EBSCO Publishing, ingenta, Munksgaard & Blackwell Science's Synergy, Swets Blackwell, Institute for Scientific Information). **Related titles:** ♦ Print ed.: Acta Ophthalmologica Scandinavica. ISSN 1395-3907.
Published by: Blackwell Munksgaard, Noerre Soegade 35, PO Box 2148, Copenhagen K 1016, Denmark. TEL 45-77-33-33-33, FAX 45-77-33-33-77, fsub@mail.munksgaard.dk, http://www.munksgaard.dk/actaophthamologica.

617.7 658 USA ISSN 1060-5991
ADMINISTRATIVE OPHTHALMOLOGY. Text in English. 1992. q. USD 60 (effective 2000). adv. **Document type:** *Academic/Scholarly.*
Published by: American Society of Ophthalmic Administrators, 4000 Legato Rd, Ste 850, Fairfax, VA 22033-4003. TEL 703-591-2222, FAX 703-591-0614. Ed. Lucy Santiago. Adv. contact Wendy Rachexo.

617.7 ITA ISSN 0390-5764
AGGIORNAMENTI DI TERAPIA OFTALMOLOGICA. Text in Italian. 1949. q. free to ophthalmologists. adv. abstr. 64 p./no. back issues avail. *Refereed.* **Document type:** *Academic/Scholarly.*
Indexed: Environ.Sci.Poll.Mgmt.
Published by: Farmigea S.p.A., Via Giovanni Carmignani, 2, Pisa, PI 56127, Italy. TEL 39-050-544000, FAX 39-050-544304, info@farmigea.it, http://www.farmigea.it. Ed., Adv. contact Renzo Canelli. Circ: 7,200 (controlled).

617.7 SWE ISSN 0348-5730
AKTUELL OPTIK OCH OPTOMETRI. Text in Swedish. 1979. 10/yr. SEK 396 domestic; SEK 495 foreign; SEK 40 newsstand/cover. adv. bk.rev. 3 cols./p. **Document type:** *Bulletin, Academic/Scholarly.*
Published by: Swedish Optometric Association SOR, Roslagsgatan 60, Stockholm 11354, Sweden. TEL 46-8-612-89-60, FAX 46-8-612-56-90. Ed., Adv. contact Johan Pohl. B&W page SEK 7,700, color page SEK 10,650; trim 265 x 185. Circ: 3,100.

618.920977 USA ISSN 1091-8531
AMERICAN ASSOCIATION FOR PEDIATRIC OPHTHALMOLOGY AND STRABISMUS. JOURNAL. Key Title: Journal of A A P O S. Text in English. 1997. bi-m. USD 119 domestic to individuals; USD 149 foreign to individuals; USD 158 domestic to institutions; USD 188 foreign to institutions; USD 67 domestic to students; USD 97 foreign to students; USD 32 per issue domestic (effective 2001). adv. **Document type:** *Journal, Academic/Scholarly.* **Description:** Presents expert information on children's eye diseases and on strabismus as it impacts all age groups.
Related titles: Online - full content ed.: ISSN 1528-3933 (from EBSCO Publishing); Online - full text ed.: (from IDEAL Online Library, Institute for Scientific Information, RoweCom Information Quest).
Indexed: Curr.Cont., Ind.Med. (1997-).
—BLDSC (4674.942000).
Published by: (American Association for Pediatric Ophthalmology and Strabismus), Mosby, Inc. (Subsidiary of: Elsevier Science), 11830 Westline Industrial Dr, St Louis, MO 63146-3318. TEL 800-325-4177, 800-654-2452, http://www.mosby.com/jaapos, http://www.mosby.com/periodicals. Ed. Dr. Sherwin J Eisenberg TEL 310-222-6447. Pub. Terrie Duhadway. Adv. contact Carol Kilzer TEL 314-453-4307. B&W page USD 740, color page USD 1,565; trim 10.88 x 8.25. Circ: 1,281.

617.7 USA ISSN 0002-9394
RE1 CODEN: AJOPAA
AMERICAN JOURNAL OF OPHTHALMOLOGY. Text in English. 1884. m. USD 96 in US & Canada to individuals; USD 190 elsewhere to individuals; USD 345 in US & Canada to institutions; USD 442 elsewhere to institutions (effective 2002). adv. bk.rev. abstr, bibl, illus. index. back issues avail.; reprint service avail. from PQC. *Refereed.* **Document type:** *Academic/Scholarly.* **Description:** Directed to ophthalmologist and visual science specialist describing clinical investigations, clinical observations and clinically relevant laboratory investigations related to ophthalmology.
Related titles: CD-ROM ed.; Microform ed.: (from PQC); Online - full text ed.: (from Gale Group, Northern Light Technology, Inc., ingenta, Swets Blackwell, ScienceDirect, Factiva, Institute for Scientific Information).
Indexed: AIM, ASCA, Agri.& Environ.Biotech.Abstr. (coverage dropped), Biodet.Abstr., Biol.Abstr., Chem.Abstr., Chem.Indus.Notes, Chem.Titles, Curr.Adv.Cancer Res., Curr.Adv.Ecol.Sci., Curr.Cont., Dent.Ind., Derwent Biotech.Abstr., Dok.Arbeitsmed., Environ.Sci.Poll.Mgmt., Excerp.Med., Helminthol.Abstr., INIS Atomind., Ind.Med. (1884-), Ind.Sci.Rev., Ind.Vet., Inpharma, Kidney, Lab.Haz.Bull., Med.& Surg.Dermat., Neurosci.Cit.Ind., Nutr.Abstr., Pharm.&Out.News, Protozool.Abstr., Psychol.Abstr., Reac., Rev.Appl.Entomol., Rev.Med.& Vet.Mycol., Risk Abstr., SSCI (coverage dropped), Sci.Cit.Ind., Trop.Dis.Bull., Vet.Bull.
—BLDSC (0828.900000), CASDDS, CISTI, EMDOCS, GNLM, IDS, ingenta, KNAW. **CCC.**
Published by: Elsevier Science, PO Box 945, New York, NY 10159-0945. t. bontemps@elsevier.com, http://www.elsevier.com/locate/ajo. Ed. Dr. B R Straatsma. R&P J E Groppi. Adv. contact Tom Meehan. B&W page USD 1,290. Circ: 15,000 (paid). **Subscr. outside the Americas to:** Elsevier Science BV, PO Box 211, Amsterdam 1000 AE, Netherlands. TEL 31-20-485-3757, FAX 31-20-485-3432.

617.7 USA ISSN 0065-9533
RE1 CODEN: TAOSAT
AMERICAN OPHTHALMOLOGICAL SOCIETY. TRANSACTIONS. Text in English. 1864. a. USD 55 (effective 2000). index. back issues avail. **Document type:** *Proceedings, Academic/Scholarly.*
Indexed: Biol.Abstr., Dent.Ind., Excerp.Med., Ind.Med. (1864-).
—BLDSC (8893.650000), CISTI, GNLM, ingenta, KNAW.
Published by: American Ophthalmological Society, PO Box 193940, San Francisco, CA 94119-3940. FAX 415-561-8531, aos@aao.org. Ed. Dr. Brooks Crawford. R&P Dr. Charles P Wilkinson. Circ: 600 (paid). **Subscr. to:** Johnson Printing, 311 NW Second Ave, Box 1177, Rochester, MN 55903. TEL 507-288-7788.

617.752 USA
AMERICAN OPTICIAN* . Text in English. 1950. q. membership only. adv. bk.rev. reprint service avail. from PQC. **Document type:** *Newsletter.*
Former titles (until Feb. 1992): O A A News; (until 1987): Dispensing Optician (0194-2174); (until (1976): Guild of Prescription Opticians. Guide; R X O - Journal of Opticianry; Guild Guide (0017-5382)
Related titles: Microform ed.: (from PQC).
Published by: Opticians Association of America, 7023 Little River Tpke Ste 207, Annandale, VA 22003-5939. TEL 703-691-8355, FAX 703-691-3929. Ed. Jacqueline Fairbarns. Circ: 7,500.

617.7 USA ISSN 0094-9620
AMERICAN OPTOMETRIC ASSOCIATION. NEWS. Text in English. 1961. s-m. USD 80 domestic to non-members; USD 95 in Canada to non-members; USD 103 elsewhere to non-members (effective 2001). adv. 24 p./no. 4 cols./p. **Document type:** *Newsletter.* **Description:** Contains news and information for members of the American Optometric Association.
—**CCC.**
Published by: American Optometric Association, 243 N Lindbergh Blvd, St. Louis, MO 63141. TEL 314-991-4100, FAX 314-991-4101, almiller@theaoa.org, http://www.aoanet.org, http://www.aoanet.org/. Ed. Robert Foster. Pub., R&P Andrew L Miller. adv.: B&W page USD 3,759, color page USD 5,297; trim 15 x 10.38. Circ: 30,000 (paid and controlled).

617.7 USA ISSN 0065-955X
CODEN: AOJTAW
AMERICAN ORTHOPTIC JOURNAL. Text in English. 1950. a. USD 27 to individuals; USD 80 to institutions (effective 2000). adv. cum.index: 1950-1960, 1971-1980. back issues avail.; reprint service avail. from PQC. *Refereed.* **Document type:** *Academic/Scholarly.*
Related titles: Microform ed.: (from PQC).
Indexed: Biol.Abstr., Excerp.Med.
—BLDSC (0847.750000), CISTI, GNLM, ingenta.
Published by: (American Association of Certified Orthoptists), University of Wisconsin Press, Journal Division, 1930 Monroe St., Madison, WI 53711. TEL 608-263-0668, FAX 608-263-1173, http://www.wisc.edu/wisconsinpress/. Ed. Dr. Thomas France. R&P Margaret Walsh TEL 608-224-3812. Adv. contact Adrienne Omen. Circ: 1,500.

617.7 ITA ISSN 0003-4665
CODEN: AOCOAG
ANNALI DI OTTALMOLOGIA E CLINICA OCULISTICA. Text in Italian; Summaries in English. 1874. bi-m. ITL 150,000; ITL 300,000 foreign (effective 1997). adv. bk.rev. charts, illus. index.
Indexed: Chem.Abstr., Excerp.Med., INIS Atomind., Ind.Med. (coverage dropped).
—BLDSC (1016.200000), CISTI, EMDOCS, GNLM, KNAW.
Published by: Casa Editrice Maccari, Via Palermo, 44, Parma, PR 43100, Italy. TEL 39-521-771268. Circ: 1,200.

617.7 USA ISSN 1530-4086
RE1 CODEN: AOPGFS
ANNALS OF OPHTHALMOLOGY. Text in English. 1994. q. USD 160 to individuals; USD 144 foreign to institutions (effective 2001). adv. bk.rev. bibl, illus. index. *Refereed.* **Document type:** *Academic/Scholarly.* **Description:** Designed to provide the practicing ophthalmologist and optometrist with new clinical knowledge and essential techniques required to deliver high-quality eye care. Articles discuss research in ophthalmology regarding diagnosis, procedures, therapies, as we as state-of-the-art management of glaucoma.
Formerly (until 1999): Annals of Ophthalmology - Glaucoma (1079-4794); Formed by the merger of (1974-1994): Glaucoma (0164-4645); (1969-1994): Annals of Ophthalmology (0003-4886); Which incorporated (1982-1985): Journal of Ocular Therapy and Surgery (0730-0883)
Related titles: Online - full text ed.: (from Institute for Scientific Information).
Indexed: ASCA, Biol.Abstr., Chem.Abstr., Curr.Cont. (coverage dropped), Dent.Ind., Dok.Arbeitsmed., Excerp.Med., Helminthol.Abstr., INIS Atomind., Ind.Med. (coverage dropped), Inpharma, Pharm.&Out.News, Reac., Sci.Cit.Ind. (coverage dropped).
—BLDSC (1043.355000), CASDDS, CISTI, EMDOCS, GNLM, Infotrieve, ingenta, KNAW. **CCC.**
Published by: American Society of Contemporary Medicine, Surgery, and Ophthalmology, 620 N. Orleans St., Ste. 208, Chicago, IL 60610-3169. TEL 800-621-4002, iaos@aol.com. Eds. Dr. David A Bellows, Dr. Randall J Bellows. R&P Deborah Pinkston. Adv. contact Mike Mason. Circ: 1,800 (controlled). **Co-sponsor:** International Association of Ocular Surgeons.

ANNUARIO OTTICO ITALIANO. see *BUSINESS AND ECONOMICS—Trade And Industrial Directories*

M

617.7 USA ISSN 0003-9950
RE1 CODEN: AROPAW
ARCHIVES OF OPHTHALMOLOGY. Text in English. 1869. m. USD 325 in North America to institutions; USD 425 to institutions Central & S. America; GBP 275 elsewhere to institutions (effective 2001). adv. bk.rev. charts, illus. index. back issues avail.; reprints avail. *Refereed.* **Document type:** *Academic/Scholarly.* **Description:** Publishes original contributions and observations on the science of vision of interest to clinicians and researchers.
Related titles: CD-ROM ed.: (from Ovid Technologies, Inc.); Microform ed.: (from PQC,PMC); Online - full text ed.: (from The Dialog Corporation, Gale Group, Ovid Technologies, Inc., EBSCO Publishing, Institute for Scientific Information); ♦ Spanish Translation: Archives of Ophthalmology (Edicion Espanola). ISSN 1130-5134.
Indexed: AIDS Abstr., AIM, ASCA, Abstr.Hyg., Abstr.Inter.Med., Agri.& Environ.Biotech.Abstr. (coverage dropped), Biol.Abstr., C.I.S. Abstr., Chem.Abstr., Chem.Indus.Notes, Chem.Titles, Curr.Adv.Cancer Res., Curr.Adv.Ecol.Sci., Curr.Cont., Dent.Ind., Derwent Biotech.Abstr., Diab.Cont., Dok.Arbeitsmed., Environ.Sci.Poll.Mgmt., Excerp.Med., HRIS, Helminthol.Abstr., INIS Atomind., Ind.Med. (1960-), Ind.Sci.Rev., Ind.Vet., Inpharma, Med.& Surg.Dermat., Neurosci.Cit.Ind., Nutr.Abstr., Pharm.&Out.News, Pollut.Abstr., Protozool.Abstr., Psychol.Abstr., Reac., Rev.Appl.Entomol., Rev.Med.& Vet.Mycol., Rev.Plant Path., Risk Abstr., Rural Recreat.Tour.Abstr., SSCI (coverage dropped), Saf.Sci.Abstr., Sci.Cit.Ind., Small Anim.Abstr., Vet.Bull., Weed Abstr.
—BLDSC (1638.450000), CASDDS, CISTI, EMDOCS, GNLM, IDS, ingenta, KNAW. **CCC.**
Published by: American Medical Association, 515 N State St, P O Box 10946, Chicago, IL 60610-0946. ama-subs@ama-assn.org, http://www.archopthalmol.com. Ed. Morton F Goldberg. Pub. Peter L Payerli. R&P Ada Jimenez Walker. Adv. contact J P Cahill. Circ: 21,500.

617.7 ESP ISSN 1130-5134
ARCHIVES OF OPHTHALMOLOGY (EDICION ESPANOLA). Text in Spanish. bi-m. USD 99. adv. **Document type:** *Academic/Scholarly.* **Description:** Contains translations of articles from the American edition, including editorials, clinical cases, laboratory technique and investigative work.
Related titles: ♦ Translation of: Archives of Ophthalmology. ISSN 0003-9950.
Indexed: Curr.Cont. (coverage dropped), Environ.Sci.Poll.Mgmt.
Published by: (American Medical Association USA), Ediciones Doyma S.A., Traversa de Gracia, 17-21, Barcelona 08021, Spain. TEL 34-93-200-0711, FAX 34-93-209-1136. Ed. J Murube del Castillo. Adv. contact Olga Gomez. color page ESP 238,000; trim 280 x 210. Circ: 2,000.

617.7 ARG ISSN 0066-6777
ARCHIVOS DE OFTALMOLOGIA DE BUENOS AIRES. Text in Spanish. 1925. q. USD 30. adv.
Indexed: Biol.Abstr., Excerp.Med.
—GNLM.
Published by: Sociedad Argentina de Oftalmologia, Viamonte, 1464-1 Dto 2, Capital Federal, Buenos Aires 1055, Argentina. Circ: 1,500.

617.7 USA ISSN 0194-8172
ARGUS (SAN FRANCISCO). Text in English. 1978. m. USD 36. adv. bk.rev. **Document type:** *Trade.* **Description:** Highlights health care reform and provides clinical news as well as advice on managed care and new health care delivery systems. Also updates members on academy news and events.
Published by: American Academy of Ophthalmology, PO Box 7424, San Francisco, CA 94120-7424. TEL 415-561-8500, FAX 415-561-8567, argus@aao.org, eyenet@aao.org. Ed., Adv. contact Stefanie Lee. R&P Pamela Beach. Circ: 21,000 (controlled).

617.7 BRA ISSN 0004-2749
CODEN: AQBOAP
ARQUIVOS BRASILEIROS DE OFTALMOLOGIA. Text in Portuguese. 1938. bi-m. USD 100 (effective 2000). adv. bk.rev. abstr, illus.
Indexed: Biol.Abstr., Excerp.Med., INIS Atomind., Ind.Med. (coverage dropped).
—BLDSC (1695.240000), CISTI, EMDOCS, GNLM.
Published by: Belfort Editora, Caixa 4086, Rua Barao de Itapetininga, 297, Centro, Sao Paulo, SP 01042-001, Brazil. Ed. Rubens Belfort Mattos. Circ: 1,500.

617.7 SGP ISSN 0129-1653
ASIA - PACIFIC JOURNAL OF OPHTHALMOLOGY. Text in English. 1987. q. USD 65 in Asia & the Pacific to individuals; USD 80 elsewhere to individuals; USD 130 in Asia & the Pacific to institutions; USD 160 elsewhere to institutions (effective 2001). adv. bk.rev. 30 p./no. *Refereed.* **Document type:** *Journal, Academic/Scholarly.* **Description:** Disseminates the latest research and development in surgical techniques, complications, management. Includes geographical and historical notes, and information on new implants and instruments.
Incorporates (in 1990): Implants in Ophthalmology (0218-0367)
Published by: Singapore National Eye Centre, 11 Third Hospital Ave, Singapore 168751, Singapore. TEL 65-227-7290, FAX 65-323-1903, TELEX SNEC RS 22842. Ed. Arthur S M Lim. Adv. contact Julie Goh. page USD 900; trim 270 x 205. Circ: 500.

617.7 USA ISSN 0273-0189
QP474
ASSOCIATION FOR RESEARCH IN VISION AND OPHTHALMOLOGY. SPRING MEETING. Text in English. a. abstr. **Document type:** *Proceedings.*
Related titles: ♦ Supplement to: Investigative Ophthalmology & Visual Science (IOVS). ISSN 0146-0404.
Published by: (Association for Research in Vision and Ophthalmology), Lippincott Williams & Wilkins (Philadelphia) (Subsidiary of: Wolters Kluwer N.V.), 530 Walnut St, Philadelphia, PA 19106-3621. TEL 301-223-2300, 800-638-3030, FAX 301-223-2400.

617.7 016 USA ISSN 0271-1281
AUDIO-DIGEST OPHTHALMOLOGY. Text in English. 1963. s-m. USD 168 (effective 2000). *Refereed.*
Media: Audio cassette/tape.
Published by: Audio-Digest Foundation (Subsidiary of: California Medical Association), 1577 E Chevy Chase Dr, Glendale, CA 91206. TEL 213-245-8505, 800-423-2308, FAX 818-240-7379, 800-845-4375. Ed. Claron L Oakley. Circ: (controlled).

617.7 DEU ISSN 0004-7902
DER AUGENARZT. Text in German. 1967. 6/yr. adv. bk.rev. abstr, illus. **Document type:** *Magazine, Trade.*
—GNLM.
Published by: (Berufsverband der Augenaerzte Deutschlands e.V.), Dr. R. Kaden Verlag, Poststr 24-26, Heidelberg 69115, Germany. TEL 49-6221-600313, FAX 49-6221-29910, marketing@kaden-verlag.de. Eds. Alexander Diehm, Gisa Kemper. adv.: B&W page DEM 4,530; trim 178 x 230. Circ: 7,800.

617.752 DEU
AUGENLICHT; das Magazin fuer gutes Sehen. Text in German. q. DEM 32 (effective 1999). adv. **Document type:** *Consumer.* **Description:** Provides information on products and services offered by ophthalmologists and opticians.
Published by: MediaWelt Produktions- und Agentur GmbH, Lintorfer Str 7-9, Ratingen 40878, Germany. TEL 49-2102-208500, FAX 49-2102-208400, media@augenspiegel.com. Pub. Heinz Juergen Hoeninger. R&P Stefanie Lemke. Adv. contact Larissa Lenz. color page DEM 10,440; trim 303 x 216. Circ: 13,000 (paid).

617.7 DEU ISSN 0004-7929
DER AUGENOPTIKER. Text in German. 1946. 13/yr. DEM 136.50 domestic; DEM 150.80 foreign; DEM 8.60 newsstand/cover (effective 2001). adv. bk.rev. bibl, charts, illus, stat. **Document type:** *Journal, Trade.*
—GNLM.
Published by: Konradin Verlag Robert Kohlhammer GmbH, Ernst Mey Str 8, Leinfelden-Echterdingen 70771, Germany. TEL 49-711-7594-0, FAX 49-711-7594-390, ao.redaktion@konradin.de, info@konradin.de, http://www.konradin.de. Ed. Stefan Zarges. Adv. contact Anna Waskala. B&W page DEM 4,980, color page DEM 7,860; trim 190 x 270. Circ: 11,872.

617.7 DEU ISSN 0004-7937
DER AUGENSPIEGEL; Forum der Augenaerzte. Text in German. 1955. m. DEM 182. adv. bk.rev. charts, illus, mkt, stat, tr.lit.
—GNLM.
Published by: Augenspiegel Verlags GmbH, Lintorfer Str 7-9, Ratingen 40878, Germany. TEL 02102-23062, FAX 02102-25488, TELEX 8589002-FOC-D. Ed. Dr. Berthold Schwab. Circ: 4,000.

AUSTRALIA. BUREAU OF STATISTICS. OPTOMETRY AND OPTICAL DISPENSING SERVICES, AUSTRALIA. see *MEDICAL SCIENCES—Abstracting, Bibliographies, Statistics*

617.75 AUS ISSN 0726-5018
AUSTRALIAN OPTOMETRY. Text in English. 1980. m. AUD 95. adv. tr.lit. **Document type:** *Newspaper, Trade.* **Description:** Provides news and features pertaining to optometry in Australia.
Published by: Optometrists Association Australia, PO Box 185, Carlton South, VIC 3053, Australia. TEL 61-3-9663-6833, FAX 61-3-9663-7478, oaanat@optometrists.asn.au. Adv. contact Sandra Shaw. B&W page USD 1,900, color page USD 3,430; trim 260 x 385. Circ: 3,100.

617.7 USA ISSN 1088-6281
CODEN: BVSQFV
BINOCULAR VISION & STRABISMUS QUARTERLY. Text in English; Abstracts in Spanish, French, German. 1985. q. USD 84 to individuals; USD 120 to institutions (effective 2001). adv. bk.rev., video rev. abstr, illus. cum.index: 1985-2000 in vol.15, no.4. 80 p./no. 3 cols./p. back issues avail.; reprints avail. *Refereed.* **Document type:** *Journal, Academic/Scholarly, Abstract/Index.* **Description:** For the professional devoting his or her practice to strabismus, amblyopia, eye movements, and other disorders of binocular vision.
Former titles (until 1996): Binocular Vision and Eye Muscle Surgery Quarterly (1073-001X); (until 1991): Binocular Vision (0749-386X)
Related titles: Online - full text ed.
Indexed: Ind.Med. (1996-).
—BLDSC (2066.654800), ingenta.
Published by: Binoculus Publishing, Summit Haus, 740 Piney Acres Cir, PO Box 3727, Dillon, CO 80435-3727. TEL 970-262-0753, FAX 970-262-0753. Ed. Dr. Paul E Romano. R&P, Adv. contact Judith Robinson. B&W page USD 270; trim 8.5 x 11. Circ: 1,000 (paid).

617.3 USA ISSN 0067-9283
BLUE BOOK OF OPTOMETRISTS. Text in English. 1912. biennial. USD 125. index. **Document type:** *Directory.*
Published by: Jobson Publishing Corporation, 5 Central St, Woodstock, VT 05091. TEL 800-238-8764, FAX 802-457-2489.

617.7 ITA ISSN 0006-677X
CODEN: BOOCAH
BOLLETTINO D'OCULISTICA. Text in Italian; Summaries in English, French, German. 1930. bi-m. ITL 90,000, USD 110 (effective 2000). adv. bk.rev. back issues avail. **Document type:** *Academic/Scholarly.*
Indexed: Chem.Abstr., Excerp.Med., Ind.Med. (coverage dropped).
—BLDSC (2239.800000), CASDDS, CISTI, GNLM.
Published by: Nuova Casa Editrice Licinio Cappelli di G.E.M. s.r.l., Via Luigi Carlo Farini, 14, Bologna, BO 40124, Italy. TEL 39-051-239060, FAX 39-051-239286. Ed. F D'Ermo. R&P Mario Musso. Adv. contact Lia Milano. Circ: 2,500.

617.7 GBR ISSN 0007-1161
CODEN: BJOPAL
BRITISH JOURNAL OF OPHTHALMOLOGY. Text in English. 1917. m. GBP 110, USD 160 combined subscription to individuals includes print & online eds.; GBP 260, USD 420 to institutions for print only (effective 2002). adv. bk.rev. abstr, bibl, charts, illus. index. reprint service avail. from PQC. *Refereed.* **Document type:** *Journal, Academic/Scholarly.* **Description:** Presents international papers from both clinicians and laboratory workers in ophthalmology to keep them abreast of trends.
Formed by the merger of: Ophthalmic Review (0266-3066); Ophthalmoscope (0266-3430); Royal London (Moorfields) Ophthalmic Hospital Reports (0266-2906)
Related titles: Microform ed.: (from PQC); Online - full text ed.: B J O Online. ISSN 1468-2079. GBP 50, USD 75 to individuals (effective 2002); Institutions contact publisher for rates. (from HighWire Pr., Ovid Technologies, Inc., Northern Light Technology, Inc., EBSCO Publishing, RoweCom Information Quest, ProQuest Information & Learning, ingenta, Swets Blackwell, SilverPlatter Information, Inc., Institute for Scientific Information).
Indexed: ASCA, Biol.Abstr., Chem.Abstr., Curr.Adv.Cancer Res., Curr.Adv.Ecol.Sci., Curr.Cont., Diab.Cont., Dok.Arbeitsmed., Environ.Sci.Poll.Mgmt., Excerp.Med., Helminthol.Abstr., INIS Atomind., Ind.Med. (1917-), Ind.Sci.Rev., Inpharma, Int.Abstr.Biol.Sci., Int.Nurs.Ind., Neurosci.Cit.Ind., Nutr.Abstr., Pharm.&Out.News, Pollut.Abstr., Protozool.Abstr., Reac., Ref.Zh., Rev.Appl.Entomol., Rev.Med.& Vet.Mycol., Rev.Plant Path., Risk Abstr., SSCI (coverage dropped), Saf.Sci.Abstr., Sci.Cit.Ind., Trop.Dis.Bull.
—BLDSC (2313.000000), ADONIS, CISTI, EMDOCS, GNLM, IDS, ingenta, KNAW. **CCC.**

M

Published by: B M J Publishing Group, B M A House, Tavistock Sq, London WC1H 9JR, United Kingdom. FAX 44-20-7383-6400, http://bjo.bmjjournals.com/. Ed. Craig Hoyt. Pub. Alex Williamson. R&P Carol Torselli TEL 44-20-7383-6674. Adv. contact Euan Currer TEL 44-20-7383-6181.

617.7 GBR ISSN 1351-6736
RE1
BRITISH JOURNAL OF OPTOMETRY AND DISPENSING. Text in English. 1993. q. GBP 40; GBP 80 foreign. adv. **Document type:** *Academic/Scholarly.*
Published by: Mark Allen Publishing Ltd., Croxted Mews, 286-288a Croxted Rd, London SE24 9BY, United Kingdom. TEL 44-208-671-7521, FAX 44-208-671-1722. Ed. Rishi Agarwal. Pub. Mark Allen. Adv. contact Ian White.

617.7 GBR ISSN 0068-2314
BRITISH ORTHOPTIC JOURNAL. Text in English. 1939. a. GBP 40 (effective 2002). adv. bk.rev. cum.index every 5 yrs. back issues avail. *Refereed.* **Document type:** *Journal, Academic/Scholarly.* **Description:** Subjects covered include orthoptics, binocular vision, ocular motility, pediatric ophthalmology, and neuro-ophthalmology.
Indexed: Biol.Abstr., Excerp.Med.
—BLDSC (2332.500000), CISTI, GNLM.
Published by: British Orthoptic Society, Tavistock House N, Tavistock Sq, London WC1H 9 HX, United Kingdom. TEL 44-20-7387-7992, FAX 44-20-7383-2584, bos@orthoptics.org.uk. Ed. Alison Y Firth TEL 44-1142-712064. Circ: 1,550.

617.7 BGR ISSN 0374-2105
CODEN: OPTMAI
BULGARIAN JOURNAL OF OPHTHALMOLOGY. Text in English. 3/yr. USD 45 foreign (effective 2002). **Document type:** *Journal.*
Indexed: INIS Atomind.
—CASDDS, CISTI.
Published by: (Bulgaria. Ministerstvo na Narodnoto Zdrave), Izdatelstvo Meditsina i Fizkultura, 11 Pl Slaveikov, Sofia 1080, Bulgaria. Ed. S Dabov. Circ: 766. **Distr. by:** Hemus, 6 Rouski blvd, Sofia 1000, Bulgaria. **Co-sponsor:** Nauchno Druzhestvo po Ophthalmologia.

BUSINESS RATIO. THE OPTICAL INDUSTRY. see *PHYSICS—Optics*

617.7 USA ISSN 0733-8902
RE977.C6 CODEN: CLAJEU
C L A O JOURNAL∗. Text in English. 1975. q. USD 76. adv. bk.rev. *Refereed.* **Document type:** *Academic/Scholarly.* **Description:** Research and review articles on contact lenses, and cornea and anterior segment of the eye for vision care professionals.
Former titles: Contact and Intraocular Lens Medical Journal (0360-1358); Contact Lens Medical Bulletin (0010-728X)
Related titles: Microform ed.: (from PQC).
Indexed: Biol.Abstr., Chem.Abstr., Excerp.Med., INIS Atomind., Ind.Med. (1983-), Protozool.Abstr.
—BLDSC (3274.311000), CASDDS, CISTI, EMDOCS, GNLM, ingenta, KNAW.
Published by: (Contact Lens Association of Ophthalmologists), Kellner-McCaffery Associates, Inc., PO Box 58, Croton on Hudson, NY 10520-0058. TEL 212-741-0280. Ed. Dr. Peter C Donshik. Circ: 3,300.

617.75 USA ISSN 0273-804X
CALIFORNIA OPTOMETRY. Text in English. 1933. s-m. USD 35 (effective 1999). adv. bk.rev. illus. *Refereed.* **Document type:** *Trade.* **Description:** Informs members on the latest economic, educational and business trends that affect the profession.
Former titles (until 1979): California Optometrist (0361-7025); California Optometrist Association. Journal (0008-1337)
Published by: California Optometric Association, 2415 K St, Sacramento, CA 95816. TEL 916-441-3990, 800-877-5738, FAX 916-448-1423, coa@coavision.org, http://www.coavision.org. Ed., Adv. contact Ian Crawford. R&P Greg Bohnstedt. Circ: 3,500.

617.7 CAN ISSN 0008-4182
CODEN: CAJOBA
CANADIAN JOURNAL OF OPHTHALMOLOGY/JOURNAL CANADIEN D'OPHTALMOLOGIE. Text in English, French. 1966. 7/yr. CND 80 domestic; USD 85 in United States; USD 95 elsewhere (effective 2001). adv. bk.rev. illus. back issues avail.; reprint service avail. from PQC. *Refereed.* **Document type:** *Academic/Scholarly.* **Description:** Contains scientific papers presented at annual meetings, and contributions from within and outside Canada.
Related titles: Microform ed.: (from PQC); Online - full text ed.: (from Institute for Scientific Information).
Indexed: ASCA, Biol.Abstr., Chem.Abstr., Curr.Cont., Excerp.Med., INIS Atomind., Ind.Med. (1966-), Ind.Sci.Rev., Inpharma, Ophthal.Lit., Pharm.&Out.News, Reac., Rev.Med.& Vet.Mycol., Rev.Plant Path., Sci.Cit.Ind.
—BLDSC (3033.700000), CASDDS, CISTI, EMDOCS, GNLM, IDS, ingenta, KNAW. **CCC.**
Published by: Canadian Ophthalmological Society, 610-1525 Carling Ave, Ottawa, ON K1Z 8R9, Canada. TEL 613-729-6779, FAX 613-729-7209, orders@allenpress.com, cos@eyesite.ca, http://www.eyesight.ca. Ed. B J MacInnis. Adv. contact Anne Keefer. B&W page CND 855, color page CND 959; trim 10.88 x 8.13. Circ: 330 (paid); 870 (controlled). **Subscr. in N. America to:** Allen Press Inc., PO Box 1897, Lawrence, KS 66044-8897.

617.7 CAN ISSN 0045-5075
CANADIAN JOURNAL OF OPTOMETRY/REVUE CANADIENNE D'OPTOMETRIE. Text in English. 1939. q. CND 45; CND 55 foreign (effective 2001). adv. bk.rev. **Document type:** *Trade.*
—CISTI.
Published by: Canadian Association of Optometrists, 234 Argyle Ave, Ottawa, ON K2P 1B9, Canada. TEL 613-235-7924, FAX 613-235-2025, cjo@opto.ca, eyedocs@opto.ca, http://www.opto.ca. Ed. Dr. Mitchell Samek. Adv. contact Ed Marriner. Circ: 4,000.

617.7 CZE ISSN 1211-9059
CESKA A SLOVENSKA OFTALMOLOGIE. Text in Czech, Slovak; Summaries in Czech, English. 1943. 6/yr. EUR 66, USD 84 (effective 2001). adv. bk.rev. abstr, bibl, illus. index. *Refereed.*
Formerly: Ceskoslovenska Oftalmologie (0009-059X)
Indexed: Chem.Abstr., Dent.Ind., Dok.Arbeitsmed., Excerp.Med., INIS Atomind., Ind.Med. (1995-).
—BLDSC (3120.258470), CISTI, EMDOCS, GNLM, Infotrieve. **CCC.**
Published by: (Ceska Lekarska Spolecnost J.E. Purkyne/Czech Medical Association), Nakladatelske Stredisko C L S J.E. Purkyne, Sokolska 31, Prague 12026, Czech Republic. TEL 42-2-24911420, FAX 42-2-24911420, nts@iol.cz, http://www.clsjep.cz, http://www.medical.cz. Ed. J Boguszakova. adv.: B&W page CZK 19,900, color page CZK 31,000; 136 x 194. Circ: 2,000. **Dist. by:** Abont s.r.o., Chlumova 17, Prague, 3 130 00, Czech Republic; **Dist. in Western countries by:** Kubon & Sagner, Hesstr 39-41, Munich 80798, Germany.

617.7 AUS ISSN 1442-6404
CODEN: ANZOEQ
CLINICAL AND EXPERIMENTAL OPHTHALMOLOGY. Text in English. 1973. bi-m. AUD 182 domestic to individuals; AUD 165 in New Zealand to individuals; USD 135 elsewhere to individuals; AUD 303 domestic to institutions; AUD 275 in New Zealand to institutions; USD 279 elsewhere to institutions; AUD 201 domestic to individuals paper & online eds. combined; AUD 182 in New Zealand to individuals paper & online eds. combined; USD 149 elsewhere to individuals paper & online eds. combined; AUD 334 domestic to institutions paper & online eds. combined; AUD 303 in New Zealand to institutions paper & online eds. combined; USD 307 elsewhere to institutions paper & online eds. combined (effective 2001). adv. reprint service avail. from ISI. **Document type:** *Academic/Scholarly.* **Description:** Reports research from around the world in all areas of ophthalmology.
Formerly: Australian and New Zealand Journal of Ophthalmology (0814-9763); Which was formed by the merger of (1947-1985): Ophthalmological Society of New Zealand (0300-8983); (1973-1985): Australian Journal of Ophthalmology; Which superseded (1960-1972): Australian College of Ophthalmologists. Transactions (0067-1789)
Related titles: Online - full text ed.: ISSN 1442-9071. AUD 164 domestic to individuals; AUD 149 in New Zealand to individuals; USD 122 elsewhere to individuals; AUD 273 domestic to institutions; AUD 248 in New Zealand to institutions; USD 252 elsewhere to institutions (effective 2001) (from EBSCO Publishing, O C L C Online Computer Library Center, Inc., RoweCom Information Quest, ingenta, Munksgaard & Blackwell Science's Synergy, Swets Blackwell, Institute for Scientific Information).
Indexed: ASCA, Biol.Abstr., Curr.Cont., Dent.Ind., Excerp.Med., Ind.Med. (coverage dropped), Ind.Sci.Rev., Inpharma, Neurosci.Cit.Ind., Pharm.&Out.News, Protozool.Abstr., Reac., Rev.Med.& Vet.Mycol., Rev.Plant Path., SSCI (coverage dropped), Sci.Cit.Ind., Sugar Ind.Abstr., Trop.Dis.Bull.
—BLDSC (3286.251920), CISTI, EMDOCS, GNLM, ingenta, KNAW. **CCC.**
Published by: (Royal Australian College of Ophthalmologists), Blackwell Science Asia Pty Ltd, PO Box 378, Carlton South, VIC 3053, Australia. TEL 61-3-9347-0300, FAX 61-3-9347-5001, info@blacksci-asia.com.au; anzjo@medeserv.com.au, http://www.blacksci.co.uk. Ed., R&P Mark Gillies TEL 61-2-9267-7006. Adv. contact Kathryn O'Brien. B&W page AUD 890, color page AUD 1,800; trim 210 x 275. Circ: 1,400. **Co-sponsor:** Ophthalmological Society of New Zealand, NZ.

617.75 AUS ISSN 0816-4622
CODEN: AJOPBB
CLINICAL AND EXPERIMENTAL OPTOMETRY. Text in English. 1913. bi-m. AUD 82; AUD 95 foreign (effective 2000). adv. bk.rev. charts, illus, stat, abstr. index. back issues avail. **Document type:** *Academic/Scholarly.* **Description:** Publishes original articles, letters to the editor and other items of educational interest.
Incorporates (1934-19??): New South Wales Journal of Optometry (0047-9918); Formerly (until 1986): Australian Journal of Optometry (0045-0642)
Indexed: Excerp.Med.
—BLDSC (3286.251940), CASDDS, GNLM, ingenta.
Published by: Optometrists Association Australia, PO Box 185, Carlton South, VIC 3053, Australia. TEL 61-3-9663-6833, FAX 61-3-9663-7478, oaanat@optometrists.asn.au. Ed. Dr. H Barry Collin. R&P, Adv. contact Sandra Shaw. Circ: 3,100.

617.7 GBR ISSN 1367-0484
RE977.C6
CONTACT LENS & ANTERIOR EYE. Text in English. 1977. q. GBP 78 in Europe to individuals for print or online ed.; USD 125 elsewhere to individuals for print or online ed.; GBP 86 combined subscription in Europe to individuals print & online; USD 138 combined subscription elsewhere to individuals print & online; GBP 135 in Europe to institutions for print or online ed.; USD 216 elsewhere to institutions for print or online ed.; GBP 148 combined subscription in Europe to institutions print & online; USD 237 combined subscription elsewhere to institutions print & online (effective 2001). charts, illus. index. back issues avail.; reprints avail. *Refereed.* **Document type:** *Journal, Trade, Academic/Scholarly.* **Description:** Publishes original and research articles on all aspects of contact lens theory and practice.
Formerly (until 1997): British Contact Lens Association. Journal (0141-7037); Which incorporated: British Contact Lens Association. Transactions
Related titles: Online - full text ed.: GBP 78, USD 125 to individuals; GBP 135, USD 216 to institutional members (effective 2001) (from EBSCO Publishing, O C L C Online Computer Library Center, Inc., RoweCom Information Quest, ingenta, Swets Blackwell).
—BLDSC (3424.971000), Infotrieve. **CCC.**
Published by: (British Contact Lens Association), Nature Publishing Group Specialist Journals (Subsidiary of: Holtzbrink Publishers), Houndmills, Basingstoke, Hants RG21 6XS, United Kingdom. TEL 44-1256-329242, FAX 44-1256-328339, subscriptions@nature.com, http://www.nature.com/clae. Ed. Richard M Pearson. Pub. Sue Deeley. R&P Trace Noel. Adv. contact Robert Sloan TEL 44-20-8882-7199.

617.75 GBR ISSN 0306-9575
CONTACT LENS JOURNAL. Text in English. 1966. m. GBP 3, USD 75. adv. bk.rev. abstr, bibl, charts, illus. index.
Formerly: Contact Lens (0010-7271)
Indexed: Curr.Adv.Ecol.Sci., Excerp.Med.
—CISTI.
Published by: Libra Publishing Ltd., 14 Fairfield Ave, Datchet, Slough, Berks SL3 9NQ, United Kingdom. Ed. Annette Whibley. Circ: 2,000.

617.752 USA ISSN 0885-9175
RE977.C6
CONTACT LENS SPECTRUM. Text in English. 1986. 20/yr. USD 43; USD 72 in Canada; USD 98 elsewhere. adv. back issues avail. **Description:** Provides contact lens professionals with clinical and technical information concerning contact lenses and solutions, guidelines for effective patient care, coverage of industry developments and new products, and analyses of market trends.
Incorporates (1976-1991): Contact Lens Forum (0363-1621)
—BLDSC (3424.984000), GNLM.
Published by: Boucher Communications, Inc., 1300 Virginia Dr, Ste 400, Ft, Washington, PA 19034. TEL 215-643-8000, FAX 215-643-8099. Ed. Joseph Barr. Adv. contact Roger Zimmer. Circ: 52,240. **Subscr. to:** Contact Lens Spectrum, PO Box 3055, Northbrook, IL 60065-3055. TEL 800-306-6332, FAX 847-564-9002.

CONTACT LENS UPDATE. see *MEDICAL SCIENCES—Abstracting, Bibliographies, Statistics*

CONTACTO. see *MEDICAL SCIENCES—Abstracting, Bibliographies, Statistics*

617.7 USA ISSN 0893-8733
CONTEMPORARY OPHTHALMIC FORUM. Text in English. 1982. q. USD 25. adv.
Formerly (until 1986): Ophthalmic Forum (0734-1652)
Published by: Silver Press, Inc., 456 Clinic Dr, Columbus, OH 43210. TEL 614-421-4960. Ed. Dr. Frederick H Davidorf. Circ: 13,600.

617.7 371.42 USA
CONTINUING EDUCATION MATTERS FOR O M P. (Opthalmic Medical Personnel) Text in English. 1980. 4/yr. USD 7; free to qualified personnel (effective 1999). **Description:** Covers current listing of continuing education courses and news related to the commission and certified opthalmic medical personnel.
Formerly (until 199?): J C A H P O Outlook
Published by: Joint Commission on Allied Health Personnel in Ophthalmology, 2025 Woodlane Dr., St. Paul, MN 55125-2995. TEL 800-284-3937, FAX 612-731-0410, jcahpo@jcahpo.org, http://www.jcahpo.org. Ed. Beverly Hagen. Circ: 16,000.

617.7 USA
CONTROVERSIES IN CLINICAL OPHTHALMOLOGY. Text in English. 1993. irreg. USD 285 to individuals; USD 350 to institutions. *Refereed.* **Document type:** *Academic/Scholarly.*
Published by: Field & Wood, Medical Periodicals, Inc., PO Box 975, Blue Bell, PA 19422. TEL 610-828-4010, FAX 610-482-0226. Ed. Dr. Joseph A Mauriello Jr.

617.7 USA ISSN 0277-3740
CODEN: CORNDB
CORNEA. Text in English. 1982. 8/yr. USD 322 domestic to individuals; USD 396 foreign to individuals; USD 543 domestic to institutions; USD 543 foreign to institutions; USD 66 newsstand/cover (effective 2002). adv. bk.rev. abstr, charts, illus. index. reprint service avail. from PQC. *Refereed.* **Document type:** *Academic/Scholarly.* **Description:** Offers the latest clinical and basic research on the cornea and the anterior segment of the eye.
Related titles: Microform ed.: (from PQC); Online - full text ed.: USD 705.90 domestic academic site license; USD 705.90 foreign academic site license; USD 787.35 domestic corporate site license; USD 787.35 foreign corporate site license (effective 2002) (from Ovid Technologies, Inc., Institute for Scientific Information).
Indexed: ASCA, Chem.Abstr., Curr.Cont., Excerp.Med., INIS Atomind., Ind.Med. (1982-), Inpharma, Nutr.Abstr., Pharm.&Out.News, Protozool.Abstr., Reac., Rev.Appl.Entomol., Rev.Med.& Vet.Mycol., Sci.Cit.Ind., Trop.Dis.Bull.
—BLDSC (3470.927500), CASDDS, CISTI, EMDOCS, GNLM, IDS, ingenta, KNAW.
Published by: (Castroviejo Cornea Society), Lippincott Williams & Wilkins (Philadelphia) (Subsidiary of: Wolters Kluwer N.V.), 530 Walnut St, Philadelphia, PA 19106-3621. TEL 215-521-8300, FAX 215-521-8902, http://www.Lww.com. Ed. Dr. Mark J Mannis. Pub. Christine Rullo. R&P Margaret Becker. Adv. contact James Nagle. B&W page USD 1,030, color page USD 2,365; trim 8.25 x 11. Circ: 1,735. **Subscr. to:** PO Box 1600, Hagerstown, MD 21740-1600. TEL 800-777-2295, FAX 301-824-7390.

617.75 646.4 ESP
COTTET MAGAZINE. Text in Spanish, Catalan. 1991. a. adv. bk.rev. bibl, mkt, maps. back issues avail. **Document type:** *Catalog, Consumer.*
Related titles: CD-ROM ed.; Online - full text ed.
Published by: S.A. Cottet, Avda. Puerta del Angel 40, Barcelona 08002, Spain. TEL 34-93-412-2060, FAX 34-93-317-0492, cottet@cottet.es, http:www.cottet.es. Ed., R&P Javier Cottet TEL 34-93-301-2232. Pub. Lourdes Mochales Aragon. adv.: color page ESP 475,000. Circ: 100,000.

617.7 CAN
COUP D'OEIL. Text in English. 1982. 5/yr.
Published by: Les Productions CT Enr., 1048 rue d' Avaugour, Chicoutimi, PQ G7H 2T1, Canada. TEL 418-696-4805, FAX 514-359-0836. adv.: B&W page CND 1,390, color page CND 1,955; trim 10.88 x 8.75. Circ: 2,492.

617.7 FRA ISSN 1251-229X
COUP D'OEIL OPHTALMOLOGIQUE. Text in French. 1985. 6/yr. FRF 450. bk.rev. *Refereed.* **Document type:** *Academic/Scholarly.* **Description:** Features in service training and post university teaching ophthalmological articles, reviews, round-ups and original papers by experts from both academic and professional circles. It spans the divide between fundamentalists and clinicians and provides a forum for debate.
Formerly (until 1992): Coup d'Oeil (0767-7634)
Published by: Editions et Regarde Attentivement, 68 bd. des Poilus, Nantes 44300, France. TEL 40-68-96-06, FAX 40-68-98-76. Ed. Jean Jacques Coulon. adv.: B&W page FRF 11,300, color page FRF 20,200. Circ: 4,000.

COURTROOM MEDICINE SERIES: THE EYE. see *LAW*

617.7 NLD ISSN 0271-3683
QP476 CODEN: CEYRDM
CURRENT EYE RESEARCH. Text in English. 1981. m., latest vol.22, 2001. ANG 511, USD 240 to individuals; ANG 1,732, USD 775, EUR 787 to institutions (effective 2001). adv. illus. index. back issues avail.; reprint service avail. from SWZ. *Refereed.* **Document type:** *Academic/Scholarly.* **Description:** Rapidly publishes clinical and basic research on anatomy, physiology, biophysics, biochemistry, developmental biology, microbiology, pharmacology and immunology of the eye.
Related titles: Online - full text ed.: (from EBSCO Publishing, O C L C Online Computer Library Center, Inc., RoweCom Information Quest, Swets Blackwell, Institute for Scientific Information).
Indexed: ASCA, Curr.Adv.Biochem., Curr.Adv.Cell & Devel.Biol., Curr.Adv.Ecol.Sci., Curr.Cont., Environ.Sci.Poll.Mgmt., Excerp.Med., INIS Atomind., Ind.Med. (1981-), Ind.Sci.Rev., Ind.Vet., Inpharma, Neurosci.Cit.Ind., Ophthal.Lit., Pharm.&Out.News, Pollut.Abstr., Protozool.Abstr., Reac., Rev.Med.& Vet.Mycol., Sci.Cit.Ind., Vet.Bull.
—BLDSC (3496.570000), ADONIS, CASDDS, CISTI, EMDOCS, GNLM, IDS, ingenta, KNAW. **CCC.**
Published by: Swets & Zeitlinger Publishers, PO Box 825, Lisse 2160 SZ, Netherlands. TEL 31-252-435111, http://www.szp.swets.nl/szp/journals/ce.htm. Pub. John R Martin TEL 31-252-435472. Adv. contact Patrick Kleian. Circ: 500.

CURRENT MEDICAL LITERATURE. OPHTHALMOLOGY. see *MEDICAL SCIENCES—Abstracting, Bibliographies, Statistics*

617.7 USA ISSN 1040-8738
CODEN: COOTEF
CURRENT OPINION IN OPHTHALMOLOGY. Text in English. 1989. bi-m. USD 320 domestic to individuals for print & online eds.; USD 320 foreign to individuals for print & online eds.; USD 721 per issue domestic to institutions; USD 721 per issue foreign to institutions; USD 111 newsstand/cover (effective 2002). adv. bibl, illus. **Document type:** *Academic/Scholarly.* **Description:** Directed toward researchers and practicing ophthalmologists. Presents review articles followed by annotated bibliographies of references consulted. A bibliography of the current world literature published during the previous year is available.
Related titles: Online - full text ed.: USD 937.30 domestic academic site license; USD 937.30 foreign academic site license; USD 1,045.45 domestic corporate site license; USD 1,045.45 foreign corporate site license (effective 2002) (from Ovid Technologies, Inc., EBSCO Publishing, Swets Blackwell); ♦ Supplement: Slide Atlas of Current Ophthalmology (Year). ISSN 1055-6575.
Indexed: CINAHL, Excerp.Med., Int.Abstr.Biol.Sci.
—BLDSC (3500.776500), ADONIS, EMDOCS, GNLM, IDS, ingenta, KNAW.
Published by: Lippincott Williams & Wilkins (Philadelphia) (Subsidiary of: Wolters Kluwer N.V.), 530 Walnut St, Philadelphia, PA 19106-3621. FAX 215-521-8902, 215-521-8902, http://www.Lww.com. Ed. George W Weinstein. Pub. Maria McMichael. R&P Tobias Weschler. Adv. contact Kelly Adamitis. **Subscr. to:** PO Box 1600, Hagerstown, MD 21740-1600.

617.7 USA ISSN 1078-7283
CURRENT TECHNIQUES IN OPHTHALMIC LASER SURGERY. Text in English. 1992. a.
Formerly (until 1994): Annual of Ophthalmic Laser Surgery (1062-4813)
—CISTI, GNLM, KNAW.
Published by: Current Science Inc., 400 Market St, Ste 700, Philadelphia, PA 19106. TEL 215-574-2200. Eds. Gabriel Coscas, Lawrence J Singerman.

617.752 DEU ISSN 0344-7103
RE1 CODEN: DDOPD4
DEUTSCHE OPTIKERZEITUNG. Text in German. 1945. m. DEM 95; DEM 130 foreign. adv. bk.rev. back issues avail. **Document type:** *Trade.*
Formerly: Sueddeutsche Optikerzeitung
Indexed: Ref.Zh.
—CASDDS.
Published by: Optische Fachveroeffentlichung GmbH, Rohrbacher Str 57, Heidelberg 69115, Germany. TEL 06221-184081, FAX 06221-183996. Ed. Dieter Baust. Adv. contact Ralf Ritter. B&W page DEM 3,680; trim 258 x 185. Circ: 9,999.

617.7 CHE ISSN 0250-3751
CODEN: DEOPDB
DEVELOPMENTS IN OPHTHALMOLOGY. Text in English. 1980. irreg., latest vol.32. CHF 200 in Europe; DEM 240 in Germany; USD 160 in United States (effective 2001). back issues avail.; reprint service avail. from ISI. *Refereed.* **Document type:** *Monographic series, Academic/Scholarly.* **Description:** Combines reviews with reports on new experimental findings.
Formed by the merger of: Advances in Ophthalmology (0065-3004); Bibliotheca Ophthalmologica (0067-8090); Modern Problems in Ophthalmology (0077-0078)
Related titles: Online - full text ed.: (from Institute for Scientific Information); ♦ Supplement to: Ophthalmologica. ISSN 0030-3755.
Indexed: Biol.Abstr., Chem.Abstr., Curr.Cont. (coverage dropped), Ind.Med. (1981-).
—BLDSC (3579.085480), CASDDS, CISTI, GNLM, Infotrieve, KNAW. **CCC.**
Published by: S. Karger AG, Allschwilerstr 10, PO Box, Basel 4009, Switzerland. TEL 41-61-306-1111, FAX 41-61-306-1234, karger@karger.ch, http://www.karger.com/bookseries/DEOPH. Ed. W Behrens Baumann.

617.7 MEX
DICCIONARIO DE ESPECIALIDADES OFTALMOLOGICAS. Text in Spanish. 1991. a.
Published by: Ediciones P L M S.A. de C.V., San BERNADINO 17, Col del Valle, Mexico City, DF 03100, Mexico. TEL 687-1766, FAX 536-5027. Ed. Dr. Emilio Rosenstein. Circ: 3,000.

617.7 MEX
DIMENSION OPTICA. Text in Spanish. bi-m. USD 350 (effective (No. 2001). adv. back issues avail. **Document type:** *Academic/Scholarly.*
Related titles: Online - full text ed.: ISSN 1605-4970. 1999.
Published by: Corporacion Optica y Publicitaria, Paseo de Mexico No. 21, Col. Jardines de Atizapan, Atizapan de Zaragoza, Estado de Mexico 52978, Mexico. TEL 52-5-8258258, dimensionoptica@usa.net, dimop@mail.com, http://www.geocities.com/HotSprings/Oasis/5181/home.htm. Ed. Rafael Balcazar Narro. Adv. contact Alejandra Moscoso Garcia.

617.7 USA
DIRECTORY OF CERTIFIED OPHTHALMIC MEDICAL PERSONNEL. Text in English. 1984. a. USD 35; free to qualified personnel (effective 1999). **Document type:** *Directory.* **Description:** Lists every person holding certification with the Commission.
Formerly: Directory of Certified Ophthalmic Medical Assistants
Published by: Joint Commission on Allied Health Personnel in Ophthalmology, 2025 Woodlane Dr., St. Paul, MN 55125-2995. TEL 800-284-3937, FAX 612-731-0410, jcahpo@jcahpo.org, http://www.jcahpo.org. Ed. Beverly Hagen.

616.7 GBR
DIRECTORY OF TRAINING POSTS IN OPHTHALMOLOGY. Text in English. a. GBP 9.50 (effective 2001). **Document type:** *Directory.*
Published by: (Royal College of Ophthalmologists), Hawker Publications Ltd., Culvert House, Culvert Rd, London SW11 5AP, United Kingdom. TEL 44-20-7720-2108, FAX 44-20-7498-3023, hawker@hawkerpubs.demon.co.uk, http://www.careinfo.org/.

617.7 IND
DOCTOR. Text in English. q. INR 60, USD 30 (effective 2000). **Document type:** *Newsletter.* **Description:** Widely-acclaimed health care public-education newsletter.
Formerly: Mini Eye Care
Published by: Dr. Narendra Kumar Ed. & Pub., C4F/216, Janakpuri, New Delhi 110 058, India. TEL 91-11-5599839, FAX 91-11-5593216.

617.7 NLD ISSN 0012-4486
RE14 CODEN: DOOPAA
DOCUMENTA OPHTHALMOLOGICA. Text in English. 1938. bi-m. EUR 590, USD 591 to institutions for print or online ed.; EUR 708, USD 709.20 to institutions for print & online eds.combined (effective 2002). adv. bk.rev. Supplement avail.; reprint service avail. from SWZ. *Refereed.* **Document type:** *Journal, Academic/Scholarly.* **Description:** Publishes studies on clinical and non-clinical ophthalmology.
Related titles: Microform ed.: (from PQC); Online - full text ed.: (from EBSCO Publishing, O C L C Online Computer Library Center, Inc., RoweCom Information Quest, Swets Blackwell, Kluwer Online, Institute for Scientific Information); ♦ Supplement: Documenta Ophthalmologica Proceedings Series. ISSN 0303-6405.
Indexed: ASCA, Biol.Abstr., Chem.Abstr., Curr.Cont. (coverage dropped), Excerp.Med., INIS Atomind., INSPEC (Jan.1985-, dropped), Ind.Med. (1938-), Ind.Sci.Rev., Ind.Vet., Inpharma, Neurosci.Cit.Ind., Nutr.Abstr., Pharm.&Out.News, Reac., SSCI (coverage dropped), Sci.Cit.Ind. (coverage dropped), Vet.Bull.
—BLDSC (3609.560000), AskIEEE, CASDDS, CISTI, GNLM, IDS, ingenta, KNAW. **CCC.**
Published by: (International Society for Clinical Electrophysiology of Vision), Kluwer Academic Publishers Group (Subsidiary of: Wolters Kluwer N.V.), Spuiboulevard 50, PO Box 17, Dordrecht 3300 AA, Netherlands. TEL 31-78-639-2392, FAX 31-78-654-2254, services@wkap.nl, http://www.wkap.nl/journalhome.htm/0012-4486. Ed. Michael F Marmor. **Subscr. in the Americas to:** Kluwer Academic - Plenum Publishers, 233 Spring St, New York, NY 10013-1578. TEL 212-620-8468, FAX 212-807-1047; **Subscr. to:** Journals Department, PO Box 322, Dordrecht 3300 AH, Netherlands. TEL 31-78-639-2392, FAX 31-78-654-6474.

617.7 NLD ISSN 0303-6405
CODEN: DOPSBP
DOCUMENTA OPHTHALMOLOGICA PROCEEDINGS SERIES. Text in English. 1973. irreg. price varies. *Refereed.* **Document type:** *Proceedings.*
Related titles: ♦ Supplement to: Documenta Ophthalmologica. ISSN 0012-4486.
Indexed: Biol.Abstr., Curr.Adv.Ecol.Sci., Nutr.Abstr., Psychol.Abstr.
—BLDSC (3609.600000), CASDDS, CISTI, GNLM, KNAW.
Published by: Kluwer Academic Publishers Group (Subsidiary of: Wolters Kluwer N.V.), Spuiboulevard 50, PO Box 17, Dordrecht 3300 AA, Netherlands. FAX 31-78-639-2254, services@wkap.nl, http://www.wkap.nl. **Dist. by:** Journals Department, PO Box 322, Dordrecht 3300 AH, Netherlands. FAX 31-78-654-6474.

617.752 ITA ISSN 1590-9638
▼ **E&F - EYEWEAR & FASHION.** Text in Italian, English. 1999. q. EUR 10.33 domestic; EUR 18.08 foreign; EUR 2.58 newsstand/cover (effective 2001). adv. music rev. back issues avail. **Document type:** *Journal, Trade.*
Published by: Edizioni Ariminum, Via Negroli, 51, Milan, MI 20133, Italy. TEL 39-02-7423727, FAX 39-02-717346, welcome@vedere.it, http://www.vedere.it. Pub., Adv. contact Isabella Morpurgo. color page XEU 2,600; 240 x 300. Circ: 12,000.

617.7 FRA ISSN 0246-0343
ENCYCLOPEDIE MEDICO-CHIRURGICALE. OPHTALMOLOGIE. Cover title: Traite d'Ophtalmologie. Variant title: Encyclopedie Medico-Chirurgicale, Instantanes Medicaux. Ophtalmologie. Text in French. 1955. 6 base vols. plus q. updates. bibl, charts, illus. *Refereed.* **Document type:** *Academic/Scholarly.* **Description:** Provides ophthalmologists with a comprehensive, up-to-date reference to diagnose and treat diseases and conditions of the eye.
Published by: Elsevier Paris, Editions Scientifiques et Medicales (Subsidiary of: Reed Elsevier plc. group), 23 rue Linois, Paris 75015, France. TEL 33-1-45589110, FAX 33-1-45589425, redaction-emc@elsevier.fr, redacion-emc@elsevier.fr, http://www.elsevier.fr, http://www.elsevier.com.

617.75 NLD ISSN 1386-1794
EURO OPTICIEN. Text in Dutch. 198?. bi-m. NLG 66.15; NLG 97.50 in Europe. adv. illus. **Document type:** *Trade.* **Description:** Informs opticians of developments in the eyeglass and contact lens arenas, both within the Netherlands and abroad. Includes news on the financial, economic, and technological aspects of the industry.
Published by: Wegener Tijdschriften Groep BV (Subsidiary of: Wegener Arcade NV), Wildenborch 5, Postbus 1860, Diemen 1112 CD, Netherlands. TEL 31-20-660-3300, FAX 31-20-660-3303, info@wtg.wegener.nl, http://www.wegener.nl. Pub. Peter Peeters. Circ: 2,500 (paid); 2,500 (controlled).

617.7 ITA ISSN 1120-6721
CODEN: EJOOEL
EUROPEAN JOURNAL OF OPHTHALMOLOGY. Text in English. 1991. q. EUR 85 in Europe to individuals; USD 109 elsewhere to individuals; EUR 120 in Europe to institutions; USD 140 elsewhere to institutions (effective 2001). adv. *Refereed.* **Document type:** *Journal, Academic/Scholarly.* **Description:** Covers clinical and basic research in ophthalmology.
Related titles: Online - full text ed.: (from Institute for Scientific Information).
Indexed: Curr.Cont., Excerp.Med. (1993-), Ind.Med. (1991-), Inpharma, Pharm.&Out.News, Reac.
—BLDSC (3829.733230), CISTI, EMDOCS, GNLM, IDS, Infotrieve, KNAW. **CCC.**
Published by: Wichtig Editore s.r.l., Via Friuli, 72, Milan, MI 20135, Italy. TEL 39-02-55195443, FAX 39-02-55195971, eur.j.ophthalmol@tin.it, http://www.eur.j.ophthalmol.com. Ed. Dr. Rosario Brancato. Pub. Dr. Diego Brancaccio. R&P Lucia Steele. Circ: 3,000 (paid); 4,500 (controlled).

617.7 BEL ISSN 0301-326X
EUROPEAN OPHTHALMOLOGICAL SOCIETY. CONGRESS ACTA✱ . Text in English, French, German. 1960. quadrennial, latest 1992, 9th, Brussels. **Document type:** *Proceedings.*
Published by: (Royal Society of Medicine, London GBR), European Ophthalmological Society, c/o Prof. Dr. L. Missotten, UZ St. Rafael, Kapucijnenvoer 33, Leuven 3000, Belgium. Ed. P D Trevor Roper. Circ: 1,500.

617.7 USA ISSN 1525-8599
EVIDENCE - BASED EYE CARE. Text in English. q. USD 93 domestic to individuals; USD 93 foreign to individuals; USD 121 per issue domestic to institutions; USD 121 per issue foreign to institutions; USD 65 to students; USD 28 newsstand/cover (effective 2002). **Description:** Presents analyses in the categories of clinical studies or trials, medical socioeconomics, and politics as it relates to healthcare. Supplies an evidence-based approach to eye care.
Related titles: Online - full text ed.: USD 157.30 domestic for academic site license; USD 157.30 foreign for academic site license; USD 175.45 domestic for corporate site license; USD 175.45 foreign for corporate site license (effective 2002).
Published by: Lippincott Williams & Wilkins (Philadelphia) (Subsidiary of: Wolters Kluwer N.V.), 530 Walnut St, Philadelphia, PA 19106-3621. TEL 301-223-2300, 800-638-3030, FAX 301-223-2320, http://www.evidence-based-eyecare.com. Eds. Dr. Gary C. Brown, Dr. Melissa M. Brown, Dr. Sanjay Sharma. **Subscr. to:** PO Box 1600, Hagerstown, MD 21740-1600.

EXCERPTA MEDICA. SECTION 12: OPHTHALMOLOGY. see *MEDICAL SCIENCES—Abstracting, Bibliographies, Statistics*

617.7 GBR ISSN 0014-4835
QP474 CODEN: EXERA6
EXPERIMENTAL EYE RESEARCH; an international journal devoted to scientific research on the eye. Text in English. 1961. m. GBP 1,250 to institutions (effective 2001). adv. charts, illus, stat. index. back issues avail.; reprint service avail. from SWZ. *Refereed.* **Document type:** *Academic/Scholarly.* **Description:** Publishes original research papers on all aspects of the anatomy, physiology, biochemistry, biophysics, molecular biology, pharmacology, developmental biology, microbiology, and immunology of the eye.
Related titles: Online - full text ed.: (from EBSCO Publishing, O C L C Online Computer Library Center, Inc., RoweCom Information Quest, ingenta, Swets Blackwell, IDEAL Online Library, Institute for Scientific Information).
Indexed: ASCA, Biol.Abstr., Chem.Abstr., Chem.Indus.Notes, Chem.Titles, Curr.Adv.Biochem., Curr.Adv.Ecol.Sci., Curr.Adv.Gen.& Molec.Biol., Curr.Cont., Dent.Ind., Eng.Ind., Excerp.Med., INIS Atomind., Ind.Med. (1961-), Ind.Sci.Rev., Inpharma, Mass Spectr.Bull., Neurosci.Cit.Ind., Nutr.Abstr., Pharm.&Out.News, Protozool.Abstr., Reac., Sci.Cit.Ind.
—BLDSC (3839.150000), ADONIS, CASDDS, CISTI, Ei, GNLM, IDS, ingenta, Linda Hall. **CCC.**
Published by: Academic Press (Subsidiary of: Harcourt Publishers Ltd.), 24 Oval Rd, London NW1 7DX, United Kingdom. TEL 44-20-7267-4466, FAX 44-20-7482-2293, apsubs@acad.com, http://www.academicpress.com/eer; http://www.europe.idealibrary.com/. Ed. J G Hollyfield. R&P Catherine John. Adv. contact Nik Screen. **Subscr. to:** Harcourt Publishers Ltd., Foots Cray High St, Sidcup, Kent DA14 5HP, United Kingdom. TEL 44-20-8300-3322, FAX 44-20-8309-0807.

617.7 GBR ISSN 0950-222X
CODEN: EYEEEC
EYE. Text in English. 1880. a. GBP 218, USD 348 (effective 1998). adv. bk.rev. index. back issues avail. *Refereed.*
Formerly (until 1979): Ophthalmological Society of the United Kingdom. Transactions (0078-5334)
Related titles: Microfiche ed.: (from BHP); Online - full text ed.: (from Institute for Scientific Information).
Indexed: AIDS Abstr., Biol.Abstr., Curr.Cont., Dent.Ind., Excerp.Med., Helminthol.Abstr., Ind.Med. (1987-), Ind.Sci.Rev., Inpharma, Int.Nurs.Ind., Pharm.&Out.News, Protozool.Abstr., Reac., Rev.Appl.Entomol., Rev.Med.& Vet.Mycol., Sci.Cit.Ind.
—BLDSC (3854.566000), CASDDS, CISTI, EMDOCS, GNLM, IDS, ingenta, KNAW.
Published by: B M J Publishing Group, B M A House, Tavistock Sq, London WC1H QJR, United Kingdom. TEL 44-171-387-4439, FAX 44-171-383-6661, http://www.bmjpg.com/. Circ: 3,250.

617.7 IND ISSN 0255-4062
EYE CARE. Text in English. 1979. a. INR 150, USD 75 (effective 2002). adv. bk.rev. **Document type:** *Academic/Scholarly.* **Description:** Annual ocular health guidebook.
Published by: (Update in Optics and Contact Lens), Dr. Narendra Kumar Ed. & Pub., C4F/216, Janakpuri, New Delhi 110 058, India. TEL 91-11-5599839, FAX 91-11-5593216. R&P Narendra Kumar. Circ: 2,000.

617.7 GBR ISSN 1368-8952
EYE NEWS. Text in English. 1995. bi-m. GBP 15 domestic; GBP 45 elsewhere (effective 2001). adv. bk.rev. back issues avail.; reprints avail. **Document type:** *Magazine, Academic/Scholarly.* **Description:** Contains editorial topics, reviews of journals and reports on new products.
—BLDSC (3854.631000).
Published by: Pinpoint Scotland Ltd., 9 Gayfield St, Edinburgh EH1 3NT, United Kingdom. TEL 44-131-557-4184, FAX 44-131-557-4701, eyenews@pinpoint-scotland.com. Ed. P I Murray. Pub., Adv. contact Cedric Chater. R&P Sophie Whiting. B&W page GBP 773, color page GBP 1,085; trim 297 x 210. Circ: 1,656 (paid); 2,954 (controlled).

617.75 USA
EYE ON OREGON. Text in English. 1934. q. USD 25. bk.rev. **Document type:** *Newsletter.*
Former titles (until vol.29, no.4, 1992): Oregon Optometry (0274-6549); Oregon Optometrist (0030-476X)
Media: Duplicated (not offset).
Published by: Oregon Optometric Association, 6901 S.E. Lake Rd., Ste. 26, Milwaukie, OR 97267-2195. TEL 503-639-5036, FAX 503-659-4189. Ed. J Gregg Mindt.

617.7 CHN ISSN 1000-4432
CODEN: YAXUE
EYE SCIENCE/YANKE XUEBAO; a view of Chinese ophthalmology. Text in Chinese, English. q. *Refereed.* **Document type:** *Academic/Scholarly.*
Indexed: Excerp.Med., Ind.Med. (1985-).
—BLDSC (3854.635000), CASDDS, GNLM.
Published by: Sun Yat-sen University of Medical Sciences, Zhongshan Ophthalmic Center, 54 Xianlie Rd, Guangzhou, Guangdong 510060, China.

617.7 USA
EYE TO EYE. Text in English. 1971. a. free per issue. **Document type:** *Newsletter.*
Former titles: International Eye Foundation - Society of Eye Surgeons. Newsletter; Eyelights
Published by: International Eye Foundation, 7801 Norfolk Ave, Bethesda, MD 20814. TEL 301-986-1830, FAX 301-986-1876, info@iefusa.org, http://www.iefusa.org. Ed. Calvin Baervelat. Circ: 1,500.

617.7 USA ISSN 0885-9167
EYECARE BUSINESS. Text in English. 1986. m. USD 90 domestic; USD 180 in Canada; USD 175 elsewhere; free to qualified personnel. adv. illus. **Document type:** *Trade.* **Description:** Provides optical dispensers the tools needed to survive the challenges of managed care and mass merchandising.
Published by: Boucher Communications, Inc., 1300 Virginia Dr, Ste 400, Ft, Washington, PA 19034. TEL 215-643-8000, FAX 215-643-8099. Ed. Stephanie Walter. Pub., Adv. contact Martin Cheifetz. Circ: 52,240. **Subscr. to:** Eyecare Business, PO Box 3055, Northbrook, IL 60065-3055. TEL 847-291-5212, FAX 847-564-9002.

617.7 USA ISSN 1097-2986
EYENET. Text in English. 1997. m. USD 128 domestic to non-members; USD 180 foreign to non-members (effective 2001); Free to members. illus. **Document type:** *Trade.* **Description:** Covers research and clinical developments in the field.
Published by: American Academy of Ophthalmology, PO Box 7424, San Francisco, CA 94120-7424. TEL 415-561-8500, FAX 415-561-8567, http:// www.eyenet.org, http://www.aao.org.

617.7 USA ISSN 1098-0946
RE939.2
EYEWEAR; for the business of dispensing. Text in English. 1997-1999; resumed 2000. m. adv. **Document type:** *Trade.* **Description:** Geared for the ophthalmic community: optometrists, opticians, and ophthalmologists. Provides eyecare professionals with the information they need to grow their business and better serve their patients.
Published by: Jobson Publishing LLC, 100 Ave of Americas, New York, NY 10013-1678. http://www.jobson.com. Pub. David Cox. Circ: 44,000.
Subscr. to: PO Box 2092, Mahopal, NY 10541.

617.7 362 USA ISSN 0899-7756
FIGHTING BLINDNESS NEWS. Text in English. 1973. 3/yr. free. bk.rev. **Document type:** *Newsletter.* **Description:** Contains articles on retinitis pigmentosa, macular degeneration, Usher syndrome and other retinal degenerations. Includes personal profiles on people affected by these diseases.
Related titles: Audio cassette/tape ed.; Braille ed.; Online - full text ed.; Large type ed. 14 pt.
Published by: Foundation Fighting Blindness, 11435 Cronhill Dr., Owings Mills, MD 21117. TEL 410-568-0150, 888-394-3937, FAX 410-363-2393, http://www.blindness.org. Ed. Robyn Miller. Circ: 70,000.

617.7 DEU ISSN 0721-1600
FOCUS (RATINGEN); Magazin fuer den erfolgreichen Augenoptiker. Text in German. 1981. m. DEM 145. bk.rev. charts, illus. **Document type:** *Trade.* **Description:** For optometrists and dispensing opticians: practice management, education and trade relations in political matters.
Published by: Spangemacher Verlags GmbH und Co. KG, Lintorfer Str 7-9, Ratingen 40878, Germany. TEL 02102-23051, FAX 02102-25488. Ed. Joerg Spangemacher. Circ: 7,500.

617.752 USA
FRAMES QUARTERLY & PRICE BOOK. Text in English. q. USD 308 domestic; USD 375 in Canada & Mexico; USD 587 elsewhere (effective 2000). adv. **Document type:** *Trade.*
Formerly: Frames
Indexed: Avery Ind.Archit.Per.
Published by: Jobson Publishing L.L.C. (Irvine), 16269 Laguna Canyon Rd, Ste 100, Irvine, CA 92618-3603. TEL 949-788-0160, FAX 949-788-0130, http://www.framesdata.com; http://www.jobson.com. Ed. Christie Walker. Pub. Skip Johnson. Adv. contact Lenor Fowler. Circ: 18,000.

617.7 JPN ISSN 0386-9601
GANKA RINSHO IHO/JAPANESE REVIEW OF CLINICAL OPHTHALMOLOGY. Text in Japanese; Summaries in English. 1906. m. JPY 15,000.
Indexed: INIS Atomind.
—BLDSC (4661.750000), CISTI.
Published by: Ganka Rinsho Ihokai/Japanese Society of Clinical Ophthalmology, Daigaku Igakubu Gankagaku Kyoshitsu, 11-1 Kaga 2-chome, Itabashi-ku, Tokyo 173-0003, Japan. TEL 03-3964-1211, FAX 03-3963-0303. Ed. Toshio Maruo.

617.7 JPN ISSN 0915-5066
GANKA SHUJUTSU KONNICHI NO KANGAEKATA/ CURRENT INSIGHTS IN OPHTHALMIC SURGERY. Text in Japanese. 1989. 4/yr.
Published by: Sutandado Makkintaiya/Standard McIntyre, 3-7 Irifune 2-chome, Chuo-ku, Tokyo 104-0042, Japan.

617.7 GBR ISSN 1465-5071
▼ **GLAUCOMA FORUM**; the IGA journal for interdisciplinary discussion. Text in English. 1999. q. GBP 12.50; GBP 3.50 newsstand/cover (effective 2001). adv. back issues avail.; reprints avail. *Refereed.* **Document type:** *Journal, Academic/Scholarly.* **Description:** Discusses professional and clinical issues relating to glaucoma.
—BLDSC (4194.280000).
Published by: International Glaucoma Association, 108c Warner Rd, London SE5 9HQ, United Kingdom. TEL 44-20-7737-3265, FAX 44-20-7733-4784, info@iga.org.uk, http://www.iga.org.uk/. Eds. Mr. David Wright, Dr. Michael Miller, Dr. Ronald Pitts Crick, Dr. S Nagusabramanian. Pub., Adv. contact Mr. David Wright. color page GBP 795, B&W page GBP 465; trim 210 x 297. Circ: 3,000.

617.7 USA ISSN 1072-7906
GLEAMS✱ . Text in English. 1982. 4/yr. free per issue. bk.rev. charts, illus. back issues avail. *Refereed.* **Document type:** *Newsletter.* **Description:** Aims to educate the public and professionals about current glaucoma diagnosis, treatment, and research.
Published by: Glaucoma Research Foundation, 200 Pine St, Ste 200, San Francisco, CA 94104-2712. TEL 415-986-3162, 800-826-6693, FAX 415-986-3763, info@glaucoma.org. Ed. Joy Guihama. R&P Lisa Wagreich. Circ: 33,000.

617.7 NLD ISSN 1386-0194
GLOBAL CONTACT. Text in English. 1992. 3/yr. free to qualified personnel. adv. illus. **Document type:** *Journal, Trade.* **Description:** Covers news affecting the contact lens industry worldwide, including new technologies, manufacturing, marketing and technical issues.
Formerly (until 1996): Contact (Hank) (1381-3676)
Related titles: E-mail ed.; Online - full content ed.
Indexed: RAPRA (1998).
Published by: E P S, Binnenhof 152, Etten-Leur 4871 BP, Netherlands. TEL 31-76-5036077, FAX 31-76-5036701, eps@euronet.nl. Ed., R&P, Adv. contact Wim Aalbers. B&W page XEU 2,650, color page XEU 2,900; trim 210 x 297. Circ: 2,750 (controlled).

617.7 DEU ISSN 0721-832X
CODEN: GACODL
GRAEFE'S ARCHIVE FOR CLINICAL AND EXPERIMENTAL OPHTHALMOLOGY. Text in English. 1854. m. EUR 1,131.10 domestic; EUR 1,120.70 in Germany; EUR 110 newsstand/cover foreign (effective 2002). adv. bibl, charts, illus. index, cum.index: vols.1-138. back issues avail.; reprint service avail. from ISI. *Refereed.* **Document type:** *Journal, Academic/Scholarly.* **Description:** Articles by leading ophthalmologists and vision research scientists provide rapid dissemination of clinical and clinically-related experimental information.
Formerly: Albrecht von Graefes Archiv fuer Klinische und Experimentelle Ophthalmologie (0065-6100)
Related titles: Microform ed.: (from PQC); Online - full text ed.: ISSN 1435-702X (from EBSCO Publishing, RoweCom Information Quest, Swets Blackwell, Springer LINK, Institute for Scientific Information).
Indexed: ASCA, Biol.Abstr., Chem.Abstr., Chem.Indus.Notes, Chem.Titles, Curr.Adv.Cell & Devel.Biol., Curr.Cont., Excerp.Med., INIS Atomind., Ind.Med. (1982-), Ind.Sci.Rev., Inpharma, Neurosci.Cit.Ind., Nutr.Abstr., Pharm.&Out.News, Protozool.Abstr., Reac., Rev.Appl.Entomol., Rev.Med.& Vet.Mycol., Sci.Cit.Ind.
—BLDSC (4207.850000), CASDDS, CISTI, EMDOCS, GNLM, IDS, ingenta, KNAW. **CCC.**
Published by: Springer-Verlag (Subsidiary of: BertelsmannSpringer), Tiergartenstr 17, Heidelberg 69121, Germany. TEL 49-6221-345-0, FAX 49-6221-345229, subscriptions@springer.de, http://link.springer.de/link/service/journals/00417/ index.htm, http://www.springer.de. Ed. G K Krieglstein.
Subscr. in N. America to: Springer-Verlag New York Inc., PO Box 2485, Secaucus, NJ 07096-2485. TEL 212-460-1500, FAX 212-473-6272.

617.7 GRC
GREEK ANNALS OF OPHTHALMOLOGY. Text in Greek; Summaries in English. 1964. q. USD 30. adv. bk.rev., film rev. abstr, bibl, charts, illus, stat, tr.lit. index.
Formerly: Ofthalmologika Chronika (0030-0683)
Indexed: Excerp.Med., Ophthal.Lit.
Published by: H. Leontiades Publishing Co., 32 Paraschou St, Athens, Greece. Ed. Dr. S Liaricos. Circ: 600.

HERPES; journal of the IHMF. see *MEDICAL SCIENCES—Communicable Diseases*

617.75 USA ISSN 0894-5810
RE1
HIGH PERFORMANCE OPTOMETRY. Text in English. 1987. m. (except May-June & Nov.-Dec. combined). USD 69 domestic to individuals; USD 79 in Canada & Mexico to individuals; USD 84 elsewhere to individuals; USD 79 domestic to institutions; USD 89 in Canada & Mexico to institutions; USD 94 elsewhere to institutions (effective 2000). index. **Document type:** *Newsletter.* **Description:** Summaries of medical and optometry journal articles about diagnosing and treating ocular disease and vision disorders.
Published by: Anadem Publishing, Inc., 3620 N High St, Columbus, OH 43214. TEL 614-262-2539, 800-633-0055, FAX 614-262-6630, anadem@erinet.com. Ed. Karla Gale. Pub. Will Kuhlmann. R&P Mike Cheadle.

617.7 JPN ISSN 0286-7486
HIKAKU GANKA KENKYU/ANIMAL'S EYE RESEARCH. Text in Japanese. 1982. s-a. membership.
Published by: Hikaku Ganka Gakkai/Japanese Society of Comparative Ophthalmology, Kokuritsu Yobo Eisei Kenkyujo, Tsukuba Igaku Jikken'yo Reichorui Senta, 1 Yahatadai, Tsukuba-shi, Ibaraki-ken 305-0000, Japan.

617.7 HKG ISSN 1021-8947
HONG KONG OPTICAL. Text in English. 1992. a. HKD 120 for 2 yrs. in Hong Kong; USD 36 for 2 yrs. in Asia except Japan; USD 54 for 2 yrs. elsewhere (effective 2000). adv. back issues avail. **Document type:** *Trade.* **Description:** Covers optometric instruments, glasses, lenses, spectacles, mountings and accessories.
Related titles: Online - full content ed.
Published by: Hong Kong Trade Development Council, 38th Fl Office Tower, Convention Plaza, 1 Harbour Rd, Wanchai, Hong Kong. TEL 852-2584-4333, publications@tdc.org.hk, hktdc@tdc.org.hk, http://www.tdc.org.hk/prodmag/optical/optical.htm. Ed. K S Chan. Adv. contact Wengi Yuen. color page HKD 1,300; 213 x 280. Circ: 15,000.

617.75 USA
I O A NEWS. Text in English. m. adv. **Document type:** *Newsletter, Trade.*
Former titles (until 1993): Observer; Iowa Journal of Optometry
Published by: Iowa Optometric Association, 1454 30th St Ste 204, West Des Moines, IA 50266-1312. TEL 515-222-5679, FAX 515-222-9073. Ed. Virgil Deering. Adv. contact Gary Ellis. Circ: 600.

617.7 DEU ISSN 0948-5627
CODEN: EJISE3
IMPLANT. Text in German. 1989. bi-m. back issues avail.; reprint service avail. from SWZ. **Document type:** *Academic/Scholarly.* **Description:** Provides a forum for original full papers and rapid communications dealing with all aspects of ocular implants, refractive surgery, and topics of related interest.
Formerly: European Journal of Implant and Refractive Surgery (0955-3681)
—CISTI, EMDOCS, GNLM, Infotrieve. **CCC.**
Published by: (European Society of Cataract and Refractive Surgeons (ESCRS)), Springer-Verlag (Subsidiary of: BertelsmannSpringer), Haber Str 7, Heidelberg 69126, Germany. TEL 49-30-8207-0, FAX 49-30-8214091, subscriptions@springer.de, http://www.springer.de, http://link.springer-ny.com.

617.7 IND ISSN 0301-4738
CODEN: IJOMBM
INDIAN JOURNAL OF OPHTHALMOLOGY. Text in English. 1953. 4/yr. bk.rev. illus. cum.index: vols. 1-5 (1953-58); vols. 11-15 (1963-67). *Refereed.* **Document type:** *Academic/Scholarly.*
Supersedes (in Sep. 1971): All India Ophthalmological Society. Journal (0044-7307)
Related titles: CD-ROM ed.
Indexed: Dent.Ind., Excerp.Med., ExtraMED, INIS Atomind., Ind.Med. (1971-), Rev.Med.& Vet.Mycol.
—BLDSC (4417.600000), CISTI, EMDOCS, GNLM, ingenta, KNAW.
Published by: All India Ophthalmological Society, c/o L.V. Prasad Eye Institute, L.V. Prasad Marg, Banjara Hills, Hyderabad, Andhra Pradesh 500 034, India. TEL 91-40-354-8267, 91-11-659-3188, FAX 91-40-354-8271, 91-11-685-2919, ijo@lvpeye.stph.net, http://www.aios.org. Ed. Taraprasad Das.

617 IND
INDIAN OPHTHALMOLOGY - YEAR BOOK. Text in English. a. **Document type:** *Proceedings.*
Formerly: All India Ophthalmological Society. Proceedings

M

Published by: All India Ophthalmological Society, c/o Karnal Eye Institute, Dyal Gingh College Rd., Karnal, Haryana 132 001, India. TEL 91-184-254040, FAX 91-184-255252, aios@aios.org, http://www.aios.org. Ed. Dr. J K Pasricha.

617.7 ESP
INFORMACION OPTICA. Text in Spanish. 12/yr.
Address: German Perez Carrasco, 81, Madrid 28027, Spain. TEL 1-377-46-40, FAX 1-377-42-86. Ed. Julio Rosas. Circ: 10,000.

617.7 610.73 USA ISSN 1060-135X
INSIGHT (ST. LOUIS). Text in English. 1991. q. USD 53 domestic to individuals; USD 65 foreign to individuals; USD 93 domestic to institutions; USD 105 foreign to institutions; USD 26 domestic to students; USD 38 foreign to students; USD 27 newsstand/cover domestic (effective 2001). adv. bk.rev. reprints avail. *Refereed.* **Document type:** *Journal, Academic/Scholarly.* **Description:** Provides information about current professional nursing issues, legislative concerns, administrative announcements, as well as offering a forum for commentaries and viewpoint articles.
Related titles: Online - full text ed.: (from IDEAL Online Library, RoweCom Information Quest).
Indexed: Int.Nurs.Ind.
—BLDSC (4518.174100), GNLM, Infotrieve. **CCC.**
Published by: (American Society of Ophthalmic Registered Nurses, Inc.), Mosby, Inc. (Subsidiary of: Elsevier Science), 11830 Westline Industrial Dr, St Louis, MO 63146-3318. TEL 314-872-8370, 800-325-4177, FAX 314-432-1380, http://www.mosby.com/insight, http://www.mosby.com/periodicals. Ed. Sarah C Smith. Pub. Terrie Duhadway. Adv. contact Gina Burkert TEL 314-453-4306. B&W page USD 1,355, color page USD 2,205; trim 10.88 x 8.25. Circ: 1,519.

617.7 USA
INSIGHT (WASHINGTON, 1990). Text in English. 1961. bi-m. (plus annual newsletter). free per issue. stat. back issues avail. **Document type:** *Newsletter.* **Description:** Covers latest issues in eye banking and corneal transplantation.
Formerly (until 1989): Foresight (Washington, 1961)
Published by: Eye Bank Association of America, 1001 Connecticut Ave, N W, Ste 601, Washington, DC 20036. TEL 202-775-4999, FAX 202-429-6036. Ed. Laura Harris. Circ: 5,000.

617.7 ESP ISSN 0020-3645
INSTITUTO BARRAQUER. ANALES. Text in English, French, Spanish. 1959. q. ESP 12,000 (effective 2000). adv. charts, illus. *Refereed.* **Document type:** *Academic/Scholarly.*
Indexed: Ophthal.Lit.
—CISTI, GNLM.
Published by: Instituto Barraquer, Laforja, 88, Barcelona 08006, Spain. TEL 34-93-2095311, FAX 34-93-2099977, centel01@sarenet.es, info@co-barraquer.es, http://www.co-barraques.es, http://www.co-barraquer.es. Ed. Rafael I Barraquer. R&P, Adv. contact Eva Luther. Circ: 2,000.

617.7 USA
INTERNATIONAL CONGRESS OF OPHTHALMOLOGY. ABSTRACTS. Text in English. quadrennial, latest 1998, 28th, Amsterdam. reprint service avail. from ISI. *Refereed.* **Document type:** *Proceedings.*
Supersedes (in 1994): Acta Concilium Ophthalmologicum (0065-115X)
Indexed: Curr.Cont. (coverage dropped), Excerp.Med.
Published by: International Federation of Ophthalmological Societies, Columbia Cornell Care, 900 3rd Ave, Ste 500, New York, NY 10022. Circ: 8,500 (controlled).

617.752 USA ISSN 0892-8967
RE977.C6 CODEN: ICCLEF
INTERNATIONAL CONTACT LENS CLINIC. Short title: I C L C. Text in English. 1973. bi-m. NLG 273, EUR 123.88 in Europe to individuals; JPY 17,200 in Japan to individuals; USD 139 elsewhere to individuals; NLG 536, EUR 243.23 in Europe to institutions; JPY 33,700 in Japan to institutions; USD 272 elsewhere to institutions (effective 2001). back issues avail. *Refereed.* **Document type:** *Academic/Scholarly.* **Description:** Provides the contact lens practitioner and researcher with clinical and research information relating to the contact lens field.
Related titles: Microform ed.: (from PQC); Online - full text ed.: (from ingenta, Swets Blackwell, ScienceDirect).
—BLDSC (4539.435000), CISTI, Infotrieve. **CCC.**
Published by: Elsevier Science, PO Box 945, New York, NY 10159-0945. TEL 212-989-5800, FAX 212-633-3990, usinfo-f@elsevier.com, http://www.elsevier.com/locate/iclc. Eds. Gerald E Lowther, N Rex Ghormley. **Subscr. in Australasia and the Far East to:** Elsevier Science (Singapore) Pte Ltd, No.1 Temasek Ave, 17-01 Millenia Tower, Singapore 039192, Singapore. TEL 65-434-3727, FAX 65-337-2230; **Subscr. in Japan to:** Elsevier Science Inc - Japan Regional Office, 9-15 Higashi-Azabu 1-chome, Minato-ku, Tokyo 106-0044, Japan. TEL 81-3-5561-5033; **Subscr. outside the Americas to:** Elsevier Science BV, PO Box 211, Amsterdam 1000 AE, Netherlands. TEL 31-20-485-3757.

INTERNATIONAL DIRECTORY OF OPTICAL GOODS AND INSTRUMENTS IMPORTERS. see *BUSINESS AND ECONOMICS—Trade And Industrial Directories*

796 612.84 USA ISSN 1071-4235
INTERNATIONAL JOURNAL OF SPORTS VISION. Text in English. 1993. a. USD 35 to members. **Document type:** *Academic/Scholarly.* **Description:** Founded by a group of ophthalmologists, optometrists, opticians, sports medicine professionals and sport science researchers, the Academy is dedicated to promoting and advancing research, development and education in the field of sports vision.
—BLDSC (4542.681320).
Published by: International Academy of Sports Vision, 200 S Progress Ave, Harrisburg, PA 17109.

617.7 NLD ISSN 0165-5701
RE1 CODEN: INOPDR
INTERNATIONAL OPHTHALMOLOGY. Text in English. 1978. bi-m. EUR 531, USD 532 to institutions for print or online ed.; EUR 637.20, USD 638.40 to institutions for print & online eds. combined (effective 2002). adv. bk.rev. illus. reprint service avail. from SWZ. *Refereed.* **Document type:** *Journal, Academic/Scholarly.* **Description:** Provides the clinician with articles on all the relevant subspecialties of ophthalmology, with a broad international scope. In addition to original research papers, the journal presents review articles, editorial comments, an international calendar of events and book reviews.
Related titles: Microform ed.: (from PQC); Online - full text ed.: (from EBSCO Publishing, O C L C Online Computer Library Center, Inc., RoweCom Information Quest, Swets Blackwell, Kluwer Online).
Indexed: ASCA, Biol.Abstr., Chem.Abstr., Curr.Cont. (coverage dropped), Excerp.Med., Helminthol.Abstr., INIS Atomind., Ind.Med. (1978-), Ind.Sci.Rev., Inpharma, Pharm.&Out.News, Protozool.Abstr., Reac., Sci.Cit.Ind. (coverage dropped).
—BLDSC (4544.804000), CASDDS, CISTI, GNLM, IDS, ingenta, KNAW. **CCC.**
Published by: Kluwer Academic Publishers Group (Subsidiary of: Wolters Kluwer N.V.), Spuiboulevard 50, PO Box 17, Dordrecht 3300 AA, Netherlands. TEL 31-78-639-2392, FAX 31-78-654-2254, services@wkap.nl, http://www.wkap.nl/journalhome.htm/0165-5701. Eds. A F Deutman, J J de Laey. **Subscr. in the Americas to:** Kluwer Academic - Plenum Publishers, 233 Spring St, New York, NY 10013-1578. TEL 212-620-8468, FAX 212-807-1047; **Subscr. to:** Journals Department, PO Box 322, Dordrecht 3300 AH, Netherlands. TEL 31-78-639-2392, FAX 31-78-654-6474.

617.7 USA ISSN 0020-8167
CODEN: IOPCAV
INTERNATIONAL OPHTHALMOLOGY CLINICS. Text in English. 1961. q. USD 245 domestic to individuals; USD 273 foreign to individuals; USD 302 domestic to institutions; USD 389 foreign to institutions; USD 91 newsstand/cover (effective 2002). adv. charts, illus, stat. index. back issues avail.; reprint service avail. from PQC. *Refereed.* **Document type:** *Academic/Scholarly.* **Description:** Covers a single, current topic in ophthalmology with a focus on diagnosis and therapy in each issue.
Related titles: Microform ed.: (from PQC); Online - full text ed.: USD 392.60 domestic academic site license; USD 479.60 foreign academic site license; USD 437.90 domestic corporate site license; USD 524.90 foreign corporate site license (effective 2002) (from Ovid Technologies, Inc., Institute for Scientific Information).
Indexed: ASCA, Biol.Abstr., Curr.Cont., Dent.Ind., Excerp.Med., Helminthol.Abstr., INIS Atomind., Ind.Med. (1961-), Inpharma, Protozool.Abstr., Reac., Rev.Appl.Entomol., Rev.Med.& Vet.Mycol.
—BLDSC (4544.805000), CISTI, GNLM, IDS, ingenta, KNAW.
Published by: Lippincott Williams & Wilkins (Philadelphia) (Subsidiary of: Wolters Kluwer N.V.), 530 Walnut St, Philadelphia, PA 19106-3621. TEL 215-521-8300, FAX 215-521-8902, http://www.Lww.com. Eds. Dr. Gilbert L Smolin, Mitchell H Friedlaender. Pub. Christine Rullo. R&P Margaret Becker. Adv. contact James Nagle. Circ: 1,048. **Subscr. to:** PO Box 1600, Hagerstown, MD 21740-1600. TEL 800-777-2295, FAX 301-824-7390.

617.7 GBR
INTERNATIONAL OPTICAL YEAR BOOK. Text in English. 1903. a. GBP 28. adv. bibl, stat. **Document type:** *Trade.*
Published by: Wilmington Publishing, Wilmington House, Church Rd, Dartford, Kent UA2 7EF, United Kingdom. TEL 44-1322-277788, FAX 44-1322-276476. Ed. Philip Mullins.

617.7 USA
THE INTERNET JOURNAL OF OPHTHALMOLOGY AND VISUAL SCIENCE. Text in English. s-a. free per issue. adv. bk.rev. back issues avail. *Refereed.* **Document type:** *Academic/Scholarly.* **Description:** Contains information from the field of ophthalmology. Original articles, reviews, case reports, streaming slide shows, streaming videos, letters to the editor, press releases, meeting information.
Media: Online - full content.
Published by: Internet Scientific Publications, L.L.C., 23 Rippling Creek Dr, Sugar Land, TX 77479. TEL 281-240-1533, FAX 281-240-1533, http://www.ispub.com/journals/ijovs.htm. Ed. Wayne Maoch. R&P Hope Morrow TEL 832-754-0335.

617.7 USA ISSN 0146-0404
RE1 CODEN: IOVSDA
INVESTIGATIVE OPHTHALMOLOGY & VISUAL SCIENCE (IOVS). Text in English. 1962. m. USD 215 to individuals; USD 335 foreign to individuals; USD 310 to institutions; USD 430 foreign to institutions (effective 1999). illus. index. *Refereed.* **Document type:** *Academic/Scholarly.* **Description:** Covers the progress in vision research and communication of resulting applications to clinical opthalmology. It containss original scientific articles concerning diagnosis, treatment, and management of diseases of the ocular complex. Papers presented before the Association for Research in Vision and Opthalmology are included regularly.
Formerly (until 1977): Investigative Ophthalmology (0020-9988)
Related titles: Microform ed.: (from PQC); Online - full text ed.: (from HighWire Pr., EBSCO Publishing, Institute for Scientific Information); Print ed.; ♦ Supplement: Association for Research in Vision and Ophthalmology. Spring Meeting. ISSN 0273-0189.
Indexed: ASCA, Biol.Abstr., Chem.Abstr., Curr.Adv.Biochem., Curr.Cont., Dent.Ind., Excerp.Med., Helminthol.Abstr., INIS Atomind., Ind.Med. (1977-), Ind.Sci.Rev., Inpharma, Int.Abstr.Biol.Sci., Pharm.&Out.News, Protozool.Abstr., Reac., Rev.Med.& Vet.Mycol., SSCI (coverage dropped), Sci.Cit.Ind., Small Anim.Abstr.
—BLDSC (4560.220000), CASDDS, CISTI, GNLM, IDS, ingenta, KNAW. **CCC.**
Published by: Association for Research in Vision and Ophthalmology, 9650 Rockville Pike, Bethesda, MD 20814-3928. TEL 301-571-5737, FAX 301-571-5719, fmarchbank@arvo.arvo.org., http://www.arvo.org/arvo. Ed. Dr. Gerald J Chader. Pub. Frances A Marchbank. R&P Sarah Sonner TEL 301-571-1860. Circ: 10,000.

JAHRBUCH FUER BLINDENFREUNDE. see *HANDICAPPED—Visually Impaired*

617.7 JPN ISSN 0370-5579
CODEN: RIGAA3
JAPANESE JOURNAL OF CLINICAL OPHTHALMOLOGY/ RINSHO GANKA. Text in Japanese; Summaries in English. 1946. m. JPY 36,800, USD 226.
Indexed: Biol.Abstr., Excerp.Med., INIS Atomind.
—BLDSC (4651.380000), CISTI, EMDOCS, GNLM.
Published by: Igaku-Shoin Ltd., 5-24-3 Hongo, Bunkyo-ku, Tokyo 113-0033, Japan. TEL 81-3-3817-5706. Circ: 5,000.

617.7 NLD ISSN 0021-5155 CODEN: JJOPA7
JAPANESE JOURNAL OF OPHTHALMOLOGY. Text in English. 1957. bi-m. EUR 178 in Europe to institutions surface mail; JPY 23,600 in Japan to institutions surface mail; USD 199 elsewhere to institutions surface mail; USD 265 elsewhere to institutions air mail; JPY 31,416 in Japan to institutions air mail; EUR 237 in Europe to institutions air mail; EUR 217 in Europe to individuals; JPY 28,700 in Japan to individuals; USD 196 in United States to individuals; USD 243 elsewhere to individuals; USD 79 in US & Canada to individuals (effective 2002). adv. bk.rev. charts, illus. back issues avail.; reprint service avail. from PQC. *Refereed.* **Document type:** *Academic/Scholarly.* **Description:** Carries papers on new developments in ophthalmology reported by authors of all nationalities.
Related titles: Microform ed.: (from PQC); Online - full text ed.: (from CompuServe, Inc., Data Arkiv A.B., JICST, ingenta, Swets Blackwell, ScienceDirect, Institute for Scientific Information).
Indexed: ASCA, Biol.Abstr., Chem.Abstr., Chem.Indus.Notes, Chem.Titles, Curr.Adv.Cell & Devel.Biol., Curr.Cont., Dent.Ind., Excerp.Med., INIS Atomind., Ind.Med. (1957-), Ind.Sci.Rev., Inpharma, Neurosci.Abstr. (coverage dropped), Neurosci.Cit.Ind., Pharm.&Out.News, Reac., Ref.Zh., Rev.Med.& Vet.Mycol., Sci.Cit.Ind., Trop.Dis.Bull.
—BLDSC (4656.770000), CASDDS, CISTI, GNLM, IDS, ingenta, KNAW.
Published by: (University of Tokyo/Tokyo Daigaku Soryushi Butsuri Kokusai Kenkyu Senta JPN, School of Medicine JPN), University of Tokyo, Graduate School of Science, Chirigaku Kyoshitsu, 3-1, Hongo 7-chome, Bunkyo-ku, Tokyo 113-0033, Japan. TEL 81-3-3815-5411, FAX 81-3-3817-0798, http://www.elsevier.com/locate/jjo. Eds. K Masuda, K Shimizu, Kanjiro Masuda. R&P Kanjiro Masuda. Circ: 1,000. **Dist. by:** Business Center for Academic Societies Japan, 5-16-9 Honkomagome, Bunkyo-ku, Tokyo 113-0021, Japan.

617.7 USA
JOINT COMMISSION ON ALLIED HEALTH PERSONNEL IN OPHTHALMOLOGY. PRESIDENT'S REPORT. Text in English. 1983. a. **Description:** Activities of the Commission.
Formerly: Joint Commission on Allied Health Personnel in Ophthalmology. Annual Report
Published by: Joint Commission on Allied Health Personnel in Ophthalmology, 2025 Woodlane Dr., St. Paul, MN 55125-2995. TEL 800-284-3837, FAX 612-731-0410. Ed. Beverly Hagen.

617.7 FRA ISSN 0181-5512
JOURNAL FRANCAIS D'OPHTALMOLOGIE. Text in French. 1881. 10/yr. FRF 1,600; FRF 1,950 foreign (effective 2000). adv. bk.rev. abstr, bibl, illus. index. reprint service avail. from ISI. *Refereed.* **Document type:** *Academic/Scholarly.* **Description:** Publishes original works, clinical or scientific facts, therapeutic notes, analyses of works, and reports on congresses.
Formed by the merger of (with vol.210, 1977): Annales d'Oculistique (0003-4371); Archives d'Ophtalmologie (0003-973X)
Related titles: Microform ed.: (from PQC); Online - full text ed.: (from Institute for Scientific Information, RoweCom Information Quest).
Indexed: ASCA, Biol.Abstr., Chem.Abstr., Curr.Cont., Dent.Ind., Excerp.Med., INIS Atomind., Ind.Med. (1978-), Inpharma, Int.Nurs.Ind., Neurosci.Cit.Ind., Pharm.&Out.News, Protozool.Abstr., Reac., Rev.Med.& Vet.Mycol.
—BLDSC (4986.410000), CISTI, GNLM, IDS, KNAW. **CCC.**
Published by: Masson - Periodiques, 120 bd. St. Germain, Paris 75006, France. TEL 33-1-40466200, FAX 33-1-40466201. Ed. J P Adenis. Circ: 3,000. **Subscr. to:** Societe de Periodiques Specialises, BP 22, Vineuil Cedex 41354, France. TEL 33-2-54504612, FAX 33-2-54504611.

617.7 FRA ISSN 0240-7914
JOURNAL FRANCAIS D'ORTHOPTIQUE. Text in French. 1969. a. FRF 100.
Indexed: Curr.Cont. (coverage dropped).
Published by: Association Francaise des Orthoptistes, Les Roussieres, St Andre de Corcy 01390, France. Ed. A P Ravault. Circ: 2,000.

617.7 USA ISSN 1045-8395
RE960
JOURNAL OF BEHAVIORAL OPTOMETRY. Text in English. 1990. bi-m. USD 50 (effective 1999). adv. index. back issues avail. *Refereed.* **Document type:** *Academic/Scholarly.* **Description:** Publishes original scholarly and clinical articles in the field of behavioral optometry, with news of issues, meetings and products of interest to the profession.
Indexed: Ref.Zh.
—BLDSC (4951.265000).
Published by: Optometric Extension Program, 1921 Carnegie Ave, Ste 3L, Santa Ana, CA 92705-5510. TEL 714-250-8070, FAX 714-250-8157. Ed. Dr. Irwin B Suchoff. R&P, Adv. contact Sally Corngold. Circ: 3,000.

617.7 USA ISSN 0886-3350 CODEN: JCSUEV
JOURNAL OF CATARACT AND REFRACTIVE SURGERY. Text in English. 1974. m. USD 139 in US & Canada to individuals; USD 234 elsewhere to individuals; USD 243 in US & Canada to institutions; USD 340 elsewhere to institutions (effective 2002). adv. back issues avail.; reprints avail. *Refereed.* **Document type:** *Journal, Academic/Scholarly.* **Description:** Publishes articles on all aspects of anterior segment surgery, including original research, as well as practical techniques and important case reports.
Formerly (until 1986): American Intra-Ocular Implant Society Journal
Related titles: Online - full text ed.: (from ingenta, Swets Blackwell, ScienceDirect, Institute for Scientific Information).
Indexed: ASCA, Chem.Abstr., Chem.Indus.Notes, Chem.Titles, Curr.Cont., Excerp.Med., INIS Atomind., Ind.Med. (1986-), Inpharma, Pharm.&Out.News, Reac., Sci.Cit.Ind.
—BLDSC (4954.900000), CASDDS, CISTI, EMDOCS, GNLM, IDS, ingenta, KNAW. **CCC.**
Published by: (American Society of Cataract and Refractive Surgery), Elsevier Science, Box 945, New York, NY 10159-0945. TEL 212-989-5800, FAX 212-633-3990, usinfo-f@elsevier.com, http://www.elsevier.com/locate/jcrs. Ed. Dr. Stephen A Obstbaum. Adv. contact Christine Ford. Circ: 7,000. **Subscr. to:** PO Box 2129, Marion, OH 43305-2129. **Co-sponsor:** European Society of Cataract and Refractive Surgeons.

617.7 362.41 GBR ISSN 0953-6833 CODEN: CEHEF2
JOURNAL OF COMMUNITY EYE HEALTH; an international journal to promote eye health worldwide. Text in English. 1988. q. GBP 25, USD 45; free in developing nations (effective 2002). adv. bk.rev. abstr, illus. 16 p./no. 3 cols./p. back issues avail. *Refereed.* **Document type:** *Academic/Scholarly.*
Formerly: Community Eye Health
Indexed: Rev.Appl.Entomol., Rev.Med.& Vet.Mycol., Trop.Dis.Bull.
Published by: International Centre for Eye Health, University College London, Institute Of Ophthalmology, Bath St, London EC1V 9EL, United Kingdom. TEL 44-20-7608-6923, 44-20-7608-6909, FAX 44-20-7250-3207, eyeresource@ucl.ac.uk, http://www.ucl.ac.uk/i00/ircpb. Ed. Dr. Murray McGavin. R&P, Adv. contact A Naughton TEL 44-20-7603-6910. Circ: 16,000.

617.7 USA
JOURNAL OF EYE TRAUMA. Text in English. 1996. q. USD 120 domestic to individuals; USD 135 in Canada to individuals; USD 150 elsewhere to individuals; USD 230 domestic to institutions; USD 245 in Canada to institutions; USD 260 elsewhere to institutions. *Refereed.* **Document type:** *Academic/Scholarly.*
Announced as: Journal of Ocular Trauma
Published by: (International Society of Ocular Trauma), Slack, Inc., 6900 Grove Rd, Thorofare, NJ 08086-9447. TEL 856-848-1000, 800-257-8290, FAX 856-853-5991, http://www.slackinc.com. Ed. Dr. Ferenc Kuhn. **Co-sponsors:** United States Eye Injury Registry; Helen Keller Eye Research Foundation, University of Alabama Medical Center.

617.741 USA ISSN 1057-0829 CODEN: JOGLES
JOURNAL OF GLAUCOMA. Text in English. 1992. bi-m. USD 228 domestic to individuals; USD 228 foreign to individuals; USD 350 domestic to institutions; USD 370 foreign to institutions (effective 2002); USD 56 newsstand/cover. adv. bk.rev. illus. back issues avail.; reprint service avail. from PQC. *Refereed.* **Document type:** *Academic/Scholarly.* **Description:** Publishes original articles on new approaches to diagnosis, innovations in pharmacological therapy and surgical technique, and basic science advances that affect clinical practice in the treatment of glaucomas.
Related titles: Online - full text ed.: USD 455 domestic for academic site license; USD 475 foreign for academic site license; USD 507.50 domestic for corporate site license; USD 527.50 foreign for corporate site license (effective 2002) (from Institute for Scientific Information).
Indexed: Curr.Cont., Excerp.Med. (1993-), Ind.Med. (1992-), Inpharma, Reac.
—BLDSC (4996.230000), EMDOCS, GNLM, IDS, KNAW.
Published by: Lippincott Williams & Wilkins (Philadelphia) (Subsidiary of: Wolters Kluwer N.V.), 530 Walnut St, Philadelphia, PA 19106-3621. TEL 215-521-8300, FAX 215-521-8902, http://www.lww.com. Ed. Dr. E Michael Van Buskirk. Pub. Christine Rullo. R&P Margaret Becker. Adv. contact Ray Thibodeau. B&W page USD 770, color page USD 1,755. Circ: 1,600. **Subscr. to:** PO Box 1600, Hagerstown, MD 21740-1600. TEL 800-777-2295, FAX 301-824-7390.

617.7 USA
RE91
JOURNAL OF LOW VISION AND NEURO-OPTOMETRIC REHABILITATION✱. Text in English. 1985. q. USD 95 domestic; USD 105 in Canada; USD 125 elsewhere (effective 2000); USD 25 newsstand/cover. adv. bk.rev. index. back issues avail.; reprints avail. **Document type:** *Trade.* **Description:** Provides news and developments that relate to the visually impaired in the fields of health, rehabilitation, and education. Focuses on new devices, diagnostic tests and industry trends.
Formerly: Journal of Vision Rehabilitation (1041-0384)
—BLDSC (5010.585000), ingenta.
Published by: (Neuro-Optometric Rehabilitation Association), Media Periodicals (Subsidiary of: Trozzolo Resources, Inc.), 802 Broadway St Ste 300, Kansas City, MO 64105-1528. TEL 816-842-8111, 808-243-5201, FAX 816-842-8188. Eds. Paul B Freeman, Randall T Jose. Circ: 500.

617.7 USA ISSN 1070-8022 CODEN: JNEOEK
JOURNAL OF NEURO-OPHTHALMOLOGY. Text in English. 1981. q. USD 231 domestic to individuals; USD 272 foreign to individuals; USD 370 domestic to institutions; USD 425 foreign to institutions; USD 101 newsstand/cover (effective 2002). adv. bk.rev. charts, illus, stat. index. back issues avail.; reprint service avail. from PQC. *Refereed.* **Document type:** *Academic/Scholarly.* **Description:** Reports on recent developments in diagnosing and treating ophthalmic, neurologic, endocrine, inflammatory, and neoplastic conditions affecting the motor and visual systems.
Formerly (until 1994): Journal of Clinical Neuro-Ophthalmology (0272-846X)
Related titles: Online - full text ed.: USD 481 domestic for academic site license; USD 536 foreign for academic site license; USD 536.50 domestic for corporate site license; USD 591.50 foreign for corporate site license (effective 2002) (from Institute for Scientific Information).
Indexed: ASCA, Curr.Cont., Dent.Ind., Excerp.Med., INIS Atomind., Ind.Med. (1994-), Inpharma, Jrnl.Watch Neuro., Neurosci.Cit.Ind., Reac., Rev.Med.& Vet.Mycol., e-psyche.
—BLDSC (5021.660000), CISTI, EMDOCS, GNLM, IDS, ingenta, KNAW.
Published by: (North American Neuro-Ophthalmology Society), Lippincott Williams & Wilkins (Philadelphia) (Subsidiary of: Wolters Kluwer N.V.), 530 Walnut St, Philadelphia, PA 19106-3621. TEL 215-521-8300, FAX 215-521-8902, http://www.lww.com. Ed. Jonathan d Trobe. Pub. Nancy Megley. R&P Margaret Becker. Adv. contact Ray Thibodeau. B&W page USD 835, color page USD 1,845. Circ: 1,289 (paid). **Subscr. to:** PO Box 1600, Hagerstown, MD 21740-1600. TEL 800-777-2295, FAX 301-824-7390.

617.7 USA ISSN 1080-7683
RE994 CODEN: JOPTFU
JOURNAL OF OCULAR PHARMACOLOGY AND THERAPEUTICS. Text in English. 1985. bi-m. USD 199 domestic to individuals; USD 299 foreign to individuals; USD 239 domestic to individuals print and online eds. combine; USD 339 foreign to individuals print and online eds. combined; USD 393 domestic to institutions; USD 509 foreign to institutions; USD 472 domestic to institutions print and online eds. combined; USD 588 foreign to institutions print and online eds. combined (effective 2002). adv. bk.rev. back issues avail.; reprints avail. *Refereed.* **Document type:** *Journal, Academic/Scholarly.* **Description:** Contains research on all aspects of therapeutic drug activity pertinent to preventing or controlling diseases of the eye.
Formerly (until 1995): Journal of Ocular Pharmacology (8756-3320)
Related titles: Online - full content ed.: USD 393 to institutions; USD 199 to individuals (effective 2002); Online - full text ed.: (from CatchWord Ltd., Institute for Scientific Information, RoweCom Information Quest).
Indexed: ASCA, Chem.Abstr., Chem.Indus.Notes, Chem.Titles, Curr.Cont., Derwent Biotech.Abstr., Excerp.Med., Ind.Med. (1995-), Inpharma, Int.Abstr.Biol.Sci., Nutr.Abstr., Ophthal.Lit., Pharm.&Out.News, Reac., Rev.Arom.& Med.Plants.
—BLDSC (5026.155020), CASDDS, CISTI, EMDOCS, GNLM, IDS, ingenta, KNAW. **CCC.**

M

Published by: Mary Ann Liebert, Inc. Publishers, 2 Madison Ave, Larchmont, NY 10538. TEL 914—834-3100, FAX 914-834-1388, info@liebertpub.com, http://www.liebertpub.com/jop. Ed. George C Y Chiou.

JOURNAL OF OPHTHALMIC NURSING & TECHNOLOGY. see *MEDICAL SCIENCES—Nurses And Nursing*

617.75 USA ISSN 0149-886X
JOURNAL OF OPTOMETRIC VISION DEVELOPMENT. Text in English. 1970. q. USD 65 to non-members; USD 25 to members (effective 2002). adv. bk.rev. abstr, charts, illus, bibl. index. back issues avail. *Refereed.* **Document type:** *Journal, Academic/Scholarly.*
Indexed: Child Devel.Abstr., Except.Child Educ.Abstr., PsycInfo, Psychol.Abstr. (1990-), e-psyche.
—CISTI, GNLM.
Published by: College of Optometrists in Vision Development, 243 N.Lindbergh Blvd. #310, St. Louis, MO 63141. TEL 314-991-4007. Ed. Dr. Sidney Groffman. Adv. contact Tammie Winkler TEL 314-991-4007. Circ: 1,800.

617.7 USA ISSN 0191-3913
CODEN: JPOSDR
JOURNAL OF PEDIATRIC OPHTHALMOLOGY AND STRABISMUS. Text in English. 1964. bi-m. USD 119 domestic to individuals (effective 2001); USD 135 in Canada to individuals; USD 168 elsewhere to individuals; USD 129 domestic to institutions (effective 2001); USD 150 in Canada to institutions; USD 178 elsewhere to institutions; USD 59 to students; USD 29 newsstand/cover (effective 2001). adv. bk.rev., film rev. abstr, bibl, charts, illus, stat. index. back issues avail.; reprint service avail. from PQC. *Refereed.* **Document type:** *Academic/Scholarly.* **Description:** Provides information useful to the pediatric ophthalmologist for the diagnosis, treatment, correction, and prevention of eye disorders in infants, children, and adolescents.
Formerly: Journal of Pediatric Ophthalmology (0022-345X)
Related titles: Microform ed.: (from PQC); Online - full text ed.: (from ProQuest Information & Learning, Institute for Scientific Information).
Indexed: ASCA, Biol.Abstr., Curr.Cont., Dent.Ind., Excerp.Med., INIS Atomind., Ind.Med. (1978-), Inpharma, Reac.
—BLDSC (5030.210000), GNLM, IDS, ingenta, KNAW. **CCC.**
Published by: Slack, Inc., 6900 Grove Rd, Thorofare, NJ 08086-9447. TEL 856-848-1000, 800-257-8290, FAX 856-853-5991, jpos@slackinc.com, http://www.slackinc.com. Eds. Dr. Leonard Nelson, Dr. Rudolph Wagner. Pub. Richard N Roash. adv.: B&W page USD 1,440, color page USD 1,900. Circ: 1,400 (paid).

JOURNAL OF REFRACTIVE SURGERY. see *MEDICAL SCIENCES—Surgery*

JOURNAL OF TOXICOLOGY. CUTANEOUS AND OCULAR TOXICOLOGY. see *PHARMACY AND PHARMACOLOGY*

617.7 JPN
KAIGAI GANKA BUNKEN JOHO/OPHTHALMOLOGY UPDATE. Text in Japanese. q.
Published by: Santen Seiyaku K.K./Santen Pharmaceutical Co., Ltd., 9-19 Shimo-Shinjo 3-chome, Higashiyodogawa-ku, Osaka-shi 533-0021, Japan.

617.75 USA ISSN 1063-1623
KANSAS OPTOMETRIC JOURNAL. Text in English. 1929. q. USD 15 (effective 1998). adv. bk.rev.
Published by: Kansas Optometric Association, 1266 S W Topeka Blvd, Topeka, KS 66612. Ed. Dr. David R Reynolds. Circ: 550.

617.7 GBR
KEY NOTE MARKET REPORT: OPHTHALMIC GOODS & SERVICES. Variant title: Ophthalmic Goods & Services. Text in English. irreg., latest vol.10, 1995. GBP 265 (effective 1999). **Document type:** *Trade.*
Formerly: Key Note Report: Ophthalmic Goods and Services (0268-9006)
Related titles: CD-ROM ed.; Online - full text ed.
Published by: Key Note Ltd., Field House, 72 Oldfield Rd, Hampton, Mddx TW12 2HQ, United Kingdom. TEL 44-20-8481-8750, FAX 44-20-8783-0049, http://www.keynote.co.uk.

617.75 USA ISSN 0886-7666
KEYSTONER. Text in English. 1947. q. membership. bk.rev. **Document type:** *Newsletter.* **Description:** Contains society news.
Published by: Pennsylvania Optometric Association, PO Box 3312, Harrisburg, PA 17105. TEL 717-233-6455. Ed. Deborah A Sohn. R&P Robert A Hall. Circ: 175.

617.7 POL ISSN 0023-2157
CODEN: KOAOAE
KLINIKA OCZNA. Text in Polish; Summaries in English. 1923. m. USD 176. adv. bk.rev. abstr, illus. index. **Document type:** *Academic/Scholarly.*
Indexed: Biol.Abstr., Chem.Abstr., Chem.Indus.Notes, Chem.Titles, Dent.Ind., Dok.Arbeitsmed., Excerp.Med., INIS Atomind., Ind.Med. (1923-).
—BLDSC (5099.300000), CASDDS, CISTI, GNLM, KNAW.
Published by: (Polskie Towarzystwo Okulistyczne/Polish Ophthalmological Society), Vesalius - Uniwersyteckie Wydawnictwo Medyczne, Ul Wislisko 1, Krakow 31538, Poland. TEL 48-12-213387. Ed. Maria Starzycka. **Co-sponsor:** Ministerstwo Zdrowia in Opieki Spolecznej.

617.7 DEU ISSN 0023-2165
CODEN: KMAUAI
KLINISCHE MONATSBLAETTER FUER AUGENHEILKUNDE UND AUGENARZTLICHE FORTBILDUNG. Text in German; Summaries in English, German. 1863. m. EUR 322.80 domestic to institutions; EUR 332.20 in Europe to institutions; EUR 353.40 elsewhere to institutions; EUR 34 newsstand/cover (effective 2002). adv. bk.rev. abstr, charts, illus. index. Supplement avail.; reprint service avail. from IRC. *Refereed.* **Document type:** *Journal, Academic/Scholarly.*
Related titles: Online - full text ed.: ISSN 1439-3999 (from Institute for Scientific Information); ♦ Supplement: Buecherei des Augenarztes. ISSN 0068-3361.
Indexed: ASCA, Biol.Abstr., Chem.Abstr., Curr.Cont., Dent.Ind., Excerp.Med., Helminthol.Abstr., INIS Atomind., Ind.Med. (1863-), Ind.Sci.Rev., Neurosci.Cit.Ind., Rev.Appl.Entomol., Rev.Med.& Vet.Mycol., SSCI (coverage dropped), Sci.Cit.Ind.
—BLDSC (5099.450000), CISTI, GNLM, IDS, KNAW. **CCC.**
Published by: Georg Thieme Verlag, Ruedigerstr 14, Stuttgart 70469, Germany. TEL 49-711-8931-0, FAX 49-711-8931298, klimo@thieme.de, kunden.service@thieme.de, http://www.thieme.de/klimo/index.html. Ed. G O Naumann. adv.: page DEM 2,850; trim 175 x 250. Circ: 2,600 (paid).

617.7 JPN
KOKURITSU KOBE SHIRYOKU SHOGAI SENTA JIGYO NENPO/KOBE VISUAL DISORDER CENTER. BUSINESS REPORT. Text in Japanese. a.
Published by: Koseisho, Kokuritsu Kobe Shiryoku Shogai Senta/Ministry of Health and Welfare, Kobe Visual Disorder Center, 1070 Akebono-cho, Nishi-ku, Kobe-shi, Hyogo-ken 651-2134, Japan.

617.75 DEU ISSN 0721-5096
DIE KONTAKTLINSE. Text in German. 1966. 10/yr. DEM 188 domestic; DEM 200 foreign; DEM 17.20 newsstand/cover (effective 2001). adv. bk.rev. **Document type:** *Journal, Trade.* **Description:** Publication for specialists devoted to contact lens technology featuring clinical articles, the latest in research and new products.
—GNLM.
Published by: (Vereinigung Deutscher Contactlinsen-Spezialisten e.V.), Konradin Verlag Robert Kohlhammer GmbH, Ernst Mey Str 8, Leinfelden-Echterdingen 70771, Germany. TEL 49-711-7594-249, FAX 49-711-7594-390, kl.redaktion@konradin.de, info@konradin.de, http://www.konradin.de. Eds. Hilmar Bussacker, Wolfgang Cagnolati. Adv. contact Anna Waskala. B&W page DEM 2,800; trim 190 x 270. Circ: 3,900.

617.7 NLD ISSN 0922-5307
CODEN: LLOPED
LASERS AND LIGHT IN OPHTHALMOLOGY. Text in English. ceased 2000; resumed 1986. q. USD 170 (effective 2000). illus. back issues avail. *Refereed.* **Document type:** *Journal, Academic/Scholarly.* **Description:** Forum covering uses of lasers and light in ophthalmology.
Formerly: Lasers in Ophthalmology (0920-3265)
—EMDOCS, GNLM.
Published by: Kugler Publications (Subsidiary of: S P B Academic Publishing b.v.), PO Box 97747, The Hague 2509 GC, Netherlands. TEL 31-70-330-0253, FAX 31-70-330-0254. Ed. Dr. J Marshall.

LIGHT (WHEATON). see *HANDICAPPED—Visually Impaired*

617.7 CHN ISSN 1000-0348
MEIGUO YIXUEHUI YANKE ZAZHI. Text in Chinese. q.
Published by: Beijing University of Medical Sciences, Affiliated No. 3 Hospital, Beijing 100083, China. TEL 2017691. Ed. Li Fengming. **Co-sponsor:** Zhonghua Yixuehui/Chinese Medical Association.

617.7 USA ISSN 0882-889X
RE46 CODEN: MPSODY
METABOLIC, PEDIATRIC AND SYSTEMIC OPHTHALMOLOGY; international journal of basic research and clinical applications. Text in English. 1977. 4/yr. USD 95 domestic to individuals; USD 85 in Canada to individuals; USD 105 foreign to individuals; USD 190 in US & Canada to libraries; USD 200 foreign to libraries; USD 50 domestic to students; USD 55 in Canada to students; USD 65 elsewhere to students (effective 2000). adv. bk.rev. charts, illus, stat. index. *Refereed.* **Document type:** *Academic/Scholarly.*
Former titles (until 1985): Metabolic Ophthalmology, Pediatric and Systemic (0883-9522); (until 1984): Metabolic, Pediatric, and Systemic Ophthalmology (0277-9382); (until 1982): Metabolic and Pediatric Ophthalmology (0191-2771); Metabolic Ophthalmology (0361-3674)
Related titles: Microform ed.: (from PQC).
Indexed: Biol.Abstr., Chem.Abstr., Curr.Adv.Ecol.Sci., Curr.Cont. (coverage dropped), Dent.Ind., Excerp.Med., INIS Atomind., Ind.Med. (1985-), Nutr.Abstr.
—BLDSC (5683.287000), CASDDS, CISTI, EMDOCS, GNLM, Infotrieve. **CCC.**
Published by: (International Society on Metabolic Eye Disease), Opto Education Corporation, 1125 Park Ave, New York, NY 10128. TEL 212-427-1246, FAX 212-289-8024. Ed. Dr. Heskel M Haddad. Circ: 1,000 (paid). **Co-sponsor:** International Society of Pediatric Ophthalmology.

617.75 USA ISSN 1071-1627
THE MICHIGAN OPTOMETRIST. Text in English. 1921. m. USD 15 (effective 2001). adv. bk.rev. charts, stat, illus. back issues avail. **Document type:** *Trade.* **Description:** Contains news for and about optometrists, their field, and related ones.
Published by: Michigan Optometric Association, 530 W Ionia St, Ste A, Lansing, MI 48933. FAX 517-482-1611, mioptoassn@aol.com, http://www.mioptassn.org. Ed. William D Dansby. Adv. contact Linda A Derose. page USD 299; 9 x 7. Circ: 850.

617.7 ITA ISSN 0026-4903
MINERVA OFTALMOLOGICA. Text in Italian; Summaries in English, Italian. 1958. q. USD 105 to individuals; USD 155 to institutions (effective 2000 - 2001). adv. bk.rev. bibl, charts, illus. index. **Document type:** *Academic/Scholarly.*
Related titles: Microform ed.: (from PQC).
Indexed: Excerp.Med., Ind.Med. (coverage dropped).
—CISTI, GNLM.
Published by: Edizioni Minerva Medica, Corso Bramante, 83-85, Turin, TO 10126, Italy. TEL 39-11-678282, FAX 39-11-674502. Pub. Alberto Oliaro. Adv. contact F Filippo. B&W page USD 1,200, color page USD 2,000; trim 270 x 190. Circ: 3,000 (paid).

617.7 NLD ISSN 0167-8612
CODEN: MPTHDI
MONOGRAPHS IN OPHTHALMOLOGY. Text in English. 1981. irreg., latest vol.15, 1994. price varies. *Refereed.* **Document type:** *Monographic series.*
Indexed: Biol.Abstr.
—CISTI, KNAW.
Published by: Kluwer Academic Publishers Group (Subsidiary of: Wolters Kluwer N.V.), Spuiboulevard 50, PO Box 17, Dordrecht 3300 AA, Netherlands. FAX 31-78-639-2254, services@wkap.nl, http://www.wkap.nl. **Dist. by:** Journals Department, PO Box 322, Dordrecht 3300 AH, Netherlands. FAX 31-78-654-6474.

NEURO-OPHTHALMOLOGY. see *MEDICAL SCIENCES—Psychiatry And Neurology*

617.75 USA ISSN 0028-4807
NEW ENGLAND JOURNAL OF OPTOMETRY. Text in English. 1949. m. (except Sep.-Jun.). USD 35 to non-members. adv. bk.rev. index. reprint service avail. from PQC. *Refereed.* **Document type:** *Academic/Scholarly.* **Description:** Publishes multidisciplinary articles on primary care, clinical co-management, clinical research, technical developments, case reports, community health and practice management.
Related titles: Microfilm ed.: (from PQC).
Indexed: PMR.
Published by: New England Council of Optometrists, 101 Tremont St, Boston, MA 02108. TEL 617-542-1233, FAX 617-542-4574. Ed. Dr. Roger Wilson. Adv. contact Jon C Lundell. Circ: 1,360.

M

NEW LITERATURE ON VISUAL IMPAIRMENT. see *HANDICAPPED—Abstracting, Bibliographies, Statistics*

617.7 USA ISSN 0077-8605
CODEN: TNOOA6
NEW ORLEANS ACADEMY OF OPHTHALMOLOGY. TRANSACTIONS. Variant title: Symposia. Text in English. a. price varies. back issues avail. **Document type:** *Academic/Scholarly.*
Indexed: Dent.Ind., Ind.Med. (coverage dropped).
Published by: (New Orleans Academy of Ophthalmology), Kugler Publications (Subsidiary of: S P B Academic Publishing b.v.), 2509 GC, P O Box 97747, The Hague, Netherlands. TEL 31-70-330-0253, FAX 31-70-330-0254, kugler.spb@wxs.nl, http://kugler.publication.com.

617.7 JPN ISSN 0374-9851
CODEN: NSIZBD
NIHON CONTACT LENS GAKKAISHI. Key Title: Nihon Kontakuto Renzu Gakkai Kaishi. Text in Japanese; Summaries in English. 1959. q. JPY 8,000 domestic; JPY 9,000 foreign (effective 2001). bk.rev. *Refereed.* **Document type:** *Proceedings, Academic/Scholarly.*
Related titles: Microform ed.; ♦ Supplement to: Nihon Ganka Kiyo. ISSN 0015-5667.
—BLDSC (4804.740000), CASDDS, GNLM.
Published by: Nihon Ganka Kiyokai, 302 Yamamoto Bldg, 3-6 Mihogaoka, Ibaraki 5670047, Japan. TEL 81-726-23-7878, FAX 81-726-23-6060, jjcls@osk.3web.ne.jp. Ed. Yuichi Ohashi. Pub., R&P, Adv. contact Keiko Miyake. Circ: 2,250.

617.7 JPN ISSN 0015-5667
CODEN: NGKYA3
NIHON GANKA KIYO/FOLIA OPHTHALMOLOGICA JAPONICA. Key Title: Nippon Ganka Kiyo. Text in Japanese; Summaries in English. 1950. m. JPY 20,000 domestic; JPY 25,000 foreign (effective 2001). adv. bk.rev. *Refereed.* **Document type:** *Proceedings, Academic/Scholarly.*
Related titles: Microform ed.; ♦ Supplement: Nihon Contact Lens Gakkaishi. ISSN 0374-9851.
Indexed: Excerp.Med., INIS Atomind., Ind.Med. (coverage dropped).
—BLDSC (3971.824000), CASDDS, CISTI, GNLM, KNAW.
Published by: Nihon Ganka Kiyokai, 302 Yamamoto Bldg, 3-6 Mihogaoka, Ibaraki 5670047, Japan. TEL 81-726-23-7878, FAX 81-726-23-6060, jjcls@osk.3web.ne.jp. Ed. Yasuo Tano. Pub., Adv. contact Keiko Miyake. Circ: 2,700 (paid).

617.7 JPN
NIHON GANKOGAKU GAKKAI YOKOSHU/ OPHTHALMOLOGICAL OPTICS SOCIETY OF JAPAN. PRELIMINARY PROGRAM. Text in Japanese. 1964. a. JPY 500.
Published by: Nihon Gankogaku Gakkai, Nikon 2-3 Marunochi 3-chome, Chiyoda-ku, Tokyo 100-0005, Japan.

617.3 JPN ISSN 0915-4302
NIHON HAKUNAISHO GAKKAISHI/JAPANESE SOCIETY FOR CATARACT RESEARCH. JOURNAL. Text in Japanese; Summaries in English, Japanese. 1989. a.
Published by: Nihon Hakunaisho Gakkai, Fujita Gakuen Hoken Eisei Daigaku Gankagaku Kyoshitsu, 1-98, Dengakugakubo, kutsukakecho, Tokoake-shi, Aichi-ken 470-11, Japan.

617.3 JPN ISSN 0289-3843
NIHON JAKUSHI SHASHI GAKKAI ZASSHI/JAPANESE ASSOCIATION OF STRABISMUS AND AMBLYOPIA. JOURNAL. Text in Japanese; Summaries in English, Japanese. 1973. a.
Published by: Nihon Jakushi Shashi Gakkai, c/o Teikyo Daigaku Igakubu Ganka Kyoshitsu, 11-1 Kaga 2-chome, Itabashi-ku, Tokyo 173-0003, Japan. **Co-sponsor:** Ganka Rinsho Ihokai - Japanese Society of Clinical Ophthalmology.

617.3 JPN ISSN 0386-4200
NIHON JAKUSHI SHASHI GAKKAIHO/JAPANESE ASSOCIATION OF STRABISMUS AND AMBLYOPIA. BULLETIN. Text in Japanese. 1964. irreg. JPY 350 per issue.
Published by: Nihon Jakushi Shashi Gakkai, c/o Teikyo Daigaku Igakubu Ganka Kyoshitsu, 11-1 Kaga 2-chome, Itabashi-ku, Tokyo 173-0003, Japan.

617.3 JPN ISSN 0285-1326
NIHON NO GANKA/JAPAN OPHTHALMOLOGISTS ASSOCIATION. JOURNAL. Text in Japanese. 1967. m. JPY 1,500 per issue.
Published by: Nihon Ganka Ikai, 4-11 Sarugaku-cho 2-chome, Chiyoda-ku, Tokyo 101-0064, Japan.

617.7 JPN ISSN 0387-5172
NIHON SHINO KUNRENSHI KYOKAISHI/JAPANESE ORTHOPTIC JOURNAL. Text in Japanese; Summaries in English, Japanese. 1972. a.
—CCC.
Published by: Nihon Shino Kenrenshi Kyokai/Japanese Association of Certified Orthoptists, 39-11 Narita-Higashi 5-chome, Suginami-ku, Tokyo 166-0015, Japan.

617.7 JPN ISSN 0029-0203
CODEN: NGZAA6
NIPPON GANKA GAKKAI ZASSHI/JAPANESE OPHTHALMOLOGICAL SOCIETY. JOURNAL. Text in Japanese; Abstracts in English, Japanese. 1897. m. JPY 15,000 domestic; JPY 20,000 foreign (effective 2000). adv. *Refereed.* **Document type:** *Academic/Scholarly.*
Indexed: Biol.Abstr., Chem.Abstr., Chem.Indus.Notes, Chem.Titles, Dent.Ind., Excerp.Med., INIS Atomind., Ind.Med. (1897-).
—BLDSC (4809.365000), CASDDS, CISTI, GNLM, KNAW.
Published by: Nippon Ganka Gakkai/Japanese Ophthalmological Society, 2-4-11-402 Sarugaku-cho, Chiyoda-ku, Tokyo 101-0064, Japan. TEL 81-3-3295-2360, FAX 81-3-3293-9384, ytano@ophthal.med.osaka-u.ac.jp. Ed., R&P Yasuo Tano. Circ: 12,000.

617.7 USA
NORTH CENTRAL OPTOMETRIC VIEWPOINT. Text in English. 1991. q. USD 50. adv. **Document type:** *Trade.* **Description:** Offers clinical articles, practice management and industry trends.
Published by: (North Central State Optometric Council), R.C. Publications, Inc. (Brookfield), PO Box 218, Cottage Grove, MN 55016-0218. TEL 651-769-0905, FAX 651-769-0907. Ed. R A Koetting. Adv. contact R W Perleberg. B&W page USD 1,200, color page USD 1,745; trim 11 x 8.5. Circ: 26,200 (controlled).

617.7 RUS
NOVOE V OFTAL'MOLOGII. Text in Russian. q. USD 89.95 in United States.
Indexed: Ref.Zh.
Published by: Reklamno-Izdatel'skii Tsentr Fedorov, Beskudnikovskii bulv 59-a, Moscow 127486, Russian Federation. TEL 7-095-4888925, FAX 7-095-4885954. **US dist. addr.:** East View Publications, 3020 Harbor Ln N, Minneapolis, MN 55447. TEL 612-550-0961.

617.7 GBR
O T; optometry today/optics today. Variant title: Optics Today. Text in English. 1961. fortn. adv. bk.rev. 60 p./no. 3 cols./p. back issues avail. *Refereed.* **Document type:** *Journal, Trade.* **Description:** Provides all optometrists, dispensing opticians, key personnel in the industry, political bodies, students in the UK and practitioners overseas with all the latest news and information in the market place. Continuing professional developments series, clinical and practice management features, conference reports, industry news, new products and opto political information.
Former titles: Optometry Today (0268-5485); Ophthalmic Optician (0030-3739); Which was formed by the union of: Association of Optometrists News; And: Dioptric News
Indexed: C.I.S. Abstr., High.Educ.Curr.Aware.Bull.
—BLDSC (6276.480000), GNLM.
Published by: Association of Optometrists, Victoria House, 178-180 Fleet Rd, Fleet, Hants GU13 8DA, United Kingdom. TEL 44-1252-816266, FAX 44-1252-816176, info@optometry.co.uk, http://www.optometry.co.uk. Ed. Maureen A Hunter. R&P Maureen Hunter TEL 44-1252-816266. Adv. contact Sarah Bradley TEL 44-1252-815350. B&W page GBP 810, color page GBP 1,950; trim 210 x 297. Circ: 14,181.

617.7 NLD ISSN 0927-3948
CODEN: OIINEN
OCULAR IMMUNOLOGY AND INFLAMMATION. Text in English. 1993. q. NLG 227 to individuals (effective 2000); USD 126 to individuals; NLG 569, USD 300 to institutions. adv. back issues avail.; reprint service avail. from PQC,SWZ. *Refereed.* **Document type:** *Academic/Scholarly.* **Description:** Publishes original research papers, reviews and short communications on all aspects of basic and clinical research pertaining to the ocular inflammatory response and its control by the immune system.
Related titles: Microform ed.: (from PQC); Online - full text ed.: (from EBSCO Publishing, O C L C Online Computer Library Center, Inc., RoweCom Information Quest, Swets Blackwell, Institute for Scientific Information).
Indexed: Curr.Cont., Excerp.Med. (1994-), Ind.Med. (1993-), Inpharma, Pharm.&Out.News, Protozool.Abstr., Reac., Sci.Cit.Ind., Trop.Dis.Bull.
—BLDSC (6235.154200), ADONIS, CASDDS, EMDOCS, GNLM, IDS, Infotrieve. **CCC.**
Published by: (International Ocular Inflammation Society), Aeolus Press (Subsidiary of: Swets & Zeitlinger BV), PO Box 825, Lisse 2160 SZ, Netherlands. FAX 31-344-572562, orders@swets.nl, http://www.swets.nl/sps/AEolus/oii1.html. Ed. A Kijlstra. Pub. J K W van Leeuwen. R&P C E van Leeuwen-Meyren. Adv. contact Patrick Kleian. B&W page NLG 600, B&W page USD 345; 175 x 240. Circ: 400. **Subscr. to:** Swets & Zeitlinger BV, PO Box 825, Lisse 2160 SZ, Netherlands. TEL 31-252-435111, FAX 31-252-415888, orders@swets.nl. **Dist. in N. America by:** Swets & Zeitlinger, PO Box 582, Downingtown, PA 19335-998. TEL 800-447-9387.

617.7 USA ISSN 1063-5114
OCULAR INFECTIOUS DISEASES. Text in English. 1995. 3/yr. USD 125 to individuals; USD 185 to institutions. *Refereed.* **Document type:** *Academic/Scholarly.*
—KNAW.
Published by: Field & Wood, Medical Periodicals, Inc., PO Box 975, Blue Bell, PA 19422. TEL 610-828-4010, FAX 215-482-0226. Eds. Dr. David M Meisler, Dr. Jeffery B Robin.

OCULAR SURGERY NEWS. see *MEDICAL SCIENCES—Surgery*

OCULAR SURGERY NEWS INTELLIGENCE REPORT. see *MEDICAL SCIENCES—Surgery*

OCULAR SURGERY NEWS INTERNATIONAL EDITION. see *MEDICAL SCIENCES—Surgery*

617.75 NLD ISSN 0029-8328
OCULUS. Text in Dutch. 1938. m. (10/yr.). NLG 125 domestic; NLG 170 foreign (effective 2000). adv. bk.rev. illus. **Document type:** *Trade.*
Published by: (Nederlandse Unie van Optiekbedrijven (NUVO)), Stichting P R & Publiciteit Optiekbranche, Postbus 677, Haarlem 2003 RR, Netherlands. TEL 31-23-531-2519, FAX 31-23-532-0192. Ed. Mariska Blokdijk. Adv. contact Erwin Cops. B&W page NLG 1,258, color page NLG 2,485; trim 297 x 210. Circ: 2,100.

617.7 FRA
CODEN: BSOFAK
OEIL ET LUMIERE. Text in French. 1949. a. USD 200. adv. bk.rev. **Document type:** *Bulletin.*
Published by: (Societes d'Ophtalmologie de France), Lamy S.A. (Marseille), 150 rue Paradis, Marseille 13006, France. Ed. Dr. Korobelnik. Circ: 2,200 (paid). **Subscr. to:** Diffusion Litteraire et Scientifique, 11 rue Moliere, Marseille 13001, France. TEL 91-33-57-91.

617.7 RUS ISSN 0235-4160
OFTAL'MOKHIRURGIYA. Text in English, Russian. 1989. q. RUR 312 domestic; USD 60 foreign (effective 2000). adv. bk.rev. abstr, bibl, charts, illus, pat, stat. *Refereed.* **Description:** Includes articles on corneal surgery, refractive surgery, surgical and laser management of glaucoma, cataract surgery and vitreoretinal surgery.
Indexed: Ref.Zh.
—BLDSC (0128.632000), East View, GNLM.
Published by: M H T K Mikrokhirurgiya Glaza/I R T C Eye Microsurgery, Beskudnikovskii bulv 59-a, Moscow 127486, Russian Federation. TEL 7-095-4888427, FAX 7-095-4888409, pcf@aha.ru. Ed. S N Fyodorov. Adv. contact L S Tumar. B&W page USD 600, color page USD 800; trim 297 x 210. Circ: 1,000 (paid and controlled). **US dist. addr.:** East View Publications, 3020 Harbor Ln N, Minneapolis, MN 55447. TEL 612-550-0961.

617.7 DNK ISSN 0108-5344
OFTALMOLOG. Text in Danish, English, Norwegian, Swedish. 1981. q. DKK 195. back issues avail. **Document type:** *Bulletin.*
Published by: (Nordiske Oftalmologiske Foreninger), Scriptor Publisher ApS, Soevangsvej 1-5, Hvidovre 2650, Denmark. TEL 45-36-77-41-13, FAX 45-36-77-41-15. Ed., R&P Hans Alroe Joergensen. **Co-sponsor:** Acta Ophthalmologica.

617.7 ROM ISSN 1220-0875
OFTALMOLOGIA. Text in Romanian; Summaries in English, French, German, Russian. 1956. q. USD 20. adv. bk.rev. bibl. charts. index. **Document type:** *Academic/Scholarly.*

M

Formerly (until 1989): Revista de Chirurgie, Oncologie, Radiologie, O.R.L., Oftalmologie, Stomatologie, Oftalmologie (1220-0859); Which superseded in part (in 1974): Oto-Rino-Laringologie si Oftalmologie (0303-5123); Which was formed by the merger of (1965-1974): Oto-Rino-Laringologie (0030-6649); (1956-1974): Oftalmologia (0030-0667)
Indexed: Chem.Abstr., Dent.Ind., Excerp.Med. (until 1992), Ind.Med. (coverage dropped).
—BLDSC (6244.700000), CISTI, GNLM.
Published by: Asociatia Medicala Romana, Societatea de Oftalmologie, Str. Progresului 8, Bucharest 70754, Romania. **Subscr. to:** ILEXIM, Str. 13 Decembrie 3, PO Box 136-137, Bucharest 70116, Romania.

617.7 UKR ISSN 0030-0675 CODEN: OFZHAV
OFTAL'MOLOGICHESKII ZHURNAL. Text in Russian; Summaries in English. 1946. 6/yr. USD 10 in Ukraine; USD 10 in Russian Federation; USD 135 elsewhere. bk.rev. bibl. index. **Description:** Publishes major clinical and laboratory reseach work from Russia, Ukraine, and other Eastern European countries related to clinical opthalmology and scientific opthalmology.
Indexed: Biol.Abstr., Chem.Abstr., Excerp.Med., INIS Atomind., Ind.Med. (coverage dropped), Int.Aerosp.Abstr., Rev.Med.& Vet.Mycol.
—CASDDS, CISTI, East View, GNLM, KNAW. **CCC.**
Published by: Naukove Tovarystvo Oftal'mologiv Ukrainy, Frantsuzskii bul 49-51, Odessa, Ukraine. TEL 380-482-603713. Ed. Ivan Logay. Pub. Valery Ponomarchuk. Adv. contact Svetlana Slobodyanik. Circ: 1,500. **US dist. addr.:** East View Publications, 3020 Harbor Ln N, Minneapolis, MN 55447. TEL 612-550-0961.

362.1 617.7 NLD ISSN 1384-0339
OP OOGHOOGTE. Text in Dutch. 1985. s-a. free per issue. illus. 6 p./no. 2 cols./p. back issues avail. **Document type:** *Newsletter.* **Description:** Reports on the foundation's activities to prevent and cure blindness in the Himalayan Central Asian region.
Published by: Stichting Oogzorg Himalaya/Foundation Eyecare Himalaya, Postbus 174, Aerdenhout 2110 AD, Netherlands. TEL 31-23-529-0073, FAX 31-23-547-1793, foundationeyecare@worldonline.nl, http://www.oogzorghimalaya.nl. Ed. Leen Parlevliet. Circ: 20,000 (controlled).

OPERATIVE TECHNIQUES IN CATARACT AND REFRACTIVE SURGERY. see *MEDICAL SCIENCES—Surgery*

617.7 FRA ISSN 0989-3105
OPHTALMOLOGIE. Text in French. 1883. bi-m. FRF 500; FRF 730 foreign (effective 1997). adv. bk.rev. illus. index. **Document type:** *Academic/Scholarly.* **Description:** Includes case reports, original articles and reviews.
Formerly (until 1987): Societe Francaise d'Ophtalmologie. Bulletins et Memoires (0081-1092)
Related titles: Online - full text ed.: (from RoweCom Information Quest).
—CISTI, EMDOCS, GNLM, Infotrieve. **CCC.**
Published by: (Societe Francaise d'Ophtalmologie), Masson - Periodiques, 120 bd. St. Germain, Paris 75006, France. TEL 33-1-40466200, FAX 33-1-40466201, http://www.sfo.asso.fr. Ed. H Offret. Circ: 8,200. **Subscr. to:** Societe de Periodiques Specialises, BP 22, Vineuil Cedex 41354, France. TEL 33-2-54504612, FAX 33-2-54504611.

617.7 FRA ISSN 0767-8959
OPHTALMOLOGISTE PRATICIEN. Text in French. 1972. 5/yr. FRF 15. adv. bk.rev.
Published by: Societe Francaise d'Ophtalmologie, 17 Villa d"Alesia, Paris 75014, France. http://www.sfo.asso.fr. Circ: 4,200.

617.75 RE939.2 GBR ISSN 0275-5408 CODEN: OPOPD5
OPHTHALMIC AND PHYSIOLOGICAL OPTICS. Text in English. 1980. 6/yr., latest vol.22, 2002. GBP 74 in Europe to individuals; USD 117 in North America to individuals; GBP 81 elsewhere to individuals; GBP 423 in Europe to institutions; USD 672 in North America to institutions; GBP 466 elsewhere to institutions (effective 2002). adv. bk.rev. charts, illus. index. *Refereed.* **Document type:** *Academic/Scholarly.* **Description:** Publishes international and interdisciplinary original research in aspects of pure and applied vision science.
Supersedes: British Journal of Physiological Optics (0007-1218)
Related titles: Microform ed.: (from PQC); Online - full text ed.: GBP 67 in Europe to individuals; USD 106 in North America to individuals; GBP 67 elsewhere to individuals; GBP 381 in Europe to institutions; USD 605 in North America to institutions; GBP 381 elsewhere to institutions (effective 2002) (from ingenta, ScienceDirect, Swets Blackwell, Institute for Scientific Information).
Indexed: ASCA, Biol.Abstr., Curr.Adv.Ecol.Sci., Curr.Cont., Dent.Ind., Ergon.Abstr., Excerp.Med., INSPEC (1983-), Ind.Med. (1981-), Inpharma, PsycInfo, Psychol.Abstr. (1981-), Reac., Sci.Cit.Ind., e-psyche.
—BLDSC (6270.870000), AskIEEE, CISTI, EMDOCS, GNLM, IDS, Infotrieve, KNAW. **CCC.**
Published by: (British College of Optometrists), Blackwell Science Ltd., PO Box 88, Oxford OX2 0NE, United Kingdom. TEL 44-1865-206180, 44-1865-206002, FAX 44-1865-206219, jnl.orders@blacksci.co.uk, http://www.elsevier.com/locate/ophopt, http://www.blackwellpublishing.com. R&P Sophie Savage. Adv. contact Jenny Applin. **Subscr. in Australasia and the Far East to:** Elsevier Science (Singapore) Pte Ltd, No.1 Temasek Ave, 17-01 Millenia Tower, Singapore 039192, Singapore**; Subscr. in the Americas to:** Elsevier Science, PO Box 945, New York, NY 10159-0945**; Subscr. to:** Elsevier Science BV, PO Box 211, Amsterdam 1000 AE, Netherlands.

617.7 615 USA ISSN 1043-1780
OPHTHALMIC DRUG FACTS. Text in English. 1990. a. USD 50; USD 57.50 foreign (effective 1999). **Description:** Provides data on ophthalmic drugs, grouped by therapeutic categories.
Published by: Facts and Comparisons, 111 W. Port Plaza, Ste. 300, St. Louis, MO 63146-3098. TEL 314-878-2515, FAX 314-878-5563. Ed. Bernie R Olin.

617.7 NLD ISSN 0928-6586 CODEN: OPEPFP
OPHTHALMIC EPIDEMIOLOGY. Text in Dutch. 1994. q. NLG 239, USD 126 to individuals; NLG 540, USD 284 to institutions (effective 2000). adv. back issues avail.; reprint service avail. from SWZ. *Refereed.* **Document type:** *Academic/Scholarly.* **Description:** Publishes research papers in ophthalmic research in the fields of epidemiology, public health, and the prevention of blindness.
Related titles: Online - full text ed.: (from EBSCO Publishing, O C L C Online Computer Library Center, Inc., RoweCom Information Quest, Swets Blackwell).
Indexed: Ind.Med. (1994-).
—BLDSC (6270.880000), ADONIS, CISTI, EMDOCS, GNLM, Infotrieve. **CCC.**
Published by: (International Society of Geographic and Epidemiological Ophthalmology (ISGEO)), Aeolus Press (Subsidiary of: Swets & Zeitlinger BV), PO Box 825, Lisse 2160 SZ, Netherlands. FAX 31-344-572562, orders@swets.nl, http://www.swets.nl/sps/AEolus/opep1.html. Ed. J P Ganley. Pub. J K W van Leeuwen. R&P C E van Leeuwen-Meyren. Adv. contact Patrick Kleian. **Subscr. to:** Swets & Zeitlinger BV, PO Box 825, Lisse 2160 SZ, Netherlands. TEL 31-252-435111, FAX 31-252-415888, orders@swets.nl. **Dist. in N. America by:** Swets & Zeitlinger, PO Box 582, Downingtown, PA 19335-998. TEL 800-447-9387.

617.7 618.92 NLD ISSN 1381-6810
OPHTHALMIC GENETICS. Text in English. 1981. q. NLG 233, USD 130 to individuals; NLG 517, USD 272 to institutions (effective 2000). adv. bk.rev. back issues avail.; reprint service avail. from SWZ. *Refereed.* **Document type:** *Academic/Scholarly.* **Description:** Contains review articles, research papers, and short communications on genetic ophthalmological problems of the newborn and of children, as well as adults.
Formerly (until 1994): Ophthalmic Paediatrics and Genetics (0167-6784)
Related titles: Microform ed.; Online - full text ed.: (from EBSCO Publishing, O C L C Online Computer Library Center, Inc., RoweCom Information Quest, Swets Blackwell).
Indexed: ASCA, Curr.Cont. (coverage dropped), Excerp.Med., Ind.Med. (1994-), Inpharma, Reac.
—BLDSC (6270.893000), ADONIS, CISTI, GNLM, IDS, ingenta, KNAW. **CCC.**
Published by: (International Society for Genetic Eye Disease USA), Aeolus Press (Subsidiary of: Swets & Zeitlinger BV), PO Box 825, Lisse 2160 SZ, Netherlands. FAX 31-344-572562, orders@swets.nl, http://www.swets.nl/sps/AEolus/og1.html. Ed. E Traboulsi. Pub. J K W van Leeuwen. R&P C E van Leeuwen-Meyren. Adv. contact Patrick Kleian. B&W page NLG 600, B&W page USD 345; 175 x 240. Circ: 500. **Subscr. to:** Swets & Zeitlinger BV, PO Box 825, Lisse 2160 SZ, Netherlands. TEL 31-252-435111, FAX 31-252-415888, orders@swets.nl. **Dist. in N. America by:** Swets & Zeitlinger, PO Box 582, Downingtown, PA 19335-998. TEL 800-447-9387. **Co-sponsor:** Ophthalmic Genetics Study Club, International Society of Paediatric Ophthalmology.

OPHTHALMIC LITERATURE. see *MEDICAL SCIENCES—Abstracting, Bibliographies, Statistics*

OPHTHALMIC NURSING; international journal of ophthalmic nursing. see *MEDICAL SCIENCES—Nurses And Nursing*

617.7 617 USA ISSN 0740-9303 CODEN: OPRSE
OPHTHALMIC PLASTIC AND RECONSTRUCTIVE SURGERY. Text in English. 1985. bi-m., latest vol.17. USD 259 domestic to individuals; USD 329 foreign to individuals; USD 398 domestic to institutions; USD 468 foreign to institutions; USD 90 newsstand/cover (effective 2002). adv. bk.rev. illus. index. back issues avail. *Refereed.* **Document type:** *Journal, Academic/Scholarly.* **Description:** Presents original articles and reviews on diagnostic techniques, surgical instruments and procedures, medical therapies, research findings, and clinical applications.
Related titles: Online - full text ed.: USD 517.40 domestic academic site license; USD 587.40 foreign academic site license; USD 577.10 domestic corporate site license; USD 647.10 foreign corporate site license (effective 2002) (from Ovid Technologies, Inc., Institute for Scientific Information).
Indexed: ASCA, Curr.Cont., Excerp.Med., INIS Atomind., Ind.Med. (1985-), Inpharma, Med.& Surg.Dermat., Reac., Sugar Ind.Abstr.
—BLDSC (6271.430000), CISTI, EMDOCS, GNLM, IDS, ingenta, KNAW.
Published by: (American Society of Ophthalmic Plastic and Reconstructive Surgery), Lippincott Williams & Wilkins (Philadelphia) (Subsidiary of: Wolters Kluwer N.V.), 530 Walnut St, Philadelphia, PA 19106-3621. TEL 215-521-8300, FAX 215-521-8902, http://www.lww.com. Eds. Dr George B Bartley, Dr Richard K Dortzbzch. Pub. Christine Rullo. R&P Margaret Becker. Adv. contact Ray Thibodeau. B&W page USD 820, color page USD 1,910. Circ: 1,230. **Subscr. to:** PO Box 1600, Hagerstown, MD 21740-1600. TEL 800-777-2295, FAX 301-824-7390.

617.7 CAN ISSN 0832-9869 CODEN: OPPRFI
OPHTHALMIC PRACTICE. Text in English. 1983. bi-m. CND 60 domestic; USD 72 in Canada; USD 94 elsewhere (effective 1999). adv. bk.rev. index. *Refereed.* **Document type:** *Trade.* **Description:** Studies ophthalmic surgery, ocular infection, intra-ocular lens implants, pediatric problems, technological advances.
Formerly: Current Canadian Ophthalmic Practice (0823-4744)
—BLDSC (6271.435000), GNLM.
Published by: Medicopea International Inc., 3333 Cote Vertu Blvd, Ste 300, St Laurent, PQ H4R 2N1, Canada. TEL 514-331-4561, FAX 514-336-1129. Ed. Leon Solomon. Pub. Laurence Goldstein. R&P Linda Armitage. Adv. contact Helen Kaplin. Circ: 1,200.

617.7 RE58 CHE ISSN 0030-3747 CODEN: OPRSAQ
OPHTHALMIC RESEARCH; journal for research in experimental and clinical ophthalmology. Text in English. 1970. bi-m. CHF 914 in Europe to institutions; CHF 931.40 elsewhere to institutions; EUR 652.80 in Europe to institutions; USD 711 elsewhere to institutions (effective 2002). adv. charts, illus, stat. index. back issues avail. *Refereed.* **Document type:** *Journal, Academic/Scholarly.* **Description:** Features original papers, reviews and short communications reporting basic and clinical experimental studies on ophthalmology.
Related titles: Microform ed.; Online - full text ed.: ISSN 1423-0259. 199?. CHF 58, EUR 42, USD 45 to institutions with print edition (effective 2001) (from EBSCO Publishing, O C L C Online Computer Library Center, Inc., RoweCom Information Quest, Swets Blackwell, Institute for Scientific Information).

M

Indexed: ASCA, Aqua.Sci.& Fish.Abstr., Biol.Abstr., Chem.Abstr., Chem.Titles, Curr.Adv.Ecol.Sci., Curr.Cont., Dent.Ind., Environ.Sci.Poll.Mgmt., Excerp.Med., Ind.Med. (1970-), Inpharma, Neurosci.Cit.Ind., Pharm.&Out.News, Pollut.Abstr., Reac., Risk Abstr., Saf.Sci.Abstr., Sci.Cit.Ind.
—BLDSC (6271.450000), CASDDS, CISTI, EMDOCS, GNLM, IDS, ingenta, KNAW. **CCC.**
Published by: S. Karger AG, Allschwilerstr 10, PO Box, Basel 4009, Switzerland. TEL 41-61-306-1111, FAX 41-61-306-1234, karger@karger.ch, http://www.online.karger.com/journals/ore, http://www.karger.com. Ed. G F Vrenseon. adv.: page USD 1,185. Circ: 850.

OPHTHALMIC SURGERY AND LASERS. see *MEDICAL SCIENCES—Surgery*

617.7 DEU ISSN 0936-2517
OPHTHALMO CHIRURGIE. Text in German. 1989. 6/yr. DEM 156 (effective 2000). adv. bk.rev. back issues avail. **Document type:** *Academic/Scholarly.*
—GNLM.
Published by: Dr. R. Kaden Verlag, Poststr 24-26, Heidelberg 69115, Germany. TEL 49-6221-600313, FAX 49-6221-29910, marketing@kaden-verlag.de. Adv. contact A Siegmann. B&W page DEM 2,575; trim 178 x 230. Circ: 1,200.

617.7 DEU ISSN 0941-293X
RE1 CODEN: OHTHEJ
DER OPHTHALMOLOGE. Text in German. 1982. m. EUR 333.92 domestic; EUR 303.72 in Germany; EUR 29 newsstand/cover foreign (effective 2002). back issues avail.; reprint service avail. from ISI. *Refereed.* **Document type:** *Journal, Academic/Scholarly.* **Description:** Covers all fields of research, science, and practice in medical conditions and treatments of the eyes.
Formerly: Fortschritte der Ophthalmologie (0723-8045)
Related titles: Microform ed.: (from PQC); Online - full text ed.: ISSN 1433-0423 (from EBSCO Publishing, RoweCom Information Quest, Swets Blackwell, Springer LINK, Institute for Scientific Information).
Indexed: Chem.Abstr., Chem.Indus.Notes, Chem.Titles, Curr.Cont., Dent.Ind., Dok.Arbeitsmed., Excerp.Med., Ind.Med. (1992-), Inpharma, Pharm.&Out.News, Reac., Rev.Med.& Vet.Mycol., Sci.Cit.Ind.
—BLDSC (6271.585000), CASDDS, CISTI, EMDOCS, GNLM, IDS, Infotrieve, KNAW. **CCC.**
Published by: Springer-Verlag (Subsidiary of: BertelsmannSpringer), Tiergartenstr 17, Heidelberg 69121, Germany. TEL 49-6221-345-0, FAX 49-6221-345229, subscriptions@springer.de, http://link.springer.de/link/service/journals/00347/index.htm, http://www.springer.de. Ed. H E Voelcker. **Subscr. in N. America to:** Springer-Verlag New York Inc., PO Box 2485, Secaucus, NJ 07096-2485. TEL 212-460-1500, FAX 212-473-6272.

617.7 CHE ISSN 0030-3755
RE1 CODEN: OPHTAD
OPHTHALMOLOGICA; international journal of ophthalmology. Text in English. 1899. bi-m. CHF 1,089 in Europe to institutions; CHF 1,106.40 elsewhere to institutions; EUR 777.80 in Europe to institutions; USD 846 elsewhere to institutions (effective 2002). adv. bk.rev. bibl, illus. index, cum.index vols.96-138. back issues avail. *Refereed.* **Document type:** *Journal, Academic/Scholarly.* **Description:** Contains a selection of patient-oriented reports covering the etiology of eye diseases, diagnostic techniques, and advances in medical and surgical treatment.
Related titles: Microform ed.; Online - full text ed.: ISSN 1423-0267. 199?. CHF 58, EUR 42, DEM 45 to institutions with print edition (effective 2002) (from EBSCO Publishing, O C L C Online Computer Library Center, Inc., RoweCom Information Quest, Swets Blackwell, Institute for Scientific Information); ♦ Supplement: Developments in Ophthalmology. ISSN 0250-3751.
Indexed: ASCA, Biol.Abstr., Chem.Abstr., Chem.Titles, Curr.Cont., Environ.Sci.Poll.Mgmt., Excerp.Med., Helminthol.Abstr., INIS Atomind., Ind.Med. (1938-), Inpharma, Neurosci.Cit.Ind., Nutr.Abstr., Pharm.&Out.News, Pollut.Abstr., Protozool.Abstr., Psychol.Abstr., Reac., Rev.Med.& Vet.Mycol., Rev.Plant Path., Risk Abstr., SSCI (coverage dropped), Saf.Sci.Abstr., Sci.Cit.Ind.
—BLDSC (6271.600000), CASDDS, CISTI, GNLM, IDS, ingenta, KNAW. **CCC.**
Published by: (Netherlands Ophthalmological Society NLD), S. Karger AG, Allschwilerstr 10, PO Box, Basel 4009, Switzerland. TEL 41-61-306-1111, FAX 41-61-306-1234, karger@karger.ch, http://www.online.karger.com/journals/oph, http://www.karger.com. Ed. C Ohrloff. adv.: page USD 1,185. Circ: 1,250.

617.7 EGY ISSN 0078-5342
OPHTHALMOLOGICAL SOCIETY OF EGYPT. BULLETIN. Text in Arabic, English, French. 1902. a. USD 10.
Indexed: Excerp.Med., Ind.Med. (coverage dropped), Ophthal.Lit.
—GNLM.
Published by: Ophthalmological Society of Egypt, Dar el Hekma, 42 Kasr el-Aini St., Cairo, Egypt.

617.7 JPN ISSN 0016-4488
OPHTHALMOLOGY/GANKA. Text in Japanese. 1959. m. JPY 2,000 per issue. bk.rev. cum.index.
Indexed: INIS Atomind., Ind.Sci.Rev., Jap.Per.Ind., Protozool.Abstr., Trop.Dis.Bull.
—CISTI, GNLM.
Published by: Kanehara Shuppan Ltd., 2-31-14 Yushima, Bunkyo-ku, Tokyo 113-0034, Japan. Circ: 5,100.

617.7 USA ISSN 0161-6420
OPHTHALMOLOGY. Text in English. 1907. m. USD 225, USD 301 elsewhere to individuals; USD 365 in US & Canada to institutions; USD 465 elsewhere to institutions (effective 2002). adv. illus. index. back issues avail. *Refereed.* **Document type:** *Academic/Scholarly.* **Description:** Publishes original articles that pertain to clinical and basic reserch in all areas of ophthalmology.
Formerly (until vol.85, 1978): American Academy of Ophthalmology. Transactions - Ophthalmology; Which superseded in part (in 1975): American Academy of Ophthalmology. Transactions (0002-7154)
Related titles: CD-ROM ed.; Microform ed.: (from PQC); Online - full text ed.: (from EBSCO Publishing, ingenta, ScienceDirect, Institute for Scientific Information).
Indexed: AIDS Abstr., ASCA, Abstr.Hyg., Aqua.Sci.& Fish.Abstr., Biol.Abstr., C.I.S. Abstr., Chem.Abstr., Curr.Adv.Cancer Res., Curr.Adv.Ecol.Sci., Curr.Cont., Dent.Ind., Dok.Arbeitsmed., Environ.Sci.Poll.Mgmt., Excerp.Med., Helminthol.Abstr., Hosp.Lit.Ind., INIS Atomind., Ind.Med. (1978-), Inpharma, Int.Nurs.Ind., Med.& Surg.Dermat., Neurosci.Cit.Ind., Pharm.&Out.News, Pollut.Abstr., Protozool.Abstr., Reac., Rev.Med.& Vet.Mycol., Risk Abstr., SSCI (coverage dropped), Saf.Sci.Abstr., Sci.Cit.Ind.
—BLDSC (6271.805000), CISTI, EMDOCS, GNLM, IDS, ingenta, KNAW.
Published by: (American Academy of Ophthalmology), Elsevier Science, PO Box 945, New York, NY 10159-0945. TEL 212-989-5800, FAX 212-633-3990, http://www.elsevier.com. Ed. Dr. Donald S Minckler. Pub. Christine Rullo. R&P Margaret Becker. Adv. contact Ray Thibodeau. B&W page USD 1,650, color page USD 3,465; trim 10.88 x 8.13. Circ: 25,498. **Subscr. outside the Americas to:** Elsevier Science BV, PO Box 211, Amsterdam 1000 AE, Netherlands. TEL 31-20-485-3757, FAX 31-20-485-3432.

617.7 USA ISSN 0896-1549
RE1 CODEN: OCNAF2
OPHTHALMOLOGY CLINICS OF NORTH AMERICA. Text in English. 1988. q. USD 159 domestic to individuals; USD 204 in Canada to individuals; USD 221 elsewhere to individuals; USD 239 domestic to institutions; USD 289 foreign to institutions; USD 73 per issue foreign (effective 2001). index. back issues avail. **Document type:** *Academic/Scholarly.* **Description:** Discusses the treatment of eye diseases and conditions.
Related titles: Microform ed.: (from PQC).
Indexed: CINAHL, Excerp.Med. (1995-).
—BLDSC (6271.816000), GNLM, Infotrieve, ingenta, KNAW. **CCC.**
Published by: W.B. Saunders Co. (Subsidiary of: Harcourt Publishers Ltd.), 11830 Westline Industrial Dr, St Louis, MO 63146. TEL 800-325-4177, http://www.wbsaunders.com. Ed. Dr. Robert L Stamper. **Subscr. to:** Periodicals Fulfillment, W B Saunders Co, 6277 Sea Harbor Dr, 4th Fl, Orlando, FL 32891-4800.

617.7 USA ISSN 1078-6392
OPHTHALMOLOGY ON C D. Text in English. 1995. a. **Document type:** *Academic/Scholarly.*
Media: CD-ROM.
Published by: (American Academy of Ophthalmology), Lippincott - Raven Publishers (Subsidiary of: Wolters Kluwer N.V.), 530 Walnut St, Philadelphia, PA 19106. TEL 215-521-8300, FAX 215-521-8902, http:/www.lrpub.com. **Subscr. to:** Box 1600, Hagerstown, MD 21741-1600. TEL 800-777-2295, FAX 301-824-7390.

OPHTHALMOLOGY PRACTICE ADVISOR. see *HEALTH FACILITIES AND ADMINISTRATION*

617.7 USA ISSN 0193-032X
OPHTHALMOLOGY TIMES; all the clinical news in sight. Text in English. 1976. 24/yr., latest vol.26. USD 190 in North America; USD 250 elsewhere; USD 10 newsstand/cover in North America (effective 2001). adv. *Refereed.* **Document type:** *Newspaper, Trade.* **Description:** Reports current clinical and non-clinical news of interest to ophthalmologists in patient care practice in the United States. Features meeting announcements and new products.
Related titles: Microform ed.: (from PQC); Online - full text ed.: (from Northern Light Technology, Inc., ProQuest Information & Learning, Gale Group, Factiva).
Indexed: Biol.Dig.
—BLDSC (6271.833000), GNLM. **CCC.**
Published by: Advanstar Communications Inc., One Park Ave 2nd Fl, New York, NY 10016. TEL 440-243-8102, ot@en.com, http://www.advanstar.com. Pub., R&P, Adv. contact Basil Scaperdas. Circ: 15,847; 18,000 (controlled).

617.7 USA
OPHTHALMOLOGY TIMES LATIN AMERICA. Abbreviated title: O T L A. Text in Portuguese, English. 1997. bi-m. USD 48 in North America; USD 90 elsewhere; USD 10 in North America; USD 19 elsewhere (effective 2001). adv. 44 p./no. 3 cols./p. back issues avail. *Refereed.* **Description:** Covers clinical news about ophthalmology in the United States and Latin America.
Published by: Advanstar Communications Inc., 201 E Sandpointe Ave Ste 600, Santa Ana, CA 92707. TEL 440-891-3103, FAX 440-891-2735, bscaperdas@advanstar.com, http://www.ophthalmologytimesamericalatina.com/. Pub. Basil Scaperdas. R&P Barbara Pritchard TEL 212-951-6600. Adv. contact Tom Pace. B&W page USD 1,300, color page USD 2,220; trim 8 x 10.75. Circ: 15,249 (controlled).

617.7 GBR ISSN 0969-0018
OPTICAL PRACTITIONER; the business magazine for optical management. Text in English. 1992. bi-m. GBP 40 domestic; GBP 45 in Europe; USD 90 in United States; GBP 50 elsewhere (effective 2000). adv. bk.rev. **Document type:** *Trade.* **Description:** Geared to the development of the optical practice as an effectively managed and successful business.
Published by: Optical World Ltd., 200 London Rd, Southend-on-Sea, Essex SS1 1PJ, United Kingdom. TEL 44-1702-345443, FAX 44-1702-431806. Ed., R&P Gerald Ward. Adv. contact Russell Ward. B&W page USD 1,100; trim 11 x 8.25. Circ: 5,000.

617.7 CAN ISSN 0824-3441
OPTICAL PRISM; Canada's optical business magazine. Text in English. 1983. 10/yr. free in Canada; free foreign (effective 1999). adv. bk.rev. back issues avail. **Document type:** *Trade.* **Description:** Provides information on practice management as well as coverage of Canada's optical industry to Canadian optometrists, opticians, ophthalmologists, suppliers and their sales personnel.
Related titles: Online - full text ed.
Published by: Nusand Publishing Inc., 250 The East Mall Ste 1113, Toronto, ON M9B 6L3, Canada. TEL 416-233-2487, FAX 416-233-1746, nusand@idirect.com, http://www.opticalprism.com. Ed., R&P Robert May. Adv. contact Monika Raepple. B&W page USD 1,353, color page USD 2,050; trim 10.88 x 8.13. Circ: 11,500 (controlled).

617.7 GBR ISSN 0969-1952
OPTICAL WORLD. Text in English. 1972. 10/yr. GBP 65 domestic; GBP 75 in Europe; GBP 95 elsewhere; GBP 150 in United States (effective 2000). adv. bk.rev. charts, illus. **Document type:** *Trade.* **Description:** International publication of interest to manufacturers, distributors and users of optical machinery and equipment.
Published by: Optical World Ltd., 200 London Rd, Southend-on-Sea, Essex SS1 1PJ, United Kingdom. TEL 44-1702-345443, FAX 44-1702-431806, TELEX 995701-9-INTCOM-G. Ed., R&P Gerald Ward. Adv. contact Russell Ward. Circ: 4,000.

617.7 GBR ISSN 0030-3968
OPTICIAN; the weekly journal for optometrists and dispensing opticians. Text in English. 1891. w. GBP 108 domestic; GBP 134, USD 201 elsewhere (effective 2000). adv. bk.rev. back issues avail.; reprints avail. **Document type:** *Trade.* **Description:** Contains exclusive news reports, clinical and technical features, practice management, new products, frames, and continuing education and training projects.
Indexed: High.Educ.Curr.Aware.Bull., INSPEC (Nov.1971-Mar.1974, dropped).
—BLDSC (6273.400000).

Published by: Reed Business Information (Subsidiary of: Reed Elsevier plc), Quadrant House, The Quadrant, Brighton Rd, Sutton, Surrey SM2 5AS, United Kingdom. TEL 44-208-652-3500, FAX 44-208-652-8977, rbp.subscriptions@rbi.co.uk, http://www.reedbusiness.com. Ed. Alison Ewbank. Pub. Trevor Parker. Adv. contact Jeff Wood. Circ: 6,717. **Subscr. to:** Quadrant Subscription Services, PO Box 302, Haywards Heath, W Sussex RH16 3YY, United Kingdom. TEL 44-1444-445566, FAX 44-1444-445447.

617.75 DNK ISSN 0900-2944
OPTIKEREN. Text in Danish. 1977. a. DKK 244, USD 35. adv. bk.rev.
Published by: Danmarks Optikerforening, Kongevejs Centret 2, Horsholm 2970, Denmark. Ed. Lis Birch. Circ: 800.

617.75 FRA ISSN 0988-3525
OPTO. Text in French. 1954. 11/yr. FRF 591. adv. bk.rev. charts, illus. **Document type:** *Newspaper.*
Formerly: Optometrie (0030-4115)
Published by: Mediacom Vision, 134 rte. de Chartres, Bures Sur Yvette 91440, France. FAX 69-28-78-06. Ed. Gerard Larnac. Pub. Jean Paul Roosen. Adv. contact Guy Moulinier. Circ: 3,650.

617.75 535 BEL
OPTOMAGAZINE. Text in French. 1970. 6/yr. BEF 2,245. adv. Supplement avail. **Document type:** *Newsletter.* **Description:** Covers optometry, contact lenses and business related matters.
Formerly: Association Professionnelle des Opticiens de Belgique. Bulletin d'Information Mensuel
Related titles: Dutch ed.
Published by: Algemene Professionele Opticiens en Optometristenbond van Belgie/Association Professionnelle des Opticiens et Optometristes de Belgique, Rue Capitaine Crespel 26, Brussels 1050, Belgium. TEL 32-2-5125526, FAX 32-2-5023402, http://www.apob.be. Ed. Ph Carlier. R&P B. Denis. Adv. contact B Denis. Circ: 2,500.

617.7 FIN ISSN 1456-7407
OPTOMETRIA. Text in Finnish. 1958. 5/yr. FIM 250 in Scandinavia; FIM 350 elsewhere (effective 2000). adv. bk.rev. **Document type:** *Trade.*
Former titles: Uusi Optikko (1455-1586); Optikko (0048-2021)
Published by: Optiikka Media Oy, Mannerheimintie 76 A, Helsinki 00250, Finland. TEL 358-09-492134, FAX 358-09-492147. Ed., R&P Ilkka Liukkonen. Adv. contact Tarja Paussoi. B&W page FIM 6,300, color page FIM 9,250; trim 260 x 188. Circ: 2,200.

617.7 USA
RE956
OPTOMETRIC EDUCATION. Text in English. 1975. q. USD 20 domestic; USD 30 foreign (effective 2001). adv. bk.rev. index. back issues avail. *Refereed.* **Document type:** *Academic/Scholarly.*
Formerly (until Fall 1991): Journal of Optometric Education (0098-6917)
Indexed: C.I.J.E.
Published by: Association of Schools and Colleges of Optometry, 6110 Executive Blvd, Ste 510, Rockville, MD 20852. TEL 301-231-5944, FAX 301-770-1828, http://www.opted.org. Ed., Adv. contact Patricia C O'Rourke. Circ: 3,000.

617.75 USA ISSN 0030-4085
OPTOMETRIC MANAGEMENT; the business and marketing magazine for optometry. Text in English. 1964. m. USD 37; USD 48 in Canada; USD 85 elsewhere (effective 2001). adv. charts, illus, tr.lit. index. reprint service avail. from PQC. **Document type:** *Trade.* **Description:** Publishes articles on practice management, financial investment and social and political problems affecting the profession of optometry.
Related titles: Microform ed.: (from PQC); Online - full text ed.: (from Northern Light Technology, Inc., ProQuest Information & Learning).
Indexed: Account.Ind. (1987-).
Published by: Cardina Business Media, Inc., 1300 Virginia Dr, Ste 400, Ft, Washington, PA 19034-3221. TEL 215-643-8138, FAX 215-643-3902. Ed., R&P Sean McKinney. Pub., Adv. contact Doug Parry. Circ: 35,000 (paid). **Subscr. to:** Optometric Management, PO Box 3055, Northbrook, IL 60065-3055. TEL 800-306-6332, FAX 847-564-9002.

617.7 CAN ISSN 0708-3173
L'OPTOMETRISTE. Text in English. 1978. 6/yr. free per issue to qualified personnel. adv. **Document type:** *Trade.* **Description:** News for French speaking optometrists in Quebec.
Published by: Association des Optometristes du Quebec, 1265 Berri St, local 740, Montreal, PQ H2L 4X4, Canada. TEL 514-288-6272, FAX 514-288-7071, aoq@login.net, http://www.login.net/assocopto/index. Ed. Dr. Jean Pierre Lagace. R&P, Adv. contact Lucie English. B&W page CND 975, color page CND 1,125; trim 10.88 x 8.13. Circ: 3,400.

617.75 USA
OPTOMETRIST'S PATIENT NEWSLETTER. Text in English. 1988. q. USD 645 per quarter for 1000 copies (effective 2001). index. **Document type:** *Newsletter, Consumer.* **Description:** Offers relationship marketing through newsletters.
Published by: Newsletters Ink, PO Box 2019, Lancaster, PA 17608-2019. TEL 717-393-1000, 800-379-5585, FAX 717-393-4702, http://www.newslettersink.com. Ed. Ann Mead Ash. Pub. Gregory A Gilson.

617.75 USA ISSN 1040-5488
RE1 CODEN: OVSCET
OPTOMETRY AND VISION SCIENCE. Text in English. 1924. m., latest vol.78. USD 201 domestic to individuals; USD 249 foreign to individuals; USD 263 domestic to institutions; USD 310 foreign to institutions; USD 27 newsstand/cover (effective 2002). adv. bk.rev. abstr, bibl, charts, illus, stat. index. *Refereed.* **Document type:** *Academic/Scholarly.* **Description:** Presents research and clinical findings in optometry, as well as case reports and instrument and technique reviews.
Former titles: American Journal of Optometry and Physiological Optics (0093-7002); (until 1974): American Journal of Optometry and Archives of American Academy of Optometry
Related titles: Microfilm ed.: (from WWS); Online - full text ed.: (from Ovid Technologies, Inc., Institute for Scientific Information).
Indexed: ASCA, Bioeng.Abstr., Biol.Abstr., Biotech.& Bioeng.Abstr., C.I.S. Abstr., Curr.Adv.Ecol.Sci., Curr.Cont., Eng.Ind., Excerp.Med., Helminthol.Abstr., INIS Atomind., INSPEC (Oct.1970-), Ind.Med. (1989-), Inpharma, Pharm.&Out.News, Protozool.Abstr., Psychol.Abstr., Reac., Ref.Zh., SSCI (coverage dropped), So.Pac.Per.Ind.
—BLDSC (6276.450000), AskIEEE, CISTI, Ei, EMDOCS, GNLM, IDS, ingenta.
Published by: (American Academy of Optometry), Williams & Wilkins (Subsidiary of: Waverly International), 351 W Camden St, Baltimore, MD 21201-2436. TEL 410-528-4068, 800-222-3790, FAX 410-528-4452, cvalton@wwilkins.com, http://www.wwilkins.com, http://www.acmq.org. Ed. Mark Bullimore. Adv. contact Christophe Valton. Circ: 3,782.

617.75 USA
RE1 CODEN: JAOPBD
OPTOMETRY: JOURNAL OF THE AMERICAN OPTOMETRIC ASSOCIATION. Text in English. 1928. m. USD 95 domestic to non-members; USD 130 in Canada to non-members; USD 145 elsewhere to non-members; free to members (effective 2001). adv. bk.rev. abstr, charts, illus, stat, tr.lit. index. back issues avail. *Refereed.* **Document type:** *Academic/Scholarly.* **Description:** Contains technical articles in the field of vision that are contributed by recognized men and women in related fields.
Formerly: American Optometric Association. Journal (0003-0244)
Indexed: AgeLine, Biol.Abstr., Curr.Cont. (coverage dropped), Dok.Arbeitsmed., Environ.Sci.Poll.Mgmt., Excerp.Med., INIS Atomind., Ind.Med. (1992-, dropped), Int.Nurs.Ind., Pollut.Abstr., PsycInfo, Psychol.Abstr. (1967-), e-psyche.
—BLDSC (6276.440000), CISTI, GNLM, KNAW. **CCC.**
Published by: American Optometric Association, 243 N Lindbergh Blvd, St. Louis, MO 63141. TEL 314-991-4100, FAX 314-991-4101, almiller@theaoa.org, http://www.aoanet.org, http://www.aoanet.org/. Ed. Paul Freeman. Pub., Adv. contact Andrew L Miller. R&P J David Kopp TEL 314-991-4100 ext 228. B&W page USD 3,920, color page USD 5,600; trim 10.88 x 8. Circ: 30,000 (paid and controlled).

617.7 IND ISSN 0048-203X
OPTOMETRY TODAY. Text in English. 1970. q. INR 400, USD 200 (effective 2002). adv. bk.rev. abstr, bibl, tr.lit. reprint service avail. from PQC. **Document type:** *Academic/Scholarly.* **Description:** Ophthalmic medicine quarterly journal.
Incorporating: Indian Optometric Association. Journal
Related titles: Microform ed.: (from PQC).
—CISTI.
Published by: Dr. Narendra Kumar Ed. & Pub., C4F/216, Janakpuri, New Delhi 110 058, India. TEL 91-11-5599839, FAX 91-11-5593216. Pub., R&P Narendra Kumar. Circ: 2,000.

617.7 616.21 NLD ISSN 0167-6830
ORBIT; the international journal on orbital disorders, oculoplastic and lacrimal surgery. Text in English. 1981. q. NLG 248, USD 135 to individuals; NLG 565, USD 297 to institutions (effective 2000). adv. bk.rev. index, cum.index. back issues avail.; reprint service avail. from SWZ. *Refereed.* **Document type:** *Academic/Scholarly.* **Description:** Contains review articles, research papers, and short communications on orbital disorders, ophthalmology, otolaryngology, reconstructive and maxillofacial surgery, endocrinology, radiology, radiotherapy, oncology, neurology, neuro-ophthalmology, neurosurgery, pathology, immunology, and hematology.
Related titles: Microform ed.; Online - full text ed.: (from EBSCO Publishing, O C L C Online Computer Library Center, Inc., RoweCom Information Quest, Swets Blackwell).
Indexed: Curr.Cont. (coverage dropped), Excerp.Med.
—BLDSC (6277.869600), ADONIS, CISTI, GNLM, Infotrieve, ingenta, KNAW. **CCC.**
Published by: (International Society on Orbital Disorders), Aeolus Press (Subsidiary of: Swets & Zeitlinger BV), PO Box 825, Lisse 2160 SZ, Netherlands. FAX 31-344-572562, orders@swets.nl, http://www.swets.nl/sps/AEolus/orbit1.html. Ed. Maarten P Mourits. Pub. J K W van Leeuwen. R&P C E van Leeuwen-Meyren. Adv. contact Patrick Kleian. B&W page NLG 600, B&W page USD 345; 175 x 240. Circ: 700. **Subscr. to:** Swets & Zeitlinger BV, PO Box 825, Lisse 2160 SZ, Netherlands. TEL 31-252-435111, FAX 31-252-415888, orders@swets.nl. **Dist. in N. America by:** Swets & Zeitlinger, PO Box 582, Downingtown, PA 19335-998. TEL 800-447-9387. **Co-sponsor:** European Society for Orbital Plastic and Reconstructive Surgery.

617.7 535 ITA ISSN 0394-0314
L'OROPTERO; rivista di scienze della visione. Text in Italian; Abstracts in English. 1986. q. ITL 50,000 domestic; ITL 60,000 foreign. bk.rev. 52 p./no. Supplement avail. *Refereed.* **Document type:** *Academic/Scholarly.*
Supersedes (after vol.2, 1983): Visione
Published by: (Istituto Regionale Studi Ottici e Optometrici), In-tersezioni, Piazza della Liberta, 17, Vinci, FI 50059, Italy. TEL 39-571-567923, FAX 39-571-56520, irsoo@leonet.it, http://www.mega.it/irsoo/. Ed. Cesare Berni. R&P Roberto Brindelli. Circ: 8,000.

617.75 ITA
OTTICA ITALIANA. Text in Italian. 12/yr.
Published by: National Federation of Opticians, Via Cenisio, 32, Milan, MI 20154, Italy. TEL 2-349-1708, FAX 2-34-91-374. Ed. Giuseppe Ricco. Circ: 9,000.

617.7 ITA
OTTICO. Text in Italian. 1975 (no.114). bi-m. ITL 3,000. adv. bk.rev. charts, illus.
Published by: Associazione Italiana Ottici, Via Giusti, 2, Sesto Fiorentino, FI 50019, Italy. TEL 55-442-090. Ed. Giuseppe Ricco. Circ: 4,000.

PERCEPTION. see *PSYCHOLOGY*

617.7 PHL ISSN 0031-7659
PHILIPPINE JOURNAL OF OPHTHALMOLOGY. Text in English. 1969. q. PHP 500, USD 20. adv. bk.rev. abstr. index. reprint service avail. from PQC. **Document type:** *Academic/Scholarly.*
Related titles: CD-ROM ed.; Microform ed.: (from PQC).
Indexed: Biol.Abstr., Chem.Abstr., Excerp.Med. (until 19??), ExtraMED, Ophthal.Lit.
—GNLM.
Published by: Philippine Academy of Ophthalmology, Philippine General Hospital, Taft Ave, Manila CPO, Manila 1000, Philippines. TEL 632-523-0421, FAX 632-523-0421. Ed. Dr. Romeo V Fajardo. Circ: 1,000.

617.7 USA ISSN 0091-6803
RE994
PHYSICIANS' DESK REFERENCE FOR OPHTHALMOLOGY. Text in English. irreg., latest vol.18, 1990. USD 39.95; USD 47.95 foreign. **Description:** Contains product information relating to optometry and ophthalmology.
Related titles: Online - full text ed.
—Infotrieve. **CCC.**
Published by: Medical Economics Co., Inc., 5 Paragon Dr, Montvale, NJ 07645-1742. TEL 201-358-7246.

617.75 CAN ISSN 1181-6058
CODEN: PROPFW
PRACTICAL OPTOMETRY. Text in English. 1990. bi-m. CND 60 domestic; USD 72 in United States; USD 94 elsewhere. adv. bk.rev. illus. index. back issues avail. *Refereed.* **Document type:** *Trade.* **Description:** Discusses diagnostic technologies, marketing techniques, co-management strategies, product news.

M

—BLDSC (6595.240000).
Published by: Medicopea International Inc., 3333 Cote Vertu Blvd, Ste 300, St Laurent, PQ H4R 2N1, Canada. TEL 514-333-4561, FAX 514-336-1129, Medicopea@netaxis.qc.ca. Ed. John Jantzi. Pub. Lawrence Goldstein. R&P Linda Armitage. Adv. contact Helen Kaplin. Circ: 2,300 (controlled).

PREVENT BLINDNESS NEWS. see *PUBLIC HEALTH AND SAFETY*

617.75 USA ISSN 1081-6437
PRIMARY CARE OPTOMETRY NEWS. Text in English. m. USD 109; USD 29 newsstand/cover (effective 2001). 44 p./no. **Document type:** *Newspaper, Academic/Scholarly.* **Description:** Provides information related to clinical and socioeconomic developments in the field of optometry.
Related titles: Online - full content ed.
Published by: Slack, Inc., 6900 Grove Rd, Thorofare, NJ 08086-9447. TEL 856-848-1000, 800-257-8290, FAX 856-853-5991, http://primarycareoptometry.com, http://www.slackinc.com. Ed. Dr. Michael Depaolis. Circ: 35,000 (paid and controlled).

617.7 GBR ISSN 1350-9462
QP479 CODEN: PRTRES
PROGRESS IN RETINAL AND EYE RESEARCH. Text in English. 1982. bi-m. EUR 694 in Europe to institutions; JPY 92,200 in Japan to institutions; USD 777 elsewhere to institutions (effective 2002). back issues avail. *Refereed.* **Document type:** *Monographic series, Academic/Scholarly.* **Description:** Reviews relevant developments and current advances in retinal science for clinicians and scientists.
Formerly (until 1994): Progress in Retinal Research (0278-4327)
Related titles: Microfilm ed.: (from PQC); Online - full text ed.: (from ingenta, Swets Blackwell, Institute for Scientific Information, ScienceDirect).
Indexed: ASCA, Chem.Abstr., Chem.Titles, Curr.Adv.Ecol.Sci., Curr.Cont., Ind.Med. (1994-), Inpharma, Int.Abstr.Biol.Sci., Neurosci.Cit.Ind., Reac., SSCI (coverage dropped), Sci.Cit.Ind.
—BLDSC (6924.525590), ADONIS, CASDDS, CISTI, EMDOCS, GNLM, IDS, KNAW. **CCC.**
Published by: Pergamon (Subsidiary of: Elsevier Science), The Boulevard, Langford Ln, East Park, Kidlington, Oxford OXB 1GB, United Kingdom. FAX 44-1865-843010, http://www.elsevier.com/locate/preteyeres. Eds. G J Chader, Neville Osborne. **Subscr. in Australasia and the Far East to:** Elsevier Science (Singapore) Pte Ltd, No.1 Temasek Ave, 17-01 Millenia Tower, Singapore 039192, Singapore. TEL 65-434-3727, FAX 65-337-2230; **Subscr. in the Americas to:** Elsevier Science, PO Box 945, New York, NY 10159-0945. TEL 212-633-3730, usinfo-f@elsevier.com; **Subscr. to:** Elsevier Science BV, PO Box 211, Amsterdam 1000 AE, Netherlands. TEL 31-20-485-3757.

617.7 CHN ISSN 1003-5141
RECENT ADVANCES IN OPHTHALMOLOGY/YANKE XIN JINZHAN. Text in Chinese; Abstracts and contents page in English. 1980. bi-m. CNY 48 domestic; USD 30 foreign (effective 2000 & 2001). adv. back issues avail. **Document type:** *Academic/Scholarly.* **Description:** Covers recent advances in Opthalmology, basic and clinical research of with columns of original articles, clinical reports, short reports, case reports and review.
Related titles: E-mail ed.; Online - full content ed.
Published by: Xinxiang Medical College/Xinxiang Yixueyuan, Xinyan Rd, Xinxiang, Henan Province 453003, China. TEL 86-373-3029404, 86-373-3029050, FAX 86-373-3027981, 86-373-3041119, ykxjza@publicz.zz.ha.cn. Ed. Rong Yu. R&P, Adv. contact Xue-Li Liu. B&W page USD 1,000, color page USD 2,000; trim 284 x 207. Circ: 4,500. **Dist. by:** China International Book Trading Corp, 35, Chegongzhuang Xilu, Haidian District, Beijing 100044, China. TEL 86-1-68413849, FAX 86-1-68412048, cibtc@mail.cibtc.com.cn, http://www.cibtc.com.cn.

617.7 GBR ISSN 0309-2437
RECENT ADVANCES IN OPHTHALMOLOGY. Text in English. 1975. irreg., latest vol.8. **Document type:** *Monographic series, Academic/Scholarly.*
—GNLM, KNAW.
Published by: Churchill Livingstone (Subsidiary of: Harcourt Publishers Ltd.), Robert Stevenson House, 1-3 Baxter's Pl, Leith Walk, Edinburgh, Midlothian EH1 3AF, United Kingdom. TEL 44-131-556-2424, FAX 44-131-459-1177, http://www.churchillmed.com. **US subscr. to:** Churchill Livingstone, 650 Ave of the Americas, New York, NY 10011. TEL 212-206-5000.

617.7 USA ISSN 0146-4582
RE22
RED BOOK OF OPHTHALMOLOGY. Text in English. biennial. USD 125. adv. **Document type:** *Directory.*
Formerly: Red Book of Eye, Ear, Nose and Throat Specialists
Published by: Jobson Publishing L.L.C. (Woodstock), 5 Central St, Woodstock, VT 05091. TEL 800-238-8764, FAX 802-457-2489, http://www.jobson.com.

REFERATOVY VYBER Z OFTALMOLOGIE/ABSTRACTS OF OPHTHALMOLOGY. see *MEDICAL SCIENCES—Abstracting, Bibliographies, Statistics*

617.7 USA ISSN 0275-004X
RE501 CODEN: RETIDX
RETINA; the journal of retinal and vitreous diseases. Text in English. 1981. bi-m., latest vol.21. USD 181 domestic to individuals; USD 260 foreign to individuals; USD 368 domestic to institutions; USD 424 foreign to institutions; USD 67 newsstand/cover (effective 2002). adv. illus. index. *Refereed.* **Document type:** *Academic/Scholarly.* **Description:** Clinically oriented to assist general ophthalmologists and vitreoretinal specialists. Features articles on surgical and other techniques for vitreoretinal disorders.
Related titles: Microform ed.: (from PQC); Online - full text ed.: (from Institute for Scientific Information).
Indexed: ASCA, Curr.Adv.Ecol.Sci., Curr.Cont., Dent.Ind., Excerp.Med. (1993-), INIS Atomind., Ind.Med. (1981-), Inpharma, Neurosci.Cit.Ind., Pharm.&Out.News, Reac., Sci.Cit.Ind.
—BLDSC (7785.510300), CISTI, EMDOCS, GNLM, IDS, ingenta, KNAW.
Published by: Lippincott Williams & Wilkins (Philadelphia) (Subsidiary of: Wolters Kluwer N.V.), 530 Walnut St, Philadelphia, PA 19106-3621. TEL 215-521-8300, FAX 215-521-8902, http://www.retinajournal.com, http://www.lww.com. Ed. Dr. Alexander J Brucker. Pub. Christine Rullo. R&P Margaret Becker. Adv. contact Ray Thibodeau. B&W page USD 1,145, color page USD 2,795; trim 11 x 8.13. Circ: 2,600. **Subscr. to:** PO Box 1600, Hagerstown, MD 21740-1600. TEL 800-777-2295, FAX 301-824-7390.

617.7 USA ISSN 1081-0226
REVIEW OF OPHTHALMOLOGY. Text in English. 1994. m. USD 72 domestic; USD 95 in Canada; USD 125 elsewhere (effective 2001). adv. cum.index. back issues avail. *Refereed.* **Document type:** *Trade.* **Description:** Magazine for office and hospital ophthalmologists, residents and staff with information and research on clinical, patient care and practice management topics.
Related titles: Online - full text ed.
—BLDSC (7793.816000). **CCC.**
Published by: Jobson Publishing LLC, 100 Ave of Americas, New York, NY 10013-1678. TEL 212-274-7000, 800-747-1652, FAX 212-431-0500, http://www.jobson.com. Ed. Stan Herrin. Pub. David Cox. Adv. contact Tom Gangemi. Circ: 18,000 (controlled). **Subscr. to:** PO Box 2092, Mahopal, NY 10541.

617.75 USA
RE1
REVIEW OF OPTOMETRY. Text in English. 1891. m. USD 42 (effective 2001). adv. bk.rev. illus. index. reprint service avail. from PQC. *Refereed.* **Document type:** *Trade.* **Description:** Targets the professionals who provide eye care services as well as ophthalmic products such as frames, ophthalmic lenses and contact lenses.
Former titles (until Aug. 1999): Chilton's Review of Optometry (0147-7633); (until Apr. 1977): Optical Journal and Review of Optometry (0030-3925)
Related titles: Microfiche ed.: (from PQC); Microfilm ed.: (from PQC); Online - full text ed.: (from Gale Group, Factiva).
—BLDSC (7793.818000), Infotrieve. **CCC.**
Published by: Jobson Publishing LLC, 100 Ave of Americas, New York, NY 10013-1678. TEL 212-274-7000, 800-747-1652, FAX 212-431-0500, http://www.jobson.com. Ed., R&P Richard Kirkner. Pub. David Cox. Adv. contact Suzanne Mouince. B&W page USD 4,160, color page USD 5,755; trim 10.75 x 8. Circ: 34,500 (controlled). **Subscr. to:** PO Box 2092, Mahopal, NY 10541.

617.7 NLD ISSN 0168-8375
CODEN: ROCREC
REVIEWS OF OCULOMOTOR RESEARCH. Text in English. 1985. irreg., latest vol.5, 1992. price varies. back issues avail. *Refereed.* **Document type:** *Monographic series, Academic/Scholarly.* **Description:** Surveys new research in the oculomotor system.
Indexed: Ind.Med. (1985-), e-psyche.
—CISTI, GNLM, Infotrieve, KNAW. **CCC.**
Published by: Elsevier Science BV, PO Box 211, Amsterdam 1000 AE, Netherlands. TEL 31-20-485-3757, 31-20-485-3911, FAX 31-20-485-3432, 31-20-485-3598, nlinfo-f@elsevier.nl; usinfo-f@elsevier.com; forinfo-kyf04035@niftyserve.or.jp, http://www.elsevier.nl/. Eds. D A Robinson, H Collewijn. **Subscr. in Australasia and the Far East to:** Elsevier Science (Singapore) Pte Ltd, No.1 Temasek Ave, 17-01 Millenia Tower, Singapore 039192, Singapore. TEL 65-434-3727, FAX 65-337-2230, asiainfo@elsevier.com.sg; **Subscr. in Japan to:** Elsevier Science Inc - Japan Regional Office, 9-15 Higashi-Azabu 1-chome, Minato-ku, Tokyo 106-0044, Japan. TEL 81-3-5561-5033, FAX 81-3-5561-5047, info@elsevier.co.jp; **Subscr. in the Americas to:** Elsevier Science, PO Box 945, New York, NY 10159-0945. TEL 212-633-3730, 888-437-4636, FAX 212-633-3680, usinfo-f@elsevier.com, http://www.elsevier.com

617.7 BRA ISSN 0034-7280
CODEN: RBOFA9
REVISTA BRASILEIRA DE OFTALMOLOGIA. Text in Portuguese; Summaries in English. 1942. q. USD 40. adv. bk.rev. abstr, bibl. index.
Indexed: Biol.Abstr., Chem.Abstr., Excerp.Med., Ind.Med. (coverage dropped).
—CISTI, GNLM.
Published by: Sociedade Brasileira de Oftalmologia, Rua Sao Salvador, 107, Zc 01, Rio De Janeiro, Brazil. Circ: 1,000.

618 CUB ISSN 0864-2176
REVISTA CUBANA DE OFTALMOLOGIA. Text in Spanish; Summaries in English, Spanish. 1987. s-a. USD 34 in North America; USD 42 in Europe; USD 50 elsewhere. **Description:** Covers ophthalmology and, in particular, the treatment of pigmentary retinosis.
Published by: (Cuba. Ministerio de Salud Publica, Centro Nacional de Informacion de Ciencias Medicas), Editorial de Ciencias Medicas, O'Reilly No. 4, Habana, Cuba. TEL 809-62-8091. Ed. Grisell Concepcion. Circ: 1,000. **Co-sponsor:** Sociedad Cubana de Oftalmologia.

617.7 MEX ISSN 0187-4519
CODEN: RMOFEM
REVISTA MEXICANA DE OFTALMOLOGIA. Text in Spanish; Abstracts in English, Spanish. 1890. bi-m. MXP 250, USD 65. adv. index. back issues avail. *Refereed.* **Document type:** *Academic/Scholarly.* **Description:** Contains original research articles and clinical studies.
Indexed: Biol.Abstr.
—GNLM.
Published by: Sociedad Mexicana de Oftalmologia, Boston No. 99, Mexico, Col. Noche Buena, Mexico City, DF 03720, Mexico. Ed. Dr. Fernando Castanon Nunez. Circ: 1,500. **Subscr. to:** Composicion Editorial Laser, S.A. de C.V., LAGO ABERTO 442-7, Col. Anahuac, Mexico City, DF 11320, Mexico. TEL 525-2600250, FAX 525-2600048.

617.7 FRA
REVUE DE L'OPHTALMOLOGIE FRANCAISE. Text in French. 5/yr. FRF 150; FRF 200 foreign. adv. Supplement avail.
Published by: O P H - Communication S.a r.1., 1 rue des Pucelles, Strasbourg 67000, France. TEL 33-3-88350109, FAX 33-3-88255190, snof@sdv.fr, http://www.snof.org. Ed. Dr. Marie Helene Robert. Adv. contact Catherine Bouvard. Circ: 4,000.

617.7 FRA
REVUE INTERNATIONALE DU TRACHOME ET DE PATHOLOGIE TROPICALE ET SUBTROPICALE ET DE SANTE PUBLIQUE. Text in French. 1923. q. free per issue. adv. bk.rev. bibl, illus.
Former titles: Revue Internationale du Trachome et de Pathologie Tropicale et Subtropicale (0301-5017); Revue Internationale du Trachome; Revue Internationale du Trachome et des Maladies Oculaires des Pays Tropicaux et Sub Tropicaux (0035-3531)
Indexed: Abstr.Hyg., Biol.Abstr., Chem.Abstr., Excerp.Med., Ind.Med. (coverage dropped), Rev.Med.& Vet.Mycol., Trop.Dis.Bull.
—CISTI, GNLM.
Published by: Ligue contre le Trachome, La Bergere, Route de Grenoble, Aspres Sur Buech 05140, France. TEL 33-4-92586560, FAX 331-45-17-52-27, TELEX 345023. Ed. Georges Cornand. **Subscr. to:** CIBA Vision Ophthalmics, B.P. 1129, Toulouse Cedex 31036, France.

617.7 JPN ISSN 0917-4338
RYOKUNAISHO/JAPAN GLAUCOMA SOCIETY. JOURNAL. Text in English, Japanese. 1990. a.

M

Published by: Nihon Ryokunaisho, Miyazaki Ika Daigaku Gankagaku Kyoshitsu, 5200 Kihara, Miyazaki-gun, Kiyotake-cho, Miyazaki-ken 889-1601, Japan.

617.7 CHE
SCHWEIZER OPTIKER. Text in German. 1925. m. CHF 118 domestic; CHF 142.50 foreign (effective 2000). adv. bk.rev. **Document type:** *Journal, Trade.*
Published by: Maihof Verlag AG, Postfach, Luzern 6002, Switzerland. TEL 41-41-4295252, FAX 41-41-4295367. Ed. Kurt Butikofer. Circ: 2,300.

617.7 GBR
SCOTTISH OPTOMETRIST. Text in English. 1976. m. GBP 28. adv. bk.rev. charts, illus.
Formerly (until Jan. 1988): Scottish Ophthalmic Practitioner (0308-7670); Supersedes: Optics (0048-2013)
Published by: Scottish Committee of Optometrist, c/o 24 Tweed Crescent, Pean Park, Pean Park, Renfred, United Kingdom. Ed. Maureen A Callender. Circ: (controlled).

617.7 USA ISSN 0882-0538 CODEN: SEOPE7
SEMINARS IN OPHTHALMOLOGY. Text in English. 1986. q. USD 148 domestic to individuals; USD 224 foreign to individuals; USD 196 domestic to institutions; USD 252 foreign to institutions; USD 89 domestic to students; USD 224 foreign to students; USD 64 newsstand/cover (effective 2000). adv. bibl, charts, illus. index. **Document type:** *Academic/Scholarly.* **Description:** Each issue focuses on a particular therapeutic or surgical technique through high-level clinical reviews geared toward trainee and practicing eye specialists.
Indexed: CINAHL, Ind.Med. (1986-).
—BLDSC (8239.456650), EMDOCS, GNLM, ingenta, KNAW. **CCC.**
Published by: W.B. Saunders Co. (Subsidiary of: Harcourt Publishers Ltd.), 11830 Westline Industrial Dr, St Louis, MO 63146. TEL 800-325-4177, http://www.wbsaunders.com. Ed. Dr. Thomas R Friberg. adv.: B&W page USD 740, color page USD 1,765; trim 10 x 7. Circ: 491. **Subscr. to:** Periodicals Fulfillment, W B Saunders Co, 6277 Sea Harbor Dr, 4th Fl, Orlando, FL 32891-4800.

617.7 JPN
SHIKAKU NO KAGAKU/JAPANESE JOURNAL OF VISUAL SCIENCE. Text in Japanese; Summaries in English. a. JPY 2,500.
Published by: Nihon Gankogaku Gakkai, Nikon 2-3 Marunochi 3-chome, Chiyoda-ku, Tokyo 100-0005, Japan.

617.7 JPN ISSN 0287-7767
SHIKAKU SHOGAI KENKYU/NIPPON LIGHTHOUSE WELFARE CENTER FOR THE BLIND. RESEARCH BULLETIN. Text in Japanese. 1973. s-a.
Published by: Nippon Raito Hausu Shokugyo Seikatsu Kunren Senta, 4-37 Imazunaka 2-chome, Tsurumi-ku, Osaka-shi 538-0042, Japan.

617.7 JPN ISSN 0289-7024
SHINKEI GANKA/NEURO-OPHTHALMOLOGY JAPAN. Text in English, Japanese. 1984. q. JPY 4,000 per issue (effective 2001). adv. bk.rev. reprints avail. *Refereed.* **Document type:** *Academic/Scholarly.*
Indexed: Excerp.Med., INIS Atomind., e-psyche.
—BLDSC (6081.511000), EMDOCS, GNLM, Infotrieve. **CCC.**
Published by: Nihon Shinkei Ganka Gakkai/Japanese Neuro-Ophthalmology Society, Kitasato University School of Allied Health Sciences, 15-1 Kitaza-To 1-chome, Sagamihara-shi, Kanagawa-ken 228-8555, Japan. TEL 81-42-778-9416, FAX 81-42-778-9417, jimukyoku@kinkeiganka.com, http://www.shinkeiganka.com. Ed. Satoshi Ishikawa. Pub. Kinko-Sha. Adv. contact M Wakakura. Circ: 1,500.

SIGHT AND SOUND NEWS. see *HEALTH FACILITIES AND ADMINISTRATION*

SKULL BASE SURGERY. see *MEDICAL SCIENCES—Surgery*

617.7 GBR ISSN 1055-6575
SLIDE ATLAS OF CURRENT OPHTHALMOLOGY (YEAR). Text in English. bi-m. USD 299.95. **Document type:** *Academic/Scholarly.* **Description:** Provides a visual review of every development in procedure and technique occurred over the previous year in the field of ophthalmology.
Related titles: ♦ Supplement to: Current Opinion in Ophthalmology. ISSN 1040-8738.
Published by: Rapid Science Publishers, 2-6 Boundary Row, London SE1 8HN, United Kingdom. TEL 44-207-865-0198, FAX 44-207-410-6600, rapid@rapidcom.co.uk. Ed. George W Weinstein.

117.7 COL ISSN 0037-8364
SOCIEDAD AMERICANA DE OFTALMOLOGIA Y OPTOMETRIA. ARCHIVOS/AMERICAN SOCIETY FOR OPHTHALMOLOGY AND OPTOMETRY. ARCHIVES. Text in Spanish. 1958. q. COP 25,000, USD 75 (effective 1995). adv. bk.rev. illus, stat. index, cum.index every 10 yrs.
Indexed: Biol.Abstr., Excerp.Med.
—CISTI.
Published by: Sociedad Americana de Oftalmologia y Optometria, Apartado Aereo 091019, Bogota, DE 8, Colombia. Ed. Dr. Angela Ma Gutierrez. Circ: 750.

617.7 ESP ISSN 0365-6691
SOCIEDAD ESPANOLA DE OFTALMOLOGIA. ARCHIVOS. Text in Spanish; Summaries in English, French, German, Spanish. 1940. m. adv. bk.rev. abstr, bibl, illus. index. back issues avail. **Document type:** *Academic/Scholarly.*
Indexed: Biol.Abstr., Excerp.Med., Ind.Med.
—BLDSC (1653.990000), CINDOC, CISTI, EMDOCS, GNLM, Infotrieve. **CCC.**
Published by: Sociedad Espanola de Oftalmologia, Donoso Cortes, 73 1o, Madrid 28015, Spain. TEL 1-5445879. Circ: 2,000.

617.7 BEL ISSN 0081-0746
SOCIETE BELGE D'OPHTALMOLOGIE. BULLETIN. Text in French. 1896. q. BEF 4,000 domestic; BEF 4,300 in Europe; BEF 4,700 elsewhere (effective 1999). adv. **Document type:** *Bulletin.*
Indexed: Biol.Abstr., Dent.Ind., Excerp.Med., Ind.Med. (1896-).
—BLDSC (2727.220000), CISTI, GNLM, KNAW.
Published by: Societe Belge d'Ophtalmologie, Marlene Verlaeckt, VZ Leuven, Kapucijnenvoer 33, Leuven 3000, Belgium. FAX 32-16-332678, http://www.bog.be/bog. Ed. M Hanssens. Circ: 900.

617.7 FRA ISSN 0081-1270 CODEN: BSOFAK
SOCIETE D'OPHTALMOLOGIE DE FRANCE. BULLETIN. Text in French. 1949. q. FRF 910, USD 170 (effective 1999). abstr.
Indexed: Biol.Abstr., Chem.Abstr., Ind.Med. (coverage dropped).
—BLDSC (2758.240000), CISTI, GNLM, KNAW.
Published by: Diffusion Generale de Librairie, 11 rue Moliere, Marseille 13001, France. TEL 33-4-91335718, FAX 33-4-91335727, BSOF@DGDDL.COM,. **Subscr. to:** B.P. 60, Marseille Cedex 20 13486, France.

617.75 ZAF ISSN 0378-9411
SOUTH AFRICAN OPTOMETRIST/SUID-AFRIKAANSE OOGKUNDIGE. Text in English. 1941. q. membership. adv. bk.rev. charts, illus. *Refereed.* **Document type:** *Academic/Scholarly.*
Indexed: Ind.S.A.Per.
Published by: South African Optometric Association, P O Box 2925, Halfway House 1685, South Africa. TEL 011-805-4517, FAX 011-805-3882, pro@saoa.co.za, http://www.saoa.co.za/. Ed. Alan Rubin. Circ: 2,000.

617.75 USA ISSN 0038-4275
RE1
SOUTHERN JOURNAL OF OPTOMETRY. Text in English. 1959. q. USD 16 (effective 1996). adv. bk.rev. abstr, illus. *Refereed.*
—CISTI.
Published by: Southern Council of Optometrists, 4661 N Shallowford Rd, Atlanta, GA 30338. TEL 770-451-8206, FAX 770-451-3156. Ed., Pub. Dr. Lyman Norden. R&P, Adv. contact Michele Middleton. B&W page USD 715, color page USD 1,465; 11 x 8.5. Circ: 6,500.

617.7 AUT ISSN 0930-4282
SPEKTRUM DER AUGENHEILKUNDE; Zeitschrift der Oesterreichischen Ophtalmologischen Gesellschaft. Text in German; Summaries in English. 1987. bi-m. EUR 156; EUR 31 newsstand/cover (effective 2002). adv. bk.rev. abstr, illus. back issues avail.; reprints avail. *Refereed.* **Document type:** *Journal, Academic/Scholarly.* **Description:** Informs ophthalmologists about developments in research and clinical practice that are relevant to their practices.
Related titles: Microform ed.: (from PQC); Online - full text ed.: (from Springer LINK).
Indexed: Excerp.Med., INIS Atomind.
—BLDSC (8411.400150), CISTI, EMDOCS, GNLM, Infotrieve, KNAW. **CCC.**
Published by: (Oesterreichische Ophthalmologische Gesellschaft), Springer-Verlag Wien (Subsidiary of: BertelsmannSpringer), Sachsenplatz 4-6, PO Box 89, Vienna, W 1201, Austria. TEL 43-1-3302415-0, FAX 43-1-330242665, journals@springer.at, http://www.springer.at. Eds. H Freyler, J Faulborn, W Goettinger. R&P Angela Foessl TEL 43-1-3302415517. Adv. contact Michael Katzenberger TEL 43-1-3302415220. B&W page XEU 790, color page XEU 1,422; 170 x 250. **N. American subscr. to:** Springer-Verlag, Journals, 175 Fifth Ave, New York, NY 10010. TEL 212-460-1500, FAX 212-473-6272, orders@springer-ny.com.

617.7 USA
ST. ANTHONY'S CODING FOR OPHTHALMOLOGY REIMBURSEMENT*. Text in English. m. USD 129. bk.rev. **Description:** Focuses on coding reimbursement issues that have economic impact on ophthalmology practices.
Published by: St. Anthony Publishing, Inc., 11410 Isaac Newton Sq N, 200, Reston, VA 22090-5012. TEL 800-632-0123. Ed. Kimberly Fullmer.

617.7 NLD ISSN 0927-3972 CODEN: SRABFL
STRABISMUS. Text in English. 1993. q. NLG 235 to individuals (effective 2000); USD 125 to individuals; NLG 506, USD 266 to institutions. adv. abstr. back issues avail.; reprint service avail. from PQC,SWZ. *Refereed.* **Document type:** *Academic/Scholarly.* **Description:** Publishes original papers and review articles on strabismus and related fields, including neurophysiology.
Related titles: Microform ed.: (from PQC); Online - full text ed.: (from EBSCO Publishing, O C L C Online Computer Library Center, Inc., RoweCom Information Quest, Swets Blackwell).
Indexed: Ind.Med. (1993-), e-psyche.
—ADONIS, Infotrieve. **CCC.**
Published by: Aeolus Press (Subsidiary of: Swets & Zeitlinger BV), PO Box 825, Lisse 2160 SZ, Netherlands. FAX 31-344-572562, orders@swets.nl, http://www.swets.nl/sps/AEolus/strabis1.html. Ed. H J Simonsz. Pub. J K W van Leeuwen. R&P C E van Leeuwen-Meyren. Adv. contact Patrick Kleian. Circ: 400. **Subscr. to:** Swets & Zeitlinger BV, PO Box 825, Lisse 2160 SZ, Netherlands. TEL 31-252-435111, FAX 31-252-415888, orders@swets.nl, http://www.swets.nl. **Dist. in N. America by:** Swets & Zeitlinger, PO Box 582, Downingtown, PA 19335-998. TEL 800-447-9387, FAX 610-524-5366.

STUDIES IN VISUAL INFORMATION PROCESSING. see *MEDICAL SCIENCES—Psychiatry And Neurology*

SUNGLASS ASSOCIATION OF AMERICA. NEWSLETTER. see *CLOTHING TRADE*

617.7 USA
SUNWEAR. Text in English. 1970. 3/yr. **Document type:** *Trade.*
Published by: Frames Data, 16269 Laguna Canyon Rd, Ste 100, Irvine, CA 92618. TEL 949-788-0150, FAX 949-788-0130, cwalker@framesdata.com, http://www.framesdata.com. Ed. Christie Walker. Circ: 30,000.

SURVEY OF OPHTHALMOLOGY. see *MEDICAL SCIENCES—Abstracting, Bibliographies, Statistics*

617.7 USA ISSN 0738-7644
TEXAS OPTOMETRY. Text in English. 1945. 3/yr. USD 12. bk.rev. charts, stat, illus.
Formerly: Texas Optometric Association. Journal
Published by: Texas Optometric Association, 1503 S I H 35, Austin, TX 78741-2502. TEL 512-451-8476. Ed. Clarke Newman. adv.: B&W page USD 365, color page USD 965; trim 10.88 x 8.13. Circ: 1,600.

TID OG SYN. see *JEWELRY, CLOCKS AND WATCHES*

617.7 TUR ISSN 1300-0659 CODEN: TOFGA
TURK OFTALMOLOJI GAZETESI/TURKISH JOURNAL OF OPHTHALMOLOGY. Text in Turkish. 1929. bi-m., latest vol.31, 2001. TRL 17,000,000 domestic; USD 45 foreign (effective 2001). *Refereed.* **Document type:** *Journal, Academic/Scholarly.*
Indexed: Excerp.Med.
—GNLM.
Published by: Turkish Ophthalmological Society, T O G Millet Cad. Gilsen Apt. B, Block No.21/9, Yusufpasa, Istanbul, Turkey. TEL 90-212-5307133, FAX 90-212-5307166, http://www.tod-tog.com/. Ed. Dr. Lale Kozer Bilgin.

M

617.7 362 USA
UPDATE (OWINGS MILLS). Text in English. 3/yr. free. **Document type:** *Newsletter.* **Description:** Contains information and research updates for those with age-related macular degeneration.
Formerly (Until 1998): Macular Update
Related titles: Audio cassette/tape ed.; Braille ed.; Online - full text ed.; Large type ed. 14 pt.
Published by: Foundation Fighting Blindness, 11435 Cronhill Dr., Owings Mills, MD 21117. TEL 410-568-0150, 888-394-3937, FAX 410-363-2393, http://www.blindness.org. Ed. Robyn Miller. Circ: 20,000.

V H L FAMILY FORUM. (Von Hippel-Lindau Disease) see *MEDICAL SCIENCES—Psychiatry And Neurology*

617.7 ITA ISSN 0302-6256
VEDERE - INTERNATIONAL; international journal on optics, frame industry and optical instruments. Text in English, French, Spanish, Italian. 1953. bi-m. (plus 2 special issues). EUR 51.65 domestic; EUR 83 foreign (effective 2001). adv. tr.lit. back issues avail. **Document type:** *Magazine, Trade.* **Description:** Covers the optical industry.
Formerly (until 1971): Vedere (0503-7565)
Published by: Edizioni Ariminum, Via Negroli, 51, Milan, MI 20133, Italy. TEL 39-02-730091, FAX 39-02-717346, welcome@vedere.it, http://www.vedere.it. Pub., Adv. contact Isabella Morpurgo. color page XEU 1,200; 210 x 290. Circ: 8,500.

617.752 ITA
VEDERE TECH INTERNATIONAL. Text in Italian, English, French, Spanish. 1992. bi-m. (plus 2 special issues). EUR 51.65 domestic; EUR 83 foreign (effective 2001). adv. back issues avail. **Document type:** *Magazine, Trade.* **Description:** Covers raw materials, machinery, equipment and components for the eyewear industry.
Published by: Edizioni Ariminum, Via Negroli, 51, Milan, MI 20133, Italy. TEL 39-02-730091, FAX 39-02-717346, welcome@vedere.it, http://www.vedere.it. Pub., Adv. contact Isabella Morpurgo. color page XEU 930; 210 x 290. Circ: 4,000.

617.7 RUS ISSN 0042-465X
RE1 CODEN: VEOFA6
VESTNIK OFTAL'MOLOGII/ANNALS OF OPHTHALMOLOGY. Text in Russian; Summaries in English. 1884. q. USD 62 foreign (effective 1999). adv. bk.rev. illus. abstr. index. **Document type:** *Journal, Academic/Scholarly.* **Description:** Publishes materials on the diagnosis and treatment of eye diseases, hygiene of vision, prevention of ophthalmic infections, ophthalmological techniques.
Indexed: Biol.Abstr., Chem.Abstr., Curr.Cont. (coverage dropped), Dent.Ind., Dok.Arbeitsmed., Excerp.Med., Helminthol.Abstr., INIS Atomind., Ind.Med. (1937-), Inpharma, Int.Aerosp.Abstr., Neurosci.Cit.Ind., Plant Sci., Reac., Ref.Zh., Sci.Cit.Ind. (coverage dropped).
—CASDDS, CISTI, East View, GNLM, IDS, Infotrieve. **CCC.**
Published by: Izdatel'stvo Meditsina, Petroverigskii per 6-8, Moscow 101000, Russian Federation. TEL 7-095-9212274, 7-095-928-86-48, FAX 7-095-9211355, meditsina@iname.com. Ed. M M Krasnov. Pub. A M Stochik. R&P V Sinitsina. Adv. contact V I Sinitsina. Circ: 2,000. **Dist. by:** Mezhdunarodnaya Kniga, B Yakimanka 39, Moscow 117049, Russian Federation. TEL 7-095-2384967, FAX 7-095-2384634.

▼ **VETERINARY OPHTHALMOLOGY.** see *VETERINARY SCIENCE*

617.7 USA
VIDEO JOURNAL OF CATARACT & REFRACTIVE SURGERY. Text in English. 1985. q. USD 220; USD 260 foreign (effective 1999). **Document type:** *Trade.* **Description:** Features new microsurgical procedures from an international cast of leaders in cataract surgery. Contains one hour of uninterrupted surgical footage recorded through the microscope. Emphasizes surgical techniques, intraocular lenses, complication management, and refractive procedures.
Formerly: Audiovisual Journal of Cataracts and Implant Surgery (1067-9812)
Media: Video.
Address: 10494 Montgomery Rd, Cincinnati, OH 45242. TEL 513-984-5133, FAX 513-984-4240. Ed. Dr. Robert Osher. R&P Elizabeth Haft.

VISION ENHANCEMENT. see *HANDICAPPED—Visually Impaired*

617.7 658.8 USA ISSN 0891-1770
VISION MONDAY. Text in English. 1987. fortn. USD 49.96. adv. **Description:** Covers news and information about the world-wide optical industry.
Published by: Jobson Publishing LLC, 100 Ave of Americas, New York, NY 10013-1678. TEL 212-274-7000, 800-747-1652, FAX 212-431-0500, http://www.jobson.com. Ed. Marge Axelrad. Circ: 12,000. **Subscr. to:** PO Box 2092, Mahopal, NY 10541.

617.7 GBR ISSN 0042-6989
QP474 CODEN: VISRAM
VISION RESEARCH; an international journal for functional aspects of vision. Text in English, French, German, Russian. 1961. 28/yr. NLG 539 in Europe to individuals (effective 2001); EUR 257 in Europe to qualified personnel; JPY 34,100 in Japan to qualified personnel (effective 2002); NLG 5,252 in Europe to institutions (effective 2001); EUR 2,538 in Europe to institutions; JPY 337,100 in Japan to institutions; USD 2,839 elsewhere to institutions; USD 2,716 With Progress in Retinal and Eye Research (effective 2002). adv. bk.rev. charts, illus. index. back issues avail. *Refereed.* **Document type:** *Academic/Scholarly.* **Description:** Publishes original research in functional aspects of the neurobiology, psychophysics and behavioral physiology of human, vertebrate and invertebrate vision, as well as computational vision research.
Incorporates (1986-1993): Clinical Vision Science (0887-6169)
Related titles: Microfilm ed.: (from PQC); Online - full text ed.: (from ingenta, Swets Blackwell, Institute for Scientific Information, ScienceDirect).
Indexed: ASCA, Apic.Abstr., Appl.Mech.Rev., Aqua.Sci.& Fish.Abstr., Biol.Abstr., Chem.Abstr., Chem.Indus.Notes, Compumath, Curr.Adv.Ecol.Sci., Curr.Cont., Curr.Ref.Fish Res., Ergon.Abstr., Excerp.Med., INIS Atomind., INSPEC (pre-1969-), Ind.Med. (1961-), Ind.Sci.Rev., Inpharma, Int.Abstr.Biol.Sci., Int.Aerosp.Abstr., Int.Build.Serv.Abstr., Neurosci.Abstr. (coverage dropped), Neurosci.Cit.Ind., Nutr.Abstr., Phys.Ber., PsycInfo, Psychol.Abstr. (1963-), Reac., SSCI (coverage dropped), Sci.Cit.Ind., Sport Fish.Abstr., Wild.Rev., e-psyche.
—BLDSC (9240.925000), ADONIS, AskIEEE, CASDDS, CISTI, EMDOCS, GNLM, IDS, ingenta, KNAW, Linda Hall. **CCC.**
Published by: (Association for Research in Vision and Ophthalmology USA), Pergamon (Subsidiary of: Elsevier Science), The Boulevard, Langford Ln, East Park, Kidlington, Oxford OXB 1GB, United Kingdom. FAX 44-1865-843010, http://www.elsevier.nl/locate/inca/263. Eds. H Speikreijse, R Blake, S M Wu, W Baehr. Circ: 2,500. **Subscr. in Australasia and the Far East to:** Elsevier Science (Singapore) Pte Ltd, No.1 Temasek Ave, 17-01 Millenia Tower, Singapore 039192, Singapore. TEL 65-434-3727, FAX 65-337-2230; **Subscr. in the Americas to:** Elsevier Science, PO Box 945, New York, NY 10159-0945. TEL 212-633-3730, FAX 212-633-3680, usinfo-f@elsevier.com; **Subscr. to:** Elsevier Science BV, PO Box 211, Amsterdam 1000 AE, Netherlands. TEL 31-20-485-3757.

VISION (SHEFFIELD). see *MEDICAL SCIENCES—Abstracting, Bibliographies, Statistics*

610 617.7 613.7 USA
VISIONARY. Text in English. 1962. 2/yr. free per issue. bk.rev. charts, illus, stat. back issues avail. **Document type:** *Newsletter.*
Published by: Illinois Society for the Prevention of Blindness, 407 S Dearborn St, Ste 1000, Chicago, IL 60605-1117. TEL 312-922-8710, FAX 312-922-8713. Ed., R&P James A McKechnie Jr. Circ: 12,000.

617.7 FRA ISSN 1149-5758
VISIONS INTERNATIONALES. Text in French. m. (10/yr). FRF 300 domestic to individuals; FRF 450 foreign to individuals; FRF 210 domestic to libraries; FRF 360 foreign to libraries (effective 2001).
Published by: L E N Medical, 15 rue des Sablons, Paris 75116, France. TEL 33-1-47553131, FAX 33-1-47553132, lenmed@club-internet.fr, http://www.webmedguide.com.

617.7 USA
VISIONS (ST. LOUIS). Text in English. bi-m. membership only. 8 p./no. **Document type:** *Newsletter, Internal.*
Published by: College of Optometrists in Vision Development, 243 N.Lindbergh Blvd. #310, St. Louis, MO 63141. TEL 314-991-4007. Ed. Dr. Stephen C Miller. Circ: 1,600.

VISUAL NEUROSCIENCE. see *MEDICAL SCIENCES—Psychiatry And Neurology*

WELCOME TO THE WORLD OF... see *SOCIAL SERVICES AND WELFARE*

617.7 DEU ISSN 0171-6417
WISSENSCHAFTLICHE VEREINIGUNG FUER AUGENOPTIK UND OPTOMETRIE. FACHVORTRAEGE DES W V A O JAHRESKONGRESSES. Text in German. 1952. a. price varies. adv. **Document type:** *Academic/Scholarly.*
Formerly: Wissenschaftliche Vereinigung der Augenoptiker. Fachvortraege der Jahrestagungen (0084-1005)
Published by: Wissenschaftliche Vereinigung fuer Augenoptik und Optometrie e.V., Adam-Karrillon-Str 32, Mainz 55118, Germany. TEL 49-6131-613061, FAX 49-6131-614872, wvao-mainz@t-online.de. Ed. Hartmut Glaser.

617.705 USA ISSN 0084-392X
RE6
THE YEAR BOOK OF OPHTHALMOLOGY. Text in English. 1958. a. USD 98 domestic; USD 104 foreign (effective 2001). illus. **Document type:** *Abstract/Index, Academic/Scholarly.* **Description:** Presents abstracts of pertinent literature with commentary by leading experts in the field.
—CISTI, GNLM.
Published by: Mosby, Inc., Continuity Division (Subsidiary of: Harcourt Health Sciences), 11830 Westline Industrial Dr, St Louis, MO 63146-3313. TEL 314-872-8370, 800-325-4177, FAX 314-432-1380, http://www.mosby.com/periodicals. Ed. Dr. Richard P Wilson.

617.7 DEU ISSN 0173-2595
CODEN: ZPAUD3
Z P A. (Zeitschrift fuer Praktische Augenheilkunde) Text in German. 1979. 11/yr. DEM 165 (effective 2000). adv. bk.rev. back issues avail. **Document type:** *Magazine, Trade.*
Indexed: Ref.Zh.
—CASDDS, GNLM.
Published by: Dr. R. Kaden Verlag, Poststr 24-26, Heidelberg 69115, Germany. TEL 49-6221-600313, FAX 49-6221-29910, marketing@kaden-verlag.de. Adv. contact A Siegmann. B&W page DEM 3,910; trim 178 x 230. Circ: 5,000.

617.752 DEU
ZEISS MARKT - MODE - MEINUNGEN; Informationen fuer Augenoptiker. Text in German. 1977. 3/yr. back issues avail.
Published by: Carl Zeiss Geschaeftsbereich Augenoptik, Postfach 1865, Aalen 73408, Germany. TEL 07361-591365. Circ: 7,500.

617.7 CHN ISSN 1006-4443
ZHONGGUO SHIYONG YANKE ZAZHI/CHINESE JOURNAL OF PRACTICAL OPHTHALMOLOGY. Text in Chinese. 1983. m. USD 40.80; USD 3.40 newsstand/cover (effective 2001). **Document type:** *Academic/Scholarly.*
Formerly (until 1993): Shiyong Yanke Zazhi (1003-5079)
Published by: China International Book Trading Corp/Zhongguo Guoji Tushu Maoyi Zonggongsi cibtc@mail.cibtc.com.cn, http://www.cibtc.com.cn. **Dist. by:** 35, Chegongzhuang Xilu, Haidian District, Beijing 100044, China.

617.7 CHN ISSN 1005-1015
CODEN: ZYAZEE
ZHONGHUA YANDIBING ZAZHI/CHINESE JOURNAL OF OCULAR FUNDUS DISEASES. Text in Chinese, English. 1985. q. USD 20.80; USD 5.20 newsstand/cover (effective 2001). adv. abstr, bibl, charts, illus, stat. index. 80 p./no. back issues avail. *Refereed.* **Document type:** *Academic/Scholarly.* **Description:** Clinical reports and research works on ocular fundus diseases relating to the infections of the interior eye and systemic involvements.
Formerly (until 1992): Yandi Bing/Ocular Fundus (1001-4071)
Published by: (West China University of Medical Sciences, First Teaching Hospital), Zhonghua Yixuehui Zazhishe, 42 Dongsi Xidajie, Beijing 100710, China. Ed. Mi Yan. Pub., R&P Chunyi Wei. Adv. contact Jian Tang. Circ: 5,000. **Dist. outside China by:** China International Book Trading Corp, 35, Chegongzhuang Xilu, Haidian District, Beijing 100044, China. TEL 86-1-68413849, FAX 86-1-68412048, cibtc@mail.cibtc.com.cn, http://www.cibtc.com.cn.

617.7 CHN ISSN 0412-4081
ZHONGHUA YANKE ZAZHI/CHINESE JOURNAL OF OPHTHALMOLOGY. Key Title: Chung-Hua Yen K'o Tsa Chih. Text in Chinese. 1951. bi-m. CNY 66 domestic; CNY 11 newsstand/cover domestic; USD 35.40 foreign; USD 5.90 newsstand/cover foreign (effective 2001). **Document type:** *Academic/Scholarly.*
Related titles: Online - full content ed.: (from WanFang Data Corp.).
Indexed: Ind.Med.

M

—BLDSC (3180.462000).
Published by: Zhonghua Yixuehui Zazhishe, 42 Dongsi Xidajie, Beijing 100710, China. cmayk@public.sti.ac.cn. Ed. Mei-Yu Li. **Dist. by:** China International Book Trading Corp, 35, Chegongzhuang Xilu, Haidian District, Beijing 100044, China. TEL 86-1-68413849, FAX 86-1-68412048, cibtc@mail.cibtc.com.cn, http://www.cibtc.com.cn.

617.7 CHN
ZHONGXIYI JIEHE YANKE ZAZHI. Text in Chinese. q.
Description: Covers the combined application of Western and traditional Chinese medicine in ophthalmology.
Published by: Wenzhou Yixueyuan/Wenzhou Institute of Medical Sciences, Wenzhou, Zhejiang 325003, China. TEL 34941. Ed. Yao Fangwei.

MEDICAL SCIENCES—Orthopedics And Traumatology

616.7 USA ISSN 1616-8747
▼ **A O RECOMMENDED LITERATURE. CRANIOMAXILLOFACIAL TRAUMA AND DISORDERS.** Text in English. 2001. 6/yr. EUR 175 in Germany to individuals; EUR 177 in Europe to individuals; EUR 181 elsewhere to individuals; EUR 358 in Germany to institutions; EUR 360 in Europe to institutions; EUR 364 elsewhere to institutions (effective 2002). **Document type:** *Journal, Academic/Scholarly.*
Related titles: Online - full text ed.: ISSN 1618-257X.
Published by: Thieme Medical Publishers, 333 Seventh Ave, New York, NY 10001. TEL 212-760-0888, 800-782-3488, FAX 212-947-1112, custserv@thieme.com, http://www.thieme.com.

616.7 USA ISSN 1616-8755
▼ **A O RECOMMENDED LITERATURE. GENERAL AND ORTHOPEDIC TRAUMA.** Text in English. 2001. 6/yr. EUR 225 in Germany to individuals; EUR 227 in Europe to individuals; EUR 231 elsewhere to individuals; EUR 558 in Germany to institutions; EUR 560 in Europe to institutions; EUR 564 elsewhere to institutions (effective 2002). **Document type:** *Journal, Academic/Scholarly.*
Related titles: Online - full text ed.: ISSN 1618-2588.
Published by: Thieme Medical Publishers, 333 Seventh Ave, New York, NY 10001. TEL 212-760-0888, 800-782-3488, FAX 212-947-1112, custserv@thieme.com, http://www.thieme.com.

616.7 USA ISSN 1616-8763
▼ **A O RECOMMENDED LITERATURE. SPINE TRAUMA AND DISORDERS.** Text in English. 2001. 6/yr. EUR 195 in Germany to individuals; EUR 197 in Europe to individuals; EUR 201 elsewhere to individuals; EUR 458 in Germany to institutions; EUR 460 in Europe to institutions; EUR 464 elsewhere to institutions (effective 2002). **Document type:** *Journal, Academic/Scholarly.*
Related titles: Online - full text ed.: ISSN 1618-2596.
Published by: Thieme Medical Publishers, 333 Seventh Ave, New York, NY 10001. TEL 212-760-0888, 800-782-3488, FAX 212-947-1112, custserv@thieme.com, http://www.thieme.com.

617.585 USA ISSN 8750-2585
A P M A NEWS. Text in English. 1980. m. USD 50 (effective 1999). adv. charts, illus, stat, tr.lit. back issues avail. **Document type:** *Trade.*
Formerly (until 1984): A P A Report (0272-7722)
Published by: American Podiatric Medical Association, 9312 Old Georgetown Rd, Bethesda, MD 20814-1698. TEL 301-571-9200, FAX 301-530-2752. Ed. David Zych. Adv. contact Jenyfer Morris. Circ: 14,000.

616.025 USA ISSN 1069-6563
CODEN: AEMEF5
ACADEMIC EMERGENCY MEDICINE. Text in English. 1994. m. USD 116 domestic to individuals; USD 126 foreign to individuals; USD 158 domestic to institutions; USD 168 foreign to institutions; USD 20 newsstand/cover domestic; USD 25 newsstand/cover foreign (effective 2001). adv. software rev., video rev., bk.rev. abstr, charts, illus, stat. index. back issues avail. *Refereed.* **Document type:** *Journal, Academic/Scholarly.* **Description:** Publishes material relevant to the practice, education, and investigation of emergency medicine, and reaches a wide audience of emergency care practitioners and educators.
Related titles: Online - full text ed.: free with paid subscription (from HighWire Pr., EBSCO Publishing, Institute for Scientific Information).
Indexed: ASCA, Crim.Just.Abstr., Curr.Cont., Excerp.Med. (1996-), Ind.Med. (1994-), Inpharma, Int.Nurs.Ind., Jrnl.Watch Emer.Med., Nutr.Abstr., Pharm.&Out.News, Reac., Rev.Appl.Entomol., Rev.Arom.& Med.Plants, Rev.Med.& Vet.Mycol., Sci.Cit.Ind., Trop.Dis.Bull.
—BLDSC (0570.511250), EMDOCS, GNLM, IDS, Infotrieve, KNAW. **CCC.**
Published by: (Society for Academic Emergency Medicine), Hanley & Belfus, Inc., 210 S 13th St, Philadelphia, PA 19107. TEL 215-546-7293, FAX 215-790-9330, LTroy@aol.com, LTroy@hanleyandbelfusl.com, http://www.aemj.org/. Ed. Dr. Michelle Biros. Adv. contact Diane R Sherel. B&W page USD 1,140; trim 11 x 8.5. Circ: 5,000 (paid). **Dist. by:** Ovid Bell Press, 1201 05 Bluff St, Fulton, MO 65251-0371. TEL 800-835-8919, FAX 573-642-0174.

617.3 BRA ISSN 0104-7795
ACTA FISIATRICA. Text in Portuguese. 1993. s-a. adv. bk.rev. back issues avail. *Refereed.* **Document type:** *Academic/Scholarly.*
Related titles: Online - full text ed.
Published by: (Academia Brasileira de Medicina de Reabilitacao), Lemos Editorial & Graficos Ltda., Rua Rui Barbosa, 70, B Vista, Sao Paulo, SP 01326-010, Brazil. TEL 55-11-251-4300, FAX 55-11-251-4300, lemospl@netpoint.com.br, http://www.lemos.com.br. Ed. Dr. Linamara Rizzo Battistella. Adv. contact Paulo Lemos. Circ: 3,000 (controlled).

617.3 BEL ISSN 0001-6462
ACTA ORTHOPAEDICA BELGICA. Text in English, French. 1945. 4/yr. EUR 75 domestic; EUR 87 foreign; EUR 19 per issue domestic; EUR 23 per issue foreign (effective 2002). bk.rev. abstr, bibl. index. **Document type:** *Journal, Academic/Scholarly.*
Related titles: ♦ Supplement: Acta Orthopaedica Belgica. Supplementum. ISSN 0772-7623.
Indexed: Bibl.Dev.Med.& Child Neur., Biol.Abstr., Excerp.Med. (1996-), Ind.Med. (1946-).
—BLDSC (0642.060000), CISTI, EMDOCS, GNLM, ingenta, KNAW.
Published by: (Association des Societes Scientifiques Medicales Belges/Vereiniging van de Belgische Wetenschappelijke Genootschappen), Acta Medica Belgica, Av Circulaire 138A, Brussels 1180, Belgium. TEL 32-2-374-5158, FAX 32-2-3749628, amb@skynet.be, http://www.ulb.ac.be/medecine/loce/amb.htm. Eds. C Coutelier, H Kinzinger.

617.3 BEL ISSN 0772-7623
ACTA ORTHOPAEDICA BELGICA. SUPPLEMENTUM. Text in English. 1946. irreg.
Related titles: ♦ Supplement to: Acta Orthopaedica Belgica. ISSN 0001-6462.
Published by: Acta Medica Belgica, Av Circulaire 138A, Brussels 1180, Belgium. TEL 32-2-374-5158, FAX 32-2-3749628, amb@skynet.be. Ed. J Dequeker.

617.3 YUG ISSN 0350-2309
ACTA ORTHOPAEDICA IUGOSLAVICA. Text mainly in Serbian; Text occasionally in English; Summaries in English. 1969. s-a. YUN 1,200; DEM 50 foreign (effective 2000). adv. bk.rev. back issues avail. *Refereed.* **Document type:** *Academic/Scholarly.* **Description:** Includes general reviews, original scientific papers, professional papers, case reports and other contributions from the fields of orthopaedic surgery, traumatology and related medical branches.
Published by: Udruzenje Ortopeda i Traumatologa/ Yugoslav Orthopaedic Association, c/o Institut za Ortopedsko-Hirurske Bolesti "Banjica", Mihajla Avramovica 28, Belgrade 11041, Yugoslavia. TEL 381-11-666447, FAX 381-11-667321. Ed., R&P, Adv. contact Zoran Vukasinovic. Circ: 200 (paid); 300 (controlled). **Co-sponsor:** Ministarstvo za Nauku i Tehnologiju Republike Srbije.

617.3 NOR ISSN 0001-6470
CODEN: AOSAAK
ACTA ORTHOPAEDICA SCANDINAVICA. Text in English. 1930. 6/yr. GBP 112, USD 184 to individuals; GBP 156, USD 258 to institutions (effective 2002). adv. bk.rev. bibl, charts, illus. index. reprint service avail. from SWZ,ISI. *Refereed.* **Document type:** *Academic/Scholarly.* **Description:** Presents original articles of basic research interest, as well as clinical studies in the field of orthopedics and related subdisciplines.
Related titles: Online - full text ed.: (from Institute for Scientific Information).
Indexed: AMED, ASCA, Bibl.Dev.Med.& Child Neur., Biol.Abstr., CINAHL, Chem.Abstr., Curr.Adv.Ecol.Sci., Curr.Cont., Dent.Ind., Excerp.Med., Focus on: Sports Sci.& Med., INIS Atomind., Ind.Med. (1930-), Ind.Sci.Rev., Inpharma, Mat.Sci.Cit.Ind. (coverage dropped), Pharm.&Out.News, Reac., Rev.Med.& Vet.Mycol., SSCI (coverage dropped), Sci.Cit.Ind.
—BLDSC (0642.100000), ADONIS, CASDDS, CISTI, EMDOCS, GNLM, IDS, ingenta, KNAW. **CCC.**
Published by: (Scandinavian Orthopaedic Association), Taylor & Francis AS (Subsidiary of: Taylor & Francis Group), Cort Adelersgt. 17, Solli, PO Box 2562, Oslo 0202, Norway. TEL 47-22-12-98-80, FAX 47-22-12-98-90, journals@tandf.no, http://www.tandf.co.uk/tfas. Eds. Anders Rydholm, Peter A Frandsen. Circ: 4,700.

617.3 NOR ISSN 0300-8827
CODEN: AOSUAC
ACTA ORTHOPAEDICA SCANDINAVICA. SUPPLEMENTUM. Text in Norwegian. irreg. free to subscribers of Acta Orthopaedica Scandinavica. adv. reprint service avail. from ISI. **Document type:** *Academic/Scholarly.*
Indexed: Biol.Abstr., CINAHL, Curr.Cont. (coverage dropped), Excerp.Med., INIS Atomind., Ind.Med. (1934-).
—BLDSC (0642.105000), ADONIS, CISTI, EMDOCS, ingenta, KNAW. **CCC.**
Published by: (Scandinavian Orthopaedic Association), Scandinavian University Press (Subsidiary of: Taylor & Francis Ltd.), Postboks 2959, Toeyen, Oslo 0608, Norway. FAX 47-22-57-53-53, journals@scup.no, http://www.scup.no/orthopaed.

616.02 USA
ADVANCED RESCUE TECHNOLOGY. Text in English. 1995. bi-m. USD 11.50 (effective 2000). adv. back issues avail. *Refereed.* **Document type:** *Magazine, Trade.* **Description:** Focuses on hands-on rescue techniques and emergency medical care of victims. For EMS personnel and first responders, including fire personnel and those involved in law enforcement and the military.
Formerly: E M S Rescue Technology
Published by: Summer Communications Inc., 7626 Densmore Ave., Van Nuys, CA 91406-2042. TEL 818-786-4367, FAX 818-786-9246, rteditor@aol.com, http://www.advancedrt.com. Ed., R&P Nancy Perry. Pub. Carol Summer. Adv. contact Judy Cohen. Circ: 30,000 (controlled).

617.1 DEU ISSN 0044-6173
CODEN: AKTRAE
AKTUELLE TRAUMATOLOGIE. Text in German; Summaries in English, German. 1971. 6/yr. EUR 219.80 domestic to institutions; EUR 224.80 in Europe to institutions; EUR 228.80 elsewhere to institutions; EUR 108 to students; EUR 44 newsstand/cover (effective 2002). bk.rev. index. reprint service avail. from PQC. **Document type:** *Journal, Academic/Scholarly.*
Related titles: Online - full text ed.
Indexed: Biol.Abstr., Curr.Cont. (coverage dropped), Dok.Arbeitsmed., Excerp.Med., Ind.Med. (coverage dropped), Sci.Cit.Ind. (coverage dropped).
—BLDSC (0785.885000), CISTI, EMDOCS, GNLM, KNAW. **CCC.**
Published by: Georg Thieme Verlag, Ruedigerstr 14, Stuttgart 70469, Germany. TEL 49-711-8931-0, FAX 49-711-8931298, trauma@thieme.de, leser.service@thieme.de, http://www.thieme.de/trauma/index.html. Ed. K Weise. R&P Michael Wachinger. Circ: 2,000.

617.585 378 USA
ALUMNUS (NEW YORK)* . Text in English. 1975. q. bk.rev. illus.
Published by: New York College of Podiatric Medicine, 52 E 124th St, New York, NY 10035. Circ: 3,000.

AMBULANCE SERVICE JOURNAL; a professional journal for ambulance and first aid personnel. see *HEALTH FACILITIES AND ADMINISTRATION*

AMBULANCE U K. see *HEALTH FACILITIES AND ADMINISTRATION*

617.3 USA ISSN 1049-9741
AMERICAN ACADEMY OF ORTHOPAEDIC SURGEONS. BULLETIN. Text in English. 1952. q. membership. back issues avail. **Document type:** *Bulletin.*
Related titles: Online - full text ed.

M

Published by: American Academy of Orthopaedic Surgeons, 6300 N. River Rd., Rosemont, IL 60018. TEL 847-384-4130, FAX 847-823-8033, nagelberg@mac.aas.org, http://www.aaos.org/wordhtml/bulletin.htm. Ed. Alvin Nagelberg. R&P Joan Golembiewsky TEL 847-384-4144. Circ: 25,000 (controlled).

617.3 USA ISSN 0516-8856
AMERICAN ACADEMY OF ORTHOPAEDIC SURGEONS. DIRECTORY. Text in English. 1933. a. membership only. **Document type:** *Directory.*
Published by: American Academy of Orthopaedic Surgeons, 6300 N. River Rd., Rosemont, IL 60018. TEL 847-384-4130, FAX 847-823-8033, winkler@aaos.org. R&P Joan Golembiewsky TEL 847-384-4144.

617.3 USA ISSN 1067-151X
AMERICAN ACADEMY OF ORTHOPAEDIC SURGEONS. JOURNAL. Text in English. 1993. 6/yr. USD 75 domestic to individuals; USD 98 foreign to individuals; USD 112 domestic to institutions; USD 123 foreign to institutions. adv. *Refereed.* **Document type:** *Academic/Scholarly, Trade.* **Description:** Covers the latest developments in the clinical practice of orthopedics, focusing on diagnosis and managementof orthopedic conditions.
Indexed: Ind.Med. (1993-), Int.Nurs.Ind.
—BLDSC (4683.732000), GNLM, KNAW.
Published by: American Academy of Orthopaedic Surgeons, 6300 N. River Rd., Rosemont, IL 60018. TEL 847-384-4130, FAX 847-823-8033, psilos@aaos.org, http://www.jaaos.org/. Ed. Paul D Psilos. R&P Joan Golembiewsky TEL 847-384-4144. Circ: 26,600.

617.585 USA ISSN 0737-5409
AMERICAN ACADEMY OF PODIATRY ADMINISTRATION NEWS-LETTER✶. Text in English. 1973 (vol.3). q. USD 15.
Formerly: American Academy of Practice Management in Podiatry. News-Letter
Published by: American Academy of Podiatry Administration, c/o John V Cicero, D P M, Sec, Ten Meadow Lane, Bloomfield, NJ 07003. **Subscr. to:** Dr. Leonard Light, 614 Central Ave, Dunkirk, NY 14048.

617.3 USA
AMERICAN COLLEGE OF FOOT AND ANKLE ORTHOPEDICS AND MEDICINE NEWSLETTER✶. Text in English. 1964. q. USD 5 to non-members. bk.rev. abstr, charts, illus. **Document type:** *Newsletter.*
Formerly (until Oct. 1993): American College of Foot Orthopedists Newsletter (0002-7987)
Published by: American College of Foot and Ankle Orthopedics and Medicine, 4603 Hwy 95 S, Box 545, Los Olivos, CA 93441-0545. TEL 208-683-3900, FAX 208-683-3700. Ed. Judith A Baerg. Circ: 1,100.

AMERICAN JOURNAL OF CRITICAL CARE. see *MEDICAL SCIENCES—Nurses And Nursing*

616.025 USA ISSN 0735-6757
CODEN: AJEMEN
AMERICAN JOURNAL OF EMERGENCY MEDICINE. Text in English. 1983. 7/yr. USD 167 domestic to individuals; USD 249 foreign to individuals; USD 242 domestic to institutions; USD 316 foreign to institutions; USD 92 domestic to students; USD 149 foreign to students; USD 46 newsstand/cover (effective 2001). adv. bk.rev. abstr, bibl, charts, illus. index. *Refereed.* **Document type:** *Journal, Academic/Scholarly.* **Description:** Covers all aspects of emergency medicine with clinical articles, case studies, reviews, worldwide news items, and editorials.
Related titles: Microform ed.: (from PQC); Online - full text ed.: (from Ovid Technologies, Inc., IDEAL Online Library, Institute for Scientific Information).
Indexed: ASCA, CINAHL, Crim.Just.Abstr., Curr.Cont., Excerp.Med., INIS Atomind., Ind.Med. (1983-), Inpharma, Med.& Surg.Dermat., Neurosci.Cit.Ind., Pharm.&Out.News, Reac., Rev.Appl.Entomol., Rev.Arom.& Med.Plants, Rev.Med.& Vet.Mycol., SSCI (coverage dropped).
—BLDSC (0824.480000), CISTI, EMDOCS, GNLM, IDS, ingenta, KNAW. **CCC.**
Published by: W.B. Saunders Co. (Subsidiary of: Harcourt Publishers Ltd.), 11830 Westline Industrial Dr, St Louis, MO 63146. TEL 800-325-4177, http://www.harcourthealth.com/amjemergmed, http://www.wbsaunders.com. Ed. Dr. J Douglas White. adv.: B&W page USD 735, color page USD 1,870; trim 10 x 7. Circ: 2,244. **Subscr. to:** Periodicals Fulfillment, W B Saunders Co, 6277 Sea Harbor Dr, 4th Fl, Orlando, FL 32891-4800.

617.3 USA ISSN 1078-4519
RD701 CODEN: AJORFL
THE AMERICAN JOURNAL OF ORTHOPEDICS. Text in English. 1972. m. USD 135 in the Americas to institutions; USD 222 elsewhere to institutions (effective 2000). adv. bk.rev. charts, illus, stat. index. back issues avail. *Refereed.* **Document type:** *Trade.*
Formerly (until 1995): Orthopaedic Review (0094-6591)
Related titles: Microform ed.: (from PQC).
Indexed: Excerp.Med., INIS Atomind., Ind.Med. (1995-), Int.Nurs.Ind.
—BLDSC (0829.190000), EMDOCS, GNLM, Infotrieve, KNAW. **CCC.**
Published by: Quadrant HealthCom, 26 Main St, Ste A, Chatham, NJ 07928-2402. TEL 973-701-8900, FAX 973-701-8892. Ed. Barbara Ready. Pub. Linda Fox. Adv. contact Denise Andrade. Circ: 25,000.

617.585 USA ISSN 8750-7315
RD563.A2 CODEN: JAPAEA
AMERICAN PODIATRIC MEDICAL ASSOCIATION. JOURNAL. Text in English. 1907. 10/yr. USD 115 domestic; USD 138 foreign (effective 2001). adv. bk.rev. bibl, illus. index, cum.index: 1973-1984. back issues avail. *Refereed.* **Document type:** *Academic/Scholarly.* **Description:** It is the oldest, most frequently cited, most authoritative, and the only monthly referred journal in the profession of foot and ankle medicine.
Incorporates: Podiatric Medicine and Surgery; Former titles (until 1984): American Podiatry Association. Journal (0003-0538); (until 1957): National Association of Chiropodists. Journal (0360-1684); (until 1921): Pedic Items
Related titles: Microfilm ed.; Online - full text ed.: (from HighWire Pr., Institute for Scientific Information).
Indexed: AMED, ASCA, AgeLine, Biol.Abstr., Curr.Adv.Ecol.Sci., Curr.Cont., Dent.Ind., Excerp.Med., Hosp.Lit.Ind., INIS Atomind., Ind.Med. (1985-), Inpharma, Int.Nurs.Ind., Med.& Surg.Dermat., Nutr.Abstr., Pharm.&Out.News, Reac., Rev.Med.& Vet.Mycol., SSCI (coverage dropped).
—BLDSC (4692.040000), CISTI, GNLM, IDS, ingenta, KNAW.
Published by: American Podiatric Medical Association, 9312 Old Georgetown Rd, Bethesda, MD 20814-1698. TEL 301-581-9200, FAX 301-530-2752, amtheuring@apma.org, http://www.japmaonline.org, http://www.apma.org. Ed. Dr. Warren S Joseph. R&P Annette Theuring. Adv. contact Gary Walchli. Circ: 14,000. **Subscr. to:** Allen Press Inc., PO Box 1897, Lawrence, KS 66044-8897.

AMERICAN PODIATRIC MEDICAL WRITERS ASSOCIATION. NEWSLETTER. see *JOURNALISM*

617.3 MEX ISSN 0044-8184
ANALES DE ORTOPEDIA Y TRAUMATOLOGIA✶. Text in Spanish; Summaries in English, Spanish. 1969 (vol.5). q. MXP 100, USD 10. adv. bibl, charts, illus.
—GNLM.
Published by: Sociedad Mexicana de Ortopedia, Ejercito Nacional 475, Primer Piso, Mexico City 17, Mexico. Ed. Dr. Carlos Hernandez Esquivel.

616.025 USA ISSN 0196-0644
RC86 CODEN: AEMED3
ANNALS OF EMERGENCY MEDICINE. Text in English. 1972. m. USD 125 domestic to individuals; USD 168 foreign to individuals; USD 221 domestic to institutions; USD 265 foreign to institutions; USD 59 domestic to students; USD 97 foreign to students; USD 23 newsstand/cover domestic (effective 2001). adv. bk.rev. back issues avail.; reprint service avail. from PQC. *Refereed.* **Document type:** *Journal, Academic/Scholarly.* **Description:** Presents pertinent information encompassing clinical studies, case reports, basic research, and discussion.
Formerly: J A C E P (0361-1124)
Related titles: Microfilm ed.; Online - full text ed.: (from Ovid Technologies, Inc., EBSCO Publishing, IDEAL Online Library, Institute for Scientific Information, RoweCom Information Quest).
Indexed: AIM, ASCA, Abstr.Health Care Manage.Stud., CINAHL, Crim.Just.Abstr., Curr.Cont., Dent.Ind., Excerp.Med., FAMLI, Helminthol.Abstr., INIS Atomind., I.P.A., Ind.Med. (1980-), Inpharma, Int.Nurs.Ind., Jrnl.Watch, Jrnl.Watch Emer.Med., Kidney, Lab.Haz.Bull., Neurosci.Cit.Ind., Pharm.&Out.News, Reac., Ref.Zh., Rev.Appl.Entomol., Rev.Med.& Vet.Mycol., Rev.Plant Path., SSCI (coverage dropped), Sci.Cit.Ind., Weed Abstr.
—BLDSC (1040.425000), CISTI, EMDOCS, GNLM, IDS, ingenta, KNAW. **CCC.**

Published by: (American College of Emergency Physicians), Mosby, Inc. (Subsidiary of: Elsevier Science), 11830 Westline Industrial Dr, St Louis, MO 63146-3318. TEL 314-872-8370, 800-325-4177, FAX 314-432-1380, http://www.mosby.com/aem, http://www.mosby.com/periodicals. Ed. Dr. Joseph F Waeckerle. Pub. Cheryl A Smart. Adv. contact Carol Kilzer TEL 314-453-4307. B&W page USD 2,655, color page USD 4,255; trim 10.88 x 8.13. Circ: 27,223.

APUNTS; medicina de l'esport. see *MEDICAL SCIENCES—Sports Medicine*

617.3 DEU ISSN 0936-8051
CODEN: AOTSEF
ARCHIVES OF ORTHOPAEDIC AND TRAUMA SURGERY. Text in English. 1903. 10/yr. EUR 1,093.50 domestic; EUR 1,087.30 in Germany; EUR 128.40 newsstand/cover foreign (effective 2002). adv. bk.rev. bibl, charts, illus. index. back issues avail.; reprint service avail. from ISI. *Refereed.* **Document type:** *Journal, Academic/Scholarly.* **Description:** Reports on the latest advances in all areas of orthopedics, including accident related injuries, experimental bone and joint surgery, and problems related to rehabilitation.
Former titles: Archives of Orthopaedic and Traumatic Surgery (0344-8444); (until 1978): Archiv fuer Orthopaedische und Unfallchirurgie (0003-9330)
Related titles: Microform ed.: (from PQC); Online - full text ed.: ISSN 1434-3916 (from EBSCO Publishing, RoweCom Information Quest, Swets Blackwell, Springer LINK, Institute for Scientific Information).
Indexed: ASCA, Biol.Abstr., Chem.Abstr., Curr.Cont., Dent.Ind., Excerp.Med., Focus on: Sports Sci.& Med., INIS Atomind., Ind.Med. (1989-), Ind.Sci.Rev., Inpharma, Mat.Sci.Cit.Ind. (coverage dropped), Pharm.&Out.News, Reac., Sci.Cit.Ind. (coverage dropped).
—BLDSC (1638.494900), CISTI, EMDOCS, GNLM, IDS, ingenta, KNAW. **CCC.**
Published by: (Deutsche Gesellschaft fuer Unfallheilkunde, Versicherungs-, Versorgungs- und Verkehrsmedizin), Springer-Verlag (Subsidiary of: BertelsmannSpringer), Tiergartenstr 17, Heidelberg 69121, Germany. TEL 49-6221-345-0, FAX 49-6221-345229, subscriptions@springer.de, http://link.springer.de/link/service/journals/00402/index.htm, http://www.springer.de. Eds. G Hierholzer, H Wagner. **Subscr. in N. America to:** Springer-Verlag New York Inc., PO Box 2485, Secaucus, NJ 07096-2485. TEL 212-460-1500, FAX 212-473-6272.

617.3 616.742 ITA ISSN 0390-7368
ARCHIVIO DI ORTOPEDIA E REUMATOLOGIA. Text in Italian; Summaries in English. 1884. q. EUR 50 foreign; EUR 15 newsstand/cover foreign (effective 2002). adv. bk.rev. abstr, bibl, illus. index. **Document type:** *Journal, Academic/Scholarly.*
Formerly: Archivio di Ortopedia (0004-0118)
Indexed: Biol.Abstr., Chem.Abstr., Ind.Med. (coverage dropped).
—CISTI, GNLM.
Published by: (Istituto Ortopedico "Gaetano Pini"), Editrice Grafiche Zanini S.r.l., Via Emilia, 41 E, Anzola Dell'Emilia, BO 40011, Italy. TEL 3951-765562, FAX 3951-766060. Ed. Luigi Parrini. Circ: 500.

617 USA ISSN 0749-8063
CODEN: ARTHE3
ARTHROSCOPY; journal of arthroscopic and related surgery. Text in English. 1985. 9/yr. USD 287 domestic to individuals Print & online eds.; USD 385 foreign to individuals Print & online eds.; USD 419 domestic to institutions Print & online eds.; USD 526 foreign to institutions Print & online eds.; USD 129 domestic to students Print & online eds.; USD 59 per issue (effective 2001). adv. bk.rev. charts, illus. index. back issues avail.; reprint service avail. from PQC. *Refereed.* **Document type:** *Academic/Scholarly.* **Description:** Explores trends and innovations in both diagnostic and operative arthroscopy.
Related titles: Online - full text ed.: (from EBSCO Publishing, IDEAL Online Library, Institute for Scientific Information).
Indexed: Curr.Cont., Excerp.Med., Focus on: Sports Sci.& Med., INIS Atomind., Ind.Med. (1985-), Inpharma, Pharm.&Out.News, Reac., Sci.Cit.Ind.
—BLDSC (1733.940000), CISTI, EMDOCS, GNLM, IDS, ingenta, KNAW.
Published by: (Arthroscopy Association of North America), W.B. Saunders Co. (Subsidiary of: Harcourt Publishers Ltd.), 11830 Westline Industrial Dr, St Louis, MO 63146. TEL 800-325-4177, http://www.arthroscopyjournal.org, http://www.wbsaunders.com. Ed. Dr. Gary G Poehling. Adv. contact Cindy Gray. B&W page USD 1,280, color page USD 2,730; trim 10 x 7. Circ: 6,254. **Subscr. to:** Periodicals Fulfillment, W B Saunders Co, 6277 Sea Harbor Dr, 4th Fl, Orlando, FL 32891-4800.
Co-sponsor: International Arthroscopy Association.

617.1 616.7 JPN ISSN 0910-223X
ARTHROSCOPY. Text in Japanese; Summaries in English. 1976. s-a. JPY 5,000, USD 50. adv. back issues avail. **Document type:** *Academic/Scholarly.* **Description:** Publishes proceedings of the annual meeting and original papers.
Published by: Japan Arthroscopy Association, c/o Dept of Orthopaedic Surgery, School of Medicine Chiba University, 1-8-1 Inohana, Chuo-ku, Chiba-shi 260-0856, Japan. TEL 81-43-226-2338, FAX 81-43-226-2369. Ed. Hideshige Moriya. Circ: 1,500.

617.3 USA ISSN 0748-8947
AUDIO-DIGEST EMERGENCY MEDICINE. Text in English. 1984. s-m. USD 168 (effective 2000). *Refereed.*
Media: Audio cassette/tape.
Published by: Audio-Digest Foundation (Subsidiary of: California Medical Association), 1577 E Chevy Chase Dr, Glendale, CA 91206. TEL 213-245-8505, 800-423-2308, FAX 818-240-7379, 800-845-4375.

617.3 USA ISSN 0271-132X
AUDIO-DIGEST ORTHOPAEDICS. Text in English. 1978. m. USD 84 (effective 2000). *Refereed.*
Media: Audio cassette/tape.
Published by: Audio-Digest Foundation (Subsidiary of: California Medical Association), 1577 E Chevy Chase Dr, Glendale, CA 91206. TEL 213-245-8505, 800-423-2308, FAX 818-240-7379, 800-845-4375. Ed. Claron L Oakley. Circ: (controlled).

616.02 NZL ISSN 1174-4707
AUSTRALASIAN JOURNAL OF DISASTER AND TRAUMA STUDIES. Text in English. 1997. irreg. (2-3/yr). bk.rev. back issues avail. *Refereed.* **Description:** Provides a forum for the publication of original research, reviews and commentaries. Includes disaster and trauma mitigation and prevention, response, support, recovery, treatment, policy formulation and planning and their implications at the individual, group, organizational and community level.
Media: Online - full text.
Published by: Massey University, School of Psychology, North Shore Mail Centre, Private Bag 102 904, Auckland, New Zealand. TEL 64-9-443-9799, http://www.massey.ac.nz/~trauma/welcome.htm.

616.02 610.73 AUS ISSN 1328-3626
AUSTRALASIAN JOURNAL OF EMERGENCY CARE. Text in English. 1977. q. AUD 40 domestic; AUD 60 foreign (effective 2000). adv. bk.rev. abstr, bibl, charts, illus. back issues avail. *Refereed.* **Document type:** *Academic/Scholarly.* **Description:** Aimed at ambulance officers, paramedics, emergency doctors, emergency nurses and other emergency care practitioners.
Former titles (until 1997): Australian Journal of Emergency Care (1322-3127); (until 1994): Ambulance World (0817-4474)
Indexed: CINAHL.
—BLDSC (1794.932000).
Published by: Australian Liquor, Hospitality & Miscellaneous Works Union, PO Box 327, North Melbourne, VIC 3051, Australia. TEL 61-3-9235-7668, FAX 61-3-9235-7680, ajec@mira.net. Ed. Andrew McDonell. R&P Fiona Lauritz. Adv. contact Justin Conlan TEL 61-3-9372-3250. Circ: 5,000.

616 USA ISSN 0894-7376
THE BACK LETTER. Key Title: Backletter. Text in English. m., latest vol.16. USD 136 domestic to individuals; USD 157 foreign to individuals; USD 170 domestic to institutions; USD 190 foreign to institutions; USD 16 newsstand/cover (effective 2002). **Document type:** *Newsletter.* **Description:** Covers all aspects of spine function, disease and injury.
Related titles: Online - full text ed.: USD 221 domestic academic site license; USD 241 foreign academic site license; USD 246.50 domestic corporate site license; USD 266.50 foreign corporate site license (effective 2002) (from Gale Group).
Published by: Lippincott Williams & Wilkins (Philadelphia) (Subsidiary of: Wolters Kluwer N.V.), 530 Walnut St, Philadelphia, PA 19106-3621. TEL 215-521-8300, FAX 215-521-8902, http://www.lww.com. Ed. Dr. Sam W Weisel. **Subscr. to:** PO Box 1600, Hagerstown, MD 21740-1600. TEL 800-777-2295, FAX 301-824-7390.

616.73 USA
THE BACKLETTER. Text in English. m. USD 125 in US & Canada; USD 145 elsewhere (effective 2000). **Description:** Sifts through more than 200 relevant specialty journals to provide focused reviews of the current literature.
Published by: Lippincott Williams & Wilkins (Philadelphia) (Subsidiary of: Wolters Kluwer N.V.), 530 Walnut St, Philadelphia, PA 19106-3621. TEL 800-638-6423, http://www.lww.com. **Subscr. to:** PO Box 1600, Hagerstown, MD 21740-1600.

617.3 JPN ISSN 0287-1645
CODEN: SEGEAW
BESSATSU SEIKEI GEKA/ORTHOPEDIC SURGERY. SPECIAL ISSUE. Text in Japanese. 1982. s-a. JPY 5,500.
Published by: Nankodo Co. Ltd., 42-6 Hongo 3-chome, Bunkyo-ku, Tokyo 113-0033, Japan. FAX 03-3811-7230.

617.3 CAN ISSN 1205-562X
BODY CAST. Text in English. 1986. q. CND 37.45, USD 42.80 in North America; USD 53.50 elsewhere. adv.
Indexed: CINAHL.
Published by: Pappin Communications, The Victoria Centre, 84 Isabella St, Pembroke, ON K8A 5S5, Canada. TEL 613-735-0952, FAX 613-735-7983. Ed. Martin McPolin. R&P Pam Smith TEL 416-292-0687. Adv. contact C B Pappin. **Subscr. to:** 4433 Sheppard Ave. E. No. 200, Agincourt, ON M1S 1V3, Canada.

617.3 JPN ISSN 0914-7047
CODEN: BONEFN
THE BONE. Text in Japanese. 1987. 4/yr. JPY 1,800 per issue (effective 1998).
—BLDSC (2247.332000), CASDDS.
Published by: Medikaru Rebyusha/Medical Review Co., Ltd., 7-3 Hirano-Machi 1-chome, Chuo-ku, Osaka-shi 541-0046, Japan. TEL 81-6-223-1556, FAX 81-6-223-1414, medrev@osk2.3web.ne.jp.

617.6 616.4 USA ISSN 8756-3282
QP88.2 CODEN: BONEDL
BONE. Text in English. 1979. m. EUR 242 in Europe to individuals; JPY 32,200 in Japan to individuals; USD 270 elsewhere to individuals; EUR 1,766 in Europe to institutions; JPY 234,600 in Japan to institutions; USD 1,975 elsewhere to institutions (effective 2002). adv. abstr, illus. back issues avail.; reprint service avail. from SWZ. *Refereed.* **Document type:** *Academic/Scholarly.* **Description:** Provides an interdisciplinary forum for rapid publication of original experimental or clinical studies and review articles on all aspects of the metabolism of bone and minerals.
Incorporates (1986-1994): Bone and Mineral (0169-6009); Formerly: Metabolic Bone Disease and Related Research (0221-8747)
Related titles: Microfilm ed.: (from PQC); Online - full text ed.: (from ingenta, Swets Blackwell, ScienceDirect, Institute for Scientific Information).
Indexed: ASCA, AgBiotech, Anim.Breed.Abstr., Biol.Abstr., Chem.Abstr., Chem.Indus.Notes, Chem.Titles, Curr.Adv.Biochem., Curr.Adv.Ecol.Sci., Curr.Cont., Dairy Sci.Abstr., Dent.Ind., Excerp.Med., INIS Atomind., Ind.Med. (1985-), Ind.Sci.Rev., Ind.Vet., Inpharma, Int.Abstr.Biol.Sci., Int.Nurs.Ind., NRN, Nutr.Abstr., Pharm.&Out.News, Pig News & Info., Poult.Abstr., Reac., Sci.Cit.Ind., Small Anim.Abstr., Vet.Bull.
—BLDSC (2247.330000), CASDDS, CISTI, EMDOCS, GNLM, IDS, ingenta, KNAW. **CCC.**
Published by: (International Bone and Mineral Society), Elsevier Science, 655 Ave of the Americas, New York, NY 10010. TEL 212-989-5800, FAX 212-633-3990, TELEX 420643 AEP UI, usinfo-f@elsevier.com, http://www.elsevier.com/locate/bone. Ed. Dr. Roland Baron. **Subscr. in Australasia and the Far East to:** Elsevier Science (Singapore) Pte Ltd, No.1 Temasek Ave, 17-01 Millenia Tower, Singapore 039192, Singapore. TEL 65-434-3727, FAX 65-337-2230; **Subscr. in Japan to:** Elsevier Science Inc - Japan Regional Office, 9-15 Higashi-Azabu 1-chome, Minato-ku, Tokyo 106-0044, Japan. TEL 81-3-5561-5033, FAX 81-3-5561-5047; **Subscr. outside the Americas to:** Elsevier Science BV, PO Box 211, Amsterdam 1000 AE, Netherlands. TEL 31-20-485-3757, FAX 31-20-485-3432, nlinfo-f@elsevier.nl, http://www.elsevier.nl.

370 USA
BRAIN INJURY ASSOCIATION. CATALOGUE OF EDUCATIONAL MATERIALS. Text in English. 1987. a. **Document type:** *Catalog.*
Formerly: National Head Injury Foundation. Catalogue of Educational Materials
Published by: Brain Injury Association, Inc., 105 N Alfred St, Alexandria, VA 22314-3010. TEL 703-236-6000, FAX 703-236-6001, publications@biausa.org, hhtp://www.biausa.org.

617.1 USA ISSN 1094-3439
BRAIN INJURY SOURCE. Text in English. 1997. q. USD 38; USD 48 foreign; USD 12.50 newsstand/cover (effective 1999). adv. bk.rev., software rev. bibl, illus. back issues avail. **Document type:** *Trade, Consumer.* **Description:** Covers issues important to the brain injury community, including scientific and research topics, epidemiologic topics, medicine, as well as pharmacological and psycho-social issues.
—BLDSC (2268.134000).
Published by: (Brain Injury Association), H D I Publishers, PO Box 131401, Houston, TX 77219. TEL 713-526-6900, FAX 713-526-7787, hdijch@hdipub.com. Ed. Larry Hoffer. Pub. Charles W Haynes. R&P Charles Haynes. Adv. contact Joyce Parker. Circ: 20,000.

617.3 USA
BRISTOL-MYERS - ZIMMER ORTHOPAEDIC SYMPOSIUM SERIES. Text in English. 1988. irreg. price varies. **Document type:** *Proceedings.*
Published by: Lippincott Williams & Wilkins (Philadelphia) (Subsidiary of: Wolters Kluwer N.V.), 530 Walnut St, Philadelphia, PA 19106-3621. TEL 301-223-2300, 800-638-3030, FAX 301-223-2400.

THE BRITISH JOURNAL OF HAND THERAPY. see *MEDICAL SCIENCES—Physical Medicine And Rehabilitation*

615.585 GBR ISSN 1460-7328
BRITISH JOURNAL OF PODIATRY. Text in English. 1998. q. GBP 55; GBP 105 in the Americas and the Middle East; GBP 135 in Australia & New Zealand; GBP 135 in Japan; GBP 6 newsstand/cover (effective 2000). adv. bk.rev. illus. index. *Refereed.* **Document type:** *Academic/Scholarly.*
Formed by the 1998 merger of part of: Journal of British Podiatric Medicine (0961-6055); Which was formerly (1914-1991): Chiropodist (0009-4706); Part of: British Journal of Podiatric Medicine and Surgery (0955-8160); Which was formerly (until 1989): Podiatric Society. Journal
Related titles: Microfilm ed.: (from PQC).
Indexed: AMED, Curr.Adv.Ecol.Sci.
—BLDSC (2319.570000).
Published by: Society of Chiropodists and Podiatrists, 53 Welbeck St, London W1M 7HE, United Kingdom. TEL 44-1714-863381, FAX 44-1719-356359, cr@scpod.org, http://www.scpod.org. Ed., R&P Clare Richards. Circ: 8,500.

617.95 GBR ISSN 0305-4179
CODEN: BURND8
BURNS; including thermal injury. Text in English. 1974. 8/yr. EUR 617 in Europe to institutions; JPY 81,900 in Japan to institutions; USD 690 elsewhere to institutions (effective 2002). adv. bk.rev. index. back issues avail. *Refereed.* **Document type:** *Academic/Scholarly.* **Description:** Focuses on the scientific, clinical and social aspects of burns. Includes clinical and scientific papers, and case reports.
Related titles: Microform ed.: (from PQC); Online - full text ed.: (from ingenta, Swets Blackwell, ScienceDirect, Institute for Scientific Information).
Indexed: ASCA, Biol.Abstr., CINAHL, Curr.Adv.Cancer Res., Curr.Adv.Ecol.Sci., Curr.Cont., Dent.Ind., Environ.Sci.Poll.Mgmt., Excerp.Med., Ind.Med. (1989-), Inpharma, Med.& Surg.Dermat., Nutr.Abstr., Pharm.&Out.News, Pollut.Abstr., Reac., Rev.Arom.& Med.Plants, Rev.Med.& Vet.Mycol., Risk Abstr., SSCI (coverage dropped), Saf.Sci.Abstr., Sugar Ind.Abstr., Trop.Dis.Bull.
—BLDSC (2931.728000), CISTI, EMDOCS, GNLM, IDS, ingenta, KNAW. **CCC.**
Published by: (International Society for Burn Injuries NLD), Pergamon (Subsidiary of: Elsevier Science), The Boulevard, Langford Ln, East Park, Kidlington, Oxford OXB 1GB, United Kingdom. FAX 44-1865-843010, nlinfo-f@elsevier/nl; usinfo-f@elsevier.com; forinfo-kyf04035@niftyserve.or.jp, http://www.elsevier.nl/locate/burns. Eds. J W L Davies, P G Shakespeare. Circ: 850. **Subscr. in Australasia and Far East to:** Elsevier Science (Singapore) Pte Ltd, No.1 Temasek Ave, 17-01 Millenia Tower, Singapore 039192, Singapore. TEL 65-434-3727, FAX 65-337-2230; **Subscr. to:** Elsevier Science BV, PO Box 211, Amsterdam 1000 AE, Netherlands. TEL 31-20-485-3757, FAX 31-20-485-3432, nlinfo-f@elsevier.nl, http://www.elsevier.nl.

M

617.1 USA
▼ **BURNS SOURCEBOOK.** Text in English. 1999. irreg., latest 1999. USD 78 per issue (effective 2001). charts. Index. **Description:** Basic consumer health information about various types of burns and scalds. Includes information on short-term and long-term treatments, tissue reconstruction, plastic surgery, prevention suggestions and first aid.
Published by: Omnigraphics, Inc., 615 Griswold St, Detroit, MI 48226. TEL 313-961-1340, 800-234-1340, FAX 313-961-1383, 800-875-1340, info@omnigraphics.com, http://www.omnigraphics.com/cgi-bin/loadpage.cgi?user_id=9112&file=0-7808-0204-7.html. Ed. Allan R Cook.

CALCIFIED TISSUE INTERNATIONAL. see *MEDICAL SCIENCES—Endocrinology*

616.02 CAN ISSN 0847-947X
CANADIAN EMERGENCY NEWS✶ . Text in English. 1978 (vol.2). 6/yr. CND 30; CND 51 foreign (effective 1998). adv. illus. *Refereed.* **Document type:** *Trade.* **Description:** For emergency medical prehospital care professionals and allied professions.
Formerly: Canadian Emergency Services News (0706-9278)
—CCC.
Published by: Pendragon Publishing Ltd., 1121 Newcastle Rd, Drumheler, AB TOJ O92, Canada. TEL 403-547-5748, FAX 403-547-5749, cen@pendragon.ab.ca, http://www.pendragon.ab.ca. Ed., R&P, Adv. contact Lyle Blumhagen. B&W page CND 1,100, color page CND 1,740; trim 10.88 x 8.25. Circ: 4,000.

616.7 CHN ISSN 1008-1275
CHINESE JOURNAL OF TRAUMATOLOGY. Text in English. 1998. q. USD 31.20; USD 7.80 newsstand/cover (effective 2001). **Document type:** *Academic/Scholarly.*
Related titles: ♦ Chinese ed.: Zhonghua Chuangshang Zazhi. ISSN 1001-8050.
Published by: Zhonghua Changshang Zazhi Bianjibu, 10 Changjiang Zhilu, Daping, Chongching 400042, China. cmachz@public.cta.cq.cn.

CHUBU NIPPON SEIKEI GEKA SAIGAI GEKA GAKKAI SHOROKU/CENTRAL JAPAN ASSOCIATION OF ORTHOPAEDIC AND TRAUMATIC SURGERY. ABSTRACTS. see *MEDICAL SCIENCES—Abstracting, Bibliographies, Statistics*

617.3 JPN ISSN 0008-9443
CHUBU NIPPON SEIKEI GEKA SAIGAI GEKA GAKKAI ZASSHI/CENTRAL JAPAN JOURNAL OF ORTHOPAEDIC SURGERY & TRAUMATOLOGY. Variant title: Central Japan Journal of Orthopaedic and Traumatic Surgery. Text in Japanese. 1958. bi-m. JPY 10,000; JPY 136,000 foreign (effective 1999). adv. **Document type:** *Academic/Scholarly.*
Indexed: INIS Atomind.
—GNLM.
Published by: Chubu Nippon Seikei Geka Saigai Geka Gakkai/Central Japan Association of Orthopaedic Surgery and Traumatology, Teramachi, Imadegawa-Sagaru, Kamigyo-ku, Kyoto-shi 602-0848, Japan. TEL 81-75-231-7599, FAX 81-75-231-7499, chubu-seisai@ma7.seikyou.ne.jp. Ed., Pub. Takashi Nakamura. R&P, Adv. contact Hiroshi Sawada. Circ: 3,600.

617.3 JPN ISSN 0915-2695
CHUGOKU SHIKOKU SEIKEI GEKA GAKKAI ZASSHI/CHUGOKU-SHIKOKU ORTHOPAEDIC ASSOCIATION. JOURNAL. Text in Japanese; Summaries in English. 1989. s-a.
Published by: Chugoku Shikoku Seikei Geka Gakkai, 7-13 Oka-Machi, Okayama-shi 700-0867, Japan.

CLINICAL BIOMECHANICS. see *MEDICAL SCIENCES—Chiropractic, Homeopathy, Osteopathy*

CLINICAL JOURNAL OF SPORT MEDICINE. see *MEDICAL SCIENCES—Sports Medicine*

617.3 USA ISSN 1069-6970
CLINICAL ORTHOPAEDIC SOCIETY. JOURNAL. Text in English. 1995. bi-m. USD 175; USD 257.50 foreign (effective 1997). back issues avail. *Refereed.* **Document type:** *Journal, Academic/Scholarly.*
Related titles: Microform ed.: (from PQC).
—CCC.
Published by: (Clinical Orthopaedic Society), John Wiley & Sons, Inc., Journals (Subsidiary of: Wiley InterScience), 605 Third Ave, New York, NY 10158. subinfo@jwiley.com, http://www.wiley.com. **Subscr. outside the Americas to:** John Wiley & Sons Ltd., Baffins Ln, Chichester, Sussex PO19 IUD, United Kingdom. TEL 44-1243-449777, FAX 44-1243-776128.

617.3 USA ISSN 0009-921X
RD701 CODEN: CORTBR
CLINICAL ORTHOPAEDICS AND RELATED RESEARCH. Text in English. 1945. m. USD 317 domestic to individuals for print & online eds.; USD 513 foreign to individuals for print & online eds.; USD 682 domestic to institutions for print & online eds.; USD 791 foreign to institutions for print & online eds.; USD 65 newsstand/cover (effective 2002). adv. illus. index. *Refereed.* **Document type:** *Academic/Scholarly.* **Description:** Publishes invited, peer-reviewed original articles on general orthopaedics and specialty topics covering the latest advances in current research and practice.
Related titles: Microform ed.: (from PQC); Online - full text ed.: USD 886.60 domestic academic site license; USD 995.60 foreign academic site license; USD 988.90 domestic corporate site license; USD 1,097.90 foreign corporate site license (effective 2002) (from Ovid Technologies, Inc., Swets Blackwell, Institute for Scientific Information).
Indexed: AIM, AMED, ASCA, Abstr.Anthropol., Aqua.Sci.& Fish.Abstr., Bibl.Dev.Med.& Child Neur., Biol.Abstr., CINAHL, Cal.Tiss.Abstr., Chem.Abstr., Curr.Adv.Cell & Devel.Biol., Curr.Adv.Ecol.Sci., Curr.Cont., Dent.Ind., Dok.Arbeitsmed., Excerp.Med., Focus on: Sports Sci.& Med., Hosp.Lit.Ind., INIS Atomind., Ind.Med. (1953-), Ind.Sci.Rev., Inpharma, Int.Nurs.Ind., Mat.Sci.Cit.Ind. (coverage dropped), Neurosci.Cit.Ind., Pharm.&Out.News, Reac., Rev.Med.& Vet.Mycol., Risk Abstr., SSCI (coverage dropped), Sci.Cit.Ind., Tox.Abstr. (coverage dropped).
—BLDSC (3286.323000), CASDDS, CISTI, EMDOCS, GNLM, IDS, ingenta, KNAW.
Published by: Lippincott Williams & Wilkins (Philadelphia) (Subsidiary of: Wolters Kluwer N.V.), 530 Walnut St, Philadelphia, PA 19106-3621. TEL 215-521-8300, FAX 215-521-8902, http://www.Lww.com. Ed. Dr. Carl T Brighton. Pub. Marcia Serepy. R&P Alice McElhinney. Adv. contact Ray Thibodeau. B&W page USD 1,670; trim 9.94 x 6.63. Circ: 9,000 (paid). **Subscr. to:** PO Box 1600, Hagerstown, MD 21740-1600. TEL 800-777-2295, FAX 301-824-7390.

▼ **CLINICAL PEDIATRIC EMERGENCY MEDICINE.** see *MEDICAL SCIENCES—Pediatrics*

617.585 USA ISSN 0891-8422
RD563
CLINICS IN PODIATRIC MEDICINE & SURGERY. Text in English. 1984. q. USD 139 domestic to individuals; USD 168 in Canada to individuals; USD 191 elsewhere to individuals; USD 195 domestic to institutions; USD 237 foreign to institutions; USD 60 per issue (effective 2001). back issues avail. **Document type:** *Journal, Academic/Scholarly.* **Description:** Each issue covers a particular topic of treating foot disorders and conditions.
Formerly (until 1986): Clinics in Podiatry (0742-0668)
Related titles: Microfilm ed.
Indexed: CINAHL, Excerp.Med., INIS Atomind., Ind.Med. (1986-).
—BLDSC (3286.590500), CISTI, EMDOCS, GNLM, ingenta, KNAW. **CCC.**
Published by: W.B. Saunders Co. (Subsidiary of: Harcourt Publishers Ltd.), 11830 Westline Industrial Dr, St Louis, MO 63146. TEL 800-325-4177, http://www.wbsaunders.com. Ed. Vincent Mandracchia. **Subscr. to:** Periodicals Fulfillment, W B Saunders Co, 6277 Sea Harbor Dr, 4th Fl, Orlando, FL 32891-4800.

COMMON DIAGNOSTIC PROCEDURES: ORTHOPEDICS AND NEUROLOGY. see *LAW*

617.3 USA ISSN 0887-1736
COMPLICATIONS IN ORTHOPEDICS. Text in English. 1986. q. **Description:** Seeks to help orthopedic surgeons maximize their clinical judgement and skill. Provides practical reports from the scientific and clinical arenas.
—Infotrieve. **CCC.**
Published by: S C P Communications, Inc., 134 W 29th St, New York, NY 10001-5304. TEL 212-631-1600, subs@scp.com, http://www.medscape.com.

▼ **CONTEMPORARY SPINE SURGERY.** see *MEDICAL SCIENCES—Surgery*

617.3 USA
CRANIAL LETTER. Text in English. 1946. q. USD 60 (effective 1998). adv. bk.rev. **Document type:** *Newsletter.*
Formerly: Cranial Academy Newsletter (0011-0825)
Published by: Cranial Academy, 8202 Clearvista Pkwy, Ste 9D, Indianapolis, IN 46256-1457. TEL 317-594-0411, FAX 317-594-9299. Ed. Patricia S Crampton. Circ: 1,200 (paid).

616.025 USA ISSN 1067-9502
CRITICAL CARE ALERT. Text in English. 1993. m. USD 199 foreign; USD 229 domestic; USD 33 newsstand/cover (effective 2001). **Document type:** *Newsletter.*
Incorporates (1993-1996): Critical Care Management (1070-4523)
Related titles: Online - full text ed.: (from Northern Light Technology, Inc.).
Published by: American Health Consultants (Subsidiary of: Medical Economics Co., Inc.), 3525 Piedmont Rd, N E, 6 Piedmont Center, Ste 400, Atlanta, GA 30305. TEL 404-262-5476, 404-262-7436, 800-688-2421, FAX 404-262-7837, 800-284-3291, custserv@ahcpub.com, http://www.ahcpub.com. Circ: 720.

616.02 AUS ISSN 1441-2772
▼ **CRITICAL CARE AND RESUSCITATION.** Text in English. 1999. q. AUD 76 domestic to individuals; AUD 90 foreign to individuals; AUD 110 domestic to institutions; AUD 150 foreign to institutions (effective 2000). **Document type:** *Trade.*
—BLDSC (3487.450670).
Published by: Australasian Academy of Critical Care Medicine, Flinders Medical Centre, Bedford Park, SA 5042, Australia. Ed. Lindsay I G Worthley.

616.025 USA
CRITICAL PATH SOURCEBOOK. Text in English. a. USD 259; USD 289 foreign (effective 1999). **Document type:** *Trade.*
Supersedes: Critical Path Manual
Published by: American Health Consultants (Subsidiary of: Medical Economics Co., Inc.), 3525 Piedmont Rd, N E, 6 Piedmont Center, Ste 400, Atlanta, GA 30305. TEL 404-262-5476, custserv@ahcpub.com, http://www.ahcpub.com.

617.3 USA ISSN 0894-2293
CURRENT EMERGENCY DIAGNOSIS AND TREATMENT. Text in English. 1983. irreg., latest vol.4. **Document type:** *Monographic series.*
Published by: Appleton & Lange, Journal Division (Subsidiary of: Simon & Schuster Company), 11 W 19th St, New York, CT 10011-4209. TEL 203-406-4500, FAX 203-406-4600.

617 USA ISSN 0739-8573
CURRENT EMERGENCY THERAPY. Text in English. 1984. irreg. **Document type:** *Monographic series.*
—CCC.
Published by: Aspen Publishers, Inc., 200 Orchard Ridge Dr, Ste 200, Gaithersburg, MD 20878. TEL 800-638-8437, FAX 301-417-7550.

CURRENT MEDICAL LITERATURE. CRITICAL CARE MONITOR. see *MEDICAL SCIENCES—Abstracting, Bibliographies, Statistics*

617 USA ISSN 1070-5295
CODEN: COCCF7
CURRENT OPINION IN CRITICAL CARE. Text in English. 1994. bi-m. USD 249 domestic to individuals for print & online eds; USD 249 foreign to individuals for print & online eds.; USD 585 per issue domestic to institutions; USD 585 per issue foreign to institutions; USD 91 newsstand/cover (effective 2002). adv. bibl. back issues avail. **Document type:** *Academic/Scholarly.*
Related titles: CD-ROM ed.; Online - full text ed.: USD 760.50 domestic academic site license; USD 760.50 foreign academic site license; USD 848.25 domestic corporate site license; USD 848.25 foreign corporate site license (effective 2002) (from Ovid Technologies, Inc., EBSCO Publishing, Swets Blackwell).
Indexed: Inpharma, Pharm.&Out.News, Reac.
—BLDSC (3500.773800), ADONIS, GNLM.
Published by: Lippincott Williams & Wilkins (Philadelphia) (Subsidiary of: Wolters Kluwer N.V.), 530 Walnut St, Philadelphia, PA 19106-3621. TEL 215-521-8300, FAX 215-521-8902, http://www.Lww.com. Ed. Dr. Jean-Louis Vincent. Pub. Maria McMichael. R&P Tobias Weschler. Adv. contact Kelly Adamitis. **Subscr. to:** PO Box 1600, Hagerstown, MD 21740-1600.

617.3 USA ISSN 1041-9918
CODEN: COORE9
CURRENT OPINION IN ORTHOPEDICS. Text in English. 1989. bi-m. USD 320 domestic to individuals print & online eds.; USD 320 foreign to individuals print & online eds.; USD 111 combined subscription per issue; USD 721 combined subscription per issue domestic to institutions; USD 721 combined subscription per issue foreign to institutions (effective 2002). adv. bibl, illus. back issues avail. **Document type:** *Academic/Scholarly.* **Description:** Directed toward researchers and practicing orthopedists. Presents review articles followed by annotated bibliographies of references consulted.
Related titles: Online - full text ed.: USD 937.30 domestic academic site license; USD 937.30 foreign academic site license; USD 1,045.45 domestic corporate site license; USD 1,045.45 foreign corporate site license (effective 2002) (from Ovid Technologies, Inc., EBSCO Publishing, Swets Blackwell); ♦ Supplement: Slide Atlas of Current Orthopaedics (Year). ISSN 1055-6583.
Indexed: Biotech.& Bioeng.Abstr. (coverage dropped), CINAHL, Cal.Tiss.Abstr., Chemorec.Abstr., Excerp.Med. (1995-), Neurosci.Abstr. (coverage dropped), Tox.Abstr. (coverage dropped).
—BLDSC (3500.776600), ADONIS, EMDOCS, GNLM, KNAW.
Published by: Lippincott Williams & Wilkins (Philadelphia) (Subsidiary of: Wolters Kluwer N.V.), 530 Walnut St, Philadelphia, PA 19106-3621. FAX 215-521-8902, 215-521-8902, http://www.Lww.com. Eds. James H Herndon, William R J Bennie. Pub. Maria McMichael. R&P Tobias Weschler. Adv. contact Kelly Adamitis. **Subscr. to:** PO Box 1600, Hagerstown, MD 21740-1600.

617.2 GBR ISSN 0268-0890
CODEN: CUOREH
CURRENT ORTHOPAEDICS. Text in English. 1986. bi-m. GBP 165 to individuals; GBP 348 to institutions (effective 2002). adv. illus. back issues avail.; reprint service avail. from PQC. *Refereed.* **Document type:** *Academic/Scholarly.* **Description:** Reviews topics in orthopedics for qualified and trainee orthopedic surgeons.
Related titles: Microfilm ed.; Online - full text ed.: (from EBSCO Publishing, O C L C Online Computer Library Center, Inc., Swets Blackwell, IDEAL Online Library, Institute for Scientific Information).
Indexed: AMED, ASCA, Excerp.Med., Ref.Zh.
—BLDSC (3500.840000), EMDOCS, GNLM, IDS, KNAW. **CCC.**
Published by: Churchill Livingstone (Subsidiary of: Harcourt Publishers Ltd.), Robert Stevenson House, 1-3 Baxter's Pl, Leith Walk, Edinburgh, Midlothian EH1 3AF, United Kingdom. TEL 44-131-556-2424, FAX 44-131-459-1177, cservice@harcourt.com, http://www.harcourt-international.com/journals/cuor. Ed. R A Dickson. Pub. Gillian Griffith. R&P Catherine John TEL 212-424-4200. Adv. contact David Dunnachie. Circ: 1,395. **Subscr. to:** Harcourt Publishers Ltd., Foots Cray High St, Sidcup, Kent DA14 5HP, United Kingdom. TEL 44-20-8308-5700, FAX 44-20-8309-0807.

CURRENT PRACTICE IN FOOT & ANKLE SURGERY; a review of state-of-the-art techniques. see *MEDICAL SCIENCES—Surgery*

617.472 USA ISSN 1068-4107
CURRENT TECHNIQUES IN ARTHROSCOPY. Text in English. 1994. a. **Document type:** *Monographic series, Academic/Scholarly.*
—CISTI.
Published by: Current Medicine, 400 Market St, Ste 700, Philadelphia, PA 19106. TEL 215-574-2257, 800-427-1796, FAX 215-574-2225. **Subscr. outside N. America to:** Current Science Ltd, Middlesex House, 34-42 Cleveland St, London W1P 6LB, United Kingdom. TEL 44-20-7323-0323.

617.752 658.8 GBR
D & A. Text in English. 1997. s-a. illus. **Document type:** *Consumer.* **Description:** Aims to put eyewear products in a stylish context for fashion-conscious customers.
Published by: (Dollond and Aitchison), Redwood Publishing, 7 St Martin's Pl, London WC2N 4HA, United Kingdom. TEL 44-207-747-0700, FAX 44-207-747-0701, gaythorne.silvester@redwood-publishing.com, http://www.redwood-publishing.com. Ed. Gaythorne Silvester. Circ: 120,000 (controlled).

D.C. TRACTS. see *MEDICAL SCIENCES—Chiropractic, Homeopathy, Osteopathy*

THE DIABETIC FOOT. see *MEDICAL SCIENCES—Endocrinology*

362.18 362 USA ISSN 1081-4507
E M S INSIDER. Text in English. 1973. m. USD 149 domestic; USD 157 in Canada; USD 174 elsewhere (effective 2001). **Document type:** *Newsletter, Trade.* **Description:** Provides the latest legislative issues, grants, new drugs and products, current trends and controversies in the field.
Formerly: E M S Communicator (0275-0716)
Published by: J E M S Communications, PO Box 2789, Carlsbad, CA 92018. TEL 760-431-9797, 800-456-JEMS, http://www.emsinsider.com, http://www.jems.com. Ed. Marion Angell Garza. Circ: 2,000 (paid).

616.02 USA ISSN 1532-1576
E M S MANAGER AND SUPERVISOR. (Emergency Medical Service) Text in English. m. USD 119 domestic to individuals; USD 127 in Canada & Mexico to individuals; USD 144 elsewhere to individuals; USD 119 domestic to institutions; USD 127 in Canada & Mexico to institutions; USD 144 elsewhere to institutions; USD 119 domestic to students; USD 127 in Canada & Mexico to students; USD 144 elsewhere to students (effective 2001). back issues avail.; reprints avail. **Document type:** *Newsletter, Trade.* **Description:** Contains practical ideas for EMS managers.
Related titles: Online - full text ed.
Published by: J E M S Communications, PO Box 2789, Carlsbad, CA 92018. TEL 800-266-JEMS, http://www.emsmanagersupervisor.com.

362.18 USA
E S C MAGAZINE. (Every Second Counts) Text in English. q. USD 44 to members; USD 50 to non-members (effective 2000).
Published by: National Safety Council, 1121 Spring Lake Dr, Itasca, IL 60143.

617.3 EGY ISSN 1110-1148
EGYPTIAN ORTHOPAEDIC JOURNAL/AL-MAJALLAH AL-MISRIYYAH LI-JIRAHAT AL-'ITHAM. Text in Arabic, English, French. 1966. q. USD 80. adv. bk.rev. abstr, bibl, charts, illus. **Document type:** *Proceedings, Academic/Scholarly.* **Description:** Publishes original research articles, news, and proceedings.
Formerly: Egyptian Orthopaedic Journal (0013-242X)
Related titles: CD-ROM ed.
Indexed: Biol.Abstr., Excerp.Med., ExtraMED.
—KNAW.
Published by: Egyptian Orthopaedic Association, P O Box 4, Alexandria 21111, Egypt. TEL 20-3-4225626. Ed. Amin M Rida. Circ: 4,000.

616.025 658 USA ISSN 1044-9167
EMERGENCY DEPARTMENT MANAGEMENT. Key Title: E D Management. Text in English. 1989. m. USD 399 domestic; USD 429 foreign; USD 67 newsstand/cover (effective 2001). **Document type:** *Newsletter.*
Incorporates (1990-1991): Reports in Emergency Nursing (1050-8759)
—BLDSC (3659.744700).
Published by: American Health Consultants (Subsidiary of: Medical Economics Co., Inc.), 3525 Piedmont Rd, N E, 6 Piedmont Center, Ste 400, Atlanta, GA 30305. TEL 404-262-5476, 404-262-7436, 800-688-2421, FAX 404-262-7837, 800-284-3291, custserv@ahcpub.com, http://www.ahcpub.com. Ed. Staci Bonner. Pub. Brenda L Mooney. Circ: 1,170.

616.02 USA ISSN 0094-6575
RA645.5
EMERGENCY MEDICAL SERVICES; the journal of emergency care, rescue and transportation. Text in English. 1972. m. USD 19.95 (effective 2001). adv. bk.rev. back issues avail.; reprints avail. *Refereed.* **Document type:** *Trade.* **Description:** Interdisciplinary publication covering critical medical, legal and psychosocial issues for emergency medical technicians, paramedics, administrators, physicians, nurses, and other emergency-care personnel.
Indexed: CINAHL, Curr.Cont. (coverage dropped), Ind.Med. (coverage dropped).
—BLDSC (3733.187000), GNLM, ingenta.
Published by: Summer Communications Inc., 7626 Densmore Ave., Van Nuys, CA 91406-2042. TEL 818-786-4367, FAX 818-786-9246, emsmag@earthlink.net, emseditor@aol.com, http://www.emsmag.com. Ed., R&P Nancy Perry. Pub. Carol Summer. Adv. contact Judy Cohen. B&W page USD 3,501, color page USD 4,341. Circ: 47,000 (paid and controlled).

616.025 USA ISSN 0013-6654
RC86
EMERGENCY MEDICINE; acute medicine for the primary-care physician. Text in English. 1969. m. USD 72 domestic to physicians; USD 96 in Canada to physicians; USD 108 elsewhere to physicians; USD 96 domestic to institutions; USD 128 in Canada to institutions; USD 145 elsewhere to institutions; USD 10 newsstand/cover domestic; USD 15 newsstand/cover in Canada; USD 20 newsstand/cover elsewhere (effective 2000). adv. bk.rev. charts, illus. index. reprint service avail. from PQC. **Document type:** *Academic/Scholarly, Trade.* **Description:** Emphasizes acute-care medicine for primary-care physicians.
Related titles: Microform ed.: (from PQC); Online - full text ed.: (from Northern Light Technology, Inc., ProQuest Information & Learning, Institute for Scientific Information).
Indexed: AgeLine, CINAHL, Curr.Cont. (coverage dropped), Helminthol.Abstr., Hosp.Lit.Ind., Inpharma, Pharm.&Out.News, Reac.
—BLDSC (3733.190000), GNLM, IDS, Infotrieve, ingenta, KNAW. **CCC.**
Published by: Quadrant HealthCom, 26 Main St, Ste A, Chatham, NJ 07928-2402. TEL 973-701-8900, FAX 973-701-8892, 973-701-8895, martindicarlantonio@qhc.com, http://www.emedmag.com. Ed. DiCarlantonio Martin. Pub. Michael Pepper. Adv. contact Denise Andrade. B&W page USD 6,865, color page USD 8,855. Circ: 150,000.

616.025 USA ISSN 1075-6914
EMERGENCY MEDICINE ALERT. Text in English. m. USD 229 domestic; USD 259 foreign; USD 38 newsstand/cover (effective 2001). *Refereed.* **Document type:** *Newsletter.* **Description:** Offers a concise review of articles and reports on advanced emergency medicine.
Incorporates (in 1997): Emergency Medicine Desk Reference; Superseded (in 1994): Advanced Cardiac Life Support Alert (1041-7974)
Related titles: Online - full text ed.: (from Northern Light Technology, Inc.).
Published by: American Health Consultants (Subsidiary of: Medical Economics Co., Inc.), 3525 Piedmont Rd, N E, 6 Piedmont Center, Ste 400, Atlanta, GA 30305. TEL 404-262-5476, 404-262-7436, 800-688-2421, FAX 404-262-7837, 800-284-3291, custserv@ahcpub.com, http://www.ahcpub.com. Circ: 920.

616.02 617.1 AUS ISSN 1035-6851
CODEN: EMEMFL
EMERGENCY MEDICINE (CARLETON SOUTH). Text in English. 1987. q. AUD 109 domestic to individuals; AUD 99 in New Zealand to individuals; USD 99 elsewhere to individuals; AUD 329 domestic to institutions; AUD 299 in New Zealand to institutions; USD 295 elsewhere to institutions; AUD 120 domestic to individuals paper & online eds combined; AUD 109 in New Zealand to individuals paper & online eds combined; USD 109 elsewhere to individuals paper & online eds combined; AUD 362 domestic to institutions paper & online eds combined; AUD 329 in New Zealand to institutions paper & online eds combined; USD 325 elsewhere to institutions paper & online eds combined (effective 2001). adv. charts, illus. back issues avail. *Refereed.* **Document type:** *Journal, Trade.* **Description:** Presents information on emergency medicine for the medical community in Australia.
Related titles: Online - full text ed.: ISSN 1442-2026. AUD 99 domestic to individuals; AUD 90 in New Zealand to individuals; USD 90 elsewhere to individuals; AUD 297 domestic to institutions; AUD 270 in New Zealand to institutions; USD 266 elsewhere to institutions (effective 2001) (from EBSCO Publishing, O C L C Online Computer Library Center, Inc., ingenta, Munksgaard & Blackwell Science's Synergy, Swets Blackwell, RoweCom Information Quest).
—BLDSC (3733.189500). **CCC.**
Published by: (Australasian College for Emergency Medicine), Blackwell Science Asia Pty Ltd, PO Box 378, Carlton South, VIC 3053, Australia. TEL 61-3-9347-0300, FAX 61-3-9347-5001, info@blacksci-asia.com.au; acem.admin@hcn.net.au, http://www.blacksci.co.uk/australi. Eds. George A Jelinek, Gerald J FitzGerald. Adv. contact Kathryn O'Brien. B&W page AUD 920, color page AUD 1,870; trim 210 x 275.

M

616.025 USA ISSN 0733-8627 CODEN: EMCAD7
EMERGENCY MEDICINE CLINICS OF NORTH AMERICA. Text in English. 1983. q. USD 140 domestic to individuals; USD 168 in Canada to individuals; USD 188 elsewhere to individuals; USD 195 domestic to institutions; USD 237 foreign to institutions; USD 60 per issue (effective 2001). **Document type:** *Academic/Scholarly.* **Description:** Delivers practical advice from experts in specialty covered as well as information on new developments in a variety of specialties with a fresh perspective on problems and controversies.
Related titles: Microform ed.: (from PQC); Online - full text ed.: (from Institute for Scientific Information); ♦ Spanish Translation: Clinicas de Medicina de Urgencias de Norteamerica; Supplement: Continuing Medical Education Supplement to Emergency Medicine Clinics of North America. USD 138 (effective 2000).
Indexed: CINAHL, Curr.Cont., Dok.Arbeitsmed., Excerp.Med., INIS Atomind., Ind.Med. (1983-), Int.Nurs.Ind., Sport Fish.Abstr.
—BLDSC (3733.190400), CISTI, EMDOCS, GNLM, IDS, ingenta, KNAW. **CCC.**
Published by: W.B. Saunders Co. (Subsidiary of: Harcourt Publishers Ltd.), Curtis Center, Independence Sq W, Philadelphia, PA 19106-3399. TEL 215-238-7800, 800-874-6418, FAX 215-238-6445, http://www.wbsaunders.com. **Subscr. to:** Periodicals Fulfillment, W B Saunders Co, 6277 Sea Harbor Dr, 4th Fl, Orlando, FL 32891-4800.

616.025 GBR ISSN 1472-0205 CODEN: JEMMEP
EMERGENCY MEDICINE JOURNAL. Abbreviated title: J A E M. Text in English. 1984. bi-m. GBP 100, USD 159 combined subscription to individuals includes print & online eds.; GBP 205, USD 324 to institutional members for print only (effective 2002). adv. bk.rev. abstr, bibl, illus. index. back issues avail. *Refereed.* **Document type:** *Journal, Academic/Scholarly.* **Description:** Acts as a major forum for education, research, and debate on all aspects of emergency medicine.
Former titles (until 2000): Journal of Accident and Emergency Medicine (1351-0622); (until 1993): Archives of Emergency Medicine (0264-4924)
Related titles: Microform ed.: (from PQC); Online - full text ed.: E M J Online. ISSN 1472-0213. 1999. GBP 65, USD 99 to individuals (effective 2002); Institutions contact publisher for online rates. (from EBSCO Publishing, O C L C Online Computer Library Center, Inc., RoweCom Information Quest, ingenta, HighWire Pr., Swets Blackwell, Ovid Technologies, Inc., Institute for Scientific Information).
Indexed: ASCA, Brit.Nur.Ind., Crim.Just.Abstr., Curr.Cont., Excerp.Med., Ind.Med. (1994-), Ind.Sci.Rev., Inpharma, Int.Nurs.Ind., Jrnl.Watch Emer.Med., Pharm.&Out.News, Reac., Rev.Appl.Entomol., SSCI (coverage dropped), Sci.Cit.Ind.
—BLDSC (3733.190420), CISTI, EMDOCS, GNLM, IDS, ingenta, KNAW. **CCC.**
Published by: (British Association for Accident and Emergency Medicine), B M J Publishing Group, B M A House, Tavistock Sq, London WC1H 9JR, United Kingdom. TEL 44-20-7387-4499, FAX 44-20-7383-6400, info.norththames@bma.org.uk, http://www.emjonline.com, http://www.bma.org.uk. Eds. Jim Wardrope, Peter Driscoll. R&P Carol Torselli TEL 44-20-7383-6674. Adv. contact Euan Currer TEL 44-20-7383-6181.

616.025 USA ISSN 1054-0725
EMERGENCY MEDICINE NEWS; reports on national news and trends in emergency medicine. Text in English. 1979. m. USD 152 domestic to individuals; USD 200 foreign to individuals; USD 212 domestic to institutions; USD 275 foreign to institutions (effective 2002); USD 18 newsstand/cover. adv. **Document type:** *Newspaper, Trade.* **Description:** Disseminates information in all areas of emergency medicine, as well as emergency departments and ambulatory care centers.
Former titles: Emergency Medicine and Ambulatory Care News; (until Aug. 1986): Emergency Department News
Published by: Lippincott Williams & Wilkins, 345 Hudson St, 16th Fl, New York, NY 10014-4502. TEL 212-840-7760, FAX 212-840-7813, http://www.lrpub.com, http://www.Lww.com. Ed. Lisa Hoffman. Pub. Nhora Cortes Comerer. R&P Kyle Booth. Adv. contact Ray Thibodeau. B&W page USD 3,775, color page USD 5,005. Circ: 23,000.

616.025 USA ISSN 0746-2506
EMERGENCY MEDICINE REPORTS; the practical journal for primary-care physicians. (Annual Emergency Medicine Reports Rapid Reference Cards also avail.) Text in English. 1980. bi-w. USD 337 domestic; USD 367 foreign; USD 26 newsstand/cover (effective 2001). **Document type:** *Newsletter.* **Description:** Features Review articles on important clinical issues in emergency medicine, with practical treatment recommendations. Topics covered include cardiology, trauma, infectious diseases, hormonal and metabolic disorders, orthopedics, etc.
Formerly (until 1983): E R Reports (Emergency Room) (0732-9628)
Related titles: CD-ROM ed.; Online - full text ed.: (from Northern Light Technology, Inc.).
Indexed: Ref.Zh.
—BLDSC (3733.190700).
Published by: American Health Consultants (Subsidiary of: Medical Economics Co., Inc.), P O Box 740056, Atlanta, GA 30374. TEL 404-262-7436, 800-688-2421, FAX 404 262-7837, 800-284-3291, custserv@ahcpub.com, http://www.emronline.com, http://www.ahcpub.com. Pub. Brenda L Mooney. Circ: 6,250.

EMERGENCY PRODUCT BUYER. see *MEDICAL SCIENCES—Surgery*

ENCYCLOPEDIE MEDICO-CHIRURGICALE. APARATO LOCOMOTOR; la referencia que necessita. see *MEDICAL SCIENCES—Rheumatology*

ENCYCLOPEDIE MEDICO-CHIRURGICALE. APPAREIL LOCOMOTEUR; vers le retour a la motricite. see *MEDICAL SCIENCES—Rheumatology*

617.585 FRA
ENCYCLOPEDIE MEDICO-CHIRURGICALE. PODOLOGIE. Cover title: Traite de Podologie. Text in French. 2 base vols. plus a. updates. bibl, charts, illus. *Refereed.* **Document type:** *Academic/Scholarly.* **Description:** Offers podiatrists a comprehensive reference for diagnosing and treating conditions affecting the feet.
Published by: Elsevier Paris, Editions Scientifiques et Medicales (Subsidiary of: Reed Elsevier plc. group), 23 rue Linois, Paris 75015, France. TEL 33-1-45589425, FAX 33-1-45589425, redaction-emc@elsevier.fr, redacion-emc@elsevier.fr, http://www.elsevier.fr, http://www.elsevier.com.

ENCYCLOPEDIE MEDICO-CHIRURGICALE. TRAITE DE RADIODIAGNOSTIC: SQUELETTE NORMAL - NEURORADIOLOGIE - APPAREIL LOCOMOTEUR. see *MEDICAL SCIENCES—Radiology And Nuclear Medicine*

ENCYCLOPEDIE MEDICO-CHIRURGICALE. TRAITE DE TECHNIQUES CHIRURGICALES. ORTHOPEDIE - TRAUMATOLOGIE. see *MEDICAL SCIENCES—Surgery*

616.02 FRA ISSN 1241-8234
ENCYCLOPEDIE MEDICO-CHIRURGICALE. URGENCES. Cover title: Traite d'Urgences. Variant title: Encyclopedie Medico-Chirurgicale, Instantanes Medicaux. Urgences. Text in French. 1939. 2 base vols. plus q. updates. bibl, charts, illus. *Refereed.* **Document type:** *Academic/Scholarly.* **Description:** Provides emergency-medicine practitioners with a comprehensive and up-to-date reference source to diagnose and treat medical conditions.
Former titles (until 1991): Encyclopedie Medico-Chirurgicale. Urgences Medicales et Chirurgicales (0246-0580); (until 1942): Encyclopedie Medico-Chirurgicale. Urgences (0246-0750)
Related titles: ♦ Italian ed.: Encyclopedie Medico-Chirurgicale. Urgenze. ISSN 1286-9341.
Published by: Elsevier Paris, Editions Scientifiques et Medicales (Subsidiary of: Reed Elsevier plc. group), 23 rue Linois, Paris 75015, France. TEL 33-1-45589110, FAX 33-1-45589425, http://www.elsevier.fr, http://www.elsevier.com.

616.02 FRA ISSN 1286-9341
ENCYCLOPEDIE MEDICO-CHIRURGICALE. URGENZE. Short title: Urgenze. Text in Italian. 2 base vols. plus q. updates. bibl, charts, illus. *Refereed.* **Document type:** *Academic/Scholarly.* **Description:** Provides emergency-medicine practitioners with a comprehensive and up-to-date reference to diagnose and treat a variety of medical conditions.
Related titles: ♦ French ed.: Encyclopedie Medico-Chirurgicale. Urgences. ISSN 1241-8234.
Published by: Elsevier Paris, Editions Scientifiques et Medicales (Subsidiary of: Reed Elsevier plc. group), 23 rue Linois, Paris 75015, France. TEL 33-1-45589110, FAX 33-1-45589425, redaction-emc@elsevier.fr, redacion-emc@elsevier.fr, http://www.elsevier.fr, http://www.elsevier.com.

617 GBR ISSN 0969-9546
EUROPEAN JOURNAL OF EMERGENCY MEDICINE. Text in English. 1994. q. USD 194 domestic to individuals; USD 194 foreign to individuals; USD 552 per issue domestic to institutions; USD 552 per issue foreign to institutions; USD 116 newsstand/cover (effective 2002). adv. reprints avail. *Refereed.* **Document type:** *Journal, Academic/Scholarly.* **Description:** Devoted to serving the European emergency medicine community and to promoting European standards of training, diagnosis and care.
Related titles: Online - full text ed.: USD 717.60 domestic academic site license; USD 717.60 foreign academic site license; USD 800.40 domestic corporate site license; USD 800.40 foreign corporate site license (effective 2002) (from EBSCO Publishing).
Indexed: Ind.Med. (1994-), Int.Nurs.Ind.
—BLDSC (3829.728600), CISTI, GNLM, KNAW.
Published by: (European Society of Emergency Medicine), Kluwer Academic & Lippencott-Raven (Subsidiary of: Wolters Kluwer N.V.), 2-6 Boundary Row, London SE1 8HN, United Kingdom. TEL 44-171-865-0198, FAX 44-171-410-6600, journal@rapidcom.co.uk, http://www.emergencymed.com, http://www.Lww.com. Ed. Herman Delooz. Adv. contact Gemma Heiser.

617.3 FRA
EUROPEAN JOURNAL OF ORTHOPAEDIC SURGERY. Text in English. 1987. q. FRF 1,643 foreign. **Document type:** *Academic/Scholarly.* **Description:** Contains original articles on orthopaedic surgery, anatomy and reconstructive surgery.
Former titles: Journal of Orthopaedic Surgery (1249-0237); French Journal of Orthopaedic Surgery (0981-1974)
Related titles: ♦ French ed.: Revue de Chirurgie Orthopedique et Reparatrice de l'Appareil Moteur. ISSN 0035-1040.
—GNLM.
Published by: Masson - Periodiques, Villa Laromiguiere, Paris 75005, France. TEL 1-40-46-62-00, FAX 1-40-46-62-01. Ed. J M Thomine.

617.3 FRA ISSN 0948-4817
EUROPEAN JOURNAL OF ORTHOPAEDIC SURGERY & TRAUMATOLOGY. Text in English; Abstracts in French. 1990. q. EUR 290 domestic; EUR 290 in Germany; EUR 106 newsstand/cover foreign (effective 2002). adv. **Document type:** *Academic/Scholarly.* **Description:** Original basic and clinical research articles on all aspects of orthopaedic surgery and traumatology.
Formerly: Orthopedie - Traumatologie (0940-3264)
Related titles: Microform ed.: (from PQC); Online - full text ed.: ISSN 1432-1068 (from EBSCO Publishing, RoweCom Information Quest, Swets Blackwell, Springer LINK).
—CISTI, GNLM, KNAW. **CCC.**
Published by: Springer-Verlag France (Subsidiary of: BertelsmannSpringer), 1 rue Paul Cezanne, Paris 75008, France. TEL 33-1-53933644, FAX 33-1-53933683, access@link.springer.de; york@springer-paris.fr, http://link.springer.de/link/service/journals/00590/index.htm. Ed. P Kehr. adv.: B&W page FRF 7,800, color page FRF 15,200; trim 210 x 275. **U.S. subscr. to:** Springer-Verlag New York Inc., PO Box 2485, Secaucus, NJ 07096-2485. **Co-sponsors:** Societe d'Orthopedie et de Traumatologie de l'Est; Group d'Etude pour la Chirurgie Osseuse European; Association of European Research Groups for Spinal Osteosynthesis.

EUROPEAN JOURNAL OF SPORTS TRAUMATOLOGY AND RELATED RESEARCH. see *MEDICAL SCIENCES—Sports Medicine*

617.1 DEU ISSN 1439-0590
EUROPEAN JOURNAL OF TRAUMA. Text in English, German; Summaries in English. 1975. bi-m. EUR 194.98 domestic; EUR 207.98 foreign; EUR 104.13 domestic to students; EUR 120.13 foreign to students; EUR 41.12 newsstand/cover (effective 2002). adv. *Refereed.* **Document type:** *Journal, Academic/Scholarly.*
Formerly (until 2000): Unfallchirurgie (0340-2649)
Related titles: Online - full text ed.: ISSN 1615-3146 (from RoweCom Information Quest, Swets Blackwell, Springer LINK).
Indexed: Ind.Med. (coverage dropped).
—BLDSC (3829.747130), CISTI, EMDOCS, GNLM, Infotrieve, KNAW. **CCC.**

Published by: Urban und Vogel Medien und Medizin Verlagsgesellschaft mbH (Subsidiary of: BertelsmannSpringer), Neumarkter Str 43, Munich 81673, Germany. TEL 49-89-43721411, FAX 49-89-43721410, ejt@urban-vogel.de, verlag@urban-vogel.de, http://www.urban-vogel.de. Ed. K H Jungbluth. R&P Oliver Renn. Adv. contact Paul Berger. Circ: 1,900. **Subscr. to:** Springer Auslieferungs Gesellschaft, Postfach 105160, Heidelberg 69041, Germany. TEL 49-6221-345244, FAX 49-6221-345244.

616.02 USA
▼ **EVERY SECOND COUNTS.** Text in English. 1999. bi-m. USD 32 to members; USD 38 to non-members (effective 2001). adv. **Document type:** *Trade.* **Description:** Contains valuable information on techniques, theory, equipment and case studies involving emergency medical response professionals.
Indexed: HRIS.
Published by: National Safety Council, 1121 Spring Lake Dr, Itasca, IL 60143. TEL 630-285-1121, 800-621-7619, FAX 630-775-2310, growj@nsc.org, http://www.nsc.org. Ed. Jennifer Grow. Circ: 30,000 (controlled).

EXCERPTA MEDICA. SECTION 19: REHABILITATION AND PHYSICAL MEDICINE. see *MEDICAL SCIENCES—Abstracting, Bibliographies, Statistics*

EXCERPTA MEDICA. SECTION 33: ORTHOPEDIC SURGERY. see *MEDICAL SCIENCES—Abstracting, Bibliographies, Statistics*

EXTRACTA ORTHOPAEDICA; Weltweit Auserlesen. see *MEDICAL SCIENCES—Abstracting, Bibliographies, Statistics*

617.752 658.8 GBR
EYEWEAR: THE INTERNATIONAL MARKET. Text in English. a. GBP 2,250, USD 4,500 (effective 1999). **Document type:** *Trade.* **Description:** Analyzes the eye-glass and contact lens market for Canada, France, Germany, Italy, Spain, the U.K., the U.S., and Japan.
Formerly (until 1995): Spectacles and Contact Lenses: The International Market
Related titles: Online - full text ed.: (from Data-Star, The Dialog Corporation).
Published by: Euromonitor, 60-61 Britton Rd, London EC1 5UX, United Kingdom. TEL 44-171-251-8024, info@euromonitor.com, http://www.euromonitor.com.

616.02 USA ISSN 1532-1568
FIRE INSIDER. Text in English. m. USD 119 domestic; USD 127 in Canada & Mexico; USD 144 foreign (effective 2001). back issues avail.; reprints avail. **Document type:** *Newsletter, Trade.* **Description:** Covers fire service personnel and events. Includes analysis of news of major fire associations, industrial fire issues, and other resources.
Related titles: Abridged ed.
Published by: J E M S Communications, 1947 Camino Vida Roble, Ste 200, Carlsbad, CA 92008. TEL 800-266-JEMS, http://www.fireinsider.com. Ed. Tim Elliott.

617.3 DNK ISSN 0901-0408
FODTERAPEUTEN✱. Text in Danish. 1932. m. (10/yr.). DKK 145. adv. bk.rev.
Published by: Landsforeningen af Statsautoriserede Fodterapeuter, Noerre Voldagde 90, Copenhagen K 1358, Denmark. Ed. Anita Ellekjaer Hansen. Circ: 1,600.

617.1 GBR ISSN 0958-2592
CODEN: FOOTEE
THE FOOT; international journal of clinical foot science. Text in English. 1991. q. GBP 65 to individuals; GBP 166 to institutions (effective 2002). adv. *Refereed.* **Document type:** *Journal, Academic/Scholarly.* **Description:** Contains primary articles and commissioned reviews on disorders of the foot and their medical or surgical treatment.
Related titles: Online - full text ed.: (from EBSCO Publishing, O C L C Online Computer Library Center, Inc., Swets Blackwell, IDEAL Online Library).
Indexed: AMED, Excerp.Med. (1993-), Ref.Zh.
—BLDSC (3984.840000), EMDOCS, GNLM, Infotrieve, KNAW. **CCC.**
Published by: Churchill Livingstone (Subsidiary of: Harcourt Publishers Ltd.), Robert Stevenson House, 1-3 Baxter's Pl, Leith Walk, Edinburgh, Midlothian EH1 3AF, United Kingdom. TEL 44-131-556-2424, FAX 44-131-558-1278, journals@harcourt.com, http://www.harcourt-international.com/journals/foot. Eds. T Duckworth, T W D Smith. Pub. Susan Young. R&P Sharon Boyle TEL 44-131-524-1747. Adv. contact David Dunnachie. Circ: 5,700. **Subscr. in the US to:** Harcourt Health Sciences, Journals Subscription Department, PO Box 156, Avenel, NJ 07001. TEL 877-839-7126; **Subscr. to:** Harcourt Publishers Ltd., Journal Sales & Marketing Dept., 32 Jamestown Rd, London NW1 7BY, United Kingdom. TEL 44-20-8308-5700.

617.3 USA ISSN 1083-7515
FOOT AND ANKLE CLINICS. Text in English. 1996. q. USD 131 domestic to individuals; USD 147 in Canada to individuals; USD 174 elsewhere to individuals; USD 171 domestic to institutions; USD 198 foreign to institutions; USD 50 per issue (effective 2001). *Refereed.* **Document type:** *Journal, Academic/Scholarly.* **Description:** Delivers practical advice from experts in specialty covered and a fresh perspective on problems and controversies.
Indexed: Ind.Med. (1996-).
Published by: W.B. Saunders Co. (Subsidiary of: Harcourt Publishers Ltd.), 11830 Westline Industrial Dr, St Louis, MO 63146. TEL 800-325-4177, wbspcs@harcourtbrace.com, http://www.wbsaunders.com. Ed. Dr. Mark Myerson. **Subscr. to:** Periodicals Dept, 6277 Sea Harbor Dr, 4th Fl, Orlando, FL 32891. TEL 800-654-2452, FAX 800-574-6418.

617.3 USA ISSN 1071-1007
RD781 CODEN: FAINE4
FOOT & ANKLE INTERNATIONAL✱. Text in English. 1980. m. USD 149 domestic to individuals; USD 197 foreign to individuals; USD 180 domestic to institutions; USD 234 foreign to institutions (effective 2000). adv. bk.rev. back issues avail. *Refereed.* **Document type:** *Academic/Scholarly.* **Description:** Focuses on new approaches to foot and ankle disorders and surgical treatment for orthopedic surgeons and podiatrists.
Formerly (until 1994): Foot and Ankle (0198-0211)
Related titles: Microfilm ed.: (from WWS); Online - full text ed.: (from Institute for Scientific Information).
Indexed: AMED, ASCA, Curr.Cont., Excerp.Med., Focus on: Sports Sci.& Med., INIS Atomind., Ind.Med. (1994-), Inpharma, Reac., Rev.Med.& Vet.Mycol., Sportsearch (1981-).
—BLDSC (3984.860000), EMDOCS, GNLM, IDS, ingenta, KNAW.
Published by: American Orthopaedic Foot and Ankle Society, 1216 Pine St, Ste 201, Seattle, WA 98101. TEL 206-223-1120, FAX 206-223-1178, aofas@aofas.org, http://www.aofas.org/. Ed. Dr. Lowell D Lutter. adv.: B&W page USD 715; trim 10.88 x 8.13. Circ: 4,062; 3,997 (paid).

617.3 USA ISSN 1068-3100
FOOT AND ANKLE QUARTERLY. Text in English. 1988. q. USD 195 domestic to individuals; USD 295 domestic to institutions; USD 330 foreign (effective 2000). adv. **Document type:** *Academic/Scholarly.* **Description:** Provides condensations of current podiatric literature accompanied by in-depth commentaries written by experts on the editorial board. Each issue also includes one 90-minute audio tape lecture and a continuing education exam.
Formerly (until 1993): Podiatry Tracts (0894-6116)
Indexed: CINAHL.
—BLDSC (3984.870000). **CCC.**
Published by: Data Trace Publishing Company, 110 West Rd, Ste 227, Baltimore, MD 21204. TEL 410-494-4994, FAX 410-494-0515, info@datatrace.com, http:.//www.datatrace.com, http://www.datatrace.com. Ed. Lawrence Lavery. R&P Cindy Lee Floyd. Adv. contact Frank Tufariello.

617.3 GBR ISSN 0266-6901
FRACTURE MAGAZINE. Text in English. 1984. q. free to customers. **Document type:** *Academic/Scholarly.*
—BLDSC (4030.759000).
Published by: Smith and Nephew Medical Ltd., Hessle Rd, PO Box 81, Hull, N Humberside HU3 2BN, United Kingdom. TEL 44-1482-225181, FAX 44-1482-328326. Ed. June Bogie. **Dist. in US by:** Smith & Nephew Casting, 2500 Distribution St, Charlotte, NC 28203.

617.3 DEU ISSN 1433-1861
CODEN: FUBEEE
DIE FUNKTIONSKRANKHEITEN DES BEWEGUNGSSYSTEMS; Zeitschrift fuer interdisziplinaere Diagnostik und Therapie. Text in German. 1986. 2/yr. EUR 85 (effective 2002). **Document type:** *Journal, Academic/Scholarly.*
Formerly (until 1998): Die Funktionskrankheiten des Bewegungsapparates (0258-2015)
—CISTI, GNLM, Infotrieve. **CCC.**
Published by: (Internationaler Arbeitskreis zur Erforschung der Funktionskrankheiten des Bewegungsapparates e.V.), Urban & Fischer Verlag, Loebdergraben 14a, Jena 07743, Germany. TEL 49-3641-626444, FAX 49-3641-626500, marketing.journals@urbanfischer.de, http://www.urbanfischer.de/journals. Ed. B Alt. R&P Martin Huber TEL 49-3641-626430. **Dist. by:** Nature Publishing Group.

GAIT AND POSTURE. see *MEDICAL SCIENCES*

617.3 RUS ISSN 1028-4427
GENII ORTOPEDII. Text in Russian. 1995. q. USD 215 in North America (effective 2000).
Indexed: Ref.Zh.
Published by: Redaktsiya Genii Ortopedii, Ul M Ul'yanovoi 6, Kurgan 640005, Russian Federation. TEL 35222-3-33-10, FAX 35222-3-60-46. Ed. V I Shevtsov. **Dist. by:** East View Publications, 3020 Harbor Ln N, Minneapolis, MN 55447. TEL 763-550-0961, FAX 763-559-2931.

617.3 ITA ISSN 0390-0134
GIORNALE ITALIANO DI ORTOPEDIA E TRAUMATOLOGIA. Text in Italian. 1975. 4/yr. USD 200 Italian ed.; USD 110 English ed.. adv. bk.rev. Supplement avail. **Description:** Covers current thought, practice and research in the science of orthopedics and traumatology.
Related titles: ♦ English ed.: Orthopaedic and Traumatology. ISSN 1129-3853.
Indexed: Biol.Abstr., Dent.Ind., Excerp.Med., Ind.Med. (coverage dropped), Rev.Med.& Vet.Mycol.
—GNLM.
Published by: Springer-Verlag Italia Srl (Subsidiary of: BertelsmannSpringer), Via Podgora, 4, Milan, MI 20122, Italy. TEL 39-2-55194656, FAX 39-2-55193360, springer@springer.it, http://link.springer.de. Circ: 4,750.

616.02 USA ISSN 0017-1565
GOLD CROSS. Text in English. 1930. q. USD 18 to non-members; USD 10 to members. adv.
Published by: (New Jersey State First Aid Council, Inc.), Leonard Publications, Inc., 10 W. Hanover Ave., Mt. Freedom, NJ 07970. TEL 973-895-9351. Ed. Julie Aberger. Circ: 6,700.

617.3 618.92 FRA ISSN 1266-7412
GROUPE D'ETUDE EN ORTHOPEDIE PEDIATRIQUE. LETTRE. Key Title: Lettre du G E O P. Text in French. 1995. 4/yr. FRF 150; FRF 150 foreign (effective 1997).
Published by: (Groupe d'Etude en Orthopedie Pediatrique), Expansion Scientifique Francaise, 31 bd. de la Tour Maubourg, Paris Cedex 7 75343, France. TEL 33-1-40626400, FAX 33-1-45556920. Circ: 6,000.

617.1 FRA
GUIDE ANNUEL DES S A M U ET S M U R DE FRANCE. (Services d'Aide Medicale Urgente) Text in French. 1988. biennial, latest 2001. FRF 450 domestic; FRF 500 foreign (effective 2002). 280 p./no. back issues avail. **Document type:** *Yearbook.*
Published by: Societe Francaise d'Editions Medicales, 22-H rue du Chateau des Rentiers, Paris 75013, France. TEL 33-01-45835054, FAX 33-01-45831354, sfem96@mail.club-internet.fr. Pub. Colette Gallula.

617 JPN ISSN 0917-365X
HAMAMATSU SEIKEI GEKA KIYO/HAMAMATSU UNIVERSITY. ANNUAL OF ORTHOPAEDIC SURGERY. Text in Japanese. 1990. a. **Document type:** *Bulletin, Academic/Scholarly.*
Published by: Hamamatsu Ika Daigaku, Seikei Gekagaku Kyoshitsu/Hamamatsu University, School of Medicine, Department of Orthopaedics, 1-20-1 Handayama, Hamamatsu-shi, Shizuoka-ken 431-3192, Japan. TEL 81-53-435-2299, FAX 81-53-435-2296.

M

617 USA ISSN 0749-0712
HAND CLINICS. Text in English. 1985. q. USD 170 domestic to individuals; USD 194 in Canada to individuals; USD 218 elsewhere to individuals; USD 234 domestic to institutions; USD 274 foreign to institutions; USD 69 per issue (effective 2001). back issues avail. *Refereed.* **Document type:** *Academic/Scholarly.*
Description: Each issue addresses a single topic in the surgical therapy of patients with disorders of the hand.
Related titles: Microfilm ed.; Online - full text ed.: (from Institute for Scientific Information).
Indexed: ASCA, CINAHL, Curr.Cont., Excerp.Med., INIS Atomind., Ind.Med. (1985-), Inpharma, Pharm.&Out.News, Reac., SSCI (coverage dropped).
—BLDSC (4241.558000), CISTI, EMDOCS, GNLM, IDS, ingenta, KNAW. **CCC.**
Published by: W.B. Saunders Co. (Subsidiary of: Harcourt Publishers Ltd.), 11830 Westline Industrial Dr, St Louis, MO 63146. TEL 800-325-4177, http://www.wbsaunders.com. Ed. Raoul Tubiana. **Subscr. to:** Periodicals Fulfillment, W B Saunders Co, 6277 Sea Harbor Dr, 4th Fl, Orlando, FL 32891-4800.

610 USA ISSN 0085-1469
CODEN: HUFHAR
HEFTE ZUR UNFALLHEILKUNDE. Text in English. irreg., latest vol.217, 1991. price varies. reprint service avail. from ISI. **Document type:** *Academic/Scholarly.*
Related titles: Microform ed.: (from PQC).
Indexed: Biol.Abstr., Excerp.Med., Ind.Med. (coverage dropped).
—CISTI, GNLM, KNAW. **CCC.**
Published by: Springer-Verlag, Journals (Subsidiary of: BertelsmannSpringer), 175 Fifth Ave, New York, NY 10010. TEL 212-460-1500, FAX 212-473-6272.

617.3 JPN ISSN 0915-8855
HIGASHINIHON RINSHO SEIKEI GEKA GAKKAI ZASSHI/EASTERN JAPAN JOURNAL OF CLINICAL ORTHOPAEDICS. Text in Japanese. 1989. irreg.
Published by: Higashinihon Rinsho Seikei Geka Gakkai/Eastern Japan Society of Clinical Orthopaedics, Nihon Daigaku Igakubu, Seikei Gekagaku Kyoshitsu, 30-1, Oyaguchi Kamicho, Itabashi-ku, Tokyo 173, Japan.

617.3 JPN ISSN 0389-3634
HIP JOINT. Text in Japanese. 1975. a. JPY 9,000 per issue.
—CISTI.
Published by: Nihon Kokansetsu Gakkai/Japanese Hip Society, Yamanashi Ika Daigaku Seikei Gekagaku Kyoshitsu, 1110 Shimo-Gato, Nakakoma-gun, Tamaho-cho, Yamanashi-ken 409-3821, Japan.

617.3 JPN ISSN 0018-3377
HOKKAIDO JOURNAL OF ORTHOPEDIC & TRAUMATIC SURGERY/HOKKAIDO SEIKEI SAIGAI GEKA ZASSHI. Text in English, Japanese. 1954. a.
Indexed: Biol.Abstr., Excerp.Med., INIS Atomind.
Published by: Hokkaido Orthopedic and Traumatic Surgery Society/Hokkaido Seikei Saigai Geka Gakkai, c/o Hokkaido Daigaku Igakubu Seikei Geka Kyoshitsu, Nishi 7-chome, Kita 15-jo, Kita-ku, Sapporo-shi, Hokkaido 060, Japan. Circ: 750.

616.02 AUS ISSN 1024-9079
HONG KONG JOURNAL OF EMERGENCY MEDICINE. Text in English. 1994. q. AUD 238 domestic; AUD 216 in New Zealand; USD 132 elsewhere; AUD 262 domestic print & online eds.; AUD 238 in New Zealand print & online eds.; USD 146 elsewhere print & online eds. (effective 2001). adv. **Document type:** *Journal, Academic/Scholarly.*
Related titles: ♦ Online - full text ed.: Hong Kong Journal of Emergency Medicine Online.
Published by: Blackwell Science Asia Pty Ltd, PO Box 378, Carlton South, VIC 3053, Australia. TEL 61-3-9347-0300, FAX 61-3-9347-5001, info@blacksci-asia.com.au, http://www.blacksci.co.uk/australi. Ed. Kim Lian Ong.

616.02 AUS
HONG KONG JOURNAL OF EMERGENCY MEDICINE ONLINE. Text in English. s-a. AUD 215 domestic; AUD 195 in New Zealand; USD 119 elsewhere (effective 2001). **Document type:** *Academic/Scholarly.*
Media: Online - full text. **Related titles:** ♦ Print ed.: Hong Kong Journal of Emergency Medicine. ISSN 1024-9079.
Published by: Blackwell Science Asia Pty Ltd, PO Box 378, Carlton South, VIC 3053, Australia. TEL 61-3-9347-0300, FAX 61-3-9347-3016, info@blacksci-asia.com.au, http://www.blacksci.co.uk/australi.

617.3 HKG ISSN 1028-2637
HONG KONG JOURNAL OF ORTHOPAEDIC SURGERY. Text in English. 1997. s-a. USD 30 (effective 2002).
Published by: Lippincott Williams & Wilkins Asia, Ste 907-910, New T&T Centre, Harbour City, 7 Canton Rd, Tsimshatsui, Kowtoon, Hong Kong. Ed. Wing-Cheung Wu.

617.3 USA ISSN 0018-5647
CODEN: BHJDEI
HOSPITAL FOR JOINT DISEASES. BULLETIN. Text in English. 1940. q. USD 72 (effective 2000). adv. bk.rev. charts, illus. cum.index: 1965-81; 1982-85; 1986-89. reprint service avail. from PQC,ISI. **Document type:** *Academic/Scholarly.*
Former titles (until 1992): Hospital for Joint Diseases Orthopaedic Institute. Bulletin (0883-9344); Hospital for Joint Diseases. Bulletin (0018-5647)
Indexed: Bioeng.Abstr., Biol.Abstr., Curr.Cont. (coverage dropped), Eng.Ind., Excerp.Med., INIS Atomind., Ind.Med. (1992-).
—BLDSC (2555.330000), CISTI, Ei, EMDOCS, GNLM, KNAW. **CCC.**
Published by: J. Michael Ryan Publishing, Inc., 24 Crescent Dr N, Andover, NJ 07821-4000. TEL 973-786-7777, FAX 973-786-7776. Ed. Dr. William Jaffe. R&P, Adv. contact James Costello. Circ: 2,500.

617.585 USA
HOSPITAL PODIATRIST. Text in English. 1976. a. membership. bk.rev. back issues avail. **Document type:** *Academic/Scholarly.*
Published by: American Association of Hospital Podiatrists, c/o Dr Earl L Cherniak, Ed, 3984 S Figueroa St, Los Angeles, CA 90037. TEL 213-747-7272, FAX 310-476-8003. Ed., R&P, Adv. contact Earl L Cherniak. Circ: 2,000.

616.025 JPN ISSN 0912-117X
IBARAKIKEN KYUKYU IGAKKAI ZASSHI/IBARAKI JOURNAL OF ACUTE MEDICINE. Text in Japanese. a. **Document type:** *Academic/Scholarly.*
Published by: Ibarakiken Ishikai, Kyukyu Iryo Kyokai, 489 Kasahara-cho, Mito-shi, Ibaraki-ken 310-0852, Japan.

617.3 IND ISSN 0019-5413
CODEN: INJOAU
INDIAN JOURNAL OF ORTHOPAEDICS. Text in English. 1967. s-a. INR 125, USD 30. adv. bk.rev. bibl, charts, illus. index.
Indexed: Excerp.Med., Indian Sci.Abstr.
—CISTI, GNLM.
Published by: (Indian Orthopaedic Association), Banaras Hindu University, Institute of Medical Sciences, Varanasi, Uttar Pradesh 221 005, India. Eds. Dr. S M Tuli, Dr. T P Srivastava. Circ: 1,600.

617 GBR ISSN 0020-1383
CODEN: INJUBF
INJURY; British journal of accident surgery. Text in English. 1969. 10/yr. EUR 114 in Europe to qualified personnel; JPY 15,100 in Japan to qualified personnel; USD 127 elsewhere to qualified personnel; EUR 631 in Europe to institutions; JPY 83,800 in Japan to institutions; USD 706 elsewhere to institutions (effective 2002). adv. bk.rev. abstr, bibl, illus. index. back issues avail. *Refereed.* **Document type:** *Academic/Scholarly.*
Description: Deals with all aspects of trauma, including fractures and soft-tissue injuries, and covers problems in the accident unit.
Related titles: Microform ed.: (from PQC); Online - full text ed.: (from ingenta, Swets Blackwell, ScienceDirect, Institute for Scientific Information).
Indexed: AMED, ASCA, Biol.Abstr., Curr.Adv.Ecol.Sci., Curr.Cont., Dent.Ind., Dok.Arbeitsmed., Environ.Sci.Poll.Mgmt., Excerp.Med., HRIS, Ind.Med. (1969-), Inpharma, Int.Nurs.Ind., Pharm.&Out.News, Pollut.Abstr., Reac., Rev.Med.& Vet.Mycol., Risk Abstr., Saf.Sci.Abstr.
—BLDSC (4514.400000), GNLM, IDS, ingenta, KNAW. **CCC.**
Published by: (Institute of Accident Surgery), Pergamon (Subsidiary of: Elsevier Science), The Boulevard, Langford Ln, East Park, Kidlington, Oxford OXB 1GB, United Kingdom. FAX 44-1865-843010, http://www.elsevier.com/locate/injury. Ed. S Krickler. **Subscr. in Australasia and the Far East to:** Elsevier Science (Singapore) Pte Ltd, No.1 Temasek Ave., No.17-01 Millenia Tower, Singapore 039192, Singapore. TEL 65-434-3727; **Subscr. in the Americas to:** Elsevier Science, PO Box 945, New York, NY 10159-0945. TEL 212-633-3730, FAX 212-633-3680, usinfo-f@elsevier.com; **Subscr. to:** Elsevier Science BV, PO Box 212, Amsterdam 1000 AE, Netherlands. TEL 31-20-485-3757, FAX 31-20-485-3432.

INTERNATIONAL JOURNAL OF TRAUMA NURSING. see *MEDICAL SCIENCES—Nurses And Nursing*

617.3 DEU ISSN 0341-2695
INTERNATIONAL ORTHOPAEDICS. Text in English, French. 1977. bi-m. EUR 592.90 domestic; EUR 583.40 in Germany; EUR 114 newsstand/cover foreign (effective 2002). adv. illus. index. reprint service avail. from ISI. *Refereed.* **Document type:** *Proceedings, Academic/Scholarly.* **Description:** Presents articles dealing with clinical orthopedic surgery or basic research directly connected with orthopedic surgery.
Supersedes (1929-1972): International Society of Orthopaedic Surgery and Traumatology. Proceedings of Congresses (0074-8552)
Related titles: Microform ed.: (from PQC); Online - full text ed.: ISSN 1432-5195 (from EBSCO Publishing, RoweCom Information Quest, Swets Blackwell, Springer LINK, Institute for Scientific Information).
Indexed: ASCA, Cal.Tiss.Abstr. (coverage dropped), Curr.Adv.Cancer Res., Curr.Cont., Excerp.Med., INIS Atomind., Ind.Med. (1977-), Ind.Sci.Rev., Inpharma, Int.Nurs.Ind., Pharm.&Out.News, Reac., Sci.Cit.Ind. (coverage dropped), Tox.Abstr. (coverage dropped).
—BLDSC (4544.856000), CISTI, EMDOCS, GNLM, IDS, ingenta, KNAW. **CCC.**
Published by: (Societe Internationale de Chirurgie Orthopedique et de Traumatologie BEL), Springer-Verlag (Subsidiary of: BertelsmannSpringer), Tiergartenstr 17, Heidelberg 69121, Germany. TEL 49-6221-345-0, FAX 49-6221-345229, subscriptions@springer.de, http://link.springer.de/link/service/journals/00264/index.htm, http://www.springer.de. Ed. K Skou-Andersen. **Subscr. in N. America to:** Springer-Verlag New York Inc., PO Box 2485, Secaucus, NJ 07096-2485. TEL 212-460-1500, FAX 212-473-6272.

616.02 USA ISSN 1092-4051
THE INTERNET JOURNAL OF EMERGENCY AND INTENSIVE CARE MEDICINE. Text in English. 1997. s-a. free per issue to qualified personnel. adv. bk.rev. back issues avail. *Refereed.* **Document type:** *Academic/Scholarly.* **Description:** Contains information from the field of critical care and intensive care medicine. Original articles, reviews, case reports, streaming slide shows, streaming videos, letters to the editor, press releases, meeting information.
Media: Online - full text.
Published by: Internet Scientific Publications, L.L.C., 23 Rippling Creek Dr, Sugar Land, TX 77479. TEL 281-240-1533, FAX 281-240-1533, jnates@anesl.med.uth.tmc.edu, http://www.ispub.com/journals/ijeicm.htm. Ed. Joseph Nates. R&P, Adv. contact Hope Morrow TEL 832-754-0335.

617.47 USA
▼ **THE INTERNET JOURNAL OF ORTHOPEDIC SURGERY.** Text in English. 2000. s-a. free per issue. adv. bk.rev. back issues avail. *Refereed.* **Document type:** *Academic/Scholarly.* **Description:** Provides information from the field of orthopedic surgery; contains original articles, reviews, case reports, streaming slide shows, streaming videos, letters to the editor, press releases, meeting information.
Media: Online - full content.
Published by: Internet Scientific Publications, L.L.C., 23 Rippling Creek Dr, Sugar Land, TX 77479. TEL 281-240-1533, FAX 281-240-1533, http://www.ispub.com/. R&P, Adv. contact Hope Morrow TEL 832-754-0335.

616.02 USA
THE INTERNET JOURNAL OF RESCUE AND DISASTER MEDICINE. Text in English. 1998. s-a. free per issue. adv. back issues avail. *Refereed.* **Document type:** *Academic/Scholarly.* **Description:** Contains information from the field of rescue medicine, traumatology, air rescue, aeromedical transportation, disaster medicine. Original articles, reviews, case reports, streaming slide shows, streaming videos, letters to the editor, press releases, meeting information.
Formed by the merger of (1997-1998): Internet Journal of Aeromedical Transportation; (1997-1998): Internet Journal of Disaster Medicine
Media: Online - full text.
Published by: Internet Scientific Publications, L.L.C., 23 Rippling Creek Dr, Sugar Land, TX 77479. TEL 281-240-1533, FAX 281-240-1533, hersche@netway.at, http://www.ispub.com/journals/ijrdm.htm. Pub., R&P, Adv. contact Hope Morrow TEL 832-754-0335.

M

617.3 USA
THE IOWA ORTHOPAEDIC JOURNAL. Text in English. 1981. a. USD 35; USD 50 foreign (effective 1998). adv. illus. *Refereed.* **Document type:** *Academic/Scholarly.* **Description:** Publishes articles relevant to orthopedic science, surgery and teaching.
Indexed: Ind.Med. (coverage dropped).
—BLDSC (4566.540000).
Published by: University of Iowa, Department of Orthopaedics, 200 Hawkins Dr, Iowa City, IA 52242-1008. TEL 319-356-2383, FAX 319-353-6754. Eds. Dennis Weigel, Matt Dobbs. Adv. contact Todd Williams. **Co-sponsor:** Iowa Orthopaedic Society.

ISOKINETICS AND EXERCISE SCIENCE. see *MEDICAL SCIENCES—Sports Medicine*

J O H N S: JOURNAL OF OTOLARYNGOLOGY, HEAD AND NECK SURGERY/JIBI INKOKA, TOKEIBU GEKA. see *MEDICAL SCIENCES—Otorhinolaryngology*

617.3 JPN
JAPAN KNEE SOCIETY. JOURNAL. Text in Japanese; Summaries in English, Japanese. s-a. USD 50 (effective 2000). adv. *Refereed.* **Document type:** *Proceedings.*
Formerly (until 1999): Tokyo Hiza Kansetsu Gakkai Kaishi
Published by: Japan Knee Society, Dept of Orthopaedic Surgery School of Medicine, University, 1-8-1 Inohana, Chuo-ku, Chiba-shi 260-0856, Japan. TEL 81-43-226-2338, FAX 81-43-226-2369, moriyati@doc.ho.chiba-u.ac.jp. Ed., R&P, Adv. contact Hideshige Moriya.

617.3 JPN
JAPANESE SOCIETY FOR STUDY OF BONE AND JOINT INFECTIONS. JOURNAL*. Text in Japanese. 1978. a. JPY 3,000. *Refereed.* **Document type:** *Academic/Scholarly.*
Former titles (until 1997): Kotsu Kansetsu Kansensho - Japanese Society for Study of Bone and Joint Infections. Proceedings of the Annual Meeting; Nihon Kotsu Kansetsu Kansensho Kenkyukai
Published by: Nihon Kotsu Kansetsu Kansensho Kenkyukai/Japanese Society of Rheumatism and Joint Surgery, Okayama University Medical School, Department of Orthopaedic Surgery, 2-5-1 Shikata-cho, Okayama 700-8558, Japan. TEL 81-86-235-7273, FAX 81-86-223-9727, orthop@md.okayama-u.ac.jp. Ed. Koichiro Hayashi.

617.3 DEU ISSN 1432-5152
JATROS ORTHO. Text in German. 1986. 12/yr. DEM 140. back issues avail. **Document type:** *Academic/Scholarly.* **Description:** Seminar papers containing summaries of orthopaedic articles, interviews and congress reports.
Former titles: Jatros Orthopaedie - Rheumatologie - Sportmedizin (0941-4770); (until 1992): Jatros Orthopaedie, Traumatologie (0941-3901); (until 1989): Jatros Orthopaedie (0930-8326)
—GNLM.
Published by: Hoffmann und Hoffmann GmbH, August-Schanz-Str 8-II, Frankfurt A.m. 60433, Germany. TEL 49-69-54800015, FAX 49-69-54800080, huhgmbh@aol.com. Ed. Peter Hoffmann. Circ: 7,000.

616.025 CHN ISSN 1006-463X
JIZHEN YIXUE/JOURNAL OF ENERGENCY MEDICINE. Text in Chinese. 1990. bi-m. USD 16.20; CNY 4.50, USD 2.70 newsstand/cover (effective 2001). **Document type:** *Academic/Scholarly.*
Related titles: Online - full content ed.: (from WanFang Data Corp.).
Published by: Zhonghua Yixuehui, Jizhen Yixue Fenhui, 68, Jiefang Lu, Hangzhou 310009, China. TEL 86-571-7077272 ext 5323, FAX 86-571-7228649, jzyx@mail.hz.zj.cn. Ed. Deyun Ding. **Dist. by:** China International Book Trading Corp, 35, Chegongzhuang Xilu, Haidian District, Beijing 100044, China. TEL 86-1-68413849, FAX 86-1-68412048, cibtc@mail.cibtc.com.cn, http://www.cibtc.com.cn.

616.7 FRA ISSN 1297-319X
JOINT BONE SPINE. Text in English. bi-m. EUR 235 in Europe to institutions; USD 324 elsewhere to institutions; EUR 185 in Europe to individuals; USD 224 elsewhere to individuals (effective 2002).
Related titles: Online - full text ed.: (from Institute for Scientific Information).
Indexed: Curr.Cont., Ind.Med., Sci.Cit.Ind.
—BLDSC (4672.250420).
Published by: Elsevier Paris, Editions Scientifiques et Medicales (Subsidiary of: Reed Elsevier plc. group), 23 rue Linois, Paris 75015, France. http://www.elsevier.com/locate/jbspin.

616 USA ISSN 1078-6260
THE JOINT LETTER. Text in English. 1995. 11/yr., latest vol.7. USD 120 domestic to individuals; USD 145 foreign to individuals; USD 185 domestic to institutions; USD 209 foreign to institutions; USD 19 newsstand/cover (effective 2002). **Document type:** *Newsletter.* **Description:** Covers joint function, disease and injury.
Related titles: Online - full text ed.: USD 240.50 domestic for academic site license; USD 264.50 foreign for academic site license; USD 268.25 domestic for corporate site license; USD 292.25 foreign for corporate site license (effective 2002).
Published by: Lippincott Williams & Wilkins (Philadelphia) (Subsidiary of: Wolters Kluwer N.V.), 530 Walnut St, Philadelphia, PA 19106-3621. TEL 215-521-8300, FAX 215-521-8902, http://www.lww.com. Eds. Dr. Joseph P Iannotti, Dr. Stanley A Herring. **Subscr. to:** PO Box 1600, Hagerstown, MD 21740-1600. TEL 800-777-2295, FAX 301-824-7390.

617.3 FRA ISSN 0242-648X
JOURNAL DE READAPTATION MEDICALE. Text in French. 4/yr. FRF 716; FRF 974 foreign (effective 2000). **Document type:** *Academic/Scholarly.* **Description:** Deals with different therapies, as well as the material problems in kinesitherapy, ergotherapy and orthophony.
Related titles: Online - full text ed.: (from RoweCom Information Quest).
—**CCC.**
Published by: Masson - Periodiques, 120 bd. St. Germain, Paris 75006, France. TEL 33-1-40466200, FAX 33-1-40466201. Ed. J M Wirotius. Circ: 1,000. **Subscr. to:** Societe de Periodiques Specialises, BP 22, Vineuil Cedex 41354, France. TEL 33-2-54504612, FAX 33-2-54504611.

616 FRA ISSN 0993-9857
CODEN: JEURE
JOURNAL EUROPEEN DES URGENCES/EUROPEAN JOURNAL OF EMERGENCIES. Variant title: J E U R. Text in English, French. 1988. 4/yr. FRF 756; FRF 957 foreign (effective 2000). adv. back issues avail. **Document type:** *Academic/Scholarly.* **Description:** Includes original articles, brief reviews, clinical cases and letters. Practical guide to emergency medicine for hospital practitioners.
Related titles: Online - full text ed.: (from RoweCom Information Quest).
Indexed: Excerp.Med.
—BLDSC (4979.640500), EMDOCS, GNLM, KNAW.
Published by: Masson - Periodiques, 120 bd. St. Germain, Paris 75006, France. TEL 33-1-40466200, FAX 33-1-40466201, TELEX 202 671 F. Ed. Patrick Barriot. Circ: 1,500. **Subscr. to:** Societe de Periodiques Specialises, BP 22, Vineuil Cedex 41354, France. TEL 33-2-54504612, FAX 33-2-54504611.

JOURNAL OF APPLIED BIOMECHANICS. see *BIOLOGY—Physiology*

617.3 USA ISSN 0883-5403
CODEN: JOAREG
JOURNAL OF ARTHROPLASTY. Text in English. 1986. 8/yr. USD 251 domestic to individuals Full text online included; USD 330 foreign to individuals Full text online included; USD 362 domestic to institutions Full text online included; USD 453 foreign to institutions Full text online included; USD 113 domestic to students Full text online included; USD 132 foreign to students Full text online included; USD 57 per issue (effective 2001). adv. charts, illus, tr.lit. index. back issues avail. *Refereed.* **Document type:** *Academic/Scholarly.* **Description:** Basic scientific and clinical information on joint replacement surgery. Covers surgical techniques, prosthetic design, biomechanics, biomaterials, metallurgy, and the biologic response to arthroplasty materials in vivo and in vitro.
Related titles: Microfilm ed.: 1986; Online - full text ed.: (from IDEAL Online Library, Institute for Scientific Information).
Indexed: ASCA, Curr.Cont., Excerp.Med., INIS Atomind., Ind.Med. (1986-), Inpharma, Int.Nurs.Ind., Mat.Sci.Cit.Ind. (coverage dropped), Pharm.&Out.News, Reac.
—BLDSC (4947.211500), EMDOCS, GNLM, IDS, ingenta, KNAW. **CCC.**
Published by: Churchill Livingstone (Subsidiary of: Harcourt Health Sciences), 11830 Westline Industrial Dr, St Louis, MO 63146. TEL 800-865-1900, http://www.arthroplastyjournal.org, http://www.churchillmed.com. Eds. Richard Rothman, M A R Freeman. adv.: B&W page USD 730, color page USD 975. Circ: 7,800. **Subscr. to:** W.B. Saunders Co., PO Box 628239, Orlando, FL 32862-8239. TEL 407-345-4000, 800-654-2452, FAX 407-363-9661, 800-225-6030, wbspcs@harcourtbrace.com, http://www.wbsaunders.com.

617.3 NLD ISSN 1053-8127
CODEN: JBMRFK
JOURNAL OF BACK AND MUSCULOSKELETAL REHABILITATION. Text in English. 1991. bi-m. EUR 296, USD 280 to institutions (effective 2002). back issues avail. *Refereed.* **Document type:** *Journal, Academic/Scholarly.* **Description:** Provides clinicians with a current guide to the assessment, diagnosis, and management of back and musculoskeletal disorders.
Related titles: Microform ed.: (from PQC); Online - full text ed.: (from ingenta, Swets Blackwell, Institute for Scientific Information, RoweCom Information Quest).
Indexed: AMED, ASCA, Excerp.Med. (1996-), Focus on: Sports Sci.& Med.
—BLDSC (4950.900000), EMDOCS, GNLM, IDS, Infotrieve, KNAW. **CCC.**
Published by: I O S Press, Nieuwe Hemweg 6B, Amsterdam 1013 BG, Netherlands. TEL 31-20-688-3355, FAX 31-20-620-3419, market@iospress.nl, http://www.iospress.nl. Ed. R N Harden TEL 312-238-6011.

617.3 USA ISSN 1094-5903
JOURNAL OF BONE AND JOINT SURGERY: AMERICAN AND BRITISH VOLUMES ON CD-ROM. Text in English. 1997. q. USD 195, GBP 119 to individuals; USD 395, GBP 186.20 to institutions (effective 2001); Subscr. for the CD-ROM containing both American & British volumes is only available though the American office.. **Document type:** *Academic/Scholarly.*
Media: CD-ROM. **Related titles:** Online - full text ed.; ♦ International ed. of: Journal of Bone and Joint Surgery: British Volume on CD-ROM. ISSN 0968-7300.
Published by: Journal of Bone and Joint Surgery, 20 Pickering St, Needham, MA 02492-3157. TEL 781-449-9780, FAX 781-449-9742, mail@jbjs.org, http://www.jbjs.org. Adv. contact Amber Howard. Circ: 1,500. **Co-publisher:** British Editorial Society of Bone and Joint Surgery.

617.3 USA ISSN 0021-9355
CODEN: JBJSA3
JOURNAL OF BONE AND JOINT SURGERY: AMERICAN VOLUME. Text in English. 1903. m. USD 125 to individuals; USD 210 to institutions (effective 2002). adv. bk.rev. bibl, charts, illus, abstr. index. back issues avail.; reprint service avail. from PQC. *Refereed.* **Document type:** *Journal, Academic/Scholarly.* **Description:** Publishes articles on orthopaedic surgery and related fields.
Supersedes in part: Journal of Bone and Joint Surgery (0375-9229)
Related titles: CD-ROM ed.: ISSN 1058-2436. 1990 (from Ovid Technologies, Inc.); Microfilm ed.: (from PQC); Online - full text ed.: (from Ovid Technologies, Inc., EBSCO Publishing, ProQuest Information & Learning, Institute for Scientific Information).
Indexed: AIM, AMED, ASCA, Abstr.Anthropol., Abstr.Health Care Manage.Stud., Bibl.Dev.Med.& Child Neur., Biol.Abstr., CINAHL, Cal.Tiss.Abstr., Chem.Abstr., Curr.Cont., Dent.Ind., Environ.Sci.Poll.Mgmt., Excerp.Med., Focus on: Sports Sci.& Med., INIS Atomind., Ind.Med. (1948-), Ind.Sci.Rev., Inpharma, Mat.Sci.Cit.Ind. (coverage dropped), Neurosci.Cit.Ind., Nutr.Abstr., Pharm.&Out.News, Pollut.Abstr., Reac., Risk Abstr., SSCI (coverage dropped), Saf.Sci.Abstr., Sci.Cit.Ind., Tox.Abstr. (coverage dropped), Vet.Bull.
—BLDSC (4954.250000), CASDDS, CISTI, GNLM, IDS, ingenta, KNAW. **CCC.**
Published by: Journal of Bone and Joint Surgery, 20 Pickering St, Needham, MA 02492-3157. TEL 781-449-9780, FAX 781-449-9742, mail@jbjs.org, http://www.jbjs.org. Ed. Dr. James D Heckman. R&P Mady issenbaum. Adv. contact Amber Howard. Circ: 30,500.

617.3 GBR ISSN 0301-620X
CODEN: JBSUAK
JOURNAL OF BONE AND JOINT SURGERY: BRITISH VOLUME. Text in English. 1948. 8/yr. USD 82 to individuals; USD 136 to institutions (effective 2001); includes supplements. adv. bk.rev. bibl, charts, illus. index. back issues avail.; reprint service avail. from PQC. *Refereed.* **Document type:** *Journal, Academic/Scholarly.* **Description:** Devoted to traumatic and orthopedic surgery and rheumatology.

M

Related titles: ♦ CD-ROM ed.: Journal of Bone and Joint Surgery: British Volume on CD-ROM. ISSN 0968-7300; Microform ed.: (from PQC); Online - full text ed.: 1997 (from Ovid Technologies, Inc., CatchWord Ltd., Institute for Scientific Information); ♦ Supplement: Journal of Bone and Joint Surgery. British Volume. Orthopaedic Proceedings. ISSN 1358-992X.

Indexed: AIDS Abstr., AIM, AMED, ASCA, Bibl.Dev.Med.& Child Neur., Biol.Abstr., Cal.Tiss.Abstr., Chem.Abstr., Curr.Adv.Cancer Res., Curr.Cont., Dent.Ind., Environ.Sci.Poll.Mgmt., Excerp.Med., Focus on: Sports Sci.& Med., INIS Atomind., Ind.Med. (1948-), Ind.Sci.Rev., Ind.Vet., Inpharma, Mat.Sci.Cit.Ind. (coverage dropped), Neurosci.Cit.Ind., Nutr.Abstr., Pharm.&Out.News, Pollut.Abstr., Reac., Risk Abstr., SSCI (coverage dropped), Saf.Sci.Abstr., Sci.Cit.Ind., Tox.Abstr. (coverage dropped), Vet.Bull.

—BLDSC (4954.255000), CASDDS, CISTI, EMDOCS, IDS, ingenta, KNAW.

Published by: British Editorial Society of Bone and Joint Surgery, 22 Buckingham St, London WC2N 6ET, United Kingdom. TEL 44-20-7782-0010, FAX 44-20-7782-0995, s.bishop@jbjs.org.uk. Ed. Frank Horan. R&P Wendy Thompson. Adv. contact Pam Noble TEL 44-1620-823383. B&W page GBP 1,180, color page GBP 2,030; trim 178 x 254. Circ: 20,000. **Subscr. in the U.S. to:** Journal of Bone and Joint Surgery, 20 Pickering St, Needham, MA 02492-3157. TEL 781-449-9780, FAX 781-449-9742.

617.3 GBR ISSN 0968-7300

JOURNAL OF BONE AND JOINT SURGERY: BRITISH VOLUME ON CD-ROM. Text in English. 1984. q. GBP 94 to individuals; GBP 247 to institutions (effective 2001). bk.rev. **Document type:** *Journal, Academic/Scholarly.* **Description:** Contains all the text and images from January 1996 onward for both the American and the British Volumes of The Journal of Bone and Joint Surgery. It provides an electronic equivalent to the print subscription, with the advantages of speed of searching and electronic facilities such as copy and paste.

Media: CD-ROM (from Ovid Technologies, Inc.). **Related titles:** Microform ed.: (from PQC); Online - full text ed.: 1997 (from Ovid Technologies, Inc., CatchWord Ltd., Institute for Scientific Information); ♦ Print ed.: Journal of Bone and Joint Surgery: British Volume. ISSN 0301-620X; ♦ International ed.: Journal of Bone and Joint Surgery: American and British Volumes on CD-ROM. ISSN 1094-5903.

Published by: British Editorial Society of Bone and Joint Surgery, 22 Buckingham St, London WC2N 6ET, United Kingdom. TEL 44-20-7782-0010, FAX 44-20-7782-0995, s.bishop@jbjs.org.uk, subs@jbjs.org.uk, http://www.jbjs.org.uk. Ed. Frank Horan. Adv. contact Pam Noble TEL 44-1620-823383.

617.3 GBR ISSN 1358-992X

JOURNAL OF BONE AND JOINT SURGERY. BRITISH VOLUME. ORTHOPAEDIC PROCEEDINGS. Text in English. irreg.

Related titles: ♦ Supplement to: Journal of Bone and Joint Surgery: British Volume. ISSN 0301-620X.

Published by: British Editorial Society of Bone and Joint Surgery, 22 Buckingham St, London WC2N 6ET, United Kingdom. TEL 44-20-7782-0010, FAX 44-20-7782-0995.

616.7 USA ISSN 0884-0431 CODEN: JBMREJ

JOURNAL OF BONE AND MINERAL RESEARCH. Text in English. 1986. m. USD 400 domestic to individuals; USD 420 in Canada to individuals; USD 470 elsewhere to individuals; USD 435 domestic to institutions; USD 455 in Canada to institutions; USD 490 elsewhere to institutions (effective 2001). adv. back issues avail.; reprints avail. *Refereed.* **Document type:** *Academic/Scholarly.* **Description:** Publishes papers on all areas of calcium regulation, skeletal physiology, and metabolic bone diseases.

Related titles: Online - full text ed.: (from EBSCO Publishing, Institute for Scientific Information).

Indexed: ASCA, BBCI, Cal.Tiss.Abstr., Chem.Abstr., Chem.Indus.Notes, Chem.Titles, Curr.Cont., Dairy Sci.Abstr., INIS Atomind., Ind.Med. (1986-), Ind.Sci.Rev., Inpharma, Int.Nurs.Ind., Kidney, Nutr.Abstr., Pharm.&Out.News, Reac., SSCI (coverage dropped), Sci.Cit.Ind., Soyabean Abstr., Tox.Abstr. (coverage dropped).

—BLDSC (4954.255530), CASDDS, CISTI, EMDOCS, GNLM, IDS, ingenta, KNAW. **CCC.**

Published by: (American Society for Bone and Mineral Research), Blackwell Science Inc., Commerce Pl, 350 Main St, Malden, MA 02148-5018. TEL 781-388-8250, FAX 781-388-8255, http://www.blackwell-science.com. R&P Tracey Davies. Adv. contact Jenny Applin. **Co-sponsor:** National Osteoporosis Foundation.

JOURNAL OF BURN CARE & REHABILITATION. see *MEDICAL SCIENCES*

610 USA ISSN 0883-9441 CODEN: JCCAER

JOURNAL OF CRITICAL CARE. Text in English. 1986 (Mar.). q. USD 157 domestic to individuals Full text online included; USD 256 foreign to individuals Full text online included; USD 260 domestic to institutions Full text online included; USD 312 foreign to institutions Full text online included; USD 73 domestic to students Full text online included; USD 154 foreign to students Full text online included; USD 79 newsstand/cover (effective 2001). adv. abstr, bibl, charts, illus. index. *Refereed.* **Document type:** *Journal, Academic/Scholarly, Trade.* **Description:** Presents multidisciplinary basic and clinical research, pertinent reviews, ethical and legal controversies, and important abstracts in all specialties and subspecialties of the field.

Related titles: Online - full text ed.: (from Institute for Scientific Information).

Indexed: ASCA, CINAHL, Chem.Abstr., Chem.Indus.Notes, Chem.Titles, Curr.Cont., Excerp.Med., Ind.Med. (1986-), Inpharma, Int.Nurs.Ind., Nutr.Abstr., Pharm.&Out.News, Reac.

—BLDSC (4965.630000), CASDDS, CISTI, EMDOCS, GNLM, IDS, ingenta, KNAW. **CCC.**

Published by: W.B. Saunders Co. (Subsidiary of: Harcourt Publishers Ltd.), 11830 Westline Industrial Dr, St Louis, MO 63146. TEL 800-325-4177, harcourthealth.com/jcritcare, http://www.wbsaunders.com. Ed. Dr. Guillermo Gutierrez. adv.: B&W page USD 785, color page USD 1,935; trim 10 x 7. Circ: 923. **Subscr. to:** Periodicals Fulfillment, W B Saunders Co, 6277 Sea Harbor Dr, 4th Fl, Orlando, FL 32891-4800. TEL 800-654-2452, FAX 800-874-6418.

616.025 USA ISSN 0736-4679

THE JOURNAL OF EMERGENCY MEDICINE. Text in English. 1983. 8/yr. EUR 136 in Europe to individuals; JPY 18,000 in Japan to individuals; USD 151 elsewhere to individuals; EUR 635 in Europe to institutions; JPY 84,400 in Japan to institutions; USD 711 elsewhere to institutions; EUR 66 in Europe residents price; JPY 8,600 in Japan residents price; USD 73 elsewhere residents price (effective 2002). adv. abstr. back issues avail. *Refereed.* **Document type:** *Academic/Scholarly.* **Description:** Publishes clinical and research articles, along with reviews, on all facets of emergency medicine practice and management.

Related titles: Microfilm ed.: (from PQC); Online - full text ed.: (from ingenta, ScienceDirect, Swets Blackwell, Institute for Scientific Information).

Indexed: CINAHL, Curr.Cont., Environ.Sci.Poll.Mgmt., Excerp.Med., INIS Atomind., Ind.Med. (1983-), Inpharma, Jrnl.Watch Emer.Med., Med.& Surg.Dermat., Pharm.&Out.News, Pollut.Abstr., Reac., Rev.Med.& Vet.Mycol., Risk Abstr., Saf.Sci.Abstr.

—BLDSC (4977.250000), CISTI, EMDOCS, GNLM, IDS, ingenta, KNAW. **CCC.**

Published by: (Canadian Association of Emergency Physicians), Elsevier Science, PO Box 945, New York, NY 10159-0945. TEL 212-989-5800, FAX 212-633-3990, usinfo-f@elsevier.com, http://www.elsevier.nl/locate/jemermed. Eds. G Sternbach, Peter Rosen. **Subscr. in Australasia and the Far East to:** Elsevier Science (Singapore) Pte Ltd, No.1 Temasek Ave, 17-01 Millenia Tower, Singapore 039192, Singapore. TEL 65-434-3727, FAX 65-337-2230; **Subscr. in Japan to:** Elsevier Science Inc - Japan Regional Office, 9-15 Higashi-Azabu 1-chome, Minato-ku, Tokyo 106-0044, Japan. TEL 81-3-5561-5033; **Subscr. outside the Americas to:** Elsevier Science BV, PO Box 211, Amsterdam 1000 AE, Netherlands. TEL 31-20-485-3757.

JOURNAL OF EYE TRAUMA. see *MEDICAL SCIENCES—Ophthalmology And Optometry*

617 USA ISSN 0885-9701

JOURNAL OF HEAD TRAUMA REHABILITATION. Text in English. 1986. bi-m. USD 155 to individuals; USD 31 newsstand/cover (effective 2002). *Refereed.* **Document type:** *Journal, Trade.* **Description:** Provides expert advice from leading practitioners involved in all disciplines of TBI and practical guidance for clinicians, administrators, and other health care professionals.

Related titles: Online - full text ed.: (from Ovid Technologies, Inc., ProQuest Information & Learning, Institute for Scientific Information).

Indexed: AMED, ASCA, AgeLine, CINAHL, Curr.Cont., Except.Child Educ.Abstr., Excerp.Med., Fam.Ind., IMFL, Ind.Med. (1986-), Int.Nurs.Ind., PsycInfo, Psychol.Abstr. (1986-), SSCI, e-psyche.

—BLDSC (4996.672000), EMDOCS, GNLM, IDS, Infotrieve, ingenta, KNAW. **CCC.**

Published by: Aspen Publishers, Inc., 200 Orchard Ridge Dr, Ste 200, Gaithersburg, MD 20878. TEL 301-417-7500, 800-638-8437, FAX 301-695-7931, customer.service@aspenpubl.com, http://www.aspenpub.com. **Dist. by:** Aspen Publishers Inc., Distribution Center, 7201 McKinney Circle, Frederick, MD 21701. TEL 301-698-7100, FAX 301-417-7550.

JOURNAL OF MANIPULATIVE AND PHYSIOLOGICAL THERAPEUTICS. see *MEDICAL SCIENCES—Chiropractic, Homeopathy, Osteopathy*

612.7 NLD ISSN 0142-4319 CODEN: JMRMD3

JOURNAL OF MUSCLE RESEARCH AND CELL MOTILITY. Text in English. 1980. 8/yr. EUR 1,360, USD 1,362 to institutions for print or online ed.; EUR 1,632, USD 1,634.40 to institutions for print & online eds.combined (effective 2002). adv. bk.rev. bibl, illus. index. reprint service avail. from PQC,ISI. *Refereed.* **Document type:** *Journal, Academic/Scholarly.* **Description:** Publishes original research on the excitation and contraction of muscle, the analysis of the processes involved, and the processes underlying cell contractility and motility.

Related titles: Online - full text ed.: (from EBSCO Publishing, O C L C Online Computer Library Center, Inc., RoweCom Information Quest, Swets Blackwell, Kluwer Online, Institute for Scientific Information).

Indexed: ASCA, Aqua.Sci.& Fish.Abstr., BBCI, Biol.Abstr., Cal.Tiss.Abstr., Chem.Abstr., Chem.Titles, Curr.Adv.Ecol.Sci., Curr.Cont., Dent.Ind., Excerp.Med., Ind.Med. (1980-), Ind.Sci.Rev., Inpharma, Int.Abstr.Biol.Sci., Neurosci.Cit.Ind., Reac., Rev.Med.& Vet.Mycol., Sci.Cit.Ind., Zoo.Rec.

—BLDSC (5021.120000), ADONIS, CASDDS, CISTI, GNLM, IDS, ingenta. **CCC.**

Published by: Kluwer Academic Publishers Group (Subsidiary of: Wolters Kluwer N.V.), Spuiboulevard 50, PO Box 17, Dordrecht 3300 AA, Netherlands. TEL 31-78-639-2392, FAX 31-78-654-2254, services@wkap.nl, http://www.wkap.nl/journalhome.htm/0142-4319. Adv. contact Gemma Heiser. **Subscr. in the Americas to:** Kluwer Academic - Plenum Publishers, 233 Spring St, New York, NY 10013-1578. TEL 212-620-8468, FAX 212-807-1047; **Subscr. to:** Journals Department, PO Box 322, Dordrecht 3300 AH, Netherlands. TEL 31-78-639-2392, FAX 31-78-654-6474.

616.7 GRC

THE JOURNAL OF MUSCULOSKELETAL AND NEURONAL INTERACTIONS. Text in English. 1990. q. *Refereed.* **Document type:** *Journal, Academic/Scholarly.* **Description:** Publishes original papers of research and clinical experience in all areas of the musculoskeletal system and its interactions with the nervous system, especially metabolic bone diseases, with particular emphasis on osteoporosis.

Former titles: Journal of Musculoskeletal Interactions (1108-7161); (until 2000): Ostoun (1106-109X)

Related titles: Online - full text ed.

Indexed: Cal.Tiss.Abstr., Neurosci.Abstr.

Published by: The International Society of Musculoskeletal and Neuronal Interactions, 7 Spiliadou Sq, Nafplion 21 100, Greece. TEL 30-752-99342, FAX 30-752-99343, jmni@ismni.org, http://www.ismni.org/jmni/index.htm. Eds. George Lyritis, Webster S. Jee. Adv. contact Susan Clarkson.

617.3 USA ISSN 0899-2517

THE JOURNAL OF MUSCULOSKELETAL MEDICINE. Text in English. 1983. m. USD 95 domestic; USD 105 foreign; USD 10 newsstand/cover domestic; USD 15 newsstand/cover foreign (effective 2001). adv. charts, illus. Index. back issues avail.; reprints avail. *Refereed.* **Document type:** *Journal, Academic/Scholarly.* **Description:** Provides practical information on diagnosis and management of a wide variety of common musculoskeletal disorders.

Related titles: Online - full text ed.: (from Gale Group, Factiva).

Indexed: CINAHL.

—BLDSC (5021.125000), GNLM, Infotrieve, KNAW. **CCC.**

Published by: Cliggott Publishing Co. (Subsidiary of: S C P Communications, Inc.), 330 Boston Post Rd, Darien, CT 06820. TEL 203-662-6400, FAX 203-662-6776, info.cliggott@scp.com, http://www.scp.com/. Ed., R&P Leo Cristofar. Pub., Adv. contact Bill Markowitz.

617 USA ISSN 1058-2452
RC927.3 CODEN: JMPAEQ
JOURNAL OF MUSCULOSKELETAL PAIN; innovations in research, theory & clinical practice. Text in English. 1993. q. USD 75 to individuals; USD 101 in Canada to individuals; USD 109 elsewhere to individuals; USD 150 to institutions; USD 203 in Canada to institutions; USD 218 elsewhere to institutions; USD 250 to libraries; USD 338 in Canada to libraries; USD 363 elsewhere to libraries (effective Aug. 2001). adv. bk.rev. charts, illus, stat. back issues avail.; reprint service avail. from HAW. *Refereed.* **Document type:** *Journal, Academic/Scholarly.* **Description:** Publishes articles by the vast array of professionals who must deal with acute and chronic musculoskeletal pain.
Related titles: Microfiche ed.: (from PQC); Microform ed.; Online - full text ed.: (from Institute for Scientific Information).
Indexed: Abstr.Anthropol., CINAHL, Cal.Tiss.Abstr., Curr.Cont., Environ.Sci.Poll.Mgmt., Ergon.Abstr., Excerp.Med. (1993-), Inpharma, Neurosci.Abstr. (coverage dropped), Per.Islam. (1992-), Pharm.&Out.News, Pollut.Abstr., PsycInfo, Reac., Ref.Zh., Risk Abstr., Saf.Sci.Abstr., e-psyche.
—BLDSC (5021.126000), EMDOCS, GNLM, Haworth, IDS, KNAW.
Published by: Haworth Press, Inc., 10 Alice St, Binghamton, NY 13904-1580. TEL 607-722-5857, 800-429-6784, FAX 607-722-6362, 800-895-0582, getinfo@haworthpressinc.com, http://www.haworthpress.com/journals/journallist.asp. Ed. I Jon Russell. Pub. William Cohen. R&P Ruthann Heath TEL 607-723-5857 ext 316. Adv. contact Jackie Blakeslee TEL 607-722-5857 ext 346. B&W page USD 315, color page USD 550; trim 6 x 8.5.

617.3 SGP ISSN 0218-9577
CODEN: JMURFZ
JOURNAL OF MUSCULOSKELETAL RESEARCH. Text in English. 1997. q. SGD 251, USD 148 to institutions (effective 2001); SGD 288 to institutions Asia Pacific & Australasia except Hong Kong and China; USD 160 elsewhere to institutions (effective 2002). *Refereed.* **Document type:** *Academic/Scholarly.* **Description:** Explores all facets of musculoskeletal disorders with emphasis on both the clinical and basic aspects of study. Also covers basic and clinical research in the fields of orthopaedics, rheumatology and rehabilitation, biomechanics, biomaterials and related areas.
Related titles: Online - full text ed.: (from ScienceDirect, Swets Blackwell).
Indexed: Aqua.Sci.& Fish.Abstr., Cal.Tiss.Abstr., Environ.Sci.Poll.Mgmt., INSPEC (Sep.1997-), Pollut.Abstr., Risk Abstr., Saf.Sci.Abstr.
—BLDSC (5021.126100).
Published by: World Scientific Publishing Co Pte Ltd, Farrer Rd, PO Box 128, Singapore 912805, Singapore. wspc@wspc.com.sg, http://www.worldscientific.com.

617.1 USA ISSN 0897-7151
CODEN: JNEUE4
JOURNAL OF NEUROTRAUMA. Text in English. 1984. m. USD 318 domestic to individuals; USD 449 foreign to individuals; USD 382 domestic to individuals print and online eds. combined; USD 513 foreign to individuals print and online eds. combined; USD 594 domestic to institutions; USD 774 foreign to institutions; USD 713 domestic to institutions print and online eds. combined; USD 893 foreign to institutions print and online eds. combined (effective 2002). adv. bk.rev. back issues avail.; reprints avail. *Refereed.* **Document type:** *Journal, Academic/Scholarly.* **Description:** Covers advances in the mechanisms and treatments of neurotrauma of the central and peripheral nervous system. Focuses on neurochemical, neurophysiological, and neuropathological research on spinal cord injury, head trauma, neural injury, and stroke.
Formerly: Central Nervous System Trauma (0737-5999)
Related titles: Online - full content ed.: USD 594 to institutions; USD 318 to individuals (effective 2002) (from Swets Blackwell); Online - full text ed.: (from CatchWord Ltd., Institute for Scientific Information, RoweCom Information Quest).
Indexed: ASCA, Curr.Cont., INIS Atomind., Ind.Med. (1988-), Ind.Sci.Rev., Inpharma, Neurosci.Cit.Ind., Reac., Sci.Cit.Ind., e-psyche.
—BLDSC (5022.270000), CISTI, EMDOCS, GNLM, IDS, ingenta, KNAW. **CCC.**
Published by: (National Neurotrauma Society), Mary Ann Liebert, Inc. Publishers, 2 Madison Ave, Larchmont, NY 10538. TEL 914—834-3100, FAX 914-834-1388, info@liebertpub.com, http://www.liebertpub.com/neu. Ed. Dr. John T Povlishock.

617.3 DEU ISSN 1434-5293
JOURNAL OF OROFACIAL ORTHOPEDICS. Text in English, German. 1931. bi-m. EUR 185.64 domestic; EUR 198.64 foreign; EUR 34.58 newsstand/cover (effective 2002). adv. bk.rev. bibl, charts, illus. index. 2 cols./p. back issues avail. *Refereed.* **Document type:** *Journal, Academic/Scholarly.*
Formerly (until 1995): Fortschritte der Kieferorthopaedie (0015-816X)
Related titles: Online - full text ed.: ISSN 1615-6714 (from RoweCom Information Quest, Swets Blackwell, Springer LINK).
Indexed: Biol.Abstr., Curr.Adv.Ecol.Sci., Curr.Tit.Dent., Dent.Ind., Excerp.Med., Ind.Med. (1996-).
—BLDSC (5027.520000), GNLM, Infotrieve. **CCC.**
Published by: (Deutsche Gesellschaft fuer Kieferorthopaedie), Urban und Vogel Medien und Medizin Verlagsgesellschaft mbH (Subsidiary of: BertelsmannSpringer), Neumarkter Str 43, Munich 81673, Germany. TEL 49-89-43721411, FAX 49-89-43721410, verlag@urban-vogel.de, http://www.urban-vogel.de. Eds. Dr. I Jonas, Dr. P Diedrich. R&P Oliver Renn. Adv. contact Paul Berger. Circ: 2,500. **Subscr. to:** Springer Auslieferungs Gesellschaft, Postfach 105160, Heidelberg 69041, Germany. TEL 49-6221-345244, FAX 49-6221-345244.

JOURNAL OF ORTHOPAEDIC AND SPORTS PHYSICAL THERAPY. see *MEDICAL SCIENCES—Sports Medicine*

JOURNAL OF ORTHOPAEDIC NURSING. see *MEDICAL SCIENCES—Nurses And Nursing*

617.3 USA ISSN 0736-0266
CODEN: JOREDR
JOURNAL OF ORTHOPAEDIC RESEARCH; a journal for musculoskeletal investigations. Text in English. 1983. bi-m. EUR 185 in Europe to individuals; JPY 24,600 in Japan to individuals; USD 207 elsewhere to individuals; EUR 261 in Europe to institutions; JPY 34,600 in Japan to institutions; USD 291 elsewhere to institutions (effective 2002). adv. illus. index. back issues avail. *Refereed.* **Document type:** *Academic/Scholarly.* **Description:** Covers experimental, theoretical and clinical aspects of orthopaedics.
Related titles: Online - full text ed.: (from Northern Light Technology, Inc., ProQuest Information & Learning, ScienceDirect, Institute for Scientific Information).
Indexed: AMED, ASCA, Bioeng.Abstr., Biotech.& Bioeng.Abstr. (coverage dropped), Cal.Tiss.Abstr., Chem.Abstr., Chem.Indus.Notes, Chem.Titles, Comput.& Info.Sys., Curr.Adv.Ecol.Sci., Curr.Cont., Dok.Arbeitsmed., Eng.Ind., Excerp.Med., INIS Atomind., ISMEC, Ind.Med. (1983-), Ind.Sci.Rev., Inpharma, Reac., Sci.Cit.Ind., Solid St.Abstr.
—BLDSC (5027.665000), CASDDS, CISTI, Ei, EMDOCS, GNLM, IDS, ingenta, KNAW.
Published by: (Orthopaedic Research Society), Journal of Bone and Joint Surgery, 20 Pickering St, Needham, MA 02492-3157. TEL 781-449-9780, http://www.elsevier.com/locate/orthres. Ed. Dr. Joseph Buckwalten. R&P Timothy Wright. Adv. contact Amber Howard. Circ: 2,500.

617.3 JPN ISSN 0949-2658
CODEN: JOSCFS
JOURNAL OF ORTHOPAEDIC SCIENCE. Text in English. 1996. bi-m. (in 1 vol., 6 nos./vol.). EUR 220.70 domestic; EUR 215 in Germany for Print & Online Eds.; EUR 38 foreign for Print & Online Eds. (effective 2002). **Document type:** *Academic/Scholarly.* **Description:** Documents the latest research and topical debates in all fields of clinical and experimental orthopedics.
Related titles: Online - full text ed.: ISSN 1436-2023 (from EBSCO Publishing, RoweCom Information Quest, Swets Blackwell, Springer LINK).
Indexed: Ind.Med. (1996-).
—BLDSC (5027.668000), CISTI, GNLM, Infotrieve, KNAW. **CCC.**
Published by: (Japanese Orthopaedic Association/Nippon Seikei Geka Gakkai), Springer-Verlag Tokyo (Subsidiary of: BertelsmannSpringer), 3-13 Hongo 3-chome, Bunkyo-ku, Tokyo 113-0033, Japan. FAX 81-3-3812-0719, orders@svt-ebs.co.jp, http://link.springer-ny.com/link/service/journals/00776/index.htm, http://www.springer.ny.com. Ed. Koichiro Hayashi. Circ: 2,800. **Subscr. in N. America to:** Springer-Verlag New York Inc., PO Box 2485, Secaucus, NJ 07096-2485. TEL 800-777-4643, 212-460-1500, 212-460-1526, FAX 201-348-4505, orders@springer-ny.com. **Dist. outside N. America & Japan by:** Springer-Verlag, Haber Str 7, Heidelberg 69126, Germany. TEL 49-20-82787-0, subscriptions@springer.de, http://link.springer.de, http://link.springer-ny.com.

617.3 HKG ISSN 1022-5536
CODEN: JOTSEC
JOURNAL OF ORTHOPAEDIC SURGERY. Text in English. 1962. s-a. USD 60. adv. bk.rev. charts, illus. reprint service avail. from PQC. **Document type:** *Academic/Scholarly.*
Formerly (until 1993): Western Pacific Orthopaedic Association. Journal (0043-4019)
Related titles: Microform ed.: (from PQC); Online - full text ed.: (from ProQuest Information & Learning).
Indexed: Excerp.Med., HongKongiana.
—BLDSC (5027.669000), CISTI, KNAW.
Published by: (Western Pacific Orthopaedic Association), Hong Kong University Press, 14-F, Hing Wai Centre, 7 Tin Wan Praya Rd, Aberdeen, Hong Kong, Hong Kong. FAX 852-2875-0734, hkupress@hkucc.hku.hk, http://www.hkupress.org. Ed. David Fang. Circ: 2,000 (controlled). **Subscr. to:** 4-F MacLehose Medical Rehabilitation Centre, 7 Sha Wan Dr, Pokfulam Rd, Sandy Bay, Hong Kong, Hong Kong.

617.3 USA ISSN 0890-5339
CODEN: JORTE5
JOURNAL OF ORTHOPAEDIC TRAUMA. Text in English. 1987. 8/yr. USD 245 domestic to individuals for print & online eds.; USD 280 foreign to individuals for print & online eds.; USD 420 domestic to institutions for print & online eds.; USD 480 foreign to institutions for print & online eds.; USD 51 newsstand/cover (effective 2002). adv. bk.rev. charts, illus. index. back issues avail.; reprint service avail. from PQC. *Refereed.* **Document type:** *Academic/Scholarly.* **Description:** Publishes original articles on the diagnosis and management of hard and soft tissue trauma.
Related titles: Online - full text ed.: USD 546 domestic academic site license; USD 606 foreign academic site license; USD 609 domestic corporate site license; USD 669 foreign corporate site license (effective 2002) (from Ovid Technologies, Inc., Institute for Scientific Information).
Indexed: ASCA, CINAHL, Curr.Cont., Focus on: Sports Sci.& Med., INIS Atomind., Ind.Med. (1987-), Inpharma, Nutr.Abstr., Reac., Sci.Cit.Ind.
—BLDSC (5027.675000), CISTI, GNLM, IDS, ingenta, KNAW.
Published by: (Orthopaedic Trauma Association), Lippincott Williams & Wilkins (Philadelphia) (Subsidiary of: Wolters Kluwer N.V.), 530 Walnut St, Philadelphia, PA 19106-3621. TEL 215-521-8300, FAX 215-521-8902, http://www.lww.com. Ed. Dr. Roy W Sanders. Pub. Kathleen Gaffney. R&P Alice McElhinney. Adv. contact Renee Artuso. B&W page USD 1,040, color page USD 2,295. Circ: 2,877 (paid). **Subscr. to:** PO Box 1600, Hagerstown, MD 21740-1600. TEL 800-777-2295, FAX 301-824-7390. **Co-sponsor:** International Society for Fracture Repair.

JOURNAL OF ORTHOPEDIC SURGICAL TECHNIQUES. see *MEDICAL SCIENCES—Surgery*

617.3 USA ISSN 0271-6798
CODEN: JPORDO
JOURNAL OF PEDIATRIC ORTHOPAEDICS. Text in English. 1981. bi-m. USD 242 domestic to individuals for print & online eds.; USD 307 foreign to individuals for print & online eds.; USD 560 domestic to institutions for print & online eds.; USD 560 foreign to institutions for print & online eds.; USD 87 newsstand/cover (effective 2002). adv. bk.rev. illus. index. back issues avail.; reprint service avail. from PQC. *Refereed.* **Document type:** *Academic/Scholarly.* **Description:** Provides answers to pediatric orthopaedic problems.
Related titles: Online - full text ed.: USD 728 domestic academic site license; USD 728 foreign academic site license; USD 812 domestic corporate site license; USD 812 foreign corporate site license (effective 2002) (from Ovid Technologies, Inc., Swets Blackwell, Institute for Scientific Information).
Indexed: ASCA, Bibl.Dev.Med.& Child Neur., Biol.Abstr., Curr.Cont., Excerp.Med., INIS Atomind., Ind.Med. (1981-), Inpharma, Neurosci.Cit.Ind., Psychol.Abstr., Reac., Rev.Med.& Vet.Mycol.
—BLDSC (5030.225000), CISTI, EMDOCS, GNLM, IDS, ingenta, KNAW.
Published by: Lippincott Williams & Wilkins (Philadelphia) (Subsidiary of: Wolters Kluwer N.V.), 530 Walnut St, Philadelphia, PA 19106-3621. TEL 215-521-8300, FAX 215-521-8902, http://www.lww.com. Eds. Dr. Lynn T Staheli, Dr. Robert N Hensinger. Pub. Kathleen Gaffney. R&P Margaret Becker. Adv. contact Ray Thibodeau. Circ: 3,771 (paid). **Subscr. to:** PO Box 1600, Hagerstown, MD 21740-1600. TEL 800-777-2295, FAX 301-824-7390.

M

617.3 USA ISSN 1060-152X
CODEN: JPOBFC

JOURNAL OF PEDIATRIC ORTHOPAEDICS, PART B. Text in English. 1992. q. USD 210 domestic to individuals for print & online eds.; USD 210 foreign to individuals for print & online eds.; USD 389 per issue domestic to institutions; USD 389 per issue foreign to institutions; USD 89 newsstand/cover (effective 2002). adv. charts, illus. *Refereed.* **Document type:** *Academic/Scholarly.* **Description:** Publishes recent developments in the treatment of musculoskeletal disorders in children, with an emphasis on advances from the European Community.

Related titles: Microform ed.: (from PQC); Online - full content ed.: USD 505.70 domestic academic site license; USD 505.70 foreign academic site license; USD 564.05 domestic corporate site license; USD 564.05 foreign corporate site license (effective 2002); Online - full text ed.: (from Institute for Scientific Information).

Indexed: ASCA, Curr.Cont., Ind.Med. (1992-), Inpharma, Reac.

—BLDSC (5030.230000), CISTI, IDS, KNAW.

Published by: (European Paediatric Orthopaedic Society), Lippincott Williams & Wilkins (Philadelphia) (Subsidiary of: Wolters Kluwer N.V.), 530 Walnut St, Philadelphia, PA 19106-3621. TEL 215-521-8300, FAX 215-521-8902, http://www.lww.com. Ed. Dr. Henri Bensahel. Pub. Kathleen Gaffney. R&P Margaret Becker. Adv. contact Ray Thibodeau. B&W page USD 1,025, color page USD 2,205. Circ: 829. **Subscr. to:** PO Box 1600, Hagerstown, MD 21740-1600. TEL 800-777-2295, FAX 301-824-7390.

JOURNAL OF PHYSIOLOGY. see *BIOLOGY—Physiology*

617.3 USA ISSN 1040-8800
RD130

JOURNAL OF PROSTHETICS AND ORTHOTICS. Variant title: J P O. Text in English. 1988. q. USD 73 domestic to individuals; USD 96 foreign to individuals; USD 93 domestic to institutions; USD 116 foreign to institutions (effective 2002). adv. bk.rev. *Refereed.* **Document type:** *Academic/Scholarly.* **Description:** Presents research articles and reports from professionals on current topics in orthotics and prosthetics.

Formed by the merger of (1947-1988): Orthotics and Prosthetics (0030-5928); Which was formerly (until 1967): Orthopedic and Prosthetic Appliance Journal; (1970-1988): Clinical Prosthetics and Orthotics (0735-0090); Which was formerly (until 1982): Newsletter, Prosthetics and Orthotics Clinic (0279-6910)

Related titles: Microfilm ed.: (from PQC); Online - full text ed.: (from Institute for Scientific Information).

Indexed: AMED, ASCA, CINAHL, SSCI (coverage dropped).

—BLDSC (5042.910000), CISTI, GNLM.

Published by: American Orthotic & Prosthetic Asssociation, 1650 King St, Ste 500, Alexandria, VA 22314. TEL 703-836-7116, FAX 703-836-0838. Ed. Thomas M Gavin. R&P Lisa L Gough. Adv. contact Amy Clontz. Circ: 4,600. **Co-sponsor:** American Orthotic and Prosthetic Association.

617.3 USA ISSN 0748-7711
RD130 CODEN: JRRDEC

JOURNAL OF REHABILITATION RESEARCH AND DEVELOPMENT. Text in English. 1964. q. free per issue to qualified personnel. bk.rev. abstr, bibl, charts, illus, pat, stat. Index. reprint service avail. from PQC. *Refereed.* **Document type:** *Government.* **Description:** Disseminates ideas in rehabilitation research and development that further efforts to meet the needs of people with disabilities.

Former titles: Journal of Rehabilitation R and D; Bulletin of Prosthetics Research (0007-506X)

Related titles: Microform ed.: (from PQC); Online - full text ed.: (from ProQuest Information & Learning, Factiva, Institute for Scientific Information).

Indexed: AMED, ASCA, AgeLine, Appl.Mech.Rev., Bioeng.Abstr., Biol.Abstr., CINAHL, Compumath, Comput.& Info.Sys., Curr.Cont., Eng.Ind., Environ.Sci.Poll.Mgmt., Except.Child Educ.Abstr., Excerp.Med., HRIS, ISMEC, Ind.Med. (1984-), Inpharma, Int.Nurs.Ind., Pollut.Abstr., Reac., Rehabil.Lit., Risk Abstr., SSCI, Saf.Sci.Abstr.

—BLDSC (5048.970000), CISTI, Ei, GNLM, ingenta, KNAW, Linda Hall.

Published by: Department of Veterans Affairs, Veterans Health Administration, Office of Research and Development, 103 S Gay St, Baltimore, MD 21202-3517. TEL 410-962-1800, FAX 410-962-9670, mail@rehab-balt.med.va.gov, http://www.va.gov. Circ: 27,000.

617.3 USA ISSN 0895-0385
CODEN: JSDIEW

JOURNAL OF SPINAL DISORDERS. Text in English. 1988. bi-m. USD 222 domestic to individuals; USD 251 foreign to individuals; USD 380 domestic to institutions; USD 405 foreign to institutions (effective 2002). adv. charts, illus. reprint service avail. from PQC. *Refereed.* **Document type:** *Journal, Academic/Scholarly.* **Description:** Features research and clinical articles on diagnosis, management, and treatment of lumbar spine disorders.

Related titles: Online - full text ed.: USD 494 domestic academic site license; USD 519 foreign academic site license; USD 551 domestic corporate academic site license; USD 576 foreign corporate site license (effective 2002) (from Ovid Technologies, Inc., Institute for Scientific Information).

Indexed: AMED, ASCA, Curr.Cont., Excerp.Med., Ind.Med. (1988-), Inpharma, Neurosci.Cit.Ind., Pharm.&Out.News, Reac.

—BLDSC (5066.182000), CISTI, EMDOCS, GNLM, IDS, KNAW.

Published by: Lippincott Williams & Wilkins (Philadelphia) (Subsidiary of: Wolters Kluwer N.V.), 530 Walnut St, Philadelphia, PA 19106-3621. TEL 215-521-8300, FAX 215-521-8902, http://www.jspinaldisorders.com, http://www.lww.com. Eds. Dr. Dan M Spengler, Dr. Thomas B Ducker. Pub. Kathleen Gaffney. R&P Margaret Becker. Adv. contact Ray Thibodeau. B&W page USD 990, color page USD 2,040. Circ: 1,851 (paid). **Subscr. to:** PO Box 1600, Hagerstown, MD 21740-1600. TEL 800-777-2295, FAX 301-824-7390.

610 JPN ISSN 0022-5274
CODEN: KOIGAU

JOURNAL OF TRANSPORTATION MEDICINE; kotsu igaku. Text in English, Japanese. 1947. bi-m. JPY 7,000. adv. **Document type:** *Academic/Scholarly.*

Indexed: C.I.S. Abstr., Excerp.Med., INIS Atomind., Ind.Med. (coverage dropped).

—BLDSC (5070.400000), CASDDS, CISTI.

Published by: Japanese Association of Transportation Medicine/Nihon Kotsu Igakkai, c/o Business Center for Academic Societies Japan, 5-16-9 Honkomagome, Bunkyo-ku, Tokyo 113-0021, Japan. TEL 03-5814-5811, FAX 03-5814-5822. Ed. Takashi Murayama. Circ: 600 (controlled).

617 USA ISSN 1079-6061
RD92 CODEN: JOTRA5

JOURNAL OF TRAUMA - INJURY, INFECTION AND CRITICAL CARE. Text in English. 1961. m. USD 262 domestic to individuals; USD 335 foreign to individuals; USD 348 domestic to institutions; USD 421 foreign to institutions (effective 2002). adv. abstr, charts, illus, stat, tr.lit. index. *Refereed.* **Document type:** *Journal, Academic/Scholarly.* **Description:** Diagnosis, management and recommendations for surgical approaches to traumatic injury for orthopedic, plastic and general surgeons.

Formerly: Journal of Trauma (0022-5282)

Related titles: CD-ROM ed.: (from Ovid Technologies, Inc.); Microfilm ed.: (from WWS); Online - full text ed.: USD 452.40 domestic academic site license; USD 525.40 foreign academic site license; USD 504.60 domestic corporate site license; USD 577.60 foreign corporate site license (effective 2002) (from Ovid Technologies, Inc., Swets Blackwell, Institute for Scientific Information).

Indexed: AIM, ASCA, Biol.Abstr., CINAHL, C.I.S. Abstr., C.L.I., Cal.Tiss.Abstr., Chem.Abstr., Chem.Indus.Notes, Chem.Titles, Crim.Just.Abstr., Curr.Adv.Ecol.Sci., Curr.Cont., Dent.Ind., Environ.Sci.Poll.Mgmt., Excerp.Med., HRIS, INIS Atomind., Ind.Med. (1961-), Ind.Sci.Rev., Ind.Vet., Inpharma, Int.Nurs.Ind., Jrnl.Watch Emer.Med., L.R.I., Neurosci.Cit.Ind., Pharm.&Out.News, Pollut.Abstr., Reac., Rev.Med.& Vet.Mycol., Risk Abstr., SSCI (coverage dropped), Saf.Sci.Abstr., Sci.Cit.Ind.

—BLDSC (5070.512000), CASDDS, CISTI, GNLM, IDS, ingenta, KNAW. **CCC.**

Published by: (American Association for the Surgery of Trauma), Lippincott Williams & Wilkins (Philadelphia) (Subsidiary of: Wolters Kluwer N.V.), 530 Walnut St, Philadelphia, PA 19106-3621. TEL 215-521-8300, FAX 215-521-8902, sisaacson@wwilkins.com, custserv@lww.com, http://www.jtrauma.com, http://www.lww.com/. Ed. Basil A Pruitt Jr. TEL 210-342-7903. adv.: B&W page USD 910; trim 10.88 x 8.5. Circ: 5,549; 5,415 (paid).

JOURNAL OF TRAUMA NURSING. see *MEDICAL SCIENCES—Nurses And Nursing*

JOURNAL OF VETERINARY EMERGENCY AND CRITICAL CARE. see *VETERINARY SCIENCE*

617.375 USA ISSN 1533-2888

▼ **JOURNAL OF WHIPLASH & RELATED DISORDERS.** Text in English. forthcoming 2002. q. USD 45, USD 61, USD 65 per vol. to individuals; USD 85, USD 115, USD 123 per vol. to institutions; USD 125, USD 169, USD 181 per vol. to libraries (effective Aug. 2001). adv. *Refereed.* **Document type:** *Journal, Academic/Scholarly.* **Description:** Dedicated to advancing the field of scientific study of the cause, veracity and treatment of whiplash and related disorders.

Published by: Haworth Press, Inc., 10 Alice St, Binghamton, NY 13904-1580. TEL 607-722-5857, 800-429-6784, FAX 607-722-6362, 800-895-0582, getinfo@haworthpressinc.com, http://www.haworthpress.com/journals/journallist.asp. Eds. Christopher J Centeno, Michael D Freeman. Pub. William Cohen. R&P Ruth Ann Heath. Adv. contact Jackie Blakeslee TEL 607-722-5857 ext 346. B&W page USD 315, color page USD 550; trim 6 x 8.5.

617.1 GBR ISSN 0969-0700

JOURNAL OF WOUND CARE. Text in English. 1992. m. GBP 37 domestic to individuals; GBP 52 in Europe to individuals; GBP 59 elsewhere to individuals; GBP 77 domestic to institutions; GBP 88 in Europe to institutions; GBP 104.50 elsewhere to institutions (effective 2000). adv. bk.rev. charts, illus, pat. cum.index. *Refereed.* **Document type:** *Academic/Scholarly, Trade.*

Indexed: Brit.Nur.Ind., CINAHL, Int.Nurs.Ind., Rev.Appl.Entomol.

—BLDSC (5072.695000), GNLM, Infotrieve. **CCC.**

Published by: Emap Healthcare Ltd. (Subsidiary of: Emap Business Communications Ltd.), Greater London House, Hampstead Rd, London NW1 7EJ, United Kingdom. TEL 44-20-7874-0200, FAX 44-20-7874-0201, http://www.emap.com. Ed. Deborah Glover. Pub. Rosemarie Finley. Adv. contact Heather Simmons. Circ: 6,000 (paid). **Subscr. to:** Macmillan Magazines Ltd, Brunel Rd, Basingstoke, Hants RG21 6XT, United Kingdom. TEL 44-1256-29242, FAX 44-1256-812358.

016.6167 USA ISSN 1521-6535

JOURNAL WATCH EMERGENCY MEDICINE. Text in English. 1997 (Sep.). m. USD 98. 8 p./no. **Document type:** *Newsletter.* **Description:** Presents concise summaries of important research appearing in the emergency medicine literature.

Published by: Massachusetts Medical Society, P O Box 9085, Waltham, MA 02254-9085.

617.3 JPN ISSN 0915-1451

KANAGAWA SEIKEI SAIGAI GEKA IKAI ZASSHI/KANAGAWA JOURNAL OF ORTHOPEDICS AND TRAUMATOLOGY. Text in Japanese. 1988. a.

Published by: Kanagawa Seikei Saigai Geka Ikai/Kanagawa Society of Orthopedics and Traumatology, Showa Daigaku Fujigaoka Byoin Seikei Geka Kyoshitsu, 1-30, Fujigaoka, Midori-ku, Yokohama-shi, Kanagawa-ken 277, Japan.

617 JPN ISSN 0915-7786

KANSAI KANSETSUKYO HIZA KENKYUKAISHI/ JOURNAL OF KANSAI ARTHROSCOPY AND KNEE. Text in Japanese. 1990. a.

Published by: Kansai Kansetsukyo Hiza Kenkyukai/Kansai Arthroscopy and Knee Society, c/o Kyoto Furitsu Ika Daigaku, Seikei Gekagaku Kyoshitsu, Kajiicho, Hirokoji, Kawaramachi, Kamigyo-ku, Kyoto-shi 602, Japan.

617.3 JPN ISSN 0286-5394

KANSETSU GEKA/JOURNAL OF JOINT SURGERY. Text in Japanese. 1981. m. JPY 33,000 (effective 1999). *Refereed.*

Published by: Medical View Co. Ltd./Mejikaru Byusha, 2-30 Ichigaya-Honmura-cho, Shinjuku-ku, Tokyo 162-0845, Japan. Circ: 8,000.

617.3 JPN ISSN 0285-6255

KANSETSU NO GEKA/JOINT SURGERY. Text in Japanese. 1974. q. JPY 1,500 per issue.

Published by: Shizen Kagakusha Co. Ltd., 1-4 Iida-Bashi 2-chome, Chiyoda-ku, Tokyo 102-0072, Japan.

617.3 JPN ISSN 0389-7087
CODEN: KSSZDW

KANTO SEIKEI SAIGAI GEKA GAKKAI ZASSHI/KANTO JOURNAL OF ORTHOPEDICS AND TRAUMATOLOGY. Text in Japanese. 1970. bi-m. membership.

Indexed: INIS Atomind.

Published by: Kanto Seikei Saigai Geka Gakkai/Kanto Society of Orthopedics and Traumatology, Jikeikai Ika Daigaku Seikei Gekagaku Kyoshitsu, 25-8 Nishi-Shinbashi 3-chome, Minato-ku, Tokyo 105-0003, Japan.

THE KNEE. see *BIOLOGY—Physiology*

617.3 JPN ISSN 0287-2285
KOSSETSU/FRACTURE. Text in Japanese. 1978. a. JPY 6,000 domestic; USD 60 foreign (effective 2001). adv. bk.rev. back issues avail. *Refereed.* **Document type:** *Abstract/Index.*
Related titles: Fax ed.
Published by: Nihon Kossetsu Chiryo Gakkai/Japan Fracture Society, Kitasato Daigaku Igakubu Seikei Geka, 15-1 Kitaza-To 1-chome, Sagamihara-shi, Kanagawa-ken 228-0829, Japan. TEL 81-42-778-9343, 81-42-778-8111, FAX 81-42-778-8050. Ed., Adv. contact Moritoshi Itoman. R&P Kumiko Akikaze. Circ: 2,000 (paid).

KOTSU KANSETSU JINTAI/JOURNAL OF MUSCULOSKELETAL SYSTEM. see *MEDICAL SCIENCES—Rheumatology*

617.3 JPN
KOTSU KEITO SHIKKAN KENKYUKAI SHOROKU/JAPANESE SOCIETY FOR SKELETAL DYSPLASIAS. PROCEEDINGS OF THE MEETING. Text in English, Japanese. 1989. a. **Document type:** *Proceedings.*
Published by: (Kotsu Keito Shikkan Kenkyukai), Kagawa Ikadaigaku Seikeigeka, 1750-1 Oaza-Ikedo, Kita-gun, Miki-cho, Kagawa-ken 761-0700, Japan. TEL 81-878-98-5111, FAX 81-878-91-0116.

616 360 GBR
L A S NEWS. Text in English. 1966. m. free per issue to qualified personnel. back issues avail. **Document type:** *Newsletter.*
Formerly: Londam
Published by: London Ambulance Service, London, 220 Waterloo Rd, London SE1 8SD, United Kingdom. TEL 071-928-0333, FAX 071-401-8969. Ed. Andrew Faith. Circ: 3,000.

617.3 617.95 HUN ISSN 1217-3231
MAGYAR TRAUMATOLOGIA, ORTHOPEDIA, KEZSEBESZET ES PLASZTIKAI SEBESZET. Text in Hungarian; Summaries in English, German, Russian. 1958. q. HUF 1,250 domestic; USD 10 foreign (effective 2000). adv. bk.rev. charts, illus, pat. index. **Document type:** *Academic/Scholarly.*
Formerly (until no.4, 1992): Magyar Traumatologia, Orthopedia es Helyreallito-Sebeszet (0025-0317)
Indexed: Biol.Abstr., Excerp.Med. (until 1992), INIS Atomind., Ind.Med. (coverage dropped).
—BLDSC (5345.850000), CISTI, GNLM.
Published by: Hungarian Traumatology Society, Karolina u 27, Budapest 1113, Hungary. Ed., Pub., R&P, Adv. contact Dr. Tibor Vizkelety TEL 36-1-4666059. Circ: 1,000. **Co-sponsor:** Hungarian Orthopaedic Society.

MEDICINE AND SPORT SCIENCE. see *MEDICAL SCIENCES—Sports Medicine*

617.11 ITA
MEDITERRANEAN CLUB FOR BURNS AND FIRE DISASTERS. ANNALS. Text in English, French; Summaries in English, French. 1987. q. ITL 30,000, USD 18 domestic; ITL 40,000 foreign (effective 1999). adv. bk.rev. bibl, illus, stat. back issues avail. *Refereed.* **Document type:** *Academic/Scholarly.* **Description:** Specializes in burns as individual pathology and in fire disaster as societal pathology (mass burns).
Formerly: Mediterranean Burns Club. Annals (1121-1539)
—BLDSC (1040.140000).
Published by: Mediterranean Club for Burns and Fire Disasters, Divisione di Chirurgia Plastica e Terapia delle Ustioni Ospedale Civico, Via C. Lazzaro, Palermo, PA 90127, Italy. TEL 39-91-6663631, FAX 39-91-596404, mbcpa@cres.it, http://www.cres.it/mbe/. Eds. M Masellis, S Gunn. R&P Michele Masellis. Adv. contact F Conte. B&W page ITL 2,000, color page ITL 3,000; trim 210 x 220. Circ: 3,200.

617.3 DEU ISSN 0340-5508
MEDIZINISCH-ORTHOPAEDISCHE TECHNIK. Text in German. 1880. bi-m. DEM 135; DEM 144.60 foreign (effective 2000). adv. bk.rev. charts, illus, pat. index. **Document type:** *Academic/Scholarly.*
—BLDSC (5535.073800), GNLM, Infotrieve. **CCC.**

Published by: Gentner Verlag Stuttgart, Forststr 131, Stuttgart 70193, Germany. TEL 49-711-63672-0, FAX 49-711-63672-11. Ed. Dr. Grifka. Adv. contact Corinna Zepter. Circ: 3,398.

617.3 USA
MEDSCAPE ORTHOPEDICS & SPORTS MEDICINE. Text in English. 1997. 6/yr. *Refereed.* **Description:** Features clinical news, full-text articles, and other features covering prevention, diagnosis, and treatment of patients with orthopedic complaints.
Media: Online - full text.
Published by: Medscape, Inc., 134 W 29th St, New York, NY 10001-5399. TEL 212-631-1600, http://www.medscape.com.

617.3 ITA CODEN: MIORA5
MINERVA ORTOPEDICA E TRAUMATOLOGICA. Text in Italian; Summaries in English, Italian. 1950. m. (10/yr.). USD 125 to individuals; USD 165 to institutions (effective 2000 - 2001). adv. bk.rev. bibl, charts, illus. index. **Document type:** *Academic/Scholarly.*
Formerly: Minerva Ortopedica (0026-4911)
Indexed: Chem.Abstr., Excerp.Med., Ind.Med. (coverage dropped).
—BLDSC (5794.315000), CISTI, GNLM.
Published by: (Societa Piemontese - Ligure - Lombarda di Ortopedia e Traumatologia), Edizioni Minerva Medica, Corso Bramante, 83-85, Turin, TO 10126, Italy. TEL 39-11-678282, FAX 39-11-674502. Ed., Pub. Alberto Oliaro. Adv. contact F Filippo. B&W page USD 1,200, color page USD 2,000; trim 270 x 190. Circ: 4,000 (paid).

617 NLD ISSN 1380-3522
N T S R. (Nederlands Tijdschrift voor Spoedeisende Medische Hulpverlening en Rampengeneeskunde) Text in Dutch. 1978. bi-m. NLG 37.50, USD 20. adv. back issues avail. **Description:** Covers topics relating to emergency medicine and ambulances.
Formerly (until 1994): Ambulance (0167-9589)
KNAW.
Published by: H H S Uitgeverij, Postbus 150, Grave 5360 AD, Netherlands. FAX 31-8860-76448. Ed. H J J Berden. Pub. A M Janssen. Adv. contact P G Hoving. Circ: 3,200.

617.1 USA ISSN 1089-2974
NATIONAL DIRECTORY OF BRAIN INJURY REHABILITATION SERVICES*. Text in English. 1985. a. USD 50 (effective 1997). **Document type:** *Directory.* **Description:** State by state listing of providers of services for people with traumatic brain injury, including rehabilitation programs and individual professionals.
Formerly: National Directory of Head Injury Rehabilitation Services (0892-6972)
Published by: Brain Injury Association, Inc., 105 N Alfred St, Alexandria, VA 22314-3010. TEL 202-296-6443, FAX 202-296-8850, publications@biausa.org.

(YEAR) NATIONAL DIRECTORY OF FIRE CHIEFS & E M S ADMINISTRATORS. see *FIRE PREVENTION*

617.1 DEU ISSN 0932-3643
NEUROORTHOPAEDIE. (Represents material presented at annual Erlangen Workshops) Text in German. 1983. irreg., latest vol.5, 1994. **Document type:** *Proceedings.*
Indexed: e-psyche.
—CISTI, KNAW.
Published by: Springer-Verlag (Subsidiary of: BertelsmannSpringer), Haber Str 7, Heidelberg 69126, Germany. FAX 49-30-82787448, subscriptions@springer.de, http://www.springer.de, http://link.springer-ny.com. **Subscr. in N. America to:** Meadowlands Pkwy., Secaucus, NJ 07094. TEL 212-460-1500, 212-473-6272.

617 USA ISSN 1063-7389
CODEN: NEHOFH
NEW HORIZONS (BALTIMORE). Variant title: New Horizons: The Science and Practice of Acute Medicine. Text in English. 1993. q. USD 110 domestic to individuals; USD 140 foreign to individuals; USD 160 domestic to institutions; USD 190 foreign to institutions. adv. back issues avail. **Document type:** *Academic/Scholarly.*
Related titles: Microform ed.; ♦ Supplement to: Critical Care Medicine. ISSN 0090-3493.
Indexed: Chem.Abstr., Chem.Indus.Notes, Chem.Titles, Curr.Cont. (coverage dropped), Excerp.Med. (1995-), Ind.Med. (1994-, dropped), Inpharma, Pharm.&Out.News, Reac., Ref.Zh.
—CASDDS, CISTI, GNLM, IDS, KNAW.

Published by: (Society of Critical Care Medicine), Williams & Wilkins (Subsidiary of: Waverly International), 351 W Camden St, Baltimore, MD 21201-2436. TEL 410-528-4068, 800-222-3790, FAX 410-528-4452, dbakerv@wwilkins.com, http://www.wwilkins.com. Ed. William C Shoemaker. Adv. contact David Baker. Circ: 8,892.

617 JPN ISSN 1340-6264
NIHON GAISHO GAKKAI ZASSHI/JAPANESE ASSOCIATION FOR THE SURGERY OF TRAUMA. JOURNAL. Text in Japanese; Abstracts in English. 1987. 4/yr. JPY 2,000. adv. *Refereed.* **Document type:** *Academic/Scholarly.*
Formerly (until 1994): Nihon Gaisho Kenkyukaishi (0914-4927)
—BLDSC (4809.095000).
Published by: Nihon Gaisho Gakkai/Japanese Association for the Surgery of Trauma, Daigaku Kyumei Kyukyu Senta, 11-1 Kaga 2-chome, Itabashi-ku, Tokyo 173-0003, Japan. TEL 81-3-3964-1211, FAX 81-3-5375-0854, jast@med.teikyo-u.ac.jp, http://www.ed.teikyo-u.ac.jp/~jast/. Ed. Kazuhiko Maekawa. Pub. Kunio Kobayashi. Adv. contact Toshio Nakatani. page JPY 30,000. Circ: 1,200 (controlled).

617.3 JPN ISSN 1340-8852
NIHON GAKU TOGAI KINO GAKKAISHI/JAPAN ASSOCIATION OF CRANIO-MANDIBULAR ORTHOPEDICS. JOURNAL. Text in Multiple languages. 1988. a. back issues avail. **Document type:** *Journal, Academic/Scholarly.*
Formerly (until 1994): Nihon Gaku Togai Kino Kenkyukaishi (0915-8766)
Published by: Nihon Gaku Togai Kino Kenkyukai, c/o Center for Academic Societies Japan, Osaka, 14th Fl, Senri Life Science Center Bldg., 1-4-2 Shinsenrihigashi-machi, Togonaka 560-0082, Japan.

617.3 JPN ISSN 0917-4648
NIHON KOTSU KEITAI KEISOKU GAKKAI ZASSHI/JAPANESE SOCIETY OF BONE MORPHOMETRY. JOURNAL. Text in Japanese; Summaries in English, Japanese. 1991. 2/yr. JPY 6,000.
Indexed: INIS Atomind.
Published by: Nihon Kotsu Keitai Keisoku Gakkai, Niigata Daigaku Igakubu Seikei Gekagaku Kyoshitsu, Asahimachi Dori 1 Bancho, Niigata-shi, Niigata-ken 951, Japan. TEL 81-25-223-6161, FAX 81-25-229-1675. Ed. Hideaki Takahashi. Circ: 1,000 (controlled).

617.3 616.89 JPN ISSN 0914-6822
NIHON PARAPUREJIA IGAKKAI ZASSHI/JAPAN MEDICAL SOCIETY OF PARAPLEGIA. JOURNAL. Text in English, Japanese; Summaries in English. 1988. a.
Indexed: e-psyche.
—BLDSC (4805.505000).
Published by: Nihon Parapurejia Igakkai, Keio Gijuku Daigaku Igakubu Seikei Gekagaku Kyoshitsu, 35 Shinano-Machi, Shinjuku-ku, Tokyo 160-0016, Japan.

617.3 616.075 JPN ISSN 0915-7107
NIHON SEIKEI GEKA CHOONPA KENKYUKAI KAISHI/JAPANESE SOCIETY OF ORTHOPEDIC ULTRASONICS. JOURNAL. Text in Japanese. 1989. a. JPY 3,000. *Refereed.* **Document type:** *Academic/Scholarly.*
Published by: Nihon Seikei Geka Choonpa Kenkyukai, Osaka Ika Daigaku Seikei Gekagaku Kyoshitsu, 2-7 Daigaku-Machi, Takatsuki-shi, Osaka-fu 569-0801, Japan. Ed. Hiromi Matsuzaki.

617 JPN ISSN 0916-1643
NIHON SEIKEI GEKA SUPOTSU IGAKKAISHI/JAPANESE JOURNAL OF ORTHOPEDIC SPORTS MEDICINE. Text in Japanese. 1982. a. membership.
Published by: Nihon Seikei Geka Supotsu Igakkai/Japanese Orthopedic Society for Sports Medicine, Yokohama Shiritsu Kowan Byoin Seikei Geka, 2-3, Shin'yamashita 3-chome, Naka-ku, Yokohama-shi, Kanagawa-ken 231, Japan.

617.3 JPN ISSN 0917-7132
NIHON SEKITSUI GEKA GAKKAI DAYORI/JAPAN SPINE RESEARCH SOCIETY. NEWS. Text in Japanese. 1991. s-a.
Published by: Nihon Sekitsui Geka Gakkai, Keio Gijuku Daigaku Igakubu Seikei Gekagaku Kyoshitsu, 35 Shinano-Machi, Shinjuku-ku, Tokyo 160-0016, Japan.

617.3 JPN ISSN 0915-6496
NIHON SEKITSUI GEKA GAKKAI ZASSHI/JAPAN SPINE RESEARCH SOCIETY. JOURNAL. Text in English, Japanese. 1990. a.

M

—BLDSC (4808.240000).
Published by: Nihon Sekitsui Geka Gakkai, Keio Gijuku Daigaku Igakubu Seikei Gekagaku Kyoshitsu, 35 Shinano-Machi, Shinjuku-ku, Tokyo 160-0016, Japan.

NIHON SHONI SEIKEI GEKA GAKKAI ZASSHI/JAPANESE PAEDIATRIC ORTHOPAEDIC ASSOCIATION. JOURNAL. see *MEDICAL SCIENCES—Pediatrics*

617.3 JPN ISSN 0915-4906
NIHON SOGAI KOTEI KENKYUKAISHI/JAPANESE SOCIETY OF EXTERNAL FIXATION. JOURNAL. Text in Japanese; Summaries in English. 1990. a.
Published by: Nihon Sogai Kotei Kenkyukai, Asahi Daigaku Murakami Kinen Byoin Seikei Geka Kyoshitsu, 3-23 Hashimoto-cho, Gifu-shi 500-8856, Japan.

617.3 JPN ISSN 0910-5700
NIHON TE NO GEKA GAKKAI ZASSHI/JAPANESE SOCIETY FOR SURGERY OF THE HAND. JOURNAL. Text in Japanese; Summaries in English. 1984. 6/yr.
Indexed: INIS Atomind.
—BLDSC (4809.518000), CISTI.
Published by: Nihon Te no Geka Gakkai, Kyusyu Daigaku Igakubu Seikei Gekagaku Kyoshitsu, 1-1, Umade 3-chome, Higashi-ku, Fukuoka-shi, Fukuoka-ken 812, Japan.

617.3 JPN ISSN 0914-6636
NIIGATA SEIKEI GEKA KENKYUKAI KAISHI/NIIGATA SOCIETY FOR ORTHOPAEDIC SURGERY. ARCHIVES. Text in Japanese. 1983. a.
Published by: Niigata Seikei Geka Kenkyukai, Niigata Daigaku Igakubu Seikei Geka Kyoshitsu, 1, Asahimachi Dori, Niigata-shi, Niigata-ken 951, Japan.

617.3 JPN ISSN 0287-1092
NISHINIHON SEKITSUI KENKYUKAISHI/WESTERN JAPANESE RESEARCH SOCIETY FOR SPINE. JOURNAL. Text in Japanese. a. JPY 6,000.
Published by: Nishinihon Sekitsui Kenkyukai, Yamaguchi Daigaku Seikei Geka Kyoshitsu, 1144 Ogushi, Ube-shi, Yamaguchi-ken 755-0000, Japan.

616.025 DEU ISSN 1434-6222
NOTFALL UND RETTUNGSMEDIZIN; german interdisciplinary journal of emergency medicine. Variant title: Notfall. Text in German. 1998. 8/yr. EUR 153.09 domestic; EUR 149.69 in Germany; EUR 21 newsstand/cover foreign (effective 2002). *Refereed.* **Document type:** *Journal, Academic/Scholarly.* **Description:** Contains new developments and information on the practices and procedures of emergency medicine.
Related titles: Online - full text ed.: ISSN 1436-0578 (from EBSCO Publishing, RoweCom Information Quest, Swets Blackwell, Springer LINK).
Published by: Springer-Verlag (Subsidiary of: BertelsmannSpringer), Tiergartenstr 17, Heidelberg 69121, Germany. TEL 49-6221-345-0, FAX 49-6221-345229, subscriptions@springer.de, http://link.springer.de/link/service/journals/10049/index.htm, http://www.springer.de. Eds. P Lemburg, W Dick. **Subscr. in N. America to:** Springer-Verlag New York Inc., PO Box 2485, Secaucus, NJ 07096-2485. TEL 212-460-1500, FAX 212-473-6272.

610 DEU ISSN 0341-2903
NOTFALLMEDIZIN. Text in German. 1975. m. EUR 86.50 domestic to institutions; EUR 100.30 in Europe to institutions; EUR 127.30 elsewhere to institutions; EUR 10.50 newsstand/cover (effective 2002). bk.rev. abstr. index. **Document type:** *Academic/Scholarly.*
Indexed: Excerp.Med.
—EMDOCS, GNLM, KNAW. **CCC.**
Published by: Demeter Verlag GmbH und Co. KG, Ruedigerstr 14, Stuttgart 70469, Germany. TEL 49-711-8931-0, FAX 49-711-8931322. Circ: 45,000.

617.3 USA ISSN 1061-4621
O & P ALMANAC; the magazine for the orthotics & prosthetics profession. Text in English. 1951. m. USD 40 domestic; USD 79 foreign (effective 2000). adv. back issues avail. **Document type:** *Trade.* **Description:** Covers professional, business, association and government activities affecting the field.
Formerly (until 1991): American Orthotic and Prosthetic Association. Almanac
Published by: American Orthotic & Prosthetic Asssociation, 1650 King St, Ste 500, Alexandria, VA 22314. TEL 703-836-7116, FAX 703-836-0838. Ed., R&P Lisa L Gough. Adv. contact Amy Clontz. B&W page USD 1,310, color page USD 2,800; bleed 8.5 x 11.125. Circ: 6,100 (paid).

617.3 DEU ISSN 0934-6694
OPERATIVE ORTHOPAEDIE UND TRAUMATOLOGIE; Standardeingriffe und neue Verfahren. Text in German. 1989. q. EUR 191.31 domestic; EUR 205.31 foreign; EUR 142.71 domestic to students; EUR 156.71 foreign to students; EUR 57.94 newsstand/cover (effective 2002). adv. bk.rev. back issues avail. *Refereed.* **Document type:** *Journal, Academic/Scholarly.*
Related titles: Online - full text ed.: ISSN 1439-0981 (from EBSCO Publishing, RoweCom Information Quest, Swets Blackwell, Springer LINK); ♦ Spanish Translation: Tecnicas Quirurgicas en Ortopedia y Traumatologia. ISSN 1132-1954.
—GNLM.
Published by: Urban und Vogel Medien und Medizin Verlagsgesellschaft mbH (Subsidiary of: BertelsmannSpringer), Neumarkter Str 43, Munich 81673, Germany. TEL 49-89-43721411, FAX 49-89-43721410, verlag@urban-vogel.de, http://www.urban-vogel.de. Ed. M Blauth. R&P Oliver Renn. Circ: 3,500. **Subscr. to:** Springer Auslieferungs Gesellschaft, Postfach 105160, Heidelberg 69041, Germany. TEL 49-6221-345244, FAX 49-6221-345244.

617 USA ISSN 1048-6666
OPERATIVE TECHNIQUES IN ORTHOPAEDICS. Text in English. 1991. q. USD 161 domestic to individuals; USD 239 foreign to individuals; USD 256 domestic to institutions; USD 290 foreign to institutions; USD 100 domestic to students; USD 145 foreign to students; USD 73 newsstand/cover (effective 2001). adv. illus. *Refereed.* **Document type:** *Academic/Scholarly.* **Description:** Treats a clinical condition or surgical procedure in detail in each issue; alternative approaches are also presented.
Indexed: CINAHL.
—BLDSC (6269.381500), CISTI, GNLM, Infotrieve, KNAW. **CCC.**
Published by: W.B. Saunders Co. (Subsidiary of: Harcourt Publishers Ltd.), 11830 Westline Industrial Dr, St Louis, MO 63146. TEL 800-325-4177, http://www.wbsaunders.com. Ed. Dr. Freddie Fu. Adv. contact Cindy Gray. B&W page USD 670, color page USD 1,600; trim 10 x 7. Circ: 2,253. **Subscr. to:** Periodicals Fulfillment, W B Saunders Co, 6277 Sea Harbor Dr, 4th Fl, Orlando, FL 32891-4800.

617.3 DEU ISSN 0085-4530
CODEN: ORHPBG
DER ORTHOPAEDE. Text in German. 1972. m. EUR 333.92 domestic; EUR 305.12 in Germany; EUR 29 newsstand/cover foreign (effective 2002). back issues avail.; reprint service avail. from ISI. *Refereed.* **Document type:** *Journal, Academic/Scholarly.* **Description:** Offers information and continuing education for the orthopedic physician. Each issue treats one leding topic from orthopedics or a neighboring discipline and gives an overview of the current state of the science and practice.
Related titles: Microform ed.: (from PQC); Online - full text ed.: ISSN 1433-0431 (from EBSCO Publishing, RoweCom Information Quest, Swets Blackwell, Springer LINK, Institute for Scientific Information).
Indexed: ASCA, Curr.Cont., Excerp.Med., INIS Atomind., Ind.Med. (1972-), Inpharma, Int.Nurs.Ind., Pharm.&Out.News, Reac.
—BLDSC (6296.114000), CISTI, IDS, Infotrieve, KNAW. **CCC.**
Published by: Springer-Verlag (Subsidiary of: BertelsmannSpringer), Tiergartenstr 17, Heidelberg 69121, Germany. TEL 49-6221-345-0, FAX 49-6221-345229, subscriptions@springer.de, http://link.springer.de/link/service/journals/00132/index.htm, http://www.springer.de. Eds. R Bauer, W Dick. **Subscr. in N. America to:** Springer-Verlag New York Inc., PO Box 2485, Secaucus, NJ 07096-2485. TEL 212-460-1500, FAX 212-473-6272.

610 JPN ISSN 0387-4095
ORTHOPAEDIC AND TRAUMATIC SURGERY/SEKEI SAIGAI GEKA. Text in English, Japanese. 1958. m. JPY 1,900 per issue. bk.rev. index.
Formerly (until 1979): Journal of Accidental Medicine (0036-2689)
Indexed: C.I.S. Abstr., INIS Atomind., Jap.Per.Ind.
—CISTI.
Published by: Kanehara Shuppan Ltd., 2-31-14 Yushima, Bunkyo-ku, Tokyo 113-0034, Japan. Ed. Dr. Yoshio Yamauchi. Circ: 7,100.

617.3 ITA ISSN 1129-3853
CODEN: IJOTD
ORTHOPAEDIC AND TRAUMATOLOGY. Text in English. 1975. 3/yr. USD 135 (effective 2000). **Document type:** *Journal, Academic/Scholarly.* **Description:** Covers current thought, practice and research in the field of orthopaedics and traumatology.
Formerly (until 2000): Italian Journal of Orthopaedics and Traumatology (0390-5489)
Related titles: Microform ed.: (from PQC); ♦ Online - full content ed.: Orthopaedic and Traumatology Online; ♦ Italian ed.: Giornale Italiano di Ortopedia e Traumatologia. ISSN 0390-0134.
Indexed: Excerp.Med. (until 1993).
—GNLM, ingenta. **CCC.**
Published by: Springer-Verlag Italia Srl (Subsidiary of: BertelsmannSpringer), Via Podgora, 4, Milan, MI 20122, Italy. TEL 39-2-55194656, FAX 39-2-55193360, springer@springer.it, http://link.springer.de. Ed. F Pipino.

617.3 ITA
▼ **ORTHOPAEDIC AND TRAUMATOLOGY ONLINE.** Text in English. 2000. 3/yr. **Document type:** *Academic/Scholarly.*
Media: Online - full content. **Related titles:** Microform ed.: (from PQC); ♦ Print ed.: Orthopaedic and Traumatology. ISSN 1129-3853.
Published by: Springer-Verlag Italia Srl (Subsidiary of: BertelsmannSpringer), Via Podgora, 4, Milan, MI 20122, Italy. TEL 39-2-55194656, FAX 39-2-55193360, springer@springer.it, http://link.springer.de.

617.3 JPN ISSN 0289-2855
ORTHOPAEDIC CERAMIC IMPLANTS. Text in English, Japanese; Summaries in English. 1981. a.
Published by: Seikei Geka Seramikku Inpuranto Kenkyukai, Kokuritsu Osaka Minami Byoin Seikei Geka, 677-2 Kido-cho, Kawachinagano-shi, Osaka-fu 586-0001, Japan.

ORTHOPAEDIC NURSING JOURNAL. see *MEDICAL SCIENCES—Nurses And Nursing*

617.3 615.82 USA ISSN 1059-1516
ORTHOPAEDIC PHYSICAL THERAPY CLINICS OF NORTH AMERICA. Text in English. 1992. q. USD 83 domestic to individuals; USD 94 in Canada to individuals; USD 114 elsewhere to individuals; USD 128 domestic to institutions; USD 169 foreign to institutions; USD 73 domestic to students; USD 43 per issue (effective 2001). index. back issues avail. **Document type:** *Academic/Scholarly.* **Description:** Publishes review articles on emerging technologies, new approaches to treatment, and other topics.
Related titles: Microform ed.: (from PQC).
Indexed: Excerp.Med. (1995-).
—BLDSC (6296.125500), GNLM, KNAW. **CCC.**
Published by: W.B. Saunders Co. (Subsidiary of: Harcourt Publishers Ltd.), 11830 Westline Industrial Dr, St Louis, MO 63146. TEL 800-325-4177, http://www.wbsaunders.com. Eds. Jan K Richardson, Z Annette Inglarsh. **Subscr. to:** Periodicals Fulfillment, 6277 Sea Harbor Dr, 4th Fl, Orlando, FL 32891-4800.

617.3 615.82 USA
ORTHOPAEDIC PHYSICAL THERAPY PRACTICE. Text in English. 1989. q. USD 30. adv. bk.rev. **Document type:** *Newsletter.*
Published by: Orthopaedic Section A P T A, 2920 East Ave S, La Crosse, WI 54601-7202. TEL 608-788-3982, FAX 608-788-3965, orthostaff@centuryinter.net. Ed. Jonathan M Cooperman. R&P Sharon L Klinski. Circ: 12,500 (paid).

617.3 GBR ISSN 0954-4755
ORTHOPAEDIC PRODUCT NEWS. Text in English. 1987. 5/yr. GBP 26 in United Kingdom; GBP 34 in Europe; GBP 48 elsewhere (effective 2000). adv. illus, tr.lit. back issues avail. **Document type:** *Catalog.* **Description:** Provides details of new products and reviews of products for orthopedic surgeons in Europe.
Related titles: Online - full text ed.
Published by: Pelican Magazines Ltd., 14 Raglan St, Harrogate HG1 1LE, United Kingdom. TEL 44-1423-569676, FAX 44-1423-569677, editor@opnews.com, http://www.opnews.com. Ed., Adv. contact Leslie Charneca. B&W page USD 960, color page USD 1,430; trim 210 x 297. Circ: 8,500.

617.3 DEU ISSN 0941-2530
ORTHOPAEDICS AND TRAUMATOLOGY; new and established surgical techniques. Text in English. 1992. q. EUR 191.31 domestic; EUR 205.31 foreign; EUR 142.71 domestic to students; EUR 156.71 foreign to students; EUR 57.94 newsstand/cover (effective 2002). **Document type:** *Journal, Academic/Scholarly.*
Related titles: Online - full text ed.: ISSN 1617-3538 (from Springer LINK).
—BLDSC (6296.128000).

M

Published by: Urban und Vogel (Subsidiary of: BertelsmannSpringer), Lindwurmstr 95, Munich 80337, Germany. TEL 49-89-53292-0, FAX 49-89-53292-100, verlag@urban-vogel.de, http://www.urban-vogel.de. Ed. H K Uhthoff. Circ: 3,000. **Subscr. in N. America to:** Springer-Verlag New York Inc., 44 Hartz Way, Secaucus, NJ 07096-2491. TEL 201-348-4033, FAX 201-348-4505. **Dist. by:** Springer-Verlag, Haber Str 7, Heidelberg 69126, Germany. TEL 49-30-8207-1, FAX 49-30-8214091.

617.3 USA
ORTHOPAEDICS TODAY INTERNATIONAL EDITION. Text in English. bi-m. USD 210 to individuals; USD 235 to institutions. *Refereed.* **Document type:** *Academic/Scholarly.* **Description:** Provides the practicing orthopaedic surgeon with practical, clinical articles.
Published by: Slack, Inc., 6900 Grove Rd, Thorofare, NJ 08086-9447. TEL 856-848-1000, 800-257-8290, FAX 856-853-5991, http://www.slackinc.com. Ed. Dr. Robert D'Ambrosia.

617.3 DEU
ORTHOPAEDIE. Text in German. bi-m. EUR 122.80 domestic to institutions; EUR 124.80 in Europe to institutions; EUR 132.80 elsewhere to institutions; EUR 24 newsstand/cover (effective 2002). **Document type:** *Journal, Academic/Scholarly.*
Published by: Georg Thieme Verlag, Ruedigerstr 14, Stuttgart 70469, Germany. TEL 49-711-8931-0, FAX 49-711-8931133, leser.service@thieme.de, http://www.thieme.de.

617.533 DEU ISSN 0941-214X
ORTHOPAEDIE MITTEILUNGEN* . Text in German. 1971. q. DEM 60. **Document type:** *Academic/Scholarly.*
Formerly (until 1990): Deutsche Gesellschaft fuer Orthopaedie und Traumatologie. Mitteilungsblatt (0723-8002)
—GNLM.
Published by: Deutsche Gesellschaft fuer Orthopaedie und Traumatologie, Wilhelm Kramm Str 61 a, Bruehl 50321, Germany. Ed. Dr. Zichney. Circ: 2,200.

617.3 DEU
ORTHOPAEDIE TECHNIK QUARTERLY. Text in English, German. q. back issues avail. *Refereed.* **Description:** Covers all aspects of prosthetics, orthotics, and rehabilitation technology.
Media: Online - full text.
Published by: Bundesinnungsverband fuer Orthopaedieschuhtechnik, Reinoldistr 7-9, Dortmund 44135, Germany. TEL 49-231-5570-5050, FAX 49-231-5570-5070, wiegard@ot-forum.de, http://www.ot-forum.de/OTQuarterly/otq-aktuell.htm. Ed. Beate Wiegard.

617.3 DEU ISSN 1435-0017
ORTHOPAEDIE UND RHEUMA. Text in German. 1998. bi-m. EUR 41.64 domestic; EUR 48.64 foreign; EUR 6.54 newsstand/cover (effective 2002). **Document type:** *Journal, Academic/Scholarly.*
Former titles: Orthopaedie und Rheuma Praxisinformation; Orthopaedie und Rheuma Nachrichten
Published by: Urban und Vogel Medien und Medizin Verlagsgesellschaft mbH (Subsidiary of: BertelsmannSpringer), Neumarkter Str 43, Munich 81673, Germany. TEL 49-89-43721411, FAX 49-89-43721410, verlag@urban-vogel.de, http://www.urban-vogel.de. Ed. Dr. Michael Piper. R&P Friederik Klein. Adv. contact Paul Berger. Circ: 5,000 (paid).

617.3 DEU ISSN 0030-588X
CODEN: OPBAAS
ORTHOPAEDISCHE PRAXIS; mit Traumatologie, Rheumatologie, physikalischer, physiotherapeutischer und balneologischer Therapie des Bewegungsapparates. Text in German. 1965. m. DEM 227 domestic; DEM 23 newsstand/cover; DEM 272 foreign; DEM 170.25 domestic to students; DEM 215.25 foreign to students (effective 2001). adv. bk.rev. charts, illus. index, cum.index. back issues avail. **Document type:** *Magazine, Academic/Scholarly.*
Indexed: Excerp.Med.
—BLDSC (6296.120000), GNLM, Infotrieve, KNAW. **CCC.**
Published by: (Vereinigung Sueddeutscher Orthopaeden e.V.), Medizinisch Literarische Verlagsgesellschaft mbH, Postfach 1151-1152, Uelzen 29501, Germany. TEL 49-581-808151, FAX 49-581-808158, mlverlag@mlverlag.de, http://www.mlverlag.de. Eds. Dr. D Clemens, Dr. G Rompe. Circ: 5,000.

617.3 USA ISSN 0030-5898
CODEN: OCLNAQ
ORTHOPEDIC CLINICS OF NORTH AMERICA. Text in English. 1970. q. USD 154 domestic to individuals; USD 178 in Canada to individuals; USD 202 elsewhere to individuals; USD 214 domestic to institutions; USD 258 foreign to institutions; USD 104 domestic to students; USD 65 per issue (effective 2001). charts, illus. index. reprint service avail. from PQC,ISI. *Refereed.* **Document type:** *Journal, Academic/Scholarly.* **Description:** Discusses the practice of orthopedic treatment.
Related titles: Microform ed.: (from PQC); Online - full text ed.: (from Institute for Scientific Information).
Indexed: AIM, AMED, ASCA, Bibl.Dev.Med.& Child Neur., Biol.Abstr., CINAHL, Curr.Adv.Ecol.Sci., Curr.Cont., Excerp.Med., INIS Atomind., Ind.Med. (1970-), Ind.Sci.Rev., Inpharma, Mat.Sci.Cit.Ind. (coverage dropped), Reac., Sci.Cit.Ind.
—BLDSC (6296.135000), CISTI, GNLM, IDS, ingenta, KNAW. **CCC.**
Published by: W.B. Saunders Co. (Subsidiary of: Harcourt Publishers Ltd.), 11830 Westline Industrial Dr, St Louis, MO 63146. TEL 800-325-4177, http://www.wbsaunders.com. **Subscr. to:** Periodicals Fulfillment, W B Saunders Co, 6277 Sea Harbor Dr, 4th Fl, Orlando, FL 32891-4800.

317.305 USA ISSN 1059-311X
ORTHOPEDIC NETWORK NEWS. Text in English. q. USD 250 (effective 1999). **Document type:** *Trade.*
Published by: Mendenhall Associates, 1500 Cedar Bend Dr, Ann Arbor, MI 48105. TEL 313-741-4710. Pub. Stan Mendenhall.

616.0754 USA
ORTHOPEDIC, NEUROLOGICAL AND CHIROPRACTIC PHYSICAL EXAMINATIONS: TECHNIQUE AND SIGNIFICANCE. Text in English. 1988. base vol. plus a. updates. USD 39.50. **Description:** Includes an alphabetical listing of the various types of examinations, a summary of different conditions and which examinations might be performed to detect them, and a diagram setting out the planes of the body.
Indexed: e-psyche.
Published by: Lexis Law Publishing (Subsidiary of: Reed Elsevier plc), PO Box 7587, Charlottesville, VA 22906-7587. TEL 804-872-7600, 800-562-1197, FAX 804-972-7666, llp.customer.support@lexis-nexis.com, http://www.lexislawpublishing.com. Ed. Barry Creighton.

ORTHOPEDIC PRACTICE ADVISOR. see *HEALTH FACILITIES AND ADMINISTRATION*

617.3 USA ISSN 1056-4543
ORTHOPEDIC RESIDENT. Text in English. 1991. q. USD 40. adv. **Document type:** *Trade.* **Description:** Acts as a guide to career, life-style, and business issues facing residents in orthopedics. Covers preparing for boards, choosing fellowships, establishing a practice, and decision-making.
Published by: Slack, Inc., 6900 Grove Rd, Thorofare, NJ 08086-9447. TEL 856-848-1000, FAX 856-853-5991, http://www.slackinc.com. Ed. Dr. G Dean MacEwen. Circ: 3,000.

617.3 USA
ORTHOPEDIC SPECIAL EDITION. Text in English. 1988. s-a. USD 50 domestic; USD 60 foreign (effective 2001). adv. **Document type:** *Trade.* **Description:** Aimed at orthopedic surgeons and rheumatologists. Covers arthroscopy, arthroplasty, pain management, braces, rheumatic disease, and orthopedic technology.
Former titles: Orthopedic and Sports Medicine News; Sports Medicine News
Published by: McMahon Group, 545 W 45th St, New York, NY 10036-3409. TEL 212-957-5300, FAX 212-957-7230, stilyou@mcmahonmed.com, http://www.mcmahonmed.com/se/indexse.htm. Ed. Sara Tilyou. adv.: B&W page USD 3,300, color page USD 1,200. Circ: 20,384.

617.3 JPN ISSN 0030-5901
ORTHOPEDIC SURGERY/SEIKEI GEKA. Text in Japanese. 1950. 15/yr. JPY 65,000. adv. charts, illus. index.
Indexed: Biol.Abstr., Ind.Med. (coverage dropped).
—CISTI, GNLM.
Published by: Nankodo Co. Ltd., 42-6 Hongo 3-chome, Bunkyo-ku, Tokyo 113-0033, Japan. FAX 03-3811-7230. Ed. Toshinobu Onomura. Circ: 8,500.

617.3 USA
▼ **ORTHOPEDIC TECHNOLOGY REVIEW.** Text in English. 1999. 10/yr. free to qualified personnel. adv. **Document type:** *Journal, Trade.* **Description:** Provides a forum for discussion of the common economic issues faced by orthopedic practitioners and health care administrators, especially those related to the development, diffusion, acquisition and utilization of medical technologies.
Related titles: Online - full text ed.
Published by: Curant Communications, Inc. (Subsidiary of: Medical World Communications), 6701 Center Drive W #450, Los Angeles, CA 90045-1556. TEL 310-306-2206, FAX 310-306-9548, mbernal@medpubs.com, http://www.orthopedictechreview.com. Ed. Kristin Trompeter. Pubs. Curtis Pickelle, Tony Ramos. Adv. contact Sharon Marsee. B&W page USD 3,520, color page USD 4,620; trim 9.125 x 13. Circ: 30,000 (controlled).

617.3 USA ISSN 0147-7447
RD701
ORTHOPEDICS. Text in English. 1978. m. USD 145 to individuals; USD 165 in Canada to individuals; USD 185 elsewhere to individuals; USD 170 to institutions; USD 190 in Canada to institutions; USD 210 elsewhere to institutions. adv. back issues avail. *Refereed.* **Document type:** *Academic/Scholarly.* **Description:** Covers the entire spectrum of orthopedic surgery and treatment.
Related titles: Online - full text ed.: (from Northern Light Technology, Inc., ProQuest Information & Learning, Institute for Scientific Information).
Indexed: ASCA, Bibl.Dev.Med.& Child Neur., CINAHL, Cal.Tiss.Abstr., Curr.Cont., Environ.Sci.Poll.Mgmt., Excerp.Med., INIS Atomind., Ind.Med. (1978-), Inpharma, Int.Nurs.Ind., Pharm.&Out.News, Pollut.Abstr., Reac., Risk Abstr., Saf.Sci.Abstr., Tox.Abstr. (coverage dropped).
—BLDSC (6296.146000), CISTI, GNLM, IDS, ingenta, KNAW. **CCC.**
Published by: Slack, Inc., 6900 Grove Rd, Thorofare, NJ 08086-9447. TEL 856-848-1000, 800-257-8290, FAX 856-853-5991, http://www.slackinc.com. Ed. Dr. Robert D'Ambrosia. Circ: 28,000.

617.3 USA ISSN 0279-5647
ORTHOPEDICS TODAY. Text in English. 1981. m. USD 170 domestic to individuals; USD 190 in Canada to individuals; USD 210 elsewhere to individuals; USD 180 domestic to institutions; USD 200 in Canada to institutions; USD 220 elsewhere to institutions. adv. illus. **Document type:** *Trade.* **Description:** Features reports from scientific meetings covering the broad spectrum of orthopedic interests.
Related titles: Online - full text ed.
—BLDSC (6296.163000). **CCC.**
Published by: Slack, Inc., 6900 Grove Rd, Thorofare, NJ 08086-9447. TEL 856-848-1000, 800-257-8290, FAX 856-853-5991, http://www.slackinc.com. Ed. Dr. John McGinty. Circ: 23,800.

617 610.73 CAN ISSN 1207-2842
ORTHOSCOPE. Text in English. 1978. q. CND 35. adv. bk.rev. index. back issues avail. **Document type:** *Newsletter.*
Former title (until 1995): C O N A Newsletter (1207-2834); (until 1994): C O N A Journal (0708-6474)
Indexed: CINAHL.
Published by: (Canadian Orthopaedic Nurses Association), Pappin Communications, The Victoria Centre, 84 Isabella St, Pembroke, ON K8A 5S5, Canada. TEL 613-735-0952, FAX 613-735-7983, http://www.nursing.ucalgary.ca/cona. Ed., R&P Bill Grudecki. Circ: 600.

617.3 BGR ISSN 0473-4378
ORTOPEDIA I TRAUMATOLOGIA. Text in Bulgarian; Summaries in English, Russian. q. BGL 15.
Indexed: Abstr.Bulg.Sci.Med.Lit., INIS Atomind.
—EMDOCS, GNLM.
Published by: (Bulgaria. Ministerstvo na Narodnoto Zdrave), Izdatelstvo Meditsina i Fizkultura, 11 Pl Slaveikov, Sofia 1080, Bulgaria. Ed. D Djerov. Circ: 815. **Distr. by:** Hemus, 6 Rouski blvd, Sofia 1000, Bulgaria. **Co-sponsor:** Nauchno Druzhestvo po Ortopedija i Traumatologija.

617.3 ITA ISSN 1123-6531
ORTOPEDIA NEWS. Text in Italian. 1995. 3/yr. adv. **Document type:** *Newsletter.*
Published by: C I C Edizioni Internazionali s.r.l., Corso Trieste 42, Rome, RM 00198, Italy. TEL 39-06-8412673, FAX 39-06-8412688, info@gruppocic.it, 1160199510. Ed. L Romanini. adv.: B&W page XEU 1,601.02, color page XEU 2,014.18; 210 x 290.

M

617.3 ITA ISSN 0030-5979
ORTOPEDICI E SANITARI. Text in Italian. 1964. m. ITL 25,000; ITL 80,000 in Europe; ITL 140,000 elsewhere (effective 1999). adv. illus, pat. **Document type:** *Trade.* **Description:** Deals with new products in orthopedic field.
Published by: Tecniche Nuove s.p.a., Via Ciro Menotti, 14, Milan, MI 20129, Italy. TEL 39-027570318, FAX 39-02-7570236, abbonamenti@tecnet.it; ortes@tecnet.it, http://www.tecnet.it/index1.html. Ed. Enzo Guaglione. Pub. Giuseppe Nardella. Adv. contact Sergio Savona. B&W page ITL 1,730,000, color page ITL 2,290,000; trim 297 x 210. Circ: 10,000.

617.3 SWE ISSN 0349-733X
ORTOPEDISKT MAGASIN; nordisk tidskrift foer ortopedi och rehabilitering. Text in Swedish. 1977. q. SEK 150 to non-members; SEK 125 to members (effective 2002). adv. **Document type:** *Magazine, Academic/Scholarly.*
Address: Everod 13, Tomelilla 27393, Sweden. TEL 46-417-31026, FAX 46-417-31261, http://www.ortopedisktmagasin.com/huvudsida.html. Ed. Boerje Ohlsson. adv.: B&W page SEK 9,200, color page SEK 12,100.

617.3 JPN ISSN 0914-8124
ORUSOPEDIKUSU/ORTHOPAEDICS. Text in Japanese. 1988. m. JPY 2,000 per issue.
Published by: (Zennihon Byoin Shuppankai), Kanehara Shuppan Ltd., 2-31-14 Yushima, Bunkyo-ku, Tokyo 113-0034, Japan.

617.3 JPN ISSN 0917-8562
OSAKA SHIDAI SEIKEI GEKA KENKYUKAISHI/OSAKA CITY UNIVERSITY ORTHOPEDIC SURGERY. BULLETIN. Text in Japanese. 1983. s-a.
Published by: Osaka Shiritsu Daigaku, Igakubu/Osaka City University, Medical School, Department of Orthopedic Surgery, Alumni Association, Seikei Gekagaku Kyoshitsu Dosokai, 5-7 Asahi-Machi 1-chome, Abeno-ku, Osaka-shi 545-0051, Japan.

OSTEOARTHRITIS AND CARTILAGE; Journal of the osteoarthritis research society international. see *MEDICAL SCIENCES—Rheumatology*

617.3 CHE ISSN 1019-1291
CODEN: OSTEFK
OSTEOLOGIE. Text in German, English. 1992. q. CHF 276 (effective 2001). adv. abstr, bibl, charts, illus. 72 p./no. **Document type:** *Journal, Academic/Scholarly.*
—GNLM.
Published by: (Deutsche Gesellschaft fuer Osteologie), Hans Huber AG, Laengassstr 76, Bern, 9 3000, Switzerland. TEL 41-31-3004500, FAX 41-31-3004591, zeitschriften@hanshuber.com, http://www.hanshuber.com. Ed. H.-G. Willert. Adv. contact Rene Waelchli. color page CHF 3,820; trim 216 x 303. Circ: 1,500.

617 USA ISSN 0889-5899
RD94
OSTOMY - WOUND MANAGEMENT; the journal of extended patient care management. Text in English. 1980. m. USD 39.95; USD 59.95 foreign (effective 1999). adv. charts, illus, stat. **Document type:** *Trade.*
Formerly: Ostomy Management
Indexed: CINAHL, Int.Nurs.Ind.
—BLDSC (6312.377000), CISTI, GNLM.
Published by: H M P Communications, LLC, 950 W Valley Rd, Ste 2800, Wayne, PA 19087. TEL 610-688-8220, 800-237-7285, FAX 610-688-1060. Ed. Kim Chesky.

OUTREACH (CHICAGO). see *HEALTH FACILITIES AND ADMINISTRATION*

616.025 GBR
OXFORD HANDBOOKS IN EMERGENCY MEDICINE. Text in English. 1991. irreg. price varies. back issues avail. **Document type:** *Monographic series.*
Published by: Oxford University Press, Oxford Journals, Walton St, Oxford OX2 6DP, United Kingdom. TEL 44-1865-56767, FAX 44-1865-56646, jnl.orders@oup.co.uk, http://www.oup.co.uk/. **Orders in N. America to:** Oxford University Press, Journals, 2001 Evans Rd, Cary, NC 27513. TEL 919-677-0977, FAX 919-677-1714.

617.1 617.3 616.992 USA
▼ **THE PAIN CLINIC: A MULTIDISCIPLINARY APPROACH TO ACUTE AND CHRONIC PAIN MANAGEMENT.** Text in English. 1999. bi-m. free (effective 2001). adv. back issues avail. *Refereed.* **Document type:** *Magazine, Academic/Scholarly.*
Published by: Odyssea Publishing, Inc., PO Box 653, Bernardsville, NJ 07924. TEL 732-805-0585, FAX 732-805-9582, pain653@aol.com, http://www.thepainclinicjournal.com/. Ed. Lloyd R Saberski, MD. Pub., R&P Susan Lusty. Adv. contact Tom Terreri TEL 973-808-1312. Circ: 36,394 (controlled).

PEDIATRIC EMERGENCY CARE. see *MEDICAL SCIENCES—Pediatrics*

616.025 618.92 USA ISSN 1082-3344
PEDIATRIC EMERGENCY MEDICINE REPORTS. Text in English. 1996. m. USD 297 domestic; USD 327 foreign; USD 50 newsstand/cover (effective 2001). **Document type:** *Newsletter.* **Description:** Contains reviews of current issues faced by physicians dealing with pediatric emergencies. Topics include airway emergencies, trauma, metabolic disorders, fevers, toxicology, and more.
Related titles: Online - full text ed.: (from Northern Light Technology, Inc.).
Published by: American Health Consultants (Subsidiary of: Medical Economics Co., Inc.), 3525 Piedmont Rd, N E, 6 Piedmont Center, Ste 400, Atlanta, GA 30305. TEL 404-262-5476, 404-262-7436, 800-688-2421, FAX 404-262-7837, 800-284-3291, custserv@ahcpub.com, http://www.ahcpub.com. Ed. Larry Mellick. Pub. Brenda L Mooney.

617.11 360 USA
PHOENIX SOCIETY NEWSLETTER. Text in English. 1980. q. USD 12; USD 20 foreign (effective 1999). adv. bk.rev. back issues avail. **Document type:** *Newsletter.* **Description:** For burn survivors, their families and professionals in fields related to burn injuries. Features news regarding prevention, treatment and rehabilitation, personal stories, listing of resource materials available.
Formerly: Icarus File (1081-4396)
Published by: Phoenix Society, Inc., 2153 Wealthy S E, Ste 215, East, Grand Rapids, MI 49506. TEL 616-458-2773, FAX 616-458-2831. Ed. Claudia Belleau. Pub., R&P Amy Acton. Adv. contact Wendy Hunt. Circ: 9,000.

617.13 USA ISSN 0890-3972
PODIATRIC PRODUCTS✶ . Text in English. 1984. 7/yr. USD 14 (effective 2000). adv. bk.rev. charts, illus. **Document type:** *Magazine, Trade.* **Description:** Provides a source for the most up-to-date news on products, services and technology for podiatrists.
Formerly (until 1986): Podiatry Products Report
Published by: Novicom, Inc. (Subsidiary of: Medical World Communications), 6701 Center Dr West, Ste 450, Los Angeles, CA 90045-1556. TEL 310-642-4400, FAX 310-641-1511, http://www.novicom.com. Ed. Miwon Seo. Adv. contacts Lisa Chose, Michael Stephenson. B&W page USD 1,453, color page USD 2,153; trim 8.125 x 10.825. Circ: 14,000 (controlled).

617.585 USA
PODIATRIST'S PATIENT NEWSLETTER. Text in English. 1983. q. USD 645 per quarter for 1000 copies (effective 2001). 4 p./no. 3 cols./p. **Document type:** *Newsletter, Consumer.*
Published by: Newsletters Ink, PO Box 2019, Lancaster, PA 17608-2019. TEL 717-393-1000, 800-379-5585, FAX 717-393-4702, http://www.newslettersink.com. Ed. Ann Mead Ash. Pub. Gregory A Gilson.

PODIATRY INDEX. see *MEDICAL SCIENCES—Abstracting, Bibliographies, Statistics*

617.585 USA ISSN 0744-3528
PODIATRY MANAGEMENT. Text in English. 1982. 9/yr. USD 30 domestic; USD 34 in Canada; USD 50 elsewhere (effective 2000). adv. bk.rev. pat, stat. back issues avail. **Document type:** *Magazine, Trade.*
Indexed: CINAHL.
—BLDSC (6541.498070).
Published by: Kane Communications, Inc., 7000 Terminal Sq, Ste 210, Upper Darby, PA 19082. TEL 610-734-2420, FAX 610-734-2423. Ed. Dr. Barry H Block. Pub., R&P Scott C Borowsky. Adv. contact David Kagan TEL 610-734-2427. color page USD 2,600, B&W page USD 1,800. Circ: 15,066.

615.585 GBR ISSN 1460-731X
PODIATRY NOW. Text in English. 1998. m. GBP 55 in Europe; GBP 70 overseas (effective 2000). *Refereed.* **Document type:** *Academic/Scholarly.*
Formed by the 1998 merger of part of: Journal of British Podiatric Medicine (0961-6055); Which was formerly (1914-1991): Chiropodist (0009-4706); Part of: British Journal of Podiatric Medicine and Surgery (0955-8160); Which was formerly (until 1989): Podiatric Society. Journal
Published by: Society of Chiropodists and Podiatrists, 53 Welbeck St, London W1M 7HE, United Kingdom. TEL 44-1714-863381, FAX 44-1719-356359, cr@scpod.org. Ed. Clare Richards.

617.3 USA ISSN 1045-7860
PODIATRY TODAY. Text in English. 1988. m. USD 36 domestic; USD 46 in Canada; USD 60 elsewhere (effective 2000). adv. **Document type:** *Magazine, Trade.*
—CCC.
Published by: H M P Communications, LLC, 950 W Valley Rd, Ste 2800, Wayne, PA 19087. TEL 610-688-8220, 800-237-7285, FAX 610-688-8050. adv.: B&W page USD 1,210, color page USD 1,810. Circ: 15,000 (controlled).

016.61 CZE ISSN 1212-4575
CODEN: POUSE
POHYBOVE USTROJI; pokroky ve vyzkumu diagnostice a terapii. Text in Czech, English. 1957. q., latest vol.7, 2000. CZK 240 domestic; USD 10 foreign (effective 2002). adv. bk.rev. abstr. *Refereed.* **Document type:** *Journal, Abstract/Index.* **Description:** Concentrates on progress in connective tissue research and its biological uses; diagnostics, pediatric orthopedic surgery and therapy, dysmorphology, bone dysplasias, congenital limb defects, plastic surgery, biomechanics and biorheology, clinical anthropology and paleopathology.
Former titles (until 1999): Pohybove Ustroji (1210-7182); (until 1993): Referatovy Vyber z Ortopedie, Traumatologie a Pribuznych Oboru (0034-2823)
Related titles: CD-ROM ed.
Indexed: Excerp.Med. (1995-).
Published by: Ortotika s.r.o., Truhlarska 8, Prague, 8 11000, Czech Republic. TEL 420-2-12314760, FAX 420-2-24816481, ambul_centrum@volny.cz, ortotika@ortotika.cz, http://www.volny.cz/ambul_centrum, http://www.ortotika.cz. Ed. Ivo Marik. Circ: 500 (controlled).

616.025 USA ISSN 1090-3127
CODEN: PEMCFS
PREHOSPITAL EMERGENCY CARE; official journal of the National Association of E M S physicians. Text in English. 1997. q., latest vol.5, 2001. USD 72 domestic to individuals; USD 82 foreign to individuals; USD 96 domestic to institutions; USD 106 foreign to institutions; USD 25 newsstand/cover (effective 2001). adv. back issues avail. *Refereed.* **Document type:** *Journal, Academic/Scholarly.* **Description:** Delivers up-to-date clinical and research information on advances in medical care in the out-of-hospital setting.
Indexed: CINAHL, Ind.Med. (1997-), Jrnl.Watch Emer.Med.
—BLDSC (6605.917000), GNLM, KNAW.
Published by: Hanley & Belfus, Inc., 210 S 13th St, Philadelphia, PA 19107. TEL 215-546-7293, FAX 215-790-9330, ltroy@aol.com. Ed. James J Menegazzi. adv.: B&W page USD 715;.

617.14 AUS ISSN 1323-2495
PRIMARY INTENTION; the Australian journal of wound management. Text in English. q. AUD 72 domestic to individuals; AUD 92 foreign to individuals; AUD 100 to membership; AUD 20 per issue domestic; AUD 25 per issue foreign (effective 2000). adv. **Document type:** *Academic/Scholarly.*
—BLDSC (6612.909295).
Published by: (Australian Wound Management Association USA), Ink Press International, 15 Northwood St, West Leederville, W.A. 6007, Australia. TEL 61-8-9388-1505, FAX 61-8-9388-1510. Eds. Jenny Prentice, Michael Stacey.

617 USA
PRINCIPLES AND TECHNIQUES IN SPINE SURGERY SERIES. Text in English. 1992. irreg. price varies. **Document type:** *Monographic series.*
Indexed: e-psyche.
Published by: Lippincott - Raven Publishers (Subsidiary of: Wolters Kluwer N.V.), 530 Walnut St, Philadelphia, PA 19106. TEL 215-521-8300, FAX 215-521-8902, http:/www.lrpub.com. R&P Alice McElhinney. **Subscr. to:** Box 1600, Hagerstown, MD 21741-1600. TEL 800-777-2295, FAX 301-824-7390.

617.3 617.58 DNK ISSN 0309-3646
CODEN: POIND7
PROSTHETICS AND ORTHOTICS INTERNATIONAL. Text in English. 1964. 3/yr. GBP 90; GBP 30 newsstand/cover (effective 2001). adv. bk.rev. illus. index. *Refereed.* **Document type:** *Journal, Academic/Scholarly.* **Description:** Publishes scientific articles on prosthetics, orthotics and related topics.
Formerly (until 1971): Prosthetics International (0555-4837)
Related titles: Online - full text ed.: (from Institute for Scientific Information).

M

Indexed: AMED, ASCA, Bibl.Dev.Med.& Child Neur., Biol.Abstr., Curr.Cont., Excerp.Med., INSPEC (1968-1971, Apr.1979-), Ind.Med. (1977-), Inpharma, Pharm.&Out.News, Reac., Ref.Zh., SSCI (coverage dropped).
—BLDSC (6935.500000), AskIEEE, CISTI, EMDOCS, GNLM, ingenta, KNAW.
Published by: International Society for Prosthetics and Orthotics, Borgervaenget 5, Copenhagen Oe 2100, Denmark. TEL 45-39-20-72-60, FAX 45-39-20-75-01. Eds. John Hughes, Norman A Jacobs TEL 44-141-552-4049. R&P, Adv. contact Norman A Jacobs TEL 44-141-552-4049. Circ: 3,300 (controlled).

616.02 ESP
▼ **PUESTA AL DIA EN URGENCIAS, EMERGENCIAS Y CATASTROFES.** Text in Spanish; Abstracts in Spanish, English. 1999. q. ESP 8,000; USD 200 foreign (effective 2000). adv. abstr, bibl, illus, stat. back issues avail. *Refereed.* **Document type:** *Academic/Scholarly.*
Published by: Aran Ediciones S.A., Castello, 128 1o, Madrid 28006, Spain. TEL 34-91-782-0030, FAX 34-91-561-5787, edita@grupoaran.com, http://www.grupoaran.com. Ed. C. Alvarez Leiva. Pub. Jose Jimenez. R&P Maria Dolores Linares TEL 34-1-7820035. Circ: 10,000.

RACHIS; revue de pathologie vertebrale. see *MEDICAL SCIENCES—Rheumatology*

REANIMATION - URGENCES. see *MEDICAL SCIENCES—Anaesthesiology*

617.3 GBR ISSN 0308-4914
RECENT ADVANCES IN ORTHOPAEDICS. Text in English. 1969. irreg., latest vol.6. **Document type:** *Monographic series, Academic/Scholarly.*
—KNAW.
Published by: Churchill Livingstone (Subsidiary of: Harcourt Publishers Ltd.), Robert Stevenson House, 1-3 Baxter's Pl, Leith Walk, Edinburgh, Midlothian EH1 3AF, United Kingdom. TEL 44-131-556-2424, FAX 44-131-459-1177, http://www.churchillmed.com. **US subscr. to:** Churchill Livingstone, 650 Ave of the Americas, New York, NY 10011. TEL 212-206-5000.

617.1 USA
RESOURCES IN WOUND CARE. Text in English. 1992. a. USD 25. adv. **Document type:** *Trade.* **Description:** Serves as a guide to wound care practitioners and purchasing agents.
Formerly: Wound Care Products Resource
Published by: Springhouse Corporation (Subsidiary of: Lippincott Williams & Wilkins (Philadelphia)), 1111 Bethlehem Tpk., Springhouse, PA 19477-0908. TEL 215-646-8700, FAX 215-646-0341, http://www.woundcarenet.com. Ed. Susan Doan Johnson. Pub. Kate Strauser. Adv. contact Janna Winans. B&W page USD 2,275; trim 10.88 x 8. Circ: 21,000.

616.02 USA ISSN 0732-2933
TL553.8
RESPONSE (FAIRFAX)* . Text in English. 1982. q. USD 12.95; USD 15.95 in Canada; USD 24.95 elsewhere. adv. bk.rev. *Refereed.* **Document type:** *Trade.* **Description:** Provides technical information to the emergency response community at the federal, state and local levels, describing new techniques, procedures, products and technology in the search, rescue and emergency services.
Published by: National Association for Search and Rescue, 4500 Southgate Pl, Ste 100, Chantilly, VA 22021-1714. TEL 703-352-1349, FAX 703-352-0309. Ed. Judi Schmitt. Adv. contact Mary Harding. B&W page USD 661, color page USD 911; trim 10.88 x 8.25. Circ: 6,000.

RESPONSE (FORTITUDE VALLEY). see *HEALTH FACILITIES AND ADMINISTRATION*

617.3 BRA ISSN 0102-3616
REVISTA BRASILEIRA DE ORTOPEDIA. Text in Portuguese. 1939-1943; resumed 1966. m. BRL 150; USD 240 foreign. adv. bibl. **Description:** Describes research in orthopedic medicine and traumatology.
Supersedes (1939-1943): Revista Brasileira de Orthopedia e Traumatologia (0102-2326)
Indexed: INIS Atomind.
Published by: (Sociedade Brasileira de Ortopedia e Traumatologia), Redprint Editora Ltda., Rua Domingos de Morais 2777, 15o cjs 151 e 154, Sao Paulo, SP 04035-001, Brazil. TEL 55-11-5724813, FAX 55-11-5711719, redprint@uol.com.br. Ed. Dr. Donato D'Angelo.

617.3 CUB
REVISTA CUBANA DE ORTOPEDIA Y TRAUMATOLOGIA. Text in Spanish; Abstracts in English, French, Spanish. 1987. s-a. USD 48 in the Americas; USD 56 in Europe; USD 64 elsewhere.
Published by: (Cuba. Ministerio de Salud Publica, Centro Nacional de Informacion de Ciencias Medicas), Editorial de Ciencias Medicas, O'Reilly No. 4, Habana, Cuba. TEL 809-62-8091. Ed. Emilio Hernandez. Circ: 1,300. **Co-sponsors:** Hospital de Ortopedia y Traumatologia "Frank Pais"; Sociedad Cubana de Ortopedia y Traumatologia.

617.3 ESP ISSN 0482-5985
REVISTA DE ORTOPEDIA Y TRAUMATOLOGIA. Text in Spanish. bi-m. ESP 14,000, USD 145 to individuals; ESP 16,900 to institutions; ESP 11,000 to students. adv. back issues avail.; reprints avail. *Refereed.* **Document type:** *Academic/Scholarly.*
Related titles: Online - full text ed.
—BLDSC (7869.340000), CINDOC, GNLM.
Published by: (Sociedad Espanola de Cirugia Ortopedica y Traumatologia), Editorial Garsi S.A. (Subsidiary of: Grupo Masson), Juan Bravo, 46, Madrid 28006, Spain. TEL 34-91-402-1212, FAX 34-91-402-0954, garsi@mad.servicom.es, http://www.masson.es. Ed. J Gonzles del Pino. adv.: B&W page ESP 122,000, color page ESP 168,000; 280 x 210. Circ: 4,000.

617.3 FRA ISSN 0035-1040
REVUE DE CHIRURGIE ORTHOPEDIQUE ET REPARATRICE DE L'APPAREIL MOTEUR. Text in French; Summaries in English. 1890. 9/yr. FRF 980; FRF 1,233 foreign (effective 2000). bk.rev. illus. index. reprint service avail. from ISI. *Refereed.* **Document type:** *Academic/Scholarly.* **Description:** Publishes original articles of clinical facts, technical notes, publication analyses, reports of meetings and congresses.
Formerly: Revue d'Orthopedie et de Chirurgie de l'Appareil Moteur (1243-2504)
Related titles: Microform ed.: (from PQC); Online - full text ed.: (from Institute for Scientific Information, RoweCom Information Quest); ♦ English ed.: European Journal of Orthopaedic Surgery.
Indexed: ASCA, Bibl.Dev.Med.& Child Neur., Curr.Cont., Dent.Ind., Excerp.Med., Ind.Med. (1951-), Inpharma, Reac., Trop.Dis.Bull.
—BLDSC (7897.150000), CISTI, EMDOCS, GNLM, IDS, KNAW. **CCC.**
Published by: (Societe Francaise de Chirurgie Orthopedique et Traumatologique), Masson - Periodiques, 120 bd. St. Germain, Paris 75006, France. TEL 33-1-40466200, FAX 33-1-40466201. Ed. J M Thomine. Circ: 6,100. **Subscr. to:** Societe de Periodiques Specialises, BP 22, Vineuil Cedex 41354, France. TEL 33-2-54504612, FAX 33-2-54504611.

617.3 JPN ISSN 0557-0433
RINSHO SEIKEI GEKA/CLINICAL ORTHOPAEDIC SURGERY. Text in Japanese. 1966. m. JPY 2,200 per issue.
Indexed: INIS Atomind.
—BLDSC (3286.319000), CISTI.
Published by: Igaku-Shoin Ltd., 5-24-3 Hongo, Bunkyo-ku, Tokyo 113-0033, Japan. TEL 81-3-3817-5704. Circ: 9,000.

617.3 ITA ISSN 0035-693X
RIVISTA ITALIANA DI ORTOPEDIA E TRAUMATOLOGIA. Text in Italian. 1961. s-a. ITL 50,000; ITL 100,000 foreign (effective 1998).
—GNLM.
Published by: Casa Editrice Maccari, Via Palermo, 44, Parma, PR 43100, Italy. TEL 39-521-771268. Circ: 1,000.

617.3 JPN ISSN 0037-1033
SEIKEI GEKA TO SAIGAI GEKA/ORTHOPEDICS AND TRAUMATOLOGY. Text in English, Japanese. 1952. s-a. JPY 10,000. adv. **Document type:** *Academic/Scholarly.*
Indexed: INIS Atomind.
Published by: Nishi Nihon Seikei Saigai Geka Gakkai/West Japan Society of Orthopedics and Traumatology, c/o Dept of Orthopedic Surgery, Kyushu University, 3-1-1 Maidashi, Higashi-ku, Fukuoka-shi 812-0054, Japan. Ed. Yoichi Sugioka. Circ: 1,000.

617.3 JPN ISSN 0911-6826
SEKICHU HENKEI/SPINAL DEFORMITY. Text in English, Japanese. 1986. a.
Published by: Nihon Sokuwansho Kenkyukai/Japanese Scoliosis Society, Chiba Daigaku Igakubu Seikei Geka Kyoshitsu, 8-1 Inohana 1-chome, Chuo-ku, Chiba-shi 260-0856, Japan.

617.3 JPN ISSN 0914-4412
SEKITSUI SEKIZUI JANARU* /SPINE AND SPINAL CORD. Text in Japanese. 1988. m. JPY 1,900 per issue.
Published by: Miwa-Shoten Ltd., 17-9 Hongo, Bunkyo-ku, Tokyo 113-0033, Japan.

617.3 JPN ISSN 0914-6024
SEKIZUI GEKA/SPINAL SURGERY. Text in English, Japanese; Summaries in English. 1987. a. JPY 3,000. **Document type:** *Academic/Scholarly.*
—BLDSC (8413.899000).
Published by: Nihon Sekizui Geka Kenkyukai Osaka/Japanese Society of Spinal Surgery, Shiritsu Daigaku Igakubu No Shinkei Gekagaku Kyoshitsu, 5-7 Asahi-Machi 1-chome, Abeno-ku, Osaka-shi 545-0051, Japan. TEL 81-6-6452157, FAX 81-6-6478065. Ed. Hiroshi Abe.

SEMINARS IN ARTHRITIS & RHEUMATISM. see *MEDICAL SCIENCES—Rheumatology*

617.3 USA ISSN 1045-4527
SEMINARS IN ARTHROPLASTY. Text in English. 1990. q. USD 145 domestic to individuals; USD 222 foreign to individuals; USD 201 domestic to institutions; USD 266 foreign to institutions; USD 98 domestic to students; USD 133 foreign to students; USD 67 newsstand/cover (effective 2001). adv. back issues avail. **Document type:** *Academic/Scholarly.* **Description:** Covers a single topic of the restorative treatment of the joints in each issue, with emphasis on developments physicians can apply directly to their practices.
—BLDSC (8239.448100), CISTI, GNLM, Infotrieve. **CCC.**
Published by: W.B. Saunders Co. (Subsidiary of: Harcourt Publishers Ltd.), 11830 Westline Industrial Dr, St Louis, MO 63146. TEL 800-325-4177, http://www.wbsaunders.com. Eds. Dr. Gerald R Williams Jr., Dr. Robert H Fitzgerald Jr. Adv. contact Cindy Gray. B&W page USD 640, color page USD 1,560; trim 10 x 7. Circ: 2,508. **Subscr. to:** Periodicals Fulfillment, W B Saunders Co, 6277 Sea Harbor Dr, 4th Fl, Orlando, FL 32891-4800.

SEMINARS IN ROENTGENOLOGY. see *MEDICAL SCIENCES—Radiology And Nuclear Medicine*

617 USA ISSN 1040-7383
CODEN: SSPSEH
SEMINARS IN SPINE SURGERY. Text in English. 1989. q. USD 154 domestic to individuals; USD 218 foreign to individuals; USD 196 domestic to institutions; USD 259 foreign to institutions; USD 98 domestic to students; USD 131 foreign to students; USD 65 newsstand/cover (effective 2001). adv. **Document type:** *Academic/Scholarly.* **Description:** Addresses a single topic in the management and care of patients with spinal injuries or conditions in each issue.
—BLDSC (8239.468000), EMDOCS, GNLM, Infotrieve, KNAW. **CCC.**
Published by: W.B. Saunders Co. (Subsidiary of: Harcourt Publishers Ltd.), 11830 Westline Industrial Dr, St Louis, MO 63146. TEL 800-325-4177, http://www.wbsaunders.com. Eds. Dr. Sam W Wiesel, Scott D Boden. Adv. contact Cindy Gray. B&W page USD 695, color page USD 1,595; trim 10 x 7. Circ: 1,509. **Subscr. to:** Periodicals Fulfillment, W B Saunders Co, 6277 Sea Harbor Dr, 4th Fl, Orlando, FL 32891-4800.

SEMINARS IN ULTRASOUND, C T AND M R. (Computerized Tomography and Magnetic Resonance) see *MEDICAL SCIENCES—Radiology And Nuclear Medicine*

617.1 FRA ISSN 0399-0265
SERVICES D'AIDE MEDICALE URGENTE. REVUE. Cover title: Revue des S A M U. Text in French. 1978. 6/yr. EUR 72 domestic; EUR 80 foreign (effective 2002). adv. bibl, charts, illus.
Indexed: Ref.Zh.
Published by: (Services d'Aide Medicale Urgente), Societe Francaise d'Editions Medicales, 22-H rue du Chateau des Rentiers, Paris 75013, France. TEL 33-01-45835054, FAX 33-01-45831354, sfem96@mail.club-internet.fr. Ed. Colette Gallula.

SHEPHARD'S AIR AMBULANCE HANDBOOK. see *TRANSPORTATION—Air Transport*

617.3 JPN
SHIN JIDAI NO SEIKEI GEKA CHIRYO/NEW ORTHOPAEDIC SURGERY NOW. Text in Japanese. 1991. q. JPY 30,000 (effective 1999).
Published by: Medical View Co. Ltd./Mejikaru Byusha, 2-30 Ichigaya-Honmura-cho, Shinjuku-ku, Tokyo 162-0845, Japan. Circ: 6,000.

M

SHINKEI GAISHO/NEUROTRAUMATOLOGY. see *MEDICAL SCIENCES—Psychiatry And Neurology*

SHOCK; molecular, cellular and systemic pathobiological aspects and therapeutic approaches. see *MEDICAL SCIENCES*

615.822 CHN ISSN 1004-6569
SHUANGZU YU BAOJIAN/CHINA REFLEXOLOGY JOURNAL. Text in Chinese. 1992. bi-m. USD 13.20; USD 2.30 newsstand/cover (effective 2001). **Document type:** *Academic/Scholarly.*
Published by: China International Book Trading Corp/Zhongguo Guoji Tushu Maoyi Zonggongsi cibtc@mail.cibtc.com.cn, http://www.cibtc.com.cn. **Dist. by:** 35, Chegongzhuang Xilu, Haidian District, Beijing 100044, China.

617.3 GBR ISSN 1055-6583
SLIDE ATLAS OF CURRENT ORTHOPAEDICS (YEAR). Text in English. bi-m. USD 299.95. **Description:** Features most timely, comprehensive presentation of all developments within the orthopedic field over the last year.
Related titles: ♦ Supplement to: Current Opinion in Orthopedics. ISSN 1041-9918.
Published by: Rapid Science Publishers, 2-6 Boundary Row, London SE1 8HN, United Kingdom. TEL 44-207-865-0198, FAX 44-207-410-6600, rapid@rapidcom.co.uk. Ed. W R J Rennie.

617.2 ESP ISSN 0212-0771
SOCIEDAD ANDALUZA DE TRAUMATOLOGIA Y ORTOPEDIA. REVISTA. Text in Spanish. 1981. s-a. ESP 6,500 to individuals; ESP 9,200 to institutions; ESP 5,200 to students (effective 2001). back issues avail.; reprints avail. *Refereed.* **Document type:** *Journal, Academic/Scholarly.*
Related titles: Online - full text ed.: 1996.
Published by: (Sociedad Andaluza de Traumatologia y Ortopedia), Ediciones Doyma S.A., Traversa de Gracia, 17-21, Barcelona 08021, Spain. TEL 34-93-200-0711, sato@doyma.es, doyma@doyma.es, http://www.doyma.es/sato. Ed. G Alvarez de Eulate. R&P Monica Barnes. Adv. contact Jose Antonio Hernandez. Circ: 1,000.

616.02 ESP
SOCIEDAD ESPANOLA DE MEDICINA DE URGENCIAS Y EMERGENCIAS. REVISTA. Short title: Emergencias. Text in Spanish. 1988. bi-m. **Document type:** *Academic/Scholarly, Trade.* **Description:** Covers various aspects of emergency medicine.
Published by: (Sociedad Espanola de Medicina de Urgencias y Emergencias), Saned S.A., Capitan Haya, 60, Madrid 28020, Spain. TEL 34-91-749-9507, FAX 34-91-749-9507, saned@meditex.es. Ed. Moya Mir. Circ: 6,500.

617.3 ITA ISSN 0394-0713
SOCIETA DI ORTOPEDIA E TRAUMATOLOGIA DELL'ITALIA MERIDIONALE ED INSULARE. ATTI E MEMORIE. Text in Italian; Summaries in English, French. 1937. s-a. ITL 40,000, USD 55 (effective 1999).
Published by: (Societa di Ortopedia e Traumatologia dell'Italia Meridionale ed Insulare), Casa Editrice Idelson, Via A. DeGasperi, 55, Naples, NA 80138, Italy. TEL 39-81-5524733, FAX 39-81-5518295, idelgno@tin.it, http://www.idelson-gnocchi.com. Ed. Nicola Misasi.

617.3 ITA
SOCIETA EMILIANA ROMAGNOLA TRIVENETA DI ORTOPEDIA E TRAUMATOLOGIA. ATTI. Text in Italian; Summaries in English. s-a. ITL 39,000. adv. back issues avail. **Document type:** *Proceedings.*
Published by: Societa Emiliana Romagnola Triveneta di Ortopedia e Traumatologia, Viale Dei Mille, 140, Parma, PR 43100, Italy. TEL 0521-290191, FAX 0521-291314, TELEX 530476 EMMEVI I. Ed. Dr. L Cugola.

617.3 FRA ISSN 0081-1033
SOCIETE FRANCAISE DE CHIRURGIE ORTHOPEDIQUE ET TRAUMATOLOGIQUE. CONFERENCES D'ENSEIGNEMENT. Text in French. 1967. a. price varies.
Published by: (Societe Francaise de Chirurgie Orthopedique et Traumatologique), Expansion Scientifique Publications, 31 bd. de la Tour Maubourg, Paris 75007, France. TEL 33-1-40626400, FAX 33-1-45556920. Ed. J Duparc.

616.02 ZAF
SOUTH AFRICAN JOURNAL OF CRITICAL CARE. Text in English. s-a. USD 10 foreign (effective 2000). illus. *Refereed.* **Document type:** *Journal, Academic/Scholarly.* **Description:** Publishes clinical and experimental research in all areas of critical care medicine.
Indexed: Ind.S.A.Per.
Published by: South African Medical Association, Health and Medical Publishing Group, 14 Central Sq, Pinelands 7430, South Africa. TEL 27-21-531-3081, FAX 27-21-531-4126, annp@samedical.org, publishing@samedical.org, http://www.samedical.org. **Subscr. to:** PO Box 74789, Lynnwood Ridge, Pretoria 0040, South Africa. TEL 27-12-481-2010, FAX 27-12-481-2061, ann@samedical.org. **Dist. by:** Private Bag X1, Pinelands 7430, South Africa. TEL 27-21-531-3081, FAX 27-21-531-4126.

617.3 USA ISSN 1059-1052
SOUTHERN ORTHOPAEDIC ASSOCIATION. JOURNAL. Spine title: J S O A. Text in English. 1992. q. USD 30 to individuals; USD 45 foreign to individuals; USD 20 to institutions; USD 35 foreign to institutions (effective 2001). adv. *Refereed.* **Document type:** *Journal, Academic/Scholarly.* **Description:** Serves as a forum to present new techniques and procedures, and contains updates about the ongoing educational activities of interest to all practicing orthopedists.
Related titles: Online - full text ed.
Indexed: Ind.Med. (1992-).
—BLDSC (4902.230000), GNLM.
Published by: (Southern Orthopaedic Association), Southern Medical Association, 35 Lakeshore Dr, Box 190088, Birmingham, AL 35219-0088. TEL 205-945-1840, 800-423-4992, FAX 205-945-1548, http://www.sma.org/soa/jsoa.htm. Ed. Dr. L Andrew Koman. Pub. William J Ranieri. R&P Cathy Galloway. Adv. contact Princess Williams. Circ: 3,500.

610.73 618.92 USA
SPINAL CONNECTION. Text in English. 1984. s-a. free per issue. adv. bk.rev. back issues avail. **Document type:** *Newsletter.* **Description:** Provides medical information on scoliosis, including an overview of the foundation's activities and services.
Published by: National Scoliosis Foundation, 5 Cabot Pl, Stoughton, MA 02072. TEL 781-341-6333, FAX 781-341-8333, scoliosis@aol.com. Circ: 25,000.

SPINAL CORD. see *MEDICAL SCIENCES—Psychiatry And Neurology*

616.7 617.06 NLD ISSN 1529-9430
▼ **THE SPINE JOURNAL.** Text in English. 2001. bi-m. EUR 85, JPY 11,800, USD 95 elsewhere to individuals; EUR 172 in Europe to institutions; JPY 22,800 in Japan to institutions; USD 192 elsewhere to institutions (effective 2002). **Description:** Publishes original articles on research and treatment related to spine and spine care, including basic science and clinical investigations.
Related titles: Online - full text ed.
Published by: (North American Spine Society USA), Elsevier Science BV, Sara Burgerhartstraat 25, Amsterdam 1055 KV, Netherlands. TEL 31-20-485-2911, FAX 31-20-485-2457, nlinfo-f@elsevier.nl, http://www.elsevier.com/locate/spinee, http://www.elsevier.nl. Ed. T G Mayer.

617.375 USA ISSN 1072-3730
SPINE LETTER. Text in English. 1994. m. USD 103 domestic to individuals; USD 131 foreign to individuals; USD 166 domestic to institutions; USD 182 foreign to institutions; USD 16 newsstand/cover (effective 2000). **Document type:** *Newsletter.*
Published by: Lippincott Williams & Wilkins (Philadelphia) (Subsidiary of: Wolters Kluwer N.V.), 530 Walnut St, Philadelphia, PA 19106-3621. TEL 301-223-2300, 800-638-3030, FAX 301-223-2400, http://www.lww.com.

617.375 USA ISSN 0362-2436
RD768 CODEN: SPINDD
SPINE (PHILADELPHIA, 1976). Text in English. 1976. 24/yr., latest vol.26. USD 404 domestic to individuals; USD 536 foreign to individuals; USD 1,015 domestic to institutions; USD 1,243 foreign to institutions; USD 47 newsstand/cover (effective 2002); Print & Online eds. combined. adv. illus. index. *Refereed.* **Document type:** *Academic/Scholarly.* **Description:** Original articles cross the entire spectrum of spinal pain, deformity and disability, and include coverage of both conservative and non-traditional treatment modalities being employed both in the U.S. and internationally.
Related titles: CD-ROM ed.; Microform ed.: (from PQC); Online - full text ed.: USD 1,319.50 domestic academic site license; USD 1,547.50 foreign academic site license; USD 1,471.75 domestic corporate site license; USD 1,699.75 foreign corporate site license (effective 2002) (from Ovid Technologies, Inc., EBSCO Publishing, Swets Blackwell, Institute for Scientific Information).
Indexed: AMED, Aqua.Sci.& Fish.Abstr., Bibl.Dev.Med.& Child Neur., Biol.Abstr., Biotech.& Bioeng.Abstr. (coverage dropped), CINAHL, Cal.Tiss.Abstr., Chem.Abstr., Chemorec.Abstr., Curr.Adv.Ecol.Sci., Curr.Cont., Dent.Ind., Dok.Arbeitsmed., Excerp.Med., Focus on: Sports Sci.& Med., Helminthol.Abstr., Hosp.Lit.Ind., INIS Atomind., Ind.Med. (1976-), Ind.Vet., Inpharma, Int.Nurs.Ind., Neurosci.Abstr. (coverage dropped), Pharm.&Out.News, Reac.
—BLDSC (8413.903000), CASDDS, CISTI, EMDOCS, GNLM, IDS, ingenta, KNAW.
Published by: Lippincott Williams & Wilkins (Philadelphia) (Subsidiary of: Wolters Kluwer N.V.), 530 Walnut St, Philadelphia, PA 19106-3621. TEL 215-521-8300, FAX 215-521-8902, http://www.spinejournal.com, http://www.lww.com. Ed. James N Weinstein. Pub. Marcia Serepy. R&P Margaret Becker. Adv. contact Ray Thibodeau. B&W page USD 1,885, color page USD 3,630; trim 10.88 x 8.13. Circ: 7,653 (paid). **Subscr. to:** PO Box 1600, Hagerstown, MD 21740-1600. TEL 800-777-2295, FAX 301-824-7390.

617 USA ISSN 1062-8592
SPORTS MEDICINE AND ARTHROSCOPY REVIEW. Text in English. 1993. q., latest vol.9. USD 164 domestic to individuals; USD 191 foreign to individuals; USD 249 domestic to institutions; USD 283 foreign to institutions; USD 64 newsstand/cover (effective 2002). adv. illus. index. back issues avail. *Refereed.* **Document type:** *Academic/Scholarly.* **Description:** Topic-oriented, invited reviews on issues and techniques in arthroscopy and sports medicine.
Related titles: Microform ed.; Online - full text ed.: USD 323.70 domestic for academic site license; USD 357.70 foreign for academic site license; USD 361.05 domestic for corporate site license; USD 395.05 foreign for corporate site license (effective 2002); (from Institute for Scientific Information).
Indexed: ASCA, Focus on: Sports Sci.& Med.
—BLDSC (8419.837370), GNLM, IDS, KNAW.
Published by: Lippincott Williams & Wilkins (Philadelphia) (Subsidiary of: Wolters Kluwer N.V.), 530 Walnut St, Philadelphia, PA 19106-3621. TEL 215-521-8300, FAX 215-521-8902, www.sportsmedarthro.com, http://www.lww.com. Eds. Kenneth E Dehaven, W Dilworth Cannon Jr. Pub. Kathleen Gaffney. R&P Margaret Becker. Adv. contact Ray Thibodeau. B&W page USD 825, color page USD 1,880. Circ: 1,022 (paid). **Subscr. to:** PO Box 1600, Hagerstown, MD 21740-1600. TEL 800-777-2295, FAX 301-824-7390.

SPORTS MEDICINE REPORTS; a physician-to-physician update on critical issues in sports medicine. see *MEDICAL SCIENCES—Sports Medicine*

616.7 USA ISSN 1091-5915
STRATEGIC ORTHOPAEDICS. Text in English. 199?. m., latest vol.5. USD 199 domestic to individuals; USD 199 foreign to individuals; USD 245 per issue domestic to institutions; USD 245 per issue foreign to institutions; USD 20 newsstand/cover (effective 2002). *Refereed.*
Related titles: Online - full text ed.: USD 318.50 domestic for academic site license; USD 318.50 foreign for academic site license; USD 355.25 domestic for corporate site license; USD 355.25 foreign for corporate site license (effective 2002).
Published by: Lippincott Williams & Wilkins (Philadelphia) (Subsidiary of: Wolters Kluwer N.V.), 530 Walnut St, Philadelphia, PA 19106-3621. TEL 301-223-2300, 800-638-3030, FAX 301-223-2400, http://www.lww.com. Ed. Thomas J Grogan.

▼ **SURGICAL THEATRE EQUIPMENT AND TECHNOLOGY (S T E T).** see *MEDICAL SCIENCES—Surgery*

SWISS SURGERY/CHIRURGIA SVIZZERA/CHIRURGIE SUISSE/SCHWEIZER CHIRURGIE. see *MEDICAL SCIENCES—Surgery*

628 USA ISSN 1071-6262
T B I CHALLENGE!. Text in English. 1982. 6/yr. membership; USD 5 to persons with brain injuries. back issues avail. **Document type:** *Consumer.* **Description:** Covers topics related to rehabilitation, prevention and legislation as they pertain to the needs and rights of persons with brain injuries and their families.
Formerly: N H I F Newsletter

M

Published by: Brain Injury Association, Inc., 105 N Alfred St, Alexandria, VA 22314-3010. TEL 703-236-6000, FAX 703-296-8850, http://www.biausa.org. Ed. Monique J Marino. R&P Rosy McGillan. Circ: 12,000.

▼ **TECHNIQUES IN FOOT & ANKLE SURGERY.** see *MEDICAL SCIENCES—Surgery*

▼ **TECHNIQUES IN KNEE SURGERY.** see *MEDICAL SCIENCES—Surgery*

617.3 USA ISSN 0885-9698
TECHNIQUES IN ORTHOPAEDICS. Text in English. 1986. q., latest vol.16. USD 209 domestic to individuals; USD 234 foreign to individuals; USD 269 domestic to institutions; USD 299 foreign to institutions; USD 68 newsstand/cover (effective 2002); Print & Online eds. combined. adv. illus. index. back issues avail. *Refereed.* **Document type:** *Journal, Academic/Scholarly.* **Description:** Publishes original, technique oriented articles covering operations, manipulations and instruments being developed and applied in such areas as arthroscopy, arthroplasty and trauma.
Related titles: Microform ed.; Online - full text ed.: USD 349.70 domestic academic site license; USD 379.70 foreign academic site license; USD 390.05 domestic corporate site license; USD 420.05 foreign corporate site license (effective 2002).
—BLDSC (8745.278000), EMDOCS, GNLM, KNAW.
Published by: Lippincott Williams & Wilkins (Philadelphia) (Subsidiary of: Wolters Kluwer N.V.), 530 Walnut St, Philadelphia, PA 19106-3621. TEL 215-521-8300, FAX 215-521-8902, www.techortho.com, http://www.lww.com. Ed. Bruce D Browner. Pub. Kathleen Gaffney. R&P Margaret Becker. Adv. contact Ray Thibodeau. B&W page USD 810. Circ: 1,989 (paid). **Subscr. to:** PO Box 1600, Hagerstown, MD 21740-1600. TEL 800-777-2295, FAX 301-824-7390.

617.1 FRA ISSN 0397-3999
TECHNIQUES ORTHOPEDIQUES. Text in French. 1976. irreg., latest 1981. FRF 875.
Published by: Expansion Scientifique, 31 bd. de la Tour Maubourg, Paris 75007, France. TEL 40-62-64-00, FAX 45-55-69-20. Eds. J Casaing, L Descamps.

617.3 ESP ISSN 0214-4352
TECNICA ORTOPEDICA INTERNACIONAL/ INTERNATIONAL ORTHOPAEDIC TECHNIQUE. Key Title: T O I. Text in English, Spanish. 1988. q. ESP 6,100, USD 65. back issues avail.; reprints avail. *Refereed.* **Document type:** *Academic/Scholarly.*
Related titles: Online - full text ed.
Published by: (Federacion Espanola de Tecnicos Ortopedicos), Editorial Garsi S.A. (Subsidiary of: Grupo Masson), Juan Bravo, 46, Madrid 28006, Spain. TEL 34-91-402-1212, FAX 34-91-402-0954, garsi@mad.servicom.es, http://www.masson.es. Ed. Oriol Cohi.

617.3 ESP ISSN 1132-1954
TECNICAS QUIRURGICAS EN ORTOPEDIA Y TRAUMATOLOGIA. Text in Spanish. 1992. q. USD 147. **Document type:** *Academic/Scholarly.*
Related titles: ♦ Translation of: Operative Orthopaedie und Traumatologie. ISSN 0934-6694.
Published by: Ediciones Doyma S.A., Traversa de Gracia, 17-21, Barcelona 08021, Spain. TEL 34-93-200-0711, FAX 34-93-209-1136. Ed. A Navarro Quilis. adv.: color page ESP 189,000. Circ: 2,500.

616.025 610.736 GBR ISSN 1360-1938
TODAY'S EMERGENCY. Text in English. 1995. q. GBP 18 domestic to individuals; GBP 30 foreign to individuals; GBP 30 domestic to institutions; GBP 50 foreign to institutions (effective 2000). adv. **Document type:** *Trade.*
Published by: Media Publishing Company, Media House, 41 Crayford Way, Dartford, Kent DA1 4JY, United Kingdom. TEL 44-1322-558029, FAX 44-1322-558524, medipub@aol.com. Ed. V Gautam. Pub., Adv. contact Terry Gardner.

617.3 JPN ISSN 0917-1789
TOGAI NAIATSU KENKYUKAI HOKOKUSHU/PROGRESS IN RESEARCH ON INTRACRANIAL PRESSURE. Text in Japanese; Summaries in English. 1990. a.
Published by: Tokai Naiatsu Kenkyukai, c/o Chugai Seiyaku K.K., Iyaku Gakujutsu Dai 3 Bu, 1-9 Kyobashi 2-chome, Chuo-ku, Tokyo 104-0031, Japan.

617.3 JPN ISSN 0915-2253
TOHKAI SEIKEI GEKA GAISHO KENKYU KAISHI/TOHKAI ORTHOPAEDIC SOCIETY OF TRAUMATOLOGY. JOURNAL. Text in Japanese. 1988. a. JPY 5,000 to non-members; JPY 1,000 per issue (effective 2000). adv. back issues avail. *Refereed.* **Document type:** *Academic/Scholarly.* **Description:** Publishes proceedings of medical meetings and original articles on traumatology, including fractures, dislocations and other injuries in the orthopaedic field.
Related titles: CD-ROM ed.; Fax ed.
Published by: Tohkai Seikei Geka Gaisho Kenkyukai/Tohkai Orthopaedic Society of Traumatology, Gifu Kenritsu Tajimi Byoin Seikei Geka, 5-161 Maebata-cho, Tajimi-shi, Gifu-ken 507-0042, Japan. TEL 81-572-22-5311, FAX 81-572-25-1246. Ed. Toshiyuki Muro. Circ: 1,000 (controlled).

617.3 JPN ISSN 0913-476X
TOHKAI SEKITSUI GEKA/JOURNAL OF TOHKAI SPINAL SURGERY. Text in Japanese; Summaries in English, Japanese. 1987. a. JPY 5,000 to non-members (effective 2000). adv. *Refereed.* **Document type:** *Academic/Scholarly.* **Description:** Contains proceedings of medical meetings, original articles, and historical reviews on spinal surgery.
Related titles: CD-ROM ed.; Online - full text ed.
Published by: Tohkai Sekitsui Geka Kenkyukai/Society of Tohkai Spinal Surgery, Gifu Kenritsu Tajimi Byoin, 5-161 Maebata-cho, Tajimi-shi, Gifu-ken 507-0042, Japan. TEL 81-3-3334-7625, FAX 81-3-3334-0497. Ed. Dr. Toshiyuki Muro. Circ: 600 (controlled).

617.3 JPN
TOHOKU ARCHIVES OF ORTHOPAEDIC SURGERY AND TRAUMATOLOGY/TOHOKU SEIKEI SAIGAI GEKA KIYO. Text in Japanese. 1957. s-a. membership. bk.rev. abstr, bibl, charts, illus. index, cum.index.
Formerly (until vol. 20, 1977): Tohoku Archivo por Orthopedia Kej Akcidenta Hirurgio (0040-8751)
Published by: Tohoku Society of Orthopaedic Surgery and Traumatology/Tohoku Seikei Saigai Geka Gakkai, c/o Dept of Orthopaedic Surgery, Tohoku University School of Medicine, 1-1 Seiryo-cho, Aoba-ku, Sendai-shi, Miyagi-ken 980-0872, Japan. Circ: 650 (controlled).

616.025 USA ISSN 0164-2340
TOPICS IN EMERGENCY MEDICINE. Text in English. 1979. q. USD 135 to individuals; USD 41 newsstand/cover (effective 2002). 90 p./no. 2 cols./p. **Document type:** *Journal, Academic/Scholarly.* **Description:** Provides in-depth coverage of information on emergency medical care, new methods in emergency medicine, advances in technology, current diagnostic techniques and lifesaving measures, procedures of choice, and instant hands-on, step-by-step guidance for quick and accurate decisions when seconds count.
Related titles: Online - full text ed.: (from Ovid Technologies, Inc., ProQuest Information & Learning).
Indexed: CINAHL, Excerp.Med.
—BLDSC (8867.437400), CISTI, GNLM, ingenta. **CCC.**
Published by: Aspen Publishers, Inc., 200 Orchard Ridge Dr, Ste 200, Gaithersburg, MD 20878. TEL 301-417-7500, 800-638-8437, FAX 301-695-7931, customer.service@aspenpubl.com, http:// www.aspenpublishers.com. Eds. Anthony Albano, Carmen G Warner. Pub. Jack Bruggeman. Circ: 2,000 (paid). **Dist. by:** Aspen Publishers Inc., Distribution Center, 7201 McKinney Circle, Frederick, MD 21701. TEL 301-698-7100, FAX 301-417-7550.

617.1 616.02 GBR ISSN 1460-4086
▼ **TRAUMA.** Text in English. 1999. q. GBP 61 in Europe to individuals; USD 90 in North America to individuals; GBP 68 rest of world to individuals; GBP 144 in Europe to institutions; USD 230 in North America to institutions; GBP 161 rest of world to institutions; GBP 48 in Europe to members basics; USD 72 in North America to members basics; GBP 54 rest of world to members basics; GBP 80 in developing nations; USD 88 newsstand/cover in North America; GBP 49 newsstand/cover rest of world (effective 2002). adv. back issues avail.; reprints avail. *Refereed.* **Document type:** *Journal, Academic/Scholarly.* **Description:** Covers all aspects of trauma care from prevention through rehabilitation.
Media: Online - full text (from EBSCO Publishing, O C L C Online Computer Library Center, Inc., RoweCom Information Quest, ingenta, Swets Blackwell).
Indexed: e-psyche.
—BLDSC (9026.856800).
Published by: Arnold Publishers (Subsidiary of: Hodder Headline plc.), 338 Euston Rd, London NW1 3BH, United Kingdom. TEL 44-20-7873-6337, FAX 44-20-7873-6325, arnoldjournals@hodder.co.uk, http://www.arnoldpublishers.com/journals/Journpages/ 14604086.htm, http://www.palliativemedjournal.com. Eds. Ian Greaves, J. M. Ryan, Keith Porter. Adv. contact Mary Attree. B&W page GBP 490, color page GBP 1,520; trim 189 x 246. **Subscr. to:** Turpin Distribution Services Ltd., Blackhorse Rd, Letchworth, Herts SG6 1HN, United Kingdom. TEL 44-1462-488900, FAX 44-1462-483011.

617.1 340 USA
TRAUMA: PERSONAL INJURY, MEDICINE, AND SURGERY. Text in English. 1959. bi-m. USD 1,787 (effective 2001).
Published by: Matthew Bender & Co., Inc. (Subsidiary of: Lexis Law Publishing), 2 Park Ave, New York, NY 10016. TEL 212-448-2000, international@bender.com, http://www.bender.com. Ed. Harold Hirsh.

TRAUMA QUARTERLY. see *MEDICAL SCIENCES—Surgery*

617 ZAF
TRAUMA REVIEW. Text in English. q. free per issue. **Document type:** *Newsletter.*
Indexed: Ind.S.A.Per.
Published by: Medical Research Council, National Trauma Research Programme, PO Box 19070, Tygerberg 7505, South Africa. TEL 27-21-9380911, FAX 27-21-9380381, http://www.mrc.ac.za/ trauma/review.htm. Ed., R&P Johan van der Spuy.

617.1 DEU ISSN 1436-6274
TRAUMA UND BERUFSKRANKHEIT. Text in German. 1998. q. DEM 210.40 domestic; DEM 215.60 foreign (effective 2001). *Refereed.* **Document type:** *Journal, Academic/Scholarly.* **Description:** Covers all aspects of trauma and emergency medicine.
Related titles: Online - full text ed.: ISSN 1436-6282 (from EBSCO Publishing, RoweCom Information Quest, Swets Blackwell, Springer LINK).
Published by: Springer-Verlag (Subsidiary of: BertelsmannSpringer), Tiergartenstr 17, Heidelberg 69121, Germany. TEL 49-6221-345-0, FAX 49-6221-345229, subscriptions@springer.de, http://link.springer.de/link/service/journals/10039/ index.htm, http://www.springer.de. Eds. A Wentzensen, M Boerner. **Subscr. to:** Springer-Verlag New York Inc., PO Box 2485, Secaucus, NJ 07096-2485. TEL 212-460-1500, FAX 212-473-6272.

617.3 USA
TRAUMAGRAM. Text in English. q. membership. **Document type:** *Newsletter.*
Published by: American Trauma Society, 8903 Presidential Pkwy, Ste 512, Upper Marlboro, MD 20772-2656. TEL 301-420-4189, FAX 301-420-0617. Ed. J J Kunkle. Circ: 4,000.

617.1 USA ISSN 1085-9373
TRAUMATOLOGY. Text in English. 1995. q. back issues avail. *Refereed.* **Document type:** *Academic/Scholarly.* **Description:** Disseminates new and original contributions to the traumatology field. Focuses on theoretical formulations, research, treatment, prevention, education, training, medical and legal and policy concerns.
Related titles: CD-ROM ed.; Online - full text ed.
Published by: Florida State University, School of Social Work. Traumatology Institute, Traumatology Forum Research Group, 2404 C University Center, Tallahassee, FL 32306-2570. TEL 850-640-2146, FAX 850-644-3967, cfigley@mailer.fsu.edu, http://www.fsu.edu/~trauma/. Ed. Charles R Figley.

TURK ANESTEZIYOLOJI VE REANIMASYON CEMIYETI DERGISI. see *MEDICAL SCIENCES—Anaesthesiology*

616.028 617.1 DEU ISSN 0177-5537
R51 CODEN: UNFAE2
DER UNFALLCHIRURG. Text in German. 1894. m. EUR 385.12 domestic; EUR 355.12 in Germany; EUR 34.10 newsstand/cover foreign (effective 2002). back issues avail.; reprint service avail. from ISI. *Refereed.* **Document type:** *Journal, Academic/Scholarly.* **Description:** Covers all aspects of trauma and emergency surgery.
Former titles: Unfallheilkunde (0341-5694); Monatsschrift fuer Unfallheilkunde (0340-1669); Monatsschrift fuer Unfallheilkunde, Versicherungs-, Versorgungs- und Verkehrsmedizin (0026-9336)

M

Related titles: Microform ed.: (from PQC); Online - full text ed.: ISSN 1433-044X (from EBSCO Publishing, RoweCom Information Quest, Swets Blackwell, Springer LINK, Institute for Scientific Information).
Indexed: ASCA, Biol.Abstr., Curr.Cont., Excerp.Med., INIS Atomind., Ind.Med. (1985-), Inpharma, Neurosci.Cit.Ind., Reac.
—BLDSC (9090.235280), CISTI, GNLM, IDS, Infotrieve, KNAW. **CCC.**
Published by: (Deutsche Gesellschaft fuer Unfallheilkunde), Springer-Verlag (Subsidiary of: BertelsmannSpringer), Tiergartenstr 17, Heidelberg 69121, Germany. TEL 49-6221-345-0, FAX 49-6221-345229, subscriptions@springer.de, http://link.springer.de/link/service/journals/00113/index.htm, http://www.springer.de. Eds. H Tscherne, L Schweiberer. **Subscr. in N. America to:** Springer-Verlag New York Inc., PO Box 2485, Secaucus, NJ 07096-2485. TEL 212-460-1500, FAX 212-473-6272.

617.3 RUS ISSN 0869-8678
VESTNIK TRAVMATOLOGII I ORTOPEDII IM. N.N. PRIOROVA. Text in Russian; Summaries in English. 1927. q. USD 113 foreign (effective 2000). bk.rev. bibl. **Document type:** *Academic/Scholarly.* **Description:** Discusses basic theoretical and practical problems of orthopedics, traumatology and prosthetics.
Formerly (until 1994): Ortopediya, Travmatologiya i Protezirovanie (0030-5987)
Indexed: Biol.Abstr., Dent.Ind., Excerp.Med., INIS Atomind., Ind.Med. (coverage dropped), Ref.Zh.
—CISTI, East View, GNLM. **CCC.**
Published by: Izdatel'stvo Meditsina, Petroverigskii per 6-8, Moscow 101000, Russian Federation. TEL 7-095-4502424, FAX 7-095-1543139, 7-095-9211355, 7-095-9286003, meditsina@iname.com, http://www.medit.ru. Ed. Yu G Shaposhnikov. R&P L Tikhomirova. Circ: 2,500. **Dist. by:** Mezhdunarodnaya Kniga, B Yakimanka 39, Moscow 117049, Russian Federation. TEL 7-095-2384967, FAX 7-095-2384634; **US dist. addr.:** East View Publications, 3020 Harbor Ln N, Minneapolis, MN 55447. TEL 612-550-0961.

VETERINARY AND COMPARATIVE ORTHOPAEDICS AND TRAUMATOLOGY. see *VETERINARY SCIENCE*

617.752 658.8 GBR
THE WORLD MARKET FOR EYEWEAR. Text in English. irreg., latest 1997. GBP 3,950, USD 7,900. **Document type:** *Trade.* **Description:** Provides a comprehensive and strategic review of the eyewear market worldwide.
Published by: Euromonitor, 60-61 Britton St, London EC1M 5UX, United Kingdom. TEL 44-20-7251-8024, info@euromonitor.com, http://www.euromonitor.com.

616.7 GBR ISSN 1369-2607
WORLD WIDE WOUNDS. Text in English. 1997. s-m. free per issue. *Refereed.* **Document type:** *Journal, Academic/Scholarly.* **Description:** Seeks to monitor and raise the standard of reference material available to professionals with an interest in wound management.
Media: Online - full text.
Published by: Surgical Materials Testing Laboratory, Princess of Wales Hospital, Coity Rd, Bridgend, S Wales CF31 1RQ, United Kingdom. TEL 44-1656-752820, FAX 44-1656-752830, www.editor@smtl.co.uk, http://www.worldwidewounds.com/. Ed., R&P Suzy Calne. **Co-sponsor:** Medical Education Partnership.

WOUND CARE. see *MEDICAL SCIENCES—Communicable Diseases*

WOUND CARE SOURCEBOOK. see *MEDICAL SCIENCES—Dermatology And Venereology*

617.1 USA ISSN 1067-1927
CODEN: WREREU
WOUND REPAIR AND REGENERATION. Text in English. 1993. bi-m. USD 130 domestic to individuals; USD 145 in Canada & Mexico to individuals; USD 155 elsewhere to individuals; USD 200 domestic to institutions; USD 215 in Canada & Mexico to institutions; USD 225 elsewhere to institutions; USD 143 to individuals print & online eds. combined; USD 220 to institutions print & online eds. combined (effective 2001). adv. abstr, illus. back issues avail.; reprints avail. *Refereed.* **Document type:** *Journal, Academic/Scholarly, Trade.* **Description:** Provides extensive international coverage of cellular and molecular biology, connective tissue, and biological mediator studies in the field of tissue repair and regeneration.
Related titles: Online - full text ed.: ISSN 1524-475X. 1999. USD 117, USD 180 to institutions (effective 2001) (from EBSCO Publishing, O C L C Online Computer Library Center, Inc., RoweCom Information Quest, ingenta, Munksgaard & Blackwell Science's Synergy, Swets Blackwell, Institute for Scientific Information).
Indexed: CINAHL, Curr.Cont., Ind.Med. (1993-), Inpharma, Int.Nurs.Ind., Pharm.&Out.News, Reac., Sci.Cit.Ind.
—BLDSC (9364.529320), CISTI, GNLM, IDS, Infotrieve, KNAW. **CCC.**
Published by: (Wound Healing Society), Blackwell Science Inc., Commerce Pl, 350 Main St, Malden, MA 02148-5018. TEL 781-388-8250, 800-759-6102, FAX 781-388-8255, journals@blacksci.com, http://www.blackwell-science.com. Eds. Dr. Thomas K Hunt, Dr. William J Lindblad. R&P Tracey Davies. Adv. contact Jenny Applin. B&W page USD 660, color page USD 1,280; trim 10.88 x 8.25. Circ: 1,400. **Co-sponsors:** European Tissue Repair Society; Japanese Society for Wound Healing; Australian Wound Management Association.

616.02 USA ISSN 1044-7946
WOUNDS; a compendium of clinical research and practice. Text in English. bi-m. USD 65.95; USD 105.95 foreign (effective 1999). *Refereed.* **Document type:** *Trade.*
Related titles: Online - full text ed.: (from Institute for Scientific Information).
Indexed: ASCA, CINAHL, Curr.Cont., Inpharma, Reac., Rev.Arom.& Med.Plants.
—BLDSC (9364.529340), GNLM, IDS.
Published by: H M P Communications, LLC, 950 W Valley Rd, Ste 2800, Wayne, PA 19087. TEL 610-688-8220, 800-237-7285, FAX 610-688-8050.

XIAOER JIJIU YIXUE/PEDIATRIC EMERGENCY MEDICINE. see *MEDICAL SCIENCES—Pediatrics*

616.025 USA ISSN 0271-7964
RC86
THE YEAR BOOK OF EMERGENCY MEDICINE. Text in English. 1981. a. USD 95 domestic; USD 101 foreign (effective 2001). **Document type:** *Abstract/Index, Academic/Scholarly.* **Description:** Presents abstracts of pertinent literature with commentary by leading experts in the field.
Related titles: CD-ROM ed.
—GNLM.
Published by: Mosby, Inc., Continuity Division (Subsidiary of: Harcourt Health Sciences), 11830 Westline Industrial Dr, St Louis, MO 63146-3313. TEL 314-872-8370, 800-325-4177, FAX 314-432-1380, http://www.mosby.com/periodicals. Ed. Dr. William P Burdick.

THE YEAR BOOK OF HAND SURGERY. see *MEDICAL SCIENCES—Surgery*

THE YEAR BOOK OF ORTHOPEDICS. see *MEDICAL SCIENCES—Abstracting, Bibliographies, Statistics*

617.3 DEU ISSN 0044-3220
CODEN: ZOIGAP
ZEITSCHRIFT FUER ORTHOPAEDIE UND IHRE GRENZGEBIETE. Text in English, German. 1891. bi-m. EUR 328.80 domestic to institutions; EUR 335.80 in Europe to institutions; EUR 348.40 elsewhere to institutions; EUR 156 to students; EUR 65 newsstand/cover (effective 2002). adv. bk.rev. bibl, charts, illus. index. reprint service avail. from IRC. *Refereed.* **Document type:** *Journal, Academic/Scholarly.*
Incorporates: Deutsche Gesellschaft fuer Orthopaedie und Ihre Grenzgebiete. Verhandlungen (0070-4091)
Related titles: Online - full text ed.: ISSN 1438-941X (from Institute for Scientific Information); ♦ Supplement: Buecherei des Orthopaeden. ISSN 0068-3388.
Indexed: ASCA, Biol.Abstr., C.I.S. Abstr., Curr.Adv.Cancer Res., Curr.Cont., Dent.Ind., Excerp.Med., INIS Atomind., Ind.Med. (1935-), Inpharma, Pharm.&Out.News, Reac., SSCI (coverage dropped), Sci.Cit.Ind. (coverage dropped).
—BLDSC (9475.670000), ADONIS, CISTI, GNLM, IDS, Infotrieve, KNAW. **CCC.**
Published by: (Deutsche Gesellschaft fuer Orthopaedie und Traumatologie), Georg Thieme Verlag, Ruedigerstr 14, Stuttgart 70469, Germany. TEL 49-711-8931-0, FAX 49-711-8931298, zfo@thieme.de, kunden.service@thieme.de, http://www.thieme.de/zfo/index.html. Ed. Dr. Juergen Kraemer. adv.: page DEM 2,700; trim 175 x 250. Circ: 2,400 (paid and controlled).

616.7 CHN ISSN 1003-0034
ZHONGGUO GUSHANG/CHINA JOURNAL OF ORTHOPAEDICS AND TRAUMATOLOGY. Text in Chinese. 1987. m. USD 44.40 domestic; CNY 6, USD 3.70 newsstand/cover domestic (effective 2001). back issues avail. **Document type:** *Academic/Scholarly.*
Related titles: Online - full content ed.: (from WanFang Data Corp.).
Published by: Zhongguo Gushang Bianji Weiyuanhui, Dongzhimen Nei, Beixincang18 Hao, Beijing 100700 , China. TEL 86-1-64014411, FAX 86-1-84036581, zggu@chinajournal.net.cn, zggszz@263.net. Ed. Tianyu Shang. **Dist. by:** China International Book Trading Corp, 35, Chegongzhuang Xilu, Haidian District, Beijing 100044, China. TEL 86-1-68413849, FAX 86-1-68412048, cibtc@mail.cibtc.com.cn, http://www.cibtc.com.cn. **Co-sponsors:** Guojia Zhongyiyao Quanliju; Zhongguo Zhongxiyi Jiehe Xuehui; Zhongguo Zhongyi Yanjiuyuan.

ZHONGGUO GUZHI SHUSONG ZAZHI/CHINESE JOURNAL OF OSTEOPOROSIS. see *GERONTOLOGY AND GERIATRICS*

617.375 CHN ISSN 1004-406X
ZHONGGUO JIZHU JISUI ZAZHI/CHINESE JOURNAL OF SPINE AND SPINAL CORD. Text in Chinese; Abstracts in Chinese, English. 1991. bi-m. USD 31.20; USD 5.20 newsstand/cover (effective 2001). adv. bibl, illus. **Document type:** *Academic/Scholarly.* **Description:** Covers clinical diagnosis, treatment techniques, rehabilitation techniques and experimental studies, osteonosus, deformation and tumors of spine and spinal cord.
Related titles: Online - full content ed.: (from WanFang Data Corp.).
Published by: Zhongri Youhao Yiyuan, Heping Jie Bei-kou, Yinghuayuan, Dongjie Zhong, Youhao Yiyuan, Beijing 100029, China. TEL 86-1-6420-6649, FAX 86-1-6421-7749, TELEX 210096 CJFH CN, cspine@public.sti.ac.cn. Ed. Guang Bo Zhang. R&P Zhu Yaming. Adv. contact Sun Jianguo. page USD 3,000. **Dist. by:** China International Book Trading Corp, 35, Chegongzhuang Xilu, Haidian District, Beijing 100044, China. TEL 86-1-68413849, FAX 86-1-68412048, cibtc@mail.cibtc.com.cn, http://www.cibtc.com.cn. **Co-sponsor:** Chinese Association of Rehabilitation Medicine, Special Board of Spine and Spinal Cord Injury.

616.02 CHN ISSN 1001-0726
ZHONGGUO SHAOSHANG CHUANGSHANG ZAZHI/CHINESE JOURNAL OF BURNS, WOUNDS & SURFACE ULCERS. Text in Chinese; Summaries in Chinese, English. 1989. q. CNY 32, USD 20 (effective 2000). adv. bk.rev. charts, abstr, illus, stat. back issues avail. *Refereed.* **Document type:** *Academic/Scholarly.* **Description:** Provides a forum to exchange information among all engaged in the treatment and care of burn injuries. Regular features include: Medical philosophy, basic medical science, case reports, burn care in practice, state of the art reviews.
Related titles: E-mail ed.
Published by: Zhongguo Shaoshang Chuangshang Keji Zhongxin/Chinese Science and Technology Center for Burns, Wounds & Surface Ulcers Society, No 54 Xibianmennei St, Xuanwu-qu, Beijing 100053, China. FAX 86-10-6304-2420, mebo@public.east.cn.net, http://www.mebo.com.cn. Ed. Rongxiang Xu. R&P, Adv. contact Mengjie Zhu TEL 86-10-6304-2423.

ZHONGGUO XIUFU CHONGJIAN WAIKE ZAZHI/CHINESE JOURNAL OF REPARATIVE AND RECONSTRUCTIVE SURGERY. see *MEDICAL SCIENCES—Surgery*

616.7 CHN ISSN 1004-745X
ZHONGGUO ZHONGYI JIZHENG/JOURNAL OF EMERGENCY SYNDROMES IN CHINESE MEDICINE. Text in Chinese. 1992. bi-m. USD 12; USD 2 newsstand/cover (effective 2001). **Document type:** *Academic/Scholarly.*
Published by: China International Book Trading Corp/Zhongguo Guoji Tushu Maoyi Zonggongsi cibtc@mail.cibtc.com.cn, http://www.cibtc.com.cn. **Dist. by:** 35, Chegongzhuang Xilu, Haidian District, Beijing 100044, China.

617.1 CHN ISSN 1001-8050
CODEN: ZCZAFD
ZHONGHUA CHUANGSHANG ZAZHI/CHINESE JOURNAL OF TRAUMATOLOGY. Text in Chinese, English. 1985. m. CNY 110.40 domestic; USD 180 foreign (effective 2001). adv. bk.rev. bibl, illus, abstr, charts, mkt, pat, stat. 80 p./no. back issues avail. *Refereed.* **Document type:** *Academic/Scholarly.*
Formerly (until 1989): Chuangshang Zazhi (1001-229X)
Related titles: CD-ROM ed.: (from Chinese Academic Journal (CD), Electronic Journals Publishing House); Online - full content ed.: (from WanFang Data Corp.); ♦ English ed.: Chinese Journal of Traumatology. ISSN 1008-1275.
Indexed: Chem.Abstr., Chem.Indus.Notes, Chem.Titles.

M

—BLDSC (3180.680900), CASDDS.
Published by: (Zhonghua Yixuehui/Chinese Medical Association, Disan Junyi Daxue Yezhan Waike Yanjiusuo/Research Institute of Surgery, 3rd Military Medical University), Zhonghua Changshang Zazhi Bianjibu, 10 Changjiang Zhilu, Daping, Chongching 400042, China. cmachz@public.cta.cq.cn, http://www.chinainfo.co.net/periodical. Ed., R&P Zhengguo Wang TEL 86-23-6875-7424. adv.: B&W page USD 420, color page USD 1,200; 210 x 290. Circ: 6,000. **Subscr. to:** Jialingqiao Xicuen No 83, Chongqing, Sichuan, China. **Dist. overseas by:** China International Book Trading Corp, 35, Chegongzhuang Xilu, Haidian District, Beijing 100044, China. TEL 86-1-68413849, FAX 86-1-68412048, cibtc@mail.cibtc.com.cn, http://www.cibtc.com.cn.

617.3 CHN ISSN 0253-2352
ZHONGHUA GUKE ZAZHI/CHINESE JOURNAL OF ORTHOPEDICS. Text in Chinese. 1981. q. CNY 117.60 domestic; USD 62.40 foreign; CNY 9.80 newsstand/cover domestic; USD 5.20 newsstand/cover foreign (effective 2001). **Document type:** *Academic/Scholarly.*
Related titles: CD-ROM ed.; Online - full content ed.: (from WanFang Data Corp.).
Indexed: ExtraMED.
—BLDSC (3180.463500).
Published by: (Zhonghua Yixuehui/Chinese Medical Association), Tianjin Yiyuan, 406, Jiefang Nanlu, Tianjin 300211, China. TEL 86-22-28334734, cjorthop@public.tjuc.com.cn. Ed. Geng-Ting Dang. **Dist. overseas by:** China International Book Trading Corp, 35, Chegongzhuang Xilu, Haidian District, Beijing 100044, China. TEL 86-1-68413849, FAX 86-1-68412048, cibtc@mail.cibtc.com.cn, http://www.cibtc.com.cn.

ZHONGHUA SHAOSHANG ZAZHI/CHINESE JOURNAL OF BURNS. see *MEDICAL SCIENCES—Dermatology And Venereology*

617.3 615.89 CHN ISSN 1001-6015
ZHONGYI ZHENGGU/JOURNAL OF TRADITIONAL CHINESE ORTHOPEDICS AND TRAUMATOLOGY. Text in Chinese. 1989. bi-m. CNY 4.80, USD 10 per issue (effective 2000). bk.rev. illus. 64 p./no. *Refereed.* **Document type:** *Academic/Scholarly.* **Description:** Covers the application of traditional Chinese medicine in orthopedics and traumatology, including diagnosis and treatment.
Published by: Luoyang Zhenggu Yanjiusuo/Luoyang Orthopedic - Traumatological Institute of Henan Province, No 1 Qiming Nanlu, Luoyang, Henan 471002, China. TEL 86-379-3953520, FAX 86-379-3953520. Ed. Guo Weihuai. **Dist. overseas by:** China International Book Trading Corp, 35 Chegongzhuang Xilu, Haidian District, Beijing 100044, China. **Co-sponsor:** Zhongguo Zhongyiyao Xuehui.

MEDICAL SCIENCES—Otorhinolaryngology

A A O A NEWS. see *MEDICAL SCIENCES—Allergology And Immunology*

616.21 USA ISSN 0149-8886
RF297
ACADEMY OF REHABILITATIVE AUDIOLOGY. JOURNAL. Short title: J A R A. Text in English. 1969. a. USD 50 domestic; USD 60 foreign (effective 2000). bk.rev. *Refereed.* **Document type:** *Trade, Academic/Scholarly.* **Description:** Forum for the exchange of ideas on, knowledge of, and experience with habilitative and rehabilitative aspects of audiology.
Indexed: AMED, C.I.J.E. (coverage dropped), CINAHL, Except.Child Educ.Abstr., Lang.& Lang.Behav.Abstr., PsycInfo, Psychol.Abstr. (1985-), SOPODA, Sociol.Abstr., e-psyche.
—BLDSC (4674.984000), GNLM, ingenta.
Published by: Academy of Rehabilitative Audiology, c/o Jennifer Basham, JARA Circ Mgr, University of Texas at Dallas, Callier Center for Communication Disorder, 1966 Inwood Rd, Dallas, TX 75235. TEL 214-905-3185. Ed. Dr. Linda D Thibodeau. R&P Robert J Dunlop. Circ: 500 (paid).

616.31 617 USA
ACOUSTIC NEUROMA ASSOCIATION NOTES. Text in English. 1981. q. USD 30 (effective 2000). **Document type:** *Newsletter.* **Description:** Provides support and information for patients who have been diagnosed with or treated for acoustic neuromas or other benign cranial nerve tumors.
Published by: Acoustic Neuroma Association, PO Box 12402, Atlanta, GA 30355. TEL 404-237-8023, FAX 404-237-2704, anausa@aol.com, http://www.anausa.org. Ed. Lois V White. Circ: 5,000.

616.21 NOR ISSN 0001-6489
CODEN: AOLAAJ
ACTA OTO-LARYNGOLOGICA. Text in English. 1918. 8/yr. GBP 127, USD 210 to individuals; GBP 248, USD 410 to institutions (effective 2002). adv. charts, illus. index. *Refereed.* **Document type:** *Academic/Scholarly.* **Description:** Presents original articles of basic research interest, as well as clinical studies in the field of otorhinolaryngology and related subdisciplines.
Related titles: Online - full text ed.: (from EBSCO Publishing, O C L C Online Computer Library Center, Inc., CatchWord Ltd., ingenta, Swets Blackwell, Institute for Scientific Information, RoweCom Information Quest); ♦ Supplement: Acta Oto-Laryngologica. Supplement. ISSN 0365-5237.
Indexed: ASCA, Agri.& Environ.Biotech.Abstr. (coverage dropped), Biol.Abstr., CINAHL, C.I.S. Abstr., Chem.Abstr., Curr.Adv.Ecol.Sci., Curr.Cont., Dairy Sci.Abstr., Dent.Ind., Derwent Biotech.Abstr., Dok.Arbeitsmed., Energy Res.Abstr., Excerp.Med., Helminthol.Abstr., Hort.Abstr., INIS Atomind., Ind.Med. (1918-), Ind.Sci.Rev., Ind.Vet., Inpharma, Int.Abstr.Biol.Sci., Lang.& Lang.Behav.Abstr., NBA, Noise Pollut.Publ.Abstr., Nutr.Abstr., Pharm.&Out.News, Psychol.Abstr., Reac., Ref.Zh., Rev.Med.& Vet.Mycol., SOPODA, SSCI (coverage dropped), Sci.Cit.Ind., Sociol.Abstr., THA.
—BLDSC (0642.250000), ADONIS, CASDDS, CISTI, EMDOCS, GNLM, IDS, ingenta, KNAW. **CCC.**
Published by: (Scandinavian Oto-Laryngological Society), Taylor & Francis AS (Subsidiary of: Taylor & Francis Group), Cort Adelersgt. 17, Solli, PO Box 2562, Oslo 0202, Norway. TEL 47-22-12-98-80, FAX 47-22-12-98-90, mail@tandf.no, http://www.tandf.co.uk/tfas. Ed. Matti Anniko. Circ: 2,100.

616.21 NOR ISSN 0365-5237
CODEN: AOLSA5
ACTA OTO-LARYNGOLOGICA. SUPPLEMENT. Text in Norwegian. 1918. irreg. adv. **Document type:** *Academic/Scholarly.*
Related titles: Online - full text ed.: (from Swets Blackwell); ♦ Supplement to: Acta Oto-Laryngologica. ISSN 0001-6489.
Indexed: CINAHL, Curr.Cont. (coverage dropped), Excerp.Med., INIS Atomind., Ind.Med. (1920-), Ind.Vet., Int.Abstr.Biol.Sci., Neurosci.Cit.Ind., Ref.Zh., Rev.Appl.Entomol., Rev.Med.& Vet.Mycol.
—BLDSC (0642.255000), ADONIS, CISTI, EMDOCS, ingenta, KNAW. **CCC.**
Published by: (Scandinavian Oto-Laryngological Society), Scandinavian University Press (Subsidiary of: Taylor & Francis Ltd.), Postboks 2959, Toeyen, Oslo 0608, Norway. FAX 47-22-57-53-53, journals@scup.no, http://www.scup.no/oto. Circ: 1,900.

616.21 BEL ISSN 0001-6497
CODEN: AORLAE
ACTA OTO-RHINO-LARYNGOLOGICA BELGICA. Text in Flemish. 1967 (vol.21). 4/yr. EUR 86.75 domestic; EUR 100 foreign; EUR 24.80 per issue domestic; EUR 28.50 per issue foreign (effective 2002). Supplement avail. **Document type:** *Journal, Academic/Scholarly.*
Indexed: Biol.Abstr., Chem.Abstr., Dent.Ind., Excerp.Med., INIS Atomind., Ind.Med. (1947-), Lang.& Lang.Behav.Abstr., NBA, Rev.Med.& Vet.Mycol., SOPODA, Sociol.Abstr.
—BLDSC (0642.270000), CISTI, EMDOCS, GNLM, KNAW.
Published by: (Association des Societes Scientifiques Medicales Belges/Vereiniging van de Belgische Wetenschappelijke Genootschappen), Acta Medica Belgica, Av Circulaire 138A, Brussels 1180, Belgium. TEL 32-2-374-5158, FAX 32-2-3749628, amb@skynet.be, http://www.ulb.ac.be/medecine/loce/amb.htm. Ed. Dr. P Hennebert.

616.21 ITA ISSN 0392-100X
CODEN: AOITDU
ACTA OTORHINOLARYNGOLOGICA ITALICA. Text in Italian. 1981. bi-m. ITL 120,000; ITL 140,000 foreign (effective 1996).
Related titles: ♦ Supplement: Acta Otorhinolaryngologica Italica. Supplement. ISSN 0393-7976.
Indexed: Excerp.Med., Ind.Med. (1981-), NBA.
—BLDSC (0642.280000), CISTI, EMDOCS, GNLM, KNAW.
Published by: Pacini Editore, Via Alessandro Gherardesca, 1, Ospedaletto, PI 56121, Italy. TEL 39-050-313011, FAX 39-050-3130300, pacini@cibernet.it, http://www.cibernet.it/pacini, http://www.pacinieditore.it. Ed. E de Campora.

616.21 ITA ISSN 0393-7976
CODEN: AOTOE
ACTA OTORHINOLARYNGOLOGICA ITALICA. SUPPLEMENT. Text in Italian. irreg.
Related titles: ♦ Supplement to: Acta Otorhinolaryngologica Italica. ISSN 0392-100X.
Indexed: Excerp.Med., Ind.Med. (coverage dropped).
—BLDSC (0642.280100), EMDOCS, KNAW.
Published by: Pacini Editore, Via A. Gherardesca 1, Ospedaletto, PI 56014, Italy. TEL 050-982439, FAX 050-983906, pacini@cibernet.it, http://www.cibernet.it/pacini, http://www.pacinieditore.it.

616.85 USA ISSN 1062-5747
ADVANCE FOR SPEECH - LANGUAGE PATHOLOGISTS AND AUDIOLOGISTS. Text in English. 1991. w. *Refereed.* **Document type:** *Trade.*
Published by: Merion Publications, Inc., 2900 Horizon Dr, PO Box 61556, King Of Prussia, PA 19406. TEL 610-278-1400, 800-355-5627, FAX 610-278-1421, advance@merion.com, http://www.advanceweb.com. Ed. Sherry Fox. Pub. Ann Kielinski. adv.: B&W page USD 2,437, color page USD 2,737; trim 10.88 x 8.38. Circ: 58,300.

617.89 CHE ISSN 0254-8747
ADVANCES IN AUDIOLOGY. Text in English. 1983. irreg., latest vol.7. CHF 200 in Europe; DEM 240 in Germany; USD 160 in United States (effective 2001); price varies. *Refereed.* **Document type:** *Monographic series, Academic/Scholarly.*
Related titles: Online - full text ed.: (from Institute for Scientific Information).
—CISTI, Infotrieve, KNAW. **CCC.**
Published by: S. Karger AG, Allschwilerstr 10, PO Box, Basel 4009, Switzerland. TEL 41-61-306-1111, FAX 41-61-306-1234, karger@karger.ch, http://www.karger.com/bookseries/ADAUD. Ed. M Hoke.

617.89 613.62 GBR
ADVANCES IN NOISE RESEARCH. Text in English. 1998. irreg., latest vol.2, 1998. price varies. back issues avail. **Document type:** *Monographic series, Proceedings, Academic/Scholarly.* **Description:** Disseminates research presented at PAN conferences and workshops, covering the medical, environmental, and social aspects of noise and its effects.
Published by: (European Commission Concerted Action on Protection Against Noise), Whurr Publishers Ltd., 19b Compton Terr, London N1 2UN, United Kingdom. TEL 44-20-7359-5979, FAX 44-20-7226-5290, info@whurr.co.uk, http://www.whurr.co.uk.

616.21 CHE ISSN 0065-3071
RF16 CODEN: ADORB9
ADVANCES IN OTO-RHINO-LARYNGOLOGY. Text in English. 1953. irreg., latest vol.58. CHF 200 in Europe; DEM 240 in Germany; USD 160 in United States (effective 2001). reprint service avail. from ISI. *Refereed.* **Document type:** *Monographic series, Academic/Scholarly.*
Related titles: Online - full text ed.
Indexed: ASCA, Biol.Abstr., Chem.Abstr., Curr.Cont. (coverage dropped), Dent.Ind., Ind.Med. (1969-).
—BLDSC (0709.570000), CASDDS, CISTI, GNLM, IDS, ingenta, KNAW. **CCC.**
Published by: S. Karger AG, Allschwilerstr 10, PO Box, Basel 4009, Switzerland. TEL 41-61-306-1111, FAX 41-61-306-1234, karger@karger.ch, http://www.karger.com/bookseries/ADORL, http://biomednet.com/karger. Ed. W Arnold.

616.21 USA ISSN 0887-6916
RF1
ADVANCES IN OTOLARYNGOLOGY - HEAD AND NECK SURGERY. Text in English. 1987. a. USD 99 domestic; USD 105 foreign (effective 2001). **Document type:** *Journal, Academic/Scholarly.* **Description:** Presents a collection of original fully referenced clinical reviews from the experts in the field.
—BLDSC (0709.569000), GNLM, KNAW.
Published by: Mosby, Inc. (Subsidiary of: Elsevier Science), 11830 Westline Industrial Dr, St Louis, MO 63146-3313. TEL 314-872-8370, 800-325-4177, FAX 314-432-1380, http://www.mosby.com/periodicals. Ed. Dr. Eugene N Myers.

617.89 CAN ISSN 1050-0545
RF286 CODEN: JAAAE3
AMERICAN ACADEMY OF AUDIOLOGY. JOURNAL. Text in English. 1989. 10/yr. USD 179 in US & Canada to individuals; USD 219 elsewhere to individuals; USD 249 in US & Canada to institutions; USD 289 elsewhere to institutions (effective 2001). adv. abstr. back issues avail. *Refereed.* **Document type:** *Journal, Academic/Scholarly.* **Description:** Features original contributions, abstracts, research reports, case studies and a clinical forum.
Related titles: Microfiche ed.; Online - full text ed.: (from ProQuest Information & Learning).
Indexed: CINAHL, Ind.Med. (1990-), Lang.& Lang.Behav.Abstr., SOPODA.
—BLDSC (4683.670000), GNLM, Infotrieve, ingenta, KNAW. **CCC.**

M

Published by: (American Academy of Audiology USA), B.C. Decker Inc., 20 Hughson St S, LCD 1, P O Box 620, Hamilton, ON L8N 3K7, Canada. TEL 905-522-7017, 800-568-7281, FAX 905-522-7839, info@bcdecker.com, http://www.bcdecker.com. Ed. James Jerger. Pub. David LeGallais. R&P Paula Presutti. Adv. contact John Birkby. Circ: 6,774 (paid).

616.21 USA ISSN 0731-8359
AMERICAN ACADEMY OF OTOLARYNGOLOGY - HEAD AND NECK SURGERY. BULLETIN. Text in English. 1982. m. USD 55 domestic to non-members; USD 65 foreign to non-members (effective 2000). adv. tr.lit. index. *Refereed.* **Document type:** *Bulletin.* **Description:** Features governmental and socioeconomic affairs plus practice management tips and information of interest to otolaryngologists. Provides information about meetings, publications, policies and activities and news. Contains employment listings and a calendar of courses, meetings and workshops.
Published by: American Academy of Otolaryngology - Head and Neck Surgery, Inc., One Prince St, Alexandria, VA 22314. TEL 703-519-1562, FAX 703-519-1587, EveG_aao@compuserve.com; entbulltn@aol.com, http://www.entnet.org. Ed., Pub. G Richard Holt. R&P Michele Finley TEL 703-519-1597. Adv. contact Lisette Bassett. B&W page USD 930, color page USD 1,900; trim 11 x 8.5. Circ: 10,100 (paid).

616.21 USA ISSN 0196-0709
RF1 CODEN: AJOTDP
AMERICAN JOURNAL OF OTOLARYNGOLOGY; head and neck medicine and surgery. Text in English. 1979. bi-m. USD 148 domestic to individuals; USD 251 foreign to individuals; USD 214 domestic to institutions; USD 303 foreign to institutions; USD 60 domestic to students; USD 150 foreign to students; USD 51 newsstand/cover (effective 2001). adv. reprint service avail. from PQC. *Refereed.* **Document type:** *Journal, Academic/Scholarly.* **Description:** Provides original reports on the developments in the fields of otology, neurotology, audiology, allergology, laryngology, speech science, bronchoesophagology, facial plastic surgery, and head and neck surgery.
Related titles: Online - full text ed.: (from IDEAL Online Library, Institute for Scientific Information).
Indexed: ASCA, CINAHL, Chem.Abstr., Chem.Indus.Notes, Chem.Titles, Curr.Cont., Dent.Ind., Excerp.Med., INIS Atomind., Ind.Med. (1979-), Inpharma, NBA, Pharm.&Out.News, Reac., Rev.Med.& Vet.Mycol., THA.
—BLDSC (0829.300000), CASDDS, CISTI, EMDOCS, GNLM, IDS, ingenta, KNAW. **CCC.**
Published by: W.B. Saunders Co. (Subsidiary of: Harcourt Publishers Ltd.), 11830 Westline Industrial Dr, St Louis, MO 63146. TEL 800-325-4177, http://www.wbsaunders.com. Ed. Dr. Jonas T Johnson. Adv. contact Cindy Gray. B&W page USD 645, color page USD 1,595; trim 7 x 10. Circ: 1,325. **Subscr. to:** Periodicals Fulfillment, W B Saunders Co, 6277 Sea Harbor Dr, 4th Fl, Orlando, FL 32891-4800.

616.21 USA ISSN 1050-6586
CODEN: AJRHE5
AMERICAN JOURNAL OF RHINOLOGY. Text in English. 1987. bi-m. USD 134 domestic to individuals; USD 164 foreign to individuals; USD 224 domestic to institutions; USD 254 foreign to institutions; USD 15 newsstand/cover domestic (effective 2001). adv. *Refereed.* **Document type:** *Academic/Scholarly.* **Description:** Clinical discussions regarding medical and surgical aspects of the nose.
Related titles: Online - full text ed.: (from Institute for Scientific Information).
Indexed: ASCA, Curr.Cont., Ind.Med. (1987-), Inpharma, Pharm.&Out.News, Reac., Ref.Zh., Rev.Med.& Vet.Mycol., Sci.Cit.Ind. (coverage dropped).
—BLDSC (0836.700000), CASDDS, EMDOCS, GNLM, IDS, Infotrieve, KNAW. **CCC.**
Published by: OceanSide Publications, Inc., 95 Pitman St, Providence, RI 02906. TEL 401-331-2510, FAX 401-331-5138. Ed., R&P Dr. Guy A Settipane. Circ: 3,000.

636.08 616.21 USA
AMERICAN LARYNGOLOGICAL ASSOCIATION. TRANSACTIONS. Text in English. 1879. a. USD 30. **Document type:** *Academic/Scholarly.* **Description:** Contains minutes of business meetings and summary of historical data relating to membership, officers, etc. No manuscripts have been published since 1995.
Published by: American Laryngological Association, Animal Scientific Program, TUFTS N E Medical Center, Dept of Otolaryngology, 750 Washington St 850, Boston, MA 02111. http://www.commercial.visi.net. Ed. Dr. Stanley Shapshay. R&P Michol Sheridan TEL 314-367-4987. Circ: 300.

617.8 USA ISSN 0096-6851
RF1 CODEN: TAOTAW
AMERICAN OTOLOGICAL SOCIETY. TRANSACTIONS. Text in English. 1868. a., latest 1998. USD 65 (effective 2000). back issues avail. *Refereed.* **Document type:** *Proceedings, Academic/Scholarly.* **Description:** Abstracts of papers and discussions presented at the meeting of the society.
—CISTI, GNLM, ingenta, Linda Hall.
Published by: American Otological Society, c/o Dr A Julianna Gulya, 1558 N Colonial Terr, Arlington, VA 22209. TEL 703-528-3436. Ed. Dr. A Julianna Gulya. R&P A J Gulya. Circ: 300 (paid).

616.21 ESP ISSN 0303-8874
CODEN: AOIAA4
ANALES OTORRINOLARINGOLOGICOS IBERO-AMERICANOS. Text in Spanish; Summaries in English, French, German. 1950. bi-m. EUR 126.87 to qualified personnel Spain and Portugal; EUR 190.33 to institutions; ESP 4,879 per issue; USD 189 in Latin America to qualified personnel; USD 202 elsewhere to institutions (effective 2002). adv. bk.rev. cum.index: 1950-1973, 1974-1983. reprint service avail. from IRC. *Refereed.* **Document type:** *Monographic series.*
Formerly (until 1973): Acta Oto-Rino-Laringologica Ibero-Americana (0001-6500)
Indexed: Biol.Abstr., Dent.Ind., Excerp.Med., Ind.Med. (1974-).
—BLDSC (0890.130000), CISTI, EMDOCS, GNLM, Infotrieve. **CCC.**
Address: Balmes, 24 pral 1a, Barcelona 08007, Spain. TEL 34-93-3173646, FAX 34-93-3173766, esmon@autovia.com. Ed. E Perello Scherdel. Pub., Adv. contact Francisco Javier Monso Lamarca. B&W page ESP 60,000, color page ESP 90,000; 240 x 165. Circ: 1,000.

616.21 FRA
ANNALES D'OTO-LARYNGOLOGIE. Text in French; Summaries in English. 1875. 8/yr. FRF 1,082; FRF 1,365 foreign (effective 1997). adv. bk.rev. bibl, illus. index. reprint service avail. from ISI. **Document type:** *Academic/Scholarly.* **Description:** Contains original works devoted to clinical studies and studies of a scientific character. Includes new techniques, reading notes, and analyses.
Former titles: Annales d'Oto-Laryngologie et de Chirurgie Cervico Faciale (0003-438X); (until 1963): Annales d'Oto-Laryngologie et de Chirurgie de la Face (0150-9713); (until 1962): Annales d'Oto-Laryngologie (0365-4931)
Related titles: Microform ed.: (from PQC); Online - full text ed.: (from RoweCom Information Quest).
Indexed: Chem.Abstr., Dent.Ind., Excerp.Med., Ind.Med. (1963-), Lang.& Lang.Behav.Abstr.
—BLDSC (0990.700000), GNLM, Infotrieve, KNAW. **CCC.**
Published by: Masson - Periodiques, 120 bd. St. Germain, Paris 75006, France. TEL 33-1-40466200, FAX 33-1-40466201. Ed. H Laccourreye. Circ: 2,000. **Subscr. to:** Societe de Periodiques Specialises, BP 22, Vineuil Cedex 41354, France. TEL 33-2-54504612, FAX 33-2-54504611.

616.21 USA ISSN 0003-4894
RF1 CODEN: AORHA2
ANNALS OF OTOLOGY, RHINOLOGY AND LARYNGOLOGY. Text in English. 1892. m. USD 170 domestic to individuals; USD 195 foreign to individuals; USD 240 domestic to institutions; USD 265 foreign to institutions (effective 2001). adv. bk.rev. charts. index. back issues avail.; reprint service avail. from PQC. *Refereed.* **Document type:** *Trade.* **Description:** Publishes original manuscripts of clinical and research importance in otolaryngology - head and neck medicine and surgery, broncho-esophagology, maxillofacial surgery, audiology, speech pathology, and related specialties.
Related titles: CD-ROM ed.: USD 175, USD 245 (effective 2001); Microfiche ed.; Online - full text ed.: (from ProQuest Information & Learning, Institute for Scientific Information).
Indexed: AIM, ASCA, Abstr.Anthropol., AgeLine, Biol.Abstr., CINAHL, Chem.Abstr., Curr.Adv.Ecol.Sci., Curr.Cont., Dent.Ind., Dok.Arbeitsmed., INIS Atomind., Ind.Med. (1897-), Ind.Sci.Rev., Inpharma, Lang.& Lang.Behav.Abstr., NBA, Neurosci.Cit.Ind., Noise Pollut.Publ.Abstr., Nutr.Abstr., Pharm.&Out.News, Protozool.Abstr., Psychol.Abstr., Reac., Rev.Med.& Vet.Mycol., SOPODA, SSCI (coverage dropped), Sci.Cit.Ind., Sociol.Abstr., THA, Trop.Dis.Bull.
—BLDSC (1043.400000), CISTI, EMDOCS, GNLM, IDS, ingenta, KNAW.
Published by: (American Laryngological Association, American Broncho-Esophagological Association), Annals Publishing Co., 4507 Laclede Ave, St. Louis, MO 63108. TEL 314-367-4987, FAX 314-367-4988, manager@annals.com, http://www.annals.com. Ed. Dr. Brian F McCabe. R&P Michol L Sheridan. Adv. contact Kenneth A Cooper Jr. B&W page USD 740; trim 11 x 8.38. Circ: 6,002.

616.21 016 USA ISSN 0886-4470
RF1 CODEN: AONSEJ
ARCHIVES OF OTOLARYNGOLOGY - HEAD & NECK SURGERY. Text in English. 1925. m. USD 350 in North America to institutions; USD 450 to institutions Central & S. America; GBP 295 elsewhere to institutions (effective 2001). adv. bk.rev. bibl, charts, illus. index. back issues avail.; reprints avail. *Refereed.* **Document type:** *Academic/Scholarly.* **Description:** Publishes original contributions and clinical observations relevant of the practice of otolaryngology.
Former titles: Archives of Otolaryngology (0003-9977); A M A Archives of Otolaryngology (0096-6894)
Related titles: CD-ROM ed.: (from Ovid Technologies, Inc.); Microform ed.: (from PQC); Online - full text ed.: (from The Dialog Corporation, Gale Group, Ovid Technologies, Inc., EBSCO Publishing, Institute for Scientific Information).
Indexed: AIM, ASCA, Abstr.Anthropol., Biol.Abstr., CINAHL, C.I.S. Abstr., Chem.Abstr., Chemorec.Abstr., Curr.Cont., Dent.Ind., Except.Child Educ.Abstr., Excerp.Med., INIS Atomind., Ind.Med. (1986-), Ind.Sci.Rev., Inpharma, Int.Nurs.Ind., Kidney, Med.& Surg.Dermat., NBA, Neurosci.Cit.Ind., Noise Pollut.Publ.Abstr., Pharm.&Out.News, Reac., Rev.Med.& Vet.Mycol., Rev.Plant Path., Sci.Cit.Ind., Trop.Dis.Bull.
—BLDSC (1638.510000), CASDDS, CISTI, EMDOCS, GNLM, IDS, Infotrieve, ingenta, KNAW. **CCC.**
Published by: American Medical Association, 515 N State St, P O Box 10946, Chicago, IL 60610-0946. ama-subs@ama-assn.org, http://www.archoto.com. Ed. Michael Johns. R&P Ada Jimenez Walker. Adv. contact Peter G Messina. Circ: 13,000.

617.8 GBR ISSN 1361-3286
CODEN: APLHFI
ASIA PACIFIC JOURNAL OF SPEECH, LANGUAGE AND HEARING. Text in English. 1996. 3/yr. USD 80 in North America to individuals; GBP 42 rest of world to individuals; GBP 21 in developing nations to individuals; USD 160 in North America to institutions; GBP 84 rest of world to institutions; GBP 42 in developing nations to institutions (effective 2001). adv. back issues avail. **Document type:** *Academic/Scholarly.* **Description:** IT is an international and interdisciplinary forum where scientists and clinicians in the field of communication disorders who are part of the Asia-Pacific community or have knowledge or experience relevant to it, can share information and expertise.
Indexed: CINAHL, Lang.& Lang.Behav.Abstr., SOPODA, Sociol.Abstr.
—BLDSC (1742.260940).
Published by: Whurr Publishers Ltd., 19b Compton Terr, London N1 2UN, United Kingdom. TEL 44-20-7359-5979, FAX 44-20-7226-5290, info@whurr.co.uk, http://www.whurrjournals.co.uk/, http://www.whurr.co.uk. Ed. Bruce Murdoch. **Subscr. in N. America to:** Whurr Publishers Ltd., PO Box 1897, Lawrence, KS 66044-8897. TEL 913-843-1221, FAX 913-843-1274, am&m@allenpress.com. **Subscr. to:** Turpin Distribution Services Ltd., Blackhorse Rd, Letchworth, Herts SG6 1HN, United Kingdom. TEL 44-1462-488900, FAX 44-1462-483011.

616.2 ITA ISSN 0066-9865
ASSOCIAZIONE ITALIANA LARINGECTOMIZZATI. ATTI (DEL) CONVEGNO NAZIONALE. Text in Italian. 1957. q. **Description:** Addresses all laryngectomees and their families with news about Association life and medical advice.
Published by: Associazione Italiana Laringectomizzati, Via Friuli, 28, Milan, MI 20135, Italy. TEL 02-5510819. Ed. Dr. Giuseppe Sapa.

616.21 USA
AUDIO-DIGEST OTOLARYNGOLOGY - HEAD AND NECK SURGERY. Text in English. 1968. s-m. USD 168 (effective 2000). *Refereed.*
Former titles: Audio-Digest Otorhinolaryngology - Head and Neck Surgery (0271-1354); Audio-Digest Otorhinolaryngology (0030-6673)
Media: Audio cassette/tape.
Published by: Audio-Digest Foundation (Subsidiary of: California Medical Association), 1577 E Chevy Chase Dr, Glendale, CA 91206. TEL 213-245-8505, 800-423-2308, FAX 818-240-7379, 800-845-4375.

M

617.8 CHE ISSN 1420-3030
RF290 CODEN: ANEOFO
AUDIOLOGY AND NEURO-OTOLOGY; basic research and clinical applications. Text in English. 1962. bi-m. CHF 798, EUR 570.80 in Europe to institutions; CHF 815.40, USD 623 overseas to institutions (effective 2002). adv. abstr, bibl, illus. index, cum.index. back issues avail. *Refereed.* **Document type:** *Journal, Academic/Scholarly.* **Description:** Provides a forum for the presentation of outstanding papers on the auditory and vestibular systems.
Former titles (until 1996): Audiology (0020-6091); International Audiology (0538-4915)
Related titles: Microfilm ed.; Online - full text ed.: ISSN 1421-9700. CHF 58, EUR 42, USD 45 with print edition (effective 2002) (from EBSCO Publishing, O C L C Online Computer Library Center, Inc., RoweCom Information Quest, ProQuest Information & Learning, Swets Blackwell, Institute for Scientific Information).
Indexed: ASCA, Acoust.Abstr., AgeLine, Aqua.Sci.& Fish.Abstr., Bibl.Dev.Med.& Child Neur., Biol.Abstr., Curr.Adv.Ecol.Sci., Curr.Cont., Dok.Arbeitsmed., Excerp.Med., Ind.Med. (1971-), Ind.Sci.Rev., Inpharma, Lang.& Lang.Behav.Abstr., NBA, Neurosci.Cit.Ind., Noise Pollut.Publ.Abstr., PsycInfo, Psychol.Abstr. (1971-), Reac., SOPODA, SSCI (coverage dropped), Sci.Cit.Ind., Sociol.Abstr., e-psyche.
—BLDSC (1789.081500), CASDDS, CISTI, EMDOCS, GNLM, IDS, Infotrieve, ingenta, KNAW. **CCC.**
Published by: (International Society of Audiology), S. Karger AG, Allschwilerstr 10, PO Box, Basel 4009, Switzerland. TEL 41-61-306-1111, 800-568-7281, FAX 41-61-306-1234, karger@karger.ch, http://www.online.karger.com/journals/aud, http://www.karger.com. Ed. M Hoke. adv.: page USD 1,185. Circ: 1,650.

617.89 USA ISSN 1535-2609
AUDIOLOGY TODAY. Text in English. 1988. bi-m. USD 35 domestic to individuals; USD 50 foreign to individuals; USD 55 domestic to institutions; USD 70 foreign to institutions (effective 2001). back issues avail.; reprints avail. **Document type:** *Magazine, Academic/Scholarly.* **Description:** Covers academy affairs and clinical practice. Includes coverage of pragmatic applications in evaluative, diagnostic and rehabilitative services.
—BLDSC (1789.084300).
Published by: American Academy of Audiology, 8300 Greensboro Dr., Ste. 750, Mclean, VA 22102. TEL 703-790-8466, info@audiology.org, http://www.audiology.org. Ed. Jerry Northern. R&P Sydney Davis. Adv. contact Rick Gabler TEL 856-256-2314.

616.21 NLD ISSN 0385-8146
CODEN: ANLADF
AURIS, NASUS, LARYNX. Text in English, French, German; Summaries in English. 1973. q. EUR 245 in Europe to institutions; JPY 32,500 in Japan to institutions; USD 274 elsewhere to institutions (effective 2002). adv. charts, illus. back issues avail. **Document type:** *Academic/Scholarly.* **Description:** Provides rapid and reviewed publications concerning the basic and clinical aspects of otorhinolaryngology and related fields such as: otology, neurotology, equilibrium sciences, bronchoesophagology, laryngology, neurolaryngology, rhinollogy, allergology, head and neck medicine and oncologic surgery, maxillofacial and plastic surgery, audiology, speech science and communication disorders.
Related titles: Online - full text ed.: (from ingenta, Swets Blackwell, ScienceDirect, Institute for Scientific Information).
Indexed: Biol.Abstr., Curr.Cont., Dent.Ind., Excerp.Med., INIS Atomind., Ind.Med. (1973-).
—BLDSC (1792.760000), CASDDS, CISTI, EMDOCS, GNLM, Infotrieve, KNAW. **CCC.**
Published by: (Society for the Promotion of International Otorhinolaryngology), Elsevier Science BV, PO Box 211, Amsterdam 1000 AE, Netherlands. nlinfo-f@elsevier.nl, http://www.elsevier.com/locate/anl, http://www.elsevier.nl. Ed. Dr. Makoto Sakai. Circ: 600. **Subscr. in Australasia and the Far East to:** Elsevier Science (Singapore) Pte Ltd, No.1 Temasek Ave, 17-01 Millenia Tower, Singapore 039192, Singapore. TEL 65-434-3727, FAX 65-337-2230; **Subscr. in Japan to:** Elsevier Science Inc - Japan Regional Office, 9-15 Higashi-Azabu 1-chome, Minato-ku, Tokyo 106-0044, Japan. TEL 81-3-5561-5033, FAX 81-3-5561-5047; **Subscr. in the Americas to:** Elsevier Science, PO Box 945, New York, NY 10159-0945. TEL 212-633-3730, FAX 212-633-3680, http://www.elsevier.com.

AUSTRALIAN JOURNAL OF AUDIOLOGY. see *HANDICAPPED—Hearing Impaired*

616.21 AUS ISSN 1037-2105
CODEN: AJOTEQ
AUSTRALIAN JOURNAL OF OTOLARYNGOLOGY. Text in English. 1962. a. AUD 47.25 domestic; AUD 51 New Zealand & Asia Pacific; AUD 54 elsewhere New Zealand & Asia Pacific (effective 2000 - 2001). adv. bk.rev. reprint service avail. from PQC. **Document type:** *Academic/Scholarly.* **Description:** Publishes research and clinical papaers in head and neck surgery.
Formerly (until 1992): Oto-Laryngological Society of Australia. Journal (0030-6614)
Related titles: Microform ed.: (from PQC); Online - full text ed.: (from ProQuest Information & Learning).
Indexed: DSH Abstr., Excerp.Med.
—BLDSC (1810.810000), EMDOCS, GNLM, KNAW.
Published by: Australian Society of Otolaryngology Head & Neck Surgery Ltd., Ste 403, 68 Alfred St, Milsons Point, NSW 2061, Australia. TEL 61-2-9954-5856, FAX 61-2-9957-6863, enquiries@asohns.org.au, http://www.asohns.org.au. Ed., R&P Dr. Marcus Atlas. Circ: 1,000.

617.89 USA
BETTER HEARING NEWS. Text in English. 1973. q. USD 10 (effective 1999). **Document type:** *Newsletter.* **Description:** Highlights of current institute activities.
Formerly: Communicator
Published by: Better Hearing Institute, 515 Kings St, Ste 420, Alexandria, VA 22314. TEL 703-684-3391, 800-327-9355, FAX 703-684-3394, mail@betterhearing.org, http://www.betterhearing.org. Ed., Pub., R&P Michele D Hartlove. Circ: 2,500.

616.21 CAN ISSN 1199-0538
C A D CHAT. Text in English, French. 1989. 10/yr. CND 25 (effective 1999). back issues avail. **Document type:** *Bulletin, Newsletter, Consumer.*
Published by: Canadian Association of the Deaf, 251 Bank St, Ste 203, Ottawa, ON K1V 7P2, Canada. TEL 613-565-2882, FAX 613-565-1207, cad@cad.ca, http://www.cad.ca, http://www.cad.co. Circ: 1,000.

616.21 FRA ISSN 0395-3971
CODEN: CCCADH
LES CAHIERS D'OTO-RHINOLARYNGOLOGIE, DE CHIRURGIE CERVICO-FACIALE ET D'AUDIOPHONOLOGIE. Variant title: Cahiers d'O R L de Chirurgie Cervico-Faciale et d'Audiophonologie. Text in French. 1966. 8/yr. FRF 530 domestic to individuals; EUR 83.75 in the European Union to individuals; FRF 570 elsewhere to individuals; FRF 370 domestic to students; EUR 60.98 in the European Union to students; FRF 420 elsewhere to students; FRF 73 newsstand/cover (effective 2001). *Refereed.* **Description:** Focuses of cervico-facial pathology and anatomy, laryngology, and otology.
Former titles (until 1976): Cahiers d'O R L et de Chirurgie Cervico-Faciale (0395-398X); (until 1973): Cahiers d'Oto-Rhinolaryngologie (0373-2827)
Indexed: NBA, Ref.Zh.
—CISTI, GNLM.
Published by: Editions la Simarre, Z.I. No. 2 - rue Joseph-Cugnot, Joue-les-Tours 37300, France. TEL 33-2-47535366, FAX 33-2-47674505. Ed. Bernard Gurrier.

616.855 JPN
CHONO GENGOGAKU KENKYU/JAPANESE JOURNAL OF COMMUNICATION DISORDERS. Text in Japanese; Summaries in English, Japanese. 1983. 3/yr. JPY 2,000 (effective 2001). **Document type:** *Academic/Scholarly.*
Published by: Nihon Chono Gengo Gakkai/Japanese Speech - Language - Hearing Association, 2-15-6-202 Minami-cho, Kokubunji-shi, Tokyo-to 185-0021, Japan. TEL 81-42-324-7397, FAX 81-42-328-7071, jslha@cd.inbox.ne.jp. Ed. Bensaku Nishimura.

616.21 GBR ISSN 0307-7772
CODEN: COTSD2
CLINICAL OTOLARYNGOLOGY AND ALLIED SCIENCES. Text in English. 1976. bi-m., latest vol.27, 2002. GBP 462 in Europe; USD 732 in North America; GBP 508 elsewhere (effective 2002). adv. bk.rev. charts, illus. index. back issues avail.; reprint service avail. from ISI. *Refereed.* **Document type:** *Academic/Scholarly.* **Description:** Devoted to clinical and clinically oriented research papers dealing with current otorhinolaryngological practice, audiology, speech pathology, and related specialties.
Related titles: Microform ed.: (from PQC); Online - full text ed.: ISSN 1365-2273. GBP 416 in Europe; USD 659 in North America; GBP 416 elsewhere (effective 2002) (from Ovid Technologies, Inc., EBSCO Publishing, O C L C Online Computer Library Center, Inc., RoweCom Information Quest, ingenta, Munksgaard & Blackwell Science's Synergy, Swets Blackwell, Institute for Scientific Information).
Indexed: ASCA, Biol.Abstr., Curr.Adv.Ecol.Sci., Curr.Cont., Excerp.Med., Ind.Med. (1976-), Inpharma, NBA, Pharm.&Out.News, Reac., Sci.Cit.Ind.
—BLDSC (3286.324000), ADONIS, CISTI, EMDOCS, GNLM, IDS, ingenta, KNAW. **CCC.**
Published by: Blackwell Science Ltd., PO Box 88, Oxford OX2 0NE, United Kingdom. TEL 44-1865-206180, 44-1865-206002, FAX 44-1865-206219, jnl.orders@blacksci.co.uk, http://www.blackwell-science.com/products/journals/cotol.htm, http://www.blackwellpublishing.com. Ed. J Hibbert. Pub. Elizabeth Whelan. R&P Sophie Savage. Adv. contact Jenny Applin. Circ: 1,735.

617.89 USA
RC423.A1
CONTEMPORARY ISSUES IN COMMUNICATION SCIENCE & DISORDERS. Text in English. 1973. a. USD 12 to non-members. adv. back issues avail. **Document type:** *Academic/Scholarly.* **Description:** Features articles and reports on a variety of current speech-language-hearing topics of special interest to students and practicing clinicians.
Formerly: National Student Speech Language Hearing Association. Journal (0736-0312)
—CCC.
Published by: National Student Speech Language Hearing Association, 10801 Rockville Pike, Rockville, MD 20852. TEL 301-897-5700, FAX 301-897-7350. Ed. Anthony J Caruso. R&P Jennifer Martinez TEL 301-897-0145. Adv. contact Pam Leppin.

CORRIERE DEI LARINGECTOMIZZATI. see *SOCIAL SERVICES AND WELFARE*

616.21 617 USA ISSN 1068-9508
CODEN: COOSFD
CURRENT OPINION IN OTOLARYNGOLOGY & HEAD AND NECK SURGERY. Text in English. 1993. bi-m. USD 210 domestic to individuals for print & online eds.; USD 210 foreign to individuals for print & online eds; USD 499 per issue domestic to institutions; USD 499 per issue foreign to institutions; USD 76 newsstand/cover (effective 2002). adv. **Document type:** *Academic/Scholarly.*
Related titles: Online - full text ed.: USD 648.70 domestic academic site license; USD 648.70 foreign academic site license; USD 723.55 domestic corporate site license; USD 723.55 foreign corporate site license (effective 2002) (from Ovid Technologies, Inc., EBSCO Publishing, Swets Blackwell).
Indexed: CINAHL, Cal.Tiss.Abstr., Excerp.Med. (1995-).
—BLDSC (3500.776700), ADONIS, GNLM, KNAW.
Published by: Lippincott Williams & Wilkins (Philadelphia) (Subsidiary of: Wolters Kluwer N.V.), 530 Walnut St, Philadelphia, PA 19106-3621. TEL 301-714-2300, 800-638-3030, http://www.Lww.com. Eds. Jack Gluckman, Richard Fabian. Pub. Maria McMichael. R&P Tobias Weschler. Adv. contact Kelly Adamitis.

617.54 616.21 NLD ISSN 1063-2581
CURRENT TOPICS IN GENERAL THORACIC SURGERY. Text in Dutch. 1985; N.S. 1991. irreg., latest vol.3, 1995. illus. *Refereed.* **Document type:** *Monographic series, Academic/Scholarly, Trade.* **Description:** Reviews clinical pre- and postoperative regimens for patients undergoing thoracic surgery.
Supersedes (in 1991): International Trends in General Thoracic Surgery (0891-3382)
—BLDSC (3504.883800), CISTI.
Published by: Elsevier Science BV, PO Box 211, Amsterdam 1000 AE, Netherlands. TEL 31-20-485-3757, 31-20-485-3911, FAX 31-20-485-3432, 31-20-485-3598, nlinfo-f@elsevier.nl, http://www.elsevier.nl. **Subscr. in Australasia and the Far East to:** Elsevier Science (Singapore) Pte Ltd, No.1 Temasek Ave, 17-01 Millenia Tower, Singapore 039192, Singapore. TEL 65-434-3727, FAX 65-337-2230, asiainfo@elsevier.com.sg; **Subscr. in Japan to:** Elsevier Science Inc - Japan Regional Office, 9-15 Higashi-Azabu 1-chome, Minato-ku, Tokyo 106-0044, Japan. TEL 81-3-5561-5033, FAX 81-3-5561-5047, info@elsevier.co.jp; **Subscr. in the Americas to:** Elsevier Science, PO Box 945, New York, NY 10159-0945. TEL 212-633-3730, 888-437-4636, FAX 212-633-3680, usinfo-f@elsevier.com, http://www.elsevier.com.

M

616.21 AUS ISSN 1120-8694
CODEN: DIESE

DISEASES OF THE ESOPHAGUS. Text in English. 1988-1992; resumed 1994. q. AUD 233 domestic to individuals; AUD 211 in New Zealand to individuals; USD 129 elsewhere to individuals; AUD 866 domestic to institutions; AUD 787 in New Zealand to institutions; USD 480 elsewhere to institutions; AUD 257 domestic to individuals paper & online eds. combined; AUD 233 in New Zealand to individuals paper & online eds. combined; USD 142 elsewhere to individuals paper & online eds. combined; AUD 953 domestic to institutions paper & online eds. combined; AUD 866 in New Zealand to institutions paper & online eds. combined; USD 528 elsewhere to institutions paper & online eds. combined (effective 2001). adv. bk.rev. abstr, bibl. **Document type:** *Journal, Academic/Scholarly.* **Description:** Explores original and review material covering all aspects of esophageal disorders, their etiology, investigation and diagnosis, and both medical and surgical treatment.
Incorporates (in July 1993): Gullet (0952-0643)
Related titles: Microform ed.: ceased (from PQC); ♦ Online - full text ed.: Diseases of the Esophagus Online. ISSN 1442-2050.
Indexed: Curr.Cont., Excerp.Med. (until 1992, 1994-), Ind.Med. (1988-).
—BLDSC (3598.210000), EMDOCS, GNLM, Infotrieve, KNAW. **CCC.**
Published by: (International Society for Diseases of the Esophagus GBR), Blackwell Science Asia Pty Ltd, PO Box 378, Carlton South, VIC 3053, Australia. TEL 61-3-9347-0300, FAX 61-3-9347-5001, info@blacksci-asia.com.au, http://www.blackwell-science.com/~cgilib/jnlpage.bin?Journal=des&File=des&Page=aims, http://www.blacksci.co.uk/australi. Ed. Rudiger J Siewert. Circ: 990.

616.21 AUS ISSN 1442-2050

DISEASES OF THE ESOPHAGUS ONLINE. Text in English. q. AUD 210 domestic to individuals; AUD 190 in New Zealand to individuals; USD 117 elsewhere to individuals; AUD 780 domestic to institutions; AUD 709 in New Zealand to institutions; USD 432 elsewhere to institutions (effective 2001). **Document type:** *Academic/Scholarly.*
Media: Online - full text (from Munksgaard & Blackwell Science's Synergy, EBSCO Publishing, O C L C Online Computer Library Center, Inc., RoweCom Information Quest, ingenta, Swets Blackwell, Institute for Scientific Information). **Related titles:** Microform ed.: ceased (from PQC); ♦ Print ed.: Diseases of the Esophagus. ISSN 1120-8694.
Published by: Blackwell Science Asia Pty Ltd, PO Box 378, Carlton South, VIC 3053, Australia. TEL 61-3-9347-0300, FAX 61-3-9347-3016, website@blacksci.com, info@blacksci-asia.com.au, http://www.blackwell-science.com/~cgilib/jnlpage.bin?Journal=des&File=des&Page=aims, http://www.blacksci.co.uk/australi.

616.21 USA ISSN 0179-051X
CODEN: DYSPE2

DYSPHAGIA; an international multidisciplinary journal devoted to swallowing and its disorders. Text in English. 1986. q. (in 1 vol., 4 nos./vol.). USD 398.40 domestic for Print & Online Eds.; USD 394.10 in Germany for Print & Online Eds.; USD 112.80 newsstand/cover foreign (effective 2002). adv. reprint service avail. from SWZ. *Refereed.* **Document type:** *Academic/Scholarly.* **Description:** Surveys all aspects of normal and dysphagic ingestion involving the mouth, pharynx, and esophagus. Draws on expertise from a variety of disciplines including gastroenterology, neurology, otolaryngology, radiology, dentistry, rehabilitation medicine, speech pathology, nursing, dietetics, medical administration and the basic biomedical sciences.
Related titles: Microform ed.: (from PQC); Online - full text ed.: ISSN 1432-0460 (from EBSCO Publishing, RoweCom Information Quest, Swets Blackwell, Springer LINK, Institute for Scientific Information).
Indexed: AMED, ASCA, Curr.Cont., Excerp.Med., INIS Atomind., Ind.Med. (1986-), Inpharma, Pharm.&Out.News, Reac.
—BLDSC (3637.270000), CISTI, GNLM, IDS, ingenta, KNAW. **CCC.**
Published by: Springer-Verlag, Journals (Subsidiary of: BertelsmannSpringer), 175 Fifth Ave, New York, NY 10010. TEL 212-460-1500, FAX 212-473-6272, orders@springer-ny.com, http://www.springer-ny.com. Ed. Bronwyn Jones. R&P Ian Gross. Adv. contact Brian Skepton. **N. American subscr. to:** Journal Fulfillment Services, PO Box 2491, Secaucus, NJ 07096-2485. TEL 800-777-4643, FAX 201-348-4505.

617.51005 GBR ISSN 1368-8944

E N T NEWS. Variant title: Ear, Nose and Throat News. Text in English. 1992. bi-m. GBP 15 in British Isles; EUR 25 in Europe; EUR 45 elsewhere (effective 2001). adv. bk.rev., software rev., video rev., Website rev. abstr, tr.lit. reprints avail. *Refereed.* **Document type:** *Magazine, Abstract/Index, Consumer.* **Description:** Features review articles from major journals of otolaryngology and audiology, as well as relavant oncology, laser, matillo-facial, speech therapy and plastic surgery journals. Reviews performed by independent medical specialists.
Related titles: E-mail ed.; Online - full text ed.
—BLDSC (3776.420900).
Published by: Pinpoint Scotland Ltd., 9 Gayfield St, Edinburgh EH1 3NT, United Kingdom. TEL 44-131-478-8401, 44-131-478-8402, FAX 44-131-557-4701, http://www.ent-news.com. Ed. Andrew McCombe. Pub. Cedric Chater. R&Ps Patricia McDonnell, Rosalean Shine. Adv. contact Rosaleen Shine. B&W page GBP 770, color page GBP 1,080; trim 210 x 297. Circ: 19,500 (controlled).

617.89 USA ISSN 0196-0202
RF286 CODEN: EAHEDS

EAR AND HEARING. Text in English. 1975. bi-m. USD 89 domestic to individuals; USD 132 foreign to individuals; USD 172 domestic to institutions; USD 215 foreign to institutions; USD 36 newsstand/cover (effective 2002). adv. illus. index. back issues avail. *Refereed.* **Document type:** *Academic/Scholarly.* **Description:** Covers assessment, diagnosis and management of auditory disorders.
Former titles: American Auditory Society. Journal (0164-5080); American Audiology Society. Journal (0360-9294)
Related titles: Microfilm ed.: (from WWS); Online - full text ed.: (from Ovid Technologies, Inc., Institute for Scientific Information).
Indexed: ASCA, Acoust.Abstr., AgeLine, CINAHL, Chic.Per.Ind., Curr.Cont., Environ.Sci.Poll.Mgmt., Excerp.Med., Ind.Med. (1980-), Ind.Sci.Rev., Inpharma, Lang.& Lang.Behav.Abstr., MLA Intl.Bibl., NBA, Neurosci.Cit.Ind., Noise Pollut.Publ.Abstr., Pollut.Abstr., Reac., Risk Abstr., SOPODA, SSCI (coverage dropped), Saf.Sci.Abstr., Sci.Cit.Ind., Sociol.Abstr.
—BLDSC (3642.866000), CISTI, GNLM, IDS, ingenta, KNAW.
Published by: (American Auditory Society), Williams & Wilkins (Subsidiary of: Waverly International), 351 W Camden St, Baltimore, MD 21201-2436. TEL 410-528-4068, 800-222-3790, FAX 410-528-4452, mricks@wwilkins.com, http://www.wwilkins.com, http://www.Lww.com. Ed. Dr. Susan Jerger. Adv. contact Melanie Ricks. B&W page USD 850; trim 10.88 x 8.13. Circ: 5,025; 4,959 (paid).

616.21 USA ISSN 0145-5613

EAR, NOSE & THROAT JOURNAL. Text in English. 1922. m. USD 60 domestic to individuals; USD 20 newsstand/cover elsewhere to individuals; USD 140 domestic to institutions; USD 40 elsewhere to institutions (effective 2002). adv. bk.rev. charts, illus. index. back issues avail.; reprints avail. *Refereed.* **Description:** Publishes recent, scientific, clinical articles and case reports in otolaryngology and head and neck surgery; provides practical hands-on information for today's busy physician.
Formerly: Eye, Ear, Nose and Throat Monthly (0014-5491)
Related titles: Microfilm ed.: (from PQC); Online - full text ed.: (from ProQuest Information & Learning, Gale Group).
Indexed: Biol.Abstr., Chem.Abstr., Dent.Ind., Environ.Sci.Poll.Mgmt., Excerp.Med., INIS Atomind., Ind.Med. (1976-), Pollut.Abstr., Rev.Med.& Vet.Mycol., Risk Abstr., Saf.Sci.Abstr., THA.
—BLDSC (3642.867000), CISTI, GNLM, ingenta, KNAW. **CCC.**
Published by: Medquest Communications, LLC, 629 Euclid Ave, Ste 1200, Cleveland, OH 44114-3003. TEL 216-522-9700, FAX 216-522-9707, editor@entjournal.com, http://primarycare.medscape.com/Medquest/ENT/public/ENT-journals.html/. Ed. Dr. Jack Pulec. Pub. Mark Goodman III. Circ: 12,300.

616.21 FRA ISSN 0246-0351

ENCYCLOPEDIE MEDICO-CHIRURGICALE. OTO-RHINO-LARYNGOLOGIE. Cover title: Traite d'Oto-Rhino-Laryngologie. Variant title: Encyclopedie Medico-Chirurgicale, Instantanes Medicaux. Oto-Rhino-Laryngologie. Text in French. 1951. 6 base vols. plus q. updates. bibl, charts, illus. *Refereed.* **Document type:** *Academic/Scholarly.* **Description:** Provides otorhinolaryngologists with a comprehensive and up-to-date reference source for diagnosing and treating disorders of the ears, nose, and throat.
Published by: Elsevier Paris, Editions Scientifiques et Medicales (Subsidiary of: Reed Elsevier plc. group), 23 rue Linois, Paris 75015, France. TEL 33-1-45589110, FAX 33-1-44589425, redaction-emc@elsevier.fr, redacion-emc@elsevier.fr, http://www.elsevier.fr, http://www.elsevier.com.

ENCYCLOPEDIE MEDICO-CHIRURGICALE. TECHNIQUES CHIRURGICALES. TETE ET COU; la reference du chirurgien. actualisee en permanence. see *MEDICAL SCIENCES—Surgery*

ENCYCLOPEDIE MEDICO-CHIRURGICALE. TECHNIQUES CHIRURGICALES. THORAX; la reference du chirurgien - actualisee en permanence. see *MEDICAL SCIENCES—Surgery*

ENCYCLOPEDIE MEDICO-CHIRURGICALE. TECNICHE CHIRURGICHE. CHIRURGIA O R L E CERVICO-FACCIALE. (Oto-Rhino-Laryngologia) see *MEDICAL SCIENCES—Surgery*

ENCYCLOPEDIE MEDICO-CHIRURGICALE. TECNICHE CHIRURGICHE. TORACE. see *MEDICAL SCIENCES—Surgery*

616.21 DEU ISSN 0937-4477
CODEN: EAOTE7

EUROPEAN ARCHIVES OF OTO-RHINO-LARYNGOLOGY. Text in English, German. 1864. 10/yr. EUR 1,733.50 domestic; EUR 1,727.30 in Germany; EUR 205.20 newsstand/cover foreign (effective 2002). adv. bibl, charts, illus. index. back issues avail.; reprint service avail. from ISI. *Refereed.* **Document type:** *Journal, Academic/Scholarly.* **Description:** Focuses on original clinical reports and clinically relevant experimental studies in the fields of oto-rhino-laryngology, and head and neck surgery.
Former titles: Archives of Oto-Rhino-Laryngology (0302-9530); Archiv fuer Klinische und Experimentelle Ohren-, Nasen- und Kehlkopfheilkunde (0003-9195)
Related titles: Microform ed.: (from PQC); Online - full text ed.: ISSN 1434-4726 (from EBSCO Publishing, RoweCom Information Quest, Swets Blackwell, Springer LINK, Institute for Scientific Information).
Indexed: ASCA, Biol.Abstr., Curr.Adv.Ecol.Sci., Curr.Cont., Dent.Ind., Excerp.Med., INIS Atomind., Ind.Med. (1990-), Ind.Sci.Rev., Inpharma, Neurosci.Cit.Ind., Nutr.Abstr., Pharm.&Out.News, Reac., Rev.Med.& Vet.Mycol., Sci.Cit.Ind.
—BLDSC (3829.488540), ADONIS, CASDDS, CISTI, EMDOCS, GNLM, IDS, ingenta, KNAW. **CCC.**
Published by: (European Federation of Oto-Rhino-Laryngological Societies), Springer-Verlag (Subsidiary of: BertelsmannSpringer), Tiergartenstr 17, Heidelberg 69121, Germany. TEL 49-6221-345-0, FAX 49-6221-345229, subscriptions@springer.de, http://link.springer.de/link/service/journals/00405/index.htm, http://www.springer.de. Eds. A D Kornblut, U Ganzer. **Subscr. in N. America to:** Springer-Verlag New York Inc., PO Box 2485, Secaucus, NJ 07096-2485. TEL 212-460-1500, FAX 212-473-6272.
Co-sponsor: European Laryngological Society.

EXCERPTA MEDICA. SECTION 11: OTORHINOLARYNGOLOGY. see *MEDICAL SCIENCES—Abstracting, Bibliographies, Statistics*

617.8 CHE ISSN 1021-7762
RC423 CODEN: FPLOEP

FOLIA PHONIATRICA ET LOGOPAEDICA; international journal of phoniatrics, speech therapy and communication pathology. Text in English, French, German; Summaries in English. 1947. bi-m. CHF 557, EUR 397.80 in Europe to institutions; CHF 574.40, USD 436 elsewhere to institutions (effective 2002). adv. bk.rev. bibl, charts, illus. index. back issues avail. *Refereed.* **Document type:** *Journal, Academic/Scholarly.* **Description:** Provides a survey of international research in physiology and pathology of speech and the voice organs.
Formerly: Folia Phoniatrica (0015-5705)
Related titles: Microform ed.; Online - full text ed.: ISSN 1421-9972. CHF 58, EUR 42, USD 45 to institutions with print edition (effective 2002) (from EBSCO Publishing, O C L C Online Computer Library Center, Inc., RoweCom Information Quest, ProQuest Information & Learning, Swets Blackwell, Institute for Scientific Information).
Indexed: AMED, ASCA, AgeLine, Arts & Hum.Cit.Ind. (coverage dropped), Bibl.Dev.Med.& Child Neur., Biol.Abstr., CINAHL, Chem.Abstr., Curr.Cont., Dent.Ind., Excerp.Med., Ind.Med. (1994-), Int.Nurs.Ind., Lang.& Lang.Behav.Abstr., M.L.A., MLA Intl.Bibl., Mid.East: Abstr.& Ind., NBA, PsycInfo, Psychol.Abstr. (1982-), Russ.Acad.Sci.Bibl., SSCI, e-psyche.
—BLDSC (3973.560000), CISTI, GNLM, IDS, ingenta, KNAW. **CCC.**

M

Published by: (International Association of Logopedics and Phoniatrics), S. Karger AG, Allschwilerstr 10, PO Box, Basel 4009, Switzerland. TEL 41-61-306-1111, FAX 41-61-306-1234, karger@karger.ch, http://www.online.karger.com/journals/fpl, http://www.karger.com. Ed. S Fex. adv.: page USD 1,185. Circ: 1,600.

616.21 DEU ISSN 0943-0121
H N O AKTUELL. (Hals - Nase - Ohren) Text in German. 1993. m. DEM 132 (effective 2000). adv. index. back issues avail. **Document type:** *Academic/Scholarly.*
—GNLM. **CCC.**
Published by: Dr. R. Kaden Verlag, Poststr 24-26, Heidelberg 69115, Germany. TEL 49-6221-600313, FAX 49-6221-29910, marketing@kaden-verlag.de. Adv. contact A Siegmann. B&W page DEM 2,625; trim 178 x 230. Circ: 4,000 (controlled).

616.21 DEU ISSN 0017-6192 CODEN: HBZHAS
H N O (BERLIN). (Hals-, Nasen-, Ohren-Heilkunde) Text in German; Summaries in English, German. 1947. m. EUR 296.34 domestic; EUR 267.84 in Germany; EUR 25.20 newsstand/cover foreign (effective 2002). adv. bk.rev. bibl, charts, illus. index. reprint service avail. from ISI. *Refereed.* **Document type:** *Journal, Academic/Scholarly.* **Description:** Contains research articles and papers on all aspects of surgery and medical treatments in the field of otorhinolaryngology.
Formerly: H N O: Wegweiser fuer Die Fachaerztliche Praxis
Related titles: Microform ed.: (from PQC); Online - full text ed.: ISSN 1433-0458 (from EBSCO Publishing, RoweCom Information Quest, Swets Blackwell, Springer LINK, Institute for Scientific Information).
Indexed: Biol.Abstr., Curr.Adv.Ecol.Sci., Curr.Cont., Excerp.Med., INIS Atomind., Ind.Med. (1947-), Inpharma, Int.Nurs.Ind., Reac.
—BLDSC (4319.500000), CISTI, GNLM, IDS, Infotrieve, KNAW. **CCC.**
Published by: Springer-Verlag (Subsidiary of: BertelsmannSpringer), Tiergartenstr 17, Heidelberg 69121, Germany. TEL 49-6221-345-0, FAX 49-6221-345229, subscriptions@springer.de, http://link.springer.de/link/service/journals/00106/index.htm, http://www.springer.de. Ed. H P Zenner. **Subscr. in N. America to:** Springer-Verlag New York Inc., PO Box 2485, Secaucus, NJ 07096-2485. TEL 212-460-1500, FAX 212-473-6272.

616.21 DEU ISSN 0341-9746
H N O (COLOGNE); Mitteilungsblatt. (Hals Nase Ohren) Text in German. 1950. bi-m. DEM 54, EUR 27.61 (effective 2000). adv. **Document type:** *Newsletter, Trade.*
Indexed: Dent.Ind., Excerp.Med.
—GNLM.
Published by: (Deutsche Berufsverband der Hals-, Nasen-, Ohrenaerzte e.V.), Deutscher Aerzte-Verlag GmbH, Dieselstr 2, Cologne 50859, Germany. TEL 49-2234-7011-0, FAX 49-2234-7011515, verlag@aerzteblatt.de, http://www.aerzteverlag.de. Circ: 4,700.

616.21 DEU ISSN 0344-9319
H N O INFORMATIONEN. (Hals - Nase - Ohren) Text in German. 1976. q. EUR 80.80 domestic to institutions; EUR 86.80 in Europe to institutions; EUR 88.80 elsewhere to institutions; EUR 23 newsstand/cover (effective 2002). **Document type:** *Journal, Academic/Scholarly.*
—GNLM.
Published by: (Deutsche Gesellschaft fuer Hals-Nasen-Ohren-Heilkunde, Kopf- und Hals-Chirurgie), Demeter Verlag GmbH und Co. KG, Ruedigerstr 14, Stuttgart 70469, Germany. TEL 49-711-8931-0, FAX 49-711-8931322, custserv@thieme.de, http://www.thieme.de.

616.21 DEU ISSN 0177-1000
H N O - NACHRICHTEN. (Hals Nase Ohren) Text in German. 1971. bi-m. EUR 41.64 domestic; EUR 48.64 foreign; EUR 6.54 newsstand/cover (effective 2002). **Document type:** *Newsletter, Academic/Scholarly.*
—GNLM.
Published by: Urban und Vogel Medien und Medizin Verlagsgesellschaft mbH (Subsidiary of: BertelsmannSpringer), Neumarkter Str 43, Munich 81673, Germany. TEL 49-89-43721411, FAX 49-89-43721410, verlag@urban-vogel.de, http://www.urban-vogel.de. Ed. Dr. Dieter Leithaeuser. R&P Friederik Klein. Adv. contact Sibylle Schurr TEL 49-89-43721353. Circ: 3,200. **Subscr. in N. America to:** Springer Auslieferungs Gesellschaft, Postfach 105160, Heidelberg 69041, Germany. TEL 49-6221-345244, FAX 49-6221-345244.

616.21 NLD ISSN 0378-5955 CODEN: HERED3
HEARING RESEARCH. Text in English. 1978. 24/yr. EUR 258 in Europe to qualified personnel; JPY 34,800 in Japan to qualified personnel; USD 289 elsewhere to qualified personnel; EUR 3,926 in Europe to institutions; JPY 520,800 in Japan to institutions; USD 4,391 elsewhere to institutions (effective 2002). adv. bk.rev. back issues avail.; reprint service avail. from SWZ. *Refereed.* **Document type:** *Academic/Scholarly.* **Description:** Publishes papers concerned with basic auditory mechanisms.
Related titles: Microform ed.: (from PQC); Online - full text ed.: (from ingenta, Swets Blackwell, ScienceDirect, Institute for Scientific Information).
Indexed: ASCA, Acoust.Abstr., Aqua.Sci.& Fish.Abstr., Biol.Abstr., Chem.Abstr., Chem.Indus.Notes, Chem.Titles, Curr.Adv.Ecol.Sci., Curr.Cont., Dent.Ind., Excerp.Med., INSPEC (Jan.1984-), Ind.Med. (1978-), Ind.Sci.Rev., Inpharma, Int.Abstr.Biol.Sci., NBA, Neurosci.Abstr. (coverage dropped), Neurosci.Cit.Ind., Noise Pollut.Publ.Abstr., Reac., Ref.Zh., SSCI (coverage dropped), Sci.Cit.Ind., Sport Fish.Abstr., Wild.Rev., Zoo.Rec.
—BLDSC (4275.286700), AskIEEE, CASDDS, CISTI, EMDOCS, GNLM, IDS, ingenta, Linda Hall. **CCC.**
Published by: Elsevier Science BV, PO Box 211, Amsterdam 1000 AE, Netherlands. TEL 31-20-485-2911, FAX 31-20-485-2457, nlinfo-f@elsevier.nl; usinfo-f@elsevier.com; forinfo-kyf04035@niftyserve.or.jp, http://www.elsevier.com/locate/heares. Ed. A R Moeller. **Subscr. in Australasia and the Far East to:** Elsevier Science (Singapore) Pte Ltd, No.1 Temasek Ave, 17-01 Millenia Tower, Singapore 039192, Singapore. TEL 65-434-3727; **Subscr. in Japan to:** Elsevier Science Inc - Japan Regional Office, 9-15 Higashi-Azabu 1-chome, Minato-ku, Tokyo 106-0044, Japan. TEL 81-3-5561-5033; **Subscr. in the Americas to:** Elsevier Science, PO Box 945, New York, NY 10159-0945. TEL 212-633-3730, usinfo-f@elsevier.com.

617.89 USA ISSN 1074-5734
THE HEARING REVIEW. Text in English. 1994. m. Free to qualified subscribers. adv. **Document type:** *Magazine, Trade.* **Description:** Covers news and trends on products and services for hearing health care professionals.
Related titles: Online - full content ed.
—BLDSC (4275.286900).
Published by: Curant Communications, Inc. (Subsidiary of: Medical World Communications), 6701 Center Drive W #450, Los Angeles, CA 90045-1556. TEL 310-642-4400, FAX 310-641-0831, http://www.hearingreview.com. Ed. Karl Strom. adv.: color page USD 4,975.

616.21 USA
HOUSE EAR INSTITUTE. REVIEW. Text in English. 1966. 3/yr. donation. *Refereed.* **Document type:** *Newsletter.* **Description:** Informs professionals and the public of new developments and current programs in our hearing research.
Formerly: Oto Review
Published by: House Ear Institute, 2100 W Third St, 5th Fl, Los Angeles, CA 90057. TEL 213-484-2642, FAX 213-483-8789, http://www.hei.org. Ed., R&P Dilys J Jones. Circ: 20,000 (controlled).

371.91 USA ISSN 0300-6883
I A L NEWS. Text in English. 1955. 3/yr. free per issue. bk.rev. illus. **Document type:** *Newsletter.*
Indexed: Rehabil.Lit.
Published by: International Association of Laryngectomees, c/o American Cancer Society, 1599 Clifton Rd N E, Atlanta, GA 30329. TEL 404-320-3333, http://www.larynxlink.com/Main/newslett.htm. Ed. Jane Del Vecchio. R&P Keith Fitzgerald. Circ: 20,000.

I F H O H JOURNAL. see *HANDICAPPED—Hearing Impaired*

616.21 IND CODEN: IJOLBJ
INDIAN JOURNAL OF OTOLARYNGOLOGY AND HEAD AND NECK SURGERY. (IJO & HNS) (Otolaryngology, Head Neck Surgery) Text in English. 1948. q. INR 800, USD 50 (effective 2001). adv. bk.rev. abstr. index. 105 p./no. 2 cols./p. *Refereed.* **Document type:** *Journal, Academic/Scholarly.*
Former titles (until 1993): Indian Journal of Otolaryngology and Head and Neck; Indian Journal of Otolaryngology (0019-5421)
Indexed: Biol.Abstr., Excerp.Med.
—BLDSC (4417.800200), CASDDS, CISTI.
Published by: Association of Otolaryngologists of India, Branch, 53 Creek Row, Kolkata, West Bengal 700 014, India. TEL 91-33-2370023, FAX 91-33-26-3598, anirbanbiswas@vsnl.com. Eds. Dr. Anirban Biswas, Santanu Banerjee. adv.: B&W page INR 8,000, color page INR 12,000. Circ: 3,500.

616.855 GBR ISSN 1368-2822
RC423.A1 CODEN: IJLDFI
INTERNATIONAL JOURNAL OF LANGUAGE AND COMMUNICATION DISORDERS. Text in English. 1966. q. GBP 104, USD 170 to individuals; GBP 208, USD 343 to institutions (effective 2002). adv. bk.rev. abstr, bibl, charts, illus, stat. index. *Refereed.* **Document type:** *Academic/Scholarly.* **Description:** Publishes papers in any area that concerns speech and language pathologists and therapists. Embraces clinical investigations, intervention and social aspects of disorders of communication.
Former titles: European Journal of Disorders of Communication (0963-7273); (until 1992): British Journal of Disorders of Communication (0007-098X); Incorporates: Speech Pathology and Therapy
Related titles: Online - full text ed.: ISSN 1460-6984. 1999 (from CatchWord Ltd., EBSCO Publishing, O C L C Online Computer Library Center, Inc., RoweCom Information Quest, Swets Blackwell, Institute for Scientific Information).
Indexed: AMED, ASCA, ASSIA, AgeLine, Bibl.Dev.Med.& Child Neur., Br.Educ.Ind., CINAHL, Curr.Adv.Ecol.Sci., Curr.Cont., Dent.Ind., ERA, Except.Child Educ.Abstr., Excerp.Med., Fam.Ind., Ind.Med. (1998-), Int.Nurs.Ind., Lang.& Lang.Behav.Abstr., Lang.Teach.& Ling.Abstr., Ling.Abstr., MLA Intl.Bibl., PsycInfo, Psychol.Abstr. (1967-), Rehabil.Lit., SOPODA, SSCI, Sociol.Abstr., e-psyche.
—BLDSC (4542.312250), ADONIS, CatchWord, EMDOCS, GNLM, IDS, ingenta, KNAW.
Published by: (Royal College of Speech and Language Therapists), Taylor & Francis Group, Taylor & Francis Ltd., 11 New Fetter Ln, London EC4P 4EE, United Kingdom. TEL 44-20-7583-9855, FAX 44-20-7842-2298, info@tandf.co.uk, http://www.tandf.co.uk. Ed. Gina Conti-Ramsden. **Subscr. in N. America to:** Taylor & Francis Ltd., 325 Chestnut St, Suite 800, Philadelphia, PA 19016. TEL 800-354-1420, FAX 215-625-8914, info@taylorandfrancis.com, http://www.taylorandfrancis.com/.

616.21 618.92 IRL ISSN 0165-5876 CODEN: IPOTDJ
INTERNATIONAL JOURNAL OF PEDIATRIC OTORHINOLARYNGOLOGY. Text in English. 1979. 15/yr. EUR 209 in Europe to individuals; JPY 27,500 in Japan to individuals; USD 233 elsewhere to individuals; EUR 1,729 in Europe to institutions; JPY 229,500 in Japan to institutions; USD 1,934 elsewhere to institutions (effective 2002). bk.rev. back issues avail. *Refereed.* **Document type:** *Academic/Scholarly.* **Description:** Provides a medium for clinical and basic contributions in all of the areas of pediatric otorhinolaryngology.
Related titles: Microform ed.: (from PQC); Online - full text ed.: (from ingenta, Swets Blackwell, ScienceDirect, Institute for Scientific Information).
Indexed: ASCA, Biol.Abstr., Curr.Adv.Cancer Res., Curr.Cont., Curr.Ind.Stat., Dent.Ind., Excerp.Med., Ind.Med. (1979-), Ind.Sci.Rev., Inpharma, Int.Abstr.Biol.Sci., NBA, Neurosci.Cit.Ind., Pharm.&Out.News, Reac., Rev.Med.& Vet.Mycol., SSCI (coverage dropped), Sci.Cit.Ind., Trop.Dis.Bull.
—BLDSC (4542.451000), CISTI, GNLM, IDS, ingenta, KNAW. **CCC.**
Published by: Elsevier Science Ireland Ltd, Elsevier House, Brookvale Plaza, E. Park, Shannon, Co. Clare, Ireland. TEL 353-61-471944, FAX 353-61-472144, http://www.elsevier.com/locate/ijporl. Ed. R J Ruben. R&P Annette Moloney. **Subscr. in Australasia and the Far East to:** Elsevier Science (Singapore) Pte Ltd, No.1 Temasek Ave, 17-01 Millenia Tower, Singapore 039192, Singapore. TEL 65-434-3727, FAX 65-337-2230; **Subscr. in the Americas to:** Elsevier Science, PO Box 945, New York, NY 10159-0945. TEL 212-633-3730, FAX 212-633-3680, usinfo-f@elsevier.com; **Subscr. to:** Elsevier Science BV, PO Box 211, Amsterdam 1000 AE, Netherlands. TEL 31-20-485-3757.

M

616.21 USA ISSN 0946-5448 CODEN: ITJOF9
INTERNATIONAL TINNITUS JOURNAL. Text in English. 1995. s-a. USD 49.50. adv. bk.rev. index. back issues avail. *Refereed.* **Document type:** *Academic/Scholarly.* **Description:** Articles provide experimental and operational reports, clinical studies, reviews, and theoretical papers relating to tinnitus. Aims to facilitate the exchange of information and ideas among interested professionals in the areas of audiology, otology, otolaryngology and neuropsychology.
Indexed: Ind.Med. (1995-).
—BLDSC (4551.030000), CASDDS.
Published by: State University of New York, Health Science Center at Brooklyn, Tinnitus Center - NES, 450 Clarkson Ave, Brooklyn, NY 11203. TEL 718-773-0888, FAX 718-465-3669. Adv. contact B Goldstein. page USD 550; trim 11 x 8.5. Circ: 1,500 (paid).

616.21 USA
▼ **THE INTERNET JOURNAL OF OTORHINOLARYNGOLOGY.** Text in English. 2000. s-a. free per issue. adv. bk.rev. back issues avail. *Refereed.* **Document type:** *Academic/Scholarly.* **Description:** Provides information from the field of ear, nose and throat medicine/surgery, otorhinolaryngology; contains original articles, reviews, case reports, streaming slide shows, streaming videos, letters to the editor, press releases and meeting information.
Media: Online - full content.
Published by: Internet Scientific Publications, L.L.C., 23 Rippling Creek Dr, Sugar Land, TX 77479. TEL 281-240-1533, FAX 281-240-1533, http://www.ispub.com/. R&P, Adv. contact Hope Morrow TEL 832-754-0335.

616.21 USA ISSN 1525-3961
▼ **J A R O.** (Journal of the Association for Research in Otolaryngology) Text in English. 2000. 4/yr. (in 1 vol., 4 nos./vol.). USD 465.90 domestic for print & online eds.; USD 233.10 in Germany for print & online eds.; USD 64.50 newsstand/cover foreign (effective 2002). **Document type:** *Journal, Academic/Scholarly.* **Description:** Publishes research findings from all disciplines related to otolaryngology and communication.
Related titles: Online - full content ed.: (from Swets Blackwell); Online - full text ed.: (from Springer LINK, Institute for Scientific Information).
Indexed: Curr.Cont.
—BLDSC (4663.110000).
Published by: Springer-Verlag (Subsidiary of: BertelsmannSpringer), Haber Str 7, Heidelberg 69126, Germany. TEL 49-30-82787-0, FAX 49-30-82787301, service@springer.de, http://www.springer.de. Ed. Eric Young.

617 JPN ISSN 0910-6820
J O H N S: JOURNAL OF OTOLARYNGOLOGY, HEAD AND NECK SURGERY/JIBI INKOKA, TOKEIBU GEKA. Text in Japanese. 1985. m. JPY 31,000; JPY 2,400 newsstand/cover (effective 1999).
Published by: Tokyo Igakusha Ltd., 35-4 Hongo 3-chome, Bunkyo-ku, Tokyo 113-0033, Japan. TEL 81-3-3811-4119, FAX 81-3-3811-6135.

616.21 JPN ISSN 0914-3491
JIBI INKOKA, TOKEIBU GEKA/OTOLARYNGOLOGY - HEAD AND NECK SURGERY. Text in Japanese; Summaries in English. 1928. m. JPY 35,600.
Related titles: Online - full text ed.: (from JICST).
Indexed: INIS Atomind., Neurosci.Cit.Ind.
—BLDSC (6313.524000), CISTI, EMDOCS, GNLM.
Published by: Igaku-Shoin Ltd., 5-24-3 Hongo, Bunkyo-ku, Tokyo 113-0033, Japan. TEL 81-3-3817-5710. Circ: 4,000.

616.21 FRA
JOURNAL FRANCAIS D'OTO-RHINO-LARYNGOLOGIE - AUDIOPHONOLOGIE - CHIRURGIE MAXILLO-FACIALE. Abbreviated title: J F O R L. Text in French. bi-m. FRF 930 domestic to qualified personnel; USD 195 foreign to qualified personnel; FRF 1,285 domestic to institutions; USD 260 foreign to institutions; FRF 550 domestic to students; USD 108 foreign to students (effective 2000).
Former titles (until 1990): Journal Francais d'Oto-Rhino-Laryngologie (0398-9771); (until 1977): J F O R L (0398-9763); (until 1972): Journal Francais d'Oto-Rhino-Laryngologie (0368-2218); (until 1967): Journal Francais d'Oto-Rhino-Laryngologie et Chirurgie Maxillo-Faciale (0021-8332); (until 1953): Journal Francais d'Oto-Rhino-Laryngologie (0398-9755)
Indexed: Biol.Abstr., Dent.Ind., INIS Atomind., Ind.Med. (coverage dropped).
—BLDSC (4986.429000), EMDOCS, GNLM.
Published by: Sedip Medical, 75 Cours Albert Thomas, Lyon Cedex 3 69447, France. TEL 33-4-72352372, FAX 33-4-72352375. Ed. Dr. C Dubreuil.

617.89 GBR ISSN 0963-7133 CODEN: JAUME3
JOURNAL OF AUDIOLOGICAL MEDICINE. Text in English. 1992. 3/yr. USD 115 in North America to individuals; GBP 60 rest of world to individuals; USD 190 in North America to institutions; GBP 105 rest of world to institutions (effective 2001). adv. bk.rev. back issues avail. *Refereed.* **Document type:** *Academic/Scholarly.* **Description:** Provides a forum for the many diverse aspects of audiological medicine: pediatric audiology, auditory electrophysiology, rehabilitation of the adult hearing and balance impaired, and neuro-otology.
Incorporates: I A P A Bulletin (0262-6853)
Indexed: ASSIA, Acoust.Abstr., CINAHL, Excerp.Med. (1993-).
—BLDSC (4949.295000), ADONIS, CISTI, EMDOCS, GNLM, KNAW.
Published by: (International Society of Physicians in Audiology), Whurr Publishers Ltd., 19b Compton Terr, London N1 2UN, United Kingdom. TEL 44-20-7359-5979, FAX 44-20-7226-5290, info@whurr.co.uk, http://www.whurr.co.uk. Ed. Linda Luxon. Adv. contact Lizzy Ewer. page GBP 250. **Subscr. in N America to:** Whurr Publishers Ltd., PO Box 1897, Lawrence, KS 66044-8897. TEL 913-843-1221, FAX 913-843-1274, am&m@allenpress.com. **Subscr. to:** Turpin Distribution Services Ltd., Blackhorse Rd, Letchworth, Herts SG6 1HN, United Kingdom. TEL 44-1462-488900, FAX 44-1462-483011, custservturpin@turpinltd.com.

JOURNAL OF BRONCHOLOGY. see *MEDICAL SCIENCES—Respiratory Diseases*

616.21 GBR ISSN 0022-2151
RF1 CODEN: JLOTAX
JOURNAL OF LARYNGOLOGY AND OTOLOGY. Text in English. 1887. m. GBP 99 rest of world to individuals; USD 227.70 in United States to individuals; GBP 150 rest of world to institutions; USD 345 in United States to institutions (effective 2000). adv. bibl, illus. index, cum.index every 10 yrs. *Refereed.* **Document type:** *Academic/Scholarly.* **Description:** Contains original scientific articles and clinical records in all fields of otology, rhinology and laryngology.
Related titles: Microform ed.: (from PQC); Online - full content ed.: (from EBSCO Publishing, O C L C Online Computer Library Center, Inc., ProQuest Information & Learning, Swets Blackwell); Online - full text ed.: (from CatchWord Ltd., Institute for Scientific Information, RoweCom Information Quest); ♦ Supplement: Journal of Laryngology and Otology. Supplement. ISSN 0144-2945.
Indexed: AIM, ASCA, Biol.Abstr., Chem.Abstr., Curr.Adv.Cancer Res., Curr.Adv.Cell & Devel.Biol., Curr.Adv.Ecol.Sci., Curr.Cont., Dent.Ind., Excerp.Med., Helminthol.Abstr., INIS Atomind., Ind.Med. (1921-), Ind.Sci.Rev., Inpharma, Int.Nurs.Ind., Lang.& Lang.Behav.Abstr., NBA, Neurosci.Cit.Ind., Nutr.Abstr., Pharm.&Out.News, Poult.Abstr., Protozool.Abstr., Reac., Rev.Med.& Vet.Mycol., Rev.Plant Path., SSCI (coverage dropped), Sci.Cit.Ind., THA.
—BLDSC (5010.100000), ADONIS, CatchWord, CISTI, GNLM, ingenta, KNAW.
Published by: Royal Society of Medicine Press Ltd, 1 Wimpole St, London W1M 8AE, United Kingdom. TEL 44-20-7290-2921, FAX 44-20-7290-2929, rsmjournals@rsm.ac.uk, http://www.roysocmed.ac.uk/pub/jlo.htm, http://www.jlo.co.uk. Eds. Guy Kenyon, Neil Weir. Circ: 2,500.

616.21 GBR ISSN 0144-2945
JOURNAL OF LARYNGOLOGY AND OTOLOGY. SUPPLEMENT. Text in English. 1978. irreg. price varies. **Document type:** *Academic/Scholarly.*
Related titles: ♦ Supplement to: Journal of Laryngology and Otology. ISSN 0022-2151.
Indexed: Ind.Med. (1978-).
—ADONIS, CISTI, KNAW.
Published by: Royal Society of Medicine Press Ltd, 1 Wimpole St, London W1M 8AE, United Kingdom. TEL 44-20-7290-2921, FAX 44-207-290-2929, http://www.roysocmed.ac.uk.

616.855 USA ISSN 1065-1438
RC423.A1 CODEN: JSLPEP
JOURNAL OF MEDICAL SPEECH - LANGUAGE PATHOLOGY. Text in English. 1993. q. USD 85 to individuals; USD 115 to institutions. *Refereed.* **Description:** Contains clinical and theoretical articles, clinical notes and dialogue covering all aspects of human communication disorders encountered in medical settings — from pediatric issues to the increasing challenges of the elderly.
Related titles: Online - full text ed.: (from Institute for Scientific Information).
Indexed: CINAHL, Lang.& Lang.Behav.Abstr., Neurosci.Cit.Ind., PsycInfo, SOPODA, Sociol.Abstr., e-psyche.
—BLDSC (5017.087500), GNLM, IDS, Infotrieve, ingenta. **CCC.**
Published by: Singular Publishing Group, Inc., 401 W A St, Ste 325, San Diego, CA 92101-7961. TEL 800-521-8545, FAX 800-774-8398, singpub@mail.cerfnet.com. Ed. Leonard L Lapointe.

616.21 CAN ISSN 0381-6605 CODEN: JOTODX
JOURNAL OF OTOLARYNGOLOGY. Text in English, French. 1972. bi-m. USD 95 in US & Canada to individuals; USD 129 elsewhere to individuals; USD 145 in US & Canada to institutions; USD 179 elsewhere to institutions (effective 2001). bk.rev. index. back issues avail. *Refereed.* **Document type:** *Journal, Academic/Scholarly.* **Description:** Devoted to all aspects of the field, as well as a broad range of related activities.
Formerly: Canadian Journal of Otolaryngology (0045-5083)
Related titles: Online - full text ed.: (from Northern Light Technology, Inc., ProQuest Information & Learning, Institute for Scientific Information).
Indexed: ASCA, Biol.Abstr., Curr.Adv.Cancer Res., Curr.Adv.Cell & Devel.Biol., Curr.Cont., Dok.Arbeitsmed., Excerp.Med., Ind.Med. (1976-), Inpharma, Lang.& Lang.Behav.Abstr., NBA, Neurosci.Cit.Ind., Pharm.&Out.News, Reac., Rev.Med.& Vet.Mycol., SOPODA, Sociol.Abstr., THA.
—BLDSC (5027.710000), CISTI, EMDOCS, GNLM, IDS, ingenta, KNAW. **CCC.**
Published by: (Canadian Society of Otolaryngology - Head and Neck Surgery), B.C. Decker Inc., 20 Hughson St S, LCD 1, P O Box 620, Hamilton, ON L8N 3K7, Canada. TEL 905-522-7017, 800-568-7281, FAX 905-522-7839, info@bcdecker.com, http://www.bcdecker.com. Ed. Dominique Dorian. Pub. David LeGallais. R&P Paula Presutti. Adv. contact Bob Sutherland. Circ: 1,200.

616.21 JPN ISSN 0030-6622
JOURNAL OF OTOLARYNGOLOGY OF JAPAN/NIHON JIBI INKOKA GAKKAI KAIHO. Text in Japanese; Summaries in English. 1890. m. JPY 15,600, USD 200 (effective 2001). adv. *Refereed.* **Document type:** *Academic/Scholarly.*
Indexed: Excerp.Med., INIS Atomind., Ind.Med. (1947-), Lang.& Lang.Behav.Abstr.
—BLDSC (5027.720000), CISTI, GNLM, KNAW.
Published by: The Oto-Rhino-Laryngological Society of Japan, Inc./Nihon Jibi Inkoka Gakkai, 3-23-14-807 Takanawa, Minato-ku, Tokyo 108-0074, Japan. TEL 81-3-3443-3085, FAX 81-3-3443-3037. Ed. Atsushi Komatsuzaki. Circ: 10,800.

616.21 USA ISSN 0892-1997
QP306 CODEN: JOVOEA
JOURNAL OF VOICE. Text in English. 1987. q. USD 109 domestic to individuals; USD 146 foreign to individuals; USD 219 domestic to institutions; USD 241 foreign to institutions (effective 1999). adv. charts, illus. back issues avail.; reprint service avail. from PQC. *Refereed.* **Document type:** *Academic/Scholarly.* **Description:** Publishes articles on the development and care of the professional voice.
Supersedes (1978-1985): Annual Symposium on Care of the Professional Voice. Transcripts
Related titles: Online - full text ed.: (from Institute for Scientific Information).
Indexed: AMED, ASCA, Acoust.Abstr., CINAHL, Curr.Cont., Excerp.Med., Ind.Med. (1987-), Inpharma, Int.Ind.Mus.Per., Music Ind., PsycInfo, RILM, Reac., SSCI (coverage dropped), e-psyche.
—BLDSC (5072.512700), EMDOCS, GNLM, IDS, Infotrieve, ingenta. **CCC.**
Published by: (Voice Foundation), Singular Publishing Group, Inc., 401 W A St, Ste 325, San Diego, CA 92101-7961. TEL 800-521-8545, FAX 800-774-8936, singpub@lmail.certnet.com. Ed. Dr. Robert T Sataloff. Adv. contact Suzann Graff. Circ: 3,000.

M

616.855 USA ISSN 0161-1461
LB3454 CODEN: LGSHA4
LANGUAGE, SPEECH AND HEARING SERVICES IN SCHOOLS. Text in English. 1970. q., latest vol.32, 2001. USD 45 to individuals (effective (No. 2002); USD 55 foreign to individuals; USD 125 to institutions; USD 160 foreign to institutions; USD 25 to members (effective 2002). adv. bibl, charts, illus. 128 p./no. back issues avail.; reprint service avail. from PQC,SCH,PSC. *Refereed.* **Document type:** *Journal, Academic/Scholarly.* **Description:** Presents up-to-date information dealing with all aspects of clinical speech, language and hearing services to children.
Related titles: Microform ed.: (from PQC); Online - full text ed.: (from H. W. Wilson, ProQuest Information & Learning, Institute for Scientific Information).
Indexed: ABSEARCH - ASHA (1945-), ASCA, C.I.J.E., CINAHL, Child Devel.Abstr., Curr.Cont., Educ.Ind. (Jan.1983-), Except.Child Educ.Abstr., Fam.Ind., Lang.& Lang.Behav.Abstr., Ling.Abstr., PsycInfo, Psychol.Abstr. (1973-), SOPODA, SSCI, Sociol.Abstr., Sp.Ed.Needs Abstr., e-psyche.
—BLDSC (5155.711900), IDS, ingenta. **CCC.**
Published by: American Speech - Language - Hearing Association, 10801 Rockville Pike, Rockville, MD 20852. TEL 301-897-5700, FAX 301-897-7358, sghoting@asha.org. Ed. Alan Kamhi. adv.: page USD 1,696. Circ: 47,000.

616.21 DEU ISSN 0935-8943
CODEN: LROTEX
LARYNGO- RHINO- OTOLOGIE; Zeitschrift fuer Hals-Nasen-Ohrenheilkunde, Kopf- und Halschirurgie. Text in German; Summaries in English, German. 1921. m. EUR 230.40 domestic to institutions; EUR 241.40 in Europe to institutions; EUR 258.80 elsewhere to institutions; EUR 126 to students; EUR 23 newsstand/cover (effective 2002). adv. bk.rev. abstr, bibl, charts, illus, stat. index. back issues avail.; reprint service avail. from PQC. *Refereed.* **Document type:** *Journal, Academic/Scholarly.*
Former titles: Laryngologie, Rhinologie, Otologie und Ihre Grenzgebiete Vereinigt mit Monatsschrift fuer Ohrenheilkunde (0340-1588); Laryngologie, Rhinologie, Otologie und Ihre Grenzgebiete (0302-9379); Zeitschrift fuer Laryngologie, Rhinologie, Otologie und Ihre Grenzgebiete (0044-3018); Incorporates (in 1974): Monatschrift fuer Ohrenheilkunde und Laryngo-Rhinologie (0026-9328)
Related titles: Online - full text ed.: ISSN 1438-8685.
Indexed: ASCA, Biol.Abstr., C.I.S. Abstr., Curr.Adv.Cancer Res., Curr.Adv.Cell & Devel.Biol., Curr.Cont., Dent.Ind., Excerp.Med., INIS Atomind., Ind.Med. (1989-), Inpharma, Lang.& Lang.Behav.Abstr., NBA, Pharm.&Out.News, Protozool.Abstr., Reac., Sci.Cit.Ind. (coverage dropped).
—BLDSC (5156.150000), CISTI, EMDOCS, GNLM, IDS, Infotrieve, KNAW. **CCC.**
Published by: (Deutsche Gesellschaft fuer Hals-, Nasen-, Ohrenheilkunde, Kopf- und Halschirurgie), Georg Thieme Verlag, Ruedigerstr 14, Stuttgart 70469, Germany. TEL 49-711-8931-0, FAX 49-711-8931298, leser.service@thieme.de, http://www.thieme.de/lary, http://www.thieme-connect.de. Ed. J Helms. R&P Peter Eich. adv.: page DEM 2,750; 175 x 250. Circ: 2,700. **Co-sponsor:** Oesterreichische Gesellschaft fuer Hals-Nasen-Ohrenheilkunde, Kopf- und Halschirurgie.

616.21 USA ISSN 0023-852X
CODEN: LARYA8
LARYNGOSCOPE. Text in English. 1896. m. USD 197 domestic to individuals for print & online eds.; USD 253 foreign to individuals for print & online eds; USD 340 domestic to institutions for print & online eds; USD 351 foreign to institutions for print & online eds; USD 29 newsstand/cover (effective 2002). adv. bk.rev. bibl, illus. index. reprint service avail. from PQC. *Refereed.* **Document type:** *Academic/Scholarly.* **Description:** Journal comprising medical, clinical and research contributions in otolaryngology, broncho-esophagology, communicative disorders, maxillofacial surgery, head and neck surgery, facial plastic and reconstructive surgery, speech and hearing defects.
Related titles: CD-ROM ed.; Microfilm ed.: (from PQC); Online - full text ed.: USD 442 domestic academic site license; USD 453 foreign academic site license; USD 493 domestic corporate site license; USD 504 foreign corporate site license (effective 2002) (from Ovid Technologies, Inc., Swets Blackwell, Institute for Scientific Information).
Indexed: ASCA, Biol.Abstr., CINAHL, Chem.Abstr., Chem.Indus.Notes, Chem.Titles, Curr.Adv.Ecol.Sci., Curr.Cont., Dairy Sci.Abstr., Dent.Ind., Dok.Arbeitsmed., Excerp.Med., INIS Atomind., Ind.Med. (1896-), Ind.Sci.Rev., Inpharma, Int.Nurs.Ind., Med.& Surg.Dermat., NBA, Neurosci.Cit.Ind., Noise Pollut.Publ.Abstr., Nutr.Abstr., Pharm.&Out.News, Reac., Rev.Med.& Vet.Mycol., Rev.Plant Path., Risk Abstr., SSCI (coverage dropped), Sci.Cit.Ind.
—BLDSC (5156.200000), CASDDS, CISTI, GNLM, IDS, ingenta, KNAW.
Published by: (American Laryngological, Rhinological and Otological Society), Lippincott Williams & Wilkins (Philadelphia) (Subsidiary of: Wolters Kluwer N.V.), 530 Walnut St, Philadelphia, PA 19106-3621. TEL 215-521-8300, FAX 215-521-8902, http://www.lww.com. Ed. Dr. Byron J Bailey. Pub. Marcia Serepy. R&P Margaret Becker. adv.: B&W page USD 875, color page USD 1,975. Circ: 7,344 (paid). **Subscr. to:** PO Box 1600, Hagerstown, MD 21740-1600. TEL 800-777-2295, FAX 301-824-7390.

616.21 FRA ISSN 0754-7188
LA LETTRE D'OTO-RHINO-LARYNGOLOGIE; et de chirurgie cervico-faciale. Text in French. 1985. m. FRF 460 domestic to individuals; FRF 580, USD 105 foreign to individuals; FRF 580 domestic to institutions; FRF 700, USD 127 foreign to institutions; FRF 290 domestic to students; USD 75 foreign to students (effective 2000). Supplement avail. **Document type:** *Academic/Scholarly.*
Published by: Edimark S.A., 62-64 rue Jean Jaures, Puteaux 92800, France. TEL 39-1-41458000, FAX 33-1-41458025, contact@edimark.fr, http://www.edimark.fr. Ed. Y Manac'h. Pub. Claudie Damour-Terrasson.

617.8 NOR ISSN 1401-5439
CODEN: LPVOF6
LOGOPEDICS PHONIATRICS VOCOLOGY. Text in English; Summaries in Danish, Finnish, Norwegian, Swedish. 1936. q. GBP 41, USD 67 to individuals; GBP 82, USD 135 to institutions (effective 2002). adv. **Document type:** *Academic/Scholarly.* **Description:** Serves as an international forum for research reports and information within the area of communication disorders.
Former titles (until 1996): Scandinavian Journal of Logopedics and Phoniatrics (0803-5032); Nordisk Tidsskrift for Logopedi og Foniatri (0105-1539); (until 1976): Nordisk Tidsskrift for Tale og Stemme (0029-1552)
Related titles: Online - full text ed.: (from EBSCO Publishing, O C L C Online Computer Library Center, Inc., RoweCom Information Quest, CatchWord Ltd., ingenta, Swets Blackwell).
Indexed: Ind.Med., Lang.& Lang.Behav.Abstr., Ling.Abstr., MLA Intl.Bibl. (coverage dropped), SOPODA, Sociol.Abstr.
—BLDSC (5292.364000). **CCC.**
Published by: (Scandinavian Cooperation Council of Logopedics and Phoniatrics), Taylor & Francis AS (Subsidiary of: Taylor & Francis Group), Cort Adelersgt. 17, Solli, PO Box 2562, Oslo 0202, Norway. TEL 47-22-12-98-80, FAX 47-22-12-98-90, journals@tandf.no, http://www.tandf.co.uk/tfas. Ed. Lena Hartelius. **Co-sponsor:** British Voice Association.

616.855 USA
MINNESOTA SPEECH - LANGUAGE - HEARING ASSOCIATION. NEWSLETTER. Text in English. 1955. s-a. USD 35 (effective 2000). adv. **Document type:** *Newsletter.*
Former titles: Minnesota Speech and Hearing Association. Newsletter; (until 1976): Minnesota Speech and Hearing Association Journal
Published by: Minnesota Speech - Language - Hearing Association, PO Box 26115, St. Louis Park, MN 55426. TEL 612-920-0787, FAX 612-920-6098. Ed. Maxine Slobof. Adv. contact Frances Laven. Circ: 650.

616.21 617 DEU ISSN 1432-9417
MUND-, KIEFER- UND GESICHTSCHIRURGIE. Text in German. 1997. bi-m. EUR 258.40 domestic; EUR 263.50 foreign; EUR 49.60 newsstand/cover (effective 2002). adv. bk.rev. abstr, charts, illus. back issues avail. *Refereed.* **Document type:** *Journal, Academic/Scholarly.* **Description:** Provides information concerning current developments in the subject fields of surgery in support of professional continuing education.
Formed by the merger of (1977-1997): Deutsche Zeitschrift fuer Mund-, Kiefer- und Gesichtschirurgie (0343-3137); (1955-1997): Fortschritte der Kiefer- und Gesichtschirurgie (0071-7916)
Related titles: Online - full text ed.: ISSN 1434-3940 (from EBSCO Publishing, RoweCom Information Quest, Swets Blackwell, Springer LINK).
Indexed: Curr.Tit.Dent., Ind.Med. (1997-).
—BLDSC (5983.754000), CISTI, GNLM, KNAW. **CCC.**
Published by: (Deutsche Gesellschaft fuer Mund-, Kiefer- und Gesichtschirurgie), Springer-Verlag (Subsidiary of: BertelsmannSpringer), Tiergartenstr 17, Heidelberg 69121, Germany. TEL 49-6221-345-0, FAX 49-6221-345229, subscriptions@springer.de, http://link.springer.de/link/service/journals/10006/index.htm, http://www.springer.de. Eds. J Muehling, P Karl. **Subscr. in N. America to:** Springer-Verlag New York Inc., PO Box 2485, Secaucus, NJ 07096-2485. TEL 212-460-1500, FAX 212-473-6272. **Co-sponsor:** Berufsverband Deutscher Aerzte fuer Mund-Kiefer-Gesichtschirurgie e.V.

617.89 USA ISSN 0887-6584
N S S L H A CLINICAL SERIES. Key Title: Clinical Series. Text in English. 1971 (no.2); N.S. 1992. biennial. price varies. adv.
Published by: National Student Speech Language Hearing Association, 10801 Rockville Pike, Rockville, MD 20852. TEL 301-897-5700, FAX 301-897-7350. Ed. Anthony J Caruso. R&P Jennifer Martinez TEL 301-897-0145. Adv. contact Pam Leppin.

616.21 USA ISSN 0077-8516
NEW JERSEY SPEECH AND HEARING ASSOCIATION. NEWSLETTER✱ . Text in English. 1969. irreg. (approx. 4/yr.). USD 5.
Published by: New Jersey Speech and Hearing Association, c/o Auriemma, 6 Crest Ln, Warren, NJ 07059-5110. Circ: 1,400.

610 NZL ISSN 1175-107X
NEW ZEALAND JOURNAL OF SPEECH-LANGUAGE THERAPY. Text in English. 1946-1997; resumed 1998. a. NZD 30 (effective 2000). adv. bk.rev. reprint service avail. from PQC. **Document type:** *Bulletin, Trade.* **Description:** Includes research papers, conference proceedings and reviews.
Former titles (until 1997): New Zealand Speech-Language Therapists Journal (0110-571X); (until May 1983): New Zealand Speech Therapists Journal (0028-8713)
Related titles: Microfilm ed.: (from PQC).
Indexed: Bibl.Engl.Lang.& Lit., DSH Abstr., Ind.N.Z.Per., Rehabil.Lit.
—**CCC.**
Published by: New Zealand Speech-Language Therapists Association, 63 Remuera Rd, Ste. 369, Newmarket, Auckland, New Zealand. TEL 3-2358257, FAX 3-2358850, nzsta@clear.net.nz. Ed. Ilsa Schwarz. Circ: 320.

617.89 613.62 GBR ISSN 1463-1741
RA772.N7
NOISE & HEALTH; an inter-disciplinary journal. Text in English. 1998. q. GBP 60 to non-members; GBP 120 to institutions (effective 2000). adv. bk.rev. abstr, illus. back issues avail.; reprints avail. *Refereed.* **Document type:** *Journal, Academic/Scholarly.* **Description:** Examines and disseminates research on all aspects of noise and its effects on human health from the perspectives of multiple disciplines. Covers a broad range of topics related to noise pollution and its medical effects, ranging from basic experimental research to clinical evaluation and treatment, along with technical aspects of noise-reduction systems and public health policy solutions to related environmental and social issues.
Related titles: Online - full text ed.: (from ingenta).
—BLDSC (6115.797000).
Published by: Institute of Laryngology & Otology, Division of Audiological Medicine (Subsidiary of: University College London), 330 Gray's Inn Rd, London WC1X 8EE, United Kingdom. TEL 44-171-915-1590, FAX 44-171-278-8041, http://www.ilo.ucl.ac.uk. Eds. Dr. Deepak Prasher, Dr. Manjula Patrick. R&P, Adv. contact Dr. Manjula Patrick. **Co-publisher:** European Commission Concerted Action on Protection Against Noise.

NOTIZIARIO BIBLIOGRAFICO DI AUDIOLOGIA O R L E FONIATRIA. see *MEDICAL SCIENCES—Abstracting, Bibliographies, Statistics*

616.21 ITA
NUOVA, CLINICA OTORINOLARINGOIATRICA. Text in Italian; Summaries in English, French, German. bi-m. ITL 40,000.
Formerly: Clinica Otorinolaringoiatrica (0009-904X)
Indexed: Biol.Abstr., Dent.Ind., Excerp.Med., Ind.Med. (coverage dropped), NBA.
—CISTI.
Published by: Universita degli Studi di Catania, Universita Ospedale Garibaldi, Otorinolaringoiatrica, Catania, CA, Italy. FAX 095-316207. Circ: 350.

616.2 FRA ISSN 0983-8201
O P A PRATIQUE. (ORL, Pneumo, Allergo) Text in French. m. (10/yr.). EUR 39 domestic to individuals; EUR 53 foreign to individuals; EUR 27 domestic to libraries; EUR 42 foreign to libraries (effective 2002). **Document type:** *Newspaper.*
Published by: L E N Medical, 15 rue des Sablons, Paris 75116, France. TEL 33-1-47553131, FAX 33-1-47553132, lenmed@club-internet.fr, http://www.webmedguide.com. Ed. Olivier de Fenoyl.

616.2 CHE ISSN 0301-1569 CODEN: ORLJAH
O R L; journal for oto-rhino-laryngology and its related specialties. Text in English. 1938. bi-m. CHF 914 in Europe to institutions; CHF 931.40 elsewhere to institutions; EUR 652.80 in Europe to institutions; USD 711 elsewhere to institutions (effective 2002). adv. bk.rev. back issues avail.; reprint service avail. from PQC. *Refereed.* **Document type:** *Journal, Academic/Scholarly.* **Description:** Contains original scientific papers of interest for both clinicians and researchers in otorhinolaryngology and head and neck surgery.
Formerly: Practica Oto-Rhino-Laryngologica (0032-6305)
Related titles: Microform ed.; Online - full text ed.: ISSN 1423-0275. FRF 58, EUR 42, USD 45 to institutions with print edition (effective 2002) (from EBSCO Publishing, O C L C Online Computer Library Center, Inc., RoweCom Information Quest, Swets Blackwell, Institute for Scientific Information).
Indexed: Biol.Abstr., Chem.Abstr., Curr.Cont., Dent.Ind., Excerp.Med., Ind.Med. (1972-), Inpharma, NBA, Noise Pollut.Publ.Abstr., Reac., SSCI (coverage dropped).
—BLDSC (6291.378000), CASDDS, CISTI, EMDOCS, GNLM, IDS, Infotrieve, ingenta, KNAW. **CCC.**
Published by: S. Karger AG, Allschwilerstr 10, PO Box, Basel 4009, Switzerland. TEL 41-61-306-1111, FAX 41-61-306-1234, karger@karger.ch, http://www.online.karger.com/journals/orl, http://www.karger.com. Ed. W Arnold. adv.: page USD 1,185. Circ: 850.

616.21 ESP ISSN 0210-7309
O.R.L. DIPS; revista internacional de otorrinolaringologia. Text in Spanish; Summaries in English, Spanish. 5/yr. ESP 6,200, USD 115 (effective 1999). adv. bibl, charts, illus, stat. index. **Document type:** *Trade.* **Description:** Original research articles in the science of otorhinolaryngology.
Indexed: Ind.Med.Esp., Ref.Zh.
Published by: Editorial Dips Rocas, Muntaner, 393 pral. 4, Barcelona 08021, Spain. TEL 39-3-2001389, FAX 39-3-2021958, edipsro@intercom.es. Ed. Dr P Quesada Marin. R&P Alvaro Trevino. Adv. contact Carlos Martin. color page ESP 105,000. Circ: 3,000.

616.21 610.73 USA
O R L - HEAD AND NECK NURSING✱. Text in English. 1982. q. *Refereed.* **Description:** Covers the practice of ORL nursing, pertinent research projects and legal issues.
Indexed: CINAHL, Int.Nurs.Ind.
—BLDSC (6291.381000).
Published by: (Society of Otorhinolaryngology and Head - Neck Nurses), Health Information Publications, Inc., 200 Valley Rd Ste 405, Mount Arlington, NJ 07856-1320. TEL 973-267-8938, FAX 973-664-3771. adv.: B&W page USD 875, color page USD 1,725; bleed 11.25 x 8.5. Circ: 970.

617.8 JPN ISSN 0030-2813
ONSEI GENGO IGAKU/JAPAN JOURNAL OF LOGOPEDICS AND PHONIATRICS. Text in Japanese; Summaries in English. 1960. 4/yr. membership. adv. bk.rev.
Indexed: Excerp.Med.
Published by: Nihon Onsei Gengo Igakkai/Japan Society of Logopedics and Phoniatrics, Hakuo Bldg, 5F, 2-3-10 Koraku, Bunkyo-ku, Tokyo 112-0004, Japan. FAX 03-5684-5954. Ed. Hiroyuki Fukuda. Circ: 1,850 (controlled).

616.21 USA ISSN 1043-1810
OPERATIVE TECHNIQUES IN OTOLARYNGOLOGY - HEAD AND NECK SURGERY. Text in English. 1990. q. USD 172 domestic to individuals; USD 218 foreign to individuals; USD 205 domestic to institutions; USD 255 foreign to institutions; USD 94 domestic to students; USD 131 foreign to students; USD 64 newsstand/cover (effective 2001). adv. illus. back issues avail. *Refereed.* **Document type:** *Academic/Scholarly.* **Description:** Presents detailed illustrations of new surgical procedures and techniques in head and neck surgery.
Indexed: CINAHL.
—BLDSC (6269.382000), GNLM, Infotrieve. **CCC.**
Published by: W.B. Saunders Co. (Subsidiary of: Harcourt Publishers Ltd.), 11830 Westline Industrial Dr, St Louis, MO 63146. TEL 800-325-4177, http://www.wbsaunders.com. Ed. Dr. Michael Friedman. Adv. contact Cindy Gray. B&W page USD 665, color page USD 1,595; trim 11 x 7.75. Circ: 2,101. **Subscr. to:** Periodicals Fulfillment, W B Saunders Co, 6277 Sea Harbor Dr, 4th Fl, Orlando, FL 32891-4800.

OPHTHALMOLOGY ON C D. see *MEDICAL SCIENCES—Ophthalmology And Optometry*

ORBIT; the international journal on orbital disorders, oculoplastic and lacrimal surgery. see *MEDICAL SCIENCES—Ophthalmology And Optometry*

616.21 610 BEL ISSN 0773-4409
OTICA; cahier des gradues en audiologie. Text in French; Summaries in English. 1977. 2/yr. BEF 600, USD 40. adv. bk.rev. abstr, bibl. back issues avail.
Published by: Groupe Otica, Av Edouard Benes 195-15, Brussels 1080, Belgium. TEL 425.57.45. Ed. Gaston Warton Madeira. Circ: 200. **Subscr. to:** Otica, Woluweveld 59, St-Stevens-Woluwe 1932, Belgium.

616.21 CHE ISSN 1014-8221 CODEN: OTNOEQ
OTO-RHINO-LARYNGOLOGIA NOVA; european journal for the practitioner, clinician and researcher. Text in English, French, German. 1992. bi-m. CHF 824 in Europe to individuals; CHF 841.40 elsewhere to institutions; EUR 588.80 in Europe to institutions; USD 642 elsewhere to institutions (effective 2002). adv. back issues avail. *Refereed.* **Document type:** *Journal, Academic/Scholarly.* **Description:** Aims to promote an exchange of scientific information between the different linguistic communities of Europe and encourage mutual understanding on a wide range of important issues.
Related titles: Microform ed.: (from PQC); Online - full text ed.: ISSN 1423-0283. CHF 58, EUR 42, USD 45 to institutions with print edition (effective 2002) (from EBSCO Publishing, O C L C Online Computer Library Center, Inc., RoweCom Information Quest, Swets Blackwell).
Indexed: ASCA, Excerp.Med. (1993-).
—BLDSC (6313.605000), EMDOCS, GNLM, IDS, KNAW.
Published by: S. Karger AG, Allschwilerstr 10, PO Box, Basel 4009, Switzerland. TEL 41-61-306-1111, FAX 41-61-306-1234, karger@karger.ch, http://www.online.karger.com/journals/orn, http://www.karger.com. Eds. P Montandon, R Haeusler. adv.: page USD 1,185.

616.21 ROM ISSN 1223-2505
OTO-RINO-LARINGOLOGIA. Text in Romanian. 1956. q. **Document type:** *Academic/Scholarly.*
Formerly: Revista de Chirurgie, Oncologie, Radiologie, ORL, Oftalmologie, Stomatologie. Oto-rino-laringologia (1220-0867); Which superseded in part (in 1974): Oto-Rino-Laringologie si Oftalmologie (0303-5123); Which was formed by the merger of (1956-1974): Oto-Rino-Laringologie (0030-6649); (1956-1974): Oftalmologia (0030-0667)
—BLDSC (6244.700000), CISTI, GNLM.
Published by: Asociatia Medicala Romana, Societatea de Otorinolaringologie, Str. Progresului 8, Bucharest 70754, Romania. Ed. M Buruiana.

616.21 POL ISSN 0030-6657 CODEN: OTPOAW
OTOLARYNGOLOGIA POLSKA. Text in Polish; Summaries in English, Russian. 1947. bi-m. USD 87. adv. bk.rev. index. **Description:** Focuses on diseases of the ear, larynx and throat.
Indexed: Biol.Abstr., Chem.Abstr., Dent.Ind., Excerp.Med., INIS Atomind., Ind.Med. (1947-).
—CASDDS, CISTI, GNLM, KNAW.
Published by: Polskie Towarzystwo Otolaryngologiczne, Ul Sklodowskiej 9, Bydgoszcz 85094, Poland. TEL 212002. Ed. Zygmunt Szmeja. **Dist. by:** Ars Polona, Krakowskie Przedmiescie 7, Warsaw, Poland.

616.21 USA ISSN 0030-6665
RF1 CODEN: OCNAB
OTOLARYNGOLOGIC CLINICS OF NORTH AMERICA. Text in English. 1968. bi-m. USD 171 domestic to individuals; USD 227 in Canada to individuals; USD 249 elsewhere to individuals; USD 258 domestic to institutions; USD 318 foreign to institutions; USD 54 per issue (effective 2001). reprint service avail. from PQC,ISI. *Refereed.* **Document type:** *Journal, Academic/Scholarly.*
Related titles: Microform ed.: (from MIM,PQC); Online - full text ed.: (from Institute for Scientific Information).
Indexed: ASCA, Biol.Abstr., CINAHL, Curr.Adv.Cancer Res., Curr.Adv.Ecol.Sci., Curr.Cont., Dent.Ind., Excerp.Med., INIS Atomind., Ind.Med. (1968-), Ind.Sci.Rev., Inpharma, Int.Nurs.Ind., Pharm.&Out.News, Reac., SSCI (coverage dropped), Sci.Cit.Ind.
—BLDSC (6313.510000), CISTI, GNLM, IDS, ingenta, KNAW. **CCC.**
Published by: W.B. Saunders Co. (Subsidiary of: Harcourt Publishers Ltd.), 11830 Westline Industrial Dr, St Louis, MO 63146. TEL 800-325-4177, http://www.wbsaunders.com. **Subscr. to:** Periodicals Fulfillment, W B Saunders Co, 6277 Sea Harbor Dr, 4th Fl, Orlando, FL 32891-4800.

617.51 USA ISSN 0194-5998 CODEN: OHNSDL
OTOLARYNGOLOGY - HEAD AND NECK SURGERY. Text in English. 1896. m. USD 195 domestic to individuals; USD 233 foreign to individuals; USD 344 domestic to institutions; USD 382 foreign to institutions; USD 96 domestic to students; USD 134 foreign to students; USD 32 newsstand/cover (effective 2001). adv. bk.rev. s-a. index. Supplement avail.; reprint service avail. from PQC. *Refereed.* **Document type:** *Journal, Academic/Scholarly.* **Description:** Scientific articles to meet the clinical and continuing educational needs of all specialists in head and neck surgery.
Former titles: Otolaryngology; Journal of Otolaryngology and Head and Neck Surgery (0161-6439); (until Vol.86, 1978): American Academy of Ophthalmology and Otolaryngology. Transactions-Otolaryngology; Which supersedes in part: American Academy of Ophthalmology and Otolaryngology. Transactions
Related titles: Microfilm ed.: (from PQC); Online - full text ed.: (from Ovid Technologies, Inc., EBSCO Publishing, IDEAL Online Library, Institute for Scientific Information, RoweCom Information Quest).
Indexed: ASCA, Biol.Abstr., CINAHL, Chem.Abstr., Curr.Adv.Cell & Devel.Biol., Curr.Cont., Excerp.Med., INIS Atomind., Ind.Med. (1981-), Ind.Sci.Rev., Inpharma, Int.Nurs.Ind., NBA, Neurosci.Abstr. (coverage dropped), Pharm.&Out.News, Reac., Rev.Med.& Vet.Mycol., Rev.Plant Path., SSCI (coverage dropped), Sci.Cit.Ind.
—BLDSC (6313.523000), CASDDS, CISTI, GNLM, IDS, ingenta, KNAW. **CCC.**
Published by: (American Academy of Otolaryngology - Head and Neck Surgery Foundation, Inc.), Mosby, Inc. (Subsidiary of: Elsevier Science), 11830 Westline Industrial Dr, St Louis, MO 63146-3318. TEL 314-872-8370, 800-325-4177, FAX 314-432-1380, http://www.mosby.com/periodicals. Ed. Dr. G Richard Holt. Pub. Terrie Duhadway. Adv. contact Michelle Kuhn. B&W page USD 1,015, color page USD 2,140; trim 10.88 x 8.13. Circ: 12,169. **Co-sponsor:** American Academy of Otolaryngic Allergy.

616.21 JPN
OTOLOGIA FUKUOKA - JIBI TO RINSHO. Text in Japanese; Summaries in English. 1955. bi-m. JPY 6,000 (effective 2001). adv. bk.rev. back issues avail. **Document type:** *Academic/Scholarly.*
Formerly: Jibi to Rinsho (0447-7227)
Indexed: Excerp.Med., INIS Atomind., Inpharma, Lang.& Lang.Behav.Abstr., Reac.
—BLDSC (6313.525000), CISTI, GNLM.
Published by: Jibi to Rinsho Co., Department of Otorhinolaryngology, Kyushu University, Fukuoka-shi 812-8582, Japan. TEL 81-92-642-5668, FAX 81-92-642-5685. Ed. Takashi Nakagawa. Pub. Sohtaro Komiyama. R&P, Adv. contact Otologia Fukuoka. Circ: 1,500.

616.21 USA ISSN 1531-7129 CODEN: AJOTBN
OTOLOGY & NEUROTOLOGY; an international forum. Text in English. 1979. bi-m., latest vol.22. USD 189 domestic to individuals; USD 215 foreign to individuals; USD 306 domestic to institutions; USD 344 foreign to institutions (effective 2002). adv. bk.rev. bibl, illus. back issues avail. *Refereed.* **Document type:** *Journal, Academic/Scholarly.* **Description:** Original articles and reviews in otology, neurology and audiology.
Formerly (until 2001): American Journal of Otology (0192-9763)
Related titles: Microform ed.: (from PQC); Online - full text ed.: USD 397.80 domestic academic site license; USD 443.70 domestic corporate site license; USD 435.80 foreign academic site license; USD 481.70 foreign corporate site license (effective 2002) (from Ovid Technologies, Inc., Institute for Scientific Information).
Indexed: ASCA, Biol.Abstr., Curr.Cont., Dent.Ind., Excerp.Med., INIS Atomind., Ind.Med. (1979-), Ind.Sci.Rev., Inpharma, Lang.& Lang.Behav.Abstr., Neurosci.Cit.Ind., Noise Pollut.Publ.Abstr., Pharm.&Out.News, Reac., Rev.Med.& Vet.Mycol., SOPODA, Sci.Cit.Ind., Sociol.Abstr.

M

—BLDSC (6313.528000), CISTI, EMDOCS, GNLM, IDS, ingenta, KNAW.
Published by: (American Otological Society), Lippincott Williams & Wilkins (Philadelphia) (Subsidiary of: Wolters Kluwer N.V.), 530 Walnut St, Philadelphia, PA 19106-3621. TEL 215-521-8300, FAX 215-521-8902, http://otology-neurotology.org/, http://www.lww.com. Ed. Dr. Robert K Jackler. Pub. Marcia Serepy. R&P Margaret Becker. Adv. contact Ray Thibodeau. B&W page USD 575, color page USD 1,695. Circ: 1,649 (paid). **Subscr. to:** PO Box 1600, Hagerstown, MD 21740-1600. TEL 800-777-2295, FAX 301-824-7390. **Co-sponsors:** American Neurotology Society; European Academy of Otology and Neurotology.

616.21 ITA ISSN 0392-6621
OTORINOLARINGOLOGIA; rivista quadrimestrale di otorinolaringologia, audiologia, foniatria, chirurgia cervico-facciale, maxillo-facciale, plastica ricostruttiva, otoneurochirurgia. Text in Italian; Summaries in English, Italian. 1951. q. USD 105 to individuals; USD 155 to institutions (effective 2000 - 2001). adv. bk.rev. bibl, charts, illus. index. *Refereed.* **Description:** Covers otorhinolaryngology, audiology, phoniatrics, maxillo-cervicofacial surgery, reconstructive plastic surgery, and otoneurosurgery.
Incorporates (in 1981): Minerva Otorinolaringologica (0026-4938); Bollettino delle Malattie dell'Orecchio, della Gola, del Naso (0392-7024); Otorinolaringologia Italiana; Nuovo Archivio Italiano di Otologia, Rinologia e Laringologia (0301-3693); Which was formerly: Archivio Italiano di Otologia, Rinologia e Laringologia (0004-0258)
Related titles: Microform ed.
Indexed: Biol.Abstr., Chem.Abstr., Excerp.Med., INIS Atomind., Ind.Med. (coverage dropped), Lang.& Lang.Behav.Abstr., NBA, SOPODA, Sociol.Abstr.
—BLDSC (6313.635000), CISTI, GNLM, KNAW.
Published by: Edizioni Minerva Medica, Corso Bramante, 83-85, Turin, TO 10126, Italy. TEL 39-11-678282, FAX 39-11-674502. Ed., Pub. Alberto Oliaro. Adv. contact F Filippo. B&W page USD 1,200, color page USD 2,000; trim 280 x 215. Circ: 3,000 (paid).

616.21 618.92 ITA ISSN 1120-3455
L'OTORINOLARINGOLOGIA PEDIATRICA. Text in Italian; Summaries in English. 1989. q. ITL 80,000, USD 70 (effective 2001).
—EMDOCS, GNLM.
Published by: (Societa Italiana di Otorinolaringologia Pediatrica), C I C Edizioni Internazionali s.r.l., Corso Trieste 42, Rome, RM 00198, Italy. TEL 39-06-8412673, FAX 39-06-8412688, info@gruppocic.it, 1160199510. Eds. D. Passali, G Motta.

616.21 BGR ISSN 0473-5609
OTORINOLARINGOLOGIJA. Text in Bulgarian; Summaries in English, Russian. q. BGL 8.
Indexed: Abstr.Bulg.Sci.Med.Lit.
—CISTI.
Published by: (Bulgaria. Ministerstvo na Narodnoto Zdrave), Izdatelstvo Meditsina i Fizkultura, 11 Pl Slaveikov, Sofia 1080, Bulgaria. Ed. V Pavlov. Circ: 765. **Distr. by:** Hemus, 6 Rouski blvd, Sofia 1000, Bulgaria. **Co-sponsor:** Nauchno Druzhestvo po Otorinolaringologia.

616.21 CZE ISSN 1210-7867
CODEN: CEOTA9
OTORINOLARYNGOLOGIE A FONIATRIE. Text in Czech, Slovak; Summaries in Czech, English. 1952. q. EUR 84, USD 112 (effective 2001). adv. bk.rev. abstr. index. *Refereed.*
Former titles (until 1994): Cesko-Slovenska Otorinolaryngologie a Foniatrie (1210-5988); (until 1991): Ceskoslovenska Otolaryngologie (0009-0603)
Indexed: C.I.S. Abstr., Dent.Ind., Excerp.Med., INIS Atomind., Ind.Med. (coverage dropped).
—CASDDS, CISTI, EMDOCS, GNLM. **CCC.**
Published by: (Ceska Lekarska Spolecnost J.E. Purkyne/Czech Medical Association), Nakladatelske Stredisko C L S J.E. Purkyne, Sokolska 31, Prague 12026, Czech Republic. TEL 42-2-24911420, FAX 42-2-24911420, nts@iol.cz, http://www.clsjep.cz, http://www.medical.cz. Ed. P Skerik. adv.: B&W page CZK 29,500, color page CZK 41,500; 244 x 166. Circ: 1,200. **Dist. by:** Abont s.r.o., Chlumova 17, Prague, 3 130 00, Czech Republic; **Dist. in Western Countries by:** Kubon & Sagner, Hesstr 39-41, Munich 80798, Germany. **Co-sponsor:** Ceskoslovanska Otolaryngologicka Spolesnost.

OTO'S SCOPE. see *BUSINESS AND ECONOMICS—Management*

616.21 PAK ISSN 0257-4985
PAKISTAN JOURNAL OF OTOLARYNGOLOGY. Text in English. 1985. q. PKR 250, USD 40, GBP 30. adv. bk.rev. **Document type:** *Academic/Scholarly.* **Description:** Publishes scientific research and articles.
Related titles: CD-ROM ed.
Indexed: Excerp.Med. (until 1992), ExtraMED, Per.Islam. (1991-).
—GNLM. **CCC.**
Published by: Pakistan Society of Otolaryngology, c/o Dr. M.H.A. Beg F.R.C.S., Modern Ear Nose and Throat Hospital, B-10 Block 13-A, Opposite PIA Planetarium, University Rd., Karachi 74400, Pakistan. TEL 92-21-4971762, FAX 92-21-4971763. Circ: 2,000.

616.21 CAN
PATIENT OF THE MONTH PROGRAM. Short title: P M P. (Also avail. in latent-image print version) Text in English. 1982. 8/yr. USD 475 to non-members; USD 340 to members (effective 2000). abstr, charts. **Description:** Aims to perfect clinical decision-making skills by simulating clinical situations with a personal computer.
Related titles: Diskette ed.
Published by: (American Academy of Otolaryngology - Head and Neck Surgery, Inc. USA), B.C. Decker, LCD 1, P O Box 620, Hamilton, ON L8N 3K7, Canada. TEL 905-522-7017, 800-568-7281, FAX 905-522-7839, info@bcdecker.com. Ed. Charles M Myer III.

616.21 JPN ISSN 0032-6313
CODEN: JIBIAG
PRACTICA OTOLOGICA KYOTO/JIBI INKOKA RINSHO. Text in Japanese; Summaries in English. 1908. m. JPY 10,000. adv. abstr, bibl, charts, illus. index. **Document type:** *Academic/Scholarly.*
Related titles: ♦ Supplement: Practica Otologica Kyoto. Supplement. ISSN 0912-1870.
Indexed: Biol.Abstr., Excerp.Med., INIS Atomind.
—BLDSC (6593.810000), GNLM, KNAW.
Published by: Kyoto University, Faculty Of Medicine, Department of Otolaryngology/Kyoto Daigaku Igakubu Jibi Inkoka Kyoshitsu, 54 Shogoin Kawara-cho, Sakyo-ku, Kyoto 606-8397, Japan. Ed. Iwao Houjo. Circ: 1,500.

616.21 JPN ISSN 0912-1870
CODEN: JIRHET
PRACTICA OTOLOGICA KYOTO. SUPPLEMENT/JIBI INKOKA RINSHO. HOSATSU. Text in Japanese; Summaries in English. 1986. irreg. **Document type:** *Academic/Scholarly.*
Related titles: ♦ Supplement to: Practica Otologica Kyoto. ISSN 0032-6313.
Indexed: Excerp.Med. (1994-).
—BLDSC (6593.812000), EMDOCS, KNAW.
Published by: Kyoto University, Faculty Of Medicine, Department of Otolaryngology/Kyoto Daigaku Igakubu Jibi Inkoka Kyoshitsu, 54 Shogoin Kawara-cho, Sakyo-ku, Kyoto 606-8397, Japan. Ed. Iwao Houjo.

617.89 ITA ISSN 1125-7210
PROGRESSI IN AUDIOLOGIA E VESTIBOLOGIA. Text in Italian. 1997. q. ITL 80,000, USD 80 (effective 2001). adv.
Published by: (Associazione Italiana di Audiologia e Vestibologia Clinica), C I C Edizioni Internazionali s.r.l., Corso Trieste 42, Rome, RM 00198, Italy. TEL 39-06-8412673, FAX 39-06-8412688, info@gruppocic.it, 1160199510. Ed. G Motta. adv.: B&W page XEU 1,239.5, color page XEU 3,300; 210 x 280.

616.21 GBR ISSN 0143-6813
RECENT ADVANCES IN OTOLARYNGOLOGY. Text in English. 1935. irreg. **Document type:** *Monographic series, Academic/Scholarly.*
—CISTI, KNAW.
Published by: Churchill Livingstone (Subsidiary of: Harcourt Publishers Ltd.), Robert Stevenson House, 1-3 Baxter's Pl, Leith Walk, Edinburgh, Midlothian EH1 3AF, United Kingdom. TEL 44-131-556-2424, FAX 44-131-459-1177, http://www.churchillmed.com. **US subscr. to:** Churchill Livingstone, 650 Ave of the Americas, New York, NY 10011. TEL 212-206-5000.

617.8 FRA ISSN 0034-222X
REEDUCATION ORTHOPHONIQUE. Text in French. 1963. q. FRF 515 domestic to non-members; FRF 595 foreign to non-members; FRF 370 to members; FRF 205 to students (effective 2000). adv. bk.rev. bibl, charts, illus, stat, tr.lit. *Refereed.* **Document type:** *Academic/Scholarly.* **Description:** Covers hearing, speech, language and voice disorders.
Published by: Federation Nationale des Orthophonistes (F N O), 2 rue des deux gares, Paris 75010, France. TEL 33-1-40346265, FAX 33-1-40374142, reeducation.orthophonique@wanadoo.fr, http://www.fno.fr. Ed., Pub. Jacques Roustit. Circ: 3,000.

616.21 BRA ISSN 0034-7299
CODEN: RBORAB
REVISTA BRASILEIRA DE OTO-RINO-LARINGOLOGIA. Text in Portuguese. 1933. bi-m. BRL 240 domestic; USD 120 foreign (effective 2000). adv. abstr, bibl, illus. index. *Refereed.* **Document type:** *Academic/Scholarly.* **Description:** Contains original papers and case reports from otolaryngology, head and neck surgery and related areas.
Indexed: Chem.Abstr., Excerp.Med., Ind.Med. (coverage dropped).
—KNAW.
Published by: Sociedade Brasileira de Otorrinolaringologia, Rua Jose Maria Lisboa, 41, 7o andar, Sao Paulo, SP 01423-000, Brazil. TEL 55-21-2870893, FAX 55-21-2870893, TELEX 55-11-3051-5044. Eds. Dr. Carlos Alberto Herrerias de Campos, Dr. Ricardo Ferreira Bento. Adv. contact Maria Szwif.

617.8 ESP ISSN 0214-4603
REVISTA DE LOGOPEDIA, FONIATRIA Y AUDIOLOGIA. Text in Spanish. 1982. q. ESP 9,700 to individuals; ESP 13,800 to institutions; ESP 7,760 to students (effective 2001). adv. bk.rev. bibl. back issues avail.; reprints avail. *Refereed.* **Document type:** *Journal, Academic/Scholarly.*
Related titles: Online - full text ed.: 1996.
Published by: (Asociacion Espanola de Logopedia, Foniatria y Audiologia), Ediciones Doyma S.A., Traversa de Gracia, 17-21, Barcelona 08021, Spain. TEL 34-93-200-0711, rlja@doyma.es, doyma@doyma.es, http://www.doyma.es/flja. Ed. Miguel Puyelo. R&P Monica Barnes. Adv. contact Jose Antonio Hernandez. B&W page ESP 122,000, color page ESP 152,000; 280 x 210. Circ: 3,000.

616.2 VEN
REVISTA OTORRINOLARINGOLOGICA. Text in Spanish; Summaries in English. 1965. q. VEB 30, USD 9. bibl. index.
Published by: Instituto Celis Perez, Apartado Postal 163, Valencia, Venezuela. Ed. Dr. A Celis Perez. Circ: 500. **Subscr. to:** Medicina Libros, Edif. Pax Cruce, Av. Avila y Caracas, Caracas, Venezuela.

616.21 FRA ISSN 0035-1334
REVUE DE LARYNGOLOGIE - OTOLOGIE - RHINOLOGIE. Text and summaries in English, French. 1880. 5/yr. FRF 810 to individuals (effective 2001). adv. bk.rev. abstr, bibl, charts, illus, stat. index.
Indexed: Biol.Abstr., Dent.Ind., Excerp.Med., Ind.Med., Lang.& Lang.Behav.Abstr., NBA, SOPODA, Sociol.Abstr.
—BLDSC (7926.450000), CISTI, GNLM, KNAW.
Published by: Revue de Laryngologie, 114 av. d'Ares, Bordeaux Cedex 33074, France. TEL 33-5-56243015, FAX 33-5-57815848, orl.bordeaux@wanadoo.fr, http://www.revue-laryngologie.com. Ed. Jacques Verhulst. Circ: 2,200.

616.21 NLD ISSN 0300-0729
CODEN: RNGYA8
RHINOLOGY. Text in English. 1963. q. NLG 233, EUR 106 (effective 2001). adv. bk.rev. index. back issues avail. *Refereed.* **Document type:** *Journal, Academic/Scholarly.* **Description:** Contains papers dealing with physiology, diagnostics, pathology, medical therapy and surgery of the nose and paranasal sinuses, including allergology.
Related titles: Online - full text ed.: (from Institute for Scientific Information).
Indexed: Biol.Abstr., Curr.Cont., Curr.Ind.Stat., Dent.Ind., Excerp.Med., Ind.Med. (1970-), Rev.Med.& Vet.Mycol.
—BLDSC (7960.743000), CISTI, EMDOCS, GNLM, KNAW.
Published by: International Rhinologic Society, c/o Journal Rhinology, Postbus 85500, Utrecht 3508 GA, Netherlands. TEL 31-30-2506644, FAX 31-30-2541922, rhinology@mail.com. Ed., Pub. Dr. E H Huizing. R&P, Adv. contact Margot Wijnen. Circ: 2,500.

616.21 617.89 ITA ISSN 0392-1360
RIVISTA ITALIANA DI OTORINOLARINGOLOGIA, AUDIOLOGIA E FONIATRIA. Text in Italian; Summaries in English. 1980. q. ITL 80,000, USD 70 (effective 2001). adv.
Indexed: Excerp.Med., NBA.
—BLDSC (7987.470000), CISTI, EMDOCS, GNLM, Infotrieve. **CCC.**

M

Published by: C I C Edizioni Internazionali s.r.l., Corso Trieste 42, Rome, RM 00198, Italy. TEL 39-06-8412673, FAX 39-06-8412688, info@gruppocic.it, 1160199510. Eds. D. Passali, T. Marullo. adv.: B&W page XEU 1,239.5, color page XEU 1,704.31; 210 x 280.

616.21 RUS ISSN 0869-5474
ROSSIISKAYA RINOLOGIYA. Text in Russian. q. USD 95 in United States.
Indexed: Ref.Zh.
—East View.
Published by: Rossiiskoe Obshchestvo Rinologov, A-ya 4, Moscow 121614, Russian Federation. TEL 7-095-4140464. Ed. G Z Piskunov. **US dist. addr.:** East View Publications, 3020 Harbor Ln N, Minneapolis, MN 55447. TEL 612-550-0961.

617.8 SWE ISSN 0105-0397
RF1 CODEN: SNADAS
SCANDINAVIAN AUDIOLOGY. Text in English. 1952. q. GBP 60, USD 99 to individuals; GBP 108, USD 179 to institutions (effective 2001). adv. bk.rev. index. *Refereed.* **Document type:** *Journal, Academic/Scholarly.*
Former titles (until 1971): Nordisk Audiologi (0105-0400); (until 1960): Nordisk Tidsskrift for Praktisk Audiologi (0105-1865)
Related titles: Online - full text ed.: (from EBSCO Publishing, O C L C Online Computer Library Center, Inc., RoweCom Information Quest, CatchWord Ltd., ingenta, Swets Blackwell, Institute for Scientific Information); ♦ Supplement: Scandinavian Audiology. Supplement. ISSN 0107-8593.
Indexed: Acoust.Abstr., Aqua.Sci.& Fish.Abstr., Biol.Abstr., CINAHL, Curr.Cont. (coverage dropped), DSH Abstr., Dok.Arbeitsmed., Environ.Sci.Poll.Mgmt., Excerp.Med., INSPEC (1979-), Ind.Med. (1972-), Inpharma, Lang.& Lang.Behav.Abstr., Neurosci.Cit.Ind., Noise Pollut.Publ.Abstr., Pollut.Abstr., PsycInfo, Psychol.Abstr. (1972-), Reac., Ref.Zh., Risk Abstr., SOPODA, SSCI (coverage dropped), Saf.Sci.Abstr., Sci.Cit.Ind. (coverage dropped), Sociol.Abstr., e-psyche.
—BLDSC (8087.469000), AskIEEE, CISTI, GNLM, IDS, KNAW, Linda Hall. **CCC.**
Published by: (Nordisk Audiologisk Selskab NOR), Taylor & Francis AS (Subsidiary of: Taylor & Francis Group), Cort Adelersgt. 17, Solli, PO Box 2562, Oslo 0202, Norway. TEL 47-22-12-98-80, FAX 47-22-12-98-90, journals@tandf.no, http://www.tandf.co.uk/tfas. Ed. Agnete Parving. adv.: B&W page SEK 6,000, color page SEK 8,000; trim 149 x 230. Circ: 1,000.

617.8 SWE ISSN 0107-8593
CODEN: SAUSBF
SCANDINAVIAN AUDIOLOGY. SUPPLEMENT. Text in English. 1971. irreg. **Document type:** *Academic/Scholarly.*
Related titles: ♦ Supplement to: Scandinavian Audiology. ISSN 0105-0397.
Indexed: CINAHL, Excerp.Med., INSPEC (1979-), Ind.Med. (1972-), PsycInfo, Ref.Zh., e-psyche.
—BLDSC (8087.471000), AskIEEE, CISTI, KNAW, Linda Hall. **CCC.**
Published by: (Nordisk Audiologisk Selskab NOR), Taylor & Francis AB (Subsidiary of: Taylor & Francis Group), Hollaendargatan 20, PO Box 3255, Stockholm 11160, Sweden. TEL 46-8-4408040, FAX 46-8-4408050, journals@scup.no, journals@se.tandf.no, http://www.scup.no/audiology.

616 USA ISSN 0734-0451
RF286 CODEN: SEMHE7
SEMINARS IN HEARING. Text in English. 1980. q. EUR 124 to individuals; EUR 328 to institutions; EUR 75 newsstand/cover (effective 2002). adv. reprint service avail. from PQC. *Refereed.* **Document type:** *Academic/Scholarly.* **Description:** Covers a topic in audiology or related area.
Supersedes in part (in 1983): Seminars in Speech, Language and Hearing (0196-108X)
Related titles: Microfilm ed.; Online - full text ed.: ISSN 1098-8955 (from EBSCO Publishing, O C L C Online Computer Library Center, Inc., RoweCom Information Quest).
Indexed: Biol.Abstr., CINAHL, Excerp.Med.
—BLDSC (8239.449800), CISTI, EMDOCS, GNLM, Infotrieve, ingenta, KNAW. **CCC.**
Published by: Thieme Medical Publishers, 333 Seventh Ave, New York, NY 10001. TEL 212-760-0888, 800-782-3488, FAX 212-947-1112, http://www.thieme.com. Ed. Dr. Jerry L Northern. Circ: 1,976. **Orders in Europe to:** Thieme International, Postfach 3001120, Stuttgart 70451, Germany. TEL 49-711-8931-0.

617.89 USA ISSN 0734-0478
RC423.A1 CODEN: SSLAEB
SEMINARS IN SPEECH AND LANGUAGE. Text in English. 1980. q. EUR 107 to individuals; EUR 328 to institutions; EUR 75 newsstand/cover (effective 2002). adv. abstr. bibl. illus. reprint service avail. from PQC. **Document type:** *Journal, Academic/Scholarly.* **Description:** Reports on clinical advances in speech and language pathology, offering diagnostic procedures, screening and assessment techniques, treatment protocols, and short- and long-term management practices.
Supersedes in part (in 1983): Seminars in Speech, Language and Hearing (0196-108X)
Related titles: Microfilm ed.; Online - full text ed.: ISSN 1098-9056 (from EBSCO Publishing, O C L C Online Computer Library Center, Inc., RoweCom Information Quest).
Indexed: AMED, Biol.Abstr., CINAHL, Ind.Med. (1983-).
—BLDSC (8239.462000), CISTI, GNLM, Infotrieve, ingenta. **CCC.**
Published by: Thieme Medical Publishers, 333 Seventh Ave, New York, NY 10001. TEL 212-760-0888, 800-782-3488, FAX 212-947-1112, http://www.thieme.com. Ed. Richard F Curlee. Circ: 2,000. **Orders in Europe to:** Thieme International, Postfach 3001120, Stuttgart 70451, Germany. TEL 49-711-8931-0.

SIGHT AND SOUND NEWS. see *HEALTH FACILITIES AND ADMINISTRATION*

SPRACHE - STIMME - GEHOER; Zeitschrift fuer Kommunikationsstoerungen. see *EDUCATION—Special Education And Rehabilitation*

616.21 USA
SPRINGER HANDBOOK OF AUDITORY RESEARCH. Text in English. irreg., latest vol.3, 1993. **Document type:** *Monographic series.*
Indexed: Zoo.Rec.
—BLDSC.
Published by: Springer-Verlag, Journals (Subsidiary of: BertelsmannSpringer), 175 Fifth Ave, New York, NY 10010. TEL 212-460-1500, FAX 212-473-6272. Eds. Arthur Popper, Richard Fay.

616.21 SWE ISSN 1400-0121
SVENSK OE N H TIDSKRIFT. Text in Swedish. 1994. q. USD 35, GBP 21 to institutions (effective 2001). adv. **Document type:** *Journal, Academic/Scholarly.*
Published by: Taylor & Francis AS (Subsidiary of: Taylor & Francis Group), Cort Adelersgt. 17, Solli, PO Box 2562, Oslo 0202, Norway. TEL 47-22-12-98-80, FAX 47-22-12-98-90, journals@tandf.no, http://www.tandf.co.uk.tfas. Ed. Tomas Gjerot. adv.: B&W page SEK 5,000, color page SEK 11,800; trim 190 x 260.

SWIAT CISZY; czasopismo polskich inwalidow sluchu. see *HANDICAPPED—Hearing Impaired*

616.21 HRV ISSN 1330-0296
SYMPOSIA OTORHINOLARYNGOLOGICA. Text in Croatian; Summaries in English. 1966. 3/yr. HRK 80 domestic to individuals; HRK 150 domestic to institutions; DEM 50 foreign (effective 2000). adv. bk.rev.
Formerly (until 1991): Symposia Otorhinolaryngologica Iugoslavica (0586-9145)
Indexed: Excerp.Med., Ind.Med. (coverage dropped).
—GNLM.
Published by: (Klinicka Bolnica "Sestre Milosrdnice", Klinika za Otorinolaringologiju i Cervikofacijalnu Kirurgiju), Zavod za Proucavanje i Zastitu Uha i Disnih Organa, Vinogradska 29, Zagreb 10000, Croatia. Ed. Boris Pegan. Circ: 300 (paid). **Co-sponsor:** Ministarstva Znanosti i Tehnologije Republike Hrvatske.

616.21 USA ISSN 0897-6368
TINNITUS TODAY. Text in English. 1975. q. USD 25 domestic; USD 40 foreign (effective 2001). adv. bk.rev. 26 p./no. 2 cols./p. back issues avail. **Document type:** *Magazine.* **Description:** Serves professionals and laypeople with scientific and anecdotal articles.
Formerly (until 1988): A T A Newsletter
Related titles: Online - full content ed.: ISSN 1530-6569.
Published by: American Tinnitus Association, PO Box 5, Portland, OR 97207. TEL 503-248-9985, 800-634-8978, FAX 503-248-0024, tinnitus@ata.org, http://www.ata.org/tinnitus_today/. Ed., R&P, Adv. contact Barbara Tabachnick Sanders TEL 503-248-9985 ext 216. Circ: 170,000.

616.21 USA ISSN 1084-7138
RF300 CODEN: TAMPFF
TRENDS IN AMPLIFICATION. Text in English. 1996. q. USD 40 domestic to individuals; USD 60 foreign to individuals; USD 75 domestic to institutions; USD 90 foreign to institutions. adv. index. back issues avail. *Refereed.* **Document type:** *Academic/Scholarly.* **Description:** For audiologists, otolaryngologists, and hearing aid dispensers. Covers current topics in amplification and hearing aids.
—BLDSC (9049.528900).
Published by: Woodland Publications, Inc., 69 Murray St, New York, NY 10007. TEL 212-566-4294, FAX 212-406-6496, woodlpub@pipeline.com. Ed. Michael Valente. Adv. contact Sue Cassidy. page USD 750; trim 11 x 8.5. Circ: 1,000 (paid).

616.21 USA
TRIOLOGISTICS✶ . Text in English. 1976. 3/yr. **Document type:** *Newsletter.* **Description:** Society information relating to the field of otolaryngology.
Published by: (American Laryngological, Rhinological and Otological Society), Triological Society, 555 N 30th St, Omaha, NE 68131-2136. TEL 314-621-6550, FAX 314-621-6688.

616.21 ITA ISSN 0042-2371
VALSALVA. Text in Italian; Summaries in English. 1923. q. USD 80 (effective 2002). adv. bk.rev. **Description:** Covers all aspects of otorhinolaryngology.
Indexed: Chem.Abstr., Dent.Ind., Excerp.Med., Ind.Med. (coverage dropped), NBA.
—CISTI, GNLM.
Published by: Edizioni Luigi Pozzi s.r.l., Via Panama, 68, Rome, RM 00198, Italy. TEL 39-06-8553548, FAX 39-06-8554105, edizioni_pozzi@tin.it. Eds. I de Vincentiis, T Marullo. Circ: 1,000.

616.21 RUS ISSN 0042-4668
CODEN: VORLA7
VESTNIK OTORINOLARINGOLOGII/ANNALS OF OTORHINOLARYNGOLOGY. Text in Russian; Summaries in English. 1936. bi-m. RUR 216 for 6 mos. to individuals; RUR 540 for 6 mos. to institutions (effective 2002). adv. bk.rev. bibl. index. **Description:** Publishes original papers of clinical, laboratory, experimental and theoretical nature dedicated to problems of etiology, pathogenesis, diagnosis of different otorhinolaryngological diseases, their relation to other infections.
Indexed: Biol.Abstr., Chem.Abstr., Dent.Ind., Dok.Arbeitsmed., Excerp.Med., Ind.Med. (1936-), Int.Aerosp.Abstr., Ref.Zh.
—CISTI, East View, GNLM, Infotrieve, KNAW. **CCC.**
Published by: (Vsesoyuznoe Nauchnoe Obshchestvo Otorinolaringologov), Media Sfera, Dmitrovskoe shosse 46, korp 2, etazh 4, P.O. Box 54, Moscow 127238, Russian Federation. TEL 7-095-4824329, FAX 7-095-4824312, mediashp@mediasphera.ru. Ed. V T Pal'chun. Adv. contact Valery Nemtsov. **Dist. by:** Mezhdunarodnaya Kniga, B Yakimanka 39, Moscow 117049, Russian Federation. TEL 7-095-2384967, FAX 7-095-2384634; **US dist. addr.:** East View Publications, 3020 Harbor Ln N, Minneapolis, MN 55447. TEL 612-550-0961. **Co-sponsor:** Ministerstvo Zdravookhraneniya.

616.21 USA ISSN 1041-892X
RF11
THE YEAR BOOK OF OTOLARYNGOLOGY - HEAD AND NECK SURGERY. Text in English. 1900. a. USD 87 domestic; USD 93 foreign (effective 2001). illus. **Document type:** *Abstract/Index, Academic/Scholarly.* **Description:** Presents abstracts of pertinent literature in the field with commentary by leading experts in the field.
Supersedes (in 1985): Year Book of Otolaryngology (0146-7247); Which was formerly (until 1975): Year Book of the Ear, Nose and Throat (0084-4055); Which superseded in part: Yearbook of the Eye, Ear, Nose and Throat
Related titles: CD-ROM ed.
Indexed: Curr.Adv.Ecol.Sci.
—CISTI, GNLM.
Published by: Mosby, Inc., Continuity Division (Subsidiary of: Harcourt Health Sciences), 11830 Westline Industrial Dr, St Louis, MO 63146-3313. TEL 314-872-8370, 800-325-4177, FAX 314-432-1380, http://www.mosby.com/periodicals. Eds. Dr. G Richard Holt, Dr. Michael Paparella, Dr. Randal Otto.

M

616.21 CHN ISSN 0412-3948
ZHONGHUA ER-BI-YANHOUKE ZAZHI/CHINESE JOURNAL OF OTORHINOLARYNGOLOGY. Key Title: Chung-Hua Erh Pi Yen Hou K'o Tsa Chih. Text in Chinese. 1953. bi-m. CNY 67.20 domestic; CNY 11.20 newsstand/cover domestic; USD 35.40 foreign; USD 5.90 newsstand/cover foreign (effective 2001). **Document type:** *Academic/Scholarly.*
Related titles: Online - full content ed.: (from WanFang Data Corp.).
Indexed: Ind.Med.
Published by: Zhonghua Yixuehui Zazhishe, 42 Dongsi Xidajie, Beijing 100710, China. TEL 86-1-65273369, ent@bnu.edu.cn, cmaebh@public.sti.ac.cn. Ed. Zi-zhong Wang.

616.21 UKR ISSN 0044-4650 CODEN: ZUNBA9
ZHURNAL USHNYKH, NOSOVYKH I GORLOVYKH BOLEZNEI*. Text in Ukrainian. 1924. bi-m. USD 110 in United States. abstr, bibl, charts, illus, stat. index. *Refereed.* **Document type:** *Academic/Scholarly.* **Description:** Concerns matters of otorhinolaryngology, and adjacent specialties; current questions of etiology, pathogenesis, diagnostics, prophylaxis and management of related diseases, ENT-head and neck surgeons, pathologists, neurologists, immunologists, radiologists, dentists, biochemists and students.
Related titles: Fax ed.; Online - full text ed.
Indexed: Biol.Abstr., Chem.Abstr., INIS Atomind., Ind.Med. (coverage dropped), Int.Aerosp.Abstr.
—CASDDS, CISTI, East View, EMDOCS, GNLM, KNAW.
Published by: Ministerstvo Zdravookhraneniya Ukraine, Vul. M Hrushevskoho 7, Kiev 252018, Ukraine. TEL 380-44-224-15-86, FAX 380-44-224-95-23. **Dist. by:** Mezhdunarodnaya Kniga, B Yakimanka 39, Moscow 117049, Russian Federation. TEL 7-095-2384967, FAX 7-095-2384634; **US dist. addr.:** East View Publications, 3020 Harbor Ln N, Minneapolis, MN 55447. TEL 612-550-0961. **Co-sponsor:** Ukrainskoe Nauchnoe Obshchestvo Otolaringolov.

MEDICAL SCIENCES—Pediatrics

618.92 USA ISSN 1099-6605
A A P GRAND ROUNDS. Text in English. m. USD 79 to members; USD 89 to non-members (effective 2001). *Refereed.* **Document type:** *Journal, Academic/Scholarly.* **Description:** Provides current updates on trends and studies in pediatric medicine.
Published by: American Academy of Pediatrics, 141 Northwest Point Blvd, Box 927, Elk Grove Village, IL 60009-0927. TEL 847-434-4000, 888-227-1773, FAX 847-434-8000, grandrounds@aap.org, kidsdocs@aap.org, http://www.aap.org/profed/grandrounds.htm. Eds. Edgar Marcuse, Lewis First.

618.92 USA ISSN 1073-0397
A A P NEWS. Text in English. 1993. m., latest vol.19. USD 60 to individuals; USD 65 to libraries; USD 15 to students (effective 2001). adv. charts, illus, stat, abstr. 40 p./no. back issues avail.; reprints avail. **Document type:** *Newspaper, Magazine, Academic/Scholarly.* **Description:** Contains news reports, clinical policy statements, legislation news, and practice management tips.
Former titles (until 1985): News and Comment - American Academy of Pediatrics (0094-8209); (until 1973): American Academy of Pediatrics. Newsletter (0094-8217)
Related titles: Online - full text ed.: AAPNews.org. 2000 (Aug) (from HighWire Pr.).
—**CCC.**
Published by: American Academy of Pediatrics, 141 Northwest Point Blvd, Box 927, Elk Grove Village, IL 60009-0927. TEL 847-434-4000, 800-433-9016, FAX 847-434-8000, aaapnews@aap.org, http://www.aap.org. Ed. Anne Hegland. R&P Kyle Ostler TEL 847-434-7892. Circ: 55,000.

ACTA DE ODONTOLOGIA PEDIATRICA; una revista internacional para la odontologia pediatrica. see *MEDICAL SCIENCES—Dentistry*

618.92 NOR ISSN 0803-5253 CODEN: APAEEL
ACTA PAEDIATRICA; an international journal of paediatrics. Text in English. 1921. m. GBP 139, USD 230 to individuals; GBP 312, USD 514 to institutions (effective 2002). adv. bk.rev. charts, illus. index, cum.index: vols.1-30 (1921-1943). *Refereed.* **Document type:** *Academic/Scholarly.* **Description:** Covers clinical and experimental research in all fields of paediatrics including developmental physiology.
Former titles (until 1991): Acta Paediatrica Scandinavica (0001-656X); Acta Paediatrica
Related titles: Online - full text ed.: (from EBSCO Publishing, O C L C Online Computer Library Center, Inc., RoweCom Information Quest, CatchWord Ltd., Swets Blackwell, Institute for Scientific Information); ♦ Supplement: Acta Paediatrica. Supplement. ISSN 0803-5326.
Indexed: ASCA, Abstr.Hyg., Bibl.Dev.Med.& Child Neur., Biol.Abstr., C.I.S. Abstr., Chem.Abstr., Curr.Adv.Ecol.Sci., Curr.Adv.Gen.& Molec.Biol., Curr.Cont., Dairy Sci.Abstr., Dent.Ind., Diab.Cont., Diar.Dis.Res., Dok.Arbeitsmed., Environ.Sci.Poll.Mgmt., Excerp.Med., Fam.Ind., GeoRef, Helminthol.Abstr., INIS Atomind., Ind.Med. (1992-), Ind.Sci.Rev., Ind.Vet., Inpharma, Int.Abstr.Biol.Sci., Int.Nurs.Ind., Kidney, Med.& Surg.Dermat., NRN, Neurosci.Cit.Ind., Nutr.Abstr., Pharm.&Out.News, Pollut.Abstr., Protozool.Abstr., Reac., Rev.Appl.Entomol., Rev.Med.& Vet.Mycol., Rice Abstr., Risk Abstr., Rural Devel.Abstr., SSCI (coverage dropped), Saf.Sci.Abstr., Sci.Cit.Ind., Sugar Ind.Abstr., Triticale Abstr., Trop.Dis.Bull.
—BLDSC (0642.400000), ADONIS, CASDDS, CISTI, EMDOCS, GNLM, IDS, ingenta, KNAW. **CCC.**
Published by: Taylor & Francis AS (Subsidiary of: Taylor & Francis Group), Cort Adelersgt. 17, Solli, PO Box 2562, Oslo 0202, Norway. TEL 47-22-12-98-80, FAX 47-22-12-98-90, journals@tandf.no, http://www.tandf.co.uk/tfas. Ed. Rolf Zetterstroem. Circ: 2,000.

618.92 ITA ISSN 0001-6551
ACTA PAEDIATRICA LATINA. Text and summaries in English, Italian. 1948. q. ITL 50,000; ITL 80,000 foreign (effective 1995). adv. bk.rev. charts, illus. back issues avail.
Indexed: Biol.Abstr., Chem.Abstr., Excerp.Med., Nutr.Abstr.
Published by: (Universita degli Studi di Padova, Clinica Pediatrica), Artigianato Grafico Editoriale s.n.c., Via Casorati, 29, Reggio Emilia, RE 42100, Italy. FAX 39-522-921169. Ed. Ernesto Sartori. Circ: 3,000.

618.92 TWN CODEN: CHEKAL
ACTA PAEDIATRICA SINICA TAIWANICA/ZHONGHUA MINGUO XIAO'ERKE YIXUEHUI ZAZHI. Text in English. 1960. bi-m. TWD 3,000 domestic; USD 100 foreign (effective 1999). adv. abstr, stat. index. *Refereed.* **Document type:** *Academic/Scholarly, Abstract/Index.*
Formerly: Acta Paediatrica Sinica (0001-6578)
Indexed: Abstr.Hyg., Biol.Abstr., Chem.Abstr., Excerp.Med., Ind.Med. (coverage dropped), Ind.Vet., Nutr.Abstr., Rev.Appl.Entomol., Rev.Med.& Vet.Mycol., Trop.Dis.Bull.
—CASDDS, CISTI, GNLM, KNAW.
Published by: Taiwan Pediatric Association, 10F-1, No 69 Sec 1, Hangchow S. Rd, Taipei, Taiwan. TEL 886-2-351-6448, FAX 886-2-351-6446, pediatr@www.pediatr.org.tw, http://www.pediatr.org.tw. Ed. Ching Yuan Lin. Pub. Tsu Fuh Yeh. Circ: 3,000.

618.92 NOR ISSN 0803-5326 CODEN: APUPEI
ACTA PAEDIATRICA. SUPPLEMENT. Text in English. irreg. **Document type:** *Academic/Scholarly.*
Formerly (until 1991): Acta Paediatrica Scandinavica. Supplement (0300-8843)
Related titles: Online - full text ed.: (from ingenta, Swets Blackwell); ♦ Supplement to: Acta Paediatrica. ISSN 0803-5253.
Indexed: Dairy Sci.Abstr., Diar.Dis.Res., Excerp.Med., INIS Atomind., Ind.Med. (1992-), Ind.Vet., Int.Abstr.Biol.Sci., Nutr.Abstr., Protozool.Abstr.
—BLDSC (0642.402000), ADONIS, CASDDS, CISTI, EMDOCS, KNAW. **CCC.**
Published by: Scandinavian University Press (Subsidiary of: Taylor & Francis Ltd.), Postboks 2959, Toeyen, Oslo 0608, Norway. FAX 47-22-57-53-53, journals@scup.no, http://www.scup.no/paed.

618.92 ESP ISSN 0001-6640
ACTA PEDIATRICA ESPANOLA. Text in Spanish. 1943. m. (11/yr.). ESP 8,500 domestic; USD 80 foreign (effective 2001). adv. *Refereed.* **Document type:** *Journal, Academic/Scholarly.* **Description:** Contains original articles on pediatric medicine and translated abstracts from prominent literature.
Indexed: Chem.Abstr., Excerp.Med., Ind.Med.Esp., Nutr.Abstr.
—BLDSC (0644.300000), CISTI, EMDOCS, GNLM, Infotrieve, KNAW. **CCC.**
Published by: Ediciones Mayo S.A., Muntaner, 374-376 4o, Barcelona 08006, Spain. TEL 34-93-2090255, FAX 34-93-2020643, edmayo@app.es, http://www.edicionesmayo.es. Ed. Dr. I Villa Elizaga. Adv. contact Jose Mayoral. Circ: 8,000 (controlled).

618.92 ITA ISSN 0393-6392
ACTA PEDIATRICA MEDITERRANEA. Text in English, Italian. 1960. 3/yr. ITL 60,000; ITL 100,000 foreign (effective 1998). adv. abstr, bibl, illus, stat. index. **Document type:** *Proceedings, Academic/Scholarly.* **Description:** Clinical cases of pediatrics and newborns are reviewed and discussed.
Formerly: Archivio Siciliano di Medicina e Chirurgia (Sezione Pediatrica)
Published by: Carbone Editore, Via Gaetano Daita, 29, Palermo, PA 90139, Italy. TEL 091-321273, FAX 091-321782. Ed. Antonino Pennino. Pub., R&P Alfonsa Carbone. Adv. contact Donatella Donato. Circ: 3,000.

618.92 USA ISSN 1041-3499
RJ550 CODEN: AMSRER
ADOLESCENT MEDICINE (PHILADELPHIA). Text in English. 1990. 3/yr., latest vol.12, 2001. USD 89 domestic to individuals; USD 99 foreign to individuals; USD 39 newsstand/cover domestic; USD 39 newsstand/cover foreign; USD 114 newsstand/cover domestic to institutions; USD 124 newsstand/cover foreign to institutions (effective 2001). abstr, charts, illus, stat. 200 p./no. 1 cols./p. back issues avail. *Refereed.* **Document type:** *Monographic series, Academic/Scholarly.*
Indexed: C.C.I.P., Ind.Med. (1990-).
—BLDSC (0696.588000), GNLM, Infotrieve. **CCC.**
Published by: Hanley & Belfus, Inc., 210 S 13th St, Philadelphia, PA 19107. TEL 215-546-7293, FAX 215-790-9330.

ADVANCES IN CHILD DEVELOPMENT AND BEHAVIOR. see *PSYCHOLOGY*

618.92 USA ISSN 0732-9598
BF719
ADVANCES IN INFANCY RESEARCH. Text in English. 1981. a. USD 73.25. reprint service avail. from ISI. *Refereed.* **Document type:** *Academic/Scholarly.*
Indexed: PsycInfo, Psychol.Abstr. (1981-), e-psyche.
—BLDSC (0709.120000), CISTI, Infotrieve, ingenta. **CCC.**
Published by: Ablex Publishing Corporation (Subsidiary of: Greenwood Publishing Group Inc.), 88 Post Rd W, Westport, CT 06881. TEL 203-323-9606, FAX 203-357-8446, http://www.jaipress.com. Eds. Carolyn Rovee Collier, Lewis P Lipsitt.

618.92 USA ISSN 0065-3101
RJ23
ADVANCES IN PEDIATRICS. Text in English. 1942. a. USD 89 domestic; USD 95 foreign (effective 2001). illus. reprint service avail. from PQC. **Document type:** *Academic/Scholarly.* **Description:** Presents a collection of original, fully referenced clinical review articles in pediatrics.
Related titles: Microfilm ed.: (from PQC).
Indexed: CINAHL, Curr.Adv.Ecol.Sci., Dent.Ind., Diar.Dis.Res., INIS Atomind., Ind.Med. (1942-).
—BLDSC (0709.590000), CISTI, GNLM, KNAW.
Published by: Mosby, Inc. (Subsidiary of: Elsevier Science), 11830 Westline Industrial Dr, St Louis, MO 63146-3313. TEL 314-872-8370, 800-325-4177, FAX 314-432-1380, http://www.mosby.com/periodicals. Ed. Dr. Lewis A Barness.

618.92 DEU ISSN 1436-2651
AERZTLICHE PRAXIS. PAEDIATRIE. Short title: Ae P Paediatrie. Text in German. 1988. 12/yr. DEM 98; DEM 126 foreign (effective 1998). adv. **Document type:** *Trade.*
Former titles (until 1998): T und E Paediatrie (1435-1099); (until 1997): T W Paediatrie (0935-3216)
Indexed: Excerp.Med.
—BLDSC (1567.785500), EMDOCS, GNLM, Infotrieve. **CCC.**
Published by: Reed Elsevier Deutschland GmbH (Subsidiary of: Reed Elsevier group), Gabrielenstr 9, Munich 80636, Germany. TEL 49-89-89817-0, FAX 49-89-89817400, http://aep.r-e.de. Ed. Gabriele Fischer V Weikersthal. Pub. Wolfram Haase. Adv. contact Kurt Wiedenhoff.

618.21 649 DEU ISSN 1430-855X
AERZTLICHER RATGEBER FUER JUNGE ELTERN. Text in German. 1982. 3/yr. adv. **Document type:** *Consumer.* **Description:** Covers medical issues relevant to children up to the age of 4.
Formerly: Elternschule (0935-0837)
Published by: (Deutsches Gruenes Kreuz e.V.), Wort und Bild Verlag Konradshoehe GmbH, Konradshoehe, Baierbrunn 82065, Germany. TEL 49-89-74433-0, FAX 49-89-74433155. Ed. Dorothee Walzel. R&P Harald Pohl TEL 49-89-74433164. Adv. contact Christine Waeninger.

M

AERZTLICHER RATGEBER FUER WERDENDE UND JUNGE MUETTER; die Schwangerschaft, Geburt und Babyzeit. see *MEDICAL SCIENCES—Obstetrics And Gynecology*

610 362.7 GBR ISSN 1355-5626 CODEN: ACHEFY

AMBULATORY CHILD HEALTH. Text in English. 1995. q. GBP 66 in Europe to individuals; USD 113 in North America to individuals; GBP 73 elsewhere to individuals; GBP 72.60 in Europe to individuals print & online eds.; USD 124.30 in North America to individuals print & online eds.; GBP 80.30 elsewhere to individuals print & online eds.; GBP 199 in Europe to institutions; USD 338 in North America to institutions; GBP 219 elsewhere to institutions; GBP 218.90 in Europe to institutions print & online eds.; USD 371.80 in North America to institutions print & online eds.; GBP 240.90 elsewhere to institutions print & online eds. (effective 2001). adv. bk.rev. **Document type:** *Journal, Academic/Scholarly.* **Description:** Aims to encourage innovation in the early detection of clinical, developmental and social problems, and to promote multidisciplinary teamwork at clinic, organization and community levels.
Related titles: ♦ Online - full text ed.: Ambulatory Child Health Online. ISSN 1467-0658.
Indexed: CINAHL, Excerp.Med. (1996-).
—BLDSC (0809.214500), CISTI, EMDOCS, GNLM, KNAW.
Published by: Blackwell Science Ltd., Osney Mead, Oxford OX2 0EL, United Kingdom. TEL 44-1865-206206, FAX 44-1865-721205, journals.cs@blacksci.co.uk, http://www.blackwell-science.com. Eds. F Page Glascoe, F Oberklaid, R C Tamnhe. Pub. Elaine Stott. R&P Sophie Savage. Adv. contact Jenny Applin. Circ: 1,250 (paid).

610 362.7 GBR ISSN 1467-0658

AMBULATORY CHILD HEALTH ONLINE. Text in English. q. USD 102 in North America to individuals; USD 305 in North America to institutions; GBP 60 elsewhere to individuals; GBP 180 elsewhere to institutions (effective 2001). *Refereed.* **Document type:** *Academic/Scholarly.*
Media: Online - full text (from EBSCO Publishing, ingenta, Munksgaard & Blackwell Science's Synergy, Swets Blackwell). **Related titles:** ♦ Print ed.: Ambulatory Child Health. ISSN 1355-5626.
Published by: Blackwell Science Ltd., Osney Mead, Oxford OX2 0EL, United Kingdom. TEL 44-1685-206206, FAX 44-1685-721205, website@blacksci.com, journals.cs@blacksci.co.uk, http://www.blackwell-science.com.

618.92 USA ISSN 1530-1567

AMBULATORY PEDIATRICS. Text in English. 1964. bi-m. USD 150 in US & Canada; USD 180 elsewhere (effective 2001). adv. *Refereed.* **Document type:** *Academic/Scholarly.* **Description:** Focuses on the education of pediatricians, child health research, emergency medicine, research methodology, complementary and alternative medicine, child health policy and adolescent medicine.
Former titles (until 2001): Ambulatory Pediatric Association. Journal; (until 1998): Ambulatory Pediatric Association. Newsletter (0002-7006)
Related titles: Online - full text ed.: (from Institute for Scientific Information).
—BLDSC (0809.215600).
Published by: (Ambulatory Pediatric Association), Allen Press Inc., PO BOx 1897, Lawrence, KS 66044. TEL 786-843-1235, FAX 785-843-1274, apa@allenpress.com, http://www.allenpress.com/catalog/pdfs/amb_ped.pdf. Ed. James M Perrin.

618.92 USA ISSN 1080-0131
RJ1

AMERICAN ACADEMY OF PEDIATRICS. COMMITTEE ON INFECTIOUS DISEASES. RED BOOK (YEAR). Text in English. 1938. irreg., latest vol.24, 1997. USD 84.95 (effective 2001). **Document type:** *Monographic series.* **Description:** Includes the latest in clinical manifestations, etiology, epidemiology, diagnostic tests, and treatments for over 200 infectious diseases.
Formerly (until 1994): American Academy of Pediatrics. Committee on Infectious Diseases. Report (Year) (0065-6909)
Related titles: CD-ROM ed.
—BLDSC (7405.555000). **CCC.**
Published by: American Academy of Pediatrics, 141 Northwest Point Blvd, Box 927, Elk Grove Village, IL 60009-0927. TEL 847-228-5005, 800-433-9016, FAX 847-228-1281, http://www.aap.org.

618.92 IND

AMERICAN ACADEMY OF PEDIATRICS. JOURNAL. INDIAN EDITION. Text in English. 1989. bi-m. (in 13 vols., 3 nos./vol.). INR 400 (effective 2001). adv. 100 p./no. back issues avail. **Document type:** *Academic/Scholarly.* **Description:** Reports on important laboratory and clinical developments in pediatrics and pediatric medicine.
Published by: Manipal Centre for Media Research & Training, C T C Bldg., Manipal 576 119, India. TEL 91-8252-71201, FAX 91-8252-70062, bmj@manipal.edu, http://www.manipal.edu. Ed. Dr. Ramdas M Pai. adv.: B&W page INR 8,000, color page INR 12,000; trim 175 x 250. Circ: 12,000 (paid).

AMERICAN ASSOCIATION FOR PEDIATRIC OPHTHALMOLOGY AND STRABISMUS. JOURNAL. see *MEDICAL SCIENCES—Ophthalmology And Optometry*

648 SWE ISSN 1102-7207

AMNINGSNYTT. Text in Swedish. 1974. q. SEK 175; SEK 225 foreign (effective 1999). adv. bk.rev. **Document type:** *Bulletin.*
Published by: Amningshjaelpen, Fack 54, Rydsgard 27403, Sweden. TEL 46-411-44-333, FAX 46-411-44-333, rikskontor@amningshjalpen.se, http://www.amningshjalpen.se. Ed. Nanna Bylund. Pub. Malin Bergstroem. Circ: 2,000.

618.92 ESP ISSN 0302-4342 CODEN: AEPEDI

ANALES ESPANOLES DE PEDIATRIA. Text in Spanish. 1968. m. **Document type:** *Academic/Scholarly.*
Related titles: Online - full text ed.: (from Institute for Scientific Information); ♦ Supplement: Anales Espanoles de Pediatria. Suplemento. ISSN 0213-9146.
Indexed: Chem.Abstr., Dairy Sci.Abstr., Dent.Ind., Excerp.Med., Helminthol.Abstr., Ind.Med. (1968-), Ind.Med.Esp., Nutr.Abstr., Protozool.Abstr., Ref.Zh., Rev.Appl.Entomol., Rev.Med.& Vet.Mycol., Sugar Ind.Abstr.
—BLDSC (0889.045000), CASDDS, CINDOC, CISTI, EMDOCS, GNLM, IDS, Infotrieve, KNAW. **CCC.**
Published by: (Asociacion Espanola de Pediatria), Ediciones Ergon S.A., Placa Josep Pallach, 10, Barcelona 08035, Spain. TEL 34-93-428-5500. Circ: 5,000.

618.92 ESP ISSN 0213-9146

ANALES ESPANOLES DE PEDIATRIA. SUPLEMENTO. Text in Spanish. 1974. irreg.
Related titles: ♦ Supplement to: Anales Espanoles de Pediatria. ISSN 0302-4342.
Published by: Ediciones Ergon S.A., Placa Josep Pallach, 10, Barcelona 08035, Spain. TEL 34-93-428-5500.

618.92 FRA ISSN 0066-2097 CODEN: APSHAE

ANNALES DE PEDIATRIE. Text in French; Summaries in English. 1954. 10/yr. FRF 1,300 domestic to individuals; FRF 1,590 foreign to individuals; FRF 650 domestic to students; FRF 795 foreign to students (effective 1999). *Refereed.* **Document type:** *Academic/Scholarly.*
Indexed: ASCA, Bibl.Dev.Med.& Child Neur., Biol.Abstr., Chem.Abstr., Curr.Adv.Gen.& Molec.Biol., Curr.Cont., Dairy Sci.Abstr., Dent.Ind., Excerp.Med., Helminthol.Abstr., INIS Atomind., Ind.Med. (coverage dropped), Inpharma, Nutr.Abstr., Pharm.&Out.News, Protozool.Abstr., Reac., Rev.Med.& Vet.Mycol., Rural Devel.Abstr., SSCI (coverage dropped), Trop.Dis.Bull.
—CASDDS, CISTI, EMDOCS, GNLM, IDS, KNAW.
Published by: (Semaine des Hopitaux), Expansion Scientifique Francaise, 31 bd. de la Tour Maubourg, Paris Cedex 7 75343, France. TEL 33-1-40626400, FAX 33-1-45556920. Ed. J L Fontaine. Circ: 5,000.

618.92 GBR ISSN 0272-4936 CODEN: ATPAD9

ANNALS OF TROPICAL PAEDIATRICS. Text in English. 1981. q. USD 217, GBP 113 to individuals; USD 586, GBP 298 to institutions (effective 2001). adv. bk.rev. back issues avail. *Refereed.* **Document type:** *Academic/Scholarly.* **Description:** Provides an international forum for problems and achievements in child health and pediatrics in the tropics and subtropics.
Related titles: Online - full text ed.: ISSN 1465-3281 (from CatchWord Ltd., EBSCO Publishing, O C L C Online Computer Library Center, Inc., RoweCom Information Quest, ProQuest Information & Learning, Swets Blackwell, Institute for Scientific Information).
Indexed: ASCA, Abstr.Anthropol., Abstr.Hyg., Curr.Adv.Ecol.Sci., Curr.Cont., Dairy Sci.Abstr., Dent.Ind., Diar.Dis.Res., ERA, Environ.Sci.Poll.Mgmt., Excerp.Med., Helminthol.Abstr., IDA, Ind.Med. (1981-), Inpharma, Int.Abstr.Biol.Sci., Int.Nurs.Ind., Microbiol.Abstr., Mult.Ed.Abstr., NRN, Nutr.Abstr., Pharm.&Out.News, Pollut.Abstr., Protozool.Abstr., Reac., Rev.Appl.Entomol., Risk Abstr., Rural Devel.Abstr., SSCI (coverage dropped), Saf.Sci.Abstr., Sp.Ed.Needs Abstr., Stud.Wom.Abstr., Trop.Dis.Bull.
—BLDSC (1045.100000), CatchWord, CISTI, EMDOCS, GNLM, IDS, Infotrieve, ingenta, KNAW. **CCC.**
Published by: Carfax Publishing Limited (Subsidiary of: Taylor & Francis Group), PO Box 25, Abingdon, Oxon OX14 3UE, United Kingdom. TEL 44-1235-401000, FAX 44-1235-401550, enquiries@carfax.co.uk, enquiry@tandf.co.uk, http://www.carfax.co.uk. Ed. R G Hendrickse.

618.92 155.4 USA

ANNUAL EDITIONS: CHILD GROWTH & DEVELOPMENT. Text in English. 1994. a. USD 12.25. **Document type:** *Academic/Scholarly.*
Indexed: e-psyche.
Published by: Dushkin - McGraw-Hill, Sluice Dock, Guilford, CT 06437-9989. TEL 203-453-4351, FAX 203-453-6000. Eds. Chris J Boyatzis, Ellen N Junn.

618.92 FRA ISSN 0929-693X CODEN: APEDE4

ARCHIVES DE PEDIATRIE. Text in French; Summaries in English, French. 1993. m. EUR 290 in Europe to institutions; USD 364 in the Americas to institutions (effective 2002). adv. bk.rev. charts, illus. index. reprint service avail. from PQC. *Refereed.* **Document type:** *Academic/Scholarly.* **Description:** Publishes clinical and research articles in all areas of pediatric medicine.
Formed by the merger of (1912-1993): Pediatrie (0031-4021); (1942-1993): Archives Francaises de Pediatrie (0003-9764)
Related titles: Microfilm ed.: (from PQC); Online - full text ed.: (from ingenta, Institute for Scientific Information).
Indexed: ASCA, Abstr.Hyg., Bibl.Dev.Med.& Child Neur., Biol.Abstr., Chem.Abstr., Curr.Adv.Cancer Res., Curr.Adv.Ecol.Sci., Curr.Cont., Dairy Sci.Abstr., Dent.Ind., Excerp.Med., Helminthol.Abstr., Ind.Med. (1994-), Ind.Sci.Rev., Inpharma, Int.Nurs.Ind., Neurosci.Cit.Ind., Nutr.Abstr., Pharm.&Out.News, Protozool.Abstr., Reac., Rev.Appl.Entomol., Rev.Med.& Vet.Mycol., SSCI (coverage dropped), Sci.Cit.Ind., Sugar Ind.Abstr., Trop.Dis.Bull.
—BLDSC (1638.965000), CASDDS, CISTI, EMDOCS, GNLM, IDS, KNAW. **CCC.**
Published by: (Societe Francaise de Pediatrie), Elsevier Paris, Editions Scientifiques et Medicales (Subsidiary of: Reed Elsevier plc. group), 23 rue Linois, Paris 75015, France. TEL 33-1-45589110, FAX 33-1-45589419, arch-ped@elsevier.fr; academic@elsevier-fr.com, http://www.elsevier.com/locate/arcped, http://www.elsevier.fr; http://www.societefrancaisepediatrie.asso.fr. Eds. L David, M Odievre. Circ: 3,200.

618.92 GBR ISSN 0003-9888 CODEN: ADCHAK

ARCHIVES OF DISEASE IN CHILDHOOD. Text in English. 1926. m. GBP 164, USD 229 combined subscription to individuals includes print & online eds.; GBP 333, USD 534 to institutions for print only (effective 2002). adv. bk.rev. charts, illus. index. back issues avail.; reprint service avail. from PQC. *Refereed.* **Document type:** *Academic/Scholarly.* **Description:** Publishes a wide range of papers on all aspects of childhood health and disease for UK pediatricians and others worldwide.
Supersedes (1904-1944): British Journal of Children's Diseases (0366-2837)
Related titles: CD-ROM ed.: (from Ovid Technologies, Inc.); Microfilm ed.; Online - full text ed.: ISSN 1468-2044. 1997. GBP 80, USD 125 to individuals (effective 2002); Institutions contact publisher for online rates. (from HighWire Pr., Ovid Technologies, Inc., EBSCO Publishing, O C L C Online Computer Library Center, Inc., RoweCom Information Quest, ProQuest Information & Learning, ingenta, Swets Blackwell, Institute for Scientific Information); ♦ Supplement: Archives of Disease in Childhood. Fetal and Neonatal Edition. ISSN 1359-2998.

M

Indexed: AIM, AMED, Abstr.Anthropol., Abstr.Health Care Manage.Stud., Abstr.Hyg., Biol.Abstr., Brit.Nur.Ind., CINAHL, Chem.Abstr., Crim.Just.Abstr., Curr.Adv.Biochem., Curr.Adv.Ecol.Sci., Curr.Cont., Curr.Lit.Fam.Plan., Dairy Sci.Abstr., Dent.Ind., Diab.Cont., Diar.Dis.Res., Dok.Arbeitsmed., Environ.Sci.Poll.Mgmt., Excerp.Med., Fam.Ind., Helminthol.Abstr., INIS Atomind., Ind.Med. (1926-), Ind.Sci.Rev., Inpharma, Int.Abstr.Biol.Sci., Int.Nurs.Ind., Kidney, Maize Abstr., Med.& Surg.Dermat., Microbiol.Abstr., NRN, Neurosci.Cit.Ind., Nutr.Abstr., Pharm.&Out.News, Pollut.Abstr., Potato Abstr., Protozool.Abstr., Psychol.Abstr., Reac., Rev.Appl.Entomol., Rev.Med.& Vet.Mycol., Rev.Plant Path., Risk Abstr., Rural Devel.Abstr., Rural Recreat.Tour.Abstr., SSCI (coverage dropped), Saf.Sci.Abstr., Sci.Cit.Ind., Sugar Ind.Abstr., THA, Triticale Abstr., Trop.Dis.Bull.
—BLDSC (1634.200000), ADONIS, CASDDS, CISTI, EMDOCS, GNLM, IDS, ingenta, KNAW. **CCC.**
Published by: (Royal College of Paediatrics and Child Health), B M J Publishing Group, B M A House, Tavistock Sq, London WC1H 9JR, United Kingdom. TEL 44-20-7387-4499, FAX 44-20-7383-6400, info.norththames@bma.org.uk, http://www.archdischild.com/, http://www.bma.org.uk. Ed. H Marcovitch. Adv. contact Euan Currer TEL 44-20-7383-6181. **Subscr. to:** PO Box 590A, Kennebunkport, ME 04046.

ARCHIVES OF DISEASE IN CHILDHOOD. FETAL AND NEONATAL EDITION. see *MEDICAL SCIENCES—Obstetrics And Gynecology*

618.92 USA ISSN 1072-4710
RJ1 CODEN: APAMEB
ARCHIVES OF PEDIATRICS & ADOLESCENT MEDICINE. Text in English. 1911. m. USD 325 in North America to institutions; USD 425 to institutions Central & S. America; GBP 275 elsewhere to institutions (effective 2001). adv. bk.rev. abstr, bibl, charts, illus. index. back issues avail.; reprints avail. *Refereed.* **Document type:** *Academic/Scholarly.* **Description:** Publishes original clinical studies, practice commentaries, updates on clinical science and practice management articles. Provides a forum for dialogue on clinical, scientific, advocacy and humanistics issues relevant to the care of pediatric patients from infancy to young adulthood.
Former titles (until Jan. 1994): A J D C - American Journal of Diseases of Children (0002-922X); A M A American Journal of Diseases of Children (0096-8994)
Related titles: CD-ROM ed.: (from Ovid Technologies, Inc.); Microform ed.: (from PQC); Online - full text ed.: (from The Dialog Corporation, Gale Group, Ovid Technologies, Inc., EBSCO Publishing, Institute for Scientific Information).
Indexed: AIDS Abstr., AIM, ASCA, Abstr.Anthropol., Abstr.Hyg., Abstr.Inter.Med., Adol.Ment.Hlth.Abstr., Agri.& Environ.Biotech.Abstr. (coverage dropped), Bibl.Dev.Med.& Child Neur., Biol.Abstr., Biol.Dig., C.C.I.P., CINAHL, Chem.Abstr., Child Devel.Abstr., Crim.Just.Abstr., Curr.Adv.Ecol.Sci., Curr.Cont., Dairy Sci.Abstr., Derwent Biotech.Abstr., Diar.Dis.Res., Dok.Arbeitsmed., Environ.Sci.Poll.Mgmt., Except.Child Educ.Abstr., Excerp.Med., FAMLI, Fam.Ind., HRIS, Helminthol.Abstr., INIS Atomind., I.P.A., Ind.Med. (1994-), Ind.Sci.Rev., Inpharma, Int.Nurs.Ind., Jrnl.Watch, Jrnl.Watch Emer.Med., Jrnl.Watch Inf.Dis., Kidney, Med.& Surg.Dermat., NRN, Nutr.Abstr., Pharm.&Out.News, Pollut.Abstr., Protozool.Abstr., Psychol.Abstr., Reac., Rev.Appl.Entomol., Rev.Arom.& Med.Plants, Rev.Med.& Vet.Mycol., Rev.Plant Path., Risk Abstr., Rural Recreat.Tour.Abstr., SSCI (coverage dropped), Saf.Sci.Abstr., Sage Race Rel.Abstr., Sci.Cit.Ind., Soyabean Abstr., THA, Trop.Dis.Bull.
—BLDSC (1638.960000), CASDDS, CISTI, EMDOCS, GNLM, IDS, ingenta, KNAW. **CCC.**
Published by: American Medical Association, 515 N State St, P O Box 10946, Chicago, IL 60610-0946. ama-subs@ama-assn.org, http://www.archpediatrics.com, http://www.ama-assn.org/public/journals/ajdc/ajdchome.htm. Ed. Catherine D Deangelis. R&P Ada Jimenez Walker. Adv. contact Phillip B Altamore. Circ: 28,500.

618.9 ESP ISSN 0402-9054
ARCHIVOS DE PEDIATRIA* ; revista de formacion medica continuada. Text in Spanish; Summaries in English. 1950. 8/yr. ESP 9,000, USD 112 (effective 1997). adv. bk.rev. bibl, illus. index. back issues avail. **Document type:** *Academic/Scholarly.*
Indexed: Ind.Med.Esp., Nutr.Abstr.
—GNLM.
Published by: Universidad de Barcelona, Departamento de Pediatria, Hospital Sant Joan de Deu, Passeig de Sant Joan de Deu, 22, Esplugues 08950, Spain. TEL 34-93-205-1557. Eds. Dr. M Cruz, Dr. R Jimenez. Circ: 2,500.

618.92 URY ISSN 0004-0584
CODEN: APURAK
ARCHIVOS DE PEDIATRIA DEL URUGUAY. Text in Spanish; Summaries in English. 1929. q. USD 50. adv. bk.rev. abstr, bibl, charts, illus. index.
Indexed: Biol.Abstr., Excerp.Med., INIS Atomind., Ind.Med. (coverage dropped), Nutr.Abstr.
—CASDDS, GNLM.
Published by: Sociedad Uruguaya de Pediatria, Casilla de Correo 10906, Montevideo, Uruguay. TEL 79-18-01, FAX 78-52-13. Ed. Dr. Leopoldo F Peluffo. Circ: 1,250.

618.92 DOM ISSN 0004-0606
ARCHIVOS DOMINICANOS DE PEDIATRIA. Text in Spanish; Summaries in English. 1965. q. DOP 400 domestic; USD 25 foreign (effective 1999). adv. bk.rev. charts, illus, bibl. index, cum.index every 10 yrs. reprints avail. **Document type:** *Bulletin.*
Indexed: Abstr.Hyg., Ind.Med. (coverage dropped), Trop.Dis.Bull.
—CISTI.
Published by: Sociedad Dominicana de Pediatricas, Fernando Valerio 7, La Julia, Santo Domingo, Dominican Republic. TEL 809-532-7663, FAX 809-532-2564, emilio.mena@codefel.net.do. Ed. Emilio Mena Castro. Circ: 700.

618.92 VEN ISSN 0004-0649
ARCHIVOS VENEZOLANOS DE PUERICULTURA Y PEDIATRIA. Text in Spanish; Summaries in English. 1939. q. VEB 30. adv. bk.rev. bibl, charts, illus. index.
Indexed: Biol.Abstr., Chem.Abstr., Excerp.Med., Nutr.Abstr.
Published by: Sociedad Venezolana de Puericultura y Pediatria, Av. Libertador-Edf. La Linca, 9 piso, Ofc. 93a, Caracas 105, Venezuela. Ed. Dr. Eduardo Urdoneta. Circ: 2,000.

618.92 USA ISSN 0271-1346
AUDIO-DIGEST PEDIATRICS. Text in English. 1955. s-m. USD 168 (effective 2000). *Refereed.*
Media: Audio cassette/tape.
—Infotrieve. **CCC.**
Published by: Audio-Digest Foundation (Subsidiary of: California Medical Association), 1577 E Chevy Chase Dr, Glendale, CA 91206. TEL 213-245-8505, 800-423-2308, FAX 818-240-7379, 800-845-4375.

AUSTRALIA. BUREAU OF STATISTICS. CHILDREN'S HEALTH SCREENING. see *MEDICAL SCIENCES—Abstracting, Bibliographies, Statistics*

AUSTRALIA. BUREAU OF STATISTICS. CHILDREN'S IMMUNISATION, AUSTRALIA. see *MEDICAL SCIENCES—Abstracting, Bibliographies, Statistics*

AUSTRALIA PAEDIATRIC NURSE JOURNAL. see *MEDICAL SCIENCES—Nurses And Nursing*

▼ **BABY (KENNESAW).** see *CHILDREN AND YOUTH—About*

618.9 649 USA
BABY MAGAZINE INFANT CARE GUIDE* . Text in English. 1989. a. free to new parents. adv. back issues avail. **Document type:** *Consumer.* **Description:** Offers new parents tips on caring for their baby.
Formerly (until Aug. 1996): Bounty Infant Care Guide
Published by: Baby Magazine, 333 E 55th St, Apt 5F, New York, NY 10022-8325. TEL 212-986-1422. Ed. Jeanne Muchnick. Pub. Suzanne Robotti. R&P Dina Kaliko. Adv. contact John Knecht. B&W page USD 78,500, color page USD 103,500; trim 7.5 x 5.25. Circ: 3,700,000 (controlled).

BABY POST. see *CHILDREN AND YOUTH—About*

BABY - UNSER GLUECK. see *CHILDREN AND YOUTH—About*

618.92 AUS ISSN 1326-1665
BABYCARE BOOK. Text in English. 1984. a. adv. **Document type:** *Consumer.* **Description:** Focuses on 1st years of a baby's life.
Published by: Bounty Services Pty. Ltd. (Subsidiary of: Emap International), 187 Thomas St., Level 6, Haymarket, NSW 2000, Australia. TEL 61-2-9581-9555. Ed. Margaret Rafferty. Pub. Mandy Key. R&P Wisal Masri. Adv. contacts Dempster Clare, Sarah Fleischer. page AUD 14,760; trim 210 x 148. Circ: 230,000.

649.1 USA
BABYFIRST. Text in English. 1996. s-a. USD 18. **Document type:** *Consumer.*
Published by: KidStuff Publication, Inc., 1080 N Delaware Ave, Ste 702, Philadelphia, PA 19125-4330. TEL 215-551-3200, FAX 215-551-3203. Ed. Nancy Lisagor. Circ: 40,000.

618.92 GBR ISSN 0963-6714
RJ1
BAILLIERE'S CLINICAL PAEDIATRICS. Text in English. 1993. q. GBP 50 to individuals; GBP 90 to institutions. *Refereed.* **Document type:** *Academic/Scholarly.*
—GNLM, Infotrieve, KNAW. **CCC.**
Published by: Bailliere Tindall (Subsidiary of: Harcourt Publishers Ltd.), 24-28 Oval Rd, London NW1 7DX, United Kingdom. TEL 44-20-7485-4752, FAX 44—20-7267-4466, http://www.hbuk.co.uk. **Subscr. in N. America to:** W.B. Saunders Co., Journal Subscription Fulfillment, 6277 Sea Harbor Dr, 4th Fl, Orlando, FL 32887-4800. TEL 800-874-6418; **Subscr. to:** Journals Subscription Fulfillment, Foots Cray High St, Sidcup, Kent DA14 5HP, United Kingdom. TEL 44-20-8300-3322, FAX 44-20-8309-0807.

618.92 610.73 SWE ISSN 0349-1994
BARNBLADET; tidskrift foer Sveriges barnsjukskoeterskor. Text in Swedish. 1976. q. SEK 150; SEK 40 newsstand/cover (effective 2000 & 2001). **Document type:** *Trade.*
Published by: (Riksfoereningen foer Barnsjukskoeterskor/ Swedish Association of Pediatric Nurses), Via Media, Fack 640, Landskrona 26125, Sweden. TEL 46-418-10780, FAX 46-418-12394, viamedia@nornemark.com, http://www.nornemark.com/viamedia. Ed. Kerstin Hedberg Nyqvist. Circ: 2,600.

BEFORE BIRTH AND BEYOND; community newsletter. see *CHILDREN AND YOUTH—About*

618.92 POL ISSN 0303-7827
BIBLIOTEKA PEDIATRY. Text in Polish. 1974. irreg.
Published by: Polskie Towarzystwo Pediatryczne, Ul Kasprzaka 17 a, Warsaw 00211, Poland. TEL 48-2-6323451, FAX 48-2-6321862. Ed. Krystyna Bozkowa.

BRAIN AND DEVELOPMENT. see *MEDICAL SCIENCES—Psychiatry And Neurology*

362.7 USA ISSN 1527-8395
BROWN UNIVERSITY CHILD & ADOLESCENT PSYCHOPHARMACOLOGY; updates on research, use of psychotropic medications and specific interventions with children & adolescents. Text in English. 1997. m., latest vol.3, 2001. USD 174 domestic to individuals; USD 217 domestic to institutions; USD 227 in Canada to institutions; USD 237 elsewhere to institutions (effective 2001). 8 p./no. back issues avail.; reprints avail. **Document type:** *Newsletter.* **Description:** Includes updates on psychotropic medication as it relates to treating children and adolescents.
Formerly: Children's Services Report (1098-5182)
Published by: Manisses Communications Group, Inc., PO Box 9758, Providence, RI 02906-9758. TEL 401-831-6020, 800-333-7771, FAX 401-861-6370, manissess@manisses.com, http://www.manisses.com. Pub. Betty R Lang. R&P Barbara Deekle.

618.92 362.7 GBR ISSN 1361-5882
C A S CADE. Text in English. 1991. q. GBP 22.50 (effective 2001). bk.rev. 12 p./no. back issues avail. *Refereed.* **Document type:** *Magazine, Consumer.* **Description:** Covers topics in the medical and social care of children with medical conditions.
Formerly (until 1992): N A W C H Update
Indexed: Brit.Nur.Ind.
—BLDSC (3058.040000).
Published by: Action for Sick Children, 300 Kingston Rd, Wimbledon, London SW20 8LX, United Kingdom. TEL 44-20-8542-4848, FAX 44-20-8542-2424, enquiries@actionforsickchildren.org, http://www.actionforsickchildren.org/. Ed., R&P, Adv. contact Polly Moreton. Pub. Cheryl Hooper.

618.92 CAN ISSN 1205-5298
C P S NEWS. Text in English. 1954. bi-m. membership only. adv. bk.rev. **Document type:** *Newsletter.* **Description:** Promotes and highlights the accomplishments and activities of the society and its members. Provides members with information on services and coming events.
Formerly: Canadian Paediatric Society. News Bulletin (0831-7682)
Related titles: French ed.: Gazette S C P. ISSN 0831-7674.

M

Published by: Canadian Paediatric Society, 2204 Walkley Rd, Ste 100, Ottawa, ON K1G 4G8, Canada. TEL 613-526-9397, FAX 613-526-3332, http://www.cps.ca. Ed. Elizabeth Moreau. Adv. contact Paige Raymond. Circ: 2,500.

618.92 USA ISSN 0882-3421
CALIFORNIA PEDIATRICIAN✱ . Text in English. 1984. s-a. **Document type:** *Trade.* **Description:** Covers pediatric health care, practice management, and doctor-patient relationships.
Published by: American Academy of Pediatrics, California District, 2929 Health Center Dr, San Diego, CA 92123-2762. TEL 619-569-5019, FAX 619-560-6340. Ed. Marvin Averback. adv.: B&W page USD 1,500, color page USD 2,500; trim 11 x 8.5. Circ: 6,500.

618.92 CAN ISSN 1199-7044
CANADIAN PAEDIATRIC SOCIETY. ANNUAL REPORT. Text in English. a. **Document type:** *Corporate.*
Related titles: French ed.: Societe Canadienne de Pediatrie. Rapport Annuel. ISSN 1191-1980.
Published by: Canadian Paediatric Society, 2204 Walkley Rd, Ste 100, Ottawa, ON K1G 4G8, Canada. TEL 613-526-9397, FAX 613-526-3332.

CANDLELIGHTERS CHILDHOOD CANCER FOUNDATION QUARTERLY NEWSLETTER. see *MEDICAL SCIENCES—Oncology*

618.92 CZE ISSN 0069-2328
CODEN: CEPEA3
CESKO-SLOVENSKA PEDIATRIE/CZECHO-SLOVAK PEDIATRICS. Key Title: Ceskoslovenska Pediatrie. Text in Czech, Slovak; Summaries in Czech, English. 1945. m. EUR 132, USD 168 (effective 2001). adv. bk.rev. abstr. *Refereed.* **Document type:** *Academic/Scholarly.*
Formerly: Pediatrice Listy
Indexed: Chem.Abstr., Child Devel.Abstr., Curr.Adv.Ecol.Sci., Dairy Sci.Abstr., Dent.Ind., Excerp.Med., INIS Atomind., Ind.Med. (coverage dropped), Nutr.Abstr., Protozool.Abstr.
—BLDSC (3122.480000), CASDDS, CISTI, EMDOCS, GNLM. **CCC.**
Published by: (Ceska Lekarska Spolecnost J.E. Purkyne/Czech Medical Association), Nakladatelske Stredisko C L S J.E. Purkyne, Sokolska 31, Prague 12026, Czech Republic. TEL 42-2-24911420, FAX 42-2-24911420, nts@iol.cz, http://www.clsjep.cz, http://www.medical.cz. Ed. L Lisa. adv.: B&W page CZK 38,700, color page CZK 50,300; 250 x 165. Circ: 4,200. **Dist. by:** Abont s.r.o., Chlumova 17, Prague, 3 130 00, Czech Republic; **Dist. in Western Countries by:** Kubon & Sagner, Hesstr 39-41, Munich 80798, Germany.

618.92 JPN
CHIBA DAIGAKU SHONI GEKA NENPO/CHIBA UNIVERSITY. SCHOOL OF MEDICINE. PEDIATRIC SURGICAL DEPARTMENT. ANNUAL REPORT. Text in Japanese. 1978. a.
Published by: Chiba Daigaku, Igakubu, 8-1 Inohana 1-chome, Chuo-ku, Chiba-shi 260-0856, Japan.

618.92 362.7 AUS ISSN 1442-4886
CHILD & ADOLESCENT HEALTH CARE. Text in English. 1998. q. AUD 25 (effective 2001). bk.rev. back issues avail. **Document type:** *Newsletter.* **Description:** Provides updates and information on pediatric health care, non-medical and psychosocial needs of children and adolescents in the health care system in Australia.
Published by: Association for the Welfare of Child Health, PO Box 113, Westmead, NSW 2122, Australia. TEL 61-3-9633-1988, FAX 61-3-9633-1180, awch@enternet.com.au, http://www.uws.edu.au/community/awch/. Ed. Anne Cutler. Circ: 400.

618.92 616.89 USA ISSN 1056-4993
RJ499.A1 CODEN: CAPAF2
CHILD AND ADOLESCENT PSYCHIATRIC CLINICS OF NORTH AMERICA. Text in English. 1992. q. USD 146 domestic to individuals; USD 168 in Canada to individuals; USD 186 elsewhere to individuals; USD 194 domestic to institutions; USD 231 foreign to institutions; USD 58 per issue (effective 2001). index. back issues avail. *Refereed.* **Document type:** *Academic/Scholarly.* **Description:** Delivers practical advice from experts in specialty covered with a fresh perspective on problems and controversies.
Related titles: Microform ed.: (from PQC); Online - full text ed.: (from Institute for Scientific Information).
Indexed: Curr.Cont., Excerp.Med. (1995-), Ind.Med. (1992-), Int.Nurs.Ind., PsycInfo, SSCI, e-psyche.
—BLDSC (3172.913600), EMDOCS, GNLM, IDS, KNAW.
Published by: W.B. Saunders Co. (Subsidiary of: Harcourt Publishers Ltd.), 11830 Westline Industrial Dr, St Louis, MO 63146. TEL 215-238-7800, 800-325-4177, http://www.wbsaunders.com. Ed. Dr. Melvin Lewis. **Subscr. to:** Periodicals Fulfillment, W B Saunders Co, 6277 Sea Harbor Dr, 4th Fl, Orlando, FL 32891-4800.

CHILD AND ADOLESCENT PSYCHOPHARMACOLOGY NEWS. see *MEDICAL SCIENCES—Psychiatry And Neurology*

618.92 155.4 616.89 USA ISSN 0193-7421
CHILD BEHAVIOR AND DEVELOPMENT✱ . Text in English. 1975. irreg.
Indexed: e-psyche.
Published by: S P Medical & Scientific Books, Inc. (Subsidiary of: Spectrum Publications, Inc.), c/o Fisher, 200 Park Ave S, New York, NY 10003-1503.

618.92 GBR ISSN 0305-1862
CODEN: CCHDDH
CHILD: CARE, HEALTH AND DEVELOPMENT. Text in English. 1975. bi-m., latest vol.28, 2002. GBP 362 in Europe; USD 575 in North America; GBP 399 elsewhere (effective 2002). adv. bk.rev. bibl, charts, illus. index. back issues avail.; reprint service avail. from ISI. *Refereed.* **Document type:** *Academic/Scholarly.* **Description:** Promotes the study of all children, but particularly those handicapped by physical, developmental, emotional, and social problems. Looks at expansion of effective programmes of health promotion, care, and treatment.
Related titles: Microform ed.: (from PQC); Online - full text ed.: ISSN 1365-2214. GBP 326 in Europe; USD 518 in North America; GBP 326 elsewhere (effective 2002) (from Ovid Technologies, Inc., EBSCO Publishing, O C L C Online Computer Library Center, Inc., RoweCom Information Quest, ingenta, Munksgaard & Blackwell Science's Synergy, Swets Blackwell, Institute for Scientific Information).
Indexed: AMED, ASCA, ASSIA, Abstr.Hyg., Bibl.Agri., Bibl.Dev.Med.& Child Neur., Br.Educ.Ind., CINAHL, Child Devel.Abstr., Curr.Adv.Ecol.Sci., Curr.Cont., ERA, Except.Child Educ.Abstr., Excerp.Med., Fam.Ind., Ind.Med. (1975-), Inpharma, Int.Nurs.Ind., Lang.& Lang.Behav.Abstr., Mult.Ed.Abstr., Nutr.Abstr., Pharm.&Out.News, PsycInfo, Psychol.Abstr. (1975-), Psycscan D.P., Reac., SOPODA, SSCI, Soc.Serv.Abstr., Sociol.Abstr., Sp.Ed.Needs Abstr., Yrbk.Assoc.Educ.& Rehab.Blind, e-psyche.
—BLDSC (3172.925000), CISTI, GNLM, IDS, ingenta, KNAW. **CCC.**
Published by: Blackwell Science Ltd., PO Box 88, Oxford OX2 0NE, United Kingdom. TEL 44-1865-206180, 44-1865-206002, FAX 44-1865-206219, jnl.orders@blacksci.co.uk, http://www.blackwell-science.com/products/journals/cchd.htm, http://www.blackwellpublishing.com. Ed. S Logan. Pub. Elaine Stott. R&P Sophie Savage. Adv. contact Jenny Applin. Circ: 720.

CHILD DEVELOPMENT. see *CHILDREN AND YOUTH—About*

618.92 USA ISSN 1064-4849
CHILD HEALTH ALERT. Text in English. 1983. 10/yr. USD 29 domestic; USD 34 in Canada & Mexico (effective 2001). illus. index. 6 p./no. 3 cols./p. back issues avail.; reprints avail. **Document type:** *Newsletter.*
Related titles: Online - full text ed.: (from Gale Group, Northern Light Technology, Inc., ProQuest Information & Learning, Factiva).
Address: PO Box 610228, Newton, MA 02461. TEL 781-239-1762, FAX 781-431-7606, alert@us@mediaoke.net. Ed. Allen A Mitchell. Pub., R&P Paula L Mitchell.

CHILD PSYCHIATRY AND HUMAN DEVELOPMENT. see *MEDICAL SCIENCES—Psychiatry And Neurology*

CHILDREN & SOCIETY. see *CHILDREN AND YOUTH—About*

618.92 USA
CHILDREN'S HOSPICE INTERNATIONAL NEWSLETTER. Text in English. q. USD 45 (effective 1998). back issues avail. **Document type:** *Newsletter.* **Description:** Pediatric hospice care issues.
Published by: Children's Hospice International, 2202 Mt Vernon Ave 3C, Alexandria, VA 22301-1314. TEL 703-684-0330, FAX 703-684-0226. Circ: 5,000.

CHILD'S NERVOUS SYSTEM. see *MEDICAL SCIENCES—Psychiatry And Neurology*

CHILD'S PLAY. see *CHILDREN AND YOUTH—About*

618.92 ITA ISSN 0009-9058
CLINICA PEDIATRICA. Text in Italian; Summaries in English, French, German, Spanish. 1930. m. adv. bk.rev. abstr, illus. index. **Document type:** *Academic/Scholarly.*
Indexed: Biol.Abstr., Chem.Abstr., Dent.Ind., Excerp.Med., e-psyche.
—CISTI, GNLM.
Address: Via Giuseppe Massarenti, 11, Bologna, BO 40138, Italy. Ed. G Salvioli.

618.92 ITA ISSN 0393-7615
CLINICA PEDIATRICA DEL NORD AMERICA. Text in Italian. 196?. bi-m. ITL 220,000, USD 180 (effective 1999). reprint service avail. from PQC. **Document type:** *Academic/Scholarly.*
Published by: Piccin Nuova Libraria, Via Altinate, 107, Padua, PD 35121, Italy. TEL 39-049-655566, FAX 39-049-8750693.

616.8 USA ISSN 0735-2530
CLINICAL INFANT REPORTS. MONOGRAPH. Text in English. irreg., latest vol.6. price varies. *Refereed.* **Document type:** *Monographic series.*
Indexed: Psychol.Abstr.
Published by: (National Center for Clinical Infant Programs), International Universities Press, Inc., 59 Boston Post Rd, Box 1524, Madison, CT 06443-1524. TEL 203-245-4000, FAX 203-245-0775, http://www.iup.com.

618.92 616.02 GBR ISSN 1522-8401
▼ **CLINICAL PEDIATRIC EMERGENCY MEDICINE.** Text in English. 2000. q. USD 103 domestic to individuals; USD 141 foreign to individuals; USD 140 domestic to institutions; USD 180 foreign to institutions; USD 75 domestic to students; USD 85 foreign to students; USD 46 per issue domestic (effective 2001). **Document type:** *Journal, Academic/Scholarly.* **Description:** Devoted to helping pediatricians and emergency physicians provide the best possible care for their young patients.
Published by: W.B. Saunders Co. Ltd. (Subsidiary of: Harcourt Publishers Ltd.), 24-28 Oval Rd, London NW1 7DX, United Kingdom. http://www.wbsaunders.com. Ed. Dr. Steven E Krug.

618.92 616.4 JPN ISSN 0918-5739
CLINICAL PEDIATRIC ENDOCRINOLOGY. Text in English, Japanese. 1989. s-a. JPY 2,000 domestic to individuals; JPY 3,000 foreign to individuals; JPY 5,000 domestic to institutions; JPY 7,000 foreign to institutions. adv. **Document type:** *Academic/Scholarly.* **Description:** Serves as the official journal for the society. Includes case reports and clinical investigations.
—BLDSC (3286.324400).
Published by: Nihon Shoninaibunpi Gakkai/Japanese Society for Pediatric Endocrinology, Department of Pediatrics, Hokkaido University School of Medicine, N-15, W-7, Kita-ku, Sapporo 060-8638, Japan. TEL 81-11-716-1161, FAX 81-11-706-7896, ken-fuji@medlhokudai.ac.jp. Ed., R&P Kenji Fujieda. **Subscr. to:** I P E C Inc., 1-24-11 Sugamo, Toshima-ku, Tokyo 170-0002, Japan.

618.92 USA ISSN 0009-9228
RJ1 CODEN: CPEDAM
CLINICAL PEDIATRICS. Text in English. 1962. m., latest vol.40. USD 129 domestic to individuals; USD 167 foreign to individuals; USD 240 domestic to institutions; USD 270 foreign to institutions (effective 2001). adv. illus. index. 3 cols./p. back issues avail.; reprints avail. *Refereed.* **Document type:** *Journal, Academic/Scholarly.* **Description:** For practitioners in all areas of child care. Contains articles on pediatric practice, clinical research, behavioral and educational problems, community health and subspecialty or affiliated specialty applications.
Related titles: Microform ed.: (from PQC); Online - full text ed.: (from LexisNexis, Ovid Technologies, Inc., Northern Light Technology, Inc., ProQuest Information & Learning, Gale Group, Institute for Scientific Information).
Indexed: AIM, ASCA, Abstr.Hyg., Bibl.Dev.Med.& Child Neur., Biol.Abstr., C.C.I.P., CINAHL, Chem.Abstr., Child Devel.Abstr., Curr.Adv.Ecol.Sci., Curr.Cont., Dairy Sci.Abstr., Dent.Ind., Diar.Dis.Res., Environ.Sci.Poll.Mgmt., Excerp.Med., Fam.Ind., Hosp.Lit.Ind., INIS Atomind., Ind.Med. (1962-), Ind.Sci.Rev., Inpharma, Int.Abstr.Biol.Sci., Int.Nurs.Ind., Med.& Surg.Dermat., NRN, Nutr.Abstr., Pharm.&Out.News, Pollut.Abstr., Protozool.Abstr., PsycInfo, Psychol.Abstr. (1982-), Reac., Rev.Appl.Entomol., Rev.Med.& Vet.Mycol., Risk Abstr., SSCI (coverage dropped), Saf.Sci.Abstr., Sci.Cit.Ind., e-psyche.

M

—BLDSC (3286.325000), CISTI, EMDOCS, GNLM, ingenta, KNAW, Linda Hall.
Published by: Westminster Publications, Inc., 708 Glen Cove Ave, Glen Head, NY 11545. TEL 516-759-0025, FAX 516-759-5524. Ed. Dr. Ben H Brouhard. Pub. Timothy R McLaughlin. adv.: B&W page USD 925, color page USD 934; trim 8 x 10.5. Circ: 4,905.

618.92 USA
CLINICAL PEDIATRICS SERIES. Text in English. 1984. irreg., latest vol.8, 1995. price varies. adv. *Refereed.* **Document type:** *Monographic series.*
Published by: Marcel Dekker, Inc., Attn: Eridania Perrez, 270 Madison Ave, New York, NY 10016-0602. TEL 212-696-9000, 800-228-1160, FAX 212-685-4540, marketing@dekker.com, http://www.dekker.com. Pub. Russell Dekker. R&P Julia Mulligan. Adv. contact Eridania Perez.

612 GBR ISSN 0069-4835
CODEN: CDVMAG
CLINICS IN DEVELOPMENTAL MEDICINE. Text in English. 1959. q. GBP 176 to individuals; USD 253 to institutions (effective 2002). **Document type:** *Monographic series.* **Description:** Covers a wide range of circumstances affecting child development. Each thematic volume provides a comprehensive study of the theoretical and clinical aspects of a specific childhood condition or disorder.
Indexed: e-psyche.
—BLDSC (3286.550000), CISTI, GNLM, ingenta, KNAW. **CCC.**
Published by: Mac Keith Press, High Holborn House 49-51, High Holborn, London WC1V 6RL, United Kingdom. TEL 44-171-405-5355, FAX 44-171-405-5365, allat@mackeith.co.uk, http://www.cup.cam.ac.uk/journals/jnlscat/cdm/cdm.html; http://www.cup.org/journals/CUPJNLS.html. Ed. Martin C.O. Bax. R&P M Pountney. **Dist. by:** Cambridge University Press, Edinburgh Bldg, Shaftesbury Rd, Cambridge CB2 2RU, United Kingdom. TEL 44-1223-312393, FAX 44—1223-315052.

618.92 TUR ISSN 0010-0161
CODEN: CSHDAO
COCUK SAGLIGI VE HASTALIKLARI DERGISI. Text in Turkish; Summaries in English. 1958. q. USD 50 (effective 1999). adv. bk.rev. abstr, bibl, charts, illus. index. *Refereed.* **Document type:** *Bulletin.*
Indexed: Abstr.Hyg., Anim.Breed.Abstr., Biol.Abstr., Excerp.Med. (1992-), Nutr.Abstr., Rev.Appl.Entomol., Rev.Med.& Vet.Mycol., Trop.Dis.Bull.
—BLDSC (3292.760800), CISTI, EMDOCS, GNLM.
Published by: International Children's Center/Uluslararasi Cocuk Sagligi Merkezi, Samanpazari, P O Box 66, Ankara 06240, Turkey. FAX 90-312-3243284. Ed. Dr. Murat Yurdakok. Adv. contact Murat Tuncer. Circ: 1,500. **Co-sponsors:** Turkish National Pediatric Society; Hacettepe University, Institute of Child Health.

618.92 CAN ISSN 1182-7076
CONTEMPORARY PEDIATRICS. Text in English. 1993. bi-m. CND 36; CND 54 foreign. adv.
—Infotrieve. **CCC.**
Published by: Thomson Healthcare Communications, 1120 Birchmount Rd, Ste 200, Scarborough, ON M1K 5G4, Canada. TEL 416-751-8900, FAX 416-751-8126. Ed. Vil Meere. Adv. contact Alexandra Hamilton. B&W page CND 1,695, color page CND 2,790; trim 10.88 x 8.13. Circ: 10,402.

618.92 USA ISSN 8750-0507
CONTEMPORARY PEDIATRICS. Text in English. 1984. m. USD 89 domestic; USD 105 foreign; USD 10 newsstand/cover (effective 2001). adv. charts, illus, stat. index. reprints avail. **Document type:** *Trade.* **Description:** Contains clinical articles on prevention, diagnosis and treatment of illness from infancy through young adulthood; also reports on important trends in pediatric practices, including innovations in practice management.
Related titles: Microform ed.: (from RPI,PQC); Online - full text ed.: (from Gale Group).
Indexed: C.C.I.P., NRN.
—BLDSC (3425.197900), GNLM, Infotrieve, KNAW. **CCC.**
Published by: Medical Economics Co., Inc., 5 Paragon Dr, Montvale, NJ 07645-1742. TEL 201-358-7200. Ed. Catherine Brown. Circ: 39,000.

CRITICAL ISSUES IN DEVELOPMENTAL & BEHAVIORAL PEDIATRICS. see *PSYCHOLOGY*

CURRENT MEDICAL LITERATURE. PAEDIATRICS. see *MEDICAL SCIENCES—Abstracting, Bibliographies, Statistics*

618.92 USA ISSN 1040-8703
RJ1 CODEN: COPEE9
CURRENT OPINION IN PEDIATRICS. Text in English. 1989. bi-m. USD 211 domestic to individuals for print & online eds.; USD 211 foreign to individuals for print & online eds; USD 479 per issue domestic to institutions; USD 479 per issue foreign to institutions; USD 74 newsstand/cover (effective 2002). adv. bibl, illus. **Document type:** *Academic/Scholarly.* **Description:** Directed toward researchers and practicing pediatricians. Presents review articles followed by annotated bibliographies of references consulted. A bibliography of the current world literature published during the previous year is available.
Related titles: Online - full text ed.: USD 622.70 domestic academic site license; USD 622.70 foreign academic site license; USD 694.55 domestic corporate site license; USD 694.55 foreign corporate site license (effective 2002) (from Ovid Technologies, Inc., EBSCO Publishing, Swets Blackwell, Institute for Scientific Information).
Indexed: CINAHL, Curr.Cont., Excerp.Med., Ind.Med. (1989-), Inpharma, Int.Nurs.Ind., Reac.
—BLDSC (3500.776800), ADONIS, EMDOCS, GNLM, KNAW.
Published by: Lippincott Williams & Wilkins (Philadelphia) (Subsidiary of: Wolters Kluwer N.V.), 530 Walnut St, Philadelphia, PA 19106-3621. FAX 215-521-8902, 215-521-8902, http://www.Lww.com. Ed. Richard B Johnston Jr. Pub. Maria McMichael. R&P Tobias Weschler. Adv. contact Kelly Adamitis. **Subscr. to:** PO Box 1600, Hagerstown, MD 21740-1600.

618.92 IND ISSN 0971-9032
CURRENT PAEDIATRIC RESEARCH. Text in English. 1997. s-a. INR 3,600 domestic; USD 100 foreign (effective 1999). adv. bk.rev. 100 p./no. back issues avail. *Refereed.* **Document type:** *Journal, Academic/Scholarly.* **Description:** Publishes original research work in all major disciplines of pediatrics.
—BLDSC (3500.870000).
Published by: Scientific Publishers of India, 6B Manzar, Sir Syed Nagar, Aligarh, Uttar Pradesh 202 002, India. TEL 91-571-703043, FAX 91-571-702678. adv.: color page USD 200, B&W page USD 100.

618.92 GBR ISSN 0957-5839
CURRENT PAEDIATRICS. Text in English. 1991. 7/yr. GBP 85 to individuals; GBP 297 to institutions (effective 2002). adv. **Document type:** *Academic/Scholarly.* **Description:** Provides concise updates on clinical practice, delivery of care, technical procedures, innovations, legal matters and basic science.
Related titles: Online - full text ed.: (from EBSCO Publishing, O C L C Online Computer Library Center, Inc., Swets Blackwell, IDEAL Online Library).
Indexed: Ref.Zh.
—BLDSC (3500.900000), GNLM, KNAW. **CCC.**
Published by: Churchill Livingstone (Subsidiary of: Harcourt Publishers Ltd.), Robert Stevenson House, 1-3 Baxter's Pl, Leith Walk, Edinburgh, Midlothian EH1 3AF, United Kingdom. TEL 44-131-556-2424, FAX 44-131-459-1177, cservice@harcourt.com, http://www.harcourt-international.com/journals/cupe. Eds. J Tyrrell, P Cartlidge. R&P Catherine John TEL 212-424-4200. Adv. contact David Dunnachie. Circ: 890. **Subscr. to:** Harcourt Publishers Ltd., Foots Cray High St, Sidcup, Kent DA14 5HP, United Kingdom. TEL 44-20-8308-5700, FAX 44-20-8309-0807.

618.92 USA ISSN 0093-8556
RJ1
CURRENT PEDIATRIC DIAGNOSIS AND TREATMENT. Text in English. 1970. irreg., latest vol.12, 1994. **Document type:** *Monographic series.*
Published by: Appleton & Lange, Journal Division (Subsidiary of: Simon & Schuster Company), 11 W 19th St, New York, CT 10011-4209. TEL 203-406-4500, FAX 203-406-4600.

618.92 USA ISSN 0045-9380
CURRENT PROBLEMS IN PEDIATRICS. Short title: C P P. Text in English. 1971. 10/yr. USD 94 domestic to individuals; USD 109 foreign to individuals; USD 153 domestic to institutions; USD 168 foreign to institutions; USD 51 domestic to students; USD 64 foreign to students; USD 17 newsstand/cover (effective 2001). illus. cum.index. back issues avail.; reprint service avail. from PQC. **Document type:** *Journal, Academic/Scholarly.* **Description:** Provides monthly monographic clinical reviews from authorities in the field, intended for practitioners.
Related titles: Microform ed.: (from PQC).
Indexed: Adol.Ment.Hlth.Abstr., Excerp.Med., INIS Atomind., Ind.Med. (1970-).
—BLDSC (3501.390000), CISTI, EMDOCS, GNLM, ingenta, KNAW. **CCC.**
Published by: Mosby, Inc. (Subsidiary of: Elsevier Science), 11830 Westline Industrial Dr, St Louis, MO 63146-3318. TEL 314-872-8370, 800-325-4177, FAX 314-432-1380, periodical.service@mosby.com, http://www.mosby.com/cppeds, http://www.mosby.com/periodicals. Ed. Virginia A Moyer. Circ: 1,907.

618.92 GBR ISSN 0268-3792
CURRENT REVIEWS IN PAEDIATRICS. Text in English. 1985. irreg., latest vol.4. **Document type:** *Monographic series, Academic/Scholarly.*
Published by: Churchill Livingstone (Subsidiary of: Harcourt Publishers Ltd.), Robert Stevenson House, 1-3 Baxter's Pl, Leith Walk, Edinburgh, Midlothian EH1 3AF, United Kingdom. TEL 44-131-556-2424, FAX 44-131-459-1177, http://www.churchillmed.com. **Subscr. to:** Harcourt Publishers Ltd., Foots Cray High St, Sidcup, Kent DA14 5HP, United Kingdom. TEL 44-20-8308-5700, FAX 44-20-8309-0807.

CYSTIC FIBROSIS. see *MEDICAL SCIENCES—Abstracting, Bibliographies, Statistics*

618.92 USA ISSN 0893-9020
DAYCARE HEALTH; review and update for early childhood group care. Text in English. 1987. bi-m. (Oct.-Jun.). USD 27 (effective 1993). abstr, bibl. index. back issues avail. **Document type:** *Trade.* **Description:** Presents current information about health issues in child care.
Published by: Mathanna Publications, PO Box 5351, Bellingham, WA 98227-9970. TEL 206-671-4350. Ed. Paula B Kobos R N.

618.92 616.8 GBR ISSN 0012-1622
RJ1 CODEN: DMCNAW
DEVELOPMENTAL MEDICINE AND CHILD NEUROLOGY. Text in English. 1958. m. (plus up to four supplements). GBP 190 to individuals; USD 253 to institutions (effective 2002). adv. bk.rev. abstr. reprint service avail. from PQC. *Refereed.* **Document type:** *Academic/Scholarly.* **Description:** Covers a wide range of clinical topics involving diseases and neurological disabilities of children.
Related titles: Microfilm ed.: (from PQC); Online - full text ed.: (from EBSCO Publishing, O C L C Online Computer Library Center, Inc., RoweCom Information Quest, Swets Blackwell, Institute for Scientific Information).
Indexed: AMED, ASCA, Abstr.Hyg., Behav.Med.Abstr., Bibl.Dev.Med.& Child Neur., Biol.Abstr., Brit.Nur.Ind., CINAHL, Cadscan, Child Devel.Abstr., Curr.Cont., DSH Abstr., Dairy Sci.Abstr., Dent.Ind., Dok.Arbeitsmed., ERA, Environ.Sci.Poll.Mgmt., Except.Child Educ.Abstr., Excerp.Med., Fam.Ind., Helminthol.Abstr., INIS Atomind., Ind.Med. (1962-), Ind.Sci.Rev., Inpharma, Int.Abstr.Biol.Sci., Lead Abstr., Med.& Surg.Dermat., Ment.Retard.Abstr., NRN, Neurosci.Cit.Ind., Nutr.Abstr., Pharm.&Out.News, PsycInfo, Psychol.Abstr. (1962-), Reac., Rehabil.Lit., Rev.Med.& Vet.Mycol., Rural Devel.Abstr., SSCI (coverage dropped), Sci.Cit.Ind., Sp.Ed.Needs Abstr., Trop.Dis.Bull., Zincscan, e-psyche.
—BLDSC (3579.055000), CISTI, GNLM, IDS, ingenta, KNAW. **CCC.**
Published by: (American Academy for Cerebral Palsy and Developmental Medicine USA), Mac Keith Press, High Holborn House 49-51, High Holborn, London WC1V 6RL, United Kingdom. TEL 44-171-405-5355, FAX 44-171-405-5365, allat@mackeith.co.uk, http://www.cup.cam.ac.uk/journals/jnlscat/dmc/dmc.html; http://www.cup.org/journals/CUPJNLS.html. Ed. Martin C.O. Bax. R&P M Pountney. adv.: page USD 520. Circ: 4,500. **Dist. by:** Cambridge University Press, Edinburgh Bldg, Shaftesbury Rd, Cambridge CB2 2RU, United Kingdom. TEL 44-1223-312393, FAX 44—1223-315052. **Co-sponsor:** British Paediatric Neurology Association.

618.92 616.6 USA ISSN 0164-9507
DIALOGUES IN PEDIATRIC UROLOGY. Text in English. 1977. m., latest vol.24, 2001. USD 65 domestic; USD 70 foreign (effective 2001). charts, illus, bibl. index. 8 p./no. back issues avail. **Document type:** *Newsletter, Academic/Scholarly.* **Description:** Publishes clinical articles on pediatric urology and surgery. Each issue devoted to a specific theme.
—BLDSC (3579.775850), GNLM.
Published by: William J. Miller Associates, Inc., 45 Villa Rd, Pearl River, NY 10965. TEL 845-735-7853, FAX 845-735-6628, wmiller969@aol.com. Ed. Dr. Richard M Ehrlich. Pub. William J Miller. Circ: 650 (paid).

618.92 DEU
DOCUMENTA PAEDIATRIE. Text in German. 1976. irreg., latest vol.21, 1994. DEM 24 (effective 2000). **Document type:** *Monographic series, Academic/Scholarly.*

M

Published by: Hansisches Verlagskontor, Mengstr 16, Luebeck 23552, Germany. TEL 49-451-7031-01, FAX 49-451-7031253. Ed. Dr. Theodor Hellbruegge.

EARLY CHILD DEVELOPMENT AND CARE. see *CHILDREN AND YOUTH—About*

EARLY HUMAN DEVELOPMENT; an international journal concerned with the continuity of fetal and post natal life. see *MEDICAL SCIENCES—Obstetrics And Gynecology*

618.92 FRA ISSN 1245-1789
ENCYCLOPEDIE MEDICO-CHIRURGICALE. PEDIATRIA/ENCYCLOPEDIE MEDICO-QUIRURGICA. PEDIATRIA. Cover title: Tratado de Pediatria. Text in Spanish. 1998. 7 base vols. plus q. updates. bibl, charts, illus. *Refereed.* **Document type:** *Academic/Scholarly.* **Description:** Offers Spanish-speaking pediatricians a comprehensive and up-to-date reference for diagnosing and treating childhood ailments.
Related titles: ♦ French ed.: Encyclopedie Medico-Chirurgicale. Pediatrie. ISSN 0246-0513.
Published by: Elsevier Paris, Editions Scientifiques et Medicales (Subsidiary of: Reed Elsevier plc. group), 23 rue Linois, Paris 75015, France. TEL 33-1-45589110, FAX 33-1-44589425, redaction-emc@elsevier.fr, redacion-emc@elsevier.fr, http://www.elsevier.fr, http://www.elsevier.com.

618.92 FRA ISSN 0246-0513
ENCYCLOPEDIE MEDICO-CHIRURGICALE. PEDIATRIE. Cover title: Traite de Pediatrie. Variant title: Encyclopedie Medico-Chirurgicale, Instantanes Medicaux. Pediatrie. Receuil Periodique de l'Encyclopedie Medico-Chirurgicale. Pediatrie. Text in French. 1960. 7 base vols. plus q. updates. bibl, charts, illus. *Refereed.* **Document type:** *Academic/Scholarly.* **Description:** Offers pediatricians a comprehensive and up-to-date reference for diagnosing and treating diseases and conditions in their young patients.
Which was formed by the merger of (1950-1960): Encyclopedie Medico-Chirurgicale. Pediatrie, La Seconde Enfance (0246-0505); (1949-1960): Encyclopedie Medico-Chirurgicale. Pediatrie, La Premiere Enfance (0246-0491); Which superseded (1934-1949): Encyclopedie Medico-Chirurgicale. Pediatrie (0246-0483)
Related titles: ♦ Spanish ed.: Encyclopedie Medico-Chirurgicale. Pediatria. ISSN 1245-1789.
Published by: Elsevier Paris, Editions Scientifiques et Medicales (Subsidiary of: Reed Elsevier plc. group), 23 rue Linois, Paris 75015, France. TEL 33-1-45589110, FAX 33-1-45589425, redaction-emc@elsevier.fr, redacion-emc@elsevier.fr, http://www.elsevier.fr, http://www.elsevier.com.

ENDOCRINE DEVELOPMENT. see *MEDICAL SCIENCES—Endocrinology*

ENFANCE; psychologie, pedagogie, neuro-psychiatrie, sociologie. see *CHILDREN AND YOUTH—About*

618.92 GBR ISSN 1090-3798
CODEN: EJPNFO
EUROPEAN JOURNAL OF PAEDIATRIC NEUROLOGY. Text in English. 1997. bi-m. GBP 87 to individuals; GBP 187 to institutions (effective 2002). **Document type:** *Academic/Scholarly.* **Description:** Multidiscipline and international publication offers articles on clinical and experimental research.
Related titles: Online - full text ed.: (from EBSCO Publishing, O C L C Online Computer Library Center, Inc., Swets Blackwell, IDEAL Online Library).
Indexed: Ind.Med. (1997-), e-psyche.
—BLDSC (3829.733370), GNLM.
Published by: W.B. Saunders Co. Ltd. (Subsidiary of: Harcourt Publishers Ltd.), 24-28 Oval Rd, London NW1 7DX, United Kingdom. TEL 44-20-7424-4200, FAX 44-20-7424-4515, cservice@harcourt.com, http://www.harcourt-international.com/journals/ejpn. Ed. Victor Dubowitz. **Subscr. to:** Harcourt Publishers Ltd., Foots Cray High St, Sidcup, Kent DA14 5HP, United Kingdom. TEL 44-20-8308-5700, FAX 44-20-8309-0807.

M

EUROPEAN JOURNAL OF PEDIATRIC DERMATOLOGY (EDIZIONE ITALIANA). see *MEDICAL SCIENCES—Dermatology And Venereology*

EUROPEAN JOURNAL OF PEDIATRIC DERMATOLOGY (ENGLISH EDITION). see *MEDICAL SCIENCES—Dermatology And Venereology*

EUROPEAN JOURNAL OF PEDIATRIC SURGERY. see *MEDICAL SCIENCES—Surgery*

EUROPEAN JOURNAL OF PEDIATRIC SURGERY. SUPPLEMENT. see *MEDICAL SCIENCES—Surgery*

618.92 DEU ISSN 0340-6199
CODEN: EJPEDT
EUROPEAN JOURNAL OF PEDIATRICS. Text in English. 1910. m. EUR 2,008.20 domestic; EUR 2,000.70 in Germany; EUR 198 newsstand/cover foreign (effective 2002). adv. charts, illus. back issues avail.; reprint service avail. from ISI. *Refereed.* **Document type:** *Journal, Academic/Scholarly.* **Description:** Covers the whole broad field of pediatrics in all its aspects.
Incorporates: Acta Paediatrica Belgica (0001-6535); Helvetica Paediatrica Acta (0018-022X); Zeitschrift fuer Kinderheilkunde
Related titles: Microform ed.: (from PQC); Online - full text ed.: ISSN 1432-1076 (from EBSCO Publishing, RoweCom Information Quest, Swets Blackwell, Springer LINK, Institute for Scientific Information); ♦ Supplement: European Journal of Pediatrics. Supplement. ISSN 0943-9676.
Indexed: ASCA, Abstr.Hyg., Agri.& Environ.Biotech.Abstr. (coverage dropped), Bibl.Dev.Med.& Child Neur., Biol.Abstr., Chem.Abstr., Chem.Indus.Notes, Chem.Titles, Curr.Adv.Biochem., Curr.Adv.Ecol.Sci., Curr.Adv.Gen.& Molec.Biol., Curr.Cont., Dairy Sci.Abstr., Dent.Ind., Derwent Biotech.Abstr., Environ.Sci.Poll.Mgmt., Excerp.Med., Helminthol.Abstr., IBR, INIS Atomind., Ind.Med. (1975-), Ind.Sci.Rev., Ind.Vet., Inpharma, Kidney, Med.& Surg.Dermat., NRN, Neurosci.Cit.Ind., Nutr.Abstr., Pharm.&Out.News, Pollut.Abstr., Protozool.Abstr., Reac., Rev.Appl.Entomol., Rev.Med.& Vet.Mycol., Risk Abstr., SSCI (coverage dropped), Saf.Sci.Abstr., Sci.Cit.Ind., Soyabean Abstr., THA, Trop.Dis.Bull.
—BLDSC (3829.733500), ADONIS, CASDDS, CISTI, EMDOCS, GNLM, IDS, Infotrieve, ingenta, KNAW. **CCC.**
Published by: (Belgian Pediatric Association), Springer-Verlag (Subsidiary of: BertelsmannSpringer), Tiergartenstr 17, Heidelberg 69121, Germany. TEL 49-6221-345-0, FAX 49-6221-345229, subscriptions@springer.de, http://link.springer.de/link/service/journals/00431/index.htm, http://www.springer.de. Eds. B Steinmann, W Proesmans. **Subscr. in N. America to:** Springer-Verlag New York Inc., PO Box 2485, Secaucus, NJ 07096-2485. TEL 212-460-1500, FAX 212-473-6272.

618.92 DEU ISSN 0943-9676
CODEN: EJPSF
EUROPEAN JOURNAL OF PEDIATRICS. SUPPLEMENT. Text in German. irreg. **Document type:** *Monographic series.*
Related titles: ♦ Supplement to: European Journal of Pediatrics. ISSN 0340-6199.
Indexed: Excerp.Med. (1996-).
—ADONIS, Infotrieve, KNAW. **CCC.**
Published by: Springer-Verlag (Subsidiary of: BertelsmannSpringer), Haber Str 7, Heidelberg 69126, Germany. FAX 49-30-8214091, orders@springer.de, http://www.springer.de, http://link.springer-ny.com. **Subscr. in N. America to:** Springer-Verlag New York Inc., PO Box 2485, Secaucus, NJ 07096-2485. TEL 212-460-1500, FAX 212-473-6272.

EXCERPTA MEDICA. SECTION 7: PEDIATRICS AND PEDIATRIC SURGERY. see *MEDICAL SCIENCES—Abstracting, Bibliographies, Statistics*

618.92 688.72 DEU ISSN 1431-9543
FAMILIE & CO. Text in German. 1996. m. DEM 48 domestic; ATS 336 in Austria; CHF 48 in Switzerland; DEM 64.80 in Europe; DEM 123 elsewhere; DEM 4.50 newsstand/cover (effective 2001). **Document type:** *Magazine, Consumer.*
Related titles: Online - full text ed.
Published by: Axel Springer Verlag AG, Axel Springer Platz 1, Hamburg 20350, Germany. TEL 49-40-34722884, FAX 49-40-34725540, redaktion@familie.de, http://www.familie.de, http://www.asv.de. Ed. Beatrix Kruse. Adv. contact Claudia Krenn. Circ: 305,318 (paid).

618.92 GBR
FAMILY MEDICINE; medical advances in practice. Text in English. 1976. m. GBP 43 domestic to individuals; GBP 63 domestic to institutions; GBP 90 foreign to institutions (effective 2000). bk.rev. charts, illus. back issues avail. **Document type:** *Trade.* **Description:** Provides doctors with practical and focused articles on conditions commonly encountered in general practice.
Former titles (until 1997): Maternal and Child Health (0262-0200); (until 1991): Journal of Maternal and Child Health (0308-4426)
Indexed: Curr.Adv.Ecol.Sci.
—BLDSC (3865.567455). **CCC.**
Published by: Medpress (Subsidiary of: Inside Communications Ltd.), 8th Fl, Tubs Hill House, London Rd, Sevenoaks, Kent TN13 1BL, United Kingdom. TEL 44-1732-464190, FAX 44-1732-740772, harriett@medpress.co.uk; petersayer@medpress.co.uk, http://www.familymedicine.co.uk. Ed. Harriett Ainley. Pub. Peter Sayer. Adv. contact Neil Hobson. Circ: 25,000 (controlled).

FETAL AND MATERNAL MEDICINE REVIEW. see *MEDICAL SCIENCES—Obstetrics And Gynecology*

618.92 ITA ISSN 0390-5845
CODEN: GSLNAG
GASLINI; rivista di pediatria e di specialita pediatriche. Text in Italian. 1969-1996; N.S. 1998. 3/yr. ITL 96,000 to individuals; ITL 120,000 to institutions. adv. **Document type:** *Academic/Scholarly.* **Description:** Covers medical and surgical issues in the field of pediatrics.
—CASDDS, GNLM.
Published by: (Istituto Pediatrico Giannina Gaslini di Genova), Masson S.p.A., Divisione Periodici, Via F.lli Bressan 2, Milan, MI 20126, Italy. TEL 39-2-270741, FAX 39-2-27074210. Ed. Francesco Perfumo. adv.: B&W page ITL 1,850,000, color page ITL 2,600,000.

618.92 USA ISSN 1069-2460
GELLIS & KAGAN'S CURRENT PEDIATRIC THERAPY*. Text in English. 1964. irreg. **Document type:** *Monographic series.*
Formerly (until 1993): Current Pediatric Therapy (0070-2021)
—CISTI.
Published by: W.B. Saunders Co. (Subsidiary of: Harcourt Publishers Ltd.), 11830 Westline Industrial Dr, St Louis, MO 63146. TEL 800-325-4177, wbspcs@harcourtbrace.com, http://www.wbsaunders.com.

GROUPE D'ETUDE EN ORTHOPEDIE PEDIATRIQUE. LETTRE. see *MEDICAL SCIENCES—Orthopedics And Traumatology*

362.1 618.92 USA
GUIDELINES FOR HEALTH SUPERVISION. Text in English. 1985. irreg., latest vol.3, 1997. USD 44.95 (effective 2001). **Document type:** *Monographic series.* **Description:** Guidelines of doctor visits for children, newborn through age 21.
Published by: American Academy of Pediatrics, 141 Northwest Point Blvd, Box 927, Elk Grove Village, IL 60009-0927. TEL 847-228-5005, 800-433-9016, FAX 847-228-1281, http://www.aap.org.

618.92 CHN ISSN 1001-3512
GUOWAI YIXUE (ERKEXUE FENCE)/FOREIGN MEDICAL SCIENCES (PEDIATRICS). Text in Chinese. 1979. bi-m. USD 16.80; USD 2.80 newsstand/cover (effective 2001).
Published by: Zhongguo Yike Daxue/Chinese University of Medical Sciences, 6, Sanhao Jie 1 Duan, Heping-qu, Shenyang, Liaoning 393501, China. Ed. Li Yongxu. **Dist. by:** China International Book Trading Corp, 35, Chegongzhuang Xilu, Haidian District, Beijing 100044, China. TEL 86-1-68413849, FAX 86-1-68412048, cibtc@mail.cibtc.com.cn, http://www.cibtc.com.cn.

618.92 USA
HANDBOOK OF COMMON POISONINGS IN CHILDREN. Text in English. 1976. irreg., latest 1994. USD 44.95 (effective 2001). **Description:** Includes essential information on poison prevention, general management of acute poisoning, drugs used in poisoned patients, toxicity calculations, and specific poisons.
Published by: American Academy of Pediatrics, 141 Northwest Point Blvd, Box 927, Elk Grove Village, IL 60009-0927. TEL 847-228-5005, 800-433-9016, FAX 847-228-1281, http://www.aap.org.

HOME CARE FAMILY NEWSLETTER. see *SOCIAL SERVICES AND WELFARE*

618.92 HND ISSN 0018-4535
HONDURAS PEDIATRICA. Text in Spanish; Summaries in English. 1963. q. free per issue to qualified personnel. adv. abstr, bibl, charts, illus. index.
Published by: Asociacion Pediatrica Hondurena, P.O. Box 105-C, Tegucigalpa D.C, Honduras. Eds. Dr. Argentina Alas de Chavez, Dr. Oscar Gonzalez Ardon. Circ: 750.

618.92 AUS ISSN 1013-9923
HONG KONG JOURNAL OF PAEDIATRICS. Text in English. 1996. s-a. AUD 238 domestic; AUD 216 in New Zealand; USD 132 elsewhere; AUD 262 domestic print & online eds.; AUD 238 in New Zealand print & online eds.; USD 146 elsewhere print & online eds. (effective 2001). adv. **Document type:** *Journal, Academic/Scholarly.*
Related titles: ♦ Online - full text ed.: Hong Kong Journal of Paediatrics Online.
Indexed: Bibl.Asian Stud. (1990).
—BLDSC (4326.385800).
Published by: Blackwell Science Asia Pty Ltd, PO Box 378, Carlton South, VIC 3053, Australia. TEL 61-3-9347-0300, FAX 61-3-9347-5001, info@blacksci-asia.com.au, http://www.blacksci.co.uk/australi. Ed. Chap Yung Yeung.

618.92 AUS
HONG KONG JOURNAL OF PAEDIATRICS ONLINE. Text in English. s-a. AUD 215 domestic; AUD 195 in New Zealand; USD 119 elsewhere (effective 2001). **Document type:** *Academic/Scholarly.*
Media: Online - full text. **Related titles:** ♦ Print ed.: Hong Kong Journal of Paediatrics. ISSN 1013-9923.
Published by: Blackwell Science Asia Pty Ltd, PO Box 378, Carlton South, VIC 3053, Australia. TEL 61-3-9347-0300, FAX 61-3-9347-3016, info@blacksci-asia.com.au, http://www.blacksci.co.uk/australi.

618.92 ARG ISSN 0521-517X
HOSPITAL DE NINOS. REVISTA. Text in Spanish. 1959. 5/yr. USD 40 (effective 1997). adv. bk.rev. *Refereed.* **Document type:** *Academic/Scholarly.*
Published by: Asociacion Medica del Hospital de Ninos, Gallo, 1330, Capital Federal, Buenos Aires 1425, Argentina. TEL 54-114-9614609, FAX 54-114-9614609, bib-guti@pccp.com.ar, http://www.pccp.com.ar/guti. Ed. Jose A Bodino. Circ: 2,000.

618.92 CAN ISSN 1494-1015
THE HOSPITAL FOR SICK CHILDREN JOURNAL. Text in English. 1984. q.
Supersedes in part (in 1999): Kaleidoscope (Toronto) (0828-2730); Which was formerly (until 1984): What's New - Hospital for Sick Children (0049-7533); (until 1970): What's New at H S C? (0827-1232)
Published by: Hospital for Sick Children, 555 University Ave, Toronto, ON M5G 1X8, Canada. FAX 416-813-5328, http://www.sickkids.on.ca. Ed. John Pires TEL 416-813-5328. Circ: 30,000.

HOSPITAL FOR SICK CHILDREN, TORONTO. RESEARCH INSTITUTE. ANNUAL REPORT. see *HEALTH FACILITIES AND ADMINISTRATION*

HOSPITAL INFANTIL DE MEXICO. BOLETIN MEDICO. see *HEALTH FACILITIES AND ADMINISTRATION*

IMAGO; giornale italiano de psicopatologia e psichiatria dell'infanzia e dell'adolescenza. see *MEDICAL SCIENCES—Psychiatry And Neurology*

618.92 IND ISSN 0019-5456
CODEN: IJPEA2
INDIAN JOURNAL OF PEDIATRICS. Text in English. 1933. bi-m. INR 600, USD 60 to individuals; INR 1,350, USD 350 to institutions; INR 500, USD 50 to students (effective 2001). adv. bk.rev. abstr, charts. index. reprint service avail. from PQC. **Document type:** *Academic/Scholarly.* **Description:** Features discussions on pediatric emergencies, current issues, clinical and technological techniques, and neonatology. Includes pharmacology and nutrition.
Related titles: Microfilm ed.: (from PQC).
Indexed: Biol.Abstr., Chem.Abstr., Child Devel.Abstr., DSH Abstr., Dairy Sci.Abstr., Dent.Ind., Diar.Dis.Res., Environ.Sci.Poll.Mgmt., Excerp.Med. (1993-), INIS Atomind., Ind.Med. (1933-), Nutr.Abstr., Pollut.Abstr., Rev.Med.& Vet.Mycol., Risk Abstr., Rural Ext.Educ.& Tr.Abstr., Saf.Sci.Abstr.
—BLDSC (4418.000000), CISTI, GNLM, KNAW.
Published by: (All India Institute of Medical Sciences, Department of Pediatrics), Scientific Publishers, 5-A New Pali Rd., P O Box 91, Jodhpur, Rajasthan 342 001, India. TEL 91-291-433323, FAX 91-291-512580, scienti@sancharnet.in, http://www.scientificpub.com. Ed. Dr. I C Verma. R&P I.C. Verma. Adv. contact Rajiv Dhir. Circ: 3,000. **Subscr. to:** c/o Dr. I.C. Verma, Editor-in-Chief, 125 (2nd Fl.), Gautam Nagar, P O Box 3875, New Delhi 110 049, India. TEL 91-11-6857587, FAX 91-11-6854434.

618.92 IND ISSN 0019-6061
RJ1 CODEN: INPDAR
INDIAN PEDIATRICS. Text in English. 1964. m. INR 250, USD 220 (effective 2001). adv. bk.rev. charts, illus. reprint service avail. from IRC.
Formed by the merger of (1952-1963): Indian Journal of Child Health (0445-7684); (1962-1963): Indian Pediatric Society. Journal (0537-2380)
Indexed: Abstr.Hyg., Biol.Abstr., Chem.Abstr., Curr.Adv.Ecol.Sci., Dairy Sci.Abstr., Dent.Ind., Diar.Dis.Res., Excerp.Med., Helminthol.Abstr., INIS Atomind., Ind.Med. (1964-), Indian Sci.Abstr., Maize Abstr., Nutr.Abstr., Protozool.Abstr., Rev.Appl.Entomol., Rev.Med.& Vet.Mycol., Rural Devel.Abstr., Triticale Abstr., Trop.Dis.Bull.
—BLDSC (4425.280000), CASDDS, CISTI, EMDOCS, GNLM, ingenta, KNAW.
Published by: (Indian Academy of Pediatrics), Scientific Publishers, 5-A New Pali Rd., P O Box 91, Jodhpur, Rajasthan 342 001, India. TEL 91-291-433323, FAX 91-291-512580, scienti@sancharnet.in, http://www.scientificpub.com. Ed. Dr. R N Srivastava. Circ: 4,800. **Dist. by:** Scientific Distribution Service, 5-A Bhagat-ko-kothi, P O Box 33, Jodhpur, Rajasthan 342 001, India.

▼ **INFANCY.** see *CHILDREN AND YOUTH—About*

INFANT BEHAVIOR AND DEVELOPMENT; an international & interdisciplinary journal. see *PSYCHOLOGY*

155.422 USA ISSN 0163-9641
RJ502.5 CODEN: IMHJDZ
INFANT MENTAL HEALTH JOURNAL. Text in English. 1980. q. USD 275 in United States; USD 323 in Canada & Mexico; USD 323 elsewhere; USD 289 combined subscription in United States for print and online eds.; USD 337 combined subscription in Canada & Mexico for print and online eds.; USD 337 combined subscription elsewhere for print and online eds. (effective 2002). adv. back issues avail.; reprint service avail. from PQC,ISI. *Refereed.* **Document type:** *Academic/Scholarly.* **Description:** Focuses on infant social-emotional development, caregiver-infant interactions, contextual and cultural influences on infant and family development, and all conditions that place infants and their families at risk for less than optimal development.
Related titles: Online - full text ed.: ISSN 1097-0355. 1996. USD 275 in United States; USD 275 in Canada & Mexico; USD 275 elsewhere (effective 2002) (from EBSCO Publishing, Wiley InterScience, Institute for Scientific Information).
Indexed: ASCA, Child Devel.Abstr., Curr.Cont., Excerp.Med., Fam.Ind., IMFL, Indian Psychol.Abstr., Lang.& Lang.Behav.Abstr., PsycInfo, Psychol.Abstr. (1980-), SSCI, Sociol.Abstr., e-psyche.
—BLDSC (4478.274000), CISTI, GNLM, IDS, ingenta. **CCC.**
Published by: (Michigan Association for Infant Mental Health), John Wiley & Sons, Inc., Journals (Subsidiary of: Wiley InterScience), 605 Third Ave, New York, NY 10158. TEL 212-850-6645, FAX 212-850-6021, subinfo@wiley.com, uscs-wis@wiley.com, http://www.wiley.com. Ed. Dr. Joy D Osofsky. adv.: B&W page GBP 640, color page GBP 1,515; trim 172 x 254. Circ: 1,050. **Subscr. outside the Americas to:** John Wiley & Sons Ltd., Baffins Ln, Chichester, Sussex PO19 IUD, United Kingdom. TEL 44-1243-779777, FAX 44-1243-843232, cs-journals@wiley.co.uk, http://www.wiley.co.uk.

618.92 GBR ISSN 1369-8036
INFANT OBSERVATION; the international journal of infant observation and its applications. Variant title: International Journal of Infant Observation. Text in English. 1997. 3/yr. GBP 30 to individuals; GBP 50 to institutions; GBP 20 to students. **Document type:** *Academic/Scholarly.* **Description:** Reflects the way in which the disciplines of psychology, psychiatry and the social sciences may be aided and enhanced by the depth of psychoanalytical infant observation.
—BLDSC (4478.277500).
Published by: Tavistock Clinic Foundation, 120 Belsize Ln, London NW3 5BA, United Kingdom. TEL 44-171-435-7111. Ed. Maureen Black. **Co-sponsor:** University of East London Press.

618.92 616.8 USA ISSN 0886-1315
INFANT SCREENING. Text in English. 1979. 4/yr. USD 15; USD 18 foreign. **Document type:** *Newsletter.*
Indexed: e-psyche.
Address: 3907 Galacia Dr, Austin, TX 78759. TEL 512-345-5685. Ed. Dr. Brad Therrell.

618.92 USA ISSN 1053-5586
RG580.D76 CODEN: IINTFZ
INFANT - TODDLER INTERVENTION; the transdisciplinary journal. Text in English. 1991. q. USD 45 to individuals; USD 90 to institutions. adv. bk.rev. *Refereed.* **Document type:** *Academic/Scholarly.* **Description:** Provides all members of the early intervention team with information that will enhance the clinical service they provide to infants and toddlers who are at risk or have disabilities.
Indexed: C.I.J.E., CINAHL, Except.Child Educ.Abstr., Lang.& Lang.Behav.Abstr., PsycInfo, SOPODA, Sociol.Abstr., e-psyche.
—BLDSC (4478.279500), Infotrieve. **CCC.**
Published by: Singular Publishing Group, Inc., 401 W A St, Ste 325, San Diego, CA 92101-7961. TEL 800-521-8545, FAX 800-774-8398, singpub@mail.cerfnet.com. Ed. Louis M Rossetti. Pub., Adv. contact Angie Singh. Circ: 1,500 (paid).

618.92 649 USA ISSN 0896-3746
RJ102 CODEN: IYCHEL
INFANTS AND YOUNG CHILDREN; an interdisciplinary journal of special care practices. Text in English. 1988. q. USD 135 to individuals; USD 41 newsstand/cover (effective 2002). *Refereed.* **Document type:** *Journal.* **Description:** Devoted to the clinical management of infants and young children (birth to three years of age) with, or at risk for, developmental disabilities. Provides current applications of educational, therapeutic, diagnostic, and family support concepts to practice settings.
Related titles: Online - full text ed.: (from ProQuest Information & Learning, Institute for Scientific Information).
Indexed: ASCA, C.I.J.E., CINAHL, Curr.Cont., Except.Child Educ.Abstr., Fam.Ind., IMFL, Lang.& Lang.Behav.Abstr., Nurs.Abstr., SOPODA, SSCI, Sociol.Abstr.
—BLDSC (4478.283000), IDS, Infotrieve, ingenta. **CCC.**
Published by: Aspen Publishers, Inc., 200 Orchard Ridge Dr, Ste 200, Gaithersburg, MD 20878. TEL 301-417-7500, 800-638-8437, FAX 301-417-7550, customer.service@aspenpul.com, http://www.aspenpub.com. **Dist. by:** Aspen Publishers Inc., Distribution Center, 7201 McKinney Circle, Frederick, MD 21701. TEL 301-698-7100, FAX 301-695-7931.

618.92 USA ISSN 1044-9779
INFECTIOUS DISEASES IN CHILDREN. Text in English. 1988. m. USD 170 domestic to individuals; USD 195 in Canada to individuals; USD 210 elsewhere to individuals; USD 180 domestic to institutions; USD 205 in Canada to institutions; USD 220 elsewhere to institutions. **Document type:** *Academic/Scholarly.* **Description:** Covers new drugs and procedures for diagnosing and treating pediatric infectious diseases.
—Infotrieve. **CCC.**
Published by: Slack, Inc., 6900 Grove Rd, Thorofare, NJ 08086-9447. TEL 856-848-1000, 800-257-8290, FAX 856-853-5991, idc@slackinc.com, http://www.slackinc.com/child/idc/. Ed. Dr. Philip A Brunell. Circ: 33,000.

614.19 USA
INFORMATION EXCHANGE. Text in English. 1983. irreg. *Refereed.* **Document type:** *Newsletter.* **Description:** Provides a national forum for exchange of information and resources on SIDS, death investigation, apnea, grief of parents and the role of professionals dealing with families suffering a SIDS loss.
Published by: National Sudden Infant Death Syndrome Resource Center, 2070 Chain Bridge Rd, Ste 450, Vienna, VA 22182-2536. TEL 703-821-8955, FAX 703-821-2098, sids@circsol.com, http://www.circsol.com/sids. Circ: 2,600.

618.92 GBR ISSN 1353-8047
HV675.72
INJURY PREVENTION. Text in English. 1995. q. GBP 81, USD 130 combined subscription to individuals includes print & online eds.; GBP 159, USD 255 to institutions (effective 2002). adv. bk.rev. charts, illus. index. reprint service avail. from PQC. *Refereed.* **Document type:** *Academic/Scholarly.* **Description:** Publishes papers that focus on the prevention of unintentional or intentional injury in the young.
Related titles: Microfilm ed.: (from PQC); Online - full text ed.: (from EBSCO Publishing, O C L C Online Computer Library Center, Inc., RoweCom Information Quest, ingenta).
Indexed: CINAHL, Ind.Med. (1995-), Int.Nurs.Ind.
—BLDSC (4514.435000), GNLM, Infotrieve, KNAW. **CCC.**

M

Published by: (International Society for Childhood and Adolescent Injury Prevention), B M J Publishing Group, B M A House, Tavistock Sq, London WC1H 9JR, United Kingdom. TEL 44-20-7387-4499, FAX 44-20-7383-6400, info.norththames@bma.org.uk, http://www.injuryprevention.com/, http://www.bma.org.uk. Ed. I B Pless. Pub. Alex Williamson. R&P Carol Torselli TEL 44-20-7383-6674. Adv. contact Euan Currer TEL 44-20-7383-6181.

618.92 USA
INJURY PREVENTION AND CONTROL FOR CHILDREN AND YOUTH. Text in English. 1987. irreg. USD 44.95 (effective 2001). **Document type:** *Monographic series.*
Formerly: Injury Control for Children and Youth
Published by: American Academy of Pediatrics, 141 Northwest Point Blvd, Box 927, Elk Grove Village, IL 60009-0927. TEL 847-228-5005, 800-433-9016, FAX 847-228-1281, http://www.aap.org.

618.92 USA ISSN 1016-8699
INTERNATIONAL CHILD HEALTH: A DIGEST OF CURRENT INFORMATION. Text in English. 1990. q. USD 48. **Document type:** *Academic/Scholarly.*
Indexed: Diar.Dis.Res.
—GNLM.
Published by: International Pediatric Association/ Association Internationale de Pediatrie, Univ of Rochester, School of Medicine, 601 Elmwood Ave, Rm 4 8104, Rochester, NY 14642-8777. TEL 716-275-0225, FAX 716-273-10387. Circ: 6,500. **Co-sponsors:** UNICEF; World Health Organization.

610 USA
INTERNATIONAL GUILD FOR INFANT SURVIVAL NEWSLETTER*. Text in English. 1965. bi-m. USD 1. stat.
Published by: International Council for Infant Survival, c/o Council of Guilds, 9178 Nadne River Circle, Fountain Valley, CA 92708. TEL 319-322-4870. Ed. Mrs. William Reuling. Circ: 500.

618.92 ISR ISSN 0334-0139
CODEN: IJAHE8
INTERNATIONAL JOURNAL OF ADOLESCENT MEDICINE AND HEALTH. Text in English. 1985. q., latest vol.14. USD 260 (effective 2002). adv. bk.rev. back issues avail. **Document type:** *Academic/Scholarly.*
Indexed: Curr.Adv.Ecol.Sci., Excerp.Med., PsycInfo, Psychol.Abstr. (1985-), e-psyche.
—BLDSC (4541.565000), EMDOCS, GNLM, KNAW.
Published by: Freund Publishing House, Ltd., P O Box 35010, Tel Aviv 61350, Israel. TEL 972-3-562-8540, FAX 972-3-562-8538, h_freund@netvision.net.il, http://www.angelfire.com/il/freund. Ed. J. Merrick. Circ: 1,000.

INTERNATIONAL JOURNAL OF CHILDBIRTH EDUCATION. see *MEDICAL SCIENCES—Obstetrics And Gynecology*

INTERNATIONAL JOURNAL OF PEDIATRIC HEMATOLOGY - ONCOLOGY. see *MEDICAL SCIENCES—Oncology*

INTERNATIONAL JOURNAL OF PEDIATRIC OTORHINOLARYNGOLOGY. see *MEDICAL SCIENCES—Otorhinolaryngology*

618.92 USA ISSN 0074-7300
INTERNATIONAL PEDIATRIC ASSOCIATION. PROCEEDINGS OF CONGRESS. Text in English. triennial, latest vol.19, 1989. **Document type:** *Proceedings.*
Published by: International Pediatric Association/ Association Internationale de Pediatrie, Univ of Rochester, School of Medicine, 601 Elmwood Ave, Rm 4 8104, Rochester, NY 14642-8777. TEL 716-275-0225, FAX 716-273-1038.

INTERNATIONAL PEDIATRICS. see *MEDICAL SCIENCES—Surgery*

INTERNATIONAL REVIEW OF CHILD NEUROLOGY SERIES. see *MEDICAL SCIENCES—Psychiatry And Neurology*

INTERNATIONAL SEMINARS IN PAEDIATRIC GASTROENTEROLOGY AND NUTRITION. see *MEDICAL SCIENCES—Gastroenterology*

618.92 USA ISSN 1528-8374
▼ **THE INTERNET JOURNAL OF PEDIATRICS AND NEONATOLOGY.** Text in English. 2000. s-a. free per issue. adv. bk.rev., Website rev. back issues avail. *Refereed.* **Document type:** *Journal, Academic/Scholarly.* **Description:** Provides information from the field of pediatrics and neonatology; contains original articles, reviews, case reports, streaming slide shows, streaming videos, letters to the editor, press releases and meeting information.
Formerly: The Internet Journal of Neonatology
Media: Online - full content.
Published by: Internet Scientific Publications, L.L.C., 23 Rippling Creek Dr, Sugar Land, TX 77479. TEL 281-240-1533, FAX 281-240-1533, http://www.ispub.com/. R&P, Adv. contact Oliver Wenker TEL 832-754-0335.

ISSUES IN COMPREHENSIVE PEDIATRIC NURSING. see *MEDICAL SCIENCES—Nurses And Nursing*

618.92 649 DEU
JA ZUM BABY; medizinischer Ratgeber fuer werdende und junge Eltern. Text in German. 3/yr. adv. **Document type:** *Magazine, Consumer.*
Published by: Marken-Verlag GmbH, Hugo-Junkers-Str 20, Cologne 50739, Germany. TEL 49-221-957427-0, FAX 49-221-95742777, marken-info@markenverlag.de, http://www.markenverlag.de. Adv. contact Frank Krauthaeuser. B&W page DEM 23,980, color page DEM 43,164. Circ: 285,000 (paid and controlled).

618.92 JPN ISSN 0021-518X
JAPANESE JOURNAL OF PEDIATRICS/SHONIKA RINSHO. Text in Japanese. 1948. m. JPY 1,900 newsstand/cover.
Indexed: Chem.Abstr., INIS Atomind.
—BLDSC (4656.950000), CISTI.
Published by: Nihon Shoni Iji Shuppansha, Wakodo, 24-18 Nishishinjuku 5-chome, Shinjuku-ku, Tokyo 100-0000, Japan.

618.92 DEU ISSN 1432-5160
JATROS PAED. Text in German. 1985. 12/yr. DEM 140 (effective 1998). back issues avail. **Document type:** *Academic/Scholarly.* **Description:** Seminar papers with summaries of pediatric articles, interviews and congress reports.
Formerly: Jatros Paediatrie (0177-9095)
—GNLM.
Published by: Hoffmann und Hoffmann GmbH, August-Schanz-Str 8-II, Frankfurt A.m. 60433, Germany. TEL 49-69-54800015, FAX 49-69-54800080, huhgmbh@aol.com. Ed. Peter Hoffmann. Circ: 5,700.

JORDMORBLADET. see *MEDICAL SCIENCES—Obstetrics And Gynecology*

618.92 BRA ISSN 0021-7557
JORNAL DE PEDIATRIA; the official journal of the Brazilian Pediatric Society. Text in Portuguese; Summaries in English, Portuguese. 1934. bi-m. USD 120 to individuals; USD 100 to institutions (effective 2001). adv. bk.rev. abstr, bibl, charts, illus, stat. index. reprint service avail. from PQC. **Document type:** *Journal, Academic/Scholarly.*
Related titles: CD-ROM ed.; Microform ed.: (from PQC); Online - full text ed.
Indexed: Biol.Abstr., Excerp.Med., INIS Atomind., Ind.Med. (until 19??, dropped), Nutr.Abstr.
—CISTI, GNLM, KNAW.
Published by: Sociedade Brasileira de Pediatria, Rua Santa Clara, 292, Copacabana, Rio De Janeiro, RJ 22041-010, Brazil. TEL 55-21-25481999, FAX 55-21-25473567, jped@sbp.com.br, http://www.jpes.com.br. Ed. Dr. Jefferson Pedro Piva. Adv. contact Yantemi Pinnerio TEL 55-11-3667-2336. page USD 1,500. Circ: 15,000.

JOURNAL OF CHILD AND ADOLESCENT PSYCHOPHARMACOLOGY. see *MEDICAL SCIENCES—Psychiatry And Neurology*

618.92 GBR ISSN 1367-4935
JOURNAL OF CHILD HEALTH CARE; for professionals working with children in the hospital and community. Text in English. 1997. q. GBP 35, USD 55 to individuals; GBP 190, USD 298 to institutions; GBP 10, USD 15 per issue to individuals; GBP 49, USD 76 per issue to institutions (effective 2002). adv. **Document type:** *Journal, Academic/Scholarly.* **Description:** A professionally focused, research-based journal which addresses child health issues from a multi-disciplinary perspective. It aims to foster critical understanding of the neonate, child and adolescent in health and illness.
Indexed: Brit.Nur.Ind., CINAHL, Int.Nurs.Ind.
—BLDSC (4957.520000).
Published by: (Association of British Paediatric Nurses), Sage Publications Ltd., 6 Bonhill St, London EC2A 4PU, United Kingdom. TEL 44-20-7374-0645, FAX 44-20-7374-8741, info@sagepub.com, http://www.sagepub.co.uk. Ed. Bernadette Carter. adv.: page GBP 200.

JOURNAL OF CHILD NEUROLOGY. see *MEDICAL SCIENCES—Psychiatry And Neurology*

JOURNAL OF CLINICAL PEDIATRIC DENTISTRY. see *MEDICAL SCIENCES—Dentistry*

618.92 JPN ISSN 0035-550X
CODEN: RSHIAY
JOURNAL OF CLINICAL PEDIATRICS/RINSHO SHONI IGAKU. Text in Japanese. 1953. bi-m. JPY 5,000, USD 6.60. adv. bk.rev. abstr, bibl, charts, illus, stat. index. **Document type:** *Trade.*
Indexed: Chem.Abstr., Excerp.Med., INIS Atomind.
—CISTI.
Published by: Association for the Care of the Child/Shoni Aiiku Kyokai, c/o Dept of Pediatrics, School of Medicine, Sapporo Medical University, Minami-1, Nishi-16-chome, Chuo-ku, Sapporo 060, Japan. Ed. Shunzo Chiba. Circ: 575.

JOURNAL OF DENTISTRY FOR CHILDREN. see *MEDICAL SCIENCES—Dentistry*

618.92 155.4 USA ISSN 0196-206X
RJ1 CODEN: JDBPD5
JOURNAL OF DEVELOPMENTAL AND BEHAVIORAL PEDIATRICS. Abbreviated title: J D B P. Text in English. 1980. bi-m. USD 215 domestic to individuals; USD 262 foreign to individuals; USD 326 domestic to institutions; USD 371 foreign to institutions (effective 2002). adv. bk.rev. *Refereed.* **Document type:** *Academic/Scholarly.* **Description:** Covers learning disabilities, behavioral reactions of children, and family dynamics. For pediatricians, child psychiatrists and special educators.
Related titles: Microfilm ed.: (from WWS); Online - full text ed.: USD 423.80 domestic for academic site license; USD 468.80 foreign for academic site license; USD 472.70 domestic for corporate site license; USD 517.70 foreign for corporate site license (effective 2002); (from Institute for Scientific Information).
Indexed: ASCA, ASSIA, Behav.Med.Abstr., Bibl.Dev.Med.& Child Neur., Chic.Per.Ind., Child Devel.Abstr., Curr.Cont., Dairy Sci.Abstr., Excerp.Med., Fam.Ind., HRIS, IMFL, INIS Atomind., Ind.Med. (1980-), Inpharma, Int.Nurs.Ind., Neurosci.Cit.Ind., Nutr.Abstr., Pharm.&Out.News, PsycInfo, Psychol.Abstr. (1980-), Psycscan D.P., Reac., SSCI, Viol.& Abuse Abstr., Yrbk.Assoc.Educ.& Rehab.Blind, e-psyche.
—BLDSC (4969.280000), CISTI, GNLM, IDS, ingenta, KNAW.
Published by: (Society for Behavioral Pediatrics), Williams & Wilkins (Subsidiary of: Waverly International), 351 W Camden St, Baltimore, MD 21201-2436. TEL 410-528-4068, 800-222-3790, FAX 410-528-4452, laibson@wwilkins.com, http://www.wwilkins.com. Ed. Dr. Paul Dworkin. Adv. contact Lynn Gibson. B&W page USD 450; trim 10.88 x 8.13. Circ: 1,612; 1,493 (paid).

618.92 NLD ISSN 0141-8955
CODEN: JIMDDP
JOURNAL OF INHERITED METABOLIC DISEASE. Text in English. 1978. 8/yr. EUR 730, USD 731 to institutions for print or online ed.; EUR 876, USD 877.20 to institutions for print & online eds.combined (effective 2002). adv. bk.rev. charts, illus. index. reprint service avail. from SWZ,ISI. *Refereed.* **Document type:** *Journal, Academic/Scholarly.* **Description:** Publishes original work, in the form of papers, short reports and case reports, covering all aspects of inherited metabolic disorderss in man and higher animals: clinical, biochemical, genetic, experimental, epidemiological and ethical.
Incorporates: Society for the Study of Inborn Errors of Metabolism. Symposia
Related titles: Microform ed.: (from PQC); Online - full text ed.: (from Ovid Technologies, Inc., EBSCO Publishing, O C L C Online Computer Library Center, Inc., RoweCom Information Quest, Swets Blackwell, Kluwer Online, Institute for Scientific Information).
Indexed: ASCA, Bibl.Dev.Med.& Child Neur., Biol.Abstr., Cal.Tiss.Abstr., Chem.Abstr., Chem.Indus.Notes, Chem.Titles, Curr.Adv.Ecol.Sci., Curr.Cont., Environ.Sci.Poll.Mgmt., Excerp.Med., Genet.Abstr. (coverage dropped), Ind.Med. (1978-), Ind.Sci.Rev., Ind.Vet., Inpharma, Int.Abstr.Biol.Sci., Mass Spectr.Bull., Neurosci.Cit.Ind., Nutr.Abstr., Pollut.Abstr., Reac., Ref.Zh., Risk Abstr., SSCI (coverage dropped), Saf.Sci.Abstr., Sci.Cit.Ind., Vet.Bull.
—BLDSC (5006.950000), CASDDS, CISTI, GNLM, IDS, ingenta, KNAW. **CCC.**

M

Published by: (Society for the Study of Inborn Errors of Metabolism), Kluwer Academic Publishers Group (Subsidiary of: Wolters Kluwer N.V.), Spuiboulevard 50, PO Box 17, Dordrecht 3300 AA, Netherlands. TEL 31-78-639-2392, FAX 31-78-654-2254, services@wkap.nl, http://www.wkap.nl/journalhome.htm/0141-8955. Ed. G T N Besley. Circ: 850. **Subscr. in the Americas to:** Kluwer Academic - Plenum Publishers, 233 Spring St, New York, NY 10013-1578. TEL 212-620-8468, FAX 212-807-1047; **Subscr. to:** Journals Department, PO Box 322, Dordrecht 3300 AH, Netherlands. TEL 31-78-639-2392, FAX 31-78-654-6474.

618.92 AUS ISSN 1034-4810
CODEN: JPCHE3

JOURNAL OF PAEDIATRICS AND CHILD HEALTH. Text in English. 1965. bi-m. AUD 165 domestic to individuals; AUD 150 in New Zealand to individuals; USD 125 elsewhere to individuals; AUD 435 domestic to institutions; AUD 395 in New Zealand to institutions; USD 525 elsewhere to institutions; AUD 182 domestic to individuals paper & online eds. combined; AUD 165 in New Zealand to individuals paper & online eds. combined; USD 138 elsewhere to individuals paper & online eds. combined; AUD 479 domestic to institutions paper & online eds. combined; AUD 435 in New Zealand to institutions paper & online eds. combined; USD 578 elsewhere to institutions paper & online eds. combined (effective 2001). adv. bk.rev. charts, illus. index. back issues avail.; reprint service avail. from PQC. *Refereed.* **Document type:** *Academic/Scholarly.* **Description:** Covers original contributions concerned with both the formal aspects of pediatric medicine and the broader fields of children's health.
Formerly (until 1990): Australian Paediatric Journal (0004-993X)
Related titles: Microfiche ed.: (from PQC); Online - full text ed.: ISSN 1440-1754. AUD 149 domestic to individuals; AUD 135 in New Zealand to individuals; USD 113 elsewhere to individuals; AUD 392 domestic to institutions; AUD 356 in New Zealand to institutions; USD 473 elsewhere to institutions (effective 2001) (from Ovid Technologies, Inc., EBSCO Publishing, O C L C Online Computer Library Center, Inc., RoweCom Information Quest, ingenta, Munksgaard & Blackwell Science's Synergy, Swets Blackwell, Institute for Scientific Information).
Indexed: ASCA, ASSIA, Abstr.Hyg., Adol.Ment.Hlth.Abstr., Bibl.Dev.Med.& Child Neur., Biol.Abstr., Chem.Abstr., Curr.Adv.Ecol.Sci., Curr.Cont., Dairy Sci.Abstr., Diar.Dis.Res., Environ.Sci.Poll.Mgmt., Excerp.Med., Helminthol.Abstr., Ind.Med. (1990-), Ind.Sci.Rev., Inpharma, Int.Nurs.Ind., NRN, Nutr.Abstr., Pharm.&Out.News, Pollut.Abstr., Reac., Rev.Med.& Vet.Mycol., Risk Abstr., Saf.Sci.Abstr., Sci.Cit.Ind., Trop.Dis.Bull., Weed Abstr.
—BLDSC (5027.778000), ADONIS, CASDDS, CISTI, EMDOCS, GNLM, IDS, ingenta, KNAW. **CCC.**
Published by: (Royal College of Physicians), Blackwell Science Asia Pty Ltd, PO Box 378, Carlton South, VIC 3053, Australia. TEL 61-3-9347-0300, FAX 61-3-9347-5001, info@blacksci-asia.com.au, http://www.blacksci.co.uk. Ed. John M Court. Adv. contact Kathryn O'Brien. B&W page AUD 935, color page AUD 2,057; trim 210 x 275. Circ: 2,100. **Co-sponsor:** Perinatal Society of Australia and New Zealand, Paediatric Research Society of Australia, Australasian Association of Paediatric Surgeons.

JOURNAL OF PAEDIATRICS, OBSTETRICS AND GYNAECOLOGY (HONG KONG EDITION). see *MEDICAL SCIENCES—Obstetrics And Gynecology*

JOURNAL OF PAEDIATRICS, OBSTETRICS AND GYNAECOLOGY (TAIWAN EDITION). see *MEDICAL SCIENCES—Obstetrics And Gynecology*

JOURNAL OF PAEDIATRICS, OBSTETRICS AND GYNAECOLOGY (THAILAND EDITION). see *MEDICAL SCIENCES—Obstetrics And Gynecology*

618.92 NLD ISSN 1083-3188
CODEN: JPAGFP

JOURNAL OF PEDIATRIC AND ADOLESCENT GYNECOLOGY. Text in Dutch. 1988. q. EUR 178 in Europe to individuals; JPY 23,700 in Japan to individuals; USD 196 elsewhere to individuals; EUR 405 in Europe to institutions; JPY 53,800 in Japan to institutions; USD 454 elsewhere to institutions (effective 2002). back issues avail.; reprints avail. *Refereed.* **Document type:** *Academic/Scholarly.* **Description:** Presents papers, case reports, reviews of literature and trends in this medical specialty.
Formerly (until 1996): Adolescent and Pediatric Gynecology (0932-8610)
Related titles: Microform ed.: (from PQC); Online - full text ed.: (from EBSCO Publishing, ingenta, ScienceDirect).
Indexed: ASCA, C.C.I.Ob.Gyn., C.C.I.P., Chic.Per.Ind., Curr.Cont. (coverage dropped), Ind.Med. (1996-), Int.Nurs.Ind., Jrnl.Watch Wom.Hlth., SSCI (coverage dropped).
—CISTI, EMDOCS, GNLM, IDS, KNAW.
Published by: (North American Society for Pediatric and Adolescent Gynecology USA), Lippincott Williams & Wilkins (Philadelphia) (Subsidiary of: Wolters Kluwer N.V.), 530 Walnut St, Philadelphia, PA 19106-3621. TEL 215-238-4200, FAX 215-521-8902, http://www.elsevier.com/locate/pedado. Eds. Joseph S Sanfilippo, P G McDonough. **Co-sponsor:** International Federation of Infantile and Juvenile Gynecology.

JOURNAL OF PEDIATRIC ENDOCRINOLOGY & METABOLISM. see *MEDICAL SCIENCES—Endocrinology*

JOURNAL OF PEDIATRIC GASTROENTEROLOGY AND NUTRITION. see *NUTRITION AND DIETETICS*

618.92 USA ISSN 0891-5245
CODEN: JPHCED

JOURNAL OF PEDIATRIC HEALTH CARE. Text in English. 1987. bi-m. USD 67 domestic to individuals; USD 83 foreign to individuals; USD 139 domestic to institutions; USD 157 foreign to institutions; USD 35 domestic to students; USD 51 foreign to students; USD 27 (effective 2001). adv. abstr, charts, illus. index. back issues avail.; reprint service avail. from PQC. *Refereed.* **Document type:** *Journal, Academic/Scholarly.* **Description:** Provides information on examination and developmental assessments, treatment, and coordination of care for various childhood illnesses.
Related titles: Microform ed.: (from PQC); Online - full text ed.: (from EBSCO Publishing, IDEAL Online Library, RoweCom Information Quest).
Indexed: CINAHL, Fam.Ind., Int.Nurs.Ind., Nurs.Abstr.
—BLDSC (5030.180000), CISTI, GNLM, ingenta. **CCC.**
Published by: (National Association of Pediatric Nurse Associates & Practitioners), Mosby, Inc. (Subsidiary of: Elsevier Science), 11830 Westline Industrial Dr, St Louis, MO 63146-3318. TEL 314-872-8370, 800-325-4177, FAX 314-432-1380, http://www.mosby.com/pedhc, http://www.mosby.com/periodicals. Ed. Bobbie Crew Nelms. Pub. Jane Ryley. Adv. contact Michelle Kuhn. B&W page USD 1,160, color page USD 2,110; trim 10.88 x 8.25. Circ: 7,024.

JOURNAL OF PEDIATRIC HEMATOLOGY - ONCOLOGY. see *MEDICAL SCIENCES—Oncology*

JOURNAL OF PEDIATRIC NURSING; nursing care of children and families. see *MEDICAL SCIENCES—Nurses And Nursing*

JOURNAL OF PEDIATRIC ORTHOPAEDICS. see *MEDICAL SCIENCES—Orthopedics And Traumatology*

JOURNAL OF PEDIATRIC ORTHOPAEDICS, PART B. see *MEDICAL SCIENCES—Orthopedics And Traumatology*

JOURNAL OF PEDIATRIC PSYCHOLOGY. see *PSYCHOLOGY*

JOURNAL OF PEDIATRIC SURGERY. see *MEDICAL SCIENCES—Surgery*

618.92 USA ISSN 0022-3476
RJ1 CODEN: JOPDAB

THE JOURNAL OF PEDIATRICS. Text in English. 1932. m. USD 148 domestic to individuals; USD 183 foreign to individuals; USD 357 domestic to institutions; USD 392 foreign to institutions; USD 78 domestic to students; USD 113 foreign to students; USD 33 newsstand/cover (effective 2001). adv. bk.rev. abstr, bibl, charts, illus. s-a. index. reprint service avail. from PQC. *Refereed.* **Document type:** *Journal, Academic/Scholarly.* **Description:** Offers practical guidance for physicians who diagnose and treat disorders in infants and children.
Related titles: CD-ROM ed.: (from Ovid Technologies, Inc.); Microfilm ed.: (from PQC,PMC); Online - full text ed.: (from Ovid Technologies, Inc., EBSCO Publishing, IDEAL Online Library, Institute for Scientific Information, RoweCom Information Quest).
Indexed: AIDS Abstr., AIM, ASCA, ASSIA, Abstr.Hyg., Agri.& Environ.Biotech.Abstr. (coverage dropped), Behav.Med.Abstr., Bibl.Agri., Bibl.Dev.Med.& Child Neur., Biol.Abstr., Biol.Dig., C.C.I.P., CINAHL, Chem.Abstr., Chem.Indus.Notes, Chem.Titles, Child Devel.Abstr., Curr.Adv.Cancer Res., Curr.Adv.Ecol.Sci., Curr.Cont., Dairy Sci.Abstr., Derwent Biotech.Abstr., Diab.Cont., Diar.Dis.Res., Dok.Arbeitsmed., Environ.Sci.Poll.Mgmt., Except.Child Educ.Abstr., Excerp.Med., Fam.Ind., Food Sci.& Tech.Abstr., Helminthol.Abstr., Hosp.Lit.Ind., IMFL, INIS Atomind., I.P.A., Ind.Med. (1932-), Ind.Sci.Rev., Ind.Vet., Inpharma, Int.Abstr.Biol.Sci., Int.Nurs.Ind., Jrnl.Watch Derm., Jrnl.Watch Emer.Med., Jrnl.Watch Inf.Dis., Kidney, Med.& Surg.Dermat., NRN, Neurosci.Cit.Ind., Nutr.Abstr., Pharm.&Out.News, Potato Abstr., Protozool.Abstr., Reac., Rev.Appl.Entomol., Rev.Arom.& Med.Plants, Rev.Med.& Vet.Mycol., Rev.Plant Path., Risk Abstr., SSCI (coverage dropped), Saf.Sci.Abstr., Sci.Cit.Ind., Soyabean Abstr., THA, Trop.Dis.Bull., Vet.Bull., Viol.& Abuse Abstr.
—BLDSC (5030.300000), ADONIS, CASDDS, CISTI, GNLM, IDS, ingenta, KNAW. **CCC.**
Published by: Mosby, Inc. (Subsidiary of: Elsevier Science), 11830 Westline Industrial Dr, St Louis, MO 63146-3318. TEL 314-872-8370, 800-325-4177, FAX 314-432-1380, http://www.mosby.com/jpeds, http://www.mosby.com/periodicals. Ed. Dr. William F Balistreri. Pub. Jane Ryley. Adv. contact Grace Williams TEL 314-453-4689. B&W page USD 1,285, color page USD 2,315; trim 10.88 x 8.13. Circ: 13,554.

JOURNAL OF PERINATOLOGY. see *MEDICAL SCIENCES—Obstetrics And Gynecology*

618.922 USA

▼ **JOURNAL OF RESPIRATORY DISEASES FOR PEDIATRICIANS.** Text in English. 1999. q. charts, illus. Index. back issues avail. *Refereed.* **Document type:** *Journal.* **Description:** Provides information about diagnosis and treatment of respiratory infections, allergies, asthmas and other illnesses that rank among the most common causes of office visits in pediatric practice.
Published by: Cliggott Publishing Co. (Subsidiary of: S C P Communications, Inc.), 330 Boston Post Rd, Darien, CT 06820. TEL 203-662-6400, FAX 203-662-6776, info.cliggott@scp.com, http://www.scp.com/. Ed., R&P Sarah Williams. Pub. Jeff Davis.

618.92 GBR ISSN 0142-6338
CODEN: JTRPAO

JOURNAL OF TROPICAL PEDIATRICS. Text in English. 1954. bi-m. GBP 60, USD 105 to individuals; GBP 180, USD 315 to institutions; GBP 43, USD 73 in developing nations to individuals; GBP 95, USD 168 in developing nations to institutions (effective Feb. 2002). adv. bk.rev. charts, illus. index. Supplement avail.; back issues avail. *Refereed.* **Document type:** *Journal, Academic/Scholarly.* **Description:** Covers all aspects of child health nutrition, including locality and quality of environment.
Formerly: Journal of Tropical Pediatrics and Environmental Child Health (0300-9920)
Related titles: Online - full text ed.: ISSN 1465-3664. GBP 162, USD 283 to institutions Online only (effective Feb. 2002) (from EBSCO Publishing, O C L C Online Computer Library Center, Inc., RoweCom Information Quest, ingenta, Swets Blackwell, Institute for Scientific Information).
Indexed: ASCA, Abstr.Anthropol., Abstr.Hyg., Abstr.Rural Dev.Trop., Cal.Tiss.Abstr., Curr.Adv.Ecol.Sci., Curr.Cont., Dairy Sci.Abstr., Dent.Ind., Diar.Dis.Res., Documentatieblad, Environ.Sci.Poll.Mgmt., Excerp.Med., Helminthol.Abstr., Ind.Med. (1980-), Ind.Sci.Rev., Inpharma, Int.Abstr.Biol.Sci., Int.Nurs.Ind., Nutr.Abstr., Pharm.&Out.News, Pollut.Abstr., Protozool.Abstr., Reac., Rev.Appl.Entomol., Rev.Med.& Vet.Mycol., Rice Abstr., Risk Abstr., Rural Devel.Abstr., SSCI (coverage dropped), Saf.Sci.Abstr., Sci.Cit.Ind., So.Pac.Per.Ind., Trop.Dis.Bull.
—BLDSC (5071.090000), CISTI, IDS, ingenta, KNAW. **CCC.**
Published by: Oxford University Press, Academic Division, Great Clarendon St, Oxford OX2 6DP, United Kingdom. TEL 44-1865-267907, FAX 44-1865-267835, jnl.info@oup.co.uk, http://tropej.oupjournals.org/, http://www.oup.co.uk/journals. Eds. E F Patrice Jeliffe, G J Ebrahim, R Moy. Pub. Mandy Sketch. R&P Fionna Willis. adv.: B&W page GBP 250, B&W page USD 450; trim 210 x 140. Circ: 500. **Affiliate:** Oxford University Press, Journals.

618.92 FRA ISSN 0399-029X
CODEN: JPPEDO

JOURNEES PARISIENNES DE PEDIATRIE. Text in French. 1966. a. price varies.
—CASDDS, GNLM.

M

Published by: (Hopital des Enfants Malades, Centre d'Etudes sur les Maladies du Metabolisme chez l'Enfant), Flammarion Medecine Sciences, 4 rue Casimir Delavigne, Paris 75006, France. Ed. P Royer. **U.S. subscr. addr.:** S.F.P.A., c/o Mr Benech, 14 E 60th St, New York, NY 10022.

618.92 688.72 DEU ISSN 0179-3489
JUNGE FAMILIE; das Baby-Journal. Text in German. 1969. bi-m. EUR 12 domestic; EUR 18 foreign (effective 2002). adv. back issues avail. **Document type:** *Magazine, Consumer.*
Published by: Junior-Verlag GmbH und Co. KG, Fehlandtstr 41, Hamburg 20354, Germany. TEL 49-40-344434, FAX 49-40-352540, info@junior-verlag.de, http://www.junior-verlag.de. Ed. Dagmar von Schweinitz. Pub. Manfred Zedler. Adv. contact Birgit Koenig. B&W page XEU 10,500, color page XEU 18,900; trim 185 x 250. Circ: 240,000 (paid and controlled).

618.92 362.3 FIN ISSN 0355-2918
KETJU; professional periodical on mental retardation. Text in Finnish. 1964. bi-m. FIM 110 (effective 1999). bk.rev. back issues avail. *Refereed.* **Document type:** *Trade.* **Description:** Concerned with medical and social services; pediatrics, mental retardation and the handicapped.
Published by: Kehitysummaliitto lRy, Viliatta 4 A, Helsinki 00700, Finland. TEL 358-9-348-090, FAX 358-9-385-3398, helena.hiila@famr.fi, http://www.famr.fi. Ed. Helena Hiila. adv.: B&W page FIM 4,500, color page FIM 9,300. Circ: 4,000 (paid).

618.92 028.5 USA
KID'S HEALTH. Text in English. 3/yr. free. back issues avail. **Document type:** *Newsletter.*
Related titles: Online - full text ed.
Published by: Children's Hospital of Orange County, PO Box 5700, Orange, CA 92668. TEL 714-997-3000, http://www.choc.org. Ed. Susan Thomas.

618.92 CAN ISSN 1493-7832
KIDS' HEALTH. Text in English. 1984. 3/yr.
Supersedes in part (in 1999): Kaleidoscope (Toronto) (0828-2730); Which was formerly (until 1984): What's New - Hospital for Sick Children (0049-7533); (until 1970): What's New at H S C? (0827-1232)
Published by: Hospital for Sick Children, 555 University Ave, Toronto, ON M5G 1X8, Canada. TEL 416-813-1500, FAX 416-813-5328, http://www.sickkids.on.ca.

618.92 NLD ISSN 0167-2436
KIND EN ADOLESCENT. Text in Dutch. 1980. q. **Document type:** *Academic/Scholarly.*
Indexed: PsycInfo, e-psyche.
—KNAW.
Published by: Bohn Stafleu van Loghum B.V. (Subsidiary of: Wolters Kluwer N.V.), Postbus 246, Houten 3990 GA, Netherlands. TEL 31-3403-95711, FAX 31-3403-50903.

618.92 NLD ISSN 0169-7072
KIND EN ZIEKENHUIS. Text in Dutch. 1977. q. NLG 60, EUR 27.27 (effective 2001). adv. bk.rev. 32 p./no. back issues avail.; reprints avail. **Document type:** *Magazine.*
Published by: (Vereniging Kind en Ziekenhuis), Landelijke Vereniging Kind en Ziekenhuis, Korte Kalkhaven 9, Dordrecht 3311 JM, Netherlands. TEL 31-78-6146361, FAX 31-78-6146361, kind.en.ziekenhuis.nl, http://www.kindenziekenhuis.nl. Ed. B van Rosendaal. Pub. M van Bergen. Circ: 2,000.

KINDER; fuer Eltern, Erzieher und Kinder. see *CHILDREN AND YOUTH—About*

618.92 DEU ISSN 1432-3605 CODEN: SKIPEJ
KINDERAERZTLICHE PRAXIS. Text in German. 1979. 8/yr. DEM 96; DEM 52 to students (effective 1999). adv. **Document type:** *Academic/Scholarly.*
Former titles: Sozialpaediatrie und Kinderaerztliche Praxis (0945-7712); (until 1993): Sozialpaediatrie in der Paediatrie fuer Praxis und Klinik (0944-2375); (until 1992): Sozial Paediatrie in Praxis und Klinik (0171-9327)
Indexed: INIS Atomind.
—EMDOCS, GNLM, Infotrieve, KNAW. **CCC.**
Published by: (Deutsche Gesellschaft fuer Sozialpaediatrie und Jugendmedizin e.V.), Verlag Kirchheim und Co. GmbH, Kaiserstr 41, Mainz 55116, Germany. TEL 49-6131-96070-0, FAX 49-6131-9607070, kirchheim@aol.com. Ed. Dr. Ruediger von Kries. Adv. contact Andreas Goerner. Circ: 8,500.

KINDERKRANKENSCHWESTER. see *MEDICAL SCIENCES—Nurses And Nursing*

KINDEROPVANG. see *CHILDREN AND YOUTH—About*

618.92 DEU ISSN 0942-5403
KINDHEIT UND ENTWICKLUNG. Text in German. q. DEM 108 (effective 2001). adv. **Document type:** *Journal, Academic/Scholarly.*
Indexed: IBR, Ind.Philos.
—GNLM.
Published by: Hogrefe Verlag GmbH und Co. KG, Rohnsweg 25, Goettingen 37085, Germany. TEL 49-551-496090, FAX 49-551-4960988, verlag@hogrefe.de, http://www.hogrefe.de.

KITA NIHON SHONIKA GAKKAI SHOROKUSHU/ PEDIATRICS SOCIETY OF NORTH JAPAN. ABSTRACTS. see *MEDICAL SCIENCES—Abstracting, Bibliographies, Statistics*

618.92 DEU ISSN 0300-8630 CODEN: KLPDB2
KLINISCHE PAEDIATRIE; Zeitschrift fuer Klinik und Praxis. Text in German; Summaries in English, German. 1880. bi-m. EUR 253.80 domestic to institutions; EUR 259.80 in Europe to institutions; EUR 267.80 elsewhere to institutions; EUR 132 to students; EUR 50 newsstand/cover (effective 2002). adv. bk.rev. abstr, charts, illus. reprint service avail. from IRC. *Refereed.* **Document type:** *Journal, Academic/Scholarly.*
Formerly: Archiv fuer Kinderheilkunde (0003-9179)
Related titles: Microfiche ed.: 1880 (from BHP); Online - full text ed.: ISSN 1439-3824; (from Institute for Scientific Information).
Indexed: ASCA, Abstr.Hyg., Agri.& Environ.Biotech.Abstr. (coverage dropped), Bibl.Dev.Med.& Child Neur., Biol.Abstr., Cal.Tiss.Abstr., Chem.Abstr., Curr.Adv.Ecol.Sci., Curr.Cont., Dairy Sci.Abstr., Derwent Biotech.Abstr., Environ.Sci.Poll.Mgmt., Excerp.Med., Helminthol.Abstr., INIS Atomind., Ind.Med. (1972-), Ind.Sci.Rev., Inpharma, Int.Nurs.Ind., Neurosci.Cit.Ind., Nutr.Abstr., Pollut.Abstr., Protozool.Abstr., Reac., Risk Abstr., Saf.Sci.Abstr., Sci.Cit.Ind., Soyabean Abstr., Trop.Dis.Bull.
—BLDSC (5099.460000), ADONIS, CASDDS, CISTI, EMDOCS, GNLM, IDS, Infotrieve, KNAW. **CCC.**
Published by: Georg Thieme Verlag, Ruedigerstr 14, Stuttgart 70469, Germany. TEL 49-711-8931-0, FAX 49-711-8931298, klinpaed@thieme.de, kunden.service@thieme.de, http://www.thieme.de/klinpaed/index.html. Eds. Dr. F Sitzmann, Dr. G Heimann. adv.: page DEM 1,800; trim 175 x 250. Circ: 900 (paid and controlled).

618.92 616.8 GBR ISSN 0969-0301 CODEN: MFPSEU
MARIANI FOUNDATION PAEDIATRIC NEUROLOGY. Text in English. 1993. irreg., latest vol.9, 2001. **Document type:** *Monographic series, Academic/Scholarly.*
Indexed: e-psyche.
—BLDSC (5373.555500), CASDDS, CISTI.
Published by: John Libbey & Co. Ltd., PO Box 276, Eastleigh SO50 5YS, United Kingdom. TEL 44-2380-650208, FAX 44-2380-650259, johnlibbey@aol.com, http://www.johnlibbey.com. Ed. Maria Majno.

MATERNAL AND CHILD HEALTH JOURNAL. see *MEDICAL SCIENCES—Obstetrics And Gynecology*

618.92 FRA ISSN 0291-0233
MEDECINE ET ENFANCE, ADOLESCENCE. Text in French. 1981. 10/yr. FRF 200; FRF 300 foreign. adv. bk.rev. *Refereed.* **Description:** A post-graduate medical journal directed at pediatricians, GP's and institutions.
Related titles: CD-ROM ed.
Indexed: INIS Atomind.
Published by: Edition et Communication Medicales, 23 rue Saint Ferdinand, Paris 75017, France. TEL 45-74-44-65, FAX 40-55-94-13. Ed. C Geselson. Circ: 10,000.

618.92 FRA ISSN 0025-6773 CODEN: MINFAW
MEDECINE INFANTILE; revue de clinique, de therapeutique et d'hygiene sociale de l'enfance. Text in French. 1894. 8/yr. FRF 460. adv. bk.rev. abstr, bibl, charts, illus.
Indexed: Biol.Abstr., Chem.Abstr., Excerp.Med., Ind.Med. (coverage dropped), Nutr.Abstr.
—CASDDS, CISTI, GNLM.
Published by: (Comite National de l'Enfance), Editions Maloine, 27 rue de l'Ecole de Medecine, Paris 75006, France. TEL 1-43-25-60-45, TELEX 203 215 F. Ed. R Perelman. Circ: 5,000.

618.92 FRA ISSN 1286-5494
MEDECINE THERAPEUTIQUE - PEDIATRIE. Key Title: M T P. Medecine Therapeutique Pediatrie. Text in French. 1998. bi-m. FRF 670 domestic to individuals; EUR 114 in Europe to individuals; FRF 790 elsewhere to individuals; FRF 1,120 domestic to institutions; EUR 183 in Europe to institutions; FRF 1,240 elsewhere to institutions; FRF 190 newsstand/cover (effective 2001). **Document type:** *Academic/Scholarly.* **Description:** Publishes only reviews and synoptic articles aimed at both practicing doctors and students.
Related titles: Online - full text ed.: FRF 670 to individuals; FRF 1,120 to institutions; FRF 420 to students (effective 2001).
—BLDSC (5487.965000).
Published by: John Libbey Eurotext, 127 av. de la Republique, Montrouge 92120, France. TEL 33-01-46730660, FAX 33-01-40840999, marketing@jle.com, http://www.john-libbey-eurotext.fr/. Eds. Christian Boitard, Pierre Bougneres. **Subscr. to:** A T E I. atei@club-internet.fr.

MEDICAL AND PEDIATRIC ONCOLOGY. see *MEDICAL SCIENCES—Oncology*

MEDICAL AND PEDIATRIC ONCOLOGY. SUPPLEMENT. see *MEDICAL SCIENCES—Oncology*

618.92 ITA
MEDICO E BAMBINO; rivista di formazione e aggiornamento professionale per il pediatra. Text in Italian. 1981. m. ITL 50,000; ITL 5,000 newsstand/cover (effective 2000). adv.
—BLDSC (5534.179000).
Published by: Edifarm S.p.A., Via P. Palagi 4, Milan, MI 20129, Italy. TEL 39-02-29520315, FAX 39-02-29520449, redazione@medicobambino.com, http://www.medicobambino.com, http://www.edifarm.com. Ed. Lori Olivieri. Adv. contact Carla Tognoni. B&W page ITL 5,800,000, color page ITL 9,300,000; trim 250 x 185. Circ: 54,000.

618.92 BGR ISSN 0324-1122
MEDITSINSKI PREGLED. DETSKI BOLESTI/MEDICAL REVIEW. CHILDREN'S DISEASES. Text in Bulgarian; Summaries in Bulgarian, English. 1972. q., latest vol.30, 2001. BGL 14 domestic; USD 38 foreign (effective 2001 - 2002). adv. bk.rev. abstr, bibl. index. 48 p./no. *Refereed.* **Document type:** *Journal, Academic/Scholarly, Abstract/Index, Bibliography.* **Description:** Presents original articles and abstracts of foreign publications in the field of pediatrics - diagnosis, treatment and prevention of children's diseases, new drugs, child health.
Indexed: Abstr.Bulg.Sci.Med.Lit.
Published by: Meditsinski Universitet - Sofia, Tsentur za Informatsiia po Meditsina/Medical University - Sofia, Medical Information Center, 1 Sv Georgi Sofiiski ul, Sofia 1431, Bulgaria. TEL 359-2-9522342, FAX 359-2-9522393, mutafov@sun.medun.acad.bg, http://www.medun.acad.bg. Ed. Dr. A Anadoliiska. R&P, Adv. contact Dr. Christo Mutafov. B&W page USD 50, color page USD 200; 12 x 18. Circ: 450.

618.92 POL
MEDYCYNA PRAKTYCZNA. PEDIATRIA. Text in Polish. 1995. bi-m. PLZ 60 (effective 2000).
Published by: Medycyna Praktyczna, Ul Skawinska 8, Krakow 31066, Poland. TEL 48-12-4305520, FAX 48-12-4305536, listy@mp.pl, http://mp.pl/czasop.htm. Ed. Jacek Mrukowicz.

METIERS DE LA PETITE ENFANCE. see *CHILDREN AND YOUTH—About*

618.92 GBR ISSN 1368-5937
MIDDLE EAST PAEDIATRICS; in support of today's children - tomorrow's adults. Text in English. 1996. q. **Document type:** *Academic/Scholarly.* **Description:** International medical journal dedicated to child care in the Middle East.
—BLDSC (5761.394000).
Published by: Pharmedia International, 1 Tamesis Gardens, Worcester Park, Surrey KT4 7JX, United Kingdom. TEL 44-20-8337-5583, FAX 44-20-8335-3932. Ed. Pat Scowen. Pub. Russ Finnerty.

MIDWIFERY. see *MEDICAL SCIENCES—Obstetrics And Gynecology*

M

618.92 ITA ISSN 0026-4946 CODEN: MIPEA5
MINERVA PEDIATRICA; rivista mensile di clinica pediatrica, puericultura, auxologia, neuropsichiatria infantile, endocrinologia, diabetologia e chirurgia pediatrica. Text in Italian; Summaries in English, Italian. 1949. m. (10/yr.). USD 125 to individuals; USD 165 to institutions (effective 2000 - 2001). adv. bk.rev. abstr, bibl, illus. index. *Refereed.* **Document type:** *Academic/Scholarly.* **Description:** Covers pediatric clinical medicine, puericulture, auxology, child psychiatry, endocrinology, diabetology and pediatric surgery.
Incorporates: Policlinico Infantile; Pediatria del Medico Pratico; Medicina Italiana; Lattante; Rivista di Clinica Pediatrica (0035-6077)
Related titles: Microform ed.: (from PQC); ♦ Supplement: Societa Italiana di Pediatria. Notiziario. ISSN 0037-8836.
Indexed: Abstr.Hyg., Biol.Abstr., Chem.Abstr., Curr.Adv.Ecol.Sci., Curr.Cont. (coverage dropped), Dairy Sci.Abstr., Dent.Ind., Excerp.Med., Helminthol.Abstr., INIS Atomind., Ind.Med. (1949-), Nutr.Abstr., Protozool.Abstr., Ref.Zh., Rev.Appl.Entomol., Rev.Med.& Vet.Mycol., Soyabean Abstr.
—BLDSC (5794.400000), CASDDS, CISTI, GNLM, KNAW.
Published by: Edizioni Minerva Medica, Corso Bramante, 83-85, Turin, TO 10126, Italy. TEL 39-11-678282, FAX 39-11-674502. Eds. G Bona, N Nigro. Pub. Alberto Oliaro. Adv. contact F Filippo. B&W page USD 1,200, color page USD 2,000; trim 270 x 190. Circ: 5,000 (paid).

618.92 DEU ISSN 0026-9298 CODEN: MOKIAY
MONATSSCHRIFT KINDERHEILKUNDE. Text in German. 1903. m. EUR 1,087 domestic; EUR 1,077.40 in Germany; EUR 104 newsstand/cover foreign (effective 2002). adv. bk.rev. bibl, charts. back issues avail.; reprint service avail. from ISI. *Refereed.* **Document type:** *Journal, Academic/Scholarly.* **Description:** Serves the continuing education of pediatricians in hospitals and practice.
Related titles: Microform ed.: (from PQC); Online - full text ed.: ISSN 1433-0474 (from EBSCO Publishing, RoweCom Information Quest, Swets Blackwell, Springer LINK, Institute for Scientific Information).
Indexed: Abstr.Hyg., Bibl.Dev.Med.& Child Neur., Biol.Abstr., Chem.Abstr., Curr.Adv.Ecol.Sci., Curr.Cont., Dairy Sci.Abstr., Excerp.Med., Helminthol.Abstr., INIS Atomind., Ind.Med. (coverage dropped), Ind.Sci.Rev., Inpharma, Nutr.Abstr., Pharm.&Out.News, Protozool.Abstr., Reac., Rev.Appl.Entomol., Rev.Arom.& Med.Plants, Rev.Med.& Vet.Mycol., Rural Recreat.Tour.Abstr., SSCI (coverage dropped), Triticale Abstr.
—BLDSC (5906.400000), CASDDS, CISTI, GNLM, IDS, Infotrieve, KNAW. **CCC.**
Published by: (Deutschen Gesellschaft fuer Kinderheilkunde und Jugendmedizin), Springer-Verlag (Subsidiary of: BertelsmannSpringer), Tiergartenstr 17, Heidelberg 69121, Germany. TEL 49-6221-345-0, FAX 49-6221-345229, subscriptions@springer.de, http://link.springer.de/link/service/journals/00112/index.htm, http://www.springer.de. Eds. F Blaeker, W Schroeter. **Subscr. in N. America to:** Springer-Verlag New York Inc., PO Box 2485, Secaucus, NJ 07096-2485. TEL 212-460-1500, FAX 212-473-6272.

618.92 ESP ISSN 0212-1603
MONOGRAFIAS DE PEDIATRIA. Text in Spanish. 1982. 6/yr. **Document type:** *Academic/Scholarly.*
Published by: Grupo Aula Medica S.A., C.I. Venecia 2 Alfa III, Isabel Colbrand, 10-12, Madrid 28050, Spain. TEL 34-1-3588657, FAX 34-1-3589067. Eds. Dr. A Nogales Espert, A Nogales.

618.92 CHE ISSN 1044-4882
MONOGRAPHS IN CLINICAL PEDIATRICS. Text in English. 1990. irreg., latest vol.10. **Document type:** *Monographic series.*
—CISTI.
Published by: Gordon and Breach - Harwood Academic (Subsidiary of: Taylor & Francis Group), PO Box 531, Lausanne 1000, Switzerland. Ed. P Lanzkowsky. **Subscr. addr. in US:** International Publishers Direct, PO Box 32160, Newark, NJ 07102. FAX 215-750-6343.

MOTHER & BABY. see *MEDICAL SCIENCES—Obstetrics And Gynecology*

N A N N CENTRAL LINES. see *MEDICAL SCIENCES—Nurses And Nursing*

617.463 USA
N O C I R C ANNUAL REPORT. Text in English. 1986. a. USD 15 (effective 2000). back issues avail.; reprints avail. **Document type:** *Newsletter.* **Description:** Provides parents, health-care professionals, and other concerned individuals with current medical and legal information on routine neonatal circumcision and female genital mutilation, and focuses on efforts to reduce the frequency of the practice, protecting the rights of infants and children.
Formerly: N O C I R C Newsletter (1070-3721)
Published by: National Organization of Circumcision Information Resource Centers, PO Box 2512, San Anselmo, CA 94979-2512. TEL 415-488-9883, FAX 415-488-9660, nocirc@concentric.net, http://www.nocirc.org. Ed., R&P Marilyn Fayre Milos. Circ: 15,000.

NATIONAL ASSOCIATION OF NEONATAL NURSES. POSITION STATEMENT. see *MEDICAL SCIENCES—Nurses And Nursing*

618.92 JPN ISSN 1341-4577
NEONATAL CARE. Text in Japanese. 1987. m. JPY 1,631 per issue.
Formerly (until vol.7, no.4, 1994): N I C U: Japanese Journal of Neonatal Care (0914-2533)
Published by: Medika Shuppan/Medicus Publishing Inc., 18-24 Hiroshiba-cho, Suita-shi, Osaka-fu 564-0052, Japan. TEL 81-6-385-6911, FAX 81-6-385-6721. Ed. Takahiko Matsui.

NEONATAL INTENSIVE CARE; the journal of perinatology - neonatology. see *MEDICAL SCIENCES—Obstetrics And Gynecology*

NEONATAL NETWORK; the journal of neonatal nursing. see *MEDICAL SCIENCES—Nurses And Nursing*

NEONATAL, PAEDIATRIC AND CHILD HEALTH NURSING. see *MEDICAL SCIENCES—Nurses And Nursing*

618.92 USA ISSN 1526-9906
▼ **NEOREVIEWS.ORG.** Text in English. 2000 (Jan.). m., latest vol.2. USD 59 to members; USD 79 to non-members and institutions (effective 2001). **Document type:** *Journal, Academic/Scholarly.* **Description:** Focuses on neonatal and perinatal topics. Delivers 3-4 reviews, case discussions, basic science insights, and "on the horizon" pieces each month.
Formerly a section of (July-Dec. 1999): Pediatrics in Review (0191-9601)
Media: Online - full content (from HighWire Pr.).
Published by: American Academy of Pediatrics, 141 Northwest Point Blvd, Box 927, Elk Grove Village, IL 60009-0927. neoreviews@aap.org, http://www.neoreviews.org, http://www.aap.org. Eds. Dr. Bill Hay, Dr. David K Stevenson.

616.8 DEU ISSN 0174-304X CODEN: NRPDDB
NEUROPEDIATRICS; journal of pediatric neurobiology, neurology and neurosurgery. Text in English. 1970. bi-m. EUR 302.80 in Europe to institutions; EUR 307.40 elsewhere to institutions; EUR 60 newsstand/cover (effective 2002). adv. *Refereed.* **Document type:** *Journal, Academic/Scholarly.*
Formerly: Neuropaediatrie (0028-3797)
Related titles: Online - full text ed.: ISSN 1439-1899 (from Institute for Scientific Information).
Indexed: ASCA, Bibl.Dev.Med.& Child Neur., Biol.Abstr., Chem.Abstr., Child Devel.Abstr., Curr.Adv.Ecol.Sci., Curr.Cont., Excerp.Med., Helminthol.Abstr., INIS Atomind., Ind.Med. (1980-), Ind.Sci.Rev., Inpharma, Neurosci.Cit.Ind., Nutr.Abstr., Pharm.&Out.News, Reac., Sci.Cit.Ind., e-psyche.
—BLDSC (6081.515500), CASDDS, CISTI, GNLM, IDS, ingenta, KNAW. **CCC.**
Published by: Georg Thieme Verlag, Ruedigerstr 14, Stuttgart 70469, Germany. TEL 49-711-8931-0, FAX 49-711-8931133, kunden.service@thieme.de, http://www.thieme.de. Circ: 1,200.

616.8 FRA ISSN 0222-9617
NEUROPSYCHIATRIE DE L'ENFANCE ET DE L'ADOLESCENCE. Text in French. 1953. 8/yr. EUR 207 in Europe to institutions; USD 254 elsewhere to institutions (effective 2002). adv. bk.rev. bibl, charts, illus. **Document type:** *Academic/Scholarly.*
Formerly: Revue de Neuropsychiatrie Infantile et d'Hygiene Mentale de l'Enfance (0035-1628)
Related titles: Microform ed.; Online - full text ed.
Indexed: Biol.Abstr., Curr.Cont. (coverage dropped), Excerp.Med., Ind.Med. (coverage dropped), Lang.& Lang.Behav.Abstr., Psychol.Abstr., Ref.Zh., SOPODA, SSCI (coverage dropped), Sociol.Abstr., e-psyche.
—BLDSC (6081.536000), CISTI, EMDOCS, GNLM, Infotrieve, KNAW. **CCC.**
Published by: (Societe Francaise de Psychiatrie de l'Enfant et de l'Adolescent), Elsevier Paris, Editions Scientifiques et Medicales (Subsidiary of: Reed Elsevier plc. group), 23 rue Linois, Paris 75015, France. TEL 33-1-45589110, FAX 33-1-45589419, http://www.elsevier.com/locate/neurenf. Circ: 5,000.

618.92 NLD
NEW CLINICAL APPLICATIONS. PAEDIATRICS. Text in English. irreg. price varies. *Refereed.* **Document type:** *Monographic series.*
Published by: Kluwer Academic Publishers Group (Subsidiary of: Wolters Kluwer N.V.), Spuiboulevard 50, PO Box 17, Dordrecht 3300 AA, Netherlands. FAX 31-78-639-2254, services@wkap.nl, http://www.wkap.nl. **Dist. by:** Journals Department, PO Box 322, Dordrecht 3300 AH, Netherlands. FAX 31-78-654-6474.

618.92 USA ISSN 0737-4216
NEW YORK PEDIATRICIAN* ; a forum on issues affecting pediatric practice in New York State. Text in English. 1983. s-a. membership. adv. bk.rev. charts, illus. **Document type:** *Academic/Scholarly.*
Formerly: Long Island Pediatrician
Related titles: Microform ed.: 1983.
Published by: American Academy of Pediatrics, District II, Queens Hospital Center, 82 68 164th St, Jamaica, NY 11432. Ed. Dr. Philip W H Eskes. Circ: 3,500.

▼ **NEWBORN AND INFANT NURSING REVIEWS.** see *MEDICAL SCIENCES—Nurses And Nursing*

618.92 NGA ISSN 0302-4660 CODEN: NJPDAK
NIGERIAN JOURNAL OF PAEDIATRICS. Text in English. 1974. q. NGN 16, USD 6. adv. charts, illus. back issues avail. **Document type:** *Journal, Academic/Scholarly.*
Related titles: CD-ROM ed.
Indexed: Abstr.Hyg., Biol.Abstr., Excerp.Med. (until 19??), ExtraMED, Trop.Dis.Bull.
—GNLM.
Published by: (Paediatric Association of Nigeria), Ibadan University Press, University of Ibadan, Ibadan, Oyo, Nigeria. Circ: 500. **Orders to:** University College Hospital, College of Medicine, PIMRAT College of Medicine, University of Ibadan, Ibadan, Oyo, Nigeria. TEL 234-2-2410088, FAX 234-2-2411768. **Co-sponsor:** University of Ibadan. Department of Paediatrics.

618.92 610 JPN ISSN 0029-0386
NIHON SHINSEIJI GAKKAI ZASSHI/ACTA NEONATOLOGICA JAPONICA. Text in Japanese; Summaries in English, Japanese. 1965. q. JPY 8,000 (effective 1999). adv. bk.rev. bibl. cum.index. back issues avail. *Refereed.* **Document type:** *Academic/Scholarly.*
Indexed: Excerp.Med., INIS Atomind.
—BLDSC (0639.757000), CISTI, EMDOCS, GNLM.
Published by: Nihon Shinseiji Gakkai/Japan Society of Neonatology, c/o Toho University School of Medicine, Department of Neonatology, 6-11-1 Omori-Nishi, Ota-ku, Tokyo 143-0015, Japan. TEL 81-3-3762-0841, FAX 81-3-3762-0842. Ed. Dr. Hiroshi Tada. Adv. contact Nihon Igaku Koukokusha. Circ: 4,000 (controlled).

618.92 JPN ISSN 0288-609X
NIHON SHONI GEKA GAKKAI ZASSHI/JAPANESE SOCIETY OF PEDIATRIC SURGEONS. JOURNAL. Text in Japanese; Summaries in English. 1965. 7/yr. JPY 2,000 per issue.
—BLDSC (4809.476000). **CCC.**
Published by: Nihon Shoni Geka Gakkai, Nihon Gakkai Jimu Senta, 16-9 Honkomagome 5-chome, Bunkyo-ku, Tokyo 113-0021, Japan.

618.92 617.3 JPN ISSN 0917-6950
NIHON SHONI SEIKEI GEKA GAKKAI ZASSHI/JAPANESE PAEDIATRIC ORTHOPAEDIC ASSOCIATION. JOURNAL. Text in English, Japanese. 1991. s-a. JPY 4,500 per issue.
Published by: Nihon Shoni Seikei Geka Gakkai, c/o Kokuritsu Shoni Byoin Seikei Geka, 35-31 Taishido 3-chome, Setagaya-ku, Tokyo 154-0004, Japan.

618.92 FRA ISSN 0765-5010
NOTES PEDIATRIQUES. Text in French. 10/yr.
Published by: Publications R C G, 23 rue Saint Ferdinand, Paris 75017, France. TEL 45-72-51-91. Ed. Dr. G Dutau. Circ: 5,000.

OPHTHALMIC GENETICS. see *MEDICAL SCIENCES—Ophthalmology And Optometry*

M

ORTHOSCOPE. see *MEDICAL SCIENCES—Orthopedics And Traumatology*

618.92 ITA ISSN 0030-6274
OSPEDALI ITALIANI - PEDIATRIA; e specialita chirurgiche. Text in Italian; Abstracts in English, French, German, Italian, Spanish. 1966. bi-m. ITL 50,000, USD 40. bk.rev. bibl, charts, illus, stat. index, cum.index. Supplement avail. **Description:** Features research papers on the science of pediatrics and specialized surgery.
Indexed: Biol.Abstr., Excerp.Med. (until 1993).
—CISTI, GNLM.
Published by: Giuseppe Caracciolo Ed. & Pub., Via Domenico Cimarosa, 180-A, Naples, NA 80127, Italy. TEL 5569280. Circ: 1,000.

L'OTORINOLARINGOLOGIA PEDIATRICA. see *MEDICAL SCIENCES—Otorhinolaryngology*

618.92 HRV ISSN 1330-1403 CODEN: PCROE6
PAEDIATRIA CROATICA; the journal for the. Text and summaries in Croatian, English. 1957. q. HRK 80 to individuals; HRK 160 to institutions; DEM 60 in Europe to institutions; USD 40 elsewhere to institutions (effective 1999). adv. bk.rev. *Refereed.*
Formerly: Arhiv za Zastitu Majke i Djeteta - Archives for Mother and Child Health (0004-1289)
Related titles: Online - full text ed.
Indexed: Excerp.Med., Ref.Zh.
—BLDSC (6333.399170), EMDOCS, GNLM.
Published by: (Hrvatsko Pedijatrijsko Drustvo), Klinika za Djecje Bolesti Zagreb, Klaiceva 16, Zagreb 10000, Croatia. TEL 385-1-4600163, FAX 385-1-4826053, vkolbas@zg.tel.hr, http://www.kdb.hr. Ed. Renata Lokar Kolbas. Circ: 1,000.

PAEDIATRIC ANAESTHESIA. see *MEDICAL SCIENCES—Anaesthesiology*

PAEDIATRIC ANAESTHESIA ONLINE. see *MEDICAL SCIENCES—Anaesthesiology*

PAEDIATRIC AND PERINATAL DRUG THERAPY. see *PHARMACY AND PHARMACOLOGY*

618.92 GBR ISSN 0269-5022
PAEDIATRIC & PERINATAL EPIDEMIOLOGY. Text in English. 1988. q., latest vol.16, 2002. GBP 115 in Europe to individuals; USD 183 in North America to individuals; GBP 127 elsewhere to individuals; GBP 322 in Europe to institutions; USD 512 in North America to institutions; GBP 355 elsewhere to institutions (effective 2002). adv. bk.rev. illus. index. back issues avail. *Refereed.* **Document type:** *Journal, Academic/Scholarly.* **Description:** Crosses the boundaries between the epidemiologist and the paediatrician, obstetrician or specialist in child health.
Related titles: Microform ed.: (from PQC); ♦ Online - full text ed.: Paediatric & Perinatal Epidemiology Online. ISSN 1365-3016.
Indexed: ASCA, Curr.Cont., Diar.Dis.Res., Excerp.Med. (1988-), Ind.Med. (1987-), Ind.Sci.Rev., Inpharma, Int.Nurs.Ind., Med.& Surg.Dermat., Pharm.&Out.News, Reac., Sci.Cit.Ind.
—BLDSC (6333.399710), EMDOCS, GNLM, IDS, Infotrieve, KNAW. **CCC.**
Published by: (Society for Paediatric Epidemiologic Research), Blackwell Science Ltd., PO Box 88, Oxford OX2 0NE, United Kingdom. TEL 44-1865-206180, 44-1865-206002, FAX 44-1865-206219, jnl.orders@blacksci.co.uk, http://www.blackwell-science.com/~cgilib/jnlpage.asp?Journal=ppe&File=ppe, http://www.blackwellpublishing.com. Ed. J Golding. Pub. Elaine Stott. R&P Jenny Applin. Adv. contact Martine Cariou Keen. Circ: 465.

618.92 GBR ISSN 1365-3016
▼ **PAEDIATRIC & PERINATAL EPIDEMIOLOGY ONLINE.** Text in English. 1999. q. GBP 104 in Europe to individuals; USD 165 in North America to individuals; GBP 104 elsewhere to individuals; GBP 290 in Europe to institutions; USD 461 in North America to institutions; GBP 290 elsewhere to institutions (effective 2002). *Refereed.* **Document type:** *Academic/Scholarly.*
Media: Online - full text (from EBSCO Publishing, ingenta, Munksgaard & Blackwell Science's Synergy, Swets Blackwell, Institute for Scientific Information, RoweCom Information Quest). **Related titles:** Microform ed.: (from PQC); ♦ Print ed.: Paediatric & Perinatal Epidemiology. ISSN 0269-5022.
Published by: Blackwell Science Ltd., Osney Mead, Oxford OX2 0EL, United Kingdom. TEL 44-1685-206206, FAX 44-1685-721205, website@blacksci.com, journals.cs@blacksci.co.uk, http://www.blackwell-science.com/~cgilib/jnlpage.bin?Journal=ppe&File=ppe&Page=aims.

▼ **PAEDIATRIC DRUGS.** see *PHARMACY AND PHARMACOLOGY*

618.92 IDN ISSN 0030-9311 CODEN: PIDOA8
PAEDIATRICA INDONESIANA; journal of the Indonesian Society of Pediatrician. Text and summaries in English. 1961. bi-m. USD 60. adv. bk.rev. abstr, bibl, charts, illus, stat. reprint service avail. from PQC. **Document type:** *Academic/Scholarly.*
Related titles: CD-ROM ed.; Microfiche ed.; Microfilm ed.: (from PQC).
Indexed: Abstr.Hyg., Biol.Abstr., Excerp.Med., Ind.Med. (coverage dropped), Nutr.Abstr., Trop.Dis.Bull.
—CISTI, GNLM.
Published by: Indonesian Society of Pediatrician, c/o Dept. of Child Health, Medical School University of Indonesia, Jalan Salemba 6, Jakarta 10430, Indonesia. TEL 62-21-314-8610, FAX 61-21-390-7743. Ed. Sudigdo Sastroasmoro. Circ: 2,000.

618.92 CAN ISSN 1205-7088
PAEDIATRICS AND CHILD HEALTH; the journal of the Canadian Paediatric Society. Text in English. 1996. 8/yr. CND 150, USD 150 to individuals; CND 190, USD 190 to institutions (effective 2000). adv. back issues avail. *Refereed.* **Document type:** *Academic/Scholarly.* **Description:** Peer-reviewed medical journal for paediatricians, family physicians, and other child health care professionals.
—BLDSC (6333.450500).
Published by: Pulsus Group Inc., 2902 S Sheridan Way, Oakville, ON L6J 7L6, Canada. TEL 905-829-4770, FAX 905-829-4799, pulsus@pulsus.com, http://www.pulsus.com. Ed. Dr. Noni MacDonald. Adv. contact Amanda Murphy. B&W page USD 2,325, color page USD 4,100. Circ: 15,500 (paid).

618.92 GBR ISSN 1352-2086
PAEDIATRICS TODAY. Text in English. 1993. q. GBP 18 domestic to individuals; GBP 30 foreign to individuals; GBP 30 domestic to institutions; GBP 50 foreign to institutions (effective 2000). **Document type:** *Trade.*
Published by: Media Publishing Company, Media House, 41 Crayford Way, Dartford, Kent DA1 4JY, United Kingdom. TEL 44-1322-558029, FAX 44-1322-558524, medipub@aol.com. Ed. M Wooldridge.

618.92 NZL ISSN 1174-5894
▼ **PAEDIATRICS TODAY.** Text in English. 1999. m. USD 95 to individuals; USD 545 to institutions (effective 2001). back issues avail. **Description:** Rapid alerts service on all aspects of drug therapy and disease management in children.
Published by: Adis International Limited, Mairangi Bay, Private Bag 65901, Auckland 1010, New Zealand. TEL 64-9-477-0700, FAX 64-9-477-0766, http://www.adis.com. **Americas subscr. to:** Adis International Inc., Attn: Subscription Dept, 860 Town Center Dr, Langhorne, PA 19047. TEL 877-872-2347.

618.92 DEU
PAEDIATRIE AKTUELL. Text in German. 1990. irreg., latest vol.4, 1993. **Document type:** *Academic/Scholarly.*
Published by: W. Zuckschwerdt Verlag GmbH, Industriestr 1, Germering 82110, Germany. TEL 49-89-894349-0, FAX 49-89-89434950.

618.92 616.5 DEU ISSN 1437-1782
PAEDIATRIE HAUTNAH. Text in German. 1989. 8/yr. EUR 70.68 domestic; EUR 81.68 foreign; EUR 55.73 domestic to students; EUR 66.73 foreign to students; EUR 15.89 newsstand/cover (effective 2002). adv. **Document type:** *Journal, Academic/Scholarly.*
Formerly (until 1998): Hautnah Paediatrie (0935-3453)
—GNLM.
Published by: Urban und Vogel Medien und Medizin Verlagsgesellschaft mbH (Subsidiary of: BertelsmannSpringer), Neumarkter Str 43, Munich 81673, Germany. TEL 49-89-43721411, FAX 49-89-43721410, verlag@urban-vogel.de, http://www.urban-vogel.de. Ed. Dr. Juergen Kerstan. R&P Friederik Klein. Adv. contact Paul Berger. Circ: 9,000 (paid). **Subscr. to:** Springer Auslieferungs Gesellschaft, Postfach 105160, Heidelberg 69041, Germany. TEL 49-6221-345244, FAX 49-6221-345244.

618.92 CHE ISSN 0030-932X CODEN: PRTPE
PAEDIATRIE UND GRENZGEBIETE/PEDIATRICS AND RELATED TOPICS. Text and summaries in English, German. 1962. 6/yr. USD 153 to individuals (effective 2001). bk.rev. charts, illus, stat. index. **Document type:** *Journal, Academic/Scholarly.*
Indexed: Curr.Adv.Ecol.Sci., Excerp.Med., INIS Atomind., Ind.Med. (coverage dropped), Nutr.Abstr.
—BLDSC (6333.200000), CISTI, GNLM, Infotrieve, KNAW. **CCC.**
Published by: Gordon and Breach - Harwood Academic (Subsidiary of: Taylor & Francis Group), PO Box 531, Lausanne 1000, Switzerland. TEL 41-21-6411280, FAX 41-21-6411281, info@gbhap.com, http://www.gbhap.com/journals/610/610-top.htm. Ed. B Schneeweiss. **Subscr. addr. in US:** International Publishers Direct, PO Box 32160, Newark, NJ 07102. FAX 215-750-6343.

618.92 AUT ISSN 0030-9338 CODEN: PAPAB5
PAEDIATRIE UND PAEDOLOGIE; oesterreichische Zeitschrift fuer Kinder- und Jugendheilkunde. Text in German. 1965. bi-m. EUR 57.70 domestic; EUR 55.10 in Germany; EUR 50.60 newsstand/cover foreign (effective 2002). adv. bk.rev. charts, illus. index. reprint service avail. from ISI. **Document type:** *Journal, Academic/Scholarly.* **Description:** Covers research in children's health and development.
Related titles: Microform ed.: (from PQC); Online - full text ed.: (from Springer LINK).
Indexed: Bibl.Dev.Med.& Child Neur., Biol.Abstr., Chem.Abstr., Curr.Adv.Cancer Res., Curr.Cont. (coverage dropped), Excerp.Med., INIS Atomind., Ind.Med. (coverage dropped), Nutr.Abstr.
—BLDSC (6333.230000), CASDDS, CISTI, GNLM. **CCC.**
Published by: Springer-Verlag Wien (Subsidiary of: BertelsmannSpringer), Sachsenplatz 4-6, PO Box 89, Vienna, W 1201, Austria. TEL 43-1-3302415-0, FAX 43-1-330242665, journals@springer.at, http://www.springer.at/paediatrie. Ed. I Mutz. R&P Angela Foessl TEL 43-1-3302415517. Adv. contact Michael Katzenberger TEL 43-1-3302415220. B&W page XEU 1,890, color page XEU 2,457; 180 x 260. **N. American subscr. to:** Springer-Verlag, Journals, 175 Fifth Ave, New York, NY 10010. TEL 212-460-1500, FAX 212-473-6272, orders@springer-ny.com, http://www.springer-ny.com.

618.92 DEU ISSN 0030-9346
PAEDIATRISCHE PRAXIS; Zeitschrift fuer Kinder- und Jugendmedizin. Text in German. 1962. 4/yr. EUR 162; EUR 45 newsstand/cover (effective 2002). bk.rev. abstr, bibl, charts, illus. index, cum.index every 5 yrs. reprint service avail. from PQC. **Document type:** *Journal, Academic/Scholarly.* **Description:** Practical information of interest to specialists in pediatrics. Features current research, questions and answers, and photographs.
Related titles: Microfilm ed.: (from PQC).
Indexed: Excerp.Med.
—BLDSC (6333.300000), CISTI, GNLM. **CCC.**
Published by: Hans Marseille Vertrieb Medizinischer Zeitschriften, Buerkleinstr 12, Munich 80538, Germany. TEL 49-89-227988, FAX 49-89-2904643, marseille-verlag@t-online.de, http://www.marseille-verlag.com. Eds. G F Wuendisch, W Stoegmann. Circ: 4,500.

618.92 PAK ISSN 0048-2722
PAKISTAN PEDIATRIC JOURNAL✱. Text in English. 1971. q. PKR 10. adv. bk.rev. bibl, charts, illus.
Published by: Association of Pediatricians of Pakistan, 111-D 27-7 Nazimabad, Karachi, 18, Pakistan. Ed. Dr. Abdul Jamil Khan.

618.92 HUN ISSN 1216-3821
PEDIATER; az apathy alapitvany gyermekorvosi folyoirata. Text in Hungarian. 1967. q. HUF 280 (effective 1996). adv. bk.rev. **Document type:** *Academic/Scholarly.*
Formerly (until 1992): Magyar Pediater (0303-5042)
Published by: Apathy Alapitvany a Gyermekek Gyogyitasaert, Ulloi ut 86, Budapest 1089, Hungary. TEL 36-1-2699398. Ed. Peter Kiss. Circ: 1,000.

618.92 FRA ISSN 0397-9180
PEDIATRE. Text in French. 1963. bi-m. FRF 460 domestic to individuals; FRF 550, EUR 83.85 foreign to individuals; FRF 300 to students (effective 2000). adv. bk.rev. reprint service avail. from ISI. **Document type:** *Bulletin, Proceedings.*
Indexed: Excerp.Med.
—CISTI, EMDOCS, GNLM.

M

Published by: (Pediatre Parisien, s.a.r.l.), Meditions Carline, 1 et 3 rue du Depart, Paris 75014, France. TEL 33-1-40640075, FAX 33-1-43222699, groupemeditions@wanadoo.fr. Ed. Dr. G. Beley. Pub. Dr. G Beley. Circ: 2,500. **Co-sponsors:** SNPF, Groupement des Pediatres; Cercle d'Etudes Pediatriques, Association Francaise Pediatre Ambulatoire.

618.92 BGR ISSN 0479-7876 CODEN: PDTAAB
PEDIATRIA. Text in Bulgarian; Summaries in English, Russian. 1962. bi-m. BGL 24, USD 7.
Indexed: Abstr.Bulg.Sci.Med.Lit., Dent.Ind., Excerp.Med. (until 1993), INIS Atomind., Ind.Med. (coverage dropped), Ref.Zh.
—CASDDS, CISTI, GNLM.
Published by: (Bulgaria. Ministerstvo na Narodnoto Zdrave), Izdatelstvo Meditsina i Fizkultura, 11 Pl Slaveikov, Sofia 1080, Bulgaria. Ed. Sh Ninjo. Circ: 1,950. **Dist. by:** Hemus, 6 Rouski blvd, Sofia 1000, Bulgaria. **Co-sponsor:** Nauchno Druzhestvo po Pediatria.

618.92 CHL ISSN 0375-9563 CODEN: PEDSAQ
PEDIATRIA*. Text in Spanish; Summaries in English. 1958. q. CLP 20,000, USD 20. adv. bk.rev. abstr, bibl, illus, stat. index. reprint service avail. from PQC. **Document type:** *Academic/Scholarly.*
Media: Microform. **Related titles:** Microfilm ed.: 1958 (from PQC).
Indexed: Dent.Ind., Excerp.Med. (until 1983), Ind.Med. (coverage dropped), Nutr.Abstr.
—GNLM.
Published by: Universidad de Chile, Departamento de Pediatria, Diag. Paraguay, 265, Torre 15, Santiago, Chile. Ed. Julio Meneghello Rivera. Circ: 1,000.

618.92 ROM ISSN 1220-580X CODEN: RPOPD
PEDIATRIA. Text in Romanian; Summaries in English, French, German, Russian. 1952. q. USD 15. adv. bk.rev. abstr, charts, illus. **Document type:** *Academic/Scholarly.*
Former titles (until 1990): Revista de Pediatrie, Obstetrica si Ginecologie. Seria Pediatrie (0303-8416); (until 1974): Pediatria (0031-3904)
Indexed: Biol.Abstr., Chem.Abstr., Excerp.Med. (until 1990), Ind.Med. (coverage dropped).
—CASDDS, CISTI, GNLM.
Published by: Romanian Medical Association, Str. Ionel Perlea Nr.10, Bucharest 70754, Romania. **Subscr. to:** ILEXIM, Str. 13 Decembrie 3, PO Box 136-137, Bucharest 70116, Romania.

618.92 ITA ISSN 0031-3890
PEDIATRIA; rivista d'igiene, medicina e chirurgia dell'infanzia. Text in Italian; Summaries in English, French, German, Italian, Spanish. 1893. q. ITL 6,000, USD 14. adv. bk.rev. abstr, illus. index.
Indexed: Chem.Abstr., Dent.Ind., Ind.Med. (coverage dropped), Nutr.Abstr.
—CISTI, GNLM.
Published by: Universita degli Studi di Napoli, Clinica Pediatrica, S. Andrea delle Dame 4, Naples, NA, Italy. Ed. Giulio Murano.

618.92 COL ISSN 0031-3882 CODEN: PEDSA
PEDIATRIA*. Text in Spanish. 1958. q.
Formerly (until 1965): Sociedad Colombiana de Pediatria y Puericultura. Revista (0120-8756)
Published by: Sociedad Colombiana de Pediatria, Avd 4 Norte, No 16-23, Apdo 3124, Coli, Colombia. TEL 2883985.

618.92 BRA ISSN 0103-2712
PEDIATRIA ATUAL. Text in Portuguese. 1988. 11/yr. USD 450 (effective 2000 - 2001). abstr, bibl. Index.
Published by: Editora de Publicacoes Cientificas Ltda., Rua Major Suckow, 30, Rocha, Rio De Janeiro, RJ 20911-160, Brazil. TEL 55-21-2013722, 55-21-5010057, FAX 55-21-2613749. Eds. Almir L de Fonseca, J M Melo. R&P, Adv. contact Ana Paula. Circ: 12,000.

618.92 ESP ISSN 1135-8831 CODEN: BSCPDR
PEDIATRIA CATALANA. Text in Spanish. 1928. bi-m. adv.
Formerly (until 1996): Butlleti de la Societat Catalana de Pediatria (0210-721X)
Indexed: Excerp.Med., Ind.Med.Esp.
—BLDSC (6417.475000), CASDDS, GNLM.
Published by: Fundacio Catalana de Pediatria, Ps Bonanova, 47 2n, Barcelona 08017, Spain. TEL 34-3-2110597, FAX 34-3-2123569. Ed. Dr. Josep Argemi I Renom. Adv. contact Jordi Mora.

618.92 BRA ISSN 0031-3920 CODEN: RBMEAU
PEDIATRIA MODERNA. Text in Portuguese; Summaries in English, Portuguese, Spanish. 1966. m. BRL 135, USD 250 (effective 2000); free to qualified personnel. adv. bk.rev., Website rev. abstr, bibl, charts, illus, stat. cum.index. back issues avail. *Refereed.* **Document type:** *Journal, Academic/Scholarly.*
Indexed: Biol.Abstr.
—CISTI.
Published by: Grupo Editorial Moreira Jr., Rua Henrique Martins, 493, Jd Paulista, Sao Paulo, SP 04504-000, Brazil. TEL 55-11-38849911, FAX 55-11-38849993, comercial@moreirajr.com.br, http://www.morelrajr.com.br/. Ed. Friederich T Simon. Pub. Americo Moreira. Adv. contact Maria Rachel Bellusci. Circ: 20,000 (controlled).

618.92 617.3 ITA ISSN 0391-898X
PEDIATRIA OGGI MEDICA E CHIRURGICA. Text in Italian; Summaries in English. 1980. q. ITL 80,000, USD 70 (effective 2001). adv.
Indexed: Excerp.Med., Ref.Zh.
—BLDSC (6417.488000), CISTI, EMDOCS, GNLM, Infotrieve. **CCC.**
Published by: C I C Edizioni Internazionali s.r.l., Corso Trieste 42, Rome, RM 00198, Italy. TEL 39-06-8412673, FAX 39-06-8412688, info@gruppocic.it, 1160199510. Pub. A Salvati. adv.: B&W page XEU 1,626.84, color page XEU 2,065.83; 210 x 290.

618.92 POL ISSN 0031-3939 CODEN: PEPOA6
PEDIATRIA POLSKA. Text in Polish; Summaries in English. 1921. m. USD 50 for 6 mos.. bk.rev. index. *Refereed.* **Document type:** *Proceedings.* **Description:** Publishes original papers on advances in pediatrics as well as clinical reports.
Indexed: Biol.Abstr., Chem.Abstr., Dent.Ind., Excerp.Med., INIS Atomind., Ind.Med. (coverage dropped), Nutr.Abstr.
—BLDSC (6417.500000), CASDDS, CISTI, GNLM, KNAW.
Published by: (Polskie Towarzystwo Pediatryczne), Wydawnictwo Medyczne Urban i Partner, Ul Marii Sklodowskiej Curie 55-61, Wroclaw 50950, Poland. TEL 48-71-225497, FAX 48-71-224391. Ed. Teresa Wyszynska. Circ: 1,500. **Co-sponsor:** Instytut Matki i Dziecka.

618.92 USA ISSN 0160-0184
PEDIATRIC ALERT. Text in English. 1976. s-m., latest vol.26, 2001. USD 76 to individuals; USD 97 to institutions; USD 51 to students (effective 2001). 6 p./no. back issues avail. **Document type:** *Newsletter.*
Published by: Medical Alert, Inc., PO Box 610228, Newton, MA 02461-0228. TEL 781-239-1762, FAX 781-239-1762, alertsrus@mediaone.net, alertsus@mediaone.net. Ed. Dr. Allen A Mitchell. R&P Katherrine Bicknell.

618.92 616.97 DNK ISSN 0905-6157 CODEN: PALUEE
PEDIATRIC ALLERGY AND IMMUNOLOGY. Text in English. 1990. bi-m. USD 300 in the Americas to institutions print & online eds. combined; GBP 208 elsewhere to institutions print & online eds. combined (effective 2002). adv. charts, illus. reprints avail. *Refereed.* **Document type:** *Journal, Academic/Scholarly.*
Related titles: Online - full text ed.: ISSN 1399-3038. GBP 179; DKK 1,755 to institutions (effective 2002) (from Ovid Technologies, Inc., EBSCO Publishing, O C L C Online Computer Library Center, Inc., RoweCom Information Quest, ingenta, Munksgaard & Blackwell Science's Synergy, Swets Blackwell, Institute for Scientific Information); ♦ Supplement: Pediatric Allergy and Immunology. Supplementum. ISSN 0906-5784.
Indexed: ASCA, Curr.Cont., Dairy Sci.Abstr., Excerp.Med., Ind.Med. (1990-), Inpharma, Int.Abstr.Biol.Sci., Nutr.Abstr., Pharm.&Out.News, Reac., Rev.Appl.Entomol., Rev.Med.& Vet.Mycol., Sci.Cit.Ind., Soyabean Abstr., Triticale Abstr.
—BLDSC (6417.527000), CISTI, EMDOCS, GNLM, IDS, Infotrieve, KNAW. **CCC.**
Published by: (European Society of Pediatric Allergy and Clinical Immunology), Blackwell Munksgaard, Noerre Soegade 35, PO Box 2148, Copenhagen K 1016, Denmark. TEL 45-77-33-33-33, FAX 45-77-33-33-77, customerservice@munksgaard.dk, http://journals.munksgaard.dk/pai, http://www.munksgaard.dk. Ed. John Warner. Adv. contact Eric Rozario TEL 45-77-33-33-01. Circ: 900.

618.92 616.97 DNK ISSN 0906-5784 CODEN: PAIUE
PEDIATRIC ALLERGY AND IMMUNOLOGY. SUPPLEMENTUM. Text in English. 1991. irreg. free with subscr. to Pediatric Allergy and Immunology. *Refereed.* **Document type:** *Academic/Scholarly.*
Related titles: Online - full text ed.: ISSN 1600-5562 (from Ovid Technologies, Inc.); ♦ Supplement to: Pediatric Allergy and Immunology. ISSN 0905-6157.
Indexed: Excerp.Med. (1994-), Int.Abstr.Biol.Sci.
—BLDSC (6417.527001), KNAW.
Published by: (European Society of Pediatric Allergy and Clinical Immunology), Blackwell Munksgaard, Noerre Soegade 35, PO Box 2148, Copenhagen K 1016, Denmark. TEL 45-77-33-33-33, FAX 45-77-33-33-77, http://www.munksgaard.dk/pai. Ed. John Warner. Adv. contact Eric Rozario TEL 45-77-33-33-01.

618.92 CHE ISSN 1017-5989 CODEN: PEAMEV
PEDIATRIC AND ADOLESCENT MEDICINE. Text in English. 1954. irreg., latest vol.9. CHF 240 in Europe; DEM 290 in Germany; USD 210 in United States (effective 2001). reprint service avail. from ISI. *Refereed.* **Document type:** *Monographic series, Academic/Scholarly.* **Description:** A problem-oriented series which seeks to clarify and evaluate difficult and evolving issues in pediatric and adolescent medicine.
Incorporates (1954-1989): Modern Problems in Paediatrics (0077-0086); (1971-1989): Monographs in Paediatrics (0077-0914); Which was formerly (1924-1971): Bibliotheca Paediatrica
Indexed: Biol.Abstr., Chem.Abstr., Curr.Cont. (coverage dropped), Ind.Med. (coverage dropped).
—BLDSC (6417.528400), CASDDS, CISTI, Infotrieve, ingenta, KNAW. **CCC.**
Published by: S. Karger AG, Allschwilerstr 10, PO Box, Basel 4009, Switzerland. TEL 41-61-306-1111, FAX 41-61-306-1234, karger@karger.ch, http://www.karger.com/bookseries/PAMED. Ed. D Branski.

618.92 616.07 USA ISSN 1093-5266 CODEN: PDPAFU
PEDIATRIC AND DEVELOPMENTAL PATHOLOGY. Text in English. 1998. bi-m. (in 1 vol., 6 nos./vol.). USD 465.90 domestic for Print & Online Eds.; USD 459.60 in Germany for Print & Online Eds.; USD 86.50 newsstand/cover foreign (effective 2002). *Refereed.* **Document type:** *Academic/Scholarly.*
Related titles: Online - full text ed.: ISSN 1615-5742 (from EBSCO Publishing, RoweCom Information Quest, Swets Blackwell, Springer LINK, Institute for Scientific Information).
Indexed: Curr.Cont., Ind.Med. (1998-), Inpharma, Pharm.&Out.News, Reac., Sci.Cit.Ind.
—BLDSC (6417.528500), CASDDS, IDS.
Published by: Springer-Verlag, Journals (Subsidiary of: BertelsmannSpringer), 175 Fifth Ave, New York, NY 10010. TEL 212-460-1500, FAX 212-473-6272, orders@springer-ny.com; dbenjam@u.washington.edu, http://www.springer-ny.com; http://link.springer.de/link/service/journals/10024/index.htm. Ed. Mugica M. Reyes. **N. American subscr. to:** Journal Fulfillment Services, PO Box 2485, Secaucus, NJ 07096-2485. TEL 800-777-4643, FAX 201-348-4505; **Subscr. outside N. America to:** Springer-Verlag, Haber Str 7, Heidelberg 69126, Germany. **Co-sponsors:** Society for Pediatric Pathology; Paediatric Pathology Society.

618.92 USA ISSN 0090-4481
RJ1
PEDIATRIC ANNALS; a journal of continuing pediatric education. Text in English. 1972. m. USD 120 to individuals; USD 140 in Canada to individuals; USD 160 elsewhere to individuals; USD 135 to institutions; USD 155 in Canada to institutions; USD 175 elsewhere to institutions. adv. bk.rev. bibl, illus, stat. index. reprint service avail. from PQC,ISI. *Refereed.* **Document type:** *Academic/Scholarly.* **Description:** Provides a thorough, practical review of a single topic in pediatrics.
Related titles: Microfilm ed.: (from PQC); Online - full text ed.: (from Northern Light Technology, Inc., ProQuest Information & Learning, Institute for Scientific Information).
Indexed: ASCA, Abstr.Hyg., Bibl.Dev.Med.& Child Neur., Biol.Abstr., C.C.I.P., CINAHL, Curr.Cont., Excerp.Med., Fam.Ind., Helminthol.Abstr., INIS Atomind., Ind.Med. (1972-), Inpharma, Int.Nurs.Ind., NRN, Pharm.&Out.News, Reac., Rev.Appl.Entomol., Rev.Med.& Vet.Mycol., SSCI (coverage dropped).
—BLDSC (6417.530000), CISTI, GNLM, IDS, ingenta, KNAW. **CCC.**
Published by: Slack, Inc., 6900 Grove Rd, Thorofare, NJ 08086-9447. TEL 856-848-1000, 800-257-8290, FAX 856-853-5991, http://www.slackinc.com/, http://www.slackinc.com/jrs.htm. Ed. Dr. William Altemeier. Circ: 33,140.

M

618.92 USA ISSN 0883-1874 CODEN: PAAIEP
PEDIATRIC ASTHMA, ALLERGY & IMMUNOLOGY. Text in English. 1987. q. USD 390 domestic to institutions; USD 505 foreign to institutions; USD 468 domestic to institutions print and online eds. combined; USD 583 foreign to institutions print and online eds. combined; USD 119 domestic to individuals; USD 217 foreign to individuals; USD 143 domestic to individuals print and online eds. combined; USD 241 foreign to individuals print and online eds. combined (effective 2002). adv. back issues avail.; reprints avail. *Refereed.* **Document type:** *Journal, Academic/Scholarly.* **Description:** Emphasizes the developmental implications of the morphologic, physiologic, and sociologic components of these problems in infants, children, and adolescents, as well as the impact of the disease processes on their families.
Related titles: Online - full content ed.: USD 390 to institutions; USD 119 to individuals (effective 2002) (from Swets Blackwell); Online - full text ed.: (from CatchWord Ltd., RoweCom Information Quest).
Indexed: ASCA, Chic.Per.Ind., Curr.Cont. (coverage dropped), Dairy Sci.Abstr., Excerp.Med. (1993-), Inpharma, Nutr.Abstr., Pharm.&Out.News, Reac., Rev.Appl.Entomol., Rev.Med.& Vet.Mycol., SSCI (coverage dropped), Triticale Abstr.
—BLDSC (6417.532000), EMDOCS, GNLM, IDS, Infotrieve, KNAW. **CCC.**
Published by: Mary Ann Liebert, Inc. Publishers, 2 Madison Ave, Larchmont, NY 10538. TEL 914—834-3100, FAX 914-834-1388, info@liebertpub.com, http://www.liebertpub.com/pai. Eds. Dr. Bettina Hilman, Dr. Robert H Schwartz.

PEDIATRIC CARDIAC SURGERY ANNUAL OF THE SEMINARS IN THORACIC AND CARDIOVASCULAR SURGERY. see *MEDICAL SCIENCES—Cardiovascular Diseases*

PEDIATRIC CARDIOLOGY. see *MEDICAL SCIENCES—Cardiovascular Diseases*

618.92 USA ISSN 1532-9798
▼ **PEDIATRIC CASE REVIEWS**; cost-effective, evidence-based diagnosis and management. Text in English. 2002. q. USD 50 to individuals; USD 150 to institutions (effective 2002). **Document type:** *Journal, Academic/Scholarly.* **Description:** Offers practical, hands-on coverage of the latest in cost-effective, evidence-based diagnostic and case management approaches.
Related titles: Online - full text ed.: USD 195 academic site license; USD 217.50 corporate site license (effective 2002).
Published by: Lippincott Williams & Wilkins (Philadelphia) (Subsidiary of: Wolters Kluwer N.V.), 530 Walnut St, Philadelphia, PA 19106-3621. TEL 215-521-8300, FAX 215-521-8902, custserv@lww.com, http://www.lww.com/. Ed. Dr. M. William Schwartz.

618.92 USA
PEDIATRIC CLINICAL PRACTICE GUIDELINES & POLICIES. Text in English. 1988. a. USD 79.95 (effective 2001). **Document type:** *Bulletin.* **Description:** Includes the full text of all AAP policy statements, practice parameters, model bills, and clinical practice guidelines for 17 pediatric conditions.
Formerly: A A P Policy Reference Guide (American Academy of Pediatrics)
Published by: American Academy of Pediatrics, 141 Northwest Point Blvd, Box 927, Elk Grove Village, IL 60009-0927. TEL 847-228-5005, 800-433-9016, FAX 847-228-1281, http://www.aap.org.

618.92 IND ISSN 0048-3133
PEDIATRIC CLINICS OF INDIA. Text in English. 1977 (vol.12). q. INR 100, USD 50. adv. charts, illus. reprint service avail. from PQC. **Document type:** *Academic/Scholarly.*
Related titles: Microfilm ed.: (from PQC).
Indexed: Nutr.Abstr.
Address: Kashyap Nursing Home, Imperial Mahal, 3 Fl., Khodadad Circle Dadar T.T., Mumbai, Maharashtra 400 014, India. TEL 91-22-412-8020, FAX 91-22-414-5056. Eds. M R Lokeshwar, Madhuri Kulkarni. Circ: 500.

618.92 USA ISSN 0031-3955
RJ23 CODEN: PCNAA8
PEDIATRIC CLINICS OF NORTH AMERICA. Text in English. 1954. bi-m. USD 116 domestic to individuals; USD 152 in Canada to individuals; USD 172 foreign to individuals; USD 179 domestic to institutions; USD 233 foreign to institutions; USD 69 domestic to students; USD 39 per issue (effective 2001). reprint service avail. from PQC,ISI. *Refereed.* **Document type:** *Journal, Academic/Scholarly.*
Related titles: Microform ed.: (from PQC); Online - full text ed.: (from Institute for Scientific Information); ♦ Spanish Translation: Clinicas Pediatricas de Norteamerica; Supplement: Continuing Medical Education Supplement to Pediatric Clinics of North America. USD 176 (effective 2000).
Indexed: AIDS Abstr., AIM, ASCA, Adol.Ment.Hlth.Abstr., Bibl.Dev.Med.& Child Neur., Biol.Abstr., C.C.I.P., CINAHL, Chem.Abstr., Curr.Adv.Cancer Res., Curr.Adv.Ecol.Sci., Curr.Cont., Dairy Sci.Abstr., Diar.Dis.Res., Environ.Sci.Poll.Mgmt., Except.Child Educ.Abstr., Excerp.Med., Fam.Ind., Helminthol.Abstr., INIS Atomind., I.P.A., Ind.Med. (1954-), Ind.Sci.Rev., Inpharma, Int.Nurs.Ind., Neurosci.Cit.Ind., Nutr.Abstr., Pharm.&Out.News, Reac., Risk Abstr., SSCI (coverage dropped), Saf.Sci.Abstr., Sci.Cit.Ind.
—BLDSC (6417.550000), CISTI, GNLM, IDS, ingenta, KNAW. **CCC.**
Published by: W.B. Saunders Co. (Subsidiary of: Harcourt Publishers Ltd.), 11830 Westline Industrial Dr, St Louis, MO 63146. TEL 800-325-4177, http://www.wbsaunders.com. **Subscr. to:** Periodicals Fulfillment, W B Saunders Co, 6277 Sea Harbor Dr, 4th Fl, Orlando, FL 32891-4800.

618.92 USA ISSN 1529-7535
▼ **PEDIATRIC CRITICAL CARE MEDICINE.** Text in English. 2000. q. USD 92 domestic to individuals; USD 112 foreign to individuals; USD 202 domestic to institutions; USD 222 foreign to institutions (effective 2002). *Refereed.* **Document type:** *Journal, Academic/Scholarly.* **Description:** Focuses exclusively on pediatric critical care medicine and critical care neonatology.
Related titles: Online - full text ed.: USD 262.60 domestic academic site license; USD 282.60 foreign academic site license; USD 292.90 domestic corporate site license; USD 312.90 foreign corporate site license (effective 2002).
Published by: (Society of Critical Care Medicine, World Federation of Pediatric Intensive and Critical Care Societies CAN), Lippincott Williams & Wilkins (Philadelphia) (Subsidiary of: Wolters Kluwer N.V.), 530 Walnut St, Philadelphia, PA 19106-3621. TEL 215-521-8300, FAX 215-521-8902, custserv@lww.com, http://www.lww.com/. **Subscr. to:** PO Box 1600, Hagerstown, MD 21740-1600. TEL 800-638-3030, FAX 310-223-2400.

PEDIATRIC DENTAL JOURNAL. see *MEDICAL SCIENCES—Dentistry*

PEDIATRIC DENTISTRY TODAY. see *MEDICAL SCIENCES—Dentistry*

PEDIATRIC DERMATOLOGY. see *MEDICAL SCIENCES—Dermatology And Venereology*

618.92 616.46 DNK ISSN 1399-543X
▼ **PEDIATRIC DIABETES.** Text in English. 2000. q. USD 202 in the Americas to institutions print & online eds. combined; GBP 140 elsewhere to institutions print & online eds. combined (effective 2002). *Refereed.* **Document type:** *Journal, Academic/Scholarly.* **Description:** Devoted to disseminating new knowledge related to the epidemiology, etiology, pathogenesis, management, complications and prevention of diabetes in childhood and adolescence.
Related titles: ♦ Online - full text ed.: Pediatric Diabetes Online. ISSN 1399-5448.
—BLDSC (6417.584000).
Published by: Blackwell Munksgaard, Noerre Soegade 35, PO Box 2148, Copenhagen K 1016, Denmark. TEL 45-77-33-33-33, FAX 45-77-33-33-77, fsub@mail.munksgaard.dk, http://www.munksgaard.dk/pediatricdiabetes. Ed. Mark Sperling. Adv. contact Eric Rozario TEL 45-77-33-33-01. Circ: 900.

618.92 616.46 DNK ISSN 1399-5448
▼ **PEDIATRIC DIABETES ONLINE.** Text in English. 2000. q. GBP 126 (effective 2002). *Refereed.* **Document type:** *Academic/Scholarly.*
Media: Online - full text (from Munksgaard & Blackwell Science's Synergy, ingenta, Swets Blackwell). **Related titles:** ♦ Print ed.: Pediatric Diabetes. ISSN 1399-543X.
—BLDSC (6417.584000).
Published by: Blackwell Munksgaard, Noerre Soegade 35, PO Box 2148, Copenhagen K 1016, Denmark. TEL 45-77-33-33-33, FAX 45-77-33-33-77, http://www.munksgaard.dk/pediatricdiabetes.

PEDIATRIC EMERGENCY & CRITICAL CARE; a clinical update for those who care for infants and children. see *MEDICAL SCIENCES—Abstracting, Bibliographies, Statistics*

618.92 616.02 USA ISSN 0749-5161 CODEN: PECAE5
PEDIATRIC EMERGENCY CARE. Text in English. 1985. bi-m., latest vol.17. USD 169 domestic to individuals; USD 199 foreign to individuals; USD 283 domestic to institutions; USD 320 foreign to institutions; USD 49 newsstand/cover (effective 2002). adv. back issues avail. *Refereed.* **Document type:** *Journal, Academic/Scholarly.* **Description:** Contains clinical information for emergency physicians and pediatricians who care for acutely ill or injured children and adolescents.
Related titles: Microfilm ed.: (from WWS); Online - full text ed.: USD 367.90 domestic accademic site license; USD 404.90 foreign accademic site license; USD 410.35 domestic corporate site license; USD 447.35 foreign corporate site license (effective 2002) (from Ovid Technologies, Inc., Institute for Scientific Information).
Indexed: ASCA, CINAHL, Curr.Cont., Ind.Med. (1985-), Inpharma, Int.Nurs.Ind., Jrnl.Watch Emer.Med., Pharm.&Out.News, Reac., Rev.Appl.Entomol., Rev.Med.& Vet.Mycol.
—BLDSC (6417.586000), EMDOCS, GNLM, IDS, ingenta, KNAW.
Published by: Lippincott Williams & Wilkins (Baltimore) (Subsidiary of: Wolters Kluwer N.V.), 351 W Camden St, Baltimore, MD 21201-2436. TEL 410-528-4068, 800-222-3790, FAX 410-528-4452, http://www.pec-online.com, http://www.wwilkins.com. Eds. Gary Fleisher, Dr. Stephen Ludwig. Adv. contact Kathleen Malamphy. Circ: 2,865.

PEDIATRIC EMERGENCY MEDICINE REPORTS. see *MEDICAL SCIENCES—Orthopedics And Traumatology*

617.98 USA ISSN 1092-6410
PEDIATRIC ENDOSURGERY & INNOVATIVE TECHNIQUES; part B of Journal of Laparoendoscopic & Advanced Surgical Techniques. Text in English. 1997. q. USD 107 domestic to individuals; USD 188 foreign to individuals; USD 128 domestic to individuals print and online eds. combined; USD 209 foreign to individuals print and online eds. combined; USD 366 domestic to institutions; USD 470 foreign to institutions; USD 439 domestic to institutions print and online eds. combined; USD 543 foreign to institutions print and online eds. combined (effective 2002). adv. back issues avail.; reprints avail. *Refereed.* **Document type:** *Journal.* **Description:** Dedicated to serving the needs of pediatric surgeons and specialists who perform diagnostic and therapeutic endoscopic procedures on infants and children.
Related titles: Online - full content ed.: USD 107 to individuals; USD 366 to institutions (effective 2002); Online - full text ed.: (from CatchWord Ltd., RoweCom Information Quest).
—BLDSC (6417.588500), GNLM, Infotrieve, KNAW. **CCC.**
Published by: Mary Ann Liebert, Inc. Publishers, 2 Madison Ave, Larchmont, NY 10538. TEL 914—834-3100, FAX 914-834-3771, info@liebertpub.com, http://www.liebertpub.com/pei. Ed. Dr. Thom E Lobe. Adv. contact Harriet Matysko.

618.92 USA ISSN 0899-8493 CODEN: PEXSFT
PEDIATRIC EXERCISE SCIENCE. Short title: P E S. Text in English. 1989. q. USD 48 to individuals; USD 144 to institutions; USD 36 to students (effective 2001). adv. bk.rev. charts, illus. back issues avail.; reprint service avail. from PSC. *Refereed.* **Document type:** *Academic/Scholarly.* **Description:** Addresses the importance of exercise during childhood and adolescence to scientists, health-care providers, and physical educators.
Related titles: Online - full text ed.: (from Institute for Scientific Information).
Indexed: AMED, ASCA, CINAHL, Child Devel.Abstr., Focus on: Sports Sci.& Med., IBZ, Phys.Ed.Ind., SSCI (coverage dropped), Sportsearch (1990-).
—BLDSC (6417.590000), GNLM, IDS, ingenta. **CCC.**
Published by: (North American Society of Pediatric Exercise Medicine), Human Kinetics Publishers, Inc., PO Box 5076, Champaign, IL 61825-5076. TEL 217-351-5076, 800-747-4457, FAX 217-351-2674, http://www.humankinetics.com. Ed. Dr. Thomas Rowland. Pub. Rainer Martens. R&P Cheri Banks TEL 217-351-5076 ext 2275. Adv. contact Patty Rodriguiz. Circ: 594 (paid and free).

618.92 USA ISSN 1067-9413
PEDIATRIC HEALTH MONITOR. Text in English. 1995. q. **Document type:** *Newsletter, Consumer.*
Published by: Data Centrum Communications, Inc., 21 W 38th St, 4th fl, New York, NY 10018.

618.92 USA ISSN 0888-0018
CODEN: PHONEN

PEDIATRIC HEMATOLOGY & ONCOLOGY. Text in English. 1984. 8/yr. GBP 201, USD 331 to individuals; GBP 456, USD 752 to institutions (effective 2002). adv. bk.rev. back issues avail.; reprint service avail. from PQC. *Refereed.* **Document type:** *Academic/Scholarly.* **Description:** Publishes experimental, biochemical and clinical articles covering immunology, pathology and pharmacology.
Formerly (until 1986): European Paediatric Haematology and Oncology (0800-2789)
Related titles: Microform ed.: (from PQC); Online - full text ed.: ISSN 1521-0669 (from CatchWord Ltd., EBSCO Publishing, O C L C Online Computer Library Center, Inc., RoweCom Information Quest, Swets Blackwell, Institute for Scientific Information).
Indexed: ASCA, Chem.Abstr., Chem.Titles, Curr.Cont., Environ.Sci.Poll.Mgmt., Excerp.Med., INIS Atomind., Ind.Med. (1986-), Ind.Sci.Rev., Inpharma, Int.Abstr.Biol.Sci., Med.& Surg.Dermat., Nutr.Abstr., Pharm.&Out.News, Pollut.Abstr., Reac., Rev.Arom.& Med.Plants, Risk Abstr., SSCI (coverage dropped), Saf.Sci.Abstr., Sci.Cit.Ind., Weed Abstr.
—BLDSC (6417.599500), CASDDS, CatchWord, CISTI, EMDOCS, GNLM, IDS, ingenta, KNAW. **CCC.**
Published by: Taylor & Francis Ltd. (Subsidiary of: Taylor & Francis Group), 325 Chestnut St, Suite 800, Philadelphia, PA 19016. TEL 215-625-8900, FAX 215-625-2940, info@tandf.co.uk, info@taylorandfrancis.com, http://www.tandf.co.uk/., http://www.taylorandfrancis.com/. Ed. Dr. Louise Parker. Circ: 600. **Subscr. to:** Taylor & Francis Group, Journals Customer Service, Rankine Rd, Basingstoke, Hants RG24 8PR, United Kingdom. TEL 44-1256-813000, FAX 44-1256-479438, enquiry@tanf.co.uk, http://www.tandf.co.uk/journals.

PEDIATRIC HEMATOLOGY - ONCOLOGY SERIES. see *MEDICAL SCIENCES—Oncology*

618.92 616.9 USA ISSN 0891-3668
CODEN: PIDJEV

THE PEDIATRIC INFECTIOUS DISEASE JOURNAL. Text in English. m., latest vol.20. USD 164 domestic to individuals Print & Online eds. combined; USD 204 foreign to individuals Print & Online eds. combined; USD 357 domestic to institutions Print & Online eds. combined; USD 357 per issue foreign to institutions; USD 28 newsstand/cover (effective 2002). adv. bk.rev. index. *Refereed.* **Document type:** *Journal, Academic/Scholarly.* **Description:** Covers the treatment of viral and bacterial illness in children.
Related titles: Microfilm ed.: (from WWS); Online - full text ed.: USD 464.10 domestic academic site license; USD 464.10 foreign academic site license; USD 517.65 domestic corporate site license; USD 517.65 foreign corporate site license (effective 2002) (from Ovid Technologies, Inc., Swets Blackwell, Institute for Scientific Information).
Indexed: ASCA, Abstr.Anthropol., Abstr.Hyg., Bibl.Dev.Med.& Child Neur., C.C.I.P., Curr.Cont., Dairy Sci.Abstr., Dent.Ind., Diar.Dis.Res., Dok.Arbeitsmed., Environ.Sci.Poll.Mgmt., Fam.Ind., Helminthol.Abstr., Ind.Med. (1987-), Ind.Sci.Rev., Ind.Vet., Inpharma, Jrnl.Watch Emer.Med., Jrnl.Watch Inf.Dis., Med.& Surg.Dermat., Microbiol.Abstr., NRN, Neurosci.Cit.Ind., Nutr.Abstr., Pharm.&Out.News, Pollut.Abstr., Protozool.Abstr., Reac., Rev.Appl.Entomol., Rev.Med.& Vet.Mycol., Risk Abstr., Rural Devel.Abstr., Rural Recreat.Tour.Abstr., Saf.Sci.Abstr., Sci.Cit.Ind., Small Anim.Abstr., Trop.Dis.Bull., Virol.Abstr. (coverage dropped).
—BLDSC (6417.601600), CISTI, EMDOCS, GNLM, IDS, ingenta, KNAW.
Published by: Lippincott Williams & Wilkins (Baltimore) (Subsidiary of: Wolters Kluwer N.V.), 351 W Camden St, Baltimore, MD 21201-2436. TEL 410-528-4068, 800-222-3790, FAX 410-528-4452, kmalamphy@wwilkins.com, http://www.pidj.com, http://www.wwilkins.com. Eds. George H McCracken Jr., Dr. John D Nelson. Adv. contact Kathleen Malamphy. Circ: 15,354.

618.92 USA ISSN 0887-8994

PEDIATRIC NEUROLOGY. Text in English. 1985. 10/yr. EUR 210 in Europe to individuals; JPY 28,000 in Japan to individuals; USD 235 elsewhere to individuals; EUR 422 in Europe to institutions; JPY 56,000 in Japan to institutions; USD 472 elsewhere to institutions (effective 2002). adv. reprints avail. *Refereed.* **Document type:** *Academic/Scholarly.* **Description:** Contains original papers, reviews, case reports, news, and professional announcements which provide current information on diseases affecting the immature nervous system.
Related titles: Microform ed.: (from PQC); Online - full text ed.: (from ingenta, ScienceDirect, Swets Blackwell, Institute for Scientific Information).
Indexed: ASCA, Curr.Cont., Excerp.Med., INIS Atomind., Ind.Med. (1985-), Inpharma, Int.Abstr.Biol.Sci., Jrnl.Watch Neuro., Neurosci.Cit.Ind., Nutr.Abstr., Pharm.&Out.News, Protozool.Abstr., Reac., Rev.Appl.Entomol., SSCI (coverage dropped), Sci.Cit.Ind., Trop.Dis.Bull., e-psyche.
—BLDSC (6417.604300), CISTI, EMDOCS, GNLM, IDS, ingenta, KNAW. **CCC.**
Published by: Elsevier Science, 655 Ave of the Americas, New York, NY 10010. FAX 212-633-3990, usinfof-@elsevier.com, usinfo-f@elsevier.com, http://www.elsevier.nl/locate/pedneu. Ed. Dr. Kenneth F Swaiman. Adv. contact Hank Blaney. B&W page USD 1,035, color page USD 1,345; 7 x 10. Circ: 1,500 (paid). **Subscr. in Australasia and the Far East to:** Elsevier Science (Singapore) Pte Ltd, No.1 Temasek Ave, 17-01 Millenia Tower, Singapore 039192, Singapore. TEL 65-434-3727, FAX 65-337-2230; **Subscr. in Japan to:** Elsevier Science Inc - Japan Regional Office, 9-15 Higashi-Azabu 1-chome, Minato-ku, Tokyo 106-0044, Japan. TEL 81-3-5561-5033, FAX 81-3-5561-5047; **Subscr. outside the Americas to:** Elsevier Science BV, PO Box 211, Amsterdam 1000 AE, Netherlands. TEL 31-20-485-3757, FAX 31-20-485-3432.

618.92 USA ISSN 0031-398X
RJ1

PEDIATRIC NEWS. Text in English. 1967. m. USD 70. adv. bk.rev. charts, illus. **Document type:** *Newspaper.*
Related titles: Microform ed.: (from PQC).
—BLDSC (6417.605000), Infotrieve. **CCC.**
Published by: International Medical News Group, 12230 Wilkins Ave, Rockville, MD 20852. TEL 301-816-8700. Ed. Phyllis Schaeffer. Circ: 35,000.

618.92 USA

PEDIATRIC NUTRITION HANDBOOK. Text in English. 1979. irreg., latest vol.4, 1998. USD 69.95 (effective 2001). **Document type:** *Monographic series.*
Published by: American Academy of Pediatrics, 141 Northwest Point Blvd, Box 927, Elk Grove Village, IL 60009-0927. TEL 847-228-5005, 800-433-9016, FAX 847-228-1281, http://www.aap.org.

618.92 USA ISSN 1522-7952
CODEN: PPMMFX

PEDIATRIC PATHOLOGY & MOLECULAR MEDICINE. Text in English. 1983. bi-m. GBP 156, USD 258 to individuals; GBP 393, USD 649 to institutions (effective 2002). adv. bk.rev. bibl, charts, illus. index. back issues avail.; reprint service avail. from PQC. *Refereed.* **Document type:** *Academic/Scholarly.* **Description:** Covers the study of disease in the developing human.
Former titles (until 1999): Pediatric Pathology & Laboratory Medicine (1077-1042); (until 1994): Pediatric Pathology (0277-0938)
Related titles: Microform ed.: (from PQC); Online - full text ed.: ISSN 1523-4525 (from CatchWord Ltd., EBSCO Publishing, O C L C Online Computer Library Center, Inc., RoweCom Information Quest, Swets Blackwell, Institute for Scientific Information).
Indexed: ASCA, Curr.Adv.Cancer Res., Curr.Adv.Ecol.Sci., Curr.Cont., Excerp.Med., INIS Atomind., Ind.Med. (until 1999, dropped), Ind.Sci.Rev., Inpharma, Neurosci.Cit.Ind., Pharm.&Out.News, Protozool.Abstr., Reac., Rev.Med.& Vet.Mycol., Sci.Cit.Ind.
—BLDSC (6417.605530), CatchWord, CISTI, EMDOCS, GNLM, IDS, ingenta, KNAW. **CCC.**
Published by: Taylor & Francis Ltd. (Subsidiary of: Taylor & Francis Group), 325 Chestnut St, Suite 800, Philadelphia, PA 19016. TEL 215-625-8900, FAX 215-625-2940, info@taylorandfrancis.com, http://www.taylorandfrancis.com/. Ed. S Tabibzadeh. Circ: 350. **Subscr. addr. in Europe:** Taylor & Francis Group, Journals Customer Service, Rankine Rd, Basingstoke, Hants RG24 8PR, United Kingdom. TEL 44-1256-813000, FAX 44-1256-479438, enquiry@tanf.co.uk, http://www.tandf.co.uk/journals. **Co-sponsor:** International Pediatric Pathology Association.

618.92 615.19 USA

PEDIATRIC PHARMACOTHERAPY; a monthly review for health care professionals. Text in English. 1995. m. *Refereed.* **Description:** Provides a brief, referenced source of continuing medication information specifically related to children. Focuses on the initiation and monitoring of medications in the primary care setting.
Related titles: Online - full text ed.
Published by: University of Virginia Health Sciences Center, Children's Medical Center, PO Box 274 11, Charlottesville, VA 22908. TEL 804-982-0921, FAX 804-982-1682, mlb3u@virginia.edu.

618.92 615.82 USA ISSN 0898-5669
CODEN: PPTHEI

PEDIATRIC PHYSICAL THERAPY. Text in English. 1989. q., latest vol.13. USD 96 domestic to individuals; USD 130 foreign to individuals; USD 159 domestic to institutions; USD 196 foreign to institutions; USD 45 newsstand/cover (effective 2002). adv. index. *Refereed.* **Document type:** *Academic/Scholarly.* **Description:** Delivers practical information on the full range of pediatric conditions, including developmental, orthopedic and respiratory concerns.
Related titles: Microfilm ed.: (from WWS); Online - full text ed.: USD 206.70 domestic for academic site license; USD 243.70 foreign for academic site license; USD 230.55 domestic for corporate site license; USD 267.55 foreign for corporate site license (effective 2002).
Indexed: AMED, CINAHL, Except.Child Educ.Abstr., IMFL.
—BLDSC (6417.605700), CISTI, EMDOCS, GNLM, KNAW.
Published by: (Section on Pediatrics, American Physical Therapy Association), Williams & Wilkins (Subsidiary of: Waverly International), 351 W Camden St, Baltimore, MD 21201-2436. TEL 410-528-4068, 800-222-3790, FAX 410-528-4452, sisaacson@wwilkins.com, http://www.wwilkins.com. Ed. Ann F Vansant. Adv. contact Sharlene Isaacson. Circ: 5,369.

PEDIATRIC PRACTICE ADVISOR. see *HEALTH FACILITIES AND ADMINISTRATION*

PEDIATRIC PRIMARY CARE; practical pediatrics for the pediatric practitioner. see *MEDICAL SCIENCES—Abstracting, Bibliographies, Statistics*

618.92 616.2 USA ISSN 8755-6863
CODEN: PEPUES

PEDIATRIC PULMONOLOGY. Text in English. 1985. m. USD 1,180 in United States; USD 1,310 in Canada & Mexico; USD 1,420 elsewhere; USD 1,239 combined subscription in United States for print and online eds.; USD 1,369 combined subscription in Canada & Mexico for print and online eds.; USD 1,479 combined subscription elsewhere for print and online eds. (effective 2002). adv. bk.rev. back issues avail. *Refereed.* **Document type:** *Academic/Scholarly.* **Description:** Covers various aspects of respiratory system disorders in infants and children.
Related titles: Online - full text ed.: ISSN 1099-0496. 1996. USD 1,180 in United States; USD 1,180 in Canada & Mexico; USD 1,180 elsewhere (effective 2002) (from EBSCO Publishing, Wiley InterScience, Institute for Scientific Information).
Indexed: ASCA, Biol.Abstr., Curr.Cont., Dairy Sci.Abstr., INIS Atomind., Ind.Med. (1985-), Ind.Sci.Rev., Inpharma, Int.Nurs.Ind., Nutr.Abstr., Pharm.&Out.News, Reac., Ref.Zh., Rev.Med.& Vet.Mycol., Sci.Cit.Ind., Trop.Dis.Bull.
—BLDSC (6417.605800), CISTI, EMDOCS, GNLM, IDS, ingenta, KNAW. **CCC.**
Published by: John Wiley & Sons, Inc., Journals (Subsidiary of: Wiley InterScience), 605 Third Ave, New York, NY 10158. TEL 212-850-6645, FAX 212-850-6021, subinfo@wiley.com, uscs-wis@wiley.com, http://www.wiley.com. Ed. Gerd J A Cropp. adv.: B&W page GBP 640, color page GBP 1,515; trim 210 x 279. Circ: 1,500. **Subscr. outside the Americas to:** John Wiley & Sons Ltd., Baffins Ln, Chichester, Sussex PO19 IUD, United Kingdom. TEL 44-1243-779777, FAX 44-1243-843232, cs-journals@wiley.co.uk.

618.92 615.842 DEU ISSN 0301-0449
CODEN: PDRYA5

PEDIATRIC RADIOLOGY; roentgenology, nuclear medicine, ultrasonics, CT, MRI. Text in English. 1973. m. EUR 860.90 domestic (effective Apr. 2002); EUR 841.70 in Germany; EUR 81.50 newsstand/cover foreign (effective 2002). adv. reprint service avail. from ISI. *Refereed.* **Document type:** *Journal, Academic/Scholarly.* **Description:** Reports on the progress and results from all areas of pediatric radiology and related fields.
Related titles: Microform ed.: (from PQC); Online - full text ed.: ISSN 1432-1998 (from EBSCO Publishing, RoweCom Information Quest, Swets Blackwell, Springer LINK, Institute for Scientific Information).
Indexed: ASCA, Bibl.Dev.Med.& Child Neur., Chem.Abstr., Curr.Adv.Cancer Res., Curr.Cont., Dairy Sci.Abstr., Dent.Ind., Excerp.Med., Helminthol.Abstr., INIS Atomind., Ind.Imag.Lit., Ind.Med. (1973-), Ind.Sci.Rev., Inpharma, Int.Nurs.Ind., Neurosci.Cit.Ind., Nutr.Abstr., Pharm.&Out.News, Protozool.Abstr., Reac., Rev.Med.& Vet.Mycol., Sci.Cit.Ind.
—BLDSC (6417.606000), CISTI, EMDOCS, GNLM, IDS, ingenta, KNAW. **CCC.**

M

Published by: (European Society of Pediatric Radiology), Springer-Verlag (Subsidiary of: BertelsmannSpringer), Tiergartenstr 17, Heidelberg 69121, Germany. TEL 49-6221-345-0, FAX 49-6221-345229, subscriptions@springer.de, http://link.springer.de/link/service/journals/00247/index.htm, http://www.springer.de. Eds. F Brunelle, W E Berdon. **Subscr. in N. America to:** Springer-Verlag New York Inc., PO Box 2485, Secaucus, NJ 07096-2485. TEL 212-460-1500, FAX 212-473-6272.

PEDIATRIC REHABILITATION. see *MEDICAL SCIENCES—Physical Medicine And Rehabilitation*

618.92 USA ISSN 0031-3998
RJ1 CODEN: PEREBL
PEDIATRIC RESEARCH; international journal of human developmental biology. Text in English. 1967. m., latest vol.50. USD 309 domestic to individuals; USD 385 foreign to individuals; USD 518 domestic to institutions; USD 594 foreign to institutions; USD 50 newsstand/cover (effective 2002); Print & Online eds. combined. adv. bk.rev. charts, illus. index. back issues avail. *Refereed.* **Document type:** *Journal, Academic/Scholarly.* **Description:** Covers advances in the understanding and management of pediatric pulmonary, endocrinological, gastroenterological, and nutritional disorders.
Related titles: Microfilm ed.: (from WWS); Online - full text ed.: USD 673.40 domestic academic site license; USD 749.40 foreign academic site license; USD 751.10 domestic corporate site license; USD 827.10 foreign corporate site license (effective 2002) (from Ovid Technologies, Inc., HighWire Pr., EBSCO Publishing, Institute for Scientific Information).
Indexed: ASCA, Abstr.Hyg., AgBiotech, Anim.Breed.Abstr., Arts & Hum.Cit.Ind. (coverage dropped), Bibl.Dev.Med.& Child Neur., Biol.Abstr., C.C.I.P., Chem.Abstr., Chem.Titles, Chic.Per.Ind., Child Devel.Abstr., Curr.Adv.Biochem., Curr.Adv.Cell & Devel.Biol., Curr.Adv.Ecol.Sci., Curr.Cont., Dairy Sci.Abstr., Dent.Ind., Diar.Dis.Res., Excerp.Med., Helminthol.Abstr., Ind.Med. (1967-), Ind.Sci.Rev., Ind.Vet., Inpharma, Kidney, Lang.& Lang.Behav.Abstr., NRN, Neurosci.Cit.Ind., Nutr.Abstr., Pharm.&Out.News, Pig News & Info., Reac., SSCI (coverage dropped), Sci.Cit.Ind., Soyabean Abstr., THA, Triticale Abstr.
—BLDSC (6417.620000), CASDDS, CISTI, GNLM, IDS, ingenta, KNAW.
Published by: (International Pediatric Research Foundation Inc.), Lippincott Williams & Wilkins (Philadelphia) (Subsidiary of: Wolters Kluwer N.V.), 530 Walnut St, Philadelphia, PA 19106-3621. TEL 215-521-8300, FAX 215-521-8902, custserv@lww.com, http://www.pedresearch.org/, http://www.lww.com/. Ed. Alvin Zipursky. Circ: 3,603. **Subscr. to:** Lippincott Williams & Wilkins (Baltimore), PO Box 1600, Hagerstown, MD 21741. TEL 301-223-2300, 81-3-5689-5400, 91-11-579-3211, 800-638-3030, FAX 301-223-2400, 81-3-5689-5402, 91-11-579-8876, customerservice@lww.com. **Co-sponsors:** American Pediatric Society; European Society for Pediatric Research; Society for Pediatric Research.

618.92 CHE ISSN 0882-9225
CODEN: PRECEA
PEDIATRIC REVIEWS AND COMMUNICATIONS. Text in English. 4/yr. (in 1 vol., 4 nos./vol.). USD 144 (effective 1998). *Refereed.*
Related titles: CD-ROM ed.; Microform ed.; Online - full text ed.
—EMDOCS, GNLM. **CCC.**
Published by: Gordon and Breach - Harwood Academic (Subsidiary of: Taylor & Francis Group), PO Box 531, Lausanne 1000, Switzerland. http://www.gbhap.com/Pediatric_Reviews_Communications/. Ed. Philip Lanzkowsky. **Subscr. addr. in US:** International Publishers Direct, PO Box 32160, Newark, NJ 07102. FAX 215-750-6343.

PEDIATRIC SURGERY INTERNATIONAL. see *MEDICAL SCIENCES—Surgery*

PEDIATRIC SURGERY UPDATE. see *MEDICAL SCIENCES—Surgery*

617.98 DNK ISSN 1397-3142
RD120.77.C45 CODEN: PETRF6
PEDIATRIC TRANSPLANTATION. Text in English. 1997. bi-m. USD 336 in the Americas to institutions print & online eds. combined; GBP 233 elsewhere to institutions print & online eds. combined (effective 2002). adv. illus. *Refereed.* **Document type:** *Academic/Scholarly.* **Description:** Deals with clinical experience and basic research in transplantation of tissues and solid organs in infants, children and adolescents.
Related titles: Online - full text ed.: ISSN 1399-3046. GBP 210 (effective 2002) (from EBSCO Publishing, O C L C Online Computer Library Center, Inc., RoweCom Information Quest, ingenta, Munksgaard & Blackwell Science's Synergy, Swets Blackwell, Institute for Scientific Information).
Indexed: Ind.Med. (1997-), Int.Nurs.Ind.
—BLDSC (6417.628330), GNLM, Infotrieve. **CCC.**
Published by: (International Pediatric Transplantation Association), Blackwell Munksgaard, Noerre Soegade 35, PO Box 2148, Copenhagen K 1016, Denmark. TEL 45-77-33-33-33, FAX 45-77-33-33-77, customerservice@munksgaard.dk, http://www.munksgaard.dk/pediatrictransplantation. Ed. Richard N Fine. Adv. contact Eric Rozario TEL 45-77-33-33-01. Circ: 800.

618.92 USA
PEDIATRICLINX. Text in English. d. adv. **Document type:** *Newsletter.* **Description:** Includes pediatric news and medical information for physicians and healthcare professionals.
Media: Online - full text. **Related titles:** E-mail ed.
Published by: MDLinx.com Inc, 316 F St NE Ste 200, Washington, DC 20002. TEL 202-543-6544, FAX 202-543-6674, info@mdlinx.com, http://www.pedriatriclinx.com. Ed. Dave Rothenberg.

648.92 ITA ISSN 1120-7507
PEDIATRICS. Text in Italian. 1989. bi-m.
Related titles: Online - full text ed.: (from Northern Light Technology, Inc.).
Indexed: Bibl.Agri., CINAHL, Crim.Just.Abstr., Curr.Cont. (coverage dropped), Ind.Sci.Rev., Jrnl.Watch Derm., Protozool.Abstr., Rev.Appl.Entomol., Sci.Cit.Ind. (coverage dropped).
Address: Viale Liguria, 20 22A, Milan, MI 20143, Italy. TEL 2-58-10-35-65, FAX 2-581-022-49. Ed. Gianni Ardito.

618.92 USA
PEDIATRICS AND THE A A P MEETING PROGRAM. Text in English. 1948. a. free per issue to members. **Description:** Lists the available courses at AAP annual meeting.
Published by: American Academy of Pediatrics, 141 Northwest Point Blvd., Box 927, Elk Grove, IL 60009-0927. TEL 708-228-5005, 888-227-1773, FAX 708-228-1281, http://www.aap.org.

618.9 ESP ISSN 0210-5721
PEDIATRICS (EDICION ESPANOLA). Text in Spanish. 1976. m. USD 129. adv. reprint service avail. from PQC. **Document type:** *Academic/Scholarly.* **Description:** Covers infectious illnesses, immunity, nutrition, community medicine, premature and newborn babies, neurology, psychiatry, cardiology, endocrinology and toxicology.
Related titles: ♦ English ed.: Pediatrics (English Edition). ISSN 0031-4005; Arabic ed.; Hungarian ed.; Russian ed.; Portuguese ed.
Indexed: Curr.Cont. (coverage dropped), Dok.Arbeitsmed., Ind.Sci.Rev., Vet.Bull.
—**CCC.**
Published by: (American Academy of Pediatrics USA), Ediciones Doyma S.A., Traversa de Gracia, 17-21, Barcelona 08021, Spain. TEL 34-93-200-0711, FAX 34-93-209-1136, http://www.aap.org. Ed. A Ballabriga Aguado. Adv. contact Olga Valls. color page ESP 292,000; trim 280 x 210. Circ: 4,000.

618.92 USA ISSN 0031-4005
RJ1 CODEN: PEDIAU
PEDIATRICS (ENGLISH EDITION). Text in English. 1948. m. USD 130 domestic to individuals; USD 145 foreign to individuals; USD 200 domestic to institutions; USD 215 foreign to institutions (effective 2001). adv. bk.rev. illus. s-a. index. back issues avail.; reprints avail. *Refereed.* **Document type:** *Academic/Scholarly.* **Description:** Contains original research and special features in the field of pediatrics. Articles cover various topics including nutrition, surgery, dentistry, public health, genetics, psychosocial development, education and nursing.
Related titles: CD-ROM ed.: (from Ovid Technologies, Inc.); Microfiche ed.; Online - full text ed.: USD 100 (effective 2001) (from HighWire Pr., LexisNexis, EBSCO Publishing, ProQuest Information & Learning, Gale Group, Factiva, Institute for Scientific Information); ♦ Spanish ed.: Pediatrics (Edicion Espanola). ISSN 0210-5721; Arabic ed.; Hungarian ed.; Russian ed.; Portuguese ed.; Regional ed.: Pediatrics (Indian Edition).
Indexed: AIDS Abstr., AIM, Abstr.Health Care Manage.Stud., Abstr.Hyg., Agri.& Environ.Biotech.Abstr. (coverage dropped), Behav.Med.Abstr., Bibl.Dev.Med.& Child Neur., Biol.Abstr., C.C.I.P., Chem.Abstr., Curr.Adv.Ecol.Sci., Curr.Cont., Dairy Sci.Abstr., Dent.Ind., Derwent Biotech.Abstr., Diab.Cont., Dok.Arbeitsmed., Except.Child Educ.Abstr., Excerp.Med., FAMLI, Food Sci.& Tech.Abstr., Helminthol.Abstr., Hosp.Lit.Ind., INIS Atomind., I.P.A., Ind.Med. (1948-), Ind.Sci.Rev., Ind.Vet., Inpharma, Int.Abstr.Biol.Sci., Int.Nurs.Ind., Jrnl.Watch, Jrnl.Watch Emer.Med., Jrnl.Watch Wom.Hlth., Kidney, L.R.I., Med.& Surg.Dermat., NRN, Nutr.Abstr., Pharm.&Out.News, Poult.Abstr., Reac., Rev.Arom.& Med.Plants, Rev.Med.& Vet.Mycol., Rev.Plant Path., Risk Abstr., Rural Recreat.Tour.Abstr., Sci.Cit.Ind., Trop.Dis.Bull., Vet.Bull.
—BLDSC (6417.650000), CASDDS, CISTI, GNLM, IDS, ingenta, KNAW. **CCC.**
Published by: American Academy of Pediatrics, 141 Northwest Point Blvd, Box 927, Elk Grove Village, IL 60009-0927. TEL 847-228-5005, 800-433-9016, FAX 847-228-5088, journals@aap.org, http://www.pediatrics.org. Ed. Dr. Jerold F Lucey. Circ: 61,000.

618.92 USA ISSN 0730-6725
PEDIATRICS FOR PARENTS; the monthly newsletter for caring adults. Text in English. 1980. m. USD 20 domestic; USD 23 in Canada; USD 26 elsewhere (effective 2000 - 2001). 12 p./no. 3 cols./p. back issues avail. **Document type:** *Newsletter.*
Related titles: Microform ed.: (from PQC); Online - full text ed.: (from Gale Group, Northern Light Technology, Inc., ProQuest Information & Learning, Factiva).
Indexed: Hlth.Ind.
—Infotrieve. **CCC.**
Published by: Pediatrics for Parents, Inc., 747 S Third St, Unit 3, Philadelphia, PA 19147-3324. TEL 215-625-9609, info@pediatricsforparents.com, pediatricsforparents@pobox.com, http://www.pedsforparents.com/, http://www.moms-refuge.com/. Ed. Dr. Richard J Sagall. Circ: 1,000 (paid).

618.92 USA ISSN 0191-9601
CODEN: PDREFI
PEDIATRICS IN REVIEW. Text in English. 1979. m. USD 175 domestic to non-members; USD 225 foreign to non-members; USD 165 domestic to members; USD 215 foreign to members (effective 2001). abstr, charts, illus. cum.index. Supplement avail.; back issues avail. *Refereed.* **Document type:** *Journal, Academic/Scholarly, Trade.*
Related titles: Online - full text ed.: (from HighWire Pr., EBSCO Publishing).
Indexed: C.C.I.P., Ind.Med. (1979-), NRN.
—BLDSC (6417.657000), GNLM, ingenta, KNAW. **CCC.**
Published by: American Academy of Pediatrics, 141 Northwest Point Blvd, Box 927, Elk Grove Village, IL 60009-0927. TEL 847-228-5005, 800-433-9016, FAX 847-228-5097, http://www.pedsinreview.org/. Ed. Dr. Robert J Haggerty. Circ: 31,000.

618.92 AUS ISSN 1328-8067
CODEN: JAMMFW
PEDIATRICS INTERNATIONAL. Text in English. 1959. bi-m. AUD 298 domestic to individuals; AUD 270 in New Zealand to individuals; USD 165 elsewhere to individuals; AUD 685 domestic to institutions; AUD 623 in New Zealand to institutions; JPY 43,550 in Japan to institutions; USD 380 elsewhere to institutions; AUD 328 domestic to individuals paper & online eds. combined; AUD 297 in New Zealand to individuals paper & online eds. combined; USD 182 elsewhere to individuals paper & online eds. combined; AUD 754 domestic to institutions paper & online eds. combined; AUD 686 in New Zealand to institutions paper & online eds. combined; JPY 47,905 in Japan to institutions paper & online eds. combined; USD 418 elsewhere to institutions paper & online eds. combined (effective 2001). adv. bk.rev. abstr, bibl, charts, illus. index. reprint service avail. from ISI. *Refereed.* **Document type:** *Academic/Scholarly.* **Description:** Contains scientific articles, clinical and laboratory studies, and case reports in the field of pediatrics and child health.
Former titles (until 1999): Acta Paediatrica Japonica. Overseas Edition (0374-5600); Paediatrica Japonica
Related titles: Microform ed.: (from PQC); Online - full text ed.: ISSN 1442-200X. AUD 269 domestic to individuals; AUD 243 in New Zealand to individuals; USD 149 elsewhere to individuals; AUD 617 domestic to institutions; AUD 561 in New Zealand to institutions; JPY 39,195 in Japan to institutions; USD 342 elsewhere to institutions (effective 2001) (from EBSCO Publishing, O C L C Online Computer Library Center, Inc., RoweCom Information Quest, ingenta, Munksgaard & Blackwell Science's Synergy, Swets Blackwell, Institute for Scientific Information); Japanese ed.: Nippon Shonika Gakkai Zasshi. ISSN 0001-6543.

Indexed: ASSIA, Biol.Abstr., Chem.Abstr., Chem.Indus.Notes, Chem.Titles, Curr.Cont., Dairy Sci.Abstr., Excerp.Med., INIS Atomind., Ind.Med. (1999-), Inpharma, Kidney, NRN, Pharm.&Out.News, Reac.
—BLDSC (6417.655800), ADONIS, CASDDS, CISTI, EMDOCS, GNLM, IDS, Infotrieve, KNAW. **CCC.**
Published by: (Japan Pediatric Society JPN), Blackwell Science Asia Pty Ltd, PO Box 378, Carlton South, VIC 3053, Australia. TEL 61-3-9347-0300, FAX 61-3-9347-5001, info@blacksci-asia.com.au, http://www.blacksci.co.uk. Ed. Shoichi Awa. Adv. contact Kathryn O'Brien. B&W page AUD 950, color page AUD 1,950; trim 210 x 275. Circ: 1,000.

618.92 FRA ISSN 0993-9717
PEDIATRIE PRATIQUE. Text in French. 1988. m. (10/yr.). EUR 39 domestic to individuals; EUR 53 foreign to individuals; EUR 27 domestic to libraries; EUR 42 foreign to libraries (effective 2002). **Document type:** *Newspaper.*
Published by: L E N Medical, 15 rue des Sablons, Paris 75116, France. TEL 33-1-47553131, FAX 33-1-47553132, lenmed@club-internet.fr, http://www.webmedguide.com. Ed. Jacques de Blic.

617 TUR ISSN 1016-5142
CODEN: PCEDE
PEDIATRIK CERRAHI DERGISI. Text in Turkish. 1987. 3/yr. adv. **Document type:** *Journal.*
Indexed: Excerp.Med.
—EMDOCS, KNAW.
Published by: Logos Yayincilik Ticaret A.S., Yildiz Posta Cad., Sinan Apt. No. 36 D 66-67, Gayrettepe, Istanbul 80280, Turkey. TEL 90-212-2880541, info@logos.com.tr, http://logos.com.tr. Ed. Dr. Tolga Dagli. Adv. contact Sukran Oznalga.

618.92 ESP ISSN 0211-3465
CODEN: PEDTDW
PEDIATRIKA. Variant title: Ciencia Pediatrika. Text in Spanish. 1981. m. (10/yr.). ESP 8,500 domestic; USD 85 in Europe; USD 105 elsewhere (effective 2001). adv. bibl, charts, illus. index. *Refereed.* **Document type:** *Journal, Academic/Scholarly.* **Description:** Publishes original clinical and research articles in all areas of pediatric medicine. Includes continuing medical education materials.
Indexed: Chem.Abstr., Excerp.Med., Ind.Med.Esp.
—BLDSC (6417.694000), CASDDS, CINDOC, GNLM. **CCC.**
Published by: Alpe Editores S.A., Pedro Rico, 27, Madrid 28029, Spain. TEL 34-91-733-8811, FAX 34-91-315-9652, alpeeditores@sistelcom.com, http://www.eol.es/buscapress/pediatrika. Ed. Dr. Isabel Polanco Allue. Pub. Angeles Alvarez Sanchez. Adv. contact Ana Jurado. color page ESP 160,000; trim 280 x 210. Circ: 4,500 (controlled).

618.92 RUS ISSN 0031-403X
CODEN: PEDTAT
PEDIATRIYA/PEDIATRICS. Text in Russian; Summaries in English. 1922. bi-m. USD 119. bk.rev. bibl. index. **Description:** Covers major problems of modern pediatrics in the Soviet Union and other countries. Includes articles and reviews devoted to the etiology, pathogenesis, clinical picture, prophylaxis and treatment of childhood diseases, surgery, neuropathology, psychiatry and other branches of pediatrics.
Indexed: Bibl.Dev.Med.& Child Neur., Biol.Abstr., Chem.Abstr., Dairy Sci.Abstr., Excerp.Med. (until 1993), Ind.Med. (coverage dropped), Ind.Sci.Rev., Nutr.Abstr., Poult.Abstr., Ref.Zh.
—CASDDS, CISTI, East View, GNLM. **CCC.**
Published by: Mezhdunarodnyi Fond Okhrany Zdorov'ya Materi i Rebenka, Novyi Arbat 5, Moscow 121019, Russian Federation. TEL 7-095-9598822, FAX 7-095-9598822. Ed. N S Kislyak. **Dist. by:** Mezhdunarodnaya Kniga, B Yakimanka 39, Moscow 117049, Russian Federation. TEL 7-095-2384967, FAX 7-095-2384634; **US dist. addr.:** East View Publications, 3020 Harbor Ln N, Minneapolis, MN 55447. TEL 612-550-0961. **Co-sponsor:** Soyuz Pediatrov Rossii.

618 UKR ISSN 0031-4048
CODEN: PDAGA2
PEDIATRIYA, AKUSHERSTVO TA GINEKOLOGIYA. Text in Ukrainian; Summaries in Russian. 1936. bi-m. USD 66 (effective 1996 & 1997). adv. bk.rev. index. **Document type:** *Academic/Scholarly.* **Description:** Provides scientific and practical information on pediatrics, obstetrics and gynecology.
Indexed: Biol.Abstr., Chem.Abstr., Ind.Med. (coverage dropped).
—CASDDS, CISTI, GNLM.
Published by: Ministerstvo Zdravookhraneniya Ukraine, Bul Shevchenko 19, Kiev 252032, Ukraine. TEL 38-44-244-2886. Ed., R&P Vitaly G Maidannik. Adv. contact Nina A Fatyushina. page USD 500. Circ: 2,000.

618.92 ZAF ISSN 1017-1711
PEDMED. Text in English. 1986. bi-m. ZAR 51.30; ZAR 84 foreign (effective 1997). adv. **Document type:** *Trade.*
Formerly: South African Paediatrics Magazine
Published by: George Warman Publications (Pty.) Ltd., PO Box 704, Cape Town 8000, South Africa. TEL 27-21-24-5320, FAX 27-21-26-1332. Ed. Dr. D Leary. Circ: 2,700.

PENNSYLVANIA SOCIETY OF DENTISTRY FOR CHILDREN NEWSLETTER. see *MEDICAL SCIENCES—Dentistry*

PERSPECTIVES IN PEDIATRIC CARDIOLOGY. see *MEDICAL SCIENCES—Cardiovascular Diseases*

618.92 PHL ISSN 0031-7667
PHILIPPINE JOURNAL OF PEDIATRICS. Text in English. 1950. bi-m. PHP 70, USD 20. adv. bk.rev. abstr. index.
Indexed: Biol.Abstr., Excerp.Med.
—CISTI, GNLM.
Published by: Philippine Pediatric Society, P.O. Box 3527, Manila, Philippines. Ed. Dr. Felix A Estrada. Circ: 2,000.

PHOENIX (BETHESDA). see *MEDICAL SCIENCES—Oncology*

618.92 615.82 USA ISSN 0194-2638
RJ53.P5 CODEN: POTPDY
PHYSICAL & OCCUPATIONAL THERAPY IN PEDIATRICS; a quarterly journal of developmental therapy. Text in English. 1980. q. USD 75 to individuals; USD 101 in Canada to individuals; USD 109 elsewhere to individuals; USD 150 to institutions; USD 203 in Canada to institutions; USD 218 elsewhere to institutions; USD 400 to libraries; USD 540 in Canada to libraries; USD 580 elsewhere to libraries (effective Aug. 2001). adv. bk.rev. back issues avail.; reprint service avail. from HAW. *Refereed.* **Document type:** *Journal, Academic/Scholarly.* **Description:** Brings information to all therapists involved in the developmental and physical rehabilitation of infants and children. Covers current clinical research and practical applications.
Related titles: Microfiche ed.: (from PQC); Microform ed.
Indexed: AMED, Biol.Abstr., CINAHL, Child Devel.Abstr., Except.Child Educ.Abstr., Excerp.Med., IMFL, Psychol.Abstr. (1980-), Rehabil.Lit., Sage Fam.Stud.Abstr., Soc.Work Res.& Abstr., Viol.& Abuse Abstr., Yrbk.Assoc.Educ.& Rehab.Blind.
—BLDSC (6475.280000), GNLM, Haworth, ingenta, KNAW.
Published by: Haworth Press, Inc., 10 Alice St, Binghamton, NY 13904-1580. TEL 607-722-5857, 800-429-6784, FAX 607-722-6362, 800-895-0582, getinfo@haworthpressinc.com, http://www.haworthpress.com/journals/journallist.asp. Eds. Irene R McEwen, Mary Law. Pub. William Cohen. R&P Ruthann Heath TEL 607-723-5857 ext 316. Adv. contact Jackie Blakeslee TEL 607-722-5857 ext 346. B&W page USD 315, color page USD 550; trim 6 x 8.5. Circ: 1,550.

618.92 POL ISSN 0079-4279
POSTEPY PEDIATRII. Text in Polish; Summaries in English, Polish, Russian. 1955. a.
Published by: Polskie Towarzystwo Pediatryczne, Ul Kasprzaka 17 a, Warsaw 00211, Poland. TEL 48-2-6323451, FAX 48-2-6321862. Ed. Jana Raszka.

618.92 MEX
PRACTICA PEDIATRICA. Text in Spanish; Summaries in English. 1929. m. MXP 350; USD 345 foreign (effective 1999). adv. bk.rev. abstr, illus. index.
Formerly (until 1993): Revista Mexicana de Pediatria (0035-0052)
Indexed: Biol.Abstr., Chem.Abstr., Excerp.Med., Ref.Zh.
—BLDSC (6593.840000), CISTI, GNLM.
Published by: Mundo Medico S.A., Ejercito Nacional 381, Mexico City, DF 11520, Mexico. TEL 52-5-2038111. Circ: 5,000.

PREGNANCY & BIRTH. see *MEDICAL SCIENCES—Obstetrics And Gynecology*

THE PREGNANCY BOOK. see *MEDICAL SCIENCES—Obstetrics And Gynecology*

PRESCRIBING REFERENCE FOR PEDIATRICIANS. see *PHARMACY AND PHARMACOLOGY*

618.92 USA ISSN 1040-2497
PRIMARY CARE REPORTS. Text in English. 1985. bi-w. USD 299 domestic; USD 329 foreign; USD 23 newsstand/cover (effective 2001). **Document type:** *Newsletter.*
Incorporates (in 1995): Women's Health Reports (1081-8588); Formerly (until 1988): Advanced Clinical Updates (0893-9837); Which was formed by the merger of (1983-1985): Family Medicine Reports (0746-2514); (1984-1985): Internal Medicine Reports (0891-835X)
Published by: American Health Consultants (Subsidiary of: Medical Economics Co., Inc.), 3525 Piedmont Rd, N E, 6 Piedmont Center, Ste 400, Atlanta, GA 30305. TEL 404-262-5476, 404-262-7436, 800-688-2421, FAX 404-262-7837, 800-284-3291, custserv@ahcpub.com, http://www.ahcpub.com. Circ: 400.

618.92 617 USA
PRINCIPLES OF PEDIATRIC NEUROSURGERY. Text in English. 1986. irreg., latest 1993. price varies. reprint service avail. from ISI. **Document type:** *Academic/Scholarly.*
Published by: Springer-Verlag, Journals (Subsidiary of: BertelsmannSpringer), 175 Fifth Ave, New York, NY 10010. TEL 212-460-1500, FAX 212-473-6272.

PROFESSION SAGE-FEMME. see *MEDICAL SCIENCES—Obstetrics And Gynecology*

618.92 CHE ISSN 0251-5601
PROGRES EN NEONATOLOGIE. Text in French. 1980. irreg., latest vol.19. CHF 190 per issue. **Document type:** *Monographic series, Academic/Scholarly.*
—CISTI.
Published by: S. Karger AG, Allschwilerstr 10, PO Box, Basel 4009, Switzerland. TEL 41-61-306-1111, FAX 41-61-306-1234, karger@karger.ch, http://www.karger.com/bookseries/PRNEO. Ed. J P Relier.

618.92 GBR ISSN 1356-7675
PROGRESS IN COMMUNITY CHILD HEALTH. Text in English. a. USD 42.95. **Description:** Aimed at community child health professionals, particularly community pediatricians and community child health nurses.
Formerly (until 1995): Progress in Child Health (0265-2013)
—BLDSC (6867.815000), GNLM.
Published by: Churchill Livingstone (Subsidiary of: Harcourt Publishers Ltd.), Robert Stevenson House, 1-3 Baxter's Pl, Leith Walk, Edinburgh, Midlothian EH1 3AF, United Kingdom. TEL 44-131-556-2424, FAX 44-131-459-1177, http://www.churchillmed.com. Ed. Nick Spencer. **Subscr. to:** Harcourt Publishers Ltd., Foots Cray High St, Sidcup, Kent DA14 5HP, United Kingdom. TEL 44-20-8308-5700, FAX 44-20-8309-0807.

PROGRESS IN PEDIATRIC CARDIOLOGY. see *MEDICAL SCIENCES—Cardiovascular Diseases*

618.92011 GBR ISSN 1363-027X
PROGRESS IN PRETERM; update on preterm birth and the immature baby. Text in English. 1996. s-a. **Document type:** *Academic/Scholarly.*
Published by: Wells Medical Ltd., Speldhurst Pl, Speldhurst Rd, Royal Tunbridge Wells, Kent TN4 0JB, United Kingdom. TEL 44-1892-511600, FAX 44-1892-511400, info@wellsmed.co.uk.

618.92 155.4 FRA ISSN 0079-726X
CODEN: PSYEAH
LA PSYCHIATRIE DE L'ENFANT. Text in French. 1958. s-a. EUR 61 domestic; EUR 72 foreign (effective 2002). cum.index. reprint service avail. from PSC. *Refereed.* **Description:** Original works in the clinical, technical and social psychological areas.
Related titles: Online - full text ed.: (from Institute for Scientific Information).
Indexed: ASCA, Curr.Cont., Excerp.Med. (until 1992), Ind.Med. (coverage dropped), PsycInfo, Psychol.Abstr. (1970-), Ref.Zh., SSCI, e-psyche.
—BLDSC (6946.243000), CISTI, GNLM, IDS, Infotrieve. **CCC.**
Published by: Presses Universitaires de France, Departement des Revues, 6 av. Reille, Paris 75685 Cedex 14, France. TEL 33-1-60873030, FAX 33-1-60792045, revues@puf.com.

QUADERNI DI PSICOTERAPIA INFANTILE. see *MEDICAL SCIENCES—Psychiatry And Neurology*

618.92 GBR ISSN 0309-0140
RECENT ADVANCES IN PAEDIATRICS. Text in English. 1954. irreg., latest vol.13. **Document type:** *Monographic series, Academic/Scholarly.*

M

—BLDSC (7303.882000), CISTI, GNLM, KNAW.
Published by: Churchill Livingstone (Subsidiary of: Harcourt Publishers Ltd.), Robert Stevenson House, 1-3 Baxter's Pl, Leith Walk, Edinburgh, Midlothian EH1 3AF, United Kingdom. TEL 44-131-556-2424, FAX 44-131-459-1177, http://www.churchillmed.com. **US subscr. to:** Churchill Livingstone, 650 Ave of the Americas, New York, NY 10011. TEL 212-206-5000.

618.92 IND
RECENT ADVANCES IN PEDIATRICS. Text in English. irreg. **Document type:** *Monographic series.*
Published by: Jaypee Brothers Medical Publishers Pvt. Ltd., G-16, EMCA House, Daryaganj, 23-3B Ansari Rd., Daryaganj, New Delhi 110 002, India. Ed. Suraj Gupte.

REFERATOVY VYBER Z PEDIATRIE/ABSTRACTS OF PEDIATRICS. see *MEDICAL SCIENCES—Abstracting, Bibliographies, Statistics*

618.92 USA ISSN 1050-964X CODEN: RPIDE7
THE REPORT ON PEDIATRIC INFECTIOUS DISEASES*. Text in English. 1991. 10/yr. USD 58 to individuals; USD 79 to institutions. **Document type:** *Academic/Scholarly.* **Description:** Includes articles on issues of importance to practicing physicians responsible for the care of infants and children.
Indexed: Excerp.Med. (1993-).
—CISTI, EMDOCS, GNLM, Infotrieve. **CCC.**
Published by: (Pediatric Infectious Diseases Society), Churchill Livingstone (Subsidiary of: Harcourt Health Sciences), 15 E 26th St, Fl 15, New York, NY 10010-1505. TEL 212-206-5040, FAX 212-727-7808, TELEX 332266, http://www.churchillmed.com. Eds. Ellen Wald, Engine Shapiro. Pub. Jane Grochowski. **Subscr. in the UK to:** Pearson Professional Ltd., Journals Subscription Department, Fourth Ave., PO Box 77, Harlow, Essex CM19 5AA, United Kingdom. TEL 44-1279-623924, FAX 44-1279-639609.

RETT SYNDROME ASSOCIATION OF AUSTRALIA NEWSLETTER. see *MEDICAL SCIENCES—Psychiatry And Neurology*

618.92 BRA ISSN 0104-1282
REVISTA BRASILEIRA DE CRESCIMENTO E DESENVOLVIMENTO HUMANO. Text in Portuguese, Spanish; Summaries in English, Portuguese. 1991. s-a., latest 2000. BRL 15. adv. bk.rev. 100 p./no. reprints avail. *Refereed.* **Document type:** *Academic/Scholarly.* **Description:** Publishes interdisciplinary works in health, education, psychology, sociology and anthropology. Observes the relationship between human growth and developmental processes, highlighting children and adolescents.
Published by: (Centro de Estudos do Crescimento e do Desenvolvimento do Ser Humano), Polo Editora Ltda., Av. Dr. Arnaldo 715, subsolo, sala 21, Sao Paulo, SP 01246-904, Brazil. TEL 55-11-30613572, FAX 55-11-3066775, cdh@fsp.usp.br, http://www.usp.br/fsp/cdh.htm. Ed. Arnaldo Augusto Franco de Siqueira. Circ: 500.

618.92 CHL ISSN 0034-7396
REVISTA CHILENA DE PEDIATRIA. Text in Spanish; Summaries in English, Spanish. 1930-1977 (no.4); resumed. bi-m. USD 150 in the Americas; USD 190 elsewhere; USD 22 newsstand/cover (effective 2000). adv. bk.rev. abstr, charts, illus. index. **Document type:** *Academic/Scholarly.* **Description:** Contains statistical, educational, and original information for professionals studying in the fields of public health and pediatrics.
Related titles: Microform ed.: (from PQC); Online - full text ed.: (from SciELO).
Indexed: Biol.Abstr., Chem.Abstr., Dent.Ind., Ind.Med. (coverage dropped).
—BLDSC.
Published by: Sociedad Chilena de Pediatria, Depto. 405, Ave. Eliodoro Yanez, 1984, Santiago, Chile. TEL 56-2-209-2924, 56-2-225-4393, 56-2-274-5001, FAX 56-2-223-2351, sochipe@reuna.cl. Eds. Dr. Francisca Ugarte, Dr. Francisco Cano. Circ: 12,000.

618.92 CUB ISSN 0034-7531
REVISTA CUBANA DE PEDIATRIA. Text in Spanish; Summaries in English, Spanish. 1928. bi-m. USD 48 in the Americas; USD 50 in Europe; USD 66 elsewhere. bibl, charts, illus. **Description:** Covers child development including infant-newborn diseases, child nutrition, respiratory tract diseases, infant mortality, airway obstruction, low birth weight, heart and congenital defects.
Formerly (until 1945): Sociedad Cubana de Pediatria. Boletin
Indexed: Abstr.Hyg., Biol.Abstr., Chem.Abstr., Excerp.Med., Ind.Med. (coverage dropped), Nutr.Abstr., Trop.Dis.Bull.
—CISTI, GNLM.
Published by: (Cuba. Ministerio de Salud Publica, Centro Nacional de Informacion de Ciencias Medicas), Editorial de Ciencias Medicas, O'Reilly No. 4, Habana, Cuba. TEL 809-62-8091. Ed. Fidel Araujo. Circ: 3,000.
Co-sponsor: Sociedad Cubana de Pediatria.

REVISTA DE PSIQUIATRIA INFANTO-JUVENIL. see *MEDICAL SCIENCES—Psychiatry And Neurology*

618.92 ESP ISSN 0034-947X CODEN: REPEAW
REVISTA ESPANOLA DE PEDIATRIA. Text in Spanish. 1946. bi-m. ESP 10,500 to individuals; ESP 15,000 to institutions; ESP 8,400 to students (effective 2001). adv. bk.rev. abstr, bibl, illus. back issues avail.; reprints avail. *Refereed.* **Document type:** *Journal, Academic/Scholarly.*
Related titles: Online - full text ed.: 1996.
Indexed: Abstr.Hyg., Biol.Abstr., Chem.Abstr., Dairy Sci.Abstr., Excerp.Med., Helminthol.Abstr., Ind.Med.Esp., Nutr.Abstr., Protozool.Abstr., Rev.Med.& Vet.Mycol., Rural Recreat.Tour.Abstr., Trop.Dis.Bull.
—BLDSC (7854.200000), CASDDS, CINDOC, CISTI, GNLM, Infotrieve, KNAW. **CCC.**
Published by: Ediciones Doyma S.A., Traversa de Gracia, 17-21, Barcelona 08021, Spain. TEL 34-93-200-0711, rep@doyma.es, doyma@doyma.es, http://www.doyma.es/rep. Ed. Manuel Hernandez. R&P Monica Barnes. Adv. contact Jose Antonio Hernandez. B&W page ESP 122,000, color page ESP 152,000; 280 x 210. Circ: 4,000.

618.92 COL ISSN 0120-6311
REVISTA INTERNACIONAL DE PEDIATRIA. Text in Spanish. 1984. irreg. (4-6/yr.).
Formerly (until Dec. 1984): Miami Children's Hospital Journal
Published by: (Miami Children's Hospital USA), Ediciones Lerner, Calle 8a, 68-A-41, Bogota, CUND, Colombia. Circ: 35,000.

618.92 PRT ISSN 0048-7880
REVISTA PORTUGUESA DE PEDIATRIA E PUERICULTURA. Text in Portuguese. m. illus.
Indexed: Ind.Med. (coverage dropped).
Published by: Clinica Pediatrica Universitaria de Lisboa, Hospital de Santa Maria, Lisbon, Portugal.

618.92 FRA ISSN 0048-8135
REVUE INTERNATIONALE DE PEDIATRIE. Text in French; Summaries in English, French. 1969. 8/yr. FRF 480 domestic to individuals; FRF 700, EUR 106.71 foreign to individuals; FRF 335 to students (effective 2001).
Indexed: Excerp.Med.
—CISTI, GNLM.
Published by: Galliena Promotion, 62 rue Amelot, Paris 75011, France. TEL 33-1-53360180, FAX 33-1-53360164.

618.92 ITA
RIVISTA ITALIANA DI PEDIATRIA. Text in Italian. 1964. bi-m. ITL 110,000; ITL 170,000 foreign (effective 1996).
Indexed: ASCA, Curr.Cont. (coverage dropped), Dairy Sci.Abstr., Excerp.Med., Protozool.Abstr., SSCI (coverage dropped).
—BLDSC.
Published by: Pacini Editore, Via Alessandro Gherardesca, 1, Ospedaletto, PI 56121, Italy. TEL 39-050-313011, FAX 39-050-3130300, pacini@cibernet.it, http://www.cibernet.it/pacini, http://www.pacinieditore.it. Ed. Nicola Principi.

618.92 RUS ISSN 1560-9561
ROSSIISKII PEDYATRICHESKII ZHURNAL/RUSSIAN JOURNAL OF PEDIATRICS. Text in Russian; Summaries in English. 1998. bi-m. USD 165 foreign (effective 2000). adv. bk.rev. abstr, bibl, illus. back issues avail. **Document type:** *Journal.* **Description:** Covers issues of experimental and clinical pediatrics; diagnosis and prevention of childhood diseases; and management of pediatric services.
Related titles: Fax ed.
Indexed: Ref.Zh.
Published by: Izdatel'stvo Meditsina, Petroverigskii per 6-8, Moscow 101000, Russian Federation. TEL 7-095-9248785, 7-095-928-86-48, FAX 7-095-9211355, 7-095-9286003, meditsina@iname.com, http://www.medit.ru. Ed. A A Baranov. Pub. A M Stochik. R&P Yu Isakov. Adv. contact O A Fadeeva TEL 7-095-923-51-40. Circ: 620. **Dist. by:** Mezhdunarodnaya Kniga, B Yakimanka 39, Moscow 117049, Russian Federation. TEL 7-095-2384967, FAX 7-095-2384634; **US dist. addr.:** East View Publications, 3020 Harbor Ln N, Minneapolis, MN 55447. TEL 612-550-0961.

ROSSIISKII VESTNIK PERINATOLOGII I PEDIATRII. see *MEDICAL SCIENCES—Obstetrics And Gynecology*

RUND UMS BABY. see *CHILDREN AND YOUTH—About*

S R C D NEWSLETTER. see *CHILDREN AND YOUTH—About*

618.92 USA
SCHOOL HEALTH: POLICY AND PRACTICE. Text in English. 1972. irreg., latest vol.5, 1993. USD 44.95 (effective 2001). **Document type:** *Monographic series.*
Formerly: School Health: A Guide for Health Professionals
Published by: American Academy of Pediatrics, 141 Northwest Point Blvd, Box 927, Elk Grove Village, IL 60009-0927. TEL 847-228-5005, 800-433-9016, FAX 847-228-1281, http://www.aap.org.

SEMINARS IN NEONATOLOGY. see *MEDICAL SCIENCES—Obstetrics And Gynecology*

618.92 616.9 USA ISSN 1045-1870
SEMINARS IN PEDIATRIC INFECTIOUS DISEASES. Text in English. 1990. q. USD 145 domestic to individuals; USD 208 foreign to individuals; USD 216 domestic to individuals; USD 262 foreign to individuals; USD 72 domestic to students; USD 125 foreign to students; USD 66 newsstand/cover (effective 2001). adv. back issues avail. **Document type:** *Academic/Scholarly.* **Description:** Provides an in-depth update on a new subject, diagnostic technique, or controversial subject in each issue.
Indexed: CINAHL.
—BLDSC (8239.456780), EMDOCS, GNLM, Infotrieve, KNAW. **CCC.**
Published by: W.B. Saunders Co. (Subsidiary of: Harcourt Publishers Ltd.), 11830 Westline Industrial Dr, St Louis, MO 63146. TEL 800-325-4177, http://www.wbsaunders.com. Ed. Dr. Ralph D Fegin. adv.: B&W page USD 715, color page USD 1,665; trim 10 x 7. Circ: 870. **Subscr. to:** Periodicals Fulfillment, W B Saunders Co, 6277 Sea Harbor Dr, 4th Fl, Orlando, FL 32891-4800.

SEMINARS IN PEDIATRIC NEUROLOGY. see *MEDICAL SCIENCES—Psychiatry And Neurology*

SEMINARS IN PEDIATRIC SURGERY. see *MEDICAL SCIENCES—Surgery*

618.92 USA ISSN 0146-0005 CODEN: SEMPDU
SEMINARS IN PERINATOLOGY. Text in English. 1977. bi-m. USD 159 domestic to individuals; USD 271 foreign to individuals; USD 259 domestic to institutions; USD 329 foreign to institutions; USD 73 domestic to students; USD 163 foreign to students; USD 55 newsstand/cover (effective 2001). adv. bibl, charts, illus. index. *Refereed.* **Document type:** *Journal, Academic/Scholarly.* **Description:** Devoted to symposia on topics of interest to obstetricians and pediatricians concerned with care of the mother, the fetus, and the newborn. Each issue is devoted to one topic and has a leading obstetrician or pediatrician serving as guest editor.
Related titles: Online - full text ed.: (from Institute for Scientific Information).
Indexed: ASCA, Bibl.Dev.Med.& Child Neur., Biol.Abstr., CINAHL, Curr.Cont., Excerp.Med., Ind.Med. (1977-), Ind.Sci.Rev., Inpharma, Pharm.&Out.News, Reac., SSCI (coverage dropped), Sci.Cit.Ind.
—BLDSC (8239.456800), CISTI, GNLM, IDS, ingenta, KNAW. **CCC.**
Published by: W.B. Saunders Co. (Subsidiary of: Harcourt Publishers Ltd.), 11830 Westline Industrial Dr, St Louis, MO 63146. TEL 800-325-4177, http://www.wbsaunders.com. Eds. Ian Gross, Dr. Mary D'Alton. adv.: B&W page USD 845, color page USD 1,945; trim 10 x 7. Circ: 1,930. **Subscr. to:** Periodicals Fulfillment, W B Saunders Co, 6277 Sea Harbor Dr, 4th Fl, Orlando, FL 32891-4800.

SHAKEN BABY ALLIANCE; dedicated to prevention, support and justice. see *CHILDREN AND YOUTH—About*

SHONI GEKA/JAPANESE JOURNAL OF PEDIATRIC SURGERY. see *MEDICAL SCIENCES—Surgery*

SHONI HOKEN KENKYU/JOURNAL OF CHILD HEALTH. see *PHYSICAL FITNESS AND HYGIENE*

M

618.92 JPN ISSN 0385-6305
SHONI NAIKA/JAPANESE JOURNAL OF PEDIATRIC MEDICINE. Text in Japanese. 1969. m. JPY 37,900; JPY 2,400 newsstand/cover (effective 1999). **Document type:** *Academic/Scholarly.*
Indexed: INIS Atomind.
Published by: Tokyo Igakusha Ltd., 35-4 Hongo 3-chome, Bunkyo-ku, Tokyo 113-0033, Japan. TEL 81-3-3811-4119, FAX 81-3-3811-6135. Ed. Naoyoshi Minami. Circ: 6,000.

618.92 JPN ISSN 0037-4121
SHONIKA/CLINICAL PEDIATRICS. Text in Japanese. 1960. m. JPY 1,600 per issue. bk.rev. index.
Indexed: CINAHL, Curr.Cont. (coverage dropped), Helminthol.Abstr., INIS Atomind., Neurosci.Cit.Ind., Nutr.Abstr.
—CISTI.
Published by: Kanehara & Co. Ltd., 2-31-14 Yushima, Bunkyo-ku, Tokyo 113-0034, Japan. Ed. Dr. Teruji Shinozuka. Circ: 6,200.

618.92 SGP ISSN 0218-9941
CODEN: SPSJBF
SINGAPORE PAEDIATRIC JOURNAL. Text in English. 1958. q. USD 50 (effective 2001). adv. bk.rev. 50 p./no. back issues avail. *Refereed.* **Document type:** *Journal, Academic/Scholarly.* **Description:** Original papers, clinical reviews and care reports.
Formerly (until Mar. 1995): Singapore Paediatric Society. Journal (0037-5683)
Indexed: Excerp.Med., Ind.Med. (until 19??, dropped).
—BLDSC, CISTI, GNLM.
Published by: Singapore Paediatric Society, c/o Department of Paediatrics, Lower Kent Ridge Rd, National University Hospital, Singapore 119074, Singapore. FAX 65-7797486, paotaysl@nus.edu.sg. Ed. H B Wong. R&P S H Quak TEL 65-7724112. Adv. contact Quak Seng Hock. Circ: 1,000.

SOCIETY OF PEDIATRIC NURSES. JOURNAL. see *MEDICAL SCIENCES—Nurses And Nursing*

SPINAL CONNECTION. see *MEDICAL SCIENCES—Orthopedics And Traumatology*

614.19 USA
SYNOPSIS (COLUMBIA). Text in English. 1990. s-a. membership. adv. bk.rev. **Document type:** *Newsletter.* **Description:** Unites families and professionals concerned about SIDS; provides up-to-date information about the syndrome to the general public, particularly to new and expectant parents. Hotline number included.
Published by: Sudden Infant Death Syndrome Alliance (SIDS), 1314 Bedford Ave, Ste 210, Baltimore, MD 21208-3737. TEL 410-653-8226, FAX 410-653-8709, sidshq@charm.net. Ed., Pub., R&P, Adv. contact Phipps Cohe.

618.92 TZA ISSN 0856-311X
RJ27.5.T43
TANZANIA JOURNAL OF PAEDIATRICS. Text in English. 1989. 2/yr. TZS 1,500, USD 3 (effective 2001). adv. **Document type:** *Newsletter, Academic/Scholarly.* **Description:** Includes information on the current situation of health in children.
Indexed: P.L.E.S.A.
Published by: Tanzania Publishing House, PO Box 65370, Dar Es Salaam, Tanzania. Ed., Adv. contact Dr. Karim P Manji. Circ: 200.

618.92 DEU
TELE-FORUM KINDERARZT. Text in German. q. DEM 205.40 (effective 2000). **Document type:** *Journal, Academic/Scholarly.*
Published by: Hansisches Verlagskontor, Mengstr 16, Luebeck 23552, Germany. TEL 49-451-7031-01, FAX 49-451-7031281.

THEIR WORLD. see *EDUCATION—Special Education And Rehabilitation*

618.92 DEU
THEMEN DER KINDERHEILKUNDE. Text in German. 1986. irreg., latest vol.13, 1999. price varies. **Document type:** *Monographic series, Academic/Scholarly.*
Published by: Schmidt-Roemhild Verlag, Mengstr 16, Luebeck 23552, Germany. TEL 49-451-7031-01, FAX 49-451-7031253, msr-luebeck@t-online.de, http://www.schmidt-roemhild.de.

618.92 NLD ISSN 0165-1870
TIJDSCHRIFT VOOR JEUGDGEZONDHEIDSZORG. Variant title: J G Z. Text in Dutch. 1968. 6/yr. NLG 72.50 (effective 1996). adv. **Document type:** *Academic/Scholarly.*
Published by: Bohn Stafleu van Loghum B.V. (Subsidiary of: Wolters Kluwer N.V.), Postbus 246, Houten 3990 GA, Netherlands. TEL 31-3403-95711, FAX 31-3403-50903. Ed. S P Verloove Vanhorick. Circ: 2,250 (paid). **Subscr. to:** Intermedia, Postbus 4, Alphen aan den Rijn 2400 MA, Netherlands. TEL 31-1720-66811, FAX 31-1720-66770.

618.92 NLD ISSN 0376-7442
CODEN: TIKID4
TIJDSCHRIFT VOOR KINDERGENEESKUNDE. Text in Dutch, English. 1932. m. NLG 138.50; NLG 69.25 to students. adv. bk.rev. charts, illus, stat. index.
Formerly: Maandschrift voor Kindergeneeskunde (0024-869X)
Indexed: Biol.Abstr., Chem.Abstr., Dent.Ind., Excerp.Med., Ind.Med. (coverage dropped).
—BLDSC (8842.300000), CISTI, EMDOCS, GNLM, KNAW.
Published by: Bohn Stafleu van Loghum B.V. (Subsidiary of: Wolters Kluwer N.V.), Postbus 246, Houten 3990 GA, Netherlands. TEL 31-3403-95711, FAX 31-3403-50903. Ed. Dr. T D Stahlie. Circ: 850.

618.92 USA ISSN 0892-0435
TOPICS IN PEDIATRICS. Text in English. 1982. 3/yr. free per issue. **Description:** For physicians, nurses, and psychosocial professionals who care for children.
Published by: Minneapolis Children's Medical Center, 2525 Chicago Ave S, Minneapolis, MN 55404. TEL 612-863-6222, FAX 612-863-6674. Ed. Dr. John MacDonald. Circ: 10,000 (controlled).

618.92 TUR ISSN 0041-4301
TURKISH JOURNAL OF PEDIATRICS. Text in English. 1958. q. USD 50 (effective 1999). adv. bk.rev. abstr, bibl, charts, illus. index. *Refereed.* **Document type:** *Bulletin.*
Related titles: Online - full text ed.: (from Institute for Scientific Information).
Indexed: ASCA, Abstr.Hyg., Biol.Abstr., Curr.Adv.Ecol.Sci., Curr.Cont. (coverage dropped), Dairy Sci.Abstr., Dent.Ind., Diar.Dis.Res., Excerp.Med., Ind.Med. (1958-), Inpharma, Nutr.Abstr., Pharm.&Out.News, Reac., Rev.Med.& Vet.Mycol., Rural Recreat.Tour.Abstr., Trop.Dis.Bull.
—BLDSC (9072.480000), CISTI, GNLM, IDS, KNAW.
Published by: International Children's Center/Uluslararasi Cocuk Sagligi Merkezi, Samanpazari, P O Box 66, Ankara 06240, Turkey. FAX 90-312-3243284. Ed. Dr. Turgay Coskun. Adv. contact Murat Tuncer. Circ: 1,500. **Co-sponsors:** Turkish National Pediatric Society; Hacettepe University, Institute of Child Health.

TWIN RESEARCH. see *BIOLOGY—Genetics*

618.92 GBR ISSN 1460-6887
VACCINES: CHILDREN & PRACTICE. Text in English. 1998. 3/yr.
—BLDSC (9138.663000).
Published by: Adis International Ltd., Chowley Oak Ln, Tattenhall, Chester, Ches CH3 9GA, United Kingdom. TEL 44-1829-771155, FAX 44-1829-770330.

649.1 DEU
WO BEKOMME ICH MEIN BABY?. Text in German. a. DEM 7.50 newsstand/cover (effective 2001). adv. **Document type:** *Magazine, Consumer.*
Published by: Buettner Medien GmbH, Westendstr 73, Frankfurt Am Main 60325, Germany. TEL 49-69-756190-0, FAX 49-69-75619041, http://www.buemed.de. Pub., Adv. contact Sven Buettner. B&W page DEM 49,781, color page DEM 79,650; trim 180 x 264. Circ: 640,000 (paid and controlled).

618.92 616.025 CHN ISSN 1007-9459
XIAOER JIJIU YIXUE/PEDIATRIC EMERGENCY MEDICINE. Text in Chinese. 1994. q. CNY 24, USD 10; CNY 6 newsstand/cover (effective 2001). 64 p./no. **Document type:** *Academic/Scholarly.*
Related titles: Online - full content ed.: (from WanFang Data Corp.).
Published by: Zhongguo Yike Daxue/Chinese University of Medical Sciences, Heping qu, 36, Sanhao Jie, Chenyang 110003, China. TEL 86-24-23893501 ext 553, 86-24-23893501 ext 6553, FAX 86-24-23926295, xejjyxz@mail.sy.ln.cn, http://www.xejjyx.com. Ed. Jianchun Sun. Circ: 7,000 (paid); 1,000 (controlled). **Dist. by:** China International Book Trading Corp, 35, Chegongzhuang Xilu, Haidian District, Beijing 100044, China. TEL 86-1-68413849, FAX 86-1-68412048, cibtc@mail.cibtc.com.cn, http://www.cibtc.com.cn.

618.92 CHN ISSN 1002-1213
XINSHENG ERKE ZAZHI/JOURNAL OF NEONATOLOGY. Text in Chinese. 1986. bi-m. **Document type:** *Academic/Scholarly.*
Published by: Beijing Medical University, First Clinical Medical College, Women and Children Hospital, Beijing 100034, China. TEL 86-1-6031122, FAX 86-1-603-7106. Ed. Huang Demin.

618.92 USA ISSN 1078-5027
YALE CHILDREN'S HEALTH LETTER. Text in English. m. USD 45; USD 60 foreign (effective 1996).
Published by: Belvoir Publications, Inc., 75 Holly Hill Ln, Box 2626, Greenwich, CT 06836-2626. TEL 203-661-6111, FAX 203-661-4802.

618.92 USA ISSN 0084-3954
RJ16
THE YEAR BOOK OF PEDIATRICS. Text in English. 1901. a. USD 82 domestic; USD 88 foreign (effective 2001). illus. reprints avail. **Document type:** *Abstract/Index, Academic/Scholarly.* **Description:** Presents abstracts of pertinent literature with commentary by leading experts in the field.
Related titles: CD-ROM ed.
Indexed: Curr.Adv.Ecol.Sci., Diar.Dis.Res.
—BLDSC (9414.800000), CISTI, GNLM.
Published by: Mosby, Inc., Continuity Division (Subsidiary of: Harcourt Health Sciences), 11830 Westline Industrial Dr, St Louis, MO 63146-3313. TEL 314-872-8370, 800-325-4177, FAX 314-432-1380, http://www.mosby.com/periodicals. Ed. Dr. James A Stockman III.

618.92 JPN
YOJI EIYO KISO CHOSA KEKKA NO GAIYO/ FUNDAMENTAL RESEARCH REPORT OF PEDIATRIC NUTRITION. Text in Japanese. 1952. every 5 yrs. **Document type:** *Government.*
Published by: Tokyo Eiseikyoku, Kenko Suishinbu/Tokyo Metropolitan Government, Bureau of Public Health, Public Health Promotion Division, 8-1 Nishi-Shinjuku 2-chome, Shinjuku-ku, Tokyo 160-0023, Japan. TEL 81-3-5320-4357, FAX 81-3-5388-1429. Circ: 1,000.

YOUR BABY. see *CHILDREN AND YOUTH—About*

618.92 CHN ISSN 1008-8830
ZHONGGUO DANGDAI ERKE ZAZHI/CHINESE JOURNAL OF CONTEMPORARY PEDIATRICS. Text in Chinese. bi-m. CNY 7.80 per issue domestic (effective 2000). back issues avail. **Document type:** *Academic/Scholarly.*
Related titles: Online - full content ed.: (from WanFang Data Corp.).
Published by: Hunan Yike Daxue, Xiangya Lu 141 Hao, Changsha, Hunan 410008, China. TEL 86-731-4327402, xycjcp@163.net, xyped@public.cs.hn.cn.

618.92 CHN ISSN 1005-2224
ZHONGGUO SHIYONG ERKE ZAZHI/CHINESE JOURNAL OF PRACTICAL PEDIATRICS. Text in Chinese; Abstracts in English. 1986. bi-m. USD 44.40; USD 3.70 newsstand/cover (effective 2001). adv. reprints avail. *Refereed.* **Document type:** *Academic/Scholarly.* **Description:** Features new developments and methods of practical diagnosis, treatment, and prevention of pediatric diseases.
Formerly: Shiyong Erke Zashi - Journal of Practical Pediatrics (1001-0866)
Published by: Zhongguo Shiyong Yixue Zazhishe/Chinese Journals' Society of Practical Medicine, 44-1, Jixian St, Heping-qu, Shenyang, Liaoning 110005, China. TEL 86-24-3394597, FAX 86-24-3391212. Eds. Ding Li Wang, Zhenxing Men. Adv. contact Jianguo Li. Circ: 35,000. **Dist. by:** China International Book Trading Corp, 35, Chegongzhuang Xilu, Haidian District, Beijing 100044, China. TEL 86-1-68413849, FAX 86-1-68412048, cibtc@mail.cibtc.com.cn, http://www.cibtc.com.cn.

ZHONGGUO YIXUE WENZHAI (ERKEXUE)/CHINA MEDICAL ABSTRACTS (PEDIATRICS). see *MEDICAL SCIENCES—Abstracting, Bibliographies, Statistics*

618.2 CHN ISSN 0578-1310
ZHONGHUA ERKE ZAZHI/CHINESE JOURNAL OF PEDIATRICS. Text in Chinese. m. CNY 93.60 domestic; USD 49.20 foreign; CNY 7.80 newsstand/cover domestic; USD 4.10 newsstand/cover foreign (effective 2001). **Document type:** *Academic/Scholarly.*
Related titles: CD-ROM ed.; Online - full content ed.: (from WanFang Data Corp.).
Indexed: ExtraMED.

Published by: Zhonghua Yixuehui Zazhishe, 42 Dongsi Xidajie, Beijing 100710, China. TEL 86-1-65273371, cibtc@mail.cibtc.com.cn, cmaek@public.sti.ac.cn, http://www.cibtc.com.cn. **Dist. by:** China International Book Trading Corp, 35 Chegongzhuang Xilu, Haidian District, Beijing 100044, China. TEL 86-1-68413849, FAX 86-1-68412048, cibtc@mail.cibtc.com.cn, http://www.cibtc.com.cn.

MEDICAL SCIENCES—Physical Medicine And Rehabilitation

A A T A NEWSLETTER. see *ART*

615.82 USA
A D T A NEWSLETTER. Text in English. 1967. q. USD 20. bk.rev. bibl. **Document type:** *Newsletter.* **Description:** Contains communications from ADTA President and membership, regional news, committee news, theory and philosophy, listing of courses, workshops, and job opportunities available.
Published by: American Dance Therapy Association, 2000 Century Plaza, Ste 108, 10632 Little Patuxent Pkwy, Columbia, MD 21044. TEL 410-997-4040, FAX 410-997-4048, info@adta.org, http://www.adta.org. Ed. Kyle Buckley.

▼ **ACTA OF BIOENGINEERING AND BIOMECHANICS.** see *BIOLOGY—Bioengineering*

615.82 613.62 USA ISSN 1099-9507
ADVANCE FOR OCCUPATIONAL THERAPY PRACTITIONERS. Text in English. 1985. w. *Refereed.* **Document type:** *Trade.*
Supersedes in part: Advance (0890-6521)
Published by: Merion Publications, Inc., 2900 Horizon Dr, PO Box 61556, King Of Prussia, PA 19406. TEL 610-265-7812, 800-355-5627, FAX 610-265-8971, advance@merion.com, http://www.advanceweb.com. Ed. E J Brown. Pub. Ann Kielinski. adv.: B&W page USD 3,500, color page USD 3,800; trim 10.88 x 8.38. Circ: 63,200.

615.8 USA ISSN 1099-9493
ADVANCE FOR PHYSICAL THERAPISTS AND P T ASSISTANTS. (Physical Therapy) Text in English. 1988. bi-w. Free to qualified subscribers. adv. *Refereed.* **Document type:** *Trade.* **Description:** Publishes advances in research, reimbursement, political and clinical news for physical therapy professionals.
Former titles: Advance for Physical Therapists (1053-7597); Which superseded in part: Advance (0890-6521)
Related titles: Online - full content ed.
Published by: Merion Publications, Inc., 2900 Horizon Dr, PO Box 61556, King Of Prussia, PA 19406. TEL 610-278-1400, 800-355-5627, FAX 610-278-1421, 610-278-1425, ljones@merion.com, advance@merion.com, http://www.advanceforpt.com/, http://www.advanceweb.com. Ed. Linda Jones. Pub. Ann Kielinski. adv.: B&W page USD 3,500, color page USD 3,800; trim 10.88 x 8.38. Circ: 74,800.

615.82 USA ISSN 0892-8878
RM735.A1
ADVANCES IN CLINICAL REHABILITATION. Text in English. 1980-1986 (vol.5); N.S. 1987. irreg. (approx. every 18 mos.). price varies. **Document type:** *Academic/Scholarly.*
Supersedes: Annual Review of Rehabilitation (0197-2251)
Indexed: Dok.Arbeitsmed., Ind.Med. (coverage dropped), Psychol.Abstr.
—CISTI.
Published by: Springer Publishing Company, 536 Broadway, New York, NY 10012. TEL 212-431-4370, FAX 212-941-7842, springer@springerpub.com, http://www.springerpub.com. Eds. M C Eisenberg, R Grzesiak. Circ: 417.

ADVANCES IN OCCUPATIONAL ERGONOMICS AND SAFETY. see *OCCUPATIONAL HEALTH AND SAFETY*

ADVANCES IN OCCUPATIONAL MEDICINE & REHABILITATION/AGGIORNAMENTI IN MEDICINA OCCUPAZIONALE E RIABILITAZIONE. see *OCCUPATIONAL HEALTH AND SAFETY*

615.82 NOR ISSN 1403-8196
RM695
▼ **ADVANCES IN PHYSIOTHERAPY.** Text in Norwegian. 1999. q. GBP 42, USD 70 to individuals; GBP 100, USD 165 to institutions (effective 2002). **Document type:** *Academic/Scholarly.* **Description:** New international journal covering all aspects of physiotherapy.
Related titles: Online - full text ed.: (from EBSCO Publishing, O C L C Online Computer Library Center, Inc., CatchWord Ltd., ingenta, Swets Blackwell, RoweCom Information Quest).
Indexed: AMED.
—BLDSC (0710.047000).
Published by: Taylor & Francis AS (Subsidiary of: Taylor & Francis Group), Cort Adelersgt. 17, Solli, PO Box 2562, Oslo 0202, Norway. TEL 47-22-12-98-80, FAX 47-22-12-98-90, journals@tandf.no, http://www.tandf.co.uk.tfas. Ed. Madeleine Abrandt Dahlgren.

613.82 USA ISSN 0065-8022
AMERICAN DANCE THERAPY ASSOCIATION. (NO.) ANNUAL CONFERENCE PROCEEDINGS*. Text in English. 1967. a., latest vol.27, 1992. USD 30 to non-members; USD 25 to members.
Published by: American Dance Therapy Association, 2000 Century Plaza, Ste 108, 10632 Little Patuxent Pkwy, Columbia, MD 21044. TEL 301-997-4040.

615.85156 USA ISSN 0007-4764
RC489.A7 CODEN: AJATA
AMERICAN JOURNAL OF ART THERAPY; art in psychotherapy, education, and rehabilitation. Text in English. 1961. q. USD 32 domestic to individuals; USD 32 in Canada to individuals; USD 38 elsewhere to individuals; USD 55.50 to libraries; USD 27 domestic to members; USD 27 in Canada to members; USD 32 elsewhere to members (effective 2000). adv. bk.rev. bibl, illus. index. reprint service avail. from PQC. *Refereed.* **Document type:** *Academic/Scholarly.* **Description:** Deals with graphic and plastic arts as they contribute to human understanding and mental health. Includes new theoretical formulations, research, and description of programs.
Formerly: Bulletin of Art Therapy
Related titles: Microform ed.: (from PQC); Online - full text ed.: (from Northern Light Technology, Inc., H. W. Wilson, ProQuest Information & Learning, Institute for Scientific Information).
Indexed: AMED, ASCA, Abstr.Soc.Geront., AgeLine, Artbibl.Mod., Arts & Hum.Cit.Ind. (coverage dropped), CINAHL, Cont.Pg.Educ., Curr.Cont., Educ.Ind. (Oct.1982-), Except.Child Educ.Abstr., Excerp.Med., Hosp.Lit.Ind., IBZ, IMFL, Ind.Med. (coverage dropped), Ind.Philos., Ment.Retard.Abstr., Mid.East: Abstr.& Ind., Psychol.Abstr., Rehabil.Lit., SSCI.
—BLDSC (0821.500000), GNLM, IDS. **CCC.**
Published by: Vermont College of Norwich University, Montpelier, VT 05602. TEL 802-828-8540, FAX 802-828-8585, mzimmerm@norwich.edu. Ed. Gladys Agell. R&P, Adv. contact Michael R Zimmerman. Circ: 1,200 (paid).

AMERICAN JOURNAL OF KNEE SURGERY. see *MEDICAL SCIENCES—Surgery*

615.8 USA ISSN 0894-9115
RM735.A1 CODEN: AJPREP
AMERICAN JOURNAL OF PHYSICAL MEDICINE AND REHABILITATION. Text in English. 1921. m. USD 163 domestic to individuals; USD 222 foreign to individuals; USD 285 domestic to institutions; USD 344 foreign to institutions; USD 27 newsstand/cover (effective 2002). adv. bk.rev. charts, illus, tr.lit. *Refereed.* **Document type:** *Journal, Academic/Scholarly.* **Description:** Covers acute and chronic clinical problems in physical medicine and rehabilitation, and their treatment utilizing the latest methods and equipment. Aims to enhance the interrelationship of practice, research, and education for the ultimate benefit of the patient.
Formerly: American Journal of Physical Medicine (0002-9491)
Related titles: Microfilm ed.: (from WWS); Online - full text ed.: USD 370.50 domestic academic site license; USD 429.50 foreign academic site license; USD 413.25 domestic corporate site license; USD 472.25 foreign corporate site license (effective 2002) (from Ovid Technologies, Inc., Institute for Scientific Information).
Indexed: AIM, AMED, ASCA, Behav.Med.Abstr., Bibl.Dev.Med.& Child Neur., Bioeng.Abstr., Biol.Abstr., CINAHL, Chem.Abstr., Curr.Cont., Eng.Ind., Ergon.Abstr., Excerp.Med., Focus on: Sports Sci.& Med., INIS Atomind., INSPEC (Aug.1973-Aug.1987, Feb.1988-), Ind.Med. (1988-), Ind.Sci.Rev., Inpharma, Int.Sci.Rev., Neurosci.Cit.Ind., Nutr.Abstr., Pharm.&Out.News, Psychol.Abstr., Reac., Rehabil.Lit., SSCI (coverage dropped), Sci.Cit.Ind., Sportsearch (1988-).
—BLDSC (0832.160000), AskIEEE, CASDDS, CISTI, Ei, EMDOCS, GNLM, IDS, ingenta, KNAW.
Published by: (Association of Academic Physiatrists), Williams & Wilkins (Subsidiary of: Waverly International), 351 W Camden St, Baltimore, MD 21201-2436. TEL 410-528-4068, 800-222-3790, FAX 410-528-4452, djones@wwilkins.com, http://www.Lww.com. Ed. Dr. Ernest W Johnson. Adv. contact David Jones. B&W page USD 730; trim 10.88 x 8.13. Circ: 4,828; 4,708 (paid).

615.8 362 FRA ISSN 0168-6054
CODEN: ARMPEQ
ANNALES DE READAPTATION ET DE MEDECINE PHYSIQUE. Text mainly in French; Summaries in English, French. 1957. 9/yr. EUR 222 in Europe to individuals; USD 292 elsewhere to individuals; EUR 307 in Europe to institutions; USD 386 in the Americas to institutions (effective 2002). adv. bk.rev. index. reprints avail. *Refereed.* **Document type:** *Academic/Scholarly.* **Description:** Publishes clinical, paraclinical and basic research papers pertaining to all aspects of the medicine of readaptation and rehabilitation.
Formerly (until 1983): Annales de Medecine Physique (0402-4621)
Related titles: Microform ed.: (from PQC); Online - full text ed.: (from ingenta, Swets Blackwell, ScienceDirect).
Indexed: Biol.Abstr., Excerp.Med.
—BLDSC (0995.170000), CISTI, EMDOCS, GNLM, Infotrieve, KNAW. **CCC.**
Published by: (Societe Francaise de Reeducation Fonctionnelle de Readaptation et de Medecine Physique), Elsevier Paris, Editions Scientifiques et Medicales (Subsidiary of: Reed Elsevier plc. group), 23 rue Linois, Paris 75015, France. TEL 33-1-45589110, FAX 33-1-45589419, armp@elsevier.fr; academic@elsevier-fr.com, http://www.elsevier.com/locate/annrmp. Ed. M Perrigot. Circ: 3,000.

615.82 JPN ISSN 0918-1431
AOMORIKEN SAGYO RYOHO KENKYU/BULLETIN OF AOMORI OCCUPATIONAL THERAPY. Text in Japanese. 1992. a. **Document type:** *Bulletin.*
Published by: Aomoriken Sagyo Ryohoshikai/Association of Aomoriken Occupational Therapists, Hirosaki Daigaku Iryo Gijutsu Tanki Daigakubu, Sagyo Ryohogakka, 66-1 Hon-cho, Hirosaki-shi, Aomori-ken 036-8203, Japan.

615.8 USA ISSN 0003-9993
RM845 CODEN: APMHAI
ARCHIVES OF PHYSICAL MEDICINE AND REHABILITATION. Text in English. 1920. m. USD 198 domestic to individuals; USD 253 foreign to individuals; USD 278 domestic to institutions; USD 333 foreign to institutions; USD 86 domestic to students; USD 141 foreign to students; USD 28 newsstand/cover (effective 2001). adv. bk.rev. charts, illus. index. reprints avail. *Refereed.* **Document type:** *Journal, Academic/Scholarly.* **Description:** Concerns the therapeutic use of physical and pharmaceutical agents in providing comprehensive care for persons with disabilities and chronic illnesses.
Related titles: Online - full text ed.: (from IDEAL Online Library, Institute for Scientific Information); Supplement: American Academy of Physical Medicine & Rehabilitation. Study Guide; American Congress of Physical Medicine & Rehabilitation. Education Issue.
Indexed: AIM, AMED, ASCA, Abstr.Health Care Manage.Stud., AgeLine, Behav.Med.Abstr., Bibl.Dev.Med.& Child Neur., Biol.Abstr., CINAHL, C.I.S. Abstr., Chem.Abstr., Curr.Cont., Dent.Ind., Environ.Sci.Poll.Mgmt., Excerp.Med., Focus on: Sports Sci.& Med., Forest Prod.Abstr., Hosp.Lit.Ind., INIS Atomind., Ind.Med. (1953-), Ind.Sci.Rev., Inpharma, Int.Nurs.Ind., Lang.& Lang.Behav.Abstr., Neurosci.Cit.Ind., Pharm.&Out.News, Phys.Ed.Ind., Reac., Rehabil.Lit., Rev.Arom.& Med.Plants, SSCI (coverage dropped), Saf.Sci.Abstr., Sci.Cit.Ind., Sportsearch (1974-).
—BLDSC (1639.000000), CISTI, EMDOCS, GNLM, IDS, ingenta, KNAW, Linda Hall. **CCC.**
Published by: (American Congress of Rehabilitation Medicine), W.B. Saunders Co. (Subsidiary of: Harcourt Publishers Ltd.), 11830 Westline Industrial Dr, St Louis, MO 63146. TEL 800-325-4177, http://www.archives-pmr.org, http://www.wbsaunders.com. Ed. Dr. Kenneth M Jaffe. adv.: B&W page USD 965, color page USD 2,200; trim 7 x 10. Circ: 10,050 (paid). **Subscr. to:** Periodicals Fulfillment, W B Saunders Co, 6277 Sea Harbor Dr, 4th Fl, Orlando, FL 32891-4800.

ARKANSAS. DIVISION OF REHABILITATION SERVICES. ANNUAL REPORT. see *EDUCATION—Special Education And Rehabilitation*

M

615.85156 USA ISSN 0742-1656
ART THERAPY. Text in English. 1983. q. USD 50, USD 74 to individuals; USD 77, USD 100 to institutions (effective 2000). adv. bk.rev. **Document type:** *Academic/Scholarly.*
Indexed: AMED, Artbibl.CT, Artbibl.Mod., C.I.J.E., CINAHL, Except.Child Educ.Abstr., PsycInfo, Psychol.Abstr., e-psyche.
—BLDSC (1733.473800), ingenta.
Published by: American Art Therapy Association, Inc., 1202 Allanson Rd, Mundelein, IL 60060. TEL 847-949-6064, FAX 847-566-4580. Ed., R&P Cathy Malchiodi. Adv. contact Karen Savage. Circ: 5,000.

ASIA PACIFIC DISABILITY REHABILITATION JOURNAL. see *SOCIAL SERVICES AND WELFARE*

▼ **ASIA PACIFIC DISABILITY REHABILITATION JOURNAL. SELECTED READINGS SERIES.** see *SOCIAL SERVICES AND WELFARE*

615.8 GBR ISSN 1368-7360
ASSOCIATION OF PAEDIATRIC CHARTERED PHYSIOTHERAPISTS. JOURNAL. Text in English. 1973. q. GBP 21; GBP 2.50 newsstand/cover (effective 2001). bk.rev. *Refereed.* **Document type:** *Journal, Academic/Scholarly.*
Formerly (until 1994): Association of Paediatric Chartered Physiotherapists. Newsletter
Published by: Association of Paediatric Chartered Physiotherapists, 14 Bedford Row, London WC1R 4ED, United Kingdom. TEL 44-20-7242-1941, FAX 44-20-7831-4509. Ed., R&P Sally Braitwaite TEL 44-121-783-4427. Circ: 1,600 (controlled). **Co-sponsor:** Chartered Society of Physiotherapy.

615.82 AUS ISSN 1440-3994
▼ **AUSTRALASIAN REHABILITATION NURSES ASSOCIATION. OFFICIAL JOURNAL.** Abbreviated title: J A R N A. Text in English. 1999 (Autumn; vol.2, no.1). q. (Jun., Sep., Dec., Mar.). AUD 60 to individuals for membership; AUD 150 to corporations for membership (effective 2001). adv. 32 p./no. back issues avail. *Refereed.* **Document type:** *Academic/Scholarly.*
Indexed: CINAHL.
—BLDSC (4662.940000).
Published by: Australasian Rehabilitation Nurses Association Inc., PO Box 3149, Putney, NSW 2112, Australia. arna@idx.com.au, http://www.arna.com.au. Eds. Joanne Lawrence, Linda Glanfield. adv.: page AUD 350.

AUSTRALIA. BUREAU OF STATISTICS. PHYSIOTHERAPY SERVICES, AUSTRALIA. see *MEDICAL SCIENCES—Abstracting, Bibliographies, Statistics*

AUSTRALIAN CONTINENCE JOURNAL. see *MEDICAL SCIENCES—Urology And Nephrology*

615.8 AUS ISSN 0004-9514
AUSTRALIAN JOURNAL OF PHYSIOTHERAPY. Text in English. 1954. q. AUD 76 domestic; AUD 110 foreign (effective 2000). adv. bk.rev., video rev. index. *Refereed.* **Document type:** *Academic/Scholarly.* **Description:** Publishes original scientific articles, news, coming events, letters.
Related titles: Online - full text ed.: (from Institute for Scientific Information).
Indexed: AMED, CINAHL, Excerp.Med., Focus on: Sports Sci.& Med.
—BLDSC (1811.100000), CISTI, EMDOCS, GNLM, KNAW.
Published by: Australian Physiotherapy Association, PO Box 6465, St Kilda Rd Central, VIC 8008, Australia. TEL 61-3-9534-9400, FAX 61-3-9534-9199, wendy.cross@physiotherapy.asn.au; elise.olney@physiotherapy.asn.au. Ed., R&P Wendy Cross. Adv. contact Elise Olney. Circ: 9,503 (controlled).

615.82 AUS ISSN 0045-0766
AUSTRALIAN OCCUPATIONAL THERAPY JOURNAL. Variant title: Australian Association of Occupational Therapists. Journal. A O T Journal. Text in English. 1951. q. AUD 209 domestic to institutions; AUD 190 in New Zealand to institutions; USD 185 elsewhere to institutions; AUD 230 domestic to institutions paper & online eds. combined; AUD 209 in New Zealand to institutions paper & online eds. combined; USD 204 elsewhere to institutions paper & online eds. combined (effective 2001). adv. bk.rev. index. back issues avail. *Refereed.* **Document type:** *Academic/Scholarly.* **Description:** Examines the practice, theory, and professional education in occupational therapy in Australia.
Related titles: Microfilm ed.: (from PQC); Online - full text ed.: ISSN 1440-1630. AUD 189 domestic to institutions; AUD 171 in New Zealand to institutions; USD 167 elsewhere to institutions (effective 2001) (from EBSCO Publishing, O C L C Online Computer Library Center, Inc., RoweCom Information Quest, ingenta, Munksgaard & Blackwell Science's Synergy, Swets Blackwell).
Indexed: AMED, ASSIA, CINAHL, Environ.Sci.Poll.Mgmt., Excerp.Med., Pollut.Abstr., PsycInfo, Psychol.Abstr. (1991-), Risk Abstr., Saf.Sci.Abstr., e-psyche.
—BLDSC (1815.950000), EMDOCS, GNLM, Infotrieve, ingenta. **CCC.**
Published by: (Australian Association of Occupational Therapists), Blackwell Science Asia Pty Ltd, PO Box 378, Carlton South, VIC 3053, Australia. TEL 61-3-9347-0300, FAX 61-3-9347-5001, info@blacksci-asia.com.au, http://www.blacksci.co.uk. Ed. Esther May. Adv. contact Kathryn O'Brien. B&W page AUD 1,012, color page AUD 2,057; trim 210 x 275. Circ: 4,100.

615.82 NLD ISSN 0168-9711
BEWEGEN EN HULPVERLENING. Text in Dutch. 1984. 4/yr. NLG 126.50. adv. **Document type:** *Academic/Scholarly.*
—GNLM, KNAW.
Published by: Bohn Stafleu van Loghum B.V. (Subsidiary of: Wolters Kluwer N.V.), Postbus 246, Houten 3990 GA, Netherlands. TEL 31-3403-95711, FAX 31-3403-50903.

BRAILLE JOURNAL OF PHYSIOTHERAPY. see *HANDICAPPED—Visually Impaired*

615.822 GBR ISSN 1369-9571
THE BRITISH JOURNAL OF HAND THERAPY. Text in English. 1996. q. GBP 40 in Europe to individual members; GBP 135 in Europe to institutions; GBP 45 rest of world to individuals; GBP 135 rest of world to institutions (effective 2000). adv. bk.rev. bibl, charts, illus. back issues avail. *Refereed.* **Document type:** *Academic/Scholarly.* **Description:** Covers hand therapy, hand injuries, occupational therapy, and physiotherapy.
—BLDSC (2309.030000).
Published by: British Association of Hand Therapists Ltd., Knights Quarter, 14 St John's Ln, London EC1M 4AJ, Chelmsford, Essex CM1 7ET, United Kingdom. TEL 44-1603-593316, FAX 44-1603-593166, c.jerosch-herold@uea.ac.uk, http://www.hea.ac.uk/baht/default/html. Ed. Christina Jerosch-Herold. R&P Christina Jerosch Herold TEL 44-1603-593316. Adv. contact Ruth Lando. Circ: 500.

615.85154 GBR
ML3919
BRITISH JOURNAL OF MUSIC THERAPY. Text in English. 1968. 2/yr. GBP 55, USD 88 (effective 2000). adv. bk.rev. index. **Document type:** *Bulletin.*
Former titles (until 1995): Journal of British Music Therapy (0951-5038); British Journal of Music Therapy (0308-244X)
Indexed: ERA, IBZ, Ind.Philos., Sp.Ed.Needs Abstr.
—BLDSC (2311.900000), GNLM, ingenta.
Published by: British Society for Music Therapy, 25 Rosslyn Ave, E. Barnet, Herts EN4 8DH, United Kingdom. Ed. Nicky Barber. R&P, Adv. contact Denize Christophers. Circ: 800. **Co-sponsor:** Association of Professional Music Therapists.

615.82 GBR ISSN 1354-8581
BRITISH JOURNAL OF THERAPY & REHABILITATION. Text in English. 1994. q. GBP 35 domestic to individuals; GBP 70 foreign to individuals; GBP 80 domestic to institutions; GBP 100 foreign to institutions. adv. **Document type:** *Academic/Scholarly.*
Indexed: AMED, Brit.Nur.Ind.
—BLDSC (2325.850000).
Published by: Mark Allen Publishing Ltd., Croxted Mews, 286-288a Croxted Rd, London SE24 9BY, United Kingdom. TEL 44-208-671-7521, FAX 44-208-671-4454. Ed. David Maskill. Pub. Mark Allen. Adv. contact Adrian Johnston.

617.1 615.53 FRA ISSN 0007-9782
CAHIERS DE KINESITHERAPIE; revue d'enseignement post-scolaire et de documentation technique. Text in French. 1962. 6/yr. FRF 596 domestic to individuals; FRF 791 foreign to individuals; FRF 745 domestic to institutions; FRF 931 foreign to institutions (effective 2000). adv. bk.rev. **Document type:** *Academic/Scholarly.* **Description:** Each issue provides thorough knowledge of a particular disease or therapy, for post-graduate learning or review.
Related titles: Microform ed.: (from PQC); Online - full text ed.: (from RoweCom Information Quest).
Indexed: Biol.Abstr., Chem.Abstr., Excerp.Med.
—BLDSC (2949.560000), CISTI, Infotrieve. **CCC.**
Published by: Masson - Periodiques, 120 bd. St. Germain, Paris 75006, France. TEL 33-1-40466200, FAX 33-1-40466201. Ed. J Barthe. Circ: 2,900. **Subscr. to:** Societe de Periodiques Specialises, BP 22, Vineuil Cedex 41354, France. TEL 33-2-54504612, FAX 33-2-54504611.

615.82 CAN
CANADIAN HEALTHCARE BUSINESS NEWS. Text in English. 1994. s-a. CND 24.50 (effective 1997). **Document type:** *Trade.* **Description:** Focusing on the business side of home healthcare, durable goods in rehabilitation, pharmacies specializing in homecare products.
Published by: B C S Communications Ltd., 101 Thorncliffe Park Dr, Toronto, ON M4H 1M2, Canada. TEL 416-421-7944, 800-798-6282, FAX 416-421-0966. Ed. Helmut Dostal. Pub. Caroline Tapp McDougall. Circ: 5,000 (controlled).

615.82 CAN ISSN 0008-4174
CANADIAN JOURNAL OF OCCUPATIONAL THERAPY/REVUE CANADIENNE D'ERGOTHERAPIE. Abbreviated title: C J O T. Text mainly in English; Text occasionally in French. 1933. 5/yr. CND 72 domestic to institutions; CND 78 in United States to institutions; CND 94 elsewhere to institutions (effective 2000). adv. bk.rev. bibl, illus. index. reprint service avail. from PQC. *Refereed.* **Document type:** *Academic/Scholarly.* **Description:** Promotes the advancement and growth of theory and practice in occupational therapy and fosters excellence in research and education.
Related titles: Online - full text ed.: (from ProQuest Information & Learning).
Indexed: AMED, AgeLine, C.I.J.E., CINAHL, Except.Child Educ.Abstr., Excerp.Med. (1994-), Ind.Med. (1939-), PsycInfo, Rehabil.Lit., e-psyche.
—BLDSC (3033.600000), CISTI, EMDOCS, GNLM, ingenta. **CCC.**
Published by: Canadian Association of Occupational Therapists, CTTC Ste 3400, 1125 Colonel By drive, Ottawa, ON K1S 5R1, Canada. TEL 613-523-2268, FAX 613-523-2552, http://www.caot.ca. Ed., R&P Geraldine Moore. Adv. contact Lisa Sheehan. B&W page CND 815; trim 9.5 x 7. Circ: 434 (paid); 8,000 (controlled).

615.8 ITA ISSN 0390-8712
CODEN: CLTM-A
CLINICA TERMALE. Text in Italian. 1941. bi-m. **Document type:** *Academic/Scholarly.*
—GNLM.
Published by: (Associazione Italiana di Idroclimatologia, Talassologia e Terapia Fisica), Societa Editrice Universo, Via Giovanni Battista Morgagni, 1, Rome, RM 00161, Italy.

613.7 USA ISSN 0896-9620
RD795 CODEN: CLKIE9
CLINICAL KINESIOLOGY. Text in English. 1947. q. USD 25 to non-members; USD 35 foreign to non-members; USD 45 to institutions; USD 55 foreign to institutions. adv. bk.rev. bibl, charts, illus. index. reprint service avail. from PSC,SCH. *Refereed.* **Document type:** *Academic/Scholarly.*
Former titles (until 1987): American Corrective Therapy Journal (0002-8088); (until 1967): Association for Physical and Mental Rehabilitation. Journal (0098-8448)
Related titles: Microform ed.: (from PQC).
Indexed: AMED, Adol.Ment.Hlth.Abstr., Biol.Abstr., CINAHL, Excerp.Med., HRIS, Hosp.Lit.Ind., Ind.Med. (coverage dropped), Phys.Ed.Ind., Psychol.Abstr., Rehabil.Lit., Sportsearch (1988-), Yrbk.Assoc.Educ.& Rehab.Blind.
—BLDSC (3286.294700), EMDOCS, GNLM, ingenta, KNAW.
Published by: American Kinesiotherapy Association, c/o Dr Geri M. Farman, Clinical Kinesiology Turnkey Publishing, 11450 Bristle Oak Trail, Austin, TX 78750. TEL 419-530-2743, FAX 419-530-4759, jdrowat@uoft02.utoledo.edu, geri@tkp.com. R&P John Drowatzky. Circ: 1,064.

M

615.82 GBR ISSN 0269-2155
CODEN: CEHAEN
CLINICAL REHABILITATION. Text in English. 1987. 6/yr. GBP 152 in Europe to individuals; USD 266 in North America to individuals; GBP 167 rest of world to individuals; GBP 429 in Europe to institutions; USD 755 in North America to institutions; GBP 470 rest of world to institutions; GBP 235 in developing nations; GBP 114 in Europe to members of qualified institutions; USD 194 in North America to members of qualified institutions; GBP 133 rest of world to members of qualified institutions; GBP 64 in Europe to members of BSRM, VRA; GBP 69 rest of world to members of BSRM, VRA; GBP 71 newsstand/cover in Europe; USD 126 newsstand/cover in North America; GBP 77 newsstand/cover rest of world (effective 2002). adv. back issues avail.; reprints avail. *Refereed.* **Document type:** *Journal, Academic/Scholarly.* **Description:** Provides a forum for ideas and information for persons concerned with rehabilitation.
Related titles: Online - full text ed.: (from EBSCO Publishing, O C L C Online Computer Library Center, Inc., RoweCom Information Quest, ingenta, Swets Blackwell, Institute for Scientific Information).
Indexed: AMED, ASSIA, CINAHL, Curr.Cont., Excerp.Med. (1993-), Ind.Med. (1987-), Inpharma, Int.Nurs.Ind., Pharm.&Out.News, PsycInfo, Psychol.Abstr. (1987-), Reac., Ref.Zh., Sci.Cit.Ind., e-psyche.
—BLDSC (3286.351500), CISTI, EMDOCS, GNLM, IDS, Infotrieve, KNAW. **CCC.**
Published by: Arnold Publishers (Subsidiary of: Hodder Headline plc.), 338 Euston Rd, London NW1 3BH, United Kingdom. TEL 44-20-7873-6337, FAX 44-20-7873-6325, arnoldjournals@hodder.co.uk, http://www.arnoldpublishers.com/journals/journtitles.htm, http://www.palliativemedjournal.com. Ed. Dr. Derick Wade. Adv. contact Mary Attree. **Subscr. to:** Turpin Distribution Services Ltd., Blackhorse Rd, Letchworth, Herts SG6 1HN, United Kingdom. TEL 44-1462-488900, FAX 44-1462-483011.

615.82 USA ISSN 1040-2217
CODEN: CPRHEZ
CONTEMPORARY PERSPECTIVES IN REHABILITATION. Text in English. 1986. irreg. price varies. **Document type:** *Monographic series.*
—CISTI.
Published by: F.A. Davis Company, 1915 Arch St, Philadelphia, PA 19103. TEL 800-323-3555, FAX 215-440-3016, orders@fadavis.com, http://www.fadavis.com. Eds. Steven L Wolf, Robert H Craven Jr.

615.82 USA ISSN 0896-2960
CRITICAL REVIEWS IN PHYSICAL & REHABILITATION MEDICINE. Text in English. 1989. q. USD 94 to individuals; USD 387 to institutions (effective 2000). adv. **Document type:** *Academic/Scholarly.* **Description:** Provides reviews of diagnostic methods, clinical modalities and techniques, and physical and rehabilitative methodologies for specific etiologies amenable to treatment by physical medicine.
Indexed: AMED, CINAHL, Excerp.Med. (1995-).
—BLDSC (3487.479800), EMDOCS, GNLM, Infotrieve, ingenta, KNAW. **CCC.**
Published by: Begell House Inc., 79 Madison Ave, Ste 1205, New York, NY 10016-7892. TEL 212-725-1999, FAX 212-213-8368, begellhouse@worldnet.att.net, orders@begellhouse.com. Eds. Ernest J Henley, Martin Grabois. Pub. William Begell. R&P, Adv. contact Jung Ra.

615.85155 USA ISSN 1089-313X
RC1220.D35
DANCE MEDICINE & SCIENCE. Text in English. 1997. q. USD 46 to members; USD 56 to non-members; USD 66 foreign; USD 66 to institutions; USD 76 foreign to institutions (effective 2000). adv. bk.rev.
—BLDSC (4967.360000), ingenta.
Published by: (International Association for Dance Medicine & Science), J. Michael Ryan Publishing, Inc., 24 Crescent Dr N, Andover, NJ 07821-4000. TEL 973-786-7777, FAX 973-786-7776. Eds. Karen S Clippinger, Scott E Brown. Pub., R&P, Adv. contact James Costello.

615.85155 USA
DANCE MEDICINE - HEALTH NEWSLETTER✶. Text in English. 1983. q. USD 15. adv. bk.rev. **Document type:** *Newsletter.*
Published by: International Center for Dance Orthopaedics and Dance Therapy, 7922 Oceanus Dr., Hollywood, CA 90046-2045. TEL 213-261-0326. Ed. Ernest L Washington M D. Circ: 200.

DISABILITY AND REHABILITATION. see *HANDICAPPED*

615.82 JPN ISSN 0919-5602
E I R E C KENKYU HOKOKUSHU. Text in Japanese; Summaries in English. 1986. a. **Document type:** *Academic/Scholarly.*
Formerly (until 1991): Rosai Rihabiriteshon Kogaku Senta Kenkyu Hokokushu (0912-7488)
Published by: Rehabilitation Engineering Center for Employment Injuries, 10-5 Komei 1-chome, Minato-ku, Nagoya-shi, Aichi-ken 455-0018, Japan. FAX 81-052-652-6275.

EDUCATIONAL THERAPY & THERAPEUTIC TEACHING. see *EDUCATION—Special Education And Rehabilitation*

615.82 FRA ISSN 1293-2965
▼ **ENCYCLOPEDIE MEDICO-CHIRURGICALE. KINESITERAPIA - MEDICINA FISICA**; como recuperar la autonomia del paciente. Cover title: Tratado de Kinesiterapia - Medicina Fisica. Variant title: Encyclopedia Medico-Quirurgica. Kinesiterapia - Medicina Fisica. Text in Spanish. 1999. 4 base vols. plus q. updates. bibl, charts, illus. *Refereed.* **Document type:** *Academic/Scholarly.* **Description:** Provides an up-to-date reference for topics in all areas of physical medicine and rehabilitation, including rheumatology, physical therapy, occupational therapy, orthopedics, and neurology.
Related titles: ♦ French ed.: Encyclopedie Medico-Chirurgicale. Kinesitherapie - Medecine Physique - Readaptation. ISSN 1283-0887; ♦ Italian ed.: Encyclopedie Medico-Chirurgicale. Medicina Riabilitativa. ISSN 1283-078X.
Published by: Elsevier Paris, Editions Scientifiques et Medicales (Subsidiary of: Reed Elsevier plc. group), 23 rue Linois, Paris 75015, France. TEL 33-1-45589110, FAX 33-1-45589110, redaction-emc@elsevier.fr, redacion-emc@elsevier.fr, http://www.elsevier.fr, http://www.elsevier.com. Ed. Jean Simonnet.

615.82 FRA ISSN 1283-0887
ENCYCLOPEDIE MEDICO-CHIRURGICALE. KINESITHERAPIE - MEDECINE PHYSIQUE - READAPTATION; de l'evaluation du handicap a la readaptation. Cover title: Traite de Kinesitherapie - Medecine Physique - Readaptation. Text in French. 1968. 4 base vols. plus q. updates. bibl, charts, illus. **Document type:** *Academic/Scholarly.* **Description:** Provides an up-to-date reference for topics in all areas of physical medicine and rehabilitation, including rheumatology, physical therapy, occupational therapy, orthopedics, and neurology.
Formerly (until 1998): Encyclopedie Medico-Chirurgicale. Kinesitherapie, Reeducation Fonctionelle (0246-0408)
Related titles: ♦ Italian ed.: Encyclopedie Medico-Chirurgicale. Medicina Riabilitativa. ISSN 1283-078X; ♦ Spanish ed.: Encyclopedie Medico-Chirurgicale. Kinesiterapia - Medicina Fisica. ISSN 1293-2965.
Published by: Elsevier Paris, Editions Scientifiques et Medicales (Subsidiary of: Reed Elsevier plc. group), 23 rue Linois, Paris 75015, France. TEL 33-1-45589110, FAX 33-1-45589110, redaction-emc@elsevier.fr, redacion-emc@elsevier.fr, http://www.elsevier.fr; http://www.emc.tm.fr. Ed. Jean Simonnet.

615.82 FRA ISSN 1283-078X
ENCYCLOPEDIE MEDICO-CHIRURGICALE. MEDICINA RIABILITATIVA; dalla valutazione dell'handicap alla rieducazione. Cover title: Trattato di Medicina Riabilitativa. Text in Italian. 1998. 4 base vols. plus q. updates. bibl, charts, illus. *Refereed.* **Document type:** *Academic/Scholarly.* **Description:** Provides an up-to-date reference for topics in all areas of physical medicine and rehabilitation, including rheumatology, physical therapy, occupational therapy, orthopedics, and neurology.
Related titles: ♦ French ed.: Encyclopedie Medico-Chirurgicale. Kinesitherapie - Medecine Physique - Readaptation. ISSN 1283-0887; ♦ Spanish ed.: Encyclopedie Medico-Chirurgicale. Kinesiterapia - Medicina Fisica. ISSN 1293-2965.
Published by: Elsevier Paris, Editions Scientifiques et Medicales (Subsidiary of: Reed Elsevier plc. group), 23 rue Linois, Paris 75015, France. TEL 33-1-45589110, FAX 33-1-45589110, redaction-emc@elsevier.fr, redacion-emc@elsevier.fr, http://www.elsevier.fr, http://www.elsevier.com. Ed. Jean Simonnet.

615.82 CHE ISSN 0258-672X
ERGOTHERAPIE. Text in French, German. 1964. m. CHF 103 (effective 2001). adv. back issues avail. **Document type:** *Journal, Academic/Scholarly.*
Indexed: IBZ.
Published by: Ergotherapeutinnen Verband Schweiz, Stauffacherstr 96, Zuerich 8026, Switzerland. TEL 41-1-2425464, FAX 41-1-2915440, evs-ase@ergotherapie.ch, http://www.ergotherapie.ch. Ed. Claudia Galli. adv.: page CHF 1,030; trim 182 x 243. Circ: 5,000 (controlled). **Dist. by:** Staempfli und Cie AG. TEL 41-31-3006699.

615.82 ITA ISSN 1125-890X
ERRE COME RIABILITAZIONE. Text in Italian. 1990. q. ITL 39,000; ITL 42,000 foreign (effective 1999). **Document type:** *Trade.*
Published by: Societa Erre s.r.l., Via Ardeatina, 306, Rome, RM 00179, Italy. TEL 39-06-5191675, FAX 39-06-5032097, info@erre.it, erre@hsantalucia.it. Ed. Giuseppe Tagliapietra.

615.82 ITA ISSN 0014-2573
CODEN: EUMPA
EUROPA MEDICOPHYSICA. Text in English, Italian. 1965. q. USD 105 to individuals; USD 155 to institutions (effective 2000 - 2001). adv. bk.rev. bibl, charts, illus. index. *Refereed.* **Document type:** *Academic/Scholarly.*
Related titles: Microform ed.: (from PQC); Online - full text ed.: (from Northern Light Technology, Inc.).
Indexed: AMED, Excerp.Med. (1995-).
—BLDSC (3829.319500), CISTI, GNLM.
Published by: (European Federation of Physical Medicine and Rehabilitation), Edizioni Minerva Medica, Corso Bramante, 83-85, Turin, TO 10126, Italy. TEL 39-11-678282, FAX 39-11-674502. Ed. P Di Benedetto. Pub. Alberto Oliaro. Adv. contact F Filippo. B&W page USD 1,200, color page USD 2,000; trim 280 x 215. Circ: 3,000 (paid). **Co-sponsor:** Italian Society of Physical Medicine and Rehabilitation.

EXCERPTA MEDICA. SECTION 19: REHABILITATION AND PHYSICAL MEDICINE. see *MEDICAL SCIENCES—Abstracting, Bibliographies, Statistics*

FISIOTERAPIA. see *MEDICAL SCIENCES—Nurses And Nursing*

615.82 ESP
FISIOTERAPIA Y CALIDAD DE VIDA. Text and summaries in Spanish. 1998. q. ESP 7,000 to individuals (effective 2000); ESP 10,000 to institutions; USD 200 foreign (effective 2000). adv. abstr, bibl, illus, stat. back issues avail. *Refereed.* **Document type:** *Academic/Scholarly.*
Published by: (Physiotherapeutics' College), Aran Ediciones S.A., Castello, 128 1o, Madrid 28006, Spain. TEL 34-91-782-0030, FAX 34-91-561-5787, edita@grupoaran.com, http://www.grupoaran.com. Pub. Jose Jimenez. R&P Maria Dolores Linares TEL 34-1-7820035. Circ: 5,000.

615.82 TUR ISSN 1300-6614
CODEN: FTRDE
FIZIK TEDAVI REHABILITASYON DERGISI. Text in Turkish. 1958. q. USD 20 (effective 1997). adv. bk.rev. *Refereed.* **Document type:** *Academic/Scholarly.* **Description:** Publishes original articles, case reports, reviews and abstract of articles published in other journals.
Indexed: Excerp.Med. (1995-).
Published by: Turkiye Fiziksel Tip ve Rehabilitasyon Dernegi, Capa, Istanbul 34390, Turkey. TEL 90-212-6330505, FAX 90-212-6328464, ftr@dernk.com.tr. Ed. Dr. Fikret Tuxun. Circ: 1,000.

FOCAL POINT; a national bulletin on family support and children's mental health. see *HANDICAPPED*

615.82 IND
FRIDAY MEETING TRANSACTIONS. Text in English. bi-m. **Document type:** *Newsletter, Academic/Scholarly.*
Related titles: Online - full content ed.
Published by: (Shree Ramana Maharishi Academy for the Blind), Asia Pacific Disability Rehabilitation Journal, J-124 Ushas Apartments, 16 th Main, 4th Block, Jayanagar, Bangalore, Karnataka 560 011, India. FAX 91-80-6633762, thomasmaya@hotmail.com, http://www.dinf.ne.jp/doc/prdl/othr/apdrj/apdrj.html. Ed. Dr. Maya Thomas.

615.8 NOR ISSN 0016-3384
FYSIOTERAPEUTEN. Text in Norwegian. 1934. 14/yr. NOK 650. adv. bk.rev. illus. *Refereed.* **Document type:** *Trade, Academic/Scholarly, Abstract/Index.*
—Infotrieve. **CCC.**
Published by: Norske Fysioterapeuters Forbund, Pilestredet 56, Postboks 7009, Majorstua, Oslo 0306, Norway. TEL 47-22-93-30-50, FAX 47-22-56-58-25, fysioterapeuten@fysio.no, http://www.fysioterapeuten.no/. Ed. Karin Helene Haugen. Circ: 7,800 (controlled).

M

615.82 DNK
FYSIOTERAPEUTEN (COPENHAGEN). Text in Danish. 1918. 22/yr. DKK 750; DKK 50 newsstand/cover (effective 2001). adv. bk.rev.
Formerly (until 2001): Danske Fysioterapeuter (0105-0648)
Published by: Danske Fysioterapeuter, Norre Voldgade 90, Copenhagen K 1358, Denmark. TEL 33-13-82-11, FAX 33-13-01-77, df@fysio.dk, http://www.fysio.dk. Ed. Michael Diepeveen. Circ: 8,612.

615.8 FIN ISSN 0789-5232
FYSIOTERAPIA. Text in Finnish; Summaries in English. 1954. 8/yr. EUR 59 domestic; EUR 64 foreign (effective 2001). adv. bk.rev. charts, illus. *Refereed.* **Document type:** *Magazine, Academic/Scholarly.* **Description:** Covers physiotherapy, movement and health, rehabilitation.
Former titles: Laakintavoimistelija (0039-5579); Suomen Laakintavoimistelija
Published by: Suomen Fysioterapeuttiliitto/Finnish Association of Physiotherapists, Asemamiehenkatu 4, Helsinki 00520, Finland. TEL 358-9-87704710, FAX 358-9-1483054, tarja.mansikkamaki@fysioterapeuttiliitto.fi, http://www.fysioterapia.net. Ed. Tarja Mansikkamaki. adv.: B&W page XEU 959, color page XEU 1,649; 175 x 260. Circ: 8,800.

615.82 GBR
GREAT BRITAIN. DEPARTMENT OF HEALTH. OCCUPATIONAL THERAPY SERVICES; summary information. Text in English. a. **Description:** Provides information about patient contacts with occupational therapy services collected from the Department of Health annual return KT26.
Published by: Department of Health, Government Statistical Service - Statistics Division 2B, Rm 430B, Skipton House, 80 London Rd, Elephant and Castle, London SE1 6LW, United Kingdom. TEL 44-171-972-5540.

615.82 GBR
GREAT BRITAIN. DEPARTMENT OF HEALTH. PHYSIOTHERAPY SERVICES; summary information. Text in English. a. **Description:** Contains information about patient contacts with physiotherapy services, collected from the Department of Health annual return KT27.
Published by: Department of Health, Government Statistical Service - Statistics Division 2B, Rm 430B, Skipton House, 80 London Rd, Elephant and Castle, London SE1 6LW, United Kingdom. TEL 44-171-972-5540.

615.892 362.29 USA ISSN 1070-8200
GUIDEPOINTS; acupuncture in recovery. Text in English. 1993. m. USD 180; USD 185 in Canada & Mexico; USD 190 elsewhere. bk.rev., software rev., video rev. charts, stat. back issues avail. **Document type:** *Newsletter, Trade.* **Description:** Provides information for professionals concerned with acupuncture in the treatment and recovery of people with addictive and mental problems.
Published by: J & M Reports, 7402 NE 58th St, Vancouver, WA 98662-5207. TEL 360-254-0186, FAX 360-260-8620, acudetox@aol.com. Ed., Pub., R&P Jay Renaud.

615.82 BGR ISSN 1311-7785
HEALED TOURIST. Text in Bulgarian; Summaries in Bulgarian, English. 1974. q. BGL 14 domestic; USD 30 foreign (effective 2001 - 2002). adv. abstr. index. 58 p./no. back issues avail. *Refereed.* **Document type:** *Academic/Scholarly.* **Description:** Presents original articles and abstracts of foreign publications on physical therapy, balneology, rehabilitation of a broad spectrum of diseases.
Formerly (until 2001): Balneoklimatologiia i Fizikalna Terapiia (0861-8569)
Indexed: Abstr.Bulg.Sci.Med.Lit.
Published by: Meditsinski Universitet - Sofia, Tsentur za Informatsiia po Meditsina/Medical University - Sofia, Medical Information Center, 1 Sv Georgi Sofiiski ul, Sofia 1431, Bulgaria. TEL 359-2-9522342, FAX 359-2-9522393, mutafov@sun.medun.acad.bg, http://www.medun.acad.bg. Ed. Sv. Grancharova. R&P, Adv. contact Dr. Christo Mutafov. B&W page USD 50, color page USD 200; 12 x 18. Circ: 150.

651.82 615.89 USA
HEALING RETREATS & SPAS. Text in English. bi-m. USD 19.95 domestic for web orders; USD 44.95 in Canada for web orders; USD 54.95 in Europe for web orders; USD 4.95 newsstand/cover; USD 6.95 newsstand/cover in Canada (effective 2001). adv. back issues avail. **Document type:** *Magazine, Consumer.* **Description:** Provides information on spas, resort hotels, and other similar destinations around the world, including information on healthy living, alternative therapy, and events coverage.
Related titles: Online - full content ed.
Published by: Healing Retreats & Spas Magazine, 24 E Cota St Ste 200, Santa Barbara, CA 93101. TEL 805-962-7107, FAX 805-962-1337, info@healingretreats.com, contact@healingretreats.com, editorial@healingretreats.com, http://www.healingretreats.com/.

615.8 JPN ISSN 0912-1455
HOKKAIDO RIGAKU RYOHO/HOKKAIDO JOURNAL OF PHYSICAL THERAPY. Text in Japanese. 1984. a. JPY 1,500.
Published by: Nihon Rigaku Ryohoshi Kyokai, Hokkaido Shikai/Japanese Physical Therapy Association, Hokkaido Chapter, Kokuritsu Ryoyojo Nishi Sapporo Byoin Rigaku Ryohoka, 7 Yamanote 5-Jo, Nishi-ku, Sapporo-shi, Hokkaido 063-0009, Japan.

615.82 JPN ISSN 0304-2081
HOKKAIDO RIHABIRITESHON GAKKAI ZASSHI/HOKKAIDO REHABILITATION ASSOCIATION. JOURNAL. Text in Japanese. 1964. a. JPY 4,000. adv. **Document type:** *Academic/Scholarly.*
Published by: Hokkaido Rehabilitation Association/ Hokkaido Rihabiriteshon Gakkai, c/o Sapporo Ika Daigaku Fuzobo Byoin Rihabilitation-bu, Nishi 17-chome, Minami 1-jo, Chuo-ku, Sapporo-shi, Hokkaido 060, Japan. Ed. Dr. Bun Ichiro Kawamura. R&P Kazutoshi Yokugushi TEL 81-11-611-2111. Adv. contact Dr. Kazutoshi Yokogushi.

615.8 JPN ISSN 0915-6429
HOKKAIDO SAGYO RYOHO GAKKAISHI/HOKKAIDO ASSOCIATION OF OCCUPATIONAL THERAPISTS. JOURNAL. Text in Japanese. 1984. a. **Document type:** *Academic/Scholarly.*
Published by: Hokkaido Sagyo Ryoho Shikai, Sapporo Ika Daigaku Eisei Tanki Daigakubu, Nishi 17-chome, Minami 3-jo, Chuo-ku, Sapporo-shi, Hokkaido 060, Japan.

I T - INVALIDITYOE. see *SOCIAL SERVICES AND WELFARE*

INDIAN JOURNAL OF OCCUPATIONAL THERAPY. see *OCCUPATIONAL HEALTH AND SAFETY*

INTERFACE (CHICAGO, 1978). see *LIBRARY AND INFORMATION SCIENCES*

617.06 USA ISSN 0342-5282
RM695 CODEN: IJRRDK
INTERNATIONAL JOURNAL OF REHABILITATION RESEARCH. Text in English, French, German; Summaries in English, French, German, Spanish. 1977. q. USD 125 domestic to individuals for print & online eds.; USD 125 foreign to individuals for print & online eds.; USD 317 per issue domestic to institutions; USD 317 per issue foreign to institutions; USD 73 newsstand/cover (effective 2002). adv. bk.rev. charts, illus. Index. reprints avail. *Refereed.* **Document type:** *Academic/Scholarly.* **Description:** Provides an interdisciplinary forum for research into disability and handicaps people in both industrial and developing nations face.
Related titles: Online - full text ed.: USD 412.10 domestic academic site license; USD 412.10 foreign academic site license; USD 459.65 domestic corporate site license; USD 459.65 foreign corporate site license (effective 2002) (from EBSCO Publishing, Institute for Scientific Information).
Indexed: AMED, ASCA, AgeLine, Bioeng.Abstr., Biol.Abstr., Biotech.& Bioeng.Abstr., C.I.J.E., CINAHL, Child Devel.Abstr., Crim.Just.Abstr., Curr.Cont., Eng.Ind., Ergon.Abstr., Except.Child Educ.Abstr., Excerp.Med., Fam.Ind., Ind.Med. (1978-), Int.Nurs.Ind., Lang.& Lang.Behav.Abstr., Psychol.Abstr., Rehabil.Lit., SSCI, Yrbk.Assoc.Educ.& Rehab.Blind.
—BLDSC (4542.526000), ADONIS, CISTI, Ei, EMDOCS, GNLM, IDS, ingenta, KNAW.
Published by: (Rehabilitation International), Lippincott Williams & Wilkins (Philadelphia) (Subsidiary of: Wolters Kluwer N.V.), 530 Walnut St, Philadelphia, PA 19106-3621. TEL 215-521-8300, FAX 215-521-8902, http://www.intjrehabilres.com, http://www.Lww.com. Ed. Juhani Wikstroem. Adv. contact Gemma Heiser. Circ: 1,000. **Subscr. to:** PO Box 1600, Hagerstown, MD 21740-1600. TEL 800-777-2295, FAX 301-824-7390.

615.8 USA ISSN 0267-0380
INTERNATIONAL PERSPECTIVES IN PHYSICAL THERAPY* . Text in English. 1985. irreg., latest vol.8. **Document type:** *Monographic series.*
—CISTI.
Published by: Churchill Livingstone (Subsidiary of: Harcourt Health Sciences), 15 E 26th St, Fl 15, New York, NY 10010-1505. TEL 212-206-5040, FAX 212-727-7808, http://www.churchillmed.com.

INTERNATIONAL SOCIETY FOR OCCUPATIONAL ERGONOMICS AND SAFETY. NEWSLETTER. see *OCCUPATIONAL HEALTH AND SAFETY*

▼ **THE INTERNET JOURNAL OF PAIN, SYMPTOM CONTROL AND PALLIATIVE CARE.** see *MEDICAL SCIENCES—Anaesthesiology*

615.8 ISR ISSN 0021-2199
ISRAEL JOURNAL OF PHYSIOTHERAPY. Text in English, Hebrew. irreg. (3-4/yr.). USD 50 to members. adv. bk.rev. charts, illus. **Document type:** *Trade.* **Description:** Publishes current research on physical therapy from around the world.
Published by: National Union of Physiotherapy in Israel, 93 Arlozorov St., Tel Aviv, Israel. TEL 972-2-722324. Eds. Mrs. Eesti Wultz, Mr. Oded Daskal. Circ: 500.

ISSUES ON AGING. see *GERONTOLOGY AND GERIATRICS*

616.07 FRA ISSN 0249-6550
JOURNAL D'ERGOTHERAPIE. Text in French. 1965. q. FRF 410 to individuals; FRF 489 foreign to individuals; FRF 584 to institutions; FRF 689 foreign to institutions (effective 2000). **Document type:** *Academic/Scholarly.* **Description:** Publishes theoretical and practical articles dealing with physiotherapy techniques.
Related titles: Microform ed.: (from PQC); Online - full text ed.: (from RoweCom Information Quest).
—GNLM, Infotrieve. **CCC.**
Published by: (Association Francaise des Ergotherapeutes), Masson - Periodiques, 120 bd. St. Germain, Paris 75006, France. TEL 33-1-40466200, FAX 33-1-40466201. Ed. O Lecluse. Circ: 2,100. **Subscr. to:** Societe de Periodiques Specialises, BP 22, Vineuil Cedex 41354, France. TEL 33-2-54504612, FAX 33-2-54504611.

JOURNAL OF BACK AND MUSCULOSKELETAL REHABILITATION. see *MEDICAL SCIENCES—Orthopedics And Traumatology*

615.8 GBR ISSN 1360-8592
CODEN: JBOTF2
JOURNAL OF BODYWORK & MOVEMENT THERAPIES. Text in English. 1997. q. GBP 48 to individuals; GBP 141 to institutions (effective 2002). adv. bk.rev. 72 p./no. 2 cols./p. back issues avail.; reprints avail. *Refereed.* **Document type:** *Journal, Academic/Scholarly.* **Description:** Covers practical approaches to musculoskeletal dysfunction applicable across all bodywork, movement and manual therapies.
Related titles: Online - full text ed.: (from Swets Blackwell, IDEAL Online Library).
Indexed: AMED, CINAHL, Cal.Tiss.Abstr., Neurosci.Abstr. (coverage dropped), Tox.Abstr. (coverage dropped).
—BLDSC (4954.235000).
Published by: Churchill Livingstone (Subsidiary of: Harcourt Publishers Ltd.), Robert Stevenson House, 1-3 Baxter's Pl, Leith Walk, Edinburgh, Midlothian EH1 3AF, United Kingdom. TEL 44-131-556-2424, FAX 44-131-558-1278, journals@harcourt.com, http://www.harcourt-international.com/journals/jbmt. Eds. Leon Chaitow, Marvin Dean. R&P Sharon Boyle TEL 44-131-524-1747. Adv. contact Deborah Watkins TEL 44-207-424-4280. Circ: 1,500 (paid). **Subsc. to:** Harcourt Publishers Ltd., Journal Sales & Marketing Dept., 32 Jamestown Rd, London NW1 7BY, United Kingdom. TEL 44-20-8308-5700; **Subscr. in the US to:** Harcourt Health Sciences, Journals Subscription Department, PO Box 156, Avenel, NJ 07001. TEL 877-839-7126.

M

615.8 USA ISSN 1533-2098
▼ **JOURNAL OF BRIEF THERAPY.** Text in English. 2001. 3/yr. USD 44 domestic to individuals; USD 52 foreign to individuals; USD 98 domestic to institutions; USD 106 foreign to institutions (effective 2001).
Published by: Springer Publishing Company, 536 Broadway, New York, NY 10012. TEL 212-431-4370, FAX 212-941-7842, springer@springerpub.com, http://www.springerjournals.com/.

617.06 USA ISSN 1062-2969
RC387.5
JOURNAL OF COGNITIVE REHABILITATION; a publication for the therapist, family and patient. Text in English. 1983. bi-m. USD 40 domestic to individuals; USD 45 in Canada to individuals; USD 55 elsewhere to individuals; USD 80 domestic to institutions; USD 85 in Canada to institutions; USD 95 elsewhere to institutions (effective 2000). adv. back issues avail.; reprint service avail. from SCH,PSC. **Document type:** *Academic/Scholarly.*
Formerly (until 1991): Cognitive Rehabilitation (0738-1069)
Indexed: AMED, CINAHL, PsycInfo, Psychol.Abstr. (1983-), e-psyche.
—BLDSC (4958.799300), CISTI, GNLM, ingenta. **CCC.**
Published by: NeuroScience Publishers, 6555 Carrollton Ave, Indianapolis, IN 46220. TEL 317-257-9672, http://www.neuroscience.cnter.com. Ed. Odie L Bracy III. Adv. contact Nancy P Bracy. Circ: 1,547.

▼ **JOURNAL OF DISABILITY AND ORAL HEALTH.** see *HANDICAPPED*

615.82 USA ISSN 0894-1130
CODEN: JHTHFX
JOURNAL OF HAND THERAPY. Text in English. 1987. q., latest vol.14, 2001. USD 76 domestic to individuals; USD 86 foreign to individuals; USD 96 domestic to institutions; USD 106 foreign to institutions; USD 25 newsstand/cover (effective 2001). adv. illus. back issues avail. *Refereed.* **Document type:** *Journal, Academic/Scholarly.* **Description:** Concerned with post-traumatic and post-surgical rehabilitation of the hand.
Indexed: CINAHL, Excerp.Med. (1996-), Ind.Med. (1987-).
—BLDSC (4996.623500), GNLM, Infotrieve, ingenta, KNAW. **CCC.**
Published by: (American Society of Hand Therapists), Hanley & Belfus, Inc., 210 S 13th St, Philadelphia, PA 19107. TEL 215-546-7293, FAX 215-790-9330. Ed. Evelyn Mackin. adv.: B&W page USD 1,360;. Circ: 4,500.

616.85154 USA ISSN 0022-2917
ML1 CODEN: JMUTA2
JOURNAL OF MUSIC THERAPY. Text in English. 1964. q. USD 120 domestic; USD 130 foreign (effective 2001). bk.rev. charts, illus. index. back issues avail.; reprint service avail. from PQC,PSC,SCH. *Refereed.* **Document type:** *Academic/Scholarly.* **Description:** Reports research in the area of music therapy and the use of music in treatment and rehabilitation settings.
Related titles: Microform ed.: (from PQC); Online - full text ed.: (from H. W. Wilson, Institute for Scientific Information).
Indexed: ASCA, AgeLine, Arts & Hum.Cit.Ind. (coverage dropped), Curr.Cont., Educ.Ind. (Jan.1983-), Except.Child Educ.Abstr., Hosp.Lit.Ind., Ind.Med., Int.Ind.Mus.Per. (1996, 1999), Music Artic.Guide, Music Ind., PsycInfo, Psychol.Abstr., RILM, SSCI, e-psyche.
—BLDSC (5021.160000), GNLM, ingenta.
Published by: American Music Therapy Association, 8455 Colesville Rd, Ste 1000, Silver Spring, MD 20910-3392. TEL 301-589-3300, FAX 301-589-5175, info@musictherapy.org, subscribe@musictherapy.org, http://www.musictherapy.org; http://www.allenpress.com. Ed. Jayne Standley. Circ: 6,000. **Subscr. to:** Allen Press Inc., PO Box 1897, Lawrence, KS 66044-8897.

M

JOURNAL OF OCCUPATIONAL REHABILITATION. see *OCCUPATIONAL HEALTH AND SAFETY*

JOURNAL OF ORTHOPAEDIC AND SPORTS PHYSICAL THERAPY. see *MEDICAL SCIENCES—Sports Medicine*

615.8 JPN ISSN 0915-5287
JOURNAL OF PHYSICAL THERAPY SCIENCE. Text in English. 1989. s-a. membership. abstr, charts, illus. index. **Document type:** *Academic/Scholarly.*
Indexed: AMED.
—BLDSC (5036.216000).
Published by: (Society of Physical Therapy Science/Rigaku Ryoho Kagakukai), I P E C Inc., 1-24-11 Sugamo, Toshima-ku, Tokyo 170-0002, Japan. TEL 81-3-5978-4067, FAX 81-3-5978-4068. Ed., R&P Hitoshi Maruyama. Circ: 1,800. **Dist. overseas by:** Japan Publications Trading Co. Ltd., Tokyo International, PO Box 5030, Tokyo 100-31, Japan. TEL 81-3-3292-3753.

615.8 362 USA ISSN 0022-4154
HD7255.A2 CODEN: JOREA
JOURNAL OF REHABILITATION. Text in English. 1935. q., latest vol.67, no.2, 2001. USD 65 in United States; USD 75 in Canada; USD 90 elsewhere (effective 2001 - 2002). adv. bk.rev. illus, pat. index. 64 p./no. back issues avail.; reprint service avail. from PSC. *Refereed.* **Document type:** *Journal, Academic/Scholarly.* **Description:** Concerned with counseling, restorative services, retraining, and placement of persons disabled by physical, mental, emotional or social disabilities. Articles deal with supervisory role, legislative concerns, consumer, current trends in rehab, etc.
Related titles: Audio cassette/tape ed.; Braille ed.; Microfilm ed.: (from PQC); Online - full text ed.: (from Gale Group, ProQuest Information & Learning, Northern Light Technology, Inc., H. W. Wilson, Factiva, Institute for Scientific Information).
Indexed: AMED, ASCA, ASSIA, Adol.Ment.Hlth.Abstr., AgeLine, Brit.Nur.Ind., C.I.J.E. (coverage dropped), CINAHL, C.I.S. Abstr., Curr.Cont., Except.Child Educ.Abstr., Excerp.Med., Fam.Ind., Hlth.Ind., Hosp.Lit.Ind., Ind.Med. (coverage dropped), P C I, Psychol.Abstr., Rehabil.Lit., SSCI, Soc.Sci.Ind. (Jan.1983-).
—BLDSC (5048.850000), GNLM, IDS, ingenta, KNAW.
Published by: National Rehabilitation Association, 633 S Washington St, Alexandria, VA 22314-4109. TEL 703-836-0850, FAX 703-836-0848, info@nationalrehab.org, http://www.nationalrehab.org. Ed. Paul Alston. R&P, Adv. contact Carol C Hamilla. B&W page USD 745, color page USD 1,805. Circ: 11,000 (controlled).

615.82 USA ISSN 0148-3846
HD7255.A2
JOURNAL OF REHABILITATION ADMINISTRATION. Text in English. q. USD 24 domestic to individuals; USD 39 foreign to individuals; USD 48 domestic to institutions; USD 63 foreign to institutions. adv. index. back issues avail. *Refereed.* **Document type:** *Academic/Scholarly.* **Description:** Publishes theoretical papers, applied research studies, and practice reports designed to improve the practice of administration, management and supervision in a wide variety of human service settings.
Formerly (until 1977): Rehabilitation Administration
Indexed: AMED, PsycInfo, Psychol.Abstr., e-psyche.
—BLDSC (5048.870000).
Published by: Elliott & Fitzpatrick, Inc., 1135 Cedar Shoals Dr, Athens, GA 30605. TEL 800-843-4977, FAX 706-546-8417. Ed. Dennis Gay. Adv. contact Tim Field. page USD 175; 7.63 x 5.38. Circ: 4,200. **Subscr. to:** PO Box 1945, Athens, GA 30603.

617 USA ISSN 1086-9654
RM930.8
JOURNAL OF REHABILITATION OUTCOMES MEASUREMENT. Text in English. 1997. q. USD 99 to individuals; USD 119 to libraries; USD 49 to students; USD 30 newsstand/cover (effective 2001). *Refereed.* **Document type:** *Academic/Scholarly.* **Description:** Publishes current and timely information on the development of validated new and existing rehabilitation outcome scales, the methodology and process of outcomes measurement used in rehabilitative care, the analysis and interpretation of data, and applications of outcome information.
Indexed: AMED, CINAHL.
—BLDSC (5048.960000), Infotrieve. **CCC.**
Published by: Aspen Publishers, Inc., 200 Orchard Ridge Dr, Ste 200, Gaithersburg, MD 20878. TEL 301-417-7500, 800-234-1660, FAX 301-417-7550, customer.service@aspenpul.com, http://www.aspenpub.com. Ed. Edward Dobrzykowski Jr. **Dist. by:** Aspen Publishers Inc., Distribution Center, 7201 McKinney Circle, Frederick, MD 21701. TEL 301-698-7100, FAX 301-695-7931.

615.82 USA ISSN 1079-0268
JOURNAL OF SPINAL CORD MEDICINE. Text in English. 1978. q. free per issue to qualified personnel. bk.rev. *Refereed.* **Document type:** *Academic/Scholarly.* **Description:** For physicians, researchers and health professionals who work in the spinal cord injury field.
Formerly: American Paraplegia Society. Journal (0195-2307)
Indexed: CINAHL, Ind.Med. (1995-), Int.Nurs.Ind., e-psyche.
—GNLM.
Published by: American Paraplegia Society, 75-20 Astoria Blvd., Jackson Heights, NY 11370-1177. TEL 718-803-3782, FAX 718-803-0414, http://www.apssci.org. Ed. Joel A DeLisa. R&P Eileen Symmons TEL 718-803-3782 ext 237. Circ: 1,500.

JOURNAL OF SPORT REHABILITATION. see *MEDICAL SCIENCES—Sports Medicine*

JOURNAL OF THERAPEUTIC HORTICULTURE. see *GARDENING AND HORTICULTURE*

615.82 FRA ISSN 0755-3951
RM695
JOURNEE DE MEDECINE PHYSIQUE ET DE REEDUCATION. Text in French. 1958. a.
Formerly: Journee de Reeducation (0075-4420)
Published by: Expansion Scientifique Publications, 31 bd. de la Tour Maubourg, Paris 75007, France. TEL 33-1-40626400, FAX 33-1-45556920. Ed. Debeyre J Samuel.

615.82 JPN
KANAGAWAKEN RIGAKU RYOHOSHIKAI NYUSU/KANAGAWA PHYSICAL THERAPY ASSOCIATION. NEWS. Text in Japanese. bi-m.
Published by: Kanagawaken Rigaku Ryohoshikai, c/o Yokohama Shiritsu Daigaku Igakubu, 3-46 Urafune-cho, Minami-ku, Yokohama-shi, Kanagawa-ken 232-0024, Japan.

615.82 JPN ISSN 0285-3477
KANAGAWAKEN SOGO RIHABIRITESHON SENTA KIYO/KANAGAWA REHABILITATION CENTER. JOURNAL. Text in Japanese; Summaries in English, Japanese. 1974. a. **Document type:** *Bulletin.*
Published by: Kanagawaken Sogo Rihabiriteshon Senta, 516 Nanasawa, Atsugi-shi, Kanagawa-ken 243-0121, Japan.

615.82 CHN
KANG FU/REHABILITATION. Text in Chinese. bi-m. CNY 7.20.
Published by: (Shanghai Yike Daxue/Shanghai University of Medical Sciences, Jiaoyu Yanjiu Zhongxin/ Educational Research Center), Kang Fu Zazhishe, No 5 Alley 733, Huaihai Zhonglu, Shanghai 200020, China. TEL 3235326. Ed. Yang Zhonghua.

616.07 FRA ISSN 0766-2262
KINE ACTUALITE. Text in French. 43/yr. FRF 750 (effective 2000). adv. **Description:** Professional news about physiotherapy, the social system, health, reports on congresses, conferences, seminars. Information on Minitel, French telematic system.
Formerly (until 1984): Kinesitherapie Actualite (0754-2038)
Published by: Societe de Presse et d'Edition de la Kinesitherapie, 24 rue des Petits Hotels, Paris 75010, France. TEL 33-1-44-83-46-46, FAX 33-1-44-83-46-47, ka@kineactu.com, http://www.kineactu.com. Ed. Franck Gougeon. R&P Gerard Colnat. Adv. contact Vincent Deperrest. Circ: 12,432.

616.822 FRA ISSN 0297-6005
KINESITHERAPEUTE PRATICIEN. Text in French. 1986. bi-m. FRF 100; FRF 160 foreign (effective 1998). adv. bibl. **Document type:** *Academic/Scholarly.* **Description:** For physiotherapists and students in physiotherapy.
Published by: Ediprosante, 1 impasse Gerard de Nerval, Toulouse 31500, France. TEL 33-5-61584752, FAX 33-5-61581976, edips@aol.com. Pub. A Garnier. R&P A. Garnier TEL 33-5-61584772. Adv. contact V Duvaux. B&W page FRF 4,300, color page FRF 5,300.

615.8 FRA ISSN 0023-1576
CODEN: KNTSAC
KINESITHERAPIE SCIENTIFIQUE. Text in French. 1965. m. FRF 725 (effective 2000). adv. charts, illus. **Description:** Clinical practice articles, research in physiotherapy, analysis, scientific information.
Formerly: Kinesitherapie
Indexed: Biol.Abstr.
—BLDSC (5096.070000), CISTI, Infotrieve. **CCC.**
Published by: Societe de Presse et d'Edition de la Kinesitherapie, 24 rue des Petits Hotels, Paris 75010, France. TEL 33-1-44-83-46-46, FAX 33-1-44-83-46-47, ks@kinephysio.com, http://www.kinephysio.com. Ed. Patrick Michaud. Adv. contact Vincent Deperrest. Circ: 6,155.

615.82 JPN ISSN 0912-5825
KOCHI RIHABIRITESHON GAKUIN SOTSUGYO RONBUNSHU/KOCHI REHABILITATION INSTITUTE. COLLEGE OF PHYSICAL THERAPY. BULLETIN OF GRADUATE STUDY. Text in Japanese. a.

Published by: Kochi Rihabiriteshon Gakuin, 292 Asahitenjin-cho, Kochi-shi 780-0955, Japan.

615.8 DEU ISSN 0023-4494
KRANKENGYMNASTIK; Zeitschrift fuer Physiotherapeuten. Text in German. 1948. m. EUR 92.40 domestic; EUR 104.40 foreign; EUR 8 newsstand/cover (effective 2002). adv. bk.rev. abstr, charts, illus. index. **Document type:** *Magazine, Academic/Scholarly.*
Indexed: AMED, Excerp.Med.
—BLDSC (5118.137000), GNLM. **CCC.**
Published by: (Deutscher Verband fuer Physiotherapie - Zentralverband der Physiotherapeuten - Krankengymnasten (ZvK) e.V.), Richard Pflaum Verlag GmbH und Co. KG, Lazarettstr 4, Munich 80636, West Germany. TEL 49-89-12607-0, FAX 49-89-12607202, richard.pflaum@pflaum.de, http://www.pflaum.de/pt.dir/kg/index.html. Ed. Antje Hueter Becker. Adv. contact Christine Keller. B&W page XEU 2,270, color page XEU 3,680; trim 185 x 256. Circ: 35,300.

615.8 JPN ISSN 0915-6739
KYOTO RIGAKU RYOHOSHIKAI KAISHI/KYOTO JOURNAL OF PHYSICAL THERAPY. Text in English, Japanese. 1971. a.
Published by: Nihon Rigaku Ryohoshi Kyokai, Kyoto Rigaku Ryohoshikai, Sei Yozefu Seishien, 6 Higashikobaicho, Kita-ku, Kyoto-shi 603-0000, Japan.

615.82 GBR ISSN 1356-689X
CODEN: MATHFH
MANUAL THERAPY. Text in English. 1996. q. GBP 70 to individuals; GBP 176 to institutions (effective 2002). adv. bk.rev. abstr, bibl. 64 p./no. 2 cols./p. back issues avail.; reprints avail. *Refereed.* **Document type:** *Journal, Academic/Scholarly.* **Description:** Serves as a resource tool for all those engaged in the many diverse aspects of manual therapy.
Related titles: Online - full text ed.: (from EBSCO Publishing, O C L C Online Computer Library Center, Inc., Swets Blackwell, IDEAL Online Library, Institute for Scientific Information).
Indexed: AMED, ASSIA, CINAHL, Focus on: Sports Sci.& Med., Ind.Med. (1995-).
—BLDSC (5365.380000), Infotrieve. **CCC.**
Published by: (Manipulation Association of Chartered Physiotherapists), Churchill Livingstone (Subsidiary of: Harcourt Publishers Ltd.), Robert Stevenson House, 1-3 Baxter's Pl, Leith Walk, Edinburgh, Midlothian EH1 3AF, United Kingdom. TEL 44-131-556-2424, FAX 44-131-558-1278, mtherapy@harcourt.com, journals@harcourt.com, http://www.harcourt-international.com/journals/math. Eds. Ann Moore, Gwendolen A Jull. R&P Sharon Boyle TEL 44-131-524-1747. Adv. contact Deborah Watkins TEL 44-207-424-4280. Circ: 5,500 (paid). **Subscr. addr. in the US:** Harcourt Health Sciences, Journals Subscription Department, PO Box 156, Avenel, NJ 07001. TEL 877-839-7126; **Subscr. to:** Harcourt Publishers Ltd., Journal Sales & Marketing Dept., 32 Jamestown Rd, London NW1 7BY, United Kingdom. TEL 44-20-8308-5700.

615.8 DEU
MANUELLE MEDIZIN UND OSTEOPATHISCHE MEDIZIN; Zeitschrift der Deutschen Gesellschaft fuer Manuelle Medizin. Text in German. 1963. bi-m. DEM 470.54 domestic; DEM 484.40 foreign (effective 2001). adv. bk.rev. index. back issues avail. *Refereed.* **Document type:** *Journal, Academic/Scholarly.* **Description:** Covers all aspects of physiotherapy and related fields.
Formerly (until 2001): Manuelle Medizin (0025-2514)
Related titles: Microform ed.: (from PQC); Online - full text ed.: ISSN 1433-0466 (from EBSCO Publishing, RoweCom Information Quest, Swets Blackwell, Springer LINK).
Indexed: AMED, Excerp.Med.
—BLDSC (5365.766000), CISTI, GNLM, Infotrieve, KNAW. **CCC.**
Published by: (Deutsche Gesellschaft fuer Manuelle Medizin), Springer-Verlag (Subsidiary of: BertelsmannSpringer), Tiergartenstr 17, Heidelberg 69121, Germany. TEL 49-6221-345-0, FAX 49-6221-345229, subscriptions@springer.de, http://link.springer.de/link/service/journals/00337/index.htm/, http://www.springer.de. Eds. E Froelich, G Gallacchi. **Subscr. in N. America to:** Springer-Verlag New York Inc., PO Box 2485, Secaucus, NJ 07096-2485. TEL 212-460-1500, FAX 212-473-6272.

615.8 DEU ISSN 1433-2671
MANUELLE THERAPIE. Text in German. 1997. q. EUR 87 domestic to institutions; EUR 88.60 in Europe to institutions; EUR 91.50 elsewhere to institutions; EUR 20 newsstand/cover (effective 2002). adv. **Document type:** *Journal, Academic/Scholarly.*
Related titles: Online - full text ed.: ISSN 1439-2348.
—GNLM.
Published by: Georg Thieme Verlag, Ruedigerstr 14, Stuttgart 70469, Germany. TEL 49-711-8931-0, FAX 49-711-8931298, leser.service@thieme.de, http://www.thieme.de. R&P Rosi Haarer Becker. Circ: 3,000 (paid).

615.82 615.53 AUS ISSN 1328-8431
MASSAGE AUSTRALIA. Text in English. 1992. q. AUD 48 domestic; AUD 70 foreign (effective 2000). adv. bk.rev. back issues avail. **Document type:** *Trade.* **Description:** Covers professional massage therapy, news and information.
Formerly: Touch Australia (1037-6801)
Published by: Massage Australia Pty. Ltd., PO Box 38, Wentworth Falls, NSW 2782, Australia. TEL 61-247573050, FAX 61-247573936. Ed., R&P Charles Carceller. Adv. contact Louisa McRay.

615.82 USA ISSN 1045-4268
MASSAGE MAGAZINE; keeping those who touch - in touch. Text in English. 1985. bi-m. USD 24 domestic; USD 28 in Canada; USD 36 elsewhere (effective 2000). adv. bk.rev., film rev. bibl, illus, stat. back issues avail. *Refereed.* **Document type:** *Trade.* **Description:** Covers the art and science of massage therapy and related healing arts, supporting readers promoting the benfits of healing touch.
Former titles: Massage and Healing Arts Magazine; Massage and Bodywork Magazine
Related titles: CD-ROM ed.
Address: 1315 W 1st, Spokane, WA 99204. TEL 509-324-8117, FAX 509-324-8606, edit@massagemag.com, http://www.massagemag.com. Ed., R&P Karen Menehan TEL 831-477-1176. Pub. Kate Spencer. Adv. contact Jeff Schmidt. Circ: 45,000 (paid).

615.82 ITA ISSN 1123-9395
MEDICINA CLINICA E TERMALE. Text in Italian; Summarics in English, Italian. 1987. q. ITL 40,000, USD 50. bibl. index. back issues avail. **Document type:** *Academic/Scholarly.* **Description:** Provides medical essays and scientific research on balneology, water cures, water therapies and more.
Published by: Tipografia la Commerciale s.n.c., Via Monte San Genesio, 7, Milan, MI 20158, Italy. TEL 39-2-6071180, FAX 39-2-66800577. Ed. Giuseppe Nappi. adv.: page ITL 1,800,000. Circ: 4,000.

615.82 ESP ISSN 0214-8714
MEDICINA DE REHABILITACION. Text in Spanish. 1986. q. ESP 6,000 domestic; USD 60 foreign (effective 2001). **Document type:** *Academic/Scholarly.*
—BLDSC (5533.662000).
Published by: (Liga para el Desarrollo de la Rehabilitacion), Editores Medicos S.A., Gabriela Mistral, 2, Madrid 28035, Spain. TEL 34-91-3768140, FAX 34-91-3739907. Circ: 3,000.

615.82 RUS
MEDIKO-SOTSYAL'NAYA EKSPRETIZA I REABILITATSIYA/MEDICOSOCIAL EXPERTISE AND REHABILITATION. Text in Russian; Contents page in English. 1998. q. USD 111 foreign (effective 2000). adv. Website rev. abstr. reprints avail. **Document type:** *Journal, Academic/Scholarly.* **Description:** Deals with social aspects of medicine.
Indexed: Ref.Zh.
Published by: Izdatel'stvo Meditsina, Petroverigskii per 6-8, Moscow 101000, Russian Federation. TEL 7-095-9248785, 7-095-928-86-48, FAX 7-095-9211355, 7-095-9286003, meditsina@name.com, http://www.medit.ru. Pub. A M Stochik. R&P V I Chissov. **US dist. addr.:** East View Publications, 3020 Harbor Ln N, Minneapolis, MN 55447. TEL 612-550-0961.

615.82 UKR
MEDITSINSKAYA REABILITATSIYA, KURORTOLOGIYA, FIZIOTERAPIYA. Text in Russian. q.
Published by: Ukrainskii N.I.I. Meditsinskoi Reabiliyatsi i Kurortologii, Per Lermontovskii 6, Odessa, Ukraine. TEL 24-23-08. **US dist. addr.:** East View Publications, 3020 Harbor Ln N, Minneapolis, MN 55447. TEL 612-550-0961.

MENTAL HEALTH ASPECTS OF DEVELOPMENTAL DISABILITIES. see *MEDICAL SCIENCES—Psychiatry And Neurology*

613.7 USA ISSN 1087-1640
QP303
MOTOR CONTROL. Text in English. 1997. q. USD 48 to individuals; USD 144 to institutions; USD 36 to students (effective 2001). adv. bk.rev., software rev., video rev. charts, illus, stat. back issues avail.; reprints avail. *Refereed.* **Document type:** *Academic/Scholarly.* **Description:** Designed to provide an internationally and multidisciplinary forum for the exchange of scientific information on the control of movement across the lifespan, including issues related to motor disorders.
Related titles: Online - full text ed.: (from Institute for Scientific Information).
Indexed: Ergon.Abstr., Focus on: Sports Sci.& Med., IBZ, Ind.Med. (1997-), Ind.Philos., e-psyche.
—BLDSC (5972.910000). **CCC.**
Published by: Human Kinetics Publishers, Inc., PO Box 5076, Champaign, IL 61825-5076. TEL 217-351-5076, 800-747-4457, FAX 217-351-2674, http://www.humankinetics.com. Ed. Mark L Latash. Pub. Rainer Martens. R&P Cheri Banks TEL 217-351-5076 ext 2275. Adv. contact Patty Rodriguiz. page USD 300; trim 9 x 6. Circ: 242.

616.85154 SWE ISSN 0349-7240
MUSIKTERAPI* . Text in Swedish. 1978. q. SEK 200 to membership.
Published by: Svenska Foerbundet foer Musikterapi (SFM), Svenska Foerbundet foe Musikterapi, c/o Anne-Sofie Panlander, Fack 812, Stockholm 10136, Sweden.

615.82 USA
N A R F REHABILITATION REPORT* . Text in English. 1982. s-m. membership. adv. **Document type:** *Newsletter.*
Formerly (until 1992): Medical Rehabilitation Review
Published by: National Association of Rehabilitation Facilities, 206 S 6th St, Springfield, IL 62701-1530. Ed. Mark W Doyon. Circ: 2,000 (controlled).

NATIONAL REHABILITATION CENTER FOR THE DISABLED. RESEARCH BULLETIN. see *HANDICAPPED*

615.82 NLD ISSN 0166-4751
NEDERLANDS TIJDSCHRIFT VOOR ERGOTHERAPIE. Text in Dutch. 1973. 6/yr. NLG 130 (effective 2000). adv. bk.rev. **Document type:** *Journal, Academic/Scholarly.*
Published by: Nederlandse Vereniging voor Ergotherapie, Kaap Hoorndreef 56B, Utrecht 3563 AV, Netherlands. TEL 31-30-262-8356, FAX 31-30-261-5967, nve@ergotheraspie.nl, nve@ergotherapie.nl. Circ: 3,000 (paid).

615.8 NZL ISSN 0303-7193
NEW ZEALAND JOURNAL OF PHYSIOTHERAPY. Text in English. 194?. 3/yr. NZD 50 (effective 2001). adv. bk.rev. abstr, charts, illus, stat. 58 p./no. back issues avail. *Refereed.* **Document type:** *Journal, Academic/Scholarly.*
Indexed: AMED, CINAHL, Ind.N.Z.Per., Inpharma, Pharm.&Out.News, Reac.
—BLDSC (6094.640000).
Published by: New Zealand Society of Physiotherapists (Inc.), PO Box 27386, Wellington, New Zealand. TEL 64-4-8016500, FAX 64-4-48015571. Ed. Sue Lord. Adv. contact Suzanne Tedder. B&W page NZD 450, color page NZD 925; 29.5 x 21. Circ: 1,900 (controlled).

615.8 NGA ISSN 0331-3735
NIGERIA SOCIETY OF PHYSIOTHERAPY. JOURNAL. Abbreviated title: J N S P. Text in English. 1972. s-a. NGN 250, USD 20. adv. *Refereed.* **Document type:** *Academic/Scholarly.* **Description:** Contains articles dealing with the pathology and research aspects of physiotherapy.
Indexed: CINAHL.
Published by: Nigeria Society of Physiotherapy, Department of Physiotherapy, College of Medicine, University of, Idi-Araba, Lagos, Lagos, Nigeria. FAX 234-1-837630, TELEX 0027636 NG. Ed., Adv. contact Dr. Isaac O Owoeye. Circ: 1,000.

615.85154 NOR ISSN 0803-9828
NORDIC JOURNAL OF MUSIC THERAPY/NORDISK TIDSSKRIFT FOR MUSIKKETERAPI. Text in English, Norwegian. 1992. s-a. EUR 9 to individuals; EUR 25 in Europe to individuals; USD 30 elsewhere to individuals; EUR 12 to institutions; EUR 35 in Europe to institutions; USD 40 elsewhere to institutions (effective 1999). adv. abstr. back issues avail. *Refereed.* **Document type:** *Academic/Scholarly.* **Description:** Covers music therapy in the nordic countries. Includes philosophical articles, qualitative and quantitative research articles, a series of classical articles, texts from practice, dialogues, reviews and overviews of the new texts in the field of music therapy.
Indexed: PsycInfo.
Published by: Sogn og Fjordane College, Faculty of Higher Education at Sandane, Sandane 6823, Norway. TEL 47-5786-6800, FAX 47-5786-6801, rune@rolvsjord@sts.hisf.no, http://www.hisf.no/njmt/. Ed. Brynjulf Stige. adv.: page USD 240.

615.8 NOR ISSN 1402-3024
NORDISK FYSIOTERAPI. Text in Norwegian. 1997. q. GBP 20, USD 33 to individuals; GBP 39, USD 65 to institutions (effective 2002). adv. **Document type:** *Academic/Scholarly.*
Indexed: AMED.
Published by: Taylor & Francis AS (Subsidiary of: Taylor & Francis Group), Cort Adelersgt. 17, Solli, PO Box 2562, Oslo 0202, Norway. TEL 47-22-12-98-80, FAX 47-22-12-98-90, journals@tandf.no, http://www.tandf.co.uk.tfas. Ed. Birgitte Bergman. adv.: B&W page NOK 8,500, color page NOK 19,000.

617.06 USA ISSN 0093-7843
HD7256.U6
NORTH DAKOTA STATE PLAN FOR REHABILITATION FACILITIES AND WORKSHOPS; annual modification. Text in English. a. free per issue. stat.
Published by: Division of Vocational Rehabilitation, State Capitol Bldg, Bismarck, ND 58505. TEL 701-224-2907.

OCCUPATIONAL ERGONOMICS. see *OCCUPATIONAL HEALTH AND SAFETY*

OCCUPATIONAL THERAPY INDEX. see *MEDICAL SCIENCES—Abstracting, Bibliographies, Statistics*

615.82 CAN
▼ **OCCUPATIONAL THERAPY NOW.** Text in English. 1999. 6/yr. CND 35 domestic to institutions; CND 50 in United States to institutions; CND 60 elsewhere to institutions (effective 2000). adv. back issues avail. **Document type:** *Academic/Scholarly, Trade.* **Description:** Provides articles on clinical applications of recent research and theory, evidence-based practice, product reviews, socio-cultural, political and economic influences on occupational therapy as well as other information relevant to the profession at large.
Related titles: Online - full text ed.
Published by: Canadian Association of Occupational Therapists, CTTC Ste 3400, 1125 Colonel By drive, Ottawa, ON K1S 5R1, Canada. TEL 613-523-2268, FAX 613-523-2552, lsheehan@caot.ca, http://www.caot.ca. Ed. Mary Clark Green. Adv. contact Lisa Sheehan.

ORTHOPAEDIC PHYSICAL THERAPY CLINICS OF NORTH AMERICA. see *MEDICAL SCIENCES—Orthopedics And Traumatology*

ORTHOPAEDIC PHYSICAL THERAPY PRACTICE. see *MEDICAL SCIENCES—Orthopedics And Traumatology*

615.82 617.087 JPN ISSN 0916-1163
OSAKA SHIRITSU SHINSHIN SHOGAISHA RIHABIRITESHON SENTA KENKYU KIYO/OSAKA MUNICIPAL REHABILITATION CENTER FOR THE DISABLED. RESEARCH REPORTS. Text in Japanese. 1986. a.
Published by: Osaka Shiritsu Shinshin Shogaisha Rehabiriteshon Senta, 2-55 Kire-Nishi 6-chome, Hirano-ku, Osaka-shi 547-0026, Japan.

615.82 CAN
OTNOW; actualites ergotherapiques. Text in English. 1979. bi-m. CND 35 domestic to institutions; USD 50 in United States to institutions; USD 60 elsewhere to institutions (effective 2000). adv. **Document type:** *Magazine.* **Description:** Reports on current professional events, issues, viewpoints and association business.
Formerly: National (Ottawa, 1979) (0820-3008)
Related titles: English ed.: ISSN 1481-5532; French ed.: ISSN 1481-5923.
Published by: Canadian Association of Occupational Therapists, CTTC Ste 3400, 1125 Colonel By drive, Ottawa, ON K1S 5R1, Canada. TEL 613-523-2268, FAX 613-523-2552, http://www.caot.ca. R&P Mary Clark Green. Adv. contact Lisa Sheehan. Circ: 6,500.

615.82 USA ISSN 1065-5077
RM695
P T - MAGAZINE OF PHYSICAL THERAPY. Text in English. 1993. m. USD 60 domestic to non-members; USD 80 foreign to non-members; USD 85 domestic to institutions; USD 110 foreign to institutions (effective 2001). adv. 96 p./no. 3 cols./p. back issues avail.; reprints avail. **Document type:** *Magazine, Trade.* **Description:** Provides legislative, health care, human interest, and association news and serves as a forum for discussion of professional issues, ideas, and innovations in clinical practice.
Related titles: Online - full text ed.: (from ProQuest Information & Learning).
Indexed: AMED, CINAHL, Gen.Sci.Ind. (Jul.1997-).
—BLDSC (6946.563020).
Published by: American Physical Therapy Association, 1111 N Fairfax St, Alexandria, VA 22314-1488. TEL 703-684-2782, FAX 703-706-3169, subscriptions@apta.org, http://www.apta.org. Ed. Donald N Tepper. Pub. Nancy Perkin Beaument. R&P Michelle Tillson TEL 703-706-3197. Adv. contact Julie Hilgenberg TEL 703-706-3197. Circ: 68,000.

615.82 RUS
PALLYATIVNAYA MEDITSINA I REABILITATSIYA. Text in Russian. bi-m. USD 165 in United States.
Indexed: Ref.Zh.
Address: A-ya 137, Moscow 127018, Russian Federation. TEL 7-095-2894348, FAX 7-095-2834348. Ed. G A Novikov. **US dist. addr.:** East View Publications, 3020 Harbor Ln N, Minneapolis, MN 55447. TEL 612-550-0961.

PEDIATRIC PHYSICAL THERAPY. see *MEDICAL SCIENCES—Pediatrics*

615.82 GBR ISSN 1363-8491
CODEN: PEREFP
PEDIATRIC REHABILITATION. Text in English. 1997. q. GBP 71, USD 117 to individuals; GBP 147, USD 242 to institutions (effective 2002). adv. **Document type:** *Academic/Scholarly.* **Description:** Encompasses issues and research involving developmental as well as acquired pediatric disabilities.
Related titles: Online - full text ed.: ISSN 1464-5270 (from CatchWord Ltd., EBSCO Publishing, O C L C Online Computer Library Center, Inc., RoweCom Information Quest, Swets Blackwell).
Indexed: AMED, Ind.Med. (1997-).
—BLDSC (6417.608000), CatchWord, CISTI.
Published by: Taylor & Francis Group, Taylor & Francis Ltd., 11 New Fetter Ln, London EC4P 4EE, United Kingdom. TEL 44-20-7583-9855, FAX 44-20-7842-2298, info@tandf.co.uk, http://www.tandf.co.uk. Eds. David Johnson, Donald Stein, Elise Rivlin. **Subscr. in N. America to:** Taylor & Francis Ltd., 325 Chestnut St, Suite 800, Philadelphia, PA 19016. TEL 800-354-1420, FAX 215-625-8914, info@taylorandfrancis.com, http://www.taylorandfrancis.com/.

615.82 USA
THE PHYSIATRIST. Text in English. 1984. 10/yr. membership. adv. **Document type:** *Newsletter.* **Description:** Covers education, research, practice and legislation issues of interest to residents and practitioners in PM&R.
Published by: American Academy of Physical Medicine and Rehabilitation, 330 N Wabash Ave, Ste 2510, Chicago, IL 60611-3514. TEL 312-464-9700, FAX 312-464-0227, info@aapmr.org, http://www.aapmr.org. Ed. Dr. Claire V Wolfe. R&P John Wilson. Adv. contact Kris Rowland. Circ: 5,700.

PHYSICAL & OCCUPATIONAL THERAPY IN PEDIATRICS; a quarterly journal of developmental therapy. see *MEDICAL SCIENCES—Pediatrics*

615.82 USA ISSN 0888-7357
RD755
PHYSICAL MEDICINE & REHABILITATION; state of the art reviews. Abbreviated title: P M & R. Text in English. 3/yr., latest vol.15, 2001. USD 89 domestic to individuals; USD 99 foreign to individuals; USD 114 domestic to institutions; USD 124 foreign to institutions; USD 39 newsstand/cover domestic; USD 39 newsstand/cover foreign (effective 2001). illus. 200 p./no. 1 cols./p. back issues avail. *Refereed.* **Document type:** *Monographic series, Academic/Scholarly.*
Indexed: AMED, CINAHL.
—BLDSC (6475.635000), CISTI, GNLM, Infotrieve. **CCC.**
Published by: Hanley & Belfus, Inc., 210 S 13th St, Philadelphia, PA 19107. TEL 215-546-7293, FAX 215-790-9330. Circ: 1,000.

615.82 USA ISSN 1047-9651
RM695 CODEN: PMRAFZ
PHYSICAL MEDICINE & REHABILITATION CLINICS OF NORTH AMERICA. Text in English. 1990. q. USD 131 domestic to individuals; USD 158 in Canada to individuals; USD 184 elsewhere to individuals; USD 175 domestic to institutions; USD 225 foreign to institutions; USD 57 per issue (effective 2001). index. back issues avail. **Document type:** *Academic/Scholarly.*
Related titles: Microform ed.: (from PQC).
Indexed: AMED, CINAHL, Excerp.Med. (1995-), Ind.Med. (1990-), Int.Nurs.Ind.
—BLDSC (6475.637000), GNLM, KNAW.
Published by: W.B. Saunders Co. (Subsidiary of: Harcourt Publishers Ltd.), 11830 Westline Industrial Dr, St Louis, MO 63146. TEL 800-325-4177, http://www.wbsaunders.com. Ed. Dr. George H Kraft. **Subscr. to:** Journal Subscription Fulfillment, 6277 Sea Harbor Dr, 4th Fl, Orlando, FL 32887-4800. TEL 800-654-2452, FAX 800-874-6418.

615.8 USA ISSN 0031-9023
RM695 CODEN: PTHEA
PHYSICAL THERAPY. Text in English. 1921. m. USD 70 domestic to individuals; USD 90 foreign to individuals; USD 95 domestic to institutions; USD 120 foreign to institutions (effective 2001). adv. bk.rev. abstr. charts, illus. index. 124 p./no. 3 cols./p. back issues avail.; reprint service avail. from PQC. *Refereed.* **Document type:** *Journal, Academic/Scholarly.* **Description:** Contributes to and documents the evolution and expansion of the scientific and professional body of knowledge in physical therapy.
Former titles (until 1962): Physiotherapy Review; (until 1926): P.T.Review
Related titles: Microform ed.: (from PQC); Online - full text ed.: (from Central Institute for Scientific & Technical Information, Northern Light Technology, Inc., EBSCO Publishing, ProQuest Information & Learning, Gale Group, Factiva, Institute for Scientific Information).
Indexed: AIM, AMED, ASCA, Abstr.Health Care Manage.Stud., AgeLine, Bibl.Dev.Med.& Child Neur., CINAHL, Curr.Cont., Except.Child Educ.Abstr., Excerp.Med., Focus on: Sports Sci.& Med., Hlth.Ind., Hosp.Lit.Ind., INIS Atomind., Ind.Med. (1964-), Ind.Sci.Rev., Inpharma, Int.Nurs.Ind., Med.& Surg.Dermat., Neurosci.Cit.Ind., Pharm.&Out.News, Phys.Ed.Ind., Reac., SSCI (coverage dropped), Sci.Cit.Ind., Sportsearch (1980-).
—BLDSC (6476.350000), CISTI, GNLM, IDS, ingenta, KNAW.
Published by: American Physical Therapy Association, 1111 N Fairfax St, Alexandria, VA 22314-1488. TEL 703-706-3124, 800-999-2782, FAX 703-684-7343, ptunderscorejournal@apta.org, http://www.ptjournal.org, http://www.apta.org. Ed. Dr. Jules Rothstein. R&P Michelle Tillson TEL 703-706-3197. Adv. contact Julie Hilgenberg TEL 703-706-3197. Circ: 77,000 (controlled).

615.82 USA ISSN 1094-0367
PHYSICAL THERAPY CASE REPORTS. Text in English. 1998. bi-m., latest vol.4. USD 57 domestic to individuals; USD 77 foreign to individuals; USD 113 domestic to institutions; USD 136 foreign to institutions; USD 24 newsstand/cover (effective 2001). adv. illus. index. *Refereed.*
Indexed: CINAHL.
—BLDSC (6476.350100).
Published by: Lippincott Williams & Wilkins (Philadelphia) (Subsidiary of: Wolters Kluwer N.V.), 530 Walnut St, Philadelphia, PA 19106-3621. TEL 301-223-2300, 800-638-3030, FAX 301-223-2400, http://www.lww.com. Ed. Darlene K Sekerak.

615.82 USA ISSN 1086-7643
PHYSICAL THERAPY IN PERSPECTIVE. Text in English. 1996. bi-m. USD 46 domestic to individuals; USD 65 foreign to individuals; USD 75 domestic to institutions; USD 93 foreign to institutions; USD 27 domestic to students; USD 43 foreign to students; USD 16 newsstand/cover (effective 2000). illus. **Description:** Topics include rehabilitation, neurologic physical therapy, orthopedics, sports medicine, pediatrics, geriatrics, pain management, biomechanics, practice issues, and more.
Published by: Mosby, Inc. (Subsidiary of: Elsevier Science), 11830 Westline Industrial Dr, St Louis, MO 63146-3318. TEL 314-872-8370, 800-453-4351, FAX 314-432-1380, http://www.mosby.com/periodicals. Ed. Carole Bernstein Lewis.

M

615.8 USA ISSN 1059-096X
PHYSICAL THERAPY PRODUCTS*. Text in English. 7/yr. USD 21 (effective 2000). adv. **Document type:** *Magazine, Trade.* **Description:** Covers the introductions of new physical therapy products, with advisory columns discussing new procedures, and other topics of interest to professionals.
Published by: Novicom, Inc. (Subsidiary of: Medical World Communications), 6701 Center Dr West, Ste 450, Los Angeles, CA 90045-1556. TEL 310-642-4400, FAX 310-641-1511, http://www.novicom.com. Ed. Greg Thompson. Adv. contacts Lisa Chose, Sharon Marsee. B&W page USD 2,338, color page USD 3,038; trim 8.125 x 10.825. Circ: 40,000.

PHYSICAL THERAPY REIMBURSEMENT NEWS. see *INSURANCE*

615.82 DEU
PHYSIKALISCHE THERAPIE HEUTE. Text in German. m. DEM 115 (effective 1996). **Document type:** *Bulletin.*
Published by: Ebert Verlag GmbH, Blankenseer Str 6-8, Luebeck 23562, Germany. TEL 49-451-501011, FAX 49-4509-2241.

615.8 ZAF
PHYSIOFORUM. Text in English. 8/yr. ZAR 120; ZAR 290 foreign (effective 1999). **Document type:** *Academic/Scholarly, Trade.*
Published by: (South African Society of Physiotherapy/Suid-Afrikaanse Fisiotherapie Vereiniging), Physiotherapy Publications, PO Box 92125, Norwood, Johannesburg 2117, South Africa. TEL 27-11-4851467, FAX 27-11-4851613.

615.8 CHE ISSN 1423-4092
PHYSIOTHERAPIE/FISIOTERAPIA. Text in French, German, Italian. 1933. m. CHF 87; CHF 111 foreign (effective 1999). adv. bk.rev. charts, illus, stat. **Document type:** *Trade.*
Formerly: Physiotherapeut (0257-7690)
Published by: Schweizerischer Physiotherapeuten-Verband, Oberstadt 8, Sempach Stadt 6204, Switzerland. TEL 41-41-4627070, FAX 41-41-4627061, info@physioswiss.ch, http://www.physioswiss.ch. Ed. Rene Huber. Pub. Hans Walker. Adv. contact Henri Haeckel. B&W page CHF 1,359, color page CHF 2,379; trim 270 x 186. Circ: 7,700.

615.8 362.41 GBR ISSN 0048-4083
PHYSIOTHERAPISTS' QUARTERLY. Text in English. 1950. q. free per issue to members. **Document type:** *Trade.* **Description:** Contains professional information for physiotherapists who are blind or visually impaired.
Media: Braille.
Published by: Royal National Institute for the Blind, PO Box 173, Peterborough, Cambs PE2 6WX, United Kingdom. TEL 44-1733-370-777, FAX 44-1733-371555, webmaster @rnib.org.uk, http://www.rnig.org.uk, http://www.rnib.org. Circ: 100. **Subscr. to:** Sarah Wynn, University of East Anglia, Maryland House, Manbey Park Rd, London E15 1EU, United Kingdom. TEL 44-181-849-3479.

615.8 GBR ISSN 0031-9406
PHYSIOTHERAPY. Text in English. 1915. m. GBP 120 in United Kingdom; GBP 175 rest of world (effective 2000). adv. bk.rev., video rev. abstr, illus. index. back issues avail. *Refereed.* **Document type:** *Academic/Scholarly.* **Description:** Contains peer-reviewed articles by national and international experts in their fields- physiotherapists, doctors, educationalists and other professionals.
Related titles: Audio cassette/tape ed.; Braille ed.
Indexed: AMED, ASSIA, Bibl.Dev.Med.& Child Neur., Brit.Nur.Ind., CINAHL, Dok.Arbeitsmed., Excerp.Med., Ind.Med. (coverage dropped).
—BLDSC (6489.000000), CISTI, GNLM, ingenta, KNAW.
Published by: Chartered Society of Physiotherapy, 14 Bedford Row, London WC1R 4ED, United Kingdom. TEL 44-207-306-6662, FAX 44-207-306-6667, membership@csphysio.org.uk, http://www.csp.org.uk. Ed., R&P Jill Whitehouse TEL 44-171-306-6660. Adv. contact Jill Fischer. B&W page GBP 1,540, color page GBP 1,840; trim 300 x 210. Circ: 34,000; 3,000 (paid); 31,000 (controlled). **Subscr. on audiocassette to:** Sarah Wynn, University of East London Maryland House, Manbey Park Rd, London E15 1EY, United Kingdom. TEL 44-181-849-3479.

615.8 GBR ISSN 1356-9791
PHYSIOTHERAPY FRONTLINE. Text in English. 1995. m. free to members. adv. **Document type:** *Trade.* **Description:** Features news, reports, course information, and employment opportunities of interest to physiotherapists.
Related titles: Audio cassette/tape ed.
Indexed: AMED, CINAHL.
—KNAW.
Published by: Chartered Society of Physiotherapy, 14 Bedford Row, London WC1R 4ED, United Kingdom. TEL 44-207-306-6662, FAX 44-207-306-6667, membership@csphysio.org.uk, http://www.csp.org.uk.

PHYSIOTHERAPY INDEX. see *MEDICAL SCIENCES—Abstracting, Bibliographies, Statistics*

615.82 AUS ISSN 1327-9599
PHYSIOTHERAPY MOVES. Text in English. 1997. q. AUD 48.30 domestic; USD 65 foreign (effective 2000). adv. **Document type:** *Newsletter.* **Description:** Aims to keep APA members, as well as politicians, health fund managers, allied health professionals, the media and general public up-to-date on current issues affecting the profession. Includes policy issues, continuing education, human interest stories etc.
Indexed: CINAHL.
Published by: Australian Physiotherapy Association, PO Box 6465, St Kilda Rd Central, VIC 8008, Australia. TEL 61-3-9534-9400, FAX 61-3-9534-9199. Ed. Wendy Cross. Adv. contact Elise Olney. Circ: 10,000.

615.8 GBR ISSN 1358-2267
PHYSIOTHERAPY RESEARCH INTERNATIONAL. Text in English. 1996. q. USD 110 in North America to individuals; GBP 60 rest of world to individuals; USD 230 in North America to institutions; GBP 125 rest of world to institutions (effective 2001). adv. back issues avail. *Refereed.* **Document type:** *Academic/Scholarly.* **Description:** Publishes original research papers on a wide range of topics in physiotherapy and other related material.
Related titles: Online - full text ed.: free (from Northern Light Technology, Inc., ProQuest Information & Learning).
Indexed: AMED, CINAHL, Ind.Med. (1996-).
—BLDSC (6489.119000).
Published by: Whurr Publishers Ltd., 19b Compton Terr, London N1 2UN, United Kingdom. TEL 44-20-7359-5979, FAX 44-20-7226-5290, info@whurr.co.uk, http://www.whurr.co.uk, http://www.whurrjournals.co.uk/. Ed. Cecily Partridge. adv.: page GBP 350. **Subscr. in N. America to:** Whurr Publishers Ltd., PO Box 1897, Lawrence, KS 66044-8897. TEL 913-843-1221, FAX 913-843-1274, am&m@allenpress.com. **Subscr. to:** Turpin Distribution Services Ltd., Blackhorse Rd, Letchworth, Herts SG6 1HN, United Kingdom. TEL 44-1462-488900, FAX 44-1462-483011, custservturpin@turpinltd.com.

615.8 USA ISSN 0959-3985
RM695 CODEN: PTHPEA
PHYSIOTHERAPY THEORY AND PRACTICE; an international journal of physical therapy. Text in English. 1985. q. GBP 90, USD 148 to individuals; GBP 199, USD 329 to institutions (effective 2002). adv. bk.rev. *Refereed.* **Document type:** *Academic/Scholarly.* **Description:** Provides a forum for recent developments and current research in physiotherapy.
Related titles: Online - full text ed.: ISSN 1532-5040 (from CatchWord Ltd., EBSCO Publishing, O C L C Online Computer Library Center, Inc., RoweCom Information Quest, Swets Blackwell).
Indexed: AMED, CINAHL.
—BLDSC (6489.140000), CatchWord, EMDOCS, GNLM, KNAW. **CCC.**
Published by: Taylor & Francis Ltd. (Subsidiary of: Taylor & Francis Group), 325 Chestnut St, Suite 800, Philadelphia, PA 19016. TEL 215-625-8900, FAX 215-625-2940, info@taylorandfrancis.com, http://www.taylorandfrancis.com/. Eds. Maureen Simmonds, Scott Hasson. **Subscr. in Europe to:** Taylor & Francis Group, Journals Customer Service, Rankine Rd, Basingstoke, Hants RG24 8PR, United Kingdom. TEL 44-1256-813000, FAX 44-1256-479438, enquiry@tanf.co.uk, http://www.tandf.co.uk/journals.

615.82 USA
PLENUM SERIES IN REHABILITATION AND HEALTH. Text in English. 1996. irreg., latest 1999. price varies. **Document type:** *Monographic series.* **Description:** Focuses on vital research issues in the field of rehabilitation, including rehabilitation and psychology, physical therapy, biofeedback, ergonomics, vocational and psychiatric rehabilitation, occupational health and therapy.
Indexed: e-psyche.
Published by: Kluwer Academic - Plenum Publishers (Subsidiary of: Wolters Kluwer N.V.), 233 Spring St, New York, NY 10013-1578. TEL 212-620-8000, 800-221-9369, FAX 212-463-0742, info@plenum.com, http://www.plenum.com. Eds. Anthony J Goreczny, Michael Feuerstein.

POST ACUTE CARE STRATEGY REPORT; the newsletter for integrating post acute services. see *MEDICAL SCIENCES—Nurses And Nursing*

615.82 POL ISSN 0860-6161
POSTEPY REHABILITACJI/ADVANCES IN REHABILITATION. Text in Polish; Summaries in English. 1987. q. USD 50 foreign (effective 2000). **Description:** Publishes papers in therapeutic rehabilitation and related disciplines, information on advances in rehabilitation of various diseases and on new rehabilitation equipment.
—GNLM.
Published by: (Akademia Wychowania Fizycznego w Warszawie), Wydawnictwo Naukowe P W Nowe, Ul Miodowa 10, Warsaw 00251, Poland. TEL 48-22-6954321, FAX 48-22-6954288. Ed. Aleksander Ronikier. **Dist. by:** Ars Polona, Krakowskie Przedmiescie 7, Warsaw, Poland.

PRAEVENTION UND REHABILITATION. see *MEDICAL SCIENCES*

615.82 DEU ISSN 0933-842X
PRAXIS DER KLINISCHEN VERHALTENSMEDIZIN UND REHABILITATION. Text in German. 1988. q. EUR 50 (effective 2001). adv. bk.rev. **Document type:** *Journal, Academic/Scholarly.*
—GNLM.
Published by: Pabst Science Publishers, Am Eichengrund 28, Lengerich 49525, Germany. TEL 35-5484-308, FAX 35-5484-550, http://www.pabst-publishers.de. Ed. Manfred Zielke. adv.: B&W page DEM 1,000; trim 242 x 175. Circ: 1,000.

615.82 DEU ISSN 0932-9692
PRAXIS ERGOTHERAPIE; Fachzeitschrift fuer Beschaeftigungs- und Arbeitstherapie. Text in German. 6/yr. DEM 59 (effective 1999). **Document type:** *Academic/Scholarly.* **Description:** Covers all subjects to occupational therapy professionals.
Indexed: IBZ.
—GNLM.
Published by: Verlag Modernes Lernen - Dortmund, Hohe Str 39, Dortmund 44139, Germany. TEL 49-231-128048, FAX 49-2311-128009. Circ: 6,600.

616.822 FRA ISSN 1258-5564
PROFESSION KINE PLUS. Text in French. 1990. q. FRF 310 domestic to individuals; FRF 440, EUR 67.08 foreign to individuals; FRF 245 to students (effective 2000).
Published by: Meditions Carline, 1 et 3 rue du Depart, Paris 75014, France. TEL 33-1-40640075, FAX 33-1-43222699, groupemeditions@wanadoo.fr.

PSYCSCAN: LEARNING DISORDERS AND MENTAL RETARDATION. see *MEDICAL SCIENCES—Abstracting, Bibliographies, Statistics*

R A D A R BULLETIN. see *HANDICAPPED*

615.85153 AUS
R D A NEWS. Text in English. 1991. s-a. AUD 20. adv. back issues avail. **Document type:** *Newsletter.* **Description:** Promotes equestrian activities for people with disability.
Published by: Riding for the Disabled Association of Australia, PO Box 424, Ascot Vale, VIC 3032, Australia. TEL 61-3-93722126, FAX 61-3-3766698. Ed., Pub., R&P, Adv. contact Susan Cusack.

615.82 ZAF
RECOMMENDED SCALES OF BENEFITS. PHYSIOTHERAPISTS. Text in English. 1994. a.
Published by: Representative Association of Medical Schemes, PO Box 2324, Parklands, Johannesburg 2121, South Africa.

615.82 362.15 CAN ISSN 1192-2508
REHAB & COMMUNITY CARE MANAGEMENT. Text in English. 1992. q. CND 25.58; USD 49.50 foreign. adv. bk.rev. *Refereed.* **Document type:** *Trade.* **Description:** Covers technological advances, therapeutic trends, management issues and government legislative changes for those dedicated to improving the quality of daily life for Canadians challenged by injury, illness or aging.
Published by: B C S Communications Ltd., 101 Thorncliffe Park Dr, Toronto, ON M4H 1M2, Canada. TEL 416-421-7944, 800-798-6282, FAX 416-421-0966. Ed. H Dostal. Pub., R&P Caroline Tapp McDougall. Adv. contact Anita Boyle Evans. B&W page CND 2,345, color page CND 3,545; trim 10.88 x 8.13. Circ: 20,000 (controlled).

REHAB REPORT. see *HANDICAPPED*

617.03 616.977 SVK ISSN 0375-0922
REHABILITACIA/REHABILITATION. Text in Slovak, Czech; Summaries in English, German, Slovak. 1967. 4/yr. USD 40 (effective 2000 - 2001). bk.rev., film rev. bibl, charts, illus. index. back issues avail. *Refereed.* **Document type:** *Bulletin.*
Indexed: Biol.Abstr., Excerp.Med.
—GNLM.
Published by: (Slovenske Postgradualna Akademie Mediciny/Academy of Further Education of Physicians and Pharmaceutists), Vydavatelsvo Liecreh Guth, Cervenova 34, Bratislava 81103, Slovakia. TEL 421-7-59545243, FAX 421-7-54414700, guth@napri.sk, http://www.rehabilitacia.sk, http://www.rehabilit@cla.sk. Ed. Anton Guth. Circ: 2,800 (paid).

615.82 ESP ISSN 0048-7120
REHABILITACION. Text in Spanish; Summaries in English, Spanish. 1967. bi-m. ESP 13,000 to individuals; ESP 18,000 to institutions; ESP 10,600 to students (effective 2001). bk.rev. abstr, bibl, illus, stat. index. back issues avail.; reprints avail. *Refereed.* **Document type:** *Journal, Monographic series, Academic/Scholarly.*
Related titles: Online - full text ed.: 1996.
Indexed: AMED, CINAHL, Excerp.Med., Ind.Med.Esp.
—BLDSC (7350.070000), CINDOC, GNLM.
Published by: (Sociedad Espanola de Rehabilitacion y Medicina Fisica), Ediciones Doyma S.A., Traversa de Gracia, 17-21, Barcelona 08021, Spain. TEL 34-93-200-0711, rh@doyma.es, doyma@doyma.es, http://www.doyma.es/rh. Eds. A Pena Arrebola, J I Ibarra Luzar. R&P Monica Barnes. Adv. contact Jose Antonio Hernandez. Circ: 2,000.

615.82 362.4 USA
REHABILITACION: PREVENCION Y INTEGRACION. Text in Spanish. 1982. s-a. bk.rev. **Description:** Covers disability and rehabilitation in Latin America, Spain and Portugal.
Published by: Rehabilitation International, 25 E 21st St, New York, NY 10010. TEL 212-420-1500, FAX 212-505-0871, TELEX 446412. Eds. Barbara Duncan, Luis Reguera. Circ: 6,000. **Co-sponsor:** I N S E R S O.

REHABILITATION INDEX. see *MEDICAL SCIENCES—Abstracting, Bibliographies, Statistics*

616.07 IND ISSN 0080-0724
REHABILITATION INDUSTRIES CORPORATION. ANNUAL REPORT*. (Report year ends Mar. 31) Text in English. 1959. a.
Published by: Rehabilitation Industries Corporation Ltd., 25 Free School St., Kolkata, West Bengal 700 016, India.

617.06 USA
REHABILITATION INTERNATIONAL. WORLD CONGRESS. PROCEEDINGS. Text in English. 1921. quadrennial, latest 1992, 17th, Nairobi. **Document type:** *Proceedings.* **Description:** Contains compendia of main papers presented at the world congress.
Published by: Rehabilitation International, 25 E 21st St, 4th Fl, New York, NY 10010. TEL 212-420-1500, FAX 212-505-0871. Circ: 3,000. **Orders to:** Association for the Physically Disabled of Kenya, APDK House, PO Box 56643, Nairobi, Kenya. TEL 254-2-332227, 254-2-219541.

REHABILITATION NURSING. see *MEDICAL SCIENCES—Nurses And Nursing*

615.82 USA
▼ **REHABILITATION SOURCEBOOK.** Text in English. 1999. irreg., latest 1999, First Edition. USD 78 per issue (effective 2001). charts. Index. **Document type:** *Consumer.* **Description:** Basic consumer health information for people recovering from heart surgery, spinal cord injury, stroke, orthopedic impairments, amputation, pulmonary impairments, traumatic injury, and more. Includes facts about physical therapy, occupational therapy, physiotherapy, speech/language therapy, massage therapy, dance therapy, art therapy, and recreational therapy; along with information on assistive and adaptive devices, a glossary, and resources for additional help and information.
Published by: Omnigraphics, Inc., 615 Griswold St, Detroit, MI 48226. TEL 313-961-1340, 800-234-1340, FAX 313-961-1383, 800-875-1340, info@omnigraphics.com, jjts@sprynet.com, http://www.omnigraphics.com. Ed. Dawn Dawn D Matthews.

615.82 BRA
REVISTA DE FISIOTERAPIA. Text in Portuguese; Abstracts in English, Portuguese. 1994. s-a. **Document type:** *Academic/Scholarly.*
Published by: Universidade de Sao Paulo, Faculdade de Medicina, Rua Cipotanea, 51, Cidade Univ. A. Salles de Oliveira, Sao Paulo, SP 05360-000, Brazil.

615.82 ESP
REVISTA DE TERAPIA OCUPACIONAL. Text in Spanish. 3/yr. ESP 5,000, USD 51 (effective 1996).
Published by: Grupo Masson, Rda General Mitre, 149, Barcelona 08022, Spain. TEL 34-93-2530200, FAX 34-93-2530515, masson@masson.es, http://www.masson.es, http://masson.es.

615.8 PRT
REVISTA FISIOTERAPIA. Text in Portuguese. 4/yr.
Address: Rua das Portas de Santo Antao, 81-1o, Lisbon 1100, Portugal. TEL 3475902, FAX 3424304, TELEX 13441 ACL. Ed. Fernando Pedro de Carvalho.

615.82 ESP ISSN 1138-6045
REVISTA IBEROAMERICANA DE FISIOTERAPIA Y KINESIOLOGIA. Text in Spanish. 1998. q. ESP 6,900, USD 75 to individuals; USD 8,200 to institutions. adv. back issues avail.; reprints avail. *Refereed.* **Document type:** *Academic/Scholarly.*
Related titles: Online - full text ed.
Published by: (Asociacion Espanola de Fisioterapeutas), Editorial Garsi S.A. (Subsidiary of: Grupo Masson), Juan Bravo, 49, Madrid 28006, Spain. TEL 34-91-402-1212, FAX 34-91-402-0954, garsi@mad.servicom.ex, http://www.masson.es. Pub. Dr. R Fernandez Cervantes. Circ: 4,000 (paid).

615.82 ITA ISSN 0557-9430
RIABILITAZIONE; rivista di medicina fisica e riabilitazione. Text in Italian. 1968. 4/yr. ITL 91,500 (effective 1999). **Document type:** *Academic/Scholarly.*
Indexed: Biol.Abstr., Excerp.Med.
—BLDSC (7963.560000), EMDOCS, GNLM, KNAW.
Published by: (Istituto di Terapia Fisica e Riabilitazione dell'Ospedale Niguarda - Ca Granda), Masson S.p.A., Divisione Periodici, Via F.lli Bressan 2, Milan, MI 20126, Italy. TEL 39-2-270741, FAX 39-2-27074210. Ed. Ivano Colombo. adv.: B&W page ITL 2,000,000, color page ITL 2,900,000; trim 240 x 170. Circ: 1,500.

615.82 ITA ISSN 0393-7518
RIABILITAZIONE E APPRENDIMENTO. Text in Italian; Summaries in English. 1980. q. ITL 90,000, USD 150 (effective 1999). **Description:** Provides a foundation for the science of rehabilitation as a growing discipline in medicine.
—BLDSC (7963.560500).
Published by: Guido Gnocchi Editore, Via Annibale De Gasperis, 55, Naples, NA 80137, Italy. TEL 39-81-5524733, FAX 39-81-5518295, idelgno@tin.it, http://www.idelson-gnocchi.com. Ed. Carlo Perfetti. Circ: 5,000.

615.82 ITA
RIABILITAZIONE OGGI. Text in Italian. 10/yr.
Published by: Editrice Spec. Riabilitazione, Via Perugino, 26, Milan, MI 20135, Italy. TEL 2-550-125-35. Ed. Dr. Romualdo Carini. Circ: 45,000.

615 ITA ISSN 1120-379X
RICERCA & PRATICA. Text in Italian. 1985. bi-m., latest vol.99, 2001. USD 117 (effective 2000). bibl. index. 48 p./no. back issues avail. **Document type:** *Academic/Scholarly.*
Related titles: Online - full text ed.
—BLDSC (7963.915000), EMDOCS, GNLM, KNAW.
Published by: (Istituto di Ricerche Farmacologiche Mario Negri), Il Pensiero Scientifico Editore s.r.l., Via Bradano, 3-C, Rome, RM 00199, Italy. TEL 39-06-862821, FAX 39-06-86282250, pensiero@pensiero.it, http://www.pensiero.it. Ed. Daniele Coen. Pub. Luca De Fiore. Adv. contact Arabella Festa. Circ: 2,000.

615.8 JPN ISSN 0915-0552
RIGAKU RYOHO JANARU/JAPANESE JOURNAL OF PHYSICAL THERAPY. Text in Japanese; Summaries in English. 1967. m. JPY 19,200, USD 123. **Document type:** *Academic/Scholarly.*
Formerly (until 1989): Rigaku Ryoho to Sagyo Ryoho - Japanese Journal of Physical Therapy and Occupational Therapy (0386-9849)
Related titles: Online - full text ed.: (from JICST).
Published by: Igaku-Shoin Ltd., 5-24-3 Hongo, Bunkyo-ku, Tokyo 113-0033, Japan. TEL 81-3-3817-5703. Circ: 7,500.

615.82 JPN ISSN 0034-351X
RIHABIRITESHON IGAKU/JAPANESE JOURNAL OF REHABILITATION MEDICINE. Text in Japanese. 1964. m. JPY 22,000, USD 66.90 (effective 2001). adv. index. 90 p./no. back issues avail. *Refereed.* **Document type:** *Academic/Scholarly.*
Related titles: Online - full text ed.: (from JICST).
—CISTI.
Published by: Japanese Association of Rehabilitation Medicine/Nippon Rihabiriteshon Igakkai, 1-1-17 Komone, Itabashi-ku, Tokyo 173-0037, Japan. TEL 81-3-5966-2031, FAX 81-3-5966-2033, http://wwwsoc.nii.ac.jp/jarm/. Ed. Hironobu Sashika. Circ: 9,700 (paid).

ROMATOLOJI VE TIBBI REHABILITASYON DERGISI/JOURNAL OF RHEUMATOLOGY AND MEDICAL REHABILITATION. see *MEDICAL SCIENCES—Rheumatology*

615.8515 USA
SENSORY INTEGRATION SPECIAL INTEREST SECTION QUARTERLY. Text in English. 1989. q. USD 20 (effective 1999). **Document type:** *Newsletter.*
Former titles (until 199?): Sensory Integration Special Interest Section Newsletter (0279-4128); American Occupational Therapy Association. Sensory Integration Specialty Section. Newsletter (0194-6358)
Published by: American Occupational Therapy Association, Inc., 4720 Montgomery Lane, Bethesda, MD 20814-3425. TEL 301-652-2682, FAX 301-652-7711.

615.82 JPN ISSN 0386-9822
SOGO REHABILITATION. Text in Japanese. 1973. m. JPY 26,800. **Description:** Studies rehabilitation medicine and related medical fields.
Published by: Igaku-Shoin Ltd., 5-24-3 Hongo, Bunkyo-ku, Tokyo 113-0033, Japan. TEL 81-3-3817-5704. Circ: 6,000.

615.8 ZAF ISSN 0379-6175
SOUTH AFRICAN JOURNAL OF PHYSIOTHERAPY. Text in English. 1925. q. ZAR 120 to non-members; ZAR 290 foreign to non-members (effective 1999). adv. bk.rev. back issues avail.
Indexed: AMED, CINAHL, Ind.S.A.Per.
—BLDSC (8339.700000), EMDOCS, GNLM, KNAW.
Published by: (South African Society of Physiotherapy/Suid-Afrikaanse Fisiotherapie Vereiniging), Physiotherapy Publications, PO Box 92125, Norwood, Johannesburg 2117, South Africa. TEL 27-11-4851467, FAX 27-11-4851613. Ed. J Beenhakker. Circ: 2,700.

▼ **THE SPINE JOURNAL.** see *MEDICAL SCIENCES—Orthopedics And Traumatology*

615.82 362.4 USA ISSN 0734-6522
SPRINGER SERIES ON REHABILITATION. Text in English. 1981. irreg., latest vol.11, 1997. price varies. **Document type:** *Monographic series.* **Description:** Covers issues in physical rehabilitation.
Published by: Springer Publishing Company, 536 Broadway, New York, NY 10012. TEL 212-431-4370, FAX 212-941-7842, springer@springerpub.com, http://www.springerpub.com. Ed. Thomas E Becker. R&P Dorothy Kouwenberg.

615.82 GBR
STROKE NEWS. Text in English. 1984. q. free per issue. adv. bk.rev. back issues avail. **Document type:** *Bulletin.*
Published by: Stroke Association, CHSA House, Whitecross St, London EC1Y 8JJ, United Kingdom. TEL 44-171-490-7999, FAX 44-171-490-2686. Ed., R&P Jo Haynes. Adv. contact Linda Aloysius. Circ: 29,000 (controlled).

TECHNOLOGY AND DISABILITY. see *HANDICAPPED*

615.82 JPN ISSN 0388-0168
TOKYO METROPOLITAN REHABILITATION CENTER FOR THE PHYSICALLY AND MENTALLY HANDICAPPED. BULLETIN. Text in English. 1987. bi-m.
Indexed: Except.Child Educ.Abstr.
Published by: Tokyo Metropolitan Rehabilitation Center for the Physically and Mentally Handicapped/Tokyoto Shinshin Shogaisha Fukushi Senta, 17-2, Toyamacho 3-chome, Shinjuku-ku, Tokyo 162, Japan.

TOPICS IN GERIATRIC REHABILITATION. see *GERONTOLOGY AND GERIATRICS*

TOPICS IN STROKE REHABILITATION. see *MEDICAL SCIENCES—Cardiovascular Diseases*

615.89 USA
TRAGER NEWSLETTER. Text in English. 1979. 3/yr. USD 45 to members (effective 1999). **Document type:** *Newsletter.* **Description:** Covers various techniques of somatics, a form of pressure therapy.
Formerly: Trager Institute Newsletter
Published by: Trager Institute, 21 Locust Ave, Mill Valley, CA 94941-2805. TEL 415-388-2688, FAX 415-388-2710, admin@trager.com, htt://www.trager.com. Ed. Don Schwartz. Circ: 2,000 (controlled).

VOCATIONAL REHABILITATION REVIEW. see *EDUCATION—Special Education And Rehabilitation*

615.82 USA ISSN 1046-5642
VOICE (FT. LAUDERDALE). Text in English. 1987. m. USD 25 (effective 2000). adv. **Document type:** *Newspaper.* **Description:** Contains rehabilitation information for case managers, managed care workers, nurses, physicians, adjusters, consumers with disabilities and caregivers.
Published by: Cary - Joy Communications, 1405 S.E. First St., Ft. Lauderdale, FL 33301. TEL 954-463-5556, FAX 954-463-2674, http://www.voicepaper.com. Ed., Pub. Ray Brasted. Adv. contact Melanie Kornblatt. page USD 1,195. Circ: 70,000 (controlled).

615.8 RUS ISSN 0042-8787
CODEN: VKFLAL
VOPROSY KURORTOLOGII, FIZIOTERAPII I LECHEBNOI FIZICHESKOI KUL'TURY/PROBLEMS OF HEALTH RESORTS, PHYSIOTHERAPY AND EXERCISE THERAPY. Text in Russian. 1923. bi-m. USD 134 foreign (effective 2000). adv. bk.rev., Website rev. illus. index. **Document type:** *Journal, Academic/Scholarly.* **Description:** Examines the mechanisms of physiological and therapeutic effects of physical and health resort factors, methods and results of their employment; also covers theoretical and practical problems involved in the use of exercise therapy in the complex treatment of different diseases.
Indexed: Biol.Abstr., Chem.Abstr., Dent.Ind., INIS Atomind., Ind.Med. (1955-), Int.Aerosp.Abstr., Int.Nurs.Ind., Ref.Zh.
—BLDSC (0043.000000), CASDDS, CISTI, East View, GNLM.
Published by: Izdatel'stvo Meditsina, Petroverigskii per 6-8, Moscow 101000, Russian Federation. TEL 7-095-9248785, 7-095-928-86-48, FAX 7-095-9211355, 7-095-9286003, meditsina@iname.cpm, http://www.medit.ru. Ed. A N Razumov. Pub. A M Stochik. R&P O Rozhenetskaya. Adv. contact S A Bugaev. Circ: 3,300. **Dist. by:** Mezhdunarodnaya Kniga, B Yakimanka 39, Moscow 117049, Russian Federation. TEL 7-095-2384967, FAX 7-095-2384634.

615.82 DEU ISSN 0939-3889
CODEN: ZMPHEJ
ZEITSCHRIFT FUER MEDIZINISCHE PHYSIK. Text in German, English, French. 1990. q. EUR 62; EUR 24 to students (effective 2002). **Document type:** *Journal, Trade, Academic/Scholarly.*
Indexed: INIS Atomind., INSPEC (1998-).
—BLDSC (9469.890000), CASDDS, GNLM.
Published by: Urban & Fischer Verlag, Loebdergraben 14a, Jena 07743, Germany. TEL 49-3641-626430, FAX 49-3641-626421, info@urbanfischer.de, http://www.urbanfischer.de/journals. Ed. K Wolschendorf. Adv. contact Sabine Schroeter.

615.82 CHN ISSN 1006-9771
ZHONGGUO KANGFU LILUN YU SHIJIAN/CHINESE JOURNAL OF REHABILITATION THEORY & PRACTICE. Text in Chinese. 1995. q. USD 8.80; CNY 4, USD 2.20 newsstand/cover (effective 2001). **Document type:** *Academic/Scholarly.*
Related titles: Online - full content ed.: (from WanFang Data Corp.).
Published by: Zhongguo Kangfu Yanjiu Zhongxin, Fengtai Qu, 10, Jiaomen Bei Lu, Beijing 100077, China. TEL 86-10-67213322 ext 6310, crrc@public.bta.net.cn, http://www.crrc.com.cn. Ed. Hong Shi Mou. **Dist. by:** China International Book Trading Corp, 35, Chegongzhuang Xilu, Haidian District, Beijing 100044, China. TEL 86-1-68413849, FAX 86-1-68412048, cibtc@mail.cibtc.com.cn, http://www.cibtc.com.cn.

615.8 CHN ISSN 0254-1408
RM695
ZHONGHUA LILIAO ZAZHI/CHINESE JOURNAL OF PHYSICAL THERAPY. Text in Chinese. 1978. q. CNY 48 domestic; USD 25.20 foreign; CNY 8 newsstand/cover domestic; USD 4.20 newsstand/cover foreign (effective 2001). **Document type:** *Academic/Scholarly.*
Related titles: CD-ROM ed.; Online - full content ed.: (from WanFang Data Corp.).
Indexed: ExtraMED.
Address: Tang Gang zi, Anshan 114048, China. TEL 86-412-2410287. Ed. Deng-Kun Nan. **Dist. by:** China International Book Trading Corp, 35, Chegongzhuang Xilu, Haidian District, Beijing 100044, China. TEL 86-1-68413849, FAX 86-1-68412048, cibtc@mail.cibtc.com.cn, http://www.cibtc.com.cn. **Co-sponsor:** Zhonghua Yixuehui/Chinese Medical Association.

610 530 CHN
ZHONGHUA WULI YU KANGFU ZAZHI/CHINESE JOURNAL OF PHYSICAL MEDICINE AND REHABILITATION. Text in Chinese. 1979. q. USD 27 foreign; CNY 8.50 newsstand/cover domestic; USD 4.50 newsstand/cover foreign (effective 2001). adv. *Refereed.* **Document type:** *Academic/Scholarly.* **Description:** Covers the latest development in physical medicine and rehabilitation.
Formerly: Zhonghua Wuli Yixue Zazhi / Chinese Journal of Physical Medicine (0254-1424)
Related titles: CD-ROM ed.
Indexed: ExtraMED.
—CISTI.
Published by: (Zhonghua Yixuehui/Chinese Medical Association), Hebei Yike Daxue/Hebei Medical University, 361 Zhongshan Donglu, Shijiazhuang, Hebei 050017, China. TEL 86-311-6044121, FAX 86-311-6059153, WL@hebmu.edu.cn. Ed. Nan Dengkun. adv.: B&W page CNY 5,000, color page CNY 8,000. Circ: 9,000. **Dist. overseas by:** China International Book Trading Corp, 35 Chegongzhuang Xilu, Haidian District, Beijing 100044, China.

MEDICAL SCIENCES—Psychiatry And Neurology

A B P CONTACT. see *HANDICAPPED*

616.8 USA
A C O NEWSLETTER. Text in English. 1968. s-a. USD 40; USD 55 foreign (effective 1999). bk.rev. **Document type:** *Newsletter.*
Related titles: Microform ed.: (from PQC).
Indexed: e-psyche.
Published by: (American College of Orgonomy), Orgonomic Publications, PO Box 490, Princeton, NJ 08542. TEL 732-821-1144, FAX 732-821-0174, http://www.orgonomy.org. Ed. Dr. Richard Schwartzman. Circ: 5,000.

616.858 USA ISSN 1084-5518
A D D - UP. (Attention Deficit Disorder) Text in English. 1995. bi-m. USD 29.95; USD 5 by e-mail. bk.rev. back issues avail. **Document type:** *Newsletter.* **Description:** Focuses on treatment of anxiety and attention deficit disorder for parents and severe anxiety disorder in adults and professionals. Also covers chronic pain disorder.
Indexed: e-psyche.
Published by: Listening Inc., 8716 Pine Ave, Gary, IN 46403. TEL 219-938-6962, FAX 219-938-7435. Ed. Patricia Work Bennett. R&P Patricia Bennett.

616.858 USA ISSN 1065-8025
A D H D REPORT. (Attention Deficit Hyperactivity Disorder) Text in English. 1993. bi-m. USD 70 domestic to individuals; USD 80 foreign to individuals; USD 105 domestic to institutions; USD 115 foreign to institutions (effective 2000). bk.rev. abstr, bibl. index. **Document type:** *Newsletter.* **Description:** Offers relevant information from research, workshops, and clinical work on ADHD, as well as from recent scientific publications and conferences from around the world.
Related titles: Online - full text ed.: (from CatchWord Ltd., RoweCom Information Quest).
Indexed: e-psyche.
Published by: Guilford Publications, Inc., 72 Spring St, New York, NY 10012. TEL 212-431-9800, 800-365-7006, FAX 212-966-6708, info@guilford.com. Ed. Russell A Barkley. R&P Kathy Kuehl. Circ: 3,500.

362.2 USA ISSN 0001-1436
A H R C CHRONICLE. Text in English. 1949. q. membership. adv. bk.rev. illus. **Document type:** *Newsletter, Consumer.* **Description:** Provides information for AHRC families and friends about news in the field and services for children who are developmentally disabled and their parents.
Indexed: e-psyche.
Published by: Association for the Help of Retarded Children, New York City Chapter, 200 Park Ave S, New York, NY 10003. TEL 212-254-8203, FAX 212-473-2225. Ed., R&P, Adv. contact Shirley Berenstein TEL 212-780-2619. Circ: 15,000.

616.83 USA
A L S NEWSLETTER. Text in English. 1996. bi-m. illus, maps. reprints avail.
Published by: Muscular Dystrophy Association, Inc., 3300 E Sunrise Dr, Tucson, AZ 85718-3208. TEL 520-529-2000, FAX 520-529-5300, publications@mdausa.org, http://www.mdausa.org. Ed. Bob Mackle. Pub. Robert Ross. R&P Carol Sowell TEL 520-529-2000. Circ: 20,000 (paid and controlled).

616.8 FRA ISSN 0999-792X
A N A E; actualites de neuropsychologie de l'enfant. (Approche Neuropsychologique des Apprentissages chez l'Enfant) Text in English, French. 5/yr., latest vol.14, 2002. EUR 35; EUR 53 foreign (effective 2002). back issues avail. *Refereed.* **Description:** For researchers and clinicians.
Related titles: Online - full text ed.: (from Institute for Scientific Information).
Indexed: Lang.& Lang.Behav.Abstr., Neurosci.Cit.Ind., PsycInfo, Psychol.Abstr. (1992-), SOPODA, Sociol.Abstr., e-psyche.
—BLDSC (1580.615000), EMDOCS.
Published by: P D G Communication, 30 rue d'Armaille, Paris 75017, France. TEL 33-1-40550595, FAX 33-1-45746567. Ed. Dr. Claude Jeanne Madelin. Pub. Patrick de Gavre.

616.89 USA
A N D I NEWS. Text in English. q. USD 20; USD 26 foreign (effective 1999). **Description:** Provides support for families implementing the diet.
Indexed: e-psyche.
Published by: Autism Network for Dietary Intervention, PO Box 17711, Rochester, NY 14617-0711. Autismndi@aol.com, http://www.members.aol.com/autismndi.

301.19 167 USA
A N R E D. Text in English. 1979. m. free per issue. bk.rev. back issues avail. *Refereed.* **Document type:** *Newsletter, Consumer.* **Description:** Causes, consequences, symptoms and treatment of anorexia nervosa and bulimia nervosa.
Formerly (until 1997): A N R E D Alert (Print)
Media: Online - full text.
Indexed: e-psyche.
Published by: Anorexia Nervosa & Related Eating Disorders, Inc., PO Box 5102, Eugene, OR 97405. TEL 541-344-1144, jarinor@rio.com, http://www.anred.com. Ed. Dr. J. Bradley Rubel. R&P Dr. J Bradley Rubel.

A P S BULLETIN. see *MEDICAL SCIENCES—Anaesthesiology*

616.8 616.2 USA
A S D A NEWS. Text in English. 1978. q. USD 40. adv. bk.rev. stat, tr.lit. back issues avail. **Document type:** *Newsletter.* **Description:** Current information on sleep disorders medicine and research.
Former titles (until 1993): A P S S Newsletter (0897-9375); (until 1986): A S D C Newsletter
Indexed: e-psyche.
Published by: American Sleep Disorders Association, 6301 Bandel Road, Ste 101, Rochester, MN 55901. TEL 507-287-6006, FAX 507-287-6008, asda@asda.org. Ed. Wolfgang Schmidt Nowara. Adv. contact Linda Freese. Circ: 2,750 (paid).

616.8 USA ISSN 0886-5620
A S E T NEWSLETTER. Text in English. 1976. q. USD 65 to members (effective 2000 - 2001). **Document type:** *Newsletter.* **Description:** Contains news of the society, educational articles, and calendar of events.
Indexed: e-psyche.
Published by: American Society of Electroneurodiagnostic Technologists, Inc., Executive Office, 204 W Seventh, Carroll, IA 51401. TEL 712-792-2978, FAX 712-792-6962, info@aset.org, http://www.aset.org. R&P Renee Yttredahl. Circ: 2,600.

616.80711 USA ISSN 1042-9670
RC336 CODEN: ACPSFE
ACADEMIC PSYCHIATRY. Text in English. 1977. q. USD 105 domestic to individuals; USD 127 foreign to individuals; USD 182 domestic to institutions; USD 192 foreign to institutions (effective 2001); Online access incl.. adv. bk.rev. bibl, charts, illus. back issues avail.; reprint service avail. from PQC,PSC,SCH,ISI. *Refereed.* **Document type:** *Journal, Consumer, Academic/Scholarly.* **Description:** Provides a forum for work which furthers knowledge in psychiatric education and stimulates improvements in academic psychiatry.
Formerly: Journal of Psychiatric Education (0363-1907)

M

Related titles: Microform ed.: (from PQC); Online - full text ed.: (from HighWire Pr., Northern Light Technology, Inc., EBSCO Publishing, RoweCom Information Quest, Institute for Scientific Information).
Indexed: ASCA, AgeLine, Behav.Med.Abstr., Chicago Psychoanal.Lit.Ind., Cont.Pg.Educ., Curr.Cont., Excerp.Med., Fam.Ind., Mid.East: Abstr.& Ind., PsycInfo, Psychol.Abstr. (1977-), Risk Abstr., SSCI, Sp.Ed.Needs Abstr., e-psyche.
—BLDSC (0570.514150), EMDOCS, GNLM, IDS, Infotrieve, ingenta. **CCC.**
Published by: (American Association of Directors of Psychiatric Residency Training), American Psychiatric Press, Inc., Journals Division, 1400 K St, N W, Ste 1101, Washington, DC 20005. TEL 800-368-5777, FAX 202-789-2648, order@appi.org, appi@psych.org, http://ap.psychiatryonline.org, http://www.psychiatryonline.org, http://www.appi.org. Ed. Dr. Samuel J Keith. R&P John McDuffie. Adv. contact Ryan Miller. Circ: 1,000. **Co-sponsor:** Association for Academic Psychiatry.

ACTA NEUROCHIRURGICA; the european journal of neurosurgery. see *MEDICAL SCIENCES—Surgery*

616.8 AUT ISSN 0065-1419
CODEN: ANCSBM
ACTA NEUROCHIRURGICA. SUPPLEMENTUM. Text in English. 1950. irreg. price varies. adv. reprint service avail. from ISI. *Refereed.* **Document type:** *Academic/Scholarly.*
Related titles: Microform ed.: (from PQC); ♦ Supplement to: Acta Neurochirurgica. ISSN 0001-6268.
Indexed: ASCA, Biol.Abstr., Curr.Cont. (coverage dropped), INIS Atomind., Ind.Med. (1994-), Inpharma, Reac., e-psyche.
—BLDSC (0639.851000), ADONIS, CISTI, KNAW. **CCC.**
Published by: Springer-Verlag Wien (Subsidiary of: BertelsmannSpringer), Sachsenplatz 4-6, PO Box 89, Vienna, W 1201, Austria. TEL 43-1-3302415-0, FAX 43-1-330242665, books@springer.at, http://www.springer.at/acta_neuro. Ed. H.-J Reulen. R&P Angela Foessl TEL 43-1-3302415517. Adv. contact Michael Katzenberger TEL 43-1-3302415220. B&W page XEU 1,000; 170 x 230. **N. American subscr. to:** Springer-Verlag, Journals, 175 Fifth Ave, New York, NY 10010. TEL 212-460-1500, FAX 212-473-6272, orders@springer-ny.com, books@springer.at.

616.8 BEL ISSN 0300-9009
RC321 CODEN: ANUBBR
ACTA NEUROLOGICA BELGICA. Text in English, French. 1900. 4/yr. EUR 54.55 domestic; EUR 62 foreign; EUR 16.10 per issue domestic; EUR 18.60 per issue foreign (effective 2002). Supplement avail. *Refereed.* **Document type:** *Journal, Academic/Scholarly.*
Supersedes in part: Acta Neurologica et Psychiatrica Belgica (0001-6284)
Related titles: Online - full text ed.: (from Institute for Scientific Information).
Indexed: ASCA, Bibl.Dev.Med.& Child Neur., Biol.Abstr., Chem.Abstr., Curr.Cont., Excerp.Med., GeoRef, INIS Atomind., Ind.Med. (1970-), Inpharma, Neurosci.Cit.Ind., Pharm.&Out.News, PsycInfo, Psychol.Abstr. (1981-), Reac., SSCI (coverage dropped), e-psyche.
—BLDSC (0639.902000), CASDDS, CISTI, EMDOCS, GNLM, IDS, ingenta, KNAW.
Published by: (Association des Societes Scientifiques Medicales Belges/Vereiniging van de Belgische Wetenschappelijke Genootschappen), Acta Medica Belgica, Av Circulaire 138A, Brussels 1180, Belgium. TEL 32-2-374-5158, FAX 32-2-3749628, amb@skynet.be, http://www.ulb.ac.be/medecine/loce/amb.htm. Ed. Dr. Andre Capon.

616.8 DNK ISSN 0001-6314
RC321 CODEN: ANRSAS
ACTA NEUROLOGICA SCANDINAVICA. Text in English. 1961. m. USD 516 in the Americas to institutions print & online eds. combines; GBP 358 elsewhere to institutions print & online eds. combined (effective 2002). adv. bk.rev. bibl, charts, illus. index. reprint service avail. from ISI. *Refereed.* **Document type:** *Journal, Academic/Scholarly.*
Supersedes in part: Acta Psychiatrica et Neurologica Scandinavica
Related titles: Online - full text ed.: ISSN 1600-0404. GBP 322 (effective 2002) (from Ovid Technologies, Inc., EBSCO Publishing, ingenta, Munksgaard & Blackwell Science's Synergy, Swets Blackwell, Institute for Scientific Information).
Indexed: ASCA, Abstr.Hyg., Agri.& Environ.Biotech.Abstr. (coverage dropped), Bibl.Dev.Med.& Child Neur., Biol.Abstr., Chem.Abstr., Chem.Indus.Notes, Chem.Titles, Curr.Adv.Ecol.Sci., Curr.Cont., Dent.Ind., Derwent Biotech.Abstr., Dok.Arbeitsmed., Excerp.Med., INIS Atomind., Ind.Med. (1961-), Ind.Sci.Rev., Inpharma, Int.Abstr.Biol.Sci., Jrnl.Watch Neuro., NRN, Neurosci.Cit.Ind., Nutr.Abstr., Pharm.&Out.News, Protozool.Abstr., PsycInfo, Psychol.Abstr. (1964-), Reac., Rev.Med.& Vet.Mycol., SSCI (coverage dropped), Sci.Cit.Ind., THA, e-psyche.
—BLDSC (0639.910000), ADONIS, CASDDS, CISTI, EMDOCS, GNLM, IDS, ingenta, KNAW. **CCC.**
Published by: Blackwell Munksgaard, Noerre Soegade 35, PO Box 2148, Copenhagen K 1016, Denmark. TEL 45-77-33-33-33, FAX 45-77-33-33-77, customerservice@munksgaard.dk, http://www.munksgaard.dk/actaneurologica. Ed. Elinor Ben-Menachem. Adv. contact Eric Rozario TEL 45-77-33-33-01. Circ: 1,100.

616.8 DNK ISSN 0065-1427
CODEN: ANSLAC
ACTA NEUROLOGICA SCANDINAVICA. SUPPLEMENTUM. Text in English. 1932. irreg. free to subscribers of Acta Neurologica Scandinavica. adv. reprint service avail. from ISI. *Refereed.* **Document type:** *Academic/Scholarly.*
Related titles: Online - full text ed.: ISSN 1600-5449 (from Ovid Technologies, Inc.).
Indexed: Biol.Abstr., Chem.Abstr., Curr.Adv.Ecol.Sci., Curr.Cont. (coverage dropped), Excerp.Med., INIS Atomind., Ind.Med. (1962-), Int.Abstr.Biol.Sci., PsycInfo, e-psyche.
—BLDSC (0639.912000), ADONIS, CASDDS, CISTI, EMDOCS, ingenta, KNAW. **CCC.**
Published by: Blackwell Munksgaard, Noerre Soegade 35, PO Box 2148, Copenhagen K 1016, Denmark. TEL 45-77-33-33-33, FAX 45-77-33-33-77, customerservice@munksgaard.dk, http://www.munksgaard.dk/actaneurologica. Ed. Elinor Ben-Menachem. Adv. contact Eric Rozario TEL 45-77-33-33-01.

626.8 TWN ISSN 1028-768X
ACTA NEUROLOGICA TAIWANICA. Text in English. 1997. q. **Document type:** *Academic/Scholarly.*
Formerly (until 1997): Acta Neurologica Sinica (1019-6099)
—BLDSC (0639.916000).
Published by: Taiwan Neurological Society, Ting Jou Lu section 3 no 8, Taipei 100, Taiwan. TEL 886-2-2364-9217, FAX 886-2-2364-9218, gant@mail.hato.com.tw, http://www.neuro.org.tw/.

616.8 DEU ISSN 0001-6322
CODEN: ANPTAL
ACTA NEUROPATHOLOGICA. Text in English. 1961. m. EUR 3,245.90 foreign; EUR 3,226.70 in Germany; EUR 320 newsstand/cover foreign (effective 2002). bibl, charts, illus. index. reprint service avail. from ISI. *Refereed.* **Document type:** *Journal, Academic/Scholarly.* **Description:** Provides information on subjects related to nerve tissue research based on modern investigative techniques, including histochemistry, electron microscopy, immunology, tissue culture, biophysics, neurochemistry, and experimental neuropathology.
Related titles: Microform ed.: (from PQC); Online - full text ed.: ISSN 1432-0533 (from EBSCO Publishing, RoweCom Information Quest, Swets Blackwell, Springer LINK, Institute for Scientific Information); ♦ Supplement: Acta Neuropathologica. Supplement. ISSN 0065-1435.
Indexed: ASCA, Abstr.Hyg., Biol.Abstr., Chem.Abstr., Chem.Indus.Notes, Chem.Titles, Curr.Adv.Ecol.Sci., Curr.Cont., Dent.Ind., Excerp.Med., Helminthol.Abstr., INIS Atomind., Ind.Med. (1961-), Ind.Sci.Rev., Ind.Vet., Inpharma, Int.Abstr.Biol.Sci., Kidney, Neurosci.Abstr. (coverage dropped), Neurosci.Cit.Ind., Nutr.Abstr., Pharm.&Out.News, Pig News & Info., Poult.Abstr., Protozool.Abstr., Reac., Rev.Appl.Entomol., Rev.Med.& Vet.Mycol., Sci.Cit.Ind., Small Anim.Abstr., Vet.Bull., Wild.Rev., e-psyche.
—BLDSC (0639.920000), CASDDS, CISTI, EMDOCS, GNLM, IDS, ingenta, KNAW. **CCC.**
Published by: (World Federation of Neurology/Federation Mondiale de Neurologie GBR), Springer-Verlag (Subsidiary of: BertelsmannSpringer), Tiergartenstr 17, Heidelberg 69121, Germany. TEL 49-6221-345-0, FAX 49-6221-345229, subscriptions@springer.de, http://link.springer.de/link/service/journals/00401/index.htm. Ed. K Jellinger. **Subscr. in N. America to:** Springer-Verlag New York Inc., PO Box 2485, Secaucus, NJ 07096-2485. TEL 212-460-1500, FAX 212-473-6272.

616.8 DEU ISSN 0065-1435
CODEN: ANLSBX
ACTA NEUROPATHOLOGICA. SUPPLEMENT. Text in English. 1962. irreg. reprint service avail. from ISI. **Document type:** *Monographic series.*
Related titles: Microform ed.: (from PQC); ♦ Supplement to: Acta Neuropathologica. ISSN 0001-6322.
Indexed: Biol.Abstr., Chem.Abstr., Ind.Med. (coverage dropped), Vet.Bull., e-psyche.
—CASDDS, CISTI, KNAW.
Published by: Springer-Verlag (Subsidiary of: BertelsmannSpringer), Haber Str 7, Heidelberg 69126, Germany. FAX 49-30-82787448, subscriptions@springer.de, http://link.springer.de.

616.89 NLD ISSN 0924-2708
CODEN: ACTNE
ACTA NEUROPSYCHIATRICA. Text in Dutch. 1989. q. USD 188 in the Americas to institutions print & online eds. combined; GBP 130 elsewhere to institutions print & online eds. combined (effective 2002). adv. *Refereed.* **Document type:** *Academic/Scholarly.* **Description:** Informs IGBP members of scientific developments in research in neuropsychiatry.
Related titles: Online - full text ed.: (from Institute for Scientific Information).
Indexed: ASCA, Excerp.Med. (1995-), Neurosci.Cit.Ind., SSCI (coverage dropped), e-psyche.
—BLDSC (0639.970000), EMDOCS, GNLM, IDS, KNAW. **CCC.**
Published by: (Dutch Interdisciplinary Society of Biological Psychiatry), Elsevier Gezondheidszorg B.V., Tijdstroom (Subsidiary of: Reed Elsevier plc Group), Planetenbaan 1, Maarssen 3600 AK, Netherlands. TEL 31-346-577577, FAX 31-346-554287, http://www.tijdstroom.nl. Ed. Dy M Maes. Adv. contact C Nieuwlands. Circ: 1,200 (controlled). **Subscr. to:** Elsevier Den Haag, Postbus 16500, The Hague 2500 BM, Netherlands. TEL 31-70-381-9900, FAX 31-70-333-8399.

616.89 ARG ISSN 0001-6896
CODEN: APQPAS
ACTA PSIQUIATRICA Y PSICOLOGICA DE AMERICA LATINA. Text in Spanish. 1954. q. USD 65 domestic to individuals; USD 75 in the Americas to individuals; USD 85 elsewhere to individuals; USD 80 domestic to institutions; USD 90 in the Americas to institutions; USD 100 elsewhere to institutions (effective 2000). adv. bk.rev. abstr, charts, illus. index. Supplement avail.; reprint service avail. from IRC,PQC,ISI. *Refereed.* **Document type:** *Academic/Scholarly.* **Description:** Devoted to psychiatry and psychology issues relevant to Latin America.
Indexed: ASCA, Biol.Abstr., Chem.Abstr., Curr.Cont. (coverage dropped), Excerp.Med., Ind.Med. (coverage dropped), PsycInfo, Psychol.Abstr. (1954-), SSCI (coverage dropped), e-psyche.
—BLDSC (0661.399000), CISTI, EMDOCS, GNLM, KNAW.
Published by: Fundacion Acta Fondo para la Salud Mental, Malabia, 2274 13 A, CC 170-Sur 25, Capital Federal, Buenos Aires 1425, Argentina. TEL 54-114-48548209, FAX 54-114-48573151, fuacta@ssdnet.com.ar. Eds. Dr. Guillermo Vidal, Fernando Lolas Stepke. R&P Dr. Guillermo Vidal. Adv. contact Dr. Diana Vidal. Circ: 3,000. **Subscr. to:** Casilla Correo 170, Succursal 25, Capital Federal, Buenos Aires 1425, Argentina.

616.89 DNK ISSN 0001-690X
CODEN: APYSA9
ACTA PSYCHIATRICA SCANDINAVICA. Text in English. 1926. m. USD 516 in the Americas to institutions print & online eds. combined; GBP 358 elsewhere to institutions print & online eds. combined (effective 2002). adv. bk.rev. charts, illus. index. reprint service avail. from ISI. *Refereed.* **Document type:** *Academic/Scholarly.*
Supersedes in part: Acta Psychiatrica et Neurologica Scandinavica
Related titles: Online - full text ed.: ISSN 1600-0447. GBP 322 (effective 2002) (from Ovid Technologies, Inc., EBSCO Publishing, O C L C Online Computer Library Center, Inc., Munksgaard & Blackwell Science's Synergy, Swets Blackwell, Institute for Scientific Information).

M

Indexed: ASCA, Abstr.Crim.& Pen., Abstr.Health Care Manage.Stud., Addic.Abstr., Adol.Ment.Hlth.Abstr., AgeLine, Agri.& Environ.Biotech.Abstr. (coverage dropped), Bibl.Dev.Med.& Child Neur., Biol.Abstr., Chem.Abstr., Chem.Indus.Notes, Chem.Titles, Crim.Just.Abstr., Curr.Adv.Ecol.Sci., Curr.Cont., Dent.Ind., Derwent Biotech.Abstr., Dok.Arbeitsmed., Environ.Sci.Poll.Mgmt., Excerp.Med., Fam.Ind., INIS Atomind., Ind.Med. (1961-), Ind.Sci.Rev., Indian Psychol.Abstr., Inpharma, Int.Abstr.Biol.Sci., Int.Nurs.Ind., Jrnl.Watch Psych., Kidney, Mid.East: Abstr.& Ind., Neurosci.Cit.Ind., Nutr.Abstr., Pharm.&Out.News, Pollut.Abstr., PsycInfo, Psychol.Abstr. (1950-), Reac., Risk Abstr., SSCI, Saf.Sci.Abstr., Sci.Cit.Ind., THA, e-psyche.
—BLDSC (0661.470000), ADONIS, CASDDS, CISTI, EMDOCS, GNLM, IDS, ingenta, KNAW. **CCC.**
Published by: Blackwell Munksgaard, Noerre Soegade 35, PO Box 2148, Copenhagen K 1016, Denmark. TEL 45-77-33-33-33, FAX 45-77-33-33-77, customerservice@munksgaard.dk, http:// www.munksgaard.dk/actapsych. Ed. Poul Munk Joergensen. Adv. contact Eric Rozario TEL 45-77-33-33-01. Circ: 1,600.

616.8 DNK ISSN 0065-1591
CODEN: ASSUA6
ACTA PSYCHIATRICA SCANDINAVICA. SUPPLEMENTUM. Text in English. 1932. irreg. free to subscribers of Acta Psychiatrica Scandinavica. adv. reprint service avail. from ISI. **Document type:** *Academic/Scholarly.*
Related titles: Online - full text ed.: ISSN 1600-5473 (from Ovid Technologies, Inc., ingenta, Swets Blackwell).
Indexed: Biol.Abstr., Chem.Abstr., Chem.Indus.Notes, Chem.Titles, Curr.Adv.Ecol.Sci., Curr.Cont. (coverage dropped), Excerp.Med., INIS Atomind., Ind.Med. (1961-), Int.Abstr.Biol.Sci., Int.Nurs.Ind., Mid.East: Abstr.& Ind., PsycInfo, e-psyche.
—BLDSC (0661.472000), ADONIS, CASDDS, CISTI, EMDOCS, ingenta, KNAW. **CCC.**
Published by: Blackwell Munksgaard, Noerre Soegade 35, PO Box 2148, Copenhagen K 1016, Denmark. TEL 871-388-8273, customerservice@munksgaard.dk, http://www.munksgaard.dk/actapsych. Ed. Poul Munk Joergensen. Adv. contact Eric Rozario TEL 45-77-33-33-01.

616.8 ESP ISSN 1139-9287
CODEN: ALNPAJ
ACTAS ESPANOLAS DE PSIQUIATRIA. Text in Spanish. 1940. bi-m. ESP 12,400 to individuals; ESP 17,700 to institutions; ESP 9,920 to students (effective 2001). back issues avail.; reprints avail. *Refereed.* **Document type:** *Journal, Academic/Scholarly.*
Former titles (until 1999): Actas Luso Espanolas de Neurologia Psiquiatria y Ciencias Afines (0300-5062); (until 1971): Actas Luso Espanolas de Neurologia y Psiquiatria (0001-7329); (until 1946): Actas Espanolas de Neurologia y Psiquiatria (0300-5054)
Related titles: Online - full text ed.: 1996 (from Institute for Scientific Information).
Indexed: ASCA, Biol.Abstr., Excerp.Med., Ind.Med. (1999-), Ind.Med.Esp., Neurosci.Cit.Ind., PsycInfo, Psychol.Abstr. (1966-), SSCI (coverage dropped), e-psyche.
—BLDSC (0615.507000), CASDDS, CINDOC, CISTI, GNLM, IDS, Infotrieve. **CCC.**
Published by: Ediciones Doyma S.A., Traversa de Gracia, 17-21, Barcelona 08021, Spain. TEL 34-93-200-0711, ale@doyma.es, doyma@doyma.es, http://www.doyma.es/. Ed. Jose Luis Carrasco. R&P Monica Barnes. Adv. contact Jose Antonio Hernandez. Circ: 2,000.

616.8 IRL ISSN 1393-7472
ACTIVITIES OF IRISH PSYCHIATRIC SERVICES (YEAR). Text in English. 1974. biennial. IEP 10 domestic; IEP 25 foreign (effective 2000). **Document type:** *Academic/Scholarly.* **Description:** Psychiatric in-patient admission, community psychiatric services, diagnosis.
Formerly (until 1995): Activities of Irish Psychiatric Hospitals and Units (Year) (0332-2602)
Indexed: e-psyche.
—BLDSC (0676.478000).
Published by: Mental Health Division, Health Research Board, 73 Lower Baggot St., Dublin 2, Ireland. TEL 353-1-676-1176, FAX 353-1-661-1856, mental_health@hrb.ie, http://www.hrb.ie. Ed. Ciaran Browne. Circ: 1,000.

616.8 362.7 CHE ISSN 0751-7696
ADOLESCENCE. Text in French. 1983. s-a. CHF 80, EUR 51.94 (effective 2002). back issues avail. **Document type:** *Journal, Academic/Scholarly.*
Related titles: Online - full text ed.: (from Northern Light Technology, Inc.).
Indexed: Addic.Abstr., Child Devel.Abstr., Commun.Abstr., THA, Wom.Stud.Ind.
—**CCC.**
Published by: Editions Medecine et Hygiene, Case Postale 456, Geneva, 4 1211, Switzerland. TEL 41-22-7029311, FAX 41-22-7029355, abonnements@medhyg.ch, http://www.medhyg.ch.

616.8 USA ISSN 0065-2008
RJ499.A1
ADOLESCENT PSYCHIATRY; annals of the American Society for Adolescent Psychiatry. Variant title: American Society for Adolescent Psychiatry. Annals. Text in English. 1971. a., latest vol.25. USD 49.95 (effective 2000). reprint service avail. from PQC. *Refereed.* **Document type:** *Monographic series, Academic/Scholarly.* **Description:** Reports on specific clinical and theoretical issues, as well as considerations of social, cultural, and political themes. Contains scholarly articles from contributors in a variety of disciplines.
Related titles: Microfilm ed.: (from PMC); Online - full text ed.: (from Northern Light Technology, Inc., ProQuest Information & Learning, Institute for Scientific Information).
Indexed: ASCA, Biol.Abstr., CINAHL, Psychol.Abstr., SSCI, e-psyche.
—BLDSC (0696.589000), GNLM, ingenta, KNAW.
Published by: (American Society for Adolescent Psychiatry), Analytic Press, Inc. (Subsidiary of: Lawrence Erlbaum Associates, Inc.), 101 West St, Hillsdale, NJ 07642. TEL 201-358-9477, FAX 201-358-4700, TAP@analyticpress.com, http://www.analyticpress.com/books/326-7.html. Ed. Aaron Esman. **Orders in the Americas, the Caribbean, China, the Far East:** Journals, 810 E 10th St, PO Box 1897, Lawrence, KS 66044-8897. **Dist. addr. in Africa:** Overseas Publications, P O Box 12292, Centrahil 6006, South Africa.; **Dist. addr. in Australia, New Zealand & Papua New Guinea:** DAInformation Services, 648 Whitehouse Rd, Mitcham, VIC 3132, Australia. TEL 61-3-9210-7788, FAX 61-3-9210-7724.; **Dist. addr. in India, Bangladesh & Sri Lanka:** VivaBooks Private Ltd, 4325/2 Ansari Rd, Darya Ganj, New Delhi 11002, India. TEL 91-11-327-9280, FAX 91-11-326-7224.; **Dist. addr. in the UK, Europe and the Middle East:** Eurospan University Press Group, Order Dept, 3 Henrietta St, London WC2E 8LU, United Kingdom. TEL 44-20-7240-0856, FAX 44-20-7379-0609, http://www.eurospan.co.uk.

616.8 SGP
ADVANCED SERIES IN NEUROSCIENCE. Text in English. 1988. irreg., latest vol.5, 1997. USD 62, GBP 39 per vol. for vol. 5 (effective 2002); price varies with each vol.. **Document type:** *Monographic series.*
Indexed: C.C.M.J., e-psyche.
Published by: World Scientific Publishing Co Pte Ltd, Farrer Rd, PO Box 128, Singapore 912805, Singapore. TEL 65-3825663, FAX 65-3825919.

616.8 AUT ISSN 0095-4829
ADVANCES AND TECHNICAL STANDARDS IN NEUROSURGERY. Text in English. 1974. irreg. price varies. reprint service avail. from ISI. *Refereed.* **Document type:** *Monographic series, Academic/Scholarly.*
Indexed: Ind.Med. (1974-), e-psyche.
—BLDSC (0698.820000), CISTI, GNLM, Infotrieve, ingenta, KNAW. **CCC.**
Published by: Springer-Verlag Wien (Subsidiary of: BertelsmannSpringer), Sachsenplatz 4-6, PO Box 89, Vienna, W 1201, Austria. TEL 43-1-3302415-0, FAX 43-1-330242665, books@springer.at, http://www.springer.at. Ed. J Pickard. R&P Angela Foessl TEL 43-1-3302415517. **Subscr. to:** Springer-Verlag, Journals. TEL 212-460-1500, FAX 212-473-6272, orders@springer-ny.com, http://www.springer-ny.com.

616.8 USA
ADVANCES (CHICAGO); progress in Alzheimer research and care. Text in English. 1981. q. free per issue. bk.rev. back issues avail. **Document type:** *Newsletter, Consumer.* **Description:** Covers trends in Alzheimer research, care, education, and professional training.
Former titles (until Aug. 1997): Alzheimer's Association Newsletter; A D R D A Newsletter
Indexed: e-psyche.
Published by: Alzheimer's Association, Inc., 919 N Michigan Ave, Ste 1000, Chicago, IL 60611-1676. TEL 312-335-8700, FAX 312-335-1110, info@alz.org, http://www.alz.org. Ed. Michele Pellissier. Circ: 160,000.

616.8 GBR ISSN 0965-1802
ADVANCES IN A L S - M N D. (Amyotrophic Lateral Sclerosis - Motor Neuron Disease) Text in English. 1991. irreg. **Document type:** *Academic/Scholarly.*
Indexed: e-psyche.
—BLDSC (0698.580000).
Published by: Smith-Gordon and Co. Ltd., 13 Shalcomb St, London SW10 0HZ, United Kingdom. TEL 44-171-351-7042, FAX 44-171-351-1250. Ed. Eldred Smith Gordon.

ADVANCES IN BIOCHEMICAL PSYCHOPHARMACOLOGY. see *PHARMACY AND PHARMACOLOGY*

616.8 CHE ISSN 0378-7354
CODEN: ABPSD5
ADVANCES IN BIOLOGICAL PSYCHIATRY. Text in English. 1978. irreg., latest vol.20. CHF 120 in Europe; DEM 140 in Germany; USD 100 in United States (effective 2001). reprint service avail. from ISI. *Refereed.* **Document type:** *Monographic series, Academic/Scholarly.*
Related titles: Online - full text ed.
Indexed: Biol.Abstr., Chem.Abstr., Chem.Indus.Notes, Chem.Titles, Curr.Cont. (coverage dropped), Psychol.Abstr., e-psyche.
—BLDSC (0700.070000), CASDDS, CISTI, Infotrieve, KNAW. **CCC.**
Published by: S. Karger AG, Allschwilerstr 10, PO Box, Basel 4009, Switzerland. TEL 41-61-306-1111, FAX 41-61-306-1234, karger@karger.ch, http://www.karger.com/bookseries/ADBIP.

ADVANCES IN CHILD NEUROPSYCHOLOGY. see *PSYCHOLOGY*

616.8 USA ISSN 0748-4410
ADVANCES IN CLINICAL NEUROPSYCHOLOGY. Text in English. 1984. irreg., latest vol.3. **Document type:** *Monographic series, Academic/Scholarly.*
Indexed: e-psyche.
Published by: Kluwer Academic - Plenum Publishers (Subsidiary of: Wolters Kluwer N.V.), 233 Spring St, New York, NY 10013-1578. TEL 212-620-8000, 800-221-9369, FAX 212-463-0742, info@plenum.com, http://www.plenum.com.

ADVANCES IN CONSCIOUSNESS RESEARCH. see *PSYCHOLOGY*

616.853 USA ISSN 0892-726X
RC372.A1 CODEN: ADEPDN
ADVANCES IN EPILEPTOLOGY. Text in English. 1980. irreg. price varies. reprint service avail. from PQC. *Refereed.* **Document type:** *Proceedings, Academic/Scholarly.*
Indexed: e-psyche.
—CASDDS, GNLM, KNAW.
Published by: Lippincott Williams & Wilkins (Philadelphia) (Subsidiary of: Wolters Kluwer N.V.), 530 Walnut St, Philadelphia, PA 19106-3621. TEL 301-223-2300, 800-638-3030, FAX 301-223-2400.

ADVANCES IN HUMAN FACTORS - ERGONOMICS. see *PSYCHOLOGY*

ADVANCES IN MENTAL RETARDATION AND DEVELOPMENTAL DISABILITIES. see *EDUCATION—Special Education And Rehabilitation*

616.8 USA ISSN 1074-7575
CODEN: ANUSED
ADVANCES IN NEURAL SCIENCE. Text in English. 1993. irreg. USD 128.50 per vol.. back issues avail. **Document type:** *Academic/Scholarly.*
Indexed: Chem.Abstr., Chem.Indus.Notes, Chem.Titles, Zoo.Rec.
—CASDDS, CISTI, GNLM.
Published by: J A I Press Inc., 100 Prospect St, Box 811, Stamford, CT 06904-0811. TEL 203-323-9606, FAX 203-357-8446, jai@jaipress.com. Ed. Sudrshan K Malhotra.

ADVANCES IN NEUROCHEMISTRY. see *BIOLOGY—Biochemistry*

616.8 USA ISSN 0091-3952
RC321 CODEN: ADNRA3
ADVANCES IN NEUROLOGY. Text in English. 1973. irreg., latest vol.69. price varies. reprint service avail. from PQC. *Refereed.* **Document type:** *Proceedings.*
Related titles: Online - full text ed.: (from Institute for Scientific Information).
Indexed: ASCA, AgeLine, Biol.Abstr., Chem.Abstr., Chem.Indus.Notes, Chem.Titles, Curr.Cont. (coverage dropped), Dent.Ind., INIS Atomind., Ind.Med. (1973-), Int.Nurs.Ind., Neurosci.Cit.Ind.
—BLDSC (0709.482000), CASDDS, CISTI, GNLM, ingenta, KNAW.

M

Published by: Lippincott Williams & Wilkins (Philadelphia) (Subsidiary of: Wolters Kluwer N.V.), 530 Walnut St, Philadelphia, PA 19106-3621. TEL 301-223-2300, 800-638-3030, FAX 301-223-2400.

615.75 616.8 USA ISSN 1057-6592 CODEN: ADNPEZ
ADVANCES IN NEUROPSYCHIATRY AND PSYCHOPHARMACOLOGY. Text in English. 1991. irreg. price varies. reprint service avail. from PQC. *Refereed.* **Document type:** *Monographic series.*
Indexed: e-psyche.
Published by: Lippincott Williams & Wilkins (Philadelphia) (Subsidiary of: Wolters Kluwer N.V.), 530 Walnut St, Philadelphia, PA 19106-3621. TEL 301-223-2300, 800-638-3030, FAX 301-223-2400.

616.8 USA ISSN 1059-1540 CODEN: ANEUE7
ADVANCES IN NEUROSCIENCE. Text in English. 1991. irreg. price varies. reprint service avail. from PQC. *Refereed.* **Document type:** *Monographic series.*
Indexed: Chem.Abstr., Chem.Indus.Notes, Chem.Titles, e-psyche.
—CISTI.
Published by: Lippincott Williams & Wilkins (Philadelphia) (Subsidiary of: Wolters Kluwer N.V.), 530 Walnut St, Philadelphia, PA 19106-3621. TEL 301-223-2300, 800-638-3030, FAX 301-223-2400.

616.8 617 JPN ISSN 0916-698X
ADVANCES IN NEUROTRAUMA RESEARCH. Text in English. 1989. a. JPY 3,500.
Indexed: e-psyche.
Published by: Japanese Society for Neurotrauma Research, Nihon Daigaku Igakubu no Shinkei Geka, Oyaguchi Kamicho, Itabashi-ku, Tokyo 173, Japan.

616.8 USA ISSN 0146-0722 CODEN: APRTDE
ADVANCES IN PAIN RESEARCH AND THERAPY. Text in English. 1976. irreg. price varies. index. reprint service avail. from PQC. *Refereed.* **Document type:** *Proceedings.*
Related titles: Online - full text ed.: (from Institute for Scientific Information).
Indexed: ASCA, Biol.Abstr., Chem.Abstr., Chem.Indus.Notes, Chem.Titles, Curr.Cont. (coverage dropped), Ind.Sci.Rev., Neurosci.Cit.Ind., Sci.Cit.Ind., e-psyche.
—BLDSC (0709.576000), CASDDS, CISTI, GNLM, ingenta, KNAW.
Published by: Lippincott Williams & Wilkins (Philadelphia) (Subsidiary of: Wolters Kluwer N.V.), 530 Walnut St, Philadelphia, PA 19106-3621. TEL 301-223-2300, 800-638-3030, FAX 301-223-2400.

616.8 GBR ISSN 1355-5146
ADVANCES IN PSYCHIATRIC TREATMENT. Text in English. 1994. bi-m. GBP 88 in Europe to individuals Print & Online eds.; USD 75 in US & Canada to individuals Print & Online eds.; GBP 95 elsewhere to individuals Print & Online eds.; GBP 99 in Europe to institutions Print & Online eds.; USD 174 in US & Canada to institutions Print & Online eds.; GBP 106 elsewhere to institutions Print & Online eds. (effective 2001). adv. **Document type:** *Academic/Scholarly.* **Description:** Promotes the continuing professional development of consultant psychiatrists.
Related titles: Online - full text ed.: Advances in Psychiatric Treatment Online. ISSN 1472-1481. 2000. GBP 68, USD 109 to individuals; GBP 90, USD 144 to institutions (effective 2001) (from HighWire Pr., EBSCO Publishing).
Indexed: e-psyche.
—BLDSC (0711.018000).
Published by: Royal College of Psychiatrists, 17 Belgrave Sq, London SW1X 8PG, United Kingdom. TEL 44-20-7235-2351, FAX 44-20-7245-1231, http://www.rcpsych.ac.uk/pub/apt.htm. Ed. Andrew Sims. Adv. contact Peter Mell. Circ: 3,200 (controlled). **Subscr. to:** Royal Society of Medicine Press Ltd, PO Box 9002, London W1A 0ZA, United Kingdom. TEL 44-20-7290-2928, FAX 44-20-7290-2924.

616.8 CHE ISSN 0065-3268
ADVANCES IN PSYCHOSOMATIC MEDICINE. Text in English. 1960. irreg., latest vol.23. CHF 120 in Europe; DEM 140 in Germany; DEM 100 in United States (effective 2001). back issues avail.; reprint service avail. from ISI. *Refereed.* **Document type:** *Monographic series, Academic/Scholarly.*
Related titles: Online - full text ed.: (from Institute for Scientific Information).
Indexed: ASCA, Biol.Abstr., Chem.Abstr., Curr.Cont. (coverage dropped), Ind.Med. (1967-), SSCI (coverage dropped), e-psyche.
—BLDSC (0711.100000), CISTI, GNLM, KNAW. **CCC.**
Published by: S. Karger AG, Allschwilerstr 10, PO Box, Basel 4009, Switzerland. TEL 41-61-306-1111, FAX 41-61-306-1234, karger@karger.ch, http://www.karger.com/bookseries/ADPSY. Ed. T N Wise.

616.8 DEU CODEN: TWNPE3
AERZTLICHE PRAXIS. NEUROLOGIE PSYCHIATRIE. Short title: Ae P Neurologie Psychiatrie. Text in German. 1987. m. DEM 98; DEM 126 foreign (effective 1998). adv. **Document type:** *Trade.*
Former titles (until 1998): T und E Neurologie Psychiatrie; (until 1997): T W Neurologie - Psychiatrie (0935-3224)
Indexed: Excerp.Med., e-psyche.
—EMDOCS, GNLM, Infotrieve. **CCC.**
Published by: Reed Elsevier Deutschland GmbH (Subsidiary of: Reed Elsevier group), Gabrielenstr 9, Munich 80636, Germany. TEL 49-89-89817-0, FAX 49-89-89817400, http://aep.r-e.de. Ed. Hans Juergen Kuntze. Pub. Wolfram Haase. Adv. contact Andrea Kroneck.

616.8 USA ISSN 1044-0534
AFTERLOSS; the monthly newsletter to comfort and care for those who mourn. Text in English. 1989. m. USD 45. index. back issues avail. **Document type:** *Newsletter, Consumer.* **Description:** Deals with the management of and education about grief following the death of a loved one. Functions to help the survivors deal with the death of a spouse, child, other relations and friends.
Indexed: e-psyche.
Published by: Afterloss, Inc., 79301 Country Club Dr, Ste 100, Indio, CA 92201-1250. TEL 760-772-7934, FAX 760-772-7390. Ed. Margie Kennedy Reeves. Pub. Barbara Lesstrang. Circ: 6,000.

AGGRESSION AND VIOLENT BEHAVIOR; a review journal. see *PSYCHOLOGY*

AGING & MENTAL HEALTH. see *GERONTOLOGY AND GERIATRICS*

612 TUR ISSN 1300-0012
AGRI/JOURNAL OF THE TURKISH SOCIETY OF ALGOLOGY; turk algoloji (agri) derneginin yayin organdir. Text in Turkish; Summaries in English. 1989. q. USD 50 (effective 1999). adv. bk.rev. abstr. *Refereed.* **Document type:** *Academic/Scholarly.* **Description:** Reports on new medical and technical issues affecting regional anesthesiologists.
Indexed: Excerp.Med. (1993-), e-psyche.
—BLDSC (0738.780000), EMDOCS, GNLM.
Published by: Turk Algoloji Dernegini/Turkish Society of Algology, Istanbul Tip Fakultesi, Agri Merkezi Capa Klinikleri, Istanbul 34390, Turkey. TEL 90-212-6350135, FAX 90-212-6310541, algotur@ibm.net. Ed., R&P Dr. Serdar Erdine. Adv. contact Dr. Suleyman Ozyalcin. page USD 500. Circ: 1,000 (paid); 500 (controlled).

AICHI IKA DAIGAKU KAREI IKAGAKU KENKYUJO KIYO/AICHI MEDICAL UNIVERSITY. INSTITUTE FOR MEDICAL SCIENCE OF AGING. BULLETIN. see *GERONTOLOGY AND GERIATRICS*

AIDS CARE; psychological and socio-medical aspects of AIDS-HIV. see *MEDICAL SCIENCES—Communicable Diseases*

616.8 DEU ISSN 0302-4350
W1 AK995GN
AKTUELLE NEUROLOGIE. Text in German; Summaries in English, German. 1974. 10/yr. EUR 252.80 domestic; EUR 268.80 in Europe; EUR 279.90 elsewhere; EUR 30 newsstand/cover (effective 2002). adv. index. back issues avail.; reprint service avail. from PQC. *Refereed.* **Document type:** *Journal, Academic/Scholarly.*
Related titles: Online - full text ed.: ISSN 1438-9428 (from Institute for Scientific Information).
Indexed: ASCA, Biol.Abstr., Curr.Adv.Gen.& Molec.Biol., Curr.Cont., Excerp.Med., INIS Atomind., Inpharma, Neurosci.Cit.Ind., Reac., Rev.Appl.Entomol., SSCI (coverage dropped), e-psyche.
—BLDSC (0785.775000), CISTI, EMDOCS, GNLM, IDS, Infotrieve, KNAW. **CCC.**
Published by: Georg Thieme Verlag, Ruedigerstr 14, Stuttgart 70469, Germany. TEL 49-711-8931-0, FAX 49-711-8931298, kunden.service@thieme.de, http://www.thieme.de/aktneu/index.html. Ed. G Kraemer. R&P Peter Eich. adv.: page DEM 2,600; 175 x 250. Circ: 4,300.

616.8 616.1 ITA ISSN 0392-9116
ALGOLOGIA. Text and summaries in English, Italian. 1982. s-a. free per issue to qualified personnel. adv. bk.rev. charts, illus. Supplement avail.; back issues avail. **Document type:** *Monographic series, Academic/Scholarly.* **Description:** Features worldwide research papers on the study of pain. Covers neurology, psychoanalysis and cardiology.
Indexed: Ind.Med. (coverage dropped), e-psyche.
—KNAW.
Published by: Institute for the Study and Therapy of Pain, Via Venezia, 10, Florence, FI 50121, Italy. TEL 39-55-577219, FAX 39-55-5417144, nuovames@pn.itnet.it. Ed., R&P Pierluigi Zucchi. Circ: 5,000.

616.8 USA
ALLIANCE (WISCONSIN). Text in English. irreg.
Media: Online - full text.
Indexed: e-psyche.
Published by: Alliance for Medical and Psychosocial Support, 10410 52nd Street South, Wisconsin Rapids, WI 54494. TEL 715-325-7537, angel@tznet.com, http://www.tznet.com/busn/advocate/. Ed. Sarah Skiba.

612.67 USA ISSN 0893-0341
RC523 CODEN: ADADE2
ALZHEIMER DISEASE AND ASSOCIATED DISORDERS. Text in English. 1987. q. USD 190 domestic to individuals; USD 234 foreign to individuals; USD 333 domestic to institutions; USD 386 foreign to institutions; USD 88 newsstand/cover (effective 2002). adv. bk.rev. charts, illus. reprint service avail. from PQC. *Refereed.* **Document type:** *Journal, Academic/Scholarly.* **Description:** Provides an international forum for reports of new research findings and approaches to diagnosis and treatment.
Related titles: Online - full text ed.: USD 432.90 domestic academic site license; USD 485.90 foreign academic site license; USD 482.85 domestic corporate site license; USD 535.85 foreign corporate site license (effective 2002) (from Ovid Technologies, Inc., Institute for Scientific Information).
Indexed: ASCA, AgeLine, Chem.Abstr., Chem.Indus.Notes, Chem.Titles, Curr.Cont., INIS Atomind., Ind.Med. (1987-), Ind.Sci.Rev., Indian Psychol.Abstr., Inpharma, Int.Abstr.Biol.Sci., Int.Nurs.Ind., Neurosci.Cit.Ind., Nutr.Abstr., Pharm.&Out.News, PsycInfo, Psychol.Abstr. (1991-), Reac., SSCI (coverage dropped), Sci.Cit.Ind., THA, e-psyche.
—BLDSC (0806.255300), CASDDS, CISTI, EMDOCS, GNLM, IDS, ingenta, KNAW.
Published by: Lippincott Williams & Wilkins (Philadelphia) (Subsidiary of: Wolters Kluwer N.V.), 530 Walnut St, Philadelphia, PA 19106-3621. TEL 215-521-8300, FAX 215-521-8902, http://www.Lww.com. Ed. Peter J Whitehouse. Pub. Nancy Megley. R&P Margaret Becker. Adv. contact Renee Artuso. B&W page USD 740, color page USD 1,875. Circ: 854 (paid). **Subscr. to:** PO Box 1600, Hagerstown, MD 21740-1600. TEL 800-777-2295, FAX 301-824-7390.

616.8 618.97 362.1 SWE ISSN 1100-0899
ALZHEIMERFOERENINGEN; et forum foer kontakt och information roerande sjukdomar av Alzheimer-typ. Text in Swedish. 1987. q. SEK 100 to members.
Indexed: e-psyche.
Published by: Alzheimerfoereningen i Sverige, Alzheimerfonden, Sunnanvaeg 14 S, Lund 22226, Sweden.

ALZHEIMER'S CARE GUIDE; published especially for those who care for people with Alzheimer's disease and related disorders. see *GERONTOLOGY AND GERIATRICS*

616.8 362.6 USA ISSN 1525-3279
▼ **ALZHEIMER'S CARE QUARTERLY.** Text in English. 2000. q. USD 135 to individuals; USD 41 newsstand/cover (effective 2002). **Document type:** *Journal.* **Description:** Reflects treatment approaches by providing clinically focused information on quality dementia care. The content is evidence- and experience-based, with a heavy focus on material that is of immediate practical use to nurses, rehabilitation professionals, administrators, and others.
Published by: Aspen Publishers, Inc., 200 Orchard Ridge Dr, Ste 200, Gaithersburg, MD 20878. TEL 301-417-7500, FAX 301-695-7931. Ed. Carol Bowlby Sifton.

M

616.8 USA
ALZHEIMER'S DISEASE REVIEW. Text in English. 1996. q. free per issue. *Refereed.* **Document type:** *Academic/Scholarly.* **Description:** Contains reviews of biomedical research on Alzheimer's disease. Topics covered include cell and molecular biology, clinical trials, epidemiology, genetics and pathology pertinent to Alzheimer's disease and aging of the nervous systems.
Media: Online - full text.
Indexed: Neurosci.Abstr., e-psyche.
Published by: University of Kentucky, Sanders - Brown Center on Aging, Lexington, KY 40536-0230. TEL 606-257-6461, FAX 606-323-2866, jwgeddes@coa.uky.edu, http://www.coa.uky.edu/ADReview. Eds. James W Geddes, William R Markesbery. R&P James Geddes. Circ: 7,000.

616.8 USA
ALZHEIMER'S DISEASE SOURCEBOOK. Text in English. 1993. irreg., latest vol.2, 1999. USD 78 per vol. (effective 2001). charts, illus, stat. Index. **Document type:** *Consumer.* **Description:** Offers basic information for the layperson on Alzheimer's disease and related neurological disorders, along with treatment and care options.
Formerly: Alzheimer's, Stroke and 29 Other Neurological Disorders
Published by: Omnigraphics, Inc., 615 Griswold St, Detroit, MI 48226. TEL 313-931-1340, 800-234-1340, FAX 313-961-1383, 800-875-1340, info@omnigraphics.com, http://www.omnigraphics.com. Ed. Karen Bellenir. Pub. Frederick G Ruffner Jr. R&P Laurie Lanzen Harris.

616.831 NZL ISSN 1173-4361
ALZHEIMERS NEWS. Text in English. 1988. q. NZD 60 (effective 2000). adv. bk.rev. back issues avail. **Document type:** *Newsletter.*
Formerly (1988-1994): A D A R D S New Zealand News (1170-5426)
Published by: Alzheimers Disease and Related Disorders Society New Zealand, P.O. Box 2808, 1st Fl., Triune House, 71 Armagh St, Christchurch, New Zealand. TEL 64-3-365-1590, FAX 64-3-379-8744. Ed., Adv. contact Tina Hartung.

616.8 618.97 GBR ISSN 1461-6130
ALZHEIMER'S REPORTS. Text in English. 1998. bi-w. GBP 90, USD 160, JPY 24,000 to individuals; GBP 180, USD 320, JPY 48,000 to institutions (effective 2001). adv. back issues avail. *Refereed.* **Document type:** *Journal.* **Description:** Publishes short communications, full length reports, case studies and commissioned reviews; and examines the publishing requirements scientists have and addresses these needs through an innovative approach to publishing.
Related titles: Online - full text ed.: (from Institute for Scientific Information).
Indexed: Curr.Cont.
—BLDSC (0806.255360).
Published by: Cardiff University, School of Biosciences, Museum Avenue, Box 911, Cardiff CF10 3US, United Kingdom. TEL 44-29-2087-5188, FAX 44-29-2087-6749, RichardsSJ@cf.ac.uk, http://www.ar-msj.demon.co.uk/alzrep.htm. Ed. Sarah-Jane Richards.

616.8 362.6 USA
ALZHEIMER'S RESEARCH REVIEW. Text in English. q. charts, illus. **Document type:** *Newsletter, Consumer.* **Description:** Describes the research sponsored by the organization into this debilitating disease.
Indexed: e-psyche.
Published by: Alzheimer's Disease Research, American Health Assistance Foundation, 15825 Shady Grove Rd, Ste 140, Rockville, MD 20850. TEL 800-437-AHAF. Ed., R&P Eve Herold TEL 301-948-3244.

616.89 USA ISSN 0890-8567
RJ499.A1 CODEN: JAAPEE
AMERICAN ACADEMY OF CHILD AND ADOLESCENT PSYCHIATRY. JOURNAL. Variant title: Journal of the American Academy of Child and Adolescent Psychiatry. Text in English. 1962. m. USD 136 domestic to individuals for print & online eds.; USD 178 foreign to individuals for print & online eds.; USD 240 domestic to institutions for print & online eds.; USD 282 foreign to institutions for print & online eds.; USD 30 newsstand/cover (effective 2002). adv. bk.rev. abstr, bibl, charts, illus. index. back issues avail.; reprint service avail. from PSC,SCH. *Refereed.* **Document type:** *Academic/Scholarly.* **Description:** Presents original papers in psychiatric research and the treatment of children and adolescents.
Formerly: American Academy of Child Psychiatry. Journal (0002-7138)
Related titles: CD-ROM ed.: (from Ovid Technologies, Inc.); Microfilm ed.: (from WWS); Online - full text ed.: USD 312 domestic academic site license; USD 354 foreign academic site license; USD 348 domestic corporate site license; USD 390 foreign corporate site license (effective 2002) (from Ovid Technologies, Inc., H. W. Wilson, Gale Group, Factiva, Institute for Scientific Information).
Indexed: ASCA, ASSIA, Adol.Ment.Hlth.Abstr., Behav.Med.Abstr., Bibl.Dev.Med.& Child Neur., C.C.I.P., Child Devel.Abstr., Crim.Just.Abstr., Curr.Cont., Dent.Ind., Dok.Arbeitsmed., Educ.Ind. (Sep.1982-Nov.1986), Excerp.Med., Fam.Ind., IMFL, Ind.Med. (1987-), Indian Psychol.Abstr., Inpharma, Int.Nurs.Ind., Jrnl.Watch Psych., Mid.East: Abstr.& Ind., NRN, Pharm.&Out.News, PsycInfo, Psychol.Abstr. (1982-), Reac., Risk Abstr., SSCI, Sci.Cit.Ind., Soc.Sci.Ind. (Jan.1987-), Soc.Work Res.& Abstr., e-psyche.
—BLDSC (4683.690000), CISTI, EMDOCS, GNLM, IDS, ingenta, KNAW.
Published by: (American Academy of Child and Adolescent Psychiatry), Williams & Wilkins (Subsidiary of: Waverly International), 351 W Camden St, Baltimore, MD 21201-2436. TEL 410-528-4068, 800-222-3790, FAX 410-528-4452, sisaacson@wwilkins.com, http://www.jaacap.com/, http://www.Lww.com. Ed. Mina K Dulcan. Adv. contact Sharlene Isaacson. B&W page USD 980; 10.88 x 8.38. Circ: 10,175; 10,090 (paid).

616.89 340 USA
RA1151
AMERICAN ACADEMY OF PSYCHIATRY AND THE LAW. JOURNAL. Text in English. 1973. q. USD 50 to individuals; USD 95 to institutions; includes Newsletter. bk.rev. bibl. reprint service avail. from PQC,WSH. **Document type:** *Academic/Scholarly.*
Formerly: American Academy of Psychiatry and the Law. Bulletin (0091-634X)
Related titles: Microfiche ed.: (from WSH); Microfilm ed.: (from WSH); Microform ed.: (from PQC,WSH).
Indexed: ASCA, Abstr.Bk.Rev.Curr.Leg.Per., Abstr.Crim.& Pen., Adol.Ment.Hlth.Abstr., AgeLine, C.L.I., Crim.Just.Abstr., Curr.Cont., Dok.Arbeitsmed., Excerp.Med., Fam.Ind., Hlth.Ind., Ind.Med. (1997-), L.R.I. (Mar.1999-), Leg.Cont., Leg.Per. (coverage dropped), PsycInfo, Psychol.Abstr. (1974-), SSCI, e-psyche.
—BLDSC (4683.732750), CISTI, EMDOCS, GNLM, IDS, ingenta.
Published by: American Academy of Psychiatry and the Law, PO Box 30, Bloomfield, CT 06002-0030. TEL 860-242-5450, FAX 860-286-0787. Ed. Dr. Seymour L Halleck. Circ: 1,750.

AMERICAN ACADEMY OF PSYCHIATRY AND THE LAW. NEWSLETTER. see *LAW*

AMERICAN ASSOCIATION OF MENTAL HEALTH PROFESSIONALS IN CORRECTIONS. MONOGRAPH SERIES. see *CRIMINOLOGY AND LAW ENFORCEMENT*

616.8 USA ISSN 0895-8033
AMERICAN ASSOCIATION ON MENTAL RETARDATION. NEWS AND NOTES. Text in English. 1988. bi-m. USD 45 (effective 1999). back issues avail. **Document type:** *Newsletter.* **Description:** For individuals with special needs in the field of mental retardation.
Indexed: e-psyche.
—CCC.
Published by: American Association on Mental Retardation, 444 N Capitol St, Washington, DC 20001-1512. TEL 202-387-1968, 800-424-3688, FAX 202-387-2193. Ed. Margaret Seiter. Pub. M Dorren Croser. R&P Stephen Stidinger. Circ: 8,247.

616.89 150 USA ISSN 0065-860X
BF173.A2 CODEN: AMIAAO
AMERICAN IMAGO; studies in psychoanalysis and culture. Text in English. 1939. q. USD 35 to individuals; USD 107 to institutions (effective 2002). adv. bk.rev. bibl, charts, illus. index. back issues avail.; reprint service avail. from PSC,SCH. *Refereed.* **Document type:** *Academic/Scholarly.* **Description:** Contributors investigate the role of psychoanalysis in culture, science, and the arts, religion, philosophy, history and education.
Related titles: Microform ed.: (from PQC,PMC); Online - full text ed.: ISSN 1085-7931. USD 84.60 (effective 2000) (from Gale Group, Project MUSE, EBSCO Publishing, O C L C Online Computer Library Center, Inc., RoweCom Information Quest, Swets Blackwell, Institute for Scientific Information).
Indexed: ASCA, Abstr.Engl.Stud., Arts & Hum.Cit.Ind., BHA, Bibl.Engl.Lang.& Lit., Biog.Ind., Chem.Abstr., Child.Lit.Abstr., Curr.Cont., Film Lit.Ind. (1974-), IBR, IBZ, Ind.Med. (coverage dropped), Ind.Philos., M.L.A., MLA Intl.Bibl., Mag.Ind., Mid.East: Abstr.& Ind., P C I, PsycInfo, Psychoanal.Abstr., Psychol.Abstr. (1939-), R.G. (coverage dropped), Rel.Ind.One, Rel.Ind.Two, SSCI (coverage dropped), e-psyche.
—BLDSC (0819.300000), GNLM, IDS, Infotrieve, ingenta. **CCC.**
Published by: (Association for Applied Psychoanalysis), Johns Hopkins University Press, Journals Publishing Division, 2715 N Charles St, Baltimore, MD 21218-4363. TEL 410-516-6988, 800-548-1784, FAX 410-516-6968, sscher@mail.press.jhu.edu, http://www.press.jhu.edu/press/journals/aim. Ed. Peter L Rudnytsky. Adv. contact Anastasia Scherr. page USD 200; 4.75 x 7.5. Circ: 728.

616.804 USA ISSN 1086-508X
RC386.5 CODEN: AJETFB
AMERICAN JOURNAL OF ELECTRONEURODIAGNOSTIC TECHNOLOGY. Text in English. 1960. q. USD 40 domestic to individuals; USD 50 foreign to individuals; USD 80 domestic to institutions; USD 90 foreign to institutions (effective 2001). adv. bk.rev. charts, illus. index, cum.index. back issues avail. *Refereed.* **Document type:** *Trade.* **Description:** Features clinical and technical aspects of electroneurodiagnostics which includes EEG, evoked potentials, polysomnography, and nerve conduction studies and specialized applications.
Formerly (until 1996): American Journal of E E G Technology (0002-9238)
Related titles: Online - full text ed.: (from Institute for Scientific Information).
Indexed: Biol.Abstr., CINAHL, Eng.Ind., Excerp.Med., INSPEC (Sep.1971-Mar.1996, Jun.1996-), Neurosci.Cit.Ind., PsycInfo, Psychol.Abstr. (1967-), Ref.Zh., SSCI (coverage dropped), e-psyche.
—BLDSC (0824.430000), AskIEEE, CISTI, Ei, EMDOCS, GNLM, IDS, ingenta, KNAW.
Published by: American Society of Electroneurodiagnostic Technologists, Inc., Executive Office, 204 W Seventh, Carroll, IA 51401. TEL 712-792-2978, FAX 712-792-6962, info@aset.org, http://www.aset.org. Ed., R&P, Adv. contact Janet Ghigo TEL 304-456-4893. Circ: 3,500. **Subscr.to:** Allen Press Inc., PO Box 1897, Lawrence, KS 66044-8897.

AMERICAN JOURNAL OF FORENSIC PSYCHIATRY. see *MEDICAL SCIENCES—Forensic Sciences*

AMERICAN JOURNAL OF GERIATRIC PSYCHIATRY; official journal of the American Association for Geriatric Psychiatry. see *GERONTOLOGY AND GERIATRICS*

616.89 USA ISSN 0002-953X
RC321 CODEN: AJPSAO
AMERICAN JOURNAL OF PSYCHIATRY. Text in English. 1844. m. USD 128 domestic to individuals; USD 194 foreign to individuals Print & online eds.; USD 340 domestic to institutions .; USD 405 foreign to institutions Print & online eds. (effective 2001). adv. bk.rev. bibl, charts, illus. index. back issues avail.; reprint service avail. from PSC,SCH. *Refereed.* **Document type:** *Journal, Academic/Scholarly.* **Description:** Presents clinical research and discussion on current psychiatric issues for psychiatrists and other mental health professionals.
Formerly (until vol.78, 1921): American Journal of Insanity (1044-4815)
Related titles: CD-ROM ed.: (from Ovid Technologies, Inc.); Microform ed.: (from PQC,PMC); Online - full text ed.: (from ProQuest Information & Learning, HighWire Pr., Ovid Technologies, Inc., Northern Light Technology, Inc., EBSCO Publishing, LexisNexis, Gale Group, Factiva, Institute for Scientific Information).

M

Indexed: AIM, ASCA, ASSIA, Abstr.Anthropol., Abstr.Crim.& Pen., Abstr.Health Care Manage.Stud., Addic.Abstr., AgeLine, Agri.& Environ.Biotech.Abstr. (coverage dropped), Arts & Hum.Cit.Ind. (coverage dropped), Behav.Med.Abstr., Bibl.Asian Stud. (1972), Bibl.Dev.Med.& Child Neur., Biol.Abstr., Brit.Nur.Ind., CINAHL, C.I.S. Abstr., Chem.Abstr., Chic.Per.Ind., Crim.Just.Abstr., Curr.Adv.Ecol.Sci., Curr.Cont., Dairy Sci.Abstr., Dent.Ind., Derwent Biotech.Abstr., Environ.Sci.Poll.Mgmt., Excerp.Med., FAMLI, Fam.Ind., HRIS, Hosp.Lit.Ind., IBZ, INIS Atomind., Ind.Med. (1921-), Ind.Per.Art.Relat.Law, Ind.Sci.Rev., Indian Psychol.Abstr., Inpharma, Int.Nurs.Ind., Jrnl.Watch, Jrnl.Watch Psych., Jrnl.Watch Wom.Hlth., Lang.& Lang.Behav.Abstr., Med.Care Rev., Mid.East: Abstr.& Ind., NRN, Neurosci.Abstr., Neurosci.Cit.Ind., Nutr.Abstr., P C I, Past.Care & Couns.Abstr., Pharm.&Out.News, Pollut.Abstr., PsycInfo, Psychol.Abstr. (1928-), Psycscan C.P., Reac., Ref.Zh., Rel.Ind.One, Rel.Ind.Two, Risk Abstr., SOPODA, SSCI, Saf.Sci.Abstr., Sci.Cit.Ind., Soc.Sci.Ind. (Nov.1982-), Soc.Work Res.& Abstr., Sociol.Abstr., Sugar Ind.Abstr., e-psyche.
—BLDSC (0835.000000), CASDDS, CISTI, EMDOCS, GNLM, IDS, ingenta, KNAW. **CCC.**
Published by: (American Psychiatric Association), American Psychiatric Press, Inc., Journals Division, 1400 K St, N W, Ste 1101, Washington, DC 20005. TEL 202-682-6020, 800-368-5777, FAX 202-789-2648, 202-682-6016, appi@psych.org, http://ajp.psychiatryonline.org, http://www.psychiatryonline.org, http://www.appi.org. Ed. Nancy C Andreasen. adv.: B&W page USD 2,700, color page USD 3,900. Circ: 44,000.

AMERICAN JOURNAL OF PSYCHOANALYSIS. see *PSYCHOLOGY*

616.8 USA ISSN 0002-9564
RC321 CODEN: AJPTAR
AMERICAN JOURNAL OF PSYCHOTHERAPY. Text in English. 1946. q. USD 64 to individuals; USD 70 in Canada to individuals; USD 76 elsewhere to individuals; USD 91 to institutions; USD 98 in Canada to institutions; USD 103 elsewhere to institutions. adv. bk.rev. abstr, bibl. index, cum.index: 1941-1965. reprint service avail. from PSC,SCH. *Refereed.* **Document type:** *Academic/Scholarly.*
Related titles: Microform ed.: (from RPI); Online - full text ed.: (from ProQuest Information & Learning, Northern Light Technology, Inc., H. W. Wilson, Gale Group, Factiva, Institute for Scientific Information).
Indexed: ASCA, Abstr.Crim.& Pen., Adol.Ment.Hlth.Abstr., AgeLine, Arts & Hum.Cit.Ind. (coverage dropped), Bibl.Asian Stud. (1970), Biol.Abstr., CINAHL, Chem.Abstr., Curr.Adv.Ecol.Sci., Curr.Cont., Excerp.Med., Fam.Ind., INIS Atomind., Ind.Med. (1947-), Ind.Sci.Rev., Indian Psychol.Abstr., Int.Nurs.Ind., Jrnl.Watch Psych., Lang.& Lang.Behav.Abstr., Mid.East: Abstr.& Ind., P C I, PsycInfo, Psychol.Abstr. (1947-), Psycscan C.P., Ref.Zh., Rel.Ind.One, Rel.Ind.Two, SOPODA, SSCI, Sage Race Rel.Abstr., Sci.Cit.Ind. (coverage dropped), Soc.Sci.Ind. (Jan.1987-), Soc.Serv.Abstr., Soc.Work Res.& Abstr., Sociol.Abstr., e-psyche.
—BLDSC (0835.600000), CISTI, EMDOCS, GNLM, IDS, ingenta, KNAW.
Published by: Association for the Advancement of Psychotherapy, Belfer Education Center, 1300 Morris Park Ave, Rm 402, Bronx, NY 10461-1602. TEL 718-430-3503, FAX 718-430-8907, info@ajp.org, http://www.ajp.org. Ed. T Byram Karasu. R&P, Adv. contact Tina Bonanno. Circ: 5,000.

AMERICAN JOURNAL ON ADDICTIONS. see *DRUG ABUSE AND ALCOHOLISM*

616.858 USA ISSN 0895-8017
RC326 CODEN: AJMREA
AMERICAN JOURNAL ON MENTAL RETARDATION. Text in English. 1876. bi-m. USD 135; USD 150 elsewhere (effective 1999). adv. bk.rev. bibl, charts, illus, stat. index. back issues avail.; reprint service avail. from PSC,SCH. *Refereed.* **Description:** Current research on biological, behavioral and educational sciences in mental retardation and related developmental disabilities.
Formerly (until 1987): American Journal of Mental Deficiency (0002-9351)
Related titles: Microform ed.: (from PQC); Online - full text ed.: (from H. W. Wilson, Institute for Scientific Information).
Indexed: ASCA, Adol.Ment.Hlth.Abstr. (1940-), AgeLine, Behav.Med.Abstr., Bibl.Dev.Med.& Child Neur., Bibl.Ind., Biol.Abstr., Bk.Rev.Ind. (1980-), Brit.Nur.Ind., C.I.J.E., Chem.Abstr., Chic.Per.Ind., Child Devel.Abstr., Child.Bk.Rev.Ind. (1980-), Curr.Adv.Ecol.Sci., Curr.Cont., Dent.Ind., Educ.Admin.Abstr., Educ.Ind. (Nov.1987-), Except.Child Educ.Abstr., Excerp.Med., Fam.Ind., INIS Atomind., Ind.Med. (1987-), Ind.Sci.Rev., Int.Nurs.Ind., Lang.& Lang.Behav.Abstr., Mid.East: Abstr.& Ind., NRN, Neurosci.Cit.Ind., PsycInfo, Psychol.Abstr., Psycscan D.P., Rehabil.Lit., SOPODA, SSCI, Sci.Cit.Ind. (coverage dropped), Soc.Serv.Abstr., Soc.Work Res.& Abstr., Sociol.Abstr., Sp.Ed.Needs Abstr., e-psyche.
—BLDSC (0828.280000), CASDDS, CISTI, EMDOCS, GNLM, IDS, ingenta, KNAW. **CCC.**
Published by: American Association on Mental Retardation, 444 N Capitol St, Washington, DC 20001-1512. TEL 202-387-1968, 800-425-3688, FAX 202-387-2193, orders@allenpress.com, http://aamr.allenpress.com/aamronline/?request=get-static&name=ajmr-info, http://www.aamr.allenpress.com. Ed. Donald Routh. Pub. M Doreen Croser. R&P, Adv. contact Stephen Stidinger. B&W page USD 520. Circ: 11,600. **Subscr.to:** Allen Press Inc., PO Box 1897, Lawrence, KS 66044-8897. FAX 785-843-1275.

616.8 USA
AMERICAN NEUROMODULATION SOCIETY. NEWSLETTER. Text in English. q. USD 200 to membership (effective 2000). back issues avail. **Document type:** *Newsletter, Academic/Scholarly.* **Description:** Discusses news and topics in neuromodulation.
Related titles: Online - full content ed.: free.
Published by: American Neuromodulation Society, 6287 Cheshire Ln N, Minneapolis, MN 55311-4245. TEL 763-559-4108, FAX 763-559-4161, american@neuromodulation.org, http://www.neuromodulation.org/index.html.

AMERICAN PARKINSON DISEASE ASSOCIATION. NEWSLETTER. see *SOCIAL SERVICES AND WELFARE*

AMERICAN PSYCHIATRIC NURSES ASSOCIATION. JOURNAL. see *MEDICAL SCIENCES—Nurses And Nursing*

AMERICAN PSYCHOANALYTIC ASSOCIATION. JOURNAL. see *PSYCHOLOGY*

616.89 USA ISSN 0091-7389
AMERICAN PSYCHOPATHOLOGICAL ASSOCIATION. PROCEEDINGS OF THE ANNUAL MEETING. Text in English. 1945. a. price varies. reprint service avail. from PQC. **Document type:** *Proceedings.*
Indexed: e-psyche.
Published by: American Psychopathological Association, c/o Dr Ellen Frank, Western Psychiatric Institute & Clinic, 3811 O Hara, Pittsburgh, PA 15213. TEL 412-624-2383.

616.8 USA
AMERICAN PSYCHOPATHOLOGICAL ASSOCIATION SERIES. Text in English. 1978. irreg. price varies. reprint service avail. from PQC. *Refereed.* **Document type:** *Proceedings.*
Indexed: e-psyche.
Published by: (American Psychopathological Association), Lippincott Williams & Wilkins (Philadelphia) (Subsidiary of: Wolters Kluwer N.V.), 530 Walnut St, Philadelphia, PA 19106-3621. TEL 301-223-2300, 800-638-3030, FAX 301-223-2400.

616.8 USA
AMERICAN SOCIETY FOR ADOLESCENT PSYCHIATRY. NEWSLETTER. Text in English. 1967. q. USD 15 to membership. adv. bk.rev. stat. **Document type:** *Newsletter.* **Description:** Covers issues related to adolescent psychiatry.
Indexed: e-psyche.
Published by: American Society for Adolescent Psychiatry, PO Box 28218, Dallas, TX 75228. TEL 972-686-6166, FAX 972-613-5532. Ed., R&P Dr. Leonard Henschel TEL 718-849-6339. Adv. contact Frances Roton. Circ: 2,700.

573.84 USA ISSN 0066-0132
QP356.3
AMERICAN SOCIETY FOR NEUROCHEMISTRY. TRANSACTIONS. Text in English. 1970. a. USD 27.75; USD 30 foreign (effective 1998). adv. back issues avail. **Document type:** *Academic/Scholarly.* **Description:** Annual meeting of investigators in the American hemisphere in neurochemistry, neurobiology, and molecular biology.
Indexed: e-psyche.
—GNLM.
Published by: American Society for Neurochemistry, c/o Dr Bernard Haber, Ed, Univ of Texas Medical Branch, 301 University Blvd, MRB 2143, Galveston, TX 77555-1069. TEL 409-772-2108, FAX 409-772-2920. Pub., R&P, Adv. contact Bernard Haber. Circ: 1,500.

AMYLOID; international journal of experimental and clinical investigation. see *MEDICAL SCIENCES—Rheumatology*

616.3995 GBR ISSN 1466-0822
▼ **AMYOTROPHIC LATERAL SCLEROSIS AND OTHER MOTOR NEURON DISORDERS.** Text in English. 1999. 4/yr. GBP 85, USD 135 to individuals; GBP 200, USD 320 to institutions (effective 2002). bk.rev. index. back issues avail. **Document type:** *Journal, Academic/Scholarly.* **Description:** Covers new treatment research and management issues in ALS and related motor neuron diseases.
Related titles: Online - full content ed.: ISSN 1471-180X; Online - full text ed.: (from CatchWord Ltd., Institute for Scientific Information).
Indexed: Curr.Cont., Neurosci.Abstr.
—BLDSC (0859.841190), CatchWord.
Published by: Martin Dunitz Ltd. (Subsidiary of: Taylor & Francis Group), 7-9 Pratt St, London NW1 0AE, United Kingdom. TEL 44-20-7482-2202, FAX 44-20-7482-7088, info@dunitzco.global.co.uk, http://www.dunitz.co.uk. Ed. Michael Swash.

616.89 ESP ISSN 0213-0599
CODEN: APSIEL
ANALES DE PSIQUIATRIA. Text in Spanish; Abstracts in Spanish, English. 1984. 10/yr. ESP 8,000; USD 200 foreign (effective 2000). adv. abstr, bibl, illus, stat. back issues avail. *Refereed.* **Document type:** *Academic/Scholarly.*
Indexed: PsycInfo, Psychol.Abstr. (1992-), e-psyche.
—BLDSC (0890.170000), EMDOCS, GNLM, KNAW.
Published by: Aran Ediciones S.A., Castello, 128 1o, Madrid 28006, Spain. TEL 34-91-782-0030, FAX 34-91-561-5787, edita@grupoaran.com, http://www.grupoaran.com. Pub. Jose Jimenez. R&P Maria Dolores Linares TEL 34-1-7820035. Circ: 3,000.

ANALGESIA. see *MEDICAL SCIENCES—Anaesthesiology*

616.8 FRA ISSN 1253-1472
▼ **ANALYSE FREUDIENNE**; revue de l'Association Analyse Freudienne. Text in French. 2000. s-a. EUR 28 domestic; EUR 34 foreign (effective 2002).
Published by: (Association Analyse Freudienne), Editions Eres, 11 rue des Alouettes, Ramonville Saint-Agne 31520, France. TEL 33-05-61751576, FAX 33-05-61735289, eres@editions-eres.com. Eds. Claude Dumezil, JJ Leconte, Chantal Garipuy.

616.8 FRA ISSN 0768-7559
▼ **ANNALES DE PSYCHIATRIE.** Text in French. 2000. q. EUR 133 in Europe to institutions; USD 168 elsewhere to institutions (effective 2002). **Document type:** *Academic/Scholarly.*
Indexed: e-psyche.
—BLDSC (0994.800000), EMDOCS, GNLM, KNAW.
Published by: Elsevier Paris, Editions Scientifiques et Medicales (Subsidiary of: Reed Elsevier plc. group), 23 rue Linois, Paris 75015, France. http://www.elsevier.com/locate/anpsy. Circ: 3,000.

616.89 ITA ISSN 0003-4606
ANNALI DI FRENIATRIA E SCIENZE AFFINI. Text in Italian. 1888; N.S. 1993. s-a. ITL 60,000 to individuals (effective 1999); USD 80; ITL 80,000 to institutions (effective 1999). adv. bk.rev. abstr, bibl, charts, illus. index. **Description:** Contains bibliographic abstracts on the most debated subjects in psychiatry, materials on the courses available at the center, and results of research at the center and other institutes.
Indexed: Excerp.Med., e-psyche.
Published by: (Centro Studi e Ricerche in Psichiatria), Guido Gnocchi Editore, Via Annibale De Gasperis, 55, Naples, NA 80137, Italy. TEL 39-81-5524733, FAX 39-81-5518295, idelgno@tin.it, http://www.idelson-gnocchi.com. Ed. Carmine Munizza. Circ: 1,000.

M

616.8 USA ISSN 1040-1237
RC321 CODEN: APSYEZ
ANNALS OF CLINICAL PSYCHIATRY. Text in English. 1989. q. USD 352, EUR 351 to institutions for print or online ed.; USD 71, EUR 71 to individuals for print or online ed.; USD 422.40, EUR 421.20 to institutions for print & online eds. (effective 2002). *Refereed.* **Document type:** *Academic/Scholarly.* **Description:** Provides clinical practitioners with the results of current research into the phenomenology and treatment of psychiatric disorders.
Related titles: Online - full text ed.: NLG 704, EUR 319.50 to institutions; NLG 844.80 to institutions for online & print edition; EUR 383.40 to institutions for online & print edition (effective 2001) (from EBSCO Publishing, O C L C Online Computer Library Center, Inc., RoweCom Information Quest, Swets Blackwell, Kluwer Online).
Indexed: Excerp.Med., Ind.Med. (1989-), Inpharma, Int.Nurs.Ind., Pharm.&Out.News, PsycInfo, Psychol.Abstr. (1989-), Reac., Sociol.Abstr., e-psyche.
—BLDSC (1040.245000), CISTI, EMDOCS, GNLM, Infotrieve, ingenta, KNAW. **CCC.**
Published by: (American Academy of Clinical Psychiatrists), Kluwer Academic - Plenum Publishers (Subsidiary of: Wolters Kluwer N.V.), 233 Spring St, New York, NY 10013-1578. TEL 212-620-8000, 800-221-9369, FAX 212-463-0742, services@wkap.nl, http://www.wkap.nl/journalhome.htm/1040-1237. Ed. Dr. Charles L Rich. R&P Rose Luongo TEL 781-871-6311.

616.8 USA ISSN 0364-5134
RC321 CODEN: ANNED3
ANNALS OF NEUROLOGY. Text in English. 1977. m. USD 370 per issue in United States; USD 370 per issue in Canada & Mexico; USD 499 per issue elsewhere; USD 389 combined subscription per issue in United States for print and online eds.; USD 389 combined subscription per issue in Canada & Mexico for print and online eds.; USD 518 combined subscription per issue elsewhere for print and online eds.; for print and online eds. (effective 2002). adv. bk.rev. abstr, charts, illus, stat. index. back issues avail.; reprint service avail. from PQC. *Refereed.* **Document type:** *Academic/Scholarly.* **Description:** Contains original articles on research and clinical advances, brief communications, neurological progress, and editorials.
Related titles: Microform ed.: (from PQC); Online - full text ed.: ISSN 1531-8249. USD 370 in United States; USD 370 in Canada & Mexico; USD 370 elsewhere (effective 2002) (from Wiley InterScience, Institute for Scientific Information).
Indexed: ASCA, Abstr.Inter.Med., Behav.Med.Abstr., Bibl.Dev.Med.& Child Neur., Biol.Abstr., Biol.Dig., Chem.Abstr., Chem.Indus.Notes, Chem.Titles, Curr.Adv.Ecol.Sci., Curr.Cont., Dent.Ind., Diab.Cont., Dok.Arbeitsmed., Excerp.Med., INIS Atomind., Ind.Med. (1977-), Ind.Sci.Rev., Inpharma, Int.Abstr.Biol.Sci., Jrnl.Watch Neuro., Neurosci.Abstr. (coverage dropped), Neurosci.Cit.Ind., Nutr.Abstr., Pharm.&Out.News, Protozool.Abstr., PsycInfo, Psychol.Abstr. (1989-), Reac., Rev.Appl.Entomol., Rev.Plant Path., Risk Abstr., SSCI (coverage dropped), Sci.Cit.Ind., THA, e-psyche.
—BLDSC (1043.140000), CASDDS, CISTI, EMDOCS, GNLM, IDS, ingenta, KNAW.
Published by: (American Neurological Association), John Wiley & Sons, Inc., Journals (Subsidiary of: Wiley InterScience), 605 Third Ave, New York, NY 10158. TEL 212-850-6645, FAX 212-850-6021, subinfo@jwiley.com, uscs-wis@wiley.com, http://www.wiley.com. adv.: B&W page USD 990, color page USD 2,235; trim 11 x 8.25. Circ: 7,372. **Subscr. addr. outside the Americas:** John Wiley & Sons Ltd., Baffins Ln, Chichester, Sussex PO19 IUD, United Kingdom. TEL 44-1243-779777, FAX 44-1243-843232, cs-journals@wiley.co.uk, http://www.wiley.co.uk. **Co-sponsor:** Child Neurology Society.

616.89 USA
ANNUAL EDITIONS: DEVIANT BEHAVIOR. Text in English. 1996. a. USD 12.25. illus. **Document type:** *Academic/Scholarly.*
Indexed: e-psyche.
Published by: Dushkin - McGraw-Hill, Sluice Dock, Guilford, CT 06437-9989. TEL 203-453-4351, FAX 203-453-6000. Ed. Lawrence M Salinger.

ANNUAL OF PSYCHOANALYSIS. see *PSYCHOLOGY*

618.928 USA ISSN 0066-4030
RJ499.A1
ANNUAL PROGRESS IN CHILD PSYCHIATRY AND CHILD DEVELOPMENT*. Text in English. 1968. a. price varies. *Refereed.* **Document type:** *Academic/Scholarly.* **Description:** New developments and trends in child psychiatry and development for professionals working with normal and disturbed children.
Indexed: Biol.Abstr., PsycInfo, Psychol.Abstr. (1976-), e-psyche.
—BLDSC (1091.400000), CISTI, GNLM, ingenta.
Published by: Brunner - Routledge (Subsidiary of: Taylor & Francis Group), 325 Chestnut St, Ste 800, Philadelphia, PA 19106. TEL 215-269-0400, FAX 215-269-0363, postmaster@bmpub.com.

616.8 USA ISSN 0147-006X
QP351 CODEN: ARNSD5
ANNUAL REVIEW OF NEUROSCIENCE. Text in English. 1978. a. USD 60 domestic to individuals; USD 65 foreign to individuals; USD 120 domestic to institutions; USD 130 foreign to institutions (effective 1999). bibl. index, cum.index. back issues avail.; reprints avail. *Refereed.* **Document type:** *Academic/Scholarly.* **Description:** Reviews filter and synthesize primary research to identify the principal contributions in neuroscience.
Related titles: Microfilm ed.: (from PQC); Online - full text ed.: (from HighWire Pr., EBSCO Publishing, Institute for Scientific Information).
Indexed: ASCA, Anim.Behav.Abstr., Aqua.Sci.& Fish.Abstr., Biol.& Agr.Ind. (Jan.1996-), Biol.Abstr., Biotech.& Bioeng.Abstr., Cal.Tiss.Abstr., Chem.Abstr., Chem.Indus.Notes, Chem.Titles, Chemorec.Abstr., Comput.Abstr., Curr.Adv.Ecol.Sci., Curr.Cont., Excerp.Med., INSPEC (coverage dropped), Ind.Med. (1978-), Ind.Sci.Rev., Inpharma, Int.Abstr.Biol.Sci., Neurosci.Abstr., Neurosci.Cit.Ind., PsycInfo, Psychol.Abstr. (1978-), Reac., SSCI (coverage dropped), Sci.Cit.Ind., Sport Fish.Abstr., THA, Zoo.Rec., e-psyche.
—BLDSC (1523.350000), ADONIS, CASDDS, CISTI, GNLM, IDS, ingenta, KNAW. **CCC.**
Published by: Annual Reviews Inc., 4139 El Camino Way, Box 10139, Palo Alto, CA 94303-0139. TEL 650-493-4400, 800-523-8635, FAX 650-424-0910, service@annurev.org; orders@allenpress.com, http://www.biomedical.annualreviews.org. Ed. Samuel Gubins. R&P Jeanne Kunz. **Subscr.to:** Allen Press Inc., PO Box 1897, Lawrence, KS 66044-8897.

616.8 JPN
ANNUAL REVIEW SHINKEI/ANNUAL REVIEW. NERVE. Text in Japanese. 1988. a. JPY 9,345 (effective 1998). adv. **Document type:** *Academic/Scholarly.*
Indexed: e-psyche.
Published by: Chugai Igakusha, 62 Yarai-cho, Shinjuku-ku, Tokyo 162-0805, Japan. R&P M Takahashi. Adv. contact M. Takahashi.

616.85 AUS ISSN 1328-7761
ANXIETY DISORDERS FOUNDATION OF AUSTRALIA. NEWSLETTER. Text in English. 1996. q. **Document type:** *Newsletter.*
Media: Online - full text.
Published by: Anxiety Disorders Foundation of Australia, NSw Branch, Shopping World, PO Box 6198, North Sydney, NSW 2060, Australia. http://www.ocs.mq.edu.au/~abaillie/adfa.html#Newsletter.

616.8 GBR ISSN 0268-7038
RC425
APHASIOLOGY. Text in English. 1987. m. GBP 331, USD 547 to individuals; GBP 786, USD 1,297 to institutions (effective 2002). adv. bk.rev. bibl, charts, illus. back issues avail. *Refereed.* **Document type:** *Academic/Scholarly.* **Description:** Information on all aspects of brain damage-related language problems for neurologists, speech therapists, psychologists in universities, and hospitals and clinics.
Related titles: Online - full text ed.: ISSN 1464-5041 (from CatchWord Ltd., EBSCO Publishing, O C L C Online Computer Library Center, Inc., RoweCom Information Quest, Swets Blackwell, Institute for Scientific Information).
Indexed: AMED, ASCA, Bibl.Ling., Curr.Cont., Excerp.Med., Inpharma, Lang.& Lang.Behav.Abstr. (1987-), Ling.Abstr., Neurosci.Cit.Ind., PsycInfo, Psychol.Abstr. (1992-), Reac., Russ.Acad.Sci.Bibl., SOPODA, SSCI (coverage dropped), Sociol.Abstr., e-psyche.
—BLDSC (1567.923000), CatchWord, EMDOCS, GNLM, IDS, Infotrieve, ingenta, KNAW. **CCC.**
Published by: Psychology Press (Subsidiary of: Taylor & Francis Group), 27 Church Rd, Hove, E Sussex BN3 2FA, United Kingdom. TEL 44-1273-207411, FAX 44-1273-205612, information@psypress.co.uk, http://www.psypress.co.uk. Eds. C Code, Robert Marshall. **Subscr. addr. in N America:** Psychology Press, Journals Customer Service, Taylor & Francis Group, 325 Chestnut St, Philadelphia, PA 19106. TEL 800-354-1420, FAX 215-625-8914, info@taylorandfrancis.com, http://www.psypress.com; **Subswcr. addr. outside N America:** Journals Customer Service, Taylor & Francis Group, Rankine Rd, Basingstoke, Hants RG24 8PR, United Kingdom. TEL 44-1256-813002, FAX 44-1256-479438, enquiry@tandf.co.uk.

616 616.8 USA ISSN 0908-4282
CODEN: ANEUF8
APPLIED NEUROPSYCHOLOGY. Text in English. 1993. q. USD 90 in US & Canada to individuals; USD 120 elsewhere to individuals; USD 340 in US & Canada to institutions; USD 370 elsewhere to institutions (effective 2002). adv. *Refereed.* **Document type:** *Journal, Academic/Scholarly.* **Description:** Publishes clinical neuropsychological articles concerning assessment, brain functioning and neuroimaging, and neuropsychological treatment and rehabilitation.
Related titles: Online - full text ed.: ISSN 1532-4826. USD 81 to individuals; USD 306 to institutions (effective 2002) (from EBSCO Publishing, O C L C Online Computer Library Center, Inc., RoweCom Information Quest, CatchWord Ltd., Swets Blackwell).
Indexed: Environ.Sci.Poll.Mgmt., Ind.Med. (1994-), Pollut.Abstr., PsycInfo, Risk Abstr., Saf.Sci.Abstr., e-psyche.
—BLDSC (1576.231000), CatchWord, GNLM, Infotrieve. **CCC.**
Published by: Lawrence Erlbaum Associates, Inc., 10 Industrial Ave, Mahwah, NJ 07430-2262. TEL 201-760-3735, 800-926-6579, FAX 201-236-0072, journals@erlbaum.com, http://www.erlbaum.com/Journals/journals/AN/an.htm. Eds. Barbara P Uzzell, Nick A DeFilippis. adv.: page USD 275; trim 7 x 10.

APPLIED PSYCHOLINGUISTICS; psychological studies of language processes. see *LINGUISTICS*

616.8 362.2 AUS
ARAFMI NEWS; providing support for carers of people with mental disorders. Text in English. 1982. q. AUD 15 (effective 2001). bk.rev. back issues avail. **Document type:** *Newsletter.*
Published by: Arafmi Queensland Inc., PO Box 248, New Farm, QLD 4005, Australia. TEL 61-7-3254-1881, FAX 61-7-3254-1736, arafmib@lrvnet.org.au. Ed. Barbara Kimber.

THE ARC INSIGHT. see *SOCIAL SERVICES AND WELFARE*

612.8 ITA ISSN 0003-9829
CODEN: AIBLAS
ARCHIVES ITALIENNES DE BIOLOGIE; journal of neuroscience. Text in English. 1882. q., latest vol.139, 2001. ITL 200,000 domestic; ITL 230,000 foreign (effective 2001). adv. bk.rev. abstr, bibl, charts, illus. index. back issues avail. *Refereed.* **Document type:** *Journal, Academic/Scholarly.* **Description:** Publishes basic research work in neuroanatomy, neurophysiology, neurobiology, neurochemistry and behavioral science.
Related titles: Microfiche ed.: (from BHP); Online - full text ed.: (from Institute for Scientific Information).
Indexed: ASCA, Anim.Behav.Abstr., Aqua.Sci.& Fish.Abstr., Biol.Abstr., Chem.Abstr., Curr.Cont., Excerp.Med., Helminthol.Abstr., Ind.Med. (1882-), Ind.Sci.Rev., Inpharma, Int.Abstr.Biol.Sci., Neurosci.Abstr. (coverage dropped), Neurosci.Cit.Ind., Nutr.Abstr., Pharm.&Out.News, Phys.Ber., Psychol.Abstr., Reac., Sci.Cit.Ind., e-psyche.
—BLDSC (1637.200000), CASDDS, CISTI, EMDOCS, GNLM, IDS, ingenta, Linda Hall.
Published by: Universita degli Studi di Pisa, Dipart. di Fisiologia e Biochimica, Via San Zeno, 31, Pisa, PI 56127, Italy. TEL 39-050-553517, FAX 39-050-552163. Ed., R&P Ottavio Pompeiano TEL 39-050-554070. Circ: 300 (paid and controlled).

M

616.8 150 GBR ISSN 0887-6177
ARCHIVES OF CLINICAL NEUROPSYCHOLOGY. Text in English. 1986. 8/yr. EUR 188 in Europe to qualified personnel; JPY 24,900 in Japan to qualified personnel; USD 210 elsewhere to qualified personnel; EUR 460 in Europe to institutions; JPY 61,100 in Japan to institutions; USD 515 elsewhere to institutions (effective 2002). back issues avail. *Refereed.* **Document type:** *Academic/Scholarly.* **Description:** Publishes original contributions dealing with psychological aspects of the etiology, diagnosis and treatment of disorders arising out of dysfunction of the central nervous system.
Related titles: Microfilm ed.: (from PQC); Online - full text ed.: (from ingenta, Swets Blackwell, ScienceDirect, Institute for Scientific Information).
Indexed: ASCA, AgeLine, Child Devel.Abstr., Curr.Cont., Excerp.Med., Fam.Ind., Neuropsych.Abstr., Neurosci.Cit.Ind., PsycInfo, Psychol.Abstr. (1986-), SSCI, e-psyche.
—BLDSC (1634.090000), CISTI, EMDOCS, GNLM, IDS, ingenta, KNAW. **CCC.**
Published by: (National Academy of Neuropsychology USA), Pergamon (Subsidiary of: Elsevier Science), The Boulevard, Langford Ln, East Park, Kidlington, Oxford OXB 1GB, United Kingdom. FAX 44-1865-843010, nlinfo-f@elsevier/nl; usinfo-f@elsevier.com; forinfo-kyf04035@niftyserve.or.jp, http://www.elsevier.com/locate/archclinneuro, http://www.elsevier.nl/. Ed. Cecil Reynolds. **Subscr. in Australasia and the Far East to:** Elsevier Science (Singapore) Pte Ltd, No.1 Temasek Ave, 17-01 Millenia Tower, Singapore 039192, Singapore. TEL 65-434-3727, FAX 65-337-2230; **Subscr. in the Americas to:** Elsevier Science, PO Box 945, New York, NY 10159-0945. TEL 212-633-3730, FAX 212-633-3680, usinfo-f@elsevier.com, http://www.elsevier.com; **Subscr. to:** Elsevier Science BV, PO Box 211, Amsterdam 1000 AE, Netherlands. TEL 31-20-485-3757, FAX 31-20-485-3432, nlinfo-f@elsevier.nl, http://www.elsevier.nl.

616.89 USA ISSN 0003-990X
RC321 CODEN: ARGPAQ
ARCHIVES OF GENERAL PSYCHIATRY. Text in English. 1959. m. USD 175 to individuals; USD 325 in North America to institutions; USD 425 to institutions Central & S. America; GBP 275 elsewhere to institutions (effective 2001). adv. bk.rev. bibl, charts, illus. index. back issues avail.; reprints avail. *Refereed.* **Document type:** *Academic/Scholarly.* **Description:** Publishes clinically relevant science in psychiatry. Includes original articles dealing with the biological origin of mental disorders and pharmaceutical therapy.
Related titles: CD-ROM ed.: (from Ovid Technologies, Inc.); Microform ed.: (from PQC); Online - full text ed.: (from The Dialog Corporation, Gale Group, Ovid Technologies, Inc., EBSCO Publishing, Institute for Scientific Information).
Indexed: AIM, AMED, ASCA, Abstr.Health Care Manage.Stud., Addic.Abstr., Adol.Ment.Hlth.Abstr., AgeLine, Agri.& Environ.Biotech.Abstr. (coverage dropped), Behav.Med.Abstr., Bibl.Dev.Med.& Child Neur., Biol.Abstr., Chem.Abstr., Chem.Indus.Notes, Chem.Titles, Chic.Per.Ind., Child Devel.Abstr., Crim.Just.Abstr., Curr.Adv.Ecol.Sci., Curr.Cont., Dent.Ind., Derwent Biotech.Abstr., Excerp.Med., Fam.Ind., IMFL, INIS Atomind., I.P.A., Ind.Med. (1960-), Ind.Per.Art.Relat.Law, Ind.Sci.Rev., Inpharma, Jrnl.Watch Psych., Med.& Surg.Dermat., Mid.East: Abstr.& Ind., NRN, Neurosci.Cit.Ind., Nutr.Abstr., Pharm.&Out.News, PsycInfo, Psychol.Abstr. (1959-), Psycscan C.P., Reac., Risk Abstr., SSCI, Sci.Cit.Ind., e-psyche.
—BLDSC (1634.350000), CASDDS, CISTI, EMDOCS, GNLM, IDS, ingenta, KNAW. **CCC.**
Published by: American Medical Association, 515 N State St, P O Box 10946, Chicago, IL 60610-0946. http://www.archgenpsychiatry.com. Ed. Jack D Barchas. R&P Ada Jimenez Walker. Circ: 38,500.

616.8 016 USA ISSN 0003-9942
RC321 CODEN: ARNEAS
ARCHIVES OF NEUROLOGY. Text in English. 1919. m. USD 350 in North America to institutions; USD 450 to institutions Central & S. America; GBP 295 elsewhere to institutions (effective 2001). adv. bk.rev. charts, illus. index. back issues avail.; reprints avail. *Refereed.* **Document type:** *Academic/Scholarly.* **Description:** Publishes original contributions on all areas of neurology.
Related titles: CD-ROM ed.: (from Ovid Technologies, Inc.); Microform ed.: (from PMC,PQC); Online - full text ed.: (from The Dialog Corporation, Gale Group, Ovid Technologies, Inc., EBSCO Publishing, Institute for Scientific Information).
Indexed: AIDS Abstr., AIM, ASCA, Abstr.Inter.Med., Agri.& Environ.Biotech.Abstr. (coverage dropped), Behav.Med.Abstr., Bibl.Dev.Med.& Child Neur., Biol.Abstr., CINAHL, Chem.Abstr., Curr.Adv.Cancer Res., Curr.Adv.Ecol.Sci., Curr.Adv.Gen.& Molec.Biol., Curr.Cont., Curr.Ind.Stat., Dent.Ind., Derwent Biotech.Abstr., Dok.Arbeitsmed., Excerp.Med., INIS Atomind., Ind.Med. (1960-), Ind.Sci.Rev., Inpharma, Int.Abstr.Biol.Sci., Jrnl.Watch Neuro., Jrnl.Watch Psych., METADEX, Med.& Surg.Dermat., Neurosci.Abstr. (coverage dropped), Neurosci.Cit.Ind., Nutr.Abstr., Pharm.&Out.News, PsycInfo, Psychol.Abstr. (1950-), Reac., Rev.Med.& Vet.Mycol., SSCI (coverage dropped), Sci.Cit.Ind., So.Pac.Per.Ind., THA, e-psyche.
—BLDSC (1638.400000), CASDDS, CISTI, EMDOCS, GNLM, IDS, ingenta, KNAW. **CCC.**
Published by: American Medical Association, 515 N State St, P O Box 10946, Chicago, IL 60610-0946. ama-subs@ama-assn.org, http://www.archneurol.com. Ed. Roger N Rosenberg. R&P Ada Jimenez Walker. Adv. contact John L Reeves. Circ: 17,500.

ARCHIVES OF PSYCHIATRIC NURSING. see *MEDICAL SCIENCES—Nurses And Nursing*

616.8 150 POL ISSN 1509-2046
▼ **ARCHIVES OF PSYCHIATRY AND PSYCHOTHERAPY.** Text and summaries in English. 1999. q. PLZ 100 domestic to individuals; USD 70 to individuals European Union and North America; USD 25 elsewhere to individuals; PLZ 200 domestic to institutions; USD 120 to institutions European Union and North America; USD 40 elsewhere to institutions (effective 2002). adv. abstr, bibl. 80 p./no. 1 cols./p. back issues avail. *Refereed.* **Document type:** *Academic/Scholarly.* **Description:** Publishes clinical, experimental, theoretical papers and case reports on psychiatry and psychotherapy.
Published by: Polskie Towarzystwo Psychiatryczne, Ul Lenartowicza 14, Krakow 31138, Poland. TEL 48-12-6331203, FAX 48-12-6334067, psych@kom-red-wyd-ptp.com.pl, http://www.kom-red-wyd-ptp.com.pl/2en.html. Ed., Pub., R&P Jerzy W Aleksandrowicz. Adv. contact Magdalena Sikora.

616.89 ITA
ARCHIVIO DI PSICHIATRIA GENERALE; l'ospedale psichiatrico. Text in Italian; Summaries in English. 1903. 3/yr. ITL 90,000, USD 150 (effective 1999).
Former titles (until 1990): Rivista l'Ospedale Psichiatrico; (until 1960): Ospedale Psichiatrico (0048-2285)
Indexed: e-psyche.
—CISTI, GNLM.
Published by: Casa Editrice Idelson, Via Annibale De Gasperis, 55, Naples, NA 80137, Italy. TEL 39-81-5524733, FAX 39-81-5518295, idelgno@tin.it, http://www.idelson-gnocchi.com. Eds. Alessandro Fiorillo, Franco Rinaldi.

616.8 364 ECU ISSN 0004-0541
ARCHIVOS DE CRIMINOLOGIA, NEURO-PSIQUIATRIA Y DISCIPLINAS CONEXAS. Text in Spanish. 1964 (vol.12). q. ECS 3,000, USD 5 per issue. bk.rev. abstr, bibl, charts, illus, stat. index.
Related titles: Microfilm ed.
Indexed: Biol.Abstr., e-psyche.
Published by: Universidad Central del Ecuador, Instituto de Criminologia, Apdo 3663, Quito, Pichincha, Ecuador. TEL 542-971. Ed. Dr. Hernando Rosero Cueva. Circ: 1,200.

616.8 MEX ISSN 1028-5938
ARCHIVOS DE NEUROCIENCIAS/ARCHIVES OF NEUROSCIENCES. Text in Spanish. 1966. q. MXP 200 to individuals; MXP 250 to institutions; USD 50 foreign; MXP 50 newsstand/cover (effective 2000). adv. bk.rev. *Refereed.* **Description:** Includes articles and research work on neurosciences.
Former titles (until 1995): Instituto Nacional de Neurologia y Neurocirugia. Archivos (0187-4705); (until 1980): Instituto Nacional de Neurologia. Revista
Indexed: Ind.Med. (coverage dropped), Ref.Zh., e-psyche.
—BLDSC (1655.451000), CISTI, KNAW.
Published by: Instituto Nacional de Neurologia y Neurocirugia, INSURGENTES SUR 3877, Col La Fama, Mexico City, DF 14269, Mexico. TEL 52-5-6064532, FAX 52-5-6063295, arcneuro@liceaga.facmed.unam.mx. Ed. Humberto Mateos Gomez. Pub., Adv. contact Yazmin Reyes Rodriguez. Circ: 2,000.

616.8 ESP ISSN 1576-0367
CODEN: ARNBBK
ARCHIVOS DE PSIQUIATRIA✱. Text in Spanish; Summaries in English. 1920. bi-m. ESP 4,500, USD 80.
Formerly (until 1999): Archivos de Neurobiologia (0004-0576)
Related titles: Supplement: Archivos de Neurobiologia. Suplemento. ISSN 1132-6166.
Indexed: Biol.Abstr., Dent.Ind., Excerp.Med., Ind.Med. (until 1992, dropped), Ind.Med.Esp., Lang.& Lang.Behav.Abstr., Neurosci.Cit.Ind., Psychol.Abstr. (1966-199?), SOPODA, SSCI (coverage dropped), Sociol.Abstr., Yrbk.Assoc.Educ.& Rehab.Blind, e-psyche.
—CINDOC, CISTI, GNLM, IDS, Infotrieve. **CCC.**
Published by: Editorial Garsi S.A. (Subsidiary of: Grupo Masson), Juan Bravo, 46, Madrid 28006, Spain. TEL 34-1-4021212. Ed. V Rodriguez Lafora. Circ: 1,000.

616.8 ITA ISSN 1120-866X
ARGOMENTI DI NEUROLOGIA. Text in Italian. 1991. 6/yr. ITL 24,000 (effective 1999). **Document type:** *Proceedings.*
Indexed: e-psyche.
Published by: Masson S.p.A., Divisione Periodici, Via F.lli Bressan 2, Milan, MI 20126, Italy. TEL 39-2-270741, FAX 39-2-27074210. Ed. Nicola Canal. adv.: B&W page ITL 4,600,000, color page ITL 6,600,000; trim 265 x 195. Circ: 6,000.

616.89 BRA ISSN 0004-282X
CODEN: ANPIAM
ARQUIVOS DE NEURO-PSIQUIATRIA. Text in Portuguese, English. 1943. q. USD 80 (effective 2001 - 2002). adv. bk.rev. abstr, bibl, charts. index, cum.index: 1943-1999. back issues avail. *Refereed.* **Document type:** *Journal, Academic/Scholarly.* **Description:** Publishes original and refereed articles on science and technology covering medical fields of neurology, neurosciences, and psychiatry.
Related titles: CD-ROM ed.; E-mail ed.; Online - full text ed.: (from SciELO, Institute for Scientific Information).
Indexed: ASCA, Biol.Abstr., Dent.Ind., Excerp.Med., INIS Atomind., Ind.Med. (1943-), Int.Nurs.Ind., Neurosci.Cit.Ind., PsycInfo, Psychol.Abstr. (1943-), Ref.Zh., e-psyche.
—BLDSC (1695.630000), CISTI, EMDOCS, GNLM, IDS, KNAW. **CCC.**
Published by: (Academia Brasileira de Neurologia/Brazilian Academy of Neurology), Associacao Arquivos de Neuro-Psiquiatria Dr. Oswaldo Lange, Praca Amadeu Amaral, 47/33, B Vista, Sao Paulo, SP 01327-010, Brazil. TEL 55-11-2876600, FAX 55-11-2898879, arqneuro@sti.com.br. Ed. Dr. Antonio Spina-Franca. R&P Adriana Machado. Adv. contact Marilia Spina-Franca. Circ: 1,700 (paid); 200 (controlled).

616.8 150 BRA ISSN 0103-0809
RA790.7.S25
ARQUIVOS DE SAUDE MENTAL DO ESTADO DE SAO PAULO. Text in Portuguese; Summaries in English. 1924. a. per issue exchange basis. bk.rev. charts, illus. *Refereed.* **Document type:** *Academic/Scholarly.*
Formerly (until 1987): Sao Paulo. Coordenadoria de Saude Mental. Arquivos (0101-1693)
Related titles: ♦ Supplement: Arquivos de Saude Mental do Estado de Sao Paulo. Suplemento. ISSN 0103-0817.
Indexed: e-psyche.
Published by: Biblioteca do Hospital de Juqueri, Franco da Rocha E.F.S.J., Franco Da Rocha, SP 07780-000, Brazil. TEL 55-11-432-5111 ext. 135, FAX 55-11-432-5444, TELEX 11-79736. Ed. Dr. Maria Tereza G Freire. Circ: 1,500.

616.5 BRA ISSN 0103-0817
ARQUIVOS DE SAUDE MENTAL DO ESTADO DE SAO PAULO. SUPLEMENTO. Text in Portuguese. 1987. a.
Related titles: ♦ Supplement to: Arquivos de Saude Mental do Estado de Sao Paulo. ISSN 0103-0809.
Published by: Biblioteca do Hospital de Juqueri, Franco da Rocha E.F.S.J., Franco Da Rocha, SP 07780-000, Brazil. TEL 55-11-432-5111 ext. 135, FAX 55-11-432-5444.

ASSESSMENT. see *PSYCHOLOGY*

ASSOCIATION FOR APPLIED PSYCHOPHYSIOLOGY AND BIOFEEDBACK. PROCEEDINGS OF THE ANNUAL MEETING. see *PSYCHOLOGY*

ASSOCIATION FOR CHILD PSYCHOANALYSIS. NEWSLETTER. see *CHILDREN AND YOUTH—About*

610 USA ISSN 0091-7443
CODEN: RPARA5
ASSOCIATION FOR RESEARCH IN NERVOUS AND MENTAL DISEASE. RESEARCH PUBLICATIONS. Text in English. a. price varies. reprint service avail. from PQC. *Refereed.* **Document type:** *Proceedings.*
Indexed: Biol.Abstr., Chem.Abstr., Chem.Indus.Notes, Chem.Titles, Curr.Cont. (coverage dropped), Dent.Ind., INIS Atomind., Ind.Med. (coverage dropped), e-psyche.

M

—BLDSC (7755.800000), CASDDS, CISTI, GNLM, ingenta, KNAW.
Published by: (Association for Research in Nervous and Mental Disease), Lippincott Williams & Wilkins (Philadelphia) (Subsidiary of: Wolters Kluwer N.V.), 530 Walnut St, Philadelphia, PA 19106-3621. TEL 301-223-2300, 800-638-3030, FAX 301-223-2400.

616.858 USA
ATTENTION!. Text in English. bi-m. USD 45 to members (effective 2000).
Indexed: e-psyche.
Published by: Children and Adults with Attention Deficit - Hyperactivity Disorders, 8181 Professional Pl., Ste. 201, Landover, MD 20785-2226. TEL 301-306-7070, 800-233-4050, FAX 301-306-7090, http://www.chadd.org.

610 016 USA ISSN 0271-1311
AUDIO-DIGEST PSYCHIATRY. Text in English. 1971. s-m. USD 168 (effective 2000). *Refereed.*
Media: Audio cassette/tape.
Indexed: e-psyche.
Published by: Audio-Digest Foundation (Subsidiary of: California Medical Association), 1577 E Chevy Chase Dr, Glendale, CA 91206. TEL 213-245-8505, 800-423-2308, FAX 818-240-7379, 800-845-4375. Ed. Claron L Oakley.

AUSTRALASIAN JOURNAL OF PSYCHOTHERAPY. see *PSYCHOLOGY*

616.8 AUS ISSN 1039-8562
RC451.A788 CODEN: AUPSF4
AUSTRALASIAN PSYCHIATRY. Text in English. 1983. q. AUD 111 domestic to individuals paper & online eds. combined; AUD 101 in New Zealand to individuals paper & online eds. combined; USD 102 elsewhere to individuals paper & online eds. combined; AUD 123 domestic to individuals paper & online eds. combined; AUD 112 in New Zealand to individuals paper & online eds. combined; USD 113 elsewhere to individuals paper & online eds. combined (effective 2001). adv. bk.rev. back issues avail.; reprints avail. **Document type:** *Academic/Scholarly, Trade.* **Description:** Discusses issues of interest to psychiatrists practicing in Australia and New Zealand and reports news of the College.
Related titles: Online - full text ed.: ISSN 1440-1665. AUD 100 domestic to individuals; AUD 91 in New Zealand to individuals; USD 92 elsewhere to individuals (effective 2001) (from EBSCO Publishing, O C L C Online Computer Library Center, Inc., RoweCom Information Quest, ingenta, Munksgaard & Blackwell Science's Synergy, Swets Blackwell).
Indexed: ASSIA, Aus.P.A.I.S. (Coverage Dropped), Excerp.Med., SOPODA, Sociol.Abstr., e-psyche.
Published by: (Royal Australian and New Zealand College of Psychiatrists), Blackwell Science Asia Pty Ltd, PO Box 378, Carlton South, VIC 3053, Australia. TEL 61-3-9347-0300, FAX 61-3-9347-5001, info@blacksci-asia.com.au, http://www.blacksci.co.uk. Ed. Harry Minas. R&P Chris Hum. Adv. contact Kathryn O'Brien. B&W page AUD 1,045, color page AUD 1,947; trim 210 x 297. Circ: 3,300.

616.8 610.73 AUS ISSN 1324-3780
AUSTRALIAN AND NEW ZEALAND JOURNAL OF MENTAL HEALTH NURSING. Text in English. 1980. q. AUD 105 domestic to individuals; AUD 95 in New Zealand to individuals; USD 95 elsewhere to individuals; AUD 264 domestic to institutions; AUD 240 in New Zealand to institutions; USD 235 elsewhere to institutions; AUD 116 domestic to individuals paper & online eds. combned; AUD 105 in New Zealand to individuals paper& online eds. combined; USD 105 elsewhere to individuals paper & online eds. combined; AUD 291 domestic to institutions paper & online eds. combined; AUD 264 in New Zealand to institutions paper & online eds. combined; USD 259 elsewhere to institutions paper & online eds. combined (effective 2001). adv. *Refereed.* **Document type:** *Journal, Academic/Scholarly, Trade.* **Description:** Examines developments and trends in mental health nursing.
Former titles (until 1992): Australian Journal of Mental Health Nursing (1035-8374); (until 1990): Australian Congress of Mental Health Nurses. Journal (0727-4173)
Related titles: Online - full text ed.: ISSN 1440-0979. AUD 95 domestic to individuals; AUD 86 in New Zealand to individuals; USD 86 elsewhere to individuals; AUD 238 domestic to institutions; AUD 216 in New Zealand to institutions; USD 212 elsewhere to institutions (effective 2001) (from EBSCO Publishing, O C L C Online Computer Library Center, Inc., RoweCom Information Quest, ingenta, Munksgaard & Blackwell Science's Synergy, Swets Blackwell).
Indexed: ASSIA, CINAHL, Environ.Sci.Poll.Mgmt., Int.Nurs.Ind., Pollut.Abstr., PsycInfo, Risk Abstr., Saf.Sci.Abstr., e-psyche.
—BLDSC (1796.889000), ingenta.
Published by: (Australian and New Zealand College of Mental Health Nurses), Blackwell Science Asia Pty Ltd, PO Box 378, Carlton South, VIC 3053, Australia. TEL 61-3-9347-0300, FAX 61-3-9347-5001, info@blacksci-asia.com.au; mclinton@ashfordhosp.com.au, http://www.blacksci.co.uk. Eds. Mike Hazelton, Michael Clinton. Adv. contact Kathryn O'Brien. B&W page AUD 935, color page AUD 2,057; trim 210 x 275.

616.89 AUS ISSN 0004-8674
RC321 CODEN: ANZPBQ
AUSTRALIAN & NEW ZEALAND JOURNAL OF PSYCHIATRY. Text in English. 1967. bi-m. AUD 187 domestic to individuals; AUD 170 in New Zealand to individuals; USD 175 elsewhere to individuals; AUD 407 domestic to institutions; AUD 370 in New Zealand to institutions; USD 350 elsewhere to institutions; AUD 206 domestic to individuals paper & online eds. combined; AUD 187 in New Zealand to individuals paper & online eds. combined; USD 193 elsewhere to individuals paper & online eds. combined; AUD 448 domestic to institutions paper & online eds. combined; AUD 407 in New Zealand to institutions paper & online eds. combined; USD 385 elsewhere to institutions paper & online eds. combined (effective 2001). adv. bk.rev. abstr, charts, illus. index. Supplement avail.; back issues avail. *Refereed.* **Document type:** *Academic/Scholarly.* **Description:** Publishes clinical and research papers and case studies in all areas of psychiatry.
Related titles: Online - full text ed.: ISSN 1440-1614. AUD 169 domestic to individuals; AUD 153 in New Zealand to individuals; USD 158 elsewhere to individuals; AUD 367 domestic to institutions; AUD 333 in New Zealand to institutions; USD 315 elsewhere to institutions (effective 2001) (from EBSCO Publishing, O C L C Online Computer Library Center, Inc., RoweCom Information Quest, ingenta, Munksgaard & Blackwell Science's Synergy, Swets Blackwell, Institute for Scientific Information).
Indexed: ASCA, ASSIA, Addic.Abstr., Adol.Ment.Hlth.Abstr., AgeLine, Arts & Hum.Cit.Ind. (coverage dropped), Biol.Abstr., CINAHL, Curr.Cont., Dok.Arbeitsmed., Environ.Sci.Poll.Mgmt., Excerp.Med., Fam.Ind., Ind.Med. (1967-), Ind.N.Z.Per., Ind.Sci.Rev., Indian Psychol.Abstr., Inpharma, Int.Nurs.Ind., Mid.East: Abstr.& Ind., Mult.Ed.Abstr., Neurosci.Cit.Ind., Nutr.Abstr., Pharm.&Out.News, Pollut.Abstr., PsycInfo, Psychol.Abstr. (1969-), Reac., Risk Abstr., SSCI, Saf.Sci.Abstr., Sci.Cit.Ind., So.Pac.Per.Ind., Sp.Ed.Needs Abstr., e-psyche.
—BLDSC (1796.893000), EMDOCS, GNLM, IDS, ingenta, KNAW. **CCC.**
Published by: (Royal Australian and New Zealand College of Psychiatrists), Blackwell Science Asia Pty Ltd, PO Box 378, Carlton South, VIC 3053, Australia. TEL 61-3-9347-0300, FAX 61-3-9347-5001, info@blacksci-asia.com.au, http://www.blacksci.co.uk. Ed. Sidney Bloch. Adv. contact Kathryn O'Brien. B&W page AUD 1,045, color page AUD 1,947; trim 210 x 275. Circ: 3,600.

616.89 155 GBR ISSN 1362-3613
RC553.A88 CODEN: AUTIFS
AUTISM; the international journal of research and practice. Text in English. 1997. q. GBP 43 to individuals; GBP 197 to institutions; GBP 12 newsstand/cover to individuals; GBP 50 newsstand/cover to institutions (effective 2002). adv. bk.rev. *Refereed.* **Document type:** *Academic/Scholarly.* **Description:** Provides a major new international forum for research of direct and practical relevance to improving the quality of life for individuals with autism or autism-related disorders.
Related titles: Online - full text ed.: (from EBSCO Publishing, O C L C Online Computer Library Center, Inc., RoweCom Information Quest, ingenta, Swets Blackwell).
Indexed: Cont.Pg.Educ., ERA, PsycInfo, e-psyche.
—BLDSC (1825.520000).
Published by: (The National Autistic Society), Sage Publications Ltd., 6 Bonhill St, London EC2A 4PU, United Kingdom. TEL 44-20-7374-0645, FAX 44-20-7374-8741, market@sagepub.co.uk, http://www.sagepub.co.uk. Eds. Mohammad Ghaziuddin, Patricia Howlin, Rita Jordan. Adv. contact Jenny Kirby. page GBP 250; trim 193 x 118. Circ: 2,300.

616.89 155 USA ISSN 0893-8474
AUTISM RESEARCH REVIEW INTERNATIONAL. Text in English. 1987. q., latest vol.15. USD 18 domestic; USD 20 foreign (effective 2001). bk.rev. back issues avail. **Document type:** *Newsletter.* **Description:** Contains summaries and reviews of world literature pertaining to autistic children, with emphasis on research pertaining to cause and treatment.
Indexed: e-psyche.
—BLDSC (1825.569000), GNLM.
Published by: Autism Research Institute, 4182 Adams Ave, San Diego, CA 92116. TEL 619-281-7165, FAX 619-563-6840, http://www.autism.com/ari/. Eds. Alison Blake, Bernard Rimland. Pub., R&P Bernard Rimland. Circ: 10,000 (paid).

AUTONOMIC NERVOUS SYSTEM. see *BIOLOGY—Physiology*

616.8 NLD ISSN 1566-0702
CODEN: JASYDS
AUTONOMIC NEUROSCIENCE: BASIC & CLINICAL. Text in English. 1979. 14/yr. EUR 2,255 in Europe to institutions; JPY 299,600 in Japan to institutions; USD 2,523 elsewhere to institutions (effective 2002). adv. bk.rev. charts, illus. back issues avail.; reprint service avail. from SWZ,ISI. *Refereed.* **Document type:** *Academic/Scholarly.* **Description:** Presents papers that deal with any aspect of the autonomic nervous system, including structure, physiology, pharmacology, biochemistry, development, evolution, aging, behavioral aspects, integrative role, and its influence on emotional and physical states of the body.
Supersedes (in 2000): Journal of the Autonomic Nervous System (0165-1838)
Related titles: Microform ed.: (from PQC); Online - full text ed.: (from ingenta, Swets Blackwell, ScienceDirect, Institute for Scientific Information).
Indexed: ASCA, Aqua.Sci.& Fish.Abstr., Biol.Abstr., Chem.Abstr., Chem.Indus.Notes, Chem.Titles, Chemorec.Abstr., Curr.Cont., Dent.Ind., Environ.Sci.Poll.Mgmt., Excerp.Med., Ind.Med. (coverage dropped), Ind.Sci.Rev., Inpharma, Int.Abstr.Biol.Sci., Neurosci.Abstr. (coverage dropped), Neurosci.Cit.Ind., Reac., Rev.Arom.& Med.Plants, Sci.Cit.Ind.
—BLDSC (1835.057000), CASDDS, CISTI, GNLM, IDS, ingenta, KNAW. **CCC.**
Published by: Elsevier Science BV, PO Box 211, Amsterdam 1000 AE, Netherlands. TEL 31-20-485-2911, FAX 31-20-485-2457, nlinfo-f@elsevier.nl, http://www.elsevier.nl/inca/publications/store/5/0/6/0/6/0/8/9/. Ed. G Burnstock. **Subscr. in Australasia and the Far East to:** Elsevier Science (Singapore) Pte Ltd, No.1 Temasek Ave, 17-01 Millenia Tower, Singapore 039192, Singapore. TEL 65-434-3727, FAX 65-337-2230; **Subscr. in Japan to:** Elsevier Science Inc - Japan Regional Office, 9-15 Higashi-Azabu 1-chome, Minato-ku, Tokyo 106-0044, Japan. TEL 81-3-5561-5033, FAX 81-3-5561-5047; **Subscr. in the Americas to:** Elsevier Science, PO Box 945, New York, NY 10159-0945. TEL 212-633-3730, FAX 212-633-3680, usinfo-f@elsevier.com.

616.8 GBR ISSN 1074-8806
RC331
BAILLIERE'S CLINICAL PSYCHIATRY; international practice and research. Text in English. 1995. q. GBP 74, USD 126 to individuals; GBP 90, USD 153 to institutions. *Refereed.* **Document type:** *Academic/Scholarly.* **Description:** Explores issues in clinical psychiatry.
Indexed: e-psyche.
—Infotrieve. **CCC.**
Published by: Bailliere Tindall (Subsidiary of: Harcourt Publishers Ltd.), 24-28 Oval Rd, London NW1 7DX, United Kingdom. TEL 44-20-7485-4752, FAX 44—20-7267-4466, http://www.hbuk.co.uk. **Subscr. in N. America to:** Periodicals Fulfillment, W B Saunders Co, 6277 Sea Harbor Dr, 4th Fl, Orlando, FL 32891-4800. TEL 800-874-6418; **Subscr. to:** Harcourt Publishers Ltd., Foots Cray High St, Sidcup, Kent DA14 5HP, United Kingdom. TEL 44-20-8300-3322, FAX 44-20-8309-0807.

159.9 DEU ISSN 1439-5142
▼ **BALINT-JOURNAL.** Text in German. 2000. q. EUR 84.80 domestic to institutions; EUR 90.80 in Europe to institutions; EUR 92.80 elsewhere to institutions; EUR 24 newsstand/cover (effective 2002). **Document type:** *Journal, Academic/Scholarly.*
Related titles: Online - full text ed.: ISSN 1439-9008.
Published by: (Deutsche Balint-Gesellschaft e.V.), Georg Thieme Verlag, Ruedigerstr 14, Stuttgart 70469, Germany. TEL 49-711-8931-0, FAX 49-711-8931298, kunden.service@thieme.de, http://www.thieme.de/balint/.

M

BEHAVIORAL AND BRAIN SCIENCES; an international journal of current research and theory with open peer commentary. see *PSYCHOLOGY*

▼ **BEHAVIORAL & COGNITIVE NEUROSCIENCE REVIEWS.** see *PSYCHOLOGY*

616.891 362.27 USA ISSN 1529-7055
BEHAVIORAL HEALTH ACCREDITATION & ACCOUNTABILITY ALERT; outcomes best practices performance measures reimburements coding. Text in English. 1996. m., latest vol.6, 2001. USD 267 domestic to individuals; USD 327 domestic to institutions; USD 337 in Canada to institutions; USD 347 elsewhere to institutions (effective 2001). 8 p./no. back issues avail.; reprints avail. **Document type:** *Newsletter, Academic/Scholarly.* **Description:** Covers outcomes, best practices, performance measures, and reimbursement, helping people get paid for behavioral health sservices.
Former titles (until 2000): Outcomes and Accountability Alert (1524-0908); (until 1999): Behavioral Health Outcomes (1090-9621); (until 1997): Outcomes (1086-444X)
Related titles: E-mail ed.
Indexed: e-psyche.
—CCC.
Published by: Manisses Communications Group, Inc., PO Box 9758, Providence, RI 02906-9758. TEL 401-831-6020, 800-333-7771, FAX 401-861-6370, manissesCS@manisses.com, http://www.manisses.com. Ed. Gary A Enos. Pub. Betty R Lang. R&P Barbara Deekle. Adv. contact Paul Newman.

BEHAVIORAL HEALTH BUSINESS NEWS. see *INSURANCE*

616.8 USA
BEHAVIORAL HEALTH SECTION NEWSLETTER. Text in English. 1983. q. USD 35. charts, stat, tr.lit. back issues avail. **Document type:** *Newsletter.* **Description:** Medical recordkeeping and documentation in mental health care facilities.
Former titles: Mental Health Section Newsletter; (until 1992): Couch..
Published by: American Health Information Management Association, Mental Health Section, 233 N Michigan Ave Ste 2150, Chicago, IL 60601. TEL 312-233-1100, FAX 312-787-9793. Ed. Laura Feste. Circ: 800.

616.8 GBR ISSN 1072-0847
RJ505.B4 CODEN: BEHIE2
BEHAVIORAL INTERVENTIONS; theory and practice in residential and community-based clinical programs. Text in English. 1986. q. USD 520 in United States; USD 520 in Canada & Mexico; USD 520 elsewhere; USD 546 combined subscription in United States for print and online eds.; USD 546 combined subscription in Canada & Mexico for print and online eds.; USD 546 combined subscription elsewhere for print and online eds. (effective 2002). adv. back issues avail.; reprint service avail. from SWZ. *Refereed.* **Document type:** *Academic/Scholarly.* **Description:** Publishes reports of research involving the utilization of behavioral techniques in applied settings.
Formerly (until 1994): Behavioral Residential Treatment (0884-5581)
Related titles: Microform ed.: (from PQC); Online - full text ed.: ISSN 1099-078X. USD 520 in United States; USD 520 in Canada & Mexico; USD 520 elsewhere (effective 2002) (from EBSCO Publishing, Wiley InterScience, Institute for Scientific Information).
Indexed: AMED, Curr.Cont., ERA, PsycInfo, Psychol.Abstr. (1988-), Psycscan B.A.& T., SSCI, e-psyche.
—BLDSC (1877.500000), EMDOCS, GNLM, Infotrieve, ingenta. **CCC.**
Published by: Wiley Europe Ltd., Baffins Ln, Chichester, W Sussex PO19 1UD, United Kingdom. TEL 44-1243-779777, FAX 44-1243-775878, cs-journals@wiley.co.uk, customer@wiley.co.uk, http://www.interscience.wiley.com/jpages/1072-0847/, http://www.wiley.co.uk. adv.: B&W page GBP 650, color page GBP 1,550; trim 165 x 248. Circ: 500. **Subscr. in the Americas to:** John Wiley & Sons, Inc., Journals, 605 Third Ave, New York, NY 10158. TEL 212-820-6021, 212-850-6645, subinfo@jwiley.com.

BEHAVIORAL MEDICINE; investigations of environmental influences on health and behavior. see *PSYCHOLOGY*

BEHAVIORAL NEUROSCIENCE. see *PSYCHOLOGY*

616.8 NLD ISSN 0166-4328
CODEN: BBREDI
BEHAVIOURAL BRAIN RESEARCH; an international journal. Text in English. 1980. 20/yr. EUR 3,492 in Europe to institutions; JPY 464,000 in Japan to institutions; USD 3,907 elsewhere to institutions (effective 2002). charts, illus. back issues avail.; reprint service avail. from SWZ,SCH,PSC,ISI. *Refereed.* **Document type:** *Academic/Scholarly.* **Description:** Publishes articles in the neurosciences, with special emphasis on neural mechanisms of behavior.
Related titles: Microform ed.: (from PQC); Online - full text ed.: (from ingenta, Swets Blackwell, ScienceDirect, Institute for Scientific Information).
Indexed: Anim.Behav.Abstr., Aqua.Sci.& Fish.Abstr., Biol.Abstr., Biotech.& Bioeng.Abstr., Chem.Abstr., Chem.Indus.Notes, Chem.Titles, Chemorec.Abstr., Curr.Cont., Dent.Ind., Excerp.Med., Ind.Med. (1980-), Ind.Sci.Rev., Indian Psychol.Abstr., Inpharma, Int.Abstr.Biol.Sci., Neurosci.Abstr., Neurosci.Cit.Ind., Nutr.Abstr., Pharm.&Out.News, PsycInfo, Psychol.Abstr. (1980-), Reac., Rev.Med.& Vet.Mycol., Sci.Cit.Ind., Soyabean Abstr., Sport Fish.Abstr., Yrbk.Assoc.Educ.& Rehab.Blind, e-psyche.
—BLDSC (1877.320000), CASDDS, CISTI, EMDOCS, GNLM, IDS, ingenta. **CCC.**
Published by: Elsevier Science BV, PO Box 211, Amsterdam 1000 AE, Netherlands. TEL 31-20-485-2911, FAX 31-20-485-2457, nlinfo-f@elsevier.nl, http://www.elsevier.com/locate/bbr, http://www.elsevier.nl. Eds. J P Huston, T E Robinson. **Subscr. in Australasia and the Far East to:** Elsevier Science (Singapore) Pte Ltd, No.1 Temasek Ave, 17-01 Millenia Tower, Singapore 039192, Singapore. TEL 65-434-3727, FAX 65-337-2230; **Subscr. in Japan to:** Elsevier Science Inc - Japan Regional Office, 9-15 Higashi-Azabu 1-chome, Minato-ku, Tokyo 106-0044, Japan. TEL 81-3-5561-5033, FAX 81-3-5561-5047; **Subscr. in the Americas to:** Elsevier Science, PO Box 945, New York, NY 10159-0945. TEL 212-633-3730, FAX 212-633-3680, usinfo-f@elsevier.com, http://www.elsevier.com.

616.8 NLD ISSN 0953-4180
CODEN: BNEUEI
BEHAVIOURAL NEUROLOGY; an international journal on the relationship between disordered human behavior and underlying biological mechanisms. Text in English. 1988. q. EUR 374, USD 342 to institutions (effective 2002). adv. bk.rev. index. *Refereed.* **Document type:** *Journal, Academic/Scholarly.* **Description:** Publishes original and review papers of a predominantly clinical nature, with emphasis on the meaning of expression of disordered human behavior.
Related titles: Online - full text ed.: (from Swets Blackwell, Institute for Scientific Information, RoweCom Information Quest).
Indexed: ASCA, Curr.Cont. (coverage dropped), Excerp.Med. (1993-), Inpharma, Int.Abstr.Biol.Sci., Neurosci.Cit.Ind., Pharm.&Out.News, PsycInfo, Psychol.Abstr., Reac., SSCI (coverage dropped), e-psyche.
—BLDSC (1877.590000), EMDOCS, GNLM, IDS, Infotrieve, ingenta, KNAW. **CCC.**
Published by: I O S Press, Nieuwe Hemweg 6B, Amsterdam 1013 BG, Netherlands. TEL 31-20-688-3355, FAX 31-20-620-3419, BNJournal@sheffield.ac.uk, market@iospress.nl, http://www.iospress.nl. Ed. Andrew Mayes TEL 44-114-271-3431. Circ: 900. **Subscr. to:** I O S Press, Inc, 5795-G Burke Centre Pkwy, Burke, VA 22015. TEL 703-323-5554, FAX 703-323-3668, iosbooks@iospress.com; Globe Publication Pvt. Ltd., C-62 Inderpuri, New Delhi 100 012, India. TEL 91-11-579-3211, 91-11-579-3212, FAX 91-11-579-8876, custserve@globepub.com, http://www.globepub.com; Kinokuniya Company Ltd, Shinjuku 3-chome, Shinjuku-ku, Tokyo 160-0022, Japan. FAX 81-3-3439-1094, journal@kinokuniya.co.jp, http://www.kinokuniya.co.jp.

619.8 NLD ISSN 0376-6357
QL750 CODEN: BPRODA
BEHAVIOURAL PROCESSES; an international journal of comparative and physiological ethology. Text in English, French, German. 1977. m. EUR 1,402 in Europe to institutions; JPY 186,000 in Japan to institutions; USD 1,569 elsewhere to institutions (effective 2002). adv. bk.rev. bibl, illus. index. back issues avail.; reprint service avail. from ISI. *Refereed.* **Document type:** *Academic/Scholarly.* **Description:** Covers comparative ethology, behavioural ecology, theoretical and quantitative ethology, neuroethology, experimental analysis and operant conditioning.
Incorporates (1981-1983): Behaviour Analysis Letters
Related titles: Microform ed.: (from PQC); Online - full text ed.: (from ingenta, Swets Blackwell, ScienceDirect, Institute for Scientific Information).
Indexed: ASCA, Anim.Behav.Abstr., Aqua.Sci.& Fish.Abstr., Bio-Contr.News & Info., Biol.Abstr., Chemorec.Abstr., Curr.Adv.Ecol.Sci., Curr.Cont., Dairy Sci.Abstr., Deep Sea Res.& Oceanogr.Abstr., Ecol.Abstr., Entomol.Abstr., Excerp.Med., Ind.Sci.Rev., Ind.Vet., Indian Psychol.Abstr., Inpharma, Int.Abstr.Biol.Sci., Neurosci.Abstr. (coverage dropped), Nutr.Abstr., Pharm.&Out.News, Pig News & Info., PsycInfo, Psychol.Abstr. (1976-), Psycscan B.A.& T., Reac., Rev.Appl.Entomol., SSCI, Sci.Cit.Ind., Sport Fish.Abstr., Vet.Bull., Zoo.Rec., e-psyche.
—BLDSC (1877.700000), CASDDS, CISTI, EMDOCS, GNLM, IDS, Infotrieve, ingenta. **CCC.**
Published by: Elsevier Science BV, PO Box 211, Amsterdam 1000 AE, Netherlands. TEL 31-20-485-2911, FAX 31-20-485-2457, nlinfo-f@elsevier.nl, http://www.elsevier.com/locate/behavproc, http://www.elsevier.nl. Eds. F Cezilly, J E R Staddon. **Subscr. in Australasia and the Far East to:** Elsevier Science (Singapore) Pte Ltd, No.1 Temasek Ave, 17-01 Millenia Tower, Singapore 039192, Singapore. TEL 65-434-3727, FAX 65-337-2230; **Subscr. in Japan to:** Elsevier Science Inc - Japan Regional Office, 9-15 Higashi-Azabu 1-chome, Minato-ku, Tokyo 106-0044, Japan. TEL 81-3-5561-5033, FAX 81-3-5561-5047; **Subscr. in the Americas to:** Elsevier Science, PO Box 945, New York, NY 10159-0945. TEL 212-633-3730, FAX 212-633-3680, usinfo-f@elsevier.com, http://www.elsevier.com.

616.89 POL ISSN 1425-0640
BIBLIOTEKA PSYCHIATRII POLSKIEJ. Text in Polish. 1995. irreg. PLZ 25 (effective 2002). 100 p./no. 1 cols./p. **Document type:** *Monographic series, Academic/Scholarly.*
Published by: Polskie Towarzystwo Psychiatryczne, Ul Lenartowicza 14, Krakow 31138, Poland. TEL 48-12-6331203, FAX 48-12-6334067, psych@kom-red-wyd-ptp.com.pl, http://www.kom-red-wyd-ptp.com.pl/bibliotekapl.html. Ed., Pub. Jerzy W Aleksandrowicz. Adv. contact Magdalena Sikora.

616.8 CHE ISSN 0067-8147
CODEN: BIBPBI
BIBLIOTHECA PSYCHIATRICA. Text in English, French, German. 1917. irreg., latest vol.169. CHF 150 in Europe; DEM 180 in Germany; USD 120 in United States (effective 2001). back issues avail.; reprint service avail. from PSC,SCH,ISI. *Refereed.* **Document type:** *Monographic series, Academic/Scholarly.*
Related titles: Online - full text ed.: (from Institute for Scientific Information).
Indexed: ASCA, Biol.Abstr., Chem.Abstr., Curr.Cont. (coverage dropped), Ind.Med. (coverage dropped), SSCI (coverage dropped).
—BLDSC (2019.390000), CISTI, GNLM, Infotrieve, KNAW. **CCC.**
Published by: S. Karger AG, Allschwilerstr 10, PO Box, Basel 4009, Switzerland. TEL 41-61-306-1111, FAX 41-61-306-1234, karger@karger.ch, http://www.karger.com/bookseries/BIBSY. Ed. B Saletu.

BIOFEEDBACK (WHEAT RIDGE). see *PSYCHOLOGY*

616.89 USA ISSN 0006-3223
RC321 CODEN: BIPCBF
BIOLOGICAL PSYCHIATRY; a journal of psychiatric research. Text in English. 1969. s-m. EUR 621 in Europe to individuals; JPY 82,400 in Japan to individuals; USD 695 elsewhere to individuals; EUR 1,667 in Europe to institutions; JPY 221,200 in Japan to institutions; USD 1,864 elsewhere to institutions; EUR 105 in Europe to students; JPY 14,000 in Japan to students; USD 140 elsewhere to students (effective 2002). adv. bk.rev. charts, illus. index. *Refereed.* **Document type:** *Academic/Scholarly.* **Description:** Covers the whole range of psychiatric research interest; presents major clinical, behavioral, epidemiological and normative studies in all subdisciplines relevant to psychiatry.
Supersedes: Recent Advances in Biological Psychiatry
Related titles: CD-ROM ed.; Microfilm ed.: (from PQC); Online - full text ed.: (from ingenta, Swets Blackwell, ScienceDirect, Institute for Scientific Information).
Indexed: ASCA, Adol.Ment.Hlth.Abstr., AgeLine, Behav.Med.Abstr., Bibl.Dev.Med.& Child Neur., Biol.Abstr., Chem.Abstr., Chem.Indus.Notes, Chem.Titles, Crim.Just.Abstr., Curr.Adv.Biochem., Curr.Adv.Ecol.Sci., Curr.Cont., Dairy Sci.Abstr., Dent.Ind., Excerp.Med., Fam.Ind., Focus on: Psychophar., INIS Atomind., Ind.Med. (1969-), Ind.Sci.Rev., Indian Psychol.Abstr., Inpharma, Int.Abstr.Biol.Sci., Jrnl.Watch Psych., Neurosci.Cit.Ind., Nutr.Abstr., Pharm.&Out.News, PsycInfo, Psychol.Abstr. (1969-), Reac., Rev.Med.& Vet.Mycol., SSCI (coverage dropped), Sci.Cit.Ind., e-psyche.

M

—BLDSC (2077.550000), ADONIS, CASDDS, CISTI, EMDOCS, GNLM, IDS, ingenta, KNAW. **CCC.**
Published by: (Society of Biological Psychiatry), Elsevier Science, 655 Ave of the Americas, New York, NY 10010. FAX 212-633-3990, usinfo-f@elsevier.com, http://www.elsevier.com/locate/biopsychiat. Ed. Dennis S Charney. adv.: B&W page USD 1,035, color page USD 2,270. Circ: 2,500 (paid). **Subscr. in Australasia and the Far East to:** Elsevier Science (Singapore) Pte Ltd, No.1 Temasek Ave, 17-01 Millenia Tower, Singapore 039192, Singapore. TEL 65-434-3727, FAX 65-337-2230**; Subscr. in Japan to:** Elsevier Science Inc - Japan Regional Office, 9-15 Higashi-Azabu 1-chome, Minato-ku, Tokyo 106-0044, Japan. TEL 81-3-5561-5033, FAX 81-3-5561-5047**; Subscr. outside the Americas to:** Elsevier Science BV, PO Box 211, Amsterdam 1000 AE, Netherlands. TEL 31-20-485-3757, FAX 31-20-485-3432, nlinfo-f@elsevier.nl.

616.89 USA ISSN 1044-422X
BIOLOGICAL THERAPIES IN PSYCHIATRY NEWSLETTER. Text in English. 1977. m. USD 65 to individuals; USD 96 to institutions; USD 50 to students (effective 2001). back issues avail. **Document type:** *Newsletter, Trade.* **Description:** Provides updates on the clinical use of psychotropic drugs to practicing psychiatrists, psychiatric house staff, residents, and students.
Former titles: Biological Therapies in Psychiatry (0895-8262); Massachusetts General Hospital Biological Therapies in Psychiatry Newsletter (0199-2716)
Related titles: Online - full content ed.
—BLDSC (2081.270000), GNLM. **CCC.**
Published by: Gelenberg Consulting & Publishing, L.L.C., PO Box 42650, Tucson, AZ 85733-2650. TEL 520-572-2039, 800-700-9589, FAX 520-626-4070, subscriptions@btpnews.com, http://www.btpnews.com/index.html. Ed. Alan J Gelenberg. Circ: 6,000 (paid).

616.895 DNK ISSN 1398-5647
▼ **BIPOLAR DISORDERS.** Text in Danish. 1999. bi-m. USD 235 in the Americas to institutions print & online eds. combined; GBP 163 elsewhere to institutions print & online eds. combined (effective 2002). **Document type:** *Trade.*
Related titles: ♦ Online - full text ed.: Bipolar Disorders Online. ISSN 1399-5618.
Indexed: Curr.Cont., e-psyche.
—BLDSC (2090.475000).
Published by: Blackwell Munksgaard, Noerre Soegade 35, PO Box 2148, Copenhagen K 1016, Denmark. TEL 45-77-33-33-33, FAX 45-77-33-33-77, customerservice@munksgaard.dk, http://journals.munksgaard.dk/bipolardisorders, http://www.munksgaard.dk. Eds. Jair C Soares, Samuel Gershon. Adv. contact Eric Rozario TEL 45-77-33-33-01. Circ: 800.

616.895 DNK ISSN 1399-5618
BIPOLAR DISORDERS ONLINE. Text in English. bi-m. GBP 147 to individuals (effective 2002). **Document type:** *Academic/Scholarly.*
Media: Online - full text (from EBSCO Publishing, O C L C Online Computer Library Center, Inc., RoweCom Information Quest, ingenta, Munksgaard & Blackwell Science's Synergy, Swets Blackwell, Institute for Scientific Information). **Related titles:** ♦ Print ed.: Bipolar Disorders. ISSN 1398-5647.
Published by: Blackwell Munksgaard, Noerre Soegade 35, PO Box 2148, Copenhagen K 1016, Denmark. TEL 45-77-33-33-33, FAX 45-77-33-33-77, fsub@mail.munksgaard.dk, http://www.munksgaard.dk/bipolardisorders.

616.8 GBR ISSN 0006-8950
RC321 CODEN: BRAIAK
BRAIN; a journal of neurology. Text in English. 1877. m. GBP 155, USD 245 to individuals; GBP 345, USD 545 to institutions (effective 2002). adv. bk.rev. bibl, illus. index. 232 p./no. back issues avail.; reprint service avail. from SWZ,PQC,PSC,SCH. *Refereed.* **Document type:** *Journal, Academic/Scholarly.* **Description:** Original papers in clinical neurology and related disciplines.
Related titles: Microfiche ed.: (from IDC); Microform ed.: (from PQC,PMC); Online - full text ed.: ISSN 1460-2156. 199?. GBP 310, USD 490 to institutions Online only (effective 2002) (from HighWire Pr., Northern Light Technology, Inc., EBSCO Publishing, O C L C Online Computer Library Center, Inc., RoweCom Information Quest, ingenta, Swets Blackwell, Institute for Scientific Information).
Indexed: AIM, AMED, ASCA, Abstr.Hyg., Agri.& Environ.Biotech.Abstr. (coverage dropped), Aqua.Sci.& Fish.Abstr., Arts & Hum.Cit.Ind. (coverage dropped), Bibl.Dev.Med.& Child Neur., Biol.Abstr., CINAHL, Chem.Abstr., Curr.Adv.Ecol.Sci., Curr.Cont., Derwent Biotech.Abstr., Diab.Cont., Ergon.Abstr., Excerp.Med., Helminthol.Abstr., INIS Atomind., Ind.Med. (1878-), Ind.Sci.Rev., Ind.Vet., Inpharma, Int.Abstr.Biol.Sci., Jrnl.Watch Neuro., Lang.& Lang.Behav.Abstr., Neurosci.Abstr., Neurosci.Cit.Ind., Nutr.Abstr., Pharm.&Out.News, PsycInfo, Psychol.Abstr., Reac., Rev.Med.& Vet.Mycol., SOPODA, SSCI (coverage dropped), Sci.Cit.Ind., So.Pac.Per.Ind., Sociol.Abstr., Vet.Bull.
—BLDSC (2268.000000), CASDDS, CISTI, EMDOCS, GNLM, IDS, ingenta, KNAW, Linda Hall. **CCC.**
Published by: Oxford University Press, Academic Division, Great Clarendon St, Oxford OX2 6DP, United Kingdom. TEL 44-1865-267907, FAX 44-1865-267835, jnl.info@oup.co.uk, http://www.oup.co.uk/brainj/, http://www.oup.co.uk/journals. Ed. J Newsom-Davies. Pub. Mandy Sketch. R&P Fionna Willis. adv.: page GBP 410, page USD 738. Circ: 2,900. **U.S. subscr. to:** Oxford University Press, Journals. TEL 800-852-7323, FAX 919-677-1714, jnlorders@oup-usa.org**; Subscr. to:** Journals Marketing, Great Clarendon St, Oxford OX2 6DP, United Kingdom.

616.8 618.92 NLD ISSN 0387-7604
RJ486 CODEN: NTHAA7
BRAIN AND DEVELOPMENT. Text in English. 1969. 8/yr. NLG 751, EUR 340.79 in Europe to institutions; JPY 47,200 in Japan to institutions; USD 381 elsewhere to institutions (effective 2001). abstr. back issues avail. *Refereed.* **Document type:** *Academic/Scholarly.* **Description:** Contains both clinical and basic studies in the field of child neurology.
Related titles: Microform ed.: (from PQC); Online - full text ed.: (from ingenta, Swets Blackwell, ScienceDirect, Institute for Scientific Information); ♦ Japanese ed.: No to Hattatsu. ISSN 0029-0831.
Indexed: ASCA, Bibl.Dev.Med.& Child Neur., Curr.Cont., Excerp.Med., INIS Atomind., Ind.Med. (1979-), Ind.Sci.Rev., Inpharma, Int.Abstr.Biol.Sci., Neurosci.Cit.Ind., Pharm.&Out.News, Reac., Rev.Med.& Vet.Mycol., Sci.Cit.Ind., e-psyche.
—BLDSC (2268.032900), CISTI, EMDOCS, GNLM, IDS, ingenta, KNAW. **CCC.**
Published by: (Japanese Society of Child Neurology/Nihon Shoni Shinkei Gakkai JPN), Elsevier Science BV, PO Box 211, Amsterdam 1000 AE, Netherlands. TEL 31-20-485-2911, FAX 31-20-485-2457, nlinfo-f@elsevier.nl, http://www.elsevier.com/locate/braindev, http://www.elsevier.nl. **Subscr. in Australasia and the Far East to:** Elsevier Science (Singapore) Pte Ltd, No.1 Temasek Ave, 17-01 Millenia Tower, Singapore 039192, Singapore. TEL 65-434-3727, FAX 65-337-2230**; Subscr. in Japan to:** Elsevier Science Inc - Japan Regional Office, 9-15 Higashi-Azabu 1-chome, Minato-ku, Tokyo 106-0044, Japan. TEL 81-3-5561-5033, FAX 81-3-5561-5047**; Subscr. in the Americas to:** Elsevier Science, PO Box 945, New York, NY 10159-0945. TEL 212-633-3730, FAX 212-633-3680, usinfo-f@elsevier.com.

616.8 NLD ISSN 1389-1987
▼ **BRAIN AND MIND**; a transdisciplinary journal of neuroscience and neurophilosophy. Text in English. 2000. 3/yr. EUR 208, USD 208 to institutions for print or online ed.; EUR 249.60, USD 249.60 to institutions for print & online eds. combined (effective 2002). **Document type:** *Academic/Scholarly.* **Description:** Examines new research in neurology, neurophysiology, neuropsychiatry, and neuropsychology.
Related titles: Online - full text ed.: (from EBSCO Publishing, O C L C Online Computer Library Center, Inc., Swets Blackwell, Kluwer Online).
Indexed: Neurosci.Abstr., e-psyche.
—BLDSC (2268.045000).
Published by: Kluwer Academic Publishers Group (Subsidiary of: Wolters Kluwer N.V.), Spuiboulevard 50, PO Box 17, Dordrecht 3300 AA, Netherlands. TEL 31-78-639-2392, FAX 31-78-654-2254, services@wkap.nl, http://www.wkap.nl/journalhome.htm/1389-1987. Ed. John Bickle. **Subscr. in N America to:** Kluwer Academic - Plenum Publishers, 233 Spring St, New York, NY 10013-1578. TEL 212-620-8468, FAX 212-807-1047**; Subscr. to:** Journals Department, PO Box 322, Dordrecht 3300 AH, Netherlands. TEL 31-78-639-2392, FAX 31-78-654-6474.

616.8 JPN ISSN 0006-8969
CODEN: BRNED8
BRAIN AND NERVE/NO TO SHINKEI. Text in Japanese; Summaries in English. 1948. m. JPY 28,800, USD 181. adv. bk.rev. abstr. cum.index.
Related titles: Online - full text ed.: (from JICST).
Indexed: Biol.Abstr., C.I.S. Abstr., Chem.Abstr., Chem.Indus.Notes, Chem.Titles, Dent.Ind., Excerp.Med., INIS Atomind., Ind.Med. (1948-), e-psyche.
—BLDSC (2268.050000), CASDDS, CISTI, EMDOCS, GNLM, KNAW.
Published by: Igaku-Shoin Ltd., 5-24-3 Hongo, Bunkyo-ku, Tokyo 113-0033, Japan. TEL 81-3-3817-5701. Circ: 4,500.

616.8 CHE ISSN 0006-8977
QL750 CODEN: BRBEBE
BRAIN, BEHAVIOR AND EVOLUTION. Text in English. 1968. m. (in 2 vol.). CHF 2,178, EUR 1,555.60 in Europe to institutions; CHF 2,212.80, USD 1,692 overseas to institutions (effective 2002). adv. bk.rev. bibl, illus. index. back issues avail.; reprint service avail. from PSC,SCH. *Refereed.* **Document type:** *Journal, Academic/Scholarly.* **Description:** Aims to understand the evolution of nervous systems and how they subserve behavior.
Related titles: Microform ed.: (from RPI); Online - full text ed.: ISSN 1421-9743. CHF 116, EUR 84, USD 90 to institutions (effective 2002) (from EBSCO Publishing, O C L C Online Computer Library Center, Inc., RoweCom Information Quest, ProQuest Information & Learning, Swets Blackwell, Institute for Scientific Information).
Indexed: ASCA, Abstr.Anthropol., Anim.Behav.Abstr., Aqua.Sci.& Fish.Abstr., Biol.Abstr., Chemorec.Abstr., Curr.Adv.Ecol.Sci., Curr.Cont., Dent.Ind., Excerp.Med., GeoRef, Ind.Med. (1968-), Ind.Sci.Rev., Inpharma, Neurosci.Abstr., Neurosci.Cit.Ind., PsycInfo, Psychol.Abstr. (1971-), Reac., Ref.Zh., Rev.Appl.Entomol., SSCI (coverage dropped), Sci.Cit.Ind., Sport Fish.Abstr., Wild.Rev., e-psyche.
—BLDSC (2268.100000), CISTI, GNLM, IDS, ingenta, KNAW, Linda Hall. **CCC.**
Published by: S. Karger AG, Allschwilerstr 10, PO Box, Basel 4009, Switzerland. TEL 41-61-306-1111, FAX 41-61-306-1234, karger@karger.ch, http://www.online.karger.com/journals/bbe. Ed. W Wilczynski. adv.: page USD 1,195. Circ: 1,000.

616.8 USA ISSN 0967-9944
BRAIN DAMAGE, BEHAVIOUR AND COGNITION. Text in English. 1989. irreg. **Document type:** *Monographic series.*
Indexed: e-psyche.
Published by: Lawrence Erlbaum Associates, Inc., 10 Industrial Ave, Mahwah, NJ 07430-2262. TEL 201-236-9500, 800-926-6579, FAX 201-236-0072, jamsel@erlbaum.com, http://www.erlbaum.com. Eds. Chris Code, Dave Mueller.

616.8 USA
▼ **BRAIN DISORDERS SOURCEBOOK.** Text in English. 1999 (Apr.). irreg. USD 78 per vol. (effective 2001). charts, bibl. master index. **Description:** Contains basic Information about non-dementing neurological disorders, including stroke and post-stroke rehabilitation, epilepsy and other seizure-inducing disorders, such as, multiple sclerosis, cerebral palsy, tourette syndrome, brain injuries and tumors, amyotrophic lateral sclerosis (ALS), and more. Also includes statistical and demographic data, treatment options, coping strategies, reports on current research initiatives, a glossary, and resource listings for additional help and information.
Published by: Omnigraphics, Inc., 615 Griswold St, Detroit, MI 48226. TEL 313-961-1340, 800-234-1340, FAX 313-961-1383, 800-875-1340, info@omnigraphics.com, http://www.omnigraphics.com. Ed. Karen Bellenir.

616.8 GBR ISSN 0269-9052
RC387.5 CODEN: BRAIEO
BRAIN INJURY. Text in English. 1987. m. GBP 346, USD 570 to individuals; GBP 690, USD 1,139 to institutions (effective 2002). adv. *Refereed.* **Document type:** *Academic/Scholarly.* **Description:** Covers all aspects of brain injury, ranging from basic scientific research to epidemiology, neuropathology, neurosurgical and other medical procedures, assessment methods, rehabilitation, and outcome.
Related titles: Online - full text ed.: ISSN 1362-301X (from CatchWord Ltd., EBSCO Publishing, O C L C Online Computer Library Center, Inc., RoweCom Information Quest, Swets Blackwell, Institute for Scientific Information).
Indexed: ASCA, Curr.Cont., Excerp.Med., Ind.Med. (1987-), Inpharma, Int.Nurs.Ind., Neurosci.Cit.Ind., Pharm.&Out.News, PsycInfo, Psychol.Abstr. (1992-), Reac., Rev.Appl.Entomol., SSCI (coverage dropped), e-psyche.
—BLDSC (2268.132000), CatchWord, CISTI, EMDOCS, GNLM, IDS, ingenta, KNAW. **CCC.**

Published by: Taylor & Francis Group, Taylor & Francis Ltd., 11 New Fetter Ln, London EC4P 4EE, United Kingdom. TEL 44-20-7583-9855, FAX 44-20-7842-2298, info@tandf.co.uk, http://www.tandf.co.uk. Eds. Jeff Kreutzer, Nathan Zasler. **Subscr. in N. America to:** Taylor & Francis Ltd., 325 Chestnut St, Suite 800, Philadelphia, PA 19016. TEL 800-354-1420, FAX 215-625-8914, info@taylorandfrancis.com, http://www.taylorandfrancis.com/.

BRAIN INJURY UPDATE. see *MEDICAL SCIENCES—Abstracting, Bibliographies, Statistics*

616.8 USA ISSN 1072-3927
BP605.N48

BRAIN - MIND; bulletin of breakthroughs. Text in English. 1975. m. USD 45; USD 55 foreign. bk.rev. illus. back issues avail. **Document type:** *Bulletin.* **Description:** Ground-breaking news from the medical, clinical, social, educational, creative and spiritual sciences.

Former titles: Brain - Mind and Common Sense (1064-671X); New Sense Bulletin (1057-0705); Incorporates: Brain - Mind Bulletin (0273-8546)

Related titles: Online - full text ed.

Indexed: New Per.Ind., e-psyche.

Published by: Interface Press, 4717 N Figueroa St, Box 42211, Los Angeles, CA 90042. TEL 213-223-2500, 800-553-6463, FAX 213-223-2519. Ed. Marilyn Ferguson. Circ: 4,000.

616.8 IND ISSN 0006-8985

BRAIN NEWS✶. Text in English. 1964. s-a. INR 30, USD 10. adv. bk.rev.

Indexed: Biol.Abstr., e-psyche.

—CISTI.

Published by: Indian Brain Research Association, Dept. of Biochemistry, 35 Ballygunge Circular Rd., Kolkata, West Bengal 700 019, India. Ed. Dr. J J Ghosh. Circ: 500.

616.8 USA ISSN 1015-6305
CODEN: BRPAE7

BRAIN PATHOLOGY. Text in English. 1990. q. USD 160 (effective 2001). adv. bk.rev. back issues avail. *Refereed.* **Document type:** *Academic/Scholarly.* **Description:** Investigates diseases of the nervous system.

Related titles: Online - full text ed.: (from Institute for Scientific Information).

Indexed: ASCA, Chem.Abstr., Chem.Indus.Notes, Chem.Titles, Curr.Cont., Excerp.Med. (1993-), Helminthol.Abstr., Ind.Med. (1990-), Ind.Sci.Rev., Inpharma, Int.Abstr.Biol.Sci., Neurosci.Cit.Ind., Pharm.&Out.News, Protozool.Abstr., Reac., Rev.Med.& Vet.Mycol., Sci.Cit.Ind., e-psyche.

—BLDSC (2268.175000), CASDDS, CISTI, EMDOCS, GNLM, IDS, KNAW.

Published by: International Society of Neuropathology, 200 Lothrop St, PUH A515, Pittsburgh, PA 15213. TEL 310-267-0543, FAX 310-267-0545, bpath@np.awing.upmc.edu, http://brainpathology.upmc.edu, http://www.brainpathology.com. Ed. Clayton A Wiley. Adv. contact Duncan A MacRae. **Subscr. to:** Allen Press Inc., PO Box 1897, Lawrence, KS 66044-8897.

616.8 NLD ISSN 0006-8993
QP376 CODEN: BRREAP

BRAIN RESEARCH; international multidisciplinary journal devoted to fundamental research in the brain sciences. Text in English. 1966. 12/yr. NLG 34,364, EUR 15,593.70 in Europe to institutions; JPY 2,158,900 in Japan to institutions; USD 17,444 elsewhere to institutions (effective 2001); Comprising 7 journals. adv. bk.rev. abstr, bibl, illus. index, cum.index: 1966-1977. back issues avail. *Refereed.* **Document type:** *Journal, Academic/Scholarly.* **Description:** Covers neuroanatomy, neurochemistry, neurophysiology, neuroendocrinology, neuropharmacology, neurotoxicology, neurocommunications, behavioral sciences, neurology and biocybernetics.

Related titles: Microform ed.: (from PQC); Online - full text ed.: (from EBSCO Publishing, ingenta, Swets Blackwell, ScienceDirect, Institute for Scientific Information).

Indexed: AIDS Abstr., ASCA, Abstr.Anthropol., Agri.& Environ.Biotech.Abstr. (coverage dropped), Anim.Behav.Abstr., Apic.Abstr., Aqua.Sci.& Fish.Abstr., Biol.Abstr., Biotech.& Bioeng.Abstr., Cal.Tiss.Abstr., Chem.Abstr., Chem.Indus.Notes, Chem.Titles, Chemorec.Abstr., Curr.Adv.Biochem., Curr.Adv.Cell & Devel.Biol., Curr.Adv.Ecol.Sci., Curr.Cont., Dairy Sci.Abstr., Dent.Ind., Derwent Biotech.Abstr., Environ.Sci.Poll.Mgmt., Excerp.Med., Helminthol.Abstr., INIS Atomind., Ind.Med. (1966-), Ind.Sci.Rev., Ind.Vet., Indian Psychol.Abstr., Inpharma, Int.Abstr.Biol.Sci., Int.Aerosp.Abstr., Neurosci.Abstr., Neurosci.Cit.Ind., Nutr.Abstr., Pharm.&Out.News, Protozool.Abstr., PsycInfo, Psychol.Abstr. (1970-), Reac., Ref.Zh., Rev.Appl.Entomol., Rev.Med.& Vet.Mycol., SSCI (coverage dropped), Sci.Cit.Ind., Sport Fish.Abstr., THA, Tox.Abstr. (coverage dropped), Vet.Bull., Weed Abstr., Wild.Rev., Zoo.Rec., e-psyche.

—BLDSC (2268.200000), ADONIS, CASDDS, CISTI, EMDOCS, GNLM, IDS, ingenta, Linda Hall. **CCC.**

Published by: Elsevier Science BV, PO Box 211, Amsterdam 1000 AE, Netherlands. TEL 31-20-485-3757, FAX 31-20-485-3432, TELEX 18582 ESPA NL, http://www.elsevier.com/locate/bri. **Subscr. in Australasia and the Far East to:** Elsevier Science (Singapore) Pte Ltd, No.1 Temasek Ave, 17-01 Millenia Tower, Singapore 039192, Singapore. TEL 65-434-3727, FAX 65-337-2230; **Subscr. in Japan to:** Elsevier Science Inc - Japan Regional Office, 9-15 Higashi-Azabu 1-chome, Minato-ku, Tokyo 106-0044, Japan. TEL 81-3-5561-5033, FAX 81-3-5561-5047; **Subscr. in the Americas to:** Elsevier Science, PO Box 945, New York, NY 10159-0945. TEL 212-633-3730, 888-437-4636, FAX 212-633-3680, usinfo-f@elsevier.com, http://www.elsevier.com.

616.89 USA ISSN 0361-9230
QP376 CODEN: BRBUDU

BRAIN RESEARCH BULLETIN. Text in English. 1976. 18/yr. EUR 437 in Europe to qualified personnel; JPY 57,900 in Japan to qualified personnel; USD 488 elsewhere to qualified personnel; EUR 2,813 in Europe to institutions; JPY 354,228 in Japan to institutions; USD 3,147 elsewhere to institutions (effective 2002). adv. bk.rev. illus. index. back issues avail.; reprint service avail. from PQC,ISI. *Refereed.* **Document type:** *Bulletin, Academic/Scholarly.* **Description:** Broad spectrum of articles in the neurosciences, emphasizing rapid communication of comprehensive articles, meeting reports and special issues.

Incorporates (1972-1987): Journal of Electrophysiological Techniques (0361-0209)

Related titles: Microfilm ed.: (from PQC); Online - full text ed.: (from ingenta, Swets Blackwell, ScienceDirect, Institute for Scientific Information).

Indexed: ASCA, Anim.Behav.Abstr., Anim.Breed.Abstr., Aqua.Sci.& Fish.Abstr., Biol.Abstr., Biotech.& Bioeng.Abstr., Cal.Tiss.Abstr. (coverage dropped), Chem.Abstr., Chem.Indus.Notes, Chem.Titles, Chemorec.Abstr., Curr.Adv.Biochem., Curr.Adv.Cancer Res., Curr.Adv.Ecol.Sci., Curr.Cont., Dairy Sci.Abstr., Dent.Ind., Excerp.Med., Helminthol.Abstr., INIS Atomind., INSPEC (1983-1987, dropped), Ind.Med. (1976-), Ind.Sci.Rev., Ind.Vet., Inpharma, Int.Abstr.Biol.Sci., Neurosci.Abstr., Neurosci.Cit.Ind., Nutr.Abstr., Pharm.&Out.News, Pig News & Info., Poult.Abstr., PsycInfo, Psychol.Abstr. (1976-), Reac., Rev.Appl.Entomol., Rev.Arom.& Med.Plants, SSCI (coverage dropped), Sci.Cit.Ind., Sugar Ind.Abstr., THA, Tox.Abstr. (coverage dropped), Vet.Bull., e-psyche.

—BLDSC (2268.201000), CASDDS, CISTI, EMDOCS, GNLM, IDS, ingenta. **CCC.**

Published by: Elsevier Science, 655 Ave of the Americas, New York, NY 10010. TEL 212-989-5800, FAX 212-633-3990, usinfo-f@elsevier.com, http://www.elsevier.nl/locate/brainresbull, http://www.elsevier.com. Ed. Stephen B Dunnett. **Subscr. in Australasia and the Far East to:** Elsevier Science (Singapore) Pte Ltd, No.1 Temasek Ave, 17-01 Millenia Tower, Singapore 039192, Singapore. TEL 65-434-3727, FAX 65-337-2230; **Subscr. in Japan to:** Elsevier Science Inc - Japan Regional Office, 9-15 Higashi-Azabu 1-chome, Minato-ku, Tokyo 106-0044, Japan. TEL 81-3-5561-5033, FAX 81-3-5561-5047; **Subscr. outside the Americas to:** Elsevier Science BV, PO Box 211, Amsterdam 1000 AE, Netherlands. TEL 31-20-485-3757, FAX 31-20-485-3432, nlinfo-f@elsevier.nl, http://www.elsevier.nl.

616.8 USA

BRAIN RESEARCH FOUNDATION ANNUAL REPORT✶. Text in English. 1983. a. **Document type:** *Corporate.* **Description:** Presents financial statement, year's activities, list of the foundation's grants to scientists at University of Chicago's Brain Research Institute, donors lists, and scientific articles highlighting a specific area of research at the institute.

Related titles: Supplement: Brainwaves Newsletter.

Indexed: e-psyche.

Published by: Brain Research Foundation, 120 S LaSalle St Ste 1300, Chicago, IL 60603-3406. TEL 312-782-4311, FAX 312-782-6437. Ed. Nancy W Hohfeler. Circ: 1,100.

616.8 NLD ISSN 1385-299X
QP376 CODEN: BRPRFP

BRAIN RESEARCH PROTOCOLS. Text in Dutch. 1997. bi-m. EUR 656 in Europe to institutions; JPY 87,200 in Japan to institutions; USD 734 elsewhere to institutions (effective 2002). abstr. back issues avail. *Refereed.*

Related titles: Online - full text ed.: (from EBSCO Publishing, ingenta, Swets Blackwell, ScienceDirect, Institute for Scientific Information).

Indexed: Derwent Biotech.Abstr., Ind.Med. (1997-), Neurosci.Cit.Ind., PsycInfo, Ref.Zh., e-psyche.

—BLDSC (2268.203000), ADONIS, CASDDS, GNLM, IDS, Infotrieve, ingenta. **CCC.**

Published by: Elsevier Science BV, Regional Sales Office, PO Box 211, Amsterdam 1000 AE, Netherlands. TEL 31-20-485-2911, nlinfo-f@elsevier.nl, http://www.elsevier.nl/locate/brp. Ed. F G Wouterlood. **Subscr. in Australasia and the Far East to:** Elsevier Science (Singapore) Pte Ltd, No.1 Temasek Ave, 17-01 Millenia Tower, Singapore 039192, Singapore. TEL 65-434-3727, FAX 65-337-2230; **Subscr. in Japan to:** Elsevier Science Inc - Japan Regional Office, 9-15 Higashi-Azabu 1-chome, Minato-ku, Tokyo 106-0044, Japan. TEL 81-3-5561-5033, FAX 81-3-5561-5047; **Subscr. in the Americas to:** Elsevier Science, PO Box 945, New York, NY 10159-0945. TEL 212-633-3730, FAX 212-633-3680, http://www.elsevier.com.

616.8 NLD ISSN 0165-0173
CODEN: BRERD2

BRAIN RESEARCH REVIEWS. Text and summaries in English. 1980. 9/yr. EUR 972 in Europe to institutions (effective 2002); JPY 129,000 in Japan to institutions; USD 1,086 elsewhere to institutions (effective 2001). adv. abstr. back issues avail.; reprint service avail. from SWZ,ISI. *Refereed.* **Document type:** *Academic/Scholarly.* **Description:** Publishes articles and research papers which give analytical surveys that define heuristic hypotheses and provide new insights into brain mechanisms.

Related titles: Microform ed.: (from PQC); Online - full text ed.: (from EBSCO Publishing, ingenta, Swets Blackwell, ScienceDirect, Institute for Scientific Information).

Indexed: ASCA, Agri.& Environ.Biotech.Abstr. (coverage dropped), Anim.Behav.Abstr., Aqua.Sci.& Fish.Abstr., Biol.Abstr., Biotech.& Bioeng.Abstr., Cal.Tiss.Abstr., Chem.Abstr., Chem.Indus.Notes, Chem.Titles, Chemorec.Abstr., Curr.Adv.Cell & Devel.Biol., Curr.Adv.Ecol.Sci., Curr.Cont., Derwent Biotech.Abstr., Excerp.Med., INIS Atomind., Ind.Med. (1989-), Ind.Sci.Rev., Inpharma, Int.Abstr.Biol.Sci., Neurosci.Abstr., Neurosci.Cit.Ind., Pharm.&Out.News, PsycInfo, Psychol.Abstr. (1979-), Reac., Ref.Zh., SSCI (coverage dropped), Sci.Cit.Ind., THA, Zoo.Rec., e-psyche.

—BLDSC (2268.205000), ADONIS, CASDDS, CISTI, GNLM, IDS, ingenta. **CCC.**

Published by: Elsevier Science BV, PO Box 211, Amsterdam 1000 AE, Netherlands. TEL 31-20-485-2911, FAX 31-20-485-2457, nlinfo-f@elsevier.nl, http://www.elsevier.nl/inca/publications/5/0/6/0/4/9/. Eds. Dr. Dominick P Purpura, P J Magistretti. **Subscr. in Australasia and the Far East to:** Elsevier Science (Singapore) Pte Ltd, No.1 Temasek Ave, 17-01 Millenia Tower, Singapore 039192, Singapore. TEL 65-434-3727, FAX 65-337-2230; **Subscr. in Japan to:** Elsevier Science Inc - Japan Regional Office, 9-15 Higashi-Azabu 1-chome, Minato-ku, Tokyo 106-0044, Japan. TEL 81-3-5561-5033, FAX 81-3-5561-5047; **Subscr. in the Americas to:** Elsevier Science, PO Box 945, New York, NY 10159-0945. TEL 212-633-3730, FAX 212-633-3680, usinfo-f@elsevier.com, http://www.elsevier.com.

616.8 USA ISSN 0896-0267
CODEN: BRTOEZ

BRAIN TOPOGRAPHY; journal of functional neurophysiology. Text in English. 1988. q. EUR 161, USD 161 to individuals for print or online ed.; EUR 806, USD 807 to institutions for print or online ed.; EUR 967.20, USD 968.40 to institutions print & online eds.combined (effective 2002). adv. *Refereed.* **Document type:** *Academic/Scholarly.* **Description:** Reviews new research in the areas of EEG, MEG, psychiatry, and neuropsychology, and explores new methodology and techniques of data analysis and manipulation.

Related titles: Microform ed.: (from PQC); Online - full text ed.: (from O C L C Online Computer Library Center, Inc., Swets Blackwell, Kluwer Online, Institute for Scientific Information, RoweCom Information Quest).

M

Indexed: Curr.Cont., Ind.Med. (1988-), Inpharma, Int.Abstr.Biol.Sci., Neurosci.Cit.Ind., Pharm.&Out.News, PsycInfo, Psychol.Abstr. (1989-), Reac., Sci.Cit.Ind., e-psyche.
—BLDSC (2268.221200), CISTI, EMDOCS, GNLM, IDS, ingenta, KNAW. **CCC.**
Published by: Kluwer Academic - Plenum Publishers (Subsidiary of: Wolters Kluwer N.V.), 233 Spring St, New York, NY 10013-1578. TEL 212-620-8000, 800-221-9369, FAX 212-463-0742, services@wkap.nl, info@plenum.com, http://www.wkap.nl/journalhome.htm/0896-0267. Ed. Dr. Peter K H Wong. **Subscr. outside N America:** Kluwer Academic Publishers Group, Journals Department, PO Box 322, Dordrecht 3300 AH, Netherlands. TEL 31-78-639-2392, FAX 31-78-654-6474.

BRAIN TUMOR PATHOLOGY. see *MEDICAL SCIENCES—Oncology*

616.8 NLD ISSN 1380-3980
BRAINSCAN; a monthly scanning service from selected Elsevier Science neuroscience journals. Text in English. 1994. m. free per issue to qualified personnel. **Document type:** *Bulletin, Abstract/Index.* **Description:** Provides abstracts of current and forthcoming articles from 20 journals, as well as information on books and congresses in the field of neuroscience.
Indexed: e-psyche.
Published by: Elsevier Science BV, PO Box 211, Amsterdam 1000 AE, Netherlands. TEL 31-20-485-2911, FAX 31-20-485-2457. Circ: (controlled). **Subscr. in Australasia and the Far East to:** Elsevier Science (Singapore) Pte Ltd, No.1 Temasek Ave, 17-01 Millenia Tower, Singapore 039192, Singapore. TEL 65-434-3727, FAX 65-337-2230; **Subscr. in Japan to:** Elsevier Science Inc - Japan Regional Office, 9-15 Higashi-Azabu 1-chome, Minato-ku, Tokyo 106-0044, Japan. TEL 81-3-5561-5033, FAX 81-3-5561-5047; **Subscr. in the Americas to:** Elsevier Science, PO Box 945, New York, NY 10159-0945. TEL 212-633-3730, FAX 212-633-3680.

616.8 BRA ISSN 0104-9275
BRAZILIAN JOURNAL OF EPILEPSY AND CLINICAL NEUROPHYSIOLOGY/JORNAL BRASILEIRO DE EPILEPSIA E NEUROFISIOLOGIA CLINICA. Text in English, Portuguese, Spanish; Summaries in English, Portuguese. 1988. q. USD 70 to non-members; USD 120 foreign to non-members. adv. reprints avail. *Refereed.* **Document type:** *Academic/Scholarly.*
Formerly (until June 1995): Liga Brasileira de Epilepsia. Jornal (0103-3212)
Indexed: Excerp.Med., e-psyche.
—BLDSC (2277.405000).
Published by: Liga Brasileira de Epilepsia, Av Ipiranga, 6690, Sala 322, Porto Alegre, RGS 90610-000, Brazil. TEL 55-51-3394936, FAX 55-51-3394936. Ed. Dr. Jaderson Costa da Costa. R&P Magda Lahorgue Nunes. Adv. contact Nurma Pereira. Circ: 700 (controlled).

BREAKTHROUGH; international mental health journal. see *PSYCHOLOGY*

BRILL'S STUDIES IN EPISTEMOLOGY, PSYCHOLOGY AND PSYCHIATRY. see *PHILOSOPHY*

BRITISH ASSOCIATION FOR PSYCHOPHARMACOLOGY. MONOGRAPH. see *PHARMACY AND PHARMACOLOGY*

BRITISH JOURNAL OF DEVELOPMENTAL DISABILITIES. see *EDUCATION—Special Education And Rehabilitation*

616.8 GBR ISSN 1354-4187
BRITISH JOURNAL OF LEARNING DISABILITIES. Text in English. 1973. q., latest vol.30, 2002. GBP 39 in Europe to individuals; USD 62 in North America to individuals; GBP 43 elsewhere to individuals; GBP 82 in Europe to institutions; USD 132 in North America to institutions; GBP 91 elsewhere to institutions (effective 2002). adv. **Document type:** *Academic/Scholarly.* **Description:** Presents original articles with multidisciplinary appeal covering all aspects of learning disabilities.
Former titles (until 1993): Mental Handicap (0261-9997); (until Mar. 1982): Apex (0141-2205)
Related titles: Online - full text ed.: ISSN 1468-3156. GBP 36 in Europe to individuals; USD 56 in North America to individuals; GBP 36 elsewhere to individuals; GBP 74 in Europe to institutions; USD 119 in North America to institutions; GBP 74 elsewhere to institutions (effective 2002) (from EBSCO Publishing, O C L C Online Computer Library Center, Inc., ingenta, Munksgaard & Blackwell Science's Synergy, Swets Blackwell).
Indexed: AMED, Br.Educ.Ind., Brit.Nur.Ind., CINAHL, Cont.Pg.Educ., Curr.Adv.Ecol.Sci., ERA, PsycInfo, Psychol.Abstr. (1993-), Rehabil.Lit., Sp.Ed.Needs Abstr., e-psyche.
—BLDSC (2311.125000).
Published by: (British Institute of Learning Disabilities), Blackwell Science Ltd., PO Box 88, Oxford OX2 0NE, United Kingdom. TEL 44-1865-206180, 44-1865-206002, FAX 44-1865-206219, journals.cs@blacksci.co.uk, jnl.orders@blacksci.co.uk, http://www.blackwell-science.com/~cgilib/jnlpage.asp?Journal=bld&File=bld, http://www.blackwellpublishing.com. Eds. Dorothy Atkinson, Jan Walmsley. Pub. Elaine Stott. R&P Sophie Savage. Adv. contact Jenny Applin. Circ: 3,700.

BRITISH JOURNAL OF MEDICAL PSYCHOLOGY. see *PSYCHOLOGY*

BRITISH JOURNAL OF PROJECTIVE PSYCHOLOGY. see *PSYCHOLOGY*

616.89 GBR ISSN 0007-1250
RC321 CODEN: BJPYAJ
BRITISH JOURNAL OF PSYCHIATRY. Text in English. 1853. m. GBP 157 to individuals; GBP 170, USD 308 foreign to individuals; GBP 185 to institutions; GBP 220, USD 429 foreign to institutions (effective 2001). adv. bk.rev. bibl, charts, illus. index. reprint service avail. from PSC,SCH. *Refereed.* **Document type:** *Academic/Scholarly.* **Description:** Covers all branches of psychiatry, with emphasis on the clinical aspects of various topics in field.
Related titles: CD-ROM ed.: (from Ovid Technologies, Inc.); Online - full text ed.: (from Ovid Technologies, Inc., HighWire Pr., EBSCO Publishing, Institute for Scientific Information).
Indexed: AMED, ASCA, ASSIA, Abstr.Health Care Manage.Stud., Abstr.Hyg., Addic.Abstr., Adol.Ment.Hlth.Abstr., AgeLine, Agri.& Environ.Biotech.Abstr. (coverage dropped), Bibl.Dev.Med.& Child Neur., Biol.Abstr., Brit.Nur.Ind., CINAHL, Chem.Abstr., Crim.Just.Abstr., Curr.Adv.Ecol.Sci., Curr.Cont., Derwent Biotech.Abstr., Diab.Cont., Dok.Arbeitsmed., Environ.Sci.Poll.Mgmt., Excerp.Med., Fam.Ind., Helminthol.Abstr., Hosp.Abstr., IMFL, I.P.A., Ind.Med. (1963-), Ind.Sci.Rev., Indian Psychol.Abstr., Inpharma, Int.Abstr.Biol.Sci., Int.Nurs.Ind., Jrnl.Watch Psych., Jrnl.Watch Wom.Hlth., Lang.& Lang.Behav.Abstr., Mid.East: Abstr.& Ind., Neurosci.Cit.Ind., Nutr.Abstr., Pharm.&Out.News, Pollut.Abstr., PsycInfo, Psychol.Abstr. (1925-), Reac., Risk Abstr., SOPODA, SSCI, Saf.Sci.Abstr., Sci.Cit.Ind., So.Pac.Per.Ind., Sociol.Abstr., Stud.Wom.Abstr., THA, Trop.Dis.Bull., e-psyche.
—BLDSC (2320.800000), ADONIS, CASDDS, CISTI, EMDOCS, GNLM, IDS, ingenta, KNAW. **CCC.**
Published by: Royal College of Psychiatrists, 17 Belgrave Sq, London SW1X 8PG, United Kingdom. TEL 44-20-7235-8857, FAX 44-20-7245-1231. Ed. Greg Wilkinson. Adv. contact Peter Mell. Circ: 13,000. **Subscr. to:** Royal Society of Medicine, 1 Wimpole St, London W1M 8AE, United Kingdom. TEL 44-20-7290-2928, FAX 44-20-7290-2924.

616.891 GBR ISSN 0265-9883
BRITISH JOURNAL OF PSYCHOTHERAPY. Text in English. 1984. q. GBP 29 domestic to individuals; GBP 41 foreign to individuals; GBP 52 domestic to institutions; GBP 66 foreign to institutions (effective 2001). adv. bk.rev. *Refereed.* **Document type:** *Journal, Academic/Scholarly.* **Description:** Covers clinical and theoretical topics relevant to the psychotherapist practising privately or in institutions. Emphasizes analytical psychotherapy, and the application of psychotherapeutic practice and theory to institutions, society and other settings.
Indexed: PsycInfo, Psychoanal.Abstr., Psychol.Abstr. (1987-), e-psyche.
—BLDSC (2321.200000), EMDOCS, GNLM, Infotrieve, KNAW. **CCC.**
Published by: Artesian Books Ltd., 18 Artesian Rd, London W2 5AR, United Kingdom. TEL 0208-287-1128, FAX 0208-287-1128, artesianbooks@fsmail.com, http://www.artesianbooks.co.uk, http://www.artesianbooks.co.uk. Ed. Jean Arundale. Adv. contact Ann Scott TEL 0207-603-6803. Circ: 2,500.

362.4 616.835 GBR ISSN 0007-1633
BRITISH POLIO FELLOWSHIP. BULLETIN. Text in English. 1939. bi-m. GBP 0.20 per issue. adv. bk.rev. illus. **Document type:** *Bulletin.*
Indexed: e-psyche.
Published by: British Polio Fellowship, 126 Radnor Ave, Bexleyheath, Welling, Kent DA16 2BY, United Kingdom. TEL 081-304-3166, FAX 081-304-3166. Ed. Kathleen M Dibley. Circ: 8,000.

BRUNNER - MAZEL INTEGRATIVE PSYCHOTHERAPY SERIES. see *PSYCHOLOGY*

612.8 JPN ISSN 0917-0898
BUREIN SAIENSU/BRAIN SCIENCE. Text in Japanese. 1990. q. JPY 1,500.
Indexed: e-psyche.
Published by: Koseisha Infomeshon Sabisu/Koseisha Information Service, 2-7 Dojima 3-chome, Kita-ku, Osaka-shi 530-0003, Japan.

612.8 JPN
BUREIN SAIENSU SAIZENSEN/FRONTIERS OF BRAIN SCIENCE. Text in Japanese. 1988. a. JPY 2,000.
Formerly (until vol.5, 1992): Burein Saiensu Kenkyu Hokokushu. Brain Science Foundation. Annual Study Report
Indexed: e-psyche.
Published by: (Burein Saiensu Shinko Zaidan), Kodansha Scientific, 9-25 Shinogawa-Machi, Shinjuku-ku, Tokyo 162-0814, Japan.

616.89 JPN ISSN 0910-4798
BYOIN, CHIIKI SEISHIN IGAKU/JAPANESE JOURNAL OF HOSPITAL AND COMMUNITY PSYCHIATRY. Text in Japanese. 1958. q. JPY 12,000. bk.rev. *Refereed.* **Document type:** *Academic/Scholarly.*
Formerly (until 1984): Byoin Seishin Igaku (0910-478X)
Indexed: e-psyche.
—BLDSC (4655.178000).
Published by: Byoin Chiiki Seishin Igakkai/Japanese Hospital and Community Psychiatry Association, National Center for Neurology & Psychiatry, 1-1 Ogawa-Higashi-cho 4-chome, Kodaira-shi, Tokyo-to 187-0031, Japan. TEL 81-423-41-2711, FAX 81-423-44-6745. Ed. Iwao Oshima.

616.8 617 USA ISSN 1068-9230
C I N N REPORT. Text in English. 1989. 2/yr. free per issue. **Document type:** *Trade.* **Description:** Contains information on neurosurgery and related considerations.
Formerly (until 1994): C N C Report
Indexed: e-psyche.
Published by: Chicago Institute of Neurosurgery and Neuroresearch, 2515 n Clark St, Ste 800, Chicago, IL 60614. TEL 773-388-7700, FAX 773-935-2132, connobd@suba.com, http://www/chicinn.com. Ed. Heather L French. Circ: 15,000.

616.8 CAN ISSN 0831-6279
C M T NEWSLETTER; published bimonthly by and for those with Charcot-Marie-Tooth disease. Text in English. 1984. bi-m. donation. illus. index. back issues avail.; reprints avail. **Document type:** *Newsletter, Academic/Scholarly.* **Description:** For people and health professionals interested in learning more about Charcot-Marie-Tooth disease, a progressive debilitating neuromuscular disorder.
Indexed: e-psyche.
Published by: (Personal Muscular Atrophy International Association, Inc.), C M T International, 1 Springbank Dr, St Catharines, ON L2S 2K1, Canada. TEL 905-687-3630, http://www.cmtint.org. Ed., Pub. Linda D Crabtree. R&P Linda Crabtree. Circ: 2,400.

616.8 NZL ISSN 1174-5908
▼ **C N S DISORDERS TODAY.** (Central Nervous System) Text in English. 1999. m. USD 95 to individuals; USD 545 to institutions (effective 2001). back issues avail. **Description:** Rapid alerts service on all aspects of drug therapy and disease management of psychiatric and neurological disorders.
Indexed: Inpharma, Pharm.&Out.News, Reac., e-psyche.
Published by: Adis International Limited, Mairangi Bay, Private Bag 65901, Auckland 1010, New Zealand. TEL 64-9-477-0700, FAX 64-9-477-0766, http://www.adis.com. **Americas subscr. to:** Adis International Inc., Attn: Subscription Dept, 860 Town Center Dr, Langhorne, PA 19047. TEL 877-872-2347.

C N S DRUG REVIEWS. see *PHARMACY AND PHARMACOLOGY*

C N S DRUGS. (Central Nervous System) see *PHARMACY AND PHARMACOLOGY*

616.8 USA ISSN 1532-8570
▼ **C N S NEWS.** (Central Nervous System) Text in English. 1999. m. USD 60 (effective 2001). adv. back issues avail. **Document type:** *Newspaper, Trade.* **Description:** Provides clinical updates, convention coverage and educational reviews in neurology and psychiatry.
Related titles: Online - full content ed.; Special ed.

Published by: McMahon Group, 545 W 45th St, 8th Fl, New York, NY 10036. TEL 212-957-5300, FAX 212-957-7230, donaldp@mcmahonmed.com, http://www.central-nervous-system.com/index.html, http://www.mcmahonmed.com. adv.: B&W page USD 4,450, color page USD 1,900.

616.89 GBR ISSN 1463-046X

▼ **C P D BULLETIN. PSYCHIATRY.** (Continuing Professional Development) Text in English. 1999. 3/yr. (1 volume per annum). GBP 45 domestic to individuals; GBP 60 foreign to individuals; GBP 60 domestic to institutions; GBP 90 foreign to institutions (effective 2000). adv. Website rev. abstr. 24 p./no. 2 cols./p. **Document type:** *Journal.*

—BLDSC (3486.192400).

Published by: Rila Publications Ltd., 73 Newman St, London W1A 4PG, United Kingdom. TEL 44-20-7631-1299, FAX 44-20-7580-7166, admin@rila.co.uk, subscriptions@rila.co.uk, http://www.nla.co.uk, http://www.rila.co.uk. Eds. Hugh Freeman, Stephen P Tyrer. Pub., Adv. contact G Da'Cambra. Circ: 2,000 (paid).

CAHIERS DE PSYCHOLOGIE CLINIQUE; une revue interdisciplinaire en psychologie clinique et psychotherapie. see *PSYCHOLOGY*

616.8 CHE ISSN 1016-9229

CAHIERS PSYCHIATRIQUES GENEVOIS. Text in French. 1987. s-a. CHF 55, EUR 35.71 domestic; CHF 65, EUR 42.20 foreign (effective 2002). **Document type:** *Journal, Academic/Scholarly.*

Indexed: e-psyche.

Published by: Editions Medecine et Hygiene, Case Postale 456, Geneva, 4 1211, Switzerland. TEL 41-22-7029311, FAX 41-22-7029355, abonnements@medhyg.ch, http://www.medhyg.ch.

616.8 GBR ISSN 1350-1461

CAMBRIDGE MEDICAL REVIEWS. NEUROLOGY AND PSYCHIATRY. Text in English. 1991. irreg. **Document type:** *Monographic series.*

Indexed: e-psyche.

Published by: Cambridge University Press, Edinburgh Bldg, Shaftesbury Rd, Cambridge CB2 2RU, United Kingdom. FAX 44-1223-315052, information@cup.cam.ac.uk, information@cambridge.org, http://www.cup.cam.ac.uk, http://www.uk.cambridge.org/journals/pmu. Ed. Robert Kerwin. R&P Linda Nicol.

616.8 CAN ISSN 0317-1671
RC321 CODEN: CJNSA2

CANADIAN JOURNAL OF NEUROLOGICAL SCIENCES. Text in English, French; Abstracts in English, French. 1974. q. CND 77 domestic; USD 75 foreign (effective 2001). adv. bk.rev. index. back issues avail.; reprint service avail. from PQC,ISI. *Refereed.* **Document type:** *Academic/Scholarly.* **Description:** Presents original work in the clinical and basic neurosciences.

Related titles: Microform ed.: (from PQC); Online - full text ed.: (from Institute for Scientific Information).

Indexed: ASCA, Aqua.Sci.& Fish.Abstr., Biol.Abstr., Chem.Abstr., Curr.Adv.Ecol.Sci., Curr.Cont., Dent.Ind., Excerp.Med., INIS Atomind., Ind.Med. (1974-), Ind.Sci.Rev., Inpharma, Int.Abstr.Biol.Sci., Jrnl.Watch Neuro., Lab.Haz.Bull., NRN, Neurosci.Abstr. (coverage dropped), Neurosci.Cit.Ind., Nutr.Abstr., Pharm.&Out.News, Reac., Sci.Cit.Ind., Weed Abstr., e-psyche.

—BLDSC (3033.300000), CASDDS, CISTI, EMDOCS, GNLM, IDS, ingenta, KNAW. **CCC.**

Published by: Canadian Journal of Neurological Sciences, Inc., P O Box 5456, Sta A, Calgary, AB T2H 1X8, Canada. TEL 403-229-9575, FAX 403-229-1661, journal@cjns.org, http://www.cjns.org. Ed., R&P Dr. Douglas W Zochodne. Pub. Sally A Gregg. Adv. contact Sally Gregg. color page CND 1,663. Circ: 1,600 (paid). **Subscr.in N. America to:** Allen Press Inc., PO Box 1897, Lawrence, KS 66044-8897. **Co-sponsors:** Canadian Neurological Society; Canadian Neurosurgical Society; Canadian Society of Clinical Neurophysiologists; Canadian Association of Child Neurology.

616.89 CAN ISSN 0706-7437
RC321 CODEN: CPAJAK

THE CANADIAN JOURNAL OF PSYCHIATRY/REVUE CANADIENNE DE PSYCHIATRIE. Text in English, French. 1956. 10/yr. CND 90; CND 110 foreign (effective 1999). adv. bk.rev. bibl, charts, illus. index. back issues avail.; reprint service avail. from PQC,PSC,SCH. *Refereed.* **Document type:** *Academic/Scholarly.* **Description:** Provides a forum for a broad spectrum of scholarly presentations, case reports, position papers, editorial contributions and current perspectives.

Formerly: Canadian Psychiatric Association Journal (0008-4824)

Related titles: Microform ed.: (from PQC); Online - full text ed.: (from EBSCO Publishing, Institute for Scientific Information).

Indexed: ASCA, ASSIA, Addic.Abstr., Adol.Ment.Hlth.Abstr., AgeLine, Bibl.Asian Stud. (1970), Bibl.Dev.Med.& Child Neur., CBCA Ref., CINAHL, Chem.Abstr., Child Devel.Abstr., Crim.Just.Abstr., Curr.Adv.Ecol.Sci., Curr.Cont., Dok.Arbeitsmed., Excerp.Med., Fam.Ind., Ind.Med. (1979-), Ind.Sci.Rev., Inpharma, Int.Nurs.Ind., Lang.& Lang.Behav.Abstr., Mid.East: Abstr.& Ind., NRN, Neurosci.Cit.Ind., Pharm.&Out.News, PsycInfo, Psychol.Abstr. (1961-), Reac., SOPODA, SSCI, Sage Fam.Stud.Abstr., Sage Urb.Stud.Abstr., Sci.Cit.Ind., So.Pac.Per.Ind., Sociol.Abstr., Sp.Ed.Needs Abstr., Yrbk.Assoc.Educ.& Rehab.Blind, e-psyche.

—BLDSC (3034.800000), CISTI, EMDOCS, GNLM, IDS, ingenta, KNAW. **CCC.**

Published by: Canadian Psychiatric Association, 260 441 MacLaren St, Ottawa, ON K2P 2H3, Canada. TEL 613-234-2815, FAX 613-234-9857, cjp@cpa-apc.org, http://www.cpa-apc.org, http://www.allenpress.com. Ed. Q Rae Grant. Pub., Adv. contact Sharon Petrie. B&W page CND 1,035, color page CND 2,010; trim 10.88 x 8.13. Circ: 3,500. **Subscr.in N.America to:** Allen Press Inc., PO Box 1897, Lawrence, KS 66044-8897.

616.89 CAN ISSN 1195-3330

CANADIAN JOURNAL OF PSYCHOANALYSIS/REVUE CANADIENNE DE PSYCHANALYSE. Text in English. 1993. s-a. CND 50 domestic to individuals; CND 60 foreign to individuals; CND 65 domestic to institutions; CND 70 foreign to institutions (effective 2001). bk.rev. *Refereed.* **Document type:** *Academic/Scholarly.*

Indexed: CBCA Ref., e-psyche.

—BLDSC (3034.850000).

Published by: (Canadian Psychoanalytic Society/Societe Canadienne de Psychanalyse), Becker Associates, P O Box 507, Sta Q, Toronto, ON M4T 2M5, Canada. TEL 416-483-7282, FAX 416-489-1713, psyanal@aei.com, http://home.ican.net/~analyst/cjp.htm. Ed., Adv. contact Donald Carveth. Circ: 500 (paid).

616.89 CAN

CANADIAN PSYCHIATRIC ASSOCIATION BULLETIN. Text in English. bi-m. **Document type:** *Journal.* **Description:** Serves as a forum for the exchange of views on current legislation and public affairs, and announces events and programs of interest to the psychiatric and mental health care community.

Related titles: Online - full text ed.

Indexed: e-psyche.

Published by: Canadian Psychiatric Association, 260 441 MacLaren St, Ottawa, ON K2P 2H3, Canada. TEL 613-234-2815, FAX 613-234-9857, bulletin@cpa-apc.org, http://www.cpa-apc.org. Ed. Dr. A G Awad. Pub. Sharon Petrie.

616.8 GBR ISSN 1357-8944

CATNAP. Text in English. 1986. q. GBP 10; GBP 15 foreign (effective 2001). back issues avail.; reprints avail. *Refereed.* **Document type:** *Bulletin.* **Description:** Aims to promote awareness of narcolepsy and provide authoritative information to narcoleptics, to health professionals, and to the public.

Formerly (until 1992): Narcolepsy Association Newsletter (1357-8936)

Indexed: e-psyche.

Published by: Narcolepsy Association (U.K.), Craven House, 121 Kingsway, London WC2B 6PA, United Kingdom. TEL 44-1273-832725, 01-322-863195, FAX 44-1273-832725, secretary@ukan.hands.com, info@narcolepsy.org.uk, http://www.narcolepsy.org.uk. Ed. W Richmond. R&P, Adv. contact M Cadwallader. Circ: 800 (controlled).

616.8 USA ISSN 0272-4340
QP351 CODEN: CMNEDI

CELLULAR & MOLECULAR NEUROBIOLOGY. Text in English. 1981. bi-m. USD 114 in the Americas to individuals for print or online ed.; EUR 114 elsewhere to individuals for print or online ed.; USD 681 in the Americas to institutions for print or online ed.; EUR 680 elsewhere to institutions for print or online ed.; USD 817.20 in the Americas to institutions for print & online eds. combined; EUR 816 elsewhere to institutions for print & online eds. combined (effective 2002). adv. back issues avail. *Refereed.* **Document type:** *Journal, Academic/Scholarly.* **Description:** Examines the anatomic, genetic, physiologic, pharmacologic, and biochemical approaches to the analysis of neuronal and brain function at the cellular and subcellular levels.

Related titles: Microfilm ed.: (from PQC); Online - full text ed.: (from EBSCO Publishing, O C L C Online Computer Library Center, Inc., RoweCom Information Quest, Swets Blackwell, Kluwer Online, Institute for Scientific Information).

Indexed: ASCA, Aqua.Sci.& Fish.Abstr., BBCI, Biol.Abstr., Biotech.& Bioeng.Abstr., Chem.Abstr., Chem.Indus.Notes, Chem.Titles, Chemorec.Abstr., Curr.Adv.Ecol.Sci., Curr.Cont., Excerp.Med., INIS Atomind., Ind.Med. (1981-), Ind.Sci.Rev., Inpharma, Int.Abstr.Biol.Sci., Neurosci.Abstr., Neurosci.Cit.Ind., Reac., Sci.Cit.Ind., e-psyche.

—BLDSC (3097.925000), CASDDS, CISTI, EMDOCS, GNLM, IDS, ingenta, KNAW. **CCC.**

Published by: Kluwer Academic - Plenum Publishers (Subsidiary of: Wolters Kluwer N.V.), 233 Spring St, New York, NY 10013-1578. TEL 212-620-8000, 800-221-9369, FAX 212-463-0742, info@plenum.com, http://www.wkap.nl/journalhome.htm/0272-4340. Ed. Dr. Juan M Saavedra. R&P Rose Luongo TEL 781-871-6311. **Subscr. outside the Americas to:** Kluwer Academic Publishers Group, Journals Department, PO Box 322, Dordrecht 3300 AH, Netherlands. TEL 31-78-639-2392, FAX 31-78-654-6474.

CELLULAR NEUROBIOLOGY. see *BIOLOGY—Cytology And Histology*

616.8 GBR ISSN 0333-1024
CODEN: CEPHDF

CEPHALALGIA; an international journal of headache. Text in English. 1981. 10/yr., latest vol.22, 2002. GBP 275 in Europe; USD 396 in North America; GBP 275 elsewhere (effective 2002). adv. index. back issues avail. *Refereed.* **Document type:** *Academic/Scholarly.* **Description:** Covers migraine and headache research.

Related titles: Microform ed.: (from PQC); Online - full text ed.: ISSN 1468-2982. GBP 248 in Europe; USD 357 in North America; GBP 248 elsewhere (effective 2002) (from EBSCO Publishing, O C L C Online Computer Library Center, Inc., RoweCom Information Quest, ingenta, Munksgaard & Blackwell Science's Synergy, Swets Blackwell, Institute for Scientific Information); ♦ Supplement: Cephalalgia. Supplement. ISSN 0800-1952.

Indexed: ASCA, Biol.Abstr., Chem.Abstr., Curr.Adv.Ecol.Sci., Curr.Cont., Dent.Ind., Excerp.Med., INIS Atomind., Ind.Med. (1981-), Ind.Sci.Rev., Inpharma, Jrnl.Watch Neuro., NRN, Neurosci.Cit.Ind., Pharm.&Out.News, Reac., SSCI (coverage dropped), Sci.Cit.Ind., e-psyche.

—BLDSC (3113.691000), ADONIS, CASDDS, CISTI, EMDOCS, GNLM, IDS, ingenta, KNAW. **CCC.**

Published by: (International Headache Society NOR), Blackwell Science Ltd., PO Box 88, Oxford OX2 0NE, United Kingdom. TEL 44-1865-206180, 44-1865-206002, FAX 44-1865-206219, jnl.orders@blacksci.co.uk, http://www.blackwell-science.com/~cgilib/jnlpage.bin?Journal=cha&File=cha&Page=aims, http://www.blackwellpublishing.com. Ed. Dr. P Goadsby. Pub. Allen Stevens. R&P Sophie Savage. Adv. contact Jenny Applin. Circ: 1,500.

616.8 GBR ISSN 0800-1952

CEPHALALGIA. SUPPLEMENT. Text in English. 1983. irreg. **Document type:** *Journal, Academic/Scholarly.*

Related titles: ♦ Supplement to: Cephalalgia. ISSN 0333-1024.

—BLDSC (3113.691100), ADONIS.

Published by: (International Headache Society NOR), Blackwell Science Ltd., Osney Mead, Oxford OX2 0EL, United Kingdom. TEL 44-1685-206206, FAX 44-1685-721205, journals.cs@blacksci.co.uk, http://www.blackwell-science.com.

616.8 GBR ISSN 1473-4222
▼ **THE CEREBELLUM.** Text in English. 2001. q. GBP 95, USD 135 to individuals; GBP 275, USD 395 to institutions (effective 2002). **Document type:** *Journal, Academic/Scholarly.* **Description:** Devoted to the science of the cerebellum and its role in ataxia and other medical disorders.
Related titles: Online - full content ed.; Online - full text ed.: (from CatchWord Ltd.).
Published by: Martin Dunitz Ltd. (Subsidiary of: Taylor & Francis Group), 7-9 Pratt St, London NW1 0AE, United Kingdom. TEL 44-20-7482-2202, FAX 44-20-7482-7088, The.Cerebellum@tandf.co.uk, info@dunitz.co.uk, http://www.dunitz.co.uk. Ed. Mario-Ubaldo Manto.

616.8 USA ISSN 1047-3211
QP383
CEREBRAL CORTEX. Text in English. 1991. m. GBP 180, USD 265 to individuals; GBP 440, USD 720 to institutions (effective 2002). adv. 116 p./no. back issues avail. *Refereed.* **Document type:** *Journal, Academic/Scholarly.* **Description:** Interdisciplinary journal publishing papers on the development, organization, plasticity, and function of the cerebral cortex.
Related titles: Online - full text ed.: ISSN 1460-2199. GBP 396, USD 648 to institutions Online only (effective 2002) (from HighWire Pr., EBSCO Publishing, O C L C Online Computer Library Center, Inc., RoweCom Information Quest, ingenta, Swets Blackwell, Institute for Scientific Information).
Indexed: ASCA, Aqua.Sci.& Fish.Abstr., Chemorec.Abstr., Compumath, Curr.Cont., Excerp.Med. (1993-), Ind.Med. (1991-), Ind.Sci.Rev., Inpharma, Int.Abstr.Biol.Sci., Neurosci.Abstr., Neurosci.Cit.Ind., Pharm.&Out.News, PsycInfo, Psychol.Abstr. (1991-), Reac., Sci.Cit.Ind., Zoo.Rec., e-psyche.
—BLDSC (3120.027550), CISTI, EMDOCS, GNLM, IDS, Infotrieve, KNAW. **CCC.**
Published by: Oxford University Press, Academic Division, Great Clarendon St, Oxford OX2 6DP, United Kingdom. TEL 44-1865-267907, FAX 44-1865-267835, jnlorders@oup-usa.org; www-admin@oup.co.uk, jnl.info@oup.co.uk, http://www.oup.co.uk/cercor/, http://www.oup.co.uk/journals. Pub. Mandy Sketch. adv.: page GBP 230, page USD 415. Circ: 760. **Subscr. outside the Americas to:** Journals Marketing, Great Clarendon St, Oxford OX2 6DP, United Kingdom.

616.8 616.15 CHE ISSN 1015-9770
CODEN: CDISE7
CEREBROVASCULAR DISEASES. Text in English. 1991. 8/yr. CHF 1,090 in Europe to institutions; CHF 1,113.20 overseas to institutions; EUR 778.40 in Europe to institutions; USD 848 overseas to institutions (effective 2002). adv. back issues avail. *Refereed.* **Document type:** *Journal, Academic/Scholarly.* **Description:** Involves a variety of specialties such as neurology, internal medicine, surgery, radiology, epidemiology, cardiology, hematology, psychology and rehabilitation. Deals with all aspects of stroke and cerebrovascular diseases. Contains original contributions, reviews of selected topics and clinical investigative studies, recent meetings reports and work-in-progress as well as discussions on controversial issues.
Related titles: Microform ed.: (from PQC); Online - full text ed.: ISSN 1421-9786. CHF 116, EUR 84, USD 90 to institutions with print edition (effective 2002) (from EBSCO Publishing, O C L C Online Computer Library Center, Inc., RoweCom Information Quest, Swets Blackwell, Institute for Scientific Information).
Indexed: Curr.Cont., Excerp.Med. (1996-), Ind.Med. (1991-), Ind.Sci.Rev., Inpharma, Jrnl.Watch Neuro., Neurosci.Cit.Ind., Pharm.&Out.News, Reac., Sci.Cit.Ind., e-psyche.
—BLDSC (3120.037790), CISTI, EMDOCS, GNLM, IDS, Infotrieve, KNAW. **CCC.**
Published by: S. Karger AG, Allschwilerstr 10, PO Box, Basel 4009, Switzerland. TEL 41-61-306-1111, FAX 41-61-306-1234, karger@karger.ch, http://www.online.karger.com/journals/ced, http://www.karger.com. Eds. J Bogousslavsky, M Hennerici. adv.: page USD 1,195.

616.8 USA ISSN 1524-6205
CEREBRUM; the Dana forum on brain science. Text in English. 1998. q. USD 30 domestic to individuals; USD 42 foreign to individuals; USD 48 to institutions; USD 7.50 newsstand/cover (effective 2000). back issues avail. **Document type:** *Academic/Scholarly, Trade.* **Description:** Interdisciplinary journal of opinion for lay readers focusing on challenging issues raised by brain research, their impact and their implications. Articles, debates, interviews, full color visual features, book reviews, book excerpts by top scientists and other thinkers.
Published by: The Dana Press, 745 Fifth Ave Ste 700, New York, NY 10151. TEL 212-223-4040, FAX 212-317-8721, cerebrum@dana.org, http://www.dana.org/cerebrum. Ed., Pub. Walter Donway. Circ: 6,000 (paid and controlled). **Subscr. to:** Cerebrum Subscriber Services, P O Box 573, Oxon Hill, MD 20745-0573. TEL 301-567-7999. **Co-sponsor:** The Charles A. Dana Foundation.

616.8 617.48 CZE ISSN 1210-7859
CODEN: CKNNAS
CESKA A SLOVENSKA NEUROLOGIE A NEUROCHIRURGIE. Text in Czech, Slovak; Summaries in Czech, English. 1937. 6/yr. EUR 84, USD 108 (effective 2001). adv. bk.rev. abstr, bibl, charts, illus. index. *Refereed.* **Document type:** *Academic/Scholarly.* **Description:** Publishes original papers from the whole range of neurology and neurosurgery.
Former titles (until 1994): Ceskoslovenska Neurologie a Neurochirurgie (0301-0597); Neurologie a Psychiatrie Ceskoslovenska
Related titles: Online - full text ed.: (from Institute for Scientific Information).
Indexed: ASCA, C.I.S. Abstr., Chem.Abstr., Curr.Adv.Ecol.Sci., Dent.Ind., Excerp.Med., INIS Atomind., Ind.Med. (until 1992, dropped), Neurosci.Cit.Ind., e-psyche.
—BLDSC (3120.258450), CASDDS, CISTI, EMDOCS, GNLM, IDS. **CCC.**
Published by: (Ceska Lekarska Spolecnost J.E. Purkyne/Czech Medical Association), Nakladatelske Stredisko C L S J.E. Purkyne, Sokolska 31, Prague 12026, Czech Republic. TEL 420-2-24911420, nts@iol.cz, http://www.clsjep.cz, http://www.medical.cz. Ed. Karel Urbanek. adv.: B&W page CZK 25,700, color page CZK 36,400; 246 x 173. Circ: 1,600. **Dist. by:** Abont s.r.o., Chlumova 17, Prague, 3 130 00, Czech Republic; **Dist. in Western countries by:** Kubon & Sagner, Hesstr 39-41, Munich 80798, Germany.

616.8 CZE ISSN 1212-0383
CESKA A SLOVENSKA PSYCHIATRIE. Text in Czech, Slovak; Summaries in Czech, English. 1904. 8/yr. EUR 112, USD 144 (effective 2001). adv. bk.rev. abstr. *Refereed.* **Document type:** *Academic/Scholarly.*
Formerly (until 1993): Cesko-Slovenska Psychiatrie (0069-2336)
Indexed: C.I.S. Abstr., Excerp.Med., Ind.Med. (coverage dropped), PsycInfo, Psychol.Abstr. (1959-), e-psyche.
—BLDSC (3120.258480), EMDOCS, GNLM, Infotrieve. **CCC.**
Published by: (Ceska Lekarska Spolecnost J.E. Purkyne/Czech Medical Association), Nakladatelske Stredisko C L S J.E. Purkyne, Sokolska 31, Prague 12026, Czech Republic. TEL 42-2-24911420, FAX 42-2-24911420, nts@iol.cz, http://www.clsjep.cz, http://www.medical.cz. Ed. Frantisek Faltus. adv.: B&W page CZK 30,100, color page CZK 42,000; 198 x 135. Circ: 2,700. **Dist. by:** Abont s.r.o., Chlumova 17, Prague, 3 130 00, Czech Republic; **Dist. in Western countries by:** Kubon & Sagner, Hesstr 39-41, Munich 80798, Germany.

CHILD AND ADOLESCENT PSYCHIATRIC CLINICS OF NORTH AMERICA. see *MEDICAL SCIENCES—Pediatrics*

616.8 615 618.92 USA ISSN 1085-0295
CHILD AND ADOLESCENT PSYCHOPHARMACOLOGY NEWS. Text in English. 1996. bi-m. USD 99 domestic to individuals; USD 109 foreign to individuals; USD 135 domestic to institutions; USD 145 foreign to institutions (effective 2000). bk.rev. abstr, bibl. index. reprint service avail. from PQC. **Document type:** *Newsletter, Academic/Scholarly.* **Description:** Addresses clinical and research information on issues related to psychopharmacology for children and adolescents, such as which drugs work, drug interactions and treatment plans.
Formerly: Child and Adolescent Psychopharmacology Newsletter
Related titles: Microform ed.: (from PQC); Online - full text ed.: (from CatchWord Ltd., RoweCom Information Quest).
Indexed: e-psyche.
Published by: Guilford Publications, Inc., 72 Spring St, New York, NY 10012. TEL 212-431-9800, 800-365-7006, FAX 212-966-6708, info@guilford.com. Ed. Stanley Kutcher. R&P Kathy Kuehl. Adv. contact Susan Pavliscak.

CHILD BEHAVIOR AND DEVELOPMENT. see *MEDICAL SCIENCES—Pediatrics*

616.89 USA ISSN 0009-398X
RJ499.A1 CODEN: CPHDA3
CHILD PSYCHIATRY AND HUMAN DEVELOPMENT. Text in English. 1970. q. USD 485 in the Americas to institutions for print or online ed.; EUR 485 elsewhere to institutions for print or online ed; USD 582 in the Americas to institutions print & online eds.combined; EUR 582 elsewhere to institutions print & online eds.combined (effective 2002). adv. bibl. index. back issues avail.; reprint service avail. from PQC,PSC,SCH,ISI. *Refereed.* **Document type:** *Journal, Academic/Scholarly.* **Description:** Serves allied professional groups of specialists in child psychiatry, social science, pediatrics, psychology, and human development.
Related titles: Microform ed.: (from PQC); Online - full text ed.: (from EBSCO Publishing, O C L C Online Computer Library Center, Inc., Swets Blackwell, Kluwer Online, Institute for Scientific Information, RoweCom Information Quest).
Indexed: ASCA, ASSIA, Abstr.Crim.& Pen., Adol.Ment.Hlth.Abstr., AgeLine, Amer.Bibl.Slavic & E.Eur.Stud., Bibl.Dev.Med.& Child Neur., Biol.Abstr., C.I.J.E. (coverage dropped), Child Devel.Abstr., Crim.Just.Abstr., Curr.Cont., Educ.Ind. (Jan.1983-Jun.1992), Except.Child Educ.Abstr., Excerp.Med., Fam.Ind., IMFL, Ind.Med. (1970-), Inpharma, Lang.& Lang.Behav.Abstr., Nutr.Abstr., Pharm.&Out.News, PsycInfo, Psychol.Abstr. (1970-), Psycscan D.P., Reac., Risk Abstr., SOPODA, SSCI, Sage Fam.Stud.Abstr., Sage Urb.Stud.Abstr., Soc.Work Res.& Abstr., Sociol.Abstr., Wom.Stud.Abstr., e-psyche.
—BLDSC (3172.945000), EMDOCS, GNLM, IDS, ingenta, KNAW. **CCC.**
Published by: (American Association of Psychiatric Services for Children), Kluwer Academic - Plenum Publishers (Subsidiary of: Wolters Kluwer N.V.), 233 Spring St, New York, NY 10013-1578. TEL 212-620-8000, 800-221-9369, FAX 212-463-0742, services@wkap.nl, info@plenum.com, http://www.wkap.nl/journalhome.htm/0009-398X. Ed. Kenneth J Tarnowski. **Subscr. outside the Americas to:** Kluwer Academic Publishers Group, Journals Department, PO Box 322, Dordrecht 3300 AH, Netherlands. TEL 31-78-639-2392, FAX 31-78-654-6474.

CHILDREN'S MENTAL HEALTH SERVICES. see *PSYCHOLOGY*

618.92 612 DEU ISSN 0256-7040
CODEN: CNSYE9
CHILD'S NERVOUS SYSTEM. Text in English. 1972. m. EUR 1,298 domestic; EUR 1,290.70 in Germany; EUR 127 newsstand/cover foreign (effective 2002). adv. bibl, charts, illus. reprint service avail. from ISI. *Refereed.* **Document type:** *Journal, Academic/Scholarly.* **Description:** Encompasses all aspects of the pediatric neurosciences including development and growth, trauma, degenerative disorders, hereditary diseases, neurophysiology, neurology and neurosurgery.
Superseded in part (in 1985): Child's Brain (0302-2803)
Related titles: Microform ed.: (from RPI); Online - full text ed.: ISSN 1433-0350 (from EBSCO Publishing, RoweCom Information Quest, Swets Blackwell, Springer LINK, Institute for Scientific Information).
Indexed: ASCA, Bibl.Dev.Med.& Child Neur., Biol.Abstr., Curr.Adv.Ecol.Sci., Curr.Cont., Dent.Ind., Excerp.Med., Helminthol.Abstr., Ind.Med. (1985-), Ind.Sci.Rev., Inpharma, Int.Nurs.Ind., Neurosci.Cit.Ind., Nutr.Abstr., Pharm.&Out.News, Protozool.Abstr., Reac., Rev.Med.& Vet.Mycol., SSCI (coverage dropped), Sci.Cit.Ind., e-psyche.
—BLDSC (3172.993080), CISTI, EMDOCS, GNLM, IDS, ingenta, KNAW. **CCC.**
Published by: (International Society for Pediatric Neurosurgery), Springer-Verlag (Subsidiary of: BertelsmannSpringer), Tiergartenstr 17, Heidelberg 69121, Germany. TEL 49-6221-345-0, FAX 49-6221-345229, subscriptions@springer.de, http://link.springer.de/link/service/journals/00381/index.htm, http://www.springer.de. Ed. A J Raimondi. Circ: 1,125. **Subscr. in N. America to:** Springer-Verlag New York Inc., PO Box 2485, Secaucus, NJ 07096-2485. TEL 212-460-1500, FAX 212-473-6272. **Co-sponsors:** European Society for Paediatric Neurosurgery; Japanese Society for Pediatric Neurosurgery.

CHOKAKU GENGO SHOGAI/COMMUNICATION DISORDER RESEARCH. see *BIOLOGY—Physiology*

616.8 ITA ISSN 0390-0088
CLINICA NEUROPSICHIATRICA. Text in Italian; Summaries in English, French, German, Italian. 1965. irreg. **Document type:** *Academic/Scholarly.*
Indexed: e-psyche.

M

Published by: Ospedale Neuropsichiatrico, Teramo, TE 64100, Italy.

616.8 GBR
CLINICAL AND NEUROBIOLOGICAL ADVANCES IN PSYCHIATRY. Text in English. irreg., latest vol.2, 1996. **Document type:** *Monographic series, Academic/Scholarly.*
Indexed: e-psyche.
—BLDSC (3286.253500).
Published by: John Wiley & Sons Ltd., Baffins Ln, Chichester, Sussex PO19 IUD, United Kingdom. http://www.wiley.co.uk. **Subscr. in US to:** John Wiley & Sons, Inc., Journals, 605 Third Ave, New York, NY 10158. http://www.wiley.co.uk.

616.891 USA ISSN 1534-6501
▼ **CLINICAL CASE STUDIES.** Text in English. 2002 (Jan). q. USD 81, GBP 56 to individuals; USD 266, GBP 183 to institutions (effective 2002). **Description:** Publishes case reports of therapeutic interventions across the age spectrum for a variety of problems and in all appropriate milieus, and covers individual therapy, couples therapy, family therapy, assessment cases and case series that present direct and systematic replications.
Related titles: Online - full text ed.
Published by: Sage Publications, Inc., 2455 Teller Rd, Thousand Oaks, CA 91320. TEL 805-499-0721, 800-818-7243, FAX 805-499-0871, 800-583-2665, info@sagepub.com, http://www.sagepub.com/. Ed. Michael Hersen. **Addr. in India:** Sage Publications India Pvt. Ltd., M-32 Market, Greater Kailash-1, PO Box 4215, New Delhi 110 024, India. TEL 91-11-6419884, 91-11-6444958, FAX 91-11-6472426, sageindia@sagepub.com, http://indiasage.com/; **Addr. in the UK:** Sage Publications Ltd., 6 Bonhill St, London EC2A 4PU, United Kingdom. TEL 44-20-7374-0645, FAX 44-20-7374-8741, info@sagepub.co.uk, http://www.sagepub.co.uk.

616.804 USA ISSN 0009-9155
CODEN: CEEGA
CLINICAL ELECTROENCEPHALOGRAPHY. Text in English. 1970. q. USD 66 domestic; USD 71 in Canada; USD 76 elsewhere (effective 2000). adv. bk.rev. charts, illus. reprint service avail. from PQC,ISI. *Refereed.* **Document type:** *Abstract/Index, Academic/Scholarly.*
Related titles: Microform ed.: 1970 (from PQC); Online - full text ed.: (from Institute for Scientific Information).
Indexed: ASCA, Bibl.Dev.Med.& Child Neur., Biol.Abstr., Curr.Cont., Excerp.Med., Ind.Med. (1970-), Ind.Sci.Rev., Inpharma, Neurosci.Cit.Ind., Pharm.&Out.News, Reac., SSCI (coverage dropped), Sci.Cit.Ind., e-psyche.
—BLDSC (3286.274000), CISTI, EMDOCS, GNLM, ingenta, KNAW.
Published by: E E G and Clinical Neuroscience Society (ECNS), Brain Research Laboratories, New York University, 550 First Avenue, New York, NY 10016. TEL 212-263-6288, 888-366-2203, FAX 212-263-6457. Ed. Miles E Drake Jr. R&P, Adv. contact Kevin Kjellberg. Circ: 2,424.

616.8 USA ISSN 0749-8047
RB127
CLINICAL JOURNAL OF PAIN. Text in English. 1985. q. USD 205 domestic to individuals; USD 205 foreign to individuals; USD 331 domestic to institutions; USD 360 foreign to institutions; USD 84 newsstand/cover (effective 2002). adv. bk.rev. charts, illus. index. back issues avail.; reprint service avail. from PQC. *Refereed.* **Document type:** *Academic/Scholarly.* **Description:** Explores all aspects of pain and pain management, including diagnostic procedures, therapeutic modalities, psychosocial dimensions, and ethical problems.
Related titles: Online - full text ed.: USD 430.30 domestic academic site license; USD 459.30 foreign academic site license; USD 479.95 domestic corporate site license; USD 508.95 foreign corporate site license (effective 2002) (from Ovid Technologies, Inc., Institute for Scientific Information).
Indexed: AMED, ASCA, Curr.Cont., Excerp.Med., Ind.Med. (1985-), Inpharma, Int.Nurs.Ind., Neurosci.Cit.Ind., Pharm.&Out.News, PsycInfo, Reac., SSCI (coverage dropped), e-psyche.
—BLDSC (3286.294200), CISTI, EMDOCS, GNLM, IDS, ingenta, KNAW.
Published by: (American Academy of Pain Medicine), Lippincott Williams & Wilkins (Philadelphia) (Subsidiary of: Wolters Kluwer N.V.), 530 Walnut St, Philadelphia, PA 19106-3621. TEL 215-521-8300, FAX 215-521-8902, http://www.Lww.com. Ed. Dennis C Turk. Pub. Shelley Johnson. R&P Margaret Becker. Adv. contact Ray Thibodeau. B&W page USD 945, color page USD 2,050. Circ: 2,447 (paid). **Subscr. to:** PO Box 1600, Hagerstown, MD 21740-1600. TEL 800-777-2295, FAX 301-824-7390.

616.8 GBR ISSN 0269-9206
RC423.A1
CLINICAL LINGUISTICS & PHONETICS. Text in English. 1987. 8/yr. GBP 144, USD 238 to individuals; GBP 366, USD 604 to institutions (effective 2002). adv. bk.rev. *Refereed.* **Document type:** *Academic/Scholarly.* **Description:** Presents articles ranging from theoretical discussions to extremely practical tutorial reviews. Language development and other psycho- or neurolinguistic areas are included where they shed light on normative behavior against which to judge the non-normal.
Related titles: Online - full text ed.: ISSN 1464-5076 (from CatchWord Ltd., EBSCO Publishing, O C L C Online Computer Library Center, Inc., RoweCom Information Quest, Swets Blackwell, Institute for Scientific Information).
Indexed: AMED, ASCA, AgeLine, Bibl.Ling., CINAHL, Curr.Cont., Excerp.Med., Lang.& Lang.Behav.Abstr. (1987-), Ling.Abstr., SOPODA, SSCI, Sociol.Abstr., e-psyche.
—BLDSC (3286.297800), CatchWord, EMDOCS, GNLM, IDS, Infotrieve, ingenta. **CCC.**
Published by: Taylor & Francis Group, Taylor & Francis Ltd., 11 New Fetter Ln, London EC4P 4EE, United Kingdom. TEL 44-20-7583-9855, FAX 44-20-7842-2298, info@tandf.co.uk, http://www.tandf.co.uk. Eds. Martin J Ball, Thomas W Powell. **Subscr. in N. America to:** Taylor & Francis Ltd., 325 Chestnut St, Suite 800, Philadelphia, PA 19016. TEL 800-354-1420, FAX 215-625-8914, info@taylorandfrancis.com, http://www.taylorandfrancis.com/.

CLINICAL NEUROCHEMISTRY. see *BIOLOGY—Biochemistry*

616.8 617 NLD ISSN 0303-8467
CODEN: CNNSBV
CLINICAL NEUROLOGY AND NEUROSURGERY; an international journal publishing papers and reports on the clinical aspects of neurology and neurosurgery. Text in English. 1975. q. EUR 298 in Europe to institutions; JPY 39,600 in Japan to institutions; USD 334 elsewhere to institutions (effective 2002). adv. bk.rev. back issues avail. *Refereed.* **Document type:** *Academic/Scholarly.* **Description:** Covers developments in the field of clinical neurology and neurosurgery, including invited reviews, original research, brief case histories of unusual clinical syndromes or diseases.
Related titles: Microform ed.: (from PQC); Online - full text ed.: (from ingenta, Swets Blackwell, ScienceDirect, Institute for Scientific Information).
Indexed: ASCA, Bibl.Dev.Med.& Child Neur., Biol.Abstr., Curr.Adv.Cancer Res., Curr.Cont., Environ.Sci.Poll.Mgmt., Excerp.Med., Ind.Med. (1974-), Inpharma, Neurosci.Abstr. (coverage dropped), Neurosci.Cit.Ind., Pharm.&Out.News, Pollut.Abstr., PsycInfo, Psychol.Abstr. (1992-), Reac., Rev.Med.& Vet.Mycol., Risk Abstr., Saf.Sci.Abstr., e-psyche.
—BLDSC (3286.310100), CISTI, EMDOCS, GNLM, IDS, ingenta. **CCC.**
Published by: Elsevier Gezondheidszorg B.V., Tijdstroom (Subsidiary of: Reed Elsevier plc Group), Planetenbaan 1, Maarssen 3600 AK, Netherlands. TEL 31-346-577577, FAX 31-346-554287, nlinfo-f@elsevier.nl; usinfo-f@elsevier.com; forinfo-kyf04035@niftyserve.or.jp, http://www.elsevier.com/locate/clineuro, http://www.tijdstroom.nl. Ed. G W Bruyn. **Subscr. in Australasia and the Far East to:** Elsevier Science (Singapore) Pte Ltd, No.1 Temasek Ave, 17-01 Millenia Tower, Singapore 039192, Singapore. TEL 65-434-3727, FAX 65-337-2230; **Subscr. in Japan to:** Elsevier Science Inc - Japan Regional Office, 9-15 Higashi-Azabu 1-chome, Minato-ku, Tokyo 106-0044, Japan. TEL 81-3-5561-5033; **Subscr. in the Americas to:** Elsevier Science, PO Box 945, New York, NY 10159-0945. TEL 212-633-3730, FAX 212-633-3680.

616.8 DEU ISSN 0722-5091
CODEN: CLNPDA
CLINICAL NEUROPATHOLOGY. Text in English. 1982. bi-m. DEM 296, EUR 151.34 to individuals; USD 180 to individual members; USD 220 to institutions; DEM 60, EUR 30.68 newsstand/cover (effective 2001). adv. *Refereed.* **Document type:** *Journal, Academic/Scholarly.* **Description:** Publishes reviews and editorials, original papers, short communications and reports on recent advances in the entire field of clinical neuropathology.
Related titles: Online - full text ed.: (from Institute for Scientific Information).
Indexed: ASCA, Curr.Adv.Ecol.Sci., Curr.Cont., Dent.Ind., Excerp.Med., Ind.Med. (1982-), Ind.Sci.Rev., Inpharma, Int.Abstr.Biol.Sci., Neurosci.Cit.Ind., Pharm.&Out.News, Protozool.Abstr., Reac., Ref.Zh., Rev.Med.& Vet.Mycol., SSCI (coverage dropped), Sci.Cit.Ind., e-psyche.
—BLDSC (3286.310400), EMDOCS, GNLM, IDS, ingenta, KNAW. **CCC.**
Published by: Dustri-Verlag Dr. Karl Feistle, Bajuwarenring 4, Oberhaching 82041, Germany. TEL 49-89-613861-0, FAX 49-89-613-5412, info@dustri.de, http://www.dustri.de. Ed. Dr. W Schlote. R&P Renate Lehmann. Adv. contact Joerg Feistle.

CLINICAL NEUROPHARMACOLOGY. see *PHARMACY AND PHARMACOLOGY*

616.8 IRL ISSN 1388-2457
RC321 CODEN: CNEUFU
CLINICAL NEUROPHYSIOLOGY. Text in English, French. 1949. m. EUR 187 in Europe to individuals; JPY 24,800 in Japan to individuals; USD 209 elsewhere to individuals; EUR 611 in Europe to institutions; JPY 81,100 in Japan to institutions; USD 684 elsewhere to institutions (effective 2002). adv. bk.rev. abstr, charts, illus. index. back issues avail. *Refereed.* **Document type:** *Journal, Academic/Scholarly.* **Description:** Fosters research and disseminates information on all aspects of clinical neurophysiology, both normal and abnormal. Publishes scholarly reports on human physiology and pathophysiology of both the central and the peripheral nervous system.
Formerly (until 1999): Electroencephalography and Clinical Neurophysiology Including Evoked Potentials and Electromyography and Motor Control; Formed by the merger of (1949-1999): Electroencephalography and Clinical Neurophysiology (0013-4694); Which incorporated: Index to Current E E G Literature (0019-3976); (1991-1999): Electroencephalography and Clinical Neurophysiology: Electromyography and Motor Control (0924-980X); (1984-1999): Electroencephalographyy and Clinical Neurophysiology: Evoked Potentials (0168-5597)
Related titles: Microform ed.: (from PQC); Online - full text ed.: (from ingenta, Swets Blackwell, ScienceDirect, Institute for Scientific Information); ♦ Supplement to: Electroencephalography and Clinical Neurophysiology. Supplements. ISSN 0424-8155.
Indexed: ASCA, AgeLine, Aqua.Sci.& Fish.Abstr., Bibl.Dev.Med.& Child Neur., Biol.Abstr., C.I.S. Abstr., Chem.Abstr., Chem.Indus.Notes, Chem.Titles, Compumath, Curr.Adv.Ecol.Sci., Curr.Cont., Dent.Ind., Ergon.Abstr., Excerp.Med., INSPEC (pre-1969-), Ind.Med. (1999-), Ind.Sci.Rev., Inpharma, Int.Abstr.Biol.Sci., Neurosci.Abstr. (coverage dropped), Neurosci.Cit.Ind., Pharm.&Out.News, PsycInfo, Psychol.Abstr. (1950-), Reac., SSCI (coverage dropped), Sci.Cit.Ind., e-psyche.
—BLDSC (3286.310645), ADONIS, AskIEEE, CASDDS, CISTI, GNLM, IDS, Infotrieve, ingenta, KNAW. **CCC.**
Published by: (International Federation of Clinical Neurophysiology), Elsevier Science Ireland Ltd, Elsevier House, Brookvale Plaza, E. Park, Shannon, Co. Clare, Ireland. TEL 353-61-709600, FAX 353-61-709100, http://www.elsevier.com/locate/clinph, http://www.elsevier.nl. Eds. F Pauri, P M Rossini. **Subscr. in Australasia and the Far East to:** Elsevier Science (Singapore) Pte Ltd, No.1 Temasek Ave, 17-01 Millenia Tower, Singapore 039192, Singapore. TEL 65-434-3727, FAX 65-337-2230, asiainfo@elsevier.com.sg; **Subscr. in the Americas to:** Elsevier Science, PO Box 945, New York, NY 10159-0945. TEL 212-633-3730, 888-437-4636, FAX 212-633-3680, usinfo-f@elsevier.com, http://www.elsevier.com; **Subscr. to:** Elsevier Science Inc - Japan Regional Office, 9-15 Higashi-Azabu 1-chome, Minato-ku, Tokyo 106-0044, Japan. TEL 81-3-5561-5033, FAX 81-3-5561-5047, info@elsevier.co.jp. **Subscr. to:** Elsevier Science BV, PO Box 211, Amsterdam 1000 AE, Netherlands. TEL 31-20-485-3757, FAX 31-20-485-3432, nlinfo-f@elsevier.nl.; **Dist. by:** Elsevier Science (Brazil).

616.8 NLD ISSN 1566-2772
▼ **CLINICAL NEUROSCIENCE RESEARCH.** Text in English. 2000. bi-m. EUR 99 in Europe to individuals; JPY 13,200 in Japan to individuals; USD 112 elsewhere to individuals; EUR 254 in Europe to institutions; JPY 33,800 in Japan to institutions; USD 285 elsewhere to institutions (effective 2002). **Document type:** *Journal, Academic/Scholarly.* **Description:** Serves as an international official journal of the Association for Research in Nervous and Mental Disease (ARNMD). The focus is on investigations in cognition, mood, behavior, and motor function of normal and abnormal brain function. Publishes articles relating to epidemiology, diagnosis, treatment, and the pathophysiology of brain disorders.
Related titles: Online - full text ed.: (from ingenta, ScienceDirect); Supplement: Clinical Neuroscience Research. Supplement.
—BLDSC (3286.310950).

M

Published by: (Association for Research in Nervous and Mental Disease USA), Elsevier Science BV, Sara Burgerhartstraat 25, Amsterdam 1055 KV, Netherlands. TEL 31-20-485-2911, FAX 31-20-485-2457, nlinfo-f@elsevier.nl, http://www.elsevier.com/locate/cnr, http://www.elsevier.nl. Eds. M F Beal, W E Bunney Jr.

617.48 USA ISSN 0069-4827
RD593.A1 CODEN: CLNEA8
CLINICAL NEUROSURGERY: PROCEEDINGS. Text in English. 1953. a. price varies. **Document type:** *Proceedings.*
Indexed: INIS Atomind., Ind.Med. (1953-), e-psyche.
—BLDSC (3286.311000), CASDDS, CISTI, GNLM, ingenta, KNAW.
Published by: (Congress of Neurological Surgeons), Lippincott Williams & Wilkins (Philadelphia) (Subsidiary of: Wolters Kluwer N.V.), 530 Walnut St, Philadelphia, PA 19106-3621. TEL 215-521-8300, FAX 215-521-8902, http://www.lww.com. **Subscr. to:** PO Box 1600, Hagerstown, MD 21740-1600. TEL 800-777-2295, FAX 301-824-7390.

616.89 USA ISSN 0270-6644
CLINICAL PSYCHIATRY NEWS. Text in English. 1973. m. USD 70. adv. bk.rev. **Document type:** *Newspaper.*
Related titles: Microform ed.: (from PQC).
Indexed: e-psyche.
—Infotrieve. **CCC.**
Published by: International Medical News Group, 12230 Wilkins Ave, Rockville, MD 20852. TEL 301-816-8700. Ed. Catherine Nellist. Circ: 32,300.

CLINICS IN DEVELOPMENTAL MEDICINE. see *MEDICAL SCIENCES—Pediatrics*

616.8 FRA ISSN 1288-6629
LA CLINIQUE LACANIENNE. Text in French. 1996. s-a. EUR 30 domestic; EUR 38 foreign (effective 2001).
Published by: Editions Eres, 11 rue des Alouettes, Ramonville Saint-Agne 31520, France. TEL 33-05-61751576, FAX 33-05-61735289, eres@editions-eres.com. Ed. Ch Lacote.

616.8 FRA ISSN 0762-7491
CLINIQUES MEDITERRANEENNES; psychanalyse et psychopathologie freudiennes. Text in French. 1984. s-a. EUR 40 domestic; EUR 45 foreign (effective 2002).
Published by: Editions Eres, 11 rue des Alouettes, Ramonville Saint-Agne 31520, France. TEL 33-05-61751576, FAX 33-05-61735289, eres@editions-eres.com. Eds. Roland Gori, Yves Poinso.

616.8 GBR ISSN 1467-5919
COGNITION AND BRAIN SCIENCES UNIT. ANNUAL REPORT. Text in English. 1960. a.
Formerly (until 1997): Human Performance Reports (0461-5905)
—BLDSC (1340.183000).
Published by: Medical Research Council, Cognition and Brain Science Unit, 15 Chaucer Rd, Cambridge CB2 2EF, United Kingdom. TEL 44-1223-355294, FAX 44-1223-359062.

616.8 NLD ISSN 0926-6410
QP360.5 CODEN: CBRREZ
COGNITIVE BRAIN RESEARCH. Text in English. 1992. 6/yr. EUR 656 in Europe to institutions; JPY 87,200 in Japan to institutions; USD 734 elsewhere to institutions (effective 2002). adv. bk.rev. back issues avail. *Refereed.* **Document type:** *Academic/Scholarly.* **Description:** Publishes original reports of research in computational neuroscience, including neural networks, brain mechanisms subserving cognition, and applications of chaos theory to the analysis of brain functions and aberrant neurobehavioral processes.
Related titles: Microform ed.: (from PQC); Online - full text ed.: (from EBSCO Publishing, ingenta, Swets Blackwell, ScienceDirect, Institute for Scientific Information).
Indexed: ASCA, Chem.Abstr., Chem.Indus.Notes, Chem.Titles, Curr.Cont., Derwent Biotech.Abstr., Excerp.Med. (1993-), Ind.Med. (1992-), Inpharma, Int.Abstr.Biol.Sci., Neurosci.Cit.Ind., Pharm.&Out.News, PsycInfo, Psychol.Abstr. (1992-), Reac., Ref.Zh., Sci.Cit.Ind., e-psyche.
—BLDSC (3292.874000), ADONIS, CASDDS, CISTI, EMDOCS, GNLM, IDS, Infotrieve, ingenta. **CCC.**
Published by: Elsevier Science BV, PO Box 211, Amsterdam 1000 AE, Netherlands. TEL 31-20-485-2911, FAX 31-20-485-2457, nlinfo-f@elsevier.nl, http://www.elsevier.com/locate/cogbrainres, http://www.elsevier.nl. Eds. D P Purpura, F E Bloom. **Subscr. in Australasia and the Far East to:** Elsevier Science (Singapore) Pte Ltd, No.1 Temasek Ave, 17-01 Millenia Tower, Singapore 039192, Singapore. TEL 65-434-3727, FAX 65-337-2230; **Subscr. in Japan to:** Elsevier Science Inc - Japan Regional Office, 9-15 Higashi-Azabu 1-chome, Minato-ku, Tokyo 106-0044, Japan. TEL 81-3-5561-5033, FAX 81-3-5561-5047; **Subscr. in the Americas to:** Elsevier Science, PO Box 945, New York, NY 10159-0945. TEL 212-633-3730, FAX 212-633-3680, usinfo-f@elsevier.com, http://www.elsevier.com.

616.8 USA ISSN 0264-3294
CODEN: COGNEP
COGNITIVE NEUROPSYCHOLOGY. Text in English. 1984. 8/yr. USD 266, GBP 161 to individuals; USD 823, GBP 499 to institutions (effective 2002). adv. bk.rev. illus. Index. reprints avail. *Refereed.* **Document type:** *Academic/Scholarly.* **Description:** Studies cognitive processes from a neuropsychological perspective.
Related titles: Online - full text ed.: ISSN 1464-0627 (from CatchWord Ltd., EBSCO Publishing, O C L C Online Computer Library Center, Inc., RoweCom Information Quest, Swets Blackwell, Institute for Scientific Information).
Indexed: AMED, ASCA, ASSIA, AgeLine, Arts & Hum.Cit.Ind. (coverage dropped), Bibl.Dev.Med.& Child Neur., Curr.Cont., Excerp.Med., Lang.& Lang.Behav.Abstr., MLA Intl.Bibl., Neuropsych.Abstr., Neurosci.Cit.Ind., PsycInfo, Psychol.Abstr. (1984-), SOPODA, SSCI, Sociol.Abstr., e-psyche.
—BLDSC (3292.879000), CatchWord, CISTI, GNLM, IDS, ingenta. **CCC.**
Published by: Psychology Press (Subsidiary of: Taylor & Francis Ltd.), 325 Chestnut St, Ste 800, Philadelphia, PA 19106. TEL 215-625-8900, FAX 215-625-2940, info@taylorandfrancis.com, http://www.psypress.com/. Ed. Alfonso Caramazza. Circ: 1,000. **Subscr. addr. outside N America:** Psychology Press, Journals Customer Service, Taylor & Francis Group, Rankine Rd, Basingstoke, Hants RG24 8PR, United Kingdom. TEL 44-1256-813002, FAX 44-1256-479438, enquiry@tandf.co.uk, http://www.psypress.co.uk.

COMMON DIAGNOSTIC PROCEDURES: ORTHOPEDICS AND NEUROLOGY. see *LAW*

COMMUNICATION OUTLOOK; focusing on communication aids and techniques. see *COMPUTERS—Artificial Intelligence*

COMMUNITY MENTAL HEALTH JOURNAL. see *SOCIAL SERVICES AND WELFARE*

616.8 GBR
COMMUNITY MENTAL HEALTH JOURNAL. Abbreviated title: C M H. Text in English. 1998. q.
Indexed: P C I, e-psyche.
Published by: Hayward Medical Communications Ltd., Covent Garden, Seven Dials Warehouse, 44 Earlham St, London WC2H 9LA, United Kingdom. TEL 44-20-7240-4493, FAX 44-20-7240-4479, admin@hayward.co.uk, http://www.hayward.co.uk. Ed. Dr. B Lewis. **Subscr. to:** Rosemary House, Lanwades Park, Kentford, Near, Newmarket, Suffolk CB8 7PW, United Kingdom. TEL 44-1638-751515, FAX 44-1638-751517.

COMMUNITY PSYCHIATRIC NURSING. see *MEDICAL SCIENCES—Nurses And Nursing*

616.8 IND
COMMUNITY PSYCHIATRY JOURNAL. Text in English.
Indexed: e-psyche.
Published by: Institute of Community Psychiatry and Mental Health, Department of Psychiatry, J. J. Group of Hospitals, Byculla, Mumbai, Maharashtra 400 008, India.

616.8 570 USA ISSN 0947-2665
COMPARATIVE BRAIN RESEARCH IN MAMMALS. Text in English. 1991. irreg. **Document type:** *Monographic series.*
Indexed: e-psyche.
Published by: Springer-Verlag, Journals (Subsidiary of: BertelsmannSpringer), 175 Fifth Ave, New York, NY 10010. TEL 212-460-1500, FAX 212-473-6272.

616.8 USA
COMPARATIVE COGNITION AND NEUROSCIENCE. Text in English. irreg. **Document type:** *Monographic series.*
Indexed: e-psyche.
Published by: Lawrence Erlbaum Associates, Inc., 10 Industrial Ave, Mahwah, NJ 07430-2262. TEL 201-236-9500, 800-926-6579, FAX 201-236-0072, orders@erlbaum.com, http://www.erlbaum.com.

616.89 USA ISSN 0010-440X
RC321 CODEN: COPYAV
COMPREHENSIVE PSYCHIATRY. Text in English. 1960. bi-m. USD 189 domestic to individuals; USD 263 foreign to individuals; USD 339 domestic to institutions; USD 383 foreign to institutions; USD 133 domestic to students; USD 159 foreign to students; USD 64 per issue (effective 2001). adv. bk.rev. abstr, bibl, charts, illus. index. reprint service avail. from SCH,PSC. *Refereed.* **Document type:** *Journal, Academic/Scholarly.* **Description:** Covers developments in clinical and basic investigations, as well as new diagnostic and therapeutic practices.
Related titles: Online - full text ed.: (from IDEAL Online Library, Institute for Scientific Information).
Indexed: ASCA, Abstr.Anthropol., Adol.Ment.Hlth.Abstr., AgeLine, Biol.Abstr., Chem.Abstr., Crim.Just.Abstr., Curr.Cont., Dent.Ind., Excerp.Med., Fam.Ind., Ind.Med. (1960-), Ind.Sci.Rev., Inpharma, Jrnl.Watch Psych., Mid.East: Abstr.& Ind., NRN, Nutr.Abstr., Pharm.&Out.News, PsycInfo, Psychol.Abstr. (1960-), Reac., SSCI, Sci.Cit.Ind., e-psyche.
—BLDSC (3366.390000), CISTI, EMDOCS, GNLM, IDS, ingenta, KNAW. **CCC.**
Published by: (American Psychopathological Association), W.B. Saunders Co. (Subsidiary of: Harcourt Publishers Ltd.), 11830 Westline Industrial Dr, St Louis, MO 63146. TEL 800-325-4177, http://www.wbsaunders.com. Ed. Dr. David L Dunner. Adv. contact Steve Gray. B&W page USD 655, color page USD 1,605; trim 10 x 7. Circ: 1,079. **Subscr. to:** Periodicals Fulfillment, W B Saunders Co, 6277 Sea Harbor Dr, 4th Fl, Orlando, FL 32891-4800.

616.8 USA ISSN 0896-1220
CONCEPTS IN NEUROSURGERY. Text in English. 1987. irreg., latest vol.6. **Document type:** *Monographic series.*
Indexed: e-psyche.
—CISTI.
Published by: Lippincott Williams & Wilkins (Philadelphia) (Subsidiary of: Wolters Kluwer N.V.), 530 Walnut St, Philadelphia, PA 19106-3621. TEL 215-521-8300, FAX 215-521-8902, http://www.lww.com. **Subscr. to:** PO Box 1600, Hagerstown, MD 21740-1600. TEL 800-777-2295, FAX 301-824-7390.

616.6 ITA ISSN 1122-0279
CONFINIA CEPHALALGICA. Text in Italian. 1992. 4/yr. ITL 80,000 (effective 1999). *Refereed.* **Document type:** *Academic/Scholarly.*
Related titles: Online - full text ed.: (from Institute for Scientific Information).
Indexed: ASCA, Excerp.Med. (1993-), Neurosci.Cit.Ind., SSCI (coverage dropped), e-psyche.
—BLDSC (3410.634500), EMDOCS, GNLM, IDS.
Published by: Masson S.p.A., Divisione Periodici, Via F.lli Bressan 2, Milan, MI 20126, Italy. TEL 39-2-270741, FAX 39-2-27074210. Ed. Gian Camillo Manzoni. adv.: B&W page ITL 2,550,000, color page ITL 3,600,000. Circ: 2,500.

616.8 USA
▼ **CONTEMPORARY CLINICAL NEUROSCIENCE.** Text in English. 2000. irreg. price varies. illus. back issues avail. *Refereed.* **Document type:** *Monographic series, Academic/Scholarly.* **Description:** Covers all aspects of clinical neuroscience and neurology.
Published by: Humana Press Inc., 999 Riverview Dr, Ste 208, Totowa, NJ 07512. TEL 973-256-1699, FAX 973-256-8341, humana@humanapr.com, http://humanapress.com. Eds. Helen Baghdoyan, Ralph Lydic. R&P Wendy A Warren.

616.8 GBR ISSN 0069-9446
CODEN: CNRSAG
CONTEMPORARY NEUROLOGY SERIES. Text in English. 1966. irreg., latest vol.48, 1996. price varies. *Refereed.* **Document type:** *Monographic series.*
Indexed: Chem.Abstr., Ind.Med. (coverage dropped), e-psyche.
—BLDSC (3425.193000), CASDDS, CISTI, GNLM, KNAW. **CCC.**
Published by: Oxford University Press, Oxford Journals, Walton St, Oxford OX2 6DP, United Kingdom. TEL 44-1865-56767, FAX 44-1865-56646, webmaster@fadavis.com, http://www.fadavis.com. Ed. Sid Gilman. **Subsc. in US to:** Oxford University Press, Journals, 2001 Evans Rd, Cary, NC 27513. TEL 919-677-0977, FAX 919-677-1714.

M

616.8 USA ISSN 1061-5954
CONTEMPORARY NEUROSCIENCE. Text in English. 1983. irreg. price varies. **Document type:** *Monographic series, Academic/Scholarly.* **Description:** Offers the latest news and concepts in neuroscience.
Indexed: e-psyche.
Published by: Humana Press Inc., 999 Riverview Dr, Ste 208, Totowa, NJ 07512. TEL 973-256-1699, FAX 973-256-8341, humana@humanapr.com, http://humanapress.com.

CONTEMPORARY NEUROSURGERY; a biweekly review of clinical neurosurgical practice. see *MEDICAL SCIENCES—Surgery*

616.8 ESP ISSN 1139-515X
CONTINUA NEUROLOGICA. Text in Spanish; Summaries in English. 1986. 3/yr. ESP 6,500 to individuals; ESP 9,200 to institutions; ESP 5,200 to students (effective 2001). adv. back issues avail.; reprints avail. *Refereed.* **Document type:** *Journal, Academic/Scholarly.* **Description:** Covers the investigative research of the Society and accredited clinics throughout the country.
Formerly (until 1998): Neurologia (0213-4853)
Related titles: Online - full text ed.: 1998.
Indexed: Ind.Med. (1986-), Ind.Med.Esp., e-psyche.
—BLDSC (6081.374900), CINDOC, EMDOCS, GNLM, Infotrieve, KNAW. **CCC.**
Published by: (Sociedad Espanola de Neurologia), Ediciones Doyma S.A., Traversa de Gracia, 17-21, Barcelona 08021, Spain. TEL 34-93-200-0711, cn@doyma.es, doyma@doyma.es, http://www.doyma.es/cn. R&P Monica Barnes. Adv. contact Jose Antonio Hernandez. Circ: 2,100.

616.89 USA ISSN 1080-2371
CONTINUUM (BALTIMORE); lifelong learning in neurology. Text in English. bi-m. USD 469 domestic to individuals; USD 505 foreign to individuals (effective 2002). **Document type:** *Academic/Scholarly.* **Description:** Provides an interactive continuing medical education program in neurology.
Indexed: e-psyche.
Published by: (American Academy of Neurology), Lippincott Williams & Wilkins (Baltimore) (Subsidiary of: Wolters Kluwer N.V.), 351 W Camden St, Baltimore, MD 21201-2436. TEL 410-528-4000, 800-787-8981, FAX 410-528-4105, custserv@wwilkins.com, custerv@lww.com, http://www.wwilkins.com, http://www.Lww.com.

616.891 ITA ISSN 1590-0223
CONTRAPPUNTO; Materiali di lavoro dell'Associazione Fiorentina di Psicoterapia Psicoanalitica. Text in Italian. 1987. 2/yr., latest vol.28, 2001. EUR 18 (effective 2001). bk.rev. **Document type:** *Bulletin, Academic/Scholarly.* **Description:** The periodical hosts a number of original studies on the problematics of psychotherapeutic techniques or psychopsychology.
Published by: Edizioni Cadmo, Casella Postale 27, Fiesole, FI 50014, Italy. TEL 39-055-50181, FAX 39-055-5018201, cadmo@casalini.it, http://www.cadmo.com. R&P Alberto Bartolomeo. **Dist. by:** Casalini Libri.

CONTRIBUICOES EM PSICOLOGIA, PSIQUIATRIA E PSICANALISE. see *PSYCHOLOGY*

616.8 USA ISSN 1042-0398
RC346
CORRELATIVE NEUROANATOMY✱. Text in English. 1952. triennial. USD 31.95 (effective 1998). **Document type:** *Academic/Scholarly.*
Supersedes (in 1988): Correlative Neuroanatomy and Functional Neurology (0892-1237)
Indexed: e-psyche.
—CISTI.
Published by: Appleton & Lange, Journal Division (Subsidiary of: Simon & Schuster Company), 11 W 19th St, New York, CT 10011-4209. TEL 203-406-4500, FAX 203-406-4600.

616.8 ITA ISSN 0010-9452
CORTEX; journal devoted to study of the nervous system and behavior. Text in English. 1964. 5/yr. ITL 164,000 to individuals; ITL 328,000 to institutions (effective 1999). adv. bk.rev. charts. index. reprint service avail. from SWZ. *Refereed.* **Document type:** *Academic/Scholarly.*
Related titles: Microform ed.: (from PQC,SWZ); Online - full text ed.: (from Institute for Scientific Information).
Indexed: AMED, ASCA, AgeLine, Bibl.Asian Stud. (1971), Bibl.Dev.Med.& Child Neur., Biol.Abstr., CINAHL, Chemorec.Abstr., Curr.Adv.Ecol.Sci., Curr.Cont., Dent.Ind., Ergon.Abstr., Excerp.Med., Ind.Med. (1964-), Ind.Sci.Rev., Inpharma, Int.Abstr.Biol.Sci., Neuropsych.Abstr., Neurosci.Abstr., Neurosci.Cit.Ind., Pharm.&Out.News, PsycInfo, Psychol.Abstr. (1964-), Reac., SSCI (coverage dropped), Sci.Cit.Ind., Yrbk.Assoc.Educ.& Rehab.Blind, e-psyche.
—BLDSC (3477.150000), CISTI, EMDOCS, GNLM, IDS, ingenta, KNAW.
Published by: Masson S.p.A., Divisione Periodici, Via F.lli Bressan 2, Milan, MI 20126, Italy. TEL 39-2-270741, FAX 39-2-27074210. Ed. Ennio De Renzi. adv.: B&W page ITL 1,850,000, color page ITL 2,600,000; trim 240 x 170. Circ: 2,000.

COUNSELLING PSYCHOLOGY QUARTERLY. see *PSYCHOLOGY*

COURTROOM MEDICINE SERIES: PSYCHIC INJURIES. see *LAW*

616.8 364 GBR ISSN 0957-9664
CODEN: CBMHEE
CRIMINAL BEHAVIOUR AND MENTAL HEALTH. Text in English. 1991. q. USD 120 in North America to individuals; GBP 70 rest of world to individuals; USD 240 in North America to institutions; GBP 140 rest of world to institutions (effective 2001). adv. bk.rev. charts, illus, stat. index. back issues avail. *Refereed.* **Document type:** *Academic/Scholarly.* **Description:** This journal is intended for psychiatrists and psychologists who work with mentally abnormal offenders, violent patients, or who are engaged in research or teaching on crime or the criminal justice system.
Related titles: Online - full content ed.: ISSN 1471-2857 (from ProQuest Information & Learning); Online - full text ed.: (from CatchWord Ltd.).
Indexed: ASSIA, Abstr.Crim.& Pen., Addic.Abstr., Crim.Just.Abstr., Excerp.Med. (1993-), Lang.& Lang.Behav.Abstr., PsycInfo, Psychol.Abstr. (1991-), SOPODA, Soc.Serv.Abstr., Sociol.Abstr., e-psyche.
—BLDSC (3487.346200), ADONIS, EMDOCS.
Published by: Whurr Publishers Ltd., 19b Compton Terr, London N1 2UN, United Kingdom. TEL 44-20-7359-5979, FAX 44-20-7226-5290, info@whurr.co.uk, http://www.whurrjournals.co.uk/, http://www.whurr.co.uk. Eds. John Gunn, Pamela J Taylor. Adv. contact Lizzy Ewer. page GBP 225. **Subscr. in N. America to:** Whurr Publishers Ltd., PO Box 1897, Lawrence, KS 66044-8897. TEL 913-843-1221, FAX 913-843-1274, am&m@allenpress.com. **Subscr. to:** Turpin Distribution Services Ltd., Blackhorse Rd, Letchworth, Herts SG6 1HN, United Kingdom. TEL 44-1462-488900, FAX 44-1462-483011, custservturpin@turpinltd.com.

612.8 USA ISSN 0892-0915
RC321 CODEN: CCNBE8
CRITICAL REVIEWS IN NEUROBIOLOGY. Text in English. 1985. q. USD 95 to individuals; USD 378 to institutions (effective 2000). adv. *Refereed.* **Document type:** *Academic/Scholarly.* **Description:** Presents comprehensive reviews, analyses, and integration of recently developed substantive observations and information which influence the understanding of normal or disturbed processes involving the nervous system.
Formerly: Critical Reviews in Clinical Neurobiology
Related titles: Online - full text ed.: (from Institute for Scientific Information).
Indexed: ASCA, Aqua.Sci.& Fish.Abstr., Cal.Tiss.Abstr., Chem.Abstr., Chem.Indus.Notes, Chem.Titles, Chemorec.Abstr., Curr.Cont., Excerp.Med., INIS Atomind., Ind.Med. (1987-), Inpharma, Int.Abstr.Biol.Sci., Neurosci.Abstr., Neurosci.Cit.Ind., Pharm.&Out.News, Reac., SSCI (coverage dropped), Sci.Cit.Ind., e-psyche.
—BLDSC (3487.478500), CASDDS, EMDOCS, GNLM, IDS, ingenta, KNAW. **CCC.**
Published by: Begell House Inc., 79 Madison Ave, Ste 1205, New York, NY 10016-7892. TEL 212-725-1999, FAX 212-213-8368, begellhouse@worldnet.att.net, orders@begellhouse.com. Eds. Charles B Nemeruff, Errol B Desouzq. Pub. William Begell. R&P, Adv. contact Jim Kelly.

CULTURE, MEDICINE AND PSYCHIATRY; an international journal of comparative cross-cultural research. see *ANTHROPOLOGY*

CURRENT ADVANCES IN NEUROSCIENCE. see *MEDICAL SCIENCES—Abstracting, Bibliographies, Statistics*

616.8 NLD ISSN 1380-7730
CURRENT ISSUES IN NEURODEGENERATIVE DISEASES✱. Text in English. 1994. irreg., latest vol.8, 1996. price varies. **Document type:** *Monographic series, Academic/Scholarly.* **Description:** Covers progress in basic science and clinical research in the fields of neurodegeneration, behavioral neurology and biological psychiatry.
Indexed: e-psyche.
—BLDSC (3499.075350).
Published by: (Research Institute Neurosciences, Vrije Universiteit Amsterdam), Academic Pharmaceutical Productions B.V., Mauritsstraat 100, Utrecht, HW 3583, Netherlands. TEL 31-30-2109521, FAX 31-30-2317907.

616.0472 NLD ISSN 0923-2354
CODEN: CMPAEH
CURRENT MANAGEMENT OF PAIN. Text in English. 1988. irreg. price varies. *Refereed.* **Document type:** *Monographic series.*
Indexed: e-psyche.
—KNAW.
Published by: Kluwer Academic Publishers Group (Subsidiary of: Wolters Kluwer N.V.), Spuiboulevard 50, PO Box 17, Dordrecht 3300 AA, Netherlands. FAX 31-78-639-2254, services@wkap.nl, http://www.wkap.nl. **Dist. by:** Kluwer Academic Publishers, PO Box 17, Dordrecht 3300 AH, Netherlands. TEL 31-78-6392392, FAX 31-78-654-6474, services@wkap.nl, http://www.wkap.nl.

CURRENT MEDICAL LITERATURE. EPILEPSY MONITOR. see *MEDICAL SCIENCES—Abstracting, Bibliographies, Statistics*

CURRENT MEDICAL LITERATURE. NEUROLOGY & NEUROSURGERY. see *MEDICAL SCIENCES—Abstracting, Bibliographies, Statistics*

CURRENT MEDICAL LITERATURE. PERSPECTIVES IN DEPRESSION. see *MEDICAL SCIENCES—Abstracting, Bibliographies, Statistics*

CURRENT MEDICAL LITERATURE. PSYCHIATRY. see *MEDICAL SCIENCES—Abstracting, Bibliographies, Statistics*

CURRENT MEDICAL LITERATURE. PSYCHIATRY REVIEWS; recent developments in psychiatric care for General Practitioners. see *MEDICAL SCIENCES—Abstracting, Bibliographies, Statistics*

616.8 NLD ISSN 0161-780X
RC321 CODEN: CNEUDS
CURRENT NEUROLOGY. Text in English. 1980. irreg., latest vol.17, 1997. price varies. illus. *Refereed.* **Document type:** *Monographic series, Academic/Scholarly.* **Description:** Presents reviews of the pertinent literature combined with original papers in neurology.
Indexed: Chem.Abstr., e-psyche.
—CASDDS, CISTI, GNLM, KNAW.
Published by: I O S Press, Van Diemenstraat 94, Amsterdam 1013 CN, Netherlands. TEL 31-20-638-2189, FAX 31-20-620-3419, market@iospress.nl, http://www.iospress.nl. **Subscr. to:** I O S Press, Inc, 5795-G Burke Centre Pkwy, Burke, VA 22015. TEL 703-323-5554, FAX 703-323-3668, iosbooks@iospress.com. **Dist. by:** Ohmsha Ltd, 3-1 Kanda-Nishiki-cho, Chiyoda-ku, Tokyo 101-0054, Japan. TEL 81-3-3233-0641, FAX 81-3-3233-2426, http://www.ohmsha.co.jp.

616.8 573.8 GBR ISSN 0959-4388
QP351 CODEN: COPUEN
CURRENT OPINION IN NEUROBIOLOGY. Text in English. 1991. bi-m. EUR 170 in Europe to individuals; JPY 20,600 in Japan to individuals; USD 184 elsewhere to individuals; EUR 213 in Europe to qualified personnel; JPY 25,700 in Japan to qualified personnel; USD 230 elsewhere to qualified personnel; EUR 908 in Europe to institutions; JPY 125,900 in Japan to institutions; USD 1,051 elsewhere to institutions (effective 2002). adv. bibl, illus. back issues avail. *Refereed.* **Document type:** *Academic/Scholarly.* **Description:** Provides infromation to researchers, educators and students of neurobiology. Presents review articles, followed by annotated bibliographies of references consulted. Includes a "Paper Alert" section, giving brief summaries of relevant papers recently published in other journals.

M

Related titles: CD-ROM ed.; Online - full text ed.: USD 227 in North America to individuals; USD 247 in North America to individuals with print ed; GBP 137 elsewhere to individuals; GBP 150 elsewhere to individuals with print ed; USD 822 in North America to institutions includes print ed; GBP 500 elsewhere to institutions includes print ed (effective 1999 & 2000) (from EBSCO Publishing, ingenta, Swets Blackwell, ScienceDirect, Institute for Scientific Information).
Indexed: ASCA, Anim.Behav.Abstr., Aqua.Sci.& Fish.Abstr., Biotech.& Bioeng.Abstr., Cal.Tiss.Abstr., Chem.Abstr., Chem.Indus.Notes, Chem.Titles, Chemorec.Abstr., Compumath, Curr.Cont., Excerp.Med. (1993-), Ind.Med. (1991-), Inpharma, Int.Abstr.Biol.Sci., Neurosci.Abstr., Neurosci.Cit.Ind., Pharm.&Out.News, PsycInfo, Reac., SSCI (coverage dropped), Sci.Cit.Ind., e-psyche.
—BLDSC (3500.775850), ADONIS, CASDDS, CISTI, EMDOCS, GNLM, IDS, ingenta, KNAW. **CCC.**
Published by: Elsevier Science Ltd., Elsevier Trends Journals, 84 Theobald's Rd, London WC1X 8RR, United Kingdom. TEL 44-20-7611-4400, FAX 44-20-7611-4468, info@current-opinion.com, http://www.elsevier.com/locate/conb, http://www.current-opinion.com. Ed. Elizabeth Westwood. Circ: 2,400. **Subscr. to:** PO Box 331, Haywards Heath, West Sussex RH16 3FG, United Kingdom. TEL 44-1444-475650, FAX 44-1444-445423. **Dist. by:** Turpin Distribution Services Ltd.

616.8 USA ISSN 1350-7540
CODEN: CONEEX
CURRENT OPINION IN NEUROLOGY. Text in English. 1987. bi-m. USD 273 domestic to individuals for print & online eds.; USD 273 foreign to individuals; USD 665 per issue domestic to institutions; USD 665 per issue foreign to institutions; USD 103 newsstand/cover (effective 2002). adv. bibl, illus. back issues avail. *Refereed.* **Document type:** *Academic/Scholarly.*
Description: Directed toward clinicians, surgeons and researchers in the field. Presents review articles followed by annotated bibliographies of references consulted. Includes a bibliography of the current world literature published during the previous year.
Formerly: Current Opinion in Neurology and Neurosurgery (0951-7383)
Related titles: CD-ROM ed.; Diskette ed.; Online - full text ed.: USD 864.50 domestic academic site license; USD 864.50 foreign academic site license; USD 964.25 domestic corporate site license; USD 964.25 foreign corporate site license (effective 2002) (from Ovid Technologies, Inc., EBSCO Publishing, Swets Blackwell, Institute for Scientific Information).
Indexed: ASCA, CINAHL, Curr.Cont., Excerp.Med., INIS Atomind., Ind.Med. (1993-), Inpharma, Int.Abstr.Biol.Sci., Neurosci.Cit.Ind., Pharm.&Out.News, Reac., Rev.Appl.Entomol., SSCI (coverage dropped), e-psyche.
—BLDSC (3500.775870), ADONIS, EMDOCS, GNLM, IDS, ingenta, KNAW.
Published by: Lippincott Williams & Wilkins (Philadelphia) (Subsidiary of: Wolters Kluwer N.V.), 530 Walnut St, Philadelphia, PA 19106-3621. TEL 215-521-8300, FAX 215-521-8902, http://www.Lww.com. Eds. Richard Frackowiak, Richard Johnson. Adv. contact Gemma Heiser. B&W page USD 775, color page USD 1,775; trim 11 x 8.5. Circ: 3,817. **Subscr. to:** PO Box 1600, Hagerstown, MD 21740-1600. TEL 800-777-2295, FAX 301-824-7390.

616.8 USA ISSN 0951-7367
CODEN: COPPE8
CURRENT OPINION IN PSYCHIATRY. Text in English. 1988. bi-m. USD 273 domestic to individuals for print online eds.; USD 273 foreign to individuals for print online eds.; USD 665 per issue domestic to institutions; USD 665 per issue foreign to institutions; USD 103 newsstand/cover (effective 2002). adv. bibl, illus. back issues avail. *Refereed.* **Document type:** *Academic/Scholarly.* **Description:** Directed toward practicing psychiatrists and researchers. Presents review articles followed by annotated bibliographies of references consulted. A bibliography of the current world literature published during the previous year is available.
Related titles: CD-ROM ed.: (from Ovid Technologies, Inc.); Diskette ed.; Online - full text ed.: USD 864.50 domestic academic site license; USD 864.50 foreign academic site license; USD 964.25 domestic corporate site license; USD 964.25 foreign corporate site license (effective 2002) (from Ovid Technologies, Inc., EBSCO Publishing, Swets Blackwell, Institute for Scientific Information).
Indexed: ASCA, Addic.Abstr., AgeLine, CINAHL, Curr.Cont., Excerp.Med., Fam.Ind., Inpharma, Reac., SSCI, e-psyche.
—BLDSC (3500.777000), ADONIS, EMDOCS, GNLM, IDS, KNAW.
Published by: Lippincott Williams & Wilkins (Philadelphia) (Subsidiary of: Wolters Kluwer N.V.), 530 Walnut St, Philadelphia, PA 19106-3621. TEL 215-521-8300, FAX 215-521-8902, http://www.Lww.com. Eds. Dr. David J Kupfer, Dr. Norman Sartorius. Adv. contact Gemma Heiser. Circ: 4,710. **Subscr. to:** PO Box 1600, Hagerstown, MD 21740-1600. TEL 800-777-2295, FAX 301-824-7390.

616 USA ISSN 1531-3433
CURRENT PAIN AND HEADACHE REPORTS. Text in English. 1994. bi-m. USD 157.50 to individuals in the US, Canada and S. America; GBP 120 elsewhere to individuals; USD 315 to institutions in the US, Canada and S. America; GBP 240 elsewhere to institutions; USD 80 to students in the US, Canada and S. America; GBP 75 elsewhere to students (effective 2001). bibl, illus. **Document type:** *Academic/Scholarly.*
Description: Covers pain management and headache; topics include: chronic visceral pain, cluster headache, neuropathic pain, migraine headache, cancer pain, uncommon headache, syndrome, fibromyalgia, cervicogenic headache, myofascial pain, tension-type headache, anesthetic techniques in, pain management, chronic daily headache.
Formerly: Current Review of Pain (1069-5850)
Related titles: Online - full content ed.
Indexed: Ind.Med. (1994-), e-psyche.
—BLDSC (3500.950000).
Published by: Current Science Inc., 400 Market St, Ste 700, Philadelphia, PA 19106. TEL 800-427-1796, FAX 215-574-2225, info@current-reports.com, http://www.current-reports.com/pa, http://www.current-science.com/. Eds. Dr. Bradley S Galer, Dr. Miroslav Backonja.

616.8 USA
CURRENT PROTOCOLS IN NEUROSCIENCE. Text in English. base vol. plus q. updates. USD 445 (effective 2001); USD 480 combined subscription for base vol. & update; USD 240 updates for base vol. & update (effective 2002). **Document type:** *Journal.*
Related titles: CD-ROM ed.: USD 490 (effective 2000); USD 520 combined subscription for base vol. & update; USD 275 renewals for base vol. & update (effective 2002).
—BLDSC (3501.543000).
Published by: John Wiley & Sons, Inc., Journals (Subsidiary of: Wiley InterScience), 605 Third Ave, New York, NY 10158. TEL 212-850-6645, FAX 212-850-6021, info@wiley.com, uscs-wis@wiley.com, http://www.wiley.com. **Subscr. outside the Americas:** John Wiley & Sons Ltd., Baffins Ln, Chichester, Sussex PO19 IUD, United Kingdom. TEL 44-1243-779777, FAX 44-1243-843232, cs-journals@wiley.co.uk, http://www.wiley.co.uk.

616.89 USA ISSN 1523-3812
CURRENT PSYCHIATRY REPORTS. Text in English. 8/yr. USD 163.95, GBP 120 to individuals; USD 327.95 to institutions; USD 85, GBP 60 to students (effective 2002); Subscr. includes both print & online eds.. **Document type:** *Journal, Academic/Scholarly.*
Related titles: Online - full content ed.: USD 85, GBP 65 (effective 2002); Online - full text ed.
Indexed: Ind.Med.
Published by: Current Science Inc., 400 Market St, Ste 700, Philadelphia, PA 19106. TEL 800-427-1796, FAX 215-574-2225, info@current-reports.com, http://www.current-reports.com/cr_jrnl_home.cfm?JournalID=PR, http://www.current-science.com/, http://www.current-science-group.com/. **Affiliate:** Current Science Ltd.

616.8 616.15 USA ISSN 1068-2252
CURRENT REVIEW OF CEREBROVASCULAR DISEASE. Text in English. 1993. irreg., latest vol.2, 1995. **Document type:** *Monographic series, Academic/Scholarly.* **Description:** Publishes important research in the field.
Indexed: e-psyche.
—GNLM.
Published by: Current Medicine, 400 Market St, Ste 700, Philadelphia, PA 19106. TEL 215-574-2257, 800-427-1796, FAX 215-574-2225. **Subscr. outside N. America to:** Current Science Ltd, Middlesex House, 34-42 Cleveland St, London W1P 6LB, United Kingdom. TEL 44-20-7323-0323.

616.8 USA ISSN 1068-4093
CURRENT TECHNIQUES IN NEUROSURGERY. Text in English. 1993. biennial. **Document type:** *Monographic series, Academic/Scholarly.*
Indexed: e-psyche.
—GNLM.
Published by: Current Medicine, 400 Market St, Ste 700, Philadelphia, PA 19106. TEL 215-574-2257, 800-427-1796, FAX 215-574-2225. **Subscr. outside N. America to:** Current Science Ltd, Middlesex House, 34-42 Cleveland St, London W1P 6LB, United Kingdom. TEL 44-20-7323-0323.

616.8 USA ISSN 0093-4747
CURRENT TOPICS IN NEUROBIOLOGY. Text in English. 1973. irreg., latest 1987. **Document type:** *Monographic series.*
Indexed: e-psyche.
—CISTI.
Published by: Kluwer Academic - Plenum Publishers (Subsidiary of: Wolters Kluwer N.V.), 233 Spring St, New York, NY 10013-1578. TEL 212-620-8000, 800-221-9369, FAX 212-463-0742, info@plenum.com, http://www.plenum.com.

616.4 USA ISSN 0723-1229
CODEN: CTNEEY
CURRENT TOPICS IN NEUROENDOCRINOLOGY. Text in English. 1982. irreg., latest vol.10, 1990. price varies. **Document type:** *Monographic series.*
Indexed: Chem.Abstr., Chem.Indus.Notes, Chem.Titles, Ind.Med. (1982-), e-psyche.
—CASDDS, CISTI, GNLM, Infotrieve. **CCC.**
Published by: Springer-Verlag, Journals (Subsidiary of: BertelsmannSpringer), 175 Fifth Ave, New York, NY 10010. TEL 212-460-1500, FAX 212-473-6272.

616.8 USA ISSN 1092-8480
CURRENT TREATMENT OPTIONS IN NEUROLOGY. Text in English. 6/yr. USD 163.95 to individual members; USD 80 to students (effective 2002); Subscr. includes both print & online eds..
Related titles: Online - full content ed.: USD 75 (effective 2002).
—BLDSC (3504.936450).
Published by: Current Science Inc., 400 Market St, Ste 700, Philadelphia, PA 19106. TEL 800-427-1796, FAX 215-574-2225, info@phl.cursci.com, http://www.treatment-options.com/cto_jrnl_homc.cfm?JournalID=NE. Ed. Steven P Ringel. **Affiliate:** Current Science Ltd.

616.8 DEU
D G S P RUNDBRIEF. Text in German. 1977. q. DEM 40. adv. bk.rev. back issues avail. **Document type:** *Bulletin.*
Indexed: e-psyche.
Published by: Deutsche Gesellschaft fuer Soziale Psychiatrie e.V., Stuppstr 14, Cologne 50823, Germany. TEL 49-221-511002. Ed. Michaela Hoffmann. Circ: 3,000.

D W D NEWSLETTER. see *GERONTOLOGY AND GERIATRICS*

616.8 GBR ISSN 1471-3012
▼ **DEMENTIA.** Text in English. 2002 (Feb.). 3/yr. GBP 34 to individuals; GBP 150 to institutions; GBP 12 newsstand/cover to individuals; GBP 51 newsstand/cover to institutions (effective 2002). *Refereed.* **Document type:** *Journal, Academic/Scholarly.* **Description:** Focuses on the social experience of dementia. It provides a forum for social research of direct relevance to improving the quality of life and care of people with dementia and their families, and will publish papers from the fields of public health, social policy, social work and sociology.
Related titles: Online - full text ed.: forthcoming.
Published by: Sage Publications Ltd., 6 Bonhill St, London EC2A 4PU, United Kingdom. TEL 44-20-7374-0645, FAX 44-20-7374-8741, market@sagepub.co.uk, http://www.sagepub.co.uk. Eds. John Keady, Phyllis Braudy Harris. **Addr in India:** Sage Publications India Pvt. Ltd., P O Box 4215, New Delhi 110 048, India. TEL 91-11-641-9884, FAX 91-11-647-2426; **Addr in US:** Sage Publications, Inc., 2455 Teller Rd, Thousand Oaks, CA 91320. TEL 805-499-0721, FAX 805-499-0871.

616.8 CHE ISSN 1420-8008
CODEN: DEMNEU
DEMENTIA AND GERIATRIC COGNITIVE DISORDERS. Text in English. 1990. bi-m. CHF 1,420 in Europe to institutions; CHF 1,443.20 overseas to institutions; EUR 1,014.40 in Europe to institutions; USD 1,104 overseas to institutions (effective 2002). adv. bibl, charts, stat. *Refereed.* **Document type:** *Journal, Academic/Scholarly.* **Description:** Examines the neural bases of cognitive dysfunction. Concentrates on neuro-degenerative diseases such as Alzheimer's and Parkinson's diseases, as well as Huntington's chorea. Covers topics of interest to professional in neurobiology, pharmacology, genetics, gerontology, and psychiatry.
Formerly (until 1996): Dementia (1013-7424)

M

Related titles: Microform ed.: (from PQC); Online - full text ed.: ISSN 1421-9824. CHF 116, EUR 84, USD 90 to institutions (effective 2002) (from EBSCO Publishing, O C L C Online Computer Library Center, Inc., RoweCom Information Quest, ProQuest Information & Learning, Swets Blackwell, Institute for Scientific Information).
Indexed: ASCA, Curr.Cont., Excerp.Med., Ind.Med. (1997-), Ind.Sci.Rev., Inpharma, Int.Nurs.Ind., METADEX, Neurosci.Cit.Ind., Pharm.&Out.News, PsycInfo, Psychol.Abstr. (1990-), Reac., Rev.Arom.& Med.Plants, SSCI (coverage dropped), Sci.Cit.Ind., e-psyche.
—BLDSC (3550.525300), CASDDS, CISTI, EMDOCS, GNLM, IDS, Infotrieve, KNAW. **CCC.**
Published by: S. Karger AG, Allschwilerstr 10, PO Box, Basel 4009, Switzerland. TEL 41-61-306-1111, FAX 41-61-306-1234, karger@karger.ch, http://www.online.karger.com/journals/dem, http://www.karger.com. Ed. V Chan Palay. adv.: page USD 1,195. **US and Canada subscr. to:** S Karger Publishers Inc.

DEPRESSION AND ANXIETY. see *PSYCHOLOGY*

616.89 USA
DEPRESSION: DISEASE STATE MANAGEMENT RESOURCE. Text in English. 1997. a. USD 269; USD 229 foreign (effective 1999). **Document type:** *Trade.*
Indexed: e-psyche.
Published by: American Health Consultants (Subsidiary of: Medical Economics Co., Inc.), 3525 Piedmont Rd, N E, 6 Piedmont Center, Ste 400, Atlanta, GA 30305. TEL 404-262-5476, custserv@ahcpub.com, http://www.ahcpub.com.

DEUTSCHE BEHINDERTENZEITSCHRIFT. see *EDUCATION—Special Education And Rehabilitation*

DEVELOPMENT AND PSYCHOPATHOLOGY. see *PSYCHOLOGY*

616.8 NLD ISSN 0165-3806
QP356.25 CODEN: DBRRDB
DEVELOPMENTAL BRAIN RESEARCH. Text in Dutch. 1981. 14/yr. EUR 2,217 in Europe to institutions; JPY 294,700 in Japan to institutions; USD 2,147 elsewhere to institutions (effective 2002). abstr. back issues avail.; reprint service avail. from ISI. *Refereed.* **Document type:** *Academic/Scholarly.* **Description:** Provides a medium for prompt publication of vitro and in vivo developmental studies concerned with the mechanism of neurogenesis, neuro migration, cell death, neuronal differentiation, synaptogenesis, myelination, the establishment of neuroglia relations and the development of various brain-barrier mechanisms.
Related titles: Online - full text ed.: (from EBSCO Publishing, ingenta, Swets Blackwell, ScienceDirect, Institute for Scientific Information).
Indexed: ASCA, Aqua.Sci.& Fish.Abstr., Bibl.Dev.Med.& Child Neur., Biol.Abstr., Biotech.& Bioeng.Abstr., Chem.Abstr., Chem.Indus.Notes, Chem.Titles, Chemorec.Abstr., Curr.Adv.Biochem., Curr.Adv.Ecol.Sci., Curr.Cont., Derwent Biotech.Abstr., Excerp.Med., INIS Atomind., Ind.Med. (1988-), Ind.Sci.Rev., Inpharma, Int.Abstr.Biol.Sci., Neurosci.Abstr., Neurosci.Cit.Ind., Pharm.&Out.News, PsycInfo, Psychol.Abstr. (1981-), Reac., Ref.Zh., Rev.Appl.Entomol., Rev.Med.& Vet.Mycol., Sci.Cit.Ind., Sport Fish.Abstr., THA, Wild.Rev., e-psyche.
—BLDSC (3579.054200), ADONIS, CASDDS, CISTI, GNLM, IDS, ingenta. **CCC.**
Published by: Elsevier Science BV, PO Box 211, Amsterdam 1000 AE, Netherlands. TEL 31-20-485-2911, FAX 31-20-485-2457, nlinfo-f@elsevier.nl; usinfo-f@elsevier.com; forinfo-kyf04035@niftyserve.or.jp, http://www.elsevier.com/inca/publications/store/5/0/6/0/5/1/, http://www.elsevier.nl. Ed. D P Purpura. **Subscr. in Australasia and the Far East to:** Elsevier Science (Singapore) Pte Ltd, No.1 Temasek Ave, 17-01 Millenia Tower, Singapore 039192, Singapore. TEL 65-434-3727, FAX 65-337-2230; **Subscr. in Japan to:** Elsevier Science Inc - Japan Regional Office, 9-15 Higashi-Azabu 1-chome, Minato-ku, Tokyo 106-0044, Japan. TEL 81-3-5561-5033; **Subscr. in the Americas to:** Elsevier Science, PO Box 945, New York, NY 10159-0945. TEL 212-633-3730, FAX 212-633-3680.

371.928 CAN ISSN 1184-0412
DEVELOPMENTAL DISABILITIES BULLETIN. Text in English. 1972. s-a. CND 19.25 domestic to individuals; USD 15 foreign to individuals; CND 32.10 domestic to institutions; USD 25 foreign to institutions. adv. bk.rev. *Refereed.* **Document type:** *Bulletin, Academic/Scholarly.* **Description:** Articles with both research and direct application to the education of, and provision of services for persons with mental retardation, learning disability and multiple handicaps.
Formerly: Mental Retardation and Learning Disability Bulletin (0822-4277)
Indexed: Except.Child Educ.Abstr., PsycInfo, Psychol.Abstr. (1972-), Yrbk.Assoc.Educ.& Rehab.Blind, e-psyche.
—BLDSC (3579.054450), GNLM. **CCC.**
Published by: University of Alberta, Developmental Disabilities Centre, 6 123D Education North, Edmonton, AB T6G 2H1, Canada. TEL 403-492-4505, FAX 403-492-1318, henny.degroot@ualberta.ca, http://www.quasar.ualberta.ca/ddc/index.html. Ed. Jack Goldberg. R&P Dick Sobsey. Adv. contact Henny Degroot. Circ: 250.

DEVELOPMENTAL MEDICINE AND CHILD NEUROLOGY. see *MEDICAL SCIENCES—Pediatrics*

616.8 CHE ISSN 0378-5866
CODEN: DENED7
DEVELOPMENTAL NEUROSCIENCE. Text in French. 1979. bi-m. CHF 1,024, DEM 731.80 in Europe to institutions; CHF 1,041.40, USD 796 overseas to institutions (effective 2002). adv. illus. index. back issues avail. *Refereed.* **Document type:** *Journal, Academic/Scholarly.* **Description:** Publishes neuroscience papers covering all stages of invertebrate, vertebrate and human development.
Related titles: Microform ed.: (from PQC); Online - full text ed.: ISSN 1421-9859. CHF 58, EUR 42, USD 45 to institutions with print edition (effective 2002) (from EBSCO Publishing, O C L C Online Computer Library Center, Inc., RoweCom Information Quest, Swets Blackwell, Institute for Scientific Information).
Indexed: ASCA, Aqua.Sci.& Fish.Abstr., Biol.Abstr., Chem.Abstr., Chem.Indus.Notes, Chem.Titles, Chemorec.Abstr., Curr.Adv.Biochem., Curr.Adv.Cell & Devel.Biol., Curr.Adv.Ecol.Sci., Curr.Cont., Excerp.Med., Helminthol.Abstr., Ind.Med. (1978-), Ind.Sci.Rev., Inpharma, Neurosci.Abstr., Neurosci.Cit.Ind., Pharm.&Out.News, Reac., Sci.Cit.Ind., e-psyche.
—BLDSC (3579.057500), CASDDS, CISTI, EMDOCS, GNLM, IDS, ingenta, KNAW. **CCC.**
Published by: S. Karger AG, Allschwilerstr 10, PO Box, Basel 4009, Switzerland. TEL 41-61-306-1111, FAX 41-61-306-1234, karger@karger.ch, http://www.online.karger.com/journals/dne, http://www.karger.com. Ed. A T Campagnoni. adv.: page USD 1,185. Circ: 800.

616.8 NLD ISSN 0166-5960
CODEN: DEVND6
DEVELOPMENTS IN NEUROLOGY. Text in Dutch. 1978. irreg., latest vol.13, 1997. illus. back issues avail. **Document type:** *Monographic series, Proceedings, Academic/Scholarly.* **Description:** Disseminates clinical and applied research in the medical specialty of neurology.
Indexed: Chem.Abstr., e-psyche.
—BLDSC (3579.085380), CASDDS, CISTI, KNAW.
Published by: Elsevier Science Publishers BV, Life Sciences Department, Molenwerf 1, Amsterdam 1014 AG, Netherlands. TEL 31-20-485-3358, FAX 31-20-485-3342, t.fischer@elsevier.nl, http://www.elsevier.nl. Ed. Tatjana Fischer-Driessen. Pub. Tatjana Fischer Driessen. R&P Jan V D Heuvel TEL 31-20-4852833. **Subscr. to:** Elsevier Science (Singapore) Pte Ltd, No.1 Temasek Ave, 17-01 Millenia Tower, Singapore 039192, Singapore. TEL 65-434-3727, FAX 65-337-2230; Elsevier Science Inc - Japan Regional Office, 9-15 Higashi-Azabu 1-chome, Minato-ku, Tokyo 106-0044, Japan. TEL 81-3-5561-5033, FAX 81-3-5561-5047, info@elsevier.co.jp; Elsevier Science, PO Box 945, New York, NY 10159-0945. FAX 212-633-3680, 212-633-3680.

616.891 615.1 USA
DI CYAN BULLETIN* . Text in English. 1950. m. bk.rev. **Document type:** *Bulletin.*
Formerly: Di Cyan and Brown Bulletin (0012-1754)
Indexed: e-psyche.
Published by: Erwin Di Cyan, Ed. & Pub., P O Box 427, Evanston, IL 60204-0427. TEL 718-252-8844.

DIALECT. see *SOCIAL SERVICES AND WELFARE*

DIGEST OF NEUROLOGY & PSYCHIATRY. see *MEDICAL SCIENCES—Abstracting, Bibliographies, Statistics*

616.891 USA ISSN 0891-3870
DIRECTIONS IN PSYCHIATRY. Text in English. 1981. q., latest vol.21, 2001. USD 377 (effective 2001). bk.rev. index. back issues avail.; reprints avail. *Refereed.* **Document type:** *Journal, Academic/Scholarly.* **Description:** Publishes scholarly, jargon-free articles on developments in psychiatry. Continuing medical education credits are available.
Indexed: e-psyche.
—BLDSC (3590.362000).
Published by: Hatherleigh Company Ltd., 5-22 46th Ave, Ste 200, Long Island City, NY 11101-5215. TEL 212-832-1584, 800-367-2550, FAX 212-832-1502, info@hatherleigh.com. Ed. Dr. Fredric F Flach. R&P Kevin Moran.

616.8 USA ISSN 0740-8250
RC459.5.U6
DIRECTORY OF PSYCHIATRY RESIDENCY TRAINING PROGRAMS. Text in English. 1982. irreg., latest vol.6. **Document type:** *Directory.*
Indexed: e-psyche.
Published by: (American Psychiatric Association), American Psychiatric Press, Inc., 1400 K St, N W, Ste 1101, Washington, DC 20005. TEL 202-682-6070, FAX 202-682-6189.

DIRECTORY OF SUICIDE PREVENTION AND CRISIS INTERVENTION CENTERS. see *PSYCHOLOGY*

▼ **DISABILITIES SOURCEBOOK.** see *HANDICAPPED—Physically Impaired*

616.748 ITA ISSN 0012-4087
DISTROFIA MUSCOLARE. Short title: D M. Text in Italian; Summaries in English, Italian. 1962. q. free per issue. adv. bk.rev. bibl, charts, illus. **Document type:** *Newsletter.* **Description:** Presents research papers from various doctors interested in the field of muscular dystrophy. Also features articles on how to deal with victims of this illness as well as how to make their lives easier and more autonomous.
Indexed: e-psyche.
Published by: Unione Italiana Lotta alla Distrofia Muscolare, Via P.P. Vergerio 19, Padua, PD 35126, Italy. TEL 39-49-8021002, FAX 39-49-8022509, dmredaz@tin.it, http://www.uildm.org. Ed. Stefano Borgato. Adv. contact Franco Bomprezzi. page ITL 975,000; trim 285 x 210. Circ: 60,000.

DOWN & UP. see *HANDICAPPED*

616.858842 USA ISSN 0161-0716
DOWN SYNDROME NEWS. Text in English. 1976. 10/yr. USD 25 domestic to membership; USD 35 foreign to membership; USD 50 parent groups; USD 75 all other organizations (effective 2001). bk.rev., film rev., video rev. bibl. index. *Refereed.* **Document type:** *Newsletter.* **Description:** Contains parent-oriented information on Down syndrome, including medical research, education issues, resources, articles by and for parents.
Indexed: e-psyche.
Published by: National Down Syndrome Congress, 7000 Peachtree Dunwoody Rd, N E 5 100, Atlanta, GA 30328-1622. TEL 770-604-9500, 800-232-NDSC, FAX 770-604-9898, ndsccenter@aol.com, http://www.ndscenter.org. Ed. Frank Murphy. R&P Gretchen Friend Jones. Circ: 10,000.

616.8 USA ISSN 1463-6212
DOWN SYNDROME NEWS AND UPDATE. Text in English. 1998. q. GBP 35 to individuals; GBP 50 to institutions (effective 2000 - 2001). back issues avail. *Refereed.* **Document type:** *Newsletter, Academic/Scholarly.* **Description:** Provides information to meet the needs of a variety of professionals and parents caring for individuals with down syndrome around the world. Read by teachers, doctors, speech and language therapists and parents.
Indexed: ERA.
—BLDSC (3620.042000).
Published by: Down Syndrome Educational Trust, Sarah Duffen Centre, Belmont St, Southsea, Hants PO5 1NA, United Kingdom. TEL 44-23-9282-4261, FAX 44-23-9282-4265, enquiries@downsnet.org, http://www.downsnet.org.

616.858 150 GBR ISSN 0968-7912
DOWN SYNDROME: RESEARCH AND PRACTICE. Text in English. 1993. 3/yr. GBP 40 to individuals; GBP 60 to institutions (effective 2000 - 2001). *Refereed.* **Document type:** *Academic/Scholarly.*
Indexed: ERA, Ind.Med. (1993-), PsycInfo, Sp.Ed.Needs Abstr., e-psyche.
—BLDSC (3620.077000), KNAW.
Published by: Down Syndrome Educational Trust, Sarah Duffen Centre, Belmont St, Southsea, Hants PO5 1NA, United Kingdom. TEL 44-23-9282-4261, FAX 44-23-9282-4265, enquiries@downsnet.org, http://www.downsnet.org. Ed. Sue Buckley. R&P Angela Byrne.

DREAMING. see *BIOLOGY—Physiology*

616.8 TUR ISSN 1018-8681
DUSUNEN ADAM. Text in Turkish. 1988. q. USD 60 (effective 2001). **Document type:** *Journal, Academic/Scholarly.*
Published by: Logos Yayincilik Ticaret A.S., Yildiz Posta Cad., Sinan Apt. No. 36 D 66-67, Gayrettepe, Istanbul 80280, Turkey. TEL 90-212-2880541, FAX 90-212-2116185, Info@logos.com.tr, http://logos.com.tr. Ed. Niyazi Alpay.

616.89 DEU ISSN 0012-740X
CODEN: DYPSAQ
DYNAMISCHE PSYCHIATRIE/DYNAMIC PSYCHIATRY; internationale Zeitschrift fuer Psychiatrie und Psychoanalyse. Text and summaries in English, German. 1968. bi-m. DEM 120; DEM 20 newsstand/cover. adv. bk.rev. bibl. index. cum.index. *Refereed.* **Document type:** *Journal, Academic/Scholarly.*
Related titles: Online - full text ed.: (from Institute for Scientific Information).
Indexed: ASCA, Abstr.Crim.& Pen., Biol.Abstr., Curr.Cont., Excerp.Med., IBZ, Ind.Philos., Psychol.Abstr., Psychol.R.G., Ref.Zh., SSCI, e-psyche.
—BLDSC (3637.140000), GNLM, IDS.
Published by: (Deutsche Akademie fuer Psychoanalyse), Pinel-Verlag fuer humanistische Psychiatrie und Philosophie, Kantstr 120-121, Berlin 10625, Germany. TEL 49-30-3132698, FAX 49-30-3136959, info@dynpsych.de, pinel@dynpsych.de, http://www.dynpsych.de/pinel/dynpsych.htm, http://www.dynpsych.de/pinel/index.htm. Ed. Dr. Guenter Ammon. Circ: 3,000.

DYSLEXIA. see *EDUCATION—Special Education And Rehabilitation*

DYSLEXIA HANDBOOK. see *EDUCATION—Special Education And Rehabilitation*

616.8 NLD ISSN 1387-9340
E P D A MAGAZINE. (European Parkinson's Disease Association) Text in Dutch. 1993. s-a.
Formerly (until 1999): Parkinson Magazine (1368-261X)
Indexed: e-psyche.
—BLDSC (3793.410000).
Published by: European Parkinson's Disease Association, Scottlaan 56, Eindhoven 5623 RB, Netherlands. TEL 31-40-2448221, FAX 31-40-2448221, http://www.shef.ac.uk/misc/groups/epda/home.html. Eds. Bridget McCall, Louise van der Valk.

616.89 AUS ISSN 1326-2610
E P P I C INFORMATION SHEET✱ . Text in English.
Description: Aimed at addressing the needs of older adolescent and young adults with emerging psychotic disorders in the Western Metropolitan region of Melbourne, Victoria.
Media: Online - full text.
Published by: Early Psychosis Prevention and Intervention Centre, Locked Bag 10, Parville, VIC 3056, Australia. TEL 61-3-9389-2403, FAX 61-3-9387-3003, iepa@vicnet.net.au, http://home.vicnet.net.au/~eppic/resources.html.

616.89 AUS ISSN 1326-0871
EARLY PSYCHOSIS NEWS. Text in English. 1994. s-a.
Media: Online - full text.
Published by: Early Psychosis Prevention and Intervention Centre, Locked Bag 10, Parville, VIC 3056, Australia. TEL 61-3-9389-2403, FAX 61-3-9387-3003, iepa@vicnet.net.au, http://www.eppic.org.au/newsletter.html.

616.8526 ITA ISSN 1124-4909
EATING AND WEIGHT DISORDERS; Studies on Anorexia, Bulimia and Obesity. Text in English. 1996. q. ITL 61.98 domestic; USD 80 foreign (effective 2002). **Document type:** *Academic/Scholarly.*
Related titles: Online - full text ed.: EUR 30.99 (effective 2002).
Indexed: Ind.Med. (1996-), e-psyche.
—BLDSC (3646.939070).
Published by: Editrice Kurtis s.r.l., Via Luigi Zoja, 30, Milan, MI 20153, Italy. TEL 39-02-48202740, FAX 39-02-4820-1219, info@kurtis.it, http://www.kurtis.it.

616.8526 USA ISSN 1048-6984
EATING DISORDERS REVIEW✱ ; current clinical information for the professional treating eating disorders. Text in English. 1990. bi-m. USD 79; USD 96 foreign (effective 1996). back issues avail. **Document type:** *Newsletter.*
Indexed: e-psyche.

Published by: Quest Publishing Co., Inc., A Division of Raven Press Ltd. (Subsidiary of: Wolters Kluwer N.V.), 345 Hudson St 36 Fl, New York, NY 10014-4502. TEL 212-930-9500. Ed. Dr. Joel Yager. Pub. Mary Waltham.

EDUCATION AND TRAINING IN MENTAL RETARDATION AND DEVELOPMENTAL DISABILITIES. see *EDUCATION—Special Education And Rehabilitation*

616.8 USA
EINSTEIN PSYCHIATRY SERIES. Text in English. irreg., latest vol.10, 1995. **Document type:** *Academic/Scholarly.*
Indexed: e-psyche.
—BLDSC (3665.634000).
Published by: (Albert Einstein College of Medicine, Yeshiva University), John Wiley & Sons, Inc., Journals (Subsidiary of: Wiley InterScience), 605 Third Ave, New York, NY 10158. subinfo@jwiley.com. Eds. Hope Conte, Robert Plutchik.

616.8 NLD ISSN 0424-8155
CODEN: EECSB3
ELECTROENCEPHALOGRAPHY AND CLINICAL NEUROPHYSIOLOGY. SUPPLEMENTS. Text in English. 1950. irreg., latest vol.52, 1999. price varies. back issues avail. *Refereed.* **Document type:** *Monographic series, Academic/Scholarly, Trade.*
Description: Offers insight in the use of electroencephalography (EEC) in a clinical neurophysiology setting.
Related titles: ♦ Supplement: Clinical Neurophysiology. ISSN 1388-2457.
Indexed: Ind.Med. (coverage dropped), Neurosci.Cit.Ind., e-psyche.
—CASDDS, CISTI, Infotrieve, KNAW. **CCC.**
Published by: (International Federation of Clinical Neurophysiology IRL), Elsevier Science BV, PO Box 211, Amsterdam 1000 AE, Netherlands. TEL 31-20-485-3757, 31-20-485-3911, FAX 31-20-485-3432, 31-20-485-3598, nlinfo-f@elsevier.nl; usinfo-f@elsevier.com; forinfo-kyf04035@niftyserve.or.jp, http://www.elsevier.nl/. **Subscr. in Australasia and the Far East to:** Elsevier Science (Singapore) Pte Ltd, No.1 Temasek Ave, 17-01 Millenia Tower, Singapore 039192, Singapore. TEL 65-434-3727, FAX 65-337-2230, asiainfo@elsevier.com.sg; **Subscr. in Japan to:** Elsevier Science Inc - Japan Regional Office, 9-15 Higashi-Azabu 1-chome, Minato-ku, Tokyo 106-0044, Japan. TEL 81-3-5561-5033, FAX 81-3-5561-5047, info@elsevier.co.jp; **Subscr. in the Americas to:** Elsevier Science, PO Box 945, New York, NY 10159-0945. TEL 212-633-3730, 888-437-4636, FAX 212-633-3680, usinfo-f@elsevier.com, http://www.elsevier.com

612.8 BEL ISSN 0301-150X
RC77.5 CODEN: EMCNA9
ELECTROMYOGRAPHY AND CLINICAL NEUROPHYSIOLOGY. Text in English. 1961. 8/yr. USD 120 (effective 2000). abstr, bibl, charts, illus. index. **Document type:** *Journal, Academic/Scholarly.*
Formerly: Electromyography (0013-4732)
Indexed: Biol.Abstr., Excerp.Med., INSPEC (Nov.1968-), Ind.Med. (1972-), Ref.Zh., e-psyche.
—BLDSC (3699.720000), AskIEEE, CISTI, EMDOCS, GNLM, ingenta, KNAW.
Published by: Editions Nauwelaerts SA, Rue de l' Eglise St Suplice 19, Beauvechain 1320, Belgium. TEL 32-10-866737, FAX 32-10-861655. Eds. F Bruyninckx, N Rosselle.

THE ELECTRONIC JOURNAL OF COMMUNICATIVE PSYCHOANALYSIS; an independent multilingual international publication. see *PSYCHOLOGY*

616.8 USA ISSN 0734-9890
CODEN: EBMOEN
EMOTIONS AND BEHAVIOR. MONOGRAPH. Text in English. irreg. price varies. *Refereed.* **Document type:** *Monographic series.*
Indexed: Psychol.Abstr., e-psyche.
Published by: (Chicago Institute for Psychoanalysis), International Universities Press, Inc., 59 Boston Post Rd, Box 1524, Madison, CT 06443-1524. TEL 203-245-4000, FAX 203-245-0775, http://www.iup.com. Ed. Dr. George H Pollock.

616.89 SWE ISSN 1102-3104
EMPATI; tidning foer information, debatt och forskning om schizofreni och andra psykiska handicapp. Text in Swedish. 1991. q. SEK 160 domestic; NOK 175 in Norway; SEK 220 Denmark & Finland; SEK 225 in Europe; SEK 230 elsewhere (effective 2001). adv. bk.rev. **Document type:** *Journal, Academic/Scholarly.*
Indexed: e-psyche.

Published by: Stiftelsen Sympatikus, Sjoevaegen 18, Solna 16955, Sweden. TEL 46-8-735-02-11, FAX 46-8-82-23-95. Ed. Kristina Hollox. Adv. contact Margarethe Weckman.

616.89 FRA ISSN 0013-7006
CODEN: ENCEAN
L'ENCEPHALE✱ ; revue de psychiatrie biologique et therapeutique. Text in French; Summaries in English, French. 1906; N.S. 1973. 6/yr. FRF 690 to individuals; FRF 790 to institutions; FRF 400 to students (effective 1999). adv. bk.rev. charts, tr.lit. index. reprint service avail. from PQC. *Refereed.* **Document type:** *Academic/Scholarly.*
Related titles: Microform ed.: (from PQC); Online - full text ed.: (from Institute for Scientific Information, RoweCom Information Quest).
Indexed: Biol.Abstr., Chem.Abstr., Chem.Indus.Notes, Chem.Titles, Curr.Cont. (coverage dropped), Excerp.Med., Ind.Med. (1906-), Int.Nurs.Ind., Lang.& Lang.Behav.Abstr., Neurosci.Cit.Ind., PsycInfo, Psychol.Abstr. (1951-), SOPODA, Sociol.Abstr., e-psyche.
—BLDSC (3738.390000), CASDDS, CISTI, GNLM, IDS, KNAW. **CCC.**
Published by: Doin Editeurs, 26 av. de l'Europe, B.P. 60, Velizy Cedex 78141, France. TEL 33-1-43265838. Ed. P Deniker. Circ: 1,200.

ENCOR RESPONDENCE. see *EDUCATION—Special Education And Rehabilitation*

ENCOUNTERER. see *PSYCHOLOGY*

616.8 FRA ISSN 0246-0378
ENCYCLOPEDIE MEDICO-CHIRURGICALE. NEUROLOGIE. Cover title: Traite de Neurologie. Variant title: Encyclopedie Medico-Chirurgicale, Instantanes Medicaux. Neurologie. Receuil Periodique de l'Encyclopedie Medico-Chirurgicale. Neurologie. Text in French. 1939. 7 base vols. plus q. updates. bibl, charts, illus. *Refereed.* **Document type:** *Academic/Scholarly.* **Description:** Offers neurologists a comprehensive, up-to-date reference for diagnosing and treating various neurological disorders.
Published by: Elsevier Paris, Editions Scientifiques et Medicales (Subsidiary of: Reed Elsevier plc. group), 23 rue Linois, Paris 75015, France. TEL 33-1-45589110, FAX 33-1-45589425, redaction-emc@elsevier.fr, redacion-emc@elsevier.fr, http://www.elsevier.fr, http://www.elsevier.com.

ENCYCLOPEDIE MEDICO-CHIRURGICALE. TRAITE DE RADIODIAGNOSTIC: SQUELETTE NORMAL - NEURORADIOLOGIE - APPAREIL LOCOMOTEUR. see *MEDICAL SCIENCES—Radiology And Nuclear Medicine*

EPIDEMIOLOGIA E PSICHIATRIA SOCIALE. see *PUBLIC HEALTH AND SAFETY*

616.853 362.196 DNK ISSN 0107-2668
EPILEPSI. Text in Danish. 1966. q. DKK 75 (effective 1998). adv. bk.rev. illus. **Document type:** *Newsletter, Consumer.* **Description:** Publishes medical and general information about epilepsy, advocacy and activities in the organization.
Formerly: Tidsskrift for Epilepsi
Indexed: e-psyche.
Published by: Dansk Epilepsiforening/Danish Eplepsy Association, Dr Sellsvej 28, Dianalund 4293, Denmark. TEL 45-58-26-44-66, FAX 45-58-26-44-51. Ed. Eva Tufte. Circ: 10,000.

616.853 USA ISSN 0013-9580
RC395 CODEN: EPILAK
EPILEPSIA. Text in English. 1960. m. USD 330 domestic to individuals; USD 350 in Canada & Mexico to individuals; USD 380 overseas to individuals; USD 625 domestic to institutions; USD 645 in Canada & Mexico to institutions; USD 675 overseas to institutions; USD 363 to individuals print & online eds. combined; USD 687.50 to institutions print & online eds. combined (effective 2001). adv. bk.rev. charts, illus. reprint service avail. from PSC. *Refereed.* **Document type:** *Journal, Academic/Scholarly.* **Description:** Provides current clinical and research results on all aspects of epilepsy.
Related titles: Online - full text ed.: USD 363 to individuals; USD 687.50 to institutions (effective 2001) (from Ovid Technologies, Inc., EBSCO Publishing, Swets Blackwell, Institute for Scientific Information).

M

Indexed: ASCA, Bibl.Dev.Med.& Child Neur., Biol.Abstr., Chem.Abstr., Chem.Indus.Notes, Chem.Titles, Curr.Adv.Ecol.Sci., Curr.Cont., Dent.Ind., Derwent Biotech.Abstr., Excerp.Med., Helminthol.Abstr., Ind.Med. (1909-), Ind.Sci.Rev., Inpharma, Int.Nurs.Ind., Jrnl.Watch Neuro., Neurosci.Abstr. (coverage dropped), Neurosci.Cit.Ind., Pharm.&Out.News, Psychol.Abstr., Reac., SSCI (coverage dropped), Sci.Cit.Ind., e-psyche.
—BLDSC (3793.700000), CASDDS, CISTI, GNLM, IDS, ingenta, KNAW.
Published by: (International League Against Epilepsy), Blackwell Science Inc., Commerce Pl, 350 Main St, Malden, MA 02148-5018. TEL 781-388-8250, FAX 781-388-8255, journals@blacksci.com, http://www.blackwell-science.com. Ed. Timothy Pedley. adv.: B&W page USD 1,195, color page USD 2,655. Circ: 3,371 (paid). **Subscr. to:** Lippincott Williams & Wilkins (Philadelphia), PO Box 1600, Hagerstown, MD 21740-1600. TEL 800-777-2295, FAX 301-824-7390.

616.853 CHE
EPILEPSIE. Text and summaries in French, German, Italian. 1983. 2/yr. CHF 20 (effective 2001). adv. bk.rev. **Document type:** *Journal, Academic/Scholarly.* **Description:** Covers medical and social aspects, featuring research in treatment, diagnosis, therapy, and heredity, as well as social and educational problems of different age groups. Includes list of events.
Indexed: e-psyche.
Published by: Schweizerische Liga gegen Epilepsie, Dorfstr 2, Postfach 233, Stafa Zurich 8712, Switzerland. TEL 41-1-926-89-71, FAX 41-1-926-89-72, slge@bluewin.ch, http://www.epi.ch. Ed. Margret Becker. R&P, Adv. contact Ernst Zweifel. Circ: 800.

616.853 FRA ISSN 1149-6576
EPILEPSIES. Text in French. bi-m. FRF 450 domestic to individuals; EUR 81 in Europe to individuals; FRF 570 elsewhere to individuals; FRF 890 domestic to institutions; EUR 148 in Europe to institutions; FRF 1,010 elsewhere to institutions; FRF 150 newsstand/cover (effective 2001). **Document type:** *Academic/Scholarly.* **Description:** Provides a forum for neurologists, specialised institutions, general practitioners, nurses, technicians and electroencephalographers.
Indexed: e-psyche.
—BLDSC (3793.740000), EMDOCS, GNLM, KNAW.
Published by: (Ligue Francaise Contre l'Epilepsie), John Libbey Eurotext, 127 av. de la Republique, Montrouge 92120, France. TEL 33-01-46730660, FAX 33-01-40840999, marketing@jle.com, http://www.john-libbey-eurotext.fr/, http://www.john-libbey-eurotext.fr. Eds. Alexis Arzimanoglou, Michele Bureau. **Subscr. to:** A T E I, 3 av. Pierre Kerautret, Romainville 92230, France. TEL 33-1-48408686, FAX 33-1-48400731, atei@club-internet.fr.

616.853 NLD ISSN 0920-1211
CODEN: EPIRE8
EPILEPSY RESEARCH. Text in English. 1987. 15/yr. EUR 1,991 in Europe to institutions; JPY 264,500 in Japan to institutions; USD 2,227 elsewhere to institutions (effective 2002). adv. bk.rev. index. back issues avail.; reprint service avail. from ISI. *Refereed.* **Document type:** *Academic/Scholarly.* **Description:** Provides for rapid publication of high-quality articles in both experimental and clinical epileptology, where the principal emphasis of the research is concerned with brain mechanisms in epilepsy.
Incorporates (1988-1999): Journal of Epilepsy (0896-6974)
Related titles: Microform ed.: (from PQC); Online - full text ed.: (from ingenta, Swets Blackwell, ScienceDirect, Institute for Scientific Information); ♦ Supplement: Epilepsy Research Supplements. ISSN 0922-9833.
Indexed: ASCA, Chem.Abstr., Chem.Indus.Notes, Chem.Titles, Curr.Cont., Excerp.Med., Ind.Med. (1987-), Inpharma, Int.Abstr.Biol.Sci., Neurosci.Cit.Ind., Pharm.&Out.News, PsycInfo, Reac., Ref.Zh., SSCI (coverage dropped), Sci.Cit.Ind., e-psyche.
—BLDSC (3793.805000), ADONIS, CASDDS, CISTI, EMDOCS, GNLM, IDS, Infotrieve, ingenta, KNAW. **CCC.**
Published by: Elsevier Science BV, PO Box 211, Amsterdam 1000 AE, Netherlands. TEL 31-20-485-2911, FAX 31-20-485-2457, http://www.elsevier.com/locate/epilepsyres. Ed. I Leppick. Circ: 850. **Subscr. in Australasia and the Far East to:** Elsevier Science (Singapore) Pte Ltd, No.1 Temasek Ave, 17-01 Millenia Tower, Singapore 039192, Singapore. TEL 65-434-3727, FAX 65-337-2230; **Subscr. in Japan to:** Elsevier Science Inc - Japan Regional Office, 9-15 Higashi-Azabu 1-chome, Minato-ku, Tokyo 106-0044, Japan. TEL 81-3-5561-5033; **Subscr. in the Americas to:** Elsevier Science, PO Box 945, New York, NY 10159-0945. TEL 212-633-3730, FAX 212-633-3680, usinfo-f@elsevier.com.

616.853 NLD ISSN 0922-9833
CODEN: ERSUED
EPILEPSY RESEARCH SUPPLEMENTS. Text in English. 1988. irreg., latest vol.12, 1996. price varies. back issues avail. *Refereed.* **Document type:** *Monographic series, Academic/Scholarly, Trade.* **Description:** Publishes research into the etiology, diagnosis, and treatment of epilepsy.
Related titles: Microform ed.; ♦ Supplement to: Epilepsy Research. ISSN 0920-1211.
Indexed: Chem.Abstr., Chem.Indus.Notes, Chem.Titles, Ind.Med. (1988-), e-psyche.
—BLDSC (3793.806000), CASDDS, CISTI, KNAW. **CCC.**
Published by: Elsevier Science BV, PO Box 211, Amsterdam 1000 AE, Netherlands. TEL 31-20-485-3757, 31-20-485-3911, FAX 31-20-485-3432, 31-20-485-3598, nlinfo-f@elsevier.nl; usinfo-f@elsevier.com; forinfo-kyf04035@niftyserve.or.jp, http://www.elsevier.nl/. **Subscr. in Australasia and the Far East to:** Elsevier Science (Singapore) Pte Ltd, No.1 Temasek Ave, 17-01 Millenia Tower, Singapore 039192, Singapore. TEL 65-434-3727, FAX 65-337-2230, asiainfo@elsevier.com.sg; **Subscr. in Japan to:** Elsevier Science Inc - Japan Regional Office, 9-15 Higashi-Azabu 1-chome, Minato-ku, Tokyo 106-0044, Japan. TEL 81-3-5561-5033, FAX 81-3-5561-5047, info@elsevier.co.jp; **Subscr. in the Americas to:** Elsevier Science, PO Box 945, New York, NY 10159-0945. TEL 212-633-3730, 888-437-4636, FAX 212-633-3680, usinfo-f@elsevier.com, http://www.elsevier.com

616.853 GBR ISSN 0958-496X
EPILEPSY TODAY. Text in English. 1976. q. GBP 12 domestic to membership; GBP 30 foreign to membership (effective 2000). adv. bk.rev. **Document type:** *Consumer.*
Former titles (until 1987): Epilepsy Now! (0262-5474); (until 1981): Epilepsy News (0308-9703); Candle (0008-5502)
Indexed: Sp.Ed.Needs Abstr., e-psyche.
Published by: British Epilepsy Association, New Anstey House, Gate Way Drive, Yeadon, Leeds LS1 1BE, United Kingdom. TEL 44-1132-108800, FAX 44-1133-910300, epilepsy@bea.org.uk, http://www.epilepsy.org.uk. Ed., R&P Sue Mitchell. Circ: 21,500.

616.853 USA ISSN 1060-9369
EPILEPSY U S A. Text in English. 1972 (vol.5). 8/yr. USD 25. bk.rev. illus. reprints avail. **Document type:** *Consumer.* **Description:** Covers medical, legal, and legislative news and features for people with epilepsy.
Formerly (until 1991): National Spokesman (0091-2387)
Indexed: Rehabil.Lit., e-psyche.
Published by: Epilepsy Foundation of America, 4351 Garden City Dr., Ste. 406, Landover, MD 20785. TEL 301-459-3700, FAX 301-577-2684, postmaster@efa.org, http://www.efa.org. Ed. Karina Barrentine. R&P Ann Scherer. Circ: 23,000.

616.853 FRA ISSN 1294-9361
▼ **EPILEPTIC DISORDERS**; international epilepsy journal with videotape. Text in English. 1999. q. FRF 1,650 domestic to individuals; USD 300 in Europe to individuals; USD 350 elsewhere to individuals; FRF 2,475 domestic to institutions; USD 450 in Europe to institutions; USD 500 elsewhere to institutions; FRF 715 domestic to students; USD 110 foreign to students (effective 2001). adv. bk.rev. back issues avail. *Refereed.* **Document type:** *Journal, Academic/Scholarly.* **Description:** Publishes clinical and review articles on all facets of epilepsy and related disorders.
Related titles: Online - full text ed.: FRF 1,650 domestic to individuals; USD 300 foreign to individuals; FRF 2,475 domestic to institutions; USD 450 foreign to institutions; FRF 715 domestic to members; USD 110 foreign to members (effective 2001) (from Institute for Scientific Information).
Indexed: Curr.Cont., Ind.Med., Neurosci.Cit.Ind.
—BLDSC (3793.807200).
Published by: (Hopital Robert-Debre, Neurologie Pediatrique), John Libbey Eurotext, 127 av. de la Republique, Montrouge 92120, France. TEL 33-01-46730660, FAX 33-01-40840999, marketing@jle.com, http://www.john-libbey-eurotext.fr. Ed. Dr. Jean Aicardi. **Subscr. to:** A T E I, 3 av. Pierre Kerautret, Romainville 92230, France. TEL 33-1-48408686, FAX 33-1-48400731, atei@club-internet.fr.

616.853 AUS ISSN 0729-7823
EPILETTER. Text in English. 1967. q. AUD 10. bk.rev. back issues avail. **Document type:** *Newsletter, Consumer.* **Description:** Covers all aspects of epilepsy, including research, human interest, medicine, fundraising and welfare.
Indexed: e-psyche.
Published by: Epilepsy Foundation of Victoria, 818 Burke Rd, Camberwell, VIC 3124, Australia. TEL 61-3-813-2866, FAX 61-3-882-7159. Ed. Gail Chrisfield. Circ: 2,500.

616.8 FRA ISSN 1287-258X
ESSAIM; revue psychanalitique. Text in French. 1998. s-a. EUR 40 domestic; EUR 45 foreign (effective 2002).
Published by: Editions Eres, 11 rue des Alouettes, Ramonville Saint-Agne 31520, France. TEL 33-05-61751576, FAX 33-05-61735289, eres@editions-eres.com. Ed. Erik Porge.

616.842 615.1 USA ISSN 1087-495X
RC483
ESSENTIAL PSYCHOPHARMACOLOGY. Text in English. 1996. q., latest vol.4, 2001. USD 95; USD 120 foreign (effective 2001). bk.rev. index. back issues avail.; reprints avail. *Refereed.* **Document type:** *Journal, Academic/Scholarly.*
Indexed: e-psyche.
—BLDSC (3811.794000).
Published by: Hatherleigh Company Ltd., 5-22 46th Ave, Ste 200, Long Island City, NY 11101-5215. TEL 212-832-1584, 800-367-2550, FAX 212-832-1502, info@hatherleigh.com. Ed. Frederic Flach. R&P Kevin J Moran.

616.8 360 USA ISSN 1523-150X
CODEN: EHSSF6
▼ **ETHICAL HUMAN SCIENCES AND SERVICES**; an international journal of critical inquiry. Text in English; Abstracts in Spanish, French. 1999. 3/yr., latest vol.3, no.1, 2001, Spring. USD 48 in United States to individuals; USD 80 for 2 yrs. in United States to individuals; USD 56 foreign to individuals; USD 96 for 2 yrs. to individuals; USD 98 in United States to institutions; USD 166 for 2 yrs. in United States to institutions; USD 108 foreign to institutions; USD 180 for 2 yrs. foreign to institutions (effective 2001). adv. bk.rev., software rev., video rev. abstr, bibl, charts, illus, stat. 120 p./no. back issues avail.; reprints avail. *Refereed.* **Document type:** *Journal, Academic/Scholarly.* **Description:** Publishes interdisciplinary and international critiques of theory and practice across the fields of health and social sciences seeking to raise the level of ethical awareness.
Indexed: Soc.Serv.Abstr., Sociol.Abstr.
—BLDSC (3814.640700).
Published by: Springer Publishing Company, 536 Broadway, New York, NY 10012. TEL 212-431-4370, FAX 212-941-7842, springer@springerpub.com, http://www.springerpub.com; http://www.icspp.org, http://www.springerjournals.com/. Ed. Peter R Breggin. Pub. Ursula Springer. R&P Dorothy Kouwenberg. adv.: B&W page USD 300; trim 10 x 7. Circ: 350 (paid).
Co-sponsor: International Center for the Study of Psychiatry and Psychology.

616.8 DEU ISSN 0940-1334
CODEN: EAPNES
EUROPEAN ARCHIVES OF PSYCHIATRY AND CLINICAL NEUROSCIENCES; official organ of the German society for biological psychiatry. (Vereinigt mit Zeitschrift fuer die Gesamte Neurologie und Psychiatrie) Text in English. 1868. bi-m. EUR 934.20 domestic; EUR 930.40 in Germany; EUR 184 newsstand/cover foreign (effective 2002). adv. bk.rev. abstr, bibl. back issues avail.; reprint service avail. from ISI. *Refereed.* **Document type:** *Journal, Academic/Scholarly.* **Description:** Covers clinical psychiatry, psychopathology, and epidemiology, as well as neuropathological, neurophysiological, and neurochemical studies of psychiatric disorders.
Former titles: European Archives of Psychiatry and Neurological Sciences (0175-758X); (until 1984): Archiv fuer Psychiatrie und Nervenkrankheiten (0003-9373)
Related titles: Microfiche ed.: (from BHP); Microform ed.: (from PQC); Online - full text ed.: ISSN 1433-8491 (from EBSCO Publishing, RoweCom Information Quest, Swets Blackwell, Springer LINK, Institute for Scientific Information).
Indexed: ASCA, Biol.Abstr., Chem.Abstr., Curr.Adv.Ecol.Sci., Curr.Adv.Gen.& Molec.Biol., Curr.Cont., Excerp.Med., Ger.J.Psych., INIS Atomind., Ind.Med. (1990-), Ind.Sci.Rev., Inpharma, Int.Nurs.Ind., Neurosci.Cit.Ind., Pharm.&Out.News, PsycInfo, Psychol.Abstr. (1971-), Reac., Risk Abstr., SSCI (coverage dropped), Sci.Cit.Ind., e-psyche.
—BLDSC (3829.488545), CASDDS, CISTI, EMDOCS, GNLM, IDS, ingenta, KNAW. **CCC.**

M

Published by: (Gesamtverband Deutscher Nervenaerzte), Dr. Dietrich Steinkopff Verlag (Subsidiary of: BertelsmannSpringer), Poststr 9, Darmstadt 64293, Germany. TEL 49-6151-82899-0, FAX 49-6151-82899-40, frey.steinkopff@springer.de, http://www.steinkopff.springer.de. R&P Dr. Maria Magdalene Nabbe. **Subscr. in N. America to:** Springer-Verlag New York Inc., PO Box 2485, Secaucus, NJ 07096-2485. TEL 212-460-1500, FAX 212-473-6272.

616.8 DEU ISSN 1018-8827

EUROPEAN CHILD & ADOLESCENT PSYCHIATRY; official journal of the European Society for Child and Adolescent Psychiatry. Text in English. 1992. q. EUR 304.20 domestic; EUR 300.40 in Germany; USD 58 newsstand/cover foreign (effective 2002). adv. bk.rev. abstr, bibl. back issues avail.; reprints avail. *Refereed.* **Document type:** *Journal, Academic/Scholarly.* **Description:** Aims to promote the growth of empirically based clinical child and adolescent psychiatry, not only in Europe but throughout the world.

Related titles: Online - full text ed.: ISSN 1435-165X (from EBSCO Publishing, RoweCom Information Quest, Swets Blackwell, Springer LINK, Institute for Scientific Information).

Indexed: ASCA, ASSIA, CINAHL, Curr.Cont., Excerp.Med. (1994-), Fam.Ind., IBZ, Ind.Med. (1992-), Int.Nurs.Ind., Lang.& Lang.Behav.Abstr., PsycInfo, Psychol.Abstr. (1992-), SOPODA, SSCI, Sociol.Abstr., e-psyche.

—BLDSC (3829.600600), CISTI, EMDOCS, GNLM, IDS, Infotrieve, KNAW. **CCC.**

Published by: (European Society for Child and Adolescent Psychiatry), Dr. Dietrich Steinkopff Verlag (Subsidiary of: BertelsmannSpringer), Poststr 9, Darmstadt 64293, Germany. TEL 49-6151-82899-0, FAX 49-6151-82899-40, frey.steinkopff@springer.de, http://www.steinkopff.springer.de. Ed. C Gillberg. Pub. Dietrich Steinkopff. R&P Sabine Ibkendanz. **Subscr. in N. America to:** Springer-Verlag, Journals; **Subscr. to:** Springer Auslieferungs Gesellschaft, Postfach 105160, Heidelberg 69041, Germany. TEL 49-6221-345244, FAX 49-6221-345244.

616.8 GBR ISSN 1351-5101
CODEN: EJNEFL

EUROPEAN JOURNAL OF NEUROLOGY. Text in English. 1994. bi-m., latest vol.9, 2002. GBP 126 in Europe to individuals; USD 195 in North America to individuals; GBP 126 elsewhere to individuals; GBP 413 in Europe to institutions; USD 595 in North America to institutions; GBP 413 elsewhere to institutions (effective 2002). adv. bk.rev. index. *Refereed.* **Document type:** *Academic/Scholarly.* **Description:** Provides a forum on the major diseases of large clinical and socioeconomic importance.

Related titles: Online - full text ed.: ISSN 1468-1331. 1994. GBP 114 in Europe to individuals; USD 176 in North America to individuals; GBP 114 elsewhere to individuals; GBP 372 in Europe to institutions; USD 536 in North America to institutions; GBP 372 elsewhere to institutions (effective 2002) (from EBSCO Publishing, O C L C Online Computer Library Center, Inc., RoweCom Information Quest, ingenta, Munksgaard & Blackwell Science's Synergy, Swets Blackwell, Institute for Scientific Information).

Indexed: ASCA, Curr.Cont., Excerp.Med. (1996-), Ind.Med. (1994-), Inpharma, Int.Abstr.Biol.Sci., Jrnl.Watch Neuro., Neurosci.Abstr. (coverage dropped), Neurosci.Cit.Ind., Nutr.Abstr., Pharm.&Out.News, Protozool.Abstr., PsycInfo, Reac., Rev.Appl.Entomol., e-psyche.

—BLDSC (3829.731680), ADONIS, CISTI, GNLM, IDS, KNAW.

Published by: Blackwell Science Ltd., PO Box 88, Oxford OX2 0NE, United Kingdom. TEL 44-1865-206180, 44-1865-206002, FAX 44-1865-206219, jnl.orders@blacksci.co.uk, http://www.blackwell-science.com/~cgilib/jnlpage.asp?Journal=ene&File=ene, http://www.blackwellpublishing.com. Eds. F Boller, P Sorensen. Pub. Allen Stevens. R&P Sophie Savage. Adv. contact Jenny Applin. Circ: 800.

616.8 GBR ISSN 0953-816X
CODEN: EJONEI

EUROPEAN JOURNAL OF NEUROSCIENCE. Text in English. 1989. m., latest vol.15, 2002. GBP 356 in Europe to individuals; USD 564 in North America to individuals; GBP 391 elsewhere to individuals; GBP 1,270 in Europe to institutions; USD 2,012 in North America to institutions; GBP 1,397 elsewhere to institutions (effective 2002). adv. *Refereed.* **Document type:** *Academic/Scholarly.* **Description:** Presents a broad scope of neuroscience, ranging from the behavioral to the molecular, with a European focus and a worldwide orientation.

Related titles: Microfiche ed.: (from PQC); Online - full text ed.: ISSN 1460-9568. GBP 321 in Europe to individuals; USD 508 in North America to individuals; GBP 321 elsewhere to individuals; GBP 172 in Europe to institutions; USD 274 in North America to institutions; GBP 172 elsewhere to institutions (effective 2002) (from Northern Light Technology, Inc., EBSCO Publishing, O C L C Online Computer Library Center, Inc., RoweCom Information Quest, ingenta, Munksgaard & Blackwell Science's Synergy, Swets Blackwell, Institute for Scientific Information); ♦ Supplement: Supplement to the European Journal of Neuroscience. ISSN 1359-5962.

Indexed: ASCA, Biol.Abstr., Curr.Cont., Excerp.Med., Ind.Med. (1989-), Ind.Sci.Rev., Inpharma, Int.Abstr.Biol.Sci., Neurosci.Abstr. (coverage dropped), Neurosci.Cit.Ind., Nutr.Abstr., Pharm.&Out.News, Reac., Rev.Med.& Vet.Mycol., SSCI (coverage dropped), Sci.Cit.Ind., e-psyche.

—ADONIS, CISTI, EMDOCS, GNLM, IDS, ingenta, KNAW. **CCC.**

Published by: Blackwell Science Ltd., PO Box 88, Oxford OX2 0NE, United Kingdom. TEL 44-1865-206180, 44-1865-206002, FAX 44-1865-206219, jnl.orders@blacksci.co.uk, http://www.blackwell-science.com/~cgilib/jnlpage.asp?Journal=ejn&File=ejn, http://www.blackwellpublishing.com. Ed. B Everitt. Pub. Amanda McLean Inglis. R&P Sophie Savage. Adv. contact Jenny Applin. Circ: 665. **Co-sponsor:** European Neuroscience Association.

EUROPEAN JOURNAL OF PAEDIATRIC NEUROLOGY. see *MEDICAL SCIENCES—Pediatrics*

616.89 ESP ISSN 0213-6163
RC321 CODEN: EJOPEO

EUROPEAN JOURNAL OF PSYCHIATRY. Text in English. 1986. q. ESP 10,800, USD 92 to individuals; ESP 13,500, USD 115 to institutions (effective 2001). adv. bk.rev. *Refereed.* **Document type:** *Academic/Scholarly.* **Description:** Reports the scientific activity of European psychiatrists. Presents an eclectic orientation in its scientific approach and is open to Psychiatry, Mental Health and all related fields.

Related titles: Online - full text ed.: (from Institute for Scientific Information).

Indexed: ASCA, AgeLine, Curr.Cont., Excerp.Med., Lang.& Lang.Behav.Abstr., PsycInfo, Psychol.Abstr. (1987-), SOPODA, SSCI, Sociol.Abstr., e-psyche.

—BLDSC (3829.737700), CINDOC, EMDOCS, GNLM, IDS, Infotrieve, KNAW. **CCC.**

Address: University of Zaragoza, Avda. S. Juan Bosco 15, P O Box 6029, Zaragoza 50009, Spain. TEL 34-976-597818, FAX 34-976-761738. Ed. A Seva.

616.891 GBR ISSN 1364-2537

EUROPEAN JOURNAL OF PSYCHOTHERAPY, COUNSELLING AND HEALTH. Text in English. 1998. 4/yr. GBP 49, USD 81 to individuals; GBP 220, USD 363 to institutions (effective 2002). **Description:** Investigates links between the different traditions of health care, counselling, and psychotherapy; the relationship of physical to mental health; and interactions among the psychotherapists, counsellors, and health care providers.

Related titles: Online - full content ed.: ISSN 1469-5901 (from EBSCO Publishing, Swets Blackwell); Online - full text ed.: (from CatchWord Ltd., RoweCom Information Quest).

Indexed: e-psyche.

—BLDSC (3829.738010), CatchWord.

Published by: Routledge (Subsidiary of: Taylor & Francis Group), 11 New Fetter Ln, London EC4P 4EE, United Kingdom. TEL 44-20-7583-9855, FAX 44-20-7842-2298, info@routledge.co.uk, http://www.tandf.co.uk/journals. Ed. Robbi Campbell. R&P Sally Sweet. **Subscr. in US & Canada:** Subscriptions, PO Box 362, Abingdon, Oxon OX14 3WB, United Kingdom. TEL 44-1235-401060, 212-216-7800, FAX 44-1235-401075, 212-564-7854.

616.8 CHE ISSN 0014-3022
CODEN: EUNEAP

EUROPEAN NEUROLOGY. Text in English. 1968. 8/yr. (in 2 vols.). CHF 1,420, EUR 1,014.40 in Europe to institutions; CHF 1,443.20, USD 1,104 elsewhere to institutions (effective 2002). adv. bk.rev. index. back issues avail. *Refereed.* **Document type:** *Journal, Academic/Scholarly.* **Description:** Covers clinical aspects of diseases of the nervous system and muscles, as well as their neuropathological, biochemical, and electrophysiological basis.

Formerly (until 1968): Psychiatria et Neurologia

Related titles: Microform ed.; Online - full text ed.: ISSN 1421-9913. CHF 116, EUR 84, USD 90 to institutions with print edition (effective 2002) (from Northern Light Technology, Inc., EBSCO Publishing, O C L C Online Computer Library Center, Inc., RoweCom Information Quest, ProQuest Information & Learning, Swets Blackwell, Institute for Scientific Information).

Indexed: ASCA, Bibl.Dev.Med.& Child Neur., Biol.Abstr., Chem.Abstr., Chem.Indus.Notes, Chem.Titles, Curr.Adv.Ecol.Sci., Curr.Cont., Dent.Ind., Excerp.Med., Helminthol.Abstr., INIS Atomind., Ind.Med. (1968-), Ind.Sci.Rev., Inpharma, Neurosci.Abstr. (coverage dropped), Neurosci.Cit.Ind., Nutr.Abstr., Pharm.&Out.News, Protozool.Abstr., PsycInfo, Psychol.Abstr. (1990-), Reac., SSCI (coverage dropped), Sci.Cit.Ind., e-psyche.

—BLDSC (3829.765000), CASDDS, CISTI, GNLM, IDS, ingenta, KNAW. **CCC.**

Published by: S. Karger AG, Allschwilerstr 10, PO Box, Basel 4009, Switzerland. TEL 41-61-306-1111, FAX 41-61-306-1234, karger@karger.ch, http://www.online.karger.com/journals/ene, http://www.karger.com. Ed. J Bogousslavsky. adv.: page USD 1,195. Circ: 1,050.

616.8 615.1 NLD ISSN 0924-977X
CODEN: EURNE8

EUROPEAN NEUROPSYCHOPHARMACOLOGY. Text in English. 1990. bi-m. EUR 569 in Europe to institutions; JPY 75,500 in Japan to institutions; USD 636 elsewhere to institutions (effective 2002). adv. bk.rev. abstr. back issues avail.; reprint service avail. from SWZ. *Refereed.* **Document type:** *Academic/Scholarly.* **Description:** Publishes clinical and basic research articles in the field of neuropsychopharmacology, with particular focus on the effects of centrally acting agents.

Related titles: Microform ed.: (from PQC); Online - full text ed.: (from ingenta, Swets Blackwell, ScienceDirect, Institute for Scientific Information).

Indexed: ASCA, Chem.Indus.Notes, Chem.Titles, Curr.Cont., Derwent Biotech.Abstr., Excerp.Med. (1993-), Focus on: Psychophar., Ind.Med. (1990-), Ind.Sci.Rev., Indian Psychol.Abstr., Inpharma, Int.Abstr.Biol.Sci., Int.Nurs.Ind., Neurosci.Cit.Ind., Pharm.&Out.News, PsycInfo, Psychol.Abstr. (1991-), Reac., SSCI (coverage dropped), Sci.Cit.Ind., e-psyche.

—BLDSC (3829.765350), CASDDS, CISTI, EMDOCS, GNLM, IDS, ingenta, KNAW. **CCC.**

Published by: (European College of Neuropsychopharmacology), Elsevier Science BV, PO Box 211, Amsterdam 1000 AE, Netherlands. TEL 31-20-485-2911, FAX 31-20-485-2457, http://www.elsevier.com/locate/euroneuro. Eds. J M van Ree, S A Montgomery. **Subscr. in Australasia and the Far East to:** Elsevier Science (Singapore) Pte Ltd, No.1 Temasek Ave, 17-01 Millenia Tower, Singapore 039192, Singapore. TEL 65-434-3727, FAX 65-337-2230; **Subscr. in Japan to:** Elsevier Science Inc - Japan Regional Office, 9-15 Higashi-Azabu 1-chome, Minato-ku, Tokyo 106-0044, Japan. TEL 81-3-5561-5033; **Subscr. in the Americas to:** Elsevier Science, PO Box 945, New York, NY 10159-0945. TEL 212-633-3730, FAX 212-633-3680, usinfo-f@elsevier.com.

616.8 FRA
CODEN: EUPSED

EUROPEAN PSYCHIATRY. Text in English. 1986. 8/yr. EUR 218 in Europe to individuals; USD 291 elsewhere to individuals; EUR 427 in Europe to institutions; EUR 537 elsewhere to institutions (effective 2002). adv. bk.rev. back issues avail. *Refereed.* **Document type:** *Academic/Scholarly.* **Description:** Presents original research in psychopathology, nosography, chemotherapy, psychotherapy, clinical methodology, biological disorders and mental pathology, psychophysiology, neuropsychology, and animal behavior.

Formerly: Psychiatry and Psychobiology (0767-399X)

Related titles: Microform ed.: (from PQC); Online - full text ed.: (from ingenta, ScienceDirect); ♦ Spanish Translation: European Psychiatry (Edicion Espanola). ISSN 1134-0665.

Indexed: ASCA, AgeLine, Biol.Abstr., Curr.Cont., Excerp.Med., Fam.Ind., Ind.Med. (coverage dropped), Inpharma, Pharm.&Out.News, PsycInfo, Psychol.Abstr. (1986-), Reac., SSCI, e-psyche.

—BLDSC (3829.842700), CINDOC, EMDOCS, GNLM, IDS, Infotrieve, ingenta, KNAW. **CCC.**

Published by: (Association of European Psychiatrists), Elsevier Paris, Editions Scientifiques et Medicales (Subsidiary of: Reed Elsevier plc. group), 23 rue Linois, Paris 75015, France. TEL 33-1-45589110, FAX 33-1-45589419, academic@elsevier-fr.com, http://www.aep.lu/. Ed. P Boyer. Circ: 3,000.

M

616.8 ESP ISSN 1134-0665
EUROPEAN PSYCHIATRY (EDICION ESPANOLA). Text in Spanish. 1994. bi-m. **Document type:** *Academic/Scholarly.* **Description:** Covers various clinical and research topics in psychiatry and psychiatric medicine.
Related titles: ♦ Translation of: European Psychiatry.
Indexed: e-psyche.
Published by: (Asociacion Europea de Psiquiatria FRA), Saned S.A., Capitan Haya, 60, Madrid 28020, Spain. TEL 34-91-749-9506, FAX 34-91-749-9507, saned@meditex.es. Ed. Dr. Carlos Ballus. adv.: page ESP 225,000. Circ: 3,000.

EUROPEAN SPINE JOURNAL. see *MEDICAL SCIENCES—Surgery*

616.8 150 GBR ISSN 1362-0347
EVIDENCE - BASED MENTAL HEALTH. Text in English. 1997. q. GBP 71, USD 100 combined subscription to individuals includes print & online eds.; GBP 149, USD 209 to institutions for print only (effective 2002). adv. back issues avail. **Document type:** *Academic/Scholarly.* **Description:** Keeps clinicians up to date by using scientific criteria to select and abstract the most reliable and important clinically relevant papers from an expanded range of journals.
Related titles: Online - full text ed.: GBP 53, USD 74 (effective 2002) (from HighWire Pr.).
Indexed: e-psyche.
Published by: B M J Publishing Group, B M A House, Tavistock Sq, London WC1H 9JR, United Kingdom. TEL 44-20-7387-4499, FAX 44-20-7383-6400, http://www.ebmentalhealth.com, http://www.evidbasedmentalhealth.com, http://www.bma.org.uk. Eds. D Streiner, J Geddes, S Reynolds. Adv. contact Steve McAuley.

616.89 FRA ISSN 0014-3855
CODEN: EVPSAG
L'EVOLUTION PSYCHIATRIQUE. Text in French. 1925. q. EUR 141 in Europe to individuals; USD 175 elsewhere to individuals; EUR 172 in Europe to institutions; USD 210 elsewhere to institutions (effective 2002). adv. bibl. *Refereed.* **Document type:** *Academic/Scholarly.* **Description:** Exposes psychiatry to the varopis currents om scientific and philosophical thought, and in clinical research and critical reflection, as they develop both in this field and in related areas.
Related titles: Online - full text ed.: (from ingenta, Institute for Scientific Information).
Indexed: ASCA, Biol.Abstr., Curr.Cont., Excerp.Med., Ind.Med. (coverage dropped), Lang.& Lang.Behav.Abstr., PsycInfo, Psychol.Abstr. (1929-), SSCI, e-psyche.
—BLDSC (3834.320000), CISTI, EMDOCS, GNLM, IDS, Infotrieve. **CCC.**
Published by: (Association Francaise d'Etudes et de Recherches Psychiatriques), Elsevier Paris, Editions Scientifiques et Medicales (Subsidiary of: Reed Elsevier plc. group), 23 rue Linois, Paris 75015, France. TEL 33-1-45589110, FAX 33-1-45589419, evolpsy@elsevier.fr; academic@elsevier-fr.com, http://www.elsevier.com/locate/evopsy. Ed. Yves Thoret. Pub. Jacques Postel.

EXCERPTA MEDICA. SECTION 32: PSYCHIATRY. see *MEDICAL SCIENCES—Abstracting, Bibliographies, Statistics*

EXCERPTA MEDICA. SECTION 8: NEUROLOGY AND NEUROSURGERY. see *MEDICAL SCIENCES—Abstracting, Bibliographies, Statistics*

616.8 AUT ISSN 1024-7033
EXISTENZANALYSE. Text in German. 1984. q. ATS 280 (effective 2000). bk.rev. **Document type:** *Academic/Scholarly.*
Formerly: Gesellschaft fuer Logotherapie und Existenzanalyse. Bulletin (0258-5383)
Indexed: e-psyche.
Published by: Gesellschaft fuer Logotherapie und Existenzanalyse, Ed.-Suess-Gasse 10, Vienna, W 1150, Austria. TEL 43-1-9859566, FAX 43-1-9824845, gle@existenzanalyse.org, http://www.existenzanalyse.org. Ed. Silvia Laengle. Circ: 1,850 (controlled).

616.8 DEU ISSN 0014-4819
QP376 CODEN: EXBRAP
EXPERIMENTAL BRAIN RESEARCH. Text in English. 1966. s-m. EUR 4,851 domestic; EUR 4,772.90 in Germany; EUR 235 newsstand/cover foreign (effective 2002). adv. bibl, charts, illus. index. back issues avail.; reprint service avail. from ISI. *Refereed.* **Document type:** *Journal, Academic/Scholarly.* **Description:** Takes an interdisciplinary approach to the study of the central and peripheral nervous systems. Covers the fields of morphology, physiology, behavior, neurochemistry, developmental neurobiology, and experimental pathology relevant to general problems of brain function.
Related titles: Microform ed.: (from PQC); Online - full text ed.: ISSN 1432-1106 (from EBSCO Publishing, RoweCom Information Quest, Swets Blackwell, Springer LINK, Institute for Scientific Information); ♦ Supplement: Experimental Brain Research Series. ISSN 0932-4011.
Indexed: ASCA, Abstr.Anthropol., Apic.Abstr., Aqua.Sci.& Fish.Abstr., Bibl.Dev.Med.& Child Neur., Biol.Abstr., Biotech.& Bioeng.Abstr., Chem.Abstr., Chem.Indus.Notes, Chem.Titles, Chemorec.Abstr., Curr.Adv.Ecol.Sci., Curr.Cont., Dairy Sci.Abstr., Dent.Ind., Excerp.Med., INIS Atomind., Ind.Med. (1966-), Ind.Sci.Rev., Inpharma, Int.Abstr.Biol.Sci., Neurosci.Abstr., Neurosci.Cit.Ind., Nutr.Abstr., Pharm.&Out.News, Psychol.Abstr., Reac., SSCI (coverage dropped), Sci.Cit.Ind., Sport Fish.Abstr., THA, Wild.Rev., Zoo.Rec., e-psyche.
—BLDSC (3838.800000), ADONIS, CASDDS, CISTI, GNLM, IDS, ingenta, Linda Hall. **CCC.**
Published by: Springer-Verlag (Subsidiary of: BertelsmannSpringer), Tiergartenstr 17, Heidelberg 69121, Germany. TEL 49-6221-345-0, FAX 49-6221-345229, subscriptions@springer.de, http://link.springer.de/link/service/journals/00221/index.htm, http://www.springer.de. Eds. R F Schmidt, V J Wilson. **Subscr. in N. America to:** Springer-Verlag New York Inc., PO Box 2485, Secaucus, NJ 07096-2485. TEL 212-460-1500, FAX 212-473-6272.

616.8 DEU ISSN 0932-4011
EXPERIMENTAL BRAIN RESEARCH SERIES. Text in English. 1986. irreg.
Related titles: ♦ Supplement to: Experimental Brain Research. ISSN 0014-4819.
Published by: Springer-Verlag (Subsidiary of: BertelsmannSpringer), Haber Str 7, Heidelberg 69126, Germany. TEL 49-30-28787-0. Ed. Dr. Beate Fruhstorfer.

616.8 USA ISSN 0172-9039
CODEN: EBRSDP
EXPERIMENTAL BRAIN RESEARCH. SUPPLEMENTA. Text in English. 1976. irreg., latest vol.18, 1989. price varies. reprint service avail. from ISI. **Document type:** *Academic/Scholarly.*
Indexed: Chem.Abstr., Ind.Sci.Rev., e-psyche.
—CASDDS, CISTI, Linda Hall.
Published by: Springer-Verlag, Journals (Subsidiary of: BertelsmannSpringer), 175 Fifth Ave, New York, NY 10010. TEL 212-460-1500, FAX 212-473-6272.

616.8 USA ISSN 0014-4886
CODEN: NEURFN
EXPERIMENTAL NEUROLOGY; a journal of neuroscience research. Text in English. 1959. m. USD 2,100 in US & Canada to institutions; USD 2,355 elsewhere to institutions (effective 2001). index. back issues avail.; reprint service avail. from SWZ. *Refereed.* **Document type:** *Academic/Scholarly.* **Description:** Publishes the results and conclusions of original research in neuroscience with emphasis on novel findings in neural development, regeneration, plasticity, and transplantation.
Incorporates (1992-1997): Neurodegeneration (1055-8330)
Related titles: Online - full text ed.: ISSN 1090-2430 (from EBSCO Publishing, O C L C Online Computer Library Center, Inc., RoweCom Information Quest, ingenta, Swets Blackwell, IDEAL Online Library, Institute for Scientific Information).
Indexed: ASCA, Aqua.Sci.& Fish.Abstr., Bibl.Dev.Med.& Child Neur., Biol.Abstr., Chem.Abstr., Chem.Indus.Notes, Chem.Titles, Curr.Adv.Biochem., Curr.Adv.Cell & Devel.Biol., Curr.Adv.Ecol.Sci., Curr.Cont., Curr.Ref.Fish Res., Dairy Sci.Abstr., Dent.Ind., Excerp.Med., Helminthol.Abstr., INIS Atomind., Ind.Med. (1959-), Ind.Sci.Rev., Inpharma, Int.Abstr.Biol.Sci., Int.Aerosp.Abstr., Neurosci.Abstr. (coverage dropped), Neurosci.Cit.Ind., Nutr.Abstr., Pharm.&Out.News, Psychol.Abstr., Reac., Sci.Cit.Ind., THA, e-psyche.
—BLDSC (3839.850000), ADONIS, CASDDS, CISTI, GNLM, IDS, Infotrieve, ingenta. **CCC.**
Published by: Academic Press, Inc., Journal Division (Subsidiary of: Harcourt Brace & Company), 525 B St, Ste 1900, San Diego, CA 92101-4495. TEL 619-230-1840, FAX 619-699-6800, apsubs@acad.com, http://www.academicpress.com/en. Ed. John R Sladek Jr.

EXPERIMENTELLE UND KLINISCHE HYPNOSE. see *MEDICAL SCIENCES—Hypnosis*

▼ **EXPERT REVIEW OF NEUROTHERAPEUTICS;** a key contribution to decision making in the treatment of neurologic and neuropsychiatric disorders. see *PHARMACY AND PHARMACOLOGY*

616.89 CAN ISSN 0834-129X
EXPRESS (MONTREAL). Text in English, French. 1983. q. CND 25. bk.rev. **Document type:** *Trade.*
Formerly (until 1986): Express de la Montagne (0821-669X)
Indexed: e-psyche.
Published by: Quebec Society for Autism/Societe Quebecoise de l'Autisme, 65 de Castelnau ouest, Montreal, PQ H2R 2W3, Canada. TEL 514-270-7386, FAX 514-270-9261.

616.8 ESP ISSN 0213-7429
FACULTAD DE MEDICINA DE BARCELONA. REVISTA DE PSIQUIATRIA. Key Title: Revista de Psiquiatria de la Facultad de Medicina de Barcelona. Text in Spanish; Summaries in English, Spanish. 1973. bi-m. (7/yr.). ESP 6,400, USD 115 (effective 1999). adv. bk.rev. illus, charts, stat. index. Supplement avail.; back issues avail. **Document type:** *Trade.* **Description:** Original research articles on various topics in psychiatry, medicine and psychology.
Formerly: Facultad de Medicina de Barcelona. Departamento de Psiquiatria. Revista (0210-1793)
Indexed: Excerp.Med., Inpharma, PsycInfo, Psychol.Abstr. (1979-), Reac., e-psyche.
—BLDSC (7870.202000), CINDOC, EMDOCS, GNLM.
Published by: (Facultad de Medicina de Barcelona, Departamento de Psiquiatria y Psicologia Medica del Hospital Clinico y Provincial de Barcelona), Editorial Dips Rocas, Muntaner, 393 pral. 4, Barcelona 08021, Spain. TEL 39-3-2001389, FAX 39-3-2021958, edipsro@intercom.es. Ed. Carlos Ballus Pascual. R&P Alvaro Trevino. Adv. contact Pilar Carreras. color page ESP 107,000; 270 x 205. Circ: 2,000.

FAMILY SUPPORT BULLETIN. see *HANDICAPPED—Physically Impaired*

616.8 USA ISSN 1070-0609
RC488.5
FAMILY SYSTEMS; a journal of natural systems thinking in psychiatry and the sciences. Text in English. 1994. s-a. USD 28 to individuals; USD 40 to institutions (effective 2000). bk.rev. *Refereed.* **Document type:** *Academic/Scholarly.* **Description:** Advances the understanding of human emotional functioning and behavior based on Bowen theory.
Indexed: e-psyche.
Published by: Georgetown Family Center, 4400 MacArthur Blvd, N W, Ste 103, Washington, DC 20007. TEL 202-965-0730, FAX 202-337-6801. Ed. Dr. Michael E Kerr. R&P Ruth Riley Sagar. Circ: 700 (paid).

616.8 USA ISSN 0091-6544
RC488.5.A1 CODEN: FATHD6
FAMILY THERAPY; the journal of the California Graduate School of Family Psychology. Text in English. 1972. 3/yr., latest vol.28, 2001. USD 72 to individuals; USD 81 to institutions (effective 2001). adv. bk.rev. charts, illus. index, cum.index. back issues avail.; reprint service avail. from PQC,PSC,SCH,ISI. **Document type:** *Journal, Academic/Scholarly.*
Related titles: CD-ROM ed.; Microform ed.: (from PQC).
Indexed: ASSIA, Adol.Ment.Hlth.Abstr., ERA, Fam.Ind., IMFL, Ind.Philos., Mid.East: Abstr.& Ind., Mult.Ed.Abstr., PsycInfo, Psychol.Abstr. (1972-), Psycscan D.P., Sage Fam.Stud.Abstr., Sage Urb.Stud.Abstr., Soc.Work Res.& Abstr., Sp.Ed.Needs Abstr., Viol.& Abuse Abstr., e-psyche.
—BLDSC (3865.576350), GNLM, ingenta. **CCC.**
Published by: (California Graduate School of Family Psychology), Libra Publishers, Inc., 3089C Clairemont Dr,, PMB 383, San Diego, CA 92117. TEL 858-571-1414. Ed. Martin Blinder. R&P Jon Kroll. Adv. contact William Kroll. page USD 150. Circ: 1,500.

616.8 FRA ISSN 1623-3883
▼ **FIGURES DE LA PSYCHANALYSE.** Text in French. 2001. s-a. EUR 38.50 domestic; EUR 43 foreign (effective 2001).

M

Published by: Editions Eres, 11 rue des Alouettes, Ramonville Saint-Agne 31520, France. TEL 33-05-61751576, FAX 33-05-61735289, eres@editions-eres.com. Ed. Ignacio Garate-Martinez.

616.89 GBR
FIRST PERSON MAGAZINE. Text in English. 1995. irreg. **Description:** Covers mental health experiences and opinions.
Related titles: Online - full text ed.
Indexed: e-psyche.
Address: 84 Townshend Terr, Richmond, Surrey TW9 1XN, United Kingdom. alex@vulliamy.demon.co.uk, http://www.vulliamt.demon.co.uk. Eds. Alex Vulliamy, Jason Lee.

FOCAL POINT; a national bulletin on family support and children's mental health. see *HANDICAPPED*

616.8982 USA ISSN 1088-3576
RJ506.A9 CODEN: FAODF5
FOCUS ON AUTISM AND OTHER DEVELOPMENTAL DISABILITIES. Text in English. 1986. q. USD 43 in North America to individuals; USD 71 elsewhere to individuals; USD 109 in North America to institutions; USD 138 elsewhere to institutions (effective 2002). adv. bk.rev. bibl. 64 p./no. back issues avail.; reprints avail. *Refereed.* **Document type:** *Journal, Academic/Scholarly.* **Description:** Publishes practitioner-oriented articles for professionals involved in the education and treatment of children and youth with autism and pervasive developmental disorders.
Formerly (until vol.11, 1996): Focus on Autistic Behavior (0887-1566)
Related titles: Microfilm ed.: (from PQC); Online - full text ed.: (from CatchWord Ltd.).
Indexed: C.I.J.E., Except.Child Educ.Abstr., IBZ, Lang.& Lang.Behav.Abstr., PsycInfo, Psychol.Abstr. (1988-), SOPODA, Sociol.Abstr., e-psyche.
—BLDSC (3964.203810), GNLM, ingenta. **CCC.**
Published by: Pro-Ed Inc., 8700 Shoal Creek Blvd, Austin, TX 78757-6897. TEL 512-451-3246, FAX 512-302-9129, proed1@aol.com, http://www.autism-society.org. Eds. John Kregel, Richard Simpson. Pub. Donald D Hammill. Adv. contact Allison Turrell. page USD 400. Circ: 3,000 (paid and free).

616.891 360 NOR ISSN 0332-5415
FOKUS PAA FAMILIEN; tidsskrift for familiebehandling. Text in Danish, Norwegian, Swedish; Summaries in English. 1972. q. NOK 340 to individuals; NOK 540, USD 95 to institutions; NOK 215 to students; NOK 150, USD 26 per issue (effective 2001). **Document type:** *Academic/Scholarly, Trade.* **Description:** Covers a wide range of topics, both theoretical and practical, in family therapy and related fields including family sociology, family education and family politics.
Indexed: IBR, IBZ, Ind.Philos., e-psyche.
—CCC.
Published by: Scandinavian University Press (Subsidiary of: Taylor & Francis Ltd.), Postboks 2959, Toeyen, Oslo 0608, Norway. FAX 47-22-57-53-53, www.universitetsforlaget.no/tidsskrifter. Eds. Astri Johnsen, Geir Lundby. Circ: 2,200.

616.8 POL
CODEN: NUPOBT
FOLIA NEUROPATHOLOGICA. Text in English; Summaries in English, Polish. 1963. q. PLZ 60; USD 120 foreign (effective 1999). bk.rev. bibl. illus. index, cum.index. back issues avail. *Refereed.* **Document type:** *Newspaper, Proceedings.* **Description:** Publishes papers devoted to achievements in experimental and clinical neuropathology.
Formerly (until vol.32, 1994): Neuropatologia Polska (0028-3894)
Related titles: E-mail ed.; Online - full text ed.: (from Institute for Scientific Information).
Indexed: ASCA, Aqua.Sci.& Fish.Abstr., Biol.Abstr., Chem.Abstr., Chem.Indus.Notes, Chem.Titles, Excerp.Med., INIS Atomind., Ind.Med. (coverage dropped), Neurosci.Cit.Ind., e-psyche.
—BLDSC (3971.636000), CASDDS, GNLM, IDS, KNAW.
Published by: Polish Association of Neuropathologists, Ul Pawinskiego 5, Warsaw 02106, Poland. TEL 48-22-6086505, FAX 48-22-6086581, radwanska@cmdik.pan.pl. Ed. Maria Dambska. **Dist. by:** Severus Publishing House, Ul Conrada 4-146, Warsaw 01922, Poland. TEL 48-22-6697401.

FOLIA PHONIATRICA ET LOGOPAEDICA; international journal of phoniatrics, speech therapy and communication pathology. see *MEDICAL SCIENCES—Otorhinolaryngology*

616.8 GBR
FORENSIC FOCUS. Text in English. irreg., latest vol.19, 2001. **Document type:** *Monographic series, Academic/Scholarly.*
Indexed: e-psyche.
—BLDSC (3987.726600).
Published by: Jessica Kingsley Publishers, 116 Pentonville Rd, London N1 9JB, United Kingdom. TEL 44-20-7883-2307, FAX 44-20-7837-2917, post@jkp.com, http://www.jkp.com. Ed. Gwen Adshead.

616.89 158 DEU ISSN 0945-2540
FORENSISCHE PSYCHIATRIE UND PSYCHOTHERAPIE. Text in English, German; Summaries in English, French, German. 1994. s-a. EUR 20, USD 30 (effective 2001). adv. bk.rev. *Refereed.* **Document type:** *Journal, Academic/Scholarly.*
Indexed: e-psyche.
—GNLM.
Published by: Pabst Science Publishers, Am Eichengrund 28, Lengerich 49525, Germany. TEL 49-5484-308, FAX 49-5484-550, pabst.publishers@t-online.de, http://www.pabst-publishers.de. Ed. Heinfried Duncker. Circ: 1,200.

616.8 DEU
FORTSCHRITTE DER NEUROLOGIE, PSYCHIATRIE. Text in German; Summaries in English, German. 1931. m. EUR 216.40 domestic to institutions; EUR 227.20 in Europe to institutions; EUR 247.80 elsewhere to institutions; EUR 21 newsstand/cover (effective 2002). adv. bk.rev. bibl, charts, illus, stat. index. Supplement avail.; back issues avail.; reprint service avail. from PQC. *Refereed.* **Document type:** *Journal, Academic/Scholarly.*
Former titles: Fortschritte der Neurologie, Psychiatrie und ihrer Grenzgebiete; Fortschritte der Neurologie - Psychiatrie (0720-4299); (until 1980): Fortschritte der Neurologie, Psychiatrie und Ihrer Grenzgebiete (0015-8194)
Related titles: Online - full text ed.: ISSN 1439-3522 (from Institute for Scientific Information).
Indexed: ASCA, Biol.Abstr., Chem.Abstr., Curr.Cont., Excerp.Med., Ger.J.Psych., INIS Atomind., Ind.Med. (1981-), Ind.Sci.Rev., Inpharma, Neurosci.Cit.Ind., Pharm.&Out.News, PsycInfo, Psychol.Abstr. (1972-), Reac., SSCI (coverage dropped), Sci.Cit.Ind., e-psyche.
—BLDSC (4022.380000), CISTI, EMDOCS, GNLM, IDS, Infotrieve, KNAW. **CCC.**
Published by: (Victor von Weizsaecker Gesellschaft), Georg Thieme Verlag, Ruedigerstr 14, Stuttgart 70469, Germany. TEL 49-711-8931-0, FAX 49-711-8931298, kunden.service@thieme.de, http://www.thieme.de/fdn. Ed. U H Peters. R&P Peter Eich. adv.: page DEM 3,200; 175 x 250. Circ: 4,300.

617.48 NLD ISSN 0922-4386
FOUNDATIONS OF NEUROLOGICAL SURGERY. Text in English. 1988. irreg. price varies. *Refereed.* **Document type:** *Monographic series.*
Indexed: e-psyche.
—KNAW.
Published by: Kluwer Academic Publishers Group (Subsidiary of: Wolters Kluwer N.V.), Spuiboulevard 50, PO Box 17, Dordrecht 3300 AA, Netherlands. FAX 31-78-639-2254, services@wkap.nl, http://www.wkap.nl. **Dist. by:** Journals Department, PO Box 322, Dordrecht 3300 AH, Netherlands. FAX 31-78-654-6474.

616.89 NLD ISSN 0924-8935
FOUNDATIONS OF NEUROLOGY. Text in English. 1990. irreg. price varies. *Refereed.* **Document type:** *Monographic series.*
Indexed: e-psyche.
—KNAW.
Published by: Kluwer Academic Publishers Group (Subsidiary of: Wolters Kluwer N.V.), Spuiboulevard 50, PO Box 17, Dordrecht 3300 AA, Netherlands. FAX 31-78-639-2254, services@wkap.nl, http://www.wkap.nl. **Dist. by:** Journals Department, PO Box 322, Dordrecht 3300 AH, Netherlands. FAX 31-78-654-6474.

616.89 NLD ISSN 0924-0179
FOUNDATIONS OF NEUROPSYCHOLOGY. Text in English. 1989. irreg. price varies. *Refereed.* **Document type:** *Monographic series.*
Indexed: e-psyche.
—CISTI.
Published by: Kluwer Academic Publishers Group (Subsidiary of: Wolters Kluwer N.V.), Spuiboulevard 50, PO Box 17, Dordrecht 3300 AA, Netherlands. FAX 31-78-639-2254, services@wkap.nl, http://www.wkap.nl. **Dist. by:** Journals Department, PO Box 322, Dordrecht 3300 AH, Netherlands. FAX 31-78-654-6474.

612.8 GBR ISSN 1353-6508
CODEN: FNEUES
FRONTIERS IN NEUROBIOLOGY. Text in English. 1994. irreg. GBP 65, USD 110.50 (effective 2002). *Refereed.* **Document type:** *Monographic series.*
Indexed: Chem.Abstr., Chem.Indus.Notes, Chem.Titles, Int.Abstr.Biol.Sci., e-psyche.
—BLDSC (4042.039500), CASDDS, CISTI, Infotrieve. **CCC.**
Published by: Portland Press Ltd., 59 Portland Pl, London W1N 3AJ, United Kingdom. TEL 44-20-7580-5530, FAX 44-20-7323-1136, sales@portland-service.com, http://www.portlandpress.com/bst/default.htm. Ed. A J Turner. R&P Adam Marshall. **Subscr. to:** Commerce Way, Colchester, Essex CO2 8HP, United Kingdom. TEL 44-1206-796351, FAX 44-1206-799331.

616.8 ITA ISSN 0393-5264
FUNCTIONAL NEUROLOGY; new trends in adaptive and behavioral disorders. Text in English. 1985. q. ITL 90,000, USD 90 (effective 2001). adv. bk.rev. back issues avail. *Refereed.* **Description:** Publishes scientific contributions dealing with all aspects of functional neurology. Focuses on the interaction of the nervous system with the environment, including neurochemistry, physiology and more.
Related titles: Online - full text ed.: (from Institute for Scientific Information).
Indexed: AMED, ASCA, Excerp.Med., Ind.Med. (1986-), Int.Abstr.Biol.Sci., Neurosci.Cit.Ind., PsycInfo, Ref.Zh., SSCI (coverage dropped), e-psyche.
—BLDSC (4055.619500), CISTI, EMDOCS, GNLM, IDS, ingenta, KNAW. **CCC.**
Published by: C I C Edizioni Internazionali s.r.l., Corso Trieste 42, Rome, RM 00198, Italy. TEL 39-06-8412673, FAX 39-06-8412688, info@gruppocic.it, 1160199510. Ed. Giuseppe Nappi. adv.: B&W page XEU 1,239.5, color page XEU 1,549.37; 210 x 270.

616.8 DEU ISSN 0931-0428
FUNDAMENTA PSYCHIATRICA; Psychiatrie und Psychotherapie in Theorie und Praxis. Text in German. 1987. 4/yr. DEM 210 to individuals; DEM 260 to institutions; DEM 100 to students (effective 2001). adv. index. **Document type:** *Journal, Academic/Scholarly.*
Indexed: P C I, e-psyche.
—GNLM, Infotrieve. **CCC.**
Published by: Schattauer GmbH, Hoelderlinstr 3, Stuttgart 70174, Germany. TEL 49-711-22987-0, FAX 49-711-2298750, info@schattauer.de, http://www.schattauer.com. Eds. A Barocka, P Joraschky. R&P Annika Schmidt TEL 49-711-2298713. Adv. contact Maria Wagner TEL 49-711-2298767. B&W page XEU 1,147.34, color page XEU 2,112.15; 183 x 227. Circ: 2,000. **Subscr. to:** CSJ, Postfach 140220, Munich 80452, Germany. TEL 49-89-20959129, schattauer@csj.de.

616.8 ISL ISSN 1022-4920
GEDVERND; arsrit Gedverndarfelags Islands. Text in Icelandic. 1966. a. ISK 500 to members (effective 1999). adv. bk.rev. *Refereed.* **Document type:** *Academic/Scholarly.*
Indexed: e-psyche.
Published by: Gedverndarfelag Islands, Hatuni 10, Reykjavik 105, Iceland. TEL 354-552-5508. Ed. Eirikur Oern Arnarson.

GENDER & PSYCHOANALYSIS; an interdisciplinary journal. see *PSYCHOLOGY*

616.8 USA ISSN 0163-8343
CODEN: GHPSDB
GENERAL HOSPITAL PSYCHIATRY; psychiatry, medicine and primary care. Text in English. 1979. bi-m. NLG 410, EUR 186.05 in Europe to individuals; JPY 25,700 in Japan to individuals; USD 208 elsewhere to individuals; NLG 1,083, EUR 491.44 in Europe to institutions; JPY 68,100 in Japan to institutions; USD 550 elsewhere to institutions (effective 2001). back issues avail. *Refereed.* **Document type:** *Academic/Scholarly.* **Description:** Emphasizes a biopsychosocial approach to illness and health, and provides a forum for communication among professionals with clinical, academic, and research interests in psychiatry.
Related titles: Microform ed.: (from PQC); Online - full text ed.: (from ingenta, Swets Blackwell, ScienceDirect, Institute for Scientific Information).
Indexed: ASCA, Abstr.Health Care Manage.Stud., AgeLine, Behav.Med.Abstr., Biol.Abstr., CINAHL, Curr.Cont., Excerp.Med., Fam.Ind., INIS Atomind., Ind.Med. (1979-), Ind.Sci.Rev., Indian Psychol.Abstr., Inpharma, Int.Nurs.Ind., Jrnl.Watch Psych., Pharm.&Out.News, PsycInfo, Psychol.Abstr. (1980-), Reac., SSCI, Sci.Cit.Ind., Soc.Work Res.& Abstr., e-psyche.
—BLDSC (4104.344000), CISTI, GNLM, IDS, ingenta, KNAW. **CCC.**

M

Published by: Elsevier Science, 655 Ave of the Americas, New York, NY 10010. TEL 212-989-5800, FAX 212-633-3990, usinfo-f@elsevier.com, http://www.elsevier.com/locate/genhospsych. Ed. Dr. Don R Lipsitt. **Subscr. in Australasia and the Far East to:** Elsevier Science (Singapore) Pte Ltd, No.1 Temasek Ave, 17-01 Millenia Tower, Singapore 039192, Singapore. TEL 65-434-3727, FAX 65-337-2230; **Subscr. in Japan to:** Elsevier Science Inc - Japan Regional Office, 9-15 Higashi-Azabu 1-chome, Minato-ku, Tokyo 106-0044, Japan. TEL 81-3-5561-5033; **Subscr. outside the Americas to:** Elsevier Science BV, PO Box 211, Amsterdam 1000 AE, Netherlands. TEL 31-20-485-3757, FAX 31-20-485-3432.

616.8 USA

GENERATIONS (WAYZATA). Text in English. 1957. q., latest vol.29. USD 25; USD 30 foreign. bk.rev. 48 p./no. back issues avail. **Document type:** *Newsletter.* **Description:** Covers meetings, current research, events and activities and other Foundation news relating to hereditary ataxias.

Indexed: Curr.Cont. (coverage dropped), Hlth.Ind., e-psyche.

Published by: National Ataxia Foundation, 2600 Fernbrook Ln., N., Ste. 119, Plymouth, MN 55447-4752. TEL 763-553-0020, FAX 763-553-0167, naf@mr.net, http://www.ataxia.org. Ed. Donna Gruetzmacher. Circ: 10,000 (controlled).

▼ **GENES, BRAIN AND BEHAVIOR.** see *BIOLOGY—Genetics*

616.89 DEU ISSN 1433-1055

GERMAN JOURNAL OF PSYCHIATRY. Text in German. 1998. irreg. back issues avail. *Refereed.* **Document type:** *Academic/Scholarly.* **Description:** Covers all fields of psychiatry.

Media: Online - full text.

Published by: University of Goettingen, Department of Psychiatry, Von-Siebold-Str 5, Goettingen 37075, Germany. TEL 49-551-392004, bbandel@gwdg.de, http://www.gwdg.de/~bbandel. Ed. Borwin Bandelow.

616.8 AUT ISSN 0258-5391

GESELLSCHAFT FUER LOGOTHERAPIE UND EXISTENZANALYSE. TAGUNGSBERICHTE. Text in German. 1985. a. ATS 140 (effective 2000). adv. back issues avail. **Document type:** *Proceedings, Academic/Scholarly.*

Indexed: e-psyche.

Published by: Gesellschaft fuer Logotherapie und Existenzanalyse, Ed.-Suess-Gasse 10, Vienna, W 1150, Austria. TEL 43-1-9859566, FAX 43-1-9824845, gle@existenzanalyse.org, http:// www.existenzanalyse.org. Circ: 2,000 (controlled).

GESTALT JOURNAL. see *PSYCHOLOGY*

GESTALT REVIEW. see *PSYCHOLOGY*

616 ITA ISSN 0391-9048

GIORNALE DI NEUROPSICOFARMACOLOGIA. Text in Italian; Summaries in Italian, English. 1979. bi-m. ITL 90,000, USD 80 (effective 2000). adv. *Refereed.*

Related titles: Online - full text ed.: (from Institute for Scientific Information).

Indexed: ASCA, Focus on: Psychophar., Neurosci.Cit.Ind., PsycInfo, Psychol.Abstr. (1989-), Ref.Zh., SSCI (coverage dropped), e-psyche.

—BLDSC (4178.475000), GNLM, IDS, Infotrieve. **CCC.**

Published by: C I C Edizioni Internazionali s.r.l., Corso Trieste 42, Rome, RM 00198, Italy. TEL 39-06-8412673, FAX 39-06-8412688, info@gruppocic.it, 1160199510. Ed. C Fieschi. Pub. A Salvati. adv.: B&W page XEU 1,626.84, color page XEU 2,065.53; 210 x 290.

616.8 ITA

GIORNALE ITALIANO DI PSICOPATOLOGIA. Text in Italian. 1995. 3/yr. ITL 100,000; USD 90 foreign.

Indexed: e-psyche.

Published by: Pacini Editore, Via Alessandro Gherardesca, 1, Ospedaletto, PI 56121, Italy. TEL 39-50-982439, FAX 39-50-983906, pacini@cibernet.it, http://www.cibernet.it/ pacini. Eds. Giovanni B Cassano, Paolo Pancheri.

616.8 USA ISSN 0894-1491
QP363.2 CODEN: GLIAEJ

GLIA. Text in English. 1988. m. USD 2,165 in United States; USD 2,305 in Canada & Mexico; USD 2,424 elsewhere; USD 2,274 combined subscription in United States for print and online eds.; USD 2,414 combined subscription in Canada & Mexico for print and online eds.; USD 2,533 combined subscription elsewhere for print and online eds. (effective 2002). adv. back issues avail. *Refereed.* **Document type:** *Academic/Scholarly.* **Description:** Devoted to the study of the form and function of neuroglial cells in health and disease.

Related titles: Microform ed.: (from PQC); Online - full text ed.: ISSN 1098-1136. USD 2,165 in United States; USD 2,165 in Canada & Mexico; USD 2,165 elsewhere (effective 2002) (from EBSCO Publishing, Wiley InterScience, Institute for Scientific Information).

Indexed: ASCA, Aqua.Sci.& Fish.Abstr., Curr.Cont., INIS Atomind., Ind.Med. (1988-), Ind.Sci.Rev., Inpharma, Int.Abstr.Biol.Sci., Neurosci.Abstr., Neurosci.Cit.Ind., Protozool.Abstr., Reac., Ref.Zh., Sci.Cit.Ind., e-psyche.

—BLDSC (4195.208000), CISTI, EMDOCS, GNLM, IDS, ingenta, KNAW. **CCC.**

Published by: John Wiley & Sons, Inc., Journals (Subsidiary of: Wiley InterScience), 605 Third Ave, New York, NY 10158. TEL 212-850-6645, FAX 212-850-6021, subinfo@wiley.com, uscs-wis@wiley.com, http://www.wiley.com. Eds. Bruce R Ransom, Helmut Hettenmann. adv.: B&W page GBP 640, color page GBP 1,515; trim 210 x 279. Circ: 700. **Subscr. outside the Americas to:** John Wiley & Sons Ltd., Baffins Ln, Chichester, Sussex PO19 IUD, United Kingdom. TEL 44-1243-779777, FAX 44-1243-843232, cs-journals@wiley.co.uk, http://www.wiley.co.uk.

GRUPPENANALYSE; Zeitschrift fuer gruppenanalytische Psychotherapie, Beratung und Supervision. see *PSYCHOLOGY*

616.89 DEU ISSN 0017-4947

GRUPPENPSYCHOTHERAPIE UND GRUPPENDYNAMIK. Text in German; Summaries in English, German. 1968. irreg. (4 nos./vol.). DEM 136; DEM 106 to students (effective 2000). *Refereed.* **Document type:** *Monographic series, Academic/Scholarly.*

Related titles: Online - full text ed.: (from Institute for Scientific Information).

Indexed: ASCA, Curr.Cont., Excerp.Med., Ger.J.Psych., IBZ, Ind.Philos., SSCI, e-psyche.

—GNLM, IDS. **CCC.**

Published by: Vandenhoeck und Ruprecht, Robert-Bosch-Breite 6, Goettingen 37079, Germany. TEL 49-551-6959-26, FAX 49-551-695917. Ed. Dr. Annelise Heigl Evers. Circ: 1,050.

616.8 CHN

GUOWAI YIXUE (NAOXIEGUAN JIBING)/FOREIGN MEDICAL SCIENCES (CEREBROVASCULAR DISEASES). Text in Chinese. bi-m. USD 21.60; USD 3.60 newsstand/cover (effective 2001). **Document type:** *Academic/Scholarly.*

Published by: China International Book Trading Corp/Zhongguo Guoji Tushu Maoyi Zonggongsi cibtc@mail.cibtc.com.cn, http://www.cibtc.com.cn. **Dist. by:** 35, Chegongzhuang Xilu, Haidian District, Beijing 100044, China.

616.891 JPN ISSN 0916-3662

HAKONIWA RYOHOGAKU KENKYU/ARCHIVES OF SANDPLAY THERAPY. Text in English, Japanese; Summaries in English. 1988. a. JPY 2,300.

Indexed: e-psyche.

Published by: Nihon Hakoniwa Ryoho Gakkai/Japan Association of Sandplay Therapy, Daigaku Kyoikugakubu, Rinsho Shinrigaku Kyoshitsu, Yoshidahon-Machi, Sakyo-ku, Kyoto-shi 606-8317, Japan.

616.8 573.8 USA ISSN 0194-0880
CODEN: HBNEEV

HANDBOOK OF BEHAVIORAL NEUROBIOLOGY. Text in English. 1978. irreg., latest vol.11, 1992. price varies. back issues avail. *Refereed.* **Document type:** *Monographic series.*

Indexed: e-psyche.

—BLDSC (4250.340000), CISTI, Infotrieve. **CCC.**

Published by: Kluwer Academic - Plenum Publishers (Subsidiary of: Wolters Kluwer N.V.), 233 Spring St, New York, NY 10013-1578. TEL 212-620-8000, 800-221-9369, FAX 212-463-0742, info@plenum.com, http://www.plenum.com. Ed. Norman T Adler.

616.8 540 NLD ISSN 0924-8196

HANDBOOK OF CHEMICAL NEUROANATOMY. Text in English. 1983. irreg., latest vol.18, 2000. price varies. illus. back issues avail. *Refereed.* **Document type:** *Monographic series, Academic/Scholarly, Trade.* **Description:** Offers medical researchers and practitioners invaluable information on the localization and function of putative transmitter substances in the nervous system.

Indexed: Neurosci.Cit.Ind., e-psyche.

—BLDSC (4250.397000).

Published by: Elsevier Science BV, PO Box 211, Amsterdam 1000 AE, Netherlands. TEL 31-20-485-3757, 31-20-485-3911, FAX 31-20-485-3432, 31-20-485-3598, nlinfo-f@elsevier.nl; usinfo-f@elsevier.com; forinfo-kyf04035@niftyserve.or.jp, http://www.elsevier.nl/. Eds. A Bjorklund, T Hokfelt. **Subscr. in Australasia and the Far East to:** Elsevier Science (Singapore) Pte Ltd, No.1 Temasek Ave, 17-01 Millenia Tower, Singapore 039192, Singapore. TEL 65-434-3727, FAX 65-337-2230, asiainfo@elsevier.com.sg; **Subscr. in Japan to:** Elsevier Science Inc - Japan Regional Office, 9-15 Higashi-Azabu 1-chome, Minato-ku, Tokyo 106-0044, Japan. TEL 81-3-5561-5033, FAX 81-3-5561-5047, info@elsevier.co.jp; **Subscr. in the Americas to:** Elsevier Science, PO Box 945, New York, NY 10159-0945. TEL 212-633-3730, 888-437-4636, FAX 212-633-3680, usinfo-f@elsevier.com, http://www.elsevier.com

616.8 NLD ISSN 0072-9752
CODEN: HACNEU

HANDBOOK OF CLINICAL NEUROLOGY; revised series. Text in English. 1969; N.S. 1985. irreg., latest vol.75, 1999. price varies. cum index: vols1-43 in vol 44, 1982. back issues avail. *Refereed.* **Document type:** *Monographic series, Academic/Scholarly, Trade.* **Description:** Provides a comprehensive reverence for understanding and treating neurologic disorders, research, and trends.

Indexed: e-psyche.

—BLDSC (4250.405000), CISTI. **CCC.**

Published by: Elsevier Science BV, PO Box 211, Amsterdam 1000 AE, Netherlands. TEL 31-20-485-3757, 31-20-485-3911, FAX 31-20-485-3432, 31-20-485-3598, nlinfo-f@elsevier.nl; usinfo-f@elsevier.com; forinfo-kyf04035@niftyserve.or.jp, http://www.elsevier.nl/. Eds. G W Bruyn, P J Vinken. **Subscr. in Australasia and the Far East to:** Elsevier Science (Singapore) Pte Ltd, No.1 Temasek Ave, 17-01 Millenia Tower, Singapore 039192, Singapore. TEL 65-434-3727, FAX 65-337-2230, asiainfo@elsevier.com.sg; **Subscr. in Japan to:** Elsevier Science Inc - Japan Regional Office, 9-15 Higashi-Azabu 1-chome, Minato-ku, Tokyo 106-0044, Japan. TEL 81-3-5561-5033, FAX 81-3-5561-5047, info@elsevier.co.jp; **Subscr. in the Americas to:** Elsevier Science, PO Box 945, New York, NY 10159-0945. TEL 212-633-3730, 888-437-4636, FAX 212-633-3680, usinfo-f@elsevier.com, http://www.elsevier.com

616.8 NLD ISSN 0304-4645

HANDBOOK OF ELECTROENCEPHALOGRAPHY AND CLINICAL NEUROPHYSIOLOGY; revised series. Text in English. 1971; N.S. 1987. irreg., latest vol.6, 1999. price varies. back issues avail. *Refereed.* **Document type:** *Monographic series, Academic/Scholarly.* **Description:** Discusses the use of electroencephalography in clinical neurophysiology settings.

Indexed: e-psyche.

Published by: Elsevier Science BV, PO Box 211, Amsterdam 1000 AE, Netherlands. TEL 31-20-485-3757, 31-20-485-3911, FAX 31-20-485-3432, 31-20-485-3598, nlinfo-f@elsevier.nl; usinfo-f@elsevier.com; forinfo-kyf04035@niftyserve.or.jp, http://www.elsevier.nl/. Ed. A Remond. **Subscr. in Australasia and the Far East to:** Elsevier Science (Singapore) Pte Ltd, No.1 Temasek Ave, 17-01 Millenia Tower, Singapore 039192, Singapore. TEL 65-434-3727, FAX 65-337-2230, asiainfo@elsevier.com.sg; **Subscr. in Japan to:** Elsevier Science Inc - Japan Regional Office, 9-15 Higashi-Azabu 1-chome, Minato-ku, Tokyo 106-0044, Japan. TEL 81-3-5561-5033, FAX 81-3-5561-5047, info@elsevier.co.jp; **Subscr. in the Americas to:** Elsevier Science, PO Box 945, New York, NY 10159-0945. TEL 212-633-3730, 888-437-4636, FAX 212-633-3680, usinfo-f@elsevier.com, http://www.elsevier.com

616.8 NLD
HANDBOOK OF NEUROPSYCHOLOGY. Text in English. 1988. irreg., latest vol.11, 1997. price varies. back issues avail. *Refereed.* **Document type:** *Monographic series, Academic/Scholarly, Trade.* **Description:** Offers a comprehensive reference of both the experimental and clinical aspects of neuropsychology.
Indexed: Neurosci.Cit.Ind., e-psyche.
—BLDSC (4250.945000).
Published by: Elsevier Science BV, PO Box 211, Amsterdam 1000 AE, Netherlands. TEL 31-20-485-3757, 31-20-485-3911, FAX 31-20-485-3432, 31-20-485-3598, nlinfo-f@elsevier.nl; usinfo-f@elsevier.com; forinfo-kyf04035@niftyserve.or.jp, http://www.elsevier.nl/. Eds. F Boller, J Grafman. **Subscr. in Australasia and the Far East to:** Elsevier Science (Singapore) Pte Ltd, No.1 Temasek Ave, 17-01 Millenia Tower, Singapore 039192, Singapore. TEL 65-434-3727, FAX 65-337-2230, asiainfo@elsevier.com.sg; **Subscr. in Japan to:** Elsevier Science Inc - Japan Regional Office, 9-15 Higashi-Azabu 1-chome, Minato-ku, Tokyo 106-0044, Japan. TEL 81-3-5561-5033, FAX 81-3-5561-5047, info@elsevier.co.jp; **Subscr. in the Americas to:** Elsevier Science, PO Box 945, New York, NY 10159-0945. TEL 212-633-3730, 888-437-4636, FAX 212-633-3680, usinfo-f@elsevier.com, http://www.elsevier.com

616.834 SWE ISSN 0348-8071
HANDIKAPP - REFLEX. Text in Swedish. 1954. bi-m. SEK 125. adv. bk.rev. illus, stat. **Description:** Deals with subjects concerned with neurological disease and disability.
Formerly: M S-Brevet (0345-8199)
Related titles: Audio cassette/tape ed.
Indexed: e-psyche.
Published by: Neurologiskt Handikappades Riksfoerbund/Swedish Association of Neurologically Disabled, Fack 3284, Stockholm 10365, Sweden. Ed. Anne Thelander. Circ: 13,500.

616.8 USA
THE HARVARD BRAIN. Variant title: Journal of Neuroscience. Text in English. 1994. a. USD 15 (effective 1998). back issues avail. **Description:** Includes interdisciplinary articles on neurosciences.
Related titles: Online - full text ed.
Indexed: e-psyche.
Published by: Harvard Undergraduate Society for Neuroscience, Leverett House Mail Center, PO Box 537, Cambridge, MA 02138-6034. husn@fas.harvard.edu, http://hcs.harvard.edu/~husn/BRAIN/. Ed. Amy Herman.

616.8 USA ISSN 0884-3783
THE HARVARD MENTAL HEALTH LETTER. Text in English. 1984. m. USD 72 domestic; USD 80 in Canada; USD 87 elsewhere (effective 2001). illus. 8 p./no. back issues avail.; reprints avail. **Document type:** *Newsletter, Consumer.* **Description:** Interprets timely mental health information for both professionals and laypeople.
Related titles: Online - full text ed.: (from Gale Group, Northern Light Technology, Inc.).
Indexed: Biol.Dig., CHNI, CINAHL, Consum.Ind. (1989-), e-psyche.
—BLDSC (4268.280000).
Published by: Harvard Health Publications Group (Subsidiary of: Harvard Medical School), 10 Shattuck St., 6th fl., Boston, MA 02115. TEL 617-432-1431, FAX 617-432-1506, hhp@hms.harvard.edu. Ed. Michael Craig Miller. Circ: 75,000 (paid). **Subscr. to:** PO Box 420448, Palm Coast, FL 32142-0448.

616.89 USA ISSN 1067-3229
CODEN: HRPSEP
HARVARD REVIEW OF PSYCHIATRY. Text in English. 1993. bi-m. GBP 80, USD 99 to individuals; GBP 133, USD 175 to institutions (effective 2002). adv. bk.rev. back issues avail.; reprints avail. *Refereed.* **Document type:** *Journal, Academic/Scholarly.* **Description:** Examines a wide variety of subjects, emphasizing the integration of research findings with clinical care. Articles cover the diagnosis and treatment of a full range of psychiatric disorders.
Incorporates (1976-1993): McLean Hospital Journal
Related titles: Online - full text ed.: ISSN 1465-7309. GBP 119, USD 157 to institutions Online only (effective 2002) (from HighWire Pr., EBSCO Publishing, O C L C Online Computer Library Center, Inc., RoweCom Information Quest, ingenta, Swets Blackwell, Institute for Scientific Information).
Indexed: ASCA, AgeLine, Biol.Abstr., Curr.Cont., Excerp.Med., Fam.Ind., Ind.Med. (1993-), Inpharma, Int.Nurs.Ind., Pharm.&Out.News, PsycInfo, Reac., SSCI, Sci.Cit.Ind. (coverage dropped), e-psyche.
—BLDSC (4270.020000), EMDOCS, GNLM, IDS, KNAW.
Published by: Oxford University Press, Academic Division, Great Clarendon St, Oxford OX2 6DP, United Kingdom. TEL 44-1865-267907, FAX 44-1865-267835, jnlorders@oup-usa.org, jnl.info@oup.co.uk, http://hrp.oupjournals.org/, http://www.oup.co.uk/journals. Ed. Dr. Joseph T Coyle. Pub. Janet Fox. adv.: B&W page GBP 385, B&W page USD 695; trim 178 x 225. Circ: 1,700. **Subscr. outside the Americas to:** Journals Marketing, Great Clarendon St, Oxford OX2 6DP, United Kingdom.

616.857 USA ISSN 0017-8748
RC392 CODEN: HEADAE
HEADACHE; the journal of head and face pain. Text in English. 1961. 10/yr. USD 115 domestic to individuals; USD 130 in Canada & Mexico to individuals; USD 145 overseas to individuals; USD 160 domestic to institutions; USD 175 in Canada & Mexico to institutions; USD 190 overseas to institutions; USD 126 to individuals print & online eds. combined; USD 176 to institutions print & online eds. combined (effective 2001). adv. bk.rev. abstr, charts, illus, stat. cum.index. back issues avail.; reprint service avail. from PQC. *Refereed.* **Document type:** *Journal, Academic/Scholarly.* **Description:** Publishes original manuscripts (clinical studies, case reports, base research), and other scientific materials concerned with the diagnosis and treatment of headache, in its many aspects, and head and face pain.
Related titles: CD-ROM ed.; Diskette ed.; Magnetic Tape ed.; Microform ed.: (from PQC); ♦ Online - full text ed.: Headache Online. ISSN 1526-4610.
Indexed: ASCA, Behav.Med.Abstr., Biol.Abstr., Chem.Abstr., Curr.Adv.Ecol.Sci., Curr.Cont., Curr.Tit.Dent., Dent.Ind., Environ.Sci.Poll.Mgmt., Excerp.Med., INIS Atomind., Ind.Med. (1961-), Ind.Sci.Rev., Inpharma, Int.Abstr.Biol.Sci., Jrnl.Watch Neuro., NRN, Neurosci.Abstr., Neurosci.Cit.Ind., Pharm.&Out.News, Pollut.Abstr., PsycInfo, Psychol.Abstr. (1983-), Reac., Ref.Zh., Risk Abstr., SSCI (coverage dropped), Saf.Sci.Abstr., Sci.Cit.Ind., THA, e-psyche.
—BLDSC (4274.640000), CASDDS, CISTI, GNLM, IDS, ingenta, KNAW. **CCC.**
Published by: (American Headache Society), Blackwell Science Inc., Commerce Pl, 350 Main St, Malden, MA 02148-5018. TEL 781-388-8250, 800-759-6102, FAX 781-388-8255, journals@blacksci.com, http://www.blackwell-science.com/~cgilib/bsinc.bin?Journal=geoscience. Ed. Dr. Keith Campbell. R&P, Adv. contact Linda McGillicuddy. B&W page USD 731; trim 10.75 x 8.25. Circ: 2,150.

616.857 USA ISSN 1526-4610
HEADACHE ONLINE. Text in English. 10/yr. USD 104 to individuals; USD 144 to institutions (effective 2001). **Document type:** *Academic/Scholarly.*
Media: Online - full text (from Munksgaard & Blackwell Science's Synergy, EBSCO Publishing, O C L C Online Computer Library Center, Inc., Northern Light Technology, Inc., RoweCom Information Quest, ProQuest Information & Learning, ingenta, Swets Blackwell, Institute for Scientific Information). **Related titles:** CD-ROM ed.; Diskette ed.; Magnetic Tape ed.; Microform ed.: (from PQC); ♦ Print ed.: Headache. ISSN 0017-8748.
Published by: (American Headache Society), Blackwell Science Inc., Commerce Pl, 350 Main St, Malden, MA 02148-5018. TEL 781-388-8250, 800-759-6102, FAX 781-388-8255, website@blacksci.com, journals@blacksci.com, http://www.blackwell-science.com/~cgilib/bsinc.bin?Journal=geoscience.

316.8588 DEU ISSN 0017-9647
HEILPAEDAGOGISCHE FORSCHUNG; Zeitschrift fuer Paedagogik und Psychologie Behinderter. Text in German. 1964. q. DEM 48 (effective 2000). bk.rev. abstr. 60 p./no. back issues avail. **Document type:** *Monographic series, Newsletter, Abstract/Index.*
Indexed: IBR, IBZ, Ind.Philos., SSCI (coverage dropped), e-psyche.
—CCC.
Published by: Universitaet Potsdam, Institut fuer Sonderpaedagogik, Postfach 601553, Potsdam 14415, Germany. TEL 49-331-9772597, FAX 49-331-9772195, goetze@rz.uni_potsdam.de, http://www.uni_potsdam.de/u/sonderpaed/spd/index/htm. Ed., Pub., Adv. contact Dr. Herbert Goetze.

616.858 USA
HILL TOPIC. Text in English. 1954. 3/yr. free per issue. **Description:** Highlights work with the mentally retarded.
Indexed: e-psyche.
Published by: Glenwood State Hospital-School, 711 Vine, Glenwood, IA 51534. TEL 712-527-4811. Ed. Stephanie Gaskill. Circ: 1,750.

612.8 JPN ISSN 0913-0241
HIRO TO KYUYO NO KAGAKU/SCIENCE OF FATIGUE AND REST. Text in Japanese; Summaries in English. 1986. a.
Indexed: e-psyche.
Published by: Hiro Kenkyukai/Society for the Study of Fatigue, Jikeikai Ika Daigaku, Dai 2 Seirigaku Kyoshitsu, 25-8 Nishi-Shinbashi 3-chome, Minato-ku, Tokyo 105-0003, Japan.

616.8 GBR ISSN 0957-154X
HISTORY OF PSYCHIATRY. Text in English. 1990. q. GBP 78 domestic to institutions; USD 160 in the Americas to institutions; GBP 80 elsewhere to institutions. back issues avail. *Refereed.* **Document type:** *Academic/Scholarly.* **Description:** Publishes research articles, analysis, information, and reviews on the history of mental illness as well as the forms of medicine, cultural response, and social policy that have evolved to understand and treat it.
Related titles: Online - full text ed.: (from Institute for Scientific Information).
Indexed: ASCA, Amer.Hist.& Life, Br.Hum.Ind., Curr.Cont., Fam.Ind., Hist.Abstr. (1990-), PsycInfo, Psychol.Abstr. (1990-), SSCI, e-psyche.
—BLDSC (4318.408000), GNLM, IDS, Infotrieve. **CCC.**
Published by: Alpha Academic (Subsidiary of: Richard Sadler Ltd.), Halfpenny Furze, Mill Ln, Chalfont St Giles, Bucks HP8 4NR, United Kingdom. TEL 44-1494-872509.

616.8 CZE ISSN 0960-7560
QP351.S65 CODEN: HOMOEB
HOMEOSTASIS; integrative brain functions in health and disease. Text in English. 1959. bi-m. USD 125 foreign (effective 1999). adv. bk.rev. illus. index. *Refereed.* **Document type:** *Academic/Scholarly.* **Description:** Devoted to understanding regulatory mechanisms ranging from molecular to systemic processes in health and disease, with emphasis on integrative functions in homeostatic control and their adaptation to environmental conditions and behavioral needs.
Formerly (until vol.33, 1991): Activitas Nervosa Superior (0001-7604)
Indexed: ASCA, Aqua.Sci.& Fish.Abstr., Biol.Abstr., C.I.S. Abstr., Chem.Abstr., Curr.Adv.Ecol.Sci., Curr.Cont. (coverage dropped), Environ.Sci.Poll.Mgmt., Excerp.Med., Ind.Med. (until 1992, dropped), Ind.Sci.Rev., Nutr.Abstr., PsycInfo, Psychol.Abstr. (1959-), Psychopharmacol.Abstr., Sci.Cit.Ind. (coverage dropped), e-psyche.
—BLDSC (4326.176430), CASDDS, CISTI, EMDOCS, GNLM, IDS, Infotrieve, KNAW. **CCC.**
Published by: Collegium Internationale Activitatis Nervosae Superioris, c/o National Institute of Public Health, Srobarova 48, Prague 10042, Czech Republic. Ed. Milan Horvath.

616.8 HKG ISSN 1026-2121
HONG KONG JOURNAL OF PSYCHIATRY. Text in Chinese. 1991. a. bk.rev. **Document type:** *Academic/Scholarly.* **Description:** Provides a medium of communication for the cultivation and advancement of psychiatry at large and for Hong Kong in particular, as well as to promote Chinese psychiatric research and practice to the world.
Formerly (until 1993): Hong Kong College of Psychiatrists. Journal (1023-0130)
Indexed: HongKongiana, Ref.Zh., e-psyche.
—BLDSC (4326.385850).
Published by: (Hong Kong College of Psychiatrists), Scientific Communications (Hong Kong) Ltd, 4/F, 11 Queen Victoria St, Central, Hong Kong, Hong Kong. http://www.medi.net.hk/users/hkjpsych/index.html. Ed., R&P, Adv. contact Chen Y.H. Eric. Circ: 5,000.

616.8 NLD ISSN 0018-4705
HOOFDLIJNEN. Text in Dutch. 1965. q. adv. bk.rev. charts, illus. **Document type:** *Trade.*
Indexed: e-psyche.
Published by: Nederlandse Vereniging van Laboranten Klinische Neurofysiologie/Dutch Association of Electro-Encephalographic Technicians, c/o I Dekker, Ed, Benesserlaan 396, Uitgeest 1911 VN, Netherlands. Circ: 600.

616.857 NLD ISSN 0920-0037
HOOFDZAKEN; nieuwsblad over migraine, hoofd- en aangezichtspijnen. Text in Dutch. 1981. 5/yr. NLG 40 (effective 2000). adv. bk.rev. back issues avail. *Refereed.* **Document type:** *Newspaper, Consumer.* **Description:** Discusses migraine and other headaches persons suffering from these disorders.
Indexed: e-psyche.

M

Published by: Nederlandse Vereniging van Migrainepatienten, PO Box 65, Elst 6660 AB, Netherlands. TEL 31-481-352391, FAX 31-481-352264, mip@wxs.nl, http://home.wxs.nl/~mip/migraine.htm. Ed., R&P Dick de Scally TEL 31-72-5333994. Circ: 8,300 (paid).

616.8 CAN ISSN 0827-7605
HORIZON (CAMBRIDGE). Text in English. 1973. q. CND 25 to members (effective 2000). back issues avail. **Document type:** *Newsletter.* **Description:** Relays items of interest about Huntington disease and the Society to families, supporters and health care professionals.
Indexed: e-psyche.
Published by: Huntington Society of Canada/Societe Huntington du Canada, 151 Frederick St, Ste 400, Kitchener, ON N2H 2M2, Canada. TEL 1-800-998-7398, info@hsc-ca.org, http://www.hsc-ca.org. Ed., R&P Mr. Shawn Mitchell. Circ: 10,000.

616.89 CUB ISSN 0138-7103
RC440
HOSPITAL PSIQUIATRICO DE LA HABANA. REVISTA. Text in Spanish; Summaries in English. 1959. 3/yr. CUP 30 domestic; USD 28 in the Americas; USD 34 in Europe; USD 42 elsewhere; USD 10 newsstand/cover (effective 2000). adv. bk.rev. abstr. back issues avail. *Refereed.* **Document type:** *Academic/Scholarly, Government.* **Description:** Covers general, pediatric, and geriatric psychiatry, rehabilitation, forensics, neurology and other topics in the field of mental health.
Indexed: Psychol.Abstr., e-psyche.
—KNAW.
Published by: Hospital Psiquiatrico de la Habana, Avenida de la Independencia No. 26520, Mazorra, Boyeros, Ciudad De La Habana CP 19220, Cuba. TEL 537-451512, FAX 537-558692, hospsig@colombus.cu, ordaz@infomed.sld.com. Ed. Dr. Luis Calzadilla Fierro. Adv. contact Eduardo Bernabe Ordaz Ducunge. Circ: 8,000.

612.8 USA ISSN 1065-9471
RC386.6.B7 CODEN: HBMAEE
HUMAN BRAIN MAPPING. Text in English. 1993. m. USD 590 in United States; USD 710 in Canada & Mexico; USD 812 elsewhere; USD 620 combined subscription in United States for print and online eds.; USD 740 combined subscription in Canada & Mexico for print and online eds.; USD 842 combined subscription elsewhere for print and online eds. (effective 2002). adv. back issues avail. *Refereed.* **Document type:** *Academic/Scholarly.* **Description:** Publishes basic, clinical, technical, and theoretical research in the interdisciplinary field of human brain mapping. Includes imaging modalities such as positron-emission tomography, single-photon emission, event-related potentials, magnetoencephalography, magnetic resonance imaging, and x-ray computed tomography.
Related titles: Microform ed.: (from PQC); Online - full text ed.: ISSN 1097-0193. 1996. USD 590 in United States; USD 590 in Canada & Mexico; USD 590 elsewhere (effective 2002) (from EBSCO Publishing, Wiley InterScience, Institute for Scientific Information).
Indexed: ASCA, Biotech.& Bioeng.Abstr., Chemorec.Abstr., Curr.Cont., Excerp.Med. (1996-), Ind.Med. (1993-), Int.Abstr.Biol.Sci., Neurosci.Abstr., Neurosci.Cit.Ind., PsycInfo, Ref.Zh., e-psyche.
—BLDSC (4336.031000), CISTI, GNLM, IDS, Infotrieve, KNAW. **CCC.**
Published by: John Wiley & Sons, Inc., Journals (Subsidiary of: Wiley InterScience), 605 Third Ave, New York, NY 10158. TEL 212-850-6645, FAX 212-850-6021, subinfo@wiley.com, uscs-wis@wiley.com, http://www.wiley.com. Ed. Peter T Fox. adv.: B&W page GBP 640, color page GBP 1,515; trim 210 x 279. Circ: 800. **Subscr. outside the Americas to:** John Wiley & Sons Ltd., Baffins Ln, Chichester, Sussex PO19 IUD, United Kingdom. TEL 44-1243-779777, FAX 44-1243-843232, cs-journals@wiley.co.uk, http://www.wiley.co.uk.

616.8 615 GBR ISSN 0885-6222
CODEN: HUPSEC
HUMAN PSYCHOPHARMACOLOGY: CLINICAL AND EXPERIMENTAL. Text in English. 1986. 8/yr. USD 985 in United States; USD 985 in Canada & Mexico; USD 985 elsewhere; USD 1,035 combined subscription in United States for print and online eds.; USD 1,035 combined subscription in Canada & Mexico for print and online eds.; USD 1,035 combined subscription elsewhere for print and online eds. (effective 2002). adv. back issues avail.; reprint service avail. from SWZ. *Refereed.* **Document type:** *Academic/Scholarly.* **Description:** Communicates the results of clinical and experimental studies relevant to the understanding of new and established psychotropic drugs.
Related titles: Microform ed.: (from PQC); Online - full text ed.: ISSN 1099-1077. 1997. USD 985 in United States; USD 985 in Canada & Mexico; USD 985 elsewhere (effective 2002) (from EBSCO Publishing, Wiley InterScience, Institute for Scientific Information).
Indexed: ASCA, Addic.Abstr., Chem.Abstr., Chem.Indus.Notes, Chem.Titles, Curr.Cont., Derwent Biotech.Abstr., Environ.Sci.Poll.Mgmt., Excerp.Med., Focus on: Psychophar., Ind.Sci.Rev., Inpharma, Int.Abstr.Biol.Sci., Neurosci.Abstr., Neurosci.Cit.Ind., Nutr.Abstr., Pharm.&Out.News, Pollut.Abstr., PsycInfo, Psychol.Abstr. (1986-), Reac., Risk Abstr., SSCI (coverage dropped), Saf.Sci.Abstr., Sci.Cit.Ind., Sugar Ind.Abstr., e-psyche.
—BLDSC (4336.380000), CASDDS, CISTI, EMDOCS, GNLM, IDS, ingenta, KNAW. **CCC.**
Published by: Wiley Europe Ltd., Baffins Ln, Chichester, W Sussex PO19 1UD, United Kingdom. TEL 44-1243-779777, FAX 44-1243-775878, customer@wiley.co.uk, http://www.wiley.co.uk. adv.: B&W page GBP 750, color page GBP 1,650; trim 200 x 260. Circ: 400. **Subscr. to:** John Wiley & Sons, Inc., Journals, 605 Third Ave, New York, NY 10158. TEL 212-850-6021, 212-850-6645, subinfo@jwiley.com.

616.858842 USA
HYDROCEPHALUS NEWS & NOTES* . Text in English. 1982. q. USD 30. bk.rev. tr.lit. back issues avail. **Document type:** *Newsletter.* **Description:** Information relating to hydrocephalus and associated problems of a medical, developmental, social and educational nature, including letters from family members.
Former titles (until 1995): Life-Line (1059-6593); National Hydro Cephalus Foundation Newsletter
Indexed: e-psyche.
Published by: National Hydrocephalus Foundation Organization, PO Box 490248, Lawrenceville, GA 30049-0005. TEL 404-995-8982. Ed. Ann Marie Liakos. Circ: 400 (paid).

HYPER ACTIVITIES. see *EDUCATION—Special Education And Rehabilitation*

I B R O HANDBOOK SERIES. see *MEDICAL SCIENCES—Surgery*

I E H REPORT ON PERINATEL DEVELOPMENTAL NEUROTOXCITY. see *ENVIRONMENTAL STUDIES—Toxicology And Environmental Safety*

616.8 USA
I T F NEWSLETTER. Text in English. 1988. q. USD 25 (effective 2001). adv. bk.rev., Website rev. charts, illus, stat. back issues avail. **Document type:** *Newsletter.* **Description:** Reports recent advances in research in layman's terms for patient and family education.
Related titles: E-mail ed.; Fax ed.
Indexed: e-psyche.
Published by: International Tremor Foundation, 7046 W 105th St, Overland, Park, KS 66212-1803. TEL 913-341-3880, FAX 913-341-1296, staff@essentialtremor.org, http://www.essentialtremor.org. Ed., Pub., R&P, Adv. contact Catherine S Rice. Circ: 6,000 (paid).

616.891 USA ISSN 0899-403X
I U P STRESS AND HEALTH SERIES. Text in English. irreg. price varies. *Refereed.*
Indexed: e-psyche.
—CISTI.
Published by: International Universities Press, Inc., 59 Boston Post Rd, Box 1524, Madison, CT 06443-1524. TEL 203-245-4000, FAX 203-245-0775, http://www.iup.com. Ed. Leo Goldberger.

616.8 618.92 ITA
IMAGO* ; giornale italiano de psicopatologia e psichiatria dell'infanzia e dell'adolescenza. Text in Italian. 3/yr. ITL 120,000, USD 180 (effective 1995).
Indexed: e-psyche.
Address: Idelson, Via de Gasperi 55, Napoli 80133, Italy. TEL 39-81-5524733, FAX 39-81-5518295. Eds. A Condini, M Bertolini.

616.89 150.19 ARG ISSN 0325-4569
IMAGO; revista de psicoanalisis, psiquiatria y psicologia. Text in Spanish. 1974. q. reprint service avail. from SCH.
Published by: Letra Viva, Coronel Diaz 1837, Buenos Aires, Argentina.

616.8 614.58 USA
IMPACT (AUSTIN). Text in English. 1971. 3/yr. free per issue. bk.rev. charts, illus, pat, stat. **Document type:** *Government.* **Description:** Informs, educates, and provides recognition to employees and friends of the agency.
Related titles: Online - full text ed.
Indexed: e-psyche.
Published by: Department of Mental Health and Mental Retardation, Public Information Office, PO Box 12668, Austin, TX 78711. TEL 512-206-4540, FAX 512-206-5093, http://www.mhmr.state.tx.us/pio/impact_magazine/main_impact_magazine.htm. Ed., R&P Laurie Lentz. Circ: 23,000 (controlled).

362.3 IND ISSN 0019-5375
HV3004
INDIAN JOURNAL OF MENTAL RETARDATION. Text in English. 1968. s-a. INR 50, USD 10. adv. bk.rev. abstr.
Indexed: Psychol.Abstr., e-psyche.
—CISTI, GNLM.
Published by: All India Association of Mental Retardation, c/o Dr. K. G. Agrawal, Ed., National Labour Institute, AB-6 Safdarjang Enclave, New Delhi 110 029, India.

616.89 IND ISSN 0019-5545
CODEN: IJRPAB
INDIAN JOURNAL OF PSYCHIATRY. Text in English. 1949. q. INR 800, USD 50 (effective 1999). adv. bk.rev. charts, illus, stat. index. *Refereed.* **Document type:** *Abstract/Index, Academic/Scholarly.* **Description:** Original articles, review articles, case reports, letter to editor in psychiatry and related disciplines.
Related titles: CD-ROM ed.
Indexed: Chem.Abstr., Excerp.Med. (until 19??), ExtraMED, Psychol.Abstr., e-psyche.
—BLDSC (4420.280000), CASDDS, CISTI, GNLM, ingenta.
Published by: (Indian Psychiatric Society), Lucknow Publishing House, 37 Cantonment Rd., Lucknow, Uttar Pradesh 224 883, India. TEL 91-522-371481, FAX 91-522-0266025, TELEX 405-202 CMCH IN. R&P, Adv. contact J.K. Trivedi. B&W page INR 2,000, color page INR 5,000; trim 25 x 16. Circ: 2,250. **Subscr. to:** Indian Psychiatric Society, c/o Dr. J.K. Trivedi, B-8, Sector-A, Mahanagar, Lucknow 226003, India.

616.8 IND ISSN 0253-7176
CODEN: IJPMEU
INDIAN JOURNAL OF PSYCHOLOGICAL MEDICINE. Text in English. 1956. s-a. USD 15. adv. bk.rev. abstr, bibl, charts, illus, stat. reprints avail. **Description:** Research and review articles, and conference papers in various areas of psychiatry and related subjects.
Formerly (until 1978): Indian Journal of Psychology (0019-5553)
Indexed: Bibl.Asian Stud. (1971-1990), Biol.Abstr., Curr.Adv.Ecol.Sci., Curr.Ind.Stat., Indian Psychol.Abstr., Indian Sci.Abstr., Lang.& Lang.Behav.Abstr., P C I, Psychol.Abstr., e-psyche.
—CISTI, ingenta.
Published by: Indian Psychiatric Society, South Zone, c/o Dr. Palaniappun M.D., Ed., D.P.M., Mnams 4A, V.P. Extension, Ayanavaran, Chennai, Tamil Nadu 600 023, India. TEL 5340. Circ: 600.

INFANT SCREENING. see *MEDICAL SCIENCES—Pediatrics*

616.8 CAN ISSN 0715-3120
INFO A L S. Text in English. 1980. a. free per issue. abstr. **Description:** Conveys latest research discoveries on the cause and cure of the A L S disease.
Indexed: e-psyche.
Published by: Amyotrophic Lateral Sclerosis Society of Canada, 220 6 Adelaide St, East, Toronto, ON M5C 1H6, Canada. TEL 416-362-0269, FAX 416-362-0414, alssoc@inforamp.net. Ed. Dr. Michael Sribney.

616.8 DEU ISSN 1437-062X
▼ **INFO NEUROLOGIE UND PSYCHIATRIE.** Text in German. 1999. bi-m. EUR 94.98 domestic; EUR 107.98 foreign; EUR 71.62 domestic to students; EUR 84.62 foreign to students; EUR 18.69 newsstand/cover (effective 2002). back issues avail. **Document type:** *Journal, Academic/Scholarly.*
Indexed: e-psyche.
Published by: Urban und Vogel Medien und Medizin Verlagsgesellschaft mbH (Subsidiary of: BertelsmannSpringer), Neumarkter Str 43, Munich 81673, Germany. TEL 49-89-43721411, FAX 49-89-43721410, verlag@urban-vogel.de, http://www.urban-vogel.de. Ed. H.C. Diener. Pub., R&P Oliver Renn. Adv. contact Peter Urban. **Subscr. to:** Springer Auslieferungs Gesellschaft, Postfach 105160, Heidelberg 69041, Germany. TEL 49-6221-345244, FAX 49-6221-345244.

616.8 BRA ISSN 0101-4331
INFORMACAO PSIQUIATRICA. Text in Portuguese; Summaries in English, Portuguese. 1980-1983 (vol.4, no.4); resumed. triennial. BRL 48, USD 72 (effective 2000). adv. bk.rev. index, cum.index. back issues avail. **Document type:** *Academic/Scholarly.* **Description:** Presents studies in clinical psychiatry.
Indexed: Excerp.Med. (1996-), Ref.Zh., e-psyche.
—BLDSC (4478.904500), EMDOCS, KNAW.
Published by: (Departamento de Psiquiatria e Psicopatologia, Universidade do Estado do Rio de Janeiro), ECN - Editora Cientifica Nacional Ltda., Rua da Gloria, 366 Andar 3, Gloria, Rio De Janeiro, RJ 20241-180, Brazil. TEL 55-21-2213235, FAX 55-21-2213235, ecn@rj.sol.com.br. Ed. Jorge Alberto Costa e Silva. R&P, Adv. contact Maria Luiza Carvalho. Circ: 5,000.

616.8 FRA ISSN 0020-0204
INFORMATION PSYCHIATRIQUE. Text in French. 1947. m., latest vol.78, 2002 (10/yr.). EUR 35; EUR 53 foreign (effective 2002). back issues avail.
Indexed: Excerp.Med., Psychol.Abstr., e-psyche.
—BLDSC (4493.920000), CISTI, GNLM.
Published by: P D G Communication, 30 rue d'Armaille, Paris 75017, France. TEL 33-1-40550595, FAX 33-1-45746567. Ed. Patrick de Gavre.

616.8 ITA ISSN 1122-8377
L'INFORMATORE S.I.N. Text in Italian. 1994. 3/yr. adv. **Document type:** *Newsletter.*
Indexed: e-psyche.
Published by: (Societa Italiana di Neurologia), C I C Edizioni Internazionali s.r.l., Corso Trieste 42, Rome, RM 00198, Italy. TEL 39-06-8412673, FAX 39-06-8412688, info@gruppocic.it, 1160199510. adv.: B&W page ITL 3,100,000, color page ITL 3,900,000; trim 210 x 290.

616.858 USA
INSIDE CHADD. Text in English. 1993. q. USD 45 to members. **Document type:** *Newsletter.*
Formerly: Chadder Box
Indexed: e-psyche.
Published by: Children and Adults with Attention Deficit - Hyperactivity Disorders, 8181 Professional Pl., Ste. 201, Landover, MD 20785-2226. TEL 301-306-7070, 800-233-4050, FAX 301-306-7090, http://www.chadd.org. Ed. Jennifer Garner.

616.834 USA ISSN 0739-9774
INSIDE M S. (Multiple Sclerosis) Text in English. 1983. q. free to members (effective 2002). adv. bk.rev. illus. **Document type:** *Consumer.* **Description:** Publishes for people with MS and their families, health professionals, counselors and others interested in solving the problems of living with the chronic disease. Also covers disability rights and reports on current research in the field.
Incorporating (in 1983): Focus on Research; M S Messenger; National Multiple Sclerosis Society. Annual Report; Patient Service News
Related titles: Microform ed.: (from PQC); Online - full text ed.: (from Gale Group, ProQuest Information & Learning, Factiva); Large type ed. 14 pt.
Indexed: Hlth.Ind., Rehabil.Lit., e-psyche.
Published by: National Multiple Sclerosis Society, 733 Third Ave, New York, NY 10017-3288. TEL 212-986-3240, FAX 212-986-7981, editor@nmss.org, http://www.nmss.org. Ed. Martha King. R&P Harry Hample TEL 212-476-0538. Adv. contact William Rosen. Circ: 680,000.

616.8914 BRA ISSN 0103-9083
INSIGHT-PSICOTERAPIA. Text in Portuguese. 1990. m. adv. bk.rev. back issues avail. *Refereed.* **Document type:** *Academic/Scholarly.*
Related titles: Online - full text ed.
Indexed: e-psyche.
Published by: Lemos Editorial & Graficos Ltda., Rua Rui Barbosa, 70, B Vista, Sao Paulo, SP 01326-010, Brazil. TEL 55-11-251-4300, FAX 55-11-251-4300, lemospl@netpoint.com.br, http://www.lemos.com.br. Ed., Adv. contact Paulo Lemos. Circ: 3,000 (controlled).

INSIGHTS (BELLE MEAD). see *HEALTH FACILITIES AND ADMINISTRATION*

612.8 USA ISSN 1053-881X
BF1 CODEN: IPBSEK
INTEGRATIVE PHYSIOLOGICAL AND BEHAVIORAL SCIENCE. Text in English. 1965. q. USD 120 to individuals; USD 240 to institutions (effective 2001). adv. index. *Refereed.* **Document type:** *Academic/Scholarly.* **Description:** Dedicated to the advancement of biological science and to interdisciplinary research and communication. Covers physiology, physiological psychology, psychopharmacology, ethology, behavioral medicine, biological psychiatry and medicine.
Former titles: Pavlovian Journal of Biological Science (0093-2213); Conditional Reflex (0010-5392)
Related titles: Microform ed.: (from PQC); Online - full content ed.; Online - full text ed.: (from CatchWord Ltd., Institute for Scientific Information).
Indexed: ASCA, Bibl.Asian Stud. (1971), Biol.Abstr., Chem.Abstr., Curr.Adv.Ecol.Sci., Curr.Cont. (coverage dropped), Curr.Ind.Stat., Curr.Ref.Fish Res., Dent.Ind., Excerp.Med., Hosp.Lit.Ind., IBZ, Ind.Med. (1991-), Ind.Philos., Neurosci.Cit.Ind., PsycInfo, Psychol.Abstr. (1966-), Psycscan B.A.& T., SSCI, Sci.Cit.Ind. (coverage dropped), e-psyche.
—BLDSC (4531.816580), CASDDS, CatchWord, CISTI, GNLM, IDS, ingenta, KNAW. **CCC.**
Published by: (Pavlovian Society), Transaction Publishers, 35 Berrue Circle, Rutgers University, Piscataway, NJ 08854-8042. TEL 732-445-2280, FAX 732-445-3138, trans@transactionpub.com, http://www.transactionpub.com. Ed. Joseph E Steinmetz. adv.: page USD 300; 5.5 x 8. Circ: 400. **Subscr. to:** Transaction Distribution Center, 390 Campus Dr, Somerset, NJ 08873. TEL 732-748-0300, FAX 732-748-1886.

616.89 GBR ISSN 0085-2007
INTERNATIONAL ASSOCIATION FOR SCIENTIFIC STUDY OF MENTAL DEFICIENCY. PROCEEDINGS OF INTERNATIONAL CONGRESS. Text in English. 1967. triennial, latest 1988, 8th, Dublin. GBP 40. **Document type:** *Proceedings.*
Indexed: e-psyche.
Published by: (International Association for Scientific Study of Mental Deficiency), Routledge (Subsidiary of: Taylor & Francis Group), 11 New Fetter Ln, London EC4P 4EE, United Kingdom. TEL 44-20-7583-9855, FAX 44-207-583-0701, info@routledge.co.uk, http://www.tandf.co.uk/journals. Ed. J Berg. Circ: 4,000.

616.855 CHE ISSN 0074-1655
INTERNATIONAL ASSOCIATION OF LOGOPEDICS AND PHONIATRICS. REPORTS OF CONGRESS. Text in English. 1947. triennial, latest 1998, 23rd, Amsterdam. USD 30. adv. bk.rev. **Document type:** *Journal, Academic/Scholarly.*
Indexed: e-psyche.
Published by: International Association of Logopedics and Phoniatrics, c/o Dr. A. Muller, 43 R Louis de Savoie, Morges 1110, Switzerland. TEL 41-21-8030800, FAX 41-21-3209300.

610 USA ISSN 0361-0462
CODEN: IBRSDZ
INTERNATIONAL BRAIN RESEARCH ORGANIZATION MONOGRAPH SERIES. Short title: I B R O Monograph Series. Text in English. 1975. irreg. price varies. reprint service avail. from PQC. **Document type:** *Monographic series.*
Indexed: Biol.Abstr., Chem.Abstr., Curr.Cont. (coverage dropped), Sci.Cit.Ind. (coverage dropped), e-psyche.
—CASDDS, CISTI, GNLM.
Published by: (International Brain Research Organization), Lippincott Williams & Wilkins (Philadelphia) (Subsidiary of: Wolters Kluwer N.V.), 530 Walnut St, Philadelphia, PA 19106-3621. TEL 301-223-2300, 800-638-3030, FAX 301-223-2400.

616.8 IRL ISSN 0074-3631
INTERNATIONAL CONGRESS OF ELECTROENCEPHALOGRAPHY AND CLINICAL NEUROPHYSIOLOGY (PROCEEDINGS). Text in English. irreg., latest 1990, 12th, Rio de Janeiro. Supplement avail. **Document type:** *Proceedings.*
Indexed: INSPEC (coverage dropped), Ind.Med. (coverage dropped), e-psyche.
Published by: (International Federation of Clinical Neurophysiology), Elsevier Science Ireland Ltd, Elsevier House, Brookvale Plaza, E. Park, Shannon, Co. Clare, Ireland. TEL 353-61-471944, FAX 353-61-472144. R&P Annette Moloney. **Subscr. in Australasia and the Far East to:** Elsevier Science (Singapore) Pte Ltd, No.1 Temasek Ave, 17-01 Millenia Tower, Singapore 039192, Singapore. TEL 65-434-3727, FAX 65-337-2230; **Subscr. in the Americas to:** Elsevier Science, PO Box 945, New York, NY 10159-0945. TEL 212-633-3730, FAX 212-633-3680; **Subscr. to:** Elsevier Science BV, PO Box 211, Amsterdam 1000 AE, Netherlands. TEL 31-20-485-3757, FAX 31-20-485-3432.

616.89 615 USA ISSN 0020-6571
INTERNATIONAL DRUG THERAPY NEWSLETTER. Text in English. 1966. m., latest vol.36. USD 160 domestic to individuals; USD 195 foreign to individuals; USD 250 domestic to institutions; USD 250 per issue foreign to institutions; USD 21 newsstand/cover (effective 2002). bk.rev. **Document type:** *Newsletter.* **Description:** Covers psychoactive drug therapy.
Related titles: Online - full text ed.: USD 325 domestic for academic site license; USD 325 foreign for academic site license; USD 362.50 domestic for corporate site license; USD 362.50 foreign for corporate site license (effective 2002).
Indexed: I.P.A., Inpharma, Pharm.&Out.News, Reac., e-psyche.
—BLDSC (4539.749000), GNLM.
Published by: Lippincott Williams & Wilkins (Philadelphia) (Subsidiary of: Wolters Kluwer N.V.), 530 Walnut St, Philadelphia, PA 19106-3621. TEL 215-521-8300, FAX 215-521-8902, http://www.lww.com. Ed. Dr. Frank J Ayd Jr. **Subscr. to:** TEL 800-777-2295, FAX 301-824-7390.

616.8 CHE
INTERNATIONAL FEDERATION FOR PSYCHOTHERAPY. CONGRESS REPORTS. Text in English. 1972. triennial, latest 1994, 16th, Seoul, S. Korea. **Document type:** *Proceedings.*
Formerly: International Federation for Medical Psychotherapy. Congress Reports (0074-5847)
Indexed: e-psyche.
Published by: International Federation for Psychotherapy, c/o Dr. Edgar Heim, Pres., Tannackerstr 3, Oberhofen Thunrsee 3653, Switzerland. TEL 033-431195.

616.89 150 USA ISSN 1062-3051
THE INTERNATIONAL JOURNAL OF COMMUNICATIVE PSYCHOANALYSIS & PSYCHOTHERAPY. Text in English. 1982. q. USD 70 to individuals; USD 80 to institutions. **Document type:** *Academic/Scholarly.* **Description:** Pertains to the activities of the Society.
Former titles (until 1992): Society for Psychoanalytic Psychotherapy. Bulletin (1052-0724); (until 1990): Society for Psychoanalytic Psychotherapy - News Letter (1048-5546)
Indexed: PsycInfo, Psychoanal.Abstr., e-psyche.
—BLDSC (4542.172530).
Published by: International Society for Communicative Psychoanalysis and Psychotherapy, c/o Muriel P Warren, 60 Dutch Hill Rd, Prel Plaza South 15, Orangeburg, NY 10962. TEL 914-365-0801, 212-595-3530. Eds. Irwing Weisberg, William Goodheart.

616.8 GBR ISSN 0736-5748
QP363.5 CODEN: IJDND6
INTERNATIONAL JOURNAL OF DEVELOPMENTAL NEUROSCIENCE. Text in English. 1983. 8/yr. EUR 1,191 in Europe to institutions; JPY 158,100 in Japan to institutions; USD 1,331 elsewhere to institutions (effective 2002). back issues avail. *Refereed.* **Document type:** *Academic/Scholarly.* **Description:** Publishes research on basic and clinical aspects of the developing nervous system.
Related titles: Microfilm ed.: (from PQC); Online - full text ed.: (from ingenta, Swets Blackwell, ScienceDirect, Institute for Scientific Information).
Indexed: ASCA, Aqua.Sci.& Fish.Abstr., Biotech.& Bioeng.Abstr., Chem.Abstr., Chem.Indus.Notes, Chem.Titles, Chemorec.Abstr., Curr.Adv.Biochem., Curr.Adv.Ecol.Sci., Curr.Adv.Gen.& Molec.Biol., Curr.Cont., Excerp.Med., Ind.Med. (1983-), Ind.Sci.Rev., Indian Psychol.Abstr., Inpharma, Int.Abstr.Biol.Sci., Neurosci.Abstr., Neurosci.Cit.Ind., PsycInfo, Psychol.Abstr. (1983-), Reac., Sci.Cit.Ind., e-psyche.
—BLDSC (4542.185100), CASDDS, CISTI, EMDOCS, GNLM, IDS, ingenta, KNAW. **CCC.**

M

Published by: (International Society for Developmental Neuroscience), Pergamon (Subsidiary of: Elsevier Science), The Boulevard, Langford Ln, East Park, Kidlington, Oxford OXB 1GB, United Kingdom. FAX 44-1865-843010, http://www.elsevier.com/locate/ijdevneu. Ed. J Regino Perez-Polo. **Subscr. in Australasia and the Far East to:** Elsevier Science (Singapore) Pte Ltd, No.1 Temasek Ave, 17-01 Millenia Tower, Singapore 039192, Singapore. TEL 65-434-3727, FAX 65-337-2230; **Subscr. in the Americas to:** Elsevier Science, PO Box 945, New York, NY 10159-0945. TEL 212-633-3730, FAX 212-633-3680, usinfo-f@elsevier.com; **Subscr. to:** Elsevier Science BV, PO Box 211, Amsterdam 1000 AE, Netherlands. TEL 31-20-485-3757.

616.8 USA ISSN 1522-4821

▼ **INTERNATIONAL JOURNAL OF EMERGENCY MENTAL HEALTH.** Text in English. 1999. q. USD 69 domestic to individuals; USD 90 foreign to individuals; USD 350 domestic to institutions; USD 410 foreign to institutions (effective 1999). *Refereed.* **Description:** Publishes manuscripts on relevant topics including psychological trauma, disaster psychology, traumatic stress, etc.
Indexed: Ind.Med.
—BLDSC (4542.232700).
Published by: Chevron Publishing Corporation, 5018 Dorsey Hall Dr., Suite 104, Ellicott City, MD 21042.

INTERNATIONAL JOURNAL OF GERIATRIC PSYCHIATRY. see *GERONTOLOGY AND GERIATRICS*

INTERNATIONAL JOURNAL OF GROUP PSYCHOTHERAPY. see *PSYCHOLOGY*

INTERNATIONAL JOURNAL OF LAW AND PSYCHIATRY. see *LAW*

▼ **THE INTERNATIONAL JOURNAL OF MENTAL HEALTH PROMOTION**; promoting mental health, preventing mental disorders. see *PUBLIC HEALTH AND SAFETY*

616.8 GBR ISSN 1049-8931
RC337 CODEN: IPSREY

INTERNATIONAL JOURNAL OF METHODS IN PSYCHIATRIC RESEARCH. Text in English. 1991-1996; N.S. 1998. q. USD 160 in North America to individuals; GBP 89 rest of world to individuals; USD 320 in North America to institutions; GBP 178 rest of world to institutions (effective 2001). adv. bk.rev. abstr. back issues avail.; reprint service avail. from SWZ. *Refereed.* **Document type:** *Academic/Scholarly.* **Description:** Contains articles pertaining to important issues in the methods of psychiatric research, the measurement of psychiatric phenomena and related biological variables.
Related titles: Microform ed.: N.S. (from PQC).
Indexed: ASCA, Curr.Cont. (coverage dropped), Psychol.Abstr. (1993-), SSCI (coverage dropped), e-psyche.
—BLDSC (4542.352300), GNLM, IDS, Infotrieve, KNAW. **CCC.**
Published by: Whurr Publishers Ltd., 19b Compton Terr, London N1 2UN, United Kingdom. TEL 44-20-7359-5979, FAX 44-20-7226-5290, info@whurr.co.uk, http://www.whurr.co.uk; http://www.whurrjournals.co.uk/. Ed. Hans Ulrich Wittchen. Adv. contact Lizzy Ewer. B&W page GBP 475, color page GBP 1,325; trim 200 x 260. Circ: 95. **Subscr. in N. America to:** Whurr Publishers Ltd., PO Box 1897, Lawrence, KS 66044-8897. TEL 913-843-1221, FAX 913-843-1274, am&m@allenpress.com. **Subscr. to:** Turpin Distribution Services Ltd., Blackhorse Rd, Letchworth, Herts SG6 1HN, United Kingdom. TEL 44-1462-488900, FAX 44-1462-483011, custservturpin@turpinltd.com.

616.8 URY ISSN 0020-7446
CODEN: IJONAO

INTERNATIONAL JOURNAL OF NEUROLOGY. Text in English. 1960. q. USD 260 to individuals; USD 320 to institutions. adv. bk.rev. bibl, charts, illus. **Document type:** *Monographic series, Academic/Scholarly.* **Description:** Focuses on specific topics in neurology, with additional sections on teaching neurology and the history of medicine.
Related titles: French ed.; German ed.; Spanish ed.
Indexed: Biol.Abstr., Chem.Abstr., Curr.Adv.Ecol.Sci., Excerp.Med., Ind.Med. (coverage dropped), e-psyche.
—CASDDS, CISTI, GNLM.
Published by: Fulton Society, Calle Buenos Aires 363, Montevideo, Uruguay. TEL 5982-95-61-07. Ed. Victor Soriano.

616.8 GBR

INTERNATIONAL JOURNAL OF NEUROPSYCHOPHARMACOLOGY. Short title: I J N P. Text in English. 1998. s-a. GBP 112, USD 190 (effective 1999). **Document type:** *Academic/Scholarly.* **Description:** Focuses on research which advances understanding of existing and new neuropsychological agents, including their mode of action and clinical application, or which provides insights into the biological basis of neuropsychiatric disorders and thereby advances their pharmacological treatment.
Indexed: Neurosci.Cit.Ind.
Published by: (Collegium Internationale Neuro-Psychopharmacologicum), Cambridge University Press, Edinburgh Bldg, Shaftesbury Rd, Cambridge CB2 2RU, United Kingdom. FAX 44-1223-315052, information@cup.cam.ac.uk, information@cambridge.org, http://www.cup.cam.ac.uk, http://www.uk.cambridge.org/journals/pmu. Ed. Bernard Lerer.

616.8 CHE ISSN 0020-7454
QP351 CODEN: IJNUB7

INTERNATIONAL JOURNAL OF NEUROSCIENCE. Text in French. 1970. 12/yr. (in 6 vols., 4 nos./vol.). GBP 1,517, USD 2,503, EUR 2,853 to individuals; GBP 3,870, USD 4,946, EUR 5,031 to institutions; GBP 8,469, USD 10,913, EUR 11,094 to corporations (effective 2002). adv. bk.rev. index. back issues avail. *Refereed.* **Document type:** *Journal, Academic/Scholarly.* **Description:** Publishes papers concerned with problems of nervous tissue, the nervous system, and behavior.
Related titles: CD-ROM ed.; Microform ed.; Online - full text ed.: (from EBSCO Publishing, RoweCom Information Quest, Institute for Scientific Information).
Indexed: ASCA, Aqua.Sci.& Fish.Abstr., Biol.Abstr., Chem.Abstr., Chemorec.Abstr., Curr.Adv.Ecol.Sci., Curr.Cont. (coverage dropped), Dent.Ind., Excerp.Med., Ind.Med. (1970-), Ind.Sci.Rev., Indian Psychol.Abstr., Int.Abstr.Biol.Sci., Neurosci.Abstr., Neurosci.Cit.Ind., PsycInfo, Psychol.Abstr. (1983-), SSCI (coverage dropped), e-psyche.
—CASDDS, CISTI, EMDOCS, GNLM, ingenta. **CCC.**
Published by: Gordon and Breach - Harwood Academic (Subsidiary of: Taylor & Francis Group), PO Box 531, Lausanne 1000, Switzerland. TEL 41-21-6411280, FAX 41-21-6411281, info@gbhap.com, http://www.gbhap.com/journals/148/148-top.htm. Ed. Dr. Sidney Weinstein. **Subscr. addr. in US:** International Publishers Direct, PO Box 32160, Newark, NJ 07102. FAX 215-750-6343.

INTERNATIONAL JOURNAL OF OFFENDER THERAPY AND COMPARATIVE CRIMINOLOGY. see *CRIMINOLOGY AND LAW ENFORCEMENT*

616.8 GBR ISSN 0968-0624

THE INTERNATIONAL JOURNAL OF PSYCHIATRIC NURSING RESEARCH. Text in English. 1994 (Aug.). 3/yr. GBP 20 in Europe to individuals; USD 32 in United States to individuals; CND 45 in Canada to individuals; GBP 22 elsewhere to individuals; GBP 50 in Europe to institutions; USD 80 in United States to institutions; CND 112 in Canada to institutions; GBP 56 elsewhere to institutions (effective 2000 - 2001). adv. bk.rev. abstr, charts, stat. back issues avail. *Refereed.* **Document type:** *Academic/Scholarly, Abstract/Index.* **Description:** Promotes the development of scholarship in the understanding of psychiatric nursing both for the academic researcher and the clinical practitioner.
Related titles: Large type ed. 12 pt.
Indexed: CINAHL, Int.Nurs.Ind., e-psyche.
—BLDSC (4542.490000).
Published by: University of Southampton, Room 1001, Building 47, Highfield, Southampton, Hamps SO17 1BJ, United Kingdom. TEL 44-1703-796549, 44-1703-794569, FAX 44-1703-796922, pws1@soton.ac.uk. Ed. William Whitfield. R&P, Adv. contact Paul Shelley.

616.89 GBR ISSN 1365-1501
CODEN: IJPCFZ

INTERNATIONAL JOURNAL OF PSYCHIATRY IN CLINICAL PRACTICE. Text in English. 1997. q. GBP 83, USD 130 to individuals; GBP 190, USD 305 to institutions (effective 2002). adv. bk.rev. index. back issues avail. **Document type:** *Academic/Scholarly.* **Description:** Covers new developments in International Cardiology.
Related titles: Online - full content ed.: ISSN 1471-1788; Online - full text ed.: (from CatchWord Ltd., Institute for Scientific Information).
Indexed: Curr.Cont., Environ.Sci.Poll.Mgmt., Excerp.Med., Pollut.Abstr., PsycInfo, Psychol.Abstr., e-psyche.
—BLDSC (4542.493000), CASDDS, CatchWord, GNLM.
Published by: Martin Dunitz Ltd. (Subsidiary of: Taylor & Francis Group), 7-9 Pratt St, London NW1 0AE, United Kingdom. TEL 44-20-7482-2202, FAX 44-20-7482-7088, info@dunitz.co.uk, http://www.dunitz.co.uk. Eds. David Baldwin, Siegfried Kasper. R&P, Adv. contact Ian Mellor. Circ: 2,500 (paid).

616.89 USA ISSN 0091-2174
RC321 CODEN: IJMEDO

INTERNATIONAL JOURNAL OF PSYCHIATRY IN MEDICINE; an international journal of medical psychology and psychiatry in the general hospital. Text in English. 1970. q. USD 60 to individuals; USD 218 to institutions (effective 2001). adv. bk.rev. bibl, charts, illus, stat. index. back issues avail.; reprints avail. *Refereed.* **Document type:** *Journal, Academic/Scholarly.* **Description:** Contains articles which apply the methods of psychiatry and psychology to the further understanding of disorders which are primarily psychiatric in nature.
Formerly: Psychiatry in Medicine (0033-278X)
Related titles: Online - full text ed.: (from Institute for Scientific Information).
Indexed: ASCA, Abstr.Anthropol., Abstr.Health Care Manage.Stud., AgeLine, Behav.Med.Abstr., Biol.Abstr., Curr.Cont., Excerp.Med., Fam.Ind., Ind.Med. (1973-), Inpharma, Mid.East: Abstr.& Ind., Nutr.Abstr., Pharm.&Out.News, PsycInfo, Psychol.Abstr. (1973-), Reac., SSCI, Soc.Work Res.& Abstr., e-psyche.
—BLDSC (4542.495000), CISTI, GNLM, IDS, Infotrieve, ingenta, KNAW. **CCC.**
Published by: Baywood Publishing Co., Inc., 26 Austin Ave, Box 337, Amityville, NY 11701. TEL 631-691-1270, FAX 631-691-1770, info@baywood.com, baywood@baywood.com, http://baywood.com/search/PreviewJournal.asp?qsRecord=7. Ed. Harold Koenig. Pub. Stuart Cohen. R&P Julie Krempa. Adv. contact Joi Tamber-Brooks.

INTERNATIONAL JOURNAL OF PSYCHOPATHOLOGY, PSYCHOPHARMACOLOGY, AND PSYCHOTHERAPY. see *PSYCHOLOGY*

616.89 GBR ISSN 1356-9082
CODEN: IJOPFZ

INTERNATIONAL JOURNAL OF PSYCHOTHERAPY. Text in English. 1996. 3/yr. GBP 57, USD 97 to individuals; GBP 172, USD 283 to institutions (effective 2002). back issues avail. **Document type:** *Academic/Scholarly.* **Description:** Publishes original research in the field, covering all orientations.
Related titles: Online - full content ed.: ISSN 1469-8498 (from Northern Light Technology, Inc., EBSCO Publishing, O C L C Online Computer Library Center, Inc., ProQuest Information & Learning, Swets Blackwell); Online - full text ed.: (from CatchWord Ltd., RoweCom Information Quest).
Indexed: Lang.& Lang.Behav.Abstr., PsycInfo, SOPODA, Sociol.Abstr., e-psyche.
—BLDSC (4542.506800), CatchWord, GNLM. **CCC.**
Published by: (European Association for Psychotherapy), Carfax Publishing Limited (Subsidiary of: Taylor & Francis Group), PO Box 25, Abingdon, Oxon OX14 3UE, United Kingdom. TEL 44-1235-401000, FAX 44-1235-401550, enquiries@carfax.co.uk, enquiry@tandf.co.uk, http://www.carfax.co.uk.

616.89 GBR ISSN 0020-7640
RC321

INTERNATIONAL JOURNAL OF SOCIAL PSYCHIATRY. (Will be published by Sage Publications Inc. from 2002, beginning with March 2002 issue. Subscr. prices GBP 37.00, US $58.00 (to individuals); GBP 195.00, US $306.00 (to institutions) (effective 2002); ad. rate GBP 200.00 per page.) Text in English. 1955. q. GBP 39 in United Kingdom to individuals; USD 165 rest of world to individuals; GBP 59 in United Kingdom to institutions incl. libraries & hospitals; USD 205 rest of world to institutions incl. libraries & hospitals (effective 2001). bk.rev. illus, stat. index. back issues avail.; reprint service avail. from PSC,SCH. *Refereed.* **Document type:** *Academic/Scholarly.* **Description:** Publishes articles on psychiatric problems, strategies for survival, drug abuse, psychiatry, social psychiatry, and psychotherapy.
Related titles: Online - full text ed.: (from Northern Light Technology, Inc., H. W. Wilson, ProQuest Information & Learning, Gale Group, Factiva, Institute for Scientific Information).
Indexed: ASCA, ASSIA, Abstr.Health Care Manage.Stud., Addic.Abstr., Adol.Ment.Hlth.Abstr., AgeLine, Bibl.Asian Stud. (1969-1998), Curr.Cont., Excerp.Med., Fam.Ind., Ind.Med. (1955-), Indian Psychol.Abstr., Int.Nurs.Ind., Intl.Bibl.Soc.Sci., Lang.& Lang.Behav.Abstr., Mid.East: Abstr.& Ind., P C I, PsycInfo, Psychol.Abstr. (1955-), SOPODA, SSCI, Sage Race Rel.Abstr., Soc.Sci.Ind. (Dec.1982-), Soc.Serv.Abstr., Sociol.Abstr., e-psyche.
—BLDSC (4542.560000), CISTI, GNLM, IDS, ingenta.

Published by: (Institute of Psychiatry), Avenue Publishing Co., 41 Georges Wood Rd, Brookmans Park, Herts AL9 7BX, United Kingdom. apublish1@aol.com, http://www.ijsp.co.uk. Ed. Dinesh Bhugra. Pub. S Bierer. R&P S. Bierer. Circ: 1,000.

616.834 GBR ISSN 1352-8963
THE INTERNATIONAL M S JOURNAL. (Multiple Sclerosis) Text in English. 1994. 3/yr. GBP 71 in United Kingdom; GBP 76 foreign (effective 2000). bk.rev. back issues avail. *Refereed.* **Document type:** *Journal, Academic/Scholarly.* **Description:** Contains review articles dealing with the biochemical, pathophysiological and clinical aspects of multiple sclerosis and related conditions. It aims to improve the awareness and understanding of MS worldwide from which will emerge clear and practical guideline for the care of people.
Related titles: Online - full text ed.: ISSN 1469-3410. 1999.
—BLDSC (4544.364500).
Published by: (Schering AG DEU), Cambridge Medical Publications Ltd., Wicker House, High St, Worthing, W Sussex BN11 1DJ, United Kingdom. TEL 44-1903-205884, FAX 44-1903-234862, cmp@hbase.com, http://www.parexel-mms.com/cmp. Pub. Robert Kasprowitz. R&P Susannah Turgoose TEL 44-1903-288249. Circ: 18,000.

616.8 GBR ISSN 1355-6177
QP360 CODEN: JINSF9
INTERNATIONAL NEUROPSYCHOLOGICAL SOCIETY. JOURNAL. Short title: J I N S. Text in English. 1995. 7/yr. GBP 126 to individuals; USD 311 to institutions (effective 2002). adv. bk.rev. Supplement avail.; back issues avail. *Refereed.* **Document type:** *Academic/Scholarly.* **Description:** Publishes primary research articles reflecting all areas of neuropsychology, including development of cognitive processes, brain-behaviour relationships, adult and child neuropsychology, developmental neuropsychology and disorders of speech and language.
Related titles: Online - full text ed.: ISSN 1469-7661. 1998 (from EBSCO Publishing, O C L C Online Computer Library Center, Inc., RoweCom Information Quest, Swets Blackwell, Institute for Scientific Information).
Indexed: Curr.Cont., Ind.Med. (1995-), Jrnl.Watch Psych., Lang.& Lang.Behav.Abstr., Neuropsych.Abstr., Neurosci.Cit.Ind., PsycInfo, SOPODA, Sci.Cit.Ind., Sociol.Abstr., e-psyche.
—BLDSC (4802.325000), GNLM, IDS, Infotrieve. **CCC.**
Published by: (International Neuropsychological Society), Cambridge University Press, Edinburgh Bldg, Shaftesbury Rd, Cambridge CB2 2RU, United Kingdom. FAX 44-1223-315052, information@cup.cam.ac.uk, information@cambridge.org, http://www.cup.org/journals/cupjnls.html. Ed. Dr. Igor Grant. R&P Linda Nicol. Adv. contact Rebecca Symons. B&W page GBP 495; trim 170 x 250. Circ: 3,400.

618.97 USA ISSN 1041-6102
CODEN: INPSE8
INTERNATIONAL PSYCHOGERIATRICS; the official journal of the Interntional Psychogeriatric Association. Text in English. 1989. q., latest vol.13, 2001. USD 88 in United States to individuals; USD 144 for 2 yrs. in United States to individuals; USD 98 foreign to individuals; USD 172 for 2 yrs. foreign to individuals; USD 188 in United States to institutions; USD 300 for 2 yrs. in United States to institutions; USD 198 foreign to institutions; USD 332 for 2 yrs. foreign to institutions (effective 2001). adv. bk.rev., software rev., video rev. abstr. 120 p./no. Supplement avail.; back issues avail.; reprints avail. *Refereed.* **Document type:** *Journal, Academic/Scholarly.* **Description:** Serves as a multidisciplinary and interdisciplinary forum for advances in psychogeriatric practice, research, service development and education worldwide.
Related titles: Online - full text ed.: (from Institute for Scientific Information).
Indexed: Abstr.Soc.Geront., AgeLine, CINAHL, Curr.Cont., Excerp.Med. (1993-), Fam.Ind., Ind.Med. (1989-), Indian Psychol.Abstr., Int.Nurs.Ind., Lang.& Lang.Behav.Abstr., PsycInfo, Psychol.Abstr. (1989-), SOPODA, SSCI, Sage Fam.Stud.Abstr., Sage Urb.Stud.Abstr., Soc.Work Res.& Abstr., Sociol.Abstr., Viol.& Abuse Abstr., e-psyche.
—BLDSC (4545.345000), EMDOCS, GNLM, Infotrieve, ingenta, KNAW. **CCC.**
Published by: (International Psychogeriatric Association), Springer Publishing Company, 536 Broadway, New York, NY 10012. TEL 212-431-4370, FAX 212-941-7842, springer@springerpub.com, http://www.springerpub.com. Ed. Robin Eastwood. R&P Dorothy Kouwenberg. Circ: 1,270 (paid).

616.8 618.92 USA ISSN 0899-3653
INTERNATIONAL REVIEW OF CHILD NEUROLOGY SERIES. Text in English. 1982. irreg. price varies. reprint service avail. from PQC. *Refereed.* **Document type:** *Monographic series.*
Indexed: e-psyche.
Published by: Lippincott Williams & Wilkins (Philadelphia) (Subsidiary of: Wolters Kluwer N.V.), 530 Walnut St, Philadelphia, PA 19106-3621. TEL 301-223-2300, 800-638-3030, FAX 301-223-2400, http://www.lww.com.

616.8 USA ISSN 0074-7742
RC341 CODEN: IRNEAE
INTERNATIONAL REVIEW OF NEUROBIOLOGY. Text in English. 1959. irreg., latest vol.42, 1998. index. back issues avail.; reprint service avail. from ISI. *Refereed.* **Document type:** *Academic/Scholarly.*
Related titles: Online - full text ed.: (from Institute for Scientific Information).
Indexed: ASCA, Aqua.Sci.& Fish.Abstr., Biol.Abstr., Biotech.& Bioeng.Abstr., Chem.Abstr., Chem.Indus.Notes, Chem.Titles, Chemorec.Abstr., Dent.Ind., Excerp.Med., Ind.Med. (1959-), Ind.Sci.Rev., Neurosci.Abstr., Neurosci.Cit.Ind., Sci.Cit.Ind., e-psyche.
—BLDSC (4547.400000), CASDDS, CISTI, GNLM, ingenta, KNAW, Linda Hall. **CCC.**
Published by: Academic Press, Inc., Journal Division (Subsidiary of: Harcourt Brace & Company), 525 B St, Ste 1900, San Diego, CA 92101-4495. TEL 619-231-0926, FAX 619-699-6715. Eds. Carl C Pfeiffer, John R Smythies. **Subscr. to:** Order Dept., 6277 Sea Harbor Dr, 4th Fl, Orlando, FL 32887. TEL 800-321-5068.

616.8 GBR ISSN 0954-0261
CODEN: IRPSE2
INTERNATIONAL REVIEW OF PSYCHIATRY. Text in English. 1989. q. GBP 153, USD 278 to individuals; GBP 473, USD 849 to institutions (effective 2002). adv. bk.rev. *Refereed.* **Document type:** *Academic/Scholarly.* **Description:** Publishes undergraduate-level reviews of topics in psychiatry.
Related titles: Microfiche ed.; Online - full text ed.: ISSN 1369-1627 (from CatchWord Ltd., Northern Light Technology, Inc., EBSCO Publishing, O C L C Online Computer Library Center, Inc., RoweCom Information Quest, ProQuest Information & Learning, Swets Blackwell, Institute for Scientific Information).
Indexed: ASCA, ASSIA, Addic.Abstr., AgeLine, Crim.Just.Abstr., Curr.Cont., ERA, Excerp.Med. (1992-), Indian Psychol.Abstr., Lang.& Lang.Behav.Abstr., Mult.Ed.Abstr., Neurosci.Cit.Ind., PsycInfo, Psychol.Abstr. (1989-), SOPODA, SSCI, Sociol.Abstr., Sp.Ed.Needs Abstr., e-psyche.
—BLDSC (4547.515000), ADONIS, CatchWord (carfax), EMDOCS, GNLM, IDS, ingenta, KNAW. **CCC.**
Published by: Carfax Publishing Limited (Subsidiary of: Taylor & Francis Group), PO Box 25, Abingdon, Oxon OX14 3UE, United Kingdom. TEL 44-1235-401000, FAX 44-1235-401550, enquiries@carfax.co.uk, enquiry@tandf.co.uk, http://www.carfax.co.uk. Ed. Paul Bebbington.

371.928 USA ISSN 0074-7750
RC570
INTERNATIONAL REVIEW OF RESEARCH IN MENTAL RETARDATION. Text in English. 1966. irreg., latest vol.21, 1997. back issues avail.; reprint service avail. from ISI. *Refereed.*
Related titles: Online - full text ed.: (from Institute for Scientific Information).
Indexed: ASCA, SSCI, e-psyche.
—CISTI, ingenta. **CCC.**
Published by: Academic Press, Inc., Journal Division (Subsidiary of: Harcourt Brace & Company), 525 B St, Ste 1900, San Diego, CA 92101-4495. TEL 619-231-0926, FAX 619-699-6715. Eds. Norman R Ellis, Norman W Bray. **Subscr. to:** Order Dept., 6277 Sea Harbor Dr, 4th Fl, Orlando, FL 32887. TEL 800-321-5068.

616.8 USA
▼ **THE INTERNET JOURNAL OF NEUROLOGY.** Text in English. 2000. s-a. free per issue. adv. bk.rev. back issues avail. *Refereed.* **Document type:** *Academic/Scholarly.* **Description:** Provides information from the field of neurology; contains original articles, reviews, case reports, streaming slide shows, streaming videos, letters to the editor, press releases and meeting information.
Media: Online - full content.
Published by: Internet Scientific Publications, L.L.C., 23 Rippling Creek Dr, Sugar Land, TX 77479. TEL 281-240-1533, FAX 281-240-1533, http://www.ispub.com/. R&P, Adv. contact Hope Morrow TEL 832-754-0335.

▼ **THE INTERNET JOURNAL OF NEUROSURGERY.** see *MEDICAL SCIENCES—Surgery*

INTUITION; a magazine for the higher potential of the mind. see *NEW AGE PUBLICATIONS*

INVERTEBRATE NEUROBIOLOGY. see *BIOLOGY—Abstracting, Bibliographies, Statistics*

616.8 IRL ISSN 0790-1186
IRISH JOURNAL OF PSYCHIATRY. Text in English. s-a. IEP 2.
Indexed: Psychol.Abstr. (1986-), e-psyche.
—GNLM.
Published by: Irish Institute of Psychiatry, 73 Lower Baggot St., Dublin 2, Ireland. Ed. Dermot Walsh.

616.89 IRL ISSN 0790-9667
CODEN: IPMEEX
IRISH JOURNAL OF PSYCHOLOGICAL MEDICINE. Text in English. 1982. q. IEP 64, EUR 107 in the European Union; USD 105, IEP 74 elsewhere (effective 2001). adv. bk.rev. charts. reprint service avail. from PQC. *Refereed.* **Document type:** *Journal, Academic/Scholarly.* **Description:** Publishes original scientific contributions in psychiatry, psychological medicine, and related basic sciences (neurosciences, biological, psychological and social sciences).
Former titles: Irish Journal of Psychotherapy and Psychosomatic Medicine (0790-0848); Irish Journal of Psychotherapy
Related titles: Microform ed.: (from PQC); Online - full text ed.: (from Institute for Scientific Information).
Indexed: ASCA, Addic.Abstr., AgeLine, Biol.Abstr., CINAHL, Curr.Cont., Excerp.Med., I.P.A., Lang.& Lang.Behav.Abstr., Neurosci.Cit.Ind., Nutr.Abstr., PsycInfo, Psychol.Abstr. (1982-), Ref.Zh., SOPODA, SSCI, Soc.Work Res.& Abstr., Sociol.Abstr., e-psyche.
—BLDSC (4572.180000), ADONIS, EMDOCS, GNLM, IDS, Infotrieve, ingenta, KNAW. **CCC.**
Published by: (Irish Institute of Psychological Medicine), MedMedia Ltd., Media House, 25 Adelaide Street, Dun Laoghaire, Co. Dublin, Ireland. TEL 353-1-2803967, FAX 353-1-2807076, niamh@medmedia.ie, http://www.ijpm.org. Ed. Brian Lawlor. Adv. contact Niamh Gleeson TEL 353-1-28003967. B&W page IEP 790, color page IEP 1,080. Circ: 3,000. **Subscr. to:** Royal Society of Medicine Services Ltd., 1 Wimpole St, London W1G 0AE, United Kingdom. TEL 44-20-7290-2927, FAX 44-20-7290-2929.

616.8 ISR ISSN 0333-7308
RC321 CODEN: IPRDAH
ISRAEL JOURNAL OF PSYCHIATRY AND RELATED SCIENCES. Text in English. 1981. q. USD 75 (effective 2001). adv. bk.rev. charts, illus. index. back issues avail.; reprint service avail. from PQC. *Refereed.* **Document type:** *Academic/Scholarly.* **Description:** Articles dealing with the bio-psycho-social aspects of mobility, relocation, acculturation, ethnicity, stress situations in war and peace, victimology and mental health in developing countries.
Supersedes (1963-1979): Israel Annals of Psychiatry and Related Disciplines (0021-1958)
Related titles: Online - full text ed.: (from ProQuest Information & Learning, Institute for Scientific Information).
Indexed: AMED, ASCA, AgeLine, Biol.Abstr., Chem.Abstr., Child Devel.Abstr., Curr.Cont., Excerp.Med., Fam.Ind., Ind.Med. (1981-), PsycInfo, Psychol.Abstr. (1963-), SSCI, e-psyche.
—BLDSC (4583.813000), EMDOCS, GNLM, IDS, ingenta, KNAW.
Published by: (Israel Psychiatric Association USA), Gefen Publishing House Ltd., Box 6056, Jerusalem 91060, Israel. Ed. Dr. David Greenberg. Circ: 950.

ISSUES IN MENTAL HEALTH NURSING. see *MEDICAL SCIENCES—Nurses And Nursing*

371.92 ITA ISSN 1123-7708
ITALIAN JOURNAL OF INTELLECTIVE IMPAIRMENT/RIVISTA ITALIANA DEL DISTURBO INTELLETTIVO. Text in English, Italian. 1988. s-a. ITL 50,000; ITL 60,000 foreign (effective 1998). bk.rev. *Refereed.* **Document type:** *Newspaper.* **Description:** Covers all areas related to intellectual disabilities from medical, psychological and educational fields.
Indexed: PsycInfo, Psychol.Abstr. (1988-), e-psyche.
—BLDSC (4588.340500).
Published by: (Gruppo Italiano per lo Studio Scientifico e Terapia dell'Insufficienza Mentale, Mongolismo e Autismo Infantili), GISSTIMMAI Editore, Via Liberta 21, S. Costanza, PS 61039, Italy. TEL 39-721-950234, mc7057@mclink.it. Ed., R&P Dr. Renato Cocchi. Circ: 150 (paid).

M

616.8 ITA ISSN 1122-2247
THE ITALIAN JOURNAL OF PSYCHIATRY AND BEHAVIOURAL SCIENCES. Text in English. 1991. q. ITL 90,000; USD 150 foreign. **Description:** Publishes the contributions of Italian researchers.
Indexed: e-psyche.
—BLDSC (4588.341250).
Published by: (Societa Italiana di Psichiatria), Casa Editrice Idelson, Via Annibale De Gasperis, 55, Naples, NA 80137, Italy. TEL 39-81-5524733, FAX 39-81-5518295, idelgno@tin.it, http://www.idelson-gnocchi.com. Ed. Carlo Lorenzo Cazzullo.

616.857 USA
J A M A MIGRAINE NEWSLINE. (Journal of the American Medical Association) Text in English. 1998. w. back issues avail. *Refereed.*
Media: Online - full text.
Published by: American Medical Association, J A M A Information Centers, 515 N State St, Chicago, IL 60610. TEL 312-464-5000, 800-262-2350, FAX 312-464-4181, migraine@ama-assn.org, http://www.ama-assn.org/special/migraine/migraine.htm.

JAMES ARTHUR LECTURE ON THE EVOLUTION OF THE HUMAN BRAIN. see *BIOLOGY—Genetics*

616.89 JPN ISSN 0289-0968
JAPANESE JOURNAL OF CHILD & ADOLESCENT PSYCHIATRY/JIDO SEINEN SEISHIN IGAKU TO SONO KINSETSU RYOIKI. Text in Japanese; Summaries in English. 1960. 5/yr. USD 30 (effective 2000). adv. bk.rev. abstr, charts. index. back issues avail. **Document type:** *Academic/Scholarly.* **Description:** Addresses problems, issues, treatments, trends, and syndromes unique to child and adolescent psychology.
Formerly: Japanese Journal of Child Psychiatry (0021-4957)
Indexed: Child Devel.Abstr., Curr.Cont. (coverage dropped), PsycInfo, Psychol.Abstr. (1960-), SSCI (coverage dropped), e-psyche.
—BLDSC (4651.358000), CISTI, GNLM, ingenta.
Published by: Japanese Society for Child and Adolescent Psychiatry, c/o Department of Neuropsychiatry, School of Medicine, Kyoto University, Sakyo-ku, Kyoto-shi 606, Japan. Ed. Dr. Sadanobu Ushizima. R&P Dr. Yoshiki Ishikawa TEL 81-75-751-3388. Adv. contact Dr. Yoshiki Ishisaka. Circ: 2,000. **Subscr. to:** Maruzen Co, Ltd., Export Dept, PO Box 605, Tokyo Central, Tokyo, Japan.

616.8 DEU ISSN 1432-5144
JATROS NEURO. Text in German. 1985. m. DEM 140 (effective 1998). back issues avail. **Document type:** *Proceedings, Academic/Scholarly.* **Description:** Publishes seminar papers containing brief summaries of original articles, interviews and congress reports.
Former titles: Jatros Neurologie, Psychiatrie und Psychotherapie (0944-4068); Jatros Neurologie - Psychiatrie (0178-7535)
Indexed: e-psyche.
—GNLM.
Published by: Hoffmann und Hoffmann GmbH, August-Schanz-Str 8-II, Frankfurt A.m. 60433, Germany. TEL 49-69-54800015, FAX 49-69-54800080, huhgmbh@aol.com. Ed. Peter Hoffmann. Circ: 4,500.

616.89 BRA ISSN 0047-2085
CODEN: JBPSAX
JORNAL BRASILEIRO DE PSIQUIATRIA. Text in Portuguese; Summaries in English, Portuguese. 1942. m. BRL 102, USD 90 (effective 2000). adv. bk.rev. bibl, charts, illus, stat. index, cum.index. back issues avail. **Document type:** *Academic/Scholarly.* **Description:** Studies in clinical psychiatry.
Related titles: Microform ed.: (from PQC).
Indexed: Biol.Abstr., Chem.Abstr., Excerp.Med., Ind.Med. (coverage dropped), PsycInfo, Psychol.Abstr. (1964-), Ref.Zh., e-psyche.
—BLDSC (4674.680000), GNLM, KNAW.
Published by: (Universidade Federal do Rio de Janeiro, Instituto de Psiquiatria), E C N - Editora Cientifica Nacional Ltda., Rua da Gloria, 366 Andar 3, Gloria, Rio De Janeiro, RJ 20241-180, Brazil. TEL 55-21-2213235, FAX 55-21-2213235, ecn@rj.sol.com.br. Eds. Joao Romildo Bueno, Marcio Versiani. R&P, Adv. contact Maria Luiza Carvalho. Circ: 5,000.

616.89 FRA ISSN 1155-1704
JOURNAL DE THERAPIE COMPORTAMENTALE ET COGNITIVE. Text in English, French. q. FRF 560 domestic to individuals; FRF 640 foreign to individuals; FRF 730 domestic to institutions; FRF 845 foreign to institutions (effective 2000). adv. bk.rev. **Document type:** *Academic/Scholarly.* **Description:** Contains a clinical section with a didactical aspect, as well as international reports on advances in behavioural science and cognition.
Related titles: Online - full text ed.: (from RoweCom Information Quest).
Indexed: e-psyche.
Published by: (Association Francaise de Therapie Comportementale et Cognitive), Masson - Periodiques, 120 bd. St. Germain, Paris 75006, France. TEL 33-1-40466200, FAX 33-1-40466201. Ed. J Cottraux. Adv. contact Frederique Baudouin. Circ: 1,500. **Subscr. to:** Societe de Periodiques Specialises, BP 22, Vineuil Cedex 41354, France. TEL 33-2-54504612, FAX 33-2-54504611.

616.8 FRA ISSN 1260-5999
JOURNAL FRANCAIS DE PSYCHIATRIE. Text in French. 1995. q., latest vol.13. EUR 45 domestic; EUR 54 foreign (effective 2001). **Document type:** *Academic/Scholarly.* **Description:** Contains articles on psychiatry.
Published by: Editions Eres, 11 rue des Alouettes, Ramonville Saint-Agne 31520, France. TEL 33-05-61751576, FAX 33-05-61735289, eres@starway.tm.fr, eres@editions-eres.com. Eds. Charles Melman, Marcel Czermak.

616.8 AUT ISSN 1608-1587
▼ **JOURNAL FUER NEUROLOGIE, NEUROCHIRURGIE UND PSYCHIATRIE;** Zeitschrift fuer Erkrankungen des Nervensystems. Text in German. 2000. q. ATS 400 (effective 2001). adv. abstr, bibl. back issues avail. *Refereed.* **Document type:** *Journal, Academic/Scholarly.* **Description:** Contains research on all aspects of neurology, neurosurgery and psychiatry.
Published by: Krause & Pachernegg GmbH, Mozartgasse 10, Gablitz 3003, Austria. TEL 43-2231-61258-0, FAX 43-2231-6125810, k_u_p@eunet.at, http://members.eunet.at/k_u_p/neuro.htm, http://members.eunet.at/k_u_p/verlag.htm. Ed. Dr. Ivo Podreka.

JOURNAL OF ABNORMAL CHILD PSYCHOLOGY. see *PSYCHOLOGY*

616.8 NLD ISSN 0165-0327
CODEN: JADID7
JOURNAL OF AFFECTIVE DISORDERS. Text in Dutch. 1979. 15/yr. EUR 187 in Europe to individuals; JPY 25,000 in Japan to individuals; USD 209 elsewhere to individuals; EUR 1,885 in Europe to institutions; JPY 250,500 in Japan to institutions; USD 2,109 elsewhere to institutions (effective 2002). illus. back issues avail.; reprints avail. *Refereed.* **Document type:** *Academic/Scholarly.* **Description:** Publishes papers concerned with affective disorders in the widest sense: depression, mania, anxiety and panic.
Related titles: Microform ed.: (from PQC); Online - full text ed.: (from ingenta, Swets Blackwell, ScienceDirect, Institute for Scientific Information).
Indexed: ASCA, Addic.Abstr., Adol.Ment.Hlth.Abstr., AgeLine, Biol.Abstr., Chem.Abstr., Curr.Cont., Excerp.Med., Fam.Ind., Ind.Med. (1979-), Ind.Sci.Rev., Indian Psychol.Abstr., Inpharma, Int.Abstr.Biol.Sci., Jrnl.Watch Psych., Neurosci.Cit.Ind., Pharm.&Out.News, PsycInfo, Psychol.Abstr. (1979-), Reac., SSCI, Sci.Cit.Ind., e-psyche.
—BLDSC (4919.986000), ADONIS, CASDDS, CISTI, GNLM, IDS, ingenta, KNAW. **CCC.**
Published by: Elsevier Science BV, PO Box 211, Amsterdam 1000 AE, Netherlands. TEL 31-20-485-2911, FAX 31-20-485-2457, http://www.elsevier.com/locate/jad. Eds. E S Paykel, G Winokur. **Subscr. in Australasia and the Far East to:** Elsevier Science (Singapore) Pte Ltd, No.1 Temasek Ave, 17-01 Millenia Tower, Singapore 039192, Singapore. TEL 65-434-3727, FAX 65-337-2230; **Subscr. in Japan to:** Elsevier Science Inc - Japan Regional Office, 9-15 Higashi-Azabu 1-chome, Minato-ku, Tokyo 106-0044, Japan. TEL 81-3-5561-5033; **Subscr. in the Americas to:** Elsevier Science, PO Box 945, New York, NY 10159-0945. TEL 212-633-3730, FAX 212-633-3680, usinfo-f@elsevier.com.

616.8 NLD ISSN 1387-2877
CODEN: JADIF9
▼ **JOURNAL OF ALZHEIMER'S DISEASE.** Abbreviated title: J A D. Text in English. 1999. q. EUR 500, USD 450 to institutions (effective 2002). *Refereed.* **Document type:** *Journal, Academic/Scholarly.* **Description:** Focuses on providing timely information for the growing number of individuals and institutions active in research on and the treatment of Alzheimer's disease.
Related titles: Online - full text ed.: (from EBSCO Publishing, Swets Blackwell, RoweCom Information Quest).
Indexed: Neurosci.Abstr., e-psyche.
—BLDSC (4927.204000), CISTI.
Published by: I O S Press, Nieuwe Hemweg 6B, Amsterdam 1013 BG, Netherlands. TEL 31-20-688-3355, FAX 31-20-620-3419, market@iospress.nl, http://www.iospress.nl; http://j-alz.com. Ed. Dr. George Perry TEL 216-368-2488. **Subscr. to:** I O S Press, Inc, 5795-G Burke Centre Pkwy, Burke, VA 22015. TEL 703-323-5554, FAX 703-323-3668, iosbooks@iospress.com; Kinokuniya Company Ltd, Shinjuku 3-chome, Shinjuku-ku, Tokyo 160-0022, Japan; Globe Publication Pvt. Ltd., C-62 Inderpuri, New Delhi 100 012, India. TEL 91-11-579-3211, 91-11-579-3212, FAX 91-11-579-8876, custserve@globepub.com, http://www.globepub.com.

JOURNAL OF ANXIETY DISORDERS. see *PSYCHOLOGY*

616.858 GBR ISSN 1360-2322
JOURNAL OF APPLIED RESEARCH IN INTELLECTUAL DISABILITIES. Text in English. 1987. q., latest vol.15, 2002. GBP 48 in Europe to individuals; USD 77 in North America to individuals; GBP 53 elsewhere to individuals; GBP 122 in Europe to institutions; USD 195 in North America to institutions; GBP 135 elsewhere to institutions (effective 2002). adv. *Refereed.* **Document type:** *Academic/Scholarly.* **Description:** Applied research in learning disabilities undertaken in the U.K. and overseas from all professional disciplines.
Formerly (until 1995): Mental Handicap Research (0952-9608)
Related titles: Online - full text ed.: ISSN 1468-3148. GBP 44 in Europe to individuals; USD 70 in North America to individuals; GBP 44 elsewhere to individuals; GBP 110 in Europe to institutions; USD 176 in North America to institutions; GBP 110 elsewhere to institutions (effective 2002) (from EBSCO Publishing, O C L C Online Computer Library Center, Inc., ingenta, Munksgaard & Blackwell Science's Synergy, Swets Blackwell, Institute for Scientific Information).
Indexed: AMED, ASCA, AgeLine, Br.Educ.Ind., Curr.Cont., ERA, P C I, PsycInfo, Psychol.Abstr. (1988-), SSCI, Soc.Work Res.& Abstr., Sp.Ed.Needs Abstr., e-psyche.
—BLDSC (4947.046000), GNLM, IDS, Infotrieve. **CCC.**
Published by: Blackwell Science Ltd., PO Box 88, Oxford OX2 0NE, United Kingdom. TEL 44-1865-206180, 44-1865-206002, FAX 44-1865-206219, journals.cs@blacksci.co.uk, jnl.orders@blacksci.co.uk, http://www.blackwell-science.com/~cgilib/jnlpage.asp?Journal=jar&File=jar, http://www.blackwellpublishing.com. Eds. D Felce, G Murphy. Pub. Elaine Stott. R&P Sophie Savage. Adv. contact Jenny Applin. Circ: 800.

616.85889 371.93 USA ISSN 1087-0547
RJ506.H9
JOURNAL OF ATTENTION DISORDERS. Text in English. 1996. q. USD 45 domestic to individuals; USD 56 foreign to individuals; USD 95 domestic to institutions; USD 106 foreign to institutions (effective 2000). adv. bk.rev. *Refereed.* **Document type:** *Academic/Scholarly.*
Indexed: PsycInfo, e-psyche.
—BLDSC (4949.240000).
Published by: Multi-Health Systems, Inc., 908 Niagara Falls Blvd, North Tonawanda, NY 14120-2060. TEL 800-268-6011, 800-456-3003, jad@mhs.com, http://www.mhs.com/jad. Ed. C Keith Conners.

JOURNAL OF AUTISM AND DEVELOPMENTAL DISORDERS. see *EDUCATION—Special Education And Rehabilitation*

M

616.89 GBR ISSN 0005-7916
RC489.B4 CODEN: JBTEAB

THE JOURNAL OF BEHAVIOR THERAPY AND EXPERIMENTAL PSYCHIATRY; an interdisciplinary journal. Text in English. 1970. q. EUR 153 in Europe to qualified personnel; JPY 20,200 in Japan to qualified personnel; USD 170 elsewhere to qualified personnel; EUR 558 in Europe to institutions; JPY 74,100 in Japan to institutions; USD 624 elsewhere to institutions (effective 2002). adv. bk.rev. index. back issues avail.; reprint service avail. from PSC,SCH. *Refereed.* **Document type:** *Academic/Scholarly.* **Description:** Covers all aspects of behavior therapy and its applications in clinical psychiatry. Includes research articles, reviews, and case studies.

Related titles: Microfilm ed.: (from PQC); Online - full text ed.: (from ingenta, Swets Blackwell, ScienceDirect, Institute for Scientific Information).

Indexed: ASCA, ASSIA, Abstr.Crim.& Pen., Addic.Abstr., Adol.Ment.Hlth.Abstr., AgeLine, Behav.Med.Abstr., Biol.Abstr., CINAHL, Child Devel.Abstr., Curr.Cont., Excerp.Med., High.Educ.Abstr., Ind.Med. (1970-), Mid.East: Abstr.& Ind., PsycInfo, Psychol.Abstr. (1970-), Psycscan B.A.& T., SSCI, THA, e-psyche.

—BLDSC (4951.250000), CISTI, GNLM, IDS, ingenta, KNAW. **CCC.**

Published by: (Behavior Therapy and Research Society), Pergamon (Subsidiary of: Elsevier Science), The Boulevard, Langford Ln, East Park, Kidlington, Oxford OXB 1GB, United Kingdom. FAX 44-1865-843010, http://www.elsevier.nl/locate/jbtep. Eds. A Arntz, M van den Hout. adv.: B&W page USD 550, color page USD 1,350. Circ: 3,100. **Subscr. in Australasia and the Far East to:** Elsevier Science (Singapore) Pte Ltd, No.1 Temasek Ave, 17-01 Millenia Tower, Singapore 039192, Singapore. TEL 65-434-3727, FAX 65-337-2230; **Subscr. in the Americas to:** Elsevier Science, PO Box 945, New York, NY 10159-0945. TEL 212-633-3730, FAX 212-633-3680, usinfo-f@elsevier.com; **Subscr. to:** Elsevier Science BV, PO Box 211, Amsterdam 1000 AE, Netherlands. TEL 31-20-485-3757.

616.8 USA ISSN 0160-7715
R726.5 CODEN: JBMEDD

JOURNAL OF BEHAVIORAL MEDICINE. Text in English. 1978. bi-m. USD 74, EUR 74 to individuals for print or online ed.; USD 638, EUR 637 to institutions for print or online ed.; USD 765.60, EUR 764.40 to institutions for print & online eds. combined (effective 2002). adv. back issues avail. *Refereed.* **Document type:** *Journal, Academic/Scholarly.* **Description:** Furthers the understanding of physical health and illness through the techniques and knowledge of the behavioral sciences. Includes papers from a wide range of disciplines.

Related titles: Microfilm ed.: (from PQC); Online - full text ed.: (from CatchWord Ltd., Ovid Technologies, Inc., EBSCO Publishing, O C L C Online Computer Library Center, Inc., RoweCom Information Quest, Swets Blackwell, Kluwer Online, Institute for Scientific Information).

Indexed: ASCA, Addic.Abstr., Adol.Ment.Hlth.Abstr., AgeLine, Behav.Med.Abstr., Biol.Abstr., CINAHL, Curr.Cont., Dent.Ind., ERA, Excerp.Med., Fam.Ind., IMFL, Ind.Med. (1978-), Lang.& Lang.Behav.Abstr., Mult.Ed.Abstr., NRN, PsycInfo, Psychol.Abstr. (1979-), Psycscan C.P., Ref.Zh., SOPODA, SSCI, Soc.Work Res.& Abstr., Sociol.Abstr., THA, e-psyche.

—BLDSC (4951.262000), CatchWord, CISTI, GNLM, IDS, ingenta, KNAW. **CCC.**

Published by: Kluwer Academic - Plenum Publishers (Subsidiary of: Wolters Kluwer N.V.), 233 Spring St, New York, NY 10013-1578. TEL 212-620-8000, 800-221-9369, FAX 212-463-0742, info@plenum.com, http://www.wkap.nl/journalhome.htm/0160-7715. Ed. W Doyle Gentry. R&P Rose Luongo TEL 781-871-6311. **Subscr. outside the Americas to:** Kluwer Academic Publishers Group, Journals Department, PO Box 322, Dordrecht 3300 AH, Netherlands. TEL 31-78-639-2392, FAX 31-78-654-6474.

616.8 USA ISSN 0748-7304
QH527 CODEN: JBRHEE

JOURNAL OF BIOLOGICAL RHYTHMS. Abbreviated title: J B R. Text in English. 1985. bi-m. USD 130 to individuals; USD 550 domestic to institutions; USD 574 elsewhere to institutions (effective 2002). adv. bibl, charts, illus. index. 88 p./no. back issues avail.; reprint service avail. from PQC. *Refereed.* **Document type:** *Journal, Academic/Scholarly.* **Description:** Reports on nature and functions of biological rhythms, using genetic, biochemical, physiological behavioral, and modeling approaches.

Related titles: Online - full text ed.: (from EBSCO Publishing, O C L C Online Computer Library Center, Inc., RoweCom Information Quest, ProQuest Information & Learning, ingenta, Swets Blackwell, Institute for Scientific Information).

Indexed: ASCA, Agricola, Anim.Behav.Abstr., Aqua.Sci.& Fish.Abstr., Biol.Abstr., Curr.Cont., Ergon.Abstr., INSPEC (Mar.1995-), Ind.Med. (1986-), Inpharma, Int.Aerosp.Abstr., Neurosci.Abstr., Neurosci.Cit.Ind., PsycInfo, Psychol.Abstr. (1986-), Reac., Sci.Cit.Ind., Zoo.Rec., e-psyche.

—BLDSC (4953.260000), AskIEEE, CASDDS, CISTI, GNLM, IDS, ingenta, KNAW, Linda Hall. **CCC.**

Published by: (Society for Research on Biological Rhythms), Sage Publications, Inc., Sage Science Press, 2455 Teller Rd, Thousand Oaks, CA 91320. TEL 805-499-0721, FAX 805-499-0871, sagescience@sagepub.com, http://www.sagepub.co.uk/journals/details/j0234.html, http://www.sagesciencepress.com. Ed. Martin Zatz. Pub. Susan Hanscom. R&P Peter Marino. Adv. contact Robert Vrooman. **Overseas subscr. to:** Sage Publications Ltd., 6 Bonhill St, London EC2A 4PU, United Kingdom. info@sagepub.com; Sage Publications India Pvt. Ltd.

616.8 JPN ISSN 1341-5301
QP376 CODEN: JBSCF5

JOURNAL OF BRAIN SCIENCE. Text in English, Japanese. 1975. q. JPY 10,000. adv. back issues avail. **Description:** Promotes integrated, interdisciplinary studies of the interaction between the neural system and the behavior and homeostasis of the living body, as well as the mental activity of the human being.

Former titles (until Mar. 1996): Neurosciences - No Kenkyukai Kaishi (0388-7448); Joken Hansha (0368-2803)

Indexed: ASCA, Biol.Abstr., Chem.Abstr., Chem.Indus.Notes, Chem.Titles, INIS Atomind., Neurosci.Cit.Ind., e-psyche.

—BLDSC (4954.293000), CASDDS, GNLM, IDS, Infotrieve. **CCC.**

Published by: Japan Neurosciences Research Association/No Kenkyukai, c/o Japan Brain Science Society Business Office, Dept of Neurochemistry Institute for Neurobiology, University Medical School, 2-5-1 Shikata-Cho, Okayama-shi 700-0914, Japan. FAX 0862-23-3569. Ed. Koichi Ishikawa. Circ: 800. **Dist. in US by:** P J D Publications Ltd, PO Box 966, Westbury, NY 11590.

▼ **JOURNAL OF CANNABIS THERAPEUTICS**; studies in endogenous, herbal, and synthetic cannabinoids. see *ALTERNATIVE MEDICINE*

616.8 USA ISSN 0271-678X
QP108.5.C4 CODEN: JCBMDN

JOURNAL OF CEREBRAL BLOOD FLOW AND METABOLISM. Text in English. 1981. m. USD 490 domestic to individuals; USD 502 foreign to individuals; USD 823 domestic to institutions; USD 823 foreign to institutions; USD 61 newsstand/cover (effective 2002). adv. bk.rev. charts, illus. index. back issues avail.; reprint service avail. from PQC. *Refereed.* **Document type:** *Journal, Academic/Scholarly.* **Description:** Gathers experimental, theoretical, and clinical information on brain circulation and metabolism.

Related titles: Online - full text ed.: USD 1,069.90 domestic academic site license; USD 1,069.90 foreign academic site license; USD 1,193.35 domestic corporate site license; USD 1,193.35 foreign corporate site license (effective 2002) (from Ovid Technologies, Inc., Institute for Scientific Information).

Indexed: ASCA, BBCI, Biol.Abstr., Chem.Abstr., Chem.Indus.Notes, Chem.Titles, Curr.Cont., Excerp.Med., INIS Atomind., Ind.Med. (1981-), Ind.Sci.Rev., Inpharma, Int.Abstr.Biol.Sci., Neurosci.Abstr. (coverage dropped), Neurosci.Cit.Ind., Pharm.&Out.News, Reac., SSCI (coverage dropped), Sci.Cit.Ind., THA, e-psyche.

—BLDSC (4955.110000), CASDDS, CISTI, EMDOCS, GNLM, IDS, ingenta, KNAW.

Published by: (International Society of Cerebral Blood Flow and Metabolism), Lippincott Williams & Wilkins (Philadelphia) (Subsidiary of: Wolters Kluwer N.V.), 530 Walnut St, Philadelphia, PA 19106-3621. TEL 215-521-8300, FAX 215-521-8902, http://www.lww.com. Ed. James McCulloch. Pub. Nancy Megley. R&P Margaret Becker. Adv. contact Ray Thibodeau. B&W page USD 865, color page USD 2,075. Circ: 1,363. **Subscr. to:** PO Box 1600, Hagerstown, MD 21740-1600. TEL 800-777-2295, FAX 301-824-7390.

616.8 NLD ISSN 0891-0618
CODEN: JCNAEE

JOURNAL OF CHEMICAL NEUROANATOMY. Text in Dutch. 1988. 8/yr. EUR 883 in Europe to institutions; JPY 117,200 in Japan to institutions; USD 987 elsewhere to institutions (effective 2002). reprint service avail. from SWZ. *Refereed.* **Document type:** *Academic/Scholarly.* **Description:** Publishes scientific reports relating to the functional and biochemical aspects of the nervous system, with emphasis on microanatomical organization.

Related titles: Microform ed.: (from PQC); Online - full text ed.: (from ingenta, Swets Blackwell, ScienceDirect, Institute for Scientific Information).

Indexed: ASCA, Aqua.Sci.& Fish.Abstr., BBCI, Chem.Abstr., Chem.Indus.Notes, Chem.Titles, Chemorec.Abstr., Curr.Adv.Cell & Devel.Biol., Curr.Cont., Excerp.Med., Ind.Med. (1988-), Ind.Sci.Rev., Inpharma, Int.Abstr.Biol.Sci., Neurosci.Abstr., Neurosci.Cit.Ind., Reac., Sci.Cit.Ind., Zoo.Rec., e-psyche.

—BLDSC (4956.850000), ADONIS, CASDDS, CISTI, EMDOCS, GNLM, IDS, ingenta. **CCC.**

Published by: Elsevier Science BV, PO Box 211, Amsterdam 1000 AE, Netherlands. TEL 31-20-485-2911, FAX 31-20-485-2457, http://www.elsevier.nl/locate/jchemneu. Eds. H W M Steinbusch, Hiroshi Kimura. **Subscr. in Australasia and the Far East to:** Elsevier Science (Singapore) Pte Ltd, No.1 Temasek Ave, 17-01 Millenia Tower, Singapore 039192, Singapore. TEL 65-434-3727, FAX 65-337-2230; **Subscr. in Japan to:** Elsevier Science Inc - Japan Regional Office, 9-15 Higashi-Azabu 1-chome, Minato-ku, Tokyo 106-0044, Japan. TEL 81-3-5561-5033; **Subscr. in the Americas to:** Elsevier Science, PO Box 945, New York, NY 10159-0945. TEL 212-633-3730, FAX 212-633-3680, usinfo-f@elsevier.com.

JOURNAL OF CHILD AND ADOLESCENT PSYCHIATRIC NURSING. see *MEDICAL SCIENCES—Nurses And Nursing*

616.8 USA ISSN 1044-5463
CODEN: JADPET

JOURNAL OF CHILD AND ADOLESCENT PSYCHOPHARMACOLOGY. Text in English. 1990. q. USD 222 domestic; USD 295 foreign; USD 266 domestic print and online eds. combined; USD 340 foreign print and online eds. combined (effective 2002). back issues avail.; reprints avail. *Refereed.* **Document type:** *Journal, Academic/Scholarly.* **Description:** Emphasizes the clinical aspects of psychotropic therapy. Includes the biological and biomedical aspects of psychiatry, behavioral aspects of pediatrics and child neurology, and the developmental aspects of the neurosciences and medicines.

Related titles: Online - full content ed.: USD 222 (effective 2002); Online - full text ed.: (from CatchWord Ltd., Institute for Scientific Information, RoweCom Information Quest).

Indexed: ASCA, Curr.Cont., Excerp.Med. (1994-), Focus on: Psychophar., Ind.Med. (1990-), Inpharma, Jrnl.Watch Psych., Pharm.&Out.News, PsycInfo, Psychol.Abstr. (1990-), Reac., Sci.Cit.Ind., e-psyche.

—BLDSC (4957.424000), CatchWord, EMDOCS, GNLM, IDS, Infotrieve, KNAW. **CCC.**

Published by: Mary Ann Liebert, Inc. Publishers, 2 Madison Ave, Larchmont, NY 10538. TEL 914—834-3100, FAX 914-834-1388, info@liebertpub.com, http://www.liebertpub.com/cap. Eds. Dr. Harold S Kopelwicz, Dr. Wayne Hugo Green.

616.8 618.92 CAN ISSN 0883-0738
CODEN: JOCNEE

JOURNAL OF CHILD NEUROLOGY. Text in English. 1985. 12/yr. USD 209 in US & Canada to individuals; USD 260 elsewhere to individuals; USD 319 in US & Canada to institutions; USD 369 elsewhere to institutions (effective 2001). back issues avail. *Refereed.* **Document type:** *Journal, Academic/Scholarly.* **Description:** Covers all aspects of nervous system disorders in children, including medical, surgical, pathological, and psychological perspectives.

Related titles: CD-ROM ed.; Online - full text ed.: (from Northern Light Technology, Inc., ProQuest Information & Learning, Institute for Scientific Information).

Indexed: ASCA, Curr.Cont., Excerp.Med., INIS Atomind., Ind.Med. (1986-), Ind.Sci.Rev., Inpharma, Jrnl.Watch Neuro., Neurosci.Cit.Ind., Nutr.Abstr., Pharm.&Out.News, PsycInfo, Psychol.Abstr. (1986-), Reac., Rev.Med.& Vet.Mycol., SSCI (coverage dropped), Sci.Cit.Ind., Trop.Dis.Bull., e-psyche.

—BLDSC (4957.625000), EMDOCS, GNLM, IDS, ingenta, KNAW. **CCC.**

M

Published by: B.C. Decker Inc., 20 Hughson St S, LCD 1, P O Box 620, Hamilton, ON L8N 3K7, Canada. TEL 905-522-7017, 800-568-7281, FAX 905-522-7839, info@bcdecker.com, http://www.bcdecker.com. Ed. Roger A Brumback. Pub. David LeGallais. R&P Paula Presutti. Adv. contact John Birkby. Circ: 2,000.

JOURNAL OF CHILD PSYCHOLOGY & PSYCHIATRY & ALLIED DISCIPLINES. see *PSYCHOLOGY*

▼ **JOURNAL OF CLINICAL ACTIVITIES, ASSIGNMENTS & HANDOUTS IN PSYCHOTHERAPY PRACTICE**; innovations in resources for treatment & intervention. see *PSYCHOLOGY*

616.8 USA ISSN 0736-0258

JOURNAL OF CLINICAL NEUROPHYSIOLOGY. Text in English. 1984. bi-m. USD 262 domestic to individuals; USD 326 foreign to individuals; USD 523 domestic to institutions; USD 598 foreign to institutions; USD 92 newsstand/cover (effective 2002). adv. bk.rev. charts, illus. index. reprint service avail. from PQC. *Refereed.* **Document type:** *Journal, Academic/Scholarly.* **Description:** Covers clinical neurology, neurosurgery, psychiatry, electroencephalography and evoked potentials, and experimental research of the central nervous system.

Related titles: Online - full text ed.: USD 679.90 domestic academic site license; USD 754.90 foreign academic site license; USD 758.35 domestic corporate site license; USD 833.35 foreign corporate site license (effective 2002) (from Ovid Technologies, Inc., Institute for Scientific Information).

Indexed: ASCA, Bibl.Dev.Med.& Child Neur., CINAHL, Curr.Cont., Excerp.Med., Ind.Med. (1984-), Ind.Sci.Rev., Inpharma, Int.Abstr.Biol.Sci., Neurosci.Abstr. (coverage dropped), Neurosci.Cit.Ind., Pharm.&Out.News, Psychol.Abstr., Reac., SSCI (coverage dropped), Sci.Cit.Ind. (coverage dropped), e-psyche.

—BLDSC (4958.578000), CISTI, EMDOCS, GNLM, IDS, ingenta, KNAW.

Published by: (American Electroencephalographic Society), Lippincott Williams & Wilkins (Philadelphia) (Subsidiary of: Wolters Kluwer N.V.), 530 Walnut St, Philadelphia, PA 19106-3621. TEL 215-521-8300, FAX 215-521-8902, http://www.lww.com. Ed. Dr. John S Ebersole. Pub. Nancy Megley. R&P Margaret Becker. Adv. contact Ray Thibodeau. B&W page USD 1,000, color page USD 2,324. Circ: 3,003 (paid). **Subscr. to:** PO Box 1600, Hagerstown, MD 21740-1600. TEL 800-777-2295, FAX 301-824-7390.

616.8 GBR ISSN 0967-5868
QP351 CODEN: PANUBL

JOURNAL OF CLINICAL NEUROSCIENCE. Text in English. 1963; N.S. 1994. bi-m. GBP 179 to individuals; GBP 308 to institutions (effective 2002). adv. bk.rev. *Refereed.* **Document type:** *Academic/Scholarly.* **Description:** Articles on clinical neurosurgery and neurology and associated neurosciences.

Former titles (until vol.31, 1994): Clinical and Experimental Neurology (0196-6383); Australian Association of Neurologists Proceedings (0084-7224)

Related titles: Microfilm ed.: N.S. (from PQC); Online - full text ed.: (from EBSCO Publishing, O C L C Online Computer Library Center, Inc., Swets Blackwell, IDEAL Online Library, Institute for Scientific Information).

Indexed: ASCA, Chem.Abstr., Chem.Indus.Notes, Chem.Titles, Curr.Cont. (coverage dropped), Excerp.Med., Helminthol.Abstr., Ind.Med. (1994-), Inpharma, Neurosci.Cit.Ind., Pharm.&Out.News, Reac., Ref.Zh., e-psyche.

—BLDSC (4958.585000), CASDDS, CISTI, GNLM, IDS, Infotrieve, ingenta, KNAW. **CCC.**

Published by: Churchill Livingstone (Subsidiary of: Harcourt Publishers Ltd.), Robert Stevenson House, 1-3 Baxter's Pl, Leith Walk, Edinburgh, Midlothian EH1 3AF, United Kingdom. TEL 44-131-556-2424, FAX 44-131-535-1704, cservice@harcourt.com, http://www.harcourt-international.com/journals/jocn. Ed. Andrew Kaye. Pub. Gillian Griffith. R&P Catherine John TEL 212-424-4200. Adv. contact David Dunnachie. Circ: 800. **Subscr. to:** Harcourt Publishers Ltd., Foots Cray High St, Sidcup, Kent DA14 5HP, United Kingdom. TEL 44-20-8308-5700, FAX 44-20-8309-0807. **Co-sponsors:** Australian Association of Neurologists; Australian and New Zealand Society for Neuropathology; Swiss Society of Neurosurgery.

616.8 USA ISSN 0160-6689
RC321 CODEN: JCLPDE

JOURNAL OF CLINICAL PSYCHIATRY. Text in English. 1940. bi-m. USD 77 domestic to individuals; USD 120 foreign to individuals; USD 97 domestic to institutions; USD 132 foreign to institutions; USD 55 to students (effective 2001). adv. bk.rev. charts, illus, stat. index. Supplement avail.; back issues avail.; reprint service avail. from PQC. *Refereed.* **Document type:** *Proceedings, Academic/Scholarly.* **Description:** Presents original material in the psychiatric, behavioral, and neural sciences, with special emphasis on papers dealing with practical and clinical subjects.

Formerly (until 1978): Diseases of the Nervous System (0012-3714)

Related titles: Microfilm ed.: (from PQC); Online - full text ed.: (from Northern Light Technology, Inc., ProQuest Information & Learning, Institute for Scientific Information).

Indexed: ASCA, ASSIA, Addic.Abstr., Adol.Ment.Hlth.Abstr., AgeLine, Agri.& Environ.Biotech.Abstr. (coverage dropped), Behav.Med.Abstr., Biol.Abstr., C.I.J.E. (coverage dropped), CINAHL, Chem.Abstr., Chem.Indus.Notes, Chem.Titles, Curr.Cont., Curr.Lit.Fam.Plan., Dairy Sci.Abstr., Dent.Ind., Derwent Biotech.Abstr., Environ.Sci.Poll.Mgmt., Excerp.Med., Fam.Ind., HRIS, IMFL, INIS Atomind., Ind.Med. (1978-), Ind.Sci.Rev., Inpharma, Int.Nurs.Ind., Jrnl.Watch Psych., Lang.& Lang.Behav.Abstr., Neurosci.Cit.Ind., Nutr.Abstr., Pharm.&Out.News, Pollut.Abstr., PsycInfo, Psychol.Abstr. (1940-), Reac., Risk Abstr., SSCI, Saf.Sci.Abstr., Sci.Cit.Ind., e-psyche.

—BLDSC (4958.688000), CASDDS, CISTI, GNLM, IDS, ingenta, KNAW. **CCC.**

Published by: Physicians Postgraduate Press, Inc., PO Box 752870, Memphis, TN 38175-2870. TEL 901-751-3800, FAX 901-751-3444, http://www.allenpress.com, http://www.psychiatrist.com. Eds. Dr. Alan J Gelenberg, John S Shelton. Pub. Irving R Shelton. Adv. contact John S Shelton. Circ: 33,000. **Subscr. to:** Allen Press Inc., PO Box 1897, Lawrence, KS 66044-8897.

616.89 USA ISSN 0742-1915

JOURNAL OF CLINICAL PSYCHIATRY MONOGRAPH SERIES. Text in English. 1984. irreg.

Indexed: PsycInfo, e-psyche.

—CISTI, GNLM, ingenta, KNAW. **CCC.**

Published by: Physicians Postgraduate Press, Inc., PO Box 752870, Memphis, TN 38175-2870. TEL 901-751-3800, FAX 901-751-3444.

612.8 153 006.3 USA ISSN 0898-929X
QP360 CODEN: JCONEO

JOURNAL OF COGNITIVE NEUROSCIENCE. Text in English. 1989. 8/yr. USD 80 in US & Canada to individuals; USD 350 in US & Canada to institutions; USD 116 elsewhere to individuals; USD 386 elsewhere to institutions (effective 2001). illus. back issues avail.; reprint service avail. from PQC. *Refereed.* **Document type:** *Academic/Scholarly.* **Description:** Provides a forum for research involving the interaction of brain and behavior. Devoted to the field of cognitive neuroscience.

Related titles: Online - full text ed.: ISSN 1530-8898. USD 77 in US & Canada to individuals; USD 315 in US & Canada to institutions (effective 2001) (from CatchWord Ltd., EBSCO Publishing, O C L C Online Computer Library Center, Inc., RoweCom Information Quest, Gale Group, Swets Blackwell, Factiva, Institute for Scientific Information).

Indexed: A.I.Abstr., ASCA, Aqua.Sci.& Fish.Abstr., Comput.Abstr., Curr.Cont., Eng.Ind., INSPEC, Ind.Med. (1989-), Ind.Sci.Rev., Inpharma, Int.Abstr.Biol.Sci., Lang.& Lang.Behav.Abstr., Neurosci.Abstr., Neurosci.Cit.Ind., Pharm.&Out.News, PsycInfo, Psychol.Abstr. (1989-), Reac., SOPODA, SSCI, Sci.Cit.Ind., Sociol.Abstr., e-psyche.

—BLDSC (4958.798500), ADONIS, CatchWord, Ei, GNLM, IDS, ingenta, KNAW.

Published by: (Cognitive Neuroscience Institute), M I T Press, 5 Cambridge Center, Cambridge, MA 02142-1407. TEL 617-253-2866, FAX 617-577-1545, journals-orders@mit.edu, http://mitpress.mit.edu/JOCN. Ed. Michael S Gazzaniga. Circ: 1,200.

JOURNAL OF COGNITIVE REHABILITATION; a publication for the therapist, family and patient. see *MEDICAL SCIENCES—Physical Medicine And Rehabilitation*

JOURNAL OF COMMUNICATION DISORDERS. see *PSYCHOLOGY*

616.8 USA ISSN 0021-9967
QL1 CODEN: JCNEAM

THE JOURNAL OF COMPARATIVE NEUROLOGY. Text in English. 1891. 52/yr. USD 16,995 in United States; USD 17,515 in Canada & Mexico; USD 17,957 elsewhere; USD 17,845 combined subscription in United States for print and online eds.; USD 18,365 combined subscription in Canada & Mexico for print and online eds.; USD 18,807 combined subscription elsewhere for print and online eds. (effective 2002). adv. abstr, bibl, charts, illus. index. back issues avail.; reprint service avail. from SWZ. *Refereed.* **Document type:** *Academic/Scholarly.* **Description:** Presents original articles about the anatomy and physiology of the nervous system, especially with regard to its structure, growth and function.

Related titles: Microfiche ed.: (from BHP,PMC,SWZ); Microform ed.: (from PQC); Online - full text ed.: ISSN 1096-9861. 1996. USD 16,995 in United States; USD 16,995 in Canada & Mexico; USD 16,995 elsewhere (effective 2002) (from EBSCO Publishing, Wiley InterScience, Institute for Scientific Information).

Indexed: ASCA, Apic.Abstr., Aqua.Sci.& Fish.Abstr., Biol.Abstr., Cal.Tiss.Abstr. (coverage dropped), Chem.Abstr., Chem.Indus.Notes, Chem.Titles, Chemorec.Abstr., Curr.Adv.Cell & Devel.Biol., Curr.Cont., Curr.Ref.Fish Res., Dent.Ind., Entomol.Abstr. (coverage dropped), Excerp.Med., Focus on: Vet.Sci.& Med., Helminthol.Abstr., INIS Atomind., Ind.Med. (1891-), Ind.Sci.Rev., Ind.Vet., Inpharma, Int.Abstr.Biol.Sci., Neurosci.Abstr., Neurosci.Cit.Ind., Poult.Abstr., Protozool.Abstr., Reac., Ref.Zh., Rev.Appl.Entomol., Sci.Cit.Ind., Small Anim.Abstr., Sport Fish.Abstr., Tox.Abstr. (coverage dropped), Vet.Bull., Wild.Rev., Zoo.Rec., e-psyche.

—BLDSC (4962.000000), CASDDS, CISTI, GNLM, IDS, ingenta, Linda Hall. **CCC.**

Published by: John Wiley & Sons, Inc., Journals (Subsidiary of: Wiley InterScience), 605 Third Ave, New York, NY 10158. TEL 212-850-6645, FAX 212-850-6021, subinfo@wiley.com, uscs-wis@wiley.com, http://www.wiley.com. Ed. Sanford L Palay. adv.: B&W page GBP 640, color page GBP 1,515; trim 210 x 279. Circ: 950. **Subscr. outside the Americas to:** John Wiley & Sons Ltd., Baffins Ln, Chichester, Sussex PO19 IUD, United Kingdom. TEL 44-1243-779777, FAX 44-1243-843232, cs-journals@wiley.co.uk, http://www.wiley.co.uk.

JOURNAL OF COMPARATIVE PHYSIOLOGY. A: SENSORY, NEURAL, AND BEHAVIORAL PHYSIOLOGY. see *BIOLOGY—Physiology*

006.32 USA ISSN 0929-5313
QP356 CODEN: JCNEFR

JOURNAL OF COMPUTATIONAL NEUROSCIENCE. Text in English. 1994. bi-m. USD 545, EUR 544 to institutions for print or online ed.; USD 654, EUR 652.80 to institutions for print & online eds.combined (effective 2002). adv. back issues avail.; reprint service avail. from SWZ. *Refereed.* **Document type:** *Journal, Academic/Scholarly.* **Description:** Publishes original papers describing theoretical and experimental work relevant to computations in the brain and nervous system.

Related titles: Online - full text ed.: (from EBSCO Publishing, O C L C Online Computer Library Center, Inc., RoweCom Information Quest, Swets Blackwell, Kluwer Online, Institute for Scientific Information).

Indexed: ASCA, Compumath, Curr.Cont., Excerp.Med. (1996-), INSPEC (Mar.1996-), Ind.Med. (1994-), Inpharma, Int.Abstr.Biol.Sci., Neurosci.Abstr., Neurosci.Cit.Ind., PsycInfo, Reac., Sci.Cit.Ind., Zent.Math., e-psyche.

—BLDSC (4963.490000), AskIEEE, CISTI, EMDOCS, GNLM, IDS, KNAW. **CCC.**

Published by: Kluwer Academic Publishers Boston, 101 Philip Dr, Assinippi Park, Norwell, MA 02061. TEL 781-871-6600, FAX 781-871-9045, services@wkap.nl, http://www.wkap.nl/journalhome.htm/0929-5313. **Subscr. outside the Americas to:** Kluwer Academic Publishers Group, Journals Department, PO Box 322, Dordrecht 3300 AH, Netherlands. TEL 31-78-639-2392, FAX 31-78-654-6474; **Subscr. to:** Kluwer Academic - Plenum Publishers, 233 Spring St, New York, NY 10013-1578. TEL 212-620-8468, FAX 212-807-1047.

JOURNAL OF CONSULTING AND CLINICAL PSYCHOLOGY. see *PSYCHOLOGY*

616.8914 USA ISSN 0894-8577
RC489.E93
JOURNAL OF CONTEMPLATIVE PSYCHOTHERAPY. Text in English. 1980. 2/yr. USD 15 to individuals; USD 25 to institutions. bk.rev. back issues avail. *Refereed.* **Document type:** *Academic/Scholarly.* **Description:** Publishes articles exploring the clinical application of contemplative disciplines in the practice of psychotherapy.
Formerly: Naropa Institute Journal of Psychology (0271-7557)
Indexed: Psychol.Abstr., e-psyche.
Published by: Naropa Institute, 2130 Arapahoe Ave, Boulder, CO 80302. TEL 303-444-0202. Ed., R&P Ms. Max Regan. Circ: 3,000.

JOURNAL OF CONTEMPORARY PSYCHOTHERAPY. see *PSYCHOLOGY*

618.97 GBR ISSN 1351-8372
THE JOURNAL OF DEMENTIA CARE; for all who work with people with dementia. Text in English. 1993. bi-m. GBP 55 domestic; GBP 25 to students; GBP 72 in Europe; GBP 98 rest of world (effective 2001). adv. *Refereed.* **Document type:** *Academic/Scholarly.* **Description:** Provides practical information, research, and networking for professionals working with people with dementia.
Indexed: Brit.Nur.Ind., e-psyche.
—BLDSC (4968.230000).
Published by: Hawker Publications Ltd., Culvert House, Culvert Rd, London SW11 5AP, United Kingdom. TEL 44-20-7720-2108, FAX 44-20-7498-3023, hawker@hawkerpubs.demon.co.uk, http://www.careinfo.org/. Ed. Sue Benson. Circ: 3,000. **Subscr. to:** ESCO Business Services, Vicarage Rd, Finchley Field, Robjohns Farm, Finchingfield, Braintree, Essex CM7 4LJ, United Kingdom. FAX 44-1371-811065.

616.8 ZAF ISSN 1560-0181
JOURNAL OF DEPRESSION AND ANXIETY. Text in English. 1998. q. USD 60 in United States (effective 2001). reprints avail. *Refereed.* **Document type:** *Journal, Academic/Scholarly.*
Published by: In House Publications, PO Box 412748, Craighall, Johannesburg 2024, South Africa. TEL 27-11-4429759, FAX 27-11-8807898, inhouse@iafrica.com, http://www.inhousepub.co.za. Eds. C P Szabo, M Berk. Pub., R&P A. Thomas. Adv. contact A Thomas. Circ: 2,000.

616.8 USA ISSN 1095-0680
CODEN: COTHE4
THE JOURNAL OF ELECTROCONVULSIVE THERAPY. Short title: E C T. Text in English. 1985. q. USD 207 domestic to individuals; USD 261 foreign to individuals; USD 442 domestic to institutions; USD 510 foreign to institutions; USD 115 newsstand/cover (effective 2002). adv. bk.rev. charts, illus. index. back issues avail.; reprint service avail. from PQC. *Refereed.* **Document type:** *Journal, Academic/Scholarly.* **Description:** Reports on major clinical and research advances worldwide on the the effects of electroconvulsive therapy, mode of seizure induction, and ethical issues.
Formerly (until 1998): Convulsive Therapy (0749-8055)
Related titles: Online - full text ed.: USD 574.60 domestic academic site license; USD 642.60 foreign academic site license; USD 640.90 domestic corporate site license; USD 708.90 foreign corporate site license (effective 2002) (from Ovid Technologies, Inc., Institute for Scientific Information).
Indexed: ASCA, Curr.Cont., Excerp.Med., Fam.Ind., Ind.Med. (1998-), Indian Psychol.Abstr., Inpharma, Jrnl.Watch Psych., Neurosci.Cit.Ind., Pharm.&Out.News, PsycInfo, Psychol.Abstr. (1988-), Reac., SSCI, e-psyche.
—BLDSC (4973.095900), CISTI, EMDOCS, GNLM, IDS, KNAW.
Published by: Lippincott Williams & Wilkins (Philadelphia) (Subsidiary of: Wolters Kluwer N.V.), 530 Walnut St, Philadelphia, PA 19106-3621. TEL 215-521-8300, FAX 215-521-8902, http://www.lww.com. Ed. Dr. Charles Horn Kellner. Pub. Maria McMichael. R&P Margaret Becker. Adv. contact Ray Thibodeau. B&W page USD 750, color page USD 1,830. Circ: 754 (paid). **Subscr. to:** PO Box 1600, Hagerstown, MD 21740-1600. TEL 800-777-2295, FAX 301-824-7390.

JOURNAL OF ELECTROPHYSIOLOGICAL TECHNOLOGY. see *BIOLOGY—Physiology*

616.89 USA ISSN 1063-4266
RJ499.A1 CODEN: JEBDFC
JOURNAL OF EMOTIONAL AND BEHAVIORAL DISORDERS. Short title: J E B D. Text in English. 1993. q. USD 43 in North America to individuals; USD 71 elsewhere to individuals; USD 109 in North America to institutions; USD 138 elsewhere to institutions (effective 2002). adv. bibl, illus. 64 p./no. back issues avail. *Refereed.* **Document type:** *Journal, Academic/Scholarly.* **Description:** Covers the diagnosis and treatment of emotional and behavioral disorders of young people, from the research and practice perspectives.
Related titles: Microfilm ed.: (from PQC); Online - full text ed.: (from ProQuest Information & Learning, Institute for Scientific Information, CatchWord Ltd.).
Indexed: ASCA, ASSIA, C.I.J.E., Crim.Just.Abstr., Curr.Cont., ERA, Except.Child Educ.Abstr., Fam.Ind., IBZ, Ind.Philos., Inpharma, Lang.& Lang.Behav.Abstr., Pharm.&Out.News, PsycInfo, Psychol.Abstr. (1993-), Reac., SOPODA, SSCI, Sociol.Abstr., Sp.Ed.Needs Abstr., e-psyche.
—BLDSC (4977.470000), IDS, Infotrieve, ingenta. **CCC.**
Published by: Pro-Ed Inc., 8700 Shoal Creek Blvd, Austin, TX 78757-6897. TEL 512-451-3246, FAX 512-302-9129, proed1@aol.com, http://www.proedinc.com. Eds. Douglas Cullinan, Michael H Epstein. Pub. Donald D Hammill. adv.: B&W page USD 400. Circ: 1,100 (paid and free).

JOURNAL OF ESTHETIC AND RESTORATIVE DENTISTRY. see *MEDICAL SCIENCES—Dentistry*

JOURNAL OF FAMILY PSYCHOTHERAPY; the official journal of the International Family Therapy Association. see *PSYCHOLOGY*

306.85 GBR ISSN 0163-4445
RC488.5
JOURNAL OF FAMILY THERAPY. Text in English. 1979. q. GBP 146 to institutions in UK & Europe; USD 230 to institutions in the Americas & Caribbean; GBP 160 elsewhere to institutions (effective 2002). adv. bk.rev. illus. index. back issues avail.; reprints avail. *Refereed.* **Document type:** *Academic/Scholarly.*
Related titles: Online - full text ed.: (from EBSCO Publishing, O C L C Online Computer Library Center, Inc., RoweCom Information Quest, ingenta, Swets Blackwell, Institute for Scientific Information).
Indexed: ASCA, ASSIA, AgeLine, C.I.J.E. (coverage dropped), Curr.Cont., ERA, Environ.Sci.Poll.Mgmt., Fam.Ind., IMFL, Lang.& Lang.Behav.Abstr., Pollut.Abstr., PsycInfo, Psychol.Abstr. (1980-), Risk Abstr., SOPODA, SSCI, Saf.Sci.Abstr., Sage Fam.Stud.Abstr., Soc.Serv.Abstr., Sociol.Abstr., Stud.Wom.Abstr., e-psyche.
—BLDSC (4983.740000), GNLM, IDS, ingenta. **CCC.**
Published by: (Association of Family Therapy), Blackwell Publishers Ltd., 108 Cowley Rd, Oxford OX4 1JF, United Kingdom. TEL 44-1865-791100, FAX 44-1865-791347, jnlinfo@blackwellpublishers.co.uk, http://www.blackwellpublishers.co.uk. Ed. Eddy Street TEL 44-1222-715593. Circ: 2,500.

616.8 USA ISSN 1521-1029
JOURNAL OF FORENSIC NEUROPSYCHOLOGY. Text in English. 1998. q. USD 60 to individuals; USD 81 in Canada to individuals; USD 87 elsewhere to individuals; USD 75 to institutions; USD 101 in Canada to institutions; USD 109 elsewhere to institutions; USD 90 to libraries; USD 122 in Canada to libraries; USD 131 elsewhere to libraries (effective Aug. 2001). adv. *Refereed.* **Document type:** *Journal, Academic/Scholarly.* **Description:** Promotes the appropriate use of clinical neuropsychology in the forensic forum.
Indexed: IBZ, Ref.Zh., e-psyche.
—BLDSC (4984.592500), Haworth.
Published by: (Neuropsychology Center, Dallas), Haworth Press, Inc., 10 Alice St, Binghamton, NY 13904-1580. TEL 607-722-5857, 800-429-6784, FAX 607-722-6362, 800-895-0582, getinfo@haworthpressinc.com; jhom@neuropsych.com, http://www.haworthpress.com/journals/journallist.asp. Ed. Jim Hom. Pub. William Cohen. R&P Ruthann Heath TEL 607-723-5857 ext 316. Adv. contact Jackie Blakeslee TEL 607-722-5857 ext 346. B&W page USD 375, color page USD 650; trim 6 x 8.5.

616.89 614 GBR ISSN 0958-5184
JOURNAL OF FORENSIC PSYCHIATRY. Text in English. 1990. 3/yr. GBP 52, USD 78 to individuals; GBP 206, USD 340 to institutions (effective 2002). adv. *Refereed.* **Document type:** *Academic/Scholarly.* **Description:** Forum for professionals working with the legal aspects of psychiatry and psychology.
Related titles: Online - full text ed.: ISSN 1469-9478 (from CatchWord Ltd., EBSCO Publishing, O C L C Online Computer Library Center, Inc., RoweCom Information Quest, Swets Blackwell, Institute for Scientific Information).
Indexed: ASCA, ASSIA, AgeLine, Biol.Dig., Crim.Just.Abstr., Curr.Cont., Excerp.Med. (1996-), Intl.Bibl.Soc.Sci., PsycInfo, SSCI, e-psyche.
—BLDSC (4984.597000), CatchWord, GNLM, IDS, Infotrieve, KNAW. **CCC.**
Published by: Routledge (Subsidiary of: Taylor & Francis Group), 11 New Fetter Ln, London EC4P 4EE, United Kingdom. TEL 44-207-842-2001, FAX 44-20-7842-2298, journals@routledge.com, http://www.routledge.com/routledge/journal/journals.html. Eds. Alec Bucanan, Paul Bowden. R&P Sally Sweet. adv.: page GBP 175; trim 190 x 115. Circ: 800. **Subscr. to:** Subscriptions, PO Box 362, Abingdon, Oxon OX14 3WB, United Kingdom. TEL 44-1235-401060, FAX 44-1235-401075.

616.8 306.4 USA ISSN 1050-5350
RC569.5.G35 CODEN: JGSTEM
JOURNAL OF GAMBLING STUDIES. Text in English. 1985. q. USD 512, EUR 511 to institutions for print or online ed.; USD 614.40, EUR 613.20 to institutions for print & online eds.combined (effective 2002). adv. reprint service avail. from PQC. *Refereed.* **Document type:** *Journal, Academic/Scholarly.* **Description:** Covers social and pathological gambling research by professionals in all disciplines, including law, psychiatry, sociology, history, and counseling.
Formerly (until 1994): Journal of Gambling Behavior (0742-0714)
Related titles: Online - full text ed.: (from EBSCO Publishing, O C L C Online Computer Library Center, Inc., Swets Blackwell, Kluwer Online, RoweCom Information Quest).
Indexed: ASSIA, Hospit.Ind., IMFL, Lang.& Lang.Behav.Abstr., PsycInfo, Psychol.Abstr. (1985-), SOPODA, Soc.Serv.Abstr., Soc.Work Res.& Abstr., Sociol.Abstr., e-psyche.
—BLDSC (4987.180000), Infotrieve, ingenta. **CCC.**
Published by: (National Council on Problem Gambling), Kluwer Academic - Plenum Publishers (Subsidiary of: Wolters Kluwer N.V.), 233 Spring St, New York, NY 10013-1578. TEL 212-620-8000, 800-221-9369, FAX 212-463-0742, info@plenum.com, http://www.wkap.nl/journalhome.htm/1050-5350. Ed. Howard J Schaffer. **Subscr. outside the Americas to:** Kluwer Academic Publishers Group, Journals Department, PO Box 322, Dordrecht 3300 AH, Netherlands. TEL 31-78-639-2392, FAX 31-78-654-6474. **Co-sponsor:** Institute for the Study of Gambling and Commercial Gaming.

618.97 USA ISSN 0022-1414
RC451.4.A5 CODEN: JGPSBZ
JOURNAL OF GERIATRIC PSYCHIATRY; official journal of the Boston Society for Gerontological Psychiatry. Text in English. 1967. s-a. USD 67.50 domestic to individuals; USD 88 foreign to individuals; USD 102 domestic to institutions; USD 128 foreign to institutions (effective 2002). adv. bk.rev. illus. back issues avail.; reprints avail. *Refereed.* **Document type:** *Journal, Academic/Scholarly.* **Description:** Presents current ideas and recent findings in the field of geriatric psychiatry. Also contains articles on Alzheimer's disease.
Indexed: ASCA, ASSIA, Abstr.Soc.Geront., AgeLine, Biol.Abstr., CINAHL, Curr.Cont. (coverage dropped), Excerp.Med., Fam.Ind., IMFL, Ind.Med. (coverage dropped), Ind.Sci.Rev., Inpharma, Lang.& Lang.Behav.Abstr., Mid.East: Abstr.& Ind., Pharm.&Out.News, PsycInfo, Psychol.Abstr. (1973-), Reac., SOPODA, SSCI (coverage dropped), Sage Fam.Stud.Abstr., Sci.Cit.Ind. (coverage dropped), Soc.Serv.Abstr., Sociol.Abstr., e-psyche.
—BLDSC (4995.080000), CISTI, GNLM, IDS, ingenta, KNAW.
Published by: (Boston Society for Gerontologic Psychiatry, Inc.), International Universities Press, Incorporated, 59 Boston Post Rd., P.O. Box 1524, Madison, CT 06443-1524. adv.: page USD 360; 4.25 x 7.

JOURNAL OF GERIATRIC PSYCHIATRY AND NEUROLOGY; an interdisciplinary forum for clinicians and scientists. see *GERONTOLOGY AND GERIATRICS*

616.857 ITA ISSN 1129-2369
▼ **THE JOURNAL OF HEADACHE AND PAIN.** Text in English. 2000. 3/yr. EUR 156.60 domestic; EUR 153.60 in Germany; USD 57.60 newsstand/cover foreign (effective 2002). **Document type:** *Journal, Academic/Scholarly.* **Description:** Dedicated to researchers involved in all aspects of headache and pain, including theory, methodology, clinical practice and care.

Related titles: ♦ Online - full content ed.: The Journal of Headache and Pain Online. ISSN 1129-2377; Online - full text ed.: (from Springer LINK, RoweCom Information Quest).
—BLDSC (4996.673000).
Published by: Springer-Verlag Italia Srl (Subsidiary of: BertelsmannSpringer), Via Podgora, 4, Milan, MI 20122, Italy. TEL 39-2-55194656, FAX 39-2-55193360, springer@springer.it, http://link.springer.de. Ed. V Gallai.

616.857 ITA ISSN 1129-2377
▼ **THE JOURNAL OF HEADACHE AND PAIN ONLINE.** Text in English. 2000. 3/yr. **Document type:** *Academic/Scholarly.* **Description:** Publishes original papers, short and rapid communications, case reports, review articles and letters pertinent to the various aspects of headache and pain.
Media: Online - full content (from Swets Blackwell).
Related titles: Online - full text ed.: (from Springer LINK, RoweCom Information Quest); ♦ Print ed.: The Journal of Headache and Pain. ISSN 1129-2369.
Published by: Springer-Verlag Italia Srl (Subsidiary of: BertelsmannSpringer), Via Podgora, 4, Milan, MI 20122, Italy. TEL 39-2-55194656, FAX 39-2-55193360, springer@springer.it, http://link.springer.de.

616.8588 GBR ISSN 1366-8250
JOURNAL OF INTELLECTUAL AND DEVELOPMENTAL DISABILITY. Text in English. 1970. q. GBP 78, USD 130 to individuals; GBP 193, USD 317 to institutions (effective 2002). adv. bk.rev. charts, illus. index. reprint service avail. from PQC. **Document type:** *Academic/Scholarly.* **Description:** Reports of research in the area of mental retardation and related disabilities.
Former titles (until 1995): Australia and New Zealand Journal of Developmental Disabilities (0726-3864); (until vol.7, 1981): Australian Journal of Developmental Disabilities (0159-9011); (until vol.6, Mar. 1980): Australian Journal of Mental Retardation (0045-0634)
Related titles: Microfilm ed.: (from PQC); Online - full text ed.: ISSN 1469-9532 (from CatchWord Ltd., Swets Blackwell, Institute for Scientific Information).
Indexed: AMED, Aus.Educ.Ind., Aus.P.A.I.S., Biol.Abstr., C.I.J.E., CINAHL, Child Devel.Abstr., ERA, Except.Child Educ.Abstr., Excerp.Med., IMFL, Ind.Med. (coverage dropped), Lang.& Lang.Behav.Abstr., Ment.Retard.Abstr., Mult.Ed.Abstr., PsycInfo, Psychol.Abstr. (1970-), Rehabil.Lit., SOPODA, Sociol.Abstr., Sp.Ed.Needs Abstr., e-psyche.
—BLDSC (5007.538430), CatchWord, EMDOCS, Infotrieve, ingenta. **CCC.**
Published by: (Australian Society for the Study of Intellectual Disability), Carfax Publishing Limited (Subsidiary of: Taylor & Francis Group), Carfax Publishing Co, PO Box 24, Abingdon, Oxon OX14 3UE, United Kingdom. FAX 44-1235-401550, enquiries@carfax.co.uk, enquiries@carfax.co.uk/, http://www.carfax.co.uk. Ed. P J Foreman. Circ: 1,400.

616.858 GBR ISSN 0964-2633
RC321 CODEN: JIDREN
JOURNAL OF INTELLECTUAL DISABILITY RESEARCH. Text in English. 1957. bi-m., latest vol.46, 2002. GBP 80 in Europe to individuals; USD 127 in North America to individuals; GBP 88 elsewhere to individuals; GBP 299 in Europe to institutions; USD 474 in North America to institutions; GBP 329 elsewhere to institutions (effective 2002). adv. bk.rev. abstr, bibl, charts, illus. index. back issues avail.; reprint service avail. from SWZ,PQC,PSC,SCH. *Refereed.* **Document type:** *Academic/Scholarly.*
Formerly (until 1991): Journal of Mental Deficiency Research (0022-264X)
Related titles: Microform ed.: (from PQC); Online - full text ed.: ISSN 1365-2788. GBP 72 in Europe to individuals; USD 115 in North America to individuals; GBP 72 elsewhere to individuals; GBP 270 in Europe to institutions; USD 427 in North America to institutions; GBP 270 elsewhere to institutions (effective 2002) (from Ovid Technologies, Inc., EBSCO Publishing, O C L C Online Computer Library Center, Inc., RoweCom Information Quest, ingenta, Munksgaard & Blackwell Science's Synergy, Swets Blackwell, Institute for Scientific Information).
Indexed: AMED, ASCA, ASSIA, Adol.Ment.Hlth.Abstr., AgeLine, Bibl.Asian Stud. (1970), Bibl.Dev.Med.& Child Neur., Biol.Abstr., Br.Educ.Ind., Brit.Nur.Ind., C.I.J.E. (coverage dropped), Chem.Abstr., Child Devel.Abstr., Curr.Adv.Ecol.Sci., Curr.Cont., Dent.Ind., ERA, Except.Child Educ.Abstr., Excerp.Med., Hosp.Abstr., Ind.Med. (1992-), Ind.Sci.Rev., Inpharma, Int.Nurs.Ind., Lang.& Lang.Behav.Abstr., Mid.East: Abstr.& Ind., Neurosci.Cit.Ind., Nutr.Abstr., Pharm.&Out.News, PsycInfo, Psychol.Abstr. (1960-), Reac., SOPODA, SSCI, Sci.Cit.Ind., Sociol.Abstr., Sp.Ed.Needs Abstr., e-psyche.
—BLDSC (5007.538440), CISTI, EMDOCS, GNLM, IDS, ingenta, KNAW. **CCC.**
Published by: (International Association for the Scientific Study of Intellectual Disability), Blackwell Science Ltd., PO Box 88, Oxford OX2 0NE, United Kingdom. TEL 44-1865-206180, 44-1865-206002, FAX 44-1865-206219, jnl.orders@blacksci.co.uk, http://www.blackwell-science.com/~cgilib/jnlpage.asp?Journal=jidr&File=jidr, http://www.blackwellpublishing.com. Ed. W I Fraser. Pub. Elaine Stott. R&P Sophie Savage. Adv. contact Jenny Applin. Circ: 1,070.

JOURNAL OF INTERPROFESSIONAL CARE. see *MEDICAL SCIENCES*

616.8 GBR ISSN 0963-8237
CODEN: JMEHEQ
JOURNAL OF MENTAL HEALTH. Text in English. 1992. bi-m. GBP 126, USD 243 to individuals; GBP 431, USD 775 to institutions (effective 2002). back issues avail. *Refereed.* **Document type:** *Academic/Scholarly.* **Description:** Presents papers of direct relevance to clinical practice including all aspects of mental health work, elderly care, and addiction. Includes topics concerning work with offenders, learning difficulties, psychiatric rehabilitation, and primary care.
Related titles: Microfiche ed.; Online - full text ed.: ISSN 1360-0567 (from CatchWord Ltd., Northern Light Technology, Inc., EBSCO Publishing, O C L C Online Computer Library Center, Inc., RoweCom Information Quest, ProQuest Information & Learning, Swets Blackwell).
Indexed: Addic.Abstr., Brit.Nur.Ind., CINAHL, ERA, Excerp.Med. (1995-), Lang.& Lang.Behav.Abstr., PsycInfo, Psychol.Abstr. (1992-), SOPODA, Soc.Serv.Abstr., Sociol.Abstr., Sp.Ed.Needs Abstr., Stud.Wom.Abstr., e-psyche.
—BLDSC (5017.670000), ADONIS, CatchWord, GNLM, Infotrieve. **CCC.**
Published by: Carfax Publishing Limited (Subsidiary of: Taylor & Francis Group), PO Box 25, Abingdon, Oxon OX14 3UE, United Kingdom. TEL 44-1235-401000, FAX 44-1235-401550, enquiries@carfax.co.uk, enquiry@tandf.co.uk, http://www.carfax.co.uk. Ed. Ian Hughes.

616.8 USA ISSN 0895-8696
QP356.2 CODEN: JMNEES
JOURNAL OF MOLECULAR NEUROSCIENCE. Text in English. 1989. bi-m. USD 435 domestic; USD 490 foreign (effective 2000). bk.rev. illus. index. *Refereed.* **Document type:** *Journal, Academic/Scholarly.* **Description:** Covers a broad range of subjects for molecular studies of neural genes through actions of the gene products to diseases caused by defects in particular genes.
Related titles: Online - full text ed.: (from O C L C Online Computer Library Center, Inc., Institute for Scientific Information).
Indexed: ASCA, Aqua.Sci.& Fish.Abstr., BBCI, Chem.Abstr., Chem.Indus.Notes, Chem.Titles, Chemorec.Abstr., Curr.Cont., INIS Atomind., Ind.Med. (1989-), Ind.Sci.Rev., Inpharma, Int.Abstr.Biol.Sci., Neurosci.Abstr., Neurosci.Cit.Ind., Reac., Sci.Cit.Ind., e-psyche.
—BLDSC (5020.717000), ADONIS, CASDDS, CISTI, GNLM, IDS, Infotrieve, KNAW. **CCC.**
Published by: Humana Press Inc., 999 Riverview Dr, Ste 208, Totowa, NJ 07512. TEL 973-256-1699, FAX 973-256-8341, humana@humanapr.com, http://humanapress.com. Eds. Ilana Gozes, Mark Mattson. R&P Richard Hruska. **Dist. in Japan by:** Maruzen Co., Ltd., International Division, Export Dept, P.O. Box 5050, Tokyo International 100-3191, Japan. TEL 81-3-3275-8591.

THE JOURNAL OF MUSCULOSKELETAL AND NEURONAL INTERACTIONS. see *MEDICAL SCIENCES—Orthopedics And Traumatology*

616.8 USA ISSN 0022-3018
RC321 CODEN: JNMDAN
JOURNAL OF NERVOUS AND MENTAL DISEASE; an educational journal of neuropsychiatry. Text in English. 1874. m. USD 233 domestic to individuals; USD 233 foreign to individuals; USD 349 domestic to institutions; USD 396 foreign to institutions; USD 31 newsstand/cover (effective 2002). adv. bk.rev. bibl, illus. index. *Refereed.* **Document type:** *Academic/Scholarly.* **Description:** Publishes studies in the social, behavioral and neurological sciences relevant to clinical psychiatry.
Related titles: Microfilm ed.: (from WWS); Online - full text ed.: USD 453.70 domestic academic site license; USD 500.70 foreign academic site license; USD 506.05 domestic corporate site license; USD 553.05 foreign corporate site license (2002) (from Ovid Technologies, Inc., Institute for Scientific Information).
Indexed: AIM, ASCA, ASSIA, Abstr.Crim.& Pen., Abstr.Health Care Manage.Stud., Abstr.Soc.Geront., Addic.Abstr., AgeLine, Agri.& Environ.Biotech.Abstr. (coverage dropped), Amer.Bibl.Slavic & E.Eur.Stud., Arts & Hum.Cit.Ind. (coverage dropped), Bibl.Asian Stud. (1971-1991), Biol.Abstr., Chem.Abstr., Chic.Per.Ind., Child Devel.Abstr., Curr.Adv.Ecol.Sci., Curr.Cont., Curr.Lit.Fam.Plan., Dent.Ind., Derwent Biotech.Abstr., Dok.Arbeitsmed., ERA, Except.Child Educ.Abstr., Excerp.Med., Fam.Ind., INIS Atomind., I.P.A., Ind.Med. (1876-), Ind.Per.Art.Relat.Law, Ind.Sci.Rev., Indian Psychol.Abstr., Inpharma, Int.Nurs.Ind., Jrnl.Watch Psych., M.L.A., MLA Intl.Bibl., Neurosci.Cit.Ind., Nutr.Abstr., Peace Res.Abstr., Pharm.&Out.News, PsycInfo, Psychol.Abstr. (1929-), Psycscan C.P., Reac., Risk Abstr., SSCI, Sage Fam.Stud.Abstr., Sci.Cit.Ind., Viol.& Abuse Abstr., e-psyche.
—BLDSC (5021.400000), CISTI, GNLM, IDS, ingenta, KNAW.
Published by: Williams & Wilkins (Subsidiary of: Waverly International), 351 W Camden St, Baltimore, MD 21201-2436. TEL 410-528-4068, 800-222-3790, FAX 410-528-4452, rezell@wwilkins.com, http://www.wwilkins.com/NMD/, http://www.Lww.com. Ed. Eugene B Brody. Adv. contact Randy Ezell. B&W page USD 465; trim 10.88 x 8.13. Circ: 2,021; 1,953 (paid).

616.8 AUT
QP364.5 CODEN: JNPSEJ
JOURNAL OF NEURAL TRANSMISSION - BASIC NEUROSCIENCES AND GENETICS - PARKINSON'S DISEASE AND ALLIED CONDITIONS - ALZHEIMER'S DISEASE AND RELATED DISORDERS - BIOLOGICAL PSYCHIATRY. Text in English. 1950. m. EUR 1,786.50 domestic; EUR 1,774.40 in Germany; EUR 172 newsstand/cover foreign (effective 2002). adv. charts, illus, abstr. index. back issues avail.; reprint service avail. from ISI. *Refereed.* **Document type:** *Journal, Academic/Scholarly.* **Description:** Publishes research in neurological disorders, including Parkinson's and Alzheimer's diseases.
Formerly: Journal of Neural Transmission - Basic Neurosciences - Neurology Section - Psychiatry Section; Which was formed by the merger of: Journal of Neural Transmission. General Section (0300-9564); Journal of Neural Transmission. Parkinson's Disease and Dementia Section (0936-3076); Which was formerly: Journal of Neuro-Visceral Relations (0022-3026)
Related titles: Microform ed.: (from PQC); Online - full text ed.: ISSN 1435-1463 (from EBSCO Publishing, RoweCom Information Quest, Swets Blackwell, Springer LINK, Institute for Scientific Information).
Indexed: ASCA, Agri.& Environ.Biotech.Abstr. (coverage dropped), Aqua.Sci.& Fish.Abstr., Biol.Abstr., Chem.Abstr., Chem.Titles, Curr.Adv.Ecol.Sci., Curr.Cont., Dairy Sci.Abstr., Derwent Biotech.Abstr., Excerp.Med., INIS Atomind., Ind.Med. (coverage dropped), Ind.Sci.Rev., Inpharma, Int.Abstr.Biol.Sci., Mass Spectr.Bull., Neurosci.Abstr., Neurosci.Cit.Ind., Nutr.Abstr., Pharm.&Out.News, Reac., SSCI (coverage dropped), Sci.Cit.Ind., Sport Fish.Abstr., THA, Weed Abstr., Wild.Rev., Zoo.Rec., e-psyche.
—BLDSC (5021.420000), ADONIS, CASDDS, CISTI, EMDOCS, GNLM, IDS, Infotrieve, ingenta, KNAW. **CCC.**
Published by: Springer-Verlag Wien (Subsidiary of: BertelsmannSpringer), Sachsenplatz 4-6, PO Box 89, Vienna, W 1201, Austria. TEL 43-1-3302415-0, FAX 43-1-330242665, journals@springer.at, http://www.springer.at/jnt. Ed. P Riederer. R&P Angela Foessl TEL 43-1-3302415517. Adv. contact Michael Katzenberger TEL 43-1-3302415220. B&W page XEU 1,000; 170 x 230. **Subscr. in N. America to:** Springer-Verlag, Journals. TEL 212-460-1500, FAX 212-473-6272, orders@springer-ny.com, http://www.springer-ny.com.

616.8 AUT ISSN 0303-6995
CODEN: JNTSD4
JOURNAL OF NEURAL TRANSMISSION. SUPPLEMENT. Text in English. 1974. irreg. adv. abstr. reprint service avail. from ISI. *Refereed.* **Document type:** *Monographic series, Academic/Scholarly.* **Description:** Publishes selected papers from conferences in applied and clinical research in neurological diseases, such as Parkinson's and Alzheimer's.
Former titles: Journal of Neuro-Visceral Relations. Supplement (0075-4323); Acta Neurovegetativa. Supplement
Related titles: Microform ed.: (from PQC); Online - full text ed.: (from Institute for Scientific Information).
Indexed: ASCA, Chem.Abstr., Chem.Indus.Notes, Chem.Titles, Curr.Cont., Excerp.Med. (1992-), INIS Atomind., Ind.Med. (1974-), Inpharma, Int.Abstr.Biol.Sci., Neurosci.Cit.Ind., Reac., Sci.Cit.Ind., e-psyche.

M

—BLDSC (5021.425000), ADONIS, CASDDS, CISTI, EMDOCS, IDS, ingenta, KNAW. **CCC.**

Published by: Springer-Verlag Wien (Subsidiary of: BertelsmannSpringer), Sachsenplatz 4-6, PO Box 89, Vienna, W 1201, Austria. TEL 43-1-3302415-0, FAX 43-1-330242665, books@springer.co.at, http://www.springer.at/jnt. Ed. P Riederer. R&P Angela Foessl TEL 43-1-3302415517. Adv. contact Michael Katzenberger TEL 43-1-3302415220. B&W page XEU 1,000; 170 x 230. **N. American subscr. to:** Springer-Verlag, Journals, 175 Fifth Ave, New York, NY 10010. TEL 212-460-1500, FAX 212-473-6272, orders@springer-ny.com, http://www.springer-ny.com.

JOURNAL OF NEURO-OPHTHALMOLOGY. see *MEDICAL SCIENCES—Ophthalmology And Optometry*

JOURNAL OF NEUROBIOLOGY; an international journal. see *BIOLOGY—Physiology*

JOURNAL OF NEUROCHEMISTRY. see *BIOLOGY—Biochemistry*

616.8 616.4 GBR ISSN 0953-8194
CODEN: JOUNE2

JOURNAL OF NEUROENDOCRINOLOGY. Text in English. 1989. m., latest vol.14, 2002. GBP 110 in Europe to individuals; USD 170 in North America to individuals; GBP 110 elsewhere to individuals; GBP 883 in Europe to institutions; USD 1,400 in North America to institutions; GBP 972 elsewhere to institutions (effective 2002); GBP 883.30 in Europe to institutions print & online eds.; GBP 121 in Europe to individuals print & online eds.; USD 1,496 in North America to institutions print & online eds.; USD 187 in North America to individuals print & online eds.; GBP 971.30 elsewhere to institutions print & online eds.; GBP 121 elsewhere to individuals print & online eds. (effective 2001). adv. bk.rev. bibl, illus. index. back issues avail. *Refereed.* **Document type:** *Journal, Academic/Scholarly.* **Description:** Integrates the fields of endocrinology and neuroscience. Covers nonvertebrate, vertebrate and clinical endocrinology.

Related titles: Microform ed.: (from PQC); ♦ Online - full text ed.: Journal of Neuroendocrinology Online. ISSN 1365-2826.

Indexed: ASCA, Chem.Abstr., Chem.Indus.Notes, Chem.Titles, Chemorec.Abstr., Curr.Cont., Excerp.Med., Ind.Med. (1989-), Ind.Sci.Rev., Inpharma, Int.Abstr.Biol.Sci., Neurosci.Abstr. (coverage dropped), Neurosci.Cit.Ind., Reac., Ref.Zh., Sci.Cit.Ind., e-psyche.

—BLDSC (5021.543000), CASDDS, CISTI, EMDOCS, GNLM, IDS, ingenta, KNAW. **CCC.**

Published by: (European Neuroendocrine Association), Blackwell Science Ltd., PO Box 88, Oxford OX2 0NE, United Kingdom. TEL 44-1865-206180, 44-1865-206002, FAX 44-1865-206219, jnl.orders@blacksci.co.uk, http://www.blackwell-science.com/products/journals/jneur.htm, http://www.blackwellpublishing.com. Ed. G Leng. Pub. Allen Stevens. R&P Sophie Savage. Adv. contact Jenny Applin. Circ: 555. **Co-sponsor:** British Neuroendocrine Group.

616.8 GBR ISSN 1365-2826

JOURNAL OF NEUROENDOCRINOLOGY ONLINE. Text in English. 1998. m. GBP 99 in Europe to individuals; USD 153 in North America to individuals; GBP 99 elsewhere to individuals; GBP 795 in Europe to institutions; USD 1,260 in North America to institutions; GBP 795 elsewhere to institutions (effective 2002). *Refereed.* **Document type:** *Academic/Scholarly.*

Media: Online - full text (from EBSCO Publishing, Munksgaard & Blackwell Science's Synergy, RoweCom Information Quest, ingenta, O C L C Online Computer Library Center, Inc., Swets Blackwell, Institute for Scientific Information). **Related titles:** Microform ed.: (from PQC); ♦ Print ed.: Journal of Neuroendocrinology. ISSN 0953-8194.

Published by: Blackwell Science Ltd., Osney Mead, Oxford OX2 0EL, United Kingdom. TEL 44-1685-206206, FAX 44-1685-721205, website@blacksci.com, journals.cs@blacksci.co.uk, http://www.blackwell-science.com/~cgilib/jnlpage.bin?Journal=jneur&File=jneur&Page=aims.

616.8 CHE ISSN 0167-7063
QP356.22 CODEN: JLNEDK

JOURNAL OF NEUROGENETICS. Text in English. 1983. 4/yr. GBP 143, USD 190, EUR 190 to individuals; GBP 525, USD 665, EUR 670 to institutions; GBP 851, USD 1,091, EUR 1,103 to corporations (effective 2002). back issues avail. *Refereed.* **Document type:** *Journal, Academic/Scholarly.* **Description:** Publishes papers in the broad field of neurogenetics, covering studies of genes and genetic variants that influence neural development and function.

Related titles: CD-ROM ed.; Microform ed.; Online - full text ed.: (from EBSCO Publishing, Institute for Scientific Information).

Indexed: AMED, ASCA, Aqua.Sci.& Fish.Abstr., Biotech.Cit.Ind., Chem.Abstr., Curr.Adv.Cell & Devel.Biol., Curr.Adv.Ecol.Sci., Curr.Adv.Gen.& Molec.Biol., Curr.Cont., Entomol.Abstr., Excerp.Med., Genet.Abstr. (coverage dropped), Ind.Med. (1983-), Inpharma, Int.Abstr.Biol.Sci., Neurosci.Abstr., Neurosci.Cit.Ind., Reac., Sci.Cit.Ind., Zoo.Rec., e-psyche.

—BLDSC (5021.545000), CASDDS, CISTI, GNLM, ingenta. **CCC.**

Published by: Gordon and Breach - Harwood Academic (Subsidiary of: Taylor & Francis Group), PO Box 531, Lausanne 1000, Switzerland. TEL 41-21-6411280, FAX 41-21-6411281, info@gbhap.com, http://www.gbhap-us.com/journals/359/359-top.htm, http://www.gbhap.com. Ed. Jeffrey C Hall. **Subscr. addr. in US:** International Publishers Direct, PO Box 32160, Newark, NJ 07102. FAX 215-750-6343.

616.8 616.07548 USA ISSN 1051-2284
CODEN: JNERET

JOURNAL OF NEUROIMAGING. Text in English. 1991. q. USD 400 domestic; USD 475 foreign (effective 2002). adv. bk.rev. abstr, charts, illus, stat. index. 96 p./no. back issues avail.; reprint service avail. from PQC. *Refereed.* **Document type:** *Journal, Academic/Scholarly.* **Description:** Includes coverage of MRI, CT, SPECT, PET, neurosonology, transcranial doppler, and carotid ultrasound, for specialists who rely on neuroimaging.

Related titles: Microform ed.: (from PQC); Online - full text ed.: (from ingenta, Swets Blackwell, Institute for Scientific Information, RoweCom Information Quest).

Indexed: ASCA, Curr.Cont., Excerp.Med. (1992-), Ind.Med. (1991-), Inpharma, Int.Abstr.Biol.Sci., Neurosci.Abstr., Neurosci.Cit.Ind., Pharm.&Out.News, Reac., e-psyche.

—BLDSC (5021.548000), CISTI, EMDOCS, GNLM, IDS, KNAW.

Published by: (American Society of Neuroimaging), Sage Publications, Inc., Sage Science Press, 2455 Teller Rd, Thousand Oaks, CA 91320. TEL 805-499-0721, FAX 805-499-0871, info@sagepub.com, http://www.sagesciencepress.com/. Ed. Lawrence R Wechsler. Pub. Susan Hanscom. R&P Peter Marino. Adv. contact Robert Vrooman. B&W page USD 790, color page USD 1,775; trim 11 x 8.25. Circ: 1,065.

616.8 616.97 NLD ISSN 0165-5728
CODEN: JNRIDW

JOURNAL OF NEUROIMMUNOLOGY. Text in English. 1981. 24/yr. EUR 3,532 in Europe to institutions; JPY 469,200 in Japan to institutions; USD 3,951 elsewhere to institutions (effective 2002). adv. charts, illus, abstr. back issues avail.; reprint service avail. from SWZ,ISI. *Refereed.* **Document type:** *Academic/Scholarly.* **Description:** Publishes both basic research and clinical problems in neuroimmunology and related neuroscientific disciplines.

Related titles: Microform ed.: (from PQC); Online - full text ed.: (from ingenta, ScienceDirect, Swets Blackwell, Institute for Scientific Information).

Indexed: AIDS & Cancer Res., ASCA, Biol.Abstr., Biotech.& Bioeng.Abstr., Chem.Abstr., Chem.Titles, Chemorec.Abstr., Curr.Adv.Cell & Devel.Biol., Curr.Adv.Ecol.Sci., Curr.Adv.Gen.& Molec.Biol., Curr.Cont., Excerp.Med., Immun.Abstr., Ind.Med. (1981-), Ind.Sci.Rev., Inpharma, Neurosci.Abstr., Neurosci.Cit.Ind., Pharm.&Out.News, Protozool.Abstr., PsycInfo, Psychol.Abstr. (1981-), Reac., Rev.Appl.Entomol., Rev.Med.& Vet.Mycol., Sci.Cit.Ind., e-psyche.

—BLDSC (5021.550000), ADONIS, CASDDS, CISTI, GNLM, IDS, ingenta, KNAW. **CCC.**

Published by: (International Society for Neuroimmunology), Elsevier Science BV, PO Box 211, Amsterdam 1000 AE, Netherlands. TEL 31-20-485-2911, FAX 31-20-485-2457, nlinfo-f@elsevier.nl; usinfo-f@elsevier.com; forinfo-kyf04035@niftyserve.or.jp, http://www.elsevier.com/locate/jneuroim. Eds. C F Brosnan, Cedric S Raine. **Subscr. in Australasia and the Far East to:** Elsevier Science (Singapore) Pte Ltd, No.1 Temasek Ave, 17-01 Millenia Tower, Singapore 039192, Singapore. TEL 65-434-3727, FAX 65-337-2230; **Subscr. in Japan to:** Elsevier Science Inc - Japan Regional Office, 9-15 Higashi-Azabu 1-chome, Minato-ku, Tokyo 106-0044, Japan. TEL 81-3-5561-5033, FAX 81-3-5561-5047; **Subscr. in the Americas to:** Elsevier Science, PO Box 945, New York, NY 10159-0945. TEL 212-633-3730, FAX 212-633-3680, usinfo-f@elsevier.com.

616.8 GBR ISSN 0911-6044

JOURNAL OF NEUROLINGUISTICS. Text in English. 1985. q. EUR 504 in Europe to institutions; JPY 66,900 in Japan to institutions; USD 564 elsewhere to institutions (effective 2002). back issues avail. *Refereed.* **Document type:** *Academic/Scholarly.* **Description:** Provides an international forum for the integration of the language sciences and the neurosciences.

Related titles: Microfilm ed.: (from PQC); Online - full text ed.: (from ingenta, ScienceDirect, Swets Blackwell, Institute for Scientific Information).

Indexed: ASCA, Arts & Hum.Cit.Ind. (coverage dropped), Bibl.Ling., ERA, Lang.& Lang.Behav.Abstr. (1985-), Ling.Abstr., Neurosci.Cit.Ind., PsycInfo, Russ.Acad.Sci.Bibl., SOPODA, SSCI, Sociol.Abstr., e-psyche.

—BLDSC (5021.553000), GNLM, IDS, Infotrieve, ingenta. **CCC.**

Published by: Pergamon (Subsidiary of: Elsevier Science), The Boulevard, Langford Ln, East Park, Kidlington, Oxford OXB 1GB, United Kingdom. FAX 44-1865-843010, http://www.elsevier.com/locate/jneuroling. Eds. John Marshall, M Paradis. **Subscr. in Australasia and the Far East to:** Elsevier Science (Singapore) Pte Ltd, No.1 Temasek Ave, 17-01 Millenia Tower, Singapore 039192, Singapore. TEL 65-434-3727, FAX 65-337-2230; **Subscr. in the Americas to:** Elsevier Science, PO Box 945, New York, NY 10159-0945. TEL 212-633-3730, FAX 212-633-3680, usinfo-f@elsevier.com; **Subscr. to:** Elsevier Science BV, PO Box 211, Amsterdam 1000 AE, Netherlands. TEL 31-20-485-3757.

616.8 TUR ISSN 1300-1817

JOURNAL OF NEUROLOGICAL SCIENCES/NOROLOJIK BILIMLER DERGISI. Text in English, Turkish. 1987. q. *Refereed.* **Description:** Publishes both experimental and clinical neuroscience articles.

Related titles: Online - full text ed.: ISSN 1302-1664. 1996.

Published by: Ege University Press, Bornova, Izmir 35100, Turkey. TEL 90-232-3881097, FAX 90-232-3881097, http://www.med.ege.edu.tr/~norolbil. Ed. Nezih Oktar.

616.8 DEU ISSN 0340-5354
CODEN: JNRYA9

JOURNAL OF NEUROLOGY/ZEITSCHRIFT FUER NEUROLOGIE; official journal of the European Neurological Society. Text in English. 1891. m. EUR 1,603.20 domestic; EUR 1,595.70 in Germany; USD 157.50 newsstand/cover foreign (effective 2002). adv. bk.rev. abstr, bibl. index. back issues avail.; reprints avail. *Refereed.* **Document type:** *Journal, Academic/Scholarly.* **Description:** Provides a source for original investigations in clinical neurology, and related basic research.

Former titles: Zeitschrift fuer Neurologie (0012-1037); Deutsche Zeitschrift fuer Nervenheilkunde

Related titles: E-mail ed.; Fax ed.; Microfiche ed.: (from BHP); Microform ed.: (from PQC); Online - full text ed.: ISSN 1432-1459 (from EBSCO Publishing, RoweCom Information Quest, Swets Blackwell, Springer LINK, Institute for Scientific Information); ♦ Supplement: Journal of Neurology. Supplement. ISSN 0939-1517.

Indexed: ASCA, Arts & Hum.Cit.Ind. (coverage dropped), Biol.Abstr., Chem.Abstr., Curr.Adv.Cancer Res., Curr.Cont., Dent.Ind., Excerp.Med., INIS Atomind., Ind.Med. (1974-), Ind.Sci.Rev., Inpharma, Jrnl.Watch Neuro., Neurosci.Abstr. (coverage dropped), Neurosci.Cit.Ind., Nutr.Abstr., Pharm.&Out.News, Reac., Rev.Appl.Entomol., Rev.Med.& Vet.Mycol., SSCI (coverage dropped), Sci.Cit.Ind., e-psyche.

—BLDSC (5021.584000), ADONIS, CASDDS, CISTI, EMDOCS, GNLM, IDS, ingenta, KNAW. **CCC.**

Published by: (European Neurological Society), Dr. Dietrich Steinkopff Verlag (Subsidiary of: BertelsmannSpringer), Poststr 9, Darmstadt 64293, Germany. TEL 49-6151-82899-0, FAX 49-6151-82899-40, frey.steinkopff@springer.de, http://www.steinkopff.springer.de. Eds. D. H. Miller, T Brandt. R&P Sabine Ibkendanz. Circ: 4,500. **Subscr. to:** Springer Verlag GmbH, Haberstr 7, Heidelberg 69126, Germany. TEL 49-6221-345200, FAX 49-6221-345229, subscriptions@springer.de. **Co-sponsor:** Deutsche Gesellschaft fuer Neurologie.

M

616.8 GBR ISSN 0022-3050
RC321 CODEN: JNNPAU
JOURNAL OF NEUROLOGY, NEUROSURGERY AND PSYCHIATRY. Text in English. 1920. m. GBP 136, USD 218 combined subscription to individuals includes print & online eds.; GBP 323, USD 518 to institutions for print only (effective 2002). adv. bk.rev. abstr, bibl, illus. index. back issues avail.; reprint service avail. from PQC. *Refereed.* **Document type:** *Academic/Scholarly.* **Description:** Focuses on clinical neurology, neurosurgery, neuropsychology, neuropsychiatry, and closely related experimental work.
Related titles: CD-ROM ed.: (from Ovid Technologies, Inc.); Microform ed.: (from PQC); Online - full text ed.: ISSN 1468-330X. 1997. GBP 80, USD 125 (effective 2002); institutions contact publisher for online rates. (from HighWire Pr., Ovid Technologies, Inc., EBSCO Publishing, O C L C Online Computer Library Center, Inc., RoweCom Information Quest, ProQuest Information & Learning, ingenta, Swets Blackwell, Institute for Scientific Information).
Indexed: AMED, ASCA, Abstr.Hyg., Behav.Med.Abstr., Bibl.Dev.Med.& Child Neur., Biol.Abstr., Chem.Abstr., Crim.Just.Abstr., Curr.Adv.Ecol.Sci., Curr.Cont., Dent.Ind., Diab.Cont., Dok.Arbeitsmed., Excerp.Med., INIS Atomind., Ind.Med. (1944-), Ind.Sci.Rev., Inpharma, Int.Abstr.Biol.Sci., Int.Nurs.Ind., Jrnl.Watch Neuro., Neurosci.Cit.Ind., Nutr.Abstr., Pharm.&Out.News, Protozool.Abstr., PsycInfo, Psychol.Abstr. (1950-), Reac., Rev.Appl.Entomol., Rev.Med.& Vet.Mycol., Risk Abstr., SSCI (coverage dropped), Sci.Cit.Ind., Trop.Dis.Bull., e-psyche.
—BLDSC (5021.600000), ADONIS, CASDDS, CISTI, GNLM, IDS, ingenta, KNAW. **CCC.**
Published by: B M J Publishing Group, B M A House, Tavistock Sq, London WC1H 9JR, United Kingdom. TEL 44-20-7387-4499, FAX 44-20-7383-6400, info.norththames@bma.org.uk, http://www.jnnp.com/, http://www.bma.org.uk. Ed. C Kennard. Adv. contact Euan Currer TEL 44-20-7383-6181.

616.8 DEU ISSN 0939-1517
CODEN: JNSUE
JOURNAL OF NEUROLOGY. SUPPLEMENT. Text in German. irreg. **Document type:** *Monographic series.*
Related titles: ♦ Supplement to: Journal of Neurology. ISSN 0340-5354.
Indexed: Excerp.Med. (1992-), e-psyche.
—ADONIS, EMDOCS, KNAW.
Published by: Springer-Verlag (Subsidiary of: BertelsmannSpringer), Haber Str 7, Heidelberg 69126, Germany. FAX 49-30-82787448, subscriptions@springer.de.

616.8 USA ISSN 0022-3069
RC321 CODEN: JNENAD
JOURNAL OF NEUROPATHOLOGY AND EXPERIMENTAL NEUROLOGY. Text in English. 1942. m. USD 155 domestic to individuals incl. print & online; USD 165 in the Americas to individuals incl. print & online; USD 175 elsewhere to individuals incl. print & online; USD 175 domestic to institutions incl. print & online; USD 185 in the Americas to institutions incl. print & online; USD 195 elsewhere to institutions incl. print & online (effective 2001). adv. bk.rev. abstr, bibl, charts, illus. index, cum.index: vol.1-15 (1942-1956); vol.16-25 (1957-1966). back issues avail.; reprint service avail. from PQC. *Refereed.* **Document type:** *Academic/Scholarly.* **Description:** Publishes original articles on neuropathology and experimental neurology, letters and news of the association.
Related titles: Microform ed.: (from PQC); Online - full text ed.: (from ProQuest Information & Learning, Institute for Scientific Information).
Indexed: ASCA, Aqua.Sci.& Fish.Abstr., Bibl.Dev.Med.& Child Neur., Biol.Abstr., Chem.Abstr., Chem.Indus.Notes, Chem.Titles, Curr.Adv.Cell & Devel.Biol., Curr.Adv.Ecol.Sci., Curr.Cont., Environ.Sci.Poll.Mgmt., Excerp.Med., INIS Atomind., Ind.Med. (1942-), Ind.Sci.Rev., Ind.Vet., Inpharma, Int.Abstr.Biol.Sci., Jrnl.Watch Neuro., Neurosci.Abstr. (coverage dropped), Neurosci.Cit.Ind., Nutr.Abstr., Pharm.&Out.News, Poult.Abstr., Protozool.Abstr., Reac., SSCI (coverage dropped), Sci.Cit.Ind., THA, Vet.Bull., e-psyche.
—BLDSC (5021.700000), CASDDS, CISTI, GNLM, IDS, ingenta, KNAW. **CCC.**
Published by: American Association of Neuropathologists, Inc., PO Box 1897, Lawrence, KS 66044-8897. TEL 785-843-1235, FAX 785-843-1274, aanp@allenpress.com, http://www.aanp-jnen.com. Ed. Dr. Michael Hart. R&P Eileen Healy. Adv. contact Michelle Kurzynski. B&W page USD 350; 9 x 7. Circ: 1,800.

JOURNAL OF NEUROPHYSIOLOGY. see *BIOLOGY—Physiology*

616.8 USA ISSN 0895-0172
RC321 CODEN: JNCNE7
JOURNAL OF NEUROPSYCHIATRY AND CLINICAL NEUROSCIENCES. Text in English. 1989. q. USD 119 domestic to individuals; USD 138 foreign to individuals; USD 252 domestic to institutions; USD 274 foreign to institutions (effective 2001). adv. bk.rev. abstr, bibl, charts, illus, stat. index. Supplement avail.; back issues avail. *Refereed.* **Document type:** *Consumer, Academic/Scholarly.* **Description:** Devoted to the relationships between the original research in psychiatry and neurology.
Related titles: Microform ed.: (from PQC); Online - full text ed.: (from HighWire Pr., EBSCO Publishing, RoweCom Information Quest, ProQuest Information & Learning, Institute for Scientific Information).
Indexed: ASCA, Chem.Abstr., Chem.Indus.Notes, Chem.Titles, Crim.Just.Abstr., Curr.Cont., Ind.Med. (1989-), Ind.Sci.Rev., Inpharma, Jrnl.Watch Psych., Neuropsych.Abstr., Neurosci.Cit.Ind., Pharm.&Out.News, PsycInfo, Psychol.Abstr. (1989-), Reac., Ref.Zh., SSCI (coverage dropped), Sci.Cit.Ind., Soc.Work Res.& Abstr., e-psyche.
—BLDSC (5022.040000), CASDDS, EMDOCS, GNLM, IDS, ingenta, KNAW. **CCC.**
Published by: (American Neuropsychiatric Association), American Psychiatric Press, Inc., Journals Division, 1400 K St, NW, Ste 1101, Washington, DC 20005. TEL 202-682-6240, 800-368-5777, FAX 202-789-2648, appi@psych.org, http://neuro.psychiatryonline.org/, http://www.psychiatryonline.org, http://www.appi.org. Ed. Dr. Stuart Yudofsky. R&P John McDuffie. Circ: 1,700.

616.8 USA ISSN 0270-6474
QP351 CODEN: JNRSDS
JOURNAL OF NEUROSCIENCE. Text in English. 1981. s-m. USD 1,495 domestic; USD 1,635 foreign (effective 1999). adv. illus. Index. back issues avail.; reprints avail. *Refereed.* **Document type:** *Academic/Scholarly.* **Description:** Offers readers rapid access to the most exciting advances occuring across the full spectrum of modern neuroscience.
Related titles: Microfiche ed.: (from PQC); Microfilm ed.: (from PQC); Online - full text ed.: USD 1,090 (effective 1999) (from HighWire Pr., EBSCO Publishing, Institute for Scientific Information).
Indexed: ASCA, Anim.Behav.Abstr., Aqua.Sci.& Fish.Abstr., Biol.& Agr.Ind. (Jan.1996-), Cal.Tiss.Abstr. (coverage dropped), Chem.Abstr., Chem.Titles, Chemorec.Abstr., Comput.Abstr., Curr.Adv.Biochem., Curr.Adv.Cell & Devel.Biol., Curr.Adv.Ecol.Sci., Curr.Adv.Gen.& Molec.Biol., Curr.Cont., Curr.Ref.Fish Res., Dent.Ind., Entomol.Abstr. (coverage dropped), Excerp.Med., INIS Atomind., Ind.Med. (1981-), Ind.Sci.Rev., Inpharma, Int.Abstr.Biol.Sci., Jrnl.Watch Psych., Neurosci.Abstr., Neurosci.Cit.Ind., Nutr.Abstr., Pharm.&Out.News, PsycInfo, Psychol.Abstr. (1993-), Reac., Ref.Zh., Rev.Appl.Entomol., Rev.Med.& Vet.Mycol., SSCI (coverage dropped), Sci.Cit.Ind., THA, Tox.Abstr. (coverage dropped), Zoo.Rec., e-psyche.
—BLDSC (5022.075000), CASDDS, CISTI, EMDOCS, GNLM, IDS, ingenta, KNAW. **CCC.**
Published by: Society for Neuroscience, 11 Dupont Circle, N W, Ste 500, Washington, DC 20036. TEL 202-462-6688, FAX 202-462-1547, jn@sfn.org; neurosci-feedback@forsythe.stanford.edu; orders@allenpress.com, http://www.jneurosci.org/; http://www.allenpress.com. Ed. David C Van Essen. Adv. contact James Cunningham. Circ: 4,100. **Subscr. to:** Allen Press Inc., PO Box 1897, Lawrence, KS 66044-8897.

616.8 NLD ISSN 0165-0270
CODEN: JNMEDT
JOURNAL OF NEUROSCIENCE METHODS. Text in English. 1979. 18/yr. EUR 3,144 in Europe to institutions; JPY 417,600 in Japan to institutions; USD 3,517 elsewhere to institutions (effective 2002). adv. charts, abstr, bibl, illus. back issues avail.; reprint service avail. from ISI. *Refereed.* **Document type:** *Academic/Scholarly.* **Description:** Publishes research papers and critical reviews addressing new methods or significant developments of recognized methods.
Related titles: Microform ed.: (from PQC); Online - full text ed.: (from ingenta, ScienceDirect, Swets Blackwell, Institute for Scientific Information).
Indexed: ASCA, Aqua.Sci.& Fish.Abstr., Biol.Abstr., Chem.Abstr., Chem.Cit.Ind., Chem.Indus.Notes, Chem.Titles, Compumath, Curr.Adv.Cell & Devel.Biol., Curr.Adv.Ecol.Sci., Curr.Cont., Excerp.Med., INIS Atomind., INSPEC (Mar.1979-), Ind.Med. (1979-), Ind.Sci.Rev., Inpharma, Int.Abstr.Biol.Sci., Mass Spectr.Bull., Neurosci.Abstr. (coverage dropped), Neurosci.Cit.Ind., Reac., Sci.Cit.Ind., e-psyche.
—BLDSC (5022.080000), AskIEEE, CASDDS, CISTI, GNLM, IDS, ingenta. **CCC.**
Published by: Elsevier Science BV, PO Box 211, Amsterdam 1000 AE, Netherlands. TEL 31-20-485-2911, FAX 31-20-485-2457, http://www.elsevier.com/locate/jneumeth. Eds. J S Kelly, Vincenzo Crunelli. **Subscr. in Australasia and the Far East to:** Elsevier Science (Singapore) Pte Ltd, No.1 Temasek Ave, 17-01 Millenia Tower, Singapore 039192, Singapore. TEL 65-434-3727, FAX 65-337-2230; **Subscr. in Japan to:** Elsevier Science Inc - Japan Regional Office, 9-15 Higashi-Azabu 1-chome, Minato-ku, Tokyo 106-0044, Japan. TEL 81-3-5561-5033; **Subscr. in the Americas to:** Elsevier Science, PO Box 945, New York, NY 10159-0945. TEL 212-633-3730, FAX 212-633-3680, usinfo-f@elsevier.com.

616.8 USA ISSN 0360-4012
QP351 CODEN: JNREDK
JOURNAL OF NEUROSCIENCE RESEARCH. Text in English. 1975. 24/yr. USD 6,500 in United States; USD 6,740 in Canada & Mexico; USD 6,944 elsewhere; USD 6,825 combined subscription in United States for print and online eds.; USD 7,065 combined subscription in Canada & Mexico for print and online eds.; USD 7,269 combined subscription elsewhere for print and online eds. (effective 2002). adv. bk.rev. charts, illus. index. back issues avail.; reprint service avail. from ISI. *Refereed.* **Document type:** *Academic/Scholarly.* **Description:** Concerned with basic research reports on molecular, cellular, and subcellular aspects of the neurosciences.
Related titles: Microform ed.: (from PQC); Online - full text ed.: ISSN 1097-4547. USD 6,500 in United States; USD 6,500 in Canada & Mexico; USD 6,500 elsewhere (effective 2002) (from EBSCO Publishing, Wiley InterScience, Institute for Scientific Information).
Indexed: ASCA, Anim.Behav.Abstr., Aqua.Sci.& Fish.Abstr., Biol.Abstr., Cal.Tiss.Abstr. (coverage dropped), Chem.Abstr., Chem.Titles, Chemorec.Abstr., Curr.Adv.Ecol.Sci., Curr.Cont., Excerp.Med., INIS Atomind., Ind.Med. (1975-), Ind.Sci.Rev., Inpharma, Int.Abstr.Biol.Sci., Neurosci.Abstr., Neurosci.Cit.Ind., Nutr.Abstr., Pharm.&Out.News, Protozool.Abstr., Reac., Sci.Cit.Ind., Sport Fish.Abstr., THA, Tox.Abstr. (coverage dropped), Wild.Rev., Zoo.Rec., e-psyche.
—BLDSC (5022.090000), CASDDS, CISTI, EMDOCS, GNLM, IDS, ingenta. **CCC.**
Published by: John Wiley & Sons, Inc., Journals (Subsidiary of: Wiley InterScience), 605 Third Ave, New York, NY 10158. TEL 212-850-6645, FAX 212-850-6021, subinfo@wiley.com, uscs-wis@wiley.com, http://www.wiley.com. Ed. Bernard Haber. adv.: B&W page GBP 640, color page GBP 1,515; trim 210 x 279. Circ: 800. **Subscr. outside the Americas to:** John Wiley & Sons Ltd., Baffins Ln, Chichester, Sussex PO19 IUD, United Kingdom. TEL 44-1243-779777, FAX 44-1243-843232, cs-journals@wiley.co.uk.

616.8 USA ISSN 0022-3085
RD1 CODEN: JONSAC
JOURNAL OF NEUROSURGERY. Text in English. 1944. m. USD 195 in US & Canada to individuals; USD 205 elsewhere to individuals; USD 215 in US & Canada to institutions; USD 225 elsewhere to institutions (effective 2000). adv. bk.rev. bibl, charts, illus. cum.index covering 50 vols. back issues avail. *Refereed.* **Document type:** *Academic/Scholarly.* **Description:** Presents medical articles relating to neurosurgery and allied specialties.
Related titles: CD-ROM ed.; Microform ed.: (from PQC,WWS); Online - full text ed.: (from EBSCO Publishing, Institute for Scientific Information).
Indexed: AIM, ASCA, Aqua.Sci.& Fish.Abstr., Biol.Abstr., Chem.Abstr., Chem.Indus.Notes, Chem.Titles, Curr.Adv.Cancer Res., Curr.Cont., Dent.Ind., Excerp.Med., Helminthol.Abstr., INIS Atomind., Ind.Med. (1944-), Ind.Sci.Rev., Inpharma, Int.Abstr.Biol.Sci., Int.Nurs.Ind., Jrnl.Watch Neuro., Neurosci.Cit.Ind., Reac., Rev.Appl.Entomol., Rev.Plant Path., Sci.Cit.Ind., e-psyche.
—BLDSC (5022.100000), CASDDS, CISTI, GNLM, IDS, ingenta, KNAW.
Published by: American Association of Neurological Surgeons, 1224 W Main St, Ste 450, Charlottesville, VA 22903. TEL 804-982-1684, FAX 804-982-1678, jneuro@virginia.edu. Ed. Dr. John A Jane. R&P Evelyn Kessler TEL 804-924-2204. Adv. contact Kathy Huntley TEL 856-848-1000. Circ: 12,500.

JOURNAL OF NEUROSURGICAL SCIENCES. see *MEDICAL SCIENCES—Surgery*

M

616.8 USA ISSN 1087-4208
JOURNAL OF NEUROTHERAPY. Text in English. 1995. q. USD 60, USD 81, USD 87 to individuals; USD 115, USD 155, USD 167 to institutions; USD 150, USD 203, USD 218 to libraries (effective Aug. 2001). adv. **Document type:** *Journal, Academic/Scholarly.* **Description:** Provides an integrated multi-disciplinary perspective on clinically relevant research, treatment, and public policy for neurotherapy.
Related titles: Online - full text ed.
Indexed: INSPEC, PsycInfo, e-psyche.
—BLDSC (5022.260000).
Published by: (Society for Neuronal Regulation), Haworth Press, Inc., 10 Alice St, Binghamton, NY 13904-1580. TEL 607-722-5857, 800-429-6784, FAX 607-722-6362, 800-895-0582, getinfo@haworthpressinc.com, http://www.haworthpress.com/journals/journallist.asp. Ed. Dr. David L Trudeau TEL 651-298-9773. adv.: B&W page USD 750, color page USD 1,000; trim 6 x 8.5.

JOURNAL OF NEUROTRAUMA. see *MEDICAL SCIENCES—Orthopedics And Traumatology*

616.8 USA ISSN 1355-0284
RC359.5 CODEN: JNVIFK
JOURNAL OF NEUROVIROLOGY. Text in English. 1995. bi-m. GBP 124, USD 205 to individuals; USD 292, USD 482 to institutions (effective 2002). adv. back issues avail. *Refereed.* **Document type:** *Academic/Scholarly.* **Description:** Studies neurotropic viruses and viral infections of the nervous system.
Related titles: Online - full text ed.: (from EBSCO Publishing, O C L C Online Computer Library Center, Inc., RoweCom Information Quest, ingenta, CatchWord Ltd., Swets Blackwell, Institute for Scientific Information).
Indexed: AIDS & Cancer Res., ASCA, Chem.Abstr., Chem.Titles, Curr.Cont., Excerp.Med. (1996-), Ind.Med. (1995-), Ind.Vet., Inpharma, Neurosci.Abstr., Neurosci.Cit.Ind., Pharm.&Out.News, Reac., Rev.Appl.Entomol., Rev.Med.& Vet.Mycol., Vet.Bull., Virol.Abstr., e-psyche.
—BLDSC (5022.285000), CASDDS, CISTI, EMDOCS, GNLM, IDS, Infotrieve, KNAW. **CCC.**
Published by: Taylor & Francis Inc, 325 Chestnut St, Ste 800, Philadelphia, PA 19106. TEL 215-625-8900, 800-354-1420, FAX 215-625-8914, info@taylorandfrancis.com, http://www.tandf.co.uk/journals/tf/13550284.html, http://www.taylorandfrancis.com. Ed. K Khalili.

616.8 USA ISSN 0022-3298
RZ460
JOURNAL OF ORGONOMY. Text in English. 1967. s-a. USD 40 domestic; USD 45 foreign; USD 20 newsstand/cover (effective 1999). bk.rev. bibl, charts, illus, stat. index, cum.index: 1967-1995. back issues avail.; reprint service avail. from PQC. *Refereed.* **Document type:** *Academic/Scholarly.* **Description:** Devoted to the study of orgone energy functions in living and nonliving nature, based on the discoveries of Wilhelm Reich.
Related titles: Microfilm ed.: (from PQC).
Indexed: e-psyche.
—ingenta.
Published by: (American College of Orgonomy), Orgonomic Publications, PO Box 490, Princeton, NJ 08542. TEL 732-821-1144, FAX 732-821-0174, http://www.orgonomy.org. Ed. Dr. Charles Konia. Pub. Dr. Peter Crist. Circ: 2,000.

616.89 CAN ISSN 0834-4825
CODEN: JORMEI
JOURNAL OF ORTHOMOLECULAR MEDICINE. Text in English. 1986. q. CND 58.85; USD 55 in United States; USD 70 elsewhere (effective 1999). adv. bk.rev. bibl, charts, illus. back issues avail.; reprint service avail. from PQC.
Former titles: Journal of Orthomolecular Psychiatry (0317-0209); (until 1973): Orthomolecular Psychiatry; (until 1972): Schizophrenia (0036-6129); (until 1969): Journal of Schizophrenia (0449-3109)
Related titles: Microform ed.: (from PQC).
Indexed: AMED, AgeLine, Biol.Abstr., Chem.Abstr., Curr.Adv.Biochem., Curr.Cont. (coverage dropped), Excerp.Med., Mid.East: Abstr.& Ind., Nutr.Abstr., PsycInfo, Psychol.Abstr. (1975-), SSCI (coverage dropped), e-psyche.
—BLDSC (5027.600000), CASDDS, CISTI, EMDOCS, GNLM, Infotrieve, ingenta, KNAW. **CCC.**
Published by: Canadian Schizophrenia Foundation, 16 Florence Ave, Toronto, ON M2N 1E9, Canada. TEL 416-733-2117, FAX 416-733-2352, centre@orthomed.org, http://www.orthomed.org. Ed. Abram Hoffer. Adv. contact Steven Carter. Circ: 1,400.

616.88 USA ISSN 0885-3924
RB127
JOURNAL OF PAIN AND SYMPTOM MANAGEMENT. Text in English. 1982. m. EUR 199 in Europe to individuals; JPY 26,400 in Japan to individuals; USD 223 elsewhere to individuals; EUR 519 in Europe to institutions; JPY 68,800 in Japan to institutions; USD 580 elsewhere to institutions; EUR 111 in Europe residents price; JPY 14,600 in Japan residents price; USD 123 elsewhere residents price (effective 2002). adv. bk.rev. index. Supplement avail.; back issues avail. *Refereed.* **Document type:** *Academic/Scholarly.* **Description:** Provides the professional with the results of important new research on pain and its clinical management.
Formerly (until 1985): P R N Forum (0743-345X)
Related titles: Microform ed.: (from PQC); Online - full text ed.: (from ingenta, ScienceDirect, Swets Blackwell, Institute for Scientific Information).
Indexed: AMED, ASCA, Behav.Med.Abstr., Brit.Nur.Ind., CINAHL, Child Devel.Abstr., Curr.Adv.Ecol.Sci., Curr.Cont., Derwent Biotech.Abstr., Excerp.Med., INIS Atomind., Ind.Med. (1986-), Inpharma, Int.Abstr.Biol.Sci., Int.Nurs.Ind., Neurosci.Cit.Ind., Nurs.Abstr., Pharm.&Out.News, PsycInfo, Psychol.Abstr. (1986-), Reac., Rev.Arom.& Med.Plants, SSCI (coverage dropped), e-psyche.
—BLDSC (5027.790000), EMDOCS, GNLM, IDS, ingenta, KNAW. **CCC.**
Published by: (Department of Anesthesiology, University of Wisconsin-Madison), Elsevier Science, PO Box 945, New York, NY 10159-0945. TEL 212-989-5800, FAX 212-633-3990, usinfo-f@elsevier.com, http://www.elsevier.com/locate/jpainsymman. Eds. George Heidrich, Dr. Russell K Portenoy. Circ: 3,200. **Subscr. in Australasia and the Far East to:** Elsevier Science (Singapore) Pte Ltd, No.1 Temasek Ave, 17-01 Millenia Tower, Singapore 039192, Singapore. TEL 65-434-3727, FAX 65-337-2230**; Subscr. in Japan to:** Elsevier Science Inc - Japan Regional Office, 9-15 Higashi-Azabu 1-chome, Minato-ku, Tokyo 106-0044, Japan. TEL 81-3-5561-5033**; Subscr. outside the Americas to:** Elsevier Science BV, PO Box 211, Amsterdam 1000 AE, Netherlands. TEL 31-20-485-3757.

JOURNAL OF PHYSIOLOGY. see *BIOLOGY—Physiology*

612.8 FRA ISSN 0928-4257
QP1 CODEN: JHYSEM
JOURNAL OF PHYSIOLOGY (PARIS); an integrative neuroscience journal. Text in English. 1899. bi-m. EUR 494 in Europe to institutions; JPY 65,500 in Japan to institutions; USD 552 elsewhere to institutions (effective 2002). bk.rev. illus. index. back issues avail.; reprint service avail. from ISI. *Refereed.* **Document type:** *Academic/Scholarly.* **Description:** Covers all aspects of neurobiology relevant to a better understanding of behavior and cognition and the integrative functions of the brain, with a focus on functional imaging, development and plasticity, cellular neurobiology, systems, behavioral and neuromuscular physiology, endocrinology, and cognition.
Formerly (until 1992): Journal de Physiologie (0021-7948)
Related titles: Microform ed.: (from PQC); Online - full text ed.: (from ingenta, ScienceDirect, Swets Blackwell, Institute for Scientific Information).
Indexed: ASCA, Anim.Breed.Abstr., Apic.Abstr., Aqua.Sci.& Fish.Abstr., Biol.Abstr., Chem.Abstr., Chem.Indus.Notes, Chem.Titles, Curr.Cont., Curr.Ref.Fish Res., Dairy Sci.Abstr., Dent.Ind., Environ.Sci.Poll.Mgmt., Ergon.Abstr., Excerp.Med., INIS Atomind., Ind.Med. (1992-), Ind.Sci.Rev., Inpharma, Int.Abstr.Biol.Sci., Neurosci.Cit.Ind., Nutr.Abstr., Pharm.&Out.News, Pollut.Abstr., Psychol.Abstr., Reac., Risk Abstr., SSCI (coverage dropped), Saf.Sci.Abstr., Sci.Cit.Ind., Sport Fish.Abstr., Wild.Rev., Zoo.Rec., e-psyche.
—BLDSC (5039.020000), CASDDS, CISTI, EMDOCS, GNLM, IDS, ingenta, KNAW, Linda Hall. **CCC.**
Published by: Elsevier Paris, Editions Scientifiques et Medicales (Subsidiary of: Reed Elsevier plc. group), 23 rue Linois, Paris 75015, France. TEL 33-1-45589110, FAX 33-1-45589419, academic@elsevier-fr.com, http://www.elsevier.com/locate/jphysparis. Ed. Y Freacutegnac. Circ: 850.

616.8 DNK ISSN 0742-3098
QP188.P55 CODEN: JPRSE9
JOURNAL OF PINEAL RESEARCH. Text in English. 8/yr. USD 766 in the Americas to institutions print & online eds. combined; GBP 532 elsewhere to institutions print & online eds. combined (effective 2002). adv. charts, illus. reprint service avail. from ISI. *Refereed.* **Document type:** *Journal, Academic/Scholarly.*
Related titles: Online - full text ed.: USD 689 (effective 2002) (from EBSCO Publishing, ingenta, Swets Blackwell, Institute for Scientific Information).
Indexed: ASCA, Anim.Breed.Abstr., Aqua.Sci.& Fish.Abstr., Biol.Abstr., Chem.Abstr., Chem.Indus.Notes, Chem.Titles, Curr.Adv.Cancer Res., Curr.Adv.Ecol.Sci., Curr.Cont., Dairy Sci.Abstr., Excerp.Med., INIS Atomind., Ind.Med. (1984-), Ind.Sci.Rev., Inpharma, Neurosci.Abstr., Neurosci.Cit.Ind., Nutr.Abstr., Pharm.&Out.News, Pig News & Info., Poult.Abstr., Protozool.Abstr., Reac., Sci.Cit.Ind., e-psyche.
—BLDSC (5040.329000), ADONIS, CASDDS, CISTI, EMDOCS, GNLM, IDS, Infotrieve. **CCC.**
Published by: Blackwell Munksgaard, Noerre Soegade 35, PO Box 2148, Copenhagen K 1016, Denmark. FAX 45-77-33-33-77, fsub@munksgaard.dk, http://www.blackwellmunksgaard.com/pinealresearch. Ed. Russel J Reiter. Circ: 250.

JOURNAL OF POLYMORPHOUS PERVERSITY. see *LITERARY AND POLITICAL REVIEWS*

THE JOURNAL OF PRIMARY PREVENTION. see *PSYCHOLOGY*

616.8 GBR ISSN 1351-0126
CODEN: JPMNE3
JOURNAL OF PSYCHIATRIC AND MENTAL HEALTH NURSING. Text in English. 1994. bi-m., latest vol.9, 2002. GBP 79 in Europe to individuals; USD 126 in North America to individuals; GBP 87 elsewhere to individuals; GBP 349 in Europe to institutions; USD 553 in North America to institutions; GBP 384 elsewhere to institutions (effective 2002). adv. bk.rev. bibl, illus. index. *Refereed.* **Document type:** *Academic/Scholarly.* **Description:** Publishes original articles that integrate the knowledge and practice of psychiatric and mental-health nursing.
Related titles: Microform ed.: (from PQC); ♦ Online - full text ed.: Journal of Psychiatric & Mental Health Nursing Online. ISSN 1365-2850.
Indexed: Brit.Nur.Ind., CINAHL, Int.Nurs.Ind., e-psyche.
—BLDSC (5043.140000), CISTI, GNLM, Infotrieve. **CCC.**
Published by: Blackwell Science Ltd., PO Box 88, Oxford OX2 0NE, United Kingdom. TEL 44-1865-206180, 44-1865-206002, FAX 44-1865-206219, jnl.orders@blacksci.co.uk, http://www.blackwell-science.com/products/journals/jpmhn.htm, http://www.blackwellpublishing.com. Ed. B Davis. Pub. Elaine Stott. R&P Sophie Savage. Adv. contact Jenny Applin. Circ: 505.

616.8 GBR ISSN 1365-2850
▼ **JOURNAL OF PSYCHIATRIC & MENTAL HEALTH NURSING ONLINE.** Text in English. 1999. bi-m. GBP 72 in Europe to individuals; USD 114 in North America to individuals; GBP 72 elsewhere to individuals; GBP 315 in Europe to institutions; USD 498 in North America to institutions; GBP 315 elsewhere to institutions (effective 2002). *Refereed.* **Document type:** *Academic/Scholarly.*
Media: Online - full text (from EBSCO Publishing, Munksgaard & Blackwell Science's Synergy, O C L C Online Computer Library Center, Inc., RoweCom Information Quest, ingenta, Swets Blackwell). **Related titles:** Microform ed.: (from PQC); ♦ Print ed.: Journal of Psychiatric and Mental Health Nursing. ISSN 1351-0126.
Published by: Blackwell Science Ltd., Osney Mead, Oxford OX2 0EL, United Kingdom. TEL 44-1685-206206, FAX 44-1685-721205, website@blacksci.com, journals.cs@blacksci.co.uk, http://www.blackwell-science.com/~cgilib/jnlpage.bin?Journal=jpmhn&File=jpmhn&Page=aims.

616.8 USA ISSN 1527-4160
JOURNAL OF PSYCHIATRIC PRACTICE. Text in English. 1997. bi-m. USD 125 domestic to individuals; USD 164 foreign to individuals; USD 206 domestic to individuals; USD 246 foreign to individuals (effective 2002). adv. **Description:** For psychiatrists, psychologists, nurses, and social workers responsible for managing psychiatric patients. Offers readable, reliable coverage on clinically applicable topics.
Formerly (until 2000): Journal of Practical Psychiatry and Behavioral Health (1076-5417)
Related titles: Online - full text ed.: USD 267.80 domestic for academic site license; USD 307.80 foreign for academic site license; USD 298.70 domestic for corporate site license; USD 338.70 foreign for corporate site license (effective 2002).
Indexed: e-psyche.
—BLDSC (5043.220000), GNLM.
Published by: Williams & Wilkins (Subsidiary of: Waverly International), 351 W Camden St, Baltimore, MD 21201-2436. TEL 410-528-4068, 800-222-3790, FAX 410-528-4452, Kmalamphy@wwilkins.com, http://www.practicalpsychiatry.com, http://www.wwilkins.com/pracpsych/. Ed. Dr. John M Oldham. Adv. contact Kathleen Malamphy. B&W page USD 770; trim 10.88 x 8.13. Circ: 6,372; 1,845 (paid).

616.89 GBR ISSN 0022-3956
RC321 CODEN: JPYRA3

JOURNAL OF PSYCHIATRIC RESEARCH. Text in English. 1961. bi-m. EUR 764 in Europe to institutions; JPY 101,400 in Japan to institutions; USD 854 elsewhere to institutions (effective 2002). adv. bk.rev. charts, illus. index. back issues avail.; reprint service avail. from PSC,SCH. *Refereed.* **Document type:** *Academic/Scholarly.* **Description:** Covers the latest developments in psychiatry and cognate disciplines.

Related titles: Microfilm ed.: (from PQC); Online - full text ed.: (from ingenta, ScienceDirect, Swets Blackwell, Institute for Scientific Information).

Indexed: ASCA, AgeLine, Bibl.Asian Stud. (1991), Biol.Abstr., Chem.Abstr., Curr.Adv.Ecol.Sci., Curr.Cont., Curr.Ind.Stat., Dent.Ind., Excerp.Med., Fam.Ind., Hosp.Lit.Ind., INIS Atomind., Ind.Med. (1961-), Ind.Sci.Rev., Inpharma, Int.Abstr.Biol.Sci., Lang.& Lang.Behav.Abstr., Mid.East: Abstr.& Ind., Neurosci.Cit.Ind., Pharm.&Out.News, PsycInfo, Psychol.Abstr. (1961-), Reac., SOPODA, SSCI, Sci.Cit.Ind., Sociol.Abstr., e-psyche.

—BLDSC (5043.250000), CASDDS, CISTI, GNLM, IDS, ingenta, KNAW. **CCC.**

Published by: Pergamon (Subsidiary of: Elsevier Science), The Boulevard, Langford Ln, East Park, Kidlington, Oxford OXB 1GB, United Kingdom. FAX 44-1865-843010, usinfo-f@elsevier.com, http://www.elsevier.com/locate/jpsychires. Eds. Joseph J Schildkraut, Merton Sandler. adv.: B&W page USD 550, color page USD 1,350. Circ: 1,250. **Subscr. in Australasia and the Far East to:** Elsevier Science (Singapore) Pte Ltd, No.1 Temasek Ave, 17-01 Millenia Tower, Singapore 039192, Singapore. TEL 65-434-3727, FAX 65-337-2230; **Subscr. in the Americas to:** Elsevier Science, PO Box 945, New York, NY 10159-0945. TEL 212-633-3730, FAX 212-633-3680; **Subscr. to:** Elsevier Science BV, PO Box 211, Amsterdam 1000 AE, Netherlands. TEL 31-20-485-3757.

JOURNAL OF PSYCHIATRY AND LAW. see *LAW*

616.8 CAN ISSN 1180-4882
RC321 CODEN: JPNEEF

JOURNAL OF PSYCHIATRY AND NEUROSCIENCE. Text in English, French. 1976. 5/yr. CND 98 to individuals; USD 77 foreign to individuals; USD 98 to institutions (effective 2000). adv. bk.rev. index. *Refereed.* **Document type:** *Academic/Scholarly.* **Description:** Publishes original research articles and review papers in clinical psychiatry (adult and child) neuroscience related to major psychiatric disorders, and neurodegenerative diseases.

Formerly: Psychiatric Journal of the University of Ottawa (0702-8466)

Related titles: Online - full text ed.: (from ProQuest Information & Learning, Institute for Scientific Information).

Indexed: ASCA, AgeLine, Arts & Hum.Cit.Ind. (coverage dropped), Biol.Abstr., CBCA Ref., Child Devel.Abstr., Crim.Just.Abstr., Curr.Cont., Excerp.Med., Ind.Med. (1991-), Neurosci.Cit.Ind., PsycInfo, Psychol.Abstr. (1976-), SSCI, Sociol.Abstr., e-psyche.

—BLDSC (5043.261000), ADONIS, CISTI, EMDOCS, GNLM, IDS, ingenta, KNAW. **CCC.**

Published by: Canadian Medical Association, 1867 Alta Vista Dr, Ottawa, ON K1H 5K9, Canada. TEL 613-731-9331, 800-663-7336 ext. 2132, FAX 613-565-2382, msproule@rohcg.on.ca, rafusj@cma.ca, http://www.cma.ca/jpn. Ed. Dr. Y D Lapierre. Adv. contact M Sproule Jones. B&W page CND 1,500, color page CND 2,700; trim 10.88 x 8.13. Circ: 7,153.

JOURNAL OF PSYCHOACTIVE DRUGS; a multidisciplinary forum. see *DRUG ABUSE AND ALCOHOLISM*

JOURNAL OF PSYCHOPHYSIOLOGY. see *PSYCHOLOGY*

JOURNAL OF PSYCHOSOMATIC OBSTETRICS AND GYNECOLOGY. see *MEDICAL SCIENCES—Obstetrics And Gynecology*

616.08 USA ISSN 0022-3999
RC52 CODEN: JPCRAT

JOURNAL OF PSYCHOSOMATIC RESEARCH. Text in English. 1956. m. EUR 281 in Europe to individuals; JPY 37,200 in Japan to individuals; USD 314 elsewhere to individuals; EUR 1,357 in Europe to institutions; JPY 180,200 in Japan to institutions; USD 1,518 elsewhere to institutions (effective 2002). adv. bk.rev. bibl, charts. index. back issues avail.; reprint service avail. from PSC,SCH. *Refereed.* **Document type:** *Journal, Academic/Scholarly.* **Description:** Reflects current research in the psychosomatic approach from both clinical and experimental perspectives, including scientific examination of theoretical topics.

Related titles: Microfilm ed.: (from PQC); Online - full text ed.: (from ingenta, ScienceDirect, Swets Blackwell, Institute for Scientific Information).

Indexed: AIDS Abstr., ASCA, ASSIA, Abstr.Hyg., Adol.Ment.Hlth.Abstr., AgeLine, Behav.Med.Abstr., Bibl.Dev.Med.& Child Neur., Biol.Abstr., Chem.Abstr., Curr.Adv.Ecol.Sci., Curr.Cont., Dent.Ind., Dok.Arbeitsmed., Excerp.Med., Fam.Ind., Ind.Med. (1956-), Ind.Sci.Rev., Ind.Vet., Inpharma, Int.Nurs.Ind., Lang.& Lang.Behav.Abstr., Mid.East: Abstr.& Ind., Neurosci.Cit.Ind., Nutr.Abstr., Pharm.&Out.News, PsycInfo, Psychol.Abstr. (1956-), Reac., Risk Abstr., SOPODA, SSCI, Sci.Cit.Ind., Sociol.Abstr., Stud.Wom.Abstr., e-psyche.

—BLDSC (5043.480000), CASDDS, CISTI, GNLM, IDS, ingenta, KNAW. **CCC.**

Published by: Elsevier Science, Box 945, New York, NY 10159-0945. TEL 212-989-5800, FAX 212-633-3990, usinfo-f@elsevier.com, http://www.elsevier.com/locate/jpsychores. Eds. Dr. Colin M Shapiro, Dr. Richard Mayou. adv.: B&W page USD 550, color page USD 1,350. Circ: 1,600. **Subscr. in Australasia and the Far East to:** Elsevier Science (Singapore) Pte Ltd, No.1 Temasek Ave, 17-01 Millenia Tower, Singapore 039192, Singapore. TEL 65-434-3727, FAX 65-337-2230; **Subscr. in Japan to:** Elsevier Science Inc - Japan Regional Office, 9-15 Higashi-Azabu 1-chome, Minato-ku, Tokyo 106-0044, Japan. TEL 81-3-5561-5033; **Subscr. outside the Americas to:** Elsevier Science BV, PO Box 211, Amsterdam 1000 AE, Netherlands. TEL 31-20-485-3757.

616.8 USA ISSN 0887-8250
TX546 CODEN: JSSDEO

JOURNAL OF SENSORY STUDIES. Text in English. 1986. bi-m., latest vol.16. USD 168 (effective 2001). bk.rev. abstr, bibl, charts, illus, stat. back issues avail.; reprints avail. *Refereed.* **Document type:** *Journal, Academic/Scholarly.* **Description:** Promotes the technical and practical advancement of sensory science, publishing a broad spectrum of papers, including observational and experimental studies in the application of sensory evaluation to the food, medical, agricultural, biological, pharmaceutical, cosmetic, consumer, and materials industries.

Related titles: Online - full text ed.: (from Institute for Scientific Information).

Indexed: Chemorec.Abstr., Curr.Cont., Dairy Sci.Abstr., Food Sci.& Tech.Abstr., Hort.Abstr., Nutr.Abstr., Sci.Cit.Ind., e-psyche.

—BLDSC (5063.600000), CASDDS, CISTI, IDS, ingenta.

Published by: Food & Nutrition Press, Inc., 6527 Main St, PO Box 374, Trumbull, CT 06611. TEL 203-261-8587, FAX 203-261-9724, foodpress@worldnetatt.net, http://www.foodscipress.com. Ed. M C Gacula Jr. Adv. contact John J O'Neil.

612.8 GBR ISSN 1350-7702
CODEN: JSRRER

JOURNAL OF SEROTONIN RESEARCH. Text in English. 1994. q. GBP 65, USD 120 to individuals; GBP 95, USD 170 to institutions. bk.rev. *Refereed.* **Document type:** *Academic/Scholarly.*

Indexed: Chem.Abstr., Chem.Indus.Notes, Chem.Titles, Excerp.Med. (1995-), e-psyche.

—CASDDS, CISTI, GNLM. **CCC.**

Published by: Euroscience Press, Euroscience Press, PO Box 3405, London N1 0NZ, United Kingdom. TEL 44-20-7601-8138, FAX 44-20-7601-7969. Ed. Dr. Ted Dinan. **Dist. by:** Royal Society of Medicine Press Ltd. TEL 44-20-7290-2900, FAX 44-20-7290-2929.

JOURNAL OF SPINAL CORD MEDICINE. see *MEDICAL SCIENCES—Physical Medicine And Rehabilitation*

JOURNAL OF SYSTEMIC THERAPIES. see *PSYCHOLOGY*

616.8 NLD ISSN 0964-704X
CODEN: JHNEFS

JOURNAL OF THE HISTORY OF THE NEUROSCIENCES; basic and clinical perspectives. Text in English. 1992. q., latest vol.10, 2001. NLG 173, USD 98 to non-members; NLG 424, USD 217 to institutions includes online ed (effective 2001). adv. back issues avail.; reprint service avail. from SWZ. *Refereed.* **Document type:** *Journal, Academic/Scholarly.* **Description:** Surveys and examines trends in the study of the neurosciences.

Related titles: Online - full content ed.: (from EBSCO Publishing, O C L C Online Computer Library Center, Inc., Swets Blackwell); Online - full text ed.: (from RoweCom Information Quest).

Indexed: Ind.Med., PsycInfo.

—BLDSC (5001.050000), GNLM, Infotrieve. **CCC.**

Published by: (International Society for the History of the Neurosciences USA), Swets & Zeitlinger BV, PO Box 825, Lisse 2160 SZ, Netherlands. TEL 31-252-435111, FAX 31-252-415888, orders@swets.nl, http://www.swets.nl/sps/journals/jhn.html. Eds. Peter Koehler, Stanley Finger. R&P J van der Valk. Adv. contact Patrick Kliean. **Dist. in N. America by:** Swets & Zeitlinger, PO Box 582, Downingtown, PA 19335-998. TEL 800-477-9387, FAX 610-524-5366. **Co-sponsors:** European Club for the History of Neurology; World Federation of Neurology/Federation Mondiale de Neurologie.

616.8 NLD ISSN 0022-510X
RC321 CODEN: JNSCAG

JOURNAL OF THE NEUROLOGICAL SCIENCES. Text and summaries in English, French, German, Spanish. 1964. 22/yr. EUR 2,647 in Europe to institutions; JPY 352,000 in Japan to institutions; USD 2,961 elsewhere to institutions (effective 2002). adv. bk.rev. bibl, charts, illus. index. back issues avail.; reprint service avail. from SWZ,ISI. *Refereed.* **Document type:** *Academic/Scholarly.* **Description:** Provides a medium for the publication of studies on the interface between clinical neurology and the basic sciences.

Related titles: Microform ed.: (from PQC); Online - full text ed.: (from ingenta, ScienceDirect, Swets Blackwell, Institute for Scientific Information).

Indexed: ASCA, Abstr.Hyg., Aqua.Sci.& Fish.Abstr., Bibl.Dev.Med.& Child Neur., Biol.Abstr., Chem.Abstr., Chem.Indus.Notes, Chem.Titles, Curr.Adv.Ecol.Sci., Curr.Cont., Excerp.Med., Helminthol.Abstr., Ind.Med. (1964-), Ind.Sci.Rev., Ind.Vet., Inpharma, Int.Abstr.Biol.Sci., Int.Nurs.Ind., Jrnl.Watch Neuro., Neurosci.Abstr., Neurosci.Cit.Ind., Nutr.Abstr., Pharm.&Out.News, Psychol.Abstr., Reac., Rev.Appl.Entomol., Rev.Arom.& Med.Plants, Rev.Med.& Vet.Mycol., SSCI (coverage dropped), Sci.Cit.Ind., Trop.Dis.Bull., Vet.Bull., e-psyche.

—BLDSC (5021.560000), CASDDS, CISTI, GNLM, IDS, ingenta, KNAW. **CCC.**

Published by: (World Federation of Neurology/Federation Mondiale de Neurologie GBR), Elsevier Science BV, PO Box 211, Amsterdam 1000 AE, Netherlands. TEL 31-20-485-3757, FAX 31-20-485-3432, TELEX 18582 ESPA NL, http://www.elsevier.com/locate/jns, http://www.elsevier.nl. Eds. R A Lewis, Robert P Lisak. **Subscr. in Australasia and the Far East to:** Elsevier Science (Singapore) Pte Ltd, No.1 Temasek Ave, 17-01 Millenia Tower, Singapore 039192, Singapore. TEL 65-434-3727, FAX 65-337-2230; **Subscr. in Japan to:** Elsevier Science Inc - Japan Regional Office, 9-15 Higashi-Azabu 1-chome, Minato-ku, Tokyo 106-0044, Japan. TEL 81-3-5561-5033, FAX 81-3-5561-5047; **Subscr. in the Americas to:** Elsevier Science, PO Box 945, New York, NY 10159-0945. TEL 212-633-3730, 888-437-4636, FAX 212-633-3680, usinfo-f@elsevier.com.

JOURNAL OF THE NEUROMUSCULOSKELETAL SYSTEM. see *MEDICAL SCIENCES—Chiropractic, Homeopathy, Osteopathy*

616.8 574.88 USA ISSN 1085-9489
CODEN: JPNSFO

JOURNAL OF THE PERIPHERAL NERVOUS SYSTEM. Text in English. 1996. q. USD 145 domestic to individuals; USD 160 in Canada & Mexico to individuals; USD 175 elsewhere to individuals; USD 205 domestic to institutions; USD 220 in Canada & Mexico to institutions; USD 235 elsewhere to institutions; USD 159.50 to individuals print & online eds. combined; USD 225.50 to institutions print & online eds. combined (effective 2001). adv. bk.rev. index, cum.index. back issues avail.; reprints avail. *Refereed.* **Document type:** *Journal, Academic/Scholarly.* **Description:** Publishes papers encompassing all topics relevant to peripheral nerves, linking molecular biology and medicine to clinical neuroscience.

Related titles: ♦ Online - full text ed.: Journal of the Peripheral Nervous System Online. ISSN 1529-8027.

M

Indexed: Curr.Cont., Ind.Med. (1996-), Inpharma, Neurosci.Cit.Ind., Pharm.&Out.News, Reac., e-psyche. —BLDSC (5073.711000), CASDDS, IDS.
Published by: Blackwell Science Inc., Commerce Pl, 350 Main St, Malden, MA 02148-5018. TEL 781-388-8250, FAX 781-388-8255, journals@blacksci.com, http://www.blackwell-science.com/~cgilib/bsinc.bin?Journal=peripheral. Pub. Carol Trumbold TEL 314-439-0365. Adv. contact David Surdel TEL 781-388-8345. page USD 750; trim 11 x 8.5. Circ: 525 (paid).

616.8 574.88 USA ISSN 1529-8027
JOURNAL OF THE PERIPHERAL NERVOUS SYSTEM ONLINE. Text in English. 4/yr. USD 131 to individuals; USD 185 to institutions (effective 2001). **Document type:** *Academic/Scholarly.*
Media: Online - full text (from EBSCO Publishing, O C L C Online Computer Library Center, Inc., ingenta, Munksgaard & Blackwell Science's Synergy, Swets Blackwell, Institute for Scientific Information). **Related titles:** ♦ Print ed.: Journal of the Peripheral Nervous System. ISSN 1085-9489.
Published by: Blackwell Science Inc., Commerce Pl, 350 Main St, Malden, MA 02148-5018. TEL 781-388-8250, 888-661-5800, FAX 781-388-8255, journals@blacksci.com, http://www.blackwell-science.com/~cgilib/bsinc.bin?Journal=peripheral.

JOURNAL OF VESTIBULAR RESEARCH: EQUILIBRIUM AND ORIENTATION; an international journal of experimental and clinical vestibular science. see *BIOLOGY—Physiology*

616.8982 CAN ISSN 1188-9136
JOURNAL ON DEVELOPMENTAL DISABILITIES/ JOURNAL SUR LES HANDICAPS DU DEVELOPPEMENT. Text in English, French. 1990. s-a.
Formerly (until 1991): BrOADD Perspectives (1196-2623)
Indexed: e-psyche.
—BLDSC (4969.290450).
Published by: Ontario Association on Developmental Disabilities/L'Association Ontarienne Sur les Handicaps du Developpement, 100 College St, Room 511, Toronto, ON M5G 1L5, Canada. TEL 416-946-3680, FAX 416-946-3680, oadd@interlog.com, http://www.interlog.com/~oadd/.

▼ **JOURNAL WATCH NEUROLOGY.** see *MEDICAL SCIENCES—Abstracting, Bibliographies, Statistics*

JOURNAL WATCH PSYCHIATRY. see *MEDICAL SCIENCES—Abstracting, Bibliographies, Statistics*

616.8 617 JPN ISSN 0918-1172
KAGAWA NO SHINKEI GEKA DANWAKAI KAISHI/KAGAWA COLLOQUIUM ON NEUROSURGERY. JOURNAL. Text in Japanese. 1985. a.
Indexed: e-psyche.
Published by: Kagawa No Shinkei Geka Danwakai, Kagawa Ika Daigaku No Shinkei Gekagaku Kyoshitsu, 1750-1 Ikedo, Kita-gun, Miki-cho, Kagawa-ken 761-0700, Japan.

616.8 JPN ISSN 0288-9617
KANAGAWA-KEN SEISHIN IGAKKAISHI/KANAGAWA ASSOCIATION OF PSYCHIATRY. JOURNAL. Text in Japanese. 1959. a. JPY 3,000 (effective 2001). adv. back issues avail. *Refereed.* **Document type:** *Academic/Scholarly.*
Indexed: e-psyche.
Published by: Kanagawa Association of Psychiatry, c/o Department of Psychiatry, University School of Medicine, Yokohama, 3-9 Fukura, Kanazawa-ku, Yokohama-shi, Kanagawa-ken 236-0004, Japan. TEL 81-45-787-2667, FAX 81-45-783-2540. Ed. Kenji Kosaka. R&P Saeko Fujikake. Adv. contact Eizo Iseki. Circ: 2,000.

616.8 AUT ISSN 0934-1420
KEY TOPICS IN BRAIN RESEARCH. Text in English. 1988. irreg. price varies. **Document type:** *Monographic series, Academic/Scholarly.*
Published by: Springer-Verlag Wien (Subsidiary of: BertelsmannSpringer), Sachsenplatz 4-6, PO Box 89, Vienna, W 1201, Austria. TEL 43-1-3302415-0, FAX 43-1-330242665, books@springer.at, http://www.springer.at. Eds. A Carlsson, P Riederer. R&P Angela Foessl TEL 43-1-3302415517. **Dist. in N. America by:** Springer-Verlag, Journals. books@springer.at, http://www.springer-ny.com.

616.8 JPN
KINOTEKI NO SHINKEI GEKA/FUNCTIONAL NEUROSURGERY. Text in English, Japanese. 1987. a. JPY 5,150, USD 33 domestic (effective 2000). adv. *Refereed.* **Document type:** *Proceedings.*
Indexed: e-psyche.
Published by: Nihon Teii No Shujutsu Kenkyukai/Japan Society for Stereotactic and Functional Neurosurgery, Department of Neurosurgery, Nihon University School of Medicine, 30-1, Oyaguchi Kamimachi, Itabashi-ku, Tokyo 173, Japan. TEL 81-3-3972-8111, FAX 81-3-3554-0425, ykatayama@med.nihon-u.ac.jp. Ed., R&P, Adv. contact Yoichi Katayama.

616.8 TUR ISSN 1017-7833
KLINIK PSIKOFARMAKOLOJI BULTENI/BULLETIN OF CLINICAL PSYCHOPHARMACOLOGY. Text in Turkish, English; Summaries in Turkish, English. 1991. q. free. Index. back issues avail. *Refereed.* **Document type:** *Bulletin, Academic/Scholarly.* **Description:** Primarily focusing on psychopharmacology, biological psychiatry and biological aspects of psychiatry.
Related titles: Online - full text ed.
Published by: Kure Iletisim Grubu A S, Siracevizler Cad 43/3, Sisli, Istanbul 80260, Turkey. TEL 90-212-2194900, FAX 90-212-2305009, kure@kure.com.tr, http://www.kure.com.tr. Ed. Mesut Cetin. Circ: 1,000.

621.3 DEU ISSN 1434-0275 CODEN: EEGEAE
KLINISCHE NEUROPHYSIOLOGIE; Zeitschrift fuer Funktionsdiagnostik des Nervensystems. Text in German; Summaries in English, German. 1970. q. EUR 213.80 domestic to institutions; EUR 213.90 in Europe to institutions; EUR 218.40 elsewhere to institutions; EUR 64 newsstand/cover (effective 2002). adv. bk.rev. abstr, bibl, charts, illus, stat. index. back issues avail.; reprint service avail. from PQC. *Refereed.* **Document type:** *Journal, Academic/Scholarly.*
Formerly: E E G - E M G (0012-7590)
Related titles: Microform ed.: (from PQC); Online - full text ed.: ISSN 1439-4081 (from Institute for Scientific Information).
Indexed: ASCA, Curr.Cont., Excerp.Med., INIS Atomind., Ind.Med. (until 1992, dropped), Neurosci.Cit.Ind., SSCI (coverage dropped), e-psyche.
—BLDSC (5099.453000), CISTI, GNLM, IDS, Infotrieve. **CCC.**
Published by: Georg Thieme Verlag, Ruedigerstr 14, Stuttgart 70469, Germany. TEL 49-711-8931-0, FAX 49-711-8931298, kunden.service@thieme.de, leser.service@thieme.de, http://www.thieme.de/klinneuro. Ed. M Stoehr. R&P Peter Eich. adv.: page DEM 1,650; 175 x 250. Circ: 1,200.

KLINISCHE NEURORADIOLOGIE. see *MEDICAL SCIENCES—Radiology And Nuclear Medicine*

616.853 CHE
KONTAKTE; Zeitung fuer Epilepsie-Betroffene. Text in German. 1986. 2/yr. CHF 15 (effective 2001). bk.rev. **Document type:** *Newspaper, Consumer.*
Indexed: e-psyche.
Published by: Schweizerische Liga gegen Epilepsie, Dorfstr 2, Postfach 233, Stafa Zurich 8712, Switzerland. TEL 41-1-926-89-71, FAX 41-1-926-89-72, slge@bluewin.ch, http://www.epi.ch. Ed. Margret Becker. Circ: 900.

616.8 KOR ISSN 1015-4817
QP351
KOREAN NEUROPSYCHIATRIC ASSOCIATION. JOURNAL. Key Title: Taehan Sin'gyong Chongsin Uihak Hoeji. Text in Korean; Summaries in English. 1962. bi-m. free per issue. adv. **Document type:** *Academic/Scholarly.*
Formerly: Neuro-Psychiatry
Indexed: e-psyche.
Published by: Korean Neuropsychiatric Association, RN.403 Osung Bd. 13-5, Youido-dong, Youngdungpo-Ku, Seoul, Korea, S.. TEL 02-786-3355. Ed. Dr. Kwang Iel Kim. Pub. Jae Ho Seok.

616.89 JPN ISSN 0023-6144 CODEN: KSSIAC
KYUSHU NEURO-PSYCHIATRY/KYUSHU SHINKEI SEISHIN IGAKU. Text in Japanese; Summaries in English. 1954. q. JPY 5,000. adv. bk.rev. bibl, charts, stat. index. **Document type:** *Proceedings, Academic/Scholarly.*
Media: Duplicated (not offset). **Related titles:** Microfilm ed.: (from PQC).
Indexed: Chem.Abstr., Curr.Ind.Stat., INIS Atomind., Psychol.Abstr., e-psyche.
—CASDDS, GNLM.
Published by: Kyushu Association of Neuro-Psychiatry/Kyushu Seishin Shinkei Gakkai, c/o Department of Neuro-Psychiatry Faculty of Medicine, Kyushu University, Maidashi, Higashi-ku, Fukuoka-shi 812-0054, Japan. TEL 81-92-642-5620, FAX 81-92-642-5644. Ed., Pub., Adv. contact Nobutada Tashiro. Circ: 1,100 (controlled).

616.8 DEU ISSN 0944-405X
RC423.A1 CODEN: LOINEW
L.O.G.O.S. INTERDISZIPLINAER. Text in English. 1994. q. EUR 68; EUR 45 to students (effective 2002). **Document type:** *Journal, Academic/Scholarly.*
Indexed: e-psyche.
—GNLM.
Published by: Urban & Fischer Verlag, Loebdergraben 14A, Jena 07743, Germany. TEL 49-3641-626444, FAX 49-3641-626421, marketing.journals@urbanfischer.de, http://www.urbanfischer.de.

616.8 USA ISSN 1470-8582
LANCET NEUROLOGY NETWORK. Text in English. 1997. bi-m. USD 75 in US & Canada to individuals; GBP 50 elsewhere to individuals; USD 220 in US & Canada to institutions; GBP 125 elsewhere to institutions (effective 2001). back issues avail. **Document type:** *Academic/Scholarly.* **Description:** Presents relevant and practice-applicable articles on the twenty subspecialty fields of neurology.
Formerly: Neurology Network Commentary (1089-4969)
Media: Online - full text. **Related titles:** Online - full text ed.
Indexed: e-psyche.
Published by: The Lancet Publishing Group (Subsidiary of: Reed Elsevier plc), 84 Theobald's Rd, London WC1X 8RR, United Kingdom. TEL 44-20-7436-4981, 44-20-7611-4102, 800-462-6198, FAX 44-20-7611-4479, 212-633-3850, custserv@lancet.com, http://www.lancetneuronet.com/. Ed. Dr. Sid Gilman.

616.8 GBR ISSN 1357-650X CODEN: LATEFV
LATERALITY. Text in English. 1996. q. GBP 68, USD 113 to individuals; GBP 149, USD 245 to institutions (effective 2002). adv. **Document type:** *Academic/Scholarly.*
Related titles: Online - full text ed.: ISSN 1464-0678 (from CatchWord Ltd., EBSCO Publishing, O C L C Online Computer Library Center, Inc., RoweCom Information Quest, Swets Blackwell, Institute for Scientific Information).
Indexed: Curr.Cont., Ergon.Abstr., Indian Psychol.Abstr., Lang.& Lang.Behav.Abstr., PsycInfo, SOPODA, SSCI, Sociol.Abstr., e-psyche.
—BLDSC (5157.679000), CatchWord.
Published by: Psychology Press (Subsidiary of: Taylor & Francis Group), 27 Church Rd, Hove, E Sussex BN3 2FA, United Kingdom. TEL 44-1273-207411, FAX 44-1273-205612, information@psypress.co.uk, http://www.psypress.co.uk. Eds. Chris McManus, Michael Corballis, Michael Peters. R&P Zoe Peden TEL 44-20-7842-2363. Adv. contact Claire Buckminster. **Subscr. addr. in N America:** Psychology Press, Journals Customer Service, Taylor & Francis Group, 325 Chestnut St, Philadelphia, PA 19106. TEL 800-354-1420, FAX 215-625-8914, info@taylorandfrancis.com, http://www.psypress.com; **Subscr. addr. outside N America:** Journals Customer Service, Taylor & Francis Group, Rankine Rd, Basingstoke, Hants RG24 8PR, United Kingdom. TEL 44-1256-813002, FAX 44-1256-479438, enquiry@tandf.co.uk.

616.8 ITA ISSN 0023-9097
LAVORO NEUROPSICHIATRICO. Text in Italian; Summaries in English, French, German, Italian. 1947. bi-m. ITL 8,000. bk.rev. bibl, charts, illus. index. Supplement avail.
Indexed: Chem.Abstr., Excerp.Med., Psychol.Abstr., e-psyche.
—CISTI.
Published by: Amministrazione Provinciale, Piazza Santa Maria Della Pieta', 5, Rome, RM 00135, Italy. Ed. Giovanni Bonfiglio. Circ: 1,200.

LAW AND MENTAL DISABILITY. see *LAW*

M

155.67 USA ISSN 1072-0502
QP406 CODEN: LEMEFO
LEARNING & MEMORY. Text in English. 1994. bi-m. USD 99 domestic to individuals; USD 125 in Canada & Mexico to individuals; USD 137 elsewhere to individuals; USD 332 domestic to institutions; USD 358 in Canada & Mexico to institutions; USD 370 elsewhere to institutions (effective 2001). adv. back issues avail. *Refereed.* **Document type:** *Journal, Academic/Scholarly.* **Description:** Publishes experimental studies in humans and animals on cognition, behavior, development, neuropsychology, neurophysiology, biochemistry, cell biology and genetics.
Related titles: Online - full text ed.: 1997 (from HighWire Pr., EBSCO Publishing, Institute for Scientific Information).
Indexed: Anim.Behav.Abstr., Aqua.Sci.& Fish.Abstr., Biotech.& Bioeng.Abstr., Chemorec.Abstr., Curr.Cont., Ind.Med. (1994-), Neurosci.Abstr., Neurosci.Cit.Ind., PsycInfo, SSCI (coverage dropped), Sci.Cit.Ind., Zoo.Rec., e-psyche.
—BLDSC (5179.325895), CISTI, GNLM, IDS, Infotrieve. **CCC.**
Published by: (Cold Spring Harbor Laboratory), Cold Spring Harbor Laboratory Press, Publications Department, 10 Skyline Dr, Plainview, NY 11803. FAX 516-349-1946, chspress@cshl.org, http://www.learnmem.org, http://www.cshl.org. Ed. L Goodman. Adv. contact Marcie Ebenstein.

616.858 GBR
LEARNING DISABILITY BULLETIN. Text in English. 1979. q. GBP 26 to individuals; GBP 38 to institutions (effective 1999). adv. **Document type:** *Bulletin.*
Formerly (until 1993): Mental Handicap Bulletin (0260-1222)
Indexed: e-psyche.
—BLDSC (2415.050000).
Published by: (British Institute of Learning Disabilities), B I L D, Wolverhampton Rd, Kidderminster, Worcs DY10 3PP, United Kingdom. TEL 44-1562-850251, FAX 44-1562-851970, bild@bild.demon.co.uk, http://www.bild.org.uk. Ed., Pub., R&P, Adv. contact Linda Averill. Circ: 1,000.

LEBENSWELTEN BEHINDERTER MENSCHEN. see *HANDICAPPED*

616.853 ITA ISSN 0394-560X
LEGA ITALIANA CONTRO L'EPILESSIA. BOLLETTINO. Text in Italian. 1973. q. ITL 250,000 to non-members (effective 1996). adv. bk.rev. **Description:** Focuses on epilepsy.
Indexed: Excerp.Med., e-psyche.
—BLDSC (2227.150000), EMDOCS, GNLM, KNAW.
Published by: Lega Italiana contro l'Epilessia, Via Antonio Fogazzaro, 37, Milan, MI 20135, Italy. TEL 39-2-5468820, FAX 39-2-8910198. Ed. Raffaele Canger. Circ: 1,100.

616.89 340 USA
LEGAL RESOURCES FOR THE MENTALLY DISABLED: A DIRECTORY OF LAWYERS AND OTHER SPECIALISTS. Text in English. 1982. a. USD 5 (effective 1998). **Document type:** *Directory.*
Formerly: Mental and Developmental Disabilities Directory of Legal Advocates
Published by: American Bar Association, 750 N Lake Shore Dr, Chicago, IL 60611. TEL 312-988-5522, FAX 312-988-5568. Ed. John Parry.

616.8 FRA ISSN 1276-9339
LA LETTRE DU NEUROLOGUE. Text in French. 1997. bi-m. FRF 300 domestic to individuals; FRF 420, USD 76 foreign to individuals; FRF 380 domestic to institutions; FRF 500, USD 91 foreign to institutions; FRF 190 domestic to students; USD 56 foreign to students (effective 2000). Supplement avail. *Refereed.* **Document type:** *Academic/Scholarly.*
Indexed: e-psyche.
Published by: Edimark S.A., 62-64 rue Jean-Jaures, Puteaux 928000, France. TEL 33-1-414-58000, FAX 33-1-41458025, contact@edimark.fr, http://www.edimark.fr. Ed. P Amarenco. Pub. Claudie Damour Terrasson.

616.8 FRA ISSN 0223-9434
LETTRE DU PSYCHIATRE; psychiatrie et medicaments. Text in French. 1979. 10/yr. FRF 297; FRF 408 foreign (effective 1997). **Document type:** *Bulletin.* **Description:** Informs on new developments of therapeutics in psychiatry.
Related titles: Microform ed.: (from PQC).
Indexed: e-psyche.
—GNLM, Infotrieve. **CCC.**

Published by: Masson - Periodiques, 120 bd. St. Germain, Paris 75006, France. TEL 33-1-40466200, FAX 33-1-40466201. Ed. H Ollat. Circ: 600. **Subscr. to:** Societe de Periodiques Specialises, BP 22, Vineuil Cedex 41354, France. TEL 33-2-54504612, FAX 33-2-54504611.

616.8 610.73 USA
LINK (WOODLAND HILLS)✱. Text in English. 1987. bi-m. free per issue. bk.rev. back issues avail.
Indexed: e-psyche.
Published by: Amyotrophic Lateral Sclerosis Association, 27001 Agoura Rd, Ste 150, Calabasas, CA 91301-5104. TEL 818-340-7500, FAX 818-340-2060. Circ: 80,000.

616.8 USA
LINKAGE (BALTIMORE). Text in English. 1991. q. free per issue. **Document type:** *Newsletter, Government.* **Description:** Keeps mental health professionals, consumers and state employees up-to-date on specific mental health issues within the state system and on general mental health issues.
Indexed: e-psyche.
Published by: Department of Health and Mental Hygiene, 201 Preston St, Rm 416A, Baltimore, MD 21201. TEL 410-767-6629, FAX 410-333-5402, jsmith@dhmh.state.md.us. Ed., R&P Jean Smith. Circ: 20,000.

616.855 SWE ISSN 1102-500X
LOGOPEDNYTT. Text in Swedish. 1979. 9/yr. SEK 200 to members (effective 1993).
Formerly (until vol.3, 1979): Logopedmeddelande
Indexed: e-psyche.
Published by: Svenska Logopedfoerbundet (SLOF), Fack 760, Nacka 13124, Sweden.

616.89 NLD ISSN 0024-8576
M G V. (Maandblad Geestelijke Volksgezondheid) Text in Dutch. 1946. 11/yr. NLG 98; NLG 112.50 foreign (effective 1999). adv. bk.rev. index. *Refereed.* **Document type:** *Academic/Scholarly, Trade.*
Indexed: e-psyche.
—BLDSC (5318.930000), GNLM, KNAW.
Published by: Trimbos Instituut, Postbus 725, Utrecht 3500 AS, Netherlands. TEL 31-30-2971119. Ed. D J Bos. Circ: 5,000 (paid).

616.834 CAN ISSN 0315-1131
M S CANADA. Text in English. 1974. q. CND 12 (effective 2000). bk.rev. **Document type:** *Newsletter.* **Description:** Provides information on M S research, how to cope with multiple sclerosis, and activities of the Society.
Indexed: e-psyche.
Published by: Multiple Sclerosis Society of Canada, 250 Bloor St E, Ste 1000, Toronto, ON M4W 3P9, Canada. TEL 416-922-6065, FAX 416-922-7538. Ed. Deanna Groetzinger. Circ: 27,000.

616.834 CAN ISSN 0707-0934
M S ONTARIO. Text in English. 1977. q. CND 10 to members (effective 2000). adv. bk.rev. **Document type:** *Newsletter.*
Related titles: E-mail ed.
Indexed: e-psyche.
Published by: Multiple Sclerosis Society of Canada, Ontario Division, 250 Bloor St E, Ste 1000, Toronto, ON M4W 3P9, Canada. TEL 416-922-6065, FAX 416-922-7538. R&P Deanna Groetzinger. Circ: 12,000.

616.834 USA
M S REALITY BYTES. (Multiple Sclerosis) Text in English. 1997. w.
Media: Online - full text.
Published by: M S World, Inc. TEL 415-242-1106, katop@msworld.org, http://www.msworld.org/realbyte/realbytes.htm/. Ed. Kathy Alberts.

MANAB MON; a journal depicting the modern trends in psychology, biology, and sociology. see *PSYCHOLOGY*

MARIANI FOUNDATION PAEDIATRIC NEUROLOGY. see *MEDICAL SCIENCES—Pediatrics*

616.8 USA ISSN 0882-3634
MARKER. Text in English. 1967. 2/yr. free per issue. bk.rev. back issues avail. **Document type:** *Magazine.* **Description:** Covers national and local news and events relevant to patients with Huntington's disease and their families. Includes medical and scientific research updates.
Formerly (until 198?): Committee to Combat Huntington's Disease Newsletter (0882-3642)
Indexed: e-psyche.

Published by: Huntington's Disease Society of America, 158 West 29th St, 7th Fl, New York, NY 10001-5300. TEL 212-239-3430, FAX 212-243-2443, hdsainfo@hdsa.org, http://www.hdsa.org/. Ed. Amy Schoenberg. Circ: 60,000.

616.89 GBR ISSN 0076-5465
MAUDSLEY MONOGRAPHS. Text in English. irreg. price varies. **Document type:** *Monographic series.*
Indexed: e-psyche.
—BLDSC (5413.271000).
Published by: (Institute of Psychiatry, University of London), Oxford University Press, Oxford Journals, Walton St, Oxford OX2 6DP, United Kingdom. TEL 44-1865-56767, FAX 44-1865-56646, jnlorders@oup.co.uk, jnl.orders@oup.co.uk, http://www.oup.co.uk. **Orders in N. America to:** Oxford University Press, Journals. TEL 919-677-0977, FAX 919-677-1714, http://www.oup.co.uk.

MEDICAL HYPNOANALYSIS JOURNAL. see *MEDICAL SCIENCES—Hypnosis*

MEDICAL MALPRACTICE: PSYCHIATRIC CARE. see *LAW—Civil Law*

618.89 USA ISSN 1082-7579
R11 CODEN: MUPSFY
MEDICAL UPDATE FOR PSYCHIATRISTS. Text in English. 1996. bi-m. NLG 278, USD 160 (effective 1998). illus. **Description:** Provides psychiatrists with up-to-date, scientifically accurate, clinically useful information on the diagnosis and treatment of non-psychiatric medical disorders.
Related titles: Online - full text ed.: (from ingenta, ScienceDirect, Swets Blackwell).
Indexed: e-psyche.
—Infotrieve. **CCC.**
Published by: Elsevier Science, PO Box 945, New York, NY 10159-0945. TEL 212-989-5800, FAX 212-633-3990, usinfo-f@elsevier.com, http://www.elsevier.nl/., http://www.elsevier.com. Ed. Dr. N L Stotland. **Subscr. in Australasia and the Far East to:** Elsevier Science (Singapore) Pte Ltd, No.1 Temasek Ave, 17-01 Millenia Tower, Singapore 039192, Singapore. TEL 65-434-3727, FAX 65-337-2230; **Subscr. in Japan to:** Elsevier Science Inc - Japan Regional Office, 9-15 Higashi-Azabu 1-chome, Minato-ku, Tokyo 106-0044, Japan. TEL 81-3-5561-5033, FAX 81-3-5561-5047; **Subscr. outside the Americas to:** Elsevier Science BV, PO Box 211, Amsterdam 1000 AE, Netherlands. TEL 31-20-485-3757, FAX 31-20-485-3432, nlinfo-f@elsevier.nl, http://www.elsevier.nl.

616.8 150.5 ITA
MEDICINA, PSICHE E ADOLESCENZA/MEDICINE, MIND AND ADOLESCENCE; semestrale di psicologia medica e di filosofia della medicina - semi-annual journal of philosophy of medicine, medical psychology and adolescentology. Text in English; Summaries in English, Italian; Text occasionally in French, Spanish. 1983. s-a. ITL 120,000 domestic; USD 120 in Europe (effective 2000). adv. bk.rev. *Refereed.* **Document type:** *Academic/Scholarly.*
Formerly: Medicina e Psiche (0394-1531)
Indexed: e-psyche.
Published by: Universita Ambrosiana, Viale Romagna, 51, Milan, MI 20133, Italy. TEL 39-2-2666880, FAX 39-2-2361226, unambro@unambro.it, http://www.adolescence.org. Ed. Giuseppe R Brera. R&P, Adv. contact Udo Ressy. Circ: 500. **Subscr. to:** Istituti Editoriali e Poligrafici Internazionali.

616.89 ITA ISSN 0025-7893
CODEN: MDPSAC
MEDICINA PSICOSOMATICA; rivista di medicina psicosomatica, psicologia clinica e psicoterapia. Text in Italian; Summaries in English, French, Italian. 1956. q. ITL 60,000; ITL 120,000 foreign. adv. bk.rev. abstr, bibl, charts. index. **Document type:** *Academic/Scholarly.*
Indexed: Biol.Abstr., Curr.Adv.Ecol.Sci., Excerp.Med., PsycInfo, Psychol.Abstr. (1972-), e-psyche.
—BLDSC (5533.650000), GNLM.
Published by: Societa Editrice Universo, Via Giovanni Battista Morgagni, 1, Rome, RM 00161, Italy. Ed. Ferruccio Antonelli.

616.8 USA
MEDICINE AND SOCIETY. Text in English. 1988. irreg., latest vol.6, 1994. price varies. back issues avail. *Refereed.* **Document type:** *Academic/Scholarly.* **Description:** Discusses psychotherapy past and present in the U.S. and Europe.
Indexed: e-psyche.
—BLDSC (5534.006900).

M

Published by: University of California Press, Journals Division, 2000 Center St, Ste 303, Berkeley, CA 94704-1223. TEL 510-642-4247, FAX 510-643-7127. Ed. Andrew Scull. **Orders to:** California-Princeton Fulfillment Services, Princeton, NJ 08618. TEL 800-777-4726, FAX 800-999-1958.

616.8 BGR ISSN 1311-6584
MEDITSINSKI PREGLED. NEVROLOGIIA I PSICHIATRIIA. Text in Bulgarian; Summaries in Bulgarian, English. 1970. q., latest vol.30, 2001. BGL 14 domestic; USD 40 foreign (effective 2001 - 2002). adv. bk.rev. abstr, bibl, illus. index. 48 p./no. back issues avail. *Refereed.* **Document type:** *Journal, Academic/Scholarly, Abstract/Index, Bibliography.* **Description:** Publishes original articles and abstracts of foreign publications in the fields of neurology and psychiatry; covers mental health services, as well as social problems related to mental disorders.
Formerly: Nervni i Psikhichni Zaboliavaniia (0204-5052)
Indexed: Abstr.Bulg.Sci.Med.Lit., e-psyche.
Published by: Meditsinski Universitet - Sofia, Tsentur za Informatsiia po Meditsina/Medical University - Sofia, Medical Information Center, 1 Sv Georgi Sofiiski ul, Sofia 1431, Bulgaria. TEL 359-2-9522342, FAX 359-2-9522393, mutafov@sun.medun.acad.bg, http://www.medun.acad.bg. Ed. Dr. E Tsvetanova. R&P, Adv. contact Dr. Christo Mutafov. B&W page USD 50, color page USD 150; trim 160 x 110. Circ: 350. **Dist. by:** Sofia Books, Ul Silivria 16, Sofia 1404, Bulgaria. TEL 359-2-9586257, sofiabooks@hotmail.com, http://www.sofiabooks.hit.bg.

616.89 USA
MEDSCAPE MENTAL HEALTH. Text in English. 1996. w. *Refereed.* **Description:** Provides clinicians with information for recognizing and managing psychiatric illnesses.
Media: Online - full text.
Indexed: e-psyche.
Published by: Medscape, Inc., 134 W 29th St, New York, NY 10001-5399. TEL 212-631-1600, http://www.medscape.com.

616.89 USA ISSN 0025-9284
RC321 CODEN: BMCLA4
MENNINGER CLINIC. BULLETIN; a journal for the mental health professions. Text in English. 1936. q. USD 60 to individuals; USD 82 foreign to individuals; USD 130 to institutions; USD 152 foreign to institutions (effective 1999). adv. bk.rev. bibl, charts, illus. index. reprint service avail. from PQC. *Refereed.* **Document type:** *Academic/Scholarly, Abstract/Index.* **Description:** Contains articles on psychiatry, psychology, psychoanalysis, child psychiatry, neuropsychology, clinical research, and related subjects, as well as clinical reports and brief communications.
Related titles: Microform ed.: (from PQC); Online - full text ed.: (from ProQuest Information & Learning, CatchWord Ltd., Institute for Scientific Information, RoweCom Information Quest).
Indexed: ASCA, Abstr.Crim.& Pen., AgeLine, Biol.Abstr., Chicago Psychoanal.Lit.Ind., Curr.Cont., Excerp.Med., Fam.Ind., Hosp.Lit.Ind., IMFL, Ind.Med. (1936-), Int.Nurs.Ind., Lang.& Lang.Behav.Abstr., Mid.East: Abstr.& Ind., P C I, PsycInfo, Psychoanal.Abstr., Psychol.Abstr. (1936-), SOPODA, SSCI, Soc.Work Res.& Abstr., Sociol.Abstr., e-psyche.
—BLDSC (2612.200000), CISTI, GNLM, IDS, ingenta, KNAW. **CCC.**
Published by: (Menninger Foundation), Guilford Publications, Inc., 72 Spring St, New York, NY 10012. TEL 212-431-9800, 800-365-7006, FAX 212-966-6708, info@guilford.com, http://www.guilford.com. Ed. Kathryn J Zerbe. Adv. contact Mary Ann Clifft. Circ: 1,500.

616.89 616.89 USA ISSN 0025-9292
RC321 CODEN: MNPVB
MENNINGER PERSPECTIVE. Text in English. 1970. q. illus. reprint service avail. from PQC. **Document type:** *Consumer.* **Description:** Articles related to mental health, mental illness, and Menninger programs.
Formerly: Menninger Quarterly
Related titles: Microform ed.: (from PQC).
Indexed: CINAHL, Intl.Mgmt.Info., Psychol.Abstr., e-psyche.
—GNLM, ingenta.
Published by: Menninger Foundation, PO Box 829, Topeka, KS 66601-0829. TEL 785-350-5000, FAX 785-273-0797, http://menninger.edu/tmc_publ_bltn.html. Circ: 66,000 (controlled).

MENTAL AND PHYSICAL DISABILITY LAW REPORTER; covers all aspects of handicapped law. see *LAW—Civil Law*

MENTAL DISABILITY LAW: CIVIL AND CRIMINAL. see *LAW*

616.858 USA
MENTAL HEALTH ASPECTS OF DEVELOPMENTAL DISABILITIES. Text in English. 1998. q. USD 63 in United States to individuals; USD 85 in United States to institutions; USD 73 in Canada & Mexico to individuals; USD 99 in Canada & Mexico to institutions; USD 81 elsewhere to individuals; USD 110 elsewhere to institutional members (effective 2000). adv. bk.rev. bibl. index. back issues avail. *Refereed.* **Document type:** *Academic/Scholarly.* **Description:** Provides clinicians and habilitative care givers with information regarding the diagnosis and treatment of neuropsychiatric disorders and therapeutic interventions that can improve the quality of psychosocial functioning of persons with developmental disabilities.
Former titles (until vol.16): Habilitative Mental Healthcare Newsletter (1057-3291); (until vol.8, 1989): Psychiatric Aspects of Mental Retardation Reviews; (until 1983): Psychiatric Aspects of Mental Retardation Newsletter (0278-9493)
Indexed: Psychol.Abstr., e-psyche.
—GNLM.
Published by: Psych-Media, Inc., PO Box 57, Bear Creek, NC 27207-0057. TEL 336-581-3700, FAX 336-581-3766, magz@emji.net, http://www.mhaspectsofdd.com. Ed. Anne Desnoyers Hurley. R&P Maggie Zwilling. Adv. contact L Vallmoeller. Circ: 1,600 (paid).

616.89 GBR ISSN 1368-1230
MENTAL HEALTH CARE. Text in English. 1997. m. GBP 32 to individuals; GBP 70 to institutions. adv. tr.lit. back issues avail. *Refereed.* **Document type:** *Academic/Scholarly.*
Indexed: CINAHL, Int.Nurs.Ind., e-psyche.
Published by: T M & D Press Ltd., United House, 41 North Rd, London N7 9DP, United Kingdom. TEL 44-20-7700-3479, FAX 44-20-7700-2049, tmd.press@btinternet.com. Ed. Catherine Jackson. Pub. Kevin Kibble. R&P Penny Stephens. Adv. contact Kavita Mohan. B&W page GBP 795, color page GBP 1,020; trim 210 x 297. Circ: 3,000 (paid); 12,000 (controlled).

MENTAL HEALTH IN CHILDREN. see *PSYCHOLOGY*

616.8 AUS
MENTAL HEALTH MATTERS. Text in English. 1974. q. AUD 28 to individual members (effective 1999). adv. bk.rev. back issues avail. **Document type:** *Newsletter.*
Supersedes (in 1993): N S W A M H News; Which was formerly: New South Wales Association for Mental Health. Newsletter (0813-1724)
Indexed: e-psyche.
Published by: New South Wales Association for Mental Health, 62 Victoria Rd, Gladesville, NSW 2111, Australia. TEL 61-2-9816-1611, FAX 61-2-9816-4056, nswamh@gpo.com.au. Ed. Gillian Church. Pub., R&P, Adv. contact Elizabeth Priestley. Circ: 500.

616.8 GBR ISSN 1353-0283
MENTAL HEALTH NURSING JOURNAL. Text in English. bi-m. GBP 47.50 in Europe to non-members; GBP 56.50 elsewhere to non-members (effective 1999). adv. bk.rev., video rev. *Refereed.* **Document type:** *Academic/Scholarly, Trade.* **Description:** Contains news of interest to CPNs including feature articles, research papers, conference reports, events listings, and association news.
Supersedes (until 1994): Community Psychiatric Nursing Journal (0265-7007); Formerly (until 1984): C P N A Journal (0264-5483); (until 1978): C P N A Newsletter
Related titles: Online - full text ed.: (from ProQuest Information & Learning).
Indexed: Brit.Nur.Ind., CINAHL, e-psyche.
Published by: Community Psychiatric Nurses Association, 50 Southwark St, London SE1 1UN, United Kingdom. TEL 44-20-7717-4000, FAX 44-20-7717-4030. Ed. Toni Turner. R&P Daniel Allen TEL 44-20-7717-4025. Adv. contact Graham Watt. Circ: 1,500. **Subscr. to:** C P N A Subscriptions, 44 Dartford Rd, Sevenoaks, Kent TN13 3TQ, United Kingdom. TEL 44-1732-455244, FAX 44-1732-457542.

616.8 GBR ISSN 1465-8720
MENTAL HEALTH PRACTICE. Text in English. 1998. 10/yr. GBP 80 in Europe to institutions; GBP 96 elsewhere to institutions (effective 2002). adv. **Document type:** *Trade.* **Description:** Up-to-date information on developments in mental health nursing.
Indexed: Brit.Nur.Ind., e-psyche.
—BLDSC (5678.583750).
Published by: (Royal College of Nursing), R C N Publishing Co. (Subsidiary of: B M J Publishing Group), R C N Direct, Copse Walk, Cardiff Gate Business Park, Cardiff CF23 8XG, United Kingdom. TEL 44-29-2054-6450, FAX 44-29-2054-6401, directjournalsteam@rcn.org.uk, http://www.rcn.org.uk/. Ed. Ian MacMillan. Adv. contact Phil Whomes. Circ: 3,100 (paid).

MENTAL HEALTH REPORT. see *SOCIAL SERVICES AND WELFARE*

360 150 GBR ISSN 1361-9322
THE MENTAL HEALTH REVIEW. Text in English. 1996. q. GBP 55 domestic to individuals; GBP 65 in Europe to individuals; GBP 70 rest of world to individuals; GBP 99 domestic to institutions; GBP 119 in Europe to institutions; GBP 125 rest of world to institutions. **Document type:** *Academic/Scholarly.* **Description:** Offers readers a medium between policy issues and innovative practice in mental health services.
Indexed: Brit.Nur.Ind.
—BLDSC (5678.584800).
Published by: (King's College London, Centre for Mental Health Services Development), Pavilion Publishing Ltd., 8 St George's Pl, Brighton, East Sussex BN1 4GB, United Kingdom. TEL 44-1273-623222, FAX 44-1273-625526, pavpub@pavilion.co.uk, http://www.pavpub.com. Ed. Elizabeth Parker.

MENTAL RETARDATION. see *EDUCATION—Special Education And Rehabilitation*

616.858 USA ISSN 1080-4013
RC569.7 CODEN: MRDRFI
MENTAL RETARDATION AND DEVELOPMENTAL DISABILITIES (NEW YORK, 1995); research reviews. Text in English. 1995. q. USD 355 in United States; USD 395 in Canada & Mexico; USD 429 elsewhere; USD 373 combined subscription in United States for print and online eds.; USD 413 combined subscription in Canada & Mexico for print and online eds.; USD 447 combined subscription elsewhere for print and online eds. (effective 2002). adv. back issues avail. *Refereed.* **Document type:** *Academic/Scholarly.*
Related titles: Microform ed.: (from PQC); Online - full text ed.: ISSN 1098-2779. 1996. USD 355 in United States; USD 355 in Canada & Mexico; USD 355 elsewhere (effective 2002) (from EBSCO Publishing, Wiley InterScience, Institute for Scientific Information).
Indexed: Child Devel.Abstr., Curr.Cont., Ind.Med., Neurosci.Cit.Ind., PsycInfo.
—BLDSC (5678.675700), CISTI, GNLM, IDS, Infotrieve, KNAW. **CCC.**
Published by: (Society for Developmental Pediatrics), John Wiley & Sons, Inc., Journals (Subsidiary of: Wiley InterScience), 605 Third Ave, New York, NY 10158. TEL 212-850-6645, FAX 212-850-6021, subinfo@wiley.com, uscs-wis@wiley.com, http://www.wiley.com. Ed. Mark Batshaw. adv.: B&W page GBP 640, color page GBP 1,515; trim 210 x 279. Circ: 850. **Subscr. outside the Americas to:** John Wiley & Sons Ltd., Baffins Ln, Chichester, Sussex PO19 IUD, United Kingdom. TEL 44-1243-779777, FAX 44-1243-843232, cs-journals@wiley.co.uk.

616.8 USA ISSN 1043-9471
QP351 CODEN: MENEE5
METHODS IN NEUROSCIENCES. Text in English. 1990. irreg., latest vol.31, 1996.
Indexed: Chem.Abstr., Chem.Titles, Neurosci.Cit.Ind., e-psyche.
—CASDDS, CISTI, Infotrieve, ingenta. **CCC.**
Published by: Academic Press, Inc., Journal Division (Subsidiary of: Harcourt Brace & Company), 525 B St, Ste 1900, San Diego, CA 92101-4495. TEL 619-231-6616, FAX 619-699-6715. Ed. P Michael Conn. **Subscr. to:** Order Dept., 6277 Sea Harbor Dr, 4th Fl, Orlando, FL 32887. TEL 800-321-5068.

362.2 616.89 FIN ISSN 0303-2558
MIELENTERVEYS/MENTAL HEALTH. Text in Finnish. 1961. bi-m. FIM 170 (effective 1996). adv. bk.rev. back issues avail. **Document type:** *Trade.*
Indexed: e-psyche.
Published by: Suomen Mielenterveysseura/Finnish Association for Mental Health, Lauttasaarentie 28-30, Helsinki 00200, Finland. TEL 358-0-615-516, FAX 358-0-692-4065. Ed. Kristina Salonen. Circ: 15,000.

616.857 GBR ISSN 0544-1153
MIGRAINE NEWS. Text in English. 1967. 3/yr. membership donation. adv. bk.rev. **Document type:** *Newsletter.*
Indexed: e-psyche.

M

Published by: Migraine Trust, 45 Great Ormond St, London WC1N 3HD, United Kingdom. TEL 44-20-7831-4818, FAX 44-20-7831-5174, migrainetrust@compuserve.com, http://www.migrainetrust.org. Ed., R&P, Adv. contact Ann Rush. Circ: 40,000.

616.89 323.4 USA
MIND FREEDOM JOURNAL; human rights in mental health. Text in English. 1988. biennial, latest vol.44. USD 20; USD 20 foreign. adv. bk.rev., video rev., film rev. illus. 64 p./no. back issues avail. **Document type:** *Journal, Consumer.* **Description:** News of human rights in mental health, especially alternatives to forced psychiatric procedures.
formerly (until Apr. 2001): Dendron News (1073-7138)
Related titles: Diskette ed.; Online - full text ed.: Digital Dendron.
Indexed: Neurosci.Cit.Ind., e-psyche.
Address: 454 Willamette St, Ste 216, Box 11284, Eugene, OR 97440-3484. TEL 541-345-9106, FAX 541-345-3737, office@mindfreedom.org, http://www.mindfreedom.org. Ed. David Oaks. Pub. Ron Unger. Adv. contacts Coquille Houshour, Matt Morrissey. page USD 250. Circ: 20,000.

616.8 ITA ISSN 0391-1772
MINERVA PSICHIATRICA. Text in Italian; Summaries in English, Italian. 1960. q. USD 105 to individuals; USD 155 to institutions (effective 2000 - 2001). adv. bk.rev. bibl, charts, illus. index. *Refereed.* **Document type:** *Academic/Scholarly.* **Description:** Covers clinical psychiatry, clinical psychology, social psychiatry, neuropsychiatry, and psychopharmacology.
Former titles (1972-1976): Minerva Psichiatrica e Psicologica (0374-9320); (1960-1972): Minerva Medicopsicologica (0026-4865)
Related titles: Microform ed.: (from PQC).
Indexed: Biol.Abstr., Excerp.Med., Ind.Med. (coverage dropped), Lang.& Lang.Behav.Abstr., PsycInfo, Psychol.Abstr. (1992-), e-psyche.
—BLDSC (5794.465000), CISTI, EMDOCS, GNLM, KNAW.
Published by: Edizioni Minerva Medica, Corso Bramante, 83-85, Turin, TO 10126, Italy. TEL 39-11-678282, FAX 39-11-674502. Ed. M De Vanna. Pub. Alberto Oliaro. Adv. contact F Filippo. B&W page USD 1,200, color page USD 2,000; trim 270 x 190. Circ: 3,000 (paid).

616.8 DEU ISSN 0946-7211
CODEN: MINUED
MINIMALLY INVASIVE NEUROSURGERY. Text in English. 1958. 4/yr. EUR 120.40 domestic to individuals; EUR 123.80 in Europe to individuals; EUR 127.80 elsewhere to individuals; EUR 336.40 domestic to institutions; EUR 339.80 in Europe to institutions; EUR 343.80 elsewhere to institutions (effective 2002). adv. bk.rev. charts, illus. reprint service avail. from PQC. *Refereed.* **Document type:** *Journal, Academic/Scholarly.*
Formerly (until 1994): Neurochirurgia (0028-3819)
Related titles: Microform ed.: (from PQC); Online - full text ed.: ISSN 1439-2291 (from Institute for Scientific Information).
Indexed: ASCA, Bibl.Dev.Med.& Child Neur., Biol.Abstr., Curr.Cont., Dent.Ind., Excerp.Med., Helminthol.Abstr., INIS Atomind., Ind.Med. (1994-), Ind.Sci.Rev., Inpharma, Int.Nurs.Ind., Neurosci.Cit.Ind., Pharm.&Out.News, Reac., Sci.Cit.Ind. (coverage dropped), Trop.Dis.Bull., e-psyche.
—BLDSC (5797.711000), GNLM, IDS, ingenta, KNAW. **CCC.**
Published by: Georg Thieme Verlag, Ruedigerstr 14, Stuttgart 70469, Germany. TEL 49-711-8931-0, FAX 49-711-8931298, min@thieme.de, leser.service@thieme.de, http://www.thieme.de/min, http://www.thieme-connect.de. Ed. Dr. Axel Perneczky. R&P Michael Wachinger. Circ: 1,000.

616.8 CHE ISSN 0077-0094
RC483 CODEN: MPPPBK
MODERN PROBLEMS OF PHARMACOPSYCHIATRY. Text in English. 1968. irreg., latest vol.25. CHF 250 in Europe; DEM 300 in Germany; CHF 220 in United States (effective 2001). reprint service avail. from ISI. *Refereed.* **Document type:** *Journal, Academic/Scholarly.* **Description:** Information on the development, evaluation and use of drugs and selected therapeutic interventions in psychiatric practice and research.
Related titles: Online - full text ed.: (from Institute for Scientific Information).
Indexed: Biol.Abstr., Chem.Abstr., Chem.Indus.Notes, Chem.Titles, Curr.Cont. (coverage dropped), Focus on: Psychophar., Ind.Med. (1968-), Psychol.Abstr., e-psyche.
—CASDDS, CISTI, GNLM, KNAW. **CCC.**

Published by: S. Karger AG, Allschwilerstr 10, PO Box, Basel 4009, Switzerland. TEL 41-61-306-1111, FAX 41-61-306-1234, karger@karger.ch, http://www.karger.com/bookseries/MOPPH.

616.8 USA ISSN 1044-7431
QP356.2 CODEN: MOCNED
MOLECULAR AND CELLULAR NEUROSCIENCES. Short title: M C N. Text in English. 1990. m. USD 635 in US & Canada to institutions; USD 700 elsewhere to institutions (effective 2001). back issues avail. *Refereed.* **Document type:** *Academic/Scholarly.* **Description:** Describes novel and original results in the areas of neurobiology, neuropharmacology, neuroendocrinology, neurochemistry, and neuroanatomy at the molecular, cellular, and tissue levels.
Related titles: Online - full text ed.: (from EBSCO Publishing, O C L C Online Computer Library Center, Inc., RoweCom Information Quest, ingenta, Swets Blackwell, IDEAL Online Library, Institute for Scientific Information).
Indexed: ASCA, Aqua.Sci.& Fish.Abstr., BBCI, Chem.Abstr., Chem.Titles, Chemorec.Abstr., Curr.Cont., Excerp.Med. (1992-), Ind.Med. (1990-), Ind.Sci.Rev., Inpharma, Neurosci.Abstr., Neurosci.Cit.Ind., Reac., Rev.Appl.Entomol., Sci.Cit.Ind., e-psyche.
—BLDSC (5900.760700), ADONIS, CASDDS, CISTI, EMDOCS, GNLM, IDS, Infotrieve, ingenta, KNAW, Linda Hall. **CCC.**
Published by: Academic Press, Inc., Journal Division (Subsidiary of: Harcourt Brace & Company), 525 B St, Ste 1900, San Diego, CA 92101-4495. TEL 619-230-1840, FAX 619-699-6800, apsubs@acad.com, http://www.academicpress.com/mcn. Eds. Frank S Walsh, Greg Lemke.

616.8 572.8 NLD ISSN 0169-328X
QP356.2 CODEN: MBREE4
MOLECULAR BRAIN RESEARCH. Text in English. 1986. 24/yr. EUR 3,589 in Europe to institutions; JPY 476,400 in Japan to institutions; USD 4,014 elsewhere to institutions (effective 2002). bibl. index. back issues avail.; reprint service avail. from SWZ,ISI. *Refereed.* **Document type:** *Academic/Scholarly.* **Description:** Provides a medium for the prompt publication of studies of molecular mechanisms of neuronal synaptic and related processes that underline the structure and function of the brain.
Related titles: Microform ed.: (from PQC); Online - full text ed.: (from EBSCO Publishing, ingenta, ScienceDirect, Swets Blackwell, Institute for Scientific Information).
Indexed: ASCA, Anim.Breed.Abstr., Aqua.Sci.& Fish.Abstr., BBCI, Biol.Abstr., Cal.Tiss.Abstr., Chem.Abstr., Chem.Indus.Notes, Chem.Titles, Chemorec.Abstr., Curr.Adv.Biochem., Curr.Adv.Cell & Devel.Biol., Curr.Adv.Gen.& Molec.Biol., Curr.Cont., Derwent Biotech.Abstr., Excerp.Med., Genet.Abstr., Hum.Gen.Abstr., Ind.Med. (1989-), Ind.Sci.Rev., Inpharma, Int.Abstr.Biol.Sci., Neurosci.Abstr., Neurosci.Cit.Ind., Nuc.Acids Abstr., Pharm.&Out.News, Reac., Ref.Zh., Sci.Cit.Ind., THA, e-psyche.
—BLDSC (5900.799000), ADONIS, CASDDS, CISTI, GNLM, IDS, ingenta. **CCC.**
Published by: Elsevier Science BV, PO Box 211, Amsterdam 1000 AE, Netherlands. TEL 31-20-485-2911, FAX 31-20-485-2457, http://www.elsevier.com/locate/molbrainres. Eds. D P Purpura, F E Bloom. **Subscr. in Australasia and the Far East to:** Elsevier Science (Singapore) Pte Ltd, No.1 Temasek Ave, 17-01 Millenia Tower, Singapore 039192, Singapore. TEL 65-434-3727, FAX 65-337-2230; **Subscr. in Japan to:** Elsevier Science Inc - Japan Regional Office, 9-15 Higashi-Azabu 1-chome, Minato-ku, Tokyo 106-0044, Japan; **Subscr. in the Americas to:** Elsevier Science, PO Box 945, New York, NY 10159-0945. TEL 212-633-3730, FAX 212-633-3680, usinfo-f@elsevier.com.

MOLECULAR NEUROBIOLOGY; a review journal. see *BIOLOGY—Biochemistry*

616.8 611.01816 GBR ISSN 1359-4184
CODEN: MOPSFQ
MOLECULAR PSYCHIATRY. Text in English. 1996. bi-m. GBP 147 in Europe to individuals for print or online; USD 221 elsewhere to individuals for print or online; GBP 162 combined subscription in Europe to individuals print & online; USD 243 combined subscription elsewhere to individuals print & online; GBP 442 in Europe to institutions for print or online; USD 663 elsewhere to institutions for print or online; GBP 486 combined subscription in Europe to institutions print & online; USD 729 combined subscription elsewhere to institutions print & online (effective 2002). adv. bk.rev. charts, illus, stat. index. back issues avail.; reprints avail. *Refereed.* **Document type:** *Journal, Academic/Scholarly.* **Description:** Aims at elucidating biological mechanisms underlying psychiatric disorders and their treatment. The empashis is on studies at the interface of pre-clinical and clinical research, including studies at the cellular, molecular, integrative, clinical, imaging and psychopharmacology levels.
Related titles: Online - full text ed.: (from EBSCO Publishing, O C L C Online Computer Library Center, Inc., RoweCom Information Quest, ingenta, Swets Blackwell, Institute for Scientific Information).
Indexed: Chem.Abstr., Chem.Indus.Notes, Chem.Titles, Curr.Cont., Excerp.Med., Focus on: Psychophar., Genet.Abstr. (coverage dropped), Ind.Med. (1996-), Inpharma, Int.Nurs.Ind., Jrnl.Watch Psych., Neurosci.Abstr., Neurosci.Cit.Ind., Nuc.Acids Abstr., Pharm.&Out.News, Reac., Sci.Cit.Ind., e-psyche.
—BLDSC (5900.826600), ADONIS, CASDDS, CISTI, GNLM, IDS, Infotrieve. **CCC.**
Published by: Nature Publishing Group Specialist Journals (Subsidiary of: Holtzbrink Publishers), Houndmills, Basingstoke, Hants RG21 6XS, United Kingdom. TEL 44-1256-329242, FAX 44-1256-328339, subscriptions@nature.com, http://www.nature.com/mp. Ed. Julio Licinio. Pub. Michael Osuch. R&P Trace Noel. Adv. contact Robert Sloan TEL 44-20-8882-7199. B&W page GBP 595, color page GBP 1,150; trim 210 x 280.

616.89 ESP ISSN 0214-4220
CODEN: MONDE4
MONOGRAFIAS DE PSIQUIATRIA. Text in Spanish. 1989. 6/yr. **Document type:** *Academic/Scholarly.*
Indexed: e-psyche.
—EMDOCS, GNLM.
Published by: Grupo Aula Medica S.A., C.I. Venecia 2 Alfa III, Isabel Colbrand, 10-12, Madrid 28050, Spain. TEL 34-1-3588657, FAX 34-1-3589067. Ed. A Nogales.

616.894 USA ISSN 0077-0620
MONOGRAPH SERIES ON SCHIZOPHRENIA. Text in English. 1950. irreg., latest vol.8, 1969. price varies. *Refereed.* **Document type:** *Monographic series.*
Indexed: e-psyche.
Published by: International Universities Press, Inc., 59 Boston Post Rd, Box 1524, Madison, CT 06443-1524. TEL 203-245-4000, FAX 203-245-0775, http://www.iup.com.

616.8 USA ISSN 0077-0671
CODEN: MGGPBE
MONOGRAPHIEN AUS DEM GESAMTGEBIETE DER PSYCHIATRIE - PSYCHIATRY SERIES. Text in English, German. 1970. irreg., latest vol.64, 1991. price varies. reprint service avail. from ISI. **Document type:** *Monographic series.*
Supersedes in part: Monographien aus dem Gesamtgebiete der Neurologie und Psychiatrie
Indexed: Ind.Med. (until 1992, dropped), Psychol.Abstr., e-psyche.
—CASDDS, GNLM, KNAW.
Published by: Springer-Verlag, Journals (Subsidiary of: BertelsmannSpringer), 175 Fifth Ave, New York, NY 10010. TEL 212-460-1500, FAX 212-473-6272.

616.8 CHE ISSN 1420-2441
CODEN: MNUSB6
MONOGRAPHS IN CLINICAL NEUROSCIENCE. Text in English. 1972. irreg., latest vol.18. CHF 180 in Europe; DEM 215 in Germany; USD 145 in United States (effective 2001). reprint service avail. from ISI. *Refereed.* **Document type:** *Monographic series, Academic/Scholarly.* **Description:** Provides a broad, interdisciplinary approach to the neural sciences, advancing current information vital for the management of various neurological diseases.
Former titles: Monographs in Neural Sciences (0300-5186); Monographs in Basic Neurology (0077-0779)
Indexed: Biol.Abstr., Chem.Abstr., Chem.Indus.Notes, Chem.Titles, Curr.Cont. (coverage dropped), Ind.Med. (until 1992, dropped), e-psyche.

M

—BLDSC (5915.411050), CASDDS, CISTI, GNLM, KNAW. **CCC.**
Published by: S. Karger AG, Allschwilerstr 10, PO Box, Basel 4009, Switzerland. TEL 41-61-306-1111, FAX 41-61-306-1234, karger@karger.ch, http://www.karger.com/bookseries/MOCLN. Ed. M Fisher.

616.8 CHE ISSN 0737-3953
MONOGRAPHS IN NEUROSCIENCE. Text in English. 1984. irreg., latest vol.5. price varies. *Refereed.* **Document type:** *Monographic series.*
Indexed: e-psyche.
—CISTI.
Published by: Gordon and Breach - Harwood Academic (Subsidiary of: Taylor & Francis Group), PO Box 531, Lausanne 1000, Switzerland. Ed. S Weinstein. **Subscr. addr. in US:** International Publishers Direct, PO Box 32160, Newark, NJ 07102. FAX 215-750-6343.

616.89 RUS ISSN 0135-2652
MOSKOVSKII PSIKHOTERAPEVTICHESKII ZHURNAL. Text in Russian. q. USD 99.95 in United States.
Indexed: Ref.Zh., e-psyche.
—East View.
Published by: Tsentr Psikhologii i Psikhoterapii, Yaroslavskaya ul 13, k 536, Moscow 129366, Russian Federation. TEL 7-095-2290716. **US dist. addr.:** East View Publications, 3020 Harbor Ln N, Minneapolis, MN 55447. TEL 612-550-0961.

MOTOR CONTROL. see *MEDICAL SCIENCES—Physical Medicine And Rehabilitation*

616.8 FRA ISSN 0245-5919
MOTRICITE CEREBRALE, READAPTATION, NEUROLOGIE DU DEVELOPPEMENT. Text in French. 1980. 4/yr. FRF 362; FRF 493 foreign (effective 1997). **Document type:** *Academic/Scholarly.* **Description:** Deals with the physiopathologic aspects of the neurology of development, and with motor or cerebral handicapped people.
Related titles: Microform ed.: (from PQC); Online - full text ed.: (from RoweCom Information Quest).
Indexed: Excerp.Med., e-psyche.
—GNLM. **CCC.**
Published by: (Cercle de Documentation et d'Information pour la Reeducation des Infirmes Moteurs Cerebraux), Masson - Periodiques, 120 bd. St. Germain, Paris 75006, France. TEL 33-1-40466200, FAX 33-1-40466201. Ed. M Le Metayer. Circ: 1,800. **Subscr. to:** Societe de Periodiques Specialises, BP 22, Vineuil Cedex 41354, France. TEL 33-2-54504612, FAX 33-2-54504611.

616.8 USA ISSN 0885-3185
CODEN: MOVDEA
MOVEMENT DISORDERS. Text in English. 1986. bi-m. USD 382 in North America to individuals; USD 442 elsewhere to individuals; USD 700 in North America to institutions; USD 790 elsewhere to institutions (effective 2001). adv. bk.rev., video rev. charts, illus. index. back issues avail.; reprint service avail. from PQC. *Refereed.* **Document type:** *Academic/Scholarly.* **Description:** Publishes original manuscripts covering diagnosis, therapeutics, pharmacology, biochemistry, physiology, etiology, genetics, and epidemiology of movement disorders; subjects include the etiology, diagnosis, management, and basic science of parkinsonism, chorea, tremors, dystonia, myoclonus, tics, tardive dyskinesia, spasticity, and ataxia.
Related titles: Online - full text ed.: (from Wiley InterScience, Institute for Scientific Information).
Indexed: ASCA, Curr.Cont., Excerp.Med., INIS Atomind., Ind.Med. (1986-), Ind.Sci.Rev., Inpharma, Int.Abstr.Biol.Sci., Int.Nurs.Ind., Jrnl.Watch Neuro., NRN, Neurosci.Cit.Ind., Pharm.&Out.News, Reac., Rev.Med.& Vet.Mycol., SSCI (coverage dropped), Sci.Cit.Ind., e-psyche.
—BLDSC (5980.317200), CISTI, EMDOCS, GNLM, IDS, ingenta, KNAW.
Published by: (Movement Disorder Society), John Wiley & Sons, Inc., Journals (Subsidiary of: Wiley InterScience), 605 Third Ave, New York, NY 10158. TEL 212-850-6645, FAX 212-850-6021, uscs-wis@wiley.com, http://www.wiley.com. Eds. Andrew J Lees, Anthony E Lang. adv.: B&W page USD 950, color page USD 2,340. Circ: 2,576 (paid). **Subscr. to:** John Wiley & Sons Ltd., Baffins Ln, Chichester, Sussex PO19 IUD, United Kingdom. TEL 44-1243-779777, FAX 44-1243-843232, cs-journals@wiley.co.uk, http://www.wiley.co.uk.

MULTIMIND - N L P AKTUELL. see *PSYCHOLOGY*

616.8 GBR ISSN 1352-4585
CODEN: MUSCFZ
MULTIPLE SCLEROSIS. Text in English. 1995. bi-m. GBP 123 in Europe to individuals; USD 232 in North America to individuals; GBP 149 rest of world to individuals; GBP 295 in Europe to institutions; USD 506 in North America to institutions; GBP 322 rest of world to institutions; USD 202 in North America to members actrims; GBP 104 in Europe to members ectrims; GBP 161 in developing nations; GBP 57 newsstand/cover in Europe; USD 97 newsstand/cover in North America; GBP 61 newsstand/cover rest of world (effective 2002). adv. back issues avail.; reprints avail. *Refereed.* **Document type:** *Journal, Academic/Scholarly.* **Description:** Covers the aetiology and pathogenesis of demyelinating and inflammatory diseases of the central nervous system.
Related titles: Online - full text ed.: (from EBSCO Publishing, O C L C Online Computer Library Center, Inc., RoweCom Information Quest, ingenta, Swets Blackwell, Institute for Scientific Information).
Indexed: AIDS & Cancer Res., Chem.Abstr., Chem.Indus.Notes, Chem.Titles, Curr.Cont., Immun.Abstr., Ind.Med. (1995-), Inpharma, Neurosci.Abstr., Neurosci.Cit.Ind., Pharm.&Out.News, Reac., Sci.Cit.Ind., Virol.Abstr. (coverage dropped), e-psyche.
—BLDSC (5983.195000), CASDDS, CISTI, GNLM, IDS, KNAW. **CCC.**
Published by: Arnold Publishers (Subsidiary of: Hodder Headline plc.), 338 Euston Rd, London NW1 3BH, United Kingdom. TEL 44-20-7873-6337, FAX 44-20-7873-6325, arnoldjournals@hodder.co.uk, http://www.arnoldpublishers.com/journals/Journpages/13524585.htm, http://www.arnoldpublishers.com/journals/journtitles.htm. Eds. Alan J Thompson, Claude Bernard, Donald Silberberg.

MUSIK-, TANZ- UND KUNSTTHERAPIE; Zeitschrift fuer kuenstlerische Therapien im Bildungs-, Sozial- und Gesundheitswesen. see *MEDICAL SCIENCES*

616.8 GBR
N A C R O POLICY PAPER*. Text in English. irreg. **Document type:** *Bulletin.*
Indexed: e-psyche.
Published by: National Association for the Care and Resettlement of Offenders, 169 Clapham Rd, London SW9 0PU, United Kingdom. TEL 44-20-7582-6500, FAX 44-20-7735-4666.

616.858 USA
N A M I ADVOCATE. Text in English. 1979. 6/yr. USD 25. adv. bk.rev. **Document type:** *Newsletter.*
Formerly: N A M I News
Indexed: e-psyche.
Published by: National Alliance for the Mentally Ill, 2107 Wilson Blvd #300, Arlington, VA 22201-3042. TEL 703-524-7600, http://www.nami.org. Ed. Frieda Eastman. Circ: 80.

362.2 USA
N A M I CALIFORNIA. JOURNAL. Text in English. 1990. q. USD 25; USD 7 newsstand/cover (effective 2001). **Document type:** *Academic/Scholarly.*
Formerly: California Alliance for the Mentally Ill. Journal (1097-802X)
Indexed: CINAHL.
—BLDSC (4828.675250).
Published by: The National Alliance for the Mentally Ill, 111 Howe Ave, Ste 475, Sacramento, CA 95825. TEL 916-567-0163, http://www.mhsource.com/hy/journal.html. Ed., Pub. Dan E Weisburd.

616.857 USA ISSN 1521-2106
N H F HEAD LINES. Text in English. 1970. bi-m. USD 20 (effective 2001). bk.rev. back issues avail. **Document type:** *Newsletter.* **Description:** Presents research and information on headache causes and treatments.
Former titles: National Headache Foundation Newsletter; National Migraine Foundation Newsletter
Indexed: CHNI, CINAHL, e-psyche.
Published by: National Headache Foundation, 428 W St James Pl, 2nd Fl, Chicago, IL 60614-2750. TEL 773-388-6395, 888-NHF-5552, FAX 773-525-7357, http://www.headaches.org. Ed. Katherine Wandersee. R&P Suzanne Simons. Circ: 45,000 (paid and controlled).

616.8 IND ISSN 0254-0886
N I M H A N S JOURNAL. Text in English. 1983. q. INR 300, USD 80. adv. bk.rev. *Refereed.* **Document type:** *Academic/Scholarly.* **Description:** Disseminates research results in mental health and neurosciences.
Indexed: ASCA, Excerp.Med., Indian Psychol.Abstr., Lang.& Lang.Behav.Abstr., Neurosci.Cit.Ind., PsycInfo, Psychol.Abstr. (1986-), SOPODA, Soc.Serv.Abstr., Sociol.Abstr., e-psyche.
—BLDSC (6113.182000), GNLM, IDS.
Published by: National Institute of Mental Health & Neuro Sciences, Bangalore, Karnataka 560 029, India. TEL 91-80-664-2121, FAX 91-80-663-1830, TELEX 0845-2186 NIMH IN, public@nimhans.rec.nic.in. Ed. S M Channabasavanna. Circ: 700.

616.8521 USA
NATIONAL CENTER FOR POST TRAUMATIC STRESS DISORDER. CLINICAL QUARTERLY. Text in English. 1990. q. USD 10 (effective 2001). **Document type:** *Government.* **Description:** Addresses the needs of practicing PTSD clinicians and program administrators, providing them with an overview of the major clinical, theoretical, and programmatic developments in the field.
Formerly: N C P (1052-7168)
Related titles: Online - full content ed.
Published by: National Center for Post Traumatic Stress Disorder (Subsidiary of: U.S. Department of Veterans Affairs), Clinical Laboratory and Education Division, VA Palo Alto Health Care System, 795 Willow Road (352E117), Menlo Park, CA 94025 . TEL 802-296-5132, bhh@icon.palo-alto.med.va.gov, ncptsd@ncptsd.org, http://www.ncptsd.org/treatment/cq/index.html. **Subscr. to:** U.S. Government Printing Office, Superintendent of Documents, PO Box 371954, Pittsburgh, PA 15250-7954. TEL 202-512-1800, FAX 202-512-2250, orders@gpo.gov, http://www.access.gpo.gov.

616.8 362.2 USA ISSN 0738-9159
NATIONAL COUNCIL NEWS. Text in English. 1977. m. USD 25. adv. bk.rev. **Document type:** *Newsletter.* **Description:** Covers issues of interest to mental health care professionals and reports Council activities.
Indexed: e-psyche.
Published by: National Community Mental Healthcare Council, 12300 Twinbrook Parkway, Ste 320, Rockville, MD 20852. TEL 301-984-6200. Ed. Joanne Petro. Circ: 3,000.

616.891 GBR
NATIONAL REGISTER OF PSYCHOTHERAPISTS. Text in English. a. **Document type:** *Directory.*
Indexed: e-psyche.
—BLDSC (6030.090000).
Published by: (U K Council for Psychotherapy), Routledge (Subsidiary of: Taylor & Francis Group), 11 New Fetter Ln, London EC4P 4EE, United Kingdom. TEL 44-20-7583-9855, FAX 44-20-7842-2298, http://www.routledge.com/routledge/journal/journals.html. **Subscr. in the US & Canada to:** 29 W 35th St, New York, NY 10001-2299. TEL 212-244-3336.

616.8 USA ISSN 1097-6256
CODEN: NANEFN
NATURE NEUROSCIENCE. Text in English. 1998. m. USD 199 domestic to individuals; GBP 185 foreign to individuals; USD 710 domestic to institutions; GBP 435 foreign to institutions (effective 2001). adv. Supplement avail.; back issues avail. *Refereed.* **Document type:** *Academic/Scholarly.* **Description:** Addresses the tremendous rate of discovery across all areas of neuroscience and provides a high-profile forum in which the most significant advances can be communicated rapidly to a wide audience.
Related titles: Online - full text ed.: (from EBSCO Publishing, ingenta, Institute for Scientific Information).
Indexed: Anim.Behav.Abstr., Aqua.Sci.& Fish.Abstr., Biotech.& Bioeng.Abstr., Cal.Tiss.Abstr., Chemorec.Abstr., Curr.Cont., Entomol.Abstr., Environ.Sci.Poll.Mgmt., Genet.Abstr., Hum.Gen.Abstr., Ind.Med. (1998-), Jrnl.Watch Psych., Neurosci.Abstr., Neurosci.Cit.Ind., Nuc.Acids Abstr., Pollut.Abstr., PsycInfo, Ref.Zh., Rev.Appl.Entomol., Saf.Sci.Abstr., Sci.Cit.Ind., Zoo.Rec., e-psyche.
—BLDSC (6047.040000), CASDDS, GNLM, Infotrieve. **CCC.**
Published by: Nature America, Inc., 345 Park Ave S, New York, NY 10010. TEL 212-726-9319, neurosci@natureny.com; subscriptions@natureny.com, http://www.nature.com/neuro/, http://www.neurosci.nature.com. Ed. Charles Jennings. Adv. contact Bill Moran. **Subscr. outside of the Americas to:** Macmillan Magazines Ltd, PO Box 5161, Brentwood, TN 37024-5161. TEL 44-1256-329242; **Subscr. to:** Allen Press Inc., PO Box 1897, Lawrence, KS 66044-8897. TEL 800-524-0384, FAX 615-377-0525.

M

616.8 GBR
▼ **NATURE REVIEWS NEUROSCIENCE.** Text in English. 2000 (Oct). m. USD 149 in United States to individuals; GBP 99 elsewhere to individuals; USD 904 in United States to institutions; GBP 565 elsewhere to institutions (effective 2001). adv. back issues avail. *Refereed.* **Document type:** *Academic/Scholarly.* **Description:** Designed to meet the needs of scientists experiencing information overload. Provides broad overviews of specific disciplines.
Related titles: Online - full content ed.
Indexed: Aqua.Sci.& Fish.Abstr., Biotech.& Bioeng.Abstr., Cal.Tiss.Abstr., Chemorec.Abstr., Curr.Cont., Neurosci.Abstr., Sci.Cit.Ind.
—BLDSC (6047.235000).
Published by: Macmillan Magazines Ltd, 4-7 Porters South, Crinan St, London N1 9XW, United Kingdom. TEL 44-20-7843-3629, 800-524-0384, FAX 44-20-7843-3601, 615-377-0525, subscriptions@natureny.com, http://www.nature.com/reviews. Ed. Peter Collins. **Subscr. to:** PO Box 5161, Brentwood, TN 37024-5161.

NEDERLANDS TIJDSCHRIFT VOOR DE PSYCHOLOGIE EN HAAR GRENSGEBIEDEN. see *PSYCHOLOGY*

NEIROFIZIOLOGIYA/NEUROPHYSIOLOGY; nauchno-teoreticheskii zhurnal. see *BIOLOGY—Physiology*

NERVE CELL BIOLOGY. see *BIOLOGY—Abstracting, Bibliographies, Statistics*

616.8 DEU ISSN 0028-2804
CODEN: NERVAF
DER NERVENARZT; Monatsschrift fuer alle Gebiete nervenaerztlicher Forschung und Praxis. (Includes: Deutsche Gesellschaft fuer Neurologie. Mitteilungsblatt and Gesellschaft Oesterreichischer Nervenaerzte und Psychiater) Text in German. 1928. m. EUR 324.57 domestic; EUR 296.07 in Germany; EUR 28 newsstand/cover foreign (effective 2002). adv. bk.rev. charts, illus. index. back issues avail.; reprint service avail. from ISI. *Refereed.* **Document type:** *Journal, Academic/Scholarly.* **Description:** Covers neurology, psychiatry, neurosurgery, and psychotherapy.
Related titles: Microform ed.: (from PQC); Online - full text ed.: ISSN 1433-0407 (from EBSCO Publishing, RoweCom Information Quest, Swets Blackwell, Springer LINK, Institute for Scientific Information).
Indexed: ASCA, Agri.& Environ.Biotech.Abstr. (coverage dropped), Biol.Abstr., Chem.Abstr., Curr.Adv.Ecol.Sci., Curr.Cont., Excerp.Med., Ger.J.Psych., INIS Atomind., Ind.Med. (1928-), Ind.Sci.Rev., Inpharma, Int.Nurs.Ind., Neurosci.Cit.Ind., Nutr.Abstr., Pharm.&Out.News, PsycInfo, Psychol.Abstr. (1929-), Reac., Rev.Appl.Entomol., Rev.Med.& Vet.Mycol., SSCI (coverage dropped), Sci.Cit.Ind., e-psyche.
—BLDSC (6076.500000), CISTI, GNLM, IDS, Infotrieve, KNAW. **CCC.**
Published by: (Deutschen Gesellschaft fuer Psychiatrie, Psychotherapie und Nervenheilkunde), Springer-Verlag (Subsidiary of: BertelsmannSpringer), Tiergartenstr 17, Heidelberg 69121, Germany. TEL 49-6221-345-0, FAX 49-6221-345229, subscriptions@springer.de, http://link.spring.de/link/service/journals/00115/index, http://www.springer.de. Eds. T Brandt, W Hacke. **Subscr. in N. America to:** Springer-Verlag New York Inc., PO Box 2485, Secaucus, NJ 07096-2485. TEL 212-460-1500, FAX 212-473-6272.

616.8 DEU ISSN 0722-1541
NERVENHEILKUNDE; Zeitschrift fuer interdisziplinaere Fortbildung. Text in German. 1982. 10/yr. DEM 220 to individuals; DEM 292 to institutions; DEM 100 to students (effective 2001). adv. *Refereed.* **Document type:** *Journal, Academic/Scholarly.*
Related titles: Online - full text ed.: (from Institute for Scientific Information).
Indexed: ASCA, Abstr.Hyg., Curr.Cont. (coverage dropped), Inpharma, Neurosci.Cit.Ind., Pharm.&Out.News, Protozool.Abstr., Reac., Rev.Med.& Vet.Mycol., SSCI (coverage dropped), e-psyche.
—BLDSC (6076.520000), EMDOCS, GNLM, IDS, Infotrieve, KNAW. **CCC.**
Published by: Schattauer GmbH, Hoelderlinstr 3, Stuttgart 70174, Germany. TEL 49-711-22987-0, FAX 49-711-2298750, info@schattauer.de, http://www.schattauer.com. Eds. D Soyka, M Spitzer. Pub. Dieter Bergemann. R&P Annika Schmidt TEL 49-711-2298713. Adv. contact Maria Wagner TEL 49-711-2298767. B&W page XEU 3,468.09, color page XEU 4,771.88; 183 x 227. Circ: 32,500. **Subscr. to:** CSJ, Postfach 140220, Munich 80452, Germany. TEL 49-89-20959129, schattauer@csj.de.

NEURAL COMPUTATION. see *COMPUTERS—Artificial Intelligence*

NEURAL NETWORK WORLD; international journal on non-standard artificial intelligence. see *COMPUTERS—Artificial Intelligence*

NEURAL NETWORKS. see *COMPUTERS—Artificial Intelligence*

616.8 ISR
CODEN: JNPLEW
NEURAL PLASTICITY. Text in English. q., latest vol.9. USD 270 (effective 2002). **Document type:** *Academic/Scholarly.*
Former titles: Journal of Neuroplasticity; (until 1998): Journal of Neural Transplantation and Plasticity (0792-8483); (until 1991): Journal of Neural Transplantation (1352-237X)
Indexed: ASCA, Curr.Cont. (coverage dropped), Excerp.Med., Ind.Med. (coverage dropped), Neurosci.Abstr. (coverage dropped), Neurosci.Cit.Ind., Psychol.Abstr., Sci.Cit.Ind. (coverage dropped), e-psyche.
—CISTI, EMDOCS, GNLM.
Published by: Freund Publishing House, Ltd., P O Box 35010, Tel Aviv 61350, Israel. TEL 972-3-562-8540, FAX 972-3-562-8538, h_freund@netvision.net.il, http://www.angelfire.com/il/freund. Ed. S Sara.

NEURAL PROCESSING LETTERS. see *COMPUTERS—Artificial Intelligence*

NEURO-CHIRURGIE. see *MEDICAL SCIENCES—Surgery*

617.7 NLD ISSN 0165-8107
NEURO-OPHTHALMOLOGY. Text in English. 1979. 8/yr. (in 2 vols.). NLG 370, USD 206 to individuals; NLG 834, USD 438 to institutions (effective 2000). adv. bk.rev. index. *Refereed.* **Document type:** *Academic/Scholarly.* **Description:** Contains review articles, research papers and short communications on diagnostic methods in neuro-ophthalmology, the visual and oculo-motor systems, the pupil, neuro-ophthalmic aspects of the orbit, migraine, and ocular manifestations of neurological diseases.
Related titles: Microform ed.; Online - full text ed.: (from EBSCO Publishing, O C L C Online Computer Library Center, Inc., RoweCom Information Quest, Swets Blackwell, Institute for Scientific Information).
Indexed: Curr.Cont., Excerp.Med., Ind.Sci.Rev., Inpharma, Neurosci.Cit.Ind., Reac., Sci.Cit.Ind., e-psyche.
—BLDSC (6081.509000), ADONIS, CISTI, GNLM, IDS, ingenta, KNAW. **CCC.**
Published by: Aeolus Press (Subsidiary of: Swets & Zeitlinger BV), PO Box 825, Lisse 2160 SZ, Netherlands. FAX 31-344-572562, orders@swets.nl, http://www.swets.nl/sps/journals/jhn.html. Ed. A Neetens. Pub. J K W van Leeuwen. R&P C E van Leeuwen-Meyeren. Adv. contact Patrick Kleian. B&W page NLG 600, B&W page USD 345; 175 x 240. Circ: 800. **Subscr. to:** Swets & Zeitlinger BV, PO Box 825, Lisse 2160 SZ, Netherlands. TEL 31-252-435111, FAX 31-252-415888, orders@swets.nl. **Dist. in N. America by:** Swets & Zeitlinger, PO Box 613, Ryersford, PA 19468. TEL 610-524-5366, 800-447-9387.

616.891 USA ISSN 1529-4145
▼ **NEURO-PSYCHOANALYSIS**; an interdisciplinary journal for psychoanalysis and the neurosciences. Text in English. 1999. s-a. USD 56 domestic to individuals; USD 73 foreign to individuals; USD 93 domestic to institutions; USD 96 foreign to institutions (effective 2002). adv. bk.rev. *Refereed.* **Document type:** *Journal, Academic/Scholarly.* **Description:** Presents original contributions from the newly converging fields of neuroscience and psychoanalysis.
Indexed: e-psyche.
—BLDSC (6081.544000).
Published by: International Universities Press, Incorporated, 59 Boston Post Rd., P.O. Box 1524, Madison, CT 06443-1524. adv.: B&W page USD 580; 6.75 x 9. Circ: 1,000 (paid).

616.8 570 MEX
R21 CODEN: BEMBA2
NEUROBIOLOGICAL RESEARCH. Text in English. 1942. q. USD 50 (effective 2000). bk.rev. **Document type:** *Academic/Scholarly.*
Former titles (until 1997): Boletin de Estudios Medicos y Biologicos (0067-9666); Instituto de Estudios Medicos y Biologicos. Boletin (0366-1695); (until 1994): Laboratorio de Estudios Medicos y Biologicos. Boletin (0020-3858)
Indexed: Biol.Abstr., Chem.Abstr., Chem.Indus.Notes, Chem.Titles, Excerp.Med., INIS Atomind., Ind.Med. (1967-), e-psyche.
—CASDDS, GNLM, KNAW.
Published by: Universidad Nacional Autonoma de Mexico, Instituto de Investigaciones Biomedicas, Centro de Neurobiologia, Apartado Postal 70-228, Cuidad Universitaria, Mexico, DF 04510, Mexico. TEL 52-5-6223838, FAX 52-5-6223839, cavaro@servidor.unam.mx. Eds. Dr. Alfonso Escobar, Flavio Mena.

NEUROBIOLOGY OF AGING; experimental and clinical research. see *BIOLOGY—Physiology*

612.8 573.8 USA ISSN 0969-9961
RC346 CODEN: NUDIEM
NEUROBIOLOGY OF DISEASE. Text in English. 1994. bi-m. USD 225 in US & Canada to institutions; USD 260 elsewhere to institutions (effective 2001). adv. bk.rev. bibl, illus. index. *Refereed.* **Document type:** *Academic/Scholarly.* **Description:** Provides a forum for top-quality research papers on such topics as molecular and cellular definitions of disease mechanisms, the neural systems underpinning behavioral disorders of higher cortical function, the genetics of inherited neurological and psychiatric diseases, aging and the central nervous system, and findings relevant to the development of new therapeutic drugs.
Related titles: Microform ed.: (from PQC); Online - full text ed.: (from EBSCO Publishing, O C L C Online Computer Library Center, Inc., RoweCom Information Quest, ingenta, Swets Blackwell, IDEAL Online Library, Institute for Scientific Information).
Indexed: ASCA, Biol.Abstr., Chem.Abstr., Chem.Indus.Notes, Chem.Titles, Curr.Cont., Excerp.Med., Ind.Med. (1994-), Inpharma, Neurosci.Cit.Ind., Pharm.&Out.News, Psychol.Abstr., Reac., Sci.Cit.Ind., e-psyche.
—BLDSC (6081.311250), ADONIS, CASDDS, CISTI, EMDOCS, GNLM, IDS, Linda Hall. **CCC.**
Published by: Academic Press, Inc., Journal Division (Subsidiary of: Harcourt Brace & Company), 525 B St, Ste 1900, San Diego, CA 92101-4495. TEL 619-230-1840, FAX 619-699-6800, apsubs@acad.com, http://www.academicpress.com/nbd. Eds. Dennis Choi, Jacques Mallet.

616.8 156 USA ISSN 1074-7427
QP406 CODEN: NLMEFR
NEUROBIOLOGY OF LEARNING AND MEMORY. Text in English. 1968. bi-m. USD 845 in US & Canada to institutions; USD 980 elsewhere to institutions (effective 2001). adv. abstr, charts, illus, stat. index. back issues avail. *Refereed.* **Document type:** *Academic/Scholarly.* **Description:** Publishes high-quality papers in all areas of neurally oriented behavioral research and emphasizes the areas of neural plasticity and of mechanisms of learning and memory.
Former titles (until 1994): Behavioral and Neural Biology (0163-1047); (until 1979): Behavioral Biology (0091-6773); Communications in Behavioral Biology (0010-3608)
Related titles: Online - full text ed.: (from EBSCO Publishing, O C L C Online Computer Library Center, Inc., RoweCom Information Quest, ingenta, Swets Blackwell, IDEAL Online Library, Institute for Scientific Information).
Indexed: ASCA, Abstr.Anthropol., Anim.Behav.Abstr., Anim.Breed.Abstr., Aqua.Sci.& Fish.Abstr., Aquacult.Abstr., Biol.& Agr.Ind. (Nov.1982-May 1989), Biol.Abstr., Biotech.& Bioeng.Abstr., Chem.Abstr., Chem.Indus.Notes, Chem.Titles, Chemorec.Abstr., Curr.Adv.Ecol.Sci., Curr.Cont., Dairy Sci.Abstr., Dent.Ind., Environ.Sci.Poll.Mgmt., Excerp.Med., INIS Atomind., Ind.Med. (1995-), Ind.Sci.Rev., Ind.Vet., Inpharma, Int.Abstr.Biol.Sci., Neurosci.Abstr., Neurosci.Cit.Ind., Nutr.Abstr., Pharm.&Out.News, Poult.Abstr., PsycInfo, Psychol.Abstr. (1972-), Reac., Russ.Acad.Sci.Bibl., SSCI, Sci.Cit.Ind., Sport Fish.Abstr., THA, Vet.Bull., Wild.Rev., Zoo.Rec., e-psyche.
—BLDSC (6081.311300), ADONIS, CASDDS, CISTI, EMDOCS, GNLM, IDS, ingenta. **CCC.**
Published by: Academic Press, Inc., Journal Division (Subsidiary of: Harcourt Brace & Company), 525 B St, Ste 1900, San Diego, CA 92101-4495. TEL 619-230-1840, FAX 619-699-6800, apsubs@acad.com, http://www.academicpress.com/nlm. Eds. James L McGaugh, William T Greenough.

616.8 GBR ISSN 1355-4794
QP360 CODEN: NROCF5
NEUROCASE. Text in English. 1995. bi-m. GBP 140, USD 260 to individuals; GBP 325, USD 495 to institutions (effective Feb. 2002). adv. bk.rev. 88 p./no. back issues avail. *Refereed.* **Document type:** *Journal, Academic/Scholarly.* **Description:** A rapid publication journal of both adult and child case studies in neuropsychology, neuropsychiatry, and behavioral neurology.

M

Related titles: CD-ROM ed.; Online - full text ed.: GBP 50, USD 80 to individuals Online only; GBP 160, USD 250 to institutions Online only (effective Feb. 2002) (from HighWire Pr., EBSCO Publishing, O C L C Online Computer Library Center, Inc., RoweCom Information Quest, ingenta, Swets Blackwell, Institute for Scientific Information).
Indexed: CINAHL, Curr.Cont., Excerp.Med. (1996-), Neurosci.Cit.Ind., PsycInfo, e-psyche.
—BLDSC (6081.311400), EMDOCS, GNLM, IDS.
Published by: Oxford University Press, Academic Division, Great Clarendon St, Oxford OX2 6DP, United Kingdom. TEL 44-1865-267907, FAX 44-1865-267835, jnl.info@oup.co.uk, http://www.oup.co.uk/neucas, http://www.oup.co.uk/journals. Eds. Branch Coslett, Ian H Robertson, J R Hodges. Pub. Mandy Sketch. R&P Fionna Willis. adv.: page GBP 180, page USD 325. Circ: 500. **Subscr. in U.S. to:** Oxford University Press, Journals, 2001 Evans Rd, Cary, NC 27513. TEL 800-852-7323, FAX 919-677-1714, jnlorders@oup-usa.org; **Subscr. to:** Journals Marketing, Great Clarendon St, Oxford OX2 6DP, United Kingdom.

619 USA ISSN 0364-3190
QP356.3 CODEN: NEREDZ
NEUROCHEMICAL RESEARCH. Text in English. 1976. m. EUR 1,371 to institutions for print or online ed.; EUR 1,645.20 to institutions print & online eds. combined (effective 2002). adv. back issues avail. *Refereed.* **Document type:** *Academic/Scholarly.* **Description:** Publishes studies using the neurochemical methodology of researching the structure and function of the nervous system.
Related titles: Microfilm ed.: (from PQC); Online - full text ed.: (from EBSCO Publishing, O C L C Online Computer Library Center, Inc., RoweCom Information Quest, Swets Blackwell, Kluwer Online, Institute for Scientific Information).
Indexed: ASCA, Aqua.Sci.& Fish.Abstr., BBCI, Biol.Abstr., Biotech.& Bioeng.Abstr., Cal.Tiss.Abstr. (coverage dropped), Chem.Abstr., Chem.Indus.Notes, Chem.Titles, Chemorec.Abstr., Curr.Adv.Biochem., Curr.Adv.Cell & Devel.Biol., Curr.Adv.Ecol.Sci., Curr.Cont., Dent.Ind., Excerp.Med., INIS Atomind., Ind.Med. (1976-), Ind.Sci.Rev., Inpharma, Int.Abstr.Biol.Sci., Neurosci.Abstr., Neurosci.Cit.Ind., Pharm.&Out.News, Reac., Ref.Zh., Rev.Med.& Vet.Mycol., Sci.Cit.Ind., THA, Tox.Abstr. (coverage dropped), Weed Abstr., e-psyche.
—BLDSC (6081.312000), CASDDS, CISTI, EMDOCS, GNLM, IDS, ingenta, KNAW. **CCC.**
Published by: Kluwer Academic - Plenum Publishers (Subsidiary of: Wolters Kluwer N.V.), 233 Spring St, New York, NY 10013-1578. TEL 212-620-8000, 800-221-9369, FAX 212-463-0742, services@wkap.nl, http://www.wkap.nl/journalhome.htm/0364-3190. Ed. Abel Lathja. R&P Rose Luongo TEL 781-871-6311.

616.8 540 GBR ISSN 0197-0186
QP356.3 CODEN: NEUIDS
NEUROCHEMISTRY INTERNATIONAL; the international journal for the rapid publication of critical reviews, original and rapid research communications in neurochemistry. Text in English. 1980. 13/yr. EUR 1,252 in Europe to institutions; JPY 166,200 in Japan to institutions; USD 1,401 elsewhere to institutions (effective 2002). back issues avail. *Refereed.* **Document type:** *Academic/Scholarly.* **Description:** Publishes papers concerned with the metabolism and function of the nervous system.
Related titles: Microfilm ed.: (from PQC); Online - full text ed.: (from ingenta, ScienceDirect, Swets Blackwell, Institute for Scientific Information).
Indexed: ASCA, Apic.Abstr., Aqua.Sci.& Fish.Abstr., BBCI, Biol.Abstr., Chem.Abstr., Chem.Indus.Notes, Chem.Titles, Chemorec.Abstr., Curr.Adv.Ecol.Sci., Curr.Cont., Excerp.Med., Ind.Med. (1980-), Ind.Sci.Rev., Indian Psychol.Abstr., Inpharma, Int.Abstr.Biol.Sci., Int.Aerosp.Abstr., Neurosci.Abstr., Neurosci.Cit.Ind., Pharm.&Out.News, PsycInfo, Psychol.Abstr. (1984-), Reac., Sci.Cit.Ind., Sport Fish.Abstr., e-psyche.
—BLDSC (6081.317000), ADONIS, CASDDS, CISTI, GNLM, IDS, ingenta, KNAW. **CCC.**
Published by: Pergamon (Subsidiary of: Elsevier Science), The Boulevard, Langford Ln, East Park, Kidlington, Oxford OXB 1GB, United Kingdom. FAX 44-1865-843010, http://www.elsevier.com/locate/neuint. Eds. Neville Osborne, W Lovenberg. **Subscr. in Australasia and the Far East to:** Elsevier Science (Singapore) Pte Ltd, No.1 Temasek Ave, 17-01 Millenia Tower, Singapore 039192, Singapore. TEL 65-434-3727, FAX 65-337-2230; **Subscr. in the Americas to:** Elsevier Science, PO Box 945, New York, NY 10159-0945. TEL 212-633-3730, FAX 212-633-3680, usinfo-f@elsevier.com; **Subscr. to:** Elsevier Science BV, PO Box 211, Amsterdam 1000 AE, Netherlands. TEL 31-20-485-3757.

616.8 617 ESP ISSN 1130-1473
NEUROCIRUGIA/NEUROSURGERY. Text in Spanish, English. 196?-197?; resumed 1989. bi-m. ESP 12,000, EUR 70 in Europe; EUR 120, USD 140 elsewhere (effective 2002). *Refereed.* **Document type:** *Journal, Academic/Scholarly.*
Supersedes: Neurocirugia Luso-Espanola (1131-3722)
Related titles: Online - full text ed.: (from Institute for Scientific Information).
Indexed: Neurosci.Cit.Ind., e-psyche.
—BLDSC (6081.352000), IDS.
Published by: Sociedad Espanola de Neurocirugia, Avenida de Pontejos 29-C, atico, Santander 39005, Spain. TEL 34-985-276518, jmizquierdo@telecable.es, http://empresas.mundivia.es/neurocirugia/, http://www.senec.org/. Ed. Dr. Diez Lobato. Pub. Dr. Izquierdo. Circ: 1,000.

616.8 USA ISSN 0047-942X
NEUROELECTRIC NEWS. Text in English. 1970. 3/yr. USD 25. bk.rev. abstr, bibl. reprint service avail. from PQC. **Description:** Emphasizes theory and clinical applications of electroneurophysiology.
Related titles: Microform ed.: (from PQC).
Indexed: e-psyche.
Published by: Neuroelectric Society, Inc., c/o Anthony Sances, Jr, Ed, Medical College of Wisconsin, 8700 W Wisconsin Ave, Milwaukee, WI 53226. Circ: 200.

616.8 CHE ISSN 1424-8522
▼ **NEUROEMBRYOLOGY.** Text in English. 2002. q. CHF 501, EUR 358.20 in Europe to institutions; CHF 512.60, USD 391 elsewhere to institutions (effective 2002). **Document type:** *Journal, Academic/Scholarly.*
Related titles: Online - full text ed.: ISSN 1424-8530. forthcoming 2002. CHF 58, EUR 42, USD 45 to institutions (effective 2002).
Published by: S. Karger AG, Allschwilerstr 10, PO Box, Basel 4009, Switzerland. TEL 41-61-3061111, FAX 41-61-3061234, karger@karger.ch, http://www.karger.com/journals/neb/neb_jh.htm.

616.8 USA ISSN 0168-0617
QP356.4 CODEN: NEPEEQ
NEUROENDOCRINE PERSPECTIVES. Text in English. 1982. irreg., latest vol.9, 1991. price varies. *Refereed.* **Document type:** *Monographic series.*
Indexed: Biol.Abstr., Chem.Abstr., Chem.Indus.Notes, Chem.Titles, e-psyche.
—CASDDS, CISTI, GNLM, Infotrieve, KNAW. **CCC.**
Published by: Springer-Verlag, Journals (Subsidiary of: BertelsmannSpringer), 175 Fifth Ave, New York, NY 10010. TEL 212-460-1500, FAX 212-473-6272. Eds. E E Mueller, R M Macleod.

NEUROENDOCRINOLOGY; international journal for basic and clinical studies on neuroendocrine relationships. see *MEDICAL SCIENCES—Endocrinology*

616.8 SWE ISSN 0172-780X
CODEN: NLETDU
NEUROENDOCRINOLOGY LETTERS. Text in English. 1979. bi-m. USD 228 to individuals; USD 380 to institutions (effective 2000). adv. bk.rev. illus. back issues avail.; reprint service avail. from ISI. *Refereed.* **Document type:** *Journal, Academic/Scholarly.* **Description:** Covers the fields of neuroendocrinology and related areas, including immunological, psychological, oncological and other aspects in normal and pathological physiology.
Related titles: Online - full text ed.: (from Institute for Scientific Information).
Indexed: ASCA, Chem.Abstr., Chem.Indus.Notes, Chem.Titles, Curr.Adv.Biochem., Curr.Adv.Ecol.Sci., Curr.Cont. (coverage dropped), Dairy Sci.Abstr., Excerp.Med., Ind.Sci.Rev., Int.Abstr.Biol.Sci., Neurosci.Cit.Ind., Sci.Cit.Ind. (coverage dropped), e-psyche.
—BLDSC (6081.371000), CASDDS, CISTI, GNLM, IDS, Infotrieve. **CCC.**
Published by: Maghira & Maas Publications, Engelbrektsgatan 19, Stockholm 114 32, Sweden. TEL 46-8-611-5565, FAX 46-8-678-0747, publisher@nel.edu, http://www.nel.edu. Ed. Dr. Peter Fedor-Freybergh.

616.8 CHE ISSN 0251-5350
CODEN: NEEPD3
NEUROEPIDEMIOLOGY. Text in English. 1982. bi-m. CHF 798, EUR 358.20 in Europe to institutions; CHF 815.40, USD 623 elsewhere to institutions (effective 2002). adv. illus. index. back issues avail. *Refereed.* **Document type:** *Journal, Academic/Scholarly.* **Description:** Devoted to descriptive analytical and experimental studies in the epidemiology of neurologic disease.
Related titles: Microform ed.: (from PQC); Online - full text ed.: ISSN 1423-0208. CHF 58, EUR 42, USD 45 to institutions with print edition (effective 2002) (from Northern Light Technology, Inc., EBSCO Publishing, O C L C Online Computer Library Center, Inc., RoweCom Information Quest, ProQuest Information & Learning, Swets Blackwell, Institute for Scientific Information).
Indexed: ASCA, Aqua.Sci.& Fish.Abstr., Biol.Abstr., Curr.Cont., Environ.Sci.Poll.Mgmt., Excerp.Med., Ind.Med. (1982-), Ind.Sci.Rev., Inpharma, Int.Nurs.Ind., NRN, Neurosci.Abstr., Neurosci.Cit.Ind., Pharm.&Out.News, Pollut.Abstr., PsycInfo, Psychol.Abstr. (1992-), Reac., Saf.Sci.Abstr., Sci.Cit.Ind., e-psyche.
—BLDSC (6081.371200), CISTI, EMDOCS, GNLM, IDS, ingenta, KNAW. **CCC.**
Published by: S. Karger AG, Allschwilerstr 10, PO Box, Basel 4009, Switzerland. TEL 41-61-306-1111, FAX 41-61-306-1234, karger@karger.ch, http://www.online.karger.com/journals/ned, http://www.karger.com. Ed. G C Roman. adv.: page USD 1,185. Circ: 800.

616.8 DEU ISSN 0947-0875
CODEN: NRFMFO
NEUROFORUM. Text in German. 1995. q. DEM 78 to individuals; DEM 158 to institutions; DEM 30 to students (effective 2000). **Document type:** *Journal, Academic/Scholarly.*
Indexed: e-psyche.
—CASDDS, GNLM, Infotrieve. **CCC.**
Published by: Spektrum Akademischer Verlag GmbH, Vangerowstr 20, Heidelberg 69115, Germany. TEL 49-6221-912645, FAX 49-6221-912638, service@mediapoly.com, http://www.spektrum-verlag.com.

NEUROGENETICS. see *BIOLOGY—Genetics*

616.8 USA ISSN 1053-8119
CODEN: NEIMEF
NEUROIMAGE. Text in English. 1992. m. USD 470 in US & Canada to institutions; USD 510 elsewhere to institutions (effective 2001). index. back issues avail. *Refereed.* **Document type:** *Academic/Scholarly.* **Description:** Focuses on the visualization of all neuroscientific data.
Related titles: Online - full text ed.: (from EBSCO Publishing, O C L C Online Computer Library Center, Inc., RoweCom Information Quest, ingenta, Swets Blackwell, IDEAL Online Library, Institute for Scientific Information).
Indexed: ASCA, Chem.Abstr., Curr.Cont., Excerp.Med. (1994-), Ind.Med. (1992-), Inpharma, Neurosci.Cit.Ind., Reac., Sci.Cit.Ind., e-psyche.
—BLDSC (6081.372200), ADONIS, CISTI, EMDOCS, GNLM, IDS, ingenta, KNAW. **CCC.**
Published by: Academic Press, Inc., Journal Division (Subsidiary of: Harcourt Brace & Company), 525 B St, Ste 1900, San Diego, CA 92101-4495. TEL 619-230-1840, FAX 619-699-6800, http://www.apnet.com/www/journal/ni.htm, http://www.academicpress.com/ni.

NEUROIMMUNOMODULATION. see *MEDICAL SCIENCES—Allergology And Immunology*

616.8 340.5 USA ISSN 1058-4706
NEUROLAW LETTER. Text in English. 1991. m. USD 96; USD 106 foreign (effective 1999). bk.rev., video rev., software rev. charts, illus. index. back issues avail. **Document type:** *Newsletter.* **Description:** For legal and health care professionals involved in traumatic brain injury litigation.
Indexed: e-psyche.
Published by: H D I Publishers, PO Box 131401, Houston, TX 77219. TEL 713-526-6900, 800-321-7037, FAX 713-526-7787, hdijch@aol.com. Ed. Ed J Sherrod Taylor. Pub. Charles Haynes. Circ: 1,100 (paid).

616.8 DEU ISSN 1616-2455
DER NEUROLOGE UND PSYCHIATER. Text in German. 1998. bi-m. EUR 58.66 domestic; EUR 63.66 foreign; EUR 46.51 domestic to students; EUR 51.51 foreign to students; EUR 6.54 newsstand/cover (effective 2002). **Document type:** *Journal, Academic/Scholarly.*
Former titles (until 2001): Neuro Praxisinformation (1435-0009); Neuro Nachrichten
Indexed: e-psyche.
Published by: Urban und Vogel Medien und Medizin Verlagsgesellschaft mbH (Subsidiary of: BertelsmannSpringer), Neumarkter Str 43, Munich 81673, Germany. TEL 49-89-43721411, FAX 49-89-43721410, verlag@urban-vogel.de, http://www.urban-vogel.de. Ed. Dr. Monika Drelmann. Adv. contact Barbara Kanters.

M

616.89 HRV ISSN 0353-8842
CODEN: NECRFZ
NEUROLOGIA CROATICA; journal of clinical neurosciences. Text in English; Summaries in Croatian. 1953. q. HRK 100 to individuals; USD 30 foreign to individuals; HRK 200 to institutions; USD 50 foreign to institutions. adv. bk.rev. illus. reprint service avail. from PQC. *Refereed.* **Document type:** *Academic/Scholarly.* **Description:** Covers advances in neurological and neurosurgical research.
Supersedes (in 1991): Neurologija (0350-9559); (in 1977): Neuropsihijatrija (0047-9438)
Related titles: Microform ed.: (from PQC); Online - full text ed.: (from Institute for Scientific Information); ♦ Supplement: Neurologia Croatica. Supplement. ISSN 1331-5196.
Indexed: ASCA, Biol.Abstr., Dent.Ind., Excerp.Med., Ind.Med. (until 1992, dropped), Neurosci.Cit.Ind., Psychol.Abstr., SSCI (coverage dropped), e-psyche.
—BLDSC (6081.377000), CASDDS, CISTI, GNLM, IDS.
Published by: University Hospital, Department of Neurology, Kispaticeva 12, Zagreb 10000, Croatia. TEL 385-1-2335505, FAX 385-1-2335595. Ed., R&P Niko Zurak. Adv. contact Vlatka Ivankovic. Circ: 1,000 (controlled). **Co-sponsor:** Department of Neuropathology.

616.89 HRV ISSN 1331-5196
NEUROLOGIA CROATICA. SUPPLEMENT. Text in English. 1994. irreg.
Related titles: ♦ Supplement to: Neurologia Croatica. ISSN 0353-8842.
Published by: University Hospital, Department of Neurology, Kispaticeva 12, Zagreb 10000, Croatia. TEL 385-1-2335505, FAX 385-1-2335595.

616.8 POL ISSN 0028-3843
CODEN: NNPOBE
NEUROLOGIA I NEUROCHIRURGIA POLSKA. Text in Polish; Summaries in English, Russian. 1951. bi-m. USD 102. adv. bk.rev. bibl, illus, stat. index, cum.index.
Indexed: Biol.Abstr., Chem.Abstr., Dent.Ind., Dok.Arbeitsmed., Excerp.Med., INIS Atomind., Ind.Med. (1967-), Ref.Zh., e-psyche.
—BLDSC (6081.380000), CASDDS, CISTI, GNLM.
Published by: Polskie Towarzystwo Neurologiczne/Polish Neurological Society, Ul Kopcinskiego 22, Lodz 90153, Poland. Ed. Dr. Jerzy Kulczycki. Circ: 1,800. **Dist. by:** Ars Polona, Krakowskie Przedmiescie 7, Warsaw, Poland. **Co-sponsor:** Polskie Towarzystwo Neurochirurgow - Polish Neurosurgeons' Society.

616.89 617.4 JPN
CODEN: NMCHBN
NEUROLOGIA MEDICO-CHIRURGICA. Text in English. 1959. m. USD 145 (effective 2001). adv. *Refereed.* **Document type:** *Academic/Scholarly.*
Former titles: Shinkei Geka (0387-2572); (until 1976): Neurologia Medico-Chirurgica (0470-8105)
Related titles: Online - full text ed.: (from Institute for Scientific Information).
Indexed: Biol.Abstr., Dent.Ind., Excerp.Med., INIS Atomind., Ind.Med. (1959-), Int.Nurs.Ind., Neurosci.Cit.Ind., e-psyche.
—BLDSC (6081.390000), IDS. **CCC.**
Published by: (Nihon No Shinkei Geka Gakkai), Japan Neurosurgical Society, c/o Editorial office, Akamon-mae Iwata Bldg, 5-27-8 Hongo, Bunkyo-ku, Tokyo 113-0033, Japan. TEL 81-3-3812-8092, FAX 81-3-3812-2090, jns@ss.iij4u.or.jp, http://www.ff.iij4u.or.jp/~neuromed/. Ed. Dr. Akira Yamaura.

616.8 USA ISSN 0733-8619
RC321
NEUROLOGIC CLINICS. Text in English. 1983. q. USD 151 domestic to individuals; USD 177 in Canada to individuals; USD 199 elsewhere to individuals; USD 212 domestic to institutions; USD 254 foreign to institutions; USD 64 per issue (effective 2001). adv. *Refereed.* **Document type:** *Journal, Academic/Scholarly.* **Description:** Each issue covers a neurologic disease in detail.
Related titles: Microform ed.: (from PQC); Online - full text ed.: (from Institute for Scientific Information).
Indexed: ASCA, CINAHL, Curr.Cont., INIS Atomind., Ind.Med. (1983-), Ind.Vet., Inpharma, Neurosci.Cit.Ind., Pharm.&Out.News, PsycInfo, Psychol.Abstr. (1987-), Reac., Rev.Med.& Vet.Mycol., SSCI (coverage dropped), e-psyche.
—BLDSC (6081.441000), CISTI, EMDOCS, GNLM, IDS, ingenta, KNAW. **CCC.**
Published by: W.B. Saunders Co. (Subsidiary of: Harcourt Publishers Ltd.), 11830 Westline Industrial Dr, St Louis, MO 63146. TEL 800-325-4177, http://www.wbsaunders.com. **Subscr. to:** Periodicals Fulfillment, W B Saunders Co, 6277 Sea Harbor Dr, 4th Fl, Orlando, FL 32891-4800.

616.8 USA
CODEN: JNRHFV
NEUROLOGIC REHABILITATION AND REPAIR. Text in English. 1987. q. USD 140 domestic to individuals; USD 160 foreign to individuals; USD 180 domestic to institutions; USD 205 foreign to institutions (effective 2000). adv. bk.rev. back issues avail. *Refereed.* **Document type:** *Academic/Scholarly.* **Description:** Deals with neurologic rehabilitation, neural repair and restoration of functions.
Formerly (until 1998): Journal of Neurologic Rehabilitation (0888-4390)
Related titles: Online - full text ed.: (from Institute for Scientific Information).
Indexed: ASCA, CINAHL, Neurosci.Cit.Ind., PsycInfo, Psychol.Abstr. (1988-), e-psyche.
—GNLM, IDS, ingenta.
Published by: (American Society of Neurorehabilitation), Demos Medical Publishing, 386 Park Ave S, Ste 201, New York, NY 10016-8804. TEL 212-683-0072, FAX 212-683-0118, info@demospub.com. Ed. Michael E Selzer. Pub. Diana Schneider. R&P Joan Wolk. Adv. contact Diana M Schneider. B&W page USD 765, color page USD 925; trim 11 x 8.25. Circ: 1,350 (paid).

616.8 USA
NEUROLOGICAL DISORDERS: D S M RESOURCE. Text in English. 1997. a. USD 269; USD 229 foreign (effective 1999). **Document type:** *Trade.*
Indexed: e-psyche.
Published by: American Health Consultants (Subsidiary of: Medical Economics Co., Inc.), 3525 Piedmont Rd, N E, 6 Piedmont Center, Ste 400, Atlanta, GA 30305. TEL 404-262-5476, custserv@ahcpub.com, http://www.ahcpub.com.

616.8 JPN
NEUROLOGICAL INSTITUTE. BULLETIN. Text in English, Japanese. 1964. a. free per issue. **Document type:** *Bulletin.*
Indexed: e-psyche.
Published by: Kyushu Daigaku, Igakubu/Kyushu University, Faculty of Medicine, Neurological Institute, Fuzoku No-Shinkeibyo Kenkyu Shisetsu, 1-1 Maidashi 3-chome, Higashi-ku, Fukuoka-shi 812-0054, Japan. TEL 81-92-641-1151, FAX 81-92-642-5545, kato@neurophy.med.kyushuu.ac.jp. Ed. Masashi Fukui. Circ: (controlled).

616.8 USA ISSN 0161-6412
RC321 CODEN: NRESDZ
NEUROLOGICAL RESEARCH; a journal of progress in neurosurgery, neurology and neurosciences. Text in English. 1979. 8/yr., latest vol.23, 2001. USD 170 to individuals; USD 825 to institutions (effective 2001). adv. bk.rev. abstr, illus, pat. index. 120 p./no. back issues avail.; reprint service avail. from PQC,ISI. *Refereed.* **Document type:** *Journal, Academic/Scholarly.* **Description:** Covers basic and clinical research in neurosurgery, neuro-oncology, neuroradiology, neuropathology and other aspects of neurological research.
Related titles: Microfilm ed.: (from PQC); Online - full text ed.: (from Northern Light Technology, Inc., ProQuest Information & Learning, Institute for Scientific Information, CatchWord Ltd.).
Indexed: ASCA, Aqua.Sci.& Fish.Abstr., Chem.Abstr., Chem.Indus.Notes, Chem.Titles, Curr.Adv.Ecol.Sci., Curr.Cont., Excerp.Med., INIS Atomind., Ind.Med. (1979-), Inpharma, Int.Abstr.Biol.Sci., Neurosci.Cit.Ind., Pharm.&Out.News, Reac., SSCI (coverage dropped), Telegen, Tox.Abstr., e-psyche.
—BLDSC (6081.442000), CASDDS, CISTI, GNLM, IDS, ingenta, KNAW. **CCC.**
Published by: Forefront Publishing Group, PMB 113, 5 River Rd., Wilton, CT 06897-4069. TEL 203-834-0631, FAX 203-834-0940, http://www.forefrontpublishing.com. Eds. Dr. George Austin, Dr. Manuel Dujovny. R&P Mary J Rawlins. Adv. contact Chris Rawlins. **Subscr. to:** Allen Press Inc., PO Box 1897, Lawrence, KS 66044-8897.

610 ITA ISSN 1590-1874
CODEN: IJNSD3
NEUROLOGICAL SCIENCES. Text in English. 1980. bi-m. EUR 145 domestic; EUR 143.30 in Germany; EUR 24.80 newsstand/cover foreign (effective 2002). adv. bk.rev. *Refereed.* **Document type:** *Academic/Scholarly.* **Description:** Provides a medium for the communication of results and ideas in the field of neuroscience.
Formerly (until 1999): The Italian Journal of Neurological Sciences (0392-0461)
Related titles: Microform ed.: (from PQC); Online - full text ed.: ISSN 1590-3478 (from EBSCO Publishing, RoweCom Information Quest, Swets Blackwell, Springer LINK, Institute for Scientific Information).
Indexed: ASCA, CINAHL, Curr.Cont., Excerp.Med., Ind.Med. (2000-), Inpharma, Neurosci.Cit.Ind., Pharm.&Out.News, PsycInfo, Psychol.Abstr. (1989-), Reac., Rev.Appl.Entomol., Rev.Med.& Vet.Mycol., Sci.Cit.Ind., e-psyche.
—BLDSC (6081.444000), CASDDS, CISTI, EMDOCS, GNLM, IDS, ingenta, KNAW.
Published by: (Societa Italiana di Neurologia), Springer-Verlag Italia S.p.A. (Subsidiary of: BertelsmannSpringer), Via Podgora, 4, Milan, MI 20122, Italy. TEL 39-02-5425971, FAX 39-02-55193360, springer@springer.it, http://www.springer.it. Ed. Giuliano Avanzini. Adv. contact A Riccardi. B&W page ITL 2,950,000, color page ITL 4,750,000; trim 245 x 177. Circ: 2,100. **N. America dist. addr.:** Springer-Verlag New York Inc., PO Box 2485, Secaucus, NJ 07096-2485. TEL 800-777-4647. **Co-sponsor:** Societa Italiana di Neurofisiologia Clinica.

NEUROLOGICAL SURGERY/NO SHINKEI GEKA. see *MEDICAL SCIENCES—Surgery*

616.8 DEU ISSN 0947-2177
NEUROLOGIE UND REHABILITATION; die Zeitschrift fuer neurologische Rehabilitation und Praevention. Text in German. 1995. q. DEM 160 (effective 1997). adv. **Document type:** *Academic/Scholarly.*
Indexed: Excerp.Med., e-psyche.
—BLDSC (6081.455000), GNLM.
Published by: (Deutsche Gesellschaft fuer Neurologische Rehabilitation), Kagerer Kommunikation, Koblenzer Str 18, Bonn 53173, Germany. TEL 49-228-95696-0, FAX 49-228-9569640. Ed. B Buelau.

616.8 USA ISSN 1074-7931
CODEN: NROLFW
THE NEUROLOGIST. Text in English. 1995. bi-m., latest vol.7. USD 175 domestic to individuals; USD 210 foreign to individuals; USD 270 domestic to institutions; USD 315 foreign to institutions; USD 48 newsstand/cover (effective 2002). *Refereed.* **Document type:** *Academic/Scholarly.* **Description:** Publishes reviews covering all major areas of neurology.
Related titles: Online - full text ed.: USD 351 domestic for academice site license; USD 396 foreign for academice site license; USD 391.50 domestic for corporate site license; USD 436.50 foreign for corporate site license (effective 2002) (from Institute for Scientific Information).
Indexed: Jrnl.Watch Neuro., Neurosci.Cit.Ind., e-psyche.
—BLDSC (6081.463500), GNLM, IDS, KNAW.
Published by: Williams & Wilkins (Subsidiary of: Waverly International), 351 W Camden St, Baltimore, MD 21201-2436. TEL 410-528-4068, 800-222-3790, FAX 410-528-4452, dbakerv@wwilkins.com, http://www.theneurologist.org, http://www.wwilkins.com. Ed. Dr. Barney Stern. Adv. contact David Baker.

616.8 USA ISSN 0028-3878
RC321 CODEN: NEURAI
NEUROLOGY. Text in English. 1951. 24/yr., latest vol.57. USD 60 domestic to individuals print & online eds.; USD 20 newsstand/cover foreign to individuals print & online eds.; USD 140 domestic to institutions print & online eds.; USD 40 foreign to institutions print & online eds. (effective 2002). adv. bk.rev. bibl, charts, illus. index. *Refereed.* **Document type:** *Trade.* **Description:** Reports, discussions, case findings and clinical findings on current research and developments in neurology. Covers neurological symptoms of diseases, diagnostic methods and treatments.
Related titles: E-mail ed.; Microform ed.: (from PQC); Online - full text ed.: USD 764.40 domestic academic site license; USD 764.40 foreign academic site license; USD 852.60 domestic corporate site license; USD 852.60 foreign corporate site license (effective 2002) (from Ovid Technologies, Inc., HighWire Pr., EBSCO Publishing, Institute for Scientific Information).
Indexed: AIDS Abstr., AIM, AMED, ASCA, AgeLine, Aqua.Sci.& Fish.Abstr., Arts & Hum.Cit.Ind. (coverage dropped), Behav.Med.Abstr., Bibl.Dev.Med.& Child Neur., Biol.Abstr., Chem.Abstr., Chem.Indus.Notes, Chem.Titles, Curr.Adv.Cancer Res., Curr.Adv.Ecol.Sci., Curr.Cont., Dent.Ind., Diab.Cont., Excerp.Med., Helminthol.Abstr., INIS Atomind., Ind.Med. (1951-), Ind.Sci.Rev., Ind.Vet., Inpharma, Int.Abstr.Biol.Sci., Int.Nurs.Ind., Jrnl.Watch, Jrnl.Watch Neuro., Jrnl.Watch Psych., Lang.& Lang.Behav.Abstr., METADEX, Neurosci.Cit.Ind., Nutr.Abstr., Pharm.&Out.News, Protozool.Abstr., PsycInfo, Psychol.Abstr. (1951-), Reac., Rev.Appl.Entomol., Rev.Med.& Vet.Mycol., SOPODA, SSCI (coverage dropped), Sci.Cit.Ind., Sociol.Abstr., Yrbk.Assoc.Educ.& Rehab.Blind, e-psyche.
—BLDSC (6081.500000), CASDDS, CISTI, GNLM, IDS, ingenta, KNAW.

M

Published by: (American Academy of Neurology), Lippincott Williams & Wilkins (Philadelphia) (Subsidiary of: Wolters Kluwer N.V.), 530 Walnut St, Philadelphia, PA 19106-3621. TEL 215-521-8300, FAX 215-521-8902, http://www.neurology.org, http://www.lww.com. Ed. Dr. Robert C Griggs. Pub. Nancy Megley. R&P Alice McElhinney. Adv. contact Roger Soderman. B&W page USD 1,335, color page USD 2,885; trim 10.88 x 8.25. Circ: 18,487 (paid). **Subscr. to:** PO Box 1600, Hagerstown, MD 21740-1600. TEL 800-777-2295, FAX 301-824-7390.

616.8 USA ISSN 0741-4234
NEUROLOGY ALERT. Text in English. 1982. m. USD 219 domestic; USD 249 foreign; USD 37 newsstand/cover (effective 2001). index. reprints avail. **Document type:** *Newsletter.*
Related titles: Audio cassette/tape ed.; Online - full text ed.: (from Northern Light Technology, Inc., Gale Group).
Indexed: e-psyche.
Published by: American Health Consultants (Subsidiary of: Medical Economics Co., Inc.), 3525 Piedmont Rd, N E, 6 Piedmont Center, Ste 400, Atlanta, GA 30305. TEL 404-262-5476, 404-262-7436, 800-688-2421, FAX 404-262-7837, 800-284-3291, custserv@ahcpub.com, http://www.ahcpub.com. Circ: 2,600.

616.8 USA ISSN 1526-8748 CODEN: JCNPFQ
NEUROLOGY AND CLINICAL NEUROPHYSIOLOGY. Text in English. 1996. a., latest vol.5, 2000. USD 30 in US & Canada to individuals; USD 150 in US & Canada to institutions (effective 2001). abstr. *Refereed.* **Document type:** *Academic/Scholarly.* **Description:** Publishes original clinical and basic science research in human neurology, neuroscience and related fields. Also publishes views and reviews, debates on controversial topics, information and news of events relevant to neurology. Accepted articles are published on an article by article basis.
Formerly: Journal of Contemporary Neurology (1081-1818); Which was announced as: Contemporary Neurology
Related titles: Online - full content ed.: (from EBSCO Publishing, Swets Blackwell); Online - full text ed.: (from CatchWord Ltd., RoweCom Information Quest).
Indexed: e-psyche.
—CatchWord.
Published by: (American Academy of Clinical Neurophysiology), M I T Press, 5 Cambridge Center, Cambridge, MA 02142-1407. TEL 617-253-2866, FAX 617-577-1545, journals-info@mit.edu, journals-orders@mit.edu/cone, http://mitpress.mit.edu/NCN, http://mitpress.mit.edu/JCN. Ed. Dr. Keith H Chiappa TEL 617-726-8737.

616.8 USA ISSN 0736-4563 CODEN: NEUND9
NEUROLOGY AND NEUROBIOLOGY. Text in English. 1982. irreg., latest vol.60, 1990. price varies. **Document type:** *Monographic series.*
Indexed: Biol.Abstr., Chem.Abstr., Chem.Indus.Notes, Chem.Titles, e-psyche.
—CASDDS, CISTI.
Published by: John Wiley & Sons, Inc., Journals (Subsidiary of: Wiley InterScience), 605 Third Ave, New York, NY 10158. TEL 212-850-6000.

616.8 GBR ISSN 1473-7086
NEUROLOGY IN PRACTICE. Text in English.
—ADONIS.
Published by: B M J Publishing Group, B M A House, Tavistock Sq, London WC1H 9JR, United Kingdom. TEL 44-20-7387-4499, FAX 44-20-7383-6400, info.norththames@bma.org.uk, http://www.bma.org.uk.

616.8 IND ISSN 0028-3886
NEUROLOGY INDIA. Text in English. 1952. q. INR 1,050, USD 145 (effective 2000). adv. bk.rev. bibl, illus. cum.index. reprint service avail. from IRC. *Refereed.* **Document type:** *Academic/Scholarly.*
Related titles: CD-ROM ed.; Online - full text ed.: (from Institute for Scientific Information).
Indexed: ASCA, Biol.Abstr., Chem.Abstr., Curr.Cont. (coverage dropped), Excerp.Med. (until 1990, 1995-), ExtraMED, INIS Atomind., Ind.Med. (1964-), Neurosci.Cit.Ind., e-psyche.
—CISTI, GNLM, IDS, ingenta, KNAW.
Published by: Neurological Society of India, Dept. of Neurology, Post-graduate Institute of Medical Education & Research, Chandigarh, Haryana 160 021, India. TEL 91-172-744568, FAX 91-172-549998, sudeshp@cpindia.com; cpni@ch1.vsnl.net.in. Ed., Pub., R&P, Adv. contact Sudesh Prabhakar. B&W page INR 10,000, color page INR 11,500; trim 25 x 165. Circ: 1,600.

616.8 DEU ISSN 0941-9500 CODEN: NPBRE4
NEUROLOGY, PSYCHIATRY AND BRAIN RESEARCH. (Supplement to: Zentralblatt Neurologie, Psychiatrie (ISSN 0722-3064)) Text in English. 1992. 4/yr. DEM 120 to individuals; DEM 358 to institutions. back issues avail. *Refereed.* **Document type:** *Journal, Academic/Scholarly.* **Description:** Publishes papers and articles on research in neurology, biologically and psychopathologically oriented psychiatry, neurosurgery and the neurosciences, including neurochemistry, neuroendocrinology, neurophysiology, neuropsychology, neuromorphology, neuroimmunology, neurogenetics, neuroepidemiology as well as therapy of neurological and psychiatric disorders.
Related titles: Online - full text ed.: (from Institute for Scientific Information).
Indexed: ASCA, Neurosci.Cit.Ind., SSCI (coverage dropped), e-psyche.
—BLDSC (6081.502500), EMDOCS, GNLM, IDS, Infotrieve, KNAW. **CCC.**
Published by: (Archiv fuer Psychiatrie und Nervenkrankheiten), Universitaetsverlag Ulm GmbH, Bahnhofstr 20, Ulm 89079, Germany. TEL 49-731-152860, FAX 49-731-152862, info@uni-verlag-ulm.de, http://www.universitaetsverlag.de/zeitschriften_npbr1.html, http://www.uni-verlag-ulm.de. Eds. Gerd Huber, Hans H Kornhuber. Adv. contact Sabine Kindermann.

616.8 USA
NEUROLOGY REPORT. Text in English. 1994. q.
Published by: American Physical Therapy Association, 1111 N Fairfax St, Alexandria, VA 22314-1488. TEL 703-706-3124, FAX 703-684-7343, http://www.apta.org.

616.8 USA ISSN 1077-4556
NEUROLOGY REVIEWS; for the primary care physician and the practicing neurologist: clinical trends & news in neurology. Text in English. 1993. m. USD 75; USD 90 foreign. adv. abstr, charts, illus. *Refereed.* **Document type:** *Trade.* **Description:** Discusses new clinical research in the treatment and diagnosis of neurological disorders and conditions.
Indexed: Inpharma, Reac., e-psyche.
Published by: Partners in Medical Communication, 2 Brighton Rd, Clifton, NJ 07012. TEL 201-913-1000, FAX 201-916-0021. Pub. Joseph J D'Onofrio. R&P Dianne Kulacz. Circ: (controlled).

616.8 USA ISSN 1533-7006
▼ **NEUROLOGY TODAY.** Text in English. 2001. m. USD 153 domestic to individuals; USD 213 foreign to individuals; USD 210 domestic to institutions; USD 264 foreign to institutions (effective 2002). **Document type:** *Journal, Academic/Scholarly.*
Published by: Lippincott Williams & Wilkins (Philadelphia) (Subsidiary of: Wolters Kluwer N.V.), 530 Walnut St, Philadelphia, PA 19106-3621. TEL 215-521-8300, FAX 215-521-8902, custserv@lww.com, http://www.lww.com/. **Subscr. to:** PO Box 1600, Hagerstown, MD 21740-1600. TEL 800-638-3030, FAX 310-223-2400.

NEUROMETHODS. see *BIOLOGY—Physiology*

616.8 USA ISSN 1094-7159 CODEN: NROMFZ
NEUROMODULATION. Text in English. 1998. q. USD 120 domestic to individuals; USD 130 in Canada & Mexico to individuals; USD 145 elsewhere to individuals; USD 195 domestic to institutions; USD 205 in Canada & Mexico to institutions; USD 220 elsewhere to institutions; USD 132 domestic to individuals print & online eds. combined; USD 143 in Canada & Mexico to individuals print & online eds. combined; USD 159.50 elsewhere to individuals print & online eds. combined; USD 214.50 domestic to institutions print & online eds. combined; USD 225.50 in Canada & Mexico to institutions print & online eds. combined; USD 242 elsewhere to institutions print & online eds. combined (effective 2001). adv. abstr. reprints avail. *Refereed.* **Document type:** *Academic/Scholarly.* **Description:** Disseminates scientific and clinical information relevant to the field of neuromodulation.
Related titles: Microform ed.; ♦ Online - full text ed.: Neuromodulation Online. ISSN 1525-1403.
Indexed: Neurosci.Cit.Ind., e-psyche.
—BLDSC (6081.504100), IDS.
Published by: (International Neuromodulation Society), Blackwell Science Inc., Commerce Pl, 350 Main St, Malden, MA 02148-5018. TEL 781-388-8250, 888-661-5800, FAX 781-388-8255, journals@blacksci.com, http://www.blackwell-science.com. Ed. Elliot S Krames. R&P Tracey Davies. Adv. contact Jenny Applin.

616.8 USA ISSN 1525-1403
NEUROMODULATION ONLINE. Text in English. q. USD 108 to individuals; USD 176 to institutions (effective 2001). **Document type:** *Academic/Scholarly.*
Media: Online - full text (from EBSCO Publishing, O C L C Online Computer Library Center, Inc., RoweCom Information Quest, ingenta, Munksgaard & Blackwell Science's Synergy, Swets Blackwell, Institute for Scientific Information). **Related titles:** Microform ed.; ♦ Print ed.: Neuromodulation. ISSN 1094-7159.
Published by: Blackwell Science Inc., Commerce Pl, 350 Main St, Malden, MA 02148-5018. TEL 781-388-8250, 800-759-6102, FAX 781-388-8255, website@blacksci.com, journals@blacksci.com, http://www.blackwell-science.com/~cgilib/bsinc.bin?Journal=geoscience.

616.8 GBR ISSN 0960-8966 CODEN: NEDIEC
NEUROMUSCULAR DISORDERS. Text in English. 1991. 8/yr. EUR 696 in Europe to institutions; JPY 92,400 in Japan to institutions; USD 779 elsewhere to institutions (effective 2002). index. *Refereed.* **Document type:** *Academic/Scholarly.* **Description:** Covers all aspects of neuromuscular disorders in childhood and adult life.
Related titles: Microfilm ed.: (from PQC); Online - full text ed.: (from ingenta, ScienceDirect, Swets Blackwell, Institute for Scientific Information).
Indexed: AMED, ASCA, Curr.Cont., Excerp.Med. (1992-), Ind.Med. (1991-), Ind.Sci.Rev., Inpharma, Int.Abstr.Biol.Sci., Neurosci.Cit.Ind., Reac., Sci.Cit.Ind., e-psyche.
—BLDSC (6081.504850), CISTI, EMDOCS, GNLM, IDS, ingenta, KNAW. **CCC.**
Published by: Pergamon (Subsidiary of: Elsevier Science), The Boulevard, Langford Ln, East Park, Kidlington, Oxford OXB 1GB, United Kingdom. FAX 44-1865-843010, http://www.elsevier.com/locate/nmd. Eds. J Miller, Victor Dubowitz. **Subscr. in Australasia and the Far East to:** Elsevier Science (Singapore) Pte Ltd, No.1 Temasek Ave, 17-01 Millenia Tower, Singapore 039192, Singapore. TEL 65-434-3727, FAX 65-337-2230; **Subscr. in the Americas to:** Elsevier Science, PO Box 945, New York, NY 10159-0945. TEL 212-633-3730, FAX 212-633-3680, usinfo-f@elsevier.com; **Subscr. to:** Elsevier Science BV, PO Box 211, Amsterdam 1000 AE, Netherlands. TEL 31-20-485-3757.

616.8 USA ISSN 0896-6273
QP356.2 CODEN: NERNET
NEURON. Text in English. 1988. 18/yr. EUR 696 in Europe to institutions; JPY 92,400 in Japan to institutions; USD 779 elsewhere to institutions (effective 2002). adv. bk.rev. abstr. *Refereed.* **Document type:** *Academic/Scholarly.* **Description:** Publishes research articles in molecular, cellular and developmental neurobiology, and also research work in systems (including visual, auditory, motor and limbic systems), neuro-imaging, learning, memory, and behavior and other cognitive studies.
Related titles: Online - full text ed.: USD 95 (effective 2001) (from HighWire Pr., ingenta, Institute for Scientific Information).
Indexed: ASCA, Aqua.Sci.& Fish.Abstr., Cal.Tiss.Abstr., Chem.Abstr., Chem.Indus.Notes, Chem.Titles, Chemorec.Abstr., Curr.Cont., Genet.Abstr., INIS Atomind., Ind.Med. (1988-), Ind.Sci.Rev., Inpharma, Int.Abstr.Biol.Sci., Neurosci.Abstr., Neurosci.Cit.Ind., Nuc.Acids Abstr., Nutr.Abstr., Pharm.&Out.News, Reac., Rev.Appl.Entomol., Sci.Cit.Ind., Sport Fish.Abstr., Tox.Abstr. (coverage dropped), Wild.Rev., Zoo.Rec., e-psyche.
—BLDSC (6081.504900), ADONIS, CASDDS, CISTI, EMDOCS, GNLM, IDS, ingenta, KNAW.
Published by: Cell Press (Subsidiary of: Reed Elsevier plc), 1100 Massachusetts Ave, Cambridge, MA 02138. TEL 617-661-7057, FAX 617-661-7061, neuron@cell.com, http://www.neuron.org/, http://www.cellpress.com. Ed. Emilie Marcus. Pub. Lynne Herndon. Adv. contact Elizabeth Wardell.

NEUROORTHOPAEDIE. see *MEDICAL SCIENCES—Orthopedics And Traumatology*

M

616.8 AUS ISSN 0919-6544
NEUROPATHOLOGY. Text in English. 1980. q. AUD 225 domestic to individuals; AUD 205 in New Zealand to individuals; USD 125 elsewhere to individuals; AUD 828 domestic to institutions; AUD 752 in New Zealand to institutions; JPY 54,780 in Japan to institutions; USD 459 elsewhere to institutions; AUD 248 domestic to individuals paper & online eds. combined; AUD 226 in New Zealand to individuals paper & online eds. combined; USD 138 elsewhere to individuals paper & online eds. combined; AUD 911 domestic to institutions paper & online eds. combined; AUD 828 in New Zealand to institutions paper & online eds. combined; JPY 60,258 in Japan to institutions paper & online eds. combined; USD 505 elsewhere to institutions paper & online eds. combined (effective 2001). adv. back issues avail. *Refereed.* **Document type:** *Academic/Scholarly.* **Description:** Explores all aspects of clinical and experimental neuropathology and related areas.
Supersedes in part (in 1993): Shinkei Byorigaku (0286-3626)
Related titles: Online - full text ed.: ISSN 1440-1789. AUD 203 domestic to individuals; AUD 185 in New Zealand to individuals; USD 113 elsewhere to individuals; AUD 746 domestic to institutions; AUD 677 in New Zealand to institutions; JPY 49,302 in Japan to institutions; USD 414 elsewhere to institutions (effective 2001) (from EBSCO Publishing, O C L C Online Computer Library Center, Inc., RoweCom Information Quest, ingenta, Munksgaard & Blackwell Science's Synergy, Swets Blackwell, Institute for Scientific Information).
Indexed: ASCA, Excerp.Med., Ind.Med., Int.Abstr.Biol.Sci., Neurosci.Abstr., Neurosci.Cit.Ind., e-psyche.
—BLDSC (6081.513800), IDS. **CCC.**
Published by: (Japanese Society of Neuropathology JPN), Blackwell Science Asia Pty Ltd, PO Box 378, Carlton South, VIC 3053, Australia. TEL 61-3-9347-0300, FAX 61-3-9347-5001, info@blacksci-asia.com.au; knagasi@med.hokudai.ac.jp, http://www.blacksci.co.uk. Eds. Kazuo Nagashima, Masato Tsukahara. Adv. contact Kathryn O'Brien. B&W page AUD 1,200, color page AUD 2,500; trim 210 x 275.

616.8 GBR ISSN 0305-1846
CODEN: NANEDL
NEUROPATHOLOGY AND APPLIED NEUROBIOLOGY. Text in English. 1975. bi-m., latest vol.28, 2002. GBP 723 in Europe; USD 1,147 in North America; GBP 796 elsewhere (effective 2002). adv. bk.rev. bibl, charts, illus. index. back issues avail.; reprint service avail. from ISI. *Refereed.* **Document type:** *Academic/Scholarly.* **Description:** Publishes papers on a range of neuropathological topics extending from experimental and molecular neuroscience to clinical papers dealing with the basic applied neurobiological aspects of human and veterinary disease.
Related titles: Microform ed.: (from PQC); Online - full text ed.: Neuropathology & Applied Neurobiology Online. ISSN 1365-2990. 1999. GBP 651 in Europe; USD 1,033 in North America; GBP 651 elsewhere (effective 2002) (from EBSCO Publishing, O C L C Online Computer Library Center, Inc., RoweCom Information Quest, ingenta, Munksgaard & Blackwell Science's Synergy, Swets Blackwell, Institute for Scientific Information); ♦ Supplement: Neuropathology and Applied Neurobiology. Supplement. ISSN 1359-1940.
Indexed: ASCA, Aqua.Sci.& Fish.Abstr., Biol.Abstr., Chem.Abstr., Chem.Indus.Notes, Chem.Titles, Curr.Adv.Cell & Devel.Biol., Curr.Adv.Ecol.Sci., Curr.Cont., Excerp.Med., Ind.Med. (1975-), Ind.Sci.Rev., Ind.Vet., Inpharma, Int.Abstr.Biol.Sci., Neurosci.Cit.Ind., Pharm.&Out.News, Reac., Rev.Med.& Vet.Mycol., Sci.Cit.Ind., Small Anim.Abstr., THA, Vet.Bull., e-psyche.
—BLDSC (6081.514000), ADONIS, CASDDS, CISTI, EMDOCS, GNLM, IDS, ingenta, KNAW. **CCC.**
Published by: (British Neuropathological Society), Blackwell Science Ltd., PO Box 88, Oxford OX2 0NE, United Kingdom. TEL 44-1865-206180, 44-1865-206002, FAX 44-1865-206219, jnl.orders@blacksci.co.uk, http://www.blackwell-science.com/~cgilib/jnlpage.asp?Journal=nan&File=nan, http://www.blackwellpublishing.com. Ed. R O Weller. Pub. Elizabeth Whelan. R&P Sophie Savage. Adv. contact Jenny Applin. Circ: 525.

M

616.8 GBR ISSN 1359-1940
NEUROPATHOLOGY AND APPLIED NEUROBIOLOGY. SUPPLEMENT. Text in English. 1995. irreg. **Document type:** *Journal, Academic/Scholarly.*
Related titles: ♦ Supplement to: Neuropathology and Applied Neurobiology. ISSN 0305-1846.
—ADONIS.
Published by: Blackwell Science Ltd., Osney Mead, Oxford OX2 0EL, United Kingdom. TEL 44-1865-206206, FAX 44-1865-721205, journals.cs@blacksci.co.uk, http://www.blackwell-science.com/.

NEUROPEDIATRICS; journal of pediatric neurobiology, neurology and neurosurgery. see *MEDICAL SCIENCES—Pediatrics*

NEUROPEPTIDES (SHEFFIELD). see *BIOLOGY—Abstracting, Bibliographies, Statistics*

NEUROPHARMACOLOGY. see *PHARMACY AND PHARMACOLOGY*

616.8 FRA ISSN 0987-7053
CODEN: NCLIE4
NEUROPHYSIOLOGIE CLINIQUE/CLINICAL NEUROPHYSIOLOGY; exploration fonctionnelle du systeme nerveux. Text in English, French. 1970. bi-m. EUR 281 in Europe to institutions; USD 338 elsewhere to institutions (effective 2002). adv. bk.rev. illus. index. reprint service avail. from ISI. *Refereed.* **Document type:** *Academic/Scholarly.* **Description:** Covers the field of neurophysiology, electroencephalography, electromyography, evoked potentials and other investigative approaches in neurology and psychiatry.
Formerly (until 1988): Revue d'Electroencephalographie et de Neurophysiologie Clinique (0370-4475)
Related titles: Microform ed.: (from PQC); Online - full text ed.: (from ingenta, ScienceDirect, Swets Blackwell, Institute for Scientific Information).
Indexed: ASCA, Bibl.Dev.Med.& Child Neur., Biol.Abstr., Curr.Cont., Excerp.Med., Ind.Med. (1988-), Inpharma, Neurosci.Cit.Ind., Pharm.&Out.News, Reac., SSCI (coverage dropped), e-psyche.
—BLDSC (6081.517800), CISTI, EMDOCS, GNLM, IDS, KNAW. **CCC.**
Published by: (Societe de Neurophysiologie Clinique de Langue Francaise), Elsevier Paris, Editions Scientifiques et Medicales (Subsidiary of: Reed Elsevier plc. group), 23 rue Linois, Paris 75015, France. TEL 33-1-45589110, FAX 33-1-45589419, neurphy@elsevier.fr; academic@elsevier-fr.com, http://www.elsevier.com/locate/neucli. Eds. C Garcia Larrea, P Genton. Circ: 3,000.

NEUROPHYSIOLOGIE - LABOR. see *MEDICAL SCIENCES—Cardiovascular Diseases*

NEUROPHYSIOLOGY. see *BIOLOGY—Abstracting, Bibliographies, Statistics*

616.8 USA ISSN 0090-2977
CODEN: NPHYBI
NEUROPHYSIOLOGY. Text in English. 1969. bi-m. EUR 2,160 to institutions for print or online ed.; EUR 2,592 to institutions print & online eds.combined (effective 2002). back issues avail. *Refereed.* **Document type:** *Academic/Scholarly.* **Description:** Explores the nature of basic nerve processes and the mechanisms of nervous system and sensory organ activity from the perspectives of multiple disciplines.
Related titles: Online - full text ed.: (from Swets Blackwell, Kluwer Online, Institute for Scientific Information, RoweCom Information Quest); ♦ Translation of: Neirofiziologiya. ISSN 0028-2561.
Indexed: Biol.Abstr., Excerp.Med., Ind.Med. (coverage dropped), Int.Abstr.Biol.Sci., Neurosci.Abstr. (coverage dropped), Neurosci.Cit.Ind., Psychol.Abstr., Sci.Cit.Ind. (coverage dropped).
—BLDSC (0416.260000), CISTI, GNLM, IDS, Infotrieve, ingenta. **CCC.**
Published by: Kluwer Academic - Plenum Publishers (Subsidiary of: Wolters Kluwer N.V.), 233 Spring St, New York, NY 10013-1578. TEL 212-620-8468, 800-221-9864, FAX 212-463-0742, info@plenum.com; kluwer@wkap.com; services@wkap.nl, http://www.plenum.com. Eds. P G Kostyuk, V I Skok.

616.8 DEU ISSN 0948-6259
NEUROPSYCHIATRIE. Text in German. 1985. q. DEM 136, EUR 69.54; DEM 40, EUR 20.45 newsstand/cover (effective 2001). adv. abstr. *Refereed.* **Document type:** *Journal, Academic/Scholarly.*
Related titles: Online - full text ed.: (from Institute for Scientific Information).
Indexed: ASCA, Excerp.Med. (1995-), Neurosci.Cit.Ind., SSCI (coverage dropped), e-psyche.
—BLDSC (6081.535700), IDS.
Published by: Dustri-Verlag Dr. Karl Feistle, Bajuwarenring 4, Oberhaching 82041, Germany. TEL 49-89-613861-0, FAX 49-89-613-5412, info@dustri.de, http://www.dustri.de. Ed. Dr. F Gerstenbrand. R&P Renate Lehmann. Adv. contact Joerg Feistle. B&W page ATS 9,400, B&W page XEU 683.12; trim 167 x 242. Circ: 1,500.

NEUROPSYCHIATRIE DE L'ENFANCE ET DE L'ADOLESCENCE. see *MEDICAL SCIENCES—Pediatrics*

616.8 USA ISSN 0894-878X
CODEN: NNNEEB
NEUROPSYCHIATRY, NEUROPSYCHOLOGY AND BEHAVIORAL NEUROLOGY. Text in English. 1989. q., latest vol.14. USD 220 domestic to individuals; USD 263 foreign to individuals; USD 356 domestic to institutions; USD 418 foreign to institutions; USD 96 newsstand/cover (effective 2002). adv. charts, illus. reprint service avail. from PQC. *Refereed.* **Document type:** *Journal, Academic/Scholarly.* **Description:** Presents original research articles on basic brain processes; includes critical review articles, case reports, and brief reports on preliminary studies and pertinent clinical issues.
Related titles: Online - full text ed.: USD 462.80 domestic for academic site license; USD 524.80 foreign for academic site license; USD 516.20 domestic for corporate site license; USD 578.20 foreign for corporate site license (effective 2002) (from Institute for Scientific Information).
Indexed: ASCA, Curr.Cont., Excerp.Med., Ind.Med. (1988-), Inpharma, Neuropsych.Abstr., Neurosci.Cit.Ind., Pharm.&Out.News, PsycInfo, Psychol.Abstr. (1988-), Reac., SSCI (coverage dropped), e-psyche.
—BLDSC (6081.543000), EMDOCS, GNLM, IDS, ingenta, KNAW.
Published by: (Behavioral Neurology Society), Lippincott Williams & Wilkins (Philadelphia) (Subsidiary of: Wolters Kluwer N.V.), 530 Walnut St, Philadelphia, PA 19106-3621. TEL 301-223-2300, 800-638-3030, FAX 301-223-2400, http://www.neuneubeneu.com, http://www.lww.com. Ed. Michael Alan Taylor. adv.: B&W page USD 615, color page USD 1,715. Circ: 854 (paid).

612.8 CHE ISSN 0302-282X
CODEN: NPBYAL
NEUROPSYCHOBIOLOGY; international journal of experimental and clinical research in biological psychiatry, pharmacopsychiatry, biological psychology, pharmacopsychology and pharmacoelectroencephalography. Text in English. 8/yr. (in 2 vols.). CHF 1,336, EUR 954.40 in Europe to institutions; CHF 1,359.20, USD 1,038 elsewhere to institutions (effective 2002). adv. bk.rev. abstr. index. back issues avail. *Refereed.* **Document type:** *Journal, Academic/Scholarly.*
Incorporates: International Pharmacopsychiatry (0020-8272)
Related titles: Microform ed.: (from PQC); Online - full text ed.: ISSN 1423-0224. CHF 116, EUR 84, USD 90 to institutions with print edition (effective 2002) (from Northern Light Technology, Inc., EBSCO Publishing, O C L C Online Computer Library Center, Inc., RoweCom Information Quest, ProQuest Information & Learning, Swets Blackwell, Institute for Scientific Information).
Indexed: ASCA, Agri.& Environ.Biotech.Abstr. (coverage dropped), Biol.Abstr., Chem.Abstr., Chem.Indus.Notes, Chem.Titles, Curr.Adv.Ecol.Sci., Curr.Cont., Dent.Ind., Derwent Biotech.Abstr., Excerp.Med., Focus on: Psychophar., Ind.Med. (1975-), Ind.Sci.Rev., Indian Psychol.Abstr., Inpharma, Neurosci.Abstr. (coverage dropped), Neurosci.Cit.Ind., Nutr.Abstr., Pharm.&Out.News, PsycInfo, Psychol.Abstr. (1975-), Reac., SSCI (coverage dropped), Sci.Cit.Ind., e-psyche.
—BLDSC (6081.545000), CASDDS, CISTI, EMDOCS, GNLM, IDS, ingenta, KNAW. **CCC.**
Published by: (International Pharmaco-EEG Group), S. Karger AG, Allschwilerstr 10, PO Box, Basel 4009, Switzerland. TEL 41-61-306-1111, FAX 41-61-306-1234, karger@karger.ch, http://www.online.karger.com/journals/nps, http://www.karger.com. adv.: page USD 1,195. Circ: 1,000.

616.8 GBR ISSN 0028-3932
RC321 CODEN: NUPSA6
NEUROPSYCHOLOGIA; an international journal in behavioural neuroscience. Text in English, French, German; Summaries in French, German. 1963. 13/yr. EUR 408 in Europe to qualified personnel; JPY 54,100 in Japan to qualified personnel; USD 456 elsewhere to qualified personnel; EUR 2,097 in Europe to institutions; JPY 278,500 in Japan to institutions; USD 2,346 elsewhere to institutions (effective 2002). adv. bk.rev. charts, illus. index. back issues avail.; reprint service avail. from PQC. *Refereed.* **Document type:** *Academic/Scholarly.* **Description:** Promotes the study of human behavior from a neurological point of view, and integrates clinical, general, and experimental contributions to the field.
Related titles: Microfilm ed.: (from PQC); Online - full text ed.: (from ingenta, ScienceDirect, Swets Blackwell, Institute for Scientific Information).

Indexed: AMED, ASCA, AgeLine, Behav.Med.Abstr., Bibl.Asian Stud. (1971), Bibl.Dev.Med.& Child Neur., Biol.Abstr., Curr.Adv.Ecol.Sci., Curr.Cont., Dent.Ind., Excerp.Med., IBR, Ind.Med. (1963-), Ind.Sci.Rev., Inpharma, Int.Abstr.Biol.Sci., Lang.& Lang.Behav.Abstr., Neuropsych.Abstr., Neurosci.Cit.Ind., Pharm.&Out.News, PsycInfo, Psychol.Abstr. (1967-), Reac., SOPODA, SSCI, Sci.Cit.Ind., Sociol.Abstr., Yrbk.Assoc.Educ.& Rehab.Blind, e-psyche.
—BLDSC (6081.550000), CISTI, GNLM, IDS, ingenta, KNAW. **CCC.**
Published by: Pergamon (Subsidiary of: Elsevier Science), The Boulevard, Langford Ln, East Park, Kidlington, Oxford OXB 1GB, United Kingdom. FAX 44-1865-843010, nlinfo-f@elsevier.nl; usinfo-f@elsevier.com; forinfo-kyf04035@niftyserve.or.jp, nlinfo-f@elsevier/nl; usinfo-f@elsevier.com; forinfo-kyf04035@niftyserve.or.jp, http://www.elsevier.com/locate/neuropsychologia. Eds. A D Milner, M Jeeves. adv.: B&W page USD 550, color page USD 1,350. Circ: 1,950. **Subscr. in Australasia and the Far East to:** Elsevier Science (Singapore) Pte Ltd, No.1 Temasek Ave, 17-01 Millenia Tower, Singapore 039192, Singapore. TEL 65-434-3727, FAX 65-337-2230; **Subscr. in the Americas to:** Elsevier Science, PO Box 945, New York, NY 10159-0945. TEL 212-633-3730, FAX 212-633-3680, usinfo-f@elsevier.com; **Subscr. to:** Elsevier Science BV, PO Box 211, Amsterdam 1000 AE, Netherlands. TEL 31-20-485-3757, FAX 31-20-485-3432, nlinfo-f@elsevier.nl.

616.8 GBR ISSN 0960-2011
RC387.5 CODEN: NREHE3
NEUROPSYCHOLOGICAL REHABILITATION; an international journal. Text in English. 1991. 5/yr. USD 177, GBP 107 to individuals; USD 371, GBP 225 to institutions (effective 2002). adv. *Refereed.* **Document type:** *Academic/Scholarly.* **Description:** Provides an international forum for the publication of well-designed and properly evaluated intervention strategies, surveys, and observational procedures that are clinically relevant and may also back up theoretical arguments or models.
Related titles: Online - full text ed.: ISSN 1464-0694 (from CatchWord Ltd., EBSCO Publishing, O C L C Online Computer Library Center, Inc., RoweCom Information Quest, Swets Blackwell, Institute for Scientific Information).
Indexed: AMED, ASCA, ASSIA, Excerp.Med. (1993-), Lang.& Lang.Behav.Abstr., Neurosci.Cit.Ind., PsycInfo, Psychol.Abstr. (1991-), SOPODA, SSCI (coverage dropped), Sociol.Abstr., e-psyche.
—BLDSC (6081.551000), CatchWord, EMDOCS, GNLM, IDS.
Published by: Psychology Press (Subsidiary of: Taylor & Francis Group), 27 Church Rd, Hove, E Sussex BN3 2FA, United Kingdom. TEL 44-1273-207411, FAX 44-1273-205612, information@psypress.co.uk, http://www.psypress.co.uk. Ed. Barbara A Wilson. **Subscr. addr. in N America:** Psychology Press, Journals Customer Service, Taylor & Francis Group, 325 Chestnut St, Philadelphia, PA 19106. TEL 800-354-1420, FAX 215-625-8914, info@taylorandfrancis.com, http://www.psypress.com; **Subscr. addr. outside N America:** Journals Customer Service, Taylor & Francis Group, Rankine Rd, Basingstoke, Hants RG24 8PR, United Kingdom. TEL 44-1256-813002, FAX 44-1256-479438, enquiry@tandf.co.uk.

616.8 150 USA ISSN 0894-4105
CODEN: NEUPEG
NEUROPSYCHOLOGY. Text in English. 1987. q. USD 92 domestic to non-members; USD 107 foreign to non-members; USD 46 domestic to members; USD 56 foreign to members; USD 146 domestic to institutions; USD 178 foreign to institutions (effective 2001). adv. illus. reprints avail. *Refereed.* **Document type:** *Academic/Scholarly.* **Description:** Features interdisciplinary contributions on assessment, treatment, and rehabilitation in clinical neuropsychology, focusing on neuropsychological measurement techniques and psychosocial adjustment of the impaired patient.
Related titles: Online - full text ed.: (from Institute for Scientific Information).
Indexed: AMED, ASCA, AgeLine, Curr.Cont., Excerp.Med. (1995-), Ind.Med. (1987-), Lang.& Lang.Behav.Abstr., Neuropsych.Abstr., Neurosci.Cit.Ind., PsycInfo, Psychol.Abstr. (1987-), Russ.Acad.Sci.Bibl., SOPODA, SSCI, Sociol.Abstr., e-psyche.
—BLDSC (6081.553000), GNLM, IDS, ingenta. **CCC.**
Published by: American Psychological Association, 750 First St., N.E., Washington, DC 20002-4242. TEL 202-336-5600, FAX 202-336-5568, http://www.apa.org/journals/neu.html, http://www.apa.org/journals/nev.html. Ed. James T Becker. Circ: 4,500.

NEUROPSYCHOLOGY ABSTRACTS. see *MEDICAL SCIENCES—Abstracting, Bibliographies, Statistics*

153.4 616.8 NLD ISSN 0927-0116
NEUROPSYCHOLOGY AND COGNITION. Text in English. 1989. irreg., latest vol.10, 1995. price varies. back issues avail. *Refereed.* **Document type:** *Monographic series.*
Indexed: e-psyche.
—BLDSC (6081.553300).
Published by: Kluwer Academic Publishers Group (Subsidiary of: Wolters Kluwer N.V.), Spuiboulevard 50, PO Box 17, Dordrecht 3300 AA, Netherlands. FAX 31-78-639-2254, services@wkap.nl, http://www.wkap.nl. **Dist. by:** Journals Department, PO Box 322, Dordrecht 3300 AH, Netherlands. FAX 31-78-654-6474.

NEUROPSYCHOLOGY, DEVELOPMENT AND COGNITION. SECTION A: JOURNAL OF CLINICAL AND EXPERIMENTAL NEUROPSYCHOLOGY. see *PSYCHOLOGY*

NEUROPSYCHOLOGY, DEVELOPMENT AND COGNITION. SECTION B: AGING, NEUROPSYCHOLOGY AND COGNITION; a journal on normal and dysfunctional development. see *PSYCHOLOGY*

NEUROPSYCHOLOGY, DEVELOPMENT, AND COGNITION. SECTION C: CHILD NEUROPSYCHOLOGY; a journal on normal and abnormal development in childhood and adolescence. see *PSYCHOLOGY*

NEUROPSYCHOLOGY, DEVELOPMENT AND COGNITION. SECTION D: THE CLINICAL NEUROPSYCHOLOGIST. see *PSYCHOLOGY*

616.8 USA ISSN 1040-7308
QP360 CODEN: NERVEJ
NEUROPSYCHOLOGY REVIEW. Text in English. 1989. q. EUR 390 to institutions for print or online ed.; EUR 468 to institutions print & online eds.combined (effective 2002). adv. back issues avail. *Refereed.* **Document type:** *Academic/Scholarly.* **Description:** Integrates and interprets topics of interest to clinical or research neuropsychologists and behavioral neurologists.
Related titles: Microfilm ed.: (from PQC); Online - full text ed.: (from EBSCO Publishing, O C L C Online Computer Library Center, Inc., Swets Blackwell, Kluwer Online, Institute for Scientific Information, RoweCom Information Quest).
Indexed: ASCA, Excerp.Med., Ind.Med. (1990-), Neuropsych.Abstr., Neurosci.Cit.Ind., PsycInfo, Psychol.Abstr. (1990-), SSCI, Soc.Work Res.& Abstr., e-psyche.
—BLDSC (6081.553600), EMDOCS, GNLM, IDS, ingenta, KNAW. **CCC.**
Published by: (University of North Carolina, Department of Psychology), Kluwer Academic - Plenum Publishers (Subsidiary of: Wolters Kluwer N.V.), 233 Spring St, New York, NY 10013-1578. TEL 212-620-8000, 800-221-9369, FAX 212-463-0742, info@plenum.com; kluwer@wkap.com; services@wkap.nl; puente@uncwil.edu, http://www.plenum.com. Ed. Antonio E Puente.

616.8 USA ISSN 0893-133X
CODEN: NEROEW
NEUROPSYCHOPHARMACOLOGY. Text in English. 1987. m. EUR 326 in Europe to individuals; JPY 43,200 in Japan to individuals; USD 365 elsewhere to individuals; EUR 947 in Europe to institutions; JPY 125,800 in Japan to institutions; USD 1,061 elsewhere to institutions (effective 2002). *Refereed.* **Document type:** *Academic/Scholarly.* **Description:** Focuses on clinical and basic science contributions to the field of neuropsychopharmacology.
Related titles: Online - full text ed.: (from EBSCO Publishing, ingenta, ScienceDirect, Institute for Scientific Information).
Indexed: ASCA, Chem.Abstr., Chem.Indus.Notes, Chem.Titles, Curr.Cont., Derwent Biotech.Abstr., Excerp.Med., Focus on: Psychophar., INIS Atomind., Ind.Med. (1987-), Ind.Sci.Rev., Inpharma, Int.Abstr.Biol.Sci., Jrnl.Watch Psych., Neurosci.Cit.Ind., Pharm.&Out.News, PsycInfo, Psychol.Abstr. (1987-), Reac., SSCI (coverage dropped), Sci.Cit.Ind., e-psyche.
—BLDSC (6081.555500), ADONIS, CASDDS, CISTI, EMDOCS, GNLM, IDS, ingenta, KNAW. **CCC.**
Published by: (American College of Neuropsychopharmacology), Elsevier Science, PO Box 945, New York, NY 10159-0945. TEL 212-989-5800, FAX 212-633-3990, usinfo-f@elsevier.com, http://www.elsevier.com/locate/neupsychopharm. Eds. H Christian Fibiger, Dr. Herbert Y Metzger. **Subscr. in Australasia and the Far East to:** Elsevier Science (Singapore) Pte Ltd, No.1 Temasek Ave, 17-01 Millenia Tower, Singapore 039192, Singapore. TEL 65-434-3727, FAX 65-337-2230; **Subscr. in Japan to:** Elsevier Science Inc - Japan Regional Office, 9-15 Higashi-Azabu 1-chome, Minato-ku, Tokyo 106-0044, Japan. TEL 81-3-5561-5033; **Subscr. outside the Americas to:** Elsevier Science BV, PO Box 211, Amsterdam 1000 AE, Netherlands. TEL 31-20-485-3757.

616.8 NLD ISSN 1053-8135
CODEN: NRORFG
NEUROREHABILITATION; an interdisciplinary journal. Text in English. 1991. bi-m. (in 2 vols., 3 nos./vol.). EUR 314, USD 287 to institutions (effective 2002). bk.rev. back issues avail. *Refereed.* **Document type:** *Journal, Academic/Scholarly.* **Description:** Provides multidisciplinary rehabilitation teams with current clinical information for treating patients who are mentally or physically handicapped because of acquired or congenital neurologic disability.
Related titles: Microform ed.: (from PQC); Online - full text ed.: (from ingenta, Swets Blackwell, Institute for Scientific Information, RoweCom Information Quest).
Indexed: AMED, ASCA, AgeLine, Curr.Cont., Excerp.Med., Fam.Ind., SSCI, e-psyche.
—BLDSC (6081.558400), ADONIS, GNLM, IDS, Infotrieve. **CCC.**
Published by: I O S Press, Nieuwe Hemweg 6B, Amsterdam 1013 BG, Netherlands. Eds. Jeffrey S Kreutzer TEL 804-828-3704, Nathan D Zasler TEL 804-270-5486. **Subscr. to:** I O S Press, Inc, 5795-G Burke Centre Pkwy, Burke, VA 22015. TEL 703-323-5554, FAX 703-323-3668, iosbooks@iospress.com; Kinokuniya Company Ltd, Shinjuku 3-chome, Shinjuku-ku, Tokyo 160-0022, Japan. FAX 81-3-3439-1094, journal@kinokuniya.co.jp, http://www.kinokuniya.co.jp; Globe Publication Pvt. Ltd., C-62 Inderpuri, New Delhi 100 012, India. TEL 91-11-579-3211, 91-11-579-3212, FAX 91-11-579-8876, custserve@globepub.com, http://www.globepub.com.

616.8 USA ISSN 0959-4965
CODEN: NERPEZ
NEUROREPORT. Text in English. 1990. 18/yr., latest vol.12. USD 699 domestic to individuals; USD 699 foreign to individuals; USD 2,664 per issue domestic to institutions; USD 2,664 per issue foreign to institutions; USD 135 newsstand/cover (effective 2002); print and online eds. combined. adv. *Refereed.* **Document type:** *Academic/Scholarly.* **Description:** Encompasses all the major fields of neuroscience while still reflecting the specialization in each given field.
Related titles: CD-ROM ed.; Online - full text ed.: USD 3,463.20 domestic academic site license; USD 3,463.20 foreign academic site license; USD 3,862.80 domestic corporate site license; USD 3,862.80 foreign corporate site license (effective 2002) (from EBSCO Publishing, Institute for Scientific Information).
Indexed: ASCA, Anim.Behav.Abstr., Aqua.Sci.& Fish.Abstr., Chem.Abstr., Chem.Indus.Notes, Chem.Titles, Chemorec.Abstr., Curr.Cont., Excerp.Med. (1992-), Ind.Med. (1990-), Inpharma, Int.Abstr.Biol.Sci., Neurosci.Abstr., Neurosci.Cit.Ind., Nutr.Abstr., Pharm.&Out.News, PsycInfo, Psychol.Abstr. (1990-), Reac., Rev.Appl.Entomol., Rev.Arom.& Med.Plants, Russ.Acad.Sci.Bibl., SSCI (coverage dropped), Sci.Cit.Ind., e-psyche.
—BLDSC (6081.558500), ADONIS, CASDDS, CISTI, EMDOCS, GNLM, IDS, ingenta, KNAW.
Published by: Lippincott Williams & Wilkins (Philadelphia) (Subsidiary of: Wolters Kluwer N.V.), 530 Walnut St, Philadelphia, PA 19106-3621. TEL 215-521-8300, FAX 215-521-8902, http://www.neuroreport.com, http://www.lww.com. Ed. David Ottoson. Adv. contact Gemma Heiser. **Subscr. to:** PO Box 1600, Hagerstown, MD 21740-1600. TEL 800-777-2295, FAX 301-824-7390.

616.8 GBR ISSN 0306-4522
QP351 CODEN: NRSCDN
NEUROSCIENCE; an international journal. Text in English. 1976. 28/yr. EUR 583 in Europe to qualified personnel; JPY 77,700 in Japan to qualified personnel; USD 652 elsewhere to qualified personnel; EUR 5,970 in Europe to institutions; JPY 793,100 in Japan to institutions; USD 6,678 elsewhere to institutions (effective 2002). adv. bk.rev. illus, stat. index. back issues avail. *Refereed.* **Document type:** *Academic/Scholarly.* **Description:** Original research on any aspect of the scientific study of the nervous system.

M

Related titles: Microfilm ed.: (from PQC); Online - full text ed.: (from ingenta, ScienceDirect, Swets Blackwell, Institute for Scientific Information).
Indexed: ASCA, Anim.Behav.Abstr., Apic.Abstr., Aqua.Sci.& Fish.Abstr., Biol.Abstr., Cal.Tiss.Abstr. (coverage dropped), Chem.Abstr., Chem.Indus.Notes, Chem.Titles, Chemorec.Abstr., Compumath, Curr.Adv.Ecol.Sci., Curr.Cont., Curr.Ref.Fish Res., Dairy Sci.Abstr., Dent.Ind., Derwent Biotech.Abstr., Excerp.Med., INIS Atomind., Ind.Med. (1976-), Ind.Sci.Rev., Ind.Vet., Inpharma, Int.Abstr.Biol.Sci., Neurosci.Abstr., Neurosci.Cit.Ind., Nutr.Abstr., Pharm.&Out.News, Protozool.Abstr., Reac., Ref.Zh., SSCI (coverage dropped), Sci.Cit.Ind., THA, Telegen, Tox.Abstr. (coverage dropped), Wild.Rev., e-psyche.
—BLDSC (6081.559000), ADONIS, CASDDS, CISTI, EMDOCS, GNLM, IDS, ingenta, KNAW. **CCC.**
Published by: (International Brain Research Organization), Pergamon (Subsidiary of: Elsevier Science), The Boulevard, Langford Ln, East Park, Kidlington, Oxford OXB 1GB, United Kingdom. FAX 44-1865-843010, http://www.elsevier.com/locate/neuroscience. Eds. A D Smith, D G Amaral. Circ: 1,500. **Subscr. in Australasia and the Far East to:** Elsevier Science (Singapore) Pte Ltd, No.1 Temasek Ave, 17-01 Millenia Tower, Singapore 039192, Singapore. TEL 65-434-3727, FAX 65-337-2230; **Subscr. in the Americas to:** Elsevier Science, PO Box 945, New York, NY 10159-0945. TEL 212-633-3730, FAX 212-633-3680, usinfo-f@elsevier.com; **Subscr. to:** Elsevier Science BV, PO Box 211, Amsterdam 1000 AE, Netherlands. TEL 31-20-485-3757.

616.8 USA ISSN 0097-0549
RC331 CODEN: NBHPBT
NEUROSCIENCE AND BEHAVIORAL PHYSIOLOGY. Text in English. 1967. bi-m. EUR 1,127 to institutions for print or online ed.; EUR 1,352.40 to institutions print & online eds. combined (effective 2002). reprint service avail. from PQC. *Refereed.* **Document type:** *Academic/Scholarly.* **Description:** Translates selected articles describing important results of studies of the nervous system from Russian neurology journals.
Formerly (until vol.5, 1972): Neuroscience Translations (0028-3959)
Related titles: Microform ed.: (from PQC,PMC); Online - full text ed.: (from Swets Blackwell, Kluwer Online, RoweCom Information Quest).
Indexed: Anim.Behav.Abstr., Aqua.Sci.& Fish.Abstr., Biol.Abstr., Chem.Abstr., Chemorec.Abstr., Curr.Cont. (coverage dropped), Excerp.Med., INIS Atomind., Ind.Med. (1972-), Neurosci.Abstr., Neurosci.Cit.Ind., Psyclnfo, Psychol.Abstr. (1973-), THA, e-psyche.
—BLDSC (6081.560000), CISTI, GNLM, ingenta. **CCC.**
Published by: (Federation of American Societies for Experimental Biology), Kluwer Academic - Plenum Publishers (Subsidiary of: Wolters Kluwer N.V.), 233 Spring St, New York, NY 10013-1578. TEL 212-620-8468, 800-221-9369, FAX 212-463-0742, info@plenum.com; kluwer@wkap.com; services@wkap.nl, http://www.plenum.com.

616.8 GBR ISSN 0149-7634
QP360 CODEN: NBREDE
NEUROSCIENCE AND BIOBEHAVIORAL REVIEWS. Text in English. 1977. 8/yr. EUR 195 in Europe to qualified personnel; JPY 25,900 in Japan to qualified personnel; USD 219 elsewhere to qualified personnel; EUR 1,329 in Europe to institutions; JPY 176,600 in Japan to institutions; USD 1,487 elsewhere to institutions (effective 2002). bk.rev. index. back issues avail.; reprint service avail. from PQC,ISI. *Refereed.* **Document type:** *Academic/Scholarly.* **Description:** Articles on anatomy, biochemistry, embryology, endocrinology, genetics, pharmacology, physiology and all aspects of biological sciences related to the problems of the nervous system.
Formerly: Biobehavioral Reviews
Related titles: Microfilm ed.: (from PQC); Online - full text ed.: (from ingenta, ScienceDirect, Swets Blackwell, Institute for Scientific Information).
Indexed: ASCA, Anim.Behav.Abstr., Aqua.Sci.& Fish.Abstr., Biol.Abstr., Biotech.& Bioeng.Abstr., Chem.Abstr., Chem.Indus.Notes, Chem.Titles, Chemorec.Abstr., Curr.Adv.Ecol.Sci., Curr.Cont., Dent.Ind., Excerp.Med., INIS Atomind., Ind.Med. (1978-), Ind.Sci.Rev., Inpharma, Int.Abstr.Biol.Sci., Neurosci.Abstr., Neurosci.Cit.Ind., Pharm.&Out.News, Psyclnfo, Psychol.Abstr. (1977-), Reac., SSCI (coverage dropped), Sci.Cit.Ind., THA, e-psyche.
—BLDSC (6081.561000), CASDDS, CISTI, GNLM, IDS, ingenta, KNAW. **CCC.**
Published by: Pergamon (Subsidiary of: Elsevier Science), The Boulevard, Langford Ln, East Park, Kidlington, Oxford OXB 1GB, United Kingdom. FAX 44-1865-843010, nlinfo-f@elsevier.nl; usinfo-f@elsevier.com; forinfo-kyf04035@niftyserve.or.jp, nlinfo-f@elsevier/nl; usinfo-f@elsevier.com; forinfo-kyf04035@niftyserve.or.jp, http://www.elsevier.com/locate/neubiorev. Eds. Ann E Kelley, Steven J Cooper. **Subscr. in Australasia and the Far East to:** Elsevier Science (Singapore) Pte Ltd, No.1 Temasek Ave, 17-01 Millenia Tower, Singapore 039192, Singapore. TEL 65-434-3727, FAX 65-337-2230; **Subscr. in the Americas to:** Elsevier Science, PO Box 945, New York, NY 10159-0945. TEL 212-633-3730, FAX 212-633-3680, usinfo-f@elsevier.com; **Subscr. to:** Elsevier Science BV, PO Box 211, Amsterdam 1000 AE, Netherlands. TEL 31-20-485-3757, FAX 31-20-485-3432, nlinfo-f@elsevier.nl.

NEUROSCIENCE COMMUNICATIONS. see *MEDICAL SCIENCES—Abstracting, Bibliographies, Statistics*

616.8 IRL ISSN 0304-3940
QP351 CODEN: NELED5
NEUROSCIENCE LETTERS; an international multidisciplinary journal devoted to the rapid publication of basic research in neurosciences. Text in English. 1975. 57/yr. EUR 5,092 in Europe to institutions; JPY 676,400 in Japan to institutions; EUR 5,696 elsewhere to institutions (effective 2002). bibl, charts, illus, abstr. reprint service avail. from SWZ. *Refereed.* **Document type:** *Academic/Scholarly.* **Description:** Publishes short reports in all areas in the fields of neuroanatomy, neurochemistry, neuroendocrinology, neuropharmacology, and neurobiology.
Related titles: Microform ed.: (from PQC); Online - full text ed.: (from ingenta, ScienceDirect, Swets Blackwell, Institute for Scientific Information).
Indexed: ASCA, Apic.Abstr., Aqua.Sci.& Fish.Abstr., Biol.Abstr., Cal.Tiss.Abstr. (coverage dropped), Chem.Abstr., Chem.Indus.Notes, Chem.Titles, Chemorec.Abstr., Curr.Adv.Biochem., Curr.Adv.Cell & Devel.Biol., Curr.Adv.Ecol.Sci., Curr.Cont., Dairy Sci.Abstr., Dent.Ind., Excerp.Med., INIS Atomind., Ind.Med. (1975-), Ind.Sci.Rev., Ind.Vet., Inpharma, Int.Abstr.Biol.Sci., Neurosci.Abstr., Neurosci.Cit.Ind., Nutr.Abstr., Pharm.&Out.News, Reac., Rev.Appl.Entomol., SSCI (coverage dropped), Sci.Cit.Ind., Sport Fish.Abstr., THA, Tox.Abstr. (coverage dropped), Vet.Bull., e-psyche.
—BLDSC (6081.562000), ADONIS, CASDDS, CISTI, EMDOCS, GNLM, IDS, ingenta, KNAW. **CCC.**
Published by: Elsevier Science Ireland Ltd, Elsevier House, Brookvale Plaza, E. Park, Shannon, Co. Clare, Ireland. TEL 353-61-471944, FAX 353-61-472144, http://www.elsevier.com/locate/neulet. Ed. M Zimmermann. R&P Annette Moloney. **Subscr. in Australasia and the Far East to:** Elsevier Science (Singapore) Pte Ltd, No.1 Temasek Ave, 17-01 Millenia Tower, Singapore 039192, Singapore. TEL 65-434-3727, FAX 65-337-2230; **Subscr. in the Americas to:** Elsevier Science, PO Box 945, New York, NY 10159-0945. TEL 212-633-3730, FAX 212-633-3680; **Subscr. to:** Elsevier Science BV, PO Box 211, Amsterdam 1000 AE, Netherlands. TEL 31-20-485-3757, nlinfo-f@elsevier.nl.

616.8 USA ISSN 1086-9956
NEUROSCIENCE-NET. Text in English. 1996. irreg. back issues avail. *Refereed.* **Document type:** *Journal, Academic/Scholarly.* **Description:** Devoted to publishing research in basic and clinical neuroscience.
Media: Online - full text.
Published by: Scientific Design & Information, 165 Cervantes Rd., Redwood City, CA 94062. http://www.beuroscience.com/main.html.

616.8 573.8 CHE ISSN 1027-6599
NEUROSCIENCE NEWS. Text in English. 1998. m. (in 2 vols., 6 nos./vol.). EUR 342 to institutions; EUR 532 to corporations (effective 2000). **Document type:** *Academic/Scholarly.*
Indexed: Neurosci.Abstr.
—BLDSC (6081.563100).
Published by: Gordon and Breach - Harwood Academic (Subsidiary of: Taylor & Francis Group), PO Box 531, Lausanne 1000, Switzerland. http://www.gbhap.com. Ed. Robert Katzman. **Subscr. addr. in US:** International Publishers Direct, PO Box 32160, Newark, NJ 07102. FAX 215-750-6343.

616.8 USA ISSN 0278-3738
NEUROSCIENCE NEWSLETTER. Text in English. 1970. bi-m. USD 50 to members. adv. back issues avail. **Document type:** *Newsletter.*
Indexed: e-psyche.
Published by: Society for Neuroscience, 11 Dupont Circle, N W, Ste 500, Washington, DC 20036. TEL 202-462-6688, FAX 202-462-2937, http://www.sfn.org/. R&P Amy M Smitherman. Adv. contact Evan Karachalios. Circ: 26,500.

616.8 IRL ISSN 0168-0102
RC337 CODEN: NERADN
NEUROSCIENCE RESEARCH. Text and summaries in English. 1984. m. EUR 999 in Europe; JPY 132,600 in Japan; USD 1,117 elsewhere (effective 2002). index. *Refereed.* **Document type:** *Academic/Scholarly.* **Description:** Covers all fields of neuroscience, from the molecular to behavioral levels.
Related titles: Microform ed.: (from PQC); Online - full text ed.: (from ingenta, ScienceDirect, Swets Blackwell, Institute for Scientific Information).
Indexed: ASCA, Apic.Abstr., Biol.Abstr., Chem.Abstr., Chem.Indus.Notes, Chem.Titles, Curr.Cont., Derwent Biotech.Abstr., Excerp.Med., Ind.Med. (1984-), Ind.Sci.Rev., Indian Psychol.Abstr., Inpharma, Int.Abstr.Biol.Sci., Neurosci.Cit.Ind., Pharm.&Out.News, Psyclnfo, Psychol.Abstr. (1984-), Reac., SSCI (coverage dropped), Sci.Cit.Ind., e-psyche.
—BLDSC (6081.563600), CASDDS, CISTI, EMDOCS, GNLM, IDS, ingenta, KNAW. **CCC.**
Published by: (Japan Neuroscience Society JPN), Elsevier Science Ireland Ltd, Elsevier House, Brookvale Plaza, E. Park, Shannon, Co. Clare, Ireland. TEL 353-61-471944, FAX 353-61-472144, http://www.elsevier.com/locate/neures. Eds. Masao Ito, T Tsumoto. R&P Annette Moloney. **Subscr. in Australasia and the Far East to:** Elsevier Science (Singapore) Pte Ltd, No.1 Temasek Ave, 17-01 Millenia Tower, Singapore 039192, Singapore. TEL 65-434-3727, FAX 65-337-2230; **Subscr. in the Americas to:** Elsevier Science, PO Box 945, New York, NY 10159-0945. TEL 212-633-3730, FAX 212-633-3680; **Subscr. to:** Elsevier Science BV, PO Box 211, Amsterdam 1000 AE, Netherlands. TEL 31-20-485-3757, FAX 31-20-485-3432.

616.8 GBR ISSN 0893-6609
RC346 CODEN: NRCOEE
NEUROSCIENCE RESEARCH COMMUNICATIONS. Text in English. 1987. 6/yr. (in 2 vols., 3 nos./vol.). USD 820 in United States; USD 880 in Canada & Mexico; USD 931 elsewhere; USD 861 combined subscription in United States for print and online eds.; USD 921 combined subscription in Canada & Mexico for print and online eds.; USD 972 combined subscription elsewhere for print and online eds. (effective 2002). adv. back issues avail.; reprint service avail. from SWZ. *Refereed.* **Document type:** *Academic/Scholarly.* **Description:** Contains international and multidisciplinary original contributions to the neurosciences.
Related titles: Online - full text ed.: ISSN 1520-6769. USD 820 in United States; USD 820 in Canada & Mexico; USD 820 elsewhere (effective 2002) (from EBSCO Publishing, Wiley InterScience, Institute for Scientific Information).
Indexed: A.I.Abstr., ASCA, Aqua.Sci.& Fish.Abstr., Chem.Abstr., Chem.Indus.Notes, Chem.Titles, Chemorec.Abstr., Curr.Cont., Excerp.Med., Ind.Sci.Rev., Inpharma, Int.Abstr.Biol.Sci., Neurosci.Abstr., Neurosci.Cit.Ind., Pharm.&Out.News, Reac., SSCI (coverage dropped), Sci.Cit.Ind., Telegen.
—BLDSC (6081.563800), CASDDS, CISTI, EMDOCS, GNLM, IDS, Infotrieve, ingenta. **CCC.**
Published by: Wiley Europe Ltd., Baffins Ln, Chichester, W Sussex PO19 1UD, United Kingdom. TEL 44-1243-779777, FAX 44-1243-775878, customer@wiley.co.uk, http://www.wiley.co.uk. adv.: B&W page GBP 595, color page GBP 1,495; trim 200 x 260. **Subscr. in the Americas to:** John Wiley & Sons, Inc., Journals, 605 Third Ave, New York, NY 10158. TEL 212-850-6021, 212-850-6645, subinfo@jwiley.com.

616.8 USA ISSN 1073-8584
RC321 CODEN: NROSFJ
THE NEUROSCIENTIST; a review journal bridging neurobiology, neurology and psychiatry. Text in English. 1995. bi-m. USD 335 domestic; USD 359 foreign (effective 2002). adv. 88 p./no. back issues avail.; reprints avail. *Refereed.* **Document type:** *Journal, Academic/Scholarly.* **Description:** Reviews laboratory and clinical research in the related fields of neurology, neurobiology, and psychiatry.
Related titles: Online - full text ed.: 1995 (from EBSCO Publishing, O C L C Online Computer Library Center, Inc., ingenta, Swets Blackwell, Institute for Scientific Information, RoweCom Information Quest).
Indexed: Cal.Tiss.Abstr., Chem.Abstr., Chem.Indus.Notes, Chem.Titles, Neurosci.Abstr., Neurosci.Cit.Ind., e-psyche.
—BLDSC (6081.578500), CASDDS, CISTI, GNLM, IDS.

M

Published by: Sage Publications, Inc., Sage Science Press, 2455 Teller Rd, Thousand Oaks, CA 91320. TEL 805-499-0721, FAX 805-499-0871, info@sagepub.com, http://www.sagesciencepress.com. Ed. Stephen Waxman. R&P Peter Marino. Adv. contact Robert Vrooman. B&W page USD 600, color page USD 1,200; bleed 8.375 x 11.125.

616.8 USA ISSN 0148-396X
RD593

NEUROSURGERY (BALTIMORE). Text in English. 1977. m., latest vol.49. USD 308 domestic to individuals Print & Online eds. combined; USD 435 foreign to individuals Print & Online eds. combined; USD 424 domestic to institutions Print & Online eds. combined; USD 550 foreign to institutions Print & Online eds. combined; USD 46 newsstand/cover (effective 2002). adv. bk.rev. abstr, bibl, charts, illus. index. back issues avail. *Refereed.* **Document type:** *Journal, Academic/Scholarly.* **Description:** Explains techniques and devices, plus pertinent research in neuroscience.

Related titles: Microfilm ed.: (from WWS); Online - full text ed.: USD 551.20 domestic academic site license; USD 677.20 foreign academic site license; USD 614.80 domestic corporate site license; USD 740.80 foreign corporate site license (effective 2002) (from Ovid Technologies, Inc., EBSCO Publishing, Institute for Scientific Information).

Indexed: Bibl.Dev.Med.& Child Neur., Curr.Adv.Cancer Res., Curr.Cont., Dent.Ind., Excerp.Med., INIS Atomind., Ind.Med. (1977-), Ind.Sci.Rev., Inpharma, Int.Nurs.Ind., Jrnl.Watch Neuro., Neurosci.Cit.Ind., Pharm.&Out.News, Reac., Rev.Med.& Vet.Mycol., Sci.Cit.Ind., e-psyche.

—BLDSC (6081.582000), CISTI, GNLM, IDS, ingenta, KNAW.

Published by: (Congress of Neurological Surgeons), Williams & Wilkins (Subsidiary of: Waverly International), 351 W Camden St, Baltimore, MD 21201-2436. TEL 410-528-4068, 800-222-3790, FAX 410-528-4452, gpessagno@wwilkins.com, http://www.wwilkins.com/neurosurgery/. Ed. Dr. Michael L J Apuzzo. Adv. contact Greg Pessagno. Circ: 9,118.

NEUROSURGERY CLINICS OF NORTH AMERICA. see *MEDICAL SCIENCES—Surgery*

▼ **NEUROSURGERY NEWS.** see *MEDICAL SCIENCES—Surgery*

616.8 USA

NEUROSURGICAL FOCUS. Text in English. m. adv. *Refereed.* **Document type:** *Academic/Scholarly.* **Description:** Provides rapid publication of original contributions. Each issue is devoted to the exploration of a topic of interest to neurosurgeons.

Media: Online - full text. **Related titles:** CD-ROM ed.

Indexed: e-psyche.

Published by: American Association of Neurological Surgeons, Park Ridge, 22 S Washington St, Park Ridge, IL 60068. TEL 847-692-9500, FAX 847-692-2589. Ed. Dr. John A Jane. R&P Evelyn Kessler.

NEUROSURGICAL REVIEW. see *MEDICAL SCIENCES—Surgery*

616.8 CHE ISSN 1029-8428

▼ **NEUROTOXICITY RESEARCH**; an international journal on processes and mechanisms in neurodegeneration, apoptosis, neuroprotection and regeneration. Text in English. 1999. 8/yr. GBP 86, USD 103, EUR 124 to individuals; GBP 338, USD 442, EUR 449 to institutions; GBP 475, USD 723, EUR 734 to corporations (effective 2002). *Refereed.* **Document type:** *Journal, Academic/Scholarly.* **Description:** Contains papers reporting on both basic and clinical research on classical neurotoxins and mechanisms associated with neurodegeneration, apoptosis, nerve regeneration, and neurotrophic actions.

Published by: Gordon and Breach - Harwood Academic (Subsidiary of: Taylor & Francis Group), PO Box 531, Lausanne 1000, Switzerland. TEL 41-21-6411280, FAX 41-21-6411281, info@gbhap.com, http:// www.gbhap.com/journals/422/422-top.htm. Ed. Richard Kostrzewa.

616.8 USA ISSN 0892-0362
CODEN: NETEEC

NEUROTOXICOLOGY AND TERATOLOGY. Text in English. 1979. 6/yr. EUR 1,280 in Europe to institutions; JPY 169,900 in Japan to institutions; USD 1,432 elsewhere to institutions (effective 2002). adv. illus, abstr. index. reprint service avail. from PQC,ISI. *Refereed.* **Document type:** *Academic/Scholarly.* **Description:** Presents original reports of systemic studies in the areas of adult neurotoxicology and developmental neurotoxicology in which the primary emphasis and theoretical context are on the nervous system and behavior.

Former titles: Neurobehavioral Toxicology and Teratology (0275-1380); Neurobehavioral Toxicology (0191-3581)

Related titles: Microfilm ed.: (from PQC); Online - full text ed.: (from ingenta, ScienceDirect, Swets Blackwell, Institute for Scientific Information).

Indexed: ASCA, Biol.Abstr., Chem.Abstr., Chem.Indus.Notes, Chem.Titles, Curr.Adv.Ecol.Sci., Curr.Cont., Dairy Sci.Abstr., Dent.Ind., Environ.Abstr., Environ.Sci.Poll.Mgmt., Excerp.Med., Helminthol.Abstr., INIS Atomind., Ind.Med. (1987-), Ind.Sci.Rev., Indian Psychol.Abstr., Inpharma, Int.Abstr.Biol.Sci., NRN, Neurosci.Abstr., Neurosci.Cit.Ind., Pharm.&Out.News, Pollut.Abstr., PsycInfo, Psychol.Abstr. (1981-), Reac., Rev.Appl.Entomol., SSCI (coverage dropped), Saf.Sci.Abstr., Sci.Cit.Ind., THA, Tox.Abstr., e-psyche.

—BLDSC (6081.586500), ADONIS, CASDDS, CISTI, EMDOCS, GNLM, IDS, ingenta, KNAW. **CCC.**

Published by: (Behavioral Toxicology Society), Elsevier Science, 655 Ave of the Americas, New York, NY 10010. TEL 212-989-5800, FAX 212-633-3990, usinfo-f@elsevier.com, http://www.elsevier.com/locate/neutera. Ed. Charles V Vorhees. **Subscr. in Australasia and the Far East to:** Elsevier Science (Singapore) Pte Ltd, No.1 Temasek Ave, 17-01 Millenia Tower, Singapore 039192, Singapore. TEL 65-434-3727, FAX 65-337-2230; **Subscr. in Japan to:** Elsevier Science Inc - Japan Regional Office, 9-15 Higashi-Azabu 1-chome, Minato-ku, Tokyo 106-0044, Japan. TEL 81-3-5561-5033; **Subscr. outside the Americas to:** Elsevier Science BV, PO Box 211, Amsterdam 1000 AE, Netherlands. TEL 31-20-485-3757. **Co-sponsor:** Neurobehavioral Teratology Society.

616.8 USA ISSN 0161-813X
RC321 CODEN: NRTXDN

NEUROTOXICOLOGY (LITTLE ROCK); an international journal. Variant title: Journal of Neurotoxicology. Text in English. 1979. 6/yr. EUR 285 in Europe to institutions; JPY 37,800 in Japan to institutions; USD 319 elsewhere to institutions (effective 2002). adv. bk.rev. abstr, bibl, charts, illus. index. Supplement avail.; back issues avail. *Refereed.* **Document type:** *Academic/Scholarly.* **Description:** Publishes original research reports and brief communications relating to neurotoxicology.

Related titles: Online - full text ed.: (from ScienceDirect, Institute for Scientific Information).

Indexed: Aqua.Sci.& Fish.Abstr., Biol.Abstr., Chem.Abstr., Curr.Cont., Environ.Sci.Poll.Mgmt., Excerp.Med., Food Sci.& Tech.Abstr., INIS Atomind., Ind.Med. (1979-), Ind.Sci.Rev., Int.Abstr.Biol.Sci., Neurosci.Abstr., Neurosci.Cit.Ind., Sci.Cit.Ind., Tox.Abstr., Weed Abstr., e-psyche.

—BLDSC (6081.585800), CASDDS, CISTI, GNLM, IDS, Infotrieve, ingenta, KNAW. **CCC.**

Published by: Elsevier Science BV, Sara Burgerhartstraat 25, Amsterdam 1055 KV, Netherlands. TEL 31-20-485-2911, FAX 31-20-485-2457, nlinfo-f@elsevier.nl, http://www.elsevier.nl/inca/publications/store/6/2/1/3/5/5/. Eds. B Garrett, J S Cranmer. Circ: 2,000. **Subscr. to:** PO Box 211, Amsterdam 1000 AE, Netherlands. TEL 31-20-485-3757, FAX 31-20-485-3432.

615.373 GBR ISSN 1357-7115

NEUROTOXINS. Text in English. 1994. a. included with Trends in Neurosciences. back issues avail. **Document type:** *Academic/Scholarly.*

Related titles: ♦ Supplement to: Trends in Neurosciences. ISSN 0166-2236.

Indexed: e-psyche.

—ADONIS.

Published by: Elsevier Science Ltd., Elsevier Trends Journals, 68 Hills Rd, Cambridge CB2 1LA, United Kingdom. TEL 44-1223-315961, FAX 44-1223-464430, TIMS@elsevier.co.uk, http://www.elsevier.nl. **Subscr. in Australasia and the Far East to:** Elsevier Science (Singapore) Pte Ltd, No.1 Temasek Ave, 17-01 Millenia Tower, Singapore 039192, Singapore. TEL 65-434-3727, FAX 65-337-2230; **Subscr. in the Americas to:** Elsevier Science, PO Box 945, New York, NY 10159-0945. TEL 212-633-3730, FAX 212-633-3680, http://www.elsevier.com; **Subscr. to:** Elsevier Current Trends Subscriptions, PO Box 331, Haywards Heath, W Sussex RH16 3FG, United Kingdom. TEL 44-1444-475650, FAX 44-1444-445423.

616.8 DEU ISSN 1436-123X

NEUROTRANSMITTER. Text in German. 1992. 11/yr. EUR 154.99 domestic; EUR 158.99 foreign; EUR 107.33 domestic to students; EUR 111.33 foreign to students; EUR 14.95 newsstand/cover (effective 2002). adv. **Document type:** *Journal, Academic/Scholarly.*

Indexed: e-psyche.

Published by: Urban und Vogel Medien und Medizin Verlagsgesellschaft mbH (Subsidiary of: BertelsmannSpringer), Neumarkter Str 43, Munich 81673, Germany. TEL 49-89-43721411, FAX 49-89-43721410, verlag@urban-vogel.de, http://www.urban-vogel.de. Ed. Dr. Albert Zacher. R&P Friederik Klein. Adv. contact Peter Urban. Circ: 6,400 (paid). **Subscr. to:** Springer Auslieferungs Gesellschaft, Postfach 105160, Heidelberg 69041, Germany. TEL 49-6221-345244, FAX 49-6221-345244.

616.8 USA

NEUROTRANSMITTER NEWSLETTER. Text in English. 199?. q. back issues avail. **Document type:** *Newsletter.*

Media: Online - full text.

Published by: Partner's Neurology Services, VBK9 Massachusetts General Hospital, Boston, MA 02129. TEL 617-726-3892, ogradys@helix.mgh.harvard.edu, http://132.183.145.103/newsletter/neurotran.html/. Ed. Sherri O'Grady.

616.8 RUS ISSN 1560-9545

NEVROLOGICHESKII ZHURNAL/JOURNAL OF NEUROLOGY. Text in Russian; Summaries in English. 1996. bi-m. USD 147 foreign (effective 2000). adv. Website rev. abstr. reprints avail. **Document type:** *Journal, Academic/Scholarly.* **Description:** Covers practical neurology, and trends and advances in the diagnosis and treatment of nervous diseases.

Indexed: Ref.Zh., e-psyche.

—BLDSC (0124.025000).

Published by: Izdatel'stvo Meditsina, Petroverigskii per 6-8, Moscow 101000, Russian Federation. TEL 7-095-9248785, 7-095-928-86-48, FAX 7-095-9211355, 7-095-9286003, meditsina@iname.com, http://www.medit.ru. Ed. N N Yakhno. Pub. A M Stochik. R&P I Izmailova. Adv. contact O A Fadeeva TEL 7-095-923-51-40. Circ: 1,500. **Dist. by:** Mezhdunarodnaya Kniga, B Yakimanka 39, Moscow 117049, Russian Federation. TEL 7-095-2384967, FAX 7-095-2384634; **US dist. addr.:** East View Publications, 3020 Harbor Ln N, Minneapolis, MN 55447. TEL 612-550-0961.

616.89 USA

THE NEW MESSAGE. Text in English. 1971. q. USD 8; USD 11 in Canada; USD 14 elsewhere. *Refereed.* **Description:** Offers people seeking emotional health and wellness stories, articles and information relating to the 12-step Emotions Anonymous Program.

Former titles: Message (St. Paul); Carrying the E A Message (1072-3765)

Indexed: e-psyche.

Published by: Emotions Anonymous, PO Box 4245, St. Paul, MN 55104-0245. TEL 651-647-9712, FAX 651-647-1593, eaisc@mtn.com, http://www.mtn.org/EA. Circ: 800 (paid).

NEW YORK (STATE). COMMISSION ON QUALITY OF CARE FOR THE MENTALLY DISABLED. ANNUAL REPORT. see *HEALTH FACILITIES AND ADMINISTRATION*

612.8 JPN

NEWSLETTER: FRONTIER RESEARCH PROGRAM. Text in Japanese. 1987. 4/yr. **Document type:** *Newsletter.* **Description:** Monitors program which conducts basic research in bio-homeostasis, frontier materials research, brain mechanisms of mind and behavior.

Indexed: e-psyche.

M

Published by: Rikagaku Kenkyusho/Institute of Physical and Chemical Research, Kokusai Furontia Kenkyu Shuishinbu, 2-1 Hirosawa, Wako shi, Saitama ken 3510106, Japan. TEL 81-48-462-1111, FAX 81-48-465-8048, mtoyoda@postman.riken.go.jp, hensan@postman.riken.go.jp.

616.8 CAN
NEWSLINK. Text in English. 1986. q. membership. adv. back issues avail. **Document type:** *Newsletter.* **Description:** Studies ALS research, fundraising and coping mechanisms and services for families with the disease.
Formerly: Communique (Vancouver)
Related titles: Diskette ed.
Indexed: e-psyche.
Published by: Amyotrophic Lateral Sclerosis Society of B.C., 1600 W 6th Ave, Ste 119, Vancouver, BC V6J 1R3, Canada. TEL 604-685-0737, FAX 604-685-0725, http://www.alsbc.ca. Ed. Sue Lewis-H'alloran. R&P, Adv. contact Judy Bonds. Circ: 6,000.

NEWSLINK (WASHINGTON). see *PSYCHOLOGY*

NIHON NO SHINKEI GEKA GAKKAI SOKAI SHOROKUSHU/JAPAN NEUROSURGICAL SOCIETY. ABSTRACTS OF THE ANNUAL MEETING. see *MEDICAL SCIENCES—Abstracting, Bibliographies, Statistics*

NIHON PARAPUREJIA IGAKKAI ZASSHI/JAPAN MEDICAL SOCIETY OF PARAPLEGIA. JOURNAL. see *MEDICAL SCIENCES—Orthopedics And Traumatology*

NO SHINKEI GEKA SOKUHO/NEUROSURGERY LETTERS. see *MEDICAL SCIENCES—Surgery*

NO SOTCHU NO GEKA/SURGERY FOR CEREBRAL STROKE. see *MEDICAL SCIENCES—Surgery*

616.8 JPN ISSN 0029-0831
CODEN: NTHAA7
NO TO HATTATSU. Text in Japanese; Summaries in English. 1969. bi-m. JPY 9,000, USD 90. adv. bk.rev. abstr. index. **Document type:** *Academic/Scholarly.*
Related titles: ♦ English ed.: Brain and Development. ISSN 0387-7604.
Indexed: Adol.Ment.Hlth.Abstr., Bibl.Dev.Med.& Child Neur., Biol.Abstr., Chem.Abstr., Curr.Adv.Ecol.Sci., Curr.Cont. (coverage dropped), Dent.Ind., Excerp.Med., Ind.Med. (coverage dropped), Ind.Sci.Rev., Int.Nurs.Ind., Nutr.Abstr., Risk Abstr., SSCI (coverage dropped), Sci.Cit.Ind. (coverage dropped), e-psyche.
—BLDSC (6113.969000), CASDDS, CISTI, GNLM, KNAW.
Published by: Japanese Society of Child Neurology/Nihon Shoni Shinkei Gakkai, Kenwado Bldg 2F, 6-13 Wakamatsu-cho, Shinjuku-ku, Tokyo 162-0056, Japan. TEL 03-33514125. Ed., R&P Toshiaki Abe. Circ: 4,000.

616.89 NOR ISSN 0803-9488
NORDIC JOURNAL OF PSYCHIATRY. Text in English, Multiple languages; Summaries in English. 1946. 6/yr. GBP 47, USD 78 to individuals; GBP 70, USD 115 to institutions (effective 2002). adv. bk.rev. index. *Refereed.* **Document type:** *Academic/Scholarly.* **Description:** Addressed to clinical psychiatrists and their co-workers as well as researchers.
Formerly: Nordisk Psykiatrisk Tidsskrift (0029-1455)
Related titles: Online - full text ed.: (from EBSCO Publishing, O C L C Online Computer Library Center, Inc., CatchWord Ltd., ingenta, Swets Blackwell, Institute for Scientific Information, RoweCom Information Quest); ♦ Supplement: Nordic Journal of Psychiatry. Supplement. ISSN 0803-9496.
Indexed: ASCA, Addic.Abstr., AgeLine, Biol.Abstr., Crim.Just.Abstr., Curr.Adv.Ecol.Sci., Curr.Cont., Excerp.Med., Fam.Ind., PsycInfo, Psychol.Abstr. (1972-), SSCI, e-psyche.
—BLDSC (6117.927050), CISTI, EMDOCS, GNLM, IDS, Infotrieve. **CCC.**
Published by: (Joint Committee of the Nordic Psychiatric Associations), Taylor & Francis AS (Subsidiary of: Taylor & Francis Group), Cort Adelersgt. 17, Solli, PO Box 2562, Oslo 0202, Norway. TEL 47-22-12-98-80, FAX 47-22-12-98-90, mail@tandf.no, http://www.tandf.co.uk/tfas. Ed. Lars von Knorring. Circ: 5,200.

616.89 NOR ISSN 0803-9496
NORDIC JOURNAL OF PSYCHIATRY. SUPPLEMENT. Text in Norwegian. 1974. irreg. adv. **Document type:** *Academic/Scholarly.*
Formerly: Nordisk Psykiatrisk Tidsskrift. Supplement (0346-8852)
Related titles: ♦ Supplement to: Nordic Journal of Psychiatry. ISSN 0803-9488.
Indexed: Excerp.Med., e-psyche.
—BLDSC (6117.927060), CISTI, EMDOCS, Infotrieve, KNAW. **CCC.**
Published by: (Joint Committee of the Nordic Psychiatric Associations), Scandinavian University Press (Subsidiary of: Taylor & Francis Ltd.), Postboks 2959, Toeyen, Oslo 0608, Norway. FAX 47-22-57-53-53, mail@scup.no, http://www.scup.no.

616.89 TUR ISSN 1300-0667
CODEN: NOPAB
NOROPSIKIYATRI ARSIVI/ARCHIVES OF NEUROPSYCHIATRY. Text in Turkish. 1964. q. TRL 400,000; USD 20 foreign. adv. *Refereed.* **Document type:** *Academic/Scholarly.* **Description:** Includes scientific research related to psychiatry, neurology, and neurosurgery.
Indexed: Excerp.Med. (1994-), e-psyche.
Published by: Turk Noropsikiyatri Dernegi, Istanbul Universitesi, Istanbul Tip Fakultesi, Topkapi - Istanbul 34390, Turkey. sercan@sim.net.tr. Ed., R&P Dr. Mustafa Sercan TEL 90-212-5436565. Adv. contact Noropsikiyatri Dernegi. B&W page TRL 150, color page TRL 200.

616.858 USA
NORTH CAROLINA MENTAL HEALTH, DEVELOPMENTAL DISABILITIES AND SUBSTANCE ABUSE LAWS. Text in English. irreg., latest 1997. USD 25. 375 p./no. Supplement avail. **Description:** Covers laws relating to mental health, developmental disabilities and substance abuse.
Indexed: e-psyche.
Published by: Lexis Law Publishing (Subsidiary of: Reed Elsevier plc), PO Box 7587, Charlottesville, VA 22906-7587. TEL 804-972-7566, 800-562-1197, FAX 800-643-1280, llp.customer.support@lexis-nexis.com, http://www.lexislawpublishing.com. Ed. George Harley.

616.8 616.15 JPN ISSN 1341-8440
NOU TO JONKAN/BRAIN AND CIRCULATION. Text in Japanese. 1996. 4/yr. JPY 2,200 (effective 1998). **Document type:** *Trade.*
Indexed: e-psyche.
Published by: Medikaru Rebyusha/Medical Review Co., Ltd., 7-3 Hirano-Machi 1-chome, Chuo-ku, Osaka-shi 541-0046, Japan. TEL 81-6-223-1556, FAX 81-6-223-1414, medrev@osk2.3web.ne.jp.

616.8 FRA ISSN 0762-6819
NOUVELLE REVUE D'ETHNOPSYCHIATRIE. Text in French; Summaries in English. 1978. 4/yr. FRF 330 to individuals; FRF 360 foreign to individuals; FRF 450 to institutions; FRF 460 foreign to institutions.
Formerly: Ethnopsychiatrica (0151-9808)
Indexed: Anthropol.Lit. (coverage dropped), e-psyche.
—GNLM.
Published by: Pensee Sauvage Editions, B.P. 141, Grenoble 38002, France. TEL 76-87-13-03, FAX 76-46-27-25. Ed. Marie Rose Noro.

616.8 ITA ISSN 1122-035X
NUOVA RIVISTA DI NEUROLOGIA. Text in Italian, English; Summaries in English. 1928. bi-m., latest vol.11, 2001. USD 117 (effective 2000). adv. bk.rev. bibl, charts, illus. 32 p./no. **Document type:** *Academic/Scholarly.*
Formerly (until 1990): Rivista di Neurologia (0035-6344)
Indexed: Biol.Abstr., Chem.Abstr., Dent.Ind., Excerp.Med., Ind.Med. (until 1992, dropped), e-psyche.
—BLDSC (6184.909100), CISTI, EMDOCS, GNLM, KNAW.
Published by: Il Pensiero Scientifico Editore s.r.l., Via Bradano, 3-C, Rome, RM 00199, Italy. TEL 39-06-862821, FAX 39-06-86282250, pensiero@pensiero.it, http://www.pensiero.it. Ed. Cristoforo Morocutti. Pub. Luca De Fiore. R&P Andrea De Fiore. Adv. contact Luciano De Fiore. Circ: 400.

616.89 CAN ISSN 1199-7699
NUTRITION & MENTAL HEALTH. Text in English. 1974. q. USD 35 domestic; USD 40 foreign (effective 1999). bk.rev. reprint service avail. from PQC. **Document type:** *Newsletter.*
Former titles (until 1993): Health and Nutrition Update (0831-8530); Huxley Institute - C S F Newsletter (0318-8272); Incorporates: Schizophrenics Anonymous International. Bulletin (0048-9360)
Indexed: Excerp.Med., e-psyche.
Published by: Canadian Schizophrenia Foundation, 16 Florence Ave, Toronto, ON M2N 1E9, Canada. TEL 416-733-2117, FAX 416-733-2352, centre@orthomed.org, http://www.orthomed.org. Ed. Steven Carter. Circ: 1,000.

616.8 614.854 CHE ISSN 1028-415X
CODEN: NNINFE
▼ **NUTRITIONAL NEUROSCIENCE**; an international journal of diet, nutrition and the nervous system. Text in English. 1999. bi-m. GBP 86, USD 105, EUR 116 to individuals; GBP 254, USD 327, EUR 338 to institutional members; GBP 419, USD 536, EUR 560 to corporations (effective 2002). **Document type:** *Journal, Academic/Scholarly.* **Description:** Provides an international, interdisciplinary broad-based forum for reporting both basic and clinical research in the field of nutrition that relates to the central and peripheral nervous system.
Related titles: Online - full text ed.: (from EBSCO Publishing, Institute for Scientific Information, RoweCom Information Quest).
Indexed: Neurosci.Abstr.
—BLDSC (6190.375000).
Published by: Gordon and Breach - Harwood Academic (Subsidiary of: Taylor & Francis Group), PO Box 531, Lausanne 1000, Switzerland. TEL 41-21-6411280, FAX 41-21-6411281, info@gbhap.com, http://www.gbhap.com/journals/416/416-top.htm. Ed. Chandan Prasad. **Subscr. addr. in US:** International Publishers Direct, PO Box 32160, Newark, NJ 07102. FAX 215-750-6343.

616.858 AUS
O C D - THE HIDDEN DISORDER. Text in English. 1992. q.
Indexed: e-psyche.
Published by: Obsessive Compulsive Disorder Support Groups of New South Wales, 60 Victoria Rd, Gladesville, NSW 2111, Australia. TEL 02-816-5688. Circ: 500. **Co-sponsor:** New South Wales Association for Mental Health.

150 361.3 610 USA ISSN 0164-212X
RC487 CODEN: OTMHDX
OCCUPATIONAL THERAPY IN MENTAL HEALTH; a journal of psychosocial practice and research. Text in English. 1980. q. USD 60 to individuals; USD 81 in Canada to individuals; USD 87 elsewhere to individuals; USD 150 to institutions; USD 203 in Canada to institutions; USD 218 elsewhere to institutions; USD 300 to libraries; USD 405 in Canada to libraries; USD 435 elsewhere to libraries (effective Aug. 2001). adv. bk.rev. bibl. back issues avail.; reprint service avail. from HAW. *Refereed.* **Document type:** *Journal, Academic/Scholarly.* **Description:** Provides current material specifically for occupational therapists in mental health clinics, psychiatric hospitals, mental health programs, hospitals, and other settings.
Related titles: Microfiche ed.: (from PQC); Microform ed.
Indexed: AMED, Abstr.Health Care Manage.Stud., Adol.Ment.Hlth.Abstr., Behav.Abstr., Biol.Abstr., CINAHL, Chicago Psychoanal.Lit.Ind., Child Devel.Abstr., Except.Child Educ.Abstr., Excerp.Med., IMFL, Past.Care & Couns.Abstr., Psychol.Abstr., Rehabil.Lit., Soc.Work Res.& Abstr., e-psyche.
—BLDSC (6231.260000), GNLM, Haworth, ingenta, KNAW.
Published by: Haworth Press, Inc., 10 Alice St, Binghamton, NY 13904-1580. TEL 607-722-5857, 800-429-6784, FAX 607-722-6362, 800-895-0582, getinfo@haworthpressinc.com, http://www.haworthpress.com/journals/journallist.asp. Eds. Mary Louise Blount, Mary Donohue. Pub. William Cohen. R&P Ruthann Heath TEL 607-723-5857 ext 316. Adv. contact Jackie Blakeslee TEL 607-722-5857 ext 346. B&W page USD 315, color page USD 550; trim 6 x 8.5. Circ: 850.

616.89 150 DNK ISSN 0105-0621
ODENSE UNIVERSITY STUDIES IN PSYCHIATRY AND MEDICAL PSYCHOLOGY. Text in Danish, English. 1973. irreg. price varies. back issues avail. **Document type:** *Monographic series, Academic/Scholarly.* **Description:** Biographies of important historical figures and how they influenced psychiatric medical history.
Indexed: Excerp.Med., e-psyche.
Published by: Odense University Press, Campusvej 55, Odense M 5230, Denmark. TEL 66-157999, FAX 66-158126, press@forlag.sdu.dk, press@forlag.ou.dk.

362.3 NLD ISSN 1382-354X
OKEE. Text in Dutch. 1993. m. NLG 55. illus. back issues avail. **Document type:** *Consumer.* **Description:** Covers all ways in which persons with mental disabilities can live as independently and productively as possible.
Related titles: Audio cassette/tape ed.
Indexed: e-psyche.
Published by: Stichting M M V H, Van Diemenstraat 182b, Amsterdam 1013 CP, Netherlands. TEL 31-20-624-0432, FAX 31-20-625-3566. Ed., Pub. Rolf Beekveldt. Circ: 4,000 (paid).

M

616.83 362.2 GBR ISSN 0265-511X
OPENMIND; the mental health magazine. Text in English. 1983. bi-m. GBP 19; GBP 37 foreign; GBP 3.50 newsstand/cover (effective 1999). adv. bk.rev., film rev., play rev. illus, tr.lit. index. back issues avail. **Document type:** *Consumer.* **Description:** Provides progressive mental health professionals, users and carers with stimulating coverage of the widest range of mental health issues.
Indexed: e-psyche.
—BLDSC (6266.325000).
Published by: Mind - The Mental Health Charity, Granta House, 15-19 Broadway, Stratford, London E15 4BQ, United Kingdom. TEL 44-20-8519-2122, FAX 44-20-8534-6399, sara@mind.org.uk, http://www.mind.org.uk. Ed., R&P, Adv. contact Sara Dunn. Pub. Anny Bracks. B&W page GBP 450; trim 210 x 297. Circ: 5,000; 5,000 (paid).

OPERATIVE TECHNIQUES IN NEUROSURGERY. see *MEDICAL SCIENCES—Surgery*

* 150.198 615.856 USA ISSN 1054-075X
ORGONOMIC FUNCTIONALISM; a journal devoted to the work of Wilhelm Reich. Text in English. 1989. a. USD 18.95 (effective 1999).
Indexed: e-psyche.
Published by: Wilhelm Reich Infant Trust, Orgonon, Box 687, Rangeley, ME 04970. TEL 207-864-3443, wreich@rangeley.org, http://www.somtel.com/-wreich/. Eds. Chester M Raphael, Dr. Mary Boyd Higgins. Circ: 200.

616.835 ITA ISSN 0030-5618
ORIZZONTI APERTI; la voce dei poliomielitici. Text in Italian. 1970 (vol.4). irreg. (3-5/yr.). free per issue. **Description:** Concerns poliomyelitis.
Indexed: e-psyche.
Published by: Associazione Nazionale Invalidi Esiti Poliomielite, Via De' Coltelli, 7-D, Bologna, BO 40124, Italy. Ed. Gianni Selleri. Circ: 16,000.

ORTHOPEDIC, NEUROLOGICAL AND CHIROPRACTIC PHYSICAL EXAMINATIONS: TECHNIQUE AND SIGNIFICANCE. see *MEDICAL SCIENCES—Orthopedics And Traumatology*

616.8 USA
P.M. NEWS (WHITE PLAINS). Text in English. 1972. bi-m. USD 15; USD 20 foreign. bk.rev. back issues avail. **Document type:** *Newsletter.* **Description:** Discusses the psychiatric specialties of anxieties, panic attacks, phobias, health anxiety, and obsessive-compulsive disorders.
Indexed: e-psyche.
Published by: White Plains Hospital Center, Anxiety and Phobia Clinic, Davis Ave at Post Rd, White Plains, NY 10601. TEL 914-681-1038, FAX 914-681-2284. Ed. Judy Chessa. Circ: 1,000.

616.89 DEU ISSN 0937-2032
P P M P. (Psychotherapie Psychosomatik Medizinische Psychologie) Text in German; Summaries in English, German. 1951. 12/yr. EUR 164.20 domestic to institutions; EUR 179.80 in Europe to institutions; EUR 184.70 elsewhere to institutions; EUR 84 to students; EUR 16 newsstand/cover (effective 2002). adv. bk.rev. abstr, bibl, charts, illus. index. back issues avail.; reprint service avail. from PQC. *Refereed.* **Document type:** *Journal, Academic/Scholarly.*
Former titles (until 1988): Psychotherapie Psychosomatik Medizinische Psychologie (0173-7937); Psychotherapie und Medizinische Psychologie (0302-8984); Zeitschrift fuer Psychotherapie und Medizinische Psychologie (0044-3417)
Related titles: Microform ed.: (from PQC); Online - full text ed.: ISSN 1439-1058 (from Institute for Scientific Information).
Indexed: ASCA, Biol.Abstr., Curr.Cont., Ger.J.Psych., Ind.Med. (1980-), PsycInfo, Psychol.Abstr. (1951-), Risk Abstr., SSCI, e-psyche.
—BLDSC (6946.558250), ADONIS, CISTI, EMDOCS, GNLM, IDS, Infotrieve, KNAW. **CCC.**
Published by: (Allgemeine Aerztliche Gesellschaft fuer Psychotherapie), Georg Thieme Verlag, Ruedigerstr 14, Stuttgart 70469, Germany. TEL 49-711-8931-0, FAX 49-711-8931298, kunden.service@thieme.de, http://www.thieme.de/ppmp. Ed. M von Rad. R&P Peter Eich. adv.: page DEM 1,850; 175 x 250. Circ: 1,500 (paid). **Co-sponsor:** Oesterreichische Aerzte-Gesellschaft fuer Psychotherapie.

616.8521 USA ISSN 1050-1835
P T S D RESEARCH QUARTERLY. Text in English. 1990. q. USD 10 (effective 2001); free to qualified personnel. bibl, abstr. **Document type:** *Government.* **Description:** Contains review articles on specific topics related to PTSD, written by guest experts.
Related titles: Online - full content ed.
Published by: National Center for Post Traumatic Stress Disorder (Subsidiary of: U.S. Department of Veterans Affairs), VA Medical and Regional Office Center (116D), 215 N Main St, White River Junction, VT 05009-0001. TEL 802-296-5132, FAX 802-296-5135, ptsd@dartmouth.edu, http://www.ncptsd.org/research/rq/rq_list.html. Ed. Dr. Matthew J Friedman. **Subscr. to:** U.S. Government Printing Office, Superintendent of Documents, PO Box 371954, Pittsburgh, PA 15250-7954. TEL 202-512-1800, FAX 202-512-2250, orders@gpo.gov, http://www.access.gpo.gov.

616.835 DNK ISSN 0901-7798
P T U NYT. Text in Danish. 1985. bi-m. DKK 175 (effective 1999). adv. **Document type:** *Academic/Scholarly.*
Formerly: Polio-Nyt (0900-5587)
Indexed: e-psyche.
Published by: Landsforeningen af Polio- Trafik og Ulykkesskadede, Fjeldhammervej 8, Rodovre 2610, Denmark. TEL 45-36-73-90-00, FAX 45-36-73-90-01, ptu-nyt@ptu.dk, http://www.ptu.dk. Ed. Charlotte Kabell. Adv. contact Stig Ulrich Jensen. Circ: 10,500.

616.8 NLD ISSN 0304-3959
RB127 CODEN: PAINDB
PAIN. Text in Dutch. 1975. 18/yr. EUR 323 in Europe to qualified personnel; JPY 42,600 in Japan to qualified personnel; USD 361 elsewhere to qualified personnel; EUR 758 in Europe to institutions; JPY 100,800 in Japan to institutions; USD 848 elsewhere to institutions (effective 2002). adv. bk.rev. abstr. back issues avail.; reprint service avail. from SWZ,ISI. *Refereed.* **Document type:** *Academic/Scholarly.* **Description:** Provides a forum for information about the nature, mechanism and treatment of pain.
Related titles: Microform ed.: (from PQC); Online - full text ed.: (from ingenta, ScienceDirect, Swets Blackwell, Institute for Scientific Information).
Indexed: AMED, ASCA, Addic.Abstr., Agri.& Environ.Biotech.Abstr. (coverage dropped), Behav.Med.Abstr., Biol.Abstr., CINAHL, Chem.Abstr., Chem.Indus.Notes, Chem.Titles, Chic.Per.Ind., Curr.Adv.Cancer Res., Curr.Adv.Ecol.Sci., Curr.Cont., Dent.Ind., Derwent Biotech.Abstr., Excerp.Med., Ind.Med. (1975-), Ind.Sci.Rev., Inpharma, Int.Abstr.Biol.Sci., Int.Nurs.Ind., Neurosci.Abstr. (coverage dropped), Neurosci.Cit.Ind., Pharm.&Out.News, PsycInfo, Psychol.Abstr. (1976-), Reac., SSCI (coverage dropped), Sci.Cit.Ind., THA, e-psyche.
—BLDSC (6333.795000), ADONIS, CASDDS, CISTI, EMDOCS, GNLM, IDS, ingenta, KNAW. **CCC.**
Published by: (International Association for the Study of Pain), Elsevier Science BV, PO Box 211, Amsterdam 1000 AE, Netherlands. TEL 31-20-485-2911, FAX 31-20-485-2457, nlinfo-f@elsevier.nl; usinfo-f@elsevier.com; forinfo-kyf04035@niftyserve.or.jp, http://www.elsevier.com/locate/painonline. Eds. Catherine Bushnell, Frances Addison, P D Wall, R Dubner. Circ: 5,000. **Subscr. in Australasia and the Far East to:** Elsevier Science (Singapore) Pte Ltd, No.1 Temasek Ave, 17-01 Millenia Tower, Singapore 039192, Singapore. TEL 65-434-3727, FAX 65-337-2230; **Subscr. in Japan to:** Elsevier Science Inc - Japan Regional Office, 9-15 Higashi-Azabu 1-chome, Minato-ku, Tokyo 106-0044, Japan. TEL 81-3-5561-5033, FAX 81-3-5561-5047; **Subscr. in the Americas to:** Elsevier Science, PO Box 945, New York, NY 10159-0945. TEL 212-633-3730, FAX 212-633-3680, usinfo-f@elsevier.com.

616.8 CHE ISSN 0255-3910
CODEN: RCSHA8
PAIN AND HEADACHE. Text in English. 1967. irreg., latest vol.13. CHF 200 in Europe; DEM 240 in Germany; USD 160 in United States (effective 2001). reprint service avail. from ISI. *Refereed.* **Document type:** *Monographic series, Academic/Scholarly.* **Description:** The latest in understanding and controlling pain.
Formerly: Research and Clinical Studies in Headache (0080-1453)
Indexed: Biol.Abstr., Chem.Abstr., Curr.Cont. (coverage dropped), Ind.Med. (until 1992, dropped), e-psyche.
—CASDDS, CISTI, GNLM, Infotrieve, KNAW. **CCC.**
Published by: S. Karger AG, Allschwilerstr 10, PO Box, Basel 4009, Switzerland. TEL 41-61-306-1111, FAX 41-61-306-1234, karger@karger.ch, http://www.karger.com/bookseries/PAHEA. Ed. H Reichmann.

THE PAIN CLINIC. see *MEDICAL SCIENCES—Anaesthesiology*

THE PAIN CLINIC (PROCEEDINGS). see *MEDICAL SCIENCES—Anaesthesiology*

616 USA ISSN 1082-3174
RB127
PAIN FORUM. Text in English. 1992. q. USD 119 domestic to individuals; GBP 100 in United Kingdom to individuals; USD 155 elsewhere to individuals; USD 165 domestic to institutions; GBP 132 in United Kingdom to institutions; USD 205 elsewhere to institutions. *Refereed.* **Document type:** *Academic/Scholarly.* **Description:** Features scholarly discussion of issues of interest to practitioners and researchers in the field of pain management. Publishes hypotheses on basic scientific and clinical topics and critiques of those hypotheses.
Formerly (until 1995): A P S Journal (1058-9139)
Indexed: ASCA, CINAHL, Excerp.Med. (1993-), Inpharma, Neurosci.Cit.Ind., Pharm.&Out.News, Reac., SSCI (coverage dropped), e-psyche.
—EMDOCS, GNLM, IDS, Infotrieve, KNAW. **CCC.**
Published by: (American Pain Society), Churchill Livingstone (Subsidiary of: Harcourt Health Sciences), 15 E 26th St, Fl 15, New York, NY 10010-1505. TEL 212-206-5040, FAX 212-206-7808, http://www.churchillmed.com. Ed. Kenneth L Casey. **UK subscr. to:** Pearson Professional Ltd., Journals Subscription Department, Fourth Ave., PO Box 77, Harlow, Essex CM19 5AA, United Kingdom. TEL 44-1279-623924, FAX 44-1279-639609; **Subscr. to:** PO Box 3217, Secaucus, NJ 07096-3217.

616.8 USA ISSN 1526-2375
▼ **PAIN MEDICINE.** Text in English. 2000. q. USD 160 domestic to individuals; USD 170 in Canada & Mexico to individuals; USD 180 elsewhere to individuals; USD 270 domestic to individuals; USD 280 in Canada & Mexico to individuals; USD 290 elsewhere to individuals; USD 176 domestic to individuals print & online eds. combined; USD 187 in Canada & Mexico to individuals print & online eds. combined; USD 198 elsewhere to individuals print & online eds. combined; USD 297 domestic to institutions print & online eds. combined; USD 308 in Canada & Mexico to institutions print & online eds. combined; USD 319 elsewhere to institutions print & online eds. combined (effective 2001). **Document type:** *Journal, Academic/Scholarly.* **Description:** Presents multi-disciplinary information dedicated to the pain clinician, teacher and researcher.
Related titles: ♦ Online - full text ed.: Pain Medicine Online. ISSN 1526-4637.
Indexed: Curr.Cont.
—BLDSC (6333.806000).
Published by: (American Academy of Pain Medicine), Blackwell Science Inc., Commerce Pl, 350 Main St, Malden, MA 02148-5018. TEL 781-388-8250, 800-759-6102, FAX 781-388-8255, journals@blacksci.com, http://www.blackwell-science.com/~cgilib/bsinc.bin?Journal=pain. Ed. Dr. Rollin Gallagher.

616.8 USA ISSN 1526-4637
PAIN MEDICINE ONLINE. Text in English. q. USD 144 to individuals; USD 243 to institutions (effective 2001). **Document type:** *Academic/Scholarly.*
Media: Online - full text (from EBSCO Publishing, O C L C Online Computer Library Center, Inc., ingenta, Munksgaard & Blackwell Science's Synergy, Swets Blackwell, Institute for Scientific Information, RoweCom Information Quest). **Related titles:** ♦ Print ed.: Pain Medicine. ISSN 1526-2375.
Published by: Blackwell Science Inc., Commerce Pl, 350 Main St, Malden, MA 02148-5018. TEL 781-388-8250, 800-759-6102, FAX 781-388-8255, website@blacksci.com, journals@blacksci.com, http://www.blackwell-science.com/~cgilib/bsinc.bin?Journal=pain.

616.8 USA ISSN 1530-7085
▼ **PAIN PRACTICE.** Text in English. 2001. q. USD 95 domestic to individuals; USD 105 in Canada & Mexico to individuals; USD 115 elsewhere to individuals; USD 195 domestic to institutions; USD 205 in Canada & Mexico to institutions; USD 215 elsewhere to institutions; USD 104.50 domestic to individuals print & online eds. combined; USD 115.50 in Canada & Mexico to individuals print & online eds. combined; USD 126.50 elsewhere to individuals print & online eds. combined; USD 214.50 domestic to institutions print & online eds. combined; USD 225.50 in Canada & Mexico to institutions print & online eds. combined; USD 236.50 elsewhere to institutions print & online eds. combined (effective 2001). adv. **Document type:** *Journal, Academic/Scholarly.* **Description:** Provides a comprehensive means of surveying developments in the various areas of importance to pain practitioners.
Related titles: ♦ Online - full text ed.: Pain Practice Online.
Published by: Blackwell Science Inc., Commerce Pl, 350 Main St, Malden, MA 02148-5018. TEL 781-388-8250, 800-759-6102, FAX 781-388-8255, journals@blacksci.com, http://www.blackwell-science.com/~cgilib/bsinc.bin?Journal=painpract. Ed. Dr. P. Prithvi Raj.

616.8 USA
▼ **PAIN PRACTICE ONLINE.** Text in English. 2001. q. USD 86 to individuals; USD 176 to institutions (effective 2001). **Document type:** *Academic/Scholarly.*
Media: Online - full text (from Swets Blackwell). **Related titles:** ♦ Print ed.: Pain Practice. ISSN 1530-7085.
Published by: Blackwell Science Inc., Commerce Pl, 350 Main St, Malden, MA 02148-5018. TEL 781-388-8250, 800-759-6102, FAX 781-388-8255, website@blacksci.com, journals@blacksci.com, http://www.blackwell-science.com/~cgilib/bsinc.bin?Journal=painpract.

612.88 616.047 CAN ISSN 1203-6765
PAIN RESEARCH & MANAGEMENT. Text in English. 1996. q. CND 95 (effective 2000). adv. bk.rev. back issues avail. *Refereed.* **Document type:** *Academic/Scholarly.* **Description:** Researches basic science and clinical apsects of pain and pain management.
Related titles: Online - full text ed.
Indexed: CBCA Ref.
—BLDSC (6333.813000).
Published by: (Canadian Pain Society), Pulsus Group Inc., 2902 S Sheridan Way, Oakville, ON L6J 7L6, Canada. TEL 905-829-4770, FAX 905-829-4799, pulsus@pulsus.com, http://www.pulsus.com. Ed. Dr. Harold Merskey. Pub. Robert B Kalina. Adv. contact Amanda Murphy. B&W page CND 2,325, color page CND 4,100; trim 10 x 7. Circ: 18,000 (controlled).

616.837 CAN ISSN 0048-2935
PARAGRAPHIC. Text in English. 1957. q. CND 10 to members. adv. bk.rev. *Refereed.* **Document type:** *Newsletter.*
Indexed: e-psyche.
Published by: Canadian Paraplegic Association, British Columbia Division, 780 S W Marine Dr, Vancouver, BC V6P 5Y7, Canada. TEL 604-324-3611, FAX 604-324-3671, vancouver@canparaplegic.org. Ed., R&P Maureen Brownlee. Circ: 4,000.

PARAPLEGIA NEWS. see *HANDICAPPED—Physically Impaired*

616.833 GBR
THE PARKINSON. Text in English. 1969. q. GBP 4 to membership (effective 2001). adv. bk.rev., software rev., Website rev. 32 p./no. **Description:** Covers matters of interest to people with Parkinson's disease.
Related titles: Audio cassette/tape ed.
Published by: Parkinson's Disease Society of the United Kingdom, 215 Vauxhall Bridge Rd, London SW1V 1EJ, United Kingdom. TEL 44-20-7931-8080, FAX 44-20-7233-9908, enquiries@parkinsons.org.uk, http://www.parkinsons.org.uk. Ed. B Cormie. adv.: color 1/2 page GBP 700. Circ: 30,000.

616.8 CAN
PARKINSON POST. Text in English. q. CND 25 to members (effective 2000). adv. back issues avail. **Document type:** *Newsletter.* **Description:** Advises readers of events, new chapters and support groups, where to get help.
Former titles: Parkinson Network (0824-7315); (until 1984): Parkinson Foundation of Canada. Bulletin (0711-236X)
Related titles: French ed.: ISSN 0845-4299.
Indexed: e-psyche.
Published by: Parkinson Foundation of Canada, 4211 Yonge St Ste 316, Toronto, ON M2P 2A9, Canada. TEL 416-227-9700, 800-565-3000, FAX 416-227-9600, http://www.parkinson.ca. Ed. Trevor Williams. Adv. contact Mara Busca. Circ: 15,000 (paid).

616.8 USA
PARKINSON REPORT. Text in English. 1957. q. membership. charts, illus. **Document type:** *Newsletter.* **Description:** Written for people affected by Parkinson's disease and explores various areas of the research.
Formerly: National Parkinson Foundation. Newsletter
Indexed: e-psyche.
Published by: National Parkinson Foundation, Inc., 1501 N W Ninth Ave Bob Hope Rd, Miami, FL 33136-9990. TEL 305-547-6666, 800-327-4545, FAX 305-548-4403. Ed. Dr. Juan Sanchez Ramos.

616.89 USA
PARKINSONIAN SPEAK-OUT. Text in English. 1987. q. USD 72. **Document type:** *Newsletter.*
Indexed: e-psyche.
Address: 55 Merrick St, Rumford, RI 02916-2520. TEL 401-435-3179. Ed. R Bernen.

616.8 GBR ISSN 1353-8020
CODEN: PRDIFO
PARKINSONISM AND RELATED DISORDERS. Text in English. 1995. q. EUR 85 in Europe to individuals; JPY 11,300 in Japan to individuals; USD 96 elsewhere to individuals; EUR 344 in Europe to institutions; JPY 41,031 in Japan to institutions; USD 385 elsewhere to institutions (effective 2002). *Refereed.* **Document type:** *Academic/Scholarly.* **Description:** Pubishes basic and clinical research that contributes to the understanding, diagnosis, and treatment of all neurodegenerative syndromes in which Parkinsonism, essential tremor, and related disorders play a part.
Related titles: Microform ed.: (from PQC); Online - full text ed.: (from ingenta, ScienceDirect, Swets Blackwell, Institute for Scientific Information).
Indexed: Curr.Cont., Inpharma, Neurosci.Cit.Ind., Pharm.&Out.News, Reac., e-psyche.
—BLDSC (6406.787000), CISTI, GNLM, Infotrieve. **CCC.**
Published by: Pergamon (Subsidiary of: Elsevier Science), The Boulevard, Langford Ln, East Park, Kidlington, Oxford OXB 1GB, United Kingdom. FAX 44-1865-843010, http://www.elsevier.nl/locate/parkreldis. Eds. Ariel Y Deutch, Donald B Calne. **Subscr. in Australasia and the Far East to:** Elsevier Science (Singapore) Pte Ltd, No.1 Temasek Ave, 17-01 Millenia Tower, Singapore 039192, Singapore. TEL 65-434-3727, FAX 65-337-2230; **Subscr. in the Americas to:** Elsevier Science, PO Box 945, New York, NY 10159-0945. TEL 212-633-3730, FAX 212-633-3680; **Subscr. to:** Elsevier Science BV, PO Box 211, Amsterdam 1000 AE, Netherlands. TEL 31-20-485-3757.

616.8 USA ISSN 0885-4807
PARKINSON'S DISEASE UPDATE. Text in English, French. 1983. m. USD 40. bk.rev. index. back issues avail. **Document type:** *Newsletter.*
Indexed: e-psyche.
Published by: Medical Publishing Co., Inc., 3917 Bluebird Rd, Huntingdon, PA 19006. TEL 215-947-6648, FAX 215-947-6638. Ed. Dr. Stuart Isaacson. Circ: 15,000. **Subscr. to:** PO Box 24622, Philadelphia, PA 19111.

616.89 NLD ISSN 0927-2658
PASSAGE; vaktijdschrift rehabilitatie. Text in Dutch. 1992. q. NLG 52.50 to individuals; NLG 68 to institutions. adv. bk.rev. abstr, charts, illus. index. back issues avail. **Document type:** *Academic/Scholarly.* **Description:** Includes information on ambulatory and residental care for people who are dependent on psychiatric care.
Incorporates (in 1994): Forum (Rotterdam) (0925-0735)
Indexed: e-psyche.
Published by: Uitgeverij S W P, Postbus 578, Utrecht 3500 AN, Netherlands. TEL 31-30-236-8060, FAX 31-30-2368140, swp@wxs.nl, http://www.swpbook.com. Ed. M Nuy. Adv. contact Hans Degraat. page NLG 350; trim 205 x 142. Circ: 1,000 (paid).

PEDIATRIC NEUROLOGY. see *MEDICAL SCIENCES—Pediatrics*

616.8 CHE ISSN 1016-2291
CODEN: PDNEEV
PEDIATRIC NEUROSURGERY. Text in English. m. (in 2 vols.). CHF 1,558 in Europe to institutions; CHF 1,592.80 elsewhere to institutions; EUR 1,113.60 in Europe to institutions; USD 1,216 elsewhere to institutions (effective 2002). adv. bk.rev. back issues avail. *Refereed.* **Document type:** *Journal, Academic/Scholarly.* **Description:** Features new information and observations in pedriatric neurosurgery and the allied fields of neuroradiology and neuropathology as they relate to the etiology of neurologic diseases and the operative care of affected patients.
Formerly (until 1991): Pediatric Neuroscience (0255-7975); Which supersedes in part (in 1985): Child's Brain (0302-2803)
Related titles: Microform ed.: (from PQC); Online - full text ed.: ISSN 1423-0305. CHF 116, EUR 84, USD 90 to institutions with print edition (effective 2002) (from EBSCO Publishing, O C L C Online Computer Library Center, Inc., RoweCom Information Quest, Swets Blackwell, Institute for Scientific Information).
Indexed: ASCA, Curr.Cont., Excerp.Med., Ind.Med. (1991-), Ind.Sci.Rev., Inpharma, Neurosci.Cit.Ind., Pharm.&Out.News, Reac., Sci.Cit.Ind., e-psyche.
—BLDSC (6417.604700), CASDDS, CISTI, EMDOCS, GNLM, IDS, ingenta, KNAW. **CCC.**
Published by: (International Society for Paediatric Neurosurgery), S. Karger AG, Allschwilerstr 10, PO Box, Basel 4009, Switzerland. TEL 41-61-306-1111, FAX 41-61-306-1234, karger@karger.ch, http://www.online.karger.com/journals/pne, http://www.karger.com. Ed. D G McLone. adv.: page USD 1,185.

PENNSYLVANIA MESSAGE. see *EDUCATION—Special Education And Rehabilitation*

616.891 DEU ISSN 1433-6308
PERSOENLICHKEITSSTOERUNGEN - THEORIE UND THERAPIE. Abbreviated title: P T T. Text in German. 1997. q. DEM 168; DEM 100 to students (effective 2001). adv. **Document type:** *Journal, Academic/Scholarly.*
Indexed: e-psyche.
Published by: Schattauer GmbH, Hoelderlinstr 3, Stuttgart 70174, Germany. TEL 49-711-22987-0, FAX 49-711-2298775, info@schattauer.de, http://www.schattauer.com. R&P Annika Schmidt TEL 49-711-2298713. Adv. contact Maria Wagner TEL 49-711-2298767. B&W page XEU 1,175.97, color page XEU 2,121.86; trim 127 x 212. **Subscr. to:** CSJ, Postfach 140220, Munich 80452, Germany. TEL 49-89-20959129, schattauer@csj.de.

616.8 ITA
PERSONALITA - DIPENDENZE. Text in Italian. 3/yr. ITL 85,000, EUR 63.90 domestic; ITL 100,000, EUR 51.65 foreign.
Indexed: e-psyche.
Published by: Mucchi Editore s.r.l., Via Emilia Est, 1527, Modena, MO 41100, Italy. TEL 39-59-374094, FAX 39-59-282628, enmucchi@tin.it. **Co-sponsors:** Federazione Italiana Operatori Tossicodipendenze; Societa di Studio per i Disturbi di Personalita, IRET.

616.8553 USA
PERSPECTIVES (BALTIMORE). Text in English. q. USD 55 to members. **Document type:** *Newsletter.*
Published by: International Dyslexia Association, 8600 LaSalle Rd, Ste 382, Chester Bldg, Baltimore, MD 21286-2044. TEL 410-296-0232. R&P Cindy Cressi. Circ: 15,000.

PERSPECTIVES IN PSYCHIATRIC CARE. see *MEDICAL SCIENCES—Nurses And Nursing*

612.8 CHE ISSN 1064-0517
QP363.5 CODEN: PDENED
PERSPECTIVES ON DEVELOPMENTAL NEUROBIOLOGY. Text in English. 1989. q. EUR 294 to institutions; EUR 460 to corporations (effective 2000). back issues avail. *Refereed.* **Document type:** *Academic/Scholarly.* **Description:** Publishes concise and authoritatively written critical reviews of recent progress in developmental neurobiology. Appeals to neuroscientists, developmental biologists, and psychobiologists, as well as those scientists interested in neuronal plasticity.
Formerly (until 1992): Comments on Modern Biology. Part D, Comments on Developmental Neurology (0896-5099)
Related titles: CD-ROM ed.; Microform ed.; Online - full text ed.: (from EBSCO Publishing, RoweCom Information Quest).

M

Indexed: ASCA, Anim.Behav.Abstr. (coverage dropped), Aqua.Sci.& Fish.Abstr., Chemorec.Abstr., Curr.Cont. (coverage dropped), Ind.Med. (1992-), Ind.Sci.Rev., Neurosci.Abstr., Neurosci.Cit.Ind., Sci.Cit.Ind. (coverage dropped), e-psyche.
—BLDSC (6428.141510), CISTI, GNLM, Infotrieve, KNAW. **CCC.**
Published by: Gordon and Breach - Harwood Academic (Subsidiary of: Taylor & Francis Group), PO Box 531, Lausanne 1000, Switzerland. http://www.gbhap.com/Perspectives_Developmental_Neurobiology/; http://biomednet.com/library/730. Eds. Alain Prochiantz, Jean Lauder. **Subscr. addr. in US:** International Publishers Direct, PO Box 32160, Newark, NJ 07102. FAX 215-750-6343.

616.89 FRA ISSN 0031-6032
PERSPECTIVES PSYCHIATRIQUES. Text in French. 1963. 5/yr. EUR 77.75 domestic; EUR 92.23 in Europe; EUR 106.41 elsewhere; EUR 52.59 domestic to students; EUR 70.13 in Europe to students; EUR 82.02 elsewhere to students (effective 2002). adv. bk.rev. **Document type:** *Academic/Scholarly.* **Description:** Presents multidisciplinary discussion and opinion on new methods of treatment and comprehension of mental illness.
Indexed: Psychol.Abstr., e-psyche.
—GNLM.
Published by: (Groupe d'Etudes de Psychiatrie Psychologie et Sciences Sociales), Editions E D K, 10 Villa d'Orleans, Paris 75014, France. TEL 33-1-48408686, FAX 33-1-48400731, martinek@francenet.fr. Ed. Dr. Jacques Fortineau. Circ: 2,500. **Subscr. to:** ATEI, 3 av. Pierre Kerautret, Romainville 93230, France. TEL 33-1-48408686, FAX 33-1-48400731.

616.89 DEU ISSN 0176-3679
RM315 CODEN: PHRMEZ
PHARMACOPSYCHIATRY; clinical pharmacology, psychiatry, psychology, neurophysiology, neurobiology, gerontopsychiatry. Text in English. 1968. bi-m. EUR 289.40 domestic to institutions; EUR 291.80 in Europe to institutions; EUR 295.40 elsewhere to institutions; EUR 58 newsstand/cover (effective 2002). adv. bibl. charts, illus, stat. index. reprint service avail. from PQC. *Refereed.* **Document type:** *Journal, Academic/Scholarly.*
Former titles: Pharmacopsychiatria (0720-4280); (until 1980): Pharmakopsychiatrie - Neuro-Psychopharmakologie (0031-7098)
Related titles: Microfiche ed.; Microfilm ed.: (from PQC); Online - full text ed.: ISSN 1439-0795 (from Institute for Scientific Information); ♦ Supplement: Pharmacopsychiatry. Supplement. ISSN 0936-9589.
Indexed: ASCA, Agri.& Environ.Biotech.Abstr. (coverage dropped), Biol.Abstr., Chem.Abstr., Chem.Titles, Curr.Adv.Ecol.Sci., Curr.Cont., Dent.Ind., Derwent Biotech.Abstr., Excerp.Med., Focus on: Psychophar., Ger.J.Psych., INIS Atomind., Ind.Med. (1984-), Ind.Sci.Rev., Inpharma, Neurosci.Cit.Ind., Pharm.&Out.News, PsycInfo, Psychol.Abstr. (1989-), Reac., Rev.Arom.& Med.Plants, SSCI (coverage dropped), Sci.Cit.Ind., e-psyche.
—BLDSC (6447.087950), ADONIS, CASDDS, CISTI, GNLM, IDS, Infotrieve, ingenta, KNAW, Linda Hall. **CCC.**
Published by: (Arbeitsgemeinschaft Neuropsychopharmakologie und Pharmakopsychiatrie), Georg Thieme Verlag, Ruedigerstr 14, Stuttgart 70469, Germany. TEL 49-711-8931-0, FAX 49-711-8931298, pharmaco@thieme.de, leser.service@thieme.de, http://www.thieme.de/pharmaco, http://www.thieme-connect.de. Ed. B Mueller Oerlinghausen. R&P Alessandra Kreibaum. Circ: 1,200.

616.89 DEU ISSN 0936-9589
PHARMACOPSYCHIATRY. SUPPLEMENT. Text in German. irreg. **Document type:** *Monographic series.*
Related titles: Online - full text ed.; ♦ Supplement to: Pharmacopsychiatry. ISSN 0176-3679.
Indexed: e-psyche.
—ADONIS, EMDOCS.
Published by: Georg Thieme Verlag, Ruedigerstr 14, Stuttgart 70469, Germany. TEL 49-711-8931-0, FAX 49-711-8931298, leser.service@thieme.de, http://www.thieme.de, http://www.thieme-connect.de.

PHILOSOPHY, PSYCHIATRY & PSYCHOLOGY. see *PHILOSOPHY*

616.8 ESP ISSN 0210-3931
PHRONESIS. Text in Spanish. 6/yr.
Indexed: e-psyche.
Address: Matematico Pedrayes, 20 1o, Oviedo, Asturias 33005, Spain. TEL 85-23-68-47. Ed. Dr. F Bueno Martinez. Circ: 50,000.

PHYSIOLOGICAL RESEARCH. see *BIOLOGY—Physiology*

PHYSIOLOGY AND BEHAVIOR; an international journal. see *BIOLOGY—Physiology*

371.928 USA ISSN 0031-9856
PINE CONE. Text in English. 1966. q. free per issue. illus. **Description:** Articles related to mental retardation.
Media: Duplicated (not offset).
Indexed: e-psyche.
Published by: Pinecrest State School, PO Box 191, Pineville, LA 71360. TEL 318-640-0754. Circ: 1,600.

616.89 NLD ISSN 1380-8095
PLUS MINUS. Text in Dutch. 1987. q. free per issue to members. bk.rev. back issues avail. **Document type:** *Newspaper.*
Indexed: e-psyche.
Published by: Nederlandse Stichting voor Manisch Depressieven, Postbus 380, Duivendrecht 1115 ZH, Netherlands. TEL 31-20-6900710. Ed. R J W Bouwens.

616.89 ITA ISSN 1591-0598
POL.IT PSYCHIATRY ONLINE ITALIA. Text in Italian, English. 1995. m.
Media: Online - full text.
Published by: Associazione Psychiatry Online Italia, Via Provana Di Leyni 13, Genoa, Italy. redazione@pol-it.org, http://www.pol-it.org/, http://www.psychiatryonline.it/. Ed. Francesco Bollorino.

616.8 DEU ISSN 0933-3851
PRAKTISCHE PSYCHIATRIE. Text in German. 1988. irreg., latest vol.3, 1991. **Document type:** *Academic/Scholarly.*
Indexed: e-psyche.
Published by: W. Zuckschwerdt Verlag GmbH, Industriestr 1, Germering 82110, Germany. TEL 49-89-894349-0, FAX 49-89-89434950. Eds. R Schuettler, R M Schulte.

616.89 150 DEU ISSN 0032-7034
CODEN: PKIKAZ
PRAXIS DER KINDERPSYCHOLOGIE UND KINDERPSYCHIATRIE. Text in German; Summaries in English, German. 1952. 10/yr. DEM 115; DEM 76 to students (effective 2000). adv. bk.rev. abstr, illus, stat. index. reprint service avail. from PSC,SCH. *Refereed.* **Document type:** *Journal, Academic/Scholarly.*
Related titles: Online - full text ed.: (from Institute for Scientific Information).
Indexed: Arts & Hum.Cit.Ind. (coverage dropped), Biol.Abstr., Curr.Cont., Excerp.Med., Ger.J.Psych., IBR, IBZ, Ind.Med. (1952-), Ind.Philos., Int.Nurs.Ind., PsycInfo, Psychol.Abstr. (1952-), SSCI, e-psyche.
—BLDSC (6603.171400), CISTI, GNLM, IDS, Infotrieve. **CCC.**
Published by: Vandenhoeck und Ruprecht, Robert-Bosch-Breite 6, Goettingen 37079, Germany. TEL 49-551-6959-26, FAX 49-551-695917. Eds. Annemarie Duehrssen, Rudolf Adam. Circ: 2,900. **Subscr. to:** Goettingen 37027, Germany.

PRAXIS DER KINDERPSYCHOLOGIE UND KINDERPSYCHIATRIE. BEIHEFTE. see *PSYCHOLOGY*

616.858 HRV ISSN 0032-7301
PREGLED PROBLEMA MENTALNO RETARDIRANIH OSOBA. Text in Serbo-Croatian. 1965. bi-m. adv. bk.rev. **Description:** Concerns mental retardation.
Indexed: Biol.Abstr., e-psyche.
Published by: Savjet Organizacija za Pomoc Mentalno Retardiranim Osobama u SFRJ, Prilaz JNA 43-III, Zagreb, Croatia. Ed. Sulejman Masovic.

616.8 USA ISSN 1522-3736
PREVENTION & TREATMENT. Text in English. 1998. irreg. adv. *Refereed.* **Document type:** *Academic/Scholarly.* **Description:** Publishes empirical and theoretical research on prevention, the outcome of psychotherapy and social and environmental interventions, biologically oriented therapy, and the combination of such interventions.
Media: Online - full text.
Published by: American Psychological Association, 211 E 70th St, New York, NY 10021. TEL 202-336-5500, 800-374-3721, admin@apa.org, http://journals.apa.org/prevention/. Ed. Martin E P Seligman.

616.89 362.2 GBR ISSN 1355-2570
CODEN: PCPSF9
PRIMARY CARE PSYCHIATRY. Text in English. 1995. q. GBP 182 to individuals; GBP 417 to institutions (effective 2001 - 2002). adv. index. *Refereed.* **Document type:** *Academic/Scholarly.* **Description:** Provides comprehensive information on all aspects of the management of psychiatric illness throughout the primary care structure.
Related titles: CD-ROM ed.; Online - full text ed.: (from CatchWord Ltd., EBSCO Publishing, Institute for Scientific Information).
Indexed: Curr.Cont., e-psyche.
—BLDSC (6612.908430), GNLM.
Published by: Librapharm Ltd, Gemini House, 162 Craven Rd, Newbury, Berks RG14 5NR, United Kingdom. TEL 44-1635-522651, FAX 44-1635-36294, journals@librapharm.com, http://www.librapharm.com. Circ: 1,200.

616.8 USA ISSN 1082-6319
PRIMARY PSYCHIATRY; first in applied psychiatric medicine. Text in English. 1994. m. USD 90 domestic; USD 145 foreign (effective 2000). adv. bk.rev. *Refereed.* **Document type:** *Academic/Scholarly.*
Indexed: Ref.Zh., e-psyche.
—BLDSC (6612.912500).
Published by: M B L Communications, 665 Broadway, New York, NY 10012-2302. TEL 212-328-0800, FAX 212-328-0600, primepsych@aol.com. Ed. Dr. Norman Sussman. Pub. James La Rossa Jr. R&P Steven Ovadia. Adv. contact Darren Brodeur. Circ: 60,000.

599.8 FRA ISSN 1279-8304
PRIMATOLOGIE. Text in Multiple languages. 1998. a. FRF 422 (effective 2000).
Indexed: Zoo.Rec.
Published by: Association pour la Diffusion des Recherches en Sciences Cognitives de Langue Francaise, CNRS - CRNC, 31 chemin Joseph Aiguier, Marseille Cedex 20 13402, France. TEL 33-4-91164279, FAX 33-4-91714938, cpc@lnf.cnrs-mrs.fr.

PRINCIPLES AND TECHNIQUES IN SPINE SURGERY SERIES. see *MEDICAL SCIENCES—Orthopedics And Traumatology*

PROBLEMS OF INDUSTRIAL PSYCHIATRIC MEDICINE SERIES. see *PSYCHOLOGY*

616.8 612.821 NLD ISSN 0079-6123
QP376 CODEN: PBRRA4
PROGRESS IN BRAIN RESEARCH. Text in Dutch. 1963. irreg., latest vol.128, 2000. price varies. back issues avail. *Refereed.* **Document type:** *Monographic series, Academic/Scholarly.* **Description:** Documents advances in the research of brain physiology.
Related titles: Online - full text ed.: (from Institute for Scientific Information).
Indexed: ASCA, BBCI, Biol.Abstr., Chem.Abstr., Chem.Indus.Notes, Chem.Titles, Dent.Ind., Excerp.Med., INIS Atomind., Ind.Med. (1963-), Ind.Sci.Rev., Neurosci.Abstr. (coverage dropped), Neurosci.Cit.Ind., SSCI (coverage dropped), Sci.Cit.Ind., Sport Fish.Abstr., Wild.Rev., Zoo.Rec., e-psyche.
—BLDSC (6866.400000), CASDDS, CISTI, GNLM, IDS, ingenta, KNAW. **CCC.**
Published by: Elsevier Science BV, PO Box 211, Amsterdam 1000 AE, Netherlands. TEL 31-20-485-3757, 31-20-485-3911, FAX 31-20-485-3432, 31-20-485-3598, nlinfo-f@elsevier.nl, http://www.elsevier.nl. **Subscr. in Australasia and the Far East to:** Elsevier Science (Singapore) Pte Ltd, No.1 Temasek Ave, 17-01 Millenia Tower, Singapore 039192, Singapore. TEL 65-434-3727, FAX 65-337-2230, asiainfo@elsevier.com.sg; **Subscr. in Japan to:** Elsevier Science Inc - Japan Regional Office, 9-15 Higashi-Azabu 1-chome, Minato-ku, Tokyo 106-0044, Japan. TEL 81-3-5561-5033, FAX 81-3-5561-5047, info@elsevier.co.jp; **Subscr. in the Americas to:** Elsevier Science, PO Box 945, New York, NY 10159-0945. TEL 212-633-3730, 888-437-4636, FAX 212-633-3680, usinfo-f@elsevier.com, http://www.elsevier.com

PROGRESS IN NEURO-PSYCHOPHARMACOLOGY AND BIOLOGICAL PSYCHIATRY. see *PHARMACY AND PHARMACOLOGY*

PROGRESS IN NEUROBIOLOGY; an international review journal. see *BIOLOGY—Physiology*

616.8 USA
PROGRESS IN NEUROINFORMATICS RESEARCH. Text in English. ceased 19??; resumed. irreg. **Document type:** *Monographic series.*
Indexed: e-psyche.

M

Published by: Lawrence Erlbaum Associates, Inc., 10 Industrial Ave, Mahwah, NJ 07430-2262. TEL 201-236-9500, FAX 201-236-0072, orders@erlbaum.com, http://www.erlbaum.com. Eds. Michael F Huerta, Stephen H Koslow.

617.48 CHE ISSN 0079-6492
PROGRESS IN NEUROLOGICAL SURGERY. Text in English. 1966. irreg., latest vol.15. CHF 190 in Europe; DEM 230 in Germany; USD 150 in United States (effective 2001). reprint service avail. from ISI. *Refereed.* **Document type:** *Monographic series, Academic/Scholarly.*
Related titles: Online - full text ed.: (from Institute for Scientific Information).
Indexed: Biol.Abstr., Chem.Abstr., Curr.Cont. (coverage dropped), Ind.Med. (coverage dropped), e-psyche.
—BLDSC (6870.340000), GNLM, Infotrieve, KNAW. **CCC.**
Published by: S. Karger AG, Allschwilerstr 10, PO Box, Basel 4009, Switzerland. TEL 41-61-306-1111, FAX 41-61-306-1234, karger@karger.ch, http://www.karger.com/bookseries/PRNES. Ed. L D Lunsford.

616.8 USA ISSN 0099-9016
RC347 CODEN: PRNPAM
PROGRESS IN NEUROPATHOLOGY. Text in English. 1971. irreg. price varies. reprint service avail. from PQC. *Refereed.* **Document type:** *Proceedings.*
Indexed: Biol.Abstr., e-psyche.
—CASDDS, CISTI, GNLM.
Published by: Lippincott Williams & Wilkins (Philadelphia) (Subsidiary of: Wolters Kluwer N.V.), 530 Walnut St, Philadelphia, PA 19106-3621. TEL 301-223-2300, 800-638-3030, FAX 301-223-2400, http://www.lww.com.

616.89 USA ISSN 1070-1443
RC455.4 CODEN: PPSHED
PROGRESS IN PSYCHIATRY. Key Title: Progress in Psychiatry Series. Text in English. 1990. irreg. price varies. back issues avail. **Document type:** *Monographic series.* **Description:** Addresses current issues in psychiatric research and practice.
Indexed: Chem.Abstr., Chem.Indus.Notes, Chem.Titles, e-psyche.
—CASDDS. **CCC.**
Published by: (American Psychiatric Association), American Psychiatric Press, Inc., 1400 K St, N W, Ste 1101, Washington, DC 20005. TEL 202-682-6020, FAX 202-682-6016.

PROGRESS IN SELF PSYCHOLOGY; conversations in self psychology. see *PSYCHOLOGY*

616.8 ITA ISSN 1591-1209
▼ **PSICHE DONNA.** Text in Italian. 2000. 3/yr. ITL 100,000, USD 100 (effective 2001). adv. **Document type:** *Journal, Academic/Scholarly.*
Published by: C I C Edizioni Internazionali s.r.l., Corso Trieste 42, Rome, RM 00198, Italy. TEL 39-06-8412673, FAX 39-06-8412688, info@gruppocic.it. Ed. E Costa. Pub. A Salvati. adv.: B&W page XEU 1,239.5, color page XEU 1,704.31; 210 x 280.

616.89 ITA ISSN 1129-0846
▼ **PSICHIATRI OGGI.** Text in Italian. 1999. m. ITL 8,000, USD 8; USD 2,000 newsstand/cover (effective 2001). adv. **Description:** Contains original articles and case reports on psychiatric diseases and correlated matters addressed to Italian psychiatrists.
Published by: C I C Edizioni Internazionali s.r.l., Corso Trieste 42, Rome, RM 00198, Italy. TEL 39-06-8412673, FAX 39-06-8412688, info@gruppocic.it, 1160199510. Ed. P L Scapicchio. adv.: B&W page ITL 4,000,000, color page ITL 5,100,000; trim 275 x 375.

616.89 ITA ISSN 0393-361X
PSICHIATRIA DELL'INFANZIA E DELL'ADOLESCENZA. Text in Italian; Summaries in English. 1907. bi-m. ITL 90,000 domestic to individuals; USD 110 foreign to individuals; ITL 110,000 domestic to institutions; USD 130 foreign to institutions. adv. bk.rev. charts, illus, stat, tr.lit. index, cum.index. **Document type:** *Academic/Scholarly.* **Description:** Encompasses all branches of psychiatry, from neonatal age to late adolescence. Comprises original research, synthetic reviews, case histories, field research, magazine reviews and more.
Former titles (until 1983): Neuropsichiatria Infantile (0028-3924); (until 1969): Infanzia Anormale
Indexed: Biol.Abstr., Excerp.Med., Lang.& Lang.Behav.Abstr., PsycInfo, Psychol.Abstr. (1993-), e-psyche.
—BLDSC (6945.843000), CISTI.
Published by: (Universita di Roma, Istituto di Neuropsichiatria Infantile), Edizioni Borla s.r.l., Via Delle Fornaci, 50, Rome, RM 00165, Italy. TEL 39-6-39376728, FAX 39-6-39376620. Ed. Giovanni Bollea. Circ: 3,000.

616.8 ITA ISSN 1127-395X
PSICHIATRIA DI CONSULTAZIONE. Text in Italian; Summaries in Italian, English. 1998. q. ITL 70,000, USD 70; ITL 20,000 newsstand/cover (effective 2001). adv. **Document type:** *Magazine.* **Description:** Contains original articles and case reports on psychiatric diseases and correlated matters addressed at Italian psychiatrists.
Published by: C I C Edizioni Internazionali s.r.l., Corso Trieste 42, Rome, RM 00198, Italy. TEL 39-06-8412673, FAX 39-06-8412688, info@gruppocic.it, 1160199510. Ed. G Invernizzi. Pub. A Salvati. adv.: B&W page ITL 2,400,000, color page ITL 3,300,000; trim 210 x 280.

616.8 150.19 ITA ISSN 0393-9774
PSICHIATRIA E PSICOTERAPIA ANALITICA/ANALYTIC PSYCHOTHERAPY AND PSYCHOPATHOLOGY. Text in English, Italian. 1982. q., latest vol.20. EUR 31 to individuals; EUR 42 to institutions (effective 2001). adv. bk.rev. charts, illus, stat. 96 p./no. back issues avail. *Refereed.* **Document type:** *Academic/Scholarly.* **Description:** Features research papers by doctors worldwide in the field of analytical psychotherapy and psychopathology. Includes articles on group psychotherapy, psychiatric rehabilitation, neuroscience, psychiatry and culture.
Indexed: Excerp.Med., PsycInfo, Psychol.Abstr. (1986-), Ref.Zh., e-psyche.
—BLDSC (6945.841000), GNLM.
Published by: Giovanni Fioriti Editore s.r.l., Via Archimede, 179, Rome, RM 00197, Italy. TEL 39-06-8072063, fioriti-wolit@tiscalinet.it, http://www.fioriti.it. Ed. Giovanni Fioriti. Pub., Adv. contact Anna Angelucci. R&P Francesca Ruffa TEL 39-6-8072069. Circ: 3,000.

616.8 ITA
PSICHIATRIA E TERRITORIO. Text in Italian; Summaries in English. 1984. q. ITL 60,000, USD 45. **Document type:** *Academic/Scholarly.* **Description:** Presents the experiences of psychiatric staff in general hospital and therapeutic community situations.
Indexed: e-psyche.
Published by: (Centro Studi Psichiatria e Territorio), Teseo Ricerche Editore, Corso Italia, 108, Pisa, PI 56125, Italy. TEL 39-50-501040, FAX 39-50-502434. Ed. Mario Di Fiorino.

616.8 ITA ISSN 0555-5299
PSICHIATRIA GENERALE E DELL'ETA EVOLUTIVA. Text in Italian. q. ITL 100,000 domestic; ITL 150,000, ITL 77 foreign (effective 2000); includes supplement.
Indexed: IBZ, Psychol.Abstr., e-psyche.
Published by: Tipografia Editrice la Garangola, Via Montona, 4, Padua, PD 35137, Italy. FAX 39-49-8751743.

616.89 ITA
LA PSICHIATRIA NELLA PRATICA MEDICA. Text in Italian. ceased 1998; resumed. q. **Document type:** *Newsletter.*
Indexed: e-psyche.
Published by: C I C Edizioni Internazionali s.r.l., Corso Trieste 42, Rome, RM 00198, Italy. TEL 39-06-8412673, FAX 39-06-8412688, info@gruppocic.it, 1160199510. Eds. C Gala, G Invernizzi.

616.89 ESP ISSN 0211-5549
CODEN: PSICE3
PSICOPATOLOGIA. Text in Spanish. 1981. q. ESP 7,100, USD 70 to individuals; ESP 8,500 to institutions; ESP 5,600 to students. adv. back issues avail.; reprints avail. *Refereed.* **Document type:** *Academic/Scholarly.*
Related titles: Online - full text ed.
Indexed: Excerp.Med., Psychol.Abstr., e-psyche.
—BLDSC (6945.864000), CINDOC, GNLM.
Published by: (Instituto de Psiquiatras de Lengua Espanola), Editorial Garsi S.A. (Subsidiary of: Grupo Masson), Juan Bravo, 46, Madrid 28006, Spain. TEL 34-91-402-1212, FAX 34-91-402-0954, garsi@mad.servicom.es, http://www.masson.es. Ed. Dr. Francisco Alonso Fernandez. adv.: B&W page ESP 107,000, color page ESP 127,000; 280 x 210. Circ: 700. **Co-sponsor:** Asociacion Espanola de Psiquiatria y Psicopatologia.

616.89 ITA ISSN 1123-766X
PSICOTERAPIA; clinica - epistemologia - ricerca. Text in Italian. 1995. 3/yr. ITL 85,000 to individuals; ITL 130,000 to institutions. **Document type:** *Academic/Scholarly.* **Description:** Covers clinical practice, epistemology and research in psychotherapy.
Indexed: e-psyche.
Published by: Moretti e Vitalli Editori, Via Betty Ambiveri 15, Bergamo, BG 24126, Italy. TEL 39-35-321588, FAX 39-35-321647. Ed. Marco Casonato.

616.891 001.3 ITA
PSICOTERAPIA E SCIENZE UMANE. Text in Italian. 1967. q. ITL 75,000; ITL 95,000 foreign (effective 1993).
Indexed: IBZ, e-psyche.
Published by: Franco Angeli Editore, Casella Postale 17175, Viale Monza, 106, Milan, MI 20127, Italy. TEL 02-2895762.

150 COL ISSN 0121-8913
PSIQUE. Text in Spanish. 1991. s-a. USD 7 newsstand/cover (effective 2000). **Document type:** *Journal, Academic/Scholarly.*
Published by: Universidad de Antioquia, Facultad de Ciencias Humanas, Apod. Aereo 1226, Medellin, ANT, Colombia. TEL 57-4-210-5763, FAX 57-4-210-5764, cspsique@antares.udea.edu.co, http://antares.udea.edu.co/~cspsique.

616.8 BRA ISSN 0104-7787
CODEN: PSBIFL
PSIQUIATRIA BIOLOGICA. Text in Portuguese, Spanish; Summaries in English, Portuguese, Spanish. 1993. q., latest vol.7, 1999. BRL 48, USD 80 (effective 2000). bk.rev. abstr, bibl, charts, illus. back issues avail. *Refereed.* **Document type:** *Magazine, Academic/Scholarly.* **Description:** Presents studies in clinical psychiatry. Biological psychiatry.
Indexed: Chem.Abstr., Ref.Zh., e-psyche.
—BLDSC (6945.933000), KNAW.
Published by: Associacao Brasileira de Psiquiatria Biologica, Rua do Ouro, 686, Serra, Belo Horizonte, MG 30220-000, Brazil. TEL 55-31-223-2389, FAX 55-31-223-2197, dacosta@ez-bh.com.br. Eds. Carlos Roberto Hojaij, Delcir da Costa. R&P, Adv. contact M. Luiza Carvalho. Circ: 5,000 (paid and controlled).

616.8 ESP ISSN 1134-5934
PSIQUIATRIA BIOLOGICA. Text in Spanish. 1994. bi-m. USD 101. **Document type:** *Academic/Scholarly.*
Indexed: e-psyche.
—**CCC.**
Published by: (Sociedad Espanola de Psiquiatria Biologica), Ediciones Doyma S.A., Traversa de Gracia, 17-21, Barcelona 08021, Spain. TEL 34-93-200-0711, FAX 34-93-209-1136. Ed. Carlos Ballus Pascual. adv.: color page ESP 238,000. Circ: 2,000.

616.89 ESP ISSN 0213-8972
PSIQUIATRIA PUBLICA. Text in Spanish; Summaries in English, French, Italian, Spanish. 1987. bi-m. ESP 3,900. adv. bk.rev. *Refereed.* **Document type:** *Trade.* **Description:** Includes reviews, original research work, clinical cases, debates, and continuous education material.
Indexed: e-psyche.
Published by: Jarpyo Editores S.A., Antonio Lopez Aguado, 4, Madrid 28029, Spain. TEL 34-913-144338, FAX 34-913-144499. Ed. Manuel Delviat. Circ: 3,000.

616.8 614.58 ESP ISSN 0210-8348
PSIQUIS; revista de psiquiatria, psicologia y psicosomatica. Text in Spanish. 1979. 6/yr. ESP 7,500 domestic; USD 80 in Europe; USD 100 elsewhere (effective 2001). adv. charts. *Refereed.* **Document type:** *Journal, Academic/Scholarly.* **Description:** Publishes original review articles in the fields of psychiatry and psychology.
Indexed: Curr.Cont. (coverage dropped), Excerp.Med. (1993-), Ind.Med.Esp., PsycInfo, Psychol.Abstr. (1981-), SSCI (coverage dropped), e-psyche.
—BLDSC (6945.935500), CINDOC, CISTI, GNLM, Infotrieve. **CCC.**
Published by: Alpe Editores S.A., Pedro Rico, 27, Madrid 28029, Spain. TEL 34-91-733-8811, FAX 34-91-315-9652, alpeeditores@sistelcom.com. Ed. Dr. J L Gonzalez de Rivera. Pub. Angeles Alvarez Sanchez. Adv. contact Ana Jurado. color page ESP 160,000; trim 280 x 210. Circ: 4,500 (controlled).

616.81 DEU ISSN 0949-1619
PSYCH. PFLEGE HEUTE; Fachzeitschrift fuer die psychiatrische Pflege. Variant title: Psychiatrische Pflege Heute. Text in German. 1995. bi-m. EUR 81.80 domestic to institutions; EUR 85.90 in Europe to institutions; EUR 90.80 elsewhere to institutions; EUR 15 newsstand/cover (effective 2002). adv. back issues avail.; reprints avail. *Refereed.* **Document type:** *Journal, Academic/Scholarly.*
Related titles: Online - full text ed.: ISSN 1439-0213.
Indexed: e-psyche.
—GNLM.
Published by: Georg Thieme Verlag, Ruedigerstr 14, Stuttgart 70469, Germany. TEL 49-711-8931-0, FAX 49-711-8931298, kunden.service@thieme.de, http://www.thieme.de/psychpflege. Ed. Hilde Schaedle Deiniger. Pub. Albrecht Hauff. R&P Peter Eich. Adv. contact Manfred Marggraf. page DEM 2,150; 175 x 250. Circ: 2,400 (paid).

616.89 HRV ISSN 0353-5053
CODEN: PSYDEI
PSYCHIATRIA DANUBINA. Text in Croatian. 1989. 4/yr. DEM 100 to individuals; DEM 150 to institutions (effective 2000). **Document type:** *Academic/Scholarly.*
Indexed: Excerp.Med., PsycInfo, Psychol.Abstr. (1991-), e-psyche.
—BLDSC (6946.124000), EMDOCS, GNLM.
Published by: University of Zagreb, School of Medicine, c/o Psychiatric University Clinic, Kispaticeva 12, Zabreb 10000, Croatia. TEL 385-1-233043. Ed. Dr. Miro Jakovljevic.

616.8 JPN ISSN 0033-2658
CODEN: SSHZAS
PSYCHIATRIA ET NEUROLOGIA JAPONICA/SEISHIN SHINKEIGAKU ZASSHI. Text in Japanese; Summaries in English, Japanese. 1962. m. adv. bibl, charts, illus. index.
Indexed: Biol.Abstr., Chem.Abstr., INIS Atomind., Ind.Med. (1935-), Inpharma, Int.Nurs.Ind., Reac., e-psyche.
—BLDSC (6946.130000), CISTI, GNLM.
Published by: Japanese Society of Psychiatry and Neurology/Nihon Seishin Shinkei Gakkai, 38-11 Hongo 3-chome, Bunkyo-ku, Tokyo 113-0033, Japan.

616.8 FIN ISSN 0079-7227
RC321 CODEN: PSFNBI
PSYCHIATRIA FENNICA. Text mainly in English. 1970. a. FIM 260 (effective 2000). adv. bk.rev. **Document type:** *Academic/Scholarly.*
Indexed: Biol.Abstr., CINAHL, Excerp.Med., PsycInfo, Psychol.Abstr. (1972-), e-psyche.
—BLDSC (6946.160000), GNLM, KNAW.
Published by: (Foundation for Psychiatric Research in Finland), Psychiatria Fennica, Arkadiankatu 21 B 20, Helsinki 00100, Finland. FAX 358-9-409663. Ed. J K Lonnqvist. R&P, Adv. contact Ani Ostamo TEL 358-9-494-077. Circ: 1,600.

616.8 FIN ISSN 0355-7707
CODEN: MPFEE8
PSYCHIATRIA FENNICA. MONOGRAFIASARJA/ PSYCHIATRIA FENNICA. MONOGRAPHS. Text in English, Finnish. 1970. irreg. price varies.
Indexed: Excerp.Med., Psychol.Abstr., e-psyche.
Published by: Psychiatria Fennica, Arkadiankatu 21 B 20, Helsinki 00100, Finland. FAX 358-9-409663. Circ: 900.

616.8 FIN ISSN 0359-3207
PSYCHIATRIA FENNICA. REPORTS. Key Title: Reports of Psychiatria Fennica. Text mainly in Finnish. 1970. irreg. price varies.
Former titles: Psychiatria Fennica. Julkaisusarja (0355-7693); Helsingin Yliopisto Keskussairaala. Psykiatrian Klinikka. Julkaisusarja (0073-1730)
Indexed: Excerp.Med., Psychol.Abstr., e-psyche.
Published by: (Foundation for Psychiatric Research in Finland), Psychiatria Fennica, Arkadiankatu 21 B 20, Helsinki 00100, Finland. FAX 358-9-409663. Ed. Marti Heikkinen. R&P, Adv. contact Ani Ostamo TEL 358-9-494-077. Circ: 400.

616.89 POL ISSN 0033-2674
CODEN: PSPOB3
PSYCHIATRIA POLSKA. Text in Polish; Summaries in English, French, German, Russian. 1923. bi-m. PLZ 60 (effective 2002). adv. bk.rev. abstr, bibl, illus. index. 150 p./no. 1 cols./p. Supplement avail.; back issues avail. *Refereed.* **Document type:** *Academic/Scholarly.* **Description:** Publishes research, clinical experimental reports and theoretical papers in the field of psychiatry.
Formerly (until 1967): Rocznik Psychiatryczny
Related titles: Online - full text ed.
Indexed: Biol.Abstr., Chem.Abstr., Excerp.Med., Ind.Med. (1967-), Int.Nurs.Ind., PsycInfo, Psychol.Abstr., e-psyche.
—BLDSC (6946.210000), CISTI, GNLM.
Published by: Polskie Towarzystwo Psychiatryczne, Ul Lenartowicza 14, Krakow 31138, Poland. TEL 48-12-6331203, FAX 48-12-6334067, psych@kom-red-wyd-ptp.com.pl, http://www.kom-red-wyd-ptp.com.pl/1en.html. Ed., Pub., R&P, Adv. contact Jerzy W Aleksandrowicz. page PLZ 1,600. Circ: 1,500.

616.89 USA ISSN 0048-5713
RC321 CODEN: PSANCS
PSYCHIATRIC ANNALS. Text in English. 1971. m. USD 120 to individuals; USD 140 in Canada to individuals; USD 160 elsewhere to individuals; USD 135 to institutions; USD 155 in Canada to institutions; USD 175 elsewhere to institutions. bk.rev. illus. index. reprint service avail. from PQC,ISI. *Refereed.* **Document type:** *Academic/Scholarly.* **Description:** Provides a thorough, multi-authored look at a single topic in psychiatry.
Related titles: Microform ed.: (from PQC); Online - full text ed.: (from Northern Light Technology, Inc., ProQuest Information & Learning, Institute for Scientific Information).
Indexed: ASCA, Adol.Ment.Hlth.Abstr., AgeLine, Biol.Abstr., Crim.Just.Abstr., Curr.Cont., Excerp.Med., Fam.Ind., Mid.East: Abstr.& Ind., Neurosci.Cit.Ind., PsycInfo, Psychol.Abstr. (1971-), SSCI, Soc.Sci.Ind. (coverage dropped), e-psyche.
—BLDSC (6946.212000), CISTI, GNLM, IDS, ingenta, KNAW. **CCC.**
Published by: Slack, Inc., 6900 Grove Rd, Thorofare, NJ 08086-9447. TEL 856-848-1000, 800-257-8290, FAX 856-853-5991, http://www.slackinc.com. Ed. Dr. Jan Fawcett. Circ: 30,035.

616.8 GBR ISSN 0955-6036
CODEN: PBULE5
PSYCHIATRIC BULLETIN. Text in English. 1971. m. GBP 55, USD 81 (effective 1999). bk.rev. *Refereed.* **Document type:** *Academic/Scholarly.*
Formerly: Royal College of Psychiatrists. Bulletin (0140-0789)
Related titles: Online - full text ed.: (from HighWire Pr., EBSCO Publishing).
Indexed: ASSIA, Abstr.Crim.& Pen., Addic.Abstr., Excerp.Med. (1995-), Hosp.Abstr., Lang.& Lang.Behav.Abstr., PsycInfo, SOPODA, Sociol.Abstr., e-psyche.
—BLDSC (6946.212400), GNLM, Infotrieve. **CCC.**
Published by: Royal College of Psychiatrists, 17 Belgrave Sq, London SW1X 8PG, United Kingdom. TEL 44-20-7235-8857, FAX 44-20-7245-1231. Ed. Tom Fuhy. Circ: 9,000. **Subscr. to:** Royal Society of Medicine Services Ltd., 1 Wimpole St, London W1G 0AE, United Kingdom. TEL 44-20-7290-2928, FAX 44-20-7290-2929.

616.89 GBR ISSN 1352-9579
PSYCHIATRIC CARE. Text in English. 1994. bi-m. GBP 45 to individuals; GBP 90 to institutions. adv. bk.rev. index. back issues avail. *Refereed.* **Document type:** *Academic/Scholarly.* **Description:** Research-based journal for all professionals concerned with the care of people with mental illness in hospital, forensic and community settings.
Related titles: Online - full text ed.: (from RoweCom Information Quest).
Indexed: Brit.Nur.Ind., CINAHL, e-psyche.
—CCC.
Published by: (Forensic Psychiatric Nurses Association), Nature Publishing Group Specialist Journals (Subsidiary of: Holtzbrink Publishers), Houndmills, Basingstoke, Hants RG21 6XS, United Kingdom. TEL 44-1256-329242, FAX 44-1256-328339, s.marshall@stockton-press.co.uk, subscriptions@nature.com, http://www.stockton-press.co.uk/pc/, http://www.nature.com. Ed. David Sallah. Pub. Katarine Hinton. Adv. contact Robert Sloan TEL 44-20-8882-7199. B&W page GBP 595, color page GBP 1,090; trim 210 x 297.

616.8 USA ISSN 1068-3178
RC483
PSYCHIATRIC CLINICS: ANNUAL OF DRUG THERAPY. Text in English. 1994. a. USD 89 domestic; USD 98 foreign (effective 2001). **Document type:** *Academic/Scholarly.* **Description:** Summarizes the year's developments in the pharmaceutical treatment of psychiatric disorders.
Indexed: Adol.Ment.Hlth.Abstr., Curr.Adv.Ecol.Sci., Curr.Cont. (coverage dropped), Ind.Med. (coverage dropped), Psychol.Abstr., SSCI (coverage dropped), e-psyche.
—GNLM.
Published by: W.B. Saunders Co. (Subsidiary of: Harcourt Publishers Ltd.), 11830 Westline Industrial Dr, St Louis, MO 63146. TEL 800-325-4177, http://www.wbsaunders.com. Eds. Dr. David L Dunner, Jerrold F Rosenbaum. **Subscr. to:** Periodicals Fulfillment, W B Saunders Co, 6277 Sea Harbor Dr, 4th Fl, Orlando, FL 32891-4800.

616.89 USA ISSN 0193-953X
RC321
PSYCHIATRIC CLINICS OF NORTH AMERICA. Text in English. 1978. q. USD 143 domestic to individuals; USD 172 in Canada to individuals; USD 199 elsewhere to individuals; USD 212 domestic to institutions; USD 256 foreign to institutions; USD 65 per issue (effective 2001). bibl, illus. index, cum.index. reprint service avail. from PQC. *Refereed.* **Document type:** *Journal, Academic/Scholarly.*
Related titles: Online - full text ed.: (from Institute for Scientific Information).
Indexed: ASCA, Adol.Ment.Hlth.Abstr., AgeLine, CINAHL, Curr.Adv.Ecol.Sci., Curr.Cont., Fam.Ind., INIS Atomind., Ind.Med. (1978-), Inpharma, Neurosci.Cit.Ind., Pharm.&Out.News, PsycInfo, Psychol.Abstr. (1982-), Reac., Rev.Appl.Entomol., SSCI, e-psyche.
—BLDSC (6946.212500), CISTI, GNLM, IDS, ingenta, KNAW. **CCC.**
Published by: W.B. Saunders Co. (Subsidiary of: Harcourt Publishers Ltd.), 11830 Westline Industrial Dr, St Louis, MO 63146. TEL 800-325-4177, http://www.wbsaunders.com. **Subscr. to:** Periodicals Fulfillment, W B Saunders Co, 6277 Sea Harbor Dr, 4th Fl, Orlando, FL 32891-4800.

616.89 USA ISSN 0033-2690
RC321 CODEN: PSYFAK
PSYCHIATRIC FORUM. Text in English. 1969. s-a. free per issue. bk.rev. **Document type:** *Academic/Scholarly.* **Description:** Contains original articles related to mental health.
Indexed: Adol.Ment.Hlth.Abstr., CINAHL, Chicago Psychoanal.Lit.Ind., Curr.Cont. (coverage dropped), Psychol.Abstr. (1971-), SSCI (coverage dropped), e-psyche.
—CISTI, GNLM.
Published by: Department of Mental Health, William S. Hall Psychiatric Institute, PO Box 202, Columbia, SC 29202. TEL 803-734-7154, FAX 803-734-4416, SRL97. Ed., R&P Lucius C Pressley. Circ: 4,000 (controlled).

PSYCHIATRIC GENETICS. see *BIOLOGY—Genetics*

616.8 USA
PSYCHIATRIC LENGTH OF STAY SERIES. Text in English. 1985. a.
Related titles: Regional ed.: Psychiatric Length of Stay Series (Northcentral Edition); Psychiatric Length of Stay Series (Northeastern Edition); Psychiatric Length of Stay Series (Southern Edition); Psychiatric Length of Stay Series (Western Edition).
Indexed: SRI, e-psyche.
Published by: H C I A Inc., 300 E Lombard St, Baltimore, MD 21202. TEL 800-568-3282, FAX 410-752-6309.

616.8 USA ISSN 0732-0868
CODEN: PSMDEQ
PSYCHIATRIC MEDICINE✱ . Text in English. 1983. q. USD 55 to individuals; USD 75 to institutions. back issues avail.
Indexed: Chem.Abstr., Psychol.Abstr., e-psyche.
—CISTI, GNLM.
Published by: S P Medical & Scientific Books, Inc. (Subsidiary of: Spectrum Publications, Inc.), c/o Fisher, 200 Park Ave S, New York, NY 10003-1503. Ed. Dr. Richard C W Hall. Circ: 500.

616.89 USA ISSN 0033-2704
RC321
PSYCHIATRIC NEWS. Text in English. 1966. bi-w. USD 62 domestic to individuals for print & online eds.; USD 159 foreign to institutions for print & online eds.; USD 109 for domestic institution or foreign individual: for print & online eds. (effective 2001). adv. bk.rev. stat. back issues avail.; reprint service avail. from PQC. **Document type:** *Journal.* **Description:** Delivers current information on everything from legislative activities to the latest developments in the drug and therapy fields.
Formerly: American Psychiatric Association. Newsletter
Related titles: Microform ed.: (from PQC); Online - full text ed.: (from EBSCO Publishing, HighWire Pr.).
Indexed: Abstr.Crim.& Pen., Ind.Per.Art.Relat.Law, Ref.Zh., Soc.Work Res.& Abstr., e-psyche.
—BLDSC (6946.215000), GNLM. **CCC.**

M

Published by: (American Psychiatric Association), American Psychiatric Press, Inc., Journals Division, 1400 K St, N W, Ste 1101, Washington, DC 20005. TEL 202-682-6210, 800-368-5777, FAX 202-789-2648, appi@psych.org, http://pn.psychiatryonline.org, http://www.psych.org/pnews/index.html, http://www.appi.org. Ed. James P Krajeski. adv.: B&W page USD 3,570, color page USD 4,820. Circ: 37,000.

616.89 USA ISSN 0033-2720 CODEN: PSQUAP
PSYCHIATRIC QUARTERLY. Text in English. 1927. q. USD 550, EUR 660 to institutions (effective 2002). adv. back issues avail.; reprint service avail. from PQC,PSC,SCH,ISI. *Refereed.* **Document type:** *Academic/Scholarly.* **Description:** Includes articles on the social, clinical, administrative, legal, political, and ethical aspects of mental illness care. Presents pertinent scientific and delivery system data.
Related titles: Microform ed.: (from PQC); Online - full text ed.: USD 445 domestic; USD 520 foreign (effective 2000) (from EBSCO Publishing, O C L C Online Computer Library Center, Inc., RoweCom Information Quest, Swets Blackwell, Kluwer Online, Institute for Scientific Information).
Indexed: ASCA, Abstr.Health Care Manage.Stud., Adol.Ment.Hlth.Abstr., AgeLine, Biol.Abstr., CINAHL, Community Ment.Health Rev., Crim.Just.Abstr., Curr.Cont., Excerp.Med., Fam.Ind., Hosp.Lit.Ind., Ind.Med. (1927-), Indian Psychol.Abstr., Lang.& Lang.Behav.Abstr., P C I, PsycInfo, Psychol.Abstr. (1977-), SOPODA, SSCI, Sociol.Abstr., e-psyche.
—BLDSC (6946.240000), CISTI, GNLM, IDS, ingenta, KNAW. **CCC.**
Published by: (New York School of Psychiatry), Human Sciences Press, Inc., 233 Spring St., New York, NY 10013-1578. TEL 212-620-8000. Ed. Stephen Rachlin. Circ: 3,400 (paid).

616.89 362.2 USA
RC439.5
PSYCHIATRIC REHABILITATION JOURNAL. Text in English. 1976. q. USD 50 to individuals; USD 60 in Canada to individuals; USD 73 elsewhere to individuals; USD 93 to institutions; USD 105 in Canada to institutions; USD 115 elsewhere to institutions. adv. bk.rev. reprint service avail. from PQC. *Refereed.* **Document type:** *Academic/Scholarly.* **Description:** Provides information relevant to the rehabilitation of persons with severe psychiatric disability. Publishes papers from mental health and rehabilitation professionals, consumers and family members.
Formed by the 1995 merger of: Psychosocial Rehabilitation Journal (0147-5622); Innovations and Research (1062-7553)
Related titles: Microfilm ed.
Indexed: ASCA, Adol.Ment.Hlth.Abstr., CINAHL, Community Ment.Health Rev., Crim.Just.Abstr., Curr.Cont., Fam.Ind., Ind.Med. (coverage dropped), Lang.& Lang.Behav.Abstr., Nurs.Abstr., PsycInfo, Psychol.Abstr. (1977-), Rehabil.Lit., SOPODA, SSCI, Sage Fam.Stud.Abstr., Soc.Work Res.& Abstr., Sociol.Abstr., Viol.& Abuse Abstr., e-psyche.
—BLDSC, IDS, Infotrieve, ingenta. **CCC.**
Published by: Boston University, Department of Rehabilitation Counseling, 930 Commonwealth Ave, Boston, MA 02215. TEL 617-353-3549, FAX 617-353-9209. Eds. Irvin Rutman, William Anthony. Pub. Dr. Leroy Spaniol. Circ: 1,300. **Co-sponsor:** International Association of Psychosocial Rehabilitation Services.

616.8 USA ISSN 1097-3435
PSYCHIATRIC REHABILITATION SKILLS. Text in English. 1996. s-a. **Document type:** *Academic/Scholarly.*
—BLDSC (6946.240800).
Published by: Recovery Press, The University of Chicago, Center for Psychiatric Rehabilitation, 7230 Arbor Dr, Tinley Part, IL 60477. TEL 708-614-4770, FAX 708-614-4780.

616.89 USA ISSN 1075-2730
RC443.A1 CODEN: PSSEFQ
PSYCHIATRIC SERVICES. Text in English. 1950. m. USD 51 domestic to individuals; USD 74 foreign to individuals; USD 85 domestic to institutions; USD 108 foreign to institutions (effective 2001). adv. bk.rev., video rev. charts, illus, stat. index. back issues avail.; reprint service avail. from PSC,SCH. *Refereed.* **Document type:** *Journal.* **Description:** Interdisciplinary journal providing coverage of all aspects of psychiatric treatment and service delivery.
Former titles (until 1994): Hospital and Community Psychiatry (0022-1597); Mental Hospitals (0096-5502)
Related titles: Microform ed.: (from MIM,PQC); Online - full text ed.: (from HighWire Pr., EBSCO Publishing, Institute for Scientific Information).
Indexed: AMED, ASCA, Abstr.Health Care Manage.Stud., AgeLine, Arts & Hum.Cit.Ind. (coverage dropped), Biol.Abstr., CINAHL, Chic.Per.Ind., Crim.Just.Abstr., Curr.Cont., Curr.Lit.Fam.Plan., Environ.Sci.Poll.Mgmt., Excerp.Med., Fam.Ind., Hosp.Lit.Ind., Ind.Med. (1995-), Ind.Sci.Rev., Indian Psychol.Abstr., Inpharma, Int.Nurs.Ind., Jrnl.Watch Psych., Jrnl.Watch Wom.Hlth., Media Rev.Dig. (Jan.1989-Dec.1990), Neurosci.Cit.Ind., Past.Care & Couns.Abstr., Pharm.&Out.News, PsycInfo, Psychol.Abstr. (1960-), Reac., Risk Abstr., SSCI, Saf.Sci.Abstr., Sci.Cit.Ind., Soc.Work Res.& Abstr., e-psyche.
—BLDSC (6946.242300), CISTI, GNLM, IDS, ingenta, KNAW. **CCC.**
Published by: (American Psychiatric Association), American Psychiatric Press, Inc., Journals Division, 1400 K St, N W, Ste 1101, Washington, DC 20005. TEL 202-682-6070, 800-368-5777, FAX 202-682-6189, psjournal@psych.org, appi@psych.org, http://psychservices.psychiatryonline.org/, http://www.psychiatryonline.org, http://www.appi.org. Ed. Dr. John A Talbott. adv.: B&W page USD 1,805, color page USD 2,805. Circ: 20,000.

616.89 USA ISSN 0893-2905
PSYCHIATRIC TIMES. Text in English. 1985. m. USD 49 domestic to individuals; USD 120 foreign to individuals. adv. bk.rev. *Refereed.* **Document type:** *Newspaper, Trade.* **Description:** Psychiatric news journal of interest to psychiatrists, mental health professionals and others in healthcare professions.
Related titles: Online - full text ed.
Indexed: CINAHL, e-psyche.
—BLDSC (6946.242600).
Published by: C M E Inc., 2801 McGaw Ave, Irvine, CA 92614-5835. TEL 949-250-1008, 800-447-4474, FAX 949-250-0445, psychtimes@aol.com, http://www.mhsource.com. Ed. Dr. John L Schwartz. Pub. David Deninno. R&P Christine Potrin. Adv. contact Rosemarie DeLuca. B&W page USD 4,515, color page USD 5,710. Circ: 42,445 (controlled).

616.89 FRA
PSYCHIATRIE. Text in French. 1983. m. FRF 460 domestic to individuals; FRF 580, USD 105 foreign to individuals; FRF 580 domestic to institutions; FRF 700, USD 127 foreign to institutions; FRF 290 domestic to students; USD 75 foreign to students (effective 2000). adv. *Refereed.* **Document type:** *Academic/Scholarly.*
Indexed: e-psyche.
—BLDSC.
Published by: Medica-Press International, 62-64 rue Jean-Jaures, Puteaux 92800, France. TEL 33-1-41458000, FAX 33-1-41458025, contact@edimark.fr, http://www.edimark.fr. Ed. C S Perletti. Pub. Claudie Damour Terrasson.

LA PSYCHIATRIE DE L'ENFANT. see *MEDICAL SCIENCES—Pediatrics*

616.8 DEU ISSN 0303-4259
PSYCHIATRISCHE PRAXIS. Text in German; Summaries in English, German. 1974. 8/yr. EUR 165.80 domestic to institutions; EUR 174.40 in Europe to institutions; EUR 183.20 elsewhere to institutions; EUR 78 to students; EUR 25 newsstand/cover (effective 2002). adv. bk.rev. bibl, charts, illus. index. back issues avail.; reprint service avail. from PQC. *Refereed.* **Document type:** *Journal, Academic/Scholarly.*
Related titles: Online - full text ed.: ISSN 1439-989X (from Institute for Scientific Information); ♦ Supplement: Psychiatrische Praxis. Supplement. ISSN 0934-3008.
Indexed: ASCA, Biol.Abstr., Curr.Cont., Excerp.Med., Ger.J.Psych., Ind.Med. (1974-), Int.Nurs.Ind., Risk Abstr., SSCI, e-psyche.
—BLDSC (6946.258000), CISTI, EMDOCS, GNLM, IDS, Infotrieve, KNAW. **CCC.**
Published by: Georg Thieme Verlag, Ruedigerstr 14, Stuttgart 70469, Germany. TEL 49-711-8931-0, FAX 49-711-8931298, leser.service@thieme.de, http://www.thieme.de/psychiat-praxis, http://www.thieme-connect.de. Ed. A Finzen. R&P Peter Eich. adv.: page DEM 1,800; 175 x 250. Circ: 1,800 (paid).

616.8 DEU ISSN 0934-3008
PSYCHIATRISCHE PRAXIS. SUPPLEMENT. Text in German. irreg. price varies. back issues avail.; reprints avail. *Refereed.* **Document type:** *Monographic series, Academic/Scholarly.*
Related titles: Online - full text ed.; ♦ Supplement to: Psychiatrische Praxis. ISSN 0303-4259.
Indexed: Excerp.Med. (1994-), e-psyche.
—EMDOCS.
Published by: Georg Thieme Verlag, Ruedigerstr 14, Stuttgart 70469, Germany. TEL 0711-8931-0, FAX 49-711-8931258, leser.service@thieme.de, http://www.thieme.de, http://www.thieme-connect.de.

616.8 CAN ISSN 0838-7982
PSYCHIATRY. Text in English. 1987. 4/yr.
Related titles: Online - full text ed.: (from Northern Light Technology, Inc.).
Indexed: Soc.Sci.Ind. (coverage dropped), e-psyche.
Published by: M P I Medical Publishing Inc., 14 Ronan Ave, Toronto, ON M4N 2X9, Canada. TEL 416-481-6384. Ed. Dr. Vivian Rakoff. Circ: 14,123.

616.89 USA ISSN 0033-2747
RC321 CODEN: PSYCAB
PSYCHIATRY; interpersonal and biological processes. Text in English. 1937. q. USD 50 domestic to individuals; USD 75 foreign to individuals; USD 185 domestic to institutions; USD 210 foreign to institutions (effective 2000). adv. bk.rev. index, cum.index: 1938-1967, 1968-1977. back issues avail.; reprint service avail. from PQC,PSC,SCH,ISI. *Refereed.* **Document type:** *Academic/Scholarly.* **Description:** New and controversial issues in psychiatry and related social and biological science disciplines.
Related titles: Microform ed.: (from MIM,PQC); Online - full text ed.: (from Northern Light Technology, Inc., ProQuest Information & Learning, Gale Group, CatchWord Ltd., Factiva, Institute for Scientific Information, RoweCom Information Quest).
Indexed: ASSIA, Abstr.Anthropol., Abstr.Crim.& Pen., Addic.Abstr., Adol.Ment.Hlth.Abstr., AgeLine, Amer.Bibl.Slavic & E.Eur.Stud., Bibl.Asian Stud. (1971), Biol.Abstr., Child Devel.Abstr., Curr.Cont., Excerp.Med., Hist.Abstr. (1970-1984, dropped), Hosp.Lit.Ind., IBZ, INIS Atomind., Ind.Med. (1938-), Int.Nurs.Ind., Lang.& Lang.Behav.Abstr., MLA Intl.Bibl., Mid.East: Abstr.& Ind., P C I, PsycInfo, Psychol.Abstr. (1938-), SOPODA, SSCI, Sage Fam.Stud.Abstr., Sage Urb.Stud.Abstr., Sci.Cit.Ind., Soc.Sci.Ind. (Feb.1982-), Soc.Work Res.& Abstr., Sociol.Abstr., e-psyche.
—BLDSC (6946.260000), CISTI, GNLM, IDS, ingenta, KNAW. **CCC.**
Published by: (Washington School of Psychiatry), Guilford Publications, Inc., 72 Spring St, 4th Fl, New York, NY 10012. TEL 212-431-9800, 800-365-7006, FAX 212-966-6708, info@guilford.com. Ed. Dr. Robert Ursano. Pub. Robert Matloff. R&P Kathy Kuehl. Adv. contact Susan Pavliscak. Circ: 2,200.

616.8 AUS ISSN 1323-1316 CODEN: PCNEFP
PSYCHIATRY AND CLINICAL NEUROSCIENCES. Text in English. 1933. 6/yr. AUD 298 domestic to individuals; AUD 270 in New Zealand to individuals; USD 165 elsewhere to individuals; AUD 1,046 domestic to institutions; AUD 951 in New Zealand to institutions; JPY 70,650 in Japan to institutions; USD 580 elsewhere to institutions; AUD 328 domestic to individuals print & online eds. combined; AUD 297 in New Zealand to individuals print & online eds. combined; USD 182 elsewhere to individuals print & online eds. combined; AUD 1,151 domestic to institutions print & online eds. combined; AUD 1,047 in New Zealand to institutions print & online eds. combined; JPY 77,715 in Japan to institutions print & online eds. combined; USD 638 elsewhere to institutions print & online eds. combined (effective 2001). adv. abstr. back issues avail. *Refereed.* **Document type:** *Journal, Academic/Scholarly.* **Description:** Publishes original resarch and reviews in all fields of psychiatry and related areas of the neurosciences.
Former titles (until 1995): Japanese Journal of Psychiatry and Neurology (0912-2036); (until 1986): Folia Psychiatrica et Neurologica Japonica (0015-5721)
Related titles: Online - full text ed.: ISSN 1440-1819. AUD 269 domestic to individuals; AUD 243 in New Zealand to individuals; USD 149 elsewhere to individuals; AUD 942 domestic to institutions; AUD 856 in New Zealand to institutions; JPY 63,585 in Japan to institutions; USD 522 elsewhere to institutions (effective 2001) (from EBSCO Publishing, O C L C Online Computer Library Center, Inc., RoweCom Information Quest, ingenta, Munksgaard & Blackwell Science's Synergy, Swets Blackwell, Institute for Scientific Information); Japanese ed.: ISSN 1341-0695.
Indexed: ASCA, ASSIA, Biol.Abstr., Chem.Abstr., Chem.Titles, Curr.Cont., Excerp.Med., INIS Atomind., Ind.Med. (1995-), Inpharma, Int.Nurs.Ind., Lang.& Lang.Behav.Abstr., Neurosci.Cit.Ind., Pharm.&Out.News, Psychol.Abstr., Reac., SOPODA, SSCI (coverage dropped), Sociol.Abstr., e-psyche.
—BLDSC (6946.260550), CASDDS, CISTI, EMDOCS, GNLM, IDS, ingenta, KNAW. **CCC.**

M

Published by: (Folia Publishing Society JPN), Blackwell Science Asia Pty Ltd, PO Box 378, Carlton South, VIC 3053, Australia. TEL 61-3-9347-0300, FAX 61-3-9347-5001, info@blacksci-asia.com.au, http://www.blacksci.co.uk. Eds. Saburo Takahishi, Yutaka Honda.

PSYCHIATRY DRUG ALERTS. see *PHARMACY AND PHARMACOLOGY*

616.8 GBR ISSN 0262-5377
PSYCHIATRY IN PRACTICE. Abbreviated title: P I P. Text in English. 1981; N.S. 1990. q. adv. bk.rev. **Document type:** *Academic/Scholarly.*
Indexed: e-psyche.
Published by: Hayward Medical Communications Ltd., Covent Garden, Seven Dials Warehouse, 44 Earlham St, London WC2H 9LA, United Kingdom. TEL 44-20-7240-4493, FAX 44-20-7240-4479, admin@hayward.co.uk, http://www.hayward.co.uk. Ed. Dr. Frank Smith. Circ: 23,000. **Subscr. to:** Rosemary House, Lanwades Park, Kentford, Near, Newmarket, Suffolk CB8 7PW, United Kingdom. TEL 44-1638-751515, FAX 44-1638-751517.

616.8 USA
PSYCHIATRY IN PROGRESS. Text in English. irreg., latest vol.3, 1996. **Document type:** *Monographic series, Academic/Scholarly.*
Indexed: e-psyche.
—BLDSC.
Published by: Hogrefe & Huber Publishers, PO Box 2487, Kirkland, WA 98083. TEL 425-820-1500, FAX 425-823-8324.

616.8 IRL
PSYCHIATRY - IRELAND. Text in English. 6/yr.
Indexed: e-psyche.
Address: 38 Albert College Park, Glasnevin, Dublin 9, Ireland. TEL 374447. Ed. Patrick O'Sullivan. Circ: 2,000.

616.89 GBR ISSN 1359-7620
PSYCHIATRY ON-LINE. Variant title: International Forum for Psychiatry. Text in English. 1994. m. free per issue. bk.rev., film rev., software rev., video rev., Website rev. *Refereed.* **Document type:** *Journal, Academic/Scholarly.* **Description:** Publishes case reports, audit, treatment protocols and review papers and research.
Media: Online - full text.
Indexed: e-psyche.
Published by: Priory Lodge Education Ltd., 2 Cornflower Way, Moreton, Wirral CH46 1SV, United Kingdom. TEL 44-151-606-1796, FAX 44-151-606-1812, ben@priory.com, solutions@priory.com, http://www.priory.co.uk/psych.htm, http://www.priory.com/. Ed. Dr. Ben Green. Circ: 60,000 (controlled).

616.8 340.6 AUS ISSN 1321-8719
CODEN: PPLAFQ
PSYCHIATRY PSYCHOLOGY AND LAW. Text in English. s-a. AUD 75 in Australia & New Zealand to individuals; AUD 90 elsewhere to individuals; AUD 100 in Australia & New Zealand to institutions; AUD 125 elsewhere to institutions (effective 2000). adv. back issues avail. *Refereed.* **Document type:** *Academic/Scholarly.* **Description:** Presents articles on topics relevant to forensic issues in psychiatry and psychology.
Related titles: Online - full text ed.: (from CatchWord Ltd.).
Indexed: ASSIA, Crim.Just.Abstr., Excerp.Med. (1995-), PsycInfo, e-psyche.
—BLDSC (6946.263650), GNLM.
Published by: (Australian and New Zealand Association of Psychiatry, Psychology and Law), Australian Academic Press Pty. Ltd., 32 Jeays St, Bowen Hills, QLD 4006, Australia. TEL 61-7-32571176, FAX 61-7-32525908, australianacademicpress@compuserve.com, http://www.australianacademicpress.com.au.

616.8 IRL ISSN 0165-1781
RC321 CODEN: PSRSDR
PSYCHIATRY RESEARCH; an international journal for rapid communication. Text in English. 1979. 15/yr. EUR 156 in Europe to individuals; JPY 21,000 in Japan to individuals; USD 175 elsewhere to individuals; EUR 1,784 in Europe to institutions; JPY 237,000 in Japan to institutions; USD 1,996 elsewhere to institutions (effective 2002). illus. back issues avail.; reprint service avail. from SWZ. *Refereed.* **Document type:** *Academic/Scholarly.* **Description:** Publishes research in biochemical, physiological, genetic, psychological and social determinants of behavior, assessment of subjective states, evaluations of somatic and non-somatic psychiatric treatments, and relevant clinically related basic studies from fields such as neuropharmacology and neurochemistry.
Related titles: Microform ed.: (from PQC); Online - full text ed.: (from ingenta, Swets Blackwell, Institute for Scientific Information, ScienceDirect).
Indexed: ASCA, AgeLine, Agri.& Environ.Biotech.Abstr. (coverage dropped), Biol.Abstr., Chem.Abstr., Chem.Indus.Notes, Chem.Titles, Curr.Cont., Derwent Biotech.Abstr., Excerp.Med., Ind.Med. (1979-), Ind.Sci.Rev., Indian Psychol.Abstr., Inpharma, Int.Abstr.Biol.Sci., Int.Nurs.Ind., Neurosci.Cit.Ind., Nutr.Abstr., Pharm.&Out.News, PsycInfo, Psychol.Abstr. (1979-), Reac., SSCI, Sci.Cit.Ind., e-psyche.
—BLDSC (6946.263700), ADONIS, CASDDS, CISTI, EMDOCS, GNLM, IDS, ingenta, KNAW. **CCC.**
Published by: Elsevier Science Ireland Ltd, Elsevier House, Brookvale Plaza, E. Park, Shannon, Co. Clare, Ireland. TEL 353-61-471944, FAX 353-61-472144, http://www.elsevier.com/locate/psychres. Eds. Frederick K Goodwin, Monte S Buchsbaum. R&P Annette Moloney. **Subscr. in Australasia and the Far East to:** Elsevier Science (Singapore) Pte Ltd, No.1 Temasek Ave, 17-01 Millenia Tower, Singapore 039192, Singapore. TEL 65-434-3727, FAX 65-337-2230; **Subscr. in the Americas to:** Elsevier Science, PO Box 945, New York, NY 10159-0945. TEL 212-633-3730, FAX 212-633-3680; **Subscr. to:** Elsevier Science BV, PO Box 211, Amsterdam 1000 AE, Netherlands. TEL 31-20-485-3757, FAX 31-20-485-3432.

616.8 IRL ISSN 0925-4927
PSYCHIATRY RESEARCH: NEUROIMAGING SECTION. Text in English. 1990. 9/yr. EUR 718 in Europe to institutions; JPY 95,400 in Japan to institutions; USD 803 elsewhere to institutions (effective 2002). back issues avail. *Refereed.* **Document type:** *Academic/Scholarly.* **Description:** Publishes manuscripts on positron emission tomography, MRI, computerized electroencephalographic topography and other imaging techniques, results in psychiatric disorders, dementias, and the effects of behavioral tasks and pharmacological treatments.
Related titles: Online - full text ed.: (from ingenta, Swets Blackwell, Institute for Scientific Information, ScienceDirect).
Indexed: ASCA, Biol.Abstr., Chem.Abstr., Curr.Cont., Derwent Biotech.Abstr., Excerp.Med., Ind.Med. (coverage dropped), Ind.Sci.Rev., Inpharma, Int.Abstr.Biol.Sci., Neurosci.Cit.Ind., Pharm.&Out.News, PsycInfo, Psychol.Abstr. (1990-), Reac., SSCI (coverage dropped), Sci.Cit.Ind., e-psyche.
—ADONIS, CISTI, EMDOCS, IDS, Infotrieve, ingenta, KNAW. **CCC.**
Published by: Elsevier Science Ireland Ltd, Elsevier House, Brookvale Plaza, E. Park, Shannon, Co. Clare, Ireland. TEL 353-61-471944, FAX 353-61-472144, http://www.elsevier.com/locate/psychresns. Ed. M S Buchsbaum. R&P Annette Moloney. **Subscr. in Australasia and the Far East to:** Elsevier Science (Singapore) Pte Ltd, No.1 Temasek Ave, 17-01 Millenia Tower, Singapore 039192, Singapore. TEL 65-434-3727, FAX 65-337-2230; **Subscr. in the Americas to:** Elsevier Science, PO Box 945, New York, NY 10159-0945. TEL 212-633-3730, FAX 212-633-3680; **Subscr. to:** Elsevier Science BV, PO Box 211, Amsterdam 1000 AE, Netherlands. TEL 31-20-485-3757, FAX 31-20-485-3432.

PSYCHNEWS INTERNATIONAL. see *PSYCHOLOGY*

616.8 DEU ISSN 0340-7845
PSYCHO; Psychiatrie, Neurologie und Psychotherapie. Text in German. 1975. m. EUR 65 domestic to institutions; EUR 78.80 in Europe to institutions; EUR 105.80 elsewhere to institutions; EUR 43 to students; EUR 8 newsstand/cover (effective 2002). adv. bk.rev. abstr. **Document type:** *Journal, Academic/Scholarly.*
Indexed: Excerp.Med., e-psyche.
—GNLM.
Published by: Demeter Verlag GmbH und Co. KG, Ruedigerstr 14, Stuttgart 70469, Germany. TEL 49-711-8931-0, FAX 49-711-8931322, http://www.demeter-verlag.de. Circ: 6,500.

PSYCHO-ONCOLOGY; journal of the psychological, social and behavioral dimensions of cancer. see *MEDICAL SCIENCES—Oncology*

PSYCHOANALYSE EN CULTUUR/PSYCHOANALYSIS AND CULTURE. see *PSYCHOLOGY*

616.9 USA ISSN 0161-5289
RC500 CODEN: PCTHDS
PSYCHOANALYSIS AND CONTEMPORARY THOUGHT; a quarterly of integrative and interdisciplinary studies. Text in English. 1978. q. USD 93 domestic to individuals; USD 118 foreign to individuals; USD 157 domestic to institutions; USD 171 foreign to institutions (effective 2002). adv. bk.rev. index. back issues avail. *Refereed.* **Document type:** *Journal, Academic/Scholarly.* **Description:** Aimed at broadening the scientific and intellectual horizon of psychoanalysis. Includes original clinical, theoretical and experimental contributions intergrating psychoanalysis with social, biological and behavioral sciences.
Incorporates (1972-1976): Psychoanalysis and Contemporary Science (0092-864X)
Indexed: Biol.Abstr., Excerp.Med., Lang.& Lang.Behav.Abstr., PsycInfo, Psychoanal.Abstr., Psychol.Abstr. (1978-), SOPODA, Sociol.Abstr., e-psyche.
—BLDSC (6946.264700), GNLM, ingenta.
Published by: (Psychoanalysis and Contemporary Science, Inc.), International Universities Press, Incorporated, 59 Boston Post Rd., P.O. Box 1524, Madison, CT 06443-1524. adv.: page USD 375; 4.25 x 7.

PSYCHOANALYSIS AND PSYCHOTHERAPY. see *PSYCHOLOGY*

PSYCHOANALYTIC BOOKS; a quarterly journal of reviews. see *PSYCHOLOGY*

PSYCHOANALYTIC PSYCHOLOGY; Journal of the Division of Psychoanalysis, American Psychological Association. see *PSYCHOLOGY*

616.8 DEU
PSYCHOANALYTISCHE BLAETTER ZU KLINIK, FORSCHUNG, ZEITGESCHEHEN. Text in German. 1994. 2/yr., latest vol.13, 1999. DEM 36 per issue. **Document type:** *Monographic series, Academic/Scholarly.*
Indexed: e-psyche.
Published by: Vandenhoeck und Ruprecht, Robert-Bosch-Breite 6, Goettingen 37079, Germany. TEL 49-551-6959-0, FAX 49-551-695917. Circ: 1,600.

616.8 GBR ISSN 1353-3339
CODEN: PSCOFA
PSYCHODYNAMIC COUNSELLING. Text in English. 1994. q. GBP 39, USD 60 to individuals; GBP 165, USD 272 to institutions (effective 2001). adv. **Document type:** *Academic/Scholarly.* **Description:** Explores the application of psychodynamic ideas through different occupational settings, techniques and theories.
Related titles: Online - full text ed.: ISSN 1470-1057 (from CatchWord Ltd., EBSCO Publishing, O C L C Online Computer Library Center, Inc., RoweCom Information Quest, Swets Blackwell).
Indexed: ASSIA, Biol.Dig., ERA, Lang.& Lang.Behav.Abstr., PsycInfo, Psychoanal.Abstr., SOPODA, Soc.Serv.Abstr., Sociol.Abstr., Stud.Wom.Abstr., e-psyche.
—BLDSC (6946.277150), CatchWord, EMDOCS, GNLM, Infotrieve. **CCC.**
Published by: Routledge (Subsidiary of: Taylor & Francis Group), 11 New Fetter Ln, London EC4P 4EE, United Kingdom. TEL 44-207-842-2001, FAX 44-20-7842-2298, journals@routledge.com, http://www.routledge.com/routledge/journal/journals.html. Ed. John Lees. R&P Sally Sweet. adv.: page GBP 175; trim 190 x 115. Circ: 2,000. **Subscr. to:** Subscriptions, PO Box 362, Abingdon, Oxon OX14 3WB, United Kingdom. TEL 44-1235-401060, FAX 44-1235-401075.

616.89 GBR ISSN 0033-2917
RC321 CODEN: PSMDCO
PSYCHOLOGICAL MEDICINE. Text in English. 1970. 6/yr. GBP 220 to individuals; USD 492 to institutions (effective 2002). adv. bk.rev. charts, illus. index. back issues avail.; reprint service avail. from SWZ. *Refereed.* **Document type:** *Academic/Scholarly.* **Description:** Contains original research in clinical psychiatry and the basic sciences relating to it.
Related titles: CD-ROM ed.: (from Ovid Technologies, Inc.); Microfilm ed.: (from PQC); Online - full text ed.: (from Ovid Technologies, Inc., EBSCO Publishing, O C L C Online Computer Library Center, Inc., RoweCom Information Quest, Swets Blackwell, Institute for Scientific Information); ♦ Supplement: Psychological Medicine. Monograph Supplement. ISSN 0264-1801.

Indexed: ASCA, ASSIA, Abstr.Health Care Manage.Stud., Abstr.Hyg., Addic.Abstr., Adol.Ment.Hlth.Abstr., AgeLine, Arts & Hum.Cit.Ind. (coverage dropped), Behav.Med.Abstr., CINAHL, Chem.Abstr., Crim.Just.Abstr., Curr.Adv.Ecol.Sci., Curr.Cont., Dok.Arbeitsmed., Environ.Sci.Poll.Mgmt., Excerp.Med., Fam.Ind., IBZ, IMFL, Ind.Med. (1970-), Ind.Sci.Rev., Inpharma, Int.Nurs.Ind., Jrnl.Watch Psych., Mid.East: Abstr.& Ind., Neurosci.Cit.Ind., Nutr.Abstr., Pharm.&Out.News, Pollut.Abstr., PsycInfo, Psychol.Abstr. (1970-), Reac., Res.High.Educ.Abstr., Risk Abstr., Rural Devel.Abstr., SSCI, Saf.Sci.Abstr., Sci.Cit.Ind., THA, e-psyche.
—BLDSC (6946.450000), CASDDS, CISTI, GNLM, IDS, ingenta, KNAW. **CCC.**
Published by: Cambridge University Press, Edinburgh Bldg, Shaftesbury Rd, Cambridge CB2 2RU, United Kingdom. FAX 44-1223-315052, information@cambridge.org, http://www.uk.cambridge.org/journals/pmu. Ed. Eugene Paykel. R&P Linda Nicol. Adv. contact Rebecca Symons.

616.8 616.4 GBR ISSN 0306-4530 CODEN: PSYCDE
PSYCHONEUROENDOCRINOLOGY. Text in English. 1976. 8/yr. EUR 1,070 in Europe to institutions; JPY 142,000 in Japan to institutions; USD 1,196 elsewhere to institutions (effective 2002). adv. bk.rev. charts, illus, stat. index. *Refereed.* **Document type:** *Academic/Scholarly.* **Description:** Addresses multidisciplinary issues in psychiatry, psychology, neurology and endocrinology.
Related titles: Microfilm ed.: (from PQC); Online - full text ed.: (from ingenta, Swets Blackwell, Institute for Scientific Information, ScienceDirect).
Indexed: ASCA, Agri.& Environ.Biotech.Abstr. (coverage dropped), Anim.Breed.Abstr., Biol.Abstr., Chem.Abstr., Chem.Indus.Notes, Chem.Titles, Curr.Adv.Ecol.Sci., Curr.Cont., Dairy Sci.Abstr., Derwent Biotech.Abstr., Excerp.Med., INIS Atomind., Ind.Med. (1975-), Ind.Sci.Rev., Ind.Vet., Inpharma, Int.Abstr.Biol.Sci., Neurosci.Abstr. (coverage dropped), Neurosci.Cit.Ind., Nutr.Abstr., Pharm.&Out.News, PsycInfo, Psychol.Abstr. (1975-), Reac., SSCI (coverage dropped), Sci.Cit.Ind., THA, e-psyche.
—BLDSC (6946.540300), ADONIS, CASDDS, CISTI, EMDOCS, GNLM, IDS, ingenta, KNAW. **CCC.**
Published by: (International Society of Psychoneuroendocrinology), Pergamon (Subsidiary of: Elsevier Science), The Boulevard, Langford Ln, East Park, Kidlington, Oxford OXB 1GB, United Kingdom. FAX 44-1865-843010, http://www.elsevier.com/locate/psyneuen. Eds. Ned H Kalin, Robert Dantzer. adv.: B&W page USD 550, color page USD 1,350. Circ: 1,000. **Subscr. in Australasia and the Far East to:** Elsevier Science (Singapore) Pte Ltd, No.1 Temasek Ave, 17-01 Millenia Tower, Singapore 039192, Singapore. TEL 65-434-3727, FAX 65-337-2230; **Subscr. in the Americas to:** Elsevier Science, PO Box 945, New York, NY 10159-0945. TEL 212-633-3730, FAX 212-633-3680, usinfo-f@elsevier.com; **Subscr. to:** Elsevier Science BV, PO Box 211, Amsterdam 1000 AE, Netherlands. TEL 31-20-485-3757.

616.89 SEN ISSN 0033-314X CODEN: PSAFB3
PSYCHOPATHOLOGIE AFRICAINE; sciences sociales et psychiatrie en Afrique. Text and summaries in English, French. 1965. 3/yr. XAF 15,000, FRF 155 in Africa to individuals; XAF 25,000, FRF 250 elsewhere to individuals; XAF 24,000, FRF 240 in Africa to institutions; XAF 36,000, FRF 360 elsewhere to institutions (effective 2000). adv. bk.rev. charts. index. *Refereed.* **Document type:** *Journal, Academic/Scholarly.* **Description:** Seeks to collect and make known works related to psychiatry, psychopathology and mental health in sub-Saharan Africa.
Related titles: CD-ROM ed.; Microfiche ed.
Indexed: Biol.Abstr., Curr.Cont. (coverage dropped), Documentatieblad, ExtraMED, Psychol.Abstr., SSCI (coverage dropped), e-psyche.
—GNLM.
Published by: Societe de Psychopathologie et d'Hygiene Mentale de Dakar, BP 5097, Dakar - Fann, Senegal. TEL 221-824-9888, FAX 221-824-9888, psyfann@ucad.refer.sn. Ed. Daouda Sow. Circ: 11,250. **Dist. by:** Librairies aux 4 Vents, Rue Felix Faure, BP 1820, Dakar, Senegal; Librairie Clairafrique, Pl de l'Independence, Rue Sadiniery, BP 1820, Dakar, Senegal; Librairie Thierry Garnier; Presence Africaine, 25 bis rue des Ecoles, Paris 75005, France; Librairie Lipsy, 25 rue des Ecoles, Paris 75005, France; L'Harmattan, 5 rue de l'Ecole Polytechnique, Paris 75005, France; Le Tiers Mythe, 21 rue Cujas, Paris 75005, France.

616.89 CHE ISSN 0254-4962 CODEN: PSYHEU
PSYCHOPATHOLOGY. Text in English. 1968. 6/yr. CHF 914 in Europe to institutions; CHF 931.40 elsewhere to institutions; EUR 652.80 in Europe to institutions; USD 711 elsewhere to institutions (effective 2002). adv. bk.rev. index. back issues avail. *Refereed.* **Document type:** *Journal, Academic/Scholarly.* **Description:** Publishes studies designed to increase the reliability and precision of explanatory concepts applied in descriptive psychopathology, phenomenology, and clinical diagnostics.
Formerly (until vol.17, 1984): Psychiatria Clinica (0033-264X)
Related titles: Microform ed.; Online - full text ed.: ISSN 1423-033X. 199?. CHF 58, EUR 42, USD 45 to institutions with print edition (effective 2002) (from Northern Light Technology, Inc., EBSCO Publishing, O C L C Online Computer Library Center, Inc., RoweCom Information Quest, ProQuest Information & Learning, Swets Blackwell, Institute for Scientific Information).
Indexed: ASCA, AgeLine, Biol.Abstr., Curr.Cont., Dent.Ind., Documentatieblad, Excerp.Med., Fam.Ind., Ind.Med. (1984-), Ind.Philos., Indian Psychol.Abstr., Inpharma, Int.Nurs.Ind., Neurosci.Cit.Ind., Pharm.&Out.News, PsycInfo, Psychol.Abstr. (1968-), Reac., Rev.Appl.Entomol., SSCI, Sci.Cit.Ind., Trop.Dis.Bull., e-psyche.
—BLDSC (6946.543700), CASDDS, CISTI, EMDOCS, GNLM, IDS, Infotrieve, ingenta, KNAW. **CCC.**
Published by: S. Karger AG, Allschwilerstr 10, PO Box, Basel 4009, Switzerland. TEL 41-61-306-1111, FAX 41-61-306-1234, karger@karger.ch, http://www.online.karger.com/journals/psp, http://www.karger.com. Eds. C Mundt, E Gabriel. adv.: page USD 1,185. Circ: 800.

PSYCHOPHARMACOLOGY. see *PHARMACY AND PHARMACOLOGY*

PSYCHOPHARMACOLOGY BULLETIN. see *PHARMACY AND PHARMACOLOGY*

PSYCHOPHARMACOLOGY UPDATE. see *PHARMACY AND PHARMACOLOGY*

612.8 GBR ISSN 0048-5772
QP351 CODEN: PSPHAF
PSYCHOPHYSIOLOGY; an international journal. Text in English. 1964. bi-m. (Plus abstracts supplement). GBP 85 to individuals; USD 235 to institutions (effective 2002). adv. bk.rev. abstr, charts, illus. index. back issues avail.; reprint service avail. from PQC,PSC,SCH. *Refereed.* **Document type:** *Academic/Scholarly.* **Description:** Concerns the relationships between human autonomic and central nervous system behavior on the one hand and cognitive performance, personality and emotions on the other. Studies effects of stress, individual differences, aging, anxiety, and psychosomatic and psychiatric disease.
Formerly: Psychophysiology Newsletter
Related titles: Microfilm ed.: (from PQC); Online - full text ed.: (from EBSCO Publishing, O C L C Online Computer Library Center, Inc., RoweCom Information Quest, Swets Blackwell, Institute for Scientific Information).
Indexed: ASCA, AgeLine, Behav.Med.Abstr., Bibl.Dev.Med.& Child Neur., Biol.Abstr., Compumath, Curr.Adv.Ecol.Sci., Curr.Cont., Curr.Ind.Stat., Ergon.Abstr., Excerp.Med., Fam.Ind., IBZ, Ind.Med. (1964-), Ind.Philos., Ind.Sci.Rev., Inpharma, Lang.& Lang.Behav.Abstr., Neurosci.Cit.Ind., Pharm.&Out.News, PsycInfo, Psychol.Abstr. (1964-), Reac., Russ.Acad.Sci.Bibl., SOPODA, SSCI, Sci.Cit.Ind., Sociol.Abstr., THA, e-psyche.
—BLDSC (6946.552000), CISTI, GNLM, IDS, ingenta, KNAW. **CCC.**
Published by: (Society for Psychophysiological Research), Cambridge University Press, Edinburgh Bldg, Shaftesbury Rd, Cambridge CB2 2RU, United Kingdom. FAX 44-1223-315052, information@cambridge.org, http://www.uk.cambridge.org/journals/pmu. Ed. Gregory A Miller. R&P Linda Nicol. Adv. contact Rebecca Symons. Circ: 2,100.

616.89 USA ISSN 0033-3174
RC49 CODEN: PSMEAP
PSYCHOSOMATIC MEDICINE. Text in English. 1938. bi-m., latest vol.63. USD 264 domestic to individuals; USD 309 foreign to individuals; USD 514 domestic to institutions; USD 560 foreign to institutions; USD 85 newsstand/cover (effective 2002). adv. bk.rev. illus. index. reprint service avail. from PSC,SCH. *Refereed.* **Document type:** *Journal, Academic/Scholarly.* **Description:** Presents research and clinical studies concerning psychosomatic disorders. Examines many disciplines, including psychiatry, psychology, and the social sciences.
Related titles: CD-ROM ed.: (from Ovid Technologies, Inc.); Microfilm ed.: (from RPI,WWS); Online - full text ed.: USD 668.20 domestic academic site license; USD 714.20 foreign academic site license; USD 745.30 domestic corporate site license; USD 791.30 foreign corporate site license (effective 2002) (from Ovid Technologies, Inc., Institute for Scientific Information).
Indexed: ASCA, AgeLine, Behav.Med.Abstr., Biol.Abstr., Brit.Nur.Ind., Chem.Abstr., Chem.Titles, Curr.Cont., Environ.Sci.Poll.Mgmt., Excerp.Med., Fam.Ind., INIS Atomind., Ind.Med. (1939-), Ind.Sci.Rev., Inpharma, Int.Nurs.Ind., Jrnl.Watch Psych., Lang.& Lang.Behav.Abstr., Med.& Surg.Dermat., Neurosci.Cit.Ind., Nutr.Abstr., Pharm.&Out.News, Pollut.Abstr., PsycInfo, Psychol.Abstr. (1939-), Reac., Risk Abstr., SOPODA, SSCI, Saf.Sci.Abstr., Sci.Cit.Ind., Sociol.Abstr., e-psyche.
—BLDSC (6946.555000), CASDDS, CISTI, GNLM, IDS, ingenta, KNAW.
Published by: (American Psychosomatic Society), Williams & Wilkins (Subsidiary of: Waverly International), 351 W Camden St, Baltimore, MD 21201-2436. TEL 410-528-4068, 800-222-3790, FAX 410-528-4452, lgibson@wwilkins.com, http://www.psychosomaticmedicine.org, http://www.wwilkins.com. Ed. Dr. J Dimsdale. Adv. contact Lynn Gibson. Circ: 2,245.

616.89 USA ISSN 0033-3182
RC49 CODEN: PSYCBC
PSYCHOSOMATICS; the journal of consultation and liaison psychiatry. Text in English. 1960. bi-m. USD 119 domestic to individuals; USD 148 foreign to individuals; USD 225 domestic to institutions; USD 254 foreign to institutions (effective 2001). bk.rev. abstr, bibl, charts, illus, stat. index. back issues avail.; reprint service avail. from PQC,PSC,SCH. *Refereed.* **Description:** Devoted to the relationship between medical and psychiatric phenomena.
Related titles: Microform ed.: (from PQC); Online - full text ed.: (from HighWire Pr., Northern Light Technology, Inc., EBSCO Publishing, RoweCom Information Quest, ProQuest Information & Learning, Institute for Scientific Information).
Indexed: ASCA, Adol.Ment.Hlth.Abstr., AgeLine, Biol.Abstr., CINAHL, Chem.Abstr., Chem.Titles, Curr.Cont., Excerp.Med., Fam.Ind., Ind.Med. (1960-), Ind.Sci.Rev., Inpharma, Int.Nurs.Ind., Jrnl.Watch Psych., Neurosci.Cit.Ind., Nutr.Abstr., Pharm.&Out.News, PsycInfo, Psychol.Abstr. (1966-), Reac., Ref.Zh., Rev.Appl.Entomol., Rev.Med.& Vet.Mycol., SSCI, Sci.Cit.Ind., Soc.Work Res.& Abstr., e-psyche.
—BLDSC (6946.557000), CASDDS, CISTI, GNLM, IDS, ingenta, KNAW. **CCC.**
Published by: (Academy of Psychosomatic Medicine), American Psychiatric Press, Inc., Journals Division, 1400 K St, N W, Ste 1101, Washington, DC 20005. TEL 202-682-6240, FAX 202-682-6341, appi@psych.org, http://psy.psychiatryonline.org/, http://www.psychiatryonline.org, http://www.appi.org. Ed. Dr. Thomas Wise. R&P John McDuffie. Circ: 2,500.

616.8 360 DEU ISSN 0930-4177
PSYCHOSOZIALE UMSCHAU. Text in German. 1985. q. DEM 40; DEM 48 foreign (effective 1999). **Document type:** *Academic/Scholarly.*
Indexed: e-psyche.
Published by: (Dachverband Psychosoziale Hilfsvereinigungen), Psychiatrie Verlag GmbH, Thomas-Mann-Str 49A, Bonn 53111, Germany. TEL 49-228-72534-0, FAX 49-228-7253420.

616.8 150 POL ISSN 0239-4170
PSYCHOTERAPIA. Text in Polish; Summaries in English. 1972. q. PLZ 40 domestic (effective 2002). bk.rev. abstr, bibl, illus. 90 p./no. 1 cols./p. back issues avail. *Refereed.* **Document type:** *Bulletin, Academic/Scholarly.* **Description:** Publishes clinical, theoretical, and experimental papers and case reports on psychotherapy and clinical psychology.
Published by: Polskie Towarzystwo Psychiatryczne, Ul Lenartowicza 14, Krakow 31138, Poland. TEL 48-12-6331203, FAX 48-12-6334067, psych@kom-red-wyd-ptp.com.pl, http://www.kom-red-wyd-ptp.com.pl/3en.html. Ed. Kazimierz Bierzynski. Pub., R&P Jerzy W Aleksandrowicz. Adv. contact Magdalena Sikora.

616.89 DEU ISSN 0935-6185
PSYCHOTHERAPEUT. Text in German. 1956. bi-m. EUR 143.50 domestic; EUR 128.70 in Germany; EUR 24.30 newsstand/cover foreign (effective 2002). adv. bk.rev. bibl, charts, illus. back issues avail.; reprint service avail. from ISI. *Refereed.* **Document type:** *Journal, Academic/Scholarly.* **Description:** Seeks to promote discussion of different approaches and psychotherapeutic schools.

M

Former titles: Praxis der Psychotherapie und Psychosomatik (0171-791X); Praxis der Psychotherapie (0032-7077)
Related titles: Microform ed.: (from PQC); Online - full text ed.: ISSN 1432-2080 (from EBSCO Publishing, RoweCom Information Quest, Swets Blackwell, Springer LINK, Institute for Scientific Information).
Indexed: ASCA, Arts & Hum.Cit.Ind. (coverage dropped), Biol.Abstr., Chem.Abstr., Curr.Cont., Excerp.Med., PsycInfo, Psychol.Abstr. (1959-), SSCI, e-psyche.
—BLDSC (6946.558210), CISTI, EMDOCS, GNLM, IDS, Infotrieve, KNAW. **CCC.**
Published by: Springer-Verlag (Subsidiary of: BertelsmannSpringer), Tiergartenstr 17, Heidelberg 69121, Germany. TEL 49-6221-345-0, FAX 49-6221-345229, subscriptions@springer.de, http://link.springer.de/link/service/journals/00278/index.htm, http://www.springer.de. Eds. J Eckert, M Cierpka. **Subscr. in N. America to:** Springer-Verlag New York Inc., PO Box 2485, Secaucus, NJ 07096-2485. TEL 212-460-1500, FAX 212-473-6272.

616.89 DEU ISSN 1438-7026
▼ **PSYCHOTHERAPIE IM DIALOG.** Abbreviated title: P i D. Text in German. 2000. q. EUR 104.10 domestic to institutions; EUR 106.30 in Europe to institutions; EUR 111.90 elsewhere to institutions; EUR 29.90 newsstand/cover (effective 2002). **Document type:** *Journal, Academic/Scholarly.*
Related titles: Online - full text ed.: ISSN 1439-913X.
Published by: Georg Thieme Verlag, Ruedigerstr 14, Stuttgart 70469, Germany. TEL 49-711-8931-0, FAX 49-711-8931298, kunden.service@thieme.de, http://www.thieme.de.

616.89 CHE ISSN 0033-3190
RC49 CODEN: PSPSBF
PSYCHOTHERAPY AND PSYCHOSOMATICS. Text in English. 1953. bi-m. CHF 914 in Europe to institutions; CHF 931.40 elsewhere to institutions; EUR 652.80 in Europe to institutions; USD 711 elsewhere to institutions (effective 2002). adv. bk.rev. charts, illus, bibl. index. back issues avail. *Refereed.* **Document type:** *Journal, Academic/Scholarly.* **Description:** Provides comprehensive coverage of the latest original research in psychotherapy and psychosomatics.
Related titles: Microform ed.; Online - full text ed.: ISSN 1423-0348. 199?. CHF 58, EUR 42, USD 45 to institutions print with edition (effective 2002) (from EBSCO Publishing, O C L C Online Computer Library Center, Inc., RoweCom Information Quest, ProQuest Information & Learning, Swets Blackwell, Institute for Scientific Information).
Indexed: ASCA, Adol.Ment.Hlth.Abstr., AgeLine, Biol.Abstr., Chem.Abstr., Curr.Cont., Dent.Ind., Documentatieblad, Excerp.Med., Fam.Ind., Ind.Med. (1965-), Ind.Sci.Rev., Indian Psychol.Abstr., Inpharma, Neurosci.Cit.Ind., Nutr.Abstr., Pharm.&Out.News, PsycInfo, Psychol.Abstr. (1953-), Reac., SSCI, Sci.Cit.Ind., Stud.Wom.Abstr., e-psyche.
—BLDSC (6946.559000), CISTI, GNLM, IDS, ingenta, KNAW. **CCC.**
Published by: (International Federation for Medical Psychotherapy), S. Karger AG, Allschwilerstr 10, PO Box, Basel 4009, Switzerland. TEL 41-61-306-1111, FAX 41-61-306-1234, karger@karger.ch, http://www.online.karger.com/journals/pps, http://www.karger.com. Ed. G Fava. adv.: page USD 1,195. Circ: 1,000.

PSYCHOTHERAPY, RECOVERY AND PERSONAL GROWTH UPDATE. see *PSYCHOLOGY*

616.89 DEU ISSN 1439-8931
▼ **PSYCHOTRAUMATOLOGIE.** Text in German. 2001. q. EUR 51 to institutions (effective 2002). **Document type:** *Academic/Scholarly.*
Media: Online - full content.
Published by: Georg Thieme Verlag, Ruedigerstr 14, Stuttgart 70469, Germany. TEL 49-711-8931-0, FAX 49-711-8931298, kunden.service@thieme.de, http://www.thieme.de.

PSYCSCAN: LEARNING DISORDERS AND MENTAL RETARDATION. see *MEDICAL SCIENCES—Abstracting, Bibliographies, Statistics*

PSYKISK HAELSA/MENTAL HEALTH. see *PSYCHOLOGY*

616.8 USA
PURE FACTS. Text in English. 1978. 10/yr. USD 28; USD 30 foreign (effective 1999). back issues avail. *Refereed.* **Document type:** *Newsletter.* **Description:** Non-profit support group helping children with learning or behavior problems and chemically-sensitive adults.
Indexed: e-psyche.
Published by: Feingold Association of the United States, 127 E Main St, Ste 106, Riverhead, NY 11901. TEL 516-369-9340, FAX 516-369-2988, orders@feingold.org, http://www.feingold.org. Ed. Jane Hersey. Circ: 6,000. **Subscr. to:** PO Box 6550, Alexandria, VA 22306.

616.89 618.92 ITA
QUADERNI DI PSICOTERAPIA INFANTILE. Text in Italian. s-a. ITL 80,000 domestic to individuals; USD 100 foreign to individuals; ITL 90,000 domestic to institutions; USD 110 foreign to institutions.
Indexed: e-psyche.
Published by: Edizioni Borla s.r.l., Via Delle Fornaci, 50, Rome, RM 00165, Italy. TEL 39-6-39376728, FAX 39-6-39376620. Eds. C Rutti, R Parlani.

616.8 ITA ISSN 0393-0645
QUADERNI ITALIANI DI PSICHIATRIA. Text in Italian. 1981. 6/yr. ITL 114,000 (effective 1999). **Document type:** *Academic/Scholarly.*
Indexed: e-psyche.
Published by: Masson S.p.A., Divisione Periodici, Via F.lli Bressan 2, Milan, MI 20126, Italy. TEL 39-2-270741, FAX 39-2-27074210. Eds. Eugenio Borgna, Vittorino Andreoli. adv.: B&W page ITL 2,550,000, color page ITL 3,600,000; trim 240 x 170. Circ: 2,000.

QUADRANT. see *PSYCHOLOGY*

616.858 USA
QUALITY OF CARE. Text in English. 1980. q. bk.rev. **Document type:** *Government.*
Indexed: e-psyche.
Published by: Commission on Quality of Care for the Mentally Disabled, 401 State St, Schenectady, NY 12305-2397. TEL 518-381-7102, FAX 518-381-7101, gigliotti@emi.com, http://www.cgc.state.ny.us. Ed. Marcus A Gigliotti. R&P Marcus A Giglotti. Circ: 13,000 (controlled).

616.89 USA ISSN 1087-1578
QUEST (TUCSON). Text in English. 1950. bi-m. USD 14 domestic; USD 22 foreign (effective 2001); free to qualified personnel. adv. bk.rev. illus. 72 p./no. reprints avail. **Document type:** *Magazine, Trade.* **Description:** Presents profiles, instructive articles, research and association news, resource listings, and helpful articles of special interest to those with neuromuscular diseases and their families.
Former titles (until 1994): M D A Reports (1061-4370); (until 1992): M D A Newsmagazine (8750-2321); M D A News - Muscular Dystrophy Association (0279-0742); Muscular Dystrophy News (0027-3759)
Related titles: Online - full text ed.: (from Gale Group).
Indexed: CHNI, Rehabil.Lit., e-psyche.
Published by: Muscular Dystrophy Association, Inc., 3300 E Sunrise Dr, Tucson, AZ 85718-3208. TEL 520-529-2000, FAX 520-529-5300, http://www.mdausa.org. Ed., R&P Carol Sowell TEL 520-529-2000. Pub. Robert Ross. Adv. contact Maureen Tuncer TEL 727-578-2734. B&W page USD 2,875. Circ: 115,000 (paid and controlled).

362.3 NLD ISSN 0166-4298
RAAKPUNT. Text in Dutch. 1957. 8/yr. NLG 45, USD 20 (effective 2001). bk.rev. illus. 28 p./no. 3 cols./p. back issues avail. **Document type:** *Newspaper.* **Description:** Contains news and information for parents and relatives of persons with mental disabilities.
Formerly: Zorgenkind (0044-5339)
Media: Duplicated (not offset). **Related titles:** Online - full text ed.
Indexed: e-psyche.
Published by: Vereniging van Ouders en Verwanten van Mensen met een Verstandelijke Handicap V O G G, Postbus 85274, Utrecht 3508 AG, Netherlands. TEL 31-30-236-3744, FAX 31-30-231-3054, utrecht@vogg.nl, http://www.fvo.nl, http://www.tro.nl. Ed. S T Overbeek. R&P S.T. Overbeek. Circ: 16,000.

RADIOSURGERY. see *MEDICAL SCIENCES—Surgery*

READING AND WRITING; an interdisciplinary journal. see *LINGUISTICS*

028.1 USA ISSN 0886-3784
READINGS; a journal of reviews and commentary in mental health. Text in English. 1986. q. USD 25 to individuals; USD 35 to institutions. adv. bk.rev. back issues avail. **Document type:** *Academic/Scholarly.* **Description:** Four to six essay reviews and 30-40 brief reviews of books that are of interest to the mental health professional.
Related titles: Microfiche ed.
Indexed: Bk.Rev.Dig. (Mar.1986-), Bk.Rev.Ind. (1990-), Child.Bk.Rev.Ind. (1990-), e-psyche.
—Infotrieve. **CCC.**
Published by: American Orthopsychiatric Association, Inc., 330 Seventh Ave, 18th Fl, New York, NY 10001. TEL 212-564-5930, FAX 212-564-6180. Ed. Ernest Herman. R&P Robert Keizer. Adv. contact Joan Adler. Circ: 11,000.

616.834 USA ISSN 1079-4220
REAL LIVING WITH MULTIPLE SCLEROSIS. Text in English. 1993. m. USD 49 domestic; USD 69 foreign; USD 6 newsstand/cover (effective 2001). **Document type:** *Consumer.* **Description:** Offers people with MS and their families information on how to cope with the clinical and personal consequences of this disease. Includes articles on alternative medicine, physical therapy, new drug therapies, initiatives to promote accessibility and more.
Related titles: Online - full text ed.: (from ProQuest Information & Learning, Gale Group, Factiva).
Indexed: e-psyche.
Published by: Springhouse Corporation (Subsidiary of: Lippincott Williams & Wilkins (Philadelphia)), 1111 Bethlehem Tpk., Springhouse, PA 19477-0908. TEL 215-646-8700, 800-783-4903, FAX 215-646-4399, http://www.springnet.com. Ed. Kimberly Callan.

616.8 GBR ISSN 0307-7403
RECENT ADVANCES IN CLINICAL NEUROLOGY. Text in English. 1975. irreg., latest vol.8. **Document type:** *Monographic series, Academic/Scholarly.*
Indexed: e-psyche.
—BLDSC (7303.803000), GNLM.
Published by: Churchill Livingstone (Subsidiary of: Harcourt Publishers Ltd.), Robert Stevenson House, 1-3 Baxter's Pl, Leith Walk, Edinburgh, Midlothian EH1 3AF, United Kingdom. TEL 44-131-556-2424, FAX 44-131-459-1177, http://www.churchillmed.com. **US subscr. to:** Churchill Livingstone, 650 Ave of the Americas, New York, NY 10011. TEL 212-206-5000.

616.8 GBR ISSN 0144-1086
RECENT ADVANCES IN CLINICAL PSYCHIATRY. Text in English. 1971. irreg., latest vol.8. **Document type:** *Monographic series, Academic/Scholarly.*
Indexed: e-psyche.
—CISTI, GNLM.
Published by: Churchill Livingstone (Subsidiary of: Harcourt Publishers Ltd.), Robert Stevenson House, 1-3 Baxter's Pl, Leith Walk, Edinburgh, Midlothian EH1 3AF, United Kingdom. TEL 44-131-556-2424, FAX 44-131-459-1177, http://www.churchillmed.com. **US subscr. to:** Churchill Livingstone, 650 Ave of the Americas, New York, NY 10011. TEL 212-206-5000.

616.853 GBR ISSN 0264-7400
RC372.A1
RECENT ADVANCES IN EPILEPSY. Text in English. 1983. irreg., latest vol.6, 1995. price varies. *Refereed.* **Document type:** *Monographic series, Academic/Scholarly.* **Description:** Publishes up-to-date reviews on topics of current interest. Highlights key points for clinical practice.
Indexed: e-psyche.
—GNLM.
Published by: Churchill Livingstone (Subsidiary of: Harcourt Publishers Ltd.), Robert Stevenson House, 1-3 Baxter's Pl, Leith Walk, Edinburgh, Midlothian EH1 3AF, United Kingdom. TEL 44-131-556-2424, FAX 44-131-459-1177, http://www.churchillmed.com. Eds. Brian S Meldrum, Timothy A Pedley. Pub. Gill Haddock. R&P Moira Trotter. Circ: 850. **Orders to:** Pearson Professional Ltd., Journals Subscription Department, Fourth Ave., PO Box 77, Harlow, Essex CM19 5AA, United Kingdom. TEL 44-1279-623924, FAX 44-1279-639609; **U.S. subscr. to:** Churchill Livingstone, 650 Ave of the Americas, New York, NY 10011. TEL 212-206-5000.

616.8 GBR ISSN 0144-0535
CODEN: RADND8
RECENT ADVANCES IN NEUROPATHOLOGY. Text in English. 1979. irreg. **Document type:** *Monographic series, Academic/Scholarly.*
Indexed: e-psyche.
—CASDDS, GNLM.
Published by: Churchill Livingstone (Subsidiary of: Harcourt Publishers Ltd.), Robert Stevenson House, 1-3 Baxter's Pl, Leith Walk, Edinburgh, Midlothian EH1 3AF, United Kingdom. TEL 44-131-556-2424, FAX 44-131-459-1177, http://www.churchillmed.com. **US subscr. to:** Churchill Livingstone, 650 Ave of the Americas, New York, NY 10011. TEL 212-206-5000.

616.8 GBR ISSN 0267-8977
RECENT ADVANCES IN PSYCHOGERIATRICS. Text in English. 1985. irreg. **Document type:** *Monographic series, Academic/Scholarly.*

M

Indexed: e-psyche.
—GNLM.
Published by: Churchill Livingstone (Subsidiary of: Harcourt Publishers Ltd.), Robert Stevenson House, 1-3 Baxter's Pl, Leith Walk, Edinburgh, Midlothian EH1 3AF, United Kingdom. TEL 44-131-556-2424, FAX 44-131-459-1177, http://www.churchillmed.com. **US subscr. to:** Churchill Livingstone, 650 Ave of the Americas, New York, NY 10011. TEL 212-206-5000.

616.8 612.015 USA
THE RECEPTORS. Text in English. 1983. irreg., latest vol.14, 1997. price varies. illus. back issues avail. *Refereed.* **Document type:** *Monographic series, Academic/Scholarly.* **Description:** Explores the biochemistry and physiology of the various neuroreceptors and how pharmacological compounds affect them.
Published by: Humana Press Inc., 999 Riverview Dr, Ste 208, Totowa, NJ 07512. TEL 973-256-1699, FAX 973-256-8341, humana@humanapr.com, http://humanapress.com. R&P Richard Hruska.

RECHT & PSYCHIATRIE. see *PSYCHOLOGY*

REFERATIVNYI ZHURNAL. PSIKHYATRIYA. see *MEDICAL SCIENCES—Abstracting, Bibliographies, Statistics*

REFERATOVY VYBER Z NEUROLOGIE/ABSTRACTS OF NEUROLOGY. see *MEDICAL SCIENCES—Abstracting, Bibliographies, Statistics*

REHABILITATION COUNSELING BULLETIN. see *HANDICAPPED*

616.831 USA
RESEARCH AND PRACTICE. Text in English. q. free per issue. **Document type:** *Trade, Academic/Scholarly.* **Description:** Disseminates new research in the detection and treatment of patients with Alzheimer's disease.
Indexed: e-psyche.
Published by: Alzheimer's Association, Inc., 1919 N Michigan Ave, Ste 1000, Chicago, IL 60611. TEL 312-335-8700, FAX 312-335-1110, http://www.alz.org. Ed. Daniela Sickanovska.

RESEARCH COMMUNICATIONS IN BEHAVIORAL PSYCHOLOGY AND PSYCHIATRY; including behavioral and neurosciences. see *PSYCHOLOGY*

616.8 GBR ISSN 0891-4222
HV1570.5.U65 CODEN: RDDIEF
RESEARCH IN DEVELOPMENTAL DISABILITIES; a multidisciplinary journal. Text in English. 1981. bi-m. EUR 160 in Europe to qualified personnel; JPY 21,200 in Japan to qualified personnel; USD 179 elsewhere to qualified personnel; EUR 442 in Europe to institutions; JPY 58,700 in Japan to institutions; USD 494 elsewhere to institutions (effective 2002). adv. back issues avail. *Refereed.* **Document type:** *Academic/Scholarly.* **Description:** Devoted to original behavioral research and theory of severe and pervasive developmental disabilities.
Formed by the 1987 merger of: Applied Research in Mental Retardation (0270-3092); Analysis and Intervention in Developmental Disabilities (0270-4684)
Related titles: Microfilm ed.: (from PQC); Online - full text ed.: (from ingenta, Swets Blackwell, Institute for Scientific Information, ScienceDirect).
Indexed: AMED, ASCA, AgeLine, Biol.Abstr., C.I.J.E., Chic.Per.Ind., Curr.Adv.Ecol.Sci., Curr.Cont., Dent.Ind., Educ.Ind. (Jun.1992-), Except.Child Educ.Abstr., Ind.Med. (1987-), Int.Nurs.Ind., Psyclnfo, Psychol.Abstr. (1987-), SSCI, Yrbk.Assoc.Educ.& Rehab.Blind, e-psyche.
—BLDSC (7738.450000), EMDOCS, GNLM, IDS, ingenta, KNAW. **CCC.**
Published by: Pergamon (Subsidiary of: Elsevier Science), The Boulevard, Langford Ln, East Park, Kidlington, Oxford OXB 1GB, United Kingdom. FAX 44-1865-843010, http://www.elsevier.com/locate/redevdis. Ed. Johnny L Matson. adv.: B&W page USD 550, color page USD 1,350. **Subscr. in Australasia and the Far East to:** Elsevier Science (Singapore) Pte Ltd, No.1 Temasek Ave, 17-01 Millenia Tower, Singapore 039192, Singapore. TEL 65-434-3727, FAX 65-337-2230; **Subscr. in the Americas to:** Elsevier Science, PO Box 945, New York, NY 10159-0945. TEL 212-633-3730, FAX 212-633-3680, usinfo-f@elsevier.com; **Subscr. to:** Elsevier Science BV, PO Box 211, Amsterdam 1000 AE, Netherlands. TEL 31-20-485-3757.

RESEARCH METHODS IN NEUROCHEMISTRY. see *BIOLOGY—Biochemistry*

▼ **RESEARCH NEWS & OPPORTUNITIES IN SCIENCE AND THEOLOGY.** see *SCIENCES: COMPREHENSIVE WORKS*

616.8 NLD ISSN 0922-6028
CODEN: RNNEEL
RESTORATIVE NEUROLOGY AND NEUROSCIENCE. Text in English. 1989. 8/yr. (in 2 vols., 4 nos./vol.). EUR 750 in Afghanistan to institutions; USD 693 to institutions (effective 2002). bk.rev. back issues avail. *Refereed.* **Document type:** *Journal, Academic/Scholarly.* **Description:** Publishes papers from an interdisciplinary perspective on the plasticity and response of the nervous system to accidental or experimental injuries, or transplantation.
Related titles: Microform ed.: (from PQC); Online - full text ed.: (from ingenta, Institute for Scientific Information, RoweCom Information Quest).
Indexed: ASCA, Chem.Abstr., Chem.Indus.Notes, Chem.Titles, Curr.Cont., Excerp.Med., Ind.Sci.Rev., Inpharma, Int.Abstr.Biol.Sci., Neurosci.Abstr. (coverage dropped), Neurosci.Cit.Ind., Pharm.&Out.News, Reac., Sci.Cit.Ind., e-psyche.
—BLDSC (7777.865100), ADONIS, CASDDS, CISTI, EMDOCS, GNLM, IDS, Infotrieve. **CCC.**
Published by: I O S Press, Nieuwe Hemweg 6B, Amsterdam 1013 BG, Netherlands. TEL 31-20-688-3355, FAX 31-20-620-3419, market@iospress.nl, http://www.chsbs.cmich.edu/psy/rnn, http://www.iospress.nl. Ed. Dr. Bernhard A Sabel TEL 49-391-611-7100. **Subscr. to:** I O S Press, Inc, 5795-G Burke Centre Pkwy, Burke, VA 22015. TEL 703-323-5554, FAX 703-323-3668, iosbooks@iospress.com; Kinokuniya Company Ltd, Shinjuku 3-chome, Shinjuku-ku, Tokyo 160-0022, Japan. FAX 81-3-3439-1094, journal@kinokuniya.co.jp, http://www.kinokuniya.co.jp; Globe Publication Pvt. Ltd., C-62 Inderpuri, New Delhi 100 012, India. TEL 91-11-579-3211, 91-11-579-3212, FAX 91-11-579-8876, custserve@globepub.com, http://www.globepub.com.

616.8 618 AUS
RETT SYNDROME ASSOCIATION OF AUSTRALIA NEWSLETTER. Text in English. 1989. q. AUD 20 (effective 2000). **Document type:** *Newsletter.*
Indexed: e-psyche.
Published by: Rett Syndrome Association of Australia, GPO Box 3497, Melbourne, VIC 3001, Australia. TEL 61-3-52433723, FAX 61-3-96157798, rettaust@bigpond.com, http://www.general.uwa.edu.au/u/hleonard/. Ed., Pub., R&P, Adv. contact Bill Callaghan. Circ: 400 (paid and controlled).

616.89 362.2 SWE ISSN 0283-7587
REVANSCH!; klientperspektivet i psykiatrin. Text in Swedish. 1980. s-m. SEK 150 (effective 1999). adv. **Document type:** *Consumer.*
Formerly (until 1985): R S M H - Information - Revansch! (0280-0187)
Indexed: e-psyche.
Published by: R S M H - Riksfoerbundet foer Social och Mental Haelsa, Fack 150 94, Stockholm 10122, Sweden. TEL 46-8-772-33-63, FAX 46-8-772-33-61, tommy.engman@rsmh.see, http://www.rsmh.se. Ed. Tommy Engman. Adv. contact Annelee Larsson.

REVIEW OF EXISTENTIAL PSYCHOLOGY AND PSYCHIATRY. see *PSYCHOLOGY*

616.8 ISR ISSN 0334-1763
CODEN: RNEUEO
REVIEWS IN THE NEUROSCIENCES. Text in English. 1986. q. USD 340 (effective 2002). adv. back issues avail. *Refereed.* **Document type:** *Academic/Scholarly.*
Related titles: Online - full text ed.: (from Institute for Scientific Information).
Indexed: ASCA, Curr.Adv.Ecol.Sci., Excerp.Med., Ind.Med. (1986-), Neurosci.Abstr. (coverage dropped), Neurosci.Cit.Ind., SSCI (coverage dropped), e-psyche.
—BLDSC (7793.571000), CASDDS, CISTI, EMDOCS, GNLM, ingenta, KNAW.
Published by: Freund Publishing House, Ltd., P O Box 35010, Tel Aviv 61350, Israel. TEL 972-3-562-8540, FAX 972-3-562-8538, h_freund@netvision.net.il, http://www.angelfire.com/il/freund. Ed. J P Huston. Circ: 1,000.

REVIEWS OF OCULOMOTOR RESEARCH. see *MEDICAL SCIENCES—Ophthalmology And Optometry*

616.8 BRA ISSN 0101-8469
CODEN: RBNEES
REVISTA BRASILEIRA DE NEUROLOGIA. Text in Portuguese; Summaries in English, Portuguese. 1949. bi-m. BRL 54, USD 72 (effective 2000). adv. charts, illus. **Document type:** *Academic/Scholarly.* **Description:** Presents studies in clinical neurology.
Formerly: Jornal Brasileiro de Neurologia (0021-7514)
Indexed: Chem.Abstr., Excerp.Med., INIS Atomind., Ind.Med. (coverage dropped), Ref.Zh., e-psyche.
—GNLM.
Published by: (Universidade Federal do Rio de Janeiro, Instituto de Neurologia), E C N - Editora Cientifica Nacional Ltda., Rua da Gloria, 366 Andar 3, Gloria, Rio De Janeiro, RJ 20241-180, Brazil. TEL 55-21-2213235, FAX 55-21-2213235, ecn@rj.sol.com.br. Eds. Eliasq Engelhardt, Jose Mauro Braz de Lima. R&P, Adv. contact Maria Luiza Carvalho. Circ: 4,000.

616.8 BRA ISSN 1414-0365
REVISTA BRASILEIRA DE NEUROLOGIA E PSIQUIATRIA. Text in Portuguese; Summaries in English, Portuguese. 1996. q. BRL 42, USD 72 (effective 1999). adv. bk.rev. abstr, bibl. back issues avail. *Refereed.* **Document type:** *Academic/Scholarly.*
Indexed: Ref.Zh.
—BLDSC (7845.370000), KNAW.
Published by: (Colegio Brasileiro de Neuropsicofarmacologia), E C N - Editora Cientifica Nacional Ltda., Rua da Gloria, 366 Andar 3, Gloria, Rio De Janeiro, RJ 20241-180, Brazil. TEL 55-21-2213235, FAX 55-21-2213235, ecn@rj.sol.com.br. Ed., Adv. contact Maria Luiza Carvalho. Pub. Jorge Alberto Costa e Silva. color page BRL 2,000; trim 210 x 280.

616.89 BRA ISSN 1516-4446
REVISTA BRASILEIRA DE PSIQUIATRIA. Abbreviated title: Revista A B P - A P A L. (2 a. supplements avail.) Text in Portuguese; Summaries in English, Spanish. 1979. q. USD 100, BRL 95 (effective 2000). adv. bk.rev. bibl, charts, stat. *Refereed.* **Document type:** *Academic/Scholarly.* **Description:** Papers on psychiatry and correlated disciplines of general interest to mental health professionals from Brazil and other Latin American countries.
Former titles (until 199?): Associacao Brasileira de Psiquiatria e Asociacion Psiquiatrica de la America Latina. Revista (0102-7646); (until 198?): Associacao Brasileira de Psiquiatria Revista (0101-5311)
Related titles: Online - full text ed.: (from SciELO).
Indexed: Biol.Abstr., Excerp.Med., Ind.Med. (coverage dropped), Psyclnfo, Psychol.Abstr. (1986-), e-psyche.
—BLDSC (7845.535000), GNLM.
Published by: Associacao Brasileira de Psiquiatria, Rua Pedro de Toledo, 967, casa 1, Vl Clementino, Sao Paulo, SP 04039-032, Brazil. TEL 55-11-549-6699, FAX 55-11-570-6210, redprint@uol.com.br, abppublicacoes@dialdata.com.br. Eds. Dr. Helena M Calil, Sergio Luis Blay. Circ: 5,000. **Co-sponsor:** Associacao Psiquiatrica da America Latina.

616.89 COL ISSN 0034-7450
CODEN: RCPSBR
REVISTA COLOMBIANA DE PSIQUIATRIA. Text in Spanish. 1964. q. USD 40. adv. bk.rev. abstr, charts, illus. index. **Document type:** *Academic/Scholarly.*
Indexed: Excerp.Med., Psychol.Abstr., e-psyche.
—GNLM.
Published by: Sociedad Colombiana de Psiquiatria, Carrera 18 No. 8487, PO Box 203, Bogota, CUND, Colombia. TEL 57-1-2561148. Ed. Roberto Chaskel. Circ: 1,500.

616.8 PER ISSN 0034-8597
REVISTA DE NEURO-PSIQUIATRIA. Text in Spanish; Summaries in English, French, German. 1938. q. USD 80. adv. bk.rev. abstr, charts, illus. index. **Document type:** *Academic/Scholarly.*
Indexed: Biol.Abstr., Excerp.Med., Ind.Med. (coverage dropped), Psychol.Abstr., e-psyche.
—CISTI, GNLM.
Published by: Propaceb, Editora de Publicaciones s.r.l., Casilla 1589, Lima 100, Peru. FAX 51-1-4385479. Eds. Javier Mariategui, Luis Trelles. Circ: 1,000.

618.8 ESP ISSN 0210-0010
REVISTA DE NEUROLOGIA. Text in Spanish. 1973. s-m. EUR 175 domestic; EUR 225 foreign (effective 2000). adv. bk.rev. *Refereed.* **Document type:** *Proceedings, Academic/Scholarly.*
Related titles: Online - full text ed.: (from Institute for Scientific Information).
Indexed: Excerp.Med., Ind.Med. (1972-), Ind.Med.Esp., Int.Nurs.Ind., Neurosci.Cit.Ind., e-psyche.
—BLDSC (7868.355000), CINDOC, GNLM, IDS, Infotrieve. **CCC.**
Address: PO Box 94121, Barcelona 08080, Spain. TEL 34-93-2478188, FAX 34-93-2317250, cvig@revneurol.com, http://www.neurologia.com. Ed. J Matias Guiu. Pub., Adv. contact Cesar Viguera. Circ: 10,000.

M

616.89 BRA ISSN 0101-6083 CODEN: RPCLF2
REVISTA DE PSIQUIATRIA CLINICA. Text in Portuguese. 1962. bi-m. adv. bk.rev. back issues avail. *Refereed.* **Document type:** *Academic/Scholarly.*
Formerly (until 1973): Universidade de Sao Paulo. Faculdade de Medicina. Hospital das Clinicas. Clinica Psiquiatrica. Boletim (0102-2814)
Related titles: Online - full text ed.
Indexed: PsycInfo, e-psyche.
Published by: (Universidade De Sao Paulo, Instituto de Psiquiatria), Lemos Editorial & Graficos Ltda., Rua Rui Barbosa, 70, B Vista, Sao Paulo, SP 01326-010, Brazil. TEL 55-11-251-4300, FAX 55-11-251-4300, lemospl@netpoint.com.br, http://www.lemos.com.br. Ed. Dr. Wagner Farid Gattaz. Adv. contact Paulo Lemos. Circ: 5,000 (controlled).

616.8 618.92 ESP ISSN 1130-9512
REVISTA DE PSIQUIATRIA INFANTO-JUVENIL. Text in Spanish. 1983. q. ESP 6,300, USD 70 (effective 1996).
Former titles (until 1990): Revista de Neuropsiquiatria Infanto-Juvenil (0214-6428); (until 1987): Revista de Neuropsiquiatria Infantil (0213-4985)
Indexed: PsycInfo, e-psyche.
—CINDOC, GNLM.
Published by: Grupo Masson, Rda General Mitre, 149, Barcelona 08022, Spain. TEL 34-93-2530200, FAX 34-93-2530515, masson@masson.es, http://www.masson.es, http://masson.es.

616.8 ECU ISSN 1019-8113
REVISTA ECUATORIANA DE NEUROLOGIA. Summaries in English, Spanish. 1992. s-a. ECS 3,000,000; USD 50 foreign. adv. bk.rev. *Refereed.* **Document type:** *Academic/Scholarly.*
Related titles: Online - full text ed.: (from Institute for Scientific Information).
Indexed: ASCA, Excerp.Med. (1993-), Neurosci.Cit.Ind., e-psyche.
—BLDSC (7852.810000), EMDOCS, GNLM, IDS, KNAW.
Published by: Sociedad Ecuatoriana de Neurologia, Apdo 09 01 3734, Guayaquil, Guayas, Ecuador. FAX 593-4285790, odbrutto@telconet.net. Ed. Dr. Oscar H Del Brutto. adv.: B&W page USD 200, color page USD 1,000. Circ: 1,000.

616.89 ESP ISSN 1137-3148
REVISTA ELECTRONICA DE PSIQUIATRIA. Variant title: Psiquiatria.Com. Text in Spanish. 1997. q. free per issue to qualified personnel. back issues avail. **Document type:** *Academic/Scholarly.* **Description:** Publishes papers on psychiatry research.
Media: Online - full text.
Published by: Internet y Salud, Apdo. de Correos 20018, Palma De Marrorca, Baleares 07080, Spain. info@intersalud.es, http://www.psiquiatria.com/noticias/archivo.htm.

616.89 FRA ISSN 0298-3850
REVUE DE MEDECINE PSYCHOSOMATIQUE. Text in French; Summaries in English. 1959. q. FRF 350 domestic to individuals; FRF 360 foreign to individuals; FRF 450 domestic to institutions; FRF 460 foreign to institutions (effective 1999).
Indexed: Excerp.Med., Ind.Med. (coverage dropped), Psychol.Abstr., e-psyche.
—CISTI, EMDOCS, GNLM.
Published by: (Societe Francaise de Medecine Psychosomatique), Pensee Sauvage Editions, B.P. 141, Grenoble 38002, France. TEL 76-87-13-03, FAX 76-46-27-25. Eds. Dr. L Chertok, Dr. M Sapir.

616.8 FRA ISSN 0035-161X
REVUE DE NEUROPSYCHIATRIE DE L'OUEST. Text in French. 1963. q. FRF 200 (effective 1999).
Indexed: e-psyche.
Published by: Societe de Neuro-Psychiatrie de l'Ouest, B.P. 226, Rennes, France.

616.8 FRA ISSN 1155-4452 CODEN: RNURER
REVUE DE NEUROPSYCHOLOGIE. Text in French. 1991. 4/yr. FRF 590 (effective 2000). adv. bk.rev. *Refereed.* **Document type:** *Academic/Scholarly.*
Related titles: Online - full text ed.: (from Institute for Scientific Information).
Indexed: ASCA, Lang.& Lang.Behav.Abstr., Neurosci.Cit.Ind., PsycInfo, Psychol.Abstr. (1991-), SOPODA, Sociol.Abstr., e-psyche.
—BLDSC (7937.880000), IDS.
Published by: Association pour la Diffusion des Recherches en Sciences Cognitives de Langue Francaise, CNRS - CRNC, 31 chemin Joseph Aiguier, Marseille Cedex 20 13402, France. TEL 33-4-91164279, FAX 33-4-91714938, cpc@lnf.cnrs-mrs.fr. Ed. Michel Habib. R&P, Adv. contact Francoise Joubaud.

REVUE EUROPEENE DE PSYCHOLOGIE APPLIQUEE/EUROPEAN REVIEW OF APPLIED PSYCHOLOGY. see *PSYCHOLOGY*

616.08 FRA ISSN 1164-4796
REVUE FRANCAISE DE PSYCHOSOMATIQUE. Text in French. 1991. s-a. FRF 295 to individuals; FRF 360 foreign to individuals (effective 2001).
Indexed: e-psyche.
—GNLM.
Published by: Presses Universitaires de France, Departement des Revues, 6 av. Reille, Paris 75685 Cedex 14, France. TEL 33-1-60873030, FAX 33-1-60792045, revues@puf.com.

616.8 FRA ISSN 0035-3787 CODEN: RENEAM
REVUE NEUROLOGIQUE. Text in French; Summaries in English. 1893. 10/yr. FRF 1,347; FRF 1,682 foreign (effective 2000). adv. bk.rev. abstr, illus. index. reprint service avail. from ISI. *Refereed.* **Document type:** *Academic/Scholarly.* **Description:** Publishes the works of the society, and French and foreign articles.
Related titles: Microfilm ed.: (from BHP); Microform ed.: (from PQC,BHP); Online - full text ed.: (from Institute for Scientific Information, RoweCom Information Quest).
Indexed: ASCA, Bibl.Dev.Med.& Child Neur., Biol.Abstr., C.I.S. Abstr., Chem.Abstr., Curr.Adv.Biochem., Curr.Adv.Cancer Res., Curr.Adv.Cell & Devel.Biol., Curr.Adv.Ecol.Sci., Curr.Cont., Excerp.Med., Helminthol.Abstr., Ind.Med. (1893-), Ind.Sci.Rev., Inpharma, Jrnl.Watch Neuro., Neurosci.Cit.Ind., Nutr.Abstr., Pharm.&Out.News, Protozool.Abstr., PsycInfo, Psychol.Abstr. (1992-), Reac., Rev.Appl.Entomol., Rev.Med.& Vet.Mycol., SSCI (coverage dropped), Sci.Cit.Ind., Trop.Dis.Bull., e-psyche.
—BLDSC (7937.750000), CISTI, EMDOCS, GNLM, IDS, KNAW. **CCC.**
Published by: (Societe Francaise de Neurologie), Masson - Periodiques, 120 bd. St. Germain, Paris 75006, France. TEL 33-1-40466200, FAX 33-1-40466201. Ed. J M Leger. Circ: 3,000. **Subscr. to:** Societe de Periodiques Specialises, BP 22, Vineuil Cedex 41354, France. TEL 33-2-54504612, FAX 33-2-54504611.

616.891 ITA ISSN 1592-8543
RICERCA IN PSICOTERAPIA. Text in Italian; Summaries in Italian, English. 1998. 3/yr. ITL 50,000 domestic; ITL 80,000 foreign (effective 2001). bibl, illus. **Document type:** *Academic/Scholarly.*
Published by: Edizioni La Vita Felice, Via Tadino, 52, Milan 20129, Italy. TEL 39-02-29524600, FAX 39-02-29401896, laviatafelice@iol.it, http://www.lavitafelice.it/pres.html. Ed. Gerardo Mastrullo.

616.8 JPN ISSN 0009-918X
RINSHO SHINKEIGAKU/CLINICAL NEUROLOGY. Text in Japanese; Summaries in English. 1960. m. JPY 13,000 (effective 2001). adv. charts, illus. index. *Refereed.* **Document type:** *Journal.*
Indexed: Biol.Abstr., Dent.Ind., Excerp.Med., INIS Atomind., Ind.Med. (1960-), Int.Nurs.Ind., e-psyche.
—BLDSC (3286.309000), CISTI, EMDOCS, GNLM, KNAW.
Published by: Japanese Society of Neurology/Nihon Shinkei Gakkai, Ichimaru Bldg, 2-31-21 Yushima, Bunkyo-ku, Tokyo 113-0034, Japan. TEL 81-3-3815-1080, FAX 81-3-3815-1931, desk@neurology-jp.org, http://www.neurology-jp.org/index.html. Ed. Nobuo Yanagisawa. Circ: 6,895.

616.8 ITA ISSN 0035-6336 CODEN: RNBLAC
RIVISTA DI NEUROBIOLOGIA. Text in Italian; Summaries in English. 1955. q. adv. bibl, charts, illus. index.
Indexed: Biol.Abstr., Chem.Abstr., Dent.Ind., Excerp.Med., Ind.Med. (coverage dropped), e-psyche.
—BLDSC, CISTI, GNLM.
Published by: Ospedale Neuropsichiatrico Provinciale, Arezzo, AR 52100, Italy. Ed. Marino Benvenuti. Circ: 300.

616.8 ITA ISSN 0035-6352
RIVISTA DI NEUROPSICHIATRIA E SCIENZE AFFINI. Text in Italian; Summaries in English. 1955. q. ITL 80,000; ITL 160,000 foreign (effective 1998). adv. bk.rev. **Document type:** *Academic/Scholarly.*
Indexed: Chem.Abstr., Excerp.Med., e-psyche.
—GNLM.
Published by: Casa Editrice Maccari, Via Palermo, 44, Parma, PR 43100, Italy. TEL 39-521-771268. Circ: 1,000.

RIVISTA DI NEURORADIOLOGIA. see *MEDICAL SCIENCES—Radiology And Nuclear Medicine*

616.89 ITA ISSN 0035-6484 CODEN: RPSID3
RIVISTA DI PSICHIATRIA. Text in Italian; Abstracts in English. 1966. bi-m. USD 117 (effective 2000). adv. bk.rev. charts, illus. index. 64 p./no. **Document type:** *Journal, Academic/Scholarly.*
Indexed: Excerp.Med., PsycInfo, Psychol.Abstr. (1966-), Ref.Zh., e-psyche.
—BLDSC (7992.731000), GNLM, KNAW.
Published by: Il Pensiero Scientifico Editore s.r.l., Via Bradano, 3-C, Rome, RM 00199, Italy. TEL 39-06-862821, FAX 39-06-86282250, pensiero@pensiero.it, http://www.pensiero.it. Eds. G C Reda, P Pancheri. Pub. Luca De Fiore. Adv. contact Luciano De Fiore. Circ: 500.

616.8 ITA ISSN 1122-2263
RIVISTA DI RIABILITAZIONE PSICHIATRICA E PSICOSOCIALE. Text in English, Italian. 1992. 3/yr. ITL 60,000 to individuals; ITL 80,000 to institutions; USD 100 foreign. **Document type:** *Academic/Scholarly.*
Related titles: ♦ Supplement: Rivista di Riabilitazione Psichiatrica e psicosociale. Supplemento. ISSN 1122-2298.
Indexed: e-psyche.
Published by: Casa Editrice Idelson, Via Annibale De Gasperis, 55, Naples, NA 80137, Italy. TEL 39-81-5524733, FAX 39-81-5518295, idelgno@tin.it, http://www.idelson-gnocchi.com. Ed. Massimo Casacchia.

616.8 ITA ISSN 1122-2298
RIVISTA DI RIABILITAZIONE PSICHIATRICA E PSICOSOCIALE. SUPPLEMENTO. Text in English, Italian. 1992. 3/yr.
Related titles: ♦ Supplement to: Rivista di Riabilitazione Psichiatrica e Psicosociale. ISSN 1122-2263.
Published by: Casa Editrice Idelson, Via Annibale De Gasperis, 55, Naples, NA 80137, Italy. TEL 39-81-5524733, FAX 39-81-5518295, idelgno@tin.it, http://www.idelson-gnocchi.com.

RIVISTA ITALIANA DI ANALISI TRANSAZIONALE E METODOLOGIE PSICOTERAPEUTICHE. see *PSYCHOLOGY*

616.8 ITA ISSN 0035-7057 CODEN: RSFMA
RIVISTA SPERIMENTALE DI FRENIATRIA; la rivista dei servizi di salute mentale. Text in Italian; Summaries in English, French. 1875. bi-m. ITL 80,000; ITL 100,000 foreign (effective 1999). adv. bk.rev. **Document type:** *Academic/Scholarly.*
Indexed: Biol.Abstr., Chem.Abstr., Excerp.Med., Ind.Med. (coverage dropped), Psychol.Abstr., e-psyche.
—BLDSC, GNLM.
Published by: (Istituti Ospedalieri Neuropsichiatrici di San Lazzaro), Centro Scientifico Editore, Via Borgone, 57, Turin, TO 10139, Italy. TEL 11-385-3656, FAX 11-385-3244. Ed. Piero Benassi.

616.8 ROM CODEN: RRNPEE
ROMANIAN JOURNAL OF NEUROLOGY: SERIE DE NEUROLOGIE ET PSYCHIATRIE. Text in English, French, German, Russian; Summaries in English. 1964. q. ROL 200, USD 55. bk.rev. charts, illus. index. **Document type:** *Academic/Scholarly.*
Former titles: Revue Roumaine de Neurologie et Psychiatrie (1017-5644); (until 1990): Revue Roumaine de Medecine. Neurologie et Psychiatrie (0259-6326); Which supersedes in part (in 1975): Revue Roumaine de Medecine (0303-822X); Which was formed by the 1974 merger of: Revue Roumaine de Medecine Interne (0035-3973); Revue Roumaine d'Endocrinologie (0035-4015); Revue Roumaine de Neurologie et de Psychiatrie (0301-7303)
Indexed: Biol.Abstr., Excerp.Med., Ind.Med. (coverage dropped), Psychol.Abstr. (1979-), e-psyche.
—BLDSC, CISTI, GNLM, KNAW, Linda Hall.
Published by: (Academia de Stiinte Medicale), Editura Academiei Romane, Calea 13 Septembrie 13, Bucharest 76117, Romania. Ed. Vlad Voiculescu. Circ: 700. **Dist. by:** Rodipet S.A.. TEL 401-618-5103, FAX 401-222-6407.

616.8 617 ROM ISSN 1220-8841
ROMANIAN NEUROSURGERY. Text in English. 1992. s-a.
Indexed: e-psyche.
Published by: (Clinica de Neurochirurgie, Academia Romana), Editura Academiei Romane, Calea 13 Septembrie 13, Bucharest 76117, Romania. Ed. Alexandru Constantinovici. **Dist. by:** Rodipet S.A.. TEL 401-618-5103, FAX 401-222-6407.

M

616.8 JPN ISSN 0914-7691
RONENKICHIHO/JOURNAL OF SENILE DEMENTIA. Text in Japanese. 1987. 4/yr. JPY 1,800 per issue (effective 1998).
Indexed: e-psyche.
Published by: Medikaru Rebyusha/Medical Review Co., Ltd., 7-3 Hirano-Machi 1-chome, Chuo-ku, Osaka-shi 541-0046, Japan. TEL 81-6-223-1556, FAX 81-6-223-1414, medrev@osk2.3web.ne.jp.

616.89 RUS
ROSSIISKII PSIKHYATRICHESKII ZHURNAL/RUSSIAN JOURNAL OF PSYCHIATRY. Text in Russian; Summaries in English. 1997. bi-m. USD 194 foreign (effective 2000). adv. bk.rev., Website rev. abstr, bibl, illus. back issues avail.; reprints avail. **Document type:** *Journal, Academic/Scholarly.* **Description:** Covers issues relevant to experimental, clinical and preventive psychiatry, as well as management of psychiatric services.
Related titles: Fax ed.
Indexed: Ref.Zh.
Published by: Izdatel'stvo Meditsina, Petroverigskii per 6-8, Moscow 101000, Russian Federation. TEL 7-095-9248785, FAX 7-095-9211355, 7-095-9286003, meditsina@iname.com, http://www.medit.ru. Ed., R&P T Dmitrieva. Pub. A M Stochik. Adv. contact O A Fadeeva TEL 7-095-923-51-40. Circ: 500. **US dist. addr.:** East View Publications, 3020 Harbor Ln N, Minneapolis, MN 55447. TEL 612-550-0961.

616.8 GBR
ROYAL COLLEGE OF PSYCHIATRISTS. COUNCIL REPORTS. Text in English. irreg., latest vol.75, 1999. **Document type:** *Monographic series.*
Indexed: e-psyche.
—BLDSC (3480.68000).
Published by: Royal College of Psychiatrists, 17 Belgrave Sq, London SW1X 8PG, United Kingdom. TEL 44-20-7235-8857, FAX 44-20-7245-1231.

S L D EXPERIENCE. see *EDUCATION—Special Education And Rehabilitation*

616.8 ITA ISSN 0390-5179
SAGGI; neuropsicologia infantile psicopedagogia riabilitazione. Text in Italian; Summaries in English. 1975. 2/yr. ITL 50,000 (effective 1999). adv. bk.rev. cum.index: 1975-1994. *Refereed.* **Document type:** *Monographic series, Academic/Scholarly.* **Description:** Covers infant neuropsychology and psychopedagogic rehabilitation.
Related titles: Online - full text ed.: (from Institute for Scientific Information).
Indexed: ASCA, Neurosci.Cit.Ind., PsycInfo, Psychol.Abstr. (1993-), SSCI (coverage dropped), e-psyche.
—IDS.
Published by: (Scientific Institute "Eugenio Medea"), Masson S.p.A., Divisione Periodici, Via F.lli Bressan 2, Milan, MI 20126, Italy. TEL 39-2-270741, FAX 39-2-27074210. Ed. Giorgio Moretti. Circ: 1,500 (controlled).

616.8 617 JPN ISSN 0385-0943
SAITAMA-KEN NO SHINKEI GEKAIKAI KAIHO/SAITAMA NEUROSURGICAL ASSOCIATION. BULLETIN. Text in Japanese. 1974. s-a. JPY 4,000 to members. **Document type:** *Bulletin.*
Indexed: e-psyche.
Published by: Saitamaken No Shinkei Gekaikai, 5-1 Naka-cho 3-chome, Urawa-shi, Saitama-ken 336-0007, Japan. Eds. Fujio Mizoguchi, Takao Ishibashi.

616.89 MEX ISSN 0185-3325
SALUD MENTAL. Text in English, Spanish. 1978. bi-m. MXP 250 domestic to individuals; USD 60 foreign to individuals; USD 90 to institutions (effective 2000). adv. bk.rev. bibl, illus, abstr. cum.index. Supplement avail.; back issues avail. *Refereed.* **Document type:** *Academic/Scholarly.* **Description:** Covers research in neurosciences, clinical psychiatry, epidemiology, mental health, psychopharmacology, history of psychiatry, problems of ethics, drug addiction and neuropsychology.
Related titles: CD-ROM ed.; Online - full text ed.: (from Institute for Scientific Information).
Indexed: ASCA, Curr.Cont., Excerp.Med. (1995-), Ind.Med. (coverage dropped), Neurosci.Cit.Ind., PsycInfo, Psychol.Abstr. (1979-), SSCI, e-psyche.
—BLDSC (8071.770000), GNLM, IDS.
Published by: (Instituto Mexicano de Psiquiatria), Editorial Laser S.A. de C.V., LAGO ALBERTO 442-7, Col Anahuac, Deleg. Miguel Hidalgo, Mexico City, DF 11320, Mexico. TEL 52-5-2600250, FAX 52-5-2600048, perezrh@imp.edu.mx. Ed. Dr. Hector Perez Rincon. Pub. Bruno Vanneuville. adv.: page USD 650. Circ: 2,000.

SAMENWERKINGSVERBAND JEUGDHULPVERLENING UTRECHT. NIEUWSBRIEF. see *CHILDREN AND YOUTH—About*

SAMIKSA. see *PSYCHOLOGY*

616.8 FRA
SANTE MENTALE. Text in French. m. FRF 290; FRF 350 foreign (effective 2000). adv.
Published by: Acte Presse, 12 rue Dupetit Thouars, Paris 75003, France. TEL 33-1-42775277, FAX 33-1-42775237, smentale@club-internet.fr. Pub. Antoine Lolivier. Adv. contact Beatrice Bertelli. B&W page FRF 14,300, color page FRF 20,700.

616.891 DNK ISSN 0106-2301
RC500
THE SCANDINAVIAN PSYCHOANALYTIC REVIEW. Text in English. 1978. s-a. USD 66 in the Americas to institutions print & online eds. combined; GBP 46 elsewhere to institutions print & online eds. combined (effective 2002). bk.rev. reprint service avail. from ISI. *Refereed.* **Document type:** *Academic/Scholarly.*
Indexed: ASCA, Curr.Cont. (coverage dropped), IMFL, PsycInfo, Psychoanal.Abstr., Psychol.Abstr. (1978-), SSCI (coverage dropped), e-psyche.
—BLDSC (8087.572800), GNLM, Infotrieve, ingenta. **CCC.**
Published by: (Psycho-Analytical Societies in Denmark, Finland, Norway and Sweden), Blackwell Munksgaard, Noerre Soegade 35, PO Box 2148, Copenhagen K 1016, Denmark. TEL 45-77-33-33-33, FAX 45-77-33-33-77, fsub@mail.munksgaard.dk, http://www.blackwellmunksgaard.com/psychoanalyticreview. Ed. Henrik Enckell. Circ: 900.

616.89 USA ISSN 0586-7614
RC514 CODEN: SCZBB3
SCHIZOPHRENIA BULLETIN. Text in English. 1969. q. USD 20 (effective 2001). abstr, bibl, charts, illus, stat. back issues avail.; reprint service avail. from PQC,PSC,SCH. *Refereed.* **Document type:** *Bulletin, Government.*
Related titles: Microform ed.: (from MIM,PQC); Online - full text ed.: (from Northern Light Technology, Inc., ProQuest Information & Learning, Institute for Scientific Information).
Indexed: ASCA, Addic.Abstr., Adol.Ment.Hlth.Abstr., AgeLine, Biol.Abstr., CINAHL, Crim.Just.Abstr., Curr.Adv.Ecol.Sci., Curr.Cont., Except.Child Educ.Abstr., Excerp.Med., Fam.Ind., IBZ, INIS Atomind., Ind.Med. (1969-), Ind.Sci.Rev., Ind.U.S.Gov.Per., Inpharma, Int.Abstr.Biol.Sci., Int.Nurs.Ind., Jrnl.Watch Psych., Neurosci.Cit.Ind., Pharm.&Out.News, PsycInfo, Psychol.Abstr. (1969-), Reac., SSCI, Sci.Cit.Ind., e-psyche.
—BLDSC (8089.400000), CISTI, EMDOCS, GNLM, IDS, ingenta, KNAW.
Published by: U.S. Public Health Service, National Institute of Mental Health, 6001 Executive Blvd, Rm 7160, Rockville, MD 20852-9663. TEL 301-443-6130, FAX 301-443-4279, lalberts@nih.gov, http://psychiatry.medscape.com/govmt/NIMH/SchizophreniaBulletin/public/journal.SB.html, http://www.nimh.nih.gov/. Eds. David Shore, John K Hsiao. R&P Lisa Alberts. Circ: 7,000. **Subscr. to:** U.S. Government Printing Office, Superintendent of Documents, PO Box 371954, Pittsburgh, PA 15250-7954. TEL 202-512-1800, FAX 202-512-2250, orders@gpo.gov, http://www.access.gpo.gov.

616.8 NLD ISSN 0920-9964
RC514 CODEN: SCRSEH
SCHIZOPHRENIA RESEARCH; an international multidisciplinary journal. Text in English. 1988. 18/yr. EUR 155 in Europe to individuals; JPY 20,400 in Japan to individuals; USD 172 elsewhere to individuals; EUR 2,462 in Europe to institutions; JPY 327,000 in Japan to institutions; USD 2,754 elsewhere to institutions (effective 2002). bk.rev. reprint service avail. from ISI. *Refereed.* **Document type:** *Academic/Scholarly.* **Description:** Presents new international research that contributes to the understanding of schizophrenic disorders.
Related titles: Microform ed.: (from PQC); Online - full text ed.: (from ingenta, Swets Blackwell, Institute for Scientific Information, ScienceDirect).
Indexed: ASCA, Addic.Abstr., AgeLine, Curr.Cont., Excerp.Med., Fam.Ind., Ind.Med. (1988-), Ind.Sci.Rev., Indian Psychol.Abstr., Inpharma, Int.Nurs.Ind., Neurosci.Cit.Ind., PsycInfo, Psychol.Abstr. (1988-), Reac., SSCI, Sci.Cit.Ind., e-psyche.
—BLDSC (8089.440000), ADONIS, CISTI, EMDOCS, GNLM, IDS, ingenta, KNAW. **CCC.**
Published by: Elsevier Science BV, PO Box 211, Amsterdam 1000 AE, Netherlands. TEL 31-20-485-2911, FAX 31-20-485-2457, http://www.elsevier.nl/locate/issn/09209964. Eds. H A Nasrallah, L E Delisi. Circ: 800. **Subscr. in Australasia and the Far East to:** Elsevier Science (Singapore) Pte Ltd, No.1 Temasek Ave, 17-01 Millenia Tower, Singapore 039192, Singapore. TEL 65-434-3727, FAX 65-337-2230; **Subscr. in Japan to:** Elsevier Science Inc - Japan Regional Office, 9-15 Higashi-Azabu 1-chome, Minato-ku, Tokyo 106-0044, Japan. TEL 81-3-5561-5033; **Subscr. in the Americas to:** Elsevier Science, PO Box 945, New York, NY 10159-0945. TEL 212-633-3730, FAX 212-633-3680, usinfo-f@elsevier.com.

616.89 CHE ISSN 0258-7661
CODEN: SANNAW
SCHWEIZER ARCHIV FUER NEUROLOGIE UND PSYCHIATRIE. Text in English, French, German, Italian. 1917. 6/yr. CHF 96; CHF 20 newsstand/cover (effective 2001). adv. bk.rev. charts, illus. index per vol. reprint service avail. from PQC. **Document type:** *Journal, Academic/Scholarly.*
Former titles (until 1985): Schweizer Archiv fuer Neurologie, Neurochirurgie und Psychiatrie (0036-7273); (until 1959): Schweizer Archiv fuer Neurologie und Psychiatrie (0370-8373)
Related titles: Microform ed.: (from PQC).
Indexed: Biol.Abstr., Chem.Abstr., Curr.Cont. (coverage dropped), Excerp.Med., Ind.Med. (coverage dropped), Ind.Vet., Nutr.Abstr., PsycInfo, Psychol.Abstr. (1970-), Ref.Zh., Vet.Bull., e-psyche.
—BLDSC (1643.185000), CASDDS, CISTI, GNLM, Infotrieve. **CCC.**
Published by: (Schweizerische Neurologische Gesellschaft), Schwabe und Co. AG, Steinentorstr 13, Basel 4010, Switzerland. TEL 41-61-2789565, FAX 41-61-2789566, verlag@schwabe.ch, http://www.schwabe.ch. Eds. Dr. A.J. Steck, Dr. D Hell, Dr. F Ferrero, Dr. J Bogousslavsky. Circ: 2,500.
Co-sponsor: Schweizerische Gesellschaft fuer Psychiatrie.

616.8 GBR ISSN 0952-2255
SCIENTIFIC BASIS OF PSYCHIATRY. Text in English. 1985. irreg. **Document type:** *Monographic series.*
Indexed: e-psyche.
—CISTI.
Published by: Cambridge University Press, Edinburgh Bldg, Shaftesbury Rd, Cambridge CB2 2RU, United Kingdom. FAX 44-1223-315052, information@cup.cam.ac.uk, information@cambridge.org, http://www.cup.cam.ac.uk, http://www.uk.cambridge.org/journals/pmu.

SCRIPT. see *PSYCHOLOGY*

616.831 AUS ISSN 1329-0940
SECRETARIAT. Text in English. 1996. bi-m.
Published by: Alzheimer's Association of Australia Inc., PO Box 108, Higgins, ACT 2615, Australia. TEL 61-2-6254-4233, FAX 61-2-6254-2522, secretariat@alzheimers.org.au, http://www.alzheimers.org.au/secretariat/index.htm.

616.8 JPN ISSN 0488-1281
SEISHIN IGAKU/CLINICAL PSYCHIATRY. Text in Japanese; Summaries in English. 1959. m. JPY 27,600, USD 272.70.
Related titles: Online - full text ed.: (from JICST).
Indexed: INIS Atomind., Inpharma, PsycInfo, Reac., Ref.Zh., e-psyche.
—BLDSC (3286.340000), CISTI, GNLM.
Published by: Igaku-Shoin Ltd., 5-24-3 Hongo, Bunkyo-ku, Tokyo 113-0033, Japan. TEL 81-3-3817-5711, FAX 81-3-3815-7802, seishin@nna.so-net.or.jp. Circ: 6,000.

616.8 JPN ISSN 0080-8547
SEISHIN IGAKU KENKYUJO, TOKYO. GYOSEKISHU/SEISHIN IGAKU INSTITUTE OF PSYCHIATRY, TOKYO. BULLETIN. Text in Japanese; Abstracts and contents page in English. 1954. a. free per issue. reprints avail.
Indexed: Biol.Abstr., Excerp.Med., e-psyche.
—BLDSC (2704.450000), CISTI, GNLM, KNAW.
Published by: Seishin Igaku Institute of Psychiatry/Seishin Igaku Kenkyujo, 11-11 Komone 4-chome, Itabashi-ku, Tokyo 173-0037, Japan. FAX 03-956-9644.

616.891 JPN ISSN 0916-8710
SEISHIN RYOHO/JAPANESE JOURNAL OF PSYCHOTHERAPY. Text in Japanese. 1975. bi-m. JPY 1,850 per issue (effective 2001). bk.rev. **Document type:** *Academic/Scholarly.*
Formerly (until 1992): Kikan Seishin Ryoho (0386-9660)
Indexed: e-psyche.

M

Published by: Kongo Shuppan, 5-16 Suido 1-chome, Bunkyo-ku, Tokyo 112-0005, Japan. TEL 81-3-3815-6661, FAX 81-3-3818-6848, kongo@kongoshuppan.co.jp, http://kongoshuppan.co.jp. Ed. Haruo Tanaka.

616.8 GBR ISSN 1059-1311
CODEN: SEIZE7
SEIZURE; European Journal of Epilepsy. Text in English. 1992. 8/yr. GBP 134 to individuals; GBP 315 to institutions (effective 2002). back issues avail.; reprint service avail. from SWZ. *Refereed.* **Document type:** *Academic/Scholarly.* **Description:** Provides an interdisciplinary forum for original research in all aspects of epilepsy, including the basic sciences, differential diagnosis and epidemiology of seizures, treatment and management of epilepsy, and related social issues.
Related titles: Online - full text ed.: (from EBSCO Publishing, RoweCom Information Quest, Swets Blackwell, IDEAL Online Library, Institute for Scientific Information).
Indexed: ASCA, Curr.Cont., Excerp.Med. (1994-), Ind.Med. (1992-), Indian Psychol.Abstr., Inpharma, Int.Nurs.Ind., Neurosci.Cit.Ind., Pharm.&Out.News, PsycInfo, Reac., Ref.Zh., Sci.Cit.Ind., e-psyche.
—BLDSC (8229.100000), EMDOCS, GNLM, IDS, Infotrieve, KNAW. **CCC.**
Published by: W.B. Saunders Co. Ltd. (Subsidiary of: Harcourt Publishers Ltd.), 24-28 Oval Rd, London NW1 7DX, United Kingdom. TEL 44-20-7424-4200, FAX 44-20-7424-4515, cservice@harcourt.com, http://www.harcourt-international.com/journals/seiz/default.cfm. Ed. T Betts. **Subscr. to:** Harcourt Publishers Ltd., Foots Cray High St, Sidcup, Kent DA14 5HP, United Kingdom. TEL 44-20-8308-5700, FAX 44-20-8309-0807.

616.8 USA ISSN 1528-9931
▼ **SEMINARS IN CEREBROVASCULAR DISEASES AND STROKE.** Text in English. 2001. q. USD 119 domestic to individuals; USD 166 domestic to institutions; USD 71 domestic to students; USD 138 foreign to individuals; USD 198 foreign to institutions; USD 138 foreign to students; USD 50 newsstand/cover (effective 2001). adv. *Refereed.* **Document type:** *Journal, Academic/Scholarly.* **Description:** Examines advances in diagnostic and management practices in the field of cerebrovascular disease.
Published by: W.B. Saunders Co. (Subsidiary of: Harcourt Publishers Ltd.), 11830 Westline Industrial Dr, St Louis, MO 63146. TEL 800-325-4177, http://www.wbsaunders.com. Ed. Dr. Jose Biller.

616.89 USA ISSN 1084-3612
SEMINARS IN CLINICAL NEUROPSYCHIATRY. Text in English. 1996. q. USD 129 domestic to individuals; USD 171 foreign to individuals; USD 175 domestic to institutions; USD 216 foreign to institutions; USD 84 domestic to students; USD 103 foreign to students; USD 55 newsstand/cover (effective 2001). **Document type:** *Journal, Academic/Scholarly.* **Description:** Reviews of developments in the understanding, assessment, and treatment of behavioral manifestations of neurobiological disorders.
Indexed: Ind.Med. (1996-).
Published by: W.B. Saunders Co. (Subsidiary of: Harcourt Publishers Ltd.), 11830 Westline Industrial Dr, St Louis, MO 63146. TEL 800-325-4177, wbspcs@harcourtbrace.com, http://www.wbsaunders.com. Ed. Dr. Gary J Tucker.

SEMINARS IN NEUROLOGICAL SURGERY. see *MEDICAL SCIENCES—Surgery*

616.8 USA ISSN 0271-8235
UNC CODEN: SEMNEP
SEMINARS IN NEUROLOGY. Text in English. 1980. q. EUR 185 to individuals; EUR 375 to institutions; EUR 87 newsstand/cover (effective 2002). adv. abstr, bibl, charts, illus, stat. index. *Refereed.* **Document type:** *Journal, Academic/Scholarly.* **Description:** Offers a broad, informed perspective on pivitol topics in contemporary neurology, along with practical tips for managing diagnostic and therapeutic problems and a reference database.
Related titles: Microform ed.: (from PQC); Online - full text ed.: ISSN 1098-9021 (from Ovid Technologies, Inc., EBSCO Publishing, O C L C Online Computer Library Center, Inc., RoweCom Information Quest, Institute for Scientific Information).
Indexed: ASCA, Abstr.Hyg., Biol.Abstr., Curr.Adv.Ecol.Sci., Curr.Cont., Excerp.Med., Ind.Med. (1981-), Inpharma, Neurosci.Cit.Ind., Pharm.&Out.News, Protozool.Abstr., Reac., e-psyche.
—BLDSC (8239.455550), CISTI, EMDOCS, GNLM, IDS, ingenta, KNAW. **CCC.**
Published by: Thieme Medical Publishers, 333 Seventh Ave, New York, NY 10001. TEL 212-760-0888, 800-782-3488, FAX 212-947-1112, http://www.thieme.com. Ed. Dr. Robert M. Pascuzzi. Circ: 3,441. **Orders in Europe to:** Thieme International, Postfach 3001120, Stuttgart 70451, Germany. TEL 49-711-8931-0.

SEMINARS IN NEUROSURGERY. see *MEDICAL SCIENCES—Surgery*

616.8 618.92 USA ISSN 1071-9091
CODEN: SPNEFD
SEMINARS IN PEDIATRIC NEUROLOGY. Text in English. 1994. q. USD 146 domestic to individuals; USD 184 foreign to individuals; USD 180 domestic to institutions; USD 221 foreign to institutions; USD 85 domestic to students; USD 110 foreign to students; USD 56 newsstand/cover (effective 2001). adv. **Document type:** *Academic/Scholarly.* **Description:** Covers topics of current importance in the field of pediatric neurology.
Indexed: CINAHL, Ind.Med. (1994-), Int.Nurs.Ind., e-psyche.
—BLDSC (8239.456785), GNLM, Infotrieve, KNAW. **CCC.**
Published by: W.B. Saunders Co. (Subsidiary of: Harcourt Publishers Ltd.), 11830 Westline Industrial Dr, St Louis, MO 63146. TEL 800-325-4177, http://www.wbsaunders.com. Ed. Dr. John B Bodensteiner. Adv. contact Steve Gray. B&W page USD 705, color page USD 1,625; trim 10 x 7. Circ: 1,028. **Subscr. to:** Periodicals Fulfillment, W B Saunders Co, 6277 Sea Harbor Dr, 4th Fl, Orlando, FL 32891-4800.

616.8 USA ISSN 1044-5765
RC321 CODEN: SNEUEZ
SEMINARS IN THE NEUROSCIENCES. Text in English. 1989. bi-m. USD 199; USD 262 foreign (effective 1998). back issues avail.; reprint service avail. from SWZ. *Refereed.* **Document type:** *Academic/Scholarly.* **Description:** For scientists in the neurological sciences and the life sciences.
Related titles: Online - full text ed.: (from EBSCO Publishing, O C L C Online Computer Library Center, Inc., ingenta, Swets Blackwell, IDEAL Online Library).
Indexed: ASCA, Anim.Behav.Abstr. (coverage dropped), Aqua.Sci.& Fish.Abstr., Biotech.& Bioeng.Abstr., Cal.Tiss.Abstr., Chem.Abstr., Chem.Indus.Notes, Chem.Titles, Chemorec.Abstr., Curr.Cont. (coverage dropped), Excerp.Med. (1993-), Ind.Sci.Rev., Neurosci.Abstr., Neurosci.Cit.Ind., SSCI (coverage dropped), Sci.Cit.Ind. (coverage dropped), Zoo.Rec., e-psyche.
—CASDDS, CISTI, EMDOCS, GNLM, IDS, ingenta. **CCC.**
Published by: Academic Press, Inc., Journal Division (Subsidiary of: Harcourt Brace & Company), 525 B St, Ste 1900, San Diego, CA 92101-4495. TEL 619-699-6800, FAX 619-230-1840, apsubs@acad.com, http://www.academicpress.com/semneuro.

612.8 NLD ISSN 1567-5157
CODEN: PRSNFC
SENSORY NEURON; the international interdisciplinary journal reporting basic and clinical research on sensory receptors and primary afferent neurons. Text in English. 1995. q. EUR 190, USD 220 includes online ed. (effective 2002). illus. back issues avail. *Refereed.* **Document type:** *Journal, Academic/Scholarly.* **Description:** Publishes research papers on all aspects of sensory receptors.
Formerly (until 2000): Primary Sensory Neuron (0929-9637)
Related titles: Online - full content ed.: 2000 (from EBSCO Publishing, Swets Blackwell); Online - full text ed.: (from CatchWord Ltd.).
Indexed: Chem.Abstr., Chem.Indus.Notes, Chem.Titles, e-psyche.
—BLDSC (8241.787800), CASDDS.
Published by: V S P (Subsidiary of: Brill Academic Publishers), PO Box 346, Zeist 3700 AH, Netherlands. TEL 31-30-692-5790, FAX 31-30-693-2081, vsppub@compuserve.com, http://www.vsppub.com/journals/jn-SenNeu.html. Ed. P W Reeh.

616.89 CHN ISSN 1002-0829
SHANGHAI JINGSHEN YIXUE/SHANGHAI ARCHIVES OF PSYCHIATRY. Text in Chinese. 1989. q. USD 13. adv. **Description:** Provides up-to-date coverage of psychiatry in China and around the world.
Indexed: e-psyche.
Published by: Shanghai Shi Jingshen Weisheng Zhongxin/Shanghai Mental Health Centre, 600 Wanping Nanlu, Shanghai 200030, China. TEL 86-21-4387250, FAX 86-21-4387986. Ed. Wenwei Yan. Adv. contact Keliang Zhan. page USD 900. Circ: 5,300.

616.8 GBR ISSN 1353-0437
SHAPING BRITISH PSYCHIATRY. Text in English. 1995. q. **Document type:** *Academic/Scholarly.*
Indexed: e-psyche.
Published by: Medical Action Communications Ltd., Medical Action Communication, PO Box 56, Egham, Surrey TW20 8QZ, United Kingdom. Ed. Jane White.

616.8 CHN ISSN 1000-7547
SHENJING JIEPOUXUE ZAZHI/CHINESE JOURNAL OF NEUROANATOMY. Text in Chinese. q. USD 25.20; USD 6.30 newsstand/cover (effective 2001). **Document type:** *Academic/Scholarly.*
Published by: China International Book Trading Corp/Zhongguo Guoji Tushu Maoyi Zonggongsi cibtc@mail.cibtc.com.cn, http://www.cibtc.com.cn. **Dist. by:** 35, Chegongzhuang Xilu, Haidian District, Beijing 100044, China.

616.8 617.7 JPN ISSN 0389-5610
SHINKEI GAISHO/NEUROTRAUMATOLOGY. Variant title: Nihon Shinkei Gaisho Gakkai Koenshu. Text in Japanese; Summaries in English. 1979. a. JPY 5,000. back issues avail. **Document type:** *Academic/Scholarly.*
Indexed: INIS Atomind., e-psyche.
Published by: Japan Society of Neurotraumatology/Nihon Shinkei Gaisho Gakkai, Tokyo Jikei University School of Medicine, Department of Neurosurgery, 3-25-8, Nishi-Shinbashi, Minato-ku, Tokyo 105-8461, Japan. TEL 81-3-3445-0358. Circ: 1,000.

SHINKEI GANKA/NEURO-OPHTHALMOLOGY JAPAN. see *MEDICAL SCIENCES—Ophthalmology And Optometry*

616.8 JPN ISSN 0037-3796
SHINKEI KAGAKU/JAPANESE NEUROCHEMICAL SOCIETY. BULLETIN. Text in Japanese. 1962. s-a. price varies. adv. bk.rev. bibl.
Formerly: Nerve Chemistry
Media: Duplicated (not offset).
Indexed: Biol.Abstr., Chem.Abstr., INIS Atomind., e-psyche.
—Linda Hall.
Published by: Japanese Neurochemical Society/Nihon Shinkei Kagakkai, Nihon Gakkai Jimu Senta, 16-9 Honkomagome 5-chome, Bunkyo-ku, Tokyo 113-0021, Japan. Ed. Yasuo Kakimoto. Circ: 1,500.

616.8 JPN ISSN 0001-8724
CODEN: SKNSAF
SHINKEI KENKYU NO SHINPO/ADVANCES IN NEUROLOGICAL SCIENCES. Text in Japanese; Summaries in Multiple languages. 1966. bi-m. JPY 33,360, USD 224.
Indexed: Apic.Abstr., Biol.Abstr., Chem.Abstr., Chem.Titles, Excerp.Med., INIS Atomind., Ind.Med. (coverage dropped), e-psyche.
—BLDSC (0709.480000), CASDDS, CISTI, GNLM.
Published by: Igaku-Shoin Ltd., 5-24-3 Hongo, Bunkyo-ku, Tokyo 113-0033, Japan. TEL 81-3-3817-5702. Circ: 3,000.

616.8 JPN ISSN 0285-9513
SHITSUGOSHO KENKYU/HIGHER BRAIN FUNCTION RESEARCH. Text in Japanese; Summaries in English, Japanese. 1981. q. JPY 2,000 per issue.
Indexed: e-psyche.
Published by: Nihon Shitsugosho Gakkai/Japanese Society of Aphasiology, Izu Nirayama Onsen Byoin, 234 Chujo, Tagata-gun, Nirayama-cho, Shizuoka-ken 410-2121, Japan.

SIGNAL'NAYA INFORMATSIYA. NEIROPEPTIDY. see *MEDICAL SCIENCES—Abstracting, Bibliographies, Statistics*

616.858842 ITA ISSN 1122-147X
SINDROME DOWN NOTIZIE. Text in Italian. 1981. q. ITL 22,500, USD 15 domestic; ITL 100,000 foreign (effective 2000). bk.rev. bibl. 80 p./no. back issues avail. **Document type:** *Magazine, Academic/Scholarly.* **Description:** Covers medical, educational, and social aspects of Down's Syndrome. For families, doctors, psychologists, social workers and teachers.
Indexed: e-psyche.
Published by: (Associazione Italiana delle Persone Down), Edizioni Junior s.r.l., Viale dell'Industria, Azzano San Paolo (BG) 24052, Italy. TEL 39-035-534123, FAX 39-035-534143, edjunior@mediacom.it, http://www.edizionijunior.it. Ed. Anna Contardi. Circ: 5,500.

M

616.8 USA ISSN 0161-8105
QP425 CODEN: SLEED6
SLEEP. Text in English. 1978. 9/yr. USD 185; USD 220 foreign (effective 1999). adv. bk.rev. index. back issues avail.; reprint service avail. from PSC,SCH. *Refereed.* **Document type:** *Trade.* **Description:** Focuses on sleep medicine and sleep research.
Related titles: Online - full text ed.: (from Institute for Scientific Information).
Indexed: ASCA, AgeLine, Aqua.Sci.& Fish.Abstr., Bibl.Dev.Med.& Child Neur., Curr.Cont., Dent.Ind., Excerp.Med., INIS Atomind., Ind.Med. (1978-), Ind.Sci.Rev., Inpharma, Neurosci.Abstr. (coverage dropped), Neurosci.Cit.Ind., Pharm.&Out.News, PsycInfo, Psychol.Abstr. (1979-), Reac., Risk Abstr., Sci.Cit.Ind., e-psyche.
—BLDSC (8309.440000), CASDDS, CISTI, GNLM, ingenta, KNAW. **CCC.**
Published by: American Sleep Disorders Association, c/o Allen Press, Box 1897, Lawrence, KS 66044. TEL 507-287-6006, FAX 507-287-6008. Ed. Thomas Roth. Circ: 5,000. **Co-publisher:** Sleep Research Society.

616.2 USA ISSN 1520-9512
SLEEP AND BREATHING. Text in English. 1997. q. EUR 103 to individuals; EUR 138 to institutions; EUR 28 newsstand/cover (effective 2002). adv. abstr. *Refereed.* **Document type:** *Journal, Academic/Scholarly.* **Description:** Discusses the newest clinical research in sleep medicine, covering topics related to the diagnosis and treatment of sleep disordered breathing, including upper airway resistance syndrome and sleep apnea.
Related titles: Online - full text ed.: ISSN 1522-1709 (from RoweCom Information Quest).
Indexed: e-psyche.
—BLDSC (8309.445000).
Published by: Thieme Medical Publishers, 333 Seventh Ave, New York, NY 10001. TEL 212-760-0888, 800-782-3488, FAX 212-947-1112, custserv@thieme.com, http://www.thieme.com. Eds. Dr. Kingman P Strohl, Dr. Nicklaus C Netzer. **Orders in Europe to:** Thieme International, Postfach 3001120, Stuttgart 70451, Germany. TEL 49-711-8931-0.

616.89 TUR ISSN 1302-1192
▼ **SLEEP AND HYPNOSIS.** Text in English. 1999. q. USD 30 domestic to individuals; USD 45 foreign to individuals; USD 75 domestic to institutions; USD 90 foreign to institutions; USD 25 to students; USD 15.50 newsstand/cover (effective 2001). Index. back issues avail. *Refereed.* **Document type:** *Journal, Academic/Scholarly.* **Description:** A multidisciplinary journal covering sleep, dream, and hypnosis research interests.
Related titles: Online - full content ed.
Published by: Kure Iletisim Grubu A S, Siracevizler Cad 43/3, Sisli, Istanbul 80260, Turkey. TEL 90-212-2194900, FAX 90-212-2305009, kure@kure.com.tr, http://www.sleepandhypnosis.com, http://www.kure.com.tr. Ed. Mehmet Yucel Agargun. Pub., R&P Nuket Dilmen Korkmaz.

616.8 NLD ISSN 1389-9457
▼ **SLEEP MEDICINE.** Text in Dutch. 2000. bi-m. EUR 75 in Europe to individuals; JPY 10,000 in Japan to individuals; USD 84 elsewhere to individuals; EUR 194 in Europe to institutions; JPY 25,800 in Japan to institutions; USD 217 elsewhere to institutions (effective 2002). adv. bk.rev. illus, abstr. reprints avail. *Refereed.* **Document type:** *Academic/Scholarly.* **Description:** Examines all human aspects of sleep, integrating the various disciplines involved in sleep medicine.
Related titles: Online - full text ed.: (from ingenta, Swets Blackwell, ScienceDirect).
—BLDSC (8309.452000).
Published by: Elsevier Science BV, Sara Burgerhartstraat 25, Amsterdam 1055 KV, Netherlands. http://www.elsevier.nl/locate/issn/13899457. Ed. Sudhansu Chokroverty. Adv. contact Carol Clark. Circ: 4,500 (paid and controlled). **in Australasia and the Far East:** Elsevier Science (Singapore) Pte Ltd, No.1 Temasek Ave, 17-01 Millenia Tower, Singapore 039192, Singapore. TEL 65-434-3727, FAX 65-337-2230; **in Japan:** Elsevier Science Inc - Japan Regional Office, 9-15 Higashi-Azabu 1-chome, Minato-ku, Tokyo 106-0044, Japan. TEL 81-3-5561-5033, FAX 81-3-5561-5047; **in the Americas:** Elsevier Science, PO Box 945, New York, NY 10159-0945. TEL 212-633-3730, 888-437-4636, FAX 212-633-3680, usinfo-f@elsevier.com, http://www.elsevier.com.

616.8 GBR ISSN 1087-0792
CODEN: SMREFC
SLEEP MEDICINE REVIEWS. Text in English. 1997. bi-m. GBP 95 to individuals; GBP 192 to institutions (effective 2002). *Refereed.* **Document type:** *Academic/Scholarly.* **Description:** Provides in-depth and up-to-date reviews of sleep disorders, including their aetiology, diagnosis, treatment and implications for related conditions at an individual and public health level.
Related titles: Online - full text ed.: (from EBSCO Publishing, O C L C Online Computer Library Center, Inc., Swets Blackwell, IDEAL Online Library, Institute for Scientific Information).
Indexed: Neurosci.Cit.Ind., Ref.Zh., e-psyche.
—BLDSC (8309.455000), IDS, Infotrieve. **CCC.**
Published by: W.B. Saunders Co. Ltd. (Subsidiary of: Harcourt Publishers Ltd.), 24-28 Oval Rd, London NW1 7DX, United Kingdom. TEL 44-20-7424-4200, FAX 44-20-7424-4515, cservice@harcourt.com, http://www.harcourt-international.com/journals/smrv. Pub. Martin Delahunty. **Subscr. to:** Harcourt Publishers Ltd., Foots Cray High St, Sidcup, Kent DA14 5HP, United Kingdom. TEL 44-20-8308-5700, FAX 44-20-8309-0807.

616.8 USA ISSN 0093-0407
SLEEP RESEARCH. Text in English. 1972. a. USD 85 (effective 1999). bk.rev. abstr, bibl. back issues avail. **Document type:** *Academic/Scholarly.* **Description:** Current claims and abstracts from the annual meeting of the Association of Professional Sleep Societies.
Indexed: e-psyche.
—GNLM.
Published by: Brain Research Institute, Brain Information Service, B R I Publications Office, 43 367 CHS, University of California at, Los Angeles, CA 90095-1746. TEL 310-825-3417, FAX 310-206-3499, bisleep@ucla.edu. Ed., R&P Michael H Chase. Circ: 2,000.

SMART DRUG NEWS. see *PHARMACY AND PHARMACOLOGY*

616.89 DEU ISSN 0933-7954
RC321 CODEN: SPPEEM
SOCIAL PSYCHIATRY AND PSYCHIATRIC EPIDEMIOLOGY; the international journal for research in social and genetic epidemiology and mental health services. Text in English. 1966. m. DEM 1,748, EUR 893.74, USD 1,064; USD 105 newsstand/cover (effective 2001). adv. bk.rev. abstr, bibl. index. back issues avail.; reprint service avail. from ISI. *Refereed.* **Document type:** *Journal, Academic/Scholarly.* **Description:** Concerned with the effects of social conditions on behavior, and the relationship between psychiatric disorders and the social environment.
Formerly: Social Psychiatry (0037-7813)
Related titles: Microform ed.: (from PQC); Online - full text ed.: ISSN 1433-9285 (from EBSCO Publishing, RoweCom Information Quest, Swets Blackwell, Springer LINK, Institute for Scientific Information).
Indexed: ASCA, Abstr.Anthropol., AgeLine, Biol.Abstr., Chic.Per.Ind., Curr.Cont., Excerp.Med., Ind.Med. (1988-), Indian Psychol.Abstr., Int.Nurs.Ind., PsycInfo, Psychol.Abstr. (1966-), Russ.Acad.Sci.Bibl., SSCI, Trop.Dis.Bull., e-psyche.
—BLDSC (8318.145700), CISTI, EMDOCS, GNLM, IDS, ingenta, KNAW. **CCC.**
Published by: Dr. Dietrich Steinkopff Verlag, Poststr 9, Darmstadt 64293, Germany. TEL 49-6151-82899-0, FAX 49-6151-82899-40, frey.steinkopff@springer.de, http://www.steinkopff.springer.de. Ed. P Bebbington. R&Ps Dr. Maria Magdalene Nabbe, Sabine Ibkendanz TEL 49-6151-82899-14. adv.: color page DEM 1,020, B&W page DEM 600; trim 210 x 277. **Subscr. to:** Springer Verlag GmbH, Haberstr 7, Heidelberg 69126, Germany. TEL 49-6221-345200, FAX 49-6221-345229, subscriptions@springer.de.

616.8 USA ISSN 0190-5295
SOCIETY FOR NEUROSCIENCE. ABSTRACTS. Text in English. 1975. irreg., latest vol.21, 1995. **Document type:** *Monographic series.*
Formerly (until 1977): Neuroscience Abstracts (0148-8791)
—BLDSC (0553.720000), GNLM. **CCC.**
Published by: Society for Neuroscience, 11 Dupont Circle, N W, Ste 500, Washington, DC 20036. TEL 202-462-6688, FAX 202-462-2937, http://www.sfn.org/.

SOCIOLOGY OF HEALTH AND ILLNESS; a journal of medical sociology. see *SOCIOLOGY*

SOINS - PSYCHIATRIE. see *MEDICAL SCIENCES—Nurses And Nursing*

SOMATOSENSORY AND MOTOR RESEARCH. see *BIOLOGY—Physiology*

616.89 RUS ISSN 0869-4893
SOTSYAL'NAYA I KLINICHESKAYA PSIKHYATRIYA. Text in Russian. 1991. q. USD 99.95 in United States. bk.rev. abstr, bibl, illus. 112 p./no. 2 cols./p. *Refereed.* **Document type:** *Journal, Academic/Scholarly.*
Indexed: Ref.Zh.
—BLDSC (0166.276500), East View.
Published by: Rossiiskoe Obshchestvo Psikhyatrov, Poteshnaya ul 3, Moscow 107258, Russian Federation. Ed. I Ya Gurovich. Circ: 3,000 (paid). **US dist. addr.:** East View Publications, 3020 Harbor Ln N, Minneapolis, MN 55447. TEL 612-550-0961.

616.8 ZAF
SOUTH AFRICAN JOURNAL OF PSYCHIATRY. Text in English. 3/yr. USD 15 foreign (effective 2000). back issues avail. *Refereed.* **Document type:** *Journal, Academic/Scholarly.* **Description:** Publishes clinical and experimental articles on all aspects of psychiatric medicine and other topics in psychiatry.
Published by: South African Medical Association, Health and Medical Publishing Group, 14 Central Sq, Pinelands 7430, South Africa. TEL 27-21-531-3081, FAX 27-21-531-4126, annp@samedical.org, publishing@samedical.org, http://www.samedical.org. R&P Peter Roberts. **Subscr. to:** PO Box 74789, Lynnwood Ridge, Pretoria 0040, South Africa. TEL 27-12-481-2010, FAX 27-12-481-2061, ann@samedical.org. **Dist. by:** Private Bag X1, Pinelands 7430, South Africa. TEL 27-21-531-3081, FAX 27-21-531-4126.

606.89 USA ISSN 1047-6334
SOUTHERN CALIFORNIA PSYCHIATRIST. Text in English. 1955. m. (11/yr.). USD 25. adv. bk.rev., film rev. **Document type:** *Newsletter.*
Formerly (until Aug. 1988): Southern California Psychiatric Society. Newsletter
Indexed: e-psyche.
Published by: Southern California Psychiatric Society, 2999 Overland Ave, Ste 116, Los Angeles, CA 90064. Ed. Dr. Nancy Rosser. R&P, Adv. contact Mindi Thelen TEL 310-815-3650. Circ: 1,350.

SOZIALPSYCHIATRISCHE INFORMATIONEN. see *PSYCHOLOGY*

616.89 ITA
LO SPECCHIO DI PSICHE. Text in Italian. 1997. irreg., latest vol.4, 1999. price varies. adv. **Document type:** *Monographic series.*
Indexed: e-psyche.
Published by: Liguori Editore srl, Via Posillipo, 394, Naples, NA 80123, Italy. TEL 39-81-7206111, FAX 39-81-7206244, http://www.liguori.it. Pub. Guido Liguori. Adv. contact Maria Liguori.

616.8 DEU ISSN 1431-3022
SPEKTRUM DER PSYCHIATRIE, PSYCHOTHERAPIE UND NERVENHEILKUNDE. Text in German. 1971. bi-m. DEM 48, EUR 24.54 (effective 2000). adv. **Document type:** *Journal, Trade.* **Description:** Clinical and scientific information for psychiatrists and neurologists.
Formerly (until 1995): Spektrum der Psychiatrie und Nervenheilkunde (0341-9738)
Indexed: e-psyche.
—GNLM.
Published by: Deutscher Aerzte-Verlag GmbH, Dieselstr 2, Cologne 50859, Germany. TEL 49-2234-7011-0, FAX 49-2234-7011515, verlag@aerzteblatt.de, http://www.aerzteverlag.de. Circ: 6,700.

616.837 617.3 GBR ISSN 1362-4393
CODEN: SPCOFM
SPINAL CORD. Text in English; Summaries in French, German. 1963. m. GBP 268 in Europe to institutions for print or online; USD 471 rest of world to institutions for print only; EUR 314 combined subscription in Europe to institutions print & online; USD 494 combined subscription elsewhere to institutions print & online (effective 2002). adv. bk.rev. abstr, charts, illus, stat. index. back issues avail.; reprints avail. *Refereed.* **Document type:** *Journal, Academic/Scholarly.*
Formerly (until 1996): Paraplegia (0031-1758)
Related titles: Online - full text ed.: USD 429 to institutions outside of Europe (effective 2001) (from EBSCO Publishing, O C L C Online Computer Library Center, Inc., RoweCom Information Quest, ingenta, Swets Blackwell, Institute for Scientific Information).
Indexed: AMED, ASCA, CINAHL, Curr.Adv.Ecol.Sci., Curr.Cont., Excerp.Med., Helminthol.Abstr., INIS Atomind., Ind.Med. (1996-), Inpharma, Int.Nurs.Ind., Neurosci.Cit.Ind., Nutr.Abstr., Pharm.&Out.News, Reac., SSCI (coverage dropped), Sp.Ed.Needs Abstr., e-psyche.

—BLDSC (8413.885000), ADONIS, CISTI, GNLM, IDS, ingenta, KNAW. **CCC.**

Published by: (International Medical Society of Paraplegia), Nature Publishing Group Specialist Journals (Subsidiary of: Holtzbrink Publishers), Houndmills, Basingstoke, Hants RG21 6XS, United Kingdom. TEL 44-1256-329242, FAX 44-1256-328339, subscriptions@nature.com, http://www.nature.com/sc. Ed. L Illis. Pub. Michael Osuch. R&P Trace Noel. Adv. contact Robert Sloan TEL 44-20-8882-7199.

SPRINGER SERIES ON BEHAVIOR THERAPY AND BEHAVIORAL MEDICINE. see *PSYCHOLOGY*

616.8 USA ISSN 0740-4212
SPRINGER SERIES ON PSYCHIATRY. Text in English. 1982. irreg., latest vol.7, 1998. price varies. **Document type:** *Monographic series.* **Description:** Explores issues in experimental and clinical psychiatry.
Indexed: e-psyche.
—BLDSC (8424.772000), CISTI.
Published by: Springer Publishing Company, 536 Broadway, New York, NY 10012. TEL 212-431-4370, FAX 212-941-7842, springer@springerpub.com, http://www.springerpub.com. Ed. Dr. Carl Eisdorfer. R&P Dorothy Kouwenberg.

DE STEM VAN DE OUDERS. see *HANDICAPPED*

STEREOTACTIC AND FUNCTIONAL NEUROSURGERY. see *MEDICAL SCIENCES—Surgery*

STRABISMUS. see *MEDICAL SCIENCES—Ophthalmology And Optometry*

616.8 GBR ISSN 1532-3005
CODEN: STMEEZ
STRESS AND HEALTH. Text in English. 1985. 5/yr. USD 1,225 in United States; USD 1,225 in Canada & Mexico; USD 1,225 elsewhere; USD 1,287 combined subscription in United States for print and online eds.; USD 1,287 combined subscription in Canada & Mexico for print and online eds.; USD 1,287 combined subscription elsewhere for print and online eds. (effective 2002). adv. back issues avail.; reprint service avail. from SWZ. *Refereed.* **Document type:** *Academic/Scholarly.* **Description:** Provides a forum for the discussion of all aspects of stress that affect the individual in both health and disease.
Formerly (until vol.18, no.5): Stress Medicine (0748-8386)
Related titles: Microform ed.: (from PQC); Online - full text ed.: ISSN 1532-2998. USD 575 in United States; USD 575 in Canada & Mexico; USD 575 elsewhere (effective 2002) (from EBSCO Publishing, ingenta, Wiley InterScience, Institute for Scientific Information).
Indexed: ASCA, AgeLine, Behav.Med.Abstr., Brit.Nur.Ind., Crim.Just.Abstr., Curr.Adv.Ecol.Sci., Curr.Cont. (coverage dropped), Environ.Sci.Poll.Mgmt., Excerp.Med., Fam.Ind., Indian Psychol.Abstr., Inpharma, Lang.& Lang.Behav.Abstr., Pharm.&Out.News, Pollut.Abstr., PsycInfo, Psychol.Abstr. (1987-), Reac., Risk Abstr., SOPODA, SSCI, Saf.Sci.Abstr., Sociol.Abstr., THA, e-psyche.
—CISTI, EMDOCS, GNLM, IDS, Infotrieve, ingenta, KNAW. **CCC.**
Published by: Wiley Europe Ltd., Baffins Ln, Chichester, W Sussex PO19 1UD, United Kingdom. TEL 44-1243-779777, FAX 44-1243-843232, customer@wiley.co.uk, http://www.wiley.co.uk. Pub. Richard Baggaley. adv.: B&W page GBP 750, color page GBP 1,650; trim 200 x 260. Circ: 400. **Subscr. in the Americas to:** John Wiley & Sons, Inc., Journals, 605 Third Ave, New York, NY 10158. TEL 212-850-6645, FAX 212-850-6021, uscs-wis@wiley.com; **Subscr. to:** John Wiley & Sons Ltd., Baffins Ln, Chichester, Sussex PO19 IUD, United Kingdom. cs-journals@wiley.co.uk.

STRESSFORSKNINGSRAPPORTER. see *PSYCHOLOGY*

616.8 SWE ISSN 1100-3278
STUDIA PSYCHOLOGICA CLINICA UPSALIENSIA. Text in English. 1989. irreg. price varies. **Document type:** *Monographic series, Academic/Scholarly.*
Published by: (Uppsala Universitet), Acta Universitatis Upsaliensis (Subsidiary of: Uppsala University), PO Box 256, Uppsala 75105, Sweden. **Dist. by:** Almqvist & Wiksell International.

616.8526 GBR
STUDIES IN EATING DISORDERS: AN INTERNATIONAL SERIES. Text in English. 1998. irreg., latest vol.2, 1998. price varies. **Document type:** *Academic/Scholarly.* **Description:** Each issue contains contributions relating to a specific topic. Includes coverage of issues faced by practicing therapists in the treatment of eating disorders, and a survey of modern approaches to the prevention of eating disorders.
Indexed: e-psyche.
Published by: Athlone Press Ltd., 1 Park Dr, London NW11 7SG, United Kingdom. TEL 44-20-8458-0888, FAX 44-20-8458-8115, athlonepress@btinternet.com. Ed. Tristan Palmer. Pub. Brian Southam. R&P Doris Southam.

616.8 GBR ISSN 1351-8194
CODEN: SNRSEQ
STUDIES IN NEUROSCIENCE. Text in English. 1985. irreg. price varies. **Document type:** *Monographic series.*
Indexed: e-psyche.
—CASDDS.
Published by: Elsevier Science Ltd., Books Division, Kidlington, PO Box 800, Oxford OX2 1DX, United Kingdom. TEL 44-1865-843000, FAX 44-1865-843010, nlinfo-f@elsevier.nl; usinfo-f@elsevier.com; forinfo-kyf04035@niftyserve.or.jp, http://www.elsevier.nl/. Ed. W Winlow. **Subscr. in Australasia and the Far East to:** Elsevier Science (Singapore) Pte Ltd, No.1 Temasek Ave, 17-01 Millenia Tower, Singapore 039192, Singapore. TEL 65-434-3727, FAX 65-337-2230; **Subscr. in the Americas to:** Elsevier Science, PO Box 945, New York, NY 10159-0945. TEL 212-633-3730, FAX 212-633-3680, usinfo-f@elsevier.com, http://www.elsevier.com; **Subscr. to:** Elsevier Science BV, PO Box 211, Amsterdam 1000 AE, Netherlands. TEL 31-20-485-3757, FAX 31-20-485-3432, nlinfo-f@elsevier.nl, http://www.elsevier.nl.

616.85 NLD ISSN 0927-1813
STUDIES IN SPEECH PATHOLOGY AND CLINICAL LINGUISTICS. Text in English. 1991. irreg., latest vol.6, 1996. price varies. *Refereed.* **Document type:** *Monographic series.* **Description:** Provides a forum for academic research in speech disorders integrating research from the related fields of speech pathology and clinical linguistics.
Indexed: Bibl.Ling., MLA Intl.Bibl., e-psyche.
—BLDSC (8491.747000).
Published by: John Benjamins Publishing Co., PO Box 36224, Amsterdam 1020 ME, Netherlands. TEL 31-20-6304747., FAX 31-20-6792956, http://www.benjamins.nl. Eds. Martin J Ball, Raymond D Kent.

152.1 NLD ISSN 0926-907X
STUDIES IN VISUAL INFORMATION PROCESSING. Text in English. 1990. irreg., latest vol.6, 1995. price varies. back issues avail. *Refereed.* **Document type:** *Monographic series, Proceedings, Academic/Scholarly.* **Description:** Publishes research in a variety of studies dealing with the acquisition, processing, and utilization of visual information.
Indexed: e-psyche.
—BLDSC (8491.846600).
Published by: Elsevier Science BV, PO Box 211, Amsterdam 1000 AE, Netherlands. TEL 31-20-485-3757, 31-20-485-3911, FAX 31-20-485-3432, 31-20-485-3598, nlinfo-f@elsevier.nl, http://www.elsevier.nl. Eds. Gery d'Yderwalle, Rudolf Groner. **Subscr. in Australasia and the Far East to:** Elsevier Science (Singapore) Pte Ltd, No.1 Temasek Ave, 17-01 Millenia Tower, Singapore 039192, Singapore. TEL 65-434-3727, FAX 65-337-2230, asiainfo@elsevier.com.sg; **Subscr. in Japan to:** Elsevier Science Inc - Japan Regional Office, 9-15 Higashi-Azabu 1-chome, Minato-ku, Tokyo 106-0044, Japan. TEL 81-3-5561-5033, FAX 81-3-5561-5047, info@elsevier.co.jp; **Subscr. in the Americas to:** Elsevier Science, PO Box 945, New York, NY 10159-0945. TEL 212-633-3730, 888-437-4636, FAX 212-633-3680, usinfo-f@elsevier.com, http://www.elsevier.com

SUICIDE AND LIFE-THREATENING BEHAVIOR; the official journal of the American Association of Suicidology . see *PSYCHOLOGY*

616.8 360 DEU ISSN 0173-458X
SUIZIDPROPHYLAXE. Text in German. 1973. q. DEM 100 (effective 2001). adv. bk.rev. back issues avail. *Refereed.* **Document type:** *Journal, Academic/Scholarly.*
Indexed: IBR, IBZ, Ind.Philos., e-psyche.
—GNLM.
Published by: (German Association of Suicide Prevention), S. Roderer Verlag, Postfach 110506, Regensburg 93018, Germany. TEL 49-941-795124, FAX 49-941-795198, roderer@donau.de, http://www.roderer-verlag.de. Circ: 1,000.

616.8 GBR ISSN 1359-5962
SUPPLEMENT TO THE EUROPEAN JOURNAL OF NEUROSCIENCE. Text in English. 1989. irreg.
Related titles: ♦ Supplement to: European Journal of Neuroscience. ISSN 0953-816X.
Indexed: Ind.Med. (1988-).
Published by: Blackwell Science Ltd., Osney Mead, Oxford OX2 0EL, United Kingdom. TEL 44-1685-206206, FAX 44-1685-721205.

SURGICAL NEUROLOGY. see *MEDICAL SCIENCES—Surgery*

616.891 362.82 SWE ISSN 1100-3421
SVENSK FAMILJETERAPI. Text in Swedish. 1988. irreg. (3-4/yr.). SEK 25 per issue (effective 1993).
Indexed: e-psyche.
Published by: Svenska Foereningen foer Familjeterapi (SFF), Sta Ursulasvej 22, Vaesteraas 72218, Sweden.

616.8 USA ISSN 0887-4476
QP364 CODEN: SYNAET
SYNAPSE (NEW YORK). Text in English. m. USD 2,595 in United States; USD 2,755 in Canada & Mexico; USD 2,891 elsewhere; USD 2,725 combined subscription in United States for print and online eds.; USD 2,885 combined subscription in Canada & Mexico for print and online eds.; USD 3,021 combined subscription elsewhere for print and online eds. (effective 2002). adv. back issues avail. *Refereed.* **Document type:** *Academic/Scholarly.* **Description:** Embraces new basic and clinical research pertaining to all aspects of synaptic structure and function, including attention to practical clinical consideration.
Related titles: Microform ed.: (from PQC); Online - full text ed.: ISSN 1098-2396. USD 2,595 in United States; USD 2,595 in Canada & Mexico; USD 2,595 elsewhere (effective 2002) (from EBSCO Publishing, Wiley InterScience, Institute for Scientific Information).
Indexed: Aqua.Sci.& Fish.Abstr., Chem.Abstr., Chem.Indus.Notes, Chem.Titles, Curr.Cont., INIS Atomind., Ind.Med. (1987-), Ind.Sci.Rev., Inpharma, Int.Abstr.Biol.Sci., Neurosci.Abstr., Neurosci.Cit.Ind., Pharm.&Out.News, Reac., Sci.Cit.Ind., e-psyche.
—BLDSC (8585.880200), CASDDS, CISTI, EMDOCS, GNLM, IDS, ingenta, KNAW. **CCC.**
Published by: John Wiley & Sons, Inc., Journals (Subsidiary of: Wiley InterScience), 605 Third Ave, New York, NY 10158. TEL 212-850-6645, FAX 212-850-6021, subinfo@wiley.com, uscs-wis@wiley.com, http://www.wiley.com. Ed. John E Johnson Jr. adv.: B&W page GBP 640, color page GBP 1,515; trim 210 x 279. Circ: 166. **Subscr. outside the Americas to:** John Wiley & Sons Ltd., Baffins Ln, Chichester, Sussex PO19 IUD, United Kingdom. TEL 44-1243-779777, FAX 44-1243-843232, cs-journals@wiley.co.uk.

616.89 DEU ISSN 1434-212X
SYNOPSIS; Zeitschrift fuer biopsychosoziale Medizin. Text in German. 1997. 4/yr. DEM 110; DEM 60 to students (effective 2001). adv. **Document type:** *Journal, Academic/Scholarly.*
Published by: Schattauer GmbH, Hoelderlinstr 3, Stuttgart 70174, Germany. TEL 49-711-2298714, FAX 49-711-2298775, info@schattauer.de, http://www.schattauer.com. Ed. Andrea Schuerg. adv.: B&W page DEM 5,442, color page DEM 7,329; trim 184 x 243. Circ: 29,850 (paid and controlled).

616.8 DEU ISSN 0933-3053
SYSTEM FAMILIE; Forschung, Beratung und Therapie. Text in German. q. DEM 210.40 domestic; DEM 214 foreign (effective 2001). *Refereed.* **Document type:** *Journal, Academic/Scholarly.* **Description:** Provides articles on the connections between family therapy practice and research.
Related titles: Online - full text ed.: ISSN 1432-2226 (from EBSCO Publishing, RoweCom Information Quest, Swets Blackwell, Springer LINK, Institute for Scientific Information).
Indexed: ASCA, Curr.Cont., IBZ, Ind.Philos., PsycInfo, SSCI, e-psyche.
—GNLM, IDS, Infotrieve. **CCC.**

M

Published by: Springer-Verlag (Subsidiary of: BertelsmannSpringer), Tiergartenstr 17, Heidelberg 69121, Germany. TEL 49-6221-345-0, FAX 49-6221-345229, subscriptions@springer.de, http://link.springer.de/link/service/journals/00491/index.htm, http://www.springer.de. Eds. B Hildenbrand, T Levold. **Subscr. in N. America to:** Springer-Verlag New York Inc., PO Box 2485, Secaucus, NJ 07096-2485. TEL 212-460-1500, FAX 212-473-6272.

SYSTEM UBW; Zeitschrift fuer klassische Psychoanalyse. see *PSYCHOLOGY*

616.89 UKR
TAVRICHESKII ZHURNAL PSIKHYATRII/ACTA PSYCHIATRICA, PSYCHOTERAPEUTICA ET ETOLOGICA TAVRICA. Text in Ukrainian. 1997. q. USD 50 foreign (effective 2000 - 2001). adv.
Description: Examines problems of psychiatry, psychotherapy, neurophysiology, ethology and psychology.
Published by: Krymskaya Respublikanskaya Assotsyatsiya Psikhyatrov Psikhoterapevtov i Psikhologov, Ul R Lyuksemburg 27, Simferopol 333000, Ukraine. TEL 380-65-255380, FAX 380-65-273806, vsam@psy.crimea.ua. Ed. Dr. Nikolai Verbenko. adv.: page USD 200. Circ: 1,000. **US dist. addr.:** East View Publications, 3020 Harbor Ln N, Minneapolis, MN 55447. TEL 612-550-0961.

TECHNIQUES IN NEUROSURGERY. see *MEDICAL SCIENCES—Surgery*

616.8 NLD ISSN 0921-0709
CODEN: TBSCEC
TECHNIQUES IN THE BEHAVIORAL AND NEURAL SCIENCES. Text in English. 1987. irreg., latest vol.13, 1999. bibl. back issues avail. *Refereed.* **Document type:** *Monographic series, Academic/Scholarly, Trade.*
Description: Describes in detail experiments in the theoretical and applied behavioral and neural sciences, discussing the merits of various experimental techniques and methods.
Indexed: Chem.Abstr., Chem.Indus.Notes, Chem.Titles, e-psyche.
—BLDSC (8743.720000), CASDDS, CISTI, Infotrieve. **CCC.**
Published by: Elsevier Science BV, PO Box 211, Amsterdam 1000 AE, Netherlands. TEL 31-20-485-3757, 31-20-485-3911, FAX 31-20-485-3432, 31-20-485-3598, nlinfo-f@elsevier.nl; usinfo-f@elsevier.com; forinfo-kyf04035@niftyserve.or.jp, http://www.elsevier.nl/. Ed. J P Huston. **Subscr. in Australasia and the Far East to:** Elsevier Science (Singapore) Pte Ltd, No.1 Temasek Ave, 17-01 Millenia Tower, Singapore 039192, Singapore. TEL 65-434-3727, FAX 65-337-2230, asiainfo@elsevier.com.sg; **Subscr. in Japan to:** Elsevier Science Inc - Japan Regional Office, 9-15 Higashi-Azabu 1-chome, Minato-ku, Tokyo 106-0044, Japan. TEL 81-3-5561-5033, FAX 81-3-5561-5047, info@elsevier.co.jp; **Subscr. in the Americas to:** Elsevier Science, PO Box 945, New York, NY 10159-0945. TEL 212-633-3730, 888-437-4636, FAX 212-633-3680, usinfo-f@elsevier.com, http://www.elsevier.com

616.8 AUT ISSN 0254-7902
TEXTE; psychoanalyse, aesthetik, kulturkritik. Text in German. 1980. q. ATS 826 (effective 2001). adv. **Document type:** *Magazine, Academic/Scholarly.*
Indexed: e-psyche.
Published by: Passagen Verlag GmbH, Walfischgasse 15-14, Vienna, W 1010, Austria. TEL 43-1-5137761, FAX 43-1-5126327, office@passagen.at. Ed., R&P Peter Engelmann. Adv. contact Thomas Szanto. **Subscr. to:** Springer Verlagsauslieferung, Postfach 89, Vienna, W 1201, Austria. TEL 43-1-3302415-249, FAX 43-1-3302426-350.

616.8 AUS ISSN 1327-9491
THERAPEUTIC GUIDELINES. NEUROLOGY. Text in English. 1997. irreg., latest version 1 (every 3-4 yrs.). AUD 31.90 newsstand/cover (effective 2001). **Document type:** *Academic/Scholarly.* **Description:** Provides up-to-date recommendations for drug therapy in treating and managing neurologic conditions and disorders and, when appropriate, alternative approaches to overall patient management.
Formerly: Neurology Guidelines
Related titles: CD-ROM ed.
Indexed: e-psyche.
Published by: Therapeutic Guidelines Ltd., Chelsea House, Level 2, 55 Flemington Rd, North Melbourne, VIC 3051, Australia. TEL 61-3-9329-1566, FAX 61-3-9326-5632, sales@tg.com.au, http://www.tg.com.au. Ed., R&P Mary Hemming. Circ: 18,000.

616.8 AUS
THERAPEUTIC GUIDELINES. PSYCHOTROPIC. Text in English. 1989. irreg., latest version 4 (every 3-4 yrs). AUD 31.90 newsstand/cover (effective 2001). bk.rev. **Document type:** *Academic/Scholarly.* **Description:** Gives concrete recommendations for rational therapy of psychotropic disease and, where necessary, justifies the choice.
Formerly: Psychotropic Guidelines (1039-1568)
Related titles: CD-ROM ed.
Indexed: e-psyche.
Published by: Therapeutic Guidelines Ltd., Chelsea House, Level 2, 55 Flemington Rd, North Melbourne, VIC 3051, Australia. TEL 61-3-9329-1566, FAX 61-3-9326-5632, sales@tg.com.au, http://www.tg.com.au. Ed., R&P Mary Hemming. Circ: 18,000. **Co-sponsor:** Victorian Drug Usage Advisory Committee.

616.8 CHE ISSN 0250-4952
THERAPIE FAMILIALE. Text in French. 1980. q. CHF 75, EUR 48.70 to individuals; CHF 155, EUR 100.64 to institutions (effective 2002). **Document type:** *Journal, Academic/Scholarly.*
Indexed: PsycInfo, Psychol.Abstr. (1991-), e-psyche.
—BLDSC (8814.754000). **CCC.**
Published by: Editions Medecine et Hygiene, Case Postale 456, Geneva, 4 1211, Switzerland. TEL 41-22-7029311, FAX 41-22-7029355, abonnements@medhyg.ch, http://www.medhyg.ch.

TIJDSCHRIFT VOOR CLIENTGERICHTE PSYCHOTHERAPIE. see *PSYCHOLOGY*

616.89 NLD ISSN 0303-7339
CODEN: TPSYB3
TIJDSCHRIFT VOOR PSYCHIATRIE. Variant title: Psychiatrie. Text in Dutch; Summaries in English. 1973 (vol.15). m. NLG 83.25 (effective 1997). adv. bk.rev. illus. index. **Document type:** *Academic/Scholarly.*
Incorporates: Tijdschrift voor Psychiatrie. Boeken (0922-0712)
Indexed: Abstr.Crim.& Pen., Excerp.Med., Nutr.Abstr., PsycInfo, Psychol.Abstr. (1985-), e-psyche.
—BLDSC (8844.180000), CISTI, EMDOCS, GNLM, KNAW.
Published by: (Nederlandse Vereniging voor Psychiatrie), Uitgeverij Boom, PO Box 400, Meppel 7940 AK, Netherlands. TEL 31-522-257012, FAX 31-522-253864. Ed. Dr. R C van der Mast. Circ: 3,800. **Co-sponsor:** Vereniging van Vlaamse Zenuwartsen.

616.89 NLD ISSN 1382-516X
TIJDSCHRIFT VOOR PSYCHOANALYSE. Text in Dutch. 1995. 4/yr. NLG 99 domestic to individuals; NLG 115 foreign to individuals; NLG 145 domestic to institutions; NLG 170 foreign to institutions. back issues avail. **Document type:** *Academic/Scholarly.* **Description:** Publishes original studies in psychoanalysis and psychoanalytical psychotherapy, including theoretical and practical subjects.
Indexed: e-psyche.
—KNAW.
Published by: (Stichting Tijdschrift voor Psychoanalyse), Uitgeverij Boom, PO Box 400, Meppel 7940 AK, Netherlands. TEL 31-522-257012, FAX 31-522-253864. Ed. Dr. Hans M Reijzer.

616.89 NLD ISSN 0165-1188
TIJDSCHRIFT VOOR PSYCHOTHERAPIE. Text in Dutch. 6/yr. NLG 122.50. adv. **Document type:** *Trade.*
Indexed: PsycInfo, Psychol.Abstr. (1977-), e-psyche.
—BLDSC (8844.250000), KNAW.
Published by: Bohn Stafleu van Loghum B.V. (Subsidiary of: Wolters Kluwer N.V.), Postbus 246, Houten 3990 GA, Netherlands. TEL 31-3403-95711, FAX 31-3403-50903.

616.8 JPN
TOKYO-TO SHINKEI KAGAKU SOGO KENKYUJO NENPO/TOKYO METROPOLITAN INSTITUTE FOR NEUROSCIENCES. ANNUAL REPORT. Text in Japanese. 1972. a.
Indexed: e-psyche.
Published by: Tokyo-to Shinkei Kagaku Sogo Kenkyujo/Tokyo Metropolitan Institute for Neurosciences, 2-6 Musashidai, Fuchu-shi, Tokyo-to 183-0042, Japan.

617.48 NLD ISSN 0924-6169
TOPICS IN NEUROSURGERY. Text in English. 1988. irreg. price varies. *Refereed.* **Document type:** *Monographic series.*
Indexed: e-psyche.
Published by: Kluwer Academic Publishers Group (Subsidiary of: Wolters Kluwer N.V.), Spuiboulevard 50, PO Box 17, Dordrecht 3300 AA, Netherlands. FAX 31-78-639-2254, services@wkap.nl, http://www.wkap.nl. **Dist. by:** Journals Department, PO Box 322, Dordrecht 3300 AH, Netherlands. FAX 31-78-654-6474.

616.8 NLD ISSN 0897-3946
TOPICS IN THE NEUROSCIENCES. Text in English. 1986. irreg. price varies. *Refereed.* **Document type:** *Monographic series.*
Indexed: e-psyche.
—CISTI, KNAW.
Published by: Kluwer Academic Publishers Group (Subsidiary of: Wolters Kluwer N.V.), Spuiboulevard 50, PO Box 17, Dordrecht 3300 AA, Netherlands. FAX 31-78-639-2254, services@wkap.nl, http://www.wkap.nl. **Dist. by:** Journals Department, PO Box 322, Dordrecht 3300 AH, Netherlands. FAX 31-78-654-6474.

616.89 FRA ISSN 0040-9375
BF173.A2
TOPIQUE - REVUE FREUDIENNE. Text in French. 1969. 2/yr. FRF 300. **Description:** Scope is to offer a place where theoretical reflection and clinical experience in psychoanalysis may enrich each other and confront their conflictual borders.
Indexed: IBR, Ind.Philos., PsycInfo, Psychoanal.Abstr., Psychol.Abstr. (1983-), e-psyche.
—Infotrieve. **CCC.**
Published by: Dunod, 5 rue Laromiguiere, Paris 75005, France. TEL 33-1-40466200, FAX 33-1-40466201, http://www.gauthier-villars.fr. Ed. S De Mijolla-Mellor.

616.89 FRA
TRAITE DE PSYCHIATRIE. Cover title: Traite de Psychiatrie. Variant title: Encyclopedie Medico-Chirurgicale, Instantanes Medicaux. Psychiatrie. Encyclopedie Medico-Chirurgicale. Psychiatrie Clinique et Therapeutique. Receuil Periodique de l'Encyclopedie Medico-Chirurgicale. Psychiatrie. Text in French. 1955. 6 base vols. plus q. updates. bibl, charts, illus. *Refereed.* **Document type:** *Academic/Scholarly.* **Description:** Offers psychiatrists an up-to-date, comprehensive reference for diagnosing and treating psychiatric disorders.
Formerly: Encyclopedie Medico-Chirurgicale. Psychiatrie (0246-1072)
Published by: Elsevier Paris, Editions Scientifiques et Medicales (Subsidiary of: Reed Elsevier plc. group), 23 rue Linois, Paris 75015, France. TEL 33-1-45589110, FAX 33-1-45589425, redaction-emc@elsevier.fr, redacion-emc@elsevier.fr, http://www.elsevier.fr, http://www.elsevier.com.

TRANSACTIONAL ANALYSIS JOURNAL. see *PSYCHOLOGY*

599.97 GBR ISSN 1363-4615
RC321 CODEN: TRPSFM
TRANSCULTURAL PSYCHIATRY. Text in English. 1956. q. INR 975 to individuals; INR 2,750 to institutions; USD 36 SAARC to individuals; USD 75 SAARC to institutions; INR 270 newsstand/cover to individuals; INR 750 newsstand/cover to institutions; USD 11 newsstand/cover SAARC to individuals; USD 20 newsstand/cover SAARC to institutions (effective 2002). adv. bk.rev. abstr, bibl, charts. index, cum.index: 1956-1972. back issues avail.; reprint service avail. from PQC. *Refereed.* **Document type:** *Journal, Academic/Scholarly.* **Description:** Provides a channel of communication for psychiatrists and social scientists around the world concerned with the relationship between culture and mental health.
Former titles (until 1997): Transcultural Psychiatric Research Review (0041-1108); (until 1969): Transcultural Psychiatric Research Review and Newsletter (0315-4386); (until 1963): Transcultural Research in Mental Health Problems. Review and Newsletter (0315-4394); Transcultural Research in Mental Health Problems. Newsletter
Related titles: Microfilm ed.: (from PQC); Online - full text ed.: (from EBSCO Publishing, O C L C Online Computer Library Center, Inc., RoweCom Information Quest, ingenta, Swets Blackwell).
Indexed: Anthropol.Lit., Excerp.Med., IBR, IBZ, Ind.Med. (coverage dropped), Lang.& Lang.Behav.Abstr., PsycInfo, Psychol.Abstr. (1987-), Soc.Serv.Abstr., Sociol.Abstr., Viol.& Abuse Abstr., e-psyche.
—BLDSC (9020.580620), GNLM, ingenta. **CCC.**

M

Published by: Sage Publications Ltd., 6 Bonhill St, London EC2A 4PU, United Kingdom. TEL 44-20-7374-0645, FAX 44-20-7374-8741, info@sagepub.co.uk, http://ww2.mcgill.ca/Psychiatry/transcultural/tprr.html, http://www.sagepub.co.uk/. Ed. L J Kirmayer. Adv. contact Jenny Kirby. page GBP 195. Circ: 600 (controlled). **Affiliates:** Sage Publications, Inc.; Sage Publications India Pvt. Ltd.

TRANSMITTERS, RECEPTORS & SYNAPSES. see *PHARMACY AND PHARMACOLOGY—Abstracting, Bibliographies, Statistics*

616.8 344.041 USA
TRAUMATIC BRAIN INJURY; evaluation and litigation. Text in English. 1994. base vol. USD 95. **Description:** Covers the medical and neuropsychological analysis of brain injury, including its causes and effects; the process of case investigation, including evaluation of liability and damages; and trial techniques, including settlement considerations.
Indexed: e-psyche.
Published by: Lexis Law Publishing (Subsidiary of: Reed Elsevier plc), PO Box 7587, Charlottesville, VA 22906-7587. TEL 804-972-7600, 800-562-1197, FAX 804-972-7666, llp.customer.support@lexis-nexis.com, http://www.lexislawpublishing.com.

616.8 USA
TRAUMATIC STRESS POINTS NEWSLETTER. Text in English. 1985. q. USD 100 (effective 2000). adv. bk.rev. *Refereed.* **Document type:** *Academic/Scholarly.* **Description:** Provides a forum for information and news on the worldwide study and treatment of traumatic stress.
Indexed: e-psyche.
Published by: International Society for Traumatic Stress Studies, 60 Revere Dr, Ste 500, Northbrook, IL 60062. TEL 847-480-9028, FAX 847-480-9282, istss@istss.org, http://www.istss.org. Ed. Dean Kilpatrick. R&P, Adv. contact Salva Jorgge TEL 212-620-8000. Circ: 2,500 (paid).

TRENDS IN COGNITIVE SCIENCES. see *PSYCHOLOGY*

616.8 GBR ISSN 0166-2236
QP351 CODEN: TNSCDR
TRENDS IN NEUROSCIENCES. Text in English. 1978. m. GBP 92, EUR 115 in Europe to individuals; JPY 14,000 in Japan to individuals; USD 126 elsewhere to individuals; EUR 908 in Europe to institutions; JPY 125,900 in Japan to institutions; USD 1,015 elsewhere to institutions; GBP 47 in Europe to students; JPY 10,100 in Japan to students; USD 78 elsewhere to students; USD 1,308 to institutions Print & online eds. combined; EUR 144 in Europe to qualified personnel; JPY 17,500 in Japan to qualified personnel; USD 157 elsewhere to qualified personnel (effective 2002). adv. bk.rev., software rev. illus. index. reprints avail. *Refereed.* **Document type:** *Academic/Scholarly.* **Description:** For research workers, teachers and students concerned with the structure and function of the brain and with the biological substrates of behavior.
Related titles: Microform ed.: (from PQC); Online - full text ed.: (from ingenta, Gale Group, Swets Blackwell, Factiva, Institute for Scientific Information, ScienceDirect); ♦ Supplement: Neurotoxins. ISSN 1357-7115.
Indexed: ASCA, Abstr.Hyg., Anim.Behav.Abstr., Aqua.Sci.& Fish.Abstr., Biol.Abstr., Cal.Tiss.Abstr., Chem.Abstr., Chemorec.Abstr., Curr.Adv.Biochem., Curr.Adv.Cell & Devel.Biol., Curr.Adv.Ecol.Sci., Curr.Adv.Gen.& Molec.Biol., Curr.Cont., Excerp.Med., Ind.Med. (1978-), Ind.Sci.Rev., Inpharma, Int.Abstr.Biol.Sci., Jrnl.Watch Neuro., Neurosci.Abstr., Neurosci.Cit.Ind., Nutr.Abstr., Pharm.&Out.News, PsycInfo, Psychol.Abstr. (1979-), Reac., Ref.Zh., Rev.Appl.Entomol., SSCI (coverage dropped), Sci.Cit.Ind., Sport Fish.Abstr., Telegen, e-psyche.
—BLDSC (9049.667000), ADONIS, CASDDS, CISTI, IDS, ingenta, KNAW. **CCC.**
Published by: Elsevier Science Ltd., Elsevier Trends Journals, 68 Hills Rd, Cambridge CB2 1LA, United Kingdom. TEL 44-1223-312961, FAX 44-1223-464430, TINS@elsevier.co.uk, TIMS@elsevier.co.uk, http://www.elsevier.com/locate/tins. Eds. Gavin Swanson, L Roberts. Adv. contact Thelma Reid. Circ: 6,000. **Subscr. in Australasia and the Far East to:** Elsevier Science (Singapore) Pte Ltd, No.1 Temasek Ave, 17-01 Millenia Tower, Singapore 039192, Singapore. TEL 65-434-3727, FAX 65-337-2230; **Subscr. in the Americas to:** Elsevier Science, PO Box 945, New York, NY 10159-0945. TEL 212-633-3730, FAX 212-633-3680, http://www.elsevier.com; **Subscr. to:** Elsevier Current Trends Subscriptions, PO Box 331, Haywards Heath, W Sussex RH16 3FG, United Kingdom. TEL 44-1444-475650, FAX 44-1444-445423.

616.858842 USA ISSN 0737-5174
TRISOMY 21✶ ; an international, multidisciplinary journal of Downs Syndrome. Text in English. 1984. q. abstr, charts, illus. index. *Refereed.*
Indexed: e-psyche.
Published by: Eterna International, Inc., PO Box 5731, Hauppauge, NY 11788-0154. Ed. Dr. Siegfried M Pueschel.

616.8 USA
U P F NEWSLETTER✶ . Text in English. 1968. q. USD 25. bk.rev.
Indexed: e-psyche.
Published by: United Parkinson Foundation, 833 W Washington Blvd, Chicago, IL 60607-2316. TEL 312-664-2344. Ed. Judy Rosner. Circ: 38,000.

616.835 USA
U.S. CENTERS FOR DISEASE CONTROL. NEUROTROPIC VIRAL DISEASES SURVEILLANCE: POLIOMYELITIS. Text in English. a. free per issue. **Document type:** *Government.*
Published by: U.S. Centers for Disease Control, 1600 Clifton Rd, Atlanta, GA 30333. TEL 404-639-3311.

616.858 USA
U.S. CONGRESS: MENTAL HEALTH✶ ; legal updates, children & youth updates, federal agencies, state reports, studies on state mental health systems. Text in English. 1972 (vol.11). irreg. (several/mo.). USD 350.
Formerly: U.S. Congress: Mental Health, Mental Retardation
Indexed: e-psyche.
Published by: National Association of State Mental Health Program Directors, 66 Canal Center Plz 302, Alexandria, VA 22314-1591. Ed. Harry Schnibbe. Circ: 135.

UNDERSTANDING STRESS, ANXIETY AND DEPRESSION. see *PSYCHOLOGY*

616.6 617.7 616.6 USA ISSN 1066-4130
V H L FAMILY FORUM. (Von Hippel-Lindau Disease) Text in English; Summaries in French, Italian, Spanish. 1993. q. USD 35; USD 50 foreign (effective 1999). adv. bk.rev. **Document type:** *Newsletter, Consumer.* **Description:** Enables physicians, patients and family members to exchange information on all aspects of the disease.
Related titles: Audio cassette/tape ed.; Online - full text ed.
Indexed: e-psyche.
Published by: V H L Family Alliance, 171 Clinton Rd, Brookline, MA 02445. TEL 617-277-5667, 800-767-4845, FAX 617-734-8233, info@vhl.org, http://www.vhl.org. Ed., Pub., Adv. contact Joyce Wilcox Graff. R&P Joyce W Graff TEL 617-232-5946. Circ: 4,000.

616.8 CHE ISSN 1016-6262
VERHALTENSTHERAPIE; Praxis - Forschung - Perspektiven. Text in German. 1991. q. CHF 178 in Europe to institutions; CHF 189.60 elsewhere to institutions; EUR 121 in Europe to institutions; USD 142 elsewhere to institutions (effective 2002). *Refereed.* **Document type:** *Journal, Academic/Scholarly.*
Related titles: Microform ed.: (from PQC); Online - full content ed.: ISSN 1423-0402. CHF 58, EUR 42, USD 45 to institutions with print edition (effective 2002) (from EBSCO Publishing, O C L C Online Computer Library Center, Inc., Swets Blackwell); Online - full text ed.: (from Institute for Scientific Information, RoweCom Information Quest).
Indexed: ASCA, Curr.Cont., PsycInfo, Psychol.Abstr. (1991-), Psycscan B.A.& T., SSCI, e-psyche.
—BLDSC (9156.600000), GNLM, IDS, KNAW.
Published by: S. Karger AG, Allschwilerstr 10, PO Box, Basel 4009, Switzerland. TEL 41-61-306-1111, FAX 41-61-306-1234, karger@karger.ch, http://www.online.karger.com/journals/ver, http://www.karger.com.

616.8 DEU
VERHALTENSTHERAPIE UND VERHALTENSMEDIZIN. Text in English, German. 1979. q. EUR 38 (effective 2001). **Document type:** *Journal, Academic/Scholarly.* **Description:** Contains specific and summary articles on the crucial questions concerning behavioural therapy.
Formerly (until 1997): Verhaltensmodifikation und Verhaltensmedizin (1013-1973)
Indexed: IBZ, e-psyche.
—GNLM.
Published by: Pabst Science Publishers, Am Eichengrund 28, Lengerich 49525, Germany. TEL 49-5484-308, FAX 49-5484-550, pabst.publishers@t-online.de, http://www.pabst-publishers.de/Psychologie/psyzeit/v_u_v/index.html. Ed. Hans Reinecker.

616.858 362.3 GBR ISSN 1358-6076
VIEWPOINT (LONDON, 1995). Text in English. 1990. 10/yr. GBP 10; GBP 12 in Europe; GBP 24.45 in the Americas; GBP 24.45 in Africa; GBP 24.45 in the Middle East; GBP 28.85 elsewhere (effective 1999). adv. bk.rev. illus. reprint service avail. from PQC. **Document type:** *Newspaper.* **Description:** Publishes features, news items and reports on services and campaigns about issues concerning people with learning disabilities. Aimed at parents, caregivers and health professionals, and people with learning disabilities.
Former titles (until 1995): Mencap News (0963-7117); (until 1992): Mencap News and Parents Voice; Incorporates: Parents Voice (0031-1936)
Indexed: ASSIA, Except.Child Educ.Abstr., e-psyche.
Published by: Royal Society for Mentally Handicapped Children and Adults, Mencap Centre, Royal Society For Mentally Handicapped Children &, 123 Golden Ln, London EC1Y 0RT, United Kingdom. TEL 44-20-7454-0454, FAX 44-20-7454-9193. Ed. Peter Mookram. Circ: 5,500.

616.858 USA
VIRGINIA MENTAL HEALTH, MENTAL RETARDATION, SUBSTANCE ABUSE AND RELATED LAW ANNOTATED. Text in English. a., latest 1996. USD 30.
Indexed: e-psyche.
Published by: Lexis Law Publishing (Subsidiary of: Reed Elsevier plc), PO Box 7587, Charlottesville, VA 22906-7587. TEL 804-972-7566, 800-562-1197, FAX 800-643-1280, llp.customer.support@lexis-nexis.com, http://www.lexislawpublishing.com. Ed. George Harley.

616.8 GBR ISSN 0952-5238
QP474 CODEN: VNEUEY
VISUAL NEUROSCIENCE. Text in English. 1988. bi-m. GBP 198 to individuals; USD 635 to institutions (effective 2002). adv. bk.rev. back issues avail.; reprint service avail. from SWZ. *Refereed.* **Description:** Theoretical and research-based articles on the neural mechanisms of vision, with primary emphasis on retinal and brain mechanisms underlying visually guided behavior and visual perception in both vertebrate and invertebrate species.
Related titles: Online - full text ed.: (from EBSCO Publishing, O C L C Online Computer Library Center, Inc., RoweCom Information Quest, Swets Blackwell, Institute for Scientific Information).
Indexed: ASCA, Apic.Abstr., Curr.Cont., Ind.Med. (1988-), Ind.Sci.Rev., Inpharma, Int.Abstr.Biol.Sci., Neurosci.Cit.Ind., PsycInfo, Psychol.Abstr. (1988-), Reac., Sci.Cit.Ind., Zoo.Rec., e-psyche.
—BLDSC (9241.296000), EMDOCS, GNLM, IDS, ingenta, KNAW. **CCC.**
Published by: Cambridge University Press, Edinburgh Bldg, Shaftesbury Rd, Cambridge CB2 2RU, United Kingdom. FAX 44-1223-315052, information@cup.cam.ac.uk, information@cambridge.org, http://www.cup.cam.ac.uk, http://www.uk.cambridge.org/journals/pmu. Ed. Peter D Spear. R&P Linda Nicol. Adv. contact Rebecca Symons.

LA VOIX DES PARENTS. see *HANDICAPPED*

WORD FROM WASHINGTON (WASHINGTON, D.C.). see *HANDICAPPED*

WORLD CONGRESS OF MUSIC THERAPY. PROCEEDINGS. see *MUSIC*

616.89 BEL ISSN 0084-1609
WORLD CONGRESS OF PSYCHIATRY. PROCEEDINGS✶
Text in English. 1950. irreg. **Document type:** *Proceedings.*
Indexed: e-psyche.
Published by: World Psychiatric Association, c/o Prof J Mendlewicz, U L B Cliniques Universite, Hopital Erasme, Service de Psych, Rte de Lennik 808, Brussels 1070, Belgium.

616.8 CHN ISSN 1005-7064
XINLI YU JIANKANG/PSYCHOLOGY AND HEALTH. Text in Chinese. 1994. m. USD 26.40; USD 2.20 newsstand/cover (effective 2001). **Document type:** *Academic/Scholarly.*
Published by: China International Book Trading Corp/Zhongguo Guoji Tushu Maoyi Zonggongsi cibtc@mail.cibtc.com.cn, http://www.cibtc.com.cn. **Dist. by:** 35, Chegongzhuang Xilu, Haidian District, Beijing 100044, China.

M

616.8 617 USA ISSN 0513-5117
RC329
THE YEAR BOOK OF NEUROLOGY & NEUROSURGERY. Text in English. 1902. a. USD 90 domestic; USD 96 foreign (effective 2001). **Document type:** *Abstract/Index, Academic/Scholarly.* **Description:** Presents abstracts of pertinent literature with commentary by leading experts in the field.
Related titles: CD-ROM ed.
Indexed: Curr.Adv.Ecol.Sci., e-psyche.
—CISTI, GNLM.
Published by: Mosby, Inc., Continuity Division (Subsidiary of: Harcourt Health Sciences), 11830 Westline Industrial Dr, St Louis, MO 63146-3313. TEL 314-872-8370, 800-325-4177, FAX 314-432-1380, http://www.mosby.com/periodicals. Eds. Dr. Ashok Verma, Dr. Scott Gibbs, Dr. Walter G Bradley.

616.89 USA ISSN 0084-3970
RC329
THE YEAR BOOK OF PSYCHIATRY AND APPLIED MENTAL HEALTH. Text in English. 1970. a. USD 85 domestic; USD 91 foreign (effective 2001). illus. **Document type:** *Abstract/Index, Academic/Scholarly.* **Description:** Presents abstracts of the pertinent literature with commentary by leading experts in the field.
Related titles: CD-ROM ed.: (from Ovid Technologies, Inc.); Online - full text ed.
Indexed: e-psyche.
—BLDSC (9415.700000), CISTI, GNLM.
Published by: Mosby, Inc., Continuity Division (Subsidiary of: Harcourt Health Sciences), 11830 Westline Industrial Dr, St Louis, MO 63146-3313. TEL 314-872-8370, 800-325-4177, FAX 314-432-1380, http://www.mosby.com/periodicals. Ed. Dr. John A Talbott.

616.8 362.7 GBR ISSN 1361-9403
YOUNGMINDS MAGAZINE. Text in English. 1989. bi-m. GBP 25 to members (effective 2002). **Document type:** *Newsletter, Academic/Scholarly.*
Formerly (until 1996): Young Minds Newsletter (1361-939X)
Indexed: e-psyche.
—BLDSC (9421.451383).
Published by: Young Minds, 102-108 Clerkenwell Rd, London EC1M 5SA, United Kingdom. TEL 44-20-7336-8445, FAX 44-20-7336-8446, young.minds@ukonline.co.uk, http://www.youngminds.org.uk. Circ: 2,600 (paid); 400 (controlled).

616.8 DEU
Z N S - ZENTRALES NERVENSYSTEM. Text in German. 1987. irreg., latest vol.2, 1988. **Document type:** *Academic/Scholarly.*
Indexed: e-psyche.
Published by: W. Zuckschwerdt Verlag GmbH, Industriestr 1, Germering 82110, Germany. TEL 49-89-894349-0, FAX 49-89-89434950. Ed. M Schirmer.

150 POL ISSN 0324-8526
ZAGADNIENIA WYCHOWAWCZE A ZDROWIE PSYCHICZNE. Text in Polish; Summaries in English, Russian. 1968. bi-m. USD 15. bibl.
Formerly (until 1973): Zagadnienia Wychowawcze w Aspekcie Zdrowia Psychicznego (0324-8690)
Indexed: e-psyche.
Published by: Polskie Towarzystwo Higieny Psychicznej/Polish Mental Hygiene Society, Ul Targowa 59-16, Warsaw 03729, Poland. TEL 48-22-186599. **Dist. by:** Ars Polona, Krakowskie Przedmiescie 7, Warsaw, Poland.

614.58 POL ISSN 0044-2003
ZDROWIE PSYCHICZNE. Text in Polish; Summaries in English, Russian. 1961. q. bk.rev. bibl. index.
Indexed: e-psyche.
Published by: Polskie Towarzystwo Higieny Psychicznej/Polish Mental Hygiene Society, Ul Targowa 59-16, Warsaw 03729, Poland. TEL 48-22-186599.

ZEITSCHRIFT FUER GERONTOPSYCHOLOGIE UND PSYCHIATRIE. see *GERONTOLOGY AND GERIATRICS*

616.89 CHE ISSN 1422-4917
ZEITSCHRIFT FUER KINDER- UND JUGENDPSYCHIATRIE UND PSYCHOTHERAPIE. Text in German. q. CHF 132 domestic; CHF 146 foreign (effective 2001). adv. 64 p./no. *Refereed.* **Document type:** *Journal, Academic/Scholarly.*
Former titles (until 1996): Zeitschrift fuer Kinder- und Jugendpsychiatrie (0301-6811); (until 1973): Jahrbuch fuer Jugendpsychiatrie und Ihre Grenzgebiete (0448-1534)
Related titles: Online - full text ed.: (from Institute for Scientific Information).
Indexed: ASCA, Biol.Abstr., Curr.Cont., Excerp.Med., Ind.Med. (1996-), PsycInfo, Psychol.Abstr. (1976-), SSCI, e-psyche.
—BLDSC (9467.490000), EMDOCS, GNLM, Infotrieve. **CCC.**
Published by: Hans Huber AG, Laengassstr 76, Bern, 9 3000, Switzerland. TEL 41-31-3004500, FAX 41-31-3004591, zeitschriften@hanshuber.com, http://www.hanshuber.com. Ed. H Remschmidt. Adv. contact Rene Waelchli. color page DEM 2,540; trim 170 x 250. Circ: 1,200.

616.8 DEU ISSN 0723-6557
BF3 CODEN: ZKPPAP
ZEITSCHRIFT FUER KLINISCHE PSYCHOLOGIE, PSYCHOPATHOLOGIE UND PSYCHOTHERAPIE. Text in German. 1951. q. DEM 112 domestic; DEM 116 foreign; DEM 30 newsstand/cover (effective 2001). adv. bk.rev. index. *Refereed.* **Document type:** *Magazine, Academic/Scholarly.*
Former titles (until 1983): Zeitschrift fuer Klinische Psychologie und Psychotherapie (0300-869X); Jahrbuch fuer Psychologie, Psychotherapie und Medizinische Anthropologie (0021-4000)
Related titles: Online - full text ed.: (from Institute for Scientific Information).
Indexed: ASCA, Biol.Abstr., Curr.Cont., Curr.Ind.Stat., Excerp.Med., Ger.J.Psych., Ind.Med. (coverage dropped), Ind.Philos., Lang.& Lang.Behav.Abstr., PsycInfo, Psychol.Abstr. (1971-), SOPODA, SSCI, Sociol.Abstr., e-psyche.
—BLDSC, GNLM, IDS, Infotrieve. **CCC.**
Published by: (Goerres-Gesellschaft), Verlag Ferdinand Schoeningh GmbH, Postfach 2540, Paderborn 33050, Germany. TEL 49-5251-127665, FAX 49-5251-127860, info@schoeningh.de, http://www.schoeningh.de. Circ: 1,000.

150 616.89 DEU
ZEITSCHRIFT FUER PSYCHOSOMATISCHE MEDIZIN UND PSYCHOANALYSE. MONOGRAPHIEN. Text in German. 1970. irreg., latest vol.23, 1999. price varies. **Document type:** *Monographic series, Academic/Scholarly.*
Formerly: Zeitschrift fuer Psychosomatische Medizin und Psychoanalyse. Beihefte (0085-8412)
Indexed: Psychol.Abstr., SSCI (coverage dropped), e-psyche.
—CISTI.
Published by: Vandenhoeck und Ruprecht, Robert-Bosch-Breite 6, Goettingen 37079, Germany. TEL 49-551-6959-0, FAX 49-551-695917.

616.89 DEU
CODEN: ZPPSB2
ZEITSCHRIFT FUER PSYCHOSOMATISCHE MEDIZIN UND PSYCHOTHERAPIE. Text in German; Summaries in English, German. 1954. q. DEM 165; DEM 132 to students (effective 2000). adv. bk.rev. abstr. index. **Document type:** *Journal, Academic/Scholarly.*
Former titles: Zeitschrift fuer Psychosomatische Medizin und Psychoanalyse (0340-5613); Zeitschrift fuer Psycho-Somatische Medizin (0375-5355)
Indexed: ASCA, Biol.Abstr., CERDIC, Curr.Cont., Ger.J.Psych., IBZ, Ind.Med. (coverage dropped), Ind.Philos., Inpharma, Nutr.Abstr., PsycInfo, Psychoanal.Abstr., Psychol.Abstr. (1956-), Reac., Risk Abstr., SSCI, Sci.Cit.Ind., e-psyche.
—BLDSC, CISTI, EMDOCS, GNLM, IDS, Infotrieve, KNAW. **CCC.**
Published by: Vandenhoeck und Ruprecht, Robert-Bosch-Breite 6, Goettingen 37079, Germany. TEL 49-551-6959-26, FAX 49-551-695917. Eds. Annemarie Duehrssen, Rudolf Adam. Circ: 1,100.

616.8 DEU ISSN 0044-4251
ZENTRALBLATT FUER NEUROCHIRURGIE. Text and summaries in English, German. 1936. 4/yr. EUR 195.90 domestic to institutions; EUR 199 in Europe to institutions; EUR 201.80 elsewhere to institutions; EUR 89 to students; EUR 52 newsstand/cover (effective 2002). adv. bk.rev. abstr, illus. index per vol. 60 p./no. *Refereed.* **Document type:** *Journal, Academic/Scholarly.* **Description:** Covers all areas of neurosurgical research and clinical practice.
Related titles: Online - full text ed.: ISSN 1438-9746 (from Institute for Scientific Information).
Indexed: ASCA, Biol.Abstr., Dent.Ind., Excerp.Med., INIS Atomind., Ind.Med. (1936-), Neurosci.Cit.Ind., e-psyche.
—BLDSC (9511.300000), CISTI, GNLM, IDS, KNAW. **CCC.**
Published by: Johann Ambrosius Barth Verlag in Medizinverlage Heidelberg GmbH & Co. KG, Ruedigerstr 14, Stuttgart 70469, Germany. TEL 49-711-8931-0, FAX 49-711-8931422, kunden.service@thieme.de, http://www.thieme.de/zblneurochir. Ed. W J Bock. Adv. contact Irmgard Mayer TEL 49-711-8931469. B&W page DEM 750; trim.

616.8 CHN ISSN 1003-2754
ZHONGFENG YU SHENJING JIBING ZAZHI/JOURNAL OF APOPLEXY AND NERVOUS DISEASES. Text in Chinese. 1984 (Mar.). bi-m. CNY 6 per issue domestic (effective 2000). back issues avail. **Document type:** *Academic/Scholarly.*
Related titles: Online - full content ed.: (from WanFang Data Corp.).
Published by: Bethune Yike Daxue, Xinming Dajie 6 Hao, Changchun 130021, China. TEL 86-431-5653531. Ed. Mingli Rao.

616.8 CHN ISSN 1005-3611
ZHONGGUO LINCHUANG XINLIXUE ZAZHI/CHINESE JOURNAL OF CLINICAL PSYCHOLOGY. Text in Chinese. 1993. q. USD 10.80; USD 2.70 newsstand/cover (effective 2001). **Document type:** *Academic/Scholarly.*
—BLDSC (3180.304000).
Published by: China International Book Trading Corp/Zhongguo Guoji Tushu Maoyi Zonggongsi cibtc@mail.cibtc.com.cn, http://www.cibtc.com.cn. **Dist. by:** 35, Chegongzhuang Xilu, Haidian District, Beijing 100044, China.

616.8 CHN ISSN 1008-0872
ZHONGGUO SHENJIN KEXUE ZAZHI/CHINESE JOURNAL OF NEUROSCIENCE. Text in Chinese, English. q. USD 88 (effective 2000). **Document type:** *Academic/Scholarly.*
Indexed: e-psyche.
Published by: Kexue Chubanshe/Science Press, 16 Donghuang Cheng Genbei Jie, Beijing 100717, China.

616.8 CHN ISSN 1006-2963
ZHONGGUO SHENJING MIANYIXUE HE SHENJINGBINGXUE ZAZHI/CHINESE JOURNAL OF NEUROIMMUNOLOGY AND NEUROLOGY. Text in Chinese. 1994. q. USD 19.60; CNY 7, USD 4.90 newsstand/cover (effective 2001).
Related titles: Online - full content ed.: (from WanFang Data Corp.).
Published by: Zhongguo Yixue Kexueyuan, Dongshan, 1, Dahua Lu, Beijing 100730, China. TEL 86-1-65132266 ext 3872, FAX 86-1-65242081, zgsm@263.net. Ed. Xian-Hao Xu. **Dist. by:** China International Book Trading Corp, 35, Chegongzhuang Xilu, Haidian District, Beijing 100044, China. TEL 86-1-68413849, FAX 86-1-68412048, cibtc@mail.cibtc.com.cn, http://www.cibtc.com.cn.

616.8 CHN ISSN 1006-7884
CODEN: CHSCA
ZHONGHUA JINGSHENKE ZAZHI/CHINESE JOURNAL OF PSYCHIATRY. Text in Chinese. 1955-1960; resumed 1996. bi-m. CNY 37.20 domestic; USD 20.40 foreign; CNY 9.30 newsstand/cover domestic; USD 5.10 newsstand/cover foreign (effective 2001). **Document type:** *Academic/Scholarly.*
Supersedes in part (1955-1960): Zhonghua Shenjing-Jingshenke Zazhi (0412-4057)
Related titles: CD-ROM ed.; Online - full content ed.: (from WanFang Data Corp.).
Indexed: Excerp.Med. (1993-), ExtraMED, Ind.Med. (coverage dropped), e-psyche.
—BLDSC (3180.605000), EMDOCS, GNLM.
Published by: Zhonghua Yixuehui Zazhishe, 42 Dongsi Xidajie, Beijing 100710, China. TEL 86-1-65271220, cmajs@public.sti.ac.cn. Ed. Yu Chen. **Dist. by:** China International Book Trading Corp, 35, Chegongzhuang Xilu, Haidian District, Beijing 100044, China. TEL 86-1-68413849, FAX 86-1-68412048, cibtc@mail.cibtc.com.cn, http://www.cibtc.com.cn.

616.8 CHN ISSN 1001-2346
ZHONGHUA SHENJING WAIKE ZAZHI/CHINESE JOURNAL OF NEUROSURGERY. Text in Chinese; Summaries in English. 1985. bi-m. USD 31.20; USD 5.20 newsstand/cover (effective 2001). adv. bk.rev. index. 64 p./no. back issues avail. *Refereed.* **Document type:** *Academic/Scholarly.*
Related titles: CD-ROM ed.
Indexed: ExtraMED, e-psyche.
—GNLM.

M

Published by: Beijing Neurosurgical Institute, 6 Tiantan Xili, Beijing 100050, China. TEL 86-1-65113169, FAX 86-1-67018349, wzjlzjmi@public.bta.net.cn. Ed. Chungcheng Wang. R&P, Adv. contact Li Li. Circ: 10,000. **Dist. overseas by:** China International Book Trading Corp, 35, Chegongzhuang Xilu, Haidian District, Beijing 100044, China. TEL 86-1-68413849, FAX 86-1-68412048, cibtc@mail.cibtc.com.cn, http://www.cibtc.com.cn. **Co-sponsor:** Zhonghua Yixuehui/Chinese Medical Association.

616.8 CHN ISSN 1006-7876
ZHONGHUA SHENJINGKE ZAZHI/CHINESE JOURNAL OF NEUROLOGY. Text in Chinese. 1955-1960; resumed 1996. bi-m. USD 30.60; CNY 9.30, USD 5.10 newsstand/cover (effective 2001). 64 p./no. *Refereed.* **Document type:** *Journal, Academic/Scholarly.*
Supersedes in part (1955-1960): Chung-Hua Shen Ching Ching Shen K'o Tsa Chih (0412-4057)
Related titles: CD-ROM ed.; Online - full content ed.: (from WanFang Data Corp.).
—BLDSC (3180.435900).
Published by: Zhonghua Yixuehui Zazhishe, 42 Dongsi Xidajie, Beijing 100710, China. TEL 86-1-65249989 ext 1440, cmasj@public.sti.ac.cn. Ed. Yalin Bao. **Dist. by:** China International Book Trading Corp, 35, Chegongzhuang Xilu, Haidian District, Beijing 100044, China. TEL 86-1-68413849, FAX 86-1-68412048, cibtc@mail.cibtc.com.cn, http://www.cibtc.com.cn.

616.8 RUS ISSN 0044-4588
RC321 CODEN: ZNPIAP
ZHURNAL NEVROPATOLOGII I PSIKHIATRII IM. S.S. KORSAKOVA/JOURNAL OF NEUROLOGY AND PSYCHIATRY. S.S. KORSAKOV. Text in Russian; Summaries in English. 1901. m. RUR 360 for 6 mos. to individuals; RUR 1,080 for 6 mos. to institutions (effective 2002). adv. bk.rev. bibl. index. *Refereed.* **Description:** Disseminates medical aid to patients by publishing original scientific investigations in etiology and pathogenesis, including the prevention and treatment of neurological and mental diseases.
Related titles: Online - full text ed.: (from Institute for Scientific Information).
Indexed: ASCA, Agri.& Environ.Biotech.Abstr. (coverage dropped), Bibl.Dev.Med.& Child Neur., Biol.Abstr., Chem.Abstr., Curr.Cont., Dent.Ind., Derwent Biotech.Abstr., Excerp.Med., INIS Atomind., Ind.Med. (coverage dropped), Inpharma, Int.Aerosp.Abstr., Neurosci.Cit.Ind., Nutr.Abstr., Pharm.&Out.News, Psychol.Abstr. (1928-), Reac., Ref.Zh., e-psyche.
—CASDDS, CISTI, East View, GNLM, IDS, KNAW. **CCC.**
Published by: (Nauchnoe Obshchestvo Nevrologov i Psikhiatrov), Media Sfera, Dmitrovskoe shosse 46, korp 2, etazh 4, P.O. Box 54, Moscow 127238, Russian Federation. TEL 7-095-4824329, FAX 7-095-4824503, mediashp@mediasphera.ru. Ed. E I Gusev. Adv. contact Valery Nemtsov. **Dist. by:** Mezhdunarodnaya Kniga, B Yakimanka 39, Moscow 117049, Russian Federation. TEL 7-095-2384967, FAX 7-095-2384634; **US dist. addr.:** East View Publications, 3020 Harbor Ln N, Minneapolis, MN 55447. TEL 612-550-0961.

ZHURNAL VOPROSY NEIROKHIRURGII IM. N.N. BURDENKO/JOURNAL OF NEUROSURGICAL PROBLEMS. see *MEDICAL SCIENCES—Surgery*

ZHURNAL VYSSHEI NERVNOI DEYATEL'NOSTI. see *BIOLOGY—Physiology*

MEDICAL SCIENCES—Radiology And Nuclear Medicine

615.842 USA ISSN 0098-6070
A C R BULLETIN. Text in English. 1942. m. USD 60 to non-members. illus. back issues avail. **Document type:** *Bulletin, Newsletter, Trade.* **Description:** Provides organization news and member information, and examines current socio-economic issues in radiology.
Former titles (until 1968): American College of Radiology. Bulletin (0002-8037); (until 1958): American College of Radiology. Monthly Newsletter
Related titles: Online - full text ed.
Indexed: Med.Care Rev.
Published by: American College of Radiology, 1891 Preston White Dr, Reston, VA 20191. TEL 703-648-8929, FAX 703-620-4730, bulletin@acr.org, http://www.acr.org/. Ed. Thomas Rogers. Circ: 30,000.

615.842 USA
A H R A LINK. Text in English. 1982. m. membership. back issues avail. **Document type:** *Newsletter.*
Formerly: A H R A Announcement
Published by: American Healthcare Radiology Administrators, 111 Boston Post Rd, Box 334, Sudbury, MA 01776-0003. TEL 978-443-7591, FAX 978-443-8046, http://www.ahraonline.org, publications@ahraonline.org, publications@ahraonline.org, http://www.ahraonline.org. Ed., R&P Holly Vietzke. Circ: 4,000.

616.075 618 USA
A I U M REPORTER. Text in English. 1985. m. USD 20 (effective 1999). adv. bk.rev. back issues avail. **Document type:** *Newsletter.* **Description:** Keeps members and ultrasound professionals up-to-date on A.I.U.M. activities, as well as on news and legislation that can affect the field. Provides educational opportunities to practitioners.
Published by: American Institute for Ultrasound in Medicine, 14750 Sweitzer Ln, Ste 100, Laurel, MD 20707-5906. TEL 301-498-4100, FAX 301-498-4450, publications@aium.org, http://www.aium.org. Ed. Steven L Edell. Adv. contact Janet Campbell. Circ: 13,000 (paid).

615.842 USA ISSN 0195-6108
RC349.R3
A J N R. (American Journal of Neuroradiology) Text in English. 1980. 10/yr. USD 230 domestic to individuals; USD 290 foreign to individuals; USD 265 domestic to institutions; USD 325 foreign to institutions (effective 2001). adv. bk.rev. back issues avail. *Refereed.* **Document type:** *Academic/Scholarly.* **Description:** Publishes original clinical articles on imaging diagnosis of the central nervous system, including the spine, for radiologists, neuroradiologists, neurosurgeons, and neurologists.
Related titles: CD-ROM ed.; Microfilm ed.: (from WWS); Online - full content ed.: (from HighWire Pr.); Online - full text ed.: (from Institute for Scientific Information).
Indexed: ASCA, Aqua.Sci.& Fish.Abstr., Curr.Cont., Dent.Ind., Excerp.Med., Helminthol.Abstr., INIS Atomind., Ind.Imag.Lit., Ind.Med. (1980-), Ind.Sci.Rev., Inpharma, Int.Nurs.Ind., Jrnl.Watch Neuro., Neurosci.Abstr. (coverage dropped), Neurosci.Cit.Ind., Pharm.&Out.News, Protozool.Abstr., Reac., Rev.Med.& Vet.Mycol., SSCI (coverage dropped), Sci.Cit.Ind., Trop.Dis.Bull.
—BLDSC (0828.400000), CISTI, EMDOCS, GNLM, IDS, ingenta, KNAW.
Published by: American Society of Neuroradiology, PO Box 3000, Denville, NJ 07834-9349. TEL 800-783-4903, FAX 973-627-5872, ajnr@asnr.org, http://www.ajnr.org. Ed. Michael S Huckman. R&P Mary Shepelak TEL 312-942-2249. Adv. contact James Pattis. Circ: 6,385. **Subscr.to:** Allen Press Inc., PO Box 1897, Lawrence, KS 66044-8897.

615.842 USA ISSN 0361-803X
RM845 CODEN: AJROAM
A J R. (American Journal of Roentgenology) Text in English. 1906. m. USD 210 domestic to individuals; USD 280 foreign to individuals; USD 375 domestic to institutions; USD 445 foreign to institutions (effective 2002). adv. bk.rev. abstr, bibl, illus. index, cum.index every 5 yrs. back issues avail. *Refereed.* **Document type:** *Academic/Scholarly.* **Description:** Original articles on all aspects of general and diagnostic radiology, covering all current modalities, including MRI.
Former titles (1952-1976): American Journal of Roentgenology, Radium Therapy and Nuclear Medicine (0002-9580); (1923-1951): American Journal of Roentgenology and Radium Therapy (0092-5632)
Related titles: Online - full text ed.: (from HighWire Pr., EBSCO Publishing, Institute for Scientific Information).
Indexed: AIDS Abstr., AIM, ASCA, Abstr.Hyg., Agri.& Environ.Biotech.Abstr. (coverage dropped), Aqua.Sci.& Fish.Abstr., Bibl.Dev.Med.& Child Neur., Biol.Abstr., C.I.S. Abstr., Chem.Abstr., Curr.Adv.Cancer Res., Curr.Adv.Ecol.Sci., Curr.Cont., Dairy Sci.Abstr., Dent.Ind., Derwent Biotech.Abstr., Excerp.Med., Helminthol.Abstr., INIS Atomind., I.P.A., Ind.Imag.Lit., Ind.Med. (1977-), Ind.Sci.Rev., Inpharma, Int.Abstr.Biol.Sci., Jrnl.Watch Emer.Med., Kidney, Med.& Surg.Dermat., Nutr.Abstr., Pharm.&Out.News, Protozool.Abstr., Reac., Rev.Appl.Entomol., Rev.Med.& Vet.Mycol., Rev.Plant Path., Risk Abstr., SSCI (coverage dropped), Sci.Cit.Ind., Trop.Dis.Bull.
—BLDSC (0836.980000), CASDDS, CISTI, EMDOCS, GNLM, IDS, ingenta, KNAW. **CCC.**
Published by: American Roentgen Ray Society, 44211 Slatestone Court, Leesburg, VA 20176-5109. TEL 703-729-3353, 800-438-2777, FAX 703-729-4839, subscribe@arrs.org, advertise@arrs.org, http://www.arrs.org. Ed. Lee F Rogers. Adv. contact Claire McConnell. B&W page USD 1,995. Circ: 24,000. **Subscr. to:** AJR, PO Box 17266, Baltimore, MD 21297-0419.

616.842 USA ISSN 0161-3863
A S R T SCANNER. Text in English. 1968. m. membership only. adv. **Document type:** *Magazine, Trade.*
Indexed: CINAHL.
Published by: American Society of Radiologic Technologists, 15000 Central Ave S E, Albuquerque, NM 87123-3917. TEL 505-298-4500, FAX 505-298-5063, randerson@asrt.org, http://www.asrt.org. Ed. Robin Anderson. Pub. Nora Tuggle. R&P Peter Gregory. Adv. contact Joan McBrayer TEL 505-298-4500 ext. 317. Circ: 84,280 (paid).

ABDOMINAL IMAGING. see *MEDICAL SCIENCES—Gastroenterology*

615.842 USA ISSN 1076-6332
ACADEMIC RADIOLOGY. Text in English. 1994. m. USD 175 to individuals; USD 240 foreign to individuals; USD 225 to institutions; USD 290 foreign to institutions (effective 2000). adv. stat. *Refereed.* **Document type:** *Academic/Scholarly.* **Description:** Publishes articles describing original investigations in new radiologic techniques and technologies; covers other clinical, theoretical, and ethical issues.
Related titles: Online - full text ed.: (from Institute for Scientific Information).
Indexed: Curr.Cont., Excerp.Med., Ind.Imag.Lit., Ind.Med. (1994-), Inpharma, Int.Nurs.Ind., Reac.
—BLDSC (0570.514240), CISTI, GNLM, IDS, Infotrieve, KNAW. **CCC.**
Published by: Association of University Radiologists, 820 Jorie Blvd., Oak Brook, IL 60523. TEL 630-571-7873, FAX 630-571-7837, http://www.aur.org. Ed. Dr. Stanley Baum. Adv. contact Jim Drew. B&W page USD 860, color page USD 2,285; trim 8.125 x 10.875. **Co-sponsors:** Society of Chairmen of Academic Radiology Departments; Association of Program Directors in Radiology; American Association of Academic Chief Residents in Radiology.

615.842 DNK ISSN 0284-1851
CODEN: ACRAE3
ACTA RADIOLOGICA. Text in English. 1921. bi-m. USD 209 in the Americas to institutions print & online eds. combined; GBP 145 elsewhere to institutions print & online eds. combined (effective 2002). adv. bk.rev. bibl, charts, illus. index, cum.index. reprint service avail. from ISI. *Refereed.* **Document type:** *Academic/Scholarly.*
Formerly (until 1986): Acta Radiologica. Diagnosis (0567-8056); Which superseded in part (in 1962): Acta Radiologica (0001-6926)
Related titles: Online - full text ed.: ISSN 1600-0455. GBP 130 (effective 2002) (from Ovid Technologies, Inc., EBSCO Publishing, ingenta, Munksgaard & Blackwell Science's Synergy, Swets Blackwell, Institute for Scientific Information); ♦ Supplement: Acta Radiologica. Supplementum. ISSN 0365-5954.
Indexed: ASCA, Agri.& Environ.Biotech.Abstr. (coverage dropped), Biol.Abstr., Chem.Abstr., Compumath, Curr.Adv.Cell & Devel.Biol., Curr.Adv.Ecol.Sci., Curr.Cont., Dent.Ind., Derwent Biotech.Abstr., Eng.Ind., Environ.Sci.Poll.Mgmt., Excerp.Med., Helminthol.Abstr., INIS Atomind., INSPEC (Jun.1973-Nov.1992, dropped), Ind.Imag.Lit., Ind.Med. (1987-), Ind.Sci.Rev., Inpharma, Kidney, Met.Abstr., Neurosci.Cit.Ind., Nutr.Abstr., Pollut.Abstr., Reac., Risk Abstr., Saf.Sci.Abstr., Sci.Cit.Ind.
—BLDSC (0662.000000), CASDDS, CISTI, GNLM, IDS, Infotrieve, ingenta, KNAW. **CCC.**
Published by: (Societies of Medical Radiology in Denmark, Finland, Iceland, Norway and Sweden), Blackwell Munksgaard, Noerre Soegade 35, PO Box 2148, Copenhagen K 1016, Denmark. TEL 45-77-33-33-33, FAX 45-77-33-33-77, customerservice@munksgaard.dk, http://www.munksgaard.dk/actaradiologica. Ed. Anders Hemmingsson. Adv. contact Eric Rozario TEL 45-77-33-33-01. Circ: 3,400.

615.847 DNK ISSN 0365-5954
CODEN: ARASA5
ACTA RADIOLOGICA. SUPPLEMENTUM. Text in English. 1921. irreg. free to subscr. of Acta Radiologica. **Document type:** *Academic/Scholarly.*
Related titles: Online - full text ed.: ISSN 1600-5481 (from Ovid Technologies, Inc., Swets Blackwell); ♦ Supplement to: Acta Radiologica. ISSN 0284-1851.
Indexed: Eng.Ind., INIS Atomind., Ind.Med. (1921-).
—BLDSC (0662.005000), CISTI, Ei, ingenta, KNAW. **CCC.**
Published by: (Societies of Medical Radiology in Denmark, Finland, Iceland, Norway and Sweden), Blackwell Munksgaard, Noerre Soegade 35, PO Box 2148, Copenhagen K 1016, Denmark. TEL 45-77-33-33-33, FAX 45-77-33-33-77, customerservice@munksgaard.dk, http://www.munksgaard.dk/actaradiologica. Ed. Anders Hemmingsson. Adv. contact Eric Rozario TEL 45-77-33-33-01.

615.842 658 USA ISSN 0738-6974
RA975.5.R3
ADMINISTRATIVE RADIOLOGY; the journal of medical imaging administration & management. Text in English. 1981. m. USD 96 domestic; USD 126 in Canada; USD 196 elsewhere (effective 2001). adv. bk.rev. illus, tr.lit. index, cum.index. back issues avail.; reprint service avail. from PQC. *Refereed.* **Document type:** *Journal, Academic/Scholarly, Trade.* **Description:** Healthcare management publication serving healthcare executives in people, business and administrative management relative to medical imaging and radiation sciences.
Related titles: Microform ed.: (from PQC).
Indexed: Int.Nurs.Ind.
—BLDSC (1583.209500), GNLM.
Published by: Glendale Publishing Corp., 934 W Glenoaks Blvd, Ste 1, Glendale, CA 91202-2755. TEL 818-500-1872. Ed. Cynthia Stout. Pub. Rick Martinez. R&P Leanne Jones. Adv. contact Harrison Jobst. Circ: 13,500 (paid).

615.842 616.07 USA ISSN 1096-6285
ADVANCE FOR ADMINISTRATORS IN RADIOLOGY AND RADIATION ONCOLOGY. Text in English. 1991. m. free per issue to qualified personnel. adv. *Refereed.* **Document type:** *Trade.*
Published by: Merion Publications, Inc., 2900 Horizon Dr, PO Box 61556, King Of Prussia, PA 19406. TEL 610-278-1400, 800-355-5627, FAX 610-278-1421, advance@merion.com, http://www.advanceweb.com. Ed. Sharon Breske. Pub. Ann Kielinski. adv.: B&W page USD 2,156, color page USD 2,956; trim 8.375 x 10.875.

616 USA
ADVANCE FOR IMAGING AND RADIATION THERAPY PROFESSIONALS. Text in English. 1988. bi-w. Free to qualified subscribers. adv. *Refereed.* **Document type:** *Magazine, Trade.* **Description:** Covers procedures and therapies used by medical imaging and radiology professionals.
Former titles: Advance for Radiologic Science Professionals (1074-231X); (until 1990): Advance for Radiologic Technologists (1042-2498)
Related titles: Online - full content ed.
Published by: Merion Publications, Inc., 2900 Horizon Dr, PO Box 61556, King Of Prussia, PA 19406. TEL 800-355-5627, FAX 610-278-1421, 610-278-1425, http://www.advanceforirt.com/, http:// www.advanceweb.com. Ed. Joe Jalkiewicz. Pub. Ann Kielinski. adv.: B&W page USD 2,156, color page USD 2,456; trim 10.88 x 8.38. Circ: 64,900.

ADVANCES IN ECHO-CONTRAST; ultrasound imaging innovations, echo-enhancing agents, clinical impact. see *MEDICAL SCIENCES—Computer Applications*

616.842 DEU
ADVANCES IN LASER MEDICINE. Text in English. irreg., latest vol.8, 1992. **Document type:** *Monographic series.*
—BLDSC (0709.255700).
Published by: (Laser-Medizin-Zentrum Berlin), Ecomed Verlagsgesellschaft AG & Co. KG, Justus-von-Liebig-Str 1, Landsberg 86899, Germany. TEL 49-8191-125-0, FAX 49-8191-125492, a.heinrich@ecomed.de, info@ecomed.de, http://www.ecomed.de.

616.075 NLD ISSN 0925-9848
ADVANCES IN M R I - CONTRAST; MRI innovations, contrast-enhancing agents, clinical impact. (Magnetic Resonance Imaging) Text in English. 1991. q. back issues avail.; reprint service avail. from SWZ. *Refereed.* **Document type:** *Academic/Scholarly.*
Related titles: Microform ed.: (from PQC).
Indexed: Aqua.Sci.& Fish.Abstr., Environ.Sci.Poll.Mgmt., Excerp.Med. (1995-).
—CISTI, EMDOCS, GNLM, Infotrieve. **CCC.**
Published by: (Schering AG DEU), Kluwer Academic Publishers Group (Subsidiary of: Wolters Kluwer N.V.), Spuiboulevard 50, PO Box 17, Dordrecht 3300 AA, Netherlands. FAX 31-78-639-2254, services@wkap.nl, http://www.wkap.nl. Circ: (controlled). **Dist. by:** Journals Department, PO Box 322, Dordrecht 3300 AH, Netherlands. FAX 31-78-654-6474.

616.07 NLD ISSN 0928-1509
ADVANCES IN X-RAY CONTRAST; x-ray enhancing agents, clinical impact and clinical research. Text in English. 1993. q. back issues avail. **Document type:** *Academic/Scholarly.* **Description:** Covers recent developments in iodinated contrast media and issues such as renal tolerance, blood clotting and pharmacokinetics, within a clinically relevant framework.
Indexed: Aqua.Sci.& Fish.Abstr.
—CISTI, GNLM, Infotrieve. **CCC.**
Published by: (Schering AG DEU), Kluwer Academic Publishers Group (Subsidiary of: Wolters Kluwer N.V.), Spuiboulevard 50, PO Box 17, Dordrecht 3300 AA, Netherlands. FAX 31-78-639-2254, services@wkap.nl, http://www.wkap.nl. Circ: (controlled). **Dist. by:** Journals Department, PO Box 322, Dordrecht 3300 AH, Netherlands. FAX 31-78-654-6474.

615.842 USA ISSN 1073-0214
AMERICAN BOARD OF NUCLEAR MEDICINE. INFORMATION POLICIES AND PROCEDURES. Text in English. 1975. a. **Document type:** *Catalog.* **Description:** Information on requirements for certifying examination in nuclear medicine.
Published by: American Board of Nuclear Medicine, 900 Veteran Ave, Los Angeles, CA 90024. TEL 310-825-6787, FAX 310-794-4821, http://www.abnm.org. Ed. William H Blahd. Circ: 1,500.

616 USA
AMERICAN INSTITUTE OF ULTRASOUND IN MEDICINE. ANNUAL SCIENTIFIC CONFERENCE. PROCEEDINGS. Text in English. a. USD 12 (effective 1999). adv. bk.rev. **Document type:** *Proceedings.*
Formerly: American Institute of Ultrasound in Medicine. Annual Scientific Conference. Program (0065-8871)
Published by: American Institute for Ultrasound in Medicine, 14750 Sweitzer Ln, Ste 100, Laurel, MD 20707-5906. TEL 301-498-4100, FAX 301-498-4450, mkalil@aium.org, http://www.aium.org. Ed. George R Leopold. R&P Maureen Kalil. Circ: 3,000.

615.842 AUT ISSN 1011-2529
ANIMAL PRODUCTION AND HEALTH NEWSLETTER. Text in English. 1976. s-a. free. **Document type:** *Newsletter, Academic/Scholarly.*
Indexed: Nutr.Abstr.
Published by: International Atomic Energy Agency/Agence Internationale de l'Energie Atomique, Division of Conference and Document Services, Wagramer Str 5, Postfach 100, Vienna, W 1400, Austria. TEL 43-1-2600-0, FAX 43-1-2600-7, sales.publications@iaea.org, http://www.iaea.org. Circ: 1,230. **Co-sponsor:** Food and Agriculture Organization.

615.842 FRA ISSN 0003-4185
CODEN: ANLRAT
ANNALES DE RADIOLOGIE; radiologie clinique, radiobiologie. Text in English, French. 1958. 6/yr. FRF 1,660 domestic to individuals; FRF 2,200 foreign to individuals; FRF 800 domestic to students; FRF 1,110 foreign to students. adv. bk.rev. abstr, charts, illus. index. **Document type:** *Academic/Scholarly.*
Indexed: Biol.Abstr., C.I.S. Abstr., Chem.Abstr., Curr.Cont. (coverage dropped), Excerp.Med., Helminthol.Abstr., INIS Atomind., Ind.Med. (until 1999, dropped), Ind.Sci.Rev., Sci.Cit.Ind. (coverage dropped).
—CASDDS, CISTI, EMDOCS, GNLM, IDS. **CCC.**
Published by: (Semaine des Hopitaux), Expansion Scientifique Francaise, 31 bd. de la Tour Maubourg, Paris Cedex 7 75343, France. TEL 33-1-40626400, FAX 33-1-45556920. Ed. J M Tubiana. Circ: 4,000.

616.07 JPN ISSN 0914-7187
CODEN: ANMEEX
ANNALS OF NUCLEAR MEDICINE. Text in English. 1987. q. JPY 1,500 per issue.
Related titles: Online - full text ed.: (from Institute for Scientific Information).
Indexed: Chem.Abstr., Chem.Indus.Notes, Chem.Titles, Curr.Cont., Excerp.Med., INIS Atomind., Ind.Med. (1987-), Inpharma, Pharm.&Out.News, Reac.
—BLDSC (1043.175000), CASDDS, CISTI, EMDOCS, GNLM, KNAW.
Published by: Japanese Society of Nuclear Medicine/Nihon Kaku Igakkai, Nihon Aisotopu Kyokai, 28-45 Honkomagome 2-chome, Bunkyo-ku, Tokyo 113-0021, Japan.

APPLIED RADIATION AND ISOTOPES. see *PHYSICS—Nuclear Physics*

615.842 USA ISSN 0160-9963
RM845
APPLIED RADIOLOGY; the journal of practical medical imaging and management. Text in English. 1972. m. USD 85 domestic; USD 100 foreign (effective 2000). adv. charts, illus, tr.lit. cum.index. *Refereed.* **Document type:** *Academic/Scholarly.*
Former titles: Applied Radiology and Nuclear Medicine (0099-2364); Applied Radiology (0044-8451)
Related titles: Online - full text ed.: (from ScienceDirect).
Indexed: Biol.Abstr., CINAHL, Excerp.Med., Hosp.Lit.Ind.
—BLDSC (1576.570000), CISTI, GNLM, ingenta, KNAW.
Published by: Anderson Publishing Ltd., 1301 W. Park Ave., Ocean, NJ 07712-3151. TEL 732-695-0600, FAX 732-695-9501, andersonpub@compuserve.com, http://www.appliedradiology.com. Eds. Jodi Harris, Theodore E Keats. Pub. Oliver O Anderson. R&P Elizabeth McDonald. Adv. contact Kieran N Anderson. Circ: 33,000. **Subscr. to:** PO Box 814, Winchester, MA 01890-9806.

615.842 363.179 ITA
ASSOCIAZIONE ITALIANA PROTEZIONE CONTRO LE RADIAZIONI. BOLLETINO. Text in Italian. 197?. bi-m. **Document type:** *Academic/Scholarly.* **Description:** Covers topics in the field of radiation protection for medical professionals and other interested groups.
Published by: Associazione Italiana Protezione contro le Radiazioni (AIRP), Laboratorio de Fisica, Istituto Superiore de Sanita, Viale Regina Elena, 299, Rome, RM 00161, Italy. Ed. F Grisanti.

615.842 AUS ISSN 0004-8461
CODEN: AURDAW
AUSTRALASIAN RADIOLOGY. Text in English. 1957. q. USD 105 elsewhere to individuals; AUD 319 domestic to institutions; AUD 290 in New Zealand to institutions; USD 280 elsewhere to institutions; USD 116 elsewhere to individuals paper & online eds. combined; AUD 351 domestic to institutions paper & online eds. combined; AUD 319 in New Zealand to institutions paper & online eds. combined; USD 308 elsewhere to institutions paper & online eds. combined (effective 2001). adv. bk.rev. charts, illus. index, cum.index. back issues avail. *Refereed.* **Document type:** *Academic/Scholarly.* **Description:** Discusses various aspects of clinical radiology.
Related titles: Microform ed.: (from PQC); Online - full text ed.: ISSN 1440-1673. USD 95 elsewhere to individuals; AUD 288 domestic to institutions; AUD 261 in New Zealand to institutions; USD 252 elsewhere to institutions (effective 2001) (from EBSCO Publishing, O C L C Online Computer Library Center, Inc., RoweCom Information Quest, ingenta, Munksgaard & Blackwell Science's Synergy, Swets Blackwell).
Indexed: Biol.Abstr., Cal.Tiss.Abstr., Chem.Abstr., Curr.Cont. (coverage dropped), Dent.Ind., Environ.Sci.Poll.Mgmt., Excerp.Med., INIS Atomind., Ind.Imag.Lit., Ind.Med. (1966-), Pollut.Abstr., Risk Abstr., Saf.Sci.Abstr., Tox.Abstr. (coverage dropped).
—BLDSC (1796.300000), ADONIS, CISTI, GNLM, ingenta, KNAW. **CCC.**
Published by: (Royal Australian and New Zealand College of Radiologists), Blackwell Science Asia Pty Ltd, PO Box 378, Carlton South, VIC 3053, Australia. TEL 61-3-9347-0300, FAX 61-3-9347-5001, info@blacksci-asia.com.au, http://www.blacksci.co.uk. Ed. Michael R Sage. Adv. contact Kathryn O'Brien. B&W page AUD 1,012, color page AUD 2,057; trim 210 x 275. Circ: 2,550.

615.842 GBR ISSN 0961-2653
B J R SUPPLEMENT. (British Journals of Radiology) Text in English. 1990. irreg.
Related titles: ♦ Supplement to: British Journal of Radiology. ISSN 0007-1285.
Indexed: Ind.Med. (1989-).
Published by: British Institute of Radiology, 36 Portland Pl, London W1B 1AT, United Kingdom. TEL 44-20-7307-1400, FAX 44-20-7307-1414, admin@bir.org.uk, http://www.bir.org.uk.

616.842 GBR ISSN 0966-1905
B M U S BULLETIN. Text in English. 1975. q. GBP 50 in United Kingdom; GBP 80 foreign (effective 2001). bk.rev. bibl, charts, illus, stat, tr.lit. back issues avail. **Document type:** *Journal, Bulletin, Academic/Scholarly.* **Description:** Analyzes current developments in ultrasound for members. Provides review articles.
—BLDSC (2116.243000).
Published by: British Medical Ultrasound Society, 36 Portland Pl, London W1B 1LS, United Kingdom. TEL 44-20-7636-3714, FAX 44-20-7323-2175, secretariat@bmus.org, http://www.bmus.org. Ed. Dr. A P Smith. Adv. contacts D A Goodall, D Scott TEL 44-20-7375-1155. Circ: 2,000 (paid).

BIOELECTROMAGNETICS. see *BIOLOGY—Biophysics*

616.82 GBR
BRITISH INSTITUTE OF RADIOLOGY REPORTS. Text in English. irreg., latest vol.22, 1991. price varies. back issues avail. **Document type:** *Monographic series.* **Description:** Covers major topics in radiation therapy and research.

M

Published by: British Institute of Radiology, 36 Portland Pl, London W1B 1AT, United Kingdom. TEL 44-20-7307-1400, FAX 44-20-7307-1414. **U.S. subscr. to:** Professional & Scientific Publications, PO Box 560B, Kennebunkport, ME 04046. **Dist. by:** Vine House Distribution Ltd.. FAX 0825-724188.

615.842 GBR ISSN 0007-1285
QC1 CODEN: BJRAAP
BRITISH JOURNAL OF RADIOLOGY. Text in English. 1896. m. GBP 360 to institutional members includes free Online access (effective 2001). adv. bk.rev. abstr, charts, illus, stat. index. back issues avail. *Refereed.* **Document type:** *Academic/Scholarly.* **Description:** Presents research covering the spectrum of radiological disciplines, including radio-diagnosis and therapy, nuclear medicine, ultrasound, NMR, radiobiology, radiation protection, and hyperthermia.
Related titles: Online - full text ed.: (from EBSCO Publishing, Swets Blackwell, Institute for Scientific Information); ♦ Supplement: B J R Supplement. ISSN 0961-2653.
Indexed: AIM, ASCA, Agri.& Environ.Biotech.Abstr. (coverage dropped), Biol.Abstr., C.I.S. Abstr., Chem.Abstr., Chem.Indus.Notes, Chem.Titles, Compumath, Curr.Adv.Cancer Res., Curr.Adv.Ecol.Sci., Curr.Cont., Dairy Sci.Abstr., Dent.Ind., Derwent Biotech.Abstr., Dok.Arbeitsmed., Excerp.Med., Helminthol.Abstr., INIS Atomind., INSPEC (pre-1969-), Ind.Imag.Lit., Ind.Med. (1928-), Ind.Sci.Rev., Inpharma, Neurosci.Cit.Ind., Nutr.Abstr., Pharm.&Out.News, Protozool.Abstr., Reac., Rev.Arom.& Med.Plants, Rev.Med.& Vet.Mycol., Risk Abstr., Sci.Cit.Ind.
—BLDSC (2323.000000), AskIEEE, CASDDS, CISTI, EMDOCS, GNLM, IDS, ingenta, KNAW. **CCC.**
Published by: British Institute of Radiology, 36 Portland Pl, London W1B 1AT, United Kingdom. TEL 44-20-7307-1400, FAX 44-20-7307-1414, admin@bir.org.uk, http://bjr.birjournals.org, http://www.bir.org.uk. Eds. J T Patton, N J McNally. Circ: 4,600. **Subscr. to:** P S P Subscriptions Direct, BMA House, Tavistock Sq, London WC1H 9JR, United Kingdom. TEL 44-20-7383-6270, FAX 44-20-7383-6402.

616.07 JPN
C Y R I C ANNUAL REPORT. (Cyclotron Radioisotope Center) Text in English. 1980. a. 225 p./no. **Document type:** *Academic/Scholarly.*
Published by: Tohoku University, Cyclotron Radioisotope Center/Tohoku Daigaku Saikurotoron Rajio Aisotopu Senta, Aoba, Aramaki, Aoba-ku, Sendai-shi, Miyagi-ken 981-0945, Japan. TEL 81-22-217-7800, FAX 81-22-217-3485. Ed. H Orihara.

615.842 CAN ISSN 0846-5371
CODEN: JCARAU
CANADIAN ASSOCIATION OF RADIOLOGISTS JOURNAL/ASSOCIATION CANADIENNE DES RADIOLOGISTES. JOURNAL. Text in English, French. 1949. 6/yr. CND 151 domestic; USD 151 foreign (effective 1999). adv. bk.rev. illus. index. back issues avail.; reprints avail. *Refereed.* **Document type:** *Academic/Scholarly.* **Description:** Concerned with medical imaging, publishing original scientific papers, case reports, reviews, articles and Residents' Corner.
Formerly (until 1985): Canadian Association of Radiologists. Journal (0008-2902)
Related titles: Microfilm ed.: (from PQC); Online - full text ed.: ISSN 1488-2361 (from LexisNexis, Institute for Scientific Information).
Indexed: ASCA, Aqua.Sci.& Fish.Abstr., Biol.Abstr., CBCA Ref., Cal.Tiss.Abstr., Chem.Abstr., Curr.Adv.Cancer Res., Curr.Cont., Environ.Sci.Poll.Mgmt., Excerp.Med., INIS Atomind., Ind.Imag.Lit., Ind.Med. (1986-), Inpharma, Neurosci.Cit.Ind., Pollut.Abstr., Reac., Rev.Med.& Vet.Mycol., Sci.Cit.Ind.
—BLDSC (4722.500000), CASDDS, CISTI, EMDOCS, GNLM. **CCC.**
Published by: Canadian Medical Association, 1867 Alta Vista Dr, Ottawa, ON K1H 5K9, Canada. TEL 613-731-9331, 800-663-7336 ext. 2132, FAX 613-565-2382, pubs@cma.ca, rafusj@cma.ca, http://www.cma.ca/carj. Ed. Craig Coblenz. Adv. contact Beverley Kirkpatrick. B&W page CND 790, color page CND 1,590; trim 10.88 x 8.13. Circ: 1,800.

615.842 CAN ISSN 0820-5930
CANADIAN JOURNAL OF MEDICAL RADIATION TECHNOLOGY/JOURNAL CANADIEN DES TECHNIQUES EN RADIATION MEDICALE. Text in English, French. 1943. q. CND 30 domestic; CND 36 in United States; CND 54 elsewhere (effective 1999). adv. bk.rev. charts, illus, stat. index, cum.index. back issues avail.; reprint service avail. from PQC. **Document type:** *Academic/Scholarly, Trade.* **Description:** Consists of a health care trade publication that features articles on recent research, new technology, professional practices, technologists' viewpoints, and book reviews.
Former titles: Canadian Journal of Radiography, Radiation Therapy, Nuclear Medicine (0382-6333); (until 1987): Canadian Journal of Radiography, Radiotherapy, Nuclear Medicine (0319-4434); Canadian Journal of Radiography, Radiotherapy, Nucleography (0015-4938); (until 1970): Focal Spot
Related titles: Microform ed.: (from PQC).
Indexed: Biol.Abstr., CINAHL, INIS Atomind.
—BLDSC (3032.300000), CISTI, GNLM, Infotrieve. **CCC.**
Published by: Canadian Association of Medical Radiation Technologists/Association Canadienne des Technologues en Radiation Medicale, Ste 1510, 130 Albert St, Ottawa, ON K1P 5G4, Canada. TEL 613-234-0012, FAX 613-234-1097, hdowns@camrt.ca, http://www.camrt.ca. Ed. Steven Brasier. R&P Heather Downs. Adv. contact Heather Downsr. Circ: 10,468 (paid).

CANCER - RADIOTHERAPIE. see *MEDICAL SCIENCES—Oncology*

616.07 616.1 USA ISSN 0174-1551
CODEN: CAIRDG
CARDIOVASCULAR AND INTERVENTIONAL RADIOLOGY. Text in English. 1978. bi-m. (in 1 vol., 6 nos./vol.). USD 417.50 domestic for Print & Online Eds.; USD 439.60 in Germany for Print & Online Eds.; USD 82.50 newsstand/cover foreign (effective 2002). adv. bk.rev. reprint service avail. from ISI. *Refereed.* **Document type:** *Academic/Scholarly.* **Description:** Examines developments in the diagnostic techniques of this specialty from all over the world.
Formerly: Cardiovascular Radiology (0342-7196)
Related titles: Microform ed.: (from PQC); Online - full text ed.: ISSN 1432-086X (from F I Z Technik, EBSCO Publishing, RoweCom Information Quest, Swets Blackwell, Springer LINK, Institute for Scientific Information).
Indexed: ASCA, Curr.Cont., Excerp.Med., Helminthol.Abstr., INIS Atomind., Ind.Imag.Lit., Ind.Med. (1980-), Inpharma, Kidney, Pharm.&Out.News, Reac., Sci.Cit.Ind. (coverage dropped).
—BLDSC (3051.438000), CISTI, GNLM, IDS, ingenta, KNAW. **CCC.**
Published by: Springer-Verlag, Journals (Subsidiary of: BertelsmannSpringer), 175 Fifth Ave, New York, NY 10010. TEL 212-460-1500, FAX 212-473-6272, orders@springer-ny.com, http://www.springer-ny.com. R&P Ian Gross. Adv. contact Jay Feinman. **N. American subscr. to:** Journal Fulfillment Services, PO Box 2485, Secaucus, NJ 07096-2485. TEL 800-777-4643, FAX 201-348-4505. **Co-sponsors:** Cardiovascular and Interventional Radiological Society of Europe; Japanese Society of Angiography and Interventional Radiology.

▼ **CARDIOVASCULAR RADIATION MEDICINE.** see *MEDICAL SCIENCES—Cardiovascular Diseases*

615.84 CZE ISSN 1210-7883
CODEN: CRADEK
CESKA RADIOLOGIE. Text in Czech, Slovak; Summaries in Czech, English. 1946. 6/yr. EUR 84, USD 108 (effective 2001). adv. bk.rev. *Refereed.* **Document type:** *Academic/Scholarly.*
Former titles: Ceskoslovenska Radiologie (0069-2344); Ceskoslovenska Roentgenologie
Indexed: Curr.Adv.Ecol.Sci., Dent.Ind., Excerp.Med., INIS Atomind., Ind.Med. (coverage dropped).
—CISTI, GNLM, Infotrieve. **CCC.**
Published by: (Ceska Lekarska Spolecnost J.E. Purkyne/Czech Medical Association), Nakladatelske Stredisko C L S J.E. Purkyne, Sokolska 31, Prague 12026, Czech Republic. TEL 420-2-24911420, FAX 420-2-24911420, nts@iol.cz, http://www.clsjep.cz, http://www.medical.cz. Ed. Dr. J Kolar. adv.: B&W page CZK 25,100, color page CZK 35,000; 245 x 167. Circ: 1,200. **Dist. by:** Abont s.r.o., Chlumova 17, Prague, 3 130 00, Czech Republic; **Dist. in Western countries by:** Kubon & Sagner, Hesstr 39-41, Munich 80798, Germany.

CHEMICAL SOCIETY OF JAPAN. SYMPOSIUM ON PHYSICAL AND CHEMICAL ASPECTS OF ULTRASOUND. PROCEEDINGS/ONPA NO BUSSEI TO KAGAKU TORONKAI KOEN RONBUNSHU. see *CHEMISTRY*

616.075 JPN ISSN 0287-0592
CHOONPA IGAKU/JAPANESE JOURNAL OF MEDICAL ULTRASONICS. Text in English, Japanese; Summaries in English. 1974. m. JPY 2,060 per issue. *Refereed.* **Document type:** *Academic/Scholarly.*
Indexed: Excerp.Med.
—EMDOCS, GNLM, Infotrieve. **CCC.**
Published by: Nihon Choonpa Igakkai/Japan Society of Ultrasonic Medicine, Hongo 3-23-1, Crosevia Hongo 3F, Bunkyo-ku, Tokyo 113, Japan. TEL 81-3-3813-5540, FAX 81-3-3816-7644. Ed. Kouichi Itoh. adv.: page JPY 400,000. Circ: 15,000.

616.075 JPN
CHOONPA KENSA GIJUTSU/JAPAN SOCIETY OF SONOGRAPHERS. JOURNAL. Text in Japanese. 1976. q.
Published by: Nihon Choonpa Igau Kensa Kenkyukai/Japan Society of Sonographers, Mitsui Kinen Byoin Chuo Kensabu, 1 Kanda-Izumi-cho, Chiyoda-ku, Tokyo 101-0024, Japan.

616.842 USA
CLINICAL DIAGNOSTIC IMAGING SERIES. Text in English. 1988. irreg. price varies. **Document type:** *Monographic series.*
Published by: Lippincott Williams & Wilkins (Philadelphia) (Subsidiary of: Wolters Kluwer N.V.), 530 Walnut St, Philadelphia, PA 19106-3621. TEL 301-223-2300, 800-638-3030, FAX 301-223-2400.

615.8 USA ISSN 0899-7071
RC78.7.T6 CODEN: CLIMEB
CLINICAL IMAGING. Text in English. 1977. bi-m. EUR 210 in Europe to individuals; JPY 27,900 in Japan to individuals; USD 235 elsewhere to individuals; EUR 635 in Europe to institutions; JPY 84,300 in Japan to institutions; USD 711 elsewhere to institutions (effective 2002). adv. bk.rev. abstr, charts, illus. index. back issues avail.; reprint service avail. from ISI. *Refereed.* **Document type:** *Academic/Scholarly.* **Description:** Provides information for radiologists, radiology residents, and radiologic technologists. Covers new technology, new applications, and important issues concerning all diagnostic imaging methods.
Former titles: C T: The Journal of Computed Tomography (0149-936X); Journal of Computed Tomography; Computed Axial Tomography (0145-7616)
Related titles: Microform ed.: (from PQC); Online - full text ed.: (from ingenta, Swets Blackwell, ScienceDirect, Institute for Scientific Information).
Indexed: ASCA, Biol.Abstr., Comput.Cont., Curr.Cont., Excerp.Med., INIS Atomind., Ind.Imag.Lit., Ind.Med. (1989-), Ind.Sci.Rev., Inpharma, Neurosci.Cit.Ind., Reac., Sci.Cit.Ind.
—BLDSC (3286.290600), CISTI, Ei, EMDOCS, GNLM, IDS, ingenta, KNAW. **CCC.**
Published by: Elsevier Science, 655 Ave of the Americas, New York, NY 10010. TEL 212-989-5800, 212-633-3686, FAX 212-633-3820, usinfo-f@elsevier.com, http://www.elsevier.com/locate/clinimag. Ed. Dr. Joseph P Whalen. Adv. contact Georgia Nikolaros. B&W page USD 985, color page USD 2,075. Circ: 2,200. **Subscr. in Australasia and the Far East to:** Elsevier Science (Singapore) Pte Ltd, No.1 Temasek Ave, 17-01 Millenia Tower, Singapore 039192, Singapore. TEL 65-434-3727, FAX 65-337-2230; **Subscr. in Japan to:** Elsevier Science Inc - Japan Regional Office, 9-15 Higashi-Azabu 1-chome, Minato-ku, Tokyo 106-0044, Japan. TEL 81-3-5561-5033, FAX 81-3-5561-5047; **Subscr. outside the Americas to:** Elsevier Science BV, PO Box 211, Amsterdam 1000 AE, Netherlands. TEL 31-20-485-3757, FAX 31-20-485-3432, nlinfo-f@elsevier.nl, http://www.elsevier.nl.

616.842 GBR ISSN 0961-9275
CLINICAL M R I; the practical journal of M R, incorporating Developments in M R. (Magnetic Resonance Imaging) Variant title: Clinical Magnetic Resonance Imaging. Text in English. 1991. q. GBP 50 domestic; USD 75 foreign; GBP 30 to MRRA members (effective 2000). adv. charts, illus. back issues avail. *Refereed.* **Document type:** *Academic/Scholarly.* **Description:** Describes the practice of medical Magnetic Resonance Imaging (MRI), as well as developments and advances in MRI.
Incorporates (1994-1996): Developments in Magnetic Resonance (1369-9504)
—BLDSC (3286.306500).
Published by: (Magnetic Resonance Radiologist's Association), Clinical Press, Redland Green Farm, Redland, Bristol BS6 7HF, United Kingdom. TEL 44-117-942-0256, kay.angell@ubht.swest.nhs.uk. Ed. Dr. Simon Blease. R&P Dr. Paul Goddard. Adv. contact Clive Booth. B&W page GBP 1,050, color page GBP 1,650. Circ: 2,500.

M

615.842 USA ISSN 0363-9762
R895.A1 CODEN: CNMEDK
CLINICAL NUCLEAR MEDICINE. Text in English. 1976. m. USD 229 domestic to individuals; USD 299 foreign to individuals; USD 400 domestic to institutions; USD 464 foreign to institutions; USD 36 newsstand/cover (effective 2002). adv. illus. index. *Refereed.* **Document type:** *Journal, Academic/Scholarly.* **Description:** Provides the most practical clinical information available in the field of nuclear medicine with original manuscripts covering all aspects of scanning and imaging.
Related titles: Microform ed.: (from PQC); Online - full text ed.: USD 520 domestic academic site license; USD 584 foreign academic site license; USD 580 domestic corporate site license; USD 644 foreign corporate site license (effective 2002) (from Ovid Technologies, Inc., Institute for Scientific Information).
Indexed: ASCA, Biol.Abstr., Curr.Adv.Cancer Res., Curr.Cont., Dairy Sci.Abstr., Dent.Ind., Excerp.Med. (1993-), INIS Atomind., Ind.Imag.Lit., Ind.Med. (1976-), Ind.Sci.Rev., Inpharma, Neurosci.Cit.Ind., Pharm.&Out.News, Protozool.Abstr., Reac., Rev.Med.& Vet.Mycol., SSCI (coverage dropped), Sci.Cit.Ind.
—BLDSC (3286.314000), CISTI, EMDOCS, GNLM, IDS, ingenta, KNAW.
Published by: Lippincott Williams & Wilkins (Philadelphia) (Subsidiary of: Wolters Kluwer N.V.), 530 Walnut St, Philadelphia, PA 19106-3621. TEL 215-521-8300, FAX 215-521-8902, http://www.Lww.com. Ed. Dr. Sheldon Baum. Pub. Karen Phillips. R&P Margaret Becker. Adv. contact Ray Thibodeau. B&W page USD 800, color page USD 1,860; trim 11 x 8.13. Circ: 2,221. **Subscr. to:** PO Box 1600, Hagerstown, MD 21740-1600. TEL 800-777-2295, FAX 301-824-7390.

615.842 616.99 GBR ISSN 0009-9260
CODEN: CLRAAG
CLINICAL RADIOLOGY. Text in English. 1949. m. GBP 84, GBP 338 to individuals (effective 2002). adv. bk.rev. index, cum.index: 1970-1979. back issues avail. *Refereed.* **Document type:** *Academic/Scholarly.* **Description:** Features original research, editorials, review articles and case reports on all aspects of diagnostic imaging, including: radiography, nuclear medicine, computed tomography, magnetic resonance imaging, ultrasonography, digital radiology and interventional radiology.
Related titles: Microform ed.: (from PQC); Online - full text ed.: (from EBSCO Publishing, O C L C Online Computer Library Center, Inc., Swets Blackwell, IDEAL Online Library, Institute for Scientific Information).
Indexed: ASCA, Biol.Abstr., C.I.S. Abstr., Cal.Tiss.Abstr., Curr.Adv.Cancer Res., Curr.Adv.Ecol.Sci., Curr.Cont., Dent.Ind., Environ.Sci.Poll.Mgmt., Excerp.Med., Helminthol.Abstr., INIS Atomind., Ind.Imag.Lit., Ind.Med. (1960-), Ind.Sci.Rev., Inpharma, Int.Abstr.Biol.Sci., Neurosci.Cit.Ind., Pharm.&Out.News, Pollut.Abstr., Reac., Ref.Zh., Rev.Med.& Vet.Mycol., Risk Abstr., SSCI (coverage dropped), Saf.Sci.Abstr., Sci.Cit.Ind., Tox.Abstr.
—BLDSC (3286.350000), CISTI, EMDOCS, GNLM, IDS, ingenta, KNAW. **CCC.**
Published by: (Royal College of Radiologists), W.B. Saunders Co. Ltd. (Subsidiary of: Harcourt Publishers Ltd.), 24-28 Oval Rd, London NW1 7DX, United Kingdom. TEL 44-20-7424-4200, FAX 44-20-7424-4515, cservice@harcourt.com, http://www.harcourt-international.com/journals/crad. Ed. A Dixon. Pub. Allen Stevens. R&P Sarah Pollard. Adv. contact Martine Cariou Keen. Circ: 4,505. **Subscr. to:** Harcourt Publishers Ltd., Foots Cray High St, Sidcup, Kent DA14 5HP, United Kingdom. TEL 44-20-8308-5700, FAX 44-20-8309-0807.

616.07 534 USA ISSN 0193-743X
CLINICS IN DIAGNOSTIC ULTRASOUND✶. Text in English. 1979. irreg., latest vol.30. **Document type:** *Monographic series, Academic/Scholarly.*
—CISTI, GNLM, Infotrieve, KNAW. **CCC.**
Published by: Churchill Livingstone (Subsidiary of: Harcourt Health Sciences), 15 E 26th St, Fl 15, New York, NY 10010-1505. TEL 212-206-5040, FAX 212-727-7808, http://www.churchillmed.com.

COMPUTERIZED MEDICAL IMAGING AND GRAPHICS; the international journal on imaging and image archiving in all medical specialties. see *MEDICAL SCIENCES—Computer Applications*

538.36 USA ISSN 1043-7347
QC762 CODEN: CMAEEM
CONCEPTS IN MAGNETIC RESONANCE; an educational quarterly. Text in English. 1989. bi-m. USD 699 in United States; USD 759 in Canada & Mexico; USD 809 elsewhere; USD 734 combined subscription in United States for print and online eds.; USD 794 combined subscription in Canada & Mexico for print and online eds.; USD 844 combined subscription elsewhere for print and online eds. (effective 2002). adv. bk.rev. charts. index, cum.index every 5 yrs. back issues avail. *Refereed.* **Document type:** *Academic/Scholarly.* **Description:** Consolidates the principle and practice of magnetic resonance for practitioners, and provides a forum for researchers to discuss fundamental aspects of magnetic resonance that relate to their research but are commonly not included in research papers.
Related titles: Online - full text ed.: ISSN 1099-0534. USD 699 in United States; USD 699 in Canada & Mexico; USD 699 elsewhere (effective 2002) (from EBSCO Publishing, Wiley InterScience, Institute for Scientific Information).
Indexed: ASCA, Anal.Abstr., Aqua.Sci.& Fish.Abstr., Chem.Abstr., Chem.Cit.Ind., Chem.Indus.Notes, Chem.Titles, Curr.Cont.
—BLDSC (3399.413400), CASDDS, CISTI, Ei, IDS, ingenta.
Published by: John Wiley & Sons, Inc., Journals (Subsidiary of: Wiley InterScience), 605 Third Ave, New York, NY 10158. TEL 212-850-6645, FAX 212-850-6021, subinfo@jwiley.com, uscs-wis@wiley.com, http://www.wiley.co.uk, http://www.wiley.com. Ed. Daniel D Traficante. adv.: B&W page GBP 640, color page GBP 1,515; trim 210 x 279. Circ: 750. **Subscr. to:** John Wiley & Sons Ltd., Baffins Ln, Chichester, Sussex PO19 IUD, United Kingdom. TEL 44-1243-779777, FAX 44-1243-843232, cs-journals@wiley.co.uk.

616.07 USA ISSN 0149-9009
CODEN: CDRAEW
CONTEMPORARY DIAGNOSTIC RADIOLOGY. Text in English. 1977. bi-w., latest vol.24. USD 315 domestic to individuals; USD 315 foreign to individuals; USD 315 domestic to institutions; USD 315 per issue foreign to institutions; USD 18 newsstand/cover (effective 2002). **Document type:** *Newsletter, Academic/Scholarly.* **Description:** Features original articles on current topics in radiology with optional Category or C.M.E. credits.
Related titles: Microfilm ed.: (from WWS); Online - full text ed.: USD 409.50 domestic for academic site license; USD 409.50 foreign for academic site license; USD 456.75 domestic for corporate site license; USD 456.75 foreign for corporate site license (effective 2002).
Published by: Lippincott Williams & Wilkins (Baltimore) (Subsidiary of: Wolters Kluwer N.V.), 351 W Camden St, Baltimore, MD 21201-2436. TEL 410-528-4000, 800-787-8981, FAX 410-528-4105, custserv@wwilkins.cm, custerv@lww.com, http://www.wwilkins.com, http://www.Lww.com. Ed. Robert E Campell. Circ: 2,800.

615.842 USA ISSN 0266-0601
CONTEMPORARY ISSUES IN COMPUTED TOMOGRAPHY✶. Text in English. 1983. irreg., latest vol.14. **Document type:** *Monographic series.*
Published by: Churchill Livingstone (Subsidiary of: Harcourt Health Sciences), 15 E 26th St, Fl 15, New York, NY 10010-1505. TEL 212-206-5040, FAX 212-727-7808, http://www.churchillmed.com.

615.842 USA ISSN 1040-8371
RC78.A1 CODEN: CRDIDF
CRITICAL REVIEWS IN DIAGNOSTIC IMAGING. Text in English. 1970. bi-m. USD 495 (effective 1998). bibl, charts, illus. back issues avail. *Refereed.* **Description:** Includes critical surveys of specific topics contributed by authors. Each author provides a review of the most significant papers from the current literature and the latest technology being used.
Former titles: C R C Critical Reviews in Diagnostic Imaging (0147-6750); C R C Critical Reviews in Clinical Radiology and Nuclear Medicine (0091-6536); C R C Critical Reviews in Radiological Sciences and Nuclear Medicine (0007-9014)
Related titles: Online - full text ed.: (from O C L C Online Computer Library Center, Inc., Swets Blackwell, ScienceDirect, Institute for Scientific Information).
Indexed: ASCA, Biol.Abstr., Curr.Cont., INIS Atomind., Ind.Med. (1980-), Ind.Sci.Rev., Inpharma, Int.Abstr.Biol.Sci., Reac., Rev.Med.& Vet.Mycol., Sci.Cit.Ind.
—BLDSC (3487.474000), CISTI, EMDOCS, GNLM, IDS, Infotrieve, ingenta, KNAW. **CCC.**
Published by: C R C Press, LLC, 2000 Corporate Blvd, N W, Boca Raton, FL 33431. TEL 561-994-0555, 800-272-7737, FAX 561-998-9784. Ed. Yen Wang. Circ: 340.

CURRENT MEDICAL LITERATURE. CARDIAC IMAGING MONITOR. see *MEDICAL SCIENCES—Abstracting, Bibliographies, Statistics*

CURRENT MEDICAL LITERATURE. MEDICAL IMAGING. see *MEDICAL SCIENCES—Abstracting, Bibliographies, Statistics*

615.842 USA ISSN 0363-0188
CODEN: CPDRDS
CURRENT PROBLEMS IN DIAGNOSTIC RADIOLOGY. Short title: C P D R. Text in English. 1972. bi-m. USD 88 domestic to individuals; USD 99 foreign to individuals; USD 142 domestic to institutions; USD 159 foreign to institutions; USD 46, USD 55 domestic to students; USD 27 per issue domestic (effective 2001). bibl, illus. cum.index. **Document type:** *Monographic series.* **Description:** Provides monographic clinical reviews written by and intended for practitioners.
Formerly: Current Problems in Radiology (0045-9399)
Related titles: Microform ed.: (from PQC).
Indexed: Biol.Abstr., Excerp.Med., INIS Atomind., Ind.Med. (1976-).
—BLDSC (3501.380000), CISTI, EMDOCS, GNLM, ingenta, KNAW. **CCC.**
Published by: Mosby, Inc. (Subsidiary of: Elsevier Science), 11830 Westline Industrial Dr, St Louis, MO 63146-3318. TEL 314-872-8370, 800-325-4177, FAX 314-432-1380, http://www.mosby.com/periodicals. Ed. Theodore E Keats. Circ: 1,030.

615.842 USA ISSN 1068-3879
CURRENT TECHNIQUES IN INTERVENTIONAL RADIOLOGY. Text in English. 1994. a. **Document type:** *Monographic series, Academic/Scholarly.* **Description:** Publishes articles on applied interventional radiology.
—CISTI, KNAW.
Published by: Current Medicine, 400 Market St, Ste 700, Philadelphia, PA 19106. TEL 215-574-2257, 800-427-1796, FAX 215-574-2225. Ed. Elizabeth Howard. **Subscr. outside N. America to:** Current Science Ltd, Middlesex House, 34-42 Cleveland St, London W1P 6LB, United Kingdom. TEL 44-20-7323-0323.

615.842 GBR
CURRENT TOPICS IN RADIOGRAPHY. Text in English. 1995. irreg. **Document type:** *Monographic series.*
—BLDSC (3504.911500).
Published by: W.B. Saunders Co. Ltd. (Subsidiary of: Harcourt Publishers Ltd.), 24-28 Oval Rd, London NW1 7DX, United Kingdom. TEL 44-20-7267-4466, FAX 44-20-7482-2293, http://www.hbuk.co.uk/hb/cat/. Eds. Audrey Paterson, Richard Price.

615.8 JPN ISSN 0914-8663
DANSO EIZO KENKYUKAI ZASSHI/JAPANESE JOURNAL OF TOMOGRAPHY. Text in Japanese; Summaries in English. 1973. a.
Indexed: INIS Atomind.
Published by: Danso Eizo Kenkyukai/Japanese Association of Tomography, Fukushima Kenritsu Ika Daigaku Hoshasenka, 1 Hiharigaoka, Fukushima-shi, Fukushima-ken 960-12, Japan.

616.07 USA ISSN 1043-1012
DECISIONS IN IMAGING ECONOMICS. Text in English. 1988. bi-m. **Document type:** *Trade.* **Description:** Concerns medical radiology and treatment through the use of nuclear medicine.
Formerly (until 1989): Decisions in Technology Economics (0898-6096)
Related titles: Online - full text ed.
Published by: Curant Communications, Inc. (Subsidiary of: Medical World Communications), 6701 Center Drive W #450, Los Angeles, CA 90045-1556. TEL 310-306-2206, FAX 310-306-9548. Ed. Cheryl Proual. Circ: 28,000.

615.842 USA ISSN 0349-490X
DENTO-MAXILLO-FACIAL RADIOLOGY. SUPPLEMENT. Text in English. irreg., latest vol.7. USD 10. **Document type:** *Proceedings, Monographic series, Academic/Scholarly.*
Related titles: ♦ Supplement to: Dentomaxillofacial Radiology. ISSN 0250-832X.
Published by: International Association of Dento-Maxillo-Facial Radiology, c/o Stuart E White, University of California, School of Dentistry, Los Angeles, CA 90024.

615.842 GBR ISSN 0250-832X
DENTOMAXILLOFACIAL RADIOLOGY. Text in English. 1971. 6/yr. GBP 102 in Europe to individuals for print or online ed.; USD 153 elsewhere to individuals for print or online ed.; GBP 112 combined subscription in Europe to individuals print & online; USD 168 combined subscription elsewhere to individuals print & online; GBP 252 in Europe to institutions for print or online ed.; USD 378 elsewhere to institutions for print or online ed.; GBP 277 combined subscription in Europe to institutions print & online; USD 416 combined subscription elsewhere to institutions print & online (effective 2002). adv. charts, illus, stat. back issues avail.; reprints avail. *Refereed.* **Document type:** *Journal, Academic/Scholarly.* **Description:** Contains research papers on radiology of the "lower third," together with clinical reports that illustrate specific uses of diagnostic imaging.
Related titles: Microform ed.: (from PQC); Online - full text ed.: (from EBSCO Publishing, O C L C Online Computer Library Center, Inc., RoweCom Information Quest, ingenta, Swets Blackwell, Institute for Scientific Information); ♦ Supplement: Dento-Maxillo-Facial Radiology. Supplement. ISSN 0349-490X.
Indexed: ASCA, Curr.Cont., INIS Atomind., Inpharma, Reac.
—BLDSC (3553.561000), GNLM, IDS, ingenta. **CCC.**
Published by: (International Association of Dento-Maxillo-Facial Radiology), Nature Publishing Group Specialist Journals (Subsidiary of: Holtzbrink Publishers), Houndmills, Basingstoke, Hants RG21 6XS, United Kingdom. TEL 44-1256-329242, FAX 44-1256-328339, subscriptions@nature.com, http://www.nature.com/dmfr. Ed. P N Hirschmann. Pub. Katy Christamanou. R&P Trace Noel. Adv. contact Robert Sloan TEL 44-20-8882-7199.

615.849 NLD ISSN 0167-9074
CODEN: DNMDDS
DEVELOPMENTS IN NUCLEAR MEDICINE. Text in English. 1981. irreg., latest vol.18, 1991. price varies. *Refereed.* **Document type:** *Monographic series.*
Indexed: Chem.Abstr., Chem.Indus.Notes, Chem.Titles.
—BLDSC (3579.085430), CASDDS, CISTI, Infotrieve, KNAW. **CCC.**
Published by: Kluwer Academic Publishers Group (Subsidiary of: Wolters Kluwer N.V.), Spuiboulevard 50, PO Box 17, Dordrecht 3300 AA, Netherlands. FAX 31-78-639-2254, services@wkap.nl, http://www.wkap.nl. **Dist. by:** Journals Department, PO Box 322, Dordrecht 3300 AH, Netherlands. FAX 31-78-654-6474.

616.0754 USA ISSN 0194-2514
RC78.7.D53
DIAGNOSTIC IMAGING. Text in English. 1979. m. USD 95; free to qualified personnel (effective 2001). adv. bk.rev. back issues avail.; reprint service avail. from PQC. **Document type:** *Journal, Trade.* **Description:** Designed for professionals in the field of radiology, nuclear medicine, and ultrasound imaging.
Related titles: Microform ed.: (from PQC); Online - full text ed.: (from ProQuest Information & Learning, Factiva).
Indexed: Dent.Ind., Ind.Sci.Rev.
—BLDSC (3579.658050), CISTI, GNLM, KNAW. **CCC.**
Published by: Miller Freeman, Inc. (Subsidiary of: United Newspapers), 600 Harrison St, San Francisco, CA 94107. TEL 415-905-2200, FAX 415-905-2233, diedit@mfi.com, http://www.dimag.com/. Ed. Peter Ogle. Pub. Sally Shankland. Circ: 31,200 (controlled). **Subscr. to:** PO Box 1064, Skokie, IL 60076-8064.

616.0754 USA
DIAGNOSTIC IMAGING AMERICA LATINA. Text in English. 2/yr. USD 40.
Published by: Miller Freeman, Inc. (Subsidiary of: United Newspapers), 600 Harrison St, San Francisco, CA 94107. TEL 415-905-2226, FAX 415-905-4967.

615.842 USA
DIAGNOSTIC IMAGING & RADIOLOGY PRODUCT COMPARISON SYSTEM. Variant title: Healthcare Product Comparison System: Diagnostic Imaging and Radiology Edition. Text in English. m. USD 1,027.40 domestic; USD 1,075.40 in Canada; USD 1,145 elsewhere (effective 2002). *Refereed.* **Description:** Covers hospital-based or freestanding radiology facilities, from MRI units to ultrasonic scanners and cardiac catheterization systems.
Related titles: CD-ROM ed.
Published by: (Emergency Care Research Institute), E C R I, 5200 Butler Pike, Plymouth, PA 19462. TEL 610-825-6000, FAX 610-834-1275, info@ecri.org, http://www.ecri.org. Ed. Nanette Bross.

616.0754 USA
DIAGNOSTIC IMAGING ASIA PACIFIC. Text in English. 4/yr. USD 65.
Published by: Miller Freeman, Inc. (Subsidiary of: United Newspapers), 600 Harrison St, San Francisco, CA 94107. TEL 415-905-2226, FAX 415-905-4967. **Subscr. to:** 100 Beach Rd, Ste 26 00, Shaw Towers, Singapore 189702, Singapore.

616.0754 USA
DIAGNOSTIC IMAGING EUROPE. Text in English. 1985. 8/yr. USD 65 in Europe; USD 120 elsewhere. **Document type:** *Trade.*
Formerly: Diagnostic Imaging International (0898-2473)
—GNLM. **CCC.**
Published by: Miller Freeman, Inc. (Subsidiary of: United Newspapers), 600 Harrison St, San Francisco, CA 94107. TEL 415-905-2200, FAX 415-905-2233. Ed. Philip Ward. Circ: 9,000.

616.075 GBR ISSN 1362-1920
DIAGNOSTIC IMAGING REVIEW. Text in English. 1996. q. free to qualified personnel. **Description:** The aim is to provide independent and impartial advice to inform purchasing decisions and encourage the safe use of medical devices based on technical assessments and when appropriate, comments from users.
—BLDSC (3579.658600).
Published by: Medical Devices Agency, Medical Devices Agency, Hannibal House, Elephant & Castle, Rm 1207, London SE1 6TQ, United Kingdom. TEL 44-20-7972-8181, FAX 44-20-7972-8105, dep@medical-devices.gov.uk, http://www.medical-devices.gov.uk. Ed. Paul Brunning.

615.842 539.2 EGY ISSN 1110-0303
EGYPTIAN JOURNAL OF RADIATION SCIENCES & APPLICATIONS. Text in Arabic, English. 1984. 2/yr. USD 77 (effective 2000). charts, illus, stat. reprint service avail. from IRC. **Document type:** *Academic/Scholarly.*
Indexed: INIS Atomind.
Published by: (National Centre for Radiation Research & Technology), National Information and Documentation Centre (NIDOC), Tahrir St., Dokki, Awqaf P.O., Cairo, Egypt. TEL 20-2-3371696. Ed. A Z El Behay. Circ: 1,000.

616.07 ITA ISSN 1121-8800
EIDO ELECTA; Mediterranean journal of radiology and imaging. Text in English, Italian; Summaries in English, French, Italian. 1989. q. ITL 80,000, USD 150 (effective 1999). **Description:** Covers radiotherapy, radiobiology, and nuclear medicine.
Published by: Casa Editrice Idelson, Via Annibale De Gasperis, 55, Naples, NA 80137, Italy. TEL 39-81-5524733, FAX 39-81-5518295, idelgno@tin.it, http://www.idelson-gnocchi.com. Ed. Elio Adelfio Cardinale.

616.07 JPN ISSN 0389-214X
EIZO JOHO MEDIKARU/IMAGE TECHNOLOGY & INFORMATION DISPLAY, MEDICAL. Text in Japanese; Summaries in English, Japanese. 1969. m. JPY 21,800. **Document type:** *Academic/Scholarly.* **Description:** Covers diagnostic imaging in medicine.
Indexed: INIS Atomind., Ref.Zh.
Published by: Sangyo Kaihatsu Kiko K.K., 1-1 Kanda-Izumi-cho, Chiyoda-ku, Tokyo 101-0024, Japan. TEL 03-3861-7051, FAX 03-5687-7744. Ed. Tsuneyoshi Sakamaki. Pub. Hiroshi Wakebe. Circ: 15,000.

616.842 DEU ISSN 1070-3004
CODEN: EMRAFG
EMERGENCY RADIOLOGY; a journal of practical imaging. Text in German. 1988. bi-m. EUR 230.50 domestic; EUR 225.40 in Germany; EUR 43 newsstand/cover foreign (effective 2002). adv. bk.rev. *Refereed.* **Document type:** *Journal, Academic/Scholarly.* **Description:** Original articles for radiologists and emergency medicine physicians treating acutely ill and injured patients. Articles deal with "first contact" decisions that need to be made immediately to optimize diagnostic accuracy and patient outcome. Emphasizes plain film procedures, but includes all imaging modalities.
Related titles: Microfiche ed.; Microfilm ed.: (from WWS); Online - full text ed.: ISSN 1438-1435 (from EBSCO Publishing, RoweCom Information Quest, Swets Blackwell, Springer LINK).
Indexed: Excerp.Med. (1995-).
—BLDSC (3733.197500), CISTI, GNLM, KNAW.
Published by: (American Society of Emergency Radiology USA), Springer-Verlag (Subsidiary of: BertelsmannSpringer), Tiergartenstr 17, Heidelberg 69121, Germany. TEL 49-6221-345-0, FAX 49-6221-345229, subscriptions@springer.de, http://link.springer.de/link/service/journals/10140/index.htm, http://www.springer.de. Ed. Dr. Theodore E Keats. Pub. Timothy Grayson. Adv. contact Aliza Rossman. B&W page USD 590; trim 10.88 x 8.13. Circ: 1,329 (paid). **Subscr. to:** Springer-Verlag New York Inc., PO Box 2485, Secaucus, NJ 07096-2485.

616.07 616.3 FRA ISSN 0246-0610
ENCYCLOPEDIE MEDICO-CHIRURGICALE. TRAITE DE RADIODIAGNOSTIC: APPAREIL DIGESTIF. Key Title: Encyclopedie Medico-Chirurgicale. Radiodiagnostic: Tome 4. Cover title: Traite de Radiodiagnostic: Appareil Digestif. Variant title: Enclyclopedie Medico-Chirurgicale. Radiodiagnostic, Tome 4: Tube Digestif, Foie, Rate, Pancreas. Encyclopedie Medico-Chirurgicale, Instantanes Medicaux, Radiodiagnostic: Tome 4. Text in French. 1954. 4 base vols. plus q. updates. bibl, charts, illus. *Refereed.* **Document type:** *Academic/Scholarly.* **Description:** Offers radiologists and gastroenterologists using radiologic techniques to diagnose gastroenterological disorders and diseases an up-to-date, comprehensive reference.
Published by: Elsevier Paris, Editions Scientifiques et Medicales (Subsidiary of: Reed Elsevier plc. group), 23 rue Linois, Paris 75015, France. TEL 33-1-45589110, FAX 33-1-45589425, redaction-emc@elsevier.fr, redacion-emc@elsevier.fr, http://www.elsevier.fr, http://www.elsevier.com.

616.07 616.2 FRA ISSN 1169-7768
ENCYCLOPEDIE MEDICO-CHIRURGICALE. TRAITE DE RADIODIAGNOSTIC: COEUR - POUMON. Key Title: Encyclopedie Medico-Chirurgicale. Radiodiagnostic. Tome 3: Coeur, Poumon. Cover title: Traite de Radiodiagnostic: Coeur - Poumon. Variant title: Encyclopedie Medico-Chirurgicale, Instantanes Medicaux. Coeur, Poumon, Larynx. Text in French. 1950. 4 base vols. plus q. updates. bibl, charts, illus. *Refereed.* **Document type:** *Academic/Scholarly.* **Description:** Offers radiologists, cardiologists, and pulmonary specialists a comprehensive, up-to-date reference for diagnosing and treating various diseases and disorders.
Former titles (until 1991): Encyclopedie Medico-Chirurgicale. Radiodiagnostic: Tome 3, Appareil Cardio-vasculaire, Appareil Pulmonaire (0246-0602); (until 1977): Encyclopedie Medico-Chirurgicale. Radiodiagnostic: Tome 3, Appareil Cardio-vasculaire, Appareil Respiratoire, Larynx (0246-1013)
Published by: Elsevier Paris, Editions Scientifiques et Medicales (Subsidiary of: Reed Elsevier plc. group), 23 rue Linois, Paris 75015, France. TEL 33-1-45589110, FAX 33-1-45589425, redaction-emc@elsevier.fr, redacion-emc@elsevier.fr, http://www.elsevier.fr, http://www.elsevier.com.

616.07 FRA
ENCYCLOPEDIE MEDICO-CHIRURGICALE. TRAITE DE RADIODIAGNOSTIC: PRINCIPES ET TECHNIQUES. Cover title: Traite de Radiodiagnostic: Principes et Techniques. Text in French. base vol. plus a. updates. bibl, charts, illus. *Refereed.* **Document type:** *Academic/Scholarly.* **Description:** Offers radiologists a comprehensive reference on principles and techniques in their field.
Published by: Elsevier Paris, Editions Scientifiques et Medicales (Subsidiary of: Reed Elsevier plc. group), 23 rue Linois, Paris 75015, France. TEL 33-1-45589110, FAX 33-1-45589425, redaction-emc@elsevier.fr, redacion-emc@elsevier.fr, http://www.elsevier.fr, http://www.elsevier.com.

616.07 FRA ISSN 1257-5143
ENCYCLOPEDIE MEDICO-CHIRURGICALE. TRAITE DE RADIODIAGNOSTIC: SQUELETTE NORMAL - NEURORADIOLOGIE - APPAREIL LOCOMOTEUR. Key Title: Encyclopedie Medico-Chirurgicale. Radiodiagnostic, 1-2. Cover title: Traite de Radiodiagnostic: Squelette Normal - Neuroradiologie - Appareil Locomoteur. Text in French. 1976. 4 base vols. plus q. updates. bibl, charts, illus. *Refereed.* **Document type:** *Academic/Scholarly.* **Description:** Provides radiologists, neuroradiologists, rheumatologists, and orthopedists with a comprehensive, up-to-date reference to diagnose disorders in their areas of specialty.

M

Former titles (until 1994): Encyclopedie Medico-Chirurgicale. Radiodiagnostic, Tomes 1 et 2: Squelette Normal, Neuroradiologie, Appareil Locomoteur (1246-9602); (until 1991): Encyclopedie Medico-Chirurgicale. Tomes 1 et 2: Neuroradiologie, Appareil Locomoteur (1155-1933); (until 1990): Encyclopedie Medico-Chirurgicale. Radiodiagnostic, Tomes 1 et 2, Squelette, Neuro-radiologie (0246-0599); Which was formed by the merger of (1956-1976): Encyclopedie Medico-Chirurgicale. Radiodiagnostic, Tome 1: Squelette Normal (0246-0998); (1953-1976): Encyclopedie Medico-Chirurgicale. Radiodiagnostic, Tome 2: Squelette Pathologique, Encephale, Moelle (0246-1005)

Published by: Elsevier Paris, Editions Scientifiques et Medicales (Subsidiary of: Reed Elsevier plc. group), 23 rue Linois, Paris 75015, France. TEL 33-1-45589110, FAX 33-1-45589425, redaction-emc@elsevier.fr, redacion-emc@elsevier.fr, http://www.elsevier.fr, http://www.elsevier.com.

616.07 616.6 618.1 FRA ISSN 1241-8218

ENCYCLOPEDIE MEDICO-CHIRURGICALE. TRAITE DE RADIODIAGNOSTIC: UROLOGIE - GYNECOLOGIE. Key Title: Encyclopedie Medico-Chirurgicale. Radiodiagnostic, 5: Urologie - Gynecologie. Cover title: Traite de Radiodiagnostic: Urologie - Gynecologie. Text in French. 1963. 3 base vols. plus q. updates. bibl, charts, illus. *Refereed.* **Document type:** *Academic/Scholarly.* **Description:** Offers radiologists, as well as urologists and gynecologists using radiology a comprehensive, up-to-date reference for diagnosing various disorders.

Former titles (until 1991): Encyclopedie Medico-Chirurgicale. Radiodiagnostic, 5: Appareil Urinaire - Appareil Genital (1154-2926); (until 1987): Encyclopedie Medico-Chirurgicale. Radiodiagnostic, Tome 5: Appareil Genito-urinaire-obstetrique (1154-2918); (until 1983): Encyclopedie Medico-Chirurgicale. Radiodiagnostic, Tome 5: Urologie, Gynecologie (0246-0629); (until 1977): Encyclopedie Medico-Chirurgicale. Radiodiagnostic, Tome 5: Appareil Genito-urinaire, Obstetrique (0246-1021)

Published by: Elsevier Paris, Editions Scientifiques et Medicales (Subsidiary of: Reed Elsevier plc. group), 23 rue Linois, Paris 75015, France. TEL 33-1-44589110, FAX 33-1-44589425, redaction-emc@elsevier.fr, redacion-emc@elsevier.fr, http://www.elsevier.fr, http://www.elsevier.com.

▼ **EUROPEAN JOURNAL OF ECHOCARDIOGRAPHY.** see *MEDICAL SCIENCES—Cardiovascular Diseases*

618 619 DEU CODEN: EJNMD9

EUROPEAN JOURNAL OF NUCLEAR MEDICINE AND MOLECULAR IMAGING. Text in English. 1976. m. EUR 1,035.90 domestic; EUR 1,016.70 in Germany; EUR 167 newsstand/cover foreign (effective 2002). reprint service avail. from ISI. *Refereed.* **Document type:** *Journal, Academic/Scholarly.* **Description:** Covers developments in nuclear medicine, including original articles on diagnosis, therapy with 'open' radionuclides, in-vitro radiobiological and radiation protection.

Formerly (until 2002): European Journal of Nuclear Medicine (0340-6997)

Related titles: Microfiche ed.: (from PQC); Online - full text ed.: (from EBSCO Publishing, RoweCom Information Quest, Swets Blackwell, Springer LINK, Institute for Scientific Information).

Indexed: ASCA, Chem.Abstr., Chem.Indus.Notes, Chem.Titles, Curr.Adv.Cancer Res., Curr.Adv.Ecol.Sci., Curr.Cont., Excerp.Med., INIS Atomind., INSPEC (1979-Dec.1993, dropped), Ind.Med. (1976-), Ind.Sci.Rev., Inpharma, Int.Nurs.Ind., Kidney, Neurosci.Cit.Ind., Pharm.&Out.News, Reac., Ref.Zh., Rev.Med.& Vet.Mycol., Sci.Cit.Ind.

—BLDSC (3829.731800), ADONIS, AskIEEE, CASDDS, CISTI, EMDOCS, GNLM, IDS, ingenta. **CCC.**

Published by: (European Association of Nuclear Medicine), Springer-Verlag (Subsidiary of: BertelsmannSpringer), Tiergartenstr 17, Heidelberg 69121, Germany. TEL 49-6221-345-0, FAX 49-6221-345229, subscriptions@springer.de, http://link.springer.de/link/service/journals/00259/index.htm, http://www.springer.de. Ed. P J Ell. **Subscr. in N. America to:** Springer-Verlag New York Inc., PO Box 2485, Secaucus, NJ 07096-2485. TEL 212-460-1500, FAX 212-473-6272.

615.842 IRL ISSN 0720-048X CODEN: EJRADR

EUROPEAN JOURNAL OF RADIOLOGY. Text in English. 1980. m. EUR 119 in Europe to individuals; JPY 15,600 in Japan to individuals; USD 132 elsewhere to individuals; EUR 1,057 in Europe to institutions; JPY 140,400 in Japan to institutions; USD 1,182 elsewhere to institutions (effective 2002). adv. bk.rev. charts, illus. index. back issues avail.; reprint service avail. from PQC. *Refereed.* **Document type:** *Academic/Scholarly.* **Description:** Serves as a medium for the exchange of information on the use of radiological and allied imaging and interventional techniques, including information on socio-economics and departmental management.

Incorporates (1987-1989): Journal of Medical Imaging (0920-5497)

Related titles: Online - full text ed.: (from ingenta, Swets Blackwell, ScienceDirect, Institute for Scientific Information).

Indexed: ASCA, Bioeng.Abstr., Chem.Abstr., Curr.Cont., Dent.Ind., Eng.Ind., Environ.Eng.Abstr., Environ.Sci.Poll.Mgmt., Excerp.Med., INIS Atomind., Ind.Imag.Lit., Ind.Med. (1981-), Inpharma, Int.Abstr.Biol.Sci., Pharm.&Out.News, Reac., Rev.Med.& Vet.Mycol.

—BLDSC (3829.738050), CASDDS, CISTI, Ei, EMDOCS, GNLM, IDS, Infotrieve, ingenta, KNAW. **CCC.**

Published by: (Netherlands Society of Radiology), Elsevier Science Ireland Ltd, Elsevier House, Brookvale Plaza, E. Park, Shannon, Co. Clare, Ireland. TEL 353-61-471944, FAX 353-61-472144, http://www.elsevier.com/locate/ejrad. Ed. H Imhof. R&P Annette Moloney. Circ: 1,500. **Subscr. in Australasia and the Far East to:** Elsevier Science (Singapore) Pte Ltd, No.1 Temasek Ave, 17-01 Millenia Tower, Singapore 039192, Singapore. TEL 65-434-3727, FAX 65-337-2230; **Subscr. in the Americas to:** Elsevier Science, PO Box 945, New York, NY 10159-0945. TEL 212-633-3730, FAX 212-633-3680, usinfo-f@elsevier.com; **Subscr. to:** Elsevier Science BV, PO Box 211, Amsterdam 1000 AE, Netherlands. TEL 31-20-485-3757.

616.075 IRL ISSN 0929-8266
R857.U48 CODEN: EJULE8

EUROPEAN JOURNAL OF ULTRASOUND. Text in English. 1994. bi-m. EUR 413 in Europe to institutions; JPY 54,800 in Japan to institutions; USD 242 elsewhere to institutions (effective 2002). bk.rev. back issues avail. *Refereed.* **Document type:** *Academic/Scholarly.* **Description:** Serves as a forum for the European scientific and clinical community working with ultrasound in the fields of medicine and biology.

Related titles: Online - full text ed.: (from ingenta, Swets Blackwell, ScienceDirect).

Indexed: Bioeng.Abstr., Eng.Ind., Excerp.Med. (1995-), Ind.Med. (1994-), Int.Nurs.Ind.

—BLDSC (3829.747200), CISTI, Ei, GNLM, Infotrieve. **CCC.**

Published by: (European Federation of Societies for Ultrasound in Medicine and Biology), Elsevier Science Ireland Ltd, Elsevier House, Brookvale Plaza, E. Park, Shannon, Co. Clare, Ireland. TEL 353-61-471944, FAX 353-61-472144, http://www.elsevier.com/locate/ejultrasou. Ed. J M Thijssen. R&P Annette Moloney. **Subscr. in Australasia and the Far East to:** Elsevier Science (Singapore) Pte Ltd, No.1 Temasek Ave, 17-01 Millenia Tower, Singapore 039192, Singapore. TEL 65-434-3727, FAX 65-337-2230; **Subscr. in the Americas to:** Elsevier Science, PO Box 945, New York, NY 10159-0945. TEL 212-633-3730, FAX 212-633-3680, usinfo-f@elsevier.com; **Subscr. to:** Elsevier Science BV, PO Box 211, Amsterdam 1000 AE, Netherlands. TEL 31-20-485-3757.

615.842 DEU ISSN 0938-7994 CODEN: EURAE3

EUROPEAN RADIOLOGY; journal of the European Congress of Radiology. Text in English. 1991. 12/yr. EUR 605.90 domestic; EUR 586.70 in Germany; EUR 56 newsstand/cover foreign (effective 2002). *Refereed.* **Document type:** *Journal, Academic/Scholarly.* **Description:** Covers all aspects of diagnostic and interventional radiology.

Incorporates (1989-1992): Diagnostic and Interventional Radiology (0998-433X)

Related titles: Online - full text ed.: ISSN 1432-1084 (from EBSCO Publishing, RoweCom Information Quest, Swets Blackwell, Springer LINK, Institute for Scientific Information).

Indexed: ASCA, Curr.Cont., INIS Atomind., Ind.Imag.Lit., Ind.Med. (1991-), Ind.Sci.Rev., Inpharma, Int.Nurs.Ind., Pharm.&Out.News, Reac., Ref.Zh., Rev.Med.& Vet.Mycol., Sci.Cit.Ind., Trop.Dis.Bull.

—BLDSC (3829.847300), CISTI, GNLM, IDS, Infotrieve, KNAW. **CCC.**

Published by: (European Association of Radiology), Springer-Verlag (Subsidiary of: BertelsmannSpringer), Tiergartenstr 17, Heidelberg 69121, Germany. TEL 49-6221-345-0, FAX 49-6221-345229, subscriptions@springer.de, http://link.springer.de/link/service/journals/00330/index.htm, http://www.springer.de. Ed. A L Baert. **Subscr. in N. America to:** Springer-Verlag New York Inc., PO Box 2485, Secaucus, NJ 07096-2485. TEL 212-460-1500, FAX 212-473-6272.

EXCERPTA MEDICA. SECTION 14: RADIOLOGY. see *MEDICAL SCIENCES—Abstracting, Bibliographies, Statistics*

EXCERPTA MEDICA. SECTION 23: NUCLEAR MEDICINE. see *MEDICAL SCIENCES—Abstracting, Bibliographies, Statistics*

616.842 JPN ISSN 0914-790X

FACIAL NERVE RESEARCH. Text in Multiple languages. 1981. a.

Indexed: INIS Atomind.

—GNLM.

Published by: Japan Society of Facial Nerve Research, Dept of Otorhinolaryngology, School of Medicine, Nihon University, 30-1 Kami-machi Oyaguchi, Itabashi-ku, Tokyo 173, Japan. TEL 03-972-8111. Ed. Jin Kanzaki.

615.8 FRA ISSN 0181-9801

FEUILLETS DE RADIOLOGIE. Text in French. 1961. 6/yr. FRF 900; FRF 1,114 foreign (effective 2000). reprint service avail. from PQC. **Document type:** *Academic/Scholarly.* **Description:** For help in the preparation of university examinations and the competitive exams of French radiology hospitals.

Related titles: Microform ed.: (from PQC); Online - full text ed.: (from RoweCom Information Quest).

Indexed: Excerp.Med., INIS Atomind.

—GNLM, Infotrieve. **CCC.**

Published by: Masson - Periodiques, 120 bd. St. Germain, Paris 75006, France. TEL 33-1-40466200, FAX 33-1-40466201. Eds. M Blery, V Bismuth. Circ: 4,000. **Subscr. to:** Societe de Periodiques Specialises, BP 22, Vineuil Cedex 41354, France. TEL 33-2-54504612, FAX 33-2-54504611.

615.842 USA ISSN 0722-7035

FRONTIERS IN EUROPEAN RADIOLOGY. Text in English. 1982. irreg., latest vol.9, 1993. price varies. reprint service avail. from ISI. **Document type:** *Academic/Scholarly.*

—CISTI, GNLM.

Published by: Springer-Verlag, Journals (Subsidiary of: BertelsmannSpringer), 175 Fifth Ave, New York, NY 10010. TEL 212-460-1500, FAX 212-473-6272.

615 616.9 CHE ISSN 0071-9676 CODEN: FRTOA7

FRONTIERS OF RADIATION THERAPY AND ONCOLOGY. Text in English. 1967. irreg., latest vol.37. CHF 230 in Europe; DEM 190 in Germany; USD 190 in United States (effective 2001). reprint service avail. from ISI. *Refereed.* **Document type:** *Journal, Academic/Scholarly.* **Description:** Covers developments in the treatment of cancer with radiation therapy.

Related titles: Online - full text ed.: (from Institute for Scientific Information).

Indexed: ASCA, Biol.Abstr., Chem.Abstr., Curr.Cont. (coverage dropped), Dent.Ind., INIS Atomind., Ind.Med. (coverage dropped).

—BLDSC (4042.060000), CASDDS, CISTI, ingenta, KNAW. **CCC.**

Published by: S. Karger AG, Allschwilerstr 10, PO Box, Basel 4009, Switzerland. TEL 41-61-306-1111, FAX 41-61-306-1234, karger@karger.ch, http://www.karger.com/bookseries/FRATO. Eds. J L Meyer, W Hinkelbein.

616.07 JPN

FUKUOKAKEN HOSHASEN GISHIKAISHI/FUKUOKA ASSOCIATION OF RADIOLOGICAL TECHNOLOGISTS. JOURNAL. Text in Japanese. bi-m.

Published by: Fukuokaken Hoshasen Gishika, Fukuoka-ken Kangoto Kenkyu Kenshu Senta, 14-5, Akasaka 1-chome, Fukuoka-shi, Fukuoka-ken 810, Japan.

616.07 615 JPN ISSN 0911-2855

GAIKOKU BUNKEN DAIJESUTO. KAKU IGAKU/FOREIGN LITERATURE DIGEST. NUCLEAR MEDICINE. Text in Japanese. 1971. bi-m.

Published by: Daiichi Rajio Aisotopu Kenkyujo/Daiichi Radioisotope Laboratories, Ltd., 19-8 Kyobashi 1-chome, Chuo-ku, Tokyo 104-0031, Japan.

M

615.842 NLD ISSN 0016-4380
CODEN: GAMMDV
GAMMA. Text in Dutch. 1950. m. NLG 136 to members (effective 2000). adv. bk.rev. illus. *Refereed.* **Document type:** *Trade.*
Indexed: Chem.Abstr., Chem.Indus.Notes, Chem.Titles.
—CASDDS, KNAW.
Published by: Nederlandse Vereniging van Radiologisch Laboranten, PO Box 19207, Utrecht 3501 DE, Netherlands. TEL 31-30-231-8842, FAX 31-30-232-1362, nvrl@wxs.nl, http://www.nvrl.nl. Ed. G J R Bos. Circ: 3,300; 3,300 (controlled).

616.0757 GEO ISSN 1512-0031
GEORGIAN JOURNAL OF RADIOLOGY. Text in Georgian. q. **Document type:** *Journal, Academic/Scholarly.*
Published by: Institute of Radiology and Interventional Diagnostics, 13 Tevdore Mgvdeli str, Tbilsi 380012, Georgia. TEL 995-32-940289, FAX 995-32-344923, radiag@access.sanet.ge.

615.842 ITA ISSN 1120-3846
GIORNALE ITALIANO DI ULTRASONOLOGIA. Text in Italian. 1990. 4/yr. ITL 120,000, USD 120 to individuals; GBP 170,000, USD 180 to institutions. adv. back issues avail.; reprints avail. **Document type:** *Academic/Scholarly.* **Description:** Disseminates the results of clinical research and stimulates scientific cooperation within the field.
Indexed: Excerp.Med. (1993-).
—EMDOCS, GNLM.
Published by: (Societa Italiana di Ultrasonologia in Medicina e Biologia), International University Press, Via Monte Delle Gioie, 22, Rome, RM 00199, Italy. TEL 39-6-86211027, FAX 39-6-86211026, univpres@tin.it. Eds. Luigi Buscarini, Tito Livraghi. R&P Giulio Bertolaccina TEL 39-6-86211028. Adv. contact Giulio Bertolaccini TEL 39-6-862110278. B&W page USD 2,800, color page USD 4,200; trim 280 x 210. Circ: 3,000.

616.07 CHN
GUOWAI YIXUE (FANGSHE YIXUE HEYIXUE FENCE)/FOREIGN MEDICAL SCIENCES (RADIOLOGY & NUCLEAR MEDICINE). Text in Chinese. bi-m. USD 20.40; USD 3.40 newsstand/cover (effective 2001). **Document type:** *Academic/Scholarly.*
Published by: China International Book Trading Corp/Zhongguo Guoji Tushu Maoyi Zonggongsi cibtc@mail.cibtc.com.cn, http://www.cibtc.com.cn. **Dist. by:** 35, Chegongzhuang Xilu, Haidian District, Beijing 100044, China.

615.842 CHN ISSN 1001-1021
GUOWAI YIXUE (LINCHUANG FANGSHEXUE FENCE)/FOREIGN MEDICAL SCIENCES (CLINICAL RADIOLOGY). Text in Chinese. 1978. bi-m.
Published by: Tianjin Fangshe Zhenliao Yanjiu Peixun Zhongxin, 123 Anshan Dao, Tianjin 300052, China. TEL 705960. Ed. Wu Enhui.

612.014 USA ISSN 0073-1498
HEALTH PHYSICS SOCIETY. NEWSLETTER. Text in English. 1959. m. membership. adv. **Document type:** *Newsletter.* **Description:** Alerts members to society events, news, and activities, both past and planned.
Indexed: INIS Atomind.
—BLDSC (4275.050070).
Published by: Health Physics Society, 1313 Dolley, Madison, VA 22101-3926. TEL 703-790-1745, FAX 703-790-2672, HPS@BurkInc.com. Ed. Genevieve S Roessler. Adv. contact Sharon Hebl. Circ: 7,000.

615.842 JPN
HOIKEN SHINPOJUMU SHIRIZU/N I R S SYMPOSIUM. PROCEEDINGS. Text in Japanese; Summaries in English. 1962. a. **Document type:** *Proceedings.*
Published by: Science and Technology Agency, National Institute of Radiological Sciences/Kagaku Gijutsucho Hoshasen Igaku Sogo Kenkyujo, 9-1 Anagawa 4-chome, Inage-ku, Chiba-shi 263-0024, Japan.

615.842 JPN ISSN 0912-0327
HOKKAIDO HOSHASEN GIJUTSU ZASSHI/JOURNAL OF HOKKAIDO RADIOLOGICAL TECHNOLOGY. Text in Japanese; Summaries in English. 1945. a. JPY 1,500 (effective 1998). adv. **Document type:** *Academic/Scholarly.*
Published by: Nihon Hoshasen Gijutsu Gakkai, Hokkaido Bukai/Japanese Society of Radiological Technology, Hokkaido Branch, 427-26, Nishi 29-chome, Kita 3-jo, Chuo-ku, Sapporo-shi, Hokkaido 060, Japan. TEL 81-11-643-2713, FAX 81-11-614-7918. Ed. Motomichi Sakata. Pub., R&P Tsutomu Kikuchi. Adv. contact Hiroshi Arai. Circ: 1,500 (controlled).

616.0757 NOR ISSN 0332-9410
HOLD PUSTEN. Text in Norwegian. 1974. 10/yr. NOK 260; NOK 290 foreign (effective 1998). adv. **Document type:** *Trade.*
—CCC.
Published by: Norsk Radiografforbund, Lakkegata 19-21, Oslo 0187, Norway. TEL 47-22-11-72-79, FAX 47-22-17-52-04, nordlid@online.no. Eds. Knut Nordlid, Per Zaring. R&P, Adv. contact Per Zarig. Circ: 1,493 (controlled).

615.842 JPN
HOSHANO CHOSA KENKYU HOKOKUSHO/NATIONAL INSTITUTE OF RADIOLOGICAL SCIENCES. SURVEY REPORT. Text in Japanese. a. **Document type:** *Government.*
Published by: Kagaku Gijutsucho, Hoshasen Igaku Sogo Kenkyujo/Science and Technology Agency, National Institute of Radiological Sciences, 9-1 Anagawa 4-chome, Inage-ku, Chiba-shi 263-0024, Japan. TEL 81-43-251-2111. Ed. Tohru Kawai.

616.07 JPN ISSN 0441-2540
CODEN: HOKAAN
HOSHASEN KAGAKU* /RADIOLOGICAL SCIENCES. Text in Japanese. 1958. m. JPY 550 per issue.
Indexed: INIS Atomind.
—CASDDS, CISTI.
Published by: Kagaku Gijutsucho, Hoshasen Igaku Sogo Kenkyujo/Science and Technology Agency, National Institute of Radiological Sciences, 1-3-1 Kasumigaseki, Chiyoda-ku, Tokyo 100-0013, Japan.

616.842 JPN
HOSHASEN RIYO KENKYUKAI HOKOKUSHO, IGAKU RIYO GURUPU/RESEARCH REPORT OF UTILIZATION OF RADIATION BY MEDICAL USER'S GROUP. Text in Japanese. a. JPY 7,000.
Published by: Nihon Genshiryoku Sangyo Kaigi/Japan Atomic Industrial Forum, Toshin Bldg, 1-1-13 Shinbashi, Minato-ku, Tokyo 105-8605, Japan. TEL 81-3-3508-2411, FAX 81-3-3508-2094, http://www.jaif.or.jp.

616.07 USA ISSN 1082-3654
QC785.5
I E E E NUCLEAR SCIENCE SYMPOSIUM AND MEDICAL IMAGING CONFERENCE. PROCEEDINGS. Text in English. 1991. a. USD 310. **Document type:** *Proceedings.*
Formerly (until 1992): I E E E Nuclear Science Symposium and Medical Imaging Conference (1078-8840)
Related titles: CD-ROM ed.
Indexed: Eng.Ind.
—BLDSC (4363.007600).
Published by: Institute of Electrical and Electronics Engineers, Inc., 3 Park Ave, 17th Fl, New York, NY 10017. TEL 800-678-4333, customer.service@ieee.org, http://www.ieee.org.

615.842 USA ISSN 0278-0062
RC78.A1 CODEN: ITMID4
I E E E TRANSACTIONS ON MEDICAL IMAGING. Text in English. 1982. m. USD 475 in North America for print or online ed.; USD 500 elsewhere for print or online ed. (effective 2002). *Refereed.* **Description:** Explores ultrasonics, x-ray imaging and tomography, image processing by computers, microwave and nuclear magnetic resonance imaging.
Related titles: CD-ROM ed.; Microfiche ed.; Online - full text ed.: (from EBSCO Publishing, Gale Group, Institute for Scientific Information).
Indexed: ASCA, Bioeng.Abstr., Biotech.& Bioeng.Abstr., Compumath, Comput.& Info.Sys., Curr.Cont., Eng.Ind., Ergon.Abstr., INIS Atomind., INSPEC (Jul.1982-), ISMEC, Ind.Med. (1982-), Ind.Sci.Rev., Inpharma, Neurosci.Cit.Ind., Reac., Ref.Zh., Sci.Cit.Ind.
—BLDSC (4363.204500), AskIEEE, CISTI, Ei, GNLM, IDS, Linda Hall. **CCC.**
Published by: Institute of Electrical and Electronics Engineers, Inc. TEL 800-701-4333, customer.service@ieee.org, subscription-service@ieee.org, http://www.ieee.org. Ed. Michael Vannier. **Subscr. to:** Maruzen Co. Ltd., 3-10 Nihonbashi 2-chome, Chuo-ku, Tokyo 103-0027, Japan. FAX 81-3-3275-0657; Universal Subscription Agency, Pvt. Ltd., 877, Udyog Vihar, V, Gurgoan 122001, India. TEL 91-124-347261, FAX 91-124-342496. **Co-sponsors:** I E E E Acoustics, Speech, and Signal Processing Society; Engineering in Medicine and Biology Society; Nuclear and Plasma Sciences Society; Ultrasonics, Ferroelectrics and Frequency Control Society.

616.842 JPN ISSN 0915-308X
IBARAKI KAKU IGAKU/IBARAKI JOURNAL OF NUCLEAR MEDICINE. Text in Japanese. 1989. s-a.
Published by: Ibarakiken Rinsho Kaku Igaku Kenkyukai/Ibaraki Association of Clinical Nuclear Medicine, Tsukuba Daigaku Fuzoku Byoin Kaku Igakushitsu, 1-1 Amakubo 2-chome, Tsukuba-shi, Ibaraki-ken 305-0005, Japan.

616.075 GBR ISSN 0965-6812
CODEN: IAGIEC
IMAGING; an international journal of clinico-radiological practice. Text in English. 1989. q. GBP 35 to members; GBP 195, USD 290 to institutions (effective 2002). **Document type:** *Academic/Scholarly.* **Description:** Provides the latest information on the integrated role of imaging modalities in diagnostic problem solving.
Formerly (until 1992): Current Imaging (0952-0619)
Indexed: Excerp.Med., Info.Media & Tech.
—BLDSC (4368.996447), EMDOCS, GNLM, Infotrieve, KNAW. **CCC.**
Published by: British Institute of Radiology, 36 Portland Pl, London W1B 1AT, United Kingdom. TEL 44-20-7307-1400, FAX 44-20-7307-1414, admin@bir.org.uk, http://imaging.birjournals.org, http://www.bir.org.uk. Ed. Philip Owen.

616.07 DEU ISSN 1433-3317
IMAGING DECISIONS M R I. Text in English. 1997. q. EUR 40 to institutions; EUR 15 newsstand/cover (effective 2001). *Refereed.* **Document type:** *Journal, Academic/Scholarly.*
Published by: Blackwell Wissenschafts Verlag GmbH, Kurfuerstendamm 57, Berlin 10707, Germany. TEL 49-30-32790635, FAX 49-30-32790610, abo@blackwis.de, http://www.blackwell.de. Eds. Dr. M Oudkerk, Dr. N Hosten.

615.842 AUS
IMAGING GUIDELINES. Text in English. irreg., latest vol.3, 1997. AUD 20 (effective 1999). **Document type:** *Trade.* **Description:** Assisting medical practitioners to make the best possible use of available imaging facilities.
Published by: Victorian Medical Postgraduate Foundation Inc., PO Box 27, Parkville, VIC 3052, Australia. TEL 61-3-9347-9633, FAX 61-3-9347-4547, vmpf@vicnet.net.au. Circ: 5,000.

INDIAN ACADEMY OF ORAL MEDICINE AND RADIOLOGY. JOURNAL. see *MEDICAL SCIENCES—Dentistry*

616.7 530 GBR
INSTITUTE OF PHYSICS AND ENGINEERING IN MEDICINE. REPORT. Text in English. 1986. irreg., latest 1996.
Former titles (until 1997): Institution of Physics and Engineering in Medicine and Biology. Report (1369-4073); (until Aug. 1996): Institute of Physical Sciences in Medicine. Report (0951-6514); (until Sep. 1995): Hospital Physicists' Association. Conference Report Series
—BLDSC, CISTI.
Published by: Institute of Physics and Engineering in Medicine., PO Box 303, York YO1 2WR, United Kingdom. TEL 44-1904-610821, FAX 44-1904-612279, office@ipem.org.uk.

613.6 GBR ISSN 0146-6453
RA1231.R2 CODEN: ANICD6
INTERNATIONAL COMMISSION ON RADIOLOGICAL PROTECTION. ANNALS. Key Title: Annals of the I C R P. Text in English. 1960. q. EUR 117 in Europe to individuals; JPY 15,500 in Japan to individuals; USD 130 elsewhere to individuals; EUR 271 in Europe to institutions; JPY 36,000 in Japan to institutions; USD 304 elsewhere to institutions (effective 2002). back issues avail. *Refereed.* **Document type:** *Academic/Scholarly.* **Description:** Covers topics in the field of radiation protection for members of the medical professions and other interested groups.
Formerly (until 1977): Advances in Radiological Protection
Related titles: Microfilm ed.: (from PQC); Online - full text ed.: (from ingenta, Swets Blackwell, ScienceDirect).
Indexed: AESIS, Abstr.Hyg., Biol.Abstr., C.I.S. Abstr., Curr.Adv.Ecol.Sci., Energy Ind., Energy Info.Abstr., Eng.Ind., Excerp.Med., INSPEC (1979-1980, dropped), Ind.Med. (1977-).
—BLDSC (4362.070000), CASDDS, CISTI, Ei, GNLM, Linda Hall. **CCC.**

M

Published by: (International Commission on Radiological Protection), Oxford University Press, Academic Division, Great Clarendon St, Oxford OX2 6DP, United Kingdom. http://www.elsevier.com/locate/icrp. **Subscr. in Australasia and the Far East to:** Elsevier Science (Singapore) Pte Ltd, No.1 Temasek Ave, 17-01 Millenia Tower, Singapore 039192, Singapore. TEL 65-434-3727, FAX 65-337-2230; **Subscr. in the Americas to:** Elsevier Science. TEL 212-633-3730, FAX 212-633-3680; **Subscr. to:** Elsevier Science BV. TEL 31-20-485-3757, FAX 31-20-485-3432.

615.84 612.014 FIN ISSN 0074-3933

INTERNATIONAL CONGRESS OF RADIOLOGY. (REPORTS). Text in Finnish. quadrennial, latest 18th, Singapore. **Document type:** *Proceedings.*

Indexed: Excerp.Med.

Published by: International Society of Radiology, c/o Prof Dr C G Standertskjoeld, Department of Radiology, Helsinki University Central Hospital, Helsinki 00290, Finland. FAX 0471-4404.

616.9897 614.4 UKR ISSN 1562-1154

▼ **INTERNATIONAL JOURNAL OF RADIATION MEDICINE/MEZHDUNARODNYI ZHURNAL RADIATSIONNOI MEDITSINYICINE.** Text in Ukrainian, Russian, English; Abstracts in English. 1999. q. UAK 20.38 domestic to individuals; RUR 620 in Russia & the CIS; USD 195 elsewhere to individuals; UAK 30.38 domestic to institutions; USD 240 elsewhere to institutions (effective 2001). bk.rev., film rev., software rev. bibl, illus. **Document type:** *Journal, Academic/Scholarly.* **Description:** Examines the mechanisms of radiation injuries development, the dose-effect relationship; assesses the risk of stochastic and deterministic effects as well as improvement of population protection against chronic internal and external irradiation (i.e. aftermath of Chernobyl accident).

Published by: (Physicians of Chernobyl), Morion LLC, a/c A-82, Kiev 01001, Ukraine. Ed., Pub. Angelina I Nyagu. Circ: 3,000 (controlled). **Subscr. to:** Physicians of Chernobyl. **Dist. by:** Physicians of Chernobyl, Kosiora ul 8, kv 49, Kiev 04135, Ukraine. TEL 380-44-2444734, FAX 380-44-4191951, kosti@morion.kiev.ua.

616.0757 USA ISSN 0360-3016
RC271.R3 CODEN: IOBPD3

INTERNATIONAL JOURNAL OF RADIATION: ONCOLOGY - BIOLOGY - PHYSICS. Text in English. 1976. 15/yr. EUR 2,539 in Europe to individuals; JPY 337,200 in Japan to individuals; USD 2,841 elsewhere to individuals; EUR 413 in Europe to institutions; JPY 54,900 in Japan to institutions; USD 462 elsewhere to institutions; EUR 43 in Europe to students; JPY 5,700 in Japan to students; USD 48 elsewhere to students (effective 2002). adv. back issues avail.; reprint service avail. from PQC. *Refereed.* **Document type:** *Journal, Academic/Scholarly.* **Description:** Provides an international forum for the latest work and developments in radiation oncology, with emphasis on the discipline's contribution to cancer management and research.

Related titles: Microfilm ed.: (from PQC); Online - full text ed.: (from ingenta, Swets Blackwell, ScienceDirect, Institute for Scientific Information); Supplement: Astro Meeting Supplement.

Indexed: ASCA, Abstr.Health Care Manage.Stud., Biol.Abstr., Biwk.Pap.Rad.Chem.& Photochem., Chem.Abstr., Chem.Indus.Notes, Chem.Titles, Curr.Adv.Cancer Res., Curr.Adv.Gen.& Molec.Biol., Curr.Cont., Dairy Sci.Abstr., Dent.Ind., Eng.Ind., Environ.Sci.Poll.Mgmt., Excerp.Med., Helminthol.Abstr., INIS Atomind., INSPEC (Nov.1976-), Ind.Imag.Lit., Ind.Med. (1975-), Ind.Sci.Rev., Ind.Vet., Inpharma, Int.Abstr.Biol.Sci., Int.Nurs.Ind., Med.& Surg.Dermat., Neurosci.Cit.Ind., Pollut.Abstr., Reac., Ref.Zh., Risk Abstr., SSCI (coverage dropped), Saf.Sci.Abstr., Sci.Cit.Ind., THA, Tox.Abstr.

—BLDSC (4542.523000), AskIEEE, CASDDS, CISTI, Ei, EMDOCS, GNLM, IDS, ingenta, KNAW. **CCC.**

Published by: Elsevier Science, 655 Ave of the Americas, New York, NY 10010. TEL 212-989-5800, FAX 212-633-3990, usinfo@elsevier.com, http://www.elsevier.com/locate/ijrobp. Eds. Dr. Philip Rubin, James D Cox. Adv. contact Georgia Nikolaros. B&W page USD 1,250, color page USD 2,565. Circ: 6,000 (paid). **Subscr. addr. in Asia and Australasia:** Elsevier Science (Singapore) Pte Ltd, No. 1 Temasek Ave, 17-01 Millenia Tower, Singapore 039192, Singapore. TEL 65-434-3727, FAX 65-337-2230, asiainfo@elsevier.com.sg; **Subscr. addr. in Europe, Middle East and Africa:** Elsevier Science BV, PO Box 211, Amsterdam 1000 AE, Netherlands. TEL 31-20-485-3757, FAX 31-20-485-3432, nlinfo-f@elsevier.nl, http://www.elsevier.nl; **Subscr. addr. in Japan:** Elsevier Science Inc - Japan Regional Office, 9-15 Higashi-Azabu 1-chome, Minato-ku, Tokyo 106-0044, Japan. TEL 81-3-5561-5033, FAX 81-3-5561-5047, info@elsevier.co.jp.

616.07 USA

▼ **THE INTERNET JOURNAL OF RADIOLOGY.** Text in English. 2000. s-a. free per issue. adv. bk.rev. back issues avail. *Refereed.* **Document type:** *Academic/Scholarly.* **Description:** Provides information from the field of radiology and nuclear medicine; contains original articles, reviews, case reports, streaming slide shows, streaming videos, letters to the editor, press releases, and meeting information.

Media: Online - full content.

Published by: Internet Scientific Publications, L.L.C., 23 Rippling Creek Dr, Sugar Land, TX 77479. TEL 281-240-1533, FAX 281-240-1533, http://www.ispub.com/. Ed. Richard Tello. R&P Hope Morrow TEL 832-754-0335.

616.075 GBR
CODEN: IRMOFA

INTERVENTION; commentary and analysis on progress in interventional radiology and endovascular technique. Text in English. 1997. q. GBP 50 in Europe; GBP 70 in US & Canada; GBP 75 elsewhere. **Document type:** *Academic/Scholarly.*

Formerly (until 1998): Interventional Radiology Monitor (1366-7130)

Published by: Remedica Publishing Ltd., 32-38 Osnaburgh St, London NW1 3ND, United Kingdom. TEL 44-171-388-7677, FAX 44-171-388-7678, info@remedica.com, http://www.remedica.com/irm/. Ed. Anthony Watkinson.

616.0757 ITA ISSN 1123-9344

INTERVENTIONAL NEURORADIOLOGY. Text in English. 1995. q. ITL 329,000 domestic; ITL 380,000 in Europe; ITL 445,000 elsewhere; ITL 80,000 per issue (effective 2001). adv. bk.rev. abstr. back issues avail. *Refereed.* **Document type:** *Academic/Scholarly.* **Description:** Examines peritherapeutic neuroradiology, surgical procedures, and related neurosciences.

Related titles: CD-ROM ed.; Diskette ed.; Fax ed.; Online - full text ed.: (from Institute for Scientific Information).

Indexed: Neurosci.Cit.Ind., Ref.Zh.

—BLDSC (4557.471854), CISTI, IDS, KNAW.

Published by: (Associazione Italiana di Neuroradiologian), Centauro SRL, Via Del Pratello, 8, Bologna, BO 40122, Italy. TEL 39-051-227634, FAX 39-051-220099, adriana.dallocca@centauro.it, http://www.centauro.it. Pub. Dr. Marco Leonardi. R&P Adriana Dall'Occa. Adv. contact Gerardo Dall'Occa. Circ: 1,800.

615.842 USA ISSN 1533-5364

▼ **THE INTERVENTIONALIST.** Text in English. 2001. bi-m. USD 83 domestic to individuals; USD 113 foreign to individuals; USD 116 domestic to institutions; USD 146 foreign to institutions (effective 2002). **Document type:** *Journal, Academic/Scholarly.*

Published by: (Society of Cardiovascular and Interventional Radiology), Lippincott Williams & Wilkins (Philadelphia) (Subsidiary of: Wolters Kluwer N.V.), 530 Walnut St, Philadelphia, PA 19106-3621. TEL 215-521-8300, FAX 215-521-8902, custserv@lww.com, http://www.lww.com/. **Subscr. to:** PO Box 1600, Hagerstown, MD 21740-1600. TEL 800-638-3030, FAX 310-223-2400.

615.842 USA ISSN 0020-9996
RC78 CODEN: INVRAV

INVESTIGATIVE RADIOLOGY. Text in English. 1966. m. USD 275 domestic to individuals; USD 367 foreign to individuals; USD 655 domestic to institutions; USD 785 foreign to institutions; USD 61 newsstand/cover (effective 2002). adv. illus. index. reprint service avail. from PQC. *Refereed.* **Document type:** *Academic/Scholarly.* **Description:** Devoted to the early publication of original reports of clinical and laboratory investigations in diagnostic imaging, the diagnostic use of radioactive isotopes, computed tomography, positron emission tomography, positron emission tomography, magnetic resonance imaging, ultrasound, digital substraction angiography and related modalities.

Related titles: Microform ed.: (from PQC); Online - full text ed.: USD 851.50 domestic academic site license; USD 981.50 foreign academic site license; USD 949.75 domestic corporate site license; USD 1,079.75 foreign corporate site license (2002) (from Ovid Technologies, Inc., Swets Blackwell, Institute for Scientific Information).

Indexed: ASCA, Agri.& Environ.Biotech.Abstr. (coverage dropped), Biol.Abstr., Chem.Abstr., Chem.Indus.Notes, Chem.Titles, Curr.Adv.Cancer Res., Curr.Cont., Derwent Biotech.Abstr., Excerp.Med., Hosp.Lit.Ind., INIS Atomind., Ind.Imag.Lit., Ind.Med. (1966-), Ind.Sci.Rev., Inpharma, Neurosci.Cit.Ind., Reac., SSCI (coverage dropped), Sci.Cit.Ind.

—BLDSC (4560.350000), CASDDS, CISTI, GNLM, IDS, ingenta, KNAW.

Published by: Lippincott Williams & Wilkins (Philadelphia) (Subsidiary of: Wolters Kluwer N.V.), 530 Walnut St, Philadelphia, PA 19106-3621. TEL 215-521-8300, FAX 215-521-8902, http://www.Lww.com. Ed. Dr. Val M Runge. Pub. Karen Phillips. R&P Margaret Becker. Adv. contact Ray Thibodeau. B&W page USD 880, color page USD 1,970; trim 11 x 8.13. Circ: 880. **Subscr. to:** PO Box 1600, Hagerstown, MD 21740-1600. TEL 800-777-2295, FAX 301-824-7390.

616.07 JPN ISSN 0917-3056

IRYO HOSHASEN BOGO NEWSLETTER/NEWSLETTER ON RADIOLOGICAL PROTECTION IN MEDICINE. Text in Japanese. 1991. 3/yr.

Published by: Iryo Hoshasen Bogo Renraku Kyogikai/Japan Association on Radiological Protection in Medicine, Nihon Aisotopu Kyokai, 28-45 Honkomagome 2-chome, Bunkyo-ku, Tokyo 113-0021, Japan.

615.842 EGY ISSN 0021-1907
CODEN: ISRRAC

ISOTOPE AND RADIATION RESEARCH. Text in English; Summaries in Arabic. 1968. s-a. USD 20. adv. bk.rev.

Indexed: Chem.Abstr., Chem.Indus.Notes, Chem.Titles, Excerp.Med. (until 1992), INIS Atomind., INSPEC (Jul.1987-), Soils & Fert.

—BLDSC (4583.325000), AskIEEE, CASDDS, CISTI.

Published by: Middle Eastern Regional Radioisotope Centre for the Arab Countries, Sh. Malaeb el Gamaa, Cairo 11321, Egypt. TELEX 2098-94381 PBDKIUN. Ed. M Mokhtar. Circ: 500.

615.842 ITA ISSN 0394-1574

ITALIAN CURRENT RADIOLOGY; trimestrale di tomografia computerizzata, ultrasuoni e nuove diagnostiche per immagini. Text in Italian. 1982. q. ITL 90,000, USD 150 (effective 1999).

—BLDSC (4588.332800), EMDOCS.

Published by: Casa Editrice Idelson, Via Annibale De Gasperis, 55, Naples, NA 80137, Italy. TEL 39-81-5524733, FAX 39-81-5518295, idelgno@tin.it, http://www.idelson-gnocchi.com. Ed. Enrico Del Vecchio. Circ: 4,000.

615 JPN ISSN 0910-1543

IYO GAZO JOHO GAKKAI ZASSHI/JAPANESE JOURNAL OF MEDICAL IMAGING AND INFORMATION SCIENCES. Text in English, Japanese; Summaries in English. 3/yr.

Published by: Iyo Gazo Joho Gakkai/Japan Society of Medical Imaging and Information Sciences, Kogei Sen i Daigaku, Kogeigakubu Denki Kogakka, Matsugasaki-Goshokaido-cho, Sakyo-ku, Kyoto-shi 606-0962, Japan.

IZOTOPTECHNIKA, DIAGNOSZTIKA/ISOTOPE TECHNICS, DIAGNOSTICS. see *CHEMISTRY*

615.842 BEL
CODEN: JBRAAN

J B R - B T R★. (Journal Belge de Radiologie - Belgisch Tijdschrift voor Radiologie) Text in Dutch, French; Summaries in Dutch, English, French, German. 1907. 6/yr. adv. charts, illus, stat. index.

M

Former titles (until 1999): Journal Belge de Radiologie (0302-7430); (until 1924): Journal de Radiologie (0302-7449); (until 1909): Journal Belge de Radiologie (0021-7646)
Indexed: Biol.Abstr., Chem.Abstr., Excerp.Med., Helminthol.Abstr., INIS Atomind., INSPEC (Jan.1973-1986, dropped), Ind.Med. (coverage dropped), Sci.Cit.Ind. (coverage dropped).
—BLDSC (4951.300000), CASDDS, CISTI, GNLM, KNAW.
Published by: Societe Royale Belge de Radiologie/Belgische Vereniging voor Radiologie, Route de Lennik 808, Brussels 1070, Belgium. TEL 32-2-5554273, FAX 32-2-5554545.

615.842 JPN
JIKI KYOMEI IGAKKAI PUROGURAMU/SOCIETY OF MAGNETIC RESONANCE IN MEDICINE. PROCEEDINGS OF ANNUAL CONFERENCE. Text in Japanese; Summaries in English. a.
Published by: Jiki Kyomei Igakkai, 465, Kajichiicho, Hirokoji Agaru, Kawaramachi Dori, Kamigyo-ku, Kyoto-shi 602, Japan.

615.842 JPN
JIKI KYOMEI TO IGAKU/MAGNETIC RESONANCE IN MEDICINE. Text in Japanese; Summaries in English. 1990. a. JPY 5,150.
Published by: Nihon Igakukan, 9-6-505 Otsuka 3-chome, Bunkyo-ku, Tokyo 112-0012, Japan. TEL 03-3942-7631, FAX 03-3942-2086. Ed. Toshiaki Kikuzawa.

615.842 FRA ISSN 0221-0363
JOURNAL DE RADIOLOGIE. Text in French; Summaries in English. 1914. m. FRF 1,701; FRF 2,205 foreign (effective 2000). adv. bk.rev. abstr, illus. index. reprint service avail. from ISI. *Refereed.* **Document type:** *Academic/Scholarly.* **Description:** Discusses radiodiagnosis and new methods of investigation. Reports on international congresses of radiology and on the section meetings of the society.
Formerly: Journal de Radiologie d'Electrologie et de Medecine Nucleaire (0021-7964)
Related titles: Microform ed.: (from PQC); Online - full text ed.: (from Institute for Scientific Information, RoweCom Information Quest).
Indexed: ASCA, Biol.Abstr., Chem.Abstr., Curr.Cont., Dent.Ind., Excerp.Med., Helminthol.Abstr., INIS Atomind., Ind.Med. (1979-), Inpharma, Int.Nurs.Ind., Reac., Rev.Med.& Vet.Mycol.
—BLDSC (5043.972000), CISTI, GNLM, IDS, KNAW, Linda Hall.
Published by: (Societe Francaise de Radiologie et Conseil des Enseignants en Radiologie de France), Masson - Periodiques, 120 bd. St. Germain, Paris 75006, France. TEL 33-1-40466200, FAX 33-1-40466201, s.mathot@masson.fr, http://www.e2med.com/display_journal.asp?journal=jr&population=im. Eds. J F Moreau, Y Menu. Circ: 5,000. **Subscr. to:** Societe de Periodiques Specialises, BP 22, Vineuil Cedex 41354, France. TEL 33-2-54504612, FAX 33-2-54504611.

616.842 FRA ISSN 0245-5552
CODEN: JEMUEF
JOURNAL D'ECHOGRAPHIE ET DE MEDECINE PAR ULTRASONS. Text in French. 1980. bi-m. FRF 905; FRF 1,085 foreign (effective 2000). **Document type:** *Academic/Scholarly.* **Description:** Publishes essentially practical articles dealing with the main fields of ultrasonic medicine.
Related titles: Microform ed.: (from PQC); Online - full text ed.: (from RoweCom Information Quest).
Indexed: Excerp.Med., INIS Atomind.
—EMDOCS, GNLM. **CCC.**
Published by: (Societe Francaise pour l'Application des Ultrasons a la Medecine et a la Biologie), Masson - Periodiques, 120 bd. St. Germain, Paris 75006, France. TEL 33-1-40466200, FAX 33-1-40466201, http://www.e2med.com/display_journal.asp?journal=jemu&population=im. Ed. J M de Bray. Circ: 2,000. **Subscr. to:** Societe de Periodiques Specialises, BP 22, Vineuil Cedex 41354, France. TEL 33-2-54504612, FAX 33-2-54504611.

617.05 USA ISSN 1044-5471
CODEN: JCLSEO
JOURNAL OF CLINICAL LASER MEDICINE & SURGERY. Text in English. 1983. bi-m. USD 177 domestic to individuals; USD 279 foreign to individuals; USD 212 domestic to individuals print and online eds. combined; USD 314 foreign to individuals print and online eds. combined; USD 376 domestic to institutions; USD 491 foreign to institutions; USD 451 domestic to institutions print and online eds. combined; USD 566 foreign to institutions print and online eds. combined (effective 2002). adv. back issues avail.; reprints avail. *Refereed.* **Document type:** *Journal, Academic/Scholarly.* **Description:** Covers advances and expanded applications and procedures, significant clinical and basic research in laser medicine, surgery and dentistry, safety programs and new instrumentation.
Formerly (until 1990): Laser Medicine and Surgery News (0736-9417)
Related titles: Online - full content ed.: USD 177 to individuals; USD 376 to institutions (effective 2002); Online - full text ed.: (from CatchWord Ltd., Institute for Scientific Information, RoweCom Information Quest).
Indexed: Bioeng.Abstr., Biotech.& Bioeng.Abstr., Curr.Cont., Eng.Ind., Excerp.Med. (1993-), Inpharma, Med.& Surg.Dermat., Pharm.&Out.News, Reac.
—BLDSC (4958.540000), CISTI, Ei, EMDOCS, GNLM, IDS, Infotrieve, KNAW. **CCC.**
Published by: (International Society for Laser Surgery and Medicine), Mary Ann Liebert, Inc. Publishers, 2 Madison Ave, Larchmont, NY 10538. TEL 914—834-3100, FAX 914-834-1388, info@liebertpub.com, http://www.liebertpub.com/lms. Ed. Dr. Raymond J Lanzafame. **Co-sponsor:** International Society for Lasers in Dentistry.

JOURNAL OF CLINICAL ONCOLOGY. see *MEDICAL SCIENCES—Oncology*

616.07 USA ISSN 0091-2751
RM862.7 CODEN: JCULDD
JOURNAL OF CLINICAL ULTRASOUND. Text in English. 1973. 9/yr. USD 815 in United States; USD 905 in Canada & Mexico; USD 981 elsewhere; USD 856 combined subscription in United States for print and online eds.; USD 946 combined subscription in Canada & Mexico for print and online eds.; USD 1,022 combined subscription elsewhere for print and online eds. (effective 2002). adv. bk.rev. abstr, charts, illus, stat. index. back issues avail.; reprint service avail. from PQC. *Refereed.* **Description:** Covers current uses of ultrasound in evaluating disorders affecting the central nervous system, fetus and placenta, gastrointestinal system, reproductive system, urinary system.
Related titles: Microform ed.: (from PQC); Online - full text ed.: ISSN 1097-0096. 1996. USD 815 in United States; USD 815 in Canada & Mexico; USD 815 elsewhere (effective 2002) (from EBSCO Publishing, Wiley InterScience, Institute for Scientific Information).
Indexed: ASCA, Acoust.Abstr., Bibl.Dev.Med.& Child Neur., Biol.Abstr., Curr.Adv.Cancer Res., Curr.Cont., Dent.Ind., Dok.Arbeitsmed., Excerp.Med., Helminthol.Abstr., INIS Atomind., INSPEC (Sep.1981-Dec.1985, dropped), Ind.Imag.Lit., Ind.Med. (1973-), Ind.Sci.Rev., Inpharma, Nutr.Abstr., Reac., Sci.Cit.Ind., Trop.Dis.Bull.
—BLDSC (4958.791000), CISTI, GNLM, IDS, ingenta, KNAW. **CCC.**
Published by: John Wiley & Sons, Inc., Journals (Subsidiary of: Wiley InterScience), 605 Third Ave, New York, NY 10158. TEL 212-850-6645, FAX 212-850-6021, subinfo@wiley.com, uscs-wis@wiley.com, http://www.wiley.com. Ed. Russell L Deter. adv.: B&W page GBP 640, color page GBP 1,515; trim 210 x 279. Circ: 3,100. **Subscr. outside the Americas to:** John Wiley & Sons Ltd., Baffins Ln, Chichester, Sussex PO19 IUD, United Kingdom. TEL 44-1243-779777, FAX 44-1243-843232, cs-journals@wiley.co.uk, http://www.wiley.co.uk.

615.842 USA ISSN 0363-8715
RC78.7.T6 CODEN: JCATD5
JOURNAL OF COMPUTER-ASSISTED TOMOGRAPHY; a radiological journal dedicated to the basic and clinical aspects of reconstructive tomography. Text in English. 1977. bi-m. USD 253 domestic to individuals; USD 313 foreign to individuals; USD 706 domestic to institutions; USD 706 foreign to institutions; USD 98 newsstand/cover (effective 2002). adv. bk.rev. index. back issues avail.; reprint service avail. from PQC. *Refereed.* **Document type:** *Academic/Scholarly.* **Description:** Articles and reports on technological advances in radiology.
Related titles: Microform ed.: (from PQC); Online - full text ed.: USD 917.80 domestic academic site license; USD 917.80 foreign academic site license; USD 1,023.70 domestic corporate site license; USD 1,023.70 foreign corporate site license (2002) (from Ovid Technologies, Inc., Swets Blackwell, Institute for Scientific Information).
Indexed: ASCA, Aqua.Sci.& Fish.Abstr., Bibl.Dev.Med.& Child Neur., Biol.Abstr., Cal.Tiss.Abstr., Curr.Cont., Dent.Ind., Excerp.Med., Helminthol.Abstr., INIS Atomind., INSPEC (Dec.1980-), Ind.Imag.Lit., Ind.Med. (1977-), Ind.Sci.Rev., Inpharma, Int.Abstr.Biol.Sci., Kidney, Neurosci.Cit.Ind., Nutr.Abstr., Protozool.Abstr., Reac., Rev.Med.& Vet.Mycol., SSCI (coverage dropped), Sci.Cit.Ind., Trop.Dis.Bull.
—BLDSC (4963.650000), AskIEEE, CISTI, EMDOCS, GNLM, IDS, ingenta, KNAW.
Published by: Lippincott Williams & Wilkins (Philadelphia) (Subsidiary of: Wolters Kluwer N.V.), 530 Walnut St, Philadelphia, PA 19106-3621. TEL 215-521-8300, FAX 215-521-8902, http://www.lww.com. Ed. Dr. Allen D Elster. Pub. Karen Phillips. R&P Margaret Becker. Adv. contact Ray Thibodeau. B&W page USD 1,150, color page USD 2,255. Circ: 3,650. **Subscr. to:** PO Box 1600, Hagerstown, MD 21740-1600. TEL 800-777-2295, FAX 301-824-7390.

616.07 USA ISSN 8756-4793
JOURNAL OF DIAGNOSTIC MEDICAL SONOGRAPHY. Text in English. 1985. bi-m. USD 270 domestic; USD 303 elsewhere (effective 2002). adv. illus. index. 56 p./no. back issues avail.; reprints avail. *Refereed.* **Document type:** *Journal, Academic/Scholarly.*
Related titles: Microform ed.; Online - full text ed.: (from ingenta, RoweCom Information Quest).
Indexed: CINAHL, Excerp.Med.
—CISTI, EMDOCS, GNLM, KNAW.
Published by: (Society of Diagnostic Medical Sonographers), Sage Publications, Inc., Sage Science Press, 2455 Teller Rd, Thousand Oaks, CA 91320. TEL 805-499-0721, FAX 805-499-0871, info@sagepub.com, http://www.sagesciencepress.com/. Ed. Jean Lea Spitz. Pub. Susan Hanscom. R&P Peter Marino. Adv. contact Diane Diamond TEL 215-675-9133. B&W page USD 1,486, color page USD 2,814; trim 8.125 x 11. Circ: 12,268.

616.075705 GBR ISSN 1460-4728
JOURNAL OF DIAGNOSTIC RADIOGRAPHY AND IMAGING. Text in English. 1998. q. GBP 60 in Europe to individuals; GBP 63 rest of world to individuals; GBP 110 in Europe to institutions; GBP 113 rest of world to institutions (effective 2000). *Refereed.* **Document type:** *Academic/Scholarly.* **Description:** Covers all of the current modalities used in diagnostic imaging. Publishes quality research from a wide range of styles and encourage debate and the exchange of information and opinion from within the field of diagnostic medical radiography.
—BLDSC (4969.430000).
Published by: Greenwich Medical Media, 137 Euston Rd, London NW1 2AA, United Kingdom. TEL 44-20-7388-5444, FAX 44-20-7383-5445, gm@greenwich-medical.co.uk, http://www.greenwich-medical.co.uk/. Eds. Martin J Benwell, Suzanne M Henwood. Pub. Gavin Jamieson.

616.842 DEU ISSN 0897-1889
CODEN: JDIMEW
JOURNAL OF DIGITAL IMAGING. Text in English. 1988 (Nov.). q. USD 413.10 domestic; USD 417.40 foreign (effective 2002). adv. index. back issues avail. *Refereed.* **Document type:** *Journal, Academic/Scholarly.* **Description:** Presents the practicing radiologist with information to enhance in the understanding, selection, and use of computer applications in everyday practice.
Related titles: Online - full text ed.: ISSN 1618-727X (from Institute for Scientific Information).
Indexed: ASCA, Bioeng.Abstr., Biotech.& Bioeng.Abstr., CINAHL, Curr.Cont., Eng.Ind., INSPEC, Ind.Imag.Lit., Ind.Med. (1988-), Inpharma, Int.Nurs.Ind., Reac., Sci.Cit.Ind.
—BLDSC (4969.610000), Ei, GNLM, IDS, KNAW. **CCC.**
Published by: (Society for Computer Applications in Radiology USA), Springer-Verlag (Subsidiary of: BertelsmannSpringer), Tiergartenstr 17, Heidelberg 69121, Germany. TEL 49-6221-345-0, FAX 49-6221-345229, subscriptions@springer.de, http://www.springer.de. Ed. S. C. Horii. adv.: B&W page USD 710, color page USD 1,810; trim 10 x 7. Circ: 1,527.

616.07 FRA ISSN 1269-1704
JOURNAL OF MAGNETIC RESONANCE ANALYSIS; applications in food science, toxicology, clinical biology, pharmacology, environmental science. Text in English. bi-m.

M

Published by: Baseline S.A.R.L., 11 rue de Brest, BP 3927, Rennes Cedex 35039, France. Eds. Gerard Martin, Jacques D de Certaines. Pub. G Pope.

616.07 USA ISSN 1053-1807
CODEN: JMRIFR

JOURNAL OF MAGNETIC RESONANCE IMAGING. Short title: J M R I. Text in English. 1990. bi-m. USD 1,040 in United States; USD 1,040 in Canada & Mexico; USD 1,184 elsewhere; USD 1,092 combined subscription in United States for print and online eds.; USD 1,092 combined subscription in Canada & Mexico for print and online eds.; USD 1,236 combined subscription elsewhere for print and online eds. (effective 2002). adv. *Refereed.* **Document type:** *Academic/Scholarly.* **Description:** Focuses on research in techniques and equipment, and clinical applications of the noninvasive diagnostic procedure.

Related titles: Online - full text ed.: ISSN 1522-2586. USD 1,040 in United States; USD 1,040 in Canada & Mexico; USD 1,040 elsewhere (effective 2002) (from National Library of Medicine, EBSCO Publishing, Wiley InterScience, Institute for Scientific Information).

Indexed: ASCA, Curr.Cont., Ind.Imag.Lit., Ind.Med. (1991-), Inpharma, Neurosci.Abstr. (coverage dropped), Neurosci.Cit.Ind., Reac.

—BLDSC (5010.791000), CISTI, GNLM, ingenta, KNAW.

Published by: (International Society for Magnetic Resonance in Medicine), John Wiley & Sons, Inc., Journals (Subsidiary of: Wiley InterScience), 605 Third Ave, New York, NY 10158. TEL 212-850-6645, FAX 212-850-6021, subinfo@wiley.com, uscs-wis@wiley.com, http://www.interscience.wiley.com/jpages/1053-1807/, http://www.wiley.com. Ed. Gary D Fullerton. adv.: B&W page USD 980; trim 10.88 x 8.13. Circ: 3,149; 2,974 (paid). **Subscr. outside the Americas to:** John Wiley & Sons Ltd., Baffins Ln, Chichester, Sussex PO19 IUD, United Kingdom. TEL 44-1243-779777, FAX 44-1243-843232, cs-journals@wiley.co.uk, http://www.wiley.co.uk.

616.07 HKG ISSN 0929-6441
CODEN: JMEUEV

JOURNAL OF MEDICAL ULTRASOUND. Text in English. 1993. q. USD 30; USD 60 foreign. **Document type:** *Academic/Scholarly.* **Description:** Covers basic, experimental, and clinical sciences in the use of medical ultrasound. Includes original articles, case reports, brief communications, review articles, association news and announcements of meetings.

Indexed: Excerp.Med. (1994-).

—BLDSC (5017.093000), EMDOCS.

Published by: (Society of Medical Ultrasound), Excerpta Medica Asia Ltd., Eight Commercial Tower 19th Fl, 8 Sun Yip St, Chai Wan, Hong Kong, Hong Kong. TEL 852-2965-1300, FAX 852-2976-0778. R&P Sindy Fok TEL 852-2965-1366. Circ: 4,800.

JOURNAL OF NEUROIMAGING. see *MEDICAL SCIENCES—Psychiatry And Neurology*

615.842 FRA ISSN 0150-9861
CODEN: JNEUD3

JOURNAL OF NEURORADIOLOGY/JOURNAL DE NEURORADIOLOGIE. Text in English, French. 1974. 4/yr. FRF 1,289; FRF 1,570 foreign (effective 2000). adv. bk.rev. illus. reprint service avail. from ISI. *Refereed.* **Document type:** *Academic/Scholarly.* **Description:** Covers all subjects common to neurology, neurosurgery, and general radiology.

Formerly (until Mar. 1978): Journal de Neuroradiologie (0335-0800)

Related titles: Microform ed.: (from PQC); Online - full text ed.: (from Institute for Scientific Information, RoweCom Information Quest).

Indexed: ASCA, Bibl.Dev.Med.& Child Neur., Biol.Abstr., Curr.Cont., Excerp.Med., Ind.Med. (1976-), Inpharma, Neurosci.Cit.Ind., Reac.

—BLDSC (5022.072000), CISTI, GNLM, IDS, KNAW. **CCC.**

Published by: (Societe Francaise de Neuroradiologie), Masson - Periodiques, 120 bd. St. Germain, Paris 75006, France. TEL 33-1-40466200, FAX 33-1-40466201, s.mathot@masson.fr, http://www.e2med.com/display_journal.asp?journal=jn&population=im. Ed. L Picard. Circ: 1,000. **Subscr. to:** Societe de Periodiques Specialises, BP 22, Vineuil Cedex 41354, France. TEL 33-2-54504612, FAX 33-2-54504611.

616.1 USA ISSN 1071-3581
CODEN: JNCAE2

JOURNAL OF NUCLEAR CARDIOLOGY. Text in English. 1994. bi-m. USD 134 domestic to individuals; USD 167 foreign to individuals; USD 188 domestic to institutions; USD 221 foreign to institutions; USD 68 domestic to students; USD 101 foreign to students; USD 37 newsstand/cover (effective 2001). adv. Supplement avail. *Refereed.* **Document type:** *Journal, Academic/Scholarly.* **Description:** Addresses all aspects of nuclear cardiology, including interpretation, diagnosis, radiopharmaceuticals, and imaging equipment. Keeps readers up-to-date on legislative and regulatory issues, as well as forthcoming events, activities and continuing education.

Related titles: Online - full text ed.: (from IDEAL Online Library, Institute for Scientific Information, RoweCom Information Quest).

Indexed: ASCA, Curr.Cont., Excerp.Med. (1995-), Ind.Med. (1994-), Ind.Sci.Rev., Inpharma, Pharm.&Out.News, Reac., Sci.Cit.Ind.

—BLDSC (5022.870000), CISTI, EMDOCS, GNLM, IDS, Infotrieve, KNAW. **CCC.**

Published by: (American Society of Nuclear Cardiology (ASNC)), Mosby, Inc. (Subsidiary of: Elsevier Science), 11830 Westline Industrial Dr, St Louis, MO 63146-3318. TEL 314-872-8370, 800-325-4177, FAX 314-432-1380, http://www.mosby.com/nuclcard, http://www.mosby.com/periodicals. Ed. Dr. Barry L Zaret. Pub. Jane Grochowski. Adv. contact Tracey Schriefer TEL 314-453-4304. B&W page USD 1,090, color page USD 2,040; trim 10.88 x 8.25. Circ: 6,728.

615.842 USA ISSN 0161-5505
RM845 CODEN: JNMEAQ

THE JOURNAL OF NUCLEAR MEDICINE. Text in English. 1960. m. USD 170 domestic to individuals; USD 180 in Canada to individuals; USD 210 elsewhere to individuals; USD 260 domestic to institutions; USD 270 in Canada to institutions; USD 290 elsewhere to institutions (effective 2001). adv. bk.rev. abstr, bibl, charts, illus. index. back issues avail.; reprint service avail. from PQC. *Refereed.* **Document type:** *Academic/Scholarly.* **Description:** Publishes papers in a wide range of areas in nuclear medicine and allied disciplines.

Incorporates: S N M Newsline; Former titles: J N M (0097-9031); Journal of Nuclear Medicine (0022-3123)

Related titles: Microform ed.: (from PQC); Online - full text ed.: J N M Online (from HighWire Pr., ProQuest Information & Learning, Institute for Scientific Information).

Indexed: ASCA, BBCI, Bibl.Asian Stud. (1971), Biol.Abstr., Chem.Abstr., Chem.Titles, Curr.Adv.Biochem., Curr.Adv.Cancer Res., Curr.Adv.Ecol.Sci., Curr.Cont., Dairy Sci.Abstr., Excerp.Med., Helminthol.Abstr., INIS Atomind., INSPEC (Dec.1968-, dropped), I.P.A., Ind.Imag.Lit., Ind.Med. (1960-), Ind.Sci.Rev., Ind.Vet., Inpharma, Kidney, Neurosci.Cit.Ind., Nutr.Abstr., Pharm.&Out.News, Protozool.Abstr., Reac., SSCI (coverage dropped), Sci.Cit.Ind., Vet.Bull.

—BLDSC (5023.300000), AskIEEE, CASDDS, CISTI, GNLM, IDS, Infotrieve, ingenta, KNAW. **CCC.**

Published by: Society of Nuclear Medicine, 1850 Samuel Morse Dr, Reston, VA 20190-5316. TEL 703-708-9000, FAX 703-708-9018, http://www.snmjournals.org/. Ed. Dr. Martin Sandler. R&P Melissa McKenna. Adv. contact Jennifer Zawacki. Circ: 14,000 (paid).

615.8 USA ISSN 0091-4916
R895.A1 CODEN: JNMTB4

JOURNAL OF NUCLEAR MEDICINE TECHNOLOGY. Text in English. 1973. q. USD 80 domestic to individuals (effective 2001); USD 85 in Canada to individuals; USD 90 elsewhere to individuals; USD 100 domestic to institutions; USD 105 in Canada to institutions; USD 110 elsewhere to institutions (effective 1999). adv. bk.rev. charts, illus. index. back issues avail.; reprint service avail. from PQC. *Refereed.* **Document type:** *Directory, Government.* **Description:** Focuses entirely on the technology crucial to nuclear medicine.

Related titles: Microform ed.: (from PQC); Online - full text ed.: (from HighWire Pr., Northern Light Technology, Inc., ProQuest Information & Learning).

Indexed: Biol.Abstr., CINAHL, Chem.Abstr., Chem.Indus.Notes, Chem.Titles, Excerp.Med. (1993-), INIS Atomind., INSPEC (Mar.1974-), I.P.A., Ind.Med. (1973-).

—BLDSC (5023.340000), AskIEEE, CASDDS, CISTI, GNLM, ingenta, KNAW. **CCC.**

Published by: Society of Nuclear Medicine, 1850 Samuel Morse Dr, Reston, VA 20190-5316. TEL 703-708-9000, FAX 703-708-9015, http://www.snmjournals.org/. Ed. Sally Spray. R&P Dawn Murphy. Adv. contact Stacey Silver. Circ: 7,000.

615 JPN ISSN 0449-3060
QH652.A1 CODEN: JRARAX

JOURNAL OF RADIATION RESEARCH. Text in English. 1960. q. JPY 8,000, USD 95 to members. adv. bk.rev. *Refereed.* **Document type:** *Academic/Scholarly.*

Formerly: Japan Radiation Research Society. Journal

Related titles: Online - full text ed.: (from Institute for Scientific Information).

Indexed: ASCA, Aqua.Sci.& Fish.Abstr., Biol.Abstr., Biwk.Pap.Rad.Chem.& Photochem., Chem.Abstr., Chem.Indus.Notes, Chem.Titles, Curr.Adv.Ecol.Sci., Curr.Cont., Dairy Sci.Abstr., Deep Sea Res.& Oceanogr.Abstr., Dent.Ind., Eng.Ind., Environ.Sci.Poll.Mgmt., Excerp.Med., INIS Atomind., INSPEC (Mar.1972-), Ind.Med. (1960-), Ind.Sci.Rev., Inpharma, Pollut.Abstr., Reac., Ref.Zh., Risk Abstr., Saf.Sci.Abstr., Sci.Cit.Ind.

—BLDSC (5043.800000), AskIEEE, CASDDS, CISTI, Ei, GNLM, IDS, Linda Hall.

Published by: Japan Radiation Research Society, 4-9-1 Anagawa, Inage-ku, Chiba-shi 263-0024, Japan. Ed. Mitsuo Ikenaga. Circ: 1,500. **Dist. by:** Business Center for Academic Societies Japan, 5-16-9 Honkomagome, Bunkyo-ku, Tokyo 113-0021, Japan. TEL 03-5814-5811.

JOURNAL OF RADIOLOGICAL PROTECTION. see *ENERGY—Nuclear Energy*

JOURNAL OF RADIOSURGERY. see *MEDICAL SCIENCES—Surgery*

616.07 GBR ISSN 1460-3969

▼ **JOURNAL OF RADIOTHERAPY IN PRACTICE.** Text in English. 1999. q. GBP 63 to individuals; GBP 116 to institutions (effective 2000). *Refereed.*

—BLDSC (5044.700000).

Published by: Greenwich Medical Media, 219 Linen Hall, Greenwich Medical Media Ltd, Flat 162, 162-168 Regent St, London W1R 5TB, United Kingdom. TEL 44-207-494-1515, FAX 44-207-494-1616, gm@greenwich-medical.co.uk, http://www.greenwich-medical.co.uk. Eds. Angela Duxbury, David Eddy.

615.842 HKG

JOURNAL OF THE HONG KONG COLLEGE OF RADIOLOGISTS. Text in English. q. **Description:** Covers diagnostic imaging, clinical oncology, and nuclear medicine. Includes articles and papers on radiological protection, quality assurance, audit in radiology, and radiological education issues.

Published by: (Hong Kong College of Radiologists), Lippincott Williams & Wilkins Asia, Ste 907-910, New T&T Centre, Harbour City, 7 Canton Rd, Tsimshatsui, Kowloon, Hong Kong.

900 USA ISSN 0883-5993
CODEN: JTIME8

JOURNAL OF THORACIC IMAGING. Text in English. 1986. q. USD 249 domestic to individuals; USD 301 foreign to individuals; USD 336 domestic to institutions; USD 386 foreign to institutions; USD 88 newsstand/cover (effective 2002). adv. illus. index. back issues avail. *Refereed.* **Document type:** *Academic/Scholarly.* **Description:** Discusses all aspects of the diagnosis of chest disease using imaging techniques.

Related titles: Microform ed.; Online - full text ed.: USD 436.80 domestic academic site license; USD 486.80 foreign academic site license; USD 487.20 domestic corporate site license; USD 537.20 foreign corporate site license (2002) (from Ovid Technologies, Inc., Institute for Scientific Information).

Indexed: ASCA, Curr.Adv.Cancer Res., Curr.Cont., Excerp.Med., INIS Atomind., Ind.Imag.Lit., Ind.Med. (1985-), Inpharma, Reac., Rev.Med.& Vet.Mycol.

—BLDSC (5069.120000), CISTI, EMDOCS, GNLM, IDS, ingenta, KNAW.

Published by: (Society of Thoracic Radiology), Lippincott Williams & Wilkins (Philadelphia) (Subsidiary of: Wolters Kluwer N.V.), 530 Walnut St, Philadelphia, PA 19106-3621. TEL 215-521-8300, FAX 215-521-8902, http://www.lww.com. Ed. Dr. Jeffrey S Klein. Pub. Karen Phillips. R&P Margaret Becker. adv.: B&W page USD 700, color page USD 1,750. **Subscr. to:** PO Box 1600, Hagerstown, MD 21740-1600. TEL 800-777-2295, FAX 301-824-7390. **Co-sponsor:** Japanese Society of Thoracic Radiology.

616.07 534 USA ISSN 0278-4297
CODEN: JUMEDA
JOURNAL OF ULTRASOUND IN MEDICINE. Text in English. 1982. m. USD 230 domestic to individuals; USD 260 in Canada & Mexico to individuals; USD 280 elsewhere to individuals; USD 255 domestic to institutions; USD 285 in Canada & Mexico to institutions; USD 305 elsewhere to institutions (effective 2001). adv. bk.rev. abstr, bibl, charts, illus. index. back issues avail.; reprint service avail. from PQC. *Refereed.* **Document type:** *Academic/Scholarly.* **Description:** Contains peer reviewed papers on basic and clinical aspects of ultrasound, advances in the field, techniques and equipment modifications.
Related titles: Microform ed.: (from PQC); Online - full text ed.: (from Institute for Scientific Information).
Indexed: ASCA, Bioeng.Abstr., Biotech.& Bioeng.Abstr., Curr.Cont., Dent.Ind., Eng.Ind., Excerp.Med., Helminthol.Abstr., INIS Atomind., Ind.Imag.Lit., Ind.Med. (1982-), Ind.Sci.Rev., Inpharma, Neurosci.Cit.Ind., Reac., Sci.Cit.Ind.
—BLDSC (5071.455000), CISTI, Ei, EMDOCS, GNLM, IDS, ingenta, KNAW. **CCC.**
Published by: American Institute for Ultrasound in Medicine, 14750 Sweitzer Ln, Ste 100, Laurel, MD 20707-5906. TEL 301-498-4100, FAX 301-498-4450, publications@aium.org, http://www.aium.org. Ed. George R Leopold. R&P Maureen Kalil. Adv. contact Lisa Sheridan. B&W page USD 1,430, color page USD 2,820; trim 10.88 x 8.25. Circ: 12,000 (paid).

615.842 USA ISSN 1051-0443
CODEN: JVIRE3
JOURNAL OF VASCULAR AND INTERVENTIONAL RADIOLOGY. Text in English. 1990. m. USD 249 domestic to individuals for print & online eds.; USD 280 foreign to individuals for print & online eds; USD 329 domestic to institutions for print & online eds; USD 329 newsstand/cover foreign to institutions; USD 26 newsstand/cover (effective 2002). adv. bk.rev. back issues avail. *Refereed.* **Document type:** *Journal, Academic/Scholarly.* **Description:** Covers clinical and laboratory studies in the field of interventional radiology.
Related titles: E-mail ed.; Microform ed.: (from PQC); Online - full text ed.: USD 427.70 domestic academic site license; USD 427.70 foreign academic site license; USD 477.05 domestic corporate site license; USD 477.05 foreign corporate site license (effective 2002) (from Ovid Technologies, Inc., HighWire Pr., Institute for Scientific Information).
Indexed: ASCA, Curr.Cont., Ind.Imag.Lit., Ind.Med. (1990-), Inpharma, Pharm.&Out.News, Reac., Sci.Cit.Ind.
—BLDSC (5072.263000), GNLM, IDS, KNAW.
Published by: (Society of Cardiovascular and Interventional Radiology), Lippincott Williams & Wilkins (Philadelphia) (Subsidiary of: Wolters Kluwer N.V.), 530 Walnut St, Philadelphia, PA 19106-3621. TEL 215-521-8300, FAX 215-521-8902, http://www.jvir.org/, http://www.lww.com. Ed. Dr. Daniel Picus. Pub. Karen Phillips. R&P Margaret Becker. Adv. contact Ray Thibodeau. Circ: 4,400. **Subscr. to:** PO Box 1600, Hagerstown, MD 21740-1600. TEL 800-777-2295, FAX 301-824-7390.

616.0754 USA ISSN 1084-824X
JOURNAL OF WOMEN'S IMAGING. Text in English. 1997. q. USD 97 domestic to individuals for print & online eds.; USD 97 foreign to individuals for print & online eds; USD 36 newsstand/cover; USD 158 per issue domestic to institutions; USD 158 per issue foreign to institutions (effective 2002). adv. back issues avail. *Refereed.* **Document type:** *Academic/Scholarly.* **Description:** Features original, peer-reviewed research articles and clinical reviews of all aspects of imaging of women during their reproductive and post-reproductive years using all available modalities, including ultrasound, radiography, tomography, nuclear and MRI.
Related titles: Online - full content ed.: USD 205.40 domestic academic site license; USD 205.40 foreign academic site license; USD 229.10 domestic corporate site license; USD 229.10 foreign corporate site license (effective 2002).
—BLDSC (5072.634600).
Published by: Lippincott Williams & Wilkins (Philadelphia) (Subsidiary of: Wolters Kluwer N.V.), 530 Walnut St, Philadelphia, PA 19106-3621. TEL 301-223-2300, 800-638-3030, FAX 301-223-2400, http:// www.jwijournal.com/, http://www.lww.com. Ed. Marcia C Javitt. adv.: B&W page USD 625, color page USD 1,500; trim 11 x 8.25. **Subscr. to:** PO Box 1600, Hagerstown, MD 21740-1600.

616.07 JPN ISSN 0075-4579
JUNTENDO UNIVERSITY. MEDICAL ULTRASONICS RESEARCH CENTER. ANNUAL REPORT✶ . Text in English. a.
Published by: Juntendo University, School of Medicine, Medical Ultrasonics Research Center, 2-1-2 Hongo, Bunkyo-ku, Tokyo 113-0033, Japan.

615.842 CAN ISSN 0022-7439
K V P NEWS. Text in English. 1964. q. membership. adv. charts, illus. **Document type:** *Newsletter.*
Media: Duplicated (not offset).
Published by: Manitoba Association of Medical Radiation Technologists Inc., 215 819 Sargent Ave, Winnipeg, MB R3E 0B9, Canada. TEL 204-774-5346. Ed. L Wills. Circ: 800.

615.8 JPN ISSN 0022-7854
CODEN: KAIGBZ
KAKU IGAKU/JAPANESE JOURNAL OF NUCLEAR MEDICINE. Variant title: Nihon Kaku Igakkai Kikanshi. Text in Japanese; Summaries in English, Japanese. 1964. 12/yr. JPY 1,500 per issue. adv. abstr, charts, illus. index.
Indexed: Biol.Abstr., Chem.Abstr., Chem.Indus.Notes, Chem.Titles, Excerp.Med., INIS Atomind., Ind.Med. (1964-), JTA.
—BLDSC (4656.650000), CASDDS, CISTI, GNLM.
Published by: Nihon Kaku Igakkai/Japanese Society of Nuclear Medicine, Nihon Aisotopu Kyokai, 2-28-45 Honkomagome, Bunkyo-ku, Tokyo 113-0021, Japan. Ed. Dr. S Hashimoto.

615.842 JPN ISSN 0912-4195
KAKU IGAKU GAZO SHINDAN/IMAGING DIAGNOSIS IN NUCLEAR MEDICINE. Text in Japanese. 1986. 3/yr.
Published by: Hokuriku Kaku Igaku Kanfarensu/Hokuriku Nuclear Medicine Conference, Kanazawa Daigaku Igakubu Kaku Igaku Kyoshitsu, 13-1 Takara-Machi, Kanazawa-shi, Ishikawa-ken 920-0934, Japan.

615.8 JPN ISSN 0289-100X
CODEN: KIGIEM
KAKU IGAKU GIJUTSU/JAPANESE JOURNAL OF NUCLEAR MEDICINE TECHNOLOGY. Text in Japanese. 1981. q.
Indexed: Chem.Abstr., Chem.Titles, INIS Atomind.
—CASDDS.
Published by: Nihon Kaku Igaku Gijutsu Gakkai/Japanese Society of Nuclear Medicine Technology, Sumitomo Byoin Aisotopu Kensabu, 2-2 Nakanoshima 5-chome, Kita-ku, Osaka-shi 530-0005, Japan.

615.8 JPN ISSN 0912-6104
KAKU IGAKU SEMINA SHOREISHU/TOKAI SEMINAR IN NUCLEAR MEDICINE. Text in Japanese. 1985. a.
Published by: (Kaku Igaku Semina Shoreishu Kenkyujo/Tokai Seminar in Nuclear Medicine), Daiichi Rajio Aisotopu Kenkyujo/Daiichi Radioisotope Laboratories, Ltd., 19-8 Kyobashi 1-chome, Chuo-ku, Tokyo 104-0031, Japan.

615.8 JPN ISSN 0910-2213
KAKU IGAKU SHOREI KENTOKAI SHOREISHU/ PROCEEDINGS OF MEETING ON CASE OF NUCLEAR MEDICINE. Text in Japanese. 1979. q.
Published by: Nihon Mejifijikkusu K.K./Japan Mediphysics Co., Ltd., 9-8 Roku-Tanji-cho, Nishinomiya-shi, Hyogo-ken 662-0918, Japan.

615.8 JPN ISSN 0461-5956
CODEN: KASHAJ
KANKO SHIKISO✶ /MEDICAL RESEARCHES FOR PHOTOSENSITIZING DYES. Text in Japanese; Summaries in English, Japanese. 1950. irreg. **Document type:** *Academic/Scholarly.*
Indexed: INIS Atomind.
—CASDDS.
Published by: (Kanko Shikiso Kenkyukai/Kyoto Daigaku Uirusu Kenkyujo), Kyoto University Press, Yoshidahon-Machi, Sakyo-ku, Kyoto-shi 606-8317, Japan.

616.075 JPN
KISO GIJUTSU KENKYU BUKAI SHIRYO/TECHNICAL REPORT OF MEDICAL ULTRASOUND ENGINEERING. Text in English, Japanese. 1986. irreg. free per issue. **Document type:** *Proceedings.*
Published by: Nihon Choonpa Igakkai/Japan Society of Ultrasonic Medicine, 23-1 Hongo 3-chome, Bunkyo-ku, Tokyo 113-0033, Japan. iin-jsum@catnet.or.jp, http://www.soc.nacsis.ac.jp/jsum. Ed. Iwaki Akiyama.

616.842 JPN ISSN 0915-0919
KITA NIHON KAKU IGAKU DANWAKAI/NORTH JAPANESE JOURNAL OF NUCLEAR MEDICINE. Text in Japanese. 1988. 2/yr.
Address: c/o Mr Mamoru Nakamura, Kokuritsu Sendai Byoin Hoshasenka, 8-8 Miyagino 2-chome, Miyagino-ku, Sendai-shi, Miyagi-ken 983-0045, Japan.

615.842 DEU ISSN 0939-7116
CODEN: KLNEFX
KLINISCHE NEURORADIOLOGIE. Text in German, English. 1991. q. EUR 176.16 domestic; EUR 182.16 foreign; EUR 109.80 domestic to students; EUR 115.80 foreign to students; EUR 50.47 newsstand/cover (effective 2002). back issues avail. *Refereed.* **Document type:** *Journal, Academic/Scholarly.*
Related titles: Online - full text ed.: ISSN 1615-6706 (from EBSCO Publishing, RoweCom Information Quest, Swets Blackwell, Springer LINK).
Indexed: Neurosci.Cit.Ind., e-psyche.
—EMDOCS, GNLM, IDS.
Published by: (Deutsche, Oesterreichische und Schweizerische Gesellschaft fuer Neuroradiologie), Urban und Vogel Medien und Medizin Verlagsgesellschaft mbH (Subsidiary of: BertelsmannSpringer), Neumarkter Str 43, Munich 81673, Germany. TEL 49-89-43721411, FAX 49-89-43721410, verlag@urban-vogel.de, http://www.urban-vogel.de. Ed. Dr. K Voigt. R&P Oliver Renn. Adv. contact Sibylle Schurr TEL 49-89-43721353. Circ: 1,100. **Subscr. to:** Springer Auslieferungs Gesellschaft, Postfach 105160, Heidelberg 69041, Germany. TEL 49-6221-345244, FAX 49-6221-345244.

616.07 JPN ISSN 0914-871X
KONIKA X REI SHASHIN KENKYU/KONICA X-RAY PHOTOGRAPHIC REVIEW. Text in Japanese. bi-m.
Published by: Konica Corp., 26-2 Nishi-Shinjuku 1-chome, Shinjuku-ku, Tokyo 160-0023, Japan.

616.075 FRA ISSN 1169-3827
L U S. (Litterature Ultra-Sonore) Text in French. m. FRF 1,775 (effective 2000). bk.rev. **Document type:** *Bulletin.*
Formerly (until 1992): Journal Francais d'Echographie
Related titles: CD-ROM ed.: FRF 1,500 base volume; FRF 200 updates (effective 2000).
Published by: Faculte de Medecine de Montpellier - Nimes, Antenne de Nimes, Av. Kennedy, Nimes 30000, France. TEL 33-2-66273177. Ed. J M Bourgeois. Circ: 2,500.

616.07 USA
M E E N CARDIOLOGY - CRITICAL CARE TECHNOLOGY. Text in English. bi-m. **Description:** Keeps users and buyers of cardiology and critical care technology apprised of the latest technology and information.
Supersedes in part (in 2000): Medical Electronics and Equipment News (0361-4174); Which was formerly: Medical Electronics News (0025-7230)
Published by: Reilly Publishing Co., 16 E Schaumburg Rd, Schaumburg, IL 60194-3536. TEL 847-882-6336, FAX 847-519-0166, rcgroup@flash.net, http:// www.rcgonline.net.

615.845 616.07 USA
CODEN: MEEQA
M E E N IMAGING TECHNOLOGY NEWS. Text in English. 1961. bi-m. free to qualified personnel. adv. bk.rev. abstr, charts, illus, stat, tr.lit. **Document type:** *Trade.* **Description:** Keeps users and buyers of medical imaging technology and services apprised of the latest technology available.
Supersedes in part (in 2000): Medical Electronics and Equipment News (0361-4174); Which was formerly: Medical Electronics News (0025-7230)
Indexed: Excerp.Med.
—GNLM.
Published by: Reilly Publishing Co., 16 E Schaumburg Rd, Schaumburg, IL 60194-3536. TEL 847-882-6336, FAX 847-519-0166, rcgroup@flash.net, http:// www.rcgonline.net. Ed. Andrea Donner. Pub. Sean Reilly. Circ: 35,000.

616.07 USA
M R I INDUSTRY REPORT. (Magnetic Resonance Imaging) Text in English. q. USD 1,097. **Document type:** *Trade.*
Published by: Miller Freeman, Inc. (Subsidiary of: United Newspapers), 600 Harrison St, San Francisco, CA 94107. TEL 415-905-2200, FAX 415-905-2233.

616.07 USA
M R TECHNOLOGIST. (Magnetic Resonance) Text in English. 12/yr. USD 85.
Published by: Miller Freeman, Inc. (Subsidiary of: United Newspapers), 600 Harrison St, San Francisco, CA 94107. TEL 415-905-2200, FAX 415-905-2233.

615.842 USA ISSN 0730-725X
RC78.7.N83 CODEN: MRIMDQ
MAGNETIC RESONANCE IMAGING; an international journal of basic research & clinical applications. Text in English. 1982. 10/yr. EUR 126 in Europe to individuals; JPY 16,600 in Japan to individuals; USD 140 elsewhere to individuals; EUR 1,052 in Europe to institutions; JPY 139,700 in Japan to institutions; USD 1,177 elsewhere to institutions (effective 2002). adv. bk.rev. back issues avail.; reprints avail. *Refereed.* **Document type:** *Academic/Scholarly.* **Description:** Covers clinical, physical and life science investigations relating to the development and use of magnetic resonance methods and instrumentation, as well as applications of imaging and spectroscopic techniques.
Incorporates (1986-1992): Reviews of Magnetic Resonance in Medicine (0883-8291)
Related titles: Microfilm ed.: (from PQC); Online - full text ed.: (from ingenta, ScienceDirect, Swets Blackwell, Institute for Scientific Information).
Indexed: ASCA, Biol.Abstr., Chem.Abstr., Chem.Indus.Notes, Chem.Titles, Curr.Adv.Cancer Res., Curr.Adv.Ecol.Sci., Curr.Cont., Food Sci.& Tech.Abstr., Hort.Abstr., INIS Atomind., INSPEC (1984-), Ind.Med. (1982-), Inpharma, Int.Abstr.Biol.Sci., Neurosci.Cit.Ind., Pharm.&Out.News, Reac., Rev.Med.& Vet.Mycol., Sci.Cit.Ind.
—BLDSC (5337.795000), AskIEEE, CASDDS, CISTI, EMDOCS, GNLM, IDS, ingenta. **CCC.**
Published by: (Society for Magnetic Resonance Imaging), Elsevier Science, 655 Ave of the Americas, New York, NY 10010. TEL 212-633-3686, FAX 212-633-3820, usinfo-f@elsevier.com, http://www.elsevier.nl/locate/mri. Ed. John Gore. Adv. contact Georgia Nikolaros. B&W page USD 945, color page USD 2,245. Circ: 1,600 (paid). **Subscr. in Australasia and the Far East to:** Elsevier Science (Singapore) Pte Ltd, No.1 Temasek Ave, 17-01 Millenia Tower, Singapore 039192, Singapore. TEL 65-434-3727, FAX 65-337-2230; **Subscr. in Japan to:** Elsevier Science Inc - Japan Regional Office, 9-15 Higashi-Azabu 1-chome, Minato-ku, Tokyo 106-0044, Japan. TEL 81-3-5561-5033; **Subscr. outside the Americas to:** Elsevier Science BV, PO Box 211, Amsterdam 1000 AE, Netherlands. TEL 31-20-485-3757.

616.842 USA ISSN 1064-9689
CODEN: MRIAFQ
MAGNETIC RESONANCE IMAGING CLINICS OF NORTH AMERICA. Spine title: M R I Clinics. Text in English. 1993. q. USD 159 domestic to individuals; USD 178 in Canada to individuals; USD 214 elsewhere to individuals; USD 213 domestic to institutions; USD 258 foreign to institutions; USD 65 per issue (effective 2001). **Document type:** *Academic/Scholarly.* **Description:** Emphasizes the conduct of examinations, interpretation of data, differential diagnosis, and pitfalls encountered in MRI practices.
Related titles: Microform ed.: (from PQC); Supplement: Continuing Medical Education Supplement to Magnetic Resonance Imaging Clinics of North America. USD 138 (effective 2000).
Indexed: CINAHL, Ind.Imag.Lit., Ind.Med. (1993-), Int.Nurs.Ind.
—BLDSC (5337.796000), CISTI, EMDOCS, GNLM, KNAW.
Published by: W.B. Saunders Co. (Subsidiary of: Harcourt Publishers Ltd.), 11830 Westline Industrial Dr, St Louis, MO 63146. TEL 800-325-4177, http://www.wbsaunders.com. Ed. Dr. Scott A Mirowitz. **Subscr. to:** Periodicals Fulfillment, W B Saunders Co, 6277 Sea Harbor Dr, 4th Fl, Orlando, FL 32891-4800. TEL 800-654-2452, FAX 800-874-6418.

615.842 GBR ISSN 0740-3194
CODEN: MRMEEN
MAGNETIC RESONANCE IN MEDICINE. Text in English. 1984. m. USD 1,295 in United States; USD 1,295 in Canada & Mexico; USD 1,439 elsewhere; USD 1,360 combined subscription in United States for print and online eds.; USD 1,360 combined subscription in Canada & Mexico for print and online eds.; USD 1,504 combined subscription elsewhere for print and online eds. (effective 2002). index. back issues avail. *Refereed.* **Document type:** *Academic/Scholarly.* **Description:** Publishes original investigations concerned with all aspects of the development and use of nuclear magnetic resonance and electron paramagnetic resonance techniques for medical applications.
Related titles: Microfilm ed.: (from WWS); Online - full text ed.: ISSN 1522-2594. USD 1,295 in United States; USD 1,295 in Canada & Mexico; USD 1,295 elsewhere (effective 2002) (from EBSCO Publishing, Wiley InterScience, Institute for Scientific Information).
Indexed: ASCA, Chem.Abstr., Chem.Cit.Ind., Chem.Indus.Notes, Chem.Titles, Curr.Adv.Cancer Res., Curr.Cont., INIS Atomind., INSPEC (Mar.1989-), Ind.Imag.Lit., Ind.Med. (1984-), Inpharma, Neurosci.Cit.Ind., Reac., Rev.Med.& Vet.Mycol., Sci.Cit.Ind.
—AskIEEE, CASDDS, CISTI, EMDOCS, GNLM, IDS, ingenta.
Published by: Wiley Europe Ltd., Baffins Ln, Chichester, W Sussex PO19 1UD, United Kingdom. TEL 44-1243-779777, FAX 44-1243-775878, customer@wiley.co.uk, http://www.interscience.wiley.com/jpages/0740-3194/, http://www.wiley.co.uk. **Subscr. in Americas to:** John Wiley & Sons, Inc., Journals, 605 Third Ave, New York, NY 10158. TEL 212-850-6021, 212-850-6645, subinfo@jwiley.com.

MAGNETIC RESONANCE MATERIALS IN PHYSICS, BIOLOGY AND MEDICINE. see *PHYSICS—Nuclear Physics*

616.07575 FRA ISSN 0928-1258
CODEN: MNIMEX
MEDECINE NUCLEAIRE; imagerie fonctionelle et metabolique. Text in French; Summaries in English, French. 1967. 9/yr. FRF 1,214, USD 232 domestic; FRF 1,390 foreign (effective 1999). adv. *Refereed.* **Document type:** *Academic/Scholarly.* **Description:** Emphasizes current nuclear medicine practices in vivo, including clinical practice, methodology and instrumentation, signal processing, and fundamental and applied biophysics.
Former titles (until 1993): Journal de Medecine Nucleaire et Biophysique (0992-3039); (until 1988): Journal de Biophysique et de Biomecanique (0766-5717); (until 1985): Journal de Biophysique et Medecine Nucleaire (0243-3354); (until 1980): Journal Francais de Biophysique et Medecine Nucleaire (0399-0435); Annales de Physique Biologique et Medicale (0029-0793)
Related titles: Online - full text ed.: (from ingenta).
Indexed: ASCA, BBCI (coverage dropped), Chem.Abstr., Curr.Cont. (coverage dropped), Excerp.Med., INIS Atomind., INSPEC (1980-), Ind.Sci.Rev., Sci.Cit.Ind. (coverage dropped).
—BLDSC (5487.920000), AskIEEE, CASDDS, CISTI, EMDOCS, GNLM, IDS, Infotrieve. **CCC.**
Published by: Societe Francaise de Biophysique et Medecine Nucleaire, 45 rue des Saints Peres, Paris Cedex 6 75270, France. Ed. X Marchandise. Circ: 1,500.

MEDICAL AND RADIOLOGICAL DEVICES GUIDANCE MANUAL. see *PUBLIC HEALTH AND SAFETY*

615 USA ISSN 0958-3947
QC795.32.R3 CODEN: MEDOEJ
MEDICAL DOSIMETRY. Text in English. 1984. q. EUR 304 in Europe to institutions; JPY 40,400 in Japan to institutions; USD 340 elsewhere to institutions (effective 2002). adv. back issues avail.; reprints avail. *Refereed.* **Document type:** *Academic/Scholarly.* **Description:** Reports on clinical and experimental developments in the field of medical dosimetry.
Formerly: American Association of Medical Dosimetrists. Journal (0739-0211)
Related titles: Microfilm ed.: (from PQC); Online - full text ed.: (from ingenta, ScienceDirect, Swets Blackwell).
Indexed: Curr.Adv.Cancer Res., INIS Atomind., INSPEC (Sum.1999-), Ind.Med. (coverage dropped), Int.Nurs.Ind.
—BLDSC (5527.130000), CISTI, GNLM, Infotrieve, ingenta, KNAW. **CCC.**
Published by: (American Association of Medical Dosimetrists), Elsevier Science, PO Box 945, New York, NY 10159-0945. TEL 212-633-3686, FAX 212-633-3820, usinfo-f@elsevier.com, http://www.elsevier.com/locate/meddos. Eds. M Tobler, P Redmond, Dr. Matt Tobler. Adv. contact Georgia Nikolaros. B&W page USD 985, color page USD 2,245. Circ: 1,700 (paid). **Subscr. in Australasia and the Far East to:** Elsevier Science (Singapore) Pte Ltd, No.1 Temasek Ave, 17-01 Millenia Tower, Singapore 039192, Singapore. TEL 65-434-3727, FAX 65-337-2230; **Subscr. in Japan to:** Elsevier Science Inc - Japan Regional Office, 9-15 Higashi-Azabu 1-chome, Minato-ku, Tokyo 106-0044, Japan. TEL 81-3-5561-5033, FAX 81-3-5561-5047; **Subscr. outside the Americas to:** Elsevier Science BV, PO Box 211, Amsterdam 1000 AE, Netherlands. TEL 31-20-485-3757, FAX 31-20-485-3432, nlinfo-f@elsevier.nl.

616.07 GBR ISSN 1361-8415
R857.O6
MEDICAL IMAGE ANALYSIS. Text in English. 1996. q. EUR 143 in Europe to individuals; JPY 19,000 in Japan to individuals; USD 160 elsewhere to individuals; EUR 417 in Europe to institutions; JPY 55,300 in Japan to institutions; USD 467 elsewhere to institutions (effective 2002). back issues avail. *Refereed.* **Document type:** *Academic/Scholarly.* **Description:** Provides a forum for the dissemination of new research results in the field of medical image analysis, with special emphasis on efforts related to the application of computer vision, virtual reality and robotics to medical imaging problems.
Related titles: Online - full text ed.: (from EBSCO Publishing, RoweCom Information Quest, ingenta, ScienceDirect, Swets Blackwell, Institute for Scientific Information).
Indexed: Curr.Cont., Ind.Med. (1996-), Sci.Cit.Ind.
—BLDSC (5527.537000), Infotrieve. **CCC.**
Published by: Elsevier Science BV, Sara Burgerhartstraat 25, Amsterdam 1055 KV, Netherlands. TEL 31-20-485-2911, FAX 31-20-485-2457, nlinfo-f@elsevier.nl, http://www.elsevier.com/locate/medima, http://www.elsevier.nl. Circ: 400.

615 JPN ISSN 0288-450X
MEDICAL IMAGING TECHNOLOGY. Text in English, Japanese. 1983. 6/yr. JPY 2,000 per issue (effective 1998). adv. *Refereed.* **Document type:** *Academic/Scholarly.* **Description:** Covers all kinds of medical image processing and pattern recognition technologies, including images of conventional X-ray, ultrasound, CT, MRI, nuclear medicine, endoscopy, microscopy, histology, cytology, telemedicine and more.
Related titles: Online - full text ed.
Indexed: INIS Atomind., INSPEC (Jan.1993-).
—BLDSC (5527.542000), AskIEEE.
Published by: (Nihon Iyo Gazo Kogakkai/Japanese Society of Medical Imaging Technology), Digital Press Inc., Texico Bldg, 9-7 Higashi-Ikebukuro, Toshima-ku, Tokyo 170-0013, Japan. TEL 81-3-3971-6702, FAX 81-3-3971-6703, homma@mel.go.jp; matsu@nirs.go.jp, http://www.crc.ricoh.com/academia/jjamit.html. Ed. Toru Matsumoto.

615.842 USA ISSN 0942-5373
CODEN: MERAED
MEDICAL RADIOLOGY. Text in English. 196?. irreg., latest 1994. price varies. reprint service avail. from ISI. **Document type:** *Academic/Scholarly.*
Formerly (until 1985): Handbuch der Medizinischen Radiologie (0085-1396)
Published by: Springer-Verlag, Journals (Subsidiary of: BertelsmannSpringer), 175 Fifth Ave, New York, NY 10010. TEL 212-460-1500, FAX 212-473-6272.

610 USA
▼ **MEDICAL TESTS SOURCEBOOK.** Text in English. 1999. irreg., latest 1999. USD 78 per issue (effective 2001). charts. Index. **Document type:** *Consumer.* **Description:** Basic consumer health information about medical tests.
Published by: Omnigraphics, Inc., 615 Griswold St, Detroit, MI 48226. TEL 313-961-1340, 800-234-1340, FAX 313-961-1383, 800-875-1340, info@omnigraphics.com, http://www.omnigraphics.com. Ed. Joyce Brennfleck Shannon.

615.842 NLD ISSN 0025-7664
CODEN: MEMUAA
MEDICAMUNDI. Text in English; Summaries in English, French, German, Spanish. 1955. q. free per issue to qualified personnel. adv. charts, illus, stat. index. *Refereed.* **Document type:** *Academic/Scholarly.* **Description:** Covers modern diagnostic imaging.
Indexed: Biol.Abstr., Chem.Abstr., Excerp.Med., INIS Atomind., INSPEC (pre-1969-), Ind.Med. (coverage dropped).
—BLDSC (5532.300000), AskIEEE, CASDDS, CISTI, GNLM.
Published by: Philips Medical Systems International B.V., PO Box 10000, Best 5680 DA, Netherlands. TEL 31-40-2763856, FAX 31-40-2762019, ovobels@best.ms.philips.com, www.philips.com/ms/clinical/index.htm. Ed. Dr. J Heinzerling. Pub. A St J Brown. Circ: 12,000 (controlled).

615.842 RUS
RM845 CODEN: MERAA9
MEDITSINSKAYA RADIOLOGIYA I RADIATSIONNAYA BEZOPASNOST'. Text in Russian; Summaries in English. 1956. bi-m. USD 109.95. bk.rev. index. **Description:** Publishes papers devoted to pathogenesis, clinical picture, prevention and treatment of radiation injuries in man. Includes information on radiological conferences and congresses held in Russia and abroad.

M

Formerly: Meditsinskaya Radiologiya (0025-8334)
Indexed: Biol.Abstr., Chem.Abstr., Chem.Indus.Notes, Chem.Titles, Dent.Ind., Derwent Biotech.Abstr., Eng.Ind., Excerp.Med., INIS Atomind., INSPEC (Jul.1981-), Ind.Med. (until 1992, dropped), Nutr.Abstr., Ref.Zh.
—BLDSC (0106.010000), AskIEEE, CASDDS, CISTI, East View, GNLM, Infotrieve, KNAW. **CCC.**
Published by: (Rossiiskaya Akademiya Meditsinskikh Nauk), Izdatel'stvo Radekon, Kashirskoe shosse 24, Moscow 115478, Russian Federation. TEL 7-095-1118375, FAX 7-095-3241670. Ed. G A Zedgenidze. **Dist. by:** Mezhdunarodnaya Kniga, B Yakimanka 39, Moscow 117049, Russian Federation. TEL 7-095-2384967, FAX 7-095-2384634; **US dist. addr.:** East View Publications, 3020 Harbor Ln N, Minneapolis, MN 55447. TEL 612-550-0961. **Co-sponsor:** Vsesoyuznoe Nauchnoe Obshchestvo Rentgenologov i Radiologov.

616.07 616.99 BGR ISSN 1310-1722
MEDITSINSKI PREGLED. RADIATSIIA I MEDITSINA. Text in Bulgarian; Summaries in Bulgarian, English. 1994. q., latest vol.8, 2001. BGL 14 domestic; USD 48 foreign (effective 2001 - 2002). adv. abstr, bibl, illus. 48 p./no. back issues avail. *Refereed.* **Document type:** *Journal, Academic/Scholarly, Abstract/Index, Bibliography.* **Description:** Covers roentgenology, nuclear medicine, radiation and protection.
Indexed: Abstr.Bulg.Sci.Med.Lit., INIS Atomind.
Published by: Meditsinski Universitet - Sofia, Tsentur za Informatsiia po Meditsina/Medical University - Sofia, Medical Information Center, 1 Sv Georgi Sofiiski ul, Sofia 1431, Bulgaria. TEL 359-2-9522342, FAX 359-2-9522393, mutafov@sun.medun.acad.bg, http://www.medun.acad.bg. Ed. St Milanov. R&P, Adv. contact Dr. Christo Mutafov. B&W page USD 50, color page USD 200; 12 x 18. Circ: 150. **Dist. by:** Sofia Books, Ul Silivria 16, Sofia 1404, Bulgaria. TEL 359-2-9586257, sofiabooks@hotmail.com, http://www.sofiabooks.hit.bg.

616.075 POL ISSN 1429-4966
MEDYCYNA PRAKTYCZNA. ULTRASONOGRAFIA. Text in Polish. 1997. q. PLZ 80 (effective 2000).
Published by: Medycyna Praktyczna, Ul Skawinska 8, Krakow 31066, Poland. TEL 48-12-4305520, FAX 48-12-4305536, listy@mp.pl, http://mp.pl/czasop.htm. Ed. Aleksandra Plichta.

MEN'EKI KAKU IGAKU/IMMUNONUCLEAR MEDICINE. see *MEDICAL SCIENCES—Allergology And Immunology*

616.842 USA ISSN 1051-1369
CODEN: MONEE7
MODERN NEURORADIOLOGY SERIES. Text in English. 1983. irreg. price varies. reprint service avail. from PQC. *Refereed.* **Document type:** *Monographic series.*
—CISTI.
Published by: Lippincott Williams & Wilkins (Philadelphia) (Subsidiary of: Wolters Kluwer N.V.), 530 Walnut St, Philadelphia, PA 19106-3621. TEL 301-223-2300, 800-638-3030, FAX 301-223-2400, http://www.lww.com.

615.842 NLD
CODEN: CPIMF6
MOLECULAR IMAGING AND BIOLOGY. Text in Dutch. 1998. bi-m. EUR 152 in Europe to individuals; JPY 21,100 in Japan to individuals; USD 171 elsewhere to individuals; EUR 306 in Europe to institutions; JPY 40,500 in Japan to institutions; USD 342 elsewhere to institutions (effective 2002). adv. back issues avail. **Description:** Provides a forum for the presentation of the latest research on clinical applications of positron imaging.
Formerly: Clinical Positron Imaging (1095-0397)
Related titles: Online - full text ed.: (from ingenta, Swets Blackwell, ScienceDirect).
—BLDSC (3286.333570). **CCC.**
Published by: (Institute for Clinical Positron Emission Tomography (PET)), Elsevier Science, 655 Ave of the Americas, New York, NY 10010. TEL 212-989-5800, FAX 212-633-3990, usinfo-f@elsevier.com. Ed. Dr. Steven Larson. Adv. contact Georgia Nikolaros. B&W page USD 985, color page USD 1,175.

615.842 USA
N C R P STATEMENTS. Text in English. 1954. irreg. free per issue.
Published by: National Council on Radiation Protection and Measurements, 7910 Woodmont Ave, Ste 800, Bethesda, MD 20814. TEL 301-657-2652. Ed. William M Beckner.

615.842 GBR ISSN 0952-3480
CODEN: NMRBEF
N M R IN BIOMEDICINE. (Nuclear Magnetic Resonance) Text in English. 1988. 8/yr. USD 1,295 in United States; USD 1,295 in Canada & Mexico; USD 1,295 elsewhere; USD 1,360 combined subscription in United States for print and online eds.; USD 1,360 combined subscription in Canada & Mexico for print and online eds.; USD 1,360 combined subscription elsewhere for print and online eds. (effective 2002). adv. back issues avail.; reprint service avail. from SWZ. *Refereed.* **Document type:** *Academic/Scholarly.* **Description:** Presents original papers in which nuclear magnetic resonance spectroscopy is used for investigating basic biochemical and clinical problems.
Related titles: Microform ed.: (from PQC); Online - full text ed.: ISSN 1099-1492. 1997. USD 1,295 in United States; USD 1,295 in Canada & Mexico; USD 1,295 elsewhere (effective 2002) (from EBSCO Publishing, Wiley InterScience, Institute for Scientific Information).
Indexed: ASCA, BBCI, Chem.Abstr., Chem.Indus.Notes, Chem.Titles, Curr.Cont., Eng.Ind., INSPEC (Feb.1990-), Ind.Med. (1988-), Ind.Sci.Rev., Inpharma, Int.Abstr.Biol.Sci., Pharm.&Out.News, Reac., Sci.Cit.Ind.
—BLDSC (6113.931000), AskIEEE, CASDDS, CISTI, Ei, EMDOCS, GNLM, IDS, Infotrieve. **CCC.**
Published by: Wiley Europe Ltd., Baffins Ln, Chichester, W Sussex PO19 1UD, United Kingdom. TEL 44-1243-779777, FAX 44-1243-775878, customer@wiley.co.uk, http://www.wiley.co.uk. adv.: B&W page GBP 650, color page GBP 1,550; trim 210 x 297. Circ: 400. **Subscr. in the Americas to:** John Wiley & Sons, Inc., Journals, 605 Third Ave, New York, NY 10158. TEL 212-850-6021, 212-850-6645, subinfo@jwiley.com.

615.842 JPN ISSN 0439-5956
R895.A1 CODEN: HISKBI
NATIONAL INSTITUTE OF RADIOLOGICAL SCIENCES. ANNUAL REPORT. Text in English. 1961. a.
—BLDSC (1364.740000), CISTI, Linda Hall.
Published by: Science and Technology Agency, National Institute of Radiological Sciences/Kagaku Gijutsucho Hoshasen Igaku Sogo Kenkyujo, 9-1 Anagawa 4-chome, Inage-ku, Chiba-shi 263-0024, Japan. TEL 0472-51-2111, FAX 0472-56-9616, TELEX 03722205-NIRS-J. Ed. T Iwakura. Circ: 1,400.

573.8 HUN ISSN 1216-8068
QP501 CODEN: NROBEZ
NEUROBIOLOGY; an international multidisciplinary journal in neuroscience. Text in English. 1966. q. USD 198 (effective 2002). adv. bk.rev. abstr, bibl. index. 120 p./no. back issues avail. **Document type:** *Journal, Academic/Scholarly.* **Description:** Publishes contributions from all subdisciplines of the neurosciences including neuroanatomy, morphology, biochemistry, physiology, pharmacology, molecular neurobiology, developmental neuroscience and more.
Former titles (until 1993): Acta Biochimica et Biophysica Hungarica (0237-6261); (until 1986): Academiae Scientiarum Hungaricae. Acta Biochimica et Biophysica (0001-5253)
Related titles: Online - full text ed.
Indexed: ASCA, Anim.Breed.Abstr., Apic.Abstr., Biol.Abstr., Chem.Abstr., Chem.Indus.Notes, Chem.Titles, Curr.Adv.Ecol.Sci., Curr.Cont. (coverage dropped), Excerp.Med., Helminthol.Abstr., INIS Atomind., Ind.Med. (1993-), Neurosci.Cit.Ind., Nutr.Abstr., SSCI (coverage dropped), Sci.Cit.Ind. (coverage dropped), e-psyche.
—BLDSC (6081.309900), CASDDS, CISTI, GNLM, IDS, Infotrieve, Linda Hall. **CCC.**
Published by: (Akademiai Kiado Rt., University of Veterinary Science), Akademiai Kiado Rt., PO Box 245, Budapest 1519, Hungary. TEL 36-1-4648233, FAX 36-1-4648297, journals@akkrt.hu. Ed. Karoly Elekes.

616.842 USA ISSN 1052-5149
CODEN: NCNAEO
NEUROIMAGING CLINICS OF NORTH AMERICA. Text in English. 1991. q. USD 159 domestic to individuals; USD 177 in Canada to individuals; USD 208 elsewhere to individuals; USD 212 domestic to institutions; USD 256 foreign to institutions; USD 65 per issue (effective 2001). adv. index. back issues avail. *Refereed.* **Document type:** *Academic/Scholarly.* **Description:** Covers a single topic in the field in each issue.
Related titles: Microform ed.: (from PQC); Online - full text ed.: (from Institute for Scientific Information); Supplement: Continuing Medical Education Supplement to Neuroimaging Clinics of North America. USD 138 (effective 2000).
Indexed: CINAHL, Excerp.Med. (1993-), Ind.Imag.Lit., Ind.Med. (1991-), Neurosci.Cit.Ind.
—BLDSC (6081.372400), CISTI, EMDOCS, GNLM, IDS, ingenta, KNAW.
Published by: W.B. Saunders Co. (Subsidiary of: Harcourt Publishers Ltd.), 11830 Westline Industrial Dr, St Louis, MO 63146. TEL 800-325-4177, http://www.wbsaunders.com. Ed. Burton P Drayer. **Subscr. to:** Periodicals Fulfillment, W B Saunders Co, 6277 Sea Harbor Dr, 4th Fl, Orlando, FL 32891-4800.

615.842 DEU ISSN 0028-3940
RC349.R3
NEURORADIOLOGY; a journal devoted to neuroimaging and interventional neuroradiology. Text in English. 1970. m. EUR 905.90 domestic; EUR 886.70 in Germany; EUR 86 newsstand/cover foreign (effective 2002). adv. charts. back issues avail.; reprint service avail. from ISI. *Refereed.* **Document type:** *Journal, Academic/Scholarly.* **Description:** Covers the diagnosis and treatment of the central nervous system, using plain X-rays, computed tomography, angiography, pneumoencephalography and isotope studies, spinal radiographs, myelography, and spinal vascular studies.
Related titles: Microform ed.: (from PQC); Online - full text ed.: ISSN 1432-1920 (from EBSCO Publishing, RoweCom Information Quest, Swets Blackwell, Springer LINK, Institute for Scientific Information).
Indexed: ASCA, Aqua.Sci.& Fish.Abstr., Bibl.Dev.Med.& Child Neur., Curr.Adv.Cancer Res., Curr.Adv.Ecol.Sci., Curr.Cont., Dent.Ind., Environ.Sci.Poll.Mgmt., Excerp.Med., Helminthol.Abstr., INIS Atomind., Ind.Imag.Lit., Ind.Med. (1970-), Ind.Sci.Rev., Inpharma, Kidney, Neurosci.Cit.Ind., Pharm.&Out.News, Reac., Rev.Appl.Entomol., Rev.Med.& Vet.Mycol., Sci.Cit.Ind., Tox.Abstr.
—BLDSC (6081.558000), CISTI, GNLM, IDS, ingenta, KNAW. **CCC.**
Published by: (European Society of Neuroradiology), Springer-Verlag (Subsidiary of: BertelsmannSpringer), Tiergartenstr 17, Heidelberg 69121, Germany. TEL 49-6221-345-0, FAX 49-6221-345229, subscriptions@springer.de, http://link.springer.de/link/service/journals/00234/index.htm, http://www.springer.de. Eds. C Manelfe, I Moseley. **Subscr. in N. America to:** Springer-Verlag New York Inc., PO Box 2485, Secaucus, NJ 07096-2485. TEL 212-460-1500, FAX 212-473-6272. **Co-sponsor:** Japanese Neuroradiological Society.

▼ **NEW ADVANCES IN NUCLEAR CARDIOLOGY**; current practice and latest developments. see *MEDICAL SCIENCES—Cardiovascular Diseases*

616.07 NLD
NEW CLINICAL APPLICATIONS. RADIOLOGY. Text in English. irreg. price varies. *Refereed.* **Document type:** *Monographic series.*
Published by: Kluwer Academic Publishers Group (Subsidiary of: Wolters Kluwer N.V.), Spuiboulevard 50, PO Box 17, Dordrecht 3300 AA, Netherlands. FAX 31-78-639-2254, services@wkap.nl, http://www.wkap.nl. **Dist. by:** Journals Department, PO Box 322, Dordrecht 3300 AH, Netherlands. FAX 31-78-654-6474.

616.07 ESP ISSN 1138-9753
NEWSLETTER DE RADIOLOGIA. Text in Spanish. 1998. q. adv. back issues avail.; reprints avail. **Document type:** *Newsletter.*
Published by: Editorial Garsi S.A. (Subsidiary of: Grupo Masson), Juan Bravo, 46, Madrid 28006, Spain. TEL 34-91-402-1212, FAX 34-91-402-0954, garsi@mad.servicom.es, http://www.masson.es.

616.07 JPN
NIHON HOSHASEN GIJUTSU GAKKAI BUNKENSHU. Text in Japanese. 1974. irreg.
Published by: Nihon Hoshasen Gijutsu Gakkai/Japanese Society of Radiological Technology, Nijo Puraza, 88, Nishinokyo Kitatsubocho, Nakagyo-ku, Kyoto-shi 604, Japan.

NIHON SEIKEI GEKA CHOONPA KENKYUKAI KAISHI/JAPANESE SOCIETY OF ORTHOPEDIC ULTRASONICS. JOURNAL. see *MEDICAL SCIENCES—Orthopedics And Traumatology*

615.8 JPN ISSN 0048-0428
CODEN: NHGZAR
NIPPON ACTA RADIOLOGICA/NIPPON IGAKU HOSHASEN GAKKAI ZASSHI. Text in Japanese; Abstracts and contents page in English. 1940. m. JPY 12,000. adv. bk.rev. illus. **Document type:** *Academic/Scholarly.*
Indexed: Biol.Abstr., Chem.Abstr., Excerp.Med., INIS Atomind., Ind.Med. (1940-), JTA.
—BLDSC (6113.254000), CASDDS, CISTI, GNLM, KNAW.
Published by: Nippon Societas Radiologica/Japan Radiological Society, Rm 301 Akamon Habitation, 5-29-13 Hongo, Bunkyo-ku, Tokyo 113-0033, Japan. FAX 03-5684-4075. Ed. Takahiro Kozuka. Circ: 6,000.

M

612.014 USA ISSN 0969-8051
R895.A1 CODEN: NMBIEO
NUCLEAR MEDICINE AND BIOLOGY. Text in English. 1973. 8/yr. EUR 266 in Europe to individuals; JPY 35,200 in Japan to individuals; USD 297 elsewhere to individuals; EUR 1,093 in Europe to institutions; JPY 145,100 in Japan to institutions; USD 1,222 elsewhere to institutions (effective 2002). adv. back issues avail.; reprint service avail. from PQC. *Refereed.* **Document type:** *Journal, Academic/Scholarly.* **Description:** Publishes papers examining and proposing new diagnostic and therapeutic procedures as well as new data obtained using established nuclear medical procedures.
Former titles (until 1993): International Journal of Radiation Applications and Instrumentation. Part B: Nuclear Medicine and Biology (0883-2897); (until 1985): International Journal of Nuclear Medicine and Biology (0047-0740)
Related titles: Microfilm ed.: (from PQC); Online - full text ed.: (from ingenta, ScienceDirect, Swets Blackwell, Institute for Scientific Information).
Indexed: ASCA, Biol.Abstr., Chem.Abstr., Chem.Cit.Ind., Chem.Indus.Notes, Chem.Titles, Curr.Adv.Ecol.Sci., Curr.Cont., Derwent Biotech.Abstr., Environ.Sci.Poll.Mgmt., Excerp.Med., INIS Atomind., INSPEC (Jan.1973-1985, dropped), Ind.Med. (1993-), Ind.Sci.Rev., Inpharma, Int.Abstr.Biol.Sci., Neurosci.Cit.Ind., Nutr.Abstr., Pharm.&Out.News, Pollut.Abstr., Reac., Sci.Cit.Ind.
—BLDSC (6180.920500), ADONIS, CASDDS, CISTI, EMDOCS, GNLM, IDS, Infotrieve, KNAW, Linda Hall. **CCC.**
Published by: Elsevier Science, 655 Ave of the Americas, New York, NY 10010. TEL 212-633-3686, FAX 212-633-3820, usinfo-f@elsevier.com, http://www.elsevier.com/locate/nucmedbio. Eds. W B Mann, W C Eckelman. Adv. contact Georgia Nikolaros. Circ: 500 (paid).

615.842 USA ISSN 0272-0108
R895.A1 CODEN: NMANDX
NUCLEAR MEDICINE ANNUAL. Text in English. a. price varies. reprint service avail. from PQC. *Refereed.* **Document type:** *Monographic series.*
Indexed: Biol.Abstr., Chem.Abstr.
—BLDSC (6180.921000), CASDDS, CISTI, GNLM, ingenta.
Published by: Lippincott Williams & Wilkins (Philadelphia) (Subsidiary of: Wolters Kluwer N.V.), 530 Walnut St, Philadelphia, PA 19106-3621. TEL 301-223-2300, 800-638-3030, FAX 301-223-2400, http://www.lww.com.

615.8 USA ISSN 0143-3636
CODEN: NMCODC
NUCLEAR MEDICINE COMMUNICATIONS. Text in English. 1980. m., latest vol.22. USD 394 domestic to individuals; USD 394 foreign to individuals; USD 1,215 per issue domestic to institutional members; USD 1,215 per issue foreign to institutional members; USD 93 newsstand/cover (effective 2002). adv. bk.rev. index. reprint service avail. from PQC. *Refereed.* **Document type:** *Academic/Scholarly.* **Description:** Promotes rapid publication of original clinical and scientific research in all aspects of nuclear medicine.
Related titles: Online - full text ed.: USD 1,579.50 domestic academic site license; USD 1,579.50 foreign academic site license; USD 1,761.75 foreign corporate site license (2002) (from Ovid Technologies, Inc., EBSCO Publishing, Institute for Scientific Information).
Indexed: ASCA, Biol.Abstr., Chem.Abstr., Chem.Titles, Curr.Adv.Cancer Res., Curr.Adv.Ecol.Sci., Curr.Cont., Environ.Sci.Poll.Mgmt., Excerp.Med., INIS Atomind., Ind.Med. (1980-), Inpharma, Int.Abstr.Biol.Sci., Neurosci.Cit.Ind., Pharm.&Out.News, Reac., Saf.Sci.Abstr.
—BLDSC (6180.923000), ADONIS, CASDDS, CISTI, GNLM, IDS, KNAW.
Published by: Lippincott Williams & Wilkins (Philadelphia) (Subsidiary of: Wolters Kluwer N.V.), 530 Walnut St, Philadelphia, PA 19106-3621. TEL 215-521-8300, FAX 215-521-8902, http://www.nuclearmedicinecomm.com, http://www.lww.com. Adv. contact Gemma Heiser. **Subscr. to:** PO Box 1600, Hagerstown, MD 21740-1600. TEL 800-777-2295, FAX 301-824-7390.

NUCLEUS. see *ENERGY—Nuclear Energy*

615.8 DEU ISSN 0029-5566
R895.A1 CODEN: NMIMAX
NUKLEARMEDIZIN/NUCLEAR MEDICINE. Text in English, French, German. 1961. 6/yr. DEM 360 to individuals; DEM 512 to institutions; DEM 100 to students (effective 2001). adv. bk.rev. abstr, bibl, charts, illus. index. *Refereed.* **Document type:** *Journal, Academic/Scholarly.* **Description:** Original material covering experimental and clinical research with radionuclides, radionuclide imaging, new concepts of functional imaging, case reports.
Related titles: Online - full text ed.: (from Institute for Scientific Information).
Indexed: ASCA, Biol.Abstr., Chem.Abstr., Chem.Titles, Curr.Cont., Excerp.Med., INIS Atomind., Ind.Med. (1976-), Inpharma, Pharm.&Out.News, Reac., Risk Abstr., Sci.Cit.Ind.
—BLDSC (6184.453000), CASDDS, CISTI, GNLM, IDS, Infotrieve. **CCC.**
Published by: (German, Austrian and Swiss Societies of Nuclear Medicine), Schattauer GmbH, Hoelderlinstr 3, Stuttgart 70174, Germany. TEL 49-711-22987-0, FAX 49-711-2298750, info@schattauer.de, http://www.schattauer.com. Pub. Dieter Bergemann. R&P Annika Schmidt TEL 49-711-2298713. Adv. contact Hans-Georg Schwarz. B&W page XEU 1,184.66, color page XEU 2,149.47; 183 x 227. Circ: 3,200. **Subscr. to:** CSJ, Postfach 140220, Munich 80452, Germany. TEL 49-89-20959129, schattauer@csj.de.

615.842 DEU ISSN 0723-7065
CODEN: NKLZD8
DER NUKLEARMEDIZINER. Text in German; Summaries in English. 1977. 4/yr. EUR 141.80 domestic to institutions; EUR 147.80 in Europe to institutions; EUR 151 elsewhere to institutions; EUR 38 to students; EUR 33.50 newsstand/cover (effective 2002). **Document type:** *Journal, Academic/Scholarly.*
Indexed: INIS Atomind., Ref.Zh.
—BLDSC (6184.485000), CASDDS, GNLM.
Published by: (Berufsverband Deutscher Nuklearmediziner), Demeter Verlag GmbH und Co. KG, Ruedigerstr 14, Stuttgart 70469, Germany. TEL 49-711-8931-0, FAX 49-711-8931322, custserv@thieme.de, http://www.demeter-verlag.de. Ed. Dr. D W Nitz. Circ: 1,800.

ORAL RADIOLOGY. see *MEDICAL SCIENCES—Dentistry*

PEDIATRIC RADIOLOGY; roentgenology, nuclear medicine, ultrasonics, CT, MRI. see *MEDICAL SCIENCES—Pediatrics*

616.07 POL ISSN 0860-1089
POLSKI PRZEGLAD RADIOLOGII. Text in Polish. 1926. q. USD 80. illus. **Document type:** *Academic/Scholarly.*
Former titles (until 1983): Polski Przeglad Radiologii i Medycyny Nucklearnej (0137-7183); (until 1961): Polski Przeglad Radiologiczny
Indexed: INIS Atomind.
—GNLM. **CCC.**
Published by: (Polskie Lekarskie Towarzystwo Radiologiczne, Zarzad Glowny), Wydawnictwo Medyczne Sanmedica Sp. z o.o., Ul Nowy Zjazd 1, Warsaw 00301, Poland. TEL 48-22-8262287, FAX 48-22-8263182. Ed. Kazimierz Niezabitowski. R&P Maria Baginska Wierzbowska. Adv. contact Jolanta Paterczyk. B&W page USD 700, color page USD 900.

PROGRESS IN NUCLEAR MAGNETIC RESONANCE SPECTROSCOPY. see *CHEMISTRY—Analytical Chemistry*

612.014 ITA
R61 CODEN: JNMSD3
THE QUARTERLY JOURNAL OF NUCLEAR MEDICINE. Text and summaries in English. 1957. q. USD 105 to individuals; USD 155 to institutions (effective 2000 - 2001). adv. bk.rev. bibl, charts, illus. index. reprint service avail. from PQC. *Refereed.* **Document type:** *Academic/Scholarly.*
Former titles (until 1995): Journal of Nuclear Biology and Medicine (1121-1075); (until 1991): Journal of Nuclear Medicine and Allied Sciences (0392-0208); Minerva Mediconucleare (0026-4857); Minerva Nuclear Medical Section
Related titles: Microform ed.: (from PQC).
Indexed: C.I.S. Abstr., Chem.Abstr., Curr.Adv.Ecol.Sci., Curr.Cont., Dairy Sci.Abstr., Excerp.Med., INIS Atomind., INSPEC (Sep.1978-Dec.1985, dropped), Ind.Med. (coverage dropped), Ind.Sci.Rev., Nutr.Abstr.
—CASDDS, CISTI, EMDOCS, GNLM, ingenta, KNAW, Linda Hall.
Published by: (Italian Association of Nuclear Medicine), Edizioni Minerva Medica, Corso Bramante, 83-85, Turin, TO 10126, Italy. TEL 39-11-678282, FAX 39-11-674502. Ed. G Lucignani. Pub. Alberto Oliaro. Adv. contact F Filippo. B&W page USD 1,200, color page USD 2,000; trim 280 x 215. Circ: 3,000 (paid). **Co-sponsor:** International Association of Radiopharmacology.

615.842 USA
R B M A BULLETIN; progress through sharing. Text in English. 1988 (vol.23, no.11). m. USD 100 domestic to non-members; USD 110 foreign to non-members (effective 2000). adv. bk.rev. **Document type:** *Bulletin.*
Published by: Radiology Business Management Association, 1550 S Coast Hwy, 201, Laguna Beach, CA 92651-3262. TEL 888-224-7262. Ed. Sharon Urch.

616.07 JPN
R E R F UPDATE. Text in English. s-a. free per issue. **Document type:** *Newsletter.*
—BLDSC.
Published by: Radiation Effects Research Foundation/Hoshasen Eiksho Kenkyujo, 5-2 Hijiyama Park, Minami-ku, Hiroshima-shi, Hiroshima-ken 732-0815, Japan. FAX 81-82-263-7279, pub-info@rerf.or.jp, http://www. rerf.or.jp/. Ed. Sheldon Wolff. Pub. Shigenobu Nagataki. R&P Reiko Sasaki. Circ: (controlled).

615.842 USA
R R S NEWS✶ . Text in English. q. membership. **Document type:** *Newsletter.*
Published by: Radiation Research Society, 820 Jorie Blvd, Oak Brook, IL 60523-2247. TEL 708-571-2881. Ed. Helen Evans. Circ: 1,500.

615.842 USA ISSN 1090-7629
R S N A ELECTRONIC JOURNAL. Text in English. 1996. irreg. back issues avail. **Description:** Aims to improve the communication of scientific and clinical research in radiology.
Media: Online - full text. **Related titles:** ♦ Supplement to: Radiographics. ISSN 0271-5333.
Published by: Radiological Society of North America, Inc., 820 Jorie Blvd., Oak Brook, IL 60523. TEL 630-571-2670, FAX 630-571-7837, http://ej.rsna.org/, http://www.rsna.org.

R S N A INDEX TO IMAGING LITERATURE. see *MEDICAL SCIENCES—Abstracting, Bibliographies, Statistics*

615.842 USA ISSN 1041-2182
R T IMAGE. (Radiologic Technology) Text in English. 1988. bi-w. USD 13. bk.rev. charts, illus. **Description:** Contains items of interest to radiology managers and radiologic science professionals in all modalities and in hospitals, free-standing centers, and schools.
Published by: Valley Forge Press, 1041 West Bridge St, Ste 6, Phoenixville, PA 19460. TEL 610-935-3302, 800-9VF-PRES, FAX 610-935-3072, vpfedit@aol.com. Ed. Deb Dellapena. Circ: 65,000.

615.842 GBR ISSN 0264-6412
RAD MAGAZINE; for medical imaging and radiotherapy professionals. Text in English. 1975. m. GBP 72 domestic; GBP 82.80 in Europe; GBP 106.80 elsewhere (effective 2001). adv. bk.rev., software rev., video rev. **Document type:** *Trade.* **Description:** Contains product news, personnel appointments, group meeting reports, and exhibition and conference reviews.
Incorporates: Consultant Radiologist and Radiotherapist
Published by: Kingsmoor Publications Ltd., Kingsmoor Publications Ltd, PO Box 3, Harlow, Essex CM19 4RF, United Kingdom. TEL 44-1279-429731, FAX 44-1279-441038. Eds. D G Messer, D J Roberts. R&P, Adv. contact D.J. Roberts. page XEU 1,465; trim 297 x 419. Circ: 8,100 (paid and controlled).

616.07 JPN
RADIATION EFFECTS RESEARCH FOUNDATION. ANNUAL REPORT/HOSHASEN EIKYO KENKYUSHO NENPO. Text in English, Japanese. a. **Document type:** *Corporate.*
Published by: Radiation Effects Research Foundation/Hoshasen Eiksho Kenkyujo, 5-2 Hijiyama Park, Minami-ku, Hiroshima-shi, Hiroshima-ken 732-0815, Japan. FAX 81-82-263-7279, pub-info@rerf.or.jp, http://www.rerf.or.jp/. Ed. Sheldon Wolff. Pub. Shigenobu Nagataki. R&P Reiko Sasaki. Circ: (controlled).

616.07 JPN
RADIATION EFFECTS RESEARCH FOUNDATION. COMMENTARY AND REVIEW SERIES/HOSHASEN EIKYO KENKYUSHO KAISETSU SOSETSU SHU. Text in English; Summaries in English, Japanese. 1989. irreg. **Document type:** *Academic/Scholarly.*
—BLDSC (3333.960000).
Published by: Radiation Effects Research Foundation/Hoshasen Eiksho Kenkyujo, 5-2 Hijiyama Park, Minami-ku, Hiroshima-shi, Hiroshima-ken 732-0815, Japan. FAX 81-82-261-7279, pub-info@rerf.or.jp, http://www.rerf.or.jp/. Ed. Sheldon Wolff. Pub. Shigenobu Nagataki. R&P Reiko Sasaki. Circ: (controlled).

M

616.07 JPN
RADIATION EFFECTS RESEARCH FOUNDATION NEWSLETTER/HOEIKEN NYUZU RETA. Text in Japanese. 1975. bi-m. free per issue. **Document type:** *Newsletter.*
Published by: Radiation Effects Research Foundation/Hoshasen Eiksho Kenkyujo, 5-2 Hijiyama Park, Minami-ku, Hiroshima-shi, Hiroshima-ken 732-0815, Japan. FAX 81-82-261-7279, pub-info@rerf.or.jp, http://www.rerf.or.jp/. Ed. Sheldon Wolff. Pub. Shigenobu Nagataki. R&P Reiko Sasaki. Circ: (controlled).

615.842 616.99 JPN ISSN 0288-2043 CODEN: RAMEER
RADIATION MEDICINE; medical imaging and radiation oncology. Text in Japanese. 1983. bi-m. JPY 12,000, USD 80. adv.
Indexed: Excerp.Med., INIS Atomind., Ind.Med. (1983-).
—BLDSC (7227.975000), CASDDS, CISTI, EMDOCS, GNLM, ingenta, KNAW.
Published by: Radiation Medicine Association, University of Faculty of Medicine, Department of Radiology, 7-3-1 Hongo, Bunkyo-ku, Tokyo 113-0033, Japan. Ed. Yasuhito Sasaki. Circ: 1,500. **Subscr. to:** Igaku-Shoin Medical Publishers Inc., 1140 Ave of the Americas, New York, NY 10036. TEL 212-944-7540.

615.842 USA
RADIATION ONCOLOGY NEWS. Text in English. 1986. 4/yr. USD 50; USD 60 foreign. bibl, tr.lit. back issues avail. **Document type:** *Newsletter.*
Formerly (until vol.4, 1990): S R O A Newsletter
Published by: Society for Radiation Oncology Administrators, 2021 Spring Rd., Ste. 600, Oak Brook, IL 60521. TEL 630-571-9065, FAX 630-571-7837, jendra@rsna.org, http://www.radonc.uchicago.edu/—ROA/. Ed., R&P Jeanne Jendra. Circ: 275.

615.842 616.992 USA ISSN 1084-1911
RADIATION THERAPIST. Text in English. 1992. s-a. USD 25 domestic; USD 50 foreign (effective 2001). adv. bk.rev. illus. index. back issues avail. *Refereed.* **Document type:** *Journal, Academic/Scholarly.*
Indexed: CINAHL.
—BLDSC (7228.016000).
Published by: American Society of Radiologic Technologists, 15000 Central Ave S E, Albuquerque, NM 87123-3917. TEL 505-298-4500, FAX 505-298-5063, kott@asrt.org, http://www.asrt.org. Ed. Katherine Ott. R&P Peter Gregory. Adv. contact Joan McBrayer TEL 505-298-4500 ext. 317. Circ: 15,000.

615.832 RUS ISSN 0869-8031 QH652.A1 CODEN: RBIREJ
RADIATSIONNAYA BIOLOGIYA, RADIOEKOLOGIYA. Text in Russian. 1961. bi-m. USD 177.50. bk.rev. index. **Document type:** *Academic/Scholarly.*
Formerly (until no.4, 1993): Radiobiologiya (0033-8192)
Indexed: Aqua.Sci.& Fish.Abstr., Biol.Abstr., Chem.Abstr., Chem.Indus.Notes, Chem.Titles, Eng.Ind., Environ.Sci.Poll.Mgmt., Excerp.Med., INIS Atomind., INSPEC (Jul.1981-), Ind.Med. (1993-), Int.Aerosp.Abstr., Pollut.Abstr., Ref.Zh., Risk Abstr., Saf.Sci.Abstr., Tox.Abstr.
—AskIEEE, CASDDS, CISTI, GNLM, Infotrieve, KNAW, Linda Hall. **CCC.**
Published by: (Otdelenie Biokhimii, Biofiziki i Khimii Fiziologicheski Aktivnykh Soedinenii, Rossiiskaya Akademiya Nauk/Russian Academy of Sciences), M A I K Nauka - Interperiodica, Mezhdunarodnyi Otdel, Profsoyuznaya ul 90, Moscow 117864, Russian Federation. TEL 7-095-3360266, FAX 7-095-420-2220. Ed. E B Burlakova. **US dist. addr.:** East View Publications, 3020 Harbor Ln N, Minneapolis, MN 55447. TEL 612-550-0961.

615.842 AUS ISSN 0033-8273 CODEN: RDGRAJ
RADIOGRAPHER. Text in English. 1948. q. adv. bk.rev. abstr, illus. index.
Indexed: Chem.Abstr., INIS Atomind., INSPEC (1982-), Ref.Zh.
—BLDSC (7236.850000), AskIEEE, CASDDS, ingenta.
Published by: Australian Institute of Radiography, c/o E.M. Hughes Sec., PO Box 1169, Collingwood, VIC 3066, Australia. TEL 61-3-94193336, FAX 61-3-94160783. Ed. E M Hughes. Adv. contacts E M Hughes, Lorraine Katramados. page AUD 550; trim 210 x 297. Circ: 4,000.

615.842 USA ISSN 0271-5333 RC78.A1
RADIOGRAPHICS. Text in English. 1981. bi-m. USD 110 domestic to non-members; USD 125 foreign to non-members (effective 2000). adv. back issues avail. *Refereed.* **Document type:** *Academic/Scholarly.* **Description:** Through extensive use of high-quality, detailed radiologic images and top quality articles, this journal delivers the very best.
Related titles: Microform ed.: (from PQC); Online - full text ed.: 1996 (from HighWire Pr., EBSCO Publishing, Institute for Scientific Information); ♦ Supplement: R S N A Electronic Journal. ISSN 1090-7629.
Indexed: ASCA, Compumath, Curr.Cont., INIS Atomind., Ind.Imag.Lit., Ind.Med. (1981-), Ind.Sci.Rev., Inpharma, Neurosci.Cit.Ind., Reac., SSCI (coverage dropped), Sci.Cit.Ind.
—BLDSC (7236.900000), CISTI, GNLM, IDS, Infotrieve, ingenta, KNAW. **CCC.**
Published by: Radiological Society of North America, Inc., 820 Jorie Blvd., Oak Brook, IL 60523. TEL 630-571-2670, FAX 630-571-7837, osborne@rsna.org, http://www.rsna.org/; http://radiographics.rsnajnls.org/. Ed. William W Olmsted. R&P Nancy Osborne. Adv. contact Jim Drew. Circ: 28,423. **Subscr. to:** Allen Press Inc., PO Box 1897, Lawrence, KS 66044-8897.

615.842 GBR ISSN 1078-8174
RADIOGRAPHY; an international journal of diagnostic imaging and radiation therapy. Text in English. 1995. q. GBP 60 to individuals; GBP 156 to institutions (effective 2002). reprint service avail. from SWZ. **Document type:** *Academic/Scholarly.* **Description:** Clinical and scientific papers on all aspects of diagnostic imaging.
Related titles: Online - full text ed.: (from EBSCO Publishing, O C L C Online Computer Library Center, Inc., Swets Blackwell, IDEAL Online Library).
Indexed: CINAHL.
—BLDSC (7237.001000), CISTI, EMDOCS, GNLM, Infotrieve, KNAW. **CCC.**
Published by: (College of Radiographers), W.B. Saunders Co. Ltd. (Subsidiary of: Harcourt Publishers Ltd.), 24-28 Oval Rd, London NW1 7DX, United Kingdom. TEL 44-20-7424-4200, FAX 44-20-7424-4515, cservice@harcourt.com, http://www.harcourt-international.com/journals/radi. **Subscr. to:** Harcourt Publishers Ltd., Foots Cray High St, Sidcup, Kent DA14 5HP, United Kingdom. TEL 44-20-8308-5700, FAX 44-20-8309-0807.

RADIOKHIMIYA. see *CHEMISTRY—Physical Chemistry*

615.842 DEU ISSN 0033-832X CODEN: RDLGBC
DER RADIOLOGE; Zeitschrift fuer diagnostische und interventionelle Radiologie, Radioonkologie, Nuklearmedizin. Text in German; Summaries in English. 1961. m. EUR 375.98 domestic; EUR 346.68 in Germany; EUR 33.20 newsstand/cover foreign (effective 2002). adv. bk.rev. charts, illus. index. back issues avail.; reprint service avail. from ISI. *Refereed.* **Document type:** *Journal, Academic/Scholarly.* **Description:** Discusses diagnostic techniques in the field of radiology.
Related titles: Microform ed.: (from PQC); Online - full text ed.: ISSN 1432-2102 (from F I Z Technik, EBSCO Publishing, RoweCom Information Quest, Swets Blackwell, Springer LINK, Institute for Scientific Information).
Indexed: ASCA, Biol.Abstr., Compumath, Curr.Cont., Dent.Ind., Excerp.Med., Helminthol.Abstr., INIS Atomind., Ind.Med. (1961-), Ind.Sci.Rev., Inpharma, Reac., Sci.Cit.Ind.
—BLDSC (7237.700000), CISTI, GNLM, IDS, Infotrieve, KNAW. **CCC.**
Published by: (Arbeitsgemeinschaft Berufsverbaende Medizinische Radiologie), Springer-Verlag (Subsidiary of: BertelsmannSpringer), Tiergartenstr 17, Heidelberg 69121, Germany. TEL 49-6221-345-0, FAX 49-6221-345229, subscriptions@springer.de, http://link.springer.de/link/service/journals/00117/index.htm, http://www.springer.de. Eds. G van Kaick, H Imhof. **Subscr. in N. America to:** Springer-Verlag New York Inc., PO Box 2485, Secaucus, NJ 07096-2485. TEL 212-460-1500, FAX 212-473-6272.

615.842 ESP ISSN 0033-8338
RADIOLOGIA. Text in Spanish. 1958. 10/yr. ESP 16,210 to individuals; USD 23,000 to institutions; USD 12,960 to students (effective 2001). bk.rev. abstr, bibl, charts, illus, stat. index. back issues avail.; reprints avail. *Refereed.* **Document type:** *Journal, Academic/Scholarly.*
Related titles: Online - full text ed.: 1996.
Indexed: Biol.Abstr., Curr.Cont. (coverage dropped), Excerp.Med., Helminthol.Abstr., INIS Atomind., Ind.Med.Esp.
—BLDSC (7237.730000), CINDOC, CISTI, KNAW.
Published by: (Sociedad Espanola de Radiologia y Electrologia Medicas y de Medicina Nuclear), Ediciones Doyma S.A., Traversa de Gracia, 17-21, Barcelona 08021, Spain. TEL 34-93-200-0711, rx@doyma.es, doyma@doyma.es, http://www.doyma.es/rx. Ed. J Fernandez Cruz. R&P Monica Barnes. Adv. contact Jose Antonio Hernandez. Circ: 3,000.

615.842 BRA ISSN 0100-3984
RADIOLOGIA BRASILEIRA. Text in Portuguese. 1958. 6/yr. USD 50. adv. *Refereed.* **Document type:** *Newspaper.* **Description:** Publishes original works in radiology, ultrasonography, nuclear medicine, radiotherapy, magnetic resonance and tomography.
Indexed: INIS Atomind.
Published by: Colegio Brasileiro de Radiologia, Departamento da Associacao Medica Brasileira, Av. Paulista, 491, 13a andar, Sao Paulo, SP 01311-909, Brazil. TEL 55-11-285-4022. Ed. Dr. Giovanni Guido Cerri. Circ: 3,000.

615.842 ITA ISSN 0033-8362
RADIOLOGIA MEDICA. Text in Italian; Summaries in English, Italian. 1914. m. (10/yr.). bk.rev. bibl, charts, illus. index. reprint service avail. from PQC. *Refereed.* **Document type:** *Academic/Scholarly.* **Description:** Covers imaging diagnostics and radiotherapy.
Formerly: Minerva Radiologica (0026-4962)
Related titles: Microform ed.: (from PQC).
Indexed: Biol.Abstr., Chem.Abstr., Dent.Ind., Excerp.Med., INIS Atomind., Ind.Med. (1914-).
—BLDSC (7237.800000), CISTI, GNLM, KNAW.
Published by: (Societa Italiana di Radiologia Medica), Edizioni Minerva Medica, Corso Bramante, 83-85, Turin, TO 10126, Italy. TEL 39-11-678282, FAX 39-11-674502. Ed. L Diguglielmo. Pub. Alberto Oliaro. Circ: 7,000.

615.842 USA ISSN 0033-8389 RM846 CODEN: RCNAAU
RADIOLOGIC CLINICS OF NORTH AMERICA. Text in English. 1963. bi-m. USD 185 domestic to individuals; USD 215 in Canada to individuals; USD 252 elsewhere to individuals; USD 243 domestic to institutions; USD 298 foreign to institutions; USD 116 domestic to students; USD 50 per issue (effective 2001). illus. reprint service avail. from PQC. *Refereed.* **Document type:** *Journal, Academic/Scholarly.*
Related titles: Microform ed.: (from MIM,PQC); Online - full text ed.: (from Institute for Scientific Information); Supplement: Continuing Medical Education Supplement to Radiologic Clinics of Norht America. USD 176 (effective 2000).
Indexed: AIM, ASCA, Biol.Abstr., CINAHL, Curr.Adv.Ecol.Sci., Curr.Cont., Dent.Ind., Excerp.Med., INIS Atomind., Ind.Imag.Lit., Ind.Med. (1963-), Ind.Sci.Rev., Inpharma, Int.Nurs.Ind., Pharm.&Out.News, Reac., Sci.Cit.Ind.
—BLDSC (7237.830000), CISTI, GNLM, IDS, ingenta, KNAW. **CCC.**
Published by: W.B. Saunders Co. (Subsidiary of: Harcourt Publishers Ltd.), 11830 Westline Industrial Dr, St Louis, MO 63146. TEL 800-325-4177, http://www.wbsaunders.com. **Subscr. to:** Periodicals Fulfillment, W B Saunders Co, 6277 Sea Harbor Dr, 4th Fl, Orlando, FL 32891-4800.

615.842 USA ISSN 0033-8397 CODEN: RATIB3
RADIOLOGIC TECHNOLOGY. Text in English. 1929. bi-m. USD 49 domestic; USD 75 foreign; USD 29.50 to students (effective 2001). adv. bk.rev. illus. cum.index. *Refereed.* **Document type:** *Academic/Scholarly.*
Related titles: Online - full text ed.: (from Northern Light Technology, Inc., Gale Group).
Indexed: Biol.Abstr., CINAHL, Chem.Abstr., Excerp.Med., Hosp.Lit.Ind., INIS Atomind., Ind.Med. (1963-), Int.Nurs.Ind.
—BLDSC (7237.850000), CISTI, GNLM, ingenta, KNAW.
Published by: American Society of Radiologic Technologists, 15000 Central Ave S E, Albuquerque, NM 87123-3917. TEL 505-298-4500, FAX 505-298-5063, http://www.asrt.org. R&P Peter Gregory. Adv. contact Joan McBrayer TEL 505-298-4500 ext. 317. Circ: 86,209 (paid).

616.842 DEU ISSN 0935-1779
RADIOLOGIE ASSISTENT. Text in German. 4/yr. DEM 29 domestic; DEM 34.50 foreign (effective 2001). adv. **Document type:** *Journal, Trade.*
—GNLM.
Published by: Schmidt-Roemhild Verlag, Mengstr 16, Luebeck 23552, Germany. TEL 49-451-7031-01, FAX 49-451-7031253, msr-luebeck@t-online.de, http://www.schmidt-roemhild.de.

M

615.842 DEU
▼ **RADIOLOGIE UP2DATE.** Text in German. 2001. 4/yr. EUR 130.10 domestic to institutions; EUR 132.90 in Europe to institutions; EUR 69 to students; EUR 32.90 newsstand/cover (effective 2002). adv. *Refereed.* **Document type:** *Journal, Academic/Scholarly.*
Related titles: Online - full text ed.
Published by: Georg Thieme Verlag, Ruedigerstr 14, Stuttgart 70469, Germany. TEL 49-711-8931-0, FAX 49-711-8931133, leser.service@thieme.de, http://www.thieme.de/rad-u2d. Ed. Dr. Ulrich Moedder.

616.07 USA ISSN 1069-1286
CODEN: RIOLEC
THE RADIOLOGIST. Text in English. 1994. bi-m., latest vol.8. USD 170 domestic to individuals; USD 195 foreign to individuals; USD 286 domestic to institutions; USD 313 foreign to institutions; USD 48 newsstand/cover (effective 2002). adv. **Document type:** *Academic/Scholarly.* **Description:** Reports on how various radiologic techniques can be used to diagnose and treat conditions.
Related titles: Online - full text ed.: USD 371.80 domestic for academic site license; USD 195 foreign for academic site license; USD 414.70 domestic for corporate site license; USD 441.70 foreign for corporate site license (effective 2002).
Indexed: Excerp.Med. (1995-).
—BLDSC (7237.996000), CISTI, EMDOCS.
Published by: Lippincott Williams & Wilkins (Baltimore) (Subsidiary of: Wolters Kluwer N.V.), 351 W Camden St, Baltimore, MD 21201-2436. TEL 410-528-4068, 800-222-3790, FAX 410-528-4452, custserv@wwilkins.com, http://www.wwilkins.com. Ed. Dr. Ronald Eisenberg. Adv. contact Kathleen Malamphy.

615.842 USA ISSN 0033-8419
RC78
RADIOLOGY; a monthly journal devoted to clinical radiology and allied sciences. Text in English. 1918. m. USD 225 domestic to non-members; USD 300 foreign to non-members; USD 80 domestic to members; USD 140 foreign to members (effective 2001). adv. bk.rev. abstr, charts, illus. index, cum.index every 3 yrs. 308 p./no. 3 cols./p. back issues avail.; reprint service avail. from PQC. *Refereed.* **Document type:** *Academic/Scholarly.* **Description:** Includes original research, reviews, commentary and expert opinion on new techniques and technology on radiology.
Related titles: Microform ed.: (from PQC); Online - full text ed.: (from HighWire Pr., EBSCO Publishing, Institute for Scientific Information).
Indexed: AIM, Agri.& Environ.Biotech.Abstr. (coverage dropped), Bibl.Dev.Med.& Child Neur., Biol.Abstr., C.I.S. Abstr., Cadscan, Cal.Tiss.Abstr., Chem.Abstr., Chem.Indus.Notes, Chem.Titles, Curr.Adv.Cancer Res., Curr.Adv.Ecol.Sci., Curr.Adv.Gen.& Molec.Biol., Curr.Cont., Dairy Sci.Abstr., Dent.Ind., Derwent Biotech.Abstr., Environ.Sci.Poll.Mgmt., Excerp.Med., Helminthol.Abstr., INIS Atomind., INSPEC (Feb.1980-), I.P.A., Ind.Imag.Lit., Ind.Med. (1923-), Ind.Sci.Rev., Inpharma, Int.Abstr.Biol.Sci., Int.Nurs.Ind., Jrnl.Watch, Jrnl.Watch Emer.Med., Kidney, Lead Abstr., Med.& Surg.Dermat., Neurosci.Abstr. (coverage dropped), Neurosci.Cit.Ind., Pharm.&Out.News, Pollut.Abstr., Protozool.Abstr., Reac., Rev.Arom.& Med.Plants, Rev.Med.& Vet.Mycol., Rev.Plant Path., SSCI (coverage dropped), Saf.Sci.Abstr., Sci.Cit.Ind., Tox.Abstr. (coverage dropped), Zincscan.
—BLDSC (7238.000000), AskIEEE, CASDDS, CISTI, GNLM, IDS, ingenta, KNAW. **CCC.**
Published by: Radiological Society of North America, Inc., 820 Jorie Blvd., Oak Brook, IL 60523. TEL 630-571-2670, FAX 630-571-7837, radiology-fb@highwire.stanford.edu, http://www.rsna.org. Ed. Dr. Anthony V Proto. R&P Nancy Osborne. Adv. contact Jim Drew. B&W page USD 2,595, color page USD 4,095. Circ: 37,038 (paid).

615.842 USA ISSN 0741-160X
RADIOLOGY AND IMAGING LETTER. Text in English. 1981. 22/yr., latest vol.21. USD 369 domestic to individuals; USD 389 foreign to individuals; USD 459 domestic to institutions; USD 459 per issue foreign to institutions; USD 21 newsstand/cover (effective 2002). bk.rev. charts, illus, tr.lit. index. back issues avail. **Document type:** *Newsletter.* **Description:** For clinical professionals. Covers latest advances in all areas of diagnostic imaging, radiation therapy and nuclear medicine, as well as safety hazards, recalls, legislation, products, legal issues and education.
Formerly (until 1984): Radiology Letter (0273-4958)
Related titles: Online - full text ed.: USD 596.70 domestic academic site license; USD 596.70 foreign academic site license; USD 665.55 domestic corporate site license; USD 665.55 foreign corporate site license (effective 2002) (from ProQuest Information & Learning).
Indexed: P.N.I.
Published by: Lippincott Williams & Wilkins (Philadelphia) (Subsidiary of: Wolters Kluwer N.V.), 530 Walnut St, Philadelphia, PA 19106-3621. TEL 215-521-8300, FAX 215-521-8902, http://www.lww.com. Ed. Linda G Huang. R&P Alice McElhinney. **Subscr. to:** PO Box 1600, Hagerstown, MD 21740-1600. TEL 800-777-2295, FAX 301-824-7390.

RADIOLOGY MANAGEMENT. see *HEALTH FACILITIES AND ADMINISTRATION*

616.0757 GBR ISSN 1461-4650
RADIOLOGY NOW. Text in English. 1982. 3/yr. back issues avail. *Refereed.* **Document type:** *Academic/Scholarly.* **Description:** Includes advances in radiology and radiological techniques.
Published by: Franklin Scientific Projects International, 516 Wandsworth Rd, London SW8 3JX, United Kingdom. TEL 44-20-7501-4085, FAX 44-20-7720-3525. Circ: 3,500.

616.6 USA
RADIONUCLIDES IN NEPHROUROLOGY. Text in English. 1996. q. USD 125 to individuals; USD 170 to institutions. *Refereed.* **Document type:** *Academic/Scholarly.*
Published by: Field & Wood, Medical Periodicals, Inc., PO Box 975, Blue Bell, PA 19422. TEL 610-828-4010, FAX 215-482-0226. Ed. Dr. O'Reilly.

615.842 IRL ISSN 0167-8140
CODEN: RAONDT
RADIOTHERAPY AND ONCOLOGY. Text in English. 1984. m. EUR 214 in Europe to individuals; JPY 28,400 in Japan to individuals; USD 240 elsewhere to individuals; EUR 1,624 in Europe to institutions; JPY 215,600 in Japan to institutions; USD 1,817 elsewhere to institutions (effective 2002). adv. index. reprint service avail. from SWZ. *Refereed.* **Document type:** *Academic/Scholarly.* **Description:** Covers areas of interest relating to radiation oncology.
Related titles: Microform ed.: (from PQC); Online - full text ed.: (from EBSCO Publishing, ingenta, Swets Blackwell, Institute for Scientific Information, ScienceDirect).
Indexed: ASCA, Aqua.Sci.& Fish.Abstr., Chem.Abstr., Chem.Indus.Notes, Chem.Titles, Curr.Adv.Cancer Res., Curr.Adv.Ecol.Sci., Curr.Cont., Environ.Sci.Poll.Mgmt., Excerp.Med., INIS Atomind., INSPEC (Jan.1996-), Ind.Med. (1983-), Ind.Sci.Rev., Inpharma, Int.Abstr.Biol.Sci., Med.& Surg.Dermat., Neurosci.Cit.Ind., Pharm.&Out.News, Reac., Ref.Zh., Risk Abstr., SSCI (coverage dropped), Saf.Sci.Abstr., Sci.Cit.Ind.
—BLDSC (7240.790000), ADONIS, AskIEEE, CASDDS, CISTI, GNLM, IDS, ingenta, KNAW. **CCC.**
Published by: (European Society for Therapeutic Radiology and Oncology), Elsevier Science Ireland Ltd, Elsevier House, Brookvale Plaza, E. Park, Shannon, Co. Clare, Ireland. TEL 353-61-471944, FAX 353-61-472144, http://www.elsevier.com/locate/radonc. Eds. H Bartelink, J Overgaard. R&P Annette Moloney. **Subscr. in Australasia and the Far East to:** Elsevier Science (Singapore) Pte Ltd, No.1 Temasek Ave, 17-01 Millenia Tower, Singapore 039192, Singapore. TEL 65-434-3727, FAX 65-337-2230; **Subscr. in the Americas to:** Elsevier Science, PO Box 945, New York, NY 10159-0945. TEL 212-633-3730, FAX 212-633-3680, usinfo-f@elsevier.com; **Subscr. to:** Elsevier Science BV, PO Box 211, Amsterdam 1000 AE, Netherlands. TEL 31-20-485-3757.

REFERATIVNYI ZHURNAL. LUCHEVAYA DIAGNOSTIKA. PART 1: ULTRAZVUKOVAYA DIAGNOSTIKA. see *MEDICAL SCIENCES—Abstracting, Bibliographies, Statistics*

REFERATIVNYI ZHURNAL. LUCHEVAYA DIAGNOSTIKA. PART 2: RENTGENODIAGNOSTIKA. MAGNITNOREZONANSNAYA TOMOGRAFIYA. see *MEDICAL SCIENCES—Abstracting, Bibliographies, Statistics*

REFERATIVNYI ZHURNAL. LUCHEVAYA DIAGNOSTIKA. PART 3: RADIONUKLIDNAYA DIAGNOSTIKA. see *MEDICAL SCIENCES—Abstracting, Bibliographies, Statistics*

REFERATOVY VYBER Z RADIODIAGNOSTIKY/ ABSTRACTS OF RADIOLOGY. see *MEDICAL SCIENCES—Abstracting, Bibliographies, Statistics*

616 615 BGR ISSN 0486-400X
CODEN: RENRAR
RENTGENOLOGIA I RADIOLOGIA. Text in Bulgarian; Summaries in Russian, English. 1962. q. BGL 16; USD 52 foreign (effective 2002). **Document type:** *Journal.* **Description:** Publishes original articles, surveys, reports, problems relating to radiation protection, scientific news, etc.
Indexed: Abstr.Bulg.Sci.Med.Lit., Chem.Abstr., Excerp.Med. (until 1993), INIS Atomind., Ref.Zh.
—CASDDS, CISTI, EMDOCS, GNLM.
Published by: (Bulgaria. Ministerstvo na Narodnoto Zdrave), Izdatelstvo Meditsina i Fizkultura, 11 Pl Slaveikov, Sofia 1080, Bulgaria. Ed. J V Nikolov. Circ: 620. **Dist. by:** Hemus, 6 Rouski blvd, Sofia 1000, Bulgaria; **Dist. by:** Sofia Books, Ul Silivria 16, Sofia 1404, Bulgaria. TEL 359-2-9586257, sofiabooks@hotmail.com, http://www.sofiabooks.hit.bg. **Co-sponsor:** Nauchno Druzhestvo po Rentgenologia i Radiologia.

616.842 BRA ISSN 0100-9699
REVISTA DA IMAGEM. Text in Portuguese; Summaries in English, Portuguese. 1978. q. USD 40. **Description:** Covers imaging methods for medical diagnosis, research, and clinical applications.
Indexed: INIS Atomind.
Published by: Sociedade Paulista de Radiologia, Av. Paulista, 491, 4o andar, Sao Paulo, SP 01311-909, Brazil. TEL 11-284-3988, FAX 11-284-3152. Ed. Antonio S Clemente Filho. Circ: 3,000.

615.842 ESP ISSN 0212-6982
REVISTA ESPANOLA DE MEDICINA NUCLEAR. Text in Spanish. 1982. bi-m. ESP 10,300 to individuals; ESP 14,700 to institutions; ESP 8,250 to students (effective 2001). adv. back issues avail.; reprints avail. *Refereed.* **Document type:** *Journal, Academic/Scholarly.*
Related titles: Online - full text ed.: 1996.
Indexed: Excerp.Med. (1992-), Ind.Med. (1982-).
—BLDSC (7854.109000), CINDOC.
Published by: (Sociedad Espanola de Medicina Nuclear), Ediciones Doyma S.A., Traversa de Gracia, 17-21, Barcelona 08021, Spain. TEL 34-93-200-0711, remn@doyma.es, doyma@doyma.es, http://www.doyma.es/remn. Ed. J M Freire Macias. R&P Monica Barnes. Adv. contact Jose Antonio Hernandez. B&W page ESP 118,000, color page ESP 145,000; 280 x 210. Circ: 1,000. **Co-sponsor:** Asociacion Latinoamericana de Sociedades de Biologia y Medicina Nuclear.

616.075 MEX ISSN 0370-6486
REVISTA MEXICANA DE RADIOLOGIA. Text in Spanish; Summaries in English. 1947. q., latest vol.53. MXP 600 domestic; MXP 60 foreign (effective 1999 - 2000). bk.rev. abstr, bibl, illus, tr.lit. back issues avail. **Document type:** *Magazine, Academic/Scholarly.* **Description:** Provides clinical and research papers to professionals in the fields of radiology and nuclear medicine.
Published by: (Federacion Mexicana de Radiologia y Images), Intersistemas S.A. de C.V., Fernando Alencastre No. 110, Col. Lomas Virreyes, Mexico City, D F 11000, Mexico. TEL 525-540-5600, FAX 525-540-3764. Ed., R&P Dr. Miguel E Stoopen. Pub. Pedro Vera Cervera. Circ: 3,000. **Subscr. to:** Federacion Mexicana de Radiologia y Images, Coahuila 35, Col. Roma, Mexico City, D F 06700, Mexico. TEL 525-584-7715, FAX 525-574-5374, tmri@compuserve.com, http://www.tmri.org.mx.

615.842 JPN ISSN 0009-9252
CODEN: JJCRA
RINSHO HOSHASEN/JAPANESE JOURNAL OF CLINICAL RADIOLOGY. Variant title: Clinical Radiology. Text in Japanese; Summaries in English. 1956. m. JPY 1,900 per issue. abstr, charts, illus. index. **Document type:** *Academic/Scholarly.*
Indexed: Dent.Ind., Excerp.Med., INIS Atomind., Ind.Med. (coverage dropped), Ind.Sci.Rev.
—BLDSC (4651.430000), CISTI, GNLM, KNAW.
Published by: Kanehara Shuppan Ltd., P.O. Box 1, Hongo Post Office, Tokyo 113-91, Japan. TEL 03-3811-7163. Ed. Dr. Katsutoshi Yoshimura. Circ: 4,700.

615.842 616.8 ITA ISSN 1120-9976
RIVISTA DI NEURORADIOLOGIA. Text in Italian, English; Summaries in English, Italian. 1988. bi-m. ITL 329,000 domestic; ITL 380,000 in Europe; ITL 50,000 per issue; ITL 445,000 elsewhere (effective 2001). adv. bk.rev. abstr. 120 p./no. back issues avail. *Refereed.* **Document type:** *Journal, Academic/Scholarly.*
Related titles: CD-ROM ed.; Diskette ed.; Fax ed.; Online - full text ed.: (from Institute for Scientific Information).
Indexed: ASCA, Excerp.Med., Neurosci.Cit.Ind., Ref.Zh., e-psyche.

M

—BLDSC (7991.435000), EMDOCS, GNLM, IDS, KNAW.
Published by: (Societa Italiana di Neuroradiologia), Centauro SRL, Via Del Pratello, 8, Bologna, BO 40122, Italy. TEL 39-051-227634, FAX 39-051-220099, adriana.dallocca@centauro.it, http://www.centauro.it. Ed. Dr. Marco Leonardi. R&P Adriana Dall'Occa. Adv. contact Gerardo Dall'Occa. page ITL 6,000,000; trim 297 x 210. Circ: 1,900.

615.842 DEU ISSN 1438-9029
CODEN: RFGVEF
ROEFO. FORTSCHRITTE AUF DEM GEBIET DER ROENTGENSTRAHLEN UND DER BILDGEBENDEN VERFAHREN. Text in German; Summaries in English, German. 1897. m. EUR 457.90 domestic to institutions; EUR 477.90 in Europe to institutions; EUR 520.90 elsewhere to institutions; EUR 46 newsstand/cover (effective 2002). adv. bk.rev. abstr, bibl, charts, illus, stat. index. reprint service avail. from PQC. *Refereed.* **Document type:** *Journal, Academic/Scholarly.*
Former titles: RoeFo. Fortschritte auf dem Gebiete der Roentgenstrahlen und der Neuen Bildgebenden Verfahren (0936-6652); Which incorporates (1948-1999): Aktuelle Radiologie (0939-267X); RoeFo. Fortschritte auf dem Gebiete der Roentgenstrahlen und der Nuklearmedizin (0340-1618); Fortschritte auf dem Gebiete der Roentgenstrahlen und der Nuklearmedizin (0015-8151)
Related titles: Microform ed.: (from PQC); Online - full text ed.: ISSN 1438-9010 (from Institute for Scientific Information).
Indexed: Biol.Abstr., C.I.S. Abstr., Chem.Abstr., Curr.Cont., Dairy Sci.Abstr., Dent.Ind., Excerp.Med., Helminthol.Abstr., INIS Atomind., INSPEC (Jul.1983-Nov.1993, dropped), Ind.Med. (1989-), Ind.Sci.Rev., Inpharma, Reac., Rev.Med.& Vet.Mycol., Sci.Cit.Ind.
—BLDSC (8019.170000), CASDDS, CISTI, EMDOCS, GNLM, IDS, Infotrieve, KNAW. **CCC.**
Published by: (Deutsche Roentgengesellschaft), Georg Thieme Verlag, Ruedigerstr 14, Stuttgart 70469, Germany. TEL 49-711-8931-0, FAX 49-711-8931298, roefo@thieme.de, leser.service@thieme.de, http://www.thieme.de/roefo, http://www.thieme-connect.de. Ed. R W Guenther. R&P Michael Wachinger. Circ: 7,000. **Co-sponsor:** Oesterreichische Roentgengesellschaft.

615.842 IND ISSN 0303-2590
ROENTGEN TECHNOLOGY. Text in English. 1974. s-a. INR 10, USD 3.
Indexed: INIS Atomind., Russ.Acad.Sci.Bibl.
—CISTI.
Published by: Indian Association of Radiological Technologists, Postgraduate Institute of Medical Education and Research, Dept. of Radiology, Chandigarh, Haryana, India.

612 USA ISSN 0739-9529
CODEN: SIRAE5
SEMINARS IN INTERVENTIONAL RADIOLOGY. Text in English. 1984. q. EUR 193 to individuals; EUR 366 to institutions; EUR 85 newsstand/cover (effective 2002). adv. abstr, bibl, illus. *Refereed.* **Document type:** *Monographic series, Academic/Scholarly.* **Description:** Each issue focuses on a a specific topic in this specialty.
Related titles: Online - full text ed.: ISSN 1098-8963 (from RoweCom Information Quest).
Indexed: ASCA, Biol.Abstr., Curr.Cont., Excerp.Med., Ind.Imag.Lit., Inpharma, Reac.
—BLDSC (8239.453000), CISTI, EMDOCS, GNLM, IDS, Infotrieve, ingenta, KNAW. **CCC.**
Published by: Thieme Medical Publishers, 333 Seventh Ave, New York, NY 10001. TEL 212-760-0888, 800-782-3488, FAX 212-947-1112, http://www.thieme.com. Ed. Dr. Peter R Mueller. Circ: 2,100. **Orders in Europe to:** Thieme International, Postfach 3001120, Stuttgart 70451, Germany. TEL 49-711-8931-0.

616.075 USA ISSN 1089-7860
CODEN: SMRAFY
SEMINARS IN MUSCULOSKELETAL RADIOLOGY. Text in English. 1997. q. EUR 142 to individuals; EUR 212 to institutions; EUR 46 newsstand/cover (effective 2002). adv. **Document type:** *Journal, Academic/Scholarly.* **Description:** Addresses advances in musculoskeletal radiology.
Related titles: Online - full text ed.: ISSN 1098-898X (from RoweCom Information Quest).
Indexed: Biol.Abstr., Curr.Cont. (coverage dropped), Excerp.Med., Ind.Med.
—BLDSC (8239.455050), GNLM.
Published by: Thieme Medical Publishers, 333 Seventh Ave, New York, NY 10001. TEL 212-760-0888, 800-782-3488, FAX 212-947-1112, http://www.thieme.com. Eds. Dr. David Karasick, Dr. Mark E Schweitzer. **Orders in Europe to:** Thieme International, Postfach 3001120, Stuttgart 70451, Germany. TEL 49-711-8931-0.

616.07575 USA ISSN 0001-2998
CODEN: SMNMAB
SEMINARS IN NUCLEAR MEDICINE. Text in English. 1971. q. USD 158 domestic to individuals; USD 229 foreign to individuals; USD 241 domestic to institutions; USD 300 foreign to institutions; USD 93 domestic to students; USD 137 foreign to students; USD 76 newsstand/cover (effective 2001). adv. abstr, bibl, charts, illus. *Refereed.* **Document type:** *Journal, Academic/Scholarly.* **Description:** Discusses new concepts and techniques developed in nuclear medicine.
Related titles: Online - full text ed.: (from Institute for Scientific Information).
Indexed: ASCA, Biol.Abstr., Chem.Abstr., Curr.Adv.Ecol.Sci., Curr.Cont., Excerp.Med., INIS Atomind., INSPEC (Jan.1971-Oct.1983, dropped), Ind.Imag.Lit., Ind.Med. (1971-), Ind.Sci.Rev., Inpharma, Pharm.&Out.News, Reac., Sci.Cit.Ind.
—BLDSC (8239.456000), CASDDS, CISTI, GNLM, IDS, ingenta. **CCC.**
Published by: W.B. Saunders Co. (Subsidiary of: Harcourt Publishers Ltd.), 11830 Westline Industrial Dr, St Louis, MO 63146. TEL 800-325-4177, http://www.wbsaunders.com. Eds. Leonard M Freeman, Dr. M Donald Blaufox. adv.: B&W page USD 1,085, color page USD 2,185; trim 10 x 7. Circ: 3,452. **Subscr. to:** Periodicals Fulfillment, W B Saunders Co, 6277 Sea Harbor Dr, 4th Fl, Orlando, FL 32891-4800.

SEMINARS IN ONCOLOGY NURSING. see *MEDICAL SCIENCES—Nurses And Nursing*

SEMINARS IN RADIATION ONCOLOGY. see *MEDICAL SCIENCES—Oncology*

616.842 USA ISSN 1070-535X
SEMINARS IN RADIOLOGIC TECHNOLOGY. Text in English. 1993. q. USD 100 combined subscription domestic to individuals Full text online inckuded; USD 160 combined subscription foreign to individuals for both print & online eds.; USD 162 combined subscription domestic to institutions for both print & online eds.; USD 208 combined subscription foreign to institutions for both print & online eds.; USD 72 combined subscription domestic to students for both print & online eds.; USD 96 combined subscription foreign to students for both print & online eds.; USD 53 newsstand/cover (effective 2001). adv. **Document type:** *Academic/Scholarly.* **Description:** Each issue covers a development in or new application of a radiologic technology.
Indexed: CINAHL.
—BLDSC (8239.457350), GNLM, Infotrieve. **CCC.**
Published by: W.B. Saunders Co. (Subsidiary of: Harcourt Publishers Ltd.), 11830 Westline Industrial Dr, St Louis, MO 63146. TEL 800-325-4177, http://www.seminarinradiologictechnology.com, http://www.wbsaunders.com. Ed. Jeffrey Papp. adv.: B&W page USD 640, color page USD 1,690; trim 10 x 7. Circ: 3,215. **Subscr. to:** Periodicals Fulfillment, W B Saunders Co, 6277 Sea Harbor Dr, 4th Fl, Orlando, FL 32891-4800.

SEMINARS IN RESPIRATORY INFECTIONS. see *MEDICAL SCIENCES—Respiratory Diseases*

615.842 USA ISSN 0037-198X
RC78 CODEN: SEROAF
SEMINARS IN ROENTGENOLOGY. Text in English. 1966. q. USD 160 domestic to individuals; USD 229 foreign to individuals; USD 257 domestic to institutions; USD 311 foreign to institutions; USD 83 domestic to students; USD 137 foreign to students; USD 78 newsstand/cover (effective 2001). adv. bibl, charts, illus. *Refereed.* **Document type:** *Journal, Academic/Scholarly.* **Description:** Designed for the practicing radiologist, each issue covers a single topic of current importance.
Related titles: Online - full text ed.: (from Institute for Scientific Information).
Indexed: ASCA, Aqua.Sci.& Fish.Abstr., Bibl.Dev.Med.& Child Neur., Biol.Abstr., CINAHL, Curr.Cont., Dent.Ind., Excerp.Med., INIS Atomind., Ind.Imag.Lit., Ind.Med. (1966-), Ind.Sci.Rev., Inpharma, Reac., Rev.Med.& Vet.Mycol., Sci.Cit.Ind.
—BLDSC (8239.460000), GNLM, IDS, ingenta, KNAW. **CCC.**
Published by: W.B. Saunders Co. (Subsidiary of: Harcourt Publishers Ltd.), 11830 Westline Industrial Dr, St Louis, MO 63146. TEL 800-325-4177, http://www.wbsaunders.com. Ed. Dr. Wallace T Miller. adv.: B&W page USD 1,000, color page USD 2,100; trim 10 x 7. Circ: 3,504. **Subscr. to:** Periodicals Fulfillment, W B Saunders Co, 6277 Sea Harbor Dr, 4th Fl, Orlando, FL 32891-4800.

615.842 USA ISSN 0887-2171
RC78.7.U4 CODEN: SEULDO
SEMINARS IN ULTRASOUND, C T AND M R. (Computerized Tomography and Magnetic Resonance) Variant title: Seminars in Ultrasound, C T and M R I. Text in English. 1980. bi-m. USD 175 domestic to individuals; USD 261 foreign to individuals; USD 254 domestic to institutions; USD 324 foreign to institutions; USD 82 domestic to students; USD 157 foreign to students; USD 55 newsstand/cover (effective 2001). adv. bibl, charts, illus. index. back issues avail. *Refereed.* **Document type:** *Journal, Academic/Scholarly.* **Description:** New concepts and research findings for physicians involved in the performance and interpretation of ultrasound.
Formerly (until 1984): Seminars in Ultrasound (0194-1720)
Related titles: Online - full text ed.: (from Institute for Scientific Information).
Indexed: ASCA, Biol.Abstr., CINAHL, Curr.Cont., Ind.Imag.Lit., Ind.Med. (1984-), Inpharma, Pharm.&Out.News, Reac., Rev.Med.& Vet.Mycol.
—BLDSC (8239.485505), CISTI, EMDOCS, GNLM, IDS, ingenta, KNAW. **CCC.**
Published by: W.B. Saunders Co. (Subsidiary of: Harcourt Publishers Ltd.), 11830 Westline Industrial Dr, St Louis, MO 63146. TEL 800-325-4177, http://www.wbsaunders.com. Eds. Dr. Howard Raymond, Dr. Joel D Schwartz, Dr. William J Zwiebel. adv.: B&W page USD 950, color page USD 2,050. Circ: 4,242. **Subscr. to:** Periodicals Fulfillment, W B Saunders Co, 6277 Sea Harbor Dr, 4th Fl, Orlando, FL 32891-4800.

616.842 NLD ISSN 0167-465X
SERIES IN RADIOLOGY. Text in English. 1979. irreg., latest vol.22, 1991. price varies. *Refereed.* **Document type:** *Monographic series.*
—BLDSC (8250.200500), CISTI, KNAW.
Published by: Kluwer Academic Publishers Group (Subsidiary of: Wolters Kluwer N.V.), Spuiboulevard 50, PO Box 17, Dordrecht 3300 AA, Netherlands. FAX 31-78-639-2254, services@wkap.nl, http://www.wkap.nl. **Dist. by:** Journals Department, PO Box 322, Dordrecht 3300 AH, Netherlands. FAX 31-78-654-6474.

615.842 NZL ISSN 1170-9758
SHADOWS; journal of the New Zealand Institute of Medical Radiation Technology. Text in English. 1958. q. NZD 67.50. adv. bk.rev. **Document type:** *Trade.* **Description:** Covers new technologies and techniques in radiology in New Zealand. Issues of importance to New Zealand MRTs are also discussed.
Published by: New Zealand Institute of Medical Radiation Technology, 637 Remuera Rd, Auckland, 5, New Zealand. TEL 64-9-5206753, FAX 64-9-5249920. Ed., R&P Coralie Christie. Circ: 800. **Subscr. to:** NZIMER, P.O. Box 4011, Nelson, New Zealand. TEL 64-3-5432097, FAX 64-3-5432273.

SHIKA HOSHASEN. see *MEDICAL SCIENCES—Dentistry*

618 DEU ISSN 0364-2348
SKELETAL RADIOLOGY; journal of radiology, pathology and orthopaedics. Text in English. 1976. m. DEM 1,337.20 domestic; DEM 1,352.80 foreign (effective 2001). adv. bk.rev. charts, illus. index. reprint service avail. from ISI. *Refereed.* **Document type:** *Journal, Academic/Scholarly.* **Description:** Covers the anatomical, pathological, physiological, clinical, metabolic, and epidemiological aspects of the many entities affecting the skeleton.
Related titles: Microfilm ed.: (from PQC); Online - full text ed.: ISSN 1432-2161 (from EBSCO Publishing, RoweCom Information Quest, Swets Blackwell, Springer LINK, Institute for Scientific Information).
Indexed: ASCA, Bibl.Dev.Med.& Child Neur., Cal.Tiss.Abstr., Curr.Adv.Cancer Res., Curr.Cont., Dent.Ind., Environ.Sci.Poll.Mgmt., Excerp.Med., INIS Atomind., Ind.Imag.Lit., Ind.Med. (1976-), Ind.Sci.Rev., Inpharma, Int.Nurs.Ind., Pollut.Abstr., Reac., Rev.Med.& Vet.Mycol., Risk Abstr., Saf.Sci.Abstr., Sci.Cit.Ind., Tox.Abstr. (coverage dropped).
—BLDSC (8295.200000), CISTI, EMDOCS, GNLM, IDS, ingenta, KNAW. **CCC.**

M

Published by: (International Skeletal Society), Springer-Verlag (Subsidiary of: BertelsmannSpringer), Tiergartenstr 17, Heidelberg 69121, Germany. TEL 49-6221-345-0, FAX 49-6221-345229, subscriptions@springer.de, http://link.springer.de/link/service/journals/00256/index.htm, http://www.springer.de. Eds. I McCall, J J Kaye. **Subscr. in N. America to:** Springer-Verlag New York Inc., PO Box 2485, Secaucus, NJ 07096-2485. TEL 212-460-1500, FAX 212-473-6272.

SOLID STATE NUCLEAR MAGNETIC RESONANCE; an international journal. see *CHEMISTRY—Analytical Chemistry*

SPECTRUM (COLLINGWOOD). see *COMMUNICATIONS—Radio*

615.842 DEU ISSN 0179-7158 CODEN: STONE4

STRAHLENTHERAPIE UND ONKOLOGIE; Zeitschrift fuer Radiologie, Strahlenbiologie, Strahlenphysik. Text and summaries in English, German. 1912. m. EUR 399.24 domestic; EUR 413.24 foreign; EUR 202.98 domestic to students; EUR 216.98 foreign to students; EUR 45.79 newsstand/cover (effective 2002). adv. bk.rev. bibl, charts, illus. index, cum.index: vols.1-125 (in 5 vols.). back issues avail. *Refereed.* **Document type:** *Journal, Academic/Scholarly.*

Formerly: Strahlentherapie; Zeitschrift fuer Radiologie und Onkologie (0039-2073)

Related titles: Microform ed.: (from PMC); Online - full text ed.: ISSN 1439-099X (from EBSCO Publishing, RoweCom Information Quest, Swets Blackwell, Springer LINK, Institute for Scientific Information).

Indexed: ASCA, Biol.Abstr., Chem.Abstr., Curr.Cont., Excerp.Med., INIS Atomind., Ind.Med. (1986-), Inpharma, Int.Nurs.Ind., Nutr.Abstr., Pharm.&Out.News, Reac.

—BLDSC (8470.010000), CASDDS, CISTI, GNLM, IDS, KNAW. **CCC.**

Published by: (Deutsche Roentgen Gesellschaft, Deutsche Gesellschaft fuer Radioonkologie), Urban und Vogel Medien und Medizin Verlagsgesellschaft mbH (Subsidiary of: BertelsmannSpringer), Neumarkter Str 43, Munich 81673, Germany. TEL 49-89-43721300, FAX 49-89-43721399, verlag@urban-vogel.de, http://www.urban-vogel.de. Ed. Dr. R Sauer. Adv. contact Sibylle Schurr TEL 49-89-43721353. Circ: 2,200. **Subscr. to:** Springer Auslieferungs Gesellschaft, Postfach 105160, Heidelberg 69041, Germany. TEL 49-6221-345244, FAX 49-6221-345244. **Co-sponsors:** Deutsche Gesellschaft fuer Medizinische Physik; Arbeitsgemeinschaft Radioonkologie (ARO) der Deutschen Krebsgesellschaft; Deutsche und Oesterreichische Gesellsch.

SURGICAL AND RADIOLOGIC ANATOMY. see *MEDICAL SCIENCES*

615.842 GBR ISSN 1360-5518 CODEN: RATOEO

SYNERGY; representing radiographers, promoting radiography. Text in English. 1988. m. GBP 56 in Europe to individuals; USD 100 elsewhere to individuals; GBP 112 in Europe to institutions; USD 200 elsewhere to institutions (effective 2000). adv. bk.rev. charts, illus. index. reprints avail. *Refereed.* **Document type:** *Academic/Scholarly.* **Description:** Reports original clinical and scientific research in all aspects of the field.

Formerly (until 1995): Radiography Today (0954-8211); Which was formed by the merger of (1935-1988): Radiography (0033-8281); (1979-1988): Radiography News (0144-5510)

Indexed: Biol.Abstr., CINAHL, Curr.Adv.Ecol.Sci., INIS Atomind., Ind.Med. (coverage dropped).

—BLDSC (8585.934600), CISTI, GNLM, ingenta, Linda Hall.

Published by: (Society and College of Radiographers), A F L Deeson Partnership Ltd., Ewell Hosue, Faversham, Kent ME13 8UP, United Kingdom. TEL 44-1795-535468, FAX 44-1795-535469, sdeeson@worldscope.co.uk. Ed. Rachel Hewitt. Adv. contact Julie Billings. Circ: 17,000.

616.07 USA ISSN 1089-2516 CODEN: TVIRFC

TECHNIQUES IN VASCULAR AND INTERVENTIONAL RADIOLOGY. Text in English. 1998. q. USD 146 domestic to individuals; USD 175 foreign to individuals; USD 188 domestic to institutions; USD 218 foreign to institutions; USD 103 domestic to students; USD 105 foreign to students; USD 55 newsstand/cover (effective 2001). adv. illus. **Document type:** *Academic/Scholarly.* **Description:** Presentations in each issue focus on a single clinical technique or problem. Illustrations and a descriptive narrative outline the steps of a particular procedure of interest to interventional surgeons and radiologists.

—BLDSC (8745.407000). **CCC.**

Published by: W.B. Saunders Co. (Subsidiary of: Harcourt Publishers Ltd.), 11830 Westline Industrial Dr, St Louis, MO 63146. TEL 800-325-4177, http://www.wbsaunders.com. Eds. Dr. Barry T Katzon, Charles P Semba. adv.: B&W page USD 690, color page USD 1,690. Circ: 1,402. **Subscr. to:** Periodicals Fulfillment, W B Saunders Co, 6277 Sea Harbor Dr, 4th Fl, Orlando, FL 32891-4800.

615.8 NLD ISSN 1381-4842 CODEN: VNGTD6

TIJDSCHRIFT VOOR NUCLEAIRE GENEESKUNDE. Text in Dutch; Text occasionally in English; Summaries in English. 1995. q. NLG 77.50 domestic to non-members; NLG 97.50 foreign to non-members (effective 2001). adv. bk.rev. abstr. *Refereed.* **Document type:** *Journal, Academic/Scholarly.* **Description:** Reports on developments in nuclear medicine and related subjects.

Formed by the merger of (1978-1995): Vangnet (0921-2574); (1979-1995): N G B (Nucleair Geneeskundig Bulletin) (0169-1279); Which incorporates: Nederlandse Vereniging voor Nucleaire Geneeskunde. Mededelingen

Indexed: INIS Atomind.

—CASDDS, KNAW.

Published by: Stichting ter Bevordering van de Nucleaire Geneeskunde, c/o Paula A Boeijen, Ouderkerkerdijk 37, Amsterdam 1096 CR, Netherlands. TEL 31-20-665-7723, paola@euronet.nl. Ed. Dr. J W van Isselt. R&P Paula A Boeijen. Adv. contact J A K Blokland TEL 31-71-526-3485. Circ: 1,300 (paid). **Co-sponsors:** Nederlandse Vereniging voor Nucleaire Geneeskunde; Vereniging voor Medisch-Nucleair (VANG); Belgisch Genootschap voor Nucleaire Geneeskunde (BGNG).

616.842 USA

TOPICS IN DIAGNOSTIC RADIOLOGY AND ADVANCED IMAGING. Text in English. 1993. s-a. USD 100 to non-members; USD 75 to members. back issues avail. **Document type:** *Academic/Scholarly.* **Description:** Contains articles on diagnostic imaging (radiology and thermology) to educate chiropractic physicians (radiologists) and others.

Formerly: Roentgenological Briefs

Published by: American Chiropractic Association, Inc., Council on Diagnostic Imaging, PO Box 25, Palatine, IL 60078-0025. FAX 708-705-1178, cdisec@aol.com, http://www.dacbr.com. Ed., R&P Dr. John Stites. Pub. Mary Ruth. Circ: 2,000 (paid). **Co-sponsor:** American Chiropractic College of Radiology, American Chiropractic College of Thermology.

616 USA ISSN 0899-3459 CODEN: TMRIEY

TOPICS IN MAGNETIC RESONANCE IMAGING. Text in English. 1989. bi-m., latest vol.12. USD 258 domestic to individuals; USD 288 foreign to individuals; USD 330 domestic to institutions; USD 380 foreign to institutions; USD 58 newsstand/cover (effective 2002). adv. illus. index. back issues avail. *Refereed.* **Document type:** *Academic/Scholarly.* **Description:** Discusses practical clinical applications of MRI to the entire body, including the brain, spine, extracranial organs, and the musculoskeletal system.

Related titles: Microform ed.; Online - full text ed.: USD 429 domestic for academic site license; USD 479 foreign for academic site license; USD 478.50 domestic for corporate site license; USD 528.50 foreign for corporate site license (effective 2002) (from Ovid Technologies, Inc.).

Indexed: ASCA, Curr.Cont. (coverage dropped), Excerp.Med., INSPEC (Feb.1998-Feb.1999, dropped), Ind.Med. (1988-), Ind.Sci.Rev., Inpharma, Reac.

—BLDSC (8867.459300), CISTI, EMDOCS, GNLM, IDS, KNAW.

Published by: Lippincott Williams & Wilkins (Philadelphia) (Subsidiary of: Wolters Kluwer N.V.), 530 Walnut St, Philadelphia, PA 19106-3621. TEL 215-521-8300, FAX 215-521-8902, http://www.topicsinmri.com, http://www.lww.com. Eds. Dr. Donald Mitchell, Dr. Michael Brant-Zawadzki, Dr. Robert Elderman. Pub. Karen Phillips. R&P Margaret Becker. Adv. contact Ray Thibodeau. B&W page USD 640, color page USD 1,665; trim 11 x 8.25. Circ: 2,482. **Subscr. to:** PO Box 1600, Hagerstown, MD 21740-1600. TEL 800-777-2295, FAX 301-824-7390.

615.842 USA ISSN 1073-0206

TRACERS. Text in English. 1985. a. back issues avail. **Document type:** *Newsletter.* **Description:** Information regarding specialty of nuclear medicine and certification.

Published by: American Board of Nuclear Medicine, 900 Veteran Ave, Los Angeles, CA 90024. TEL 310-825-6787, FAX 310-794-4821. Ed. William H Blahd. Circ: 3,900.

616.07 USA

U.S. NUCLEAR REGULATORY COMMISSION. RULES AND REGULATIONS FOR MEDICAL LICENSEES. Text in English. base vol. plus irreg. updates. USD 354 (effective 2001). **Document type:** *Government.* **Description:** Contains information from "Nuclear Regulatory Commission Rules and Regulations", Parts 19, 20, 30, 32, 33, and 35.

Published by: U.S. Nuclear Regulatory Commission, 1 White Flint North Bldg, 11555 Rockville Pike, Rockville, MD 20852-2738. http://www.nrc.gov/. **Subscr. to:** U.S. Government Printing Office, Superintendent of Documents, PO Box 371954, Pittsburgh, PA 15250-7954. TEL 202-512-1800, FAX 202-512-2250, orders@gpo.gov, http://www.access.gpo.gov.

616.07 UKR

UKRAINS'KYI RADIOLOHICHNYI ZHURNAL. Text in Ukrainian; Abstracts in English, Russian; Contents page in English, Ukrainian. 1993. q. USD 30 for 2 yrs. domestic; USD 75 foreign (effective 2000). adv. *Refereed.* **Document type:** *Academic/Scholarly.* **Description:** Includes articles on diagnostic and therapeutic radiology, radiation oncology, radiobiology, and radiation protection, including related problems at Chernobyl.

Published by: Instytut Medychnoi Radiologii im. S.P. Hrihor'eva, Vul Pushkins'ka 82, Kharkov, Ukraine. TEL 380-572-431542, 380-572-430557, 380-572-454028, FAX 380-572-431125, imr@online.kharkiv.net. Ed. Mykola I Pylypenko. Adv. contact Dr. Natalia Mitryayeva. page USD 100. **US dist. addr.:** East View Publications, 3020 Harbor Ln N, Minneapolis, MN 55447. TEL 612-550-0961.

616.07 500 USA ISSN 0161-7346
RC78.7.U4 CODEN: ULIMD4

ULTRASONIC IMAGING; an international journal. Text in English. 1979. q. USD 182 in US & Canada; USD 232 elsewhere. adv. index. back issues avail. *Refereed.* **Document type:** *Academic/Scholarly.* **Description:** Covers the development and application of ultrasonic techniques, with emphasis on medical diagnosis.

Related titles: Online - full text ed.: (from EBSCO Publishing, ingenta, IDEAL Online Library, Institute for Scientific Information).

Indexed: ASCA, CINAHL, Curr.Cont., INSPEC (Jul.1979-), Ind.Med. (1979-), Sci.Cit.Ind.

—BLDSC (9082.787000), AskIEEE, CISTI, GNLM, IDS, ingenta. **CCC.**

Published by: Dynamedia, Inc., 2 Fulham Court, Silver Spring, MD 20902. TEL 301-649-3447, 800-468-4680, FAX 301-649-3447. Ed. Melvin Linzer.

616.07 POL

ULTRASONOGRAFIA. Text in Polish. 1991. irreg. *Refereed.* **Document type:** *Academic/Scholarly.*

Formerly (until 1998): Ultrasonografia Polska (0867-3845)

Published by: Polskie Towarzystwo Ultrasonograficzne, c/o Zaklad Diagnostyki Obrazowej, Woj. Szpital Brodnowski, Ul Kondratowicza 8, Warsaw 03242, Poland. TEL 48-22-8119677, FAX 48-22-8119591, usgptuwj@euroson.edu.pl. Eds. Wieslaw Jakubovski, Zbigniew Kalina.

ULTRASOUND IN OBSTETRICS & GYNECOLOGY. see *MEDICAL SCIENCES—Obstetrics And Gynecology*

615.842 USA ISSN 0894-8771
RC78.7.U4 CODEN: ULQUEZ
ULTRASOUND QUARTERLY. Text in English. 1983. q., latest vol.17. USD 185 domestic to individuals; USD 226 foreign to individuals; USD 273 domestic to institutions; USD 305 foreign to institutions; USD 70 newsstand/cover (effective 2002). adv. charts, illus. reprint service avail. from PQC. *Refereed.* **Document type:** *Academic/Scholarly.* **Description:** Publishes original articles on diagnostic information obtained by recent technological advances, and discussions of fundamental or controversial subjects.
Formerly (until 1989): Ultrasound Annual (0888-8264)
Related titles: Online - full text ed.: USD 354.90 domestic for academic site license; USD 386.90 foreign for academic site license; USD 395.85 domestic for corporate site license; USD 427.85 foreign for corporate site license (effective 2002).
—BLDSC (9082.815550), EMDOCS, GNLM, KNAW.
Published by: Lippincott Williams & Wilkins (Philadelphia) (Subsidiary of: Wolters Kluwer N.V.), 530 Walnut St, Philadelphia, PA 19106-3621. TEL 215-521-8300, FAX 215-521-8902, http://www.ultrasound-quarterly.com, http://www.lww.com. Ed. Dr. Matthew Rifkin. Pub. Karen Phillips. R&P Margaret Becker. Adv. contact Ray Thibodeau. B&W page USD 700, color page USD 1,750. Circ: 1,000. **Subscr. to:** PO Box 1600, Hagerstown, MD 21740-1600. TEL 800-777-2295, FAX 301-824-7390.

UNIVERSITY OF TEXAS. M.D. ANDERSON CANCER CENTER. RESEARCH REPORT. see *MEDICAL SCIENCES—Oncology*

615.842 RUS ISSN 0042-4676
CODEN: VRRAAT
VESTNIK RENTGENOLOGII I RADIOLOGII/ANNALS OF ROENTGENOLOGY AND RADIOLOGY. Text in Russian; Summaries in English. 1920. bi-m. USD 159. adv. bk.rev. bibl. index. **Description:** Publishes original papers devoted to elaboration on new methods of X-ray examination and updating the existing ones, their clinical use, problems of computer diagnosis in roentgenology, and more.
Indexed: Biol.Abstr., Chem.Abstr., Dent.Ind., Eng.Ind., Excerp.Med., INIS Atomind., Ind.Med. (1920-), Ref.Zh.
—CISTI, East View, GNLM, Infotrieve. **CCC.**
Published by: Nauchnoe Obshchestvo Rentgenologov i Radiologov, Cherepkovskaya 3-ya ul 15a, k 4, Moscow 121552, Russian Federation. TEL 7-095-4146314. Ed. A P Savchenko. Adv. contact L N Druzhinina. **Dist. by:** Mezhdunarodnaya Kniga, B Yakimanka 39, Moscow 117049, Russian Federation. TEL 7-095-2384967, FAX 7-095-2384634; **US dist. addr.:** East View Publications, 3020 Harbor Ln N, Minneapolis, MN 55447. TEL 612-550-0961.

615.842 618 USA ISSN 1052-2182
VIDEO JOURNAL OF COLOR FLOW IMAGING. Text in English. 1987. q. USD 250; USD 275 in Canada; USD 295 in Japan; USD 335 elsewhere. adv. back issues avail. *Refereed.* **Document type:** *Academic/Scholarly.* **Description:** Covers ultrasound imaging. Consists of tutorials, reviews, case reports and original research.
Supersedes in part (in 1991): Dynamic Cardiovascular Imaging (0891-9313)
—GNLM, Infotrieve. **CCC.**
Published by: Dynamedia, Inc., 2 Fulham Court, Silver Spring, MD 20902. TEL 301-649-6886, FAX 301-649-3447. Eds. C R B Merritt, D E Strandness. Circ: 1,000.

615.84 612.014 USA
VIEWBOX. Text in English. 4/yr.
Formerly: American Osteopathic College of Radiology. Newsletter. (0065-9576)
Published by: American Osteopathic College of Radiology, 119 E 2nd St, Milan, MO 63556. TEL 800-258-2627. Circ: 400.

618 570 RUS ISSN 0302-556X
VOPROSY RADIOBIOLOGII I BIOLOGICHESKOGO DEISTVIYA TSITOSTATICHESKIKH PREPARATOV. Text in Russian. 1969. irreg. bibl, illus.
Published by: (Tomskii Meditsinskii Institut, Tsentral'naya Nauchno-Issledovatel'skaya Laboratoriya), Izdatel'stvo Tomskii Universitet, Pr-t Lenina 36, Tomsk, 10, Russian Federation.

WOMEN'S IMAGING; the journal of breast imaging. see *MEDICAL SCIENCES—Obstetrics And Gynecology*

615.84 USA ISSN 0098-1672
RC78 CODEN: YBDRE3
THE YEAR BOOK OF DIAGNOSTIC RADIOLOGY. Text in English. 1932. a. USD 95 domestic; USD 101 foreign (effective 2001). illus. reprints avail. **Document type:** *Academic/Scholarly, Abstract/Index.* **Description:** Presents abstracts of pertinent literature with commentary by leading experts in the field.
Formerly (until 1975): Year Book of Radiology (0084-3989)
Related titles: CD-ROM ed.
Indexed: Curr.Adv.Ecol.Sci.
—BLDSC (9411.629000), CISTI, GNLM.
Published by: Mosby, Inc., Continuity Division (Subsidiary of: Harcourt Health Sciences), 11830 Westline Industrial Dr, St Louis, MO 63146-3313. TEL 314-872-8370, 800-325-4177, FAX 314-432-1380, http://www.mosby.com/periodicals. Ed. Dr. Anne G Osborn.

615.8 USA ISSN 0084-3903
RC93.A1 CODEN: YNUMAH
THE YEAR BOOK OF NUCLEAR MEDICINE. Text in English. 1966. a. USD 99 domestic; USD 105 foreign (effective 2001). illus. **Document type:** *Abstract/Index, Academic/Scholarly.* **Description:** Presents abstracts of pertinent literature with commentary by leading experts in the field.
Related titles: CD-ROM ed.
Indexed: Curr.Adv.Ecol.Sci.
—CISTI, GNLM.
Published by: Mosby, Inc., Continuity Division (Subsidiary of: Harcourt Health Sciences), 11830 Westline Industrial Dr, St Louis, MO 63146-3313. TEL 314-872-8370, 800-325-4177, FAX 314-432-1380, http://www.mosby.com/periodicals. Ed. Dr. Alexander Gottschalk.

615.842 CHN ISSN 1001-6384
YINGXIANG YIXUE/MEDICAL IMAGING. Text in Chinese. 1988. s-a. USD 10. adv. bk.rev.
Published by: Tianjin Di'er Yixueyuan/Tianjin No. 2 Medical Academy, 1 Guangdong Lu, Tianjin 300203, China. TEL 395086. Ed. Wu Enhui. **Co-sponsor:** Japan Association of Radiological Technologists.

615.842 DEU ISSN 0722-5067
ZEITSCHRIFT FUER CHEMOTHERAPIE. Text in German. 1980. 6/yr. DEM 54 (effective 2000). back issues avail. **Document type:** *Magazine, Academic/Scholarly.*
—GNLM.
Address: c/o Prof. Hartmut Lode, Eichenallee 36A, Berlin 14050, Germany. TEL 49-30-3125059, FAX 49-30-3124742. Ed. Dr. Ralf Stahlmann.

616.075 CHN ISSN 1002-0101
CODEN: ZCYZEE
ZHONGGUO CHAOSHENG YIXUE ZAZHI/CHINESE JOURNAL OF ULTRASOUND IN MEDICINE. Text in Chinese; Summaries in English. 1985. m. USD 180, USD 216 (effective 2001). bk.rev. illus. *Refereed.* **Document type:** *Academic/Scholarly.* **Description:** Discusses issues of interest to ultrasound radiologists in all areas of medicine.
Related titles: E-mail ed.
—BLDSC (3180.687000).
Published by: Chinese Information Center of Ultrasound Diagnosis, No.9 xiao Ying Rd, Chao Yang District, Beijing 100101, China. TEL 86-10-64935887, FAX 86-10-64941874, caume@public.bta.net.cn. Ed., R&P Wanxue Guo TEL 86-1-64902637. Adv. contact Jianxun Wang. **Dist. overseas by:** China International Book Trading Corp, 35, Chegongzhuang Xilu, Haidian District, Beijing 100044, China. TEL 86-1-68413849, FAX 86-1-68412048, cibtc@mail.cibtc.com.cn, http://www.cibtc.com.cn.

615.842 CHN ISSN 1003-3289
ZHONGGUO YIXUE YINGXIANG JISHU/CHINESE JOURNAL OF MEDICAL IMAGING TECHNOLOGY. Text in Chinese. 1985. bi-m. CNY 120 domestic; USD 75.60 foreign; CNY 10 newsstand/cover domestic; USD 6.30 newsstand/cover foreign (effective 2001). adv. back issues avail. **Document type:** *Academic/Scholarly.* **Description:** Contains research papers on the new developments of medical equipments in the field of medical imaging technology.
Related titles: Online - full content ed.: (from WanFang Data Corp.).
Indexed: INSPEC (2000-).
Published by: (Zhongguo Kexueyuan/Chinese Academy of Sciences, Zhongguo Kejian Youxian Gongsi), Zhongguo Yixue Yingxiang Jishu Bianjibu, PO Box 2712, Beijing 100080, China. TEL 86-1-6253-6197, FAX 86-1-6254-2307. Ed. Zhuchun Tao. **Dist. by:** China International Book Trading Corp, 35, Chegongzhuang Xilu, Haidian District, Beijing 100044, China. TEL 86-1-68413849, FAX 86-1-68412048, cibtc@mail.cibtc.com.cn, http://www.cibtc.com.cn.

616.075 CHN ISSN 1004-4477
ZHONGHUA CHAOSHENG YINGXIANGXUE ZAZHI/CHINESE JOURNAL OF ULTRASONOGRAPHY. Text in Chinese; Abstracts in English. 1992. bi-m. CNY 27 (effective 1999). 56 p./no. *Refereed.* **Document type:** *Academic/Scholarly.* **Description:** Covers new developments in theories and applications of ultrasonic diagnosis.
Related titles: CD-ROM ed.
Published by: (Zhonghua Yixuehui/Chinese Medical Association), Hebei Yike Daxue/Hebei Medical University, 361 Zhongshan Donglu, Shijiazhuang, Hebei 050017, China. TEL 86-311-6059153, FAX 86-311-6059153, hebydqks@public.sj.he.cn, WL@hebmu.edu.cn. Ed. Jinxi Zhang. adv.: B&W page CNY 6,000, color page CNY 12,000. Circ: 12,000. **Dist. overseas by:** China International Book Trading Corp, 35 Chegongzhuang Xilu, Haidian District, Beijing 100044, China.

616.07 CHN ISSN 0254-5098
ZHONGHUA FANGSHE YIXUE YU FANGHU ZAZHI/CHINESE JOURNAL OF RADIOLOGICAL MEDICINE AND PROTECTION. Text in Chinese. 1981. bi-m. CNY 60 domestic; USD 50 foreign; CNY 10 newsstand/cover domestic; USD 4.20 newsstand/cover foreign (effective 2001). **Document type:** *Academic/Scholarly.*
Related titles: Online - full content ed.: (from WanFang Data Corp.).
—BLDSC (3180.650000).
Address: 2, Dewai Xinkang Jie, Beijing 100088, China. TEL 86-1-62389620, eoj@mail.nrmpin.ac.cn. Pub. Hanmin Zhu. **Dist. by:** China International Book Trading Corp, 35, Chegongzhuang Xilu, Haidian District, Beijing 100044, China. TEL 86-1-68413849, FAX 86-1-68412048, cibtc@mail.cibtc.com.cn, http://www.cibtc.com.cn.

616.07 CHN ISSN 1005-1201
ZHONGHUA FANGSHEXUA ZAZHI/CHINESE JOURNAL OF RADIOLOGY. Text in Chinese. m. USD 75.60 foreign; CNY 141.60 domestic; USD 6.30 newsstand/cover foreign; CNY 11.80 newsstand/cover domestic (effective 2001). adv. 80 p./no. *Refereed.* **Document type:** *Academic/Scholarly.*
Related titles: Online - full content ed.: (from WanFang Data Corp.).
—BLDSC.
Published by: Zhonghua Yixuehui Zazhishe, 42 Dongsi Xidajie, Beijing 100710, China. TEL 86-1-65271225, cmazzs@public.sti.ac.cn, cnjr.editor@bj.col.com.cn, cmafs@public.sti.ac.cn. Ed. Yuji Gao. adv.: page USD 1,700; 200 x 290. Circ: 30,000 (paid); 100 (controlled).
Co-sponsor: Chinese Medical Association.

MEDICAL SCIENCES—Respiratory Diseases

616.2 USA ISSN 0893-8520
CODEN: AATIEN
A A R C TIMES. Text in English. 1977. m. USD 65. adv. reprints avail. **Description:** Presents news and features for the cardiorespiratory care profession.
Formerly: A A R Times (0195-1777)
Related titles: Microfilm ed.: (from PQC).
Indexed: CINAHL.
—BLDSC (0537.535500), CISTI, Infotrieve. **CCC.**
Published by: (American Association for Respiratory Care), Daedalus Enterprises, Inc., 11030 Ables Lane, Dallas, TX 75229. TEL 972-243-2272, FAX 972-484-6010. Ed. Marsha Cathcart. Circ: 37,000.

A S D A NEWS. see *MEDICAL SCIENCES—Psychiatry And Neurology*

616.2 USA ISSN 0892-8916
A T S NEWS. Text in English. 1975. m. membership only. cum.index. **Document type:** *Newsletter.*
Published by: American Thoracic Society, 1740 Broadway, New York, NY 10019-4374. TEL 212-315-6440, FAX 212-315-6455, http://www.thoracic.org. Ed. Lori Atkins. R&P Christina Shephard. Circ: 13,000.

615.64 USA ISSN 1096-6307
ADVANCE FOR MANAGERS OF RESPIRATORY CARE. Text in English. 1992. m. free to qualified professionals. adv. bk.rev., software rev., video rev. charts, illus, tr.lit. index. *Refereed.* **Description:** Reports regularly to management on news in staffing, clinical practice and theory, financial issues, restructuring managed care and disease management.

M

Published by: Merion Publications, Inc., 2900 Horizon Dr, PO Box 61556, King Of Prussia, PA 19406. TEL 610-265-7812, 800-355-5627, FAX 610-278-1421, advance@merion.com, http://www.advanceweb.com. Ed. Sharlene Sephton. Pub. Ann Kielinski. Adv. contact Judy Thwaite. B&W page USD 2,437, color page USD 2,737; trim 10.88 x 8.38.

615 USA ISSN 1074-2301
ADVANCE FOR RESPIRATORY CARE PRACTITIONERS. Text in English. bi-w. *Refereed.* **Document type:** *Trade.*
Published by: Merion Publications, Inc., 2900 Horizon Dr, PO Box 61556, King Of Prussia, PA 19406. TEL 610-278-1400, 800-355-5627, FAX 610-278-1421, advance@merion.com, http://www.advanceweb.com. Ed. Vern Enge. Pub. Ann Kielinski. adv.: B&W page USD 2,437, color page USD 2,737; trim 10.88 x 8.38. Circ: 42,900.

616.2 CAN ISSN 1187-9106
AIRWAVE✻. Text in English. 1974. 3/yr. free per issue. adv. stat. back issues avail. **Document type:** *Newsletter.* **Description:** Keeps MLA program users, donors and volunteers up-to-date regarding organization activities.
Formerly (until 1989): Easy Breathing (0315-2421)
Published by: (Manitoba Lung Association), Idea Marketing Group, 629 McDermot Ave, Winnipeg, MB R3A 1P6, Canada. TEL 204-774-5501, FAX 204-772-5083. Ed. Linda Sawchuk. Circ: 5,000.

ALLERGY & ASTHMA ADVOCATE. see *MEDICAL SCIENCES—Allergology And Immunology*

616.2 USA ISSN 1073-449X
RC306 CODEN: AJCMED
AMERICAN JOURNAL OF RESPIRATORY AND CRITICAL CARE MEDICINE. Text in English. 1917. m. USD 160 to individuals; USD 290 to institutions (effective 2001). adv. bk.rev. abstr, bibl, charts, illus, stat. index, cum.index. back issues avail.; reprint service avail. from PQC. *Refereed.* **Document type:** *Academic/Scholarly.* **Description:** Original articles, case reports and notes on significant work in every aspect of disease of the respiratory tract.
Former titles (until 1994): American Review of Respiratory Disease (0003-0805); (until 1959): American Review of Tuberculosis and Pulmonary Diseases (0096-039X); (until 1955): American Review of Tuberculosis (0096-0381)
Related titles: Microform ed.: (from PQC,PMC); Online - full text ed.: (from HighWire Pr., EBSCO Publishing, Institute for Scientific Information).
Indexed: AIDS Abstr., AIM, AMED, ASCA, Abstr.Hyg., Abstr.Inter.Med., Agri.& Environ.Biotech.Abstr. (coverage dropped), Behav.Med.Abstr., Biol.Abstr., Biol.Dig., CINAHL, C.I.S. Abstr., Chem.Abstr., Curr.Adv.Cell & Devel.Biol., Curr.Adv.Ecol.Sci., Curr.Adv.Gen.& Molec.Biol., Curr.Cont., Dairy Sci.Abstr., Dent.Ind., Derwent Biotech.Abstr., Energy Ind., Energy Info.Abstr., Environ.Sci.Poll.Mgmt., Excerp.Med., Forest Prod.Abstr., Helminthol.Abstr., Hosp.Lit.Ind., INIS Atomind., Ind.Med. (1994-), Ind.Sci.Rev., Ind.Vet., Inpharma, Int.Abstr.Biol.Sci., Int.Nurs.Ind., Jrnl.Watch, Jrnl.Watch Inf.Dis., Lab.Haz.Bull., Microbiol.Abstr., Neurosci.Cit.Ind., Nutr.Abstr., Ocean.Abstr. (coverage dropped), Pharm.&Out.News, Pollut.Abstr., Protozool.Abstr., Reac., Rev.Appl.Entomol., Rev.Med.& Vet.Mycol., Rev.Plant Path., Risk Abstr., SSCI (coverage dropped), Saf.Sci.Abstr., Sci.Cit.Ind., THA, Trop.Dis.Bull., Vet.Bull., Weed Abstr.
—BLDSC (0836.590000), ADONIS, CASDDS, CISTI, EMDOCS, GNLM, IDS, Infotrieve, ingenta, KNAW. **CCC.**
Published by: (American Thoracic Society), American Lung Association, 1740 Broadway, New York, NY 10019-4374. TEL 212-315-8700, ajrccm-feedback@forsythe.stanford.edu, http://www.ajrccm.org/. Ed. Alan R Leff. Circ: 20,000 (paid and controlled).

616.2 USA ISSN 1044-1549
QP121.A1 CODEN: AJRBEL
AMERICAN JOURNAL OF RESPIRATORY CELL AND MOLECULAR BIOLOGY. Text in English. 1989. m. USD 125; USD 145 foreign (effective 1999). back issues avail. *Refereed.* **Description:** Publishes papers that report significant and original observations in the area of pulmonary biology.
Related titles: Online - full text ed.: (from HighWire Pr., EBSCO Publishing, ProQuest Information & Learning, Institute for Scientific Information).
Indexed: ASCA, BBCI, Chem.Abstr., Chem.Indus.Notes, Chem.Titles, Curr.Cont., INIS Atomind., Ind.Med. (1989-), Ind.Sci.Rev., Inpharma, Nutr.Abstr., Pharm.&Out.News, Reac., Rev.Med.& Vet.Mycol., Sci.Cit.Ind., THA.
—BLDSC (0836.600000), ADONIS, CASDDS, CISTI, GNLM, IDS, ingenta, KNAW. **CCC.**
Published by: (American Thoracic Society), American Lung Association, 1740 Broadway, New York, NY 10019-4374. TEL 212-315-8771, FAX 212-315-6498, cshepherd@lungusa.org, http://www.ajrcmb.org/.

616.2 JPN
ANNUAL REVIEW KOKYUKI/ANNUAL REVIEW. RESPIRATORY ORGAN. Text in Japanese. 1988. a. JPY 8,610 (effective 1998). adv. **Document type:** *Academic/Scholarly.*
Published by: Chugai Igakusha, 62 Yarai-cho, Shinjuku-ku, Tokyo 162-0805, Japan. R&P M Takahashi. Adv. contact M. Takahashi.

APPLIED CARDIOPULMONARY PATHOPHYSIOLOGY; the interface between laboratory and clinical practice. see *BIOLOGY—Physiology*

616.2 ARG ISSN 0004-0509
ARCHIVOS ARGENTINOS DE TISIOLOGIA Y NEUMONOLOGIA. Text in Spanish. 1924. q.
Formerly: Archivos de Tisiologia
Indexed: Biol.Abstr., Chem.Abstr.
Published by: Hospital Municipal Dr. Enrique Tornu, Sociedad de Tisiologia y Neumonologia, Hospital Tornu, Buenos Aires, Argentina.

616.2 ESP ISSN 0300-2896
CODEN: ARBRDA
ARCHIVOS DE BRONCONEUMOLOGIA. Text in Spanish; Summaries in English. m. (9/yr.). USD 113. adv. bk.rev. reprint service avail. from PQC. **Document type:** *Academic/Scholarly.* **Description:** Covers broncho-pneumology, respiratory immunology, biochemical studies of secretions, and pulmonary surgery.
Related titles: Online - full text ed.: (from Institute for Scientific Information).
Indexed: Excerp.Med., Ind.Med. (1964-), Ind.Med.Esp., Int.Nurs.Ind.
—CINDOC, EMDOCS, GNLM, Infotrieve, KNAW. **CCC.**
Published by: (Sociedad Espanola de Neumologia y Cirugia Toracica), Ediciones Doyma S.A., Traversa de Gracia, 17-21, Barcelona 08021, Spain. TEL 34-93-200-0711, FAX 34-93-209-1136. Ed. J Ruiz Manzano. Adv. contact Anna Pahissa. color page ESP 238,000; trim 280 x 210. Circ: 3,100.

616.246 BRA ISSN 0004-2765
ARQUIVOS BRASILEIROS DE TUBERCULOSE E DOENCAS DO TORAX. Summaries in English. 1938-1982; resumed 1987. q. per issue exchange basis. adv. bk.rev. bibl, charts, illus.
Formerly: I B I T Arquivos
Indexed: Biol.Abstr., Chem.Abstr.
—GNLM.
Published by: Instituto Brasileiro para Investigacao do Torax, Caixa Postal 635, Salvador, BA, Brazil. Ed. Jose Silveira. Circ: 1,000.

616.238 NZL
ASTHMA AND RESPIRATORY NEWS. Text in English. 1989. q. NZD 15 (effective 2001). 8 p./no. **Document type:** *Consumer.* **Description:** Provides the latest news and research on respiratory-tract diseases.
Former titles: Asthma in New Zealand; (until Sep. 1999): Asthma New Zealand (1170-1846)
Published by: Asthma and Respiratory Foundation of New Zealand, PO Box 1459, Wellington, New Zealand. TEL 64-4-499-4593, FAX 64—4-499-4594, arf@asthmanz.co.nz, http://www.asthmanz.co.nz. Ed. Kerry Hines. Circ: 12,000.

616.2 USA
ASTHMA: DISEASE STATE MANAGEMENT RESOURCE. Text in English. 1996. a., latest vol.4, 2000. USD 295 domestic; USD 325 foreign (effective 2001). **Document type:** *Trade.*
Published by: American Health Consultants (Subsidiary of: Medical Economics Co., Inc.), 3525 Piedmont Rd, N E, 6 Piedmont Center, Ste 400, Atlanta, GA 30305. TEL 404-262-5476, 404-262-7436, 800-688-2421, FAX 404-262-7837, 800-284-3291, custserv@ahcpub.com, http://www.ahcpub.com.

616.23 AUS
ASTHMA MATTERS. Text in English. 1964. q. AUD 20 (effective 2001). adv. bk.rev. back issues avail. **Document type:** *Newsletter, Consumer.* **Description:** Contains text published by the Asthma Foundation of N.S.W., a voluntary organization involved in research, welfare and education to assist people with asthma, their caregivers and the general community.
Formerly: Asthma Welfarer (0044-9776)
Published by: Asthma Foundation of New South Wales, Unit 1, 82-86 Pacific Hwy, St Leonards, NSW 2065, Australia. TEL 61-2-9906-3233, FAX 61-2-9906-4493. Ed. Richie Willcocks. R&P, Adv. contact Susie Lough. Circ: 5,000.

616.2 DEU ISSN 0341-3055
CODEN: ATLUDF
ATEMWEGS- UND LUNGENKRANKHEITEN. Text in German. 1975. m. DEM 258, EUR 131.91; DEM 28, EUR 14.32 newsstand/cover (effective 2001). adv. abstr. **Document type:** *Journal, Academic/Scholarly.*
Indexed: Biol.Abstr., Chem.Abstr., Chem.Indus.Notes, Chem.Titles, Curr.Adv.Ecol.Sci., Curr.Cont. (coverage dropped), Derwent Biotech.Abstr., Dok.Arbeitsmed., Excerp.Med., INIS Atomind., Ind.Sci.Rev., Inpharma, Reac., Ref.Zh., Sci.Cit.Ind. (coverage dropped).
—BLDSC (1765.856000), CASDDS, EMDOCS, GNLM, Infotrieve, KNAW. **CCC.**
Published by: Dustri-Verlag Dr. Karl Feistle, Bajuwarenring 4, Oberhaching 82041, Germany. TEL 49-89-613861-0, FAX 49-89-613-5412, info@dustri.de, http://www.dustri.de. Ed. Dr. D Nolte. R&P Renate Lehmann. Adv. contact Joerg Feistle. B&W page DEM 2,900, B&W page XEU 1,482.75; trim 167 x 242. Circ: 3,900.

AUSTRALIA. BUREAU OF STATISTICS. DEATHS DUE TO DISEASES AND CANCERS OF THE RESPIRATORY SYSTEM, AUSTRALIA. see *MEDICAL SCIENCES—Abstracting, Bibliographies, Statistics*

AUSTRALIA. BUREAU OF STATISTICS. NATIONAL HEALTH SURVEY: ASTHMA AND OTHER RESPIRATORY CONDITIONS, AUSTRALIA. see *MEDICAL SCIENCES—Abstracting, Bibliographies, Statistics*

616.2 USA ISSN 0005-6367
BATTING THE BREEZE✻. Text in English. 1965. bi-m. USD 15. adv. **Description:** Educational articles for patients with emphysema and other respiratory diseases.
Published by: Emphysema Anonymous, Inc., 327 34th Ave. N., Apt. 202, St. Petersburg, FL 33704-1352. TEL 813-391-9977. Ed. William E Jaeckle. Circ: 3,500.

616.2 USA
BRONCHIAL MUCOLOGY SERIES. Text in English. 1988. irreg. price varies. reprint service avail. from PQC. *Refereed.* **Document type:** *Monographic series.*
Published by: Lippincott Williams & Wilkins (Philadelphia) (Subsidiary of: Wolters Kluwer N.V.), 530 Walnut St, Philadelphia, PA 19106-3621. TEL 301-223-2300, 800-638-3030, FAX 301-223-2400.

616.2 RUS
BRONKHYAL'NAYA ASTMA I DRUGIE ALLERGICHESKIE ZABOLEVANIYA. Text in Russian. m. USD 175 in the Americas (effective 2000).
Published by: Vserossiiskii Institut Nauchnoi i Tekhnicheskoi Informatsii (VINITI), Usievicha ul 20-a, Moscow 125315, Russian Federation. TEL 7-095-1526441, FAX 7-095-943-0060. **Dist. by:** East View Publications, 3020 Harbor Ln N, Minneapolis, MN 55447. TEL 763-550-0961, FAX 763-559-2931.

616.2 378 USA
C C H S NEWS. Text in English. 1979. q. **Document type:** *Newsletter.* **Description:** Highlights current events at the college and in the field of respiratory care.
Related titles: Online - full text ed.
Published by: California College for Health Services, 222 W 24th St, National City, CA 91950-6605. TEL 619-477-4800, FAX 619-477-4360, cchsinfo@cchs.edu, http://www.cchs.edu. Ed. Cheryl Latif. Pub., R&P Scott Croydon. Circ: 8,000.

615.64 CAN ISSN 1205-9838
CODEN: CJRTFU
CANADIAN JOURNAL OF RESPIRATORY THERAPY/REVUE CANADIENNE DE LA THERAPIE RESPIRATOIRE. Short title: C J R T - R C T R. Text in English, French. 1965. 5/yr. CND 37 domestic to institutions (effective 1999); CND 15 newsstand/cover; USD 37 newsstand/cover foreign to institutions (effective 1999). adv. bk.rev. charts, illus, stat, bibl. back issues avail.; reprints avail. *Refereed.* **Document type:** *Academic/Scholarly.* **Description:** Official publication of Canadian Society of Respiratory Therapists. Contains feature articles, new product news, history, editorials and abstracts.
Former titles (1985-1996): Registered Respiratory Therapist (0831-2478); (1971-1985): Respiratory Technology (0319-1494); (1965-1971): Canadian Inhalation Therapy (0008-3852)

M

Related titles: Online - full text ed.: (from LexisNexis).
Indexed: CINAHL.
—CISTI, GNLM, Infotrieve. **CCC.**
Published by: Canadian Society of Respiratory Therapists, 1785 Alta Vista Dr Ste 102, Ottawa, ON K1G 3Y6, Canada. TEL 613-731-3164, FAX 613-521-4314, pubs@cma.ca, http://www.cma.ca/cjrt. Ed. Norman Tiffin. R&P Marie Claire Bedard. Adv. contact Beverley Kirkpatrick. B&W page CND 1,060, color page CND 1,650; trim 10.88 x 8.38. Circ: 2,900.

615.64 CAN ISSN 1198-2241
CANADIAN RESPIRATORY JOURNAL. Text in English, French. q. CND 145 domestic; USD 190 foreign (effective 2000). adv. bk.rev. *Refereed.* **Document type:** *Academic/Scholarly.* **Description:** Publishes original research in all areas of respiratory research and therapy, reviews, case reports, letters to the editor, industry news, meeting announcements and reports.
Indexed: Excerp.Med. (1996-), Ind.Med. (1994-).
—BLDSC (3044.615000), CISTI, GNLM, Infotrieve, KNAW. **CCC.**
Published by: (Canadian Thoracic Society), Pulsus Group Inc., 2902 S Sheridan Way, Oakville, ON L6J 7L6, Canada. TEL 905-829-4770, FAX 905-829-4799, pulsus@pulsus.com, http://www.pulsus.com. Ed. Dr. Norman Jones. Pub. Robert B Kalina. adv.: B&W page CND 2,325, color page CND 4,100. Circ: 15,500.

616.2 PER ISSN 0069-2166
CENTRO DE SALUD "MAX ARIAS SCHREIBER", LIMA. CONGRESO NACIONAL DE TUBERCULOSIS Y ENFERMEDADES RESPIRATORIAS* . Text in Spanish. irreg., latest vol.9, 1970.
Published by: Dispensario Antituberculoso "Max Arias Schreiber", Raymondi 2da Cuadra, La Victoria, Lima 13, Peru.

616.246 PAK ISSN 0528-7944
THE CHALLENGE. Text in English. 1959. q. PKR 60, USD 16. adv. bk.rev. charts, stat, bibl, illus. *Refereed.* **Document type:** *Academic/Scholarly.* **Description:** Covers news, views and new methods relating to global TB control.
Related titles: CD-ROM ed.; Online - full text ed.: (from Northern Light Technology, Inc.).
Indexed: Acad.Ind., ExtraMED, Ind.Med. (coverage dropped).
—GNLM.
Published by: Pakistan Anti-Tuberculosis Association, Block No. 55, Rm. 8, Secretariat, Karachi, Pakistan. TEL 92-21-5688011. Adv. contact M Z Baig. Circ: 2,000.

616.2 616.12 USA ISSN 0012-3692
RC705 CODEN: CHETBF
CHEST; the cardiopulmonary and critical care journal. Text in English. 1935. m. USD 132 domestic to individuals; USD 162 foreign to individuals; USD 174 domestic to institutions; USD 210 foreign to institutions (effective 2001). adv. bk.rev. bibl, illus. s-a. index. back issues avail.; reprints avail. *Refereed.* **Document type:** *Academic/Scholarly.* **Description:** Features original manuscripts dealing with continuing medical education in the medical or surgical aspects of pulmonary and cardiologic diseases.
Formerly: Diseases of the Chest
Related titles: CD-ROM ed.: (from Ovid Technologies, Inc.); Microform ed.: (from PQC); Online - full text ed.: (from Gale Group, Ovid Technologies, Inc., HighWire Pr., Northern Light Technology, Inc., EBSCO Publishing, ProQuest Information & Learning, Factiva, Institute for Scientific Information).
Indexed: AIDS Abstr., AIM, AMED, ASCA, Abstr.Hyg., Abstr.Inter.Med., Behav.Med.Abstr., Biol.Abstr., CINAHL, C.I.S. Abstr., Chem.Abstr., Chem.Indus.Notes, Chem.Titles, Curr.Adv.Ecol.Sci., Curr.Cont., Dairy Sci.Abstr., Dent.Ind., Dok.Arbeitsmed., Environ.Sci.Poll.Mgmt., Excerp.Med., Helminthol.Abstr., INIS Atomind., Ind.Med. (1970-), Ind.Sci.Rev., Ind.Vet., Inpharma, Int.Abstr.Biol.Sci., Int.Nurs.Ind., Jrnl.Watch, Jrnl.Watch Emer.Med., Jrnl.Watch Inf.Dis., Kidney, Neurosci.Cit.Ind., Nutr.Abstr., Pharm.&Out.News, Pig News & Info., Pollut.Abstr., Protozool.Abstr., Reac., Rev.Appl.Entomol., Rev.Med.& Vet.Mycol., Rev.Plant Path., Risk Abstr., SSCI (coverage dropped), Sci.Cit.Ind., Small Anim.Abstr., THA, Trop.Dis.Bull., Weed Abstr.
—BLDSC (3172.530000), ADONIS, CASDDS, CISTI, EMDOCS, GNLM, IDS, ingenta, KNAW, Linda Hall. **CCC.**
Published by: American College of Chest Physicians, 3300 Dundee Rd, Northbrook, IL 60062. TEL 847-498-1400, FAX 847-498-5460, registration@chestnet.org, http://www.chestnet.org. Ed. Dr. A Jay Block. Pub. Alvin Lever. R&P Steve Welch. Adv. contact Pat Micek. B&W page USD 1,400. Circ: 22,000. **Subscr. to:** Allen Press Inc., PO Box 1897, Lawrence, KS 66044-8897.

616.2 GBR
CHEST MEDICINE ON-LINE. Text in English. m. free per issue. bk.rev., software rev., video rev. *Refereed.* **Document type:** *Academic/Scholarly.* **Description:** Publishes case reports, audits, treatments, protocols, review papers and research on chest problems.
Media: Online - full text.
Published by: Priory Lodge Education Ltd., 2 Cornflower Way, Moreton, Wirral CH46 1SV, United Kingdom. TEL 44-151-606-1796, FAX 44-151-606-1812, solutions@priory.com, http://www.priory.com/chest.htm. Ed. Dr. Peter Davies. Circ: 25,000 (controlled).

616.2 USA ISSN 1068-0640
CODEN: CPMEF2
CLINICAL PULMONARY MEDICINE. Text in English. 1994. bi-m. USD 150 domestic to individuals; USD 186 foreign to individuals; USD 235 domestic to institutions; USD 277 foreign to institutions; USD 43 newsstand/cover (effective 2002). adv. **Document type:** *Academic/Scholarly.* **Description:** Disseminates research on the diagnosis and treatment of lung diseases.
Indexed: Excerp.Med. (1995-).
—BLDSC (3286.347000), EMDOCS, GNLM, KNAW.
Published by: Lippincott Williams & Wilkins (Baltimore) (Subsidiary of: Wolters Kluwer N.V.), 351 W Camden St, Baltimore, MD 21201-2436. TEL 410-528-4068, 800-222-3790, FAX 410-528-4452, apessagno@wwilkins.com, http://www.Lww.com. Ed. Dr. Michael S Niederman. Pub. Nancy Collins. Adv. contact Greg Pessagno. B&W page USD 715; trim 10.88 x 8.13. Circ: 2,496; 2,216 (paid).

616.2 USA ISSN 0272-5231
RC941
CLINICS IN CHEST MEDICINE. Text in English. 1980. q. USD 158 domestic to individuals; USD 175 in Canada to individuals; USD 198 elsewhere to individuals; USD 207 domestic to institutions; USD 247 foreign to institutions; USD 158 domestic to students; USD 62 per issue (effective 2001). *Refereed.* **Document type:** *Journal, Academic/Scholarly.* **Description:** Delivers practical advice from specialty covered with a fresh perspective on problems and controversies.
Related titles: Online - full text ed.: (from Institute for Scientific Information).
Indexed: ASCA, CINAHL, Curr.Cont., Dok.Arbeitsmed., Excerp.Med., INIS Atomind., Ind.Med. (1980-), Ind.Sci.Rev., Inpharma, Pharm.&Out.News, Reac., SSCI (coverage dropped), Sci.Cit.Ind.
—BLDSC (3286.545000), CISTI, EMDOCS, GNLM, IDS, ingenta, KNAW. **CCC.**
Published by: W.B. Saunders Co. (Subsidiary of: Harcourt Publishers Ltd.), 11830 Westline Industrial Dr, St Louis, MO 63146. TEL 800-325-4177, http://www.wbsaunders.com. **Subscr. to:** Periodicals Fulfillment, W B Saunders Co, 6277 Sea Harbor Dr, 4th Fl, Orlando, FL 32891-4800.

616.2 USA
COPING WITH ALLERGIES AND ASTHMA. Text in English. 1998. 5/yr. USD 13.95 domestic; USD 20 foreign (effective 2001). reprints avail. *Refereed.* **Document type:** *Magazine, Consumer.* **Description:** Targets those fighting asthma and/or allergies, allergists and immunologists, pulmonologists, and support groups. Challenges readers to develop a positive proactive approach and improve their quality of life by becoming allergy and asthma fighters, rather than sufferers. Provides readers with treatment options, offering practical "how-to" information as well as personal accounts.
Published by: Media America, PO Box 682268, Franklin, TN 37068-2268. TEL 615-790-2400, FAX 615-794-0179, copingmag@aol.com. Ed. Irene Wood. Pub. Michael D Holt. R&P Marsha Moore TEL 615-790-2400 ext 27. Adv. contact Paula K Chadwell. Circ: 30,000 (paid and controlled).

CURRENT MEDICAL LITERATURE. RESPIRATORY MEDICINE. see *MEDICAL SCIENCES—Abstracting, Bibliographies, Statistics*

616.7 USA ISSN 1070-5287
CURRENT OPINION IN PULMONARY MEDICINE. Text in English. 1995. bi-m. USD 239 domestic to individuals for print & online eds.; USD 239 foreign to individuals for print & online eds.; USD 84 newsstand/cover; USD 539 per issue domestic to institutions; USD 539 per issue foreign to institutions (effective 2002). adv. bibl, illus. **Document type:** *Academic/Scholarly.* **Description:** Keeps readers abreast of clinical and research advances in the field.
Related titles: CD-ROM ed.; Online - full text ed.: USD 700.70 domestic academic site license; USD 700.70 foreign academic site license; USD 781.55 domestic corporate site license; USD 781.55 foreign corporate site license (effective 2002) (from Swets Blackwell, Ovid Technologies, Inc.).
Indexed: CINAHL, Excerp.Med., Ind.Med. (1995-), Inpharma, Pharm.&Out.News, Reac.
—BLDSC (3500.777200), ADONIS.
Published by: Lippincott Williams & Wilkins (Philadelphia) (Subsidiary of: Wolters Kluwer N.V.), 530 Walnut St, Philadelphia, PA 19106-3621. FAX 215-521-8902, 215-521-8902, http://www.Lww.com. Ed. M P Sharma. Pub. Maria McMichael. R&P Tobias Weschler. Adv. contact Kelly Adamitis. Circ: 401. **Subscr. to:** PO Box 1600, Hagerstown, MD 21740-1600.

616.2 AUT ISSN 1609-2961
▼ **DIFFICULT AIRWAY.** Text in English. 2000. q. USD 75 domestic; USD 115 foreign; USD 35 newsstand/cover (effective 2001). adv. back issues avail. *Refereed.* **Document type:** *Journal, Academic/Scholarly.* **Description:** Publishes articles, case reports, reviews, and letters that aim to improve communication in understanding difficult airway management.
Related titles: Online - full text ed.: ISSN 1609-297X.
Published by: V I C E R Publishing, PO Box 14, Vienna A-1097, Austria. TEL 43-676-9568085, FAX 43-676-9568086, vicer@vicer.org, http://www.vicer.org. Ed., R&P Roland Hofbauer. adv.: B&W page USD 1,700, color page USD 2,200. Circ: 1,000 (paid and controlled).

616.2 GBR
DIRECTORY OF TRAINING POSTS AND SERIES IN ADULT AND PAEDIATRIC RESPIRATORY MEDICINE. Text in English. 1996. a. GBP 9.50 (effective 2001). **Document type:** *Directory.*
Published by: (British Thoracic Society), Hawker Publications Ltd., Culvert House, Culvert Rd, London SW11 5AP, United Kingdom. TEL 44-20-7720-2108, FAX 44-20-7498-3023, hawker@hawkerpubs.demon.co.uk, http://www.careinfo.org/.

616.2 JPN
DOUBLE - BARRED CROSS/FUKUJUJI. Text in Japanese. 1955. bi-m. free per issue. adv. bk.rev. charts, illus, stat. 32 p./no.
Formerly: Red Double-Barred Cross (0016-2531)
Published by: Japan Anti-Tuberculosis Association/Kekkaku Yobokai, 1-3-12 Misaki-cho, Chiyoda-ku, Tokyo 101-0061, Japan. TEL 81-3-3292-9211, FAX 81-3-3292-9208, jata@jatahq.org, http://www.jatahq.org. Ed., Pub. Mutsuo Sato. Circ: 18,000.

616.2 FRA ISSN 1155-195X
ENCYCLOPEDIE MEDICO-CHIRURGICALE. PNEUMOLOGIE. Cover title: Traite de Pneumologie. Variant title: Encyclopedie Medico-Chirurgicale, Instantanes Medicaux. Pneumologie. Text in French. 4 base vols. plus q. updates. bibl, charts, illus. *Refereed.* **Document type:** *Academic/Scholarly.* **Description:** Provides specialists in diagnosing and treating respiratory-tract diseases with a comprehensive and up-to-date reference.
Formerly (until 1991): Encyclopedie Medico-Chirurgicale. Poumon, Plevre, Mediastin (0246-036X)
Published by: Elsevier Paris, Editions Scientifiques et Medicales (Subsidiary of: Reed Elsevier plc. group), 23 rue Linois, Paris 75015, France. TEL 33-1-45589110, FAX 33-1-45589425, redaction-emc@elsevier.fr, redacion-emc@elsevier.fr, http://www.elsevier.fr, http://www.elsevier.com.

ENCYCLOPEDIE MEDICO-CHIRURGICALE. TRAITE DE RADIODIAGNOSTIC: COEUR - POUMON. see *MEDICAL SCIENCES—Radiology And Nuclear Medicine*

616.2 CHE ISSN 0903-1936
CODEN: ERJOEI
THE EUROPEAN RESPIRATORY JOURNAL. Text in English; Summaries in French. 1924. m. GBP 383, USD 654 (effective 2001). adv. bk.rev. illus. index. reprint service avail. from ISI. *Refereed.* **Document type:** *Academic/Scholarly.*
Formed by the merger of: European Journal of Respiratory Diseases (0106-4339); Which was formerly: Acta Tuberculosa et Pneumologica Belgica (0001-7078); Clinical Respiratory Physiology (0271-9983); Which was formerly: Bulletin Europeen de Physiopathologie Respiratoire (0395-3890)

Related titles: Online - full text ed.: (from EBSCO Publishing, O C L C Online Computer Library Center, Inc., RoweCom Information Quest, Munksgaard & Blackwell Science's Synergy, Swets Blackwell, Institute for Scientific Information); ♦ Supplement: European Respiratory Journal. Supplement. ISSN 0904-1850.
Indexed: AESIS, AMED, ASCA, Abstr.Hyg., Agri.& Environ.Biotech.Abstr. (coverage dropped), Agri.Eng.Abstr., Biol.Abstr., CINAHL, C.I.S. Abstr., Chem.Abstr., Chem.Indus.Notes, Chem.Titles, Curr.Adv.Ecol.Sci., Curr.Cont., Dent.Ind., Derwent Biotech.Abstr., Dok.Arbeitsmed., Environ.Sci.Poll.Mgmt., Excerp.Med., Helminthol.Abstr., INIS Atomind., Ind.Med. (1988-), Ind.Sci.Rev., Ind.Vet., Inpharma, Int.Abstr.Biol.Sci., Int.Nurs.Ind., Neurosci.Cit.Ind., Nutr.Abstr., Pharm.&Out.News, Pig News & Info., Reac., Rev.Appl.Entomol., Rev.Med.& Vet.Mycol., Rev.Plant Path., Risk Abstr., SSCI (coverage dropped), Saf.Sci.Abstr., Sci.Cit.Ind., THA, Triticale Abstr., Trop.Dis.Bull., Vet.Bull., Weed Abstr.
—BLDSC (3829.924200), CASDDS, CISTI, EMDOCS, GNLM, IDS, Infotrieve, ingenta, KNAW. **CCC.**
Published by: European Respiratory Society, 1 Bd de Grancy, Lausanne 1006, Switzerland. TEL 41-21-6130202, FAX 41-21-6172865, info@ersnet.org. Circ: 5,500.

616.2 CHE ISSN 0904-1850
CODEN: ERJSEU
EUROPEAN RESPIRATORY JOURNAL. SUPPLEMENT. Text in English. 1934. irreg. adv. reprint service avail. from ISI. **Document type:** *Monographic series, Academic/Scholarly.*
Former titles (until 1987): European Journal of Respiratory Diseases. Supplementum (0106-4347); (until 1979): Scandinavian Journal of Respiratory Diseases. Supplementum (0080-6730); (until 1965): Acta Tuberculosea et Pneumologica Scandinavica, Supplementum (0365-7612); (until 1961): Acta Tuberculosea Scandinavica. Supplementum (0365-7604)
Related titles: ♦ Supplement to: The European Respiratory Journal. ISSN 0903-1936.
Indexed: Biol.Abstr., Curr.Adv.Ecol.Sci., Curr.Cont. (coverage dropped), Excerp.Med. (1992-), INIS Atomind., Ind.Med. (1988-), Ind.Sci.Rev., Int.Abstr.Biol.Sci.
—CASDDS, CISTI, EMDOCS, KNAW. **CCC.**
Published by: European Respiratory Society, 1 Bd de Grancy, Lausanne 1006, Switzerland. TEL 41-21-6130202, FAX 41-21-6172865, info@ersnet.org.

616.2 CHE ISSN 1025-448X
EUROPEAN RESPIRATORY MONOGRAPH. Text in English. 1996. irreg. (3-4/yr.). GBP 25 per issue; USD 40 per issue with European Respiratory Review. **Document type:** *Monographic series, Academic/Scholarly.*
Published by: European Respiratory Society, 1 Bd de Grancy, Lausanne 1006, Switzerland. TEL 41-21-6130202, FAX 41-21-6172865, info@ersnet.org, http://www.ersnet.org. **Subscr. to:** Maney Publishing, Hudson Rd, Leeds, W Yorks LS9 7DL, United Kingdom. TEL 44-113-249-7481, FAX 44-113-248-6983.

616.2 CHE ISSN 0905-9180
CODEN: EREWEH
EUROPEAN RESPIRATORY REVIEW. Text in English. 1991. irreg. (5-6/yr.). GBP 115, USD 196. adv. bk.rev. reprints avail. *Refereed.* **Document type:** *Monographic series, Academic/Scholarly.*
Indexed: Excerp.Med. (1992-), Inpharma, Int.Abstr.Biol.Sci., Pharm.&Out.News, Reac.
—BLDSC (3829.924400), EMDOCS, GNLM, Infotrieve, KNAW. **CCC.**
Published by: European Respiratory Society, 1 Bd de Grancy, Lausanne 1006, Switzerland. TEL 41-21-6130202, FAX 41-21-6172865, info@ersnet.org, http://www.ersnet.org. Circ: 2,500. **Subscr. to:** Maney Publishing, Hudson Rd, Leeds, W Yorks LS9 7DL, United Kingdom. TEL 44-113-249-7481, FAX 44-113-248-6983.

EXCERPTA MEDICA. SECTION 15: CHEST DISEASES, THORACIC SURGERY AND TUBERCULOSIS. see *MEDICAL SCIENCES—Abstracting, Bibliographies, Statistics*

616.2 USA ISSN 0190-2148
QP121.A1 CODEN: EXLRDA
EXPERIMENTAL LUNG RESEARCH. Text in English. 1979. 8/yr. GBP 287, USD 473 to individuals; GBP 760, USD 1,254 to institutions (effective 2002). adv. back issues avail.; reprint service avail. from PQC. *Refereed.* **Document type:** *Academic/Scholarly.* **Description:** Explores mechanisms of pulmonary biology and pathobiology, investigated at biochemical, subcellular, cellular, and tissue levels.
Related titles: Online - full text ed.: ISSN 1521-0499 (from CatchWord Ltd., EBSCO Publishing, O C L C Online Computer Library Center, Inc., RoweCom Information Quest, Swets Blackwell, Institute for Scientific Information).
Indexed: ASCA, Aqua.Sci.& Fish.Abstr., Biol.Abstr., Chem.Abstr., Chem.Indus.Notes, Chem.Titles, Curr.Adv.Cell & Devel.Biol., Curr.Adv.Ecol.Sci., Curr.Cont., Environ.Sci.Poll.Mgmt., Excerp.Med., INIS Atomind., Ind.Med. (1980-), Ind.Sci.Rev., Ind.Vet., Inpharma, Int.Abstr.Biol.Sci., Microbiol.Abstr., Pharm.&Out.News, Reac., Sci.Cit.Ind., THA, Vet.Bull.
—BLDSC (3839.440000), ADONIS, CASDDS, CatchWord, CISTI, GNLM, IDS, ingenta. **CCC.**
Published by: Taylor & Francis Ltd. (Subsidiary of: Taylor & Francis Group), 325 Chestnut St, Suite 800, Philadelphia, PA 19016. TEL 215-625-8900, FAX 215-625-2940, info@taylorandfrancis.com, http://www.taylorandfrancis.com/. Ed. Paul Nettesheim. Circ: 400. **Subscr. addr. in Europe:** Taylor & Francis Group, Journals Customer Service, Rankine Rd, Basingstoke, Hants RG24 8PR, United Kingdom. TEL 44-1256-813000, FAX 44-1256-479438, enquiry@tanf.co.uk, http://www.tandf.co.uk/journals.

FOCUS ON PULMONARY PHARMACOLOGY AND TOXICOLOGY. see *ENVIRONMENTAL STUDIES—Toxicology And Environmental Safety*

616.2 VEN ISSN 0798-3719
FOUNDATION - INTERNATIONAL SEMINAR THE RESPIRATORY PULSE. SCIENTIFIC REVIEW. Key Title: Scientific Review - Foundation International Seminar the Respiratory Pulse. Text in English, Spanish. 1992. a. USD 5. **Description:** Includes articles related to respiratory system and different human organs related.
Published by: Fundacion Seminario Internacional "El Pulso Respiratorio", Ed. Caribana Apto. 43, Cruce Avda. Universitaria y P. Los Ilustres, Valle Abajo, Caracas, DF 1040, Venezuela. TEL 58-2-6627366, respulse@reacciun.ve. Ed. Dr. Americo Gonzalez Bogen. Circ: 1,000.

616.2 CHN ISSN 1001-1064
GUOWAI YIXUE (HUXI XITONG FENCE)/FOREIGN MEDICAL SCIENCES (RESPIRATORY SYSTEMS). Text in Chinese. 1981. q. USD 6; USD 1.50 newsstand/cover (effective 2001). 56 p./no. *Refereed.* **Document type:** *Academic/Scholarly.* **Description:** Covers the latest development in the field of respiratory diseases.
Published by: (Ministry of Hygiene, Management Committee of Medical Information), Hebei Yike Daxue/Hebei Medical University, 361 Zhongshan Donglu, Shijiazhuang, Hebei 050017, China. TEL 86-311-6059153, FAX 86-311-6059153, hebydqks@public.sj.he.cn, WL@hebmu.edu.cn. Ed. Ling Yiling. adv.: B&W page CNY 5,000, color page CNY 7,000. Circ: 9,000. **Dist. overseas by:** China International Book Trading Corp, 35, Chegongzhuang Xilu, Haidian District, Beijing 100044, China. TEL 86-1-68413849, FAX 86-1-68412048, cibtc@mail.cibtc.com.cn, http://www.cibtc.com.cn.

H L B NEWSLETTER; reporting on heart, lung and blood disease research policy development. see *MEDICAL SCIENCES—Experimental Medicine, Laboratory Technique*

HJAERT-LUNGFONDENS KVARTALSSKRIFT. see *MEDICAL SCIENCES—Cardiovascular Diseases*

616.2 JPN
HOKKAIDO UNIVERSITY. INSTITUTE OF IMMUNOLOGICAL SCIENCE. BULLETIN. Text in Japanese; Summaries in English, Japanese. 1953. a. per issue exchange basis.
Formerly (until 1975): Kekkaku No Kenkyu (0075-5354)
Indexed: Biol.Abstr.
Published by: Hokkaido University, Institute of Immunological Science, North 15, West 7, Sapporo 060, Japan. Ed. Ken Ichi Yamamoto. Circ: 300.

616.246 FRA ISSN 1019-9853
I U A T L D NEWSLETTER (EDITION ESPANOLA). Text in Spanish. 3/yr.
Related titles: ♦ French ed.: International Union against Tuberculosis and Lung Disease. Newsletter. ISSN 1021-7754; ♦ French ed.: I U A T L D Newsletter (Edition Francaise). ISSN 1019-4924.
Published by: International Union against Tuberculosis and Lung Disease/Union Internationale contre la Tuberculose et les Maladies Respiratoires, 68 bd. Saint-Michel, Paris 75006, France.

616.246 FRA ISSN 1019-4924
I U A T L D NEWSLETTER (EDITION FRANCAISE). Text in French. 3/yr.
Related titles: ♦ French ed.: International Union against Tuberculosis and Lung Disease. Newsletter. ISSN 1021-7754; ♦ Spanish ed.: I U A T L D Newsletter (Edition Espanola). ISSN 1019-9853.
Published by: International Union against Tuberculosis and Lung Disease/Union Internationale contre la Tuberculose et les Maladies Respiratoires, 68 bd. Saint-Michel, Paris 75006, France.

616.2 IND ISSN 0019-5707
CODEN: IJTBAD
INDIAN JOURNAL OF TUBERCULOSIS. Text in English. 1953. q. INR 350, USD 30 (effective 2000). adv. bk.rev. abstr, bibl, charts, illus, stat. index, cum.index. *Refereed.* **Document type:** *Academic/Scholarly.* **Description:** Contains original papers, review articles, case reports in all aspects of tuberculosis and other chest diseases.
Indexed: Abstr.Hyg., Biol.Abstr., Chem.Abstr., Excerp.Med., Protozool.Abstr., Rev.Med.& Vet.Mycol., Trop.Dis.Bull.
—BLDSC (4421.700000), CISTI, GNLM, KNAW.
Published by: Tuberculosis Association of India, 3 Red Cross Rd., New Delhi 110 001, India. TEL 91-11-3711303. Ed. D R Nagpaul. Circ: 3,000 (paid).

616.2 MEX ISSN 0187-7585
INSTITUTO NACIONAL DE ENFERMEDADES RESPIRATORIAS. REVISTA. Short title: Revista I N E R. Text in Spanish; Summaries in English, Spanish. 1988. q. MXP 200 domestic; USD 40 foreign; MXP 55 newsstand/cover. adv. bk.rev. illus, stat. back issues avail. *Refereed.* **Document type:** *Academic/Scholarly.* **Description:** Contains original articles, research reports, review articles, clinical cases and notices related to the pathology of the respiratory tract.
Related titles: CD-ROM ed.; Online - full text ed.
—EMDOCS.
Published by: Instituto Nacional de Enfermedades Respiratorias, CLZ TLALPAN 4502, Col Seccion XVI, Mexico City, DF 14080, Mexico. TEL 52-5-6664539, FAX 52-5-6663187, iner@cenids.ssa.gob.mx. Ed., R&P Celso Garcia Espinosa. Circ: 3,000; 3,000 (controlled).

616.246 FRA ISSN 1027-3719
CODEN: IJTDFO
INTERNATIONAL JOURNAL OF TUBERCULOSIS AND LUNG DISEASE. Text in English; Summaries in French, Spanish. 1997. m. USD 180 to individuals; USD 250 to institutions (effective 2000). adv. Supplement avail. *Refereed.* **Document type:** *Academic/Scholarly.* **Description:** Aims to encourage continuing education of physicians and other health personnel. Contains the most up-to-date information in the field of tuberculosis and lung health. Includes original articles and commissioned reviews on clinical, biological and epidemiological research. Also covers implementation and assessment of field projects and action programs for tuberculosis control and the promotion of lung health.
Related titles: Online - full text ed.: (from Institute for Scientific Information).
Indexed: AIDS & Cancer Res., Abstr.Hyg., Curr.Cont., Dairy Sci.Abstr., Derwent Biotech.Abstr., Environ.Sci.Poll.Mgmt., Ind.Med. (1997-), Ind.Vet., Inpharma, Int.Nurs.Ind., Microbiol.Abstr., Pharm.&Out.News, Pollut.Abstr., Reac., Ref.Zh., Rev.Med.& Vet.Mycol., Risk Abstr., Rural Devel.Abstr., Saf.Sci.Abstr., Sci.Cit.Ind., Trop.Dis.Bull., Vet.Bull., Virol.Abstr.
—BLDSC (4542.696180), GNLM, KNAW.
Published by: International Union against Tuberculosis and Lung Disease/Union Internationale contre la Tuberculose et les Maladies Respiratoires, 68 bd. Saint-Michel, Paris 75006, France. TEL 33-1-44320360, FAX 33-1-43-29-90-87, union@iuatld.org, http://www.iuatld.org. Ed. Michael D Iseman. Adv. contact Clare Pierard. Circ: 2,000.

616.2 613.62 620 USA ISSN 0892-6298
INTERNATIONAL SOCIETY FOR RESPIRATORY PROTECTION. JOURNAL. Variant title: Journal of the I S R P. Text in English. 1983. q. USD 45 to members (effective 1997). *Refereed.* **Description:** A forum for open and responsible discussion in the field of respiratory protection.

—BLDSC (4802.508000).
Published by: International Society for Respiratory Protection, Fission Energy and System Safety Program, Hazards Control Dept, Lawrence Livermore National Laboratory, Box 808, L 379, Livermore, CA 94550. TEL 510-422-5215, FAX 510-422-5176. Ed. James S Johnson. **Subscr. to:** Bradley S. Squibb, Aerojet Ordnance, Box 158, Jonesborough, TN 37659. TEL 615-753-1388, FAX 615-753-8645.

616.246 FRA
INTERNATIONAL UNION AGAINST TUBERCULOSIS AND LUNG DISEASE. CONFERENCE PROCEEDINGS. Text in French. quadrennial. **Document type:** *Proceedings.*
Supersedes: International Union against Tuberculosis. Conference Proceedings (0074-9257)
Published by: International Union against Tuberculosis and Lung Disease/Union Internationale contre la Tuberculose et les Maladies Respiratoires, 68 bd. Saint-Michel, Paris 75006, France. TEL 33-1-46-33-08-30, FAX 33-1-43-29-90-87. Ed. Dr Nils E Billo.

616.246 FRA ISSN 1021-7754
INTERNATIONAL UNION AGAINST TUBERCULOSIS AND LUNG DISEASE. NEWSLETTER. Text in French. 1991. 3/yr.
Related titles: ♦ French ed.: I U A T L D Newsletter (Edition Francaise). ISSN 1019-4924; ♦ Spanish ed.: I U A T L D Newsletter (Edition Espanola). ISSN 1019-9853.
—BLDSC (6107.478000).
Published by: International Union against Tuberculosis and Lung Disease/Union Internationale contre la Tuberculose et les Maladies Respiratoires, 68 bd. Saint-Michel, Paris 75006, France. TEL 33-1-44320360, FAX 33-1-43-29-90-87, IUATLDParis@compuserve.com. Ed. Nils Billo.

616.2 USA
THE INTERNET JOURNAL OF PULMONARY MEDICINE. Text in English. 1997. s-a. free per issue. adv. bk.rev. back issues avail. *Refereed.* **Document type:** *Academic/Scholarly.* **Description:** Contains information from the field of pulmonary medicine and respiratory diseases. Original articles, reviews, case reports, streaming slide shows, streaming videos, letters to the editor, press releases, meeting information.
Media: Online - full text.
Published by: Internet Scientific Publications, L.L.C., 23 Rippling Creek Dr, Sugar Land, TX 77479. TEL 281-240-1533, FAX 281-240-1533, scherer@ispub.com, http://www.ispub.com/journals/ijpm.htm. Ed. Armando Huaringa. R&P, Adv. contact Hope Morrow TEL 832-754-0335.

616.202 USA
▼ **J A M A ASTHMA NEWSLINE.** (Journal of the American Medical Association) Text in English. 1999. w. adv. back issues avail. *Refereed.*
Media: Online - full text.
Published by: American Medical Association, J A M A Information Centers, 515 N State St, Chicago, IL 60610. TEL 312-464-5000, 800-262-2350, FAX 312-464-4181, sdthma@ama-assn.org, http://www.ama-assn.org/special/asthma/asthma.htm. Adv. contact Crystal Wells.

616.2 BRA ISSN 0102-3586
JORNAL DE PNEUMOLOGIA. Text in English, Portuguese, Spanish; Summaries in English, Portuguese. 1974. q. BRL 60 domestic; USD 50 foreign (effective 2000 & 2001). adv. bk.rev. *Refereed.* **Document type:** *Proceedings, Academic/Scholarly, Corporate.* **Description:** Publishes original research articles and case studies.
Indexed: INIS Atomind.
—GNLM.
Published by: Sociedade Brasileira de Pneumologia e Tisiologia, Departamento de Clinica Medica, Centro, Caixa Postal 595, Botucatu, SP 18603-971, Brazil. TEL 55-14-8216530, FAX 55-14-8216530, jpneumo@laser.com.br, http://www.ricpropaganda.com.br. Ed., R&P Thais Helena A T Queluz. Adv. contact Mr Katayama TEL 55-11-5711719. Circ: 3,000 (paid and controlled).

616.2 USA ISSN 0894-2684
CODEN: JAEMEP
JOURNAL OF AEROSOL MEDICINE; deposition, clearance, and effects in the lung. Text in English. 1988. q. USD 139 domestic to individuals; USD 248 foreign to individuals; USD 167 domestic to individuals print and online eds. combined; USD 276 foreign to individuals print and online eds. combined; USD 388 domestic to institutions; USD 492 foreign to institutions; USD 466 domestic to institutions print and online eds. combined; USD 570 foreign to institutions print and online eds. combined (effective 2002). back issues avail.; reprints avail. *Refereed.* **Document type:** *Journal, Academic/Scholarly.* **Description:** Contains original articles and reviews that apply aerosols to the delivery of medication and the investigation for physiologic, pharmacologic, and toxicologic phenomena in the lung.
Related titles: Online - full content ed.: USD 139 to individuals; USD 388 to institutions (effective 2002) (from Swets Blackwell); Online - full text ed.: (from CatchWord Ltd., Institute for Scientific Information, RoweCom Information Quest).
Indexed: ASCA, Curr.Cont., Environ.Sci.Poll.Mgmt., Excerp.Med. (1993-), I.P.A., Inpharma, Pollut.Abstr., Reac., Rev.Med.& Vet.Mycol.
—BLDSC (4919.054000), CISTI, EMDOCS, GNLM, IDS, Infotrieve, ingenta, KNAW. **CCC.**
Published by: Mary Ann Liebert, Inc. Publishers, 2 Madison Ave, Larchmont, NY 10538. TEL 914—834-3100, FAX 914-834-1388, info@liebertpub.com, http://www.liebertpub.com/jam. Ed. Dr. Gerald C Smaldone.

616.97 USA ISSN 0277-0903
RC591 CODEN: JOUADU
JOURNAL OF ASTHMA (NEW YORK). Text in English. 1964. 8/yr. USD 145 to individuals print & online eds.; USD 1,050 to institutions print only (effective 2002). adv. bk.rev. bibl, charts, illus, stat. index, cum. index: 1963-1965. reprints avail. *Refereed.* **Document type:** *Academic/Scholarly.* **Description:** Provides information on new developments in the understanding and management of asthma.
Formerly (until vol.18, 1981): Journal of Asthma Research (0021-9134)
Related titles: Microfilm ed.; Online - full text ed.: (from Institute for Scientific Information, RoweCom Information Quest).
Indexed: ASCA, Biol.Abstr., Chem.Abstr., Curr.Cont., Dent.Ind., Excerp.Med., INIS Atomind., Ind.Med. (1981-), Inpharma, Int.Abstr.Biol.Sci., Lab.Haz.Bull., NRN, Pharm.&Out.News, PsycInfo, Psychol.Abstr. (1963-), Reac., Rev.Appl.Entomol., Rev.Arom.& Med.Plants, Rev.Med.& Vet.Mycol., SSCI (coverage dropped), THA, Trop.Dis.Bull., e-psyche.
—BLDSC (4947.295000), CASDDS, EMDOCS, GNLM, IDS, ingenta, KNAW. **CCC.**
Published by: (Association for the Care of Asthma), Marcel Dekker Inc., 270 Madison Ave, New York, NY 10016. TEL 212-696-9000, 800-228-1160, FAX 212-685-4540, journals@dekker.com, http://www.dekker.com/servlet/product/productid/JAS. Ed. David Tinkelman. R&P Julia Mulligan. Adv. contact Tony Di Biase. B&W page USD 1,160. Circ: 8,400.

616.2 USA ISSN 1070-8030
CODEN: JBROF2
JOURNAL OF BRONCHOLOGY. Text in English. 1994. q. USD 165 domestic to individuals; USD 198 foreign to individuals; USD 241 domestic to institutions; USD 269 foreign to institutions (effective 2002); USD 61 newsstand/cover. adv. charts, illus. *Refereed.* **Document type:** *Academic/Scholarly.* **Description:** Examines all aspects of the prevention, diagnosis and treatment of disorders affecting the respiratory system.
Related titles: Online - full text ed.: USD 313.30 domestic for academic site license; USD 341.30 foreign for academic site license; USD 349.45 domestic for corporate site license; USD 377.45 foreign for corporate site license (effective 2002).
—BLDSC (4954.552500), GNLM, KNAW.
Published by: (World Association for Bronchology), Lippincott Williams & Wilkins (Philadelphia) (Subsidiary of: Wolters Kluwer N.V.), 530 Walnut St, Philadelphia, PA 19106-3621. TEL 215-521-8300, FAX 215-521-8902, http://www.Lww.com. Ed. Udaya B S Prakash. Pub. Christine Rullo. R&P Alice McElhinney. Adv. contact Ray Thibodeau. B&W page USD 710, color page USD 1,715. Circ: 835. **Subscr. to:** PO Box 1600, Hagerstown, MD 21740-1600. TEL 800-777-2295, FAX 301-824-7390. **Co-sponsor:** American Association for Bronchology.

JOURNAL OF CHEMOTHERAPY. see *MEDICAL SCIENCES—Oncology*

616.2 USA ISSN 0194-259X
RC705 CODEN: JRDIFQ
THE JOURNAL OF RESPIRATORY DISEASES. Text in English. 1979. m. USD 95 domestic; USD 105 foreign; USD 10 newsstand/cover domestic; USD 15 newsstand/cover foreign (effective 2001). adv. charts, illus. Index. back issues avail.; reprints avail. *Refereed.* **Document type:** *Journal, Academic/Scholarly.* **Description:** Provides practical information about diagnosis and treatment pertaining to the respiratory system, both as the site of primary disease and as a complication of other clinical problems.
Related titles: Online - full text ed.: (from Gale Group).
Indexed: CINAHL, Excerp.Med. (1996-).
—BLDSC (5052.038200), CISTI, EMDOCS, GNLM, KNAW. **CCC.**
Published by: Cliggott Publishing Co. (Subsidiary of: S C P Communications, Inc.), 330 Boston Post Rd, Darien, CT 06820. TEL 203-662-6400, FAX 203-662-6776, info.cliggott@scp.com, http://www.scp.com/. Ed., R&P Sarah Williams. Pub. Jeff Davis. Circ: 86,966.

▼ **JOURNAL OF RESPIRATORY DISEASES FOR PEDIATRICIANS.** see *MEDICAL SCIENCES—Pediatrics*

616.246 JPN ISSN 0022-9776
CODEN: KEKKAG
KEKKAKU/TUBERCULOSIS. Text in Japanese; Abstracts in English. 1923. m. adv. abstr, bibl, charts, illus. index. **Document type:** *Academic/Scholarly.* **Description:** Publishes articles which are devoted to understanding and improving studies in tuberculosis and related fields, including original reports, reviews, case reports and short reports.
Indexed: Biol.Abstr., Chem.Abstr., Chem.Indus.Notes, Chem.Titles, Excerp.Med., INIS Atomind., Ind.Med. (1923-), Inpharma, Int.Nurs.Ind., Reac.
—BLDSC (5089.250000), CASDDS, CISTI, GNLM.
Published by: Japanese Society for Tuberculosis, c/o Research Institute of Tuberculosis, Matsuyama 3-chome, Kiyose-shi, Tokyo-to 204-0022, Japan. TEL 81-424-92-2091, FAX 81-424-91-8315. Ed. Nobukatsu Ishikawa. Circ: 3,000. **Subscr. to:** Tonggang Shudian, Export Dept, Rm 106 NKB Azeria Bldg, 7-7 Shinogawa-Machi, Shinjuku-ku, Tokyo 162-0814, Japan. TEL 81-3-3269-2131, FAX 81-3-3269-8655.

616.2 JPN ISSN 0452-3458
CODEN: KOJUA9
KOKYU TO JUNKAN/RESPIRATION AND CIRCULATION. Text in Japanese; Summaries in English. 1953. m. JPY 2,400 per issue.
Related titles: Online - full text ed.: (from JICST).
Indexed: Biol.Abstr., Chem.Abstr., Chem.Titles, Excerp.Med., INIS Atomind., Ind.Med. (coverage dropped), Inpharma, Reac.
—CASDDS, EMDOCS, GNLM, KNAW.
Published by: Igaku-Shoin Ltd., 5-24-3 Hongo, Bunkyo-ku, Tokyo 113-0033, Japan. TEL 81-3-3817-5703. Circ: 4,500.

KOKYUKI GEKA/JAPANESE ASSOCIATION FOR CHEST SURGERY. JOURNAL. see *MEDICAL SCIENCES—Surgery*

KOSANKINBYO KENKYUSHO ZASSHI. see *MEDICAL SCIENCES—Communicable Diseases*

L M S ALERT. OBSTRUCTIVE AIRWAYS DISEASE. (Literature Monitoring and Evaluation Service) see *MEDICAL SCIENCES—Abstracting, Bibliographies, Statistics*

616.2 FRA
LA LETTRE DU PNEUMOLOGUE. Text in French. bi-m. FRF 300 domestic to individuals; FRF 420, USD 76 foreign to individuals; FRF 380 domestic to institutions; FRF 500, USD 91 foreign to institutions; FRF 190 domestic to students; USD 56 foreign to students (effective 2000). *Refereed.* **Document type:** *Academic/Scholarly.*
Published by: Edimark S.A., 62-64 rue Jean Jaures, Puteaux 92800, France. TEL 33-1-414-58000, FAX 33-1-41458025, contact@edimark.fr, http://www.edimark.fr. Ed. Philippe Godard. Pub. Claudie Damour-Terrasson.

LIVEWELL. see *PHYSICAL FITNESS AND HYGIENE*

M

616.2 ITA ISSN 0368-7546
CODEN: LCTMAU
LOTTA CONTRO LA TUBERCOLOSI E LE MALATTIE POLMONARI SOCIALI. Text in Italian. 1930. q. ITL 60,000. adv. bk.rev. bibl, charts, illus, stat. index, cum.index: 1943-1944. **Document type:** *Bulletin, Academic/Scholarly.* **Description:** Covers the study and research of tuberculosis and respiratory diseases.
Formerly (until 1972): Lotta contro la Tubercolosi (0024-6638)
Indexed: Abstr.Hyg., Biol.Abstr., C.I.S. Abstr., Chem.Abstr., Dairy Sci.Abstr., Excerp.Med., Helminthol.Abstr., Ind.Med. (coverage dropped), Trop.Dis.Bull.
—BLDSC (5294.890000), CISTI, EMDOCS, GNLM, KNAW.
Published by: Federazione Italiana contro la Tubercolosi e le Malattie Polmonari Sociali, Via Giovanni Da Procida, 7-D, Rome, RM 00162, Italy. TEL 39-6-44240682. Circ: 3,000.

616.2 USA ISSN 0341-2040
CODEN: LUNGD9
LUNG; an international journal on lungs, airways and breathing. Text in English. 1903. bi-m. (in 1 vol., 6 nos./vol.). USD 388.90 domestic for Print & Online Eds.; USD 382.60 in Germany for Print & Online Eds.; USD 71.10 newsstand/cover foreign (effective 2002). adv. back issues avail.; reprint service avail. from ISI. *Refereed.* **Document type:** *Academic/Scholarly.* **Description:** Contains original articles on all aspects of basic and clinical research dealing with the lungs, airways, and breathing, including epidemiological, clinical, pathophysiological, biochemical and pharmacological studies.
Former titles: Pneumonologie - Pneumonology (0033-4073); Beitraege zur Klinik und Erforschung der Tuberkulose und der Lungenkrankheiten
Related titles: Microform ed.: (from PQC); Online - full text ed.: ISSN 1432-1750 (from EBSCO Publishing, RoweCom Information Quest, Swets Blackwell, Springer LINK, Institute for Scientific Information).
Indexed: ASCA, Agri.& Environ.Biotech.Abstr. (coverage dropped), Biol.Abstr., C.I.S. Abstr., Chem.Abstr., Chem.Indus.Notes, Chem.Titles, Curr.Adv.Ecol.Sci., Curr.Cont., Derwent Biotech.Abstr., Environ.Sci.Poll.Mgmt., Excerp.Med., INIS Atomind., Ind.Med. (1976-), Ind.Sci.Rev., Ind.Vet., Inpharma, Pharm.&Out.News, Pollut.Abstr., Reac., Rev.Med.& Vet.Mycol., Risk Abstr., Saf.Sci.Abstr., Sci.Cit.Ind., Vet.Bull.
—BLDSC (5307.160000), ADONIS, CASDDS, CISTI, EMDOCS, GNLM, IDS, ingenta, KNAW. **CCC.**
Published by: Springer-Verlag, Journals (Subsidiary of: BertelsmannSpringer), 175 Fifth Ave, New York, NY 10010. TEL 212-460-1500, FAX 212-473-6272, orders@springer-ny.com, http://www.springer-ny.com. Ed. M H Williams Jr. R&P Ian Gross. Adv. contact Jay Feinman. **N. American subscr. to:** Journal Fulfillment Services, PO Box 2485, Secaucus, NJ 07096-2485. TEL 800-777-4643, FAX 201-348-4505.

LUNG BIOLOGY IN HEALTH AND DISEASE. see *BIOLOGY—Physiology*

616.2 JPN ISSN 0919-5742
CODEN: LUPEFF
THE LUNG PERSPECTIVES. Text in Japanese. 1993. 4/yr. JPY 2,100 per issue (effective 1998).
Indexed: Chem.Abstr., Chem.Indus.Notes, Chem.Titles.
—BLDSC (5307.275000), CASDDS.
Published by: Medikaru Rebyusha/Medical Review Co., Ltd., 7-3 Hirano-Machi 1-chome, Chuo-ku, Osaka-shi 541-0046, Japan. TEL 81-6-223-1667, FAX 81-6-223-1338, meview@osk3.3web.ne.jp.

616.2 JPN ISSN 0917-1363
MAKUGATA HAI/MEMBRANE OXYGENATOR. Text in English, Japanese. 1978. a.
Published by: Makugata Jinko Hai Kenkyukai Jimukyoku, c/o Okayama Daigaku Dai 2 Geka, 2-51 Shikata-cho, Okayama-shi 700-0914, Japan.

M

616.2 JPN
MEDICAL CONFERENCE SERIES. Text in Japanese. 1961. a. JPY 2,835 newsstand/cover (effective 2001). 50 p./no. **Document type:** *Proceedings.*
Published by: Japan Anti-Tuberculosis Association/Kekkaku Yobokai, 1-3-12 Misaki-cho, Chiyoda-ku, Tokyo 101-0061, Japan. TEL 81-3-3292-9211, FAX 81-3-3292-9208, jata@jatahq.org, http://www.jatahq.org. Pub. Toru Mori. Circ: 15,000.

616.2 USA
MEDICAL SCIENTIFIC UPDATE. Text in English. 1982. m. free per issue. **Description:** Informs physicians about clinical programs and research activities conducted at the center.
Published by: National Jewish Medical and Research Center, 1400 Jackson St, Denver, CO 80206. TEL 303-398-1000. Ed. Cherilynn Castleman. Circ: 26,000 (controlled).

616.2 ITA ISSN 0393-8506
MEDICINA TORACICA. Text in Italian. 1978. 4/yr. ITL 90,000 (effective 1999). *Refereed.* **Document type:** *Academic/Scholarly.*
Published by: Masson S.p.A., Divisione Periodici, Via F.lli Bressan 2, Milan, MI 20126, Italy. TEL 39-2-270741, FAX 39-2-27074210. Ed. E Pozzi. adv.: B&W page ITL 2,550,000, color page ITL 3,600,000; trim 285 x 210. Circ: 3,000.

616.2 USA
MEDSCAPE RESPIRATORY CARE. Text in English. 1997. 6/yr. *Refereed.* **Description:** Provides both primary care physicians and specialists with information for the prevention, diagnosis, and management of respiratory diseases.
Media: Online - full text.
Published by: Medscape, Inc., 134 W 29th St, New York, NY 10001-5399. TEL 212-631-1600, http://www.medscape.com.

616.2 USA ISSN 0047-7060
MICHIGAN SOCIETY FOR RESPIRATORY THERAPY. JOURNAL. Text in English. 1965. s-a. membership. adv. bk.rev. abstr.
Formerly (until spring 1975): Michigan Airway
Indexed: CINAHL.
Published by: Michigan Society for Respiratory Therapy, 120 W Saginaw St, E, PO Box 950, Lansing, MI 48823. Ed. John Darin. Circ: 2,000.

616.2 ITA ISSN 0026-4954
MINERVA PNEUMOLOGICA; rivista trimestrale di fisiopatologia e clinica delle malattie dell'apparato respiratorio. Text in Italian; Summaries in English, Italian. 1962. q. USD 105 to individuals; USD 155 to institutions (effective 2000 - 2001). adv. bibl, charts, illus. index. *Refereed.* **Description:** Covers pathophysiology and clinical medicine of the diseases of the respiratory system.
Related titles: Microform ed.: (from PQC).
Indexed: Biol.Abstr., Excerp.Med.
—BLDSC (5794.450000), CISTI, GNLM, KNAW.
Published by: Edizioni Minerva Medica, Corso Bramante, 83-85, Turin, TO 10126, Italy. TEL 39-11-678282, FAX 39-11-674502. Ed. O Orlandi. Pub. Alberto Oliaro. Adv. contact F Filippo. B&W page USD 1,200, color page USD 2,000; trim 270 x 190. Circ: 2,900 (paid).

616.2 ITA ISSN 1122-0643
CODEN: MACDE
MONALDI ARCHIVES FOR CHEST DISEASE. Text and summaries in English. 1945. bi-m. ITL 185,000, USD 140 (effective 2000). adv. bk.rev. *Refereed.* **Document type:** *Academic/Scholarly.* **Description:** Publishes original work, editorials, and reviews on matters of clinical respiratory medicine and rehabilitation.
Former titles (until 1994): Archivio Monaldi per le Malattie del Torace (1120-0391); (until 1987): Archivio di Tisiologia e delle Malattie dell'Aparato Respiratorio (0004-0185)
Indexed: Biol.Abstr., Chem.Abstr., Dent.Ind., Excerp.Med., Ind.Med. (1993-), Int.Nurs.Ind.
—BLDSC (5901.590800), CASDDS, CISTI, EMDOCS, GNLM, KNAW.
Published by: PI-ME Tipografia Editrice s.r.l., Viale Sardegna, 64, Pavia, PV 27100, Italy. TEL 39-0322-884973, FAX 39-0322-884776, monaldi.veruno@fsm.it. Eds. Ciro Rampulla, Claudio F Donner TEL 39-0322-1884811. R&P Claudio F Donner TEL 39-0322-1884811. Circ: 3,500.

MUCOSAL IMMUNOLOGY UPDATE. see *MEDICAL SCIENCES—Allergology And Immunology*

616.246 614 IND
N T I BULLETIN. Text in English. 1964. q. free per issue. bk.rev. abstr, bibl, illus. **Document type:** *Bulletin.* **Description:** Contains original research articles, field reports, TB programmes, and discussions on current problems in the field.
Formerly (until vol.29, 1993): N T I Newsletter (0047-9136)
Published by: National Tuberculosis Institute, 8 Bellary Rd., Bangalore, Karnataka 560 003, India. TEL 361192-93. Circ: 1,000.

NATIONAL ASTHMA CAMPAIGN'S ASTHMA JOURNAL. see *MEDICAL SCIENCES—Allergology And Immunology*

NATIONAL CENTRE FOR OCCUPATIONAL HEALTH. ANNUAL REPORT. see *OCCUPATIONAL HEALTH AND SAFETY*

616.2 NLD ISSN 0925-1944
NEDERLANDSE CYSTIC FIBROSIS STICHTING. C F NIEUWS. Text in Dutch. 1969. q. NLG 30 (effective 2001). adv. 2 p./no. 2 cols./p. **Document type:** *Journal, Abstract/Index, Academic/Scholarly.*
Formerly: Nederlandse Cystic Fibrosis Stichting. Bericht
Published by: Nederlandse Cystic Fibrosis Stichting, Dr A Schweitzerweg 3, Baarn 3744 MG, Netherlands. TEL 31-35-6479257, FAX 31-35-6479489, info@ncfs.nl, htpp://www.info@ncfs.nl. Ed. J. Noordhoek. R&P J Noordhoek TEL 31-35-5429503. Adv. contact J Noordhork. Circ: 2,000.

616.2 USA
NEW DIRECTIONS (DENVER). Text in English. 1986. q. free per issue. **Document type:** *Newsletter.* **Description:** Assistance for patients coping with respiratory and immune system problems.
Formerly: Lung Line Letter
Published by: National Jewish Medical and Research Center, 1400 Jackson St, Denver, CO 80206. TEL 303-398-1080, FAX 303-398-1125. Ed. Li Gwatkin. Circ: 200,000 (controlled).

616.2 JPN ISSN 0029-0645
NIHON KIKAN SHOKUDOKA GAKKAI KAIHO/JAPAN BRONCHO-ESOPHAGOLOGICAL SOCIETY. JOURNAL. Text in Japanese, English; Summaries in English. 1950. bi-m. JPY 12,000 domestic; JPY 13,000 foreign (effective 2001). adv. bk.rev. abstr. cum.index. back issues avail. *Refereed.* **Document type:** *Academic/Scholarly.* **Description:** Reports on branchoesophagological from basic and clinical points of view.
Indexed: Biol.Abstr., Excerp.Med., INIS Atomind.
—CISTI.
Published by: Nihon Kikan Shokudoka Gakkai/Japan Broncho-Esophagological Society, Hakuo Bldg, 2-3-10 Koraku, Bunkyo-ku, Tokyo 112-0004, Japan. TEL 81-3-3818-3030, FAX 81-3-3815-2810, kishoku@hi-ho.ne.jp. Ed., R&P Koshu Nagao. adv.: B&W page JPY 60,000; trim 233 x 142. Circ: 3,700.

613 USA
NOVA REPORT ON LUNG HEALTH AND WELLNESS. Text in English. 1964. bi-m. free per issue. film rev. stat.
Former titles (until 1983): Potomac View on Lung Health; Potomac View (0032-5643)
Media: Duplicated (not offset).
Published by: American Lung Association of Northern Virginia, 9735 Main St, Fairfax, VA 22031. TEL 703-591-4131. Ed. Kurt Gregory Erickson. Circ: 6,000.

616.2 USA
NUCLEAR AND SPACE RADIATION EFFECTS CONFERENCE. PROCEEDINGS. Text in English. a. USD 116. **Document type:** *Proceedings.*
Published by: Institute of Electrical and Electronics Engineers, Inc., 3 Park Ave, 17th Fl, New York, NY 10017. TEL 800-678-4333, customer.service@ieee.org, http://www.ieee.org.

O E D A NEWSLETTER. see *OCCUPATIONAL HEALTH AND SAFETY*

O P A PRATIQUE. (ORL, Pneumo, Allergo) see *MEDICAL SCIENCES—Otorhinolaryngology*

616.2 CAN
ONTARIO THORACIC REVIEWS. Text in English. 1985. 3/yr. free per issue to members. adv. **Document type:** *Trade.* **Description:** Covers advances in treatment and prevention of respiratory disease.
Published by: Ontario Thoracic Society, 573 King St E, Toronto, ON M5A 4L3, Canada. TEL 416-864-9911, FAX 416-864-9916. Ed. Dr. Robert Hyland. R&P Sheila Bussmann. Circ: 6,000.

616.2 GBR ISSN 1526-0542
▼ **PAEDIATRIC RESPIRATORY REVIEWS.** Text in English. 2000 (Mar.). q. GBP 66 to individuals; GBP 142 to institutions (effective 2002). **Document type:** *Academic/Scholarly.* **Description:** Articles relevant to the continuing medical and professional development of paediatricians specializing in the diagnosis, treatment, and management of respiratory disease.
Related titles: Online - full text ed.: ISSN 1526-0550 (from EBSCO Publishing, O C L C Online Computer Library Center, Inc., Swets Blackwell, IDEAL Online Library).

Published by: Churchill Livingstone (Subsidiary of: Harcourt Publishers Ltd.), Robert Stevenson House, 1-3 Baxter's Pl, Leith Walk, Edinburgh, Midlothian EH1 3AF, United Kingdom. TEL 44-131-556-2424, FAX 44-131-489-1177, cservice@harcourt.com, http://www.harcourt-international.com/journals/prrv. **Subscr. to:** Harcourt Publishers Ltd., Foots Cray High St, Sidcup, Kent DA14 5HP, United Kingdom. TEL 44-20-8308-5700, FAX 44-20-8309-0807.

PEDIATRIC PULMONOLOGY. see *MEDICAL SCIENCES—Pediatrics*

616.2 USA
PNEUMOGRAM✱. Text in English. 1980. q. free per issue. adv.
Published by: Cigna Health Care, c/o Equicor Health Plan, 400 N Brand Blvd, 400, Glendale, CA 91203-2311. TEL 818-995-7338, FAX 818-995-0878. Ed. Chuck Swanson. Circ: 2,623.

616.995 616.2 ROM
PNEUMOLOGIA. Text in Romanian; Summaries in English, French, German, Russian. 1952. 4/yr. USD 20. adv. bk.rev. abstr, charts, illus.
Former titles (until 1999): Pneumoftiziologie (0377-5011); Ftiziologia (0016-2329)
Indexed: Biol.Abstr., Chem.Abstr., Ind.Med. (coverage dropped).
—BLDSC (6541.112100), CISTI, GNLM.
Published by: Romanian Medical Association, Str. Ionel Perlea Nr.10, Bucharest 70754, Romania. TEL 401-3141062. **Subscr. to:** ILEXIM, Str. 13 Decembrie 3, PO Box 136-137, Bucharest 70116, Romania.

616.2 BGR ISSN 0324-1491
CODEN: PNFTD3
PNEUMOLOGIA I FTIZIATRIA. Text in Bulgarian; Summaries in Bulgarian, English. 1964. 3/yr., latest vol.35, 2001. BGL 9 domestic; USD 40 foreign (effective 2001 - 2002). adv. abstr, bibl. 64 p./no. *Refereed.* **Document type:** *Academic/Scholarly, Abstract/Index, Bibliography.* **Description:** Publishes original articles on lung diseases with emphasis on tuberculosis.
Formerly: Ftiziatria
Indexed: Abstr.Bulg.Sci.Med.Lit., C.I.S. Abstr., Excerp.Med. (until 1993).
—CISTI, GNLM.
Published by: Meditsinski Universitet - Sofia, Tsentur za Informatsiia po Meditsina/Medical University - Sofia, Medical Information Center, 1 Sv Georgi Sofiiski ul, Sofia 1431, Bulgaria. TEL 359-2-9522342, FAX 359-2-9522393, mutafov@sun.medun.acad.bg, http://www.medun.acad.bg. Ed. St Ivanov. R&P, Adv. contact Dr. Christo Mutafov. Circ: 300. **Co-sponsor:** Nauchno Druzhestvo po Pneumologia i Ftiziatria.

616.2 DEU ISSN 0934-8387
CODEN: PNEMEC
PNEUMOLOGIE. Text in German; Summaries in English, German. 1945. m. EUR 219.80 domestic to institutions; EUR 231.80 in Europe to institutions; EUR 247.80 elsewhere to institutions; EUR 22 newsstand/cover (effective 2002). adv. bk.rev. charts, illus, stat. index. back issues avail.; reprint service avail. from PQC. *Refereed.* **Document type:** *Journal, Academic/Scholarly.*
Former titles: Praxis und Klinik der Pneumologie (0342-7498); Praxis der Pneumologie (0032-7069); Incorporates: Tuberkulosearzt
Related titles: Microfilm ed.: (from PQC); Online - full text ed.: ISSN 1438-8790.
Indexed: Biol.Abstr., C.I.S. Abstr., Chem.Abstr., Curr.Cont. (coverage dropped), Dent.Ind., Derwent Biotech.Abstr., INIS Atomind., Ind.Med. (1989-), Ind.Vet., Int.Nurs.Ind., Sci.Cit.Ind. (coverage dropped), Vet.Bull.
—BLDSC (6541.113200), ADONIS, CASDDS, CISTI, EMDOCS, GNLM, Infotrieve, KNAW. **CCC.**
Published by: (Deutsche Gesellschaft fuer Pneumologie), Georg Thieme Verlag, Ruedigerstr 14, Stuttgart 70469, Germany. TEL 49-711-8931-0, FAX 49-711-8931298, leser.service@thieme.de, http://www.thieme.de/pneumologie. Ed. H Magnussen. R&P Peter Eich. adv.: page DEM 2,950; 175 x 250. Circ: 3,200.

616.2 POL ISSN 0867-7077
CODEN: PAPKE4
PNEUMONOLOGIA I ALERGOLOGIA POLSKA. Text in Polish; Summaries in English. 1926. bi-m. PLZ 60 domestic; PLZ 120 foreign (effective 2000). adv. bk.rev. abstr, illus, stat. *Refereed.* **Document type:** *Academic/Scholarly.* **Description:** Discusses diseases of the lungs, epidemiology, physiology of respiration and clinical pneumonology, allergic diseases of the respiratory system.
Former titles (until 1991): Pneumonologia Polska (0376-4761); Gruzlica i Choroby Pluc (0017-4955)
Indexed: Chem.Abstr., Chem.Titles, Dok.Arbeitsmed., Excerp.Med., INIS Atomind., Ind.Med. (1991-).
—BLDSC (6541.112200), CASDDS, CISTI, EMDOCS, GNLM.
Published by: Instytut Gruzlicy i Chorob Pluc/Institute of Tuberculosis and Pulmonary Diseases, Ul Plocka 26, Warsaw 01138, Poland. TEL 48-22-6912108, FAX 48-22-6912452, u.demkow@igichp.edu.pl. Ed. Elzbieta Wiatr. Adv. contact Miroslawa Kostek. Circ: 1,100. **Co-sponsors:** Polish Society of Allergology; Polish Society of Phtysiopneunomology.

616.238 GBR ISSN 1471-4418
PRIMARY CARE RESPIRATORY JOURNAL. Text in English. q.
Formerly (until 2000): Asthma in General Practice (0968-039X)
Related titles: Online - full text ed.
—BLDSC (6612.908442).
Published by: (General Practice Airways Group (GPIAG)), Strategic Medical Publishing, Action International House, Crabtree Office Village, Eversley Way, Thorpe, Egham, Surrey TW20 8RY, United Kingdom. Ed. Dr. Mark Levy.

616.246 RUS ISSN 0032-9533
CODEN: PRTUAX
PROBLEMY TUBERKULEZA/PROBLEMS OF TUBERCULOSIS. Text in Russian; Summaries in English. 1923. bi-m. USD 152 foreign (effective 2000). adv. bk.rev. index. **Document type:** *Journal.* **Description:** Deals with problems of epidemiology and organization of tuberculosis control, as well as prophylaxis, clinical diagnosis and treatment of tuberculosis. Includes data on the theoretical and practical achievements in phthisis and pulmonology.
Indexed: Biol.Abstr., Chem.Abstr., Chem.Indus.Notes, Chem.Titles, Dent.Ind., Dok.Arbeitsmed., Excerp.Med., Ind.Med. (1935-), Ind.Vet., Ref.Zh., Vet.Bull.
—BLDSC (0133.840000), CASDDS, CISTI, East View, GNLM. **CCC.**
Published by: Izdatel'stvo Meditsina, Petroverigskii per 6-8, Moscow 101000, Russian Federation. TEL 7-095-2681441, 7-095-928-86-48, FAX 7-095-9211355, meditsina@iname.com, http://www.medit.ru. Ed. A G Khomenko. Pub. A M Stochik. R&P G Postnikova. Adv. contact O A Fadeeva TEL 7-095-923-51-40. Circ: 1,550. **Dist. by:** Mezhdunarodnaya Kniga, B Yakimanka 39, Moscow 117049, Russian Federation. TEL 7-095-2384967, FAX 7-095-2384634.

616.2 CHE ISSN 1422-2140
QP121.A1 CODEN: PGRRB6
PROGRESS IN RESPIRATORY RESEARCH. Text in English. 1963. irreg., latest vol.31. CHF 230 in Europe; DEM 275 in Germany; USD 185 in United States (effective 2001). reprint service avail. from ISI. *Refereed.* **Document type:** *Monographic series, Academic/Scholarly.* **Description:** Surveys of new knowledge on normal and impaired respiratory function.
Formerly: Progress in Respiration Research (0079-6751)
Related titles: Online - full text ed.: (from Institute for Scientific Information).
Indexed: Biol.Abstr., Chem.Abstr., Curr.Adv.Ecol.Sci., Curr.Cont. (coverage dropped), Ind.Med. (coverage dropped).
—BLDSC (6924.525540), CASDDS, CISTI, GNLM, KNAW. **CCC.**
Published by: S. Karger AG, Allschwilerstr 10, PO Box, Basel 4009, Switzerland. TEL 41-61-306-1111, FAX 41-61-306-1234, karger@karger.ch, http://www.karger.com/bookseries/PRRER. Ed. C T Bolliger.

616.2 USA
PULMONARY DISORDERS: D S M RESOURCE. (Disease State Management) Text in English. 1997. a. USD 269; USD 229 foreign (effective 1999). **Document type:** *Trade.*
Published by: American Health Consultants (Subsidiary of: Medical Economics Co., Inc.), 3525 Piedmont Rd, N E, 6 Piedmont Center, Ste 400, Atlanta, GA 30305. TEL 404-262-5476, custserv@ahcpub.com, http://www.ahcpub.com.

616.2 USA
PULMONARY PERSPECTIVES. Text in English. q. adv. *Refereed.* **Document type:** *Academic/Scholarly.* **Description:** Contains brief articles with editorial commentary for practicing physicians in the chest disciplines.
Published by: American College of Chest Physicians, 3300 Dundee Rd, Northbrook, IL 60062. TEL 847-498-1400, FAX 847-498-5460, editor@chestnet.org. Ed. Deborah Shure. Pub. Alvin Lever. R&P Pam Goorsky. Adv. contact Pat Micek. Circ: 16,000.

616.2 GBR ISSN 1094-5539
CODEN: PPTHFJ
PULMONARY PHARMACOLOGY & THERAPEUTICS. Text in English. 1988. bi-m. GBP 315 to institutions (effective 2001). bk.rev. reprint service avail. from SWZ. *Refereed.* **Document type:** *Academic/Scholarly.* **Description:** Concerned with lung pharmacology from molecular to clinical aspects.
Formerly (until 1997): Pulmonary Pharmacology (Edinburgh) (0952-0600)
Related titles: Online - full text ed.: (from EBSCO Publishing, O C L C Online Computer Library Center, Inc., RoweCom Information Quest, ingenta, Swets Blackwell, IDEAL Online Library, Institute for Scientific Information).
Indexed: Biol.Abstr., Chem.Abstr., Chem.Indus.Notes, Chem.Titles, Curr.Cont. (coverage dropped), Derwent Biotech.Abstr., Excerp.Med., Ind.Med. (1997-), Sci.Cit.Ind. (coverage dropped).
—BLDSC (7156.978500), ADONIS, CASDDS, CISTI, EMDOCS, GNLM, IDS, Infotrieve, KNAW. **CCC.**
Published by: Academic Press (Subsidiary of: Harcourt Publishers Ltd.), 24 Oval Rd, London NW1 7DX, United Kingdom. TEL 44-20-7267-4466, FAX 44-20-7482-2293, apsubs@acad.com, http://www.academicpress.com/ppt. **Subscr. to:** Harcourt Publishers Ltd., Foots Cray High St, Sidcup, Kent DA14 5HP, United Kingdom. TEL 44-20-8300-3322, FAX 44-20-8309-0807.

616.2 USA ISSN 1086-4423
PULMONARY REVIEWS; trends in pulmonary and critical care medicine. Text in English. 1996. 9/yr. USD 75; USD 90 foreign. adv. abstr, charts, illus. *Refereed.* **Document type:** *Trade.* **Description:** Discusses research in the diagnosis and treatment of pulmonary conditions.
Published by: Partners in Medical Communication, 2 Brighton Rd, Clifton, NJ 07012. TEL 201-916-1000, FAX 201-916-0021, pulmorev@aol.com. Ed. Alfred J Saint Jacques. Pub. Susan Panetta. R&P Steve Svec. Circ: (controlled).

616.2 RUS ISSN 0869-0189
PUL'MONOLOGIYA. Text in Russian; Summaries in English. 1991. q. RUR 35; USD 4 foreign (effective 2000). adv. bibl, charts, illus, stat. back issues avail. *Refereed.* **Document type:** *Academic/Scholarly.* **Description:** Publishes experimental and clinical works on all aspects of respiratory medicine. Includes original studies, lectures, reviews and data on pharmacological products.
Related titles: Online - full text ed.
Indexed: INIS Atomind., Ref.Zh.
Published by: Institut Pulmonologii, 11-ya Parkovaya ul 32-36, korp 4, Moscow 105077, Russian Federation. TEL 7-095-4654877, FAX 7-095-4654877, pulmo@dol.ru, http://wildcat.ili.rssi.ru/pulmo. Ed. Alexander G Chuchalin. Adv. contact Dimitry Soldatov. color page USD 1,200. Circ: 2,000. **Dist. by:** Agentsiya Rospechat, Pr-t Marshala Zhukova 4, Moscow 128837, Russian Federation.

616.2 USA ISSN 1040-6050
R T; the journal for respiratory care practitioners. Variant title: R T Magazine. Text in English. 1988. bi-m. free to qualified personnel. adv. **Document type:** *Magazine, Trade.* **Description:** Features literature reviews of clinical topics, articles on respiratory care department management, legislative and regulatory news, case reports, profiles of outstanding facilities and practitioners, and departments containing news, industry news, and new product information.
Indexed: CINAHL.
—BLDSC (8037.002000).
Published by: Curant Communications, Inc. (Subsidiary of: Medical World Communications), 6701 Center Drive W #450, Los Angeles, CA 90045-1556. TEL 310-306-2206, FAX 310-306-9548, psmith@medpubs.com, http://www.rtmagazine.com. Ed. Paige Smith. Pubs. Curtis Pickelle, Tony Ramos. R&P Tammy Reynolds. Adv. contact Renee Luttrell. B&W page USD 2,790, color page USD 3,590; trim 10.88 x 8.38. Circ: 20,000 (controlled).

616.2 USA
R T INTERNATIONAL. (Respiratory Therapy) Text in English. 1992. a. free to qualified personnel. adv. **Document type:** *Journal, Trade.*
Related titles: Online - full text ed.

M

Published by: Curant Communications, Inc. (Subsidiary of: Medical World Communications), 6701 Center Drive W #450, Los Angeles, CA 90045-1556. TEL 310-306-2206, FAX 310-306-9548, psmith@medpubs.com, http://www.rtmagazine.com/. Pub. Tony Ramos. Adv. contact Sharon Marsee. B&W page USD 2,930; trim 10.88 x 8.38.

616.2 USA
R T SOLUTIONS E - ZINE. Text in English. 1996. bi-m. **Document type:** *Trade.* **Description:** Web-based interactive forum for respiratory care professionals.
Media: Online - full text.
Address: wjb@beachweb.win.net, http://www.win.net/~beachweb/rtsolut1.html. Ed. William Beach.

616.2 ITA ISSN 0033-9563
RASSEGNA DI PATOLOGIA DELL'APPARATO RESPIRATORIO. Text in Italian. 1951. bi-m. ITL 120,000; ITL 150,000 foreign (effective 1996). adv. bk.rev. bibl, charts, illus. index.
Indexed: Chem.Abstr., Excerp.Med.
—GNLM.
Published by: (Associazione Italiana Pneumologi Ospedalieri), Pacini Editore, Via Alessandro Gherardesca, 1, Ospedaletto, PI 56121, Italy. TEL 39-050-313011, FAX 39-050-3130300, pacini@cibernet.it, http://www.cibernet.it/pacini, http://www.pacinieditore.it. Ed. Benito Leoncini. Circ: 1,000.

616.2 GBR ISSN 0308-6623
RECENT ADVANCES IN RESPIRATORY MEDICINE. Text in English. 1976. irreg., latest vol.5. **Document type:** *Monographic series, Academic/Scholarly.*
—CISTI, GNLM, KNAW.
Published by: Churchill Livingstone (Subsidiary of: Harcourt Publishers Ltd.), Robert Stevenson House, 1-3 Baxter's Pl, Leith Walk, Edinburgh, Midlothian EH1 3AF, United Kingdom. TEL 44-131-556-2424, FAX 44-131-459-1177, http://www.churchillmed.com. **US subscr. to:** Churchill Livingstone, 650 Ave of the Americas, New York, NY 10011. TEL 212-206-5000.

REFERATIVNYI ZHURNAL. TUBERKULEZ. see *MEDICAL SCIENCES—Abstracting, Bibliographies, Statistics*

616.2 ARG ISSN 0326-9116
RESPIRACION; revista de enfermedades respiratorias y tuberculosis. Text in Spanish. 1986. q., latest vol.11, 1996.
Published by: Fundacion Ayuda al Enfermo Respiratorio, Avda. Sarsfield Velez, 405, Capital Federal, Buenos Aires 1281, Argentina. TEL 54-11-44318374, FAX 54-11-44333742, contacto@contactounido.com.ar, http://www.contactounido.com.ar. Ed. Luis Julio Gonzalez Montaner.

617.54 616.995 CHE ISSN 0025-7931
RC705 CODEN: RESPBD
RESPIRATION; international journal of thoracic medicine. Text in English. 1944. bi-m. CHF 1,024, EUR 731.80 in Europe to institutions; CHF 1,041.40, USD 796 elsewhere to institutions (effective 2002). adv. charts, illus. back issues avail. *Refereed.* **Document type:** *Journal, Academic/Scholarly.* **Description:** Provides the results of both clinical and experimental investigations on all aspects of the respiratory system in health and disease.
Formerly: Medicina Thoracalis
Related titles: Microform ed.; Online - full text ed.: ISSN 1423-0356. 1997. CHF 58, EUR 42, USD 45 to institutions with print edition (effective 2002) (from EBSCO Publishing, O C L C Online Computer Library Center, Inc., RoweCom Information Quest, Swets Blackwell, Institute for Scientific Information).
Indexed: AMED, ASCA, Biol.Abstr., C.I.S. Abstr., Chem.Abstr., Chem.Indus.Notes, Chem.Titles, Curr.Adv.Ecol.Sci., Curr.Cont., Dok.Arbeitsmed., Excerp.Med., Helminthol.Abstr., INIS Atomind., Ind.Med. (1968-), Ind.Sci.Rev., Inpharma, Nutr.Abstr., Pharm.&Out.News, Reac., Rev.Appl.Entomol., Rev.Plant Path., Sci.Cit.Ind., THA.
—BLDSC (7777.620000), CASDDS, CISTI, GNLM, IDS, ingenta, KNAW. **CCC.**
Published by: S. Karger AG, Allschwilerstr 10, PO Box, Basel 4009, Switzerland. TEL 41-61-306-1111, FAX 41-61-306-1234, karger@karger.ch, http://www.online.karger.com/journals/res, http://www.karger.com. Ed. C T Bolliger. adv.: page USD 1,185. Circ: 1,200.

RESPIRATION PHYSIOLOGY. see *BIOLOGY—Physiology*

615.64 USA ISSN 0020-1324
RESPIRATORY CARE; a monthly science journal. Short title: R C. Text in English, Italian, Japanese, French. 1956. m. USD 50. adv. bk.rev. abstr, charts, illus. index. reprints avail. **Description:** Disseminates information, viewpoints, and questions about respiratory disease, research, clinical and laboratory practice, education, and patient care science.
Formerly (until 1971): Inhalation Therapy
Related titles: Microform ed.: (from PQC); Online - full text ed.
Indexed: Biol.Abstr., CINAHL, Excerp.Med., Hosp.Lit.Ind., Ind.Med. (1971-), Nurs.Abstr., THA.
—BLDSC (7777.660000), CISTI, GNLM, ingenta, KNAW. **CCC.**
Published by: (American Association for Respiratory Care), Daedalus Enterprises, Inc., 11030 Ables Lane, Dallas, TX 75229. TEL 972-243-2272, FAX 972-484-6010, http://www.rcjournal.com. Ed. David J Pierson. Circ: 38,000.

615.64 USA ISSN 1078-5337
RESPIRATORY CARE CLINICS. Text in English. 1995. q. USD 68 domestic to individuals; USD 94 in Canada to individuals; USD 102 foreign to individuals; USD 98 domestic to institutions; USD 137 foreign to institutions; USD 49 domestic to students; USD 35 per issue (effective 2001). **Document type:** *Academic/Scholarly.* **Description:** Contains clinical and experimental reviews aimed primarily at respiratory therapists, as well as physicians and nurses involved in this area of care.
Indexed: Ind.Med. (1995-).
—BLDSC (7777.660050), CISTI, GNLM, KNAW.
Published by: W.B. Saunders Co. (Subsidiary of: Harcourt Publishers Ltd.), 11830 Westline Industrial Dr, St Louis, MO 63146. TEL 800-325-4177, http://www.wbsaunders.com. Eds. Dr. Neil MacIntyre, Richard D Branson. **Subscr. to:** Periodicals Fulfillment, W B Saunders Co, 6277 Sea Harbor Dr, 4th Fl, Orlando, FL 32891-4800.

616.2 658 USA ISSN 1076-6030
RESPIRATORY CARE MANAGER. Text in English. 1992. m. USD 167. **Document type:** *Newsletter.* **Description:** Provides information and guidance for managers in respiratory care, including coverage of regulatory issues, quality improvement, patient-focused care, budget and staff management techniques.
—CCC.
Published by: Opus Communications, PO Box 1168, Marblehead, MA 01945. TEL 781-639-1872, FAX 781-639-2982, customer_service@opuscomm.com, http://www.opuscomm.com.

616.2 GBR ISSN 0262-7043
RESPIRATORY DISEASE IN PRACTICE. Abbreviated title: R D I P. Text in English. 1982. q. adv. bk.rev. **Document type:** *Academic/Scholarly.*
—BLDSC (7777.661000).
Published by: Hayward Medical Communications Ltd., Covent Garden, Seven Dials Warehouse, 44 Earlham St, London WC2H 9LA, United Kingdom. TEL 44-20-7240-4493, FAX 44-20-7240-4479, admin@hayward.co.uk, http://www.hayward.co.uk. Ed. Dr. Phillip Ind. Circ: 14,000. **Subscr. to:** Rosemary House, Lanwades Park, Kentford, Near, Newmarket, Suffolk CB8 7PW, United Kingdom. TEL 44-1638-751515, FAX 44-1638-751517.

616.246 KEN
RESPIRATORY DISEASES RESEARCH CENTRE. ANNUAL REPORT. Text in English. 1974. a. free per issue. back issues avail. **Document type:** *Corporate.*
Former titles: Kenya Tuberculosis and Respiratory Diseases Research Center. Annual Report; Kenya Tuberculosis Investigation Centre. Annual Report; Supersedes in part: East African Tuberculosis Investigation Centre. Annual Report
Indexed: Biol.Abstr.
Published by: Kenya Medical Research Institute, Kenya Tuberculosis & Respiratory Diseases Research Centre, PO Box 47855, Nairobi, Kenya. Circ: 200.

616.2 USA ISSN 1067-9324
RESPIRATORY HEALTH MONITOR. Text in English. 1993. m. **Document type:** *Newsletter, Consumer.*
Published by: Data Centrum Communications, Inc., 21 W 38th St, 4th fl, New York, NY 10018.

616.2 GBR ISSN 0954-6111
CODEN: RMEDEY
RESPIRATORY MEDICINE. Text in English. 1907. m. GBP 128 to individuals; GBP 309 to institutions (effective 2002). adv. bk.rev. charts, illus, stat. index. back issues avail.; reprint service avail. from SWZ. *Refereed.* **Document type:** *Academic/Scholarly.* **Description:** Provides an international forum for new information of relevance to the physician working in the field of respiratory medicine.
Formerly: British Journal of Diseases of the Chest (0007-0971)
Related titles: Microform ed.: (from PQC); Online - full text ed.: (from EBSCO Publishing, O C L C Online Computer Library Center, Inc., Swets Blackwell, IDEAL Online Library, Institute for Scientific Information).
Indexed: AIDS Abstr., AMED, ASCA, Abstr.Hyg., Agri.& Environ.Biotech.Abstr. (coverage dropped), Biol.Abstr., C.I.S. Abstr., Chem.Abstr., Curr.Adv.Ecol.Sci., Curr.Cont., Derwent Biotech.Abstr., Environ.Sci.Poll.Mgmt., Excerp.Med., Helminthol.Abstr., Ind.Med. (1989-), Ind.Sci.Rev., Inpharma, Int.Nurs.Ind., Nutr.Abstr., Pharm.&Out.News, Pig News & Info., Pollut.Abstr., Protozool.Abstr., Reac., Ref.Zh., Rev.Appl.Entomol., Rev.Med.& Vet.Mycol., Rev.Plant Path., Risk Abstr., SSCI (coverage dropped), Saf.Sci.Abstr., Sci.Cit.Ind., THA, Trop.Dis.Bull.
—BLDSC (7777.661900), CASDDS, CISTI, EMDOCS, GNLM, IDS, ingenta, KNAW. **CCC.**
Published by: W.B. Saunders Co. Ltd. (Subsidiary of: Harcourt Publishers Ltd.), 24-28 Oval Rd, London NW1 7DX, United Kingdom. TEL 44-20-7424-4200, FAX 44-20-7424-4515, cservice@harcourt.com, http://www.harcourt-international.com/journals/rmed. Eds. J Fish, R Dahl. **Subscr. to:** Harcourt Publishers Ltd., Foots Cray High St, Sidcup, Kent DA14 5HP, United Kingdom. TEL 44-20-8308-5700, FAX 44-20-8309-0807.

RESPIRATORY PHARMACOLOGY AND PHARMACOTHERAPY. see *PHARMACY AND PHARMACOLOGY*

616.2 USA ISSN 0895-0881
RESPIRATORY PRACTITIONER✱ . Text in English. 1986. q. USD 25. adv. **Description:** For individuals and institutions involved in the services and technologies of respiratory care and its associated diseases.
Published by: Reliable Multi-Media Productions, 5705 Sepulveda Blvd, Culver City, CA 90230-6405. Eds. James B Fink, Stephan W Ruesh. Circ: 20,000.

616.2 GBR ISSN 1465-9921
▼ **RESPIRATORY RESEARCH.** Text in English. 2000. bi-m. GBP 200 in United Kingdom; USD 300 elsewhere (effective 2001). **Document type:** *Journal, Academic/Scholarly.* **Description:** Aims to ensure that researchers and clinicians have easy access to the latest mechanism-defining research and analysis, particularly in the areas of genetics, biochemistry and cell biology.
Published by: Current Science Ltd, Middlesex House, 34-42 Cleveland St, London W1P 6LB, United Kingdom. TEL 44-20-7323-0323, FAX 44-20-7580-1938, info@respiratory-research.com, http://respiratory-research.com/, http://www.currentsciencegroup.com. Eds. Kenneth L Brigham, Peter J Barnes.

616.2 USA ISSN 1068-963X
RESPIRATORY THERAPY PRODUCTS. Text in English. 1993. s-a. **Document type:** *Journal, Trade.* **Description:** Contains information on new and existing products from the manufacturers of respiratory care equipment and supplies.
Published by: Curant Communications, Inc. (Subsidiary of: Medical World Communications), 6701 Center Drive W #450, Los Angeles, CA 90045-1556. TEL 310-306-2206, FAX 310-306-9548, psmith@medpubs.com, http://www.rtmagazine.com. Pub. Tony Ramos. Adv. contact Sharon Marsee.

616.2 AUS ISSN 1323-7799
CODEN: RSPIFB
RESPIROLOGY. Text in English. 1996. q. AUD 577 domestic to institutions; AUD 525 in New Zealand to institutions; USD 320 elsewhere to institutions; AUD 635 domestic to institutions paper & onlline eds. combined; AUD 578 in New Zealand to institutions paper & onlline eds. combined; USD 352 elsewhere to institutions paper & onlline eds. combined (effective 2001). adv. back issues avail. **Document type:** *Academic/Scholarly.* **Description:** Publishes articles of scientific excellence in clinical and experimental respiratory biology and disease, and related fields of research.

Related titles: Online - full text ed.: ISSN 1440-1843. AUD 520 domestic to institutions; AUD 473 in New Zealand to institutions; USD 288 elsewhere to institutions (effective 2001) (from EBSCO Publishing, O C L C Online Computer Library Center, Inc., RoweCom Information Quest, ingenta, Munksgaard & Blackwell Science's Synergy, Swets Blackwell).
Indexed: Environ.Sci.Poll.Mgmt., Ind.Med. (1996-), Inpharma, Pharm.&Out.News, Pollut.Abstr., Reac., Rev.Appl.Entomol., Rev.Med.& Vet.Mycol., Risk Abstr., Saf.Sci.Abstr.
—BLDSC (7777.666000), CISTI, GNLM, Infotrieve, KNAW. **CCC.**
Published by: (Asian Pacific Society of Respirology JPN), Blackwell Science Asia Pty Ltd, PO Box 378, Carlton South, VIC 3053, Australia. TEL 61-3-9347-0300, FAX 61-3-9347-5001, info@blacksci-asia.com.au, http://www.blacksci.co.uk. Ed. Philip J Thompson. Adv. contact Kathryn O'Brien. B&W page AUD 1,012, color page AUD 2,057; trim 210 x 275.

616.2 615.8 IRL ISSN 0300-9572 CODEN: RSUSBS
RESUSCITATION; an interdisciplinary journal for the dissemination of clinical and basic science research relating to acute care medicine and cardiopulmonary resuscitation. Text in English. 1972. m. EUR 126 in Europe to individuals; JPY 16,800 in Japan to individuals; USD 141 elsewhere to individuals; EUR 959 in Europe to institutions; JPY 127,200 in Japan to institutions; USD 1,074 elsewhere to institutions (effective 2002). adv. bk.rev. charts, illus. index. reprints avail. *Refereed.* **Document type:** *Academic/Scholarly.* **Description:** Covers the etiology, pathophysiology, diagnosis and treatment of acute diseases.
Related titles: Microform ed.: (from PQC); Online - full text ed.: (from ingenta, Swets Blackwell, Institute for Scientific Information, ScienceDirect).
Indexed: ASCA, Biol.Abstr., Chem.Abstr., Chem.Indus.Notes, Chem.Titles, Curr.Adv.Ecol.Sci., Curr.Cont., Excerp.Med., Ind.Med. (1972-), Inpharma, Int.Nurs.Ind., Jrnl.Watch Emer.Med., Pharm.&Out.News, Reac., Ref.Zh., SSCI (coverage dropped), Sci.Cit.Ind.
—BLDSC (7785.420000), ADONIS, CASDDS, CISTI, EMDOCS, GNLM, IDS, ingenta, KNAW. **CCC.**
Published by: (European Resuscitation Council), Elsevier Science Ireland Ltd, Elsevier House, Brookvale Plaza, E. Park, Shannon, Co. Clare, Ireland. TEL 353-61-471944, FAX 353-61-472144, http://www.elsevier.nl/locate/resuscitation. Eds. J Ornato, P J F Baskett. **Subscr. in Australasia and the Far East to:** Elsevier Science (Singapore) Pte Ltd, No.1 Temasek Ave, 17-01 Millenia Tower, Singapore 039192, Singapore. TEL 65-434-3727, FAX 65-337-2230; **Subscr. in the Americas to:** Elsevier Science, PO Box 945, New York, NY 10159-0945. TEL 212-633-3730, FAX 212-633-3680; **Subscr. to:** Elsevier Science BV, PO Box 211, Amsterdam 1000 AE, Netherlands. TEL 31-20-485-3757, FAX 31-20-485-3432.

616.2 616.1 FRA ISSN 0761-8417 CODEN: RPCLEZ
REVUE DE PNEUMOLOGIE CLINIQUE; le poumon et le coeur. Text in French; Summaries in English. 1945. 6/yr. FRF 865; FRF 1,058 foreign (effective 2000). adv. bk.rev. abstr, bibl, charts, illus, stat. index. reprint service avail. from PQC,ISI. **Document type:** *Academic/Scholarly.* **Description:** Devoted to the pathology and therapy of afflictions of the respiratory tract.
Formerly: Poumon et le Coeur (0032-5821)
Related titles: Microform ed.: (from PQC); Online - full text ed.: (from RoweCom Information Quest).
Indexed: Biol.Abstr., C.I.S. Abstr., Chem.Abstr., Dent.Ind., Dok.Arbeitsmed., Excerp.Med., Ind.Med. (1984-), Rev.Med.& Vet.Mycol., Rev.Plant Path.
—BLDSC (7942.535000), CASDDS, CISTI, GNLM, Infotrieve, KNAW. **CCC.**
Published by: Masson - Periodiques, 120 bd. St. Germain, Paris 75006, France. TEL 33-1-40466200, FAX 33-1-40466201. Eds. C Mayaud, M Milleron. Circ: 1,500. **Subscr. to:** Societe de Periodiques Specialises, BP 22, Vineuil Cedex 41354, France. TEL 33-2-54504612, FAX 33-2-54504611.

616.2 FRA ISSN 0761-8425 CODEN: RMREEY
REVUE DES MALADIES RESPIRATOIRES. Text in French. 1893. 6/yr. FRF 998; FRF 1,370 foreign (effective 2000). adv. bk.rev. abstr, illus. index. reprint service avail. from ISI. *Refereed.* **Document type:** *Academic/Scholarly.* **Description:** Publishes original articles on clinical and laboratory work in the field of respiratory diseases.
Former titles (until 1983): Revue Francaise des Maladies Respiratoires (0301-0279); (until 1973): Revue de Tuberculose et de Pneumologie (0035-1792)
Related titles: Microfilm ed.; Online - full text ed.: (from Institute for Scientific Information, RoweCom Information Quest).
Indexed: ASCA, Biol.Abstr., C.I.S. Abstr., Chem.Abstr., Curr.Adv.Ecol.Sci., Curr.Cont., Dairy Sci.Abstr., Dok.Arbeitsmed., Excerp.Med., Helminthol.Abstr., Ind.Med. (1984-), Inpharma, Int.Nurs.Ind., Pharm.&Out.News, Protozool.Abstr., Reac., Rev.Med.& Vet.Mycol., Rev.Plant Path., SSCI (coverage dropped).
—BLDSC (7926.824000), CASDDS, CISTI, EMDOCS, GNLM, IDS, Infotrieve, KNAW. **CCC.**
Published by: (Societe de Pneumologie de Langue Francaise), Masson - Periodiques, 120 bd. St. Germain, Paris 75006, France. TEL 33-1-40466200, FAX 33-1-40466201. Ed. B Housset. Circ: 3,000. **Subscr. to:** Societe de Periodiques Specialises, BP 22, Vineuil Cedex 41354, France. TEL 33-2-54504612, FAX 33-2-54504611. **Co-sponsor:** Comite National de Defense Contre la Tuberculose.

616.2 JPN ISSN 0911-1182
RINSHO KOKYU SEIRI/JOURNAL OF CLINICAL RESPIRATORY PHYSIOLOGY. Text in Japanese. 1968. s-a. JPY 2,000 per issue.
Published by: (Rinsho Kokyu Seiri Kenkyukai/Society of Clinical Respiratory Physiology), Faiza Seiyaku K.K./Pfizer Pharmaceuticals, Inc., 1-1 Nishi-Shinjuku 2-chome, Shinjuku-ku, Tokyo 160-0023, Japan.

616.2 ITA ISSN 0302-4717
RIVISTA DI PATOLOGIA E CLINICA DELLA TUBERCOLOSI E DI PNEUMOLOGIA. Text in Italian; Summaries in English, French. 1927. bi-m. ITL 40,000, USD 70. adv. bk.rev. abstr. index, cum.index.
Formerly: Rivista di Patologia e Clinica della Tubercolosi (0035-6425)
Indexed: Biol.Abstr., Excerp.Med. (until 1993).
—CISTI, GNLM.
Published by: Associazione Emilia Romagna Contro la Tubercolosi e le Malatie Polmonari Sociali, Via Giovanni Brugnoli, 5, Bologna, BO 40122, Italy. Ed. Enrico Fasano. Circ: 1,000.

616.2 ZAF ISSN 0081-2501
S.A.N.T.A. ANNUAL REPORT. Text in English. 1949. a. free per issue. **Document type:** *Corporate.* **Description:** Features SANTA's financial statements, review of the year's activities, history of investments made, as well as the present status of TB containment.
Published by: South African National Tuberculosis Association/Suid-Afrikaanse Nasionale Tuberkulose Vereniging, Private Bag X10030, Edenvale 1610, South Africa. TEL 27-11-454-0260, FAX 27-11-454-0096, santa@santa.org.za, http://www.santa.org.za. Ed. Eve Stubbs. R&P Jacqui van Rensburg. Circ: 2,000.

616.246 ZAF
S.A.N.T.A. T B AND HEALTH NEWS. Text in English. 1953. q. donation. adv. charts, illus, stat. **Document type:** *Newsletter.* **Description:** Informs readers of news and events involving the association, and discusses issues relating to tuberculosis in South Africa.
Formerly (until vol.33, no.9, 1994): S.A.N.T.A. T B News (0036-0872)
Published by: South African National Tuberculosis Association/Suid-Afrikaanse Nasionale Tuberkulose Vereniging, Private Bag X10030, Edenvale 1610, South Africa. TEL 27-11-454-0260, FAX 27-11-454-0096, santa@santa.org.za, http://www.santa.org.za. Ed. Eve Stubbs. R&P, Adv. contact Jacqui van Rensburg. Circ: 9,000.

616.2 USA ISSN 1069-3424 CODEN: SRCCEX
SEMINARS IN RESPIRATORY AND CRITICAL CARE MEDICINE. Text in English. 1979. bi-m. EUR 206 to individuals; EUR 410 to institutions; EUR 62 newsstand/cover (effective 2002). adv. index. reprint service avail. from PQC. *Refereed.* **Document type:** *Journal, Academic/Scholarly.* **Description:** Contains clinical articles written by pulmonary clinicians providing an overview of principles and practice of modern respiratory care.
Formerly (until 1994): Seminars in Respiratory Medicine (0192-9755)
Related titles: Microform ed.: (from PQC); Online - full text ed.: ISSN 1098-9048 (from Ovid Technologies, Inc., EBSCO Publishing, O C L C Online Computer Library Center, Inc., RoweCom Information Quest, Institute for Scientific Information).
Indexed: ASCA, Biol.Abstr., Curr.Adv.Ecol.Sci., Curr.Cont., Excerp.Med., Helminthol.Abstr., Ind.Sci.Rev., Inpharma, Nutr.Abstr., Pharm.&Out.News, Reac., Rev.Med.& Vet.Mycol., SSCI (coverage dropped), Sci.Cit.Ind., THA.
—BLDSC (8239.457750), CISTI, EMDOCS, GNLM, IDS, ingenta, KNAW. **CCC.**
Published by: Thieme Medical Publishers, 333 Seventh Ave, New York, NY 10001. TEL 212-760-0888, 800-782-3488, FAX 212-947-1112, http://www.thieme.com. Ed. Dr. Joseph P Lynch III. Circ: 2,615. **Orders in Europe to:** Georg Thieme Verlag, Postfach 301120, Stuttgart 70451, Germany. TEL 49-711-8931-0, 49-711-8931-298.

616.2 USA ISSN 0882-0546 CODEN: SRINES
SEMINARS IN RESPIRATORY INFECTIONS. Text in English. 1986. q. USD 146 domestic to individuals; USD 209 foreign to individuals; USD 210 domestic to institutions; USD 263 foreign to institutions; USD 97 domestic to students; USD 125 foreign to students; USD 66 newsstand/cover (effective 2001). adv. abstr, bibl, charts, illus. index. **Document type:** *Academic/Scholarly.* **Description:** Each issue treats a type of infection relative to lung disorders in depth.
Indexed: CINAHL, INIS Atomind., Ind.Med. (1986-), Int.Nurs.Ind.
—BLDSC (8239.457800), CISTI, EMDOCS, GNLM, ingenta, KNAW. **CCC.**
Published by: W.B. Saunders Co. (Subsidiary of: Harcourt Publishers Ltd.), 11830 Westline Industrial Dr, St Louis, MO 63146. TEL 800-325-4177, http://www.wbsaunders.com. Ed. Dr. George A Sarosi. adv.: B&W page USD 805, color page USD 1,880; trim 10 x 7. Circ: 675. **Subscr. to:** Periodicals Fulfillment, W B Saunders Co, 6277 Sea Harbor Dr, 4th Fl, Orlando, FL 32891-4800.

616.246 614.49 USA ISSN 1082-8664
T B MONITOR. (Tuberculosis) Text in English. 1994. m. USD 527 domestic; USD 557 foreign; USD 88 newsstand/cover (effective 2001). **Document type:** *Newsletter.*
Incorporates (1993-1994): Correctional Health Care Management
Indexed: CINAHL.
—BLDSC (8612.371000).
Published by: American Health Consultants (Subsidiary of: Medical Economics Co., Inc.), 3525 Piedmont Rd, N E, 6 Piedmont Center, Ste 400, Atlanta, GA 30305. TEL 404-262-5476, 404-262-7436, 800-688-2421, FAX 404-262-7837, 800-284-3291, custserv@ahcpub.com, http://www.ahcpub.com.

616.246 614.49 USA
T B SOURCEBOOK. (Tuberculosis) Text in English. 1997. a. USD 269; USD 269 foreign (effective 1999). **Document type:** *Trade.*
Published by: American Health Consultants (Subsidiary of: Medical Economics Co., Inc.), 3525 Piedmont Rd, N E, 6 Piedmont Center, Ste 400, Atlanta, GA 30305. TEL 404-262-5476, custserv@ahcpub.com, http://www.ahcpub.com.

616.2 USA ISSN 8756-8616
TECHNOLOGY FOR RESPIRATORY THERAPY. Text in English. m. USD 205.80 domestic; USD 221 in Canada; USD 249.60 elsewhere (effective 2001). *Refereed.* **Document type:** *Newsletter.* **Description:** Contains technology-related information for respiratory specialists.
Formerly: Health Devices Update: Respiratory Therapy
—CCC.
Published by: (Emergency Care Research Institute), E C R I, 5200 Butler Pike, Plymouth, PA 19462. TEL 610-825-6000, FAX 610-834-1275, info@ecri.org, http://www.ecri.org. Ed. Beth Richardson.

616.2 NLD ISSN 0040-2125
TEGEN DE TUBERCULOSE. Text in Dutch. 1904. q. free. adv. bk.rev. illus. **Document type:** *Journal, Academic/Scholarly.*
Published by: Koninklijke Nederlandse Centrale Vereniging tot Bestrijding der Tuberculose, PO Box 146, The Hague 2501 CC, Netherlands. TEL 31-70-4167222, FAX 31-70-3584004, kncvtbc@kncvtbc.nl. Ed. J F Broekmans. R&P M J Havermans. Circ: 5,000.

616.2 AUS ISSN 1441-516X
THERAPEUTIC GUIDELINES. RESPIRATORY. Text in English. 1994. irreg., latest version 2 (every 3-4 yrs.). AUD 31.90 newsstand/cover (effective 2001). **Document type:** *Academic/Scholarly.* **Description:** Gives concrete recommendations for rational therapy of respiratory disease and, where necessary, justifies the choice of therapy.
Formerly (until 1999): Respiratory Drug Guidelines
Published by: Therapeutic Guidelines Ltd., Chelsea House, Level 2, 55 Flemington Rd, North Melbourne, VIC 3051, Australia. TEL 61-3-9329-1566, FAX 61-3-9326-5632, sales@tg.com.au, http://www.tg.com.au. Ed., R&P Mary Hemming. Circ: 18,000.

M

616.2 USA ISSN 1042-2846
TODAY IN MEDICINE. RESPIRATORY DISEASE. Text in English. 198?. bi-m.
Published by: Data Centrum Communications, Inc., 21 W 38th St, 4th fl, New York, NY 10018.

616.2 URY ISSN 0049-4143
TORAX. Text in Spanish; Summaries in English. 1952. q. UYP 15, USD 20. adv. bibl, charts, illus. index.
Supersedes: Revista de Tuberculosis del Uruguay
Indexed: Biol.Abstr., Excerp.Med., Ind.Med. (coverage dropped).
—GNLM.
Published by: Sociedad de Tisiologia y Enfermedades del Torax de Uruguay, Av. Dieciocho De Julio, 2175, Casilla de Correos 10724, Montevideo 11208, Uruguay. Ed. Dante Tomalino. **Co-sponsor:** Sociedad de Cardiologia.

616.246 GBR ISSN 1472-9792
CODEN: TLDIEP
TUBERCULOSIS. Text in English. 1992. bi-m. GBP 106 to individuals; GBP 353 to institutions (effective 2002). adv. abstr, bibl, illus. index. Supplement avail.; back issues avail.; reprints avail. *Refereed.* **Document type:** *Journal, Academic/Scholarly.* **Description:** Publishes primary articles and commissioned reviews on both research and clinical work in tuberculosis and other lung diseases.
Formerly (until 2001): Tubercle and Lung Disease (0962-8479); Which was formed by the merger of (1919-1992): Tubercle (0041-3879); (1986-1992): International Union against Tuberculosis and Lung Disease. Bulletin (1011-789X); Which was formerly (1924-1986): International Union against Tuberculosis. Bulletin (0074-9249)
Related titles: Online - full text ed.: (from EBSCO Publishing, RoweCom Information Quest, Swets Blackwell, IDEAL Online Library, Institute for Scientific Information).
Indexed: ASCA, Abstr.Hyg., Agri.& Environ.Biotech.Abstr. (coverage dropped), Biol.Abstr., Chem.Abstr., Curr.Adv.Ecol.Sci., Curr.Cont., Dairy Sci.Abstr., Derwent Biotech.Abstr., Environ.Sci.Poll.Mgmt., Excerp.Med., Ind.Med. (1992-), Ind.Sci.Rev., Ind.Vet., Inpharma, Int.Abstr.Biol.Sci., Microbiol.Abstr., Pharm.&Out.News, Pollut.Abstr., Reac., Ref.Zh., Rev.Med.& Vet.Mycol., Risk Abstr., Saf.Sci.Abstr., Sci.Cit.Ind. (coverage dropped), THA, Trop.Dis.Bull., Vet.Bull.
—BLDSC (9068.125000), ADONIS, CISTI, EMDOCS, GNLM, IDS, Infotrieve, ingenta, KNAW. **CCC.**
Published by: Churchill Livingstone (Subsidiary of: Harcourt Publishers Ltd.), Robert Stevenson House, 1-3 Baxter's Pl, Leith Walk, Edinburgh, Midlothian EH1 3AF, United Kingdom. TEL 44-131-556-2424, FAX 44-131-459-1177, http://www.harcourt-international.com/journals/tube. Eds. Douglas Young, Jerrold J Ellner, Patrick J Brennan. Pub. Pub Gillian Griffith. Adv. contact Fiona Nacnab. Circ: 3,000. **Subscr. to:** Harcourt Publishers Ltd., Foots Cray High St, Sidcup, Kent DA14 5HP, United Kingdom. TEL 44-20-8308-5700, FAX 44-20-8309-0807.

616.2 613.1 RUS
TUBERKULEZ I EKOLOGIYA. Text in Russian. q. USD 95 in United States.
Published by: Izdatel'stvo Interkhim, Ul Dostoevskogo 4, Moscow 103030, Russian Federation. TEL 7-095-2819603. **US dist. addr.:** East View Publications, 3020 Harbor Ln N, Minneapolis, MN 55447. TEL 612-550-0961.

616.246 614 USA
RC313
U.S. CENTERS FOR DISEASE CONTROL. REPORTED TUBERCULOSIS IN THE UNITED STATES. Text in English. 1974. irreg., latest 1995. free per issue. charts, illus. **Document type:** *Government.*
Formerly: U.S. Centers for Disease Control. Tuberculosis Statistics in the United States; Which was formed by the merger of: U.S. Centers for Disease Control. Tuberculosis in the United States (0149-2616); U.S. Centers for Disease Control. Tuberculosis Statistics. States and Cities; Which was formerly: U.S. Centers for Disease Control. Tuberculosis Statistics: States and Cities; Which was formed by the merger of: U.S. Centers for Disease Control. Reported Tuberculosis Data; U.S. Centers for Disease Control. Tuberculosis Program Reports
Published by: U.S. Centers for Disease Control, Division of Tuberculosis Elimination, 1600 Clifton Rd, Atlanta, GA 30333. TEL 404-634-2512. Circ: 7,000.

616.995 ARG ISSN 0301-8911
UNIVERSIDAD DE BUENOS AIRES. CATEDRA DE PATOLOGIA Y CLINICA DE LA TUBERCULOSIS. ANALES. Text in Spanish. 1970 (vol.29). irreg.
Indexed: Biol.Abstr.
—GNLM.
Published by: Universidad de Buenos Aires, Catedra de Patologia y Clinica de la Tuberculosis, Avda. Sarsfield Velez, 405, Capital Federal, Buenos Aires 1281, Argentina.

616.2 USA
UPDATE (BIRMINGHAM). Text in English. q. free.
Published by: American Lung Assoc. of Alabama, 900 S. 18th St., Birmingham, AL 35205. TEL 205-933-8821, FAX 205-930-1717, http://www.alabamalung.org.

616.2 USA
VOICE FOUNDATION. NEWSLETTER. Text in English. 3/yr. USD 50. **Document type:** *Newsletter.*
Published by: Voice Foundation, 1721 Pine St, Philadelphia, PA 19103. Ed. Charlotte Cathcart.

616.2 USA ISSN 8756-3452
RC705
THE YEAR BOOK OF PULMONARY DISEASE. Text in English. 1986. a. USD 88 domestic; USD 94 foreign (effective 2001). illus. **Document type:** *Abstract/Index, Academic/Scholarly.* **Description:** Presents abstracts of pertinent literature with commentary by leading experts in the field.
Related titles: CD-ROM ed.
—GNLM.
Published by: Mosby, Inc., Continuity Division (Subsidiary of: Harcourt Health Sciences), 11830 Westline Industrial Dr, St Louis, MO 63146-3313. TEL 314-872-8370, 800-325-4177, FAX 314-432-1380, http://www.mosby.com/periodicals. Ed. Dr. James Jett.

616.2 ZMB ISSN 0084-5000
ZAMBIA. PNEUMOCONIOSIS MEDICAL AND RESEARCH BUREAU AND PNEUMOCONIOSIS COMPENSATION BOARD. ANNUAL REPORT. Text in English. 1964. a. ZMK 100. **Document type:** *Government.*
Published by: (Zambia. Pneumoconiosis Medical and Research Bureau and Pneumoconiosis Compensation Board), Government Printing Department, PO Box 30136, Lusaka, Zambia.

616.23 JPN ISSN 0914-7683
ZENSOKU/ASTHMA. Text in Japanese. 1988. 4/yr. JPY 1,800 per issue (effective 1998).
Published by: Medikaru Rebyusha/Medical Review Co., Ltd., 7-3 Hirano-Machi 1-chome, Chuo-ku, Osaka-shi 541-0046, Japan. TEL 81-6-223-1667, FAX 81-6-223-1338, meview@osk3.3web.ne.jp.

616.2 CHN ISSN 1000-6621
ZHONGGUO FANGLAO TONGXUN/CHINESE ANTITUBERCULOSIS ASSOCIATION. BULLETIN. Text in English. q. CNY 5 per issue domestic (effective 2000). back issues avail. **Document type:** *Academic/Scholarly.* **Description:** Covers the treatment of tuberculosis, discussions, reports, and other related issues.
Related titles: Online - full content ed.: (from WanFang Data Corp.).
Published by: Zhongguo Fanglao Xuehui Zhuban, Dong 4 Xibei Daijie 42 Hao, Beijing 100710, China. Ed. Lixing Zhang.

616.99424 CHN ISSN 1009-3419
ZHONGGUO FEIYAN ZAZHI/CHINESE JOURNAL OF LUNG CANCER. Text in Chinese. 1998 (Jul.). bi-m. back issues avail. **Document type:** *Academic/Scholarly.*
Related titles: Online - full content ed.: (from WanFang Data Corp.).
Published by: Zhongguo Kanguan Xiehui, Guoxuehang 37 Hao, Chengdu, Sichuan, China. TEL 86-28-5422587, FAX 86-28-5422743, cnlungca@mail.sc.cninfo.net. Ed. Yan Sun. **Co-sponsor:** Zhongguo Fanglao Xuehui.

616.995 CHN ISSN 1001-0939
ZHONGHUA JIEHE HE HUXI ZAZHI/CHINESE JOURNAL OF TUBERCULOSIS AND RESPIRATORY DISEASES. Text in Chinese. 1978. m. CNY 108 domestic; USD 56.40 foreign; CNY 9 newsstand/cover domestic; USD 4.70 newsstand/cover foreign (effective 2001). abstr, charts, illus. 64 p./no. *Refereed.* **Document type:** *Academic/Scholarly.*
Formerly (until 1986): Zhonghua Jiehe he Huxiji Jibing Zazhi (0253-2689)
Related titles: ♦ CD-ROM ed.: Chinese Academic Journal. Medicine & Hygiene. ISSN 1007-8053; Online - full content ed.: 1998 (from WanFang Data Corp.).
Indexed: Ind.Med.
Published by: Zhonghua Yixuehui Zazhishe, 42 Dongsi Xidajie, Beijing 100710, China. cmahx@public.sti.ca.cn. Ed. Nanshan Zhong. **Dist. by:** China International Book Trading Corp, 35, Chegongzhuang Xilu, Haidian District, Beijing 100044, China. TEL 86-1-68413849, FAX 86-1-68412048, cibtc@mail.cibtc.com.cn, http://www.cibtc.com.cn.

MEDICAL SCIENCES—Rheumatology

616.742 PRT ISSN 0303-464X
CODEN: ARUPB
ACTA REUMATOLOGICA PORTUGUESA. Text in Portuguese; Summaries in English, Portuguese. 1973. q. PTE 2,000 in Portugal; USD 30 in United States; PTE 500 newsstand/cover in Portugal; USD 3 newsstand/cover in United States (effective 2000). adv. bk.rev. abstr, bibl, charts, illus, stat. **Document type:** *Academic/Scholarly.*
Indexed: Excerp.Med. (1994-).
—BLDSC (0662.561000), EMDOCS, GNLM.
Published by: Sociedade Portuguesa de Reumatologia, Rua de Dona Estefania, 177 1o D, Lisbon 1000, Portugal. TEL 351-21-3534395. Circ: 6,000 (controlled).

616.7 YUG ISSN 0351-7217
ACTA RHEUMATOLOGICA BELGRADENSIA✶ **.** Text in Serbo-Croatian. 1971. s-a. YUN 100 domestic; DEM 50 foreign (effective 2000). *Refereed.* **Document type:** *Academic/Scholarly.*
—GNLM.
Published by: Reumatoloski Institut/Institute of Rheumatology, c/o Srpsko Lekarsko Drustvo, Dzordza Vasingtona 19, Belgrade 11000, Yugoslavia. TEL 381-11-3612376, FAX 381-11-3612376. Ed. Nada Pilipovic. Adv. contact Nemanja Damjanov.

616.742 FRA ISSN 0065-1818
ACTUALITE RHUMATOLOGIQUE PRESENTEE AU PRATICIEN; cahier annuel d'informations et de renseignements. Text in French. a. price varies.
—GNLM, Infotrieve. **CCC.**
Published by: Expansion Scientifique Publications, 31 bd. de la Tour Maubourg, Paris 75007, France. TEL 33-1-40626400, FAX 33-1-45556920.

616.72 DEU ISSN 0341-051X
CODEN: AKRHDB
AKTUELLE RHEUMATOLOGIE. Text in German; Summaries in English, German. 1976. bi-m. EUR 171.80 domestic to institutions; EUR 176.80 in Europe to institutions; EUR 180.80 elsewhere to institutions; EUR 96 to students; EUR 34 newsstand/cover (effective 2002). index. reprint service avail. from PQC. *Refereed.* **Document type:** *Journal, Academic/Scholarly.*
Related titles: Online - full text ed.: ISSN 1438-9940 (from Institute for Scientific Information).
Indexed: ASCA, Curr.Adv.Ecol.Sci., Curr.Cont. (coverage dropped), Excerp.Med., INIS Atomind., Inpharma, Reac.
—BLDSC (0785.873000), CISTI, EMDOCS, GNLM, IDS, Infotrieve, KNAW. **CCC.**
Published by: Georg Thieme Verlag, Ruedigerstr 14, Stuttgart 70469, Germany. TEL 49-711-8931-0, FAX 49-711-8931298, rheuma@thieme.de, leser.service@thieme.de, http://www.thieme.de/rheuma/index.html. Ed. W Miehle. R&P Michael Wachinger. Circ: 3,200.

616.7 GBR ISSN 1350-6129
CODEN: AIJIET
AMYLOID; international journal of experimental and clinical investigation. Text in English. 1994. q. GBP 115, USD 185 to individuals; GBP 170, USD 275 to institutions (effective 2000). adv. back issues avail. *Refereed.* **Document type:** *Academic/Scholarly.*
Related titles: Online - full text ed.: (from Institute for Scientific Information).
Indexed: ASCA, BBCI, Chem.Indus.Notes, Chem.Titles, Curr.Cont., Ind.Med. (1994-), Ind.Sci.Rev., Inpharma, Int.Abstr.Biol.Sci., Mass Spectr.Bull., Nutr.Abstr., Pharm.&Out.News, Reac., Sci.Cit.Ind., e-psyche.
—BLDSC (0859.841173), ADONIS, CASDDS, CISTI, GNLM, IDS, KNAW.
Published by: (International Society of Amyloidosis), Parthenon Publishing Group (Subsidiary of: C R C Press (New York)), Casterton Hall, Casterton, Carnforth, Lancs LA6 2LA, United Kingdom. TEL 44-1524-272084, 44-1524-272084, mail@parthpub.com, http://www.parthpub.com/. Ed. Jean Wright. Adv. contact Julia Tissington.

M

616.742 GBR ISSN 0003-4967
CODEN: ARDIAO
ANNALS OF THE RHEUMATIC DISEASES; the EULAR journal. Text in English. 1939. m. GBP 162, USD 260 combined subscription to individuals includes print & online eds.; GBP 346, USD 554 to institutions for Print only (effective 2002). adv. bk.rev. charts, illus. index. back issues avail.; reprint service avail. from PQC. *Refereed.* **Document type:** *Academic/Scholarly.* **Description:** Contains work on all aspects of rheumatology and disorders of connective tissue.
Related titles: CD-ROM ed.: (from Ovid Technologies, Inc.); Microform ed.: (from PQC); Online - full text ed.: A R D Online. ISSN 1468-2060. GBP 80, USD 125 to individuals (effective 2002); Institutions contact publisher for rates. (from HighWire Pr., Ovid Technologies, Inc., EBSCO Publishing, RoweCom Information Quest, ProQuest Information & Learning, ingenta, Gale Group, Swets Blackwell, SilverPlatter Information, Inc., Institute for Scientific Information).
Indexed: AMED, ASCA, Abstr.Inter.Med., Behav.Med.Abstr., Biol.Abstr., CINAHL, C.I.S. Abstr., Cal.Tiss.Abstr., Chem.Abstr., Chem.Indus.Notes, Chem.Titles, Curr.Cont., Dent.Ind., Derwent Biotech.Abstr., Environ.Sci.Poll.Mgmt., Excerp.Med., Helminthol.Abstr., INIS Atomind., Ind.Med. (1939-), Ind.Sci.Rev., Inpharma, Int.Abstr.Biol.Sci., Kidney, Med.& Surg.Dermat., Nutr.Abstr., Pharm.&Out.News, Pollut.Abstr., Reac., Ref.Zh., Rev.Appl.Entomol., Rev.Med.& Vet.Mycol., Risk Abstr., SSCI (coverage dropped), Saf.Sci.Abstr., Sci.Cit.Ind., Tox.Abstr. (coverage dropped).
—BLDSC (1043.800000), ADONIS, CASDDS, CISTI, EMDOCS, GNLM, IDS, Infotrieve, ingenta, KNAW. **CCC.**
Published by: B M J Publishing Group, B M A House, Tavistock Sq, London WC1H 9JR, United Kingdom. TEL 44-20-7387-4499, FAX 44-20-7383-6400, info.norththames@bma.org.uk, http://www.annrheumdis.com/, http://ard.bmjjournals.com/, http://www.bma.org.uk. Ed. Leo van de Putte. Pub. Alex Williamson. R&P Carol Torselli TEL 44-20-7383-6674. Adv. contact Euan Currer TEL 44-20-7383-6181. **Subscr. to:** PO Box 4590A, Kennebunkport, ME 04046.

ARCHIVIO DI ORTOPEDIA E REUMATOLOGIA. see *MEDICAL SCIENCES—Orthopedics And Traumatology*

616.742 USA ISSN 0004-3591
RC927.A1 CODEN: ARHEAW
ARTHRITIS AND RHEUMATISM. Text in English. 1958. m. USD 610 in United States; USD 790 in Canada & Mexico; USD 943 elsewhere; USD 641 combined subscription in United States for print and online eds.; USD 821 combined subscription in Canada & Mexico for print and online eds.; USD 974 combined subscription elsewhere for print and online eds. (effective 2002). adv. bk.rev. bibl, charts, illus. back issues avail. *Refereed.* **Document type:** *Academic/Scholarly.* **Description:** Publishes original research, progress reports, clinical rounds, and review articles related to the diagnosis and treatment of all forms of arthritis and rheumatic diseases.
Incorporates: Arthritis Care and Research (0893-7524)
Related titles: Microform ed.: (from PQC); Online - full text ed.: ISSN 1529-0131. USD 610 in United States; USD 610 in Canada & Mexico; USD 610 elsewhere (effective 2002) (from Ovid Technologies, Inc., EBSCO Publishing, Wiley InterScience, Institute for Scientific Information).
Indexed: AIM, ASCA, Abstr.Anthropol., Agri.& Environ.Biotech.Abstr. (coverage dropped), Behav.Med.Abstr., Biol.Abstr., CINAHL, C.I.S. Abstr., Cal.Tiss.Abstr., Chem.Abstr., Chem.Indus.Notes, Chem.Titles, Curr.Adv.Ecol.Sci., Curr.Cont., Dent.Ind., Derwent Biotech.Abstr., Environ.Sci.Poll.Mgmt., Excerp.Med., Helminthol.Abstr., INIS Atomind., I.P.A., Immun.Abstr. (coverage dropped), Ind.Med. (1958-), Ind.Sci.Rev., Inpharma, Int.Abstr.Biol.Sci., Int.Nurs.Ind., Jrnl.Watch, Kidney, Med.& Surg.Dermat., Neurosci.Cit.Ind., Pharm.&Out.News, Pollut.Abstr., Protozool.Abstr., Reac., Rev.Appl.Entomol., Rev.Med.& Vet.Mycol., Risk Abstr., SSCI (coverage dropped), Saf.Sci.Abstr., Sci.Cit.Ind., THA, Tox.Abstr. (coverage dropped).
—BLDSC (1733.800000), CASDDS, CISTI, EMDOCS, GNLM, IDS, ingenta, KNAW.
Published by: (American College of Rheumatology), John Wiley & Sons, Inc., Journals (Subsidiary of: Wiley InterScience), 605 Third Ave, New York, NY 10158. TEL 212-850-6645, FAX 212-850-6021, uscs-wis@wiley.com, http://www.wiley.com. Ed. Dr. David S Pisetsky. adv.: B&W page USD 1,995, color page USD 3,880; trim 11 x 8.5. Circ: 9,357. **Subscr. to:** John Wiley & Sons Ltd., Baffins Ln, Chichester, Sussex PO19 IUD, United Kingdom. TEL 44-1243-779777, FAX 44-1243-843232, cs-journals@wiley.co.uk, http://www.wiley.co.uk.

616.742 USA
ARTHRITIS: DISEASE STATE MANAGEMENT RESOURCE. Text in English. 1997. a. USD 295 domestic; USD 325 foreign (effective 2001). **Document type:** *Trade.*
Published by: American Health Consultants (Subsidiary of: Medical Economics Co., Inc.), 3525 Piedmont Rd, N E, 6 Piedmont Center, Ste 400, Atlanta, GA 30305. TEL 404-262-5476, 404-262-7436, 800-688-2421, FAX 404-262-7837, 800-284-3291, custserv@ahcpub.com, http://www.ahcpub.com. **Subscr. to:** PO Box 530161, Atlanta, GA 30353-0161.

616.7 USA ISSN 0191-2836
ARTHRITIS FOUNDATION ANNUAL REPORT* . Text in English. 1948. a.
Published by: Arthritis Foundation, 1330 W Peach Tree St, Atlanta, GA 30309. TEL 404-872-7100, FAX 404-872-0457.

616.722 USA ISSN 1067-9421
ARTHRITIS HEALTH MONITOR. Text in English. 1994. m. **Document type:** *Newsletter, Consumer.*
Published by: Data Centrum Communications, Inc., 21 W 38th St, 4th fl, New York, NY 10018.

616.7 USA
ARTHRITIS HOTLINE. Text in English. 1993. 3/yr. USD 12 (effective 2000). back issues avail. **Document type:** *Newsletter, Consumer.* **Description:** Keeps patients, family members, and medical professionals informed on recent advances in arthritis and related conditions.
Address: 8230 Walnut Hill, 11, Dallas, TX 75231. TEL 214-363-2812, FAX 214-692-8591. Ed., R&P Dr. Scott Zashin. Adv. contact Terri Groom. Circ: 1,000.

616.742 NZL ISSN 1171-8986
ARTHRITIS NEWS. Text in English. 1983. q. adv. index. **Document type:** *Newsletter.* **Description:** Covers arthritis care, management and news.
Published by: Arthritis Foundation of N Z Inc., P.O. Box 10020, Wellington, New Zealand. TEL 64-4-4721427, FAX 64-4-4727066. Ed., Adv. contact Carol Culling. page NZD 550. Circ: 15,000.

616.742 CAN ISSN 0820-9006
ARTHRITIS NEWS. Text in English. 1979. q. USD 14.95 domestic; USD 25.50 foreign. adv. bk.rev. **Document type:** *Consumer.* **Description:** Provides articles on arthritis, its treatment, the latest research and coping strategies.
Formerly: C.A.R. Scope (0068-8258)
Related titles: French ed.: Arthro Express. ISSN 1198-7669.
Published by: Arthritis Society, 250 Bloor St E Ste 901, Toronto, ON M4W 3P2, Canada. TEL 410-967-1414, FAX 416-967-7171, bthompson@mhpublishing.com. Ed. Beth Thompson. Pub. Marc Thibodeau. R&P Sharon McConnell. Adv. contact Norm Cook. Circ: 20,000 (paid). **Subscr. to:** Maclean Hunter Healthcare, Maclean Hunter Bldg, 777 Bay St, 5th Fl, Toronto, ON M5W 1A7, Canada. TEL 416-596-2791, FAX 416-596-3499.

616.742 USA
ARTHRITIS SELF-MANAGEMENT. Text in English. m. USD 30 (effective 2001). Index. back issues avail. **Document type:** *Newsletter.* **Description:** Publsihes practical and intructive information for people with arthritis.
Published by: R.A. Rapaport Publishing, Inc., 150 W 22nd St, New York, NY 10011. TEL 212-989-0200, FAX 212-989-4786, staff@rapaportpublishing.com, http://www.arthritis-self-mgmt.com. Ed. Christine Grove. Pub. Richard A Rapaport.

616.7 USA ISSN 0890-1120
RC933.A1
ARTHRITIS TODAY; the magazine for help and hope. Text in English. 1980. bi-m. USD 20 to membership; USD 4.95 newsstand/cover (effective 2001). adv. illus. back issues avail.; reprints avail. **Document type:** *Magazine, Consumer.* **Description:** Offers persons suffering from arthritis hope and help in a wide variety of areas.
Formerly (until 1987): National Arthritis News (0882-9705)
Related titles: Online - full text ed.: (from Gale Group, Factiva).
Indexed: CHNI, Hlth.Ind.
—BLDSC (1733.877900).
Published by: Arthritis Foundation, 1330 W Peach Tree St,, Atlanta, GA 30309. TEL 404-872-7100, 800-933-0032, FAX 404-872-9559, atmail@arthritis.org, http://www.arthritis.org. Ed. Cindy McDaniel. Pub. William M Otto. Adv. contact Terry Earley. B&W page USD 17,250, color page USD 25,409. Circ: 650,000 (paid).

616.742 GBR ISSN 0969-7039
ARTHRITIS TODAY. Text in English. 1965. q. GBP 15 (effective 2000). charts, illus. **Document type:** *Consumer.* **Description:** Offers the general reader reviews of ARC-funded research and its progress, along with advice for coping with arthritis from day-to-day.
Formerly (until 1992): Arthritis Research Today (0960-4499)
—BLDSC (1733.878000).
Published by: Arthritis Research Campaign, PO Box 177, Chesterfield, Derbys S41 7TQ, United Kingdom. TEL 44-1264-558033, FAX 44-1264-558007, info@arc.org.uk. Circ: 125,000.

ARTHROSCOPY. see *MEDICAL SCIENCES—Orthopedics And Traumatology*

AUTOIMMUNE DISEASES. see *MEDICAL SCIENCES—Abstracting, Bibliographies, Statistics*

616.7 GBR ISSN 1521-6942
CODEN: BBPRFF
BAILLIERE'S BEST PRACTICE & RESEARCH IN CLINICAL RHEUMATOLOGY. Text in English. 1975. 5/yr. GBP 112 to individuals; GBP 196 to institutions (effective 2002). *Refereed.* **Document type:** *Academic/Scholarly.*
Formerly (until 1999): Bailliere's Clinical Rheumatology (0950-3579); Which superseded in part (in 1987): Clinics in Rheumatic Diseases (0307-742X)
Related titles: Online - full text ed.: (from EBSCO Publishing, O C L C Online Computer Library Center, Inc., Swets Blackwell, IDEAL Online Library, Institute for Scientific Information, RoweCom Information Quest).
Indexed: ASCA, Biol.Abstr., Curr.Adv.Ecol.Sci., Curr.Cont., Excerp.Med., Ind.Med. (1999-), Ind.Sci.Rev., Inpharma, Pharm.&Out.News, Reac., SSCI (coverage dropped), Sci.Cit.Ind.
—BLDSC (1856.716950), CASDDS, CISTI, EMDOCS, GNLM, IDS, Infotrieve, ingenta, KNAW. **CCC.**
Published by: Bailliere Tindall (Subsidiary of: Harcourt Publishers Ltd.), 24-28 Oval Rd, London NW1 7DX, United Kingdom. TEL 44-20-7424-4200, FAX 44-20-7424-4515, cservice@harcourt.com, http://www.harcourt-international.com/journals/berh. **Subscr. to:** Harcourt Publishers Ltd., Foots Cray High St, Sidcup, Kent DA14 5HP, United Kingdom. TEL 44-20-8308-5700, FAX 44-20-8309-0807.

616.7 DEU
BECHTEREW-BRIEF. Text in German. 1980. q. EUR 28.63 to membership (effective 2002). adv. bk.rev. charts, illus. cum.index: 1980-1999. 100 p./no. 2 cols./p. back issues avail. *Refereed.* **Document type:** *Newsletter, Trade.*
Published by: Deutsche Vereinigung Morbus Bechterew, Metzgergasse 16, Schweinfurt 97421, Germany. TEL 49-9721-22033, FAX 49-9721-22955, dvmb@talknet.de. Ed. Ernst Feldtkeller. R&P, Adv. contact Ludwig Hammel. page DEM 1,200; trim 126 x 180. Circ: 18,000 (controlled).

616.7 CZE ISSN 1210-7905
CODEN: CRVMEG
CESKA REVMATOLOGIE. Text in Czech, Slovak; Summaries in Czech, English. 1923. q. EUR 64, USD 80 (effective 2001). adv. *Refereed.* **Document type:** *Academic/Scholarly.* **Description:** Publishes novelties in the diagnosis and treatment of rheumatic diseases. Focuses on pharmacotherapy of rheumatic diseases and surgical treatment.
Supersedes in part (in 1993): Fysiatricky a Reumatologicky Vestnik (0072-0038)
—BLDSC (3120.319000), CASDDS, CISTI, GNLM, Infotrieve. **CCC.**
Published by: (Ceska Lekarska Spolecnost J.E. Purkyne/Czech Medical Association), Nakladatelske Stredisko C L S J.E. Purkyne, Sokolska 31, Prague 12026, Czech Republic. TEL 42-2-24911420, FAX 42-2-24911420, nts@iol.cz, http://www.clsjep.cz, http://www.medical.cz. Ed. Jiri Vencovsky. adv.: B&W page CZK 29,300, color page CZK 41,200; 244 x 166. Circ: 850. **Dist. by:** Abont s.r.o., Chlumova 17, Prague, 3 130 00, Czech Republic; **Dist. in Western countries by:** Kubon & Sagner, Hesstr 39-41, Munich 80798, Germany.

616.7 ITA ISSN 0392-856X
CODEN: CERHDP
CLINICAL AND EXPERIMENTAL RHEUMATOLOGY. Text in English. 1983. bi-m. EUR 164 in Europe to individuals; USD 140 elsewhere to individuals; ITL 188 in Europe to institutions; USD 160 elsewhere to institutions; ITL 82, USD 70 to students (effective 2001). Supplement avail.; back issues avail. *Refereed.* **Document type:** *Academic/Scholarly.*

Related titles: Online - full text ed.: (from Institute for Scientific Information).
Indexed: ASCA, Curr.Cont., Ind.Med. (1983-), Ind.Sci.Rev., Inpharma, Int.Abstr.Biol.Sci., Kidney, Med.& Surg.Dermat., Neurosci.Cit.Ind., Pharm.&Out.News, Protozool.Abstr., Reac., Rev.Med.& Vet.Mycol., SSCI (coverage dropped), Sci.Cit.Ind.
—BLDSC (3286.252700), CASDDS, CISTI, EMDOCS, GNLM, IDS, ingenta, KNAW.
Published by: Pacini Editore, Via Alessandro Gherardesca, 1, Ospedaletto, PI 56121, Italy. TEL 39-050-982439, FAX 39-050-983905, pacini@cibernet.it, http://www.clinexprheumatol.org. **Subscr. to:** Via Santa Maria, 31, Pisa, PI 56126, Italy.

616.742 BEL ISSN 0770-3198
CODEN: CLRHD6
CLINICAL RHEUMATOLOGY. Text in English. 1946. 6/yr. EUR 280 domestic; EUR 277.10 in Germany; EUR 52.80 newsstand/cover foreign (effective 2002). adv. abstr, illus. Supplement avail. *Refereed.* **Document type:** *Academic/Scholarly.*
Formerly: Journal Belge de Rhumatologie et de Medecine Physique (0021-7654)
Related titles: Online - full text ed.: (from EBSCO Publishing, RoweCom Information Quest, Swets Blackwell, Springer LINK, Institute for Scientific Information).
Indexed: AMED, ASCA, Biol.Abstr., Chem.Abstr., Curr.Cont., Excerp.Med., Ind.Med. (1982-), Inpharma, Int.Abstr.Biol.Sci., Nutr.Abstr., Pharm.&Out.News, Reac., Rev.Med.& Vet.Mycol., SSCI (coverage dropped).
—BLDSC (3286.374600), CASDDS, CISTI, EMDOCS, GNLM, IDS, ingenta, KNAW.
Published by: (Association des Societes Scientifiques Medicales Belges/Vereiniging van de Belgische Wetenschappelijke Genootschappen), Acta Medica Belgica, Av Circulaire 138A, Brussels 1180, Belgium. TEL 32-2-374-5158, FAX 32-2-3749628. Ed. J Dequeker.

616.748 CAN ISSN 0828-301X
CONNECTIONS. Text in English. 1984. q. free per issue. bk.rev. illus. back issues avail. **Document type:** *Newsletter.* **Description:** Covers research news, fund raising, client profiles and disability issues.
Related titles: French ed.: Connexions.
Published by: Muscular Dystrophy Association of Canada, 2345 Yonge St, 9th Fl, Toronto, ON M4P 2E5, Canada. TEL 416-488-0030, FAX 416-488-7523. Ed. M W Thompson. Circ: 16,000 (controlled).

616.7 ITA ISSN 0394-0748
CONNECTIVE TISSUE DISEASES/MALATTIE DEL TESSUTO CONNETTIVO. Text in English, Italian. 1981. s-a. ITL 50,000, USD 70 (effective 1999). stat. **Description:** Presents research papers on the study of connective tissue diseases.
—EMDOCS.
Published by: (Societa Neopolitana Mario Giordano), Casa Editrice Idelson, Via Annibale De Gasperis, 55, Naples, NA 80137, Italy. TEL 39-81-5524733, FAX 39-81-5518295, idelgno@tin.it, http://www.idelson-gnocchi.com. Ed. Giuseppe Tirri.

CURRENT MEDICAL LITERATURE. RHEUMATOLOGY. see *MEDICAL SCIENCES—Abstracting, Bibliographies, Statistics*

616.7 USA ISSN 1040-8711
RC925.A1 CODEN: CORHES
CURRENT OPINION IN RHEUMATOLOGY. Text in English. 1989. bi-m. USD 239 domestic to individuals for print and online eds.; USD 239 foreign to individuals for print and online eds.; USD 84 newsstand/cover; USD 539 per issue domestic to institutions; USD 539 per issue foreign to institutions (effective 2002). adv. bibl, illus. **Document type:** *Academic/Scholarly.* **Description:** Directed toward researchers and practicing rheumatologists. Presents review articles followed by annotated bibliographies of references consulted. A bibliography of the current world literature published during the previous year is available.
Related titles: Online - full text ed.: USD 700.70 domestic academic site license; USD 700.70 foreign academic site license; USD 781.55 domestic corporate site license; USD 781.55 foreign corporate site license (effective 2002) (from Ovid Technologies, Inc., EBSCO Publishing, Swets Blackwell, Institute for Scientific Information).
Indexed: CINAHL, Cal.Tiss.Abstr., Chem.Abstr., Chem.Indus.Notes, Chem.Titles, Chemorec.Abstr., Curr.Cont., Environ.Sci.Poll.Mgmt., Excerp.Med., Ind.Med. (1989-), Inpharma, Int.Abstr.Biol.Sci., Neurosci.Abstr. (coverage dropped), Pharm.&Out.News, Reac., Risk Abstr., Saf.Sci.Abstr., Sci.Cit.Ind., Tox.Abstr. (coverage dropped).
—BLDSC (3500.778000), ADONIS, CASDDS, CISTI, EMDOCS, GNLM, ingenta, KNAW.
Published by: Lippincott Williams & Wilkins (Philadelphia) (Subsidiary of: Wolters Kluwer N.V.), 530 Walnut St, Philadelphia, PA 19106-3621. FAX 215-521-8902, 215-521-8902, http://www.Lww.com. Ed. G G Hunder. Pub. Maria McMichael. R&P Tobias Weschler. Adv. contact Kelly Adamitis. **Subscr. to:** PO Box 1600, Hagerstown, MD 21740-1600.

616.723 GBR ISSN 1523-3774
▼ **CURRENT RHEUMATOLOGY REPORTS.** Text in English. 1999. 8/yr. USD 163.95, GBP 120 to individuals; USD 327.95 to institutions; USD 80, GBP 60 to students (effective 2002); Subscr. includes both print & online eds.. **Document type:** *Journal, Academic/Scholarly.*
Related titles: Online - full content ed.: USD 85, GBP 60 (effective 2002).
Indexed: Ind.Med.
—BLDSC (3502.660000).
Published by: Current Science Inc., 400 Market St, Ste 700, Philadelphia, PA 19106. TEL 800-427-1796, FAX 215-574-2225, info@current-reports.com, http://www.current-reports.com/cr_jrnl_home.cfm?JournalID=RR. Ed. Bruce N Cronstein. **Affiliate:** Current Science Ltd.

616.7 617.3 FRA ISSN 1286-935X
ENCYCLOPEDIE MEDICO-CHIRURGICALE. APARATO LOCOMOTOR; la referencia que necessita. Text in Spanish. 1998. 6 base vols. plus q. updates. bibl, illus. *Refereed.* **Document type:** *Academic/Scholarly.* **Description:** Offers an up-to-date reference in topics concerning locomotor dysfunctions.
Related titles: ♦ French ed.: Encyclopedie Medico-Chirurgicale. Appareil Locomoteur. ISSN 0246-0521.
Published by: Elsevier Paris, Editions Scientifiques et Medicales (Subsidiary of: Reed Elsevier plc. group), 23 rue Linois, Paris 75015, France. TEL 33-1-45589110, FAX 33-1-45589110, redaction-emc@elsevier.fr, redacion-emc@elsevier.fr, http://www.elsevier.fr; http://www.emc.tm.fr. Ed. Henri Dorfman.

616.7 617.3 FRA ISSN 0246-0521
ENCYCLOPEDIE MEDICO-CHIRURGICALE. APPAREIL LOCOMOTEUR; vers le retour a la motricite. Cover title: Traite d'Appareil Locomoteur. Variant title: Encyclopedie Medico-Chirurgicale, Instantanes Medicaux. Appareil Locomoteur. Receuil de l'Encyclopedie Medico-Chirurgicale. Appareil Locomoteur. Text in French. 1961. 6 base vols. plus q. updates. bibl, illus. *Refereed.* **Document type:** *Academic/Scholarly.* **Description:** Offers an up-to-date reference in topics concerning rheumatology.
Formed by the merger of (1937-1960): Encyclopedie Medico-Chirurgicale. Os, Articulations, Fractures, Luxations (0246-0645); (1938-1960): Encyclopedie Medico-Chirurgicale. Pathologie des Membres (0246-0718)
Related titles: ♦ Spanish ed.: Encyclopedie Medico-Chirurgicale. Aparato Locomotor. ISSN 1286-935X.
Published by: Elsevier Paris, Editions Scientifiques et Medicales (Subsidiary of: Reed Elsevier plc. group), 23 rue Linois, Paris 75015, France. TEL 33-1-45589110, FAX 33-1-45589119, redaction-emc@elsevier.fr, redacion-emc@elsevier.fr, http://www.elsevier.fr, http://www.elsevier.com. Ed. Henri Dorfman.

ENCYCLOPEDIE MEDICO-CHIRURGICALE. TRAITE DE RADIODIAGNOSTIC: SQUELETTE NORMAL - NEURORADIOLOGIE - APPAREIL LOCOMOTEUR. see *MEDICAL SCIENCES—Radiology And Nuclear Medicine*

EXCERPTA MEDICA. SECTION 31: ARTHRITIS AND RHEUMATISM. see *MEDICAL SCIENCES—Abstracting, Bibliographies, Statistics*

616.74 USA
FIBROMYALGIA HEALTH LETTER. Text in English. bi-m. USD 24.95. **Document type:** *Newsletter.* **Description:** Provides information, advice and research news about fibromyalgia, the second-most commonly diagnosed musculoskeletal disorder.
Published by: Arthritis Foundation, Box 921907, Norcross, GA 30010-1907. http://www.arthritis.org.

616.7 USA
FIBROMYALGIA NETWORK NEWSLETTER. Text in English. 1988. q. USD 25; USD 27 in Canada; USD 30 elsewhere (effective 2000). bk.rev. back issues avail. **Document type:** *Newsletter, Consumer.* **Description:** Provides information for patients and physicians on fibromyalgia syndrome (FMS) and chronic fatigue syndrome (CFS), major disabling, chronic conditions characterized by multiple areas of pain plus fatigue.
Published by: (Fibromyalgia Network), Health Information Network, Inc., PO Box 31750, Tucson, AZ 85751-1750. TEL 520-290-5508, 800-853-2929, FAX 520-290-5550, http://www.fmnetnews.com. Ed., Pub. Kristin Thorson. R&P Sonja Diaz. Circ: 40,000.

616.7 CHE
FORUM R. Text in French, German, Italian. q. **Document type:** *Newsletter.*
Published by: Schweizer Rheumaliga, Renggerstr 71, Zuerich 8038, Switzerland. TEL 01-4825600, FAX 01-4826439. Ed. Gisela Dalvit. Circ: 30,000.

616.7 ESP
FUNDACION ESPANOLA DE REUMATOLOGIA. SEMINARIOS. Text in Spanish; Abstracts in Spanish, English. bi-m. adv. abstr, bibl, illus, stat. back issues avail. *Refereed.* **Document type:** *Academic/Scholarly.*
Published by: (Sociedad Espanola de Reumatologia), Aran Ediciones S.A., Castello, 128 1o, Madrid 28006, Spain. TEL 34-91-782-0030, FAX 34-91-561-5787, edita@grupoaran.com, http://www.grupoaran.com. Ed. A. Laffon Roca. Pub. Jose Jimenez. R&P Maria Dolores Linares TEL 34-1-7820035. Circ: 3,000.

DIE FUNKTIONSKRANKHEITEN DES BEWEGUNGSSYSTEMS; Zeitschrift fuer interdisziplinaere Diagnostik und Therapie. see *MEDICAL SCIENCES—Orthopedics And Traumatology*

INTERNATIONAL JOURNAL OF GASTROENTEROLOGY. see *MEDICAL SCIENCES—Gastroenterology*

616.7 USA
▼ **THE INTERNET JOURNAL OF RHEUMATOLOGY.** Text in English. 2000. s-a. free per issue. adv. bk.rev. back issues avail. *Refereed.* **Document type:** *Academic/Scholarly.* **Description:** Provides information from the field of rheumatology; contains original articles, reviews, case reports, streaming slide shows, streaming videos, letters to the editor, press releases and meeting information.
Media: Online - full content.
Published by: Internet Scientific Publications, L.L.C., 23 Rippling Creek Dr, Sugar Land, TX 77479. TEL 281-240-1533, FAX 281-240-1533, http://www.ispub.com/. R&P, Adv. contact Hope Morrow TEL 832-754-0335.

616.7 USA ISSN 1076-1608
CODEN: JCRHFM
J C R: JOURNAL OF CLINICAL RHEUMATOLOGY; practical reports on rheumatic & musculoskeletal disease. Text in English. 1995. bi-m. USD 135 domestic to individuals; USD 167 foreign to individuals; USD 250 domestic to institutions; USD 250 foreign to institutions; USD 42 newsstand/cover (effective 2002). adv. **Document type:** *Academic/Scholarly.* **Description:** Reviews and reports on clinical and laboratory research in rheumatology.
Formerly: Journal of Clinical Rheumatology (1076-1608)
Related titles: Online - full text ed.: USD 325 domestic for academic site license; USD 325 foreign for academic site license; USD 362.50 domestic for corporate site license; USD 362.50 foreign for corporate site license (effective 2002) (from Institute for Scientific Information).
Indexed: Curr.Cont., Excerp.Med. (1996-), Inpharma, Pharm.&Out.News, Reac.
—BLDSC (4958.730000), GNLM, IDS, KNAW.
Published by: Lippincott Williams & Wilkins (Baltimore) (Subsidiary of: Wolters Kluwer N.V.), 351 W Camden St, Baltimore, MD 21201-2436. TEL 410-528-4000, 800-638-6423, FAX 410-528-4452, apessagno@wwilkins.com, htt://www.Lww.com. Ed. Dr. H Ralph Schumacher. Adv. contact Greg Pessagno. B&W page USD 800; trim 10.88 x 8.13. Circ: 1,799; 1,624 (paid).

THE JOURNAL OF MUSCULOSKELETAL MEDICINE. see *MEDICAL SCIENCES—Orthopedics And Traumatology*

JOURNAL OF MUSCULOSKELETAL PAIN; innovations in research, theory & clinical practice. see *MEDICAL SCIENCES—Orthopedics And Traumatology*

JOURNAL OF MUSCULOSKELETAL RESEARCH. see *MEDICAL SCIENCES—Orthopedics And Traumatology*

616.742 CAN ISSN 0315-162X CODEN: JRHUA9
JOURNAL OF RHEUMATOLOGY. Text in English. 1974. m. CND 240 domestic to individuals; USD 230 foreign to individuals; CND 270 domestic to institutions; USD 260 foreign to institutions (effective 2001); Includes full text online. adv. bk.rev. index. back issues avail. *Refereed.* **Document type:** *Academic/Scholarly.* **Description:** Includes original research on rheumatology and related fields. Covers case studies, editorials on new therapies, epidemiology. economics and ethics.
Related titles: Microform ed.: (from PQC); Online - full text ed.: (from Institute for Scientific Information).
Indexed: ASCA, Behav.Med.Abstr., Biol.Abstr., Chem.Abstr., Chem.Indus.Notes, Chem.Titles, Chic.Per.Ind., Curr.Adv.Cancer Res., Curr.Adv.Ecol.Sci., Curr.Adv.Gen.& Molec.Biol., Curr.Cont., Dairy Sci.Abstr., Dent.Ind., Derwent Biotech.Abstr., Dok.Arbeitsmed., Excerp.Med., INIS Atomind., Ind.Med. (1974-), Ind.Sci.Rev., Inpharma, Int.Abstr.Biol.Sci., Int.Nurs.Ind., Kidney, Med.& Surg.Dermat., Neurosci.Cit.Ind., Nutr.Abstr., Pharm.&Out.News, Protozool.Abstr., Reac., Ref.Zh., Rev.Appl.Entomol., Rev.Arom.& Med.Plants, Rev.Med.& Vet.Mycol., SSCI (coverage dropped), Sci.Cit.Ind.
—BLDSC (5052.070000), CASDDS, CISTI, EMDOCS, GNLM, IDS, ingenta, KNAW. **CCC.**
Published by: Journal of Rheumatology Publishing Co. Ltd., 920 Yonge St, Ste 115, Toronto, ON M4W 3C7, Canada. TEL 416-967-5155, FAX 416-967-7556, jrheum@jrheumcom, http://www.jrheum.com. Ed. D A Gordon. Adv. contact Bill McCausland. Circ: 3,500. **Subscr. in US to:** Allen Press Inc., PO Box 1897, Lawrence, KS 66044-8897.

616.7 617.3 JPN ISSN 0915-1125
KOTSU KANSETSU JINTAI/JOURNAL OF MUSCULOSKELETAL SYSTEM. Text in Japanese. m. JPY 2,400 per issue.
Published by: Kokusai Isho Shuppan, 42-4 Hongo 3-chome, Bunkyo-ku, Tokyo 113-0033, Japan.

L M S ALERT. PAIN CONTROL. (Literature Monitoring and Evaluation Service) see *MEDICAL SCIENCES—Abstracting, Bibliographies, Statistics*

L M S ALERT. RHEUMATIC DISEASE. (Literature Monitoring and Evaluation Service) see *MEDICAL SCIENCES—Abstracting, Bibliographies, Statistics*

616.7 FRA ISSN 0761-5027
LA LETTRE DU RHUMATOLOGUE. Text in French. 1983. m. FRF 460 domestic to individuals; FRF 580, USD 105 foreign to individuals; FRF 580 domestic to institutions; FRF 700, USD 127 foreign to institutions; USD 290 domestic to students; USD 75 foreign to students (effective 2000). Supplement avail. *Refereed.* **Document type:** *Academic/Scholarly.*
Published by: Edimark S.A., 62-64 rue Jean Jaures, Puteaux 92800, France. TEL 33-1-414-58000, FAX 33-1-41458025, contact@edimark.fr, http://www.edimark.fr. Ed. B Combe. Pub. Claudie Damour-Terrasson.

LOOSE CONNECTIONS. see *SOCIAL SERVICES AND WELFARE*

616.7 GBR ISSN 0961-2033 CODEN: LUPUES
LUPUS. Text in English. 1991. 12/yr. GBP 149 in Europe to individuals; USD 293 in North America to individuals; GBP 184 rest of world to individuals; GBP 384 in Europe to institutions; USD 677 in North America to institutions; GBP 435 rest of world to institutions; GBP 217 in developing nations; GBP 57 newsstand/cover in Europe; USD 97 newsstand/cover in North America; GBP 61 newsstand/cover rest of world (effective 2002). adv. back issues avail.; reprints avail. *Refereed.* **Document type:** *Journal, Academic/Scholarly.* **Description:** Comprehensive information on all aspects of lupus care and research.
Related titles: Online - full text ed.: (from EBSCO Publishing, O C L C Online Computer Library Center, Inc., RoweCom Information Quest, ingenta, Swets Blackwell, Institute for Scientific Information).
Indexed: AIDS & Cancer Res., ASCA, Chem.Abstr., Chem.Indus.Notes, Chem.Titles, Curr.Cont., Excerp.Med. (1993-), Genet.Abstr. (coverage dropped), Immun.Abstr., Ind.Med. (1991-), Inpharma, Int.Abstr.Biol.Sci., Nuc.Acids Abstr., Pharm.&Out.News, Protozool.Abstr., Reac., Sci.Cit.Ind.
—BLDSC (5307.422000), CASDDS, CISTI, EMDOCS, GNLM, IDS, Infotrieve, KNAW. **CCC.**
Published by: Arnold Publishers (Subsidiary of: Hodder Headline plc.), 338 Euston Rd, London NW1 3BH, United Kingdom. TEL 44-20-7873-6337, FAX 44-20-7873-6325, arnoldjournals@hodder.co.uk, http://www.arnoldpublishers.com/journals/Journpages/09612033.htm, http://www.arnoldpublishers.com/journals/journtitles.htm. Ed. Dr. Graham R V Hughes.

616.7 AUS ISSN 1033-2480
LUPUS ASSOCIATION OF NEW SOUTH WALES. NEWSLETTER. Text in English. 1979. 5/yr. AUD 20 (effective 2001). bk.rev. back issues avail. **Document type:** *Newsletter.* **Description:** News and educational articles from the association, a self-help organization for sufferers of Systemic Lupus Erythematosus and related diseases.
Published by: Lupus Association of New South Wales Inc., PO Box 89, North Ryde, NSW 2113, Australia. TEL 61-2-98786055. Ed., R&P Leslie McAllister. Circ: 1,600.

616.7 USA
LUPUS BEACON. Text in English. 1984. 5/yr. USD 20 domestic; USD 22 in Canada & Mexico; USD 26 elsewhere (effective 1999). bk.rev. back issues avail. *Refereed.* **Document type:** *Newsletter.* **Description:** Educational and medical news for patients with systemic lupus erythematosus.
Formerly: L E Beacon
Published by: L.E. Support Club, 8039 Nova Ct, N, Charleston, SC 29420. TEL 843-764-1769, FAX 843-572-9909, hmesic@awod.com, http://www.galaxymall.com/commerce/lupus. Ed., R&P Harriet B Mesic. Circ: 1,500.

616.77 USA ISSN 0732-0280
LUPUS NEWS. Text in English. 1979. q. USD 25 domestic; USD 35 foreign (effective 2000). bk.rev. illus. reprints avail. *Refereed.* **Document type:** *Newsletter.* **Description:** Addresses the many facets of systemic lupus erythematosus - physical, emotional, psychological.
Published by: Lupus Foundation of America, Inc., 1300 Piccard Dr, Ste 200, Rockville, MD 20850. TEL 301-670-9292, FAX 301-670-9486, lupusnews@aol.com, http://www.lupus.org. Ed., R&P, Adv. contact Jenny Allan. Circ: 55,000.

616.742 GBR
MATHILDA AND TERENCE KENNEDY INSTITUTE OF RHEUMATOLOGY TRUST. ANNUAL REPORT. Text in English. 1967. a. free per issue. **Document type:** *Corporate.*
Formerly (until 2001): Mathilda and Terence Kennedy Institute of Rheumatology. Annual Report
Published by: Mathilda and Terence Kennedy Institute of Rheumatology Trust, 1 Aspenlea Rd, London W6 8LH, United Kingdom. TEL 44-181-383-4444, FAX 44-181-383-4499, kir-enquiries-dl@ic.ac.uk. Circ: 1,000 (controlled).

616.7 JPN ISSN 1439-7595
MODERN RHEUMATOLOGY. Text in English. q. EUR 194.40 domestic; EUR 190.80 in Germany; EUR 84 newsstand/cover foreign to individuals includes online ed. (effective 2002). adv. back issues avail. *Refereed.* **Document type:** *Journal, Academic/Scholarly.* **Description:** Publishes current Japanese research in rheumatology and associated areas (pathology, physiology, clinical immunology).
Formerly (until 1999): Japanese Journal of Rheumatology (0169-1163); Supersedes in part (in 1986): Ryumachi (0300-9157)
Related titles: Online - full text ed.: (from Springer LINK, RoweCom Information Quest).
Indexed: Inpharma, Pharm.&Out.News, Reac.
—BLDSC (5895.300000), CISTI, GNLM.
Published by: (Nihon Ryumachi Gakkai/Japan Rheumatism Association), Springer-Verlag Tokyo (Subsidiary of: BertelsmannSpringer) TEL 81-3-3812-0617, FAX 81-3-3812-4699, orders@svt-ebs.co.jp, http://link.springer-ny.com/link/service/journals/10165/index.htm, http://www.springer.de. **Subscr. to:** Springer-Verlag New York Inc., PO Box 2485, Secaucus, NJ 07096-2485. TEL 800-777-4643, 212-460-1526, FAX 201-348-4505, orders@springer-ny.com; Springer-Verlag, c/o Gabriele Kubitza, Haberstrasse 7, Heidelberg 69126, Germany. TEL 49-6221-345242, FAX 49-6221-345229, subscriptions@springer.de, http://link.springer.de, http://link.springer-ny.com.

616.7 NLD ISSN 0924-4506
NEW CLINICAL APPLICATIONS. RHEUMATOLOGY. Text in English. 1989. irreg. price varies. **Document type:** *Monographic series.*
Published by: Kluwer Academic Publishers Group (Subsidiary of: Wolters Kluwer N.V.), Spuiboulevard 50, PO Box 17, Dordrecht 3300 AA, Netherlands. FAX 31-78-639-2254, services@wkap.nl, http://www.wkap.nl. **Dist. by:** Journals Department, PO Box 322, Dordrecht 3300 AH, Netherlands. FAX 31-78-654-6474.

616.7 JPN ISSN 0287-3214
NIHON RYUMACHI KANSETSU GEKA GAKKAI ZASSHI/JAPANESE JOURNAL OF RHEUMATISM AND JOINT SURGERY. Text in English, Japanese. 1982. q.
Indexed: INIS Atomind.
Published by: Nihon Ryumachi Kansetsu Geka Gakkai, Shiga Ika Daigaku Seikei Gekagaku Kyoshitsu, Seta Tsukiwacho, Otsu-shi, Shiga-ken 520-21, Japan.

616.7 JPN
NIHON RYUMACHI KANSETSU GEKA GEKKAI/JAPANESE SOCIETY OF RHEUMATISM AND JOINT SURGERY. CONGRESS. Text in English, Japanese. 1984. a.
Published by: Nihon Ryumachi Kansetsu Geka Gakkai, Shiga Ika Daigaku Seikei Gekagaku Kyoshitsu, Seta Tsukiwacho, Otsu-shi, Shiga-ken 520-21, Japan.

NIHON SEKITSUI GEKA GAKKAI DAYORI/JAPAN SPINE RESEARCH SOCIETY. NEWS. see *MEDICAL SCIENCES—Orthopedics And Traumatology*

NIHON SEKITSUI GEKA GAKKAI ZASSHI/JAPAN SPINE RESEARCH SOCIETY. JOURNAL. see *MEDICAL SCIENCES—Orthopedics And Traumatology*

616.7 DNK ISSN 0108-2841
NYT OM GIGT. Text in Danish. 1982. q. DKK 84 (effective 1999). adv. illus.
Published by: Gigtforeningen, Gentoftegade 118, Gentofte 2820, Denmark. TEL 45-39-77-80-00, FAX 45-39-65-11-96. Ed. Ingrid Due Pedersen. Pub., Adv. contact Orskov Gruppen.

616.7 AUS
ON THE MOVE (ASHFORD)✶. Text in English. 1983. q. AUD 10. adv. bk.rev. back issues avail. **Document type:** *Consumer.* **Description:** News of foundation activities, information on self-help courses, researches on arthritis and treatments.
Former titles: Arthritis Action; Arthritis News
Published by: Arthritis Foundation of South Australia, c/o Arthritis & Rheumatism Council, Wynyard House, 291 George St., Sydney, NSW, NSW 2000, Australia. TEL 61-8-2972488, FAX 61-8-2931177. Ed., R&P, Adv. contact Sharon Rose. Circ: 8,000.

616.7 GBR ISSN 1063-4584 CODEN: OSCAEO
OSTEOARTHRITIS AND CARTILAGE; Journal of the osteoarthritis research society international. Text in English. 1993. 12/yr. GBP 138 to individuals; GBP 354 to institutions (effective 2002). adv. back issues avail.; reprint service avail. from SWZ. *Refereed.* **Document type:** *Academic/Scholarly.* **Description:** Publishes original articles on clinical, laboratory, and therapeutic research in osteoarthritis and related concerns, including cartilage, collagen, and orthopedics.
Related titles: Online - full text ed.: (from EBSCO Publishing, RoweCom Information Quest, Swets Blackwell, IDEAL Online Library, Institute for Scientific Information).
Indexed: AMED, ASCA, Curr.Cont., Excerp.Med. (1994-), Ind.Med. (1993-), Inpharma, Pharm.&Out.News, Reac., Ref.Zh., Sci.Cit.Ind.
—BLDSC (6303.858870), CISTI, EMDOCS, GNLM, IDS, Infotrieve, ingenta, KNAW. **CCC.**
Published by: (Osteoarthritis Research Society), W.B. Saunders Co. Ltd. (Subsidiary of: Harcourt Publishers Ltd.), 24-28 Oval Rd, London NW1 7DX, United Kingdom. TEL 44-20-7424-4200, FAX 44-20-7424-4515, cservice@harcourt.com, http://www.harcourt-international.com/journals/joca/. Ed. R D Altman. **Subscr. to:** Harcourt Publishers Ltd., Foots Cray High St, Sidcup, Kent DA14 5HP, United Kingdom. TEL 44-20-8308-5700, FAX 44-20-8309-0807.

▼ **THE PAIN CLINIC: A MULTIDISCIPLINARY APPROACH TO ACUTE AND CHRONIC PAIN MANAGEMENT.** see *MEDICAL SCIENCES—Orthopedics And Traumatology*

PRACTICAL GASTROENTEROLOGY; for the busy gastroenterologist. see *MEDICAL SCIENCES—Gastroenterology*

M

616.7 617.3 FRA ISSN 0997-7503
RACHIS; revue de pathologie vertebrale. Text in French. 1989. bi-m. FRF 800 domestic; FRF 1,000 foreign. adv. bk.rev. charts, illus. index.
Indexed: Bio-Contr.News & Info., Crop Physiol.Abstr., Field Crop Abstr., Food Sci.& Tech.Abstr., Herb.Abstr., Irr.& Drain.Abstr., Plant Breed.Abstr., Plant Gen.Res.Abstr., Rev.Appl.Entomol., Rev.Plant Path., Seed Abstr., Soils & Fert., Triticale Abstr., Weed Abstr.
—BLDSC (7225.976000).
Published by: Edimedica, 149 bd. Voltaire, Asniers 92600, France. TEL 33-47-935603, FAX 33-47-931728. Ed. F Vidal. Circ: 4,000.

616.7 GBR ISSN 0309-2283
RECENT ADVANCES IN RHEUMATOLOGY. Text in English. 1976. irreg., latest vol.4. **Document type:** *Monographic series, Academic/Scholarly.*
—CISTI.
Published by: Churchill Livingstone (Subsidiary of: Harcourt Publishers Ltd.), Robert Stevenson House, 1-3 Baxter's Pl, Leith Walk, Edinburgh, Midlothian EH1 3AF, United Kingdom. TEL 44-131-556-2424, FAX 44-131-459-1177, http://www.churchillmed.com. **US subscr. to:** Churchill Livingstone, 650 Ave of the Americas, New York, NY 10011. TEL 212-206-5000.

REFERATOVY VYBER Z REVMATOLOGIE/ABSTRACTS OF RHEUMATOLOGY. see *MEDICAL SCIENCES—Abstracting, Bibliographies, Statistics*

616.742 CZE ISSN 1211-2658 CODEN: FYRVAX
REHABILITACE A FYZIKALNI LEKARSTVI. Text in Czech, Slovak; Summaries in Czech, English. 1923. q. EUR 84, USD 112 (effective 2001). adv. bk.rev. *Refereed.* **Document type:** *Academic/Scholarly.*
Supersedes in part (in 1993): Fysiatricky a Reumatologicky Vestnik (0072-0038)
Indexed: Biol.Abstr., Excerp.Med., Ind.Med. (coverage dropped).
—CASDDS, CISTI, EMDOCS, GNLM, Infotrieve. **CCC.**
Published by: (Ceska Lekarska Spolecnost J.E. Purkyne/Czech Medical Association), Nakladatelske Stredisko C L S J.E. Purkyne, Sokolska 31, Prague 12026, Czech Republic. TEL 42-2-24911420, FAX 42-2-24911420, nts@iol.cz, http://www.clsjep.cz, http://www.medical.cz. Ed. V Janda. adv.: B&W page CZK 23,200, color page CZK 36,400; 245 x 167. Circ: 2,400. **Dist. by:** Abont s.r.o., Chlumova 17, Prague, 3 130 00, Czech Republic; **Dist. in Western Countries by:** Kubon & Sagner, Hesstr 39-41, Munich 80798, Germany.

616.742 SWE ISSN 1104-0696
REUMATIKERTIDNINGEN. Text in Swedish. 1949. bi-m. SEK 200 to members (effective 2001). adv. bk.rev. back issues avail. **Document type:** *Magazine, Consumer.*
Formerly (until 1994): Reuma (0034-6209)
Related titles: Audio cassette/tape ed.; Online - full text ed.
Published by: Reumatiker Foerbundet/Swedish National Association Against Rheumatism, Alstroemergatan 39, Fack 12851, Stockholm 11298, Sweden. TEL 46-8-692-58-00, FAX 46-8-650-64-15, brev@rmr.se, http://www.rmr.se, http://www.geocidies.rmr.se. Ed., Pub. Anders Arhammar. adv.: B&W page SEK 14,900, color page SEK 14,900; trim 250 x 180. Circ: 53,000; 54,900 (controlled).

616.7 ITA ISSN 0048-7449
REUMATISMO. Text in Italian. 1949. 4/yr. USD 115 to non-members (effective 1994). adv. bk.rev. illus. Supplement avail.; back issues avail. *Refereed.* **Document type:** *Bulletin.*
Indexed: Biol.Abstr., Chem.Abstr., Excerp.Med., Ind.Med. (coverage dropped), Inpharma, Reac.
—BLDSC (7785.544100), CISTI, GNLM.
Published by: Societa Italiana di Reumatologia (S.I.R.), Corso Plebisciti, 9, Milan, MI 20129, Italy. TEL 39-2-7382330, FAX 39-2-7385763, TELEX 33215 BOFFIS I. Ed. Claudio Cervini. adv.: B&W page ITL 1,550,000, color page ITL 2,800,000; trim 230 x 135. Circ: 2,500.

616.7 HRV ISSN 0374-1338
REUMATIZAM. Text in Croatian; Summaries in English. 1954. bi-m. adv. bk.rev. index. back issues avail.
Indexed: Biol.Abstr., Ind.Med. (1954-).
—CISTI, GNLM.
Published by: Croatian League Against Rheumatism, Lovcenska 100, Zagreb 41000, Croatia. TEL 041-572-440. Ed. Ivo Jajic. Circ: 1,000. **Subscr. to:** Jurjevska 25-I, Zagreb 41000, Croatia.

616.742 POL ISSN 0034-6233 CODEN: RMTOA2
REUMATOLOGIA. Text in Polish; Summaries in English. 1963. q. PLZ 50, USD 150 (effective 2002). adv. bk.rev. bibl, charts, illus. index. 110 p./no. 1 cols./p. back issues avail. *Refereed.* **Document type:** *Academic/Scholarly.* **Description:** Publishes original and clinical reports, review papers, case reports, conference reports and announcements.
Indexed: Biol.Abstr., Chem.Abstr., Dent.Ind., Excerp.Med., Ind.Med. (coverage dropped).
—BLDSC (7785.548000), CASDDS, GNLM, KNAW.
Published by: Instytut Reumatologiczny/Institute of Rheumatology, Ul Spartanska 1, Warsaw 02637, Poland. TEL 48-1033-22-8444241, FAX 48-1033-22-8449522. Ed. Jacek Pazdur. Circ: 1,000 (paid). **Co-sponsor:** Polskie Towarzystwo Reumatologiczne/Polish Rheumatological Society.

616.7 ITA ISSN 0391-8963
IL REUMATOLOGO. Text in Italian; Summaries in English. 1980. q. ITL 30,000, USD 30 (effective 2000). adv.
Published by: C I C Edizioni Internazionali s.r.l., Corso Trieste 42, Rome, RM 00198, Italy. TEL 39-06-8412673, FAX 39-06-8412688, info@gruppocic.it, 1160199510. Ed. C Cervini. adv.: B&W page XEU 1,601.02, color page XEU 2,014.18; 210 x 290.

616.7 BRA ISSN 0482-5004 CODEN: RBREBM
REVISTA BRASILEIRA DE REUMATOLOGIA/BRAZILIAN JOURNAL OF RHEUMATOLOGY. Text in Portuguese; Summaries in English. 1957. bi-m. abstr.
Indexed: Chem.Abstr., INIS Atomind.
—BLDSC (7845.700000), CASDDS.
Published by: (Sociedade Brasileira de Reumatologia/Brazilian Society of Rheumatology), Redprint Editora Ltda., Rua Domingos de Morais 2777, 15o cjs 151 e 154, Sao Paulo, SP 04035-001, Brazil. TEL 55-11-5724813, FAX 55-11-5711719, redprint@uol.com.br. Ed. Luis Eduardo Coelho Andrade.

616.7 ESP ISSN 0304-4815
REVISTA ESPANOLA DE REUMATOLOGIA. Text in Spanish; Summaries in English, Spanish. 1974. 10/yr. USD 113 to non-members. adv. charts, illus, stat. index. reprint service avail. from PQC. **Document type:** *Academic/Scholarly.* **Description:** Contains investigative work in the field of rheumatology done in Spain. Serves to continue the education of internists and physicians.
Indexed: Excerp.Med., Ind.Med.Esp., Inpharma, Reac.
—BLDSC (7854.310000), CINDOC, EMDOCS, GNLM, KNAW. **CCC.**
Published by: (Sociedad Espanola de Reumatologia), Ediciones Doyma S.A., Traversa de Gracia, 17-21, Barcelona 08021, Spain. TEL 34-93-200-0711, FAX 34-93-209-1136. Ed. M Figueroa Pedrosa. Adv. contact Julio Esteva. color page ESP 238,000; trim 280 x 210. Circ: 2,000.

616.7 615.533 BGR ISSN 1310-0505
REVMATOLOGIIA. Text in Bulgarian; Summaries in Bulgarian, English. 1993. q., latest vol.9, 2001. BGL 20 domestic; USD 55 foreign (effective 2001 - 2002). adv. bk.rev. abstr, bibl, illus. index. 56 p./no. back issues avail. *Refereed.* **Document type:** *Journal, Academic/Scholarly, Abstract/Index, Bibliography.* **Description:** Presents original articles in the field of rheumatology and related diseases for medical researchers and practitioners.
Indexed: Abstr.Bulg.Sci.Med.Lit., Ref.Zh.
—BLDSC (0140.585780).
Published by: Meditsinski Universitet - Sofia, Tsentur za Informatsiia po Meditsina/Medical University - Sofia, Medical Information Center, 1 Sv Georgi Sofiiski ul, Sofia 1431, Bulgaria. TEL 359-2-9522342, FAX 359-2-9522393, mutafov@sun.medun.acad.bg, http://www.medun.acad.bg. Ed. Dr. J Sheitanov. R&P, Adv. contact Dr. Christo Mutafov. B&W page USD 70, color page USD 170; trim 230 x 170. Circ: 300. **Co-sponsor:** Bulgarsko Nauchno Druzhestvo po Revmatologiia.

616.742 FRA ISSN 1169-8330 CODEN: RRMOA2
REVUE DU RHUMATISME (EDITION FRANCAISE). Text in French. 1933. 12/yr. EUR 279 in Europe to individuals; USD 336 elsewhere to individuals; EUR 313 in Europe to institutions; USD 375 elsewhere to institutions (effective 2002). adv. bk.rev. abstr, bibl, charts, illus. index. reprint service avail. from PQC. **Document type:** *Academic/Scholarly.*
Supersedes in part (in 1993): Revue du Rhumatisme et des Maladies Osteoarticulaires (0035-2659); Which was formerly (until 1946): Revue du Rhumatisme (0301-8474)
Related titles: Microform ed.: (from PQC); Online - full text ed.: (from ScienceDirect).
Indexed: Biol.Abstr., C.I.S. Abstr., Chem.Abstr., Curr.Cont. (coverage dropped), Excerp.Med. (until 1994), Helminthol.Abstr., Ind.Med. (until 1994, dropped), Ind.Sci.Rev., Nutr.Abstr., Ref.Zh., Sci.Cit.Ind. (coverage dropped).
—BLDSC (7945.590000), CASDDS, CISTI, GNLM, Infotrieve. **CCC.**
Published by: (Societe Francaise de Rhumatologie), Elsevier Paris, Editions Scientifiques et Medicales (Subsidiary of: Reed Elsevier plc. group), 23 rue Linois, Paris 75015, France. TEL 33-1-45589110, FAX 33-1-45589419, http://www.elsevier.com/locate/rhum. Circ: 5,000.

616.742 FRA ISSN 1169-8446 CODEN: RRHUE
REVUE DU RHUMATISME (ENGLISH EDITION). Text in French. 1933. 10/yr. USD 1,300 domestic to individuals; USD 1,500 foreign to individuals; USD 650 domestic to students; USD 750 foreign to students. *Refereed.* **Document type:** *Academic/Scholarly.*
Supersedes in part (in 1993): Revue du Rhumatisme et des Maladies Osteoarticulaires (0035-2659); Which was formerly (until 1946): Revue du Rhumatisme (0301-8474)
Indexed: ASCA, Cal.Tiss.Abstr., Chemorec.Abstr., Curr.Cont. (coverage dropped), Excerp.Med. (1994-), Ind.Med. (1994-, dropped), Inpharma, Neurosci.Abstr. (coverage dropped), Pharm.&Out.News, Pollut.Abstr., Reac., Rev.Med.& Vet.Mycol., Sci.Cit.Ind. (coverage dropped), Trop.Dis.Bull.
—CASDDS, CISTI, GNLM, IDS, Infotrieve, KNAW. **CCC.**
Published by: (Societe Francaise de Rhumatologie), Expansion Scientifique Francaise, 31 bd. de la Tour Maubourg, Paris Cedex 7 75343, France. TEL 33-1-40626400, FAX 33-1-45556920. Ed. T Bardin.

616.7 ESP ISSN 0211-7274
RHEUMA. Text in Spanish. 8/yr. ESP 6,000 (effective 2001). back issues avail.; reprints avail. **Document type:** *Journal.*
Published by: Jarpyo Editores S.A., Antonio Lopez Aguado, 4, Madrid 28029, Spain. TEL 34-913-144338, FAX 34-913-144499, editorial@jarpyo.es, http://www.jarpyo.es. Ed. Juan Torres. Circ: 2,096.

616.7 DEU ISSN 0945-7178
RHEUMA JOURNAL. Text in German. 4/yr. DEM 28.25; DEM 30 foreign (effective 1999). adv. **Document type:** *Newsletter.*
Published by: P. Keppler Verlag GmbH und Co. KG, Industriestr 2, Heusenstamm 63150, Germany. TEL 49-6104-606313, FAX 49-6104-606334, pkepplerverlag@t-online.de, info@kepplermediengruppe.de. Ed. Herta Koehler. Adv. contact R Nandkisore. Circ: 20,000.

616.742 GBR ISSN 1469-3089
RHEUMATIC DISEASE: IN PRACTICE (SERIES 4). Text in English. 1959; N.S. 1985; N.S. 1994. 3/yr. free per issue. **Document type:** *Academic/Scholarly, Trade.* **Description:** Intended to provide succinct and practical advice for general practitioners and hospital doctors about the diagnosis and management of common rheumatic conditions.
Supersedes (in 2000): Reports on Rheumatic Diseases. Series 3. Practical Problems (1351-4873); (in 1994): Reports on Rheumatic Diseases. Series 2. Practical Problems (1351-3060); Which superseded in part: Reports on Rheumatic Diseases (0957-0381); Which superseded (in 1985): Rheumatic Diseases Report; (in 1983): Reports on Rheumatic Diseases (0048-7279)
—BLDSC.
Published by: Arthritis Research Campaign, Copeman House, St. Mary's Ct, St. Mary's Gate, Chesterfield, Derbys S41-7TD, United Kingdom. TEL 44-2146-558033, FAX 44-1246-558007. Circ: 40,000.

616.742 GBR ISSN 1469-3097
RHEUMATIC DISEASE TOPICAL REVIEWS. Text in English. 1959; N.S. 1985; N.S. 1994. 3/yr. free per issue. **Document type:** *Academic/Scholarly, Trade.* **Description:** Offers advice on the diagnosis and treatment of common problems, topical research findings, and theories. Aimed at physicians and other health care professionals.
Supersedes (in 2000): Reports on Rheumatic Diseases. Series 3. Topical Reviews (1351-4881); (in 1994): Reports on Rheumatic Diseases. Series 2. Topical Reviews (1351-3508); Which superseded in part: Reports on Rheumatic Diseases (0957-0381); Which superseded (in 1985): Rheumatic Diseases Report; (in 1983): Reports on Rheumatic Diseases (0048-7279)
—BLDSC, GNLM.

M

Published by: Arthritis Research Campaign, Copeman House, St. Mary's Ct, St. Mary's Gate, Chesterfield, Derbys S41-7TD, United Kingdom. TEL 44-1264-558033, FAX 44-1246-558007, info@arc.org.uk, http://www.arc.org.uk. Ed. Robert Cooper.

616.742 USA ISSN 0007-5248
RC927 CODEN: BRDIAZ
RHEUMATIC DISEASES. BULLETIN. Text in English. 1950. bi-m. USD 15; free in US. bibl. cum.index.every 4 yrs. reprint service avail. from PQC. *Refereed.*
Related titles: Microform ed.: (from PQC); Online - full text ed.: (from Northern Light Technology, Inc., ProQuest Information & Learning, Institute for Scientific Information).
Indexed: ASCA, Biol.Abstr., Chem.Abstr., Curr.Cont., Excerp.Med., Ind.Med. (1950-), Ind.Sci.Rev., Inpharma, Pharm.&Out.News, Reac., Rev.Med.& Vet.Mycol., Sci.Cit.Ind.
—BLDSC (2885.200000), CASDDS, CISTI, GNLM, IDS, ingenta, KNAW. **CCC.**
Published by: Arthritis Foundation, 1330 W Peach Tree St, Atlanta, GA 30309. TEL 404-872-7100, FAX 404-872-9559, http://www.arthritis.org. Ed. Dr. John S Sergent. Circ: 26,000.

616.7 USA ISSN 0889-857X
RC927 CODEN: CRHDDK
RHEUMATIC DISEASES CLINICS OF NORTH AMERICA. Text in English. 1987. q. USD 151 domestic to individuals; USD 181 in Canada to individuals; USD 199 elsewhere to individuals; USD 214 domestic to institutions; USD 260 foreign to institutions; USD 66 per issue (effective 2001). index. back issues avail. *Refereed.* **Document type:** *Academic/Scholarly.* **Description:** Discusses topics in the diagnosis and treatment of rheumatic conditions.
Supersedes in part (in 1987): Clinics in Rheumatic Diseases (0307-742X)
Related titles: Online - full text ed.: (from Institute for Scientific Information).
Indexed: ASCA, CINAHL, Curr.Cont., INIS Atomind., Ind.Med. (1987-), Ind.Sci.Rev., Inpharma, Int.Nurs.Ind., Neurosci.Cit.Ind., Nutr.Abstr., Pharm.&Out.News, Reac., Rev.Appl.Entomol., SSCI (coverage dropped), Sci.Cit.Ind.
—BLDSC (7960.618000), CASDDS, CISTI, EMDOCS, GNLM, IDS, ingenta, KNAW. **CCC.**
Published by: W.B. Saunders Co. (Subsidiary of: Harcourt Publishers Ltd.), 11830 Westline Industrial Dr, St Louis, MO 63146. TEL 800-325-4177, http://www.wbsaunders.com. **Subscr. to:** Periodicals Fulfillment, W B Saunders Co, 6277 Sea Harbor Dr, 4th Fl, Orlando, FL 32891-4800.

616.742 IND ISSN 0035-4546
RHEUMATISM. Text and summaries in English, Hindi. 1965. q. INR 32, USD 12. adv. bk.rev. abstr, charts, illus. index.
Indexed: AMED, Biol.Abstr.
—BLDSC, CISTI.
Published by: M M L Centre for Rheumatic Diseases, Sanskriti Bhawan, Jhandewalan, New Delhi 110 055, India. TEL 011-3313306. Ed. Kaviraj A Majumdar. Circ: 200.

616.7 SVK ISSN 1210-1931
CODEN: RHEUE
RHEUMATOLOGIA. Text in Slovak. 1987. 4/yr. USD 40 (effective 2002).
Indexed: Excerp.Med. (1994-).
—BLDSC (7960.719000), EMDOCS, GNLM, KNAW.
Published by: Slovak Academic Press Ltd., Nam Slobody 6, PO Box 57, Bratislava 81005, Slovakia. TEL 427-2-55421729, vs.t@vurch.sk, http://www.elis.sk.

616.742 GBR ISSN 1462-0324
CODEN: RUMAFK
RHEUMATOLOGY. Text in English. 1952. m. GBP 365, USD 610 (effective 2002). adv. bk.rev. bibl, illus. index. 132 p./no. back issues avail.; reprint service avail. from PQC. *Refereed.* **Document type:** *Journal, Academic/Scholarly.* **Description:** Devoted to clinical and laboratory rheumatology, treatment therapy, immunology, and new-drug developments worldwide.
Former titles (until 1999): British Journal of Rheumatology (0263-7103); (until 1983): Rheumatology and Rehabilitation (0300-3396); (until 1973): Rheumatology and Physical Medicine (0003-4908); (until 1970): Annals of Physical Medicine (0365-5547)
Related titles: Microform ed.: (from PQC); Online - full text ed.: ISSN 1460-2172. GBP 325, USD 545 to institutions online only (effective 2002) (from EBSCO Publishing, Northern Light Technology, Inc., O C L C Online Computer Library Center, Inc., RoweCom Information Quest, ingenta, Swets Blackwell, Institute for Scientific Information).
Indexed: AIM, AMED, ASCA, Abstr.Inter.Med., Agri.& Environ.Biotech.Abstr. (coverage dropped), Behav.Med.Abstr., Biol.Abstr., Biol.Dig., CINAHL, Chem.Abstr., Chem.Indus.Notes, Chem.Titles, Curr.Adv.Ecol.Sci., Curr.Cont., Dent.Ind., Derwent Biotech.Abstr., Excerp.Med., Helminthol.Abstr., INIS Atomind., Ind.Med. (1999-), Ind.Sci.Rev., Inpharma, Int.Abstr.Biol.Sci., Med.& Surg.Dermat., Neurosci.Cit.Ind., Nutr.Abstr., Pharm.&Out.News, Reac., Rev.Appl.Entomol., SSCI (coverage dropped), Sci.Cit.Ind.
—BLDSC (7960.731900), CASDDS, CISTI, EMDOCS, GNLM, IDS, ingenta, KNAW. **CCC.**
Published by: (British Society of Rheumatology), Oxford University Press, Academic Division, Great Clarendon St, Oxford OX2 6DP, United Kingdom. TEL 44-1865-267907, FAX 44-1865-267835, jnl.info@oup.co.uk, http://rheumatology.oupjournals.org/, http://www.oup.co.uk/journals. Ed. David L Scott. Pub. Mandy Sketch. R&P Fiona Willis. adv.: B&W page GBP 430, B&W page USD 774; trim 165 x 243. Circ: 3,000. **US subscr. to:** Oxford University Press, Journals, 2001 Evans Rd, Cary, NC 27513. TEL 800-852-7323, FAX 919-677-1714, jnlorders@oup-usa.org; **Subscr. to:** Journals Marketing, Great Clarendon St, Oxford OX2 6DP, United Kingdom.

616.742 CHE ISSN 0080-2727
RC927.A1 CODEN: RHEUBD
RHEUMATOLOGY; the interdisciplinary concept. Text in English. 1966. irreg., latest vol.18. CHF 200 in Europe; DEM 240 in Germany; USD 180 in United States (effective 2001). reprint service avail. from ISI. *Refereed.* **Document type:** *Monographic series, Academic/Scholarly.*
Related titles: Online - full text ed.: (from Northern Light Technology, Inc.).
Indexed: Biol.Abstr., Chem.Abstr., Curr.Cont. (coverage dropped), Ind.Med. (coverage dropped).
—BLDSC (7960.730000), CASDDS, CISTI, GNLM, KNAW. **CCC.**
Published by: S. Karger AG, Allschwilerstr 10, PO Box, Basel 4009, Switzerland. TEL 41-61-306-1111, FAX 41-61-306-1234, karger@karger.ch, http://www.karger.com/bookseries/RHEUM. Ed. F Hiepe.

616.7 GBR
RHEUMATOLOGY IN PRACTICE. Text in English. 1990. 2/yr. **Document type:** *Academic/Scholarly.*
Supersedes in part (in 1991): Gastroenterology and Rheumatology in Practice (0959-3314); Which was formed by the merger of (1981-1990): Rheumatology in Practice (0262-5512); (1983-1990): Gastroenterology in Practice (0264-7478)
Published by: Hayward Medical Communications Ltd., Covent Garden, Seven Dials Warehouse, 44 Earlham St, London WC2H 9LA, United Kingdom. TEL 44-20-7240-4493, FAX 44-20-7240-4479, admin@hayward.co.uk, http://www.hayward.co.uk. Ed. Paul Emery. Circ: 16,000. **Subscr. to:** Rosemary House, Lanwades Park, Kentford, Near, Newmarket, Suffolk CB8 7PW, United Kingdom. TEL 44-1638-751515, FAX 44-1638-751517.

616.7 DEU ISSN 0172-8172
CODEN: RHINDE
RHEUMATOLOGY INTERNATIONAL; clinical and experimental investigations. Text in English. 1981. bi-m. EUR 426.20 domestic; EUR 422.40 foreign; EUR 82.40 newsstand/cover foreign (effective 2002). adv. reprint service avail. from ISI. *Refereed.* **Document type:** *Journal, Academic/Scholarly.* **Description:** Reflects world-wide progress in the research, diagnosis, and treatment of various rheumatic diseases.
Related titles: Microform ed.: (from PQC); Online - full text ed.: ISSN 1437-160X (from EBSCO Publishing, RoweCom Information Quest, Swets Blackwell, Springer LINK, Institute for Scientific Information).
Indexed: ASCA, Chem.Abstr., Chem.Titles, Curr.Adv.Ecol.Sci., Curr.Cont., Dent.Ind., Excerp.Med., Ind.Med. (1981-), Inpharma, Pharm.&Out.News, Reac., Sci.Cit.Ind.
—BLDSC (7960.738300), ADONIS, CASDDS, CISTI, GNLM, IDS, KNAW. **CCC.**
Published by: Springer-Verlag (Subsidiary of: BertelsmannSpringer), Tiergartenstr 17, Heidelberg 69121, Germany. TEL 49-6221-345-0, FAX 49-6221-345229, subscriptions@springer.de, http://link.springer.de/link/service/journals/00296/index.htm, http://www.springer.de. Ed. J R Kalden. **Subscr. in N. America to:** Springer-Verlag New York Inc., PO Box 2485, Secaucus, NJ 07096-2485. TEL 212-460-1500, FAX 212-473-6272.

616.7 FRA ISSN 0295-5261
RHUMATOLOGIE PRATIQUE. Text in French. 1986. m. (10/yr). EUR 23 domestic to individuals; EUR 31 foreign to individuals; EUR 16 domestic to libraries; EUR 25 foreign to libraries (effective 2002). **Document type:** *Newspaper.*
Published by: L E N Medical, 15 rue des Sablons, Paris 75116, France. TEL 33-1-47553131, FAX 33-1-47553132, lenmed@club-internet.fr, http://www.webmedguide.com. Ed. Dr. Gerald Ratzbaum.

616.99105 615.82 TUR ISSN 1300-0691
ROMATOLOJI VE TIBBI REHABILITASYON DERGISI/JOURNAL OF RHEUMATOLOGY AND MEDICAL REHABILITATION. Text and summaries in English, Turkish. 1990. q., latest vol.9, 1998. TRL 15,000,000, USD 50; USD 200 foreign. adv. bk.rev. back issues avail. *Refereed.* **Document type:** *Academic/Scholarly.* **Description:** Contains original articles and case reports are published in topics related with rheumatology, physical medicine, sports medicine and medical rehabilitation of all kinds.
Indexed: Excerp.Med. (1994-).
—BLDSC (8020.400000).
Published by: Turk Tibbi Rehabilitasyon Kurumu Dernegi/Turkish Society of Rehabilitational Medicine, Hacettepe Universitesi, Tip Fakultesi, Hacettepe - Ankara 06100, Turkey. TEL 90-312-309-4142, FAX 90-312-3105769, hufftr@tr-net.net.tr. Ed., Pub., R&P, Adv. contact Zafer Hascelik. B&W page USD 200, color page USD 300; trim 210 x 290. Circ: 500 (paid); 250 (controlled).

616.742 NLD ISSN 1566-6018
ROND REUMA. Text in Dutch. q. NLG 35 (effective 2000). **Document type:** *Journal, Academic/Scholarly.* **Description:** Contains general (non-medical) information on activities against rheumatism.
Former titles (until 1999): Reuma Nu (1385-7169); (until 1996): Reuma Bulletin (0034-6217)
Published by: Nationaal Reumafonds, Postbus 59091, Amsterdam 1040 KB, Netherlands. TEL 31-20-5896464, FAX 31-20-5896444, info@reumafonds.nl, http://www.reumafonds.nl. Ed. Margret Westhoff.

616.7 JPN ISSN 0300-9157
RYUMACHI. Text in Japanese. q. **Document type:** *Academic/Scholarly.*
Indexed: Ind.Med.
—BLDSC (8053.596000).
Published by: Nihon Ryumachi Gakkai/Japan Rheumatism Association, 2-39-7, Minami-Otsuka, Toshima-ku, Tokyo 170-0005, Japan. TEL 81-3-3946-5661, FAX 81-3-3946-7600.

616.742 NOR ISSN 0300-9742
RC927 CODEN: SJRHAT
SCANDINAVIAN JOURNAL OF RHEUMATOLOGY. Text in Norwegian. 6/yr. GBP 93, USD 145 to individuals; GBP 148, USD 245 to institutions (effective 2002). adv. *Refereed.* **Document type:** *Academic/Scholarly.* **Description:** Covers clinical and experimental aspects of rheumatic diseases.
Formerly: Acta Rheumatologica Scandinavica (0001-6934)
Related titles: Online - full text ed.: (from EBSCO Publishing, O C L C Online Computer Library Center, Inc., RoweCom Information Quest, CatchWord Ltd., Swets Blackwell, Institute for Scientific Information); ♦ Supplement: Scandinavian Journal of Rheumatology. Supplement. ISSN 0301-3847.
Indexed: ASCA, Agri.& Environ.Biotech.Abstr. (coverage dropped), Behav.Med.Abstr., Biol.Abstr., Chem.Abstr., Curr.Adv.Ecol.Sci., Curr.Cont., Dent.Ind., Derwent Biotech.Abstr., Energy Res.Abstr., Excerp.Med., INIS Atomind., Ind.Med. (1972-), Ind.Sci.Rev., Inpharma, Int.Abstr.Biol.Sci., Med.& Surg.Dermat., Nutr.Abstr., Pharm.&Out.News, Reac., SSCI (coverage dropped), Sci.Cit.Ind., THA.
—BLDSC (8087.546000), ADONIS, CASDDS, CISTI, EMDOCS, GNLM, IDS, Infotrieve, ingenta, KNAW. **CCC.**

M

Published by: (Scandinavian Society for Rheumatology), Taylor & Francis AS (Subsidiary of: Taylor & Francis Group), Cort Adelersgt. 17, Solli, PO Box 2562, Oslo 0202, Norway. TEL 47-22-12-98-80, FAX 47-22-12-98-90, journals@tandf.no, http://www.tandf.co.uk/tfas. Ed. Gunnar Husby. Circ: 1,800.

617.742 NOR ISSN 0301-3847
CODEN: SJRSAS

SCANDINAVIAN JOURNAL OF RHEUMATOLOGY. SUPPLEMENT. Text in English. 1958. irreg. **Document type:** *Academic/Scholarly.*
Formerly (until 1973): Acta Rheumatologica Scandinavica. Supplementum (0065-163X)
Related titles: Online - full text ed.: (from ingenta, Swets Blackwell); ♦ Supplement to: Scandinavian Journal of Rheumatology. ISSN 0300-9742.
Indexed: AMED, Excerp.Med., Ind.Med. (1973-), Int.Abstr.Biol.Sci.
—BLDSC (8087.546300), ADONIS, CASDDS, CISTI, EMDOCS, Infotrieve, KNAW. **CCC.**
Published by: (Scandinavian Society for Rheumatology), Scandinavian University Press (Subsidiary of: Taylor & Francis Ltd.), Postboks 2959, Toeyen, Oslo 0608, Norway. FAX 47-22-57-53-53, journals@scup.no, http://www.scup.no/rheumatology.

616.7 USA ISSN 0049-0172
RC933.A1 CODEN: SAHRBF

SEMINARS IN ARTHRITIS & RHEUMATISM. Text in English. 1971. bi-m. USD 183 domestic to individuals; USD 283 foreign to individuals; USD 304 domestic to institutions; USD 374 foreign to institutions; USD 82, USD 169 domestic to students; USD 63 newsstand/cover (effective 2001). adv. bibl, charts, illus. index. *Refereed.* **Document type:** *Journal, Academic/Scholarly.* **Description:** Provides clinical expositions of topics of current importance to practicing physicians, including inflammatory and degenerative disorders of bone, joints, and connective tissue; arthritis; gout; and collagen diseases.
Related titles: Online - full text ed.: (from IDEAL Online Library, Institute for Scientific Information).
Indexed: ASCA, Behav.Med.Abstr., Biol.Abstr., CINAHL, Chem.Abstr., Chem.Indus.Notes, Chem.Titles, Curr.Adv.Ecol.Sci., Curr.Cont., Dent.Ind., Excerp.Med., INIS Atomind., Ind.Med. (1971-), Ind.Sci.Rev., Inpharma, Med.& Surg.Dermat., Nutr.Abstr., Pharm.&Out.News, Protozool.Abstr., Reac., Rev.Med.& Vet.Mycol., SSCI (coverage dropped), Sci.Cit.Ind.
—BLDSC (8239.448000), CASDDS, CISTI, GNLM, IDS, ingenta, KNAW. **CCC.**
Published by: W.B. Saunders Co. (Subsidiary of: Harcourt Publishers Ltd.), 11830 Westline Industrial Dr, St Louis, MO 63146. TEL 800-325-4177, http://www.wbsaunders.com. Eds. Norman L Gottlieb, Dr. Roy D Altman. Adv. contact Steve Gray. B&W page USD 1,080, color page USD 2,050; trim 10 x 7. Circ: 2,906. **Subscr. to:** Periodicals Fulfillment, W B Saunders Co, 6277 Sea Harbor Dr, 4th Fl, Orlando, FL 32891-4800.

616.7 USA ISSN 1048-6763

TODAY IN MEDICINE. MUSCULOSKELETAL MEDICINE. Text in English. 199?. bi-m.
Published by: Data Centrum Communications, Inc., 21 W 38th St, 4th fl, New York, NY 10018.

YEAR BOOK OF RHEUMATOLOGY, ARTHRITIS, AND MUSCULOSKELETAL DISEASE. see *MEDICAL SCIENCES—Abstracting, Bibliographies, Statistics*

616.742 DEU ISSN 0340-1855
CODEN: ZRHMBQ

ZEITSCHRIFT FUER RHEUMATOLOGIE. Text and summaries in English, German. 1938. bi-m. EUR 375.31 domestic; EUR 370.21 in Germany; EUR 72 foreign (effective 2002). adv. bk.rev. abstr, bibl, charts, illus, pat. back issues avail.; reprints avail. *Refereed.* **Document type:** *Journal, Academic/Scholarly.*
Formerly: Zeitschrift fuer Rheumaforschung (0044-345X)
Related titles: Microform ed.: (from PQC); Online - full text ed.: ISSN 1435-1250 (from EBSCO Publishing, RoweCom Information Quest, Swets Blackwell, Springer LINK, Institute for Scientific Information).
Indexed: ASCA, Agri.& Environ.Biotech.Abstr. (coverage dropped), Biol.Abstr., Chem.Abstr., Chem.Indus.Notes, Chem.Titles, Curr.Adv.Ecol.Sci., Curr.Cont., Dent.Ind., Derwent Biotech.Abstr., INIS Atomind., Ind.Med. (1974-), Ind.Sci.Rev., Inpharma, Int.Nurs.Ind., Reac., Rev.Appl.Entomol., SSCI (coverage dropped), Sci.Cit.Ind.
—BLDSC (9485.455000), ADONIS, CASDDS, CISTI, EMDOCS, GNLM, IDS, Infotrieve, KNAW. **CCC.**
Published by: Dr. Dietrich Steinkopff Verlag (Subsidiary of: BertelsmannSpringer), Poststr 9, Darmstadt 64293, Germany. TEL 49-6151-82899-0, FAX 49-6151-82899-40, frey.steinkopff@springer.de, http://www.steinkopff.springer.de. Circ: 1,500. **Subscr. in N. America to:** Springer-Verlag, Journals; **Subscr. to:** Springer GmbH Auslieferungsgesellschaft, Haberstr 7, Heidelberg 69126, Germany. TEL 49-6221-345239, FAX 49-6221-345249, subscriptions@springer.de. **Co-sponsors:** Deutsche Gesellschaft fuer Rheumatologie; Oesterreichische Gesellschaft fuer Rheumatologie; Schweizerische Gesellschaft fuer Rheumatologie; Berufsverband Deutscher Rheumatologen; Gesellschaft fuer Psychosomatik in der Rheumatologie.

616.7 CHN ISSN 1007-7480

ZHONGHUA FENGSHIBINGXUE ZAZHI/CHINESE JOURNAL OF RHEUMATOLOGY. Text in Chinese. 1997. bi-m. CNY 48, USD 25.20; CNY 8, USD 4.20 newsstand/cover (effective 2001). **Document type:** *Journal, Academic/Scholarly.* **Description:** Reports on the leading clinical experiments and studies with a theoretical basis. Contains editorials, original articles, reviews, lectures, clinical studies, clinicopathological discussions, academic trends in China and abroad, case reporting, technical exchanges, and other columns.
Related titles: Online - full content ed.: (from WanFang Data Corp.).
Published by: Zhonghua Yixuehui/Chinese Medical Association, 23 Donghuamen, Taiyuan, Shanxi 030013, China. TEL 86-351-3071551 ext 2153, cmafsb@public.sti.ac.cn. Ed. Dong Yi. R&P, Adv. contact Haiyuan Dong. Circ: 15,500 (paid); 200 (controlled). **Dist. overseas by:** China International Book Trading Corp, 35, Chegongzhuang Xilu, Haidian District, Beijing 100044, China. TEL 86-1-68413849, FAX 86-1-68412048, cibtc@mail.cibtc.com.cn, http://www.cibtc.com.cn.

MEDICAL SCIENCES—Sports Medicine

A C S M'S HEALTH & FITNESS JOURNAL. see *PHYSICAL FITNESS AND HYGIENE*

A S M A NEWS. (American Sports Medicine Association) see *SPORTS AND GAMES*

617.1 MEX

A T P ENERGIA Y MOVIMIENTO. Text in Spanish. 1988. bi-m. MXP 300, USD 55 (effective 1996 & 1997). *Refereed.* **Document type:** *Academic/Scholarly.* **Description:** Contains original articles in sports medicine and coaching, review articles, research reports, clinical cases and notices.
Published by: Obsidiana Editores S.A., CZDA DE TLALPAN 2365, Col Ciudad Jardin, Mexico City, DF 04370, Mexico. TEL 52-5-689-9133. Ed. Dr. Eva Franco. Circ: 5,000. **Dist. by:** Distribuidora Editorial de Mexico SA de CV, P.O. Box 76-026, Mexico City, DF 04201, Mexico. TEL 52-5-544-7953, FAX 52-5-689-6545.

ABILITY BALLROOM DANCE JOURNAL. see *DANCE*

612.044 617.1027 CZE ISSN 1212-1428

ACTA UNIVERSITATIS CAROLINAE: KINANTHROPOLOGICA. Text in Czech. 1965. s-a. CZK 100, USD 5 (effective 1999). **Document type:** *Academic/Scholarly.* **Description:** Covers sport science, psychology, pedagogy, physiology, sports medicine, biomechanics.
Formerly (until 1995): Acta Universitatis Carolinae: Gymnica (0323-0511)
Published by: (Univerzita Karlovo), Vydavatelstvi Karolinum, Ovocny trh 5, Prague 116 36, Czech Republic. TEL 42-2-24491270, FAX 42-2-24212041, edice@cuni.cz; rychtecky@ftvs.cuni.cz. Ed., R&P Antonin Rychtecki. Circ: 250. **Subscr. to:** Knihovna FTVS UK, J Martiho 31, Prague 16262, Czech Republic. TEL 42-2-20172019, FAX 42-2-364075.

617.1 USA

AMERICAN ACADEMY OF PODIATRIC SPORTS MEDICINE NEWSLETTER*✱*. Text in English. 1982. q. USD 30. adv. **Document type:** *Newsletter.*
Formerly: American Academy of Podiatric Sports Medicine Journal
Indexed: Sportsearch (1988-).
Published by: American Academy of Podiatric Sports Medicine, PO Box 880187, Boca Raton, FL 33488-0187. TEL 301-424-7440. Ed., Adv. contact Larry Shane. Circ: 8,000.

617.1 USA ISSN 1056-9677

AMERICAN COLLEGE OF SPORTS MEDICINE. CERTIFIED NEWS. Text in English. 3/yr. **Document type:** *Newsletter.* **Description:** Provides continuing education credits (CECs) and information to those certified by ACSM.
Published by: American College of Sports Medicine, Certification Committee, PO Box 1440, Indianapolis, IN 46206-1440. TEL 317-637-9200, FAX 317-634-7817.

AMERICAN JOURNAL OF KNEE SURGERY. see *MEDICAL SCIENCES—Surgery*

617.1027 USA ISSN 1524-2196

▼ **AMERICAN JOURNAL OF MEDICINE AND SPORTS.** Text in English. 1999. bi-m. USD 90 domestic to individuals; USD 105 foreign to individuals; USD 105 domestic to institutions; USD 120 foreign to institutions (effective 2001). adv. bk.rev. abstr, charts, illus. back issues avail.; reprints avail. *Refereed.* **Document type:** *Journal, Academic/Scholarly.*
Published by: LeJacq Communications, Inc., 777 W Putnam Ave, Greenwich, CT 06830-5014. TEL 209-531-0450, FAX 203-531-0533, showell@lejacq.com. Ed. Barry Franklin. Pub. Louis Lejacq. R&P Andrea Townsend. Adv. contact Joann Kalaka-Adams TEL 732-747-6525. B&W page USD 4,650, color page USD 1,235; trim 10.75 x 8. Circ: 90,000 (controlled).

617 USA ISSN 0363-5465
RC1200 CODEN: AJSMDO

AMERICAN JOURNAL OF SPORTS MEDICINE. Text in English. 1972. bi-m. USD 95 to individuals; USD 115 to institutions (effective 2001). adv. illus. cum.index: 1972-1996. back issues avail.; reprints avail. *Refereed.* **Document type:** *Journal, Academic/Scholarly.* **Description:** Presents original scientific research directed to orthopaedic surgeons specializing in sports medicine.
Formerly (until 1976): Journal of Sports Medicine (0090-4201)
Related titles: CD-ROM ed.; Microfilm ed.: (from PQC); Microform ed.; Online - full text ed.: (from Gale Group, ProQuest Information & Learning, Northern Light Technology, Inc., Factiva, Institute for Scientific Information).
Indexed: AMED, ASCA, Abstr.Anthropol., Behav.Med.Abstr., CINAHL, Curr.Cont., Educ.Ind. (Jul.1983-Jun.1992), Environ.Sci.Poll.Mgmt., Excerp.Med., Focus on: Sports Sci.& Med., Gen.Sci.Ind. (Jun.1992-), Hlth.Ind., INIS Atomind., Ind.Med. (1976-), Inpharma, NRN, Pharm.&Out.News, Phys.Ed.Ind., Pollut.Abstr., Reac., Risk Abstr., Saf.Sci.Abstr., Sci.Cit.Ind., Sportsearch (1976-).
—EMDOCS, GNLM, IDS, ingenta, KNAW. **CCC.**
Published by: American Orthopaedic Society for Sports Medicine, 6300 North River Rd, Ste 200, Rosemont, IL 60018. TEL 847-292-4900, 877-321-3500, FAX 847-292-4905, aossm@aossm.org, http://journal.ajsm.org/, http://www.aossm.org. Ed. Dr. Robert E Leach. Adv. contact Gary Walchli. Circ: 10,754 (paid).

615.8 FRA ISSN 0302-427X

ANNALES DE KINESITHERAPIE. Text in French. 1974. 8/yr. FRF 827; FRF 1,034 foreign (effective 2000). adv. bk.rev. charts, illus. reprint service avail. from ISI. **Document type:** *Academic/Scholarly.* **Description:** Focuses on physical therapy and rehabilitation. Contains original articles, new developments, practical suggestions and technical articles.
Formed by the merger of: Revue de Kinesitherapie (0035-1172); Journal de Kinesitherapie (0021-7751)
Related titles: Microform ed.: (from PQC); Online - full text ed.: (from RoweCom Information Quest).
Indexed: Biol.Abstr., Curr.Cont. (coverage dropped), Sportsearch (1974-).
—BLDSC (0981.040000), CISTI, Infotrieve. **CCC.**
Published by: (Societe de Kinesitherapie), Masson - Periodiques, 120 bd. St. Germain, Paris 75006, France. TEL 33-1-40466200, FAX 33-1-40466201. Ed. E Viel. Circ: 3,500. **Subscr. to:** Societe de Periodiques Specialises, BP 22, Vineuil Cedex 41354, France. TEL 33-2-54504612, FAX 33-2-54504611.

617.1 JPN ISSN 0918-0257

AOMORIKEN SUPOTSU IGAKU KENKYUKAISHI/ AOMORI SOCIETY OF SPORTS MEDICINE. JOURNAL. Text in Japanese. 1989. s-a. abstr, bibl, charts, illus, stat. back issues avail. **Document type:** *Proceedings, Academic/Scholarly.*
Formerly: Aomoriken Supotsu Igaku Kenkyukai Koenshu
Published by: Aomoriken Supotsu Igaku Kenkyukai/Aomori Society of Sports Medicine, c/o Mr Yoshihisa Okamura, Hirosaki Daigaku Igakubu Seikei Geka Kyoshitsu, 5 Zaifu-cho, Hirosaki-shi, Aomori-ken 036-8216, Japan.

M

617.3 ESP ISSN 0212-4009
APUNTS; medicina de l'esport. Text in Catalan, Spanish. 1986. q. ESP 2,500; ESP 3,000 foreign (effective 1998). adv. bibl, illus. index. back issues avail.
Formerly: Apuntes de Medicina Deportiva
Indexed: Ind.Med.Esp.
—CINDOC.
Published by: Centro d'Estudis de l'Alt Rendiment Esportiu, Direccio General de l'Esport, Ave. PAISOS CATALAN, 12, Esplugues De Llobregat, Barcelona 08950, Spain. TEL 54-93-480-4900, FAX 54-93-480-4910, TELEX 54845 GCDE. Circ: 2,000. **Dist. by:** Les Punxes, Sardenya, 75-81 08018, Barcelona 08013, Spain.

617.1 USA ISSN 1078-7895
RC1200 CODEN: ATTOF5
ATHLETIC THERAPY TODAY. Text in English. 1996. bi-m. USD 36 to individuals; USD 108 to institutions; USD 30 to students (effective 2001). adv. illus. Index. back issues avail.; reprints avail. *Refereed.* **Document type:** *Journal, Academic/Scholarly.* **Description:** Designed to provide insights into professional practice issues, highlight sports health care techniques, share experiential knowledge and provide practical applications of current research.
Related titles: Online - full text ed.: (from Institute for Scientific Information).
Indexed: AMED, CINAHL, Focus on: Sports Sci.& Med.
—BLDSC (1765.879690), Infotrieve, ingenta. **CCC.**
Published by: Human Kinetics Publishers, Inc., PO Box 5076, Champaign, IL 61825-5076. TEL 217-351-5076, FAX 217-351-2674, clydew@hkusa.com, http://www.humankinetics.com/products/journals/journal.cfm?id=ATT. Ed. Richard Ray. Pub. Rainer Martens. R&P Cheri Banks TEL 217-351-5076 ext 2275. Adv. contact Patty Rodriguiz. Circ: 2,099 (paid).

612.044 POL ISSN 0860-021X
BIOLOGY OF SPORT; a quarterly journal of sport and exercise sciences. Text in English. 1984. q. *Refereed.* **Description:** Publishes reports of methodological and experimental work on science of sport, natural sciences, medicine and pharmacology, technical sciences, biocybernetics and applications of statistics and psychology, with priority for inter-disciplinary papers.
Related titles: Online - full text ed.: (from Institute for Scientific Information).
Indexed: Focus on: Sports Sci.& Med.
—BLDSC (2087.247000).
Published by: Instytut Sportu/Institute of Sport, ul. Trylogoo 2/16, Warsaw 01-982, Poland. TEL 48-22-8340812, FAX 48-22-8350977, insp@insp.waw.pl, http://www.insp.pl/bos/. Ed. Ryszard Grucza.

617 GBR ISSN 0306-3674
CODEN: BJSMDZ
BRITISH JOURNAL OF SPORTS MEDICINE. Text in English. 1968. q. GBP 95, USD 153 combined subscription to individuals includes print & online eds.; GBP 205, USD 329 to institutions print only (effective 2002). adv. bk.rev. illus, stat. Supplement avail.; back issues avail.; reprints avail. *Refereed.* **Document type:** *Journal, Academic/Scholarly.* **Description:** Covers management of injuries and physiotherapy, physiological evaluations of sports performance, psychology, nutrition, and the role of medical personnel.
Incorporates: British Association of Sport and Medicine. Bulletin
Related titles: Microform ed.: (from PQC); Online - full text ed.: B J S M Online. ISSN 1473-0480. 2000. GBP 65, USD 99 to individuals (effective 2002); Institutions contact publisher for online rates. (from EBSCO Publishing, RoweCom Information Quest, ingenta, Swets Blackwell, HighWire Pr., SilverPlatter Information, Inc., Ovid Technologies, Inc., Institute for Scientific Information).
Indexed: AMED, ASCA, CINAHL, Crim.Just.Abstr., Curr.Adv.Ecol.Sci., Curr.Cont., Environ.Sci.Poll.Mgmt., Ergon.Abstr., Focus on: Sports Sci.& Med., Ind.Med. (1969-), Ind.Sci.Rev., Inpharma, Int.Nurs.Ind., NRN, Nutr.Abstr., Pharm.&Out.News, Phys.Ed.Ind., Pollut.Abstr., Reac., Ref.Zh., Risk Abstr., SSCI (coverage dropped), Saf.Sci.Abstr., Sci.Cit.Ind., Sportsearch (1975-).
—BLDSC (2324.900000), ADONIS, CASDDS, EMDOCS, GNLM, IDS, ingenta, KNAW. **CCC.**
Published by: (British Association of Sport and Medicine), B M J Publishing Group, B M A House, Tavistock Sq, London WC1H 9JR, United Kingdom. TEL 44-20-7387-4499, FAX 44-20-7383-6400, info.norththames@bma.org.uk, http://bjsm.bmjjournals.com/, http://www.bma.org.uk. Ed. Paul McCrory. Pub. Alex Williamson. R&P Carol Torselli TEL 44-20-7383-6674. Adv. contact Euan Currer TEL 44-20-7383-6181.

CAHIERS DE KINESITHERAPIE; revue d'enseignement post-scolaire et de documentation technique. see *MEDICAL SCIENCES—Physical Medicine And Rehabilitation*

CANADIAN JOURNAL OF APPLIED PHYSIOLOGY/ REVUE CANADIENNE DE PHYSIOLOGIE APPLIQUEE. see *SPORTS AND GAMES*

617.1 USA ISSN 1050-642X
RC1200 CODEN: CJSMED
CLINICAL JOURNAL OF SPORT MEDICINE. Text in English. 1975. q. USD 195 domestic to individuals; USD 195 foreign to individuals; USD 340 domestic to institutions; USD 340 foreign to institutions; USD 78 newsstand/cover (effective 2002). adv. bk.rev. charts, illus. reprint service avail. from PQC. *Refereed.* **Document type:** *Academic/Scholarly.* **Description:** Features original research articles, clinical reviews, case reports, new techniques and procedures in physical examination, exercise testing, diagnostic imaging, and other developments relevant to the clinical practice of sports medicine.
Former titles (until 1990): Canadian Academy of Sport Medicine Review (0831-2893); Canadian Academy of Sport Medicine Newsletter
Related titles: Online - full text ed.: USD 442 domestic academic site license; USD 442 foreign academic site license; USD 493 domestic corporate site license; USD 493 foreign corporate site license (2002) (from Ovid Technologies, Inc., Institute for Scientific Information).
Indexed: ASCA, Curr.Cont., Excerp.Med. (1993-), Focus on: Sports Sci.& Med., Ind.Med. (1991-), Inpharma, Reac., Sci.Cit.Ind., Sportsearch (1991-).
—BLDSC (3286.294300), EMDOCS, GNLM, IDS, ingenta, KNAW.
Published by: (Canadian Academy of Sport Medicine CAN), Lippincott Williams & Wilkins (Philadelphia) (Subsidiary of: Wolters Kluwer N.V.), 530 Walnut St, Philadelphia, PA 19106-3621. TEL 301-223-2300, FAX 301-223-2400, http://www.cjsportmed.com/, http://www.Lww.com. Eds. Andrew Pipe, Willem Meeuwisse. adv.: B&W page USD 930, color page USD 2,030. Circ: 2,170 (paid). **Subscr. to:** PO Box 1600, Hagerstown, MD 21740-1600. **Co-sponsor:** American Medical Society for Sports Medicine.

617 USA ISSN 0278-5919
CLINICS IN SPORTS MEDICINE. Text in English. 1982. q. USD 150 domestic; USD 172 in Canada; USD 199 elsewhere; USD 204 domestic; USD 244 foreign; USD 62 per issue (effective 2001). *Refereed.* **Document type:** *Journal, Academic/Scholarly.* **Description:** Delivers practical advice from experts in specialty covered as well as information on new developments in a variety of specialties with a fresh perspective on problems and controversies.
Related titles: Microform ed.: (from PQC); Online - full text ed.: (from Institute for Scientific Information); ♦ Spanish Translation: Clinicas de Medicina Deportiva de Norteamerica.
Indexed: AMED, ASCA, CINAHL, Curr.Cont., Dent.Ind., Excerp.Med., Focus on: Sports Sci.& Med., INIS Atomind., Ind.Med. (1982-), Inpharma, Int.Nurs.Ind., Nutr.Abstr., Pharm.&Out.News, Reac., Sportsearch (1982-).
—BLDSC (3286.595500), EMDOCS, GNLM, IDS, ingenta, KNAW. **CCC.**
Published by: W.B. Saunders Co. (Subsidiary of: Harcourt Publishers Ltd.), 11830 Westline Industrial Dr, St Louis, MO 63146. TEL 800-325-4177, http://www.wbsaunders.com. Ed. Dr. Mark D Miller. **Subscr. to:** Periodicals Fulfillment, W B Saunders Co, 6277 Sea Harbor Dr, 4th Fl, Orlando, FL 32891-4800.

617.1 USA ISSN 1069-5842
CURRENT REVIEW OF SPORTS MEDICINE. Text in English. 1994. irreg. **Document type:** *Monographic series, Academic/Scholarly.*
—GNLM.
Published by: Current Medicine, 400 Market St, Ste 700, Philadelphia, PA 19106. TEL 215-574-2257, 800-427-1796, FAX 215-574-2225. **Subscr. outside N. America to:** Current Science Ltd, Middlesex House, 34-42 Cleveland St, London W1P 6LB, United Kingdom. TEL 44-20-7323-0323.

617.102 DEU ISSN 0344-5925
CODEN: DZSPD8
DEUTSCHE ZEITSCHRIFT FUER SPORTMEDIZIN. Text in German. 1949. 11/yr. DEM 167 (effective 2002). adv. **Document type:** *Journal, Trade.*
Formerly: Sportarzt und Sportmedizin
Indexed: Chem.Abstr., Chem.Indus.Notes, Chem.Titles, IBR, IBZ, Nutr.Abstr., Sportsearch (1978-).
—CASDDS, GNLM, Infotrieve. **CCC.**
Published by: W W F Verlagsgesellschaft mbH, Am Eggenkamp 37-39, Greven 48257, Germany. TEL 49-2571-937630, FAX 49-2571-937650, verlag@wwf-medien.de. Ed. Dr. Urte Kuenstlinger. Circ: 14,867.

617 ITA ISSN 1592-3894
EUROPEAN JOURNAL OF SPORTS TRAUMATOLOGY AND RELATED RESEARCH. Text and summaries in English, Italian. 1979. q. EUR 82.63 domestic; USD 105 foreign (effective 2002). *Refereed.* **Description:** Contains original studies on experimental and clinical research. Includes case reports, short communications, interviews and conferences.
Former titles (until 2001): Journal of Sports Traumatology and Related Research (1120-3137); (until 1990): Italian Journal of Sports Traumatology (0391-4089)
Related titles: Online - full text ed.: EUR 41.31 (effective 2002) (from Institute for Scientific Information).
Indexed: ASCA, Excerp.Med., Focus on: Sports Sci.& Med., Ref.Zh., Sportsearch (1989-).
—BLDSC (5066.400000), EMDOCS, GNLM, IDS, KNAW.
Published by: Editrice Kurtis s.r.l., Via Luigi Zoja, 30, Milan, MI 20153, Italy. TEL 39-02-48202740, FAX 39-02-4820-1219, info@kurtis.it, http://www.kurtis.it. Ed. Paolo Aglietti.

613.7 USA ISSN 0091-6331
RC1200 CODEN: ESSRB8
EXERCISE AND SPORT SCIENCES REVIEWS. Text in English. 1973. q. USD 74 domestic to individuals; USD 86 foreign to individuals; USD 86 domestic to institutions; USD 98 foreign to institutions; USD 24 newsstand/cover (effective 2002). adv. charts, illus. back issues avail. *Refereed.* **Document type:** *Academic/Scholarly.* **Description:** Includes brief reviews for readers with a broad interest in scientific issues related to exercise, movement, physical activity and/or sports.
Indexed: AMED, ASCA, Biol.Abstr., Focus on: Sports Sci.& Med. (coverage dropped), Ind.Med. (1973-), Ind.Sci.Rev., Sci.Cit.Ind. (coverage dropped), Sportsearch (1973-).
—BLDSC (3836.233000), CASDDS, CISTI, GNLM, ingenta, KNAW, Linda Hall.
Published by: (American College of Sports Medicine), Lippincott Williams & Wilkins (Baltimore) (Subsidiary of: Wolters Kluwer N.V.), 351 W Camden St, Baltimore, MD 21201-2436. TEL 410-528-4000, 410-528-4185, FAX 800-447-8438, bschrame@lww.com, http://www.acsm-essr.com, http:/www.lww.com/acsmcrc. Ed. Douglas R Seals. Pub. Susan Harris. Adv. contact Sharlene Isaacson. B&W page USD 735, color page USD 1,180; trim 8.125 x 10.875. Circ: 11,772 (paid).

616.07 612.7 USA ISSN 1077-5552
QP301 CODEN: EIREFY
EXERCISE IMMUNOLOGY REVIEW. Text in English. 1995. a. USD 26 to individuals; USD 60 to institutions; USD 20 to students (effective 2001). adv. back issues avail.; reprints avail. *Refereed.* **Document type:** *Journal, Trade.* **Description:** Committed to developing and enriching knowledge in all aspects of immunology that relate to sport, exercise, and regular physical activity.
Related titles: Online - full text ed.: (from Institute for Scientific Information).
Indexed: CINAHL, Focus on: Sports Sci.& Med., Ind.Med. (1995-), Phys.Ed.Ind.
—BLDSC (3836.235700), GNLM, IDS, Infotrieve. **CCC.**
Published by: Human Kinetics Publishers, Inc., PO Box 5076, Champaign, IL 61825-5076. TEL 217-351-5076, FAX 217-351-2674, orders@hkusa.com, http://www.humankinetics.com/products/journals/journal.cfm?id=EIR. Ed. Hinnak Northoff. Pub. Rainer Martens. R&P Cheri Banks TEL 217-351-5076 ext 2275. Adv. contact David Kotarba TEL 800-747-4457 x 2389. Circ: 550 (paid).

EXERCISE STANDARDS AND MALPRACTICE REPORTER. see *LAW*

FOOT & ANKLE INTERNATIONAL. see *MEDICAL SCIENCES—Orthopedics And Traumatology*

FUJIAN TIYU KEJI/FUJIAN SPORTS SCIENCE AND TECHNOLOGY. see *SPORTS AND GAMES*

613.711 617.1027 NLD ISSN 0016-6448
CODEN: GESPBS
GENEESKUNDE EN SPORT. Text in Dutch; Abstracts in English. 1968. bi-m., latest 2001. NLG 94.50 domestic to non-members; NLG 125 domestic to institutions; NLG 67.40, NLG 54.50 domestic to members (effective 2001). adv. bk.rev. illus, stat, abstr. 40 p./no. 2 cols./p. back issues avail. *Refereed.* **Document type:** *Journal, Academic/Scholarly.*
Indexed: Biol.Abstr.

M

—BLDSC (4096.443000), GNLM, KNAW.
Published by: (Vereniging voor Sportgeneeskunde), Geneeskunde en Sport, Postbus 52, Bilthoven 3720 AB, Netherlands. TEL 31-30-225-2290, FAX 31-30-225-2498, gens@sportgeneeskunde.com, usg@sportgeneeskunde.com, http://www.sportgeneeskunde.com. Eds. A van der Lccix, R Stoecucit. Adv. contact Anjo Bruinsmc. Circ: 3,000.

617.1 HKG ISSN 1027-7323
THE HONG KONG JOURNAL OF SPORTS MEDICINE AND SPORTS SCIENCE. Text in English. 1995. s-a. HKD 80, USD 10 newsstand/cover (effective 2001). 100 p./no. back issues avail. **Document type:** *Journal, Academic/Scholarly.*
Indexed: CINAHL.
—BLDSC (4326.386500).
Published by: Hong Kong Association of Sports Medicine & Sports Science, c/o Dr. Stephen Hui Research Centre of Physical Recreation and Wellness, The Hong Kong Baptist University, Kowloon Tong, Hong Kong. TEL 852-2339-7127, FAX 852-2339-5777, http://fsmhk.com.hk/hkasmass. Ed., Adv. contact Frank Fu.

INTERNATIONAL JOURNAL OF SPORT NUTRITION & EXERCISE METABOLISM. see *NUTRITION AND DIETETICS*

616.8 ITA ISSN 0047-0767
GV706.4 CODEN: ISPYAN
INTERNATIONAL JOURNAL OF SPORT PSYCHOLOGY. Text in English. 1970. q. USD 120 (effective 2002). adv. bk.rev. reprint service avail. from SWZ. *Refereed.* **Document type:** *Academic/Scholarly.* **Description:** Covers sports medicine.
Related titles: Microform ed.: (from SWZ); Online - full text ed.: (from Institute for Scientific Information).
Indexed: AMED, ASCA, AgeLine, Curr.Cont., Focus on: Sports Sci.& Med., Ind.Philos., Phys.Ed.Ind., PsycInfo, Psychol.Abstr. (1970-), Rural Devel.Abstr., Rural Recreat.Tour.Abstr., SSCI, Sportsearch (1974-), e-psyche.
—BLDSC (4542.681000), IDS, ingenta.
Published by: (International Society of Sports Psychology), Edizioni Luigi Pozzi s.r.l., Via Panama, 68, Rome, RM 00198, Italy. TEL 39-06-8553548, FAX 39-06-8554105, edizioni_pozzi@tin.it. Circ: 1,500.

610 DEU ISSN 0172-4622
CODEN: IJSMDA
INTERNATIONAL JOURNAL OF SPORTS MEDICINE. Text in English. 1980. 8/yr. EUR 345.80 domestic to institutions; EUR 348.60 in Europe to institutions; EUR 357.80 elsewhere to institutions; EUR 52 newsstand/cover (effective 2002). bk.rev. abstr, bibl, charts, illus. reprints avail. *Refereed.* **Document type:** *Journal, Academic/Scholarly.*
Related titles: Online - full text ed.: ISSN 1439-3964 (from Institute for Scientific Information); ♦ Supplement: International Journal of Sports Medicine. Supplement. ISSN 0943-917X.
Indexed: AMED, ASCA, Chem.Abstr., Chem.Indus.Notes, Chem.Titles, Curr.Cont., Dok.Arbeitsmed., Excerp.Med., Focus on: Sports Sci.& Med., Ind.Med. (1980-), Ind.Sci.Rev., Inpharma, NRN, Nutr.Abstr., Pharm.&Out.News, Reac., Rev.Arom.& Med.Plants, Rural Recreat.Tour.Abstr., SSCI (coverage dropped), Sci.Cit.Ind., Sportsearch (1980-), Sugar Ind.Abstr.
—BLDSC (4542.681300), ADONIS, CASDDS, CISTI, GNLM, IDS, Infotrieve, ingenta, KNAW. **CCC.**
Published by: Georg Thieme Verlag, Ruedigerstr 14, Stuttgart 70469, Germany. TEL 49-711-8931-0, FAX 49-711-8931298, sportsmed@thieme.de, kunden.service@thieme.de, leser.service@thieme.de, http://www.thieme.de/sportsmed. Eds. Maria Hopman, W M Sherman. R&P Michael Wachinger. Circ: 1,500 (paid and controlled).

610 DEU ISSN 0943-917X
INTERNATIONAL JOURNAL OF SPORTS MEDICINE. SUPPLEMENT. Text in English. 1982. irreg. **Document type:** *Monographic series, Academic/Scholarly.*
Related titles: ♦ Supplement to: International Journal of Sports Medicine. ISSN 0172-4622.
—ADONIS.
Published by: Georg Thieme Verlag, Ruedigerstr 14, Stuttgart 70469, Germany. TEL 49-711-8931-0, FAX 49-711-8931298, kunden.service@thieme.de, http://www.thieme.de.

INTERNATIONAL JOURNAL OF SPORTS VISION. see *MEDICAL SCIENCES—Ophthalmology And Optometry*

617 613 NLD ISSN 0959-3020
RM727.I76 CODEN: IESCEE
ISOKINETICS AND EXERCISE SCIENCE. Text in English. 1991-1996; resumed 1997. q. EUR 304, USD 282 to institutions (effective 2002). illus. back issues avail. *Refereed.* **Document type:** *Journal, Academic/Scholarly.* **Description:** Meets the needs of the contemporary exercise scientist and medical practitioner through a consolidated focus on the field of isokinetics.
Related titles: Microform ed.: (from PQC); Online - full text ed.: (from ingenta, Swets Blackwell, Institute for Scientific Information, RoweCom Information Quest).
Indexed: AMED, ASCA, Excerp.Med. (1996-), Focus on: Sports Sci.& Med., SSCI (coverage dropped).
—BLDSC (4583.269000), EMDOCS, IDS, Infotrieve, ingenta, KNAW. **CCC.**
Published by: I O S Press, Nieuwe Hemweg 6B, Amsterdam 1013 BG, Netherlands. TEL 31-20-688-3355, FAX 31-20-620-3419, market@iospress.nl, http://www.iospress.nl. Ed. Zeevi Dvir TEL 972-3-640-9019. **Subscr. to:** I O S Press, Inc, 5795-G Burke Centre Pkwy, Burke, VA 22015. TEL 703-323-5554, FAX 703-323-3668, iosbooks@iospress.com; Kinokuniya Company Ltd, Shinjuku 3-chome, Shinjuku-ku, Tokyo 160-0022, Japan. FAX 81-3-3439-1094, journal@kinokuniya.co.jp, http://www.kinokuniya.co.jp; Globe Publication Pvt. Ltd., C-62 Inderpuri, New Delhi 100 012, India. TEL 91-11-579-3211, 91-11-579-3212, FAX 91-11-579-8876, custserve@globepub.com, http://www.globepub.com.

JAPANESE JOURNAL OF PHYSICAL FITNESS AND SPORTS MEDICINE. see *PHYSICAL FITNESS AND HYGIENE*

617.1 FRA ISSN 0762-915X
JOURNAL DE TRAUMATOLOGIE DU SPORT. Text in French. 1983. 4/yr. FRF 599; FRF 769 foreign (effective 2000). **Document type:** *Academic/Scholarly.* **Description:** For all specialists concerned with bone, visceral, urological, and neurological traumatology, and reconstructive surgery, and for intensive care anaesthesists.
Related titles: Online - full text ed.: (from RoweCom Information Quest).
—BLDSC (5070.525100), CISTI, GNLM, Infotrieve. **CCC.**
Published by: Masson - Periodiques, 120 bd. St. Germain, Paris 75006, France. TEL 33-1-40466200, FAX 33-1-40466201. Eds. G Saillant, J Rodineau. Circ: 2,100. **Subscr. to:** Societe de Periodiques Specialises, BP 22, Vineuil Cedex 41354, France. TEL 33-2-54504612, FAX 33-2-54504611.

617.1 USA ISSN 1041-3200
GV706.4
JOURNAL OF APPLIED SPORT PSYCHOLOGY. Text in English. 1989. q. GBP 39, USD 65 to individuals; GBP 102, USD 169 to institutions (effective 2002). adv. *Refereed.* **Document type:** *Academic/Scholarly.* **Description:** Promotes quality research in the field of sport psychology.
Related titles: Online - full text ed.: (from CatchWord Ltd., Institute for Scientific Information).
Indexed: ASCA, AgeLine, Curr.Cont., Focus on: Sports Sci.& Med., Mark.Res.Abstr. (1963-), PsycInfo, Psychol.Abstr. (1989-), SSCI, e-psyche.
—BLDSC (4947.105000), IDS, ingenta. **CCC.**
Published by: Association for the Advancement of Applied Sport Psychology, c/o Faculty of Kinesiology, University of Western Ontario, London, ON N6A 3K7, Canada. TEL 519-661-4118, FAX 519-661-2008, jasp@julian.uwo.ca; orders@allenpress.com, http://spot.colorado.edu/~aaasp; http://www.allenpress.com. Ed. Albert V Carron. Circ: 1,000. **Subscr. in US to:** Allen Press Inc., PO Box 1897, Lawrence, KS 66044-8897.

796 USA ISSN 1062-6050
RC1200 CODEN: JATTEJ
JOURNAL OF ATHLETIC TRAINING. Text in English. 1956. q. USD 32; USD 40 foreign (effective 2001). adv. bk.rev. bibl, illus. index, cum.index. back issues avail.; reprint service avail. from PQC. *Refereed.* **Document type:** *Academic/Scholarly.*
Former titles (until 1992): Athletic Training (0160-8320); National Athletic Trainers Association. Journal (0027-8718)
Related titles: Microfiche ed.: (from PQC); Online - full text ed.: (from Northern Light Technology, Inc., ProQuest Information & Learning, Gale Group, Factiva, Institute for Scientific Information).
Indexed: AMED, ASCA, C.I.J.E., CINAHL, Excerp.Med., Focus on: Sports Sci.& Med., Phys.Ed.Ind., Russ.Acad.Sci.Bibl., Sports Per.Ind., Sportsearch (1974-).
—BLDSC (4947.850000), IDS, ingenta.
Published by: National Athletic Trainers Association, Inc., 2952 N Stemmons Fwy, Dallas, TX 75247. TEL 800-879-6282, FAX 214-637-2206, http://www.journalofathletictraining.org, http://www.nata.org/. Ed., R&P David Perrin. Circ: 29,000 (paid and controlled).

JOURNAL OF BACK AND MUSCULOSKELETAL REHABILITATION. see *MEDICAL SCIENCES—Orthopedics And Traumatology*

THE JOURNAL OF MUSCULOSKELETAL MEDICINE. see *MEDICAL SCIENCES—Orthopedics And Traumatology*

JOURNAL OF MUSCULOSKELETAL RESEARCH. see *MEDICAL SCIENCES—Orthopedics And Traumatology*

617 615.82 USA ISSN 0190-6011
RD701 CODEN: JOSPDV
JOURNAL OF ORTHOPAEDIC AND SPORTS PHYSICAL THERAPY. Text in English. 1971. m. USD 180 domestic to institutions; USD 228 foreign to institutions (effective 2001). adv. bk.rev. illus. Index. back issues avail.; reprints avail. *Refereed.* **Document type:** *Academic/Scholarly.* **Description:** Clinical developments in sports medicine for practicing physical therapists, athletic trainers and orthopedic surgeons.
Related titles: Microfilm ed.: (from WWS); Online - full text ed.: (from Institute for Scientific Information).
Indexed: AMED, ASCA, Behav.Med.Abstr., CINAHL, Curr.Cont., Environ.Sci.Poll.Mgmt., Excerp.Med., Focus on: Sports Sci.& Med., Ind.Med. (1979-), Inpharma, Phys.Ed.Ind., Reac., Rehabil.Lit., Saf.Sci.Abstr., Sportsearch (1980-).
—BLDSC (5027.660000), GNLM, IDS, ingenta, KNAW.
Published by: (Orthopaedic and Sports Physical Therapy Sections, American Physical Therapy Association), Allen Press Inc., PO Box 1897, Lawrence, KS 66044-8897. TEL 785-843-1235, 800-627-0932, FAX 785-843-1274, jospt@allenpress.com, http://www.allenpress.com; http://www.orthopt.org. Ed. Richard P Difabio. Pub. Theresa Pickel. R&P Gerald Cook TEL 608-788-2554. Adv. contact Martha Chapin. B&W page USD 1,055, color page USD 1,070; trim 10.88 x 8.13. Circ: 19,255 (paid).

617.1 AUS ISSN 1440-2440
GV557 CODEN: JSMSF6
JOURNAL OF SCIENCE AND MEDICINE IN SPORT. Text in English. 1961. q. AUD 30; AUD 45 foreign (effective 1999). adv. bk.rev. charts, illus, stat. back issues avail. *Refereed.* **Document type:** *Academic/Scholarly.* **Description:** Focuses on sports science and medicine.
Formerly (until Dec. 1997): Australian Journal of Science and Medicine in Sport (0813-6289); Which was formed by the 1983 merger of: Australian Journal of Sport Sciences (0725-4679); Australian Journal of Sports Medicine and Exercise Sciences (0811-6377); Which was formerly (until 1982): Australian Journal of Sports Medicine (0045-0650)
Indexed: AMED, Abstr.Anthropol., Environ.Sci.Poll.Mgmt., Ergon.Abstr., Excerp.Med., Geotech.Abstr., Ind.Med. (1998-), Inpharma, NRN, Pharm.&Out.News, Phys.Ed.Ind., Pollut.Abstr., Reac., Risk Abstr., Saf.Sci.Abstr., Sportsearch (1984-).
—BLDSC (5054.840000), EMDOCS, GNLM, ingenta.
Published by: (Australian Council for Health, Physical Education and Recreation Inc.), Sports Medicine Australia, PO Box 897, Belconnen, ACT 2616, Australia. TEL 61-2-6251-6944, FAX 61-2-6253-1489, TELEX AUSIS 62400. Ed. Bruce Abernethy. Circ: 3,500.

JOURNAL OF SMOOTH MUSCLE RESEARCH/NIHON HEIKATSUKIN GAKKAI KIKANSHI. see *MEDICAL SCIENCES*

JOURNAL OF SPORT AND EXERCISE PSYCHOLOGY. see *PSYCHOLOGY*

617.1 USA ISSN 1056-6716
RD97 CODEN: JSRHEV
JOURNAL OF SPORT REHABILITATION. Short title: J S R. Text in English. 1992. q. USD 45 to individuals; USD 135 to institutions; USD 30 to students (effective 2001). adv. bk.rev. abstr, bibl, charts, stat, illus. index. back issues avail.; reprint service avail. from PSC. *Refereed.* **Document type:** *Academic/Scholarly.* **Description:** Investigates the process of rehabilitation of sport and exercise injuries regardless of age, gender, athletic ability, level of fitness or health status of the participant.
Related titles: Online - full text ed.: (from Institute for Scientific Information).
Indexed: AMED, ASCA, CINAHL, Curr.Cont., Excerp.Med. (1993-), Focus on: Sports Sci.& Med., IBZ, Inpharma, Pharm.&Out.News, Reac.
—BLDSC (5066.189000), EMDOCS, GNLM, IDS, Infotrieve, ingenta, KNAW. **CCC.**

M

Published by: Human Kinetics Publishers, Inc., PO Box 5076, Champaign, IL 61825-5076. TEL 217-351-5076, FAX 217-351-2674, http://www.humankinetics.com. Ed. Christopher Ingersoll. Pub. Rainer Martens. R&P Cheri Banks TEL 217-351-5076 ext 2275. Adv. contact Patty Rodriguiz. Circ: 566 (paid).

JOURNAL OF SPORTS CHIROPRACTIC AND REHABILITATION. see *MEDICAL SCIENCES—Chiropractic, Homeopathy, Osteopathy*

610 613.7 ITA ISSN 0022-4707 CODEN: JMPFA3
THE JOURNAL OF SPORTS MEDICINE AND PHYSICAL FITNESS. Text in English. 1961. q. ITL 120,000, USD 126 to individuals; USD 198 to institutions (effective 2000 - 2001). adv. bk.rev. bibl, charts, illus. index. back issues avail.; reprint service avail. from SWZ. *Refereed.* **Document type:** *Academic/Scholarly.* **Description:** Covers applied physiology, preventive medicine, sports medicine and traumatology, and sports psychology.
Related titles: Microform ed.: (from SWZ); Online - full text ed.: (from Institute for Scientific Information).
Indexed: AMED, ASCA, CINAHL, Chem.Abstr., Chem.Indus.Notes, Chem.Titles, Curr.Cont., Excerp.Med., Focus on: Sports Sci.& Med., Ind.Med. (1961-), Inpharma, Mid.East: Abstr.& Ind., NRN, Nutr.Abstr., Pharm.&Out.News, Phys.Ed.Ind., Reac., SSCI (coverage dropped), Sportsearch (1975-).
—BLDSC (5066.200000), CASDDS, CISTI, GNLM, IDS, ingenta, KNAW.
Published by: Edizioni Minerva Medica, Corso Bramante, 83-85, Turin, TO 10126, Italy. TEL 39-11-678282, FAX 39-11-674502. Eds. A Del Monte, A Ljungqvist, F La Cava, G Santilli. Pub. Alberto Oliaro. Adv. contact F Filippo. B&W page USD 1,200, color page USD 2,000; trim 280 x 215. Circ: 5,000 (paid).

JOURNAL OF SPORTS SCIENCES. see *SPORTS AND GAMES*

617.1 USA ISSN 1064-8011
GV711
JOURNAL OF STRENGTH AND CONDITIONING RESEARCH; the research journal of the National Strength and Conditioning Association. Text in English. 1987. q. USD 90 domestic to institutions; USD 98 foreign to institutions (effective 2001). adv. charts, illus. Index. back issues avail.; reprints avail. *Refereed.* **Document type:** *Academic/Scholarly.* **Description:** Publishes original research dealing with strength and conditioning in sports and exercise.
Formerly: Journal of Applied Sports Research
Related titles: Online - full text ed.: (from Institute for Scientific Information).
Indexed: ASCA, CINAHL, Focus on: Sports Sci.& Med., IBZ, SSCI (coverage dropped), Sportsearch (1987-).
—BLDSC (5066.873700), IDS, Infotrieve, ingenta. **CCC.**
Published by: National Strength and Conditioning Association, 1955 N Union Blvd, Colorado Springs, CO 80905. acg@allenpress.com; nsca@nsca-lift.org, scunningham@allenpress.com, http://www.nsca-lift.org. Eds. Sarah Cunningham, William J Kraemer. adv.: B&W page USD 550; trim 11 x 8.5. Circ: 16,780 (paid).

JUOKSIJA. see *PHYSICAL FITNESS AND HYGIENE*

617.1 DEU ISSN 0942-2056 CODEN: KSSAEQ
KNEE SURGERY, SPORTS TRAUMATOLOGY, ARTHROSCOPY. Text in English. 1993. bi-m. EUR 355.50 domestic; EUR 350.40 in Germany; EUR 68 foreign (effective 2002). *Refereed.* **Document type:** *Journal, Academic/Scholarly.* **Description:** Covers various aspects of knee surgery, arthroscopy and sports traumatology.
Related titles: Microform ed.: (from PQC); Online - full text ed.: ISSN 1433-7347 (from EBSCO Publishing, RoweCom Information Quest, Swets Blackwell, Springer LINK, Institute for Scientific Information).
Indexed: Curr.Cont., Focus on: Sports Sci.& Med., Ind.Med. (1993-), Sci.Cit.Ind.
—BLDSC (5099.864200), CISTI, IDS, Infotrieve, KNAW. **CCC.**
Published by: (European Society of Sports Traumatology, Knee Surgery and Arthroscopy), Springer-Verlag (Subsidiary of: BertelsmannSpringer), Tiergartenstr 17, Heidelberg 69121, Germany. TEL 49-6221-345-0, FAX 49-6221-345229, subscriptions@springer.de, http://link.springer.de/link/service/journals/00167/index.htm, http://www.springer.de. Ed. E Eriksson. **Subscr. in N. America to:** Springer-Verlag New York Inc., PO Box 2485, Secaucus, NJ 07096-2485. TEL 212-460-1500, FAX 212-473-6272.

610 613.7 FRA ISSN 0025-6722 CODEN: MNSPBL
MEDECINE DU SPORT. Text in French; Summaries in English, German. 1925. bi-m. FRF 550; FRF 700 foreign; FRF 440 to students (effective 2000). adv. bk.rev. abstr, bibl, charts, illus, stat. index.
Formerly: Medecine Education Physique et Sport
Indexed: Aqua.Sci.& Fish.Abstr., Aquacult.Abstr., Biol.Abstr., Environ.Sci.Poll.Mgmt., Russ.Acad.Sci.Bibl., Sportsearch (1971-).
—GNLM. **CCC.**
Published by: Meditions Carline, 1 et 3 rue du Depart, Paris 75014, France. TEL 33-1-40640075, FAX 33-1-43222699, groupemeditions@wanadoo.fr. Circ: 1,500.

617.102 ITA ISSN 0025-7826
MEDICINA DELLO SPORT. Text and summaries in English, Italian, Spanish. 1947. q. USD 105 to individuals; USD 155 to institutions (effective 2000 - 2001). adv. bk.rev. bibl, charts, illus. index. *Refereed.* **Document type:** *Academic/Scholarly.*
Related titles: Online - full text ed.: (from Institute for Scientific Information).
Indexed: ASCA, Biol.Abstr., Chem.Abstr., Excerp.Med., Focus on: Sports Sci.& Med., Ind.Med. (coverage dropped), SSCI (coverage dropped), Sportsearch (1974-).
—BLDSC (5533.700000), CISTI, GNLM, IDS.
Published by: (Federazione Medico-Sportiva Italiana), Edizioni Minerva Medica, Corso Bramante, 83-85, Turin, TO 10126, Italy. TEL 39-11-678282, FAX 39-11-674502. Eds. G Tuccimei, T Lubich. Pub. Alberto Oliaro. Adv. contact F Filippo. B&W page USD 1,400, color page USD 2,300; trim 270 x 190. Circ: 6,000.

617.1 ESP
MEDICINA Y DEPORTE. Text in Spanish. 1986. q. bibl, illus.
Published by: Asociacion Asturiana de Medicina de la Educacion Fisica y el Deporte, Catedratico Gimeno, Oviedo, Asturias 33007, Spain.

617.102 USA ISSN 0195-9131
RC1200 CODEN: MSPEDA
MEDICINE AND SCIENCE IN SPORTS AND EXERCISE. Text in English. 1969. m. USD 270 domestic to individuals; USD 328 foreign to individuals; USD 460 domestic to institutions; USD 517 foreign to institutions; USD 33 newsstand/cover (effective 2002). adv. bk.rev. abstr, bibl, charts, illus. index. back issues avail.; reprints avail. *Refereed.* **Document type:** *Academic/Scholarly.* **Description:** Research in sports medicine topics for exercise physiologists, physiatrists, physical therapists and athletic trainers.
Formerly: Medicine and Science in Sports (0025-7990)
Related titles: Microfilm ed.: (from PQC,WWS); Online - full text ed.: USD 598 domestic for academic site license; USD 655 foreign for academic site license; USD 667 domestic for corporate site license; USD 724 foreign for corporate site license (effective 2002) (from Ovid Technologies, Inc., H. W. Wilson, Gale Group, Swets Blackwell, Institute for Scientific Information).
Indexed: AMED, ASCA, Abstr.Anthropol., AgeLine, Biol.Abstr., CINAHL, Chem.Abstr., Chem.Indus.Notes, Chem.Titles, Curr.Adv.Biochem., Curr.Adv.Ecol.Sci., Curr.Cont., Educ.Ind. (Jul.1992-), Environ.Sci.Poll.Mgmt., Excerp.Med., Focus on: Sports Sci.& Med., Gen.Sci.Ind. (Jul.1997-), INIS Atomind., Ind.Med. (1980-), Ind.Sci.Rev., Inpharma, Int.Abstr.Biol.Sci., Int.Aerosp.Abstr., Neurosci.Cit.Ind., Nutr.Abstr., Pharm.&Out.News, Phys.Ed.Ind., Pollut.Abstr., PsycInfo, Psychol.Abstr. (1983-), Reac., Risk Abstr., Russ.Acad.Sci.Bibl., SSCI (coverage dropped), Saf.Sci.Abstr., Sci.Cit.Ind., Sportsearch (1980-), Sugar Ind.Abstr., Wom.Stud.Abstr., e-psyche.
—BLDSC (5534.006700), CASDDS, GNLM, IDS, ingenta, KNAW.
Published by: American College of Sports Medicine, PO Box 1440, Indianapolis, IN 46206-1440. TEL 317-637-9200, FAX 317-634-7817, http://www.ms-se.com/, http://www.Lww.com. Ed. Kent B Pandolf. R&P Debbie Heisse TEL 410-528-4050. Adv. contact Sharlene Isaacson. Circ: 13,148. **Subscr. to:** Williams & Wilkins, 351 W Camden St, Baltimore, MD 21201-2436. TEL 800-638-6423, 800-486-5643, 410-528-4185, FAX 800-447-8438, bschrame@lww.com, http://www.lww.com/acsmcrc.

617.102 CHE ISSN 0254-5020 CODEN: MSPOB4
MEDICINE AND SPORT SCIENCE. Text in English. 1966. irreg., latest vol.44. CHF 200 in Europe; DEM 240 in Germany; USD 160 in United States (effective 2001). back issues avail.; reprint service avail. from ISI. *Refereed.* **Document type:** *Monographic series, Academic/Scholarly.* **Description:** Provides information on the development of sports medicine as a dynamic scientific discipline.
Formerly: Medicine and Sport (0076-6070)
Indexed: Biol.Abstr., Chem.Abstr., Curr.Cont. (coverage dropped), Ind.Med. (coverage dropped).
—BLDSC (5534.007300), CASDDS, CISTI, Infotrieve, KNAW. **CCC.**
Published by: S. Karger AG, Allschwilerstr 10, PO Box, Basel 4009, Switzerland. TEL 41-61-306-1111, FAX 41-61-306-1234, karger@karger.ch, http://www.karger.com/bookseries/MSPSC. Eds. J Borms, L J Micheli, M Hebbelinck.

MEDSCAPE ORTHOPEDICS & SPORTS MEDICINE. see *MEDICAL SCIENCES—Orthopedics And Traumatology*

MODERN ATHLETE AND COACH. see *SPORTS AND GAMES—Outdoor Life*

MOTOR CONTROL. see *MEDICAL SCIENCES—Physical Medicine And Rehabilitation*

MOVIMENTO. see *MEDICAL SCIENCES*

617.1 NZL ISSN 0110-6384
NEW ZEALAND JOURNAL OF SPORTS MEDICINE. Text in English. 1969. q. NZD 85, USD 46, AUD 73 to individuals (effective 2000). bk.rev. *Refereed.* **Document type:** *Academic/Scholarly.* **Description:** Covers all aspects of sports medicine amd sports science research.
Formerly (until 1973): Sports Medicine Bulletin
Indexed: Ind.N.Z.Per., Inpharma, Pharm.&Out.News, Reac.
—BLDSC (6095.100000), ingenta.
Published by: Sports Medicine New Zealand, 96 Anzac Ave, P.O. Box 6398, Dunedin, New Zealand. TEL 64-3-4777887, FAX 64-3-4777882. Ed. Dale Speedy. Adv. contact Brenda Allum. Circ: 1,000 (controlled).

NIHON SEIKEI GEKA SUPOTSU IGAKKAISHI/JAPANESE JOURNAL OF ORTHOPEDIC SPORTS MEDICINE. see *MEDICAL SCIENCES—Orthopedics And Traumatology*

617.1027 BEL
OLYMPIC HEALTH NEWS (EDITION FRANCAISE). Text in French. q. illus. **Document type:** *Newsletter, Trade.*
Related titles: Dutch ed.: Olympic Health News (Nederlandse Editie).
Published by: Comite Olympique et Interfederal Belge/Belgian Olympic and Interfederal Committee, Av de Bouchout 9, Brussels 1020, Belgium. TEL 32-2-474-5150, FAX 32-2-479-4656, info@olympic.be, info@olympic.org, http://www.olympic.be. Ed., R&P Guido de Bondt.

617.1 USA ISSN 1060-1872
OPERATIVE TECHNIQUES IN SPORTS MEDICINE. Text in English. 1993. q. USD 161 domestic to individuals; USD 219 foreign to individuals; USD 250 domestic to institutions; USD 299 foreign to institutions; USD 96 domestic to students; USD 131 foreign to students; USD 75 newsstand/cover (effective 2001). adv. illus. *Refereed.* **Document type:** *Academic/Scholarly.* **Description:** Discusses a new clinical condition or surgical procedure in each issue.
Related titles: Online - full text ed.: (from Institute for Scientific Information).
Indexed: CINAHL, Focus on: Sports Sci.& Med.
—BLDSC (6269.382500), GNLM, IDS, Infotrieve. **CCC.**
Published by: W.B. Saunders Co. (Subsidiary of: Harcourt Publishers Ltd.), 11830 Westline Industrial Dr, St Louis, MO 63146. TEL 800-325-4177, http://www.wbsaunders.com. Eds. Dr. David Drez Jr., Jesse C Delee. Adv. contact Cindy Gray. B&W page USD 660, color page USD 1,570; trim 11 x 7.75. Circ: 2,645. **Subscr. to:** Periodicals Fulfillment, W B Saunders Co, 6277 Sea Harbor Dr, 4th Fl, Orlando, FL 32891-4800.

ORTHOPAEDIC AND TRAUMATIC SURGERY/SEKEI SAIGAI GEKA. see *MEDICAL SCIENCES—Orthopedics And Traumatology*

PEDIATRIC EXERCISE SCIENCE. see *MEDICAL SCIENCES—Pediatrics*

PERSONAL FITNESS. see *PHYSICAL FITNESS AND HYGIENE*

617.102 GBR ISSN 1466-853X
PHYSICAL THERAPY IN SPORT. Text in English. 1978. q. GBP 50 to individuals; GBP 107 to institutions (effective 2002). adv. bk.rev. abstr. 48 p./no. 2 cols./p. back issues avail.; reprints avail. *Refereed.* **Document type:** *Journal, Academic/Scholarly.* **Description:** Aims to provide a forum for the publication of material that is indispensable for the day-to-day practices and continuing professional development of all healthcare professionals involved in sports medicine.
Formerly (until 2000): Physiotherapy in Sport (0954-0741)
Related titles: Online - full text ed.: (from Swets Blackwell, IDEAL Online Library).
Indexed: AMED.
—BLDSC (6476.350650).
Published by: (Association of Chartered Physiotherapists in Sports Medicine), Churchill Livingstone (Subsidiary of: Harcourt Publishers Ltd.), Robert Stevenson House, 1-3 Baxter's Pl, Leith Walk, Edinburgh, Midlothian EH1 3AF, United Kingdom. TEL 44-131-556-2424, FAX 44-131-558-1278, journals@harcourt.com, http://www.harcourt-international.com/journals/ptsp. Eds. Gregory Kolt, Kevin Foreman, Marvin Dean, Zoe Hudson. R&P Sharon Boyle TEL 44-131-524-1747. Adv. contact Deborah Watkins TEL 44-207-424-4280. Circ: 2,000 (paid). **Subscr. addr. in the US to:** Harcourt Health Sciences, Journals Subscription Department, PO Box 156, Avenel, NJ 07001; **Subscr. to:** Harcourt Publishers Ltd., Journal Sales & Marketing Dept., 32 Jamestown Rd, London NW1 7BY, United Kingdom.

610 617.102 USA ISSN 0091-3847
RC1200
THE PHYSICIAN AND SPORTSMEDICINE; a peer reviewed journal of medical aspects of sports, exercise and fitness. Text in English. 1973. m. USD 46 to individuals; USD 53 in Canada to individuals; USD 130 elsewhere to individuals (effective 2000). adv. bk.rev. illus. cum.index: 1973-1986. reprint service avail. from PQC. *Refereed.* **Document type:** *Academic/Scholarly.* **Description:** Serves health care professionals' interests in the medical aspects of sports, exercise and fitness.
Related titles: Microform ed.: (from PQC); Online - full text ed.: (from The Dialog Corporation, Dow Jones Interactive, Gale Group, NewsNet, LexisNexis, ProQuest Information & Learning, Institute for Scientific Information).
Indexed: AMED, ASCA, AgeLine, Bus.Ind., C.I.J.E., CINAHL, Curr.Cont., Environ.Sci.Poll.Mgmt., Excerp.Med., Focus on: Sports Sci.& Med., Gen.Sci.Ind. (Jun.1984-), Hlth.Ind., Inpharma, L.R.I., NRN, Pharm.&Out.News, Phys.Ed.Ind., Pollut.Abstr., Protozool.Abstr., Reac., Risk Abstr., SSCI (coverage dropped), Saf.Sci.Abstr., Sportsearch (1974-), Tr.& Indus.Ind.
—BLDSC (6476.357000), CISTI, GNLM, IDS, ingenta, KNAW. **CCC.**
Published by: McGraw-Hill Companies, 4530 W 77th St Ste 350, Minneapolis, MN 55435. TEL 952-835-3222, http://www.physsportsmed.com. Ed. Susan Hawthorne. Pub. Gary Gyss. R&P Grace Voss. Adv. contact Terri Minni. B&W page USD 5,616, color page USD 7,516. Circ: 114,100. **Subscr. to:** PO Box 462, Hightstown, NJ 08520-9205.

617.1 CHE ISSN 1424-3814
PLUSPORT NEWS. Text and summaries in French, German. 1962. bi-m. CHF 32 (effective 2001). adv. bk.rev. **Document type:** *Journal, Trade.*
Former titles (until 2000): Behindertensport (1422-0210); (until 1978): Invalidensport (0020-9880)
Published by: Schweizerischer Verband fuer Behindertensport, Chriesbaumstr 6, Volketswil 8604, Switzerland. TEL 41-1-9460860, FAX 41-1-9460870. Ed., R&P Elvira Jaeger. Circ: 8,847.

PSYCHOLOGY AND SOCIOLOGY OF SPORT: CURRENT SELECTED RESEARCH. see *PSYCHOLOGY*

QUEST (CHAMPAIGN). see *EDUCATION—Teaching Methods And Curriculum*

617.1 BRA ISSN 1517-8692
REVISTA BRASILEIRA DE MEDICINA DO ESPORTE. Text in Portuguese; Abstracts in English, Portuguese. 1995. bi-m. BRL 50.
Formerly: Revista Brasileira de Medicina Esportiva
Published by: (Sociedade Brasileira de Medicina do Esporte), Redprint Editora Ltda., Rua Domingos de Morais 2777, 15o cjs 151 e 154, Sao Paulo, SP 04035-001, Brazil. TEL 55-11-5724813, FAX 55-11-5711719, redprint@uol.com.br. Ed. Antonio Claudio Lucas da Nobrega.

617.1 ZAF
S A SPORTS MEDICINE. Text in English. 1984. q. USD 20 foreign (effective 2000). adv. illus. *Refereed.* **Document type:** *Academic/Scholarly.* **Description:** Examines clinical and experimental topics in all areas of sports medicine.
Former titles (until 1994): South African Journal of Sports Medicine (1015-5163); (unitl 1989): S A Sports Medicine Association. Journal (0259-4870); (until 1986): S A Journal of Sports Medicine (0257-9308)
—BLDSC (8340.230000).
Published by: South African Medical Association, Health and Medical Publishing Group, 14 Central Sq, Pinelands 7430, South Africa. TEL 27-21-531-3081, FAX 27-21-5314126, publishing@samedical.org, http://www.samedical.org. R&P Peter Roberts. **Subscr. to:** PO Box 74789, Lynnwood Ridge, Pretoria 0040, South Africa. TEL 27-12-481-2010, FAX 27-12-481-2061, ann@samedical.org. **Dist. by:** Private Bag X1, Pinelands 7430, South Africa. TEL 27-21-531-3081, FAX 27-21-531-4126.

617.1 FRA ISSN 1278-4516
S M S. LE SPECIALISTE DE MEDECINE DU SPORT. Text in French. 1979. 6/yr. FRF 350 domestic to individuals; FRF 500, EUR 76.22 foreign to individuals; FRF 220 to students (effective 2001). adv. **Description:** Contains sports medicine information for the general practitioner.
Former titles (until 1996): Actualites Sport et Medecine (1151-3195); (until 1990): Sport Medicine Actualites (0753-2814); (until 1985): Sport Medicine (0245-5021)
Published by: Meditions Carline, 1 et 3 rue du Depart, Paris 75014, France. TEL 33-1-40640075, FAX 33-1-43222699. Circ: 12,000.

617.1 613.7 FRA ISSN 0247-106X
S T A P S; Review STAPS & bulletin de Liaison. (Sciences et Techniques des Activites Physiques et Sportives) Text in French; Summaries in Italian, German, English, Spanish. 1980. 3/yr. FRF 200 to individuals; FRF 280 to institutions. 80 p./no. **Document type:** *Bulletin.*
Published by: Association Francophone pour la Recherche en Activites Physiques et Sportives, AFRAPS, UFR STAPS, 700 Av. du Pic St Loup, Jontpellien 34090, France. TEL 33-04-67415733, FAX 33-04-67415733, htpp://www.afraps.asso.fr.

617.1 DNK ISSN 0905-7188
RC1200 CODEN: SMSSEO
SCANDINAVIAN JOURNAL OF MEDICINE & SCIENCE IN SPORTS. Text in English. 1979. bi-m. USD 251 in the Americas to institutions print & online eds. combined; GBP 174 elsewhere to institutions print & online eds. combined (effective 2002). *Refereed.* **Document type:** *Journal, Academic/Scholarly.* **Description:** Publishes original articles in the fields of traumatology and orthopedics, physiology, biomechanics, and cardiology, as well as sociological, pedagogic, historical and philosophical contributions to the study of sports.
Formerly (until 1990): Scandinavian Journal of Sports Sciences (0357-5632)
Related titles: ♦ Online - full text ed.: Scandinavian Journal of Medicine & Science in Sports Online. ISSN 1600-0838.
Indexed: AMED, ASCA, Biol.Abstr., Curr.Cont., Excerp.Med., Focus on: Sports Sci.& Med., Ind.Med. (1991-), Inpharma, Lang.& Lang.Behav.Abstr., Nutr.Abstr., Pharm.&Out.News, Reac., SOPODA, SSCI (coverage dropped), Sci.Cit.Ind., Sociol.Abstr., Sportsearch (1979-).
—BLDSC (8087.517400), EMDOCS, GNLM, IDS, Infotrieve, ingenta, KNAW. **CCC.**
Published by: (Scandinavian Foundation of Medical Science in Sports), Blackwell Munksgaard, Noerre Soegade 35, PO Box 2148, Copenhagen K 1016, Denmark. TEL 45-77-33-33-33, FAX 45-77-33-33-77, fsub@munksgaard.dk, http://www.munksgaard.dk/sportsmedicine. Ed. M. Kjaer. Adv. contact Eric Rozario TEL 45-77-33-33-01. Circ: 4,000.

617.1 DNK ISSN 1600-0838
SCANDINAVIAN JOURNAL OF MEDICINE & SCIENCE IN SPORTS ONLINE. Text in English. bi-m. GBP 157 (effective 2002). *Refereed.* **Document type:** *Academic/Scholarly.*
Media: Online - full text (from EBSCO Publishing, ingenta, Swets Blackwell, Institute for Scientific Information). **Related titles:** ♦ Print ed.: Scandinavian Journal of Medicine & Science in Sports. ISSN 0905-7188.
Published by: Blackwell Munksgaard, Noerre Soegade 35, PO Box 2148, Copenhagen K 1016, Denmark. TEL 45-77-33-33-33, FAX 45-77-33-33-77, fsub@mail.munksgaard.dk, http://www.munksgaard.dk.

617.102 CHE ISSN 1022-6699
RC1200
SCHWEIZERISCHE ZEITSCHRIFT FUER SPORTMEDIZIN UND SPORTTRAUMATOLOGIE/REVISTA SVIZZERA PER MEDICINA E TRAUMATOLOGIA DELLO SPORT/REVUE SUISSE POUR MEDECINE ET TRAUMATOLOGIE DE SPORTS. Text in French, German, Italian; Summaries in English, French. 1963. 4/yr. CHF 55; CHF 75 in United States; CHF 16 newsstand/cover (effective 2001). adv. bk.rev. bibl, charts, illus. index. **Document type:** *Journal, Academic/Scholarly.*
Formerly (until 1993): Schweizerische Zeitschrift fuer Sportmedizin (0036-7885)
Indexed: Biol.Abstr., Chem.Abstr., Excerp.Med., Ind.Med. (coverage dropped), Sportsearch.
—BLDSC, EMDOCS, GNLM, Infotrieve. **CCC.**
Published by: (Schweizerische Gesellschaft fuer Sportmedizin), Paul Haupt AG, Falkenplatz 14, Bern 3001, Switzerland. TEL 41-31-3012434, FAX 41-31-3015469, verlag@haupt.ch, http://www.haupt.ch.

617.1 FRA ISSN 0765-1597
CODEN: SCSPED
SCIENCE & SPORTS; journal de la medecine, des sciences et des techniques des activites physiques, sportives et des pratiques corporelles. Text in French; Summaries in English, French. 1986. bi-m. EUR 225 in Europe to institutions; USD 264 elsewhere to institutions (effective 2002). *Refereed.* **Document type:** *Academic/Scholarly.* **Description:** Covers central topics related to sports medicine, connected with internal medicine, traumatology, psychology, physiology, biochemistry, biomechanics or technology. Includes original articles, letters to the editor and technical notes.
Related titles: Online - full text ed.: (from ingenta, Institute for Scientific Information).
Indexed: AMED, ASCA, Biol.Abstr., Excerp.Med., Focus on: Sports Sci.& Med.
—BLDSC (8142.998000), CASDDS, EMDOCS, GNLM, IDS, Infotrieve, ingenta. **CCC.**
Published by: (Societe Francaise de Medecine du Sport), Elsevier Paris, Editions Scientifiques et Medicales (Subsidiary of: Reed Elsevier plc. group), 23 rue Linois, Paris 75015, France. TEL 33-1-45589110, FAX 33-1-45589419, s&s@elsevier.fr; academic@elsevier-fr.com, http://www.elsevier.com/locate/scispo. Ed. Pierre C Pesquies. Circ: 2,000.

617.1 ESP ISSN 0214-8927
SELECCION. Text in Spanish. 1990. q. ESP 5,000 domestic; USD 55 in Europe; USD 65 elsewhere (effective 2001). adv. charts. *Refereed.* **Document type:** *Journal, Academic/Scholarly.* **Description:** Offers original clinical and applied research articles, as well as reviews in the field of sports medicine.
Published by: (Asociacion Espanola de Escuelas de Medicina de la Educacion Fisica y el Deporte), Alpe Editores S.A., Pedro Rico, 27, Madrid 28029, Spain. TEL 34-91-733-8811, FAX 34-91-315-9652, alpeeditores@sistelcom.com. Ed. Fernando Santonja. Pub. Angeles Alvarez Sanchez. Adv. contact Ana Jurado. B&W page ESP 95,000, color page ESP 160,000; trim 280 x 210. Circ: 4,000 (controlled).

SOCIOLOGY OF SPORT JOURNAL. see *SOCIOLOGY*

SOMATICS; magazine - journal of the mind - body arts and sciences. see *PHYSICAL FITNESS AND HYGIENE*

617.102 TUR ISSN 1300-0551
SPOR HEKIMLIGI DERGISI/TURKISH JOURNAL OF SPORTS MEDICINE. Text in Turkish; Summaries in English. 1966. q. TRL 1,500,000, USD 35 (effective 1998). adv. bk.rev. abstr. **Document type:** *Academic/Scholarly.* **Description:** Covers physiological, cardiologic, biochemical, and anthropometric aspects of sports medicine, as well as orthopedic, traumatological and physical therapy and rehabilitation.
Indexed: Sportsearch (1979-).
—BLDSC (9072.496000).
Published by: (Turkish Association of Sports Medicine), Ege University Press, Bornova, Izmir 35100, Turkey. TEL 90-232-3881097, FAX 90-232-3881097, http://medicine.ege.edu.tr/spor_hek. Eds. Dr. Fikret Durusoy, Necati Akgun. Circ: 350.

617.1 TUR ISSN 1300-5278
SPOR VE TIP. Text in Turkish. 1993. 6/yr. USD 70 (effective 2001). **Document type:** *Journal, Academic/Scholarly.*
Published by: Lodos Yayincilik Ticaret A.S., Yildiz Posta Cad., Sinan Apt.no. 36 D 66-67, Gayrettepe - Instanbul 80280, Turkey. TEL 90-212-2880541, FAX 90-212-2116185, info@logos.com.tr, http://logos.com.tr.

M

617.1027 616.12 ITA ISSN 1591-1195
▼ **SPORT CARDIOLOGY.** Text in Italian; Summaries in English. 2000. 3/yr. ITL 100,000, USD 100 (effective 2001). adv. **Document type:** *Journal, Academic/Scholarly.*
Published by: C I C Edizioni Internazionali s.r.l., Corso Trieste 42, Rome, RM 00198, Italy. TEL 39-06-8412673, FAX 39-06-8412688, info@gruppocic.it, http://www.gruppocic.it. Ed. Armando Dagianti. Pub. A Salvati. adv.: B&W page XEU 1,239.5, color page XEU 1,704.31; 210 x 280.

617.1 ITA ISSN 0392-9647
SPORT & MEDICINA. Text in Italian. 1984. bi-m. ITL 30,000; ITL 60,000 foreign. adv. bk.rev. cum.index. back issues avail.; reprints avail. **Description:** Features articles in fields of sports and medicine. Includes articles on pharmaceutical aids and physical fitness.
Published by: Edi. Ermes, Viale Enrico Forlanini, 65, Milan, MI 20134, Italy. TEL 02-70209911, FAX 02-70209919. Ed. Raffaele Grandi. Circ: 18,000.

617.1 AUS ISSN 1032-5662
SPORT HEALTH. Text in English. 1983. q. AUD 30 domestic; AUD 45 foreign (effective 1999). bk.rev., video rev. charts, illus, stat. index. back issues avail. **Description:** Education and news in sports medicine and science.
Indexed: Sportsearch (1983-).
—BLDSC.
Published by: Sports Medicine Australia, PO Box 897, Belconnen, ACT 2616, Australia. TEL 61-6-2516944, FAX 61-6-2531489, TELEX AUSUS 62400. Ed. Peter Brukner.

617.1 FRA ISSN 0993-1252
SPORT MED. Text in French. 1988. 10/yr. FRF 420 domestic; FRF 645, EUR 98.33 foreign; FRF 265 to students (effective 2001). adv. bk.rev.
Published by: Meditions Carline, 1 et 3 rue du Depart, Paris 75014, France. TEL 33-1-40640075, FAX 33-1-43222699. Ed. Patrick Borg. Pub. Christian de Vaublanc. Adv. contact Sonzyk Brault. Circ: 16,000.

617.1 DEU ISSN 0949-328X
SPORT-ORTHOPAEDIE - SPORT-TRAUMATOLOGIE. Text in German, English. 1991. q. EUR 68 (effective 2002). **Document type:** *Journal, Academic/Scholarly.*
Former titles (until 1995): Praktische Sport-Traumatologie, -Medizin (0949-3271); (until 1992): Praktische Sport-Traumatologie und Sportmedizin (0177-0438)
—GNLM.
Published by: Urban & Fischer Verlag, Loebdergraben 14a, Jena 07743, Germany. TEL 49-3641-626430, FAX 49-3641-626421, info@urbanfischer.de, http://www.urbanfischer.de.

SPORT SCIENCES INTERNATIONAL. see *SPORTS AND GAMES*

617.1 ESP ISSN 1130-0183
SPORT & MEDICINA. Text in Spanish. bi-m.
Published by: Ediciones Eseuve S.A., c/o Oficina de Justificacion de la Difusion (OJD), Plaza Marques de Salamanca, 9-4D, Madrid 28006, Spain. TEL 34-91-539-0103, FAX 34-91-528-8759. Ed. Alberto Munoz Soler. Circ: 21,000.

617.1 GBR ISSN 1353-2693
SPORTCARE; the journal for professionals in sport. Text in English. 1994. bi-m. GBP 32; GBP 47 foreign (effective 2000). **Document type:** *Trade.*
Published by: National Sports Medicine Institute, Medical College of St Bartholomew's Hospital, Charterhouse Sq, London EC1M 6BQ, United Kingdom. TEL 44-20-7251-0583, FAX 44-20-7251-0774, enquiry@nsmi.org.uk, http://www.nsmi.org.uk. Ed. Lee Willis. **Subscr. in Americas to:** Quintessence Publishing Co., Inc., 551 Kimberly Dr, Carol Stream, IL 60188-1881. TEL 708-682-3223, FAX 708-682-3288.

617.102 DEU ISSN 0075-8655
SPORTMEDIZINISCHE SCHRIFTENREIHE. Text in German. 1967. irreg., latest vol.29, 1993. price varies. back issues avail. **Document type:** *Monographic series.*
—GNLM.
Published by: Johann Ambrosius Barth Verlag in Medizinverlage Heidelberg GmbH & Co. KG, Postfach 102869, Heidelberg 69018, Germany. TEL 49-6221-489437, FAX 49-711-8931422, fuchsm@huethig.de, http://www.huethig.de, http://www.thieme.de. Ed. K Tittel.

SPORTS AND RECREATIONAL INJURIES. see *LAW*

617.1027 USA
▼ **SPORTS IN PRIMARY CARE.** Text in English. 2001. m. USD 95 domestic; USD 105 foreign; USD 40 to students; USD 10 newsstand/cover domestic; USD 15 newsstand/cover foreign (effective 2001). charts, illus. Index. back issues avail. *Refereed.* **Document type:** *Journal, Trade.* **Description:** Provides primary care physicians with news analysis and practical reviews on sports medicine.
Published by: Cliggott Publishing Co. (Subsidiary of: S C P Communications, Inc.), 330 Boston Post Rd, Darien, CT 06820. TEL 203-662-6400, FAX 203-662-6776, info.cliggott@scp.com. Ed., R&P Leo Cristofar. Pub. Bill Markowitz.

610 NZL ISSN 0112-1642
CODEN: SPMEE7
SPORTS MEDICINE; reviews of applied medicine and science in sport and exercise. Text in English. 1984. m. USD 165 to individuals for print or online ed.; USD 795 to institutions for print or online ed.; USD 198 combined subscription to individuals for both print & online eds.; USD 954 combined subscription to institutions for both print & online eds. (effective 2001). abstr, bibl, illus. back issues avail. *Refereed.* **Document type:** *Academic/Scholarly.* **Description:** Provides comprehensive reviews of the latest research in applied medicine and science in sport and exercise.
Related titles: Online - full text ed.: (from Ovid Technologies, Inc., EBSCO Publishing, O C L C Online Computer Library Center, Inc., RoweCom Information Quest, ingenta, Swets Blackwell, Institute for Scientific Information).
Indexed: AMED, ASCA, Cal.Tiss.Abstr., Curr.Adv.Ecol.Sci., Curr.Cont., Environ.Sci.Poll.Mgmt., Excerp.Med., Focus on: Sports Sci.& Med., Ind.Med. (1984-), Inpharma, NRN, Nutr.Abstr., Pharm.&Out.News, Pollut.Abstr., Reac., Risk Abstr., Rural Recreat.Tour.Abstr., Saf.Sci.Abstr., Sci.Cit.Ind., Sportsearch (1984-).
—BLDSC (8419.837340), ADONIS, CASDDS, CISTI, GNLM, IDS, ingenta, KNAW. **CCC.**
Published by: Adis International Limited, Mairangi Bay, Private Bag 65901, Auckland 1010, New Zealand. TEL 64-9-477-0700, FAX 64-9-477-0766, sportsmed@adis.co.nz, http://www.adis.com; http://biomednet.com/llbrary/jspm. Ed. Jeremy N Shanahan. Pub. Paul Chrisp. R&P Will Charles. Circ: 930. **Subscr. in the Americas to:** Adis International Inc., Attn: Subscription Dept, 860 Town Center Dr, Langhorne, PA 19047. TEL 877-872-2347.

617.1027 USA ISSN 1521-8333
SPORTS MEDICINE ALERT; the clinician's practical guide to diagnosis, treatment, rehabilitation and prevention of injury and disease. Text in English. 1992. m. USD 187 domestic; USD 207 in Canada; USD 227 elsewhere (effective 2000). adv. abstr. *Refereed.* **Document type:** *Newsletter.* **Description:** Helps physicians keep up with clinical developments in sports medicine, primary care, recent research studies, and related issues, including medicolegal updates.
Former titles (until 1998): Sports Medicine in Primary Care; (until 1995): Phys Ed. Journal of Sports Medicine (1062-9297)
—BLDSC (8419.837365).
Published by: Mountainview Publishing, L.L.C., 235 Mountainview St, Decatur, GA 30030-2027. TEL 404-377-0300, 800-685-TEAM, FAX 404-377-0604, mdsport@aol.com. Ed. Dr. Rob Johnson. Pub., Adv. contact Elizabeth Medley-Wilson. R&P Elizabeth Medley Wilson.

SPORTS MEDICINE AND ARTHROSCOPY REVIEW. see *MEDICAL SCIENCES—Orthopedics And Traumatology*

617.1 613.7 USA ISSN 0746-9306
SPORTS MEDICINE BULLETIN. Text in English. 1966. q. membership only. **Document type:** *Newsletter.* **Description:** Newsmagazine to inform members about ACSM issues, upcoming events, future plans and member news.
Published by: American College of Sports Medicine, PO Box 1440, Indianapolis, IN 46206-1440. TEL 317-637-9200, FAX 317-634-7817, pub2acsm@acsm.org. Ed. Virginia Rogers. Circ: 16,000.

617.1 GBR ISSN 0952-4630
SPORTS MEDICINE BULLETIN. Text in English. 1980. m. GBP 48 in United Kingdom to individuals; GBP 55 to individuals rest of Europe; GBP 60 rest of world to individuals; GBP 60 in United Kingdom to institutions; GBP 65 to institutions rest of Europe; GBP 75 rest of world to institutions (effective 2000). adv. back issues avail. **Document type:** *Bibliography.* **Description:** Contains details of articles on all aspects of sports medicine and exercise science.
—GNLM.
Published by: National Sports Medicine Institute, Medical College of St Bartholomew's Hospital, Charterhouse Sq, London EC1M 6BQ, United Kingdom. TEL 44-20-7251-0583, FAX 44-20-7251-0774, enquiry@nsmi.org.uk, http://www.nsmi.org.uk. Adv. contact Kathryn Walter.

617.102 USA ISSN 0731-9770
RC1200
SPORTS MEDICINE DIGEST. Key Title: Sportsmedicine Digest. Text in English. 1979. m., latest vol.23. USD 125 domestic to individuals; USD 145 foreign to individuals; USD 155 domestic to institutions; USD 175 foreign to institutions; USD 15 newsstand/cover (effective 2002). bk.rev. back issues avail. **Document type:** *Newsletter.*
Related titles: Online - full text ed.: USD 201.50 domestic for academic site license; USD 221.50 foreign for academic site license; USD 224.75 domestic for corporate site license; USD 244.75 foreign for corporate site license (effective 2002).
Indexed: Sportsearch (1980-).
—BLDSC (8419.837530), GNLM, ingenta.
Published by: Lippincott Williams & Wilkins (Philadelphia) (Subsidiary of: Wolters Kluwer N.V.), 530 Walnut St, Philadelphia, PA 19106-3621. TEL 215-521-8300, FAX 215-521-8902, http://www.lww.com. Eds. Dr. James C Puffer, Dr. John A Gergfeld. R&P Tobias Weschler. Circ: 1,017. **Subscr. to:** PO Box 1600, Hagerstown, MD 21740-1600. TEL 800-777-2295, FAX 301-824-7390.

617.1027 USA
SPORTS MEDICINE REPORTS; a physician-to-physician update on critical issues in sports medicine. Text in English. 1998. q. USD 100 (effective 1999). adv. back issues avail. **Document type:** *Newsletter.* **Description:** Provides clinicians with the latest research on sports medicine practices and quality of care issues.
Published by: Mountainview Publishing, L.L.C., 235 Mountainview St, Decatur, GA 30030-2027. TEL 404-377-0300, FAX 404-377-0604, mdsport@aol.com. Ed. Dr. Rob Johnson. Pub., R&P Liz Medley-Wilson. Adv. contact Liz Medley Wilson.

SPORTS MEDICINE STANDARDS & MALPRACTICE REPORTER. see *LAW*

617.1 CHE ISSN 1057-8315
RC1200 CODEN: SMTJE2
SPORTS MEDICINE, TRAINING AND REHABILITATION; an international journal. Text in English. 1988. 4/yr. GBP 119, USD 144, EUR 158 to individuals; GBP 536, USD 640, EUR 685 to institutions; GBP 809, USD 976, EUR 1,049 to corporations (effective 2002). *Refereed.* **Document type:** *Academic/Scholarly.*
Formerly: Sports Training, Medicine and Rehabilitation (0893-102X)
Related titles: CD-ROM ed.; Microform ed.; Online - full text ed.: (from RoweCom Information Quest).
Indexed: AMED, Environ.Sci.Poll.Mgmt., Excerp.Med. (1993-), Pollut.Abstr., Risk Abstr., Saf.Sci.Abstr.
—BLDSC (8419.837568), EMDOCS, GNLM, ingenta. **CCC.**
Published by: Gordon and Breach - Harwood Academic (Subsidiary of: Taylor & Francis Group), PO Box 531, Lausanne 1000, Switzerland. http://www.gbhap.com/Sports_Medicine/. Ed. Eric Banister. **Subscr. addr. in US:** International Publishers Direct, PO Box 32160, Newark, NJ 07102. FAX 215-750-6343.

SPORTS TRAINERS DIGEST. see *SPORTS AND GAMES*

STRATEGIES (RESTON); a journal for physical and sport educators. see *EDUCATION—Teaching Methods And Curriculum*

SUID-AFRIKAANSE TYDSKRIF VIR NAVORSING IN SPORT, LIGGAAMLIKE OPVOEDKUNDE EN ONTSPANNING/SOUTH AFRICAN JOURNAL FOR RESEARCH IN SPORT, PHYSICAL EDUCATION AND RECREATION. see *PHYSICAL FITNESS AND HYGIENE*

TENNISPRO MAGAZINE. see *SPORTS AND GAMES—Ball Games*

613.7 CHN ISSN 1006-1207
TIYU KEYAN/SPORTS SCIENCE RESEARCH. Text in Chinese. 1962. q. *Refereed.* **Document type:** *Journal, Academic/Scholarly.*
Published by: Shanghai Research Institute of Sports Science, 87 Wuxing Rd, Shanghai 200030, China. Eds. Bishuang Situ, Guosheng Wei. Pub. Wenyu Chen.

610 613.7 JPN ISSN 0914-4285
TOKYO JIKEIKAI IKA DAIGAKU TAIRYOKU IGAKU KENKYUSHITSU NENPO/JIKEI UNIVERSITY. SCHOOL OF MEDICINE. ANNUAL REPORT OF LABORATORY SPORTS MEDICINE. Text in English, Japanese. irreg.
Published by: Tokyo Jikeikai Ika Daigaku, Tairyoku Igaku Kenkyushitsu, 3-1 Kokuryo-cho 8-chome, Chofu-shi, Tokyo-to 182-0022, Japan.

DER UNFALLCHIRURG. see *MEDICAL SCIENCES—Orthopedics And Traumatology*

617.1 USA ISSN 0162-0908
RC1200
THE YEAR BOOK OF SPORTS MEDICINE. Text in English. 1979. a. USD 89 domestic; USD 95 foreign (effective 2001). illus. reprints avail. **Document type:** *Abstract/Index, Academic/Scholarly.* **Description:** Presents abstracts of the pertinent literature with commentary by leading experts in the field.
Related titles: CD-ROM ed.
—BLDSC (9416.417000), GNLM.
Published by: (American College of Sports Medicine), Mosby, Inc., Continuity Division (Subsidiary of: Harcourt Health Sciences), 11830 Westline Industrial Dr, St Louis, MO 63146-3313. TEL 314-872-8370, 800-325-4177, FAX 314-432-1380, http://www.mosby.com/periodicals. Ed. Dr. Roy J Shephard.

617.1 CHN ISSN 1000-6710
ZHONGGUO YUNDONG YIXUE ZAZHI/CHINESE JOURNAL OF SPORTS MEDICAL SCIENCE. Text in Chinese. 1982. q. USD 20.80; CNY 10, USD 5.20 newsstand/cover (effective 2001). **Document type:** *Academic/Scholarly.*
Related titles: Online - full content ed.: (from WanFang Data Corp.).
—BLDSC (3180.676800).
Published by: (Zhongguo Tiyu Kexue Xuehui/China Sports Science Society), Renmin Tiyu Chubanshe/People's Sports Publishing House, c/o Guojia Tiweike Yanjiusuo, 11, Beijing Tiyuguan Lu, Beijing 100061, China. TEL 86-1-67112233. Eds. Bingpu Zhao, Lu Shaozhong. **Dist. by:** China International Book Trading Corp, 35, Chegongzhuang Xilu, Haidian District, Beijing 100044, China. TEL 86-1-68413849, FAX 86-1-68412048, cibtc@mail.cibtc.com.cn, http://www.cibtc.com.cn. **Co-sponsor:** Yundong Yixue Xuehui/Sports Medical Science Association.

MEDICAL SCIENCES—Surgery

617.95 USA
A A A A S F NEWS. Text in English. s-a. membership only. adv. back issues avail. **Document type:** *Newsletter.* **Description:** Covers topics of interest to member plastic surgeons, specifically concerning ambulatory surgery facilities.
Formerly: Plastic Surgery Accreditation News (1066-8128)
Published by: American Association for Accreditation of Ambulatory Surgery Facilities, 1202 Allanson Rd, Mundelein, IL 60060. TEL 708-949-6058. Ed. Robert Hamas. Adv. contact Edward Stygar. Circ: 500 (controlled).

617 USA
A C O M S REVIEW. Text in English. 1975. q. back issues avail.; reprints avail. **Document type:** *Newsletter.*
Published by: American College of Oral & Maxillofacial Surgeons, 1100 N W Loop 410, Ste 506, San Antonio, TX 78213-2266. TEL 210-344-5674, FAX 210-344-9754. Ed. Dr. John R Westine. Circ: 6,000.

617 USA ISSN 0001-0790
A C O S NEWS. Text in English. 1962. m. members only. adv. abstr. **Document type:** *Newsletter.*
Published by: American College of Osteopathic Surgeons, 123 N Henry St, Alexandria, VA 22314. TEL 703-684-0416. Ed. Sharon H Cool. Circ: 1,450.

617 AUS ISSN 1445-1433
CODEN: ANZJA7
A N Z JOURNAL OF SURGERY. Text in English. 1931. m. AUD 193 domestic to individuals; AUD 175 in New Zealand to individuals; USD 175 elsewhere to individuals; AUD 578 domestic to institutions; AUD 525 in New Zealand to institutions; USD 710 elsewhere to institutions; AUD 213 domestic to individuals paper & online eds. combined; AUD 193 in New Zealand to individuals paper & online eds. combined; USD 193 elsewhere to individuals paper & online eds. combined; AUD 636 domestic to institutions paper & online eds. combined; AUD 578 in New Zealand to institutions paper & online eds. combined; USD 781 elsewhere to institutions paper & online eds. combined (effective 2001). adv. bk.rev. bibl. illus. index. back issues avail.; reprint service avail. from PQC. *Refereed.* **Document type:** *Academic/Scholarly.* **Description:** Covers original contributions related to clinical practice and research in all fields of surgery and related disciplines.
Formerly (until 2001): Australian and New Zeland Journal of Surgery (0004-8682)
Related titles: Microform ed.: (from PQC); Online - full text ed.: ISSN 1440-1622. AUD 174 domestic to individuals; AUD 158 in New Zealand to individuals; USD 158 elsewhere to individuals; AUD 521 domestic to institutions; AUD 473 in New Zealand to institutions; USD 639 elsewhere to institutions (effective 2001) (from Ovid Technologies, Inc., EBSCO Publishing, O C L C Online Computer Library Center, Inc., RoweCom Information Quest, ingenta, Munksgaard & Blackwell Science's Synergy, Swets Blackwell, Institute for Scientific Information).
Indexed: ASCA, Biol.Abstr., Curr.Adv.Cancer Res., Curr.Cont., Dent.Ind., Excerp.Med., Helminthol.Abstr., INIS Atomind., Ind.Med. (1931-), Ind.Sci.Rev., Inpharma, Int.Nurs.Ind., Neurosci.Cit.Ind., Nutr.Abstr., Pharm.&Out.News, Reac., Rev.Med.& Vet.Mycol., SSCI (coverage dropped), Sci.Cit.Ind.
—BLDSC (1566.878000), ADONIS, CISTI, EMDOCS, GNLM, IDS, ingenta, KNAW. **CCC.**
Published by: (Royal Australasian College of Surgeons), Blackwell Science Asia Pty Ltd, PO Box 378, Carlton South, VIC 3053, Australia. TEL 61-3-9347-0300, FAX 61-3-9347-5001, info@blacksci-asia.com.au, http://www.blacksci.co.uk. Ed. Robert Thomas. adv.: B&W page AUD 1,012, color page AUD 2,057; trim 275 x 210. Circ: 6,300.

ACOUSTIC NEUROMA ASSOCIATION NOTES. see *MEDICAL SCIENCES—Otorhinolaryngology*

617.95 CZE ISSN 0001-5423
ACTA CHIRURGIAE PLASTICAE; international journal of plastic surgery. Text in English; Summaries in Czech, English. 1959. q. EUR 92, USD 120 (effective 2001). adv. bk.rev. charts, illus. index. *Refereed.* **Document type:** *Academic/Scholarly.* **Description:** Publishes clinical, experimental and theoretical work from the field of plastic, reconstructive and aesthetic surgery.
Indexed: Biol.Abstr., Dent.Ind., Excerp.Med., INIS Atomind., Ind.Med. (1959-).
—BLDSC (0611.100000), CISTI, KNAW.
Published by: (Ceska Lekarska Spolecnost J.E. Purkyne/Czech Medical Association), Nakladatelske Stredisko C L S J.E. Purkyne, Sokolska 31, Prague 12026, Czech Republic. TEL 42-2-24911420, FAX 42-2-24911420, http://www.clsjep.cz. Ed. M Tvredek. R&P A Leblova TEL 42-2-71747230. adv.: B&W page CZK 21,100, color page CZK 31,600; 245 x 167. Circ: 550. **Dist. by:** Abont s.r.o., Chlumova 17, Prague, 3 130 00, Czech Republic; **Dist. in Western countries by:** Kubon & Sagner, Hesstr 39-41, Munich 80798, Germany.

617 AUT ISSN 0001-544X
CODEN: ACAUB9
ACTA CHIRURGICA AUSTRIACA. Text in German, English; Summaries in English. 1968. 6/yr. ATS 3,715 in Europe; ATS 3,921.68 elsewhere; ATS 4,086.83 in Europe print & online eds. combined; ATS 4,313.85 elsewhere print & online eds. combined (effective 2001). reprint service avail. from ISI. **Document type:** *Academic/Scholarly.*
Related titles: ♦ Online - full text ed.: Acta Chirurgica Austriaca Online. ISSN 1563-2563.
Indexed: ASCA, Biol.Abstr., Curr.Cont. (coverage dropped), Excerp.Med. (until 1992, 1994-), INIS Atomind.
—BLDSC (0611.128000), ADONIS, CISTI, EMDOCS, GNLM, Infotrieve, KNAW. **CCC.**
Published by: (Oesterreichische Gesellschaft fuer Chirurgie), Blackwell Wissenschafts-Verlag Vienna, Firmiangasse 7-1, Vienna, W 1130, Austria. TEL 43-1-8779351-0, FAX 43-1-877935124, verlag@blackwis.at, http://www.blackwell.de/aca.htm. Ed. Dr. B Niederle. Circ: 1,500.

617 AUT ISSN 1563-2563
ACTA CHIRURGICA AUSTRIACA ONLINE. Text in German. 6/yr. ATS 3,344 (effective 2001). **Document type:** *Academic/Scholarly.*
Media: Online - full text (from Munksgaard & Blackwell Science's Synergy). **Related titles:** ♦ Print ed.: Acta Chirurgica Austriaca. ISSN 0001-544X.
Published by: Blackwell Wissenschafts-Verlag Vienna, Firmiangasse 7-1, Vienna, W 1130, Austria. TEL 43-1-8779351-0, FAX 43-1-877935124, verlag@blackwis.at, http://www.blackwell.de/aca.htm.

617 BEL ISSN 0001-5458
CODEN: ACBEAX
ACTA CHIRURGICA BELGICA. Text in French; Summaries in English. 1901. 6/yr. EUR 54.55 domestic; EUR 62 foreign; EUR 11.15 per vol. domestic; EUR 12.40 per vol. foreign (effective 2002). adv. bk.rev. charts, illus. index. *Refereed.* **Document type:** *Journal, Academic/Scholarly.*
Related titles: Online - full text ed.: (from Institute for Scientific Information); ♦ Supplement: Acta Chirurgica Belgica. Supplementum. ISSN 0515-2763.
Indexed: ASCA, Biol.Abstr., C.I.S. Abstr., Chem.Abstr., Curr.Cont., Dent.Ind., Excerp.Med., Helminthol.Abstr., Ind.Med. (1946-), Inpharma, Nutr.Abstr., Pharm.&Out.News, Reac., Rev.Med.& Vet.Mycol.
—BLDSC (0611.130000), CASDDS, CISTI, GNLM, IDS, ingenta, KNAW.
Published by: (Association des Societes Scientifiques Medicales Belges/Vereiniging van de Belgische Wetenschappelijke Genootschappen), Acta Medica Belgica, Av Circulaire 138A, Brussels 1180, Belgium. TEL 32-2-374-5158, FAX 32-2-3749628, amb@skynet.be, http://www.ulb.ac.be/medecine/loce/amb.htm.

617 BEL ISSN 0515-2763
ACTA CHIRURGICA BELGICA. SUPPLEMENTUM. Text in English. 1950. irreg.
Related titles: ♦ Supplement to: Acta Chirurgica Belgica. ISSN 0001-5458.
Indexed: INIS Atomind.
Published by: Acta Medica Belgica, Av Circulaire 138A, Brussels 1180, Belgium. TEL 32-2-374-5158, FAX 32-2-3749628. Ed. J Dequeker.

617 ITA ISSN 0001-5466
CODEN: ACHIA7
ACTA CHIRURGICA ITALICA. Text in Italian; Summaries in English. 1944. 3/yr. ITL 80,000 domestic; ITL 150,000, EUR 77 foreign (effective 2000). bk.rev. index. back issues avail.
Related titles: Online - full text ed.: (from Institute for Scientific Information).
Indexed: Biol.Abstr., Chem.Abstr., Dent.Ind., Excerp.Med., Ind.Med. (coverage dropped), Ref.Zh.
—BLDSC (0611.140000), CISTI, EMDOCS, GNLM, IDS.
Published by: (Societa Italiana di Fisiopatologia Chirurgica), Tipografia Editrice la Garangola, Via Montona, 4, Padua, PD 35137, Italy. FAX 39-49-8751743. Ed. R Vecchioni. **Co-sponsor:** Societa Triveneta di Chirurgia.

617 ITA ISSN 0393-6376
ACTA CHIRURGICA MEDITERRANEA. Text in English, Italian. 1960. bi-m. ITL 60,000; ITL 100,000 foreign (effective 1998). adv. abstr, bibl, illus, stat. index. **Document type:** *Proceedings, Academic/Scholarly.* **Description:** Clinical cases in the surgical field are reviewed and discussed.
Formerly: Archivio Siciliano di Medicina e Chirurgia (Sezione Chirurgica)
Indexed: Helminthol.Abstr., Nutr.Abstr., Ref.Zh.
Published by: Carbone Editore, Via Gaetano Daita, 29, Palermo, PA 90139, Italy. TEL 39-91-321-273, FAX 39-91-321782. Ed. Antonino Pennino. Pub., R&P Alfonsa Carbone. Adv. contact Donatella Donato. Circ: 6,000.

617 BRA ISSN 0102-8650
ACTA CIRURGICA BRASILEIRA. Text in Portuguese. 1986. q. BRL 120 (effective 1999). back issues avail. **Document type:** *Academic/Scholarly.*
Related titles: Online - full text ed.: (from SciELO); ♦ Supplement: Acta Cirurgica Brasileira. Suplemento. ISSN 0102-9592.
Indexed: INIS Atomind.
Published by: Sociedade Brasileira para o Desenvolvimento da Pesquisa em Cirurgia/Brazilian Society for the Development of Research in Surgery, Av Doutor Dante Pazzanese, 50 Andar 14, VI Mariana, Sao Paulo, SP 04012-180, Brazil. TEL 55-11-5756433, golden@ruralsp.bom.br, http://www.scielo.br. Ed. Saul Goldenber.

617 BRA ISSN 0102-9592
ACTA CIRURGICA BRASILEIRA. SUPLEMENTO. Text in Portuguese. 1986. a. back issues avail. **Document type:** *Academic/Scholarly.*
Related titles: ♦ Supplement to: Acta Cirurgica Brasileira. ISSN 0102-8650.
Published by: Sociedade Brasileira para o Desenvolvimento da Pesquisa em Cirurgia/Brazilian Society for the Development of Research in Surgery, Av Doutor Dante Pazzanese, 500 Andar 14, VI Mariana, Sao Paulo, SP 04012-180, Brazil. TEL 55-11-5756433, golden@ruralsp.com.br, http://www.scielo.br. Ed. Saul Goldenber.

616 AUT ISSN 0001-6268
CODEN: ACNUA5
ACTA NEUROCHIRURGICA; the european journal of neurosurgery. Text in English. 1950. m. EUR 2,016.80; EUR 2,011.10 in Germany; EUR 198 newsstand/cover (effective 2002). adv. abstr. back issues avail.; reprint service avail. from ISI. *Refereed.* **Document type:** *Journal, Academic/Scholarly.* **Description:** Papers dealing with clinical neurosurgery - diagnosis and diagnostic techniques, operative surgery and results, postoperative treatment, and research work in neurosciences.
Related titles: Microfilm ed.: (from PQC); Online - full text ed.: ISSN 0942-0940 (from EBSCO Publishing, RoweCom Information Quest, Swets Blackwell, Springer LINK, Institute for Scientific Information); ♦ Supplement: Acta Neurochirurgica. Supplementum. ISSN 0065-1419.
Indexed: ASCA, Bibl.Dev.Med.& Child Neur., Curr.Adv.Cancer Res., Curr.Adv.Ecol.Sci., Curr.Cont., Excerp.Med., INIS Atomind., Ind.Med. (1950-), Ind.Sci.Rev., Inpharma, Int.Nurs.Ind., Neurosci.Cit.Ind., Pharm.&Out.News, Reac., Rev.Med.& Vet.Mycol., Sci.Cit.Ind., e-psyche.
—BLDSC (0639.850000), ADONIS, CISTI, EMDOCS, GNLM, IDS, ingenta, KNAW. **CCC.**
Published by: Springer-Verlag Wien (Subsidiary of: BertelsmannSpringer), Sachsenplatz 4-6, PO Box 89, Vienna, W 1201, Austria. TEL 43-1-3302415-0, FAX 43-1-330242665, journals@springer.at, http://www.springer.at/acta_neuro. Ed. L Calliauw. R&P Angela Foessl TEL 43-1-3302415517. Adv. contact Michael Katzenberger TEL 43-1-3302415220. B&W page XEU 1,000; 170 x 230. **Subscr. in N. America to:** Springer-Verlag, Journals, 175 Fifth Ave, New York, NY 10010. TEL 212-460-1500, FAX 212-473-6272, orders@springer-ny.com, http://www.springer-ny.com.

ACTA NEUROCHIRURGICA. SUPPLEMENTUM. see *MEDICAL SCIENCES—Psychiatry And Neurology*

617 ITA ISSN 0392-3088
ACTA PHONIATRICA LATINA. Text in Italian. 1978. q. ITL 80,000 domestic; ITL 150,000, EUR 77 foreign (effective 2000). back issues avail.
Indexed: Excerp.Med., Lang.& Lang.Behav.Abstr., NBA, SOPODA, Sociol.Abstr.
—BLDSC (0648.600000).
Published by: Tipografia Editrice la Garangola, Via Montona, 4, Padua, PD 35137, Italy. FAX 39-49-8751743.

617.3 ESP
ACTUALIDAD EN CIRUGIA ORAL Y MAXILOFACIAL. Text in Spanish. bi-m. ESP 5,000; USD 200 foreign (effective 2000). adv. abstr, bibl, illus, stat. back issues avail. *Refereed.* **Document type:** *Academic/Scholarly.*
Published by: (Sociedad Espanola de Cirugia Oral y Maxilofacial), Aran Ediciones S.A., Castello, 128 1o, Madrid 28006, Spain. TEL 34-91-782-0030, FAX 34-91-561-5787, edita@grupoaran.com, http://www.grupoaran.com. Ed. F. Garcia Marin. Pub. Jose Jimenez. R&P Maria Dolores Linares TEL 34-1-7820035. Circ: 10,000.

ADVANCES AND TECHNICAL STANDARDS IN NEUROSURGERY. see *MEDICAL SCIENCES—Psychiatry And Neurology*

ADVANCES IN CARDIAC SURGERY. see *MEDICAL SCIENCES—Cardiovascular Diseases*

ADVANCES IN NEUROTRAUMA RESEARCH. see *MEDICAL SCIENCES—Psychiatry And Neurology*

ADVANCES IN OTOLARYNGOLOGY - HEAD AND NECK SURGERY. see *MEDICAL SCIENCES—Otorhinolaryngology*

ADVANCES IN RENAL REPLACEMENT THERAPY. see *MEDICAL SCIENCES—Urology And Nephrology*

617.082 USA ISSN 0065-3411
RD1
ADVANCES IN SURGERY. Text in English. 1966. a. USD 85 domestic; USD 91 foreign (effective 2001). illus. reprint service avail. from PQC. **Document type:** *Academic/Scholarly.* **Description:** Presents a collection of original, fully referenced review articles in selected clinical topics important in all areas of surgery.
Related titles: Microfilm ed.: (from PQC).
Indexed: Ind.Med. (1965-).
—BLDSC (0711.595000), GNLM, KNAW.
Published by: Mosby, Inc. (Subsidiary of: Elsevier Science), 11830 Westline Industrial Dr, St Louis, MO 63146-3313. TEL 314-872-8370, 800-325-4177, FAX 314-432-1380, http://www.mosby.com/periodicals. Ed. Dr. John L Cameron.

617.4 USA ISSN 1069-7292
RD598.5
ADVANCES IN VASCULAR SURGERY. Text in English. 1993. a. USD 95 domestic; USD 101 foreign (effective 2001). **Document type:** *Academic/Scholarly.* **Description:** Presents original, fully referenced review articles on selected clinical topics in the field of vascular surgery.
—BLDSC (0711.730000). **CCC.**
Published by: Mosby, Inc. (Subsidiary of: Elsevier Science), 11830 Westline Industrial Dr, St Louis, MO 63146-3313. TEL 314-872-8370, 800-325-4177, FAX 314-432-1380, http://www.mosby.com/periodicals. Ed. Dr. Anthony D Whittemore.

617.95 USA ISSN 0364-216X
RD119
AESTHETIC PLASTIC SURGERY. Text in English. 1977. bi-m. (in 1 vol., 6 nos./vol.). USD 400.30 domestic for Print & Online Eds.; USD 373.60 in Germany for Print & Online Eds.; USD 69.30 newsstand/cover foreign (effective 2002). adv. reprints avail. *Refereed.* **Document type:** *Academic/Scholarly.* **Description:** Devoted to the aesthetic surgery of the entire body surface, including facial surgery, body surgery, and extremity surgery. Provides a forum for original articles dealing with techniques advancing the art of aesthetic plastic surgery.
Related titles: Microform ed.: (from PQC); Online - full text ed.: ISSN 1432-5241; (from EBSCO Publishing, RoweCom Information Quest, Swets Blackwell, Springer LINK, Institute for Scientific Information).
Indexed: ASCA, Curr.Cont., Excerp.Med., INIS Atomind., Ind.Med. (1976-), Inpharma, Jrnl.Watch Derm., Med.& Surg.Dermat., Pharm.&Out.News, Reac., Sci.Cit.Ind. (coverage dropped).
—CISTI, EMDOCS, GNLM, IDS, ingenta, KNAW. **CCC.**
Published by: Springer-Verlag, Journals (Subsidiary of: BertelsmannSpringer), 175 Fifth Ave, New York, NY 10010. TEL 212-460-1500, FAX 212-473-6272, orders@springer-ny.com, http://www.springer-ny.com. Ed. Blair O Rogers. R&P Ian Gross. Adv. contact Brian Skepton. **N. America subscr. to:** Journal Fulfillment Services, PO Box 2485, Secaucus, NJ 07096-2485. TEL 800-777-4643, FAX 201-348-4505. **Co-sponsors:** International Society of Aesthetic Plastic Surgery; Lipoplasty Society of North America.

617.95 USA ISSN 1090-820X
AESTHETIC SURGERY JOURNAL. Text in English. 1988. bi-m. USD 106 domestic to individuals; USD 126 per issue foreign to individuals; USD 150 per issue domestic to institutions; USD 170 per issue foreign to institutions; USD 59 per issue domestic to students; USD 79 per issue foreign to students; USD 29 newsstand/cover domestic (effective 2001). adv. *Refereed.* **Document type:** *Journal, Academic/Scholarly.* **Description:** Covers topics of current interest to keep practitioners of aesthetic plastic surgery up-to-date with the changing trends and developments in the field.
Formerly (until 1997): Aesthetic Surgery Quarterly (1084-0761)
Related titles: Online - full text ed.: (from EBSCO Publishing, IDEAL Online Library, RoweCom Information Quest).
—BLDSC (0730.384000), Infotrieve. **CCC.**
Published by: (American Society for Aesthetic Plastic Surgery), Mosby, Inc. (Subsidiary of: Elsevier Science), 11830 Westline Industrial Dr, St Louis, MO 63146-3318. TEL 314-872-8370, 800-325-4177, FAX 314-432-1380, customerservice@mosby.com, http://www.mosby.com/aesthetic, http://www.mosby.com/periodicals. Ed. Dr. Stanley A Klatsky. Pub. Terrie Duhadway. Adv. contact Steve Gray TEL 610-293-1722. B&W page USD 2,100, color page USD 2,925; trim 11 x 8.25. Circ: 4,748.

617 DEU ISSN 0944-5943
AMBULANT OPERIEREN. Text in German. 1994. q. EUR 118.80 domestic to institutions; EUR 122.40 in Europe to institutions; EUR 126.80 elsewhere to institutions; EUR 35 newsstand/cover (effective 2002). adv. **Document type:** *Journal, Academic/Scholarly.*
Related titles: Online - full text ed.
—GNLM.
Published by: Georg Thieme Verlag, Ruedigerstr 14, Stuttgart 70469, Germany. TEL 49-711-8931-0, FAX 49-711-8931298, leser.service@thieme.de, http://www.thieme.de/fachzeitschriften/09445943.html. Ed. Georg Feldkamp. R&P Michael Wachinger. Circ: 2,000.

617 NLD ISSN 0966-6532
CODEN: AMSUF3
AMBULATORY SURGERY. Text in English. 1993. q. EUR 286 in Europe to institutions; JPY 37,900 in Japan to institutions; USD 320 elsewhere to institutions (effective 2002). back issues avail. *Refereed.* **Document type:** *Academic/Scholarly.* **Description:** Promotes and develops this system of patient management by providing a multidisciplinary international forum for health care professionals involved in day-care surgery. Publishes peer-reviewed original articles relating to the practice of ambulatory surgery.
Related titles: Microform ed.: (from PQC); Online - full text ed.: (from ingenta, Swets Blackwell, ScienceDirect).
—BLDSC (0809.215700), CISTI, GNLM, Infotrieve, KNAW. **CCC.**
Published by: Elsevier Science BV, PO Box 211, Amsterdam 1000 AE, Netherlands. nlinfo-f@elsevier.nl, http://www.elsevier.com/ambsur. Eds. Bernard V Wetchler, Paul E M Jarrett. **Subscr. in Australasia and the Far East to:** Elsevier Science (Singapore) Pte Ltd, No.1 Temasek Ave, 17-01 Millenia Tower, Singapore 039192, Singapore. TEL 65-434-3727, FAX 65-337-2230; **Subscr. in Japan to:** Elsevier Science Inc - Japan Regional Office, 9-15 Higashi-Azabu 1-chome, Minato-ku, Tokyo 106-0044, Japan. TEL 81-3-5561-5033, FAX 81-3-5561-5047; **Subscr. in the Americas to:** Elsevier Science, PO Box 945, New York, NY 10159-0945. TEL 212-633-3730, FAX 212-633-3680, usinfo-f@elsevier.com.

617 USA ISSN 0002-8045
RD1
AMERICAN COLLEGE OF SURGEONS. BULLETIN. Text in English. 1916. m. free per issue. charts, illus. index. back issues avail.; reprint service avail. from PQC. **Document type:** *Bulletin.*
Related titles: Microform ed.: (from PQC).
Indexed: Chem.Abstr., Int.Nurs.Ind., Med.Care Rev.
—BLDSC (2386.540000), CISTI, GNLM, ingenta, KNAW. **CCC.**
Published by: American College of Surgeons, Communications Department, 633 N Saint Clair St, Chicago, IL 60611-3211. TEL 312-202-5000, FAX 312-202-5001, http://www.focs.org. Ed. Stephen J Regnier. R&P Linn Meyer TEL 312-202-5311. Circ: 67,850 (controlled).

617 NLD ISSN 1072-7515
RD1 CODEN: JACSEX
AMERICAN COLLEGE OF SURGEONS. JOURNAL. Key Title: Journal of the American College of Surgeons. Text in English. 1905. m. USD 139 in US & Canada to individuals; USD 52 elsewhere to individuals; USD 225 in US & Canada to institutions; USD 406 elsewhere to institutions (effective 2002). adv. bk.rev. bibl, charts, illus. s-a. index. back issues avail.; reprint service avail. from PQC. *Refereed.* **Document type:** *Academic/Scholarly.* **Description:** Contains original manuscripts of leading surgical articles from throughout the world.
Formerly (until 1994): Surgery, Gynecology and Obstetrics (0039-6087)
Related titles: Microform ed.: (from PQC,PMC); Online - full text ed.: (from ProQuest Information & Learning, ingenta, ScienceDirect, Swets Blackwell, Institute for Scientific Information).
Indexed: AIM, ASCA, Abstr.Hyg., Biol.Abstr., Chem.Abstr., Curr.Adv.Ecol.Sci., Curr.Cont., Dent.Ind., Excerp.Med., Helminthol.Abstr., Hosp.Lit.Ind., INIS Atomind., Ind.Med. (1994-), Ind.Sci.Rev., Ind.Vet., Inpharma, Int.Abstr.Biol.Sci., Int.Nurs.Ind., Jrnl.Watch Emer.Med., Kidney, Med.& Surg.Dermat., Nutr.Abstr., Pharm.&Out.News, Reac., Rev.Med.& Vet.Mycol., Rev.Plant Path., Sci.Cit.Ind., Trop.Dis.Bull., Vet.Bull.
—BLDSC (4685.784000), CASDDS, CISTI, EMDOCS, GNLM, IDS, ingenta, KNAW. **CCC.**

M

Published by: (American College of Surgeons USA), Elsevier Science BV, PO Box 211, Amsterdam 1000 AE, Netherlands. TEL 31-20-485-3757, FAX 31-20-485-3432, nlinfo-f@elsevier.nl, http://www.elsevier.com/locate/jamcollsurg. Eds. Seymour I Schwartz, Seymour Schwatrz, Wendy Cowles Husser. Adv. contact Frank Cox. Circ: 15,532. **Subscr. addr. in Asia & Australasia:** Elsevier Science (Singapore) Pte Ltd, No. 1 Temasek Ave, 17-01 Millenia Tower, Singapore 039192, Singapore. TEL 65-434-3727, FAX 65-337-2230, asiainfo@elsevier.com.sg; **Subscr. addr. in Japan:** Elsevier Science Inc - Japan Regional Office, 9-15 Higashi-Azabu 1-chome, Minato-ku, Tokyo 106-0044, Japan. TEL 81-3-5561-5033, FAX 81-3-5561-5047; **Subscr. addr. in Latin America:** Elsevier Science (Brazil), Regional Sales Office, Rua Sete de Setembro 111/16 andar, Rio de Janeiro, RJ 20050-002 Centro, Brazil. TEL 55-21-509-5340, FAX 55-21-507-1991, elsevier@campus.com.br; **Subscr. addr. in N America:** Elsevier Science, PO Box 945, New York, NY 10159-0945. TEL 212-633-3730, 888-437-4636, FAX 212-633-3680, usinfo-f@elsevier.com, http://www.elsevier.com.

617.95 USA ISSN 0748-8068
AMERICAN JOURNAL OF COSMETIC SURGERY. Text in English. 1984. q. USD 128 domestic; USD 154 foreign (effective 2001). adv. bk.rev. back issues avail.; reprints avail. *Refereed.* **Document type:** *Academic/Scholarly.* **Description:** Covers thought, experience, opinion, technique, research, legal aspects, patient relations, office protocol and any other subject relating to cosmetic surgery.
Indexed: Jrnl.Watch Derm.
—GNLM.
Published by: American Academy of Cosmetic Surgery, Inc., 401 N Michigan Ave, Ste 2400, Chicago, IL 60611-4212. FAX 312-644-1815, aacs@sba.com; orders@allenpress.com, http://www.allenpress.com. Ed. Dr. Melvin A Shiffman. adv.: B&W page USD 900, color page USD 1,725. Circ: 8,500. **Dist. by:** Allen Press Inc.. TEL 785-843-1235, FAX 785-843-1274, orders@allenpress.com, http://www.cosmeticsurgery.org.

617 USA ISSN 0899-7403
AMERICAN JOURNAL OF KNEE SURGERY. Abbreviated title: A J K S. Text in English. 1988. q. USD 120 domestic to individuals; USD 135 in Canada to individuals; USD 150 elsewhere to individuals; USD 140 domestic to institutions; USD 155 in Canada to institutions; USD 170 elsewhere to institutions. adv. back issues avail.; reprints avail. *Refereed.* **Document type:** *Academic/Scholarly.* **Description:** Provides a forum for practical, clinical information in such areas as arthroscopy, arthroplasty, magnetic resonance imaging, and reconstructive surgery.
Related titles: Microform ed.: (from PQC); Online - full text ed.: (from Northern Light Technology, Inc., ProQuest Information & Learning).
Indexed: Ind.Med. (1988-).
—BLDSC (0826.870000), CISTI, GNLM, Infotrieve, KNAW. **CCC.**
Published by: Slack, Inc., 6900 Grove Rd, Thorofare, NJ 08086-9447. TEL 856-848-1000, 800-257-8290, FAX 856-853-5991, http://www.slackinc.com. Ed. Dr. John McGinty. Pub. John C. Carter. adv.: B&W page USD 1,450, color page USD 2,890. Circ: 1,000 (paid).

617 USA ISSN 0002-9610
RD1 CODEN: AJSUAB
AMERICAN JOURNAL OF SURGERY. Text in English. 1891. m. USD 112 in US & Canada to individuals; USD 257 elsewhere to individuals; USD 226 in US & Canada to institutions; USD 378 elsewhere to institutions; USD 58 in US & Canada to qualified personnel; USD 163 elsewhere to qualified personnel (effective 2002). adv. bk.rev. bibl, charts, illus. reprint service avail. from PQC. *Refereed.* **Document type:** *Academic/Scholarly.* **Description:** Specializes in clinical papers on general surgery, including latest operative techniques and procedures. The official publication of record of eight major surgical associations in the US.
Related titles: CD-ROM ed.: (from Ovid Technologies, Inc.); Microform ed.: (from RPI,PMC); Online - full text ed.: (from Ovid Technologies, Inc., ingenta, Gale Group, Swets Blackwell, ScienceDirect, Institute for Scientific Information).
Indexed: AIM, ASCA, Abstr.Inter.Med., Biol.Abstr., C.I.S. Abstr., Chem.Abstr., Chem.Indus.Notes, Chem.Titles, Curr.Adv.Cancer Res., Curr.Adv.Ecol.Sci., Curr.Cont., Dairy Sci.Abstr., Dent.Ind., Excerp.Med., Helminthol.Abstr., INIS Atomind., I.P.A., Ind.Med. (1905-), Ind.Sci.Rev., Inpharma, Int.Abstr.Biol.Sci., Int.Nurs.Ind., Kidney, Med.& Surg.Dermat., Nutr.Abstr., Pharm.&Out.News, Reac., Rev.Med.& Vet.Mycol., Rev.Plant Path., Risk Abstr., SSCI (coverage dropped), Sci.Cit.Ind.
—BLDSC (0838.500000), ADONIS, CASDDS, CISTI, EMDOCS, GNLM, IDS, ingenta, KNAW. **CCC.**
Published by: Elsevier Science, 655 Ave of the Americas, New York, NY 10010. FAX 212-633-3990, usinfo@elsevier.com, http://www.elsevier.com/locate/amjsurg. Ed. Hiram Polk. Adv. contact Hank Blaney. B&W page USD 2,315, color page USD 4,080. Circ: 13,100 (paid).

AMERICAN JOURNAL OF SURGICAL PATHOLOGY. see *MEDICAL SCIENCES*

617 DNK ISSN 1600-6135
▼ **AMERICAN JOURNAL OF TRANSPLANTATION.** Text in English. 2001 (May). 10/yr. USD 400 in the Americas to institutions print & online eds. combined; GBP 278 elsewhere to institutions print & online eds. combined (effective 2002). *Refereed.* **Document type:** *Journal, Academic/Scholarly.* **Description:** Provides a forum for the rapid publication of new high quality data in organ and tissue transplantation and the related sciences.
Related titles: ♦ Online - full text ed.: American Journal of Transplantation Online. ISSN 1600-6143.
Published by: (American Society of Transplant Surgeons USA, American Society of Transplantation USA), Blackwell Munksgaard, Noerre Soegade 35, PO Box 2148, Copenhagen K 1016, Denmark. TEL 45-77-33-33-33, FAX 45-77-33-33-77, amjtrans@ualberta.ca, fsub@mail.munksgaard.dk, http://journals.munksgaard.dk/ajt, http://www.munksgaard.dk. Ed. Dr. Philip Halloran. Adv. contact Eric Rozario TEL 45-77-33-33-01. Circ: 2,600.

617 DNK ISSN 1600-6143
▼ **AMERICAN JOURNAL OF TRANSPLANTATION ONLINE.** Text in English. 2001 (May). 10/yr. GBP 250 (effective 2002). *Refereed.* **Document type:** *Academic/Scholarly.*
Media: Online - full text (from Munksgaard & Blackwell Science's Synergy, Swets Blackwell). **Related titles:** ♦ Print ed.: American Journal of Transplantation. ISSN 1600-6135.
Published by: (American Society of Transplantation USA, American Society of Transplant Surgeons USA), Blackwell Munksgaard, Noerre Soegade 35, PO Box 2148, Copenhagen K 1016, Denmark. TEL 45-77-33-33-33, FAX 45-77-33-33-77, fsub@mail.munksgaard.dk, http://www.munksgaard.dk.

616 USA ISSN 1531-0914
▼ **AMERICAN SOCIETY FOR SURGERY OF THE HAND. JOURNAL.** Text in English. 2001. q. USD 110 domestic to individuals; USD 139 domestic to institutions; USD 79 domestic to students; USD 130 foreign to individuals; USD 159 foreign to institutions; USD 40 newsstand/cover (effective 2001). adv. *Refereed.* **Document type:** *Journal, Consumer.* **Description:** Contains information on the latest advances and techniques in hand surgery.
Related titles: Online - full text ed.: ISSN 1532-852X.
Published by: (American Society for Surgery of the Hand), W.B. Saunders Co. (Subsidiary of: Harcourt Publishers Ltd.), 11830 Westline Industrial Dr, St Louis, MO 63146. TEL 800-325-4177, http://www.clinicalhandjournal.org, http://www.wbsaunders.com. Ed. Dr. Arnold-Peter Weiss.

617 USA ISSN 0003-1348
RD1 CODEN: AMSUAW
AMERICAN SURGEON. Text in English. 1935. m. USD 95 to individuals; USD 120 foreign to individuals; USD 180 to institutions; USD 205 foreign to institutions. adv. illus. index. reprints avail. *Refereed.* **Document type:** *Academic/Scholarly.*
Related titles: Microform ed.: (from PQC); Online - full text ed.: (from Northern Light Technology, Inc., ProQuest Information & Learning, Institute for Scientific Information).
Indexed: ASCA, AgeLine, Biol.Abstr., Chem.Abstr., Curr.Cont., Excerp.Med., Helminthol.Abstr., Hosp.Lit.Ind., INIS Atomind., Ind.Med. (1951-), Ind.Sci.Rev., Ind.Vet., Inpharma, Int.Nurs.Ind., Med.& Surg.Dermat., Nutr.Abstr., Reac., Rev.Appl.Entomol., Rev.Med.& Vet.Mycol., SSCI (coverage dropped), Sci.Cit.Ind., Small Anim.Abstr.
—BLDSC (0857.750000), CISTI, EMDOCS, GNLM, IDS, ingenta, KNAW. **CCC.**
Published by: Southeastern Surgical Congress, 141 W Wienca Rd, No B100, Atlanta, GA 30342. TEL 404-255-4549, FAX 404-255-5442, sesc@mindspring.com; deptsurg.mlast@mail.mcg.edu, http://www.sesc.org. Ed., R&P Talmadge A Bowden TEL 706-721-4686. Pub. Jannette Crosby. Adv. contact Marc Wilson. Circ: 4,600. **Co-sponsor:** American College of Surgeons - Southern California Chapter and the Midwest Surgical Association.

617 617 BRA ISSN 0003-245X
ANAIS PAULISTAS DE MEDICINA E CIRURGIA. Text in Portuguese. 1913. q. BRL 5,000, USD 30. adv. bk.rev. bibl, illus. index.
Indexed: Biol.Abstr., Chem.Abstr., Excerp.Med., Ind.Med. (coverage dropped).
—CISTI, GNLM.
Published by: Real e Benerita Sociedade Portuguesa de Sao Paulo, Rua Maestro Cardim, 769, Liberdade, Sao Paulo, SP 01323-001, Brazil. Ed. Abrahao Kerzner. Circ: 2,000.

617 ARG ISSN 0066-1465
ANALES DE CIRUGIA. Text in Spanish. 1935. irreg.
Indexed: Biol.Abstr., Excerp.Med.
Address: Calle Paraguay, 40, Rosario, Santa Fe 2000, Argentina.

ANALES DE CIRUGIA CARDIACA Y CIRUGIA VASCULAR. see *MEDICAL SCIENCES—Cardiovascular Diseases*

ANESTEZIOLOGIYA I REANIMATOLOGIYA/ ANESTHESIOLOGY AND INTENSIVE CARE. see *MEDICAL SCIENCES—Anaesthesiology*

617 RUS
ANGIOLOGIYA I SOSUDISTAYA KHIRURGIYA. Text in Russian. q. USD 139.95 in United States.
Indexed: Ref.Zh.
Published by: Info-Media, Barrikadnaya ul 2, str 3, Moscow 123836, Russian Federation. TEL 7-095-1202581, FAX 7-095-2521162. Ed. A V Pokrovskii. **US dist. addr.:** East View Publications, 3020 Harbor Ln N, Minneapolis, MN 55447. TEL 612-550-0961.

617 618.1 FIN ISSN 0355-9521
CODEN: ACGYDJ
ANNALES CHIRURGIAE ET GYNAECOLOGIAE. Text in English. 1946. q. FIM 400 in Scandinavia to individuals; FIM 600 in Europe to individuals; FIM 800 elsewhere to individuals; FIM 700 in Scandinavia to institutions; FIM 1,100 in Europe to institutions; FIM 1,200 elsewhere to institutions; FIM 150 newsstand/cover in Scandinavia; FIM 250 newsstand/cover in Scandinavia special issues (effective 2000). adv. bibl, charts, illus. Supplement avail.; back issues avail. *Refereed.* **Document type:** *Academic/Scholarly.*
Formerly (until 1976): Annales Chirurgiae et Gynaecologiae Fenniae (0003-3855)
Related titles: Microform ed.: (from PQC); Online - full text ed.: (from Institute for Scientific Information).
Indexed: ASCA, Biol.Abstr., Chem.Abstr., Curr.Adv.Ecol.Sci., Curr.Cont., Excerp.Med., INIS Atomind., Ind.Med. (1976-), Inpharma, Int.Nurs.Ind., Pharm.&Out.News, Reac., Ref.Zh.
—BLDSC (0970.510000), CASDDS, CISTI, EMDOCS, GNLM, ingenta, KNAW.
Published by: Finnish Surgical Society, ACG Editorial Office, PL 79, Helsinki 00501, Finland. TEL 358-9-393-091, FAX 358-9-393-0801, http://www.fimnet.fi/acg. Ed. Peter Roberts. R&P Anja Maaskola. Circ: 2,000. **Co-sponsor:** Scandinavian Surgical Society.

617 FRA ISSN 0003-3944
ANNALES DE CHIRURGIE. Text in French. 1947. 10/yr. EUR 274 in Europe to institutions; USD 347 elsewhere to institutions (effective 2002). *Refereed.* **Document type:** *Academic/Scholarly.*
Incorporates (in 2000): Chirurgie (0001-4001); Which was formerly (until 1969): Academie de Chirurgie. Memoires (0368-8291); (until 1935): Societe Nationale de Chirurgie. Bulletins et Memoires (0366-4503); (until 1923): Societe de Chirurgie de Paris. Bulletins et Memoires (0366-466X); Which was formed by the merger of (1847-1874): Societe de Chirurgie de Paris. Memoires (0150-9659); (1871-1874): Societe de Chirurgie de Paris. Bulletin (0150-9802); Which was formerly: Societe Imperiale de Chirurgie de Paris (0150-9675); (1851-1865): Societe de Chirurgie de Paris. Bulletin (0150-9667)
Related titles: Online - full text ed.: (from Institute for Scientific Information); ♦ Supplement: Annales de Chirurgie Thoracique et Cardio-Vasculaire. ISSN 0066-2054.
Indexed: ASCA, Biol.Abstr., Chem.Abstr., Curr.Adv.Cancer Res., Curr.Cont., Excerp.Med., Ind.Med. (1947-), Inpharma, Int.Nurs.Ind., Pharm.&Out.News, Protozool.Abstr., Reac., Ref.Zh., SSCI (coverage dropped), Trop.Dis.Bull.
—BLDSC (0970.532000), CISTI, EMDOCS, GNLM, IDS, Infotrieve, KNAW. **CCC.**

M

Published by: (Semaine des Hopitaux), Elsevier Paris, Editions Scientifiques et Medicales (Subsidiary of: Reed Elsevier plc. group), 23 rue Linois, Paris 75015, France. http://www.elsevier.com/locate/anchir. Circ: 3,000.

617.95 FRA ISSN 0294-1260
CODEN: ACESE
ANNALES DE CHIRURGIE PLASTIQUE ET ESTHETIQUE. Text in French; Summaries in English. 1956. 6/yr. EUR 292 in Europe to institutions; USD 343 elsewhere to institutions (effective 2002). adv. abstr, charts, illus. **Document type:** *Academic/Scholarly.*
Formerly: Annales de Chirurgie Plastique (0003-3960)
Indexed: Biol.Abstr., Chem.Abstr., Curr.Cont. (coverage dropped), Excerp.Med., INIS Atomind., Ind.Med. (1983-), Med.& Surg.Dermat., Ref.Zh.
—BLDSC (0970.541000), CISTI, EMDOCS, GNLM, Infotrieve, KNAW. **CCC.**
Published by: (Semaine des Hopitaux), Elsevier Paris, Editions Scientifiques et Medicales (Subsidiary of: Reed Elsevier plc. group), 23 rue Linois, Paris 75015, France. http://www.elsevier.com/locate/anplas. Circ: 3,000.

ANNALES DE CHIRURGIE THORACIQUE ET CARDIO-VASCULAIRE. see *MEDICAL SCIENCES—Cardiovascular Diseases*

617 ITA ISSN 0003-469X
CODEN: AICHAL
ANNALI ITALIANI DI CHIRURGIA. Text in Italian. 1922. bi-m. ITL 90,000 domestic; USD 110 foreign (effective 2000). adv. bk.rev. abstr, charts, illus. index. back issues avail. **Document type:** *Academic/Scholarly.*
Related titles: Fax ed.
Indexed: Biol.Abstr., Chem.Abstr., Dent.Ind., Excerp.Med., Ind.Med. (1922-).
—BLDSC (1014.300000), CISTI, GNLM, KNAW.
Published by: Nuova Casa Editrice Licinio Cappelli di G.E.M. s.r.l., Via Luigi Carlo Farini, 14, Bologna, BO 40124, Italy. TEL 39-051-239060, FAX 39-051-239286. Ed. Nicola Picardi. R&P Mario Musso. Adv. contact Lia Milano. Circ: 3,000.

617.95 USA ISSN 0148-7043
RD118.AI CODEN: APCSD4
ANNALS OF PLASTIC SURGERY. Text in English. 1978. m. USD 293 domestic to individuals; USD 393 foreign to individuals; USD 470 domestic to institutions; USD 575 foreign to institutions; USD 49 newsstand/cover (effective 2002). adv. bk.rev. abstr, charts, illus, stat. index. back issues avail.; reprint service avail. from PQC. *Refereed.* **Document type:** *Academic/Scholarly.* **Description:** Forum for the latest in surgical techniques, interesting cases, and practical briefs on surgical devices. Includes articles, case reports, hypotheses, and letters to the editor.
Related titles: Microform ed.: (from PQC); Online - full text ed.: (from Institute for Scientific Information).
Indexed: ASCA, Biol.Abstr., CINAHL, Curr.Cont., Dent.Ind., Excerp.Med., INIS Atomind., Ind.Med. (1978-), Ind.Sci.Rev., Inpharma, Med.& Surg.Dermat., Pharm.&Out.News, Reac., Rev.Med.& Vet.Mycol., Sci.Cit.Ind.
—BLDSC (1043.525000), EMDOCS, GNLM, IDS, ingenta, KNAW.
Published by: Lippincott Williams & Wilkins (Philadelphia) (Subsidiary of: Wolters Kluwer N.V.), 530 Walnut St, Philadelphia, PA 19106-3621. TEL 215-521-8300, FAX 215-521-8902, http://www.annalsplasticsurgery.com, http://www.Lww.com. Ed. Dr. William D Morain. Pub. Marcia Serepy. R&P Margaret Becker. Adv. contact Ray Thibodeau. B&W page USD 900, color page USD 1,925; trim 8.25 x 11. Circ: 3,134. **Subscr. to:** PO Box 1600, Hagerstown, MD 21740-1600. TEL 800-777-2295, FAX 301-824-7390.

617 USA ISSN 0003-4932
RD1 CODEN: ANSUA5
ANNALS OF SURGERY. Text in English. 1885. m. USD 168 domestic to individuals print and online eds. combined; USD 259 foreign to individuals print and online eds. combined; USD 426 domestic to institutions print and online eds. combined; USD 544 foreign to institutions print and online eds. combined; USD 47 newsstand/cover print and online eds. combined (effective 2002). adv. bk.rev. illus. index. reprint service avail. from PQC. *Refereed.* **Document type:** *Academic/Scholarly.*
Related titles: Microform ed.: (from PQC,PMC); Online - full text ed.: USD 553.80 domestic academic site license; USD 671.80 foreign academic site license; USD 617.70 domestic corporate site license; USD 735.70 foreign corporate site license (effective 2002) (from Ovid Technologies, Inc., EBSCO Publishing, Swets Blackwell, Institute for Scientific Information).
Indexed: AIM, ASCA, Abstr.Health Care Manage.Stud., Abstr.Inter.Med., Biol.Abstr., Chem.Abstr., Curr.Adv.Cancer Res., Curr.Adv.Ecol.Sci., Curr.Cont., Dairy Sci.Abstr., Excerp.Med., Helminthol.Abstr., Hosp.Lit.Ind., INIS Atomind., Ind.Med. (1885-), Ind.Sci.Rev., Inpharma, Jrnl.Watch, Jrnl.Watch Emer.Med., Kidney, Med.& Surg.Dermat., Nutr.Abstr., Pharm.&Out.News, Reac., Risk Abstr., SSCI (coverage dropped), Sci.Cit.Ind.
—BLDSC (1044.500000), CASDDS, CISTI, EMDOCS, GNLM, IDS, ingenta, KNAW.
Published by: Lippincott Williams & Wilkins (Philadelphia) (Subsidiary of: Wolters Kluwer N.V.), 530 Walnut St, Philadelphia, PA 19106-3621. TEL 215-521-8300, FAX 215-521-8902, http://www.annalsofsurgery.com, http://www.Lww.com. Ed. Dr. Layton F Rikkers. Pub. Marcia Serepy. R&P Margaret Becker. Adv. contact Ray Thibodeau. B&W page USD 2,415, color page USD 4,014. Circ: 12,047. **Subscr. to:** PO Box 1600, Hagerstown, MD 21740-1600. TEL 800-777-2295, FAX 301-824-7390. **Co-sponsors:** Philadelphia Academy of Surgery; New York Surgical Society; Southern Surgical Association; American Surgical Association.

617 USA ISSN 1068-9265
RD651 CODEN: ASONF4
ANNALS OF SURGICAL ONCOLOGY. Text in English. 1994. 10/yr. USD 331 domestic to individuals; USD 384 foreign to individuals; USD 470 domestic to institutions; USD 523 foreign to institutions (effective 2002); USD 54 newsstand/cover. adv. charts, illus. *Refereed.* **Document type:** *Academic/Scholarly.* **Description:** Presents significant developments involving multidisciplinary cancer care and research, for practicing surgeons in all specialties.
Related titles: Microform ed.: (from PQC); Online - full text ed.: USD 611 domestic academic site license; USD 664 foreign academic site license; USD 681.50 domestic corporate site license; USD 734.50 foreign corporate site license (2002) (from Ovid Technologies, Inc., Institute for Scientific Information).
Indexed: ASCA, Curr.Cont., Ind.Med. (1994-), Ind.Sci.Rev., Inpharma, Pharm.&Out.News, Reac., Sci.Cit.Ind.
—BLDSC (1044.550000), CISTI, GNLM, IDS, KNAW.
Published by: (Society of Surgical Oncology), Lippincott Williams & Wilkins (Philadelphia) (Subsidiary of: Wolters Kluwer N.V.), 530 Walnut St, Philadelphia, PA 19106-3621. TEL 215-521-8300, FAX 215-521-8902, http://www.annalssurgicaloncology.com, http://www.Lww.com. Ed. Dr. Charles M Balch. Pub. Christine Rullo. R&P Margaret Becker. Adv. contact Ray Thibodeau. B&W page USD 930, color page USD 1,980. Circ: 1,958. **Subscr. to:** PO Box 1600, Hagerstown, MD 21740-1600. TEL 800-777-2295, FAX 301-824-7390.

617.54 JPN ISSN 1341-1098
ANNALS OF THORACIC AND CARDIOVASCULAR SURGERY. Text in English. 1981. bi-m. USD 175.
Formerly (until 1995): Rinsho Kyobu Geka - Japanese Annals of Thoracic Surgery (0389-7893)
Indexed: INIS Atomind., Ind.Med. (1995-).
—BLDSC (1044.700000), CISTI, GNLM.
Published by: (Association of Thoracic and Cardiovascular Surgeons of Asia, Editorial Committee of A T C S), Nihon Akuseru Shupuringa Shuppan K.K./Axel Springer, Japan Publishing Inc., 2-1 Niban-cho, Chiyoda-ku, Tokyo 102-0084, Japan. FAX 81-3-3239-9388. Ed. Yukiyasu Sezai.

617.54 USA ISSN 0003-4975
RD536 CODEN: ATHSAK
ANNALS OF THORACIC SURGERY. Text in English. 1965. m. EUR 240 in Europe to individuals; JPY 33,180 in Japan to individuals; USD 239 in United States to individuals; USD 269 elsewhere to individuals; EUR 397 in Europe to institutions; JPY 52,600 in Japan to institutions; USD 405 in United States to institutions; USD 443 elsewhere to institutions (effective 2002). adv. bk.rev. charts, illus, abstr. index. back issues avail. *Refereed.* **Document type:** *Journal, Academic/Scholarly.* **Description:** Presents original papers on topics in thoracic and cardiovascular surgery, featuring case reports, "how-to-do-it" articles, classics in thoracic surgery, collective and current reviews, and correspondence.
Related titles: Microform ed.: (from PQC); Online - full text ed.: (from HighWire Pr., EBSCO Publishing, ingenta, Swets Blackwell, ScienceDirect, Institute for Scientific Information).
Indexed: AIM, ASCA, Abstr.Hyg., Abstr.Inter.Med., Biol.Abstr., CINAHL, Curr.Adv.Cancer Res., Curr.Cont., Excerp.Med., Helminthol.Abstr., INIS Atomind., Ind.Med. (1965-), Ind.Sci.Rev., Inpharma, Int.Nurs.Ind., Kidney, Mat.Sci.Cit.Ind. (coverage dropped), Neurosci.Cit.Ind., Nutr.Abstr., Pharm.&Out.News, Reac., Rev.Med.& Vet.Mycol., Sci.Cit.Ind.
—BLDSC (1044.750000), ADONIS, CISTI, EMDOCS, GNLM, IDS, ingenta, KNAW. **CCC.**
Published by: (Society of Thoracic Surgeons), Elsevier Science, Box 945, New York, NY 10159-0945. TEL 212-989-5800, FAX 212-633-3990, usinfo-f@elsevier.com, http://www.elsevier.com/locate/athoracsur. Eds. Dr. L Henry Edmunds Jr., Dr. Thomas Ferguson. Circ: 8,100. **Subscr. in Australasia and the Far East to:** Elsevier Science (Singapore) Pte Ltd, No.1 Temasek Ave, 17-01 Millenia Tower, Singapore 039192, Singapore. TEL 65-434-3727, FAX 65-337-2230; **Subscr. in Japan to:** Elsevier Science Inc - Japan Regional Office, 9-15 Higashi-Azabu 1-chome, Minato-ku, Tokyo 106-0044, Japan. TEL 81-3-5561-5033, FAX 81-3-5561-5047; **Subscr. outside the Americas to:** Elsevier Science BV, PO Box 211, Amsterdam 1000 AE, Netherlands. TEL 31-20-485-3757, FAX 31-20-485-3432. **Co-sponsor:** Southern Thoracic Surgical Association.

617 616.1 USA ISSN 0890-5096
CODEN: AVSUEV
ANNALS OF VASCULAR SURGERY; international journal of vascular surgery. Text in English. 1986. bi-m. (in 1 vol., 6 nos./vol.). USD 456.30 in Germany for Print & Online Eds.; USD 429.60 elsewhere for Print & Online Eds.; USD 80.50 newsstand/cover in Germany (effective 2002). adv. *Refereed.* **Document type:** *Academic/Scholarly.* **Description:** Worldwide coverage of all clinical or research-oriented work going on today in vascular surgery.
Related titles: Online - full text ed.: ISSN 1615-5947 (from Northern Light Technology, Inc., EBSCO Publishing, RoweCom Information Quest, ProQuest Information & Learning, Swets Blackwell, Springer LINK, Institute for Scientific Information).
Indexed: ASCA, Curr.Cont., Excerp.Med., INIS Atomind., Ind.Med. (1986-), Ind.Sci.Rev., Inpharma, Pharm.&Out.News, Reac., Sci.Cit.Ind.
—BLDSC (1045.350000), CISTI, EMDOCS, GNLM, IDS, ingenta, KNAW. **CCC.**
Published by: Springer-Verlag, Journals (Subsidiary of: BertelsmannSpringer), 175 Fifth Ave, New York, NY 10010. TEL 212-460-1500, FAX 212-473-6272, orders@springer-ny.com; helpdesk@link.springer.de, http://link.springer.de/link/service/journals/10016/index.htm. Eds. Dr. Edouard Kieffer, Dr. Ramon Berguer. Adv. contact Jay Feinman.

617 RUS
ANNALY KHIRURGICHESKOI GEPATOLOGII. Text in Russian. q. USD 95 in United States.
Published by: Assotsiatsiya Khirurgov-Gepatologov, Kolomenskii pr-t 4, Klinich b-tsa 7, Moscow 115446, Russian Federation. TEL 7-095-1188238, FAX 7-095-1188238. Ed. E I Gal'perin. **US dist. addr.:** East View Publications, 3020 Harbor Ln N, Minneapolis, MN 55447. TEL 612-559-0961.

617 RUS
ANNALY KHIRURGII. Text in Russian. bi-m. USD 199 foreign (effective 2000).
Published by: Izdatel'stvo Meditsina, Petroverigskii per 6-8, Moscow 101000, Russian Federation. TEL 7-095-4244044, FAX 7-095-4244188. Ed. L A Bockeria. **US dist. addr.:** East View Publications, 3020 Harbor Ln N, Minneapolis, MN 55447. TEL 612-550-0961.

617 RUS
ANNALY KHIRURGII/ANNALS OF SURGERY. Text in Russian; Summaries in English. 1996. bi-m. USD 237 foreign (effective 2000). adv. bk.rev., Website rev. abstr. reprints avail. **Document type:** *Journal, Academic/Scholarly.* **Description:** Covers all aspects of general and special surgery, training of specialists, latest advances in the field, and information from leading surgical centers world-wide.
Published by: Izdatel'stvo Meditsina, Petroverigskii per 6-8, Moscow 101000, Russian Federation. TEL 7-095-9248785, 7-095-928-86-48, FAX 7-095-9211355, 7-095-9286003, meditsina@iname.com, http://www.medit.ru. Ed. L A Bockeria. Pub. A M Stochik. R&P T Ivanova. Adv. contact O A Fadeeva TEL 7-095-923-51-40. Circ: 1,500. **Dist. by:** Mezhdunarodnaya Kniga, B Yakimanka 39, Moscow 117049, Russian Federation. TEL 7-095-2384967, FAX 7-095-2384634.

ANNUAL OF CARDIAC SURGERY. see *MEDICAL SCIENCES—Abstracting, Bibliographies, Statistics*

M

617 IND ISSN 0003-5998
R97
THE ANTISEPTIC; monthly journal of medicine and surgery. Text in English. 1904. m. INR 240; INR 1,920 foreign (effective 1999). adv. bk.rev. abstr, bibl, illus. index. reprint service avail. from PQC. **Document type:** *Trade.*
Indexed: Chem.Abstr., Excerp.Med., INIS Atomind., Ind.Med. (coverage dropped).
—CISTI, GNLM.
Published by: Professional Publications Ltd., Satya Sai Nagar, P O Box 2, Madurai, Tamil Nadu 625 003, India. TEL 0452-673701, FAX 0452-674602. Pub. R Lakshmipathy. Circ: 26,760.

617 JPN ISSN 0003-9152
CODEN: NIGHAE
ARCHIV FUER JAPANISCHE CHIRURGIE/NIHON GEKA HOKAN. Text in Multiple languages. 1924. bi-m. JPY 6,000; or exchange basis. abstr, charts, illus. index.
Indexed: Biol.Abstr., Chem.Abstr., Chem.Indus.Notes, Chem.Titles, Curr.Cont. (coverage dropped), Excerp.Med., INIS Atomind., Ind.Med. (1924-).
—BLDSC (1615.400000), CASDDS, CISTI, EMDOCS, GNLM.
Published by: Kyoto University, Faculty Of Medicine, Department of Surgery, 54 Shogoin Kawara-sho, Sakyo-ku, Kyoto 606-8397, Japan. Ed. Kazae Ozawa. Circ: 1,000.

617.95 USA ISSN 1521-2491
▼ **ARCHIVES OF FACIAL PLASTIC SURGERY.** Text in English. 1999. q. USD 195 in North America to institutions; USD 245 to institutions Central and S. America; GBP 145 elsewhere to institutions (effective 2001). adv. back issues avail. *Refereed.* **Description:** Publishes articles on all aspects of reconstructive and cosmetic surgery of the head and neck.
Related titles: Online - full text ed.: (from Ovid Technologies, Inc.).
Indexed: Ind.Med., Jrnl.Watch Derm.
—BLDSC (1634.278050).
Published by: American Medical Association, 515 N State St, P O Box 10946, Chicago, IL 60610-0946. ama@subscription.co.uk, http://www.ama-assn.org, http://www.archfacial.com.

617 USA ISSN 0004-0010
CODEN: ARSUAX
ARCHIVES OF SURGERY. Text in English. 1920. m. USD 325 in North America to institutions; USD 425 to institutions Central & S. America; GBP 275 elsewhere to institutions (effective 2001). adv. bk.rev. charts, illus. index. back issues avail.; reprints avail. *Refereed.* **Document type:** *Academic/Scholarly.* **Description:** Publishes original contributions and papers from surgical societies. Clinical observations and commentaries provide current information useful to the practicing general surgeon.
Related titles: CD-ROM ed.: (from Ovid Technologies, Inc.); Microform ed.: (from PQC,PMC); Online - full text ed.: (from The Dialog Corporation, Gale Group, Ovid Technologies, Inc., EBSCO Publishing, Institute for Scientific Information).
Indexed: AIM, ASCA, Abstr.Inter.Med., Arts & Hum.Cit.Ind. (coverage dropped), Biol.Abstr., CINAHL, C.I.S. Abstr., Chem.Abstr., Chem.Indus.Notes, Chem.Titles, Curr.Adv.Cancer Res., Curr.Adv.Cell & Devel.Biol., Curr.Adv.Ecol.Sci., Curr.Cont., Dairy Sci.Abstr., Dent.Ind., Environ.Sci.Poll.Mgmt., Excerp.Med., Helminthol.Abstr., INIS Atomind., Ind.Med. (1960-), Ind.Sci.Rev., Inpharma, Int.Nurs.Ind., Med.& Surg.Dermat., Nutr.Abstr., Pharm.&Out.News, Pollut.Abstr., Protozool.Abstr., Reac., Rev.Med.& Vet.Mycol., Risk Abstr., SSCI (coverage dropped), Saf.Sci.Abstr., Sci.Cit.Ind.
—BLDSC (1643.200000), CASDDS, CISTI, EMDOCS, GNLM, IDS, ingenta, KNAW. **CCC.**
Published by: American Medical Association, 515 N State St, P O Box 10946, Chicago, IL 60610-0946. ama-subs@ama-assn.org, http://www.archsurg.com. Ed. Claude H Organ. R&P Ada Jimenez Walker. Adv. contact J P Cahill. Circ: 39,000.

617.54 616.1 ITA ISSN 0391-7029
ARCHIVIO DI CHIRURGIA TORACICA E CARDIOVASCOLARE. Text in English, Italian. 1979. bi-m., latest vol.2, 2001. USD 120 (effective 2002). adv. bk.rev. *Refereed.* **Document type:** *Journal, Academic/Scholarly.* **Description:** Articles on thoracic and cardiovascular surgery.
—GNLM.
Published by: Edizioni Luigi Pozzi s.r.l., Via Panama, 68, Rome, RM 00198, Italy. TEL 39-06-8553548, FAX 39-06-8554105, edizioni_pozzi@tin.it. Ed. B Marino. Circ: 1,200. **Co-sponsor:** Italian Society of Thoracic Surgery.

ARQUIVOS BRASILEIROS DE CIRURGIA DIGESTIVA. see *MEDICAL SCIENCES—Gastroenterology*

617 BRA ISSN 0066-7846
ARQUIVOS DE CIRURGIA CLINICA E EXPERIMENTAL*. Abstracts occasionally in English. 1937. irreg. USD 35. index, cum.index. Supplement avail.
Indexed: Biol.Abstr.
Published by: Universidade de Sao Paulo, Hospital das Clinicas, Centro, Caixa Postal 8091, Sao Paulo, SP 01065-970, Brazil. Ed. Ruy G Bevilacqua. Circ: 10,000.

617 PRT ISSN 0872-2226
CODEN: APCIFA
ARQUIVOS PORTUGUESES DE CIRURGIA. Text in English, Portuguese. 1990. q. PTE 2,000. adv. **Document type:** *Academic/Scholarly.*
Published by: A E F M U P, Alameda Prof. H. Montiero, Piso 1, Apdo. 4514, Porto Codex 4008, Portugal. TEL 351-2-5509355, FAX 351-2-5509096. Ed. Amarante Junior. Adv. contact Fernando Araujo. B&W page PTE 150,000. Circ: 2,500. **Co-sponsor:** Hospital de S. Joao, Faculdade de Medicina do Porto.

ARTHROSCOPY; journal of arthroscopic and related surgery. see *MEDICAL SCIENCES—Orthopedics And Traumatology*

ARTHROSCOPY. see *MEDICAL SCIENCES—Orthopedics And Traumatology*

ARTIFICIAL ORGANS. see *MEDICAL SCIENCES—Experimental Medicine, Laboratory Technique*

ASIAN JOURNAL OF ORAL AND MAXILLOFACIAL SURGERY. see *MEDICAL SCIENCES—Dentistry*

617 HKG ISSN 1015-9584
CODEN: AJSUEF
ASIAN JOURNAL OF SURGERY. Text in English. 1978. 4/yr. USD 356 foreign; USD 352.30 in Germany; USD 100.50 newsstand/cover foreign (effective 2002). adv. 120 p./no. *Refereed.* **Document type:** *Journal, Academic/Scholarly.*
Formerly (until 1989): Southeast Asian Journal of Surgery (0258-3186)
Related titles: Online - full text ed.: ISSN 0219-3108 (from Swets Blackwell, Springer LINK, RoweCom Information Quest).
Indexed: Excerp.Med.
—BLDSC (1742.578000), CISTI, EMDOCS, GNLM, KNAW.
Published by: (Asian Surgical Association CHN), Springer-Verlag Hong Kong Ltd. (Subsidiary of: BertelsmannSpringer), Unit 1702, Tower 1, Enterprise Square, 9 Sheung Yuet Rd, Kowloon Bay, Kowloon, Hong Kong. TEL 852-2723-9698, FAX 852-2724-2366, springer@springer.com.hk, http://link.springer.de/link/service/journals/. Ed. Edward Lai. adv.: B&W page USD 2,000, color page USD 4,000. Circ: 1,800 (controlled).

617 USA ISSN 1082-3131
ATLAS OF THE HAND CLINICS. Text in English. 1996. s-a. USD 123 domestic; USD 149 foreign; USD 75 per issue (effective 2001); for subscribers to Hand Clinics only. **Document type:** *Academic/Scholarly.* **Description:** Delivers practical advice from experts in specialty covered with a fresh perspective on problems and controversies.
—BLDSC (1767.025200).
Published by: W.B. Saunders Co. (Subsidiary of: Harcourt Publishers Ltd.), Curtis Center, 3rd Fl, Independence Sq W, Philadelphia, PA 19106-3399. TEL 215-238-7800, FAX 215-238-6445, wbspcs@harcourtbrace.com, http://www.wbsaunders.com. Ed. Dr. A Lee Osterman. **Subscr. to:** Periodicals Fulfillment, W B Saunders Co, 6277 Sea Harbor Dr, 4th Fl, Orlando, FL 32891-4800.

ATLAS OF THE ORAL AND MAXILLOFACIAL SURGERY CLINICS OF NORTH AMERICA. see *MEDICAL SCIENCES—Dentistry*

616.21 USA ISSN 1047-6954
AUDIO-DIGEST GENERAL SURGERY. Text in English. 1954. s-m. USD 168 (effective 2000). *Refereed.*
Formerly: Audio-Digest Surgery (0271-1273)
Media: Audio cassette/tape.
Published by: Audio-Digest Foundation (Subsidiary of: California Medical Association), 1577 E Chevy Chase Dr, Glendale, CA 91206. TEL 213-245-8505, 800-423-2308, FAX 818-240-7379, 800-845-4375. Ed. Claron L Oakley.

AUSTRALASIAN JOURNAL OF EMERGENCY CARE. see *MEDICAL SCIENCES—Orthopedics And Traumatology*

AUSTRALIAN JOURNAL OF OTOLARYNGOLOGY. see *MEDICAL SCIENCES—Otorhinolaryngology*

616 AUS ISSN 0157-5821
AUSTRALIAN SURGEON. Text in English. 1977. q. membership only. adv. **Document type:** *Newsletter, Bulletin.*
Related titles: Supplement: Australian Surgeon News.
—ingenta.
Published by: Australian Association of Surgeons, Ste. 1, 2 A Mona Rd, Darling Point, NSW 2027, Australia. FAX 61-2-3635001, aas@enternet.com.au. Ed., Adv. contact Christopher Thomas. R&P John Wansbrough TEL 61-2-9363-4411. Circ: 2,000.

617 ESP
BARCELONA QUIRURGICA. Text in Spanish. 1957. 4/yr. ESP 5,300, USD 115 (effective 1999). adv. bk.rev. **Document type:** *Trade.* **Description:** Covers all the specialties of surgery.
Published by: Editorial Dips Rocas, Muntaner, 393 pral. 4, Barcelona 08021, Spain. TEL 39-3-2001389, FAX 39-3-2021958, edipsro@intercom.es. Ed. G Gili Cirera. R&P Alvaro Trevino. Adv. contact Carles Martin. color page ESP 110,000. Circ: 3,000.

617 CHE ISSN 1013-7459
CODEN: BBCHEL
BASLER BEITRAEGE ZUR CHIRURGIE; Aktuelle Entwicklungen und neue Verfahren aus der chirurgischen Praxis kompakt vermittelt. Text in German. 1989. irreg., latest vol.7, 1995. CHF 68 (effective 2000). abstr, bibl, charts. **Document type:** *Magazine, Trade.* **Description:** Discusses developments in surgery and its techniques.
—GNLM, KNAW.
Published by: (University of Basel, Department of Surgery), Schwabe und Co. AG, Steinentorstr 13, Basel 4010, Switzerland. TEL 41-61-2789565, FAX 41-61-2789566, TELEX CH-962652, verlag@schwabe.ch, http://www.schwabe.ch. Eds. M Duerig, U Laffer.

617 USA
BODY CONTOURING SURGERY. Text in English. 1996. 2/yr. USD 265 to individuals; USD 350 to institutions. back issues avail. *Refereed.* **Document type:** *Academic/Scholarly.*
Published by: Field & Wood, Medical Periodicals, Inc., PO Box 975, Blue Bell, PA 19422. TEL 610-828-4010, FAX 215-482-0226. Ed. Dr. Ricardo Baroudi.

617.95 GBR
BODY LANGUAGE. Text in English. q. GBP 19 in the European Union; GBP 22 elsewhere (effective 2000). adv. **Document type:** *Magazine, Consumer, Trade.* **Description:** Provides independent information on all procedures and treatments as well as news and views of modern cosmetic surgery products and techniques.
Published by: New Millennium Publishing Ltd., PO Box 222, Tring, Herts HP23 5TT, United Kingdom. TEL 44-1442-827208, http://www.bodylanguage.net. Ed. David Williams.

617.6 GBR ISSN 1356-3807
BRITISH DENTAL NURSES' JOURNAL. Text in English. 1973 (vol.32). q. GBP 35; GBP 40 foreign (effective 1999). adv. bk.rev. illus. **Document type:** *Academic/Scholarly.*
Formerly (until 1995): British Dental Surgery Assistant (0007-0629)
Indexed: Dent.Ind.
—GNLM.
Published by: British Association of Dental Nurses, 11 Pharos St, Fleetwood, Lancs FY7 6BG, United Kingdom. TEL 44-1253-778631, FAX 44-1253-773266. Ed. Pamela A Swain. R&P, Adv. contact Pamela Swain. Circ: 3,500.

617 GBR ISSN 0268-8697
CODEN: BJNEEL
BRITISH JOURNAL OF NEUROSURGERY. Text in English. 1987. bi-m. GBP 189, USD 312 to individuals; GBP 544, USD 924 to institutions (effective 2002). adv. bk.rev. abstr. index. back issues avail. *Refereed.* **Document type:** *Academic/Scholarly.*
Related titles: Microfiche ed.; Online - full text ed.: ISSN 1360-046X (from CatchWord Ltd., Northern Light Technology, Inc., EBSCO Publishing, O C L C Online Computer Library Center, Inc., RoweCom Information Quest, ProQuest Information & Learning, Swets Blackwell, Institute for Scientific Information).

M

Indexed: ASCA, Abstr.Hyg., Abstr.Soc.Geront., Curr.Cont., Excerp.Med., Helminthol.Abstr., Ind.Med. (1987-), Inpharma, Neurosci.Cit.Ind., Peace Res.Abstr., Pharm.&Out.News, Reac., Rev.Med.& Vet.Mycol., Viol.& Abuse Abstr.
—BLDSC (2311.940000), ADONIS, CatchWord, CISTI, EMDOCS, GNLM, IDS, ingenta, KNAW. **CCC.**
Published by: Carfax Publishing Limited (Subsidiary of: Taylor & Francis Group), PO Box 25, Abingdon, Oxon OX14 3UE, United Kingdom. TEL 44-1235-401000, FAX 44-1235-401550, enquiries@carfax.co.uk, enquiry@tandf.co.uk, http://www.carfax.co.uk. Ed. Robert Maurice Williams. adv.: B&W page GBP 250.

617.3 GBR ISSN 0266-4356
BRITISH JOURNAL OF ORAL AND MAXILLOFACIAL SURGERY. Text in English. 1963. bi-m. GBP 110 to individuals; GBP 280 to institutions (effective 2002). adv. bk.rev. charts, illus. index. *Refereed.* **Document type:** *Journal, Academic/Scholarly.* **Description:** Provides contemporary information on developments within the scope of oral and maxillofacial surgery.
Formerly: British Journal of Oral Surgery (0007-117X)
Related titles: Microform ed.: (from PQC); Online - full text ed.: (from EBSCO Publishing, O C L C Online Computer Library Center, Inc., Swets Blackwell, IDEAL Online Library, Institute for Scientific Information).
Indexed: ASCA, Biol.Abstr., Cal.Tiss.Abstr., Curr.Adv.Ecol.Sci., Curr.Cont., Curr.Tit.Dent., Dent.Abstr., Dent.Ind., Environ.Sci.Poll.Mgmt., Excerp.Med., Ind.Med. (1984-), Ind.Sci.Rev., Inpharma, Microbiol.Abstr., Pharm.&Out.News, Pollut.Abstr., Reac., Res.High.Educ.Abstr., Rev.Med.& Vet.Mycol., Risk Abstr., SSCI (coverage dropped), Saf.Sci.Abstr., Sci.Cit.Ind.
—BLDSC (2314.200000), CISTI, EMDOCS, GNLM, IDS, Infotrieve, ingenta, KNAW. **CCC.**
Published by: (British Association of Oral and Maxillofacial Surgeons), Churchill Livingstone (Subsidiary of: Harcourt Publishers Ltd.), Robert Stevenson House, 1-3 Baxter's Pl, Leith Walk, Edinburgh, Midlothian EH1 3AF, United Kingdom. TEL 44-131-556-2424, FAX 44-131-459-1177, cservice.harcourt.com, http://www.harcourt-international.com/journals/bjom. Ed. Glenn Lello. Pub. Gillian Griffith. R&P Catherine John TEL 212-424-4200. Adv. contact David Dunnachie. Circ: 1,970. **Subscr. to:** Harcourt Publishers Ltd., Foots Cray High St, Sidcup, Kent DA14 5HP, United Kingdom. TEL 44-20-8308-5700, FAX 44-20-8309-0807.

BRITISH JOURNAL OF PERIOPERATIVE NURSING. see *MEDICAL SCIENCES—Nurses And Nursing*

617.95 GBR ISSN 0007-1226
CODEN: BJPSAZ
BRITISH JOURNAL OF PLASTIC SURGERY. Text in English. 1948. 8/yr. GBP 159 to individuals; GBP 240 to institutions (effective 2002). adv. bk.rev. abstr, illus. index. back issues avail.; reprint service avail. from SWZ. *Refereed.* **Document type:** *Journal, Academic/Scholarly.* **Description:** Discusses techniques and developments in plastic surgery.
Related titles: Microform ed.: (from PQC); Online - full text ed.: (from EBSCO Publishing, RoweCom Information Quest, Swets Blackwell, IDEAL Online Library, Institute for Scientific Information).
Indexed: ASCA, Biol.Abstr., Chem.Abstr., Curr.Adv.Ecol.Sci., Curr.Cont., Dent.Ind., Environ.Sci.Poll.Mgmt., Excerp.Med., INIS Atomind., Ind.Med. (1948-), Ind.Sci.Rev., Inpharma, Int.Nurs.Ind., Jrnl.Watch Derm., Med.& Surg.Dermat., Pharm.&Out.News, Reac., Risk Abstr., Rural Devel.Abstr., Sci.Cit.Ind., Trop.Dis.Bull.
—BLDSC (2319.500000), CISTI, EMDOCS, GNLM, IDS, ingenta, KNAW. **CCC.**
Published by: (British Association of Plastic Surgeons), Churchill Livingstone (Subsidiary of: Harcourt Publishers Ltd.), Robert Stevenson House, 1-3 Baxter's Pl, Leith Walk, Edinburgh, Midlothian EH1 3AF, United Kingdom. TEL 44-131-556-2424, FAX 44-131-459-1177, cservice.harcourt.com, http://www.harcourt-international.com/journals/bjps. Ed. N Parkhouse. Pub. Gillian Griffith. R&P Catherine John TEL 212-424-4200. Adv. contact David Dunnachie. Circ: 4,800. **Subscr. to:** Harcourt Publishers Ltd., Foots Cray High St, Sidcup, Kent DA14 5HP, United Kingdom. TEL 44-20-8308-5700, FAX 44-20-8309-0807.

617 GBR ISSN 0007-1323
RD1 CODEN: BJSUAM
BRITISH JOURNAL OF SURGERY. Text in English. 1913. m., latest vol.89, 2002. GBP 90 in Europe to individuals; USD 156 in North America to individuals; GBP 104 elsewhere to individuals; GBP 175 in Europe to institutions; USD 300 in North America to institutions; GBP 193 elsewhere to institutions (effective 2002). adv. bk.rev. abstr, illus. index. back issues avail. *Refereed.* **Document type:** *Academic/Scholarly.* **Description:** Publishes original papers and reviews covering the latest techniques, treatment, and advances in surgery. Includes abstracts of the Surgical Research and the Vascular Societies.
Related titles: CD-ROM ed.: (from Ovid Technologies, Inc.); Microform ed.: (from PQC); Online - full text ed.: ISSN 1365-2168. 1997. GBP 81 in Europe to individuals; USD 141 in North America to individuals; GBP 81 elsewhere to individuals; GBP 158 in Europe to institutions; USD 270 in North America to institutions; GBP 158 elsewhere to institutions (effective 2002) (from Ovid Technologies, Inc., EBSCO Publishing, O C L C Online Computer Library Center, Inc., RoweCom Information Quest, ingenta, Munksgaard & Blackwell Science's Synergy, Swets Blackwell, Institute for Scientific Information); Supplement: British Journal of Surgery. Supplement. ISSN 1355-7688.
Indexed: AIM, ASCA, Abstr.Hyg., Abstr.Inter.Med., Agri.& Environ.Biotech.Abstr. (coverage dropped), Biol.Abstr., Chem.Abstr., Curr.Adv.Ecol.Sci., Curr.Cont., Dairy Sci.Abstr., Dent.Ind., Derwent Biotech.Abstr., Dok.Arbeitsmed., Environ.Sci.Poll.Mgmt., Excerp.Med., Helminthol.Abstr., INIS Atomind., Ind.Med. (1913-), Ind.Sci.Rev., Ind.Vet., Inpharma, Int.Abstr.Biol.Sci., Int.Nurs.Ind., Kidney, Med.& Surg.Dermat., Neurosci.Cit.Ind., Nutr.Abstr., Pharm.&Out.News, Pig News & Info., Pollut.Abstr., Protozool.Abstr., Reac., Rev.Med.& Vet.Mycol., Risk Abstr., SSCI (coverage dropped), Saf.Sci.Abstr., Sci.Cit.Ind., Small Anim.Abstr., Sugar Ind.Abstr., Triticale Abstr., Trop.Dis.Bull., Vet.Bull.
—BLDSC (2325.000000), ADONIS, CISTI, EMDOCS, GNLM, IDS, ingenta, KNAW. **CCC.**
Published by: (Surgery Research Society), Blackwell Science Ltd., PO Box 88, Oxford OX2 0NE, United Kingdom. TEL 44-1865-206180, 44-1865-206002, FAX 44-1865-206219, jnl.orders@blacksci.co.uk, http://www.blackwell-science.com/~cgilib/jnlpage.asp?Journal=bjs&File=bjs, http://www.blackwellpublishing.com. Eds. J Farndon, J Murie. Pub. Allen Stevens. R&P Sophie Savage. Adv. contact Jenny Applin. Circ: 8,800.

C I N N REPORT. see *MEDICAL SCIENCES—Psychiatry And Neurology*

617 TUR ISSN 1016-5118
CAGDAS CERRAHI DERGISI. Text in Turkish; Summaries in English. 1987. q. USD 60 (effective 2001). **Document type:** *Journal, Academic/Scholarly.*
Published by: Logos Yayincilik Ticaret A.S., Yildiz Posta Cad., Sinan Apt. No. 36 D 66-67, Gayrettepe, Istanbul 80280, Turkey. TEL 90-212-2885022, FAX 90-212-2116185, info@logos.com.tr, http://logos.com.tr. Ed. A Vedat Durgun.

617 FRA ISSN 0301-0791
CAHIERS DE CHIRURGIE. Text in French. 1972. 4/yr. FRF 550 to non-members; FRF 600 foreign to non-members; FRF 270 to members; FRF 300 foreign to members. adv. bk.rev.
Indexed: Biol.Abstr.
Published by: College National des Chirurgiens Francais, 7 av. Theophile Gautier, Paris 75016, France. TEL 46-47-71-04, FAX 45-27-15-39. Ed. Dr. J Meurette. adv.: B&W page FRF 3,900, color page FRF 9,800; 297 x 210. Circ: 4,000.

CANADIAN JOURNAL OF CARDIOLOGY. see *MEDICAL SCIENCES—Cardiovascular Diseases*

617.95 CAN ISSN 1195-2199
CANADIAN JOURNAL OF PLASTIC SURGERY. Text in English. 1993. bi-m. CND 90 domestic to individuals; USD 90 in United States to individuals; USD 100 elsewhere to individuals; CND 110 domestic to institutions; USD 110 in United States to institutions; USD 120 elsewhere to institutions (effective 2000). adv. **Document type:** *Academic/Scholarly.*
Indexed: CBCA Ref.
—BLDSC (3034.520000), CISTI, GNLM.
Published by: Pulsus Group Inc., 2902 S Sheridan Way, Oakville, ON L6J 7L6, Canada. TEL 905-829-4770, FAX 905-829-4799, pulsus@pulsus.com, http://www.pulsus.com. Ed. Dr. Peter Wyshynski. Pub. Robert B Kalina. adv.: B&W page CND 1,530, color page CND 2,840; trim 10.88 x 8.13. Circ: 5,200.

617 CAN ISSN 0008-428X
CODEN: CJSUAX
CANADIAN JOURNAL OF SURGERY/JOURNAL CANADIEN DE CHIRURGIE. Short title: C J S - J C C. Text in English, French. 1957. 6/yr. CND 160 domestic to institutions; CND 121 foreign to institutions (effective 1999). adv. bk.rev. bibl, charts, illus. index. back issues avail.; reprints avail. *Refereed.* **Document type:** *Academic/Scholarly.* **Description:** Presents high quality original articles, symposia reports and reviews, contributions on social issues, surgical practice, surgical biology for the clinician, radiology for surgeons and book reviews.
Related titles: Microform ed.: (from PQC); Online - full text ed.: (from ProQuest Information & Learning, LexisNexis, Institute for Scientific Information).
Indexed: ASCA, Biol.Abstr., CBCA Ref., Chem.Abstr., Curr.Cont., Dent.Ind., Environ.Sci.Poll.Mgmt., Excerp.Med., Helminthol.Abstr., INIS Atomind., Ind.Med. (1957-), Ind.Sci.Rev., Inpharma, NRN, Nutr.Abstr., Pharm.&Out.News, Pollut.Abstr., Reac., Ref.Zh., Rev.Med.& Vet.Mycol., Risk Abstr., Saf.Sci.Abstr., Sci.Cit.Ind.
—BLDSC (3035.800000), CISTI, GNLM, IDS, ingenta, KNAW. **CCC.**
Published by: Canadian Medical Association, 1867 Alta Vista Dr, Ottawa, ON K1H 5K9, Canada. TEL 613-731-9331, FAX 613-523-0937, pubs@cma.ca, http://www.cma.ca/cjs. Ed. Dr. Jonathan L Meakins. adv.: B&W page CND 1,300, color page CND 2,725; trim 10.88 x 8.13. Circ: 2,839.

CANADIAN OPERATING ROOM NURSING JOURNAL. see *MEDICAL SCIENCES—Nurses And Nursing*

617 616.1 USA ISSN 1072-9798
CARDIAC SURGERY. Text in English. 1992. irreg., latest vol.4, 1995. price varies. **Document type:** *Monographic series.*
—CISTI, KNAW.
Published by: Kluwer Academic - Plenum Publishers (Subsidiary of: Wolters Kluwer N.V.), 233 Spring St, New York, NY 10013-1578. TEL 212-620-8000, 800-221-9369, FAX 212-463-0742, info@plenum.com, http://www.plenum.com. Eds. A C Cernaianu, A J Delrossi.

CARDIOVASCULAR SURGERY. see *MEDICAL SCIENCES—Cardiovascular Diseases*

CARDIOVASCULAR SURGERY. see *MEDICAL SCIENCES—Cardiovascular Diseases*

CESKA A SLOVENSKA NEUROLOGIE A NEUROCHIRURGIE. see *MEDICAL SCIENCES—Psychiatry And Neurology*

617 USA ISSN 1052-3359
CODEN: CSCAFT
CHEST SURGERY CLINICS OF NORTH AMERICA. Text in English. 1991. q. USD 143 domestic to individuals; USD 161 in Canada to individuals; USD 187 elsewhere to individuals; USD 188 domestic to institutions; USD 232 foreign to institutions; USD 59 per issue (effective 2001). index. back issues avail. **Document type:** *Academic/Scholarly.* **Description:** Covers a single specific topic in the diagnosis or surgical treatment of lung, heart, and throat diseases in each issue.
Related titles: Microform ed.: (from PQC).
Indexed: Excerp.Med. (1995-), Ind.Med. (1991-).
—BLDSC (3172.604300), CISTI, EMDOCS, GNLM, KNAW.
Published by: W.B. Saunders Co. (Subsidiary of: Harcourt Publishers Ltd.), 11830 Westline Industrial Dr, St Louis, MO 63146. TEL 800-325-4177, http://www.wbsaunders.com. Ed. Dr. L Penfield Faber. **Subscr. to:** Periodicals Fulfillment, 6277 Sea Harbor Dr, 4th Fl, Orlando, FL 32891-4800. TEL 800-654-2452, FAX 800-874-6418.

CHINA MEDICAL ABSTRACTS (SURGERY). see *ABSTRACTING AND INDEXING SERVICES*

615.534 GBR ISSN 0009-4714
CHIROPODY REVIEW. Text in English. 1939. bi-m. GBP 15 domestic; GBP 25 foreign (effective 2000). adv. bk.rev. *Refereed.* **Document type:** *Trade, Academic/Scholarly.* **Description:** Features innovations in the field of podiatry.
Published by: Institute of Chiropodists, 27 Wright St, Southport, Merseyside PR9 0TL, United Kingdom. TEL 44-2392-768000, FAX 44-2392-504823. Ed. R H S Henry. R&P R.H.S. Henry. Adv. contact Jill Burnett Hurst. Circ: 2,500.

617 DEU ISSN 0009-4722
DER CHIRURG; Zeitschrift fuer alle Gebiete der operativen Medizin. Text in German. 1928. m. EUR 332.74 domestic; EUR 319.34 in Germany; EUR 30.40 newsstand/cover foreign (effective 2002). adv. bk.rev. abstr, bibl, charts, illus. index. back issues avail.; reprint service avail. from ISI. *Refereed.* **Document type:** *Journal, Academic/Scholarly.* **Description:** Covers all aspects of surgery and related fields of medicine.
Related titles: Microform ed.: (from PQC); Online - full text ed.: ISSN 1433-0385 (from EBSCO Publishing, RoweCom Information Quest, Swets Blackwell, Springer LINK, Institute for Scientific Information).
Indexed: ASCA, Abstr.Hyg., Agri.& Environ.Biotech.Abstr. (coverage dropped), Biol.Abstr., Chem.Abstr., Curr.Adv.Cancer Res., Curr.Cont., Derwent Biotech.Abstr., Dok.Arbeitsmed., Excerp.Med., Helminthol.Abstr., INIS Atomind., Ind.Med. (1928-), Ind.Sci.Rev., Inpharma, Int.Nurs.Ind., Nutr.Abstr., Pharm.&Out.News, Reac., Rev.Med.& Vet.Mycol., Sci.Cit.Ind.
—BLDSC (3181.150000), CISTI, GNLM, IDS, Infotrieve, KNAW. **CCC.**
Published by: (Berufsverband der Deutschen Chirurgen e.V.), Springer-Verlag (Subsidiary of: BertelsmannSpringer), Tiergartenstr 17, Heidelberg 69121, Germany. TEL 49-6221-345-0, FAX 49-6221-345229, subscriptions@springer.de, http://link.springer.de/link/service/journals/00104/index.htm, http://www.springer.de. Eds. C Herfarth, V Schumpelick. **Subscr. in N. America to:** Springer-Verlag New York Inc., PO Box 2485, Secaucus, NJ 07096-2485. TEL 212-460-1500, FAX 212-473-6272. **Co-sponsor:** Deutsche Gesellschaft fuer Chirurgie.

617 ROM ISSN 1221-9118
CODEN: RCOCDA
CHIRURGIA. Text in Romanian; Summaries in English, French, German, Russian. 1952. bi-m. USD 25. adv. bk.rev. abstr, charts, illus.
Supersedes in part (in 1990): Revista de Chirurgie, Oncologie, Radiologie, O.R.L., Oftalmologie, Stomatologie, Chirurgia (0377-5003); Formerly (until 1975): Chirurgia (0009-4730)
Indexed: Biol.Abstr., Chem.Abstr., Excerp.Med., Ind.Med. (1990-).
—CISTI, GNLM.
Published by: Uniunea Societatilor de Stiinte Medicale din Rumania, Str. Progresului 8, Bucharest 70754, Romania. **Subscr. to:** ILEXIM, Str. 13 Decembrie 3, PO Box 136-137, Bucharest 70116, Romania.

617 BGR ISSN 0450-2167
CODEN: KHIGAF
CHIRURGIA. Text in Bulgarian; Summaries in English, Russian. 1948. bi-m. BGL 24; USD 72 foreign (effective 2002). **Document type:** *Journal.*
Indexed: Chem.Abstr., Dent.Ind., Excerp.Med., Helminthol.Abstr., INIS Atomind., Ind.Med. (1951-).
—BLDSC (0394.790000), CASDDS, CISTI, GNLM.
Published by: (Bulgaria. Ministerstvo na Narodnoto Zdrave), Izdatelstvo Meditsina i Fizkultura, 11 Pl Slaveikov, Sofia 1080, Bulgaria. Ed. N Vasilev. Circ: 1,200. **Co-sponsor:** Nauchno Druzhestvo po Chirurgia.

617 ITA ISSN 0394-9508
CHIRURGIA. Text in Italian; Summaries in English. 1988. bi-m. USD 125 to individuals; USD 165 to institutions (effective 1999). adv. bk.rev. bibl, charts, illus. back issues avail. *Refereed.* **Document type:** *Academic/Scholarly.* **Description:** Original articles on clinical and experimental surgery.
Indexed: Excerp.Med.
—BLDSC (3181.183000), CISTI, EMDOCS, GNLM, KNAW.
Published by: (Societa Italiana di Chirurgia), Edizioni Minerva Medica, Corso Bramante, 83-85, Turin, TO 10126, Italy. TEL 39-11-678282, FAX 39-11-674502. Ed. Giuseppe Pezzuoli. Pub. Alberto Oliaro. Adv. contact F Filippo. B&W page USD 1,400, color page USD 2,300; trim 280 x 215. Circ: 5,000 (paid).

617 ITA ISSN 0009-4749
CODEN: CHOMA9
CHIRURGIA DEGLI ORGANI DI MOVIMENTO. Text in Italian, English. 1917. q. ITL 90,000, USD 110 (effective 2000). adv. bk.rev. abstr, bibl, illus. **Document type:** *Academic/Scholarly.*
Indexed: Biol.Abstr., Chem.Abstr., Dent.Ind., Excerp.Med., Ind.Med. (1917-).
—BLDSC (3181.300000), CISTI, GNLM, KNAW.
Published by: Nuova Casa Editrice Licinio Cappelli di G.E.M. s.r.l., Via Luigi Carlo Farini, 14, Bologna, BO 40124, Italy. TEL 39-051-239060, FAX 39-051-239286. Ed. Nicola Milana. Circ: 3,000.

616 ITA ISSN 0392-0771
CHIRURGIA DEL PIEDE. Text and summaries in English, Italian. 1977. 3/yr. USD 105 to individuals; USD 155 to institutions (effective 2000 - 2001). adv. *Refereed.* **Document type:** *Academic/Scholarly.* **Description:** Covers the anatomy, physiology, pathology and clinical medicine of the foot.
Formerly: Rivista di Chirurgia del Piede
Indexed: AMED, Excerp.Med.
—BLDSC (3181.360000), CISTI, EMDOCS.
Published by: Edizioni Minerva Medica, Corso Bramante, 83-85, Turin, TO 10126, Italy. TEL 39-11-678282, FAX 39-11-674502. Ed. Giacomo Pisani. Pub. Alberto Oliaro. Adv. contact F Filippo. B&W page USD 1,200, color page USD 2,000; trim 280 x 215. Circ: 2,000 (paid).

617 ITA ISSN 0009-4757
CODEN: CHPAAC
CHIRURGIA E PATOLOGIA SPERIMENTALE✶. Text in Italian. 1953. q. ITL 47,000, USD 59. adv.
Indexed: Biol.Abstr., Chem.Abstr., Dent.Ind., Excerp.Med., Ind.Med. (coverage dropped).
—CISTI, GNLM.
Published by: Universita Cattolica del Sacro Cuore, Clinica Chirurgica, Via Della Pineta Sacchetti, 526, Rome, RM 00168, Italy. Circ: 500.

CHIRURGIA GASTROENTEROLOGICA; rassegna trimestrale di chirurgia dell'apparato digerente e degli organi addominali. see *MEDICAL SCIENCES—Gastroenterology*

617 ITA ISSN 0009-4773
CHIRURGIA ITALIANA. Text in Italian; Summaries in English. 1947. bi-m. ITL 270,000; ITL 330,000 foreign (effective 1998). adv. bk.rev. index, cum.index.
Indexed: Biol.Abstr., Chem.Abstr., Excerp.Med., Ind.Med. (1947-).
—CISTI, GNLM.
Published by: Bi & Gi Editori, Via Ca' Di Cozzi, 41, Verona, VR 37124, Italy. TEL 39-45-8300968, FAX 39-45-8300970, bi&gi.editori@alice.it.

617.95 HRV ISSN 0009-4781
CODEN: CMXPAU
CHIRURGIA MAXILLOFACIALIS ET PLASTICA/ MAXILLOFACIAL AND PLASTIC SURGERY. Text in Croatian, English; Abstracts in English. 1957. 3/yr. USD 30. adv. bk.rev. reprint service avail. from IRC. **Description:** Publishes articles on maxillofacial, plastic and reconstructive surgery, as well as related disciplines.
Related titles: Online - full text ed.
Indexed: Dent.Ind., Excerp.Med., Ind.Med. (1956-).
—CISTI, GNLM.
Published by: Hrvatski Lijecnicki Zbor, Drustvo za Maksilofacijalnu i Plasticnu Kirurgiju/Croatian Medical Association, Society for Maxillofacial and Plastic Surgery, Subiceva 9, Zagreb, Croatia. TEL 385-41-420-470, FAX 385-41-425-629. Ed. Darco Mocan. Circ: 500.

617 FRA ISSN 1297-3203
CODEN: AMSPEL
▼ **CHIRURGIE DE LA MAIN.** Text in English, French. 2000. bi-m. EUR 165 in Europe to individuals; USD 211 elsewhere to individuals; EUR 172 in Europe to institutions; USD 224 elsewhere to institutions (effective 2002). **Document type:** *Academic/Scholarly.*
Formed by the merger of (1996-2000): Main (1262-3601); (1990-2000): Annales de Chirurgie de la Main et du Membre Superieur (1153-2424); Which was formerly (1982-1989): Annales de Chirurgie de la Main (0753-9053)
Indexed: Biol.Abstr., Excerp.Med., Ind.Med. (coverage dropped).
—BLDSC (3181.466000), CISTI, EMDOCS, GNLM, KNAW. **CCC.**
Published by: (Societes de Chirurgie de la Main), Elsevier Paris, Editions Scientifiques et Medicales (Subsidiary of: Reed Elsevier plc. group), 23 rue Linois, Paris 75015, France. http://www.elsevier.com/locate/main. Circ: 4,000. **Co-sponsors:** Societe Belge de Chirurgie de la Main; Groupe d'Etude de la Main; Societe Francaise de Chirurgie de la Main.

617 DEU ISSN 0009-4846
CODEN: CHPXBE
CHIRURGISCHE PRAXIS; taegliche Praxis der gesamten Chirurgie. Text in German. 1957. 4/yr. EUR 162 (effective 2002). bk.rev. abstr, charts, illus. index, cum.index every 5 yrs. **Document type:** *Journal, Academic/Scholarly.* **Description:** Articles about orthopedic, internal and plastic surgery, featuring new techniques. Includes questions and answers, detailed photographs.
Related titles: Microfilm ed.: (from PQC).
Indexed: Biol.Abstr., Excerp.Med.
—CISTI, GNLM, Infotrieve. **CCC.**
Published by: Hans Marseille Vertrieb Medizinischer Zeitschriften, Buerkleinstr 12, Munich 80538, Germany. TEL 49-89-227988, FAX 49-89-2904643, marseille-verlag@t-online.de, http://www.marseille-verlag.com. Circ: 5,000.

617 JPN
CHUBU GEKA GAKKAI SOKAIGO/CHUBU SURGICAL SOCIETY. PROCEEDINGS OF ANNUAL MEETING. Text in Japanese. 1965. a. **Document type:** *Proceedings.*
Published by: Chubu Geka Gakkai, Nagoya Daigaku Igakubu Dai 1 Gekagaku Kyoshitsu, 65 Tsurumai-cho, Showa-ku, Nagoya-shi, Aichi-ken 466-0065, Japan.

617 ESP ISSN 0213-5353
CIRUGIA DE URGENCIA. Text in Spanish. 1986. 10/yr.
Address: Antonio Lopez Aguado, 4, Madrid 28029, Spain. TEL 1-314-43-38, FAX 1-314-44-99. Circ: 5,184.

617 URY ISSN 0009-7381
CODEN: CRGUAT
CIRUGIA DEL URUGUAY. Abbreviated title: C U. Contents page in English, Spanish. 1920. bi-m. USD 35 to non-members (effective 1996). adv. abstr, bibl, illus. index. Supplement avail. **Document type:** *Academic/Scholarly.*
Formerly (1965-1969): Revista de Cirugia del Uruguay; Supersedes (1930-1964): Sociedad de Cirugia del Uruguay. Boletines
Indexed: Biol.Abstr., Excerp.Med., INIS Atomind.
—BLDSC (3267.623000).
Published by: Sociedad de Cirugia del Uruguay, Casilla de Correos 10972, Montevideo, Uruguay. Circ: 1,000 (controlled). **Co-sponsor:** Congresos Uruguayos de Cirugia.

617 ESP ISSN 0009-739X
CODEN: CRESAD
CIRUGIA ESPANOLA. Text in English, French, Spanish; Abstracts in English. 1946. m. USD 129. adv. bk.rev. abstr, bibl, illus, charts. index. **Document type:** *Academic/Scholarly.*
Formerly (until 1969): Cirugia, Ginecologia y Urologia (0412-5878)
Indexed: Biol.Abstr., Chem.Abstr., Excerp.Med., Helminthol.Abstr., Ind.Med.Esp.
—CASDDS, CINDOC, CISTI, GNLM.
Published by: (Asociacion Espanola de Cirujanos), Ediciones Doyma S.A., Traversa de Gracia, 17-21, Barcelona 08021, Spain. TEL 34-93-200-0711, FAX 34-93-209-1136, TELEX 51964 INK E. Ed. J L Balibrea Cantero. Adv. contact Julio Esteva. color page ESP 238,000; trim 180 x 210. Circ: 2,800.

617.95 ESP ISSN 0376-7892
CIRUGIA PLASTICA IBERO LATINOAMERICANA. Text in Spanish; Summaries in English, Spanish. 1975. q. ESP 6,000, USD 60 (effective 1999 & 2000). adv. bk.rev. charts, illus. cum.index: 1968-1998. reprint service avail. from PQC. **Document type:** *Academic/Scholarly.*
Formed by the merger of: Revista Latinoamericana de Cirugia Plastica (0034-9755); (1968-1975): Revista Espanola de Cirugia Plastica (0034-9364)
Related titles: Diskette ed.; Microform ed.: (from PQC).
Indexed: Biol.Abstr., Excerp.Med., Ind.Med.Esp.
—BLDSC (3267.610000), EMDOCS, GNLM.
Published by: Sociedad Espanola de Cirugia Plastica, Casilla 10059, Madrid 28080, Spain. TEL 34-91-4454934, FAX 34-91-4454934, cirplast@teleline.es. Ed. F Rodriguez Duran. R&P, Adv. contact Juan Quetglas. B&W page USD 300. Circ: 1,000. **Co-sponsor:** Federacion Ibero Latinoamericana de Cirugia Plastica.

617.95 URY ISSN 0009-7403
CIRUGIA PLASTICA URUGUAYA. Text in Spanish; Summaries in English, Spanish. 1960. q.
Formerly: Cirugia Plastica del Uruguay
Published by: (Sociedad de Cirugia Plastica del Uruguay), Hospital de Clinicas "Dr. Manuel Quintela", Universidad de la Republica, Avda. Italia s-n, Montevideo, Uruguay.

617 MEX ISSN 0009-7411
CIRUGIA Y CIRUJANOS. Text in Spanish. 1933. bi-m. USD 100 (effective 1995). adv. bk.rev. abstr, bibl, illus. **Document type:** *Academic/Scholarly.* **Description:** Publishes surgical and medical articles.
Indexed: Biol.Abstr., Chem.Abstr., Excerp.Med., Ind.Med. (coverage dropped).
—CISTI, GNLM, KNAW.

M

Published by: Academia Mexicana de Cirugia/Mexican Academy of Surgery, Col. Centro, Deleg. Cuauhtemoc, Apartado Postal 7994, Mexico City, DF 06080, Mexico. TEL 52-5-588-0458, FAX 52-5-761-2581. Ed. Dr. Humberto Hurtado. Adv. contact Francisco Tenorio Gonzalez. Circ: 3,000.

617.522 USA ISSN 1055-6656
RD525 CODEN: CPJOEG
CLEFT PALATE - CRANIOFACIAL JOURNAL; Official Publication of the American Cleft Palate-Craniofacial Association. Text in English. 1964. bi-m. USD 210 domestic to institutions; USD 245 foreign to institutions; USD 235 domestic to institutions print & online eds.; USD 270 foreign to institutions print & online eds. (effective 2001). adv. bk.rev. abstr, charts, illus, stat. cum.index: 1964-1988. back issues avail. *Refereed.* **Document type:** *Academic/Scholarly.* **Description:** International interdisciplinary professional journal on clinical and research activities in cleft palate and other craniofacial anomalies.
Formerly: Cleft Palate Journal (0009-8701)
Related titles: Microform ed.: (from MIM,WWS); Online - full text ed.: (from Northern Light Technology, Inc., Institute for Scientific Information).
Indexed: ASCA, CINAHL, Chic.Per.Ind., Child Devel.Abstr., Curr.Adv.Ecol.Sci., Curr.Cont., Dent.Ind., Excerp.Med., INIS Atomind., Ind.Med. (1991-), Ind.Sci.Rev., Ind.Vet., Inpharma, Lang.& Lang.Behav.Abstr., Reac., Rehabil.Lit., SOPODA, SSCI (coverage dropped), Sci.Cit.Ind., Sociol.Abstr.
—BLDSC (3278.559800), CISTI, EMDOCS, GNLM, IDS, ingenta, KNAW. **CCC.**
Published by: (American Cleft Palate - Craniofacial Association), Allen Press, Inc., Division Alliance Communications Group, PO Box 1897, Lawrence, KS 66044. TEL 785-843-1235, FAX 785-843-1274, cpcj@allenpress.com, cpcj @allenpress.com, http://cpcj.allenpress.com, http://www.allenpress.com. Ed. Jerald B Moon. R&P Debbie Ogle TEL 412-369-4032. Adv. contact Gigi Gallinger. B&W page USD 1,100, color page USD 1,050; trim 10.88 x 8.13. Circ: 3,240 (paid).

616 ITA ISSN 0393-7577
CLINICA CHIRURGICA DEL NORD AMERICA. Text in Italian. 1968. bi-m. ITL 220,000, USD 180 (effective 1999). reprint service avail. from PQC. **Document type:** *Academic/Scholarly.*
Published by: Piccin Nuova Libraria, Via Altinate, 107, Padua, PD 35121, Italy. TEL 39-49-655566, FAX 39-49-8750693.

CLINICAL NEUROLOGY AND NEUROSURGERY; an international journal publishing papers and reports on the clinical aspects of neurology and neurosurgery. see *MEDICAL SCIENCES—Psychiatry And Neurology*

CLINICAL NEUROSURGERY: PROCEEDINGS. see *MEDICAL SCIENCES—Psychiatry And Neurology*

617 GBR ISSN 0263-4422
CLINICAL SURGERY INTERNATIONAL. Text in English. 1981. irreg., latest vol.19. adv. **Document type:** *Monographic series, Academic/Scholarly.*
—KNAW.
Published by: Churchill Livingstone (Subsidiary of: Harcourt Publishers Ltd.), Robert Stevenson House, 1-3 Baxter's Pl, Leith Walk, Edinburgh, Midlothian EH1 3AF, United Kingdom. TEL 44-131-556-2424, FAX 44-131-459-1177, http://www.churchillmed.com. R&P Catherine John TEL 212-424-4200. Adv. contact David Dunnachie. **Subscr. to:** Harcourt Publishers Ltd., Foots Cray High St, Sidcup, Kent DA14 5HP, United Kingdom. TEL 44-20-8308-5700, FAX 44-20-8309-0807.

617 DNK ISSN 0902-0063
CODEN: CLTRED
CLINICAL TRANSPLANTATION. Text in English. 1987. bi-m. USD 384 in the Americas to institutions print & online eds. combined; GBP 267 elsewhere to institutions print & online eds. combined (effective 2002). bk.rev. reprint service avail. from ISI. *Refereed.* **Document type:** *Academic/Scholarly.*
Related titles: Online - full text ed.: ISSN 1399-0012. GBP 240 (2002) (from Ovid Technologies, Inc., EBSCO Publishing, O C L C Online Computer Library Center, Inc., RoweCom Information Quest, ingenta, Munksgaard & Blackwell Science's Synergy, Swets Blackwell, Institute for Scientific Information).
Indexed: ASCA, Curr.Cont., Excerp.Med., INIS Atomind., Ind.Med. (1987-), Inpharma, Int.Abstr.Biol.Sci., Pharm.&Out.News, Protozool.Abstr., Reac., Rev.Med.& Vet.Mycol., SSCI (coverage dropped).
—BLDSC (3286.399780), CISTI, EMDOCS, GNLM, IDS, Infotrieve, ingenta, KNAW. **CCC.**
Published by: Blackwell Munksgaard, Noerre Soegade 35, PO Box 2148, Copenhagen K 1016, Denmark. TEL 45-77-33-33-33, FAX 45-77-33-33-77, customerservice@munksgaard.dk, http://journals.munksgaard.dk/clinicaltransplantation, http://www.munksgaard.dk/journals/transplantation/index.htmt. Ed. John S Najarian. Adv. contact Eric Rozario TEL 45-77-33-33-01. Circ: 800.

CLINICAL UPDATE. see *MEDICAL SCIENCES—Oncology*

617 USA ISSN 1531-0043
CLINICS IN COLON & RECTAL SURGERY. Text in English. 1988. s-a. EUR 162 to individuals; EUR 304 to institutions; EUR 76 newsstand/cover (effective 2002). adv. index. *Refereed.* **Document type:** *Journal, Academic/Scholarly.* **Description:** Explores the most pertinent clinical and research topics in this specialty.
Formerly (until 2001): Perspectives in Colon & Rectal Surgery (0894-8054)
Related titles: Online - full text ed.: ISSN 1521-5741 (from RoweCom Information Quest); ♦ Supplement: Colon and Rectal Surgery Outlook. ISSN 0894-8062.
—GNLM, Infotrieve. **CCC.**
Published by: Thieme Medical Publishers, 333 Seventh Ave, New York, NY 10001. TEL 212-760-0888, 800-782-3488, FAX 212-947-1112, http://www.thieme.com. Ed. Dr. Theodore R Schrock. Adv. contact Sally Kahn. **Orders in Europe to:** Thieme International, Postfach 301120, Stuttgart 70451, Germany. TEL 49-711-8931-0.

617 USA ISSN 0094-1298
CLINICS IN PLASTIC SURGERY. Text in English. 1974. q. USD 200 domestic to individuals; USD 231 in Canada to individuals; USD 254 elsewhere to individuals; USD 279 domestic to institutions; USD 319 foreign to institutions; USD 80 per issue (effective 2001). reprint service avail. from PQC,ISI. *Refereed.* **Document type:** *Journal, Academic/Scholarly.* **Description:** Delivers practical advice from experts in each specialty covered as well as information on new developments in a variety of specialties with a fresh perspective on problems and controversies.
Related titles: Microform ed.; Online - full text ed.: (from Institute for Scientific Information).
Indexed: ASCA, Curr.Cont., Dent.Ind., Excerp.Med., INIS Atomind., Ind.Med. (1974-), Ind.Sci.Rev., Inpharma, Int.Nurs.Ind., Med.& Surg.Dermat., Reac., SSCI (coverage dropped), Sci.Cit.Ind. (coverage dropped).
—BLDSC (3286.590000), CISTI, EMDOCS, GNLM, IDS, ingenta, KNAW. **CCC.**
Published by: W.B. Saunders Co. (Subsidiary of: Harcourt Publishers Ltd.), 11830 Westline Industrial Dr, St Louis, MO 63146. TEL 800-325-4177, http://www.wbsaunders.com. **Subscr. to:** Periodicals Fulfillment, W B Saunders Co, 6277 Sea Harbor Dr, 4th Fl, Orlando, FL 32891-4800.

617 GBR ISSN 1467-0100
▼ **COCHLEAR IMPLANTS INTERNATIONAL.** Text in English. 2000. s-a. USD 76 in North America to individuals; GBP 42 rest of world to individuals; USD 135 in North America to institutions; GBP 75 rest of world to institutions (effective 2001). **Document type:** *Journal.* **Description:** Aimed at all those involved with cochlear implants: surgery, pre- and post-operative care, research or manufacture of the implants themselves.
—BLDSC (3292.724200).
Published by: Whurr Publishers Ltd., 19b Compton Terr, London N1 2UN, United Kingdom. TEL 44-20-7359-5979, FAX 44-20-7226-5290, info@whurr.co.uk, http://www.whurrjournals.co.uk/, http://www.whurr.co.uk. Ed. John Graham. **Subscr. in N. America to:** Whurr Publishers Ltd., PO Box 1897, Lawrence, KS 66044-8897. TEL 913-843-1221, FAX 913-843-1274, am&m@allenpress.com. **Dist. by:** Turpin Distribution Services Ltd., Blackhorse Rd, Letchworth, Herts SG6 1HN, United Kingdom. TEL 44-1462-488900, FAX 44-1462-483011, custservturpin@turpinltd.com.

617 BRA ISSN 0100-6991
COLEGIO BRASILEIRO DE CIRURGIOES. REVISTA. Text in Portuguese; Abstracts in English. 1944. bi-m. BRL 270 to non-members (effective 2000). adv. bk.rev. back issues avail. *Refereed.* **Document type:** *Academic/Scholarly.* **Description:** Includes reports of original investigations, review papers, editorials, case reports, letters to the editor and proceedings of meetings.
Indexed: INIS Atomind.
Published by: Colegio Brasileiro de Cirurgioes, Rua Visconde de Silva, 52 Andar 3, Rio De Janeiro, RJ 22271-090, Brazil. TEL 55-21-5379164, FAX 55-21-2862595. Ed. Jose Antonio Gomes de Souza. Circ: 7,000.

617 AUS ISSN 1028-4001
COLLEGE OF SURGEONS HONG KONG. ANNALS. Text in English. 1997. q. AUD 397 domestic to institutions; AUD 361 in New Zealand to institutions; USD 220 elsewhere to institutions; AUD 437 domestic to institutions paper & online eds. combined; AUD 398 in New Zealand to institutions paper & online eds. combined; USD 242 elsewhere to institutions paper & online eds. combined (effective 2001). back issues avail.; reprints avail. *Refereed.* **Document type:** *Academic/Scholarly.* **Description:** Publishes clinical and research papers in all areas of surgery and related disciplines.
Related titles: Online - full text ed.: ISSN 1442-2034. AUD 358 domestic to institutions; AUD 325 in New Zealand to institutions; USD 198 elsewhere to institutions (effective 2001) (from EBSCO Publishing, O C L C Online Computer Library Center, Inc., RoweCom Information Quest, ingenta, Munksgaard & Blackwell Science's Synergy, Swets Blackwell).
—BLDSC (1022.750000). **CCC.**
Published by: (College of Surgeons Hong Kong HKG, United Christian Hospital HKG), Blackwell Science Asia Pty Ltd, PO Box 378, Carlton South, VIC 3053, Australia. TEL 61-3-9347-0300, FAX 61-3-9347-5001, info@blacksci-asia.com.au; kwokphys@ha.org.hk, http://www.blacksci.co.uk. Eds. Lyn Clearihan, Samuel P Y Kwok. R&P Chris Hum.

COLON AND RECTAL SURGERY OUTLOOK. see *MEDICAL SCIENCES—Abstracting, Bibliographies, Statistics*

617 USA ISSN 1053-749X
CODEN: CSURE
COMPLICATIONS IN SURGERY. Text in English. 1982. m. adv.
Formerly (until 1991): Infections in Surgery (0277-7746)
Media: Online - full text.
Indexed: ASCA, Curr.Cont. (coverage dropped), Excerp.Med., Rev.Med.& Vet.Mycol.
—CISTI, EMDOCS, GNLM, IDS, Infotrieve. **CCC.**
Published by: S C P Communications, Inc., 134 W 29th St, New York, NY 10001-5304. TEL 212-631-1600, editor@scp.com, http://www.medscape.com. Ed. Katherine Rice.

617.02854 USA ISSN 1092-9088
CODEN: JIGSF8
COMPUTER AIDED SURGERY. Text in English. 1995. bi-m. USD 430 in United States; USD 430 in Canada & Mexico; USD 430 elsewhere; USD 452 combined subscription in United States for print and online eds.; USD 452 combined subscription in Canada & Mexico for print and online eds.; USD 452 combined subscription elsewhere for print and online eds. (effective 2002). adv. back issues avail. *Refereed.* **Document type:** *Academic/Scholarly.* **Description:** Covers all aspects of surgery performed in conjunction with imaging, and includes the latest applications in neurosurgery, orthopedics, and other surgical subspecialties.
Formerly: Journal of Image Guided Surgery (1078-7844)
Related titles: Online - full text ed.: ISSN 1097-0150. USD 430 in United States; USD 430 in Canada & Mexico; USD 430 elsewhere (effective 2002) (from EBSCO Publishing, Wiley InterScience).
Indexed: Ergon.Abstr., Ind.Med. (1997-), Int.Nurs.Ind.
—BLDSC (3393.542410), CISTI, GNLM, Infotrieve, KNAW. **CCC.**
Published by: John Wiley & Sons, Inc., Journals (Subsidiary of: Wiley InterScience), 605 Third Ave, New York, NY 10158. TEL 212-850-6645, FAX 212-850-6021, mmchugh@wiley.com, uscs-wis@wiley.com, http://journals.wiley.com/cas/, http://www.wiley.com. Ed. Richard Bucholz. adv.: B&W page GBP 640, color page GBP 1,515; trim 210 x 279. Circ: 855. **Subscr. outside the Americas to:** John Wiley & Sons Ltd., Baffins Ln, Chichester, Sussex PO19 IUD, United Kingdom. TEL 44-1243-779777, FAX 44-1243-843232, cs-journals@wiley.co.uk, http://www.wiley.co.uk.

CONCEPTS IN NEUROSURGERY. see *MEDICAL SCIENCES—Psychiatry And Neurology*

CONTEMPORARY ISSUES IN SURGICAL PATHOLOGY. see *MEDICAL SCIENCES*

617 616.8 USA ISSN 0163-2108
CODEN: CNEUET
CONTEMPORARY NEUROSURGERY; a biweekly review of clinical neurosurgical practice. Text in English. 1978. 27/yr., latest vol.23. USD 345 domestic to individuals; USD 345 foreign to individuals; USD 345 domestic to institutions; USD 345 foreign to institutions; USD 17 newsstand/cover (effective 2002). **Document type:** *Academic/Scholarly.* **Description:** Features original articles on current topics in neurosurgery with optional Category or C.M.E. credits.
Related titles: Online - full text ed.: USD 448.50 domestic for academic site license; USD 448.50 foreign for academic site license; USD 500.25 foreign for corporate site license (effective 2002).
Indexed: e-psyche.
—BLDSC (3425.195300).
Published by: Lippincott Williams & Wilkins (Baltimore) (Subsidiary of: Wolters Kluwer N.V.), 351 W Camden St, Baltimore, MD 21201-2436. TEL 800-787-8981, FAX 410-528-4105, custerv@lww.com, http://www.Lww.com. Ed. Dr. Ali Krisht. Circ: 1,400.

617.95 USA ISSN 1527-4268
▼ **CONTEMPORARY SPINE SURGERY.** Text in English. 2000. m. USD 159 to individuals; USD 209 to institutions (effective 2002). **Document type:** *Newsletter, Academic/Scholarly.* **Description:** Each issue contains up-to-date information on a single topic of vital importance in spine surgery.
Related titles: Online - full text ed.: USD 271.70 academic site license; USD 303.05 corporate site license (effective 2002).
Published by: Lippincott Williams & Wilkins (Philadelphia) (Subsidiary of: Wolters Kluwer N.V.), 530 Walnut St, Philadelphia, PA 19106-3621. TEL 215-521-8300, FAX 215-521-8902, custserv@lww.com, http://www.lww.com/. Ed. Dr. Gunnar Andersson.

617 USA ISSN 0045-8341
RD1 CODEN: CSGYA
CONTEMPORARY SURGERY. Text in English. 1972. m. USD 79 domestic to individuals; USD 89 in Canada to individuals; USD 109 elsewhere to individuals; USD 92 domestic to institutions; USD 104 in Canada to institutions; USD 122 elsewhere to institutions; USD 39 domestic to students (effective 2001). adv. bk.rev. bibl, charts, illus. index. back issues avail.; reprint service avail. from PQC. *Refereed.* **Document type:** *Academic/Scholarly.* **Description:** Original clinical information covering the latest developments and techniques in surgery.
Related titles: Microform ed.: (from PQC); Online - full text ed.: (from ProQuest Information & Learning).
Indexed: Biol.Abstr., Excerp.Med.
—GNLM, ingenta, KNAW. **CCC.**
Published by: Dowden Health Media, Inc, 110 Summit Ave, Montvale, NJ 07645. TEL 201-391-9100, FAX 201-391-2778, contemporarysurgery@dowdenhealth.com, http://www.contemporarysurgery.com, http://www.dowdenpub.com. Ed. Gary A Soucie. Pub. Laura Dowden TEL 201-782-5737. Circ: 50,000 (controlled).

617.95 USA ISSN 1094-6810
COSMETIC SURGERY TIMES; a magazine for the innovative cosmetic surgery practice. Text in English. 1997. 10/yr., latest vol.4. USD 95 United States & Possessions; USD 140 in Canada & Mexico; USD 185 elsewhere; USD 10 newsstand/cover United States & Possessions (effective 2001). adv. tr.lit. back issues avail. *Refereed.* **Document type:** *Trade.* **Description:** Covers cosmetic surgery, research, and meetings for dermatology surgeons, plastic surgeons, facial plastic surgeons, oculoplastic surgeons, and oromaxillofacial surgeons.
—**CCC.**
Published by: Advanstar Communications Inc., Healthcare Group, 7500 Old Oak Blvd, Cleveland, OH 44130-3369. TEL 440-243-8100, FAX 440-891-2735, cosmetictimes@advanstar.com, http://www.cosmeticsurgerytimes.com; http://www.advanstar.com. Eds. Sue Guard, Tim Troy. adv.: B&W page USD 2,685, color page USD 4,185; trim 14.5 x 10. Circ: 10,340.

617.4 USA ISSN 1052-4436
RD598.5
CURRENT CRITICAL PROBLEMS IN VASCULAR SURGERY. Text in English. 1989. a. **Document type:** *Academic/Scholarly.*
—GNLM.
Published by: Quality Medical Publishing, Inc., 11970 Borman Dr., Ste. 222, St. Louis, MO 63146. TEL 314-878-7808, 800-348-7808, FAX 314-878-9937. R&P Michelle Leamon TEL 800-423-6865.

CURRENT MEDICAL LITERATURE. GENERAL SURGERY. see *MEDICAL SCIENCES—Abstracting, Bibliographies, Statistics*

CURRENT MEDICAL LITERATURE. SURGICAL INFECTION. see *MEDICAL SCIENCES—Abstracting, Bibliographies, Statistics*

CURRENT OPINION IN OTOLARYNGOLOGY & HEAD AND NECK SURGERY. see *MEDICAL SCIENCES—Otorhinolaryngology*

617.5 USA ISSN 1074-1224
RD781.C87
CURRENT PRACTICE IN FOOT & ANKLE SURGERY; a review of state-of-the-art techniques. Text in English. 1993. irreg. USD 55. back issues avail. **Document type:** *Monographic series.*
Published by: McGraw-Hill Companies, Professional & Reference Division, Engineering and Science Group, 11 W 19th St, New York, NY 10011. TEL 212-337-6017. Eds. Dr. Carol C Frey, Dr. Glenn B Pfeffer.

617 USA ISSN 0011-3840
RD1 CODEN: CPSUA
CURRENT PROBLEMS IN SURGERY. Short title: C P S. Text in English. 1964. m. USD 115 domestic to individuals; USD 132 foreign to individuals; USD 186 domestic to institutions; USD 206 foreign to institutions; USD 57 domestic to students; USD 73 foreign to students; USD 18 per issue domestic (effective 2001). charts, illus. cum.index. back issues avail.; reprint service avail. from PQC. *Refereed.* **Description:** Written by recognized surgical experts. CPS is a monographic journal which provides current fully referenced information to practicing surgeons.
Related titles: Microfilm ed.: (from PQC); Online - full text ed.: (from Institute for Scientific Information).
Indexed: AIM, ASCA, Curr.Cont., Dent.Ind., Excerp.Med., Ind.Med. (1964-), Ind.Sci.Rev., Inpharma, Pharm.&Out.News, Reac., Sci.Cit.Ind.
—BLDSC (3501.450000), CISTI, EMDOCS, GNLM, IDS, ingenta, KNAW. **CCC.**
Published by: Mosby, Inc. (Subsidiary of: Elsevier Science), 11830 Westline Industrial Dr, St Louis, MO 63146-3318. TEL 314-872-8370, 800-325-4177, FAX 314-432-1380, http://www.mosby.com/cpsurg, http://www.mosby.com/periodicals. Ed. Dr. Samuel A Wells Jr. Circ: 9,691.

617 USA ISSN 0149-7944
RD1 CODEN: CUSUDB
CURRENT SURGERY. Text in English. 1943. bi-m. EUR 158 in Europe to individuals; JPY 21,000 in Japan to individuals; USD 132 elsewhere to individuals; EUR 202 in Europe to institutions; JPY 26,800 in Japan to institutions; USD 176 elsewhere to institutions (effective 2002). adv. illus. index. *Refereed.* **Document type:** *Academic/Scholarly.* **Description:** Publishes surveys and reports on significant articles on general surgery, surgical subspecialties and nonsurgical medicine.
Formerly (until 1978): Review of Surgery (0034-6780)
Related titles: Microfilm ed.: (from PQC,WWS); Online - full text ed.: (from ingenta, Swets Blackwell, ScienceDirect).
Indexed: Biol.Abstr., Chem.Abstr., Dent.Ind., INIS Atomind., Ind.Med. (coverage dropped).
—BLDSC (3504.047000), CASDDS, CISTI, EMDOCS, GNLM, IDS, Infotrieve, ingenta. **CCC.**
Published by: (Association of Program Directors in Surgery), Elsevier Science, 655 Ave of the Americas, New York, NY 10010. FAX 212-633-3990, usinfo-f@elsevier.com, http://www.elsevier.com/locate/cursur. Ed. Dr. Walter J Pories. Pub. Lisa Berger. Adv. contact Hank Blaney. B&W page USD 860, color page USD 1,855. Circ: 1,600 (paid). **Subscr. in Australasia and the Far East to:** Elsevier Science (Singapore) Pte Ltd, No.1 Temasek Ave, 17-01 Millenia Tower, Singapore 039192, Singapore. TEL 65-434-3727, FAX 65-337-2230; **Subscr. in Japan to:** Elsevier Science Inc - Japan Regional Office, 9-15 Higashi-Azabu 1-chome, Minato-ku, Tokyo 106-0044, Japan. TEL 81-3-5561-5033; **Subscr. outside the Americas to:** Elsevier Science BV, PO Box 211, Amsterdam 1000 AE, Netherlands. TEL 31-20-485-3757, FAX 31-20-485-3432.

617 USA ISSN 0894-2277
CURRENT SURGICAL DIAGNOSIS & TREATMENT*. Text in English. 1980. irreg., latest vol.10, 1993. USD 45 (effective 1998). **Document type:** *Academic/Scholarly.*
Related titles: CD-ROM ed.
—**CCC.**
Published by: Appleton & Lange, Journal Division (Subsidiary of: Simon & Schuster Company), 11 W 19th St, New York, CT 10011-4209. TEL 203-406-4500, FAX 203-406-4600. Ed. Lawrence W Way.

CURRENT TECHNIQUES IN ARTHROSCOPY. see *MEDICAL SCIENCES—Orthopedics And Traumatology*

CURRENT TECHNIQUES IN NEUROSURGERY. see *MEDICAL SCIENCES—Psychiatry And Neurology*

617 USA ISSN 1051-8452
CURRENT THERAPY IN VASCULAR SURGERY. Text in English. 1987. irreg. **Document type:** *Monographic series.*
—**CCC.**
Published by: Mosby, Inc. (Subsidiary of: Elsevier Science), 11830 Westline Industrial Dr, St Louis, MO 63146-3318. TEL 314-872-8370, 800-325-4177, FAX 314-432-1380, http://www.mosby.com/periodicals.

CURRENT TOPICS IN GENERAL THORACIC SURGERY. see *MEDICAL SCIENCES—Otorhinolaryngology*

617 TUR ISSN 1301-1839
DAMAR CERRAHISI DERGISI/TURKISH JOURNAL OF VASCULAR SURGERY. Text in Turkish; Summaries in English, Turkish. 1992. 3/yr. membership. adv. back issues avail. **Document type:** *Academic/Scholarly.* **Description:** Covers vascular surgery, diseases and treatment.
Published by: Nobel Tip Kitapevleri Ltd., Millet Cad 82-1, Capa Topkapi, Istanbul, Turkey. TEL 90-212-5856746. Ed., R&P, Adv. contact Murat Kayabali TEL 90-212-531-2082. Circ: 500.

617 DNK ISSN 0900-4041
DANSK KIRURGISK SELSKAB. NYHEDSBREV. Text in Danish. 1982. q. membership. adv. bk.rev. **Document type:** *Newsletter, Proceedings, Academic/Scholarly.* **Description:** Information on the activities of the society, with programs and abstracts of meetings held by the society.
Published by: Dansk Kirurgisk Selskab/Danish Surgical Society, Kirurgisk Afd D, Amtssygehuset, Gentofte, Hellerup 2900, Denmark. TEL 45-39-77-33-68, FAX 45-39-77-76-29. Ed. Dr. Niels Baekgaard.

DENTO-MAXILLO-FACIAL RADIOLOGY. SUPPLEMENT. see *MEDICAL SCIENCES—Radiology And Nuclear Medicine*

DENTOMAXILLOFACIAL RADIOLOGY. see *MEDICAL SCIENCES—Radiology And Nuclear Medicine*

617 USA ISSN 1076-0512
CODEN: DESUFE
DERMATOLOGIC SURGERY. Text in English. 1975. m. USD 140 domestic to individuals; USD 160 in Canada & Mexico to individuals; USD 190 elsewhere to individuals; USD 295 domestic to institutions; USD 315 in Canada & Mexico to institutions; USD 345 elsewhere to institutions; USD 154 to individuals print & online eds. combined; USD 324.50 to institutions print & online eds. combined (effective 2001). adv. bk.rev. index. reprints avail. *Refereed.* **Document type:** *Journal, Academic/Scholarly.* **Description:** Publishes information on new research, methods and instruments used in performing all types of cutaneous surgery.
Former titles (until 1995): Journal of Dermatologic Surgery and Oncology (0148-0812); (until 1976): Journal of Dermatologic Surgery (0097-9716)
Related titles: Microform ed.: (from PQC); ♦ Online - full text ed.: Dermatologic Surgery Online. ISSN 1524-4725.
Indexed: ASCA, Biol.Abstr., Curr.Adv.Cancer Res., Curr.Cont., Dent.Ind., Excerp.Med., Helminthol.Abstr., INIS Atomind., Ind.Med. (1995-), Ind.Sci.Rev., Inpharma, Int.Abstr.Biol.Sci., Jrnl.Watch Derm., Med.& Surg.Dermat., Nutr.Abstr., Pharm.&Out.News, Reac., Rev.Med.& Vet.Mycol., Sci.Cit.Ind.
—BLDSC (3555.140000), CISTI, GNLM, IDS, ingenta, KNAW. **CCC.**
Published by: (American Society for Dermatologic Surgery), Blackwell Science Inc., Commerce Pl, 350 Main St, Malden, MA 02148-5018. TEL 781-388-8250, 800-759-6102, FAX 781-388-8255, TELEX 420643 AEP UI, journals@blacksci.com, http://www.blackwell-science.com. Ed. Dr. R L Moyo. R&P Tracey Davies. Adv. contact Jenny Applin. Circ: 13,015. **Co-sponsors:** American College of Mohs Micrographic Surgery and Cutaneous Oncology; International Society for Dermatologic Surgery; North American Society of Phlebology; International Society of Hair Restoration Surgery; International Society of Cosmetic.

M

617 USA ISSN 1524-4725
DERMATOLOGIC SURGERY ONLINE. Text in English. m. USD 126 to individuals; USD 266 to institutions (effective 2001). **Document type:** *Academic/Scholarly.*
Media: Online - full text (from EBSCO Publishing, Munksgaard & Blackwell Science's Synergy, O C L C Online Computer Library Center, Inc., RoweCom Information Quest, ingenta, Swets Blackwell, Institute for Scientific Information). **Related titles:** Microform ed.: (from PQC); ♦ Print ed.: Dermatologic Surgery. ISSN 1076-0512.
Published by: Blackwell Science Inc., Commerce Pl, 350 Main St, Malden, MA 02148-5018. TEL 781-388-8250, 888-661-5800, FAX 781-388-8255, journals@blacksci.com, http://www.blackwell-science.com/~cgilib/bsinc.bin?Journal=practice.

617 RUS ISSN 1560-9510
DETSKAYA KHIRURGIYA. Text in Russian; Summaries in English. 1997. bi-m. USD 150 foreign (effective 2000). adv. bk.rev., Website rev. abstr, bibl, illus. back issues avail. **Document type:** *Journal, Academic/Scholarly.* **Description:** Provides experimental and clinical data for pediatric surgical treatment, anesthesiology. Also examines management.
Related titles: Fax ed.
Indexed: Ref.Zh.
Published by: Izdatel'stvo Meditsina, Petroverigskii per 6-8, Moscow 101000, Russian Federation. TEL 7-095-9248785, 7-095-928-86-48, FAX 7-095-9211355, 7-095-9286003, http://www.medit.ru. Ed. Yu F Isakov. Pub. A M Stochik. R&P Yu Isakov. Adv. contact O A Fadeeva TEL 7-095-923-51-40. Circ: 500. **Dist. by:** Mezhdunarodnaya Kniga, B Yakimanka 39, Moscow 117049, Russian Federation. TEL 7-095-2384967, FAX 7-095-2384634; **US dist. addr.:** East View Publications, 3020 Harbor Ln N, Minneapolis, MN 55447. TEL 612-550-0961.

617 DEU
DEUTSCHE GESELLSCHAFT FUER CHIRURGIE. ZEITSCHRIFT. Text in German. 1972. 5/yr. EUR 70.80 domestic to institutions; EUR 79.80 in Europe to institutions; EUR 82.80 elsewhere to institutions; EUR 19 newsstand/cover (effective 2002). **Document type:** *Journal, Academic/Scholarly.*
Published by: (Deutsche Gesellschaft fuer Chirurgie), Demeter Verlag GmbH und Co. KG, Ruedigerstr 14, Stuttgart 70469, Germany. TEL 49-711-8931-0, FAX 49-711-8931322, custserv@thieme.de, http://www.demeter-verlag.de.

617 NLD ISSN 0167-5079
DEVELOPMENTS IN SURGERY. Text in English. 1979. irreg. price varies. *Refereed.* **Document type:** *Monographic series.*
—CISTI.
Published by: Kluwer Academic Publishers Group (Subsidiary of: Wolters Kluwer N.V.), Spuiboulevard 50, PO Box 17, Dordrecht 3300 AA, Netherlands. FAX 31-78-639-2254, services@wkap.nl, http://www.wkap.nl. **Dist. by:** Journals Department, PO Box 322, Dordrecht 3300 AH, Netherlands. FAX 31-78-654-6474.

617 616.3 CHE ISSN 0253-4886
DIGESTIVE SURGERY. Text in English. 1984. bi-m. CHF 1,310, EUR 935.80 in Europe to institutions; CHF 1,327.40, USD 1,016 overseas to institutions (effective 2002). adv. illus. index. back issues avail. *Refereed.* **Document type:** *Journal, Academic/Scholarly.* **Description:** Answers the complete information needs of surgeons concerned with diseases of the alimentary tract. Keeps the specialist aware of advances in all fields contributing to improvements in the diagnosis and treatment of gastrointestinal disease.
Incorporates: Surgical Gastroenterology
Related titles: Microform ed.: (from PQC); Online - full text ed.: ISSN 1421-9883. CHF 58, EUR 42, USD 45 to institutions with print edition (effective 2002) (from EBSCO Publishing, O C L C Online Computer Library Center, Inc., RoweCom Information Quest, Swets Blackwell, Institute for Scientific Information).
Indexed: ASCA, Curr.Cont., Excerp.Med., Ind.Med. (1984-), Int.Nurs.Ind.
—BLDSC (3588.346900), CISTI, EMDOCS, GNLM, IDS, Infotrieve, KNAW. **CCC.**
Published by: (Collegium Internationale Chirurgiae Digestivae), S. Karger AG, Allschwilerstr 10, PO Box, Basel 4009, Switzerland. TEL 41-61-306-1111, FAX 41-61-306-1234, karger@karger.ch, http://www.online.karger.com/journals/dsu, http://www.karger.com. Eds. E H Farthmann, M W Buechler. adv.: page USD 1,205. Circ: 1,000.

DIRECTORY OF OPERATING THEATRES AND DEPARTMENTS OF SURGERY (YEAR). see *HEALTH FACILITIES AND ADMINISTRATION*

617.0029 GBR
DIRECTORY OF SURGICAL SPECIALISTS. Text in English. 1997. a. GBP 95 (effective 1998). adv. **Document type:** *Directory.* **Description:** Aims to assist medical professionals in referring patients to consultants. Entries identify surgeons main areas of surgical activity and their most frequently performed procedures.
Published by: Financial Times Healthcare, Maple House, 149 Tottenham Ct Rd, London W1P 9LL, United Kingdom. TEL 44-207-896-2066, FAX 44-20-7896-2213, lizg@pearson-pro.com, http://www.fthealthcare.com. Adv. contact Liz Godden.

617 USA ISSN 0012-3706
CODEN: DICRAG
DISEASES OF THE COLON AND RECTUM. Text in English. 1958. m. USD 263 domestic to individuals; USD 316 foreign to individuals; USD 387 domestic to institutions; USD 440 foreign to institutions; USD 34 newsstand/cover (effective 2002). adv. illus. index. *Refereed.* **Document type:** *Academic/Scholarly.* **Description:** Contains original articles on the surgical management of lower gastrointestinal tract disorders.
Related titles: Microfilm ed.: (from PQC,WWS); Online - full text ed.: USD 503.10 domestic for academic site license; USD 556.10 foreign for academic site license; USD 561.15 domestic for corporate site license; USD 614.15 foreign for corporate site license (effective 2002) (from Ovid Technologies, Inc., LexisNexis, Institute for Scientific Information).
Indexed: ASCA, Behav.Med.Abstr., Biol.Abstr., Chem.Abstr., Curr.Adv.Cancer Res., Curr.Adv.Ecol.Sci., Curr.Cont., Dent.Ind., Excerp.Med., Helminthol.Abstr., Hosp.Lit.Ind., INIS Atomind., Ind.Med. (1958-), Ind.Sci.Rev., Inpharma, Int.Abstr.Biol.Sci., Int.Nurs.Ind., Jrnl.Watch Gastr., NRN, Nutr.Abstr., Pharm.&Out.News, Protozool.Abstr., Reac., Rev.Med.& Vet.Mycol., SSCI (coverage dropped), Sci.Cit.Ind., THA.
—BLDSC (3598.200000), GNLM, IDS, ingenta, KNAW.
Published by: (American Society of Colon and Rectal Surgeons), Williams & Wilkins (Subsidiary of: Waverly International), 351 W Camden St, Baltimore, MD 21201-2436. TEL 410-528-4000, FAX 410-528-4312, sreed@wwilkins.com, http://www.wwilkins.com, http://www.Lww.com. Ed. Dr. Victor Fazio. Adv. contact Sherry Reed. B&W page USD 1,215; 11.13 x 8.38. Circ: 5,642; 5,271 (paid).

617 ZMB ISSN 1024-297X
EAST AND CENTRAL AFRICAN JOURNAL OF SURGERY. Text and summaries in English. 1978. a. ZMK 10 in Africa; GBP 20 elsewhere. adv. bk.rev. cum.index. back issues avail. *Refereed.* **Document type:** *Academic/Scholarly.* **Description:** Publishes original papers on surgery with special relevance for Africa.
Supersedes (in 1994): Association of Surgeons of East Africa. Proceedings (0253-8466)
—GNLM.
Published by: Association of Surgeons of East Africa, Woodlands, PO Box 320159, Lusaka, Zambia. TEL 260-1-230710, FAX 260-1-250753, medorth@zamnet.zm. Ed., R&P John E Jellis. Circ: 800.

617 EGY ISSN 0013-2454
EGYPTIAN SURGICAL SOCIETY QUARTERLY REVIEW. Text in English. 1966. q. EGP 1. adv. bk.rev. bibl, charts, illus.
Published by: Egyptian Surgical Society, Dar el Hekma, 42 Kasr el-Aini St., Cairo, Egypt. Ed. Ahmed Abu Zikry.

617 ITA ISSN 1128-3270
ELECTRONIC JOURNAL OF SURGERY AND SPECIALISTIC MEDICINE. Text in English. s-a.
Media: Online - full text.
Address: PO Box 481, Rome 00187, Italy. ejs@galactica.it, http://www.galactica.it/ejs/. Eds. Cosimo Nave, Marcelo Della Corte.

617 616.025 CAN ISSN 1195-0897
EMERGENCY PRODUCT BUYER. Text in English. 1986. bi-m. USD 35; CND 45 foreign. adv. bk.rev. abstr, charts, illus, stat, tr.lit. back issues avail. *Refereed.* **Document type:** *Trade.* **Description:** Provides a source of continuing medical, business education and professional news for ambulance officers, paramedics, emergency physicians and nurses, and EMS management and training officers in Canada.
Former titles: Emergency Prehospital Medicine (0836-7272); (until 1987): Canadian Journal of Prehospital Medicine (0829-5603)
Published by: C M E Communications, Inc., 20854 Dalton Rd, P O Box 507, Sutton W., ON L0E 1L0, Canada. TEL 416-722-9839, FAX 416-722-9687. Ed. Michael Roschette. Adv. contact John W Moir. Circ: 6,200.

ENCYCLOPEDIE MEDICO-CHIRURGICALE. ANESTESIA - RIANIMAZIONE. see *MEDICAL SCIENCES—Anaesthesiology*

ENCYCLOPEDIE MEDICO-CHIRURGICALE. ANESTHESIE - REANIMATION. see *MEDICAL SCIENCES—Anaesthesiology*

617.5 616.3 FRA ISSN 0246-0424
ENCYCLOPEDIE MEDICO-CHIRURGICALE. TECHNIQUES CHIRURGICALES. APPAREIL DIGESTIF; la reference du chirurgien - actualisee en permanence. Cover title: Techniques Chirurgicales - Appareil Digestif. Variant title: Encyclopedie Medico-Chirurgicale, Instantanes Medicaux. Techniques Chirurgicales - Appareil Digestif. Receuil Periodique de L'Encyclopedie Medico-Chirurgicale. Techniques Chirurgicales - Appareil Digestif. Text in French. 1964. 4 base vols. plus q. updates. bibl, charts, illus. *Refereed.* **Document type:** *Academic/Scholarly.* **Description:** Provides an up-to-date reference to topics concerning GI-tract and abdominal surgery.
Related titles: ♦ Italian ed.: Encyclopedie Medico-Chirurgicale. Tecniche Chirurgiche. Chirurgia Addominale. ISSN 1283-0798.
Published by: Elsevier Paris, Editions Scientifiques et Medicales (Subsidiary of: Reed Elsevier plc. group), 23 rue Linois, Paris 75015, France. TEL 33-1-45589110, FAX 33-1-45589425, redaction-emc@elsevier.fr, redacion-emc@elsevier.fr, http://www.elsevier.fr, http://www.elsevier.com. Ed. Pascal Horay.

617.5 616.13 FRA ISSN 0246-0459
ENCYCLOPEDIE MEDICO-CHIRURGICALE. TECHNIQUES CHIRURGICALES. CHIRURGIE VASCULAIRE; la reference du chirurgien - actualisee en permanence. Cover title: Techniques Chirurgicales - Chirurgie Vasculaire. Variant title: Encyclopedie Medico-Chirurgicale, Instantanes Medicaux. Techniques Chiruirgicales - Chirurgie Vasculaire. Text in French. 1966. 2 base vols. plus q. updates. bibl, charts, illus. *Refereed.* **Document type:** *Academic/Scholarly.* **Description:** Provides an up-to-date reference tool for topics in vascular surgery.
Related titles: ♦ Italian ed.: Encyclopedie Medico-Chirurgicale. Tecniche Chirurgiche. Chirurgia Vascolare. ISSN 1283-0801.
Published by: Elsevier Paris, Editions Scientifiques et Medicales (Subsidiary of: Reed Elsevier plc. group), 23 rue Linois, Paris 75015, France. TEL 33-1-45589110, FAX 33-1-45589425, redaction-emc@elsevier.fr, redacion-emc@elsevier.fr, http://www.elsevier.fr, http://www.elsevier.com. Ed. Pascal Horay.

617.5 616.21 FRA
ENCYCLOPEDIE MEDICO-CHIRURGICALE. TECHNIQUES CHIRURGICALES. TETE ET COU; la reference du chirurgien. actualisee en permanence. Cover title: Techniques Chirgicales. Tete et Cou. Text in French. 2 base vols. plus a. updates. bibl, charts, illus. **Document type:** *Academic/Scholarly.* **Description:** Provides an up-to-date reference for surgeons in otolaryngology.
Supersedes in part (in 1991): Encyclopedie Medico-Chirurgicale. Techniques Chirurgicales. Cou et Tete (1155-570X)
Related titles: ♦ Italian ed.: Encyclopedie Medico-Chirurgicale. Tecniche Chirurgiche. Chirurgia O R L e Cervico-facciale. ISSN 1292-3036.
Published by: Elsevier Paris, Editions Scientifiques et Medicales (Subsidiary of: Reed Elsevier plc. group), 23 rue Linois, Paris 75015, France. TEL 33-1-45589425, FAX 31-1-45589425, redaction-emc@elsevier.fr, redacion-emc@elsevier.fr, http://www.elsevier.fr, http://www.elsevier.com. Ed. Pascal Horay.

617.5 616.21 FRA ISSN 1241-8226
ENCYCLOPEDIE MEDICO-CHIRURGICALE. TECHNIQUES CHIRURGICALES. THORAX; la reference du chirurgien - actualisee en permanence. Cover title: Techniques Chirurgicales. Thorax. Variant title: Encyclopedie Medico-Chirurgicale, Instantanes Medicaux. Techniques Chirurgicales - Thorax. Text in French. 2 base vols. plus q. updates. bibl, charts, illus. *Refereed.* **Document type:** *Academic/Scholarly.* **Description:** Presents surgeons in otorhinolaryngology with an up-to-date reference on thoracic surgery.
Supersedes in part (in 1991): Encyclopedie Medico-Chirurgicale. Techniques Chirurgicales. Cou - Thorax (1155-570X)
Related titles: ♦ Italian ed.: Encyclopedie Medico-Chirurgicale. Tecniche Chirurgiche. Torace. ISSN 1288-3336.

M

Published by: Elsevier Paris, Editions Scientifiques et Medicales (Subsidiary of: Reed Elsevier plc. group), 23 rue Linois, Paris 75015, France. TEL 33-1-45589110, FAX 33-1-45589425, redaction-emc@elsevier.fr, redacion-emc@elsevier.fr, http://www.elsevier.fr, http://www.elsevier.com. Ed. Pascal Horay.

617.5 616.3 FRA ISSN 1283-0798
ENCYCLOPEDIE MEDICO-CHIRURGICALE. TECNICHE CHIRURGICHE. CHIRURGIA ADDOMINALE. Variant title: Tecniche Chirurgiche Addominale. Text in Italian. 1998. 3 base vols. plus s-a. updates. bibl, charts, illus. *Refereed.* **Document type:** *Academic/Scholarly.* **Description:** Provides an up-to-date reference on topics in abdominal and GI-tract surgery.
Related titles: ♦ French ed.: Encyclopedie Medico-Chirurgicale. Techniques Chirurgicales. Appareil Digestif. ISSN 0246-0424.
Published by: Elsevier Paris, Editions Scientifiques et Medicales (Subsidiary of: Reed Elsevier plc. group), 23 rue Linois, Paris 75015, France. TEL 33-1-45589110, FAX 33-1-45589425, redaction-emc@elsevier.fr, redacion-emc@elsevier.fr, http://www.elsevier.fr, http://www.elsevier.com. Ed. Pascal Horay.

617.5 616.21 FRA ISSN 1292-3036
ENCYCLOPEDIE MEDICO-CHIRURGICALE. TECNICHE CHIRURGICHE. CHIRURGIA O R L E CERVICO-FACCIALE. (Oto-Rhino-Laryngologia) Cover title: Tecniche Chirurgiche. Chirurgia O R L e Cervico-Facciale. Text in Italian. 1998. base vol. plus a. updates. bibl, charts, illus. **Document type:** *Academic/Scholarly.* **Description:** Provides an up-to-date source for topics in otorhinolaryngologic surgery.
Related titles: ♦ French ed.: Encyclopedie Medico-Chirurgicale. Techniques Chirurgicales. Tete et Cou.
Published by: Elsevier Paris, Editions Scientifiques et Medicales (Subsidiary of: Reed Elsevier plc. group), 23 rue Linois, Paris 75015, France. TEL 33-1-45589110, FAX 33-1-45589425, redaction-emc@elsevier.fr, redacion-emc@elsevier.fr, http://www.elsevier.fr, http://www.elsevier.com. Ed. Pascal Horay.

617.5 616.13 FRA ISSN 1283-0801
ENCYCLOPEDIE MEDICO-CHIRURGICALE. TECNICHE CHIRURGICHE. CHIRURGIA VASCOLARE. Cover title: Tecniche Chirurgiche. Chirurgia Vascolare. Text in Italian. 1998. 2 base vols. plus s-a. updates. bibl, charts, illus. *Refereed.* **Document type:** *Academic/Scholarly.* **Description:** Provides an up-to-date reference tool for topics in vascular surgery.
Related titles: ♦ French ed.: Encyclopedie Medico-Chirurgicale. Techniques Chirurgicales. Chirurgie Vasculaire. ISSN 0246-0459.
Published by: Elsevier Paris, Editions Scientifiques et Medicales (Subsidiary of: Reed Elsevier plc. group), 23 rue Linois, Paris 75015, France. TEL 33-1-45589110, FAX 33-1-45589425, redaction-emc@elsevier.fr, redacion-emc@elsevier.fr, http://www.elsevier.fr, http://www.elsevier.com. Ed. Pascal Horay.

617.5 616.21 FRA ISSN 1288-3336
ENCYCLOPEDIE MEDICO-CHIRURGICALE. TECNICHE CHIRURGICHE. TORACE. Cover title: Tecniche Chirurgicale. Torace. Text in Italian. 1989. base vol. plus a. updates. bibl, charts, illus. *Refereed.* **Document type:** *Academic/Scholarly.* **Description:** Presents surgeons in otorhinolaryngology with an up-to-date reference on topics on surgery of the thorax.
Related titles: ♦ French ed.: Encyclopedie Medico-Chirurgicale. Techniques Chirurgicales. Thorax. ISSN 1241-8226.
Published by: Elsevier Paris, Editions Scientifiques et Medicales (Subsidiary of: Reed Elsevier plc. group), 23 rue Linois, Paris 75015, France. TEL 33-1-45589110, FAX 33-1-44589425, redaction-emc@elsevier.fr, redacion-emc@elsevier.fr, http://www.elsevier.fr, http://www.elsevier.com. Ed. Pascal Horay.

617 618 FRA
ENCYCLOPEDIE MEDICO-CHIRURGICALE. TRAITE DE TECHNIQUES CHIRURGICALES. GYNECOLOGIE. Text in French. 1966. base vol. plus a. updates. bibl, charts, illus. *Refereed.* **Document type:** *Academic/Scholarly.* **Description:** Provides ob-gyns with a comprehensive reference on surgical techniques.
Supersedes in part (in 1997): Encyclopedie Medico-Chirurgicale. Traite de Techniques Chirurgicales - Urologie - Gynecologie (0246-0432)
Published by: Elsevier Paris, Editions Scientifiques et Medicales (Subsidiary of: Reed Elsevier plc. group), 23 rue Linois, Paris 75015, France. TEL 33-1-45589110, FAX 33-1-45589425, redaction-emc@elsevier.fr, redacion-emc@elsevier.fr, http://www.elsevier.fr, http://www.elsevier.com.

617.1 FRA ISSN 0246-0467
ENCYCLOPEDIE MEDICO-CHIRURGICALE. TRAITE DE TECHNIQUES CHIRURGICALES. ORTHOPEDIE - TRAUMATOLOGIE. Cover title: Traite de Techniques Chirurgicales - Orthopedie - Traumatologie. Text in French. 1966. 4 base vols. plus q. updates. bibl, charts, illus. *Refereed.* **Document type:** *Academic/Scholarly.* **Description:** Offers orthopedic surgeons a comprehensive, up-to-date reference.
Published by: Elsevier Paris, Editions Scientifiques et Medicales (Subsidiary of: Reed Elsevier plc. group), 23 rue Linois, Paris 75015, France. TEL 33-1-45589110, FAX 33-1-45589425, redaction-emc@elsevier.fr, redacion-emc@elsevier.fr, http://www.elsevier.fr, http://www.elsevier.com.

617 616.6 FRA ISSN 1283-0879
ENCYCLOPEDIE MEDICO-CHIRURGICALE. TRAITE DE TECHNIQUES CHIRURGICALES. UROLOGIE. Cover title: Traite de Techniques Chirurgicales - Urologie. Text in French. 1966. 2 base vols. plus q. updates. bibl, charts, illus. *Refereed.* **Document type:** *Academic/Scholarly.* **Description:** Offers urologists a comprehensive, up-to-date reference on surgical techniques.
Supersedes in part (in 1997): Encyclopedie Medico-Chirurgicale. Techniques Chirurgicales - Urologie - Gynecologie
Published by: Elsevier Paris, Editions Scientifiques et Medicales (Subsidiary of: Reed Elsevier plc. group), 23 rue Linois, Paris 75015, France. TEL 33-1-45589110, FAX 33-1-45589425, redaction-emc@elsevier.fr, redacion-emc@elsevier.fr, http://www.elsevier.fr, http://www.elsevier.com.

617 RUS
ENDOSKOPICHESKAYA KHIRURGIYA. Text in Russian. 1995. bi-m. RUR 216 for 6 mos. to individuals; RUR 540 for 6 mos. to institutions (effective 2002).
Indexed: Ref.Zh.
Published by: (Rossiiskaya Assotsyatsiya Endoskopicheskoi Khirurgii), Media Sfera, Dmitrovskoe shosse 46, korp 2, etazh 4, P.O. Box 54, Moscow 127238, Russian Federation. TEL 7-095-4824329, FAX 7-095-4824312, mediashp@mediasphera.ru. Ed. Sergey Yemelyanov. **Dist. by:** East View Publications, 3020 Harbor Ln N, Minneapolis, MN 55447. TEL 763-550-0961, FAX 763-559-2931.

617 DEU ISSN 0939-7248
CODEN: EPSUEX
EUROPEAN JOURNAL OF PEDIATRIC SURGERY. Text in German. 1960. bi-m. EUR 324.80 domestic to institutions; EUR 327.80 in Europe to institutions; EUR 332.80 elsewhere to institutions; EUR 67 newsstand/cover to institutions (effective 2002). adv. bk.rev. abstr, charts, illus. index. reprint service avail. from ISI. *Refereed.* **Document type:** *Journal, Academic/Scholarly.* **Description:** Aims to integrate and coordinate all endeavors in pediatric surgery and related disciplines in accordance with European standards, to widen the scope and variety of published papers in the specialty and to provide a European forum for pediatric surgery and specialties.
Formed by the 1991 merger of: Zeitschrift fuer Kinderchirurgie (0174-3082); Which was formerly (until 1981): Zeitschrift fuer Kinderchirurgie und Grenzgebiete (0044-2909); Chirurgie Pediatrique (0180-5738); Which was formerly (until vol.18, 1977): Annales de Chirurgie Infantile (0003-3952)
Related titles: Microform ed.: (from PQC); Online - full text ed.: (from Institute for Scientific Information); Print ed.: ISSN 1439-359X; ♦ Supplement: European Journal of Pediatric Surgery. Supplement. ISSN 0939-6764.
Indexed: ASCA, Bibl.Dev.Med.& Child Neur., Biol.Abstr., Curr.Adv.Cell & Devel.Biol., Curr.Adv.Ecol.Sci., Curr.Cont., Dent.Ind., Excerp.Med., Helminthol.Abstr., INIS Atomind., Ind.Med. (1991-), Ind.Sci.Rev., Inpharma, Neurosci.Cit.Ind., Nutr.Abstr., Pharm.&Out.News, Protozool.Abstr., Reac., Ref.Zh., Sci.Cit.Ind.
—BLDSC (3829.733450), CISTI, EMDOCS, GNLM, IDS, Infotrieve. **CCC.**
Published by: Hippokrates Verlag GmbH, Postfach 300504, Stuttgart 70445, Germany. TEL 49-711-8931-0, FAX 49-711-8931706, kunden.service@thieme.de, http://www.thieme.de. Eds. A M Holschneider, Y Revillon. Circ: 2,000. **Subscr. to:** Societe de Periodiques Specialises, BP 22, Vineuil Cedex 41354, France. **Co-publisher:** Masson - Periodiques, FR.

617 DEU ISSN 0939-6764
EUROPEAN JOURNAL OF PEDIATRIC SURGERY. SUPPLEMENT. Text in German. 1966. irreg. **Document type:** *Academic/Scholarly.*
Former titles (until 1991): Zeitschrift fuer Kinderchirurgie. Supplement (0932-5654); (until 1981): Zeitschrift fuer Kinderchirurgie und Grenzgebiete (0932-5638)
Related titles: ♦ Supplement to: European Journal of Pediatric Surgery. ISSN 0939-7248.
Indexed: Excerp.Med. (1993-).
—EMDOCS, KNAW.
Published by: Hippokrates Verlag GmbH, Postfach 300504, Stuttgart 70445, Germany. TEL 0711-8931-0, FAX 0711-891453. Ed. Guenther Buck. **Co-publisher:** Masson.

617.95 DEU ISSN 0930-343X
EUROPEAN JOURNAL OF PLASTIC SURGERY. Text in English. 1971. 8/yr. EUR 500.70 domestic; EUR 493.80 in Germany; EUR 72 newsstand/cover foreign (effective 2002). back issues avail.; reprint service avail. from ISI. *Refereed.* **Document type:** *Journal, Academic/Scholarly.* **Description:** Covers developments in microsurgery, tissue expansion, craniofacial surgery, and the spin-offs of these techniques into the areas of trauma, the treatment of malignancy, and aesthetic surgery.
Formerly: Chirurgia Plastica (0340-5664)
Related titles: Microform ed.: (from PQC); Online - full text ed.: ISSN 1435-0130 (from EBSCO Publishing, RoweCom Information Quest, Swets Blackwell, Springer LINK).
Indexed: ASCA, Biol.Abstr., Curr.Adv.Cancer Res., Curr.Cont., Excerp.Med., Inpharma, Med.& Surg.Dermat., Reac., Rev.Appl.Entomol., Rev.Arom.& Med.Plants, Rev.Med.& Vet.Mycol., Sci.Cit.Ind. (coverage dropped).
—BLDSC (3829.736300), CISTI, EMDOCS, GNLM, IDS, Infotrieve, ingenta. **CCC.**
Published by: (European Association of Plastic Surgeons), Springer-Verlag (Subsidiary of: BertelsmannSpringer), Tiergartenstr 17, Heidelberg 69121, Germany. TEL 49-6221-345-0, FAX 49-6221-345229, subscriptions@springer.de, http://link.springer.de/link/service/journals/00238/index.htm, http://www.springer.de. Eds. D E Tolhurst, I T Jackson. **Subscr. in N. America to:** Springer-Verlag New York Inc., PO Box 2485, Secaucus, NJ 07096-2485. TEL 212-460-1500, FAX 212-473-6272. **Co-sponsors:** Association of German Plastic Surgeons; Austrian Society for Plastic and Reconstructive Surgery; Belgian Society for Plastic, Reconstructive and Aesthetic Surgery.

617 NOR ISSN 1102-4151
CODEN: ACHIEB
EUROPEAN JOURNAL OF SURGERY. Text in English. 1869. 12/yr. GBP 108, USD 178 to individuals; GBP 227, USD 375 to institutions (effective 2002). adv. index, cum.index every 10-15 yrs. *Refereed.* **Document type:** *Academic/Scholarly.* **Description:** Focuses on promoting clinical progress, research and the exchange of research information within the field of surgery.
Incorporates (in 1996): Theoretical Surgery (0179-8669); Former titles (until 1992): Acta Chirurgica (1102-1101); (until 1991): Acta Chirurgica Scandinavica (0001-5482); Incorporates (in 1992): Netherlands Journal of Surgery (0167-2487); Which was formerly (1949-1979): Archivum Chirurgicum Neerlandicum (0004-0657)
Related titles: Online - full text ed.: (from EBSCO Publishing, O C L C Online Computer Library Center, Inc., RoweCom Information Quest, CatchWord Ltd., ingenta, Swets Blackwell, Institute for Scientific Information); ♦ Supplement: European Journal of Surgery. Supplement. ISSN 1102-416X.
Indexed: ASCA, Biol.Abstr., Chem.Abstr., Curr.Adv.Ecol.Sci., Curr.Cont., Energy Res.Abstr., Excerp.Med., Helminthol.Abstr., INIS Atomind., Ind.Med. (1991-), Ind.Sci.Rev., Ind.Vet., Inpharma, Nutr.Abstr., Pharm.&Out.News, Pig News & Info., Protozool.Abstr., Reac., Rev.Med.& Vet.Mycol., SSCI (coverage dropped), Sci.Cit.Ind., Sportsearch.
—BLDSC (3829.745300), ADONIS, CASDDS, CISTI, EMDOCS, GNLM, IDS, Infotrieve, ingenta, KNAW. **CCC.**
Published by: Taylor & Francis AS (Subsidiary of: Taylor & Francis Group), Cort Adelersgt. 17, Solli, PO Box 2562, Oslo 0202, Norway. TEL 47-22-12-98-80, FAX 47-22-12-98-90, journals@tandf.no, http://www.tandf.co.uk/tfas. Ed. Sten Lennquist. Circ: 4,500.

617 NOR ISSN 1102-416X
CODEN: ACSSAO
EUROPEAN JOURNAL OF SURGERY. SUPPLEMENT. Text in English. 1922. irreg. **Document type:** *Monographic series.*
Former titles (until 1992): Acta Chirurgica. Supplement (1102-3309); (until 1991): Acta Chirurgica Scandinavica. Supplement (0301-1860)
Related titles: Online - full text ed.: (from Swets Blackwell); ♦ Supplement to: European Journal of Surgery. ISSN 1102-4151.
Indexed: Excerp.Med. (1992-), Ind.Med. (coverage dropped).

M

—BLDSC (3829.745320), ADONIS, CASDDS, CISTI, EMDOCS, KNAW. **CCC.**
Published by: Scandinavian University Press (Subsidiary of: Taylor & Francis Ltd.), Postboks 2959, Toeyen, Oslo 0608, Norway. FAX 47-22-57-53-53, journals@scup.no, http://www.scup.no/surgery.

617 ITA
THE EUROPEAN JOURNAL OF TRAUMA AND EMERGENCY SURGERY. Text in Multiple languages. 1978. 4/yr. ITL 92,000 (effective 1999). **Document type:** *Academic/Scholarly.*
Former titles (until 199?): European Journal of Emergency Surgery and Intensive Care; (until vol.19, no.2, 1996): Journal of Emergency Surgery and Intensive Care (1120-8708); Urgentis Chirurgiae Commentaria (0392-8101)
—ingenta.
Published by: (European Association of Trauma and Emergency Surgery (E.A.T.E.S.)), Masson, Divisione Periodici, Via Flli. Bressan 2, Milan, MI 20126, Italy. TEL 39-2-270741, FAX 39-2-27074210. Ed. E Caviha. adv.: B&W page ITL 2,550,000, color page ITL 3,600,000; trim 275 x 210. Circ: 2,000.

EUROPEAN JOURNAL OF VASCULAR AND ENDOVASCULAR SURGERY. see *MEDICAL SCIENCES—Cardiovascular Diseases*

617 DEU ISSN 0940-6719
CODEN: ESJOEP
EUROPEAN SPINE JOURNAL. Text in English. 1992. bi-m. EUR 493.20 domestic; EUR 490.40 in Germany; EUR 96 newsstand/cover foreign (effective 2002). *Refereed.* **Document type:** *Journal, Academic/Scholarly.* **Description:** Devoted to spine surgery and all related disciplines, including functional and surgical anatomy, biomechanics and pathophysiology, neurology, as well as basic sciences, diagnostic procedures and alternative methods.
Related titles: Online - full text ed.: ISSN 1432-0932 (from EBSCO Publishing, RoweCom Information Quest, Swets Blackwell, Springer LINK, Institute for Scientific Information).
Indexed: AMED, Curr.Cont., Excerp.Med. (1993-), Ind.Med. (1992-), Inpharma, Pharm.&Out.News, Reac., e-psyche.
—BLDSC (3830.232200), ADONIS, CISTI, EMDOCS, GNLM, IDS, Infotrieve, KNAW. **CCC.**
Published by: (European Spine Society), Springer-Verlag (Subsidiary of: BertelsmannSpringer), Tiergartenstr 17, Heidelberg 69121, Germany. TEL 49-6221-345-0, FAX 49-6221-345229, subscriptions@springer.de, http://link.springer.de/link/service/journals/00586/index.htm, http://www.springer.de. Ed. M Aebi. **Subscr. in N. America to:** Springer-Verlag New York Inc., PO Box 2485, Secaucus, NJ 07096-2485. TEL 212-460-1500, FAX 212-473-6272.

617 CHE ISSN 0014-312X
CODEN: EUSRBM
EUROPEAN SURGICAL RESEARCH; clinical and experimental surgery. Text in English. 1969. bi-m. CHF 956, EUR 682.80 in Europe to institutions; CHF 973.40, USD 744 elsewhere to institutions (effective 2002). adv. back issues avail. *Refereed.* **Document type:** *Journal, Academic/Scholarly.* **Description:** Features original clinical and experimental papers and short technical notes in various fields of operative medicine. Coverage includes surgery, surgical pathophysiology, drug usage, and new surgical techniques.
Related titles: Microform ed.; Online - full text ed.: ISSN 1421-9921. CHF 58, EUR 42, USD 45 to institutions with print edition (effective 2002) (from EBSCO Publishing, O C L C Online Computer Library Center, Inc., RoweCom Information Quest, Swets Blackwell, Institute for Scientific Information).
Indexed: ASCA, Biol.Abstr., Chem.Abstr., Chem.Indus.Notes, Chem.Titles, Curr.Adv.Ecol.Sci., Curr.Cont., Excerp.Med., INIS Atomind., Ind.Med. (1969-), Ind.Sci.Rev., Ind.Vet., Inpharma, Pharm.&Out.News, Reac., Sci.Cit.Ind., Vet.Bull.
—BLDSC (3830.235000), CASDDS, CISTI, GNLM, IDS, ingenta, KNAW. **CCC.**
Published by: S. Karger AG, Allschwilerstr 10, PO Box, Basel 4009, Switzerland. TEL 41-61-306-1111, FAX 41-61-306-1234, karger@karger.ch, http://www.online.karger.com/journals/esr, http://www.karger.com. Ed. K Messmer. adv.: page USD 1,185. Circ: 800.

EXCERPTA MEDICA. SECTION 18: CARDIOVASCULAR DISEASES AND CARDIOVASCULAR SURGERY. see *MEDICAL SCIENCES—Abstracting, Bibliographies, Statistics*

EXCERPTA MEDICA. SECTION 33: ORTHOPEDIC SURGERY. see *MEDICAL SCIENCES—Abstracting, Bibliographies, Statistics*

EXCERPTA MEDICA. SECTION 7: PEDIATRICS AND PEDIATRIC SURGERY. see *MEDICAL SCIENCES—Abstracting, Bibliographies, Statistics*

EXCERPTA MEDICA. SECTION 8: NEUROLOGY AND NEUROSURGERY. see *MEDICAL SCIENCES—Abstracting, Bibliographies, Statistics*

EXCERPTA MEDICA. SECTION 9: SURGERY. see *MEDICAL SCIENCES—Abstracting, Bibliographies, Statistics*

EXTRACTA DERMATOLOGICA; weltweit Auserlesen. see *MEDICAL SCIENCES—Abstracting, Bibliographies, Statistics*

EXTRACTA ORTHOPAEDICA; Weltweit Auserlesen. see *MEDICAL SCIENCES—Abstracting, Bibliographies, Statistics*

617.95 USA ISSN 0736-6825
CODEN: FPSUEA
FACIAL PLASTIC SURGERY; international quarterly monographs. Text in English. 1983. q. EUR 171 to individuals; EUR 311 to institutions (effective 2002). adv. *Refereed.* **Document type:** *Journal, Academic/Scholarly.* **Description:** Publishes clinically oriented articles examining a specific topic in facial plastic surgery in each issue.
Formerly (until 1983): Seminars in Facial Plastic Surgery
Related titles: Microfilm ed.; Online - full text ed.: ISSN 1098-8793 (from RoweCom Information Quest).
Indexed: Biol.Abstr., Excerp.Med., INIS Atomind.
—BLDSC (3863.421000), CISTI, EMDOCS, GNLM, ingenta. **CCC.**
Published by: Thieme Medical Publishers, 333 Seventh Ave, New York, NY 10001. TEL 212-760-0888, 800-782-3488, FAX 212-947-1112, http://www.thieme.com. Eds. Dr. M Eugene Tardy, Tony Bull. Circ: 2,173. **Orders in Europe to:** Thieme International, Postfach 301120, Stuttgart 70451, Germany. TEL 49-711-8931-0.

617.5 USA ISSN 1064-7406
FACIAL PLASTIC SURGERY CLINICS OF NORTH AMERICA. Text in English. 1993. q. USD 164 to individuals; USD 190 in Canada to individuals; USD 224 elsewhere to individuals; USD 225 to institutions; USD 269 foreign to institutions; USD 68 per issue (effective 2001). illus. back issues avail. **Document type:** *Academic/Scholarly.* **Description:** Reviews a single topic in the field in each issue, with emphasis on techniques and procedures.
Related titles: Microform ed.: (from PQC).
—BLDSC (3863.421700), CISTI, GNLM, KNAW.
Published by: W.B. Saunders Co. (Subsidiary of: Harcourt Publishers Ltd.), 11830 Westline Industrial Dr, St Louis, MO 63146. TEL 800-325-4177, http://www.wbsaunders.com. Eds. J Regan Thomas, Dr. Wayne F Larrabee Jr. **Subscr. to:** Periodicals Fulfillment, W B Saunders Co, 6277 Sea Harbor Dr, 4th Fl, Orlando, FL 32891-4800.

FIBRIN SEALING IN SURGICAL AND NONSURGICAL FIELDS. see *MEDICAL SCIENCES*

617 GBR ISSN 1268-7731
CODEN: FASUF8
FOOT AND ANKLE SURGERY. Text in English. 1992. q., latest vol.8, 2002. GBP 105 in Europe to individuals; USD 178 in North America to individuals; GBP 116 elsewhere to individuals; GBP 204 in Europe to institutions; USD 323 in North America to institutions; GBP 224 elsewhere to institutions (effective 2002). adv. *Refereed.* **Document type:** *Academic/Scholarly.* **Description:** Presents a broad approach to foot and ankle disorders, from basic to clinical management. Explores trauma and chronic diseases in both children and adults.
Formerly: European Journal of Foot and Ankle Surgery
Related titles: Online - full text ed.: ISSN 1460-9584. GBP 95 in Europe to individuals; USD 161 in North America to individuals; GBP 95 elsewhere to individuals; GBP 184 in Europe to institutions; USD 291 in North America to institutions; GBP 184 elsewhere to institutions (effective 2002) (from EBSCO Publishing, O C L C Online Computer Library Center, Inc., RoweCom Information Quest, ingenta, Munksgaard & Blackwell Science's Synergy, Swets Blackwell).
—BLDSC (3984.875000), Infotrieve, KNAW. **CCC.**
Published by: Blackwell Science Ltd., PO Box 88, Oxford OX2 0NE, United Kingdom. TEL 44-1865-206180, 44-1865-206002, FAX 44-1865-206219, jnl.orders@blacksci.co.uk, http://www.blackwell-science.com/~cgilib/jnlpage.asp?Journal=fas&File=fas, http://www.blackwellpublishing.com. Eds. N Wulker, S Giannini. Pub. Aileen Boyd Squires. R&P Sophie Savage. Adv. contact Jenny Applin. Circ: 1,500. **Co-sponsor:** European Foot and Ankle Society.

617 TWN
FORMOSAN JOURNAL OF SURGERY. Text in Chinese, English. 1968. bi-m. TWD 200 (effective 2001). illus. back issues avail. *Refereed.* **Document type:** *Journal, Academic/Scholarly.* **Description:** Publishes scholarly research in all clinical and experimental areas of surgery and related fields.
Formerly (until 1999): Surgical Association R O C. Journal (1011-6788)
—BLDSC (4008.425000).
Published by: Surgical Association, c/o National Taiwan University Hospital, Dept of Surgery, No 7, Chung-Shan Rd, Taipei 100, Taiwan. TEL 886-2-2397-0800 ext 5640, 886-2-2356-2120, FAX 886-2-2393-0877, journal@surgery.org.tw, http://www.surgery.org.tw. Ed. Chun-Jean Lee. Pub. Shen-Long Howng. Circ: 5,000. **Co-sponsors:** Association of Thoracic and Cardiovascular Surgeons of Asia; Surgical Society of Gastroenterology R O C; Chinese Association of Endocrine Surgeons; Chinese Association of Pediatric Surgeons; Transplantation Society of Taiwan, R O C.

617 DEU ISSN 0930-8245
FORTSCHRITTE IN DER CHIRURGIE. Text in German. 1986. irreg., latest vol.10, 1996. **Document type:** *Academic/Scholarly.*
Published by: W. Zuckschwerdt Verlag GmbH, Industriestr 1, Germering 82110, Germany. TEL 49-89-894349-0, FAX 49-89-89434950. Eds. F P Gall, P Hermanek.

FOUNDATIONS OF NEUROLOGICAL SURGERY. see *MEDICAL SCIENCES—Psychiatry And Neurology*

617 JPN
FUKUOKAKEN RINSHO GEKA IGAKKAI KAISHI/FUKUOKA SOCIETY FOR CLINICAL SURGERY. JOURNAL. Text in Japanese. 1976. a. membership.
Published by: Fukuokaken Rinsho Geka Igakkai, 9-30 Hakataeki-Minami 2-chome, Hakata-ku, Fukuoka-shi 812-0016, Japan.

617 ITA ISSN 0016-5662
GAZZETTA INTERNAZIONALE DI MEDICINA E CHIRURGIA*. Text in Italian. 1971 (vol.76). s-m. ITL 12,320.
Indexed: Chem.Abstr.
—CISTI, GNLM.
Published by: Edizioni Mediche e Scientifiche, Largo A.Ravizza 17, Rome, RM, Italy. Eds. C Bazzicalupo, G Marcozzi.

616.1 DEU ISSN 0948-7034
GEFAESSCHIRURGIE; Zeitschrift fuer vaskulaere und endovaskulaere Chirurgie. Text in German. 1996. q. EUR 167.98 domestic; EUR 165.48 in Germany; EUR 47.70 newsstand/cover foreign (effective 2002). back issues avail. *Refereed.* **Document type:** *Journal, Academic/Scholarly.* **Description:** Supplies information on current developments in vascular surgery with a view to supporting continuing professional education.
Related titles: Online - full text ed.: ISSN 1434-3932 (from EBSCO Publishing, RoweCom Information Quest, Swets Blackwell, Springer LINK).
—BLDSC (4095.788000), GNLM, KNAW.
Published by: (Deutsche Gesellschaft fuer Gefaesschirurgie), Springer-Verlag (Subsidiary of: BertelsmannSpringer), Tiergartenstr 17, Heidelberg 69121, Germany. TEL 49-6221-345-0, FAX 49-6221-345229, subscriptions@springer.de, http://link.springer.de/link/service/journals/00772/index.htm, http://www.springer.de. Ed. J.-R. Allenberg. **Subscr. in N. America to:** Springer-Verlag New York Inc., PO Box 2485, Secaucus, NJ 07096-2485. TEL 212-460-1500, FAX 212-473-6272. **Co-sponsors:** Oesterreichische Gesellschaft fuer Gefaesschirurgie; Schweizerische Gesellschaft fuer Gefaesschirurgie.

617 JPN ISSN 0433-2644
CODEN: GECYA8
GEKA CHIRYO/SURGICAL THERAPY. Text in Japanese. 1959. m. USD 354 (effective 2000).
Indexed: INIS Atomind.
—CASDDS, CISTI, GNLM.
Published by: Nagai Shoten Co. Ltd., 21-15 Fukushima 8-chome, Fukushima-ku, Osaka-shi 553-0003, Japan. Ed. Tadao Nagai.

M

GEKA SHUDANKAI SHOROKUSHU/TOKYO SURGICAL SOCIETY. ABSTRACTS. see *MEDICAL SCIENCES—Abstracting, Bibliographies, Statistics*

617 JPN ISSN 0389-5564
CODEN: GTEIDA
GEKA TO TAISHA EIYO/JAPANESE JOURNAL OF SURGICAL METABOLISM AND NUTRITION. Text in Japanese; Summaries in English, Japanese. 1968. 5/yr. JPY 2,000 per issue.
Indexed: Chem.Abstr., Chem.Indus.Notes, Chem.Titles.
—BLDSC (4658.863000), CASDDS, CISTI, KNAW.
Published by: Nihon Geka Taisha Eiyo Gakkai/Japanese Academy of Surgical Metabolism and Nutrition, Nihon Gakkai Jimu Senta, 16-9 Honkomagome 5-chome, Bunkyo-ku, Tokyo 113-0021, Japan.

617 USA ISSN 1099-4122
GENERAL SURGERY NEWS. Text in English. m. USD 60; USD 75 foreign (effective 1999).
Former title (until 1997): General Surgery and Laparoscopy News (1065-7088)
Related titles: Online - full text ed.
Published by: McMahon Group, 545 W 45th St, 8th Fl, New York, NY 10036. TEL 212-957-5300, FAX 212-957-7230. Ed. Devon Schuyler. Circ: 36,862.

616 ITA ISSN 0391-9005
IL GIORNALE DI CHIRURGIA. Text in Italian; Summaries in English. 1980. 10/yr. ITL 110,000, USD 100 (effective 2001). adv.
Indexed: Excerp.Med., Ind.Med. (1980-).
—BLDSC (4177.350000), GNLM, Infotrieve. **CCC.**
Published by: (Societa Italiana di Ricerche in Chirurgia), C I C Edizioni Internazionali s.r.l., Corso Trieste 42, Rome, RM 00198, Italy. TEL 39-06-8412673, FAX 39-06-8412688, info@gruppocic.it, 1160199510. Ed. G Dimatteo. Pub. A Salvati. adv.: B&W page XEU 1,239.5, color page XEU 1,704.31; 210 x 280.

617 ITA ISSN 1122-8679
GIORNALE ITALIANO DI CHIRURGIA VASCOLARE. Text in English, Italian. 1994. q. USD 105 to individuals; USD 155 to institutions. adv. *Refereed.* **Document type:** *Academic/Scholarly.*
—CISTI, GNLM.
Published by: Edizioni Minerva Medica, Corso Bramante, 83-85, Turin, TO 10126, Italy. TEL 011-67-82-82, FAX 39-11-674502. Ed. M D'Addato. Pub. A Oliaro. Adv. contact F Filippo. B&W page USD 1,400, color page USD 2,300; trim 280 x 215. Circ: 2,900 (paid).

617 USA ISSN 1522-1628
GRAFT; organ & cell transplantation. Text in English. 1998. 8/yr. USD 620 domestic; USD 652 foreign (effective 2002). adv. charts, illus. 56 p./no. back issues avail.; reprints avail. *Refereed.* **Document type:** *Journal, Academic/Scholarly.* **Description:** Publishes reviews, literature reviews, commentaries, meeting reports, and industry news. Topics include surgical techniques, organ allocation, graft versus host disease, immunosuppression, acute rejection, immunobiology, and clinical management of transplant patients.
Related titles: Online - full text ed.: (from Swets Blackwell, RoweCom Information Quest).
—BLDSC (4208.116000).
Published by: (Transplantation Society), Sage Publications, Inc., Sage Science Press, 2455 Teller Rd, Thousand Oaks, CA 91320. TEL 805-499-0721, FAX 805-499-0871, info@sagepub.com, http://www.sagesciencepress.com. Eds. Dr. Camillo Ricordi, Dr. Mohamed H Sayegh. Pub. Susan Hanscom. R&P Peter Marino. Adv. contact Robert Vrooman. B&W page USD 600, color page USD 1,600; bleed 8.375 x 11.125. Circ: 300 (paid). **Co-sponsors:** American Society of Transplantation; International Pancreas and Islet Transplantation Association.

617 RUS ISSN 0236-2791
CODEN: GSKHEV
GRUDNAYA I SERDECHNO-SOSUDISTAYA KHIRURGIYA/CHEST AND CARDIOVASCULAR SURGERY. Text in Russian; Summaries in English. 1959. bi-m. USD 237 foreign (effective 2000). adv. bk.rev., Website rev. bibl. index. reprints avail. **Document type:** *Journal, Academic/Scholarly.* **Description:** Publishes original articles, reviews on new trends in the field of chest and cardiovascular surgery and related subjects.
Formerly: Grudnaya Khirurgiya (0017-4866)
Indexed: Biol.Abstr., Excerp.Med., Ind.Med. (coverage dropped), Ref.Zh.
—CISTI, East View, GNLM.
Published by: Izdatel'stvo Meditsina, Petroverigskii per 6-8, Moscow 101000, Russian Federation. TEL 7-095-9248785, 7-095-928-86-48, FAX 7-095-9211355, 7-095-9286003. Ed. V S Saveliev. Pub. A M Stochik. R&P T Ivanova. Adv. contact O A Fadeeva TEL 7-095-923-51-40. Circ: 700. **Dist. by:** Mezhdunarodnaya Kniga, B Yakimanka 39, Moscow 117049, Russian Federation. TEL 7-095-2384967, FAX 7-095-2384634; **US dist. addr.:** East View Publications, 3020 Harbor Ln N, Minneapolis, MN 55447. TEL 612-550-0961.

GYNAECOLOGICAL ENDOSCOPY. see *MEDICAL SCIENCES—Obstetrics And Gynecology*

GYNAECOLOGICAL ENDOSCOPY. SUPPLEMENT. see *MEDICAL SCIENCES—Obstetrics And Gynecology*

GYNECOLOGIC SURGERY SOCIETY. MEMBERSHIP NEWSLETTER. see *MEDICAL SCIENCES—Obstetrics And Gynecology*

617 CHE ISSN 0894-8569
CODEN: HPBSE9
H P B SURGERY; a world journal of hepatic, pancreatic, and biliary surgery. Text in English. 6/yr. EUR 524 to institutions; EUR 819 to corporations (effective 2000). *Refereed.* **Document type:** *Academic/Scholarly.*
Related titles: Microform ed.; Online - full text ed.: (from EBSCO Publishing, ingenta, RoweCom Information Quest).
Indexed: Ind.Med. (1988-).
—BLDSC (4335.262350), CISTI, EMDOCS, GNLM, Infotrieve. **CCC.**
Published by: Gordon and Breach - Harwood Academic (Subsidiary of: Taylor & Francis Group), PO Box 531, Lausanne 1000, Switzerland. Ed. Malcolm Puntis. **Subscr. addr. in US:** International Publishers Direct, PO Box 32160, Newark, NJ 07102. FAX 215-750-6343.

HAMAMATSU SEIKEI GEKA KIYO/HAMAMATSU UNIVERSITY. ANNUAL OF ORTHOPAEDIC SURGERY. see *MEDICAL SCIENCES—Orthopedics And Traumatology*

617 SGP ISSN 0218-8104
HAND SURGERY. Text in English. 1996. s-a. SGD 131, USD 77 (effective 2001); SGD 139 in Asia Pacific & Australasia except Hong Kong and China; USD 77 (effective 2002). **Document type:** *Academic/Scholarly.* **Description:** An international journal devoted to hand and upper limb surgery and related research.
Related titles: Online - full text ed.: (from Swets Blackwell).
Indexed: Cal.Tiss.Abstr., Ind.Med.
—BLDSC (4241.595500).
Published by: (Asia-Pacific Federation of Societies for Surgery of the Hand), World Scientific Publishing Co Pte Ltd, Farrer Rd, PO Box 128, Singapore 912805, Singapore. TEL 65-3825663, FAX 65-3825919, TELEX RS-28561-WSPC, wspcsl@singnet.com.sg.; sales@wspc2.demon.co.uk; wspc@wspc.com, http://www.singnet.com.sg/~wspclib.

617.95 DEU ISSN 0722-1819
CODEN: HMPCD9
HANDCHIRURGIE - MIKROCHIRURGIE - PLASTISCHE CHIRURGIE. Text in German. 1982. bi-m. EUR 231.80 domestic to institutions; EUR 236.40 in Europe to institutions; EUR 241.80 elsewhere to institutions; EUR 45 newsstand/cover (effective 2002). **Document type:** *Journal, Academic/Scholarly.*
Formed by the merger of (1969-1982): Handchirurgie (0046-6794); (1977-1982): Zeitschrift fuer Plastische Chirurgie (0342-7978)
Indexed: Biol.Abstr., Dent.Ind., Excerp.Med., Ind.Med. (1982-).
—BLDSC (4254.577000), CISTI, EMDOCS, GNLM, Infotrieve, KNAW. **CCC.**
Published by: Hippokrates Verlag GmbH, Postfach 300504, Stuttgart 70445, Germany. TEL 49-711-8931-0, FAX 49-711-8931706, kunden.service@thieme.de. Circ: 1,600. **Co-sponsors:** Deutschsprachige Arbeitsgemeinschaft fuer Handchirurgie; Deutschsprachige Arbeitsgemeinschaft fuer Mikrochirurgie der Peripheren Nerven; Verein der Deutschen Plastischen Chirurgie; Deutsche Gesellschaft fuer Handchirurgie; Oesterreichischen.

617 USA ISSN 1043-3074
RD523 CODEN: HEANEE
HEAD & NECK; journal for the sciences and specialities of the head and neck. Text in English. 1978. m., latest vol.23, 2001, Dec. USD 920 in United States; USD 1,040 in Canada & Mexico; USD 1,142 elsewhere; USD 966 combined subscription in United States for print and online eds.; USD 1,086 combined subscription in Canada & Mexico for print and online eds.; USD 1,188 combined subscription elsewhere for print and online eds. (effective 2002). adv. bk.rev. abstr, charts, illus, stat. index. 90 p./no. 2 cols./p. back issues avail.; reprint service avail. from PQC. *Refereed.* **Document type:** *Journal, Academic/Scholarly.* **Description:** Examines the management and prevention of all diseases in the head and neck area, including benign and malignant tumors, congenital deformities, and trauma.
Formerly (until 1989): Head and Neck Surgery (0148-6403)
Related titles: Microform ed.: (from PQC); Online - full text ed.: ISSN 1097-0347. USD 920 in United States; USD 920 in Canada & Mexico; USD 920 elsewhere (effective 2002) (from EBSCO Publishing, Wiley InterScience, Institute for Scientific Information).
Indexed: ASCA, Curr.Cont., Excerp.Med., INIS Atomind., Ind.Med. (1989-), Ind.Sci.Rev., Inpharma, Pharm.&Out.News, Reac., Rev.Med.& Vet.Mycol., Sci.Cit.Ind.
—BLDSC (4274.608500), CISTI, GNLM, IDS, ingenta, KNAW.
Published by: John Wiley & Sons, Inc., Journals (Subsidiary of: Wiley InterScience) subinfo@wiley.com, http://www.interscience.wiley.com. Ed. Dr. Randal S Weber. Adv. contact Roberta Frederick. B&W page GBP 640, color page GBP 1,515; trim 210 x 279. Circ: 2,500 (paid). **Subscr. outside the Americas to:** John Wiley & Sons Ltd., Baffins Ln, Chichester, Sussex PO19 IUD, United Kingdom. TEL 44-1243-779777, FAX 44-1243-843232, cs-journals@wiley.co.uk, http://www.wiley.co.uk.

617 DEU ISSN 1265-4906
CODEN: HERNFW
HERNIA; the journal of hernias and abdominal wall surgery. Text in English. 1997. q. EUR 300 domestic to individuals; EUR 300 in Germany to institutions; EUR 96 foreign to institutions (effective 2002). adv. **Document type:** *Academic/Scholarly.* **Description:** Promotes research and fundamental studies on groin hernias as well as on surgery of the anterior and postero-lateral walls of the abdominal cavity, diaphragm and perineum.
Related titles: Online - full text ed.: (from EBSCO Publishing, RoweCom Information Quest, Swets Blackwell, Springer LINK).
—BLDSC (4300.154100), CISTI, Infotrieve. **CCC.**
Published by: (Groupe de Recherche Europien de la Paroi Abdominale), Springer-Verlag France (Subsidiary of: BertelsmannSpringer), 1 rue Paul Cezanne, Paris 75008, France. TEL 33-1-53933644, FAX 33-1-53933683, york@springer-paris.fr, http://link.springer.de/link/service/journals/10029/index.htm. adv.: B&W page FRF 11,000, color page FRF 19,400; trim 210 x 275. **Subscr. in N. America to:** Springer-Verlag New York Inc., PO Box 2485, Secaucus, NJ 07096-2485. TEL 212-460-1500, FAX 212-473-6272. **Co-sponsor:** American Hernia Society.

617 JPN ISSN 0288-7509
HOKKAIDO GEKA ZASSHI/HOKKAIDO JOURNAL OF SURGERY. Text in Japanese; Summaries in English, Japanese. 1952. s-a.
Indexed: INIS Atomind.
Published by: Hokkaido Geka Gakkai/Hokkaido Surgical Society, Hokkaido Daigaku Igakubu, Nishi 7-chome, Kita 5-jo, Kita-ku, Sapporo-shi, Hokkaido 060, Japan.

617 JPN ISSN 0913-7629
HOKURIKU GEKA GAKKAI ZASSHI/HOKURIKU JOURNAL OF SURGERY. Text in Japanese; Summaries in English. 1982. a. JPY 3,000 (effective 2001). reprints avail. *Refereed.* **Document type:** *Academic/Scholarly.*
Published by: Hokuriku Geka Gakkai/Hokuriku Surgical Society, Kanazawa University School of Medicine, Department of Surgery, 13-1, Takaramachi, Kanazawa-shi, Ishikawa-ken 920-8641, Japan. TEL 81-76-265-2354, FAX 81-76-222-6833, go@med.kanazawa-u.ac.jp. Ed., R&P Go Watanabe. Circ: 1,000.

617 USA ISSN 0362-0727
RD701
HOSPITAL FOR SPECIAL SURGERY. JOURNAL. Text in English. 1975. irreg.
Published by: Hospital for Special Surgery, Public Relations Department, 535 E 70th St, New York, NY 10021.

M

617 JPN ISSN 0385-5325
HYOGOKEN ZENGEKAIKAI KAISHI/HYOGO ASSOCIATION OF SURGEONS. JOURNAL. Text in Japanese. 1962. irreg.
Published by: Hyogoken Zengeka Ikai, 1-30 Nakayamatedori 6-chome, Chuo-ku, Kobe-shi, Hyogo-ken 650-0004, Japan.

617 616.8 GBR ISSN 0742-504X CODEN: IHSED6
I B R O HANDBOOK SERIES. Text in English. 1982. irreg., latest vol.17, 1996. **Document type:** *Monographic series, Academic/Scholarly.*
Indexed: e-psyche.
—BLDSC (4360.160500), CASDDS, CISTI.
Published by: (International Brain Research Organization USA), John Wiley & Sons Ltd., Baffins Ln, Chichester, Sussex PO19 IUD, United Kingdom. FAX 44-1243-775878, cs-books@wiley.co.uk, http://www.wiley.co.uk. Ed. Z Henderson.

I S C T S - WORLD SOCIETY OF CARDIO - THORACIC SURGEONS. ANNUAL MEETING. see *MEDICAL SCIENCES—Cardiovascular Diseases*

617 JPN ISSN 0917-9070
ICHIGE/JUNTENDO UNIVERSITY. CLINICAL SURGERY SOCIETY. JOURNAL. Text in Japanese. 2/yr.
Published by: Juntendo Daigaku, Igakubu, Daiichi Geka Rinsho Kenkyukai, 1-1 Hongo 2-chome, Bunkyo-ku, Tokyo 113-0033, Japan.

INDIAN JOURNAL OF COLO-PROCTOLOGY. see *MEDICAL SCIENCES—Gastroenterology*

617.95 IND ISSN 0970-0358
INDIAN JOURNAL OF PLASTIC SURGERY. Text in English. 1967. 2/yr. INR 700; USD 15.25 foreign (effective 1999). adv. bk.rev. abstr, bibl, illus. back issues avail.; reprint service avail. from IRC. *Refereed.* **Document type:** *Academic/Scholarly.* **Description:** Deals with topics in plastic surgery.
—CISTI.
Published by: Association of Plastic Surgeons of India, Ganga Hospital, Swarnambika Layout, Coimbatore, Tamil Nadu 641 009, India. TEL 91-422-235050, FAX 91-422-235608, rajahand@md3.vsnl.net.in. Ed., Pub., R&P S Raja Sabapathy. adv.: B&W page INR 6,000, color page INR 12,500; trim 280 x 210. Circ: 750.

617 IND ISSN 0019-5650
RD1 CODEN: IJSUAV
INDIAN JOURNAL OF SURGERY. Text in English. 1970 (vol.32). bi-m. INR 50, USD 15. adv. bk.rev. charts, illus.
Indexed: Biol.Abstr., Chem.Abstr., Excerp.Med., INIS Atomind.
—BLDSC (4421.350000), CISTI, GNLM.
Published by: (Association of Surgeons in India), Popular Prakashan Pvt. Ltd., 35-C Tardeo Rd., Mumbai, Maharashtra 400 034, India. Ed. Dr. R K Gandhi. Circ: 2,400.

617 IND ISSN 0019-5863 CODEN: IMGAAY
INDIAN MEDICAL GAZETTE*. Text in English. 1961. m. INR 150. bk.rev. abstr, bibl, illus. **Description:** Promotes the development of modern medicine and surgery in India.
Indexed: Chem.Abstr., Excerp.Med., Nutr.Abstr.
—CASDDS, CISTI, GNLM.
Published by: Martin & Harris Private Ltd., Savory Chambers, Wallace St., Mumbai, Maharashtra 400 001, India. Ed. L K Pandeya. Circ: 27,689.

INTERNATIONAL JOURNAL OF ADULT ORTHODONTICS AND ORTHOGNATHIC SURGERY. see *MEDICAL SCIENCES—Dentistry*

INTERNATIONAL JOURNAL OF ANGIOLOGY. see *MEDICAL SCIENCES—Cardiovascular Diseases*

617 DEU ISSN 0179-1958 CODEN: IJCDE6
INTERNATIONAL JOURNAL OF COLORECTAL DISEASE. Text in English. 1986. bi-m. EUR 414.20 domestic; EUR 410.40 in Germany; EUR 80 newsstand/cover foreign (effective 2002). *Refereed.* **Document type:** *Journal, Academic/Scholarly.* **Description:** Includes clinical and laboratory research in the field with sections devoted to symposia and reviews of subjects of topical interest.
Related titles: Online - full text ed.: ISSN 1432-1262 (from EBSCO Publishing, RoweCom Information Quest, Swets Blackwell, Springer LINK, Institute for Scientific Information).
Indexed: ASCA, Curr.Cont., Excerp.Med., Ind.Med. (1986-), Inpharma, Nutr.Abstr., Pharm.&Out.News, Reac.
—BLDSC (4542.172400), CISTI, GNLM, IDS, KNAW. **CCC.**
Published by: (Association of Coloproctology of Great Britain and Ireland), Springer-Verlag (Subsidiary of: BertelsmannSpringer), Tiergartenstr 17, Heidelberg 69121, Germany. TEL 49-6221-345-0, FAX 49-6221-345229, subscriptions@springer.de, http://link.springer.de/link/service/journals/00384/index.htm, http://www.springer.de. Ed. H J Buhr. **Subscr. in N. America to:** Springer-Verlag New York Inc., PO Box 2485, Secaucus, NJ 07096-2485. TEL 212-460-1500, FAX 212-473-6272.

▼ **INTERNATIONAL JOURNAL OF COSMETIC SURGERY AND AESTHETIC DERMATOLOGY.** see *MEDICAL SCIENCES—Dermatology And Venereology*

617 USA
THE INTERNATIONAL JOURNAL OF COSMETIC SURGERY AND AESTHETIC DERMATOLOGY. Text in English. 1993. q. USD 179 (effective 2001). adv. *Refereed.*
Former titles: The International Journal of Cosmetic and Restorative Surgery; International Journal of Aesthetic and Restorative Surgery (1069-5249)
—GNLM.
Published by: Maryann Liebert, Publisher, 2 Madison Ave, Larchmont, NY 10537. TEL 610-896-6677, info@liebert.com. Eds. Howard Sobel, Melvin Shiffman. Circ: 5,000; 500 (paid).

INTERNATIONAL JOURNAL OF ORAL & MAXILLOFACIAL SURGERY. see *MEDICAL SCIENCES—Dentistry*

INTERNATIONAL JOURNAL OF PERIODONTICS & RESTORATIVE DENTISTRY. see *MEDICAL SCIENCES—Dentistry*

617 CHE ISSN 1028-5229
▼ **INTERNATIONAL JOURNAL OF SURGICAL INVESTIGATION.** Text in English. 2000. bi-m. USD 106 to individuals (effective 2001). **Document type:** *Journal, Academic/Scholarly.* **Description:** Contains articles involving all aspects of surgical investigation limited to prospective clinical trials, large retrospective outcome research and basic science research involving all surgical disciplines.
Related titles: Online - full text ed.: (from EBSCO Publishing, RoweCom Information Quest).
Published by: Gordon and Breach - Harwood Academic (Subsidiary of: Taylor & Francis Group), PO Box 531, Lausanne 1000, Switzerland. TEL 41-21-6411280, FAX 41-21-6411281, info@gbhap.com, http://www.gbhap.com/journals/417/417-top.htm. Ed. Walter Longo. **Subscr. addr. in US:** International Publishers Direct, PO Box 32160, Newark, NJ 07102. FAX 215-750-6343.

617 USA ISSN 1066-8969 CODEN: IJSPFL
INTERNATIONAL JOURNAL OF SURGICAL PATHOLOGY. Text in English. 1993. q., latest vol.9. USD 145 domestic to individuals; USD 175 foreign to individuals; USD 220 domestic to institutions; USD 245 foreign to institutions (effective 2001). adv. bk.rev. back issues avail.; reprints avail. *Refereed.* **Document type:** *Journal, Academic/Scholarly.* **Description:** Forum for the communication of scientific information in the field of surgical pathology. Includes studies that emphasize diagnostic and prognostic features involving human tissue.
Related titles: Microfiche ed.: (from PQC); Microfilm ed.: (from PQC); Online - full text ed.: (from Ovid Technologies, Inc., Northern Light Technology, Inc., ProQuest Information & Learning, Institute for Scientific Information).
Indexed: Curr.Cont., Excerp.Med. (1995-), Int.Abstr.Biol.Sci., Trop.Dis.Bull.
—BLDSC (4542.685300), CASDDS, GNLM, KNAW.
Published by: (Australasian, Hong Kong, Spanish, Korean Divisions, International Academy of Pathology), Westminster Publications, Inc., 708 Glen Cove Ave, Glen Head, NY 11545. TEL 516-759-0025, FAX 516-759-5524. Ed. Juan Rosai, MD. Pub. Timothy R McLaughlin. adv.: B&W page USD 1,050, color page USD 1,035; trim 8.5 x 11. Circ: 2,241 (paid).

617 618.92 USA ISSN 0885-6265
INTERNATIONAL PEDIATRICS. Text in English. 1984. q. USD 25 domestic to individuals; USD 45 foreign to individuals (effective 2001). adv. **Document type:** *Magazine, Trade.* **Description:** Provides an international forum for the exchange of information and ideas encompassed in the field of pediatrics, and provides both general pediatricians and specialists with a single source practical reference. Each issue presents a review of some of the most recent developments in pediatrics and addresses rapidly evolving topics.
—BLDSC (4544.896500).
Published by: Miami Children's Hospital, 3100 S W 62nd Ave, Miami, FL 33155-3009. TEL 305-663-6824, FAX 305-663-8446, journals@mch.com, http://www.int-pediatrics.org. Ed. Fima Lifshitz.

617.005 GBR ISSN 1465-8747
▼ **THE INTERNATIONAL REVIEW OF MODERN SURGERY.** Text in English. 1999. a. adv. **Document type:** *Journal, Trade.* **Description:** Provides an analysis of the latest trends and highlights the specific management, technology and drug developments that are essential to patient treatment and recovery.
Published by: Sterling Publications Ltd. (Subsidiary of: Sterling Publishing Group Plc.), Brunel House, 55-57 North Wharf Rd, London W2 1LA, United Kingdom. TEL 44-20-7915-9660, FAX 44-20-7724-2089, rms@sterlingpublications.com, info@sterlingpublications.com, http://www.sterlingpublications.com/publications/reviewmodernsurgery.html. Pub. Sarah Woddis. Circ: 10,000 (controlled).

617 ITA ISSN 0020-8868 CODEN: INTSAO
INTERNATIONAL SURGERY. Text in English. 1913. q. USD 105 to individuals; USD 155 to institutions. adv. bk.rev. abstr, illus. index. reprint service avail. from PQC. *Refereed.* **Document type:** *Academic/Scholarly.* **Description:** Publishes original scientific articles covering important clinical observations, surgical techniques, experimental surgery and research.
Formerly: International College of Surgeons. Journal
Related titles: Microform ed.: 1913 (from PQC); Online - full text ed.: (from Institute for Scientific Information).
Indexed: ASCA, Biol.Abstr., Chem.Abstr., Curr.Cont., Excerp.Med., Helminthol.Abstr., Hosp.Lit.Ind., INIS Atomind., Ind.Med. (1966-), Inpharma, Pharm.&Out.News, Reac., Sci.Cit.Ind. (coverage dropped).
—BLDSC (4550.020000), GNLM, IDS, ingenta, KNAW.
Published by: International College of Surgeons, 1516 North Lake Shore Drive, Chicago, IL 60160-1607. TEL 312-642-3555, FAX 312-787-1624, info@icsglobal.org, http://www.icsglobal.org/. adv.: B&W page USD 1,500, color page USD 2,400; trim 280 x 215. Circ: 10,000.

617 USA
INTERNATIONAL U S SURGEON. Text in English. 1940. q. membership.
Former titles: News and Notes (Chicago); U S News and Notes
Published by: International College of Surgeons, United States Section, 1516 N Lake Shore Dr, Chicago, IL 60610-1694. TEL 312-787-6274, FAX 312-787-9289. Circ: 6,000.

617.48 USA
▼ **THE INTERNET JOURNAL OF NEUROSURGERY.** Text in English. 2000. s-a. free per issue. bk.rev. back issues avail. **Document type:** *Academic/Scholarly.* **Description:** Contains information from the field of neurosurgery and spine orthopedic surgery. Original articles, reviews, case reports, streaming slide shows, streaming videos, letters to the editor, press releases, meeting information.
Media: Online - full content.
Published by: Internet Scientific Publications, L.L.C., 23 Rippling Creek Dr, Sugar Land, TX 77479. TEL 281-240-1533, FAX 281-240-1533, http://www.ispub.com/. Ed. Ziya Gokaslan. R&P, Adv. contact Hope Morrow TEL 832-754-0335.

▼ **THE INTERNET JOURNAL OF ORTHOPEDIC SURGERY.** see *MEDICAL SCIENCES—Orthopedics And Traumatology*

▼ **THE INTERNET JOURNAL OF PERFUSIONISTS.** see *MEDICAL SCIENCES—Cardiovascular Diseases*

M

617.95 USA
▼ **THE INTERNET JOURNAL OF PLASTIC SURGERY.** Text in English. 2000. s-a. free per issue. adv. bk.rev. back issues avail. *Refereed.* **Document type:** *Academic/Scholarly.* **Description:** Provides information from the field of plastic and reconstructive surgery; contains original articles, reviews, case reports, streaming slide shows, streaming videos, letters to the editor, press releases, meeting information.
Media: Online - full content.
Published by: Internet Scientific Publications, L.L.C., 23 Rippling Creek Dr, Sugar Land, TX 77479. TEL 281-240-1533, FAX 281-240-1533, http://www.ispub.com/. Ed. Howard Langstein. R&P, Adv. contact Hope Morrow TEL 832-754-0335.

617 USA
▼ **THE INTERNET JOURNAL OF POLISH ANESTHESIOLOGY AND SURGERY.** Text in English. ceased; resumed 1999. irreg. adv. *Refereed.* **Document type:** *Academic/Scholarly.*
Media: Online - full text.
Published by: Internet Scientific Publications, L.L.C., 23 Rippling Creek Dr, Sugar Land, TX 77479. wojcie@enramp.net, http://www.ispub.com/journals/ijpas.htm. Ed. Zbigniew J Wojciechowski.

617 USA
▼ **THE INTERNET JOURNAL OF SURGERY.** Text in English. 2000. s-a. free per issue. adv. bk.rev. back issues avail. *Refereed.* **Document type:** *Academic/Scholarly.* **Description:** Contains information from the field of surgery. Original articles, reviews, case reports, streaming slide shows, streaming videos, letters to the editor, press releases, meeting information.
Media: Online - full content.
Published by: Internet Scientific Publications, L.L.C., 23 Rippling Creek Dr, Sugar Land, TX 77479. TEL 281-240-1533, FAX 281-240-1533, http://www.ispub.com/journals/ijs.htm. R&P, Adv. contact Hope Morrow TEL 832-754-0335.

617.6 616.1 USA ISSN 1524-0274
THE INTERNET JOURNAL OF THORACIC AND CARDIOVASCULAR SURGERY. Text in English. 1997. s-a. free per issue. adv. bk.rev. back issues avail. *Refereed.* **Document type:** *Academic/Scholarly.* **Description:** Covers the field of thoracic, cardiac and vascular surgery. Original articles, reviews, case reports, streaming slide shows, streaming videos, letters to the editor, press releases, meeting information.
Media: Online - full text.
Published by: Internet Scientific Publications, L.L.C., 23 Rippling Creek Dr, Sugar Land, TX 77479. TEL 281-240-1533, FAX 281-240-1533, http://www.ispub.com/journals/ijtcvs.htm. Ed. Peter Oberwalder. Pub., R&P, Adv. contact Hope Morrow TEL 832-754-0335.

INTERVENTIONAL CARDIOLOGY NEWSLETTER. see *MEDICAL SCIENCES—Cardiovascular Diseases*

617 DEU ISSN 0935-6517
JAHRBUCH DER CHIRURGIE. Text in German; Summaries in English, German. 1988. a. DEM 126.40. back issues avail. **Document type:** *Academic/Scholarly.*
—GNLM.
Published by: Biermann Verlag GmbH, Nideggenerstr 18, Zuelpich 53909, Germany. TEL 49-2252-9410-0, FAX 49-2252-941015. Eds. H Buente, T Junginger.

JAPANESE JOURNAL OF INTERVENTIONAL CARDIOLOGY. see *MEDICAL SCIENCES—Cardiovascular Diseases*

617.95 JPN ISSN 0021-5228
JAPANESE JOURNAL OF PLASTIC & RECONSTRUCTIVE SURGERY/KEISEI GEKA. Text mainly in Japanese; Text occasionally in English. m. JPY 39,660. adv. bk.rev. charts, illus. index. **Document type:** *Academic/Scholarly.*
Indexed: Biol.Abstr., Excerp.Med., INIS Atomind.
—BLDSC (4658.100000), CISTI, GNLM.
Published by: Kokuseido Publishing Co. Ltd., 23-5-202 Hongo 3-chome, Bunkyo-ku, Tokyo 113-0033, Japan. TEL 81-3-3811-0995, FAX 81-3-3813-1866. Ed., R&P Akira Imai. Circ: 3,500.

617.54 JPN ISSN 1344-4964
CODEN: NKZAAY
THE JAPANESE JOURNAL OF THORACIC AND CARDIOVASCULAR SURGERY. Text in Japanese; Summaries in English, Japanese. 1953. m. JPY 1,000 per issue.
Formerly (until 1998): Nihon Kyobu Geka Gakkai Zasshi / Japanese Association for Thoracic Surgery. Journal (0369-4739)
Indexed: Biol.Abstr., Excerp.Med., INIS Atomind., Ind.Med. (1998-).
—EMDOCS, GNLM, IDS, KNAW.
Published by: Nihon Kyobu Geka Gakkai, 3-10 Koraku 2-chome, Bunkyo-ku, Tokyo 112-0004, Japan.

617.54 JPN ISSN 0021-5252
JAPANESE JOURNAL OF THORACIC SURGERY/KYOBU GEKA. Text in Japanese; Abstracts and contents page in English. 1948. 13/yr. JPY 46,000. adv. charts, illus. index. **Document type:** *Academic/Scholarly.*
Indexed: Curr.Cont. (coverage dropped), Excerp.Med., INIS Atomind., Ind.Med. (1948-).
—BLDSC (4658.900000), CISTI, GNLM, KNAW.
Published by: Nankodo Co. Ltd., 42-6 Hongo 3-chome, Bunkyo-ku, Tokyo 113-0033, Japan. FAX 03-3811-7230. Eds. Akira Furuse, Shigefumi Fujimura. Circ: 3,000.

617 JPN ISSN 0915-9118
JIN ISHOKU KEKKAN GEKA/RENAL TRANSPLANTATION, VASCULAR SURGERY. Text in English, Japanese. 1989. 2/yr. JPY 2,000 (effective 1998). **Document type:** *Academic/Scholarly.*
Published by: Jin Ishoku Kekkan Geka Kenkyukai/Japanese Society of Renal Transplantation and Vascular Surgery, Women s Medical College, Department of Urology, 8-1 Kawada-cho, Shinjuku-ku, Tokyo 162-0054, Japan. Ed. Hiroshi Toma.

617 FRA ISSN 0021-7697
CODEN: JOCHAQ
JOURNAL DE CHIRURGIE. Text in French. 1908. 10/yr. FRF 1,285; FRF 1,542 foreign (effective 2000). adv. bk.rev. abstr, bibl, illus. index. reprint service avail. from PQC. *Refereed.* **Document type:** *Academic/Scholarly.* **Description:** Provides original articles, and clinical cases on the main surgical specialities. Includes a regular section on experimental surgery and a review of the international publications in surgery.
Related titles: Microform ed.: (from PQC); Online - full text ed.: (from Institute for Scientific Information, RoweCom Information Quest).
Indexed: ASCA, Biol.Abstr., C.I.S. Abstr., Curr.Cont., Excerp.Med., Helminthol.Abstr., Ind.Med. (1908-), Ind.Sci.Rev., Inpharma, Int.Nurs.Ind., Pharm.&Out.News, Reac., Rev.Med.& Vet.Mycol., Sci.Cit.Ind. (coverage dropped).
—BLDSC (4958.200000), CISTI, GNLM, IDS, Infotrieve. **CCC.**
Published by: Masson - Periodiques, 120 bd. St. Germain, Paris 75006, France. TEL 33-1-40466200, FAX 33-1-40466201. Ed. Ph Detrie. Circ: 3,500. **Subscr. to:** Societe de Periodiques Specialises, BP 22, Vineuil Cedex 41354, France. TEL 33-2-54504612, FAX 33-2-54504611.

617 FRA ISSN 0021-7913
JOURNAL DE MEDECINE ET DE CHIRURGIE PRATIQUES✶. Text in French. 1830. s-m. FRF 250.
Indexed: Excerp.Med.
—CISTI, GNLM.
Published by: Association des Amis de Just Lucas Championniere, c/o Expansion Scientifique, 15 rue Saint-Benoit, Paris Cedex 6 75278, France.

617 USA ISSN 0021-8421
JOURNAL OF ABDOMINAL SURGERY. Variant title: Abdominal Surgery. Text in English. 1959. m. USD 15. adv. bk.rev. abstr, charts, illus, stat. index. *Refereed.*
Indexed: Biol.Abstr., Excerp.Med.
—GNLM.
Published by: American Society of Abdominal Surgeons, 675 Main St, Melrose, MA 02176. TEL 617-665-6102. Eds. John M Langone, Dr. Meyer O Cantor. Circ: 13,900.

617 USA ISSN 0885-3282
R856.A1 CODEN: JBAPEL
JOURNAL OF BIOMATERIALS APPLICATIONS. Text in English. 1986. q. USD 425 for print or electronic eds.; USD 485 for print and electronic eds. (effective 2001). back issues avail.; reprints avail. *Refereed.* **Document type:** *Journal, Academic/Scholarly.* **Description:** Covers research and development of biomaterials used in surgical products and medical devices.
Related titles: E-mail ed.; Online - full content ed.; Online - full text ed.: (from Institute for Scientific Information).
Indexed: ASCA, Alloys Ind., Bioeng.Abstr., Biotech.& Bioeng.Abstr., Chem.Abstr., Chem.Indus.Notes, Chem.Titles, Eng.Ind., Eng.Mat.Abstr., INIS Atomind., Ind.Med. (1986-), METADEX, Mat.Sci.Cit.Ind., Met.Abstr., Met.Abstr.Ind., Nonfer.Met.Alert, PCC Alert, RAPRA (1996-), Steels Alert, World Alum.Abstr.
—BLDSC (4953.515000), CASDDS, CISTI, Ei, GNLM, IDS, Infotrieve. **CCC.**
Published by: Sage Publications, Inc., 2111 W Hillcrest Dr, Thousand Oaks, CA 91320. info@sagepub.com, http://www.sagepub.com. Circ: 180 (paid).

JOURNAL OF BONE AND JOINT SURGERY: AMERICAN AND BRITISH VOLUMES ON CD-ROM. see *MEDICAL SCIENCES—Orthopedics And Traumatology*

JOURNAL OF BONE AND JOINT SURGERY: BRITISH VOLUME. see *MEDICAL SCIENCES—Orthopedics And Traumatology*

JOURNAL OF BONE AND JOINT SURGERY. BRITISH VOLUME. ORTHOPAEDIC PROCEEDINGS. see *MEDICAL SCIENCES—Orthopedics And Traumatology*

THE JOURNAL OF CARDIOVASCULAR SURGERY. see *MEDICAL SCIENCES—Cardiovascular Diseases*

JOURNAL OF CATARACT AND REFRACTIVE SURGERY. see *MEDICAL SCIENCES—Ophthalmology And Optometry*

JOURNAL OF CLINICAL LASER MEDICINE & SURGERY. see *MEDICAL SCIENCES—Radiology And Nuclear Medicine*

617 GBR ISSN 1010-5182
CODEN: JCMSET
JOURNAL OF CRANIO-MAXILLO-FACIAL SURGERY. Text in English. 1973. bi-m. GBP 107 to individuals; GBP 239 to institutions (effective 2002). adv. illus. index. reprint service avail. from PQC. *Refereed.* **Document type:** *Journal, Academic/Scholarly.* **Description:** Covers all aspects of surgery of the head, face and jaw.
Former titles: Journal of Cranio and Maxillofacial Surgery; Journal of Maxillofacial Surgery (0301-0503)
Related titles: Microform ed.: (from PQC); Online - full text ed.: (from EBSCO Publishing, O C L C Online Computer Library Center, Inc., Swets Blackwell, IDEAL Online Library, Institute for Scientific Information).
Indexed: ASCA, Biol.Abstr., Curr.Adv.Cancer Res., Curr.Cont., Curr.Tit.Dent., Dent.Ind., Excerp.Med., INIS Atomind., Ind.Med. (1987-), Ind.Sci.Rev., Inpharma, Reac., Rev.Med.& Vet.Mycol., Sci.Cit.Ind.
—BLDSC (4965.482000), CISTI, EMDOCS, GNLM, IDS, ingenta, KNAW. **CCC.**
Published by: (European Association for Cranio Maxillo-Facial Surgery), Churchill Livingstone (Subsidiary of: Harcourt Publishers Ltd.), Robert Stevenson House, 1-3 Baxter's Pl, Leith Walk, Edinburgh, Midlothian EH1 3AF, United Kingdom. TEL 44-131-556-2424, FAX 44-131-459-1177, cservice@harcourt.com, http://www.harcourt-international.com/journals/jcms. Ed. Dr. Karsten Gundlach. R&P Catherine John TEL 212-424-4200. Adv. contact David Dunnachie. Circ: 1,775. **Subscr. to:** Harcourt Publishers Ltd., Foots Cray High St, Sidcup, Kent DA14 5HP, United Kingdom. TEL 44-20-8308-5700, FAX 44-20-8309-0807.

617 USA ISSN 1074-3219
CODEN: JCTRFS
JOURNAL OF CRANIO-MAXILLOFACIAL TRAUMA. Variant title: J C M T. Text in English. 1995. q. USD 161 domestic to individuals; USD 227 foreign to individuals (effective 2000). adv. abstr, charts, illus. index. back issues avail.; reprints avail. *Refereed.* **Document type:** *Academic/Scholarly.* **Description:** Publishes clinical, technical and review articles concerning cranio-maxillofacial trauma patient care for neurosurgeons, ophthalmologists, oral and maxillofacial surgeons, otolaryngologists, plastic and reconstructive surgeons.
Indexed: Excerp.Med. (1996-).
—EMDOCS, GNLM.
Published by: Montage Media Corp., 1000 Wyckoff Ave, Mahwah, NJ 07430. TEL 201-891-3200, FAX 201-891-2626, jcmt@montagemedia.com, http://www.montagemedia.com. Ed. Dr. Paul N Manson. Pub. Stephen E Sweeney. R&P Laura K Franklin TEL 201-891-3200 ext 115. Adv. contact Jim King. B&W page USD 1,396, color page USD 2,596; trim 10.88 x 8.13. Circ: 11,800.

M

617.95 USA ISSN 1049-2275
CODEN: JSURE8
JOURNAL OF CRANIOFACIAL SURGERY. Text in English. 1990. bi-m. USD 484 domestic to individuals; USD 484 foreign to individuals; USD 695 domestic to institutions; USD 775 foreign to institutions (effective 2002); USD 118 newsstand/cover. adv. bk.rev. abstr, charts, illus, stat. index. back issues avail.; reprint service avail. from PQC. *Refereed.* **Document type:** *Academic/Scholarly.* **Description:** Covers all areas of craniofacial surgery, including treatment of congenital malformation, repair of posttraumatic deformation, treatment of oncological deformities, and resection of tumors in the skull base.
Related titles: Microform ed.: (from PQC); Online - full text ed.: USD 903.50 domestic academic site license; USD 983.50 foreign academic site license; USD 1,007.75 domestic corporate site license; USD 1,087.75 foreign corporate site license (2002); (from Institute for Scientific Information).
Indexed: ASCA, Curr.Cont., Curr.Tit.Dent., Excerp.Med. (1993-), Ind.Sci.Rev., Inpharma, Reac., Sci.Cit.Ind.
—BLDSC (4965.476000), CISTI, EMDOCS, GNLM, IDS, ingenta, KNAW.
Published by: (American Association of Pediatric Plastic Surgeons), Lippincott Williams & Wilkins (Philadelphia) (Subsidiary of: Wolters Kluwer N.V.), 530 Walnut St, Philadelphia, PA 19106-3621. TEL 215-521-8300, FAX 215-521-8902, http://www.lww.com. Ed. Dr. Mutaz B Habal. Pub. Terri Monturano. R&P Margaret Becker. Adv. contact James Nagle. B&W page USD 705; trim 11 x 8.25. Circ: 496. **Subscr. to:** PO Box 1600, Hagerstown, MD 21740-1600. TEL 800-777-2295, FAX 301-824-7390. **Co-sponsors:** International Society of Craniofacial Surgery; European Society of Craniofacial Surgery.

▼ **JOURNAL OF CUTANEOUS LASER THERAPY.** see *MEDICAL SCIENCES—Dermatology And Venereology*

JOURNAL OF CUTANEOUS MEDICINE AND SURGERY. see *MEDICAL SCIENCES—Dermatology And Venereology*

617.4 616.1 USA ISSN 1526-6028
CODEN: JESUFC
JOURNAL OF ENDOVASCULAR THERAPY. Text in English. 1994. bi-m. USD 100 domestic to individuals; USD 125 foreign to individuals; USD 150 domestic to institutions; USD 175 foreign to institutions (effective 2000). adv. bk.rev. charts, illus. *Refereed.* **Document type:** *Academic/Scholarly.* **Description:** Presents interesting, difficult or unusual case reports representing all topics related to international vascular diagnosis and therapy.
Formerly (until 2000): Journal of Endovascular Surgery (1074-6218); Which supersedes (in 1995): Vascular Surgery (Armonk) (1067-5051)
Related titles: Online - full text ed.: (from Institute for Scientific Information).
Indexed: ASCA, CINAHL, Curr.Cont., Excerp.Med. (1996-), Ind.Med. (2000-), Inpharma, Reac., Sci.Cit.Ind.
—BLDSC (4978.230000), CISTI, GNLM, IDS, Infotrieve, KNAW. **CCC.**
Published by: (International Society for Endovascular Surgery), Alliance Communications Group (Subsidiary of: Allen Press Inc.), 810 East 10th St, Lawrence, KS 66044. adv.: B&W page USD 800, color page USD 1,735; trim 10.88 x 8.25. Circ: 3,300.

▼ **JOURNAL OF FELINE MEDICINE AND SURGERY.** see *VETERINARY SCIENCE*

617 USA ISSN 1067-2516
CODEN: JFSUEI
JOURNAL OF FOOT AND ANKLE SURGERY. Text in English. 1963. bi-m. USD 109 to individuals; USD 162 to institutions (effective 2000). adv. *Refereed.* **Document type:** *Academic/Scholarly.* **Description:** Clinical advances in foot surgery for podiatrists and orthopedic foot surgeons. Each issue includes a 10 question continuing education exam.
Former titles (until 1993): Journal of Foot Surgery (0449-2544); (until 1967): American College of Foot Surgeons. Journal (0517-0591)
Related titles: CD-ROM ed.
Indexed: AMED, CINAHL, Excerp.Med., INIS Atomind., Ind.Med. (1993-), Int.Nurs.Ind.
—BLDSC (4984.572000), EMDOCS, GNLM, ingenta, KNAW.
Published by: (American College of Foot and Ankle Surgeons), Data Trace Publishing Company, 110 West Rd, Ste 227, Baltimore, MD 21204. TEL 410-494-4994, FAX 410-494-0515, info@datatrace.com, http://www.datatrace.com. Ed. Dr. Lowell Scott Weil. R&P Cindy Lee Floyd. Adv. contact Frank Tufariello. Circ: 6,553.

617 USA ISSN 1091-255X
JOURNAL OF GASTROINTESTINAL SURGERY. Text in English. 1997. bi-m. EUR 134 in Europe to individuals; JPY 17,800 in Japan to individuals; USD 150 elsewhere to individuals; EUR 174 in Europe to institutions; JPY 23,100 in Japan to institutions; USD 195 elsewhere to institutions (effective 2002). adv. *Refereed.* **Document type:** *Academic/Scholarly.* **Description:** Designed to furnish the surgeon with the latest developments in gastrointestinal surgery.
Related titles: Online - full text ed.: (from Institute for Scientific Information).
Indexed: Curr.Cont., Ind.Med. (1997-).
—BLDSC (4987.625000), Infotrieve. **CCC.**
Published by: (Society for Surgery of the Alimentary Tract, Inc.), Quality Medical Publishing, Inc., 11970 Borman Dr., Ste. 222, St. Louis, MO 63146. TEL 314-878-7808, 800-348-7808, FAX 314-878-9937, qmp@qmp.com, http://www.qmp.com. Eds. Dr. John L Cameron, Dr. Keith A Kelly. R&P Michelle Leamon TEL 800-423-6865. Adv. contact Cindy Meilink. B&W page USD 1,000, color page USD 2,050. Circ: 4,774.

JOURNAL OF GYNECOLOGIC SURGERY. see *MEDICAL SCIENCES—Obstetrics And Gynecology*

616 USA ISSN 0363-5023
RD559 CODEN: JHSUDV
JOURNAL OF HAND SURGERY: AMERICAN VOLUME. Text in English. 1976. bi-m. USD 157 combined subscription domestic to individuals for both print & online eds.; USD 231 combined subscription foreign to individuals for both print & online eds.; USD 272 combined subscription domestic to institutions for both print & online eds.; USD 346 combined subscription foreign to institutions for both print & online eds.; USD 72 combined subscription domestic to students for both print & online eds.; USD 139 combined subscription foreign to students for both print & online eds.; USD 58 per issue (effective 2001). adv. bk.rev. charts, illus. index. reprint service avail. from PQC. *Refereed.* **Document type:** *Journal, Academic/Scholarly.* **Description:** Edited for hand, orthopedic, plastic and reconstructive, and general surgeons who seek to restore function to the hand and upper extremity.
Related titles: CD-ROM ed.: USD 195 per issue to individuals; USD 350 per issue to institutions (effective 2000); Microfilm ed.: 1976 (from PQC); Online - full content ed.: (from EBSCO Publishing, O C L C Online Computer Library Center, Inc., ProQuest Information & Learning, Swets Blackwell); Online - full text ed.: (from IDEAL Online Library, Institute for Scientific Information); ♦ Regional ed.: Journal of Hand Surgery: British and European Volume. ISSN 0266-7681.
Indexed: ASCA, Bibl.Dev.Med.& Child Neur., Biol.Abstr., Curr.Adv.Ecol.Sci., Curr.Cont., Dok.Arbeitsmed., Excerp.Med., INIS Atomind., Ind.Med. (1976-), Inpharma, Neurosci.Cit.Ind., Reac., Rev.Med.& Vet.Mycol.
—BLDSC (4996.620000), CISTI, EMDOCS, GNLM, IDS, ingenta, KNAW. **CCC.**
Published by: (American Society for Surgery of the Hand), W.B. Saunders Co. (Subsidiary of: Harcourt Publishers Ltd.), P.O. Box 628239, Orlando, FL 32862-8239. TEL 407-345-4000, FAX 215-238-6445, 407-363-9661, 800-225-6030, wbspcs@harcourtbrace.com, http://www.jhandsurg.org. Ed. Paul R Manske. Circ: 7,900.

617 GBR ISSN 0266-7681
JOURNAL OF HAND SURGERY: BRITISH AND EUROPEAN VOLUME. Text in English. 1969. bi-m. GBP 170 to individuals; GBP 260 to institutions (effective 2002). adv. back issues avail. *Refereed.* **Document type:** *Journal, Academic/Scholarly.* **Description:** Dedicated to the needs of hand, plastic, reconstructive and orthopaedic surgeons.
Formerly: Hand (0072-968X)
Related titles: CD-ROM ed.: USD 190 per issue to individuals; USD 350 per issue to institutions (effective 2000); Microform ed.: (from PQC); Online - full text ed.: (from EBSCO Publishing, O C L C Online Computer Library Center, Inc., RoweCom Information Quest, Swets Blackwell, IDEAL Online Library, Institute for Scientific Information); ♦ Regional ed.: Journal of Hand Surgery: American Volume. ISSN 0363-5023.
Indexed: ASCA, Curr.Cont., Excerp.Med., INIS Atomind., Ind.Med. (1984-), Inpharma, Neurosci.Cit.Ind., Reac., Rev.Med.& Vet.Mycol.
—BLDSC (4996.623000), EMDOCS, GNLM, IDS, Infotrieve, KNAW. **CCC.**
Published by: (British Society for Surgery of the Hand), Churchill Livingstone (Subsidiary of: Harcourt Publishers Ltd.), Robert Stevenson House, 1-3 Baxter's Pl, Leith Walk, Edinburgh, Midlothian EH1 3AF, United Kingdom. TEL 44-131-556-2424, FAX 44-131-459-1177, cservice@harcourt.com, http://www.harcourt-international.com/journals/jhsb. Ed. T Davis. Adv. contact David Dunnachie. Circ: 3,100. **Subscr. in the US to:** W B Saunders Company, 6277 Sea Harbor Dr, Orlando, FL 32887-4800. TEL 407-345-4000, FAX 407-363-9661; **Subscr. to:** Harcourt Publishers Ltd., Foots Cray High St, Sidcup, Kent DA14 5HP, United Kingdom. TEL 44-20-8308-5700, FAX 44-20-8309-0807.

617 GBR ISSN 1053-2498
RD598 CODEN: JHLTES
THE JOURNAL OF HEART AND LUNG TRANSPLANTATION. Text in English. 1981. m. EUR 198 in Europe to individuals; JPY 27,510 in Japan to individuals; USD 134 in US & Canada to individuals; USD 222 elsewhere to individuals; EUR 282 in Europe to institutions; JPY 37,400 in Japan to institutions; USD 224 in US & Canada to institutions; USD 315 elsewhere to institutions; EUR 111 in Europe residents price; JPY 15,330 in Japan residents price; USD 79 in US & Canada residents price; USD 123 elsewhere residents price (effective 2002). adv. charts, illus. index. back issues avail.; reprint service avail. from PQC. *Refereed.* **Document type:** *Academic/Scholarly.* **Description:** Presents the latest clinical information on the rapidly evolving field of intrathoracic transplantation, support and replacement.
Former titles (until 1991): Journal of Heart Transplantation (0887-2570); Heart Transplantation
Related titles: Microfilm ed.: (from PQC); Online - full text ed.: (from EBSCO Publishing, ingenta, ScienceDirect, Swets Blackwell, Institute for Scientific Information).
Indexed: ASCA, Curr.Cont., Excerp.Med., INIS Atomind., Ind.Med. (1991-), Inpharma, Pharm.&Out.News, Reac., Rev.Med.& Vet.Mycol., Sci.Cit.Ind.
—BLDSC (4996.874000), CISTI, EMDOCS, GNLM, IDS, ingenta, KNAW. **CCC.**
Published by: (International Society for Heart and Lung Transplantation, European Society of Cardiology FRA), Elsevier Science, Box 945, New York, NY 10159-0945. TEL 212-989-5800, 888-437-4636, http://www.elsevier.com/locate/healun. Eds. J K Kirklin, P Holmes. adv.: B&W page USD 845, color page USD 1,560; trim 10.88 x 8.25. Circ: 3,682.

617 JPN ISSN 0944-1166
CODEN: JHBSFA
JOURNAL OF HEPATO - BILIARY - PANCREATIC SURGERY. Text in English. 1993. bi-m. (in 1 vol., 6 nos./vol.). EUR 260.70 domestic; EUR 255 in Germany; EUR 46 newsstand/cover foreign for Print & Online Eds. (effective 2001). **Document type:** *Academic/Scholarly.* **Description:** Deals with clinical investigations of and basic research on all aspects of the field of hepatic, biliary, and pancreatic surgery. Also presents case studies and descriptions of surgical techniques.
Related titles: Online - full content ed.: ISSN 1436-0691 (from EBSCO Publishing, Swets Blackwell); Online - full text ed.: (from Springer LINK, RoweCom Information Quest).
Indexed: Ind.Med. (1993-).
—BLDSC (4997.670000), CISTI, GNLM, Infotrieve. **CCC.**
Published by: (Japanese Society of Hepato-Biliary-Pancreatic Surgery), Springer-Verlag Tokyo, Eastern Book Service, Inc. (Subsidiary of: BertelsmannSpringer), 3-13 Hongo 3-chome, Bunkyo-ku, Tokyo 113-0033, Japan. FAX 81-3-3812-0719, orders@svt-ebs.co.jp, http://link.springer-ny.com/link/service/journals/00534/index.htm. Ed. T Takada. **Subscr. in N. America to:** Springer-Verlag New York Inc., PO Box 2485, Secaucus, NJ 07096-2485. TEL 800-777-4643, 212-460-1500, 212-460-1526, FAX 201-348-4505, 212-473-6272, orders@springer-ny.com; **Subscr. to:** Eastern Book Service, Inc., 3-13 Hongo 3-chome, Bunkyo-ku, Tokyo 113-8480, Japan. TEL 81-3-3818-0861, FAX 81-3-3818-0864, orders@svt-ebs.co.jp. **Dist. outside Japan by:** Springer-Verlag, Haber Str 7, Heidelberg 69126, Germany. TEL 49-30-82787-0, subscriptions@springer.de, http://link.springer.de, http://link.springer-ny.com.

617 USA ISSN 0894-1939
CODEN: JISUE5
JOURNAL OF INVESTIGATIVE SURGERY. Text in English. 1988. bi-m. GBP 181, USD 298 to individuals; GBP 418, USD 690 to institutions (effective 2002). *Refereed.* **Document type:** *Academic/Scholarly.* **Description:** Discusses the development of novel surgical concepts and the development of surgical models, devices, and instruments.

M

Related titles: Online - full text ed.: ISSN 1521-0553 (from CatchWord Ltd., EBSCO Publishing, O C L C Online Computer Library Center, Inc., RoweCom Information Quest, Swets Blackwell, Institute for Scientific Information).
Indexed: ASCA, Curr.Cont., INIS Atomind., Ind.Med. (1988-), Inpharma, Pharm.&Out.News, Reac.
—BLDSC (5008.020000), CatchWord, EMDOCS, GNLM, IDS, Infotrieve, KNAW. **CCC.**
Published by: Taylor & Francis Ltd. (Subsidiary of: Taylor & Francis Group), 325 Chestnut St, Suite 800, Philadelphia, PA 19016. TEL 215-625-8900, FAX 215-625-2940, info@taylorandfrancis.com, http://www.taylorandfrancis.com/. Ed. A Karim Qayumi. **Subscr. addr. in Europe:** Taylor & Francis Group, Journals Customer Service, Rankine Rd, Basingstoke, Hants RG24 8PR, United Kingdom. TEL 44-1256-813000, FAX 44-1256-479438, enquiry@tanf.co.uk, http://www.tandf.co.uk/journals.

617 USA ISSN 1092-6429 CODEN: JLSUEQ
JOURNAL OF LAPAROENDOSCOPIC & ADVANCED SURGICAL TECHNIQUES. Text in English. 1990. bi-m. USD 209 domestic to individuals; USD 318 foreign to individuals; USD 251 domestic to individuals print and online eds. combined; USD 360 foreign to individuals print and online eds. combined; USD 450 domestic to institutions; USD 568 foreign to institutions; USD 540 domestic to institutions print and online eds. combined; USD 658 foreign to institutions print and online eds. combined (effective 2002). adv. back issues avail.; reprints avail. *Refereed.* **Document type:** *Journal, Academic/Scholarly.* **Description:** Disseminates information on the surgical techniques that encompass laparoscopy and endoscopy.
Formerly (until 1997): Journal of Laparoendoscopic Surgery (1052-3901)
Related titles: Online - full content ed.: USD 450 to institutions; USD 209 to individuals (effective 2002) (from Swets Blackwell); Online - full text ed.: (from CatchWord Ltd., Institute for Scientific Information, RoweCom Information Quest).
Indexed: ASCA, Curr.Cont., Excerp.Med. (1992-), Ind.Med. (1997-), Inpharma, Reac., Sci.Cit.Ind.
—BLDSC (5010.098500), CatchWord, CISTI, EMDOCS, GNLM, IDS, ingenta, KNAW. **CCC.**
Published by: Mary Ann Liebert, Inc. Publishers, 2 Madison Ave, Larchmont, NY 10538. TEL 914—834-3100, FAX 914-834-1388, info@liebertpub.com, http://www.liebertpub.com/lap. Ed. Dr. Bruce Shirmer.

617 USA ISSN 1050-6934 CODEN: JLEIEM
JOURNAL OF LONG-TERM EFFECTS OF MEDICAL IMPLANTS. Text in English. q. USD 96 to individuals; USD 416 to institutions (effective 2000). adv. *Refereed.* **Document type:** *Academic/Scholarly.* **Description:** Aims to better understand the mechanism of failure of pre-clinically tested medical implants during long-term in vivo service, both in appropriate animal models and in humans, and establishing an effective linkage between pre-clinical and clinical studies.
Indexed: ASCA, Alloys Ind., Bioeng.Abstr., Biotech.& Bioeng.Abstr., Cal.Tiss.Abstr., Chem.Indus.Notes, Chem.Titles, Curr.Cont. (coverage dropped), Eng.Ind., Eng.Mat.Abstr., Environ.Sci.Poll.Mgmt., Excerp.Med. (1993-), Ind.Sci.Rev., Inpharma, METADEX, Mat.Sci.Cit.Ind. (coverage dropped), Med.& Pharm.Biotech.Abstr., Met.Abstr., Met.Abstr.Ind., Microbiol.Abstr., Nonfer.Met.Alert, PCC Alert, Pollut.Abstr., Reac., Risk Abstr., Saf.Sci.Abstr., Sci.Cit.Ind. (coverage dropped), Steels Alert, Tox.Abstr., World Alum.Abstr.
—BLDSC (5010.560500), CASDDS, CISTI, Ei, EMDOCS, GNLM, IDS, Infotrieve, KNAW. **CCC.**
Published by: Begell House Inc., 79 Madison Ave, Ste 1205, New York, NY 10016-7892. TEL 212-725-1999, FAX 212-213-8368, begellhouse@worldnet.att.net, orders@begellhouse.com. Ed. Stephen D Bruck. Pub. William Begell. R&P, Adv. contact Jung Ra.

617 JPN ISSN 0917-7728
JOURNAL OF MICROWAVE SURGERY. Text in English, Japanese. 1988. a. JPY 3,000 (effective 1998).
Formerly (until 1991): Maikurowebu Sajeri (0917-1231)
Published by: Medikaru Rebyusha/Medical Review Co., Ltd., 7-3 Hirano-Machi 1-chome, Chuo-ku, Osaka-shi 541-0046, Japan. TEL 81-6-223-1556, FAX 81-6-223-1414, medrev@osk2.3web.ne.jp. Ed. Hatsuoka Jabuse.

JOURNAL OF NEUROLOGY, NEUROSURGERY AND PSYCHIATRY. see *MEDICAL SCIENCES—Psychiatry And Neurology*

JOURNAL OF NEUROSURGERY. see *MEDICAL SCIENCES—Psychiatry And Neurology*

JOURNAL OF NEUROSURGICAL ANESTHESIOLOGY. see *MEDICAL SCIENCES—Anaesthesiology*

617 616.8 ITA ISSN 0390-5616
JOURNAL OF NEUROSURGICAL SCIENCES. Text in English. 1957. q. USD 105 to individuals; USD 155 to institutions (effective 2000 - 2001). adv. bk.rev. bibl, charts, illus. index. *Refereed.* **Document type:** *Academic/Scholarly.*
Incorporates: Journal of Pediatric Neurosciences; Formerly (until 1973): Minerva Neurochirurgica (0026-4881)
Related titles: Microform ed.: (from RPI,PQC); Online - full text ed.: (from Northern Light Technology, Inc., ProQuest Information & Learning).
Indexed: Bibl.Dev.Med.& Child Neur., Biol.Abstr., Curr.Adv.Cancer Res., Curr.Adv.Gen.& Molec.Biol., Curr.Cont. (coverage dropped), Excerp.Med., Ind.Med. (1973-), Ind.Vet., Nutr.Abstr., Ref.Zh., e-psyche.
—BLDSC (5022.250000), CISTI, GNLM, ingenta, KNAW.
Published by: (Societa Italiana di Neurochirurgia), Edizioni Minerva Medica, Corso Bramante, 83-85, Turin, TO 10126, Italy. TEL 39-11-678282, FAX 39-11-674502. Ed. R M Villani. Pub. Alberto Oliaro. Adv. contact F Filippo. B&W page USD 1,200, color page USD 2,000; trim 270 x 190. Circ: 3,000 (paid).

617 GBR
THE JOURNAL OF ONE-DAY SURGERY. Text in English. 1991. q. GBP 20 domestic; GBP 22 foreign (effective 2000). adv. bk.rev. abstr. 28 p./no. 2 cols./p. back issues avail. *Refereed.* **Document type:** *Journal, Academic/Scholarly.*
Indexed: Brit.Nur.Ind.
—BLDSC (5026.314600).
Published by: (British Association of Day Surgery), Newton Mann Ltd., Stretton Rd, Tansley, Matlock, Derbys DE4 5GE, United Kingdom. TEL 44-1629-583941, FAX 44-1629-580479, ods@newtonmann.co.uk. Ed. Ian Jackson. Adv. contact Valerie Greaves TEL 01455-558635. B&W page GBP 345, color page GBP 595; trim 210 x 297.

JOURNAL OF ORAL AND MAXILLOFACIAL SURGERY. see *MEDICAL SCIENCES—Dentistry*

617.3 GBR ISSN 0334-0236 CODEN: JOSTEA
JOURNAL OF ORTHOPEDIC SURGICAL TECHNIQUES. Text in English. 1985. q. USD 85 to individuals; USD 145 to institutions. adv. bk.rev. **Document type:** *Academic/Scholarly.* **Description:** International forum dealing mainly with the techniques of orthopaedic surgery, operative and conservative, and with clinical basic research on the techniques themselves.
Indexed: Curr.Adv.Ecol.Sci., Excerp.Med.
—CISTI, EMDOCS, GNLM.
Published by: Medical Advance of Technique & Research Ltd., 48 Aylestone Ave, London NW6 7AA, United Kingdom. FAX 0181-960-8901. Ed. Dan Herness. Circ: 1,000.

617 USA ISSN 0022-3468
RD137.A1 CODEN: JPDSA3
JOURNAL OF PEDIATRIC SURGERY. Text in English. 1966 (Feb.). m. USD 275 combined subscription domestic to individuals for both print & online eds.; USD 396 combined subscription foreign to individuals for both print & online eds.; USD 436 combined subscription domestic to institutions for both print & online eds.; USD 499 combined subscription foreign to institutions for both print & online eds.; USD 187 combined subscription domestic to students for both print & online eds.; USD 223 combined subscription foreign to students for both print & online eds.; USD 42 newsstand/cover (effective 2001). adv. bk.rev. abstr, bibl, charts, illus. index. *Refereed.* **Document type:** *Journal, Academic/Scholarly.* **Description:** Disseminates original articles that address the need to improve the surgical care of infants and children, through advances in physiology and pathology, as well as surgical techniques.
Related titles: Online - full text ed.: (from IDEAL Online Library, Institute for Scientific Information).
Indexed: ASCA, Bibl.Dev.Med.& Child Neur., Biol.Abstr., C.C.I.P., Curr.Adv.Cancer Res., Curr.Adv.Gen.& Molec.Biol., Curr.Cont., Dent.Ind., Environ.Sci.Poll.Mgmt., Excerp.Med., INIS Atomind., Ind.Med. (1966-), Ind.Sci.Rev., Inpharma, Int.Nurs.Ind., Neurosci.Cit.Ind., Nutr.Abstr., Pharm.&Out.News, Pollut.Abstr., Protozool.Abstr., Reac., Risk Abstr., SSCI (coverage dropped), Saf.Sci.Abstr., Sci.Cit.Ind.
—BLDSC (5030.275000), CISTI, GNLM, IDS, ingenta, KNAW. **CCC.**
Published by: (Surgical Section, American Academy of Pediatrics), W.B. Saunders Co. (Subsidiary of: Harcourt Publishers Ltd.), 11830 Westline Industrial Dr, St Louis, MO 63146. TEL 800-325-4177, http://www.jpedsurg.org, http://www.wbsaunders.com. Ed. Jay L Grosfeld. adv.: B&W page USD 1,020, color page USD 2,020; trim 10 x 7. Circ: 3,424. **Subscr. to:** Periodicals Fulfillment, W B Saunders Co, 6277 Sea Harbor Dr, 4th Fl, Orlando, FL 32891-4800. **Co-sponsors:** British Association of Paediatric Surgeons; American Pediatric Surgical Association; Canadian Association of Paediatric Surgeons, Pacific Association of Pediatric Surgeons.

617.5 USA ISSN 1077-2847
JOURNAL OF PELVIC SURGERY. Text in English. 1995. bi-m. USD 158 domestic to individuals; USD 218 foreign to individuals; USD 281 domestic to institutions; USD 297 foreign to institutions; USD 45 newsstand/cover (effective 2002). adv. back issues avail. *Refereed.* **Document type:** *Academic/Scholarly.* **Description:** Publishes original articles, reviews and case reports covering all areas of the surgical treatment of pelvic disease, including diagnosis, pre- and post-operative care, surgical complications, imaging and critical care of pelvic surgery patients.
Related titles: Online - full text ed.: USD 365.30 domestic for academic site license; USD 381.30 foreign for academic site license; USD 407.45 domestic for corporate site license; USD 423.45 foreign for corporate site license (effective 2002).
—BLDSC (5030.430000), CISTI, GNLM.
Published by: Lippincott Williams & Wilkins (Philadelphia) (Subsidiary of: Wolters Kluwer N.V.), 530 Walnut St, Philadelphia, PA 19106-3621. TEL 215-521-8300, FAX 215-521-8902, http://www.lww.com. Ed. Dr. Raymond A Lee. Pub. Marjorie Spraycar. R&P Margaret Becker. Adv. contact Ray Thibodeau. B&W page USD 520, color page USD 1,420; trim 11 x 8.5. Circ: 1,149. **Subscr. to:** PO Box 1600, Hagerstown, MD 21740-1600. TEL 800-777-2295, FAX 301-824-7390.

617 USA ISSN 1096-4053 CODEN: JRADFU
JOURNAL OF RADIOSURGERY. Text in English. 1998. q. USD 225, NLG 495, EUR 224.50 to institutions for print or online ed.; USD 270 to institutions for print & online eds,combined; NLG 594 to institutions for print & online eds.combined; EUR 269.40 to institutions for print & online eds,combined (effective 2001). *Refereed.* **Document type:** *Journal, Academic/Scholarly.* **Description:** Covers technical and clinical innovations, radiography, and pathologic reports, as well as scientific studies related to the field.
Related titles: Online - full text ed.: (from EBSCO Publishing, O C L C Online Computer Library Center, Inc., RoweCom Information Quest, Swets Blackwell, Kluwer Online).
—BLDSC (5044.500000), GNLM. **CCC.**
Published by: Kluwer Academic - Plenum Publishers (Subsidiary of: Wolters Kluwer N.V.), 233 Spring St, New York, NY 10013-1578. TEL 212-620-8000, 800-221-9369, FAX 212-463-0742, info@plenum.com, http://www.wkap.nl/journalhome.htm/1096-4053. Eds. Ehud Arbit, Dr. Gil Lederman. R&P Rose Luongo TEL 781-871-6311. **Subscr. outside the Americas to:** Kluwer Academic Publishers Group, Journals Department, PO Box 322, Dordrecht 3300 AH, Netherlands. TEL 31-78-639-2392, FAX 31-78-654-6474.

616 USA ISSN 0743-684X CODEN: JRMIE2
JOURNAL OF RECONSTRUCTIVE MICROSURGERY. Text in English. 1984. 8/yr. EUR 255 to individuals; EUR 536 to institutions; EUR 62 newsstand/cover (effective 2002). adv. illus. *Refereed.* **Document type:** *Journal, Academic/Scholarly.* **Description:** Discusses the latest microsurgical procedures, technologies, innovations, materials, and significant problem cases.
Related titles: Microfilm ed.; Online - full text ed.: ISSN 1098-8947 (from RoweCom Information Quest, Institute for Scientific Information).
Indexed: ASCA, Curr.Cont., Excerp.Med., INIS Atomind., Ind.Med. (1984-), Inpharma, Int.Nurs.Ind., Reac.
—BLDSC (5048.157000), CISTI, EMDOCS, GNLM, IDS, ingenta, KNAW. **CCC.**
Published by: (International Society of Reconstructive Microsurgery), Thieme Medical Publishers, 333 Seventh Ave, New York, NY 10001. TEL 212-760-0888, 800-782-3488, FAX 212-947-1112, http://www.thieme.com. Ed. Dr. Berish Strauch. Circ: 1,945. **Orders in Europe to:** Thieme International, Postfach 301120, Stuttgart 70451, Germany. TEL 49-711-8931-0. **Co-sponsor:** American Society of the Peripheral Nerve.

M

617.7 USA ISSN 1081-597X CODEN: JRSUFZ
JOURNAL OF REFRACTIVE SURGERY. Text in English. 1983. bi-m. USD 149 domestic to individuals; USD 198 foreign to individuals; USD 179 domestic to institutions; USD 228 foreign to institutions (effective 2001). adv. bk.rev. abstr, charts, illus, stat, tr.lit. index. back issues avail.; reprints avail. *Refereed.* **Document type:** *Academic/Scholarly.* **Description:** Forum for original research, review, and evaluation of refractive and corneal surgical procedures.
Former titles (until Jan. 1995): Journal of Refractive and Corneal Surgery (1081-0803); (until 1994): Refractive and Corneal Surgery (1042-962X); (until 1989): Journal of Refractive Surgery (0883-0444)
Related titles: Online - full text ed.: (from Institute for Scientific Information).
Indexed: ASCA, Curr.Cont., Ind.Med. (1995-), Inpharma, Ophthal.Lit., Pharm.&Out.News, Reac., Sci.Cit.Ind.
—BLDSC (5048.290000), CISTI, EMDOCS, GNLM, IDS, Infotrieve, ingenta, KNAW. **CCC.**
Published by: (International Society of Refractive Keratoplasty), Slack, Inc., 6900 Grove Rd, Thorofare, NJ 08086-9447. TEL 856-848-1000, 800-257-8290, FAX 856-853-5991, http://www.slackinc.com, http://www.slackinc.com/jrs.htm. Ed. Dr. George Waring. Pub. Richard N Roash. Adv. contact Theresa Dempsey. Circ: 2,000. **Subscr. in Japan to:** Woodbell Inc., 4-22-11 Kitaka-Sai, Edogawa-ku, Tokyo 134-0081, Japan. **Co-sponsor:** European Refractive Surgery Society.

617.57 USA ISSN 1058-2746
JOURNAL OF SHOULDER AND ELBOW SURGERY. Text in English. 1992. bi-m. USD 133 domestic to individuals; USD 161 foreign to individuals; USD 172 domestic to institutions; USD 200 foreign to institutions; USD 69 domestic to students; USD 97 foreign to students; USD 34 newsstand/cover (effective 2001). adv. back issues avail.; reprints avail. *Refereed.* **Document type:** *Journal, Academic/Scholarly.* **Description:** For orthopedic surgeons who seek to restore form and function of the shoulder girdle, arm, and elbow by medical and surgical means. Provides an international forum for the exchange of information on new techniques, instruments, and materials.
Related titles: Online - full text ed.: (from IDEAL Online Library, Institute for Scientific Information, RoweCom Information Quest).
Indexed: Alloys Ind., Curr.Cont., Focus on: Sports Sci.& Med., Ind.Med. (1992-), Met.Abstr., Met.Abstr.Ind., Nonfer.Met.Alert, PCC Alert, Sci.Cit.Ind., Steels Alert.
—BLDSC (5064.435000), CISTI, GNLM, IDS, Infotrieve, KNAW. **CCC.**
Published by: (American Shoulder and Elbow Surgeons), Mosby, Inc. (Subsidiary of: Elsevier Science), 11830 Westline Industrial Dr, St Louis, MO 63146-3318. TEL 314-872-8370, 800-325-4177, FAX 314-432-1380, http://www.mosby.com/periodicals. Ed. Dr. Robert J Neviaser. Pub. Cynthia Baudendistel. Adv. contacts Gina Burkert TEL 314-453-4306, Michelle Kuhn. B&W page USD 1,080, color page USD 2,080; trim 10.88 x 8.25. Circ: 3,097. **Co-sponsors:** European Society for Surgery of Shoulder and Elbow; Japan Shoulder Society; Brazilian Orthopaedic and Traumatologic Society, Shoulder and Elbow Committee; Shoulder and Elbow Society of Australia; South African Shoulder and Elbow Surgeons; In.

JOURNAL OF SPINAL DISORDERS. see *MEDICAL SCIENCES—Orthopedics And Traumatology*

617 616.994 USA ISSN 0022-4790
RD651 CODEN: JSONAU
JOURNAL OF SURGICAL ONCOLOGY. Text in English. 1969. 12/yr. (in 3 vols., 4 nos./vol.). USD 2,295 in United States; USD 2,415 in Canada & Mexico; USD 2,517 elsewhere; USD 2,410 combined subscription in United States for print and online eds.; USD 2,530 combined subscription in Canada & Mexico for print and online eds.; USD 2,632 combined subscription elsewhere for print and online eds. (effective 2002). adv. charts, illus, stat. index. back issues avail.; reprint service avail. from ISI. *Refereed.* **Description:** Encompasses surgical approaches and presents studies of related topics such as radiotherapy, chemotherapy, and immunotherapy.
Related titles: Microform ed.: (from PQC); Online - full text ed.: ISSN 1096-9098. USD 2,295 in United States; USD 2,295 in Canada & Mexico; USD 2,295 elsewhere (effective 2002) (from EBSCO Publishing, Wiley InterScience, Institute for Scientific Information).
Indexed: ASCA, Biol.Abstr., Chem.Abstr., Chem.Indus.Notes, Chem.Titles, Curr.Adv.Ecol.Sci., Curr.Cont., Dent.Ind., Excerp.Med., INIS Atomind., Ind.Med. (1969-), Ind.Sci.Rev., Inpharma, Int.Nurs.Ind., Med.& Surg.Dermat., Pharm.&Out.News, Reac., Ref.Zh., Sci.Cit.Ind.
—BLDSC (5067.380000), CASDDS, CISTI, GNLM, IDS, ingenta, KNAW. **CCC.**
Published by: John Wiley & Sons, Inc., Journals (Subsidiary of: Wiley InterScience), 605 Third Ave, New York, NY 10158. TEL 212-850-6645, FAX 212-850-6021, subinfo@wiley.com, uscs-wis@wiley.com, http://www.wiley.com. Ed. Gerald P Murphy. adv.: B&W page GBP 640, color page GBP 1,515; trim 210 x 279. Circ: 1,000. **Subscr. outside the Americas to:** John Wiley & Sons Ltd., Baffins Ln, Chichester, Sussex PO19 IUD, United Kingdom. TEL 44-1243-779777, FAX 44-1243-843232, cs-journals@wiley.co.uk.

617 USA ISSN 1095-7340
JOURNAL OF SURGICAL OUTCOMES. Text in English. 1998. q. USD 104 domestic to individuals; USD 127 foreign to individuals; USD 168 domestic to institutions; USD 193 foreign to institutions; USD 58 domestic to students; USD 127 foreign to students; USD 49 newsstand/cover (effective 2000). *Refereed.* **Document type:** *Journal, Academic/Scholarly.*
Published by: W.B. Saunders Co. (Subsidiary of: Harcourt Publishers Ltd.), 11830 Westline Industrial Dr, St Louis, MO 63146. TEL 800-325-4177, wbspcs@harcourtbrace.com, http://www.wbsaunders.com.

JOURNAL OF SURGICAL PATHOLOGY. see *MEDICAL SCIENCES*

617 USA ISSN 0161-9721
RD1
JOURNAL OF SURGICAL PRACTICE*. Text in English. 1972. bi-m. adv.
Formerly: Surgical Team (0091-6277)
Published by: McMahon Publishing Co., 83 Peaceable St, West, Redding, CT 06896. Ed. Kenneth J Zeserson. Circ: 90,000.

617 USA ISSN 0022-4804
RD1 CODEN: JSGRA2
JOURNAL OF SURGICAL RESEARCH; clinical and laboratory investigation. Text in English. 1961. 14/yr. USD 1,110 in US & Canada to institutions; USD 1,279 elsewhere to institutions (effective 2001). adv. bk.rev. charts, illus. index. back issues avail. *Refereed.* **Document type:** *Academic/Scholarly.* **Description:** Publishes original articles concerned with clinical and laboratory investigations relevant to surgical practice and teaching.
Related titles: Online - full text ed.: (from EBSCO Publishing, O C L C Online Computer Library Center, Inc., RoweCom Information Quest, ingenta, Swets Blackwell, IDEAL Online Library, Institute for Scientific Information).
Indexed: ASCA, Biol.Abstr., Chem.Abstr., Chem.Indus.Notes, Chem.Titles, Curr.Cont., Environ.Sci.Poll.Mgmt., Excerp.Med., INIS Atomind., Ind.Med. (1961-), Ind.Sci.Rev., Ind.Vet., Inpharma, Med.& Surg.Dermat., Neurosci.Cit.Ind., Nutr.Abstr., Pharm.&Out.News, Pollut.Abstr., Reac., Rev.Med.& Vet.Mycol., Risk Abstr., Saf.Sci.Abstr., Sci.Cit.Ind., Vet.Bull.
—BLDSC (5067.400000), ADONIS, CASDDS, CISTI, GNLM, IDS, ingenta, KNAW. **CCC.**
Published by: (Association for Academic Surgery), Academic Press, Inc., Journal Division (Subsidiary of: Harcourt Brace & Company), 525 B St, Ste 1900, San Diego, CA 92101-4495. TEL 619-230-1840, FAX 619-699-6800, apsubs@acad.com, http://www.academicpress.com/jsr. Eds. Bruce L Gerwertz, Wiley Souba.

617 USA ISSN 0022-5223
RD536 CODEN: JTCSAQ
THE JOURNAL OF THORACIC AND CARDIOVASCULAR SURGERY. Text in English. 1931. m. USD 206 domestic to individuals; USD 246 foreign to individuals; USD 381 domestic to institutions; USD 422 foreign to institutions; USD 105 domestic to students; USD 145 foreign to students; USD 36 newsstand/cover (effective 2001). adv. bibl, illus. s-a. index. reprint service avail. from PQC. *Refereed.* **Document type:** *Journal, Academic/Scholarly.* **Description:** Devoted to conditions of the heart, lungs, chest and great vessels where surgical intervention is indicated.
Formerly: Journal of Thoracic Surgery
Related titles: Microfilm ed.: (from PQC); Online - full text ed.: (from Ovid Technologies, Inc., HighWire Pr., EBSCO Publishing, IDEAL Online Library, Institute for Scientific Information, RoweCom Information Quest).
Indexed: AIM, ASCA, Abstr.Hyg., Biol.Abstr., Chem.Abstr., Chem.Indus.Notes, Chem.Titles, Curr.Adv.Cancer Res., Curr.Cont., Excerp.Med., Helminthol.Abstr., INIS Atomind., Ind.Med. (1959-), Ind.Sci.Rev., Inpharma, Int.Abstr.Biol.Sci., Jrnl.Watch Card., Nutr.Abstr., Pharm.&Out.News, Reac., Rev.Med.& Vet.Mycol., Rev.Plant Path., SSCI (coverage dropped), Sci.Cit.Ind.
—BLDSC (5069.100000), CASDDS, CISTI, GNLM, IDS, ingenta, KNAW. **CCC.**
Published by: (American Association for Thoracic Surgery), Mosby, Inc. (Subsidiary of: Elsevier Science), 11830 Westline Industrial Dr, St Louis, MO 63146-3318. TEL 314-872-8370, 800-325-4177, FAX 314-432-1380, http://www.mosby.com/periodicals. Ed. Dr. John A Waldhausen. Pub. Cynthia Baudendistel. Adv. contact Carol Kilzer TEL 314-453-4307. B&W page USD 1,070, color page USD 2,245; trim 10.88 x 8.13. Circ: 8,815. **Co-sponsor:** Western Thoracic Surgical Association.

617.4 USA ISSN 0741-5214
RD598.5
JOURNAL OF VASCULAR SURGERY. Text in English. 1984. m. USD 192 domestic to individuals; USD 230 foreign to individuals; USD 371 domestic to institutions; USD 409 foreign to institutions; USD 99 domestic to students; USD 137 foreign to students; USD 35 newsstand/cover (effective 2001). adv. bk.rev. s-a. index. reprint service avail. from PQC. *Refereed.* **Document type:** *Journal, Academic/Scholarly.* **Description:** Presents latest advances in the knowledge of the peripheral vascular system and vascular surgery.
Related titles: Microfilm ed.: (from PQC); Online - full text ed.: (from Ovid Technologies, Inc., EBSCO Publishing, IDEAL Online Library, Institute for Scientific Information, RoweCom Information Quest).
Indexed: ASCA, Curr.Adv.Cancer Res., Curr.Cont., Excerp.Med., INIS Atomind., Ind.Med. (1984-), Inpharma, Int.Nurs.Ind., Jrnl.Watch Card., Neurosci.Cit.Ind., Pharm.&Out.News, Reac., Rev.Med.& Vet.Mycol., SSCI (coverage dropped), Sci.Cit.Ind.
—BLDSC (5072.270000), CISTI, EMDOCS, GNLM, IDS, ingenta, KNAW. **CCC.**
Published by: (Society for Vascular Surgery), Mosby, Inc. (Subsidiary of: Elsevier Science), 11830 Westline Industrial Dr, St Louis, MO 63146-3318. TEL 314-872-8370, 800-325-4177, FAX 314-432-1380, http://www.mosby.com/periodicals. Eds. Dr. K Wayne Johnston, Robert B Rutherford. Pub. Cynthia Baudendistel. Adv. contact Gale Schlogl TEL 314-453-4337. B&W page USD 1,435, color page USD 2,660; trim 10.88 x 8.25. Circ: 7,465. **Co-sponsor:** International Society for Cardiovascular Surgery, North American Chapter.

617.554 USA ISSN 1071-5754
RD540.6
JOURNAL OF W O C N. Key Title: Journal of Wound, Ostomy, and Continence Nursing. Text in English. 1974. bi-m. USD 63 domestic to individuals; USD 79 foreign to individuals; USD 190 domestic to institutions; USD 206 foreign to institutions; USD 36 domestic to students; USD 52 foreign to students; USD 35 newsstand/cover (effective 2001). adv. charts, illus, stat. index. reprint service avail. from PQC. *Refereed.* **Document type:** *Journal, Academic/Scholarly.* **Description:** Serves enterostomal therapy practitioners with data relating to the care of persons with stomas, draining wounds, fistulas, dermal ulcers and incontinence.
Former titles (until 1994): Journal of E T Nursing (1055-3045); (until 1991): Journal of Enterostomal Therapy (0270-1170); (until 1979): E T Journal (0195-9883)
Related titles: Microfilm ed.: (from PQC); Online - full text ed.: (from EBSCO Publishing, IDEAL Online Library, RoweCom Information Quest).
Indexed: CINAHL, INIS Atomind., Int.Nurs.Ind., Nurs.Abstr.
—BLDSC (5072.632700), GNLM, Infotrieve, KNAW. **CCC.**
Published by: (Wound, Ostomy and Continence Nurses Society), Mosby, Inc. (Subsidiary of: Elsevier Science), 11830 Westline Industrial Dr, St Louis, MO 63146-3318. TEL 314-872-8370, 800-325-4177, FAX 314-432-1380, http://www.mosby.com/jwocn, http://www.mosby.com/periodicals. Ed. Mikel Gray. Pub. Nathania Sawyer. Adv. contact Gale Schlogl TEL 314-453-4337. B&W page USD 1,195, color page USD 2,120; trim 10.88 x 8.25. Circ: 5,383.

KAGAWA NO SHINKEI GEKA DANWAKAI KAISHI/KAGAWA COLLOQUIUM ON NEUROSURGERY. JOURNAL. see *MEDICAL SCIENCES—Psychiatry And Neurology*

617 JPN ISSN 0913-459X
KAGOSHIMAKEN RINSHO GEKA IKAISHI/KAGOSHIMA SOCIETY FOR CLINICAL SURGERY. JOURNAL. Text in Japanese. 1985. a.

M

Published by: Kagoshimaken Rinsho Geka Ikai, 8-1 Chuo-cho, Kagoshima-shi 890-0053, Japan.

617 JPN ISSN 0912-0904
KANAGAWA KANSETSU GEKA KENKYUKAISHI/JOINT. Text in English, Japanese. 1986. s-a.
Published by: Kanagawa Kansetsu Geka Kenkyukai/Kanagawa Society of Joint Surgery, Showa Daigaku Igakubu, Fuzoku Fujigaoka Byoin Seikei Geka, 1-30, Fujigaoka, Midori-ku, Yokohama-shi, Kanagawaken 227, Japan.

KANSAI KANSETSUKYO HIZA KENKYUKAISHI/ JOURNAL OF KANSAI ARTHROSCOPY AND KNEE. see *MEDICAL SCIENCES—Orthopedics And Traumatology*

617.95 CHE ISSN 1422-8408
RD118.A1
KEY ISSUES IN PLASTIC AND COSMETIC SURGERY. Text in English. 1984. a. USD 200 (effective 2001). illus. *Refereed.* **Document type:** *Journal, Academic/Scholarly.* **Description:** Presents a collection of original, fully referenced review articles written by experts in plastic and cosmetic surgery.
Formerly (until 1999): Advances in Plastic and Reconstructive Surgery (0748-5212)
—BLDSC (5091.823370), GNLM, KNAW.
Published by: S. Karger AG, Allschwilerstr 10, PO Box, Basel 4009, Switzerland. TEL 41-61-3061111, FAX 41-61-3061234, karger@karger.ch, http://www.karger.com/bookseries/KEYIP.

617 GBR
KEY NOTE MARKET REPORT: COSMETIC SURGERY. Text in English. 1995. irreg., latest vol.2, 1997. GBP 265 (effective 1999). **Document type:** *Bulletin.*
Published by: Key Note Ltd., Field House, 72 Oldfield Rd, Hampton, Mddx TW12 2HQ, United Kingdom. TEL 44-20-8481-8750, FAX 44-20-8783-0049, http://www.keynote.co.uk. Ed. Donna Jones.

617 RUS ISSN 0023-1207
CODEN: KHIRAE
KHIRURGIYA. ZHURNAL IM. N.I. PIROGOVA/SURGERY. Text in Russian; Summaries in English. 1925. bi-m. RUR 360 for 6 mos. to individuals; RUR 1,080 for 6 mos. to institutions (effective 2002). adv. bk.rev. index. **Description:** Discusses general and abdominal surgery, oncology, traumatology, endocrinology, pediatric surgery, problems of chest surgery and anesthesiology.
Indexed: Biol.Abstr., Chem.Abstr., Curr.Cont. (coverage dropped), Dent.Ind., Excerp.Med., Helminthol.Abstr., Ind.Med. (1937-), Neurosci.Cit.Ind., Nutr.Abstr., Ref.Zh., SSCI (coverage dropped).
—BLDSC (0394.785000), CISTI, East View, GNLM, IDS, Infotrieve. **CCC.**
Published by: (Assotsiatsiya Khirurgov im. N.I. Pirogova), Media Sfera TEL 7-095-4824329, mediashp@mediasphera.ru. Ed. N N Malinovskii. Adv. contact T A Roshe. **Dist. by:** Mezhdunarodnaya Kniga, B Yakimanka 39, Moscow 117049, Russian Federation. TEL 7-095-2384967, FAX 7-095-2384634; **US dist. addr.:** East View Publications, 3020 Harbor Ln N, Minneapolis, MN 55447. TEL 612-550-0961. **Co-sponsor:** Ministerstvo Zdravookhraneniya.

617 UKR
CODEN: KLKHAM
KLINICHNA KHIRURHIYA. Text in Ukrainian. 1961. m. USD 175. bk.rev. abstr. bibl. index. *Refereed.* **Document type:** *Academic/Scholarly.*
Former titles (until 1993): Klinicheskaya Khirurgiya (0023-2130); Novyi Khirurgicheskii Arkhiv
Indexed: Biol.Abstr., Chem.Abstr., Dent.Ind., Excerp.Med., INIS Atomind., Ind.Med. (coverage dropped).
—BLDSC (0089.258100), CASDDS, CISTI, East View, GNLM, IDS, KNAW. **CCC.**
Published by: (Ministerstvo Okhrany Zdorov'ia Ukrainy), Nauchnoe Obshchestvo Khirurgov Ukrainy, Ul Geroev Sebastopoliya 30, Kiev 252180, Ukraine. TEL 380-44-488-1811. **US dist. addr.:** East View Publications, 3020 Harbor Ln N, Minneapolis, MN 55447. TEL 612-550-0961.

KNEE SURGERY, SPORTS TRAUMATOLOGY, ARTHROSCOPY. see *MEDICAL SCIENCES—Sports Medicine*

617 JPN
KOKYUKI GEKA/JAPANESE ASSOCIATION FOR CHEST SURGERY. JOURNAL. Text in English, Japanese. 1987. bi-m. adv. **Document type:** *Academic/Scholarly.*
Published by: Nihon Kokyuki Geka Gakkai, Kyoto Daigaku Kyobu Shikkan Kenkyujo Kyobu Geka, 53, Shogoin Kawaracho, Sakyo-ku, Kyoto-shi 606, Japan. Ed., R&P Hiromi Wada. Adv. contact Yasumasa Monden.

617 JPN ISSN 0914-4463
KOTSU TO IRYO/TRAFFIC ACCIDENTS AND MEDICAL CARE. Text in Japanese. 1987. bi-m. JPY 1,000 per issue.
Published by: Nihon Kotsu Iryo Kyogikai/Japan Traffic Accidents Litigation's Medical Expert Association, 20-go Toranomon, Minato-ku, Tokyo 105-0001, Japan. TEL 03-5473-8883. Ed. Mitsutaka Matsuo.

L M S ALERT. IMMUNOTHERAPEUTICS. TRANSPLANT REJECTION. (Literature Monitoring and Evaluation Service) see *MEDICAL SCIENCES—Abstracting, Bibliographies, Statistics*

617 DEU ISSN 1435-2443
CODEN: LAACBS
LANGENBECKS ARCHIVES OF SURGERY. Text in English. 1860. 8/yr. EUR 728.20 domestic; EUR 720.70 in Germany; EUR 84 newsstand/cover foreign (effective 2002). back issues avail.; reprint service avail. from ISI. *Refereed.* **Document type:** *Journal, Academic/Scholarly.* **Description:** Provides an international forum for the controlled results of clinical surgery.
Formerly (until 1997): Langenbecks Archiv fuer Chirurgie (0023-8236); Which incorporates (in 1975): Bruns' Beitraege fuer Klinische Chirurgie (0007-2680)
Related titles: Microform ed.: (from PQC); Online - full text ed.: ISSN 1435-2451 (from EBSCO Publishing, RoweCom Information Quest, Swets Blackwell, Springer LINK, Institute for Scientific Information).
Indexed: ASCA, Biol.Abstr., Chem.Abstr., Curr.Cont., Dent.Ind., Excerp.Med., INIS Atomind., Ind.Med. (1998-), Ind.Sci.Rev., Inpharma, Int.Nurs.Ind., Reac., Trop.Dis.Bull.
—BLDSC (5155.680500), CISTI, GNLM, IDS, KNAW. **CCC.**
Published by: (Deutsche Gesellschaft fuer Chirurgie), Springer-Verlag (Subsidiary of: BertelsmannSpringer), Tiergartenstr 17, Heidelberg 69121, Germany. TEL 49-6221-345-0, FAX 49-6221-345229, subscriptions@springer.de, http://link.springer.de/service/journals/00423/index.htm, http://www.springer.de. Ed. H G Beger. **Subscr. in N. America to:** Springer-Verlag New York Inc., PO Box 2485, Secaucus, NJ 07096-2485. TEL 212-460-1500, FAX 212-473-6272.

617 535.58 USA ISSN 0196-8092
CODEN: LSMEDI
LASERS IN SURGERY AND MEDICINE. Text in English. 1980. 11/yr. USD 1,310 in United States; USD 1,420 in Canada & Mexico; USD 1,513 elsewhere; USD 1,376 combined subscription in United States for print and online eds.; USD 1,486 combined subscription in Canada & Mexico for print and online eds.; USD 1,579 combined subscription elsewhere for print and online eds. (effective 2002). adv. abstr, bibl, charts, illus. index. back issues avail.; reprint service avail. from ISI. *Refereed.* **Document type:** *Academic/Scholarly.* **Description:** Covers all aspects of biomedical applications of lasers. Presents research regarding clinical trials, new therapeutic techniques, laser biophysics and bioengineering, and photobiology.
Related titles: Microform ed.: (from PQC); Online - full text ed.: ISSN 1096-9101. 1996. USD 1,310 in United States; USD 1,310 in Canada & Mexico; USD 1,310 elsewhere (effective 2002) (from EBSCO Publishing, Wiley InterScience, Institute for Scientific Information).
Indexed: ASCA, Curr.Cont., Dent.Ind., Excerp.Med., INIS Atomind., INSPEC (1999-), Ind.Med. (1980-), Inpharma, Jrnl.Watch Derm., Med.& Surg.Dermat., Pharm.&Out.News, Reac., Ref.Zh., Sci.Cit.Ind.
—BLDSC (5156.683000), CASDDS, CISTI, GNLM, IDS, ingenta, KNAW. **CCC.**
Published by: John Wiley & Sons, Inc., Journals (Subsidiary of: Wiley InterScience), 605 Third Ave, New York, NY 10158. TEL 212-850-6645, FAX 212-850-6021, subinfo@wiley.com, uscs-wis@wiley.com, http://www.wiley.com. Ed. Robert H Ossof. adv.: B&W page GBP 640, color page GBP 1,515; trim 210 x 279. Circ: 3,750. **Subscr. outside the Americas to:** John Wiley & Sons Ltd., Baffins Ln, Chichester, Sussex PO19 IUD, United Kingdom. TEL 44-1243-779777, FAX 44-1243-843232, cs-journals@wiley.co.uk.

617 FRA ISSN 0024-3493
CODEN: LICHA6
LILLE CHIRURGICAL✱. Text in French. 1945. q. FRF 160. adv. bk.rev. illus. index.
Indexed: Biol.Abstr., Excerp.Med., Ind.Med. (coverage dropped).
—CISTI, GNLM.
Published by: (Societe de Chirurgie de Lille), Editions Morel et Corduant, 11 rue des Bouchers, Lille 59000, France. Circ: 1,000.

LIVER TRANSPLANTATION. see *MEDICAL SCIENCES—Gastroenterology*

617 USA
MANAGEMENT AND AVOIDANCE OF COMPLICATIONS IN EYELID SURGERY. Text in English. 1993. irreg., latest vol.3. USD 295 to individuals; USD 355 to institutions. *Refereed.* **Document type:** *Academic/Scholarly.*
Published by: Field & Wood, Medical Periodicals, Inc., PO Box 975, Blue Bell, PA 19422. TEL 610-828-4010, FAX 215-482-0226. Ed. Dr. Joseph A Mauriello Jr.

617 FRA ISSN 0759-2280
MEDECINE ET CHIRURGIE DU PIED. Text in French. 1984. 4/yr. EUR 192 domestic to institutions; EUR 58 newsstand/cover foreign to institutions (effective 2002). **Document type:** *Academic/Scholarly.*
—BLDSC (5487.729300). **CCC.**
Published by: (Societe Francaise de Medecine et Chirurgie du Pied), Elsevier Paris, Editions Scientifiques et Medicales (Subsidiary of: Reed Elsevier plc. group), 23 rue Linois, Paris 75015, France. http://www.elsevier.com/locate/pied. Circ: 2,500.

617 USA
RD27.42
MEDICAL ECONOMICS GENERAL SURGERY - ORTHOPEDIC SURGERY. Text in English. 1982. m. USD 65; USD 109 foreign (effective 1998). adv. **Document type:** *Trade.* **Description:** Covers non-clinical aspects of a surgeon's practice, including investments, taxes, office management and family spending.
Formerly (until 1995): Medical Economics for Surgeons (0744-4206)
Related titles: Microform ed.: (from RPI,PQC).
Indexed: Ind.Med. (coverage dropped).
—CCC.
Published by: Medical Economics Co., Inc., 5 Paragon Dr, Montvale, NJ 07645-1742. TEL 201-358-7200. Ed. Barbara Weiss. Circ: 48,000.

617 CRI ISSN 0377-1253
MEDICINA Y CIRUGIA. Text in Spanish; Summaries in English, Spanish. 1974.
Indexed: Biol.Abstr.
Published by: Colegio de Medicos y Cirujanos, Apdo 4054, San Jose 1000, Costa Rica.

617 BGR ISSN 0204-5389
MEDITSINSKI PREGLED. KHIRURGICHNI ZABOLIAVANIIA. Variant title: Surgical Diseases. Text in Bulgarian; Summaries in Bulgarian, English. 1970. q., latest vol.32, 2001. BGL 14 domestic; USD 48 foreign (effective 2002). adv. abstr, bibl, illus. index. 48 p./no. back issues avail. *Refereed.* **Document type:** *Journal, Academic/Scholarly, Abstract/Index, Bibliography.* **Description:** Presents original articles and abstracts of foreign publications on surgery, covering special surgical conditions, operative surgery, and surgical equipment.
Indexed: Abstr.Bulg.Sci.Med.Lit.
Published by: Meditsinski Universitet - Sofia, Tsentur za Informatsiia po Meditsina/Medical University - Sofia, Medical Information Center, 1 Sv Georgi Sofiiski ul, Sofia 1431, Bulgaria. TEL 359-2-9522342, FAX 359-2-9522393, mutafov@sun.medun.acad.bg, http://www.medun.acad.bg. Ed. Dr. G Zlatarski. R&P, Adv. contact Dr. Christo Mutafov. B&W page USD 50, color page USD 150; trim 160 x 110. Circ: 300. **Dist. by:** Sofia Books, Ul Silivria 16, Sofia 1404, Bulgaria. TEL 359-2-9586257, sofiabooks@hotmail.com, http://www.sofiabooks.hit.bg.

617 USA ISSN 1092-0811
RD99.A1
MEDSURG NURSING. Text in English. 1992. bi-m. USD 28 domestic to individuals; USD 43 foreign to individuals; USD 40 domestic to institutions; USD 55 foreign to institutions (effective 2000). back issues avail. *Refereed.* **Document type:** *Academic/Scholarly.*
Related titles: Online - full text ed.: (from Northern Light Technology, Inc., Gale Group).
Indexed: CINAHL, Fam.Ind., Int.Nurs.Ind.
—BLDSC (5535.589000), CISTI, Infotrieve, ingenta. **CCC.**
Published by: Jannetti Publications, Inc., East Holly Ave, Box 56, Pitman, NJ 08071-0056. TEL 856-256-2300, FAX 856-589-7463, MSJRNL@ajj.com, http://www.cinahl.com/jrnls/MEDN/medn.htm.

617 POL ISSN 1428-2712
MEDYCYNA PRAKTYCZNA. CHIRURGIA. Text in Polish. 1997. bi-m. PLZ 80 (effective 2000).
Published by: Medycyna Praktyczna, Ul Skawinska 8, Krakow 31066, Poland. TEL 48-12-4305520, FAX 48-12-4305536, listy@mp.pl, http://mp.pl/czasop.htm. Ed. Marcin Zielinski.

617 681 USA ISSN 0738-1085
RD33.6
MICROSURGERY. Text in English. 1983. m. USD 520 in United States; USD 600 in Canada & Mexico; USD 668 elsewhere; USD 546 combined subscription in United States for print and online eds.; USD 626 combined subscription in Canada & Mexico for print and online eds.; USD 694 combined subscription elsewhere for print and online eds. (effective 2002). adv. bk.rev. bibl, charts, illus. index. back issues avail.; reprint service avail. from ISI. *Refereed.* **Document type:** *Academic/Scholarly.* **Description:** Acts as a multidisciplinary forum for original ideas regarding the use of the operating microscope in a variety of areas.
Formed by the merger of (1979-1982): Journal of Microsurgery (0191-3239); (1979-1981): International Journal of Microsurgery (0222-5069)
Related titles: Microform ed.: (from PQC); Online - full text ed.: ISSN 1098-2752. 1996. USD 520 in United States; USD 520 in Canada & Mexico; USD 520 elsewhere (effective 2002) (from EBSCO Publishing, Wiley InterScience, Institute for Scientific Information).
Indexed: ASCA, Biol.Abstr., Curr.Cont., Excerp.Med., INIS Atomind., Ind.Med. (1983-), Inpharma, Neurosci.Cit.Ind., Reac., Ref.Zh.
—BLDSC (5760.770000), CISTI, EMDOCS, GNLM, IDS, ingenta, KNAW. **CCC.**
Published by: John Wiley & Sons, Inc., Journals (Subsidiary of: Wiley InterScience), 605 Third Ave, New York, NY 10158. TEL 212-850-6645, FAX 212-850-6021, subinfo@wiley.com, uscs-wis@wiley.com, http://www.wiley.com. Ed. A Bowen. adv.: B&W page GBP 640, color page GBP 1,515; trim 210 x 279. Circ: 950. **Subscr. outside the Americas to:** John Wiley & Sons Ltd., Baffins Ln, Chichester, Sussex PO19 IUD, United Kingdom. TEL 44-1243-779777, FAX 44-1243-843232, cs-journals@wiley.co.uk.

617 ITA ISSN 0026-4733
MINERVA CHIRURGICA. Text in Italian; Summaries in English, Italian. 1946. m. (10/yr.). USD 140 to individuals; USD 170 to institutions (effective 2000 - 2001). adv. bk.rev. bibl, charts, illus. index. *Refereed.* **Document type:** *Academic/Scholarly.*
Related titles: Microform ed.: (from PQC); Online - full text ed.: (from Institute for Scientific Information); ♦ Supplement: Notiziario Chirurgico. ISSN 0392-3584.
Indexed: Biol.Abstr., Chem.Abstr., Dent.Ind., Excerp.Med., INIS Atomind., Ind.Med. (1946-), Nutr.Abstr., Ref.Zh.
—CISTI, GNLM, IDS, KNAW.
Published by: Edizioni Minerva Medica, Corso Bramante, 83-85, Turin, TO 10126, Italy. TEL 39-11-678282, FAX 39-11-674502. Ed. P A Giudice. Pub. Alberto Oliaro. Adv. contact F Filippo. B&W page USD 1,200, color page USD 2,000; trim 270 x 190. Circ: 5,000 (paid).

617 DEU ISSN 0941-455X
MINIMAL INVASIVE CHIRURGIE. Text in German, English. 1991. q. EUR 68 (effective 2002). **Document type:** *Journal, Academic/Scholarly.*
Published by: Urban & Fischer Verlag, Loebdergraben 14a, Jena 07743, Germany. TEL 49-3641-626430, FAX 49-3641-626421, info@urbanfischer.de, http://www.urbanfischer.de. Ed. H-P Bruch. R&P Martin Huber TEL 49-3641-626430. Adv. contact Sabine Schroeter.

MINIMALLY INVASIVE NEUROSURGERY. see *MEDICAL SCIENCES—Psychiatry And Neurology*

616 USA ISSN 0723-0990
MODERN NEUROSURGERY. Text in English. 1982. quadrennial. price varies. **Document type:** *Proceedings.*
Published by: Springer-Verlag, Journals (Subsidiary of: BertelsmannSpringer), 175 Fifth Ave, New York, NY 10010. TEL 212-460-1500, FAX 212-473-6272. Ed. M Brock.

MUND-, KIEFER- UND GESICHTSCHIRURGIE. see *MEDICAL SCIENCES—Otorhinolaryngology*

NAIBUNPI GEKA/ENDOCRINE SURGERY. see *MEDICAL SCIENCES—Endocrinology*

617.54 MEX ISSN 1405-2938
NEUMOLOGIA Y CIRUGIA DE TORAX. Variant title: Revista de Neumologia y Cirugia de Torax. Text in Spanish; Summaries in English. 1939. q. MXP 210, USD 40 (effective 1996 & 1997). bk.rev. bibl, charts, illus. index. *Refereed.* **Document type:** *Academic/Scholarly.* **Description:** Includes original articles, research reports, review articles, clinical cases and notices.
Indexed: Ind.Med. (coverage dropped).
Published by: (Sociedad Mexicana de Neumologia y Cirugia de Torax), Obsidiana Editores S.A., CZDA DE TLALPAN 2365, Col Ciudad Jardin, Mexico City, DF 04370, Mexico. TEL 52-5-689-9133. Eds. Dr. Juan Urueta, Dr. Mario H Vargas. Pub. Jorge Godoy-Gutierrez. Circ: 2,000. **Dist. by:** Distribuidora Editorial de Mexico SA de CV, P.O. Box 76-026, Mexico City, DF 04201, Mexico. TEL 52-5-544-7953, FAX 52-5-689-6545.

617 616.8 FRA ISSN 0028-3770
CODEN: NUREB9
NEURO-CHIRURGIE. Text in French. 1955. 7/yr. FRF 1,557; FRF 1,814 foreign (effective 2000). adv. bk.rev. illus. index. reprint service avail. from ISI. *Refereed.* **Document type:** *Academic/Scholarly.* **Description:** The scope goes beyond neurosurgery into neuro-anaesthesiology, neuroradiology, electro-encephalography, gamma-encephalography, echo-encephalography, neuro-ophthalmology, oto-neurology, neuro-endocrinology and more.
Related titles: Microform ed.: (from PQC); Online - full text ed.: (from Institute for Scientific Information, RoweCom Information Quest).
Indexed: Biol.Abstr., Curr.Cont., Excerp.Med., Helminthol.Abstr., Ind.Med. (1955-), Ind.Sci.Rev., Inpharma, Neurosci.Cit.Ind., Pharm.&Out.News, Reac., Rev.Med.& Vet.Mycol., Sci.Cit.Ind., Trop.Dis.Bull., e-psyche.
—BLDSC (6081.350000), CISTI, GNLM, IDS, KNAW. **CCC.**
Published by: (Societe Francaise de Neurochirurgie), Masson - Periodiques, 120 bd. St. Germain, Paris 75006, France. TEL 33-1-40466200, FAX 33-1-40466201. Ed. P M Hurth. Circ: 1,500. **Subscr. to:** Societe de Periodiques Specialises, BP 22, Vineuil Cedex 41354, France. TEL 33-2-54504612, FAX 33-2-54504611.

NEUROCIRUGIA/NEUROSURGERY. see *MEDICAL SCIENCES—Psychiatry And Neurology*

NEUROLOGIA I NEUROCHIRURGIA POLSKA. see *MEDICAL SCIENCES—Psychiatry And Neurology*

NEUROLOGIA MEDICO-CHIRURGICA. see *MEDICAL SCIENCES—Psychiatry And Neurology*

NEUROLOGICAL RESEARCH; a journal of progress in neurosurgery, neurology and neurosciences. see *MEDICAL SCIENCES—Psychiatry And Neurology*

617.4 616.8 JPN ISSN 0301-2603
CODEN: NOKGB6
NEUROLOGICAL SURGERY/NO SHINKEI GEKA. Text in Japanese; Summaries in English. 1973. m. JPY 2,400 per issue. adv. bk.rev. *Refereed.*
Related titles: Online - full text ed.: (from JICST, Institute for Scientific Information).
Indexed: ASCA, Biol.Abstr., Chem.Abstr., Chem.Indus.Notes, Chem.Titles, Dent.Ind., Excerp.Med., Ind.Med. (1973-), Neurosci.Cit.Ind., e-psyche.
—BLDSC (6081.445000), CASDDS, CISTI, EMDOCS, GNLM, IDS, KNAW.
Published by: Igaku-Shoin Ltd., 5-24-3 Hongo, Bunkyo-ku, Tokyo 113-0033, Japan. TEL 81-3-3817-5702. Circ: 6,000.

NEUROPEDIATRICS; journal of pediatric neurobiology, neurology and neurosurgery. see *MEDICAL SCIENCES—Pediatrics*

NEUROSURGERY (BALTIMORE). see *MEDICAL SCIENCES—Psychiatry And Neurology*

617 616.8 USA ISSN 1042-3680
CODEN: NCNAFP
NEUROSURGERY CLINICS OF NORTH AMERICA. Text in English. 1989. q. USD 172 domestic to individuals; USD 194 in Canada to individuals; USD 221 elsewhere to individuals; USD 232 domestic to institutions; USD 281 foreign to institutions; USD 71 per issue (effective 2001). adv. *Refereed.* **Document type:** *Journal, Academic/Scholarly.* **Description:** Each issue addresses a single topic in the diagnosis and therapy of patients with neurological disorders.
Related titles: Microform ed.: (from PQC); Online - full text ed.: (from Institute for Scientific Information).
Indexed: ASCA, CINAHL, Curr.Cont., Excerp.Med. (1995-), Ind.Med. (1990-), Inpharma, Int.Nurs.Ind., Neurosci.Cit.Ind., Pharm.&Out.News, Reac., e-psyche.
—BLDSC (6081.582500), GNLM, IDS, Infotrieve, ingenta, KNAW. **CCC.**
Published by: W.B. Saunders Co. (Subsidiary of: Harcourt Publishers Ltd.), 11830 Westline Industrial Dr, St Louis, MO 63146. TEL 800-325-4177, http://www.wbsaunders.com. Eds. Dr. H Richard Winn, Dr. Marc R Mayberg. **Subscr. to:** Periodicals Fulfillment, W B Saunders Co, 6277 Sea Harbor Dr, 4th Fl, Orlando, FL 32891-4800.

617 USA ISSN 1525-819X
▼ **NEUROSURGERY NEWS.** Text in English. 2000. bi-m. USD 79 domestic to institutions; USD 114 foreign to institutions (effective 2002). **Document type:** *Newsletter, Academic/Scholarly.* **Description:** Provides neurosurgeons with an informal and easily read compendium of information.
Published by: (Congress of Neurological Surgeons), Lippincott Williams & Wilkins (Philadelphia) (Subsidiary of: Wolters Kluwer N.V.), 530 Walnut St, Philadelphia, PA 19106-3621. TEL 215-521-8300, FAX 215-521-8902, custserv@lww.com, http://www.lww.com/. Ed. Dr. Michael Levy.

617 USA ISSN 1050-6438
CODEN: NEQUEB
NEUROSURGERY QUARTERLY. Text in English. 1991. q., latest vol.11. USD 186 domestic to individuals; USD 229 foreign to individuals; USD 270 domestic to institutions; USD 320 foreign to institutions; USD 72 newsstand/cover (effective 2002). adv. charts, illus. reprint service avail. from PQC. *Refereed.* **Document type:** *Academic/Scholarly.* **Description:** Presents comprehensive reviews by international authorities on the surgical management and treatment of neurological disorders.
Related titles: Online - full text ed.: USD 351 domestic for academic site license; USD 401 foreign foracademic site license; USD 391.50 domestic for corporate site license; USD 441.50 foreign for corporate site license (effective 2002) (from Institute for Scientific Information).
Indexed: ASCA, Excerp.Med. (1992-), Neurosci.Cit.Ind.
—BLDSC (6081.582800), EMDOCS, GNLM, IDS, KNAW.
Published by: Lippincott Williams & Wilkins (Philadelphia) (Subsidiary of: Wolters Kluwer N.V.), 530 Walnut St, Philadelphia, PA 19106-3621. TEL 215-521-8300, FAX 215-521-8902, http://www.neurosurgery-quarterly.com, http://www.lww.com. Ed. Dr. Donlin M Long. Pub. Marjorie Spraycar. R&P Margaret Becker. Adv. contact Ray Thibodeau. B&W page USD 740, color page USD 1,830. Circ: 1,085 (paid).

NEUROSURGICAL FOCUS. see *MEDICAL SCIENCES—Psychiatry And Neurology*

616 DEU ISSN 0344-5607
CODEN: NSREDV
NEUROSURGICAL REVIEW. Text in German. 1978. 4/yr. EUR 282.40 domestic; EUR 278.60 in Germany; EUR 80.40 newsstand/cover foreign (effective 2002). *Refereed.* **Document type:** *Journal, Academic/Scholarly.* **Description:** Provides a forum for comprehensive reviews on current issues in neurosurgery.
Related titles: Online - full text ed.: ISSN 1437-2320 (from EBSCO Publishing, RoweCom Information Quest, Swets Blackwell, Springer LINK, Institute for Scientific Information).
Indexed: ASCA, Curr.Adv.Ecol.Sci., Curr.Cont. (coverage dropped), Dent.Ind., Excerp.Med., Ind.Med. (1978-), Inpharma, Neurosci.Cit.Ind., Pharm.&Out.News, Reac., Rev.Med.& Vet.Mycol., e-psyche.
—BLDSC (6081.585000), CISTI, EMDOCS, GNLM, IDS, ingenta, KNAW. **CCC.**
Published by: Springer-Verlag (Subsidiary of: BertelsmannSpringer), Tiergartenstr 17, Heidelberg 69121, Germany. TEL 49-6221-345-0, FAX 49-6221-345229, subscriptions@springer.de, http://link.springer.de/link/service/journals/10143/index.htm, http://www.springer.de. Eds. D Voth, K Sano. **Subscr. to:** Springer-Verlag New York Inc., PO Box 2485, Secaucus, NJ 07096-2485. TEL 212-460-1500, FAX 212-473-6272.

617.95 USA
NEW YOU. Text in English. q. **Document type:** *Magazine, Consumer.* **Description:** Contains in-depth information on cosmetic surgery procedures as well as feature stories and news articles.

M

Published by: PersonalSurgeon.com, 292 Madison Ave, 23rd Fl, New York, NY 10017. TEL 212-561-8779, 877-561-8781, info@personalsurgeon.com, http://personalsurgeon.com.

NEWS REVIEW; a journal for theatre personnel nationwide. see *MEDICAL SCIENCES—Anaesthesiology*

617 JPN ISSN 0914-9058
NIHON ASHI NO GEKA KENKYUKAI ZASSHI/JAPAN SOCIETY FOR SURGERY OF THE FOOT. JOURNAL. Text in Japanese. 1980. a.
Published by: Nihon Ashi no Geka Kenkyukai, Sei Marianna Ika Daigaku Seikei Gekagaku Kyoshitsu, 16-1 Sugao 2-chome, Miyamae-ku, Kawasaki-shi, Kanagawa-ken 216-0015, Japan.

617.95 JPN ISSN 0288-2027
NIHON BIYO GEKA GAKKAI KAIHO/JAPAN SOCIETY OF AESTHETIC PLASTIC SURGERY. JOURNAL. Text in Japanese; Summaries in English. 1979. q.
Published by: Nihon Geka Taisha Eiyo Gakkai/Japanese Academy of Surgical Metabolism and Nutrition, Nihon Gakkai Jimu Senta, 16-9 Honkomagome 5-chome, Bunkyo-ku, Tokyo 113-0021, Japan.

NIHON GEKAKEI RENGO GAKKAI GAKUJUTSU SHUKAI SHOROKUGO/JAPANESE COLLEGE OF SURGEONS. ABSTRACTS OF MEETING. see *MEDICAL SCIENCES—Abstracting, Bibliographies, Statistics*

NIHON GEKAKEI RENGO GAKKAISHI/JAPANESE COLLEGE OF SURGEONS. JOURNAL. see *MEDICAL SCIENCES—Abstracting, Bibliographies, Statistics*

362.19795 JPN ISSN 0578-7947
NIHON ISHOKU GAKKAI ZASSHI/JAPANESE JOURNAL OF TRANSPLANTATION. Text in Japanese. 1965. bi-m. *Refereed.* **Document type:** *Academic/Scholarly.*
Address: c/o Dr. Kikuo Nomoto, Nihon Gakkai Jimu Center, 5-16-9 Honkomagome, Bunkyo-ku, Tokyo 113-8622, Japan.

617.95 JPN
NIHON KEISEI GEKA GAKKAI GAKUJUTSU SHUKAI/JAPAN SOCIETY OF PLASTIC AND RECONSTRUCTIVE SURGERY. ANNUAL MEETING. Text in English, Japanese. a.
Published by: Nihon Keisei Geka Gakkai, Nihon Gakkai Jimu Senta, 16-9 Honkomagome 5-chome, Bunkyo-ku, Tokyo 113-0021, Japan.

617.95 JPN ISSN 0389-4703
CODEN: NKGKE7
NIHON KEISEI GEKA GAKKAI KAISHI/JAPAN SOCIETY OF PLASTIC AND RECONSTRUCTIVE SURGERY. JOURNAL. Text in Japanese; Summaries in English. 1981. m. JPY 3,000 per issue.
—BLDSC (4808.060000).
Published by: Nihon Keisei Geka Gakkai, Nihon Gakkai Jimu Senta, 16-9 Honkomagome 5-chome, Bunkyo-ku, Tokyo 113-0021, Japan.

616 JPN ISSN 0916-4936
NIHON MAIKURO SAJARI GAKKAI KAISHI/JAPANESE SOCIETY OF RECONSTRUCTIVE MICROSURGERY. JOURNAL. Text in Japanese; Summaries in English. 1988. s-a. JPY 8,000 (effective 2001). **Document type:** *Journal, Academic/Scholarly.*
Published by: Nihon Maikuro Sajari Gakkai, Keio Daigaku Igakubu Maikuro Sajarishitsu, 35 Shinano-Machi, Shinjuku-ku, Tokyo 160-8582, Japan. TEL 81-3-3353-1211, FAX 81-3-3226-0989.

NIHON NO SHINKEI GEKA GAKKAI SOKAI SHOROKUSHU/JAPAN NEUROSURGICAL SOCIETY. ABSTRACTS OF THE ANNUAL MEETING. see *MEDICAL SCIENCES—Abstracting, Bibliographies, Statistics*

617 JPN ISSN 0386-9776
NIHON RINSHO GEKA IGAKKAI ZASSHI/JAPANESE SOCIETY FOR CLINICAL SURGERY. JOURNAL. Text in English, Japanese. 1937. m. JPY 1,000 per issue. **Document type:** *Academic/Scholarly.*
Indexed: INIS Atomind.
—CISTI.
Published by: Nihon Rinsho Geka Igakkai, Eregansu Iidabashi 402, 4-3 Iida-Bashi 3-chome, Chiyoda-ku, Tokyo 102-0072, Japan. Ed. Junichi Ishii. Circ: 16,000.

NIHON RYUMACHI KANSETSU GEKA GAKKAI ZASSHI/JAPANESE JOURNAL OF RHEUMATISM AND JOINT SURGERY. see *MEDICAL SCIENCES—Rheumatology*

NIHON RYUMACHI KANSETSU GEKA GEKKAI/JAPANESE SOCIETY OF RHEUMATISM AND JOINT SURGERY. CONGRESS. see *MEDICAL SCIENCES—Rheumatology*

617 JPN ISSN 0285-1474
NIHON SHINZO KEKKAN GEKA GAKKAI ZASSHI/JAPANESE JOURNAL OF CARDIOVASCULAR SURGERY. Text in Japanese. 1972. bi-m. *Refereed.* **Document type:** *Journal, Academic/Scholarly.*
Incorporates: Nihon Shinzo Kekkan Geka Gakkai Gakujutsu Sokai Nittei to Endai Shorokushu/Japanese Society for Cardiovascular Surgery. Abstracts of Meeting; Formerly (until 1948): Kyobu geka (0021-5252)
Indexed: INIS Atomind.
—CISTI, Infotrieve. **CCC.**
Published by: Nihon Shinzo Kekkan Geka Gakkai/Japanese Society for Cardiovascular Surgery, c/o Business Center of Academic Societies Japan, 5-16-9 Honkomagome, Bunkyo-ku, Tokyo 113-8622, Japan. TEL 81-3-5814-5810, FAX 81-3-5814-5820, http://square.umin.ac.jp/jscvs/. Ed. Shiaki Kawada.

NIHON SHONI GEKA GAKKAI ZASSHI/JAPANESE SOCIETY OF PEDIATRIC SURGEONS. JOURNAL. see *MEDICAL SCIENCES—Pediatrics*

617 JPN ISSN 1340-8593
NIHON SHUJUTSU IGAKKAISHI/JAPANESE ASSOCIATION FOR OPERATIVE MEDICINE. JOURNAL. Text in Japanese; Summaries in English. 1980. q. **Document type:** *Academic/Scholarly.*
Formerly (until 1993): Nihon Shujutsubu Igakkaishi - Japanese Association for Operating Room Technology. Journal (0914-4498)
Published by: Nihon Shujutsubu Igakkai, c/o Surgical Center, University of Hospital, 7-3-1 Hongo, Bunkyo-ku, Tokyo 113-0033, Japan. TEL 81-3-5800-8674, FAX 81-3-5689-8217. Ed. Toyoki Kugimiya. Pub. Ooya Shokai. R&P Y Kakehashi.

617 JPN ISSN 0914-594X
NIHON TOGAI GAKU GANMEN GEKA GAKKAISHI/JAPAN SOCIETY OF CRANIO-MAXILLO-FACIAL SURGERY. JOURNAL. Text in Japanese; Summaries in English, Japanese. 1984. a.
Indexed: INIS Atomind.
Published by: Nihon Togai Gaku Ganmen Geka Gakkai, c/o Nagasaki Daigaku Igakubu Fuzoku Byoin Keisei Geka, 7-1, Sakamotomachi, Nagasaki-shi, Nagasaki-ken 852, Japan.

617.95 JPN ISSN 0387-9194
NIPPON BIYO GEKA GAKKAISHI/JAPAN SOCIETY OF AESTHETIC SURGERY. JOURNAL. Text and summaries in English, Japanese. 1962. q. USD 50. adv.
Description: Publishes scientific papers relating to medicine and aesthetic/cosmetic surgery.
Published by: Nippon Biyo Geka Gakkai, 12-5 Shinbashi 1-chome, Minato-ku, Tokyo 105-0004, Japan. TEL 81-3-3571-1270, FAX 81-3-3573-2113, jujinfu@white.plala.or.jp, http://www.jujin.com. Ed. Takashi Akamatsu. Pub. Fumihiko Umezawa. R&P, Adv. contact Junichiro Taguchi. page JPY 30,000. Circ: 750 (paid); 400 (controlled).

617 JPN ISSN 0301-4894
CODEN: NGGZAK
NIPPON GEKA GAKKAI ZASSHI/JAPAN SURGICAL SOCIETY. JOURNAL. Text in Japanese; Summaries in English, Japanese. 1899. m. JPY 900 per issue (effective 2000). **Document type:** *Academic/Scholarly.*
Formerly (until 1907): Nippon Geka Gakkaishi (0301-4886)
Indexed: Chem.Abstr., Chem.Titles, INIS Atomind., Ind.Med. (1907-).
—BLDSC (4808.350000), CASDDS, CISTI, GNLM.
Published by: Nihon Geka Gakkai, Hakuoh Bldg 3-10 Koraku, Bunkyo-ku, Tokyo 112-0004, Japan. Ed. Seiki Matsuno.

NO SHINKEI GEKA JANARU/JAPANESE JOURNAL OF NEUROSURGERY. see *PSYCHOLOGY*

617.4 616.8 JPN ISSN 0917-1495
NO SHINKEI GEKA SOKUHO/NEUROSURGERY LETTERS. Text in Japanese. 1990. m. JPY 1,223 per issue.
Indexed: e-psyche.
Published by: Medika Shuppan/Medicus Publishing Inc., 18-24 Hiroshiba-cho, Suita-shi, Osaka-fu 564-0052, Japan. TEL 81-6-385-6911, FAX 81-6-385-6721. Ed. Takahiko Matsui.

617.3 616.89 JPN ISSN 0914-5508
NO SOTCHU NO GEKA/SURGERY FOR CEREBRAL STROKE. Text in Japanese; Summaries in English. 1973. q. JPY 2,200 per issue.
Indexed: INIS Atomind., e-psyche.
Published by: (Nihon No Sotchu no Geka Kenkyukai/Japanese Conference on Surgery of Cerebral Stroke), Nyuronsha, 21-19-305 Higashi-Gotanda 5-chome, Shinagawa-ku, Tokyo 141-0022, Japan.

617 ITA ISSN 0392-3584
NOTIZIARIO CHIRURGICO. Text in Italian. 1980. q. adv. **Document type:** *Academic/Scholarly.*
Related titles: ♦ Supplement to: Minerva Chirurgica. ISSN 0026-4733.
Indexed: Excerp.Med., Ind.Med. (coverage dropped).
—CISTI.
Published by: Edizioni Minerva Medica, Corso Bramante, 83-85, Turin, TO 10126, Italy. TEL 39-11-678282, FAX 39-11-674502. Pub. A Oliaro. Adv. contact F Filippo. B&W page USD 1,200, color page USD 2,000; trim 270 x 190.

617 DEU ISSN 0178-1715
O P JOURNAL; wissenschaftlich - medizinische informationen fuer das O P personal. Text in German. 1985. 3/yr. EUR 61.10 domestic to institutions; EUR 72.40 in Europe to institutions; EUR 77 elsewhere to institutions; EUR 22 newsstand/cover (effective 2002). **Document type:** *Journal, Academic/Scholarly.*
Related titles: Online - full text ed.
—GNLM.
Published by: Georg Thieme Verlag, Ruedigerstr 14, Stuttgart 70469, Germany. TEL 49-711-8931-0, FAX 49-711-8931298, leser.service@thieme.de, http://www.thieme.de. Eds. G Hierholzer, S Weller. R&P Michael Wachinger.

O R REPORTS. (Operating Room) see *HEALTH FACILITIES AND ADMINISTRATION—Abstracting, Bibliographies, Statistics*

617 USA ISSN 0960-8923
CODEN: OBSUEB
OBESITY SURGERY; including Laparoscopy and Allied Care. Text in English. 1991. bi-m., latest vol.11, 2001. USD 240 to non-members; USD 137 to members; USD 476 to institutions (effective 2002). adv. bibl, abstr, stat. 150 p./no. back issues avail.; reprints avail. *Refereed.* **Document type:** *Journal, Academic/Scholarly.*
Description: Aims to provide an international and interdisciplinary opportunity for publishing and communicating important research and techniques for treatment of massive obesity.
Related titles: Online - full text ed.: 1990 (from EBSCO Publishing, Institute for Scientific Information).
Indexed: ASCA, Curr.Cont., Environ.Sci.Poll.Mgmt., Excerp.Med. (1992-), Ind.Med. (1991-), Inpharma, Int.Nurs.Ind., Pollut.Abstr., Reac., Risk Abstr., SSCI (coverage dropped), Saf.Sci.Abstr.
—BLDSC (6196.953000), ADONIS, CISTI, EMDOCS, GNLM, IDS, ingenta, KNAW.
Published by: (Councils of the International Federation for the Surgery of Obesity), F D Communications Inc., 5863 Leslie St., Box 1002, Toronto, ON M2H 1J8, Canada. TEL 416-224-5055, FAX 416-224-5455, medicine@sympatico.ca, http://www.obesitysurgery.com. Ed., R&P Dr. Mervyn Deitel TEL 416-750-9608. Pub., Adv. contact Fran Deitel. B&W page USD 625, color page USD 755; trim 8.25 x 11.125. Circ: 1,475.

617.7 USA ISSN 8750-3085
OCULAR SURGERY NEWS. Text in English. bi-w. USD 295 domestic to individuals; USD 340 in Canada to individuals; USD 380 elsewhere to individuals; USD 315 domestic to institutions; USD 360 in Canada to institutions; USD 400 elsewhere to institutions. adv. **Document type:** *Newspaper, Academic/Scholarly.*
Description: Provides coverage of scientific meetings and events in ophthalmology as well as current practice management issues.
Formerly: I O L and Ocular Surgery News
—BLDSC (6235.154600). **CCC.**
Published by: Slack, Inc., 6900 Grove Rd, Thorofare, NJ 08086-9447. TEL 856-848-1000, 800-257-8290, FAX 856-853-5991, http://www.slackinc.com. Ed. Dr. Donald R Sanders.

617.7 USA ISSN 1079-3267
OCULAR SURGERY NEWS INTELLIGENCE REPORT. Text in English. 1994. w. USD 37 to individuals; USD 57 to institutions. **Document type:** *Newsletter, Academic/Scholarly.* **Description:** Offers news on health care reform, new technologies, legal issues and more.
Media: Fax. **Related titles:** Fax ed.

M

Published by: Slack, Inc., 6900 Grove Rd, Thorofare, NJ 08086-9447. TEL 856-848-1000, 800-257-8290, FAX 856-853-5991, http://www.slackinc.com. Ed. Dr. Donald Sanders.

617.7 USA ISSN 1047-9120
OCULAR SURGERY NEWS INTERNATIONAL EDITION. Abbreviated title: O S N I E. Text in English. 1990. m. USD 210 domestic to individuals; USD 230 in Canada to individuals; USD 250 elsewhere to individuals; USD 230 domestic to institutions; USD 250 in Canada to institutions; USD 270 elsewhere to institutions. **Document type:** *Newspaper, Academic/Scholarly.* **Description:** Provides coverage of scientific meetings and developments in all subspecialties in ophthalmology.
—**CCC.**
Published by: Slack, Inc., 6900 Grove Rd, Thorofare, NJ 08086-9447. TEL 856-848-1000, 800-257-8290, FAX 856-853-5991, http://www.slackinc.com. Ed. Dr. Donald R Sanders. Circ: 17,000.

OFTAL'MOKHIRURGIYA. see *MEDICAL SCIENCES—Ophthalmology And Optometry*

617 USA
OPERATING ROOM RISK MANAGEMENT. Text in English. bi-m. USD 635.80 domestic; USD 651 in Canada; USD 805 elsewhere (effective 2002). *Refereed.* **Document type:** *Trade.* **Description:** Covers operating room risk management and quality assurance issues.
Published by: (Emergency Care Research Institute), E C R I, 5200 Butler Pike, Plymouth, PA 19462. TEL 610-825-6000, FAX 610-834-1275, info@ecri.org, http://www.ecri.org. Ed. Andrea Zarod.

617 USA ISSN 1092-4469
OPERATIVE TECHNIQUES IN CATARACT AND REFRACTIVE SURGERY. Text in English. 1998. q. USD 130 domestic to individuals; USD 158 foreign to individuals; USD 160 domestic to institutions; USD 193 foreign to institutions; USD 92 domestic to students; USD 158 foreign to students; USD 49 newsstand/cover (effective 2000). illus. **Document type:** *Academic/Scholarly.* **Description:** Details the latest advances in cataract and refractive surgery.
—BLDSC (6269.381270). **CCC.**
Published by: W.B. Saunders Co. (Subsidiary of: Harcourt Publishers Ltd.), Curtis Center, 3rd Fl, Independence Sq W, Philadelphia, PA 19106-3399. TEL 215-238-7800, FAX 215-238-6445, wbspcs@harcourtbrace.com, http://www.wbsaunders.com; http://www.customerservice.wbsaunders.com. Ed. Dr. Richard Elander. **Subscr. to:** Periodicals Fulfillment, W B Saunders Co, 6277 Sea Harbor Dr, 4th Fl, Orlando, FL 32891-4800. TEL 800-654-5452.

617 USA ISSN 1524-153X
▼ **OPERATIVE TECHNIQUES IN GENERAL SURGERY.** Text in English. 2000. q. USD 126 domestic to individuals; USD 149 foreign to individuals; USD 177 domestic to institutions; USD 199 foreign to institutions; USD 75 domestic to students; USD 89 foreign to students; USD 50 newsstand/cover (effective 2001). illus. **Document type:** *Journal, Academic/Scholarly.* **Description:** Highly illustrated review articles on surgical techniques with step-by-step descriptions of procedures.
Published by: W.B. Saunders Co. (Subsidiary of: Harcourt Publishers Ltd.), 11830 Westline Industrial Dr, St Louis, MO 63146. TEL 800-325-4177, wbspcs@harcourtbrace.com, http://www.wbsaunders.com. Eds. Dr. David Farley, Dr. Jon Van Heerden.

617 USA ISSN 1085-5610
OPERATIVE TECHNIQUES IN GYNECOLOGIC SURGERY. Text in English. q. USD 129 domestic to individuals; USD 174 foreign to individuals; USD 204 domestic to institutions; USD 253 foreign to institutions; USD 87 domestic to students; USD 104 foreign to students; USD 64 newsstand/cover (effective 2001). illus. **Document type:** *Academic/Scholarly.* **Description:** Provides highly illustrated articles on state-of-the-art surgical techniques written by leading surgeons in the specialty.
—**CCC.**
Published by: W.B. Saunders Co. (Subsidiary of: Harcourt Publishers Ltd.), Curtis Center, 3rd Fl, Independence Sq W, Philadelphia, PA 19106-3399. TEL 215-238-7800, FAX 215-238-6445, wbspcs@harcourtbrace.com, http://www.wbsaunders.com; http://customerservice.wbsaunders.com. Ed. Dr. David M Gershenson. **Subscr. to:** Periodicals Fulfillment, W B Saunders Co, 6277 Sea Harbor Dr, 4th Fl, Orlando, FL 32891-4800.

617 USA ISSN 1092-440X
OPERATIVE TECHNIQUES IN NEUROSURGERY. Text in English. 1998. q. USD 159 domestic to individuals; USD 185 foreign to individuals; USD 199 domestic to institutions; USD 225 foreign to institutions; USD 76 domestic to students; USD 111 foreign to students; USD 57 newsstand/cover (effective 2001). illus. **Document type:** *Academic/Scholarly.* **Description:** Provides a comprehensive and current overview of procedures in neurosurgery by combining the usefulness of color atlas, the authority of a textbook, and the timeliness of a journal.
—BLDSC (6269.381400). **CCC.**
Published by: W.B. Saunders Co. (Subsidiary of: Harcourt Publishers Ltd.), Curtis Center, 3rd Fl, Independence Sq W, Philadelphia, PA 19106-3399. TEL 215-238-7800, FAX 215-238-6445, wbspcs@harcourtbrace.com, http://www.wbsaunders.com; http://www.customerservice.wbsaunders.com. Ed. Dr. Robert F Spetzler. **Subscr. to:** Periodicals Fulfillment, W B Saunders Co, 6277 Sea Harbor Dr, 4th Fl, Orlando, FL 32891-4800. TEL 800-654-5452.

OPERATIVE TECHNIQUES IN OTOLARYNGOLOGY - HEAD AND NECK SURGERY. see *MEDICAL SCIENCES—Otorhinolaryngology*

617 USA ISSN 1071-0949
OPERATIVE TECHNIQUES IN PLASTIC AND RECONSTRUCTIVE SURGERY. Text in English. 1994. q. USD 171 domestic to individuals; USD 218 foreign to individuals; USD 239 domestic to institutions; USD 275 foreign to institutions; USD 123 domestic to students; USD 131 foreign to students; USD 69 newsstand/cover (effective 2001). adv. illus. *Refereed.* **Document type:** *Academic/Scholarly.* **Description:** Each issue focuses on a particular restorative surgical procedure or clinical condition.
—BLDSC (6269.382300), GNLM, Infotrieve. **CCC.**
Published by: W.B. Saunders Co. (Subsidiary of: Harcourt Publishers Ltd.), 11830 Westline Industrial Dr, St Louis, MO 63146. TEL 800-325-4177, http://www.wbsaunders.com. Eds. Dr. Glyn Jones, John H Culbertson Jr. Adv. contact Cindy Gray. color page USD 1,540, B&W page USD 630; trim 11 x 7.75. Circ: 1,782. **Subscr. to:** Periodicals Fulfillment, W B Saunders Co, 6277 Sea Harbor Dr, 4th Fl, Orlando, FL 32891-4800. TEL 800-654-5452.

617 USA ISSN 1522-2942
OPERATIVE TECHNIQUES IN THORACIC AND CARDIOVASCULAR SURGERY. Text in English. q. USD 154 domestic to individuals; USD 179 foreign to individuals; USD 199 domestic to institutions; USD 223 foreign to institutions; USD 96 domestic to students; USD 107 foreign to students; USD 56 newsstand/cover (effective 2001). illus. **Document type:** *Academic/Scholarly.* **Description:** Provides highly illustrated review articles on techniques in cardiovascular and thoracic surgery written by renowned surgeons.
—BLDSC (6269.382520).
Published by: W.B. Saunders Co. (Subsidiary of: Harcourt Publishers Ltd.), Curtis Center, 3rd Fl, Independence Sq W, Philadelphia, PA 19106-3399. TEL 215-238-7800, FAX 215-238-6445, wbspcs@harcourtbrace.com, http://www.wbsaunders.com; http://www.customerservice.wbsaunders.com. Ed. Dr. James L Cox. **Subscr. to:** Periodicals Fulfillment, W B Saunders Co, 6277 Sea Harbor Dr, 4th Fl, Orlando, FL 32891-4800. TEL 800-654-5452.

OPHTHALMIC PLASTIC AND RECONSTRUCTIVE SURGERY. see *MEDICAL SCIENCES—Ophthalmology And Optometry*

617.7 USA ISSN 1082-3069
RE80 CODEN: OSLAF2
OPHTHALMIC SURGERY AND LASERS. Text in English. 1968. m. USD 69 in US & Canada to individuals; USD 118 rest of world to individuals; USD 99 in US & Canada to institutions; USD 148 rest of world to institutions; USD 29 newsstand/cover (effective 2001). adv. bk.rev. charts, illus. back issues avail.; reprint service avail. from PQC. **Document type:** *Academic/Scholarly.* **Description:** Covers the entire spectrum of ophthalmic surgery and treatment. Also presents the latest applications for laser surgery as well as potential indications and treatment modalities in regularly featured experimental science articles.
Formerly (until 1995): Ophthalmic Surgery (0022-023X); Which supersedes: Journal of Cryosurgery
Related titles: Microform ed.: (from PQC); Online - full text ed.: (from ProQuest Information & Learning, Institute for Scientific Information).
Indexed: ASCA, Biol.Abstr., Curr.Cont., Dent.Ind., Environ.Sci.Poll.Mgmt., Excerp.Med., Helminthol.Abstr., INIS Atomind., Ind.Med. (1995-), Inpharma, Med.& Surg.Dermat., Neurosci.Cit.Ind., Pharm.&Out.News, Pollut.Abstr., Reac., Rev.Med.& Vet.Mycol., Risk Abstr., SSCI (coverage dropped), Saf.Sci.Abstr., Sci.Cit.Ind.
—BLDSC (6271.510000), CISTI, GNLM, IDS, ingenta, KNAW. **CCC.**
Published by: Slack, Inc., 6900 Grove Rd, Thorofare, NJ 08086-9447. TEL 856-848-1000, FAX 856-853-5991, osl@slackinc.com, http://www.slackinc.com/eye/os/oshome.htm. Ed. Dr. Carmen A Puliafito. adv.: B&W page USD 1,390, color page USD 3,710. Circ: 1,800 (paid).

OPHTHALMO CHIRURGIE. see *MEDICAL SCIENCES—Ophthalmology And Optometry*

OPPORTUNITIES FOR THEATRE STAFF & OTHER SPECIALISTS. see *MEDICAL SCIENCES—Nurses And Nursing*

617.6 USA ISSN 1042-3699
ORAL AND MAXILLOFACIAL SURGERY CLINICS OF NORTH AMERICA. Text in English. 1989. q. USD 147 domestic to individuals; USD 172 in Canada to individuals; USD 195 elsewhere to individuals; USD 205 domestic to institutions; USD 245 foreign to institutions; USD 62 per issue (effective 2001). **Document type:** *Academic/Scholarly.* **Description:** Aimed at oral maxillofacial surgeons and discusses surgical procedures, including orthroscopy, cosmetic oral, maxillofacial surgery, and surgery of cleft palette.
Related titles: Microform ed.: (from PQC).
—BLDSC (6277.442000), GNLM.
Published by: W.B. Saunders Co. (Subsidiary of: Harcourt Publishers Ltd.), 11830 Westline Industrial Dr, St Louis, MO 63146. TEL 800-325-4177, http://www.wbsaunders.com. **Subscr. to:** Periodicals Fulfillment, W B Saunders Co, 6277 Sea Harbor Dr, 4th Fl, Orlando, FL 32891-4800.

ORAL SURGERY, ORAL MEDICINE, ORAL PATHOLOGY, ORAL RADIOLOGY, AND ENDODONTICS. see *MEDICAL SCIENCES—Dentistry*

ORBIT; the international journal on orbital disorders, oculoplastic and lacrimal surgery. see *MEDICAL SCIENCES—Ophthalmology And Optometry*

ORTHOPAEDIC AND TRAUMATIC SURGERY/SEKEI SAIGAI GEKA. see *MEDICAL SCIENCES—Orthopedics And Traumatology*

617 ITA ISSN 0030-6266
OSPEDALI D'ITALIA - CHIRURGIA. Summaries in English. 1959. bi-m. ITL 100,000. adv. bk.rev. abstr, bibl, charts, illus. index.
Indexed: Biol.Abstr., Excerp.Med. (until 1995), Ind.Med. (coverage dropped).
—CISTI, GNLM.
Published by: Editrice Sedicesimo, Via Mannelli, 29 r, Florence, Fl 50136, Italy. TEL 055-2476781, FAX 055-2478568. Ed. Carlo Massimo. Circ: 3,000.

OSTOMY - WOUND MANAGEMENT; the journal of extended patient care management. see *MEDICAL SCIENCES—Orthopedics And Traumatology*

OTOLARYNGOLOGY - HEAD AND NECK SURGERY. see *MEDICAL SCIENCES—Otorhinolaryngology*

617 USA
CODEN: SUFOAX
OWEN H. WANGENSTEEN SURGICAL FORUM. Variant title: Surgical Forum. Text in English. 1950. a. USD 30 (effective 2001). charts, illus. back issues avail. **Document type:** *Proceedings, Abstract/Index.*
Formerly: Forum on Fundamental Surgical Problems (0071-8041)
Related titles: CD-ROM ed.
Indexed: ASCA, Biol.Abstr., Chem.Abstr., Chem.Indus.Notes, Chem.Titles, Curr.Adv.Ecol.Sci., Curr.Cont. (coverage dropped), Excerp.Med. (until 1993), INIS Atomind.
—BLDSC (8548.220000), CASDDS, GNLM, IDS, KNAW. **CCC.**
Published by: American College of Surgeons, Communications Department, 633 N Saint Clair St, Chicago, IL 60611-3211. TEL 312-202-5000, FAX 312-202-5001, http://www.facs.org. R&P Linn Meyer TEL 312-202-5311. Circ: 2,000.

PEDIATRIA OGGI MEDICA E CHIRURGICA. see *MEDICAL SCIENCES—Pediatrics*

PEDIATRIC CARDIOLOGY. see *MEDICAL SCIENCES—Cardiovascular Diseases*

PEDIATRIC ENDOSURGERY & INNOVATIVE TECHNIQUES; part B of Journal of Laparoendoscopic & Advanced Surgical Techniques. see *MEDICAL SCIENCES—Pediatrics*

617 618.92 DEU ISSN 0179-0358
CODEN: PSUIED
PEDIATRIC SURGERY INTERNATIONAL. Text in English. 8/yr. EUR 542.60 domestic; EUR 529.90 foreign; EUR 76.80 newsstand/cover foreign (effective 2002). *Refereed.* **Document type:** *Journal, Academic/Scholarly.* **Description:** Devoted to publishing new and important information from the entire spectrum of pediatric surgery.
Related titles: Microform ed.: (from PQC); Online - full text ed.: (from EBSCO Publishing, RoweCom Information Quest, Swets Blackwell, Springer LINK, Institute for Scientific Information).
Indexed: ASCA, Curr.Cont., Ind.Med. (1986-), Inpharma, Pharm.&Out.News, Reac., Trop.Dis.Bull.
—BLDSC (6417.628000), CISTI, GNLM, IDS, Infotrieve, KNAW. **CCC.**
Published by: Springer-Verlag (Subsidiary of: BertelsmannSpringer), Tiergartenstr 17, Heidelberg 69121, Germany. TEL 49-6221-345-0, FAX 49-6221-345229, subscriptions@springer.de, http://link.springer.de/link/service/journals/00383/index.htm, http://www.springer.de. Ed. A F Schaerli. **Subscr. in N. America to:** Springer-Verlag New York Inc., PO Box 2485, Secaucus, NJ 07096-2485. TEL 212-460-1500, FAX 212-473-6272.

617 618.92 PRI ISSN 1089-7739
PEDIATRIC SURGERY UPDATE. Text in English. 1993. m. free per issue. *Refereed.* **Document type:** *Newsletter.* **Description:** Covers current issues and reviews in the practice of pediatric surgery for primary physicians, pediatricians, surgeons, residents, medical students, and other health-related professionals.
Related titles: Online - full text ed.
Address: PO Box 10426, Caprra Heighys Sta, San Juan 00922-0426, Puerto Rico. TEL 787-786-3495, titolugo@coqui.net, http://home.coqui.net/titolugo/. Ed. Dr. Humberto Lugo-Vicente. R&P Dr. Humberto Lugo Vicente.

PEDIATRIC TRANSPLANTATION. see *MEDICAL SCIENCES—Pediatrics*

PEDIATRIK CERRAHI DERGISI. see *MEDICAL SCIENCES—Pediatrics*

PERIANESTHESIA AND AMBULATORY SURGERY NURSING UPDATE. see *MEDICAL SCIENCES—Nurses And Nursing*

PERIOPERATIVE SERVICES MANAGEMENT RESOURCE. see *MEDICAL SCIENCES—Nurses And Nursing*

617 USA ISSN 1531-0035
RD598.5
PERSPECTIVES IN VASCULAR SURGERY AND ENDOVASCULAR THERAPY. Text in English. 1988. s-a. EUR 273 to individuals; EUR 381 to institutions; EUR 158 newsstand/cover (effective 2002). adv. back issues avail. *Refereed.* **Document type:** *Journal, Academic/Scholarly.* **Description:** Features detailed clinical discussions and reports of new procedures in this specialty, along with notes, commentary, and dialogues.
Formerly: Perspectives in Vascular Surgery (0894-8046)
Related titles: Online - full text ed.: ISSN 1521-5768 (from RoweCom Information Quest); ♦ Supplement: Vascular Surgery Outlook. ISSN 0894-8038.
—GNLM.
Published by: Thieme Medical Publishers, 333 Seventh Ave, New York, NY 10001. TEL 212-760-0888, 800-782-3488, FAX 212-947-1112, http://www.thieme.com. Ed. Dr. Jerry Goldstone. Adv. contact Sally Kahn. **Orders in Europe to:** Thieme International, Postfach 3001120, Stuttgart 70451, Germany. TEL 49-711-8931-0.

617 PHL ISSN 0031-7691
PHILIPPINE JOURNAL OF SURGICAL SPECIALITIES. Text in English. 1946. q. PHP 50 to non-members; PHP 40 to members (effective 2001). adv. charts, illus, stat, abstr, bibl. 50 p./no. back issues avail. *Refereed.* **Document type:** *Journal, Academic/Scholarly.*
Formerly: Philippine Journal of Surgery and Surgery Specialties
Related titles: CD-ROM ed.: 1970 (vol.25); Online - full content ed.
Indexed: Biol.Abstr., Chem.Abstr., ExtraMED, Ind.Med. (until 19??, dropped).
Published by: Philippine College of Surgeons, 3F PCS Bldg, 992 Edsa, Quezon City, Philippines. TEL 632-929-4047, FAX 632-929-2297, pcs@pcs.org.ph, http://www.pcs.org.ph. Ed. Adriano V Laudico. Circ: 1,000.

617.95 USA ISSN 0032-1052
CODEN: PRSUAS
PLASTIC AND RECONSTRUCTIVE SURGERY. Text in English. 1946. 14/yr., latest vol.108. USD 414 domestic to individuals Print & Online eds. combined; USD 527 foreign to individuals Print & Online eds. combined; USD 492 domestic to institutions Print & Online eds. combined; USD 605 foreign to institutions Print & Online eds. combined; USD 40 newsstand/cover (effective 2002). adv. bk.rev. abstr, charts, illus. index, cum.index vols.59-72, 1985. *Refereed.* **Document type:** *Academic/Scholarly.* **Description:** Examines plastic and reconstructive surgery techniques.
Related titles: Microfilm ed.: (from WWS); Online - full text ed.: USD 639.60 domestic academic site license; USD 752.60 foreign academic site license; USD 713.40 domestic corporate site license; USD 826.40 foreign corporate site license (2002) (from Ovid Technologies, Inc., Swets Blackwell, Institute for Scientific Information).
Indexed: AIM, ASCA, Biol.Abstr., Chem.Abstr., Curr.Adv.Cancer Res., Curr.Adv.Cell & Devel.Biol., Curr.Cont., Dairy Sci.Abstr., Dent.Ind., Excerp.Med., INIS Atomind., Ind.Med. (1946-), Ind.Sci.Rev., Inpharma, Int.Nurs.Ind., Jrnl.Watch Derm., Mat.Sci.Cit.Ind. (coverage dropped), Med.& Surg.Dermat., Neurosci.Cit.Ind., Pharm.&Out.News, Reac., Rev.Med.& Vet.Mycol., SSCI (coverage dropped), Sci.Cit.Ind.
—BLDSC (6528.924000), CISTI, GNLM, IDS, ingenta, KNAW.
Published by: (American Society of Plastic and Reconstructive Surgeons), Williams & Wilkins (Subsidiary of: Waverly International), 351 W Camden St, Baltimore, MD 21201-2436. TEL 410-528-4068, 800-222-3790, FAX 410-528-4452, jmichael@wwilkins.com, http://www.plasreconsurg.com, http://www.wilkins.com. Ed. Dr. Robert M Goldwyn. Adv. contact Joyce Michael. Circ: 13,555.

617.95 USA ISSN 1043-4119
PLASTIC SURGERY NEWS. Text in English. 1989. m. USD 75 (effective 2000). adv. **Document type:** *Newsletter.*
Published by: American Society of Plastic Surgeons, 444 E Algonquin Rd, Arlington, IL 60005-4664. TEL 847-228-9900, FAX 847-229-9131, psnews@aol.com, http://www.plastic surgery.org, http://www.plasticsurgery.org. Ed., R&P John Everson. Circ: 5,700.

PLASTIC SURGERY OUTLOOK. see *MEDICAL SCIENCES—Abstracting, Bibliographies, Statistics*

617.95 USA
PLASTIC SURGERY PRODUCTS*. Text in English. 1991. m. USD 36 (effective 2000). adv. **Document type:** *Magazine, Trade.* **Description:** Offers the latest news in products and services as well as informational articles for plastic surgery professionals.
Published by: Novicom, Inc. (Subsidiary of: Medical World Communications), 6701 Center Dr West, Ste 450, Los Angeles, CA 90045-1556. TEL 310-642-4400, FAX 310-641-1511, http://www.novicom.com. Ed. Rashida Syed. Adv. contacts April Hyatt, Lisa Chose. B&W page USD 1,566, color page USD 2,266; trim 8.125 x 10.825. Circ: 12,000.

PLASTIC SURGICAL NURSING. see *MEDICAL SCIENCES—Nurses And Nursing*

617.585 DEU ISSN 1430-8886
PODOLOGIE. Text in German. 1948. m. DEM 117.35, EUR 60; DEM 142.78, EUR 73 foreign; DEM 11.73, EUR 6 newsstand/cover; DEM 15.65, EUR 8 newsstand/cover foreign (effective 2001). adv. bk.rev. charts, illus. index. **Document type:** *Magazine, Academic/Scholarly.*
Formerly: Fuss (0427-7783)
Published by: Verlag Neuer Merkur GmbH, Anton-Ditt-Bogen 23, Munich 80939, Germany. TEL 49-89-318905-0, FAX 49-89-31890538, info@vnm-gmbh.de, info@vnmonline.de, http://www.vnm-gmbh.de, http://www.vnmonline.de. Circ: 9,166.

617 ITA ISSN 0032-2636
POLICLINICO. SEZIONE CHIRURGICA. Text in Italian, English; Summaries in English. 1897. q. USD 80 (effective 2002). adv. charts, illus, stat.
Indexed: Chem.Abstr., Excerp.Med., Ind.Med. (coverage dropped).
—CISTI, GNLM.
Published by: Edizioni Luigi Pozzi s.r.l., Via Panama, 68, Rome, RM 00198, Italy. TEL 39-06-8553548, FAX 39-06-8554105, edizioni_pozzi@tin.it. Eds. G F Fegiz, S Stipa. Circ: 1,850.

617 POL ISSN 0032-373X
POLSKI PRZEGLAD CHIRURGICZNY. Text in Polish; Summaries in English. 1922. m. USD 16. adv. bk.rev. index. *Refereed.* **Document type:** *Journal, Academic/Scholarly.*
Indexed: Biol.Abstr., Chem.Abstr., Dent.Ind., Ind.Med. (coverage dropped), Ref.Zh.
—CISTI, GNLM.
Published by: (Towarzystwo Chirurgow Polskich), Fundacja Polski Przeglad Chirurgiczny, Ul Nowiniarska 1 m 28, Warsaw 00235, Poland. FAX 48-22-6354531, ppch@amwaw.edu.pl. Ed. Wojciech Noszczyk. R&P, Adv. contact Regina Nowicka. Circ: 2,100.

617.0956 GBR ISSN 0959-6674
POSTGRADUATE SURGERY: MIDDLE EAST*. Text in English. 1990. q. GBP 20 in Europe; GBP 30 elsewhere. adv. bk.rev. charts, illus. **Document type:** *Academic/Scholarly.* **Description:** Contains specially commissioned review articles written at the postgraduate level on surgical and anaesthetic techniques for specialists in the Middle East.
Published by: George Warman Publications Ltd., Unit 2, Riverview Business Park, Walnut Tree Close, Guildford, Surrey GU1 4QT, United Kingdom. TEL 44-1483-304944, FAX 44-1483-303191. Ed. Christopher Wastell. Circ: 6,200.

617.96 DEU ISSN 0079-4899
PRAKTISCHE CHIRURGIE. Text in German. 1936. irreg., latest vol.103, 1991. price varies. adv. reprint service avail. from IRC. **Document type:** *Monographic series.*
Supersedes: Vortraege aus der Praktischen Chirurgie (0083-6931)
—GNLM.
Published by: Ferdinand Enke Verlag, Postfach 300366, Stuttgart 70443, Germany. TEL 49-711-25520-0, FAX 49-711-2552030. Eds. A Encke, K Kremer. R&P, Adv. contact Babette Kehrenberg.

617 DEU
PRAXIS NAH. Text in German. 1970. m. DEM 106. back issues avail.
Formerly: Arzthelferin Aktuell (0176-1897)
—GNLM.
Published by: (Berufsverband der Arzthelferinnen), Verlag Johann August Koch, Postfach 1829, Marburg 35007, Germany. Circ: 32,000.

PRINCIPLES AND TECHNIQUES IN GYNECOLOGIC SURGERY SERIES. see *MEDICAL SCIENCES—Obstetrics And Gynecology*

PRINCIPLES OF PEDIATRIC NEUROSURGERY. see *MEDICAL SCIENCES—Pediatrics*

617 USA ISSN 0739-8328
RD98
PROBLEMS IN GENERAL SURGERY. Text in English. 1984. q., latest vol.18. USD 158 domestic to individuals; USD 207 foreign to individuals; USD 238 domestic to institutions; USD 294 foreign to institutions; USD 66 newsstand/cover (effective 2002). adv. illus. *Refereed.* **Document type:** *Academic/Scholarly.*
Related titles: Microform ed.: (from PQC); Online - full text ed.: USD 309.40 domestic for academic site license; USD 365.40 foreign for academic site license; USD 345.10 domestic for corporate site license; USD 401.10 foreign for corporate site license (effective 2002).
Indexed: Excerp.Med. (1993-).
—BLDSC (6617.885000), EMDOCS, GNLM, KNAW.
Published by: Lippincott Williams & Wilkins (Philadelphia) (Subsidiary of: Wolters Kluwer N.V.), 530 Walnut St, Philadelphia, PA 19106-3621. TEL 215-521-8300, FAX 215-521-8902, http://www.problemsgeneralsurgery.com, http://www.lww.com. Ed. Dr. Nathaniel J Sopher. R&P Margaret Becker. Adv. contact Suzann Graff. Circ: 4,000. **Subscr. to:** PO Box 1600, Hagerstown, MD 21740-1600. TEL 800-777-2295, FAX 301-824-7390.

PROGRESS IN NEUROLOGICAL SURGERY. see *MEDICAL SCIENCES—Psychiatry And Neurology*

617 CHE ISSN 0079-6824
RD11 CODEN: PSURA2
PROGRESS IN SURGERY. Text in English. 1961. irreg., latest vol.26. CHF 210 in Europe; DEM 250 in Germany; USD 180 in United States (effective 2001). reprint service avail. from ISI. *Refereed.* **Document type:** *Monographic series, Academic/Scholarly.*
Related titles: Online - full text ed.: (from Institute for Scientific Information).
Indexed: ASCA, Biol.Abstr., Chem.Abstr., Curr.Cont. (coverage dropped), Ind.Med. (coverage dropped), Ind.Sci.Rev.
—CISTI, GNLM, Infotrieve, KNAW. **CCC.**
Published by: S. Karger AG, Allschwilerstr 10, PO Box, Basel 4009, Switzerland. TEL 41-61-306-1111, FAX 41-61-306-1234, karger@karger.ch, http://www.karger.com/bookseries/PRSUR. Eds. E H Farthmann, M W Buechler.

PROGRESS IN SURGICAL PATHOLOGY. see *MEDICAL SCIENCES*

617.4 USA ISSN 1526-9248
RD129.5 CODEN: JTCOEI
PROGRESS IN TRANSPLANTATION; the journal for procurement and clinical transplant professionals. Text in English. 1991. q. USD 55 domestic to non-members; USD 90 foreign to non-members; USD 110 domestic to institutions; USD 120 foreign to institutions; USD 20 newsstand/cover domestic (effective 2000). adv. illus. reprints avail. *Refereed.* **Document type:** *Academic/Scholarly.*
Formerly (until 1999): Journal of Transplant Coordination (0905-9199)
Indexed: CINAHL, Excerp.Med. (1993-), Ind.Med. (coverage dropped), Int.Nurs.Ind.
—BLDSC (6924.608580), CISTI, EMDOCS, GNLM, Infotrieve. **CCC.**
Published by: (North American Transplant Coordinators Organization), InnoVision Communications, 101 Columbia, Aliso Viejo, CA 92656. TEL 949-448-7370, FAX 949-362-2049. Ed. Linda Ohler. R&P Beth Wos TEL 800-899-1712. Circ: 2,400 (paid). **Subscr. to:** PO Box 627, Holmes, PA 19403. TEL 800-899-1712, FAX 714-362-2022.

QUADERNI DI MEDICINA E CHIRURGIA. see *MEDICAL SCIENCES*

617 IND ISSN 0033-5657
CODEN: QJSSAB
QUARTERLY JOURNAL OF SURGICAL SCIENCES. Text in English. 1965. q. INR 40, USD 10. charts, illus, stat. reprint service avail. from PQC.
Related titles: Microform ed.: (from PQC).
Indexed: Chem.Abstr., INIS Atomind., Ind.Med. (coverage dropped).
—CASDDS, CISTI.
Published by: Banaras Hindu University, Institute of Medical Sciences, Surgical Research Laboratory, Varanasi, Uttar Pradesh 221 005, India. Ed. K N Udupa. Circ: 1,200.

617 CHE ISSN 1024-2651
RADIOSURGERY. Text in English. 1995. biennial, latest vol.3. CHF 200 in Europe; DEM 240 in Germany; USD 175 in United States (effective 2001). **Document type:** *Monographic series, Academic/Scholarly.* **Description:** Summarizes the most up-to-date information on stereotactic radiosurgery.
Indexed: e-psyche.
—BLDSC (7240.470000), KNAW.
Published by: (International Stereotactic Radiosurgery Society), S. Karger AG, Allschwilerstr 10, PO Box, Basel 4009, Switzerland. TEL 41-61-306-1111, FAX 41-61-306-1234, karger@karger.ch, http://www.karger.com/bookseries/RADIO.

617 ITA ISSN 0033-9776
CODEN: RMSAAN
RASSEGNA MEDICA SARDA. Text in Italian; Summaries in English. 1882. bi-m. ITL 30,000. adv. bk.rev. charts, illus. index, cum.index.
Indexed: Biol.Abstr., C.I.S. Abstr., Chem.Abstr., Excerp.Med., Rev.Plant Path.
—CASDDS, CISTI, GNLM.
Published by: Universita degli Studi di Cagliari, Facolta di Medicina Chirurgia, Casella Postale 287, Cagliari, CA 09100, Italy. Ed. A Cabitza. Circ: 550.

617 RUS
REANIMATOLOGIYA I INTENSIVNAYA TERAPIYA. Text in Russian. q. USD 85 in United States.
Published by: Vserossiiskii Institut Nauchnoi i Tekhnicheskoi Informatsii (VINITI), Usievicha ul 20-a, Moscow 125315, Russian Federation. TEL 7-095-1526441, FAX 7-095-943-0060. **US dist. addr.:** East View Publications, 3020 Harbor Ln N, Minneapolis, MN 55447. TEL 612-550-0961.

RECENT ADVANCES IN OPHTHALMOLOGY/YANKE XIN JINZHAN. see *MEDICAL SCIENCES—Ophthalmology And Optometry*

617.95 GBR ISSN 0309-2674
RECENT ADVANCES IN PLASTIC SURGERY. Text in English. 1976. irreg., latest vol.4. **Document type:** *Monographic series, Academic/Scholarly.*
—KNAW.
Published by: Churchill Livingstone (Subsidiary of: Harcourt Publishers Ltd.), Robert Stevenson House, 1-3 Baxter's Pl, Leith Walk, Edinburgh, Midlothian EH1 3AF, United Kingdom. TEL 44-131-556-2424, FAX 44-131-459-1177, http://www.churchillmed.com. **US subscr. to:** Churchill Livingstone, 650 Ave of the Americas, New York, NY 10011. TEL 212-206-5000.

617 GBR ISSN 0143-8395
RECENT ADVANCES IN SURGERY. Text in English. 1928. irreg., latest vol.18. **Document type:** *Monographic series, Academic/Scholarly.*
—BLDSC (7303.995000), CISTI, GNLM, KNAW.
Published by: Churchill Livingstone (Subsidiary of: Harcourt Publishers Ltd.), Robert Stevenson House, 1-3 Baxter's Pl, Leith Walk, Edinburgh, Midlothian EH1 3AF, United Kingdom. TEL 44-131-556-2424, FAX 44-131-459-1177, http://www.churchillmed.com. **US subscr. to:** Churchill Livingstone, 650 Ave of the Americas, New York, NY 10011. TEL 212-206-5000.

RESPIRATION; international journal of thoracic medicine. see *MEDICAL SCIENCES—Respiratory Diseases*

617 BRA ISSN 0034-7124
CODEN: RBCHAN
REVISTA BRASILEIRA DE CIRURGIA. Text in Portuguese; Summaries in English, Portuguese. 1932. bi-m. USD 200. adv. bk.rev. charts, illus. index.
Indexed: Biol.Abstr., Chem.Abstr., Excerp.Med., INIS Atomind., Ind.Med. (coverage dropped).
—CISTI, GNLM.
Published by: Cidade - Editora Cientifica Ltda., Rua Mexico, 90-Andar 2, Centro, Rio De Janeiro, RJ 20031-141, Brazil. Ed. Fernando Moyses. R&P Jose Soly Torres. Adv. contact Sergio Hardy. Circ: 7,000.

REVISTA BRASILEIRA DE CIRURGIA CARDIOVASCULAR. see *MEDICAL SCIENCES—Cardiovascular Diseases*

617 CUB ISSN 0034-7493
REVISTA CUBANA DE CIRUGIA. Text in Spanish; Summaries in English, Spanish. 1962. 3/yr. USD 34 in the Americas; USD 42 in Europe; USD 50 elsewhere. bibl, charts, illus. index.
Indexed: Biol.Abstr., Chem.Abstr., Excerp.Med., INIS Atomind., Ind.Med. (coverage dropped).
—CISTI.
Published by: Ministerio de Salud Publica, Centro Nacional de Informacion de Ciencias Medicas, O'Reilly No. 4, Havana, Cuba. TEL 809-62-8091. Ed. Ulises Barnet. Circ: 2,000. **Co-sponsor:** Sociedad Cubana de Cirurgia.

REVISTA DE ORTOPEDIA Y TRAUMATOLOGIA. see *MEDICAL SCIENCES—Orthopedics And Traumatology*

617.6 ESP ISSN 1130-0558
REVISTA ESPANOLA DE CIRUGIA ORAL Y MAXILOFACIAL*. Text in Spanish; Summaries in English. 1979. 3/yr. ESP 3,000, USD 40.
Formerly (until 1977): Revista Iberoamericana de Cirugia Oral y Maxilofacial (0210-5926)
—CINDOC.
Published by: (Sociedad Espanola de Cirugia Oral y Maxilofacial), Ediciones Ergon S.A., Pza. Josep Pallach 10, 1o, Barcelona 08035, Spain. TEL 2010911, FAX 2015911. **Subscr. to:** Cempro, Plaza Conde Valle Suchil 20, Madrid 28015, Spain.

617 ESP ISSN 1132-6336
REVISTA ESPANOLA DE TRASPLANTES. Text in Spanish. 1992. q. **Document type:** *Academic/Scholarly.* **Description:** Publishes research and clinical articles concerning organ transplant surgery.
—CINDOC.
Published by: (Organizacion Nacional de Trasplantes), Saned S.A., Capitan Haya, 60, Madrid 28020, Spain. TEL 34-91-749-9507, FAX 34-91-749-9507, saned@meditex.es. Ed. Rafael Matesanz. adv.: page ESP 225,000. Circ: 2,000.

REVISTA INTERNACIONAL DE DERMATOLOGIA Y DERMOCOSMETICA CLINICA. see *MEDICAL SCIENCES—Dermatology And Venereology*

REVISTA MEDICO-CHIRURGICALA. see *MEDICAL SCIENCES*

REVISTA PORTUGUESA DE ESTOMATOLOGIA E CIRURGIA MAXILO-FACIAL. see *MEDICAL SCIENCES—Dentistry*

617 VEN ISSN 0378-6420
REVISTA VENEZOLANA DE CIRUGIA*. Text in Spanish. bi-m. VEB 13.50.
Former titles (until 1976): Sociedad Venezolana de Cirugia. Revista (0378-6412); (until 1975): Sociedad Venezolana de Cirugia. Boletin
Published by: Sociedad Venezolana de Cirugia, Torre del Colegio 150, Of. A, Avde. Jose Maria Vargas, Urb. Santa Fe, Caracas 1080, Venezuela.

617 FRA ISSN 0336-7525
REVUE DE CHIRURGIE ESTHETIQUE DE LANGUE FRANCAISE. Text in French; Summaries in English, French. 1975. q. FRF 950 domestic; FRF 1,100 foreign (effective 2000). adv. bk.rev. bibl.
Published by: Societe Francaise de Chirurgie Esthetique, 54 av. Lefevre, Le Plessis-Trevise 94420, France. TEL 33-1-45941664, FAX 33-1-40549972. Ed. Dr. Jacques Bassot.

617.6 FRA ISSN 0035-1768
CODEN: RSCMAL
REVUE DE STOMATOLOGIE ET DE CHIRURGIE MAXILLO-FACIALE. Text in French. 1894. 6/yr. FRF 1,409; FRF 1,664 foreign (effective 2000). adv. bk.rev. illus. index. reprint service avail. from ISI. **Document type:** *Academic/Scholarly.* **Description:** Presents general reviews on topical subjects, original articles concerning maxillofacial pathology and surgery, and practical notes concerning topical therapeutics or techniques.
Formerly: Revue de Stomatologie
Related titles: Microform ed.: (from PQC); Online - full text ed.: (from RoweCom Information Quest).
Indexed: Biol.Abstr., Curr.Adv.Cancer Res., Curr.Adv.Ecol.Sci., Curr.Cont. (coverage dropped), Curr.Tit.Dent., Dent.Ind., Excerp.Med., Ind.Med. (1969-).
—BLDSC (7953.325000), CISTI, GNLM, Infotrieve, KNAW. **CCC.**
Published by: Masson - Periodiques, 120 bd. St. Germain, Paris 75006, France. TEL 33-1-40466200, FAX 33-1-40466201. Ed. M Grellet. Circ: 1,600. **Subscr. to:** Societe de Periodiques Specialises, BP 22, Vineuil Cedex 41354, France. TEL 33-2-54504612, FAX 33-2-54504611.

617 JPN ISSN 0386-9857
CODEN: RIGEBG
RINSHO GEKA/JOURNAL OF CLINICAL SURGERY. Text in Japanese. 1945. m. JPY 2,300 per issue.
Indexed: INIS Atomind.
—CASDDS, CISTI, GNLM.
Published by: Igaku-Shoin Ltd., 5-24-3 Hongo, Bunkyo-ku, Tokyo 113-0033, Japan. TEL 81-3-3817-5708.

RIVISTA DI MEDICINA E CHIRURGIA. see *MEDICAL SCIENCES*

617 ITA ISSN 0035-6689
RIVISTA GENERALE ITALIANA DI CHIRURGIA. Text in Italian; Summaries in English. 1950. bi-m. ITL 80,000; ITL 160,000 foreign (effective 1998). adv. bk.rev.
Indexed: Excerp.Med., Psychol.Abstr.
—GNLM.
Published by: Casa Editrice Maccari, Via Palermo, 44, Parma, PR 43100, Italy. TEL 39-521-771268. Ed. F Morino. Circ: 1,200.

617.95 ITA ISSN 0391-2221
RIVISTA ITALIANA DI CHIRURGIA PLASTICA. Text in Italian. 1968. q. ITL 100,000 domestic; ITL 180,000, EUR 92.40 foreign (effective 2000); includes supplement. back issues avail.
Indexed: Excerp.Med.
—BLDSC (7987.293000), CISTI, EMDOCS, GNLM.
Published by: (Societa Italiana di Chirurgia Plastica), Tipografia Editrice la Garangola, Via Montona, 4, Padua, PD 35137, Italy. FAX 39-49-8751743.

M

ROMANIAN NEUROSURGERY. see *MEDICAL SCIENCES—Psychiatry And Neurology*

617 GBR ISSN 0035-8835 CODEN: JRCSAC
ROYAL COLLEGE OF SURGEONS OF EDINBURGH. JOURNAL. Text in English. 1955. bi-m. GBP 160 in the European Union to individuals; USD 300 in North America to individuals; GBP 178 elsewhere to individuals (effective 2000). adv. bk.rev. charts, illus. index, cum.index every 5 yrs. back issues avail. *Refereed.* **Document type:** *Academic/Scholarly.*
Related titles: Microform ed.: (from PQC); Online - full text ed.: (from EBSCO Publishing, O C L C Online Computer Library Center, Inc., Institute for Scientific Information).
Indexed: Biol.Abstr., CINAHL, Curr.Adv.Ecol.Sci., Curr.Cont., Dent.Ind., Excerp.Med., Helminthol.Abstr., INIS Atomind., Ind.Med. (1955-), Inpharma, Int.Nurs.Ind., Nutr.Abstr., Pharm.&Out.News, Reac., Rev.Med.& Vet.Mycol., THA.
—BLDSC (4856.200000), CISTI, GNLM, IDS, ingenta, KNAW. **CCC.**
Published by: (Royal College of Surgeons of Edinburgh), Edinburgh University Press, 22 George Sq, Edinburgh, Midlothian EH8 9LF, United Kingdom. TEL 44-131-650-1000, FAX 44-131-662-0053, journals@eup.ed.ac.uk, http://www.eup.ed.ac.uk/journals. Ed. A Cuschieri. Pub. Allen Stevens. R&P Sarah Pollard. Adv. contact Douglas McNaughton. Circ: 9,650.

617 GBR ISSN 0035-8843 CODEN: ARCSAF
ROYAL COLLEGE OF SURGEONS OF ENGLAND. ANNALS. Text in English. 1947. bi-m. GBP 115 in Europe to individuals; USD 211 in United States to individuals; GBP 126 elsewhere to individuals; GBP 132 in Europe to institutions; USD 246 in United States to institutions; GBP 144 elsewhere to institutions (effective 2002). adv. bk.rev., Website rev. abstr, bibl. annual article index. back issues avail. *Refereed.* **Document type:** *Bulletin, Journal, Academic/Scholarly.* **Description:** Scientific journal covering aspects of surgery and dental surgery.
Related titles: Microform ed.: (from PQC); Online - full text ed.: (from Institute for Scientific Information).
Indexed: ASCA, Biol.Abstr., Chem.Abstr., Curr.Adv.Ecol.Sci., Curr.Cont., Dent.Ind., Environ.Sci.Poll.Mgmt., Excerp.Med., GeoRef, Helminthol.Abstr., INIS Atomind., Ind.Med. (1947-), Ind.Sci.Rev., Inpharma, Int.Nurs.Ind., NRN, Nutr.Abstr., Pharm.&Out.News, Pollut.Abstr., Reac., Risk Abstr., Saf.Sci.Abstr., Sci.Cit.Ind., THA.
—BLDSC (1031.550000), CISTI, GNLM, ingenta, KNAW.
Published by: (Royal College of Surgeons of England), Royal Society of Medicine Press Ltd, 1 Wimpole St, London W1M 8AE, United Kingdom. TEL 44-20-7290-2921, FAX 44-20-7290-2929, http://www.roysocmed.ac.uk/pub/arcs.htm. Ed. John Lumley.

617 CZE ISSN 0035-9351
ROZHLEDY V CHIRURGII. Text in Czech, Slovak; Summaries in Czech, English. 1922. m. EUR 144, USD 180 (effective 2001). adv. bk.rev. *Refereed.*
Indexed: Curr.Adv.Ecol.Sci., INIS Atomind., Ind.Med. (1937-).
—BLDSC (8033.480000), CISTI, GNLM, Infotrieve, KNAW. **CCC.**
Published by: (Ceska Lekarska Spolecnost J.E. Purkyne/Czech Medical Association), Nakladatelske Stredisko C L S J.E. Purkyne, Sokolska 31, Prague 12026, Czech Republic. TEL 420-2-24911420, FAX 420-2-24911420, nts@iol.cz, http://www.clsjep.cz, http://www.medical.cz. Ed. M Hajek. adv.: B&W page CZK 28,600, color page CZK 40,200; 250 x 170. Circ: 1,800. **Dist. by:** Abont s.r.o., Chlumova 17, Prague, 3 130 00, Czech Republic.

SAITAMA-KEN NO SHINKEI GEKAIKAI KAIHO/SAITAMA NEUROSURGICAL ASSOCIATION. BULLETIN. see *MEDICAL SCIENCES—Psychiatry And Neurology*

658 USA ISSN 0190-5066
SAME-DAY SURGERY. Text in English. 1977. m. USD 499 domestic; USD 529 foreign; USD 83 newsstand/cover (effective 2001). bk.rev. back issues avail.; reprints avail. **Document type:** *Newsletter, Academic/Scholarly.*
Incorporates (1989-1997): Advanced Technology in Surgical Care; Which was formerly (until 199?): Clinical Laser Monthly (0746-469X); (until 1996): Surgery Alert (0748-1942); (until 1995): Same-Day Surgery Manual; (until 1995): Anesthesiology Malpractice Protection Report (1050-8775); Which incorporated (in 1991): Anesthesiology Alert (1040-7774)
Related titles: Microfilm ed.: (from PQC); Online - full text ed.
Indexed: CINAHL.
—BLDSC (8071.966000).
Published by: American Health Consultants (Subsidiary of: Medical Economics Co., Inc.), 3525 Piedmont Rd, N E, 6 Piedmont Center, Ste 400, Atlanta, GA 30305. TEL 404-262-3291, 404-262-7436, 800-688-2421, FAX 404-262-7837, 800-284-3291, custserv@ahcpub.com, http://www.ahcpub.com. Circ: 1,960.

617 BRA ISSN 0036-4258
SANATORIO SAO LUCAS. BOLETIM✱. Text in Portuguese. 1939. bi-m. free per issue. adv. bk.rev. illus. index.
Related titles: Microfilm ed.: 1939 (from PQC).
Indexed: Excerp.Med., Ind.Med. (coverage dropped).
Published by: Fundacao para o Progresso da Cirurgia, Rua Pirapitingui, 80, Liberdade, Sao Paulo, SP 01508-020, Brazil. Ed. R Ney Penteado De Castro. Circ: 2,000 (controlled).

SANFUJINKA MAIKURO SAJARI GAKKAI ZASSHI/JAPANESE JOURNAL OF GYNECOLOGICAL MICROSURGERY. see *MEDICAL SCIENCES—Obstetrics And Gynecology*

SANFUJINKA SHUJUTSU/GYNECOLOGIC AND OBSTETRIC SURGERY. see *MEDICAL SCIENCES—Obstetrics And Gynecology*

617.54 617.41 SWE ISSN 1401-7431 CODEN: SCJOFY
SCANDINAVIAN CARDIOVASCULAR JOURNAL. Text in English. 1967. 6/yr. GBP 70, USD 115 to individuals; GBP 155, USD 255 to institutions (effective 2002). adv. *Refereed.* **Document type:** *Journal, Academic/Scholarly.* **Description:** Promotes cardiovascular research that crosses disciplinary boundaries.
Formerly (until 1997): Scandinavian Journal of Thoracic and Cardiovascular Surgery (0036-5580)
Related titles: Online - full text ed.: (from EBSCO Publishing, O C L C Online Computer Library Center, Inc., RoweCom Information Quest, CatchWord Ltd., ingenta, Swets Blackwell, Institute for Scientific Information); ♦ Supplement: Scandinavian Cardiovascular Journal. Supplementum. ISSN 1401-7458.
Indexed: ASCA, Biol.Abstr., Curr.Cont., Excerp.Med., INIS Atomind., Ind.Med. (1997-), Ind.Sci.Rev., Inpharma, Int.Nurs.Ind., Pharm.&Out.News, Reac., Sci.Cit.Ind.
—BLDSC (8087.472600), CISTI, GNLM, IDS, Infotrieve, ingenta, KNAW. **CCC.**
Published by: (Scandinavian Association for Thoracic and Cardiovascular Surgery NOR), Taylor & Francis AS (Subsidiary of: Taylor & Francis Group), Cort Adelersgt. 17, Solli, PO Box 2562, Oslo 0202, Norway. TEL 47-22-12-98-80, FAX 47-22-12-98-90, journals@tandf.no, http://www.tandf.co.uk/tfas. Ed. Rolf Ekroth. adv.: B&W page SEK 14,000, color page SEK 20,000; trim 190 x 260. Circ: 2,600.

617.54 617.41 SWE ISSN 1401-7458 CODEN: SCJSFC
SCANDINAVIAN CARDIOVASCULAR JOURNAL. SUPPLEMENTUM. Text in English. 1969. irreg. **Document type:** *Monographic series.*
Formerly (until 1997): Scandinavian Journal of Thoracic and Cardiovascular Surgery. Supplementum (0586-9587)
Related titles: ♦ Supplement to: Scandinavian Cardiovascular Journal. ISSN 1401-7431.
Indexed: Ind.Med. (1997-).
—BLDSC (8087.472605), CISTI, KNAW. **CCC.**
Published by: (Scandinavian Association for Thoracic and Cardiovascular Surgery NOR), Taylor & Francis AB (Subsidiary of: Taylor & Francis Group), Hollaendargatan 20, PO Box 3255, Stockholm 11160, Sweden. TEL 46-8-4408040, FAX 46-8-4408050, journals@se.tandf.no, http://www.tandf.co.uk/journals/tfas.html.

617.95 NOR ISSN 0284-4311 CODEN: SJPSEM
SCANDINAVIAN JOURNAL OF PLASTIC AND RECONSTRUCTIVE SURGERY AND HAND SURGERY. Text in English. 1967. bi-m. GBP 75, USD 124 to individuals; GBP 173, USD 286 to institutions (effective 2002). adv. *Refereed.* **Document type:** *Academic/Scholarly.* **Description:** Intended to serve as a forum for plastic surgery, hand surgery and related research in Scandinavia. Interest is focused on original articles on basic research and clinical evaluation.
Formerly (until 1987): Scandinavian Journal of Plastic and Reconstructive Surgery (0036-5556)
Related titles: Online - full text ed.: (from EBSCO Publishing, O C L C Online Computer Library Center, Inc., RoweCom Information Quest, CatchWord Ltd., ingenta, Swets Blackwell, Institute for Scientific Information); ♦ Supplement: Scandinavian Journal of Plastic and Reconstructive Surgery and Hand Surgery. Supplement. ISSN 1235-662X.
Indexed: ASCA, Biol.Abstr., Curr.Adv.Cell & Devel.Biol., Curr.Cont., Dent.Ind., Excerp.Med., INIS Atomind., Ind.Med. (1987-), Ind.Sci.Rev., Inpharma, Med.& Surg.Dermat., Nutr.Abstr., Reac., Sci.Cit.Ind.
—BLDSC (8087.518500), ADONIS, CASDDS, CISTI, EMDOCS, GNLM, IDS, ingenta, KNAW. **CCC.**
Published by: (Scandinavian Association of Plastic Surgeons), Taylor & Francis AS (Subsidiary of: Taylor & Francis Group), Cort Adelersgt. 17, Solli, PO Box 2562, Oslo 0202, Norway. TEL 47-22-12-98-80, FAX 47-22-12-98-90, journals@tandf.no, http://www.tandf.co.uk/tfas. Ed. Jan Lilja. Circ: 4,600.

617.95 NOR ISSN 1235-662X
SCANDINAVIAN JOURNAL OF PLASTIC AND RECONSTRUCTIVE SURGERY AND HAND SURGERY. SUPPLEMENT. Text in English. 1967. irreg. **Document type:** *Academic/Scholarly.*
Supersedes (1967-1984): Scandinavian Journal of Plastic and Reconstructive Surgery. Supplementum (0581-9474)
Related titles: ♦ Supplement to: Scandinavian Journal of Plastic and Reconstructive Surgery and Hand Surgery. ISSN 0284-4311.
Indexed: Excerp.Med. (1993-), Ind.Med. (coverage dropped).
—BLDSC (8087.519000), CISTI, EMDOCS, Infotrieve, KNAW. **CCC.**
Published by: (Scandinavian Hand Surgery Foundation), Scandinavian University Press (Subsidiary of: Taylor & Francis Ltd.), Postboks 2959, Toeyen, Oslo 0608, Norway. FAX 47-22-57-53-53, journals@scup.no, http://www.scup.no/primhealth.

SCHWEIZER ARCHIV FUER NEUROLOGIE UND PSYCHIATRIE. see *MEDICAL SCIENCES—Psychiatry And Neurology*

617.585 CHE
SCHWEIZER PODOLOGE✱. Text in French, German. 1943. m. adv.
Formerly (until 1980): Schweizer Pedicure (0036-7435)
Published by: Schweizerischer Podologenverband, Grundstr 14, Postfach 212, Rotkreuz 6343, Switzerland. Ed. Wilhelm Heiz. Circ: 600.

617 USA
SCIENTIFIC AMERICAN SURGERY. Text in English. 1988. base vol. plus q. updates. USD 250 to individuals; USD 310 to institutions; includes supplements. adv. **Document type:** *Academic/Scholarly.* **Description:** Contains current information for surgeons on all aspects of perioperative care and surgical technique and disease.
Formerly (until 1995): Care of the Surgical Patient
Published by: Scientific American, Inc., 415 Madison Ave, New York, NY 10017-1111. TEL 212-754-0550, FAX 212-754-1138. Ed. Douglas Wilmore. Circ: 10,000.

617.6 USA ISSN 1044-7032
SELECTED READINGS IN ORAL AND MAXILLOFACIAL SURGERY. Text in English. 1988. bi-m. USD 185 domestic per 8-issue vol.; USD 210 foreign per 8-issue vol. (effective 2000). **Document type:** *Academic/Scholarly.*
—BLDSC (8234.855000).
Published by: University of Texas at Dallas, Southwestern Medical Center at Dallas, 5323 Harry Hines Blvd, Dallas, TX 75390-9109. TEL 214-648-3548, FAX 214-648-2918. Ed., R&P Dr. Douglas P Sinn. Circ: 1,000.

617.95 USA ISSN 0739-5523
SELECTED READINGS IN PLASTIC SURGERY. Text in English. 1980. 20/yr., latest vol.9. USD 200 domestic to individuals; USD 220 foreign to individuals; USD 210 domestic to institutions; USD 230 foreign to institutions (effective 2000). bibl. **Document type:** *Monographic series.*
—GNLM.
Address: 411 N Washington Ave, Ste 6900, Dallas, TX 75246. TEL 214-824-0154, FAX 214-824-0463, darlingg@airmail.net. Ed. Dr. Fritz E Barton Jr. R&P Grace Darling. Circ: 1,500 (controlled).

SEMINARS IN ANESTHESIA, PERIOPERATIVE MEDICINE AND PAIN. see *MEDICAL SCIENCES—Anaesthesiology*

616.3 USA ISSN 1043-1489
SEMINARS IN COLON AND RECTAL SURGERY. Text in English. 1990. q. USD 146 domestic to individuals; USD 195 foreign to individuals; USD 194 domestic to institutions; USD 239 foreign to institutions; USD 76 domestic to students; USD 117 foreign to students; USD 60 newsstand/cover (effective 2001). adv. **Document type:** *Academic/Scholarly.* **Description:** Each issue focuses on a single topic on the surgical treatment of patients with disorders of the colon or rectum.
Indexed: CINAHL.
—BLDSC (8239.448400), CISTI, GNLM, Infotrieve. **CCC.**
Published by: W.B. Saunders Co. (Subsidiary of: Harcourt Publishers Ltd.), 11830 Westline Industrial Dr, St Louis, MO 63146. TEL 800-325-4177, http://www.wbsaunders.com. Ed. Dr. David J Schoetz Jr. adv.: B&W page USD 765, color page USD 1,815; trim 10 x 7. Circ: 900. **Subscr. to:** Periodicals Fulfillment, W B Saunders Co, 6277 Sea Harbor Dr, 4th Fl, Orlando, FL 32891-4800.

617 618 USA ISSN 1071-5517
SEMINARS IN LAPAROSCOPIC SURGERY. Text in English. 1994 (Mar.). q. USD 126 domestic to individuals; USD 180 foreign to individuals; USD 169 domestic to institutions; USD 219 foreign to institutions; USD 70 domestic to students; USD 108 foreign to students; USD 55 newsstand/cover (effective 2001). adv. illus. back issues avail. **Document type:** *Academic/Scholarly.* **Description:** Each issue focuses on a current application of this minimally invasive surgery; also covers surgical techniques and technological advances.
Indexed: Ind.Med. (1994-).
—BLDSC (8239.453500), GNLM, Infotrieve, KNAW. **CCC.**
Published by: W.B. Saunders Co. (Subsidiary of: Harcourt Publishers Ltd.), 11830 Westline Industrial Dr, St Louis, MO 63146. TEL 800-325-4177, http://www.wbsaunders.com. Eds. Dr. Alfred Cuschieri, Bruce V MacFayden Jr. adv.: B&W page USD 745, color page USD 1,820; trim 10 x 7. Circ: 1,025. **Subscr. to:** Periodicals Fulfillment, W B Saunders Co, 6277 Sea Harbor Dr, 4th Fl, Orlando, FL 32891-4800.

616 USA ISSN 0160-2489
SEMINARS IN NEUROLOGICAL SURGERY. Text in English. 1978. irreg. reprint service avail. from PQC. *Refereed.* **Document type:** *Monographic series, Academic/Scholarly.*
Indexed: ASCA, Excerp.Med., e-psyche.
Published by: Lippincott Williams & Wilkins (Philadelphia) (Subsidiary of: Wolters Kluwer N.V.), 530 Walnut St, Philadelphia, PA 19106-3621. TEL 301-223-2300, 800-638-3030, FAX 301-223-2400, http://www.lww.com.

617 USA ISSN 1526-8012
SEMINARS IN NEUROSURGERY. Text in English. 1990. 3/yr. (in May, August & November). EUR 165 to individuals; EUR 210 to institutions; EUR 61 newsstand/cover (effective 2002). adv. **Document type:** *Journal, Academic/Scholarly.* **Description:** Presents an insightful coverage of the latest trends in neurosurgical techniques, equipment, and patient management, guest edited by top international authorities.
Formerly: Perspectives in Neurological Surgery (1045-3733)
Related titles: Online - full text ed.: ISSN 1526-4572 (from RoweCom Information Quest).
Indexed: ASCA, Neurosci.Cit.Ind., e-psyche.
—BLDSC (8239.455600), IDS, Infotrieve. **CCC.**
Published by: Thieme Medical Publishers, 333 Seventh Ave, New York, NY 10001. TEL 212-760-0888, 800-782-3488, FAX 212-947-1112, http://www.thieme.com//onGJMFKAEJLKFFK/display/768. Ed. Dr. Winfield S Fisher III. Adv. contact Sally Kahn. **Orders in Europe to:** Thieme International, Postfach 301120, Stuttgart 70451, Germany. TEL 49-711-8931-0.

618.92 USA ISSN 1055-8586
CODEN: SPSUEH
SEMINARS IN PEDIATRIC SURGERY. Text in English. 1992 (Feb.). q. USD 158 domestic to individuals; USD 200 foreign to individuals; USD 208 domestic to institutions; USD 266 foreign to institutions; USD 98 domestic to students; USD 120 foreign to students; USD 67 newsstand/cover (effective 2001). adv. back issues avail. **Document type:** *Academic/Scholarly.* **Description:** Addresses a single topic of the specialty in each issue.
Indexed: Excerp.Med. (1994-), Ind.Med. (1992-).
—BLDSC (8239.456790), EMDOCS, GNLM, Infotrieve, KNAW. **CCC.**
Published by: W.B. Saunders Co. (Subsidiary of: Harcourt Publishers Ltd.), 11830 Westline Industrial Dr, St Louis, MO 63146. TEL 800-325-4177, http://www.wbsaunders.com. Ed. Jay L Grosfeld. adv.: B&W page USD 645, color page USD 1,595; trim 10 x 7. Circ: 1,093. **Subscr. to:** Periodicals Fulfillment, W B Saunders Co, 6277 Sea Harbor Dr, 4th Fl, Orlando, FL 32891-4800.

SEMINARS IN PERINATOLOGY. see *MEDICAL SCIENCES—Pediatrics*

SEMINARS IN PERIOPERATIVE NURSING. see *MEDICAL SCIENCES—Nurses And Nursing*

617 USA ISSN 1535-2188
RD118.A1 CODEN: PPSUEI
SEMINARS IN PLASTIC SURGERY. Text in English. 1987. q. EUR 204 to individuals; EUR 352 to institutions; EUR 81 newsstand/cover (effective 2002). adv. cum.index: vols.1-5. *Refereed.* **Document type:** *Journal, Academic/Scholarly.* **Description:** Covers developments and all other aspects of plastic, aesthetic, and reconstructive surgery.
Formerly (until 2001): Perspectives in Plastic Surgery (0892-3957)
Related titles: Online - full text ed.: ISSN 1521-575X (from RoweCom Information Quest); ♦ Supplement: Plastic Surgery Outlook. ISSN 0892-3965.
—GNLM, Infotrieve. **CCC.**
Published by: Thieme Medical Publishers, 333 Seventh Ave, New York, NY 10001. TEL 212-760-0888, 800-782-3488, FAX 212-947-1112, http://www.thieme.com. Ed. Dr. Saleh M Shenaq. Adv. contact Sally Kahn. **Orders in Europe to:** Thieme International, Postfach 301120, Stuttgart 70451, Germany. TEL 49-711-8931-0.

SEMINARS IN SPINE SURGERY. see *MEDICAL SCIENCES—Orthopedics And Traumatology*

SEMINARS IN SURGICAL ONCOLOGY. see *MEDICAL SCIENCES—Oncology*

617.54 616.1 USA ISSN 1043-0679
SEMINARS IN THORACIC AND CARDIOVASCULAR SURGERY. Text in English. 1989. q. USD 158 domestic to individuals; USD 217 foreign to individuals; USD 212 domestic to institutions; USD 269 foreign to institutions; USD 85 domestic to students; USD 130 foreign to students; USD 68 newsstand/cover (effective 2001). adv. **Document type:** *Journal, Academic/Scholarly.* **Description:** Offers original articles that provide a current perspective on a relevant new topic in thoracic and cardiovascular surgery.
Indexed: Ind.Med. (1989-), Int.Nurs.Ind.
—BLDSC (8239.475000), CISTI, GNLM, Infotrieve, KNAW. **CCC.**
Published by: W.B. Saunders Co. (Subsidiary of: Harcourt Publishers Ltd.), 11830 Westline Industrial Dr, St Louis, MO 63146. TEL 800-325-4177, http://www.wbsaunders.com. Ed. Dr. James L Cox. adv.: B&W page USD 775, color page USD 1,900; trim 10 x 7. Circ: 2,020. **Subscr. to:** Periodicals Fulfillment, W B Saunders Co, 6277 Sea Harbor Dr, 4th Fl, Orlando, FL 32891-4800.

616 USA ISSN 0895-7967
CODEN: SVSUEP
SEMINARS IN VASCULAR SURGERY. Text in English. 1988. q. USD 155 domestic to individuals; USD 205 foreign to individuals; USD 229 domestic to institutions; USD 274 foreign to institutions; USD 79 domestic to students; USD 123 foreign to students; USD 69 newsstand/cover (effective 2001). adv. back issues avail. **Document type:** *Academic/Scholarly.* **Description:** Provides clinical information to keep specialists in the field up to date.
Indexed: Excerp.Med., Ind.Med. (1988-).
—BLDSC (8239.486500), CISTI, EMDOCS, GNLM, Infotrieve, ingenta, KNAW. **CCC.**
Published by: W.B. Saunders Co. (Subsidiary of: Harcourt Publishers Ltd.), 11830 Westline Industrial Dr, St Louis, MO 63146. TEL 800-325-4177, http://www.wbsaunders.com. Ed. Dr. Robert B Rutherford. adv.: B&W page USD 785, color page USD 1,885; trim 10 x 7. Circ: 2,004. **Subscr. to:** Periodicals Fulfillment, W B Saunders Co, 6277 Sea Harbor Dr, 4th Fl, Orlando, FL 32891-4800.

617 JPN ISSN 0917-7175
SHINSHU TO MEN'EKI/SURGICAL TRAUMA & IMMUNOLOGICAL RESPONSES. Text in Japanese. 1991. q. JPY 2,000 per issue.
Published by: Medical View Co. Ltd./Mejikaru Byusha, 2-30 Ichigaya-Honmura-cho, Shinjuku-ku, Tokyo 162-0845, Japan. Circ: 8,000.

617 JPN ISSN 0385-6313
SHONI GEKA/JAPANESE JOURNAL OF PEDIATRIC SURGERY. Text in Japanese; Summaries in English. 1969. m. JPY 2,500; JPY 38,000 newsstand/cover (effective 1999).
Indexed: INIS Atomind.
—CISTI.
Published by: Tokyo Igakusha Ltd., 35-4 Hongo 3-chome, Bunkyo-ku, Tokyo 113-0033, Japan. TEL 81-3-3811-4119, FAX 81-3-3811-4119.

617 JPN ISSN 0037-4423
SHUJUTSU/OPERATION. Text in Japanese. 1947. m. JPY 1,750 per issue. bk.rev. cum.index.
Indexed: INIS Atomind., Ind.Med. (coverage dropped).
—CISTI, GNLM.
Published by: Kanehara & Co. Ltd., 2-31-14 Yushima, Bunkyo-ku, Tokyo 113-0034, Japan. Ed. Dr. Tokuji Ichikawa. Circ: 9,500.

617 USA ISSN 1052-1453
CODEN: SBSUEL
SKULL BASE SURGERY. Text in English. 1991. q. EUR 189 to individuals; EUR 375 to institutions; EUR 87 newsstand/cover (effective 2002). adv. *Refereed.* **Document type:** *Journal, Academic/Scholarly.* **Description:** Takes a multidisciplinary approach, using original research articles.
Related titles: Online - full text ed.: ISSN 1098-9072 (from Ovid Technologies, Inc., EBSCO Publishing, O C L C Online Computer Library Center, Inc., RoweCom Information Quest).
Indexed: ASCA, Curr.Cont. (coverage dropped), Excerp.Med. (1993-), Inpharma, Neurosci.Cit.Ind., Reac., Rev.Med.& Vet.Mycol.
—EMDOCS, GNLM, IDS, Infotrieve, KNAW. **CCC.**
Published by: Thieme Medical Publishers, 333 Seventh Ave, New York, NY 10001. TEL 212-760-0888, 800-782-3488, FAX 212-947-1112, http://www.thieme.com. Eds. Dr. Douglas E Mattox, Dr. Madjid Samii. Circ: 1,100. **Orders in Europe to:** Thieme International, Postfach 3001120, Stuttgart 70451, Germany. TEL 49-711-8931-0.

617 BRA
SOCIEDADE DE MEDICINA E CIRURGIA DE SAO JOSE DO RIO PRETO. REVISTA. Text and summaries in English, Portuguese. 1968. q. BRL 100, USD 15. adv. bk.rev. illus. index.
Related titles: Microform ed.
Indexed: Biol.Abstr.
Published by: Sociedade de Medicina e Cirurgia de Sao Jose do Rio Preto, Rua Spinola s-n, Sao Jose Da Rio Preto 15100, Brazil. Ed. Dr. Jorge Paulete. Circ: (controlled).

617 ITA ISSN 1121-1342
SOCIETA MEDICO-CHIRURGICA DELLA PROVINCIA DI CREMONA. BOLLETTINO. Text in Italian; Summaries in English. 1946. s-a. ITL 30,000, USD 20. adv. abstr, bibl, charts, illus. index.
Former titles (until 1982): Societa Medico-Chirurgica e Ospedali Provincia de Cremona. Bollettino (0391-5999); (until 1975): Societa Medico-Chirurgica di Cremona. Bollettino (0037-8852)
Indexed: Biol.Abstr., Ind.Med. (coverage dropped).
—CISTI.
Published by: Societa Medico-Chirurgica di Cremona, Ordine dei Medici, Via Palestro, 66, Cremona, CR 26100, Italy. TEL 0372-35224. Ed. Luciano Boari. Circ: 400.

616 ITA
SOCIETA MEDICO-CHIRURGICA DI MODENA. BOLLETTINO. Text in Italian; Summaries in English. 1982 (vol.82). fortn. ITL 10,000, USD 7.
Indexed: Biol.Abstr.
Published by: Societa Medico-Chirurgica di Modena, Policlinico, Via del Pozzo, Modena, MO 41100, Italy. Circ: 500.

617 USA ISSN 1086-8089
SOCIETY OF LAPAROENDOSCOPIC SURGEONS. JOURNAL. Abbreviated title: J S L S. Text in English. 1997. q. **Document type:** *Trade.*
Indexed: Ind.Med. (coverage dropped).
—BLDSC (4889.800000).
Published by: Society of Laparoendoscopic Surgeons, Incorporated, 7330 SW 62nd Pl., Suite 410, Miami, FL 33143-4825. Ed. Michael S Kavic TEL 330-480-3124.

SOINS - CHIRURGIE. see *MEDICAL SCIENCES—Nurses And Nursing*

617 ZAF ISSN 0038-2361
CODEN: SAJSBS
SOUTH AFRICAN JOURNAL OF SURGERY/SUID-AFRIKAANSE JOERNAAL VIR CHIRURGIE. Text in Afrikaans, English. 1963. q. USD 40 foreign (effective 2000). adv. bk.rev. bibl, charts, illus. index. reprint service avail. from PQC,ISI. *Refereed.* **Document type:** *Academic/Scholarly.* **Description:** Publishes clinical and research articles in all areas of surgery.
Related titles: Microform ed.: (from PQC); Online - full text ed.: (from Institute for Scientific Information).
Indexed: ASCA, Abstr.Hyg., Biol.Abstr., Curr.Cont., Excerp.Med., Helminthol.Abstr., INIS Atomind., Ind.Med. (1963-), Ind.S.A.Per., Inpharma, Pharm.&Out.News, Reac., Trop.Dis.Bull.
—BLDSC (8340.300000), CISTI, GNLM, IDS, ingenta, KNAW.
Published by: (Association of Surgeons of South Africa), South African Medical Association, Health and Medical Publishing Group, 14 Central Sq, Pinelands 7430, South Africa. Ed. M R Q Davies. R&P Peter Roberts. Adv. contact Andre Botes TEL 27-11-706-2088. Circ: 1,000. **Subscr. to:** PO Box 74789, Lynnwood Ridge, Pretoria 0040, South Africa. **Dist. by:** Private Bag X1, Pinelands 7430, South Africa.

617 USA
SOUTHERN SURGICAL ASSOCIATION. TRANSACTIONS. Text in English. 1991. a. **Document type:** *Academic/Scholarly.*
Related titles: Microform ed.: (from PQC).
Published by: (Southern Surgical Association), Lippincott Williams & Wilkins (Philadelphia) (Subsidiary of: Wolters Kluwer N.V.), 530 Walnut St, Philadelphia, PA 19106-3621. TEL 301-223-2300, 800-638-3030, FAX 301-223-2400, http://www.lww.com.

SPOR HEKIMLIGI DERGISI/TURKISH JOURNAL OF SPORTS MEDICINE. see *MEDICAL SCIENCES—Sports Medicine*

617 USA
ST. ANTHONY'S CODING FOR GENERAL SURGERY REIMBURSEMENT✱. Text in English. m. USD 129. **Description:** Focuses on day-to-day coding and reimbursement issues faced by general surgery practitioners.
Published by: St. Anthony Publishing, Inc., 11410 Isaac Newton Sq N, 200, Reston, VA 22090-5012. TEL 800-632-0123. Ed. Kimberly Fullmer.

617 CHE ISSN 1011-6125
CODEN: SFUNE4
STEREOTACTIC AND FUNCTIONAL NEUROSURGERY. Text in English. 1938. 8/yr. (in 2 vols.). CHF 854 in Europe to institutions; CHF 877.20 elsewhere to institutions; EUR 610.40 in Europe to institutions; USD 668 elsewhere to institutions (effective 2002). adv. bibl, illus, charts. index. back issues avail. *Refereed.* **Document type:** *Journal, Academic/Scholarly.* **Description:** Provides a single source for the reader to keep abreast of developments in the most rapidly advancing subspecialty within neurosurgery.
Former titles: Applied Neurophysiology (0302-2773); Confinia Neurologia (0010-5678)
Related titles: Microform ed.: (from RPI); Online - full text ed.: ISSN 1423-0372. CHF 116, EUR 84, USD 90 to institutions with print edition (effective 2002) (from EBSCO Publishing, O C L C Online Computer Library Center, Inc., RoweCom Information Quest, Swets Blackwell, Institute for Scientific Information).
Indexed: ASCA, Bibl.Dev.Med.& Child Neur., Biol.Abstr., Chem.Abstr., Compumath, Curr.Adv.Ecol.Sci., Curr.Cont. (coverage dropped), Dent.Ind., Excerp.Med., Helminthol.Abstr., Ind.Med. (1989-), Ind.Sci.Rev., Neurosci.Cit.Ind., Psychol.Abstr., Sci.Cit.Ind. (coverage dropped), e-psyche.
—BLDSC (8464.368000), CASDDS, CISTI, EMDOCS, GNLM, IDS, ingenta, KNAW. **CCC.**
Published by: (World and American Society for Stereotactic and Functional Neurosurgery), S. Karger AG, Allschwilerstr 10, PO Box, Basel 4009, Switzerland. TEL 41-61-306-1111, FAX 41-61-306-1234, karger@karger.ch, http://www.online.karger.com/journals/sfn, http://www.karger.com. Ed. P L Gildenberg. adv.: page USD 1,195. Circ: 1,000.

617 JPN ISSN 0016-593X
SURGERY/GEKA. Text in Japanese. 1937. 13/yr. JPY 47,000. adv. charts, illus. index. **Document type:** *Academic/Scholarly.*
Indexed: INIS Atomind.
—CISTI.
Published by: Nankodo Co. Ltd., 42-6 Hongo 3-chome, Bunkyo-ku, Tokyo 113-0033, Japan. FAX 03-3811-7230. Ed. Kenji Sakurai. Circ: 6,000.

617 USA ISSN 0039-6060
RD1 CODEN: SURGAZ
SURGERY. Text in English. 1937. m. USD 195 domestic to individuals; USD 233 foreign to individuals; USD 344 domestic to institutions; USD 382 foreign to institutions; USD 96 domestic to students; USD 134 foreign to students; USD 32 newsstand/cover (effective 2001). adv. illus. s-a. index. reprint service avail. from PQC. *Refereed.* **Document type:** *Journal, Academic/Scholarly.* **Description:** Contains information on developments in clinical and experimental surgery.
Related titles: Microfilm ed.: (from PQC,PMC); Online - full text ed.: (from Ovid Technologies, Inc., EBSCO Publishing, IDEAL Online Library, Institute for Scientific Information, RoweCom Information Quest).
Indexed: AIM, ASCA, Abstr.Health Care Manage.Stud., Biol.Abstr., Cal.Tiss.Abstr., Chem.Abstr., Chemorec.Abstr., Curr.Adv.Cancer Res., Curr.Adv.Ecol.Sci., Curr.Adv.Gen.& Molec.Biol., Curr.Cont., Dairy Sci.Abstr., Environ.Sci.Poll.Mgmt., Excerp.Med., Helminthol.Abstr., INIS Atomind., Ind.Med. (1937-), Ind.Sci.Rev., Int.Abstr.Biol.Sci., Kidney, Med.& Surg.Dermat., Neurosci.Abstr. (coverage dropped), Nutr.Abstr., Pig News & Info., Pollut.Abstr., Rev.Med.& Vet.Mycol., Risk Abstr., Saf.Sci.Abstr., Sci.Cit.Ind.
—BLDSC (8548.125000), ADONIS, CASDDS, CISTI, GNLM, IDS, ingenta, KNAW. **CCC.**
Published by: (Society of University Surgeons), Mosby, Inc. (Subsidiary of: Elsevier Science), 11830 Westline Industrial Dr, St Louis, MO 63146-3318. TEL 314-872-8370, 800-325-4177, FAX 314-432-1380, customerservice@mosby.com, http://www.mosby.com/periodicals. Eds. George Zuidema, Dr. Walter F Ballinger. Pub. Cynthia Baudendistel. Adv. contact Carole Kilzer. B&W page USD 1,165, color page USD 2,090; trim 10.88 x 8.13. Circ: 5,943. **Co-sponsors:** American Association of Endocrine Surgeons; Central Surgical Association.

617 GBR ISSN 0263-9319
SURGERY. Text in English. m. GBP 79.20; GBP 84 foreign. adv. **Document type:** *Academic/Scholarly.*
—BLDSC (8548.123600), CISTI.
Published by: The Medicine Group (Journals) Ltd., Publishing House, 62 Stert St, Abingdon, Oxon OX14 3UQ, United Kingdom. TEL 44-1235-555770, FAX 44-1235-554691. Eds. John Craven, John Lumley. Adv. contact Christian Benzing.

617 JPN ISSN 1340-5594
SURGERY FRONTIER. Text in Japanese. 1994. 4/yr. JPY 2,400 per issue (effective 1998).
Published by: Medikaru Rebyusha/Medical Review Co., Ltd., 7-3 Hirano-Machi 1-chome, Chuo-ku, Osaka-shi 541-0046, Japan. TEL 81-6-223-1468, FAX 81-6-223-1245, medrev@osk2.3web.ne.jp.

617 JPN ISSN 0941-1291
CODEN: SUTOE
SURGERY TODAY. Text in English. 1899. m. (in 1 vol., 12 nos./vol.). JPY 50,000 domestic; USD 614 in North America; DEM 948 elsewhere; DEM 1,038, EUR 530.72 in Germany for Print & Online Eds.; DEM 1,052.40, EUR 538.08 elsewhere for Print & Online Eds. (effective 2001). bk.rev. *Refereed.* **Document type:** *Academic/Scholarly.* **Description:** Covers recent advances and new developments in all fields of surgery, both clinical and experimental.
Formerly (until 1991): Japanese Journal of Surgery (0047-1909)
Related titles: Online - full text ed.: ISSN 1436-2813 (from EBSCO Publishing, RoweCom Information Quest, Swets Blackwell, Springer LINK, Institute for Scientific Information).
Indexed: ASCA, Biol.Abstr., Chem.Abstr., Curr.Cont., Excerp.Med., INIS Atomind., Ind.Med. (1992-), Inpharma, Pharm.&Out.News, Reac., SSCI (coverage dropped), So.Pac.Per.Ind.
—BLDSC (8548.164500), ADONIS, CASDDS, CISTI, EMDOCS, GNLM, IDS, ingenta, KNAW.
Published by: (Japan Surgical Society/Nihon Gan Chiryo Gakkai), Springer-Verlag Tokyo (Subsidiary of: BertelsmannSpringer), 3-13 Hongo 3-chome, Bunkyo-ku, Tokyo 113-0033, Japan. TEL 81-3-3812-0617, FAX 81-3-3812-4699, orders@svt-ebs.co.jp, http://link.springer-ny.com/link/service/journals/00595/index.htm. Ed. Morito Monden. Circ: 1,500. **Subscr. in N. America to:** Springer-Verlag New York Inc., PO Box 2485, Secaucus, NJ 07096-2485. TEL 800-777-4643, 212-460-1526, FAX 201-348-4505, orders@springer-ny.com; **Subscr. to:** Springer-Verlag, c/o Gabriele Kubitza, Haberstrasse 7, Heidelberg 69126, Germany. TEL 49-6221-345242, FAX 49-6221-345229, subscriptions@springer.de, http://link.springer.de, http://link.springer-ny.com.

SURGICAL AND RADIOLOGIC ANATOMY. see *MEDICAL SCIENCES*

617 USA ISSN 0039-6109
RD34 CODEN: SCNAA7
SURGICAL CLINICS OF NORTH AMERICA. Text in English. 1912. bi-m. USD 158 domestic to individuals; USD 185 in Canada to individuals; USD 215 elsewhere to individuals; USD 220 domestic to institutions; USD 269 foreign to institutions; USD 104 domestic to students; USD 45 per issue (effective 2001). adv. bibl, illus. index, cum.index every 3 yrs. reprint service avail. from PQC,ISI. *Refereed.* **Document type:** *Journal, Academic/Scholarly.* **Description:** Discusses various surgical techniques and procedures.
Related titles: Microform ed.: (from PQC); Online - full text ed.: (from Institute for Scientific Information); ♦ Spanish Translation: Clinicas Quirurgicas de Norteamerica.
Indexed: AIM, ASCA, Biol.Abstr., CINAHL, Chem.Abstr., Curr.Adv.Ecol.Sci., Curr.Cont., Excerp.Med., Helminthol.Abstr., INIS Atomind., Ind.Med. (1921-), Ind.Sci.Rev., Inpharma, Int.Nurs.Ind., Nutr.Abstr., Pharm.&Out.News, Reac., Sci.Cit.Ind.
—BLDSC (8548.200000), CASDDS, CISTI, GNLM, IDS, ingenta, KNAW. **CCC.**
Published by: W.B. Saunders Co. (Subsidiary of: Harcourt Publishers Ltd.), 11830 Westline Industrial Dr, St Louis, MO 63146. TEL 800-325-4177, http://www.wbsaunders.com. **Subscr. to:** Periodicals Fulfillment, W B Saunders Co, 6277 Sea Harbor Dr, 4th Fl, Orlando, FL 32891-4800.

617 USA ISSN 0930-2794
CODEN: SUREEX
SURGICAL ENDOSCOPY; ultrasound and interventional techniques. Text in English. 1987. m. (in 1 vol., 12 nos./vol.). USD 437.80 in Germany for Print & Online Eds.; USD 481.60 elsewhere for Print & Online Eds.; USD 88.60 newsstand/cover in Germany; USD 132.40 newsstand/cover elsewhere (effective 2001). adv. reprints avail. *Refereed.* **Document type:** *Academic/Scholarly.* **Description:** Represents the surgical aspects of interventional endoscopy, ultrasound and other techniques in the fields of gastroenterology, obstetrics, gynecology, and urology, as well as gastroenterologic, thoracic, traumatic, orthopedic and pediatric surgery.
Related titles: Microform ed.: (from PQC); Online - full text ed.: ISSN 1432-2218 (from EBSCO Publishing, RoweCom Information Quest, Swets Blackwell, Springer LINK, Institute for Scientific Information).
Indexed: ASCA, Biol.Abstr., Curr.Cont., Ergon.Abstr., Ind.Med. (1987-), Inpharma, Reac., Sci.Cit.Ind., Trop.Dis.Bull.
—BLDSC (8548.215000), CISTI, GNLM, IDS, Infotrieve, KNAW. **CCC.**
Published by: Springer-Verlag, Journals (Subsidiary of: BertelsmannSpringer), 175 Fifth Ave, New York, NY 10010. TEL 212-460-1500, FAX 212-473-6272, orders@springer-ny.com, http://www.springer-ny.com. Eds. A Cuschieri, B MacFadyen. R&P Ian Gross. Adv. contact Jay Feinman. **N. American subscr. to:** Journal Fulfillment Services, PO Box 2485, Secaucus, NJ 07096-2485. TEL 800-777-4643, FAX 201-348-4505. **Co-sponsors:** Society of American Gastrointestinal Endoscopic Surgeons; European Association for Endoscopic Surgery.

617.22 616.01 USA ISSN 1096-2964
▼ **SURGICAL INFECTIONS.** Text in English. 2000. q. USD 149 domestic to individuals; USD 199 foreign to individuals; USD 179 domestic to individuals; USD 229 foreign to individuals; USD 237 domestic to institutions; USD 299 foreign to institutions; USD 284 domestic to institutions; USD 346 foreign to institutions (effective 2002). back issues avail.; reprints avail. *Refereed.* **Document type:** *Journal, Academic/Scholarly.* **Description:** Covers all aspects of surgical infections and the latest advances in the development of new pharmaceuticals and new treatment modes.
Related titles: Online - full content ed.: USD 237 to institutions; USD 149 to individuals (effective 2002) (from EBSCO Publishing, O C L C Online Computer Library Center, Inc., Swets Blackwell); Online - full text ed.: (from CatchWord Ltd., RoweCom Information Quest).
—BLDSC (8548.227000), CatchWord. **CCC.**
Published by: Mary Ann Liebert, Inc. Publishers, 2 Madison Ave, Larchmont, NY 10538. TEL 914—834-3100, FAX 914-834-1388, info@liebertpub.com, http://www.liebertpub.com/sur. Ed. Dr. Philip S Barie.

617 616.3 618 USA
CODEN: SLENEY
SURGICAL LAPAROSCOPY, ENDOSCOPY AND PERCUTANEOUS TECHNIQUES. Text in English. 1991. bi-m., latest vol.11. USD 215 to individuals; USD 372 to institutions (effective 2002). adv. charts, illus. reprint service avail. from PQC. *Refereed.* **Document type:** *Journal, Academic/Scholarly.* **Description:** Publishes reports on major developments in laparoscopic and endoscopic techniques and procedures, current clinical and basic science research, patient management, surgical complications, and new developments in instrumentation and technology.
Formerly (until 1999): Surgical Laparoscopy and Endoscopy (1051-7200)
Related titles: Microform ed.: (from PQC); Online - full text ed.: USD 483.60 academic site license; USD 539.40 corporate site license (effective 2002) (from Ovid Technologies, Inc., Institute for Scientific Information).
Indexed: ASCA, Curr.Cont., Excerp.Med. (1992-), Ind.Med. (1993-, dropped), Inpharma, Reac., Sci.Cit.Ind.
—BLDSC, CISTI, EMDOCS, GNLM, IDS.
Published by: Lippincott Williams & Wilkins (Philadelphia) (Subsidiary of: Wolters Kluwer N.V.), 530 Walnut St, Philadelphia, PA 19106-3621. TEL 215-521-8300, FAX 215-521-8902, http://www.surgical-laparoscopy.com, http://www.lww.com. Eds. Carol E.H. Scott Connor, Dr. Maurice E. Arrequi. Pub. Marjorie Spraycar. R&P Margaret Becker. Adv. contact Ray Thibodeau. B&W page USD 955, color page USD 2,035. Circ: 2,222. **Subscr. to:** PO Box 1600, Hagerstown, MD 21740-1600. TEL 800-777-2295, FAX 301-824-7390.

617 IND
SURGICAL MEMOIRS; Biological Memoris. Text in English. s-a. USD 75 (effective 2001). **Document type:** *Academic/Scholarly.*
Published by: H P C Publishers Distributors Pvt. Ltd., 1st Fl., Flats 1 & 2, Darya Ganj, 4805-24 Bharat Ram Rd., New Delhi 110 002, India. FAX 91-11-619-3511, hpcpd@nda.vsnl.net.in, hpcpd@hpc.cc, http://www.hpc.cc, http://www.bizdelhi.com/publisher/hpc.

617 616.8 USA ISSN 0090-3019
RD593 CODEN: SGNRAI
SURGICAL NEUROLOGY. Text in English. 1973. m. EUR 296 in Europe to individuals; JPY 39,200 in Japan to individuals; USD 331 elsewhere to individuals; EUR 605 in Europe to institutions; JPY 80,200 in Japan to institutions; USD 676 elsewhere to institutions (effective 2002). adv. bk.rev. index. reprints avail. *Refereed.* **Document type:** *Academic/Scholarly.* **Description:** Provides neurosurgeons with timely and comprehensive coverage of important clinical and research advances in neurosurgery.
Related titles: Microform ed.: (from PQC); Online - full text ed.: (from ingenta, Swets Blackwell, Institute for Scientific Information, ScienceDirect).
Indexed: ASCA, Bibl.Dev.Med.& Child Neur., Biol.Abstr., Curr.Adv.Cancer Res., Curr.Adv.Ecol.Sci., Curr.Cont., Dent.Ind., Excerp.Med., Helminthol.Abstr., INIS Atomind., Ind.Med. (1973-), Ind.Sci.Rev., Inpharma, Int.Abstr.Biol.Sci., Int.Nurs.Ind., Neurosci.Cit.Ind., Pharm.&Out.News, Reac., Rev.Med.& Vet.Mycol., Sci.Cit.Ind., e-psyche.
—BLDSC (8548.240000), CISTI, GNLM, IDS, ingenta, KNAW. **CCC.**
Published by: Elsevier Science, 655 Ave of the Americas, New York, NY 10010. FAX 212-633-3990, usinfo-f@elsevier.com, http://www.elsevier.nl/locate/issn/00903019. Ed. Dr. James I Ausman. Adv. contact Hank Blaney. B&W page USD 870, color page USD 1,970. Circ: 2,500 (paid). **Subscr. in Australasia and the Far East to:** Elsevier Science (Singapore) Pte Ltd, No.1 Temasek Ave, 17-01 Millenia Tower, Singapore 039192, Singapore. TEL 65-434-3727, FAX 65-337-2230; **Subscr. in Japan to:** Elsevier Science Inc - Japan Regional Office, 9-15 Higashi-Azabu 1-chome, Minato-ku, Tokyo 106-0044, Japan. TEL 81-3-5561-5033; **Subscr. outside the Americas to:** Elsevier Science BV, PO Box 211, Amsterdam 1000 AE, Netherlands. TEL 31-20-485-3757, FAX 31-20-485-3432.

SURGICAL ONCOLOGY CLINICS OF NORTH AMERICA. see *MEDICAL SCIENCES—Oncology*

SURGICAL PATHOLOGY. see *MEDICAL SCIENCES*

617 USA ISSN 1080-6393
SURGICAL PHYSICIAN ASSISTANT. Text in English. 1995. 12/yr. USD 60 to individuals; USD 98 to institutions (effective 2000). adv. illus. **Document type:** *Academic/Scholarly.* **Description:** Provides information on all aspects of surgery, including pre- and post-operative care, sedation, pain management, and surgical techniques.
Published by: Odyssea Publishing, Inc., PO Box 653, Bernardsville, NJ 07924. TEL 732-805-0585, 800-315-1490, FAX 732-805-9582, surgicalpa@aol.com, http://www.surgicalpa.com. Ed. Douglas Condit. Pub., Adv. contact Susan Lusty. R&P Linda Kotrba. 1/2 page USD 2,705; trim 10.75 x 7.875. Circ: 15,000. **Co-sponsors:** Association of Physician Assistants in Cardiovascular Surgery; American Association of Surgical Physician Assistants; Physician Assistants in Orthopaedic Surgery; Association of Neurosurgical Physician Assistants.

617 USA
SURGICAL PRODUCT COMPARISON SYSTEM. Variant title: Healthcare Product Comparison System: Surgical Edition. Text in English. m. USD 561.40 domestic; USD 625.40 in Canada; USD 645 elsewhere (effective 2002). **Document type:** *Trade.* **Description:** Covers ambulatory surgery facilities, from arthroscopes to operating tables.
Related titles: CD-ROM ed.
Published by: (Emergency Care Research Institute), E C R I, 5200 Butler Pike, Plymouth, PA 19462. TEL 610-825-6000, FAX 610-834-1275, info@ecri.org, http://www.ecri.org. Ed. Nanette Bross.

617 CHE ISSN 0882-9233
CODEN: SRCOEZ
SURGICAL RESEARCH COMMUNICATIONS. Text in English. 1986. 4/yr. USD 131 (effective 1999). *Refereed.*
Related titles: CD-ROM ed.; Microform ed.; Online - full text ed.
—CISTI, EMDOCS, GNLM, Infotrieve. **CCC.**
Published by: Gordon and Breach - Harwood Academic (Subsidiary of: Taylor & Francis Group), PO Box 531, Lausanne 1000, Switzerland. http://www.gbhap.com/Surgical_Research_Communications/. Ed. D J Leaper. **Subscr. addr. in US:** International Publishers Direct, PO Box 32160, Newark, NJ 07102. FAX 215-750-6343.

616 USA ISSN 0161-1372
RD1
SURGICAL ROUNDS. Text in English. 1978. m. USD 57 (effective 2000). adv. back issues avail. **Document type:** *Magazine, Trade.* **Description:** Provides timely, practical, well-illustrated, how-to articles of interest to office- and hospital-based surgeons.
Related titles: Microform ed.: (from PQC).
Indexed: CINAHL.
—BLDSC (8548.249000), GNLM, KNAW.
Published by: Romaine Pierson Publishing Co. (Subsidiary of: Medical World Communications), 1065 Old Country Rd, Ste 213, Westbury, NY 11590-5628. TEL 516-883-6350, FAX 516-883-6609. Ed. Dr. Bernard M Jaffe. Pub. Robert Grant. Adv. contact Grace Cass. Circ: 53,530.

617 658 USA ISSN 1079-8269
SURGICAL SERVICES MANAGEMENT. Text in English. 1995. m. USD 35 domestic to members; USD 39.50 domestic to non-members; USD 65 foreign to individuals; USD 6 newsstand/cover domestic; USD 8 newsstand/cover foreign (effective 2000). adv. bk.rev. illus. back issues avail.; reprint service avail. from PQC. *Refereed.* **Document type:** *Academic/Scholarly, Trade.* **Description:** Provides up-to-date information to managers who interact within the surgical services environment.
Related titles: Online - full text ed.: (from Northern Light Technology, Inc., ProQuest Information & Learning).
Indexed: CINAHL.
—Infotrieve. **CCC.**
Published by: Association of periOperative Registered Nurses, Inc., 2170 S Parker Rd, Ste 300, Denver, CO 80231-5711. TEL 303-755-6304, FAX 303-750-3441, ssm@aorn.org, http://www.aorn.org. Ed. Suzanne F Ward. Pub. Warren Kolber. Adv. contact Janet Mongeon. Circ: 14,000. **Subscr. to:** Customer Service, PO Box 3000, Denville, NJ 07834-9807. TEL 973-627-5872.

617 USA ISSN 0164-4238
SURGICAL TECHNOLOGIST. Text in English. 1969. m. USD 36 domestic to non-members; USD 48 foreign to non-members; USD 4 newsstand/cover (effective 2001). adv. bk.rev. illus. **Document type:** *Academic/Scholarly.* **Description:** Emphasis is given to surgical procedures and equipment, legislative-regulatory issues, aseptic techniques and professional development.
Formerly (until 1978): O R Tech
Indexed: CINAHL, Hosp.Lit.Ind.
—BLDSC (8548.259000).
Published by: Association of Surgical Technologists, Inc., 7108 C S Alton Way, Englewood, CO 80112-2106. TEL 303-694-9130, 303-694-9169, ast@ast.org, http://www.ast.ogr. Ed., R&P Kathy Poppen. Pub. William Teutsch. Adv. contact Sheila Vanderpool. B&W page USD 1,396. Circ: 17,371.

617 GBR ISSN 1466-4828
▼ **SURGICAL THEATRE EQUIPMENT AND TECHNNOLOGY (S T E T).** Text in English. 1999. s-a. GBP 60; GBP 67 foreign (effective 2000). adv. illus, tr.lit. back issues avail. *Refereed.* **Document type:** *Directory, Trade.*
Related titles: E-mail ed.; Online - full text ed.
Published by: Ballantyne Ross Ltd., 16 Hampden Gurney St, London W1H 5AL, United Kingdom. TEL 44-1717-245444, FAX 44-1717-242632, info@ballentyneross.com, http://www.balross.com. Pub. Anthony Theodorou. Adv. contact Darren Higham. color page GBP 3,250. Circ: 8,800 (controlled).

617 GBR ISSN 0039-6125
SURGO. Text in English. 1933. 3/yr. GBP 5; GBP 7.50 foreign. adv. bk.rev. bibl, charts, illus. **Document type:** *Academic/Scholarly.*
Published by: University of Glasgow, Medico-Chirurgical Society, University Union, 32 University Ave, Glasgow, Lanarkshire G12 8LX, United Kingdom. 9355031g@student.gla.ac.uk. Ed., R&P Paul Glen. Circ: 1,000.

617 USA
SUTURELINE. Text in English. q. membership. adv.
Published by: American Association of Surgical Physician Assistants, P O Box 867, Bernardsville, NJ 07924. TEL 888-882-2772, FAX 732-805-9582, http://www.aaspa.com. Circ: 500.

617 NOR ISSN 0346-847X
SVENSK KIRURGI. Text in Swedish. 1974; N.S. 1994. 6/yr. GBP 21, USD 35 to institutions (effective 2002). **Document type:** *Academic/Scholarly.*
Published by: Taylor & Francis AS (Subsidiary of: Taylor & Francis Group), Cort Adelersgt. 17, Solli, PO Box 2562, Oslo 0202, Norway. TEL 47-22-12-98-80, FAX 47-22-12-98-90, journals@tandf.no, http://www.tandf.co.uk.tfas. Ed. Martin Bjoerk.

617 CHE ISSN 1023-9332
RD92 CODEN: SWSUFX
SWISS SURGERY/CHIRURGIA SVIZZERA/CHIRURGIE SUISSE/SCHWEIZER CHIRURGIE. Text in English, French, German. 1995. bi-m. CHF 190 domestic; CHF 203 foreign (effective 2001). adv. index. 48 p./no. Supplement avail. *Refereed.* **Document type:** *Journal, Academic/Scholarly.*
Formed by the merger of (1945-1995): Helvetica Chirurgica Acta (0018-0181); (1990-1995): Zeitschrift fuer Unfallchirurgie und Versicherungsmedizin (1017-1584); Which was formerly: Zeitschrift fuer Unfallchirurgie, Versicherungsmedizin und Berufskrankheiten (0254-6310); (until 1982): Zeitschrift fuer Unfallmedizin und Berufskrankheiten (0044-3603); (until 1935): Schweizerische Zeitschrift fuer Unfallmedizin und Berufskrankheiten (0640-3603); (1907-1928): Revue Suisse des Accidents de Travail (1420-2115)
Indexed: Abstr.Hyg., Biol.Abstr., C.I.S. Abstr., Chem.Abstr., Curr.Cont. (coverage dropped), Dent.Ind., Excerp.Med., Helminthol.Abstr., Ind.Med. (1995-), Int.Nurs.Ind., Trop.Dis.Bull.
—BLDSC (8576.790000), CISTI, GNLM, IDS, KNAW. **CCC.**
Published by: (Schweizerische Gesellschaft fuer Traumatologie und Versicherunsmedizin), Hans Huber AG, Laengassstr 76, Bern, 9 3000, Switzerland. TEL 41-31-3004500, FAX 41-31-3004591, zeitschriften@hanshuber.com, http://www.hanshuber.com. Ed. Dr. Adrian Leutenegger. Adv. contact Rene Waelchli. color page CHF 2,852; trim 216 x 303. Circ: 2,000 (controlled). **Co-sponsor:** Schweizerische Gesellschaft fuer Chirurgie.

617.95 USA ISSN 1536-0644
▼ **TECHNIQUES IN FOOT & ANKLE SURGERY.** Text in English. forthcoming 2002. q. USD 99 to individuals; USD 139 to institutions (effective 2002). illus. **Document type:** *Journal, Academic/Scholarly.* **Description:** Contains detailed information on the most innovative and successful surgical techniques for the correction of foot and ankle disorders.
Related titles: Online - full text ed.: USD 180.70 academic site license; USD 201.55 corporate site license (effective 2002).

Published by: Lippincott Williams & Wilkins (Philadelphia) (Subsidiary of: Wolters Kluwer N.V.), 530 Walnut St, Philadelphia, PA 19106-3621. TEL 215-521-8300, FAX 215-521-8902, custserv@lww.com, http://www.lww.com/. Eds. Dr. Bruce E. Cohen, Dr. Robert B. Anderson, Dr. W. Hodges Davis. **Subscr. to:** PO Box 1600, Hagerstown, MD 21740-1600. TEL 800-638-3030, FAX 310-223-2400.

617.57059 USA ISSN 1089-3393

TECHNIQUES IN HAND & UPPER EXTREMITY SURGERY. Text in English. 1997. q., latest vol.5. USD 129 domestic to individuals; USD 129 foreign to individuals; USD 199 per issue domestic to institutions; USD 199 per issue foreign to institutions; USD 47 newsstand/cover (effective 2002); Print & Online eds. combined. adv. **Document type:** *Academic/Scholarly.* **Description:** Presents information on the latest surgical techniques, updates on the newest equipment and progress in therapies for rehabilitation of the hand, shoulder and elbow.

Related titles: Online - full text ed.: USD 258.70 domestic academic site license; USD 258.70 foreign academic site license; USD 288.55 domestic corporate site licens; USD 288.55 foreign corporate site licens (2002).

—BLDSC (8745.101000).

Published by: Lippincott Williams & Wilkins (Philadelphia) (Subsidiary of: Wolters Kluwer N.V.), 530 Walnut St, Philadelphia, PA 19106-3621. TEL 301-223-2300, 800-638-3030, FAX 301-223-2400, http://www.tech-handsurgery.com, http://www.lww.com. Ed. Andrew J Weiland. adv.: B&W page USD 700, color page USD 1,350; trim 10.88 x 8.13. Circ: 738 (paid).

617.95 USA ISSN 1536-0636

▼ **TECHNIQUES IN KNEE SURGERY.** Text in English. forthcoming 2002. q. USD 99 to individuals; USD 139 to institutions (effective 2002). illus. **Document type:** *Journal, Academic/Scholarly.* **Description:** Contains step-by-step details on reconstructive knee surgery techniques and points out the advantages and limitations of new equipment and technology.

Related titles: Online - full text ed.: USD 180.70 academic site license; USD 201.55 corporate site license (effective 2002).

Published by: Lippincott Williams & Wilkins (Philadelphia) (Subsidiary of: Wolters Kluwer N.V.), 530 Walnut St, Philadelphia, PA 19106-3621. TEL 215-521-8300, FAX 215-521-8902, custserv@lww.com, http://www.lww.com/. Eds. Dr. Peter T. Simonian, Dr. Russell E. Windsor, Dr. Thomas L. Wickiewicz. **Subscr. to:** PO Box 1600, Hagerstown, MD 21740-1600. TEL 800-638-3030, FAX 310-223-2400.

617 USA ISSN 1077-2855

TECHNIQUES IN NEUROSURGERY. Text in English. 1995. q., latest vol.7. USD 169 domestic to individuals; USD 169 foreign to individuals; USD 254 per issue domestic to individuals; USD 254 per issue foreign to individuals; USD 58 newsstand/cover (effective 2002). adv. back issues avail. **Document type:** *Academic/Scholarly.* **Description:** Provides complete reviews of neurosurgical procedures, relevant instrumentation and anatomy.

Related titles: Online - full text ed.: USD 330.20 domestic for academic site license; USD 330.20 foreign for academic site license; USD 368.30 foreign for corporate site license; USD 368.30 domestic for corporate site license (effective 2002) (from Institute for Scientific Information).

Indexed: Neurosci.Cit.Ind., e-psyche.

—GNLM, IDS.

Published by: Lippincott Williams & Wilkins (Philadelphia) (Subsidiary of: Wolters Kluwer N.V.), 530 Walnut St, Philadelphia, PA 19106-3621. TEL 215-521-8300, FAX 215-521-8902, www.techs-neurosurgery.com, http://www.lww.com. Eds. Dr. Christopher M Loftus, Dr. H Hunt Batjer. Pub. Marjorie Spraycar. R&P Margaret Becker. Adv. contact Ray Thibodeau. B&W page USD 700, color page USD 1,675. Circ: 860. **Subscr. to:** PO Box 1600, Hagerstown, MD 21740-1600. TEL 800-777-2295, FAX 301-824-7390.

617 USA ISSN 1523-9896

▼ **TECHNIQUES IN SHOULDER AND ELBOW SURGERY.** Text in English. 2000. q. USD 129 domestic to individuals; USD 129 foreign to individuals; USD 199 domestic to institutions; USD 199 foreign to institutions (effective 2002). **Document type:** *Academic/Scholarly.*

Related titles: Online - full text ed.: USD 258.70 domestic for academic site license; USD 258.70 foreign for academic site license; USD 288.55 domestic for corporate site license; USD 288.55 foreign for corporate site license (effective 2002).

—BLDSC (8745.346000).

Published by: Lippincott Williams & Wilkins (Baltimore) (Subsidiary of: Wolters Kluwer N.V.), 12107 Insurance Way, Hagerstown, MD 21740. http://www.shoulderelbowsurgery.com. Ed. Russell F Warren.

617 DEU ISSN 0171-6425
CODEN: TCSUD4

THE THORACIC AND CARDIOVASCULAR SURGEON. Text in English. 1952. bi-m. EUR 257.80 domestic to institutions; EUR 261.80 in Europe to institutions; EUR 272.40 elsewhere to institutions; EUR 50 newsstand/cover (effective 2002). adv. bk.rev. abstr, bibl, charts, illus, stat. index. reprint service avail. from PQC. *Refereed.* **Document type:** *Journal, Academic/Scholarly.*

Formerly (until 1978): Thoraxchirurgie - Vaskulaere Chirurgie (0040-6384)

Related titles: Online - full text ed.: ISSN 1439-1902 (from Institute for Scientific Information).

Indexed: ASCA, Chem.Abstr., Curr.Cont., Excerp.Med., INIS Atomind., Ind.Med. (1979-), Inpharma, Pharm.&Out.News, Reac., Rev.Med.& Vet.Mycol., Sci.Cit.Ind.

—BLDSC (8820.240000), CASDDS, CISTI, GNLM, IDS, Infotrieve, ingenta, KNAW. **CCC.**

Published by: (Deutsche Gesellschaft fuer Thorax-, Herz- und Gefaesschirurgie), Georg Thieme Verlag, Ruedigerstr 14, Stuttgart 70469, Germany. TEL 49-711-8931-0, FAX 49-711-8931298, thoracic@thieme.de, leser.service@thieme.de, http://www.thieme.de/thoracic, http://www.thieme-connect.de. Ed. P Kloevekorn. R&P Alessandra Kreibaum. Circ: 1,600.

TOPICS IN NEUROSURGERY. see *MEDICAL SCIENCES—Psychiatry And Neurology*

TRANSPLANT CHRONICLES. see *MEDICAL SCIENCES—Urology And Nephrology*

617.4 DNK ISSN 1398-2273
CODEN: TIDSFZ

▼ **TRANSPLANT INFECTIOUS DISEASE.** Text in English. 1999. q. USD 252 in the Americas to institutions print & online eds. combined; GBP 175 elsewhere to institutions print & online eds. combined (effective 2002). *Refereed.* **Document type:** *Journal, Academic/Scholarly.* **Description:** Provides a forum for presenting the most current information on the prevention and treatment of infection complicating organ and bone marrow transplantation.

Related titles: ♦ Online - full text ed.: Transplant Infectious Disease Online. ISSN 1399-3062.

—BLDSC (9024.988700).

Published by: (Transplantation Society USA), Blackwell Munksgaard, Noerre Soegade 35, PO Box 2148, Copenhagen K 1016, Denmark. FAX 45-77-33-33-77, fsub@munksgaard.dk, http://journals.munksgaard.dk/transplantinfectious, http://www.muksgaard.dk. Ed. Robert Rubin. Adv. contact Eric Rozario TEL 45-77-33-33-01. Circ: 500 (paid and free).

617.4 DNK ISSN 1399-3062

TRANSPLANT INFECTIOUS DISEASE ONLINE. Text in English. q. GBP 158 (effective 2002). *Refereed.* **Document type:** *Academic/Scholarly.*

Media: Online - full text (from EBSCO Publishing, O C L C Online Computer Library Center, Inc., RoweCom Information Quest, ingenta, Munksgaard & Blackwell Science's Synergy, Swets Blackwell). **Related titles:** ♦ Print ed.: Transplant Infectious Disease. ISSN 1398-2273.

Published by: Blackwell Munksgaard, Noerre Soegade 35, PO Box 2148, Copenhagen K 1016, Denmark. TEL 45-77-33-33-33, FAX 45-77-33-33-77, fsub@mail.munksgaard.dk, http://www.munksgaard.dk.

TRANSPLANT NURSES JOURNAL. see *MEDICAL SCIENCES—Nurses And Nursing*

617 USA ISSN 0041-1337
QP89 CODEN: TRPLAU

TRANSPLANTATION. Text in English. 1963. s-m., latest vol.72. USD 523 domestic to individuals; USD 629 foreign to individuals; USD 832 domestic to institutions; USD 938 foreign to institutions; USD 37 newsstand/cover (effective 2002). adv. bk.rev. illus. index. back issues avail. *Refereed.* **Document type:** *Journal, Academic/Scholarly.* **Description:** Publishes original papers and abstracts from pertinent specialties: immunology, hematology, endocrinology and embryology.

Related titles: Microfilm ed.: (from WWS); Online - full text ed.: USD 1,081.60 domestic for academic site license; USD 1,187.60 foreign for academic site license; USD 1,206.40 domestic for corporate site license; USD 1,312.40 foreign for corporate site license (effective 2002) (from Ovid Technologies, Inc., EBSCO Publishing, Institute for Scientific Information).

Indexed: AIDS & Cancer Res., ASCA, Anim.Breed.Abstr., Biol.Abstr., Chem.Abstr., Chem.Indus.Notes, Curr.Adv.Cancer Res., Curr.Adv.Ecol.Sci., Curr.Cont., Dairy Sci.Abstr., Diab.Cont., Excerp.Med., INIS Atomind., Immun.Abstr., Ind.Med. (1963-), Ind.Sci.Rev., Ind.Vet., Inpharma, Int.Abstr.Biol.Sci., Jrnl.Watch Gastr., Kidney, Med.& Surg.Dermat., Neurosci.Cit.Ind., Pharm.&Out.News, Poult.Abstr., Protozool.Abstr., Reac., Rev.Med.& Vet.Mycol., Risk Abstr., SSCI (coverage dropped), Sci.Cit.Ind., Telegen, Vet.Bull.

—BLDSC (9024.990000), CASDDS, CISTI, GNLM, IDS, ingenta, KNAW, Linda Hall.

Published by: (Transplantation Society), Williams & Wilkins (Subsidiary of: Waverly International), 351 W Camden St, Baltimore, MD 21201-2436. TEL 410-528-4068, 800-222-3790, FAX 410-528-4452, sreed@wwilkins.com, http://www.wwilkins.com. Ed. Dr. A P Monaco. Adv. contact Sherry Reed. Circ: 3,818.

617 USA ISSN 0041-1345
RD120.7 CODEN: TRPPA8

TRANSPLANTATION PROCEEDINGS. Text in English. 1969. 8/yr. EUR 348 in Europe to individuals; JPY 49,455 in Japan to individuals; USD 390 in North America to individuals; USD 371 elsewhere to individuals; EUR 636 in Europe to institutions; JPY 84,500 in Japan to institutions; USD 564 in North America to institutions; USD 668 elsewhere to institutions (effective 2002). adv. bibl, charts, illus. index. back issues avail.; reprints avail. *Refereed.* **Document type:** *Proceedings, Academic/Scholarly.* **Description:** Includes reviews and original reports in current problems in transplantation biology and medicine.

Related titles: Microform ed.: (from PQC); Online - full text ed.: (from EBSCO Publishing, ingenta, Swets Blackwell, Institute for Scientific Information, ScienceDirect).

Indexed: ASCA, Anim.Breed.Abstr., Biol.Abstr., Chem.Abstr., Chem.Titles, Curr.Adv.Cancer Res., Curr.Adv.Ecol.Sci., Curr.Cont., Excerp.Med., INIS Atomind., Ind.Med. (1969-), Ind.Sci.Rev., Ind.Vet., Inpharma, Int.Abstr.Biol.Sci., Int.Nurs.Ind., Med.& Surg.Dermat., Neurosci.Cit.Ind., Pharm.&Out.News, Protozool.Abstr., Reac., Rev.Med.& Vet.Mycol., SSCI (coverage dropped), Sci.Cit.Ind.

—BLDSC (9025.100000), CASDDS, CISTI, GNLM, IDS, ingenta, KNAW. **CCC.**

Published by: (Transplantation Society), Elsevier Science, Box 945, New York, NY 10159-0945. TEL 212-989-5800, 888-437-4636, FAX 212-633-3990, usinfo-f@elsevier.com, http://www.elsevier.com/locate/issn/00411345. Eds. Dr. Felix T Rapaport, J Dausset, P R Casson. Circ: 2,600.

617 USA ISSN 0955-470X

TRANSPLANTATION REVIEWS. Text in English. q. USD 175 domestic to individuals; USD 235 foreign to individuals; USD 234 domestic to institutions; USD 273 foreign to institutions; USD 91 domestic to students; USD 141 foreign to students; USD 69 newsstand/cover (effective 2001). adv. back issues avail. *Refereed.* **Document type:** *Academic/Scholarly.* **Description:** Contains review articles on the latest developments in both clinical and experimental transplantation surgery.

—BLDSC (9025.220000), GNLM, Infotrieve, ingenta, KNAW. **CCC.**

Published by: W.B. Saunders Co. (Subsidiary of: Harcourt Publishers Ltd.), 11830 Westline Industrial Dr, St Louis, MO 63146. TEL 800-325-4177, http://www.wbsaunders.com. Eds. Dr. Nicholas J Tilney, Peter J Morris. adv.: B&W page USD 715, color page USD 1,815; trim 10 x 7. Circ: 663. **Subscr. to:** Periodicals Dept, 6277 Sea Harbor Dr, 4th Fl, Orlando, FL 32891. TEL 800-654-2452, FAX 800-874-6418.

617 DEU ISSN 0946-9648

TRANSPLANTATIONSMEDIZIN. Text and summaries in English, German. 1989. q. DEM 64 domestic; DEM 70 foreign (effective 2001). adv. bk.rev. abstr. *Refereed.* **Document type:** *Journal, Academic/Scholarly.* **Description:** Contains original articles and case reports on transplantation in surgery, immunology, internal medicine, urology, nephrology.

Formerly (until 1994): Zeitschrift fuer Transplantationsmedizin (0935-1965)

Indexed: Excerp.Med. (1994-).

—BLDSC (9025.255000), CISTI, EMDOCS, GNLM, Infotrieve, KNAW. **CCC.**

Published by: (Deutsche Transplantationsgesellschaft), Pabst Science Publishers, Am Eichengrund 28, Lengerich 49525, Germany. TEL 49-5484-308, FAX 49-5484-550, pabst.publishers@t-online.de, http://www.pabst-publishers.de/txmed. Ed. A E Lison. Circ: 1,300.

617.95 RUS
TRANSPLANTOLOGIYA I ISKUSSTVENNYE ORGANY. Text in Russian. irreg. USD 120 in United States. **Document type:** *Journal, Academic/Scholarly, Trade.*
Published by: Assotsiatsiya Medinvest, Shchukinskaya 1, Moscow 123182, Russian Federation. TEL 7-095-1938605. **US dist. addr.:** East View Publications, 3020 Harbor Ln N, Minneapolis, MN 55447. TEL 612-550-0961.

617 ESP ISSN 1134-315X CODEN: TANSE
TRANSPLANTOLOGY; journal of cell and organ transplantation. Text and summaries in Spanish. 1989. q. ESP 7,000; USD 200 foreign (effective 2000). adv. abstr, bibl, illus, stat. back issues avail. *Refereed.* **Document type:** *Academic/Scholarly.*
Formerly (until 1992): Trasplante of Organs and Tissues (0214-820X)
Indexed: Excerp.Med.
—BLDSC (9025.260000), GNLM.
Published by: (Sociedad Espanola de Transplante/Spanish Transplantation Society), Aran Ediciones S.A., Castello, 128 1o, Madrid 28006, Spain. TEL 34-91-782-0030, FAX 34-91-561-5787, edita@grupoaran.com, http://www.grupoaran.com. Ed. V. Cuevas-Mons. Pub. Jose Jimenez. R&P Maria Dolores Linares TEL 34-1-7820035. Circ: 3,000.

617.3 NLD ISSN 0743-6637 CODEN: TRAUEK
TRAUMA QUARTERLY. Text in English. 1984-1993; resumed 1995. q. EUR 99, USD 115 to individuals includes online ed.; EUR 206, USD 239 to institutions includes online ed. (effective 2002). adv. illus. index. back issues avail. *Refereed.* **Document type:** *Journal, Academic/Scholarly.* **Description:** Provides for surgically oriented discussion of clinical care in the trauma care setting.
Related titles: Online - full content ed.: 2000 (from EBSCO Publishing, Swets Blackwell); Online - full text ed.: (from CatchWord Ltd.).
Indexed: CINAHL, Hlth.Ind.
—BLDSC (9026.857300), CASDDS, GNLM, ingenta.
Published by: V S P (Subsidiary of: Brill Academic Publishers), PO Box 346, Zeist 3700 AH, Netherlands. TEL 31-30-692-5790, FAX 31-30-693-2081, vsppub@compuserve.com, http://www.vsppub.com/journals/jn-TraQua.html. Ed. Thomas M. Scalea.

617 JPN ISSN 0917-0197
TRENDS & TOPICS IN TRANSPLANTATION. Text in Japanese. 1992. q.
Published by: Standard McIntyre/Sutandado Makkintaiya, 3-7 Irifune 2-chome, Chuo-ku, Tokyo 104-0042, Japan.

617 TUR ISSN 1300-0705 CODEN: UCDEE
ULUSAL CERRAHI DERGISI/TURKISH JOURNAL OF SURGERY. Text in Turkish. 1985. bi-m. USD 30 (effective 2001). adv. bk.rev. back issues avail. *Refereed.* **Document type:** *Journal, Academic/Scholarly.* **Description:** Publishes research and clinical articles relating to general surgery, including gastrointestinal, endocrine, breast and endoscopic surgery, surgical physiology and surgical oncology.
Indexed: Excerp.Med. (1994-).
—GNLM.
Published by: Turkish Surgical Society, Guzelbahce Sok. 35-7, Nisantasi - Istanbul 80200, Turkey. TEL 90-212-2475295, FAX 90-212-2470835, ctopuzlu@superonline.com. Ed. Dr. Cemalettin Topuzlu. Adv. contact A. S. Eksel. page USD 500. Circ: 1,000 (controlled).

617 ITA ISSN 0014-648X
UNIVERSITA DEGLI STUDI DI PERUGIA. FACOLTA DI MEDICINA E CHIRURGIA. ANNALI. (Includes: Accademia Anatomico Chirurgica. Atti) Text in Italian. 1885. q. ITL 30,000.
Indexed: Apic.Abstr., Chem.Abstr., Excerp.Med., Hort.Abstr.
Published by: Universita degli Studi di Perugia, Facolta di Medicina e Chirurgia, Perugia, PG, Italy. Ed. Giovanni Bolis. Circ: 500.

616 USA ISSN 0042-2835
RD598 CODEN: VASUA9
VASCULAR SURGERY (GLEN HEAD). Text in English. 1967. bi-m., latest vol.35. USD 178 domestic to individuals; USD 198 foreign to individuals; USD 298 domestic to institutions; USD 318 foreign to institutions (effective 2001). adv. 3 cols./p. back issues avail.; reprints avail. *Refereed.* **Document type:** *Journal, Academic/Scholarly.* **Description:** Contains original papers relating to any phase of vascular diseases, operative procedures, clinical or laboratory research and case reports.
Related titles: Online - full text ed.: (from Ovid Technologies, Inc., ProQuest Information & Learning, Institute for Scientific Information).
Indexed: ASCA, Biol.Abstr., Curr.Adv.Cancer Res., Curr.Cont. (coverage dropped), Excerp.Med., Inpharma, Pharm.&Out.News, Reac.
—BLDSC (9148.900000), CISTI, GNLM, ingenta, KNAW.
Published by: Westminster Publications, Inc., 708 Glen Cove Ave, Glen Head, NY 11545. TEL 516-759-0025, FAX 516-759-5524. Ed. D Eugene Strandness. Pub. Timothy R McLaughlin. adv.: B&W page USD 1,050, color page USD 1,035; trim 8.5 x 11. Circ: 4,418.

VASCULAR SURGERY OUTLOOK. see *MEDICAL SCIENCES—Abstracting, Bibliographies, Statistics*

617.95 DEU ISSN 1436-3682
VEREINIGUNG DER DEUTSCHEN PLASTISCHEN CHIRURGEN. ZEITSCHRIFT. Text in German. 1994. s-a. DEM 60 to institutions (effective 2000). **Document type:** *Academic/Scholarly.*
Published by: (Vereinigung der Deutschen Plastischen Chirurgen), Demeter Verlag GmbH und Co. KG, Ruedigerstr 14, Stuttgart 70469, Germany. TEL 49-711-8931-0, FAX 49-711-89311322, custserv@thieme.de, http://www.demeter-verlag.de.

617 RUS ISSN 0042-4625 CODEN: VKHGAG
VESTNIK KHIRURGII IM. I.I. GREKOVA/I.I. GREKOV ANNALS OF SURGERY. Text in Russian; Summaries in English, Russian. 1885. m. RUR 46 (effective 1999). adv. bk.rev. illus. index. back issues avail. *Refereed.* **Document type:** *Abstract/Index.* **Description:** Carries articles touching on various problems of clinical and experimental surgery, anesthesiology and reanimatology.
Related titles: E-mail ed.; Fax ed.; Online - full text ed.
Indexed: Biol.Abstr., Chem.Abstr., Dent.Ind., Dok.Arbeitsmed., Excerp.Med., INIS Atomind., Ind.Med. (1935-), Int.Nurs.Ind., Ref.Zh.
—BLDSC (0036.700000), CISTI, GNLM, IDS, Infotrieve, KNAW. **CCC.**
Published by: Aesculapius, B Zelenina ul 43, St Petersburg 197110, Russian Federation. TEL 7-812-2353009, FAX 7-812-2350986, aeseulapmail.wplus.net, http://www.aeseulap.ru. Ed. F G Uglov. Pub. Catherine Tkalenko. R&P, Adv. contact Alexei Belkin TEL 7-812-235-1719. B&W page USD 600, color page USD 2,000; trim 295 x 210. Circ: 2,000 (paid). **Dist. by:** Mezhdunarodnaya Kniga, B Yakimanka 39, Moscow 117049, Russian Federation. TEL 7-095-2384967, FAX 7-095-2384634; **US dist. addr.:** East View Publications, 3020 Harbor Ln N, Minneapolis, MN 55447. TEL 612-550-0961.

VIDEO JOURNAL OF CATARACT & REFRACTIVE SURGERY. see *MEDICAL SCIENCES—Ophthalmology And Optometry*

617 ESP ISSN 0212-7695
VIDEO REVISTA DE CIRUGIA/VIDEO REVIEW OF SURGERY. Text in English, French, Italian, Spanish. 1984. 6/yr. ESP 22,500 to individuals; ESP 32,000 to institutions. adv. **Document type:** *Trade.*
Media: Video.
Published by: (Asociacion Europea de Video Cirugia), Video Medica S.L., Badal, 102 Bis Loc 1, Barcelona 08014, Spain. TEL 34-3-4319666, FAX 34-3-4219942. Ed. Carlos Ballesta Lopez. Adv. contact G Fourtanier. Circ: 5,000.

617 DEU ISSN 1435-3067 CODEN: VISZFH
VISZERALCHIRURGIE. Text in German; Summaries in English, German. 1966. bi-m. EUR 212.90 domestic to institutions; EUR 219.80 in Europe to institutions; EUR 229.60 elsewhere to institutions; EUR 108 to students; EUR 44 newsstand/cover (effective 2002). adv. bibl, charts, illus, stat. index. reprint service avail. from PQC. **Document type:** *Journal, Academic/Scholarly.*
Formerly (until 1998): Aktuelle Chirurgie (0001-785X)
Related titles: Online - full text ed.: ISSN 1439-1643.
Indexed: Excerp.Med.
—BLDSC (9241.570000), CISTI, EMDOCS, GNLM, Infotrieve. **CCC.**
Published by: Georg Thieme Verlag, Ruedigerstr 14, Stuttgart 70469, Germany. TEL 49-711-8931-0, FAX 49-711-8931298, viszeral@thieme.de, leser.service@thieme.de, http://www.thieme.de/viszeral. Ed. H Becker. Circ: 1,700.

617 USA ISSN 0364-2313 CODEN: WJSUDI
WORLD JOURNAL OF SURGERY. Text in English. 1936. m. USD 661.70 domestic for Print & Online Eds.; USD 608.30 in Germany for Print & Online Eds.; USD 55.40 newsstand/cover foreign (effective 2002). bk.rev. reprint service avail. from ISI. *Refereed.* **Document type:** *Academic/Scholarly.* **Description:** Provides rapid dissemination of new and important information about the science and art of surgery throughout the world.
Supersedes (in 1976): Societe Internationale de Chirurgie. Bulletin (0037-945X); Formerly: Journal International de Chirurgie
Related titles: CD-ROM ed.; Microform ed.: (from PQC); Online - full text ed.: ISSN 1432-2323 (from EBSCO Publishing, RoweCom Information Quest, Swets Blackwell, Springer LINK, Institute for Scientific Information).
Indexed: ASCA, Biol.Abstr., Chem.Abstr., Curr.Cont., Excerp.Med., INIS Atomind., Ind.Med. (1977-), Ind.Sci.Rev., Inpharma, Int.Nurs.Ind., Protozool.Abstr., Reac., SSCI (coverage dropped), Sci.Cit.Ind., Trop.Dis.Bull.
—BLDSC (9356.074300), CASDDS, CISTI, EMDOCS, GNLM, IDS, ingenta, KNAW. **CCC.**
Published by: Springer-Verlag, Journals (Subsidiary of: BertelsmannSpringer), 175 Fifth Ave, New York, NY 10010. TEL 212-460-1500, FAX 212-473-6272, orders@springer-ny.com, http://www.springer-ny.com; http://link.springer.de/link/service/journals/00268/index.htm. Ed. Ronald K Tompkins. R&P Ian Gross. Adv. contact Brian Skepton. **N. American subscr. to:** Journal Fulfillment Services, PO Box 2485, Secaucus, NJ 07096-2485. TEL 800-777-4643, FAX 201-348-4505.

617 USA ISSN 1075-3931
WORLDPLAST; the world journal of plastic surgery. Text in English. 1995. q. USD 165 to individuals; USD 210 to institutions. *Refereed.* **Document type:** *Academic/Scholarly.*
—BLDSC (9360.485000), GNLM.
Published by: Field & Wood, Medical Periodicals, Inc., PO Box 975, Blue Bell, PA 19422. TEL 610-828-4010, FAX 215-482-0226. Ed. Dr. Jose Guerrerosantos.

617.95 DNK ISSN 0908-665X CODEN: XENOFL
XENOTRANSPLANTATION. Text in Danish. 1994. q. USD 348 in the Americas to institutions print & online eds. combined; GBP 242 elsewhere to institutions print & online eds. combined (effective 2002). *Refereed.* **Document type:** *Academic/Scholarly.* **Description:** Reports new findings in the field of organ and tissue transplantation across species barriers.
Related titles: Online - full text ed.: ISSN 1399-3089. GBP 218 (effective 2002) (from Ovid Technologies, Inc., EBSCO Publishing, O C L C Online Computer Library Center, Inc., RoweCom Information Quest, ingenta, Munksgaard & Blackwell Science's Synergy, Swets Blackwell, Institute for Scientific Information).
Indexed: Curr.Cont., Ind.Med. (1994-), Inpharma, Int.Abstr.Biol.Sci., Reac., Sci.Cit.Ind.
—BLDSC (9367.026000), CISTI, GNLM, IDS, Infotrieve, KNAW. **CCC.**
Published by: Blackwell Munksgaard, Noerre Soegade 35, PO Box 2148, Copenhagen K 1016, Denmark. TEL 45-77-33-33-33, FAX 45-77-33-33-77, fsub@munksgaard.dk, http://journals.munksgaard.dk/xenotransplantation, http://www.munksgaard.dk. Ed. David K C Cooper. Adv. contact Eric Rozario TEL 45-77-33-33-01. Circ: 600.

617 USA ISSN 0739-5949
RD559 CODEN: YBHSEQ
THE YEAR BOOK OF HAND SURGERY. Text in English. 1985. a. USD 95 domestic; USD 101 foreign (effective 2001). illus. **Document type:** *Abstract/Index, Academic/Scholarly.* **Description:** Presents abstracts of pertinent literature with commentary by leading experts in the field.
Related titles: CD-ROM ed.
—CISTI, GNLM.
Published by: Mosby, Inc., Continuity Division (Subsidiary of: Harcourt Health Sciences), 11830 Westline Industrial Dr, St Louis, MO 63146-3313. TEL 314-872-8370, 800-325-4177, FAX 314-432-1380, http://www.mosby.com/periodicals. Ed. Dr. Peter C Amadio.

M

THE YEAR BOOK OF NEUROLOGY & NEUROSURGERY. see *MEDICAL SCIENCES—Psychiatry And Neurology*

617.95 USA ISSN 1040-175X
RD118.A1 CODEN: YPRSA
THE YEAR BOOK OF PLASTIC, RECONSTRUCTIVE, AND AESTHETIC SURGERY. Text in English. 1970. a. USD 97 domestic; USD 103 foreign (effective 2001). illus. reprints avail. **Document type:** *Abstract/Index, Academic/Scholarly.* **Description:** Presents abstracts of pertinent literature with commentary by leading experts in the field.
Formerly (until 1989): Year Book of Plastic and Reconstructive Surgery (0084-3962)
Related titles: CD-ROM ed.; Online - full text ed.
—CISTI, GNLM.
Published by: Mosby, Inc., Continuity Division (Subsidiary of: Harcourt Health Sciences), 11830 Westline Industrial Dr, St Louis, MO 63146-3313. TEL 314-872-8370, 800-325-4177, FAX 314-432-1380, http://www.mosby.com/periodicals. Ed. Dr. Stephen Miller.

617.005 USA ISSN 0090-3671
RD9
THE YEAR BOOK OF SURGERY. Text in English. 1901. a. USD 88 domestic; USD 94 foreign (effective 2001). illus. **Document type:** *Abstract/Index, Academic/Scholarly.* **Description:** Presents abstracts of pertinent literature with commentary by leading experts in the field.
Incorporates in part (1933-1970): Year Book of General Surgery (0084-3776)
Related titles: CD-ROM ed.
—BLDSC (9416.450000), CISTI, GNLM.
Published by: Mosby, Inc., Continuity Division (Subsidiary of: Harcourt Health Sciences), 11830 Westline Industrial Dr, St Louis, MO 63146-3313. TEL 314-872-8370, 800-325-4177, FAX 314-432-1380, http://www.mosby.com/periodicals. Ed. Dr. Edward M Copeland III.

THE YEAR BOOK OF VASCULAR SURGERY. see *MEDICAL SCIENCES—Cardiovascular Diseases*

617 NLD
YEARBOOK OF CELL AND TISSUES TRANSPLANTATION (YEARS). Text in Dutch. biennial. **Document type:** *Academic/Scholarly.*
Published by: Kluwer Academic Publishers Group (Subsidiary of: Wolters Kluwer N.V.), Spuiboulevard 50, PO Box 17, Dordrecht 3300 AA, Netherlands. FAX 31-78-639-2254, services@wkap.nl, http://www.wkap.nl. Eds. Robert P Lanza, William L Chick. **Dist. by:** Journals Department, PO Box 322, Dordrecht 3300 AH, Netherlands. FAX 31-78-654-6474.

ZEITSCHRIFT FUER HERZ, THORAX- UND GEFAESSCHIRURGIE. see *MEDICAL SCIENCES—Cardiovascular Diseases*

617 DEU ISSN 0044-409X
CODEN: ZECHAU
ZENTRALBLATT FUER CHIRURGIE. Text in German. 1874. m. EUR 239.80 domestic to institutions; EUR 250.80 in Europe to institutions; EUR 255.30 elsewhere to institutions; EUR 106 to students; EUR 23 newsstand/cover (effective 2002). adv. bk.rev. abstr, charts, illus. index. 80 p./no. back issues avail. *Refereed.* **Document type:** *Journal, Academic/Scholarly.*
Related titles: Microfiche ed.: (from BHP); Online - full text ed.: ISSN 1438-9592; (from Institute for Scientific Information).
Indexed: ASCA, Chem.Abstr., Curr.Cont., Dent.Ind., Excerp.Med., INIS Atomind., Ind.Med. (1903-), Inpharma, Int.Nurs.Ind., Nutr.Abstr., Reac., Rev.Med.& Vet.Mycol.
—BLDSC (9504.700000), CISTI, GNLM, IDS, Infotrieve, KNAW. **CCC.**
Published by: (Vereinigung Mittelrheinischer Chirurgen), Johann Ambrosius Barth Verlag in Medizinverlage Heidelberg GmbH & Co. KG, Ruedigerstr 14, Stuttgart 70469, Germany. TEL 49-711-8931-0, FAX 49-711-8931422, zblchir@medizinverlage.de, kunden.service@thieme.de, http://www.thieme.de/zblchir. Eds. A Encke, E H Farthmann. Adv. contact Irmgard Mayer TEL 49-711-8931469. B&W page DEM 2,700; trim 210 x 280. Circ: 2,000. **Co-sponsors:** Thueringische Gesellschaft fuer Chirurgie; Saechsische Chirurgenvereinigung; Vereinigung der Bayerischen Chirurgen.

617 DEU ISSN 0940-9599
ZENTRALBLATT FUER KINDERCHIRURGIE. Text in German. 1992. q. EUR 134.90 domestic to institutions; EUR 138 in Europe to institutions; EUR 140.80 elsewhere to institutions; EUR 60 to students; EUR 37 newsstand/cover (effective 2002). 40 p./no. **Document type:** *Journal, Academic/Scholarly.*
Related titles: Online - full text ed.: ISSN 1438-9770.
—GNLM.
Published by: (Deutsche Gesellschaft fuer Kinderchirurgie), Johann Ambrosius Barth Verlag in Medizinverlage Heidelberg GmbH & Co. KG, Ruedigerstr 14, Stuttgart 70469, Germany. TEL 49-711-8931-0, FAX 49-711-8931422, zblkichir@medizinverlage.de, kunden.service@thieme.de, http://www.thieme.de/zblkichir. Ed. S Hofmann von Kap-herr. Circ: 900.

ZENTRALBLATT FUER NEUROCHIRURGIE. see *MEDICAL SCIENCES—Psychiatry And Neurology*

617 CHN ISSN 1005-2208
ZHONGGUO SHIYONG WAIKE ZAZHI/CHINESE JOURNAL OF PRACTICAL SURGERY. Text in Chinese; Abstracts in English. 1981. m. CNY 48, USD 60 (effective 1997 & 1998). adv. *Refereed.* **Document type:** *Academic/Scholarly.* **Description:** Features new developments and methods of practical diagnosis, treatment, and prevention of surgical diseases.
Formerly: Shiyong Waike Zazhi - Journal of Practical Surgery (1001-0831)
Published by: Zhongguo Shiyong Yixue Zazhishe/Chinese Journals' Society of Practical Medicine, 44-1, Jixian St, Heping-qu, Shenyang, Liaoning 110005, China. TEL 86-24-3395362, FAX 96-24-3391212. Eds. Qingli Wang, Sanguang He. R&P Qingli Wang. Adv. contact Jianguo Li. page USD 1,500. Circ: 50,000.

617.95 CHN ISSN 1002-1892
CODEN: ZXCZEH
ZHONGGUO XIUFU CHONGJIAN WAIKE ZAZHI/CHINESE JOURNAL OF REPARATIVE AND RECONSTRUCTIVE SURGERY. Text in Chinese; Summaries in English. 1987. bi-m. CNY 45 (effective 2000). illus. 64 p./no. *Refereed.* **Document type:** *Academic/Scholarly.* **Description:** Contains original research articles and clinical reviews on reparative and reconstructive surgery. Also covers new instruments, materials and techniques.
Formerly (until 1991): Xiufu Chongjian Waike Zazhi
Indexed: Ind.Med. (199?-), Ref.Zh.
—BLDSC (3180.674200), GNLM.
Published by: (Xiufu Chongjian Waike Zhuanye Weiyuanhui, Zhongguo Kangfu Yixuehui/Chinese Association of Rehabilitation Medicine), Zhongguo Xiufu Chongjian Waike Zazhi Bianjibu, Huaxi Yike Daxue Fushu Diyi Yiyuan Nei, 37 Guoxue Xiang, Chengdu, Sichuan 610041, China. TEL 86-28-5422431, 86-28-5422432, FAX 86-28-5422432, orthop@public.cd.sc.cn. Ed., Pub. Zhiming Yang. R&P, Adv. contact Jun Yu. Circ: 6,000. **Dist. overseas by:** China International Book Trading Corp, 35 Chegongzhuang Xilu, Haidian District, Beijing 100044, China.

617 CHN ISSN 1007-6948
ZHONGGUO ZHONGXIYI JIEHE WAIKE ZAZHI/CHINESE JOURNAL OF SURGERY OF INTEGRATED TRADITIONAL CHINESE AND WESTERN MEDICINE. Text in Chinese. bi-m. USD 25.20; USD 4.20 newsstand/cover (effective 2001). **Document type:** *Academic/Scholarly.*
Published by: China International Book Trading Corp/Zhongguo Guoji Tushu Maoyi Zonggongsi cibtc@mail.cibtc.com.cn, http://www.cibtc.com.cn. **Dist. by:** 35, Chegongzhuang Xilu, Haidian District, Beijing 100044, China.

617 CHN ISSN 0254-1785
ZHONGHUA QIGUAN YIZHI ZAZHI/CHINESE JOURNAL OF ORGAN TRANSPLANTATION. Text in Chinese. 1980. bi-m. (q. before 2000). CNY 48 domestic; USD 18 foreign; CNY 8 newsstand/cover domestic; USD 4.50 newsstand/cover foreign (effective 2001). **Document type:** *Academic/Scholarly.*
Related titles: Online - full content ed.: (from WanFang Data Corp.).
—BLDSC (3180.463000).
Published by: Zhonghua Yixueyuan (Wuhan Fenhui)/Chinese Medical Association (Wuhan Branch), Hankou Shenglijie #177, Wuhan 430014, China. TEL 86-27-2806143, zhqgyzzz@pubic.wh.hb.cn. Ed. Yong-Shang Zhang. **Dist. by:** China International Book Trading Corp, 35, Chegongzhuang Xilu, Haidian District, Beijing 100044, China. TEL 86-1-68413849, FAX 86-1-68412048, cibtc@mail.cibtc.com.cn, http://www.cibtc.com.cn.

ZHONGHUA SHAOSHANG ZAZHI/CHINESE JOURNAL OF BURNS. see *MEDICAL SCIENCES—Dermatology And Venereology*

ZHONGHUA SHENJING WAIKE ZAZHI/CHINESE JOURNAL OF NEUROSURGERY. see *MEDICAL SCIENCES—Psychiatry And Neurology*

617 CHN ISSN 1005-054X
ZHONGHUA SHOUWAIKE ZAZHI/CHINESE JOURNAL OF HAND SURGERY. Text in Chinese. 1985. q. USD 20.80; USD 5.20 newsstand/cover (effective 2001). **Document type:** *Academic/Scholarly.*
Formerly: Shouwaike Zazhi/ Journal of Hand Surgery (1003-9457)
Published by: Zhonghua Yixuehui Zazhishe, 42 Dongsi Xidajie, Beijing 100710, China. **Dist. by:** China International Book Trading Corp, 35, Chegongzhuang Xilu, Haidian District, Beijing 100044, China. TEL 86-1-68413849, FAX 86-1-68412048, cibtc@mail.cibtc.com.cn, http://www.cibtc.com.cn.

617 CHN ISSN 0529-5815
ZHONGHUA WAIKE ZAZHI/CHINESE JOURNAL OF SURGERY. Text in Chinese. m. CNY 73 domestic; USD 61.20 foreign; CNY 5.10 newsstand/cover domestic; USD 6.10 newsstand/cover foreign (effective 2001). **Document type:** *Academic/Scholarly.*
Related titles: CD-ROM ed.; Online - full content ed.: (from WanFang Data Corp.).
Indexed: ExtraMED, Ind.Med. (1953-).
—BLDSC (3180.680000).
Published by: Zhonghua Yixuehui Zazhishe, 42 Dongsi Xidajie, Beijing 100710, China. TEL 86-1-65273361, cmawk@public.sti.ac.cn. **Dist. by:** China International Book Trading Corp, 35, Chegongzhuang Xilu, Haidian District, Beijing 100044, China. TEL 86-1-68413849, FAX 86-1-68412048, cibtc@mail.cibtc.com.cn, http://www.cibtc.com.cn.

617.95 CHN ISSN 1000-7806
CODEN: ZZSZE9
ZHONGHUA ZHENGXING SHAOSHANG WAIKE ZAZHI/CHINESE JOURNAL OF PLASTIC SURGERY AND BURNS. Text in Chinese; Summaries in English. 1985. bi-m. CNY 48 domestic; USD 34.80 foreign; CNY 8 newsstand/cover domestic; USD 6.80 newsstand/cover foreign (effective 2001). adv. bk.rev. back issues avail. **Document type:** *Academic/Scholarly.*
Related titles: CD-ROM ed.; Online - full content ed.: (from WanFang Data Corp.).
Indexed: ExtraMED, Ind.Med. (coverage dropped).
—GNLM.
Published by: Zhongguo Yixue Kexueyuan, Zhengxing Shaoshang Waike Yanjiusuo, Beijing 100041, China. TEL 86-1-68862233 ext 3029, hexm@cdm.imicams.ac.cn. Ed. Ye-Guang Song. Circ: 6,200. **Dist. overseas by:** China International Book Trading Corp, 35, Chegongzhuang Xilu, Haidian District, Beijing 100044, China. TEL 86-1-68413849, FAX 86-1-68412048, cibtc@mail.cibtc.com.cn, http://www.cibtc.com.cn.

616.89 RUS ISSN 0042-8817
CODEN: ZVNBDJ
ZHURNAL VOPROSY NEIROKHIRURGII IM. N.N. BURDENKO/JOURNAL OF NEUROSURGICAL PROBLEMS. Text in Russian; Summaries in English. 1937. q. USD 108 foreign (effective 2000). adv. bk.rev. index. **Description:** Discusses theoretical, practical and organization problems of modern neurosurgery. Informs of the advances in the treatment of neurosurgical diseases of the central, peripheral and vegetative nervous system.
Indexed: Biol.Abstr., Chem.Abstr., Excerp.Med., Ind.Med. (1977-), Int.Aerosp.Abstr., Ref.Zh.
—CISTI, East View, GNLM.
Published by: Izdatel'stvo Meditsina, Petroverigskii per 6-8, Moscow 101000, Russian Federation. TEL 7-095-9286255, FAX 7-095-9211355, meditsina@iname.com, http://www.medit.ru. Ed. A N Konovalov. Pub. A M Stochik. R&P V Ivannikova. Adv. contact O A Fadeeva TEL 7-095-923-51-40. Circ: 750. **Dist. by:** Mezhdunarodnaya Kniga, B Yakimanka 39, Moscow 117049, Russian Federation. TEL 7-095-2384967, FAX 7-095-2384634.

M

MEDICAL SCIENCES—Urology And Nephrology

616.6 USA ISSN 1088-7350
A U A NEWS. Text in English. 1987. 8/yr., latest vol.6. USD 86 domestic to individuals; USD 112 foreign to individuals; USD 107 domestic to institutions; USD 133 foreign to institutions (effective 2002). adv. **Document type:** *Trade.* **Description:** Issues news and developments in urology, including clinical information, case studies, and reports on economic policies and legislation.
Formerly (until 1996): A U A Today (1046-1051)
Published by: (American Urological Association), Williams & Wilkins, Newsletters (Subsidiary of: Waverly International), 351 W Camden St, Baltimore, MD 21201-2436. TEL 410-528-4068, 800-222-3790, FAX 410-528-4452, kmalamphy@wilkins.com, http://www.wwilkins.com. Ed. Debbie Polly. Adv. contact Kathleen Malamphy. Circ: 11,189.

666 CAN
A U A PATIENT MANAGEMENT PROGRAM. Text in English. q. USD 279 to non-members; USD 249 to members (effective 2000). **Document type:** *Academic/Scholarly.* **Description:** Interactive series of programs dealing with all aspects of urological problems. Offers 5 category 1 AMA credits, for a total of 20 per volume.
Media: CD-ROM. **Related titles:** Diskette ed.
Published by: B.C. Decker, LCD 1, P O Box 620, Hamilton, ON L8N 3K7, Canada. TEL 905-522-7017, 800-568-7281, FAX 905-522-7839, info@bcdecker.com. Ed. George Drach.

616.6 BEL ISSN 0001-7183
CODEN: AUBEAN
ACTA UROLOGICA BELGICA. Text in English, French. 1927. 4/yr. BEF 3,100; BEF 4,200 foreign (effective 1999). adv. bk.rev. abstr, bibl, charts, illus. index. **Document type:** *Academic/Scholarly.*
Indexed: Biol.Abstr., Chem.Abstr., Excerp.Med., INIS Atomind., Ind.Med. (1955-).
—BLDSC (0670.415000), CISTI, GNLM, KNAW.
Published by: (Association des Societes Scientifiques Medicales Belges/Vereiniging van de Belgische Wetenschappelijke Genootschappen), Acta Medica Belgica, Av Circulaire 138A, Brussels 1180, Belgium. TEL 32-2-374-5158, FAX 32-2-3749628, amb@skynet.be, http://www.ulb.ac.be/medecine/loce/amb.htm. Ed. Ch Bouffioux.

616.6 JPN ISSN 0018-1994
CODEN: HIKYAJ
ACTA UROLOGICA JAPONICA/HINYOKIKA KIYO. Text in Japanese; Summaries in English. 1955. m. JPY 10,000, USD 50. adv. index.
Indexed: Biol.Abstr., Excerp.Med., INIS Atomind., Ind.Med. (1955-), Inpharma, Reac., Ref.Zh.
—BLDSC (0670.420000), CISTI, EMDOCS, GNLM, KNAW.
Published by: Kyoto University, Faculty Of Medicine, Department of Urology/Kyoto Daigaku Igakubu Hinyokikagaku Kyoshitsu, 54 Shogoin Kawara-cho, Sakyo-ku, Kyoto 606-8397, Japan. TEL 81-75-751-3326, FAX 81-75-761-3441. Ed. Osamu Yoshida. Circ: 2,500.

616.6 FRA ISSN 0073-3326
ACTUALITES NEPHROLOGIQUES. Text in French. 1960. a. price varies. cum.index: 1960-69.
Indexed: Chem.Abstr., Excerp.Med.
—**CCC.**
Published by: (Hopital Necker, Clinique Nephrologique), Flammarion Medecine Sciences, 4 rue Casimir Delavigne, Paris 75006, France. Ed. J P Grunfeld. **U.S. subscr. address:** S.F.P.A., c/o Mr Benech, 14 E 60th St, New York, NY 10022.

616.6 USA
CODEN: ANGYBQ
ADVANCES IN NEPHROLOGY. Text in English. 1971. a. USD 96 domestic; USD 102 foreign (effective 2001). reprint service avail. from PQC. **Document type:** *Academic/Scholarly.* **Description:** Presents original topical review articles of importance in nephrology.
Formerly: Advances in Nephrology from the Necker Hospital (0084-5957)
Related titles: Microfilm ed.: (from PQC).
Indexed: Biol.Abstr., Chem.Abstr., Chem.Indus.Notes, Chem.Titles, Ind.Med. (1971-), e-psyche.
—BLDSC (0709.470000), CASDDS, CISTI, GNLM, ingenta, KNAW.
Published by: Mosby, Inc. (Subsidiary of: Elsevier Science), 11830 Westline Industrial Dr, St Louis, MO 63146-3313. TEL 314-872-8370, 800-325-4177, FAX 314-432-1380. Ed. Dr. Jean Pierre Grunfeld.

616.6 617 USA ISSN 1073-4449
ADVANCES IN RENAL REPLACEMENT THERAPY. Text in English. 1994. q. USD 144 domestic to individuals; USD 177 foreign to individuals; USD 174 domestic to institutions; USD 211 foreign to institutions; USD 103 domestic to students; USD 126 foreign to students; USD 53 newsstand/cover (effective 2001). adv. reprints avail. **Document type:** *Journal, Academic/Scholarly.* **Description:** Reports on advancements in the treatment and care of patients with kidney failure. Contains material also of interest to medical technicians, nurses, and social workers.
Related titles: Online - full text ed.: (from EBSCO Publishing, Institute for Scientific Information).
Indexed: CINAHL, Curr.Cont., Excerp.Med. (1996-), Ind.Med. (1994-), Int.Nurs.Ind.
—BLDSC (0711.318000), EMDOCS, GNLM, IDS, Infotrieve, KNAW. **CCC.**
Published by: (National Kidney Foundation), W.B. Saunders Co. (Subsidiary of: Harcourt Publishers Ltd.), 11830 Westline Industrial Dr, St Louis, MO 63146. TEL 800-325-4177, http://www.wbsaunders.com. Ed. James F Winchester. adv.: B&W page USD 695, color page USD 1,775; trim 10 x 7. Circ: 2,669. **Subscr. to:** Periodicals Fulfillment, W B Saunders Co, 6277 Sea Harbor Dr, 4th Fl, Orlando, FL 32891-4800.

ADVANCES IN REPRODUCTIVE HEALTH CARE. see *MEDICAL SCIENCES—Obstetrics And Gynecology*

616.6 DEU ISSN 1435-1080
CODEN: TWUNE
AERZTLICHE PRAXIS. UROLOGIE, NEPHROLOGIE. Short title: Ae P Urologie, Nephrologie. Text in German. 1989. 6/yr. DEM 89 domestic; DEM 112 foreign; DEM 44.50 domestic to students; DEM 56 foreign to students (effective 2001). adv. **Document type:** *Journal, Trade.*
Former titles (until 1998): Therapie und Erfolg. Urologie, Nephrologie (1435-1072); (until 1997): Therapie Woche - Urologie, Nephrologie (0936-2002)
Indexed: Excerp.Med.
—EMDOCS, GNLM, KNAW.
Published by: Reed Elsevier Deutschland GmbH (Subsidiary of: Reed Elsevier group), Gabrielenstr 9, Munich 80636, Germany. TEL 49-89-89817162, FAX 49-89-89817400, aep-anzeigen@r-e.de, http://aep.r-e.de. Ed. Hans Juergen Kuntze. Pub. Wolfram Haase. Adv. contact Andrea Kroneck.

616.6 DEU ISSN 0001-7868
CODEN: ZURNAV
AKTUELLE UROLOGIE. Text in German; Summaries in English, German. 1970. 7/yr. EUR 248.80 domestic to institutions; EUR 258.80 in Europe to institutions; EUR 281.80 elsewhere to institutions; EUR 118 to students; EUR 46 newsstand/cover (effective 2002). adv. bk.rev. abstr, bibl, charts, illus, stat. index. reprint service avail. from PQC. *Refereed.* **Document type:** *Journal, Academic/Scholarly.*
Incorporates (1907-1991): Zeitschrift fuer Urologie und Nephrologie (0044-3611)
Related titles: Online - full text ed.: ISSN 1438-8820 (from Institute for Scientific Information).
Indexed: ASCA, Biol.Abstr., Chem.Abstr., Curr.Adv.Cancer Res., Curr.Cont., Excerp.Med. (until 1992), INIS Atomind., Ind.Med. (coverage dropped), Inpharma, Reac., Sci.Cit.Ind. (coverage dropped).
—BLDSC (0785.887000), CASDDS, CISTI, GNLM, IDS, Infotrieve. **CCC.**
Published by: Georg Thieme Verlag, Ruedigerstr 14, Stuttgart 70469, Germany. TEL 49-711-8931-0, FAX 49-711-8931298, aktuelle-urologie@thieme.de, leser.service@thieme.de, http://www.thieme.de/uro/index.html. Ed. J Thueroff. R&P Alessandra Kreibaum. Circ: 2,700.

616.6 USA ISSN 0272-6386
CODEN: AJKDDP
AMERICAN JOURNAL OF KIDNEY DISEASES. Text in English. 1981 (Jul.). m. USD 298 domestic to individuals; USD 484 foreign to individuals; USD 497 domestic to institutions; USD 565 foreign to institutions; USD 175 domestic to students; USD 231 foreign to students; USD 48 newsstand/cover (effective 2001). adv. bk.rev. abstr. index. *Refereed.* **Document type:** *Journal, Academic/Scholarly.* **Description:** Official journal of the NKF includes research papers, position papers and proceedings of National Kidney Foundation scientific symposia.
Related titles: Online - full text ed.: (from HighWire Pr., EBSCO Publishing, IDEAL Online Library, Institute for Scientific Information).
Indexed: ASCA, Abstr.Inter.Med., CINAHL, Chem.Abstr., Chem.Indus.Notes, Chem.Titles, Curr.Adv.Ecol.Sci., Curr.Cont., Excerp.Med., INIS Atomind., Ind.Med. (1981-), Ind.Sci.Rev., Inpharma, Int.Nurs.Ind., Kidney, Nutr.Abstr., Pharm.&Out.News, Reac., Rev.Arom.& Med.Plants, Rev.Med.& Vet.Mycol., SSCI (coverage dropped), Sci.Cit.Ind., So.Pac.Per.Ind., THA.
—BLDSC (0826.860000), CASDDS, CISTI, EMDOCS, GNLM, IDS, ingenta, KNAW. **CCC.**
Published by: (National Kidney Foundation), W.B. Saunders Co. (Subsidiary of: Harcourt Publishers Ltd.), 11830 Westline Industrial Dr, St Louis, MO 63146. TEL 800-325-4177, http://www.ajkd.org, http://www.wbsaunders.com. Ed. Neil A Kurtzmann. Adv. contact Valerie Marvin. B&W page USD 1,050, color page USD 2,250; trim 10 x 7. Circ: 6,868. **Subscr. to:** Periodicals Fulfillment, W B Saunders Co, 6277 Sea Harbor Dr, 4th Fl, Orlando, FL 32891-4800.

616.6 CHE ISSN 0250-8095
CODEN: AJNED9
AMERICAN JOURNAL OF NEPHROLOGY. Text in English. 1981. 6/yr. CHF 1,180, EUR 842.80 in Europe to institutions; CHF 1,197.40, USD 916 overseas to institutions (effective 2002). adv. illus. index. back issues avail. *Refereed.* **Document type:** *Journal, Academic/Scholarly.* **Description:** Aims to provide the clinical care of adult and pediatric nephrology patients. The editorial scope ranges from studies on the biochemistry and immunology of kidney diseases to new knowledge on such established clinical problems as dialysis, transplantation, and hypertension.
Related titles: Microform ed.: (from PQC); Online - full text ed.: ISSN 1421-9670. CHF 58, EUR 42, USD 45 with print edition (effective 2002) (from Northern Light Technology, Inc., EBSCO Publishing, O C L C Online Computer Library Center, Inc., RoweCom Information Quest, ProQuest Information & Learning, Swets Blackwell, Institute for Scientific Information).
Indexed: ASCA, Biol.Abstr., Chem.Abstr., Curr.Adv.Ecol.Sci., Curr.Cont., Dent.Ind., Derwent Biotech.Abstr., Excerp.Med., Ind.Med. (1981-), Ind.Sci.Rev., Inpharma, Kidney, Nutr.Abstr., Pharm.&Out.News, Protozool.Abstr., Reac., Rev.Appl.Entomol., Rev.Arom.& Med.Plants, Rev.Med.& Vet.Mycol., SSCI (coverage dropped), Sci.Cit.Ind.
—BLDSC (0828.370000), CASDDS, CISTI, EMDOCS, GNLM, IDS, ingenta, KNAW. **CCC.**
Published by: S. Karger AG, Allschwilerstr 10, PO Box, Basel 4009, Switzerland. TEL 41-61-306-1111, FAX 41-61-306-1234, karger@karger.ch, http://www.online.karger.com/journals/ajn. Ed. S G Massry. adv.: page USD 1,205. Circ: 2,900.

AMERICAN JOURNAL OF PHYSIOLOGY: RENAL PHYSIOLOGY. see *BIOLOGY—Physiology*

616.6 USA
AMERICAN KIDNEY FUND. ANNUAL REPORT. Text in English. 1971. a. free per issue. **Document type:** *Corporate.*
Published by: American Kidney Fund, 6110 Executive Blvd, Ste 1010, Rockville, MD 20852-3903. TEL 301-881-3052, FAX 301-881-0898, permann@akfinc.org, http://www.akfinc.org. Ed. Phylis Ermann. R&P Anna Monsef. Circ: 3,000.

616.6 USA ISSN 1046-6673
CODEN: JASNEU
AMERICAN SOCIETY OF NEPHROLOGY. JOURNAL. Abbreviated title: J A S N. Text in English. 1990. m. USD 413 domestic to individuals for print & online eds.; USD 496 foreign to individuals for print & online eds; USD 567 domestic to institutions for print & online eds; USD 650 foreign to institutions for print & online eds; USD 50 newsstand/cover (effective 2002). adv. abstr. back issues avail. *Refereed.* **Document type:** *Academic/Scholarly.* **Description:** Contains original articles for nephrologists and other specialists who study kidney function and renal diseases.
Related titles: Microfilm ed.: (from WWS); Online - full text ed.: USD 737.10 domestic academic site license; USD 820.10 foreign academic site license; USD 822.15 domestic corporate site license; USD 905.15 foreign corporate site license (effective 2002) (from HighWire Pr., EBSCO Publishing, Institute for Scientific Information).
Indexed: ASCA, Chem.Abstr., Chem.Indus.Notes, Chem.Titles, Curr.Cont., Excerp.Med. (1995-), Ind.Med. (1990-), Ind.Sci.Rev., Inpharma, Kidney, Nutr.Abstr., Pharm.&Out.News, Reac., Rev.Appl.Entomol., SSCI (coverage dropped), Sci.Cit.Ind., Soyabean Abstr.
—BLDSC (4693.005000), CASDDS, CISTI, GNLM, IDS, ingenta, KNAW.

Published by: (American Society of Nephrology), Williams & Wilkins (Subsidiary of: Waverly International), 351 W Camden St, Baltimore, MD 21201-2436. TEL 410-528-4068, 800-222-3790, FAX 410-528-4452, sreed@wwilkins.com, http://www.jasn.org/, http://www.Lww.com. Ed. Dr. C Craig Fisher. Adv. contact Sherry Reed. B&W page USD 1,020; trim 10.88 x 8.13. Circ: 7,390; 7,133 (paid).

616.6 FRA ISSN 0003-4401 CODEN: AUROAV

ANNALES D'UROLOGIE. Text in French; Summaries in English. 1967. 6/yr. EUR 294 in Europe to institutions; USD 380 elsewhere to institutions (effective 2002). bk.rev. *Refereed.* **Document type:** *Academic/Scholarly.*

Related titles: Online - full text ed.: (from Institute for Scientific Information).

Indexed: ASCA, Biol.Abstr., Curr.Cont., Excerp.Med., Helminthol.Abstr., Ind.Med. (1969-), Ind.Sci.Rev., Inpharma, Pharm.&Out.News, Reac., Rev.Med.& Vet.Mycol., Sci.Cit.Ind. (coverage dropped).

—BLDSC (1003.500000), CASDDS, CISTI, EMDOCS, GNLM, IDS, Infotrieve, KNAW. **CCC.**

Published by: (Semaine des Hopitaux), Elsevier Paris, Editions Scientifiques et Medicales (Subsidiary of: Reed Elsevier plc. group), 23 rue Linois, Paris 75015, France. http://www.elsevier.com/locate/anuro. Circ: 3,900.

616.6 JPN

ANNUAL REVIEW JINZO/ANNUAL REVIEW. KIDNEY. Text in Japanese. 1988. a. JPY 8,925 (effective 1998). adv. **Document type:** *Academic/Scholarly.*

Published by: Chugai Igakusha, 62 Yarai-cho, Shinjuku-ku, Tokyo 162-0805, Japan. R&P M Takahashi. Adv. contact M. Takahashi.

616.6 ITA

ARCHIVIO ITALIANO DI UROLOGIA E ANDROLOGIA. Text in English, Italian; Summaries in English. 1924. 5/yr. ITL 98,000 (effective 1999). bk.rev. charts, illus. back issues avail. **Document type:** *Proceedings, Academic/Scholarly.*

Former titles: Archivio Italiano di Urologia e Nefrologia, Andrologia (1120-8538); Archivio Italiano di Dermatologia, Sifilografia, Venereologia e Sessuologia; Archivio Italiano di Urologia e Nefrologia (0004-0460)

Indexed: Biol.Abstr., Excerp.Med., Ind.Med. (coverage dropped).

—BLDSC (1647.510000), CISTI, EMDOCS, GNLM, KNAW.

Published by: (Universita di Milano), Masson S.p.A., Divisione Periodici, Via F.lli Bressan 2, Milan, MI 20126, Italy. TEL 39-2-270741, FAX 39-2-27074210. Ed. P Pegoraro. adv.: B&W page ITL 2,400,000, color page ITL 3,450,000; trim 240 x 170. Circ: 2,500. **Co-sponsor:** Societa Italiana di Ecografia Urologica e Nefrologica.

616.6 ESP ISSN 0004-0614 CODEN: AEURAB

ARCHIVOS ESPANOLES DE UROLOGIA. Text in Spanish; Summaries in English. 1944. m. ESP 14,000 to individuals; ESP 19,000 to institutions; USD 160 in Europe; USD 165 elsewhere (effective 2001). adv. bk.rev. bibl, charts, illus, stat, tr.lit. index. back issues avail.; reprints avail. *Refereed.* **Document type:** *Academic/Scholarly.* **Description:** Includes original research and clinical case studies.

Related titles: Online - full text ed.

Indexed: Biol.Abstr., Chem.Abstr., Excerp.Med., Ind.Med. (1944-), Ind.Med.Esp., Ref.Zh.

—BLDSC (1654.960000), CASDDS, CISTI, GNLM, Infotrieve, KNAW. **CCC.**

Published by: Iniestares S.A., 3o Pta. 4, San Gregorio, 8, Madrid 28004, Spain. TEL 34-91-9196001, FAX 34-91-9197768, urologia@arch-espanoles-de-urologia.es, http://www.arch_espanoles_de_urologia.es, http://www.arch-espanoles-de-urologia.es. Ed. Dr. E Perez Castro Ellendt. Adv. contact Concha Martin. Circ: 1,500.

616.6 YUG ISSN 0354-7760

ARCHIVUM UROLOGICUM. Text in English, Serbian. 1974. q. YUN 600; EUR 100 foreign. adv. bk.rev. back issues avail. *Refereed.* **Document type:** *Academic/Scholarly.* **Description:** Covers urology, nephrology and surgery.

Formerly: Uroloski Arhiv (0351-093X)

Published by: Uroloska Klinika, Univerzetskog Klinickog Centra, Gen Zdanova 51, Belgrade 1000, Yugoslavia. TEL 381-11-656277, FAX 381-11-659460, savamira@eunet.yu. Ed. Sava Micic. R&P G. Arizanovic. Adv. contact G Arizanovic. B&W page XEU 500, color page XEU 1,500. Circ: 500.

616.6 USA ISSN 1063-5777

ATLAS OF THE UROLOGIC CLINICS OF NORTH AMERICA. Text in English. 1993. s-a. USD 143 domestic; USD 183 foreign; USD 92 per issue (effective 2001). illus. back issues avail. **Document type:** *Journal, Academic/Scholarly.* **Description:** Contains line drawings and photographs, along with articles, on a specific urologic surgical technique or problem.

Related titles: Microform ed.: (from PQC).

—BLDSC (1767.087500).

Published by: W.B. Saunders Co. (Subsidiary of: Harcourt Publishers Ltd.), 11830 Westline Industrial Dr, St Louis, MO 63146. TEL 800-325-4177, http://www.wbsaunders.com. Ed. Dr. Martin I Resnick. **Subscr. to:** Periodicals Fulfillment, W B Saunders Co, 6277 Sea Harbor Dr, 4th Fl, Orlando, FL 32891-4800.

616.6 USA ISSN 0271-1338

AUDIO-DIGEST UROLOGY. Text in English. 1978. m. USD 84 (effective 2000). *Refereed.*

Media: Audio cassette/tape.

Published by: Audio-Digest Foundation (Subsidiary of: California Medical Association), 1577 E Chevy Chase Dr, Glendale, CA 91206. TEL 213-245-8505, 800-423-2308, FAX 818-240-7379, 800-845-4375. Ed. Claron L Oakley. Circ: (controlled).

616.6 615.82 AUS ISSN 1324-2989

AUSTRALIAN CONTINENCE JOURNAL. Text in English. 1995. q. AUD 60.

Published by: Continence Foundation of Australia, 293 Royal Parade, Parkville, VIC 3052, Australia. TEL 03-93472522, FAX 03-93472533, info@contfound.org.au, http://www.contfound.org.au. Ed. Dr. Kate Moore. Pub. Gary Davidson. Circ: 2,000.

616.6 GBR ISSN 1464-4096 CODEN: BJURAN

B J U INTERNATIONAL. (British Journal of Urology) Text in English. 1929. 18/yr., latest vol.89, 2002. GBP 109 in Europe to individuals; USD 175 in North America to individuals; GBP 119 elsewhere to individuals; GBP 295 in Europe to institutions; USD 466 in North America to institutions; GBP 323 elsewhere to institutions (effective 2002). adv. bk.rev. abstr, bibl, illus. index, cum.index. back issues avail. *Refereed.* **Document type:** *Journal, Academic/Scholarly.* **Description:** Presents coverage of contemporary urological opinion, clinical reports and studies, innovations and developments.

Formerly (until 1999): British Journal of Urology (0007-1331)

Related titles: Microform ed.: (from PQC); Online - full text ed.: ISSN 1464-410X. GBP 99 in Europe to individuals; USD 158 in North America to individuals; GBP 99 elsewhere to individuals; GBP 266 in Europe to institutions; USD 420 in North America to institutions; GBP 266 elsewhere to institutions (effective 2002) (from Ovid Technologies, Inc., EBSCO Publishing, O C L C Online Computer Library Center, Inc., RoweCom Information Quest, ingenta, Munksgaard & Blackwell Science's Synergy, Swets Blackwell, Institute for Scientific Information); ♦ Supplement: B J U International. Supplement. ISSN 1465-5101.

Indexed: ASCA, Biol.Abstr., Chem.Abstr., Chem.Indus.Notes, Chem.Titles, Curr.Adv.Cancer Res., Curr.Adv.Ecol.Sci., Curr.Cont., Environ.Sci.Poll.Mgmt., Excerp.Med., Helminthol.Abstr., INIS Atomind., Ind.Med. (1999-), Ind.Sci.Rev., Ind.Vet., Inpharma, Int.Abstr.Biol.Sci., Int.Nurs.Ind., Microbiol.Abstr., NRN, Neurosci.Cit.Ind., Nutr.Abstr., Pharm.&Out.News, Reac., Rev.Med.& Vet.Mycol., Rev.Plant Path., SSCI (coverage dropped), Sci.Cit.Ind., Small Anim.Abstr., THA, Triticale Abstr., Trop.Dis.Bull.

—BLDSC (2105.758000), ADONIS, CASDDS, CISTI, EMDOCS, GNLM, IDS, ingenta, KNAW. **CCC.**

Published by: (British Association of Urological Surgeons), Blackwell Science Ltd., PO Box 88, Oxford OX2 0NE, United Kingdom. TEL 44-1865-206180, 44-1865-206002, FAX 44-1865-206219, jnl.orders@blacksci.co.uk, http://www.blackwell-science.com/products/journals/bju.htm, http://www.blackwellpublishing.com. Ed. H Whitfield. Pub. Allen Stevens. R&P Sophie Savage. Adv. contact Jenny Applin. Circ: 4,560. **Co-sponsor:** European Society of Paediatric Urology.

616.6 GBR ISSN 1465-5101

B J U INTERNATIONAL. SUPPLEMENT. Text in English. **Document type:** *Journal, Academic/Scholarly.*

Related titles: Online - full text ed.: (from Ovid Technologies, Inc.); ♦ Supplement to: B J U International. ISSN 1464-4096.

—ADONIS.

Published by: Blackwell Science Ltd., Osney Mead, Oxford OX2 0EL, United Kingdom. TEL 44-1865-206206, FAX 44-1865-721205, journals.cs@blacksci.co.uk, http://www.blackwell-science.com/.

616.6 CAN

BLADDERTALK. Text in English. 1992. q. CND 35; USD 35 foreign. **Document type:** *Newsletter.* **Description:** Features testimonials by patients, research information, news from urology conferences, coping tips, information on pharmaceuticals.

Formerly (until Sep. 1996): Helpline

Published by: Canadian Interstitial Cystitis Society, 406 S Willingdon Ave, P O Box 28625, Burnaby, BC V5C 6J4, Canada. TEL 250-758-4894, FAX 250-758-3207, smcnical@pacificcoast.net. Circ: 1,000.

616.6 GBR ISSN 1365-5604

BRITISH JOURNAL OF RENAL MEDICINE. Abbreviated title: B J R M. Text in English. 1996. q. bk.rev. **Document type:** *Academic/Scholarly.*

—BLDSC (2324.250000).

Published by: Hayward Medical Communications Ltd., Covent Garden, Seven Dials Warehouse, 44 Earlham St, London WC2H 9LA, United Kingdom. TEL 44-20-7240-4493, FAX 44-20-7240-4479, admin@hayward.co.uk, http://wwww.hayward.co.uk, http://www.ejpc.co.uk. Ed. Dr. John Bradley. Circ: 2,000. **Subscr. to:** Rosemary House, Lanwades Park, Kentford, Near, Newmarket, Suffolk CB8 7PW, United Kingdom. TEL 44-1638-751515, FAX 44-1638-751517.

C A N N T JOURNAL. see *MEDICAL SCIENCES—Nurses And Nursing*

616.6 USA

C N N T NEWSLETTER. Text in English. q. free per issue. *Refereed.* **Document type:** *Newsletter.* **Description:** Includes technological, legislative, medical, and education-related articles of interest to nephrology nurses and technicians.

Formerly: Renal Nursing and Technology Today

Published by: National Kidney Foundation, Council of Nephrology Nurses & Technicians, 30 East 33rd St, New York, NY 10016. TEL 212-889-2210, FAX 212-689-9261, http://www.kidney.org. Circ: 700.

616.6 USA

C R N NEWS AND BRIEFS NEWSLETTER. Text in English. q. **Document type:** *Newsletter.* **Description:** Includes a calendar of events, regional news, legislative updates, committee/project updates and educational resources.

Published by: National Kidney Foundation, 30 East 33rd St, New York, NY 10016. TEL 212-889-2210, http://www.kidney.org. Circ: 2,000.

616.6 CAN ISSN 1195-9479

CANADIAN JOURNAL OF UROLOGY. Text in English. 1994. bi-m. CND 140 to individuals; USD 200 foreign to individuals; CND 280 to institutions; USD 380 foreign to institutions (effective 2001). adv. charts, abstr, bibl. *Refereed.* **Document type:** *Journal, Academic/Scholarly.*

Indexed: Ind.Med.

—BLDSC (3036.600000).

Address: 2330 Ward St. Ste. 604, St. Laurent, PQ H4M 2V6, Canada. TEL 514-744-1184, FAX 514-744-1138. Ed. Dr. Laurence H Klotz. adv.: B&W page CND 1,925, color page CND 3,255.

616.6 JPN ISSN 1342-1751 CODEN: CENPFV

CLINICAL AND EXPERIMENTAL NEPHROLOGY. Text in English. 1997. q. (in 1 vol., 4 nos./vol.). EUR 190 domestic for Print & Online Eds.; EUR 186.80 in Germany for Print & Online Eds; EUR 51 newsstand/cover foreign for Print & Online Eds (effective 2002). *Refereed.* **Document type:** *Journal, Academic/Scholarly.* **Description:** Covers the biology, physiology of the kidney, and the basic & clinical science of kidney diseases.

Related titles: ♦ Online - full text ed.: Clinical and Experimental Nephrology Online. ISSN 1437-7799.

—BLDSC (3286.251550), CASDDS, CISTI, GNLM.

M

Published by: (Japanese Society of Nephrology), Springer-Verlag Tokyo, Eastern Book Service, Inc. (Subsidiary of: BertelsmannSpringer), 3-13 Hongo 3-chome, Bunkyo-ku, Tokyo 113-0033, Japan. TEL 81-3-3812-0617, FAX 81-3-3812-4699, http://link.springer-ny.com/link/service/journals/10157/about.htm. Ed. Masashi Imai. **Subscr. in N. America to:** Springer-Verlag New York Inc., PO Box 2485, Secaucus, NJ 07096-2485. TEL 800-777-4643, 212-460-1526, FAX 201-348-4505, orders@springer-ny.com; **Subscr. outside N. America & Japan to:** Springer-Verlag, c/o Gabriele Kubitza, Haberstrasse 7, Heidelberg 69126, Germany. TEL 49-6221-345242, FAX 49-6221-345229, subscriptions@springer.de, http://www.link.springer.de, http://link.springer-ny.com. **Dist. by:** Eastern Book Service, Inc.. TEL 81-3-3818-0861, FAX 81-3-3818-0864, orders@svt-ebs.co.jp.

616.6 JPN ISSN 1437-7799
CLINICAL AND EXPERIMENTAL NEPHROLOGY ONLINE. Text in English. 4/yr. *Refereed.* **Document type:** *Journal, Academic/Scholarly.*
Media: Online - full text (from EBSCO Publishing, RoweCom Information Quest, Swets Blackwell, Springer LINK). **Related titles:** ♦ Print ed.: Clinical and Experimental Nephrology. ISSN 1342-1751.
Published by: (Japanese Society of Nephrology), Springer-Verlag Tokyo (Subsidiary of: BertelsmannSpringer), 3-13 Hongo 3-chome, Bunkyo-ku, Tokyo 113-0033, Japan.

616.6 DEU ISSN 0301-0430
CODEN: CLNHBI
CLINICAL NEPHROLOGY. Text in English. 1973. m. DEM 380, EUR 194.29, USD 198 to individuals; USD 244 to institutions; DEM 425, EUR 217.30, USD 228 to individuals print & online eds.; USD 284 to institutions print & online eds.; DEM 40 newsstand/cover (effective 2001). adv. reprint service avail. from SWZ. *Refereed.* **Document type:** *Journal, Academic/Scholarly.*
Related titles: Online - full text ed.: (from Institute for Scientific Information).
Indexed: ASCA, Biol.Abstr., Chem.Abstr., Chem.Indus.Notes, Chem.Titles, Curr.Adv.Ecol.Sci., Curr.Cont., Excerp.Med., INIS Atomind., Ind.Med. (1973-), Ind.Sci.Rev., Inpharma, Int.Abstr.Biol.Sci., Int.Nurs.Ind., Kidney, Nutr.Abstr., Pharm.&Out.News, Reac., Ref.Zh., Rev.Med.& Vet.Mycol., Rev.Plant Path., Sci.Cit.Ind., Trop.Dis.Bull.
—BLDSC (3286.307100), CASDDS, EMDOCS, GNLM, IDS, ingenta, KNAW. **CCC.**
Published by: Dustri-Verlag Dr. Karl Feistle, Bajuwarenring 4, Oberhaching 82041, Germany. TEL 49-89-613861-0, FAX 49-89-613-5412, info@dustri.de, http://www.clinnephrol.com, http://www.dustri.de. Ed. Dr. K M Koch. R&P Renate Lehmann. Adv. contact Joerg Feistle. B&W page USD 765, color page USD 1,590; bleed 8.5 x 11.75. Circ: 4,900.

616.1 USA ISSN 0177-8994
CLINICAL PRACTICE IN UROLOGY. Text in English. 1982. irreg., latest 1991. price varies. **Document type:** *Monographic series.*
Published by: Springer-Verlag, Journals (Subsidiary of: BertelsmannSpringer), 175 Fifth Ave, New York, NY 10010. TEL 212-460-1500, FAX 212-473-6272. Ed. Geoffrey D Chisholm.

616.6 USA
CLINICAL STRATEGIES: A K F NEWSLETTER FOR NEPHROLOGY PROFESSIONALS. Text in English. 1984. 2/yr. free per issue. index. back issues avail. **Description:** Offers current information to health professionals in the renal community. Reports on developments in the renal field as well as the AKF services and programs.
Formerly (until 1993): A K F Newsletter for Health Professionals
Published by: American Kidney Fund, 6110 Executive Blvd, Ste 1010, Rockville, MD 20852-3903. TEL 301-881-3052, 800-638-8299, FAX 301-881-0898, permann@akfinc.org, http://www.akfinc.org. Ed., Pub., R&P Phylis Ermann. Circ: 12,000.

616.6 USA ISSN 0899-837X
CONTEMPORARY DIALYSIS & NEPHROLOGY; the news and issues journal of the renal care field. Text in English. 1979. m. USD 42 domestic; USD 47 in Canada & Mexico; USD 67 elsewhere (effective 2001). adv. bk.rev. charts, illus, stat. back issues avail. **Document type:** *Magazine, Trade.* **Description:** Deals with news and issues regarding renal care.
Formerly: Contemporary Dialysis (0273-6535)
Indexed: Chem.Abstr.
—BLDSC (3425.178410), GNLM, Infotrieve, ingenta. **CCC.**
Published by: Ashlee Publishing Co., Inc., 18 E 41st St, 20th Fl, New York, NY 10017-6222. TEL 212-376-7722, FAX 212-376-7723. Ed. Gordon Lore. Pub. Jordan Wright. Adv. contact Karen Glasser TEL 818-704-5555. B&W page USD 2,310; 8.25 x 10.875. Circ: 19,900 (controlled).

616.6 USA ISSN 0161-9934
CODEN: CISND8
CONTEMPORARY ISSUES IN NEPHROLOGY*. Text in English. 1978. irreg., latest vol.30. **Document type:** *Monographic series.*
Indexed: Chem.Abstr., Chem.Indus.Notes, Chem.Titles.
—CASDDS, CISTI, KNAW.
Published by: Churchill Livingstone (Subsidiary of: Harcourt Health Sciences), 15 E 26th St, Fl 15, New York, NY 10010-1505. TEL 212-206-5040, FAX 212-727-7808, http://www.churchillmed.com.

616.6 USA ISSN 0278-1700
CODEN: CONHD7
CONTEMPORARY NEPHROLOGY. Text in English. 1981. biennial, latest vol.5, 1989. price varies. back issues avail. *Refereed.* **Document type:** *Monographic series.*
—CASDDS, GNLM, Infotrieve, KNAW. **CCC.**
Published by: Kluwer Academic - Plenum Publishers (Subsidiary of: Wolters Kluwer N.V.), 233 Spring St, New York, NY 10013-1578. TEL 212-620-8000, 800-221-9369, FAX 212-463-0742, info@plenum.com, http://www.plenum.com. Eds. Saulo Klahr, Shaul G Massry.

616.6 USA ISSN 1042-2250
CONTEMPORARY UROLOGY. Text in English. 1989. m. USD 99 domestic; USD 126 foreign; USD 10 newsstand/cover (effective 2001). adv. charts, illus. index. reprints avail. **Document type:** *Trade.* **Description:** Contains articles and departments regarding practical solutions to clinical problems in urology.
Related titles: Microform ed.: (from PQC).
Indexed: CINAHL.
—BLDSC (3425.314500), GNLM, Infotrieve. **CCC.**
Published by: Medical Economics Co., Inc., 5 Paragon Dr, Montvale, NJ 07645-1742. TEL 201-358-7200. Ed. Mark Zacharia. Circ: 5,075.

616.6 CHE ISSN 0302-5144
CODEN: CNEPDD
CONTRIBUTIONS TO NEPHROLOGY. Text in English. 1975. irreg., latest vol.135. CHF 210 in Europe; DEM 250 in Germany; USD 180 in United States (2001). reprint service avail. from ISI. *Refereed.* **Document type:** *Monographic series, Academic/Scholarly.*
Related titles: Online - full text ed.: (from Institute for Scientific Information).
Indexed: ASCA, Biol.Abstr., CINAHL, Chem.Abstr., Chem.Indus.Notes, Chem.Titles, Curr.Cont. (coverage dropped), Ind.Med. (1975-).
—BLDSC (3461.035000), CASDDS, CISTI, EMDOCS, GNLM, IDS, Infotrieve, ingenta, KNAW. **CCC.**
Published by: S. Karger AG, Allschwilerstr 10, PO Box, Basel 4009, Switzerland. TEL 41-61-306-1111, FAX 41-61-306-1234, karger@karger.ch, http://www.karger.com/bookseries/CONEP, http://www.karger.ch. Eds. C Ronco, G M Berlyne.

616.6 USA
▼ **CURRENT CLINICAL UROLOGY.** Text in English. 1999. irreg. price varies. illus. back issues avail. *Refereed.* **Document type:** *Journal, Academic/Scholarly.* **Description:** Covers all aspects of urology and related internal medicine and surgery.
Published by: Humana Press Inc., 999 Riverview Dr, Ste 208, Totowa, NJ 07512. TEL 973-256-1699, FAX 973-256-8341, humana@humanapr.com, http://humanapress.com. Ed. Eric Klein. R&P Wendy A Warren.

CURRENT MEDICAL LITERATURE. NEPHROLOGY AND HYPERTENSION. see *MEDICAL SCIENCES—Abstracting, Bibliographies, Statistics*

CURRENT MEDICAL LITERATURE. PROSTATIC DISEASE. see *MEDICAL SCIENCES—Abstracting, Bibliographies, Statistics*

CURRENT MEDICAL LITERATURE. UROLOGY. see *MEDICAL SCIENCES—Abstracting, Bibliographies, Statistics*

610 USA ISSN 1062-4821
CODEN: CNHYEM
CURRENT OPINION IN NEPHROLOGY & HYPERTENSION. Text in English. 1992. bi-m. USD 273 domestic to individuals for Print & Online eds.; USD 273 foreign to individuals for Print & Online eds.; USD 665 per issue domestic to institutions; USD 665 per issue foreign to institutions; USD 103 newsstand/cover (effective 2002). adv. bibl, illus. back issues avail. *Refereed.* **Document type:** *Academic/Scholarly.* **Description:** Presents review articles directed toward clinicians and practicing kidney and hypertension specialists.
Related titles: CD-ROM ed.; Diskette ed.; Online - full text ed.: USD 864.50 domestic academic site license; USD 864.50 foreign academic site license; USD 964.25 domestic corporate site license; USD 964.25 foreign corporate site license (effective 2002) (from Ovid Technologies, Inc., EBSCO Publishing, Swets Blackwell, Institute for Scientific Information).
Indexed: CINAHL, Curr.Cont., Excerp.Med. (1995-), Ind.Med. (1992-), Inpharma, Int.Abstr.Biol.Sci., Pharm.&Out.News, Reac., Sci.Cit.Ind.
—BLDSC (3500.775830), ADONIS, CISTI, EMDOCS, IDS, Infotrieve. **CCC.**
Published by: Lippincott Williams & Wilkins (Philadelphia) (Subsidiary of: Wolters Kluwer N.V.), 530 Walnut St, Philadelphia, PA 19106-3621. TEL 215-521-8300, FAX 215-521-8902, http://www.Lww.com. Ed. Dr. Barry M Brenner. Adv. contact Gemma Heiser. Circ: 3,670. **Subscr. to:** PO Box 1600, Hagerstown, MD 21740-1600. TEL 800-777-2295, FAX 301-824-7390.

616.6 USA ISSN 0963-0643
CODEN: CUOUEQ
CURRENT OPINION IN UROLOGY. Text in English. 1992. bi-m. USD 273 domestic to individuals for print & online eds.; USD 273 foreign to individuals for print & online eds.; USD 665 per issue domestic to institutions; USD 665 per issue foreign to institutions; USD 103 newsstand/cover (effective 2002). adv. bibl, illus. index. back issues avail. **Document type:** *Academic/Scholarly.* **Description:** Presents review articles directed toward clinicians and practicing urologists.
Related titles: CD-ROM ed.; Diskette ed.; Online - full text ed.: USD 864.50 domestic academic site license; USD 864.50 foreign academic site license; USD 964.25 domestic corporate site license; USD 964.25 foreign corporate site license (effective 2002) (from Ovid Technologies, Inc., EBSCO Publishing, Swets Blackwell).
Indexed: Excerp.Med. (1993-), Ind.Med. (1991-), Int.Abstr.Biol.Sci.
—BLDSC (3500.779500), ADONIS, CISTI, EMDOCS, GNLM, KNAW.
Published by: Lippincott Williams & Wilkins (Philadelphia) (Subsidiary of: Wolters Kluwer N.V.), 530 Walnut St, Philadelphia, PA 19106-3621. FAX 215-521-8902, 215-521-8902, http://www.Lww.com. Eds. David F Paulson, Michael Marberger. Adv. contact Gemma Heiser. color page GBP 1,210. Circ: 3,165. **Subscr. to:** PO Box 1600, Hagerstown, MD 21740-1600.

616.6 DEU ISSN 0941-0406
DEUTSCHE ARBEITSGEMEINSCHAFT FUER KLINISCHE NEPHROLOGIE. MITTEILUNGEN. Text in German. a. DEM 68 (effective 2000). **Document type:** *Academic/Scholarly.*
Formerly (until 1993): Arbeitsgemeinschaft fuer Klinische Nephrologie. Mitteilungen (0172-7311)
—GNLM.
Published by: (Deutsche Arbeitsgemeinschaft fuer Klinische Nephrologie e.V.), Vandenhoeck und Ruprecht, Robert-Bosch-Breite 6, Goettingen 37079, Germany. TEL 49-551-6959-0, FAX 49-551-695917. Ed. E Quellhorst.

616.6 DEU ISSN 0178-4625
DEUTSCHE GESELLSCHAFT FUER UROLOGIE. MITTEILUNGEN*. Text in German. 1985. q. DEM 96. **Document type:** *Academic/Scholarly.*
—GNLM.
Published by: (Deutsche Gesellschaft fuer Urologie), Demeter Verlag GmbH und Co. KG, Ammonitenstr 1, Balingen 72336, Germany. Circ: 4,400.

616.6 USA
DEUTSCHE GESELLSCHAFT FUER UROLOGIE. VERHANDLUNGEN. Text in English. 1962 (19th session). irreg., latest 1988 (39th session). price varies. reprint service avail. from ISI. **Document type:** *Monographic series.*
Formerly: Deutsche Gesellschaft fuer Urologie. Verhandlungsbericht (0070-413X)
—CISTI, GNLM.
Published by: Springer-Verlag, Journals (Subsidiary of: BertelsmannSpringer), 175 Fifth Ave, New York, NY 10010. TEL 212-460-1500, FAX 212-473-6272.

M

616.6 NLD ISSN 0167-8205 CODEN: DNEPDO
DEVELOPMENTS IN NEPHROLOGY. Text in English. 1981. irreg., latest vol.34, 1993. price varies. back issues avail. *Refereed.* **Document type:** *Monographic series.*
Indexed: Chem.Abstr., Chem.Indus.Notes, Chem.Titles. —BLDSC (3579.085360), CASDDS, CISTI, KNAW. **CCC.**
Published by: Kluwer Academic Publishers Group (Subsidiary of: Wolters Kluwer N.V.), Spuiboulevard 50, PO Box 17, Dordrecht 3300 AA, Netherlands. FAX 31-78-639-2254, services@wkap.nl, http://www.wkap.nl. **Dist. by:** Journals Department, PO Box 322, Dordrecht 3300 AH, Netherlands. FAX 31-78-654-6474.

616.6 610.73 SWE ISSN 1104-4616
DIALAESEN; tidningen foer personal inom nyursyukvaard. Text in Swedish. 1993. q. adv. **Document type:** *Magazine, Academic/Scholarly.* **Description:** For all medical personnel involved with nephrology.
Address: Bjoernbaersvaegen 10, Upplands Vaesby 19465, Sweden. TEL 46-8-59420313, FAX 46-8-59420313, pia.dialasen@telia.com. Ed. Karin Johansson. Pub., Adv. contact Pia Lundstroem. page SEK 12,300.

DIALOGUES IN PEDIATRIC UROLOGY. see *MEDICAL SCIENCES—Pediatrics*

616.6 DEU ISSN 0932-190X
DIALYSE JOURNAL. Text in German; Summaries in English, German. 1983. q. EUR 15 (effective 2001). adv. bk.rev. *Refereed.* **Document type:** *Journal, Academic/Scholarly.* **Description:** Contains practice-oriented summary articles for physicians involved with dialysis.
Indexed: Ref.Zh. —GNLM.
Published by: Pabst Science Publishers, Am Eichengrund 28, Lengerich 49525, Germany. TEL 49-5484-308, FAX 49-5484-550, pabst.publishers@t-online.de, http://www.pabst-publishers.de. Ed. Petra Reinke. Circ: 7,200.

616.6 DEU ISSN 0724-0252
DER DIALYSEPATIENT; Zeitschrift fuer chronisch Nierenkranke. Text in German. 1976. q. DEM 37.20 (effective 1999). adv. bk.rev. **Document type:** *Academic/Scholarly.* **Description:** Covers nephrology in the areas of medicine, law, social services and welfare for doctors, patients and medical personnel.
Published by: (Dialysepatienten Deutschlands e.V.), Verlag Kirchheim und Co. GmbH, Kaiserstr 41, Mainz 55116, Germany. TEL 49-6131-96070-0, FAX 49-6131-9607070, kirchheim@aol.com. Ed. Alexander Schulz. Adv. contact Andreas Goerner. Circ: 20,000.

616.61 USA ISSN 0090-2934 CODEN: DITRD2
DIALYSIS & TRANSPLANTATION. Text in English. 1972. m. USD 35 domestic; USD 60 foreign (effective 2000). adv. charts, illus. *Refereed.* **Document type:** *Trade.* **Description:** For nephrology professionals; publishes clinical application articles on new techniques and technologies, as well as coverage of pertinent legislative and economic issues.
Related titles: Online - full text ed.: (from Institute for Scientific Information).
Indexed: ASCA, Biol.Abstr., Curr.Adv.Ecol.Sci., Curr.Cont., Excerp.Med., Inpharma, Nutr.Abstr., Pharm.&Out.News, Reac., Ref.Zh., Rev.Med.& Vet.Mycol. —BLDSC (3579.785000), CASDDS, CISTI, GNLM, IDS, ingenta, KNAW.
Published by: Creative Age Publications, Inc., 7628 Densmore Ave, Van Nuys, CA 91406-2042. TEL 818-782-7328, FAX 818-782-7450. Ed., R&P Joseph G Herman. Pub. Deborah Carver. Adv. contact Tom S Blackstone. B&W page USD 3,034, color page USD 3,884. Circ: 22,731.

616.6 DEU ISSN 0940-5623
DIATRA JOURNAL. Text in German. 1991. q. DEM 35. bk.rev. **Description:** Covers nephrology and transplantation in the areas of medicine, law and social welfare.
Published by: Diatra Verlag GmbH, Balduinstr 2, Eltville 65332, Germany. TEL 6123-1007, FAX 6123-1220. Ed. S K Hammers Kaplan. adv.: B&W page DEM 1,636; trim 170 x 260. Circ: 19,000.

616.6 616.4 ITA
▼ **E D NEWS.** Text in Italian. 2001. 3/yr. adv. **Document type:** *Newsletter, Academic/Scholarly.*
Published by: C I C Edizioni Internazionali s.r.l., Corso Trieste 42, Rome, RM 00198, Italy. TEL 39-06-8412673, FAX 39-06-8412688, info@gruppocic.it, http://www.gruppocic.it. Ed. V Mirone. Pub. A Salvati.

616.6 CHE ISSN 1019-083X
E D T N A - E R C A JOURNAL. Text in English. 1983. q. CHF 60. bk.rev. back issues avail.; reprints avail. *Refereed.* **Document type:** *Journal, Academic/Scholarly.*
Formerly (until 1985): E D T N A Journal (0265-3133)
Related titles: Dutch ed.: ISSN 1019-0864; French ed.: ISSN 1019-0848; German ed.: ISSN 1019-0856; Italian ed.: ISSN 1019-0880; Spanish ed.: ISSN 1019-0872; Greek ed.
Indexed: Brit.Nur.Ind., CINAHL, Excerp.Med. (1994-), Int.Nurs.Ind. —BLDSC (3661.116725), EMDOCS.
Published by: European Dialysis and Transplant Nurses Association, European Renal Care Association, PO Box 3052, Luzern 6002, Switzerland. TEL 41-41-4407555, FAX 41-41-4403962, edtna_erca@compuserve.com, http://edtna-erca.org. Ed. Anna Marti I Munros. R&P Terrance Balkan. Adv. contact Wolfgang Pabst TEL 49-5484-308. Circ: 4,000.

616.6 FRA ISSN 1155-1917
ENCYCLOPEDIE MEDICO-CHIRURGICALE. NEPHROLOGIE - UROLOGIE. Cover title: Traite de Nephrologie - Urologie. Variant title: Encyclopedie Medico-Chirurgicale, Instantanes Medicaux. Nephrologie - Urologie. Text in French. 1939. 4 base vols. plus q. updates. bibl, charts, illus. *Refereed.* **Document type:** *Academic/Scholarly.* **Description:** Provides urologists with a comprehensive, up-to-date reference for diagnosing and treating kidney and other urinary-tract diseases, disorders, and conditions.
Former titles (until 1991): Encyclopedie Medico-Chirurgicale. Rein, Organes Genito-urinaires (0246-0572); (until 1957): Encyclopedie Medico-Chirurgicale. Rein (0246-0742)
Published by: Elsevier Paris, Editions Scientifiques et Medicales (Subsidiary of: Reed Elsevier plc. group), 15 rue Linois, Paris Cedex 15 75015, France. TEL 33-1-45589110, FAX 33-1-45589425, redaction-emc@elsevier.fr, redacion-emc@elsevier.fr, http://www.elsevier.fr, http://www.elsevier.com.

ENCYCLOPEDIE MEDICO-CHIRURGICALE. TRAITE DE RADIODIAGNOSTIC: UROLOGIE - GYNECOLOGIE. see *MEDICAL SCIENCES—Radiology And Nuclear Medicine*

ENCYCLOPEDIE MEDICO-CHIRURGICALE. TRAITE DE TECHNIQUES CHIRURGICALES. UROLOGIE. see *MEDICAL SCIENCES—Surgery*

616.6 CHE ISSN 0302-2838 CODEN: EUURAV
EUROPEAN UROLOGY. Text in English. m. EUR 695 in Europe to individuals; JPY 92,200 in Japan to individuals; USD 778 elsewhere to individuals; EUR 1,359 in Europe to institutions; JPY 180,400 in Japan to institutions; USD 1,521 elsewhere to institutions (effective 2002). abstr. index. back issues avail. *Refereed.* **Document type:** *Journal, Academic/Scholarly.* **Description:** Publishes original research articles on a wide range of urological disorders. Covers oncology, impotence, infertility, pediatrics, lithiasis, and endourology.
Related titles: Microform ed.; Online - full text ed.: ISSN 1421-993X. CHF 116 in Europe with print edition; CHF 116 overseas with print edition; DEM 156 in Germany with print edition; USD 90 in United States with print edition (effective 2001) (from EBSCO Publishing, O C L C Online Computer Library Center, Inc., RoweCom Information Quest, Swets Blackwell, Institute for Scientific Information).
Indexed: ASCA, Biol.Abstr., Cal.Tiss.Abstr., Chem.Abstr., Curr.Adv.Cell & Devel.Biol., Curr.Adv.Ecol.Sci., Curr.Cont., Environ.Sci.Poll.Mgmt., Excerp.Med., Helminthol.Abstr., Ind.Med. (1975-), Ind.Sci.Rev., Inpharma, Int.Nurs.Ind., NRN, Nutr.Abstr., Pharm.&Out.News, Reac., Risk Abstr., Rural Devel.Abstr., Saf.Sci.Abstr., Sci.Cit.Ind., Tox.Abstr. (coverage dropped). —BLDSC (3830.370500), CASDDS, CISTI, EMDOCS, GNLM, IDS, ingenta, KNAW. **CCC.**
Published by: (European Association of Urology), Elsevier Science BV, PO Box 211, Amsterdam 1000 AE, Netherlands. TEL 31-20-485-3757, FAX 31-20-485-3432, european.urology@uroweb.nl, nlinfo-f@elsevier.nl, http://www.elsevier.nl. Circ: 3,200. **Co-sponsors:** European Organization for Research and Treatment of Cancer, Genito Urinary Group; European Society for Urological Oncology and Endocrinology.

616.6 NLD ISSN 0968-7645
EUROPEAN UROLOGY UPDATE SERIES. Text in Dutch. 1992. bi-m. **Document type:** *Academic/Scholarly.*
Published by: European Board of Urology, Education Committee - Office of Education, PO Box 25285, Rotterdam 3001 HG, Netherlands. TEL 31-10-4366665, FAX 31-10-4366669. Ed. H N Whitfield.

EXCERPTA MEDICA. SECTION 28: UROLOGY AND NEPHROLOGY. see *MEDICAL SCIENCES—Abstracting, Bibliographies, Statistics*

616.6 CHE ISSN 1018-7782 CODEN: EXNEEG
EXPERIMENTAL NEPHROLOGY; a journal of renal cell biology and functional genomics. Text in English. 1993. 6/yr. CHF 1,037 in Europe to institutions; CHF 1,054.40 elsewhere to institutions; EUR 740.80 in Europe to institutions; USD 806 elsewhere to institutions (effective 2002). adv. back issues avail. *Refereed.* **Document type:** *Journal, Academic/Scholarly.* **Description:** Devoted to the biology of the kidney, including developmental, cellular and molecular aspects, and to the scientific basis of renal diseases.
Related titles: Microform ed.: (from PQC); Online - full text ed.: ISSN 1421-9956. CHF 58, EUR 42, USD 45 to institutions with print edition (effective 2002) (from EBSCO Publishing, O C L C Online Computer Library Center, Inc., RoweCom Information Quest, Swets Blackwell, Institute for Scientific Information).
Indexed: ASCA, Chem.Abstr., Chem.Indus.Notes, Chem.Titles, Curr.Cont., Excerp.Med. (1994-), Ind.Med. (1993-), Inpharma, Mass Spectr.Bull., Pharm.&Out.News, Reac., Sci.Cit.Ind. —BLDSC (3839.830000), CASDDS, EMDOCS, GNLM, IDS, Infotrieve, KNAW. **CCC.**
Published by: S. Karger AG, Allschwilerstr 10, PO Box, Basel 4009, Switzerland. TEL 41-61-306-1111, FAX 41-61-3061235, karger@karger.ch, http://www.online.karger.com/journals/exn, http://www.karger.com. Ed. L G Fine. adv.: page USD 1,195.

616.6 DEU ISSN 0344-5038
EXTRACTA UROLOGICA. Text in German. 1978. bi-m. DEM 99. back issues avail. **Document type:** *Academic/Scholarly.* —GNLM.
Published by: Selecta Verlagsgesellschaft mbH, Postfach 4240, Wiesbaden 65032, Germany. TEL 0611-1705-0, FAX 0611-1705379. Ed. Dr. Juergen Boedeker. Circ: 2,400.

616.6 USA
FAMILY FOCUS. Text in English. q. free per issue. **Document type:** *Newspaper.* **Description:** Information for dialysis and transplant patients and their families.
Published by: National Kidney Foundation, 30 East 33rd St, New York, NY 10016. TEL 212-889-2210, FAX 212-689-9261, http://www.kidney.org. Ed. Karen King. Circ: 135,000 (controlled and free).

616.6 USA ISSN 1525-9471
FOR PATIENTS ONLY. Text in English. 1988. bi-m. USD 17 domestic; USD 22 in Canada & Mexico; USD 32 elsewhere (effective 2001). adv. **Document type:** *Magazine, Trade.* **Description:** Brings professional understanding to patients living with chronic kidney disease. Covers patient-caregiver relationships, psychological issues, homecare and rehabilitation.
Published by: Ashlee Publishing Co., Inc., 18 E 41st St, 20th Fl, New York, NY 10017-6222. TEL 212-376-7722, FAX 212-376-7723. Pub. Jordan Wright. Adv. contact Karen Glasser TEL 818-704-5555. B&W page USD 2,150, color page USD 3,000; trim 10.875 x 8.25. Circ: 11,500.

616.6 360 USA
FOR THOSE WHO GIVE AND GRIEVE; a quarterly newsletter for donor families. Text in English. 1991. q. free per issue. **Document type:** *Newsletter.* **Description:** Discusses grief among families of organ donors, programs for these families, and support organizations to assist families.
Published by: National Kidney Foundation, 30 East 33rd St, New York, NY 10016. TEL 212-889-2210, FAX 212-689-9261. Circ: 30,000.

616.6 ITA ISSN 0394-9362
GIORNALE DI TECNICHE NEFROLOGICHE E DIALITICHE. Text in Italian. 1989. q. EUR 52 in Europe to individuals; USD 78 elsewhere to individuals; EUR 67 in Europe to institutions; USD 92 elsewhere to institutions (effective 2001). bibl, charts, illus. 48 p./no. back issues avail.; reprints avail. *Refereed.* **Document type:** *Journal, Academic/Scholarly.*

M

Published by: Wichtig Editore s.r.l., Via Friuli, 72, Milan, MI 20135, Italy. TEL 39-02-55195443, FAX 39-02-55195971, info@wichtig-publisher.com. Eds. Dr. N Di Paolo, Dr. V Buoncristiani. Pub. Dr. Diego Brancaccio. Adv. contact Nella Bini. Circ: 500 (controlled).

616.6 ITA ISSN 0393-5590
GIORNALE ITALIANO DI NEFROLOGIA. Text in Italian; Summaries in English. 1984. bi-m. EUR 83 in Europe to individuals; USD 117 elsewhere to individuals; EUR 109 in Europe to institutions; USD 140 elsewhere to institutions (effective 2001). abstr, bibl, charts, illus. Index. 128 p./no. back issues avail.; reprints avail. *Refereed.* **Document type:** *Journal, Academic/Scholarly.*
Indexed: Inpharma, Reac.
—BLDSC (4178.233000), EMDOCS, GNLM, KNAW.
Published by: Wichtig Editore s.r.l., Via Friuli, 72, Milan, MI 20135, Italy. TEL 39-02-55195443, FAX 39-02-55195971, info@wichtig-publisher.com. Ed. Dr. G Maschio. Pub. Dr. Diego Brancaccio. R&P Lucia Steele. Adv. contact Nella Bini. Circ: 2,000 (controlled).

616.6 BRA
▼ **GLOSSARIUM UROLOGIA.** Text in Portuguese. 2000. a. BRL 40 (effective 2000). adv. illus. *Refereed.* **Document type:** *Consumer, Trade.*
Published by: Elea Ciencia Editorial Ltda., Rua Haddock Lobo, 86 Andar 6, Estacio, Rio De Janeiro, RJ 20260-132, Brazil. TEL 55-21-293-2112, FAX 55-21-293-7818, elea@openlink.com.br. Ed., Pub. Luiz Augusto Rodrigues. R&P, Adv. contact Alexandre Augusto Rodrigues. color page BRL 4,375; trim 15 x 21. Circ: 3,000. **Subscr. to:** Rua Haddock Lobo, 86 17o andar, Rio de Janeiro, RJ 20260-132, Brazil. TEL 55-21-5028317, FAX 55-21-5022737, alanmarketing@openlink.com.br.

616.6 DEU ISSN 0935-8234
HAEUSLICHE PFLEGE; Organisieren - Betreuen - Kompetent beraten. Text in German. 1992. m. EUR 69 domestic; EUR 71 foreign (effective 2002). **Document type:** *Journal, Trade.*
—GNLM.
Published by: Vincentz Verlag, Schiffgraben 43, Hannover 30175, Germany. TEL 49-511-9910000, FAX 49-511-9910099, info@vincentz.de, http://www.vincentz.de. Ed. Stefan Neumann. Circ: 8,254.

616.6 USA ISSN 0932-2329
HANDBOOK OF UROLOGY. Text in English. 1959. irreg. **Document type:** *Monographic series.*
Formerly (until 1985): Handbuch der Urologie (0374-8006)
Published by: Springer-Verlag, Journals (Subsidiary of: BertelsmannSpringer), 175 Fifth Ave, New York, NY 10010. TEL 212-460-1500, FAX 212-473-6272.

616.6 360 AUS
HARICOT; newsletter for the renal patients of Australia. Text in English. 1983. q. free per issue. bk.rev. back issues avail.
Address: PO Box 3, Diamond Creek, VIC 3089, Australia. Eds. J Coleman, S Evans. Circ: 1,500.

HOKKAIDO TOSEKI RYOHO GAKKAI PUROGURAMU ENDAI SHOROKU/HOKKAIDO SOCIETY FOR DIALYSIS THERAPY. PROGRAM AND ABSTRACTS. see *MEDICAL SCIENCES—Abstracting, Bibliographies, Statistics*

616.6 JPN
HOKKAIDO TOSEKI RYOHO GAKKAI SHINPOJUMU/HOKKAIDO SOCIETY FOR DIALYSIS THERAPY. PROCEEDINGS OF SYMPOSIUM. Text in Japanese. 1988. a. **Document type:** *Proceedings.*
Published by: Hokkaido Toseki Ryoho Gakkai, 3, Nishi 7-chome, Kita 1-jo, Chuo-ku, Sapporo-shi, Hokkaido 090, Japan.

616.6 HKG ISSN 1561-5413
HONG KONG JOURNAL OF NEPHROLOGY. Text in English. biennial. HKD 100; USD 25 in United States (effective 2002). **Document type:** *Journal, Academic/Scholarly.* **Description:** Promotes research in the field of nephrology and a forum for the discussion of key issues in nephrology for Hong Kong and Southeast Asia. Also serves as a source of communication between nephrologists of Hong Kong and China and the international community.
Published by: (Hong Kong Society of Nephrology USA), Lippincott Williams & Wilkins Asia, Ste 907-910, New T&T Centre, Harbour City, 7 Canton Rd, Tsimshatsui, Kowtoon, Hong Kong. TEL 822-26323129, FAX 852-26489864, hkjn@hkjn.org, http://www.hkjn.org. Ed. Dr. Philip T K Li. Adv. contact Dr. Francine Wong TEL 852-29588888.

616.6 USA
I C A UPDATE (NEW YORK)* . Text in English. 1984. 4/yr. USD 40 to membership; USD 60 foreign to membership. **Document type:** *Newsletter.* **Description:** Creates public awareness and provides information about IC research and ICA activities to patients and the medical community.
Published by: Interstitial Cystitis Association, 51 Monroe St, Ste 1402, Rockville, MD 20050-2408. TEL 212-979-6057, FAX 212-677-6139, icinfo@aol.com, http://www.ichelp.com. Ed., R&P Debra Slade.

616.6 USA ISSN 0896-9647
INFECTIONS IN UROLOGY. Text in English. 1988. bi-m. USD 60 domestic to individuals; USD 78 foreign to individuals; USD 110 domestic to institutions; USD 128 foreign to institutions; USD 40 domestic to students; USD 58 foreign to students. *Refereed.*
—GNLM, IDS, Infotrieve. **CCC.**
Published by: S C P Communications, Inc., 134 W 29th St, New York, NY 10001-5304. TEL 212-631-1600, subs@scp.com, http://www.medscape.com.

616.65 GBR ISSN 0105-6263 CODEN: IJANDP
INTERNATIONAL JOURNAL OF ANDROLOGY. Text in English. bi-m., latest vol.25, 2002. GBP 275 in Europe; USD 431 in North America; GBP 299 elsewhere (effective 2002). adv. bk.rev. abstr, bibl, illus. index. back issues avail. *Refereed.* **Document type:** *Academic/Scholarly.*
Related titles: Microform ed.: (from PQC); Online - full text ed.: ISSN 1365-2605. GBP 248 in Europe; USD 388 in North America; GBP 248 elsewhere (effective 2002) (from Ovid Technologies, Inc., EBSCO Publishing, O C L C Online Computer Library Center, Inc., RoweCom Information Quest, ingenta, Munksgaard & Blackwell Science's Synergy, Swets Blackwell, Institute for Scientific Information).
Indexed: ASCA, AgBiotech, Anim.Breed.Abstr., Biol.Abstr., Chem.Abstr., Chem.Indus.Notes, Chem.Titles, Curr.Adv.Ecol.Sci., Curr.Cont., Dent.Ind., Excerp.Med., Ind.Med. (1978-), Ind.Vet., Inpharma, Int.Abstr.Biol.Sci., Pharm.&Out.News, Pig News & Info., Protozool.Abstr., Reac., Sci.Cit.Ind., Small Anim.Abstr., THA, Vet.Bull.
—BLDSC (4542.080000), ADONIS, CASDDS, CISTI, EMDOCS, GNLM, IDS, ingenta, KNAW. **CCC.**
Published by: (European Academy of Andrology), Blackwell Science Ltd., PO Box 88, Oxford OX2 0NE, United Kingdom. TEL 44-1865-206180, 44-1865-206002, FAX 44-1865-206219, jnl.orders@blacksci.co.uk, http://www.blackwell-science.com/~cgilib/jnlpage.asp?Journal=ija&File=ija, http://www.blackwellpublishing.com. Ed. R Sharpe. Pub. Allen Stevens. R&P Sophie Savage. Adv. contact Jenny Applin. Circ: 465.

616.65 GBR ISSN 0106-1607 CODEN: IJSPDJ
INTERNATIONAL JOURNAL OF ANDROLOGY. SUPPLEMENT. Text in English. 1978. irreg. price varies. adv. illus. **Document type:** *Academic/Scholarly.*
Related titles: Online - full text ed.: (from Ovid Technologies, Inc.).
Indexed: Biol.Abstr., Chem.Abstr., Curr.Cont. (coverage dropped).
—ADONIS, CASDDS, CISTI.
Published by: Blackwell Science Ltd., Osney Mead, Oxford OX2 0EL, United Kingdom. TEL 44-1865-206206, FAX 44-1865-721205, journals.cs@blacksci.co.uk, http://www.blackwell-science.com. Pub. Allen Stevens. R&P Sophie Savage. Adv. contact Jenny Applin.

616.6 GBR ISSN 0955-9930 CODEN: IJIRFB
INTERNATIONAL JOURNAL OF IMPOTENCE RESEARCH. Text in English. 1989. bi-m. GBP 90 in Europe to individuals for print or online ed.; USD 135 elsewhere to individuals for print or online ed.; GBP 99 combined subscription in Europe to individuals print & online; USD 149 combined subscription elsewhere to individuals print & online; GBP 220 in Europe to institutions for print or online ed.; USD 220 elsewhere to institutions for print or online ed.; GBP 242 combined subscription in Europe to institutions print & online; USD 363 combined subscription elsewhere to institutions print & online (effective 2000). adv. charts, illus, stat. back issues avail. *Refereed.* **Document type:** *Journal, Academic/Scholarly.* **Description:** Devoted exclusively to impotence research, including methods of assessing normal and abnormal erectile dysfunction methods of delivery to create erection.
Related titles: Online - full text ed.: (from EBSCO Publishing, O C L C Online Computer Library Center, Inc., RoweCom Information Quest, ingenta, Swets Blackwell, Institute for Scientific Information).
Indexed: Curr.Cont., Ind.Med. (1989-), Inpharma, Pharm.&Out.News, Reac., Sci.Cit.Ind.
—BLDSC (4542.302700), CISTI, GNLM, IDS, Infotrieve, KNAW. **CCC.**
Published by: (International Society for Impotence Research), Nature Publishing Group Specialist Journals (Subsidiary of: Holtzbrink Publishers), Houndmills, Basingstoke, Hants RG21 6XS, United Kingdom. TEL 44-1256-329242, FAX 44-1256-328339, subscriptions@nature.com, http://www.nature.com/ijir. Eds. A Melman, G Wagner. Pub. Sue Deeley. R&P Trace Noel. Adv. contact Robert Sloan TEL 44-20-8882-7199.

616.6 AUS ISSN 0919-8172 CODEN: IJURF3
INTERNATIONAL JOURNAL OF UROLOGY. Text in English. 1994. m. AUD 352 domestic to individuals; AUD 320 in New Zealand to individuals; USD 195 elsewhere to individuals; AUD 1,172 domestic to institutions; AUD 1,066 in New Zealand to institutions; JPY 67,500 in Japan to institutions; USD 650 elsewhere to institutions; AUD 388 domestic to individuals paper & online eds. combined; AUD 352 in New Zealand to individuals paper & online eds. combined; USD 215 elsewhere to individuals paper & online eds. combined; AUD 1,290 domestic to institutions paper & online eds. combined; AUD 1,173 in New Zealand to institutions paper & online eds. combined; JPY 74,250 in Japan to institutions paper & online eds. combined; USD 715 elsewhere to institutions paper & online eds. combined (effective 2001). adv. *Refereed.* **Document type:** *Academic/Scholarly.* **Description:** Covers the latest clinical and experimental developments in the field of urology.
Related titles: Online - full text ed.: ISSN 1442-2042. 1999. AUD 317 domestic to individuals; AUD 288 in New Zealand to individuals; USD 176 elsewhere to individuals; AUD 1,055 domestic to institutions; AUD 960 in New Zealand to institutions; JPY 60,750 in Japan to institutions; USD 585 elsewhere to institutions (effective 2001) (from EBSCO Publishing, O C L C Online Computer Library Center, Inc., RoweCom Information Quest, ingenta, Munksgaard & Blackwell Science's Synergy, Swets Blackwell, Institute for Scientific Information).
Indexed: Curr.Cont., Excerp.Med. (1996-), INIS Atomind., Ind.Med. (1994-), Inpharma, Int.Abstr.Biol.Sci., Nutr.Abstr., Pharm.&Out.News, Reac., Rev.Med.& Vet.Mycol.
—BLDSC (4542.697100), ADONIS, CISTI, GNLM, IDS, ingenta, KNAW.
Published by: (Japanese Urological Association/Shadan Hojin, Nihon Hinyokika Gakkai JPN), Blackwell Science Asia Pty Ltd, PO Box 378, Carlton South, VIC 3053, Australia. TEL 61-3-9347-0300, FAX 61-3-9347-5001, info@blacksci-asia.com.au; jpurol@mb.infoweb.ne.jp, http://www.blacksci.co.uk. Ed. As Yoshio. R&P Chris Hum. Adv. contact Kathryn O'Brien. Circ: 4,027 (paid).

616.6 USA ISSN 0276-2315
INTERNATIONAL PERSPECTIVES IN UROLOGY. Text in English. 1981. irreg., latest vol.14. **Document type:** *Monographic series.*
—CISTI.
Published by: Lippincott Williams & Wilkins (Philadelphia) (Subsidiary of: Wolters Kluwer N.V.), 530 Walnut St, Philadelphia, PA 19106-3621. TEL 215-521-8300, FAX 215-521-8902, http://services.lww.com/websites/journalsites.cfm. **Subscr. to:** PO Box 1600, Hagerstown, MD 21740-1600. TEL 800-777-2295, FAX 301-824-7390.

M

616.6 GRC
INTERNATIONAL SATELLITE SYMPOSIUM ON ACUTE RENAL FAILURE. PROCEEDINGS. Text in Greek. 1960. biennial. USD 100 (effective 1995-1996). *Refereed.* **Document type:** *Proceedings, Academic/Scholarly.*
Formerly: International Congress of Nephrology. Abstracts of Reports and Communications (0074-3771)
Indexed: Chem.Abstr.
Published by: International Society of Nephrology, Commission on Acute Renal Failure, Hippokration General Hospital, 50 Papanastasiou St, Thessaloniki 543 42, Greece. TEL 30-31-835955, FAX 30-31-861111. Ed. Menelaos Papadimitriou. **Co-sponsors:** Hellenic Society of Nephrology; Aristotelian University.

616.6 FRA ISSN 0074-8579
INTERNATIONAL SOCIETY OF UROLOGY. REPORTS OF CONGRESS. (Reports published in host country) Text in French. irreg., latest 1975, 17th, Madrid. **Document type:** *Proceedings.*
Published by: International Society of Urology, c/o Prof. Rene Kuess, 63 av. Niel, Paris 75017, France.

INTERNATIONAL UROGYNECOLOGY JOURNAL. see *MEDICAL SCIENCES—Obstetrics And Gynecology*

616.6 NLD ISSN 0301-1623
CODEN: IURNAE
INTERNATIONAL UROLOGY AND NEPHROLOGY. Text in English. 1969. bi-m. EUR 570, USD 571 to institutions for print or online ed.; EUR 684, USD 682.20 to institutions for print & online eds.combined (effective 2002). adv. bk.rev. back issues avail. *Refereed.* **Document type:** *Journal, Academic/Scholarly.* **Description:** Publishes original papers, preliminary reports and reviews which contribute to progress in urological surgery, nephrology and andrology.
Incorporates (1991-2000): Geriatric Nephrology and Urology (0924-8455); Formerly (until 1970): Urology and Nephrology (0042-1162)
Related titles: Online - full text ed.: (from EBSCO Publishing, O C L C Online Computer Library Center, Inc., RoweCom Information Quest, Swets Blackwell, Kluwer Online).
Indexed: Biol.Abstr., Chem.Abstr., Curr.Cont. (coverage dropped), Excerp.Med., INIS Atomind., Ind.Med. (1970-).
—BLDSC (4551.568000), CASDDS, CISTI, EMDOCS, GNLM, ingenta, KNAW. **CCC.**
Published by: Kluwer Academic Publishers Group (Subsidiary of: Wolters Kluwer N.V.), Spuiboulevard 50, PO Box 17, Dordrecht 3300 AA, Netherlands. TEL 31-78-639-2392, FAX 31-78-654-2254, services@wkap.nl, http://www.wkap.nl/journalhome.htm/0301-1623. Eds. Dimitrios G Oreopoulos, Jozsef Kondas. **Subscr. in the Americas to:** Kluwer Academic - Plenum Publishers, 233 Spring St, New York, NY 10013-1578. TEL 212-620-8468, FAX 212-807-1047; **Subscr. to:** Journals Department, PO Box 322, Dordrecht 3300 AH, Netherlands. TEL 31-78-639-2392, FAX 31-78-654-6474.

616.6 DEU ISSN 0921-9862
RC902.A1
INTERNATIONAL YEARBOOK OF NEPHROLOGY. Text in English. 1989. a., latest 1993. back issues avail. **Document type:** *Academic/Scholarly.*
Related titles: Online - full text ed.: (from Institute for Scientific Information).
Indexed: ASCA, Sci.Cit.Ind.
—BLDSC (4552.334000), GNLM.
Published by: Springer-Verlag (Subsidiary of: BertelsmannSpringer), Haber Str 7, Heidelberg 69126, Germany. FAX 49-30-82787448, subscriptions@springer.de, http://www.springer.de, http://link.springer-ny.com. **Subscr. in N. America to:** Springer-Verlag New York Inc., PO Box 2485, Secaucus, NJ 07096-2485. TEL 212-460-1500.

616.6 USA
▼ **THE INTERNET JOURNAL OF UROLOGY.** Text in English. 2000. s-a. free per issue. adv. bk.rev. back issues avail. *Refereed.* **Document type:** *Academic/Scholarly.* **Description:** Provides information from the field of urology; contains original articles, reviews, case reports, streaming slide shows, streaming videos, letters to the editor, press releases and meeting information.
Published by: Internet Scientific Publications, L.L.C., 23 Rippling Creek Dr, Sugar Land, TX 77479. TEL 281-240-1533, FAX 281-240-1533, http://www.ispub.com/. Ed. Chris Wood. R&P Hope Morrow TEL 832-754-0335.

616.6 ITA ISSN 1121-8428
J N: JOURNAL OF NEPHROLOGY. Text in English. 1988. bi-m. EUR 184 in Europe to individuals; USD 210 elsewhere to individuals; EUR 227 in Europe to institutions; USD 250 elsewhere to institutions (effective 2001). adv. abstr, bibl, charts, illus. Index. 64 p./no. back issues avail.; reprints avail. *Refereed.* **Document type:** *Journal, Academic/Scholarly.*
Formerly (until 1992): Journal of Nephrology (1120-3625)
Related titles: Online - full text ed.: (from Institute for Scientific Information).
Indexed: ASCA, Curr.Cont., Excerp.Med. (1994-), Ind.Med. (1988-), Inpharma, Kidney, Pharm.&Out.News, Reac., Ref.Zh.
—BLDSC (5021.399400), CISTI, EMDOCS, GNLM, IDS, Infotrieve, KNAW. **CCC.**
Published by: Wichtig Editore s.r.l., Via Friuli, 72, Milan, MI 20135, Italy. TEL 39-02-55195443, FAX 39-02-55195971, info@wichtig-publisher.com, http://www.wichtig-publisher.com/jn. Ed. Dr. G D'Amico. Pub. Dr. Diego Brancaccio. R&P, Adv. contact Lucia Steele. color page USD 1,450; trim 21 x 28. Circ: 2,000 (paid); 2,600 (controlled).

616.6 DEU ISSN 0932-1624
JAHRBUCH DER UROLOGIE (YEAR). Text in German. 1986. a. **Document type:** *Academic/Scholarly.*
—BLDSC (4632.650120).
Published by: Med. Hochschule Hannover, Klinik und Poliklinik fuer Urologie, Konstanty-Gutschow-Str 8, Hannover 30625, Germany. Ed. M Truss.

616.6 JPN ISSN 0914-6180
JAPANESE JOURNAL OF UROLOGICAL SURGERY. Text in Japanese. 1988. m.
Published by: Igaku Tosho Shuppan Co. Ltd., 2-28-1 Tohgane Bldg, Hongo, Bunkyo-ku, Tokyo 113-0033, Japan.

616.6 JPN ISSN 0021-5287
CODEN: NGKZA6
THE JAPANESE JOURNAL OF UROLOGY/NIHON HINYOKIKA GAKKAI ZASSHI. Text in Japanese; Summaries in English. 1911. m. JPY 20,000. adv. reprint service avail. from PQC.
Related titles: Microform ed.: (from PQC).
Indexed: C.I.S. Abstr., Curr.Cont. (coverage dropped), Excerp.Med., INIS Atomind., Ind.Med. (1917-).
—BLDSC (4659.050000), CASDDS, CISTI, GNLM, IDS, KNAW.
Published by: Japanese Urological Association, Faculty of Medicine/Nihon Hinyokika Gakkai, Taisei Bldg, 3-14-10 Hongo, Bunkyo-ku, Tokyo 113-0033, Japan. FAX 81-3-3814-4117. Ed., Pub. Kazuki Kawabe. Circ: 5,500.

616.6 DEU ISSN 1432-5179
JATROS URO. Text in German. 1986. 12/yr. DEM 140 (effective 1998). back issues avail. **Document type:** *Academic/Scholarly.* **Description:** Seminar papers with summaries of original articles, interviews and congress reports.
Former titles: Jatros Urologie, Nephrologie und Andrologie (0941-4789); (until 1992): Jatros Urologie - Nephrologie (0941-391X); (until 1989): Jatros Urologie (0178-7527)
—GNLM. **CCC.**
Published by: Hoffmann und Hoffmann GmbH, August-Schanz-Str 8-II, Frankfurt A.m. 60433, Germany. TEL 49-69-54800015, FAX 49-69-54800080, huhgmbh@aol.com. Ed. Peter Hoffmann. Circ: 2,500.

JIN TO TOSEKI/KIDNEY AND DIALYSIS. see *MEDICAL SCIENCES*

616.6 FRA ISSN 0248-0018
CODEN: JOURDD
JOURNAL D'UROLOGIE. Text in French. 1912. 6/yr. FRF 990; FRF 1,197 foreign (effective 1997). adv. bk.rev. abstr, illus. index. reprint service avail. from ISI. *Refereed.* **Document type:** *Academic/Scholarly.* **Description:** Publishes original articles, topical outlines, clinical and therapeutic data and meeting reports.
Formerly: Journal d'Urologie et de Nephrologie (0021-8200)
Related titles: Microform ed.: (from PQC).
Indexed: ASCA, Chem.Abstr., Curr.Adv.Cancer Res., Curr.Cont. (coverage dropped), Excerp.Med., Helminthol.Abstr., INIS Atomind., Ind.Med. (coverage dropped), Ind.Sci.Rev., Inpharma, Nutr.Abstr., Reac., Sci.Cit.Ind. (coverage dropped).
—CISTI, EMDOCS, GNLM, IDS, Infotrieve. **CCC.**
Published by: Masson - Periodiques, 120 bd. St. Germain, Paris 75006, France. TEL 33-1-40466200, FAX 33-1-40466201. Ed. B Debre. Circ: 2,100. **Subscr. to:** Societe de Periodiques Specialises, BP 22, Vineuil Cedex 41354, France. TEL 33-2-54504612, FAX 33-2-54504611.

616.6 DEU
JOURNAL FUER DAS NEPHROLOGISCHE TEAM. Text in German; Summaries in English, German. 1983. q. EUR 20; EUR 7.50 newsstand/cover (effective 2001). adv. bk.rev. back issues avail. *Refereed.* **Document type:** *Journal, Academic/Scholarly.* **Description:** Contains original articles and case reports on nephrology and dialysis.
Formerly: Nierenpatient (0176-5183)
—GNLM.
Published by: Pabst Science Publishers, Am Eichengrund 28, Lengerich 49525, Germany. TEL 49-5484-308, FAX 49-5484-550, pabst.publishers@t-online.de, http://www.pabst-publishers.de/jai/. Ed. Wolfgang Pabst. Circ: 12,600.

616.6 AUT ISSN 1023-6090
JOURNAL FUER UROLOGIE UND UROGYNAEKOLOGIE; Zeitschrift fuer Urologie und Urogynaekologie in Klinik und Praxis. Text in German. 1994. q. ATS 400; ATS 120 newsstand/cover (effective 2001). adv. abstr, bibl. back issues avail. *Refereed.* **Document type:** *Journal, Academic/Scholarly.* **Description:** Contains research articles on various aspects of urology.
—BLDSC (5071.875000).
Published by: Krause & Pachernegg GmbH, Mozartgasse 10, Gablitz 3003, Austria. TEL 43-2231-61258-0, FAX 43-2231-6125810, k_u_p@eunet.at, http://members.eunet.at/k_u_p/uro.htm, http://members.eunet.at/k_u_p/verlag.htm. Ed. Dr. Franz Fischl.

JOURNAL OF ANDROLOGY. see *MEDICAL SCIENCES*

616.6 USA ISSN 0892-7790
CODEN: JENDE3
JOURNAL OF ENDOUROLOGY. Text in English. 1987. 10/yr., latest vol.16, 2002. USD 187 domestic to individuals; USD 278 foreign to individuals; USD 224 domestic to individuals print and online eds. combined; USD 315 foreign to individuals print and online eds. combined; USD 477 domestic to institutions; USD 588 foreign to institutions; USD 572 domestic to institutions print and online eds. combined; USD 683 foreign to institutions print and online eds. combined (effective 2002). back issues avail.; reprints avail. *Refereed.* **Document type:** *Journal, Academic/Scholarly.* **Description:** Covers topics, including percutaneous renal and ureteral procedures, ureteroscopy for diagnostic and therapeutic indications, endoscopic use of lasers, and extracorporeal lithotripsy of renal and uretheral stones.
Related titles: Online - full content ed.: USD 477 to institutions; USD 187 to individuals (effective 2002) (from Swets Blackwell); Online - full text ed.: (from CatchWord Ltd., Institute for Scientific Information, RoweCom Information Quest).
Indexed: ASCA, Curr.Cont., Excerp.Med. (1993-), Ind.Med. (1987-), Inpharma, Pharm.&Out.News, Reac., Sci.Cit.Ind.
—BLDSC (4978.210000), CISTI, EMDOCS, GNLM, IDS, ingenta, KNAW. **CCC.**
Published by: (Endourological Society), Mary Ann Liebert, Inc. Publishers, 2 Madison Ave, Larchmont, NY 10538. TEL 914—834-3100, FAX 914-834-1388, info@liebertpub.com, http://www.liebertpub.com/end. Eds. Dr. Arthur D Smith, Dr. Ralph V Clayman.

JOURNAL OF LOWER GENITAL TRACT DISEASE. see *MEDICAL SCIENCES—Obstetrics And Gynecology*

JOURNAL OF LOWER GENITAL TRACT DISEASE ONLINE. see *MEDICAL SCIENCES—Obstetrics And Gynecology*

616.6 360 USA
JOURNAL OF NEPHROLOGY SOCIAL WORK. Text in English. 1977. a. USD 10 to non-members (effective 2000); free to members. **Document type:** *Journal, Academic/Scholarly.* **Description:** Official journal of the Council of Nephrology Social Workers of the NKF compiles significant original and recently published articles relating to the practice of nephrology social work.
Formerly: C N S W Perspectives
Published by: National Kidney Foundation, Council of Nephrology Social Workers, 30 E 33rd St, New York, NY 10016. TEL 212-889-2210, http://www.kidney.org. Circ: 900.

JOURNAL OF RENAL NUTRITION. see *NUTRITION AND DIETETICS*

M

616.6 USA ISSN 1054-8734
CODEN: JUPAEE
JOURNAL OF UROGENITAL PATHOLOGY. Text in English. 1991. q. USD 125 to individuals; USD 155 to institutions. bk.rev. *Refereed.* **Document type:** *Academic/Scholarly.*
Indexed: Excerp.Med. (1993-1995).
—EMDOCS, GNLM.
Published by: Field & Wood, Medical Periodicals, Inc., PO Box 975, Blue Bell, PA 19422. TEL 610-828-4010, FAX 215-482-0226. Ed. Dr. Ivan Damjanov.

616.6 USA ISSN 1067-1919
JOURNAL OF UROLOGIC PATHOLOGY. Text in English. 1993. bi-m. USD 440 domestic; USD 490 foreign (effective 2000). adv. bk.rev. illus. index. *Refereed.* **Document type:** *Journal, Academic/Scholarly.* **Description:** Provides the latest information on pathology of the genitourinary tract. The primary emphasis is on diseases that clinically fall under the domain of urologists, urologic oncologists, and andrologists.
Indexed: Curr.Cont. (coverage dropped), Sci.Cit.Ind. (coverage dropped).
—BLDSC (5071.730000), CISTI, GNLM, KNAW. **CCC.**
Published by: (International Society of Urological Pathology), Humana Press Inc., 999 Riverview Dr, Ste 208, Totowa, NJ 07512. TEL 973-256-1699, FAX 973-256-8341, humana@humanapr.com, http://humanapress.com. Ed. Dr. John N Eble. R&P Richard Hruska. Adv. contact Thomas B Lanigan Jr. **Dist. in Japan by:** Maruzen Co., Ltd., International Division, Export Dept, P.O. Box 5050, Tokyo International 100-3191, Japan. TEL 81-3-3275-8591.

616.6 USA ISSN 0022-5347
RC870 CODEN: JOURAA
JOURNAL OF UROLOGY. Text in English. 1917. m. USD 462 domestic to individuals for print & online eds.; USD 619 foreign to individuals for print & online eds; USD 510 domestic to institutions for print & online eds; USD 667 foreign to institutions for print & online eds; USD 55 newsstand/cover (effective 2002). adv. abstr, bibl, illus. index. *Refereed.* **Document type:** *Academic/Scholarly.* **Description:** Publishes clinical papers, commentary, research and new techniques for the urologist.
Incorporates (in Jan. 1982): Investigation Urology (0021-0005); Urological Survey (0042-1146)
Related titles: CD-ROM ed.: (from Ovid Technologies, Inc.); Microfilm ed.: (from WWS); Online - full text ed.: USD 663 domestic academic site license; USD 820 foreign academic site license; USD 739.50 domestic corporate site license; USD 896.50 foreign corporate site license (effective 2002) (from Ovid Technologies, Inc., EBSCO Publishing, Swets Blackwell, Institute for Scientific Information); ♦ Spanish Translation: Journal of Urology (Edicion Espanola). ISSN 1133-8245.
Indexed: AIM, ASCA, Agri.& Environ.Biotech.Abstr. (coverage dropped), Biol.Abstr., C.I.S. Abstr., Cal.Tiss.Abstr. (coverage dropped), Chem.Abstr., Chem.Indus.Notes, Chem.Titles, Curr.Adv.Cancer Res., Curr.Adv.Cell & Devel.Biol., Curr.Adv.Ecol.Sci., Curr.Adv.Gen.& Molec.Biol., Curr.Cont., Derwent Biotech.Abstr., Excerp.Med., Helminthol.Abstr., INIS Atomind., Ind.Med. (1917-), Ind.Sci.Rev., Ind.Vet., Inpharma, Int.Abstr.Biol.Sci., Int.Nurs.Ind., Kidney, Med.& Surg.Dermat., NRN, Neurosci.Cit.Ind., Nutr.Abstr., Pharm.&Out.News, Protozool.Abstr., Reac., Rev.Med.& Vet.Mycol., Rev.Plant Path., SSCI (coverage dropped), Sci.Cit.Ind., THA.
—BLDSC (5071.900000), CASDDS, CISTI, GNLM, IDS, ingenta, KNAW.
Published by: (American Urological Association), Williams & Wilkins (Subsidiary of: Waverly International), 351 W Camden St, Baltimore, MD 21201-2436. TEL 410-528-4068, 800-222-3790, FAX 410-528-4452, stauber@wwilkins.com, http://www.Lww.com. Ed. Dr. Jay T Gillenwater. Adv. contact Steve Tauber. B&W page USD 2,275; trim 10.88 x 8.13. Circ: 19,008; 18,571 (paid).

616.6 ESP ISSN 1133-8245
JOURNAL OF UROLOGY (EDICION ESPANOLA). Text in Spanish. 1994. bi-m. **Document type:** *Academic/Scholarly.* **Description:** Explores clinical and research topics in urology.
Related titles: ♦ Translation of: Journal of Urology. ISSN 0022-5347.
Indexed: Tox.Abstr. (coverage dropped).
Published by: (American Urology Association USA), Saned S.A., Capitan Haya, 60, Madrid 28020, Spain. TEL 34-91-749-9507, FAX 34-91-749-9507, saned@meditex.es. Ed. Dr. Resel Estevez. adv.: page ESP 245,000. Circ: 3,000.

616.6 CHE ISSN 1420-4096
CODEN: RPBIEL
KIDNEY AND BLOOD PRESSURE RESEARCH. Text in French. 1979. bi-m. CHF 999, EUR 713.80 in Europe to institutions; CHF 1,016.40, USD 777 elsewhere to institutions (effective 2002). adv. bk.rev. illus. index. back issues avail. *Refereed.* **Document type:** *Journal, Academic/Scholarly.* **Description:** Comprises both clinical and basic studies at the interface of nephrology and cardiovascular research.
Former titles (until 1996): Renal Physiology and Biochemistry (1011-6524); (until 1989): Renal Physiology (0378-5858)
Related titles: Microfilm ed.; Microform ed.: (from PQC); Online - full text ed.: ISSN 1423-0143. CHF 58, EUR 42, USD 45 to institutions with print edition (effective 2002) (from EBSCO Publishing, O C L C Online Computer Library Center, Inc., RoweCom Information Quest, ProQuest Information & Learning, Swets Blackwell, Institute for Scientific Information).
Indexed: ASCA, Biol.Abstr., Chem.Abstr., Chem.Titles, Curr.Adv.Ecol.Sci., Curr.Cont., Excerp.Med., Ind.Med. (1996-), Inpharma, Nutr.Abstr., Pharm.&Out.News, Reac., Rev.Med.& Vet.Mycol., Sci.Cit.Ind.
—BLDSC (5094.207500), CASDDS, CISTI, EMDOCS, GNLM, IDS, Infotrieve, ingenta, KNAW. **CCC.**
Published by: (Gesellschaft fuer Nephrologie), S. Karger AG, Allschwilerstr 10, PO Box, Basel 4009, Switzerland. TEL 41-61-306-1111, FAX 41-61-306-1234, karger@karger.ch, http://www.online.karger.com/journals/kbr, http://www.karger.com. Eds. C Bauer, K H Rahn, W H Hoerl. adv.: page USD 1,205. Circ: 800.
Co-sponsors: Deutsche Liga zur Bekaempfung des hohen Blutdruckes e.V.; Deutsche Hypertonie Gesellschaft.

616.6 USA ISSN 0270-062X
CODEN: KIDID6
KIDNEY DISEASES. Text in English. 1979. irreg., latest vol.10, 1992. price varies. adv. *Refereed.* **Document type:** *Monographic series.*
Indexed: Chem.Abstr.
—BLDSC (5094.230000), CASDDS, CISTI. **CCC.**
Published by: Marcel Dekker, Inc., Attn: Eridania Perrez, 270 Madison Ave, New York, NY 10016-0602. TEL 212-696-9000, 800-228-1160, FAX 212-685-4540, marketing@dekker.com, http://www.dekker.com. Pub. Russell Dekker. R&P Julia Mulligan. Adv. contact Eridania Perez.

616.6 GBR ISSN 1369-3050
KIDNEY FORUM. Text in English. 1998. quadrennial. GBP 60, USD 100 to individuals; GBP 210, USD 350 to institutions; GBP 30, USD 50 to students (2001). *Refereed.* **Document type:** *Academic/Scholarly.*
—BLDSC (5094.280000). **CCC.**
Published by: Sheffield Academic Press Ltd, Mansion House, 19 Kingfield Rd, Sheffield, S Yorks S11 9AS, United Kingdom. TEL 44-114-255-4433, FAX 44-114-255-4626, SSanderson@sheffac.demon.co.uk.

616.6 USA ISSN 0085-2538
RC902.A1 CODEN: KDYIA5
KIDNEY INTERNATIONAL. Text in English. 1972. m. (in 2 vols.). USD 700 domestic to individuals; USD 700 foreign to individuals; USD 1,050 domestic to institutions; USD 1,050 foreign to institutions; USD 770 to individuals print & online eds. combined; USD 1,155 to institutions print & online eds. combined (effective 2001). adv. back issues avail.; reprint service avail. from ISI. *Refereed.* **Document type:** *Academic/Scholarly.* **Description:** Provides current information on renal physiology, biochemistry, pathology, immunology and morphology.
Related titles: Microform ed.: (from PQC); Online - full text ed.: Kidney International Online. ISSN 1523-1755. USD 630 to individuals; USD 945 to institutions (effective 2001) (from Ovid Technologies, Inc., EBSCO Publishing, O C L C Online Computer Library Center, Inc., RoweCom Information Quest, ingenta, Munksgaard & Blackwell Science's Synergy, Swets Blackwell, Institute for Scientific Information); ♦ Supplement: Kidney International. Supplement. ISSN 0098-6577.
Indexed: ASCA, Abstr.Hyg., Biol.Abstr., Chem.Abstr., Chem.Indus.Notes, Chem.Titles, Curr.Adv.Ecol.Sci., Curr.Cont., Dairy Sci.Abstr., Diab.Cont., Excerp.Med., INIS Atomind., Ind.Med. (1972-), Ind.Sci.Rev., Inpharma, Int.Abstr.Biol.Sci., Kidney, Neurosci.Cit.Ind., Nutr.Abstr., Pharm.&Out.News, Reac., Sci.Cit.Ind., THA, Trop.Dis.Bull.
—BLDSC (5094.300000), ADONIS, CASDDS, CISTI, GNLM, IDS, ingenta, KNAW. **CCC.**
Published by: (International Society of Nephrology), Blackwell Science Inc., Commerce Pl, 350 Main St, Malden, MA 02148-5018. TEL 781-388-8250, 800-759-6102, FAX 781-388-8255, journals@blacksci.com, http://www.blackwell-science.com. Ed. Dr. Thomas E Andreoli. R&P Tracey Davies. Adv. contact Jenny Applin. Circ: 9,000.

616.6 USA ISSN 0098-6577
CODEN: KISUDF
KIDNEY INTERNATIONAL. SUPPLEMENT. Text in English. 1974. irreg. price varies. reprint service avail. from ISI. **Document type:** *Academic/Scholarly.*
Related titles: Online - full text ed.: (from Ovid Technologies, Inc., Swets Blackwell); ♦ Supplement to: Kidney International. ISSN 0085-2538.
Indexed: Biol.Abstr., Chem.Abstr., Chem.Titles, Excerp.Med. (1993-), INIS Atomind., Ind.Med. (1974-), Int.Abstr.Biol.Sci., Nutr.Abstr.
—BLDSC (5094.301000), ADONIS, CASDDS, CISTI, ingenta, KNAW. **CCC.**
Published by: (International Society of Nephrology), Blackwell Science Inc., Commerce Pl, 350 Main St, Malden, MA 02148-5018. TEL 781-388-8250, 800-759-6102, FAX 781-388-8255, journals@blacksci.com, http://www.blackwell-science.com. R&P Tracey Davies.

KIDNEY (NEW YORK, 1992); a current survey of world literature. see *MEDICAL SCIENCES—Abstracting, Bibliographies, Statistics*

616.6 DEU ISSN 0174-2752
CODEN: KEURDM
KLINISCHE UND EXPERIMENTELLE UROLOGIE. Text in German. 1980. irreg., latest vol.25, 1995. back issues avail. **Document type:** *Academic/Scholarly.*
Indexed: Chem.Abstr., Chem.Titles.
—CASDDS, CISTI.
Published by: W. Zuckschwerdt Verlag GmbH, Industriestr 1, Germering 82110, Germany. TEL 49-89-894349-0, FAX 49-89-89434950. Eds. A Hofstetter, M Kriegmair. Circ: 1,500.

616.6 JPN ISSN 0919-5491
KONYOUSANKESSHO TO TSUFU/HYPERURICEMIA AND GOUT. Text in Japanese. 1993. 2/yr. JPY 1,900 per issue (effective 1998).
Published by: Medikaru Rebyusha/Medical Review Co., Ltd., 7-3 Hirano-Machi 1-chome, Chuo-ku, Osaka-shi 541-0046, Japan. TEL 81-6-223-1667, FAX 81-6-223-1338, meview@osk3.3web.ne.jp.

616.6 ITA
LETTERA DI UROLOGIA. Text in Italian. 1989. bi-m. adv.
Formerly (until 1989): Lettera di Uroginecologia (1120-0456)
Published by: C I C Edizioni Internazionali s.r.l., Corso Trieste 42, Rome, RM 00198, Italy. TEL 39-06-8412673, FAX 39-06-8412688, info@gruppocic.it, 1160199510. Ed. A Salvati. adv.: B&W page ITL 3,100,000, color page ITL 3,900,000; trim 210 x 290.

616.6 HUN ISSN 0864-8921
MAGYAR UROLOGIA. Text in Hungarian. 1974. 4/yr. **Document type:** *Academic/Scholarly.*
Formerly (until 1989): Urologiai es Nephrologiai Szemle (0133-3127)
Indexed: Excerp.Med., INIS Atomind.
—BLDSC (5351.015000), EMDOCS, GNLM.
Published by: Society of Hungarian Urological Surgeons, Nagyerdei korut 98, PO Box 29, Debrecen 4012, Hungary.

616.6 ITA ISSN 0393-2249
CODEN: MINEAT
MINERVA UROLOGICA E NEFROLOGICA; rivista trimestrale di fisiopatologia e clinica delle malattie renali e di urologia medica e chirurgica. Text in Italian; Summaries in English, Italian. 1949. q. USD 105 to individuals; USD 155 to institutions (effective 2000 - 2001). adv. bk.rev. bibl, charts, illus. index. *Refereed.* **Description:** Covers pathophysiology and clinical medicine of renal disease and medical and surgical urology.
Formed by the merger of (1949-1983): Minerva Urologica (0026-4989); (1954-1983): Minerva Nefrologica (0026-4873)
Related titles: Microform ed.: (from PQC).
Indexed: Biol.Abstr., Chem.Abstr., Excerp.Med., Ind.Med. (1984-).
—BLDSC (5794.720000), CASDDS, CISTI, EMDOCS, GNLM, KNAW.

Published by: Edizioni Minerva Medica, Corso Bramante, 83-85, Turin, TO 10126, Italy. TEL 39-11-678282, FAX 39-11-674502. Eds. A Tizzani, P Stratta. Pub. Alberto Oliaro. Adv. contact F Filippo. B&W page USD 1,200, color page USD 2,000; trim 270 x 190. Circ: 3,000 (paid).

616.6 JPN ISSN 0910-2329
NAGANOKEN JINKO TOSEKI KENKYUKAISHI/NAGANO PREFECTURAL SOCIETY OF DIALYSIS THERAPY. JOURNAL. Text in English, Japanese; Summaries in English. 1978. a.
Published by: Naganoken Jinko Toseki Kenkyukai, Koseiren Saku Sogo Byoin, 197, Usuda, Usudamachi, Minamisaku-gun, Nakano-shi, Nagano-ken 384-03, Japan.

616.6 USA
NATIONAL KIDNEY FOUNDATION. ANNUAL MEETING PROGRAM. Text in English. a. free per issue to qualified personnel. **Document type:** *Proceedings.* **Description:** Contains the agenda of all sessions of the NKF annual meeting, including scientific council programs, and summaries of papers submitted for presentation.
Formerly: National Kidney Foundation. Programs and Abstracts Book
Published by: National Kidney Foundation, 30 East 33rd St, New York, NY 10016. TEL 212-889-2210.

616.6 USA ISSN 0077-5096
NATIONAL KIDNEY FOUNDATION. ANNUAL REPORT. Text in English. 1957. a. free per issue.
Published by: National Kidney Foundation, 30 East 33rd St, New York, NY 10016. TEL 212-889-2210.

616.6 USA
NATIONAL KIDNEY FOUNDATION. PROCEEDINGS BOOK. Text in English. a. USD 10 (effective 2000). abstr. **Document type:** *Proceedings.* **Description:** Contains agendas of all clinical nephrology meetings including consultative nephrology; primary care nephrology; dietitian, social worker and nurses and technicians' sessions. Also includes summary papers of presentations.
Published by: National Kidney Foundation, 30 East 33rd St, New York, NY 10016. TEL 212-889-2210, http://www.kidney.org.

616.6 USA
NATIONAL KIDNEY FOUNDATION. RESEARCH PROGRAM. Text in English. a. free per issue. **Document type:** *Directory.* **Description:** Lists information on research projects supported by the NKF, with biographies of investigators and summaries of research reports.
Published by: National Kidney Foundation, 30 East 33rd St, New York, NY 10016. TEL 212-889-2210.

616.6 NLD ISSN 0929-0184
CODEN: NTURE
NEDERLANDS TIJDSCHRIFT VOOR UROLOGIE. Text in Dutch. 1993. q. NLG 75 foreign to members. adv. *Refereed.* **Document type:** *Academic/Scholarly, Trade.* **Description:** Informs urologists and urologists in training of developments in their field and alerts members to association news and forthcoming congresses and symposia.
Indexed: Excerp.Med. (1995-).
—BLDSC (6072.470000), GNLM, KNAW.
Published by: (Nederlandse Vereniging voor Urologie), Elsevier Gezondheidszorg B.V., Tijdstroom (Subsidiary of: Reed Elsevier plc Group), Planetenbaan 1, Maarssen 3600 AK, Netherlands. TEL 31-346-577577, FAX 31-346-554287, http://www.tijdstroom.nl. Ed. E Boeve. Adv. contact C Nieuwlands. Circ: 500. **Subscr. to:** Elsevier Den Haag, Postbus 16500, The Hague 2500 BM, Netherlands. TEL 31-70-381-9900, FAX 31-70-333-8399.

616.6 ESP ISSN 0211-6995
NEFROLOGIA. Text in Spanish. 6/yr. *Refereed.*
Related titles: Online - full text ed.: (from Institute for Scientific Information).
Indexed: ASCA, Curr.Cont., Excerp.Med., Ind.Med. (1981-), Inpharma, Pharm.&Out.News, Reac., SSCI (coverage dropped).
—BLDSC (6075.150500), CISTI, GNLM, IDS, Infotrieve, KNAW. **CCC.**
Published by: Grupo Aula Medica S.A., C.I. Venecia 2 Alfa III, Isabel Colbrand, 10-12, Madrid 28050, Spain. TEL 34-1-3588657, FAX 34-1-3589067. Eds. Dr. Rafael Matesanz, J M Culebras.

616.6 BGR ISSN 0204-6105
NEFROLOGIIA, HEMODIALIZA I TRANSPLANTATSIIA. Text in Bulgarian; Summaries in Bulgarian, English. 1995. q., latest vol.6, 2000. BGL 6 domestic; USD 60 foreign (effective 2001). bk.rev. abstr, bibl. 56 p./no. *Refereed.* **Document type:** *Journal, Bibliography, Abstract/Index.* **Description:** Publishes original articles by Bulgarian authors in the fields of nephrology, hemodialysis and kidney transplantation.
Indexed: Ref.Zh.
Published by: Meditsinski Universitet - Sofia, Tsentur za Informatsiia po Meditsina/Medical University - Sofia, Medical Information Center, 1 Sv Georgi Sofiiski ul, Sofia 1431, Bulgaria. TEL 359-2-9522342, FAX 359-2-9522393, mutafov@sun.medun.acad.bg, http://www.medun.acad.bg. Ed. Dr. Z Kiriakov. R&P, Adv. contact Dr. Christo Mutafov. Circ: 500.

616.6 CHE ISSN 0250-4960
CODEN: NEPHDY
NEPHROLOGIE. Text in French. 1980. 6/yr. CHF 120, EUR 77.92 to individuals; CHF 180, EUR 116.88 to institutions (effective 2002). adv. bk.rev. *Refereed.* **Document type:** *Journal, Academic/Scholarly.*
Related titles: Online - full text ed.: (from Institute for Scientific Information).
Indexed: ASCA, Biol.Abstr., Chem.Abstr., Chem.Indus.Notes, Chem.Titles, Curr.Cont., Excerp.Med., Ind.Med. (1980-), Inpharma, Int.Nurs.Ind., Pharm.&Out.News, Reac.
—BLDSC (6075.677000), CASDDS, CISTI, EMDOCS, GNLM, IDS, Infotrieve, KNAW. **CCC.**
Published by: Editions Medecine et Hygiene, Case Postale 456, Geneva, 4 1211, Switzerland. TEL 41-22-7029311, FAX 41-22-7029355, abonnements@medhyg.ch, http://www.medhyg.ch. Circ: 1,100.

616.6 AUS ISSN 1320-5358
CODEN: NEPHF2
NEPHROLOGY. Text in English. 1995. q. AUD 720 domestic to institutions; AUD 654 in New Zealand to institutions; USD 399 elsewhere to institutions; AUD 792 domestic to institutions paper & online eds. combined; AUD 720 in New Zealand to institutions paper & online eds. combined; USD 439 elsewhere to institutions paper & online eds. combined (effective 2001). adv. back issues avail. *Refereed.* **Document type:** *Academic/Scholarly.* **Description:** Publishes research covering the clinical and experimental aspects of nephrology.
Related titles: Online - full text ed.: Nephrology Online. ISSN 1440-1797. AUD 648 domestic to institutions; AUD 589 in New Zealand to institutions; USD 360 elsewhere to institutions (effective 2001) (from EBSCO Publishing, ingenta, Munksgaard & Blackwell Science's Synergy, Swets Blackwell, Institute for Scientific Information, RoweCom Information Quest).
Indexed: Chem.Abstr., Chem.Indus.Notes, Chem.Titles, Curr.Cont., Inpharma, Pharm.&Out.News, Reac.
—BLDSC (6075.684400), ADONIS, CASDDS, CISTI, GNLM, IDS, Infotrieve, KNAW. **CCC.**
Published by: Blackwell Science Asia Pty Ltd, PO Box 378, Carlton South, VIC 3053, Australia. TEL 61-3-9347-0300, FAX 61-3-9347-5001, nfo@blacksci-asia.com.au, http://www.blacksci.co.uk. Ed. Gavin Becker. Adv. contact Kathryn O'Brien. B&W page AUD 1,000, color page AUD 2,050; trim 210 x 275.

616.6 GBR ISSN 0931-0509
CODEN: NDTREA
NEPHROLOGY, DIALYSIS AND TRANSPLANTATION. Text in English. 1986. m. GBP 180, USD 320 to individuals; GBP 430, USD 775 to institutions (effective 2002). adv. bk.rev. 228 p./no. back issues avail. *Refereed.* **Document type:** *Journal, Academic/Scholarly.* **Description:** Clinical and laboratory investigation of relevance to nephrology, dialysis and transplantation.
Related titles: Online - full text ed.: ISSN 1460-2385. GBP 385, USD 695 to institutions Online only (effective 2002) (from HighWire Pr., EBSCO Publishing, O C L C Online Computer Library Center, Inc., RoweCom Information Quest, ingenta, Swets Blackwell, Institute for Scientific Information).
Indexed: ASCA, Abstr.Hyg., Chem.Abstr., Chem.Indus.Notes, Chem.Titles, Curr.Cont., Excerp.Med., Helminthol.Abstr., Ind.Med. (1986-), Ind.Sci.Rev., Inpharma, Int.Nurs.Ind., Kidney, Nutr.Abstr., Pharm.&Out.News, Protozool.Abstr., Reac., Rev.Appl.Entomol., Rev.Med.& Vet.Mycol., Sci.Cit.Ind., Trop.Dis.Bull.
—BLDSC (6075.685300), CASDDS, EMDOCS, GNLM, IDS, ingenta, KNAW. **CCC.**
Published by: (European Dialysis and Transplant Association), Oxford University Press, Academic Division, Great Clarendon St, Oxford OX2 6DP, United Kingdom. TEL 44-1865-267907, FAX 44-1865-267835, jnl.info@oup.co.uk, http://www.oup.co.uk/ndt/, http://www.oup.co.uk/journals. Ed. Tilman B Drueke. Pub. Mandy Sketch. R&P Fionna Willis. adv.: page GBP 900, page USD 1,620. Circ: 5,750. **U.S. subscr. to:** Oxford University Press, Journals, 2001 Evans Rd, Cary, NC 27513. TEL 800-852-7323, FAX 919-677-1714, jnlorders@oup-usa.org; **Subscr. to:** Journals Marketing, Great Clarendon St, Oxford OX2 6DP, United Kingdom. **Co-sponsor:** European Renal Association.

616.6 USA ISSN 0896-1263
CODEN: NNISES
NEPHROLOGY NEWS & ISSUES✱. Text in English. 1987. m. USD 50; USD 80 foreign. adv. bk.rev. illus, stat. *Refereed.* **Document type:** *Trade.* **Description:** Serves the nephrology and renal care community, including nephrologists, surgeons, nurses, technicians and administrators in transplant centers, private practice, in-hospital and free standing clinics. Reports news and information on new techniques, issues, products, government actions and other developments.
Incorporates: Nephrology News and Issues - Europe
Indexed: Int.Nurs.Ind.
—BLDSC (6075.685600), GNLM.
Published by: Nephrology News & Issues, Inc., 13880 N Northsight Blvd #101, Scottsdale, AZ 85260-3666. TEL 602-443-4635, FAX 602-443-4528, http://www.medicalnews.com/nephrology. Ed., R&P Mark E Neumann. Pub., Adv. contact Lawrence R Coutts. B&W page USD 2,755, color page USD 3,605; trim 10.88 x 8.13. Circ: 3,300 (paid); 16,400 (controlled).

NEPHROLOGY NURSING JOURNAL. see *MEDICAL SCIENCES—Nurses And Nursing*

616.6 CHE ISSN 0028-2766
CODEN: NPRNAY
NEPHRON. Text in English. 1964. m. (3 vols./yr.). CHF 1,929, EUR 1,377.60 in Europe to institutions; CHF 1,963.80, USD 1,500 elsewhere to institutions (effective 2002). adv. charts, illus. index. back issues avail. *Refereed.* **Document type:** *Journal, Academic/Scholarly.* **Description:** Provides extensive coverage to important developments concerning the structure, functions and diseases of the kidneys. Contains practice-oriented findings from many fields, including anatomy, pathophysiology, biochemistry, microbiology, endocrinology, immunology and pharmacology.
Related titles: Microform ed.: (from RPI); Online - full text ed.: ISSN 1423-0186. CHF 174, EUR 126, USD 135 to institutions with print edition (effective 2002) (from Northern Light Technology, Inc., EBSCO Publishing, O C L C Online Computer Library Center, Inc., RoweCom Information Quest, ProQuest Information & Learning, Swets Blackwell, Institute for Scientific Information).
Indexed: AIDS Abstr., ASCA, Biol.Abstr., Chem.Abstr., Chem.Indus.Notes, Chem.Titles, Curr.Adv.Cancer Res., Curr.Adv.Ecol.Sci., Curr.Cont., Dent.Ind., Diab.Cont., Excerp.Med., Helminthol.Abstr., Ind.Med. (1964-), Ind.Sci.Rev., Inpharma, Int.Abstr.Biol.Sci., Kidney, Nutr.Abstr., Pharm.&Out.News, Protozool.Abstr., Reac., Rev.Med.& Vet.Mycol., SSCI (coverage dropped), Sci.Cit.Ind., Weed Abstr.
—BLDSC (6075.690000), CASDDS, CISTI, GNLM, IDS, ingenta, KNAW. **CCC.**
Published by: S. Karger AG, Allschwilerstr 10, PO Box, Basel 4009, Switzerland. TEL 41-61-306-1111, FAX 41-61-306-1234, karger@karger.ch, http://www.online.karger.com/journals/nef, http://www.karger.com. Eds. G M Berlyne, S Ito. adv.: page USD 1,205. Circ: 3,000.

616.1 USA ISSN 0733-2467
CODEN: NEUREM
NEUROUROLOGY AND URODYNAMICS. Text in English. 1982. bi-m. USD 1,310 in United States; USD 1,370 in Canada & Mexico; USD 1,421 elsewhere; USD 1,376 combined subscription in United States for print and online eds.; USD 1,436 combined subscription in Canada & Mexico for print and online eds.; USD 1,487 combined subscription elsewhere for print and online eds. (effective 2002). adv. bk.rev. back issues avail. *Refereed.* **Document type:** *Academic/Scholarly.* **Description:** Provides multidisciplinary coverage of recent developments in the study of the urinary tract function.
Related titles: Microform ed.: (from PQC); Online - full text ed.: ISSN 1520-6777. 1996. USD 1,310 in United States; USD 1,310 in Canada & Mexico; USD 1,310 elsewhere (effective 2002) (from EBSCO Publishing, Wiley InterScience, Institute for Scientific Information).

M

Indexed: ASCA, Biol.Abstr., Chem.Abstr., Chem.Indus.Notes, Chem.Titles, Curr.Adv.Ecol.Sci., Curr.Cont., Excerp.Med., Ind.Med. (1982-), Inpharma, Neurosci.Cit.Ind., Pharm.&Out.News, Reac., Ref.Zh., Sci.Cit.Ind.
—BLDSC (6081.589000), CASDDS, EMDOCS, GNLM, IDS, Infotrieve, ingenta, KNAW. **CCC.**
Published by: John Wiley & Sons, Inc., Journals (Subsidiary of: Wiley InterScience), 605 Third Ave, New York, NY 10158. TEL 212-850-6645, FAX 212-850-6021, subinfo@wiley.com, uscs-wis@wiley.com, http://www.wiley.com. Ed. Jerry G Blaivas. adv.: B&W page GBP 640, color page GBP 1,515; trim 174 x 254. Circ: 2,150. **Subscr. outside the Americas to:** John Wiley & Sons Ltd., Baffins Ln, Chichester, Sussex PO19 IUD, United Kingdom. TEL 44-1243-779777, FAX 44-1243-843232, cs-journals@wiley.co.uk.

616.6 NLD ISSN 0924-4999
NEW CLINICAL APPLICATIONS. DERMATOLOGY. Text in English. 1986. irreg. price varies. *Refereed.* **Document type:** *Monographic series.*
Published by: Kluwer Academic Publishers Group (Subsidiary of: Wolters Kluwer N.V.), Spuiboulevard 50, PO Box 17, Dordrecht 3300 AA, Netherlands. FAX 31-78-639-2254, services@wkap.nl, http://www.wkap.nl. **Dist. by:** Journals Department, PO Box 322, Dordrecht 3300 AH, Netherlands. FAX 31-78-654-6474.

616.6 NLD ISSN 0924-4514
NEW CLINICAL APPLICATIONS. NEPHROLOGY. Text in English. 1988. irreg. price varies. *Refereed.* **Document type:** *Monographic series.*
Published by: Kluwer Academic Publishers Group (Subsidiary of: Wolters Kluwer N.V.), Spuiboulevard 50, PO Box 17, Dordrecht 3300 AA, Netherlands. FAX 31-78-639-2254, services@wkap.nl, http://www.wkap.nl. **Dist. by:** Journals Department, PO Box 322, Dordrecht 3300 AH, Netherlands. FAX 31-78-654-6474.

616.61 JPN
NIHON TOSEKI IGAKKAI ZASSHI/JAPANESE SOCIETY OF DIALYSIS THERAPY. JOURNAL. Text in English, Japanese. 1968. m. JPY 1,000 per issue.
Former titles (until 1994): Nihon Toseki Ryoho Gakkai Zasshi (0911-5889); (until 1985): Jinko Toseki Kenkyukai Kaishi (0288-7045)
Published by: Nihon Toseki Ryoho Gakkai, 38-11 Hongo 3-chome, Bunkyo-ku, Tokyo 113-0033, Japan.

616.61 JPN ISSN 0914-7136
NIHON TOSEKI IKAI ZASSHI/JOURNAL OF JAPAN CLINICAL DIALYSIS. Text in Japanese. 1985. 3/yr. **Document type:** *Academic/Scholarly.*
Published by: Nihon Toseki Ikai, 15-2 Kanda-Suda-cho 1-chome, Chiyoda-ku, Tokyo 101-0041, Japan. TEL 81-3-3255-6471, FAX 81-3-3255-6471. Ed. Nobutshi Iida.

616.6 JPN ISSN 0029-0726
NISHINIHON JOURNAL OF UROLOGY/NISHI NIHON HINYOKIKA. Text in Japanese; Summaries in English. 1969. m. JPY 10,000. adv. bk.rev. **Document type:** *Academic/Scholarly.*
Supersedes in part: Dermatology and Urology - Hifu to Hinyo (0011-9091)
Indexed: Biol.Abstr., Excerp.Med., INIS Atomind.
—BLDSC (6113.604000), CISTI, GNLM, KNAW.
Published by: Kyushu University, Faculty of Medicine, Department of Urology, Department of Dermatology, 3-1-1 Maidashi, Higashi-ku, Fukuoka-shi 812-0054, Japan. TEL 81-92-641-1151, FAX 81-92-651-0165. Ed. Joichi Kumazawa. Circ: 3,000.

616.61060489 DNK ISSN 0108-2388
NYRENYT; medlemsblad. Text in Danish. 1981. 6/yr. DKK 100. adv. bk.rev. illus. **Document type:** *Bulletin.*
Formerly: Dialyse og Transplantation (0108-2779)
Published by: Nyreforeningen/Danish Kidney Association, Oesterparken 9, Taastrup 2630, Denmark. TEL 45-43-52-42-52, FAX 45-43-71-00-96. Ed. Poul B Joergensen. adv.: B&W page USD 500. Circ: 4,600.

616.61 JPN ISSN 0912-6937
OSAKA TOSEKI KENKYUKAI KAISHI/OSAKA SOCIETY FOR DIALYSIS THERAPY. JOURNAL. Text in Japanese. 1983. s-a. JPY 1,000 (effective 1999). adv. *Refereed.* **Document type:** *Academic/Scholarly.*
Published by: Osaka Toseki Kenkyukai, Shiritsu Daigaku Igakubu Hinyokika Kyoshitsu, 5-7 Asahi-Machi 1-chome, Abeno-ku, Osaka-shi 545-0051, Japan. TEL 81-6-645-2166, FAX 81-6-647-4426. Ed., Adv. contact Mitsushige Nishikawa. Pub., R&P Taketoshi Kishimoto. Circ: 3,000.

616.6 USA
PAN AMERICAN JOURNAL OF ORGAN REPLACEMENT THERAPIES; dialysis & transplantation. Text in English. 1996. q. USD 99 to individuals; USD 145 to institutions. *Refereed.* **Document type:** *Academic/Scholarly.*
Announced as: Pan American Journal of Dialysis and Transplantation
Published by: (Pan American Society for Dialysis & Transplantation), Field & Wood, Medical Periodicals, Inc., PO Box 975, Blue Bell, PA 19422. TEL 610-828-4010, FAX 215-482-0226. Ed. Dr. Alejandro Trevino Beccera.

616.6 DEU ISSN 0931-041X
CODEN: PEDNEF
PEDIATRIC NEPHROLOGY. Text in English. 1987. 12/yr. EUR 1,895.90 domestic; EUR 1,876.70 in Germany; EUR 185 newsstand/cover foreign (effective 2002). *Refereed.* **Document type:** *Journal, Academic/Scholarly.* **Description:** Laboratory and clinical research of acute and chronic diseases that affect renal function in children.
Related titles: Online - full text ed.: ISSN 1432-198X (from EBSCO Publishing, RoweCom Information Quest, Swets Blackwell, Springer LINK, Institute for Scientific Information).
Indexed: ASCA, Curr.Cont., Ind.Med. (1987-), Kidney, Sci.Cit.Ind.
—BLDSC (6417.603000), CASDDS, CISTI, EMDOCS, GNLM, IDS, ingenta, KNAW. **CCC.**
Published by: (International Pediatric Nephrology Association), Springer-Verlag (Subsidiary of: BertelsmannSpringer), Tiergartenstr 17, Heidelberg 69121, Germany. TEL 49-6221-345-0, FAX 49-6221-345229, subscriptions@springer.de, http://link.springer.de/link/service/journals/00467/index.htm, http://www.springer.de. Eds. M Broyer, R W Chesney. **Subscr. in N. America to:** Springer-Verlag New York Inc., PO Box 2485, Secaucus, NJ 07096-2485. TEL 212-460-1500, FAX 212-473-6272.

PERITONEAL DIALYSIS INTERNATIONAL. see *MEDICAL SCIENCES*

616.6 FRA ISSN 1166-7087
PROGRES EN UROLOGIE. Text in French. 1991. bi-m. FRF 875; FRF 155 newsstand/cover (effective 1998). adv. *Refereed.* **Document type:** *Newspaper.* **Description:** Contains one or two review articles, ten original articles, four clinical cases, one surgical technique paper, and an international bibliographical survey.
Related titles: Online - full text ed.: (from Institute for Scientific Information).
Indexed: Curr.Cont., Ind.Med. (1991-), Inpharma, Pharm.&Out.News, Reac., Ref.Zh.
—BLDSC (6864.938800), CISTI, GNLM, KNAW.
Published by: (Association Francaise d'Urologie), Progres en Urologie S.A.R.L., 7 bd. Flandrin, Paris 75116, France. TEL 33-1-45033196, FAX 33-1-45047289. Ed. Bernard Gattegno. Pub., R&P, Adv. contact Saad Khoury. Circ: 2,500. **Co-sponsors:** Societe Francaise d'Urologie; Association des Urologues du Quebec.

PROSTATE CANCER. see *MEDICAL SCIENCES—Oncology*

PROSTATE CANCER AND PROSTATIC DISEASES. see *MEDICAL SCIENCES—Oncology*

RADIONUCLIDES IN NEPHROUROLOGY. see *MEDICAL SCIENCES—Radiology And Nuclear Medicine*

616.6 GBR ISSN 0264-3081
RECENT ADVANCES IN RENAL MEDICINE. Text in English. 1975. irreg. **Document type:** *Monographic series, Academic/Scholarly.*
Formerly (until 1982): Recent Advances in Renal Disease (0309-2429)
—CISTI.
Published by: Churchill Livingstone (Subsidiary of: Harcourt Publishers Ltd.), Robert Stevenson House, 1-3 Baxter's Pl, Leith Walk, Edinburgh, Midlothian EH1 3AF, United Kingdom. TEL 44-131-556-2424, FAX 44-131-459-1177, http://www.churchillmed.com. **US subscr. to:** Churchill Livingstone, 650 Ave of the Americas, New York, NY 10011. TEL 212-206-5000.

616.6 GBR ISSN 0261-8788
RECENT ADVANCES IN UROLOGY, ANDROLOGY. Text in English. 1957. irreg., latest vol.6. **Document type:** *Monographic series, Academic/Scholarly.*
Formerly (until 1981): Recent Advances in Urology (0309-2739)
—CISTI, GNLM.
Published by: Churchill Livingstone (Subsidiary of: Harcourt Publishers Ltd.), Robert Stevenson House, 1-3 Baxter's Pl, Leith Walk, Edinburgh, Midlothian EH1 3AF, United Kingdom. TEL 44-131-556-2424, FAX 44-131-459-1177, http://churchillmed.com. **US subscr. to:** Churchill Livingstone, 650 Ave of the Americas, New York, NY 10011. TEL 212-206-5000.

616.6 USA ISSN 0886-022X
RC918.R4 CODEN: REFAE8
RENAL FAILURE. Text in English. 1979. bi-m. USD 145 to individuals print & online eds.; USD 1,025 to institutions print only (effective 2002). adv. *Refereed.* **Document type:** *Academic/Scholarly.* **Description:** Addresses advances in the fields of chronic renal failure, hypertension, and renal transplantation.
Former titles: Uremia Investigation; Clinical and Experimental Dialysis and Apheresis (0276-5497); (until 1981): Journal of Dialysis (0362-8558)
Related titles: Microform ed.: (from RPI); Online - full text ed.: (from EBSCO Publishing, O C L C Online Computer Library Center, Inc., RoweCom Information Quest, Swets Blackwell, Institute for Scientific Information).
Indexed: ASCA, Biol.Abstr., Chem.Abstr., Chem.Indus.Notes, Chem.Titles, Curr.Cont., Excerp.Med., INIS Atomind., Ind.Med. (1987-), Ind.Sci.Rev., Inpharma, Nutr.Abstr., Pharm.&Out.News, Protozool.Abstr., Reac., Ref.Zh., Rev.Appl.Entomol., SSCI (coverage dropped), Sci.Cit.Ind. (coverage dropped), Soyabean Abstr.
—BLDSC (7356.869800), CASDDS, CISTI, EMDOCS, GNLM, IDS, Infotrieve, KNAW. **CCC.**
Published by: Marcel Dekker Inc., 270 Madison Ave, New York, NY 10016. TEL 212-696-9000, 800-228-1160, FAX 212-685-4540, http://www.dekker.com/servlet/product/productid/JDI. Ed. William F Finn. R&P Julia Mulligan. Adv. contact Anne Mullins. Circ: 425.

616.6 360 USA
RENALINK. Text in English. 1977. q. membership. bibl. **Document type:** *Newsletter.* **Description:** Covers professional, legislative and regional issues of concern to social workers, nurses, technicians, and dietitians who specialize in working with renal patients.
Formerly (until 2000): C N S W Newsletter (0164-7032)
Published by: National Kidney Foundation, 30 East 33rd St, New York, NY 10016. TEL 212-889-2210, FAX 212-689-9261. Circ: 2,500.

616.6 ARG ISSN 0327-3326
REVISTA ARGENTINA DE UROLOGIA. Text in Spanish. 1932-1988; resumed 1990. q. adv. illus.
Former titles (until 1988): Revista Argentina de Urologia y Nefrologia (0048-7627); (until 1966): Revista Argentina de Urologia (0325-2531)
Indexed: Biol.Abstr., Ind.Med. (coverage dropped).
—GNLM.
Published by: Sociedad Argentina de Urologia, Pasaje De la Carcova 3526, Buenos Aires, Argentina. TEL 54-11-4963-4336, urolog@infovia.com.ar.

616.6 BOL ISSN 1018-5321
REVISTA BOLIVIANA DE NEFROLOGIA. Text in Spanish. 1990. s-a. free per issue. adv. charts, illus, stat.
Published by: Sociedad Boliviana de Nefrologia, Casilla de Correos 6, Sucre, Bolivia. TEL 591-064-23282, FAX 591-064-25559. Ed. Antonio Dubravcic L. Circ: 500.

616.6 JPN ISSN 0385-2393
RINSHO HINYOKIKA/JAPANESE JOURNAL OF CLINICAL UROLOGY. Text in Japanese; Summaries in English. 1946. m. JPY 35,300.
Indexed: INIS Atomind.
—BLDSC (4651.450000), CISTI, EMDOCS, GNLM.
Published by: Igaku-Shoin Ltd., 5-25-3 Hongo, Bunkyo-ku, Tokyo 113-0033, Japan. TEL 81-3-3817-5709. Circ: 4,000.

616.61 JPN ISSN 0910-5808
RINSHO TOSEKI/JAPANESE JOURNAL OF CLINICAL DIALYSIS. Text in Japanese. 1985. m. JPY 1,960 per issue.
Published by: Nihon Medikaru Senta/Japan Medical Center Inc., 1-64 Kanda-Jinbo-cho, Chiyoda-ku, Tokyo 101-0051, Japan.

616.6 SAU ISSN 1319-2442
SAUDI JOURNAL OF KIDNEY DISEASES AND TRANSPLANTATION. Text in English. 1990. q. SAR 150 (effective 2001). *Refereed.* **Document type:** *Academic/Scholarly.* **Description:** Includes editorial reviews from experts worldwide, original articles, case reports, review articles, practical procedures, letters, and country reports on renal replacement therapy.
Formerly: Saudi Kidney Disease and Transplantation

—BLDSC (8076.974300), GNLM.
Published by: Saudi Center for Organ Transplantation, Publication Office, P O Box 27049, Riyadh 11417, Saudi Arabia. TEL 966-1-4451100, FAX 966-1-4453934, TELEX 406310 KIDNEY SJ, scot@naseej.com.sa. Ed. Hassan Abu Aisha. R&P Faissal A.M. Shaheen. Adv. contact Faissal A M Shaheen. Circ: 3,500.

616.6 SWE ISSN 0036-5599
CODEN: SJUNAS
SCANDINAVIAN JOURNAL OF UROLOGY AND NEPHROLOGY. Text in English. 1967. 6/yr. GBP 75, USD 124 to individuals; GBP 167, USD 275 to institutions (effective 2002). adv. charts, illus. *Refereed.* **Document type:** *Journal, Academic/Scholarly.* **Description:** Focuses on basic and clinical research work in the two fields of medicine within the five Nordic countries.
Related titles: Online - full text ed.: (from EBSCO Publishing, O C L C Online Computer Library Center, Inc., RoweCom Information Quest, CatchWord Ltd., ingenta, Swets Blackwell, Institute for Scientific Information); ♦ Supplement: Scandinavian Journal of Urology and Nephrology. Supplement. ISSN 0300-8886.
Indexed: ASCA, Agri.& Environ.Biotech.Abstr. (coverage dropped), Anim.Breed.Abstr., Biol.Abstr., Chem.Abstr., Chem.Indus.Notes, Chem.Titles, Curr.Adv.Ecol.Sci., Curr.Cont., Derwent Biotech.Abstr., Excerp.Med., Helminthol.Abstr., INIS Atomind., Ind.Med. (1967-), Ind.Sci.Rev., Int.Abstr.Biol.Sci., Nutr.Abstr., SSCI (coverage dropped), Sci.Cit.Ind., THA.
—BLDSC (8087.560000), ADONIS, CASDDS, CISTI, GNLM, IDS, ingenta, KNAW. **CCC.**
Published by: (Scandinavian Association of Urology NOR), Taylor & Francis AS (Subsidiary of: Taylor & Francis Group), Cort Adelersgt. 17, Solli, PO Box 2562, Oslo 0202, Norway. TEL 47-22-12-98-80, FAX 47-22-12-98-90, journals@tandf.no, http://www.tandf.co.uk.tfas. Ed. Jan Adolfson. adv.: B&W page SEK 5,400, color page SEK 12,800; trim 190 x 260. Circ: 2,600.

616.6 SWE ISSN 0300-8886
CODEN: SJUNBT
SCANDINAVIAN JOURNAL OF UROLOGY AND NEPHROLOGY. SUPPLEMENT. Text in English. 1968. irreg. **Document type:** *Academic/Scholarly.*
Related titles: Online - full text ed.: (from Swets Blackwell); ♦ Supplement to: Scandinavian Journal of Urology and Nephrology. ISSN 0036-5599.
Indexed: Chem.Abstr., Excerp.Med. (1993-), INIS Atomind., Ind.Med. (1968-), Int.Abstr.Biol.Sci.
—BLDSC (8087.565000), ADONIS, CASDDS, CISTI, EMDOCS, ingenta, KNAW. **CCC.**
Published by: Taylor & Francis AB (Subsidiary of: Taylor & Francis Group), Hollaendargatan 20, PO Box 3255, Stockholm 11160, Sweden. TEL 46-8-4408040, FAX 46-8-4408050, journals@se.tandf.no, http://www.tandf.co.uk/journals/tfas.html.

616.6 USA ISSN 0894-0959
SEMINARS IN DIALYSIS. Text in English. 1988. bi-m. USD 135 domestic to individuals; USD 150 in Canada & Mexico to individuals; USD 170 elsewhere to individuals; USD 245 domestic to institutions; USD 260 in Canada & Mexico to institutions; USD 280 elsewhere to institutions; USD 148.50 domestic to individuals print & online eds. combined; USD 165 in Canada & Mexico to individuals print & online eds. combined; USD 187 elsewhere to individuals print & online eds. combined; USD 269.50 domestic to institutions print & online eds. combined; USD 286 in Canada & Mexico to institutions print & online eds. combined; USD 308 elsewhere to institutions print & online eds. combined (effective 2001). adv. reprints avail. *Refereed.* **Document type:** *Academic/Scholarly.* **Description:** Clinical journal devoted to research and practice of dialysis.
Related titles: Online - full text ed.: ISSN 1525-139X. USD 122 to individuals; USD 221 to institutions (effective 2001) (from Ovid Technologies, Inc., EBSCO Publishing, O C L C Online Computer Library Center, Inc., RoweCom Information Quest, ingenta, Munksgaard & Blackwell Science's Synergy, Swets Blackwell, Institute for Scientific Information).
Indexed: ASCA, Curr.Cont., Ind.Med. (1988-), Inpharma, Pharm.&Out.News, Reac., SSCI (coverage dropped), Sci.Cit.Ind.
—BLDSC (8239.448930), GNLM, IDS, Infotrieve. **CCC.**
Published by: Blackwell Science Inc., Commerce Pl, 350 Main St, Malden, MA 02148-5018. TEL 781-388-8250, 800-759-6102, FAX 781-388-8255, journals@blacksci.com, http://www.blackwell-science.com. Ed. Dr. Richard Sherman. R&P Tracey Davies. Adv. contact Jenny Applin. Circ: 3,000.

616.6 USA ISSN 0270-9295
CODEN: SNEPDJ
SEMINARS IN NEPHROLOGY. Text in English. 1981 (Mar.). bi-m. USD 192 domestic to individuals; USD 281 foreign to individuals; USD 283 domestic to institutions; USD 349 foreign to institutions; USD 86 domestic to students; USD 168 foreign to students; USD 59 newsstand/cover (effective 2001). adv. bibl, charts, illus. index. *Refereed.* **Document type:** *Journal, Academic/Scholarly.* **Description:** Each issue covers new concepts and original research into one particular kidney disorder.
Related titles: Online - full text ed.: (from Institute for Scientific Information).
Indexed: ASCA, Chem.Abstr., Chem.Titles, Curr.Cont., Ind.Med. (1981-), Ind.Sci.Rev., Inpharma, Pharm.&Out.News, Reac., Sci.Cit.Ind.
—BLDSC (8239.455200), CASDDS, EMDOCS, GNLM, IDS, ingenta, KNAW. **CCC.**
Published by: W.B. Saunders Co. (Subsidiary of: Harcourt Publishers Ltd.), 11830 Westline Industrial Dr, St Louis, MO 63146. TEL 800-325-4177, http://www.wbsaunders.com. Ed. Dr. Neil A Kurtzman. adv.: B&W page USD 885, color page USD 1,960; trim 10 x 7. Circ: 2,044. **Subscr. to:** Periodicals Fulfillment, W B Saunders Co, 6277 Sea Harbor Dr, 4th Fl, Orlando, FL 32891-4800.

SEMINARS IN UROLOGIC ONCOLOGY. see *MEDICAL SCIENCES—Oncology*

SEX & HEALTH. see *MEN'S HEALTH*

635 GBR
ST PETER'S NEWS. Text in English. q.
Published by: (University College London), St. Peter's Trust for Kidney, Bladder & Prostate Research (Subsidiary of: University College London), 48 Riding House St, London W1W 7EY, United Kingdom. TEL 44-20-76799369, FAX 44-20-76377006, spt@ucl.ac.uk, http://www.ucl.ac.uk/uro-neph/spt/news/. Ed. Anne Campling. **Co-sponsor:** H R H The Duchess of Gloucester G C V O.

616.6 USA ISSN 1079-3259
RD571 CODEN: TEURFL
TECHNIQUES IN UROLOGY. Text in English. 1995. q., latest vol.7. USD 155 domestic to individuals; USD 250 foreign to institutions; USD 62 newsstand/cover (effective 2001). adv. *Refereed.* **Document type:** *Academic/Scholarly.* **Description:** Provides expert knowledge and guidance on the most advanced procedures for the treatment of urologic disorders.
Indexed: Ind.Med. (1995-).
—BLDSC (8745.405000), CISTI, EMDOCS, GNLM, KNAW.
Published by: Lippincott Williams & Wilkins (Philadelphia) (Subsidiary of: Wolters Kluwer N.V.), 530 Walnut St, Philadelphia, PA 19106-3621. TEL 215-521-8300, FAX 215-521-8902, www.techniquesinurology.com, http://www.lww.com. Eds. Dr. David Albala, Dr. Leonard G Gomellay. Pub. Jim Merritt. R&P Margaret Becker. Adv. contact Ray Thibodeau. B&W page USD 775, color page USD 1,700. Circ: 985. **Subscr. to:** PO Box 1600, Hagerstown, MD 21740-1600. TEL 800-777-2295, FAX 301-824-7390.

616.1 USA ISSN 1091-6660
CODEN: THAPF4
THERAPEUTIC APHERESIS. Text in English. 1997. bi-m. USD 155 domestic to individuals; USD 165 in Canada & Mexico to individuals; USD 180 elsewhere to individuals; USD 210 domestic to institutions; USD 220 in Canada & Mexico to institutions; USD 235 elsewhere to institutions; USD 170.50 domestic to individuals print & online eds. combined; USD 181.50 in Canada & Mexico to individuals print & online eds. combined; USD 198 elsewhere to individuals print & online eds. combined; USD 231 domestic to institutions print & online eds. combined; USD 242 in Canada & Mexico to institutions print & online eds. combined; USD 258.50 elsewhere to institutions print & online eds. combined (effective 2001). adv. back issues avail.; reprints avail. *Refereed.* **Document type:** *Journal, Academic/Scholarly.* **Description:** Covers the development of new devices and techniques of apheresis in the treatment of severe refractory diseases.
Related titles: ♦ Online - full text ed.: Therapeutic Apheresis Online. ISSN 1526-0968.
Indexed: Chem.Abstr., Ind.Med. (1997-), Int.Nurs.Ind.
—BLDSC (8814.642650), CASDDS, CISTI, Infotrieve. **CCC.**
Published by: (International Society for Apheresis), Blackwell Science Inc., Commerce Pl, 350 Main St, Malden, MA 02148-5018. TEL 781-388-8250, FAX 781-388-8255, journals@blacksci.com, http://www.blackwell-science.com. Ed. Tadao Akizawa. R&P Tracey Davies. Adv. contact Jenny Applin. **Co-sponsor:** Japanese Society for Apherisis.

616.1 USA ISSN 1526-0968
THERAPEUTIC APHERESIS ONLINE. Text in English. bi-m. USD 140 to individuals; USD 189 to institutions (effective 2001). **Document type:** *Academic/Scholarly.*
Media: Online - full text (from EBSCO Publishing, O C L C Online Computer Library Center, Inc., RoweCom Information Quest, ingenta, Munksgaard & Blackwell Science's Synergy, Swets Blackwell). **Related titles:** ♦ Print ed.: Therapeutic Apheresis. ISSN 1091-6660.
Published by: Blackwell Science Inc., Commerce Pl, 350 Main St, Malden, MA 02148-5018. TEL 781-388-8250, 800-759-6102, FAX 781-388-8255, website@blacksci.com, journals@blacksci.com, http://www.blackwell-science.com/~cgilib/bsinc.bin?Journal=apheresis.

616.6 NLD ISSN 0924-6177
TOPICS IN RENAL MEDICINE. Text in English. 1986. irreg. price varies. *Refereed.* **Document type:** *Monographic series.*
—KNAW.
Published by: Kluwer Academic Publishers Group (Subsidiary of: Wolters Kluwer N.V.), Spuiboulevard 50, PO Box 17, Dordrecht 3300 AA, Netherlands. FAX 31-78-639-2254, services@wkap.nl, http://www.wkap.nl. Ed. Vittorio E Andreucci. **Dist. by:** Journals Department, PO Box 322, Dordrecht 3300 AH, Netherlands. FAX 31-78-654-6474.

616.6 JPN
TOSEKI/DIALYSIS. Text in Japanese. 1972. a. JPY 4,000.
Published by: Nihon Toseki Ryoho Gakkai, 38-11 Hongo 3-chome, Bunkyo-ku, Tokyo 113-0033, Japan.

616.6 JPN ISSN 0917-2114
TOSEKI FURONTIA/QUARTERLY JOURNAL OF DIALYSIS. Text in Japanese. 1991. 4/yr. JPY 500 per issue (effective 1998).
Published by: (Fuso Yakuhin Kogyo K.K./Fuso Pharmaceutical Industries, Ltd.), Medikaru Rebyusha/Medical Review Co., Ltd., 7-3 Hirano-Machi 1-chome, Chuo-ku, Osaka-shi 541-0046, Japan. TEL 81-6-223-1556, FAX 81-6-223-1414, medrev@osk2.3web.ne.jp.

616.6 617 USA
TRANSPLANT CHRONICLES. Text in English. q. free per issue. **Document type:** *Newsletter.* **Description:** News and information for transplant patients and their families.
Published by: National Kidney Foundation, 30 East 33rd St, New York, NY 10016. TEL 212-889-2210. Circ: 45,000.

616.6 GBR ISSN 1362-5306
TRENDS IN UROLOGY, GYNAECOLOGY & SEXUAL HEALTH. Text in English. 1996. bi-m. GBP 65 (effective 1999).
—BLDSC (9049.688730).
Published by: A & M Publishing Ltd., Alexandra House, First Fl, 1-5 Alexandra Terr., Guilford, Surrey GU1 4BX, United Kingdom. TEL 44-1483-534888, FAX 44-1483-533316, ampublishing@am-publishing.co.uk.

616.6 ESP ISSN 1133-0414
UNIVERSIDAD COMPLUTENSE. CLINICAS UROLOGICAS. Text in Spanish. 1993. a. ESP 4,000, USD 45 (effective 2001). back issues avail. **Document type:** *Academic/Scholarly.* **Description:** Presents monographic issues on urologic topics.
—CINDOC.
Published by: Universidad Complutense de Madrid, Hospital Universitario San Carlos, Catedra de Urologia, Servicio de Publicaciones, C. Isaac Peral s/n, Madrid 28040, Spain. TEL 34-1-3946934, FAX 34-1-3946978, lresel@hcsc.insalud.es, http://www.ucm.es/info/extensio/publicaciones/sepindex.htm. Ed. Luis Resel.

616.6 USA ISSN 1074-8687
URO-GRAM. Text in English. 1976. bi-m. USD 60 to members. adv. bk.rev. *Refereed.* **Document type:** *Newsletter.* **Description:** Provides urology health care workers with information, news and events of the association as well as items affecting urologic practice in general.
Published by: Society of Urologic Nurses and Associates, PO Box 56, Pitman, NJ 08071-0056. TEL 856-256-2335, FAX 856-589-7463, suna@ajj.com, http://www.suna.org. Ed., R&P Glenda Wilkinson. Adv. contact Cheryl Underhill. Circ: 2,500.

616.6 DEU ISSN 1432-9026
URO NEWS. Text in German. 1997. 6/yr. EUR 41.64 domestic; EUR 48.64 foreign; EUR 32.30 domestic to students; EUR 39.30 foreign to students; EUR 7.48 newsstand/cover (effective 2002). adv. **Document type:** *Journal, Academic/Scholarly.*
Published by: Urban und Vogel Medien und Medizin Verlagsgesellschaft mbH (Subsidiary of: BertelsmannSpringer), Neumarkter Str 43, Munich 81673, Germany. TEL 49-89-43721411, FAX 49-89-43721410, niemann@urban-vogel.de, http://www.urban-vogel.de. Ed. Dr. Walther Grohmann. R&P Friederik Klein. Adv. contact Paul Berger. Circ: 3,200. **Subscr. to:** Springer Auslieferungs Gesellschaft, Postfach 105160, Heidelberg 69041, Germany. TEL 49-6221-345244, FAX 49-6221-345244.

616.6 ITA ISSN 1120-5989
CODEN: UNUCFG
URODINAMICA; neurology, continence and pelvic floor. Text in English. 1991. q. EUR 61.98 domestic; USD 80 (effective 2002). **Description:** Publishes original articles on urodynamics and related research.
Related titles: Online - full text ed.: EUR 30.99 (effective 2002).
—BLDSC (9124.395500).
Published by: Editrice Kurtis s.r.l., Via Luigi Zoja, 30, Milan, MI 20153, Italy. TEL 39-02-48202740, FAX 39-2-48201219, info@kurtis.it, http://www.kurtis.it. Ed. W Artibani.

UROGYNAECOLOGIA INTERNATIONAL JOURNAL. see *MEDICAL SCIENCES—Obstetrics And Gynecology*

616.6 DEU ISSN 0340-2592
CODEN: URGABW
DER UROLOGE. SECTION A; Zeitschrift fuer klinische und praktische Urologie. Key Title: Urologe. Ausgabe A. Text in German; Summaries in English, German. 1962. 12/yr. EUR 353.78 domestic; EUR 339.68 in Germany; EUR 66.40 newsstand/cover foreign (effective 2002). adv. bk.rev. abstr, charts, illus. index, cum.index: 1962-1969. back issues avail.; reprint service avail. from ISI. *Refereed.* **Document type:** *Journal, Academic/Scholarly.* **Description:** Covers new developments and techniques in urology.
Formerly (until 1970): Urologe (0375-4685)
Related titles: Microform ed.: (from PQC); Online - full text ed.: ISSN 1433-0563 (from EBSCO Publishing, RoweCom Information Quest, Swets Blackwell, Springer LINK, Institute for Scientific Information).
Indexed: ASCA, Curr.Cont., Excerp.Med., Helminthol.Abstr., INIS Atomind., Ind.Med. (1970-), Ind.Sci.Rev., Inpharma, Pharm.&Out.News, Reac., Sci.Cit.Ind.
—BLDSC (9124.410000), CISTI, EMDOCS, GNLM, IDS, Infotrieve, KNAW. **CCC.**
Published by: (Deutsche Gesellschaft fuer Urologie), Springer-Verlag (Subsidiary of: BertelsmannSpringer), Tiergartenstr 17, Heidelberg 69121, Germany. TEL 49-6221-345-0, FAX 49-6221-345229, subscriptions@springer.de, http://link.springer.de/link/service/journals/00120/index.htm, http://www.springer.de. Eds. H Huland, R Hautmann. **Subscr. in N. America to:** Springer-Verlag New York Inc., PO Box 2485, Secaucus, NJ 07096-2485. TEL 212-460-1500, FAX 212-473-6272.

616.6 DEU ISSN 0042-1111
DER UROLOGE. SECTION B. Key Title: Urologe. Ausgabe B. Text in German. 1961. bi-m. EUR 353.78 domestic; EUR 340.18 in Germany; EUR 66.40 newsstand/cover foreign (effective 2002). adv. charts, illus. index. back issues avail.; reprint service avail. from ISI. *Refereed.* **Document type:** *Journal, Academic/Scholarly.*
Formerly (until 1970): Urologische Facharzt (0301-1410)
Related titles: Microform ed.: (from PQC); Online - full text ed.: ISSN 1433-0571 (from EBSCO Publishing, RoweCom Information Quest, Swets Blackwell, Springer LINK).
Indexed: Curr.Cont. (coverage dropped), Excerp.Med., Helminthol.Abstr., INIS Atomind.
—BLDSC (9124.420000), CISTI, Infotrieve, KNAW. **CCC.**
Published by: (Berufsverband der Deutschen Urologen), Springer-Verlag (Subsidiary of: BertelsmannSpringer), Tiergartenstr 17, Heidelberg 69121, Germany. TEL 49-6221-345-0, FAX 49-6221-345229, subscriptions@springer.de, http://link.springer.de/link/service/journals/00131/index.htm, http://www.springer.de. Eds. H Jonitz, P May. **Subscr. in N. America to:** Springer-Verlag New York Inc., PO Box 2485, Secaucus, NJ 07096-2485. TEL 212-460-1500, FAX 212-473-6272.

616.6 ITA ISSN 0391-5603
UROLOGIA/UROLOGY; rivista internazionale di cultura urologica. Text in English, Italian. 1934. q. USD 150 in Europe; USD 170 elsewhere. adv. bk.rev. charts, illus. index. back issues avail. **Document type:** *Journal, Academic/Scholarly, Abstract/Index.*
Indexed: Biol.Abstr., Chem.Abstr., Excerp.Med., Sci.Cit.Ind. (coverage dropped).
—CISTI.
Published by: (Society of Urology of Northern Italy), Libreria Editrice Canova, Viale della Liberazione 40, Dosson Di Casier, TV 31030, Italy. TEL 39-0422-322393, FAX 39-0422-322305, rivistaurologia@medicinaitaliana.net, http://www.rivistaurologia.net, http://www.medicinaitaliana.net/urologia. Ed. Giuseppe Anselmo. Circ: 1,300 (controlled).

616.6 BRA ISSN 1413-0351
UROLOGIA CONTEMPORANEA. Text and summaries in Portuguese. 1995. q. adv. bk.rev. back issues avail. *Refereed.* **Document type:** *Academic/Scholarly.*
Related titles: Online - full text ed.
Published by: (Associacao Paulista de Medicina, Departamento Urologia), Lemos Editorial & Graficos Ltda., Rua Rui Barbosa, 70, B Vista, Sao Paulo, SP 01326-010, Brazil. TEL 55-11-251-4300, FAX 55-11-251-4300, lemospl@netpoint.com.br, http://www.lemos.com.br. Eds. Eric Roger Wroclawski, Dr. Nelson Rodrigues Netto Jr. Adv. contact Paulo Lemos. Circ: 3,500 (controlled).

616.6 ESP ISSN 1136-7172
UROLOGIA INTEGRADA Y DE INVESTIGACION. Text in Spanish. 1996. q. ESP 14,600 to individuals; ESP 20,000 to institutions; ESP 11,680 to students (effective 2001). adv. back issues avail.; reprints avail. *Refereed.* **Document type:** *Academic/Scholarly.*
Related titles: Online - full text ed.: 1996.
Published by: Ediciones Doyma S.A., Traversa de Gracia, 17-21, Barcelona 08021, Spain. TEL 34-93-200-0711, uii@doyma.es, doyma@doyma.es, http://www.doyma.es/uii. Ed. Jesus Salinas Casado. R&P Monica Barnes. Adv. contact Jose Antonio Hernandez. B&W page ESP 122,000, color page ESP 152,000; 280 x 210.

616.6 CHE ISSN 0042-1138
CODEN: URINAC
UROLOGIA INTERNATIONALIS. Text in English. 1955. 8/yr. (in 2 vols.). CHF 1,594 in Europe to institutions; CHF 1,617.20 elsewhere to institutions; EUR 1,138.40 in Europe to institutions; USD 1,238 elsewhere to institutions (effective 2002). adv. bk.rev. bibl, charts, illus. index. back issues avail. *Refereed.* **Document type:** *Journal, Academic/Scholarly.* **Description:** Presents original papers and reports of practice-oriented research into the etiology, pathophysiology and management of diseases of the urinary and urogenital tract.
Incorporates (Jan. 2000): Acta Urologica Italica (0394-2511)
Related titles: Microform ed.; Online - full text ed.: ISSN 1423-0399. 199?. CHF 116, EUR 84, USD 90 to institutions with print edition (effective 2002) (from EBSCO Publishing, O C L C Online Computer Library Center, Inc., RoweCom Information Quest, Swets Blackwell, Institute for Scientific Information).
Indexed: ASCA, Biol.Abstr., Chem.Abstr., Chem.Indus.Notes, Chem.Titles, Curr.Cont., Excerp.Med., Helminthol.Abstr., INIS Atomind., Ind.Med. (1955-), Inpharma, Pharm.&Out.News, Reac., Rev.Med.& Vet.Mycol., SSCI (coverage dropped).
—BLDSC (9124.480000), CASDDS, CISTI, GNLM, IDS, ingenta, KNAW. **CCC.**
Published by: S. Karger AG, Allschwilerstr 10, PO Box, Basel 4009, Switzerland. TEL 41-61-306-1111, FAX 41-61-306-1234, karger@karger.ch, http://www.online.karger.com/journals/uin, http://www.karger.com. Eds. D Hauri, M.P. Wirth. adv.: page USD 1,195. Circ: 1,000.

616.6 USA ISSN 0094-0143
CODEN: UCNADW
UROLOGIC CLINICS OF NORTH AMERICA. Text in English. 1974. q. USD 159 domestic to individuals; USD 190 in Canada to individuals; USD 219 elsewhere to individuals; USD 225 domestic to institutions; USD 272 foreign to institutions; USD 69 per issue (effective 2001). reprint service avail. from PQC,ISI. *Refereed.* **Document type:** *Journal, Academic/Scholarly.*
Related titles: Microform ed.: (from PQC); Online - full text ed.: (from Institute for Scientific Information); Supplement: Continuing Medical Education Supplement to Urologic Clinics of North America. USD 138 (effective 2000).
Indexed: AIM, ASCA, Biol.Abstr., CINAHL, Curr.Cont., Dent.Ind., Excerp.Med., INIS Atomind., Ind.Med. (1974-), Ind.Sci.Rev., Inpharma, Neurosci.Cit.Ind., Pharm.&Out.News, Reac., SSCI (coverage dropped), Sci.Cit.Ind.
—BLDSC (9124.620000), CISTI, GNLM, IDS, ingenta, KNAW. **CCC.**
Published by: W.B. Saunders Co. (Subsidiary of: Harcourt Publishers Ltd.), 11830 Westline Industrial Dr, St Louis, MO 63146. TEL 800-325-4177, http://www.wbsaunders.com. **Subscr. to:** Periodicals Fulfillment, W B Saunders Co, 6277 Sea Harbor Dr, 4th Fl, Orlando, FL 32891-4800.

616.6 610.736 USA ISSN 1053-816X
CODEN: URNUES
UROLOGIC NURSING. Text in English. 1980. bi-m. USD 40 domestic to individuals; USD 60 foreign to individuals; USD 60 domestic to institutions; USD 80 foreign to institutions (effective 2000). adv. reprints avail. *Refereed.* **Document type:** *Academic/Scholarly.* **Description:** For nurses, technicians, and allied health care professionals.
Formerly (until 1989): A U A A Journal (0882-9594)
Related titles: Online - full text ed.: (from Northern Light Technology, Inc., ProQuest Information & Learning).
Indexed: CINAHL, Int.Nurs.Ind.
—BLDSC (9124.625000), CISTI, GNLM, Infotrieve, ingenta. **CCC.**
Published by: (Society of Urologic Nurses and Associates, Inc. (SUNA)), Jannetti Publications, Inc., East Holly Ave, Box 56, Pitman, NJ 08071-0056. TEL 856-256-2300, FAX 856-689-7463. Ed. Patricia Bates. adv.: B&W page USD 955, color page USD 1,730; trim 10.88 x 8.25. Circ: 5,000. **Co-sponsor:** Urology Nurses of Canada (UNC).

UROLOGIC ONCOLOGY. see *MEDICAL SCIENCES—Oncology*

616.6 DEU ISSN 0300-5623
CODEN: URLRA5
UROLOGICAL RESEARCH; journal of clinical and laboratory investigation. Text and summaries in English. 1973. bi-m. EUR 720 domestic; EUR 715.40 in Germany; EUR 141 newsstand/cover foreign (effective 2002). adv. charts. index. back issues avail.; reprint service avail. from ISI. *Refereed.* **Document type:** *Journal, Academic/Scholarly.* **Description:** Covers research in the fields of clinical medicine, animal experimentation, and laboratory techniques. Contributions are designed to increase understanding of the functions of the genitourinary system in normal and diseased states.
Related titles: Microform ed.: (from PQC); Online - full text ed.: ISSN 1434-0879 (from EBSCO Publishing, RoweCom Information Quest, Swets Blackwell, Springer LINK, Institute for Scientific Information).
Indexed: ASCA, Chem.Abstr., Chem.Indus.Notes, Curr.Adv.Cancer Res., Curr.Cont., Excerp.Med., INIS Atomind., Ind.Med. (1973-), Inpharma, Kidney, Pharm.&Out.News, Reac., Rev.Arom.& Med.Plants, Rev.Med.& Vet.Mycol., Sci.Cit.Ind.
—BLDSC (9124.650000), CASDDS, CISTI, EMDOCS, GNLM, IDS, ingenta, KNAW. **CCC.**
Published by: Springer-Verlag (Subsidiary of: BertelsmannSpringer), Tiergartenstr 17, Heidelberg 69121, Germany. TEL 49-6221-345-0, FAX 49-6221-345229, subscriptions@springer.de, http://link.springer.de/link/service/journals/00240/index.htm, http://www.springer.de. Ed. F H Schroeder. **Subscr. in N. America to:** Springer-Verlag New York Inc., PO Box 2485, Secaucus, NJ 07096-2485. TEL 212-460-1500, FAX 212-473-6272.

616.6 RUS
CODEN: URNEAA
UROLOGIYA/UROLOGY. Text in Russian; Summaries in English. 1923. bi-m. USD 150 foreign (effective 2000). adv. bk.rev. bibl, abstr. **Document type:** *Journal, Academic/Scholarly.* **Description:** Reports on the advances of Russian and foreign medicine in the domain of urology and nephrology.
Former titles (until 1999): Urologiya i Nefrologiya (0042-1154); (until 1965): Urologiya (0258-8404)
Indexed: Biol.Abstr., Chem.Abstr., Excerp.Med., Ind.Med. (coverage dropped), Ref.Zh.
—CASDDS, CISTI, East View, GNLM, Infotrieve. **CCC.**
Published by: Izdatel'stvo Meditsina, Petroverigskii per 6-8, Moscow 101000, Russian Federation. TEL 7-095-9248785, 7-095-928-86-48, FAX 7-095-9211355, 7-095-9286003, meditsina@iname.com. Ed. N A Lopatkin. Pub. A M Stochik. R&P L Sladkova. Adv. contact O A Fadeeva TEL 7-095-923-51-40. Circ: 2,000. **Dist. by:** Mezhdunarodnaya Kniga, B Yakimanka 39, Moscow 117049, Russian Federation. TEL 7-095-2384967, FAX 7-095-2384634.

616.6 USA ISSN 0090-4295
RC870
UROLOGY. Text in English. 1973. m. USD 149 in US & Canada to individuals; USD 249 elsewhere to individuals; USD 304 in US & Canada to institutions; USD 404 elsewhere to institutions; USD 45 in US & Canada to students; USD 145 elsewhere to students (effective 2001). adv. bk.rev. abstr, bibl, charts, stat. back issues avail.; reprint service avail. from PQC,ISI. *Refereed.* **Document type:** *Academic/Scholarly.*
Description: For hospital based and private practice physicians. Contains original scientific reports, case reports and review updates.
Related titles: Microform ed.; Online - full text ed.: (from ingenta, Swets Blackwell, Institute for Scientific Information, ScienceDirect).
Indexed: ASCA, Abstr.Hyg., Biol.Abstr., Curr.Adv.Cancer Res., Curr.Adv.Ecol.Sci., Curr.Cont., Dent.Ind., Excerp.Med., INIS Atomind., Ind.Med. (1973-), Ind.Sci.Rev., Inpharma, Int.Abstr.Biol.Sci., NRN, Neurosci.Cit.Ind., Nutr.Abstr., Pharm.&Out.News, Protozool.Abstr., Reac., Rev.Med.& Vet.Mycol., Rev.Plant Path., SSCI (coverage dropped), Sci.Cit.Ind., THA, Trop.Dis.Bull.
—BLDSC (9124.703000), CISTI, GNLM, IDS, ingenta, KNAW. **CCC.**
Published by: Excerpta Medica, Inc. (Subsidiary of: Reed Elsevier Medical group), 105 Raider Blvd., Belle Mead, NJ 08502. TEL 908-874-8550, FAX 908-874-8419, http://www.elsevier.nl/locate/issn/00904295. Eds. Dr. Joseph E Oesterling, Mary Politano. Circ: 7,500.
Subscr. to: PO Box 10673, Riverton, NJ 08076.

616.6 USA ISSN 0197-7709
UROLOGY DIGEST. Text in English. 1962. 10/yr. USD 27.50. adv. bk.rev. abstr, charts, illus. reprint service avail. from PQC.
Former titles: Journal of Continuing Education in Urology (0148-5172); Urology Digest (0042-1170); Incorporating: Urology Abstracts, Modern Urology
Related titles: Microform ed.: 1962 (from PQC).
—GNLM.
Published by: Medical Digest, Inc., 445 Central Ave., Northfield, IL 60093. TEL 312-446-4400. Ed. Thomas A Stamey M D. Circ: 6,131.

616.6 GBR ISSN 1368-8960
UROLOGY NEWS. Text in English. 1996. bi-m. GBP 15 domestic; GBP 45 elsewhere (effective 2001). adv. bk.rev. back issues avail. *Refereed.* **Document type:** *Trade.* **Description:** Reviews current literature in urology and related fields.
Related titles: Online - full text ed.
—BLDSC (9124.707150).
Published by: Pinpoint Scotland Ltd., 9 Gayfield St, Edinburgh EH1 3NT, United Kingdom. TEL 44-131-478-8404, FAX 44-131-557-4701, urologynews@pinpoint-scotland.com. Ed. Robyn Webber. Pub. Cedric Chater. R&P, Adv. contact Jennifer Park. B&W page GBP 687, color page GBP 974; trim 297 x 210. Circ: 4,500; 41,000 (controlled).

616.6 USA ISSN 0093-9722
UROLOGY TIMES. Text in English. 1973. m., latest vol.28. USD 95 United States & Possessions; USD 140 in Canada & Mexico; USD 185 elsewhere; USD 10 newsstand/cover United States & Possessions (effective 2001). **Document type:** *Trade.* **Description:** News for office-based and hospital-based urologists and osteopathic urologists.
Related titles: Microform ed.: (from PQC); Online - full text ed.: (from The Dialog Corporation, Gale Group, Northern Light Technology, Inc., ProQuest Information & Learning, Factiva).
—Infotrieve. **CCC.**
Published by: Advanstar Communications Inc., 201 E Sandpointe Ave Ste 600, Santa Ana, CA 92707. TEL 440-891-2767, FAX 440-891-2735, http://www.urologytimes.com, http://www.urologytimes.com; http://www.advanstar.com. Ed. Richard R Kerr. Circ: 9,600.

UROONCOLOGY. see *MEDICAL SCIENCES—Oncology*

V H L FAMILY FORUM. (Von Hippel-Lindau Disease) see *MEDICAL SCIENCES—Psychiatry And Neurology*

616.6 DEU ISSN 0724-4983
CODEN: WJURDJ
WORLD JOURNAL OF UROLOGY. Text in English. 1983. bi-m. EUR 499.20 domestic; EUR 495.40 in Germany; EUR 97 newsstand/cover foreign (effective 2002). adv. bk.rev. charts, illus. reprint service avail. from ISI. *Refereed.* **Document type:** *Journal, Academic/Scholarly.* **Description:** Conveys the essential results of urological research and their practical and clinical relevance.
Related titles: Microform ed.: (from PQC); Online - full text ed.: ISSN 1433-8726 (from EBSCO Publishing, RoweCom Information Quest, Swets Blackwell, Springer LINK, Institute for Scientific Information).
Indexed: ASCA, Curr.Adv.Ecol.Sci., Curr.Cont., Ind.Med. (1983-), Ind.Sci.Rev., Inpharma, Int.Nurs.Ind., NRN, Reac., Sci.Cit.Ind.
—BLDSC (9356.074500), CASDDS, CISTI, EMDOCS, GNLM, IDS, Infotrieve, ingenta, KNAW. **CCC.**
Published by: (Urological Research Society), Springer-Verlag (Subsidiary of: BertelsmannSpringer), Tiergartenstr 17, Heidelberg 69121, Germany. TEL 49-6221-345-0, FAX 49-6221-345229, subscriptions@springer.de, http://link.springer.de/link/service/journals/000345/index.htm, http://www.springer.de. Eds. R J Krane, U Jonas. **Subscr. in N. America to:** Springer-Verlag New York Inc., PO Box 2485, Secaucus, NJ 07096-2485. TEL 212-460-1500, FAX 212-473-6272.

616.6 USA ISSN 1086-7139
RC902.A1
YEAR BOOK OF NEPHROLOGY, HYPERTENSION, AND MINERAL METABOLISM. Text in English. 1991. a. USD 89 domestic; USD 95 foreign (effective 2001). illus. **Document type:** *Academic/Scholarly.*
Formerly (until 1996): Year Book of Nephrology (1046-6266)
Related titles: CD-ROM ed.
—GNLM.
Published by: Mosby, Inc. (Subsidiary of: Elsevier Science), 11830 Westline Industrial Dr, St Louis, MO 63146-3313. TEL 314-872-8370, 800-325-4177, FAX 314-432-1380, http://www.mosby.com/periodicals. Ed. Dr. Steve J Schwab.

616.6 USA ISSN 0084-4071
THE YEAR BOOK OF UROLOGY. Text in English. 1922. a. USD 96 domestic; USD 102 foreign (effective 2001). illus. **Document type:** *Abstract/Index, Academic/Scholarly.* **Description:** Presents abstracts of the pertinent literature with commentary by experts in the field.
Related titles: CD-ROM ed.
Indexed: Curr.Adv.Ecol.Sci.
—CISTI, GNLM.
Published by: Mosby, Inc., Continuity Division (Subsidiary of: Harcourt Health Sciences), 11830 Westline Industrial Dr, St Louis, MO 63146-3313. TEL 314-872-8370, 800-325-4177, FAX 314-432-1380, http://www.mosby.com/periodicals. Ed. Dr. Douglas L Coplen Jr.

616.6 CHN ISSN 1000-6702
ZHONGHUA MINIAO WAIKE ZAZHI/CHINESE JOURNAL OF UROLOGY. Text in Chinese. 1980. m. CNY 105.60 domestic; USD 55.20 foreign; CNY 8.80 newsstand/cover domestic; USD 4.60 newsstand/cover foreign (effective 2001). **Document type:** *Academic/Scholarly.*
Published by: Zhonghua Yixuehui (Beijing Fenhui)/Chinese Medical Association (Beijing Branch), Dongdan 3 Tiaojia 7 Hao, Beijing 0253-9713, China. TEL 86-1-6522347, cmamnw@public.sti.ac.cn. Ed. Fang-Liu Gu. **Dist. by:** China International Book Trading Corp, 35, Chegongzhuang Xilu, Haidian District, Beijing 100044, China. TEL 86-1-68413849, FAX 86-1-68412048, cibtc@mail.cibtc.com.cn, http://www.cibtc.com.cn.

MEETINGS AND CONGRESSES

A S D A NEWS. see *MEDICAL SCIENCES—Psychiatry And Neurology*

AERZTE ZEITUNG. see *MEDICAL SCIENCES*

610.6 USA ISSN 1083-8104
BIOMEDICAL MEETINGS INDEX✶ . Text in English. 1994. q. USD 80; USD 100 foreign. adv. back issues avail. **Document type:** *Directory.* **Description:** A comprehensive guide to meetings, symposia, congresses, and short-courses in all areas of the biomedical sciences. Audience includes researchers, physicians, biomedical communications experts and journalists.
Related titles: Diskette ed.: 1994.
Published by: Wallace and Associates, 532 Laguardia Place, 510, New York, NY 10012-1428. RobWallace@Delphi.com. Ed. Robert W Wallace. Adv. contact Robert Wallace. page USD 250.

610 011 CHE ISSN 0301-2891
CALENDAR OF CONGRESSES OF MEDICAL SCIENCES. Text in English, French. 1949. a. CHF 10, USD 5.50. adv. **Document type:** *Directory.*
Formed by the merger of: Calendar of International Congresses of Medical Sciences (0589-915X); Calendar of Regional Congresses of Medical Sciences (0574-248X)
Published by: Council for International Organizations of Medical Sciences/Conseil des Organisations Internationales des Sciences Medicales, c/o World Health Organization, 20 Ave Appia, Geneva, 27 1211, Switzerland. TEL 41-22-7913406, FAX 41-22-7910746, TELEX 415416. Ed. Dr. Zbigniew Bankowski. Circ: 2,000.

011 610 CAN ISSN 1193-6452
CANADIAN DIRECTORY OF HEALTH CARE CONFERENCES/REPERTOIRE CANADIEN DES CONFERENCES DE SOINS DE SANTE. Text in English. 1991. m. free per issue. **Document type:** *Directory.* **Description:** Lists all Canadian health care conferences currently scheduled to the year 2000. Listings are organized by month and year and include location, theme, sponsoring organization and contact person.
Media: Online - full text.
Published by: Canadian Nurses Association/Association des Infirmieres et Infirmiers du Canada, 50 Drway, Ottawa, ON K2P 1E2, Canada. TEL 613-237-2133, FAX 613-237-3520, pubs@cna-nurses.ca, http://www.cna-nurses.ca.

CLINICAL CONGRESS NEWS. see *MEDICAL SCIENCES*

011 DEU ISSN 0933-9760
DEMETER KONGRESS KALENDER MEDIZIN✶ . Text in German. 1961. a. DEM 43. **Document type:** *Catalog.*
—GNLM.
Published by: Demeter Verlag GmbH und Co. KG, Ammonitenstr 1, Balingen 72336, Germany.

617.6 011 CAN
DENTAL GUIDE (SCARBOROUGH); the CE planner for the dental profession. Text in English. 1993. q. CND 35; CND 55 foreign. adv. **Description:** Lists dental conferences, meetings and seminars around the world, with a focus on travel combined with dental education.
Published by: Thomson Healthcare Communications, 1120 Birchmount Rd, Ste 200, Scarborough, ON M1K 5G4, Canada. TEL 416-750-8900, FAX 416-751-8126. Ed. Heather Howie. Adv. contact Peter Greenhough. B&W page CND 1,595, color page CND 2,685; trim 10.75 x 8.13. Circ: 16,000.

011 617.6 DEU
DEUTSCHER KONGRESS KALENDER ZAHNMEDIZINER✶ . Text in German. 1980. a. DEM 25. **Document type:** *Catalog.*
Published by: Demeter Verlag GmbH und Co. KG, Ammonitenstr 1, Balingen 72336, Germany.

610 011 ESP ISSN 0210-5578
DIARIO DE CONGRESOS MEDICOS. Text in Spanish. 1972. irreg. (approx. 40/yr.). free per issue to qualified personnel. reprint service avail. from PQC. **Document type:** *Academic/Scholarly.* **Description:** Publishes the best and most interesting papers from national and international medical conferences.
—**CCC.**
Published by: Ediciones Doyma S.A., Traversa de Gracia, 17-21, Barcelona 08021, Spain. TEL 34-93-200-0711, FAX 34-93-209-1136. Ed. Pedro Espinosa Bravo. adv.: page ESP 270,000; trim 420 x 305. Circ: 3,000.

FEDERAZIONE DELLE SOCIETA MEDICO-SCIENTIFICHE ITALIANE. CONGRESSI (YEAR). see *MEDICAL SCIENCES*

FRANCE. INSTITUT NATIONAL DE LA SANTE ET DE LA RECHERCHE MEDICALE. COLLOQUES. see *MEDICAL SCIENCES*

GENETICS SOCIETY OF CANADA BULLETIN. see *BIOLOGY—Genetics*

GIORNALE DEI CONGRESSI MEDICI. see *MEDICAL SCIENCES*

610 USA
H C E A ASSOCIATION ALERT; The newsletter for the healthcare exhibition & meeting organizer. Text in English. 1998. 2/yr. free to members. 4 p./no. 2 cols./p. back issues avail. **Document type:** *Newsletter, Trade.* **Description:** Includes critical analysis of association related issues, advocacy for healthcare conventions and exhibitions as an industry, and needs oriented articles.

Published by: Healthcare Convention & Exhibitors Association, 5775 Peachtree Dunwoody Rd, Ste 500 G, Atlanta, GA 30342. TEL 404-252-3663, FAX 404-252-0774, hcea@kellencompany.com, hcea@assnhq.com, http://www.hcea.org. Eds. Jane Boyle TEL 404-252-3663, Mary Anderson. Adv. contact Jane Boyle TEL 404-252-3663. Circ: 4,000 (controlled).

060 610 USA
H C E A DIRECTORY; a directory of healthcare meetings and conventions. Text in English. 2/yr., latest vol.99. USD 245 to non-members (effective 2000). 600 p./no. 2 cols./p. **Document type:** *Directory, Trade.* **Description:** Lists more than 6000 healthcare meetings.
Formerly: H C E A Handbook
Published by: Healthcare Convention & Exhibitors Association, 5775 Peachtree Dunwoody Rd, Ste 500 G, Atlanta, GA 30342. TEL 404-252-3663, FAX 404-252-0774, kellercompany.com, hcea@asshq.com, http://www.hcea.org. R&P Lavay Sheldon. Adv. contact Gretta Hall TEL 404-252-3663. Circ: 1,000 (paid).

610 011 USA
INSIGHT (ATLANTA). Text in English. 2/yr. free to members. 24 p./no. 2 cols./p. back issues avail. **Document type:** *Magazine, Trade.*
Published by: Healthcare Convention & Exhibitors Association, 5775 Peachtree Dunwoody Rd, Ste 500 G, Atlanta, GA 30342. TEL 404-252-3663, FAX 404-252-0774, hcea@kellencompany.com, hcea@assnhq.com, http://www.hcea.org. Ed. Mary Anderson. Circ: 2,000.

INTERNATIONAL COLLEGE OF DENTISTS. KEY; journal of events. see *MEDICAL SCIENCES—Dentistry*

INTERNATIONAL CONGRESS SERIES. see *SCIENCES: COMPREHENSIVE WORKS*

MEDICAL EXPRESS REPORTS. see *MEDICAL SCIENCES*

MEDICAL FORUM REPORTER. see *MEDICAL SCIENCES*

011 DEU ISSN 0175-3053
MEDIZINISCHE KONGRESSE; national - international. Text in German. 1957. a. DEM 35; DEM 60 in Europe; DEM 75 elsewhere (effective 2000). adv. back issues avail. **Document type:** *Directory, Trade.*
Published by: M, K & K Verlagsgesellschaft mbH, Mitteldicker Weg 1, Neu-Isnburg 63263, Germany. TEL 49-69-69500845, FAX 49-69-69500850. Ed., Pub. Ingrid Haack. R&P Dieter Haack. Adv. contact Monika Schmidt. B&W page DEM 7,300, color page DEM 10,300; trim 131 x 187. Circ: 32,000.

PHYSICIANS' TRAVEL & MEETING GUIDE. see *TRAVEL AND TOURISM*

616.07 ZAF
SOUTH AFRICAN SOCIETY OF PATHOLOGISTS. CONGRESS BROCHURE. Text in Afrikaans, English. a. free per issue. adv. *Refereed.* **Document type:** *Proceedings.*
Published by: South Africa Society of Pathologists, PO Box 2034, Pretoria 0001, South Africa. TEL 27-12-3283600. Circ: 300.

616.994 011 CHE
U I C C INTERNATIONAL CALENDAR OF MEETINGS ON CANCER. Text in English. biennial. free per issue. **Document type:** *Proceedings.*
Formerly: U I C C Calendar of International Meetings on Cancer
Published by: Union Internationale Contre le Cancer/International Union Against Cancer, 3 rue de Conseil General, Geneva 1205, Switzerland. TEL 41-22-8091811, FAX 41-22-8091810, info@uicc.org, http://www.uicc.org/calendars/.

011 610 USA ISSN 0161-2875
CODEN: WMMEDT
WORLD MEETINGS: MEDICINE. Text in English. 1978. q. USD 175 (effective 2000). **Document type:** *Journal, Trade.*
—BLDSC (9356.655750), GNLM.
Published by: Gale Group (Subsidiary of: The Thomson Corporation), PO Box 159, Thorndike, ME 04986-0159. TEL 207-948-2962 ext 239, FAX 207-948-2863, http;//www.galegroup.com. Ed. Susan Drummond.

MEETINGS AND CONGRESSES—Abstracting, Bibliographies, Statistics

016 GBR ISSN 0959-4906
Z7403
BRITISH LIBRARY. DOCUMENT SUPPLY CENTRE. INDEX OF CONFERENCE PROCEEDINGS. Text in English. 1964. m. (plus a. cumulation). GBP 95 in United Kingdom to institutions; GBP 99 rest of world to institutions (effective 2001); GBP 120 in United Kingdom to institutions; GBP 130 rest of world to institutions (effective 2002). cum.index: 1964-1988. back issues avail. **Document type:** *Proceedings, Abstract/Index.*
Formerly: British Library. Lending Division. Index of Conference Proceedings Received (0305-5183)
Related titles: Online - full text ed.
Indexed: AESIS, Dairy Sci.Abstr., Rev.Appl.Entomol., Rev.Plant Path., Russ.Acad.Sci.Bibl.
—BLDSC (4377.416600), CISTI, GNLM, Linda Hall.
Published by: British Library, Document Supply Centre, c/o Mike Marcus, British Library, Boston Spa, Wetherby, W Yorkshir LS23 7BQ, United Kingdom. TEL 44-1937-546080, FAX 44-1937-546286, http://www.bl.uk/services/bsds/nbs. **Subscr. to:** Turpin Distribution Services Ltd., Blackhorse Rd, Letchworth, Herts SG6 1HN, United Kingdom. TEL 44-1462-488900, FAX 44-1462-483011.

DIRECTORY OF PUBLISHED PROCEEDINGS. SERIES S E M T - SCIENCE, ENGINEERING, MEDICINE AND TECHNOLOGY. see *SCIENCES: COMPREHENSIVE WORKS—Abstracting, Bibliographies, Statistics*

MEN'S HEALTH

96 INC. see *LITERATURE*

ADVANCES IN HEALTH EDUCATION AND PROMOTION. see *PHYSICAL FITNESS AND HYGIENE*

612.67 GBR ISSN 1368-5538
CODEN: AGMAF7
THE AGING MALE. Text in English. 1998. q. GBP 75, USD 130 to individuals; GBP 135, USD 220 to institutions (effective 2000). adv. bk.rev. illus. reprints avail. *Refereed.* **Document type:** *Academic/Scholarly.*
Related titles: Online - full text ed.: ISSN 1473-0790 (from CatchWord Ltd.).
—BLDSC (0736.363500), ADONIS.
Published by: Parthenon Publishing Group (Subsidiary of: C R C Press (New York)), Casterton Hall, Casterton, Carnforth, Lancs LA6 2LA, United Kingdom. TEL 44-1524-272084, FAX 44-1524-271587, mail@parthpub.com, http://www.parthpub.com/. Ed., R&P Jean Wright. Adv. contact Julia Tissington.

THE AKWA LETTER. see *PHYSICAL FITNESS AND HYGIENE*

AXIOM; living life to the full. see *HOMOSEXUALITY*

CARERS IN VICTORIA. see *SOCIAL SERVICES AND WELFARE*

613.081 USA
CHROME - DOME. Text in English. 1972. s-a. USD 10. bk.rev. **Document type:** *Newsletter.*
Published by: Baldheaded Men of America, 102 Bald Dr, Morehead City, NC 28557. TEL 252-726-1855, FAX 252-726-6061. Ed. John T Capps. Circ: 15,000.

CITY WOMAN. see *WOMEN'S HEALTH*

CONTEMPORARY SEXUALITY; the international resource for educators, researchers and therapists. see *PSYCHOLOGY*

EQUAL TIME: OUTREACH NEWSLETTER. see *HOMOSEXUALITY*

613.081 USA ISSN 1086-1122
EXERCISE & HEALTH; the complete fitness guide for men. Text in English. 1996. q. USD 4.50 newsstand/cover; CND 5.95 newsstand/cover in Canada; GBP 2.95 newsstand/cover in United Kingdom. adv. illus. **Document type:** *Consumer.*
Published by: Harris Publications, Inc., 1115 Broadway, New York, NY 10010. TEL 212-807-7100, FAX 212-627-4678, exercisehealth@harris-pub.com. Ed. Michael Catarevas. Pub. Stanley Harris. Adv. contact Melissa Cianciulli. **Dist. in UK by:** Comag, Tavistock Works, Tavistock Rd, W Drayton, Middx UB7 7QX, United Kingdom. TEL 44-1895-444055, FAX 44-1895-433602.

EXERCISE FOR MEN ONLY. see *PHYSICAL FITNESS AND HYGIENE*

613.081 GBR ISSN 1468-974X
▼ **F H M BIONIC**; we can rebuild you. (For Him Magazine) Text in English. 1999. m. GBP 27.75; GBP 3 newsstand/cover (effective 2001). adv. **Document type:** *Magazine, Consumer.* **Description:** Provides practical health and fitness information and advice for men.
Related titles: Online - full text ed.
Published by: Emap Metro Ltd. (Subsidiary of: Emap Consumer Magazines Ltd.), Mappin House, 4 Winsley St, London W1W 8HF, United Kingdom. TEL 44-20-7436-1515, FAX 44-20-7636-5792, http://www.fhm.com/bionic/, http://www.emap.com. Adv. contact Dan Reeves.

▼ **GYM**; for the physical man. see *PHYSICAL FITNESS AND HYGIENE*

613.081 USA ISSN 1089-1102
HARVARD MEN'S HEALTH WATCH. Variant title: Men's Health Watch. Text in English. 1996. m. USD 24 domestic; USD 40 in Canada; USD 47 elsewhere (effective 2000). 8 p./no. 3 cols./p. back issues avail. **Document type:** *Newsletter, Consumer.* **Description:** Helps the general reader interpret important issues in men's health in a timely and accurate manner.
—BLDSC (4268.275000).
Published by: Harvard Health Publications Group (Subsidiary of: Harvard Medical School), 164 Longwood Ave, Boston, MA 02115. TEL 617-432-1485, FAX 617-432-1506, harvardmen@palmcoastd.com, hhp@hms.harvard.edu, http://www.health.harvard.edu/newsletters/mntext.html. **Subscr. to:** PO Box 420099, Palm Coasat, FL 32142-0099. TEL 800-829-9045.

HEALTH & FITNESS MAGAZINE FOR HEALTHY, SOUND LIVING. see *PHYSICAL FITNESS AND HYGIENE*

HEALTH AND STRESS; the newsletter of the American Institute of Stress. see *MEDICAL SCIENCES*

HEALTH EDUCATION. see *PHYSICAL FITNESS AND HYGIENE*

HOOFDZAKEN; nieuwsblad over migraine, hoofd- en aangezichtspijnen. see *MEDICAL SCIENCES—Psychiatry And Neurology*

610 USA ISSN 1532-6306
▼ **INTERNATIONAL JOURNAL OF MEN'S HEALTH.** Text in English. 2002 (Jan). 3/yr. USD 50 domestic to individuals; USD 65 foreign to individuals; USD 150 domestic to institutions; USD 165 foreign to institutions (effective 2001). adv. bk.rev. Index. back issues avail.; reprints avail. *Refereed.* **Document type:** *Journal, Academic/Scholarly.* **Description:** Covers all aspects of men's health.
Related titles: Online - full content ed.
Published by: Men's Studies Press, P O Box 32, Harriman, TN 37748-0032. TEL 423-369-2375, FAX 423-369-1125, editor@mensstudies.com, http://www.mensstudies.com/mspjournals.html. Pub. James A Doyle. adv.: B&W page USD 150; 4.75 x 7.875.

613.081 USA ISSN 1529-1197
▼ **JOURNAL OF MEN'S HEALTH.** Text in English. 2000. q. USD 89 domestic to individuals; USD 135 foreign to individuals .; USD 107 domestic to individuals for Print & Online eds.; USD 153 foreign to individuals for Print & Online eds.; USD 165 domestic to institutions .; USD 215 foreign to institutions; USD 198 domestic to institutions for Print & Online eds.; USD 248 foreign to institutions for Print & Online eds. (effective 2002). back issues avail.; reprints avail. *Refereed.* **Document type:** *Journal, Consumer.* **Description:** Provides information on current medical and therapeutic issues of concern to men, including sexual dysfunction, gender-related surgery, studies on testosterone, male metabolism and stress, and mental health.
Related titles: Online - full content ed.: USD 102 to individuals; USD 190 to institutions (effective 2002); Online - full text ed.: (from CatchWord Ltd.).
Published by: Mary Ann Liebert, Inc. Publishers, 2 Madison Ave, Larchmont, NY 10538. TEL 914–834-3100, FAX 914-834-1388, info@liebertpub.com, http://www.liebertpub.com/jmh. Ed. Dr. Gary Onik. R&P Esther Bicovany. Adv. contact Harriet Matysko.

JOURNAL OF SPIRITUAL BODYWORK. see *ALTERNATIVE MEDICINE*

MAENNER AKTUELL. see *HOMOSEXUALITY*

613.7 USA ISSN 0893-4460
GV481
MEN'S FITNESS; when performance counts. Variant title: Joe Weider's Men's Fitness. Text in English. 1985. m. USD 14.97 domestic; USD 29.97 foreign; USD 3.99; USD 4.99 in Canada (effective 2001). adv. bk.rev. illus. reprints avail. **Document type:** *Magazine, Consumer.* **Description:** Discusses health and nutrition for active men.
Formerly (until 1987): Joe Weider's Sports Fitness (0885-0763)
Related titles: Online - full text ed.: (from America Online, Inc., Gale Group).
Indexed: Phys.Ed.Ind., Sports Per.Ind.
—ingenta.
Published by: Weider Publications, 21100 Erwin St, Woodland Hills, CA 91367. TEL 818-884-6800, FAX 818-704-5734, http://www.mensfitness.com. Ed. Jerry Kindela. Pub. Joseph Weider. R&P Anne Byron. adv.: B&W page USD 29,430, color page USD 39,150; trim 10.5 x 7.88. Circ: 550,000 (paid). **Subscr. to:** PO Box 37211, Boone, IA 50037. **Dist. in the UK by:** Comag, Tavistock Works, Tavistock Rd, W Drayton, Middx UB7 7QX, United Kingdom. TEL 44-1895-444055, FAX 44-1895-433602.

613.081 USA ISSN 1531-457X
▼ **MEN'S FITNESS EN ESPANOL.** Variant title: Joe Weider's Men's Fitness en Espanol. Text in Spanish. 2000. m. USD 26; USD 2.95 newsstand/cover (effective 2001). adv. **Document type:** *Magazine, Consumer.* **Description:** Presents articles and features on the latest in exercise, health sports training and adventures travel.
Published by: Ideas Publishing Group, 1101 Brickell Ave, 15th Fl, Miami, FL 33131. TEL 305-371-9393, 800-792-5999, FAX 305-371-9392, mensfitness@ideaspublishinggroup.com, newsesp@gate.net, http://www.ideaspublishinggroup.com/magazines/mensfitness.html. Ed. Jose Forteza. Pub. Joe Weider. adv.: color page USD 17,100. Circ: 280,000 (paid).

610 FRA ISSN 1294-971X
▼ **MEN'S HEALTH.** Text in French. 1999. bi-m. adv. **Document type:** *Magazine, Consumer.*
Published by: Media Mag Editions 83 (Subsidiary of: Axel Springer Verlag AG), 28 rue Jean Jaures, Puteaux 92800, France. TEL 33-1-47626003, FAX 33-1-47759914, editions.83.francis.morel@wanadoo.fr. Circ: 80,000 (paid and controlled).

613.081 RUS ISSN 1562-5117
MEN'S HEALTH. Text in Russian. 1998. m. adv. **Document type:** *Magazine, Consumer.*
Published by: Independent Media, Vyborgskaya ul 16, Moscow 125212, Russian Federation. TEL 7-095-232-3200, FAX 7-095-232-1761, rec4floor@imedia.ru, http://www.mhealth.ru, http://www.independentmedia.ru. Ed. Ilya Bezugly. Pub. Karen Dukess. Adv. contact Arkadi Tsimbler. Circ: 50,000.

610 DEU ISSN 1432-3818
MEN'S HEALTH (GERMANY EDITION); das Magazin fuer Maenner. Text in German. 1996. m. DEM 64.80; DEM 6 newsstand/cover (effective 2001). adv. back issues avail. **Document type:** *Magazine, Consumer.*
Related titles: E-mail ed.; Fax ed.; Online - full text ed.; ♦ Regional ed.: Men's Health (United States Edition). ISSN 1054-4836; ♦ Men's Health (United Kingdom Edition); ♦ Men's Health (South Africa Edition).
Published by: Rodale Motor Presse GmbH und Co. KG, Leuschnerstr 1, Stuttgart 70174, Germany. TEL 49-711-1822590, FAX 49-711-1822550, abo@menshealth.de, http://www.menshealth.de. Ed. Dr. Frank Hofman. Pub. Dr. Thomas Garms. R&P Christine Juergensen TEL 49-853-30331. Adv. contact Corinna Weiss. B&W page DEM 31,800, color page DEM 31,800. Circ: 268,469 (paid). **Subscr. to:** P M S GmbH & Co. KG, Postfach 20080, Hamburg, Germany. TEL 49-203-76908-0, FAX 49-203-7690830.

610 PRT
▼ **MEN'S HEALTH (PORTUGAL EDITION).** Text in Portuguese. 2001. m. PTE 250 newsstand/cover (effective 2001). adv. **Document type:** *Magazine, Consumer.*
Published by: Motorpress Lisboa, SA, Rua Policarpio Anjos No. 4, Cruz Quebrada 1495-742, Portugal. TEL 351-21-4154500, FAX 351-21-4154501. Ed. Paulo Sousa Costa. Pub. Montse Sala. Adv. contact Rita Vidreiro. Circ: 72,000 (paid).

613.081 ZAF
MEN'S HEALTH (SOUTH AFRICA EDITION). Text in English. m. ZAR 182; ZAR 18.95 newsstand/cover. adv. **Document type:** *Magazine, Consumer.*
Related titles: Print ed.: Men's Health Online. ISSN 1563-5783; ♦ Regional ed.: Men's Health (United States Edition). ISSN 1054-4836; ♦ Men's Health (Germany Edition). ISSN 1432-3818; ♦ Men's Health (United Kingdom Edition).
Published by: Touchline Media, PO Box 16368, Vlaeberg, Cape Town 8018, South Africa. TEL 27-21-217810, FAX 27-21-215118, http://www.touchline.co.za. Circ: 70,000.

610 ESP
▼ **MEN'S HEALTH (SPAIN EDITION).** Text in Spanish. 2001. m. ESP 400 newsstand/cover (effective 2001). adv. **Document type:** *Magazine, Consumer.*
Published by: Motorpress-Iberica, S.A., Ancora, 40, Madrid 28045, Spain. TEL 34-1-91-3470100, FAX 34-1-91-3470152, marketing@mpib.es, http://www.autopistaonline.com/htm_apo/corporat/corporat2.htm. Ed. Antonio Orti. Pub. Joaquim Oliveira. Adv. contact Alicia Martinez-Pereda. Circ: 230,000 (paid).

610 GBR
MEN'S HEALTH (UNITED KINGDOM EDITION); tons of useful stuff. Text in English. 10/yr. GBP 37; GBP 3 newsstand/cover (effective 1999). adv. **Document type:** *Consumer.*
Related titles: ♦ Regional ed.: Men's Health (United States Edition). ISSN 1054-4836; ♦ Men's Health (Germany Edition). ISSN 1432-3818; ♦ Men's Health (South Africa Edition).
Published by: Rodale Ltd., Rodale Press, 7-10 Chandos St, London W1M 0AD, United Kingdom. TEL 44-171-291-6000, FAX 44-171-291-6060, sgeller1@rodale.co.uk. Ed. Simon Geller. Pub. Tony Long. Adv. contact Lorraine Kaye. Circ: 188,264 (paid). **Subscr. to:** FREEPOST MID06177, Market Harborough, Leicester, Leics LE87 4ET, United Kingdom. **Dist. by:** MarketForce (UK), 247 Tottenham Court Rd, London W1P 0AU, United Kingdom. TEL 44-20-7261-6996, FAX 44-20-7261-6951.

610 USA ISSN 1054-4836
RA777.8 CODEN: MEHEE9
MEN'S HEALTH (UNITED STATES EDITION). Text in English. 1986. 10/yr. USD 24.97 domestic; USD 39.50 in Canada; USD 49.07 elsewhere; USD 3.50 newsstand/cover domestic; USD 4.95 newsstand/cover in Canada (effective 2000). adv. illus. reprints avail. **Document type:** *Magazine, Consumer.* **Description:** Tells men how to look good and how to live better and longer.
Related titles: Online - full text ed.: (from ProQuest Information & Learning, Gale Group); ♦ Regional ed.: Men's Health (Germany Edition). ISSN 1432-3818; ♦ Men's Health (United Kingdom Edition); ♦ Men's Health (South Africa Edition).
Indexed: CHNI, CINAHL, Hlth.Ind., R.G. (Jan.1991-), R.G.Abstr. (Jan.1991-).
—ingenta. **CCC.**
Published by: Rodale, 33 E Minor St, Emmaus, PA 18098. TEL 610-967-5171, FAX 610-967-8963, customer_service@rodale.com, http://www.menshealth.com, http://www.rodale.com. Ed. Greg Gutfeld. Pub. Paul Turcotte. adv.: B&W page USD 91,790, color page USD 104,900; trim 10.88 x 8.25. Circ: 1,700,000 (paid). **Subscr. to:** PO Box 7318, Red Oak, IA 51591-2380.

613 305.31 USA ISSN 1058-3041
MEN'S WORKOUT. Text in English. 1990. 8/yr. USD 17.97; USD 4.50 newsstand/cover; GBP 2.95 newsstand/cover in United Kingdom; CND 5.95 newsstand/cover in Canada (effective 1999). **Document type:** *Consumer.*
Published by: Harris Publications, Inc., 1115 Broadway, New York, NY 10010. TEL 212-807-7100. Ed. Michael Catareva. Pub. Stanley R Harris. **UK dist. addr.:** Comag, Tavistock Works, Tavistock Rd, W Drayton, Middx UB7 7QX, United Kingdom. TEL 44-1895-433600, FAX 44-189-543-3606.

MENSTUFF, THE NATIONAL MEN'S RESOURCE. see *MEN'S STUDIES*

613.081 USA
▼ **MUSCLE ELEGANCE.** Text in English. 2000. q. USD 7.95 newsstand/cover domestic; CND 9.95 newsstand/cover in Canada (effective 2002). adv. **Document type:** *Magazine, Consumer.*
Published by: Muscle Elegance Magazine, Inc., PMB No.409, 13300-56 Cleveland Ave, Ft. Myers, FL 33907. http://www.muscleelegancemag.com/. Ed. Denise Masino.

OUTLOOK (SEATTLE); reproductive health. see *PUBLIC HEALTH AND SAFETY*

613.7 USA ISSN 1097-4717
SEX & HEALTH. Text in English. 1985. m. USD 48. adv. bk.rev. charts, illus. index. back issues avail. **Document type:** *Newsletter.* **Description:** Delivers current medical advice on health subjects unique to men with ways to improve health, "slow down" the aging process, reduce stress, plus information on nutrition.
Former titles (until 1997): Men's Confidential Newsletter (1066-5706); (until 1993): Men's Health Newsletter (0747-8461)
Indexed: CHNI.
Published by: (Men's Health Institute), Rodale, 33 E Minor St, Emmaus, PA 18098. TEL 610-967-7627, FAX 610-967-7725, http://www.rodale.com. Ed. Michael Lafavore. Pub. John Griffin. Circ: 110,000 (paid). **Subscr. to:** PO Box 7315, Red Oak, IA 51591-0315.

613.081 155 USA ISSN 0277-3422
SPRINGER SERIES: FOCUS ON MEN. Text in English. 1980. irreg., latest vol.10, 1998. price varies. **Document type:** *Monographic series.* **Description:** Focuses on men's issues from a psychological perspective.
Indexed: e-psyche.
Published by: Springer Publishing Company, 536 Broadway, New York, NY 10012. TEL 212-431-4370, FAX 212-941-4370, springer@springerpub.com, http://www.springerpub.com. R&P Dorothy Kouwenberg.

▼ **TODAY'S HEALTH AND WELLNESS.** see *PHYSICAL FITNESS AND HYGIENE*

VENEREOLOGY; the interdisciplinary international journal of sexual health. see *MEDICAL SCIENCES—Dermatology And Venereology*

MEN'S INTERESTS

AMERICAN CROSSDRESSER. see *HOMOSEXUALITY*

BEAU. see *HOMOSEXUALITY*

306.772 USA
CELEBRATE THE SELF; the magazine of solo sex. Text in English. ceased; resumed 1993. bi-m. USD 24.95 domestic; USD 28.95 in Canada & Mexico; USD 39.95 elsewhere (effective 2000). bk.rev., video rev. illus. **Document type:** *Consumer.* **Description:** Covers men and masturbation. Includes personal narratives and letters, techniques, sex and health, and news.
Address: PO Box 8888, Mobile, AL 36689. TEL 334-380-0606, FAX 334-380-0606, factorpress@zebra.net. Ed. Allan Erich. Pub. Robert Bahr. R&P Allen Metzqar. Circ: 1,500 (paid).

EXERCISE FOR MEN ONLY. see *PHYSICAL FITNESS AND HYGIENE*

305.31 USA
FEMME MIRROR. Text in English. 1976. q. USD 36. adv. bk.rev. *Refereed.* **Document type:** *Newsletter.* **Description:** Contains information of interest to heterosexual transvestites and cross-dressers.
Published by: Tri Ess, PO Box 194, Tulane, CA 93275. TEL 209-688-9246, jeftris@aol.com. Ed., R&P, Adv. contact Jane Ellen Fairfax TEL 713-349-8969. Circ: 1,200.

052 GBR ISSN 0015-833X
FORUM (LONDON, 1967); the international journal of human relations. Text in English. 1967. m. GBP 28.75; GBP 3.75 newsstand/cover (effective 2000). adv. bk.rev. illus. index. **Document type:** *Consumer.*
Indexed: Can.Per.Ind., Res.High.Educ.Abstr., Russ.Acad.Sci.Bibl., e-psyche.
Published by: (Forum International), Northern & Shell Publications, Northern & Shell Tower, City Harbour, PO Box 381, London E14 9GL, United Kingdom. TEL 44-20-7308-5090, FAX 44-20-7308-5078, forum@norshell.co.uk. Ed. Elizabeth Coldwell. Adv. contact Amanda Keer. B&W page GBP 2,050, color page GBP 2,250; trim 148 x 210. Circ: 40,000 (paid). **Subscr. to:** 43 Millharbour, London E14 9TR, United Kingdom. TEL 44-20-7538-8288.

▼ **GYM**; for the physical man. see *PHYSICAL FITNESS AND HYGIENE*

▼ **JOURNAL OF COUPLE & RELATIONSHIP THERAPY.** see *PSYCHOLOGY*

MEN'S WORKOUT. see *MEN'S HEALTH*

M

MENSTUFF, THE NATIONAL MEN'S RESOURCE. see *MEN'S STUDIES*

NATURAL BODYBUILDING AND FITNESS. see *PHYSICAL FITNESS AND HYGIENE*

NATURAL MUSCLE MAGAZINE. see *PHYSICAL FITNESS AND HYGIENE*

ONTARIO WRESTLER MAGAZINE. see *SPORTS AND GAMES*

SEX & HEALTH. see *MEN'S HEALTH*

MEN'S STUDIES

305.31 613.081 USA
MENSTUFF, THE NATIONAL MEN'S RESOURCE. Text in English. 1985. q. free per issue. bk.rev. illus. **Document type:** *Newsletter.* **Description:** Publishes information, events listings, resources and reviews concerning a positive change in male roles and relationships.
Former titles: Menstuff (Print) (1074-7842); (until 1993): National Men's Resource Calendar
Media: Online - full text.
Published by: National Men's Resource Center, PO Box 800, San Anselmo, CA 94979-0800. menstuff@menstuff.org, http://www.menstuff.org. Ed., Pub. Gordon Clay.

▼ **PSYCHOLOGY OF MEN & MASCULINITY.** see *PSYCHOLOGY*

305.3 USA
WINGSPAN (LA JOLLA)✱ ; journal of the male spirit. Text in English. 1986. q. USD 16. adv. **Document type:** *Newsletter.* **Description:** Covers issues pertaining to male psychology and spirituality, with think pieces from leaders of the men's movement, workshop profiles and extensive listings of nationwide men's events.
Indexed: e-psyche.
Address: 2333 Camino Del Rio S Ste 200, San Diego, CA 92108-3600. TEL 619-454-4622, wingspanj@aol.com. Ed. Christopher Harding. Adv. contact Randall Mount. B&W page USD 1,960. Circ: 25,000.

METALLURGY

see also MINES AND MINING INDUSTRY

I E H REPORT ON FACTORS AFFECTING THE ABSORPTION OF TOXIC METALS FROM THE DIET. see *ENVIRONMENTAL STUDIES—Toxicology And Environmental Safety*

MAGNESIUM RESEARCH. see *MEDICAL SCIENCES*

PARTICULATE SCIENCE AND TECHNOLOGY; an international journal. see *ENGINEERING—Chemical Engineering*

661.0724 BEL ISSN 1024-4204
SELENIUM - TELLURIUM DEVELOPMENT ASSOCIATION. BULLETIN. Text in English. irreg. (3-4/yr.). bibl, illus. **Document type:** *Bulletin.* **Description:** Promotes knowledge about applications of selenium and tellurium in metallurgy, pharmaceuticals, feed additives, pigments, chemicals and electronics.
Indexed: AESIS, Alloys Ind., Eng.Mat.Abstr., METADEX, Met.Abstr., Met.Abstr.Ind., Nonfer.Met.Alert, PCC Alert, Steels Alert, World Alum.Abstr.
Published by: Selenium - Tellurium Development Association, Borgtstraat 301, Grimbergen 1850, Belgium. TEL 32-2-252-1490, FAX 32-2-252-2775, info@stda.be, http://www.stda.be. Ed. Yves Palmieri. Circ: 2,000.

METALLURGY—Abstracting, Bibliographies, Statistics

C A SELECTS. INORGANIC & ORGANOMETALLIC REACTION SYSTEMS. see *CHEMISTRY—Abstracting, Bibliographies, Statistics*

C A SELECTS. METALLO ENZYMES & METALLO COENZYMES. see *CHEMISTRY—Abstracting, Bibliographies, Statistics*

METEOROLOGY

ADVANCES IN NATURAL AND TECHNOLOGICAL HAZARDS RESEARCH. see *PUBLIC HEALTH AND SAFETY*

570 USA ISSN 0067-8902
QH543
BIOMETEOROLOGY; proceedings of the International Congress of Biometeorology. Text in English. triennial, latest 1996, 14th, Ljibljana, Slovenia. USD 75 to non-members; USD 50 to members. **Document type:** *Proceedings.*
Formerly: International Biometeorology Congress. Summaries and Reports Presented to the Congress (0074-2082)
Indexed: Biol.Abstr., Curr.Cont. (coverage dropped). —GNLM.
Published by: International Society of Biometeorology, c/o Dr Wayne L Decker, Treas, Dept of Soil & Atmospheric Sciences, University of Missouri, 116 Gentry Hall, Columbia, MO 65211. Circ: 1,200.

570 AUS ISSN 1022-9205
BIOMETEOROLOGY BULLETIN. Text in English. s-a. membership. adv. **Document type:** *Bulletin.*
Published by: International Society of Biometeorology, c/o Dr. Paul J. Beggs, Ed., Department of Physical Geography, Macquarie University, NSW 2109, Australia. TEL 61-2-9850-8399, FAX 61-2-9850-8420, pbeggs@ocs1.ocs.mq.edu.au, http://www.es.mq.edu.au/ISB/. Ed., R&P, Adv. contact Dr. Paul J Beggs. Circ: 300 (controlled).

551.5 570 DEU ISSN 0020-7128
QH543 CODEN: IJBMAO
INTERNATIONAL JOURNAL OF BIOMETEOROLOGY; the description, causes, and implications of climatic change. Text in English. 1957. q. EUR 469.40 domestic; EUR 466.90 in Germany; EUR 138 newsstand/cover foreign (effective 2002). adv. abstr, bibl, charts, illus. index. reprints avail. *Refereed.* **Document type:** *Journal, Academic/Scholarly.* **Description:** Covers research in plant, animal, human and general biometeorology in the areas of plant-weather interaction, ecological modeling, animal-weather interaction, and the effects of electric, magnetic and electromagnetic fields on biological functions.
Related titles: Online - full text ed.: ISSN 1432-1254 (from EBSCO Publishing, RoweCom Information Quest, Swets Blackwell, Springer LINK, Institute for Scientific Information).
Indexed: ASCA, Agri.Eng.Abstr., Agricola, Anim.Breed.Abstr., Aqua.Sci.& Fish.Abstr., BBCI, Biol.Abstr., Cal.Tiss.Abstr., Chem.Abstr., Crop Physiol.Abstr., Curr.Adv.Ecol.Sci., Curr.Cont., Dairy Sci.Abstr., Environ.Sci.Poll.Mgmt., Excerp.Med., Field Crop Abstr., Forest.Abstr., GeoRef, Helminthol.Abstr., Herb.Abstr., Hort.Abstr., Ind.Med. (1961-), Ind.Sci.Rev., Ind.Vet., Meteor.& Geoastrophys.Abstr., Ornam.Hort., Pig News & Info., Pollut.Abstr., Postharvest, Ref.Zh., Rev.Appl.Entomol., Rev.Med.& Vet.Mycol., Rev.Plant Path., SSCI (coverage dropped), Sci.Cit.Ind., Sel.Water Res.Abstr., Sport Fish.Abstr., Vet.Bull., Weed Abstr., Wild.Rev., Zoo.Rec.
—BLDSC (4542.154000), CASDDS, CISTI, GNLM, IDS, ingenta, Linda Hall. **CCC.**
Published by: (International Society of Biometeorology), Springer-Verlag (Subsidiary of: BertelsmannSpringer), Tiergartenstr 17, Heidelberg 69121, Germany. TEL 49-6221-345-0, FAX 49-6221-345229, subscriptions@springer.de, http://link.springer.de/link/service/journals/00484/index.htm, http://www.springer.de. Ed. M Iriki. Circ: 1,300. **Subscr. in N. America to:** Springer-Verlag New York Inc., PO Box 2485, Secaucus, NJ 07096-2485. TEL 212-460-1500, FAX 212-473-6272.

METROLOGY AND STANDARDIZATION

389.6 CHE ISSN 1424-6074
RS189 CODEN: DVBSA3
DEVELOPMENTS IN BIOLOGICALS. Text in English. 1973. irreg., latest vol.104. price varies. back issues avail. *Refereed.* **Document type:** *Monographic series, Proceedings, Academic/Scholarly.* **Description:** Reports on the development and use of standardized biologicals.
Formerly (until 1999): Developments in Biological Standardization (0301-5149); Which was formed by the merger of (1964-1973): Progress in Immunobiological Standardization (0079-6344); (1966-1973): Symposia Series in Immunobiological Standardization (0082-0768)
Indexed: ASCA, Biol.Abstr., Chem.Abstr., Chem.Indus.Notes, Chem.Titles, Curr.Cont. (coverage dropped), Dairy Sci.Abstr., Eng.Ind., Excerp.Med., Ind.Med. (coverage dropped), Ind.Sci.Rev., Ind.Vet., Rev.Plant Path., Sci.Cit.Ind. (coverage dropped), Vet.Bull.
—BLDSC (3579.067010), CASDDS, CISTI, GNLM, Infotrieve, ingenta, KNAW. **CCC.**
Published by: (International Association for Biologicals), S. Karger AG, Allschwilerstr 10, PO Box, Basel 4009, Switzerland. TEL 41-61-3061111, FAX 41-61-3061234, karger@karger.ch, http://www.karger.com/bookseries/DEBIS.

F D C CONTROL NEWSLETTER. (Food, Drug, and Cosmetics) see *FOOD AND FOOD INDUSTRIES*

JOURNAL OF OUTCOME MEASUREMENT; dedicated to health, education, and social science. (JOM) see *EDUCATION*

MICROBIOLOGY

see BIOLOGY—Microbiology

MICROCOMPUTERS

see COMPUTERS—Microcomputers

MICROSCOPY

see BIOLOGY—Microscopy

MILITARY

see also CIVIL DEFENSE

▼ **ARMED FORCES MEDICAL DEVELOPMENTS.** see *MEDICAL SCIENCES*

610.6 GBR
ARMY MEDICAL SERVICES MAGAZINE. Text in English. 1927. 3/yr. GBP 3.30 (effective 1999). adv. bk.rev. *Refereed.* **Document type:** *Newsletter, Government.* **Description:** Unit news of organizations within the Army Medical Services.
Published by: R A M C Historical Museum, Keogh Barracks, Ash Vale, Aldershot, Hants GU12 5RQ, United Kingdom. TEL 44-1252-340212, FAX 44-1252-340224. Ed. P H Starling. R&P P.H. Starling TEL 44-1252-340250. Circ: 2,500.

THE B V A BULLETIN. (Blinded Veterans Association) see *HANDICAPPED—Visually Impaired*

DI SI JUNYI DAXUE XUEBAO/FOURTH MILITARY MEDICAL UNIVERSITY. JOURNAL. see *MEDICAL SCIENCES*

355 GBR ISSN 0956-2400
FALLING LEAF. Text in English. 1958. q. GBP 10, USD 17 (effective 2000). adv. bk.rev. illus. **Document type:** *Bulletin.* **Description:** Primarily concerns the dissemination and effects of aerial propaganda leaflets in wars and conflicts.
Indexed: Russ.Acad.Sci.Bibl., e-psyche.
Published by: Psywar Society, c/o K.B. Moore, 7 N. Park Ave., Leeds LS8 1DN, United Kingdom. TEL 44-113-266-3976, keith@kaymoore.demon.co.uk, http://www.kaymoore.demon.co.uk. Ed., R&P David Minshall. Pub., Adv. contact K.B. Moore. Circ: 150.

353.538 USA ISSN 0883-3370
UB357
FEDERAL BENEFITS FOR VETERANS AND DEPENDENTS. Text in English. 1961. a. USD 5 (effective 1999). **Document type:** *Government.* **Description:** Outlines and describes benefits and services available to US veterans and their dependents. Also lists V.A. facilities nationwide.
Formerly: U.S. Veterans Administration. V A Fact Sheets (0083-3576)
Related titles: Online - full text ed.
Published by: (Office of Public Affairs), U.S. Department of Veterans Affairs, 810 Vermont Ave, N W 008C2, Washington, DC 20420. TEL 202-273-5730, http://www.va.gov/benefits.htm/. Ed. Bonner H Day. **Subscr. to:** U.S. Government Printing Office, Superintendent of Documents.

FLYING SAFETY. see *AERONAUTICS AND SPACE FLIGHT*

GULHANE MEDICAL JOURNAL. see *MEDICAL SCIENCES*

J M N R. (Journal of Military Nursing & Research) see *MEDICAL SCIENCES—Nurses And Nursing*

JIEFANGJUN JIANKANG/P L A HEALTH. see *PHYSICAL FITNESS AND HYGIENE*

JIEFANGJUN YIXUE ZAZHI/MEDICAL JOURNAL OF CHINESE PEOPLE'S LIBERATION ARMY. see *MEDICAL SCIENCES*

JUNSHI YIXUE KEXUEYUAN YUANKAN/ACADEMY OF MILITARY MEDICAL SCIENCES. BULLETIN. see *MEDICAL SCIENCES*

MEDICINE, CONFLICT AND SURVIVAL; international medical concerns on global security issues. see *MEDICAL SCIENCES*

355 CHE ISSN 0026-3907
MILITAER-KUECHENCHEF. Text in German. 1971 (vol.15). bi-m. adv. charts, illus.
Published by: Verband Schweizerischer Militaerkuechenchefs, Muehleweg 10, Langnau-Gattikon 8135, Switzerland. TEL 01-7201462. Ed. Major Qm Stampfli Pius.

355 NOR ISSN 0801-8960
MILITAERPSYKOLOGISKE MEDDELELSER. Text in Norwegian. 1955. irreg. free. **Document type:** *Journal, Trade.*
Published by: Norwegian Armed Forces, Chief Psychologist, Oslo Mil, Huseby, K-P, Oslo 0016, Norway. Ed. Ivar Hansen.

MILITARY PSYCHOLOGY. see *PSYCHOLOGY*

355 USA
UC333
THE MOBILITY FORUM; journal of the Air Mobility Command. Text in English. 1954. m. USD 25 (effective 2001). bk.rev. stat. reprint service avail. from PQC. **Document type:** *Magazine, Government.* **Description:** Safety publication.
Formerly (until 1991): M A C Flyer (0024-788X)
Related titles: Microform ed.: (from MIM,PQC).
Indexed: Air Un.Lib.Ind., Ind.U.S.Gov.Per.
—ingenta.
Published by: U.S. Air Force, Air Mobility Command, Directorate of Safety, Headquarters AMC-SER, 510 B St., Rm. E117, Scott Air Force Base, IL 62225-5020. TEL 618-256-3534, FAX 618-256-8174, http://public.scott.af.mil/hqamc/tmf/themobil.htm, http://www.safb.af.mil/hqamc/pa/tmf/themobil.htm. Ed. Maj John Ward. R&P David Rubelcaba. Circ: 12,000. **Orders to:** U.S. Government Printing Office, Superintendent of Documents, PO Box 371954, Pittsburgh, PA 15250-7954. TEL 202-512-1800, FAX 202-512-2250, orders@gpo.gov, http://www.access.gpo.gov.

NATIONAL CENTER FOR POST TRAUMATIC STRESS DISORDER. CLINICAL QUARTERLY. see *MEDICAL SCIENCES—Psychiatry And Neurology*

NEDERLANDS MILITAIR GENEESKUNDIG TIJDSCHRIFT. see *MEDICAL SCIENCES*

P T S D RESEARCH QUARTERLY. see *MEDICAL SCIENCES—Psychiatry And Neurology*

REVISTA CUBANA DE MEDICINA MILITAR. see *MEDICAL SCIENCES*

REVISTA DE MEDICINA MILITARA. see *MEDICAL SCIENCES*

REVISTA MEDICA DA AERONAUTICA DO BRASIL. see *MEDICAL SCIENCES*

355 CAN ISSN 1208-9400
SAFETY DIGEST (OTTAWA)/DIGEST DE SECURITE. Text in English. 1973. 4/yr. CND 11, USD 13.40. illus. **Document type:** *Government.*
Formerly (until 1996): General Safety Digest (0707-0403)
Related titles: French ed.
Published by: Department of National Defence, Directorate of General Safety, National Defence Headquarters, Major General George Pearkes Bldg, 101 Colonel By Dr, Ottawa, ON K1A 0K2, Canada. TEL 613-995-3291, FAX 613-992-5484, http://www.vcds.dnd.ca/vcds/dsafeg/digest/index_e.htm. Ed., R&P Bob Britton. Circ: 10,000. **Dist. by:** Canada Communication Group, Ottawa, ON K1A 0S9, Canada.

363.286 USA
U.S. COAST GUARD. MARINE SAFETY MANUAL. VOLUME 1: ADMINISTRATION AND MANAGEMENT. Text in English. base vol. plus irreg. updates. USD 16 (effective 2001). **Document type:** *Academic/Scholarly.* **Description:** Presents the authority, background and rationale for the various marine safety activities of the Coast Guard and prescribes the essential functions which must be performed to attain the overall marine safety objectives of the Coast Guard.
Published by: U.S. Coast Guard, 2100 Second St, S W, Washington, DC 20593. http://www.uscg.mil/hq/g-m/nmc/pubs/msm/. **Subscr. to:** U.S. Government Printing Office, Superintendent of Documents, PO Box 371954, Pittsburgh, PA 15250-7954. TEL 202-512-1800, FAX 202-512-2250, orders@gpo.gov, http://www.access.gpo.gov.

363.286 USA
U.S. COAST GUARD. MARINE SAFETY MANUAL. VOLUME 10: INTERAGENCY AGREEMENTTS AND ACRONYMS. Text in English. base vol. plus irreg. updates. USD 48 (effective 2001). **Document type:** *Government.* **Description:** Presents the authority, background and rationale for the various marine safety activities of the Coast Guard and prescribes the essential functions which must be performed to attain the overall marine safety objectives of the Coast Guard.
Published by: U.S. Coast Guard, 2100 Second St, S W, Washington, DC 20593. http://www.uscg.mil/hq/g-m/nmc/pubs/msm/. **Subscr. to:** U.S. Government Printing Office, Superintendent of Documents, PO Box 371954, Pittsburgh, PA 15250-7954. TEL 202-512-1800, FAX 202-512-2250, orders@gpo.gov, http://www.access.gpo.gov.

363.286 USA
U.S. COAST GUARD. MARINE SAFETY MANUAL. VOLUME 2: MATERIEL INSPECTION. Text in English. base vol. plus irreg. updates. USD 84 (effective 2001). **Document type:** *Government.* **Description:** Presents the authority, background and rationale for the various marine safety activities of the Coast Guard and prescribes the essential functions which must be performed to attain the overall marine safety objectives of the Coast Guard.
Published by: U.S. Coast Guard, 2100 Second St, S W, Washington, DC 20593. http://www.uscg.mil/hq/g-m/nmc/pubs/msm/. **Subscr. to:** U.S. Government Printing Office, Superintendent of Documents, PO Box 371954, Pittsburgh, PA 15250-7954. TEL 202-512-1800, FAX 202-512-2250, orders@gpo.gov, http://www.access.gpo.gov.

363.286 USA
U.S. COAST GUARD. MARINE SAFETY MANUAL. VOLUME 3: MARINE INDUSTRY PERSONNEL. Text in English. base vol. plus irreg. updates. USD 54 (effective 2001). **Document type:** *Government.* **Description:** Presents the authority, background and rationale for the various marine safety activities of the Coast Guard and prescribes the essential functions which must be performed to attain the overall marine safety objectives of the Coast Guard.
Published by: U.S. Coast Guard, 2100 Second St, S W, Washington, DC 20593. http://www.uscg.mil/hq/g-m/nmc/pubs/msm/. **Subscr. to:** U.S. Government Printing Office, Superintendent of Documents, PO Box 371954, Pittsburgh, PA 15250-7954. TEL 202-512-1800, FAX 202-512-2250, orders@gpo.gov, http://www.access.gpo.gov.

363.286 USA
U.S. COAST GUARD. MARINE SAFETY MANUAL. VOLUME 4: TECHNICAL. Text in English. base vol. plus irreg. updates. USD 73 (effective 2001). **Document type:** *Government.* **Description:** Presents the authority, background and rationale for the various marine safety activities of the Coast Guard and prescribes the essential functions which must be performed to attain the overall marine safety objectives of the Coast Guard.
Published by: U.S. Coast Guard http://www.uscg.mil/hq/g-m/nmc/pubs/msm/. **Subscr. to:** U.S. Government Printing Office, Superintendent of Documents, PO Box 371954, Pittsburgh, PA 15250-7954. TEL 202-512-1800, FAX 202-512-2250, orders@gpo.gov, http://www.access.gpo.gov.

363.286 USA
U.S. COAST GUARD. MARINE SAFETY MANUAL. VOLUME 5: INVESTIGATIONS. Text in English. base vol. plus irreg. updates. USD 50 (effective 2001). **Document type:** *Government.* **Description:** Presents the authority, background and rationale for the various marine safety activities of the Coast Guard and prescribes the essential functions which must be performed to attain the overall marine safety objectives of the Coast Guard.
Published by: U.S. Coast Guard, 2100 Second St, S W, Washington, DC 20593. http://www.uscg.mil/hq/g-m/nmc/pubs/msm/. **Subscr. to:** U.S. Government Printing Office, Superintendent of Documents, PO Box 371954, Pittsburgh, PA 15250-7954. TEL 202-512-1800, FAX 202-512-2250, orders@gpo.gov, http://www.access.gpo.gov.

363.286 USA
U.S. COAST GUARD. MARINE SAFETY MANUAL. VOLUME 6: PORTS AND WATERWAYS ACTIVITIES. Text in English. base vol. plus irreg. updates. USD 76 (effective 2001). **Document type:** *Government.* **Description:** Presents the authority, background and rationale for the various marine safety activities of the Coast Guard and prescribes the essential functions which must be performed to attain the overall marine safety objectives of the Coast Guard.
Related titles: Online - full content ed.
Published by: U.S. Coast Guard, 2100 Second St, S W, Washington, DC 20593. http://www.uscg.mil/hq/g-m/nmc/pubs/msm/. **Subscr. to:** U.S. Government Printing Office, Superintendent of Documents, PO Box 371954, Pittsburgh, PA 15250-7954. TEL 202-512-1800, FAX 202-512-2250, orders@gpo.gov, http://www.access.gpo.gov.

363.286 USA
U.S. COAST GUARD. MARINE SAFETY MANUAL. VOLUME 7: PORT SECURITY. Text in English. base vol. plus irreg. updates. USD 74 (effective 2001). **Document type:** *Government.* **Description:** Presents the authority, background and rationale for the various marine safety activities of the Coast Guard and prescribes the essential functions which must be performed to attain the overall marine safety objectives of the Coast Guard.
Published by: U.S. Coast Guard, 2100 Second St, S W, Washington, DC 20593. http://www.uscg.mil/hq/g-m/nmc/pubs/msm/. **Subscr. to:** U.S. Government Printing Office, Superintendent of Documents, PO Box 371954, Pittsburgh, PA 15250-7954. TEL 202-512-1800, FAX 202-512-2250, orders@gpo.gov, http://www.access.gpo.gov.

363.286 USA
U.S. COAST GUARD. MARINE SAFETY MANUAL. VOLUME 9: ENVIRONMENTAL PROTECTION. Text in English. base vol. plus irreg. updates. **Document type:** *Government.* **Description:** Presents the authority, background and rationale for the various marine safety activities of the Coast Guard and prescribes the essential functions which must be performed to attain the overall marine safety objectives of the Coast Guard.
Published by: U.S. Coast Guard, 2100 Second St, S W, Washington, DC 20593. http://www.uscg.mil/hq/g-m/nmc/pubs/msm/. **Subscr. to:** U.S. Government Printing Office, Superintendent of Documents, PO Box 371954, Pittsburgh, PA 15250-7954. TEL 202-512-1800, FAX 202-512-2250, orders@gpo.gov, http://www.access.gpo.gov.

U.S. DEFENSE LOGISTICS AGENCY. D O D HAZARDOUS MATERIALS INFORMATION SYSTEM: HAZARDOUS ITEM LISTING. see *PUBLIC HEALTH AND SAFETY*

UNION DES AVEUGLES DE GUERRE. BULLETIN BIMESTRIEL. see *HANDICAPPED—Visually Impaired*

UNITED ARAB EMIRATES. AL-QIYADAH AL-AAMAH LIL-QUWWAT AL-MUSALLIHAH. MAJALLAH AL-TIBBIYYAH/UNITED ARAB EMIRATES. GENERAL COMMAND FOR THE ARMED FORCES. MEDICAL JOURNAL. see *MEDICAL SCIENCES*

VITAL SIGNS (CAMBRIDGE). see *PUBLIC HEALTH AND SAFETY*

VOJNOSANITETSKI PREGLED/MILITARY MEDICAL AND PHARMACEUTICAL; casopis lekara i farmaceuta vojske Jugoslavije. see *MEDICAL SCIENCES*

WEHRMEDIZIN UND WEHRPHARMAZIE. see *MEDICAL SCIENCES*

M

WOUND BALLISTICS REVIEW. see *MEDICAL SCIENCES—Forensic Sciences*

MINES AND MINING INDUSTRY

see also METALLURGY

622.8 631.62 DEU ISSN 0949-7234
A S VORORT; Fachmagazin fuer die Arbeitssicherheit und den Gesundheitsschutz in Bergbau. (Arbeit und Sicherheit) Text in German. 1947. 10/yr. DEM 44 (effective 2001). adv. **Document type:** *Journal, Trade.*
Former titles: Arbeit und Sicherheit (0344-239X); Grubensicherheit (0017-4858)
—CCC.
Published by: (Nordrhein-Westfalen. N R W, Abteilung Bergbau und Energie), Verlag Glueckauf GmbH, Postfach 185620, Essen 45206, Germany. TEL 49-2054-924-0, FAX 49-2054-924129, asvorort@aol.com, vge-vertrieb@t-online.de, vge-anzeigen@t-online.de, http://www.vge.de. Ed. Bernd Litke. R&P Eckart Pasche TEL 49-2054-924120. Adv. contact Ute Perkovic TEL 49-2054-924130. B&W page DEM 6,400, color page DEM 7,720; trim 182 x 269. Circ: 36,000 (controlled). **Co-sponsor:** Bergbau-Berufsgenossenschaft.

338.2 662 CAN ISSN 0008-4492
CODEN: CAMJA9
CANADIAN MINING JOURNAL. Text in English. 1879. bi-m. CND 39.95 domestic; USD 51.95 in United States; USD 62.95 elsewhere (effective 1999). adv. illus, mkt. index. *Refereed.* **Document type:** *Trade.* **Description:** Provides technical oriented information and on-site coverage of mine and mill operations.
Incorporates: Mining in Canada (0047-7494)
Related titles: Microfiche ed.: (from MML); Microfilm ed.: (from PMC,MML); Microform ed.: (from MML); Online - full text ed.: (from Gale Group, Infomart Dialog, Northern Light Technology, Inc., ProQuest Information & Learning, Factiva, Institute for Scientific Information).
Indexed: ABI Inform. (Feb.1993-), AESIS, ASCA, Bus.& Indus. (Apr.1995-), CBCA Bus. (1993-), CBCA Ref., C.I.S. Abstr., Cadscan, Can.B.P.I., Can.Per.Ind. (Feb.1996-), Chem.Abstr., Curr.Cont., Eng.Ind., Environ.Eng.Abstr., Environ.Per.Bibl., Environ.Sci.Poll.Mgmt., Excerp.Med., Fuel & Energy Abstr., GeoRef, I.M.M.Abstr., INIS Atomind., INSPEC (Oct.1975-May 1978, dropped), Key to Econ.Sci., Lead Abstr., Met.Abstr., Petrol.Abstr. (coverage dropped), Zincscan.
—BLDSC (3042.000000), CASDDS, CISTI, Ei, IDS, Infotrieve, ingenta, Linda Hall. **CCC.**
Published by: Southam Magazine Group, 1450 Don Mills Rd, Don Mills, ON M3B 2X7, Canada. TEL 416-445-6641, FAX 416-442-2272. Ed. Jane Werniuk. Pub. Ray Perks. adv.: B&W page CND 2,350. Circ: 8,495.

FEDERAL MINE SAFETY AND HEALTH REVIEW COMMISSION DECISIONS. see *OCCUPATIONAL HEALTH AND SAFETY*

622 610 USA
GOLD INSTITUTE. INTERNATIONAL CONFERENCE ON GOLD & SILVER IN MEDICINE. PROCEEDINGS. Text in English. irreg., latest 1998. USD 75 (effective 1999). **Document type:** *Proceedings.* **Description:** Reports on new clinical research on gold in England, Canada, the Netherlands and the United States.
Published by: Gold Institute, Administrative Office/Institut de l'Or, Bureau Administratif, 1112 16th St, NW, Ste 240, Washington, DC 20036-4823. TEL 202-835-0185, FAX 202-835-0155, info@goldinstitute.org, http://www.goldinstitute.org. **Co-sponsor:** Silver Institute.

INJURY EXPERIENCE IN SAND AND GRAVEL MINING. see *OCCUPATIONAL HEALTH AND SAFETY—Abstracting, Bibliographies, Statistics*

INTERNATIONAL PEAT JOURNAL. see *BIOLOGY—Botany*

622 351.823 USA ISSN 1051-533X
LEGAL QUARTERLY DIGEST OF MINE SAFETY AND HEALTH DECISIONS. Text in English. 1990. q. USD 475 (effective 1999 & 2000). index. **Document type:** *Abstract/Index, Trade.* **Description:** Summarizes legal decisions, mine safety issues and health cases.
Published by: Legal Publication Services, 888 Pittsford Mendon Center Rd, Pittsford, NY 14534. TEL 716-582-3211, FAX 716-582-2879, MineSafety@aol.com. Ed. Nicole Dejeet. R&P Ellen Smith.

622.8 ZAF
MINE SAFETY DIGEST. Text in English. bi-m. ZAR 64 domestic; ZAR 129 elsewhere (effective 2000). charts, illus, stat. **Document type:** *Trade.* **Description:** Discusses all aspects of mine safety.
Published by: T M L Business Publishing (Subsidiary of: Times Media Ltd.), PO Box 182, Pinegowrie, Gauteng 2123, South Africa. TEL 27-11-789-2144, FAX 27-11-789-3196. Ed. Roy Bennetts.

622 ZAF ISSN 0368-3206
MINE VENTILATION SOCIETY OF SOUTH AFRICA. JOURNAL. Text in English. 1948. q. ZAR 220 domestic; ZAR 550 foreign (effective 2001). bk.rev. charts, illus. index, cum.index every 10 yrs. back issues avail.; reprint service avail. from PQC. *Refereed.* **Document type:** *Journal, Academic/Scholarly.* **Description:** Presents technical papers and notes.
Related titles: Microform ed.: (from PQC).
Indexed: C.I.S. Abstr., Eng.Ind., Environ.Sci.Poll.Mgmt., Fluidex, Fuel & Energy Abstr., I.M.M.Abstr., INIS Atomind., ISMEC, Ind.S.A.Per., Pollut.Abstr., Risk Abstr., Saf.Sci.Abstr.
—BLDSC (4826.500000), CISTI, ingenta.
Published by: Mine Ventilation Society of South Africa, PO Box 93480, Yeoville, Johannesburg 2143, South Africa. TEL 27-11-487-1073, minevent@global.co.za. Ed. Marco Biffi. R&P, Adv. contact Sue Moseley. Circ: 1,250.

622 613.62 BEL ISSN 0588-702X
MINES SAFETY AND HEALTH COMMISSION. REPORT/ORGANE PERMANENT POUR LA SECURITE DANS LES MINES DE HOUILLE. RAPPORT. Text in English. 1959. a. free per issue. **Document type:** *Corporate.*
Formerly (until 1966): European Coal and Steel Community. Organe Permanent pour la Securite dans les Mines de Houille. Rapport
Published by: Commission of the European Communities, Rue de la Loi - Wetstraat 200, Brussels 1049, Belgium. **Dist. in the U.S. by:** Bernan Associates, 4611 F Assembly Dr, Lanham, MD 20706. TEL 301-459-0056, 800-274-4447.

RESSOURCE EN SANTE ET EN SECURITE. see *OCCUPATIONAL HEALTH AND SAFETY*

SEGURIDAD. see *OCCUPATIONAL HEALTH AND SAFETY*

MINES AND MINING INDUSTRY—Abstracting, Bibliographies, Statistics

622 USA ISSN 1072-768X
MINE SAFETY AND HEALTH NEWS. Text in English. 1994. 24/yr. USD 625 (effective 2000). index. **Document type:** *Newsletter.* **Description:** Covers proposed and final rules, policies of the Mine Safety and Health Administration and court cases of the Federal Mine Safety and Health Review Commission.
Related titles: Diskette ed.: USD 625 (effective 2000).
Published by: Legal Publication Services, 888 Pittsford Mendon Center Rd, Pittsford, NY 14534. TEL 716-582-3211, FAX 716-582-2879, MineSafety@aol.com. Ed. Nicole Dejeet. R&P Ellen Smith.

MOTION PICTURES

PSYCHOLOGICAL CINEMA REGISTER; films and video in the behavioral sciences. see *PSYCHOLOGY—Abstracting, Bibliographies, Statistics*

MOTION PICTURES—Abstracting, Bibliographies, Statistics

011.37 USA ISSN 0093-7215
HV2395
CATALOG OF CAPTIONED FILMS FOR THE DEAF*. Text in English. a. **Document type:** *Catalog.*
Published by: Associations for Education of the Deaf, Special Materials Project, c/o Assoc Builder Contra, 4061 Powder Mill Rd, Beltsville, MD 20705-3149.

MUNICIPAL GOVERNMENT

see PUBLIC ADMINISTRATION—Municipal Government

MUSEUMS AND ART GALLERIES

ADLER MUSEUM BULLETIN. see *MEDICAL SCIENCES*

613.075 AUS ISSN 1442-1283
HEALTH AND MEDICINE MUSEUMS NEWSLETTER. Text in English. 1991. s-a. AUD 11 in Australia to individuals; AUD 15 in New Zealand to individuals; AUD 20 elsewhere to individuals; AUD 28.50 in Australia to institutions; AUD 30 in New Zealand to institutions; AUD 35 elsewhere to institutions (effective 2001). **Document type:** *Newsletter.* **Description:** Each issue contains: a main article on some aspect of acquiring, managing or utilizing collections, news of health and medicine museums and exhibitions around Australia, notices of new publications and journal articles.
Formerly (until 1993): Museums Association of Australia. Health and Medicine Museums Section. Newsletter (1036-3041)
Related titles: Online - full text ed.
Published by: Health and Medicine Museums, PO Box K346, Haymarket, NSW 1238, Australia. TEL 61-2-9217-0254, FAX 61-2-9217-0355, maganh@phm.gov.au, http://amol.org.au/hmm/Latest_Newsletter/latest_newsletter.html. Ed. Megan Hicks.

ZOO - NACHRICHTEN; Allwetterzoo - Nachrichten. see *BIOLOGY—Zoology*

MUSIC

see also DANCE; SOUND RECORDING AND REPRODUCTION

▼ **ARTS THERAPIES RESEARCH LIBRARY.** see *MEDICAL SCIENCES*

BRAILLE MUSIC MAGAZINE. see *HANDICAPPED—Visually Impaired*

BRITISH JOURNAL OF MUSIC THERAPY. see *MEDICAL SCIENCES—Physical Medicine And Rehabilitation*

780 616.89 GBR ISSN 0953-7511
ML3919
BRITISH SOCIETY FOR MUSIC THERAPY. BULLETIN. Text in English. 1987. 3/yr. **Document type:** *Bulletin.*
Indexed: e-psyche.
—BLDSC (2425.300000), GNLM.
Published by: British Society for Music Therapy, 25 Rosslyn Ave, E. Barnet, Herts EN4 8DH, United Kingdom. Ed. Denize Christophers. Circ: 800.

780 158 CAN
CANADIAN JOURNAL OF MUSIC THERAPY/REVUE CANADIENNE DE MUSICOTHERAPIE. Text in English, French. 1993. a. bk.rev. bibl, charts, illus, stat. back issues avail. *Refereed.* **Document type:** *Academic/Scholarly.* **Description:** Covers the therapeutic application of music for clients and patients. Serves children with disabilities, including emotional behavior delays, individuals with psychiatric diagnoses, and the elderly.
Indexed: Can.Mus.Per.Ind. (1973-1979), PsycInfo, e-psyche.
Published by: Canadian Association for Music Therapy/Association de Musicotherapie du Canada, c/o Linda Tracy, Administrative Assistant, Wilfrid Lauria University, Waterloo, ON N2L 3C5, Canada. TEL 519-884-1970, FAX 519-884-8853, camt@musictherapy.ca, ltracy@mach1.wlu.ca. Ed. Carolyn Bereznak Kenny. Circ: 430 (paid).

780 USA ISSN 0193-9041
CONTRIBUTIONS TO THE STUDY OF MUSIC AND DANCE. Text in English. 1981. irreg. price varies.
—BLDSC (3461.454100).
Published by: Greenwood Press, Inc. (Subsidiary of: Greenwood Publishing Group Inc.), 88 Post Rd W, Box 5007, Westport, CT 06881. TEL 203-226-3571, FAX 203-226-1502.

GOOD VIBRATIONS. see *HANDICAPPED—Visually Impaired*

JOURNAL OF MUSIC THERAPY. see *MEDICAL SCIENCES—Physical Medicine And Rehabilitation*

MEDICAL PROBLEMS OF PERFORMING ARTISTS. see *MEDICAL SCIENCES*

M

N

780 150 USA ISSN 0734-6875
ML3920
MUSIC THERAPY PERSPECTIVES. Text in English. 1983. 2/yr. USD 110 domestic; USD 120 foreign (effective 2001). adv. back issues avail. *Refereed.* **Document type:** *Academic/Scholarly.* **Description:** Focuses on the theory, practice and administration of music therapy.
Indexed: Int.Ind.Mus.Per., Music Ind., PsycInfo, Psychol.Abstr. (1987-), e-psyche.
—BLDSC (5990.435100), ingenta.
Published by: American Music Therapy Association, 8455 Colesville Rd, Ste 1000, Silver Spring, MD 20910-3392. TEL 301-589-3300, FAX 301-589-5175, subscribe@musictherapy.org; orders@allenpress.com, http://www.musictherapy.org; http://www.allenpress.com. Ed. Brian Wilson. **Subscr. to:** Allen Press Inc., PO Box 1897, Lawrence, KS 66044-8897.

780 DEU ISSN 0177-350X
ML3830
MUSIKPSYCHOLOGIE. Text in German. 1984. irreg. DEM 54. back issues avail. **Document type:** *Monographic series.*
Indexed: IBR, IBZ, Ind.Philos., Music Ind., RILM, e-psyche.
Published by: (Deutsche Gesellschaft fuer Musikpsychologie), Florian Noetzel Verlag, Heinrichshofen Buecher, Valoisstr 11, Wilhelmshaven 26382, Germany. Circ: 1,000.

MUSIKTERAPI. see *MEDICAL SCIENCES—Physical Medicine And Rehabilitation*

NORDIC JOURNAL OF MUSIC THERAPY/NORDISK TIDSSKRIFT FOR MUSIKKETERAPI. see *MEDICAL SCIENCES—Physical Medicine And Rehabilitation*

PIANO-TUNERS QUARTERLY. see *HANDICAPPED—Visually Impaired*

781.15 GBR ISSN 0305-7356
ML5
PSYCHOLOGY OF MUSIC. Text in English. 1973. s-a. GBP 30 domestic; USD 55 foreign; GBP 12 to students (effective 2000). adv. bk.rev. illus. cum.index every 5 vols. reprints avail. *Refereed.* **Document type:** *Academic/Scholarly.*
Indexed: Br.Educ.Ind., Documentatieblad, Indian Psychol.Abstr., Int.Ind.Mus.Per. (1996), Music Ind., PsycInfo, Psychol.Abstr. (1976-), RILM, e-psyche.
—BLDSC (6946.536000), ingenta. **CCC.**
Published by: Society for Research in Psychology of Music and Music Education, Department of Music, The University, Sheffield, S Yorks S10 2TN, United Kingdom. TEL 44-114-222-0475, FAX 44-114-266-8053, j.w.davidson@sheffield.ac.uk; uncover@carl.org, http://www.personal.leeds.ac.uk/~muswlw/srpmme/. Ed., R&P, Adv. contact Jane Davidson TEL 44-303-758-3030. Circ: 700.

780.01 USA ISSN 0275-3987
ML3830
PSYCHOMUSICOLOGY; a journal of research in music cognition. Text in English. 1981. s-a., latest vol.16. USD 27 domestic; USD 33 foreign (effective 2001). bk.rev. bibl, charts, stat. back issues avail. *Refereed.* **Document type:** *Academic/Scholarly.* **Description:** Serves as a journal of research in music cognition, providing a forum for reports of experimental research, reviews of research and theoretical papers that are based on experimental research.
Indexed: Educ.Ind. (coverage dropped), Int.Ind.Mus.Per. (1994-1997), Music Ind., PsycInfo, Psychol.Abstr. (1981-), RILM, e-psyche.
—BLDSC (6946.540070), ingenta.
Published by: Florida State University, Center for Music Research, 214 KMU, Tallahassee, FL 32306-1180. TEL 850-644-5786, FAX 850-644-6100, taylor_k@cmr.fsu.edu. Ed., R&P Jack A Taylor. Adv. contact Jerry P Wood. Circ: 300.

780 616.89 ZAF ISSN 1012-2850
SOUTH AFRICAN JOURNAL OF MUSIC THERAPY/SUID-AFRIKAANSE TYDSKRIF VIR MUSIEKTERAPIE. Text in English. 1982. 2/yr. ZAR 40 (effective 1998). adv. bk.rev. bibl, charts. cum.index. back issues avail. *Refereed.* **Document type:** *Academic/Scholarly.* **Description:** Music for therapeutic purposes.
Indexed: Ind.S.A.Per., RILM, e-psyche.
Published by: Music Therapy Society of Southern Africa, 2 Shaw Rd, Rondebosch, Cape Town 7700, South Africa. TEL 27-21-7623523, FAX 27-21-7977575. R&P S Woodward TEL 27-11-6851054. Adv. contact G Buckley. Circ: 250. **Co-sponsor:** Southern African Music Rights Organization.

780 616.8 ITA
WORLD CONGRESS OF MUSIC THERAPY. PROCEEDINGS. Text in Italian. 1990. irreg. ITL 73,000. **Document type:** *Proceedings.*
Indexed: e-psyche.
Published by: Associazione Italiana Studi di Musicoterapia, Via Brignole De Ferrari, 6-2, Genoa, GE 16125, Italy. TEL 39-10-2512393. Ed. Giovanna Mutti.

NATIVE AMERICAN STUDIES

see also HISTORY—History Of North And South America

305.897 USA ISSN 0893-5394
RC451.5.I5
AMERICAN INDIAN AND ALASKA NATIVE MENTAL HEALTH RESEARCH. Text in English. 1978. 3/yr. USD 35; USD 44 foreign (effective 1997). adv. illus. index. back issues avail.; reprints avail. *Refereed.* **Document type:** *Academic/Scholarly.* **Description:** Provides empirical research, program evaluation, case studies and unpublished dissertations.
Former titles (until 1986): White Cloud Journal of American Indian Mental Health (0886-5027); (until 1982): White Cloud Journal of American Indian - Alaska Native Mental Health (0190-2482)
Related titles: Online - full text ed.: (from ProQuest Information & Learning, Institute for Scientific Information).
Indexed: ASCA, Abstr.Health Care Manage.Stud., Anthropol.Lit. (coverage dropped), C.I.J.E., Crim.Just.Abstr., Curr.Cont., Fam.Ind., Ind.Med. (1997-), Lang.& Lang.Behav.Abstr., Psychol.Abstr. (1987-), SOPODA, SSCI, Soc.Work Res.& Abstr., Sociol.Abstr., e-psyche.
—GNLM, IDS, ingenta.
Published by: (National Center for American Indian Mental Health Research), University Press of Colorado, PO Box 849, Niwot, CO 80544. TEL 303-530-5337, FAX 303-530-5306, billie.greene@uchsc.edu, http://www.uchsc.edu/ai/ncaianmhr/journal/jover2.htm, http://www.press.uchicago.edu/cgi-bin/hfs.cgi/66/colorado/aian.ctl. R&P Laura Furney. Adv. contact Pete Hammond. Circ: 1,000.

ASSOCIATION OF AMERICAN INDIAN PHYSICIANS NEWSLETTER. see *MEDICAL SCIENCES*

333.72 USA
COUNTRY ROAD CHRONICLES. Text in English. 1993. m. USD 27 domestic; USD 57 foreign (effective 1999). adv. bk.rev., music rev., video rev. 24 p./no. back issues avail. **Document type:** *Newspaper, Consumer.* **Description:** Dedicated to Native American Culture. Deals with Mother Earth news, about living with her animals, environment, universe and her people.
Formerly: Country Road Gazette
Published by: Van Raper Productions, 101 Meadow Ridge Ct, Dingmans Ferry, PA 18328. TEL 570-828-1778, FAX 570-828-7959, cherokee@countryroadschronicles.com, http://www.countryroadchronicles.com/. Ed., Pub. Elaine V Raper. Adv. contact Lenny Raper. B&W page USD 963.97; trim 15 x 11.5. Circ: 27,135 (paid).

NEEDLEWORK

see also ARTS AND HANDICRAFTS; HOBBIES

NEW AGE PUBLICATIONS

see also ASTROLOGY; PARAPSYCHOLOGY AND OCCULTISM

APPLIED PSYCHOPHYSIOLOGY AND BIOFEEDBACK. see *PSYCHOLOGY*

BEYOND P E. (Physical Education) see *PHYSICAL FITNESS AND HYGIENE*

181.45 USA
BODYWORK SERIES. Text in English. irreg., latest vol.3. adv. **Document type:** *Magazine, Consumer.* **Description:** Features unique exercises that benefit the health of the nervous system.
Indexed: e-psyche.
Published by: Himalayan International Institute (HII), RR 1 Box 407, Honesdale, PA 18431-9718. TEL 570-253-4929, FAX 570-253-6360, yimag@yimag.org, http://www.yimag.org. Ed. Deborah Willoughby. R&P Irene Petryszal. Adv. contact Jim McGinley.

181.45 USA
BREATH SERIES; a progression of pranayama practices. Text in English. irreg., latest vol.4. adv. **Document type:** *Consumer.* **Description:** Helps readers learn the importance of proper breathing.
Indexed: e-psyche.
Published by: Himalayan International Institute (HII), RR 1 Box 407, Honesdale, PA 18431-9718. TEL 570-253-4929, FAX 570-253-6360, yimag@yimag.org, http://www.yimag.org. Ed. Deborah Willoughby. R&P Irene Petryszak. Adv. contact Jim McGinley.

COLOURAMA; world's premier colour magazine & directory. see *ALTERNATIVE MEDICINE*

110 USA
COMMON GROUND (SAN ANSELMO); resources for personal transformation. Text in English. 1973. q. USD 15 (effective 2000). adv. bk.rev. illus. **Document type:** *Directory.* **Description:** Lists resources for personal growth, with interviews and feature articles on topics relating to personal development.
Indexed: e-psyche.
Published by: Baha'uddin Andy Alpine, Ed. & Pub., 305 San Anselmo Ave, Ste 313, San Anselmo, CA 94960. TEL 415-459-4900, FAX 415-459-4974, TELEX 428701, info@commongroundmag.com, http://www.commongroundmag.com. R&P Baha'uddin Andy Alpine TEL 415-455-1644. Adv. contact Donna Simonson. B&W page USD 1,390, color page USD 2,060; trim 13.25 x 10.5. Circ: 105,000.

135.3 154.63 USA ISSN 1054-6707
BF1074
DREAM NETWORK; a quarterly journal exploring dreams and myth. Text in English. 1982. q. USD 22 domestic; USD 32 in Canada & Mexico; USD 38 elsewhere (effective 2002). adv. bk.rev., film rev., music rev., tel.rev., video rev., Website rev. illus. cum.index: 1982-1991. 52 p./no. back issues avail.; reprints avail. **Document type:** *Journal, Magazine, Consumer, Academic/Scholarly.* **Description:** Provides a forum for exchange of ideas among individuals interested in understanding the symbologic language of dreams, with a focus on dream sharing and exploring relationships between dream and mythology.
Formerly (until 1989): Dream Network Bulletin
Related titles: E-mail ed.; Online - full content ed.
Indexed: e-psyche.
Address: P O Box 1026, Moab, UT 84532-1026. TEL 435-259-5936, FAX 435-259-5936, dreamkey@lasal.net, http://dreamnetwork.net. Ed., Pub., Adv. contact H Roberta Ossana. page USD 300; 7.25 x 9.5. Circ: 4,000.

261.513 USA
FOUR CORNERS. Text in English. bi-m. USD 20; USD 30 foreign (effective 1999). adv. illus. back issues avail. **Document type:** *Consumer.* **Description:** Includes articles and news about paranormal, occult phenomena, astrology and alternative medicine in the Southwest.
Address: PO Box 1776, Sedona, AZ 86339-1776. TEL 520-282-7233, FAX 520-204-9698, badger@sedona.net, http://www.fourcornersmag.com. Ed. Lane Masterson Badger. Pub. Samantha Ruckman.

158 USA ISSN 1067-1366
GOING BONKERS; a magazine for our times. Cover title: Bonkers. Text in English. 1993. q. USD 11 domestic; USD 17 in Canada; USD 22 elsewhere; USD 3.99 newsstand/cover. adv. illus. index. reprints avail. **Document type:** *Consumer.* **Description:** Examines psychological issues through humor. Features excerpts of works by well-known authors.
Indexed: e-psyche.
Published by: Harold Publications, 333 Royal Poinciana Plaza, Palm Beach, FL 33480-9875. TEL 561-659-0975, 800-777-1999, FAX 561-659-2295, bonkers@goingbonkers.com, http://www.goingbonkers.com. Ed., Pub. Margaret Harold Roberts.

613.2 USA
GOOD LIFE TIMES✱ ; choices in health, education and the arts. Text in English. 1978. m. USD 20. adv. bk.rev.
Formerly: Wholistic Living News
Published by: Association for Wholistic Living, 6970 Central Ave, Lemon Grove, CA 91945-2110. Ed. Dr. Mark Solomon. Circ: 50,000.

615.89 USA
HOLISTIC HEALTH DIRECTORY. Text in English. 1992. a. USD 5.95. **Document type:** *Directory.* **Description:** Lists holistic health care practitioners throughout the U.S., including physicians, physical and occupational therapists, chiropractors, acupuncturists, and natural healers.

Related titles: Microfiche ed.: (from PQC).
Published by: New Age Publishing, Inc., 42 Pleasant St, Watertown, MA 02172. TEL 617-926-0200, FAX 617-926-5021, http://www.spdcc.com/home/newage/hhd.html. Ed. Joan Oliver. Pub. David H Thorne. Circ: 200,000.

133.9 USA
HOLISTIC HEALTH SOURCEBOOK. Text in English. 1997. irreg. USD 39.95. **Document type:** *Directory.* **Description:** Provides source information on holistic health related topics.
Published by: Reference Press International, PO Box 4126, Greenwich, CT 06830. TEL 203-629-4900, FAX 203-622-5983, ml2626@aol.com. Ed., Pub., R&P Cheryl Klein Lacoff.

INTERNATIONAL JOURNAL OF AROMATHERAPY. see *ALTERNATIVE MEDICINE*

133 158 USA ISSN 1091-2851
THE INTERNATIONAL JOURNAL OF SELF-HELP AND SELF-CARE. Text in English. 1998. q. USD 49 to individuals; USD 150 to institutions (effective 2001). bk.rev. reprints avail. **Document type:** *Journal, Consumer.* **Description:** Contains articles of a scientific character - presentations of theory and research on self-help, as well as notices of current literature and other materials of value in the field.
Indexed: Soc.Serv.Abstr., Sociol.Abstr., e-psyche.
—BLDSC (4542.544645).
Published by: Baywood Publishing Co., Inc., 26 Austin Ave, Box 337, Amityville, NY 11701. TEL 631-691-1270, 800-638-7819, FAX 631-691-1770, info@baywood.com, baywood@baywood.com, http://baywood.com/search/PreviewJournal.asp?qsRecord=9, http://www.baywood.com. Ed. Alfred Katz. R&P Julie Krempa. Adv. contact Joi Tamber-Brooks.

155 USA ISSN 1085-3529
INTUITION; a magazine for the higher potential of the mind. Text in English. 1988. bi-m. USD 19.95; USD 24.95 in Canada & Mexico; USD 29.95 elsewhere; USD 4.95 newsstand/cover (effective 2000). adv. bk.rev. illus. back issues avail.; reprints avail. **Document type:** *Consumer.* **Description:** Publishes articles discussing intuition and creativity, including profiles, interviews and news of issues relating to the development and application of intuition in all fields of endeavor.
Indexed: Alt.Press Ind., e-psyche.
Published by: Intuitive Media, Inc., 275 Brannan St, 3d Fl, San Francisco, CA 94107-2016. TEL 415-538-8171, FAX 415-538-8175, intuitmag@aol.com, http://www.intuitionmagazine.com. Ed., Pub., R&P Colleen Mauro. Adv. contact Jody Stathakis. page USD 778; trim 9.5 x 7.25. Circ: 25,000. **Subscr. to:** PO Box 460773, San Francisco, CA 94146-9804.

JOURNAL OF REGRESSION THERAPY. see *PSYCHOLOGY*

▼ **L O H A S JOURNAL.** see *BUSINESS AND ECONOMICS*

156 DEU ISSN 0177-3852
MERIDIAN✶ ; Zeitschrift fuer Kosmobiologie, Astrologie und angewandte Psychologie. Text in German. 1979. 6/yr. DEM 52.
Incorporates: Kosmobiologie (0023-4214); Kosmischer Beobachter (0177-3844)
Indexed: e-psyche.
Published by: Ebertin-Verlag, Kronenstr 2, Postfach 167, Freiburg 79001, Germany.

NATURAL HEALTH. see *ALTERNATIVE MEDICINE*

NATURE AND HEALTH. see *ALTERNATIVE MEDICINE*

110 613.7 USA
NEW AGE JOURNAL SOURCEBOOK. Text in English. a. USD 4.95. adv. **Document type:** *Consumer.*
Published by: New Age Publishing, Inc., 42 Pleasant St, Watertown, MA 02172. TEL 617-926-0200.

613 USA ISSN 1088-1441
NEW LIFE; for those who are changing. Text in English. bi-m. USD 20 (effective 1999). illus. **Description:** Reference and resource guide for holistic health, environment and New Age. Examines consciousness and the human potential, and provides information on products and services.
Formerly: Serenity's New Life (1051-2195)
Published by: Serenity Health Organization, Inc., 218 W 72nd St, Ste 2FE, New York, NY 10023. TEL 212-787-1600. Ed. Mark Becker. Circ: 60,000.

NEXUS (BOULDER); Colorado's holistic journal. see *ALTERNATIVE MEDICINE*

100 USA
ON COURSE; inspiration for the inner journey. Text in English. 1983. bi-m. USD 6 newsstand/cover. adv. bk.rev. bibl, illus. back issues avail. **Description:** A course in miracles orientation and attitudinal healing helps bring people of different faiths together. Includes daily meditations, quotations, jokes, parables, prayers, poems, and seasonal perspectives.
Formerly: Mustard Seed
Published by: Interfaith Fellowship, 25 South St, Washingtonville, NY 10992-0250. TEL 914-496-9089, FAX 914-496-1450. Ed., Pub. Jon Mundy. Circ: 9,000.

133 615.89 NLD ISSN 0165-5027
ONKRUID; voor aarde, lichaam en geest. Text in Dutch. 1978. bi-m. NLG 39, EUR 17.73 domestic; NLG 60, EUR 27.27 foreign (effective 2000). adv. bk.rev. illus. back issues avail. **Document type:** *Magazine, Consumer.* **Description:** Covers alternative health, environmental and spiritual concerns.
Related titles: Online - full text ed.
Published by: Stichting Onkruid, West 32, Avenhorn 1633 JC, Netherlands. TEL 31-229-542800, FAX 31-229-542315, onkruid@onkruid.nl, http://www.onkruid.nl. Ed., Pub., R&P Paul Breekveldt. Adv. contact Ali Bree. Circ: 30,000 (paid).

ORGANICA; a magazine of arts & activism. see *LITERATURE*

THE PANIC RELIEF NEWS. see *PSYCHOLOGY*

PULSAR; Zeitschrift fuer Gesundheit, Therapie und Innere Entwicklung. see *ALTERNATIVE MEDICINE*

RADIANCE TECHNIQUE JOURNAL. see *ALTERNATIVE MEDICINE*

RAINBOW NEWS; the spirit of aotearoa. see *ALTERNATIVE MEDICINE*

100 133 USA ISSN 0886-036X
REALITY CHANGE; the global Seth journal. Text in English. 1980. q. USD 29.95 domestic; USD 36.95 in Canada & Mexico; USD 49.95 elsewhere. adv. bk.rev. back issues avail. **Document type:** *Consumer.* **Description:** Explores the concepts and ideas outlined in the 22-volume system of philosophy written by Seth, Jane Roberts, and Robert Butts.
Indexed: e-psyche.
Published by: Seth Network International, PO Box 1620, Eugene, OR 97440-1620. TEL 541-686-0803, FAX 541-683-1084, sethnet@efn.org, http://www.efn.org/~sethweb. Ed., R&P, Adv. contact Katharine Newcomb. Pubs. Lynda Dahl, Stan Ulkowski. B&W page USD 285; 11 x 8.5. Circ: 1,500.

SELF & SOCIETY; European journal of humanistic psychology. see *PSYCHOLOGY*

SOMATICS; magazine - journal of the mind - body arts and sciences. see *PHYSICAL FITNESS AND HYGIENE*

SPIRITUALITY & HEALTH; the soul body connection. see *ALTERNATIVE MEDICINE*

100 152 USA
TAROT NETWORK NEWS. Text in English. 1981. s-a. USD 10. adv. bk.rev. back issues avail. **Document type:** *Newsletter.* **Description:** Provides a guide to the content and application of the Tarot.
Indexed: e-psyche.
Published by: Taroco, PO Box 104, Sausalito, CA 94966. TEL 415-332-9254. Ed. Gary W Ross. Pub. Jack Hurley. Adv. contact Geri Kepler. Circ: 350.

158 USA
TRANSFORMATION TIMES; new age journal. Text in English. 1982. 10/yr. USD 8 (effective 2001). adv. bk.rev. **Document type:** *Newspaper.*
Published by: (Christ Light Community Church), Life Resources Unlimited, PO Box 425, Beavercreek, OR 97004. TEL 503-632-7141. Ed. Connie L Faubel. Circ: 8,000.

VITALITY MAGAZINE; Toronto's monthly wellness journal. see *ALTERNATIVE MEDICINE*

WEGETARIANIN; zdrowie, ekologia, mistycyzm. see *NUTRITION AND DIETETICS*

613.2 USA ISSN 0279-5590
CODEN: CMMOD9
WHOLE LIFE TIMES✶ . Text in English. 1979. 8/yr. USD 11.95. adv. bk.rev.
Related titles: Online - full text ed.: (from Gale Group).
Indexed: ABI Inform., Alt.Press Ind., B.P.I., Hlth.Ind.
Published by: Whole Life Company, Inc., 12 Jacob Amsden Rd, Westborough, MA 01581-1766. Ed. Kimberly French. Circ: 140,000.

WINGSPAN (LA JOLLA); journal of the male spirit. see *MEN'S STUDIES*

181.45 USA ISSN 1055-7911
B132.Y6
YOGA INTERNATIONAL. Text in English. 1991. bi-m. USD 18 domestic; USD 26 in Canada; USD 30 elsewhere; USD 4.99 newsstand/cover (effective 2000). adv. bk.rev., video rev. illus. back issues avail. *Refereed.* **Document type:** *Consumer.* **Description:** Brings information on the practice of yoga and yoga' sister science Ayurveda.
Supersedes (in July 1991): Dawn (Honesdale) (0277-4461)
Related titles: Online - full text ed.
Indexed: e-psyche.
Published by: Himalayan International Institute (HII), RR 1 Box 407, Honesdale, PA 18431-9718. TEL 570-253-4929, 800-253-6243, FAX 570-253-6360, yimag@yimag.org, http://www.yimag.org. Ed. Deborah Willoughby. R&P Irene Petryszak. Adv. contact Jim McGinley. B&W page USD 810, color page USD 1,000; trim 10.88 x 8.13. Circ: 24,500 (controlled).

NUCLEAR ENERGY

see ENERGY—Nuclear Energy

NUCLEAR PHYSICS

see PHYSICS—Nuclear Physics

NUMISMATICS

see also HOBBIES

NURSES AND NURSING

see MEDICAL SCIENCES—Nurses And Nursing

NUTRITION AND DIETETICS

see also FOOD AND FOOD INDUSTRIES; HEALTH FACILITIES AND ADMINISTRATION; PHARMACY AND PHARMACOLOGY; PHYSICAL FITNESS AND HYGIENE

A N D I NEWS. see *MEDICAL SCIENCES—Psychiatry And Neurology*

ACTIVE MAGAZINE. see *WOMEN'S HEALTH*

614.854 DEU ISSN 0940-2098
ADIPOSITAS. Text in German. 1991. s-a. DEM 60 to institutions (effective 2000). **Document type:** *Academic/Scholarly.*
—GNLM.
Published by: (Deutsche Adipositas-Gesellschaft), Demeter Verlag GmbH und Co. KG, Ruedigerstr 14, Stuttgart 70469, Germany. TEL 49-711-8931-0, FAX 49-711-8931322, custserv@thieme.de, http://www.demeter-verlag.de.

613.2 USA ISSN 1043-4526
TX537 CODEN: AFNREL
ADVANCES IN FOOD AND NUTRITION RESEARCH. Text in English. 1948. irreg., latest vol.42, 1998. index. reprint service avail. from ISI.
Formerly (until 1990): Advances in Food Research (0065-2628)
Indexed: Abstr.Hyg., Agricola, Aqua.Sci.& Fish.Abstr., Aquacult.Abstr., Biol.& Agr.Ind. (Jan.1984-Jan.1989), Biol.Abstr., Chem.Abstr., Chem.Indus.Notes, Chem.Titles, Dairy Sci.Abstr., Environ.Sci.Poll.Mgmt., Excerp.Med., Food Sci.& Tech.Abstr., INIS Atomind., Ind.Med. (1989-), Nutr.Abstr., Ocean.Abstr. (coverage dropped), Seed Abstr., Sport Fish.Abstr., Trop.Dis.Bull.
—BLDSC (0706.850000), CASDDS, CISTI, GNLM, Infotrieve, ingenta, Linda Hall. **CCC.**

N

Published by: Academic Press, Inc., Journal Division (Subsidiary of: Harcourt Brace & Company), 525 B St, Ste 1900, San Diego, CA 92101-4495. TEL 619-231-0926, FAX 619-699-6715. Eds. E M Mrak, George F Stewart. **Subscr. to:** Order Dept., 6277 Sea Harbor Dr, 4th Fl, Orlando, FL 32887. TEL 800-321-5068.

613.2 USA ISSN 0149-9483
QP141.A1 CODEN: ANURD9
ADVANCES IN NUTRITIONAL RESEARCH. Text in English. 1977. irreg., latest vol.9, 1994. price varies. back issues avail. *Refereed.* **Document type:** *Monographic series.* **Description:** Provides authoritative accounts of the current state of knowledge regarding major topics of research in the nutritional sciences.
Related titles: Online - full text ed.: (from Institute for Scientific Information).
Indexed: ASCA, Chem.Abstr., Chem.Indus.Notes, Chem.Titles, Ind.Med. (1977-), Ind.Sci.Rev., Sci.Cit.Ind.
—CASDDS, CISTI, GNLM, ingenta, KNAW, Linda Hall. **CCC.**
Published by: Kluwer Academic - Plenum Publishers (Subsidiary of: Wolters Kluwer N.V.), 233 Spring St, New York, NY 10013-1578. TEL 212-620-8000, 800-221-9369, FAX 212-463-0742, info@plenum.com, http://www.plenum.com. Ed. Harold H Draper.

613.26 051 USA ISSN 1521-1118
AHIMSA. Text in English. 1960. 4/yr. USD 18 domestic; USD 25 foreign (effective 2000). bk.rev. index, cum.index. **Document type:** *Newsletter.* **Description:** Presents Vegan (total-vegetarian) diet, lifestyle, and philosophies.
Published by: American Vegan Society, 56 Dinshah Ln,, P O Box 369, Malaga, NJ 08328-0908. TEL 856-694-2887, FAX 856-694-2288. Ed. H Jay Dinshah. R&P Jay Dinshah.

AKTIV; Magazin fuer Gesundheit, Ernaehrung und Schoenheit. see *PHYSICAL FITNESS AND HYGIENE*

612.3 DEU ISSN 0341-0501
CODEN: AEKPDQ
AKTUELLE ERNAEHRUNGSMEDIZIN; Zeitschrift fuer Stoffwechselforschung, klinische Ernaehrung und Diaetetik. Text in German. 1976. bi-m. EUR 155.80 domestic to institutions; EUR 160.80 in Europe to institutions; EUR 164.80 elsewhere to institutions; EUR 30 newsstand/cover (effective 2002). index. reprint service avail. from PQC. **Document type:** *Journal, Academic/Scholarly.*
Related titles: Online - full text ed.: ISSN 1438-9916.
Indexed: Chem.Abstr., Curr.Cont. (coverage dropped), Dairy Sci.Abstr., Excerp.Med., INIS Atomind., Ind.Vet., Nutr.Abstr., Potato Abstr., Rev.Med.& Vet.Mycol., Sugar Ind.Abstr., Triticale Abstr.
—BLDSC (0785.735000), CASDDS, CISTI, EMDOCS, GNLM, Infotrieve. **CCC.**
Published by: (Deutsche Gesellschaft fuer Ernaehrungsmedizin), Georg Thieme Verlag, Ruedigerstr 14, Stuttgart 70469, Germany. TEL 49-711-8931-0, FAX 49-711-8931298, akternmed@thieme.de, leser.service@thieme.de, http://www.thieme.de/akternmed/index.html. Ed. G Wolfram. Circ: 3,100. **Co-sponsors:** Oesterreichischen Arbeitsgemeinschaft fuer klinische Ernaehrung; Gesellschaft fuer klinische Ernaehrung der Schweiz; Deutsche Akademie fuer Ernaehrungsmedizin.

616.39 ESP ISSN 1139-6903
ALIMARKET. NO ALIMENTACION. Text in Spanish. 1993. a. adv.
Published by: Publicaciones Alimarket S.A., Albasanz, 14 3o, Madrid 28037, Spain. TEL 34-91-3274340, FAX 34-91-3274522, informa@alimarket.es, http://www.alimarket.es. R&P Carlos Guerrero.

613.2 ESP ISSN 1136-4815
ALIMENTACION, NUTRICION Y SALUD. Text in Spanish. 1994. irreg., latest vol.6, no.2.
Indexed: Food Sci.& Tech.Abstr.
—BLDSC (0787.866000), CINDOC.
Published by: Instituto Danone, Buenos Aires, 21, Barcelona 08029, Spain. TEL 34-3-2912000, FAX 34-3-4196592. Ed. M Serrano Rios.

613.2 FRA
CODEN: ALLVAR
ALIMENTATION ET LA VIE - NOUVELLE PRESENTATION. Text in French. 1942. q. FRF 65. adv. bibl, charts, stat.
Formerly: Alimentation et la Vie (0065-6267)
Indexed: Dairy Sci.Abstr., INIS Atomind., Ind.Vet., Nutr.Abstr., Vet.Bull.
—CASDDS, CISTI, GNLM.
Published by: Societe Scientifique d'Hygiene Alimentaire, 16 rue de l'Estrapade, Paris 75005, France. Ed. Georges Le Moan. **Co-sponsor:** Association Francaise des Techniciens de l'Alimentation Animale.

613.2 ITA ISSN 0392-7512
CODEN: ANMTD9
ALIMENTAZIONE NUTRIZIONE METABOLISMO; rivista trimestrale di studi nutrizionali ed endocrino-metabolici. Text in English, French, Italian; Summaries in English, Italian. 1979. q. ITL 64,000, USD 35.70. adv. bk.rev. bibl, charts, illus. index. back issues avail.
Indexed: Biol.Abstr., Chem.Abstr.
—CASDDS, CISTI.
Published by: Societa Editrice Universo, Via Giovanni Battista Morgagni, 1, Rome, RM 00161, Italy. Ed. Michelangelo Cairella. Circ: 500.

613.2 BRA ISSN 0103-4235
CODEN: ALNUE4
ALIMENTOS E NUTRICAO. Text in Portuguese; Abstracts in English, Portuguese. 1989. a. USD 30 or exchange basis (effective 2001). abstr, bibl, charts. back issues avail. *Refereed.* **Document type:** *Journal, Academic/Scholarly.*
Indexed: Chem.Abstr., Chem.Indus.Notes, Chem.Titles, Dairy Sci.Abstr., Field Crop Abstr., Food Sci.& Tech.Abstr., Hort.Abstr., Maize Abstr., Nutr.Abstr., Plant Breed.Abstr., Postharvest, Ref.Zh., Rev.Med.& Vet.Mycol.
—CASDDS, CISTI, KNAW.
Published by: Universidade Estadual Paulista, Ave. VICENTE FERREIRA, 1278, Centro, Caixa Postal 71, Marilia, SP 17515-901, Brazil. TEL 55-144-222504, FAX 55-144-222504, cgb@marilia.unesp.br. Ed. Thais Borges Cesar.

ALIVE; Canadian journal of health and nutrition. see *PHYSICAL FITNESS AND HYGIENE*

613.2 USA ISSN 0731-5724
RC620.A1 CODEN: JONUDL
AMERICAN COLLEGE OF NUTRITION. JOURNAL. Text in English. 1982. 6/yr. USD 90 domestic to individuals; USD 130 foreign to individuals; USD 180 domestic to institutions; USD 220 foreign to institutions (effective 2001). adv. bk.rev. abstr, bibl, illus. index. back issues avail.; reprints avail. *Refereed.* **Document type:** *Academic/Scholarly.* **Description:** Covers nutrition research as it applies to patient care.
Related titles: Microform ed.; Online - full text ed.: (from Institute for Scientific Information).
Indexed: ASCA, Agricola, Bibl.Agri., Biol.Abstr., Chem.Abstr., Chem.Indus.Notes, Chem.Titles, Curr.Adv.Biochem., Curr.Adv.Ecol.Sci., Curr.Cont., Dairy Sci.Abstr., Excerp.Med., INIS Atomind., Ind.Med. (1982-), Ind.Sci.Rev., Inpharma, Int.Abstr.Biol.Sci., Maize Abstr., NRN, Nutr.Abstr., Pharm.&Out.News, Reac., Rev.Arom.& Med.Plants, SSCI (coverage dropped), Sci.Cit.Ind., Soyabean Abstr., Sugar Ind.Abstr., THA, Triticale Abstr.
—BLDSC (4685.780000), CASDDS, CISTI, EMDOCS, GNLM, IDS, ingenta, KNAW, Linda Hall. **CCC.**
Published by: American College of Nutrition, c/o Hospital for Joint Disease, 301 E. 17th St., New York, NY 10003. TEL 212-777-1037, 313-993-5226, FAX 212-777-1103, 313-577-8616, http://www.am-coll-nutr.org/jacn/jacn.htm. Ed. David Klurfeld. Circ: 1,600 (paid).

613.26 USA ISSN 0002-8223
RM214 CODEN: JADAAE
AMERICAN DIETETIC ASSOCIATION. JOURNAL. Text in English. 1925. m. USD 125; USD 150 in Canada; USD 205 elsewhere (effective 2000). adv. bk.rev. abstr, bibl, charts, illus. index. back issues avail.; reprint service avail. from PQC. *Refereed.* **Document type:** *Academic/Scholarly.* **Description:** Publishes reports of original research and other papers covering all aspects of dietetics, including nutrition and diet therapy, community nutrition, education, and administration.
Formerly: American Dietetic Association. Bulletin
Related titles: Microform ed.: (from PMC,PQC); Online - full text ed.: (from Gale Group, ProQuest Information & Learning, Factiva, Institute for Scientific Information).
Indexed: AIM, ASCA, Abstr.Health Care Manage.Stud., Abstr.Hyg., AgeLine, Agricola, Art.Hosp.& Tour., Behav.Med.Abstr., Bibl.Agri., Biol.& Agr.Ind. (Jan.1983-), Biol.Abstr., CINAHL, C.I.S. Abstr., Cal.Tiss.Abstr., Chem.Abstr., Chem.Indus.Notes, Chem.Titles, Chic.Per.Ind., Curr.Adv.Biochem., Curr.Adv.Ecol.Sci., Curr.Cont., Dairy Sci.Abstr., Dent.Ind., Diar.Dis.Res., Dok.Arbeitsmed., Environ.Per.Bibl., Environ.Sci.Poll.Mgmt., Excerp.Med., Food Sci.& Tech.Abstr., Gen.Sci.Ind. (Apr.1984-), Helminthol.Abstr., Hlth.Ind., Hosp.Lit.Ind., INIS Atomind., Ind.Med. (1925-), Ind.Sci.Rev., Inpharma, Int.Nurs.Ind., NRN, Nutr.Abstr., Pharm.&Out.News, Pollut.Abstr., Potato Abstr., Poult.Abstr., Psychol.Abstr., Reac., Risk Abstr., SSCI (coverage dropped), Saf.Sci.Abstr., Sci.Cit.Ind., Soc.Work Res.& Abstr., Sugar Ind.Abstr., THA, Triticale Abstr.
—BLDSC (4686.130000), CASDDS, CISTI, GNLM, IDS, ingenta, KNAW, Linda Hall.
Published by: American Dietetic Association, 216 W Jackson Blvd, Ste 800, Chicago, IL 60606-6995. TEL 312-899-0040, FAX 312-899-1757, journal@eatright.org, http://www.eatright.org/journaltoc.html. Ed. Elaine R Monsen. Adv. contact Vicki Guinta. B&W page USD 3,650; trim 10.88 x 8.13. Circ: 67,000 (paid).

AMERICAN INSTITUTE FOR CANCER RESEARCH NEWSLETTER. see *MEDICAL SCIENCES—Oncology*

613.2 USA ISSN 0002-9165
RC584 CODEN: AJCNAC
AMERICAN JOURNAL OF CLINICAL NUTRITION; a journal reporting the practical application of our world-wide knowledge of nutrition. Text in English. 1952. m. USD 140 domestic to individuals Print & online eds.; USD 160 foreign to individuals Print & online eds.; USD 220 domestic to institutions Print & online eds.; USD 240 foreign to institutions Print & online eds.; USD 85 domestic to students Print & online eds.; USD 105 foreign to students Print & online eds. (effective 2001). adv. bk.rev. bibl, charts, illus. index. Supplement avail.; back issues avail.; reprints avail. *Refereed.* **Document type:** *Academic/Scholarly.* **Description:** Publishes original research contributed by scientists throughout the world, editorials, reviews, special articles, meeting reports. Special supplements are devoted to symposia, workshops, and other long reports.
Related titles: Microfilm ed.: (from PMC,PQC); Online - full text ed.: USD 55 to students (effective 2001) (from HighWire Pr., EBSCO Publishing, ProQuest Information & Learning, Gale Group, Factiva, Institute for Scientific Information).
Indexed: AIM, AMED, A.S.& T.Ind. (coverage dropped), ASCA, Abstr.Hyg., Abstr.Inter.Med., AgeLine, Agricola, Amer.Bibl.Slavic & E.Eur.Stud., Anim.Breed.Abstr., Behav.Med.Abstr., Bibl.Agri., Bibl.Dev.Med.& Child Neur., Biol.& Agr.Ind. (Nov.1982-), Biol.Abstr., CINAHL, Chem.Abstr., Chem.Indus.Notes, Chem.Titles, Curr.Adv.Biochem., Curr.Cont., Dairy Sci.Abstr., Derwent Biotech.Abstr., Diar.Dis.Res., Dok.Arbeitsmed., Energy Rev., Environ.Per.Bibl., Environ.Sci.Poll.Mgmt., Excerp.Med., Fam.Ind., Food Sci.& Tech.Abstr., Helminthol.Abstr., INIS Atomind., Ind.Med. (1954-), Ind.Sci.Rev., Ind.Vet., Inpharma, Int.Abstr.Biol.Sci., Int.Nurs.Ind., Kidney, Maize Abstr., NRN, Neurosci.Cit.Ind., Nutr.Abstr., Pharm.&Out.News, Pig News & Info., Pollut.Abstr., Potato Abstr., Protozool.Abstr., Psychol.Abstr., Reac., Rev.Arom.& Med.Plants, Rev.Plant Path., Rice Abstr., Risk Abstr., Rural Recreat.Tour.Abstr., SSCI (coverage dropped), Saf.Sci.Abstr., Sci.Cit.Ind., So.Pac.Per.Ind., Soyabean Abstr., Sugar Ind.Abstr., Triticale Abstr., Trop.Dis.Bull., Vet.Bull., World Ag.Econ.& Rur.Soc.Abstr.
—BLDSC (0823.000000), CASDDS, CINDOC, CISTI, EMDOCS, GNLM, IDS, Infotrieve, ingenta, Linda Hall. **CCC.**
Published by: American Society for Clinical Nutrition, Inc., 9650 Rockville Pike, Rm L-2310, Bethesda, MD 20814-3998. TEL 301-530-7029, 800-433-2732, FAX 301-571-5728, journal@ascn.faseb.org; staff@dues.faseb.org; orders@allenpress.com, http://www.ajcn.org/. Ed. Charles Halsted. R&P Lorali Barber. Adv. contact Susan Mergenhagen. Circ: 7,000. **Subscr.to:** Allen Press Inc., PO Box 1897, Lawrence, KS 66044-8897.

AMERICAN JOURNAL OF HEALTH PROMOTION. see *PUBLIC HEALTH AND SAFETY*

ANIMAL NUTRITION ASSOCIATION OF CANADA. EASTERN NUTRITION CONFERENCE. PROCEEDINGS. see *AGRICULTURE—Poultry And Livestock*

612.3 CHE ISSN 0250-6807
CODEN: ANUMDS
ANNALS OF NUTRITION AND METABOLISM; European journal of nutrition, metabolic diseases and dietetics. Text in English, French, German. 1959. bi-m. CHF 779 in Europe to institutions; CHF 796.40 overseas to institutions; EUR 556.80 in Europe to institutions; USD 608 overseas to institutions (effective 2002). adv. bibl, charts, illus. index. back issues avail.; reprints avail. *Refereed.* **Document type:** *Journal, Academic/Scholarly.* **Description:** Reports of basic research, primarily on the biochemical and physiological aspects of nutrition.
Incorporates (1947-1980): Annales de la Nutrition et de l'Alimentation (0003-4037); Former titles (until 1980): Nutrition and Metabolism (0029-6678); (until 1970): Nutritio et Dieta
Related titles: Microform ed.; Online - full text ed.: ISSN 1421-9697. CHF 58, EUR 42, USD 45 with print only (effective 2002) (from EBSCO Publishing, O C L C Online Computer Library Center, Inc., RoweCom Information Quest, Swets Blackwell, Institute for Scientific Information); ♦ Supplement: Annals of Nutrition & Metabolism. Supplement. ISSN 1018-9688.
Indexed: Abstr.Hyg., Agri.& Environ.Biotech.Abstr. (coverage dropped), Agricola, Anim.Breed.Abstr., Bibl.Agri., Biol.Abstr., Cadscan, Chem.Abstr., Chem.Indus.Notes, Chem.Titles, Curr.Adv.Ecol.Sci., Curr.Cont., Dairy Sci.Abstr., Dent.Ind., Derwent Biotech.Abstr., Excerp.Med., Food Sci.& Tech.Abstr., INIS Atomind., Ind.Med. (1981-), Ind.Sci.Rev., Inpharma, Int.Abstr.Biol.Sci., Lead Abstr., Maize Abstr., NRN, Nutr.Abstr., Pharm.&Out.News, Potato Abstr., Poult.Abstr., Reac., Sci.Cit.Ind., Soyabean Abstr., Triticale Abstr., Zincscan.
—BLDSC (1043.250000), CASDDS, CISTI, EMDOCS, GNLM, IDS, Infotrieve, ingenta, KNAW, Linda Hall. **CCC.**
Published by: (Federation of European Nutrition Societies), S. Karger AG, Allschwilerstr 10, PO Box, Basel 4009, Switzerland. TEL 41-61-306-1111, FAX 41-61-306-1234, karger@karger.ch, http://www.online.karger.com/journals/anm, http://www.karger.com. Ed. I Elmdfa. adv.: page USD 1,185. Circ: 1,250.

612.3 CHE ISSN 1018-9688
ANNALS OF NUTRITION & METABOLISM. SUPPLEMENT. Text in English, French, German. 1982. irreg.
Related titles: ♦ Supplement to: Annals of Nutrition and Metabolism. ISSN 0250-6807.
Published by: S. Karger AG, Allschwilerstr 10, PO Box, Basel 4009, Switzerland. FAX 41-61-30161234.

613.2 USA ISSN 1055-6990
TX341
ANNUAL EDITIONS: NUTRITION. Text in English. 1988. a. USD 12.25. illus. *Refereed.* **Document type:** *Academic/Scholarly.*
Indexed: Sugar Ind.Abstr.
Published by: Dushkin - McGraw-Hill, Sluice Dock, Guilford, CT 06437-9989. TEL 203-453-4351, FAX 203-453-6000. Eds. Charlotte Cook Fuller, Stephen Barrett. Pub. Ian Nielsen. R&P Cheryl Greenleaf.

613.2 USA ISSN 0199-9885
QP141.A1 CODEN: ARNTD8
ANNUAL REVIEW OF NUTRITION. Text in English. 1981. a. USD 60 domestic to individuals; USD 65 foreign to individuals; USD 120 domestic to institutions; USD 130 foreign to institutions (effective 1999). adv. bibl, charts. index, cum.index. back issues avail.; reprints avail. *Refereed.* **Document type:** *Academic/Scholarly.* **Description:** Synthesizes and filters primary research to identify the principal contributions in the field of physiology.
Related titles: Microform ed.: (from PQC); Online - full text ed.: (from HighWire Pr., EBSCO Publishing, H. W. Wilson, Institute for Scientific Information).
Indexed: ASCA, Abstr.Hyg., AgBiotech, Agricola, Aqua.Sci.& Fish.Abstr., Biol.& Agr.Ind. (Jan.1989-), Biol.Abstr., CINAHL, Cal.Tiss.Abstr., Chem.Abstr., Chem.Indus.Notes, Chem.Titles, Curr.Adv.Ecol.Sci., Curr.Cont., Dairy Sci.Abstr., Dent.Ind., Diar.Dis.Res., Environ.Sci.Poll.Mgmt., Food Sci.& Tech.Abstr., Ind.Med. (1981-), Ind.Sci.Rev., Inpharma, Int.Abstr.Biol.Sci., Microbiol.Abstr., Nutr.Abstr., Pig News & Info., Pollut.Abstr., Potato Abstr., Poult.Abstr., Reac., Sci.Cit.Ind., Sugar Ind.Abstr., Triticale Abstr.
—BLDSC (1524.300000), ADONIS, CASDDS, CISTI, EMDOCS, GNLM, IDS, ingenta, KNAW, Linda Hall. **CCC.**
Published by: Annual Reviews Inc., 4139 El Camino Way, Box 10139, Palo Alto, CA 94303-0139. TEL 650-493-4400, 800-523-8635, FAX 650-424-0910, service@annurev.org; orders@allenpress.com, http://www.biomedical.annualreviews.org. Ed. Samuel Gubins. R&P, Adv. contact Swati Aneja TEL 650-843-6634. **Subscr.to:** Allen Press Inc., PO Box 1897, Lawrence, KS 66044-8897.

ANTHROPOLOGY OF FOOD AND NUTRITION. see *FOOD AND FOOD INDUSTRIES*

ANTROPO-EKOLOGIIA. see *ENVIRONMENTAL STUDIES*

613.26 GBR ISSN 0195-6663
QP136 CODEN: APPTD4
APPETITE; the journal for research on intake, and dietary practices, their control and consequences. Text in English. 1980. bi-m. GBP 435 to institutions (effective 2001). adv. bk.rev. illus. index. reprint service avail. from SWZ. *Refereed.* **Document type:** *Academic/Scholarly.* **Description:** Specializes in behavioural nutrition and the cultural, sensory, and physiological influences on choices and intakes of foods and drinks.
Related titles: Online - full text ed.: ISSN 1095-8304 (from EBSCO Publishing, O C L C Online Computer Library Center, Inc., RoweCom Information Quest, ingenta, Swets Blackwell, IDEAL Online Library, Institute for Scientific Information).
Indexed: ASCA, Agricola, Anim.Behav.Abstr. (coverage dropped), Biotech.& Bioeng.Abstr., Chem.Abstr., Chem.Indus.Notes, Chem.Titles, Chemorec.Abstr., Curr.Adv.Ecol.Sci., Curr.Cont., Dairy Sci.Abstr., Dent.Ind., Excerp.Med., Food Sci.& Tech.Abstr., Ind.Med. (1980-), Ind.Sci.Rev., Inpharma, NRN, Neurosci.Cit.Ind., Nutr.Abstr., Potato Abstr., Poult.Abstr., PsycInfo, Psychol.Abstr. (1980-), Reac., SSCI (coverage dropped), Sci.Cit.Ind., Sugar Ind.Abstr., THA, Triticale Abstr., e-psyche.
—BLDSC (1570.200000), ADONIS, CASDDS, CISTI, EMDOCS, GNLM, IDS, ingenta. **CCC.**
Published by: Academic Press (Subsidiary of: Harcourt Publishers Ltd.), 24 Oval Rd, London NW1 7DX, United Kingdom. TEL 44-20-7267-4466, FAX 44-20-7482-2293, apsubs@acad.com, http://www.academicpress.com/appetite; http://www.europe.idealibrary.com/. Eds. B Hoebel, D A Booth. R&P Catherine John. Adv. contact Nik Screen. **Subscr. to:** Harcourt Publishers Ltd., Foots Cray High St, Sidcup, Kent DA14 5HP, United Kingdom. TEL 44-20-8300-3322, FAX 44-20-8309-0807.

613.2 VEN ISSN 0004-0622
TX341 CODEN: ALANBH
ARCHIVOS LATINOAMERICANOS DE NUTRICION. Text in English, French, Portuguese, Spanish. 1966. q. USD 60 to individuals in Western Hemisphere; USD 100 elsewhere to individuals; USD 165 to institutions in Western Hemisphere; USD 185 elsewhere to institutions (effective 2001). adv. bk.rev. abstr, bibl, charts. index. back issues avail.; reprint service avail. from ISI. *Refereed.* **Document type:** *Journal.* **Description:** Presents results of research in the fields of food and nutrition conducted in the Americas.
Formerly: Archivos Venezolanos de Nutricion
Related titles: Online - full text ed.: (from Institute for Scientific Information).
Indexed: ASCA, Anim.Breed.Abstr., Biol.Abstr., Chem.Abstr., Chem.Indus.Notes, Chem.Titles, Curr.Adv.Ecol.Sci., Curr.Cont., Dairy Sci.Abstr., Dent.Ind., Excerp.Med., Field Crop Abstr., Food Sci.& Tech.Abstr., Helminthol.Abstr., Hort.Abstr., Ind.Med. (1966-), Ind.Vet., Int.Nurs.Ind., Maize Abstr., NRN, Nutr.Abstr., Pig News & Info., Plant Breed.Abstr., Plant Grow.Reg.Abstr., Postharvest, Potato Abstr., Poult.Abstr., Rev.Arom.& Med.Plants, Rice Abstr., Rural Devel.Abstr., SSCI (coverage dropped), Seed Abstr., Soyabean Abstr., Sugar Ind.Abstr., Triticale Abstr., World Ag.Econ.& Rur.Soc.Abstr.
—BLDSC (1655.300000), CASDDS, CISTI, GNLM, IDS, Infotrieve, Linda Hall. **CCC.**
Published by: Sociedad Latinoamericana de Nutricion/Latin American Nutrition Society, Chacao, Apartado Postal 62778, Caracas, DF 1060, Venezuela. FAX 58-212-2860061, josefelizchavez@cantv.net. Ed. Dr. Jose Felix Chavez P. Circ: 1,000.

613.2 AUS ISSN 0964-7058
CODEN: APJNFQ
ASIA PACIFIC JOURNAL OF CLINICAL NUTRITION. Text in English. 1992. q. AUD 216 domestic to individuals; AUD 197 in New Zealand to individuals; USD 120 elsewhere to individuals; AUD 415 domestic to institutions; AUD 377 in New Zealand to institutions; USD 230 to institutions; AUD 238 domestic to individuals paper & online eds. combined; AUD 217 in New Zealand to individuals paper & online eds. combined; USD 132 elsewhere to individuals paper & online eds. combined; AUD 457 domestic to institutions paper & online eds. combined; AUD 415 in New Zealand to institutions paper & online eds. combined; USD 253 elsewhere to institutions paper & online eds. combined (effective 2001). adv. bk.rev. *Refereed.* **Document type:** *Academic/Scholarly.* **Description:** Promotes the education and training of clinical nutritionists in the region and enhances the practice of human nutrition and related disciplines in their application to health and the prevention of disease.
Related titles: Online - full text ed.: ISSN 1440-6047. AUD 195 domestic to individuals; AUD 178 in New Zealand to individuals; USD 108 elsewhere to individuals; AUD 374 domestic to institutions; AUD 340 in New Zealand to institutions; USD 207 elsewhere to institutions (effective 2001) (from EBSCO Publishing, O C L C Online Computer Library Center, Inc., RoweCom Information Quest, ingenta, Munksgaard & Blackwell Science's Synergy, Swets Blackwell, Institute for Scientific Information).
Indexed: Curr.Cont., Dairy Sci.Abstr., Food Sci.& Tech.Abstr., Nutr.Abstr., Rev.Arom.& Med.Plants, Rice Abstr., Rural Devel.Abstr., Soyabean Abstr., Triticale Abstr., World Ag.Econ.& Rur.Soc.Abstr.
—BLDSC (1742.260680), CASDDS, CISTI, Infotrieve. **CCC.**
Published by: (Asia Pacific Clinical Nutrition Society), Blackwell Science Asia Pty Ltd, PO Box 378, Carlton South, VIC 3053, Australia. TEL 61-3-9347-0300, FAX 61-3-9347-5001, info@blacksci-asia.com.au; mark.wahlqvist@med.monash.edu.au, http://www.blacksci.co.uk. Ed. Mark Wahlqvist. Adv. contact Kathryn O'Brien.

614.854 USA
▼ **ATKINS: A PASSION FOR HEALTHY LIVING.** Text in English. 2000 (June). q. free. illus. **Document type:** *Magazine, Consumer.* **Description:** Offers advice on better health through nutrition. Includes articles, news, and recipes.
Published by: Atkins Center for Complementary Medicine, 152 E 55th St, New York, NY 10022. TEL 212-758-2110, 888-ATKINS8, http://www.atkinsmag.com, http://atkinscenter.com.

AUSTRALASIAN COLLEGE OF NUTRITIONAL AND ENVIRONMENTAL MEDICINE. JOURNAL. see *MEDICAL SCIENCES*

AUSTRALIA. BUREAU OF STATISTICS. INFORMATION PAPER: NATIONAL NUTRITION SURVEY, CONFIDENTIALISED UNIT RECORD FILE. see *NUTRITION AND DIETETICS—Abstracting, Bibliographies, Statistics*

613.26 AUS
AUSTRALIAN VEGETARIAN. Text in English. 1962. bi-m. AUD 4. adv. bk.rev. **Description:** Covers cooking methods and philosophies.
Published by: Vegetarian Society South Australia, Rundle Sta., PO Box 46, Adelaide, SA 5000, Australia. Eds. E M Fearnside, T Allen. Circ: 1,000.

613.2 GBR
B N F ANNUAL CONFERENCE PROCEEDINGS. Text in English. a. GBP 27; GBP 36 foreign. back issues avail. **Document type:** *Academic/Scholarly.* **Description:** Presents papers on diet, nutrition, and health.
Published by: British Nutrition Foundation, High Holborn House, 52-54 High Holborn, London WC1V 6RQ, United Kingdom. TEL 44-20-7404-6504, FAX 44-20-7404-6747, 100634.445@compuserve.com. R&P Ursula Arens. Circ: 800.

613.2 GBR ISSN 1350-6854
B N F BRIEFING PAPERS. Text in English. 1980. irreg. GBP 5. back issues avail. **Document type:** *Academic/Scholarly.* **Description:** Covers nutrition during pregnancy, salt intake, obesity, dental health, sports nutrition, food labeling, food fortification, heart disease, cancer, vegetarianism, nutrition in older people, nutrition in infancy, food processing, meat in the diet, and related topics.
—BLDSC (2283.958220).

N

Published by: British Nutrition Foundation, High Holborn House, 52-54 High Holborn, London WC1V 6RQ, United Kingdom. TEL 44-20-7404-6504, FAX 44-20-7404-6747. R&P Maxine Ide. Circ: 800.

613.2 GBR
B N F TASK FORCE REPORTS. Text in English. 1983. irreg., latest 1999. back issues avail. **Document type:** *Academic/Scholarly.* **Description:** Provides detailed overview reports on sugars and syrups, trans-fatty acids, calcium, complex carbohydrates, unsaturated fatty acids, iron, oral health and obesity.
Published by: British Nutrition Foundation, High Holborn House, 52-54 High Holborn, London WC1V 6RQ, United Kingdom. british_nutrition@compuserve.com.

613.2 305.42 GBR ISSN 1461-0523
BEST DIET. Text in English. 1998. m. GBP 1.15 newsstand/cover (effective 2000). adv. **Document type:** *Consumer.* **Description:** Provides advice and information on losing weight in a healthy and nutritious manner.
Published by: Gruner & Jahr (UK), 197 Marsh Wall, London E14 9SG, United Kingdom. TEL 44-171-519-5500, FAX 44-171-519-5521, best@grunerandjahr.co.uk.

613.26 USA
BETTER HOMES AND GARDENS LIFESTYLE. Text in English. 1982. q. USD 3.99 newsstand/cover domestic; CND 4.99 newsstand/cover in Canada (effective 2000). adv. illus. **Document type:** *Consumer.* **Description:** Compiles recipes for nutritious, low-calorie and low-fat dishes. Provides easy-to-follow diet plans and special tips for cutting calories from everyday favorite foods.
Former titles: Better Homes and Gardens Low Calorie, Low Fat Recipes; Better Homes and Gardens Low Calorie Recipes; Diet and Exercise (0163-0334)
Published by: Meredith Corporation, 1716 Locust St, Des Moines, IA 50309-3023. TEL 515-284-2532, FAX 515-284-2877, http://www.betterhomesandgardens.com. Pub. Steve Levinson. Adv. contact Diane Claude. B&W page USD 20,925, color page USD 28,560; trim 10.5 x 8. Circ: 400,000 (paid).

613.2 USA
BETTER LIFE. Text in English. 1981. q. USD 19; USD 22 foreign (effective 1997). bk.rev. **Document type:** *Consumer.*
Formerly (until 1997): Wellness Notes
Published by: (Circle of Life), Lifecircle Publications, 566 White Pond Dr, C 113, Akron, OH 44320. TEL 330-865-9225, 800-542-1923, http://www.healthyreferral.com/natural. Ed. Jonathon Miller. Circ: 2,000.

613.2 USA
TX341
BETTER NUTRITION. Text in English. 1938. m. USD 34 domestic (effective 2001). adv. illus. reprint service avail. from PQC. **Document type:** *Trade.* **Description:** Educates consumers on the latest industry research and on natural methods for achieving optimal health and enhanced longevity.
Former titles: Better Nutrition for Today's Living; (until 1990): Better Nutrition (0405-668X); Incorporates (in 1990): Today's Living (0743-7285)
Related titles: Microform ed.: (from PQC); Online - full text ed.: (from Gale Group, Factiva).
Indexed: Hlth.Ind., PMR.
—BLDSC (1947.085000). **CCC.**
Published by: Sabot Publishing, 9 River Bend Dr S Ste 41, Stamford, CT 06907. TEL 203-328-7040, 800-829-3340, FAX 230-328-7079, jamesg@cowles.com, http://www.betternutrition.com. Ed. James J Gormley. adv.: B&W page USD 9,995, color page USD 12,145. Circ: 486,000 (paid).

BIO NACHRICHTEN. see *AGRICULTURE—Crop Production And Soil*

BLUEBOOK UPDATE. see *AGRICULTURE—Crop Production And Soil*

613.262 USA
BOVINE VETERINARIAN. Text in English. 1993. 8/yr. USD 49.94 (effective 2000). adv. **Document type:** *Trade.* **Description:** Focuses on business management information for bovine veterinarians so they can better assist their beef and dairy clients.
Published by: Vance Publishing Corporation (Lenexa), Livestock Division, 10901 W. 84th Terr., Lenexa, KS 66214-1631. TEL 913-438-8700, FAX 913-438-0695. Ed., R&P Geni Wren. Pub. Bill Newham. Adv. contact Cliff Becker. Circ: 7,500.

BRAZILIAN JOURNAL OF FOOD TECHNOLOGY. see *FOOD AND FOOD INDUSTRIES*

612.3 AUS ISSN 0729-2759
BREASTFEEDING REVIEW. Text in English. 1982. 3/yr. AUD 35 domestic; AUD 45 foreign; AUD 20 newsstand/cover (effective 1999). adv. bk.rev., video rev. back issues avail. *Refereed.* **Document type:** *Academic/Scholarly.* **Description:** For medical, nursing and allied health professionals, contains current research and developments in all aspects of human lactation, original papers, summaries of research, reviews and clinical comment.
Indexed: CINAHL, Int.Nurs.Ind.
—ingenta.
Published by: Nursing Mothers' Association of Australia, PO Box 4000, Glen Iris, VIC 3146, Australia. TEL 61-3-98850855, FAX 61-3-98850866, nursingm@nmaa.asn, http://www.nmaa.asn.au. Ed., R&P, Adv. contact Kim Boyd TEL 61-3-5332-8886. B&W page AUD 600. Circ: 1,500 (paid).

613.2 USA ISSN 1057-6606
CODEN: BMNSEG
BRISTOL-MYERS SQUIBB - MEAD JOHNSON NUTRITION SYMPOSIA. Text in English. 1983. a. **Document type:** *Monographic series, Academic/Scholarly.*
Formerly (until 1979): Bristol-Myers Nutrition Symposia (0742-8405)
Indexed: Chem.Abstr., Chem.Indus.Notes, Chem.Titles.
—CASDDS, CISTI, KNAW.
Published by: (Bristol-Myers Squibb), Lippincott Williams & Wilkins (Philadelphia) (Subsidiary of: Wolters Kluwer N.V.), 530 Walnut St, Philadelphia, PA 19106-3621. TEL 301-223-2300, 800-638-3030, FAX 301-223-2400.

612.3 GBR ISSN 0007-1145
TX501 CODEN: BJNUAV
THE BRITISH JOURNAL OF NUTRITION; an international journal of nutritional science. Text in English. 1947. m. GBP 475 to institutions; USD 830 in the Americas to institutions; GBP 490 to institutions print & online; USD 860 in the Americas to institutions print & online (effective 2002). adv. bk.rev. bibl, charts, illus, abstr. index. back issues avail.; reprints avail. *Refereed.* **Document type:** *Journal, Academic/Scholarly.* **Description:** Devoted to the advancement of the scientific study of nutrition and its application to the maintenance of human and animal health. Includes papers on clinical and human nutrition, as well as general nutrition.
Related titles: Microform ed.: (from PQC,PMC,SWZ); Online - full text ed.: GBP 465 to institutions; USD 815 in the Americas to institutions (effective 2002) (from EBSCO Publishing, H. W. Wilson, RoweCom Information Quest, ingenta, Swets Blackwell, Institute for Scientific Information); ♦ Supplement: Nutrition Research Reviews. ISSN 0954-4224.
Indexed: ASCA, Abstr.Hyg., Agri.& Environ.Biotech.Abstr. (coverage dropped), Agricola, Agroforest.Abstr., Anal.Abstr., Anim.Breed.Abstr., Behav.Med.Abstr., Bibl.Agri., Biol.& Agr.Ind. (Jan.1983-), Biol.Abstr., CINAHL, Chem.Abstr., Chem.Indus.Notes, Chem.Titles, Curr.Adv.Biochem., Curr.Adv.Ecol.Sci., Curr.Cont., Dairy Sci.Abstr., Dent.Ind., Derwent Biotech.Abstr., Diar.Dis.Res., Environ.Per.Bibl. (1977-1994), Excerp.Med., Fam.Ind., Food Sci.& Tech.Abstr., Helminthol.Abstr., Herb.Abstr., INIS Atomind., Ind.Med. (1947-), Ind.Sci.Rev., Ind.Vet., Inpharma, Int.Abstr.Biol.Sci., Maize Abstr., Mass Spectr.Bull., NRN, Nutr.Abstr., Pharm.&Out.News, Pig News & Info., Postharvest, Potato Abstr., Poult.Abstr., Protozool.Abstr., Reac., Rev.Arom.& Med.Plants, Rice Abstr., Rural Devel.Abstr., Sci.Cit.Ind., Small Anim.Abstr., Sorghum & Millets Abstr., Soyabean Abstr., Sport Fish.Abstr., Sugar Ind.Abstr., THA, Triticale Abstr., Trop.Dis.Bull., Vet.Bull., Weed Abstr.
—BLDSC (2312.000000), CASDDS, CISTI, EMDOCS, GNLM, IDS, ingenta, Linda Hall. **CCC.**
Published by: (Nutrition Society), CABI Publishing, Wallingford, Oxon OX10 8DE, United Kingdom. TEL 44-1491-832111, FAX 44-1491-829-292, publishing@cabi.org, http://www.cabi.org/primjour/BJN/bjn.htm, http://www.ingenta.com. Ed. P Trayhurn. Adv. contact S Harris. B&W page GBP 550; 170 x 240. **N. American office:** 10 E 40th St, Ste 3203, New York, NY 10016. TEL 212-481-7018, 800-528-4841, FAX 212-686-7993, cabi-nao@cabi.org.

613.2 USA ISSN 0007-7364
BUXOM BELLE COURIER✱. Text in English. 1959. m. USD 1. charts, illus, stat.
Media: Duplicated (not offset).
Published by: Buxom Belles International, Inc., 619 Spencer, Ferndale, MI 48220. Ed. Dee Phillips. Circ: 2,800.

BWINO: HEALTH CARE NEWS. see *PHYSICAL FITNESS AND HYGIENE*

C M U JOURNAL OF SCIENCE. see *AGRICULTURE*

CAB INTERNATIONAL. BUREAU OF NUTRITION. ANNOTATED BIBLIOGRAPHIES. see *NUTRITION AND DIETETICS—Abstracting, Bibliographies, Statistics*

613.2 FRA ISSN 0007-9960
CODEN: CNDQA8
CAHIERS DE NUTRITION ET DE DIETETIQUE. Text in French. 1966. 6/yr. FRF 526; FRF 601 foreign (effective 2000). adv. bk.rev. charts, illus. **Document type:** *Academic/Scholarly.* **Description:** Establishes a relationship between the medical world and the food industry. Publishes original articles and general reviews.
Related titles: Online - full text ed.: (from RoweCom Information Quest).
Indexed: AgBiotech, Biol.Abstr., Chem.Abstr., Chem.Indus.Notes, Chem.Titles, Curr.Adv.Biochem., Curr.Adv.Ecol.Sci., Curr.Adv.Gen.& Molec.Biol., Curr.Cont. (coverage dropped), Dairy Sci.Abstr., Excerp.Med. (1994-), Food Sci.& Tech.Abstr., Ind.Vet., Nutr.Abstr., Potato Abstr., Poult.Abstr., Rural Recreat.Tour.Abstr., Soyabean Abstr., Sugar Ind.Abstr., World Ag.Econ.& Rur.Soc.Abstr.
—BLDSC (2950.200000), CASDDS, CISTI, EMDOCS, GNLM, Infotrieve, Linda Hall. **CCC.**
Published by: Masson - Periodiques, 120 bd. St. Germain, Paris 75006, France. TEL 33-1-40466200, FAX 33-1-40466201. Ed. Claude Sautier. Circ: 3,500 (controlled). **Subscr. to:** Societe de Periodiques Specialises, BP 22, Vineuil Cedex 41354, France. TEL 33-2-54504612, FAX 33-2-54504611.

613.2 JAM ISSN 0376-7655
TX360.C35
CAJANUS. Text in English. 1968. q. USD 6 in developing nations; USD 12 in United States (effective 1999). bk.rev. bibl, charts. index. **Document type:** *Newsletter.* **Description:** Research articles on nutrition and dietary intake, focusing on the population of the Caribbean.
Indexed: Dairy Sci.Abstr., Food Sci.& Tech.Abstr., Nutr.Abstr., Rural Ext.Educ.& Tr.Abstr.
—CISTI, Linda Hall.
Published by: Caribbean Food and Nutrition Institute, University of the West Indies, U.W.I. Mona Campus, PO Box 140, Kingston 7, Jamaica. TEL 876-927-1540-1, FAX 876-927-1927, TELEX 3705. Ed. Clare A Forrester. Circ: 2,028. **Co-sponsor:** Pan American Health Organization, World Health Organization.

613.26 USA ISSN 1049-1791
CALORIE CONTROL COMMENTARY. Text in English. 1979. 2/yr. free in United States; USD 10 foreign (effective 2000). charts, illus, stat. back issues avail. **Document type:** *Newsletter.* **Description:** Newsletter summarizing scientific, regulatory and other developments relating to sweeteners, fat replacers, dieting, weight control and low-calorie - reduced fat foods and beverages.
Published by: Calorie Control Council, 5775 Peachtree Dunwoody Rd, Ste 500 G, Atlanta, GA 30342. TEL 404-252-3663, FAX 404-252-0774, ccc@assnhq.com, http://www.caloriecontrol.org. Ed. Keith C Keeney. R&P Keith Keeney. Circ: 12,000 (controlled).

613.2 CAN ISSN 1486-3847
CODEN: JCDTAH
CANADIAN JOURNAL OF DIETETIC PRACTICE AND RESEARCH/REVUE CANADIENNE DE LA PRACTIQUE ET DE LA RECHERCHE EN DIETETIQUE. Text in English, French. 1939. q. CND 75, USD 75 (effective 2000); (foreign $55). adv. bk.rev. abstr, charts, illus. index. *Refereed.* **Document type:** *Academic/Scholarly.* **Description:** Publishes articles and research reports in nutrition, dietetics, food administration and management.
Formerly (until 1998): Canadian Dietetic Association. Journal (0008-3399)
Related titles: Microfilm ed.: (from PQC); Online - full text ed.: (from ProQuest Information & Learning, Institute for Scientific Information).
Indexed: ASCA, AgBiotech, Agricola, Biol.Abstr., CINAHL, Chem.Abstr., Curr.Cont., Dairy Sci.Abstr., Food Sci.& Tech.Abstr., NRN, Nutr.Abstr., SSCI (coverage dropped).
—BLDSC (3031.138000), CASDDS, CISTI, GNLM, IDS, Infotrieve, ingenta. **CCC.**
Published by: Dietitians of Canada, 480 University Ave, Ste 604, Toronto, ON M5G 1V2, Canada. TEL 416-596-0857, FAX 416-596-0603. Ed. Dawna Royall. Adv. contact Joan Embury. Circ: 6,000.

613.2 VIR
CARIBBEAN DIET DIGEST. Cover title: Dr. Carter's Caribbean Diet Digest. Text in English. q. USD 18.
Published by: Caribbean Diet Institute, PO Box 191, Frederiksted, St. Croix, Virgin Isl., US.

613.2 USA ISSN 1049-4901 CODEN: CNSEEH
CARNATION NUTRITION EDUCATION SERIES. Text in English. 1989. irreg. price varies. **Document type:** *Proceedings.*
—CISTI.
Published by: Lippincott Williams & Wilkins (Philadelphia) (Subsidiary of: Wolters Kluwer N.V.), 530 Walnut St, Philadelphia, PA 19106-3621. TEL 301-223-2300, 800-638-3030, FAX 301-223-2400.

613.26 ITA ISSN 0392-7318 CODEN: CLDID7
LA CLINICA DIETOLOGICA. Text in Italian. 1974. q. ITL 60,000; ITL 120,000 foreign. **Document type:** *Academic/Scholarly.*
Indexed: Biol.Abstr., Dairy Sci.Abstr., Nutr.Abstr., Soyabean Abstr., Sugar Ind.Abstr.
—BLDSC (3286.201000), GNLM.
Published by: Societa Editrice Universo, Via Giovanni Battista Morgagni, 1, Rome, RM 00161, Italy. Ed. Michelangelo Cairella.

613.2 GBR ISSN 0261-5614 CODEN: CLNUDP
CLINICAL NUTRITION. Text in English. 1982. bi-m. GBP 155 to individuals; GBP 456 to institutions (effective 2002). adv. bk.rev. back issues avail. *Refereed.* **Document type:** *Journal, Academic/Scholarly.* **Description:** Provides essential scientific information on nutritional and metabolic care and the relationship between nutrition and disease both in the setting of basic science and clinical practice.
Related titles: Microform ed.: (from PQC); Online - full text ed.: (from EBSCO Publishing, O C L C Online Computer Library Center, Inc., Swets Blackwell, IDEAL Online Library, Institute for Scientific Information).
Indexed: ASCA, Aqua.Sci.& Fish.Abstr., Aquacult.Abstr., Chem.Abstr., Chem.Indus.Notes, Chem.Titles, Curr.Adv.Ecol.Sci., Curr.Cont., Dairy Sci.Abstr., Excerp.Med., Ind.Med. (1982-), Inpharma, Int.Abstr.Biol.Sci., Int.Nurs.Ind., NRN, Nutr.Abstr., Pharm.&Out.News, Reac., Ref.Zh., SSCI (coverage dropped), Soyabean Abstr.
—BLDSC (3286.314500), CASDDS, EMDOCS, GNLM, IDS, ingenta, KNAW. **CCC.**
Published by: (European Society of Parenteral and Enteral Nutrition), Churchill Livingstone (Subsidiary of: Harcourt Publishers Ltd.), Robert Stevenson House, 1-3 Baxter's Pl, Leith Walk, Edinburgh, Midlothian EH1 3AF, United Kingdom. TEL 44-131-556-2424, FAX 44-131-459-1177, http://www.harcourt-international.com/journals/clnu, http://www.churchillmed.com. Ed. M A Gassull. Pub. Gillian Griffith. R&P Catherine John TEL 212-424-4200. Adv. contact David Dunnachie. Circ: 1,125. **Subscr. to:** Harcourt Publishers Ltd., Foots Cray High St, Sidcup, Kent DA14 5HP, United Kingdom. TEL 44-20-8308-5700, FAX 44-20-8309-0807.

CO-OP NEWS (HANOVER). see *FOOD AND FOOD INDUSTRIES—Grocery Trade*

052 GBR
THE COMPLETE FAT UNIT GUIDE. Text in English. a. GBP 1.95 newsstand/cover. **Document type:** *Consumer.*
Published by: Emap Elan Ltd. (Subsidiary of: Emap Consumer Magazines Ltd.), Endeavour House, 189 Shaftesbury Ave, London WC2H 8JG, United Kingdom. TEL 44-207-437-9011, FAX 44-207-208-3709, http://www.emap.com. **Subscr. to:** Tower Publishing Services Ltd., Tower House, Sovereign Park, Lathkill St, Market Harborough, Leics LE16 9EF, United Kingdom. TEL 44-1858-435339, FAX 44-1858-434958.

613.2 GBR
THE COMPOSITION OF FOODS. Text in English. irreg., latest vol.7, 2000. GBP 39.95 per vol. (effective 2002). Supplement avail. **Document type:** *Trade.* **Description:** Contains revised and updated nutrient data on nearly 1,200 foods.
Published by: Royal Society of Chemistry, Thomas Graham House, Science Park, Milton Rd, Cambridge CB4 4WF, United Kingdom. TEL 44-1223-432360, FAX 44-1223-423429, sales@rsc.org, http://www.rsc.org/. Ed. B Holland. **Dist. by:** Turpin Distribution Services Ltd., Blackhorse Rd, Letchworth, Herts SG6 1HN, United Kingdom. TEL 44-1462-488900, FAX 44-1462-483011.

613.2 USA
CONNELLY REPORT*. Text in English. m. USD 48. **Document type:** *Newsletter.* **Description:** Covers health, nutrition, life extension and related topics.
Published by: Met-Rx U S A, Inc., 17861 Von Karman Ave, Irvine, CA 92614-6213. Ed. Dr. Scott Connelly. Circ: 56,000.

CONSCIOUS CHOICE; the journal of ecology and natural living. see *ENVIRONMENTAL STUDIES*

COOKING LIGHT; the magazine of food and fitness. see *HOME ECONOMICS*

612.3 USA
COOKING NEWS. Text in English. fortn. free per issue. **Document type:** *Newsletter.*
Media: Online - full text.
Published by: E G W Publishing Co., 1041 Shary Circle, Concord, CA 94518. TEL 925-671-9852, FAX 510-671-0692, hstevens@egw.com, http://www.naturalland.com/cv/cnc.htm.

613.2 MEX ISSN 0186-3274
CUADERNOS DE NUTRICION. Text in Spanish. 1981. bi-m. MXP 150, USD 50; MXP 25 newsstand/cover (effective 1999). adv. bk.rev. illus. cum.index: 1992-1997. *Refereed.* **Document type:** *Academic/Scholarly.* **Description:** Includes articles on basic nutrition, economics, production, food technology, and social aspects like food habits and traditions.
Published by: (Fomento de Nutricion y Salud), Cuadernos de Nutricion A.C., ALTATA 51 P.B., Col Hipodromo de la Condesa, Mexico City, DF 06170, Mexico. TEL 52-5-5151939, FAX 52-5-2726207, cuadernos@fns.org.mx. Ed., R&P Dr. Hector Bourges Rodriguez. Adv. contact Enrique Rios. page MXP 11,500; trim 275 x 210. Circ: 10,000 (controlled). **Dist. by:** Publicaciones CITEM, S.A. de C. V. Mier y Pesado 126 y 128, Col Del Valle, Mexico City, DF 03100, Mexico. TEL 52-5-6874699.

CURRENT MEDICAL LITERATURE. CLINICAL NUTRITION. see *NUTRITION AND DIETETICS—Abstracting, Bibliographies, Statistics*

612.3 USA ISSN 1363-1950 CODEN: COCMF3
CURRENT OPINION IN CLINICAL NUTRITION AND METABOLIC CARE. Text in English. 1998. bi-m. USD 265 domestic to individuals for print & online eds.; USD 265 foreign to individuals for print & online eds; USD 665 per issue domestic to institutions; USD 665 per issue foreign to institutions; USD 103 newsstand/cover (effective 2002). adv. back issues avail. *Refereed.* **Document type:** *Academic/Scholarly.* **Description:** Keeps up-to-date with the expanding volume of information in the fields of clinical nutrition and metabolic care.
Related titles: Online - full text ed.: USD 864.50 domestic academic site license; USD 864.50 foreign academic site license; USD 964.25 domestic corporate site license; USD 964.25 foreign corporate site license (effective 2002) (from Ovid Technologies, Inc., EBSCO Publishing, Swets Blackwell).
Indexed: Abstr.Hyg., Ind.Med. (1998-), Nutr.Abstr.
—BLDSC (3500.773530), CASDDS, Infotrieve.
Published by: Lippincott Williams & Wilkins (Philadelphia) (Subsidiary of: Wolters Kluwer N.V.), 530 Walnut St, Philadelphia, PA 19106-3621. TEL 215-521-8300, FAX 215-521-8902, http://www.Lww.com. Eds. John M Kinney, Luc A Cynober, Yvon A Carpentier. Adv. contact Gemma Heiser. **Subscr. to:** PO Box 1600, Hagerstown, MD 21740-1600. TEL 800-777-2295, FAX 301-824-7390.

616.39 USA ISSN 0191-2453 CODEN: CTNDDU
CURRENT TOPICS IN NUTRITION AND DISEASE. Text in English. 1977. irreg., latest vol.22, 1990. price varies. bibl. illus. index. *Refereed.*
Indexed: Biol.Abstr., Chem.Abstr., Chem.Indus.Notes, Chem.Titles.
—CASDDS, CISTI.
Published by: John Wiley & Sons, Inc., Journals (Subsidiary of: Wiley InterScience), 605 Third Ave, New York, NY 10158. TEL 212-475-7700.

613.2 USA ISSN 0011-5568 CODEN: DACDAK
DAIRY COUNCIL DIGEST; an interpretive review of recent nutrition research. Text in English. 1929. bi-m. free per issue. illus. index. back issues avail.; reprints avail. **Document type:** *Academic/Scholarly.* **Description:** Covers recent research information for nutrition professionals. Each issue examines a single topic.
Media: Online - full text (from Northern Light Technology, Inc., ProQuest Information & Learning). **Related titles:** Microform ed.: (from PQC).
Indexed: CHNI, Dairy Sci.Abstr., Hlth.Ind., Nutr.Abstr.
—CASDDS, CISTI, Linda Hall.
Published by: National Dairy Council, O'Hare International Center, 10255 W. Higgins Rd., Ste. 900, Rosemont, IL 60018-5616. TEL 847-803-2000, FAX 847-803-2077, http://www.nationaldairycouncil.org. Circ: 25,000.

613.2 USA ISSN 1073-8436
DELICIOUS!; guide to natural living. Text in English. 1985. m. USD 24 domestic; USD 44 foreign; USD 2.75 newsstand/cover (effective 2001). back issues avail. **Document type:** *Magazine, Consumer.* **Description:** Provides natural health and natural food information in a practical, clear, easy-to-understand format that motivates readers to make healthy choices for themselves and their families.
Related titles: Online - full text ed.
Published by: New Hope Natural Media (Subsidiary of: Penton Media, Inc.), 1401 Pearl St, Boulder, CO 80302. TEL 303-939-8440, FAX 303-440-8884, sales@newhope.com, http://www.healthwell.com. Ed. Karen Raterman. Pub. Maurice Lluch.

DIABETES, NUTRITION & METABOLISM, CLINICAL AND EXPERIMENTAL. see *MEDICAL SCIENCES—Endocrinology*

DIET & FITNESS MAGAZINE. see *PHYSICAL FITNESS AND HYGIENE*

613.2 613.7 USA
DIET & NUTRITION SOURCEBOOK. Text in English. 1996. irreg., latest vol.2, 1999. USD 78 per vol. (effective 2002). charts, illus, stat. master index. **Document type:** *Consumer.* **Description:** Offers consumers advice on nutrition and weight control.
Published by: Omnigraphics, Inc., 615 Griswold St, Detroit, MI 48226. TEL 313-961-1340, 800-234-1340, FAX 313-961-1383, 800-875-1340, info@omnigraphics.com, http://www.omnigraphics.com. Ed. Karen Bellenir. Pub. Frederick G Ruffner Jr.

613.26 USA
DIETARY GUIDELINES FOR AMERICANS. Text in English. irreg. **Document type:** *Consumer, Government.*
Formerly: U S D A Dietary Guidelines
Published by: U.S. Department of Agriculture, Center for Nutrition Policy and Promotion, 1120 20th St, N W, Ste 200, North Lobby, Washington, DC 20036. TEL 202-418-2312, FAX 202-208-2321, http://www.usda.gov/fcs/cnpp.htm. **Dist. by:** U.S. Government Printing Office, Superintendent of Documents, PO Box 371954, Pittsburgh, PA 15250-7954. TEL 202-512-1800, FAX 202-512-2250, orders@gpo.gov, http://www.access.gpo.gov.

613.26 USA ISSN 1062-1121
DIETARY MANAGER MAGAZINE. Text in English. 1992. 10/yr. USD 35. adv. bk.rev. **Document type:** *Trade.* **Description:** A valuable management and training tool for professionals in non-commercial food service.
Published by: Dietary Managers Association, 406 Surrey Woods Dr., St. Charles, IL 60174-2386. TEL 630-587-6336, 800-323-1908, FAX 630-587-6308, http://www.dmaonline.org. Ed. Diane Everett. Adv. contact Susan Wrona. page USD 647; trim 10.88 x 8.13. Circ: 16,750.

613.26 CAN ISSN 0834-3160
DIETETIQUE EN ACTION. Text in English, French. 1986. 3/yr. CND 58.85 (effective 1998). bk.rev. **Document type:** *Bulletin.*
Indexed: Pt.de Rep. (1989-).
Published by: Ordre Professionel des Dietetistes du Quebec, 1425 bd Rene Levesque O, Bur 703, Montreal, PQ H3G 1T7, Canada. TEL 514-393-3733, FAX 514-393-3582, opdq@opdq.org. Ed. Annie Langlois. adv.: B&W page CND 615, color page CND 1,345; trim 11 x 8.5. Circ: 2,500.

613.26 SWE ISSN 0348-0674
DIETISTEN; kostekonomi, dietetik. Text in Swedish. 1949. 6/yr. SEK 585 (effective 2000). adv. **Document type:** *Magazine, Consumer.*
Former titles (until vol.3, 1977): Svenska Ekonomifoerestaandares Tidskrift (0346-2293); (until vol.3, 1968): Svenska Ekonomifoerestaandarinnors Tidskrift; (until vol.7, 1950): Meddelande fraan Svenska Ekonomifoerestaandarinnors Foerening

N

Published by: S D F - Svensk Dietist och Kostekonomfoerening, Fack 45148, Stockholm 10430, Sweden. TEL 46-8-38-38-29, FAX 46-8-38-38-29, annika.elias@orgryte.goteborg.se, http://www.dietist-kostekonomforening.a.se. Ed. Inger Lagerman. Pub. Annika Elias. adv.: B&W page SEK 9,000, color page SEK 15,000; trim 194 x 270. Circ: 2,000.

613.2 USA
DIETITIAN'S EDGE. Text in English. bi-m. USD 20; USD 5 newsstand/cover (effective 2001). adv.
Published by: Dietitian's Edge LLC, 70 Hilltop Rd, 3rd fl, Ramsey, NJ 07446. TEL 201-825-2552, FAX 201-825-0553. Ed. Tamara Schryver. Adv. contact Heather Shanley.

613.2 SWE ISSN 0348-9361
DROPPJOURNALEN; tidskrift om nutrition och vaetsketerapi. Text in Swedish. 1979-1981; resumed 1984. q.
Published by: Kabi Pharmacia AB, Stockholm 11287, Sweden.

EATING AND WEIGHT DISORDERS; Studies on Anorexia, Bulimia and Obesity. see *MEDICAL SCIENCES—Psychiatry And Neurology*

EATING DISORDERS REVIEW; current clinical information for the professional treating eating disorders. see *MEDICAL SCIENCES—Psychiatry And Neurology*

ECOLE NATIONALE SUPERIEURE DE BIOLOGIE APPLIQUEE A LA NUTRITION ET A L'ALIMENTATION. CAHIERS. see *FOOD AND FOOD INDUSTRIES*

613.2 CHE ISSN 0367-0244
TX341 CODEN: ECFNBN
ECOLOGY OF FOOD AND NUTRITION. Text in French. 1971. 6/yr. GBP 85, USD 103, EUR 114 to individuals; GBP 523, USD 651, EUR 667 to institutions; GBP 817, USD 1,016, EUR 1,058 to corporations (effective 2002). adv. bk.rev. bibl, charts, illus, stat. index. back issues avail.; reprints avail. *Refereed.* **Document type:** *Academic/Scholarly.* **Description:** Emphasizes foods and their utilization in satisfying the nutritional needs of mankind, but also extends to nonfood contributions, to obesity and leanness, malnutrition, vitamin requirements, and mineral needs.
Related titles: Microform ed.; Online - full text ed.: (from Institute for Scientific Information).
Indexed: A.I.C.P., ASCA, Abstr.Anthropol., Abstr.Hyg., Abstr.Rural Dev.Trop., Agricola, Agroforest.Abstr., Anthropol.Lit. (coverage dropped), Bibl.Agri., Biol.Abstr., Cadscan, Chem.Abstr., Curr.Adv.Ecol.Sci., Curr.Cont., Dairy Sci.Abstr., Ecol.Abstr., Energy Ind., Energy Info.Abstr., Environ.Per.Bibl. (1991-), Excerp.Med., Field Crop Abstr., Food Sci.& Tech.Abstr., Forest Prod.Abstr., Forest.Abstr., Herb.Abstr., Hort.Abstr., IBZ, IDA, Ind.Sci.Rev., Intl.Bibl.Soc.Sci., Lead Abstr., Maize Abstr., NRN, Nutr.Abstr., Plant Gen.Res.Abstr., Postharvest, Potato Abstr., Rice Abstr., Rural Devel.Abstr., SSCI (coverage dropped), Sci.Cit.Ind., Seed Abstr., So.Pac.Per.Ind., Soils & Fert., Soyabean Abstr., Triticale Abstr., Trop.Dis.Bull., Weed Abstr., World Ag.Econ.& Rur.Soc.Abstr., Zincscan.
—BLDSC (3650.043000), CISTI, Infotrieve, ingenta, Linda Hall. **CCC.**
Published by: Gordon and Breach - Harwood Academic (Subsidiary of: Taylor & Francis Group), PO Box 531, Lausanne 1000, Switzerland. http://www.gbhap-us.com/journals/126/126-top.html. Ed. Peter L Pellett. **Subscr. addr. in US:** International Publishers Direct, PO Box 32160, Newark, NJ 07102. FAX 215-750-6343.

613.2 BEL ISSN 0004-5144
EDUCATION SANITAIRE ET NUTRITIONNELLE D'AFRIQUE CENTRALE. Text in French. 1927. q. BEF 150.
Formerly: Assistance aux Maternites et Dispensaires en Afrique Centrale
Published by: Centre d'Education Sanitaire et Nutritionnelle d'Afrique Centrale, 11 Rue Brialmont, Brussels 1030, Belgium. TEL 32-2-2170497. Ed. M M Moeremans d'Emaus. Circ: 1,000.

613.2 JPN
EIYO KANRI NO KENKYU/STUDY ON NUTRITION CONTROL. Text in Japanese. a. JPY 1,900.
Published by: Zenkoku Jichitai Byoin Kyogikai/Japan Municipal Hospital Association, Godo Kaikan, 3-27 Kioi-cho, Chiyoda-ku, Tokyo 102-0094, Japan.

613.2 JPN ISSN 0013-6492
EIYO NIPPON/NUTRITION OF JAPAN. Text in Japanese. 1958. m. JPY 850 per issue.
—CISTI.
Published by: Nihon Eiyoshikai/Japan Dietetic Association, 1-39 Kanda-Jinbo-cho, Chiyoda-ku, Tokyo 101-0051, Japan.

613.2 JPN ISSN 0915-759X
CODEN: EHCHES
EIYOU HYOKA TO CHIRYO/JAPANESE JOURNAL OF NUTRITIONAL ASSESSMENT. Text in Japanese. 1987. 4/yr. JPY 1,900 (effective 1998).
—CASDDS.
Published by: Medikaru Rebyusha/Medical Review Co., Ltd., 7-3 Hirano-Machi 1-chome, Chuo-ku, Osaka-shi 541-0046, Japan. TEL 81-6-223-1556, FAX 81-6-223-1414, medrev@osk2.3web.ne.jp.

ENCUESTA NACIONAL DE NUTRICION. see *NUTRITION AND DIETETICS—Abstracting, Bibliographies, Statistics*

ENCYCLOPEDIE MEDICO-CHIRURGICALE. ENDOCRINOLOGIE - NUTRITION. see *MEDICAL SCIENCES—Endocrinology*

613.2 051 USA
ENERGY TIMES; enhancing your life through proper nutrition. Text in English. 10/yr. USD 2.50 newsstand/cover (effective 2001). adv. **Document type:** *Magazine, Consumer.* **Description:** Educates consumers looking to lead a healthy lifestyle. Includes information on nutrition, natural foods, herbs, natural products, recipes, fitness, alternative health care and more.
Published by: Energy Times Inc, 548 Broadhollow Rd, Melville, NY 11747. TEL 631-777-7773, FAX 631-755-1064, advertising@energytimes.com. Ed., Pub. Gerard McIntee.

613.2 USA ISSN 0893-4452
ENVIRONMENTAL NUTRITION; the newsletter of food, nutrition and health. Text in English. 1977. m. USD 30 domestic to libraries; USD 49 foreign to libraries. bk.rev. illus. index. back issues avail.; reprints avail. **Document type:** *Consumer.*
Formerly: Environmental Nutrition Newsletter (0195-4024)
Related titles: Online - full text ed.: (from Gale Group, Northern Light Technology, Inc., Factiva).
Indexed: Agricola, CHNI, Hlth.Ind.
—BLDSC (3791.527600). **CCC.**
Published by: Environmental Nutrition, Inc., 52 Riverside Dr, Ste 15A, New York, NY 10024-6599. TEL 212-362-0424, FAX 212-362-2066, 76521.2250@compuserve.com. Ed. Susan Male Smith. Pub., R&P Betty Ivie Goldblatt. Circ: 85,000. **Subscr. to:** PO Box 420451, Palm Coast, FL 32142-0451.

ENVIRONMENTAL OPPORTUNITIES. see *ENVIRONMENTAL STUDIES*

613.2 ITA
ERBORISTERIA DOMANI. Text in Italian. 1978. m. (11/yr.). ITL 86,000. **Document type:** *Consumer.*
Indexed: Apic.Abstr.
Published by: Demetrio Benelli Ed. & Pub., Piazza Riccardo Wagner, 1, Milan, MI 20145, Italy. TEL 39-2-4816742, FAX 39-2-4817843. adv.: B&W page ITL 1,400,000, color page ITL 2,400,000. Circ: 20,000.

613.2 DEU
HC290.5.C6
ERNAEHRUNG IM FOKUS; Zeitschrift fuer Fach-, Lehr- und Beratungskraefte im Bereich Ernaehrung. Text in German. 1956. m. DEM 48 (effective 2001). bk.rev. *Refereed.* **Document type:** *Journal, Academic/Scholarly, Government.*
Former titles (until 2001): A I D Verbraucherdienst (0720-7522); (until 1979): Verbraucherdienst (0720-650X); (until 1978): Verbraucherdienst. Ausgabe B (0505-2432)
Indexed: Food Sci.& Tech.Abstr.
—BLDSC (9155.778000).
Published by: Auswertungs- und Informationsdienst fuer Ernaehrung Landwirtschaft und Forsten e.V., Friedrich-Ebert-Str 3, Bonn 53177, Germany. TEL 49-228-84990, FAX 49-228-8499177, TELEX 886323-AIDNB-D, aid@aid.de, http://www.aid.de. Ed. Birgit Jaehnig. Circ: 8,500.

613.2 DEU ISSN 0367-0899
ERNAEHRUNGS - LEHRE UND PRAXIS. Text in German. 1964. m.
Related titles: ♦ Supplement: Ernaehrungs Umschau. ISSN 0174-0008.
Published by: Umschau Zeitschriftenverlag Breidenstein GmbH, Stuttgarter Str 18-24, Frankfurt Am Main 60329, Germany. TEL 49-69-2600-621, FAX 49-69-2600-609. Ed. Werner Stark.

613.2 DEU ISSN 0174-0008
CODEN: ERUMAT
ERNAEHRUNGS UMSCHAU; Forschung und Praxis. Text in German. 1954. m. DEM 141; DEM 102 to students (effective 2000). adv. bk.rev. charts, illus, stat. index. back issues avail. *Refereed.* **Document type:** *Consumer.*
Formed by the merger of (1964-1977): Ernaehrungs - Umschau. Ausgabe B (0340-2371); (1964-1977): Ernaehrungs - Umschau. Ausgabe M (0340-2320); Which was formerly (until 1964): Ernaehrungs - Umschau (0014-021X)
Related titles: Online - full text ed.: (from Institute for Scientific Information); ♦ Supplement to: Ernaehrungs - Lehre und Praxis. ISSN 0367-0899.
Indexed: Abstr.Hyg., Biol.Abstr., Chem.Abstr., Chem.Indus.Notes, Chem.Titles, Curr.Adv.Ecol.Sci., Curr.Cont., Dairy Sci.Abstr., Excerp.Med., Food Sci.& Tech.Abstr., INIS Atomind., Nutr.Abstr., Pig News & Info., Plant Breed.Abstr., Postharvest, Rev.Appl.Entomol., Rev.Med.& Vet.Mycol., Sugar Ind.Abstr., Triticale Abstr., Vet.Bull.
—BLDSC (3810.730000), CASDDS, GNLM, Infotrieve. **CCC.**
Published by: (Deutsche Gesellschaft fuer Ernaehrung), Umschau Zeitschriftenverlag Breidenstein GmbH, Stuttgarter Str 18-24, Frankfurt Am Main 60329, Germany. TEL 49-69-2600-670, FAX 49-69-2600-619. Ed. Sabine Fankhaenel. adv.: B&W page DEM 5,260, color page DEM 8,380; trim 257 x 176. Circ: 11,277.
Co-sponsor: Guetegemeinschaft Diaetverpflegung.

ERNAEHRUNGSDIENST; unabhaengige Handels- und Boersenzeitung. see *AGRICULTURE—Feed, Flour And Grain*

613.2 CHE ISSN 0071-1179
TX341 CODEN: ERNFA7
ERNAEHRUNGSFORSCHUNG/NUTRITION RESEARCH; aktuelle Informationen aus Wissenschaft und Praxis. Text in German. 1956. 4/yr. GBP 63, USD 76, EUR 84 to individuals; GBP 254, USD 327, EUR 338 to institutions; GBP 410, USD 536, EUR 547 to corporations (effective 2002). charts, illus. index. **Document type:** *Journal, Academic/Scholarly.*
Indexed: Biol.Abstr., Chem.Abstr., Dairy Sci.Abstr., Excerp.Med., Food Sci.& Tech.Abstr., Maize Abstr., Nutr.Abstr., Pig News & Info., Soyabean Abstr.
—BLDSC (3810.700000), CASDDS, CISTI, GNLM, Infotrieve, Linda Hall. **CCC.**
Published by: (Akademie der Wissenschaften DDR, Zentralinstitut fuer Ernaehrung), Gordon and Breach - Harwood Academic (Subsidiary of: Taylor & Francis Group), PO Box 531, Lausanne 1000, Switzerland. TEL 41-21-6411280, FAX 41-21-6411281, info@gbhap.com, http://www.gbhap.com. Ed. Hans Albrecht Ketz. **Subscr. addr. in US:** International Publishers Direct, PO Box 32160, Newark, NJ 07102. FAX 215-750-6343.

612.3 DEU ISSN 0721-5118
ERNAEHRUNGSRUNDBRIEF. Text in German. 1970. q. DEM 32 domestic; DEM 36 foreign (effective 2001). adv. bk.rev. index. 64 p./no. 1 cols./p. back issues avail. **Document type:** *Bulletin, Consumer, Academic/Scholarly.*
Published by: Arbeitskreis fuer Ernaehrungsforschung e.V., Niddastr 14, Bad Vilbel 61118, Germany. TEL 49-6101-521825, FAX 49-6101-521886, ak-ernaehrung@t-online.de. Ed., Adv. contact Petra Kuehne. Circ: 4,000.

613.2 GBR ISSN 0954-3007
CODEN: EJCNEQ
EUROPEAN JOURNAL OF CLINICAL NUTRITION. Text in English. 1976. m. GBP 150 in Europe to individuals for print or online ed.; USD 225 elsewhere to individuals for print or online ed.; GBP 165 combined subscription in Europe to individuals print & online; USD 248 combined subscription elsewhere to individuals print & online; GBP 330 in Europe to institutions for print or online ed.; USD 495 elsewhere to institutions for print or online ed.; GBP 363 combined subscription in Europe to institutions print & online; USD 545 combined subscription elsewhere to institutions print & online (effective 2002). adv. bk.rev. illus, charts, stat. reprints avail. *Refereed.* **Document type:** *Journal, Academic/Scholarly.*
Formerly (until 1987): Human Nutrition. Clinical Nutrition (0263-8290); Which superseded in part (in 1981): Journal of Human Nutrition (0308-4329); Which was formerly (until 1976): Nutrition (0029-6600)
Related titles: Online - full text ed.: (from EBSCO Publishing, O C L C Online Computer Library Center, Inc., RoweCom Information Quest, ingenta, Gale Group, Swets Blackwell, Factiva, Institute for Scientific Information).

Indexed: ASCA, Agricola, Bibl.Agri., Curr.Cont., Dairy Sci.Abstr., Diar.Dis.Res., Excerp.Med., Gen.Sci.Ind. (Jan.1988-Jun.1992), Helminthol.Abstr., Ind.Med. (1988-), Inpharma, Int.Abstr.Biol.Sci., Maize Abstr., NRN, Nutr.Abstr., Pharm.&Out.News, Potato Abstr., Protozool.Abstr., Reac., Rice Abstr., Rural Devel.Abstr., SSCI (coverage dropped), Sci.Cit.Ind., Soyabean Abstr., Sugar Ind.Abstr., Triticale Abstr., Trop.Dis.Bull.
—BLDSC (3829.728000), CASDDS, CISTI, EMDOCS, GNLM, IDS, ingenta, KNAW, Linda Hall. **CCC.**
Published by: Nature Publishing Group Specialist Journals (Subsidiary of: Holtzbrink Publishers), Houndmills, Basingstoke, Hants RG21 6XS, United Kingdom. TEL 44-1256-329242, FAX 44-1256-328339, subscriptions@nature.com, http://www.nature.com/ejcn. Ed. J C Seidell. Pub. Michael Osuch. R&P Trace Noel. Adv. contact Robert Sloan TEL 44-20-8882-7199.

613.2 DEU ISSN 1436-6207
QP141.A1 CODEN: ZERNAL
EUROPEAN JOURNAL OF NUTRITION. Text and summaries in English, German. 1960. 6/yr. EUR 332.90 domestic (effective 2002); EUR 323.40 in Germany (effective 2001); EUR 62 newsstand/cover foreign (effective 2002). adv. bk.rev. charts, illus, abstr. index. back issues avail.; reprints avail. *Refereed.* **Document type:** *Journal, Academic/Scholarly.*
Formerly (until 1999): Zeitschrift fuer Ernaehrungswissenschaft (0044-264X)
Related titles: Microform ed.: (from PQC); Online - full text ed.: ISSN 1436-6215 (from EBSCO Publishing, RoweCom Information Quest, Swets Blackwell, Springer LINK, Institute for Scientific Information).
Indexed: ASCA, Biol.Abstr., Chem.Abstr., Chem.Indus.Notes, Chem.Titles, Curr.Adv.Biochem., Curr.Adv.Cell & Devel.Biol., Curr.Adv.Ecol.Sci., Curr.Cont., Dairy Sci.Abstr., Excerp.Med., Food Sci.& Tech.Abstr., INIS Atomind., Ind.Med. (1999-), Int.Nurs.Ind., Maize Abstr., Nutr.Abstr., Pig News & Info., Poult.Abstr., Soyabean Abstr., Triticale Abstr.
—BLDSC (3829.731900), CASDDS, CISTI, GNLM, IDS, Infotrieve, ingenta, Linda Hall. **CCC.**
Published by: Dr. Dietrich Steinkopff Verlag (Subsidiary of: BertelsmannSpringer), Platz der deutschen Einheit 25, Darmstadt 64293, Germany. TEL 49-6151-82899-0, FAX 49-6151-82899-40, frey.steinkopff@springer.de, http://www.steinkopff.springer.de. Ed. G Rechkemmer. R&P Dr. Maria Magdalene Nabbe. Circ: 1,500. **Subscr. to:** Springer GmbH Auslieferungsgesellschaft, Haberstr 7, Heidelberg 69126, Germany. TEL 49-6221-345239, FAX 49-6221-345249, subscriptions@springer.de.

EXERCISE PHYSIOLOGY: CURRENT SELECTED RESEARCH. see *PHYSICAL FITNESS AND HYGIENE*

EXTENDED CARE PRODUCT NEWS. see *PHYSICAL FITNESS AND HYGIENE*

613.2 USA ISSN 1014-3181
F A O FOOD AND NUTRITION SERIES. Text in English, French, Spanish. 1948. irreg., latest no.29, 1997. price varies. **Document type:** *Monographic series.*
Formerly: F A O Nutritional Study (0071-7088)
Related titles: Spanish ed.: Coleccion F A O, Alimentacion y Nutricion. ISSN 1014-3173; French ed.: Collection F A O, Alimentation et Nutrition. ISSN 0253-2549.
Indexed: Food Sci.& Tech.Abstr., Ind.Med. (coverage dropped), Ind.Vet., Nutr.Abstr., Pig News & Info., Vet.Bull., World Ag.Econ.& Rur.Soc.Abstr.
—CISTI.
Published by: Food and Agriculture Organization of the United Nations, c/o Bernan Associates, 4611 F Assembly Dr, Lanham, MD 20706-4391. TEL 301-459-7666, FAX 301-459-0056.

613.26 USA
F A R M REPORT. Text in English. 1981. irreg. (3-4/yr.). USD 20 to members (effective 2000). bk.rev. **Document type:** *Newsletter, Trade.* **Description:** Promotes vegetarianism and exposes the adverse impacts of factory farming. Includes articles on eating trends and developments in the meat industry.
Published by: Farm Animal Report Movement, PO Box 30654, Bethesda, MD 20824. TEL 301-530-1737, FAX 301-530-5747, farm@farmusa.org, http://www.farmusa.org. Ed., Pub. Alex Hershaft. Circ: 12,000 (controlled).

FAMILY ECONOMICS AND NUTRITION REVIEW. see *HOME ECONOMICS*

613.2 USA ISSN 0895-0040
FELIX LETTER; a commentary on nutrition. Text in English. 1981. 6/yr. USD 12 in North America; USD 20 in Europe (effective 2001). bk.rev. back issues avail. **Document type:** *Newsletter, Academic/Scholarly.* **Description:** Critical review and commentary on nutrition research. Promotes nutrition as an alternative to or adjunctive to medical approaches to illness.
Published by: Clara Felix, Ed. & Pub., PO Box 7094, Berkeley, CA 94707. TEL 510-526-6268, FAX 510-524-1735, felixltr81@aol.com. Ed., Pub., R&P Clara Felix. Circ: 2,000 (paid and free).

613.2 DEU ISSN 0720-8731
CODEN: FPEREX
FETT IN DER PARENTERALEN ERNAEHRUNG. Text in German. 1981. irreg., latest vol.5, 1998. **Document type:** *Academic/Scholarly.*
—CASDDS.
Published by: W. Zuckschwerdt Verlag GmbH, Industriestr 1, Germering 82110, Germany. TEL 49-89-894349-0, FAX 49-89-89434950.

FOEDEVARENYT. see *FOOD AND FOOD INDUSTRIES*

613.2 CHE ISSN 0740-9710
TX341 CODEN: FOFWEC
FOOD AND FOODWAYS; explorations in the history and culture of human nutrition. Text in English. q. GBP 96, USD 140, EUR 160 to individuals; GBP 396, USD 549, EUR 551 to institutions; GBP 613, USD 852, EUR 859 to corporations (effective 2002). adv. *Refereed.*
Related titles: Microform ed.
Indexed: Amer.Hist.& Life, Food Sci.& Tech.Abstr., Hist.Abstr. (1992-), IBZ, Intl.Bibl.Soc.Sci., P C I.
—BLDSC (3977.038450), ingenta. **CCC.**
Published by: Gordon and Breach - Harwood Academic (Subsidiary of: Taylor & Francis Group), PO Box 531, Lausanne 1000, Switzerland. Ed. Steven L Kaplan. **Subscr. addr. in US:** International Publishers Direct, PO Box 32160, Newark, NJ 07102. FAX 215-750-6343.

613.2 JPN ISSN 0379-5721
TX341 CODEN: FNBPDV
FOOD AND NUTRITION BULLETIN. Text in English. q. USD 40 (effective 1999). adv. bk.rev. cum.index: vols.1-3. back issues avail. *Refereed.* **Document type:** *Bulletin.*
Supersedes (in 1978): Protein-Calorie Advisory Group of the United Nations System. P A G Bulletin
Related titles: Microfiche ed.: (from CIS).
Indexed: Agroforest.Abstr., Chem.Abstr., Dairy Sci.Abstr., Diar.Dis.Res., Food Sci.& Tech.Abstr., Forest Prod.Abstr., Forest.Abstr., Helminthol.Abstr., IDA, IIS, Maize Abstr., Nutr.Abstr., Postharvest, Potato Abstr., Rev.Med.& Vet.Mycol., Rice Abstr., Rural Devel.Abstr., Russ.Acad.Sci.Bibl., Seed Abstr., Sorghum & Millets Abstr., Triticale Abstr., Trop.Dis.Bull., World Ag.Econ.& Rur.Soc.Abstr.
—BLDSC (3977.043200), CISTI, ingenta.
Published by: International Nutrition Foundation, 53-70 Jingu-Mae 5-chome, Shibuya-ku, Tokyo 150-0001, Japan. TEL 81-3-3499-2828, FAX 81-3-3499-2828, TELEX J25442 UNATUNIV, unucpo@zork.tiac.net. Ed., R&P Nevin S Scrimshaw TEL 03-5467-1319. Adv. contact Marc Kaufman. Circ: 2,400. **Dist. by:** Charles St Sta Box 500, Boston, MA 02114-0500.

613.2 CHE ISSN 0275-5769
FOOD AND NUTRITION IN HISTORY AND ANTHROPOLOGY. Text in English. 1980. irreg., latest vol.13. *Refereed.* **Document type:** *Monographic series.*
Indexed: Anthropol.Lit.
—CISTI.
Published by: Gordon and Breach - Harwood Academic (Subsidiary of: Taylor & Francis Group), PO Box 531, Lausanne 1000, Switzerland. Ed. Solomon Katz. **Subscr. addr. in US:** International Publishers Direct, PO Box 32160, Newark, NJ 07102. FAX 215-750-6343.

613.2 USA
FOOD & NUTRITION NEWSLETTER. Text in English. w. **Document type:** *Newsletter.* **Description:** Provides dietary guidelines, food product information, nutrition education and other health issues.
Media: Online - full content. **Related titles:** E-mail ed.
Published by: Virginia Cooperative Extension http://www.ext.vt.edu/news/periodicals/foods.

613.2 USA
FOOD & NUTRITION RESEARCH BRIEFS. Text in English. 1995. q. back issues avail. **Document type:** *Bulletin, Government.*
Media: Online - full text.
Published by: U.S. Department of Agriculture, Agricultural Research Service, Whitten Bldg, 14th and Independence Ave, S W, Washington, DC 20250-9410. TEL 202-720-2600, jmcbride@asrr.arsusda.gov, http://www.ars.usda.gov/is/np/fnrb/.

FOOD HYGIENIC SOCIETY OF JAPAN. JOURNAL/SHOKUHIN EISEIGAKU ZASSHI. see *PUBLIC HEALTH AND SAFETY*

613.2 USA
FOOD, NEUTRACEUTICALS AND NUTRITION. Text in English. 1977. m., latest vol.25. USD 76 (effective Apr. 2001). bk.rev. charts, illus, stat. back issues avail. **Document type:** *Newsletter, Academic/Scholarly.* **Description:** Covers food, nutrition and health research, education, and policy issues.
Formerly (until Apr. 1999): Food, Nutrition & Health Newsletter (0160-8053)
Published by: Food & Nutrition Press, Inc., 6527 Main St, PO Box 374, Trumbull, CT 06611. TEL 203-261-8587, FAX 203-261-9724, foodpress@worldnetatt.net, http://www.foodscipress.com. Eds. Michele C Fisher, Paul A Lachance.

613.2 ITA ISSN 1014-806X
RA601
FOOD NUTRITION AND AGRICULTURE/ALIMENTACION NUTRICION Y AGRICULTURA/ALIMENTATION NUTRITION ET AGRICULTURE. Text in English, French, Spanish. 1974. 3/yr. free per issue. bk.rev. charts, stat, illus. cum.index. **Description:** FAO world review of food policy and nutrition. Each issue covers a specific theme, in addition to regular reports of committees and updates on food laws.
Formed by the 1991 merger of: Food and Nutrition (0304-8942); Alimentation et Nutrition (0251-1452); Alimentacion y Nutricion (0251-1428); Supersedes: Nutrition Newsletter (0428-9447)
Related titles: Online - full text ed.: (from Gale Group).
Indexed: Abstr.Hyg., Biol.& Agr.Ind. (coverage dropped), Curr.Adv.Ecol.Sci., Dairy Sci.Abstr., Diar.Dis.Res., Documentatieblad, Field Crop Abstr., Food Sci.& Tech.Abstr., Herb.Abstr., IIS, Ind.Med. (coverage dropped), Mag.Ind., Maize Abstr., Nutr.Abstr., Postharvest, Poult.Abstr., Rural Devel.Abstr., Rural Recreat.Tour.Abstr., Russ.Acad.Sci.Bibl., Trop.Dis.Bull., World Ag.Econ.& Rur.Soc.Abstr.
—BLDSC (3981.304500), CISTI, GNLM, Infotrieve, ingenta, Linda Hall. **CCC.**
Published by: Food and Agriculture Organization of the United Nations (Rome), Sales and Marketing Group, Viale delle Terme di Caracalla, Rome 00100, Italy. TEL 39-06-57054350, FAX 39-06-57053360, publications-sales@fao.org. Ed. Kim Atkinson. Circ: 10,000.

664 USA ISSN 1046-705X
TX543 CODEN: FSTUE2
FOOD STRUCTURE. Text in English. 1982. q. USD 100; USD 120 foreign. bk.rev. illus. cum.index. back issues avail. *Refereed.* **Document type:** *Academic/Scholarly.* **Description:** Covers the structure of foods and feeds with special emphasis on the relation between processing, molecular properties, microstructure and macroscopic behavior.
Formerly (until vol.8, no.2, 1989): Food Microstructure (0730-5419)
Indexed: ASCA, Biol.Abstr., Chem.Abstr., Chem.Indus.Notes, Chem.Titles, Curr.Adv.Ecol.Sci., Curr.Cont. (coverage dropped), Dairy Sci.Abstr., Food Sci.& Tech.Abstr., Ind.Sci.Rev., SSCI (coverage dropped), Sci.Cit.Ind. (coverage dropped).
—CASDDS, CISTI, IDS, Infotrieve, ingenta, Linda Hall. **CCC.**
Published by: Scanning Microscopy International, Inc., AMF O Hare, PO Box 66507, Chicago, IL 60666-0507. TEL 312-529-6677, FAX 312-980-6698. Ed. Om Johari. Circ: 300.

613.2 ESP
FORMACION CONTINUADA EN NUTRICION Y OBESIDAD. Text in Spanish. bi-m. **Document type:** *Academic/Scholarly.*
Published by: (Sociedad Espanola de Nutricion Basica y Aplicada), Ediciones Doyma S.A., Traversa de Gracia, 17-21, Barcelona 08021, Spain. TEL 34-93-200-0711, FAX 34-93-209-1136, comercial@doymanet.es, http://www.doyma.es/, http://www.doyma.es/. Ed. Carlos Herrera. adv.: page ESP 259,000; trim 280 x 210. Circ: 4,000. **Co-sponsor:** Sociedad Espanola para el Estudio de la Obesidad.

N

613.2 CHE ISSN 1660-0347
TX341 CODEN: BNDSA3
FORUM OF NUTRITION. Text in English. 1960. irreg., latest vol.55. CHF 200 in Europe; DEM 240 in Germany; USD 170 in United States (effective 2001). back issues avail.; reprint service avail. from ISI. *Refereed.* **Document type:** *Monographic series, Academic/Scholarly.*
Formerly: Bibliotheca Nutritio et Dieta (0067-8198)
Related titles: Online - full text ed.: (from Institute for Scientific Information).
Indexed: ASCA, Biodet.Abstr., Biol.Abstr., Chem.Abstr., Curr.Cont. (coverage dropped), Dairy Sci.Abstr., Food Sci.& Tech.Abstr., Ind.Med. (1960-), Nutr.Abstr.
—BLDSC (2019.200000), CASDDS, CISTI, GNLM, KNAW. **CCC.**
Published by: S. Karger AG, Allschwilerstr 10, PO Box, Basel 4009, Switzerland. TEL 41-61-306-1111, FAX 41-61-306-1234, karger@karger.ch, http://www.karger.com. Eds. J C Somogyi, P Walter.

FRISCH GEKOCHT; ist halb gewonnen. see *HOME ECONOMICS*

FRONTIERS IN FOODS AND FOOD INGREDIENTS. see *FOOD AND FOOD INDUSTRIES*

613.2 JPN ISSN 0385-5880
FUKUYAMA AKENOHOSHI GAKUIN EIYO SENMON GAKKO KENKYU KIYO/FUKUYAMA AKENOHOSHI GAKUIN SCHOOL OF DIETETICS. BULLETIN. Text in Japanese. 1973. irreg.
Published by: Fukuyama Akenohoshi Gakuin Eiyo Senmon Gakko, 4-1 Nishi-Fukatsu-cho 3-chome, Fukuyama-shi, Hiroshima-ken 721-0975, Japan.

613.2 USA ISSN 1470-0336
FUNCTIONAL FOODS AND NUTRACEUTICALS; the magazine for the global supply market. Text in English. 1998. bi-m. adv. **Document type:** *Magazine, Trade.*
Formerly (until 1999): Functional Foods (1462-0286)
Published by: New Hope Natural Media (Subsidiary of: Penton Media, Inc.), 1401 Pearl St, Boulder, CO 80302. TEL 303-939-8440, FAX 303-939-9886, sales@newhope.com, http://www.healthwell.com.

612.3 USA ISSN 0890-507X
G I G NEWSLETTER✱ . Text in English. 1974. q. USD 30 domestic; USD 40 foreign (effective 2000). bk.rev. index. back issues avail. **Document type:** *Newsletter, Academic/Scholarly.* **Description:** Contains research reports, food product and drug information, seminar-meeting announcements, activities of national and local interest, and recipes.
Published by: Gluten Intolerance Group of North America, 15110 10th Ave SW No A, Seattle, WA 98166-1820. TEL 206-246-6652, FAX 206-246-6531. Ed., R&P, Adv. contact Cynthia R Kupper. Circ: 2,000.

612.3 NCL ISSN 1022-9221
GARDEN TO KITCHEN NEWSLETTER. Text in French. 1992. s-a. **Document type:** *Newsletter.*
Published by: Secretariat of the Pacific Community, PO Box D5, Noumea Cedex 98848, New Caledonia. TEL 687-262000, FAX 687-263818, spc@spc.int, http://www.spc.int.

613.2 USA
GARLIC TIMES✱ ; the newsletter of lovers of the stinking rose. Text in English. 1976. a. USD 21 for 2 yrs.. adv. bk.rev. back issues avail. **Document type:** *Newsletter.*
Published by: (Lovers of the Stinking Rose), Harris Publishing, 1563 Solan Ave, Ste 201, Berkeley, CA 94707-2116. Ed. L John Harris. Circ: 5,000.

GATHERED VIEW; national newsletter of the Prader-Willi syndrome Assn. (USA). see *MEDICAL SCIENCES*

613.2 ITA ISSN 1122-2239
GIORNALE ITALIANO DI NUTRIZIONE CLINICA E METABOLISMO. Text in English, Italian. 1991. 3/yr. ITL 90,000, USD 100 (effective 1999). **Description:** Presents original data and discusses theoretical and practical aspects of clinical and preventive nutrition.
Former titles: Giornale Italiano di Nutrizione Clinica e Preventiva; Rivista Italiana di Nutrizione Clinica e Preventiva
Published by: Casa Editrice Idelson, Via Annibale De Gasperis, 55, Naples, NA 80137, Italy. TEL 39-81-5524733, FAX 39-81-5518295, idelgno@tin.it, http://www.idelson-gnocchi.com. Ed. Franco Contaldo.

613.2 IDN ISSN 0436-0265
GIZI INDONESIA. Text in English, Indonesian. q. IDR 1,200. adv. bk.rev. illus.
Published by: (Indonesian Nutrition Association), Akedemi Gizi, J1. Hang Jebat III/F3, Kebayoran Baru, P.O. Box 8 KBB, Jakarta, Indonesia. Ed. Ig Tarnotjo.

GOOD HEALTH MAGAZINE. see *PHYSICAL FITNESS AND HYGIENE*

GOOD LIFE TIMES; choices in health, education and the arts. see *NEW AGE PUBLICATIONS*

GOOD MEDICINE. see *PHYSICAL FITNESS AND HYGIENE*

613.2 USA
GOOD-NEWS-LETTER (WASHINGTON, 1990). Text in English. 1990. bi-m. free per issue. **Document type:** *Newsletter.* **Description:** For children ages 7-10. Contains games and puzzles that teach children about good nutrition in an entertaining manner.
Published by: American Institute for Cancer Research (AICR), 1759 R St, N W, Washington, DC 20009. TEL 202-328-7744, FAX 202-328-7226, aicrweb@aicr.org, htt://www.aicr.org. Ed. Christine Murray. R&P Susan Simolunas. Circ: 11,000.

612.3 USA
GREAT BODY. Text in English. 1989. bi-m. USD 2.95 per issue. adv. **Description:** Provides information on healthy eating and dieting, as well as work-out routines and fitness programs to improve health and stamina.
Published by: Harris Publications, Inc., 1115 Broadway, New York, NY 10010. TEL 212-807-7100. Ed. Mary Greenberg. Circ: 30,000.

613.2 USA ISSN 1097-5756
GREATLIFE✱ . Text in English. 1998. m. **Document type:** *Magazine, Consumer.*
Published by: Fairfax Publications, Inc., 320 N Larchmont Blvd, Los Angeles, CA 90004-3012. grtlife@aol.com. Ed. Lynn Prowitt-Smith.

▼ **GUSTO!.** see *HOME ECONOMICS*

613.2 615 USA
H S R: HEALTH SUPPLEMENT RETAILER. Text in English. 1995. m. USD 50 in United States; USD 75 in Canada; USD 115 elsewhere (effective 2000). adv. charts, pat, tr.lit. back issues avail. **Document type:** *Magazine, Trade.* **Description:** Serves the dietary supplement industry with news, market information, analyses, and new product information. Aimed at owners of retail stores and manufacturers.
Related titles: Online - full text ed.
Published by: Virgo Publishing, Inc., 3300 N Central Ave, Ste 2500, Phoenix, AZ 85012. TEL 480-990-1101, FAX 480-990-0819, hsrmag@vpico.com, virgopub@vpico.com, http://www.hsrmagazine.com, http://www.vpico.com. adv.: B&W page USD 2,860, color page USD 3,935; trim 7 x 10. Circ: 19,570.

613.2 SWE ISSN 0345-4797
HAELSA. Variant title: Tidskrift foer Haelsa. Text in Swedish. 1940. m. (11/yr.). SEK 365 (effective 2001). adv. bk.rev. *Refereed.* **Document type:** *Magazine, Consumer.* **Description:** Focuses on health, physical fitness, hygiene, consumer education and protection.
Former titles (until vol.10, 1971): Tidskrift Foer Haelsa; (until 1956): Waerlands Maanads-Magasin; (until vol.5, 1944): Solvikingen
Related titles: Audio cassette/tape ed.
Published by: Haelsa & Helhet Foerlags AB, Fack 33, Orsa 79421, Sweden. TEL 46-250-42423, FAX 46-250-431-91, per.frisk@health.se. Ed., Pub. Per Frisk. Adv. contact Renee Linden. color page SEK 21,900; trim 190 x 265. Circ: 44,700 (paid and controlled).

613.2 PAK ISSN 0259-3734
HAMDARD NAUNEHAL. Text in English. 1952. m. USD 30 (effective 2000). **Document type:** *Academic/Scholarly.*
Published by: Hamdard Foundation, Nazimabad No.3, Karachi 74600, Pakistan. TEL 92-21-6616001, FAX 92-21-6611755. Ed. Masood Ahmed Barakaatee.

613.2 KOR ISSN 1226-3311
HAN'GUG SIGPUM YEONG'YANG GWAHAG HOEJI/KOREAN SOCIETY OF FOOD SCIENCE AND NUTRITION. JOURNAL. Text in Korean; Summaries in English. 1972. q. KRW 30,000 elsewhere to individuals; USD 50 foreign; KRW 5,000 newsstand/cover (effective 2001). adv. 200 p./no. reprints avail. *Refereed.* **Document type:** *Journal, Academic/Scholarly.*
Formerly (until 1996): Han'gug Yeong'yang Sigryang Haghoeji/Korean Society of Food and Nutrition. Journal (0253-3154)
Media: Large Type (10 pt.). **Related titles:** CD-ROM ed.; Online - full content ed.
Indexed: Food Sci.& Tech.Abstr.
—BLDSC (4812.344700).
Published by: Korean Society of Food Science and Nutrition, 424-12 Jangjun 2-dong, Keumjung-go, Pusan 609-840, Korea, S.. TEL 82-51-512-3168, FAX 82-51-557-1428, kfn@chollian.net, http://society.kordic.re.kr/~kfn/. Eds. Kwang-Soo Oh, Mihyang Kim, Woo-Po Park, Young-Jun Cha. Pub. Eul-Sang Kim. adv.: page KRW 500,000; 210 x 280.

HEALTH AND FITNESS; all you need for life!. see *PHYSICAL FITNESS AND HYGIENE*

613.2 ZAF
HEALTH COUNTER NEWS. Text in English. 1976. m. ZAR 3.20. adv.
Address: PO Box 961, Noordwyk 1686, South Africa.

613.2 USA ISSN 1055-8241
HEALTH DIET & NUTRITION✱ . Text in English. 1991. q. USD 29.99. adv. Supplement avail. **Document type:** *Consumer.* **Description:** Covers basic nutrition information, dietary habits, and personal health care.
Published by: Publishing & Business Consultants, 4427 W Slauson Ave, Los Angeles, CA 90043-2717. TEL 213-732-3477, FAX 213-732-9123. Ed. Andeson Napoleon Atia. Circ: 120,000.

613.2 USA
HEALTH EXPRESS (LAS VEGAS)✱ . Text in English. 12/yr. USD 12. adv.
Published by: International Academy of Nutritional Consultants, 2375 Tropicana, Ste 270, Las Vegas, NV 90109. TEL 702-454-1665.

613.2 IND ISSN 0970-8685
HEALTH FOR THE MILLIONS. Text in English. 1975. bi-m. INR 150 domestic; USD 35 foreign; INR 35 newsstand/cover domestic (effective 2000). adv. bk.rev. bibl, illus. **Document type:** *Academic/Scholarly, Consumer.* **Description:** Aims to influence decision making and disseminates practical information on health policies and programs affecting the public.
Indexed: Curr.Adv.Ecol.Sci., Pub.Admin.Abstr.
Published by: Health for the Millions Trust, Voluntary Health Association of India, Tong Swasthya Bhawan, South of IIT, 40 Institutional Area, New Delhi 110 016, India. TEL 91-11-6518071, FAX 91-11-6853708, vhai@del2.vsnl.net.in. Ed. Mathew Nampudakam. Pub., R&P Alok Mukhopadhyay. Adv. contact P K Kaul. B&W page INR 6,000. Circ: 3,000.

612.3 613.7 USA
HEALTH NEWS. Text in English. fortn. free per issue. **Document type:** *Newsletter.*
Media: Online - full text.
Indexed: CINAHL.
Published by: E G W Publishing Co., 1041 Shary Circle, Concord, CA 94518. TEL 925-671-9852, FAX 510-671-0692, hstevens@egw.com, http://www.naturalland.com/hv/hnc.htm.

613.7 USA ISSN 0883-8216
RA776.5
HEALTH SCIENCE; living in harmony with nature. Text in English. 1978. bi-m. USD 25; USD 45 foreign (effective 1998). adv. bk.rev. charts, illus. cum.index: 1978-1983. back issues avail.
Former titles (until vol.8, no.2): Vegetarian Health Science (8750-1643); Health Science (0161-5874)
Published by: American Natural Hygiene Society, Inc., PO Box 30630, Tampa, FL 33630. TEL 813-855-6607. Ed. James Michael Lennon. Circ: 7,500.

HEALTHCARE NEW ORLEANS. see *PHYSICAL FITNESS AND HYGIENE*

613.2 305.896 USA ISSN 1077-5668
HEALTHQUEST; total wellness for body, mind and spirit. Text in English. 1993. bi-m. USD 12 (effective 2001). adv. bk.rev. illus. back issues avail.; reprints avail. **Document type:** *Magazine, Consumer.* **Description:** Covers holistic health and allopathic and natural medicine issues important to Black Americans and addresses mind, body, and spiritual health issues. Also covers fitness, diet, disease, public health issues, travel, self-image, and other health-related issues.
Indexed: ENW, Ind.Per.Blacks.
Published by: Levas, Inc., 200 Highpoint Dr, Ste 215, Chalfont, PA 18914. TEL 215-822-7935, FAX 215-997-9582, editor@healthquestmag.com, http://www.healthquestmag.com. Ed. Hilary Beard. R&P Sara Lomax Reese. Adv. contact Joan Horvath. Circ: 500,000.

613.2 USA ISSN 0897-9251
HEALTHWAYS. Text in English. 1987. 3/yr. USD 25 domestic; USD 30 foreign (effective 2000). bk.rev.
Document type: *Newsletter.*
Published by: International Macrobiotic Shiatsu Society, 1410 Oneco Avenue, Winter Park, FL 32789. TEL 707-444-8620, FAX 707-445-2391. Ed. Patrick McCarty. Circ: 600.

613.4 GBR
HEALTHY EATING. Text in English. 1990. m. GBP 25; GBP 2.50 newsstand/cover (effective 1999). adv.
Document type: *Consumer.* **Description:** Articles on food, health and fitness, eating for health, recipes, food allergy and intolerance, vitamins and supplements.
Published by: Market Link Publishing plc, The Mill, Bearwalden Business Park, Wendens Ambro, Saffron Walden, Saffron Walden, Essex CB11 4JX, United Kingdom. TEL 44-1799-544200, FAX 44-1799-544202. Ed. Cathering Custace. Pub. Charlotte House. **Dist. by:** Seymour, 86 Newman St, London W1P 3EX, United Kingdom. TEL 44-20-7396-8000, FAX 44-207-396-8002.

613.2 USA
HEALTHY HOME COOKIN' NEWSLETTER. Text in English. w. free per issue. **Document type:** *Newsletter.*
Media: Online - full text. **Related titles:** E-mail ed.
Published by: Greg Landry, Ed. & Pub., 2805 Newkirk Ave, Wilmington, NC 28412. greg@landry.com, http://www.landry.com.

HEALTHY TIMES (NORTH BERGEN). see *PHYSICAL FITNESS AND HYGIENE*

613.2 CAN ISSN 1075-0169
CODEN: HWJOFJ
HEALTHY WEIGHT JOURNAL; research, news and commentary across the weight spectrum. Text in English. 1986. bi-m. USD 65 in US & Canada to individuals; USD 85 elsewhere to individuals; USD 99 in US & Canada to individuals; USD 135 elsewhere to individuals (effective 2001). adv. bk.rev. abstr. index. back issues avail. **Document type:** *Journal, Academic/Scholarly.* **Description:** Reports research and information on weight including causes, prevalence, treatment, prevention, health risks of obesity and eating disorders, impact on individuals, social and political issues and the weight loss industry.
Former titles (until 1994): Obesity and Health (1044-1522); (until 1989): International Obesity Newsletter (0893-2204); Obesity Newsletter (0891-4028)
Related titles: Online - full text ed.: (from ProQuest Information & Learning, Factiva).
Indexed: Agricola, C.I.J.E. (coverage dropped), Consum.Ind. (1989-), Environ.Sci.Poll.Mgmt., NRN, Nurs.Abstr., Pollut.Abstr., Risk Abstr., Saf.Sci.Abstr., Soc.Work Res.& Abstr.
—Infotrieve. **CCC.**
Published by: B.C. Decker Inc., 20 Hughson St S, LCD 1, P O Box 620, Hamilton, ON L8N 3K7, Canada. TEL 905-522-7017, 800-568-7281, FAX 905-522-7839, info@bcdecker.com, http://www.bcdecker.com. Ed. Frances M Berg. Pub. David LeGallais. R&P Paula Presutti. Adv. contact John Birkby. Circ: 1,600.

HERE'S HEALTH; a monthly guide to health, nutrition, natural food and natural therapy. see *PHYSICAL FITNESS AND HYGIENE*

613.25 JPN
HIMAN CHIRYO KENKYUKAI KOENSHU/JAPANESE SOCIETY FOR OBESITY THERAPY. PROCEEDINGS. Text in Japanese. a.
Published by: Himan Chiryo Kenkyukai, Daigaku Igakubu Dai 2 Geka, 8-1 Inohana 1-chome, Chuo-ku, Chiba-shi 260-0856, Japan.

613.2 JPN ISSN 0289-5137
CODEN: HBSKE6
HIROSHIMA BUNKYO SHOKUMOTSU EIYO KENKYUKAISHI/HIROSHIMA BUNKYO WOMEN'S COLLEGE. SOCIETY FOR FOOD NUTRITION. JOURNAL. Text in Japanese. 1983. a.
—KNAW.
Published by: Hiroshima Bunkyo Shokumotsu, Eiyo Kenkyukai, Hiroshima Bunkyo Joshi Daigaku Tanki Daigakubu, 2-1 Kabe-Higashi 1-chome, Asakita-ku, Hiroshima-shi 731-0222, Japan.

613.2 USA ISSN 0886-6848
QP141.A1 CODEN: HNUTEP
HUMAN NUTRITION. Text in English. 1979. irreg., latest vol.8, 1993. price varies. back issues avail. *Refereed.*
Document type: *Monographic series.*
Indexed: AgeLine.
—CISTI.
Published by: Kluwer Academic - Plenum Publishers (Subsidiary of: Wolters Kluwer N.V.), 233 Spring St, New York, NY 10013-1578. TEL 212-620-8468, 800-221-9369, FAX 212-463-0742, TELEX 23-421139, info@plenum.com, http://www.plenum.com. Eds. David Kritchev, Roslyn B Alfin Slater.

HUNGER NOTES. see *SOCIAL SERVICES AND WELFARE*

HYGIENE AND NUTRITION IN FOOD SERVICE AND CATERING; an international journal. see *FOOD AND FOOD INDUSTRIES*

616.39 USA ISSN 0936-4072
I L S I HUMAN NUTRITION REVIEWS. Text in English. 1986. irreg., latest 1989. price varies. reprint service avail. from ISI. **Document type:** *Academic/Scholarly.*
Published by: Springer-Verlag, Journals (Subsidiary of: BertelsmannSpringer), 175 Fifth Ave, New York, NY 10010. TEL 212-460-1500, FAX 212-473-6272.

613.2 DEU
I L S I MONOGRAPH. Text in German. irreg., latest 1993.
Document type: *Monographic series.*
Published by: (International Life Sciences Institute), Springer-Verlag (Subsidiary of: BertelsmannSpringer), Haber Str 7, Heidelberg 69126, Germany. FAX 49-30-82787448, subscriptions@springer.de, http://www.springer.de, http://link.springer-ny.com. **Subscr. in N. America to:** Meadowlands Pkwy., Secaucus, NJ 07094. TEL 212-460-1500.

613.2 IND ISSN 0022-3174
TX341 CODEN: IJNDAN
INDIAN JOURNAL OF NUTRITION AND DIETETICS. Text in English. 1964. m. INR 150, USD 60 (effective 2001). adv. bk.rev. bibl, charts, stat. index. *Refereed.*
Document type: *Academic/Scholarly.* **Description:** Research papers and review articles in the fields of nutrition and dietetics.
Formerly (until vol.7, 1970): Journal of Nutrition and Dietetics
Related titles: CD-ROM ed.
Indexed: Abstr.Hyg., Biol.Abstr., Chem.Abstr., Curr.Cont. (coverage dropped), Dairy Sci.Abstr., Diar.Dis.Res., ExtraMED, Field Crop Abstr., Food Sci.& Tech.Abstr., Helminthol.Abstr., Hort.Abstr., INIS Atomind., Maize Abstr., Nutr.Abstr., Plant Breed.Abstr., Postharvest, Poult.Abstr., Rev.Appl.Entomol., Rev.Arom.& Med.Plants, Rev.Med.& Vet.Mycol., Rice Abstr., Seed Abstr., Sorghum & Millets Abstr., Soyabean Abstr., Sugar Ind.Abstr., Triticale Abstr., Trop.Dis.Bull., Trop.Oil Seeds Abstr.
—CASDDS, CISTI, GNLM, ingenta, Linda Hall.
Published by: (Avinashilingam Institute for Home Science and Higher Education for Women), Scientific Publishers, 5-A New Pali Rd., P O Box 91, Jodhpur, Rajasthan 342 001, India. TEL 91-291-433323, FAX 91-291-512580, scienti@sancharnet.in, http://www.scientificpub.com.

613.2 GBR ISSN 1464-0074
INGREDIENTS, HEALTH & NUTRITION. Text in English. 1998. q. GBP 150 (effective 1999). **Document type:** *Trade.*
—BLDSC (4513.304550).
Published by: Turret R A I plc, Armstrong House, 38 Market Sq, Uxbridge, Middx UB8 1TG, United Kingdom. TEL 44-1895-454545, FAX 44-1895-454647, agrifood@turret-rai.co.uk, http://www.turret-rai.com. Ed. Rajiv Desai.

613.2 GBR ISSN 1369-8664
INSIDE STORY; on food and health. Text in English. 1992. m. GBP 29.95 domestic; GBP 45 foreign (effective 2000). adv.
Formerly (1992-1997): Berrydales Special Diet News (1363-2426)
Published by: Berrydales Books, 5 Lawn Road, London NW3 2XS, United Kingdom. TEL 44-20-7722-2866, FAX 44-20-7722-7685, berrydales@compuserve.com. Ed., Pub. Michelle Berriedale-Johnson. adv.: page GBP 2,135. Circ: 24,000.

613.2 GTM ISSN 0533-4179
INSTITUTO DE NUTRICION DE CENTRO AMERICA Y PANAMA (INCAP). INFORME ANUAL. Text in English. 1950. a. per issue exchange basis.
Related titles: Spanish ed.
Indexed: Biol.Abstr., Nutr.Abstr.
Published by: Institute of Nutrition of Central America and Panama (INCAP)/Instituto de Nutricion de Centro America y Panama, Carretera ROOSEVELT ZONA, 11, Apartado Postal 1188, Guatemala City 01901, Guatemala. TEL 723762, FAX 715658, TELEX 5696 INCAP GU, delgado@uclvmz. Ed. Carlos Cipriani. Circ: 1,100.

N

INSTITUTO DE TECNOLOGIA DE ALIMENTOS. INSTRUCOES PRATICAS. see *FOOD AND FOOD INDUSTRIES*

INSTITUTO DE TECNOLOGIA DE ALIMENTOS. INSTRUCOES TECNICAS. see *FOOD AND FOOD INDUSTRIES*

613.2 NER ISSN 0534-4700
INTER-AFRICAN CONFERENCE ON FOOD AND NUTRITION. PROGRAMA E INFORMACOES*. Text in English, French, Portuguese. irreg. **Document type:** *Proceedings.*
Published by: (Commission for Technical Co-Operation in Africa South of the Sahara), Maison de l'Afrique, BP 878, Niamey, Niger.

613.2 NER ISSN 0538-2785
INTER-AFRICAN CONFERENCE ON FOOD AND NUTRITION. REPORT*. Text in Niger-Congo. 1949. irreg. **Document type:** *Proceedings.*
Published by: (Commission for Technical Co-Operation in Africa South of the Sahara), Maison de l'Afrique, BP 878, Niamey, Niger.

613.2 AUS ISSN 0813-9008
CODEN: ICNRDJ
INTERNATIONAL CLINICAL NUTRITION REVIEW. Text in English. 1981. q. AUD 59 domestic; AUD 69 in Australia & New Zealand; AUD 79 elsewhere (effective 1999). bk.rev. **Document type:** *Academic/Scholarly.*
Description: Reports recent nutritional research from journals worldwide with original articles emphasizing potential clinical applications.
Incorporates: Orthomolecular Review (0725-7090)
Indexed: Chem.Abstr., Curr.Adv.Ecol.Sci., Dairy Sci.Abstr., NRN, Nutr.Abstr.
—BLDSC (4538.673500), CASDDS, CISTI, GNLM, Infotrieve. **CCC.**
Published by: Integrated Therapies Pty. Ltd., PO Box 370, Manly, NSW 2095, Australia. TEL 61-2-9977-0771, FAX 61-2-9977-0267. Ed. Robert A Buist. Circ: 2,000.

INTERNATIONAL JOURNAL FOR VITAMIN AND NUTRITION RESEARCH. see *PHARMACY AND PHARMACOLOGY*

INTERNATIONAL JOURNAL OF ALTERNATIVE & COMPLEMENTARY MEDICINE. see *ALTERNATIVE MEDICINE*

156 USA ISSN 1044-811X
BF1 CODEN: IJMREU
INTERNATIONAL JOURNAL OF BIOSOCIAL AND MEDICAL RESEARCH; bridging the gap between the natural and social sciences to better understand human behavior. Text in English. 1979. s-a. USD 25 domestic to individuals; USD 50 foreign to individuals; USD 50 to institutions. adv. bk.rev. back issues avail. *Refereed.*
Description: Publishes studies on behavior as it relates to nutrition, neurotoxicology and environmental health.
Formerly (until 1989): International Journal for Biosocial Research (0731-9169)
Indexed: Excerp.Med., Food Sci.& Tech.Abstr., Lang.& Lang.Behav.Abstr., Neurosci.Abstr. (coverage dropped), Nutr.Abstr., Psychol.Abstr., SOPODA, Sociol.Abstr., e-psyche.
—GNLM, Infotrieve, ingenta. **CCC.**
Published by: (Foundation for Biosocial Research), Life Sciences Press, PO Box 1174, Tacoma, WA 98401-1174. TEL 253-922-0448, FAX 253-922-0479. Ed. Alexander G Schauss. Circ: 3,500.

N

616.39 616.852 155.633 USA ISSN 0276-3478
RC552.A72 CODEN: INDIDJ

INTERNATIONAL JOURNAL OF EATING DISORDERS. Text in English. 1981. 8/yr. USD 1,215 in United States; USD 1,295 in Canada & Mexico; USD 1,363 elsewhere; USD 1,276 combined subscription in United States for print and online eds.; USD 1,356 combined subscription in Canada & Mexico for print and online eds.; USD 1,424 combined subscription elsewhere for print and online eds. (effective 2002). adv. bk.rev. bibl, stat. Cum. Index. back issues avail.; reprint service avail. from PSC,SCH. *Refereed.* **Document type:** *Academic/Scholarly.* **Description:** Publishes basic research, clinical and theoretical articles of scholarly substance on a variety of aspects of anorexia nervosa, bulimia, obesity and other atypical patterns of eating behavior and body weight regulation.

Related titles: Microform ed.: (from PQC); Online - full text ed.: ISSN 1098-108X. 1996. USD 1,215 in United States; USD 1,215 in Canada & Mexico; USD 1,215 elsewhere (effective 2002) (from EBSCO Publishing, Gale Group, Wiley InterScience, Institute for Scientific Information).

Indexed: ASCA, Abstr.Anthropol., Adol.Ment.Hlth.Abstr., AgeLine, Agricola, Biol.Abstr., CINAHL, Curr.Adv.Ecol.Sci., Curr.Cont., Dairy Sci.Abstr., ERA, Environ.Sci.Poll.Mgmt., Excerp.Med., Fam.Ind., Food Sci.& Tech.Abstr., Ind.Med. (1981-), Inpharma, Jrnl.Watch Psych., Mult.Ed.Abstr., NRN, Nutr.Abstr., Pharm.&Out.News, Pollut.Abstr., PsycInfo, Psychol.Abstr. (1981-), Reac., Risk Abstr., SSCI, Saf.Sci.Abstr., Soc.Sci.Ind. (Jan.1994-), Sp.Ed.Needs Abstr., Stud.Wom.Abstr., THA, e-psyche.

—BLDSC (4542.195500), CISTI, EMDOCS, GNLM, IDS, ingenta, KNAW. **CCC.**

Published by: John Wiley & Sons, Inc., Journals (Subsidiary of: Wiley InterScience), 605 Third Ave, New York, NY 10158. TEL 212-850-6645, FAX 212-850-6021, subinfo@wiley.com, uscs-wis@wiley.com, http://www.wiley.com. Ed. Dr. Michael Strober. adv.: B&W page GBP 640, color page GBP 1,515; trim 178 x 254. Circ: 1,200. **Subscr. outside the Americas to:** John Wiley & Sons Ltd., Baffins Ln, Chichester, Sussex PO19 IUD, United Kingdom. TEL 44-1243-779777, FAX 44-1243-843232, cs-journals@wiley.co.uk, http://www.wiley.co.uk.

612.3 GBR ISSN 0963-7486
CODEN: IJFNEH

INTERNATIONAL JOURNAL OF FOOD SCIENCES AND NUTRITION. Text in English. 1973. 6/yr. GBP 167, USD 274 to individuals; GBP 405, USD 670 to institutions (effective 2002). back issues avail. *Refereed.* **Document type:** *Academic/Scholarly.* **Description:** Analyzes the common elements of food science and nutrition. Examines biotechnological, nutritional, and physiological issues.

Former titles: Food Sciences and Nutrition (0954-3465); Human Nutrition. Food Sciences and Nutrition (0952-8954); Journal of Plant Foods (0142-968X); Plant Foods for Man (0306-2686)

Related titles: Online - full text ed.: ISSN 1465-3478 (from CatchWord Ltd., EBSCO Publishing, O C L C Online Computer Library Center, Inc., RoweCom Information Quest, ProQuest Information & Learning, Gale Group, Swets Blackwell, Factiva, Institute for Scientific Information).

Indexed: AMED, ASCA, Abstr.Hyg., Agricola, Agroforest.Abstr., Anim.Breed.Abstr., Chem.Abstr., Chem.Indus.Notes, Chem.Titles, Crop Physiol.Abstr., Curr.Cont., Curr.Pack.Abstr., Dairy Sci.Abstr., Diar.Dis.Res., Excerp.Med. (1996-), Field Crop Abstr., Food Sci.& Tech.Abstr., Forest Prod.Abstr., Forest.Abstr., Gen.Sci.Ind. (Jan.1992-), Helminthol.Abstr., Hort.Abstr., Ind.Med. (1992-), Int.Abstr.Biol.Sci., Int.Packag.Abstr., Maize Abstr., Nutr.Abstr., Plant Breed.Abstr., Postharvest, Potato Abstr., Ref.Zh., Rev.Appl.Entomol., Rev.Arom.& Med.Plants, Rev.Med.& Vet.Mycol., Rice Abstr., Rural Devel.Abstr., Seed Abstr., Soyabean Abstr., Sugar Ind.Abstr., Triticale Abstr., Trop.Dis.Bull.

—BLDSC (4542.254000), CASDDS, CatchWord, CISTI, GNLM, IDS, ingenta. **CCC.**

Published by: Carfax Publishing Limited (Subsidiary of: Taylor & Francis Group), PO Box 25, Abingdon, Oxon OX14 3UE, United Kingdom. TEL 44-1235-401000, FAX 44-1235-401550, enquiries@carfax.co.uk, enquiry@tandf.co.uk, http://www.carfax.co.uk. Ed. C J K Henry. Circ: 1,000 (controlled).

613.25 GBR ISSN 0307-0565
RC628 CODEN: IJOBDP

INTERNATIONAL JOURNAL OF OBESITY. Text in English. 1977. m. GBP 170 in Europe to individuals; GBP 185, USD 290 elsewhere to individuals; GBP 375 in Europe to institutions; GBP 385 elsewhere to institutional members; USD 604 elsewhere to institutions; GBP 187 in Europe to individuals Print & Online eds.; GBP 203, USD 319 elsewhere to individuals Print & Online eds.; GBP 413 in Europe to institutions Print & Online eds.; GBP 440, USD 691 elsewhere to institutions Print & Online eds. (effective 2000). adv. bk.rev. cum.index. back issues avail. *Refereed.* **Document type:** *Academic/Scholarly.* **Description:** Reports about animal and human studies in the areas of basic, clinical and applied biochemistry, physiology, and genetics together with the molecular, metabolic, psychological and epidemiological aspects of obesity and related disorders.

Related titles: Online - full text ed.: (from EBSCO Publishing, O C L C Online Computer Library Center, Inc., RoweCom Information Quest, ingenta, Swets Blackwell, Institute for Scientific Information).

Indexed: Abstr.Hyg., Agricola, Anim.Breed.Abstr., Chem.Abstr., Chem.Indus.Notes, Chem.Titles, Curr.Adv.Ecol.Sci., Curr.Cont., Dairy Sci.Abstr., Dent.Ind., Environ.Sci.Poll.Mgmt., Excerp.Med., Fam.Ind., Food Sci.& Tech.Abstr., Ind.Med. (1992-), Ind.Sci.Rev., Inpharma, Int.Abstr.Biol.Sci., NRN, Neurosci.Cit.Ind., Nutr.Abstr., Pharm.&Out.News, Pollut.Abstr., Poult.Abstr., Reac., Ref.Zh., Risk Abstr., Rural Recreat.Tour.Abstr., SSCI (coverage dropped), Saf.Sci.Abstr., Sci.Cit.Ind., Soyabean Abstr., Sugar Ind.Abstr., THA, Trop.Dis.Bull.

—BLDSC (4542.410000), ADONIS, CASDDS, CISTI, EMDOCS, GNLM, IDS, ingenta, KNAW. **CCC.**

Published by: (International Association for the Study of Obesity), Nature Publishing Group Specialist Journals (Subsidiary of: Holtzbrink Publishers), Houndmills, Basingstoke, Hants RG21 6XS, United Kingdom. TEL 44-1256-329242, FAX 44-1256-328339, c.morton@stockton-press.co.uk, subscriptions@nature.com, http://www.stockton-press.co.uk, http://www.nature.com. Eds. Ian Macdonald, Jean-Pierre Despres. Pub. Sue Deeley. R&P Pat Blowers. Adv. contact Robert Sloan TEL 44-20-8882-7199. B&W page GBP 595, color page GBP 1,150; trim 210 x 297.

613.2 USA
RC1235 CODEN: ISNUE5

INTERNATIONAL JOURNAL OF SPORT NUTRITION & EXERCISE METABOLISM. Short title: I J S N. Text in English. 1991. q. USD 42 to individuals; USD 126 to institutions; USD 30 to students (effective 2001). adv. bk.rev. abstr, bibl, charts, stat, illus. index. back issues avail.; reprint service avail. from PSC. *Refereed.* **Document type:** *Journal, Academic/Scholarly.* **Description:** Advances understanding of nutritional aspects of human physical and athletic performance.

Formerly: International Journal of Sport Nutrition (1050-1606)

Related titles: Online - full text ed.: (from Gale Group, Institute for Scientific Information).

Indexed: ASCA, Agricola, CINAHL, Chem.Abstr., Chem.Indus.Notes, Chem.Titles, Curr.Cont., Dairy Sci.Abstr., Excerp.Med. (1995-), Focus on: Sports Sci.& Med., Gen.Sci.Ind. (Mar.2000-), IBZ, Ind.Med. (1993-, dropped), Inpharma, Int.Abstr.Biol.Sci., Nutr.Abstr., Phys.Ed.Ind., Reac., Ref.Zh., Rural Recreat.Tour.Abstr., Sportsearch.

—BLDSC (4542.680800), CASDDS, GNLM, IDS, Infotrieve, ingenta, KNAW. **CCC.**

Published by: Human Kinetics Publishers, Inc., PO Box 5076, Champaign, IL 61825-5076. TEL 217-351-5076, 800-747-4457, FAX 217-351-2674, http://www.humankinetics.com/products/journals/journal.cfm?id=IJSNEM. Ed. Priscilla M Clarkson. Pub. Rainer Martens. R&P Cheri Banks TEL 217-351-5076 ext 2275. Circ: 1,228 (paid).

INTERNATIONAL SEMINARS IN PAEDIATRIC GASTROENTEROLOGY AND NUTRITION. see *MEDICAL SCIENCES—Gastroenterology*

615.9 GBR

ISSUES IN NUTRITION AND TOXICOLOGY SERIES. Text in English. 1994 (no.2). irreg. price varies. **Document type:** *Monographic series.*

Published by: Chapman & Hall Ltd. (Subsidiary of: International Thomson Publishing Group), Journals Department, Chapman & Hall, 2-6 Boundary Row, London SE1 8HN, United Kingdom. TEL 44-20-75860066, FAX 44-20-7522-9623.

613.2 JPN ISSN 0388-127X

J P E N: JAPANESE JOURNAL OF PARENTERAL AND ENTERAL NUTRITION/YUEKI EIYO JANARU. Text in Japanese. 1979. m. JPY 24,000. adv. *Refereed.* **Document type:** *Academic/Scholarly.*

Indexed: CINAHL, Int.Nurs.Ind.

Published by: Medikaru Koa/Medical Core Co., Ltd., 8-1 Haccho-Bori 3-chome, Chuo-ku, Tokyo 104-0032, Japan. TEL 81-3-3553-7741, FAX 81-3-3553-7745, medical@mail5.alpha-net.ne.jp, http://www.alpha-net.ne.jp/users2/medical. Ed., Adv. contact Sansetsu Hyashi. Pub. Sansetsu Hayashi. Circ: 3,000 (paid); (controlled).

613.2 JPN ISSN 0485-1412
CODEN: RNEYAW

JAPANESE JOURNAL OF CLINICAL NUTRITION/ RINSHO EIYO. Text in Japanese. 1952. m. JPY 930 per issue. adv. bk.rev. charts, illus.

Indexed: Chem.Abstr.

—CASDDS, CISTI.

Published by: Ishiyaku Publishers Inc., 7-10 Honkomagome 1-chome, Bunkyo-ku, Tokyo 113-0021, Japan. Ed. Hiroshi Miura. Circ: 16,500.

613.2 JPN ISSN 0021-5147
RA784 CODEN: EYGZAD

JAPANESE JOURNAL OF NUTRITION/EIYOGAKU ZASSHI. Text in Japanese. 1941. bi-m. JPY 5,670 (effective 1999). adv. bk.rev. **Document type:** *Academic/Scholarly.*

Indexed: Biol.Abstr., Chem.Abstr., Chem.Indus.Notes, Chem.Titles, Dairy Sci.Abstr., Field Crop Abstr., Food Sci.& Tech.Abstr., INIS Atomind., Maize Abstr., Nutr.Abstr., Rice Abstr., Seed Abstr., Soyabean Abstr.

—BLDSC (4656.750000), CASDDS, CISTI, ingenta, Linda Hall.

Published by: (Japan Dietetics Society), Daiichi Shuppan K.K., 1-39 Kanda-Jinbo-cho, Chiyoda-ku, Tokyo 101-0051, Japan. TEL 81-3-3291-4576, FAX 81-3-3291-4579. Ed. Shuhei Kobayashi. **Subscr. to:** Japan Publications Trading Co. Ltd., Tokyo International, PO Box 5030, Tokyo 100-31, Japan.

613.2 JPN ISSN 0287-3516
RM214 CODEN: NESGDC

JAPANESE SOCIETY OF NUTRITION AND FOOD SCIENCE. JOURNAL/NIPPON EIYO SHOKURYO GAKKAISHI. Text in Japanese; Summaries in English. 1947. 6/yr. JPY 18,000 to non-members; JPY 4,200 to students; JPY 6,300 to members. adv. bk.rev. **Document type:** *Academic/Scholarly.*

Formerly: Food and Nutrition - Eiyo to Shokuryo (0021-5376)

Indexed: Biol.Abstr., Chem.Abstr., Chem.Indus.Notes, Chem.Titles, Dairy Sci.Abstr., Eng.Ind., Field Crop Abstr., Food Sci.& Tech.Abstr., Hort.Abstr., INIS Atomind., Maize Abstr., Nutr.Abstr., Postharvest, Rev.Arom.& Med.Plants, Rice Abstr., Seed Abstr., So.Pac.Per.Ind., Soyabean Abstr., Sugar Ind.Abstr., Triticale Abstr.

—BLDSC (4809.474000), CASDDS, CISTI, Ei, Infotrieve, ingenta, Linda Hall. **CCC.**

Published by: Japanese Society of Nutrition and Food Science/Nippon Eiyo Shokuryo Gakkai, c/o Business Center for Academic Societies Japan, 5-16-9 Honkomagome, Bunkyo-ku, Tokyo 113-0021, Japan. TEL 03-5814-5801, FAX 03-5814-5820. Ed. Yousuke Seyama. Circ: 4,300.

613.262 GBR ISSN 0021-681X

JEWISH VEGETARIAN. Text in English. 1965. q. GBP 10, USD 18 (effective 2001). adv. bk.rev. **Document type:** *Consumer.*

Published by: International Jewish Vegetarian Society, 855, Finchley Rd, London NW11 7NU, United Kingdom. TEL 44-20-8455-0692, FAX 44-20-8455-1465. Ed., R&P, Adv. contact Shirley Labelda. Circ: 8,000.

613.262 USA
TX392

JEWISH VEGETARIAN NEWSLETTER. Text in English. 1983. q. USD 12; USD 15 foreign (effective 1999). bk.rev. **Document type:** *Newsletter.* **Description:** Discusses Judaism and vegetarianism. Topics include health, ecology, world hunger, animal rights and Jewish holidays.

Formerly: Jewish Vegetarians of North America (0883-1904)

Published by: Jewish Vegetarians of North America, 6938 Reliance Rd, Federalsburg, MD 21632. TEL 410-754-5550, imossman@skipjack.bluecrab.org, http://www.orbyss.com. Ed. Eva R Mossman. R&P Israel Mossman. Circ: 600; 900 (paid); 520 (controlled).

JIANKANG BAO/HEALTH NEWS. see *PHYSICAL FITNESS AND HYGIENE*

613.2 JPN ISSN 0286-0511
CODEN: JEDKD7
JOSHI EIYO DAIGAKU KIYO/KAGAWA NUTRITION COLLEGE. JOURNAL. Text in English, Japanese. 1970. a. adv. *Refereed.* **Document type:** *Academic/Scholarly.* **Description:** Contains reviews and original papers on natural sciences, humanities and social sciences.
Indexed: Chem.Abstr., Chem.Indus.Notes, Chem.Titles, Jap.Per.Ind.
—BLDSC (4810.190000), CASDDS.
Published by: Joshi Eiyo Daigaku, 24-3 Komagome 3-chome, Toshima-ku, Tokyo 170-0003, Japan. Ed. Yoshiko Kagawa. R&P, Adv. contact Masaru Tsujimura. Circ: 900.

613.2 AUT ISSN 1563-2873
▼ **JOURNAL FUER ERNAEHRUNGSMEDIZIN**; interdisziplinaeres Organ fuer Praevention und Therapie von Krankheiten durch Ernaehrung. Text in German. 1999. q. ATS 400 (effective 2001). bk.rev. abstr, bibl. back issues avail. *Refereed.* **Document type:** *Journal, Academic/Scholarly.* **Description:** Presents an interdisciplinary forum for research into the prevention of nutritional deficiencies and diseases.
Published by: Krause & Pachernegg GmbH, Mozartgasse 10, Gablitz 3003, Austria. TEL 43-2231-61258-0, FAX 43-2231-6125810, k_u_p@eunet.at, http://members.eunet.at/k_u_p/nahr.htm, http://members.eunet.at/k_u_p/verlag.htm. Ed. Dr. Kurt Widhalm.

JOURNAL OF CLINICAL BIOCHEMICAL AND NUTRITION. see *BIOLOGY—Biochemistry*

613.26 ZAF
CODEN: TDHUDO
JOURNAL OF FAMILY ECOLOGY AND CONSUMER SCIENCE/TYDSKRIF VIR GESINEKOLOGIE EN VERBRUIKERSWETENSKAPPE. Text in Afrikaans, English. 1973. 2/yr. ZAR 45. adv. bk.rev. **Document type:** *Academic/Scholarly.*
Formerly: Journal of Dietetics and Home Economics (0378-5254)
Indexed: INIS Atomind., Ind.S.A.Per., Nutr.Abstr.
—CASDDS.
Published by: Home Economics Association of Southern Africa, PO Box 35269, Menlo Park, Pretoria 0102, South Africa. TEL 27-12-4202854, FAX 27-12-436867. Ed. E Boshoff.

613.2 KOR ISSN 1226-332X
JOURNAL OF FOOD SCIENCE AND NUTRITION. Text in English. 1996. q. KRW 30,000 domestic to individuals; USD 50 foreign to individuals; USD 100,000 domestic to libraries; KRW 5,000 newsstand/cover (effective 2001). adv. 80 p./no. reprints avail. *Refereed.* **Document type:** *Academic/Scholarly.*
Related titles: CD-ROM ed.; Online - full content ed.
—BLDSC (4984.560500).
Published by: Korean Society of Food Science and Nutrition, 424-12 Jangjun 2-dong, Keumjung-go, Pusan 609-840, Korea, S.. TEL 82-51-512-3168, FAX 82-51-557-1428, kfn@chollian.net, http://society.kordic.re.kr/~kfn/. Eds. Cherl Kim, Myung-Sook Choi, Taesum Park. Pub. Eul-Sang Kim. adv.: page KRW 500,000; 210 x 280.

612.3 USA
JOURNAL OF HEALTH SCIENCE* . Text in English. 1981. q. USD 10. adv. illus.
Indexed: AESIS, Anal.Abstr., Aqua.Sci.& Fish.Abstr., Environ.Sci.Poll.Mgmt., Mass Spectr.Bull., Microbiol.Abstr., Nutr.Abstr., Pollut.Abstr., Risk Abstr., Saf.Sci.Abstr., Sel.Water Res.Abstr., Soyabean Abstr., Tox.Abstr. (coverage dropped).
Published by: Health News Network, Inc., 6323 Saw Flower St, Portland, OR 97221-1071. Ed. Cameron Stauth.

613.2 GBR ISSN 0952-3871
CODEN: JHNDEO
JOURNAL OF HUMAN NUTRITION AND DIETETICS. Text in English. 1988. bi-m., latest vol.15, 2002. GBP 75 in Europe to individuals; USD 120 in North America to individuals; GBP 83 elsewhere to individuals; GBP 254 in Europe to institutions; USD 404 in North America to institutions; GBP 280 elsewhere to institutions (effective 2002). adv. bk.rev. abstr, bibl, illus. index. back issues avail. *Refereed.* **Document type:** *Academic/Scholarly.*
Formerly (until 1987): Human Nutrition. Applied Nutrition (0263-8495); Which superseded in part (in 1981): Journal of Human Nutrition (0308-4329); Which was formerly (until 1976): Nutrition (0029-6600)
Related titles: Microform ed.: (from PQC); Online - full text ed.: ISSN 1365-277X. GBP 68 in Europe to individuals; USD 108 in North America to individuals; GBP 68 elsewhere to individuals; GBP 229 in Europe to institutions; USD 364 in North America to institutions; GBP 229 elsewhere to institutions (effective 2002) (from Ovid Technologies, Inc., EBSCO Publishing, O C L C Online Computer Library Center, Inc., RoweCom Information Quest, ingenta, Munksgaard & Blackwell Science's Synergy, Swets Blackwell, Institute for Scientific Information).
Indexed: ASCA, Agricola, Art.Hosp.& Tour., CINAHL, Curr.Cont., Dairy Sci.Abstr., Diab.Cont., Food Sci.& Tech.Abstr., Gen.Sci.Ind. (1984-1987, dropped), Inpharma, Nutr.Abstr., Potato Abstr., Reac., SSCI (coverage dropped), Sci.Cit.Ind., Sugar Ind.Abstr., World Ag.Econ.& Rur.Soc.Abstr.
—BLDSC (5003.419300), CASDDS, CISTI, EMDOCS, GNLM, IDS, Infotrieve, ingenta, KNAW, Linda Hall. **CCC.**
Published by: (British Dietetic Association), Blackwell Science Ltd., PO Box 88, Oxford OX2 0NE, United Kingdom. TEL 44-1865-206180, 44-1865-206002, FAX 44-1865-206219, jnl.orders@blacksci.co.uk, http://www.blackwell-science.com/~cgilib/jnlpage.asp?Journal=jhnd&File=jhnd, http://www.blackwellpublishing.com. Ed. Jane Thomas. Pub. Elaine Stott. R&P Sophie Young. Adv. contact Jenny Applin. Circ: 4,325.

JOURNAL OF MUSCLE FOODS. see *FOOD AND FOOD INDUSTRIES*

JOURNAL OF NUTRACEUTICALS, FUNCTIONAL & MEDICAL FOODS; innovations in research, practice, commercialization & policy. see *PHARMACY AND PHARMACOLOGY*

613.2 USA ISSN 0022-3166
RM214 CODEN: JONUAI
JOURNAL OF NUTRITION. Text in English. 1928. m. USD 105 domestic to individuals; USD 125 foreign to individuals; USD 390 domestic to institutions; USD 410 foreign to institutions; USD 30 to students (effective 2001). adv. bk.rev. abstr, bibl, charts, illus. index. back issues avail.; reprint service avail. from PQC. *Refereed.* **Document type:** *Academic/Scholarly.* **Description:** Publishes reports of original research in all aspects of nutrition.
Related titles: Microform ed.: (from PQC,PMC); Online - full text ed.: (from HighWire Pr., Northern Light Technology, Inc., EBSCO Publishing, RoweCom Information Quest, ProQuest Information & Learning, Gale Group, Factiva, Institute for Scientific Information).
Indexed: ASCA, Abstr.Anthropol., Abstr.Hyg., AgBiotech, Agri.& Environ.Biotech.Abstr. (coverage dropped), Agricola, Anim.Breed.Abstr., Aqua.Sci.& Fish.Abstr., Behav.Med.Abstr., Biol.& Agr.Ind. (Jan.1983-), Biol.Abstr., Biol.Dig., Cadscan, Chem.Abstr., Chem.Indus.Notes, Chem.Titles, Curr.Adv.Cancer Res., Curr.Adv.Ecol.Sci., Curr.Cont., Curr.Ref.Fish Res., Dairy Sci.Abstr., Dent.Ind., Derwent Biotech.Abstr., Diar.Dis.Res., Environ.Per.Bibl., Environ.Sci.Poll.Mgmt., Excerp.Med., Food Sci.& Tech.Abstr., Gen.Sci.Ind. (Aug.1983-), Helminthol.Abstr., INIS Atomind., Ind.Med. (1928-), Ind.Sci.Rev., Ind.Vet., Inpharma, Int.Abstr.Biol.Sci., Int.Nurs.Ind., Lead Abstr., Maize Abstr., NRN, Neurosci.Cit.Ind., Nutr.Abstr., Pharm.&Out.News, Pig News & Info., Plant Breed.Abstr., Potato Abstr., Poult.Abstr., Protozool.Abstr., Reac., Rev.Appl.Entomol., Rev.Arom.& Med.Plants, Rev.Med.& Vet.Mycol., Rice Abstr., Risk Abstr., Rural Devel.Abstr., SSCI (coverage dropped), Saf.Sci.Abstr., Sci.Cit.Ind., Sorghum & Millets Abstr., Soyabean Abstr., Sport Fish.Abstr., Sugar Ind.Abstr., THA, Triticale Abstr., Trop.Dis.Bull., Trop.Oil Seeds Abstr., Vet.Bull., Wild.Rev., Zincscan, Zoo.Rec.
—BLDSC (5024.000000), CASDDS, CINDOC, CISTI, GNLM, IDS, ingenta, KNAW, Linda Hall. **CCC.**
Published by: American Institute of Nutrition, 9650 Rockville Pike, Bethesda, MD 20814. TEL 301-530-7050, FAX 301-571-1892, jnutri@uiuc.edu; orders@allenpress.com, http://www.nutrition.org. Ed. Dr. Willard Visek. Circ: 4,430. **Subscr. to:** Allen Press Inc., PO Box 1897, Lawrence, KS 66044-8897.

613.2 CAN ISSN 0022-3182
QP141.A1
JOURNAL OF NUTRITION EDUCATION. Text in English. 1969. bi-m. USD 149 in US & Canada to individuals; USD 179 elsewhere to individuals; USD 215 in US & Canada to institutions; USD 249 elsewhere to institutions (effective 2001). adv. bk.rev. index. back issues avail.; reprint service avail. from SCH,PSC. *Refereed.* **Document type:** *Academic/Scholarly.* **Description:** Designed to stimulate interest and research in applied nutritional sciences and to disseminate information to educators and others concerned about positive nutritional practices and policies.
Related titles: Online - full text ed.: (from Northern Light Technology, Inc., ProQuest Information & Learning, Gale Group, Factiva, Institute for Scientific Information).
Indexed: ASCA, AgeLine, Agricola, Art.Hosp.& Tour., Behav.Med.Abstr., C.I.J.E. (coverage dropped), CINAHL, Chic.Per.Ind., Cont.Pg.Educ., Curr.Cont., Dairy Sci.Abstr., ERA, Educ.Ind. (Jun.1983-), Educ.Tech.Abstr., Environ.Per.Bibl., Food Sci.& Tech.Abstr., Gen.Sci.Ind. (Jun.1984-), Mult.Ed.Abstr., NRN, Nutr.Abstr., Rev.Appl.Entomol., SSCI (coverage dropped), Sp.Ed.Needs Abstr., Stud.Wom.Abstr., Tech.Educ.Abstr.
—BLDSC (5024.700000), GNLM, IDS, ingenta. **CCC.**
Published by: (Society for Nutrition Education), B.C. Decker Inc., 20 Hughson St S, LCD 1, P O Box 620, Hamilton, ON L8N 3K7, Canada. TEL 905-522-7017, 800-568-7281, FAX 905-522-7839, info@bcdecker.com, http://www.bcdecker.com. Ed. Jane Voichick. Pub. David LeGallais. R&P Paula Presutti. Adv. contact John Birkby. Circ: 2,856.

JOURNAL OF NUTRITION FOR THE ELDERLY. see *GERONTOLOGY AND GERIATRICS*

JOURNAL OF NUTRITION, HEALTH AND AGING. see *MEDICAL SCIENCES—Internal Medicine*

613.2 USA ISSN 1055-1379
TX341 CODEN: JNMDFS
JOURNAL OF NUTRITION IN RECIPE & MENU DEVELOPMENT; innovations in nutritional issues for food product development. Text in English. 1994. q. USD 40 to individuals; USD 54 in Canada to individuals; USD 58 elsewhere to individuals; USD 75 to institutions; USD 101 in Canada to institutions; USD 109 elsewhere to institutions; USD 140 to libraries; USD 189 in Canada to libraries; USD 203 elsewhere to libraries (effective Aug. 2001). adv. bk.rev. reprint service avail. from HAW. *Refereed.* **Document type:** *Journal, Academic/Scholarly.* **Description:** Publishes research and practice papers relating directly to new recipe and menu concepts aimed at health promotion.
Related titles: Microfiche ed.: (from PQC); Microform ed.
Indexed: Dairy Sci.Abstr., Environ.Sci.Poll.Mgmt., Food Sci.& Tech.Abstr., Lod.Restr.& Tour.Ind., Nutr.Abstr., Per.Islam. (1993-).
—BLDSC (5024.720000), Haworth.
Published by: Haworth Hospitality Press (Subsidiary of: Haworth Press, Inc.), 10 Alice St, Binghamton, NY 13904-1580. TEL 607-722-5857, 800-429-6784, FAX 607-722-6362, 800-895-0582, getinfo@haworthpressinc.com, http://www.haworthpress.com/journals/journallist.asp. Ed. Barbara Almanza. Pub. William Cohen. R&P Ruthann Heath TEL 607-722-5857 ext 316. Adv. contact Jackie Blakeslee TEL 607-722-5857 ext 346. B&W page USD 315, color page USD 550; trim 6 x 8.5.

613.2 GBR ISSN 1359-0847
CODEN: JNEMFF
JOURNAL OF NUTRITIONAL & ENVIRONMENTAL MEDICINE. Text in English. 1990. q. GBP 143, USD 152 to individuals; GBP 531, USD 698 to institutions (effective 2002). *Refereed.* **Document type:** *Academic/Scholarly.* **Description:** Aimed at physicians, surgeons, dietitians, nutritionists, clinical biochemists, clinical psychologists, as well as students in these fields. Covers the field of nutrition and its relationship to clinical medicine.
Formerly: Journal of Nutritional Medicine (0955-6664)
Related titles: Online - full text ed.: ISSN 1364-6907 (from CatchWord Ltd., Northern Light Technology, Inc., EBSCO Publishing, O C L C Online Computer Library Center, Inc., RoweCom Information Quest, ProQuest Information & Learning, Swets Blackwell).
Indexed: AMED, Agricola, Aqua.Sci.& Fish.Abstr., CINAHL, Cal.Tiss.Abstr., Chem.Abstr., Chem.Titles, Crim.Just.Abstr., Dairy Sci.Abstr., ERA, Environ.Sci.Poll.Mgmt., Excerp.Med. (1993-), Food Sci.& Tech.Abstr., Mult.Ed.Abstr., Nutr.Abstr., Ref.Zh., Rev.Appl.Entomol., Rev.Med.& Vet.Mycol., Risk Abstr., Saf.Sci.Abstr., Stud.Wom.Abstr., Triticale Abstr., Trop.Dis.Bull.

N

—BLDSC (5024.725000), ADONIS, CASDDS, CatchWord, CISTI, EMDOCS, GNLM, Infotrieve, ingenta, KNAW. **CCC.**

Published by: Carfax Publishing Limited (Subsidiary of: Taylor & Francis Group), PO Box 25, Abingdon, Oxon OX14 3UE, United Kingdom. TEL 44-1235-401000, FAX 44-1235-401550, enquiries@carfax.co.uk, enquiry@tandf.co.uk, http://www.carfax.co.uk. Eds. Damien Downing, Stephen Davies.

612.3 USA ISSN 0955-2863
QP141.A1 CODEN: JNBIEL

JOURNAL OF NUTRITIONAL BIOCHEMISTRY. Text in English. 1970. m. EUR 188 in Europe to individuals; JPY 25,000 in Japan to individuals; USD 211 elsewhere to individuals; EUR 679 in Europe to institutions; JPY 90,200 in Japan to institutions; USD 760 elsewhere to institutions (effective 2002). adv. charts, illus. index. back issues avail.; reprints avail. *Refereed.* **Document type:** *Academic/Scholarly.* **Description:** Forum for advances and issues in nutrition, nutritional biochemistry and food sciences.

Supersedes (in 1990): Nutrition Reports International (0029-6635)

Related titles: Microfilm ed.: (from PQC); Online - full text ed.: (from ingenta, ScienceDirect, Swets Blackwell, Institute for Scientific Information).

Indexed: ASCA, AgeLine, Agricola, Anim.Breed.Abstr., BBCI, Bibl.Agri., Biol.Abstr., Cadscan, Chem.Abstr., Chem.Indus.Notes, Chem.Titles, Curr.Adv.Biochem., Curr.Adv.Ecol.Sci., Curr.Cont., Dairy Sci.Abstr., Diar.Dis.Res., Environ.Per.Bibl., Excerp.Med., Food Sci.& Tech.Abstr., Helminthol.Abstr., Herb.Abstr., Ind.Sci.Rev., Ind.Vet., Inpharma, Int.Abstr.Biol.Sci., Maize Abstr., Mass Spectr.Bull., NRN, Nutr.Abstr., Pig News & Info., Poult.Abstr., Protozool.Abstr., Reac., Rev.Arom.& Med.Plants, Rev.Med.& Vet.Mycol., Rice Abstr., Risk Abstr., Sci.Cit.Ind., Sorghum & Millets Abstr., Soyabean Abstr., Sport Fish.Abstr., Sugar Ind.Abstr., Triticale Abstr., Trop.Oil Seeds Abstr., Vet.Bull., Weed Abstr., Wild.Rev., Zincscan, Zoo.Rec.

—BLDSC (5024.730000), CASDDS, CISTI, EMDOCS, GNLM, IDS, ingenta, Linda Hall. **CCC.**

Published by: Elsevier Science, PO Box 945, New York, NY 10159-0945. TEL 212-989-5800, FAX 212-633-3990, usinfo-f@elsevier.com, http://www.elsevier.com/locate/jnutbio. Eds. C E Greenwood, Dr. Steven H Zeisel. **Subscr. in Australasia and the Far East to:** Elsevier Science (Singapore) Pte Ltd, No.1 Temasek Ave, 17-01 Millenia Tower, Singapore 039192, Singapore. TEL 65-434-3727, FAX 65-337-2230; **Subscr. in Japan to:** Elsevier Science Inc - Japan Regional Office, 9-15 Higashi-Azabu 1-chome, Minato-ku, Tokyo 106-0044, Japan. TEL 81-3-5561-5033; **Subscr. outside the Americas to:** Elsevier Science BV, PO Box 211, Amsterdam 1000 AE, Netherlands. TEL 31-20-485-3757.

613.2 JPN ISSN 0301-4800
CODEN: JNSVA5

JOURNAL OF NUTRITIONAL SCIENCE AND VITAMINOLOGY. Text in Japanese. 1954. bi-m. USD 145 (effective 1996). bk.rev. bibl, charts, illus. index. *Refereed.* **Document type:** *Academic/Scholarly.*

Formerly (until 1972): Journal of Vitaminology (0022-5398)

Related titles: Online - full text ed.: (from Institute for Scientific Information).

Indexed: ASCA, Agri.& Environ.Biotech.Abstr. (coverage dropped), Aqua.Sci.& Fish.Abstr., Biol.Abstr., Chem.Abstr., Chem.Indus.Notes, Chem.Titles, Curr.Adv.Ecol.Sci., Curr.Cont., Dairy Sci.Abstr., Derwent Biotech.Abstr., Environ.Sci.Poll.Mgmt., Excerp.Med., Field Crop Abstr., Food Sci.& Tech.Abstr., INIS Atomind., Ind.Med. (1973-), Ind.Sci.Rev., Ind.Vet., Inpharma, Int.Abstr.Biol.Sci., NRN, Nutr.Abstr., Plant Breed.Abstr., Postharvest, Poult.Abstr., Reac., Rev.Arom.& Med.Plants, Rice Abstr., Risk Abstr., Saf.Sci.Abstr., Sci.Cit.Ind., Seed Abstr., Soyabean Abstr., Sugar Ind.Abstr., Triticale Abstr., Vet.Bull.

—BLDSC (5024.750000), CASDDS, CINDOC, CISTI, EMDOCS, GNLM, IDS, ingenta, Linda Hall. **CCC.**

Published by: (Japanese Society of Nutrition and Food Science/Nippon Eiyo Shokuryo Gakkai), Center for Academic Publications Japan, 2-4-16 Yayoi, Bunkyo-ku, Tokyo 113-0032, Japan. TEL 81-3-3817-5821, FAX 81-3-3817-5830, capj@crisscross.com. Circ: 1,500. **Dist. by:** Business Center for Academic Societies Japan, 5-16-9 Honkomagome, Bunkyo-ku, Tokyo 113-0021, Japan. TEL 81-3-5814-5811. **Co-sponsor:** Vitamin Society of Japan.

612.3 USA ISSN 0148-6071
RM224 CODEN: JPENDU

JOURNAL OF PARENTERAL AND ENTERAL NUTRITION. Key Title: J P E N: Journal of Parenteral and Enteral Nutrition. Text in English. 1979. bi-m. USD 90 domestic to individuals; USD 105 in Canada & Mexico to individuals; USD 125 elsewhere to individuals; USD 151 domestic to institutions; USD 166 in Canada & Mexico to institutions; USD 186 elsewhere to institutions (effective 2001). adv. bk.rev. back issues avail.; reprint service avail. from ISI. *Refereed.* **Document type:** *Journal, Academic/Scholarly.* **Description:** Research on nutritional deficiency and its treatment, including administration, risks and complications.

Related titles: Microform ed.: (from PQC); Online - full text ed.: (from ProQuest Information & Learning, Institute for Scientific Information).

Indexed: ASCA, CINAHL, Curr.Cont., Dairy Sci.Abstr., INIS Atomind., I.P.A., Ind.Med. (1977-), Ind.Sci.Rev., Ind.Vet., Inpharma, NRN, Nutr.Abstr., Pig News & Info., Protozool.Abstr., Reac., SSCI (coverage dropped), Sci.Cit.Ind., Soyabean Abstr., Triticale Abstr., Trop.Dis.Bull.

—BLDSC (5029.100000), CASDDS, CISTI, GNLM, IDS, ingenta, KNAW. **CCC.**

Published by: American Society for Parenteral and Enteral Nutrition, 8630 Fenton St, Ste 412, Silver Spring, MD 20910-3805. TEL 301-587-6315, FAX 301-587-2365, aspen@nutr.org, http://www.nutritioncare.org. Ed. Dr. Charles Van Way. R&P Carolyn Kohagura. Adv. contact Adrian S Nickel. B&W page USD 1,325. Circ: 10,113.

612.3 USA ISSN 0277-2116
CODEN: JPGND6

JOURNAL OF PEDIATRIC GASTROENTEROLOGY AND NUTRITION. Text in English. 1982. 10/yr. USD 358 domestic to individuals; USD 358 foreign to individuals; USD 677 domestic to institutions; USD 763 foreign to institutions; USD 71 newsstand/cover (effective 2002). adv. bk.rev. charts, illus. index. back issues avail.; reprint service avail. from PQC. *Refereed.* **Document type:** *Academic/Scholarly.* **Description:** Reports of studies on nutrition, normal and abnormal functions of the alimentary tract and associated organs, with emphasis on development and its relation to infant and childhood nutrition.

Related titles: Online - full text ed.: USD 880.10 domestic for academic site license; USD 966.10 foreign for academic site license; USD 981.65 domestic for corporate site license; USD 1,067.65 foreign for corporate site license (effective 2002) (from Ovid Technologies, Inc., Institute for Scientific Information).

Indexed: ASCA, Agricola, Bibl.Agri., C.C.I.P., Chem.Abstr., Chem.Indus.Notes, Chem.Titles, Curr.Adv.Ecol.Sci., Curr.Cont., Dairy Sci.Abstr., Dent.Ind., Diar.Dis.Res., Excerp.Med., Food Sci.& Tech.Abstr., INIS Atomind., Ind.Med. (1982-), Ind.Sci.Rev., Ind.Vet., Inpharma, Int.Abstr.Biol.Sci., Jrnl.Watch Gastr., Maize Abstr., NRN, Nutr.Abstr., Pharm.&Out.News, Pig News & Info., Protozool.Abstr., Reac., Rev.Med.& Vet.Mycol., Rice Abstr., Rural Devel.Abstr., Sci.Cit.Ind., Soyabean Abstr., Sugar Ind.Abstr., Triticale Abstr.

—BLDSC (5030.175000), CASDDS, CISTI, EMDOCS, GNLM, IDS, ingenta, KNAW.

Published by: Lippincott Williams & Wilkins (Philadelphia) (Subsidiary of: Wolters Kluwer N.V.), 530 Walnut St, Philadelphia, PA 19106-3621. TEL 215-521-8300, FAX 215-521-8902, http://www.lww.com. Eds. Dr. John A Walker Smith, William Walker. Pub. Shelley Johnson. R&P Margaret Becker. Adv. contact Ray Thibodeau. B&W page USD 1,020, color page USD 2,465. Circ: 2,408 (paid). **Subscr. to:** PO Box 1600, Hagerstown, MD 21740-1600. TEL 800-777-2295, FAX 301-824-7390. **Co-sponsors:** North American Society for Pediatric Gastroenterology and Nutrition; European Society for Pediatric Gastroenterology and Nutrition.

616.39 USA ISSN 1051-2276

JOURNAL OF RENAL NUTRITION. Text in English. 1991. q. USD 106 domestic to individuals; USD 144 foreign to individuals; USD 142 domestic to institutions; USD 170 foreign to institutions; USD 63 domestic to students; USD 107 foreign to students; USD 43 newsstand/cover (effective 2001). adv. bk.rev. back issues avail. *Refereed.* **Document type:** *Journal, Academic/Scholarly.* **Description:** Official journal of the Council on Renal Nutrition of the NKF. Includes research papers related renal nutrition, as well as program updates and symposia proceedings of the NKF.

Related titles: Online - full text ed.: (from IDEAL Online Library).

Indexed: CINAHL, Ind.Med. (1991-).

—BLDSC (5049.460000), GNLM, Infotrieve. **CCC.**

Published by: (Council on Renal Nutrition, National Kidney Foundation), W.B. Saunders Co. (Subsidiary of: Harcourt Publishers Ltd.), 11830 Westline Industrial Dr, St Louis, MO 63146. TEL 800-325-4177, http://www.wbsaunders.com. Ed. Dr. Jordi Goldstein. adv.: B&W page USD 680, color page USD 1,780; trim 10 x 7. Circ: 2,143. **Subscr. to:** Periodicals Fulfillment, W B Saunders Co, 6277 Sea Harbor Dr, 4th Fl, Orlando, FL 32891-4800.

JOURNAL OF SENSORY STUDIES. see *MEDICAL SCIENCES—Psychiatry And Neurology*

JOURNEY TO HEALTH. see *PHYSICAL FITNESS AND HYGIENE*

613.262 USA

JUST EAT AN APPLE. Abbreviated title: J E A A. Text in English. bi-m. USD 30 domestic; USD 40 in Canada & Mexico; USD 45 elsewhere (effective 2001). adv. back issues avail. **Document type:** *Magazine, Consumer.* **Description:** Features articles on raw food & natural living.

Published by: Nature's First Law, PO Box 900202, San Diego, CA 92190. TEL 619-645-7282, http://www.rawfood.com, 888-729-3663, nature@rawfood.com. Ed. Frederic Patenaude.

613.2 USA

K D A COMMUNICATOR. Text in English. 1946. 6/yr. USD 25; USD 75 foreign (effective 1997). bk.rev. **Document type:** *Newsletter.* **Description:** Covers professional and educational activities of the association's members.

Formerly: Sunflower (0039-5382)

Published by: Kansas Dietetic Association, c/o Department of Hotel, Restaurant, Institution Management and Dietetics, Justin Hall 104, Kansas State University, Manhattan, KS 66103. TEL 913-532-5521, FAX 913-532-5504, cws@ksuvm.edu. Ed. Karen A Miller. Circ: 750.

613.2 DEU ISSN 0174-2469
CODEN: KLEREQ

KLINISCHE ERNAEHRUNG. Text in German. 1980. irreg., latest vol.38, 1994. **Document type:** *Academic/Scholarly.*

Indexed: Chem.Abstr., Chem.Titles.

—BLDSC (5099.366000), CASDDS, CISTI.

Published by: W. Zuckschwerdt Verlag GmbH, Industriestr 1, Germering 82110, Germany. TEL 49-89-894349-0, FAX 49-89-89434950.

613.2 JPN ISSN 0911-565X

KOBE GAKUIN DAIGAKU EIYOGAKUBU RONBUNSHU/KOBE GAKUIN UNIVERSITY. FACULTY OF NUTRITION. JOURNAL. Text in English, German, Japanese; Summaries in English. 1969. a.

Published by: Kobe Gakuin Daigaku, Eiyogakubu, 518 Ikawadanichoarise, Nishi-ku, Kobe-shi, Hyogo-ken 651-2113, Japan.

613.2 JPN

KOKUMIN EIYO NO GENJO/REPORT OF NATIONAL NUTRITIVE CONDITIONS. Text in Japanese. 1947. s-a. JPY 2,575 (effective 1999). **Document type:** *Government.*

Published by: (Japan. Koseisho, Japan. Hoken Iryokyoku), Daiichi Shuppan K.K., 1-39 Kanda-Jinbo-cho, Chiyoda-ku, Tokyo 101-0051, Japan. TEL 81-3-3291-4567, FAX 81-3-3291-4579.

612.3 JPN ISSN 0368-5209
TX341

KOKURITSU KENKO EIYO KENKYUJO HOKOKU/NATIONAL INSTITUTE OF HEALTH AND NUTRITION. ANNUAL REPORT. Text in Japanese; Summaries in English. 1949. a. per issue exchange basis. **Document type:** *Government.*

Formerly: Kokuritsu Eiyo Kenkyujo Hokoku - National Institute of Nutrition. Annual Report

Indexed: Biol.Abstr., Nutr.Abstr.

—BLDSC (1364.711000), CISTI, GNLM, Linda Hall.

Published by: Kosei-sho, Kokuritsu Kenko Eiyo Kenkyujo/National Institute of Health and Nutrition, 1-23-1 Toyama-cho, Shinjuku-ku, Tokyo 162-8636, Japan. TEL 81-3-3203-5721, FAX 81-3-3202-3278. Ed. S. Kobayashi. R&P S Kobayashi.

613.2 JPN ISSN 0913-5537
CODEN: KDKAEH

KOSHIEN DAIGAKU KIYO. A, EIYOGAKUBU HEN/KOSHIEN UNIVERSITY. FACULTY OF NUTRITION. BULLETIN. Text in Japanese; Summaries in English, Japanese. 1970. a.

Published by: Koshien Daigaku, 10-1 Momijigaoka, Takarazuka-shi, Hyogo-ken 665-0006, Japan. TEL 0797-87-5111. Ed. Hiroyuki Masutani. Circ: 500.

KRAUT UND RUEBEN; biologisches Gaertnern und naturgemaesses Leben. see *GARDENING AND HORTICULTURE*

KUCHNIA; magazyn dla smakoszy. see *HOME ECONOMICS*

LET'S LIVE; America's foremost health & preventive medicine magazine. see *PHYSICAL FITNESS AND HYGIENE*

613.26 NLD ISSN 1567-3502
LEVEN. Text in Dutch. bi-m. NLG 39.50 (effective 2000). adv. bk.rev. *Refereed.* **Document type:** *Magazine, Consumer.* **Description:** Covers topics relating to vegetarianism, nutrition, animal welfare and related matters.
Former titles (until 2000): Leven en Laten Leven (0166-0802); (until 1971): Vegetische Bode
Published by: Nederlandse Vegetariersbond, Larenseweg 26, Hilversum 1221 CM, Netherlands. TEL 31-35-6834796, FAX 31-35-6836152. Ed. Hans van Boven. Circ: 10,000 (paid and controlled).

LIFE FORCE NEWS. see *LIFESTYLE*

613.2 USA
LIFELINELETTER. Text in English. 1977. bi-m. USD 35 (effective 2000). bk.rev. back issues avail. **Document type:** *Newsletter.* **Description:** Provides support, education and information on research in the field of home parenteral or enteral nutrition.
Published by: Oley Foundation for Home Parenteral & Enteral Nutrition, 214 Hun Memorial A 28, Albany Medical Center, Albany, NY 12208-3478. TEL 518-262-5079, FAX 518-262-5528, bishopj@mail.amc.edu, http://www.oley.org. Ed., Adv. contact Roslyn Scheib Dahl. Circ: 4,500.

613.262 CAN ISSN 0834-3543
LIFELINES (TORONTO); the voice of Toronto's vegetarian community. Text in English. 1987. bi-m. CND 20 (effective 2000). adv. bk.rev. illus. back issues avail. *Refereed.* **Document type:** *Newsletter.* **Description:** Publishes a range of articles and news items geared toward vegetarian lifestyles. Includes recipes. Target audience is Toronto and vegetarians, however the publications aims at broader appeal to vegetarians and would-be vegetarians around the world.
Formerly: Toronto Vegetarian Association. Newsletter (0049-4232)
Published by: Toronto Vegetarian Association, 2300 Yonge St, Ste 1101, P O Box 2307, Toronto, ON M4P 1E4, Canada. TEL 416-544-9800, FAX 416-544-9094, lifelines@veg.on.ca, http://www.tva@veg.on.ca. Ed., R&P, Adv. contact Lisa Rogers. Circ: 3,000.

613.26 642 USA ISSN 1094-9143
LOW-FAT & FAST. Text in English. s-a. USD 3.99 newsstand/cover. illus. **Document type:** *Consumer.* **Description:** Provides readers with a broad range of meatless recipes and features stories focusing on various themes.
Published by: Cowles Enthusiast Media, 4 Highridge Park, Stamford, CT 06905. TEL 203-322-2900, 800-829-3340, FAX 203-322-1966, donnas@cowles.com, http://www.cowles.com. Ed. Donna Sapolin. Pub. Susan Tauster.

613.26 USA
LOW FAT - NO FAT COOKING. Text in English. bi-m. USD 3.99 newsstand/cover; CND 4.99 newsstand/cover in Canada. bk.rev. back issues avail. **Document type:** *Consumer.* **Description:** Provides assistance and guidelines in maintaining a healthy lifestyle through sensible cooking and eating habits.
Published by: Goodman Media Group, Inc., 1700 Broadway, 34th Fl, New York, NY 10019. TEL 212-541-7100, FAX 212-245-1241, http://www.goodmanmediagroup.com. Ed. Liz George. **Dist. by:** Curtis Circulation Co., 730 River Rd, New, Milford, CA 90210. TEL 201-634-7400, FAX 201-634-7499.

MAA BRA; specialtidningen foer kropp & sjael. see *PHYSICAL FITNESS AND HYGIENE*

613.2 USA
MACROBIOTICS TODAY. Text in English. 1960. 6/yr. USD 20 domestic to non-members; USD 30 foreign to non-members (effective 2000). adv. bk.rev. **Document type:** *Consumer.* **Description:** Contains articles, interviews and news events concerning macrobiotics and alternative health care.
Formerly (until 1984): G O M F News
Published by: George Ohsawa Macrobiotic Foundation, PO Box 3998, Chico, CA 95927-3998. TEL 530-566-9765, FAX 530-566-9768, gomf@2xtreme.net, http://www.gomf.macrobiotic.net. Ed., Adv. contact Bob Ligon. Pub. Carl Ferre. Circ: 5,000.

MEALEY'S LITIGATION REPORT: FEN-PHEN - REDUX. see *PHARMACY AND PHARMACOLOGY*

613.2 FRA ISSN 0398-7604
CODEN: MENUDI
MEDECINE ET NUTRITION. Text in French. 1965. 6/yr. FRF 450 domestic to individuals; EUR 71.65 in the European Union to individuals; FRF 500 elsewhere to individuals; FRF 340 domestic to students; EUR 54.88 in the European Union to students; FRF 380 elsewhere to students; FRF 83 newsstand/cover (effective 2001). adv. bibl, charts, illus. **Description:** Publishes original studies on the fundamental and applied aspects of food and nutrition.
Former titles (until 1975): Annales d'Hygiene de Langue Francaise. Medecine et Nutrition (0398-7582); Annales d'Hygiene de Langue Francaise (0003-4363)
Indexed: Biol.Abstr., C.I.S. Abstr., Chem.Abstr., Chem.Titles, Dairy Sci.Abstr., Excerp.Med., Food Sci.& Tech.Abstr., Nutr.Abstr., Potato Abstr., Rev.Med.& Vet.Mycol., Soyabean Abstr.
—BLDSC (5487.732500), CASDDS, CISTI, EMDOCS, GNLM, Infotrieve. **CCC.**
Published by: (Societe d'Hygiene de Langue Francaise), Editions la Simarre, Z.I. No. 2 - rue Joseph-Cugnot, Joue-les-Tours 37300, France. TEL 33-2-47535366, FAX 33-2-47674505. Circ: 10,000.

613.2 IND ISSN 0971-4219
CODEN: MNRCFF
MEDICAL AND NUTRITIONAL RESEARCH COMMUNICATIONS. Text in English. 1993. 3/yr. INR 60 domestic to individuals; USD 20 foreign to individuals; INR 75 domestic to institutions; USD 75 foreign to institutions. **Document type:** *Academic/Scholarly.* **Description:** Publishes papers on all aspects of medicine and nutrition, yoga, meditation, and health care, including various Indian systems of medicine and homeopathy.
Indexed: Chem.Abstr., Chem.Indus.Notes, Chem.Titles.
—CASDDS, CISTI.
Published by: Kunneth Institute of Medical Sciences, Medical Research Centre, Madichal, Tamil Nadu 629 163, India. TEL 04651-6432, FAX 04651-7400. Ed. S Krishnamurthy.

MEDITSINSKI PREGLED. DETSKI BOLESTI/MEDICAL REVIEW. CHILDREN'S DISEASES. see *MEDICAL SCIENCES—Pediatrics*

MEMPHIS HEALTH CARE NEWS. see *PHYSICAL FITNESS AND HYGIENE*

MILITAER-KUECHENCHEF. see *MILITARY*

613.2 USA
MINNESOTA NUTRITION CONFERENCE. Text in English. a. USD 25 in North America; USD 37.50 elsewhere. **Document type:** *Proceedings.*
—BLDSC (5810.413000).
Published by: University of Minnesota, Coffey Hall, 1420 Eckles Ave., St. Paul, MN 55108-6068. TEL 612-625-8173.

616.39 CHE ISSN 0026-6841
RA421 CODEN: MGLHAE
MITTEILUNGEN AUS DER GEBIETE DER LEBENSMITTELUNTERSUCHUNG UND HYGIENE/TRAVAUX DE CHIMIE ALIMENTAIRE ET D'HYGIENE. Text mainly in French, German; Text occasionally in English, Italian. 1910. 6/yr. CHF 66. adv. bk.rev. bibl, illus. index. **Document type:** *Trade.*
Indexed: AgBiotech, Agri.& Environ.Biotech.Abstr. (coverage dropped), Anal.Abstr., Biol.Abstr., Chem.Abstr., Chem.Titles, Dairy Sci.Abstr., Derwent Biotech.Abstr., Excerp.Med., Field Crop Abstr., Food Sci.& Tech.Abstr., GeoRef, Hort.Abstr., Ind.Med. (coverage dropped), Ind.Vet., Mass Spectr.Bull., Nutr.Abstr., Packag.Sci.Tech., Postharvest, Potato Abstr., Poult.Abstr., Protozool.Abstr., Rev.Appl.Entomol., Rev.Med.& Vet.Mycol., Rev.Plant Path., Soils & Fert., Soyabean Abstr., Sugar Ind.Abstr., Triticale Abstr., VITIS, Vet.Bull., Weed Abstr.
—CASDDS, CISTI, Linda Hall.
Published by: Bundesamt fuer Gesundheit, Bern 3003, Switzerland. Circ: 1,700. **Co-sponsors:** Schweizerische Gesellschaft fuer Lebensmittel- und Umweltchemie; Schweizerische Gesellschaft fuer Lebensmittelhygiene.

613.2 USA
N A A F A NEWSLETTER. Text in English. 1969. 6/yr. USD 40 to members. adv. bk.rev. back issues avail. **Document type:** *Newsletter.* **Description:** Provides information regarding obesity research, size discrimination, and advances in the size acceptance movement.
Published by: National Association to Advance Fat Acceptance, Inc., P O Box 188620, Sacramento, CA 95818. TEL 916-558-6880, FAX 916-558-6881, naafa@naafa.org.com. Ed. Sally E Smith. Circ: 5,000.

612.3 ITA ISSN 0939-4753
CODEN: NMCDEE
N M C D. (Nutrition, Metabolism and Cardiovascular Diseases) Text in English. 1991. bi-m. EUR 61.98 domestic; USD 10 foreign (effective 2002). adv. bk.rev. *Refereed.* **Document type:** *Academic/Scholarly.*
Related titles: Online - full text ed.: EUR 30.99 (effective 2002) (from Institute for Scientific Information).
Indexed: ASCA, Chem.Abstr., Chem.Indus.Notes, Chem.Titles, Curr.Cont., Ind.Med. (1991-), Inpharma, Nutr.Abstr., Pharm.&Out.News, Reac., Sci.Cit.Ind.
—BLDSC (6188.440000), CASDDS, CISTI, GNLM, IDS, Infotrieve, KNAW. **CCC.**
Published by: Medikal Press s.r.l., Via Luigi Zoja, 30, Milan, MI 20153, Italy. TEL 39-2-48202740, FAX 39-2-48201219. Ed. Mario Mancini.

N N F A TODAY. see *FOOD AND FOOD INDUSTRIES*

613.2 USA
N O H A NEWS. Text in English. 1976. q., latest vol.26, no.3. USD 10 to non-members; free to members (effective 2000). bk.rev. back issues avail. **Document type:** *Newsletter.* **Description:** Reports on nutritional information and research findings culled from a wide range of scientific sources; includes a column written by members of the professional advisory board.
Indexed: Ref.Zh.
Published by: Nutrition for Optimal Health Association, PO Box 380, Winnetka, IL 60093. TEL 708-786-5326, 847-604-3258, FAX 847-604-3358, nohainfo@aol.com, http://www.nutrition4health.org. Ed. Marjorie Fisher. Circ: 700.

613.2 DEU ISSN 0027-769X
TX341 CODEN: NAHRAR
NAHRUNG/FOOD. Text in English, German. 1957. 6/yr. EUR 578 in Europe; CHF 958 in Switzerland & Liechtenstein; USD 768 elsewhere; EUR 607 combined subscription in Europe for print and online eds.; CHF 1,006 combined subscription in Switzerland & Liechtenstein, for print and online eds.; USD 807 combined subscription elsewhere for print and online eds. (effective 2002). adv. charts, illus, abstr, bibl. index. back issues avail.; reprints avail. *Refereed.* **Document type:** *Journal, Academic/Scholarly.*
Related titles: Online - full text ed.: ISSN 1521-3803. EUR 578 in Europe; CHF 958 in Switzerland & Liechtenstein; USD 768 elsewhere (effective 2002) (from EBSCO Publishing, Wiley InterScience, Institute for Scientific Information).
Indexed: ASCA, Agri.Eng.Abstr., Anal.Abstr., Anim.Breed.Abstr., Apic.Abstr., Biol.Abstr., Cadscan, Chem.Abstr., Chem.Indus.Notes, Chem.Titles, Crop Physiol.Abstr., Curr.Adv.Ecol.Sci., Curr.Cont., Curr.Pack.Abstr., Dairy Sci.Abstr., Excerp.Med., Field Crop Abstr., Food Sci.& Tech.Abstr., Herb.Abstr., Hort.Abstr., INIS Atomind., Ind.Med. (1957-), Ind.Vet., Lead Abstr., Maize Abstr., Mass Spectr.Bull., Nutr.Abstr., Pig News & Info., Plant Breed.Abstr., Plant Grow.Reg.Abstr., Postharvest, Potato Abstr., Poult.Abstr., Ref.Zh., Rev.Appl.Entomol., Rev.Arom.& Med.Plants, Rev.Med.& Vet.Mycol., Rev.Plant Path., SSCI (coverage dropped), Sci.Cit.Ind., Seed Abstr., Soils & Fert., Soyabean Abstr., Sugar Ind.Abstr., Triticale Abstr., Vet.Bull., Zincscan.
—BLDSC (6015.300000), CASDDS, CINDOC, CISTI, GNLM, IDS, Infotrieve, Linda Hall. **CCC.**
Published by: Wiley - V C H, Postfach 101161, Weinheim 69451, Germany. TEL 49-6201-606-147, FAX 49-6201-606-117, subservice@wiley-vch.de, http://www.interscience.wiley.com. Ed. Thomas Henle. R&P Claudia Rutz. Adv. contact I Sinhoff. Circ: 450. **Subscr. in the Americas to:** John Wiley & Sons, Inc., Journals. TEL 44-1243-779777, 212-850-6645, FAX 212-850-6021; **Subscr. outside Germany, Austria & Switzerland to:** John Wiley & Sons Ltd., Baffins Ln, Chichester, Sussex PO19 IUD, United Kingdom. TEL 44-1243-779777, FAX 44-1243-843232.

N

613.2 338.1771 GBR
NATIONAL DAIRY COUNCIL. QUARTERLY REVIEW. Text in English. 1975. a. free per issue. abstr, charts, stat. **Document type:** *Academic/Scholarly.* **Description:** Reports research on the nutritional issues of milk and other dairy products.
Related titles: Online - full text ed.
Indexed: Food Sci.& Tech.Abstr.
—BLDSC.
Published by: The Dairy Council, National Dairy Council, 5-7 John Princes St, London W1G OJN, United Kingdom. TEL 44-171-499-7822, i.wakeling@ndc.uk.com, i.wakeling@dairycouncil.org.uk, http://www.milk.co.uk. Eds. Ian Wakeling, Lynn Pickett. Circ: 20,000 (controlled).

613.2 IND ISSN 0377-3744
NATIONAL INSTITUTE OF NUTRITION. ANNUAL REPORT. Text in English. 1946. a. free per issue. **Document type:** *Academic/Scholarly.*
Formerly: Nutrition Research Laboratories. Annual Report
Published by: National Institute of Nutrition, Indian Council of Medical Research, Jamai-Osmania, Hyderabad, Andhra Pradesh 500 007, India. Circ: 1,000.

613.262 DEU ISSN 1437-0735
NATUERLICH VEGETARISCH. Text in German. 1949. bi-m. DEM 42 domestic; DEM 51 foreign (effective 2001). adv. bk.rev. 52 p./no. back issues avail. *Refereed.* **Document type:** *Magazine, Consumer.* **Description:** Contains information on all aspects of vegetarianism.
Formerly: Vegetarier (0178-9104)
Published by: Vegetarier Bund Deutschlands e.V., Blumenstr 3, Hannover 30159, Germany. TEL 49-511-3632050, FAX 49-511-3632007, info@vegetarierbund.de, http://www.vegetarierbund.de. R&P Hildegund Scholvien TEL 49-6305-993108. Adv. contact Norbert Moch. B&W page DEM 1,200, color page DEM 1,400. Circ: 4,500.

613.2 DEU ISSN 0932-3503
NATUR UND HEILEN; die Monatszeitschrift fuer gesundes Leben. Text in German. 1924. m. EUR 40.80 domestic; EUR 47.55 foreign (effective 2001). adv. bk.rev. back issues avail. **Document type:** *Magazine, Consumer.* **Description:** For people who are interested in healthy life and natural healing.
Indexed: AMED.
—BLDSC (6033.868000), GNLM.
Published by: Verlag Natur und Heilen, Nikolaistr 5, Munich 80802, Germany. TEL 49-89-38015910, FAX 49-89-38015916, natur-und-heilen@t-online.de, http://www.naturundheilen.de. Ed., Pub., R&P Hansjoerg Volkhardt. Adv. contact Eva Ziervogel. B&W page XEU 2,000, color page XEU 3,375; trim 124 x 224. Circ: 50,200; 71,000 (paid).

613.2 GBR
NATURAL FOOD TRADER. Text in English. 1960. m. GBP 36; GBP 48 foreign. adv. bk.rev. illus. **Document type:** *Trade.* **Description:** For health food store professionals.
Formerly: Health Food Trader (0046-7049)
Indexed: Pollut.Abstr.
—CCC.
Published by: I B T M Ltd., Queensway House, 2 Queensway, Redhill RH1 1QS, United Kingdom. TEL 0737-768611, FAX 0737-760425. Ed. Paul Rouse. Circ: 4,500 (controlled).

NATURAL FOODS MERCHANDISER; new ideas, trends, products for the natural and organic foods industry. see *BUSINESS AND ECONOMICS—Marketing And Purchasing*

612.3 AUS ISSN 0816-2751
NATURAL HEALTH. Text in English. 1961. bi-m. AUD 32; AUD 44 foreign. adv. bk.rev. back issues avail. **Description:** To promote health and well-being through a more natural way of living, recognizing that prevention is far better than cure.
Published by: Natural Health Society of Australia Ltd., Ste. 28, 541 High St, Penrith, NSW 2750, Australia. TEL 047-215068. Ed. Roger French. Circ: 6,000.

613.2 USA
NATURAL HYGIENE SOCIETY OF NEW JERSEY. NEWSLETTER. Text in English. 1981. 8/yr. USD 15. abstr. back issues avail. **Document type:** *Newsletter.* **Description:** Covers various issues in health and hygiene, includes exercise, diet and behavior.
Formerly: American Natural Hygiene Society. New Jersey Chapter. Newsletter
Published by: Natural Hygiene of New Jersey, Inc., PO Box 142, Pompton Plains, NJ 07444. TEL 201-839-5919. Ed. John R Chorba. Circ: 350.

NATURAL LAND NEWS. see *PHYSICAL FITNESS AND HYGIENE*

613.2 658 USA ISSN 1525-5301
NATURAL PRODUCTS INDUSTRY INSIDER. Text in English. 1996. 13/yr. USD 249 domestic; USD 349 foreign (effective 2000). adv. **Document type:** *Magazine, Trade.* **Description:** Contains coverage of marketing, manufacturing, regulatory and financial news that affects the dietary supplement industry.
Published by: Virgo Publishing, Inc., 3300 N Central Ave, Ste 2500, Phoenix, AZ 85012. TEL 480-990-1101, FAX 480-990-0819, hgranato@vpico.com, virgopub@vpico.com, http://www.naturalproductsinsider.com, http://www.vpico.com. Ed. Heather Granato. Adv. contact Russ Titsch. B&W page USD 2,960, color page USD 4,035; bleed 8.375 x 11.125. Circ: 9,000 (paid and controlled).

613.26 NLD ISSN 0166-7203
NEDERLANDS TIJDSCHRIFT VOOR DIETISTEN. Text in Dutch. 1970. 10/yr. NLG 1,536 to non-members; BEF 1,536 in Belgium to non-members. bk.rev. **Document type:** *Academic/Scholarly.* **Description:** Informs society members of developments in the field of dietetics.
Published by: (Nederlandse Vereniging voor Dietisten), Elsevier Gezondheidszorg B.V., Tijdstroom (Subsidiary of: Reed Elsevier plc Group), Planetenbaan 1, Maarssen 3600 AK, Netherlands. TEL 31-346-577577, FAX 31-346-554287, http://www.tijdstroom.nl. Ed. M A Donker Willenborg. Circ: 3,717. **Subscr. to:** Elsevier Den Haag, Postbus 16500, The Hague 2500 BM, Netherlands. TEL 31-70-381-9900, FAX 31-70-333-8399.

613.2 CHE
NESTLE FOUNDATION. ANNUAL REPORT. Text in English. 1969. a. free. **Document type:** *Corporate.*
Indexed: Dairy Sci.Abstr., Nutr.Abstr., Rural Devel.Abstr.
Published by: Nestle Foundation, 4 Place de la Gare, Lausanne 1003, Switzerland. FAX 41-21-3203392. Ed. B Schuerch. Circ: 1,500.

613.2 USA ISSN 0742-2806
CODEN: NNWSDT
NESTLE NUTRITION SERIES. Key Title: Nestle Nutrition Workshop. Text in English. 1982. irreg. price varies. reprint service avail. from PQC. *Refereed.* **Document type:** *Proceedings.*
Indexed: Chem.Abstr., Chem.Indus.Notes, Chem.Titles, Dairy Sci.Abstr.
—BLDSC (6076.609000), CASDDS, CISTI.
Published by: Lippincott Williams & Wilkins (Philadelphia) (Subsidiary of: Wolters Kluwer N.V.), 530 Walnut St, Philadelphia, PA 19106-3621. TEL 301-223-2300, 800-638-3030, FAX 301-223-2400, http://www.lww.com. **Subscr. to:** PO Box 1600, Hagerstown, MD 21740-1600.

613.2 CHE ISSN 1422-7584
▼ **NESTLE NUTRITION WORKSHOP SERIES CLINICAL AND PERFORMANCE PROGRAMME.** Text in English. 1999. irreg., latest vol.5. DEM 160 in Europe; DEM 190 in Germany; DEM 140 in United States (effective 2001). **Document type:** *Journal, Academic/Scholarly.*
Indexed: Chem.Abstr., Chem.Titles.
—BLDSC (6076.609500).
Published by: S. Karger AG, Allschwilerstr 10, PO Box, Basel 4009, Switzerland. TEL 41-61-306-1111, FAX 41-61-306-1234, karger@karger.ch, http://www.karger.com/bookseries/NNWOS.

NEW CUISINE ALTERNATIVE SERIES. see *HOME ECONOMICS*

613.2 USA
NEW PRODUCT REVIEW. Text in English. 1994. q. adv. **Document type:** *Magazine, Trade.* **Description:** Provides information on the latest natural products and ingredients available.
Published by: New Hope Natural Media (Subsidiary of: Penton Media, Inc.), 1401 Pearl St, Boulder, CO 80302. TEL 303-939-8440, FAX 303-939-9886, sales@newhope.com, http://www.healthwell.com. adv.: B&W page USD 5,150, color page USD 8,060; trim 10.75 x 14.75.

613.26 NZL ISSN 0110-635X
NEW ZEALAND DIETETIC ASSOCIATION. JOURNAL. Text in English. 1946. 2/yr. NZD 45 domestic; NZD 53 in Australasia; NZD 63 elsewhere (effective 2000). adv. bk.rev. *Refereed.* **Document type:** *Academic/Scholarly.* **Description:** Presents research, reviews and conference papers of relevance to New Zealand dietitians.
Formerly: New Zealand Dietetic Association. Bulletin
Indexed: Ind.N.Z.Per., Nutr.Abstr.
Published by: New Zealand Dietetic Association Inc., P.O. Box 5065, Wellington, New Zealand. TEL 64-4-473-7885. Circ: 450.

613.2 NGA ISSN 0189-0913
CODEN: NJNSEP
NIGERIAN JOURNAL OF NUTRITIONAL SCIENCES. Text in English. 1980. s-a. NGN 10. **Document type:** *Academic/Scholarly.*
Related titles: CD-ROM ed.
Indexed: ExtraMED.
—CASDDS.
Published by: (Nutritional Society of Nigeria), Ibadan University Press, University of Ibadan, Ibadan, Oyo, Nigeria. Ed. Dr. Tola Atinmo. Circ: 2,000. **Co-sponsor:** University of Ibadan. Department of Human Nutrition.

613.2 JPN ISSN 0912-9405
NIHON JOMYAKU KEICHO EIYO KENKYUKAISHI/ JAPANESE SOCIETY OF PARENTERAL AND ENTERAL NUTRITION. JOURNAL. Text in English, Japanese. 1986. a.
Published by: Nihon Jomyaku Keicho Eiyo Kenkyukai, Jikeikai Ika Daigaku Dai 2 Geka, 25-8 Nishi-Shinbashi 3-chome, Minato-ku, Tokyo 105-0003, Japan.

613.2 JPN ISSN 0286-8202
CODEN: NREZEN
NIHON RINSHO EIYO GAKKAI ZASSHI/JAPANESE SOCIETY OF CLINICAL NUTRITION. JOURNAL. Text in Japanese; Summaries in English. 1982. 3/yr. JPY 5,000. adv. *Refereed.* **Document type:** *Academic/Scholarly.*
Published by: Nihon Rinsho Eiyo Gakkai, c/o Nihon Gakkai Jimu Senta, 16-9 Honkomagome 5-chome, Bunkyo-ku, Tokyo 113-0021, Japan. TEL 81-3-5814-5801. Ed. Yoshiya Hata. Adv. contact Nobuhiko Takeda.

613.2 JPN ISSN 0029-0572
NINGEN IGAKU/HUMAN MEDICINE. Text in Japanese. 1938. m. JPY 2,000, USD 7. adv. bk.rev. illus, tr.lit.
Published by: Ningen Igakusha, 5-16-23 Senrioka, Settsu-shi, Osaka-fu 566-0001, Japan. Ed. Takaaki Oura. Circ: 20,000.

NISARG ANE AROGYA. see *PHYSICAL FITNESS AND HYGIENE*

NUTRACEUTICALS INTERNATIONAL. see *PHARMACY AND PHARMACOLOGY*

362.176 USA
NUTRACEUTICALS WORLD; serving the dietary supplement, functional food and nutritional beverage industries. Text in English. 8/yr. adv. **Document type:** *Magazine, Trade.* **Description:** Showcases the latest products and trends and tracks the global nutraceuticals industry. Also covers market and technology developments, dissects regulatory issues and provides new product and market sourcing information as well as covering all the major trade shows and conferences in the nutritional supplement and food and beverage industries.
Published by: Rodman Publications, Inc., 17 S Franklin Tpke, Ramsey, NJ 07446. TEL 201-825-2552, FAX 201-825-0553, nutraceuticals@rodpub.com, http://www.nutraceuticalsworld.com. Ed. Ellen Schutt. Pub. Robin Pask-Donkersloot. Adv. contact Stephen Lipscomb. B&W page USD 2,400, color page USD 3,300; bleed 8.375 x 11.125.

613.2 NLD ISSN 0167-4587
CODEN: NUSYD8
NUTRICIA SYMPOSIA. Text in English. 1964. irreg. price varies. *Refereed.* **Document type:** *Proceedings.*
—CASDDS.
Published by: Kluwer Academic Publishers Group (Subsidiary of: Wolters Kluwer N.V.), Spuiboulevard 50, PO Box 17, Dordrecht 3300 AA, Netherlands. FAX 31-78-639-2254, services@wkap.nl, http://www.wkap.nl. **Dist. by:** Journals Department, PO Box 322, Dordrecht 3300 AH, Netherlands. FAX 31-78-654-6474.

612.3 ESP ISSN 0211-6057
CODEN: NUTCDF
NUTRICION CLINICA; dietetica hospitalaria. Text in Spanish. 1981. bi-m. ESP 6,000 domestic; USD 65 in Europe; USD 70 elsewhere (effective 2001). adv. charts. *Refereed.* **Document type:** *Journal, Academic/Scholarly.* **Description:** Offers original research and review articles in nutrition and dietetics.
Indexed: Chem.Abstr., Excerp.Med., Ind.Med.Esp., Triticale Abstr.
—CASDDS, CINDOC, CISTI, GNLM, Infotrieve. **CCC.**

Published by: (Sociedad Espanola de Nutricion (S.E.N.)), Alpe Editores S.A., Pedro Rico, 27, Madrid 28029, Spain. TEL 34-91-733-8811, FAX 34-91-315-9652, alpeeditores@sistelcom.com. Ed. Dr. Alfredo Entrala Bueno. Pub. Angeles Alvarez Sanchez. Adv. contact Ana Jurado. color page ESP 160,000; 280 x 210. Circ: 3,500 (controlled).

613.2 AUS ISSN 1320-9701
NUTRIDATE. Text in English. 1990. q. AUD 49.95 (effective 2000). back issues avail. **Document type:** *Academic/Scholarly.* **Description:** Presents recent developments in nutrition, health and physical education for 12th grade students.
Indexed: WMB.
Published by: Warringal Publications, 114 Argyle St, Fitzroy, VIC 3065, Australia. TEL 61-3-9416-0200, FAX 61-3-9416-0402. Ed. Dorothy Carey. Pub. Jane Arter. Circ: 1,500.

613.2 IND ISSN 0550-404X
NUTRITION. Text in English. 1966. q. INR 8. **Document type:** *Academic/Scholarly.* **Description:** Popular magazine concerning food and nutrition.
Indexed: Curr.Cont. (coverage dropped), Ind.Sci.Rev., Soyabean Abstr., Sugar Ind.Abstr.
Published by: National Institute of Nutrition, Indian Council of Medical Research, Jamai-Osmania, Hyderabad, Andhra Pradesh 500 007, India. Ed. M Mohanram. Circ: 4,000.

616.39 USA ISSN 0899-9007
QP141.A1 CODEN: NUTRER
NUTRITION; the international journal of applied and basic nutritional sciences. Text in English. 1985. m. EUR 214 in Europe to individuals; JPY 28,300 in Japan to individuals; USD 239 elsewhere to individuals; EUR 380 in Europe to institutions; JPY 50,500 in Japan to institutions; USD 425 elsewhere to institutions; EUR 1,790.16 in Europe to institutions Nutrition Package; JPY 252,700 in Japan to institutions Nutrition Package; USD 2,003 elsewhere to institutions Nutrition Package (effective 2002). adv. back issues avail. *Refereed.* **Document type:** *Academic/Scholarly.* **Description:** Publishes news of current research and practice in the field of applied and basic nutrition.
Formerly (until 1987): Nutrition International (0888-1294)
Related titles: Online - full text ed.: (from ingenta, ScienceDirect, Swets Blackwell, Institute for Scientific Information).
Indexed: ASCA, CINAHL, Chem.Abstr., Chem.Titles, Curr.Cont., Dairy Sci.Abstr., Excerp.Med., Food Sci.& Tech.Abstr., Ind.Med. (1987-), Ind.Sci.Rev., Inpharma, Int.Nurs.Ind., NRN, Nutr.Abstr., Pharm.&Out.News, Reac., Rev.Arom.& Med.Plants, Sci.Cit.Ind.
—BLDSC (6187.930000), CASDDS, CISTI, GNLM, IDS, Infotrieve, KNAW. **CCC.**
Published by: Elsevier Science, PO Box 945, New York, NY 10159-0945. TEL 212-989-5800, FAX 212-633-3990, usinfo-f@elsevier.com, http://www.elsevier.com/locate/nut. Eds. D Labadarios, Dr. Michael Meguid. Circ: 20,112. **Subscr. in Australasia and the Far East to:** Elsevier Science (Singapore) Pte Ltd, No.1 Temasek Ave, 17-01 Millenia Tower, Singapore 039192, Singapore. TEL 65-434-3727, FAX 65-337-2230; **Subscr. in Japan to:** Elsevier Science Inc - Japan Regional Office, 9-15 Higashi-Azabu 1-chome, Minato-ku, Tokyo 106-0044, Japan. TEL 81-3-5561-5033; **Subscr. outside the Americas to:** Elsevier Science BV, PO Box 211, Amsterdam 1000 AE, Netherlands. TEL 31-20-485-3757.

NUTRITION ABSTRACTS AND REVIEWS. SERIES A: HUMAN AND EXPERIMENTAL. see *NUTRITION AND DIETETICS—Abstracting, Bibliographies, Statistics*

613.2 USA ISSN 0885-7792
CODEN: NAHLED
NUTRITION ACTION HEALTHLETTER. Text in English. 1974. 10/yr. USD 24 domestic; CND 36 in Canada; USD 32 elsewhere; USD 2.50 newsstand/cover (effective 2001). bk.rev. abstr, bibl, illus, charts. Index. 16 p./no. 2 cols./p. back issues avail.; reprints avail. **Document type:** *Newsletter.* **Description:** Deals with news, commentary, features, letters, and advocacy on nutrition and food policy, in order to promote good health.
Formerly: Nutrition Action (0199-5510); Incorporating (1976-1980): Intake (New Hyde Park) (0732-6920)
Related titles: Microform ed.: (from PQC); Online - full text ed.: (from Gale Group, ProQuest Information & Learning, Factiva).
Indexed: Agricola, Alt.Press Ind., Biol.Dig., CHNI, CINAHL, Consum.Ind. (1993-1997), Hlth.Ind.
—BLDSC (6188.025100).
Published by: Center for Science in the Public Interest, 1875 Connecticut Ave, N W, Ste 300, Washington, DC 20009-5728. TEL 202-332-9110, FAX 202-265-4954, civc@cspinet.org, cspi@cspinet.org, http://www.cspinet.org/nah/. Ed. Stephen B Schmidt. Pub. Michael Jacobson. R&P Adam Pearson TEL 202-332-9110 Ext 316. Circ: 800,000 (paid).

613.2 USA ISSN 0163-5581
CODEN: NUCADQ
NUTRITION AND CANCER; an international journal. Text in English. 1978. bi-m. USD 225 in US & Canada to individuals; USD 280 elsewhere to individuals; USD 995 in US & Canada to institutions; USD 1,050 elsewhere to institutions (effective 2002). adv. bk.rev. charts, illus. back issues avail. *Refereed.* **Document type:** *Journal, Academic/Scholarly.* **Description:** Reports and reviews current findings on the effect of nutrition on the etiology, therapy, and prevention of cancer.
Related titles: Online - full text ed.: ISSN 1532-7914. USD 202.50 to individuals; USD 895.50 to institutions (effective 2002) (from CatchWord Ltd., EBSCO Publishing, O C L C Online Computer Library Center, Inc., RoweCom Information Quest, Swets Blackwell, Institute for Scientific Information).
Indexed: ASCA, Agricola, Bibl.Agri., Biol.Abstr., Chem.Abstr., Chem.Indus.Notes, Chem.Titles, Curr.Cont., Dairy Sci.Abstr., Dent.Ind., Environ.Sci.Poll.Mgmt., Excerp.Med., Food Sci.& Tech.Abstr., INIS Atomind., Ind.Med. (1978-), Ind.Sci.Rev., Inpharma, Int.Abstr.Biol.Sci., Maize Abstr., Microbiol.Abstr., NRN, Nutr.Abstr., Pharm.&Out.News, Pollut.Abstr., Poult.Abstr., Reac., Rev.Med.& Vet.Mycol., Risk Abstr., Saf.Sci.Abstr., Sci.Cit.Ind., Soyabean Abstr., Sugar Ind.Abstr., THA, Tox.Abstr., Triticale Abstr.
—BLDSC (6188.045000), CASDDS, CatchWord, CISTI, GNLM, ingenta, KNAW. **CCC.**
Published by: Lawrence Erlbaum Associates, Inc., 10 Industrial Ave, Mahwah, NJ 07430-2262. TEL 201-760-3735, 800-926-6579, FAX 201-236-0072, journals@erlbaum.com, http://www.erlbaum.com/Journals/journals/NC/nc.htm. Ed. Leonard A Cohen. adv.: page USD 300; trim 7 x 10. Circ: 500.

613.2 USA ISSN 8750-8370
NUTRITION & DIETARY CONSULTANT; America's only journal for the practicing professional. Text in English. 1979. m. USD 15.96. adv. back issues avail. **Document type:** *Trade.* **Description:** For the nutritional consultant and dietitian in private practice; covers health maintenance, vitamin, mineral, and herbal therapies, food evaluation and diet management.
Former titles: Your Nutritional Consultant (8750-3395); (until 1984): Nutritional Consultant and Health Express (0746-9799); (until 1981): Nutritional Consultant; Incorporates: Herald of Holistic Health Newsletter
Published by: American Association of Nutritional Consultants, 1641 E Sunset Rd, B 117, Las Vegas, NV 89119. TEL 702-361-1132, FAX 702-739-7225. Ed. Myra E Zelikovics. Circ: 43,000.

613.2 GBR ISSN 0034-6659
CODEN: NFSCD7
NUTRITION AND FOOD SCIENCE. Text in English. 1966. bi-m. USD 2,099 in North America; EUR 2,229 in Europe; AUD 2,409 in Australasia; GBP 1,309 in the UK & rest of the world (effective 2002); Subscr. includes print & online access.. adv. bk.rev. abstr, charts, stat. index. reprint service avail. from SWZ. **Document type:** *Academic/Scholarly.* **Description:** Keeps you informed about new initiatives, the latest research findings and innovative ways of responding to changes in public attitudes.
Formerly: Review of Nutrition and Food Science
Related titles: Online - full text ed.: (from EBSCO Publishing, O C L C Online Computer Library Center, Inc., RoweCom Information Quest, ingenta, Gale Group, Swets Blackwell).
Indexed: AgBiotech, Agricola, Anim.Breed.Abstr., Aqua.Sci.& Fish.Abstr., Aquacult.Abstr., Art.Hosp.& Tour., Br.Tech.Ind., Chem.Abstr., Curr.Adv.Ecol.Sci., Dairy Sci.Abstr., Emrld.Intell., Environ.Sci.Poll.Mgmt., Food Sci.& Tech.Abstr., Maize Abstr., Nutr.Abstr., Pollut.Abstr., Postharvest, Rev.Appl.Entomol., Rev.Plant Path., Rural Recreat.Tour.Abstr., Soyabean Abstr., Sugar Ind.Abstr., Weed Abstr., World Ag.Econ.& Rur.Soc.Abstr.
—BLDSC (6188.070000), CASDDS, CISTI, Infotrieve, Linda Hall. **CCC.**
Published by: Emerald, 60-62 Toller Ln, Bradford, W Yorks BD8 9BY, United Kingdom. TEL 44-1274-777700, FAX 44-1274-785200, info@emeraldinsight.com, http://www.emeraldinsight.com/nfs.htm, http://www.emeraldinsight.com/journals/. Ed. Dilys Wells. Adv. contact Jeremy Wright. Circ: 3,500.

613.2 USA
NUTRITION AND HEALTH. Text in English. 1997. irreg., latest vol.3, 1999. price varies. illus. back issues avail. *Refereed.* **Document type:** *Monographic series, Academic/Scholarly.* **Description:** Examines a wide variety of topics in the ways in which good nutrition can maintain health. Also covers procedures physicians can take to ensure the good nutrition of their patients, including managing obesity and eating disorders.
Published by: Humana Press Inc., 999 Riverview Dr, Ste 208, Totowa, NJ 07512. TEL 973-256-1699, FAX 973-256-8341, humana@humanapr.com, http://humanapress.com. R&P Richard Hruska.

613.2 GBR ISSN 0260-1060
CODEN: NUHEDT
NUTRITION AND HEALTH. Text in English. 1982. 4/yr. GBP 139, USD 219 (effective 2001). adv. bk.rev. **Document type:** *Academic/Scholarly.* **Description:** Covers preventive medical and nutrition education.
Related titles: Microform ed.
Indexed: ASSIA, Chem.Abstr., Chem.Titles, Curr.Adv.Ecol.Sci., Dairy Sci.Abstr., Environ.Per.Bibl. (1985-1994), Excerp.Med., Food Sci.& Tech.Abstr., Ind.Med. (1982-), Ind.Vet., Lang.& Lang.Behav.Abstr., Maize Abstr., NRN, Nutr.Abstr., Rural Devel.Abstr., Rural Recreat.Tour.Abstr., SOPODA, Soc.Serv.Abstr., Sociol.Abstr., Trop.Dis.Bull., Vet.Bull.
—BLDSC (6188.073000), CASDDS, CISTI, GNLM, Infotrieve, ingenta, KNAW. **CCC.**
Published by: (McCarrison Society), A B Academic Publishers, PO Box 42, Bicester, Oxon OX26 6NW, United Kingdom. jrnls@abapubl.demon.co.uk. Ed. Edward Kirby.

613.2 USA ISSN 0149-2667
CODEN: NUBRD4
NUTRITION AND THE BRAIN. Text in English. 1975. irreg. price varies. reprint service avail. from PQC. *Refereed.* **Document type:** *Monographic series.*
Indexed: Biol.Abstr., Curr.Cont. (coverage dropped), Sci.Cit.Ind. (coverage dropped).
—CASDDS, CISTI, KNAW.
Published by: Lippincott Williams & Wilkins (Philadelphia) (Subsidiary of: Wolters Kluwer N.V.), 530 Walnut St, Philadelphia, PA 19106-3621. TEL 301-223-2300, 800-638-3030, FAX 301-223-2400, http://www.lww.com. **Subscr. to:** PO Box 1600, Hagerstown, MD 21740-1600.

613.2 USA ISSN 0732-0167
NUTRITION & THE M.D.; a continuing education service for physicians and nutritionists. Text in English. 1974. m., latest vol.27. USD 84 domestic to individuals; USD 104 foreign to individuals; USD 135 domestic to institutions; USD 155 foreign to institutions; USD 14 newsstand/cover (effective 2002). back issues avail. **Document type:** *Newsletter.* **Description:** Each issue covers a single topic from several aspects.
Related titles: Online - full text ed.: USD 175.50 domestic for academic site license; USD 195.50 foreign for academic site license; USD 195.75 domestic for corporate site license; USD 215.75 foreign for corporate site license (effective 2002).
Published by: Lippincott Williams & Wilkins (Philadelphia) (Subsidiary of: Wolters Kluwer N.V.), 530 Walnut St, Philadelphia, PA 19106-3621. TEL 215-521-8300, FAX 215-521-8902, http://www.lww.com. Ed. Dr. Russell Merritt. R&P Margaret Becker. Circ: 4,108. **Subscr. to:** PO Box 1600, Hagerstown, MD 21740-1600. TEL 800-777-2295, FAX 301-824-7390.

613.2 GBR ISSN 1471-9827
CODEN: BNUBD6
NUTRITION BULLETIN. Text in English. 1968. 4/yr., latest vol.27, 2002. GBP 65 in Europe to individuals; USD 104 in North America to individuals; GBP 72 elsewhere to individuals; GBP 210 in Europe to institutions; USD 333 in North America to institutions; GBP 231 elsewhere to institutions (effective 2002). index. back issues avail. *Refereed.* **Document type:** *Journal, Academic/Scholarly.* **Description:** Contains overview articles and covers the current state of knowledge in clinical nutrition, food processing, and food policy. Highlights areas of controversy and debate, summarizes concepts and methods, and discusses recently published scientific papers and newsworthy issues.
Former titles (until 1993): B N F Nutrition Bulletin (0141-9684); (until 1977): B N F Bulletin (0307-3548); (until 1972): British Nutrition Foundation. Information Bulletin (0142-0151)

N

Related titles: Online - full text ed.: Nutrition Bulletin Online. ISSN 1467-3010. 2000. GBP 59 in Europe to individuals; USD 94 in North America to individuals; GBP 59 elsewhere to individuals; GBP 189 in Europe to institutions; USD 300 in North America to institutions; GBP 189 elsewhere to institutions (effective 2002) (from EBSCO Publishing, O C L C Online Computer Library Center, Inc., ingenta, Munksgaard & Blackwell Science's Synergy, Swets Blackwell).
Indexed: Abstr.Hyg., AgBiotech, Agricola, Art.Hosp.& Tour., Biol.Abstr., Cal.Tiss.Abstr., Chem.Abstr., Curr.Adv.Ecol.Sci., Dairy Sci.Abstr., Food Sci.& Tech.Abstr., Nutr.Abstr., Packag.Sci.Tech., Ref.Zh., Tox.Abstr., Trop.Dis.Bull.
—BLDSC (6188.120000), CASDDS, CISTI.
Published by: (British Nutrition Foundation), Blackwell Science Ltd., PO Box 88, Oxford OX2 0NE, United Kingdom. TEL 44-1865-206180, 44-1865-206002, FAX 44-1865-206219, jnl.orders@blacksci.co.uk, http://www.blackwell-science.com/~cgilib/jnlpage.asp?Journal=nbu&File=nbu, http://www.blackwellpublishing.com. Ed. G Goldberg. Pub. Elaine Stott. R&P Sophie Savage. Adv. contact Jenny Applin. Circ: 1,000.

613.2 USA
NUTRITION BUSINESS JOURNAL. Text in English. 1996. m. USD 795 domestic; USD 845 foreign (effective 2001). back issues avail. **Document type:** *Journal, Trade.* **Description:** Provides a strategic business overview of the nutrition, natural health and natural products for executives within the industry.
Related titles: Online - full text ed.
Published by: Nutrition Business International, Inc., 4452 Park Blvd, Ste 301, San Diego, CA 92116. TEL 619-295-7685 ext.12, FAX 619-295-5743, info@nutritionbusiness.com, http://www.nutritionbusiness.com. Ed., R&P Jill Martens TEL 619-295-7685 ext.13.

613.2 USA ISSN 1093-4545
NUTRITION FORUM. Text in English. 1984. bi-m. USD 35 to individuals; USD 50 to institutions (effective 1999). adv. bk.rev. illus. Index. reprints avail. **Document type:** *Newsletter.* **Description:** Publishes investigative journalism concerning health-related nutritional methods and products. Reports news about alternative health care, quackery, food science and related subjects.
Former titles (until 1997): Nutrition and Health Forum (1091-2428); (until 1996): Nutrition Forum (0748-8165)
Related titles: Online - full text ed.: (from Gale Group, Northern Light Technology, Inc., ProQuest Information & Learning, Factiva).
Indexed: CHNI, Consum.Ind. (1989-1998), Hlth.Ind.
—BLDSC (6188.282500).
Published by: Prometheus Books Incorporated, 59 John Glenn Dr., Amherst, NY 14228. TEL 716-691-0133, FAX 716-691-0137, http://www.quackwatch.com/04consumereducation/nf.html. Ed., Adv. contact Lewis Vaughn. Pub. Paul Kurtz. R&P Gretchen Kurtz. Circ: 2,000.

613.2 CAN ISSN 0318-4501
NUTRITION FORUM/FORUM DE NUTRITION. Text in English. 1966. s-a. membership. bk.rev.
Formerly (until 1973): Newsletter - Nutrition (0318-4498)
Related titles: Online - full text ed.: (from Northern Light Technology, Inc.).
—CISTI. **CCC.**
Published by: Canadian Society for Nutritional Sciences, Department of Foods and Nutrition, University of Manitoba, Winnipeg, MB R3T 2N2, Canada. TEL 613-993-4484. Ed. Vivian Bruce. Circ: (controlled). **Dist. by:** Department de Nutrition, Universite de Manitoba, Montreal, PQ H30 3J7, Canada.

613.2 USA ISSN 0892-1474
THE NUTRITION FUNDING REPORT; a monthly guide to locating resources. Text in English. 1986. m., latest vol.17, 2002. USD 45 (effective 2001). **Document type:** *Newsletter.* **Description:** Itemizes available resources for food, nutrition and other health-related activities: grants, contracts, scholarships, fellowships, and publications, all from charities, corporations, foundations, government and other sources.
Related titles: Online - full text ed.: USD 65 includes print ed. (effective 2000).
Published by: Nutrition Legislation Services, PO Box 75035, Washington, DC 20013. TEL 202-488-8879, FAX 202-554-3116, http://www.nutritionservices.com. Ed., Pub., R&P Lenora Moragne.

613.2 USA ISSN 0164-7202
NUTRITION HEALTH REVIEW; The Consumer's Medical Journal. Text in English. 1975. q. USD 24 for 2 yrs. domestic; USD 36 for 2 yrs. in Canada; USD 66 for 2 yrs. foreign; USD 3 newsstand/cover (effective 2001). bk.rev., video rev. charts, illus, stat. **Document type:** *Newspaper, Consumer.* **Description:** Provides information on nutrition, health and medicine for consumers and related health professionals.
Related titles: CD-ROM ed.; Microfilm ed.; Microform ed.: (from PQC); Online - full text ed.: (from Gale Group, Northern Light Technology, Inc., ProQuest Information & Learning).
Indexed: Hlth.Ind., e-psyche.
Published by: Vegetus Publications, 27 Tunbridge Rd., Haverford, PA 19041-0000. TEL 610-896-1853, FAX 610-896-1857. Ed., R&P Andrew Rifkin. Pub. Frank Ray Rifkin. Circ: 280,800 (controlled).

613.2 USA ISSN 1096-6781
NUTRITION IN CLINICAL CARE. Text in English. bi-m. USD 65 domestic to individuals; USD 80 in Canada & Mexico to individuals; USD 95 elsewhere to individuals; USD 150 domestic to institutions; USD 165 in Canada & Mexico to institutions; USD 180 elsewhere to institutions; USD 71.50 domestic to individuals print & online eds. combined; USD 88 in Canada & Mexico to individuals print & online eds. combined; USD 104.50 elsewhere to individuals print & online eds. combined; USD 165 domestic to institutions print & online eds. combined; USD 181.50 in Canada & Mexico to institutions print & online eds. combined; USD 198 elsewhere to institutions print & online eds. combined (effective 2001). adv. reprints avail. *Refereed.* **Document type:** *Academic/Scholarly.* **Description:** Dedicated to the exchange and enhancement of knowledge in clinical nutrition through the rapid, accurate publication of practical, analytic reviews of major topics in nutrition.
Related titles: ♦ Online - full text ed.: Nutrition in Clinical Care Online. ISSN 1523-5408.
—BLDSC (6188.125000).
Published by: (Tufts University), Blackwell Science Inc., Commerce Pl, 350 Main St, Malden, MA 02148-5018. TEL 781-388-8250, FAX 781-388-8255, journals@blacksci.com, http://www.blackwell-science.com. Ed. Dr. Robert M Russell. R&P Tracey Davies. Adv. contact Jenny Applin.

613.2 USA ISSN 1523-5408
NUTRITION IN CLINICAL CARE ONLINE. Text in English. bi-m. USD 59 to individuals; USD 135 to institutions (effective 2001). **Document type:** *Academic/Scholarly.*
Media: Online - full text (from EBSCO Publishing, O C L C Online Computer Library Center, Inc., RoweCom Information Quest, ingenta, Munksgaard & Blackwell Science's Synergy, Swets Blackwell). **Related titles:** ♦ Print ed.: Nutrition in Clinical Care. ISSN 1096-6781.
Published by: Blackwell Science Inc., Commerce Pl, 350 Main St, Malden, MA 02148-5018. TEL 781-388-8250, 800-759-6102, FAX 781-388-8255, website@blacksci.com, journals@blacksci.com, http://www.blackwell-science.com/~cgilib/bsinc.bin?Journal=geoscience.

613.2 USA ISSN 0884-5336
CODEN: NCPREH
NUTRITION IN CLINICAL PRACTICE. Short title: N C P. Text in English. 1986. bi-m. USD 42 domestic to individuals; USD 57 in Canada & Mexico to individuals; USD 72 elsewhere to individuals; USD 88 domestic to institutions; USD 103 in Canada & Mexico to institutions; USD 116 elsewhere to institutions (effective 2001). adv. back issues avail. *Refereed.* **Document type:** *Academic/Scholarly.* **Description:** Multidisciplinary clinical journal providing information on clinical nutrition for health care personnel. Publishes articles, clinical observations, case reports, techniques and procedures.
Related titles: Microform ed.: (from PQC); Online - full text ed.: (from Northern Light Technology, Inc., ProQuest Information & Learning).
Indexed: CINAHL, I.P.A., Nutr.Abstr.
—BLDSC (6188.130000), CISTI, GNLM, ingenta, KNAW. **CCC.**
Published by: American Society for Parenteral and Enteral Nutrition, 8630 Fenton St, Ste 412, Silver Spring, MD 20910-3805. TEL 301-587-6315, FAX 301-587-3323, 301-587-2365, aspen@nutr.org, http://www.nutritioncare.org. Ed. Dr. Charles Van Way. R&P Carolyn Kohagura. Adv. contact Adrian S Nickel. B&W page USD 1,060. Circ: 8,152.

613.2 GBR ISSN 1470-4730
NUTRITION IN PRACTICE. Text in English. 1992. 3/yr. **Document type:** *Trade.*
Formerly (until 2000): Practice Nutrition (0965-9722)
—BLDSC (6188.595000).
Published by: Advisa Medica, Gordon House, Station Rd, Mill Hill, London NW7 2HZ, United Kingdom. TEL 44-20-8906-2767, FAX 44-20-8906-0261, info@advisa.co.uk. Ed. Jonathan Levy.

613.2 USA
NUTRITION JOURNAL✶. Text in English. bi-m.
Published by: Dimon Creative Communications, 3099 N Lima St, Burbank, CA 91504-2013. TEL 818-845-3748, FAX 818-954-8916. Ed. Michael Meguid. Circ: 12,000.

613.2 USA
NUTRITION LEGISLATION AND REGULATORY NEWS; a twice-monthly report of United States legislative, executive, and regulatory activities. Text in English. 1985. s-m., latest vol.16, 2002. USD 150 in North America; USD 175 elsewhere (effective 2000). bk.rev. **Document type:** *Newsletter.* **Description:** Offers legislative and regulatory information covering all aspects of nutrition: research, education, international, food assistance, manpower training, monitoring, and food quality and safety.
Formerly: Nutrition Legislation News (8756-6060)
Related titles: Online - full text ed.: USD 175 in North America includes print ed.; USD 200 elsewhere includes print ed. (effective 2000).
Published by: Nutrition Legislation Services, PO Box 75035, Washington, DC 20013. TEL 202-488-8879, FAX 202-554-3116, lmoragne@erols.com, http://www.nutritionservices.com. Pub. Lenora Moragne. R&P Nora Champion.

613.2 USA
NUTRITION NEWS (CONCORD). Text in English. fortn. free per issue. **Document type:** *Newsletter.*
Media: Online - full text.
Published by: E G W Publishing Co., 1041 Shary Circle, Concord, CA 94518. TEL 925-671-9852, FAX 510-671-0692, hstevens@egw.com, http://www.naturalland.com/nv/nnc.htm.

613.2 USA
NUTRITION NEWS FOCUS. Text in English. d. free per issue. **Document type:** *Newsletter, Consumer.* **Description:** Offers non-experts unbiased information on nutrition, enabling them to make sense of the huge amount of information on the subject published in the news media.
Media: Online - full text.
Published by: Nutrition News Focus Inc., 4426 St. Clair Ave, Studio City, CA 91604. TEL 818-761-8074, FAX 818-761-7025, ken@nutritionnewsfocus.com, http://www.nutritionnewsfocus.com/. Ed. Dr. David Klurfeld. Adv. contact Ken Deifik.

NUTRITION NEWS IN ZAMBIA. see *FOOD AND FOOD INDUSTRIES*

613.2 USA ISSN 8756-5919
NUTRITION NEWS (RIVERSIDE). Text in English. 1976. m. USD 18 domestic; USD 22 in Canada & Mexico; USD 29 elsewhere (effective 2001). bk.rev. back issues avail. **Document type:** *Newsletter.* **Description:** Reviews health and nutrition related topics, primarily on dietary, herbal and vitamin supplements, for a general audience.
Published by: Nutrition News, 4108 Watkins Dr, Riverside, CA 92507-4701. TEL 909-784-7500, FAX 909-784-7555, nutenews@earthlink.net. Ed., R&P Siri Khalsa. Pub. Gurumantra Khalsa. Circ: 50,000 (paid).

613.2 USA
NUTRITION NOTES. Text in English. 1965. q. USD 30. back issues avail. **Document type:** *Newsletter.* **Description:** Information on awards, publications, reports, meetings; updates readers (nutrition scientists) on legislation.
Published by: American Institute of Nutrition, 9650 Rockville Pike, Bethesda, MD 20814. TEL 301-530-7050, FAX 301-571-1892. Ed. Carolyn Berdanier. Circ: 2,750.

612.3 USA ISSN 0740-8684
NUTRITION REPORT✶. Text in English. 1983. m. USD 54. abstr, bibl. **Document type:** *Newsletter.* **Description:** Provides concise summaries of recently published scientific research on vitamins and minerals.
Published by: Health Media Communications, PO Box 17630, San Diego, CA 92177-7630. TEL 619-688-0377, FAX 619-688-9370. Ed. Andrea Harrison. Circ: 4,000.

613.2 USA ISSN 0271-5317
QP141.A1 CODEN: NTRSDC
NUTRITION RESEARCH; the international medium for rapid publication of communications in the nutritional sciences . Text in English. 1981. 122/yr. EUR 246 in Europe to individuals; JPY 32,700 in Japan to individuals; USD 274 elsewhere to individuals; EUR 1,090 in Europe to institutions; JPY 144,800 in Japan to institutions; USD 1,220 elsewhere to institutions (effective 2002). adv. bk.rev. illus. index. back issues avail.; reprints avail. *Refereed.* **Document type:** *Academic/Scholarly.* **Description:** Reports on basic and applied research on all aspects of food and nutrition, including relevant topics from the social sciences.
Incorporates (1975-1993): Progress in Food and Nutrition Science (0306-0632); Which was formerly: International Encyclopedia of Food and Nutrition (0074-4700)
Related titles: Microfilm ed.: (from PQC); Online - full text ed.: (from ingenta, ScienceDirect, Swets Blackwell, Institute for Scientific Information).
Indexed: ASCA, Abstr.Hyg., Agricola, Bibl.Agri., Biol.& Agr.Ind. (Sep.1989-), Biol.Abstr., Chem.Abstr., Chem.Titles, Curr.Adv.Ecol.Sci., Curr.Cont., Dairy Sci.Abstr., Diar.Dis.Res., Energy Ind., Energy Info.Abstr., Environ.Sci.Poll.Mgmt., Excerp.Med., Food Sci.& Tech.Abstr., Forest Prod.Abstr., Ind.Med. (coverage dropped), Ind.Sci.Rev., Ind.Vet., Inpharma, Int.Abstr.Biol.Sci., Maize Abstr., NRN, Nutr.Abstr., Pharm.&Out.News, Pig News & Info., Poult.Abstr., Protozool.Abstr., Reac., Rev.Appl.Entomol., Rev.Arom.& Med.Plants, Rice Abstr., SSCI (coverage dropped), Saf.Sci.Abstr., Sci.Cit.Ind., Soyabean Abstr., Sugar Ind.Abstr., Triticale Abstr., Trop.Dis.Bull., Trop.Oil Seeds Abstr., Vet.Bull.
—BLDSC (6188.950000), CASDDS, CISTI, EMDOCS, GNLM, IDS, Infotrieve, ingenta. **CCC.**
Published by: Elsevier Science, 655 Ave of the Americas, New York, NY 10010. FAX 212-633-3990, usinfo-f@elsevier.com, http://www.elsevier.com/locate/nutres. Ed. Ranjit K Chandra. Adv. contact Hank Blaney. B&W page USD 985, color page USD 2,160. Circ: 580 (paid). **Subscr. in Australasia and the Far East to:** Elsevier Science (Singapore) Pte Ltd, No.1 Temasek Ave, 17-01 Millenia Tower, Singapore 039192, Singapore. TEL 65-434-3727, FAX 65-337-2230; **Subscr. in Japan to:** Elsevier Science Inc - Japan Regional Office, 9-15 Higashi-Azabu 1-chome, Minato-ku, Tokyo 106-0044, Japan. TEL 81-3-5561-5033; **Subscr. outside the Americas to:** Elsevier Science BV, PO Box 211, Amsterdam 1000 AE, Netherlands. TEL 31-20-485-3757.

613.2 USA ISSN 0736-0037
CODEN: GTNEEA
NUTRITION RESEARCH NEWSLETTER; a monthly update for food, nutrition, and health professionals. Text in English. 1983. m. USD 149 in North America to institutions; USD 169 elsewhere to institutions (effective 2001). abstr. index. reprint service avail. from ISI. **Document type:** *Newsletter, Abstract/Index.* **Description:** Presents an overview of all aspects of nutrition. Aims to provide a broad-based knowledge of the role that food and food supplements can play in health.
Incorporates (1981-1998): Food Safety Notebook (1050-1843)
Related titles: Online - full text ed.: (from Northern Light Technology, Inc., Gale Group, Factiva).
—CASDDS, CISTI.
Published by: Technical Insights (Subsidiary of: John Wiley & Sons, Inc., Journals), 605 3rd Ave, New York, NY 10158-0012. TEL 212-850-8600, FAX 212-850-8800, insights@wiley.com, http://www.wiley.com/technical_insights. Circ: 1,100.

612.3 GBR ISSN 0954-4224
QP141.A1 CODEN: NREREX
NUTRITION RESEARCH REVIEWS. Text in English. 1988. s-a. GBP 120 to institutions; USD 215 in the Americas to institutions; GBP 130 to institutions includes single-site online access; USD 230 in the Americas to institutions includes single-site online access (effective 2002). adv. back issues avail. *Refereed.* **Document type:** *Academic/Scholarly.* **Description:** Reviews research on a variety of nutritional problems.
Related titles: Microform ed.: (from PQC); Online - full text ed.: GBP 110, USD 195 to institutions (effective 2002) (from EBSCO Publishing, H. W. Wilson, RoweCom Information Quest, ingenta, Swets Blackwell, Institute for Scientific Information); ♦ Supplement to: The British Journal of Nutrition. ISSN 0007-1145.
Indexed: Agricola, Biol.& Agr.Ind. (Jan.1996-), Chem.Abstr., Chem.Indus.Notes, Chem.Titles, Curr.Cont., Dairy Sci.Abstr., Environ.Per.Bibl. (1990-1994), Ind.Vet., Nutr.Abstr., Pig News & Info., Poult.Abstr., Rev.Arom.& Med.Plants, Rural Devel.Abstr., Sci.Cit.Ind., Soyabean Abstr., Sugar Ind.Abstr.
—BLDSC (6188.975000), CASDDS, CISTI, GNLM, IDS, Infotrieve, ingenta, KNAW, Linda Hall. **CCC.**
Published by: (Nutrition Society), CABI Publishing, Wallingford, Oxon OX10 8DE, United Kingdom. TEL 44-1491-832111, FAX 44 1491 826 090, publishing@cabi.org, http://www.cabi.org/Publishing/Products/Journals/Primary/NRR/Index.asp, http://www.ingenta.com. Ed. M I Gurr. Adv. contact S Harris. B&W page GBP 550; 135 x 205. **N. American subscr. to:** 10 E 40th St, Ste 3203, New York, NY 10016. TEL 212-481-7018, 800-528-4841, FAX 212-686-7993, cabi-nao@cabi.org.

613.2 CAN
NUTRITION RESOURCES BULLETIN. Text in English. 1996. bi-m. **Description:** Covers normal nutrition such as healthy eating, life cycle nutrition, sports nutrition, vegetarianism, and cultural and ethnic resources; medical nutrition, including special diets; quantity food preparation; food service management; food safety; food science and food security.
Media: Online - full content.
Published by: Simon Fraser University, School of Kinesiology, Burnaby, BC V5A 1S6, Canada. http://www.sfu.ca/~jfremont/resbul.html.

NUTRITION REVIEW. see *MEDICAL SCIENCES*

612.3 USA ISSN 0029-6643
TX341 CODEN: NUREA8
NUTRITION REVIEWS. Text in English. 1942. m. USD 185 in North America to institutions; USD 220 elsewhere to institutions (effective 2001). adv. bk.rev. abstr. bibl. illus. index. back issues avail.; reprint service avail. from PQC. *Refereed.* **Document type:** *Academic/Scholarly.* **Description:** International journal of authoritative and critical reviews of significant developments in all areas of nutrition science and policy.
Related titles: Microfilm ed.: (from PQC); Online - full text ed.: (from ProQuest Information & Learning, Ovid Technologies, Inc., Northern Light Technology, Inc., Gale Group, Factiva, Institute for Scientific Information).
Indexed: ASCA, Abstr.Hyg., Acad.Ind., AgBiotech, Agricola, Aqua.Sci.& Fish.Abstr., Bibl.Agri., Biol.& Agr.Ind. (Jan.1983-), Biol.Abstr., CINAHL, Cadscan, Chem.Abstr., Crop Physiol.Abstr., Curr.Adv.Biochem., Curr.Adv.Ecol.Sci., Curr.Cont., Dairy Sci.Abstr., Dent.Ind., Diar.Dis.Res., Environ.Per.Bibl., Environ.Sci.Poll.Mgmt., Excerp.Med., Field Crop Abstr., Food Sci.& Tech.Abstr., Gen.Sci.Ind. (Sep.1983-), Helminthol.Abstr., Hlth.Ind., INIS Atomind., Ind.Med. (1942-), Ind.Sci.Rev., Ind.Vet., Inpharma, Int.Abstr.Biol.Sci., Lead Abstr., Maize Abstr., NRN, Nutr.Abstr., Pharm.&Out.News, Plant Breed.Abstr., Pollut.Abstr., Protozool.Abstr., Reac., Rev.Med.& Vet.Mycol., Rev.Plant Path., Rice Abstr., Risk Abstr., Rural Devel.Abstr., SSCI (coverage dropped), Saf.Sci.Abstr., Sci.Cit.Ind., Soyabean Abstr., Trop.Dis.Bull., Vet.Bull., World Ag.Econ.& Rur.Soc.Abstr.
—BLDSC (6189.000000), CASDDS, CISTI, GNLM, IDS, ingenta, Linda Hall. **CCC.**
Published by: International Life Sciences Institute, 1126 16th St N W, 110, Washington, DC 20036-4810. TEL 202-659-0074, FAX 202-659-8654, ilsi@allenpress.com, http://www.ilsi.org. Ed. Dr. Irwin H Rosenberg. R&P Joe Albrecht. Circ: 4,400. **Subscr. to:** Allen Press Inc., PO Box 7055, Lawrence, KS 66044-7055. ilsi@allenpress.com, http:/www.ilsi.org.

613.2 USA
NUTRITION SCIENCE NEWS. Text in English. m. USD 79 domestic; USD 91 in Canada; USD 106 elsewhere (effective 2001). **Document type:** *Magazine, Trade.* **Description:** Comprehensive information resource on vitamins, minerals, herbs, homeopathy, nutraceuticals, and other supplements.
Related titles: Online - full text ed.
Published by: New Hope Natural Media (Subsidiary of: Penton Media, Inc.), 1401 Pearl St, Boulder, CO 80302. TEL 303-939-8440, FAX 303-473-0519, sales@newhope.com, http://www.nutritionsciencenews.com/.

613.2 NLD ISSN 0924-4557
CODEN: NUTSDT
NUTRITION SCIENCES. Text in English. 1982. irreg. price varies. **Document type:** *Monographic series.*
—BLDSC.
Published by: Kluwer Academic Publishers Group (Subsidiary of: Wolters Kluwer N.V.), Spuiboulevard 50, PO Box 17, Dordrecht 3300 AA, Netherlands. FAX 31-78-639-2254, services@wkap.nl, http://www.wkap.nl. **Dist. by:** Journals Department, PO Box 322, Dordrecht 3300 AH, Netherlands. FAX 31-78-654-6474.

613.2 AUS ISSN 0314-1004
CODEN: PNSADB
NUTRITION SOCIETY OF AUSTRALIA. PROCEEDINGS. Text in English. 1976. a. AUD 55 in Australia & New Zealand; AUD 60 elsewhere (effective 1999). index. back issues avail. **Document type:** *Proceedings.*
Indexed: Agricola, Anim.Breed.Abstr., Biol.Abstr., Chem.Abstr., Chem.Indus.Notes, Chem.Titles, Curr.Cont. (coverage dropped), Dairy Sci.Abstr., Food Sci.& Tech.Abstr., Ind.Vet., Nutr.Abstr., Postharvest, Rev.Med.& Vet.Mycol., Rice Abstr., Soyabean Abstr., Sugar Ind.Abstr., Triticale Abstr.
—BLDSC (6779.400000), CASDDS, CISTI, GNLM, KNAW, Linda Hall.
Published by: Nutrition Society of Australia, 13 Jeffrey St, Mount Waverley, VIC 3149, Australia. TEL 09-368-3365, FAX 09-474-1881, ca@netwide.com.au. Ed. J R Mercer. Circ: 1,000.

613.2 IND ISSN 0253-7567
NUTRITION SOCIETY OF INDIA. PROCEEDINGS. Text in English. 1967. a. (in 46 vols.), latest vol.46. INR 150, USD 7 (effective 2001). back issues avail. **Document type:** *Proceedings.*
Indexed: Agroforest.Abstr., Nutr.Abstr., Rice Abstr., Soyabean Abstr., Trop.Oil Seeds Abstr.
—BLDSC (6779.600000), CISTI.
Published by: Nutrition Society of India, c/o National Institute of Nutrition, Jamai Osmania P.O., Hyderabad, Andhra Pradesh 500 007, India. TEL 91-40-7018909, FAX 91-40-7019074, icmrnin@ren.nic.in; nsihyderabad@yahoo.com. Circ: 1,500.

613.2 GBR ISSN 0029-6651
TX501 CODEN: PNUSA4
NUTRITION SOCIETY. PROCEEDINGS. Text in English. 1941. bi-m. GBP 295 to institutions; USD 495 in the Americas to institutions; GBP 310 to institutions includes single-site online access; USD 520 in the Americas to institutions includes single-site online access (effective 2002). abstr, bibl, charts. index. back issues avail. *Refereed.* **Document type:** *Proceedings.* **Description:** Publishes papers presented by invitation at symposia of the society, and abstracts of original communications presented at other meetings.
Related titles: Microform ed.: (from PQC,PMC,SWZ); Online - full text ed.: GBP 285 to institutions; USD 480 in the Americas to institutions (effective 2002) (from EBSCO Publishing, RoweCom Information Quest, ingenta, Swets Blackwell, Institute for Scientific Information).
Indexed: ASCA, Abstr.Hyg., AgBiotech, Agri.& Environ.Biotech.Abstr. (coverage dropped), Agricola, Anim.Breed.Abstr., Bibl.Agri., Biol.& Agr.Ind. (Jan.1983-Jan.1989), Biol.Abstr., CINAHL, Cadscan, Chem.Abstr., Chem.Indus.Notes, Chem.Titles, Curr.Adv.Ecol.Sci., Curr.Cont., Dairy Sci.Abstr., Derwent Biotech.Abstr., Diar.Dis.Res., Energy Ind., Energy Info.Abstr., Field Crop Abstr., Food Sci.& Tech.Abstr., Helminthol.Abstr., Herb.Abstr., INIS Atomind., Ind.Med. (1944-), Ind.Sci.Rev., Ind.Vet., Inpharma, Lead Abstr., NRN, Nutr.Abstr., Pharm.&Out.News, Poult.Abstr., Reac., Rev.Appl.Entomol., Risk Abstr., Rural Recreat.Tour.Abstr., SSCI (coverage dropped), Sci.Cit.Ind., Triticale Abstr., Trop.Dis.Bull., Vet.Bull., World Ag.Econ.& Rur.Soc.Abstr., Zincscan.
—BLDSC (6780.000000), CASDDS, CISTI, GNLM, IDS, ingenta, Linda Hall. **CCC.**
Published by: (Nutrition Society), CABI Publishing, Wallingford, Oxon OX10 8DE, United Kingdom. TEL 44-1491-832111, FAX 44-1491-829198, publishing@cabi.org, http://www.cabi.org/Publishing/Products/Journals/Primary/PNS/Index.asp. **U.S. subscr. to:** 10 E 40th St, Ste 3203, New York, NY 10016. TEL 212-481-7018, 800-528-4841, FAX 212-686-7993, cabi-nao@cabi.org.

613.2 USA ISSN 0029-666X
RA784
NUTRITION TODAY. Text in English. 1985. bi-m., latest vol.36. USD 67 domestic to individuals; USD 97 foreign to individuals; USD 157 domestic to institutions; USD 197 foreign to institutions; USD 33 newsstand/cover (effective 2002). adv. bk.rev. illus. index. reprints avail. **Document type:** *Journal, Academic/Scholarly.* **Description:** Presents articles on developments in nutrition for dieticians, nutritionists, and physicians.
Related titles: Microfilm ed.: (from WWS); Online - full text ed.: USD 204.10 domestic for academic site license; USD 244.10 foreign for academic site license; USD 227.65 domestic for corporate site license; USD 267.65 foreign for corporate site license (effective 2002) (from Gale Group, Northern Light Technology, Inc., H. W. Wilson, Factiva).

N

Indexed: A.S.& T.Ind. (Sep.1983-), Agricola, Bibl.Agri., Biol.Abstr., CHNI, Curr.Cont. (coverage dropped), Dairy Sci.Abstr., Environ.Per.Bibl. (1991-), Fam.Ind., Food Sci.& Tech.Abstr., Gen.Sci.Ind. (Mar.1984-), Hlth.Ind., NRN, Nutr.Abstr.
—BLDSC (6190.100000), CISTI, GNLM, ingenta, Linda Hall.
Published by: Lippincott Williams & Wilkins (Philadelphia) (Subsidiary of: Wolters Kluwer N.V.), 530 Walnut St, Philadelphia, PA 19106-3621. TEL 215-521-8300, FAX 215-521-8902, cvalton@wwilkins.com, custserv@lww.com, http://www.wwilkins.com/productdetailresults/1,2265,53238582,00.html, http://www.lww.com/. Ed. Helen Guthrie. Adv. contact Christophe Valton. Circ: 4,780.

613.2 USA ISSN 0736-0096
NUTRITION WEEK. Text in English. 1970. w. (48/yr.). USD 85. bk.rev. bibl. index. **Document type:** *Newsletter.* **Description:** Offers an independent up-to-date examination of events in food and nutrition policy, be they specific reports on congressional action, or in-depth analyses about the trends shaping nutrition policymaking.
Former titles: C N I Weekly Report (0191-0833); C N I Report
Indexed: Bibl.Agri.
Published by: Community Nutrition Institute, 910 17th St N W, No 413, Washington, DC 20006. TEL 202-776-0595, FAX 202-776-0599, cni@unidial.com. Ed., R&P Pam Muha. Pub. Rodney E Leonard. Circ: 2,000.

NUTRITIONAL ANTHROPOLOGY. see *ANTHROPOLOGY*

▼ **NUTRITIONAL NEUROSCIENCE**; an international journal of diet, nutrition and the nervous system. see *MEDICAL SCIENCES—Psychiatry And Neurology*

613.2 JAM ISSN 0255-8203
TX360.C35
NYAM NEWS. Text in English. 1975. m. free per issue. **Document type:** *Newsletter.* **Description:** Feature service directed mainly at students, teachers and the mass media in the English-speaking Caribbean, giving sample information on topical and pertinent food and nutrition issues.
Indexed: Nutr.Abstr.
Published by: Caribbean Food and Nutrition Institute, University of the West Indies, U.W.I. Mona Campus, PO Box 140, Kingston 7, Jamaica. TEL 876-927-1540-1, FAX 876-927-1927. Ed. Clare A Forrester. R&P Clare Forrester. Circ: 700. **Co-sponsor:** Pan American Health Organization, World Health Organization.

613.26 JPN ISSN 0910-7258
NYU DAIETTO SERAPI/NEW DIET THERAPY. Text in Japanese. 1985. q. JPY 1,400 per issue.
Published by: Nihon Rinsho Eiyo Kyokai/Japanese Clinical Nutrition Association, Toho Daigaku Igakubu Fuzoku Omori Byoin Eiyobu, 11-1 Omori-Nishi 6-chome, Ota-ku, Tokyo 143-0015, Japan.

613.25 GBR ISSN 1462-1819
OBESITY MATTERS. Text in English. 1998. 2/yr. GBP 25 domestic; GBP 42.50 foreign; GBP 15 newsstand/cover. adv. bk.rev. tr.lit. back issues avail. *Refereed.* **Document type:** *Academic/Scholarly.* **Description:** Contains research results and activities involved in the study of obesity and its causes.
Published by: (European Association for the Study of Obesity), Mediscript Ltd., 1 Mountview Ct, 310 Friern Barnet Ln, London N20 0LD, United Kingdom. TEL 44-20-8446-8898, FAX 44-20-8446-9194, 101607.3205@compuserve.com. Ed., R&P, Adv. contact Linda Lazarus. Pub. Fatima Patel.

613.2 GBR ISSN 1467-7881
▼ **OBESITY REVIEWS.** Text in English. 2000. q., latest vol.3, 2002. GBP 63 in Europe to individuals; USD 100 in North America to individuals; GBP 69 elsewhere to individuals; GBP 163 in Europe to institutions; USD 258 in North America to institutions; GBP 179 elsewhere to institutions (effective 2002). adv. *Refereed.* **Document type:** *Journal, Academic/Scholarly.* **Description:** Provides a forum for publishing updated reviews in all disciplines related to obesity.
Related titles: ♦ Online - full text ed.: Obesity Reviews Online. ISSN 1467-789X.
—BLDSC (6196.952700).
Published by: Blackwell Science Ltd., PO Box 88, Oxford OX2 0NE, United Kingdom. TEL 44-1865-206180, 44-1865-206002, FAX 44-1865-206219, jnl.orders@blacksci.co.uk, http://www.blackwell-science.com/obr, http://www.blackwellpublishing.com. R&P Sophie Savage. Adv. contact Jenny Applin.

613.2 GBR ISSN 1467-789X
▼ **OBESITY REVIEWS ONLINE.** Text in English. 2000. q. GBP 57 in Europe to individuals; USD 90 in North America to individuals; GBP 57 elsewhere to individuals; GBP 147 in Europe to institutions; USD 233 in North America to institutions; GBP 147 elsewhere to institutions (effective 2002). *Refereed.* **Document type:** *Academic/Scholarly.*
Media: Online - full text (from EBSCO Publishing, O C L C Online Computer Library Center, Inc., ingenta, Munksgaard & Blackwell Science's Synergy, Swets Blackwell, RoweCom Information Quest). **Related titles:** ♦ Print ed.: Obesity Reviews. ISSN 1467-7881.
Published by: Blackwell Science Ltd., Osney Mead, Oxford OX2 0EL, United Kingdom. TEL 44-1685-206206, FAX 44-1685-721205, website@blacksci.com, journals.cs@blacksci.co.uk, http://www.blackwell-science.com/~cgilib/jnlpage.bin?Journal=obr&File=obr&Page=aims.

THE OILY PRESS LIPID LIBRARY. see *BIOLOGY—Biochemistry*

ONTARIO WRESTLER MAGAZINE. see *SPORTS AND GAMES*

613.2 USA ISSN 0195-0924
ORGANIC CONSUMER REPORT. Text in English. w. USD 5. bk.rev.
—CCC.
Published by: Eden Ranch, PO Box 370, Topanga, CA 90290. TEL 213-455-2065. Ed. Judith Eagan. Circ: (controlled).

612.3 CAN
ORGANIC LIVING. Text in English. 1997 (Dec.). bi-m. free. **Document type:** *Newsletter.*
Media: Online - full text.
Published by: Pro Organics Marketing Inc., 4535 Still Creek Ave., Burnaby, BC V5C 5V1, Canada. sboyle@proorganics.com, http://www.proorganics.com/newsletter/. Ed. Steve Boyle.

612.3 NLD ISSN 0920-9166
DE ORTHOMOLECULAIRE KOERIER; Nederlands - Vlaams tijdschrift voor nutritionele geneeskunde. Text and summaries in Dutch. 1986. bi-m. NLG 64.80; NLG 85.80 foreign. adv. back issues avail. **Document type:** *Bulletin.* **Description:** Covers orthomolecular medicine and nutrition, micronutrients and food supplementation.
—KNAW.
Published by: Orthos Media B.V., Antwerpsestraat 1 A, The Hague 2587 AE, Netherlands. TEL 31-70-358-5673, FAX 31-70-358-7504, http://www.soe.nl. Ed. W Diekstra. Pub. R Nieuwenhuis. R&P R. Nieuwenhuis. Adv. contact R van den Ent. B&W page NLG 1,100, color page NLG 2,050; trim 265 x 185. Circ: 2,250.

613.2 USA ISSN 0748-8394
OUTPOST EXCHANGE; Milwaukee's food and wellness magazine. Text in English. 1971. m. USD 12. adv. bk.rev. **Document type:** *Consumer.*
Published by: (Outpost Natural Foods), Outpost Exchange, 204 E Capitol Dr, Milwaukee, WI 53212. TEL 414-964-7789, FAX 414-964-0317, exchange@execpc.com. Ed. Malcolm Woods. R&P Kristine Lorentzsen. Adv. contact Margee Foolke. B&W page USD 360. Circ: 20,000; 4,800 (paid).

613.2 USA
P C C SOUND CONSUMER. Text in English. 1974. m. USD 12 to non-members (effective 1999). adv. bk.rev. illus. back issues avail. **Document type:** *Newsletter.*
Formerly: Puget Consumers Co-op Newsletter
Published by: Puget Consumers Co-op, 4201 Roosevelt Way, N E, Seattle, WA 98105-6008. TEL 206-547-1222, FAX 206-545-7131, http://www.pugetcoop.com. Ed. Kim Runciman. Adv. contact Nancy Gagnat. Circ: 36,000.

613.26 NCL ISSN 1023-9197
PACIFIC DIET ADVISORY LEAFLET. Text in English. 1995. irreg., latest vol.8, 1995. **Document type:** *Monographic series.*
Related titles: French ed.: Fiches Techniques sur l'Alimentation et la Sante dans le Pacifique.
Published by: Secretariat of the Pacific Community, PO Box D5, Noumea Cedex 98848, New Caledonia. TEL 687-262000, FAX 687-263818, spc@spc.int, http://www.spc.int.

612.3 NCL ISSN 1022-2782
PACIFIC ISLANDS NUTRITION. Text in English. 1989. q. **Document type:** *Newsletter.*
Related titles: French ed.: Nutrition en Oceanie. ISSN 1022-2790.
Published by: Secretariat of the Pacific Community, PO Box D5, Noumea Cedex 98848, New Caledonia. TEL 687-262000, FAX 687-263818, spc@spc.int, http://www.spc.int.

PERSONAL CARE NEWS. see *PHYSICAL FITNESS AND HYGIENE*

PERSONAL FITNESS. see *PHYSICAL FITNESS AND HYGIENE*

PHARMA UND FOOD; Hygiene - Produktion - Ausruestung. see *PHARMACY AND PHARMACOLOGY*

613.2 PHL ISSN 0031-7640
TX501 CODEN: PJNUAF
PHILIPPINE JOURNAL OF NUTRITION. Text in English. 1949. q. USD 12. adv. bk.rev. abstr, charts, illus. index. reprint service avail. from PQC.
Formerly: Nutrition News
Related titles: CD-ROM ed.; Microform ed.: (from PQC).
Indexed: Biol.Abstr., Chem.Abstr., Dairy Sci.Abstr., ExtraMED, Food Sci.& Tech.Abstr., Nutr.Abstr., Philip.Abstr., Rural Recreat.Tour.Abstr., World Ag.Econ.& Rur.Soc.Abstr.
—BLDSC (6188.458000), CASDDS, CISTI, GNLM.
Published by: Philippine Association of Nutrition, c/o Nutrition Foundation of the, 107 E. Rodriguez., Sr. Blvd., Quezon City, Philippines. Ed. Velona A Corpus. Circ: 2,000.

613.2 PHL
PHILIPPINES. FOOD AND NUTRITION RESEARCH INSTITUTE. ANNUAL REPORT. Text in English. 1950. a. **Document type:** *Corporate, Academic/Scholarly.* **Description:** Offers a detailed compilation of the institute's various projects and activities. Includes completed research, research in progress, public services, staff papers and publications, staff development, cooperative activities, foreign visitors, financial resources, and technical staff.
Formerly: Philippines. Food and Nutrition Research Center. Annual Report (0071-7142)
Published by: Food and Nutrition Research Institute, Science Complex, Bicutan, Tagiug Mm 1631, Philippines. TEL 63-2-837-2071, FAX 63-2-837-2934. Ed., R&P Catherine Q Castaneda TEL 837-81-13. Circ: (controlled).

PHYSICAL. see *PHYSICAL FITNESS AND HYGIENE*

613.2 USA
PLANETARY HEALTH. Text in English. 1989. 4/yr. USD 30 to individuals; USD 50 families (effective 2000). adv. bk.rev. **Document type:** *Magazine.*
Former titles: One Peaceful World; Return to Paradise
Published by: One Peaceful World, Inc., PO Box 10, Becket, MA 01223. TEL 413-623-2322, FAX 413-623-6042, opw@macrobiotics.org, http://www.macrobiotics.org. Ed., Pub., R&P Alex Jack. Adv. contact Laura Wepman. Circ: 10,000.

612.3 NLD ISSN 0921-9668
TX341 CODEN: PFHNE8
PLANT FOODS FOR HUMAN NUTRITION. Text in English. 1952. q. EUR 432 to institutions for print or online ed. (effective 2001); EUR 518.40 to institutions print & online eds.combined (effective 2002). adv. bk.rev. bibl, charts, illus. reprint service avail. from SWZ. *Refereed.* **Document type:** *Academic/Scholarly.* **Description:** Publishes reports of original research concerned with the improvement and evaluation of the nutritional quality of plant foods for humans, as they are influenced by biotechnology, plant breeding, cooking and processing, plant and soil ecology, and plant production practices.
Former titles (until 1987): Qualitas Plantarum (0377-3205); (until 1973): Qualitas Plantarum et Materiae Vegetabiles (0033-5134)
Related titles: Microform ed.: (from PQC); Online - full text ed.: (from EBSCO Publishing, O C L C Online Computer Library Center, Inc., RoweCom Information Quest, Swets Blackwell, Kluwer Online, Institute for Scientific Information).
Indexed: ASCA, Agricola, Agroforest.Abstr., Bibl.Agri., Biol.Abstr., Chem.Abstr., Chem.Indus.Notes, Chem.Titles, Curr.Adv.Biochem., Curr.Adv.Ecol.Sci., Curr.Adv.Plant Sci., Curr.Cont., Dairy Sci.Abstr., Excerp.Med., Field Crop Abstr., Food Sci.& Tech.Abstr., Forest.Abstr., Herb.Abstr., Hort.Abstr., INIS Atomind., I.P.A., Ind.Med. (1987-), Int.Abstr.Biol.Sci., Maize Abstr., Nutr.Abstr., Plant Breed.Abstr., Plant Grow.Reg.Abstr., Plant Sci., Postharvest, Potato Abstr., Poult.Abstr., Rev.Appl.Entomol., Rev.Plant Path., Rice Abstr., SSCI (coverage dropped), Seed Abstr., Soils & Fert., Soyabean Abstr., Sugar Ind.Abstr., Triticale Abstr., Trop.Dis.Bull., Trop.Oil Seeds Abstr., VITIS.

—BLDSC (6517.500000), CASDDS, CISTI, EMDOCS, GNLM, IDS, Infotrieve, ingenta, Linda Hall. **CCC.**
Published by: Kluwer Academic Publishers Group (Subsidiary of: Wolters Kluwer N.V.), Spuiboulevard 50, PO Box 17, Dordrecht 3300 AA, Netherlands. FAX 31-78-639-2254, services@wkap.nl, http://www.wkap.nl. Ed. H A Bock. **Dist. by:** Journals Department, PO Box 322, Dordrecht 3300 AH, Netherlands. TEL 781-871-6600, FAX 31-78-654-6474.

613.2 664 GBR
POSITIVE EATING. Text in English. biennial, latest 1995. GBP 1,250. **Document type:** *Trade.* **Description:** Investigates the role food plays in modern lifestyles and studies the interface between food, health and nutrition.
Published by: Seymour - Cooke Ltd. Food Research International, 42 Colebrooke Row, London N1 8AF, United Kingdom. TEL 44-171-704-9951, FAX 44-171-226-5298.

POSITIVE HEALTH; integrated medicine for the 21st century. see *PHYSICAL FITNESS AND HYGIENE*

POTRAVINARSKE AKTUALITY. VYZIVA A LEGISLATIVA. see *FOOD AND FOOD INDUSTRIES*

PROFESSIONEALLEVATORE. see *AGRICULTURE—Poultry And Livestock*

613.2 GBR ISSN 1368-9800
CODEN: PHNUF6
PUBLIC HEALTH NUTRITION. Text in English. 1998. q. GBP 275 to institutions; USD 480 in the Americas to institutions; GBP 285 to institutions includes online access; USD 500 in the Americas to institutions includes online access (effective 2002). adv. *Refereed.* **Document type:** *Academic/Scholarly.*
Related titles: Online - full text ed.: GBP 265, USD 465 to institutions (effective 2002) (from EBSCO Publishing, RoweCom Information Quest, ingenta, Swets Blackwell).
Indexed: Agricola, Dairy Sci.Abstr., Food Sci.& Tech.Abstr., Ind.Med. (1998-), Nutr.Abstr., Rev.Arom.& Med.Plants, Soyabean Abstr., Trop.Dis.Bull., Weed Abstr., World Ag.Econ.& Rur.Soc.Abstr.
—BLDSC (6964.770000), ingenta.
Published by: (Nutrition Society), CABI Publishing, Wallingford, Oxon OX10 8DE, United Kingdom. TEL 44-1491-832111, 212-686-7993, FAX 44-1491-829198, publishing@cabi.org, http://www.cabi.org/Publishing/Products/Journals/Primary/PHN/Index.asp. Adv. contact S Harris. B&W page GBP 550; 170 x 240. Circ: 250. **U.S. subscr. to:** 10 E 40th St, Ste 3203, New York, NY 10016. TEL 212-481-7018, 800-528-4841, FAX 212-686-7993, cabi-nao@cabi.org.

613.2 CHL ISSN 0716-1549
REVISTA CHILENA DE NUTRICION. Text in Spanish. 1980. 3/yr.
Supersedes (1961-1968): Nutricion, Bromatologia y Toxicologia (0550-4023)
Indexed: Food Sci.& Tech.Abstr.
—BLDSC (7848.910000).
Published by: Sociedad Chilena de Nutricion Bromatologia y Toxicologia, Universidad de Chile, Fac. de Medicina Depto. Nutricion, Independencia, 1027, Santiago, Chile. Ed. Hector Araya.

613.2 CUB ISSN 0864-2133
REVISTA CUBANA DE ALIMENTACION Y NUTRICION. Text in Spanish; Summaries in English, Spanish. 1987. s-a. USD 30 in North America; USD 38 in Europe; USD 46 elsewhere. **Description:** Covers nutrition and food hygiene.
Published by: (Cuba. Ministerio de Salud Publica, Centro Nacional de Informacion de Ciencias Medicas), Editorial de Ciencias Medicas, O'Reilly No. 4, Habana, Cuba. TEL 62-8091, FAX 338187. Ed. Ana Dolores del Campo. Circ: 1,000. **Co-sponsors:** Instituto Nacional de Alimentacion y Nutricion; Sociedad Cubana de Alimentacion y Nutricion.

REVISTA DE INVESTIGACION CLINICA. see *MEDICAL SCIENCES*

363.8 BRA ISSN 1415-5273
REVISTA DE NUTRICAO. Text in Portuguese, English, Spanish; Summaries in Portuguese, English, Spanish. 1988. 3/yr., latest vol.14, 2001. BRL 40 domestic; BRL 40 foreign (effective 2001). bk.rev. abstr. 95 p./no. back issues avail. *Refereed.* **Document type:** *Magazine, Academic/Scholarly.* **Description:** Publishes research and works that deal with the study and development of nutritional science for academics and professionals.
Supersedes (in 1998): Revista de Nutricao da PUCCAMP (0103-1627)
Related titles: E-mail ed.; Fax ed.
Indexed: Dairy Sci.Abstr., Nutr.Abstr., Triticale Abstr., Trop.Dis.Bull.
Published by: Pontificia Universidade Catolica de Campinas, Faculdade de Ciencias Medicas, Av. John Boyd Dunlop, s/n, Bloco C, Jd. Ipaussurama, Campinas, SP 13020-904, Brazil. TEL 55-19-37298349, FAX 55-19-37298576, femrev@puc-campinas.br, http://www.puccamp.br. Eds., Pubs. Rosa Wanda Diez Garcia, Semiramis Martins Alvares Domene. Circ: 1,200.

REVUE DE L'INDUSTRIE ALIMENTAIRE. see *FOOD AND FOOD INDUSTRIES*

613.2 ITA ISSN 0393-5582
RIVISTA ITALIANA DI NUTRIZIONE PARENTERALE ED ENTERALE. Text in Italian; Summaries in English. 1983. 4/yr. EUR 52 in Europe to individuals; USD 78 elsewhere to individuals; EUR 67 in Europe to institutions; USD 92 elsewhere to institutions (effective 2001). abstr, bibl, charts, illus. 64 p./no. back issues avail.; reprints avail. **Document type:** *Journal, Academic/Scholarly.*
—BLDSC (7987.442500), EMDOCS, GNLM, KNAW.
Published by: Wichtig Editore s.r.l., Via Friuli, 72, Milan, MI 20135, Italy. TEL 39-02-55195443, FAX 39-02-55195971, info@wichtig-publisher.com. Ed. Dr. Maurizio Muscaritoli. R&P Lucia Steele. Adv. contact Nella Bini. Circ: 1,000 (paid); 1,200 (controlled).

ROSEMARY CONLEY DIET & FITNESS. see *PHYSICAL FITNESS AND HYGIENE*

636.089 GBR ISSN 0952-7222
ROWETT RESEARCH INSTITUTE ANNUAL REPORT. Text in English. 1922. a. free per issue. *Refereed.* **Document type:** *Academic/Scholarly, Corporate.*
Indexed: Nutr.Abstr.
—BLDSC (1416.900000).
Published by: Rowett Research Institute, Greenburn Rd, Bucksburn, Aberdeen AB21 9SB, United Kingdom. TEL 44-1224-712751, FAX 44-1224-715349, enquiries@rri.sari.ac.uk, http://www.rri.sari.ac.uk. Ed. John C Macrae. R&P Hilary Robertson. Circ: 2,000 (controlled).

RUNNING & FITNEWS. see *PHYSICAL FITNESS AND HYGIENE*

613.2 ITA
SALVALINEA/WEIGHT WATCHERS. Text in Italian. 1978. m. ITL 40,000; ITL 64,000 foreign.
Published by: Salvalinea s.r.l., Foro Buonaparte, 51, Milan, MI 20121, Italy. TEL 39-2-86454190, FAX 39-2-86454209. Ed. Fiammetta Fadda. adv.: B&W page ITL 5,870,000, color page ITL 10,565,000. Circ: 75,000.

363.7 USA
SATYA; magazine of vegetarianism, environmentalism, and animal advocacy. Text in English. 1993. m. USD 15. adv. bk.rev. illus. **Description:** Committed to teaching people about compassionate living in New York City. Issues focus on a single topic related to vegetarianism, environmentalism, or animal rights.
Related titles: Online - full text ed.
Published by: Stealth Technologies, Inc., PO Box 138, Prince St Sta, New York, NY 10012. TEL 212-674-0952, FAX 212-598-1856, stealth@interport.net, http://www.montelis.com/satya/. Ed. Martin Rowe. Pub. Beth Gould. R&P Julie Hughes. Adv. contact Linda Scoville. Circ: 20,000.

612.3 SWE ISSN 1102-6480
CODEN: SJNUEI
SCANDINAVIAN JOURNAL OF NUTRITION/NAERINGSFORSKNING. Text in English; Summaries in English. 1957. q. SEK 450; SEK 230 to students (effective 2000). bk.rev. back issues avail. *Refereed.* **Document type:** *Journal, Academic/Scholarly.* **Description:** Directed to present state of the art in the various fields within nutrition. Provides readers with information through original and review articles and reports.
Formerly (until vol.36, 1992): Naeringsforskning (0027-7878)
Related titles: Online - full text ed.; ♦ Supplement: Scandinavian Journal of Nutrition. Supplement. ISSN 1102-6510.
Indexed: Dairy Sci.Abstr., Excerp.Med. (1993-), Food Sci.& Tech.Abstr., Nutr.Abstr., Rev.Appl.Entomol., Sugar Ind.Abstr., Triticale Abstr.
—BLDSC (6015.349000), EMDOCS, GNLM, Linda Hall.
Published by: Swedish Nutrition Foundation, Ideon, Lund 22370, Sweden. TEL 46-46-2862280, FAX 46-46-2862281, info@snf.ideon.se, http://www.snf.ideon.se/sjn/index.htm. Ed. Goesta Samuelson. Circ: 2,500 (controlled).

612.3 SWE ISSN 1102-6510
SCANDINAVIAN JOURNAL OF NUTRITION. SUPPLEMENT. Text in English. 1958. irreg.
Formerly (until 1990): Naringsforskning. Supplement (0346-7104)
Related titles: ♦ Supplement to: Scandinavian Journal of Nutrition. ISSN 1102-6480.
Indexed: Food Sci.& Tech.Abstr., Nutr.Abstr.
—BLDSC (6015.349100), Linda Hall.
Published by: Swedish Nutrition Foundation, Ideon, Lund 22370, Sweden. TEL 46-46-2862280, FAX 46-46-2862281.

613.26 DEU
SCHLANK UND FIT. Text in German. 2/yr. DEM 4.95 newsstand/cover (effective 2000). adv. **Document type:** *Magazine, Consumer.* **Description:** Contains articles on losing weight in a healthy and nutritious manner.
Published by: Marken-Verlag GmbH, Hugo-Junkers-Str 20, Cologne 50739, Germany. TEL 49-221-957427-0, FAX 49-221-95742777, marken-info@markenverlag.de, http://www.markenverlag.de. Adv. contact Frank Krauthaeuser. page DEM 7,500; trim 210 x 285. Circ: 70,000 (paid and controlled).

613.2 DEU ISSN 0931-1068
SCHROT UND KORN. Text in German. m. adv. **Document type:** *Bulletin.*
Published by: Verlag Gesund Essen GmbH, Am Eichwald 24, Schaafheim 64850, Germany. TEL 06073-80057, FAX 06073-9548. Ed. Renee Herrnkind Galuschka. Adv. contact Sabine Kauffmann. Circ: 145,583.

613.2 USA
SEA BREEZE. Text in English. 1977. bi-m. USD 25. bk.rev. **Document type:** *Newsletter.*
Published by: Wachters' Organic Sea Products, 360 Shaw Rd, South San Francisco, CA 94080. FAX 650-875-1626. Circ: 50,000 (controlled).

613.2 JPN ISSN 0286-6366
CODEN: KSTDD5
SEITOKU EIYO TANKI DAIGAKU KIYO/SEITOKU JUNIOR COLLEGE OF NUTRITION. MEMOIRS. Text in English, Japanese. 1965. a.
Indexed: Chem.Abstr., Chem.Indus.Notes, Chem.Titles, Jap.Per.Ind.
—BLDSC (5634.815000), CASDDS.
Published by: Seitoku Eiyo Tanki Daigaku, 4-6 Nishi-Shinkoiwa 1-chome, Katsushika-ku, Tokyo 124-0025, Japan.

SEMEINYI DOKTOR; prakticheskie sovety po meditsine. see *MEDICAL SCIENCES*

613.2 JPN
SHIGAKEN KOSHU EIYO KATSUDO NO GAIYO/ANNUAL REPORT OF PUBLIC NUTRITION IN SHIGA PREFECTURE. Text in Japanese. a. **Document type:** *Government.*
Published by: Shigaken Kenko Fukushibu/Shiga Prefectural Government, Health and Welfare Division, 1-1 Kyomachi 4-chome, Otsu-shi, Shiga-ken 520-0044, Japan.

613.2 CHN
SHIPIN KE-JI/FOOD SCIENCE. Text in Chinese. m. USD 0.40 per issue.
Indexed: Food Sci.& Tech.Abstr.
Published by: China International Book Trading Corp/Zhongguo Guoji Tushu Maoyi Zonggongsi, 35 Chegongzhuang Xilu, Haidian District, Beijing 100044, China. TEL 86-1-68413849, FAX 86-1-68412048, cibtc@mail.cibtc.com.cn, http://www.cibtc.com.cn.

▼ **SIMPLYLITE**; low-fat food - no-fuss fitness. see *PHYSICAL FITNESS AND HYGIENE*

613.2 GBR ISSN 0955-758X
SLIMMER. Text in English. 198?. 10/yr. GBP 15.60 in United Kingdom; GBP 22 newsstand/cover rest of Europe; GBP 27 newsstand/cover in United States; GBP 32 newsstand/cover rest of world; GBP 1.95 newsstand/cover (effective 2000). **Document type:** *Consumer.* **Description:** Provides readers with information on how to achieve and maintain a healthy lifestyle with proper nutrition, exercise and beauty tips.
Published by: Aceville Publications Ltd., Castle House, 97 High St, Colchester, Essex CO1 1TH, United Kingdom. TEL 44-1206-505900, FAX 44-1206-505905, shooting@maze.u-net.com. Circ: 90,000 (paid). **Dist. by:** Seymour, 86 Newman St, London W1P 3EX, United Kingdom. TEL 44-20-7396-8000, FAX 44-20-7396-8002.

N

052 AUS ISSN 1321-8824
SLIMMING. Text in English. 1992. m. **Document type:** *Consumer.*
Formerly (until 1993): Slimming Australia (1321-8840)
Published by: Emap Australia Pty. Ltd. (Subsidiary of: Emap International), 187 Thomas St., Level 6, Haymarket, NSW 2000, Australia. TEL 61-2-9581-9400, FAX 61-2-9331-9570.

613.2 GBR ISSN 0144-8129
SLIMMING. Text in English. 1969. 11/yr. GBP 21.45; GBP 1.95 newsstand/cover (effective 2000). adv. bk.rev. **Document type:** *Magazine, Consumer.* **Description:** Encourages safe and steady weight loss and weight maintenance through healthy eating and an active lifestyle. Provides practical guide to individuals to help them reach and maintain their target weight.
Formerly (until Mar. 1979): Slimming and Nutrition (0049-075X)
Published by: Emap Esprit Ltd. (Subsidiary of: Emap Consumer Magazines Ltd.), Greater London House, Hampstead, London NW1 7EJ, United Kingdom. TEL 44-207-8740200, FAX 44-207-8740570, gill.mond@emap.com, http://www.emap.com. Ed. Juliette Kellow. adv.: B&W page GBP 4,450, color page GBP 4,450; trim 210 x 297. Circ: 98,489. **Subscr. to:** Tower Publishing Services Ltd., Tower House, Sovereign Park, Lathkill St, Market Harborough, Leics LE16 9EF, United Kingdom. TEL 44-1858-435339, FAX 44-1858-432164.

362.176 ZAF ISSN 1011-8578
SOUTH AFRICAN JOURNAL OF CLINICAL NUTRITION. Text in English. 1988. q. USD 20 foreign (effective 2000). back issues avail. *Refereed.* **Document type:** *Journal, Academic/Scholarly.* **Description:** Publishes clinical and experimental research in nutrition.
Indexed: Ind.S.A.Per.
Published by: South African Medical Association, Health and Medical Publishing Group, 14 Central Sq, Pinelands 7430, South Africa. TEL 27-21-531-3081, FAX 27-21-531-4126, annp@samedical.org, publishing@samedical.org, http://www.samedical.org. R&P Peter Roberts. **Subscr. to:** PO Box 74789, Lynnwood Ridge, Pretoria 0040, South Africa. TEL 27-12-481-2010, FAX 27-12-481-2061, ann@samedical.org. **Dist. by:** Private Bag X1, Pinelands 7430, South Africa. TEL 27-21-531-3081, FAX 27-21-531-4126.

SOUTH PACIFIC FOODS LEAFLET. see *FOOD AND FOOD INDUSTRIES*

613.2 JPN ISSN 0919-9535
CODEN: DTKKEE
SOY PROTEIN RESEARCH COMMITTEE. REPORT. Text in Japanese; Summaries in English. 1980. a.
Formerly (until 1993): Nutritional Science of Soy Protein (0288-6219)
Indexed: Chem.Abstr., Field Crop Abstr., Food Sci.& Tech.Abstr., Nutr.Abstr., Plant Breed.Abstr., Rice Abstr., Seed Abstr., Soyabean Abstr., Sugar Ind.Abstr.
—CASDDS.
Published by: Soy Protein Research Committee, c/o Fuji Oil Co, Ltd., 1 Sumiyoshi-cho, Izumisano-shi, Osaka-fu 598-0061, Japan. TEL 0724-63-1120, FAX 0724-0491.

613.2 USA ISSN 1048-8413
SPECIALTY COOKING; cookbook magazine. Text in English. 1989. q. USD 5.99 (effective 2000). **Document type:** *Consumer.* **Description:** Covers diabetic and low-cholesterol cooking and cooking to prevent cancer, heart disease and obesity.
Incorporates: Cookbook Series; Good Cooking Series
Published by: Lifetime Periodicals, Inc., 2131 Hollywood Blvd, Hollywood, FL 33020. TEL 954-925-5242, FAX 954-925-5244, FELLPUB@aol.com, http://www.lifetimebooks.com. Ed. Callie Ruckner. Pub. Donald Lessne. Circ: 65,000.

SPECTRUM (PETERBOROUGH). see *PHYSICAL FITNESS AND HYGIENE*

613.2 USA
SPOTLIGHT ON FOOD. Text in English. 1986. m.
Media: Online - full content.
Address: 604 E Pitkin, Fort Collins, CO 80524. http://linden.fortnet.org/~fivstar/spot.htm. Ed. Kathrynne Holden.

613.26 USA ISSN 0744-9860
SPROUTLETTER. Text in English. 1980. q. USD 12 (effective 2001). adv. bk.rev. charts, illus, tr.lit. cum.index. back issues avail. **Document type:** *Newsletter.* **Description:** Explores nutrition, holistic health, vegetarianism, sprouting, live foods, blue-green algae, probiotics, enzymes, Amazonian healing herbs, indoor food gardening. Also includes recipes and product listings.
Published by: Sprouting Publications, PO Box 62, Ashland, OR 97520. TEL 541-488-2326, 800-569-2363, FAX 707-667-1841, lolaroja@mail.com. Ed., Pub. Michael Linden. R&P, Adv. contact Mark Nobel. Circ: 3,000 (paid and controlled).

STUDIES IN EATING DISORDERS: AN INTERNATIONAL SERIES. see *MEDICAL SCIENCES—Psychiatry And Neurology*

613.26 USA ISSN 1067-3768
SUPPORT LINE. Text in English. 1984. bi-m. USD 25 to individuals; USD 48 to institutions (effective 2000). adv. *Refereed.* **Document type:** *Newsletter.*
Former titles (until 1992): Dietitians in Nutritional Support (0892-5879); (until 1987): Dietitians in Critical Care (0892-5860)
Indexed: CINAHL.
—BLDSC (8547.638310).
Published by: American Dietetic Association, Dietitians in Nutrition Support, 216 W Jackson Blvd, Ste 800, Chicago, IL 60606-6995. TEL 919-684-4278. Eds. Jeanette Hasse, Mary Marian TEL 520-626-4948. R&P Mary Marian TEL 520-626-4948. Circ: 3,700 (paid).

TETSU TAISHA KENKYUKAI PUROGURAMU SHOROKUSHU/CONFERENCE ON CURRENT TOPICS FOR IRON METABOLISM. PROGRAM AND ABSTRACTS. see *BIOLOGY—Biochemistry*

613.2 JPN
TOKYO TOMIN NO EIYO JOKYO/REPORT ON NUTRITIVE CONDITIONS IN TOKYO. Text in Japanese. 1968. a. **Document type:** *Government.*
Published by: Tokyo Eiseikyoku, Kenko Suishinbu/Tokyo Metropolitan Government, Bureau of Public Health, Public Health Promotion Division, 8-1 Nishi-Shinjuku 2-chome, Shinjuku-ku, Tokyo 160-0023, Japan. TEL 81-3-5320-4357, FAX 81-3-5388-1429. Circ: 1,000.

613.2 USA ISSN 0883-5691
QP141.A1
TOPICS IN CLINICAL NUTRITION. Text in English. 1986. q. USD 135 to individuals; USD 41 newsstand/cover (effective 2002). *Refereed.* **Document type:** *Journal.* **Description:** Provides current information regarding the multitude of changes taking place in nutrition today. Offers practical hands-on tips as well as strategies for motivating clients and their families.
Related titles: Online - full text ed.: (from ProQuest Information & Learning).
Indexed: AMED, Agricola, CINAHL, Dairy Sci.Abstr., Food Sci.& Tech.Abstr., Nutr.Abstr., Sugar Ind.Abstr.
—BLDSC (8867.432800), GNLM, Infotrieve, ingenta. **CCC.**
Published by: Aspen Publishers, Inc., 200 Orchard Ridge Dr, Ste 200, Gaithersburg, MD 20878. TEL 301-695-7931, 800-638-8437, FAX 301-417-7550, customer.service@aspenpul.com, http://www.aspenpub.com. **Dist. by:** Aspen Publishers Inc., Distribution Center, 7201 McKinney Circle, Frederick, MD 21701. TEL 301-698-7100, FAX 301-695-7931.

TOPS NEWS. see *PHYSICAL FITNESS AND HYGIENE*

613.2 USA ISSN 0274-6743
TOTAL HEALTH; for longevity. Text in English. 1979. bi-m. USD 16 domestic; USD 21 foreign (effective 1999). adv. bk.rev. **Document type:** *Consumer.* **Description:** Presents preventive health care life-style articles covering nutrition, diet, fitness, travel, psychological-spiritual health encompassing mind, body, and spirit. Emphasis on anti-aging.
Formerly: Trio
Related titles: Microform ed.: (from PQC); Online - full text ed.: (from Gale Group, ProQuest Information & Learning, Northern Light Technology, Inc., Factiva).
Indexed: Hlth.Ind., e-psyche.
Published by: Total Health Holdings LLC, 165 N 100 St E, Ste 2, Saint George, UT 84770-2505. TEL 435-673-1789, 888-316-6051, FAX 435-634-9336, thm@infowest.com, http:///www.totalhelathmagazine.com. Ed., Pub., R&P Lyle Hurd Jr. Adv. contact Richard Hurd. Circ: 95,000.

641.5 USA ISSN 1523-4045
▼ **TRADITIONAL KITCHENS PRESENT;** Mary Dee's quick and tasty recipes. Text in English. 1999. USD 3.99 newsstand/cover; CND 4.99 newsstand/cover in Canada. adv. illus. back issues avail. **Document type:** *Consumer.* **Description:** Presents a warm, friendly, guilt-free aproach to better living that fits in with today's hectic, jam-packed, fast-paced, plan-ahead lifestyles.
Published by: Roxbury Media, LLC, 27 Glen Rd, PO Box 140, Sandy Hook, CT 06482. TEL 203-426-6533, FAX 203-426-9533. **Subscr. to:** Sunbelt Fulfillment Services, 307 Southgate Ct, Brentwood, TN 37027. **Dist. by:** Curtis Circulation Co., 730 River Rd, New, Milford, CA 90210. TEL 201-634-7400, FAX 201-634-7499.

TRENDS IN FOOD SCIENCE AND TECHNOLOGY (REFERENCE EDITION). see *FOOD AND FOOD INDUSTRIES*

TROPHOS - MEDIZIN UND ERNAEHRUNG. see *MEDICAL SCIENCES*

613.2 USA
CODEN: TUDLET
TUFTS UNIVERSITY HEALTH & NUTRITION LETTER. Text in English. 1983. m. USD 28 domestic; USD 33 foreign (effective 2001). bk.rev. illus. back issues avail.; reprints avail. **Document type:** *Newsletter.*
Formerly (until 1997): Tufts University Diet and Nutrition Letter (0747-4105)
Related titles: Microfilm ed.; Microform ed.: (from PQC); Online - full text ed.: (from Gale Group).
Indexed: Agricola, Biol.Dig., CHNI, CINAHL, Consum.Ind. (1991-1997), Hlth.Ind.
Published by: W H White Publications, 50 Broadway, 15th Fl, New York, NY 10004-1607. FAX 212-668-0421, tuftshnltr@aol.com, http://www.healthletter.tufts.edu. Ed. Dr. Stanley N Gershoff. R&P T Nemeth TEL 212-668-0411. Circ: 200,000. **Subscr. to:** PO Box 420914, Palm Coast, FL 32142-824580322.

UNIVERSITY OF CALIFORNIA, BERKELEY. WELLNESS LETTER; the newsletter of nutrition, fitness, and stress management. see *PHYSICAL FITNESS AND HYGIENE*

THE UNIVERSITY OF TEXAS LIFETIME HEALTH LETTER; useful news about health, fitness, nutrition, and mental well-being. see *PHYSICAL FITNESS AND HYGIENE*

613.2 ZAF
V I C MEDICAL UPDATE. Text in English. 3/yr. free per issue to qualified personnel. *Refereed.* **Document type:** *Bulletin, Academic/Scholarly.* **Description:** Provides an accurate, scientific, timely review of current vitamin related issues and research.
Indexed: Nutr.Abstr.
Published by: Vitamin Information Centre, PO Box 182, Isando, Transvaal 1600, South Africa. TEL 27-11-3934794, FAX 27-11-3934790. R&P Mrs. H L Robertson. **Co-sponsor:** Roche Products (Pty) Ltd.

613.2 SWE ISSN 0042-2657
TX341 CODEN: VAFOAS
VAAR FOEDA. Text in Swedish; Summaries in English. 1949. 6/yr. SEK 350; SEK 430 foreign (effective 1999). bk.rev. charts, illus. *Refereed.* **Document type:** *Government.* **Description:** Covers activities in food control projects, new regulations and current research.
Indexed: Chem.Abstr., Chem.Indus.Notes, Dairy Sci.Abstr., Food Sci.& Tech.Abstr., Hort.Abstr., INIS Atomind., Ind.Vet., Nutr.Abstr., Postharvest, Rev.Appl.Entomol., Sugar Ind.Abstr., Triticale Abstr., Vet.Bull.
—CASDDS, CISTI, Linda Hall.
Published by: Statens Livsmedelsverk/National Food Administration, Fack 622, Uppsala 75126, Sweden. TEL 46-18-17-55-00, FAX 46-18-10-58-48, TELEX 76121 SLVUPS, var.foda@slv.se, http://www.slv.se. Ed. Lena Boija. Circ: 5,500.

613.26 GBR ISSN 0307-4811
THE VEGAN. Text in English. 1946. q. GBP 7.80 domestic; GBP 9.80 overseas; GBP 1.95 newsstand/cover (effective 1999). adv. bk.rev. illus. back issues avail.; reprints avail. **Document type:** *Consumer.* **Description:** Supplies information on animal rights, vegan nutrition, health and ecology.
Published by: Vegan Society, 7 Battle Rd, St Leonards-on-Sea, E Sussex TN37 7AA, United Kingdom. TEL 44-1424-427393, FAX 44-1424-717064, info@vegansociety.com, http://www.vegansociety.com/. Ed., R&P Richard Farhall. Adv. contact Jenny Sawyer. Circ: 7,000.

613.262 179.3 USA ISSN 1084-9289
THE VEGAN NEWS. Text in English. 1993. q. USD 15; USD 20 foreign. adv. bk.rev. **Document type:** *Newsletter.* **Description:** Reports organization news and covers vegetarian diets and lifestyles.
Formerly (until Oct. 1994): East Bay Vegan News
Related titles: Online - full text ed.
Published by: Vegan Action, PO Box 4353, Berkeley, CA 94704. TEL 510-654-6297, FAX 510-595-7569, info@veganorg, http://www.vegan.org. Ed., Adv. contact Leor Jacobi. page USD 300. Circ: 10,000 (controlled).

613.2 SWE
VEGETAR. Text in Swedish. 1903. 4/yr. SEK 180 to membership; SEK 210 in Europe to membership; SEK 235 elsewhere to membership (effective 2001).
(until 1997): Nya Vegetar; (until 1995): Vegetar (1102-0199); (until vol.4, 1989): Haelsonytt (0345-4827); (until vol.6, 1967): Vegetarianen
Published by: Svenska Vegetariska Foereningen (SVF), Saagargatan 4, Stockholm 11636, Sweden. TEL 46-8-702-11-16, FAX 46-8-702-11-17, svf@vegetarian.se, http://www.vegetarian.se. Ed. Monica Engstroem.

VEGETARIAN ASTROLOGER. see *ASTROLOGY*

613.262 USA ISSN 0885-7636
VEGETARIAN JOURNAL. Text in English. 1982. bi-m. USD 20 domestic to members; USD 30 in Canada & Mexico to members; USD 42 elsewhere to members; USD 3.50 newsstand/cover domestic; CND 4.50 newsstand/cover in Canada (effective 2001). bk.rev., film rev. illus. Index. reprint service avail. from PQC. **Document type:** *Consumer.* **Description:** Covers various aspects of vegetarianism and veganism, including health, recipes, ethics, ecology, world hunger, and animal rights. Contains information about restaurants, new products carried by supermarkets, and results of the latest medical research. Aims to present nutritional information based on current scientific literature in an easy and practical fashion.
Formerly: Baltimore Vegetarians (0883-1165)
Related titles: CD-ROM ed.
Published by: Vegetarian Resource Group, PO Box 1463, Baltimore, MD 21203. TEL 410-366-8343, vrg@vrg.org, http://www.vrg.org. Ed. Debra Wasserman. Circ: 25,000.

613.262 USA ISSN 1072-0820
VEGETARIAN JOURNAL'S FOODSERVICE UPDATE; healthy tips and recipes for institutions. Text in English. 1993. q. USD 20 domestic; USD 30 foreign (effective 2001). bk.rev. back issues avail. **Document type:** *Newsletter.* **Description:** For food service personnel and others working for healthier food in schools, restaurants, hospitals and other institutions. Contains quantity recipes, tips, product reviews, and educational resources. Spotlights leaders in the industry who are providing healthy options.
Published by: Vegetarian Resource Group, PO Box 1463, Baltimore, MD 21203. TEL 410-366-8343, vrg@vrg.org, http://www.vrg.org. Ed. Debra Wasserman.

613.26 GBR ISSN 1364-3150
QP144.V44 CODEN: VNUTFA
VEGETARIAN NUTRITION; an international journal. Text in English. 3/yr. GBP 139, USD 219 (effective 1998). **Document type:** *Academic/Scholarly.*
Indexed: Nutr.Abstr.
—BLDSC (9152.775000), CASDDS.
Published by: Emerald, 60-62 Toller Ln, Bradford, W Yorks BD8 9BY, United Kingdom. FAX 44-1274-785200, editorial@mcb.co.uk, info@emeraldinsight.com, http://www.mcb.co.uk, http://www.emeraldinsight.com/journals/. Ed. Mark Messina.

613.26 USA ISSN 0164-8497
TX392 CODEN: VETIFB
VEGETARIAN TIMES. Text in English. 1974. m. USD 24 domestic; USD 36 foreign (effective 2001). adv. bk.rev. illus, tr.lit. reprint service avail. from PQC. **Document type:** *Magazine, Consumer.* **Description:** Contains vegetarian recipes, dietary information, advice on buying whole foods and preparing foods for maximum nutritional value, and articles on nutritional approaches to disease, information for travelers and profiles of prominent vegetarians.
Incorporates: Vegetarian World
Related titles: Microform ed.: (from PQC); Online - full text ed.: (from Gale Group, Northern Light Technology, Inc., ProQuest Information & Learning, Factiva).
Indexed: CHNI, Hlth.Ind., New Per.Ind., WMB.
—ingenta.
Published by: Sabot Publishing, 9 River Bend Dr S Ste 41, Stamford, CT 06907. TEL 203-328-7040, 800-829-3340, FAX 203-328-7008, donnas@cowles.com, http://www.vegetariantimes.com. Ed. Suzanne Berber. Pub. Susan Tauster. R&P Terry Christofferson. adv.: B&W page USD 8,485, color page USD 10,880. Circ: 340,000 (paid).

613.26 USA ISSN 0271-1591
VEGETARIAN VOICE. Text in English. 1974. q. USD 23 to individuals. bk.rev. illus. **Document type:** *Consumer.* **Description:** Information on nutrition, cooking, health, animal and environmental protection for people interested in vegetarianism, with organization news and reports on annual conferences.
Indexed: Alt.Press Ind. (1992-), Art.Hosp.& Tour.
Published by: North American Vegetarian Society, PO Box 72, Dolgeville, NY 13329. TEL 518-568-7970, navs@telenet.net, http://www.cyberveg.org/navs. Ed. Jennie O Collura. Circ: 11,000.

613.262 DNK ISSN 0109-8861
VEGETARISK TIDSSKRIFT. Text in Danish. irreg., latest vol.77, 1983 (1-2/yr.). DKK 30. illus.
Formerly: V F (0109-8845)
Published by: Dansk Vegetar-og Raakostforening, Ny Vestergaardsvej 6, Vaerlose 3500, Denmark.

613.262 USA ISSN 1085-763X
VEGGING OUT; devoted to vegetarian food, nutrition and families. Text in English. 6/yr. USD 15.
Address: PO Box 17385, Milwaukee, WI 53217-0385. veggie@execpc.com, http://www.execpc.com/~veggie. Eds. Debra A Kasprzak, Lisa Rivero. Pub. Lisa Rivero.

VIBRANT LIFE; abundant living for you and your family. see *PHYSICAL FITNESS AND HYGIENE*

VIE ET SANTE; le mensuel du mieux-etre. see *PHYSICAL FITNESS AND HYGIENE*

613.2 ITA ISSN 1120-4591
VITALITY. Text in Italian. 1989. m. ITL 52,800; ITL 80,000 foreign. adv. back issues avail. **Document type:** *Consumer.*
Published by: Rusconi Editore S.p.A., Servizio Abbonamenti, Viale Sarca, 235, Milan, MI 20126, Italy. TEL 39-2-66191, FAX 39-2-6619-2480. Ed. M Picollo. Adv. contact Eduardo Giliberti. color page ITL 14,000,000. Circ: 121,727.

613.262 FRA ISSN 0042-7608
VIVRE EN HARMONIE. Text in French. 1952. m. FRF 140 (effective 2000). bk.rev. bibl, charts, illus. **Description:** Discusses cures with plants and clay, ecology, recipes and information about vegetarian food.
Published by: (Centre Fraternel Vivre en Harmonie), Editions Vivre en Harmonie, 26 rue Remy, Auvers sur Oise 95430, France. TEL 33-1-34480942, FAX 33-1-34480932. Ed., R&P Pascal Labbe.

613.2 NLD ISSN 0168-8901
VLEES IN VOEDING. Text in Dutch. 1983. q. illus. **Document type:** *Academic/Scholarly.* **Description:** Discusses issues relating to meat and nutrition and related research.
Published by: Voorlichtingsbureau Vlees, Postbus 39, Rijswijk (ZH) 2280 AA, Netherlands. TEL 31-70-3991155, FAX 31-70-3906830, http://www.vleesinfo.nl. Ed. Marleen H Essenberg.

613.2 NLD
TX341
VOEDING NU; Netherlands journal of nutrition. Text in Dutch; Text occasionally in English. 1998. 11/yr. NLG 76.50 domestic to individuals; BEF 1,585 in Belgium to individuals; NLG 49.50 domestic to students; BEF 1,045 in Belgium to students (effective 2000). adv. bk.rev. charts, illus. index. back issues avail. **Document type:** *Journal, Trade.* **Description:** Reviews research and information in all areas of nutrition.
Formed by the merger of (1939-1998): Voeding (0042-7926); (1990-1998): Voeding en Voorlichting (0924-6045); Which was formed by the merger of (1978-1989): Voedingsinformatie (0165-7496); (1985-1989): Groepsvoeding Informatie (0923-1099); Which was formerly (1974-1985): Groepsvoeding Informatiekrant (0923-1080)
Indexed: Biol.Abstr., Chem.Abstr., Chem.Indus.Notes, Dairy Sci.Abstr., Food Sci.& Tech.Abstr., INIS Atomind., Ind.Med. (coverage dropped), Nutr.Abstr., Rural Recreat.Tour.Abstr., Sugar Ind.Abstr., World Ag.Econ.& Rur.Soc.Abstr.
—BLDSC, CASDDS, CISTI, GNLM.
Published by: (Voedingscentrum), Keesing Noordervliet BV, De Molen 82, Houten 3995 AX, Netherlands. TEL 31-30-635-8585, FAX 31-30-635-8500, voedingnu@keesing.nl, http://www.voedingnu.nl, http://www.keesing.nl. Ed. Dr. W J Gerritsen. Pub. P T Both. Adv. contact P Scholten. B&W page NLG 2,900, color page NLG 4,850. Circ: 6,798 (paid). **Subscr. to:** Abonneeservice, Antwoordnummer 10299, Amsterdam 1000 PA, Netherlands. TEL 31-20-564-1222, FAX 31-20-697-0305, service@keesing.nl.

613.2 NLD ISSN 0922-8012
VOEDINGSMAGAZINE. Text in Dutch. 1988. bi-m. free. back issues avail. **Document type:** *Magazine, Trade.* **Description:** Contains information on nutrition and health matters for general practitioners, registered dieticians, medical specialists in food-related disciplines, and educators in nutrition and health.
Indexed: Dairy Sci.Abstr., Nutr.Abstr., Rev.Plant Path., Weed Abstr., World Ag.Econ.& Rur.Soc.Abstr.
—KNAW.
Published by: Stichting Zuivel Voeding en Gezondheid, Postbus 6017, Maarssen 3600 HA, Netherlands. TEL 31-30-241-2241, FAX 31-30-241-1840. Ed. G J Hiddink. Circ: 31,000.

612.3 RUS ISSN 0042-8833
CODEN: VPITAR
VOPROSY PITANIYA/PROBLEMS OF NUTRITION. Text in Russian. 1932. bi-m. USD 60 foreign (effective 2002). adv. index. 48 p./no. **Document type:** *Journal, Academic/Scholarly.* **Description:** Publishes original and survey articles that reflect joint work done by physiologists, biochemists, hygienists, pathophysiologists, clinicians and technologists dealing with nutrition problems.
Indexed: Abstr.Hyg., AgBiotech, Aqua.Sci.& Fish.Abstr., Aquacult.Abstr., Biol.Abstr., Chem.Abstr., Chem.Indus.Notes, Dairy Sci.Abstr., Dent.Ind., Dok.Arbeitsmed., Environ.Sci.Poll.Mgmt., Food Sci.& Tech.Abstr., INIS Atomind., Ind.Med. (1932-), Int.Aerosp.Abstr., Maize Abstr., Nutr.Abstr., Postharvest, Poult.Abstr., Ref.Zh., Russ.Acad.Sci.Bibl., Seed Abstr., Soyabean Abstr., Triticale Abstr., Trop.Dis.Bull., World Ag.Econ.& Rur.Soc.Abstr.
—CASDDS, CISTI, East View, GNLM, Infotrieve, Linda Hall. **CCC.**
Published by: (Institut Pitaniya, Rossiiskaya Akademiya Nauk/Russian Academy of Sciences), Nutritec, Dmitrovskoe shosse 46-2, Moscow 127238, Russian Federation. TEL 7-095-4824118, FAX 7-095-4844312. Ed. V A Tutelyan. Pub. M N Solovova. Adv. contact G O Marchik. Circ: 1,700. **Dist. by:** Mezhdunarodnaya Kniga, B Yakimanka 39, Moscow 117049, Russian Federation. **Co-sponsor:** Ministerstvo Zdravookhraneniya.

613.2 CZE ISSN 1211-846X
TX341
VYZIVA A POTRAVINY. Text in Czech; Summaries in English. 1946. bi-m., latest vol.55, 2001. CZK 48 per issue (effective 2001). adv. bk.rev. 36 p./no. back issues avail. *Refereed.* **Document type:** *Bulletin, Newsletter.* **Description:** Provides nutrition news, recommendations, nutrition and food policy, new raw materials and food, catering, food processing, market information, food safety and food security, hygienic standards, etc.
Former titles (until 1994): Vyziva; (until 1991): Vyziva Lidu (0042-9414)
Related titles: ♦ Supplement: Vyziva a Spotreba Potravin v Cislech. ISSN 1212-0022.
Indexed: Biol.Abstr., Chem.Abstr., Dairy Sci.Abstr., Food Sci.& Tech.Abstr., Rural Recreat.Tour.Abstr., World Ag.Econ.& Rur.Soc.Abstr.
—CCC.
Published by: Spolecnost pro Vyzivu/Czech Nutrition Society, Sobeslavska 40, Prague, 3 130 00, Czech Republic. TEL 420-2-67311280, FAX 420-2-71732669, vyziva.spv@volny.cz. Ed. Ctibor Perlin. Pub., R&P Jan Susta. Adv. contact Marie Voldanova. page CZK 27,000; 210 x 295. Circ: 5,500 (controlled). **Dist. by:** PNS a.s., Hvozdanska 5-7, Prague 14831, Czech Republic.

613.2 CZE ISSN 1212-0022
VYZIVA A SPOTREBA POTRAVIN V CISLECH. Text in Czech. 1995. a. CZK 48 (effective 2001). Website rev. 24 p./no. *Refereed.* **Document type:** *Yearbook.*
Related titles: ♦ Supplement to: Vyziva a Potraviny. ISSN 1211-846X.
Published by: Spolecnost pro Vyzivu/Czech Nutrition Society, Sobeslavska 40, Prague, 3 130 00, Czech Republic. TEL 420-2-67311280, FAX 420-2-71732669. Ed. Ctibor Perlin. Circ: 5,500 (paid).

N

613.2 SVK ISSN 0042-9406
VYZIVA A ZDRAVIE/NUTRITION AND HEALTH; journal for rational nutrition. Text in Slovak; Abstracts occasionally in English, Russian. 1956. m. USD 38 (effective 2000). adv. bk.rev. charts, illus.
Indexed: Chem.Abstr.
Published by: Slovenska Spolecnost pre Racionalnu Vyzivu/Slovak Society for Rational Nourishment, Krizna 52 III, Bratislava 82108, Slovakia. Ed. Vojtech Spanko. Circ: 9,000. **Subscr. to:** Slovart, Gottwaldovo nam 48, Bratislava 805 32, Czechoslovakia.

WARM EARTH; organic growing - healthy living. see *GARDENING AND HORTICULTURE*

WARSAW AGRICULTURAL UNIVERSITY. S G G W. ANNALS. FOOD TECHNOLOGY AND NUTRITION. see *FOOD AND FOOD INDUSTRIES*

613.26 POL ISSN 1230-7890
WEGETARIANIN; zdrowie, ekologia, mistycyzm. Text in Polish. 1993. m. USD 8.40 (effective 1998). bk.rev. bibl, illus. **Description:** Publishes articles translated mainly from US sources about all aspects of vegetarianism, natural hygiene, alternative medicine, ecology.
Published by: Wydawnictwo Vegan, Ul Hutnicza 18-44, Lublin 20218, Poland. TEL 48-81-7464811, FAX 48-81-7464811. Ed. Tomasz Nocun. adv.: page USD 350. Circ: 30,000.

613.25 USA
WEIGHT LOSS NEWS. Text in English. fortn. free per issue. **Document type:** *Newsletter.*
Media: Online - full text.
Published by: E G W Publishing Co., 1041 Shary Circle, Concord, CA 94518. TEL 925-671-9852, FAX 510-671-0692, hstevens@egw.com, http://www.naturalland.com/wlv/wlnc.htm.

613.26 USA ISSN 0043-2180
RM222.2
WEIGHT WATCHERS MAGAZINE. Text in English. 1968. bi-m. USD 14.95 (effective 2001). adv. bk.rev. illus. Index. reprints avail. **Document type:** *Consumer.* **Description:** For women who want to change their lives for the better. Provides "how-to" tips on smart eating, beauty, fashion, fitness, health and nutrition.
Related titles: Microfiche ed.: (from NRP); Microform ed.: (from PQC); Online - full text ed.: (from Gale Group).
Indexed: CHNI, Mag.Ind.
—ingenta.
Published by: Weight Watchers Publishing Group (Subsidiary of: Weight Watchers International, Inc.), 360 Lexington ave, Woodbury, NY 10017. TEL 212-370-0644, 800-978-2400, FAX 212-687-4398, http://www.weightwatchers.com/. Ed. Nancy Galiardi. Adv. contact Kay Parmenter. B&W page USD 12,250, color page USD 17,500; trim 10.88 x 8. Circ: 1,060,000 (paid).

WELLBEING MAGAZINE; personal and planetary healing. see *PHYSICAL FITNESS AND HYGIENE*

WHOLE LIFE TIMES. see *NEW AGE PUBLICATIONS*

613.2 CHE ISSN 0084-2230
QP141.A1 CODEN: WRNDAT
WORLD REVIEW OF NUTRITION AND DIETETICS. Text in English. 1964. irreg., latest vol.90. CHF 230 in Europe; DEM 275 in Germany; USD 185 in United States (effective 2001). reprint service avail. from ISI. *Refereed.* **Document type:** *Monographic series, Academic/Scholarly.*
Related titles: Online - full text ed.
Indexed: Abstr.Hyg., Biol.Abstr., Chem.Abstr., Chem.Indus.Notes, Chem.Titles, Curr.Cont. (coverage dropped), Dairy Sci.Abstr., Dent.Ind., Food Sci.& Tech.Abstr., Ind.Med. (1959-), Nutr.Abstr., Rice Abstr., Triticale Abstr., Trop.Dis.Bull.
—BLDSC (9359.180000), CASDDS, CISTI, GNLM, ingenta, KNAW, Linda Hall. **CCC.**
Published by: S. Karger AG, Allschwilerstr 10, PO Box, Basel 4009, Switzerland. TEL 41-61-306-1111, FAX 41-61-306-1234, karger@karger.ch, http://www.karger.com/bookseries/WRUND. Ed. A P Simopoulos.

Y M C A WEEKLY NEWS. (Young Men's Christian Association) see *PHYSICAL FITNESS AND HYGIENE*

YAOWU SHIPIN FENXI/JOURNAL OF FOOD AND DRUG ANALYSIS. see *FOOD AND FOOD INDUSTRIES*

613.2 CHN ISSN 0512-7955
QP141 CODEN: YYHPA4
YINGYANG XUEBAO/JOURNAL OF NUTRITION. Text in Chinese. 1956-1958; resumed 1982. q. USD 27.20; USD 6.80 newsstand/cover (effective 2001). **Document type:** *Academic/Scholarly.*
Related titles: Online - full content ed.: (from WanFang Data Corp.).
Indexed: Chem.Abstr., Chem.Indus.Notes, Chem.Titles.
—CASDDS.
Published by: Zhongguo Yingyang Xuehui/Chinese Nutrition Society, 1 Dali Dao, Heping-qu, Tianjin 300050, China. TEL 86-22-3322197, FAX 86-22-3314818. Ed. Gu Jingfan. **Dist. by:** China International Book Trading Corp, 35, Chegongzhuang Xilu, Haidian District, Beijing 100044, China. TEL 86-1-68413849, FAX 86-1-68412048, cibtc@mail.cibtc.com.cn, http://www.cibtc.com.cn.

YOGA AND HEALTH. see *PHYSICAL FITNESS AND HYGIENE*

613.2 GBR ISSN 0955-4211
YOUR GREATEST GUIDE TO CALORIES. Text in English. q. GBP 1.95 (effective 1999). **Document type:** *Consumer.*
Published by: Emap Elan Ltd. (Subsidiary of: Emap Consumer Magazines Ltd.), Endeavour House, 189 Shaftesbury Ave, London WC2H 8JG, United Kingdom. TEL 44-207-437-9011, FAX 44-207-208-3709, http://www.emap.com. **Subscr. to:** Tower Publishing Services Ltd., Tower House, Sovereign Park, Lathkill St, Market Harborough, Leics LE16 9EF, United Kingdom. TEL 44-1858-438833, FAX 44-1858-434958.

ZAMBIA. NATIONAL FOOD AND NUTRITION COMMISSION. ANNUAL REPORT. see *FOOD AND FOOD INDUSTRIES*

613.26 JPN
ZEN EISHIKYO GEPPO/JAPANESE ASSOCIATION OF DIETITIAN TRAINING INSTITUTE. MONTHLY BULLETIN. Text in Japanese. m.
Published by: Zenkoku Eiyoshi Yosei Shisetsu Kyokai, 16-6 Kita-Otsuka, Toshima-ku, Tokyo 170-0004, Japan.

613.2 CHN ISSN 1004-7484
ZHONGGUO BAOJIAN YINGYANG/CHINA HEALTH NUTRITION. Text in Chinese. 1989. bi-m. USD 28.80; USD 2.40 newsstand/cover (effective 2001). **Document type:** *Academic/Scholarly.*
Published by: China International Book Trading Corp/Zhongguo Guoji Tushu Maoyi Zonggongsi cibtc@mail.cibtc.com.cn, http://www.cibtc.com.cn. **Dist. by:** 35, Chegongzhuang Xilu, Haidian District, Beijing 100044, China.

612.3 POL ISSN 0209-164X
CODEN: ZCMEDQ
ZYWIENIE CZLOWIEKA I METABOLIZM/POLISH JOURNAL OF HUMAN NUTRITION AND METABOLISM. Text in Polish; Summaries in English. 1973. 4/yr. PLZ 60; PLZ 60 foreign; PLZ 15 newsstand/cover (effective 2000). bk.rev. **Document type:** *Academic/Scholarly.* **Description:** Contains articles on physiology and biochemistry of nutrition, assessment of dietary habits and nutritional status of different population groups.
Formerly (until 1983): Zywienie Czlowieka (0303-7851)
Indexed: AgroAgen, AgroLibrex, Chem.Abstr., Chem.Indus.Notes, Chem.Titles, Dairy Sci.Abstr., Food Sci.& Tech.Abstr., Nutr.Abstr., Postharvest, Seed Abstr.
—BLDSC (9538.941000), CASDDS, CISTI, GNLM, KNAW.
Published by: Instytut Zywnosci i Zywienia/National Food and Nutrition Institute, Ul Powsinska 61-63, Warsaw 02903, Poland. TEL 48-22-8422171, FAX 48-22-8421103, TELEX 816854. Ed., R&P Swiatoslaw Ziemlanski. Circ: 500. **Dist. by:** Ars Polona, Krakowskie Przedmiescie 7, Warsaw, Poland.

NUTRITION AND DIETETICS—Abstracting, Bibliographies, Statistics

50 TITRES SUR... see *POPULATION STUDIES—Abstracting, Bibliographies, Statistics*

613.2021 AUS
AUSTRALIA. BUREAU OF STATISTICS. AUSTRALIA'S FOOD AND NUTRITION. Text in English. 1994. irreg., latest 1994. AUD 27 (effective 2001). **Document type:** *Government.* **Description:** Examines the structure of the food supply and the effects of the political, physical and social nature of Australia on nutrition.
Published by: Australian Bureau of Statistics, PO Box 10, Belconnen, ACT 2616, Australia. TEL 61-2-6252-5249, FAX 61-2-6252-6778, http://www.abs.gov.au. **Co-sponsor:** Australian Institute of Health and Welfare.

613.2021 AUS
AUSTRALIA. BUREAU OF STATISTICS. INFORMATION PAPER: NATIONAL NUTRITION SURVEY, CONFIDENTIALISED UNIT RECORD FILE. Text in English. 1995. irreg. AUD 10 (effective 2001).
Published by: Australian Bureau of Statistics, PO Box 10, Belconnen, ACT 2616, Australia. TEL 61-2-6252-5249, FAX 61-2-6252-6778, http://www.abs.gov.au.

613.2021 AUS
AUSTRALIA. BUREAU OF STATISTICS. NATIONAL NUTRITION SURVEY: FOODS EATEN, AUSTRALIA. Text in English. 1998. irreg., latest 1995. AUD 32 (effective 2001). **Document type:** *Government.*
Published by: Australian Bureau of Statistics, PO Box 10, Belconnen, ACT 2616, Australia. TEL 61-2-6252-5249, FAX 61-2-6252-6778, http://www.abs.gov.au. **Co-sponsor:** Department of Health and Family Services.

613.2021 AUS
AUSTRALIA. BUREAU OF STATISTICS. NATIONAL NUTRITION SURVEY: NUTRIENT INTAKES AND PHYSICAL MEASUREMENTS, AUSTRALIA. Text in English. 1998. irreg. AUD 35 (effective 2001). **Document type:** *Government.*
Formerly: Australia. Bureau of Statistics. National Nutrition Survey: Nutrient Intake, Australia
Published by: Australian Bureau of Statistics, PO Box 10, Belconnen, ACT 2616, Australia. TEL 61-2-6252-5249, FAX 61-2-6252-6778, http://www.abs.gov.au. **Co-sponsor:** Department of Health and Family Services.

613.2021 AUS
AUSTRALIA. BUREAU OF STATISTICS. WESTERN AUSTRALIAN OFFICE. HOME SAFETY DEVICES, WESTERN AUSTRALIA. Text in English. 1996. irreg., latest 1996. AUD 14.50 (effective 2001). **Document type:** *Government.*
Published by: Australian Bureau of Statistics, Western Australian Office, PO Box K 881, Perth, W.A. 6001, Australia. TEL 61-8-9360-5307, FAX 61-8-9360-5955, http://www.abs.gov.au.

016.6132 GBR
CAB INTERNATIONAL. BUREAU OF NUTRITION. ANNOTATED BIBLIOGRAPHIES. Text in English. irreg. GBP 35, USD 60. bk.rev. **Document type:** *Abstract/Index, Bibliography.*
Formerly: Commonwealth Bureau of Nutrition. Annotated Bibliographies (0069-6935)
Related titles: Online - full text ed.: (from CISTI, DIMDI, The Dialog Corporation, European Space Agency).
Indexed: Nutr.Abstr.
Published by: CAB International, Bureau of Nutrition, C A B International, Mongewell, Wallingford, Oxon OX10 8DE, United Kingdom. TEL 44-1491-832111, FAX 44-1491-833508, TELEX 847964 COMAGG G. Ed. Elizabeth Dodsworth. R&P Wendy Davies. **U.S. subscr. to:** CAB International, North American Office, 845 N Park Ave, Tucson, AZ 85719. TEL 800-528-4841.

016.6123 GBR ISSN 0965-7126
CODEN: CLCNEI
CURRENT MEDICAL LITERATURE. CLINICAL NUTRITION. Text in English. 1992. q. USD 60 to individuals; USD 20 newsstand/cover to individuals; USD 140 to institutions; USD 40 newsstand/cover to institutions (2002). back issues avail. **Document type:** *Abstract/Index.*
—**CCC.**
Published by: (Royal Society of Medicine), Current Medical Literature Ltd., 40-42 Osnaburgh St, London NW1 3ND, United Kingdom. TEL 44-20-7465-8377, FAX 44-20-7465-8380, enquiries@curmedlit.co.uk. **Dist. by:** Cassis Publishing Ltd., Realpage House, Abingdon Science Park, Barton Ln., Abingdon, Oxon OX13 3NB, United Kingdom. TEL 44-1235-537352, FAX 44-1235-537353.

613.2021 HND
ENCUESTA NACIONAL DE NUTRICION. (In 8 regional editions) Text in Spanish. a. **Document type:** *Government.*
Published by: Ministerio de Salud Publica, 4a Avda 3a Calle, Tegucigalpa D.C., Honduras.

016.616398 NZL ISSN 1174-5746
L M S ALERT. OBESITY. (Literature Monitoring and Evaluation Service) Text in English. 1998. m. *Refereed.* **Document type:** *Abstract/Index.*
Related titles: CD-ROM ed.; Online - full text ed.
Published by: Adis International Limited, Mairangi Bay, Private Bag 65901, Auckland 1010, New Zealand. TEL 64-9-477-0700, FAX 64-9-977-0784, monique.curran@adis.com, http://www.adis.com. Ed. Monique Curran. Pub. Christopher J Mellor.

016.6132 GBR ISSN 0309-1295
QP141.A1
NUTRITION ABSTRACTS AND REVIEWS. SERIES A: HUMAN AND EXPERIMENTAL. Text in English. 1977. m. GBP 980 to institutions; USD 1,660 in the Americas to institutions; GBP 995 to institutions Includes single site online access; USD 1,740 in the Americas to institutions Includes single site online access (effective 2002). adv. bk.rev. illus. index, cum.index: vols.1-10 (in 2 vols.). back issues avail.; reprint service avail. from SCH,PSC. **Document type:** *Abstract/Index.* **Description:** Aimed at research workers, consultants, public health specialists, advisors, and general practitioners.
Incorporates: Reviews in Clinical Nutrition; Supersedes in part: Nutrition Abstracts and Reviews (0029-6619)
Related titles: Online - full text ed.: GBP 820 to institutions; USD 1,430 in the Americas to institutions (effective 2002) (from DIMDI, The Dialog Corporation, S T N International).
Indexed: Nutr.Abstr.
—CISTI, GNLM, Infotrieve, Linda Hall. **CCC.**
Published by: CABI Publishing, Wallingford, Oxon OX10 8DE, United Kingdom. TEL 44-1491-832111, FAX 44-1491-829198, publishing@cabi.org, http://www.cabi.org/Publishing/Products/Journals/Abstract/NARA/Index.asp, http://www.ingenta.com. Adv. contact S Harris. B&W page GBP 200; 170 x 267. **U.S. subscr. to:** 10 E 40th St, Ste 3203, New York, NY 10016. TEL 212-481-7018, 800-528-4841, FAX 212-686-7993, cabi-nao@cabi.org.

OBSTETRICS AND GYNECOLOGY

see MEDICAL SCIENCES—Obstetrics And Gynecology

OCCUPATIONAL HEALTH AND SAFETY

613.62 USA
RC963 CODEN: AIHAAP
A I H A J; journal for the science of occupational and environmental health and safety. Text in English. 1940. bi-m. USD 160 to institutions; USD 175 in Canada & Mexico to institutions; USD 235 elsewhere to institutions (effective 1999). adv. bk.rev. bibl, charts, illus. index, cum.index. back issues avail.; reprints avail. *Refereed.* **Document type:** *Trade, Academic/Scholarly.* **Description:** Offers a broad spectrum of technical articles together with literature, new products, and other AIHA news.
Former titles (until 2000): American Industrial Hygiene Association Journal (0002-8894); (until 1957): American Industrial Hygiene Association Quarterly (0096-820X); (until 1946): Industrial Hygiene
Related titles: Microfiche ed.; Microfilm ed.; Online - full text ed.: USD 150 to institutions; USD 165 in Canada & Mexico to institutions (effective 1999) (from EBSCO Publishing, H. W. Wilson).
Indexed: ABI Inform. (Jan.1993-), API Abstr., API Catal., API Hlth.& Environ., API Oil., API Pet.Ref., API Pet.Subst., API Transport., A.S.& T.Ind. (Sep.1983-Dec.1999), ASCA, Abstr.Hyg., Acoust.Abstr., Agri.Eng.Abstr., Alloys Ind., Anal.Abstr., B.C.I.R.A., Bibl.Ind., Biodet.Abstr., Biol.Abstr., Br.Ceram.Abstr., C.I.S. Abstr., Cadscan, Chem.Abstr., Chem.Indus.Notes, Chem.Titles, Curr.Adv.Ecol.Sci., Curr.Cont., Dairy Sci.Abstr., Energy Ind., Energy Info.Abstr., Eng.Mat.Abstr., Environ.Abstr., Environ.Sci.Poll.Mgmt., Ergon.Abstr., Excerp.Med., Forest Prod.Abstr., Fuel & Energy Abstr., IBZ, INIS Atomind., Ind.Hyg.Dig., Ind.Med. (2000-), Ind.Sci.Rev., Ind.Vet., Intl.Polym.Sci.& Tech., Lab.Haz.Bull., Lead Abstr., METADEX, Maize Abstr., Mass Spectr.Bull., Med.& Surg.Dermat., Met.Abstr., Met.Abstr.Ind., NRN, Noise Pollut.Publ.Abstr., Nonfer.Met.Alert, Nutr.Abstr., Ocean.Abstr. (coverage dropped), PCC Alert, Pig News & Info., Pollut.Abstr., Poult.Abstr., Protozool.Abstr., RAPRA (1979-), Rev.Appl.Entomol., Rev.Med.& Vet.Mycol., Rev.Plant Path., Rice Abstr., Risk Abstr., SSCI (coverage dropped), Saf.Sci.Abstr., Sci.Cit.Ind., Steels Alert, Sugar Ind.Abstr., THA, Tox.Abstr., Trop.Dis.Bull., Vet.Bull., Weed Abstr., World Alum.Abstr., World Surf.Coat., Zincscan.
—BLDSC (0819.995000), CASDDS, CISTI, EMDOCS, GNLM, IDS, ingenta, Linda Hall. **CCC.**
Published by: American Industrial Hygiene Association, 2700 Prosperity Ave, Ste 250, Fairfax, VA 22031-4307. TEL 703-849-8888, FAX 703-207-3561, infonet@aiha.org, http://aiha.allenpress.com/aihaonline/?request=index-html, http://www.aiha.org. Ed. Howard Cohen. R&P Deborah Williams. Circ: 13,000.

613.62 USA ISSN 1059-1753
A O T A SELF STUDY SERIES. Text in English. 1990. m.
Published by: American Occupational Therapy Association, Inc., 4720 Montgomery Lane, Bethesda, MD 20814-3425. TEL 301-652-2682, FAX 301-652-7711.

A S VORORT; Fachmagazin fuer die Arbeitssicherheit und den Gesundheitsschutz in Bergbau. (Arbeit und Sicherheit) see *MINES AND MINING INDUSTRY*

614.85 DEU ISSN 0938-7226
ABWEHR BETRIEBLICHER STOERFAELLE. Text in German. 1990. irreg. DEM 168 (effective 2000). **Document type:** *Journal, Trade.*
Published by: Erich Schmidt Verlag GmbH & Co. (Berlin), Genthiner Str 30G, Berlin 10785, Germany. TEL 49-30-250085-0, FAX 49-30-25008521, vertrieb@esvmedien.de, htttp://www.erich-schmidt-verlag.de.

363.11 CAN ISSN 0044-5878
ACCIDENT PREVENTION. Text in English. 1952. bi-m. CND 18 domestic; CND 24 in United States; CND 33 elsewhere. bk.rev. abstr, illus, charts. **Document type:** *Trade.*
Indexed: C.I.S. Abstr., CSNB.
—BLDSC (0573.200000).
Published by: Industrial Accident Prevention Association, 250 Yonge St, 28th Fl, Toronto, ON M5B 2N4, Canada. TEL 416-506-8888, FAX 416-506-8880. Circ: 35,000.

613.62 658 USA
ADMINISTRATION & MANAGEMENT SPECIAL INTEREST SECTION QUARTERLY. Text in English. 1985. q. USD 20 (effective 1999). adv. **Document type:** *Newsletter.*
Formerly (until 199?): Administration and Management Special Interest Section Newsletter (8756-629X)
Published by: American Occupational Therapy Association, Inc., 4720 Montgomery Lane, Bethesda, MD 20814-3425. TEL 301-652-2682, FAX 301-652-7711. Ed. Amy L Eutsey. R&P Lynne Andrews. Adv. contact Stephanie Abrams TEL 301-652-6611 ext. 2715.

ADVANCE FOR OCCUPATIONAL THERAPY PRACTITIONERS. see *MEDICAL SCIENCES—Physical Medicine And Rehabilitation*

ADVANCES IN NOISE RESEARCH. see *MEDICAL SCIENCES—Otorhinolaryngology*

363.11 NLD ISSN 1384-2269
ADVANCES IN OCCUPATIONAL ERGONOMICS AND SAFETY. Text in English. 1997. irreg., latest vol.3, 1999. price varies. back issues avail. **Document type:** *Journal, Proceedings, Academic/Scholarly.* **Description:** Disseminates research in the field of occupational health and safety; covers ergonomics.
—BLDSC (0709.530550).
Published by: I O S Press, Van Diemenstraat 94, Amsterdam 1013 CN, Netherlands. TEL 31-20-638-2189, FAX 31-20-620-3419, market@iospress.nl, http://www.iospress.nl. **Subscr. to:** I O S Press, Inc, 5795-G Burke Centre Pkwy, Burke, VA 22015. TEL 703-323-5554, FAX 703-323-3668, iosbooks@iospress.com. **Dist. by:** Ohmsha Ltd, 3-1 Kanda-Nishiki-cho, Chiyoda-ku, Tokyo 101-0054, Japan. TEL 81-3-3233-0641, FAX 81-3-3233-2426, http://www.ohmsha.co.jp.

613.62 615.82 ITA ISSN 1123-8364
ADVANCES IN OCCUPATIONAL MEDICINE & REHABILITATION/AGGIORNAMENTI IN MEDICINA OCCUPAZIONALE E RIABILITAZIONE. Text in Italian. 1995. 3/yr. **Document type:** *Academic/Scholarly, Trade.* **Description:** Covers important advances in occupational and physical therapy.
—BLDSC (0709.530600).
Published by: (Fondazione Salvatore Maugeri), PI-ME Press, Viale Sardegna, 64, Pavia, PV 27100, Italy. TEL 39-0382-539124, FAX 39-0382-22485. Ed. Dr. Narcello Imbriani. **Subscr. to:** Via P Azzario, 19, Pavia, PV 27100, Italy.

613.62 FIN ISSN 0788-4877
AFRICAN NEWSLETTER ON OCCUPATIONAL HEALTH AND SAFETY. Text in English. 1987. 3/yr. free (effective 2001). 28 p./no. Supplement avail.; back issues avail. **Document type:** *Newsletter.* **Description:** Reviews issues of concern to persons involved in occupational health and safety in African countries.
Formerly (until 1991): East African Newsletter on Occupational Health and Safety (0783-6201)
Related titles: Online - full text ed.: African Newsletter on Occupational Health and Safety - Online. ISSN 1239-4386. 1995.
Indexed: Saf.Sci.Abstr.
—BLDSC (0732.902500).
Published by: Finnish Institute of Occupational Health, Topeliuksenkatu 41a A, Helsinki 00250, Finland. TEL 358-9-4747-2694, FAX 358-9-4747-2548, http://www.occuphealth.fi/e/info/anl/index.htm. Ed. Suvi Lehtinen.

620.8 NLD ISSN 1389-1316
AGEING AND ERGONOMICS SERIES. Key Title: Series Ageing and Ergonomics. Text in English. 1998. irreg. price varies. illus. **Document type:** *Monographic series.*
Published by: Delft University Press, PO Box 98, Delft 2600 MG, Netherlands. TEL 31-15-278-3254, FAX 31-15-2781661, DUP@DUP.TUDelft.nl. Ed. J M Dirken.

363.1 NOR ISSN 0808-6567
AKTUELL SIKKERHET. Text in Norwegian. 1997. 6/yr. NOK 380 domestic; NOK 410 foreign (effective 2001). adv. **Document type:** *Trade, Consumer.*
Published by: Vanebo Forlag AS, Postboks 130, Kirkenaer 2260, Norway. TEL 47-62-94-10-00, FAX 47-62-94-10-10, firmapost@vanebo.no. Eds. Jan Tveita TEL 47-62-82-32-30, Ove Hansrud TEL 47-62-82-91-00. Adv. contact Rolf Goplen. B&W page NOK 12,500, color page NOK 16,500; 190 x 265. Circ: 8,416.

614.85 ITA ISSN 0393-7054
AMBIENTE E SICUREZZA SUL LAVORO. Text in Italian. m. (11/yr.). ITL 200,000 domestic; ITL 220,000 in Europe; ITL 240,000 elsewhere (effective 2000). adv. illus. **Document type:** *Trade.*
Published by: E P C s.r.l., Via Dell' Acqua Traversa, 187-189, Rome, RM 00135, Italy. TEL 39-06-3313000, FAX 39-06-3313212, amsl@epcinforma.com. Ed. Michele Lepore. Pub. Pier Roberto Pais. Adv. contact Roberto Barberini. Circ: 10,000.

613.62 USA ISSN 0271-3586
CODEN: AJIMD8
AMERICAN JOURNAL OF INDUSTRIAL MEDICINE. Text in English. 1980. m. USD 2,995 in United States; USD 3,115 in Canada & Mexico; USD 3,217 elsewhere; USD 3,145 combined subscription in United States for print and online eds.; USD 3,265 combined subscription in Canada & Mexico for print and online eds.; USD 3,367 combined subscription elsewhere for print and online eds. (effective 2002). adv. bk.rev. bibl, charts, illus. index. back issues avail.; reprints avail. *Refereed.* **Document type:** *Academic/Scholarly.* **Description:** Presents both clinical and laboratory findings, as well as general academic and scientific contributions in the fundamental or applied study of occupational disease.
Related titles: Microform ed.: (from PQC); Online - full text ed.: ISSN 1097-0274. USD 2,995 in United States; USD 2,995 in Canada & Mexico; USD 2,995 elsewhere (effective 2002) (from EBSCO Publishing, Wiley InterScience, Institute for Scientific Information).
Indexed: AESIS, ASCA, Abstr.Hyg., Acoust.Abstr., Biol.Abstr., Br.Ceram.Abstr., CSNB, Cadscan, Chem.Abstr., Chem.Indus.Notes, Chem.Titles, Chic.Per.Ind., Crim.Just.Abstr., Curr.Adv.Ecol.Sci., Curr.Cont., Dairy Sci.Abstr., Dent.Ind., Environ.Sci.Poll.Mgmt., Ergon.Abstr., Excerp.Med., Forest Prod.Abstr., INIS Atomind., Ind.Med. (1980-), Ind.Sci.Rev., Inpharma, Int.Nurs.Ind., Lab.Haz.Bull., Lead Abstr., METADEX, Med.& Surg.Dermat., Microbiol.Abstr., NRN, Pharm.&Out.News, Pollut.Abstr., Reac., Ref.Zh., Rev.Appl.Entomol., Rev.Med.& Vet.Mycol., Rev.Plant Path., Risk Abstr., SSCI (coverage dropped), Saf.Sci.Abstr., Sci.Cit.Ind., THA, Tox.Abstr., Weed Abstr., Zincscan.
—BLDSC (0826.750000), CASDDS, CISTI, EMDOCS, GNLM, IDS, Infotrieve, ingenta. **CCC.**
Published by: John Wiley & Sons, Inc., Journals (Subsidiary of: Wiley InterScience), 605 Third Ave, New York, NY 10158. TEL 212-850-6645, FAX 212-850-6021, uscs-wis@wiley.com, http://www.wiley.com. Ed. P J Landrigan. adv.: B&W page GBP 614, color page GBP 1,515; trim 174 x 254. Circ: 1,150. **Subscr. outside the Americas to:** John Wiley & Sons Ltd., Baffins Ln, Chichester, Sussex PO19 IUD, United Kingdom. TEL 44-1243-779777, FAX 44-1243-843232, cs-journals@wiley.co.uk, http://www.wiley.co.uk.

615.851 USA ISSN 0272-9490
RM735.A1 CODEN: AJOTAM
AMERICAN JOURNAL OF OCCUPATIONAL THERAPY. Text in English. 1947. 6/yr. USD 50 domestic to individuals; USD 120 domestic to institutions; USD 130 foreign (effective 2001). adv. bk.rev. abstr, bibl, charts, illus. index. back issues avail.; reprints avail. *Refereed.* **Document type:** *Academic/Scholarly.*
Former titles (until 1978): A J O T: The American Journal of Occupational Therapy (0161-326X); (until 1977): American Journal of Occupational Therapy (0002-9386)
Related titles: Microform ed.: (from PQC); Online - full text ed.: (from Institute for Scientific Information).
Indexed: AMED, ASCA, ASSIA, Abstr.Soc.Geront., AgeLine, Bibl.Dev.Med.& Child Neur., Biol.Abstr., C.I.J.E. (coverage dropped), CINAHL, Curr.Cont., Dent.Ind., Dok.Arbeitsmed., Except.Child Educ.Abstr., Excerp.Med., Fam.Ind., Hosp.Lit.Ind., IMFL, Ind.Med. (1947-), Int.Nurs.Ind., Neurosci.Cit.Ind., PsycInfo, Psychol.Abstr. (1950-), Rehabil.Lit., SSCI, e-psyche.
—BLDSC (0828.750000), CISTI, GNLM, ingenta, KNAW.
Published by: American Occupational Therapy Association, Inc., 4720 Montgomery Lane, Bethesda, MD 20814-3425. TEL 301-652-2682, FAX 301-652-7711, http://www.aota.org/nonmembers/area7/links/LINK03.asp. Ed. Betty Hasselkus. Circ: 58,000.

613.62 USA ISSN 0145-8922
AMERICAN OCCUPATIONAL THERAPY ASSOCIATION. ANNUAL REPORT. Text in English. 1972. a. **Document type:** *Corporate.*
Published by: American Occupational Therapy Association, Inc., 4720 Montgomery Lane, Bethesda, MD 20814-3425. TEL 301-652-2682, FAX 301-652-7711.

AMERICANS WITH DISABILITIES ACT LAW AND REGULATIONS. see *LAW—Civil Law*

AMERISURE SAFETY NEWS. see *PUBLIC HEALTH AND SAFETY*

ANGEWANDTE ARBEITSWISSENSCHAFT. see *BUSINESS AND ECONOMICS—Labor And Industrial Relations*

363.11 948.9 DNK ISSN 1396-6715
ANMELDTE ARBEJDSULYKKER OG ARBEJDSBETINGEDE LIDELSER. Text in Danish. 1979. a. price varies. adv. **Document type:** *Trade.* **Description:** Contains statistics on reported occupational accidents and diseases.
Formed by the 1994 merger of: Anmeldte Arbejdsbetingede Lidelser. Aarsopgoerelse (0901-9197); Anmeldte Arbejdsulykker. Yearbook (0905-1902); Which was formerly (until 1984): Arbejdsulykker. Aarsstatistik (0106-9683)
Published by: Danish Working Environment Service, Analysis and Documentation Office, Landskronagade 33, Copenhagen Oe 2100, Denmark. TEL 45-39-15-20-00, FAX 45-39-15-25-60. Ed. Kirsten Joergensen. Adv. contact Annegrethe Rasmussen. Circ: 1,000.

613.62 GBR ISSN 0003-4878
RC963 CODEN: AOHYA3
ANNALS OF OCCUPATIONAL HYGIENE. Text in English. 1958. 8/yr. GBP 525, USD 910 to individuals; GBP 525, USD 910 to institutions (effective 2002). adv. bk.rev. charts, illus. index. 72 p./no. back issues avail.; reprints avail. *Refereed.* **Document type:** *Journal, Academic/Scholarly.* **Description:** Aims to promote a healthy working environment through publication of research papers and reviews on health hazards and risks resulting from work - specially their recognition, quantification, management and control.
Related titles: Microfilm ed.: (from PQC); Online - full text ed.: (from ingenta, Swets Blackwell, ScienceDirect, Institute for Scientific Information).
Indexed: ASCA, Abstr.Hyg., Acoust.Abstr., Bioeng.Abstr., Biol.Abstr., Biol.Dig., Br.Ceram.Abstr., C.I.S. Abstr., CSNB, Chem.Abstr., Chem.Indus.Notes, Chem.Titles, Compumath, Comput.& Info.Sys., Curr.Adv.Ecol.Sci., Curr.Cont., Electron.& Communic.Abstr.J., Eng.Ind., Environ.Sci.Poll.Mgmt., Ergon.Abstr., Excerp.Med., Helminthol.Abstr., I.M.M.Abstr., INIS Atomind., ISMEC, Ind.Hyg.Dig., Ind.Med. (1958-), Ind.Sci.Rev., Ind.Vet., Inpharma, Int.Abstr.Biol.Sci., Intl.Polym.Sci.& Tech., Lab.Haz.Bull., METADEX, Mass Spectr.Bull., Med.& Surg.Dermat., Noise Pollut.Publ.Abstr., Pollut.Abstr., RAPRA (1975-1984, 1989-), Reac., Rev.Appl.Entomol., Rev.Med.& Vet.Mycol., Risk Abstr., SSCI (coverage dropped), Saf.Sci.Abstr., Sci.Cit.Ind., THA, Tox.Abstr., Trop.Dis.Bull.
—BLDSC (1043.300000), CASDDS, CISTI, Ei, EMDOCS, GNLM, IDS, ingenta. **CCC.**
Published by: (British Occupational Hygiene Society), Oxford University Press, Academic Division, Great Clarendon St, Oxford OX2 6DP, United Kingdom. TEL 44-1865-267907, FAX 44-1865-267835, jnl.info@oup.co.uk, http://www3.oup.co.uk/annhyg/, http://www.oup.co.uk/journals. Eds. Stephen M Rappaport, Trevor L Ogden. Pub. Mandy Sketch. R&P Fionna Willis. Adv. contact Helen Pearson TEL 44-1235-201904. Circ: 1,700. **Subscr. to:** Journals Marketing, Great Clarendon St, Oxford OX2 6DP, United Kingdom.

ANTROPO-EKOLOGIIA. see *ENVIRONMENTAL STUDIES*

AOMORIKEN SAGYO RYOHO KENKYU/BULLETIN OF AOMORI OCCUPATIONAL THERAPY. see *MEDICAL SCIENCES—Physical Medicine And Rehabilitation*

613.62 USA ISSN 1047-322X
RC963.A1 CODEN: AOEHE9
APPLIED OCCUPATIONAL & ENVIRONMENTAL HYGIENE. Text in English. 1986. m. GBP 127, USD 210 to individuals; GBP 239, USD 395 to institutions (effective 2002). adv. bk.rev. abstr, charts, illus. Index. back issues avail.; reprints avail. *Refereed.* **Document type:** *Academic/Scholarly.* **Description:** Articles of interest to the occupational and environmental safety and health professional.
Formerly (until vol.5, no.1, 1990): Applied Industrial Hygiene (0882-8032)
Related titles: Online - full text ed.: ISSN 1521-0898 (from CatchWord Ltd., EBSCO Publishing, O C L C Online Computer Library Center, Inc., RoweCom Information Quest, ingenta, Swets Blackwell).
Indexed: CSNB, Chem.Abstr., Chem.Indus.Notes, Chem.Titles, Curr.Cont. (coverage dropped), Environ.Abstr., Environ.Per.Bibl. (1993-), Environ.Sci.Poll.Mgmt., Ergon.Abstr., Excerp.Med., Ind.Hyg.Dig., Ind.Med. (1990-), Lab.Haz.Bull., Mass Spectr.Bull., Pollut.Abstr., Risk Abstr., Saf.Sci.Abstr., Tox.Abstr., World Surf.Coat.
—BLDSC (1576.239000), CASDDS, CatchWord, CISTI, EMDOCS, GNLM, Infotrieve, ingenta. **CCC.**
Published by: (American Conference of Governmental Industrial Hygienists, Inc.), Taylor & Francis Inc, 325 Chestnut St, Ste 800, Philadelphia, PA 19106. TEL 215-625-8900, 800-354-1420, FAX 215-625-8914, info@taylorandfrancis.com, http://www.tandf.co.uk/journals/tf/1047322x.html, http://www.taylorandfrancis.com. Ed. J Thomas Pierce. Circ: 5,000 (paid).

614.8 NOR ISSN 0332-7124
HD7200
ARBEIDERVERN; working environment journal. Text in Norwegian. 1973. 6/yr. NOK 120 (effective 2000). adv. illus. **Document type:** *Trade.*
Indexed: C.I.S. Abstr., INIS Atomind., Lab.Haz.Bull.
—CCC.
Published by: Direktoratet for Arbeidstilsynet/Directorate of Labour Inspection, Fr Nansens vei 14, Postboks 8103, Dep, Oslo 0032, Norway. TEL 47-22-95-70-00, FAX 47-22-60-77-72. Ed. Lise Ekern. Circ: 28,300.

363.1 NOR ISSN 0800-2088
ARBEIDSMILJOE. Text in Norwegian. 1951. 8/yr. NOK 380 (effective 2001). adv. bk.rev. **Document type:** *Bulletin, Academic/Scholarly.* **Description:** Concentrates on work environment, occupational health and safety. Contains research articles and general information about safety and health.
Former titles (until 1982): Vern og Velferd Arbejdsmiljoe (0332-9127); (until 1980): Vern og Velferd (0049-5964)
—CCC.
Published by: Arbeidsmiljoesenteret, Chr. Krogsgate 1, Postboks 9326, Groenland, Oslo 0135, Norway. TEL 47-22-05-78-00, FAX 47-22-05-78-39, paul.norberg@arbeidsmiljosenteret.no, http://www.arbeidsmiljosenteret.no. Ed. Paul Norberg TEL 46-22-05-78-07. Adv. contact Heidi Olafsen TEL 46-22-09-69-10. B&W page NOK 10,300, color page NOK 14,900; trim 185 x 260. Circ: 9,000.

363.11 NLD ISSN 0929-1105
ARBEIDSOMSTANDIGHEDEN CONCREET. Text in Dutch. 1992. 11/yr. NLG 140 (effective 1998). adv. **Document type:** *Trade.*
Formerly (until 1993): Arbeidsomstandigheden-actueel (0927-4480)
Published by: (Nederlands Instituut voor Arbeidsomstandigheden), Uitgeverij Kluwer BV (Subsidiary of: Wolters Kluwer N.V.), Postbus 23, Deventer 7400 GA, Netherlands. TEL 31-570-633155, FAX 31-570-633834. Ed. E Pennekamp. Circ: 6,600.

614.85 BEL ISSN 0770-7649
ARBEIDSVEILIGHEID. Text in Flemish. 1982. s-m. BEF 5,380. index. **Description:** Focuses on latest developments in workers' safety.
Published by: C E D Samsom (Subsidiary of: Wolters Samsom Belgie n.v.), Kouterveld 14, Diegem 1831, Belgium. TEL 32-2-7231111.

613.62 DEU ISSN 0946-7599
ARBEIT UND GESUNDHEIT; Zeitschrift fuer Sicherheit und Gesundheit bei der Arbeit. Text in German. 1949. m. DEM 16.32 (effective 2001). adv. **Document type:** *Journal, Trade.*
Published by: (Hauptverband der gewerblichen Berufsgenossenschaften e.V.), Universum Verlagsanstalt GmbH KG, Taunusstr 54, Wiesbaden 65183, Germany. TEL 49-611-9030-0, FAX 49-611-9030382, uv@universum.de, http://www.universum.de. Circ: 431,728 (controlled).

ARBEITSMEDIZIN, SOZIALMEDIZIN, UMWELTMEDIZIN; Zeitschrift fuer Praxis, Klinik, Forschung, Begutachtung. see *PUBLIC HEALTH AND SAFETY*

ARBEITSMEDIZIN, SOZIALMEDIZIN, UMWELTMEDIZIN. SUPPLEMENT. see *PUBLIC HEALTH AND SAFETY*

363.11 DNK ISSN 0905-5010
ARBEJDSMILJOE. Text in Danish. 1982. m. (11/yr.). DKK 337.60 (effective 1998). adv. *Refereed.*
Formerly (until 1982): Pas Paa (0105-6239)
Published by: Arbejdsmiljoefondet, Vermundsgade 38, Copenhagen O 2100, Denmark. TEL 45-39-16-05-00, FAX 45-39-16-05-80. Ed. Jim Jaeger. Adv. contact Gorm Bjaerring. Circ: 17,500.

363.11 SWE ISSN 0346-7805
ARBETARSKYDD. Text in Swedish. 1972. 15/yr. SEK 475. adv. 20 p./no. 5 cols./p. **Document type:** *Newspaper, Trade.*
Former titles (until 1975): Aktuell Information (0345-0244); (until 1974): Aktuellt fraan Arbetarskyddsverket (0345-0252)
Published by: Arbetarskyddsstyrelsen, Ekelundsvaegen 16-20, Solna 17184, Sweden. TEL 46-8-730-99-00, FAX 46-8-730-90-68, hansolof.wiklund@arbsky.se, http://www.arbsky.se. Ed., Pub. Hans Olof Wiklund. Adv. contact Torbjoern Jonsson. B&W page SEK 25,000, color page SEK 27,000; trim 252 x 360. Circ: 23,300 (controlled).

614.85 SWE ISSN 0348-2138
ARBETARSKYDDSSTYRELSENS FOERFATTNINGSSAMLING. Text in Swedish. 1978. irreg. SEK 730 (effective 1997). **Document type:** *Government.*
Formed by the merger of: Arbetarskyddsstyrelsens Meddelanden; Arbetarskyddsstyrelsens Anvisningar
Published by: Arbetarskyddsstyrelsen, Ekelundsvaegen 16-20, Solna 17184, Sweden. TEL 46-8-730-90-00, FAX 46-8-730-90-10, karina.harjula@arbsky.se, http://www.arbsky.se. Circ: 14,000. **Subscr. to:** STK-Distribution, Fack 84, Vallingby 16212, Sweden.

363.11 NLD ISSN 0169-9237
ARBO BULLETIN. Text in Dutch. 1986. 6/yr. NLG 238 (effective 1999). adv. **Document type:** *Bulletin, Trade.*
Published by: (Nederlands Instituut voor Arbeidsomstandigheden), Uitgeverij Kluwer BV (Subsidiary of: Wolters Kluwer N.V.), Postbus 23, Deventer 7400 GA, Netherlands. TEL 31-570-633155, FAX 31-570-633834. Ed. H J van Zwam.

363.11 NLD
ARBO JAARBOEK. Text in Dutch. 1959. a. NLG 130 (effective 1999). adv. bk.rev. **Document type:** *Trade.* **Description:** Constitutes a yearbook for those professionally occupied with the working environment.
Formerly: Veiligheidsjaarboek (0083-534X)
Published by: (Nederlands Instituut voor Arbeidsomstandigheden), Uitgeverij Kluwer BV (Subsidiary of: Wolters Kluwer N.V.), Postbus 23, Deventer 7400 GA, Netherlands. FAX 31-570-633834. Circ: 4,000.

363.11 690 NLD ISSN 1382-7197
ARBOUW JOURNAAL. Text in Dutch. 1991. 4/yr. NLG 55 (effective 1999). adv. **Document type:** *Trade.* **Description:** Covers issues relating to the improvement of working conditions in the construction industry.
Published by: (Stichting Arbouw), Uitgeverij Kluwer BV (Subsidiary of: Wolters Kluwer N.V.), Postbus 23, Deventer 7400 GA, Netherlands. TEL 31-570-633155, FAX 31-570-633834.

ARCHIVES BELGES DE SANTE PUBLIQUE. see *PUBLIC HEALTH AND SAFETY*

362.1 613.6 FRA ISSN 1250-3274 CODEN: AMPMAR
ARCHIVES DES MALADIES PROFESSIONNELLES; organe officiel des societes de medecine du travail. Text in French; Summaries in English. 1938. 8/yr. FRF 1,214; FRF 1,516 foreign (effective 2000). adv. bk.rev. illus. index. reprint service avail. from ISI. **Document type:** *Academic/Scholarly.* **Description:** Supplies technical, scientific and practical information to practitioners devoted to occupational medicine or professional pathology.
Formerly (until 1992): Archives des Maladies Professionnelles de Medecine du Travail et de Securite Sociale (0003-9691)
Related titles: Microform ed.: (from PQC); Online - full text ed.: (from RoweCom Information Quest).
Indexed: Abstr.Hyg., Biol.Abstr., C.I.S. Abstr., CSNB, Chem.Abstr., Curr.Adv.Ecol.Sci., Ergon.Abstr., Excerp.Med., Helminthol.Abstr., Hort.Abstr., INIS Atomind., Ind.Med. (coverage dropped), Ind.Vet., Lab.Haz.Bull., Nutr.Abstr., Protozool.Abstr., Rev.Appl.Entomol., Rev.Plant Path., Trop.Dis.Bull.
—BLDSC (1637.390000), CASDDS, CISTI, EMDOCS, GNLM, Infotrieve, KNAW. **CCC.**
Published by: (Societes de Medecine du Travail), Masson - Periodiques, 120 bd. St. Germain, Paris 75006, France. TEL 33-1-40466200, FAX 33-1-40466201. Ed. Patrick Hadengue. Circ: 3,500. **Subscr. to:** Societe de Periodiques Specialises, BP 22, Vineuil Cedex 41354, France. TEL 33-2-54504612, FAX 33-2-54504611.

613.62 ITA
ARCHIVIO DI SCIENZE DEL LAVORO. Text in Italian. 1993 (vol.9, no.1). q. ITL 66,000; ITL 99,000 foreign. **Document type:** *Journal, Academic/Scholarly.*
Indexed: Chem.Abstr., Chem.Indus.Notes, Chem.Titles.
Published by: Istituto Poligrafico e Zecca dello Stato, Via Nomentana 2, Rome, RM 00161, Italy. TEL 39-06-8559648, FAX 39-06-8559648. Ed. Carmelo Bellocco.

613.62 620.8 ESP
ARCHIVOS DE PREVENCION DE RIESGOS LABORALES. Text in Spanish. 1998. q. ESP 9,200 to individuals; ESP 13,100 to institutions (effective 2001). adv. back issues avail.; reprints avail. *Refereed.* **Document type:** *Journal, Academic/Scholarly.*
Related titles: Online - full text ed.: 1998.
Published by: (Societat Catalana de Medicina i Securetat en el Treball), Ediciones Doyma S.A., Traversa de Gracia, 17-21, Barcelona 08021, Spain. TEL 34-93-200-0711, doyma@doyma.es, http://www.doyma.es/. Ed. F Garcia Benavides. R&P Monica Barnes. Adv. contact Jose Antonio Hernandez. B&W page ESP 75,000, color page ESP 100,000; 280 x 210. Circ: 1,000 (paid).

ARHIV ZA HIGIJENU RADA I TOKSIKOLOGIJU/ ARCHIVES OF INDUSTRIAL HYGIENE AND TOXICOLOGY. see *ENVIRONMENTAL STUDIES—Toxicology And Environmental Safety*

613.62 USA ISSN 0197-7903 N1
ART HAZARDS NEWS. Text in English. 1978. q. USD 24; USD 26.50 in Canada; USD 29 elsewhere. adv. bk.rev. illus. index. reprints avail. **Document type:** *Newsletter.* **Description:** News on research and education pertaining to hazards in the arts (including visual and performing arts, and museums and educational facilities), covering such topics as precautions, legislation and regulations, lawsuits, and calendars of events.
Published by: Center for Safety in the Arts, 2124 Broadway, 310, New York, NY 10023-1722. csa@artswire.org, http://www.tmn.com:70/1/Artswire/csa. Ed., Pub., Adv. contact Angela Babin. Circ: 2,500.

ASIAN ENVIRONMENT; journal of environmental science and technology for balanced development. see *ENVIRONMENTAL STUDIES*

363.11 613.62 FIN ISSN 1237-0843
ASIAN - PACIFIC NEWSLETTER ON OCCUPATIONAL HEALTH AND SAFETY. Text in English. 1994. 3/yr. free (effective 2001). back issues avail. **Document type:** *Newsletter.* **Description:** Covers issues of occupational health and safety in the Asia-Pacific region.
Related titles: Online - full text ed.: Asian - Pacific Newsletter on Occupational Health and Safety - Online. ISSN 1564-4790.
Indexed: Environ.Sci.Poll.Mgmt., Pollut.Abstr., Saf.Sci.Abstr.
Published by: Finnish Institute of Occupational Health, Topeliuksenkatu 41a A, Helsinki 00250, Finland. TEL 358-9-4747-2470, FAX 358-9-241-3804, http://www.occuphealth.fi/e/info/asian/asindex.htmm. Ed. Inkeri Haataja. **Co-sponsor:** International Labour Organization, Asian-Pacific Regional Programme on Occupational Health and Safety, SZ.

613.62 FRA ISSN 0066-927X
ASSOCIATION FRANCAISE DES TECHNICIENS ET INGENIEURS DE SECURITE ET DES MEDECINS DU TRAVAIL. ANNUAIRE. Text in French. 1965. a. FRF 360. adv.
Published by: Association Francaise des Techniciens et Ingenieurs de Securite et des Medecins du Travail (AFTIM), 1 pl. Uranie, Joinville le Pont 94340, France. TEL 33-1-48-85-70-59, FAX 33-1-48-85-02-99.

613.62 POL ISSN 1230-4700
ATEST. Text in Polish; Summaries in English, Russian. 1947. m. USD 96 foreign (effective 1999). adv. bk.rev. bibl, illus, pat. index. **Document type:** *Trade.* **Description:** Covers work safety and hygiene, and labor medicine.
Former titles (until 1992): Ochrona Pracy (0029-8220); (until 1952): Bezpieczenstwo i Higiena Pracy (1230-4727)
Indexed: AgroLibrex, C.I.S. Abstr., Chem.Abstr., INIS Atomind.
Published by: (Naczelna Organizacja Techniczna), Wydawnictwo SIGMA - N O T Sp. z o.o., Ul Mazowiecka 12, PO Box 1004, Warsaw 00950, Poland. TEL 48-22-8180918, FAX 48-22-6192187. Ed. Jerzy Knyziak. adv.: B&W page DEM 900. Circ: 7,000. **Dist. by:** SIGMA NOT Ltd., Ul Bartycka 20, Warsaw 00716, Poland. **Co-sponsor:** Panstwowa Inspekcja Pracy.

614.85 AUS ISSN 1328-9071
AUSTRALIAN OCCUPATIONAL HEALTH & SAFETY FILE. Text in English. 1993. q. price varies. **Document type:** *Trade.*
Related titles: CD-ROM ed.; Online - full text ed.
Published by: I H S Australian Pty. Ltd., Level 3, 33 Rowe St, Eastwood, NSW 2122, Australia. TEL 61-2-9804-1200, FAX 61-2-9804-0200, ihs@ihs.com.au, http://www.ihs.com.au.

614.85 AUS
AUSTRALIAN OCCUPATIONAL HEALTH & SAFETY YEARBOOK. Text in English. 1993. a. AUD 125 (effective 2001). adv. **Document type:** *Trade.*
Related titles: CD-ROM ed.; Online - full text ed.
Published by: I H S Australian Pty. Ltd., Level 3, 33 Rowe St, Eastwood, NSW 2122, Australia. TEL 61-2-9804-1200, FAX 61-2-9804-0200, ihs@ihs.com.au, http://www.ihs.com.au.

614.85 USA
B C S P NEWSLETTER. Text in English. 1975. 2/yr. membership only. back issues avail. **Document type:** *Newsletter.* **Description:** Professional certification in safety, demographics of safety professionals and credentialling activities.
Published by: Board of Certified Safety Professionals, 208 Burwash, Savoy, IL 61874. TEL 217-359-9263, http://www.bcsp.org. Ed. Roger L Brauer.

B F S - BERICHTE. (Bundesamt fuer Strahlenschutz) see *ENERGY—Nuclear Energy*

B F S - E T. (Bundesamt fuer Strahlenschutz - Entsorgung und Transport) see *ENERGY—Nuclear Energy*

B F S - I A R. (Bundesamt fuer Strahlenschutz - Atmosphaerische Radioaktivitaet) see *ENERGY—Nuclear Energy*

B F S - I S H BERICHTE. see *ENERGY—Nuclear Energy*

B F S - K T. (Bundesamt fuer Strahlenschutz - Kerntechnische Sicherheit) see *ENERGY—Nuclear Energy*

B F S - S T. (Bundesamt fuer Strahlenschutz - Strahlenschutz) see *ENERGY—Nuclear Energy*

B F S - SCHRIFTEN. (Bundesamt fuer Strahlenschutz) see *ENERGY—Nuclear Energy*

613.62 DEU
B G W JAHRESBERICHT. Text in German. a. **Document type:** *Bulletin, Government.*
Formerly: B G W Verwaltungsbericht
Published by: Berufsgenossenschaft fuer Gesundheitsdienst und Wohlfahrtspflege, Pappelallee 35-37, Hamburg 22089, Germany. TEL 49-40-20207-0, FAX 49-40-20207-525.

614.85 DEU ISSN 0933-4629
B I A HANDBUCH. Text in German. 1985. irreg. DEM 168 (effective 2000). **Document type:** *Bulletin, Trade.*
Published by: (Berufsgenossenschaftliches Institut fuer Arbeitssicherheit), Erich Schmidt Verlag GmbH & Co. (Berlin), Genthiner Str 30G, Berlin 10785, Germany. TEL 49-30-250085-0, FAX 49-30-25008511, esv@esvmedien.de, http://www.erich-schmidt-verlag.de.

614.85 USA
B N A'S SAFETY LIBRARY ON C D. Text in English. 1994. m. USD 795 (effective 1999). **Description:** Collection of resources including the laws, regulations, related documents and analysis covering occupational safety and health issues.
Media: CD-ROM.
Published by: The Bureau of National Affairs, Inc., 1231 25th St, N W, Washington, DC 20037. TEL 202-452-4200, FAX 202-822-8092.

658.3 USA ISSN 1091-2894
B N A'S SAFETYNET. Text in English. 1977. bi-w. USD 335 (effective 2001). index. 8 p./no. back issues avail. **Document type:** *Newsletter.* **Description:** Review of workplace safety and health regulations, policies and trends.
Formerly (until 1996): Job Safety and Health (Washington) (0149-7510)
Related titles: Online - full text ed.: (from Human Resources Information Network, Bureau of National Affairs, Inc., (BNA), The).
—**CCC.**
Published by: The Bureau of National Affairs, Inc., 1231 25th St, N W, Washington, DC 20037. TEL 202-452-4200, 800-372-1033, 800-452-7773, FAX 202-822-8092, customercare@bna.com, bnaplus@bna.com, http://www.bna.com/. Pub. Gregory McCaffery.

617.03 CAN
BACK TO WORK. Text in English. 1997. m. CND 249 (effective 2000). adv. **Document type:** *Trade.* **Description:** Dedicated to providing cost-effective strategies for managing employee rehabilitation and return-to-work.
Published by: Southam Information Products Ltd., 1450 Don Mills Rd, Don Mills, ON M3B 2X7, Canada. TEL 416-445-6641, 800-668-2374, FAX 416-442-2200. Ed. Cindy Moser. Pub., R&P, Adv. contact Peter Boxer.

363.11 613.62 FIN ISSN 1455-8459
BARENTS NEWSLETTER ON OCCUPATIONAL HEALTH AND SAFETY. Text in English, Russian. 1998. 3/yr. back issues avail. *Refereed.* **Document type:** *Newsletter, Academic/Scholarly.* **Description:** Reports on issues of concern to persons involved in occupational safety and health.
Related titles: Online - full text ed.
Published by: Finnish Institute of Occupational Health, Topeliuksenkatu 41a A, Helsinki 00250, Finland. TEL 358-9-4747-2344, FAX 358-9-878-3326, http://www.occuphealth.fi/e/info/barents/index/html. Eds. Marjanna Mattila, Suvi Lehtinen.

363.7 FRA
BATIMENT - ENTRETIEN. Text in French. 1968. bi-m. FRF 72. adv.
Address: 91 rue du Faubourg Saint Denis, Paris 75010, France. TEL 42-46-55-24, FAX 48-00-05-03. Ed. Bernard Abenesdra. Circ: 10,500.

613.62 DEU ISSN 0341-096X
BAU; Mitteilungsblatt. Text in German. 1949. q. **Document type:** *Newsletter.*
Published by: Bau-Berufsgenossenschaft Wuppertal, Eulenbergstr 15-21, Cologne 51065, Germany. TEL 0221-6703175.

614.85 DEU ISSN 0931-2862
BAU-BERUFSGENOSSENSCHAFT HANNOVER. MITTEILUNGSBLATT. Text in German. 1976. q. free per issue. adv. bk.rev. back issues avail. **Document type:** *Newspaper, Trade.*
Published by: Bau-Berufsgenossenschaft Hannover, Hildesheimer Str 309, Hannover 30519, Germany. TEL 49-511-987-0, FAX 49-511-9872440. Ed. Rolf Schaper. Adv. contact Bernhard Foerster. Circ: 76,000.

BERUFSGENOSSENSCHAFT FUER GESUNDHEITSDIENST UND WOHLFAHRTSPFLEGE. MITTEILUNGEN. see *INSURANCE*

O

613.62 DEU ISSN 0933-4289
BERUFSKRANKHEITENVERORDNUNG. Text in German. 1977. irreg. DEM 128 (effective 2000). **Document type:** *Bulletin, Trade.*
Published by: Erich Schmidt Verlag GmbH & Co. (Berlin), Genthiner Str 30G, Berlin 10785, Germany. TEL 49-30-250085-0, FAX 49-30-25008521, vertrieb@esvmedien.de, http://www.erich-schmidt-verlag.de.

614.85 USA
T55.A1
BEST'S SAFETY AND SECURITY DIRECTORY; safety-industrial hygiene-security. Text in English. 1946. a. USD 95 (effective 2000). adv. **Document type:** *Directory.*
Formerly (until 1998): Best's Safety Directory (0090-7480)
Related titles: Online - full text ed.
—Infotrieve. **CCC.**
Published by: A.M. Best Co., Ambest Rd, Oldwick, NJ 08858. TEL 908-439-2200, FAX 908-439-3296, http://www.ambest.com/safety/index.html. Ed. Renee Herb.

O

613.62 RUS ISSN 0409-2961
TN295 CODEN: BZTPAM
BEZOPASNOST' TRUDA V PROMYSHLENNOSTI/ LABOUR SAFETY IN INDUSTRY. Text in Russian. 1932. m. RUR 50 domestic (effective 1999); USD 127 foreign. adv. *Refereed.* **Description:** Covers a wide variety of themes relevant to industrial production and safety.
Indexed: Chem.Abstr., Chem.Indus.Notes, Chem.Titles, GeoRef, INIS Atomind., Ref.Zh., Russ.Acad.Sci.Bibl.
—CASDDS, East View.
Published by: Nauchno-Tekhnicheskii Tsentr po Bezopasnosti v Promyshlennosti Gosgortekhnazdora Rossii, Luk'yanova ul 4, korp 8, kom 310, Moscow 107066, Russian Federation. TEL 7-095-2639874, FAX 7-095-2612189. Ed. S N Buinovskii. Pub. V I Sidorov. Adv. contact N Yu Solenikova. **US dist. addr.:** East View Publications, 3020 Harbor Ln N, Minneapolis, MN 55447. TEL 612-550-0961.

614.85 SVK ISSN 0322-8347
BEZPECNA PRACA. Text in Czech, Slovak; Summaries in English, German, Russian. 1969. bi-m. SKK 294 domestic; USD 45 newsstand/cover foreign (effective 2001). adv. **Document type:** *Monographic series.* **Description:** Deals with theory and praxis of occupational safety.
Related titles: CD-ROM ed.; E-mail ed.; Fax ed.
Indexed: C.I.S. Abstr., Russ.Acad.Sci.Bibl.
Published by: Vyskumny a Vzdelavaci Ustav Bezpecnosti Prace/Research Institute of Work Security, Stefanikova 47, Bratislava 81435, Slovakia. TEL 421-7-43330666, FAX 421-7-43330666. Pub. Anastazia Bezakova. adv.: B&W page SKK 13,000, color page SKK 35,000. **Dist. by:** Messrs. L.K. Permanent Ltd., PO Box 4, Bratislava 83414, Slovakia.

613.62 POL ISSN 0137-7043
BEZPIECZENSTWO PRACY. Text in Polish. 1971. m. PLZ 27 per quarter. adv. bk.rev. **Document type:** *Academic/Scholarly.* **Description:** Covers occupational safety and ergonomics.
Indexed: AgroLibrex.
Published by: Centralny Instytut Ochrony Pracy/Central Institute for Labour Protection, Ul Czerniakowska 16, Warsaw 00701, Poland. TEL 48-22-6233675, FAX 48-22-6233693, oinip@ciop.waw.pl, oinip@ciop.pl. Ed. Barbar Malczewska. Adv. contact Barbara Malczewska. Circ: 4,500 (controlled).

614.85 DEU ISSN 0935-9451
BILAG BRIEF. Text in German. 1982. 2/yr. DEM 15. adv. bk.rev. bibl, illus. back issues avail. **Document type:** *Newsletter.*
Published by: Berliner Infoladen fuer Arbeit und Gesundheit e.V., Gneisenaustr 2A, Berlin 10961, Germany. TEL 49-30-6932090. Ed. Eberhard Goebel Beate Guthke. Adv. contact Beate Guthke. Circ: 1,200.

613.62 DEU ISSN 0930-195X
BIOLOGISCHE ARBEITSSTOFF TOLERANZ WERTE UND EXPOSITIONSAEQUIVALENTE FUER KREBSERZEUGENDE ARBEITSSTOFFE. Text in German. 1983. irreg., latest 1998. **Document type:** *Monographic series, Academic/Scholarly.*
Published by: (Deutsche Forschungsgemeinschaft), Wiley - V C H, Postfach 101161, Weinheim 69451, Germany. TEL 49-6201-606-0, FAX 49-6201-606-328, subservice@wiley-vch.de, http://www.wiley-vch.de. Circ: 600 (controlled).

614.85 ISR
BITECHUT. Text in Hebrew. bi-m.
Published by: Safety and Hygiene Institute, 22 Mazeh St., Tel Aviv, Israel. TEL 03-297311.

613.7 USA ISSN 0275-9101
BODY BULLETIN NEWSLETTER. Text in English. 1981. m. **Document type:** *Newsletter.* **Description:** Introduces employees to safe and sensible ways to deal with common health problems.
Related titles: Online - full text ed.: (from ProQuest Information & Learning, Gale Group).
—CCC.
Published by: Rodale, 33 E Minor St, Emmaus, PA 18098. TEL 610-967-5171, FAX 610-967-7725, http://www.rodale.com.

658.382 GBR
BRITISH SAFETY COUNCIL GUIDES. Text in English. m. (11/yr.). **Document type:** *Monographic series, Trade.*
Published by: British Safety Council, 70 Chancellors Rd, London W6 9RS, United Kingdom. TEL 44-20-8741-1231, FAX 44-20-8741-4555, bsc1@mail.britishsafetycouncil.co.uk, mail@britsafe.org, http://www.britishsafetycouncil.co.uk/bsc, http://www.britsafe.org/.

613 IRL ISSN 1393-8797
BUSINESS HEALTH. Text in English. m.
Former titles (until 2000): Health & Safety (0791-8380); (until 1988): Sciath (0791-1602)
Published by: Jude Publications Ltd., 9 Nth Frederick St, Dublin 2, Ireland. TEL 353-1-6713500, FAX 353-1-6713074. Pub. Anne-Marie Moran.

613.62 620 USA
C S P DIRECTORY AND INTERNATIONAL REGISTRY OF CERTIFIED SAFETY PROFESSIONALS. Text in English. 1975. biennial. USD 60 (effective 2000). adv. **Document type:** *Directory.* **Description:** Lists certified individuals by location, examination passed, services offered and areas of expertise.
Formerly: C S P Directory
Related titles: CD-ROM ed.: USD 250 (effective 2000).
Published by: Board of Certified Safety Professionals, 208 Barwash Ave, Savoy, IL 61874. TEL 217-359-9263. Circ: 13,000.

613.63 614.85 USA ISSN 1062-6743
C T D NEWS✱. Text in English. 1991. m. USD 173. adv. index. back issues avail. **Document type:** *Newsletter.* **Description:** Deals with occupational health and computer injury issues.
Related titles: Diskette ed.: 1991; Online - full text ed.: 1991 (from Gale Group).
Indexed: CSNB.
—CCC.
Published by: Center for Workplace Health, PO Box 980, Horsham, PA 19044-0980. TEL 610-896-2770, 800-554-4283, FAX 610-896-2762. Ed. Michael Gauf. Pub. James Kinsella. R&P Isabelle Vesey. Adv. contact Bradley Aronson. Circ: 4,365.

613.62 USA ISSN 1054-1209
CAL - O S H A REPORTER. (Occupational Safety and Health Administration) Text in English. 1973. w. USD 337 (effective 1998). adv. bk.rev. index. back issues avail. **Document type:** *Newsletter.* **Description:** Written for occupational safety and health practitioners primarily in California. Covers job safety and health, workers' compensation, toxics, risk management and other related issues. Provides detailed coverage of laws, regulations and complete summaries of all related court cases.
Former titles: California - O S H A Reporter; Cal - O S H A Reporter
Related titles: Online - full text ed.: (from LexisNexis).
Published by: Commanon Corporation, PO Box 1100, Grass Valley, CA 95945-1100. TEL 530-477-8500, FAX 530-477-8600, creator@content.com, http://www.cal-osha.com. Ed. Anne Bell. Pub. J Dale Debber. R&P J. Dale Debber TEL 530-470-7500. Adv. contact Terry Boyer. Circ: 2,956 (paid).

613.62 USA
KFC584.A15
CALIFORNIA SAFETY & HEALTH MONITOR✱. Text in English. 1992. bi-w. USD 387. index. back issues avail. **Description:** Notification service providing comprehensive coverage of state and local job safety and health developments and related workplace developments.
Formerly: B N A California Safety and Health Report (1065-3104)
Published by: M. Lee Smith Publishers LLC, 5201 Virginia Way, PO Box 5094, Brentwoood, TN 37024-5094. TEL 615-373-7517, FAX 615-373-5183. Ed. Jeffrey Tanenbaum.

344 613.62 CAN
CANADIAN EMPLOYMENT SAFETY AND HEALTH GUIDE. Text in English. m. CND 860. **Document type:** *Trade.* **Description:** Reports on federal and provincial legislation on employment safety and health plus relevant case law.
Indexed: CBCA Bus. (1996-).
Published by: C C H Canadian Ltd., 90 Sheppard Ave E, Ste 300, North York, ON M2N 6X1, Canada. TEL 416-224-2248, 800-268-4522, FAX 416-224-2243, http://camelot.ca.cch.com.

CANADIAN MINING JOURNAL. see *MINES AND MINING INDUSTRY*

614.8 CAN ISSN 0709-5252
CANADIAN OCCUPATIONAL HEALTH & SAFETY NEWS. Text in English. 1978. w. CND 399 (effective 2000). adv. q. index. **Document type:** *Newsletter.* **Description:** Contains the latest legislative and regulatory changes, new techniques and technology, calendars of forthcoming conferences and workshops and WHMIS updates.
Formerly: Canadian Industrial Health and Safety News (0701-8983)
Related titles: ♦ Supplement: Review of O H & S Legislation in (Year). ISSN 1207-0661.
Indexed: INIS Atomind.
—CISTI.
Published by: Southam Information Products Ltd., 1450 Don Mills Rd, Don Mills, ON M3B 2X7, Canada. TEL 416-445-6641, 800-668-2374, FAX 416-442-2200. Ed. Angela Stelmakowich. Pub., Adv. contact Peter Boxer.

363.1 340 CAN ISSN 0704-3724
CANADIAN OCCUPATIONAL SAFETY & HEALTH LAW. Text in English. 1978. m. CND 1,149 (effective 2000). adv. bk.rev. cum.index. **Description:** A guide to all federal and provincial health and safety acts, including all regulations.
Related titles: ♦ Supplement: Canadian Occupational Safety and Health Law Monthly Report. ISSN 0825-608X.
Published by: Southam Information Products Ltd., 1450 Don Mills Rd, Don Mills, ON M3B 2X7, Canada. TEL 416-445-6641, 800-668-2374, FAX 416-442-2200. Ed. Lidia Lubka. Pub. Todd Latham. Adv. contact Ian Rhind.

363.1 340 CAN ISSN 0825-608X
CANADIAN OCCUPATIONAL SAFETY AND HEALTH LAW MONTHLY REPORT. Text in English. 1984. m. **Description:** Keeps up with new draft legislation, judicial decisions and enforcement activities.
Related titles: ♦ Supplement to: Canadian Occupational Safety & Health Law. ISSN 0704-3724.
Published by: Southam Information Products Ltd., 1450 Don Mills Rd, Don Mills, ON M3B 2X7, Canada. TEL 416-445-6641, 800-668-2374, FAX 416-442-2200. Ed. Lidia Lubka. Pub. Todd Latham.

CHEMICAL SAFETY SHEETS. see *CHEMISTRY*

613.62 USA ISSN 0073-7488
CHEMICAL-TOXICOLOGICAL SERIES. BULLETINS. Text in English. 1947. irreg., latest vol.8, 1969. price varies. **Document type:** *Bulletin, Monographic series.*
Formerly: Industrial Hygiene Foundation. Chemical-Toxicological Series. Bulletin (0537-5215)
Published by: Industrial Health Foundation, Inc., 34 Penn Circle W, Pittsburgh, PA 15206. TEL 412-363-6600, FAX 412-363-6605, IHFincorp@aol.com, http://members.aol.com/ihfincorp/ihf.htm. R&P Marianne C Kaschak.

613.62 614.85 NLD
CHEMIEKAARTEN; gegevens voor veilig werken met chemicalien. Text in Dutch. 1977. a. NLG 189.50. **Description:** Standard work on the effects of chemicals on the human being and prevention possibilities.
Published by: (Nederlandse Instituut voor Arbeidsomstandigheden/Dutch Institute for the Working Environment), Samsom H.D. Tjeenk Willink B.V. (Subsidiary of: Wolters Kluwer N.V.), Postbus 316, Alphen aan den Rijn 2400 AH, Netherlands. TEL 31-1720-66822, FAX 31-1720-66639. Circ: 10,000.
Co-sponsors: Nederlandse Vereniging voor Veiligheidskunde; Vereniging van de Nederlandse Chemische Industrie/Association of the Dutch Chemical Industry.

CHILD LABOR MONITOR. see *CHILDREN AND YOUTH—About*

613.62 338 FRA
CLEANER PRODUCTION. Text in English. 2/yr. illus. *Refereed.* **Document type:** *Newsletter.* **Description:** Provides information on cleaner technologies and products, actions by governments and organizations to promote cleaner production and the UNEP IEPAC Cleaner Production activities and network.
Related titles: ♦ Supplement to: Industry and Environment. ISSN 0378-9993; ♦ Supplement to: Comite Francais pour l'Environnement. Lettre. ISSN 0999-6249.
Published by: United Nations Environment Programme, Industry and Environment Programme Activity Centre, 39-43 quai Andre Citroen, Paris Cedex 15 73739, France. TEL 33-1-44371450, FAX 33-1-44371474, unep.tie@unep.fr, unepie@unep.fr, http://www.uneptie.org. Ed. G Clark.

CLEANROOM TECHNOLOGY. see *ENGINEERING*

▼ **CLINICS IN OCCUPATIONAL AND ENVIRONMENTAL MEDICINE.** see *MEDICAL SCIENCES*

COATINGS, REGULATIONS AND THE ENVIRONMENT. see *PAINTS AND PROTECTIVE COATINGS*

613.62 USA
COMMUNITY AND WORKER RIGHT-TO-KNOW NEWS. Text in English. fortn. USD 479. index. **Document type:** *Newsletter.* **Description:** Publishes articles on right-to-know and emergency planning, health and safety with a focus on explosions, fires, and spills. Aimed at environmental managers seeking information on compliance.
Related titles: Online - full text ed.: (from Gale Group).
Published by: Thompson Publishing Group, 1725 K St, N W, Ste 700, Washington, DC 20006. TEL 202-739-9698. Ed. Felicia Day. Pub. Daphne Musselwhite.

658.3 344.73 613.62 USA ISSN 1077-5889
COMPLIANCE MAGAZINE; workplace safety, health & environment. Text in English. 1994. 10/yr., latest vol.8, no.1, 2001. USD 55 in North America; USD 140 elsewhere; USD 10 newsstand/cover domestic; USD 13 newsstand/cover foreign (effective 2001). adv. software rev., Website rev. illus, stat, tr.lit. 48 p./no. 4 cols./p. back issues avail. **Document type:** *Magazine, Trade.* **Description:** Aims to inform and educate industry professionals responsible for workplace safety, health and environment about existing regulations, significant new laws and recent compliance product developments that affect their operations.
Indexed: Eng.Ind., Environ.Sci.Poll.Mgmt., Pollut.Abstr., Risk Abstr., Saf.Sci.Abstr.
—Ei.
Published by: Douglas Publications, Inc., 2807 N Parham Rd, Ste 200, Richmond, VA 23294. TEL 804-762-9600, FAX 804-217-8999, bhintch@douglaspublications.com, info@douglaspublications.com, http://www.compliancemag.com. Ed. Betty Hintch. Adv. contact Russell Lindsay TEL 254-867-1011. B&W page USD 8,347, color page USD 9,397; trim 10 x 14.75. Circ: 60,000 (controlled). **Subscr. to:** Compliance, P O Box 811, Winchester, MA 01890. TEL 888-246-8484.

614 MEX ISSN 0185-2353
CONDICIONES DE TRABAJO. Text in Spanish. 1976. 3/yr. free per issue. bibl, charts, illus, stat. **Document type:** *Government.* **Description:** Presents recommendations from the government on health insurance, hygiene, and work conditions in the work force.
Published by: Secretaria del Trabajo y Prevision Social, Direccion General de Seguridad e Higiene en el Trabajo, Calzada Azcapotzalco-La Villa No. 209, Junto Metro Ferreria, Mexico City, DF 02020, Mexico. TEL 52-5-3943344, FAX 52-5-3942644. Ed. Juan .Antonio Legaspi Velasco. Circ: 3,000.

352.14 USA ISSN 1533-1490
▼ **CONSTRUCTION & ENGINEERING MAGAZINE**; OSHA news, legal issues, workers' comp, safety issues, products, services. Text in English. 2001. bi-m. USD 34 domestic; USD 49 in Canada & Mexico; USD 84 elsewhere; USD 6 newsstand/cover domestic; USD 9 newsstand/cover elsewhere (effective 2001). adv. Website rev. illus, tr.lit. back issues avail.; reprints avail. **Document type:** *Magazine, Trade.* **Description:** Focuses on on-the-job hazards, safety, and compliance, and practical information on construction safety. Targets construction industry safety professionals.
Published by: Douglas Publications, Inc., 2807 N Parham Rd, Ste 200, Richmond, VA 23294. info@douglaspublications.com, http://www.cesmag.com. Ed. Betty Hintch. Pub., Adv. contact Russell Lindsay TEL 254-867-1011. B&W page USD 3,075, color page USD 4,065; trim 8.175 x 10.875. Circ: 20,000 (controlled). **Subscr. to:** CES, PO Box 833, Winchester, MA 23294.

614.85 GBR
CRONER'S DANGEROUS SUBSTANCES. Text in English. 1983. base vol. plus bi-m. updates. EUR 441.21 (effective 2001). **Description:** Covers European requirements for dangerous substance classification, packaging, and labeling, with emphasis on the U.K.
Related titles: CD-ROM ed.
Published by: Croner Publications Ltd. (Subsidiary of: Wolters Kluwer N.V.), Croner Publications Ltd, Croner House, 100 London Rd, Kingston Upon Thames, Surrey KT2 6SR, United Kingdom. TEL 44-208-547-3333, FAX 44-20-8547-2638, hs@croner.cch.co.uk, info@croner.cch.co.uk, http://www.croner.cch.co.uk. Ed. K Mitchell.

614.85 340.5 GBR
CRONER'S HEALTH AND SAFETY CASE LAW. Text in English. 1984. base vol. plus q. updates. GBP 213; GBP 136.50 updates. **Description:** Deals with all areas of U.K. health and safety case law. Compiles and interprets recent and important legal decisions in the health and safety field.
Related titles: Diskette ed.
Published by: Croner Publications Ltd. (Subsidiary of: Wolters Kluwer N.V.), Croner House, 173 Kingston Rd, New Malden, Surrey KT3 3SS, United Kingdom. TEL 44-208-547-3333, FAX 44-20-8547-2637, info@croner.co.uk, info@croner.cch.co.uk, http://www.croner.co.uk. Ed. Claire Beresford.

613.62 614.85 GBR ISSN 1352-5611
CRONER'S HEALTH & SAFETY MANAGER. Variant title: Health & Safety Manager. Text in English. 1994. base vol. plus m. updates. GBP 399; GBP 355 updates. **Document type:** *Trade.* **Description:** Provides information to assist with building and maintaining an effective safety culture within organizations.
Published by: Croner Publications Ltd. (Subsidiary of: Wolters Kluwer N.V.), Croner House, 173 Kingston Rd, New Malden, Surrey KT3 3SS, United Kingdom. TEL 44-208-547-3333, FAX 44-20-8547-2637, info@croner.co.uk, info@croner.cch.co.uk, http://www.croner.co.uk.

613.62 614.85 GBR
CRONER'S OFFICE HEALTH & SAFETY. Variant title: Croner's Office Health & Safety. Text in English. base vol. plus bi-m. updates. EUR 359.72 (effective 2001). **Document type:** *Trade.* **Description:** Provides information on health and safety legislation within the office environment, giving necessary practical advice.
Formerly: Office Health & Safety Briefing (0968-6606); Formerly: Croner's Health and Safety at Work
Related titles: CD-ROM ed.; Diskette ed.
Indexed: World Surf.Coat.
Published by: Croner Publications Ltd. (Subsidiary of: Wolters Kluwer N.V.), Croner Publications Ltd, Croner House, 100 London Rd, Kingston Upon Thames, Surrey KT2 6SR, United Kingdom. TEL 44-208-547-3333, FAX 44-20-8547-2638, hs@croner.cch.co.uk, info@croner.cch.co.uk, http://www.croner.cch.co.uk, http://www.croner.co.uk. Ed. S Harding.

613.62 GBR
CRONER'S SUBSTANCES HAZARDOUS TO HEALTH. Text in English. 1986. base vol. plus q. updates. EUR 716.69 (effective 2001). **Document type:** *Trade.* **Description:** Provides a practical guide to the assessment, measurement, and control of specific hazardous substances.
Related titles: CD-ROM ed.
Published by: Croner Publications Ltd. (Subsidiary of: Wolters Kluwer N.V.), Croner Publications Ltd, Croner House, 100 London Rd, Kingston Upon Thames, Surrey KT2 6SR, United Kingdom. TEL 44-208-547-3333, FAX 44-20-8547-2638, hs@croner.cch.co.uk, info@croner.cch.co.uk, http://www.croner.cch.co.uk, http://www.croner.co.uk. Ed. L Parker.

CURRENT ISSUES IN FOOD SAFETY. see *FOOD AND FOOD INDUSTRIES*

613.62 USA ISSN 0270-3777
T55.3.H3 CODEN: DPIRDU
DANGEROUS PROPERTIES OF INDUSTRIAL MATERIALS REPORT*. Text in English. 1980. bi-m. USD 210 domestic; USD 250 in Canada. adv. bk.rev. bibl, charts, illus, stat. cum.index. back issues avail.
Indexed: Abstr.Bull.Inst.Pap.Chem., CAD CAM Abstr., C.I.S. Abstr., Chem.Abstr., Chem.Indus.Notes, Chem.Titles, Corros.Abstr., Dent.Ind., Environ.Abstr., Environ.Sci.Poll.Mgmt., GeoRef, Lab.Haz.Bull., Text.Tech.Dig. (1981-1990), Tox.Abstr.
—CASDDS, CISTI, ingenta, Linda Hall.
Published by: Van Nostrand Reinhold Co., 605 3rd Ave, New York, NY 10158-0180. TEL 212-254-3232, FAX 212-673-1239. Ed. N Irving Sax. Circ: 2,000 (controlled).

DELO + VARNOST; revija za varstvo pri delu. see *BUSINESS AND ECONOMICS—Labor And Industrial Relations*

DEVELOPMENTAL DISABILITIES SPECIAL INTEREST SECTION QUARTERLY. see *PSYCHOLOGY*

DICTIONNAIRE PERMANENT: SECURITE ET CONDITIONS DE TRAVAIL. see *BUSINESS AND ECONOMICS—Labor And Industrial Relations*

614.85 FRA ISSN 0339-6517
DOCUMENTS POUR LE MEDECIN DU TRAVAIL. Text in French. 1973. q. FRF 380. bk.rev. index, cum.index. **Document type:** *Newspaper, Corporate, Government.* **Description:** Scientific and medical publication for occupational medical practitioners.
Indexed: C.I.S. Abstr.
—BLDSC (3609.113080), GNLM.
Published by: Institut National de Recherche et de Securite pour la Prevention des Accidents du Travail et des Maladies Professionnelles, Ministere du Travail, 30 rue Olivier Noyer, Paris Cedex 14 75680, France. TEL 40-44-30-00, FAX 40-44-30-99. Ed. A Leprince. Circ: 10,000.

614.85 SWE ISSN 1403-9710
DU & JOBBET; arbetsmiljoetidningen. Text in Swedish. 1912. 11/yr. SEK 495; SEK 48 newsstand/cover (effective 2000). adv. bk.rev. charts, illus. back issues avail. **Document type:** *Magazine, Trade.*
Former titles (until 1999): Arbetsmiljoe (0003-7834); (until 1970): Arbetarskyddet
Indexed: C.I.S. Abstr.
—BLDSC (3630.577000).
Published by: Foereningen foer Arbetarskydd/Swedish Work Environment Association, Fack 17550, Stockholm 11891, Sweden. TEL 46-8-442-46-00, FAX 46-8-442-96-07, redaktionen@duochjobbet.com, http://www.duochjobbet.com. Ed., Pub. Eva Berlin. Adv. contact Peter Linden. B&W page SEK 30,600, color page SEK 34,000; trim 190 x 244. Circ: 120,000.

613.62 363.73 USA
E H & S PRODUCTS. (Environmental, Health & Safety) Text in English. s-a. Free to qualified subscribers. adv. **Document type:** *Trade.* **Description:** Publishes new product information for environmental, health and safety professionals.
Related titles: Online - full content ed.
Published by: Stevens Publishing Corporation, 5151 Beltline Rd, 10th fl, Dallas, TX 75240. TEL 972-687-6700, FAX 972-687-6770, http://www.ehs-online.com/, http://www.stevenspublishing.com/. adv.: color page USD 6,605.

613.62 USA ISSN 1062-5526
E M F HEALTH & SAFETY DIGEST. (Electric and Magnetic Field) Text in English. 1983. 10/yr. USD 450; USD 300 to non-profit organizations. bk.rev. bibl, charts. back issues avail. **Document type:** *Newsletter, Trade.* **Description:** Covers international communications on research and risk of electric and magnetic fields.
Former titles: Transmission - Distribution Health and Safety Report (0737-5743); T and D Health and Safety Report (0736-5047)
Indexed: Hist.Abstr. (coverage dropped), Sociol.Abstr.
Published by: Robert S. Banks Associates, PO Box 141049, University Sta, Minneapolis, MN 55414-6049. TEL 612-623-4600, FAX 612-623-3645, digest@rsba.com. Ed., R&P Janet Lathrop. Circ: 500 (paid).

613.62 USA ISSN 1070-4027
E M F HEALTH REPORT. (Electric and Magnetic Field) Text in English. 1993. bi-m. USD 285 domestic to institutions; USD 315 foreign to institutions (effective 2002). back issues avail. **Document type:** *Newsletter, Academic/Scholarly.* **Description:** covers health effects of powerlines, cell phones and medical applications of electric and magnetic field.
Published by: Information Ventures, Incorporated, 42 S. 15th St., Suite 700, Philadelphia, PA 19102-2299. TEL 215-569-2300, FAX 215-569-2575, http://infoventures.com/emf/hrpt. Ed. Robert B. Goldberg. Pub. Bruce Kleinstein.

O

EDUCATION SPECIAL INTEREST SECTION QUARTERLY. see *EDUCATION—Adult Education*

ELECTRICAL SENSITIVITY NEWS. see *PUBLIC HEALTH AND SAFETY*

613.62 613.85 USA
▼ **EMPLOYER HEALTH REGISTER.** Text in English. 2000. a. USD 125 per issue (effective 2000). **Description:** Guide to products and services for employers to improve the health and productivity of their employees.
Published by: Work - Loss Data Institute LLC, 500 N Shoreline Blvd, Ste 1101 N, Corpus Christi, TX 70471. TEL 361-883-5000, FAX 361-883-7025, http://www.employerhealth.com. Ed. Philip L Denniston.

613 CAN
EMPLOYER'S HEALTH & SAFETY MANUAL - ONTARIO. Text in English. 1989. 6/yr. CND 235. back issues avail. **Description:** Provides a complete text of the Occupational Health and Safety Act and amendments, as well as vital information on how to meet its responsibilities and obligations. Includes checklists and sample forms for supervisors and front-line managers.
Published by: Carswell, One Corporate Plaza, 2075 Kennedy Rd, Scarborough, ON M1T 3V4, Canada. TEL 416-609-8000, FAX 416-298-5094. Eds. Charles Humphrey, Cheryl Eduards. Circ: 2,800.

363.1 613.62 AUS ISSN 0728-635X
EMPLOYERS' REVIEW. Text in English. 1928. 23/yr. membership only. adv. bk.rev. **Document type:** *Newsletter.*
Published by: Employers' Federation of New South Wales, 313 Sussex St, Sydney, NSW 2001, Australia. FAX 61-2-261-1968. Ed. Jill Allen. Circ: 3,300.

331 313.62 USA ISSN 0093-1535
EMPLOYMENT SAFETY AND HEALTH GUIDE. Text in English. 1971. w. USD 1,139 (effective 2001). **Description:** Full text of standards, regulations, laws, and executive orders issued by OSHA and MSHA. Includes analysis, official forms and OSHA Field Inspection Reference Manual.
Related titles: CD-ROM ed.
—CCC.
Published by: C C H Incorporated, 2700 Lake Cook Rd., Riverwoods, IL 60015. TEL 847-267-7000, 800-449-9525, FAX 773-866-3895, http://www.cch.com. Ed. Paul Gibson. Pub. Catherine Wolfe.

ENCYCLOPEDIE MEDICO-CHIRURGICALE. TRAITE DE TOXICOLOGIE - PATHOLOGIE PROFESSIONELLE. see *ENVIRONMENTAL STUDIES—Toxicology And Environmental Safety*

ENVIRONMENTAL HEALTH BRIEFING. see *PUBLIC HEALTH AND SAFETY*

ERGA. see *OCCUPATIONAL HEALTH AND SAFETY—Abstracting, Bibliographies, Statistics*

363.11 613.62 EST
ESTONIAN NEWSLETTER ON OCCUPATIONAL HEALTH AND SAFETY. Text in English, Estonian, Russian. 1997. irreg. (3-4/yr.). **Document type:** *Newsletter, Academic/Scholarly.* **Description:** Discusses issues concerning the medical and clinical aspects of occupational health and safety.
Related titles: Online - full text ed.
Published by: Estonian Centre of Experimental and Clinical Medicine, Hiiu 42, Tallin 0016, Estonia. TEL 372-6-670-6820, http://www.occuphealth.fi/eng/info/estonia/index.htm. **Co-sponsors:** Estonian Centre of Occupational Health; Finnish Institute of Occupational Health, FI.

016.7 GBR ISSN 1357-2628
EURO O S H. (Occupational Safety & Health) Text in English. 1996. a. GBP 1,500, USD 2,400 for single user. **Description:** Database of EU and member state legislation pertaining to occupational safety and health, with ILO conventions and recommendations.
Media: CD-ROM.
Published by: Chapman & Hall Ltd. (Subsidiary of: International Thomson Publishing Group), Journals Department, Chapman & Hall, 2-6 Boundary Row, London SE1 8HN, United Kingdom. TEL 44-20-7865-0066, FAX 44-207-5220101, cust.serv@chall.co.uk. Eds. Alan C Neal, Frank B Wright.

363.11 USA ISSN 0743-6149
HD7269.B92
EVALUATING YOUR FIRM'S INJURY & ILLNESS RECORD. CONSTRUCTION INDUSTRIES. Text in English. a. **Document type:** *Government.*
Published by: U.S. Department of Labor, Bureau of Labor Statistics, 441 G St N W, Washington, DC 20212. TEL 202-655-4000. **Subscr. to:** U.S. Government Printing Office, Superintendent of Documents.

363.11 USA ISSN 0742-339X
HD8051
EVALUATING YOUR FIRM'S INJURY & ILLNESS RECORD. SERVICE INDUSTRIES. Text in English. a. **Document type:** *Government.*
Published by: U.S. Department of Labor, Bureau of Labor Statistics, 441 G St N W, Washington, DC 20212. TEL 202-655-4000. **Subscr. to:** U.S. Government Printing Office, Superintendent of Documents.

363.11 USA ISSN 0742-3403
HD8051
EVALUATING YOUR FIRM'S INJURY & ILLNESS RECORD. TRANSPORTATION & PUBLIC UTILITIES INDUSTRIES. Text in English. a. **Document type:** *Government.*
Published by: U.S. Department of Labor, Bureau of Labor Statistics, 441 G St N W, Washington, DC 20212. TEL 202-655-4000. **Subscr. to:** U.S. Government Printing Office, Superintendent of Documents.

363.11 USA ISSN 0742-3411
EVALUATING YOUR FIRM'S INJURY & ILLNESS RECORD. WHOLESALE & RETAIL TRADE INDUSTRIES. Text in English. a. **Document type:** *Government.*
Published by: U.S. Department of Labor, Bureau of Labor Statistics, 441 G St N W, Washington, DC 20212. TEL 202-655-4000. **Subscr. to:** U.S. Government Printing Office, Superintendent of Documents.

EVERYONE'S BACKYARD. see *ENVIRONMENTAL STUDIES—Waste Management*

FAKTOR ARBEITSSCHUTZ. see *INSURANCE*

622.8 USA
FEDERAL MINE SAFETY AND HEALTH REVIEW COMMISSION DECISIONS. Text in English. 1978. m. USD 110 (effective 2001). **Document type:** *Government.*
Related titles: Online - full content ed.
Indexed: MEDOC.
Published by: U.S. Federal Mine Safety and Health Review Commission, 1730 K St N W, 6th Fl, Washington, DC 20006. TEL 202-653-5633, FAX 202-653-5030, info@fmshrc.gov, http://www.fmshrc.gov/. Ed. Jean Ellen. Circ: 300. **Subscr. to:** U.S. Government Printing Office, Superintendent of Documents, PO Box 371954, Pittsburgh, PA 15250-7954. TEL 202-512-1800, FAX 202-512-2250, orders@gpo.gov, http://www.access.gpo.gov.

613 USA ISSN 1057-994X
FOCUS ON FEDERAL EMPLOYEE HEALTH AND ASSISTANCE PROGRAMS. Text in English. 1989. bi-m. USD 6. **Document type:** *Newsletter, Government.* **Description:** Provides news and developments in federal employee health and fitness programs, counseling, work and family AIDS and drug-free workplace programs.
Published by: (U.S. Office of Personnel Management, Office of Public Policy), U.S. Office of Personnel Management, Employee Health Services Branch, 1900 E St, NW, No 7412, Washington, DC 20415. TEL 202-606-1638, FAX 202-606-0967. Ed. Tracey Long. Circ: 2,900 (paid). **Subscr. to:** Supt. of Documents, Govt Printing Office, Washington, DC 20402.

614.85 664 GBR ISSN 0964-9158
FOOD SAFETY BRIEFING. Text in English. 1991. m. GBP 99. bk.rev. **Document type:** *Bulletin, Abstract/Index.* **Description:** Provides summaries of newly published U.K. and E.C. legislation, reports, and other authoritative and official publications on food safety and hygiene and related issues.
Related titles: Diskette ed.; Online - full text ed.: GBP 150.
Published by: Barbour Index, New Lodge, Drift Rd, Winkfield, Windsor, Berks SL4 4RQ, United Kingdom. TEL 44-1344-884121, FAX 44-1344-884112. Ed. D Denton.

363.11 613.6 FRA ISSN 0007-9952
CODEN: CNDIBJ
FRANCE. INSTITUT NATIONAL DE RECHERCHE ET DE SECURITE POUR LA PREVENTION DES ACCIDENTS DU TRAVAIL ET DES MALADIES PROFESSIONNELLES. CAHIERS DE NOTES DOCUMENTAIRES; securite et hygiene du travail. Text in French. 1956. q. FRF 420; FRF 570 foreign (effective 1998). abstr, charts, illus. index, cum.index. **Document type:** *Academic/Scholarly.* **Description:** Scientific and technical publication in the field of occupational safety and health.
Indexed: C.I.S. Abstr., CSNB, Chem.Abstr., Chem.Indus.Notes, INIS Atomind., Lab.Haz.Bull.
—BLDSC (2950.000000), CASDDS, CISTI, GNLM.
Published by: Institut National de Recherche et de Securite pour la Prevention des Accidents du Travail et des Maladies Professionnelles, 30 rue Olivier Noyer, Paris Cedex 14 75680, France. TEL 33-1-40443000, FAX 33-1-40443099, thanh@inrs.fr. Circ: 10,000.

614.85 DEU
G I T SPEZIAL SICHERHEIT UND MANAGEMENT. Text in German. 1992. 6/yr. DEM 78. adv. **Document type:** *Trade.*
Formerly: G I T Spezial Arbeitsschutz - Arbeitssicherheit
Published by: G I T Verlag GmbH, Roesslerstr 90, Darmstadt 64293, Germany. TEL 49-6151-8090-0, FAX 49-6151-8090144, gitverlaggmbh@gitverlag.com, http://www.gitverlag.com. Adv. contact Markus Gelbert. B&W page DEM 9,490, color page DEM 12,670; trim 260 x 185. Circ: 30,000.

613.62 ESP
GACETA DE LA PROTECCION LABORAL. Text in Spanish. q. ESP 4,640 (effective 1999). **Document type:** *Trade.*
Published by: Prensa Tecnica S.A., Casp, 118-120 6o, Barcelona 08013, Spain. TEL 34-3-2455190, FAX 34-3-2322773.

613.62 DEU
GEGENGIFT; Hamburger Hefte fuer Arbeit und Gesundheit. Text in German. 1986. 2/yr. DEM 50 for 5 nos.. adv. bk.rev. back issues avail. **Document type:** *Newsletter.* **Description:** Covers all areas of occupational health; aimed at safety activists and employees.
Published by: Gruppe Arbeit und Gesundheit, Informationsstelle Arbeit und Gesundheit, Schanzenstr 75, Hamburg 20357, Germany. TEL 49-40-4392858, FAX 49-40-4392818. Ed. Henning Wriedt. Circ: 1,500.

613.62 JPN
GENERAL GUIDEBOOK ON INDUSTRIAL SAFETY. Text in Japanese. a. JPY 520 (effective 2000). **Description:** Educational and promotional booklet for Japan's annual National Safety Week.
Formerly: Guidebook on Industrial Safety
Published by: Japan Industrial Safety and Health Association, Publishing and Sales Department, 5-35-1 Shiba, Minato-ku, Tokyo 108-0014, Japan. TEL 81-3-3452-6841, FAX 81-3-3454-8043. Ed. Toru Sasaki.

614.85 DEU
GERMANY. BUNDESANSTALT FUER ARBEITSSCHUTZ UND ARBEITSMEDIZIN. AMTLICHE MITTEILUNGEN. Text in German. 1984. q. bk.rev. 20 p./no. 2 cols./p. **Document type:** *Government.*
Formerly: Germany. Bundesanstalt fuer Arbeitsschutz. Amtliche Mitteilungen
Published by: Bundesanstalt fuer Arbeitsschutz und Arbeitsmedizin/Federal Institute for Occupational Safety and Health, Friedrich-Henkel-Weg 1-25, Dortmund 44149, Germany. TEL 49-231-9071-0, FAX 49-231-9071454, poststelle@baua.bund.de, http://www.baua.de. Eds. Angelika Limbach, Wolfgang Dicke. Circ: 105,000.

GERONTOLOGY SPECIAL INTEREST SECTION QUARTERLY. see *GERONTOLOGY AND GERIATRICS*

614.85 DEU
GESUNDHEITSSCHUTZ AM ARBEITSPLATZ CD-ROM. Text in German. base vol. plus irreg. updates. EUR 140 base vol(s). per vol.; EUR 50 updates per issue (effective 2002). **Document type:** *Trade.*
Media: CD-ROM.
Published by: Verlag C.H. Beck, Wilhelmstr 9, Munich 80791, Germany. TEL 49-89-38189-338, FAX 49-89-38189-398, abo.service@beck.de, http://www.beck.de.

616.98 ITA ISSN 0391-9889
CODEN: GIMLDG
GIORNALE ITALIANO DI MEDICINA DEL LAVORO. Text in English, Italian; Summaries in English. 1979. bi-m. ITL 80,000, USD 100. adv. bk.rev. index, cum.index. back issues avail. **Description:** Features research papers on various topics of occupational health.
Indexed: Biol.Abstr., Chem.Abstr., Dent.Ind., Excerp.Med., Ind.Hyg.Dig., Ind.Med. (coverage dropped).
—CASDDS, CISTI, GNLM.
Published by: Giardini Editori e Stampatori, Via Santa Bibbiana, 28, Pisa, PI 56127, Italy. TEL 050-502531. Ed. Francesco Candura. Circ: 1,500.

631.62 CHN ISSN 1000-7164
CODEN: GWZHEW
GONGYE WEISHENG YU ZHIYEBIN/INDUSTRIAL HEALTH AND OCCUPATIONAL DISEASES. Text in Chinese. 1983. bi-m. **Document type:** *Trade.*
Indexed: Chem.Abstr., Chem.Indus.Notes, Chem.Titles, Lab.Haz.Bull.
—BLDSC (4454.740000), CASDDS.
Published by: (Angang Laodong Weisheng Yanjiusuo), Gongye Weisheng yu Zhiyebin Zazhi Bianweihui, No 29, 219 Gongyuan, Anshan, Liaoning 114001, China. TEL 86-412-537140. Ed. Xu Mengren. **Dist. overseas by:** China International Book Trading Corp, 35 Chegongzhuang Xilu, Haidian District, Beijing 100044, China.

GREAT BRITAIN. HEALTH & SAFETY EXECUTIVE. TECHNOLOGY AND HEALTH SCIENCES DIVISION. SPECIALIST INSPECTOR REPORTS. see *PUBLIC HEALTH AND SAFETY*

613.62 ISR
HABITECHUT. Text in Arabic. q.
Published by: Safety and Hygiene Institute, 7 Solomon St, Tel Aviv 66023, Israel. TEL 03-374933.

614.85 USA
HAZARD CONTROL MANAGER. Text in English. s-a. adv. **Document type:** *Newsletter, Directory.* **Description:** Covers the management of safety programs.
Published by: Board of Certified Hazard Control Management, 8009 Carita Ct, Bethesda, MD 20817. TEL 301-770-2540. Ed., Pub., R&P, Adv. contact Harold M Gordon.

613.62 GBR ISSN 0964-962X
HAZARDOUS SUBSTANCES. Text in English. 1990. 10/yr. GBP 196; GBP 221, USD 442 foreign (effective 2000). back issues avail. **Document type:** *Newsletter.* **Description:** Covers the storage, transportation, processing, disposal, and laboratory research use of hazardous substances.
Indexed: Euro.LJI, Intl.Polym.Sci.& Tech., LJI, RAPRA (1990-1999), World Surf.Coat.
—BLDSC (4274.451150).
Published by: Monitor Press Ltd. (Subsidiary of: Informa Group PLC), Suffolk House, Church Field Rd, Sudbury, Suffolk CO10 2YA, United Kingdom. TEL 44-1787-378607, FAX 44-1787-880201, http://www.monitorpress.co.uk. Ed. Lawrence Waterman. Pub. Zoe Turner. R&P Liz Dittner.

614.85 GBR ISSN 0267-7296
HAZARDS MAGAZINE. Text in English. 1976. q. GBP 10 in Europe to individuals; GBP 15 elsewhere to individuals; GBP 22 in Europe to institutions; GBP 27 elsewhere to institutions (effective 1999). adv. bk.rev. abstr, charts, illus, stat. index. back issues avail. **Document type:** *Bulletin.* **Description:** Aims to help workers organize health and safety concerns through their unions.
Formerly (until 1984): Hazards Bulletin (0140-0525)
Indexed: Br.Tech.Ind., CSNB, INIS Atomind.
—BLDSC (4274.451570).
Published by: Hazards Publications Ltd., Hazards Publications Ltd, PO Box 199, Sheffield, S Yorks S1 4YL, United Kingdom. TEL 44-114-276-5695, FAX 44-114-276-7257, editor@hazards.org; sub@hazards.org. Ed. Rory O'Neill. Adv. contact Jawad Qasrawi. Circ: 7,000.

613.62 USA
HEALTH AND SAFETY AT WORK. Variant title: Croner's Health and Safety at Work. Text in English. GBP 299.05 (effective 2001). **Document type:** *Newsletter, Trade.*
Related titles: CD-ROM ed.: GBP 375 (effective 2001); Online - full text ed.: GBP 340 (effective 2001).
Published by: Croner.C C H Group Ltd., 145 London Rd, Kingston, Surrey KT2 6SR, United Kingdom. TEL 44-20-8247-1176, FAX 44-20-8547-2637, info@croner.cch.co.uk, http://www.croner.cch.co.uk.

614 GBR ISSN 0141-8246
HEALTH & SAFETY AT WORK. Text in English. 1978. m. GBP 65 in United Kingdom; GBP 101 overseas (effective 2000). adv. bk.rev. reprint service avail. from PQC. **Document type:** *Trade.* **Description:** For safety management.
Related titles: Microform ed.: (from PQC); Online - full text ed.: (from Gale Group, Factiva).
Indexed: ABI Inform. (Jan.1992-Win.1992), Account.& Data Proc.Abstr., Alloys Ind., BMT, Br.Ceram.Abstr., Br.Rail.Bd., Br.Tech.Ind., Build.Manage.Abstr., CBNB (1989-), C.I.S. Abstr., CSNB, Cadscan, Ergon.Abstr., Excerp.Med., INIS Atomind., Intl.Polym.Sci.& Tech., Lab.Haz.Bull., Lead Abstr., Met.Abstr., Met.Abstr.Ind., Mgmt.& Market.Abstr., Nonfer.Met.Alert, PCC Alert, RAPRA (1978-), Steels Alert, W.R.C.Inf., World Alum.Abstr., World Surf.Coat., World Text.Abstr., Zincscan.
—BLDSC (4274.869800), CISTI, GNLM. **CCC.**
Published by: Tolley Publishing Co Ltd (Subsidiary of: Butterworths), Tolley House, 2 Addiscombe Rd, Croydon, Surrey CR9 5AF, United Kingdom. TEL 44-20-8686—9141, FAX 44-20-8686-3155, http://www.tolley.co.uk. Ed. Isobel Allen. Adv. contact Philip Woodgate. B&W page GBP 980. Circ: 11,500.

344.204 GBR ISSN 0966-8365
HEALTH & SAFETY AT WORK ACT NEWSLETTER. Short title: H A S W A Newsletter. Text in English. 1992. m. GBP 133 (effective 1999). **Document type:** *Newsletter.*
Published by: British Safety Council, 70 Chancellors Rd, London W6 9RS, United Kingdom. TEL 44-20-8741-1231, FAX 44-20-8741-4555, bsc1.mail@britishsafetycouncil.co.uk, mail@britsafe.org, http://www.britishsafetycouncil.co.uk/bsc, http://www.britsafe.org/.

613.62 614.85 GBR
HEALTH AND SAFETY AT WORK DIRECTORY. Variant title: Croner's Health and Safety at Work Directory. Text in English. a. **Document type:** *Directory, Trade.* **Description:** Lists a wide range of health and safety based industry bodies and training organisations.
Media: Online - full content.
Published by: Croner.C C H Group Ltd., 145 London Rd, Kingston, Surrey KT2 6SR, United Kingdom. TEL 44-20-8247-1176, FAX 44-20-8547-2637, info@croner.cch.co.uk, http://www.croner.cch.co.uk.

613.62 GBR ISSN 0963-5351
HEALTH AND SAFETY BRIEFING. Variant title: Croner's Health and Safety Briefing. Text in English. 1991. fortn. GBP 299.05 (effective 2001). **Document type:** *Newsletter, Trade.* **Description:** Provides timely information on issues affecting health and safety at work.
Published by: Croner.C C H Group Ltd., 145 London Rd, Kingston, Surrey KT2 6SR, United Kingdom. TEL 44-20-8247-1176, FAX 44-20-8547-2637, info@croner.cch.co.uk, http://www.croner.cch.co.uk.

613.62 GBR
HEALTH & SAFETY COMMISSION ANNUAL REPORT AND THE HEALTH & SAFETY COMMISSION EXECUTIVE ACCOUNTS. Text in English. a. **Document type:** *Government.*
Formerly: Health & Safety Commission. Annual Report and Accounts
—BLDSC (4274.846020).
Published by: (Great Britain. Health & Safety Commission), Stationery Office Ltd, PO Box 276, London SW8 5DT, United Kingdom. TEL 44-870-600-5522, FAX 44-20-7873-8200.

340 613.62 GBR ISSN 0140-8534
KD3168.A13 CODEN: HSMOE5
HEALTH & SAFETY MONITOR. Text in English. 1977. m. GBP 192, USD 434, HKD 3,386 (effective 2001). back issues avail. **Document type:** *Newsletter, Trade.* **Description:** Advisory service on Codes of Practice and the changing legal and technical requirements of Health and Safety at Work.
Indexed: Cadscan, Euro.LJI, LJI, Lead Abstr., Mgmt.& Market.Abstr., Zincscan.
—BLDSC (4274.865500).
Published by: Informa Global Pharmaceuticals & Healthcare (Subsidiary of: Financial Times Business.), Mortimer House, 37-41 Mortimer St, London W1N 7RJ, United Kingdom. TEL 44-1206-772113, FAX 44-20-7453-2386, enquiries@informa.com, http://www.informapharma.com/LS0323, http://www.informapharma,com. Ed. Peter Mansell.

614 GBR ISSN 0954-5972
HEALTH AND SAFETY OFFICER'S HANDBOOK*. Text in English. 1983. a. GBP 25. adv. charts, illus. **Document type:** *Trade.*

—BLDSC (4274.866250).
Published by: Millbank Publications Ltd., 25 Catherine St, London WC2B 5JS, United Kingdom. TEL 44-171-813-3180, FAX 44-171-813-3184. Ed. R E Rynsley. R&P R E Aboud. Adv. contact J Darcy. Circ: 2,000.

HEALTH & SAFETY RESOURCE. see *FORESTS AND FORESTRY*

613.62 IRL
HEALTH & SAFETY REVIEW. Text in English. 1996. 10/yr. EUR 145 (effective 2001). **Document type:** *Journal, Trade.* **Description:** Covers all aspects of health, safety and environmental issues which impact on the workplace.
Related titles: Online - full content ed.
Published by: IRN Publishing, 123 Ranelagh, Dublin 6, Ireland. TEL 353-1-4972711, FAX 353-1-4972799, orlae.irn.ie, irn@irn.ie, http://www.healthandsafetyreview.ie, http://www.irn.ie. Ed. Herbert Mulligan. Pub. Martin Macdonnell. Adv. contact Orla McAleer.

HEALTH & SAFETY SPECIFIERS; health, safety and environmental safety. see *PUBLIC HEALTH AND SAFETY*

613.62 CAN
HEALTH IN THE WORKPLACE. Text in English. 12/yr. CND 175. **Document type:** *Newsletter.* **Description:** Covers complex, work-related health problems in straightforward language. Studies precedent-setting court cases in Canada, the US and the world.
Published by: Carswell, One Corporate Plaza, 2075 Kennedy Rd, Scarborough, ON M1T 3V4, Canada. TEL 416-609-8000, FAX 416-298-5094. Ed. Laurie Blake.

HEALTH STREAM NEWSLETTER. see *PUBLIC HEALTH AND SAFETY*

HEALTHCARE HAZARD MANAGEMENT MONITOR. see *MEDICAL SCIENCES*

HOPE HEALTH LETTER. see *PHYSICAL FITNESS AND HYGIENE*

613.62 JPN ISSN 0911-3363
HOPPO SANGYO EISEI/JOURNAL OF NORTHERN OCCUPATIONAL HEALTH. Text in English, Japanese; Summaries in English. 1938. biennial. free per issue. back issues avail. **Document type:** *Academic/Scholarly.*
Formerly: Hoppo Sangyo Eisei Kyoukai Kaishi
Published by: Association of Northern Occupational Health/Hoppo Sangyo Eisei Kyoukai, c/o Department of Hygiene and Preventive Medicine, Hokkaido University School of Medicine, Kita-15 nishi-7, Kita-ku, Sapporo 060, Japan. TEL 011-706-5066, FAX 011-717-1140. Ed. Naoki Sugawara.

HOSPITAL EMPLOYEE HEALTH. see *HEALTH FACILITIES AND ADMINISTRATION*

HUMAN FACTORS AND ERGONOMICS IN MANUFACTURING. see *ENGINEERING—Industrial Engineering*

331 USA
HUMAN RESOURCES MANAGEMENT - O S H A COMPLIANCE. Text in English. base vol. plus m. updates. USD 459 (effective 2001). **Description:** Provides practical guidance on compliance issues arising under federal OSHA and state OSHA Acts. Offers the guidelines and examples needed to establish an effective company safety program.
Formerly: C C H - O S H A Compliance Guide
Related titles: CD-ROM ed.: USD 479 (effective 2000).
Published by: C C H Incorporated, 2700 Lake Cook Rd., Riverwoods, IL 60015. TEL 847-267-7000, 800-449-9525, FAX 773-866-3895, http://www.cch.com. Ed. Paul Gibson.

▼ **I E H REPORT ON APPROACHES TO PREDICTING TOXICITY FROM OCCUPATIONAL EXPOSURE TO DUSTS.** see *ENVIRONMENTAL STUDIES—Toxicology And Environmental Safety*

614.8 628 331.8 CHE ISSN 0376-9410
I Z A. (Illustrierte Zeitschrift fuer Arbeitssicherheit) Text and summaries in German. 1953. s-m. CHF 39; CHF 50 foreign (effective 1998). **Document type:** *Trade.*
Indexed: Ref.Zh.

O

Published by: Ott Verlag und Druck AG, Laenggasse 57, Postfach 802, Thun, 7 3607, Switzerland. TEL 41-33-2253939, FAX 41-33-2253933. Ed. Alfred Lauchli Wyss. adv.: B&W page CHF 920; trim 265 x 185. Circ: 5,500.

613.62 614.85 ITA
IGIENE, SICUREZZA, CONTROLLI. Text in Italian. 9/yr. ITL 120,000 domestic; ITL 140,000 in Europe; ITL 160,000 elsewhere (effective 2000).
Published by: E P C s.r.l., Via Dell' Acqua Traversa, 187-189, Rome, RM 00135, Italy. TEL 39-06-3313000, FAX 39-06-3313212, alibe@epcinforma.com.

INDIAN JOURNAL OF INDUSTRIAL MEDICINE. see *MEDICAL SCIENCES*

615.8 IND ISSN 0445-7706
INDIAN JOURNAL OF OCCUPATIONAL THERAPY. Text in English. 1956. 4/yr. USD 20. adv. bk.rev. **Document type:** *Academic/Scholarly.*
Indexed: Indian Psychol.Abstr.
Published by: All India Occupational Therapists' Association, 136 Sunlight Colony-2, Didharth Enclave, New Delhi 110 014, India. TEL 6832232. Ed. M S Warhade. Circ: 750.

613 614 331 IDN ISSN 0126-0987
INDONESIAN JOURNAL OF INDUSTRIAL HYGIENE, OCCUPATIONAL HEALTH-SAFETY AND SOCIAL SECURITY/MAJALAH HIGENE PERUSAHAAN, KESEHATAN-KESELAMATAN KERJA, DAN JAMINAN SOSIAL. Text in English, Indonesian. 1969. q. charts, stat. reprint service avail. from PQC.
Related titles: Microfilm ed.: (from PQC).
Published by: National Institute of Industrial Hygiene and Occupational Health/Lembaga Nasional Higene Perusahaan dan Kesehatan Kerja, Jl. Jend. A. Yani 69-70, Jakarta, Indonesia.

614.85 CAN ISSN 0712-774X
INDUSTRIAL ACCIDENT PREVENTION ASSOCIATION. ANNUAL REVIEW. Text in English. 1918. a. **Document type:** *Corporate.*
Formerly: Industrial Accident Prevention Association. Annual Report (0073-7305)
Published by: Industrial Accident Prevention Association, 250 Yonge St, 28th Fl, Toronto, ON M5B 2N4, Canada. TEL 416-506-8888. Circ: 7,500.

613.62 JPN ISSN 0019-8366
RC963 CODEN: INHEAO
INDUSTRIAL HEALTH. Text in English. 1963. q. membership. charts, illus. index. reprints avail. *Refereed.* **Document type:** *Academic/Scholarly.*
Description: Contains research articles in the area of industrial health.
Related titles: Online - full text ed.: (from The Dialog Corporation, JICST, Institute for Scientific Information).
Indexed: ASCA, Abstr.Hyg., Acoust.Abstr., Art & Archaeol.Tech.Abstr., Biol.Abstr., C.I.S. Abstr., CSNB, Chem.Abstr., Curr.Cont. (coverage dropped), Dairy Sci.Abstr., Dent.Ind., Environ.Sci.Poll.Mgmt., Ergon.Abstr., Excerp.Med., Forest Prod.Abstr., INIS Atomind., Ind.Hyg.Dig., Ind.Med. (1963-), Int.Abstr.Biol.Sci., Int.Nurs.Ind., Lab.Haz.Bull., Med.& Surg.Dermat., Nutr.Abstr., Pollut.Abstr., Risk Abstr., SSCI (coverage dropped), Saf.Sci.Abstr., Sci.Cit.Ind. (coverage dropped), Tox.Abstr., Trop.Dis.Bull.
—BLDSC (4454.700000), CASDDS, CISTI, GNLM, IDS, ingenta, KNAW.
Published by: National Institute of Industrial Health/Rodo-sho Sangyo Igaku Sogo Kenkyujo, 21-1 Nagao 6-chome, Tama-ku, Kawasaki-shi, Kanagawa-ken 214-0023, Japan. TEL 81-044-865-6111, FAX 81-044-865-6116, http://www.niih.go.jp. Ed., R&P Haruhiko Sakurai. Circ: 1,100.

613.62 340 USA ISSN 0890-3018
INDUSTRIAL HEALTH & HAZARDS UPDATE. Text in English. 1984. m. USD 369 domestic; USD 409 in Canada; USD 479 elsewhere (effective 2001). back issues avail.; reprints avail. **Document type:** *Newsletter.* **Description:** Covers occupational health, safety, hazards, and related subjects. Designed for busy executives in the health, medical, environmental, legal, management, and technological fields of industry, government, commerce, and academia.
Incorporates (1994-200?): Environmental Problems & Remediation (1077-1395)
Related titles: Online - full text ed.: (from Data-Star, Human Resources Information Network, Gale Group, NewsNet, Northern Light Technology, Inc., Factiva).
—CCC.
Published by: Merton Allen Associates, InfoTeam Inc., PO Box 15640, Plantation, FL 33318-5640. TEL 954-473-9560, FAX 954-473-0544. Eds. David R Allen, Merton Allen.

613.2 USA ISSN 0073-7496
INDUSTRIAL HEALTH FOUNDATION. ENGINEERING SERIES. BULLETINS. Text in English. 1936. irreg., latest vol.8, 1971. price varies. **Document type:** *Bulletin, Monographic series.*
Published by: Industrial Health Foundation, Inc., 34 Penn Circle W, Pittsburgh, PA 15206. TEL 412-363-6600, FAX 412-363-6605, IHFincorp@aol.com, http://members.aol.com/ihfincorp/ihf.htm. R&P Marianne C Kaschak.

331.8 613.62 USA ISSN 0073-750X
INDUSTRIAL HEALTH FOUNDATION. LEGAL SERIES BULLETINS. Text in English. 1936. irreg., latest vol.9, 1972. price varies. **Document type:** *Bulletin.*
Formerly: Industrial Hygiene Foundation of America. Legal Series Bulletin
Published by: Industrial Health Foundation, Inc., 34 Penn Circle W, Pittsburgh, PA 15206. TEL 412-363-6600, FAX 412-363-6605, IHFincorp@aol.com, http://members.aol.com/ihf. R&P Marianne C Kaschak.

331 614 USA
INDUSTRIAL HEALTH FOUNDATION. MANAGEMENT SERIES. Text in English. 1971. irreg., latest vol.2, 1978. price varies. back issues avail. **Document type:** *Monographic series.*
Published by: Industrial Health Foundation, Inc., 34 Penn Circle W, Pittsburgh, PA 15206. TEL 412-363-6600, FAX 412-363-6605, IHFincorp@aol.com, http://members.aol.com/ihfincorp/ihf.htm. R&P Marianne C Kaschak.

613.62 USA ISSN 0073-7518
HD7260
INDUSTRIAL HEALTH FOUNDATION. MEDICAL SERIES. BULLETINS. Text in English. 1937. irreg., latest vol.21, 1982. price varies. **Document type:** *Monographic series.*
Published by: Industrial Health Foundation, Inc., 34 Penn Circle W, Pittsburgh, PA 15206. TEL 412-363-6600, FAX 412-363-6605, IHFincorp@aol.com, http://members.aol.com/ihfincorp/ihf.htm. R&P Marianne C Kaschak.

613.62 USA ISSN 0073-7526
INDUSTRIAL HEALTH FOUNDATION. NURSING SERIES. BULLETINS. Text in English. 1965. irreg., latest vol.3, 1971. price varies. **Document type:** *Bulletin, Monographic series.*
Published by: Industrial Health Foundation, Inc., 34 Penn Circle W, Pittsburgh, PA 15206. TEL 412-363-6600, FAX 412-363-6605, IHFincorp@aol.com, http://members.aol.com/ihfincorp/ihf. R&P Marianne C Kaschak.

331 USA ISSN 0147-5401
INDUSTRIAL HYGIENE NEWS. Text in English. 1978. 7/yr. free to qualified personnel. adv. bk.rev. tr.lit. back issues avail. **Document type:** *Trade.* **Description:** Information on occupational health and safety. Persons responsible for the industrial hygiene function, nurses and physicians, management, insurance executives, industrial hygienists, safety directors, plant engineers.
Related titles: Online - full text ed.
Published by: Rimbach Publishing, Inc., 8650 Babcock Blvd, Pittsburgh, PA 15237-5821. TEL 412-364-5366, FAX 412-369-9720, info@rimbach.com, http://www.rimbach.com. Ed. David C Lavender. Pub. Norberta Rimbach. Adv. contact Raquel Rimbach. page USD 4,450; trim 16 x 11. Circ: 62,000 (controlled).

614.85 USA
CODEN: CIHNEM
INDUSTRIAL SAFETY AND HYGIENE NEWS; news of safety, health and hygiene, environmental, fire, security and emergency protection equipment. Text in English. 1967. m. USD 120; free to qualified personnel. adv. charts, illus, tr.lit. back issues avail.; reprint service avail. from PQC. **Document type:** *Newspaper, Trade.* **Description:** Publication directed toward heavy industry that offers news, how-to features and product coverage for safety professionals.
Former titles: Chilton's Industrial Safety and Hygiene News (8755-2566); (until 1982): Industrial Safety and Hygiene News; (until 1981): Industrial Safety Product News (0192-8325); (until 1978): Safety Products News (0278-8217)
Related titles: Microform ed.: (from PQC); Online - full text ed.
Indexed: Curr.Pack.Abstr., Environ.Sci.Poll.Mgmt., Ind.Hyg.Dig., Pollut.Abstr.
—CCC.
Published by: Business News Publishing Co., 755 W Big Beaver, Ste 1000, Troy, MI 48084. TEL 248-362-3700, FAX 248-362-0317, djsafe@bellatlantic.net, http://www.ishn.com/. Ed., Pub. Dave Johnson. Circ: 62,000.

614.85 IND ISSN 0301-4746
T55.A1
INDUSTRIAL SAFETY CHRONICLE. Text in English. 1969. q. INR 40, USD 8. adv. bk.rev. illus.
Indexed: C.I.S. Abstr., INIS Atomind.
Published by: National Safety Council, Central Labour Institute Bldg., Sion, Mumbai, Maharashtra 400 022, India. Ed. A A Krishnan. Circ: 1,500.

363.11 GBR ISSN 0262-3226
INDUSTRIAL SAFETY DATA FILE. Text in English. 1982. m. GBP 90, USD 257. illus. s-a. index. **Document type:** *Trade.*
Supersedes: Industrial Safety (0019-8757)
Indexed: Br.Tech.Ind., C.I.S. Abstr., INIS Atomind.
—CISTI, Linda Hall.
Published by: Wilmington Business Publishing, Apex House, London Rd, Northfleet, Kent DA11 9JA, United Kingdom. TEL 44-1322-277788, FAX 44-1474-569418, wbp@wilmington.co.uk. Ed. Dina Chase. Circ: 2,500.

628.5 NLD ISSN 0921-9110
INDUSTRIAL SAFETY SERIES. Text in Dutch. 1987. irreg., latest vol.5, 1995. price varies. back issues avail. *Refereed.* **Document type:** *Monographic series.*
—BLDSC (4462.440000). **CCC.**
Published by: Elsevier Science BV, Books Division, PO Box 211, Amsterdam 1000 AE, Netherlands. TEL 31-20-485-2911, nlinfo-f@elsevier.nl; usinfo-f@elsevier.com; forinfo-kyf04035@niftyserve.or.jp, http://www.elsevier.nl/. **Subscr. in Australasia and the Far East to:** Elsevier Science (Singapore) Pte Ltd, No.1 Temasek Ave, 17-01 Millenia Tower, Singapore 039192, Singapore. TEL 65-434-3727, FAX 65-337-2230; **Subscr. in Japan to:** Elsevier Science Inc - Japan Regional Office, 9-15 Higashi-Azabu 1-chome, Minato-ku, Tokyo 106-0044, Japan. TEL 81-3-5561-5033, FAX 81-3-5561-5047; **Subscr. in the Americas to:** Elsevier Science, PO Box 945, New York, NY 10159-0945. TEL 212-633-3730, FAX 212-633-3680, usinfo-f@elsevier.com, http://www.elsevier.com.

INDUSTRIAL VENTILATION; A MANUAL OF RECOMMENDED PRACTICE. see *HEATING, PLUMBING AND REFRIGERATION*

363.11 USA
INSIDE O S H A. (Occupational Safety and Health Administration) Text in English. bi-w. USD 725 in US & Canada; USD 775 elsewhere (effective 2001). **Document type:** *Newsletter.*
Related titles: E-mail ed.
Published by: Inside Washington Publishers, PO Box 7167, Ben Franklin Sta, Washington, DC 20044-7167. TEL 703-416-8500, FAX 703-416-8543, service@iwpnews.com.

613.6 363.11 GBR ISSN 0968-4999
INSPECTOR. Text in English. 1954. bi-m. GBP 40; GBP 50 foreign. adv. bk.rev. illus, tr.lit. index. back issues avail. **Document type:** *Trade.* **Description:** Covers occupational health and safety in both the private and public sectors.
Published by: Institute of Safety & Public Protection, PO Box 1381, Rugby, Warks CV21 2ZF, United Kingdom. TEL 44-1788-536389, FAX 44-1788-550152613, info@assocnbureau.demon.co.uk. Ed., R&P John Saunders. Adv. contact John Corfield. page GBP 200. Circ: 350 (paid).

613.62 GBR
INSTITUTE OF OCCUPATIONAL HEALTH. PROCEEDINGS. Text in English. irreg. **Document type:** *Proceedings.*
Published by: University of Birmingham, Institute of Occupational Health, University Of Birmingham, Edgbaston, PO Box 363, Birmingham, Worcs B15 2TT, United Kingdom. TEL 44-121-414-6030, FAX 44-121-414-6217, institute-of-occupational-health@bham.ac.uk.

363.11 613.62 GBR ISSN 1366-1965
INSTITUTION OF OCCUPATIONAL SAFETY AND HEALTH. JOURNAL. Text in English. 1997. s-a. GBP 30 to non-members; GBP 20 to members. **Document type:** *Academic/Scholarly.* **Description:** Publishes research in the field of occupational safety and health.
—BLDSC (4799.300000).
Published by: (Institution of Occupational Safety and Health), I O S H Publishing Ltd., The Grange, Highfield Dr, Wigston, Leics LE18 1NN, United Kingdom. TEL 44-116-257-3100, FAX 44-116-257-3101, ioshpubs@iosh.co.uk, http://www.iosh.co.uk.

613.62 DEU ISSN 0340-0131
RC963.A1 CODEN: IAEHDW
INTERNATIONAL ARCHIVES OF OCCUPATIONAL AND ENVIRONMENTAL HEALTH. Text in English. 1930. 8/yr. EUR 1,620.70 domestic; EUR 1,613.80 in Germany; EUR 240 newsstand/cover foreign (effective 2002). adv. bibl, charts, illus. index. back issues avail.; reprint service avail. from ISI. *Refereed.* **Document type:** *Journal, Academic/Scholarly.* **Description:** Covers occupational, environmental, and social medicine, and their subdisciplines.
Former titles (until 1975): International Archives of Occupational Health (0020-5923); (until 1970): Internationales Archiv fuer Gewerbepathologie und Gewerbehygiene; (until 1962): Archiv fuer Gewerbepathologie und Gewerbehygiene
Related titles: Microform ed.: (from PQC); Online - full text ed.: ISSN 1432-1246 (from EBSCO Publishing, RoweCom Information Quest, Swets Blackwell, Springer LINK, Institute for Scientific Information).
Indexed: ASCA, Abstr.Hyg., Acoust.Abstr., Aqua.Sci.& Fish.Abstr., Biol.Abstr., CINAHL, C.I.S. Abstr., CSNB, Cadscan, Chem.Abstr., Chem.Indus.Notes, Chem.Titles, Curr.Adv.Cancer Res., Curr.Adv.Ecol.Sci., Curr.Cont., Dent.Ind., Environ.Sci.Poll.Mgmt., Ergon.Abstr., Excerp.Med., INIS Atomind., Ind.Med. (1975-), Ind.Sci.Rev., Inpharma, Int.Abstr.Biol.Sci., Int.Nurs.Ind., Lab.Haz.Bull., Lead Abstr., Med.& Surg.Dermat., NRN, Nutr.Abstr., Pollut.Abstr., Reac., Risk Abstr., SSCI (coverage dropped), Saf.Sci.Abstr., Sci.Cit.Ind., Sugar Ind.Abstr., Tox.Abstr., Trop.Dis.Bull., Zincscan.
—BLDSC (4536.128000), CASDDS, CISTI, EMDOCS, GNLM, IDS, ingenta. **CCC.**
Published by: Springer-Verlag (Subsidiary of: BertelsmannSpringer), Tiergartenstr 17, Heidelberg 69121, Germany. TEL 49-6221-345-0, FAX 49-6221-345229, subscriptions@springer.de, http://link.springer.de/link/service/journals/00420/index.htm, http://www.springer.de. Ed. G Lehnert. **Subscr. in N. America to:** Springer-Verlag New York Inc., PO Box 2485, Secaucus, NJ 07096-2485. TEL 212-460-1500, FAX 212-473-6272.

INTERNATIONAL COMMISSION ON RADIOLOGICAL PROTECTION. ANNALS. see *MEDICAL SCIENCES—Radiology And Nuclear Medicine*

613.62 AUS ISSN 0074-3828
INTERNATIONAL CONGRESS OF OCCUPATIONAL THERAPY. PROCEEDINGS. Text in English. 1974. irreg., latest 1978, 7th, Jerusalem. **Document type:** *Proceedings.*
Published by: World Federation of Occupational Therapists, 20 Syree Court, Marmion, W.A. 6020, Australia. Circ: 1,500.

INTERNATIONAL HOSPITAL & AGED CARE JOURNAL. see *HEALTH FACILITIES AND ADMINISTRATION*

613.62 USA ISSN 1077-3525
RC963.A1 CODEN: IOEHFU
INTERNATIONAL JOURNAL OF OCCUPATIONAL AND ENVIRONMENTAL HEALTH. Text in English. 1995. q., latest vol.7, 2001. USD 86 domestic to individuals; USD 106 domestic to institutions; USD 25 newsstand/cover; USD 96 per issue foreign to individuals; USD 116 per issue foreign to institutions (effective 2001). adv. charts, illus. Index. back issues avail.; reprints avail. *Refereed.* **Document type:** *Journal, Academic/Scholarly.* **Description:** Authoritative resource delivering up-to-date clinical and research information on promotion of health in the workplace and the wider issue of the relationship between human health and the environment.
Indexed: Abstr.Hyg., CINAHL, CSNB, Ergon.Abstr., Ind.Med. (1995-), Rev.Appl.Entomol.
—BLDSC (4542.410800), CISTI, GNLM, Infotrieve. **CCC.**
Published by: Hanley & Belfus, Inc., 210 S 13th St, Philadelphia, PA 19107. TEL 215-546-4995, 800-962-1892, FAX 215-790-9330. Pub. Sandra Lovegrove. Adv. contact Diane R Sherel. B&W page USD 590; trim 11 x 8.25. Circ: 1,000.

613.85 POL ISSN 1232-1087
INTERNATIONAL JOURNAL OF OCCUPATIONAL MEDICINE AND ENVIRONMENTAL HEALTH. Text in English. 1988. q. USD 160 to individuals; USD 200 to institutions (effective 2002). bk.rev. abstr, bibl, illus. index. 90 p./no. 2 cols./p. back issues avail.; reprints avail. *Refereed.* **Document type:** *Journal, Academic/Scholarly.* **Description:** Publishes papers concerning industrial hygiene, preventive medicine, diagnosis and treatment of occupational diseases, physiology and psychology of work, toxicological research, environmental toxicology, environmental epidemiology, and epidemiological studies devoted to occupational problems.
Former titles (until 1993): Polish Journal of Occupational Medicine and Environmental Health (0867-8383); (until 1991): Polish Journal of Occupational Medicine (0860-6536)
Related titles: CD-ROM ed.
Indexed: Abstr.Hyg., Aqua.Sci.& Fish.Abstr., Environ.Sci.Poll.Mgmt., Ergon.Abstr., Excerp.Med., INIS Atomind., Ind.Med. (1994-), Pollut.Abstr., Ref.Zh., Rev.Med.& Vet.Mycol., Rev.Plant Path., Risk Abstr., Saf.Sci.Abstr., Tox.Abstr., Trop.Dis.Bull.
—BLDSC (4542.412000), CISTI, EMDOCS, GNLM.
Published by: Instytut Medycyny Pracy im. Jerzego Nofera/Nofer Institute of Occupational Medicine, Ul Sw. Teresy 8, PO Box 199, Lodz 90950, Poland. TEL 48-42-6314745, FAX 48-42-6314719, redakcja@porta.imp.lodz.pl. Ed. Konrad Rydzynski. R&P, Adv. contact Wieslaw Sulkowski. Circ: 400. **Co-sponsor:** Polish Association of Occupational Medicine.

363.11 620.8 613.62 POL ISSN 1080-3548
T59.7 CODEN: IJOEF2
INTERNATIONAL JOURNAL OF OCCUPATIONAL SAFETY AND ERGONOMICS. Variant title: J O S E. Text in English. 1995. q. USD 50 domestic to individuals; USD 70 foreign to individuals; USD 170 domestic to institutions; USD 190 foreign to institutions; USD 40 to members (effective 2001). adv. bk.rev. index. back issues avail. *Refereed.* **Document type:** *Journal, Academic/Scholarly.* **Description:** Covers occupational safety and ergonomics for research workers from experts in the United States, Canada, Central and Eastern Europe. Includes studies of hazardous chemicals, physical and biological agents, new technologies for protection, criteria and requirements of occupational safety and ergonomics as well as the information about seminars and conferences organized in Poland and abroad.
Indexed: Environ.Sci.Poll.Mgmt., Ergon.Abstr., Excerp.Med. (1996-), INSPEC (1995-1997, dropped), Ind.Med. (1995-), Pollut.Abstr., Risk Abstr., Saf.Sci.Abstr.
—BLDSC (4542.414000), AskIEEE, GNLM, Infotrieve. **CCC.**
Published by: Centralny Instytut Ochrony Pracy/Central Institute for Labour Protection, Ul Czerniakowska 16, Warsaw 00701, Poland. TEL 48-22-6233698, FAX 48-22-6233693, oinip@ciop.pl. Ed. Danuta Koradecka. Circ: 200. **Co-sponsors:** International Ergonomics Association; International Labour Office.

363.11 USA
INTERNATIONAL SOCIETY FOR OCCUPATIONAL ERGONOMICS AND SAFETY. NEWSLETTER. Text in English. 1997. s-a. membership. back issues avail. **Document type:** *Newsletter, Academic/Scholarly.* **Description:** Informs members of important news and events.
Published by: International Society for Occupational Ergonomics and Safety, ISOES c/o Biz-comm, 1503 Inlet Ct, Reston, VA 20190. TEL 703-689-9619, FAX 703-689-9637, yearout@unca.edu, biz@biz-comm.com, http://isoes.org/newsletter.htm. Ed. Robert Yearout TEL 828-251-6854.

INTERNATIONAL SOCIETY FOR RESPIRATORY PROTECTION. JOURNAL. see *MEDICAL SCIENCES—Respiratory Diseases*

IRISH SECURITY NEWS. see *CRIMINOLOGY AND LAW ENFORCEMENT—Security*

614.85 JPN
JAPAN INDUSTRIAL SAFETY AND HEALTH ASSOCIATION. ANNUAL REPORT. Text in Japanese. a.
Published by: Japan Industrial Safety and Health Association, International Cooperation Department, 5-35-1, Shiba, Minato-ku, Tokyo 108-0014, Japan. TEL 81-3-3452-6841, FAX 81-3-3454-4596.

614.85 690 CHN ISSN 1004-552X
JIANZHU ANQUAN/CONSTRUCTION SAFETY. Text in Chinese, English. 1986. m. CNY 48. 48 p./no. **Document type:** *Trade.* **Description:** Covers comprehensive safety science and technology which caters the need of national contruction industry; contains safety scientific technology, safety administration, electrical safety, mechanical safety, scaffold safety, accident analysis.
Published by: Jianzhu Anquan Zazhishe, 95 Jiefang Lu, Er(2) Duan, Chengdu, Sichuan 610081, China. TEL 86-28-3373856, FAX 86-28-3331029. Ed. Yan Zhou. Adv. contact Min Wu. Circ: 40,000. **Dist. overseas by:** China International Book Trading Corp, 35 Chegongzhuang Xilu, Haidian District, Beijing 100044, China.

JITSUMU TENBO/SAFETY NEWS ON BOILER AND CRANE ENGINEERING. see *MACHINERY*

614.85 USA ISSN 1057-5820
HD7260
JOB SAFETY AND HEALTH QUARTERLY. Text in English. 1989. q. USD 17 (effective 2001). illus. Index. back issues avail.; reprints avail. **Document type:** *Government.* **Description:** Features articles on job safety and health topics and contains current information on O.S.H.A. activities.
Related titles: Online - full content ed.; Online - full text ed.: (from H. W. Wilson).
Indexed: B.P.I. (Jul.1995-).
—ingenta.
Published by: U.S. Occupational Safety and Health Administration, Office of Public Affairs, Rm N3647, 200 Constitution Ave, N W, Washington, DC 20210. TEL 202-523-8148, http://www.osha-slc.gov/html/jshq-index.html. Ed. Kerri Lawrence. R&P Anne Cye TEL 206-693-1999. **Subscr. to:** U.S. Government Printing Office, Superintendent of Documents, PO Box 371954, Pittsburgh, PA 15250-7954. TEL 202-512-1800, FAX 202-512-2250, orders@gpo.gov, http://www.access.gpo.gov.

613.62 USA ISSN 1059-924X
RC965.A5
JOURNAL OF AGROMEDICINE; interface of human health & agriculture. Text in English. 1993. q. USD 60 to individuals; USD 81 in Canada to individuals; USD 87 elsewhere to individuals; USD 95 to institutions; USD 128 in Canada to institutions; USD 138 elsewhere to institutions; USD 150 to libraries; USD 203 in Canada to libraries; USD 218 elsewhere to libraries (effective Aug. 2001). adv. bk.rev. back issues avail.; reprint service avail. from HAW. *Refereed.* **Document type:** *Journal, Academic/Scholarly.* **Description:** Focuses on the health effects of agricultural operations on workers and their families, consumers, and the environment.
Related titles: Microfiche ed.: (from PQC); Microform ed.
Indexed: Abstr.Anthropol., Abstr.Hyg., Agricola, Aqua.Sci.& Fish.Abstr., Biostat., CINAHL, Environ.Per.Bibl. (1993-), Environ.Sci.Poll.Mgmt., Food Sci.& Tech.Abstr., Geo.Abstr.H.G., Geo.Abstr.P.G., Helminthol.Abstr., IDA, Nutr.Abstr., Pig News & Info., Pollut.Abstr., Ref.Zh., Rev.Appl.Entomol., Rev.Med.& Vet.Mycol., Risk Abstr., Rural Devel.Abstr., Saf.Sci.Abstr.
—BLDSC (4926.240000), CISTI, Haworth.
Published by: Haworth Press, Inc., 10 Alice St, Binghamton, NY 13904-1580. TEL 607-722-5857, 800-429-6784, FAX 607-722-6362, 800-895-0582, getinfo@haworthpressinc.com, http://www.haworthpress.com/journals/journallist.asp. Ed. Stanley H Schuman. Pub. William Cohen. R&P Ruthann Heath TEL 607-723-5857 ext 316. Adv. contact Jackie Blakeslee TEL 607-722-5857 ext 346. B&W page USD 315, color page USD 550; trim 6 x 8.5.

613.62 GBR ISSN 0954-576X
JOURNAL OF HEALTH AND SAFETY. Text in English. 1988. 3/yr. GBP 10; GBP 12.50 foreign. adv. bk.rev. back issues avail. **Document type:** *Academic/Scholarly.* **Description:** Contains articles, conference papers, and more relating to all aspects of occupational health and safety.
Formed by the 1988 merger of: British Health and Safety Society. Newsletter (0268-0580); British Health and Safety Society. Reviews Bulletin (0268-0572)
Indexed: Lab.Haz.Bull.
Published by: British Health and Safety Society, c/o Health & Safety Unit, Aston University, Aston Triangle, Birmingham, W Mids B4 7ET, United Kingdom. TEL 44-121-359-3621, FAX 44-121-333-5809, bhss@aston.ac.uk. Ed. Roger C Clarke. Circ: 400.

613.62 616.9 USA ISSN 1096-3707
JOURNAL OF HEALTHCARE SAFETY, COMPLIANCE & INFECTION CONTROL. Text in English. 1997. 10/yr. USD 160 domestic; USD 198 in Canada; USD 253 elsewhere (effective 2000). *Refereed.* **Document type:** *Academic/Scholarly, Trade.* **Description:** Provides news, information, and peer-reviewed articles of importance and interest to those responsible for the physical and environmental safety of all in healthcare settings.
—BLDSC (4996.873000). **CCC.**
Published by: Prime National Publishing Corp., 470 Boston Post Rd, Weston, MA 02493. TEL 781-899-2702, FAX 781-899-4900, jhscic@pnpco.com, http://www.pnpco.com. Ed. Peter E Senne. Pub. Richard A DeVito Sr. TEL 781-899-2702 ext. 107. R&P Dennis N Ricci.

▼ **JOURNAL OF HUMAN FACTORS AND AEROSPACE SAFETY.** see *AERONAUTICS AND SPACE FLIGHT*

JOURNAL OF OCCUPATIONAL AND ENVIRONMENTAL MEDICINE. see *MEDICAL SCIENCES*

613.6 JPN ISSN 1341-9145
CODEN: JOCHFV
JOURNAL OF OCCUPATIONAL HEALTH. Text in English. 1996. q. JPY 10,000; JPY 12,000 foreign (effective 1999). *Refereed.* **Document type:** *Academic/Scholarly.*
Related titles: Online - full text ed.: (from Institute for Scientific Information); ♦ Japanese ed.: Sangyo Eiseigaku Zasshi. ISSN 1341-0725.
Indexed: Chem.Abstr., Chem.Indus.Notes, Chem.Titles, Int.Abstr.Biol.Sci., Mass Spectr.Bull., Ref.Zh.
—BLDSC (5026.088000), CASDDS, CISTI, GNLM, IDS, Infotrieve. **CCC.**
Published by: Japan Society for Occupational Health/Nihon Sangyo Eisei Gakkai, Public Health Bldg, 1-29-8 Shinjuku, Shinjuku-ku, Tokyo 160-0022, Japan. TEL 81-3-3356-1536, FAX 81-3-5362-3746, http://wshiivx.med.uoeh-u.ac.jp/sannei/index.html. Ed. Kazuyuki Omae. Pub. Yukio Fujiki. Circ: 8,000. **Subscr. to:** International Press Editing Center, 1-2-3 Sugamo, Toshima-ku, Tokyo 170-0002, Japan. TEL 81-3-5978-467, FAX 81-3-5978-4068.

158.7 USA ISSN 1076-8998
RC967.5 CODEN: JOHPFC
JOURNAL OF OCCUPATIONAL HEALTH PSYCHOLOGY. Text in English. 1996. q. USD 40 domestic to non-members; USD 55 foreign to non-members; USD 32 domestic to members; USD 42 foreign to members; USD 92 domestic to institutions; USD 124 foreign to institutions (effective 2001). *Refereed.* **Document type:** *Journal, Academic/Scholarly.* **Description:** Publishes research, theory, and public policy articles that concern the application of psychology to improving the quality of worklife and to protecting and promoting the safety, health and well-being of workers.
Indexed: AgeLine, Ind.Med. (1996-), Int.Nurs.Ind., PsycInfo, Soc.Work Res.& Abstr.
—BLDSC (5026.095000), Infotrieve. **CCC.**
Published by: American Psychological Association, 750 First St., N.E., Washington, DC 20002-4242. TEL 202-336-5600, 800-374-2721, FAX 202-336-5568, subscriptions@apa.org, http://www.apa.org/journals/ohp.html. Ed. Julian Barling. Circ: 500.

615.8 USA ISSN 1053-0487
RC964 CODEN: JOCTEW
JOURNAL OF OCCUPATIONAL REHABILITATION. Text in English. 1991. q. USD 517, EUR 516 to institutions for print or online ed.; USD 620.40, EUR 619.20 to institutions for print & online eds.combined (effective 2002). adv. bk.rev. back issues avail. *Refereed.* **Document type:** *Journal, Academic/Scholarly.* **Description:** Provides a multidisciplinary forum for the publication of original research, theoretical papers, review articles, and case studies related to the mechanism and management of work-related disabilities.
Related titles: Online - full text ed.: (from EBSCO Publishing, O C L C Online Computer Library Center, Inc., Swets Blackwell, Kluwer Online, Institute for Scientific Information, RoweCom Information Quest).
Indexed: AMED, ASCA, Abstr.Soc.Geront., AgeLine, CINAHL, Curr.Cont., Environ.Sci.Poll.Mgmt., Excerp.Med. (1996-), Human Resour.Abstr., Pollut.Abstr., PsycInfo, Psychol.Abstr. (1991-), Risk Abstr., SSCI, Saf.Sci.Abstr., e-psyche.
—BLDSC (5026.125000), IDS, Infotrieve, ingenta. **CCC.**
Published by: Kluwer Academic - Plenum Publishers (Subsidiary of: Wolters Kluwer N.V.), 233 Spring St, New York, NY 10013-1578. TEL 212-620-8000, 800-221-9369, FAX 212-463-0742, info@plenum.com, http://www.wkap.nl/journalhome.htm/1053-0487. Ed. Michael Feuerstein. R&P Rose Luongo TEL 781-871-6311. **Subscr. outside the Americas to:** Kluwer Academic Publishers Group, Journals Department, PO Box 322, Dordrecht 3300 AH, Netherlands. TEL 31-78-639-2392, FAX 31-78-654-6474.

363.7 GBR ISSN 0022-4375
HV675.A1 CODEN: JSFRAV
JOURNAL OF SAFETY RESEARCH. Text in English. 1982. q. EUR 537 in Europe to institutions; JPY 71,300 in Japan to institutions; USD 601 elsewhere to institutions (effective 2002). adv. bk.rev. illus. Index. back issues avail.; reprints avail. *Refereed.* **Document type:** *Academic/Scholarly.* **Description:** Provides a forum for the exchange of ideas and data developed through research experience in all areas of safety including traffic, industry, farm, home, school and public.
Related titles: Microfilm ed.: (from PQC); Online - full text ed.: (from ingenta, Gale Group, ScienceDirect, Swets Blackwell, Factiva, Institute for Scientific Information).
Indexed: ASCA, AgeLine, Aqua.Sci.& Fish.Abstr., Biol.Abstr., C.I.S. Abstr., Curr.Cont., Curr.Ind.Stat., Eng.Ind., Environ.Sci.Poll.Mgmt., Ergon.Abstr., HRIS, Pollut.Abstr., PsycInfo, Psychol.Abstr. (1969-), Psycscan A.P., Risk Abstr., SSCI, Saf.Sci.Abstr., e-psyche.
—BLDSC (5052.130000), CISTI, Ei, IDS, Infotrieve, ingenta, Linda Hall. **CCC.**
Published by: (National Safety Council), Pergamon (Subsidiary of: Elsevier Science), The Boulevard, Langford Ln, East Park, Kidlington, Oxford OXB 1GB, United Kingdom. FAX 44-1865-843010, nlinfo-f@elsevier/nl; usinfo-f@elsevier.com; forinfo-kyf04035@niftyserve.or.jp, http://www.elsevier.com/locate/jsr. Eds. Mei-Li Lin, Thomas Planek. **Subscr. in Australasia and the Far East to:** Elsevier Science (Singapore) Pte Ltd, No.1 Temasek Ave, 17-01 Millenia Tower, Singapore 039192, Singapore. TEL 65-434-3727, FAX 65-337-2230; **Subscr. in the Americas to:** Elsevier Science, PO Box 945, New York, NY 10159-0945. TEL 212-633-3730, FAX 212-633-3680, usinfo-f@elsevier.com; **Subscr. to:** Elsevier Science BV, PO Box 211, Amsterdam 1000 AE, Netherlands. TEL 31-20-485-3757, FAX 31-20-485-3432, nlinfo-f@elsevier.nl.

614.85 NLD ISSN 1052-2263
HD7255.A2 CODEN: JVREFA
JOURNAL OF VOCATIONAL REHABILITATION. Text in English. 1991. bi-m. (in 2 vols., 3 nos./vol.). EUR 200, USD 252 to institutions (effective 2002). bk.rev. abstr, illus. back issues avail. *Refereed.* **Document type:** *Journal, Academic/Scholarly.* **Description:** Topics range from supported employment to psychiatric impairment, vocational training, and physical disability.
Related titles: Microform ed.: (from PQC); Online - full text ed.: (from ingenta, Swets Blackwell, RoweCom Information Quest).
Indexed: AMED, Except.Child Educ.Abstr., Excerp.Med. (1996-), PsycInfo, e-psyche.
—BLDSC (5072.512400), EMDOCS, GNLM, Infotrieve. **CCC.**
Published by: I O S Press, Nieuwe Hemweg 6B, Amsterdam 1013 BG, Netherlands. TEL 31-20-688-3355, FAX 31-20-620-3419, market@iospress.nl, http://www.iospress.nl. Ed. Paul H Wehman TEL 804-828-1851. **Subscr. to:** I O S Press, Inc, 5795-G Burke Centre Pkwy, Burke, VA 22015. TEL 703-323-5554, FAX 703-323-3668, iosbooks@iospress.com; Kinokuniya Company Ltd, Shinjuku 3-chome, Shinjuku-ku, Tokyo 160-0022, Japan. FAX 81-3-3439-1094, journal@kinokuniya.co.jp, http://www.kinokuniya.co.jp; Globe Publication Pvt. Ltd., C-62 Inderpuri, New Delhi 100 012, India. TEL 91-11-579-3211, 91-11-579-3212, FAX 91-11-579-8876, custserve@globepub.com, http://www.globepub.com.

614.85 USA ISSN 1087-853X
KELLER'S COMPLIANCE FOCUS. Text in English. 1992. s-m. USD 149 (effective 2001). **Description:** Provides OSHA, EPA, DOT, EEOC, and SBA developments. Includes how-to articles on topics such as: hazmat training, driver safety and confined spaces.
Formerly: Keller's Regulatory Update (1063-4479)
Published by: J.J. Keller & Associates, Inc., 3003 W Breezewood Lane, Box 368, Neenah, WI 54957-0368. TEL 920-722-2848, 800-327-6868, FAX 920-727-7526, http://www.jjkeller.com.

614.85 USA ISSN 1053-3826
KELLER'S INDUSTRIAL SAFETY REPORT. Text in English. 1980. m. USD 125 (effective 2001). **Description:** Reports on state and federal regulations dealing with the manufacture, distribution, disposal, transport of and exposure to hazardous substances.
Formerly: Hazardous Substance Advisor
Published by: J.J. Keller & Associates, Inc., 3003 W Breezewood Lane, Box 368, Neenah, WI 54957-0368. TEL 920-722-2848, 800-327-6868, FAX 920-727-7526, http://www.jjkeller.com.

614.85 USA ISSN 1077-7008
KELLER'S O S H A SAFETY TRAINING NEWSLETTER. Text in English. 1994. m. USD 125 (effective 2001). **Document type:** *Newsletter.* **Description:** Provides OSHA regulatory updates with training tips, how-to-comply information and training program assessment methods.
Formerly: Keller's O S H A Safety Training Guide
Published by: J.J. Keller & Associates, Inc., 3003 W Breezewood Lane, Box 368, Neenah, WI 54957-0368. TEL 920-722-3848, 800-327-6868, FAX 920-727-7526, http://www.jjkeller.com.

614.85 USA ISSN 1090-3445
KELLER'S SAFETY MANAGEMENT TODAY NEWSLETTER. Text in English. 1996. m. USD 125 (effective 2001). **Document type:** *Newsletter.* **Description:** Includes articles on ways to improve worker safety, selling safety, and what to do when employees bring problems to work. Included are questions and answers on how to save time and money.
Published by: J.J. Keller & Associates, Inc., 3003 W Breezewood Lane, Box 368, Neenah, WI 54957-0368. TEL 920-722-2848, 800-327-6868, FAX 920-727-7526, http://www.jjkeller.com.

KELLER'S TRANSPORTATION SAFETY TRAINING NEWSLETTER. see *TRANSPORTATION*

614.85 JPN
KENSETSU KOJI SAIGAI BOSHI TEIANSHU/ PROPOSALS FOR INDUSTRIAL SAFETY OF CONSTRUCTION. Text in Japanese. 1982. s-a.
Published by: (Kanto Shibu), Nihon Doboku Kogyo Kyokai/Japan Civil Engineering Contractors' Association, Inc., 5-1 Haccho-Bori 2-chome, Chuo-ku, Tokyo 104-0032, Japan.

KOKUTETSU CHUO HOKEN KANRIJOHO; health control. see *PUBLIC HEALTH AND SAFETY*

614.85 ITA ISSN 0390-2528
LAVORO SICURO; uomo, ambiente, macchine. Text in Italian. 1973. m. (9/yr.). ITL 125,000 (effective 2000). adv. **Description:** Provides information about work accident prevention, health problems at work, and safety environment.
Published by: Gruppo Editoriale J C E, Via Ferri, 6, Cinisello Balsamo, MI 20092, Italy. TEL 39-02-660251, FAX 39-02-6127620, info@jce.it, http://www.jce.it. Ed. Vittorio Vedolato. Pub. Jacopo Castelfranchi. adv.: B&W page ITL 1,990,000, color page ITL 3,190,000; trim 280 x 210. Circ: 5,000.

LEGAL QUARTERLY DIGEST OF MINE SAFETY AND HEALTH DECISIONS. see *MINES AND MINING INDUSTRY*

614.82 FRA
LETTRE D'INFORMATION SUR LA RECHERCHE HYGIENE ET SECURITE. Text in French. 1982. irreg. free per issue. bk.rev. **Document type:** *Newsletter.*
Formerly: I N R S Lettre d'Information sur la Recherche
Related titles: English ed.: Safety Research News. ISSN 0765-913X.
Published by: Institut National de Recherche et de Securite pour la Prevention des Accidents du Travail et des Maladies Professionnelles, 30 rue Olivier Noyer, Paris Cedex 14 75680, France. TEL 33-1-40443000, FAX 33-1-40443099, TELEX 203-594 INSPAR. Ed. B Moncelon. **Co-sponsors:** International Social Security Association; International Section for Research on Prevention of Occupational Risks.

LINYE LAODONG ANQUAN/FORESTRY LABOUR SAFETY. see *FORESTS AND FORESTRY*

LOSS PREVENTION BULLETIN. see *ENGINEERING—Chemical Engineering*

614.85 GBR
LOSS PREVENTION COUNCIL. REPORT S H E. Text in English. irreg., latest vol.9, 1993. GBP 20. adv.
Document type: *Monographic series.*
—BLDSC.
Published by: Loss Prevention Council, Melrose Ave, Borehamwood, Herts WD6 2BJ, United Kingdom. TEL 44-181-207-2345, FAX 44-181-207-6305, info@lpc.co.uk. Ed. Liz Catchpole. R&P Michael Gale. Adv. contact Paulette Elgie.

613.62 USA
M I O S H A NEWS. (Michigan Occupational Safety and Health Act) Text in English. 1952. q. free. charts, illus.
Document type: *Newsletter, Government.* **Description:** Contains articles pertaining to occupational safety and health, engineering controls and interpretations of federal and state occupational health standards.
Formerly (until 1997): Michigan's Health (0026-2501)
Related titles: Online - full text ed.
Published by: Department of Consumer and Industry Services, Bureau of Safety and Regulation, PO Box 30643, Lansing, MI 48909-8143. TEL 517-322-1791, FAX 517-372-1374, http://www.cis.state.mi.us/bsr/mionews.htm. Ed., R&P Judith Simons. Circ: 8,500.

613.62 USA
MAINE. BUREAU OF LABOR STANDARDS. SAFETY WORKS. Text in English. 1994. q. free per issue.
Document type: *Newsletter.* **Description:** Contains articles concerning safety and health issues in Maine.
Formerly: Maine. Bureau of Labor Standards. Safety and Health Monitor
Published by: Department of Labor, Bureau of Labor Standards, 45 State House Station, Augusta, ME 04333-0045. TEL 207-624-6440, FAX 207-624-6449, webmaster_bls@state.me.us. Ed., R&P Lynne Lamstein. Circ: 1,749.

363.11 USA
MAINE. DEPARTMENT OF LABOR. BUREAU OF LABOR STANDARDS. CHARACTERISTICS OF WORK-RELATED INJURIES & ILLNESSES. Text in English. a. free per issue. **Document type:** *Government.* **Description:** Summary of data collected from workers' compensation reports of injury or illness.
Published by: Department of Labor, Bureau of Labor Standards, Technical Services Division, 45 State House Station, Augusta, ME 04333-0045. TEL 207-624-6440, FAX 207-624-6449, webmaster_bls@state.me.us. Ed., R&P Janet Austin. Circ: 533.

363.7 GBR
MANAGEMENT O H S & E. Text in English. 1997. m. free to qualified personnel; GBP 55 in Europe; GBP 150 elsewhere (effective 2000). adv. bk.rev. back issues avail. **Document type:** *Academic/Scholarly, Trade.*
Description: Presents news, features and legislation updates relating to workplace health, safety and environment aimed at professionals and management.
Formerly: Occupational Health, Safety and Environment (1369-1236)
Related titles: CD-ROM ed.; Online - full text ed.
Published by: Angel Business Communications Ltd., Kingsland House, 361-373 City Rd, London EC1V 1PQ, United Kingdom. TEL 44-1926-512424, FAX 44-1926-512948, helene@angelbc.co.uk, http://www.angelbc.com/. Ed., R&P Helene Ashe Roy. Adv. contact Stephen Whitehurst. B&W page GBP 1,794, color page GBP 2,394; trim 210 x 297. Circ: 20,000.

614.8 ESP ISSN 0212-1050
MAPFRE SEGURIDAD. Text in Spanish; Summaries in English. 1981. q. free per issue. adv. cum.index: 1981-1991. back issues avail. **Document type:** *Trade.*
Description: Covers accident and fire prevention, industrial hygiene, occupational medicine, and safety at work.
Indexed: Ind.SST, World Surf.Coat.
—CINDOC.
Published by: (Fundacion Mapfre), Editorial Mapfre, Ctra. Majadahonda a Pozuelo km. 3500, Majadahonda, (Madrid) 28220, Spain. TEL 91-626-55-17, FAX 91-581-21-42. Adv. contact Javier Delbusto. Circ: 21,226 (controlled).

613.62 FRA ISSN 0025-6757
MEDECINE ET TRAVAIL. Text in French. 1961. q. FRF 1,200. adv. bk.rev. **Description:** Publishes articles on occupational medicine, industrial health, hygienics, and safety at work.
Indexed: C.I.S. Abstr., Excerp.Med.
—BLDSC (5487.733200).
Published by: Syndicat National Professionnel des Medecins du Travail, 12 impasse Mas, Toulouse 31000, France. TEL 61-99-20-77, FAX 61-62-75-66. Eds. Dr. F Blanc, M C Remesy. Circ: 1,250.

613.62 ESP
MEDICINA DE LA EMPRESA; publicacion dedicada a la seguridad y medicina del trabajo. Text in Spanish. 1963. q. ESP 500, USD 8. adv. bk.rev. illus.
Indexed: C.I.S. Abstr.
Published by: Sociedad Catalana de Seguridad y Medicina del Trabajo, Tapineria, 10 pral, Barcelona 08002, Spain. Ed. Dr. B Gardoqui. Circ: (controlled).

613.62 ITA
RC963 CODEN: MELAAD
MEDICINA DEL LAVORO ED ERGONOMIA. Text in Italian; Summaries in English, Italian. 1901. bi-m. ITL 90,000. adv. bk.rev. illus, stat. index.
Former titles: Medicina del Lavoro (0025-7818); (until 1925): Il Lavoro (1125-3460)
Indexed: Abstr.Hyg., Biol.Abstr., C.I.S. Abstr., CSNB, Chem.Abstr., Chem.Titles, Ergon.Abstr., Excerp.Med., Helminthol.Abstr., INIS Atomind., Ind.Hyg.Dig., Ind.Med. (1925-), Ind.Vet., Int.Nurs.Ind., Lab.Haz.Bull., Nutr.Abstr., Rev.Appl.Entomol., Trop.Dis.Bull., Weed Abstr.
—BLDSC (5533.600000), CASDDS, CISTI, GNLM, KNAW.
Published by: (Istituti Clinici di Perfezionamento), PI-ME Press, Viale Sardegna, 64, Pavia, PV 27100, Italy. TEL 39-0382-539124, FAX 39-0382-22485, pime@mbox.systemy.it. Ed. Francesco Candura. Circ: 1,200.

613.6 RUS
CODEN: GTPZAB
MEDITSINA TRUDA I PROMYSHLENNAYA EKOLOGIYA. Text in Russian. 1957. m. RUR 360; USD 156 foreign (effective 1999). adv. bk.rev. index. *Refereed.*
Document type: *Academic/Scholarly.* **Description:** Covers hygiene in industry and agriculture, physiology of labor, industrial toxicology, clinical picture of occupational diseases.
Formerly (until 1993): Gigiena Truda i Professional'nye Zabolevaniya (0016-9919)
Indexed: Abstr.Hyg., Bioeng.Abstr., Biol.Abstr., CEABA, C.I.S. Abstr., Chem.Abstr., Chem.Indus.Notes, Chem.Titles, Dent.Ind., Eng.Ind., Excerp.Med., INIS Atomind., Ind.Hyg.Dig., Ind.Med. (coverage dropped), Int.Aerosp.Abstr., Ref.Zh., Rev.Med.& Vet.Mycol., Russ.Acad.Sci.Bibl., Trop.Dis.Bull., World Bibl.Soc.Sec.
—BLDSC (0103.294000), CASDDS, CISTI, East View, GNLM, Infotrieve. **CCC.**
Published by: Institut Meditsiny Truda, Pr-t Budennogo 31, Moscow 105275, Russian Federation. TEL 7-095-3661110, FAX 7-095-3660583. Ed. N.F. Izmerov. Pub. N F Izmerov. R&P G A Suvorov. Adv. contact N A Kalashnikova. Circ: 600. **US dist. addr.:** East View Publications, 3020 Harbor Ln N, Minneapolis, MN 55447. TEL 612-550-0961.

MEDYCYNA PRACY. see *MEDICAL SCIENCES*

MENTAL HEALTH SPECIAL INTEREST SECTION QUARTERLY. see *PSYCHOLOGY*

614.85 DEU ISSN 0936-1197
MERKBLAETTER GEFAEHRLICHE ARBEITSSTOFFE. Text in German. 1974. irreg. DEM 890. **Document type:** *Bulletin.*
Published by: Ecomed Verlagsgesellschaft AG & Co. KG, Justus-von-Liebig-Str 1, Landsberg 86899, Germany. TEL 49-8191-125-0, FAX 49-8191-125492. Eds. K Birett, R Kuehn. Circ: 10,500 (controlled).

MINE SAFETY DIGEST. see *MINES AND MINING INDUSTRY*

MINE VENTILATION SOCIETY OF SOUTH AFRICA. JOURNAL. see *MINES AND MINING INDUSTRY*

MINES SAFETY AND HEALTH COMMISSION. REPORT/ORGANE PERMANENT POUR LA SECURITE DANS LES MINES DE HOUILLE. RAPPORT. see *MINES AND MINING INDUSTRY*

MOTOR CARRIER SAFETY REPORT. see *TRANSPORTATION—Trucks And Trucking*

613.6 363.11 HUN ISSN 0027-3619
T55.A1 CODEN: MMUZDM
MUNKAVEDELEM/LABOR SAFETY. Text in Hungarian; Summaries in English, German, Russian. 1955. q. USD 20. adv. bk.rev.
Indexed: Abstr.Hyg., Chem.Abstr., Russ.Acad.Sci.Bibl., Trop.Dis.Bull.
—CASDDS.
Published by: (Munkavedelmi Tudomanyos Kutatointezet, Szakszervezetek Orszagos Tanacsa), Nepszava Lapkiado Vallalat, Rakoczi ut 54, Budapest 1964, Hungary. TEL 222-408. Ed. Gyula Nagy. Circ: 5,000.
Subscr. to: Kultura, PO Box 149, Budapest 1389, Hungary. **Co-sponsor:** Orszagos Munkaegeszsegugyi Intezet.

613.62 USA
N I O S H MANUAL OF ANALYTICAL METHODS. Variant title: N M A M. Text in English. latest 4th Edition, base vol. plus irreg. updates. USD 64 for basic manual vols. 1, 2 & 3 and updates of indeterminate period (effective 2001). **Description:** A compilation of methods for sampling and analysis of the contaminants in workplace air, and in the blood and urine of workers who are occupationally exposed to that air.
Related titles: Diskette ed.
Published by: U.S. National Institute for Occupational Safety and Health, Attn: Publications, 4676 Columbia Pkwy, Cincinnati, OH 45226. TEL 800-356-4674, FAX 513-533-8573, pubstaft@cdc.gov. **Subscr. to (for diskette):** U.S. Government Printing Office, Superintendent of Documents, PO Box 371954, Pittsburgh, PA 15250-7954. TEL 202-512-1800, FAX 202-512-2250, orders@gpo.gov, http://www.access.gpo.gov.

615.902 USA
N I O S H POCKET GUIDE TO CHEMICAL HAZARDS. Variant title: N P G. Text in English. irreg., latest 1997.
Description: Intended as a source of general industrial hygiene information for workers, employers, and occupational health professionals. Aims to help users recognize and control occupational chemical hazards. Includes information about substances found in the work environment including chemical structures or formulas, properties, measurement methods, signs and symptoms of exposure, and procedures for emergency treatment.
Related titles: CD-ROM ed.; Diskette ed.
Published by: U.S. National Institute for Occupational Safety and Health, Attn: Publications, 4676 Columbia Pkwy, Cincinnati, OH 45226. TEL 800-356-4674, FAX 703-605-6900, pubstaft@cdc.gov. **Subscr. (for diskette) to:** Industrial Hygiene Services Inc., 11760 Westline Industrial Drive, St. Louis, MO 63146; **Subscr. to:** National Technical Information Service, Government Research Center. TEL 703-605-6000, FAX 703-321-8547.

614.85 613.62 USA
N I O S H T I C. Text in English. q. bibl. **Document type:** *Bibliography, Government.* **Description:** Contains information from a wide variety of sources in addition to those with a primary occupational safety and health orientation in order to aid the examination of all aspects of adverse effects experienced by workers.
Media: Online - full text (from Canadian Centre for Occupational Health & Safety, The Dialog Corporation, European Space Agency, NISC, National Library of Medicine, Telesystemes-Questel). **Related titles:** CD-ROM ed.: (from SilverPlatter Information, Inc.).
Published by: U.S. National Institute for Occupational Safety and Health, Technical Information Center, Attn: Publications, 4676 Columbia Pkwy, Cincinnati, OH 45226. TEL 800-356-4674, FAX 513-533-8573, pubstaft@niosdtl.em.cdc.gov.

N P R A NATIONAL SAFETY CONFERENCE. PROCEEDINGS. see *PETROLEUM AND GAS*

363.11 NLD ISSN 0928-4923
N V V K INFO. Text in Dutch. 1987. 5/yr. adv. **Document type:** *Trade.*
Formerly (until 1992): N V V K Nieuws (0929-1245)
Published by: (Nederlandse Vereniging voor Veiligheidskunde), Uitgeverij Kluwer BV (Subsidiary of: Wolters Kluwer N.V.), Postbus 23, Deventer 7400 GA, Netherlands. TEL 31-570-633155, FAX 31-570-633834. Circ: 1,500 (controlled).

615.8 JPN ISSN 0917-3617
NAGANOKEN SAGYO RYOHOSHIKAI GAKUJUTSUSHI/NAGANO ASSOCIATION OF OCCUPATIONAL THERAPISTS. JOURNAL. Text in Japanese. 1982. a. adv. **Document type:** *Academic/Scholarly.*
Published by: Naganoken Sagyo Ryohoshikai, Kakeyu Byoin, 1308 Nishi-Uchi, Chiisagata-gun, Maruko-machi, Nagano-ken 386-0322, Japan. Ed. Yoko Sato. Adv. contact Shigeru Aketa.

O

O

614.85 616.2 ZAF ISSN 0374-9800
NATIONAL CENTRE FOR OCCUPATIONAL HEALTH. ANNUAL REPORT. Text in English. 1957. irreg. free per issue. **Document type:** *Government.*
Formerly: National Institute for Occupational Diseases. Annual Report
Published by: Department of Health, National Centre for Occupational Health, PO Box 4788, Johannesburg 2000, South Africa. FAX 27-11-720-6608. Ed. Dr. A C Cantrell. Circ: 400 (controlled).

614.85 JPN
NATIONAL INSTITUTE OF INDUSTRIAL SAFETY. ANNUAL REPORT. Text in Japanese. 1968. a. free per issue. back issues avail. **Document type:** *Corporate.*
Formerly (until 1992): Research Institute of Industrial Safety. Annual Report
—BLDSC (1364.716700).
Published by: National Institute of Industrial Safety/Sangyo Anzen Kenkyujo, Umezono 1-4-6, Tokyo 108, Kiyose 204-0024, Japan. Circ: 2,000.

613.6 AUT ISSN 1016-0515
NEUE B S. (Betriebs Sicherheit) Variant title: Sicherheitsmagazin. Text in German. 1965. 10/yr. ATS 210. adv. bk.rev. abstr, illus, stat. index. **Document type:** *Consumer.*
Formerly (until 1988): Betriebssicherheit - B S (0005-3287)
Indexed: C.I.S. Abstr., INIS Atomind.
—BLDSC (6077.321200).
Published by: (Allgemeine Unfallversicherungsanstalt), Elbemuehl Druck- und Verlagsgesellschaft mbH, Altmannsdorferstrasse 154-156, Vienna, W 1231, Austria. TEL 43-1-66232966236, FAX 43-1-66232966385. Ed. Ilse Zembaty. Adv. contact Margot Weidner. B&W page ATS 55,000, color page ATS 65,000; 242 x 185. Circ: 280,000.

363.7 USA ISSN 1048-2911
RA566.3 CODEN: NESLES
NEW SOLUTIONS; a journal of environmental and occupational health policy. Text in English. 1990. q. USD 53 to individuals; USD 138 to institutions (effective 2001). back issues avail.; reprints avail. **Document type:** *Journal.* **Description:** Investigated problems of occupational and environmental health with the people at risk - the workers and the community.
Indexed: Alt.Press Ind., Environ.Abstr., Environ.Per.Bibl. (1991-), Environ.Sci.Poll.Mgmt., P.A.I.S., Pollut.Abstr., Ref.Zh., Risk Abstr., Saf.Sci.Abstr., Sel.Water Res.Abstr., Soc.Serv.Abstr., Sociol.Abstr.
—BLDSC (6088.645000), CIS, GNLM, ingenta.
Published by: (Oil, Chemical & Atomic Workers Union), Baywood Publishing Co., Inc., 26 Austin Ave, Box 337, Amityville, NY 11701. TEL 631-691-1270, 800-638-7819, FAX 631-691-1770, info@baywood.com, baywood@baywood.com, http://baywood.com/search/PreviewJournal.asp?qsRecord=20, http://www.baywood.com. Ed. Charles Levenstein. R&P Julie Krempa. Adv. contact Joi Tamber-Brooks.
Co-publisher: University of Massachusetts at Lowell.

NOISE & HEALTH; an inter-disciplinary journal. see *MEDICAL SCIENCES—Otorhinolaryngology*

313.620711 NOR
NORWAY. DIREKTORATET FOR ARBEIDSTILSYNET. FORSKRIFTER/REGULATIONS. Text in Norwegian. irreg. price varies. charts, illus. **Document type:** *Trade.*
Formerly: Norway. Statens Arbeidstilsyn Direktoratet. Verneregler
Published by: Direktoratet for Arbeidstilsynet/Directorate of Labour Inspection, Fr Nansens vei 14, Postboks 8103, Dep, Oslo 0032, Norway. TEL 47-22-95-70-00, FAX 47-22-60-77-72. **Subscr. to:** Tiden Norsk Forlag, Youngstorget, Postboks 8813, Oslo 0181, Norway.

613.62 USA ISSN 0888-1626
NOTICIAS DE SEGURIDAD✶. Text in Spanish. 1938. m. USD 32. adv. **Document type:** *Trade.*
Published by: Inter-American Safety Council, 80 Commerce Way, Ste B, Totowa, NJ 07512-1154. TEL 201-871-0004, FAX 201-871-2074, TELEX 135407. Circ: 10,000.

613.62 GBR
O E D A NEWSLETTER. Text in English. 1996. irreg. GBP 10 domestic; GBP 25 foreign (effective 2000). bk.rev. illus. **Document type:** *Newsletter.* **Description:** Discusses cases of individuals and groups of workers who have been exposed to asbestos on the job. Provides support for families affected by the disease.
Formerly (until 1998): S P A I D News (0144-4301)
Published by: Occupational and Environmental Diseases Association, Bush Hill Park, Mitre House, 66 Abbey Rd, Enfield, Mddx EN1 2QN, United Kingdom. TEL 44-181-360-8490. Circ: 2,000.

613.6 616.9 362 USA ISSN 0894-2811
THE O E M REPORT. (Occupational and Environmental Medicine) Text in English. 1987. m. USD 185 in US & Canada; USD 205 elsewhere. bk.rev. *Refereed.* **Document type:** *Newsletter.* **Description:** Provides scientific information and opinion to occupational and environmental health professionals in a timely fashion.
—BLDSC (6235.495000).
Published by: O E M Health Information Inc., 8 West St, Beverly, MA 01915. TEL 978-921-7300, FAX 978-921-0304, oem@oempress.com, http://www.oempress.com. Ed. Dr. Robert J McCunney. Pub., R&P Curtis R Vouwie.

613.62 363.11 CAN ISSN 0827-4576
O H S CANADA. (Occupational Health & Safety) Text in English. 1985. 8/yr. CND 90 (effective 2000). adv. bk.rev. charts, illus, stat, tr.lit. index. back issues avail. **Description:** Provides information on accident prevention, occupational hygiene, laws and standards, workers' compensation.
Related titles: Online - full text ed.: (from ProQuest Information & Learning, Factiva).
Indexed: ABI Inform. (Jan.1992-), Can.B.P.I., Can.Per.Ind. (Jan.1988-).
—BLDSC (6228.859000), CISTI, Infotrieve. **CCC.**
Published by: Southam Information Products Ltd., 1450 Don Mills Rd, Don Mills, ON M3B 2X7, Canada. TEL 416-445-6641, 800-668-2374, FAX 416-442-2200. Ed. David Dehaas. Pub., R&P, Adv. contact Peter Boxer. Circ: 7,000.

O H S DIRECTORY. (Occupational Health & Safety) see *PUBLIC HEALTH AND SAFETY*

O O H N A JOURNAL. see *MEDICAL SCIENCES—Nurses And Nursing*

636.11 GBR ISSN 1462-4958
O S & H BULLETIN. (Occupational Safety and Health) Text in English. 1971. m. GBP 30.59 to non-members; GBP 26 to members; GBP 35.94 foreign to members (effective 2000). **Document type:** *Bulletin.*
Former titles (until 1997): R O S P A Bulletin (0143-3377); Which incorporated (in 1979): O S & H Bulletin (0309-1155); Which was formerly (until 1976): Occupational Safety & Health. Supplement (0029-7992); Occupational Safety Bulletin; Industrial Accident Prevention Bulletin
Indexed: Br.Tech.Ind., CSNB.
—BLDSC (8024.700000).
Published by: Royal Society for the Prevention of Accidents, Edgbaston Park, 353 Bristol Rd, Edgbaston, Birmingham, Worcs B5 7ST, United Kingdom. TEL 44-121-248-2000, FAX 44-121-248-2001, help@rospa.com.uk, http://www.rospa.com.uk. Ed. Jacky Steemson. Adv. contacts Amanda Walker TEL 44-1753-670888, Sue Philo TEL 44-1367-820181.

613.62 362.1 USA
O S H A AND SAFETY MEETINGS HANDBOOK. (Occupational Safety and Health Administration) Text in English. q. USD 295 (effective 1999). **Document type:** *Trade.* **Description:** Contains 30 complete OSHA training meetings, training materials on every OSHA required topic, over 60 reproducible handouts, training exercises, quizzes and a "train the trainer" section with helpful hints.
Formerly: Safety Meetings Handbook
Published by: Business & Legal Reports, Inc., Attn: Tom Picinich, 39 Academy St, Madison, CT 06443. TEL 203-245-7448, FAX 203-245-0483, service@blr.com, http://www.blr.com. Ed. Judy Ruddy. Pub. Robert L Brady.

363.11 USA
O S H A FASTSEARCH; Occupational Safety and Health Administration regulations. Text in English. 1992. q. (plus m. updates). USD 399.
Published by: FastSearch Corporation, PO Box 12427, Scottsdale, AZ 85267-2427. TEL 800-232-4590, FAX 612-595-0229. Ed. Alan Rosenauer. Circ: 1,600.

363.11 USA
O S H A NEWS. (Occupational Safety and Health Administration) Text in English. 1996. bi-w. USD 187 (effective 1997). **Document type:** *Newsletter.* **Description:** Contains information and news about developments in the field of occupational safety and health, with a focus on developments regarding OSHA and CFR 1910 and 1926 regulations.
Formed by the 1996 merger of: O S H A News for Construction; O S H A News for General Industry
Published by: Merritt Publishing, P O Box 955, Santa Monica, CA 90406. TEL 310-450-7234, FAX 310-396-4563, cnitzschner@merrittpublishing.com. Ed. Connie Nitzschner. Circ: 4,000.

614.85 USA
O S H A REGULATIONS, DOCUMENTS, AND TECHNICAL INFORMATION ON CD-ROM. (CD-ROM can be used with both Windows and Macintosh systems) Text in English. q. USD 45 (effective 2001). **Document type:** *Government.* **Description:** Contains the text of all OSHA regulations (standards), selected documents, and technical information from the OSHA Computerized Information System. Includes Mine Safety and Health Regulations.
Media: CD-ROM.
Published by: U.S. Occupational Safety and Health Administration, Office of Public Affairs, Rm N3647, 200 Constitution Ave, N W, Washington, DC 20210. **Subscr. to:** U.S. Government Printing Office, Superintendent of Documents, PO Box 371954, Pittsburgh, PA 15250-7954. TEL 202-512-1800, FAX 202-512-2250, orders@gpo.gov, http://www.access.gpo.gov.

O S H A REQUIRED SAFETY TRAINING FOR SUPERVISORS. (Occupational Safety and Health Administration) see *ENVIRONMENTAL STUDIES*

613.62 USA
O S H A UP TO DATE NEWSLETTER. (U.S. Occupational Safety & Health Administration) Text in English. m. USD 40 to members; USD 46 to non-members (effective 2001). **Document type:** *Newsletter.*
Published by: National Safety Council, Periodicals Department, 1121 Spring Lake Dr, Itasca, IL 60143. TEL 630-285-1121, FAX 630-775-2310. Ed. Jennifer Grow. Pub. Suzanne Powills. Circ: 30,000.

614.85 GBR ISSN 1352-0334
O S H BRIEFING. (Occupational Safety and Health) Text in English. 1993. m. GBP 99. bk.rev. **Document type:** *Bulletin, Abstract/Index.* **Description:** Provides concise summaries of newly published U.K. and E.C. legislation, reports, and other documents of an official and authoritative nature. Covers health, safety, fire safety, and related topics.
Related titles: Diskette ed.; Online - full text ed.: GBP 150.
Published by: Babour Index plc., New Lodge Drift Rd, Winkfield, Windsor, Berks SL4 4RQ, United Kingdom. TEL 44-1344-884121, FAX 44-1344-884112, dd@ehas.demon.co.uk. Ed. D Denton.

615.851 USA ISSN 1084-4902
O T PRACTICE. (Occupational Therapy) Text in English. 1995. bi-w. USD 75 domestic to individuals; USD 140 foreign to individuals; USD 135 domestic to institutions; USD 195 foreign to institutions (effective 2001). adv. bk.rev., software rev. charts, illus, stat, tr.lit. index. back issues avail. **Document type:** *Trade.* **Description:** Provides professional information and news on all aspects of occupational therapy practice and covers topics such as managed care, assistive technology, aquatic therapy, geriatrics, and visual impairments.
Indexed: CINAHL.
—BLDSC (6313.177000), ingenta.
Published by: American Occupational Therapy Association, Inc., 4720 Montgomery Lane, Bethesda, MD 20814-3425. TEL 301-652-2682, FAX 301-652-7711, otpractice@aota.org, http://www.aota.org. Ed. Laura Farr Collins. Adv. contact Stephanie Abrams TEL 301-652-6611 ext. 2715. B&W page USD 2,627, color page USD 3,352; trim 10.88 x 8.13. Circ: 55,000.

613.62 USA ISSN 0893-1712
O T WEEK. (Occupational Therapy) Text in English. 1939. m. USD 80 to individuals; USD 175 to institutions; USD 200 foreign to institutions (effective 1999). adv. charts, illus.
Former titles (until 1985): Occupational Therapy Newspaper; Occupational Therapy; American Occupational Therapy Association. Newsletter
Indexed: Rehabil.Lit.
—ingenta.
Published by: American Occupational Therapy Association, Inc., 4720 Montgomery Lane, Bethesda, MD 20814-3425. TEL 301-652-2682, FAX 301-652-7711. Ed. Paula Steib. Circ: 42,000.

613.62 BEL ISSN 0771-2634
OBJECTIF PREVENTION. Text in French. 1964. m. BEF 880.
Related titles: ♦ Dutch ed.: Operatie Veiligheid. ISSN 0771-2588.
Published by: Association Nationale pour la Prevention des Accidents du Travail (ANPAT), Rue Gachard 88, Bte 4, Brussels 1050, Belgium. TEL 32-2-648-03-37, FAX 32-2-648-68-67. Circ: 27,000.

613.62 616.98 GBR ISSN 1351-0711
RC963 CODEN: OEMEEM
OCCUPATIONAL AND ENVIRONMENTAL MEDICINE. Text in English. 1944. m. GBP 129, USD 206 combined subscription to individuals includes print & online eds.; GBP 218, USD 350 to institutions for print only (effective 2002). adv. bk.rev. abstr, charts, illus. index, cum.index: 1944-1960. back issues avail.; reprint service avail. from PQC. *Refereed.* **Document type:** *Academic/Scholarly.* **Description:** Focuses on current interest in the whole field of occupational medicine.
Formerly (until 1993): British Journal of Industrial Medicine (0007-1072)
Related titles: CD-ROM ed.: (from Ovid Technologies, Inc.); Microform ed.: (from PQC); Online - full text ed.: O E M Online. ISSN 1470-7926. GBP 65, USD 99 to individuals (effective 2002); Institutions please contact publisher for online rates. (from Ovid Technologies, Inc., HighWire Pr., EBSCO Publishing, O C L C Online Computer Library Center, Inc., ProQuest Information & Learning, ingenta, Swets Blackwell, SilverPlatter Information, Inc., Institute for Scientific Information).
Indexed: AESIS, API Abstr., API Catal., API Hlth.& Environ., API Oil., API Pet.Ref., API Pet.Subst., API Transport., ASCA, Abstr.Hyg., Acoust.Abstr., Arts & Hum.Cit.Ind. (coverage dropped), B.C.I.R.A., Biol.Abstr., Br.Ceram.Abstr., Br.Tech.Ind., CAD CAM Abstr., C.I.S. Abstr., CSNB, Cadscan, Chem.Abstr., Chem.Titles, Cott.& Trop.Fibr.Abstr., Curr.Adv.Ecol.Sci., Curr.Cont., Dent.Ind., Energy Rev., Environ.Abstr., Environ.Per.Bibl. (1981-), Environ.Sci.Poll.Mgmt., Ergon.Abstr., Excerp.Med., Forest Prod.Abstr., GeoRef, Helminthol.Abstr., INIS Atomind., Ind.Hyg.Dig., Ind.Med. (1994-), Ind.Sci.Rev., Ind.Vet., Inpharma, Int.Abstr.Biol.Sci., Lab.Haz.Bull., Lead Abstr., METADEX, Med.& Surg.Dermat., NRN, Neurosci.Cit.Ind., Nutr.Abstr., Pharm.&Out.News, Plant Breed.Abstr., Pollut.Abstr., Poult.Abstr., Reac., Ref.Zh., Rev.Appl.Entomol., Risk Abstr., SSCI (coverage dropped), Saf.Sci.Abstr., Sci.Cit.Ind., THA, Trop.Dis.Bull., Vet.Bull., Weed Abstr., World Surf.Coat., World Text.Abstr., Zincscan.
—BLDSC (6227.833000), ADONIS, CASDDS, CISTI, EMDOCS, GNLM, IDS, ingenta, KNAW. **CCC.**
Published by: B M J Publishing Group, B M A House, Tavistock Sq, London WC1H 9JR, United Kingdom. TEL 44-20-7387-4499, FAX 44-20-7383-6400, info.norththames@bma.org.uk, http://www.occenvmed.com, http://www.bma.org.uk. Ed. Anne Cockcroft. Pub. Alex Williamson. R&P Carol Torselli TEL 44-20-7383-6674. Adv. contact Euan Currer TEL 44-20-7383-6181.

363.11 USA ISSN 1359-9364
T59.7
OCCUPATIONAL ERGONOMICS. Text in English. 1998. q. NLG 180, USD 90 to individuals; NLG 484, USD 242 to institutions (effective 2000). adv. bk.rev. illus. back issues avail.; reprints avail. *Refereed.* **Document type:** *Journal, Academic/Scholarly.* **Description:** Takes an application-oriented approach to the occupational and engineering aspects of ergonomics, safety and health care, and rehabilitation issues.
Announced as: Occupational Ergonomics and Safety
Related titles: Online - full text ed.: (from Swets Blackwell, RoweCom Information Quest).
Indexed: Curr.Cont. (coverage dropped), Environ.Sci.Poll.Mgmt., Ergon.Abstr., Pollut.Abstr., Risk Abstr., SSCI (coverage dropped), Saf.Sci.Abstr., Sci.Cit.Ind. (coverage dropped).
—BLDSC (6227.970000).
Published by: (International Society for Occupational Ergonomics and Safety), I O S Press, Nieuwe Hemweg 6B, Amsterdam 1013 BG, Netherlands. Ed. Biman Das TEL 902-494-3296. R&P C Koolbergen TEL 31-20-638-2189. Adv. contact M Janmaat. **Subscr. to:** Kinokuniya Company Ltd, Shinjuku 3-chome, Shinjuku-ku, Tokyo 160-0022, Japan. FAX 81-3-3439-1094, journal@kinokuniya.co.jp, http://www.kinokuniya.co.jp; Globe Publication Pvt. Ltd., C-62 Inderpuri, New Delhi 100 012, India. TEL 91-11-579-3211, 91-11-579-3212, FAX 91-11-579-8876, custserve@globepub.com, http://www.globepub.com.

613.62 USA
OCCUPATIONAL EXPOSURE SOURCEBOOK. Text in English. 1997. a. USD 269; USD 269 foreign (effective 1999). **Document type:** *Trade.*
Published by: American Health Consultants (Subsidiary of: Medical Economics Co., Inc.), 3525 Piedmont Rd, N E, 6 Piedmont Center, Ste 400, Atlanta, GA 30305. TEL 404-262-5476, custserv@ahcpub.com, http://www.ahcpub.com.

363.7 USA ISSN 0029-7909
CODEN: OCHAAZ
OCCUPATIONAL HAZARDS; magazine of health & environment. Text in English. 1938. m. USD 50 domestic; USD 70 in Canada; USD 100 elsewhere (effective 2001). adv. bk.rev. charts, illus, stat, tr.lit. index. reprint service avail. from PQC. **Document type:** *Trade.* **Description:** News on industrial safety, occupational health, environmental control, insurance, first aid, medical care, and hazardous material control.
Related titles: Microform ed.: (from PQC); Online - full text ed.: O H Online (from Gale Group, ProQuest Information & Learning, Northern Light Technology, Inc., H. W. Wilson, Factiva).
Indexed: ABI Inform. (Aug.1979-), Aqua.Sci.& Fish.Abstr., B.P.I. (Jul.1989-), BPIA, Bus.Ind., C.I.S. Abstr., CSNB, Chem.Abstr., Environ.Sci.Poll.Mgmt., Hlth.Ind., Ind.Hyg.Dig., L.R.I., Lab.Haz.Bull., PROMT, Pers.Manage.Abstr., Pollut.Abstr., Risk Abstr., Saf.Sci.Abstr., Tox.Abstr., Tr.& Indus.Ind., Work Rel.Abstr.
—BLDSC (6228.000000), CISTI, IDS, Infotrieve, Linda Hall. **CCC.**
Published by: Penton Media, Inc. (Subsidiary of: Pittway Company), 1300 E 9th St, Cleveland, OH 44114-1503. TEL 216-696-7000, FAX 216-696-8765, information@penton.com, http://www.occupationalhazards.com/, http://www.penton.com. Ed. Stephen Minter. Adv. contact Gina Pisarek TEL 216-931-9534. B&W page USD 7,400. Circ: 60,000 (controlled). **Subscr. to:** PO Box 901979, Cleveland, OH 44190-1979.

613.62 USA ISSN 0362-4064
RC963 CODEN: OHSADQ
OCCUPATIONAL HEALTH & SAFETY. Text in English. 1932. m. USD 99 in United States; USD 109 in Canada; USD 119 elsewhere (effective 2001). adv. bk.rev. charts, illus. Index. 108 p./no. 3 cols./p. reprint service avail. from PQC. *Refereed.* **Document type:** *Journal, Trade.* **Description:** Helps professionals understand and control injury, illness and hazardous exposures in the workplace.
Former titles (until 1976): The International Journal of Occupational Health & Safety (0093-2205); (until 1974): International Industrial Medicine and Surgery (0163-934X); (until 1969): The International Journal of Industrial Medicine & Surgery (0093-2191); (until 1967): Industrial Medicine and Surgery (0019-8536); (until 1949): Industrial Medicine and Surgery Trauma (0163-9331); (until 1949): Industrial Medicine (0093-2183)
Related titles: Microform ed.: (from PQC); Online - full text ed.: (from ProQuest Information & Learning, Northern Light Technology, Inc., Factiva).
Indexed: ABI Inform. (Jan.1991-), Abstr.Hyg., AgeLine, B.P.I. (Jul.1989-), Biol.Abstr., CINAHL, C.I.S. Abstr., Chem.Abstr., Dent.Ind., Environ.Sci.Poll.Mgmt., Ergon.Abstr., Hosp.Lit.Ind., INIS Atomind., INSPEC (May 1972-Oct.1973, Nov.1974-Jan.1983, dropped), Ind.Hyg.Dig., Ind.Med. (1976-), Lab.Haz.Bull., Noise Pollut.Publ.Abstr., P.A.I.S., Pers.Lit., Pollut.Abstr., Risk Abstr., Saf.Sci.Abstr., Tr.& Dev.Alert, Trop.Dis.Bull.
—BLDSC (6228.858000), CISTI, GNLM, ingenta, KNAW, Linda Hall. **CCC.**
Published by: Stevens Publishing Corporation, 5151 Beltline Rd, 10th fl, Dallas, TX 75240. TEL 972-687-6700, FAX 972-687-6770, http://www.ohsonline.com/, http://www.stevenspublishing.com/. Ed. Jerry Laws. Pub. Dana Corbin. Circ: 93,000 (paid and free).

OCCUPATIONAL HEALTH AND SAFETY LAW. see *LAW*

OCCUPATIONAL HEALTH AND SAFETY LAW NEW SOUTH WALES. see *LAW*

352.67 AUS
OCCUPATIONAL HEALTH & SAFETY LEGISLATION SERVICE. Text in English. irreg., latest 1995, Mar. price varies. **Document type:** *Government.*
Published by: Law Press (Victoria), 52-58 Chetwynd St, West Melbourne, VIC 3003, Australia. TEL 61-3-93208686, FAX 61-3-93208699.

613.62029 USA ISSN 0896-3835
CODEN: OHSDE2
OCCUPATIONAL HEALTH & SAFETY NEWS. Text in English. m. USD 399. adv. **Document type:** *Newsletter.* **Description:** Discusses industry news and legislative updates, ergonomics, drug testing, corporate liability and O S H A compliance. Includes case studies and checklists.
Published by: Stevens Publishing Corporation, 5151 Beltline Rd, 10th fl, Dallas, TX 75240. TEL 972-687-6700, FAX 972-687-6770. Ed. Darla Bean.

613.62 614.85 USA ISSN 1524-0622
OCCUPATIONAL HEALTH & SAFETY WEEK. Text in English. w. USD 491. **Document type:** *Newsletter.* **Description:** Discusses government policy on occupational health and safety, OSHA Commission review, legislative updates, and tips on workplace health..
Formerly: OSHAWeek (1057-1485)
—**CCC.**
Published by: Stevens Publishing Corporation, 5151 Beltline Rd, 10th fl, Dallas, TX 75240. TEL 972-687-6700, FAX 972-687-6770. Ed. Darla Bean.

613.62 GBR ISSN 0969-708X
OCCUPATIONAL HEALTH BULLETIN. Text in English. 1986. s-a. back issues avail. **Document type:** *Bulletin.*
Formerly: University of Birmingham. Institute of Occupational Health. Bulletin (0958-6040)
Indexed: Lab.Haz.Bull.
Published by: University of Birmingham, Institute of Occupational Health, University Of Birmingham, Edgbaston, PO Box 363, Birmingham, Worcs B15 2TT, United Kingdom. TEL 44-121-414-6030, FAX 44-121-414-6217, institute-of-occupational-health@bham.ac.uk.

613.62 USA ISSN 1082-5339
OCCUPATIONAL HEALTH MANAGEMENT. Text in English. 1991. m. USD 399 domestic; USD 429 foreign; USD 67 newsstand/cover (effective 2001). **Document type:** *Newsletter.*
Published by: American Health Consultants (Subsidiary of: Medical Economics Co., Inc.), 3525 Piedmont Rd, N E, 6 Piedmont Center, Ste 400, Atlanta, GA 30305. TEL 404-262-5476, 404-262-7436, 800-688-2421, FAX 404-262-7837, 800-284-3291, custserv@ahcpub.com, http://www.ahcpub.com. Circ: 1,220.

613 AUS ISSN 1441-144X
OCCUPATIONAL HEALTH NEWS. Text in English. 1984. fortn. AUD 450; includes Inside O H S. **Document type:** *Newsletter.* **Description:** Provides information on occupational health and safety. Alerts employers and unions to key developments in work place safety and health from Australia and throughout the world.
Formerly (until 1998): Occupational Health Newsletter (1320-1514)
Published by: Newsletter Information Services, PO Box 693, Manly, NSW 2095, Australia. TEL 61-2-9977-7500, FAX 61-2-9977-3310, customer.support@newsinfo.com.au, http://www.newsinfo.com.au. Ed. Sheena Frost.

613.62 GBR ISSN 0951-4600
OCCUPATIONAL HEALTH REVIEW. Short title: O H R. Text in English. 1987. bi-m. GBP 200 domestic; GBP 210 foreign (effective 1999). back issues avail. **Document type:** *Trade.* **Description:** For specialists and nonspecialists in the area of occupational medicine and employee welfare.
Indexed: Brit.Nur.Ind., INIS Atomind., Intl.Polym.Sci.& Tech., Mgmt.& Market.Abstr., RAPRA (1991-), World Surf.Coat.
—BLDSC (6228.990000), GNLM.
Published by: Eclipse Group Ltd., Industrial Relations Services, 18 Highbury Park, London N5 2AB, United Kingdom. TEL 44-20-7354-5858, FAX 44-207-226-8618. Ed. John Ballard.

363.11 CHE ISSN 1061-0251
CODEN: OCHYE9
OCCUPATIONAL HYGIENE; risk management of occupational hazards. Text in English. 1993. 6/yr. EUR 278 to institutions; EUR 428 to corporations (effective 2000). back issues avail. **Document type:** *Academic/Scholarly.* **Description:** Presents recent developments in the science of anticipation, recognition, evaluation and control of occupational hazards.
Related titles: CD-ROM ed.; Microform ed.; Online - full text ed.: (from RoweCom Information Quest).
Indexed: Environ.Abstr., Environ.Sci.Poll.Mgmt., Ind.Med. (1994-), METADEX, Pollut.Abstr., RAPRA (1998-), Risk Abstr., Saf.Sci.Abstr., Sel.Water Res.Abstr.
—BLDSC (6229.080000). **CCC.**
Published by: Gordon and Breach - Harwood Academic (Subsidiary of: Taylor & Francis Group), PO Box 531, Lausanne 1000, Switzerland. http://www.gbhap.com/Occupational_Hygiene/; http://biomednet.com/library/225. Ed. Michel Guillemin. **Subscr. addr. in US:** International Publishers Direct, PO Box 32160, Newark, NJ 07102. FAX 215-750-6343.

613.62 GBR
CODEN: OHMOD4
OCCUPATIONAL HYGIENE HANDBOOKS. Text in English. 1978. irreg. price varies. back issues avail. **Document type:** *Monographic series.*

O

Formerly: Occupational Hygiene Monographs (0141-7568) —CISTI, Infotrieve. **CCC.**
Published by: H & H Scientific Consultants Ltd., PO Box MT27, Leeds, W Yorks LS17 8QP, United Kingdom. TEL 44-113-268-7189, FAX 44-113-268-7191, hhsc@hhsc.co.uk, http://www.hhsc.co.uk. Ed. Dr. Donald Hughes. Circ: 5,000.

363.11 USA
OCCUPATIONAL INJURIES AND ILLNESSES. Text in English. 1992. irreg. (in 3 vols.). USD 365 (effective 1999). **Description:** Provides information on work-related illnesses and injuries, including information on injuries to the head, neck, shoulder, hand, wrist, lower back, and the effects of known toxic substances.
Related titles: CD-ROM ed.
Published by: Matthew Bender & Co., Inc. (Subsidiary of: Lexis Law Publishing), 2 Park Ave, New York, NY 10016. TEL 212-448-2000, international@bender.com, http://www.bender.com. Ed. Daniel Stone.

O

363.11 USA ISSN 0198-7771
HD7262.5.U62
OCCUPATIONAL INJURIES & ILLNESSES IN MAINE. Text in English. a. free. **Document type:** *Government.* **Description:** Data collected from the survey of occupational injuries and illnesses.
Published by: Department of Labor, Bureau of Labor Standards, Techical Services Division, 45 State House Station, Augusta, ME 04333-0045. TEL 207-624-6440, FAX 207-624-6449, webmaster_bls@state.me.us. Ed., R&P Robert W Leighton Jr. Circ: 615.

613.62 616.98 GBR ISSN 0962-7480
CODEN: OCMEE8
OCCUPATIONAL MEDICINE. Text in English. 1951. 8/yr. GBP 125, USD 210 to individuals; GBP 295, USD 500 to institutions (effective Feb. 2002). adv. bk.rev. illus. index. 72 p./no. back issues avail. *Refereed.* **Document type:** *Journal, Academic/Scholarly.* **Description:** Covers original and review articles on all aspects of occupational health.
Former titles (until 1991): Society of Occupational Medicine. Journal (0301-0023); Society of Occupational Medicine Transactions (0037-9972)
Related titles: Microform ed.: (from PQC); Online - full text ed.: GBP 265, USD 450 to institutions Online only (effective Feb. 2002) (from EBSCO Publishing, Swets Blackwell, HighWire Pr., Ovid Technologies, Inc., Institute for Scientific Information).
Indexed: ASCA, Biol.Abstr., C.I.S. Abstr., CSNB, Chem.Abstr., Crim.Just.Abstr., Curr.Adv.Ecol.Sci., Curr.Cont., Environ.Sci.Poll.Mgmt., Ergon.Abstr., Excerp.Med., INIS Atomind., Ind.Med. (1992-), Inpharma, Int.Abstr.Biol.Sci., Int.Nurs.Ind., L.R.I., Lab.Haz.Bull., Nutr.Abstr., Pharm.&Out.News, Pollut.Abstr., Reac., Rev.Appl.Entomol., Rev.Med.& Vet.Mycol., Risk Abstr., SSCI (coverage dropped), Saf.Sci.Abstr., Trop.Dis.Bull.
—BLDSC (6229.610000), ADONIS, CASDDS, CISTI, EMDOCS, GNLM, IDS, ingenta, KNAW.
Published by: Oxford University Press, Academic Division, Great Clarendon St, Oxford OX2 6DP, United Kingdom. TEL 44-1865-267907, FAX 44-1865-267835, jnl.info@oup.co.uk, http://occmed.oupjouranls.org/, http://www.oup.co.uk/journals, http://www3.oup.co.uk/occmed/. Ed. Dr. J R Beach. Pub. Mandy Sketch. R&P Fionna Willis. Adv. contact Gemma Heiser. Circ: 2,650. **Subscr. in the US to:** Oxford University Press, Journals, 2001 Evans Rd, Cary, NC 27513. TEL 919-677-0977, 800-852-7323, FAX 919-677-1714, jnlorders@oup-usa.org, http://www.oup-usa.org; **Subscr. to:** Journals Marketing, Great Clarendon St, Oxford OX2 6DP, United Kingdom.

613.62 USA ISSN 0885-114X
RC963.A1 CODEN: SAOME4
OCCUPATIONAL MEDICINE (PHILADELPHIA); state of the art reviews. Text in English. q., latest vol.16, 2001. USD 99 domestic to individuals; USD 109 foreign to individuals; USD 106 domestic to institutions; USD 136 foreign to institutions; USD 39 newsstand/cover domestic; USD 39 newsstand/cover foreign (effective 2001). illus. 200 p./no. 1 cols./p. back issues avail. *Refereed.* **Document type:** *Monographic series, Academic/Scholarly.*
Related titles: Online - full text ed.: (from Institute for Scientific Information).
Indexed: Abstr.Hyg., CINAHL, Curr.Cont., INIS Atomind., Ind.Med. (1986-), Ind.Vet., Int.Nurs.Ind., Pig News & Info., Poult.Abstr.
—BLDSC (6229.620000), CASDDS, CISTI, GNLM, IDS, KNAW. **CCC.**
Published by: Hanley & Belfus, Inc., 210 S 13th St, Philadelphia, PA 19107. TEL 215-546-7293, FAX 215-790-9330. Circ: 1,600.

363.7 ZAF
OCCUPATIONAL SAFETY & ENVIRONMENTAL NEWS. Text in English. 1993. m. adv. illus. **Document type:** *Trade.*
Published by: Complete Publishing (Pty.) Ltd., PO Box 87745, Houghton, Johannesburg 2041, South Africa. TEL 27-11-7892112, FAX 27-11-789-5347.

363.11 613.6 GBR ISSN 0143-5353
T55.A1
OCCUPATIONAL SAFETY AND HEALTH. Text in English. 1946. m. GBP 58.82 to non-members; GBP 50 to members; GBP 66.11 foreign to members (effective 2000). adv. bk.rev. abstr, charts, illus, tr.lit. index.
Formerly: British Journal of Occupational Safety
Related titles: Online - full text ed.: (from Gale Group).
Indexed: Abstr.Hyg., Account.& Data Proc.Abstr., Agri.Eng.Abstr., Art.Hosp.& Tour., B.C.I.R.A., BMT, Br.Ceram.Abstr., Br.Rail.Bd., Br.Tech.Ind., C.I.S. Abstr., CSNB, Cadscan, Emerald, INIS Atomind., Lab.Haz.Bull., Lead Abstr., Mgmt.& Market.Abstr., RAPRA, Ref.Zh., Repindex, Trop.Dis.Bull., World Text.Abstr., Zincscan.
—CISTI, Linda Hall.
Published by: Royal Society for the Prevention of Accidents, Edgbaston Park, 353 Bristol Rd, Edgbaston, Birmingham, Worcs B5 7ST, United Kingdom. TEL 44-121-248-2000, FAX 44-121-248-2001, help@rospa.com.uk, http://www.rospa.com.uk. Ed. Jacky Steemson. Adv. contacts Amanda Walker TEL 44-1753-670888, Sue Philo TEL 44-1367-820181. Circ: 10,000.

614.85 JPN
OCCUPATIONAL SAFETY & HEALTH. Text in Japanese. m. JPY 9,480 (effective 1998). **Description:** Magazine for occupational safety managers, specialists and practitioners.
Formerly: Safety
Published by: Japan Industrial Safety and Health Association, Publishing and Sales Department, 5-35-1 Shiba, Minato-ku, Tokyo 108-0014, Japan. TEL 81-3-3452-6841, FAX 81-3-3453-8034. Ed. Noriyuki Okano.

613.62 614.85 USA
OCCUPATIONAL SAFETY AND HEALTH ACT. Text in English. 1978. 3 base vols. plus s-a. updates. USD 460; USD 326 updates. **Description:** A comprehensive analysis of OSHA, its regulations, and its enforcement.
Related titles: CD-ROM ed.
Published by: Matthew Bender & Co., Inc. (Subsidiary of: Lexis Law Publishing), 2 Park Ave, New York, NY 10016. TEL 212-448-2000, international@bender.com, http://www.bender.com. Eds. R Ben Hogan, Robert Moran.

613.62 346.066 USA
OCCUPATIONAL SAFETY & HEALTH DAILY. Text in English. d. back issues avail. **Document type:** *Newsletter, Trade.* **Description:** Covers legislative, regulatory, and judicial developments affecting job safety and health.
Media: Online - full text.
Published by: The Bureau of National Affairs, Inc., 1231 25th St, N W, Washington, DC 20037. TEL 800-372-1033, 800-452-7773, FAX 800-253-0332, customercare@bna.com, http://www.bna.com/products/ens/ohdm.htm. **Subscr. to:** 9435 Key West Ave, Rockville, MD 20850.

344.043 USA
OCCUPATIONAL SAFETY AND HEALTH HANDBOOK; an employer's guide to OSHA laws, regulations, and practices. Text in English. 1993. base vol. (1-2/yr.). USD 95.
Published by: Lexis Law Publishing (Subsidiary of: Reed Elsevier plc), PO Box 7587, Charlottesville, VA 22906-7587. TEL 804-972-7600, 800-562-1197, FAX 804-972-7666, llp.customer.support@lexis-nexis.com, http://www.lexislawpublishing.com. Ed. Jeffrey L Hirsch.

613.62 AUS
OCCUPATIONAL SAFETY AND HEALTH HANDBOOK. Text in English. base vol. plus irreg. updates. AUD 400 to non-members; AUD 200 to members (effective 2000). stat. back issues avail. **Document type:** *Academic/Scholarly.* **Description:** Provides a easy to use reference guide for achieving workplace safety. The handbook explains critical areas of OSH law and helps employers create and implement an effective OSH management system.
Published by: Chamber of Commerce and Industry of Western Australia, 190 Hay St, East Perth, W.A. 6004, Australia. TEL 61-8-9365-7555, FAX 61-8-9365-7550, info@cciwa.asn.au. Ed. Sophia Cochrane.

613.62 AUS
OCCUPATIONAL SAFETY AND HEALTH PROCEDURES MANUAL. Text in English. base vol. plus irreg. updates. AUD 450 base vol(s). per issue (effective 2000). **Document type:** *Academic/Scholarly.* **Description:** Includes a range of practical, proven procedures, consistent with industry standards.
Published by: Chamber of Commerce and Industry of Western Australia, 190 Hay St, East Perth, W.A. 6004, Australia. TEL 61-8-9365-7555, FAX 61-8-9365-7550, info@cciwa.asn.au. Ed. Greg Richards.

331 USA ISSN 0095-3237
KF3570.A1
OCCUPATIONAL SAFETY & HEALTH REPORTER; a weekly review of workplace health and safety. Text in English. 1971. w. USD 1,419 (effective 2001). charts, stat. index. 30 p./no. back issues avail. **Description:** Notification and reference service which provides information on federal and state regulation of occupational safety and health, standards, legislation, enforcement activities, research, and legal decisions.
Related titles: Online - full text ed.: ISSN 1522-4082 (from The Dialog Corporation, Human Resources Information Network, Bureau of National Affairs, Inc., (BNA), The).
Indexed: Environ.Abstr., Ind.Hyg.Dig., Lab.Haz.Bull.
—BLDSC (6231.205000), Infotrieve. **CCC.**
Published by: The Bureau of National Affairs, Inc., 1231 25th St, N W, Washington, DC 20037. TEL 202-452-4200, 800-372-1033, 800-452-7773, FAX 202-822-8092, customercare@bna.com, bnaplus@bna.com, http://www.bna.com/. Pub. Gregory McCaffery.

613.62 CHE ISSN 0078-3129
CODEN: OSHSDY
OCCUPATIONAL SAFETY AND HEALTH SERIES. Text in English. 1963. irreg., latest vol.70, 1993. price varies. **Document type:** *Monographic series.*
Related titles: Microform ed.: (from ILO); French ed.; Spanish ed.
Indexed: I.M.M.Abstr.
—BLDSC (6231.210000), GNLM, Infotrieve, KNAW, Linda Hall. **CCC.**
Published by: (International Labour Office), I L O Publications, Geneva, 22 1211, Switzerland. TEL 41-22-799-6111, FAX 41-22-799-6358. **Dist. in US by:** I L O Publications Center, 9 Jay Gould Court, Ste. CT, PO Box 753, Waldorf, MD 20602. TEL 301-638-3152, FAX 301-843-0159, ilopubs@tasco1.com.

613.62 GBR ISSN 0966-7903
OCCUPATIONAL THERAPY INTERNATIONAL. Text in English. 1994. q. USD 115 in North America to individuals; GBP 60 rest of world to individuals; USD 220 in North America to institutions; GBP 120 rest of world to institutions (effective 2001). adv. back issues avail. *Refereed.* **Document type:** *Academic/Scholarly.* **Description:** Covers clinical research, current practices, technology, professional issues, education, trends in health care, industrial health and other areas of interest to occupational therapists throughout the world.
Related titles: Online - full text ed.: (from Northern Light Technology, Inc., ProQuest Information & Learning).
Indexed: AMED, ASSIA, CINAHL.
—BLDSC (6231.254800), CISTI.
Published by: Whurr Publishers Ltd., 19b Compton Terr, London N1 2UN, United Kingdom. TEL 44-20-7359-5979, FAX 44-20-7226-5290, info@whurr.co.uk, http://www.whurr.co.uk; http://www.whurrjournals.co.uk/. Ed. Frank Stein. Adv. contact Lizzy Ewer. page GBP 150. **Subscr. in N. America to:** Whurr Publishers Ltd., PO Box 1897, Lawrence, KS 66044-8897. TEL 913-843-1221, FAX 913-843-1274, am&m@allenpress.com. **Subscr. to:** Turpin Distribution Services Ltd., Blackhorse Rd, Letchworth, Herts SG6 1HN, United Kingdom. TEL 44-1462-488900, FAX 44-1462-483011, custservturpin@turpinltd.com.

613.62 613.85 USA
OFFICIAL DISABILITY GUIDELINES. Text in English. 1996. a. USD 165 per issue (effective 2000). *Refereed.* **Description:** Provides length of disability data with codes from CDC and OSHA. Audience includes case managers, physical therapists, nurses, risk managers, and insurance personnel.
Related titles: CD-ROM ed.
Published by: Work - Loss Data Institute LLC, 500 N Shoreline Blvd, Ste 1101 N, Corpus Christi, TX 70471. TEL 361-883-5000, FAX 361-883-7025, http://odg-disability.com. Ed. Philip L Denniston.

614.8 USA ISSN 0198-7208
HD7260
OHIO MONITOR. Text in English. 1928. m. free per issue to qualified personnel. bk.rev. abstr, charts, illus, stat.

Formerly: Monitor (0026-9751)
Indexed: Alloys Ind., Met.Abstr., Met.Abstr.Ind., Nonfer.Met.Alert, PCC Alert, Steels Alert.
—CCC.
Published by: Industrial Commission, Division of Safety and Hygiene, 246 N High St, Columbus, OH 43215. TEL 614-466-3385. Ed. Robert L McCullough. Circ: 75,000.

ONTARIO HEALTH AND SAFETY LAW; a complete guide to the law and procedures, with digest of cases. see *LAW*

613.62 658 USA ISSN 1086-0266
HD49 CODEN: ORENFX
ORGANIZATION & ENVIRONMENT. Text in English. 1987. q. INR 1,200 to individuals; INR 3,500 to institutions; USD 43 SAARC to individuals; USD 100 SAARC to institutions; INR 330 newsstand/cover to individuals; INR 975 newsstand/cover to institutions; USD 12 newsstand/cover SAARC to individuals; USD 29 newsstand/cover SAARC to institutions (effective 2002). bk.rev. back issues avail. *Refereed.* **Document type:** *Journal, Academic/Scholarly.* **Description:** Provides an international forum featuring work on the social causes and consequences of environmental damage, restoration, and sustainability, centering on patterns of organizing human production and consumption.
Former titles (until 1996): Industrial and Environmental Crisis Quarterly; Industrial Crisis Quarterly (0921-8106)
Related titles: Microfilm ed.: (from PQC); Online - full text ed.: (from EBSCO Publishing, O C L C Online Computer Library Center, Inc., RoweCom Information Quest, ingenta, Swets Blackwell, Institute for Scientific Information); Special ed.: The Organization Dimentions of Global Enviornmental Change.
Indexed: ABI Inform., Curr.Cont., Ecol.Abstr., Educ.Admin.Abstr., Environ.Abstr., Environ.Sci.Poll.Mgmt., Geol.Abstr., Human Resour.Abstr., IBZ, Indian Psychol.Abstr., Intl.Bibl.S.S.Soc.Cult.Anthro., Intl.Bibl.Soc.Sci., J.of Econ.Lit., Lang.& Lang.Behav.Abstr., Left Ind., Peace Res.Abstr., Pollut.Abstr., SOPODA, Sage Urb.Stud.Abstr., Soc.Serv.Abstr., Sociol.Abstr., Wild.Rev.
—BLDSC (6289.122000), Infotrieve, ingenta. **CCC.**
Published by: (Industrial Crisis Institute Inc., New York), Sage Publications, Inc., 2455 Teller Rd, Thousand Oaks, CA 91320. TEL 805-499-0721, FAX 805-499-0871, info@sagepub.com, http://www.coba.usf.edu/jermier/journal.htm, http://www.sagepub.com/. Eds. John Bellamy Foster, John M Jermier. R&P Tanya Udin. Adv. contact DeAnna Vega Hammersley. Circ: 250. **Affiliates:** Sage Publications Ltd.; Sage Publications India Pvt. Ltd.

PHYSICAL DISABILITIES SPECIAL INTEREST SECTION QUARTERLY. see *HANDICAPPED*

PRACOVNI LEKARSTVI. see *MEDICAL SCIENCES*

363.11 613.6 FRA ISSN 0982-443X
PREVENIR LES RISQUES DU METIER. Text in French. 1959. q. **Document type:** *Newspaper, Consumer.*
Formerly (until 1984): Risques du Metier (0048-8321)
Indexed: C.I.S. Abstr.
Published by: Institut National de Recherche et de Securite pour la Prevention des Accidents du Travail et des Maladies Professionnelles, 30 rue Olivier Noyer, Paris Cedex 14 75680, France. TEL 33-1-40443000, FAX 33-1-40443099, richez@inrs.fr, thanh@inrs.fr. Ed. Didier Gout. Circ: 143,000.

363.11 NLD ISSN 0169-0884
PREVENTIE. Text in Dutch. 1975. m. adv. **Document type:** *Trade.*
Former titles (until 1983): Stip (0166-3259); (until 1977): Beveiliging (0920-0991)
Published by: (Stichting Informatie Preventie), Samsom Bedrijfsinformatie BV (Subsidiary of: Wolters Kluwer N.V.), Postbus 4, Alphen aan den Rijn 2400 MA, Netherlands. TEL 31-172-466775, FAX 31-172-440681.

613.6 HTI
PREVOYANCE. Text in French. 1981. s-a. free per issue. charts, illus, stat.
Formerly (until 1980): Prevention (0048-5241)
Published by: Office d'Assurance Accidents du Travail Maladie et Maternite, B.P. 1324, Port-au-Prince, Haiti. Ed. Gerson Alexis. Circ: 2,000.

620.8 USA ISSN 0099-0027
T55.A1 CODEN: PRSAD5
PROFESSIONAL SAFETY. Text in English. 1956. m. USD 60 to non-members; USD 17.50 to members (effective 2001). adv. bk.rev. charts, illus, tr.lit. index. back issues avail.; reprint service avail. from PQC. *Refereed.* **Document type:** *Academic/Scholarly.* **Description:** For safety professionals. Features information on developments in the research and technology of accident prevention, safety management and program development.
Formerly (until 1974): American Society of Safety Engineers. Journal (0003-1208)
Related titles: Online - full text ed.: (from ProQuest Information & Learning, Northern Light Technology, Inc., H. W. Wilson, Factiva).
Indexed: ABI Inform. (Jan.1985-), A.S.& T.Ind. (Aug.1983-), AgeLine, Alloys Ind., C.I.S. Abstr., Eng.Ind., Environ.Per.Bibl., Environ.Sci.Poll.Mgmt., Ergon.Abstr., INIS Atomind., ISMEC, Met.Abstr., Met.Abstr.Ind., Mgmt.& Market.Abstr., Nonfer.Met.Alert, PCC Alert, Risk Abstr., Saf.Sci.Abstr., Steels Alert, Tox.Abstr.
—BLDSC (6864.215000), CISTI, Ei, Infotrieve, ingenta, Linda Hall. **CCC.**
Published by: American Society of Safety Engineers, 1800 E Oakton St, Des Plaines, IL 60018-2187. TEL 847-768-3433, FAX 847-296-3769, http://www.asse.org/bprofe1.htm. Ed. Sue Trebswether. Adv. contact Tina Ellingsen. B&W page USD 2,445, color page USD 4,025. Circ: 30,000 (paid).

363.11 USA ISSN 1086-6353
R S O MAGAZINE. (Radiation Safety Officer) Text in English. 1996. bi-m., latest vol.6. USD 39 in North America to individuals; USD 74 elsewhere to individuals; USD 125 in North America to institutions; USD 160 elsewhere to institutions (effective 2001). adv. bk.rev., software rev. tr.lit. 32 p./no. 2 cols./p. back issues avail. *Refereed.* **Document type:** *Journal, Trade.* **Description:** Presents practical, work-related information to licensed users of radioactive materials, including training topics, NRC and other guidelines and procedures, and topics relating to the use, storage and disposal of nuclear materials. For radiation safety officers at laboratories, medical facilities, in industry, and at power plants.
Published by: R S A Publications, 19 Pendleton Dr, Box 19, Hebron, CT 06248. TEL 860-228-0824, FAX 860-228-4402, publish@radpro.com, http://www.radpro.com. Ed. K Paul Steinmeyer. R&P, Adv. contact Sharyn Mathews TEL 860-228-0487. Circ: 1,200 (paid).

614.8 539.2 USA ISSN 0740-0640
R895.A1 CODEN: RPMAEI
RADIATION PROTECTION MANAGEMENT; the journal of applied health physics. Text in English. 1983. bi-m., latest vol.18. USD 49 in North America to individuals; USD 84 elsewhere to individuals; USD 399 in North America to institutions; USD 434 elsewhere to institutions (effective 2001). adv. bk.rev., Website rev., software rev. index. Supplement avail.; back issues avail. *Refereed.* **Document type:** *Journal, Trade.* **Description:** Presents practical, work-related information on applied radiation protection programs at nuclear power plants, fuel facilities, laboratories and waste disposal facilities. Covers the entire spectrum of industrial health physics topics, as well as respiratory protection, technical management, and relevant computer applications.
Indexed: Chem.Abstr., Chem.Indus.Notes, Chem.Titles, Eng.Ind., INIS Atomind., Mass Spectr.Bull.
—BLDSC (7227.994000), CASDDS, Ei.
Published by: R S A Publications, 19 Pendleton Dr, Box 19, Hebron, CT 06248. TEL 860-228-0824, FAX 860-228-4402, publish@radpro.com, http://www.radpro.com. Ed. K Paul Steinmeyer. R&P, Adv. contact Sharyn Mathews TEL 860-228-0487. Circ: 1,200 (paid).

362.104 NOR ISSN 0805-5238
RAMAZZINI/NORWEGIAN JOURNAL OF OCCUPATIONAL MEDICINE. Text in Norwegian. 1969. 4/yr. NOK 250 (effective 1998). adv. bk.rev. **Document type:** *Academic/Scholarly.* **Description:** Covers industrial and occupational medicine, as well as general preventive medicine.
Former titles (until 1994): Norsk Tidsskrift for Arbeidsmedisin (0803-2394); (until 1991): Norsk Bedriftshelsetjeneste (0333-0249); (until 1980): Norsk Fretagshaelsovaerd (0332-8910); (until 1978): N I R - Nytt (0358-4909)
—CCC.
Published by: Norsk Arbeidsmedisinsk Forening, Postboks 1152, Sentrum, Oslo 0107, Norway. TEL 47-23-10-90-00, FAX 47-23-10-91-00. Ed. Dr. Aud Nistov. R&P Eli M Berrg Hansen. Circ: 1,783.

REFERATIVNYI ZHURNAL. MEDITSINA TRUDA. see *MEDICAL SCIENCES—Abstracting, Bibliographies, Statistics*

REPETITIVE STRESS INJURY LITIGATION REPORTER. see *LAW*

614.85 622.8 CAN ISSN 1198-1237
RESSOURCE EN SANTE ET EN SECURITE. Text in French. 1955. bi-m. free per issue. bk.rev. back issues avail. **Document type:** *Trade.* **Description:** For the mining, forestry, and pulp and paper industries of Ontario.
Supersedes in part (in 1994): Tallyboard (0712-3094)
Related titles: ♦ English ed.: Health & Safety Resource. ISSN 1198-1229.
Published by: Ontario Natural Resource Safety Association, 690 Mc Keown Ave, P O Box 2050, North Bay, ON P1B 9P1, Canada. TEL 705-474-SAFE, FAX 705-472-5800. Ed. Susan Haldane. Circ: 10,000 (controlled).

614.8 CAN ISSN 1207-0661
REVIEW OF O H & S LEGISLATION IN (YEAR). (Occupational Health & Safety) Text in English. 1993. a. adv. **Document type:** *Newsletter.* **Description:** Publishes new, revised health and safety legislation which came into force during the year.
Related titles: ♦ Supplement to: Canadian Occupational Health & Safety News. ISSN 0709-5252.
Published by: Southam Information Products Ltd., 1450 Don Mills Rd, Don Mills, ON M3B 2X7, Canada. TEL 416-445-6641, 800-668-2374, FAX 416-442-2200. Ed. Cindy Gardiner. Pub., R&P, Adv. contact Doug Finley.

613.62 BRA ISSN 0303-7657
RC963.7.B6 CODEN: RBSOEQ
REVISTA BRASILEIRA DE SAUDE OCUPACIONAL. Text in Portuguese, Spanish. 1973. q. BRL 60. adv. bk.rev. **Document type:** *Trade.* **Description:** Presents articles on occupational health, hygiene and safety.
Indexed: C.I.S. Abstr., CSNB, INIS Atomind., Ind.Med. (coverage dropped), Lab.Haz.Bull., Repindex.
Published by: Fundacao Jorge Duprat Figueiredo de Seguranca e Medicina do Trabalho (Fundacentro), Rua Capote Valente, 710, Pinheiros, Sao Paulo, SP 05409-002, Brazil. TEL 55-11-853-5895, FAX 55-11-306666258. Ed. Jose Carlos Castilha Crozera. Circ: 5,000.

614.85 BRA
REVISTA DE TERAPIA OCUPACIONAL. Text in Portuguese. 1990. s-a. per issue exchange basis. bk.rev. bibl. **Document type:** *Academic/Scholarly.*
Published by: Universidade de Sao Paulo, Curso de Terapia Ocupacional, Rua Cipotanea 51, Cidade Universitaria Armando Salles de Oliveira, Sao Paulo, SP 05508-900, Brazil. TEL 011-818-4061.

REVISTA DE TERAPIA OCUPACIONAL. see *MEDICAL SCIENCES—Physical Medicine And Rehabilitation*

613.62 BRA ISSN 0102-4884
REVISTA FUNDACENTRO. Key Title: Fundacentro. Text in Portuguese. 1980. m. free per issue. **Document type:** *Academic/Scholarly.*
Published by: Fundacao Jorge Duprat Figueiredo de Seguranca e Medicina do Trabalho (Fundacentro), Rua Capote Valente, 710, Pinheiros, Sao Paulo, SP 05409-002, Brazil. TEL 55-11-853-5895, FAX 55-11-30666258.

613.62 FRA ISSN 0300-0559
REVUE DE MEDECINE DU TRAVAIL. Summaries in English, French. 1972. bi-m. FRF 500, USD 100 (effective 1995). adv. bk.rev. index. back issues avail. **Document type:** *Bulletin.* **Description:** Covers all subjects concerning occupational health, medicine, and ergonomics industrial toxicologies.
—BLDSC (7931.800000), GNLM.
Published by: Groupement National des Medecins du Batiment et des Travaux Publics, 7 rue la Perouse, Paris 75116, France. TEL 40-69-53-77, FAX 45-53-58-77. Eds. M Amphoux, M Blaizot. Circ: 2,000.

613.62 368 363 ITA ISSN 0035-5836
HD7816.I8 CODEN: RIMPAA
RIVISTA DEGLI INFORTUNI E DELLE MALATTIE PROFESSIONALI. Text in Italian. 1914. bi-m. ITL 42,000. adv. bk.rev. abstr, bibl, charts, illus, stat. index, cum.index.
Indexed: C.I.S. Abstr., Chem.Abstr., INIS Atomind., World Bibl.Soc.Sec.
—CASDDS, CISTI.

O

Published by: Istituto Nazionale per l'Assicurazione Contro gli Infortuni sul Lavoro, Via Quattro Novembre, 144, Rome, RM 00187, Italy. Circ: 8,000.

610 JPN ISSN 0022-443X
HD4811 CODEN: ROKAAV
RODO KAGAKU (KAWASAKI, 1924)/JOURNAL OF SCIENCE OF LABOUR. Text in English, Japanese. 1924. m. JPY 8,800. adv. bk.rev. abstr, bibl. index. **Document type:** *Academic/Scholarly.*
Related titles: Microfilm ed.
Indexed: Abstr.Hyg., C.I.S. Abstr., Chem.Abstr., Chem.Titles, Environ.Sci.Poll.Mgmt., Ergon.Abstr., Forest Prod.Abstr., Forest.Abstr., INIS Atomind., Ind.Hyg.Dig., Nutr.Abstr., Psychol.Abstr., Rev.Appl.Entomol., Rev.Med.& Vet.Mycol., Saf.Sci.Abstr., Trop.Dis.Bull., Weed Abstr.
—BLDSC (5056.230000), CASDDS, CISTI, GNLM, ingenta.
Published by: Institute for Science of Labour/Rodo Kagaku Kenkyujo, 2-8-14 Sugao, Miyamae-ku, Kawasaki-shi, Kanagawa-ken 216-0015, Japan. FAX 81-44-977-7504. Ed., R&P Kazutaka Kogi TEL 81-44-977-2121. Circ: 2,500.

610 JPN ISSN 0035-7774
CODEN: ROKAAV
RODO NO KAGAKU (KAWASAKI, 1946)/DIGEST OF SCIENCE OF LABOUR. Text in Japanese. 1946. m. JPY 11,000. adv. bk.rev. **Document type:** *Academic/Scholarly.*
Indexed: Chem.Abstr., Russ.Acad.Sci.Bibl.
Published by: Institute for Science of Labour/Rodo Kagaku Kenkyujo, 2-8-14 Sugao, Miyamae-ku, Kawasaki-shi, Kanagawa-ken 216-0015, Japan. FAX 81-44-97-7504. Ed. Kazutaka Kogi TEL 81-44-977-2121. Circ: 3,000.

613.62 614.85 USA ISSN 1084-578X
S S A JOURNAL. Text in English. 1985. q. USD 125 domestic; USD 140 foreign (effective 2001). adv. bk.rev. back issues avail. *Refereed.* **Document type:** *Academic/Scholarly.* **Description:** Dedicated to communication and education concerning environmental, health and safety issues relating to the electronic and high technology industries.
Related titles: Online - full text ed.: (from Institute for Scientific Information).
Indexed: Curr.Cont., Eng.Ind.
—BLDSC (8425.202500), IDS.
Published by: (Semiconductor Safety Association), Cognizant Communication Corporation, 3 Hartsdale Rd, Elmsford, NY 10523-3701. TEL 914-592-7720, FAX 914-592-8981, cogcomm@aol.com, http://www.cognizantcommunication.com. Ed. Lee Neil. Pub., R&P Robert N Miranda. Adv. contact Lori Miranda.

331 USA
SAFE WORKER. Text in English. m. USD 27 to members; USD 19 to non-members (effective 2001). illus. **Description:** On-the-job safety information for non-supervisory personnel.
Published by: National Safety Council, 1121 Spring Lake Dr, Itasca, IL 60143. TEL 630-285-1121, FAX 630-775-2310, http://www.nsc.org. Ed. Laura Coyne. Pub. Suzanne Powills. Circ: 190,000.

SAFEGUARD (AUCKLAND); the magazine for better safety and health at the workplace. see *PUBLIC HEALTH AND SAFETY*

SAFEGUARD - BUYERS GUIDE. see *PUBLIC HEALTH AND SAFETY*

363.72 USA ISSN 0891-1797
HD7260
SAFETY AND HEALTH; the international safety, health and environmental magazine. Text in English. 1919. m. USD 80 to members; USD 91 to non-members (effective 2000). adv. bk.rev. abstr, bibl, charts, illus, stat, tr.lit. index, cum.index. reprint service avail. from PQC. **Document type:** *Trade.* **Description:** For occupational safety, health and environmental professionals. Provides extensive coverage of international safety, health and environmental issues, including occupational health, traffic safety, environmental health and industrial hygiene.
Former titles (until 1986): National Safety and Health News (8756-5366); (until May 1985): National Safety News (0028-0100)
Related titles: Microform ed.: (from PQC); Online - full text ed.: (from Gale Group, Factiva).
Indexed: Abstr.Bull.Inst.Pap.Chem., AgeLine, Aqua.Sci.& Fish.Abstr., B.P.I. (Jan.1987-), Bus.Ind., C.I.S. Abstr., CSNB, Chem.Abstr., Environ.Sci.Poll.Mgmt., Hlth.Ind., Ind.Hyg.Dig., L.R.I., Pollut.Abstr., Risk Abstr., Saf.Sci.Abstr., Tr.& Dev.Alert, Tr.& Indus.Ind.
—BLDSC (8065.709600), IDS, ingenta, Linda Hall.

Published by: National Safety Council, Periodicals Department, 1121 Spring Lake Dr, Itasca, IL 60143. TEL 630-285-1121, FAX 630-775-2310, http://www.nsc.org. Ed. John Dyslin. Pub., Adv. contact Suzanne Powills. Circ: 26,000.

363.11 613.6 JPN
SAFETY & HEALTH IN JAPAN. Text in English. irreg., latest vol.27, 1999. **Document type:** *Newsletter.* **Description:** Provides information about the Association's activities, including awards, conferences and conventions relating to occupational health and safety. Also covers government activities and initiatives, and information from recent papers on topics such as disaster prevention, traffic safety, and public health.
Indexed: CSNB, Lab.Haz.Bull.
—BLDSC.
Published by: Japan Industrial Safety and Health Association, International Cooperation Department, 5-35-1, Shiba, Minato-ku, Tokyo 108-0014, Japan. TEL 81-3-3452-6841, FAX 81-3-3454-4596.

614.85 USA ISSN 1077-9787
SAFETY COMPLIANCE ALERT. Abbreviated title: S C A. Text in English. 1994. s-m. USD 299. charts. **Document type:** *Newsletter.* **Description:** Aims to keep safety professionals current on safety rules and worker compliance.
Published by: Progressive Business Publications, 370 Technology Dr, Malvern, PA 19355-1315. TEL 610-695-8600, 800-220-5000, FAX 610-647-8089, editor@pbp.com, http://www.pbp.com. Ed. Maureen Hennessy. R&P Curt Brown. Circ: 18,114 (paid).

614.8 USA ISSN 1069-2037
SAFETY COMPLIANCE LETTER; with OSHA highlights. Text in English. s-m. USD 179 to individuals; USD 9 newsstand/cover (effective 2002). index. **Document type:** *Newsletter.* **Description:** Provides managers responsible for the environmental, health, and safety function with the leading edge information they need to ensure compliance with federal and state regulations, maintain a safe workplace, and control related costs.
Formerly (until 1986): O S H A Compliance Letter (0092-5799)
Published by: Bureau of Business Practice (Subsidiary of: Aspen Publishers, Inc.), 125 Eugene O'Neill Dr, Ste 103, New London, CT 06320. TEL 860-442-4365, 800-243-0876, rebecca_armitage@prenhall.com, http://www.bppnews.com. Ed. Michele S Rubin. Pub. Peter Garabedian.

SAFETY DIGEST (OTTAWA)/DIGEST DE SECURITE. see *MILITARY*

636.11 GBR
SAFETY EXPRESS. Text in English. 1995. bi-m. GBP 18.82 to non-members; GBP 16 to members; GBP 22.11 foreign to members (effective 2000). adv. video rev. stat, tr.lit. back issues avail. **Document type:** *Consumer.*
Published by: Royal Society for the Prevention of Accidents, Edgbaston Park, 353 Bristol Rd, Edgbaston, Birmingham, Worcs B5 7ST, United Kingdom. TEL 44-121-248-2000, FAX 44-121-248-2001, help@rospa.com.uk, http://www.rospa.com.uk. Ed. Jacky Steemson. Adv. contacts Amanda Walker TEL 44-1753-670888, Sue Philo TEL 44-1367-820181. Circ: 5,000 (paid).

614.85 USA
SAFETY FOCUS NEWSLETTER. Text in English. bi-m. USD 24 to members; USD 29 to non-members (effective 1999). **Document type:** *Newsletter, Consumer, Trade.* **Description:** Aims to promote the public's awareness of good safety and health practices.
Published by: National Safety Council, 1121 Spring Lake Dr, Itasca, IL 60143. TEL 630-775-2276, FAX 630-775-2185, http://www.nsc.org. Ed. Laura Coyne. Pub. John H Kennedy.

614.85 GBR
SAFETY GUIDE. Text in English. 1994. m. GBP 240 (effective 1998). **Document type:** *Trade.*
Published by: British Safety Council, 70 Chancellors Rd, London W6 9RS, United Kingdom. TEL 44-20-8741-1231, FAX 44-20-8741-4555, bsc1@mailbritishsafetycouncil.co.uk, mail@britsafe.org, http://www.britishsafetycouncil.co.uk/bsc, http://www.britsafe.org/.

621.95 363.11 ZAF
SAFETY, HEALTH & PROTECTIVE EQUIPMENT BUYER'S GUIDE. Text in English. 1993. a. illus. **Document type:** *Directory.*

Published by: Delinds Publications, PO Box 72366, Parkview, Johannesburg 2122, South Africa.

363.11 354.7 ZAF ISSN 0377-8592
T55.A1
SAFETY MANAGEMENT; the bigger picture in occupational safety, health and environmental risk management. Text in English. 1958. m., latest 2001 (11/yr.). ZAR 130 domestic; USD 200 foreign (effective 2001 - 2002). adv. bk.rev., Website rev., software rev., video rev. illus, stat, tr.lit, pat, abstr. Supplement avail. **Document type:** *Magazine, Trade.* **Description:** Explores the various echelons of management and the workforce in industrial, commercial, financial and governmental undertakings. Emphasis on all aspects of occupational health, safety, and environment.
Formerly: Safety in Industry (0036-2484); Incorporates: Safety Digest (0036-2468)
Indexed: C.I.S. Abstr., CSNB, INIS Atomind., Lab.Haz.Bull.
Published by: National Occupational Safety Association, PO Box 26434, Arcadia, Pretoria 0007, South Africa. TEL 27-12-3039700, FAX 27-12-3039870, taniam@nosa.co.za, http://www.nosa.co.za. Ed. Ed Furter. Adv. contact Eugene Howell TEL 27-12-3039717. B&W page ZAR 170, color page ZAR 980. Circ: 6,300 (paid and controlled). **Co-sponsor:** Association of Societies for Occupational Safety and Health.

613.62 658 USA
SAFETY MANAGEMENT. Text in English. 1975. m. USD 149 to individuals; USD 15 newsstand/cover (effective 2002). index. **Document type:** *Newsletter.* **Description:** Provides guidelines for developing far-reaching safety programs and reduces workers' compensation costs by reducing accidents. Includes dramatized OSHA cases with analysis.
Indexed: Br.Tech.Ind.
Published by: Bureau of Business Practice (Subsidiary of: Aspen Publishers, Inc.), 125 Eugene O'Neill Dr, Ste 103, New London, CT 06320. TEL 860-442-4365, 800-243-0876, FAX 860-437-3555, rebecca_armitage@prenhall.com, http://www.bbpnews.com. Ed. Jane Winkler. Pub. Peter Garabedian. R&P Kathryn Mennone.

658.382 GBR ISSN 0951-2624
SAFETY MANAGEMENT MAGAZINE. Key Title: Safety Management. Text in English. 1959. m. (11/yr.). GBP 44 domestic; GBP 66 foreign; GBP 3.75 newsstand/cover. adv. bk.rev., video rev. **Document type:** *Trade.* **Description:** Aims to provide objective reporting on news, as well as in-depth features on issues in the field of occupational health and safety. Includes listings of forthcoming events, an information section, and important helplines.
Former titles (until 1986): Safety & Risk Management (0267-8624); (until 1984): Safety & Fire News (0953-1157); Which was formed by the merger of (1981-1983): Fire News (0262-4451); Safety
Indexed: CSNB, Ref.Zh.
—BLDSC (8066.201000).
Published by: British Safety Council, 70 Chancellors Rd, London W6 9RS, United Kingdom. TEL 44-20-8741-1231, FAX 44-20-8741-4555, bsc1@mail.britishsafetycouncil.co.uk, mail@britsafe.org, http://www.britishsafetycouncil.co.uk, http://www.britsafe.org/. Ed. Robert Jarvis. R&P Ian Fraser. Adv. contact Brian Carter. B&W page GBP 1,122, color page GBP 1,446; trim 210 x 297. Circ: 22,973.

613.62 362.1 USA
SAFETY MEETING REPROS. Text in English. q. USD 295 (effective 1999). **Document type:** *Trade.* **Description:** Contains everything needed to teach and motivate safe work, habits from the assembly line to the front office. Includes detailed meeting plans, OSHA requirements, reproducible handouts, safety procedures and practical exercises.
Published by: Business & Legal Reports, Inc., Attn: Tom Picinich, 39 Academy St, Madison, CT 06443. TEL 203-245-7448, FAX 203-245-0483, service@blr.com, http://www.blr.com. Ed. April Katz. Pub. Robert L Brady.

SAFETY NEWS. see *WATER RESOURCES*

363.11 USA ISSN 1078-0114
SAFETY NOW; putting safety into practice. Text in English. 1994. m. USD 159 to individuals; USD 16 newsstand/cover (effective 2002). index. **Document type:** *Newsletter.* **Description:** Trains supervisors and team leaders throughout the plant to make safety an integral part of their jobs. Includes monthly safety meeting planner and reproducible employee quiz.

Published by: Bureau of Business Practice (Subsidiary of: Aspen Publishers, Inc.), 125 Eugene O'Neill Dr, Ste 103, New London, CT 06320. TEL 860-442-4365, 800-243-0876, FAX 860-437-3555, rebecca_armitage@prenhall.com, http://www.bbpnews.com. Ed. Jane Winkler. Pub. Peter Garabedian. R&P Kathryn Mennone.

613 USA
SAFETY ONLINE; virtual community for the safety industry. Text in English. d.
Media: Online - full text.
Address: 1287 W 108th St, Cleveland, OH 44102. info@safetyonline.com, http://safetyonline.net. Ed. Sandy Smith.

614.8 USA
SAFETY REMINDER. Text in English. 1973. m. price varies. **Document type:** *Newsletter.* **Description:** Includes safety checklists, case decisions covering the legal problems of safety and security, "Questions and Answers" that probe all aspects of industrial safety and security, and safety and security ideas that work.
Formerly: Safety & Security for Supervisors (1040-4236)
Published by: Business & Legal Reports, Inc., PO Box 6001, Old Saybrook, CT 06475-6001. TEL 860-510-0100, 800-727-5257, FAX 860-510-7224. Ed. Judy Ruddy.

363.7 USA
SAFETY RESOURCES* ; middle management to CEO issues. Text in English. 1990. q. USD 30 to non-members; USD 12 to members. adv. *Refereed.* **Document type:** *Trade.* **Description:** Focuses on workers' compensation issues. Addresses safety, health and environmental issues.
Published by: (Florida Employers Safety Association), Gulf Atlantic Communications Corporation, Inc., 15565 Highway 441, Delray Beach, FL 33446-2736. TEL 954-489-4070, FAX 954-489-4079, sozker@emi.net. Ed., R&P Susan Ozker. Pub. David R Sanz. adv.: B&W page USD 1,500. Circ: 10,000 (controlled).

331 613 NLD ISSN 0925-7535
HD7262 CODEN: SSCIEO
SAFETY SCIENCE. Text in English, French, German. 1977. 9/yr. EUR 793 in Europe to institutions; JPY 105,300 in Japan to institutions; USD 886 elsewhere to institutions (effective 2002). adv. bk.rev. charts, illus. index. reprints avail. *Refereed.* **Document type:** *Academic/Scholarly.* **Description:** For safety engineers and inspectors, industrial engineers, research scientists, industrial psychologists and ergonomists. Presents research papers on aspects of work-related risks of various occupations.
Formerly (until 1992): Journal of Occupational Accidents (0376-6349)
Related titles: Microform ed.: (from PQC); Online - full text ed.: (from ingenta, Swets Blackwell, Institute for Scientific Information, ScienceDirect).
Indexed: AESIS, ASCA, Abstr.Hyg., Agri.Eng.Abstr., Alloys Ind., Aqua.Sci.& Fish.Abstr., Biol.Abstr., C.I.S. Abstr., CSNB, Curr.Cont., Eng.Ind., Eng.Mat.Abstr., Environ.Sci.Poll.Mgmt., Ergon.Abstr., Excerp.Med., HRIS, INIS Atomind., METADEX, Met.Abstr., Met.Abstr.Ind., Nonfer.Met.Alert, P.A.I.S., PCC Alert, Pollut.Abstr., Risk Abstr., SSCI (coverage dropped), Saf.Sci.Abstr., Steels Alert, Trop.Dis.Bull., World Alum.Abstr.
—BLDSC (8069.124900), Ei, EMDOCS, GNLM, IDS, Infotrieve, ingenta, Linda Hall. **CCC.**
Published by: Elsevier Science BV, PO Box 211, Amsterdam 1000 AE, Netherlands. TEL 31-20-485-2911, FAX 31-20-485-2457, nlinfo-f@elsevier.nl, http://www.elsevier.nl/locate/issn/09257535. Ed. A R Hale. **Subscr. in Australasia and the Far East to:** Elsevier Science (Singapore) Pte Ltd, No.1 Temasek Ave, 17-01 Millenia Tower, Singapore 039192, Singapore. TEL 65-434-3727, FAX 65-337-2230; **Subscr. in Japan to:** Elsevier Science Inc - Japan Regional Office, 9-15 Higashi-Azabu 1-chome, Minato-ku, Tokyo 106-0044, Japan. TEL 81-3-5561-5033, FAX 81-3-5561-5047; **Subscr. in the Americas to:** Elsevier Science, PO Box 945, New York, NY 10159-0945. TEL 212-633-3730, FAX 212-633-3680, usinfo-f@elsevier.com.

SAFETY SCIENCE MONITOR. see *PUBLIC HEALTH AND SAFETY*

614 USA
SAFETY SIGNALS. Text in English. 1974. bi-m. free per issue. bk.rev. **Document type:** *Newsletter.* **Description:** Contains information about the safety equipment industry, member companies, association activities and upcoming meetings and events.
Published by: Industrial Safety Equipment Association, 1901 N Moore St, Ste 808, Arlington, VA 22209. TEL 703-525-1695, FAX 703-528-2148, isea@safetycentral.org, http://www.safetycentral.org. Ed., Pub., R&P Bruce R Clash. Circ: 450 (controlled).

614.85 DEU
SAFETY UND SECURITY. Text in German. a. adv.
Document type: *Directory.*
Published by: G I T Verlag GmbH, Roesslerstr 90, Darmstadt 64293, Germany. TEL 49-6151-8090-0, FAX 49-6151-8090183, gitverlaggmbh@gitverlag.com, http://www.gitverlag.com. Adv. contact Steffen Ebert.

614.85 AUS ISSN 1321-9553
SAFETY W A; West Australian journal of occupational safety and health. Text in English. 1972. bi-m. AUD 55 (effective 2000). bk.rev. charts, stat, tr.lit. *Refereed.* **Document type:** *Bulletin.* **Description:** For safety personnel managers and human resources people detailing the latest occupational safety and health issues on a local, national and international level.
Former titles: I F A P Bulletin; I F A P News (0311-0311)
Related titles: Online - full text ed.
Published by: Industrial Foundation for Accident Prevention, PO Box 339, Willetton, W.A. 6155, Australia. TEL 61-9-3103760, FAX 61-9-3323511, ageorge@ifap.asn.au, http://www.ifap.asn.au. Ed. David Leith. R&P Arianne George TEL 61-9-4306611. Circ: 1,700.

SAFETYEXCHANGE; railway safety is everyone's business. see *TRANSPORTATION—Railroads*

620.8 JPN ISSN 0911-8063
SANGYO ANZEN KENKYUJO GIJUTSU SHISHIN/NATIONAL INSTITUTE OF INDUSTRIAL SAFETY. TECHNICAL RECOMMENDATION. Text in Japanese. 1972. irreg. back issues avail.
Published by: National Institute of Industrial Safety/Sangyo Anzen Kenkyujo, 1-4-6 Ume-Zono, Kiyose-shi, Tokyo-to 204-0024, Japan. Circ: 450.

613.62 614.7 JPN ISSN 0911-6923
T55.A1
SANGYO ANZEN KENKYUJO KENKYU HOKOKU/NATIONAL INSTITUTE OF INDUSTRIAL SAFETY. RESEARCH REPORT. Text in Japanese; Summaries in English. 1968. a. back issues avail.
Document type: *Academic/Scholarly.*
Formerly: Sangyo Anzen Kenkyujo Hokoku (0911-6915)
Indexed: Ref.Zh.
—BLDSC (7762.851000).
Published by: National Institute of Industrial Safety/Sangyo Anzen Kenkyujo, 1-4-6 Ume-Zono, Kiyose-shi, Tokyo-to 204-0024, Japan. Circ: 450.

613.6 JPN ISSN 1341-0725
CODEN: SEZAFI
SANGYO EISEIGAKU ZASSHI. Text in Japanese; Summaries in English. 1959. 6/yr. JPY 12,000 (effective 1997). adv. bk.rev. illus. index. **Document type:** *Academic/Scholarly.*
Formerly (until 1995): Japanese Journal of Industrial Health - Sangyo Igaku (0047-1879)
Media: Duplicated (not offset). **Related titles:** ♦ English ed.: Journal of Occupational Health. ISSN 1341-9145.
Indexed: Abstr.Hyg., C.I.S. Abstr., Chem.Abstr., Chem.Titles, Curr.Cont. (coverage dropped), Environ.Sci.Poll.Mgmt., Excerp.Med., INIS Atomind., Ind.Hyg.Dig., Ind.Med. (1995-), Lab.Haz.Bull., Saf.Sci.Abstr., Trop.Dis.Bull.
—BLDSC (8073.242000), CASDDS, CISTI, GNLM, KNAW, Linda Hall. **CCC.**
Published by: Japan Society for Occupational Health/Nihon Sangyo Eisei Gakkai, Public Health Bldg, 1-29-8 Shinjuku, Shinjuku-ku, Tokyo 160-0022, Japan. TEL 81-3-3356-1536, FAX 81-3-3356-1536. Ed., R&P, Adv. contact Akio Sato. Pub. Shogo Shima. Circ: 5,300.

613.6 FIN ISSN 0355-3140
RC963.A1 CODEN: SWEHDO
SCANDINAVIAN JOURNAL OF WORK, ENVIRONMENT & HEALTH. Text in English. 1975. bi-m. EUR 170 in Scandinavia; EUR 190 elsewhere; EUR 590 combined subscription paper and online versions (effective 2002). bk.rev. abstr, illus. index. back issues avail. *Refereed.*
Document type: *Journal, Academic/Scholarly.*
Description: Seeks to promote and disseminate research in the fields of occupational health and safety and the work environment.
Formed by the merger of: Nordisk Hygienisk Tidskrift (0029-1374); Work - Environment - Health (0300-3221)
Related titles: Online - full text ed.: FIM 3,000 (effective 2000) (from Institute for Scientific Information); ♦ Supplement: Scandinavian Journal of Work, Environment and Health. Supplement. ISSN 0356-6528.
Indexed: ASCA, ASSIA, Abstr.Hyg., AgeLine, Biol.Abstr., C.I.S. Abstr., CSNB, Chem.Abstr., Chem.Titles, Curr.Adv.Cancer Res., Curr.Cont., Curr.Ind.Stat., Dent.Ind., Environ.Abstr., Environ.Sci.Poll.Mgmt., Ergon.Abstr., Excerp.Med., Forest Prod.Abstr., Geo.Abstr.H.G., Geo.Abstr.P.G., INIS Atomind., Ind.Hyg.Dig., Ind.Med. (1975-), Ind.Sci.Rev., Inpharma, Int.Abstr.Biol.Sci., Int.Nurs.Ind., Lab.Haz.Bull., METADEX, NRN, Nutr.Abstr., Pollut.Abstr., PsycInfo, Psychol.Abstr. (1984-), Reac., Ref.Zh., Rev.Appl.Entomol., Risk Abstr., SSCI (coverage dropped), Saf.Sci.Abstr., Sci.Cit.Ind., Sel.Water Res.Abstr., THA, Tox.Abstr., Trop.Dis.Bull., World Surf.Coat., e-psyche.
—BLDSC (8087.568000), CASDDS, CISTI, EMDOCS, GNLM, IDS, Infotrieve, ingenta. **CCC.**
Published by: Finnish Institute of Occupational Health, Topeliuksenkatu 41a A, Helsinki 00250, Finland. TEL 358-9-4747-2482, FAX 358-9-878-3326, terja.paananen@occuphealth.fi, terja.pehkonen@occuphealth.fi, http://www.occuphealth.fi/eng/dept/sjweh/index.htm. Ed. Dr. Mikko Harma. R&P Terja Paananen. Circ: 1,600.
Co-sponsor: National Institutes of Occupational Health for Sweden, Norway and Denmark.

613.6 FIN ISSN 0356-6528
SCANDINAVIAN JOURNAL OF WORK, ENVIRONMENT AND HEALTH. SUPPLEMENT. Text in English. 1976. irreg.
Related titles: ♦ Supplement to: Scandinavian Journal of Work, Environment & Health. ISSN 0355-3140.
Published by: Finnish Institute of Occupational Health, Topeliuksenkatu 41a A, Helsinki 00250, Finland. TEL 358-9-4747-2482, FAX 358-9-878-3326, terja.paananen@occuhealth.fi, http://www.occuphealth.fi/eng/dept/sjweh/index.htm.

614 FRA ISSN 0755-2386
SECURITE ET MEDECINE DU TRAVAIL. Text in French. 1969. q. FRF 100. adv. bibl, charts, illus.
Indexed: C.I.S. Abstr.
—CISTI.
Published by: Association Francaise des Techniciens et Ingenieurs de Securite et des Medecins du Travail (AFTIM), 1 pl. Uranie, Joinville le Pont 94340, France. Ed. Jacky Bellaguet.

614.85 622 ESP ISSN 0378-9551
SEGURIDAD. Text in Spanish. 1960. q. ESP 800.
Document type: *Trade.*
—CINDOC.
Published by: Comision de Seguridad en la Industria Siderometalurgica, JOSE CUETO, 40 1 Izda, Apartado 195, Aviles, Asturias 33400, Spain. TEL 85-56-29-59, FAX 85-56-28-02. Ed. J L Poyal Costa.

620.8 NLD
SERIES IN PHYSICAL ERGONOMICS. Text in English. 1993. irreg., latest vol.5, 1995. back issues avail.
Document type: *Monographic series.* **Description:** Discusses ways in which products can be made to better accommodate the human body.
Published by: Delft University Press, PO Box 98, Delft 2600 MG, Netherlands. TEL 31-15-278-3254, FAX 31-15-2781661, dup@dup.tudelft.nl. Ed. J M Dirken.

613.62 USA ISSN 0732-7722
KF3568.15
SHEPARD'S FEDERAL OCCUPATIONAL SAFETY AND HEALTH CITATIONS. Text in English. 1981. base vol. plus q. updates. USD 380. **Description:** Analysis of federal occupational safety and health cases and statutes.
Published by: Shepard's (Subsidiary of: Reed Elsevier plc), 555 Middle Creek Pkwy, Colorado Springs, CO 80921. TEL 800-743-7393, customer_service@shepards.com, http://www.shepards.com.

SHEPARD'S O S H A CITATIONS. (Occupational Safety and Health) see *LAW—Judicial Systems*

614.85 613.62 CHN
SHIJIE LAODONG ANQUAN WEISHENG DONGTAI* /WORLD INDUSTRIAL SAFETY AND HYGIENE DEVELOPMENT. Text in Chinese. m.
Published by: Zhongguo Laodong Anquan Weisheng Qingbao Zhongxin/China Industrial Safety and Hygiene Information Center, A-1 Xibahe, Chaoyang-qu, Beijing 100028, China. TEL 4219190.

O

613.6 368.5 AUT ISSN 0037-4512
SICHERE ARBEIT; Zeitschrift fuer Arbeitsschutz. Text in German. 1947. bi-m. ATS 555 domestic; ATS 645 foreign (effective 2000). adv. bk.rev. charts, illus, stat. index. **Document type:** *Magazine, Consumer.*
Indexed: C.I.S. Abstr., INIS Atomind., Ref.Zh.
Published by: (Allgemeine Unfallversicherungsanstalt), Bohmann Druck und Verlag GmbH & Co. KG, Leberstrasse 122, Vienna, W 1110, Austria. TEL 43-1-74095-0, FAX 43-1-74095-183, sichere-arbeit.zv@bohmann.co.at, http://www.bohmann.co.at. Ed. Regina Ender. Adv. contact Gabriele Krotz. B&W page ATS 32,000, color page ATS 44,000; trim 185 x 250. Circ: 13,000.

613.62 DEU
SICHERHEIT AM ARBEITSPLATZ. Text in German. 1971. q. adv. **Document type:** *Bulletin.*
Published by: Lederindustrie-Berufsgenossenschaft, Postfach 310180, Mainz 55062, Germany. TEL 49-6131-7851, FAX 49-6131-785271. Ed., Adv. contact Joerg Meyer. R&P Bernhard Brandt.

363.1 CAN ISSN 0228-9091
SIGNAL. Text in English, French. 1989. q. free per issue. adv. **Document type:** *Newsletter.* **Description:** Covers road safety, home and occupational safety, accident prevention instructions and research data.
Related titles: Online - full text ed.: (from Northern Light Technology, Inc.).
Published by: Ligue Securite du Quebec/Quebec Safety League, Quebec, PQ H8N 2W9, Canada. TEL 514-595-9110, FAX 514-595-3398. Ed., R&P Diane Des Autels. Circ: 10,000.

SIMPLY BETTER. see *LIFESTYLE*

614 USA ISSN 1043-1721
RA399.A1
SOCIETY FOR HEALTH SYSTEMS. JOURNAL. Key Title: Journal of the Society for Health Systems. Text in English. q. **Document type:** *Academic/Scholarly.*
Formerly (until 1989): I E News: Health Services
Indexed: Ind.Med. (1989-), Int.Nurs.Ind.
—CISTI, GNLM, Infotrieve. **CCC.**
Published by: (Society for Health Systems), Institute of Industrial Engineers, 25 Technology Parkway South, Norcross, GA 30092. TEL 770-449-0460, 800-494-0460, FAX 770-263-8532. Circ: 1,000.

614.85 USA ISSN 1080-0395
STAYING SAFE ON THE JOB. Text in English. 1979. m. USD 24 (effective 1999). **Document type:** *Newsletter.* **Description:** Provides helpful safety information to employees that can help reduce on-the-job accidents, saving company money on costly insurance and workers' compensation claims.
Former titles (until 1994): Safety Pays on the Job (1077-3649); On the Safety Side
Published by: Bureau of Business Practice (Subsidiary of: Aspen Publishers, Inc.), 125 Eugene O'Neill Dr, Ste 103, New London, CT 06320. TEL 860-442-4365, 800-243-0876, FAX 860-437-3555, rebecca_armitage@prenhall.com, http://www.bbpnews.com. Ed. Michele Rubin. Pub. Peter Garabedian. R&P Kathryn Mennone.

614.85 DEU ISSN 0935-4905
STRAHLENSCHUTZ. Text in German. 1973. irreg. DEM 186 (effective 2000). **Document type:** *Bulletin, Trade.*
Published by: Erich Schmidt Verlag GmbH & Co. (Berlin), Genthiner Str 30G, Berlin 10785, Germany. TEL 49-30-250085-0, FAX 49-30-25008521, vertrieb@esvmedien.de, http://www.erich-schmidt-verlag.de.

614.85 DEU ISSN 0947-434X
TK9152 CODEN: STPRFM
STRAHLENSCHUTZPRAXIS; Zeitschrift fuer den sicheren Umgang mit ionisierender und nichtionisierender Strahlung. Text in German. 1995. q. DEM 98; DEM 28 newsstand/cover (effective 2000). adv. **Document type:** *Trade.*
Indexed: Chem.Abstr., Chem.Indus.Notes, Chem.Titles, GeoRef, INIS Atomind.
—CASDDS. **CCC.**
Published by: (Fachverband fuer Strahlenschutz e.V.), T Ue V Verlag GmbH, Am Grauen Stein 1, Cologne 51105, Germany. TEL 49-221-80635350, FAX 49-221-8063510, verlag@tuev-rheinland.de, http://www.tuev-rheinland.de. Ed. Dr. Rupprecht Maushart. Adv. contact Gudrun Karafiol. B&W page DEM 1,850; trim 254 x 160.

613.62 DEU
SUEDDEUTSCHE METALL-BERUFSGENOSSENSCHAFT. MITTEILUNGEN. Text in German. 1947. q. membership. **Document type:** *Bulletin.*
Formerly (until 1993): Sueddeutsche Eisen- und Stahl-Berufsgenossenschaft. Mitteilungen (0178-0182)
Published by: Sueddeutsche Metall-Berufsgenossenschaft, Wilhelm-Theodor-Roemheld-Str 15, Mainz 55130, Germany. TEL 06131-802-1, FAX 06131-802-232.

363.11 SWE
SWEDISH WORK ENVIRONMENT AUTHORITY. NEWSLETTER. Text in English, Swedish. 1975. biennial. free per issue. back issues avail. *Refereed.* **Document type:** *Newsletter.* **Description:** Provides articles on specific work environment issues.
Former titles (until 2000): National Board of Occupational Safety and Health. Newsletter (Online) (1403-9672); (until 1996): National Board of Occupational Safety and Health. Newsletter (Print) (0348-7598)
Media: Online - full content.
Indexed: CSNB, Ergon.Abstr., RAPRA (1992-).
Published by: Swedish Work Environmental Authority, Solna 17184, Sweden. TEL 46-8-730-9000, FAX 46-8-730-1967, http://www.av.se/english. Ed. Elisabet Delang. Pub. Bertil Remaeus.

613.62 613.62 USA ISSN 1066-7660
SYNERGIST (FAIRFAX). Text in English. 1989. m. USD 65; USD 90 foreign (effective 1999). charts, stat, tr.lit. back issues avail. **Description:** Provides information on issues affecting the profession and the association. Includes meeting announcements and conference updates.
Indexed: AgeLine, CSNB.
Published by: American Industrial Hygiene Association, 2700 Prosperity Ave, Ste 250, Fairfax, VA 22031-4307. TEL 703-849-8888, FAX 703-207-3561, infonet@aiha.org, http://www.aiha.org. Ed. Debbie Williams. Circ: 11,000.

613 GBR
SYSTEM CONCEPTS LTD; ergonomics in practice. Text in English. m.
Media: Online - full text.
Address: 2 Savoy Court, The Strand, London WC2R 0EZ, United Kingdom. helpdesk@system-concepts.com, http://www.system-concepts.com.

613.6 DEU
CODEN: TUSZA6
TECHNISCHE UEBERWACHUNG. Text in German. 1960. 9/yr. EUR 192 (effective 2002). adv. bk.rev. charts, illus, pat, tr.mk. index. back issues avail.; reprints avail. **Document type:** *Magazine, Trade.*
Former titles (until 1996): T Ue - Technische Ueberwachung. Sicherheit Zuverlaessigheit und Umweltschutz in Wirtschaft und Verkehr (0376-1185); (until 1970): Technische Ueberwachung (0372-2457); Which was formed by the merger of (1955-1960): Technische Ueberwachung (Munich) (0173-9883); (1955-1960): B T U - Betrieb und Technische Ueberwachung (0404-5696); Which was formerly (until 1956): Betrieb und Technische Ueberwachung (0173-9891)
Indexed: Alloys Ind., CEABA, Chem.Abstr., IBR, INIS Atomind., INSPEC (Jan.1969-Sep.1972, dropped), Met.Abstr., Met.Abstr.Ind., Nonfer.Met.Alert, PCC Alert, Steels Alert.
—BLDSC (8753.500000), CASDDS, CISTI, Ei, Linda Hall. **CCC.**
Published by: (Verband der Technischen Ueberwachungsvereine e.V.), Springer V D I Verlag, Heinrichstr 24, Duesseldorf 40239, Germany. TEL 49-211-6103-0, FAX 49-211-6103414, anzeigen@technikwissen.de, info@technikwissen.de, http://www.technikwissen.de. Ed. E Zimmermann. Adv. contact Karin Assig TEL 49-211-6103312. B&W page XEU 2,208; trim 185 x 270. Circ: 4,500.

TECHNOLOGY SPECIAL INTEREST SECTION QUARTERLY. see *TECHNOLOGY: COMPREHENSIVE WORKS*

▼ **TIDSSKRIFT FOR ARBEJDSLIV.** see *BUSINESS AND ECONOMICS—Labor And Industrial Relations*

363.11 613.6 GBR
TOLLEY'S HEALTH AND SAFETY AT WORK HANDBOOK. Text in English. a., latest 2000. GBP 65 (effective 2000). **Document type:** *Trade.* **Description:** Covers key aspects of health and safety as well as related environmental and employment information.
—BLDSC.
Published by: (Royal Society for the Prevention of Accidents), Tolley Publishing Co Ltd (Subsidiary of: Butterworths), Tolley House, 2 Addiscombe Rd, Croydon, Surrey CR9 5AF, United Kingdom. TEL 44-20-8686—9141, FAX 44-20-8686-3155, http://www.tolley.co.uk. Ed. Malcolm Dewis.

613.62 USA
TOPHEALTH∗ ; the health promotion and wellness letter. Text in English. 1987. m. price varies. **Document type:** *Newsletter.* **Description:** Promotes the good health of members and employees of organizations and corporations.
Related titles: Spanish ed.: 1987.
Published by: Dreyfuss Hunt, Inc., PO Box 381116, Birmingham, AL 35238-1116. TEL 617-244-6965. Ed. Dr. Arnon I Dreyfuss.

613.62 USA
TOPHEALTH EN ESPANOL∗ ; the health promotion and wellness letter. Text in Spanish. 1990. m. price varies. **Document type:** *Newsletter.* **Description:** Promotes the good health of members and employees of organizations and corporations.
Published by: Dreyfuss Hunt, Inc., PO Box 381116, Birmingham, AL 35238-1116. Ed. Dr. Arnon I Dreyfuss.

614.85 NLD
TOPICS IN SAFETY, RISK, RELIABILITY AND QUALITY. Text in English. 1991. irreg. price varies. *Refereed.* **Document type:** *Monographic series.* **Description:** Publishes studies covering the spectrum of disciplines required to deal with safety, quality and reliability of products, processes and services.
Formerly (until vol.4, 1995): Topics in Safety, Reliability and Quality (0927-1015)
—BLDSC, CISTI.
Published by: Kluwer Academic Publishers Group (Subsidiary of: Wolters Kluwer N.V.), Spuiboulevard 50, PO Box 17, Dordrecht 3300 AA, Netherlands. FAX 31-78-639-2254, services@wkap.nl, http://www.wkap.nl. Ed. A Z Keller. **Dist. by:** Journals Department, PO Box 322, Dordrecht 3300 AH, Netherlands. FAX 31-78-654-6474.

TOXICOLOGY AND INDUSTRIAL HEALTH; an international journal. see *ENVIRONMENTAL STUDIES—Toxicology And Environmental Safety*

TRANSPORTATION SAFETY SPECIAL REPORTS. see *PUBLIC HEALTH AND SAFETY*

TRAUMA UND BERUFSKRANKHEIT. see *MEDICAL SCIENCES—Orthopedics And Traumatology*

613.62 CAN ISSN 0829-0369
TRAVAIL ET SANTE; revue francophone pour la sante du travail et de l'environnement. Text in English. 1985. 4/yr. CND 30; CND 45 foreign (effective 1997). adv.
Indexed: Agri.Eng.Abstr., Ergon.Abstr., Pt.de Rep. (1989-).
Published by: Group de Communication Sansectra Inc., P O Box 1089, Napierville, PQ J0J 1L0, Canada. TEL 514-245-7285, FAX 514-245-0593. Ed. Robert Richards. Adv. contact Jean Yves Martel. Circ: 1,904.

614 331 FRA ISSN 0373-1944
HD7262
TRAVAIL ET SECURITE. Text in French. 1949. m. FRF 250; FRF 340 foreign (effective 1998). bk.rev., film rev. bibl, illus. cum.index. **Document type:** *Newspaper.*
Indexed: C.I.S. Abstr., INIS Atomind., World Surf.Coat.
—BLDSC (9027.000000).
Published by: Institut National de Recherche et de Securite pour la Prevention des Accidents du Travail et des Maladies Professionnelles, 30 rue Olivier Noyer, Paris Cedex 14 75680, France. TEL 33-1-40443000, FAX 33-1-40443099, thanh@inrs.fr. Ed. Didier Gout. Circ: 65,000.

TREEWORKER. see *FORESTS AND FORESTRY*

363.11 345.0242 USA ISSN 1081-4140
TRIODYNE SAFETY BULLETIN. Text in English. 1995. irreg. free. **Document type:** *Bulletin.*
Published by: Triodyne Inc., 5950 W Touhy Ave, Niles, IL 60714-4610. TEL 847-677-4730, FAX 847-647-2047, infoserv@triodyne.com, http://www.triodyne.com.

613.62 FIN ISSN 0041-4816
TYO - TERVEYS - TURVALLISUUS/WORK - HEALTH - SAFETY. Text in Finnish. 1971. 12/yr. FIM 380 (effective 2000). adv. bk.rev. illus. **Document type:** *Academic/Scholarly.*
Indexed: C.I.S. Abstr., Ergon.Abstr., Pollut.Abstr., Ref.Zh., Risk Abstr., Saf.Sci.Abstr.

Published by: Finnish Institute of Occupational Health, Topeliuksenkatu 41a A, Helsinki 00250, Finland. TEL 358-9-47471, FAX 358-9-4747-2548. Ed., R&P Matti Tapiainen. Adv. contact Ingmar Qvist TEL 358-9-2213-246. B&W page FIM 15,900, color page FIM 26,500; 211 x 248. Circ: 69,923.

U.S. COAST GUARD. MARINE SAFETY MANUAL. VOLUME 1: ADMINISTRATION AND MANAGEMENT. see *MILITARY*

U.S. COAST GUARD. MARINE SAFETY MANUAL. VOLUME 10: INTERAGENCY AGREEMENTTS AND ACRONYMS. see *MILITARY*

U.S. COAST GUARD. MARINE SAFETY MANUAL. VOLUME 2: MATERIEL INSPECTION. see *MILITARY*

U.S. COAST GUARD. MARINE SAFETY MANUAL. VOLUME 3: MARINE INDUSTRY PERSONNEL. see *MILITARY*

U.S. COAST GUARD. MARINE SAFETY MANUAL. VOLUME 4: TECHNICAL. see *MILITARY*

U.S. COAST GUARD. MARINE SAFETY MANUAL. VOLUME 5: INVESTIGATIONS. see *MILITARY*

U.S. COAST GUARD. MARINE SAFETY MANUAL. VOLUME 6: PORTS AND WATERWAYS ACTIVITIES. see *MILITARY*

U.S. COAST GUARD. MARINE SAFETY MANUAL. VOLUME 7: PORT SECURITY. see *MILITARY*

U.S. COAST GUARD. MARINE SAFETY MANUAL. VOLUME 9: ENVIRONMENTAL PROTECTION. see *MILITARY*

363.1 USA
RC965.R25
U.S. NUCLEAR REGULATORY COMMISSION. OCCUPATIONAL RADIATION AT COMMERCIAL NUCLEAR POWER REACTORS AND OTHER FACILITIES. ANNUAL REPORT. Key Title: Occupational Radiation Exposure, Annual Report. Text in English. 1970. a.
Former titles: U.S. Nuclear Regulatory Commission. Occupational Radiation Exposure. Annual Report (0198-8360); U.S. Nuclear Regulatory Commission. Annual Occupational Radiation Exposure Report
Published by: U.S. Nuclear Regulatory Commission, Office of Nuclear Regulatory Research, Washington, DC 20555. TEL 301-492-7000. Circ: 2,000.

344 USA ISSN 0094-7776
KF3568.3.A2
U.S. OCCUPATIONAL SAFETY AND HEALTH REVIEW COMMISSION. ADMINISTRATIVE LAW JUDGE AND COMMISSION DECISIONS. Key Title: O S A H R C Reports. Text in English. 1975. m. USD 43. **Document type:** *Government.*
Related titles: CD-ROM ed.: USD 27 (effective 2001).
Published by: U.S. Occupational Safety and Health Review Commission, 1 S LaFayette Ctr, 1120 20th St, N W 9th Fl, Washington, DC 20036-3419. TEL 202-606-5100, FAX 202-606-5050. Ed. Linda A Whitsett. Circ: 700. **Orders to:** U.S. Government Printing Office, Superintendent of Documents, PO Box 371954, Pittsburgh, PA 15250-7954. TEL 202-512-1800, FAX 202-512-2250, orders@gpo.gov, http://www.access.gpo.gov.

UMWELTMEDIZIN IN FORSCHUNG UND PRAXIS. see *MEDICAL SCIENCES*

DER UNFALLCHIRURG. see *MEDICAL SCIENCES—Orthopedics And Traumatology*

UNION MATTERS. see *LABOR UNIONS*

363.11 GBR
UNITED KINGDOM OFFSHORE HEALTH & SAFETY MANAGEMENT GUIDE. Text in English. 1980. q. GBP 225 (effective 1999). **Document type:** *Trade.*
Former titles (until 1995): Whitehead's United Kingdom Offshore Legislation Guide; (until 1994): United Kingdom Offshore Legislation Guide (0260-6135)
Published by: O C B Germanischer Lloyd, Bon Accord House, Riverside Dr, Aberdeen AB11 7SL, United Kingdom. sean_cotter@tolley.ccmail.compuserve.com. Ed. Sean Cotter. Pub. Carol Doyle Linden. R&P Rowena Watts. Circ: 500 (paid).

363.11 GBR
UNITED KINGDOM OFFSHORE HEALTH & SAFETY MANAGEMENT NEWSLETTER. Text in English. 1994. bi-m. GBP 75 (effective 1999). **Document type:** *Newsletter.*
Published by: O C B Germanischer Lloyd, Bon Accord House, Riverside Dr, Aberdeen AB11 7SL, United Kingdom. sean_cotter@tolley.ccmail.compuserve.com. Ed. Sean Cotter. Pub. Carol Doyle Linden. R&P Rowena Watts.

613.62 JPN ISSN 0387-821X
CODEN: JOUOD4
UNIVERSITY OF OCCUPATIONAL AND ENVIRONMENTAL HEALTH. JOURNAL. Key Title: Journal of U O E H. Text in English, Japanese; Summaries in English. 1979. q. USD 48. bk.rev. back issues avail. **Document type:** *Academic/Scholarly.*
Description: Focuses on occupational and environmental health sciences, but includes articles in other fields of medicine and humanities.
Indexed: Abstr.Hyg., Biol.Abstr., C.I.S. Abstr., Excerp.Med., INIS Atomind., Ind.Med. (1979-), Nutr.Abstr., Trop.Dis.Bull.
—BLDSC (4912.250000), CASDDS, CISTI, EMDOCS, GNLM.
Published by: University of Occupational and Environmental Health Japan, 1-1 Iseigaoka, Yahatanishi-ku, Kitakyushu-shi, Fukuoka-ken 807-0804, Japan. FAX 093-692-4876. Ed. Toshiji Koboyashi. Circ: 900 (controlled).

363.11 NLD ISSN 0926-4205
VOORKOMEN. Text in Dutch. 1951. bi-m. pat.
Description: For workers and scholars; seeks to increase interest and motivation concerning the working environment.
Formed by the merger of (1970-1990): Techniek en Veiligheid (0924-4441); Doen en Laten (0926-4191); Which was formerly (until 1983): Veilig Werken (0042-3130)
Published by: Nederlands Instituut voor Arbeidsomstandigheden, Postbus 75665, Amsterdam 1070 AR, Netherlands. TEL 31-20-5498425, FAX 31-20-6462310. Circ. 160,000.

614.85 CAN
W H M I S COMPLIANCE MANUAL. (Workplace Hazardous Materials Information Systems) Text in English. 1989. 3/yr. CND 195. **Description:** For companies developing and maintaining a program to comply with WHMIS requirements throughout Canada.
Published by: Carswell, One Corporate Plaza, 2075 Kennedy Rd, Scarborough, ON M1T 3V4, Canada. TEL 416-609-8000, FAX 416-298-5094. Ed. R Ferguson.

363.11 NLD ISSN 1051-9815
RM735.A1 CODEN: WORKFK
WORK; a journal of prevention, assessment & rehabilitation. Text in English. 1990. bi-m. (in 2 vols., 3 nos./vol.). EUR 330, USD 303 to institutions (effective 2002). back issues avail. *Refereed.* **Document type:** *Journal, Academic/Scholarly.* **Description:** Each issue is devoted to one topic within the scope of work practice, such as injury prevention, work assessment, and the older worker.
Related titles: Online - full text ed.: (from ingenta, RoweCom Information Quest).
Indexed: AMED, CINAHL, Environ.Sci.Poll.Mgmt., Ergon.Abstr., Excerp.Med., Pollut.Abstr., Risk Abstr., Saf.Sci.Abstr.
—BLDSC (9348.040100), GNLM, Infotrieve. **CCC.**
Published by: I O S Press, Nieuwe Hemweg 6B, Amsterdam 1013 BG, Netherlands. TEL 31-20-688-3355, FAX 31-20-620-3419, market@iospress.nl, http://www.iospress.nl. Ed. Karen Jacobs TEL 978-688-1554. **Subscr. to:** I O S Press, Inc, 5795-G Burke Centre Pkwy, Burke, VA 22015. TEL 703-323-5554, FAX 703-323-3668, iosbooks@iospress.com; Kinokuniya Company Ltd, Shinjuku 3-chome, Shinjuku-ku, Tokyo 160-0022, Japan. FAX 81-3-3439-1094, journal@kinokuniya.co.jp, http://www.kinokuniya.co.jp; Globe Publication Pvt. Ltd., C-62 Inderpuri, New Delhi 100 012, India. TEL 91-11-579-3211, 91-11-579-3212, FAX 91-11-579-8876, custserve@globepub.com, http://www.globepub.com.

WORK AND STRESS. see *PSYCHOLOGY*

WORK PROGRAMS SPECIAL INTEREST SECTION QUARTERLY. see *OCCUPATIONS AND CAREERS*

WORKERS' COMPENSATION - BUSINESS MANAGEMENT GUIDE. see *INSURANCE*

WORKER'S COMPENSATION GUIDE. see *BUSINESS AND ECONOMICS—Personnel Management*

613.62 GBR ISSN 1351-4792
WORKERS' HEALTH INTERNATIONAL NEWSLETTER. Text in English. s-a. GBP 15 (effective 1999). adv. **Document type:** *Newsletter.*
Related titles: Spanish ed.: W H I N en Espanol. ISSN 1130-8575.
Indexed: CSNB, Lab.Haz.Bull.
Published by: Hazards Publications Ltd., Hazards Publications Ltd, PO Box 199, Sheffield, S Yorks S1 4YL, United Kingdom. TEL 44-114-276-5695, FAX 44-114-276-7257, editor@hazards.org: sub@hazards.org. Eds. Rory O'Neill, Simon Pickvance. Adv. contact Jawad Qasrawi.

363.11 ZAF
WORKERS LIFE (PRETORIA). Text in English, Sotho, Northern, Sotho, Southern, Zulu; Summaries in English. 1985. m. ZAR 660 per month domestic for 10 copies; USD 200 per month foreign for 1 copy (effective 2001 - 2002). adv. bk.rev., Website rev., video rev., software rev. abstr, pat, stat, tr.lit. **Document type:** *Magazine, Government, Trade.*
Published by: National Occupational Safety Association, PO Box 26434, Arcadia, Pretoria 0007, South Africa. TEL 27-12-3039700, FAX 27-12-3039870, taniam@nosa.co.za, http://www.nosa.co.za. Ed. Sipho Siso. R&P Ed Furter. Adv. contact Eugene Howell TEL 27-12-3039717. page ZAR 640; 297 x 418. Circ: 13,800 (paid and controlled).

WORKLIFE REPORT. see *BUSINESS AND ECONOMICS—Labor And Industrial Relations*

614.85 USA ISSN 1528-8013
▼ **WORKPLACE ERGONOMICS NEWS.** Text in English. 1999. m. USD 197 (effective 2001). **Document type:** *Newsletter, Trade.* **Description:** Publishes information on government regulations, prevention and treatment strategies and trends within the industry.
Published by: Stevens Publishing Corporation, 5151 Beltline Rd, 10th fl, Dallas, TX 75240. TEL 972-687-6700, FAX 972-687-6770, custserv@stevenspublishing.com, http://www.stevenspublishing.com/news.html. Pub. Ralph Jensen.

363.11 CAN ISSN 1494-7412
WORKSAFE MAGAZINE. Text in English. 1995. 6/yr. free. back issues avail. **Document type:** *Newspaper, Government.* **Description:** Provides information on workplace health and safety in BC, as well as information on policies and operations of the WCB.
Formerly (until 2000): Prevention at Work (1208-882X); Which was formed by 1995 the merger of: W C B News (0709-9428); Which was formerly (1958-1974): Workmen's Compensation Board of British Columbia. News Bulletin (0524-5621); (1991-1995): Your Workplace Health & Safety (1191-1263); Which was formerly: Health and Safety Digest (0714-8429); (1967-1975): Safety Digest (Vancouver) (0714-8488)
Related titles: Online - full text ed.
Published by: Workers' Compensation Board, Communications Department, P O Box 5350,, Sta Terminal, Vancouver, BC V6B 5L5, Canada. TEL 604-279-7572, FAX 604-279-7406, http://www.worksafebc.ca, http://www.wcb.bc.ca. Ed. Diane Bentley. R&P Dawn Knoll. Circ: 25,000.

613.62 614.85 CAN ISSN 1203-3774
WORKSITE NEWS. Text in English. 1992. 10/yr. CND 65 domestic (effective 2001). adv. **Document type:** *Magazine, Trade.* **Description:** Covers occupational safety, health and environmental issues for the industrial and commericial sectors across North America.
Published by: Morrow Communications, Inc., 3216-108A St, Edmonton, AB T6J 3E2, Canada. TEL 888-430-6405, worksite@worldgate.com, http://www.worksite-news.com.

614.8 CHE ISSN 0084-165X
WORLD CONGRESS ON THE PREVENTION OF OCCUPATIONAL ACCIDENTS AND DISEASES. PROCEEDINGS. (Proceedings published by national organizing committee) Text in Multiple languages. 1955. triennial, latest 1993, 13th, New Delhi. **Document type:** *Proceedings.* **Description:** Presents issues concerning concepts, scope, organization, financing and implementation of occupational health services, with the aim of education and training.
Published by: International Social Security Association, Case Postale 1, Geneva, 22 1211, Switzerland. FAX 41-22-799-85-09, iisa@ilo.org.

WUERTTEMBERGISCHE BAU-BERUFSGENOSSENSCHAFT. MITTEILUNGEN. see *BUILDING AND CONSTRUCTION*

614.85 JPN
YEARBOOK OF INDUSTRIAL SAFETY AND HEALTH. Text in Japanese. a. JPY 4,000 (effective 2001). **Description:** Covers activities and relevant information in the field of industrial safety and health in Japan.
Formerly: Yearbook of Industrial Safety
Published by: Japan Industrial Safety and Health Association, Publishing and Sales Department, 5-35-1 Shiba, Minato-ku, Tokyo 108-0014, Japan. TEL 81-3-3452-6841, FAX 81-3-3453-8034. Ed. Toru Sasaki.

613.62 DEU ISSN 0944-2502
CODEN: ZAAEE
ZENTRALBLATT FUER ARBEITSMEDIZIN, ARBEITSSCHUTZ UND ERGONOMIE. Text in German. 1951. m. EUR 143.46 domestic; EUR 162.18 foreign; EUR 12.84 newsstand/cover (effective 2002). adv. bk.rev. abstr, bibl, charts, illus, pat. index. **Document type:** *Journal, Trade.*
Former titles (until 1992): Zentralblatt fuer Arbeitsmedizin, Arbeitsschutz, Prophylaxe und Ergonomie (0173-3338); (until 1980): Zentralblatt fuer Arbeitsmedizin, Arbeitsschutz und Prophylaxe (0340-7047); Which was formed by the 1976 merger of: Zentralblatt fuer Arbeitsmedizin und Arbeitsschutz (0044-4049); Prophylaxe (Heidelberg) (0033-1368)
Indexed: Abstr.Hyg., Biol.Abstr., C.I.S. Abstr., Chem.Abstr., Chem.Indus.Notes, Chem.Infd., Chem.Titles, Ergon.Abstr., Excerp.Med., IBZ, INIS Atomind., Ind.Med. (coverage dropped).
—BLDSC (9500.799500), CASDDS, CISTI, EMDOCS, GNLM, Infotrieve. **CCC.**
Published by: Dr. Curt Haefner Verlag GmbH, Bachstr 14-16, Heidelberg 69121, Germany. TEL 49-6221-6446-0, FAX 49-6221-644640, info@haefner-verlag.de, http://www.haefner-verlag.de. Circ: 3,500.

613.62 CHN ISSN 1003-3033
ZHONGGUO ANQUAN KEXUE XUEBAO/CHINESE SAFETY SCIENCE JOURNAL. Text in Chinese. 1991. bi-m. CNY 10 per issue domestic (effective 2000). back issues avail. **Document type:** *Academic/Scholarly.*
Published by: Zhongguo Laodong Baohu Kexue Jishu Xuehui Bianji Chubanbu, Zhaoyang-qu, Huixin Xi Jie 17 Hao, Beijing 100029, China. TEL 86-1-64915341, 86-1-64915566 ext 2717. Ed. Deshu Xu.

613.62 CHN ISSN 1002-221X
ZHONGGUO GONGYE YIXUE ZAZHI/CHINESE JOURNAL OF INDUSTRIAL MEDICINE. Text in Chinese. 1988 (Oct.). bi-m. USD 17.40; USD 2.90 newsstand/cover (effective 2001). bk.rev. abstr, pat, stat. 64 p./no. back issues avail. **Document type:** *Journal, Academic/Scholarly.*
Related titles: Online - full content ed.: (from WanFang Data Corp.).
—BLDSC (3180.354500).
Published by: Shenyang Institute of Occupational Health and Medicine, Tiexi-qu, Nan 11 Xi Lu 18 Hao, Shenyang 110024, China. TEL 86-24-25732571, FAX 86-24-25731482, sycpcc@pub.sy.ln.cn. Eds. Feng Sheng He, Jin Duo Zhao. Circ: 2,000 (paid). **Dist. by:** China International Book Trading Corp, 35, Chegongzhuang Xilu, Haidian District, Beijing 100044, China. TEL 86-1-68413849, FAX 86-1-68412048, cibtc@mail.cibtc.com.cn, http://www.cibtc.com.cn. **Co-sponsor:** Zhonghua Yufangyi Xuehui/China Preventive Medical Association.

613.62 CHN ISSN 1001-9391
CODEN: ZLWZEX
ZHONGHUA LAODONG WEISHENG ZHIYEBING ZAZHI* /CHINESE JOURNAL OF INDUSTRIAL HYGIENE AND OCCUPATIONAL DISEASES. Text in Chinese. 1983. bi-m. USD 22.20; USD 3.70 newsstand/cover (effective 2001). **Document type:** *Academic/Scholarly.* **Description:** Contains epidemiological investigation on industrial hygiene and occupational medicine, and studies on prevention, diagnosis and treatment of occupational diseases.
Indexed: Chem.Abstr., Chem.Indus.Notes, Chem.Titles, Lab.Haz.Bull.
—BLDSC (3180.354000), CASDDS, CISTI.
Published by: (Tianjin Shi Laodong Weisheng Zhiyebing Yanjiusuo/Tianjin Institute of Industrial Hygiene and Occupational Diseases), China International Book Trading Corp/Zhongguo Guoji Tushu Maoyi Zonggongsi cibtc@mail.cibtc.com.cn, http://www.cibtc.com.cn. Ed. Gang Baoqi. Circ: 4,000 (paid); 400 (controlled). **Dist. by:** 35, Chegongzhuang Xilu, Haidian District, Beijing 100044, China.

OCCUPATIONAL HEALTH AND SAFETY—Abstracting, Bibliographies, Statistics

613.62 USA
AMERICAN INDUSTRIAL HYGIENE ASSOCIATION. CONFERENCE ABSTRACTS. Text in English. bi-m. USD 20 to individuals; USD 160 to institutions. **Document type:** *Proceedings.* **Description:** Abstracts of papers presented at the annual meeting of the American Industrial Hygiene Conference.
Published by: American Industrial Hygiene Association, 2700 Prosperity Ave, Ste 250, Fairfax, VA 22031-4307. TEL 703-849-8888. **Subscr. to:** AIHA Journal, Dept 796, Alexandria, VA 22334-0796.

613.62 011 USA ISSN 1047-8124
CODEN: CSOHE7
C A SELECTS. OCCUPATIONAL EXPOSURE & HAZARDS. Text in English. 1988. s-w. USD 275 (effective 2001). **Document type:** *Abstract/Index.* **Description:** Covers occupational exposure and related hazards. Includes epidemiological studies on workplace exposure of humans to chemicals, biological agents, radiation, and noise.
Formerly (until 1989): BIOSIS CAS Selects: Occupational Exposure
Published by: Chemical Abstracts Service (Subsidiary of: American Chemical Society), 2540 Olentangy River Rd, Box 3012, Columbus, OH 43210-0012. TEL 614-447-3600, 800-753-4227, FAX 614-447-3751.

613.62 USA ISSN 1083-2769
CODEN: CSPSFC
C A SELECTS PLUS. CHEMICAL HAZARDS, HEALTH & SAFETY. Text in English. s-w. USD 275 (effective 2001). **Document type:** *Abstract/Index.* **Description:** Covers safety in chemical laboratories and in the chemical and nuclear industries; health and safety of personnel working in these areas or working with hazardous substances.
Formerly: C A Selects. Chemical Hazards, Health and Safety (0190-9398)
Published by: Chemical Abstracts Service (Subsidiary of: American Chemical Society), 2540 Olentangy River Rd, Box 3012, Columbus, OH 43210-0012. TEL 614-447-3600, 800-753-4227, FAX 614-447-3751.

016.61362 GBR ISSN 0265-5721
CODEN: CHINEK
CHEMICAL HAZARDS IN INDUSTRY. Text in English. 1984. m. GBP 761, USD 1,196 to individuals (effective 2002). abstr. reprints avail. **Document type:** *Journal, Abstract/Index.* **Description:** Provides current awareness of such topics as health and safety, chemical and biological hazards, plant safety, legislation, protective equipment and storage relating to the chemical and allied industries.
Related titles: CD-ROM ed.: (from The Dialog Corporation); E-mail ed.; Online - full text ed.: price varies (from Data-Star, The Dialog Corporation, Questel Orbit Inc., S T N International).
—CCC.
Published by: Royal Society of Chemistry, Thomas Graham House, Science Park, Milton Rd, Cambridge CB4 4WF, United Kingdom. TEL 44-1223-432360, FAX 44-1223-423429, sales@rsc.org, http://www.rsc.org/csnb. Ed. Janet Crombie. **Subscr. to.:** Turpin Distribution Services Ltd., Blackhorse Rd, Letchworth, Herts SG6 1HN, United Kingdom. TEL 44-1462-672555.

016.61362 GBR
CHEMICAL SAFETY NEWSBASE. Text in English. m. price varies. abstr. back issues avail. **Document type:** *Abstract/Index.* **Description:** Provides information on the hazards of chemicals used in industry, and all health and safety matters relevant to the laboratory and office environment. Contains information from over 200 journals and includes over 45,000 items with coverage dating back to 1981.
Media: Online - full text (from Data-Star, The Dialog Corporation, Questel Orbit Inc., S T N International, F I Z Technik). **Related titles:** CD-ROM ed.: Environmental Chemistry, Health & Safety. USD 1,695 (from The Dialog Corporation).
Published by: Royal Society of Chemistry, Thomas Graham House, Science Park, Milton Rd, Cambridge CB4 4WF, United Kingdom. TEL 44-1223-432360, FAX 44-1223-423429, sales@rsc.org, http://www.rsc.org/csnb.

E & P HEALTH, SAFETY AND ENVIRONMENT. (Exploration and Production) see *PETROLEUM AND GAS—Abstracting, Bibliographies, Statistics*

016.614 ESP ISSN 0213-943X
Z6675.I5
ERGA. Text in Spanish. 1973. m. ESP 4,240 (effective 2000). adv. bk.rev. index, cum.index: 1975-1988. **Document type:** *Bibliography, Government.*
Former titles (until 1988): Instituto Nacional de Seguridad e Higiene en el Trabajo. Boletin Bibliografico (0212-2359); (until 1981): Spain. Servicio Social de Higiene y Seguridad del Trabajo. Boletin Bibliografico (0210-069X)
Published by: Instituto Nacional de Seguridad e Higiene en el Trabajo, Ministerio de Trabajo y Seguridad Social, Dulcet, 2-10, Barcelona 08034, Spain. FAX 34-3-2803642, cnctinsht@mtas.es, http://www.mtas.es/insht. Ed. Emilio Castejon. Adv. contact Irene Cabanas. Circ: 2,000.

EXCERPTA MEDICA. SECTION 35: OCCUPATIONAL HEALTH AND INDUSTRIAL MEDICINE. see *MEDICAL SCIENCES—Abstracting, Bibliographies, Statistics*

614.85 USA
FATAL OCCUPATIONAL INJURIES IN MAINE. Text in English. 1991. a. **Document type:** *Government.* **Description:** Provides statistics concerning work-related fatalities in Maine.
Published by: Department of Labor, Bureau of Labor Standards, Technical Services Division, 45 State House Station, Augusta, ME 04333-0045. TEL 207-624-6440, FAX 207-624-6449, webmaster-bls@state.me.us, webmaster_bls@state.me.us. Ed., R&P Robert W Leighton Jr. Circ: 524.

016.61362 GBR ISSN 0966-906X
HAZARDS IN THE OFFICE. Text in English. 1993. bi-m. GBP 169, USD 266 to individuals (effective 2002). **Document type:** *Abstract/Index.* **Description:** Source of information on the hidden hazards in the office environment and the vital safety procedures to be adopted to prevent injury.
Related titles: CD-ROM ed.: (from The Dialog Corporation); Online - full text ed.: price varies (from Data-Star, The Dialog Corporation, S T N International).
Published by: Royal Society of Chemistry, Thomas Graham House, Science Park, Milton Rd, Cambridge CB4 4WF, United Kingdom. TEL 44-1223-432360, FAX 44-1223-423429, acquisitions@rsc.org, sales@rsc.org, advertising@rsc.org, http://www.rsc.org/csnb. Ed. Janet Bingham. **Subscr. to:** Turpin Distribution Services Ltd., Blackhorse Rd, Letchworth, Herts SG6 1HN, United Kingdom. TEL 44-1462-672555, FAX 44-1462-480947.

HEALTH AND SAFETY SCIENCE ABSTRACTS. see *PUBLIC HEALTH AND SAFETY—Abstracting, Bibliographies, Statistics*

614.85 ITA ISSN 0021-2539
I N A I L NOTIZIARIO STATISTICO. Text in Italian. 1951. q. ITL 16,200. charts. index. **Description:** Contains statistics of injuries and diseases obtained during professional activities.
Published by: Istituto Nazionale per l'Assicurazione Contro gli Infortuni sul Lavoro, Viale Stefano Gradi, 55, Rome, RM 00143, Italy. TEL 39-6-54872217, FAX 39-6-51957270. Circ: 2,500 (paid). **Subscr. to:** Via Quattro Novembre, 144, Rome, RM 00187, Italy. **Co-sponsor:** Consulenza Statistico Attuariale.

613.62 FRA ISSN 0335-0274
I N R S BULLETIN DE DOCUMENTATION. Text in French. 7/yr. FRF 320 (effective 1999). index, cum.index. **Document type:** *Bibliography.* **Description:** Contains bibliographic information about occupational safety and health.
Published by: Institut National de Recherche et de Securite pour la Prevention des Accidents du Travail et des Maladies Professionnelles, 30 rue Olivier Noyer, Paris Cedex 14 75680, France. TEL 33-1-40443000, FAX 33-1-40443099, thanh@inrs.fr. Circ: 2,500.

613.62 016 USA ISSN 0019-8382
CODEN: IHYDA
INDUSTRIAL HYGIENE DIGEST. Text in English. 1937. m. USD 225 to non-members; USD 240 foreign to non-members. bk.rev. index, cum.index every 10 yrs. **Document type:** *Abstract/Index.*
—GNLM, Linda Hall.
Published by: Industrial Health Foundation, Inc., 34 Penn Circle W, Pittsburgh, PA 15206. TEL 412-363-6600, FAX 412-363-6605, IHFincorp@aol.com, http://members.aol.com/ihfincorp/ihf.htm. R&P Marianne C Kaschak. Circ: 1,000.

363.11 622 USA ISSN 0270-2053
TN295
INJURY EXPERIENCE IN SAND AND GRAVEL MINING. Text in English. a. **Document type:** *Government.*
Former titles (until 1978): Injury Experience in the Sand and Gravel Industry (0191-6645); (until 1973): Injury Experience and Worktime Data for the Sand and Gravel Industry (0364-3131)
Published by: U.S. Department of Labor, Mine Safety and Health Administration, 4015 Wilson Blvd, Arlington, VA 22203. TEL 703-235-1452. **Subscr. to:** U.S. Government Printing Office, Superintendent of Documents. TEL 202-783-3238.

331.8 016 613 CHE ISSN 0074-2147
INTERNATIONAL CATALOGUE OF OCCUPATIONAL SAFETY AND HEALTH FILMS. Text in English, French, Spanish. 1969. irreg. **Document type:** *Catalog.*
Published by: (International Labour Office), I L O Publications, Geneva, 22 1211, Switzerland. TEL 41-22-799-6111, FAX 41-22-798-6358. **Dist. in US by:** I L O Publications Center, 9 Jay Gould Court, Ste. CT, PO Box 753, Waldorf, MD 20602. TEL 301-638-3152, FAX 301-843-0159, ilopubs@tasco1.com.

016.61485 016.661 GBR ISSN 0261-2917
CODEN: LHBUD2
LABORATORY HAZARDS BULLETIN. Text in English. 1981. m. GBP 436, USD 622 to individuals (effective 2002). adv. index. cum.index. **Document type:** *Bulletin, Abstract/Index.* **Description:** Reports on safety measures, potential hazards and new legislation affecting the well-being of employees working in laboratories.
Related titles: CD-ROM ed.: (from The Dialog Corporation); Online - full text ed.: (from Data-Star, The Dialog Corporation, Questel Orbit Inc., S T N International).
Indexed: INIS Atomind.
—CCC.
Published by: Royal Society of Chemistry, Thomas Graham House, Science Park, Milton Rd, Cambridge CB4 4WF, United Kingdom. TEL 44-1223-432360, FAX 44-1223-423429, acquisitions@rsc.org, sales@rsc.org, advertising@rsc.org, http://www.rsc.org/csnb. Ed. Janet Crombie. **Subscr. to:** Turpin Distribution Services Ltd., Blackhorse Rd, Letchworth, Herts SG6 1HN, United Kingdom. TEL 44-1462-672555, FAX 44-1462-480947.

613.62 ESP
LANEKO LESIOEN ESTATISTIKAK (YEAR)/ ESTADISTICAS DE LA LESIONES PROFESIONALES. Text in Spanish. a., latest 1996.
Published by: (Basque Region. Lan eta Gizarte Segurantza Saila/Departamento de Trabajo y Seguridad Social), Eusko Jaurlaritzaren Argitalpen-Zerbitzu Nagusia/Servicio Central de Publicaciones del Gobierno Vasco, Donostia-San Sebastian, 1, Vitoria-gasteiz, Alava 01010, Spain. TEL 34-945-018561, FAX 34-945-018709, hac-sabd@ej-gv.es, http://www.ej-gv.net/publicaciones. Circ: 2,000.

338.47665 USA
N P R A STATISTICAL REPORT. ANNUAL SURVEY OF OCCUPATIONAL INJURIES & INJURIES. Text in English. a. back issues avail. **Document type:** *Trade.* **Description:** Provides a statistical overview of injuries at petrochemical plants and refineries.
Published by: National Petroleum Refiners Association, 1899 L St, NW, Ste 1000, Washington, DC 20036-3896. TEL 202-457-0480, FAX 202-457-0486, http://www.npradc.org.

NETHERLANDS. CENTRAAL BUREAU VOOR DE STATISTIEK. LEEFSITUATIE VAN DE NEDERLANDSE BEVOLKING, DEEL 1: GEZONDHEID EN KWALITEIT VAN DE ARBEID. see *PUBLIC HEALTH AND SAFETY—Abstracting, Bibliographies, Statistics*

614.85 USA
OCCUPATIONAL HEALTH. Text in English. irreg. price varies.
Published by: (Nuclear Regulatory Commission), U.S. National Technical Information Service, 5825 Port Royal Rd, Springfield, VA 22161. TEL 703-605-6060.

016.61362 AUS ISSN 1324-8715
OCCUPATIONAL HEALTH & SAFETY CURRENT CONTENTS. Short title: O H & S Current Contents. Text in English. 1986. bi-m. AUD 60 domestic; AUD 90 foreign (effective 2000). back issues avail. **Document type:** *Abstract/Index.* **Description:** Includes listing of all new publications in OH&S received in VIOSH Australia and the E.J. Barker University Library.
Published by: V I O S H Australia, c/o University of Ballarat, University Dr, Mt. Helen, PO Box 663, Ballarat, VIC 3353, Australia. TEL 61-3-53279160, FAX 61-3-53279151, d.elshaug@ballarat.edu.au. Ed. Dianne Elshang. R&P Dianne Elshaug.

613.62 310 USA ISSN 1063-3820
HD7262.5.U62
OCCUPATIONAL INJURY & ILLNESS INFORMATION. Text in English. a. free per issue. **Document type:** *Government.* **Description:** Statistical report on work-related injuries and illnesses in Alaska's work force.
Related titles: Online - full text ed.
Published by: Department of Labor, Research and Analysis Section, PO Box 25501, Juneau, AK 99802-5501. TEL 907-465-4939, FAX 907-465-2101, http://www.labor.state.ak.us/research/cfoi/cfoihome.htm.

614.8 016 CHE ISSN 1010-7053
T55.A1 CODEN: SHWOEV
SAFETY AND HEALTH AT WORK. Text in English. 1974. bi-m. CHF 350 (effective 2001). adv. bk.rev. abstr. index, cum.index. **Document type:** *Abstract/Index.*
Former titles: C I S Abstracts (0302-7651); Occupational Safety and Health Abstracts (0029-7984)
Related titles: CD-ROM ed.: 1987 (from SilverPlatter Information, Inc.); Online - full text ed.: (from Questel Orbit Inc., Canadian Centre for Occupational Health & Safety); ♦ French ed.: Securite et Sante au Travail. ISSN 1010-7061.
Indexed: Ergon.Abstr.
—CASDDS, GNLM, Linda Hall.
Published by: International Labour Office, International Occupational Safety and Health Information Centre/Bureau International du Travail, Centre International d'Informations de Securite et de Sante au Travail, 4 route des Morillons, Geneva, 22 1211, Switzerland. TEL 41-22-799-6111, FAX 41-22-799-8516, cis@ilo.org, http://www.ilo.org. Circ: 1,500.

614.8 016 CHE ISSN 1010-7061
SECURITE ET SANTE AU TRAVAIL. Text in French. 1974. bi-m. CHF 350 (effective 2001). adv. bk.rev. **Document type:** *Bulletin, Abstract/Index.*
Former titles: Bulletin C I S (0250-4235); Bulletin Bibliographique de la Prevention (0045-3498)
Related titles: CD-ROM ed.: (from SilverPlatter Information, Inc.); Online - full text ed.: (from Questel Orbit Inc.); ♦ English ed.: Safety and Health at Work. ISSN 1010-7053.
Indexed: C.I.S. Abstr., Ergon.Abstr., Lab.Haz.Bull.
Published by: International Labour Office, International Occupational Safety and Health Information Centre/Bureau International du Travail, Centre International d'Informations de Securite et de Sante au Travail, 4 route des Morillons, Geneva, 22 1211, Switzerland. TEL 41-22-799-6111, FAX 41-22-799-8516, cis@ilo.org, http://www.ilo.org. Circ: 500 (paid).

613.62 016 RUS ISSN 0202-8905
SIGNAL'NAYA INFORMATSIYA. TEKHNIKA BEZOPASNOSTI. SANITARNAYA TEKHNIKA. Text in Russian. 1971. s-m. **Document type:** *Abstract/Index.*
Published by: Vserossiiskii Institut Nauchnoi i Tekhnicheskoi Informatsii (VINITI), Usievicha ul 20-a, Moscow 125315, Russian Federation. TEL 7-095-1526441. **Dist. by:** Mezhdunarodnaya Kniga, B Yakimanka 39, Moscow 117049, Russian Federation. TEL 7-095-2384967, FAX 7-095-2384634.

614.852 310 USA ISSN 0195-9344
WESTERN WOOD PRODUCTS ASSOCIATION. QUARTERLY INJURY & ILLNESS INCIDENCE REPORT. Text in English. q. USD 18 (effective 2001). back issues avail. **Document type:** *Trade.* **Description:** Supplies a year-to-date injury-control index and annual summary of injuries sustained by lumberjacks in Western timber forests.
Published by: Western Wood Products Association, 512 S W Fifth Ave Ste 500, Portland, OR 97236. TEL 503-224-3930, FAX 503-224-3935, info@wwpa.org, http://www.wwpa.org. R&P Robert Bernardt Jr.

OCCUPATIONS AND CAREERS

see also BUSINESS AND ECONOMICS—Labor And Industrial Relations

371.42 150 GBR
A E P APPOINTMENTS BROADSHEET. Text in English. 1978. w. membership. adv. back issues avail. **Document type:** *Newsletter.* **Description:** Contains advertisements for vacant positions in educational psychology.
Indexed: e-psyche.
Published by: Association of Educational Psychologists, 26 The Avenue, Durham, Durham DH1 4ED, United Kingdom. TEL 44-191-3849512, FAX 44-191-3865287. Ed. K S Brown. Adv. contact Lynn Flowers. Circ: 2,200.

A S P B NEWS; the newsletter of the American Society of Plant Biologists. see *BIOLOGY—Botany*

370.15 USA
ALABAMA COUNSELING ASSOCIATION. JOURNAL. Text in English. 1974. s-a. USD 10 to non-members (effective 1999). adv. bk.rev. charts. *Refereed.*
Former titles: Alabama Association for Counseling and Development Journal; Alabama Personnel and Guidance Journal
Published by: Alabama Counseling Association, c/o Dr Ervin L Wood, Sta 36, UWA, Livingston, AL 35470. TEL 205-652-3578, FAX 205-652-3522. R&P Dr. Ervin L Wood. Circ: 2,300.

371.42 DEU ISSN 0931-8895
BERUFLICHE REHABILITATION. Text in German. 1987. bi-m. EUR 27; EUR 7.20 newsstand/cover. adv. bk.rev. **Document type:** *Journal, Trade.*
Published by: (Bundesarbeitsgemeinschaft der Berufsbildungswerke), Lambertus-Verlag GmbH, Mitscherlichstr 56, Freiburg Im Breisgau 79108, Germany. TEL 49-761-36825-0, FAX 49-761-3682533, info@lambertus.de, http://www.lambertus.de. Ed. Philibert Magin. Circ: 1,600.

371.4 GBR ISSN 0306-9885
LB1027.5 CODEN: BJGCDD
BRITISH JOURNAL OF GUIDANCE AND COUNSELLING. Text in English. 1973. q. GBP 93, USD 167 to individuals; GBP 223, USD 399 to institutions (effective 2002). adv. bk.rev. abstr. index. back issues avail. *Refereed.* **Document type:** *Academic/Scholarly.*
Related titles: Microfiche ed.; Online - full content ed.: ISSN 1469-3534 (from EBSCO Publishing, O C L C Online Computer Library Center, Inc., ProQuest Information & Learning, Swets Blackwell); Online - full text ed.: (from CatchWord Ltd., Institute for Scientific Information, RoweCom Information Quest).
Indexed: ASSIA, Br.Educ.Ind., Brit.Nur.Ind., C.I.J.E., Cont.Pg.Educ., Curr.Cont., ERA, Educ.Tech.Abstr., FAMLI, High.Educ.Curr.Aware.Bull., IBZ, Ind.Philos., Indian Psychol.Abstr., Lang.& Lang.Behav.Abstr., Mult.Ed.Abstr., PsycInfo, Psychol.Abstr. (1973-), Res.High.Educ.Abstr., SOMA, SOPODA, SSCI, Sociol.Abstr., Sociol.Educ.Abstr., Sp.Ed.Needs Abstr., Stud.Wom.Abstr., Tech.Educ.Abstr., WMB, e-psyche.
—BLDSC (2308.700000), CatchWord, Infotrieve. **CCC.**
Published by: (Careers Research and Advisory Centre), Carfax Publishing Limited (Subsidiary of: Taylor & Francis Group), PO Box 25, Abingdon, Oxon OX14 3UE, United Kingdom. TEL 44-1235-401000, FAX 44-1235-401550, enquiries@carfax.co.uk, enquiry@tandf.co.uk, http://www.carfax.co.uk. Ed. Tony Watts. Circ: 750.

CAREER DEVELOPMENT FOR EXCEPTIONAL INDIVIDUALS. see *EDUCATION—Special Education And Rehabilitation*

371.42 USA ISSN 0889-4019
HF5381.A1
THE CAREER DEVELOPMENT QUARTERLY. Text in English. 1952. q. USD 45 domestic to individuals; USD 57 foreign to individuals; USD 80 domestic to institutions; USD 92 foreign to institutions (effective 2001). adv. bibl, charts, illus, abstr. index. 96 p./no. back issues avail.; reprint service avail. from PQC. *Refereed.* **Document type:** *Journal, Academic/Scholarly.* **Description:** Concerned with research, theory, and practice in career development, career counseling, occupational resources, labor market dynamics, and career education.
Formerly (until 1986): Vocational Guidance Quarterly (0042-7764)
Related titles: Microform ed.: 1952 (from PQC); Online - full text ed.: 1952 (from ProQuest Information & Learning, Northern Light Technology, Inc., H. W. Wilson, Factiva, Institute for Scientific Information).
Indexed: ASCA, AgeLine, Amer.Bibl.Slavic & E.Eur.Stud., BPIA, C.I.J.E., Cont.Pg.Educ., Curr.Cont., Educ.Ind. (Nov.1982-Jun.1986), High.Educ.Abstr., High.Educ.Curr.Aware.Bull., Int.Lab.Doc., Mult.Ed.Abstr., PsycInfo, Psychol.Abstr. (1954-), Psycscan A.P., SSCI, Soc.Work Res.& Abstr., Stud.Wom.Abstr., Tr.& Dev.Alert, Yrbk.Assoc.Educ.& Rehab.Blind, e-psyche.
—BLDSC (3051.706000), IDS, ingenta. **CCC.**

Published by: (National Career Development Association), American Counseling Association, 5999 Stevenson Ave, Alexandria, VA 22304-3300. TEL 703-823-9800, 800-347-6647, FAX 703-823-0252, http://www.counseling.org. Ed. Spencer Niles. R&P Cynthia Peay TEL 703-823-9800 x 249. Adv. contact Kathy Maguire TEL 703-823-9800 ext 207. Circ: 5,900.

CAREER PLANNING AND ADULT DEVELOPMENT JOURNAL. see *EDUCATION—Adult Education*

CAREER PLANNING AND ADULT DEVELOPMENT NETWORK NEWSLETTER; a newsletter for career counselors, educators, and human resource specialists. see *EDUCATION—Adult Education*

CONTINUING EDUCATION MATTERS FOR O M P. (Opthalmic Medical Personnel) see *MEDICAL SCIENCES—Ophthalmology And Optometry*

COUNSELING TODAY. see *PSYCHOLOGY*

331.702 USA ISSN 0884-4291
CREATIVE CHILD AND ADULT QUARTERLY. Text in English. 1975. q. USD 55; USD 65 foreign. adv. bk.rev. abstr, bibl, charts, illus, tr.lit. reprint service avail. from PQC. **Description:** Includes research studies, reviews, reports on programs and in-depth career guidance interviews with functioning creative individuals.
Formerly (until 1976): Creative Child and Adult (0098-7565)
Related titles: Microform ed.: (from PQC); Online - full text ed.: (from H. W. Wilson).
Indexed: C.I.J.E. (coverage dropped), Child Devel.Abstr., Curr.Cont. (coverage dropped), Educ.Ind. (Jun.1992-), Except.Child Educ.Abstr., Psychol.Abstr.
—ingenta.
Published by: National Association for Creative Children and Adults, 8080 Springvalley Dr, Cincinnati, OH 45236-1395. TEL 513-631-1777. Ed. Ann F Isaacs. Circ: 6,000.

DIMENSIONS (RIMROCK). see *PARAPSYCHOLOGY AND OCCULTISM*

DIRECTORY OF INTERNSHIPS, RESIDENCIES AND REGISTRARSHIPS AVAILABLE IN VICTORIAN HOSPITALS. see *HEALTH FACILITIES AND ADMINISTRATION*

DIRECTORY OF OSTEOPATHIC POSTDOCTORAL EDUCATION. see *MEDICAL SCIENCES—Chiropractic, Homeopathy, Osteopathy*

HEALTH CAREER POST. see *HEALTH FACILITIES AND ADMINISTRATION*

HEALTHCARE EMPLOYMENT JOURNAL; serving healthcare professionals. see *MEDICAL SCIENCES*

371.42 610 USA ISSN 1047-7276
HEALTHCARE TRENDS AND TRANSITION. Text in English. bi-m. adv. **Document type:** *Trade.*
Published by: Nex, Inc., PO Box 48, Eden, MD 21822. TEL 800-541-9129, FAX 301-749-8769. Ed. Karen Flynn. Pub. Walter Moore. R&P Patty Stille Lederman. Adv. contact Cary Lederman.

JAPANESE NURSING ASSOCIATION RESEARCH REPORT. see *MEDICAL SCIENCES—Nurses And Nursing*

371.42 USA ISSN 1099-0208
RA977
THE JOBBANK GUIDE TO HEALTH CARE COMPANIES; includes hospitals, medical centers, clinical labs, pharmaceutical manufacturers, biotechnology firms and more. Text in English. biennial. USD 17.95 (effective 2000). adv. **Document type:** *Directory, Trade.* **Description:** Constitutes an up-to-date career directory for 10,500 companies in the health care, biotechnology and pharmaceutical industries. Includes hospitals, medical centers, clinical labs, pharmaceutical manufacturers, biotechnology firms and more.
Published by: Adams Media Corporation, 260 Center St, Holbrook, MA 02343. TEL 781-767-8100, 800-872-5627, FAX 781-767-2055, reference@adamsmedia.com, http://www.adamsmedia.com. Ed. Steven Graber. Pub. Bob Adams. R&P, Adv. contact Nancy True TEL 781-607-5260.

JOURNAL OF CAREER ASSESSMENT. see *PSYCHOLOGY*

JOURNAL OF COUNSELING & DEVELOPMENT. see *PSYCHOLOGY*

JOURNAL OF EMPLOYMENT COUNSELING. see *PSYCHOLOGY*

331.1 610 USA
MEDICAL INDUSTRY EMPLOYMENT OPPORTUNITIES. Text in English. s-m. USD 145 (effective 1998 & 1999). **Document type:** *Newsletter.* **Description:** Each issue profiles a new group of approximately 100 job openings nationwide, in almost all key medical manufacturing industry sectors.
Published by: Biomedical Market Newsletter, Inc., 3237 Idaho Pl, Costa Mesa, CA 92626-2207. TEL 714-434-9500, 800-875-8181, FAX 714-434-9755. Pub., R&P David G Anast.

371.42 610.73 USA ISSN 1076-7223
MINORITY NURSE. Text in English. 1993. s-a. USD 35 (effective 2000). adv. **Description:** Addresses career concerns of minority nursing professionals and the unique challenges and opportunities for these professionals.
Indexed: CINAHL.
—BLDSC (5810.553734).
Published by: C A S S Recruitment Media, 1800 Sherman Ave Ste 404, Evanston, IL 60201-3769. Eds. Paula Lipp TEL 215-269-8190, Tim Clancy. Pub. Tim Clancy. R&P Paula Lipp TEL 215-269-8190. adv.: B&W page USD 5,950, color page USD 7,145; trim 8 x 10.75. Circ: 30,000.

OPPORTUNITIES FOR MINORITY STUDENTS IN THE U.S. DENTAL SCHOOLS. see *EDUCATION—Higher Education*

331.1 610 USA ISSN 1071-0671
R690
PETERSON'S JOB OPPORTUNITIES IN HEALTH CARE. Text in English. a. USD 21.95. **Document type:** *Directory, Trade.* **Description:** Identifies hiring organizations in the healthcare field, including medical equipment and supply companies, pharmaceutical firms, health insurance and managed care companies, skilled nursing care facilities, hospitals, and medical laboratories.
Published by: Peterson's Magazine Group, 202 Carnegie Center, PO Box 2123, Princeton, NJ 08543-2123. TEL 609-243-9111, FAX 609-243-9150, http://www.petersons.com. Ed. Barbara Lawrence.

371.42 613 USA
RECRUITMENT DIRECTIONS. Text in English. 1985. 6/yr. USD 200. adv. bk.rev.
Published by: National Association for Healthcare Recruitment, PO Box 531107, Orlando, FL 32853-1107. TEL 407-843-6981, FAX 407-423-4648. Ed. Cathy Allman. R&P Karen Hart. Circ: 1,600.

REHABILITATION COUNSELING BULLETIN. see *HANDICAPPED*

331.1 360 USA
SOCIAL SERVICE JOBS. Text in English. 1975. fortn. USD 118; USD 142 foreign (effective 1999). adv. back issues avail. **Document type:** *Newsletter.* **Description:** List current jobs nationally in the areas of social work, psychology, and counseling.
Published by: Employment Listings for the Social Services, 10 Angela Dr, Framingham, MA 01701. TEL 508-626-8644, FAX 508-626-9389. Ed., R&P, Adv. contact M.B. Sack. Pub. M B Sack. Circ: 5,250 (paid).

UNIQUE OPPORTUNITIES; the physician's resource. see *MEDICAL SCIENCES*

371.42 USA ISSN 0740-8501
WASHINGTON COUNSELETTER. Text in English. 1963. m. (Oct.-May). USD 32.55 (effective 2000). bk.rev., film rev. **Document type:** *Newsletter.* **Description:** Publishes articles, events, programs, activities, and reviews of the professional literature of interest to counselors and educators.
Published by: Chronicle Guidance Publications, Inc., PO Box 1190, Moravia, NY 13118. TEL 315-497-0330, 800-622-7284, FAX 315-497-3359, customerservice@chronicleguidance.com, http://www.chronicleguidance.com. Circ: 5,250.

331.1 613.62 USA
WORK PROGRAMS SPECIAL INTEREST SECTION QUARTERLY. Text in English. 1987. q. USD 20 (effective 1999). **Document type:** *Newsletter.*
Formerly (until 199?): Work Programs Special Interest Section Newsletter (1043-1462)
Published by: American Occupational Therapy Association, Inc., 4720 Montgomery Lane, Bethesda, MD 20814-3425. TEL 301-652-2682, FAX 301-652-7711.

OCCUPATIONS AND CAREERS— Abstracting, Bibliographies, Statistics

FINLAND. TILASTOKESKUS. TERVEYS. see *PUBLIC HEALTH AND SAFETY—Abstracting, Bibliographies, Statistics*

OCEANOGRAPHY

see EARTH SCIENCES—Oceanography

OFFICE EQUIPMENT AND SERVICES

see BUSINESS AND ECONOMICS—Office Equipment And Services

ONCOLOGY

see MEDICAL SCIENCES—Oncology

DRUG RESISTANCE UPDATE. see *MEDICAL SCIENCES*

OPHTHALMOLOGY AND OPTOMETRY

see MEDICAL SCIENCES—Ophthalmology And Optometry

OPTICS

see PHYSICS—Optics

ORGANIC CHEMISTRY

see CHEMISTRY—Organic Chemistry

ORIENTAL STUDIES

see also HISTORY—History Of Asia; LINGUISTICS; LITERATURE; PHILOSOPHY

MERIDIANS (COLUMBIA); redefining health. see *ALTERNATIVE MEDICINE*

SHAMAN; journal of the international society for shamanistic research. see *ALTERNATIVE MEDICINE*

950 GBR ISSN 1355-8307
TAI CHI & ALTERNATIVE HEALTH. Text in English. q. GBP 12 domestic; GBP 16 in Europe; GBP 20 elsewhere; GBP 2.70 newsstand/cover; USD 6 newsstand/cover in United States (effective 2001). **Document type:** *Magazine, Consumer.* **Description:** Features in-depth articles on all aspects of Tai Chi Chuan - history, theory, martial applications as well as interviews with leading Tai Chi masters.
Address: PO Box 6404, London E18 1EX, United Kingdom. TEL 44-20-85029307, FAX 44-20-85517553, tcah@taichiwl.demon.co.uk, http://www.taichiwl.demon.co.uk. **Dist. by:** International Publishers Direct, 674 Via de la Valle, Ste 200, Solana Beach, CA 92075. TEL 619-481-5928, FAX 619-259-7580.

ORNITHOLOGY

see BIOLOGY—Ornithology

ORTHOPEDICS AND TRAUMATOLOGY

see MEDICAL SCIENCES—Orthopedics And Traumatology

OTORHINOLARYNGOLOGY

see MEDICAL SCIENCES—Otorhinolaryngology

OUTDOOR LIFE

see SPORTS AND GAMES—Outdoor Life

P

PACKAGING

658.7 664.09 USA ISSN 1085-2077
TP368
FOOD & DRUG PACKAGING. Text in English. 1959. m. USD 65; USD 75 in Canada; USD 140 elsewhere (effective 1999). adv. charts, illus, tr.lit. index. **Document type:** *Magazine, Trade.* **Description:** Industry journal covering new products, marketing trends and regulatory developments in packaging for the food, drug, pharmaceutical and cosmetic industries.
Former titles (until 1995): New Food and Drug Packaging (1075-3028); (until 1993): Food and Drug Packaging (0015-6272)
Related titles: Microform ed.; Online - full text ed.: (from Gale Group, Northern Light Technology, Inc., Factiva).
Indexed: Alloys Ind., Bus.& Indus. (Jun.1994-), Int.Packag.Abstr., Met.Abstr., Met.Abstr.Ind., Nonfer.Met.Alert, PCC Alert, PROMT, Steels Alert.
—BLDSC (3977.033000).
Published by: Stagnito Communications, Inc. (Subsidiary of: Medical World Communications), Stagnito Packaging Group, 210 S Fifth St, St. Charles, IL 60174. TEL 630-377-0100, FAX 630-377-1678, comments@packaginginfo.com, info@stagnito.com, http://www.packaginginfo.com, http://www.stagnito.com. adv.: B&W page USD 7,330. Circ: 74,833.

688.8 615 USA ISSN 1081-5481
PHARMACEUTICAL & MEDICAL PACKAGING NEWS. Text in English. 1993. m. USD 150 (effective 2001); free to qualified personnel. adv. **Document type:** *Trade.*
Indexed: Alloys Ind., I.P.A., Int.Packag.Abstr., Met.Abstr., Met.Abstr.Ind., Nonfer.Met.Alert, PCC Alert, Steels Alert.
—BLDSC (6442.755000).
Published by: Canon Communications LLC, 11444 W Olympic Blvd, Ste 900, Los Angeles, CA 90064-1549. TEL 310-445-4200, FAX 310-445-4299, feedback@devicelink.com, http://www.devicelink.com/pmpn. Ed. Daphne Allen. Pub. William F Cobert. Adv. contact Patricia Spinner. B&W page USD 3,895, color page USD 4,990. Circ: 20,040 (controlled).

PHARMACEUTICAL MANUFACTURING & PACKING SOURCER. see *PHARMACY AND PHARMACOLOGY*

PAINTS AND PROTECTIVE COATINGS

667.6 614.85 GBR ISSN 0967-2508
COATINGS, REGULATIONS AND THE ENVIRONMENT. Abbreviated title: C O R E. Text in English. 1981. m. GBP 220 to non-members; GBP 200 to members (effective Jan. 2000). abstr. index. **Document type:** *Abstract/Index.* **Description:** Provides up-to-date information on safety, health and environmental issues relevant to the coatings industry.
Former titles (until 1992): Survey on Hazards, Pollution and Legislation in the Coating Field (0953-8801); (until 1986): Hazards, Pollution and Legislation in the Coatings Field (0262-7116)
Indexed: CSNB, Curr.Cont. (coverage dropped), Lab.Haz.Bull.
—BLDSC (3292.608400), Infotrieve. **CCC.**
Published by: Paint Research Association, 8 Waldgreave Rd, Teddington, Middx TW11 8EP, United Kingdom. TEL 44-20-8614-4800, FAX 44-208-943-4705, coatings@pra.org.uk, http://www.pra.org.uk. Ed. Yvonne Kershaw.

667.6 DEU ISSN 0945-8409
RADCURELETTER. Text in English. bi-m. DEM 168, USD 116 (effective 1998). adv. **Document type:** *Trade.*
Indexed: World Surf.Coat.
Published by: (European Association for the Advancement of Radiation Curing), Vincentz Verlag, Schiffgraben 43, Hannover 30175, Germany. TEL 49-511-9910235, FAX 49-511-9910299, info@coatings.de, info@vincentz.de, http://www.coatings.de, http://www.vincentz.de. Ed. Dr. Frank Rothbarth. Adv. contact Frauke Hallwass. Circ: 1,096.

363.7 GBR
S H E ALERT. (Safety, Health and the Environment) Text in English. m. GBP 500 to non-members; GBP 430 to members (effective Jan. 2000). **Document type:** *Bulletin.*
Published by: Paint Research Association, 8 Waldegrave Rd, Teddington, Middx TW11 8LD, United Kingdom. TEL 44-20-8977-4427, coatings@pra.org.uk, http://www.pra.org.uk. Ed. Yvonne Kershaw.

PALEONTOLOGY

ALTENBURGER NATURWISSENSCHAFTLICHE FORSCHUNGEN. see *BIOLOGY*

AMERICAN MUSEUM NOVITATES. see *BIOLOGY—Zoology*

CARNEGIE MUSEUM OF NATURAL HISTORY. ANNALS. see *SCIENCES: COMPREHENSIVE WORKS*

CARNEGIE MUSEUM OF NATURAL HISTORY. BULLETIN. see *SCIENCES: COMPREHENSIVE WORKS*

595.33 591 USA ISSN 0886-3806
CYPRIS; international ostracoda newsletter. Text in English. 1983. a. membership. bk.rev. bibl. **Document type:** *Newsletter.* **Description:** To improve international contacts between ostracode workers.
Related titles: Online - full text ed.
Indexed: GeoRef.
Published by: International Research Group on Ostracoda, U S Geological Survey, Federal Center, MS 300, PO Box 25046, Denver, CO 80225. TEL 303-236-5440, FAX 303-236-5448, http://ncgmp.cr.usgs.gov/ncgmp/ostracodes. Ed. Elizabeth Brouers. Circ: 400 (controlled).

DORTMUNDER BEITRAEGE ZUR LANDESKUNDE. see *BIOLOGY*

560 579 DEU ISSN 0932-4739
QH274 CODEN: EJPREZ
EUROPEAN JOURNAL OF PROTISTOLOGY. Text in English. 1964. 4/yr. EUR 153 domestic to individuals; GBP 106 foreign to individuals; EUR 368 domestic to institutions; GBP 327 foreign to institutions (effective 2002). abstr, bibl, charts, illus. *Refereed.* **Document type:** *Journal, Academic/Scholarly.*
Formerly: Protistologica (0033-1821)
Related titles: Online - full text ed.: (from Institute for Scientific Information).
Indexed: ASCA, Abstr.Hyg., Aqua.Sci.& Fish.Abstr., Bio-Contr.News & Info., Biol.Abstr., Chem.Abstr., Curr.Adv.Ecol.Sci., Curr.Adv.Plant Sci., Curr.Cont., Deep Sea Res.& Oceanogr.Abstr., Entomol.Abstr., Environ.Sci.Poll.Mgmt., GeoRef, Helminthol.Abstr., Ind.Sci.Rev., Ind.Vet., Int.Abstr.Biol.Sci., Microbiol.Abstr., Nutr.Abstr., Plant Sci., Protozool.Abstr., Rev.Appl.Entomol., Sci.Cit.Ind., Sel.Water Res.Abstr., Soils & Fert., Sport Fish.Abstr., Trop.Dis.Bull., Vet.Bull., Zoo.Rec.
—BLDSC (3829.737600), CASDDS, CISTI, IDS, Infotrieve, ingenta, Linda Hall. **CCC.**
Published by: (France. Centre National de la Recherche Scientifique FRA), Urban & Fischer Verlag, Loebdergraben 14a, Jena 07743, Germany. TEL 49-3641-626444, FAX 49-3641-626500, journals@urbanfischer.de, http://www.urbanfischer.de/journal. Ed. M A Sleigh. R&P Martin Huber TEL 49-3641-626430. Circ: 450. **Subscr. to:** Nature Publishing Group, Brunel Rd, Basingstoke RG21 6XS, United Kingdom. TEL 44-1256-302629, FAX 44-1256-463570, j.stephens@macmillan.com.

FLORIDA MUSEUM OF NATURAL HISTORY. BULLETIN. see *BIOLOGY*

GORTANIA; atti del Museo Friulano di Storia Naturale. see *SCIENCES: COMPREHENSIVE WORKS*

570.9 CHE ISSN 0891-2963
QE701 CODEN: HIBIEW
HISTORICAL BIOLOGY; an international journal of paleobiology. Text in English. 1988. 4/yr. GBP 79, USD 96, EUR 106 to individuals; GBP 391, USD 510, EUR 520 to institutions; GBP 645, USD 836, EUR 859 to corporations (effective 2002). illus. back issues avail.; reprints avail. *Refereed.* **Document type:** *Academic/Scholarly.* **Description:** Provides a vehicle for developments in the sciences concerned with the history of life through geological time and the biology of past organism.
Related titles: CD-ROM ed.; Microform ed.; Online - full text ed.: (from RoweCom Information Quest).
Indexed: Ecol.Abstr., GeoRef, Geol.Abstr., Zoo.Rec.
—BLDSC (4316.155000), CISTI. **CCC.**
Published by: Gordon and Breach - Harwood Academic (Subsidiary of: Taylor & Francis Group), PO Box 531, Lausanne 1000, Switzerland. http://www.gbhap.com/Historical_Biology/; http://biomednet.com./library/357. Eds. A Hallam, R Thomas. **Subscr. addr. in US:** International Publishers Direct, PO Box 32160, Newark, NJ 07102. FAX 215-750-6343.

560 CHE ISSN 1042-0940
QE720.5 CODEN: ICHSER
ICHNOS; the study of plant and animal traces. Text in English. 1990. 4/yr. GBP 86, USD 127, EUR 127 to individuals; GBP 421, USD 599, EUR 604 to institutions; GBP 647, USD 932, EUR 943 to corporations (effective 2002). *Refereed.* **Document type:** *Academic/Scholarly.*
Related titles: CD-ROM ed.; Microform ed.; Online - full text ed.: (from RoweCom Information Quest).
Indexed: AESIS, Geo.Abstr.P.G., GeoRef, Geol.Abstr., Zoo.Rec.
—BLDSC (4361.843000), CISTI, Infotrieve, ingenta. **CCC.**
Published by: Gordon and Breach - Harwood Academic (Subsidiary of: Taylor & Francis Group), PO Box 531, Lausanne 1000, Switzerland. http://www.gbhap.com/Ichnos/. Eds. George Pemberton, Ronald Pickerill. **Subscr. addr. in US:** International Publishers Direct, PO Box 32160, Newark, NJ 07102. FAX 215-750-6343.

NATURWISSENSCHAFTLICHER VEREIN IN HAMBURG. ABHANDLUNGEN. see *BIOLOGY—Zoology*

NATURWISSENSCHAFTLICHER VEREIN ZU BREMEN. ABHANDLUNGEN. see *BIOLOGY*

NATUURHISTORISCH GENOOTSCHAP IN LIMBURG. PUBLICATIES. see *BIOLOGY*

NEUROTOXINS. see *MEDICAL SCIENCES—Psychiatry And Neurology*

SOUTH AFRICAN MUSEUM. ANNALS/SUID-AFRIKAANSE MUSEUM. ANNALE. see *BIOLOGY*

STUDI PER L'ECOLOGIA DEL QUATERNARIO. see *ANTHROPOLOGY*

PAPER AND PULP

see also FORESTS AND FORESTRY—Lumber And Wood; PACKAGING

PARAPSYCHOLOGY AND OCCULTISM

see also NEW AGE PUBLICATIONS

133 150 AUS ISSN 1035-9621
AUSTRALIAN PARAPSYCHOLOGICAL REVIEW. Text in English. 1983. 2/yr. AUD 20. bk.rev. charts, illus. back issues avail. **Document type:** *Newsletter, Academic/Scholarly.* **Description:** Promotes scientific study of parapsychological and related phenomena. Emphasis on Australian studies.
Former titles: Australian Institute of Parapsychological Research Bulletin; Australian Institute of Psychic Research Bulletin (0813-2194)
Indexed: e-psyche.
Published by: Australian Institute of Parapsychological Research Inc., PO Box 176, Annandale, NSW 2038, Australia. TEL 61-2-95163291, M.Hough@cchs.usyd.edu.au. Ed. Harvey Irwin. Circ: 400.

133 370.15 150 371.42 USA
DIMENSIONS (RIMROCK). Text in English. 1980. bi-m. USD 20. adv. bk.rev. **Document type:** *Newsletter.*
Indexed: e-psyche.
Published by: Delphi Publications, 654 S 12th St, Cottonwood, AZ 86326-4511. TEL 520-634-2390, FAX 520-539-3689. Ed., R&P Jay Harris. Adv. contact Dean Jeffries. Circ: 10,000.

IMAGINATION, COGNITION AND PERSONALITY. see *PSYCHOLOGY*

130 USA ISSN 0022-3387
BF1001 CODEN: JPRPAU
JOURNAL OF PARAPSYCHOLOGY; a scientific quarterly dealing with extrasensory perception, the psychokinetic effect and related topics. Text in English. 1937. q. USD 40 to individuals; USD 46 foreign to individuals; USD 25 to students; USD 31 foreign to students (effective 2000). adv. bk.rev. abstr, bibl, charts, illus. index. back issues avail.; reprint service avail. from PQC,PSC,SCH,ISI. *Refereed.* **Document type:** *Academic/Scholarly.*
Related titles: Microform ed.: (from PQC); Online - full text ed.: (from Gale Group, ProQuest Information & Learning, Northern Light Technology, Inc., H. W. Wilson, Factiva, Institute for Scientific Information).

P

Indexed: ASCA, ASSIA, Biol.Abstr., Curr.Cont., Excerp.Med., IBZ, Ind.Philos., Mid.East: Abstr.& Ind., Psyclnfo, Psychol.Abstr. (1937-), Ref.Zh., Russ.Acad.Sci.Bibl., SSCI, Soc.Sci.Ind. (Mar.1982-), e-psyche.
—BLDSC (5028.800000), IDS, Infotrieve, ingenta. **CCC.**
Published by: (Rhine Research Center), Parapsychology Press, 402 N Buchanan Blvd, Durham, NC 27701-1728. TEL 919-688-8241, FAX 919-683-4338, journal@rhine.org, http://www.rhine.org. Ed. John Palmer. R&P, Adv. contact Paul Blue. Circ: 1,000 (paid).

REALITY CHANGE; the global Seth journal. see *NEW AGE PUBLICATIONS*

SUBTLE ENERGIES AND ENERGY MEDICINE; an interdisciplinary journal of energetic and informational interactions. see *PHYSICS*

TRANSFORMATION TIMES; new age journal. see *NEW AGE PUBLICATIONS*

PATENTS, TRADEMARKS AND COPYRIGHTS

EXPERT OPINION ON THERAPEUTIC PATENTS; authoritative analysis of patenting trends. see *PHARMACY AND PHARMACOLOGY*

608.7 DEU ISSN 0941-0031
EXTRACTS FROM EUROPEAN PATENT SPECIFICATIONS. PART 2. ELECTRICITY, PHYSICS, PRECISION ENGINEERING, OPTICS AND ACOUSTICS. Text in English. w. DEM 1,746 (effective 2000). **Document type:** *Journal, Abstract/Index.*
Related titles: ♦ German ed.: Auszuege aus den Europaeischen Patentschriften. Teil 2. Elektrotechnik, Physik, Feinmechanik und Optik, Akustik. ISSN 0941-0015.
Published by: Wila Verlag Wilhelm Lampl GmbH, Landsberger Str 191A, Munich 80687, Germany. TEL 49-89-547560, FAX 49-89-54756309, info@wila-verlag.de, http://www.wila-verlag.de. Ed. Michael Lipp. Adv. contact Petra Benesch.

FEDERAL BIO-TECHNOLOGY TRANSFER DIRECTORY. see *BIOLOGY—Biotechnology*

GUIDE TO MEDICAL DEVICE REGISTRATION IN JAPAN. see *MEDICAL SCIENCES*

608.7 DEU
INFORMATION SOURCES IN PATENTS. Text in English. 1992. irreg. GBP 56 (effective 2001). **Document type:** *Directory, Trade.* **Description:** Enables information professionals and librarians to evaluate information sources on patents.
Published by: K.G. Saur Verlag (Subsidiary of: Gale Group), Ortlerstr 8, Munich 81373, Germany. TEL 49-89-76902-0, FAX 49-89-76902150, info@saur.de, http://www.saur.de. Ed. C P Auger.

PATENT FAST-ALERT. see *PHARMACY AND PHARMACOLOGY*

PATENTS, TRADEMARKS AND COPYRIGHTS—Abstracting, Bibliographies, Statistics

C A SELECTS. PHARMACEUTICAL CHEMISTRY (PATENTS). see *PHARMACY AND PHARMACOLOGY—Abstracting, Bibliographies, Statistics*

PEDIATRICS

see MEDICAL SCIENCES—Pediatrics

PERFUMES AND COSMETICS

see BEAUTY CULTURE—Perfumes And Cosmetics

PERSONAL COMPUTERS

see COMPUTERS—Personal Computers

PERSONNEL MANAGEMENT

see BUSINESS AND ECONOMICS—Personnel Management

PETROLEUM AND GAS

C O N C A W E REVIEW. see *ENVIRONMENTAL STUDIES*

CHEMICALS, DRUGS, PHARMACEUTICALS, PETROLEUM, PETROCHEMICALS, FERTILIZERS. see *ENGINEERING—Chemical Engineering*

665.5 661.804 USA
N P R A NATIONAL SAFETY CONFERENCE. PROCEEDINGS. Text in English. a. USD 10 per issue to non-members (effective 1999 & 2000). back issues avail. **Document type:** *Proceedings, Academic/Scholarly.* **Description:** Presents research into petrochemical plant and refinery safety.
Indexed: API Abstr.
Published by: National Petroleum Refiners Association, 1899 L St, NW, Ste 1000, Washington, DC 20036-3896. TEL 202-457-0480, FAX 202-457-0486, http://www.npradc.org.

UNITED KINGDOM OFFSHORE HEALTH & SAFETY MANAGEMENT GUIDE. see *OCCUPATIONAL HEALTH AND SAFETY*

UNITED KINGDOM OFFSHORE HEALTH & SAFETY MANAGEMENT NEWSLETTER. see *OCCUPATIONAL HEALTH AND SAFETY*

PETROLEUM AND GAS—Abstracting, Bibliographies, Statistics

016.3637 USA ISSN 1067-1013
E & P HEALTH, SAFETY AND ENVIRONMENT. (Exploration and Production) Text in English. 1993. m. USD 190 (effective 2000). **Document type:** *Abstract/Index.* **Description:** Covers petroleum-related literature and patents relevant to environmental, health and safety issues, including remediation, pollution control, incident response, and spill recovery.
Related titles: Online - full text ed.
Published by: University of Tulsa, Information Services Division, 600 S College Ave, Tulsa, OK 74104-3189. TEL 918-631-2297, 800-247-8678, FAX 918-599-9361, TELEX 497543, question@tured.pa.utulsa.edu, http://www.pa.utulsa.edu/. Ed. Rafael E Ubico.

INDEX AND ABSTRACTS OF A P I HEALTH-RELATED RESEARCH (YEARS). see *PUBLIC HEALTH AND SAFETY—Abstracting, Bibliographies, Statistics*

N P R A STATISTICAL REPORT. ANNUAL SURVEY OF OCCUPATIONAL INJURIES & INJURIES. see *OCCUPATIONAL HEALTH AND SAFETY—Abstracting, Bibliographies, Statistics*

PETS

see also ANIMAL WELFARE

636.7 USA
AMERICAN KENNEL CLUB PUPPIES. Text in English. a. **Description:** Contains information for new puppy owners.
Published by: American Kennel Club, Inc., 260 Madison Ave, New York, NY 10016. TEL 212-696-8260, FAX 212-696-8217. Pub. George Berger TEL 212-696-8282. Adv. contact Gina Lash TEL 212-696-8260.

636 ESP ISSN 0214-3151
ANIMALIA; revista especializada en animales de compania. Text in Spanish. m. (11/yr.). ESP 15,000; ESP 17,500 foreign (effective 1999). adv. **Document type:** *Trade.* **Description:** Dedicated to pets, including health care, medicines, diet, show activities and more.
Indexed: Anim.Behav.Abstr., Aqua.Sci.& Fish.Abstr., Aquacult.Abstr., Entomol.Abstr., Environ.Sci.Poll.Mgmt., Pollut.Abstr., Zoo.Rec.
Published by: Elsevier Informacion Profesional, SA (Subsidiary of: Reed Elsevier plc), Entenca 28, Apdo. No. 350 F.D., Barcelona 08015, Spain. TEL 34-3-292-4638, FAX 34-3-425-2880. Ed. Antoni Prats I Esteve. Pub., Adv. contact Manuel Masip. Circ: 7,000.

636.7 179.3 POL ISSN 1231-6857
ASKO; dwumiesiecznik kynologiczny. Key Title: As. Text in Polish. 1991. bi-m. PLZ 20, USD 20. adv. bk.rev. charts, illus, tr.lit. back issues avail. **Document type:** *Academic/Scholarly, Consumer.* **Description:** Concentrates on animal welfare, especially dogs. Provides description of dog races, short essays concerning dog shows.
Published by: Wydawnictwo As, Ul Kozielska 120 a, Raciborz 47411, Poland. TEL 48-36-4157932. Ed. Elzbieta Boruch Priebe. adv.: page PLZ 800. Circ: 10,000.

636 SWE ISSN 0006-4076
BLAA STJAERNAN; djurvaard inom totalfoersvaret. Text in Swedish. 1965. 6/yr. SEK 180 to non-members. adv. bk.rev. illus. **Document type:** *Newsletter.*
Published by: Svenska Blaa Stjaernan, Linneg 89, Fack 5435, Stockholm 11484, Sweden. TEL 46-8-788-76-97, FAX 46-8-788-76-97. Eds. Karin Wiebe, Nina von Krusenstierna. Circ: 9,000.

636 GBR
BUDGERIGAR WORLD. Text in English. 1974. m. GBP 30, USD 60 (effective 2001). adv. bk.rev. 48 p./no. back issues avail. **Document type:** *Magazine.*
Published by: Budgerigar World Ltd., County Press Buildings, Station Rd, Bala, Gwynedd LL23 7PG, United Kingdom. TEL 44-1678-521251, budgerigarworld@msn.com. Ed. T A Tuxford. Pub. G. Evans. Adv. contact G Evans.

COMPANION ANIMAL PRACTICE. see *VETERINARY SCIENCE*

F A B JOURNAL. see *ANIMAL WELFARE*

636.7 362.41 USA
GUIDE LINES (YORKTOWN HEIGHTS). Text in English. 1954. q. free per issue. **Document type:** *Newsletter.*
Published by: Guiding Eyes for the Blind, 611 Granite Springs Rd, Yorktown Heights, NY 10598-3499. Ed. Karen McClure.

HENSTON VETERINARY VADE MECUM (SMALL ANIMAL). see *VETERINARY SCIENCE*

636 GBR
KENNEL AND CATTERY MANAGEMENT. Text in English. 1983. m. GBP 14; GBP 18 foreign (effective 2002). bk.rev. back issues avail. **Document type:** *Trade.* **Description:** Covers nutrition, hygiene, veterinary advice, breeding, and management.
Published by: Albatross Publications, Albatross Publications, PO Box 523, Horsham, West Sussex, Surrey RH12 4WL, United Kingdom. TEL 44-1293-871201. Ed., Pub., Adv. contact Carol Andrews. Circ: 3,500.

179.3 USA ISSN 1090-3992
N A C A NEWS. Text in English. 1978. bi-m. USD 25 domestic; USD 30 foreign (effective 2001). adv. bk.rev., film rev. charts, stat, tr.lit. 44 p./no. **Document type:** *Trade.*
Indexed: Aquacult.Abstr.
Published by: National Animal Control Association, PO Box 480851, Kansas City, MO 64148-0851. TEL 913-768-1319, FAX 913-768-1378, naca@interserv.com, http://www.nacanet.org. Ed., Pub., R&P, Adv. contact John Mays. Circ: 4,500.

PARTNERS (SYLMAR). see *SOCIAL SERVICES AND WELFARE*

636.7 362.41 USA
PILOT DOGS. Text in English. 1950. q. free per issue.
Published by: Pilot Light, 625 W Town St, Columbus, OH 43215.

PRATIQUE MEDICALE ET CHIRURGICALE DE L'ANIMAL DE COMPAGNIE. see *VETERINARY SCIENCE*

636 FRA ISSN 0768-8733
SANS LAISSE; magazine de l'education et des sports canins. Text in French. 1978. m. FRF 290 domestic; FRF 350 foreign. adv. bk.rev. index. *Refereed.* **Document type:** *Bulletin.* **Description:** Publishes articles on dog ownership as sport.
Formerly (until 1987): Berger Allemand (0183-3197)
Published by: S A R L Sans Laisse, 76 rue Jules Ferry, Lunel 34400, France. TEL 46-7715569, FAX 46-7910089, sans.laisse@wanadoo.fr. Ed., R&P Alain Dupont. Adv. contact Cathy Hugon. Circ: 18,000.

636.089 GBR ISSN 0268-991X
YOU & YOUR VET. Text in English. 1985. q. adv. bk.rev. **Document type:** *Consumer.* **Description:** Discusses pet care and veterinary topics of interest to the general public.

Published by: British Veterinary Association, 7 Mansfield St, London W1M 0AT, United Kingdom. TEL 0171-636-6541, FAX 0171-637-0620. Ed. Martin Alder. Adv. contact Gillian Notton. Circ: 50,000.

PHARMACY AND PHARMACOLOGY

see also DRUG ABUSE AND ALCOHOLISM; MEDICAL SCIENCES

1199 NEWS. see *LABOR UNIONS*

615 378 USA
A A C P NEWS. Text in English. 1972. m. USD 25 (effective 1998). adv. bibl, illus. **Document type:** *Newsletter.*
Published by: American Association of Colleges of Pharmacy, 1426 Prince St, Alexandria, VA 22314-2815. TEL 703-739-2330. Ed. C Edwin Webb. Circ: 2,500.

615 SWE ISSN 1103-1255
A A F - TIDNINGEN. Text in Swedish. 1955. q. SEK 175 to members. adv. **Document type:** *Magazine, Trade.*
Former titles (until 1992): Medlemsblad - A A F; (until 1984): A S F Medlemsblad; (until 1963): Apoteksstaederskefoerbundets Medlemsblad
Published by: Apoteksanstaelldas Foerbund (AAF), Fack 176, Stockholm 10123, Sweden. TEL 46-8-7231625, FAX 46-8-7231624. Ed. Eva Ruden. adv.: B&W page SEK 2,800, color page SEK 4,800; 217 x 280.

615 USA
A A P S NEWS* . Text in English. 1986. m. (except Nov.). membership. adv. **Document type:** *Newsletter.*
Formerly: A A P S Newsletter
Published by: American Association of Pharmaceutical Scientists, 2107 Wilson Blvd #700, Arlington, VA 22201-3042. TEL 703-548-3000, FAX 703-684-7349. Ed., R&P, Adv. contact Jon Bowen TEL 703-518-8413. Circ: 9,000 (controlled).

615 USA ISSN 1063-8792
CODEN: ADINE4
A H F S DRUG INFORMATION. Text in English. 1959. base vol. updates 3/yr. USD 169.95 domestic; USD 258.95 foreign (effective 2001). 3720 p./no. reprint service avail. from PQC. **Document type:** *Academic/Scholarly.* **Description:** Contains detailed monographs on virtually every drug entity available in the US. Includes information on uses, cautions, drug interactions, chemistry, stability, pharmacology, pharmaco-kinetics, toxicity, dosage and administration.
Formerly (until 1984): American Hospital Formulary Service (8756-6028)
Related titles: CD-ROM ed.: A H F Sfirst Professional and Enterprise. 1996. USD 375 (effective 2001); Online - full text ed.: Drug Information. 1984 (from Data-Star, The Dialog Corporation).
—Infotrieve. **CCC.**
Published by: (American Hospital Formulary Service), American Society of Health-System Pharmacists, 7272 Wisconsin Ave, Bethesda, MD 20814. TEL 301-657-3000, FAX 301-657-1251, 301-657-8857, ahfs@ashp.org, pdiso@ashp.org, http://www.ashp.org. Ed. Gerald K McEvoy.

615.19 USA
A I H P NOTES. Text in English. 1955. q. membership. back issues avail. **Document type:** *Newsletter.* **Description:** News and information on the history of pharmacy and about activities of the institute.
Published by: American Institute of the History of Pharmacy, Pharmacy Bldg, Madison, WI 53706. TEL 608-262-5635. Ed. Beth D Fisher. Circ: 1,000.

A P S BULLETIN. see *MEDICAL SCIENCES—Anaesthesiology*

615 DEU
A P V NEWS. (Arbeitsgemeinschaft fuer Pharmazeutische Verfahrenstechnik) Text in German. q. **Document type:** *Journal, Trade.*
Published by: Arbeitsgemeinschaft fuer Pharmazeutische Verfahrenstechnik e. V., Kurfuerstenstr 59, Mainz 55118, Germany. TEL 49-6131-97690, FAX 49-6131-976969, apv@apv-mainz.de, http://www.apv-mainz.de. Circ: 21,000 (controlled). **Co-publisher:** Editio Cantor Verlag.

615 USA ISSN 1050-5725
A S C P UPDATE. Text in English. 1969. bi-m., latest vol.31. USD 24. bk.rev. 8 p./no. 3 cols./p. back issues avail. **Document type:** *Newsletter, Government, Trade.* **Description:** News on issues and legislation relevant to members of the American Society of Consultant Pharmacists.
Related titles: Online - full text ed.
Published by: American Society of Consultant Pharmacists, 1321 Duke St, Alexandria, VA 22314-3563. TEL 703-739-1300, FAX 703-739-1321, http://www.ascp.com/public/pubs/update/. Ed., R&P Jill F Johnson TEL 703-739-1300. Pub. Robert D Appel. Circ: 6,500.

615.1 USA ISSN 0001-2483
A S H P NEWSLETTER. Text in English. 1968. m. membership. illus. **Document type:** *Newsletter.* **Description:** Contains articles on pharmacy and member news.
—Infotrieve. **CCC.**
Published by: American Society of Health-System Pharmacists, 7272 Wisconsin Ave, Bethesda, MD 20814. TEL 301-657-3000, FAX 301-657-1615. Circ: 30,000.

615.1 370.58 USA
ACCREDITED PROFESSIONAL PROGRAMS OF COLLEGES AND SCHOOLS OF PHARMACY. Variant title: American Council on Pharmaceutical Education Annual Directory (Years). Text in English. 1940. a. free. *Refereed.* **Document type:** *Directory.*
Formerly: Accredited Colleges of Pharmacy (0065-7980)
Published by: American Council on Pharmaceutical Education, 311 W Superior St, Ste 512, Chicago, IL 60610. TEL 312-664-3575, FAX 312-664-4652. Ed. Dr. Peter H Vlasses. Circ: 10,000.

ACTA BIOLOGICA IUGOSLAVICA. SERIJA C: IUGOSLAVICA PHYSIOLOGICA ET PHARMACOLOGICA ACTA. see *BIOLOGY*

615.1 HRV ISSN 1330-0075
RS1 CODEN: ACPHEE
ACTA PHARMACEUTICA. Text in English. 1951. q. USD 40 (effective 1998). adv. bk.rev. charts, illus. index, cum.index. reprint service avail. from ISI. *Refereed.* **Document type:** *Academic/Scholarly.* **Description:** Publishes review articles, original papers and preliminary communications dealing with pharmacy and related fields.
Formerly (until 1992): Acta Pharmaceutica Iugoslavica (0001-6667)
Related titles: Online - full text ed.
Indexed: ASCA, Agri.& Environ.Biotech.Abstr. (coverage dropped), Anal.Abstr., Biol.Abstr., Chem.Abstr., Chem.Indus.Notes, Chem.Titles, Curr.Adv.Ecol.Sci., Curr.Cont. (coverage dropped), Derwent Biotech.Abstr., Excerp.Med., Hort.Abstr., INIS Atomind., I.P.A., Ind.Sci.Rev., MOS, NPU, Plant Breed.Abstr., Ref.Zh., Sci.Cit.Ind. (coverage dropped).
—BLDSC (0645.650000), CASDDS, CISTI, EMDOCS, GNLM, IDS, KNAW, Linda Hall.
Published by: Hrvatsko Farmaceutsko Drustvo/Croatian Pharmaceutical Society, Masarykova 2, Zagreb 10000, Croatia. TEL 385-1-427944, FAX 385-1-431301. Ed. Svjetlana Luterotti. Adv. contact Marina Carevic. Circ: 600.

615.1 HUN ISSN 0001-6659
CODEN: APHGAO
ACTA PHARMACEUTICA HUNGARICA. Text mainly in Hungarian; Summaries in English. 1925. bi-m. HUF 2,100; HUF 350 newsstand/cover (effective 1999). adv. bk.rev. charts, illus. back issues avail.; reprint service avail. from IRC. **Document type:** *Academic/Scholarly.*
Related titles: Online - full text ed.
Indexed: Agri.& Environ.Biotech.Abstr. (coverage dropped), Anal.Abstr., Aqua.Sci.& Fish.Abstr., Biol.Abstr., Chem.Abstr., Chem.Indus.Notes, Chem.Titles, Dent.Ind., Derwent Biotech.Abstr., Environ.Sci.Poll.Mgmt., Excerp.Med., Hort.Abstr., INIS Atomind., I.P.A., Ind.Med. (1953-), NPU, Pollut.Abstr., Risk Abstr., Tox.Abstr.
—BLDSC (0645.000000), CASDDS, CISTI, GNLM, KNAW, Linda Hall.
Published by: Magyar Gyogyszereszeti Tarsasag/Hungarian Pharmaceutical Association, Gyomroi ut 19-21, PO Box 27, Budapest 1475, Hungary. TEL 36-1-4314620, FAX 36-1-2605604, TELEX 22-5067, s.gorog@richter.hu. Ed., R&P Sandor Gorog. Pub. Z Vincze. Adv. contact Zoltan Hanko. Circ: 2,900. **Subscr. to:** Kultura, PO Box 149, Budapest 1389, Hungary.

615.19 TUR ISSN 1300-638X
CODEN: APTUES
ACTA PHARMACEUTICA TURCICA. Text in English, French, German; Summaries in English, Turkish. 1954. q., latest vol.43. USD 10 domestic; USD 30 foreign (effective 2001). bk.rev. abstr. back issues avail. *Refereed.* **Document type:** *Proceedings, Academic/Scholarly.* **Description:** Publishes original research and reviews concerning pharmacy, pharmacology, cosmetics, medicine, chemistry, environment, microbiology, biology and biotechnology.
Formerly (until 1984): Eczacilik Bulteni (0367-0236)
Indexed: Anal.Abstr., Biol.Abstr., Chem.Abstr., Chem.Indus.Notes, Chem.Titles, Dairy Sci.Abstr., Excerp.Med., Food Sci.& Tech.Abstr., Herb.Abstr., Hort.Abstr., I.P.A., NPU, Protozool.Abstr., Rev.Arom.& Med.Plants, Rev.Med.& Vet.Mycol.
—BLDSC (0646.619000), CASDDS, EMDOCS, GNLM, KNAW.
Published by: ETAM A.S. Matbaa Tesisleri, Anadolu Universitesi Eczacilik Fakultesi, Eczacilik Teknolojisi Bolumu, Eskisehir 26470, Turkey. TEL 90-222-2360051, 90-222-3350581, FAX 90-222-3350750, lgenc@anadolu.edu.tr, http://www.anadolu.edu.tr. Ed., Pub., R&P, Adv. contact Erden Guler. Circ: 1,125; 1,125 (controlled).

615 CHN
ACTA PHARMACOLOGICA SINICA. Text in English. m. back issues avail. **Document type:** *Academic/Scholarly.*
Related titles: Online - full content ed.: (from WanFang Data Corp.); ♦ Chinese ed.: Zhongguo Yaoli Xuebao. ISSN 0253-9756.
Indexed: Anim.Breed.Abstr., Ind.Med. (2000-), Inpharma, Nutr.Abstr., Pharm.&Out.News, Protozool.Abstr., Reac., Rev.Appl.Entomol., Rev.Arom.& Med.Plants, Sugar Ind.Abstr.
Published by: (Zhongguo Yaoli Xueyuan/Chinese Pharmacological Society), Shanghai Institute of Materia Medica (Subsidiary of: Chinese Academy of Sciences/Zhongguo Kexueyuan), 294 Taiyuan Rd, Shanghai 200031, China. Ed. Dr. Guang-Sheng Ding.

ACTA PHYSIOLOGICA ET PHARMACOLOGICA BULGARICA. see *BIOLOGY—Physiology*

ACTA PHYSIOLOGICA HUNGARICA. see *BIOLOGY—Physiology*

ACTA PHYSIOLOGICA PHARMACOLOGICA ET THERAPEUTICA LATINOAMERICANA; fisiologia, farmacologia, bioquimica y ciencias afines. see *BIOLOGY—Physiology*

615.1 POL ISSN 0001-6837
CODEN: APPHAX
ACTA POLONIAE PHARMACEUTICA; drug research. Text and summaries in English. 1937. bi-m. USD 180 (effective 1998). charts, illus. index. *Refereed.* **Document type:** *Academic/Scholarly.* **Description:** Publishes scientific papers on pharmaceutical analysis, natural drugs, pharmacology, and drug synthesis.
Indexed: ASCA, Agri.& Environ.Biotech.Abstr. (coverage dropped), Biol.Abstr., Chem.Abstr., Chem.Indus.Notes, Chem.Titles, Curr.Adv.Ecol.Sci., Curr.Chem.React. (coverage dropped), Derwent Biotech.Abstr., Excerp.Med., Helminthol.Abstr., Hort.Abstr., INIS Atomind., I.P.A., Ind.Chem. (coverage dropped), Ind.Med. (1937-), Ind.Sci.Rev., MOS, NPU, Nutr.Abstr., Sci.Cit.Ind. (coverage dropped).
—BLDSC (0659.000000), CASDDS, CISTI, EMDOCS, GNLM, Linda Hall.
Published by: Polskie Towarzystwo Farmaceutyczne/Polish Pharmaceutical Society, Ul Dluga 16, Warsaw 00238, Poland. TEL 48-22-0310241, FAX 48-22-8310243. Ed. Aleksander P Mazurek.

ACTA TOXICOLOGICA ET THERAPEUTICA; international journal of toxicology, pharmacology and therapy. see *ENVIRONMENTAL STUDIES—Toxicology And Environmental Safety*

615.1 CAN ISSN 1195-2857
L'ACTUALITE PHARMACEUTIQUE. Text in French. 1929. m. CND 29. adv. illus. **Document type:** *Magazine, Trade.* **Description:** For French-speaking pharmacists in retail and hospital locations.
Formerly: Pharmacien (0031-692X)
Related titles: Microfiche ed.: (from MML); Microform ed.: (from MML); ♦ English ed.: Pharmacist News.
Indexed: I.P.A.
—Linda Hall.
Published by: Rogers Media Publishing Ltd, 1001 boul de Maisonneuve Ouest, Rm 1100, Montreal, PQ H3A 3E1, Canada. TEL 514-843-2581, FAX 514-845-7503, http://www.medalliance.ca, http://www.rogers.com. Ed. Michel Legault. Circ: 4,109.

P

615 FRA ISSN 0515-3700
ACTUALITES PHARMACEUTIQUES. Text in French. 1961. m. (11/yr). EUR 157 in Europe to institutions; USD 199 elsewhere to institutions (effective 2002). adv. **Document type:** *Academic/Scholarly.* **Description:** Provides practical and scientific information; offers clarifications on categories of medicines or illnesses and articles on pharmaceutical and socio-professional news; summarizes all the medicines put on the market in the preceding year as well as less recent medicines that may have undergone modifications.
Supersedes: Officine et Techniques Pharmaceutiques
Related titles: Online - full text ed.
Indexed: Agri.& Environ.Biotech.Abstr. (coverage dropped), Chem.Abstr., INIS Atomind., I.P.A., Ref.Zh.
—BLDSC (0677.324000), GNLM.
Published by: Elsevier Paris, Editions Scientifiques et Medicales (Subsidiary of: Reed Elsevier plc. group), 23 rue Linois, Paris 75015, France. TEL 33-1-45589110, FAX 33-1-45589419, s.delarue@elsevier.fr; academic@elsevier-fr.com, http://www.elsevier.com/locate/actpha. Ed. J Buxeraud.

615.19 NLD ISSN 0169-409X
CODEN: ADDREP
ADVANCED DRUG DELIVERY REVIEWS. Text in English. 1987. 21/yr. EUR 3,153 in Europe to institutions; JPY 418,700 in Japan to institutions; USD 3,527 elsewhere to institutions (effective 2002). adv. bk.rev. index. back issues avail.; reprint service avail. from SWZ. *Refereed.* **Document type:** *Academic/Scholarly.* **Description:** Publishes critical review articles on current and emerging aspects of research into the design and development of advanced drug delivery systems and their application to experimental and clinical therapeutics.
Related titles: Microform ed.: (from PQC); Online - full text ed.: (from ingenta, Swets Blackwell, ScienceDirect, Institute for Scientific Information).
Indexed: ASCA, Bioeng.Abstr., Biol.Abstr., Biotech.& Bioeng.Abstr., Chem.Abstr., Chem.Cit.Ind., Chem.Indus.Notes, Chem.Titles, Curr.Cont., Derwent Biotech.Abstr., Eng.Ind., Excerp.Med., I.P.A., Ind.Med., Ind.Sci.Rev., Inpharma, Int.Abstr.Biol.Sci., Mat.Sci.Cit.Ind. (coverage dropped), Pharm.&Out.News, Protozool.Abstr., Reac., Sci.Cit.Ind.
—BLDSC (0696.845000), ADONIS, CASDDS, CISTI, Ei, EMDOCS, GNLM, IDS, Infotrieve, KNAW. **CCC.**
Published by: Elsevier Science BV, PO Box 211, Amsterdam 1000 AE, Netherlands. TEL 31-20-485-2911, FAX 31-20-485-2457, nlinfo-f@elsevier.nl, http://www.elsevier.com/locate/drugdeliv. Eds. K. L. R. Brouwer, V. H. L. Lee. **Subscr. in Australasia and the Far East to:** Elsevier Science (Singapore) Pte Ltd, No.1 Temasek Ave, 17-01 Millenia Tower, Singapore 039192, Singapore. TEL 65-434-3727, FAX 65-337-2230; **Subscr. in Japan to:** Elsevier Science Inc - Japan Regional Office, 9-15 Higashi-Azabu 1-chome, Minato-ku, Tokyo 106-0044, Japan. TEL 81-3-5561-5033, FAX 81-3-5561-5047; **Subscr. in the Americas to:** Elsevier Science, PO Box 945, New York, NY 10159-0945. TEL 212-633-3730, FAX 212-633-3680.

615.19 USA ISSN 1075-8593
CODEN: AADDEU
ADVANCES IN ANTIVIRAL DRUG DESIGN. Text in English. 1993. irreg., latest vol.3. USD 109.50. **Document type:** *Monographic series, Academic/Scholarly.* **Description:** Provides a comprehensive account on the inception of antiviral drugs, their design, synthesis, and demonstration of therapeutic potential.
Indexed: Chem.Abstr., Chem.Indus.Notes, Chem.Titles.
—BLDSC (0698.920000), CASDDS, CISTI, GNLM. **CCC.**
Published by: J A I Press Inc., 100 Prospect St, Box 811, Stamford, CT 06904-0811. TEL 203-323-9606, FAX 203-357-8446, jai@jaipress.com. Ed. Erik De Clercq.

615 616.8 USA ISSN 0065-2229
RM315 CODEN: ABPYBL
ADVANCES IN BIOCHEMICAL PSYCHOPHARMACOLOGY. Text in English. 1969. irreg. price varies. reprint service avail. from PQC. *Refereed.* **Document type:** *Monographic series.*
Related titles: Online - full text ed.: (from Institute for Scientific Information).
Indexed: ASCA, BBCI, Biol.Abstr., Chem.Abstr., Chem.Indus.Notes, Chem.Titles, Curr.Cont. (coverage dropped), Focus on: Psychophar., INIS Atomind., Ind.Med. (until 1999, dropped), Ind.Sci.Rev., Neurosci.Cit.Ind., Sci.Cit.Ind. (coverage dropped), e-psyche.
—CASDDS, CISTI, GNLM, ingenta, KNAW, Linda Hall.
Published by: Lippincott Williams & Wilkins (Philadelphia) (Subsidiary of: Wolters Kluwer N.V.), 530 Walnut St, Philadelphia, PA 19106-3621. TEL 301-223-2300, 800-638-3030, FAX 301-223-2400.

615 USA
ADVANCES IN CLINICAL PHARMACOLOGY. Text in English. 1994. irreg. price varies. *Refereed.* **Document type:** *Monographic series.*
Published by: Lippincott Williams & Wilkins (Philadelphia) (Subsidiary of: Wolters Kluwer N.V.), 530 Walnut St, Philadelphia, PA 19106-3621. TEL 301-223-2300, 800-638-3030, FAX 301-223-2400.

ADVANCES IN COMBUSTION TOXICOLOGY. see *ENVIRONMENTAL STUDIES—Toxicology And Environmental Safety*

615.1 USA ISSN 0065-2490
RS1 CODEN: ADRRAN
ADVANCES IN DRUG RESEARCH. Text in English. 1964. irreg., latest vol.30, 1997. index. reprint service avail. from ISI. *Refereed.* **Document type:** *Academic/Scholarly.*
Indexed: Agri.& Environ.Biotech.Abstr. (coverage dropped), Aqua.Sci.& Fish.Abstr., Biol.Abstr., Chem.Abstr., Chem.Indus.Notes, Chem.Titles, Derwent Biotech.Abstr., Environ.Sci.Poll.Mgmt., Excerp.Med., Ind.Med. (1964-), Ind.Vet., Pollut.Abstr., Risk Abstr., Saf.Sci.Abstr., Vet.Bull.
—BLDSC (0704.300000), CASDDS, CISTI, EMDOCS, GNLM, ingenta, KNAW, Linda Hall. **CCC.**
Published by: Academic Press, Inc., Journal Division (Subsidiary of: Harcourt Brace & Company), 525 B St, Ste 1900, San Diego, CA 92101-4495. TEL 619-231-0926, FAX 619-699-6715. Ed. B Testa. **Subscr. to:** Order Dept., 6277 Sea Harbor Dr, 4th Fl, Orlando, FL 32887. TEL 800-321-5068.

ADVANCES IN NEUROPSYCHIATRY AND PSYCHOPHARMACOLOGY. see *MEDICAL SCIENCES—Psychiatry And Neurology*

615 USA ISSN 0065-3136
RS1 CODEN: APHMA8
ADVANCES IN PHARMACEUTICAL SCIENCES. Text in English. 1964. irreg., latest vol.7, 1995. index. reprint service avail. from ISI. *Refereed.* **Document type:** *Academic/Scholarly.*
Related titles: Online - full text ed.
Indexed: Agri.& Environ.Biotech.Abstr. (coverage dropped), Biol.Abstr., Chem.Abstr., Chem.Indus.Notes, Chem.Titles, I.P.A., Ind.Med. (coverage dropped).
—BLDSC (0709.740000), CASDDS, CISTI, GNLM, Infotrieve, ingenta, KNAW, Linda Hall. **CCC.**
Published by: Academic Press, Inc., Journal Division (Subsidiary of: Harcourt Brace & Company), 525 B St, Ste 1900, San Diego, CA 92101-4495. TEL 619-231-0926, FAX 619-699-6715. Eds. A H Beckett, H S Bean. **Subscr. to:** Order Dept., 6277 Sea Harbor Dr, 4th Fl, Orlando, FL 32887. TEL 800-321-5068.

615 CHE
ADVANCES IN PHARMACOLOGICAL SCIENCES. Text in English. 1990. irreg. price varies. **Document type:** *Monographic series, Academic/Scholarly.*
Published by: Birkhaeuser Verlag AG (Subsidiary of: BertelsmannSpringer), Klosterberg, Postfach 133, Basel 4010, Switzerland. TEL 41-61-2050707, FAX 41-61-2050792, orders@birkhauser.ch.

615.1 USA ISSN 1054-3589
RM30 CODEN: ADPHEL
ADVANCES IN PHARMACOLOGY. Text in English. 1962. irreg., latest vol.44, 1998. index. reprint service avail. from ISI. *Refereed.* **Document type:** *Academic/Scholarly.*
Former titles (until 1991): Advances in Pharmacology and Chemotherapy (0065-3144); Advances in Pharmacology; Advances in Chemotherapy
Indexed: Agri.& Environ.Biotech.Abstr. (coverage dropped), Biol.Abstr., Chem.Abstr., Chem.Indus.Notes, Chem.Titles, Derwent Biotech.Abstr., Ind.Med. (1990-), Ind.Sci.Rev., Ind.Vet., Sci.Cit.Ind. (coverage dropped), Vet.Bull.
—BLDSC (0709.760000), CASDDS, CISTI, GNLM, ingenta, KNAW, Linda Hall. **CCC.**
Published by: Academic Press, Inc., Journal Division (Subsidiary of: Harcourt Brace & Company), 525 B St, Ste 1900, San Diego, CA 92101-4495. TEL 619-231-0926, FAX 619-699-6715. Ed. S Garattini. **Subscr. to:** Order Dept., 6277 Sea Harbor Dr, 4th Fl, Orlando, FL 32887. TEL 800-321-5068.

615 USA ISSN 0732-8141
QP801.P68 CODEN: ATLRD6
ADVANCES IN PROSTAGLANDIN, THROMBOXANE, AND LEUKOTRIENE RESEARCH. Text in English. 1976. irreg., latest vol.23. price varies. reprint service avail. from PQC. *Refereed.* **Document type:** *Proceedings.*
Formerly (until 1982): Advances in Prostaglandin and Thromboxane Research (0361-5952)
Related titles: Online - full text ed.: (from Institute for Scientific Information).
Indexed: ASCA, Anim.Breed.Abstr., BBCI, Biol.Abstr., Chem.Abstr., Curr.Adv.Ecol.Sci., Curr.Cont. (coverage dropped), Derwent Biotech.Abstr., INIS Atomind., Ind.Med. (coverage dropped), Ind.Sci.Rev., Sci.Cit.Ind.
—CASDDS, CISTI, GNLM, KNAW.
Published by: Lippincott Williams & Wilkins (Philadelphia) (Subsidiary of: Wolters Kluwer N.V.), 530 Walnut St, Philadelphia, PA 19106-3621. TEL 301-223-2300, 800-638-3030, FAX 301-223-2400.

615.1 615 USA ISSN 0044-6394
CODEN: ADRBBA
ADVERSE DRUG REACTION BULLETIN. Text in English. 1966. bi-m., latest vol.211. USD 61 domestic to individuals; USD 61 foreign to individuals; USD 99 domestic to institutions; USD 99 foreign to institutions (effective 2002). index. back issues avail.; reprints avail. *Refereed.* **Document type:** *Academic/Scholarly.* **Description:** Provides comprehensive coverage on adverse drug reactions.
Related titles: Microfilm ed.: (from PQC); Online - full text ed.: (from EBSCO Publishing); Italian ed.
Indexed: Biol.Abstr., Curr.Adv.Ecol.Sci., Environ.Sci.Poll.Mgmt., Excerp.Med., INIS Atomind., I.P.A., Ind.Med. (coverage dropped), Inpharma, Pharm.&Out.News, Pollut.Abstr., Reac., Risk Abstr., Saf.Sci.Abstr., Tox.Abstr.
—BLDSC (0712.232000), CISTI, EMDOCS, GNLM, KNAW.
Published by: Lippincott Williams & Wilkins (Philadelphia) (Subsidiary of: Wolters Kluwer N.V.), 530 Walnut St, Philadelphia, PA 19106-3621. TEL 215-521-8300, FAX 215-521-8902, http://www.lww.com. Ed. R E Ferner. Circ: 1,799. **Subscr. to:** PO Box 1600, Hagerstown, MD 21740-1600. TEL 800-777-2295, FAX 301-824-7390.

615.9 GBR ISSN 0964-198X
RM302.5 CODEN: ADRRER
ADVERSE DRUG REACTIONS AND TOXICOLOGICAL REVIEWS. Text in English. 1982. q. GBP 185, USD 330 to institutions (effective Mar. 2001). adv. bk.rev. 64 p./no. back issues avail. *Refereed.* **Document type:** *Academic/Scholarly.* **Description:** Covers developments in the field of adverse drug reactions and toxicology.
Formerly (until 1991): Adverse Drug Reactions and Acute Poisoning Reviews (0260-647X)
Related titles: Online - full text ed.: (from Institute for Scientific Information).
Indexed: ASCA, Biol.Abstr., Chem.Abstr., Curr.Adv.Ecol.Sci., Curr.Cont. (coverage dropped), Environ.Sci.Poll.Mgmt., Excerp.Med., Ind.Med. (1991-), Ind.Sci.Rev., Inpharma, Int.Abstr.Biol.Sci., NRN, Pollut.Abstr., Reac., Ref.Zh., Risk Abstr., SSCI (coverage dropped), Saf.Sci.Abstr., Sci.Cit.Ind. (coverage dropped).
—BLDSC (0712.233000), CASDDS, CISTI, EMDOCS, GNLM, IDS, ingenta, KNAW. **CCC.**
Published by: Oxford University Press, Academic Division, Great Clarendon St, Oxford OX2 6DP, United Kingdom. TEL 44-1865-267907, FAX 44-1865-267835, jnl.info@oup.co.uk, http://www3.oup.co.uk/drugsj/, http://www.oup.co.uk/journals. Ed. J P Griffin. Pub. Mandy Sketch. R&P Fionna Willis. Circ: 350. **US subscr. to:** Oxford University Press, Journals, 2001 Evans Rd, Cary, NC 27513. TEL 800-852-7323, FAX 919-677-1714, jnlorders@oup-usa.org.

615 DEU ISSN 0942-2242
CODEN: AEHDFB
ADVERSE EFFECTS OF HERBAL DRUGS. Text in German. 1992. a. **Document type:** *Monographic series.*
—CASDDS, GNLM, Infotrieve. **CCC.**
Published by: Springer-Verlag (Subsidiary of: BertelsmannSpringer), Haber Str 7, Heidelberg 69126, Germany. TEL 49-30-8207-0, FAX 49-30-8214091, subscriptions@springer.de, http://www.springer.de, http://link.springer-ny.com.

615 DNK ISSN 0900-3142
AFHAENGING. Text in Danish. 1984. q. free per issue.
Published by: Landsforeningen for Human Narkobehandling, Lundtofteparken 32, Kgs Lyngby 2800, Denmark. Ed. P T Pedersen.

615 NGA ISSN 0044-6564
AFRICAN JOURNAL OF PHARMACY AND PHARMACEUTICAL SCIENCES. Text in English. 1970. q. USD 100, NGN 60, USD 120. adv. bk.rev. illus. **Document type:** *Academic/Scholarly.* **Description:** Reviews and reports the research and other aspects of those sciences that contribute to the discovery, evaluation, and development of medicinal substances.
Indexed: Excerp.Med., I.P.A.

P

Address: 21 Wharf Rd., PO Box 399, Apapa, Lagos State, Nigeria. Ed. Bode Ladejobi. Circ: 40,000.

615.1 GBR ISSN 1465-3745
THE AGRICULTURAL AND VETERINARY PHARMACIST. Text in English. 1998. q. **Document type:** *Newsletter, Trade.* **Description:** Provides a means of promoting agricultural and veterinary pharmacy.
Published by: Royal Pharmaceutical Society of Great Britain, Agricultural and Veterinary Pharmacists Group, 1 Lambeth High St, London SE1 7JN, United Kingdom. TEL 44-20-7735-9141, pharmpress@rpsgb.org.uk. Ed. Steven Kayne.

AIDS ORGANISATIONS WORLDWIDE. see *MEDICAL SCIENCES—Communicable Diseases*

AIDS REFERENCE MANUAL. see *MEDICAL SCIENCES—Communicable Diseases*

AIDS TREATMENT UPDATE. see *MEDICAL SCIENCES—Communicable Diseases*

AKTUELLT. see *DRUG ABUSE AND ALCOHOLISM*

THE ALKALOIDS; chemistry and biology. see *CHEMISTRY—Organic Chemistry*

615.1 USA ISSN 0002-5690
ALLEGHENY COUNTY PHARMACIST* . Text in English. 1947. m. membership. adv. illus.
Published by: Allegheny County Pharmaceutical Association, PO Box 16528, Pittsburgh, PA 15242-1028. TEL 412-922-2440. Ed. Carole F Ladik. Circ: 800.

615 USA
AMERICAN ASSOCIATION OF COLLEGES OF PHARMACY. (YEAR) PROFILE OF PHARMACY FACULTY. Text in English. 1980. a. USD 25 (effective 1999). **Document type:** *Monographic series.* **Description:** Offers information on the faculty members of the AACP.
Formerly: American Association of Colleges of Pharmacy. Annual Survey of Faculty Salaries
Published by: American Association of Colleges of Pharmacy, Office of Academic Affairs, 1426 Prince St, Alexandria, VA 22314-2815. FAX 703-836-8982, smeyer@aacp.org. Ed. Susan M Meyer. R&P Richard Penna. Circ: 2,500.

615.1 USA ISSN 0190-5279
RS1 CODEN: AMDREK
AMERICAN DRUGGIST. Text in English. 1871. m. USD 44. adv. charts, illus, mkt, stat, tr.lit. reprints avail. **Document type:** *Trade.* **Description:** Covering professional and business topics, and providing news analysis for pharmacists practicing in retail, hospital, and managed care settings.
Formerly: American Druggist Merchandising (0090-6638)
Related titles: Microform ed.: (from PQC); Online - full text ed.: (from Gale Group, Northern Light Technology, Inc., ProQuest Information & Learning, Factiva).
Indexed: B.P.I. (coverage dropped), Bus.Ind., Excerp.Med., Hlth.Ind., I.P.A., L.R.I., PROMT, Tr.& Indus.Ind.
—CISTI, EMDOCS, GNLM, ingenta, KNAW.
Published by: Press Corps, American Druggist, 444 Park Ave S, Ste 402, New York, NY 10016-7321. TEL 212-686-8584, FAX 212-686-9098, AmDruggist@aol.com. Ed., R&P Janice Zoeller. Adv. contact Gordon Duncan. Circ: 104,000.

615 USA
AMERICAN HEALTH CONSULTANTS. PHASE III REPORT. Text in English. 1995. q. USD 437 domestic; USD 467 foreign; USD 219 newsstand/cover (effective 2001). **Document type:** *Newsletter.*
Published by: American Health Consultants (Subsidiary of: Medical Economics Co., Inc.), 3525 Piedmont Rd, N E, 6 Piedmont Center, Ste 400, Atlanta, GA 30305. TEL 404-262-5476, 404-262-7436, 800-688-2421, FAX 404-262-7837, 800-284-3291, custserv@ahcpub.com, http://www.ahcpub.com.

AMERICAN HERB ASSOCIATION NEWSLETTER. see *GARDENING AND HORTICULTURE*

615.1 USA ISSN 0270-0611
AMERICAN INSTITUTE OF THE HISTORY OF PHARMACY. PUBLICATIONS. Text in English. 1972. irreg. **Document type:** *Monographic series.*
Published by: American Institute of the History of Pharmacy, Pharmacy Bldg, Madison, WI 53706. TEL 608-262-5378.

▼ **AMERICAN JOURNAL OF CARDIOVASCULAR DRUGS.** see *MEDICAL SCIENCES—Cardiovascular Diseases*

615.1 USA ISSN 1079-2082
RS1 CODEN: AHSPEK
AMERICAN JOURNAL OF HEALTH-SYSTEM PHARMACY. Text in English. 1943. s-m. USD 195 domestic; USD 225 foreign (effective 2001). adv. bk.rev. abstr, bibl, charts, illus, tr.lit. index. back issues avail.; reprint service avail. from PQC,ISI. *Refereed.* **Document type:** *Academic/Scholarly.* **Description:** Covers all facets of pharmacy in components of health systems. Provides current information on the clinical use of new drugs - current thinking on drug therapy in selected diseases and clinical trials evaluating drug effects and adverse drug reactions.
Formerly (until 1995): American Journal of Hospital Pharmacy (0002-9289); Incorporates (1982-1993): Clinical Pharmacy (0278-2677)
Related titles: CD-ROM ed.: (from Ovid Technologies, Inc.); Microform ed.: (from PQC); Online - full text ed.: (from Ovid Technologies, Inc., EBSCO Publishing, Institute for Scientific Information).
Indexed: ASCA, Abstr.Health Care Manage.Stud., AgeLine, Agri.& Environ.Biotech.Abstr. (coverage dropped), Biol.Abstr., CINAHL, Chem.Abstr., Chem.Indus.Notes, Chem.Titles, Curr.Adv.Cancer Res., Curr.Adv.Ecol.Sci., Curr.Cont., Dairy Sci.Abstr., Dent.Ind., Derwent Biotech.Abstr., Excerp.Med., Helminthol.Abstr., Hosp.Lit.Ind., INIS Atomind., I.P.A., Ind.Med. (1995-), Ind.Sci.Rev., Inpharma, Int.Nurs.Ind., Kidney, Med.& Surg.Dermat., Med.Care Rev., Nutr.Abstr., Pharm.&Out.News, Protozool.Abstr., Reac., Rev.Arom.& Med.Plants, Rev.Med.& Vet.Mycol., SSCI (coverage dropped), Sci.Cit.Ind.
—BLDSC (0824.770000), CASDDS, CISTI, EMDOCS, GNLM, IDS, ingenta, KNAW, Linda Hall. **CCC.**
Published by: American Society of Health-System Pharmacists, 7272 Wisconsin Ave, Bethesda, MD 20814. TEL 301-657-3000, FAX 301-657-1251, 301-657-8857, ajhp@ashp.org, http://www.ashp.org. Ed. C Richard Talley. R&P Jill A Sellers. adv.: B&W page USD 3,100, color page USD 4,870. Circ: 39,232.

615.10711 USA ISSN 0002-9459
RS110 CODEN: AJPDAD
AMERICAN JOURNAL OF PHARMACEUTICAL EDUCATION. Text in English. 1937. q. USD 40 to individuals; USD 65 foreign to individuals; USD 100 to libraries. bk.rev. bibl, charts, illus. index, cum.index every 10 yrs. back issues avail. *Refereed.* **Document type:** *Academic/Scholarly.*
Related titles: Microfilm ed.: (from PQC,PMC); Online - full text ed.: (from Northern Light Technology, Inc., ProQuest Information & Learning, Institute for Scientific Information).
Indexed: ASCA, Biol.Abstr., C.I.J.E., Chem.Abstr., Cont.Pg.Educ., Curr.Adv.Ecol.Sci., Curr.Cont., Excerp.Med., High.Educ.Curr.Aware.Bull., Hosp.Lit.Ind., INIS Atomind., I.P.A., Ind.Sci.Rev., Inpharma, Pharm.&Out.News, Reac., Rev.Med.& Vet.Mycol., SSCI (coverage dropped), Sci.Cit.Ind.
—BLDSC (0830.000000), CASDDS, CISTI, GNLM, IDS, ingenta.
Published by: American Association of Colleges of Pharmacy, 1426 Prince St, Alexandria, VA 22314-2815. TEL 703-739-2330. Ed. George H Cocolas. Circ: 2,300.

AMERICAN JOURNAL OF THERAPEUTICS. see *MEDICAL SCIENCES*

615.1 USA
RS1 CODEN: AMPHDF
AMERICAN PHARMACEUTICAL ASSOCIATION. JOURNAL. Text in English. 1912. bi-m. USD 50 to non-members (effective 2000). adv. bk.rev. charts, illus. index. *Refereed.*
Former titles: American Pharmacy (0160-3450); American Pharmaceutical Association. Journal (0003-0465)
Related titles: Microform ed.: (from PQC,PMC); Online - full text ed.
Indexed: AgeLine, Biol.Abstr., Chem.Abstr., Curr.Adv.Ecol.Sci., Curr.Cont. (coverage dropped), Excerp.Med., Helminthol.Abstr., INIS Atomind., I.P.A., Ind.Med. (coverage dropped), Int.Nurs.Ind., MEDSOC, Med.Care Rev., Nutr.Abstr.
—CASDDS, CISTI, EMDOCS, GNLM, ingenta, Linda Hall. **CCC.**
Published by: American Pharmaceutical Association, 2215 Constitution Ave, N W, Washington, DC 20037. TEL 202-628-4410. Ed. Marlene Bloom. Circ: 48,800.

615.1 USA ISSN 1093-5401
HD9666.1
AMERICA'S PHARMACIST. Text in English. 1893. m. USD 50 (effective 2001). adv. charts, illus, tr.lit. **Document type:** *Trade.* **Description:** Features on activities of independent pharmacists and issues to which they relate: legislative, regulatory, clinical, and marketing.
Formerly (until 1997): N A R D Journal (0027-5972)
Indexed: I.P.A., Search.
—ingenta, Linda Hall.
Published by: National Community Pharmacists Association, 205 Daingerfield Rd, Alexandria, VA 22314. TEL 703-683-8200, FAX 703-683-3619. Ed. Robert Malone. Circ: 35,000 (controlled).

615 658.8 GBR
ANALGESICS: THE INTERNATIONAL MARKET. Text in English. a. GBP 2,250, USD 4,500 (effective 1999). **Document type:** *Trade.* **Description:** Analyzes the market for nonprescription pain relievers in France, Germany, Italy, Spain, the U.K., the U.S., and Japan.
Related titles: Online - full text ed.: (from Data-Star, The Dialog Corporation).
Published by: Euromonitor, 60-61 Britton St, London EC1M 5UX, United Kingdom. TEL 44-20-7251-8024, info@euromonitor.com, http://www.euromonitor.com.

615.19 USA ISSN 0099-5428
RS189 CODEN: APDSB7
ANALYTICAL PROFILES OF DRUG SUBSTANCES. Text in English. 1972. irreg., latest vol.25, 1998. reprint service avail. from ISI. *Refereed.*
Indexed: Chem.Abstr.
—CASDDS, CISTI, GNLM, KNAW. **CCC.**
Published by: Academic Press, Inc., Journal Division (Subsidiary of: Harcourt Brace & Company), 525 B St, Ste 1900, San Diego, CA 92101-4495. TEL 619-231-0926, FAX 619-699-6715. Ed. Klaus Florey. **Subscr. to:** Order Dept., 6277 Sea Harbor Dr, 4th Fl, Orlando, FL 32887. TEL 800-321-5068.

615.1 FRA ISSN 0003-4509
RS1 CODEN: APFRAD
ANNALES PHARMACEUTIQUES FRANCAISES. Text in French; Summaries in English. 1943. 6/yr. FRF 1,650; FRF 1,975 foreign (effective 2000). adv. bk.rev. bibl, illus. index. reprint service avail. from ISI. **Document type:** *Academic/Scholarly.* **Description:** Publishes original articles, technical notes of interest to practitioners, and meeting reports of the Academy.
Indexed: Agri.& Environ.Biotech.Abstr. (coverage dropped), Anal.Abstr., Apic.Abstr., Biol.Abstr., C.I.S. Abstr., Chem.Abstr., Chem.Indus.Notes, Chem.Titles, Curr.Adv.Ecol.Sci., Curr.Chem.React. (coverage dropped), Curr.Cont. (coverage dropped), Derwent Biotech.Abstr., Excerp.Med., Helminthol.Abstr., INIS Atomind., I.P.A., Ind.Chem. (coverage dropped), Ind.Med. (1943-), Ind.Sci.Rev., MOS, NPU, Rev.Med.& Vet.Mycol., Sci.Cit.Ind. (coverage dropped).
—BLDSC (0992.000000), CASDDS, CISTI, EMDOCS, GNLM, Infotrieve, KNAW, Linda Hall. **CCC.**
Published by: (Academie Nationale de Pharmacie), Masson - Periodiques, 120 bd. St. Germain, Paris 75006, France. TEL 33-1-40466200, FAX 33-1-40466201. Ed. G Deysson. Circ: 1,500. **Subscr. to:** Societe de Periodiques Specialises, BP 22, Vineuil Cedex 41354, France. TEL 33-2-54504612, FAX 33-2-54504611.

615.1 POL ISSN 0867-0609
ANNALES UNIVERSITATIS MARIAE CURIE-SKLODOWSKA. SECTIO DDD. PHARMACIA. Text in English, Polish; Summaries in English. 1988. a. price varies. **Document type:** *Academic/Scholarly.*
Indexed: Hort.Abstr., Nutr.Abstr., Plant Gen.Res.Abstr.
Published by: Uniwersytet Marii Curie-Sklodowskiej, Wydawnictwo, Pl M Curie Sklodowskiej 5, Lublin 20031, Poland. TEL 48-81-375304, FAX 48-81-336699. Ed. Romuald Langwinski. Circ: 600.

615.1 USA ISSN 1060-0280
RM300 CODEN: APHRER
THE ANNALS OF PHARMACOTHERAPY. Text in English; Summaries in French, Spanish. 1967. m. (July-Aug. combined). USD 92 domestic to individuals; USD 117 foreign to individuals; USD 249 domestic to institutions; USD 274 foreign to institutions (effective 2001). adv. bk.rev., software rev. abstr, bibl, charts, illus. index. 128 p./no. 2 cols./p. back issues avail.; reprints avail. *Refereed.* **Document type:** *Journal, Academic/Scholarly.* **Description:** Aimed at health care professionals involved in drug therapy. Provides an interdisciplinary approach to the study of pharmacotherapy.

P

Former titles (until 1992): D I C P - The Annals of Pharmacotherapy (1042-9611); (until 1988): Drug Intelligence and Clinical Pharmacy (0012-6578); (until 1969): Drug Intelligence
Related titles: Microform ed.: (from PQC); Online - full text ed.: (from Institute for Scientific Information).
Indexed: Abstr.Health Care Manage.Stud., AgeLine, Agri.& Environ.Biotech.Abstr. (coverage dropped), Biol.Abstr., CINAHL, Chem.Abstr., Chem.Indus.Notes, Chem.Titles, Curr.Adv.Ecol.Sci., Curr.Cont., Dairy Sci.Abstr., Dent.Ind., Derwent Biotech.Abstr., Environ.Sci.Poll.Mgmt., Helminthol.Abstr., Hosp.Lit.Ind., INIS Atomind., I.P.A., Ind.Med. (1992-), Ind.Sci.Rev., Inpharma, Int.Nurs.Ind., Kidney, Nutr.Abstr., Pharm.&Out.News, Pollut.Abstr., Reac., Ref.Zh., Rev.Med.& Vet.Mycol., Risk Abstr., Saf.Sci.Abstr., Sci.Cit.Ind., THA.
—BLDSC (1043.417500), CASDDS, CISTI, EMDOCS, GNLM, IDS, ingenta, KNAW.
Published by: Harvey Whitney Books Company, PO Box 42696, Cincinnati, OH 45242. TEL 513-793-3555, 877-742-7631, FAX 513-793-3600, customerserv@theannals.com, http://www.theannals.com. Ed., Pub. Harvey Whitney Jr. R&P, Adv. contact Greg J Johnson. Circ: 6,000 (paid). **Subscr. to:** Allen Press Inc., PO Box 1897, Lawrence, KS 66044-8897.

615 FRA ISSN 1285-7599
L'ANNUAIRE DU PHARMACIEN. Text in French. 1932. a. FRF 1,695 (effective 1999). adv. **Document type:** *Directory.*
Formerly (until 1997): Annuaire General de la Pharmacie Francaise (0066-3158)
Published by: (Association Generale des Syndicats Pharmaceutiques), Rosenwald, 10 rue Vineuse, Paris 75116, France. TEL 33-1-44308100, FAX 33-1-44308111, rosenwal@wanadoo.fr. Circ: 6,000.

P

ANNUAIRE FOURNI-LABO PHARMACIE (YEAR); cosmetique et alimentaire. see *BUSINESS AND ECONOMICS—Trade And Industrial Directories*

615.19 GBR ISSN 0260-955X
ANNUAL REGISTER OF PHARMACEUTICAL CHEMISTS. Text in English. 1869. a. GBP 110 in United Kingdom; GBP 120 elsewhere (effective 2001). index. **Document type:** *Directory.* **Description:** Contains an alphabetical list of names and addresses of all registered pharmacists; corporate bodies operating retail pharmacy businesses with the names of their superintendents; and the business titles and addresses of all registered retail pharmacies in country, county and town order.
—BLDSC (1094.500000).
Published by: Euromed Communications Ltd., Pharmaceutical Press, 1 Lambeth High St, London SE1 7JN, United Kingdom. TEL 44-20-7735-9141, http://www.euromed.uk.com. Pub. Charles Fry. Circ: 1,000. **Dist. by:** Pharmaceutical Press, PO Box 151, Wallingford, Oxford OX10 8QU, United Kingdom. TEL 44-1491-829272, FAX 44-1491-829292, rpsgb@cabi.org.

615.1 USA ISSN 0065-7743
RS402 CODEN: ARMCBI
ANNUAL REPORTS IN MEDICINAL CHEMISTRY. Text in English. 1966. irreg., latest vol.32, 1997. reprint service avail. from ISI. *Refereed.*
Related titles: Online - full text ed.: (from Institute for Scientific Information).
Indexed: ASCA, BBCI, Biol.Abstr., Chem.Abstr., Chem.Indus.Notes, Chem.Titles, Curr.Cont. (coverage dropped), Dairy Sci.Abstr., Ind.Sci.Rev., Sci.Cit.Ind.
—BLDSC (1513.050000), CASDDS, CISTI, GNLM, ingenta, KNAW, Linda Hall. **CCC.**
Published by: (Division of Medicinal Chemistry, American Chemical Society), Academic Press, Inc., Journal Division (Subsidiary of: Harcourt Brace & Company), 525 B St, Ste 1900, San Diego, CA 92101-4495. TEL 619-231-0926, FAX 619-699-6715. Ed. Denis M Bailey. **Subscr. to:** Order Dept., 6277 Sea Harbor Dr, 4th Fl, Orlando, FL 32887. TEL 800-321-5068.

615.1 USA ISSN 0362-1642
RM16 CODEN: ARPTDI
ANNUAL REVIEW OF PHARMACOLOGY AND TOXICOLOGY. Text in English. 1961. a. USD 60 domestic to individuals; USD 65 foreign to individuals; USD 120 domestic to institutions; USD 130 foreign to institutions (effective 1999). adv. bibl, charts. index, cum.index. back issues avail.; reprints avail. *Refereed.* **Document type:** *Academic/Scholarly.* **Description:** Reviews, filters and synthesizes primary research to identify the principal contributions in the fields of pharmacology and toxicology.
Formerly (until vol.15, 1975): Annual Review of Pharmacology (0066-4251)
Related titles: Microfilm ed.: (from PQC); Online - full text ed.: (from HighWire Pr., EBSCO Publishing, Institute for Scientific Information).
Indexed: ASCA, Agri.& Environ.Biotech.Abstr. (coverage dropped), Aqua.Sci.& Fish.Abstr., Biol.Abstr., Chem.Abstr., Chem.Indus.Notes, Chem.Titles, Curr.Adv.Ecol.Sci., Curr.Cont., Derwent Biotech.Abstr., Environ.Sci.Poll.Mgmt., Excerp.Med., Helminthol.Abstr., INIS Atomind., Ind.Med. (1976-), Ind.Sci.Rev., Ind.Vet., Inpharma, Int.Abstr.Biol.Sci., Media Rev.Dig., Neurosci.Abstr., PsycInfo, Psychol.Abstr. (1976-), Reac., SSCI (coverage dropped), Sci.Cit.Ind., THA, Tox.Abstr., Vet.Bull., e-psyche.
—BLDSC (1525.880000), ADONIS, CASDDS, CINDOC, CISTI, EMDOCS, GNLM, IDS, ingenta, KNAW, Linda Hall. **CCC.**
Published by: Annual Reviews Inc., 4139 El Camino Way, Box 10139, Palo Alto, CA 94303-0139. TEL 650-493-4400, 800-523-8635, FAX 650-424-0910, service@annurev.org, http://www.annualreviews.org. Ed. Samuel Gubins. R&P, Adv. contact Swati Aneja TEL 650-843-6634. **Subscr.to:** Allen Press Inc., PO Box 1897, Lawrence, KS 66044-8897.

615.329 NZL ISSN 1174-5924
▼ **ANTI-INFECTIVES TODAY.** Text in English. 1999. m. USD 95 to individuals; USD 545 to institutions (effective 2001). back issues avail. **Document type:** *Academic/Scholarly.* **Description:** Rapid alerts service on all aspects of drug therapy and disease management of infections.
Published by: Adis International Limited, Mairangi Bay, Private Bag 65901, Auckland 1010, New Zealand. TEL 64-9-477-0700, FAX 64-9-477-0766, http://www.adis.com. **Americas subscr. to:** Adis International Inc., Attn: Subscription Dept, 860 Town Center Dr, Langhorne, PA 19047. TEL 877-872-2347.

615 GBR
ANTIBACTERIAL PRODUCTS AND MARKETS. Text in English. irreg. GBP 495, USD 1,040, JPY 119,000 (effective 2000). **Document type:** *Bulletin, Monographic series, Academic/Scholarly, Trade.* **Description:** Provides updates on the latest trends in the research & development of antibacterial products market.
Formerly: Scrip's Antibacterial Report
—BLDSC (8211.859365).
Published by: Scrip Reports (Subsidiary of: P J B Publications Ltd.), 18/20 Hill Rise, Richmond, Surrey TW10 6UA, United Kingdom. TEL 44-20-8332-8964, FAX 44-20-8332-8992, 44-20-8948-6866, custserv@repsinfo.demon.co.uk, http://www.pjbpubs.com/scriprep/index.html. **Dist. in US by:** Pharmabooks Ltd., 1775 Broadway, Ste 511, New York, NY 10019. TEL 212-262-8234.

615.329 USA
ANTIBIOTIC RESISTANCE SOURCEBOOK. Text in English. 1996. a. USD 269; USD 185 foreign (effective 1999). **Document type:** *Trade.*
Published by: American Health Consultants (Subsidiary of: Medical Economics Co., Inc.), 3525 Piedmont Rd, N E, 6 Piedmont Center, Ste 400, Atlanta, GA 30305. TEL 404-262-5476, custserv@ahcpub.com, http://www.ahcpub.com.

615.1 CHE ISSN 0066-4758
RM260 CODEN: ANBCB3
ANTIBIOTICS AND CHEMOTHERAPY. Text in English. 1954. irreg., latest vol.50. CHF 220 in Europe; DEM 260 in Germany; USD 180 in United States (effective 2001). reprint service avail. from ISI. *Refereed.* **Document type:** *Journal, Academic/Scholarly.*
Indexed: Biol.Abstr., Chem.Abstr., Chem.Indus.Notes, Chem.Titles, Curr.Adv.Ecol.Sci., Curr.Cont. (coverage dropped), Ind.Med. (1971-).
—BLDSC (1546.980000), CASDDS, CINDOC, CISTI, GNLM, ingenta, KNAW. **CCC.**
Published by: S. Karger AG, Allschwilerstr 10, PO Box, Basel 4009, Switzerland. TEL 41-61-306-1111, FAX 41-61-306-1234, karger@karger.ch, http://www.karger.com/bookseries/ANCHE. Ed. H Schoenfeld.

615.329 RUS ISSN 0235-2990
RM265 CODEN: ANKHEW
ANTIBIOTIKI I KHIMIOTERAPIYA/ANTIBIOTICS AND CHEMOTHERAPY. Text in Russian. 1956. m. RUR 288 for 6 mos. to individuals; RUR 720 for 6 mos. to institutions (effective 2000). adv. **Document type:** *Academic/Scholarly.* **Description:** Covers research and chemical transformation of antibiotics, relation between structure and function, experimental and clinical antibiotic therapy, molecular mechanisms of action of antimicrobial antibiotics, antibiotic resistance mechanisms, antitumour, and more.
Former titles: Antibiotiki i Meditsinskaya Biotekhnologiya (0233-7525); Antibiotiki (0003-5637)
Indexed: Agri.& Environ.Biotech.Abstr. (coverage dropped), Anal.Abstr., Biol.Abstr., Chem.Abstr., Chem.Indus.Notes, Chem.Titles, Curr.Biotech.Abstr., Curr.Chem.React. (coverage dropped), Curr.Cont. (coverage dropped), Dairy Sci.Abstr., Derwent Biotech.Abstr., Excerp.Med., Helminthol.Abstr., INIS Atomind., Ind.Chem. (coverage dropped), Ind.Med. (1988-), Ind.Sci.Rev., NPU, Nutr.Abstr., Ref.Zh., Rev.Med.& Vet.Mycol., Rev.Plant Path., Sci.Cit.Ind. (coverage dropped), Sugar Ind.Abstr.
—CASDDS, CINDOC, CISTI, East View, EMDOCS, GNLM, KNAW, Linda Hall. **CCC.**
Published by: Media Sfera, Dmitrovskoe shosse 46, korp 2, etazh 4, P.O. Box 54, Moscow 127238, Russian Federation. TEL 7-095-4820604, 7-095-4824329, FAX 7-095-4824312, mediashp@mediasphera.ru. Ed. Aleksey Yegorov. Adv. contact Valery Nemtsov. **Dist. by:** Mezhdunarodnaya Kniga, B Yakimanka 39, Moscow 117049, Russian Federation. TEL 7-095-2384967, FAX 7-095-2384634; **US dist. addr.:** East View Publications, 3020 Harbor Ln N, Minneapolis, MN 55447. TEL 612-550-0961.

616.9 615 USA ISSN 0897-9871
ANTIVIRAL AGENTS BULLETIN; antiviral drug and vaccine development information. Text in English. 1988. m. USD 350 domestic; USD 410 foreign (effective 2000). adv. bk.rev. pat. index. back issues avail. **Document type:** *Bulletin.* **Description:** Covers news, federal activities, patents, and technology transfer information concerning HIV and antiviral drug and vaccine development.
Related titles: Online - full text ed.: (from Northern Light Technology, Inc., Factiva).
Indexed: Bus.& Indus. (Feb.1995-).
—BLDSC (1552.825000), GNLM.
Published by: Biotechnology Information Institute, 1700 Rockville Pike, Ste 400, Rockville, MD 20852. TEL 301-424-0255, FAX 301-424-0257, biotech@bioinfo.com, http://www.bioinfo.com. Ed., Adv. contact Ronald A Rader.

ANTIVIRAL CHEMISTRY AND CHEMOTHERAPY. see *BIOLOGY—Biochemistry*

615 SWE ISSN 0349-2516
APOTEKET; tidning foer apotekens kunder. Text in Swedish. 1980. 5/yr. free per issue. **Document type:** *Magazine, Consumer.*
Related titles: Audio cassette/tape ed.
Published by: Apoteket AB, Stockholm 13188, Sweden. TEL 46-8-466-10-00, FAX 46-8-466-15-10, tidningin.apoteket@apoteket.se. Ed. Gudrun Tawlo Lindskug. Circ: 525,000.

615.1 USA ISSN 0003-6560
APOTHECARY; the business journal for pharmacy. Text in English. 1888. q. USD 16; free to qualified personnel. adv. bk.rev. charts, illus. index. reprint service avail. from PQC. *Refereed.* **Document type:** *Trade.*
Incorporates: Mid-Atlantic Apothecary (0026-2943)
Related titles: Microform ed.: (from PQC); Online - full text ed.
Indexed: I.P.A.
—Linda Hall.
Published by: (Massachusetts College of Pharmacy and Allied Health Sciences), Health Care Marketing Services, H C M S Inc., PO Box AP, Los Altos, CA 94023-0179. TEL 415-941-3955, 800-462-4546, FAX 415-941-2303. Ed. Jerold K Karabensh. Pub. Janet L Goodman. R&P Vicki Cooper. Adv. contact Dale C Osborne. Circ: 65,000 (controlled).

615 NLD ISSN 0921-0288
APOTHEEKMANAGEMENT. Text in Dutch. 1987. 8/yr. NLG 101. adv. *Refereed.* **Document type:** *Trade.*
Published by: Mediselect B.V., Postbus 63, Leusden 3830 AB, Netherlands. TEL 31-33-4229900, FAX 31-33-4229922, info@mediselect.nl. Ed. P B Mertens. Circ: 2,300 (controlled).

615 AUT
DIE APOTHEKE. Text in German. bi-m.
Published by: Apotheke, Spitalgasse 31, Postfach 75, Vienna, W 1094, Austria. TEL 01-423588, FAX 01-4085355. Ed. H Jakesz. Circ: 98,500.

615 DEU
APOTHEKE AKTUELL. Text in German. bi-m. **Document type:** *Magazine, Trade.* **Description:** Contains information and advice for pharmacists and their clients.

Published by: (Bundesverband Deutscher Apotheker e.V.), Yukom Medien GmbH (Subsidiary of: Axel Springer Verlag AG), Schleissheimer Str 141, Munich 80797, Germany. TEL 49-89-30620-0, FAX 49-89-30620102, info@yukom.de, http://www.yukom.de. Circ: 10,000 (controlled).

APOTHEKE HEUTE; Schaufenster - Werbung - Einrichtung - Marketing. see *ADVERTISING AND PUBLIC RELATIONS*

615.19 DEU ISSN 0177-9591
APOTHEKE UND KRANKENHAUS. Text in German. 1985. q. EUR 62.28 domestic; EUR 65.04 foreign; EUR 18 newsstand/cover (effective 2002). **Document type:** *Journal, Trade.* **Description:** For hospital pharmacists.
—GNLM, Infotrieve. **CCC.**
Published by: (Bundesverband Krankenhausversorgender Apotheker e.V.), Deutscher Apotheker Verlag, Postfach 101061, Stuttgart 70009, Germany. TEL 49-711-2582-0, FAX 49-711-2582290, service@deutscher-apotheker-verlag.de, http://www.deutscher-apotheker-verlag.de. Ed. Klaus Grimm. Circ: 1,000.

615.19 DEU
APOTHEKEN JOURNAL REISE UND PHARMAZIE. Text in German. 1979. m. DEM 90. adv. bk.rev. **Document type:** *Trade.*
Formerly: Apotheker Journal (0720-1028)
—GNLM.
Published by: Otto Hoffmanns Verlag GmbH, Arnulfstr 10, Munich 80335, Germany. TEL 49-89-545845-0, FAX 49-89-54584520. Ed. Dr. Helmut Becker. Circ: 20,000.

615.19 DEU
APOTHEKEN KURIER. Text in German. 1985. m. **Document type:** *Trade.*
Published by: Pharma-Kurier Verlagsgesellschaft mbH, Borsigstr 1-3, Heusenstamm 63150, Germany. TEL 49-6104-606331, FAX 49-6104-606333, pkvpharma@t-online.de, ak@keplermediengruppe.de, http://www.kepplermedien.de. adv.: B&W page DEM 14,000, color page DEM 19,600; trim 210 x 280.

615 DEU ISSN 0724-9950
APOTHEKEN-MAGAZIN. Text in German. 1983. m. adv. **Document type:** *Magazine, Trade.*
Published by: Gebr. Storck GmbH, Bebelstr 102, Oberhausen 46049, Germany. TEL 49-208-848020, FAX 49-208-8480242. adv.: page DEM 6,200. Circ: 21,980 (controlled).

615.1 DEU ISSN 0721-8370
APOTHEKEN-PRAXIS; Forum fuer Marketing und Management. Text in German. 1979. 8/yr. **Document type:** *Journal, Trade.*
Published by: Deutscher Apotheker Verlag, Postfach 101061, Stuttgart 70009, Germany. TEL 49-711-2582-0, FAX 49-711-2582290, daz@deutscher-apotheker-verlag.de, http://www.deutscher-apotheker-verlag.de.

615 DEU ISSN 0720-549X
DER APOTHEKER-BERATER. Text in German. 1980. m. EUR 162 in Germany; EUR 162 foreign (effective 2002). **Document type:** *Journal, Trade.*
Published by: (Institut fuer Wirtschaftspublizistik), Vogel Verlag und Druck GmbH & Co. KG, Max-Planck-Str 7-9, Wuerzburg 97064, Germany. TEL 49-931-418-0, FAX 49-931-4182905, http://www.vogel-medien.de. **Subscr. to:** DataM-Services GmbH, Fichtestr 9, Wuerzburg 97074, Germany. TEL 49-931-417001, FAX 49-931-4170499, swestenberger@datam-services.de, http://www.datam-services.de.

615.1 DEU ISSN 0066-5347
APOTHEKER - JAHRBUCH. Text in German. 1915. a. EUR 39.90 (effective 2001); price varies. adv. index, cum.index. **Document type:** *Yearbook, Trade.* **Description:** Focuses on new pharmaceutical laws and decrees, jurisdiction, statistical data and important addresses.
—GNLM, Linda Hall.
Published by: (Deutscher Apotheker Verlag), Wissenschaftliche Verlagsgesellschaft mbH, Postfach 101061, Stuttgart 70009, Germany. TEL 49-711-2582-0, FAX 49-711-2582-290, service@wissenschaftliche-verlagsgesellschaft.de, http://www.wissenschaftliche-verlagsgesellschaft.de. Eds. Gert Schorn, Peter Ditzel.

615.1 DEU ISSN 0178-4862
APOTHEKER-ZEITUNG; Politik, Wirtschaft, Management, Recht. Text in German. 1985. w. **Document type:** *Newspaper, Trade.*
Related titles: ♦ Supplement to: Deutsche Apotheker Zeitung. ISSN 0011-9857.
Published by: Deutscher Apotheker Verlag, Postfach 101061, Stuttgart 70009, Germany. TEL 49-711-2582-0, 49-711-2582234, service@deutscher-apotheker-verlag.de, http://www.deutscher-apotheker-verlag.de. Eds. Dr. Klaus Brauer, Peter Ditzel.

615.1 BEL ISSN 0003-6579
APOTHEKERSBLAD. Text in Dutch. 1950. 10/yr. BEF 3,233 domestic; BEF 4,050 foreign (effective 2000). adv. bk.rev. index. **Document type:** *Bulletin.* **Description:** For Belgian community pharmacists.
Indexed: I.P.A.
Published by: Algemene Pharmaceutische Bond, Archimedesstraat 11, Brussels 1000, Belgium. TEL 32-2-2854200, FAX 32-2-2854285. Ed. D Broeckx. Circ: 4,500.

615.9 USA
APPROVED BIOEQUIVALENCY CODES. Text in English. 1992. m. USD 150; USD 1,150 foreign (effective 1999). **Description:** Lists FDA approved drug substitution information.
Published by: Facts and Comparisons, 111 W. Port Plaza, Ste. 300, St. Louis, MO 63146-3098. TEL 800-223-0554, FAX 314-878-5563. Ed. Bernie R Olin.

615.7 USA ISSN 1048-5996
RM301.45 .A66
APPROVED DRUG PRODUCTS WITH THERAPEUTIC EQUIVALENCE EVALUATIONS. Text in English. 1980. base vol. plus irreg. updates. USD 101 (effective 2001). **Document type:** *Government.* **Description:** Contains information required to identify a particular drug product. Includes N.D.A. and A.N.D.A. number for each entry.
Formerly (until 1985): Approved Prescription Drug Products with Therapeutic Equivalence Evaluations (0733-4036)
Related titles: Diskette ed.: USD 388 in North America; USD 766 elsewhere.
—CISTI.
Published by: U.S. Food and Drug Administration, Office of Public Affairs, 5600 Fishers Ln, Rockville, MD 20857. TEL 301-443-5315, http://www.ntis.gov. **Subscr. to:** U.S. Government Printing Office, Superintendent of Documents, PO Box 371954, Pittsburgh, PA 15250-7954. TEL 202-512-1800, FAX 202-512-2250, orders@gpo.gov, http://www.access.gpo.gov. **Dist. by:** National Technical Information Center, 5285 Port Royal Rd, Springfield, VA 22161. TEL 703-487-4650, FAX 703-321-5847.

615.10715 USA
APPROVED PROVIDERS OF CONTINUING PHARMACEUTICAL EDUCATION. Text in English. a. free. **Document type:** *Directory.*
Published by: American Council on Pharmaceutical Education, 311 W Superior St, Ste 512, Chicago, IL 60610. TEL 312-664-3575, FAX 312-664-4652. Ed. Dr. Peter H Vlasses.

615 UKR
APTEKA. Text in Ukrainian. w. USD 450 in United States.
Published by: Marion Ltd., Vladimirskaya ul 42, Kiev, Russian Federation. TEL 380-44-221-1523. **US dist. addr.:** East View Publications, 3020 Harbor Ln N, Minneapolis, MN 55447. TEL 612-550-0961.

615.1 GRC ISSN 0003-8148
CODEN: APKTAA
ARCHEIA TES PHARMAKEUTIKES (ATHENS). Text in English, French, Greek. 1932. irreg. GRD 150, USD 3. adv. bk.rev. bibl, charts, illus. index.
Indexed: Biol.Abstr., Chem.Abstr.
—CASDDS.
Published by: Greek Pharmaceutical Society, Emm. Benakis 30, Athens 106 78, Greece. Ed. N H Choulis. Circ: 1,000.

615.1 DEU ISSN 0365-6233
RS1 CODEN: ARPMAS
ARCHIV DER PHARMAZIE. Text in English. 1822. m. EUR 818 in Europe; CHF 1,398 in Switzerland & Liechtenstein; USD 1,068 elsewhere; EUR 859 combined subscription in Europe for print and online eds.; CHF 1,468 combined subscription in Switzerland & Liechtenstein, for print and online eds.; USD 1,122 combined subscription elsewhere for print and online eds. (effective 2002). bk.rev. charts, illus. index. reprint service avail. from ISI. *Refereed.* **Document type:** *Journal, Academic/Scholarly.* **Description:** Devoted to research and development in all fields of pharmaceutical chemistry.
Related titles: Microfiche ed.: (from BHP); Microfilm ed.: (from VCI); Online - full text ed.: ISSN 1521-4184. EUR 818 in Europe; CHF 1,398 in Switzerland & Liechtenstein; USD 1,068 elsewhere (effective 2002) (from EBSCO Publishing, Wiley InterScience, Institute for Scientific Information).
Indexed: ASCA, Anal.Abstr., Biol.Abstr., Chem.Abstr., Chem.Cit.Ind., Chem.Indus.Notes, Chem.Titles, Crop Physiol.Abstr., Curr.Adv.Ecol.Sci., Curr.Chem.React., Curr.Cont., Derwent Biotech.Abstr., Excerp.Med., Helminthol.Abstr., Hort.Abstr., I.P.A., Ind.Chem., Ind.Med. (1972-), Ind.Sci.Rev., Inpharma, MOS, Mass Spectr.Bull., NPU, Pharm.&Out.News, Protozool.Abstr., RCI, Reac., Ref.Zh., Rev.Med.& Vet.Mycol., Rev.Plant Path., Sci.Cit.Ind.
—BLDSC (1622.800000), CASDDS, CINDOC, CISTI, EMDOCS, GNLM, IDS, Infotrieve, ingenta, Linda Hall. **CCC.**
Published by: (Deutsche Pharmazeutische Gesellschaft), Wiley - V C H, Postfach 101161, Weinheim 69451, Germany. TEL 49-6201-606-147, FAX 49-6201-606-117, subservice@wiley-vch.de, http://www.interscience.wiley.com/archivderpharmazie, http://www.wiley-vch.de. Ed. R W Hartmann. R&P Claudia Rutz. Circ: 800. **Subscr. in the Americas to:** John Wiley & Sons, Inc., Journals, 605 Third Ave, New York, NY 10158. TEL 212-850-6645, FAX 212-850-6021; **Subscr. outside Germany, Austria & Switzerland to:** John Wiley & Sons Ltd., Baffins Ln, Chichester, Sussex PO19 IUD, United Kingdom. FAX 44-143-843232, 44-1243-843232.

615 KOR ISSN 0253-6269
CODEN: APHRDQ
ARCHIVES OF PHARMACAL RESEARCH. Text in English. 1978. bi-m. USD 120 (effective 2000). adv. back issues avail. *Refereed.* **Document type:** *Academic/Scholarly.*
Related titles: Online - full text ed.: (from Institute for Scientific Information).
Indexed: ASCA, BBCI, Biol.Abstr., Chem.Abstr., Chem.Indus.Notes, Chem.Titles, Curr.Cont., Excerp.Med., Forest.Abstr., Helminthol.Abstr., Hort.Abstr., I.P.A., Ind.Med. (1978-), Inpharma, Maize Abstr., Mass Spectr.Bull., Nutr.Abstr., Pharm.&Out.News, Reac., Hev.Arom.& Med.Plants, Rev.Med.& Vet.Mycol., Weed Abstr.
—BLDSC (1638.975000), CASDDS, EMDOCS, GNLM, IDS, KNAW.
Published by: Pharmaceutical Society of Korea, 1489-3 Suhcho 3 dong, Suhcho-gu, Seoul 137073, Korea, S.. TEL 82-2-584-3257, FAX 82-2-521-1781, pskor@thrunet.com, pskor@chollian.net, http://www.psk.or.kr, http://www.apr.psk.or.kr, http://www.pharmbiomed.org. Ed. Uhtaek Oh. Pub. Chang Jong Kim. R&P, Adv. contact Young Choong Kim. Circ: 1,500.

P

615.9 YUG ISSN 0354-3854
ARCHIVES OF TOXICOLOGY, KINETICS AND XENOBIOTIC METABOLISM; official journal of the toxicology section of the serbian medical society. Text in English; Summaries in English, Serbian. 1993. q. YUN 70 to individuals; YUN 700 to institutions (effective 2000). adv. bk.rev., software rev. back issues avail. *Refereed.* **Document type:** *Academic/Scholarly.* **Description:** Devoted to the evaluation of data, methods and opinions in the areas of toxicology, pharmacology, clinical pharmacology and xenobiotic metabolism.
Related titles: E-mail ed.
Published by: Serbian Medical Society, Toxicology Section, Dzordza Vasingtona 19, Belgrade 11000, Yugoslavia. TEL 381-11-3246090, FAX 381-11-3246090, ncktvma@unet.yu, http://www.solair.eunet.yu/~drmik/. Ed. Bogdan Boskovic. R&P, Adv. contact Matej Maksimovic TEL 381-11-543690. B&W page DEM 500, color page DEM 1,000. Circ: 200. **Subscr. to:** Nikolaja Gogolja 86, Belgrade 11030, Yugoslavia. **Distr. by:** National Poison Control Centre, Military Medical Academy, Crnotravska 17, Belgrade 110, Yugoslavia. TEL 381-11-3672187.

615.9 DEU ISSN 0171-9750
RA1190 CODEN: ATSUDG
ARCHIVES OF TOXICOLOGY. SUPPLEMENT. Text in English. 1978. irreg. reprint service avail. from ISI. **Document type:** *Monographic series.*
Related titles: Microform ed.: (from PQC).
Indexed: Chem.Abstr., Chem.Indus.Notes, Chem.Titles, Dent.Ind., Ind.Med. (1978-), NRN, Nutr.Abstr.
—BLDSC (1643.510100), CASDDS, CISTI, KNAW, Linda Hall. **CCC.**
Published by: Springer-Verlag (Subsidiary of: BertelsmannSpringer), Haber Str 7, Heidelberg 69126, Germany. FAX 49-30-82787448, subscriptions@springer.de, http://www.springer.de, http://link.springer-ny.com.

ARHIV ZA HIGIJENU RADA I TOKSIKOLOGIJU/ ARCHIVES OF INDUSTRIAL HYGIENE AND TOXICOLOGY. see *ENVIRONMENTAL STUDIES—Toxicology And Environmental Safety*

615.9 JPN
ARIS. Text in Japanese. 1991. m. JPY 3,000.
Indexed: Avery Ind.Archit.Per., BHA.
Published by: Odashima Iyaku Joho Senta/Odashima Pharmaceutical Information Center, 68 Oroshi-Machi, Hanamaki-shi, Iwate-ken 025-0311, Japan.

615.1 USA
ARIZONA PHARMACIST. Text in English. 1921. q. USD 30 to non-members (effective 2001); Free to members. adv. illus. 36 p./no. back issues avail. **Document type:** *Journal, Trade.* **Description:** Covers issues relevant to pharmacists and others working in that field. Includes new products, continuing education, alternative therapies, and patient care.
Former titles: New Arizona Pharmacist; Arizona Pharmacist (0004-1602)
Related titles: Supplement: Pharmacy Post (Tempe).
Indexed: I.P.A.
Published by: Arizona Pharmaceutical Association, 1845 E. Southern Ave, Tempe, AZ 85282-5831. TEL 480-838-3385, FAX 480-838-3557, azpa@azpharmacy.org, http://www.azpharmacy.org. Ed. Brenda Halbert. adv.: B&W page USD 425. Circ: 919 (paid and free).

P

615.9 610 USA
ARIZONA POISON CONTROL SYSTEM NEWSLETTER. Text in English. 1980. q. free per issue. **Document type:** *Newsletter.* **Description:** Updates and reviews about clinical toxicology and poisonings, for physicians, pharmacists and pharmacologists.
Published by: Arizona Poison Control System, University of Arizona, College of Pharmacy, Tucson, AZ 85721. TEL 602-626-1587, FAX 602-626-4063. Ed. Dr. Theodore G Tong. Circ: 3,000.

615.1 ESP ISSN 0004-2927
CODEN: APHRAN
ARS PHARMACEUTICA. Text in Spanish; Summaries in English. 1960. 4/yr. ESP 3,500 (effective 2001). adv. bk.rev. bibl, charts, illus. index.
Related titles: Online - full text ed.
Indexed: Aqua.Sci.& Fish.Abstr., Biol.Abstr., Chem.Abstr., Chem.Indus.Notes, Chem.Titles, Environ.Sci.Poll.Mgmt., Excerp.Med., INIS Atomind., I.P.A., Ind.Med.Esp., Ind.SST, Microbiol.Abstr., Pollut.Abstr., Ref.Zh., Risk Abstr., Saf.Sci.Abstr.
—BLDSC (1697.700000), CASDDS, CINDOC, CISTI, EMDOCS, GNLM, Infotrieve, KNAW. **CCC.**
Published by: (Facultad de Farmacia, Universidad de Granada), Editorial Universidad de Granada, Antiguo Colegio Maximo, Campus de Cartuja, Granada 18071, Spain. TEL 34-58-243930, FAX 34-58-243931. Ed. Jesus Cabo Torres. Circ: 1,000.

ARTERE. see *HEALTH FACILITIES AND ADMINISTRATION*

615 DEU ISSN 0066-8192
ARZNEI-TELEGRAMM. Text in German. 1970. m. DEM 104.64 to individuals; DEM 198.52 to institutions (effective 1999). bk.rev. **Document type:** *Academic/Scholarly.*
—GNLM.
Published by: Arzneimittel Information Berlin GmbH (A.T.I.), Bismarckstr 63, Berlin 10627, Germany. TEL 49-30-7949020, FAX 49-30-79490220, ati@berlin.snafu, http://www.arznei-telegramm.de. Ed. W Becker Brueser. Circ: 29,000.

615.1 DEU ISSN 0004-4172
RM301.25 CODEN: ARZNAD
ARZNEIMITTEL-FORSCHUNG/DRUG RESEARCH. Text in English, German. 1951. m. DEM 567.19, EUR 290 domestic; DEM 641.51, EUR 328 foreign; DEM 652.27, EUR 333.50 domestic print & online eds. combined; DEM 737.74, EUR 377.20 foreign print & online eds. combined (effective 2001). adv. bk.rev. charts, illus, tr.lit. index. reprint service avail. from IRC. *Refereed.* **Document type:** *Journal, Trade.* **Description:** Presents the results of research in novel drug molecules and the evaluation of new drugs in development.
Related titles: Online - full text ed.: (from Institute for Scientific Information).
Indexed: ASCA, Agri.& Environ.Biotech.Abstr. (coverage dropped), Anal.Abstr., Apic.Abstr., Biol.Abstr., CEABA, Chem.Abstr., Chem.Cit.Ind., Chem.Infd., Curr.Adv.Biochem., Curr.Adv.Ecol.Sci., Curr.Adv.Gen.& Molec.Biol., Curr.Biotech.Abstr., Curr.Chem.React., Curr.Cont., Curr.Ind.Stat., Dairy Sci.Abstr., Derwent Biotech.Abstr., Excerp.Med., Helminthol.Abstr., Hort.Abstr., INIS Atomind., I.P.A., Ind.Chem., Ind.Med. (1951-), Ind.Sci.Rev., Ind.Vet., Inpharma, Int.Abstr.Biol.Sci., Int.Nurs.Ind., Mass Spectr.Bull., Neurosci.Cit.Ind., Nutr.Abstr., Pharm.&Out.News, Protozool.Abstr., RCI, Reac., Ref.Zh., Rev.Appl.Entomol., Rev.Arom.& Med.Plants, Rev.Med.& Vet.Mycol., Rev.Plant Path., SSCI (coverage dropped), Sci.Cit.Ind., Vet.Bull., Weed Abstr.
—BLDSC (1738.000000), ADONIS, CASDDS, CINDOC, CISTI, EMDOCS, GNLM, IDS, KNAW, Linda Hall. **CCC.**
Published by: Editio Cantor Verlag, Postfach 1255, Aulendorf 88322, Germany. TEL 49-7525-940135, FAX 49-7525-940180, info@ecv.de, http://www.ecv.de/afhome.htm. Eds. H G Classen, V Schramm. adv.: B&W page DEM 3,189, color page DEM 5,172; trim 192 x 270. Circ: 5,200.

615.19 DEU ISSN 0933-1859
ARZNEIMITTEL, REZEPTPRUEFUNG, REGRESS. Text in German. 1978. irreg. DEM 178 (effective 2000). **Document type:** *Bulletin, Trade.*
Published by: Erich Schmidt Verlag GmbH & Co. (Berlin), Genthiner Str 30G, Berlin 10785, Germany. TEL 49-30-250085-0, FAX 49-30-25008521, vertrieb@esvmedien.de, http://www.erich-schmidt-verlag.de.

615.19 DEU ISSN 0935-2767
ARZNEIMITTEL ZEITUNG. Text in German. 1988. fortn. DEM 90. adv. bk.rev. **Document type:** *Newspaper.* **Description:** Information for employers in the pharmaceutical industry.
Published by: Aerzte Zeitung Verlagsgesellschaft mbH (Subsidiary of: BertelsmannSpringer), Am Forsthaus Gravenbruch 5, Neu-Isenburg 63263, Germany. TEL 49-6102-5060, FAX 49-6102-58740. Ed. Dieter Eschenbach. Pub. Gerald Kosaris. Adv. contact Ute Krille. Circ: 8,000.

615 DEU
DER ARZNEIMITTELBRIEF; unabhaengiges Informationsblatt fuer den Arzt. Text in German. 1967. m. DEM 76 (effective 2000). **Document type:** *Magazine, Academic/Scholarly.*
—BLDSC (1738.080000).
Published by: Westkreuz Druckerei und Verlag, Toepchiner Weg 198-200, Berlin 12309, Germany. TEL 49-30-7452047, FAX 49-30-7453066.

615.19 DEU ISSN 0723-6913
ARZNEIMITTELTHERAPIE; Informationen zur Pharmakotherapie fuer Aerzte und Arzneimittelkommissionen. Abbreviated title: A M T. Text in German. 1983. m. EUR 41.88 domestic; EUR 29.88 domestic to students; EUR 57 foreign; EUR 6 newsstand/cover (effective 2002). adv. bk.rev. **Document type:** *Journal, Academic/Scholarly, Trade.*
Indexed: Chem.Abstr., Ref.Zh.
—BLDSC (1738.120000), GNLM. **CCC.**
Published by: Wissenschaftliche Verlagsgesellschaft mbH, Postfach 101061, Stuttgart 70009, Germany. TEL 49-711-2582-0, FAX 49-711-2582-290, sheinzl@wissenschaftliche-verlagsgesellschaft.de, http://www.wissenschaftliche-verlagsgesellschaft.de. Ed. Susanne Heinzl. Adv. contact Klaus Graef TEL 49-711-2582245. Circ: 18,000.

615.19 SGP ISSN 0217-9687
CODEN: APJPEV
ASIA PACIFIC JOURNAL OF PHARMACOLOGY. Text in English. q. SGD 160 to individuals; SGD 250 to institutions (effective 1999). **Document type:** *Academic/Scholarly.* **Description:** Covers all aspects of experimental and clinical research on synthetic and natural drugs.
Related titles: Online - full text ed.: (from Institute for Scientific Information).
Indexed: ASCA, Chem.Abstr., Chem.Indus.Notes, Chem.Titles, Curr.Cont. (coverage dropped), Dairy Sci.Abstr., Inpharma, Neurosci.Cit.Ind., Nutr.Abstr., Pharm.&Out.News, Protozool.Abstr., Psychol.Abstr. (1992-), Reac., Rev.Arom.& Med.Plants, Rev.Med.& Vet.Mycol., Soyabean Abstr.
—BLDSC (1742.260800), CASDDS, EMDOCS, GNLM, IDS, KNAW.
Published by: Singapore University Press, Ground Floor Yusof Ishak House, 10 Kent Ridge Crescent, Singapore 119260, Singapore. TEL 65-7761148, FAX 65-7740652, supbooks@nus.edu.sg, http://www.nus.sg/sup. Ed. K Hashimoto.

615.19 FRA
ASSOCIATION DES PHARMACIENS DE L'INDUSTRIE. BULLETIN. Text in French. 6/yr. **Document type:** *Bulletin.*
Published by: Association des Pharmaciens de l'Industrie, 12 av. Victor Hugo, Paris 75116, France. TEL 45-00-78-18. Circ: 3,000.

615.1 CAN ISSN 0066-9555
ASSOCIATION OF FACULTIES OF PHARMACY OF CANADA. PROCEEDINGS. Text in English. 1970. a. membership. **Document type:** *Proceedings.*
Formerly (until vol.26, 1969): Canadian Conference of Pharmaceutical Faculties. Proceedings
Published by: Association of Faculties of Pharmacy, c/o J. Blackburn, 2609 Eastview, Saskatoon, SK S7J 3G7, Canada. FAX 604-822-4451, jblackburn@sk.sympatico.ca, http://www.pharmacy.ualberta.ca. Ed. J Blackburn. Circ: 200.

615.9 JPN ISSN 0914-7268
ATARASHII YAKUGAKU O MEZASHITE. Text in Japanese. 1965. a. JPY 1,000.
Published by: Shin'yakugaku Kenkyusha Gijutsusha Shudan/Japanese Youthful Group for Pharmaceutical Science and Technology, Komatsu Byoin Yakuzaika, 11-6 Kawakatsu-cho, Neyagawa-shi, Osaka-fu 572-0015, Japan.

615 ESP ISSN 1139-7357
CODEN: FACLE2
ATENCION FARMACEUTICA; European journal of clinical pharmacy. Text in English, Spanish. 1983. bi-m. ESP 9,500 domestic; EUR 144.24 in Europe; USD 175 elsewhere (effective 2000). **Document type:** *Academic/Scholarly.*
Formerly (until 1999): Farmacia Clinica (0212-6583)
Indexed: Chem.Abstr., Chem.Indus.Notes, Chem.Titles, Excerp.Med., I.P.A., Ind.SST, Inpharma, Reac.
—BLDSC (1765.858350), CASDDS, CINDOC, GNLM, Infotrieve, KNAW. **CCC.**
Published by: Rasgo Editorial S.A., Llaca, 16, Ent. 4a, Barcelona 08015, Spain. TEL 34-93-223-9982, FAX 34-93-211-7561, revista@farmclin.com, http://www.farmclin.com. Ed. Manuela Velazquez.

615 AUS ISSN 1325-8540
AUSTRALIAN ADVERSE DRUG REACTIONS BULLETIN. Text in English. 1995. q. free. Index. back issues avail. **Document type:** *Bulletin, Government.*
Media: Online - full text.
Indexed: Inpharma, Pharm.&Out.News, Reac.
—BLDSC (1796.773000).
Published by: Therapeutic Goods Administration, PO Box 100, Woden, ACT 2606, Australia. TEL 61-2-6232-8610, 61-2-6232-8444, FAX 61-2-6232-8222, tga-information-officer@health.gov.au, http://www.anzfa.gov.au/.

615 AUS ISSN 0706-3202
AUSTRALIAN INSTITUTE OF PHARMACY MANAGEMENT NEWSLETTER✶. Text in English. 1981. bi-m. free per issue to members. **Document type:** *Newsletter.*
—CISTI.
Published by: Pharmacy Guild of Australia, PO Box 2036, Canberra Mail Centre, ACT 2600, Australia. TEL 61-2-6270-1888, FAX 61-2-6270-1800, guild.nat@guild.org.au. Circ: 5,000.

615 AUS ISSN 0310-6810
CODEN: AUHPAI
AUSTRALIAN JOURNAL OF HOSPITAL PHARMACY. Text in English. 1966. q. AUD 94.50 domestic; AUD 115 foreign (effective 2000). adv. bk.rev. abstr, illus, stat. *Refereed.* **Document type:** *Academic/Scholarly.* **Description:** Aims to assist in the development of the practice of hospital pharmacy in Australia.
Indexed: Biol.Abstr., Chem.Abstr., Chem.Indus.Notes, Chem.Titles, Derwent Biotech.Abstr., Excerp.Med., I.P.A., Inpharma, Pharm.&Out.News, Reac.
—BLDSC (1808.700000), CASDDS, CISTI, EMDOCS, GNLM, Infotrieve, ingenta, KNAW, Linda Hall. **CCC.**
Published by: Society of Hospital Pharmacists of Australia, Level 11, 114 Albert Rd, South Melbourne, VIC 3205, Australia. TEL 61-3-9690-6733, FAX 61-3-9696-7634, ajhp@shpa.org.au, http://www.shpa.org.au. Ed. John Low. R&P Jennifer Johnstone. Adv. contact Noelle Hutchison. B&W page AUD 1,600, color page AUD 2,300; trim 297 x 210. Circ: 2,200.

615.1 AUS ISSN 0004-8399
AUSTRALIAN JOURNAL OF PHARMACY. Text in English. 1886. m. AUD 80; AUD 120 foreign (effective 1999). adv. bk.rev. illus, mkt. index. back issues avail. **Document type:** *Trade.*

Related titles: Microfilm ed.: (from PQC).
Indexed: Agri.& Environ.Biotech.Abstr. (coverage dropped), Aus.Sci.Ind., Biol.Abstr., Chem.Abstr., Excerp.Med., I.P.A., Inpharma, Pharm.&Out.News, Reac.
—BLDSC (1810.850000), CISTI, GNLM, Linda Hall.
Published by: Australian Pharmaceutical Publishing Co. Ltd., 40 Burwood Rd, Hawthorn, VIC 3122, Australia. TEL 61-3-9810-9800, FAX 61-3-9819-1706, http:appco@hcn.net.au, http://www.appco.com.au. Ed. Snezna Kerekovic. Circ: 7,600.

615 AUS ISSN 0728-4632
AUSTRALIAN PHARMACIST. Text in English. 1982. m. (11/yr.). AUD 70; AUD 100 foreign (effective 1999). adv. bk.rev. *Refereed.* **Document type:** *Trade.* **Description:** Contains continuing education material, news and information, research papers, therapeutic management reviews.
—ingenta.
Published by: Pharmaceutical Society of Australia, PO Box 21, Curtin, ACT 2605, Australia. TEL 61-2-6288-4777, FAX 61-2-6285-2869, australian.pharmacist@psa.org.au, http://www.psa.org.au. Ed., R&P Julie Wissmann. Adv. contact Jonathan Tremain. B&W page AUD 1,770, color page AUD 2,970. Circ: 9,482.

AUSTRALIAN PHYSIOLOGICAL AND PHARMACOLOGICAL SOCIETY. PROCEEDINGS (ONLINE EDITION). see *BIOLOGY—Physiology*

615 AUS ISSN 0312-8008
AUSTRALIAN PRESCRIBER. Text in English. 1975. 6/yr. free per issue to qualified personnel. bk.rev. *Refereed.* **Document type:** *Academic/Scholarly, Government.* **Description:** Provides an independent review of drugs and therapeutics.
Formerly: Prescriber's Journal (0085-5103)
Related titles: Online - full text ed.
Indexed: Diar.Dis.Res., Excerp.Med. (1995-), I.P.A., Inpharma, Pharm.&Out.News, Reac.
—BLDSC (1818.260000), EMDOCS, GNLM, ingenta, KNAW.
Address: GPO Box 9848, Canberra City, ACT 2601, Australia. TEL 61-2-6289-1555, 61-2-6289-7777, 800-020-103, FAX 61-2-62898641, info@australianprescriber.com, http://www.australianprescriber.com, http://www.health.gov.au. Ed. Dr. J. S. Dowden. Circ: 60,000 (controlled). **Co-sponsor:** Commonwealth Department of Health & Aged Care.

615.7 AUS ISSN 1321-9758
AUSTRALIAN PRESCRIPTION PRODUCTS GUIDE. Text in English. 1959. base vol. plus s-a. updates. AUD 165 domestic; AUD 270 foreign (effective 1999). **Document type:** *Trade.*
Formerly: Prescription Products Guide (0818-4445); Incorporates: Non-Prescription Products Guide (0818-4453); Formerly (until 1986): Prescription Proprietaries Guide (0729-2333)
Related titles: CD-ROM ed.: E A P P G. AUD 300 domestic; AUD 365 foreign (effective 1999).
Published by: Australian Pharmaceutical Publishing Co. Ltd., 40 Burwood Rd, Hawthorn, VIC 3122, Australia. TEL 61-3-9810-9800, FAX 61-3-9819-1706, appco@hcn.net.au, http://www.appco.com.au. Ed. J Thomas. Circ: 5,000.

615 GBR ISSN 1474-8665
CODEN: JAPHDU
AUTONOMIC & AUTACOID PHARMACOLOGY. Text in English. 1980. bi-m., latest vol.22, 2002. GBP 123 in Europe to individuals; USD 195 in North America to individuals; GBP 135 elsewhere to individuals; GBP 475 in Europe to institutions; USD 752 in North America to institutions; GBP 522 elsewhere to institutions (effective 2002). adv. abstr, bibl, illus. index. back issues avail. *Refereed.* **Document type:** *Academic/Scholarly.*
Formerly: Journal of Autonomic Pharmacology (0144-1795)
Related titles: Microform ed.: (from PQC); Online - full text ed.: ISSN 1474-8673. 1999. GBP 111 in Europe to individuals; USD 176 in North America to individuals; GBP 111 elsewhere to individuals; GBP 428 in Europe to institutions; USD 677 in North America to institutions; GBP 428 elsewhere to institutions (effective 2002) (from EBSCO Publishing, Munksgaard & Blackwell Science's Synergy, O C L C Online Computer Library Center, Inc., RoweCom Information Quest, ingenta, Swets Blackwell, Institute for Scientific Information).
Indexed: ASCA, Apic.Abstr., Aqua.Sci.& Fish.Abstr., Biol.Abstr., Chem.Abstr., Chem.Indus.Notes, Chem.Titles, Curr.Cont., Derwent Biotech.Abstr., Excerp.Med., Ind.Med. (1980-), Ind.Sci.Rev., Inpharma, Int.Abstr.Biol.Sci., Neurosci.Abstr. (coverage dropped), Neurosci.Cit.Ind., Pharm.&Out.News, Reac., Sci.Cit.Ind.
—BLDSC (4949.900000), ADONIS, CASDDS, CISTI, GNLM, IDS, ingenta, KNAW. **CCC.**
Published by: Blackwell Science Ltd., PO Box 88, Oxford OX2 0NE, United Kingdom. TEL 44-1865-206180, 44-1865-206002, FAX 44-1865-206219, jnl.orders@blacksci.co.uk, http://www.blackwellpublishing.com. Ed. K J Broadley. Pub. Allen Stevens. R&P Sophie Savage. Adv. contact Jenny Applin. Circ: 200.

615.19 USA
AZOAN. Text in English. 1923. a. free per issue. back issues avail. **Description:** Fraternity news, officers' reports, chapter reports, and professional articles.
Published by: Alpha Zeta Omega Pharmaceutical Fraternity, c/o Bruce Strell, 4422 Porpoise Dr, Tampa, FL 33617-8316. Circ: 2,000.

615.9 CAN ISSN 1203-214X
B C PHARMACY. Text in English. 1987. q. adv.
Formerly (until 1992): B C Pharmacist (0843-168X)
Published by: Canada Wide Magazines & Communications Ltd., 4180 Lougheed Hwy, 4th Fl, Burnaby, BC V5C 6A7, Canada. TEL 604-299-7311, FAX 604-299-9188. Pub. Peter Legge. Circ: 2,703.

615 DEU
B P I JAHRESBERICHT. Text in German. a. **Document type:** *Corporate.*
Published by: Bundesverband der Pharmazeutischen Industrie e.V., Karlstr 21, Frankfurt Am Main 60329, Germany. TEL 49-69-2556-1261, FAX 49-69-1603. Ed. Thomas Postina.

615 BHS
BAHAMAS PHARMACEUTICAL ASSOCIATION. NEWSLETTER. Text in English. m. **Document type:** *Newsletter.*
Published by: Bahamas Pharmaceutical Association, P.O. Box 3730, Nassau Np, Bahamas.

615 BGD ISSN 0301-4606
CODEN: BPJLAQ
BANGLADESH PHARMACEUTICAL JOURNAL. Text in English. 1972. q.
Related titles: Online - full text ed.
Indexed: Chem.Abstr., Excerp.Med., I.P.A.
—CASDDS, Linda Hall.
Published by: Bangladesh Pharmaceutical Society, University of Dhaka, Ramna, Dhaka 2, Bangladesh.

615 ITA
CODEN: GCMTEX
LE BASI RAZIONALI DELLA TERAPIA; Farmacologia Sperimentale e Clinica. Short title: G e B. Text in Italian; Summaries in English, French. 1971. q., latest vol.30, 2000. ITL 98,000 domestic; USD 130 foreign; ITL 24,500 per issue (effective 2001). adv. bk.rev. charts, illus. index. back issues avail. *Refereed.* **Document type:** *Journal, Academic/Scholarly.*
Supersedes: Giornale di Clinica Medica e Basi Razionali della Terapia (1120-8392); Which was formed by the merger of (1920-1991): Giornale di Clinica Medica (0017-0275); (1971-1991): Le Basi Razionali della Terapia (0393-7569)
Indexed: Biol.Abstr., Chem.Abstr., Excerp.Med., Ind.Med. (coverage dropped).
—CASDDS, CISTI, GNLM.
Published by: Piccin Editore, Via Altinate, 107, Padua, PD 35121, Italy. TEL 39-049-655566, FAX 39-049-8750693, info@piccinonline.com, http://www.piccinonline.com. Eds. Mariano Ferrari, Pier Luigi Canonico. Pub., R&P Massimo Piccin. adv.: B&W page ITL 6,000,000, color page ITL 9,900,000; trim 195 x 270. Circ: 64,300.

615 USA ISSN 0891-2033
BASIC AND CLINICAL PHARMACOLOGY*. Text in English. 1982. irreg., latest vol.6, 1994. **Document type:** *Monographic series.*
—Infotrieve. **CCC.**
Published by: Appleton & Lange, Journal Division (Subsidiary of: Simon & Schuster Company), 11 W 19th St, New York, CT 10011-4209. TEL 203-406-4500, FAX 203-406-4600.

615 540 DEU
BAYER REPORT. Text in German. 1958. 2/yr. free to stockholders. abstr, bibl, charts, illus, stat. back issues avail. **Document type:** *Magazine, Corporate.*
Formerly: Bayer Berichte (0005-6960)
Related titles: French ed.: ISSN 1438-0056; Italian ed.: ISSN 1437-8191; Japanese ed.; Portuguese ed.; Spanish ed.: ISSN 1437-8183; English ed.: ISSN 0343-1630.
Indexed: Intl.Polym.Sci.& Tech., RAPRA (1974-), Text.Tech.Dig. (1958-1991).
Published by: Bayer AG, Corporate Communications, Kaiser-Wilhelm-Allee, Leverkusen 51368, Germany. TEL 49-214-3058992, FAX 49-214-30571985, ute.bode.ub@bayer-ag.de, http://www.bayer.com. Ed. Ute Bode. Circ: 350,000.

615 150 USA ISSN 0955-8810
CODEN: BPHAEL
BEHAVIOURAL PHARMACOLOGY. Text in English. 1990. 8/yr. USD 222 domestic to individuals; USD 222 foreign to individuals; USD 735 domestic to institutions; USD 735 foreign to institutions; USD 84 newsstand/cover (effective 2002). adv. index. back issues avail.; reprints avail. *Refereed.* **Document type:** *Academic/Scholarly.* **Description:** Covers areas ranging from ethopharmacology to the pharmacology of schedule-controlled operant behavior.
Related titles: CD-ROM ed.; Online - full text ed.: USD 955.50 domestic for academic site license; USD 955.50 foreign for academic site license; USD 1,065.75 domestic for corporate site license; USD 1,065.75 foreign for corporate site license (effective 2002) (from Ovid Technologies, Inc., Institute for Scientific Information).
Indexed: ASCA, Addic.Abstr., Chem.Indus.Notes, Chem.Titles, Curr.Cont., Excerp.Med. (1993-), Focus on: Psychophar., Ind.Med. (1989-), Ind.Sci.Rev., Inpharma, Int.Abstr.Biol.Sci., Neurosci.Cit.Ind., Pharm.&Out.News, PsycInfo, Psychol.Abstr. (1989-), Psycscan B.A.& T., Reac., Rev.Med.& Vet.Mycol., SSCI (coverage dropped), Sci.Cit.Ind., e-psyche.
—BLDSC (1877.630000), ADONIS, CASDDS, CISTI, EMDOCS, GNLM, IDS, KNAW.
Published by: Lippincott Williams & Wilkins (Philadelphia) (Subsidiary of: Wolters Kluwer N.V.), 530 Walnut St, Philadelphia, PA 19106-3621. TEL 215-521-8300, FAX 215-521-8902, http://www.Lww.com. Ed. Paul Wilner. Adv. contact Gemma Heiser. Circ: 700. **Subscr. to:** PO Box 1600, Hagerstown, MD 21740-1600. TEL 800-777-2295, FAX 301-824-7390.

P

615.1 USA
RA975.5.P5
BEST PRACTICES FOR HEALTH-SYSTEM PHARMACY. Text in English. 1983. a. USD 49 (effective 2001). **Document type:** *Academic/Scholarly.* **Description:** Includes ASHP statements, guidelines, technical assistance bulletins, technician training program accreditation regulations and standards, residency accreditation regulations and standards, therapeutic positions statements, and therapeutic guidelines.
Formerly: Practice Standards of A S H P (Year) (0898-6738)
—CCC.
Published by: American Society of Health-System Pharmacists, 7272 Wisconsin Ave, Bethesda, MD 20814. TEL 301-657-4383, 301-657-3000, FAX 301-657-1251, http://www.ashp.org. Ed. Joseph Deffenbaugh Jr. R&P Jill Sellers. Circ: 15,000.

615 FRA ISSN 0154-893X
BIEN-ETRE ET SANTE. Text in French. 1977. m. (10/yr). FRF 145; FRF 14.50 newsstand/cover (effective 2000). adv. **Document type:** *Magazine, Consumer.* **Description:** Published by pharmacists offering practical advice and recommendations to acquire well-being.
Published by: SANTECOM, 75 rue des Vignes, Paris 75016, France. TEL 33-1-53925300, FAX 33-1-53925309, bienetresante@santecom.fr. Ed. Helene Vinon. Pub. Louis Robert Porte. adv.: color page FRF 120,000; trim 205 x 285. Circ: 530,164 (controlled).

615.1 USA ISSN 0006-2952
QP901 CODEN: BCPCA6
BIOCHEMICAL PHARMACOLOGY. Text in English. 1958. s-m. EUR 5,156 in Europe to institutions; JPY 684,800 in Japan to institutions; USD 5,767 elsewhere to institutions; EUR 519 in Europe to qualified personnel; JPY 69,000 in Japan to qualified personnel; USD 581 elsewhere to qualified personnel (effective 2002). adv. bk.rev. charts, illus, abstr. index. back issues avail.; reprint service avail. from PQC. *Refereed.* **Document type:** *Journal, Academic/Scholarly.* **Description:** Publishes research findings in biochemical pharmacology, with particular emphasis on molecular and structural biology and genetics.
Related titles: Microfilm ed.: (from PQC); Online - full text ed.: (from EBSCO Publishing, ingenta, Swets Blackwell, ScienceDirect, Institute for Scientific Information).

Indexed: ASCA, Abstr.Inter.Med., AgBiotech, Agri.& Environ.Biotech.Abstr. (coverage dropped), Anal.Abstr., Anim.Breed.Abstr., Apic.Abstr., BBCI, Biol.Abstr., Biotech.Cit.Ind., C.I.S. Abstr., Cal.Tiss.Abstr. (coverage dropped), Chem.Abstr., Chem.Cit.Ind., Chem.Indus.Notes, Chem.Titles, Chemorec.Abstr., Curr.Adv.Biochem., Curr.Adv.Cancer Res., Curr.Adv.Cell & Devel.Biol., Curr.Adv.Ecol.Sci., Curr.Adv.Gen.& Molec.Biol., Curr.Cont., Dairy Sci.Abstr., Dent.Ind., Derwent Biotech.Abstr., Environ.Sci.Poll.Mgmt., Excerp.Med., Helminthol.Abstr., Hort.Abstr., INIS Atomind., I.P.A., Ind.Med. (1958-), Ind.Sci.Rev., Ind.Vet., Inpharma, Int.Abstr.Biol.Sci., Mass Spectr.Bull., Neurosci.Abstr. (coverage dropped), Neurosci.Cit.Ind., Nuc.Acids Abstr., Nutr.Abstr., Pharm.&Out.News, Protozool.Abstr., Psychol.Abstr., Reac., Ref.Zh., Rev.Appl.Entomol., Rev.Arom.& Med.Plants, Rev.Med.& Vet.Mycol., Rev.Plant Path., SSCI (coverage dropped), Sci.Cit.Ind., Soyabean Abstr., Sugar Ind.Abstr., Tox.Abstr. (coverage dropped), Vet.Bull., Weed Abstr.
—BLDSC (2067.700000), ADONIS, CASDDS, CINDOC, CISTI, EMDOCS, GNLM, IDS, ingenta, KNAW, Linda Hall. **CCC.**
Published by: Elsevier Science, Box 945, New York, NY 10159-0945. TEL 212-989-5800, FAX 212-633-3990, usinfo-f@elsevier.com, http://www.elsevier.com/locate/biochempharm. Eds. Alan C Sartorelli, Jacques E Gielen. Circ: 1,150. **Subscr. in Australasia and the Far East to:** Elsevier Science (Singapore) Pte Ltd, No.1 Temasek Ave, 17-01 Millenia Tower, Singapore 039192, Singapore. TEL 65-434-3727, FAX 65-337-2230; **Subscr. in Japan to:** Elsevier Science Inc - Japan Regional Office, 9-15 Higashi-Azabu 1-chome, Minato-ku, Tokyo 106-0044, Japan. TEL 81-3-5561-5033, FAX 81-3-5561-5047; **Subscr. outside the Americas to:** Elsevier Science BV, PO Box 211, Amsterdam 1000 AE, Netherlands. TEL 31-20-485-3757, FAX 31-20-485-3432.

▼ **BIOCOMMERCE DATA'S BUSINESS PROFILE SERIES. VOLUME 1: THE U S BIOTECHNOLOGY DIRECTORY.** see *BIOLOGY—Biotechnology*

▼ **BIOCOMMERCE DATA'S BUSINESS PROFILE SERIES. VOLUME 2. THE EUROPEAN BIOTECHNOLOGY DIRECTORY.** see *BIOLOGY—Biotechnology*

▼ **BIOCOMMERCE DATA'S BUSINESS PROFILE SERIES. VOLUME 3: THE INTERNATIONAL BIOTECHNOLOGY DIRECTORY.** see *BIOLOGY—Biotechnology*

BIOCOMMERCE DATA'S BUSINESS PROFILE SERIES. VOLUME 4: THE U K BIOTECHNOLOGY DIRECTORY. see *BIOLOGY—Biotechnology*

615 616.97 NZL ISSN 1173-8804
CODEN: BIDRF4
BIODRUGS; clinical immunotherapeutics, biopharmaceuticals and gene therapy. Text in English. 1994. m. USD 165 to individuals Print or Online ed.; USD 198 to individuals Print and Online combined eds.; USD 1,095 to institutions Print or Online ed.; USD 1,314 to institutions Print and Online combined eds. (effective 2001). back issues avail. *Refereed.* **Document type:** *Academic/Scholarly.* **Description:** Covers clinical aspects of immunopharmacology, immune disorder treatments, clinical use of immunomodulating agents and cytokines.
Formerly: Clinical Immunotherapeutics (1172-7039)
Related titles: Online - full text ed.: (from Ovid Technologies, Inc., EBSCO Publishing, O C L C Online Computer Library Center, Inc., RoweCom Information Quest, ingenta, Swets Blackwell, Institute for Scientific Information).
Indexed: ASCA, Curr.Cont., Excerp.Med. (1995-), Focus on: Mol.Med., Ind.Sci.Rev., Inpharma, Nutr.Abstr., Pharm.&Out.News, Reac., Sci.Cit.Ind.
—BLDSC (2071.900000), ADONIS, CASDDS, CISTI, EMDOCS, GNLM, IDS, Infotrieve, KNAW. **CCC.**
Published by: Adis International Limited, Mairangi Bay, Private Bag 65901, Auckland 1010, New Zealand. TEL 64-9-477-0700, FAX 64-9-477-0766, biodrugs.adis.co.nz, http://www.adis.com; http://biomednet.com/library/jbod. Ed. Anne Bardsley-Elliot. Pub. Paul Chrisp. R&P Will Charles. Circ: 120. **Americas subscr. to:** Adis International Inc., Attn: Subscription Dept, 860 Town Center Dr, Langhorne, PA 19047. TEL 877-872-2347.

615.1 JPN ISSN 0918-6158
QP501 CODEN: BPBLEO
BIOLOGICAL & PHARMACEUTICAL BULLETIN. Text in English. 1978. m. JPY 10,300, USD 125 (effective 2001); includes Chemical & Pharmaceutical Bulletin. adv. charts, stat. index. 130 p./no. *Refereed.* **Document type:** *Bulletin, Academic/Scholarly.*
Formerly (until 1993): Journal of Pharmacobio-Dynamics (0386-846X)
Related titles: Online - full text ed.: (from Institute for Scientific Information).
Indexed: ASCA, Abstr.Hyg., AgBiotech, Agri.& Environ.Biotech.Abstr. (coverage dropped), Agroforest.Abstr., Anal.Abstr., Anim.Breed.Abstr., Aqua.Sci.& Fish.Abstr., Biol.Abstr., Chem.Abstr., Chem.Cit.Ind., Chem.Indus.Notes, Chem.Titles, Crop Physiol.Abstr., Curr.Adv.Cell & Devel.Biol., Curr.Adv.Ecol.Sci., Curr.Cont., Dairy Sci.Abstr., Dent.Ind., Derwent Biotech.Abstr., Environ.Sci.Poll.Mgmt., Excerp.Med., Field Crop Abstr., Forest Prod.Abstr., Hort.Abstr., INIS Atomind., Ind.Med. (1993-), Ind.Sci.Rev., Ind.Vet., Inpharma, Mass Spectr.Bull., Microbiol.Abstr., NPU, Neurosci.Abstr. (coverage dropped), Neurosci.Cit.Ind., Nutr.Abstr., Pharm.&Out.News, Plant Breed.Abstr., Plant Gen.Res.Abstr., Plant Grow.Reg.Abstr., Protozool.Abstr., Reac., Ref.Zh., Rev.Appl.Entomol., Rev.Arom.& Med.Plants, Rev.Med.& Vet.Mycol., Rev.Plant Path., Rice Abstr., Sci.Cit.Ind., Seed Abstr., Soyabean Abstr., Sport Fish.Abstr., Sugar Ind.Abstr., Triticale Abstr., Vet.Bull., Weed Abstr.
—BLDSC (2074.650000), CASDDS, CINDOC, CISTI, EMDOCS, GNLM, IDS, ingenta, KNAW, Linda Hall. **CCC.**
Published by: Pharmaceutical Society of Japan/Nihon Yakugakkai, 2-12-15, Shibuya, Shibuya-ku, Tokyo 150-0002, Japan. TEL 81-3-3406-3321, FAX 81-3-3498-1835, ronb@pharm.or.jp, http://bpb.pharm.or.jp. Ed. Tatsuya Takano. Circ: 3,650. **Subscr. to:** Japan Publications Trading Co. Ltd., P.O. Box 5030, Tokyo 100-33191, Japan. FAX 81-3-3292-0410.

BIOLOGY OF SPORT; a quarterly journal of sport and exercise sciences. see *MEDICAL SCIENCES—Sports Medicine*

BIOMEDICAL AND ENVIRONMENTAL SCIENCES. see *MEDICAL SCIENCES*

BIOMEDICAL MEETINGS INDEX. see *MEETINGS AND CONGRESSES*

BIOMEDICINE AND PHARMACOTHERAPY. see *MEDICAL SCIENCES*

615 USA ISSN 1040-8304
CODEN: BPRME5
BIOPHARM; the applied technologies of biopharmaceutical development. Text in English. 1987. m., latest vol.14. USD 64 domestic; USD 84 in Canada & Mexico; USD 124 elsewhere (effective 2001). adv. back issues avail.; reprints avail. *Refereed.* **Document type:** *Trade.* **Description:** Focuses on the science and industry of developing biotechnology-derived pharmaceutical products and biotherapeutic methods. Covers scientific and technical applications as well as issues, regulatory affairs, and business matters for scientists, engineers, managers, technicians, and corporate management.
Formerly: Biopharm Manufacturing (1040-8045)
Related titles: Online - full text ed.: (from Northern Light Technology, Inc., ProQuest Information & Learning, Gale Group, Factiva, Institute for Scientific Information).
Indexed: Aqua.Sci.& Fish.Abstr., Biotech.& Bioeng.Abstr., Biotech.Cit.Ind., Bus.& Indus. (Nov.1996-), Derwent Biotech.Abstr., Environ.Sci.Poll.Mgmt., Med.& Pharm.Biotech.Abstr., Telegen, Virol.Abstr.
—BLDSC (2089.353500), CASDDS, GNLM, IDS, Infotrieve, KNAW. **CCC.**
Published by: Advanstar Communications Inc., 7500 Old Oak Blvd, Cleveland, OH 44130. TEL 440-891-2767, 800-364-0085, FAX 440-891-2726, fulfill@superfill.com, http://www.biopharm-mag.com. Ed. Anne Montgomery. Circ: 20,500.

BIOPHARM. see *VETERINARY SCIENCE*

615 GBR ISSN 0142-2782
CODEN: BDDID8
BIOPHARMACEUTICS & DRUG DISPOSITION. Text in English. 1980. 9/yr. USD 1,775 in United States; USD 1,775 in Canada & Mexico; USD 1,775 elsewhere; USD 1,864 combined subscription in United States for print and online eds.; USD 1,864 combined subscription in Canada & Mexico for print and online eds.; USD 1,864 combined subscription elsewhere for print and online eds. (effective 2002). adv. back issues avail.; reprint service avail. from SWZ,PQC,ISI. *Refereed.* **Document type:** *Academic/Scholarly.* **Description:** Presents original reports of studies in biopharmaceutics, drug disposition and pharmacokinetics, especially those which have a direct relation to the therapeutic use of drugs.
Related titles: Microform ed.: (from PQC); Online - full text ed.: ISSN 1099-081X. 1997. USD 1,775 in United States; USD 1,775 in Canada & Mexico; USD 1,775 elsewhere (effective 2002) (from EBSCO Publishing, Wiley InterScience, Institute for Scientific Information).
Indexed: ASCA, Agri.& Environ.Biotech.Abstr. (coverage dropped), Anal.Abstr., Aqua.Sci.& Fish.Abstr., BBCI, Chem.Abstr., Chem.Indus.Notes, Chem.Titles, Curr.Adv.Ecol.Sci., Curr.Cont., Dairy Sci.Abstr., Derwent Biotech.Abstr., Environ.Sci.Poll.Mgmt., Excerp.Med., I.P.A., Ind.Med. (1979-), Ind.Sci.Rev., Inpharma, Mass Spectr.Bull., Pharm.&Out.News, Pollut.Abstr., Reac., Ref.Zh., Risk Abstr., Saf.Sci.Abstr., Sci.Cit.Ind.
—BLDSC (2089.355000), CASDDS, CISTI, EMDOCS, GNLM, IDS, Infotrieve, KNAW. **CCC.**
Published by: Wiley Europe Ltd., Baffins Ln, Chichester, W Sussex PO19 1UD, United Kingdom. TEL 44-1243-779777, FAX 44-1243-775878, customer.wiley.co.uk, customer@wiley.co.uk, http://www.interscience.wiley.com/jpages/0142-2782/, http://www.wiley.co.uk. adv.: B&W page GBP 650, color page GBP 1,550; trim 210 x 297. Circ: 550. **Subscr. in the Americas to:** John Wiley & Sons, Inc., Journals, 605 Third Ave, New York, NY 10158. TEL 212-850-6021, 212-850-6645, subinfo@jwiley.com.

BIOPHOENIX DATABASE ON CD-ROM. see *MEDICAL SCIENCES*

BIOTECHNOLOGY IN THE U.S. PHARMACEUTICAL INDUSTRY. see *BIOLOGY—Biotechnology*

615.328 JPN ISSN 0911-9477
BITAMIN B KENKYU IIKAI KIJI/VITAMIN B RESEARCH COMMITTEE. REPORT. Text in Japanese. irreg.
Published by: Bitamin B Kenkyu Iinkai/Vitamin B Research Committee, Nihon Itaria Kaikan, 4 Yoshidaushinomiya-cho, Sakyo-ku, Kyoto-shi 606-8302, Japan.

615.328 JPN
BITAMIN B KENKYU IINKAI HOKOKUSHO/VITAMIN B RESEARCH COMMITTEE. SHORT NOTE. Text in Japanese. a.
Published by: Bitamin B Kenkyu Iinkai/Vitamin B Research Committee, Nihon Itaria Kaikan, 4 Yoshidaushinomiya-cho, Sakyo-ku, Kyoto-shi 606-8302, Japan.

615.1 USA ISSN 0006-503X
BLUE AND GOLD TRIANGLE OF LAMBDA KAPPA SIGMA. Text in English. 1926. irreg. (4 nos. every 2 yrs.). USD 10 (effective 1997). adv. bk.rev. illus. **Document type:** *Newsletter.*
Published by: Lambda Kappa Sigma International Pharmaceutical Fraternity, 20110 Glenoaks Dr, Brookfield, WI 53045. TEL 262-784-8405, FAX 262-784-8406, lks@lks.org, http://www.lks.org. Ed. Nancy Horst. Circ: 12,000.

BLUEPRINT (NOTTINGHAM). see *BUSINESS AND ECONOMICS—Personnel Management*

615.1 ITA ISSN 0006-6648
CODEN: BCFAAI
BOLLETTINO CHIMICO FARMACEUTICO. Text in French, German, Italian; Summaries in English. 1861. m. ITL 452,000; USD 425 foreign (effective 2000). adv. bk.rev. pat. index. **Document type:** *Bulletin, Academic/Scholarly.* **Description:** Covers biopharmaceutics, pharmaceutical technology, pharmacokinetics, and industrial pharmacy.
Indexed: Agri.& Environ.Biotech.Abstr. (coverage dropped), Biol.Abstr., Chem.Abstr., Chem.Indus.Notes, Chem.Titles, Derwent Biotech.Abstr., Excerp.Med., I.P.A., Ind.Med. (1892-), Mass Spectr.Bull.
—BLDSC (2236.000000), CASDDS, CISTI, EMDOCS, GNLM, KNAW, Linda Hall.
Published by: Societa Editoriale Farmaceutica s.r.l., Via Ausonio, 12, Milan, MI 20123, Italy. TEL 02-89404545, FAX 02-89401168. Ed. G C Lubner. Adv. contact F Lubner. Circ: 3,000.

615.19 ITA ISSN 1120-8678
BOLLETTINO DI FARMACOSORVEGLIANZA. Text in Italian. 1990. 10/yr. free per issue. **Document type:** *Bulletin.*
Published by: (Societa Italiana per la Verifica e lo Sviluppo dei Farmaci Post-registrazione), Masson S.p.A., Divisione Periodici, Via F.lli Bressan 2, Milan, MI 20126, Italy. TEL 39-2-270741, FAX 39-2-27074210. Ed. Ettore Ambrosioni. Circ: 25,000.

615 DEU ISSN 0722-7159
BRAUNSCHWEIGER VEROEFFENTLICHUNGEN ZUR GESCHICHTE DER PHARMAZIE UND NATURWISSENSCHAFTEN. Text in German. 1957. irreg., latest vol.42, 1999. price varies. **Document type:** *Monographic series, Academic/Scholarly.*
Formerly: Technische Universitaet Braunschweig. Pharmaziegeschichtlichen Seminar. Veroeffentlichungen (0068-0729)
Published by: (Technische Universitaet Braunschweig), Deutscher Apotheker Verlag, Postfach 101061, Stuttgart 70009, Germany. TEL 49-711-2582-0, FAX 49-711-2582290. Ed. Erika Hickel.

BRIGGS UPDATE: DRUGS IN PREGNANCY AND LACTATION. see *MEDICAL SCIENCES—Obstetrics And Gynecology*

615 616.8 GBR ISSN 0264-2689
CODEN: BAPMEQ
BRITISH ASSOCIATION FOR PSYCHOPHARMACOLOGY. MONOGRAPH. Text in English. 1979. irreg. price varies. **Document type:** *Monographic series.*
Indexed: Chem.Abstr., Chem.Indus.Notes, Chem.Titles, e-psyche.
—CASDDS, CISTI, KNAW.
Published by: (British Association for Psychopharmacology), Oxford University Press, Oxford Journals, Walton St, Oxford OX2 6DP, United Kingdom. FAX 44-1865-267485, jnlorders@oup.co.uk, jnl.orders@oup.co.uk, http://www.oup.co.uk. **Orders in N. America to:** Oxford University Press, Journals. TEL 919-677-0977, FAX 919-677-1714, http://www.oup.co.uk.

617.96 GBR ISSN 0306-5251
CODEN: BCPHBM
BRITISH JOURNAL OF CLINICAL PHARMACOLOGY. Text in English. 1974. m., latest vol.53, 2002. GBP 109 in Europe to individuals; USD 185 in North America to individuals; GBP 120 elsewhere to individuals; GBP 550 in Europe to institutions; USD 872 in North America to institutions; GBP 605 elsewhere to institutions (effective 2002). adv. bk.rev. abstr, bibl, charts, illus. index. Supplement avail.; back issues avail. *Refereed.* **Document type:** *Academic/Scholarly.* **Description:** Contains papers and reports on all aspects of drug action in humans.
Related titles: Microform ed.: (from PQC); Online - full text ed.: ISSN 1365-2125. 1997. GBP 99 in Europe to individuals; USD 167 in North America to individuals; GBP 99 elsewhere to individuals; GBP 495 in Europe to institutions; USD 785 in North America to institutions; GBP 495 elsewhere to institutions (effective 2002) (from Ovid Technologies, Inc., EBSCO Publishing, O C L C Online Computer Library Center, Inc., RoweCom Information Quest, ingenta, Munksgaard & Blackwell Science's Synergy, Swets Blackwell, Institute for Scientific Information); ♦ Supplement: British Journal of Clinical Pharmacology. Supplement. ISSN 0264-3774.
Indexed: ASCA, Abstr.Inter.Med., Addic.Abstr., Agri.& Environ.Biotech.Abstr. (coverage dropped), Biol.Abstr., Chem.Abstr., Chem.Indus.Notes, Chem.Titles, Curr.Adv.Ecol.Sci., Curr.Cont., Dairy Sci.Abstr., Dent.Ind., Derwent Biotech.Abstr., Environ.Sci.Poll.Mgmt., Excerp.Med., Helminthol.Abstr., INIS Atomind., I.P.A., Ind.Med. (1974-), Ind.Sci.Rev., Inpharma, Int.Abstr.Biol.Sci., Int.Nurs.Ind., Kidney, Med.& Surg.Dermat., Neurosci.Cit.Ind., Nutr.Abstr., Pharm.&Out.News, Pollut.Abstr., Protozool.Abstr., Reac., Ref.Zh., Rev.Med.& Vet.Mycol., Risk Abstr., SSCI (coverage dropped), Saf.Sci.Abstr., Sci.Cit.Ind., Sugar Ind.Abstr., THA, Trop.Dis.Bull.
—BLDSC (2307.180000), ADONIS, CASDDS, CISTI, EMDOCS, GNLM, IDS, ingenta, KNAW. **CCC.**
Published by: (British Pharmacological Society), Blackwell Science Ltd., PO Box 88, Oxford OX2 0NE, United Kingdom. TEL 44-1865-206180, 44-1865-206002, FAX 44-1865-206219, journals.cs@blacksci.co.uk, jnl.orders@blacksci.co.uk, http://www.blackwell-science.com/products/journals/bjcp.htm, http://www.blackwellpublishing.com. Ed. G T Tucker. Pub. Elizabeth Whelan. R&P Sophie Savage. Adv. contact Jenny Applin. Circ: 1,570.

617.96 GBR ISSN 0264-3774
BRITISH JOURNAL OF CLINICAL PHARMACOLOGY. SUPPLEMENT. Text in English. 1976. irreg. **Document type:** *Journal, Academic/Scholarly.*
Related titles: ♦ Supplement to: British Journal of Clinical Pharmacology. ISSN 0306-5251.
—ADONIS.
Published by: Blackwell Science Ltd., Osney Mead, Oxford OX2 0EL, United Kingdom. TEL 44-1685-206206, FAX 44-1685-721205, journals.cs@blacksci.co.uk, http://www.blackwell-science.com.

615 GBR ISSN 0007-1188
CODEN: BJPCBM
BRITISH JOURNAL OF PHARMACOLOGY. Text in English. 1946. 24/yr. USD 310 in United States to individuals for print or online ed.; USD 341 combined subscription in United States to individuals print & online; GBP 1,027 combined subscription in Europe to institutions print & online; USD 1,764 elsewhere to institutions for print only; GBP 1,130 combined subscription in Europe to institutions print & online; USD 1,941 combined subscription elsewhere to institutions print & online (effective 2001); individual rates are for US subscribers. adv. charts, illus, stat. index. back issues avail. *Refereed.* **Document type:** *Journal, Academic/Scholarly.* **Description:** Presents original papers in experimental pharmacology.
Formerly: British Journal of Pharmacology and Chemotherapy
Related titles: Online - full text ed.: USD 1,643 to institutions outside Europe (effective 2001) (from HighWire Pr., EBSCO Publishing, O C L C Online Computer Library Center, Inc., RoweCom Information Quest, Institute for Scientific Information).
Indexed: ASCA, Agri.& Environ.Biotech.Abstr. (coverage dropped), Anim.Behav.Abstr. (coverage dropped), Anim.Breed.Abstr., Aqua.Sci.& Fish.Abstr., BBCI, Biol.Abstr., C.I.S. Abstr., Cal.Tiss.Abstr., Chem.Abstr., Chem.Indus.Notes, Chem.Titles, Curr.Adv.Cancer Res., Curr.Adv.Cell & Devel.Biol., Curr.Adv.Ecol.Sci., Curr.Chem.React., Curr.Cont., Dairy Sci.Abstr., Dent.Ind., Derwent Biotech.Abstr., Environ.Sci.Poll.Mgmt., Excerp.Med., Helminthol.Abstr., INIS Atomind., I.P.A., Ind.Chem., Ind.Med. (1968-), Ind.Sci.Rev., Ind.Vet., Inpharma, Int.Abstr.Biol.Sci., Jrnl.Watch Psych., Mass Spectr.Bull., Neurosci.Abstr. (coverage dropped), Neurosci.Cit.Ind., Nutr.Abstr., Pharm.&Out.News, Protozool.Abstr., RCI, Reac., Rev.Appl.Entomol., Rev.Arom.& Med.Plants, Rev.Med.& Vet.Mycol., SSCI (coverage dropped), Sci.Cit.Ind., THA, Tox.Abstr. (coverage dropped), Vet.Bull.
—BLDSC (2314.700000), ADONIS, CASDDS, CINDOC, CISTI, EMDOCS, GNLM, IDS, ingenta, KNAW, Linda Hall. **CCC.**
Published by: (British Pharmacological Society), Nature Publishing Group Specialist Journals (Subsidiary of: Holtzbrink Publishers), Houndmills, Basingstoke, Hants RG21 6XS, United Kingdom. TEL 44-1256-329242, FAX 44-1256-328339, subscriptions@nature.com, http://www.nature.com/bjp. Eds. P K Moore, R A North. Pub. Sue Deeley. R&P Trace Noel. Adv. contact Robert Sloan TEL 44-20-8882-7199.

615.1 GBR ISSN 0260-535X
BRITISH NATIONAL FORMULARY. Text in English. 1981. 2/yr. GBP 35 in United Kingdom; GBP 39 elsewhere (effective 2001). adv. index. **Document type:** *Academic/Scholarly.* **Description:** Gives information for prescribers in the National Health Service and other health care professionals about drugs and medicines available on prescriptions in the UK.
Related titles: CD-ROM ed.: GBP 70 (effective 2001); Single user only; other prices on application; Online - full text ed.
—BLDSC (2331.060000), Infotrieve. **CCC.**
Published by: (Euromed Communications Ltd.), Pharmaceutical Press (Subsidiary of: Euromed Communications Ltd.), 1 Lambeth High St, London SE1 7JN, United Kingdom. http://bnf.org/. Ed. D Mehta. Pub. Charles Fry. **Co-sponsor:** British Medical Association.

615.11941 GBR ISSN 1354-6643
BRITISH PHARMACOPOEIA. Key Title: British Pharmacopoeia and British Pharmacopoeia (Veterinary). Text in English. 1864. irreg., latest 1998. GBP 595 (effective 1998). **Document type:** *Government.* **Description:** Compiles official UK standards for medicines.
Incorporates (1977-1994): British Pharmacopoeia: Veterinary Edition
Related titles: Online - full text ed.
—BLDSC (2336.300000).
Published by: Stationery Office, 51 Nine Elms Ln, London SW8 5DA, United Kingdom. TEL 44-20-7873-0011, FAX 44-20-7873-8247, book.orders@theso.co.uk, http://www.national-publishing.co.uk.

615.1 GBR ISSN 0068-2519
BRITISH SOCIETY FOR THE HISTORY OF PHARMACY. TRANSACTIONS. Text in English. 1970. irreg. price varies. **Document type:** *Academic/Scholarly.*
Published by: British Society for the History of Pharmacy, 36 York Pl, Edinburgh, Midlothian EH1 3HU, United Kingdom. TEL 44-131-556-4386. Ed. Dr. J G L Burnby.

615.9 615.19 POL ISSN 0365-9445
RA1258 CODEN: BCTKAG
BROMATOLOGIA I CHEMIA TOKSYKOLOGICZNA. Text in Polish; Summaries in English. q. USD 100 (effective 1998). *Refereed.* **Document type:** *Academic/Scholarly.* **Description:** Deals with bromatology and toxicological chemistry. Contains scientific papers.
Indexed: AgroLibrex, Apic.Abstr., Aqua.Sci.& Fish.Abstr., Biol.Abstr., Chem.Abstr., Chem.Indus.Notes, Chem.Titles, Dairy Sci.Abstr., Environ.Sci.Poll.Mgmt., Excerp.Med., Food Sci.& Tech.Abstr., INIS Atomind., Maize Abstr., Nutr.Abstr., Pig News & Info., Poult.Abstr., Ref.Zh., Soils & Fert., Soyabean Abstr., Sugar Ind.Abstr., Tox.Abstr., Triticale Abstr., Weed Abstr., Zoo.Rec.
—CASDDS, GNLM, Linda Hall.
Published by: Polskie Towarzystwo Farmaceutyczne/Polish Pharmaceutical Society, Ul Dluga 16, Warsaw 00238, Poland. TEL 48-22-8310241, FAX 48-22-8310243.

BROWN UNIVERSITY GERIATRIC PSYCHOPHARMACOLOGY UPDATE; updates on use of psychotropic medications in geriatrics and pertinent regulatory issues. see *GERONTOLOGY AND GERIATRICS*

615 340 USA
BUREAU OF VOLUNTARY COMPLIANCE NEWSLETTERS. (Avail. in 35 state editions each with a national news section.) Text in English. 1979. q. USD 100. **Document type:** *Newsletter.*
Published by: National Association of Boards of Pharmacy, 700 Busse Hwy, Park Ridge, IL 60068-2402. TEL 708-698-6227, FAX 708-698-0124. Ed. Janice D Teplitz. Circ: 145,000.

789.56 658.8 GBR ISSN 1470-7012
BUSINESS RATIO. PHARMACEUTICAL MANUFACTURERS & DEVELOPERS. Text in English. 1973. a. GBP 275 (effective 2001). charts, stat. **Document type:** *Trade.*
Former titles (until 2000): Business Ratio Plus: Pharmaceutical Manufacturers and Developers (1358-8435); (until 1994): Business Ratio Plus. Pharmaceutical Manufacturers; (until 1992): Business Ratio Report. Pharmaceutical Manufacturers (0261-9350)
Published by: The Prospect Shop Ltd., Field House, 72 Oldfield Rd, Hampton, Middx TW12 2HQ, United Kingdom. TEL 44-20-8461-8730, 44-20-8481-8720, FAX 44-20-8783-1940, info@theprospectshop.co.uk.

615 658.8 GBR ISSN 1467-8926
BUSINESS RATIO. RETAIL AND WHOLESALE CHEMISTS. Text in English. 1981. a. GBP 275 (effective 2001). charts, stat. **Document type:** *Trade.*
Former titles (until 1999): Business Ratio Plus: Retail & Wholesale Chemists (1356-6067); (until 1994): Business Ratio Report. Retail and Wholesale Chemists (0261-9482)
Published by: The Prospect Shop Ltd., Field House, 72 Oldfield Rd, Hampton, Middx TW12 2HQ, United Kingdom. TEL 44-20-8461-8730, 44-20-8481-8720, FAX 44-20-8783-1940, info@theprospectshop.co.uk.

615.9 JPN ISSN 0389-9098
CODEN: BYYADW
BYOIN YAKUGAKU/JAPANESE JOURNAL OF HOSPITAL PHARMACY. Text in English, Japanese; Summaries in English. 1975. bi-m. JPY 1,500 per issue.
Indexed: Chem.Abstr., Chem.Indus.Notes, Chem.Titles, Excerp.Med., I.P.A.
—CASDDS, GNLM.
Published by: Nihon Byoin Yakuzaishikai/Japanese Society of Hospital Pharmacists, 12-15-304 Shibuya 2-chome, Shibuya-ku, Tokyo 150-0002, Japan.

C A SELECTS. ALKOXYLATED OLEOCHEMICALS. see *PHARMACY AND PHARMACOLOGY—Abstracting, Bibliographies, Statistics*

C A SELECTS. CALCIUM CHANNEL BLOCKERS. see *PHARMACY AND PHARMACOLOGY—Abstracting, Bibliographies, Statistics*

C A SELECTS. DRUG ANALYSIS BIOLOGICAL FLUIDS & TISSUES. see *PHARMACY AND PHARMACOLOGY—Abstracting, Bibliographies, Statistics*

P

615.1 USA ISSN 1080-563X
CODEN: CDREF
C N S DRUG REVIEWS. Text in English. 1995. q., latest vol.7, 2001. USD 168 domestic to individuals; USD 198 foreign to individuals; USD 285 domestic to institutions; USD 310 foreign to institutions (effective 2001). adv. index. back issues avail. *Refereed.* **Document type:** *Academic/Scholarly.* **Description:** Reviews of pharmacology, toxicology, pharmacokinetics, clinical trials with new drugs affecting the central nervous system, and reports on current scientific meetings.
Related titles: Online - full content ed.: ISSN 1527-3458; Online - full text ed.: (from Institute for Scientific Information).
Indexed: Chem.Abstr., Chem.Indus.Notes, Chem.Titles, Excerp.Med. (1996-), Focus on: Psychophar., Inpharma, Pharm.&Out.News, PsycInfo, Reac., e-psyche.
—BLDSC (3287.314343), CASDDS, CISTI, EMDOCS, GNLM, Infotrieve, KNAW. **CCC.**
Published by: Neva Press Inc., PO Box 347, Branford, CT 06405. TEL 203-272-5338, FAX 203-272-5338, nevapress@snet.net, http://www.nevapress.com. Eds. Alexander Scriabine, Israel Hanin. R&P, Adv. contact Barbara Botti. page USD 500; 5 x 7.5. Circ: 90 (paid); 110 (controlled).

615.1 616.8 NZL ISSN 1172-7047
CODEN: CNDREF
C N S DRUGS. (Central Nervous System) Text in English. 1994. m. USD 165 to individuals Print or Online ed.; USD 198 to individuals Print and Online combined eds.; USD 1,095 to institutions Print or Online ed.; USD 1,314 to institutions Print and Online combined eds. (effective 2001). bk.rev. back issues avail. *Refereed.* **Document type:** *Academic/Scholarly.* **Description:** Covers clinical aspects of psychiatric and neurological pharmacology.
Related titles: Online - full text ed.: (from Ovid Technologies, Inc., EBSCO Publishing, O C L C Online Computer Library Center, Inc., RoweCom Information Quest, ingenta, Swets Blackwell, Institute for Scientific Information).
Indexed: ASCA, Chem.Abstr., Chem.Indus.Notes, Chem.Titles, Curr.Cont., Excerp.Med. (1995-), Focus on: Psychophar., Forest Prod.Abstr., Helminthol.Abstr., Ind.Sci.Rev., Inpharma, Neurosci.Abstr., Neurosci.Cit.Ind., Pharm.&Out.News, Protozool.Abstr., PsycInfo, Reac., Rev.Arom.& Med.Plants, Rev.Med.& Vet.Mycol., Sci.Cit.Ind., Tox.Abstr., e-psyche.
—BLDSC (3287.314345), ADONIS, CASDDS, CISTI, EMDOCS, GNLM, IDS, Infotrieve, KNAW. **CCC.**
Published by: Adis International Limited, Mairangi Bay, Private Bag 65901, Auckland 1010, New Zealand. TEL 64-9-477-0700, FAX 64-9-477-0766, cnsdrugs@adis.co.nz, http://www.adis.com; http://biomednet.com/library/jcnd. Ed. Katharine Palmer. Pub. Paul Chrisp. R&P Will Charles. Circ: 250. **Americas subscr. to:** Adis International Inc., Attn: Subscription Dept, 860 Town Center Dr, Langhorne, PA 19047. TEL 877-872-2347.

615.1 USA
C P F I NEWSLETTER. Text in English. 1984. q. free per issue. bk.rev. back issues avail. **Document type:** *Newsletter.* **Description:** Communication link and network of Christian pharmacists around the world.
Published by: Christian Pharmacists Fellowship International, PO Box 1717, Bristol, TN 37621-1717. Ed. James E Thompson. Circ: 2,000.

615.19 USA
CALIFORNIA JOURNAL OF HEALTH - SYSTEM PHARMACY. Text in English. 1989. m. USD 75. adv. back issues avail. *Refereed.* **Document type:** *Trade.* **Description:** Reports news and legislature updates.
Formerly: California Journal of Hospital Pharmacy (1072-7809)
Indexed: I.P.A.
—GNLM.
Published by: California Society of Health - System Pharmacists, 725 30th St, Ste 208, Sacramento, CA 95816-3842. TEL 916-447-1033, FAX 916-447-2396, susan.trembly@cshp.org. Ed. Teresa Ann Miller. R&P Susan Trembly. Adv. contact Diana Granger. Circ: 3,800.

615.1 USA ISSN 0739-0483
CALIFORNIA PHARMACIST. Text in English. 1954. q. USD 25 domestic to non-members (effective 2001); free to members. adv. bk.rev. charts, illus, stat. index. *Refereed.* **Document type:** *Trade.* **Description:** Contains inofmation for pharmacists to enable them to serve the public health and welfare. Includes continuing education articles. Readers California pharmacists, professors of pharmacy and pharmacy students.
Formerly: California Pharmacy (0008-1388)
Indexed: I.P.A.
—BLDSC (3015.180000).
Published by: California Pharmacists Association, 1112, I St, Ste 300, Sacramento, CA 95814. TEL 916-444-7811, FAX 916-444-7929, pubs@cpha.com, cpha1@sna.com, http://www.cpha.com. R&P, Adv. contact Jamie Keswedet. B&W page USD 1,070, color page USD 1,800; trim 11 x 8.5. Circ: 5,500 (controlled).

615 CAN ISSN 1198-581X
CODEN: CJCPFB
CANADIAN JOURNAL OF CLINICAL PHARMACOLOGY/ JOURNAL CANADIEN DE PHARMACOLOGIE CLINIQUE. Text in English. 1994. q. CND 95 domestic; USD 130 foreign (effective 2000). adv. **Document type:** *Academic/Scholarly.*
Indexed: Excerp.Med. (1996-), Ind.Med. (1994-).
—BLDSC (3031.035000), CISTI, GNLM, Infotrieve, KNAW. **CCC.**
Published by: (Canadian Society for Clinical Pharmacology), Pulsus Group Inc., 2902 S Sheridan Way, Oakville, ON L6J 7L6, Canada. TEL 905-829-4770, FAX 905-829-4799, pulsus@pulsus.com, http://www.pulsus.com. Ed. Dr. Neil H Shear. Pub. Robert B Kalina. adv.: B&W page CND 1,530, color page CND 2,840; trim 10.88 x 8.13. Circ: 7,000.

CANADIAN JOURNAL OF HERBALISM. see *ALTERNATIVE MEDICINE*

615.1 CAN ISSN 0008-4123
CODEN: CJHPAV
CANADIAN JOURNAL OF HOSPITAL PHARMACY. Text in English, French. 1948. bi-m. CND 50 domestic; CND 57.20 in United States; CND 62.10 foreign (effective 2000). adv. bk.rev. abstr, charts, illus, pat, tr.lit. index. reprint service avail. from PQC. *Refereed.* **Document type:** *Academic/Scholarly.* **Description:** Publishes original research, clinical reviews, case reports, and topical discussions on pharmacy practice that are of use and interest to pharmacists engaged in institutional practice.
Formerly: Hospital Pharmacist
Related titles: Microform ed.: (from PQC); Online - full text ed.
Indexed: Agri.& Environ.Biotech.Abstr. (coverage dropped), Biol.Abstr., Chem.Abstr., Derwent Biotech.Abstr., Excerp.Med., Hosp.Lit.Ind., I.P.A., Inpharma, Pharm.&Out.News, Reac.
—BLDSC (3031.700000), CISTI, EMDOCS, GNLM, Infotrieve, ingenta, KNAW. **CCC.**
Published by: Canadian Society of Hospital Pharmacists, 1145 Hunt Club Rd, Ste 350, Ottawa, ON K1V 0Y3, Canada. TEL 613-736-9733, FAX 613-736-5660. Ed. Scott Walker. Adv. contact Marnie Boggs Reach. Circ: 3,300.

CANADIAN JOURNAL OF PHYSIOLOGY AND PHARMACOLOGY/JOURNAL CANADIEN DE PHYSIOLOGIE ET PHARMACOLOGIE. see *BIOLOGY—Physiology*

615.1 CAN ISSN 0828-6914
CODEN: CPJOAC
CANADIAN PHARMACEUTICAL JOURNAL/REVUE PHARMACEUTIQUE CANADIENNE. Short title: C P J - R P C. Text in English. 1868. 10/yr. CND 74.90 to non-members; CND 66 to members. adv. bk.rev. *Refereed.* **Document type:** *Trade.*
Related titles: Microfiche ed.: (from MML); Microform ed.: (from MML); Online - full text ed.: (from LexisNexis).
Indexed: Agri.& Environ.Biotech.Abstr. (coverage dropped), Biol.Abstr., CBCA Bus. (1998-), CBCA Ref., Can.B.P.I., Derwent Biotech.Abstr., Excerp.Med., I.P.A., Inpharma, Reac.
—BLDSC (3043.800000), CISTI, EMDOCS, GNLM, Infotrieve, KNAW. **CCC.**
Published by: (Canadian Pharmaceutical Association), Keith Healthcare Communications, 1785 Alta Vista Dr, Ottawa, ON K1G 3Y6, Canada. TEL 613-727-1364, FAX 613-739-7765, cpj@cyberus.ca. Ed., R&P Andrew Reinboldt. Pub. Clifford K Goodman. Adv. contact Deb Hopper. Circ: 20,000.

CANCER BIOTHERAPY & RADIOPHARMACEUTICALS. see *MEDICAL SCIENCES—Oncology*

CANCER CHEMOTHERAPY AND PHARMACOLOGY. see *MEDICAL SCIENCES—Oncology*

CANCER CHEMOTHERAPY AND PHARMACOLOGY. SUPPLEMENT. see *MEDICAL SCIENCES—Oncology*

615 USA ISSN 0897-5957
CODEN: CDREEA
CARDIOVASCULAR DRUG REVIEWS. Text in English. 1983. 4/yr., latest vol.19, 2001. USD 168 in US & Canada to individuals; USD 198 elsewhere to individuals; USD 285 in US & Canada to institutions; USD 310 elsewhere to institutions (effective 2001). adv. back issues avail. *Refereed.* **Document type:** *Journal, Academic/Scholarly.* **Description:** Reviews of pharmacology, pharmacokinetics, toxicology, clinical trials of new cardiovascular drugs, and reports on current scientific meetings.
Former titles (until 1988): New Cardiovascular Drugs (0891-3692); (until 1985): New Drugs Annual, Cardiovascular Drugs (0742-387X)
Related titles: Online - full content ed.: ISSN 1527-3466; Online - full text ed.: (from Institute for Scientific Information).
Indexed: ASCA, Chem.Abstr., Chem.Indus.Notes, Chem.Titles, Excerp.Med., Ind.Sci.Rev., Inpharma, Reac., Sci.Cit.Ind.
—BLDSC (3051.461500), CASDDS, CISTI, EMDOCS, GNLM, IDS, Infotrieve, KNAW. **CCC.**
Published by: Neva Press Inc., PO Box 347, Branford, CT 06405. TEL 203-272-5338, FAX 203-272-5338, nevapress@snet.net, http://www.nevapress.com. Ed. Alexander Scriabine. R&P, Adv. contact Barbara Botti. page USD 500; 5 x 7.5. Circ: 130 (paid); 120 (controlled).

CARDIOVASCULAR DRUGS AND THERAPY. see *MEDICAL SCIENCES—Cardiovascular Diseases*

615 USA ISSN 0528-1725
CAROLINA JOURNAL OF PHARMACY. Text in English. 1915. bi-m. USD 60. adv. back issues avail. **Document type:** *Trade.* **Description:** Covers issues related to pharmacy practice with emphasis on North Carolina pharmacy.
Indexed: I.P.A.
—Linda Hall.
Published by: North Carolina Pharmaceutical Association, PO Box 151, Chapel Hill, NC 27514. TEL 919-967-2237, FAX 919-968-9430. Ed. Fred Eckel. R&P, Adv. contact Brent Spodek. Circ: 3,000.

CATEGORY REPORT - HEALTH & BEAUTY AIDS. see *BEAUTY CULTURE—Perfumes And Cosmetics*

CATEGORY REPORT - HOUSEHOLD, PET & MISCELLANEOUS PRODUCTS. see *BEAUTY CULTURE—Perfumes And Cosmetics*

615.19 USA
THE CATHOLIC PHARMACIST. Short title: T.C.P. Text in English. 1968. q., latest vol.34, 2001. USD 20 to members (effective 2000). adv. bk.rev. 8 p./no. back issues avail. **Document type:** *Newsletter, Trade.* **Description:** Acquaints members with the latest developments in their church affecting their profession, as well as feature articles and membership news.
Published by: National Catholic Pharmacists Guild of the United States, 1012 Surrey Hills Dr., St. Louis, MO 63117-1438. TEL 314-645-0085. Ed., R&P, Adv. contact John Paul Winkelmann. Circ: 375.

CELLULAR AND MOLECULAR MECHANISMS OF INFLAMMATION; receptors of inflammatory cells: structure-function relationships. see *BIOLOGY*

615 NLD
CENTRE FOR MEDICINES RESEARCH WORKSHOP. Variant title: C M R Workshop. Text in English. irreg., latest vol.4, 1994. price varies. *Refereed.* **Document type:** *Proceedings.*
Published by: (Centre for Medicines Research GBR), Kluwer Academic Publishers Group (Subsidiary of: Wolters Kluwer N.V.), Spuiboulevard 50, PO Box 17, Dordrecht 3300 AA, Netherlands. FAX 31-78-639-2254, services@wkap.nl, http://www.wkap.nl. **Dist. by:** Journals Department, PO Box 322, Dordrecht 3300 AH, Netherlands. FAX 31-78-654-6474.

615.19 MDG
CENTRE NATIONAL DE RECHERCHES PHARMACEUTIQUES. ARCHIVES. Text in French. a. MGF 8,000, USD 5. back issues avail.
Indexed: P.L.E.S.A.
Published by: Centre National de Recherches Pharmaceutiques, BP 694, Antananarivo 101, Madagascar. TEL 33288. **Affiliate:** Centre d'Information et de Documentation Scientifique et Technique.

615 CZE ISSN 1210-7816
RS1 CODEN: CSLFEK
CESKA A SLOVENSKA FARMACIE/CZECH AND SLOVAK PHARMACY. Text in Czech, Slovak; Summaries in Czech, English. 1952. 6/yr. EUR 84, USD 108 (effective 2001). adv. bk.rev. index. *Refereed.* **Document type:** *Academic/Scholarly.* **Description:** Publishes original papers, reviews and short communications form the field of pharmacy and allied disciplines. Provides information on research dealing with synthetic and natural drugs, pharmacokinetics, technology of new drug forms, cultivation of medicinal plants, pharmaceutical care, dispensing, etc.
Formerly (until 1994): Ceskoslovenska Farmacie (0009-0530)
Related titles: Online - full text ed.
Indexed: Agri.& Environ.Biotech.Abstr. (coverage dropped), Anal.Abstr., Biol.Abstr., C.I.S. Abstr., Chem.Abstr., Chem.Indus.Notes, Chem.Titles, Curr.Adv.Ecol.Sci., Derwent Biotech.Abstr., Excerp.Med., INIS Atomind., I.P.A., Ind.Med. (1994-), Protozool.Abstr.
—BLDSC (3120.258380), CASDDS, CISTI, EMDOCS, GNLM, Infotrieve, Linda Hall. **CCC.**
Published by: (Ceska Lekarska Spolecnost J.E. Purkyne/Czech Medical Association), Nakladatelske Stredisko C L S J.E. Purkyne, Sokolska 31, Prague 12026, Czech Republic. TEL 42-2-24911420, FAX 42-2-24911420, nts@iol.cz, http://www.clsjep.cz, http://www.medical.cz. Ed. P Komarek. adv.: B&W page CZK 29,300, color page CZK 41,000; 246 x 180. Circ: 900. **Dist. by:** Abont s.r.o., Chlumova 17, Prague, 3 130 00, Czech Republic; **Dist. in Western countries by:** Kubon & Sagner, Hesstr 39-41, Munich 80798, Germany.

CHEMICAL & PHARMACEUTICAL BULLETIN. see *CHEMISTRY*

CHEMICAL RESEARCH IN TOXICOLOGY. see *ENVIRONMENTAL STUDIES—Toxicology And Environmental Safety*

CHEMICALS, DRUGS, PHARMACEUTICALS, PETROLEUM, PETROCHEMICALS, FERTILIZERS. see *ENGINEERING—Chemical Engineering*

CHEMISCHE RUNDSCHAU; Zeitung fuer Chemie, Lebensmitteltechnologie, Pharmazie und Biotechnologie. see *CHEMISTRY*

615.1 GBR ISSN 0009-3033
RS1.C54 CODEN: CHDRA3
CHEMIST & DRUGGIST; for retailer, wholesaler, manufacturer. Text in English. 1859. w. GBP 140 (effective 2001). adv. bk.rev. charts, illus, mkt, pat, tr.mk. s-a. index. **Document type:** *Magazine, Trade.*
Incorporates: Retail Chemist (0034-6020)
Related titles: Microform ed.: (from PQC); Online - full text ed.: (from Gale Group, ProQuest Information & Learning); ♦ Supplement: Chemist & Druggist Price List. ISSN 0266-3023; ♦ O T C - Over the Counter.
Indexed: Br.Tech.Ind., Bus.& Indus. (Feb.1995-), Chem.Abstr., I.P.A., PROMT.
—BLDSC (3167.000000), CASDDS, Infotrieve, ingenta, KNAW, Linda Hall. **CCC.**
Published by: (Pharmaceutical Society of Northern Ireland), C M P Information (Subsidiary of: United Business Media), Riverbank House, Angel Ln., Tonbridge, Kent TN9 1SE, United Kingdom. TEL 44-1732-364422, FAX 44-1732-361534, TELEX 95132 BENTON G, chemdrug@dotpharmacy.com, http://www.dotpharmacy.com. Ed. Patrick Grice. Adv. contact Ian Gerrard. Circ: 15,413.

615.1029 GBR ISSN 0262-5881
CHEMIST & DRUGGIST DIRECTORY. Text in English. 1868. a. GBP 129 (effective 2002). adv. **Document type:** *Directory.* **Description:** Lists the pharmaceutical and affiliated trades. Coverage includes tablet and capsule identification guide. Lists multiple retail outlets, wholesalers, pharmaceutical organizations, and drug contraindications.
—BLDSC (3167.500000).
Published by: C M P Information (Subsidiary of: United Business Media), Sovereign House, Sovereign Way, Tonbridge, Kent TN9 1RW, United Kingdom. TEL 44-1732-362666, FAX 44-1732-367301, enquiries@cmpinformation.com, http://www.mfplc.com, http://www.cmpinformation.com. Ed. Gwen Young. R&P Sarah Walker. Adv. contact Elaine Soni TEL 44-1732-377423. Circ: 2,900.

615.1 IND ISSN 0009-3041
CHEMIST & DRUGSTORE NEWS. Text in English. m. INR 20. bk.rev.
Published by: India Publications Co., Denabank House, 2nd Fl., 31 Hamam St., Mumbai, Maharashtra 400 001, India. Ed. Eric Martin. Circ: (controlled).

615.1 PAK ISSN 0009-3149
CHEMISTS REVIEW. Text in English, Urdu. 1957. m. PKR 250. adv. bk.rev. charts, illus.
Address: P O Box 376, Karachi, Pakistan. Ed. M Y Ansari. Circ: 5,000.

615.1 CHE ISSN 0009-3157
RM260 CODEN: CHTHBK
CHEMOTHERAPY; international journal of experimental and clinical chemotherapy. Text in English. 1960. bi-m. CHF 891 in Europe to institutions; CHF 908.40 overseas to institutions; EUR 636.80 in Europe to institutions; USD 694 overseas to institutions (effective 2002). adv. bk.rev. bibl, charts, illus. back issues avail. *Refereed.* **Document type:** *Journal, Academic/Scholarly.* **Description:** Publishes the results of investigations into the mode of action and pharmacologic properties of antibacterial, antiviral and antitumor substances.
Formerly (until 1967): Chemotherapia (0366-7170)
Related titles: Microfilm ed.; Online - full text ed.: ISSN 1421-9794. CHF 58, EUR 42, USD 45 to institutions (effective 2002) (from EBSCO Publishing, O C L C Online Computer Library Center, Inc., RoweCom Information Quest, Swets Blackwell, Institute for Scientific Information).
Indexed: ASCA, Abstr.Hyg., Agri.& Environ.Biotech.Abstr. (coverage dropped), Biodet.Abstr., Biol.Abstr., Chem.Abstr., Chem.Indus.Notes, Chem.Titles, Curr.Adv.Cancer Res., Curr.Cont., Dairy Sci.Abstr., Derwent Biotech.Abstr., Diar.Dis.Res., Environ.Sci.Poll.Mgmt., Excerp.Med., Helminthol.Abstr., I.P.A., Ind.Med. (1968-), Ind.Sci.Rev., Inpharma, Med.& Pharm.Biotech.Abstr., Microbiol.Abstr., Pharm.&Out.News, Protozool.Abstr., Reac., Rev.Med.& Vet.Mycol., Rev.Plant Path., Sci.Cit.Ind., Trop.Dis.Bull., Vet.Bull.
—BLDSC (3172.304000), CASDDS, CISTI, GNLM, IDS, Infotrieve, ingenta, KNAW. **CCC.**
Published by: S. Karger AG, Allschwilerstr 10, PO Box, Basel 4009, Switzerland. TEL 41-61-306-1111, FAX 41-61-306-1234, karger@karger.ch, http://www.online.karger.com/journals/che, http://www.karger.com. Ed. H Schoenfeld. adv.: page USD 1,185. Circ: 1,300.

615 920 ITA
CHI E CHI SANITA E SALUTE. Text in Italian. 1992. a. ITL 40,000 (effective 1998). **Document type:** *Directory.*
Published by: Crisalide Press, Via Brusuglio, 66, Milan, MI 20161, Italy. TEL 39-2-6464663, FAX 39-2-6461622. Ed. Bianca Carretto. Circ: 10,000.

615.9 JPN
CHIBA DAIGAKU YAKUGAKUBU KENKYU GYOSEKI MOKUROKU/CHIBA UNIVERSITY. FACULTY OF PHARMACEUTICAL SCIENCES. LIST OF RESEARCH ACTIVITIES. Text in Japanese. 1984. biennial. **Document type:** *Academic/Scholarly.*
Published by: Chiba Daigaku, Yakugakubu/Chiba University, Faculty of Pharmaceutical Sciences, 1-33 Yayoi-cho, Inage-ku, Chiba-shi 263-0022, Japan. TEL 81-43-290-2981, FAX 81-43-290-2974. Circ: 300.

615.9 617.6 JPN ISSN 0300-029X
CHIKEN ISHIYAKU JOHO/INVESTIGATIONAL DRUG INFORMATION. MEDICAL AND DENTAL. Text in Japanese. 1970. a. JPY 25,000.
Published by: Iji Shuppansha, 2-8 Shinkawa 1-chome, Chuo-ku, Tokyo 104-0033, Japan.

CHILD AND ADOLESCENT PSYCHOPHARMACOLOGY NEWS. see *MEDICAL SCIENCES—Psychiatry And Neurology*

CHIMICA OGGI/CHEMISTRY TODAY. see *CHEMISTRY*

615.9 USA
CHINA DISTRIBUTOR SALES AUDIT. Text in English. 1995. q. USD 40 (effective 1998). index. back issues avail. **Document type:** *Trade.* **Description:** Contains data on sales by 20 large Chinese distributors of Western-type pharmaceuticals.
Related titles: Chinese ed.
Published by: ChinaMetrik, 1010 Wisconsin Ave N W, Ste 310, Washington, DC 20007-3603. TEL 202-331-9370, FAX 202-337-4498, cmetrik@aol.com. Ed. A Wolters. R&P J Ebersole.

615.9 USA
CHINA DRUG PURCHASE AUDIT. Text in English. 1985. q. USD 19,750. index. back issues avail. **Document type:** *Trade.* **Description:** Contains data on purchases of Western-type drugs by sample of 50 major Chinese hospitals.
Related titles: Chinese ed.
Published by: ChinaMetrik, 1010 Wisconsin Ave N W, Ste 310, Washington, DC 20007-3603. TEL 202-331-9370, FAX 202-337-4498, cmetrik@aol.com. Ed. A Wolters. R&P J Ebersole.

CHINA PHARMACEUTICAL AND MEDICAL INSTRUMENTS. see *MEDICAL SCIENCES*

CHINESE MEDICAL SCIENCES JOURNAL. see *MEDICAL SCIENCES*

615.19 ESP ISSN 1575-3409
CODEN: CIPHEA
CIENCIA Y TECNOLOGIA PHARMACEUTICA; revista espanola del medicamento y del producto sanitario. Text in Spanish. 1987. every 3 mos. ESP 6,000 domestic; USD 65 in Europe; USD 70 elsewhere (effective 2001). adv. charts. *Refereed.* **Document type:** *Academic/Scholarly.* **Description:** Publishes research and reviews in pharmacology.
Former titles: Ciencia Pharmaceutica (1131-5253); (until 1990): Pharmaklinik (1011-4386)
Indexed: Chem.Abstr., Chem.Indus.Notes, Chem.Titles, Excerp.Med., I.P.A.
—BLDSC (3198.095000), CASDDS, CINDOC, CISTI, EMDOCS, GNLM, Infotrieve. **CCC.**
Published by: Alpe Editores S.A., Pedro Rico, 27, Madrid 28029, Spain. TEL 34-91-733-8811, FAX 34-91-315-9652, alpeeditores@sistelcom.com. Ed. Dr. Jose Maria Sune Arbussa. Pub. Angeles Alvarez Sanchez. Adv. contact Ana Jurado. color page ESP 160,000; trim 210 x 280. Circ: 3,500 (controlled).

CLINICAL AND EXPERIMENTAL PHARMACOLOGY & PHYSIOLOGY. see *BIOLOGY—Physiology*

CLINICAL AND EXPERIMENTAL PHARMACOLOGY & PHYSIOLOGY. SUPPLEMENT. see *BIOLOGY—Physiology*

615.9 USA
CLINICAL CONSULT. Text in English. 1982. m., latest vol.16. free per issue to members. back issues avail.; reprints avail. **Document type:** *Newsletter, Academic/Scholarly.* **Description:** Focuses on geriatric drug therapy and, or clinical illness and offers guidance to readers on drug therapy monitoring criteria.
Related titles: Online - full text ed.
Published by: American Society of Consultant Pharmacists, 1321 Duke St, Alexandria, VA 22314-3563. TEL 703-739-1300, FAX 703-739-1321, http://www.ascp.com/public/pubs/cc. Ed. H Edward Davidson. Pub. R Tim Webster. R&P David K Buerger TEL 703-739-1300. Circ: 7,000 (controlled).

615 NZL ISSN 1173-2563
CODEN: CDINFR
CLINICAL DRUG INVESTIGATION. Text in English. 1989. m. USD 95 to individuals Print or Online ed.; USD 114 to individuals Print and Online combined eds.; USD 295 to institutions Print or Online ed.; USD 354 to institutions Print and Online combined eds. (effective 2001). back issues avail. *Refereed.* **Document type:** *Academic/Scholarly.* **Description:** Publishes original research covering all phases of clinical drug development and therapeutic use of drugs.
Formerly (until 1995): Drug Investigation (0114-2402)
Related titles: Online - full text ed.: (from Ovid Technologies, Inc., EBSCO Publishing, O C L C Online Computer Library Center, Inc., RoweCom Information Quest, ingenta, Swets Blackwell, Institute for Scientific Information).
Indexed: ASCA, Abstr.Hyg., Chem.Abstr., Chem.Indus.Notes, Chem.Titles, Curr.Cont., Derwent Biotech.Abstr., Excerp.Med., I.P.A., Ind.Med. (coverage dropped), Inpharma, Int.Abstr.Biol.Sci., Nutr.Abstr., Pharm.&Out.News, Protozool.Abstr., Reac., Rev.Arom.& Med.Plants, Rev.Med.& Vet.Mycol., Sci.Cit.Ind., Sugar Ind.Abstr., Trop.Dis.Bull.
—BLDSC (3286.273600), ADONIS, CASDDS, CISTI, EMDOCS, GNLM, IDS, Infotrieve, ingenta, KNAW, Linda Hall. **CCC.**
Published by: Adis International Limited, Mairangi Bay, Private Bag 65901, Auckland 1010, New Zealand. TEL 64-9-477-0700, FAX 64-9-477-0766, clindruginvest@adis.co.nz, http://www.adis.com. Ed. Paul Battershill. Pub. Paul Chrisp. R&P Will Charles. Circ: 3,000. **Americas subscr. to:** Adis International Inc., Attn: Subscription Dept, 860 Town Center Dr, Langhorne, PA 19047. TEL 877-872-2347.

P

615 USA ISSN 1208-6495
CLINICAL HANDBOOK OF PSYCHOTROPIC DRUGS. Text in English. 1988. irreg., base vol. plus q. updates. USD 89.50. **Document type:** *Monographic series, Academic/Scholarly.*
Published by: Hogrefe & Huber Publishers, PO Box 2487, Kirkland, WA 98083. TEL 425-820-1500, FAX 425-823-8324, hh@hhpub.com, http://www.hhpub.com/journals. Eds. J Joel Jeffries, Kalyna Bezchlibnyk-Butler.

570 615 USA ISSN 1068-1191
CLINICAL INVESTIGATOR NEWS. Text in English. 1993. m. USD 563 in US & Canada; USD 593 elsewhere (effective 2001). bibl, pat, stat, tr.lit. back issues avail. **Document type:** *Newsletter.* **Description:** Covers new drug study opportunities, which companies are targeting, what compounds, when they plan to begin trials, and where they stand in their research.
Indexed: Inpharma, Pharm.&Out.News, Reac.
—**CCC.**
Published by: C T B International Publishing Inc., PO Box 218, Maplewood, NJ 07040-0218. TEL 973-379-7749, FAX 973-379-1158, info@ctbintl.com, http://www.ctbintl.com. Ed., R&P Christopher Brogna. Pub. Oykue Brogna.

615 USA ISSN 0362-5664
RM315 CODEN: CLNEDB
CLINICAL NEUROPHARMACOLOGY. Text in English. 1978. bi-m. USD 243 domestic to individuals; USD 310 foreign to individuals; USD 460 domestic to institutions; USD 545 foreign to institutions; USD 82 newsstand/cover (effective 2002). adv. charts, illus. index. back issues avail.; reprint service avail. from PQC. *Refereed.* **Document type:** *Academic/Scholarly.* **Description:** Features reviews and original investigations on the pharmacology of central nervous system dysfunction.
Related titles: Online - full text ed.: USD 598 domestic for academic site license; USD 683 foreign for academic site license; USD 667 domestic for corporate site license; USD 752 foreign for corporate site license (effective 2002) (from Ovid Technologies, Inc., Institute for Scientific Information).
Indexed: ASCA, Biol.Abstr., Chem.Abstr., Chem.Indus.Notes, Chem.Titles, Curr.Adv.Ecol.Sci., Curr.Cont., Derwent Biotech.Abstr., Excerp.Med., Focus on: Psychophar., Ind.Med. (1976-), Ind.Sci.Rev., Inpharma, Int.Abstr.Biol.Sci., Neurosci.Cit.Ind., Nutr.Abstr., Pharm.&Out.News, PsycInfo, Psychol.Abstr. (1990-), Reac., SSCI (coverage dropped), Sci.Cit.Ind., e-psyche.
—BLDSC (3286.310600), CASDDS, CISTI, EMDOCS, GNLM, IDS, ingenta, KNAW.
Published by: Lippincott Williams & Wilkins (Philadelphia) (Subsidiary of: Wolters Kluwer N.V.), 530 Walnut St, Philadelphia, PA 19106-3621. TEL 215-521-8300, FAX 215-521-8902, http://www.Lww.com. Ed. Dr. Christopher E Goetz. Pub. Nancy Megley. R&P Margaret Becker. Adv. contact Ray Thibodeau. B&W page USD 655, color page USD 1,795. Circ: 731 (paid). **Subscr. to:** PO Box 1600, Hagerstown, MD 21740-1600. TEL 800-777-2295, FAX 301-824-7390.

615.19 USA ISSN 0886-7879
CLINICAL PHARMACOKINETIC NEWSLETTER. Text in English. 1984. q. USD 10. bk.rev. bibl, charts, illus. cum.index.
Published by: Rhode Island Hospital, Department of Pharmacy, 593 Eddy St, Providence, RI 02902. TEL 401-277-5050. Ed. Dr. Louis P Jeffrey. Circ: 1,000.

615 NZL ISSN 0312-5963
CODEN: CPKNDH
CLINICAL PHARMACOKINETICS. Text in English. 1976. m. USD 1,095 Print or Online ed.; USD 1,314 Print and Online combined eds. (effective 2001). back issues avail. *Refereed.* **Document type:** *Academic/Scholarly.* **Description:** Provides clinically relevant pharmacokinetic knowledge to aid in the delivery of rational drug therapy.
Related titles: Online - full text ed.: (from Ovid Technologies, Inc., EBSCO Publishing, O C L C Online Computer Library Center, Inc., RoweCom Information Quest, ingenta, Swets Blackwell, Institute for Scientific Information).
Indexed: ASCA, Agri.& Environ.Biotech.Abstr. (coverage dropped), Biol.Abstr., Chem.Abstr., Chem.Indus.Notes, Chem.Titles, Curr.Adv.Cancer Res., Curr.Adv.Ecol.Sci., Curr.Cont., Dairy Sci.Abstr., Dent.Ind., Derwent Biotech.Abstr., Excerp.Med., I.P.A., Ind.Med. (1976-), Ind.Sci.Rev., Inpharma, Kidney, Nutr.Abstr., Pharm.&Out.News, Protozool.Abstr., Reac., Rev.Med.& Vet.Mycol., SSCI (coverage dropped), Sci.Cit.Ind., THA.
—BLDSC (3286.327000), ADONIS, CASDDS, CISTI, EMDOCS, GNLM, IDS, ingenta, KNAW. **CCC.**
Published by: Adis International Limited, Mairangi Bay, Private Bag 65901, Auckland 1010, New Zealand. TEL 64-9-477-0700, FAX 64-9-477-0766, cpk@adis.co.nz, http://www.adis.com; http://biomednet.com/library/jclp. Ed. Nick Holford. Pub. Paul Chrisp. R&P Will Charles. Circ: 1,200. **Americas subscr. to:** Adis International Inc., Attn: Subscription Dept, 860 Town Center Dr, Langhorne, PA 19047. TEL 877-872-2347.

615 USA ISSN 0009-9236
RM1 CODEN: CLPTAT
CLINICAL PHARMACOLOGY & THERAPEUTICS. Text in English. 1960. m. USD 172 domestic to individuals; USD 205 foreign to individuals; USD 356 domestic to institutions; USD 393 foreign to institutions; USD 86 domestic to students; USD 119 foreign to students; USD 33 newsstand/cover (effective 2001). adv. charts, illus. s-a. index. reprint service avail. from PQC. *Refereed.* **Document type:** *Journal, Academic/Scholarly.* **Description:** Devoted to the study of the nature, action, disposition, efficacy and total evaluation of drugs as they are used in man.
Related titles: Microform ed.: (from PQC); Online - full text ed.: (from Ovid Technologies, Inc., IDEAL Online Library, Institute for Scientific Information, RoweCom Information Quest).
Indexed: AIM, ASCA, Abstr.Inter.Med., AgeLine, Agri.& Environ.Biotech.Abstr. (coverage dropped), Behav.Med.Abstr., Biol.Abstr., CINAHL, Chem.Abstr., Chem.Indus.Notes, Chem.Titles, Curr.Adv.Ecol.Sci., Curr.Cont., Curr.Ind.Stat., Dairy Sci.Abstr., Dent.Ind., Derwent Biotech.Abstr., Excerp.Med., INIS Atomind., I.P.A., Ind.Med. (1960-), Ind.Sci.Rev., Inpharma, Jrnl.Watch Derm., Jrnl.Watch Psych., Kidney, Med.& Surg.Dermat., NRN, Neurosci.Cit.Ind., Nutr.Abstr., Pharm.&Out.News, Protozool.Abstr., Reac., Rev.Arom.& Med.Plants, Rev.Med.& Vet.Mycol., Sci.Cit.Ind., Sugar Ind.Abstr., THA, Trop.Dis.Bull.
—BLDSC (3286.330000), ADONIS, CASDDS, CISTI, EMDOCS, GNLM, IDS, ingenta, KNAW, Linda Hall. **CCC.**
Published by: (American Society for Pharmacology and Experimental Therapeutics), Mosby, Inc. (Subsidiary of: Elsevier Science), 11830 Westline Industrial Dr, St Louis, MO 63146-3318. TEL 314-872-8370, 800-325-4177, FAX 314-432-1380, http://www.mosby.com/cpt, http://www.mosby.com/periodicals. Ed. Dr. Marcus M Reidenberg. Pub. Nathania Sawyer. Adv. contact Carol Kilzer TEL 314-453-4307. B&W page USD 1,090, color page USD 1,990; trim 10.88 x 8.25. Circ: 4,340. **Co-sponsor:** American Society for Clinical Pharmacology and Therapeutics.

615.19 USA
CLINICAL PHARMACOLOGY SERIES. Text in English. 1983. irreg., latest vol.18, 1993. price varies. adv. **Document type:** *Monographic series.*
Published by: Marcel Dekker, Inc., Attn: Eridania Perrez, 270 Madison Ave, New York, NY 10016-0602. TEL 212-696-9000, 800-228-1160, FAX 212-685-4540, marketing@dekker.com, http://www.dekker.com. Pub. Russell Dekker. R&P Julia Mulligan. Adv. contact Eridania Perez.

615.1072 USA ISSN 1060-1333
RS122 CODEN: CRRAES
CLINICAL RESEARCH AND REGULATORY AFFAIRS; a journal devoted to documentation of the clinical research process in the pharmaceutical industry. Text in English. 1984. q. USD 95 to individuals print & online eds.; USD 750 to institutions print only (effective 2002). adv. bk.rev. illus, charts, stat. index. *Refereed.* **Document type:** *Academic/Scholarly.* **Description:** For rapid communication of new and significant data pertaining to the documentation of the industrial clinical research process.
Formerly (until 1992): Clinical Research Practices and Drug Regulatory Affairs (0735-7915)
Related titles: Microform ed.: (from RPI); Online - full text ed.: (from Institute for Scientific Information, RoweCom Information Quest).
Indexed: ASCA, Biol.Abstr., Curr.Adv.Ecol.Sci., Environ.Sci.Poll.Mgmt., Excerp.Med., I.P.A., Pollut.Abstr., Ref.Zh., Risk Abstr., Saf.Sci.Abstr.
—BLDSC (3286.372100), CISTI, EMDOCS, GNLM, IDS, Infotrieve, ingenta, KNAW. **CCC.**
Published by: Marcel Dekker Inc., 270 Madison Ave, New York, NY 10016. TEL 212-696-9000, 800-228-1160, FAX 212-685-4540, http://www.dekker.com/servlet/product/productid/CRP. Ed. Barry Bleidt. R&P Julia Mulligan. Adv. contact Diane Saulon. page USD 800. Circ: 225.

CLINICAL TRIALS MONITOR. see *MEDICAL SCIENCES*

615.7 ITA ISSN 0390-8739
COLLEGAMENTO. Text in Italian. 1957. m. (10/yr.). ITL 50,000. adv.
Related titles: Online - full text ed.
Indexed: I.P.A.
Published by: (Unione Tecnica Italiana Farmacisti), U T E T SpA, Corso Raffaello 28, Turin 10125, Italy. TEL 39-02-29003555, FAX 39-02-6599049. Ed. Luigi Casanova. Adv. contact Corrado Trevisan. B&W page ITL 3,340,000, color page ITL 5,000,000; trim 246 x 185. Circ: 18,500.

615.1 USA ISSN 0010-163X
COLORADO JOURNAL OF PHARMACY. Text in English. 1958. q. USD 5. illus.
Indexed: Biol.Abstr.
Published by: University of Colorado, School of Pharmacy, PO Box 297, Boulder, CO 80309-0297. TEL 303-492-6278. Ed. James A Roth. Circ: 1,500.

COMMENTS ON TOXICOLOGY. see *ENVIRONMENTAL STUDIES—Toxicology And Environmental Safety*

COMMUNICATOR (ATHENS). see *CLUBS*

615.1 USA ISSN 1096-9179
COMMUNITY PHARMACIST; meeting the professional and educational needs of today's practitioner. Text in English. 1908. bi-m. USD 25 domestic; USD 60 foreign; USD 5 newsstand/cover (effective 2001). adv. bk.rev. back issues avail.; reprints avail. **Document type:** *Journal, Trade.* **Description:** Addresses the professional and business needs, concerns, and continuing education of retail pharmacists.
Formed by the merger of: Southern Pharmacy Journal (0192-5792); Which was formerly (until 1979): Southeastern Drug - Southern Pharmaceutical Journal (0095-2354); and: Pharmacy West (0191-6394); Which was formerly: West Coast - Rocky Mountain Druggist; Which was formed by the merger of: West Coast Druggist (0043-3101); and: Rocky Mountain Druggist (0035-757X); Southeastern Drug - Southern Pharmaceutical Journal was formed by the merger of: Southeastern Drug Journal (0038-3651); and: Southern Pharmaceutical Journal (0038-4410)
Indexed: I.P.A.
Published by: E L F Publications, 5285 W Louisiana Ave, Ste 112, Lakewood, CO 80232-5976. TEL 303-975-0075, 800-922-8513, FAX 303-975-0132, 603-507-0443, elfedit@qwest.net, elfpub@qwest.net. Pubs. Judith D Lane, Ronald R Quam. R&P Judith D Lane. Adv. contact Jerry Lester. B&W page USD 4,900; trim 8.375 x 10.825. Circ: 56,000 (controlled).

615.19 658.8 GBR ISSN 0960-376X
COMMUNITY PHARMACY. Text in English. 1980. m. GBP 58 domestic; GBP 48 foreign. adv. illus. **Document type:** *Magazine, Trade.* **Description:** For persons involved with pharmacies and pharmaceuticals. Discusses product news, nonprescription medications, and pharmacy in business.
Formerly (until 1986): O T C Medication (0260-518X)
Related titles: Online - full text ed.: (from Gale Group, ProQuest Information & Learning, LexisNexis).
Indexed: Bus.& Indus. (Sep.1995-).
—BLDSC (3363.647500).
Published by: C M P Information (Subsidiary of: United Business Media), Sovereign House, Sovereign Way, Tonbridge, Kent TN9 1RW, United Kingdom. TEL 44-1732-364422, FAX 44-1732-361534, enquiries@cmpinformation.com, http://www.dotpharmacy.com, http://www.cmpinformation.com. Ed. Ailsa Colquhoun. Adv. contact Julian Debruxelles. Circ: 13,813 (controlled).

COMPARATIVE BIOCHEMISTRY AND PHYSIOLOGY. TOXICOLOGY & PHARMACOLOGY. see *BIOLOGY—Biochemistry*

615 CAN ISSN 0069-7966
COMPENDIUM OF PHARMACEUTICALS AND SPECIALTIES. Text in English, French. 1960. a. CND 127; CND 131 French ed. (effective 2000). bk.rev. **Document type:** *Catalog.*
Related titles: CD-ROM ed.; English ed.; French ed.: Compendium des Produits et Specialites Pharmaceutiques. ISSN 0317-2813.
—BLDSC (3363.971000), CISTI, Infotrieve. **CCC.**
Published by: Canadian Pharmacists Association, 1785 Alta Vista Dr, Ottawa, ON K1G 3Y6, Canada. TEL 613-523-7877, FAX 613-523-0445, cpha@cdnpharm.ca, http://www.cdnpharm.ca. Pub. Leesa Bruce. Circ: 100,000.

615.329 USA
CONNECTICUT PHARMACIST. Text in English. 1943. q. USD 12. adv. **Document type:** *Trade.*

P

Indexed: I.P.A.
Published by: Connecticut Pharmacists Association, 35 Cold Spring Rd, Ste 125, Rocky Hill, CT 06067-3167. TEL 860-563-4619, FAX 860-257-8241. Ed., Adv. contact Marc S McQuaid. B&W page USD 450, color page USD 650; trim 11 x 8.5. Circ: 1,500.

615.328 USA ISSN 0888-5109
THE CONSULTANT PHARMACIST. Text in English. 1986. m., latest vol.16. USD 45 domestic to individuals; USD 65 foreign to individuals; USD 75 domestic to institutions; USD 95 foreign to institutions (effective 1999). adv. Website rev. index. back issues avail.; reprints avail. *Refereed.* **Document type:** *Journal, Academic/Scholarly.* **Description:** Publishes articles, news and information relevant to pharmacy practice in long-term care facilities, prisons, hospices, adult day care centers, home health care, and other related extended care facilities and settings.
Related titles: Online - full text ed.
Indexed: Abstr.Soc.Geront., I.P.A.
—BLDSC (3423.763000), GNLM.
Published by: American Society of Consultant Pharmacists, 1321 Duke St, Alexandria, VA 22314-3563. TEL 703-739-1300, FAX 703-739-1321, http://www.ascp.com/public/pubs/tcp/. Ed. H Edward Davidson. Pub. R Tim Webster. R&P David K Buerger TEL 703-739-1300. Adv. contact Don Dougherty TEL 215-348-4351. B&W page USD 2,745, color page USD 4,070; bleed 8.375 x 11.175. Circ: 11,000.

615.9 USA ISSN 0738-0615
CONSUMER PHARMACIST; drug information newsletter. Text in English. 1982. bi-m. USD 48 (effective 2001). adv. bk.rev. **Document type:** *Newsletter, Consumer.*
Published by: Elba Medical Foundation, 4924 Folse Dr., Box 1403, Metairie, LA 70004-1403. TEL 504-833-3600. Ed. John F Dimaggio. Circ: 6,000.

615 USA
CONTRACT PHARMA. Text in English. bi-m. adv. **Document type:** *Magazine, Trade.* **Description:** Provides a mix of industry news, technical features, and association event coverage for the pharmaceutical and biopharmaceutical industries.
Published by: Rodman Publications, Inc., 17 S Franklin Tpke, Ramsey, NJ 07446. TEL 201-825-2552, FAX 201-825-0553, gil@rodpub.com, http://www.contractpharma.com. Ed. Gil Roth. Pub. Gary Durr. adv.: B&W page USD 4,475, color page USD 5,625; bleed 8.375 x 11.125. Circ: 20,000.

CONTROLLED RELEASE SOCIETY. INTERNATIONAL SYMPOSIUM ON CONTROLLED RELEASE OF BIOACTIVE MATERIALS. PROCEEDINGS. see *CHEMISTRY—Organic Chemistry*

615.1 ITA ISSN 0010-9207
CORRIERE DEL FARMACISTA. Text in Italian. 1945. m. ITL 2,500, USD 4. adv. abstr.
Indexed: Chem.Abstr., Ind.Med. (coverage dropped).
Published by: Armando Giordano Ed. & Pub., Piazza d Aosta, 37, San Giuseppe Vesuviano, NA 80047, Italy.

615 658.8 GBR
COUGH AND COLD REMEDIES: THE INTERNATIONAL MARKET. Text in English. a. GBP 2,250, USD 4,500. **Document type:** *Trade.* **Description:** Analyzes the market for nonprescription cough and cold remedies for France, Germany, Italy, Spain, the U.K., the U.S., and Japan.
Related titles: Online - full text ed.: (from Data-Star, The Dialog Corporation).
Published by: Euromonitor, 60-61 Britton St, London EC1M 5UX, United Kingdom. TEL 44-20-7251-8024, info@euromonitor.com, http://www.euromonitor.com.

615.19 USA ISSN 0743-4863
RS201.V43 CODEN: CRTSEO
CRITICAL REVIEWS IN THERAPEUTIC DRUG CARRIER SYSTEMS. Text in English. 1985. bi-m. USD 132 to individuals; USD 586 to institutions (effective 2000). adv. *Refereed.* **Document type:** *Academic/Scholarly.* **Description:** Publishes comprehensive, multidisciplinary critical review papers encompassing the basic biological, medical, pharmaceutical, and physical sciences with emphasis on clinical applications.
Related titles: Online - full text ed.: (from Institute for Scientific Information).
Indexed: ASCA, Chem.Abstr., Chem.Indus.Notes, Chem.Titles, Curr.Cont., Excerp.Med. (1995-), INIS Atomind., Ind.Med. (1984-), Ind.Sci.Rev., Inpharma, Pharm.&Out.News, Reac., SSCI (coverage dropped), Sci.Cit.Ind.
—BLDSC (3487.483700), CASDDS, CISTI, EMDOCS, GNLM, IDS, Infotrieve, ingenta, KNAW, Linda Hall. **CCC.**

Published by: Begell House Inc., 79 Madison Ave, Ste 1205, New York, NY 10016-7892. TEL 212-725-1999, FAX 212-213-8368, begellhouse@worldnet.att.net, orders@begellhouse.com. Ed. Stephen D Bruck. Pub. William Begell. R&P, Adv. contact Jung Ra.

CRITICAL REVIEWS IN TOXICOLOGY. see *ENVIRONMENTAL STUDIES—Toxicology And Environmental Safety*

615.1 ITA ISSN 0011-1783
CODEN: CRFMAY
CRONACHE FARMACEUTICHE. Text in English, French, Italian. 1958. bi-m. EUR 60 domestic; EUR 80 foreign; EUR 12 per issue (effective 2002). adv. bk.rev. abstr, bibl, illus. index. back issues avail. **Document type:** *Bulletin.*
Indexed: Agri.& Environ.Biotech.Abstr. (coverage dropped), Biol.Abstr., Chem.Abstr., Excerp.Med., I.P.A., Ref.Zh.
—CASDDS, GNLM.
Published by: Societa Italiana di Scienze Farmaceutiche, Viale Abruzzi, 32, Milan, MI 20131, Italy. TEL 39-2-29513303, FAX 39-2-29520179, sisf@comm2000.it. Ed. Piero Sensi. adv.: B&W page XEU 220; 280 x 210. Circ: 1,200.

CUBA. CENTRO DE INFORMACION Y DOCUMENTACION AGROPECUARIO. BOLETIN DE RESENAS. SERIE: PLANTAS MEDICINALES. see *BIOLOGY—Botany*

CURRENT CARDIOVASCULAR DRUGS (YEAR). see *MEDICAL SCIENCES—Cardiovascular Diseases*

615.9 JPN ISSN 0911-2847
CURRENT CONCEPTS IN HOSPITAL PHARMACY/BYOIN YAKKYOKU. Text in Japanese. 1985. 3/yr.
Published by: Standard McIntyre/Sutandado Makkintaiya, 3-7 Irifune 2-chome, Chuo-ku, Tokyo 104-0042, Japan.

615 GBR
▼ **CURRENT DRUG DISCOVERY.** Text in English. 2001. m. GBP 66, USD 99 to individuals; GBP 133, USD 199 to corporations (effective 2001). **Document type:** *Journal, Academic/Scholarly, Trade.* **Description:** Provides intelligence for members of the pharmaceutical R&D industry, covering areas such as: investigational drugs, enabling technologies, industry activity, patent insight, regulatory issues, analyst comments, conference coverage, and features from opinion leaders, advertorials.
Published by: Current Drugs Ltd., 34-42 Cleveland St, Middlesex House, London W1P 6LB, United Kingdom. TEL 44-207-580-8393, FAX 44-207-580-5646, info@current-drugs.com, http://www.current-drugs.com.

615 USA ISSN 1389-2002
▼ **CURRENT DRUG METABOLISM.** Text in English. 2000 (Jun.). q. USD 110, USD 600 to institutions (effective 2000). adv. *Refereed.* **Document type:** *Academic/Scholarly.* **Description:** Features reviews in drug metabolism, disposition and related areas.
Related titles: Online - full text ed.: (from Swets Blackwell, Institute for Scientific Information).
Indexed: BBCI, Biotech.& Bioeng.Abstr., Med.& Pharm.Biotech.Abstr., Tox.Abstr.
—BLDSC (3496.400200).
Published by: Bentham Science Publishers, 102 N.E. 2nd St, Mail Box 135, Boca Raton, FL 33432. FAX 561-393-7229, m.bentham@inter.nl.net. Ed. Chandran Prakash. Adv. contact Tom Lucas.

615 USA ISSN 1389-4501
▼ **CURRENT DRUG TARGETS.** Text in English. 2000 (Jun.). q. USD 110 to individuals; USD 600 to institutions (effective 2000). adv. *Refereed.* **Document type:** *Academic/Scholarly.* **Description:** Features reviews on the discovery, characterization, and validation of novel human drug targets for drug discovery.
Related titles: Online - full text ed.: (from Swets Blackwell).
Indexed: Biotech.& Bioeng.Abstr., Med.& Pharm.Biotech.Abstr., Neurosci.Abstr.
Published by: Bentham Science Publishers, 102 N.E. 2nd St, Mail Box 135, Boca Raton, FL 33432. FAX 561-393-7229, m.bentham@inter.nl.net. Adv. contact Tom Lucas.

CURRENT INFECTIOUS DISEASE DRUGS. see *MEDICAL SCIENCES—Communicable Diseases*

CURRENT ISSUES IN TOXICOLOGY. see *ENVIRONMENTAL STUDIES—Toxicology And Environmental Safety*

CURRENT MEDICAL LITERATURE. INTERNATIONAL HOSPITAL PHARMACY. see *PHARMACY AND PHARMACOLOGY—Abstracting, Bibliographies, Statistics*

615 NLD ISSN 1568-0142
▼ **CURRENT MEDICINAL CHEMISTRY - ANTI-INFLAMMATORY & ANTI-ALLERGY AGENTS.** Text in English. forthcoming 2002 (Mar.). **Document type:** *Journal.* **Description:** Covers developments in medicinal chemistry and rational drug design for the discovery of new anti-inflammatory and anti-allergy agents.
Related titles: Online - full text ed.: forthcoming (from Swets Blackwell).
Published by: Bentham Science Publishers, 102 N.E. 2nd St, Mail Box 135, Boca Raton, FL 33432. FAX 561-393-7229, shidding@worldonline.nl, http://www.bentham.org/cmcaiaa/index.html. Ed. Mark J. Suto TEL 858-625-6555.

615.19 GBR ISSN 1367-6733
CURRENT OPINION IN DRUG DISCOVERY & DEVELOPMENT. Text in English. 1998. bi-m. GBP 1,655, USD 2,700 (effective 2002). **Document type:** *Journal, Trade.* **Description:** Covers all of the chemical aspects involved in the drug discovery and development process.
—BLDSC (3500.774100).
Published by: Current Drugs Ltd., 34-42 Cleveland St, Middlesex House, London W1P 6LB, United Kingdom. TEL 44-207-580-8393, FAX 44-207-580-5646, info@current-drugs.com, http://www.current-drugs.com. Ed. Tara Dyson. **Subscr. to:** Current Drugs Ltd., 400 Market St, Ste 700, Philadelphia, PA 19106.

615 GBR ISSN 1472-4472
CURRENT OPINION IN INVESTIGATIONAL DRUGS. Text in English. m. GBP 1,655, USD 2,700 (effective 2001). **Document type:** *Journal, Academic/Scholarly, Trade.* **Description:** Provides comprehensive coverage of all therapeutic areas, including a general section containing patent and paper alerts, individual therapeutic chapters provide short, focused overviews, reviews and evaluations on the latest drug developments. Also contains a critical overivew per issue in each therapeutic area, and short mini-reviews containing critical commentary on all areas of current interest.
Incorporates (1999-2000): Current Opinion in Anti-Inflammatory & Immunomodulatory Investigational Drugs (1464-8474)
Published by: Current Drugs Ltd., 34-42 Cleveland St, Middlesex House, London W1P 6LB, United Kingdom. TEL 44-207-580-8393, FAX 44-207-580-5646, info@current-drugs.com, http://www.current-drugs.com/products/COID/COID.HTM. Ed. Mike Williams.

615.7 GBR ISSN 1464-8431
▼ **CURRENT OPINION IN MOLECULAR THERAPEUTICS.** Text in English. 1999. bi-m. GBP 1,655, USD 2,700 (effective 2002). **Document type:** *Journal, Trade.* **Description:** Covers all aspects of molecular medicine research while focusing on clinical developments in gene transfer therapeutics and the utilization of recombinant technologies.
Related titles: Online - full text ed.: (from Institute for Scientific Information).
Indexed: Biotech.Cit.Ind.
Published by: Current Drugs Ltd., 34-42 Cleveland St, Middlesex House, London W1P 6LB, United Kingdom. TEL 44-207-580-8393, FAX 44-207-580-5646, info@current-drugs.com, http://www.current-drugs.com. Ed. Tara Dyson. **Subscr. to:** Current Drugs Ltd., 400 Market St, Ste 700, Philadelphia, PA 19106. TEL 215-721-9700, FAX 215-721-9287.

615 GBR ISSN 1471-4892
▼ **CURRENT OPINION IN PHARMACOLOGY.** Text in English. 2001. bi-m. EUR 170 in Europe to individuals; JPY 20,600 in Japan to individuals; USD 184 elsewhere to individuals; EUR 213 in Europe to qualified personnel; JPY 25,700 in Japan to qualified personnel; USD 230 elsewhere to qualified personnel; EUR 908 in Europe to institutions; JPY 125,900 in Japan to institutions; USD 1,015 elsewhere to institutions (effective 2002).
Related titles: Online - full text ed.: (from ScienceDirect).
—BLDSC (3500.776920).
Published by: Elsevier Science Ltd., Elsevier Trends Journals, 84 Theobald's Rd, London WC1X 8RR, United Kingdom. TEL 44-20-7611-4400, FAX 44-20-7611-4401, info@current-opinion.com, http://www.elsevier.com/locate/coph, http://www.elsevier.nl, http://www.current-opinion.com. Ed. Caroline P J Ash.

P

▼ **CURRENT PHARMACEUTICAL BIOTECHNOLOGY.** see *BIOLOGY—Biotechnology*

615 USA ISSN 1381-6128
RS420 CODEN: CPDEFP
CURRENT PHARMACEUTICAL DESIGN. Text in English. 1995. 18/yr. USD 490 to individuals; USD 2,100 to institutions (effective 2000). adv. *Refereed.* **Document type:** *Academic/Scholarly.* **Description:** Publishes reviews in therapeutic areas of drug design, including CNS agents, anticancer agents, anti-inflammatory and anti-allergy agents, cardiovascular, hematological, endocrine, metabolic, and anti-infection agents.
Related titles: Online - full text ed.: (from ingenta, Swets Blackwell, Institute for Scientific Information).
Indexed: BBCI, Chem.Abstr., Chem.Indus.Notes, Chem.Titles, Curr.Cont., Environ.Sci.Poll.Mgmt., Ind.Med. (1995-), Inpharma, Med.& Pharm.Biotech.Abstr., Microbiol.Abstr., Pharm.&Out.News, Reac., Sci.Cit.Ind.
—BLDSC (3501.280460), CASDDS, CISTI, GNLM, IDS, Infotrieve. **CCC.**
Published by: Bentham Science Publishers, 102 N.E. 2nd St, Mail Box 135, Boca Raton, FL 33432. FAX 561-393-7229, m.bentham@inter.nl.net, http://www.bcipubl.demon.co.uk/cpd. Adv. contact Tom Lucas.

615 USA
CURRENT PROTOCOLS IN PHARMACOLOGY. Text in English. base vol. plus q. updates. USD 500 (effective 2001); USD 535 combined subscription for base vol. & update; USD 255 updates (effective 2002). **Document type:** *Journal.*
Related titles: CD-ROM ed.: USD 490 (effective 2001); USD 520 combined subscription for base vol. & update; USD 275 renewals for base vol. & update (effective 2002).
Published by: John Wiley & Sons, Inc., Journals (Subsidiary of: Wiley InterScience), 605 Third Ave, New York, NY 10158. TEL 212-850-6645, FAX 212-850-6021, info@wiley.com, uscs-wis@wiley.com, http://www.wiley.com. **Subscr. addr. outside the Amesricas:** John Wiley & Sons Ltd., Baffins Ln, Chichester, Sussex PO19 IUD, United Kingdom. TEL 44-1243-779777, FAX 44-1243-843232, cs-journals@wiley.co.uk.

CURRENT THERAPEUTICS; Australia's journal of disease management and drug treatment. see *MEDICAL SCIENCES*

CURRENT TOPICS IN ENVIRONMENTAL AND TOXICOLOGICAL CHEMISTRY. see *ENVIRONMENTAL STUDIES—Toxicology And Environmental Safety*

CURRENT TOXICOLOGY AND THERAPY. see *MEDICAL SCIENCES*

615.1 USA
D C A T DIGEST✶. Text in English. 1960. 9/yr. membership only. stat. **Document type:** *Bulletin.*
Formerly: D C A T Bulletin (0300-7340)
Published by: Drug, Chemical and Allied Trades Association, 510 US Highway 130 No B1, Hightstown, NJ 08520-2649. TEL 516-496-3317, FAX 516-496-2231. Ed. Art Cavaler. Pub. Richard J Lerman. Circ: 2,000.

615 JPN ISSN 0917-3099
D I NYUSU/DRUG INFORMATION NEWS. Text in Japanese. 1989. bi-m.
Published by: Komaki Shimin Byoin Iyakuhin Johoshitsu/Komaki City Hospital, Drug Information Room, 1-20 Jobushi, Komaki-shi, Aichi-ken 485-0044, Japan.

615.1 NLD ISSN 0165-6112
D W: DROGISTEN WEEKBLAD; onafhankelijk vakblad voor drogisterij, parfumerie, reformzaak. Text in Dutch. 1968. w. (Thu.). NLG 96 (effective 2000). adv. bk.rev., film rev. abstr, charts, illus, mkt, pat, stat. **Document type:** *Newspaper, Trade.*
Former titles: Drogisten Weekblad; (until 1975): Drogistenblad de Vergulde Gaper (0012-6349)
Indexed: Key to Econ.Sci.
Published by: Van der Weij Periodieken B.V., Postbus 285, Hilversum 1200 AG, Netherlands. TEL 31-35-6249741, FAX 31-35-6214354, vdweij@euronet.nl. Ed. Jolanda van Hoek. adv.: B&W page NLG 5,450, color page NLG 7,750; trim 278 x 394. Circ: 7,800 (paid and controlled).

615.9 JPN ISSN 0286-8016
CODEN: DYDNDM
DAIICHI YAKKA DAIGAKU KENKYU NENPO/DAIICHI COLLEGE OF PHARMACEUTICAL SCIENCES. ANNUAL REPORT. Text in English, Japanese. 1971. a.
Indexed: Chem.Abstr., Chem.Indus.Notes, Chem.Titles, Jap.Per.Ind.
—CASDDS.
Published by: Daiichi Yakka Daigaku/Daiichi College of Pharmaceutical Sciences, 22-1 Tamagawa-Machi, Minami-ku, Fukuoka-shi 815-0037, Japan.

615 354.489 DNK
DANISH MEDICINES AGENCY. ANNUAL REPORT. Text in Danish. 1981. a. free per issue. **Document type:** *Government.*
Formerly (until 1997): Denmark. Sundhedsstyrelsen. Laegemiddelafdelingen. Aarsberetning (0109-9930)
Published by: Danish Medicines Agency, Frederikssundsvej 378, Broenshoej 2700, Denmark. TEL 45-44-88—91-11, FAX 45-44-91-73-73, dkma@dkma.dk. Ed. Torben Moeller Nielsen. R&P Torben Moeller-Nielsen TEL 45-44-88-93-40. **Subscr. to:** Statens Informationstjeneste, PO Box 1103, Copenhagen K 1009, Denmark.

615.1 DNK ISSN 0105-7480
DANSKE LAEGEMIDDELSTANDARDER. Text in Danish. 1978. a. DKK 198.40 domestic (effective 2000). **Document type:** *Government.*
Published by: (Denmark. Farmaceutiske Laboratorium, Denmark. Sundhedsstyrelsen), Nyt Nordisk Forlag-Arnold Busck A-S, Koebmagergade 49, Copenhagen K 1150, Denmark. TEL 45-33-73-35-75, FAX 45-33-73-35-76, nnf@nytnordiskforlag.dk.

615 IRN ISSN 1560-8115
DARU. Text in Persian, Modern; Summaries in English. 1972. 4/yr. USD 50 to individuals; USD 100 to institutions; USD 25 to students (effective 1999). adv. bk.rev. **Document type:** *Academic/Scholarly.* **Description:** Covers broad range of topics including pharmaceutics, pharmacokinetics, pharmacotherapy, medical chemistry, drug analysis, pharmacognosy and natural products, toxicology and pharmacology, biotechnology, clinical investigations and social aspects of pharmacy.
Formerly: University of Teheran. School of Pharmacy. Journal
Indexed: Chem.Abstr., Chem.Indus.Notes, Chem.Titles, I.P.A.
Published by: Tehran University of Medical Sciences, Faculty of Pharmacy, Shahreza Ave., Teheran 14155-645, Iran. TEL 98-21-6112324, FAX 98-21-6461178. Ed., R&P Ali Khalaj. Adv. contact Abbas Shafiee.

DE TEXTOS. see *SOCIOLOGY*

615 610.73 USA ISSN 1088-8276
DELMAR'S DRUG GUIDE FOR NURSES. Text in English. 1996. a. **Document type:** *Trade.*
Published by: Delmar Publishers Inc., 3 Columbia Cir, PO Box 125 19, Albany, NY 12212-2519. TEL 518-464-3569, 800-998-7498, FAX 518-464-0358.

DEMENTIA AND GERIATRIC COGNITIVE DISORDERS. see *MEDICAL SCIENCES—Psychiatry And Neurology*

615 JPN ISSN 0916-1147
DENSHO TO IGAKU/TRADITION AND MEDICINE. Text in Japanese. 1988. s-a. JPY 800. adv. bk.rev. **Document type:** *Academic/Scholarly.* **Description:** Focuses on holistic traditional medicine.
Published by: Tokyo Yakka Daigaku, Doitsugo Kenkyushitsu/Tokyo College of Pharmacy, Department of German Language, 1432-1 Horinochi, Hachioji-shi, Tokyo-to 192-0355, Japan. TEL 0426-76-5842, FAX 0426-76-5825. Ed. Nobuo Shida. Adv. contact Noriko Miyamoto.

615.1 DEU ISSN 0011-9849
DER DEUTSCHE APOTHEKER; die aktuelle Zeitschrift fuer pharmazeutische Berufe. Text in German. 1949. m. DEM 104 domestic; DEM 120 foreign (effective 2001). adv. bk.rev. bibl, charts, illus. index. **Document type:** *Magazine, Trade.*
Related titles: Online - full text ed.
Indexed: Biol.Abstr., Chem.Abstr., I.P.A., Int.Packag.Abstr.
—Infotrieve. **CCC.**
Published by: Verlag Der Deutsche Apotheker, Hans Thoma Str 1, Oberursel 61440, Germany. TEL 49-6171-55012, FAX 49-6171-55142. Ed., Adv. contact Siegfried Beyer Enke. Circ: 18,000.

615.1 DEU ISSN 0011-9857
CODEN: DAZEA2
DEUTSCHE APOTHEKER ZEITUNG; vereinigt mit Sueddeutsche Apotheker-Zeitung. Unabhaengige pharmazeutische Zeitschrift fuer Wissenschaft und Praxis. Abbreviated title: D A Z. Text in German. 1861. w. EUR 169 domestic; EUR 120.12 domestic to students; EUR 294.32 foreign; EUR 8 newsstand/cover (effective 2002). adv. bk.rev. charts, illus. index. **Document type:** *Newspaper, Trade.*
Related titles: CD-ROM ed.: EUR 129.48 plus postage (effective 2002); Online - full text ed.; ♦ Supplement: Geschichte der Pharmazie. ISSN 0939-334X; ♦ P K A Aktuell. ISSN 0944-7032; ♦ Neue Arzneimittel. ISSN 0724-567X; ♦ Apotheker und Kunst. ISSN 0341-0110; ♦ Apotheke Heute. ISSN 0173-1882; ♦ Pharmazie Heute. ISSN 0369-979X; ♦ Student und Praktikant. ISSN 0721-8672; ♦ Apotheker-Zeitung. ISSN 0178-4862.
Indexed: Agri.& Environ.Biotech.Abstr. (coverage dropped), Anal.Abstr., Biol.Abstr., Chem.Abstr., Chem.Indus.Notes, Chem.Titles, Derwent Biotech.Abstr., Excerp.Med., I.P.A.
—BLDSC (3563.000000), CASDDS, CISTI, GNLM, Infotrieve, KNAW. **CCC.**
Published by: Deutscher Apotheker Verlag, Postfach 101061, Stuttgart 70009, Germany. TEL 49-711-2582-0, FAX 49-711-2582290, daz@deutscher-apotheker-verlag.de, http://www.deutscher-apotheker-verlag.de/daz. Eds. Dr. Klaus Brauer, Peter Ditzel. Adv. contact Klaus Graef TEL 49-711-2582245. Circ: 37,500.

615.19 DEU ISSN 0174-0164
DEUTSCHE DROGISTEN ZEITUNG. Short title: D D Z. Text in German. 1945. m. DEM 75 (effective 1999). **Document type:** *Trade.*
Published by: E S Fachschriften Verlag GmbH, Paul-Gerhardt-Allee 24, Munich 81245, Germany. TEL 49-89-8347077, FAX 49-89-8341962. Circ: 15,000.

615 NLD ISSN 0167-6431
CODEN: DEPHDQ
DEVELOPMENTS IN PHARMACOLOGY. Text in English. 1980. irreg. price varies. *Refereed.* **Document type:** *Monographic series.*
—CASDDS, CISTI.
Published by: (Commission of the European Communities BEL), Kluwer Academic Publishers Group (Subsidiary of: Wolters Kluwer N.V.), Spuiboulevard 50, PO Box 17, Dordrecht 3300 AA, Netherlands. FAX 31-78-639-2254, services@wkap.nl, http://www.wkap.nl. **Dist. by:** Journals Department, PO Box 322, Dordrecht 3300 AH, Netherlands. FAX 31-78-654-6474.

DI CYAN BULLETIN. see *MEDICAL SCIENCES—Psychiatry And Neurology*

615.19 610 USA ISSN 1054-9609
CODEN: DIINF5
DIAGNOSTICS INTELLIGENCE. Text in English. 1990. m. USD 492 in US & Canada; USD 514 foreign (effective 2001). illus. back issues avail. **Document type:** *Newsletter.* **Description:** For executives in the medical in vitro diagnostics business. Covers the latest in research, new markets, new product launches, regulatory affairs, litigation, business opportunities, finance and patents.
Related titles: Supplement: In Vitro Diagnostics Industry Directory; Emerging Infectious Disease Test Markets; Commercial Opportunities in Cardiovascular Diagnosis; Commercial Opportunities in Pharmacogenomics.
Indexed: CBNB (1994-), Chem.Abstr., Chem.Indus.Notes, Chem.Titles.
—CASDDS. **CCC.**
Published by: C T B International Publishing Inc., PO Box 218, Maplewood, NJ 07040-0218. TEL 973-379-7749, FAX 973-379-1158, info@ctbintl.com, http://www.ctbintl.com. Ed. Christopher Brogna. Pub. Oykue Brogna.

615 MEX
DICCIONARIO DE ESPECIALIDADES FARMACEUTICAS. Text in Spanish. 1944. a. USD 70. adv.
Published by: Ediciones P L M S.A. de C.V., San BERNADINO 17, Col del Valle, Mexico City, DF 03100, Mexico. TEL 687-1766, FAX 536-5027, TELEX 1772912 EPLMME. Ed. Dr. Rogelio Silis. Circ: 60,000.

615 BRA
DICIONARIO DE ESPECIALIDADES FARMACEUTICAS. Text in Portuguese. 1971. a. USD 70 (effective 2000 - 2001). adv.
Published by: Editora de Publicacoes Cientificas Ltda., Rua Major Suckow, 30, Rocha, Rio De Janeiro, RJ 20911-160, Brazil. TEL 55-21-2013722, 55-21-5010057, FAX 55-21-2613749. Eds. Jose Maria de Sousa e Melo, J M Melo. R&P, Adv. contact Ana Paula. Circ: 60,000.

615 610.28 USA ISSN 1073-4414
DICKINSON'S F D A REVIEW; human & animal drugs - biologics - medical devices. (U.S. Food and Drug Administration) Text in English. 1994. m. USD 760 in North America; USD 815 elsewhere. bk.rev. charts, bibl. Supplement avail.; back issues avail. **Document type:** *Newsletter.* **Description:** Reviews F.D.A. policy, litigation issues, and enforcement of regulations of drugs, biologics, medical devices and veterinary medicines.
Formed by the merger of (1985-1994): Dickinson's F D A (0885-159X); (1992-1994): Dickinson's F D A Inspection (1063-2433)
Published by: Ferdic Inc., PO Box 28, Camp Hill, PA 17011. TEL 717-731-1426, FAX 717-731-1427, ferdic@ezonline.com. Ed., Pub., R&P James G Dickinson TEL 520-684-3112.

547.7 GBR ISSN 0966-2146
DICTIONARY OF NATURAL PRODUCTS ON CD-ROM. Text in English. 1991. s-a. GBP 3,500; GBP 950 renewals. **Document type:** *Trade.* **Description:** Provides a database of more than 120,000 natural products and related compounds with full-text retrieval and substructure searching.
Media: CD-ROM.
Published by: Chapman & Hall, Electronic Publishing Division, Chapman & Hall, 2-6 Boundary Row, London SE1 8HN, United Kingdom. TEL 44-20-7865-0066, FAX 44-20-7522-0101, cust.serv@chall.co.uk, http://www.epd.chapmanhall.com. **Dist. by:** Cheriton House, North Way, Andover, Hamps SP10 5BE, United Kingdom. TEL 44-1264-332424, FAX 44-1264-342787.

615 FRA ISSN 0419-1153
DICTIONNAIRE VIDAL* . Text in French. 1914. a. (plus updates 3/yr.). FRF 515; FRF 670 foreign. **Description:** Directory to ethical pharmaceuticals, diagnostic products and OTC products.
Supersedes: Dictionnaire des Specialites Pharmaceutiques
Related titles: CD-ROM ed.: 1914.
Published by: O.V.P. - Editions du Vidal, 33 av. de Wagram, Paris Cedex 17 75854, France. TEL 47-23-90-91, FAX 47-20-72-89, TELEX OVP 603 506 F. Circ: 185,000.

615 658.8 GBR
DIGESTIVE REMEDIES: THE INTERNATIONAL MARKET. Text in English. a. GBP 2,250, USD 4,500 (effective 1999). **Document type:** *Trade.* **Description:** Analyzes the market for nonprescription digestive remedies in France, Germany, Italy, Spain, the U.K., the U.S., and Japan.
Related titles: Online - full text ed.: (from Data-Star, The Dialog Corporation).
Published by: Euromonitor, 60-61 Britton St, London EC1M 5UX, United Kingdom. TEL 44-20-7251-8024, info@euromonitor.com, http://www.euromonitor.com.

DIRECTORY OF HIGH VOLUME INDEPENDENT DRUG STORES (YEAR). see *BUSINESS AND ECONOMICS—Trade And Industrial Directories*

615 BRA ISSN 0070-6612
DIRETORIO BRASILEIRO DA INDUSTRIA FARMACEUTICA. Text in Portuguese. 1968. biennial. free per issue. adv. **Document type:** *Directory.*
Published by: Associacao Brasileira da Industria Farmaceutica, Rua Beira Rio, 57 7o, VI Olimpia, Sao Paulo, SP 04548-050, Brazil. TEL 011-820-3775, TELEX 011-822-6628. Ed. Jose Eduardo Bandeira de Mello.

615 GBR
DIURETIC AGENTS. Text in English. irreg. **Document type:** *Monographic series.*
Published by: Marius Press, Marius Press, Over Kellet, PO Box 15, Carnforth, Lancs LA6 1HW, United Kingdom. TEL 44-1524-733027, FAX 44-1524-736659. Ed. S Johnson. R&P F N Johnson.

DOJIN NYUSU/DOJIN NEWS. see *CHEMISTRY—Analytical Chemistry*

DONJINDO NEWSLETTER. see *CHEMISTRY—Analytical Chemistry*

615 JPN ISSN 0389-746X
DORAGGU MAGAJIN/DRUG MAGAZINE. Text in Japanese. 1958. m.
Address: 3-15 Nihonbashihoncho 2-chome, Chuo-ku, Tokyo 103-0023, Japan.

615.1 FIN ISSN 0783-4233
DOSIS. Text in Finnish; Summaries in English. 1985. q. FIM 300 domestic; FIM 330 foreign (effective 2000). adv. **Document type:** *Newspaper, Academic/Scholarly.* **Description:** Publishes scientific articles and reports in pharmacology.
Published by: Suomen Farmasialiitto/Finish Pharmacists' Association, Iso Roobertinkatu 7A, Helsinki 00510, Finland. TEL 358-9-605219, FAX 358-9-605112, harri.ovaskainen@farmasialiitto.fi, http://www.farmasialiitto.fi. Ed. Jukka Monkkonen. Adv. contact Harri Ovaskainen. B&W page FIM 6,800, color page FIM 12,200. Circ: 6,500.

DR. MED. MABUSE; Zeitschrift fuer Gesundheitswesen. see *MEDICAL SCIENCES*

615 CHE
DROGA INFORMATIONS* . Text in German. m.
Published by: Gebr. Aeschbacher AG, Worb 3076, Switzerland. Ed. T Waegli. Circ: 1,100.

615.4 DEU ISSN 0945-4500
DROGERIE & PARFUEMERIE. Text in German. 1930. m. DEM 7.50 newsstand/cover (effective 2000). adv. **Document type:** *Magazine, Trade.*
Formerly (until 1993): Deutsche Drogerie (0722-9518); Which incorporated (in 1991): D D F - Journal (0720-633X); Which was formerly (until 1981): D D F. Drogeriewaren - Fachenmagazin (0720-6348); (1965-1977): D D F - Das Drogisten Fachblatt (0011-4804)
Published by: Marken-Verlag GmbH, Hugo-Junkers-Str 20, Cologne 50739, Germany. TEL 49-221-957427-0, FAX 49-221-95742777, marken-info@markenverlag.de, http://www.markenverlag.de. adv.: B&W page DEM 4,280, color page DEM 8,200. Circ: 8,200 (paid and controlled).

615 CHE
DROGISTENSTERN. Text in German. 10/yr. free per issue. **Document type:** *Bulletin.*
Published by: Drogerie Marketing Zentrale, Postfach 924, Biel Fd 2501, Switzerland. TEL 41-32-3425055, FAX 41-32-3425058. Eds. Meta Zweifel, Rudi Koller. adv.: B&W page CHF 18,895, color page CHF 18,895. Circ: 429,040.

615 ESP
DROGUERIA ACTUALIDAD. Text in Spanish. 6/yr.
Address: Via Agusta 59, 8o 812, Barcelona 08006, Spain. TEL 3-2378865, FAX 3-415-86-88. Ed. Salvador Beltran Nunez. Circ: 15,000.

▼ **DROIT & DISPOSITIFS MEDICAUX ACTUALITES.** see *MEDICAL SCIENCES—Experimental Medicine, Laboratory Technique*

615 FRA ISSN 1165-5372
DROIT & PHARMACIE ACTUALITES. Text in French. 1993. 48/yr. EUR 3,811.22 (effective 2001). **Document type:** *Journal, Trade.* **Description:** Contains in-depth analyses of the latest French and European regulatory news on drugs and other healthcare products.
Published by: Droit & Pharmacie, 12 rue de Lorraine, Levallois-Perret Cedex 92309, France. TEL 33-1-55-46-91-00, FAX 33-1-55-46-91-01, info@droit-et-pharmacie.fr, http://www.droit-et-pharmacie.fr.

DROPPJOURNALEN; tidskrift om nutrition och vaetsketerapi. see *NUTRITION AND DIETETICS*

615.1 USA ISSN 0148-0545
RA1190 CODEN: DCTODJ
DRUG AND CHEMICAL TOXICOLOGY; an international journal for rapid communication. Text in English. 1978. q. USD 95 to individuals print & online eds.; USD 875 to institutions (effective 2002). adv. *Refereed.* **Document type:** *Journal, Academic/Scholarly.* **Description:** Features full-length research papers, review articles, and short notes. Presents findings on a broad range of topics related to the safety evaluation of drugs, chemicals, and medical products.
Related titles: Microform ed.: (from RPI); Online - full text ed.: (from EBSCO Publishing, O C L C Online Computer Library Center, Inc., RoweCom Information Quest, Swets Blackwell, Institute for Scientific Information).
Indexed: ASCA, Agri.& Environ.Biotech.Abstr. (coverage dropped), BBCI, Biol.Abstr., Chem.Abstr., Chem.Indus.Notes, Chem.Titles, Curr.Adv.Ecol.Sci., Curr.Cont., Derwent Biotech.Abstr., Environ.Abstr., Environ.Per.Bibl. (1981-), Environ.Sci.Poll.Mgmt., Excerp.Med., INIS Atomind., I.P.A., Ind.Med. (1977-), Ind.Sci.Rev., Ind.Vet., Inpharma, Int.Abstr.Biol.Sci., Mass Spectr.Bull., Nutr.Abstr., Pharm.&Out.News, Pig News & Info., Pollut.Abstr., Reac., Ref.Zh., Rev.Med.& Vet.Mycol., Sci.Cit.Ind., Tox.Abstr., Vet.Bull., Weed Abstr.
—BLDSC (3627.985000), CASDDS, CISTI, GNLM, IDS, ingenta, KNAW, Linda Hall. **CCC.**
Published by: Marcel Dekker Inc., 270 Madison Ave, New York, NY 10016. TEL 212-696-9000, 800-228-1160, FAX 212-685-4540, journals@dekker.com, custserv@dekker.com, http://www.dekker.com/servlet/product/productid/DCT. Ed. Gerald L Kennedy Jr. R&P Julia Mulligan. Adv. contact Diane Saulon. B&W page USD 800. Circ: 350. **Dist. addr. in Europe, Far East, Middle East & Africa:** Marcel Dekker AG, Hutgasse 4, PO Box 812, Basel 4001, Switzerland. TEL 41-61-261-8482, FAX 41-61-261-8896, intlcustserv@dekker.com.

615.9 USA
DRUG AND CHEMICAL TOXICOLOGY SERIES. Text in English. 1984. irreg., latest vol.10, 1995. price varies. adv. *Refereed.* **Document type:** *Monographic series.*
Published by: Marcel Dekker, Inc., Attn: Eridania Perrez, 270 Madison Ave, New York, NY 10016-0602. TEL 212-696-9000, 800-228-1160, FAX 212-685-4540, marketing@dekker.com, http://www.dekker.com. Eds. F W Oehme, Francesco J Dicarlo. R&P Julia Mulligan. Adv. contact Eridania Perez.

DRUG AND MARKET DEVELOPMENT NEWSLETTER. see *MEDICAL SCIENCES*

P

615.5 GBR ISSN 0012-6543
DRUG AND THERAPEUTICS BULLETIN. Text in English. 1963. m. GBP 41. cum.index. reprint service avail. from PQC. **Document type:** *Bulletin.* **Description:** Provides impartial and expert information for doctors and pharmacists on the clinical use of drugs.
Related titles: CD-ROM ed.; Online - full text ed.: (from Institute for Scientific Information).
Indexed: Brit.Nur.Ind., Dent.Ind., Diab.Cont., Excerp.Med., FAMLI, INIS Atomind., I.P.A., Ind.Med. (1963-), Inpharma, Pharm.&Out.News, Reac.
—BLDSC (3629.100000), GNLM, KNAW.
Published by: (Consumers' Association), Which? Ltd., 2 Marylebone Rd, London NW1 4DF, United Kingdom. TEL 44-20-7830-6171, FAX 44-20-7830-6220, http://www.which.net. Ed. Dr. J Collier. R&P Gill Rowley. Circ: 99,000. **Subscr. to:** Consumers' Association, Castlemead, Gascoyne Way, Hertford, Herts SG14 1LH, United Kingdom. TEL 44-207-830-8500.

615 JPN ISSN 0289-9922
DRUG APPROVAL AND LICENSING PROCEDURES IN JAPAN. Text in English. 1973. a. JPY 56,000. **Description:** Explains Japanese pharmaceutical approval procedures.
Related titles: ♦ Japanese ed.: Iyakuhin Seizo Shishin. ISSN 0911-9329.
Published by: (Society of Japanese Pharmacopoeia), Yakugyo Jiho Co. Ltd., 2-36 Kanda-Jinbo-cho, Chiyoda-ku, Tokyo 101-0051, Japan.

615 USA ISSN 1080-5826
CODEN: DBTRFN
DRUG BENEFIT TRENDS; for pharmacy managers and managed health care professionals. Text in English. 1988. m. USD 95 domestic; USD 105 foreign; USD 120 to libraries; USD 40 to students; USD 10 newsstand/cover domestic; USD 15 newsstand/cover foreign (effective 2001). charts, illus. Index. back issues avail. *Refereed.* **Document type:** *Journal.* **Description:** Provides practical information to improve management of the drug benefit.
Indexed: I.P.A.
—BLDSC (3629.103100). **CCC.**
Published by: Cliggott Publishing Co. (Subsidiary of: S C P Communications, Inc.), 330 Boston Post Rd, Darien, CT 06820. editor@scp.com. Ed. Ken Moss. Pub. Hillary Ford.

615.1 330 USA ISSN 1530-3438
▼ **DRUG COST MANAGEMENT REPORT.** Text in English. 2000. m. **Document type:** *Newsletter.* **Description:** Includes data and information gathered from HMOs and PBMs, coupled with information on what's working in efforts to control drug costs.

Published by: Atlantic Information Services, Inc., 1100 17th St, N W, Ste 300, Washington, DC 20036. TEL 202-775-9008, FAX 202-331-9542, http://www.aishealth.com. Ed. Susan Namovicz-Peat. Pub. Richard Biehl.

615 ESP
DRUG DATA REPORT. Text in English. 1979. m. USD 1,100 (effective 2000). adv. back issues avail. **Description:** Contains essential drug information in a condensed monograph form. Publishes about 10,000 new compounds each year.
Formerly: Annual Drug Data Report (0379-4121)
Related titles: Online - full text ed.: (from The Dialog Corporation).
Indexed: Inpharma, Pharm.&Out.News, Reac.
—GNLM, Infotrieve. **CCC.**
Published by: Prous Science, PO Box 540, Barcelona 08080, Spain. TEL 34-93-4592220, FAX 34-93-4581535, service@prous.com. R&P A Graul.

615.19 USA ISSN 1071-7544
RS199.5 CODEN: DDELEB
DRUG DELIVERY; journal of delivery and targeting of therapeutic agents. Text in English. 1992. q. GBP 134, USD 221 to individuals; GBP 278, USD 458 to institutions (effective 2002). index. back issues avail. *Refereed.* **Document type:** *Academic/Scholarly.* **Description:** Focuses on drug delivery technology at the theoretical as well as practical level. Includes basic research, development, and application principles on the molecular, cellular, and higher levels of targeting sites, as well as physical, chemical and immunokinetic modes of delivery.
Formerly (until 1993): Drug Targeting and Delivery (1058-241X)
Related titles: Online - full text ed.: ISSN 1521-0464 (from CatchWord Ltd., EBSCO Publishing, O C L C Online Computer Library Center, Inc., RoweCom Information Quest, Swets Blackwell, Institute for Scientific Information).
Indexed: BBCI, Chem.Abstr., Excerp.Med. (1995-), Ind.Med. (1993-), Inpharma, Pharm.&Out.News, Reac., Tox.Abstr.
—BLDSC (3629.417000), CASDDS, CatchWord, CISTI, GNLM, IDS, Infotrieve, KNAW. **CCC.**
Published by: Taylor & Francis Ltd. (Subsidiary of: Taylor & Francis Group), 325 Chestnut St, Suite 800, Philadelphia, PA 19016. TEL 215-625-8900, FAX 215-625-2940, info@taylorandfrancis.com, http://www.taylorandfrancis.com/. Eds. Alfred Stracher, Dr. Tony L Whateley. **Subscr. aadr. in Europe:** Taylor & Francis Group, Journals Customer Service, Rankine Rd, Basingstoke, Hants RG24 8PR, United Kingdom. TEL 44-1256-813000, FAX 44-1256-479438, enquiry@tanf.co.uk, http://www.tandf.co.uk/journals.

615 JPN ISSN 0913-5006
CODEN: DDSYEI
DRUG DELIVERY SYSTEM. Short title: D D S. Text in Japanese; Summaries in English. 1986. bi-m. JPY 1,500 per issue.
Indexed: Chem.Abstr., Chem.Indus.Notes, Chem.Titles.
—BLDSC (3629.104800), CASDDS.
Published by: Nihon D D S Gakkai/Japan Society of Drug Delivery System, Seimarianna Daigaku Nanbyo Chiryo Kenkyu Senta, 16-1 Sugao 2-chome, Miyamae-ku, Kawasaki-shi, Kanagawa-ken 216-0015, Japan.

615 GBR ISSN 1472-4715
▼ **DRUG DELIVERY SYSTEMS AND SCIENCES.** Text in English. 2001. q. GBP 48 in Europe; GBP 60 elsewhere (effective 2001). bk.rev. back issues avail.; reprints avail. *Refereed.* **Document type:** *Journal, Academic/Scholarly.* **Description:** Contains primarily original work resulting from research and technological developments in the drug delivery field.
Published by: Euromed Scientific Ltd., The Old Surgery, Liphook Rd, Haslemere, Surrey GU27 1NL, United Kingdom. TEL 44-1428-656665, FAX 44-1428-656643, info@euromed.uk.com, http://www.euromed.uk.com/ddss.htm. Pub. Joel Ridge. Adv. contact Allan Andrews TEL 44-1621-851007. Circ: 6,000 (paid).

615.19 USA
▼ **DRUG DELIVERY TECHNOLOGY.** Text in English. 2001 (Oct.). 8/yr. free domestic; USD 88 in Canada & Mexico; USD 136 elsewhere (effective 2002). adv. *Refereed.* **Document type:** *Magazine, Trade.* **Description:** Contains technical articles that describe practical solutions to drug delivery challenges.
Related titles: Online - full text ed.
Address: 350 Main Rd, Montville, NJ 07045. TEL 973-299-1200, FAX 973-299-7937, info@drugdeliverytech.com, http://www.drugdeliverytech.com. Ed. Dan Marino. Pub. Ralph Vitaro. Adv. contact Warren DeGraff. B&W page USD 4,875, color page USD 6,210; trim 8.125 x 10.875. Circ: 20,000 (paid and controlled).

615.19 CHE ISSN 1055-9612
RS420 CODEN: DDDIEV
DRUG DESIGN AND DISCOVERY. Text in English. 1986. q. GBP 177, USD 235, EUR 235 to individuals; GBP 716, USD 920, EUR 925 to institutions; GBP 1,119, USD 1,413, EUR 1,463 to corporations (effective 2002). *Refereed.* **Document type:** *Journal, Academic/Scholarly.*
Formerly: Drug Design and Delivery (0884-2884)
Related titles: CD-ROM ed.; Microform ed.; Online - full text ed.: (from EBSCO Publishing, RoweCom Information Quest).
Indexed: Aqua.Sci.& Fish.Abstr., Biotech.& Bioeng.Abstr., Derwent Biotech.Abstr., Environ.Sci.Poll.Mgmt., Excerp.Med., I.P.A., Ind.Med. (1991-), Inpharma, Med.& Pharm.Biotech.Abstr., Reac.
—BLDSC (3629.115420), CISTI, EMDOCS, GNLM, ingenta, KNAW. **CCC.**
Published by: Gordon and Breach - Harwood Academic (Subsidiary of: Taylor & Francis Group), PO Box 531, Lausanne 1000, Switzerland. TEL 41-21-6411280, FAX 41-21-6411281, info@gbhap.com, http://www.gbhap.com/Drug_Design_Discovery/. Ed. G L Olson. **Subscr. addr. in US:** International Publishers Direct, PO Box 32160, Newark, NJ 07102. FAX 215-750-6343.

615 USA ISSN 0363-9045
RS402 CODEN: DDIPD8
DRUG DEVELOPMENT AND INDUSTRIAL PHARMACY. Text in English. 1975. 10/yr. USD 255 to individuals for print & online eds.; USD 2,175 to institutions for print only (effective 2002). adv. *Refereed.* **Document type:** *Academic/Scholarly.* **Description:** Covers aspects of the development, production, and evaluation of drugs and pharmaceutical products.
Formerly: Drug Development Communications (0095-5183)
Related titles: Microform ed.: (from RPI); Online - full text ed.: (from EBSCO Publishing, O C L C Online Computer Library Center, Inc., RoweCom Information Quest, Swets Blackwell, Institute for Scientific Information).
Indexed: ASCA, Agri.& Environ.Biotech.Abstr. (coverage dropped), Anal.Abstr., Anim.Breed.Abstr., Biol.Abstr., Biotech.& Bioeng.Abstr., Chem.Abstr., Chem.Cit.Ind., Chem.Indus.Notes, Chem.Titles, Curr.Adv.Ecol.Sci., Curr.Cont., Derwent Biotech.Abstr., Environ.Sci.Poll.Mgmt., Excerp.Med., Helminthol.Abstr., I.P.A., Ind.Med. (1977-), Ind.Sci.Rev., Inpharma, Mat.Sci.Cit.Ind. (coverage dropped), Microbiol.Abstr., Pharm.&Out.News, Pollut.Abstr., Reac., Ref.Zh., Rev.Arom.& Med.Plants, Rev.Med.& Vet.Mycol., Risk Abstr., Saf.Sci.Abstr., Sci.Cit.Ind., Sugar Ind.Abstr.
—BLDSC (3629.116000), CASDDS, CINDOC, CISTI, EMDOCS, GNLM, IDS, Infotrieve, KNAW, Linda Hall. **CCC.**
Published by: Marcel Dekker Inc., 270 Madison Ave, New York, NY 10016. TEL 212-696-9000, FAX 212-685-4540, journals@dekker.com, http://www.dekker.com/servlet/product/productid/DDC. Ed. Robert O Williams III. R&P Julia Mulligan. Adv. contact Anne Mullins. B&W page USD 800. Circ: 875. **Dist. addr. in Europe, Far East, Middle East & Africa:** Marcel Dekker AG, Hutgasse 4, PO Box 812, Basel 4001, Switzerland. TEL 41-61-261-8482, FAX 41-61-261-8896, intlcustserv@dekker.com.

615.1 USA ISSN 1088-5447
DRUG DEVELOPMENT PIPELINE. Text in English. m. USD 175 domestic; USD 198 foreign (effective 2001). back issues avail. **Document type:** *Newsletter.* **Description:** Summarizes changes in the drug development plans of U.S. and Canadian pharmaceutical companies.
Published by: C T B International Publishing Inc., PO Box 218, Maplewood, NJ 07040-0218. TEL 973-379-7749, FAX 973-379-1158, info@ctbintl.com, http://www.ctbintl.com. Ed., R&P Christopher Brogna. Pub. Oykue Brogna.

615.19 USA ISSN 0272-4391
CODEN: DDREDK
DRUG DEVELOPMENT RESEARCH. Text in English. 1981. m. USD 3,995 in United States; USD 4,115 in Canada & Mexico; USD 4,217 elsewhere; USD 4,195 combined subscription in United States for print and online eds.; USD 4,315 combined subscription in Canada & Mexico for print and online eds.; USD 4,417 combined subscription elsewhere for print and online eds. (effective 2002). adv. bibl, charts, illus. index. back issues avail. *Refereed.* **Document type:** *Academic/Scholarly.* **Description:** Reflects original research reports and comprehensive reviews about systematic studies in pharmacology and toxicology, as related to the development of safe and efficacious drugs.
Related titles: Microform ed.: (from PQC); Online - full text ed.: ISSN 1098-2299. USD 3,995 in United States; USD 3,995 in Canada & Mexico; USD 3,995 elsewhere (effective 2002) (from EBSCO Publishing, Wiley InterScience, Institute for Scientific Information).
Indexed: ASCA, Agri.& Environ.Biotech.Abstr. (coverage dropped), Aqua.Sci.& Fish.Abstr., Biol.Abstr., Chem.Abstr., Chem.Indus.Notes, Chem.Titles, Curr.Adv.Cell & Devel.Biol., Curr.Adv.Ecol.Sci., Curr.Cont., Derwent Biotech.Abstr., Environ.Sci.Poll.Mgmt., Excerp.Med., I.P.A., Ind.Sci.Rev., Inpharma, Neurosci.Cit.Ind., Pharm.&Out.News, Reac., Rev.Med.& Vet.Mycol., SSCI (coverage dropped), Sci.Cit.Ind., Sugar Ind.Abstr.
—BLDSC (3629.119000), CASDDS, CISTI, EMDOCS, GNLM, IDS, ingenta, KNAW. **CCC.**
Published by: John Wiley & Sons, Inc., Journals (Subsidiary of: Wiley InterScience), 605 Third Ave, New York, NY 10158. TEL 212-850-6645, FAX 212-850-6021, subinfo@wiley.com, uscs-wis@wiley.com, http://www.wiley.com. Eds. David J Triggle, Michael Williams. adv.: B&W page GBP 640, color page GBP 1,515; trim 174 x 254. Circ: 550. **Subscr. outside the Americas to:** John Wiley & Sons Ltd., Baffins Ln, Chichester, Sussex PO19 IUD, United Kingdom. TEL 44-1243-779777, FAX 44-1243-843232, cs-journals@wiley.co.uk, http://www.wiley.co.uk.

615.1 USA ISSN 1524-783X
▼ **DRUG DISCOVERY & DEVELOPMENT.** Text in English. 1999. 8/yr. USD 81.90 domestic; USD 118.90 in Canada; USD 113.90 in Mexico; USD 174.90 elsewhere; USD 12 newsstand/cover domestic; USD 14 newsstand/cover foreign (effective 2001). adv. illus, tr.lit. reprints avail. **Document type:** *Journal, Trade.* **Description:** Provides the pharmaceutical and biotech research community with the latest drug discovery developments.
Related titles: Online - full text ed.: (from H. W. Wilson).
Indexed: B.P.I. (Jan.2001-).
—CCC.
Published by: Cahners Business Information, 2000 Clearwater Dr, Oak Brook, IL 60523. TEL 630-320-7171, FAX 630-320-7160, http://www.dddmag.com. Eds. Tim Studt TEL 630-320-7168, Robert Cassidy TEL 630-320-7172. Pub. Robert Cassidy TEL 630-320-7172. adv.: B&W page USD 5,440; trim 10.5 x 7.88. Circ: 50,000 (controlled).

615 USA
DRUG DISCOVERY - TECHNOLOGY NEWS. Text in English. 1998. m. USD 425 (effective 2001). back issues avail.; reprints avail. **Document type:** *Newsletter.* **Description:** Covers the latest news on drug discovery, new compounds, bulk manufacturing, drug delivery, compounding, and new regulations.
Published by: Business Communications Co., Inc. (Norwalk), 25 Van Zant St, Ste 13, Norwalk, CT 06855-1781. TEL 203-853-4266, FAX 203-853-0348, sales@bccresearch.com, http://www.bccresearch.com. Eds. Steve Edwards, Alan Hall.

615.1 660 GBR ISSN 1359-6446
RS420 CODEN: DDTOFS
DRUG DISCOVERY TODAY. Text in English. 1996. s-m. EUR 180 in Europe to individuals; JPY 21,400 in Japan to individuals; USD 192 elsewhere to individuals; EUR 225 in Europe to qualified personnel; JPY 26,700 in Japan to qualified personnel; USD 240 elsewhere to qualified personnel; EUR 1,407 in Europe to institutions; JPY 195,800 in Japan to institutions; USD 1,575 elsewhere to institutions (effective 2002). adv. back issues avail.; reprints avail. *Refereed.* **Document type:** *Academic/Scholarly, Trade.* **Description:** Offers pharmacists and physicians news in pharmacologic research.
Incorporates (1998-2001): Pharmaceutical Science and Technology Today (1461-5347)
Related titles: Online - full text ed.: (from ingenta, Swets Blackwell, ScienceDirect, Institute for Scientific Information).

Indexed: BBCI, Chem.Abstr., Chem.Indus.Notes, Chem.Titles, Curr.Cont., Environ.Sci.Poll.Mgmt., Excerp.Med., I.P.A., Inpharma, Med.& Pharm.Biotech.Abstr., Microbiol.Abstr., Pharm.&Out.News, Protozool.Abstr., Reac., Rev.Med.& Vet.Mycol., Sci.Cit.Ind.
—BLDSC (3629.120500), CASDDS, GNLM, IDS, Infotrieve. **CCC.**
Published by: Elsevier Science Ltd., Elsevier Trends Journals, 68 Hills Rd, Cambridge CB2 1LA, United Kingdom. TEL 44-1223-315961, FAX 44-1223-464430, DDT@elsevier.co.uk, http://www.elsevier.com/locate/drugdiscov. Eds. Debbie Tanter, Rebecca Lawrence. **Subscr. in Australasia and the Far East to:** Elsevier Science (Singapore) Pte Ltd, No.1 Temasek Ave, 17-01 Millenia Tower, Singapore 039192, Singapore. TEL 65-434-3727, FAX 65-337-2230; **Subscr. in the Americas to:** Elsevier Science, PO Box 945, New York, NY 10159-0945. TEL 212-633-3730, FAX 212-633-3680; **Subscr. to:** Elsevier Current Trends Subscriptions, PO Box 331, Haywards Heath, W Sussex RH16 3FG, United Kingdom. TEL 44-1444-675650, FAX 44-1444-445423.

615.5 SWE ISSN 0282-5783
DRUG EFFECTS IN CLINICAL CHEMISTRY✶ . Text in Swedish. 1977. triennial. SEK 300 (effective 1996). **Document type:** *Academic/Scholarly.*
Former titles (until 1992): Drug Interference and Drug Effects in Clinical Chemistry; (until 1986): Drug Interference and Effects in Clinical Chemistry; (until 1984): Drug Effects in Clinical Chemistry; (until 1978): Laekemedels Paaverkan paa Laboratorieundersoekningar
Published by: Apoteksbolaget AB/National Corporation of Swedish Pharmacies, c/o Svenska Tidningsutgivarefoereningen, Kungsholmstorg 5, Fack 22500, Stockholm 10422, Sweden. Ed. Nils Tryding.

615.1 USA ISSN 0277-9714
RM300
DRUG FACTS AND COMPARISONS. Text in English. 1947. m. USD 260; USD 299 foreign (effective 1999). index. **Description:** Reference guide listing over 16,000 drugs, including Rx and OTC, arranged by therapeutic class. Facilitates comparisons of costs, brands, and drugs.
Formerly: Facts and Comparisons (0014-6617)
Related titles: Online - full text ed.
Indexed: Inpharma, Reac.
—BLDSC (3629.126000).
Published by: Facts and Comparisons, 111 W. Port Plaza, Ste. 300, St. Louis, MO 63146-3098. TEL 800-223-0554, FAX 314-878-5563. Ed. Bernie R Olin.

615 614.4 USA ISSN 1061-2335
DRUG G M P REPORT. (Good Manufacturing Practices) Text in English. 1992. m. USD 627 in North America; USD 642 elsewhere (effective Nov. 2001). 8 p./no. back issues avail. **Document type:** *Newsletter.* **Description:** Reports on good manufacturing practices as they relate to the pharmaceutical industry.
Related titles: E-mail ed.: (from Data-Star, The Dialog Corporation).
—CCC.
Published by: Washington Business Information, Inc., 300 N Washington St, Ste 200, Falls Church, Arlington, VA 22046. TEL 703-538-7600, FAX 703 538-7676, ddouglass@fdanews.com, http://www.fdanews.com. Ed. Dennis Melamed.

615.06 NLD ISSN 0921-2582
CODEN: DRDIER
DRUG INDUCED DISORDERS. Text in Dutch. 1985. irreg., latest vol.5, 1992. NLG 395 domestic for vol 5; EUR 179.24 in Europe for vol 5; USD 227 elsewhere for vol 5. back issues avail. *Refereed.* **Document type:** *Monographic series, Academic/Scholarly, Trade.* **Description:** Discusses disorders caused by the side-effects of drugs.
Indexed: Chem.Abstr., Chem.Indus.Notes, Chem.Titles.
—CASDDS, CISTI, KNAW.
Published by: Elsevier Science BV, PO Box 211, Amsterdam 1000 AE, Netherlands. TEL 31-20-485-3757, 31-20-485-3911, FAX 31-20-485-3432, 31-20-485-3598, nlinfo-f@elsevier.nl, http://www.elsevier.nl. Ed. B H C Stricker. **Subscr. in Australasia and the Far East to:** Elsevier Science (Singapore) Pte Ltd, No.1 Temasek Ave, 17-01 Millenia Tower, Singapore 039192, Singapore. TEL 65-434-3727, FAX 65-337-2230, asiainfo@elsevier.com.sg; **Subscr. in Japan to:** Elsevier Science Inc - Japan Regional Office, 9-15 Higashi-Azabu 1-chome, Minato-ku, Tokyo 106-0044, Japan. TEL 81-3-5561-5033, FAX 81-3-5561-5047, info@elsevier.co.jp; **Subscr. in the Americas to:** Elsevier Science, PO Box 945, New York, NY 10159-0945. TEL 212-633-3730, 888-437-4636, FAX 212-633-3680, usinfo-f@elsevier.com, http://www.elsevier.com

615.1 USA ISSN 0092-8615
RM1 CODEN: DGIJB9
DRUG INFORMATION JOURNAL. Text in English. 1966. q. USD 225; USD 65 to libraries. adv. index. back issues avail. *Refereed.* **Document type:** *Academic/Scholarly.*
Formerly: Drug Information Bulletin (0012-656X)
Related titles: CD-ROM ed.; Microfilm ed.: (from PQC); Online - full text ed.: (from Northern Light Technology, Inc., ProQuest Information & Learning, Institute for Scientific Information).
Indexed: AgeLine, Aqua.Sci.& Fish.Abstr., Biol.Abstr., Chem.Abstr., Curr.Adv.Ecol.Sci., Environ.Sci.Poll.Mgmt., Excerp.Med., I.P.A., Inform.Sci.Abstr., Inpharma, LISA, Microbiol.Abstr., Nutr.Abstr., Pharm.&Out.News, Pollut.Abstr., Reac., Ref.Zh., Rev.Appl.Entomol., Rev.Arom.& Med.Plants, Weed Abstr.
—BLDSC (3629.160000), CASDDS, CISTI, GNLM, IDS, Infotrieve, ingenta, Linda Hall. **CCC.**
Published by: Drug Information Association, 501 Office Center Dr, Ste 450, Fort Washington, PA 19034-3211. TEL 215-628-2288, FAX 215-641-1229, dia@diahome.org, http://www.diahome.org. Ed. Thomas Teal. Circ: 22,000.

615.7 USA
DRUG INTERACTION FACTS. Text in English. q. USD 59.95 domestic; USD 68.90 foreign (effective 1999). Supplement avail. **Description:** Reference for drug and food interactions of clinical significance, suspected but unsubstantiated interactions, with concise synopsis of onset, severity and documentation.
Related titles: CD-ROM ed.
Published by: Facts and Comparisons, 111 W. Port Plaza, Ste. 300, St. Louis, MO 63146-3098. TEL 800-223-0554, FAX 314-878-5563. Ed. David S Tatro.

615.19 USA ISSN 1527-1498
DRUG MARKETING. Text in English. w. USD 797 in North America; USD 847 elsewhere (effective Nov. 2001). 8 p./no. back issues avail. **Document type:** *Newsletter.*
Published by: Washington Business Information, Inc., 300 N Washington St, Ste 200, Falls Church, Arlington, VA 22046. TEL 703-538-7660, FAX 703-538-7676, http://www.fdanews.com. Ed. Peter Riebling.

615 USA ISSN 0090-9556
RM301 CODEN: DMDSAI
DRUG METABOLISM AND DISPOSITION. Text in English. 1973. m. USD 112, USD 157 to individuals; USD 214, USD 259 to institutions (effective 2000); includes online access. adv. bk.rev. illus. index. back issues avail. *Refereed.* **Document type:** *Academic/Scholarly.* **Description:** Covers metabolism of pharmacological agents or drugs and environmental chemicals, reactants and preservatives for pharmacologists, toxicologists and medical chemists.
Related titles: Microfilm ed.: (from WWS); Online - full text ed.: ISSN 1521-009X. USD 90 to individuals; USD 171 to institutions (effective 2000) (from HighWire Pr., EBSCO Publishing, Institute for Scientific Information).
Indexed: ASCA, Agri.& Environ.Biotech.Abstr. (coverage dropped), Aqua.Sci.& Fish.Abstr., BBCI, Biol.Abstr., Chem.Abstr., Chem.Cit.Ind., Chem.Indus.Notes, Chem.Titles, Curr.Adv.Ecol.Sci., Curr.Cont., Dairy Sci.Abstr., Derwent Biotech.Abstr., Environ.Sci.Poll.Mgmt., Excerp.Med., Helminthol.Abstr., INIS Atomind., Ind.Med. (1973-), Ind.Sci.Rev., Ind.Vet., Inpharma, Int.Abstr.Biol.Sci., Mass Spectr.Bull., Nutr.Abstr., Pharm.&Out.News, Pollut.Abstr., Protozool.Abstr., Reac., Ref.Zh., Rev.Med.& Vet.Mycol., Risk Abstr., Saf.Sci.Abstr., Sci.Cit.Ind., Tox.Abstr., Vet.Bull.
—BLDSC (3629.325000), CASDDS, CISTI, GNLM, IDS, ingenta, KNAW, Linda Hall.
Published by: American Society for Pharmacology and Experimental Therapeutics (ASPET), 9650 Rockville Pike, Bethesda, MD 20814-3998. TEL 301-530-7024, FAX 301-571-5728, staff@dues.faseb.org, http://www.dmd.org. Ed. James R Halpert. R&P Richard Dodenhoff TEL 301-571-5754. Adv. contact Frances Yates. Circ: 1,004; 944 (paid).

615.19 ISR ISSN 0792-5077
RM302 CODEN: DMDIEQ
DRUG METABOLISM AND DRUG INTERACTIONS. Text in English. 1972. q., latest vol.19. USD 300 (effective 2002). adv. bk.rev. index. back issues avail. **Document type:** *Academic/Scholarly.*
Former titles (until 1988): Reviews on Drug Metabolism and Drug Interactions (0334-2190); (until vol. 3): Reviews on Drug Interactions (0048-7546)
Indexed: Chem.Abstr., Chem.Indus.Notes, Chem.Titles, Curr.Adv.Ecol.Sci., Derwent Biotech.Abstr., Excerp.Med., I.P.A., Ind.Med. (1988-).
—BLDSC (3629.326000), CASDDS, EMDOCS, GNLM, KNAW.
Published by: Freund Publishing House, Ltd., P O Box 35010, Tel Aviv 61350, Israel. TEL 972-3-562-8540, FAX 972-3-562-8538, h_freund@netvision.net.il, http://www.angelfire.com/il/freund. Ed. N Kingsley.

DRUG METABOLISM REVIEWS. see *MEDICAL SCIENCES*

615.1 IND ISSN 0026-8194
DRUG NEWS. Text in English. 1937. m. INR 25.
Indexed: PROMT.
Published by: India Publications Co., Denabank House, 2nd Fl., 31 Hamam St., Mumbai, Maharashtra 400 001, India. Ed. Eric Martin.

615.19 ESP ISSN 0214-0934
CODEN: DNPEED
DRUG NEWS & PERSPECTIVES; the international drug newsmagazine. Text in English. 1988. 10/yr. USD 750 (effective 2000). adv. bk.rev. back issues avail. *Refereed.* **Description:** For scientists and managers in pharmaceutical research and development.
Related titles: Online - full text ed.: (from The Dialog Corporation, Gale Group, Factiva, Institute for Scientific Information).
Indexed: BBCI, I.P.A., Inpharma, Pharm.&Out.News, Reac.
—CASDDS, CISTI, EMDOCS, GNLM, IDS, Infotrieve, KNAW. **CCC.**
Published by: Prous Science, PO Box 540, Barcelona 08080, Spain. TEL 34-93-4592220, FAX 34-93-4581535, service@prous.com. R&P Ann Wescott.

615 USA
DRUG OUTCOMES SOURCEBOOK. Text in English. a.
Published by: Thompson Financial / I M G Media, Healthcare Information Center (Subsidiary of: Thompson Publishing Group), 11 Penn Plaza, 17th Fl, New York, NY 10001-2006. TEL 212-967-7000, FAX 212-967-7155. Pub. Spencer Vibbert.

DRUG PRODUCT LIABILITY. see *LAW*

DRUG RESISTANCE UPDATE. see *MEDICAL SCIENCES*

615 NZL ISSN 0114-5916
CODEN: DRSAEA
DRUG SAFETY. Text in English. 1986. 15/yr. USD 165 to individuals Print or Online ed.; USD 198 to individuals Print and Online combined eds.; USD 1,250 to institutions Print or Online ed.; USD 1,500 to institutions Print and Online combined eds. (effective 2001). bk.rev. back issues avail. *Refereed.* **Document type:** *Academic/Scholarly.* **Description:** Provides evaluations of adverse drug experience and risk-benefit. Articles are designed to assist in the correct, safe utilization of today's drugs.
Former titles (until 1990): Medical Toxicology and Adverse Drug Experience (0113-5244); (until 1987): Medical Toxicology (0112-5966)
Related titles: Online - full text ed.: (from Ovid Technologies, Inc., EBSCO Publishing, O C L C Online Computer Library Center, Inc., RoweCom Information Quest, ingenta, Swets Blackwell, Institute for Scientific Information).
Indexed: Chem.Abstr., Chem.Indus.Notes, Chem.Titles, Curr.Cont., Dairy Sci.Abstr., Derwent Biotech.Abstr., Environ.Sci.Poll.Mgmt., Excerp.Med., I.P.A., Ind.Med. (1990-), Inpharma, Int.Abstr.Biol.Sci., Med.& Surg.Dermat., NRN, Neurosci.Abstr. (coverage dropped), Nutr.Abstr., Pharm.&Out.News, Pollut.Abstr., Protozool.Abstr., Reac., Rev.Med.& Vet.Mycol., Risk Abstr., SSCI (coverage dropped), Saf.Sci.Abstr., Sci.Cit.Ind.
—BLDSC (3629.395000), ADONIS, CASDDS, CISTI, GNLM, IDS, ingenta, KNAW. **CCC.**

P

Published by: Adis International Limited, Mairangi Bay, Private Bag 65901, Auckland 1010, New Zealand. TEL 64-9-477-0700, FAX 64-9-477-0766, drugsafety@adis.co.nz, http://www.adis.com; http://biomednet.com/library/jdrs. Ed. Rosie Stather. Pub. Paul Chrisp. R&P Will Charles. Circ: 600. **Subscr. in the Americas to:** Adis International Inc., Attn: Subscription Dept, 860 Town Center Dr, Langhorne, PA 19047. TEL 877-872-2347.

615.5 381.456151 USA
DRUG STORE NEWS. CONTINUING EDUCATION QUARTERLY. Text in English. 1986. q. USD 59.95 domestic; USD 69.95 in Canada; USD 199 elsewhere; USD 15 newsstand/cover (effective 2001). adv. illus. **Document type:** *Journal, Trade.*
Former titles: Drug Store News. Chain Pharmacy; (until 1997): Drug Store News for the Pharmacist (1055-2952); (until 1991): Drug Store News, Inside Pharmacy (0891-9828)
Indexed: I.P.A.
—**CCC.**
Published by: Lebhar-Friedman, Inc., 425 Park Ave, New York, NY 10022. TEL 212-756-5000. Ed. Kimberly Werner. Pub. John Kerlon. Circ: 56,537. **Affiliate:** Pub. Jill Manee.

DRUG TARGETING. see *PHARMACY AND PHARMACOLOGY—Abstracting, Bibliographies, Statistics*

615.1 USA ISSN 0012-6616
DRUG TOPICS. Text in English. 1857. s-m. (23/yr). USD 61 domestic; USD 109 foreign; USD 10 newsstand/cover domestic; USD 15 newsstand/cover foreign (effective 2001). adv. bk.rev. charts, illus, mkt, pat, tr.lit. **Document type:** *Trade.* **Description:** Publishes current trends and developments affecting the pharmacy field. Includes merchandising, government affairs, management, professional and clinical news, and continuing education.
Related titles: Microform ed.: (from RPI,PQC); Online - full text ed.: (from ProQuest Information & Learning, Gale Group, Northern Light Technology, Inc., Factiva).
Indexed: ABI Inform. (Apr.1974-), B.P.I. (Jul.1989-), Bus.& Indus. (Jul.1995-), Bus.Ind., Hlth.Ind., I.P.A., PROMT, Tr.& Indus.Ind.
—BLDSC (3629.450000), CISTI, EMDOCS, GNLM, Infotrieve, ingenta. **CCC.**
Published by: Medical Economics Co., Inc., 5 Paragon Dr, Montvale, NJ 07645-1742. TEL 800-526-4870, customer_service@medec.com, http://crugtopics.com. Ed. Val Cardinale. Pub. Carol Jaxel. Adv. contact Liz Gevers. B&W page USD 8,160, color page USD 10,680. Circ: 110,793. **Subscr. to:** Medical Economics Co, Inc, P D R, PO Box 162, Montvale, NJ 07645-1742. TEL 800-232-7379, 201-722-2680.

615.1 338 USA ISSN 1072-1142
HD9666.1
DRUG TOPICS REDBOOK. Text in English. 1897. a. USD 54.95 (effective 1999). **Document type:** *Trade.* **Description:** Works as reference book for pharmacists; lists pricing and packaging information on more than 100,000 prescription and over-the-counter products, including forms, strength, size, N.D.C., and price. Includes reference section on hard-to-find information.
Related titles: Magnetic Tape ed.; ♦ Supplement: Drug Topics Redbook Update. ISSN 0731-8596.
—**CCC.**
Published by: Medical Economics Co., Inc., 5 Paragon Dr, Montvale, NJ 07645-1742. TEL 201-358-7200, FAX 201-573-4956. Ed. Valentine Cardinale. Circ: 60,000.

615.1 USA ISSN 0731-8596
DRUG TOPICS REDBOOK UPDATE. Text in English. m. USD 99 (effective 1999). **Description:** Covers monthly price changes of prescription and over-the-counter drugs, pricing and packaging information on top-volume products and newly introduced drugs.
Related titles: ♦ Supplement to: Drug Topics Redbook. ISSN 1072-1142.
—**CCC.**
Published by: Medical Economics Co., Inc., 5 Paragon Dr, Montvale, NJ 07645-1742. TEL 201-358-7200.

615.7 USA ISSN 0884-8998
DRUG UTILIZATION REVIEW. Text in English. 1985. m. USD 399 domestic; USD 429 foreign; USD 67 newsstand/cover (effective 2001). back issues avail.; reprints avail. **Document type:** *Newsletter.*
Related titles: Online - full text ed.: (from Northern Light Technology, Inc., Gale Group).
Published by: American Health Consultants (Subsidiary of: Medical Economics Co., Inc.), 3525 Piedmont Rd, N E, 6 Piedmont Center, Ste 400, Atlanta, GA 30305. TEL 404-262-5476, 404-262-7436, 800-688-2421, FAX 404-262-7837, 800-284-3291, custserv@ahcpub.com, http://www.ahcpub.com. Circ: 1,485.

615.7 USA ISSN 1089-5590
DRUGLINK. Text in English. m. USD 99.95 (effective 2001). **Document type:** *Newsletter.* **Description:** Summarizes new findings and recent developments in drug therapy. Information on investigational drugs, OTCs, actions, reactions and interactions and more.
Formerly (until 1997): Drug Newsletter (0731-5163)
Published by: Facts and Comparisons, 111 W. Port Plaza, Ste. 300, St. Louis, MO 63146-3098. TEL 800-223-0554, FAX 314-878-5563.

615.1 NZL ISSN 0012-6667
RM1 CODEN: DRUGAY
DRUGS. Text in English. 1971. m. USD 1,995 Print or Online ed.; USD 2,394 Print and Online eds. (effective 2001). adv. abstr, bibl, charts, illus. back issues avail. *Refereed.* **Document type:** *Academic/Scholarly.* **Description:** Features comprehensive drug evaluations on new and established drugs, review articles on all aspects of drugs and drug therapy and disease management articles.
Related titles: Online - full text ed.: (from Ovid Technologies, Inc., EBSCO Publishing, O C L C Online Computer Library Center, Inc., RoweCom Information Quest, ingenta, Swets Blackwell, Institute for Scientific Information).
Indexed: Agri.& Environ.Biotech.Abstr. (coverage dropped), Biol.Abstr., Chem.Abstr., Chem.Indus.Notes, Chem.Titles, Curr.Adv.Cancer Res., Curr.Cont., Dent.Ind., Derwent Biotech.Abstr., Environ.Sci.Poll.Mgmt., Excerp.Med., Helminthol.Abstr., I.P.A., Ind.Med. (1971-), Ind.Sci.Rev., Int.Abstr.Biol.Sci., Med.& Surg.Dermat., Microbiol.Abstr., Neurosci.Abstr. (coverage dropped), Pollut.Abstr., Protozool.Abstr., Risk Abstr., Saf.Sci.Abstr., Sci.Cit.Ind., Tox.Abstr.
—BLDSC (3629.600000), ADONIS, CASDDS, CISTI, GNLM, IDS, Infotrieve, ingenta, KNAW, Linda Hall. **CCC.**
Published by: Adis International Limited, Mairangi Bay, Private Bag 65901, Auckland 1010, New Zealand. TEL 64-9-477-0700, FAX 64-9-477-0766, drugs@adis.co.nz, http://www.adis.com; http://biomednet.com/library/jdrg. Ed. Dene J Peters. Pub. Paul Chrisp. R&P Will Charles. Circ: 2,500. **Americas subscr. to:** Adis International Inc., Attn: Subscription Dept, 860 Town Center Dr, Langhorne, PA 19047. TEL 877-872-2347, 877-234-7329.

615.58 NZL ISSN 1170-229X
RC953.7 CODEN: DRAGE6
DRUGS & AGING. Text in English. 1991. m. USD 165 to individuals Print or Online ed.; USD 198 to individuals Print and Online combined eds.; USD 1,095 to institutions Print or Online ed.; USD 1,314 to institutions Print and Online combined eds. (effective 2001). back issues avail. *Refereed.* **Document type:** *Academic/Scholarly.* **Description:** Promotes rational, safe pharmacotherapy in elderly population.
Related titles: Online - full text ed.: (from Ovid Technologies, Inc., EBSCO Publishing, O C L C Online Computer Library Center, Inc., RoweCom Information Quest, ingenta, Swets Blackwell, Institute for Scientific Information).
Indexed: ASCA, Chem.Abstr., Chem.Indus.Notes, Chem.Titles, Curr.Cont., Derwent Biotech.Abstr., Excerp.Med. (1996-), Ind.Med. (1991-), Ind.Sci.Rev., Inpharma, Int.Abstr.Biol.Sci., Int.Nurs.Ind., Pharm.&Out.News, Reac., Rev.Arom.& Med.Plants, Rev.Med.& Vet.Mycol., SSCI (coverage dropped), Sci.Cit.Ind.
—BLDSC (3629.612000), ADONIS, CASDDS, CISTI, GNLM, IDS, ingenta, KNAW. **CCC.**
Published by: Adis International Limited, Mairangi Bay, Private Bag 65901, Auckland 1010, New Zealand. TEL 64-9-477-0700, FAX 64-9-477-0766, drugs.aging@adis.co.nzz, http://www.adis.com; http://biomednet.com/library/jdag. Ed. Rachel Foster. Pub. Paul Chrisp. R&P Will Charles. Circ: 400. **Americas subscr. to:** Adis International Inc., Attn: Subscription Dept, 860 Town Center Dr, Langhorne, PA 19047. TEL 877234-73291, 877-872-2347.

DRUGS AND BIOLOGY GUIDANCE MANUAL. see *PUBLIC HEALTH AND SAFETY*

615.9 614 USA ISSN 8756-5935
DRUGS AND DEVICE RECALL BULLETIN. Text in English. 1985. m. USD 55 (effective 2001). back issues avail. **Document type:** *Bulletin.* **Description:** Current data on FDA recalls.
Published by: Rx-Data-Pac Service, 8907 Terwilliger s Tr, Cincinnati, OH 45249. TEL 513-489-0943, FAX 513-489-0943. Ed. Dr. I H Goodman.

615.7 USA ISSN 0360-2583
CODEN: DPHSDS
DRUGS AND THE PHARMACEUTICAL SCIENCES. Text in English. 1975. irreg., latest vol.97, 1999. price varies. adv. *Refereed.* **Document type:** *Monographic series.*
Indexed: Chem.Abstr., Chem.Indus.Notes, Chem.Titles.
—BLDSC (3629.630000), CASDDS, CISTI, KNAW. **CCC.**
Published by: Marcel Dekker, Inc., Attn: Eridania Perrez, 270 Madison Ave, New York, NY 10016-0602. TEL 212-696-9000, 800-228-1160, FAX 212-685-4540, marketing@dekker.com, http://www.dekker.com. Ed. J Swarbrick. R&P Julia Mulligan. Adv. contact Eridania Perez.

615 NZL ISSN 1172-0360
CODEN: DTHPEE
DRUGS & THERAPY PERSPECTIVES. Text in English. 1993. bi-w. USD 150 to individuals Print or Online ed.; USD 180 to individuals Print and Online combined eds.; USD 350 to institutions Print or Online ed.; USD 420 to institutions Print and Online combined eds. (effective 2001). back issues avail. *Refereed.* **Document type:** *Academic/Scholarly.* **Description:** Provides reviews of new drugs, disease treatment algorithms, brief economic evaluations of new drugs.
Related titles: Online - full text ed.: (from Institute for Scientific Information).
Indexed: Excerp.Med. (1995-), Inpharma, Pharm.&Out.News, Reac.
—BLDSC (3629.665000), GNLM, Infotrieve, KNAW. **CCC.**
Published by: Adis International Limited, Mairangi Bay, Private Bag 65901, Auckland 1010, New Zealand. TEL 64-9-477-0700, FAX 64-9-477-0766, dtp@adis.co.nzdis.co.nz, http://www.adis.com; http://biomednet.com/library/jdtp. Ed. Alison Forbes. Pub. Paul Chrips. R&P Will Charles. Circ: 1,600. **Subscr. in the Americas to:** Adis International Inc., Attn: Subscription Dept, 860 Town Center Dr, Langhorne, PA 19047. TEL 877-872-2347.

DRUGS CASES; including narcotics cases. see *LAW*

615.9 JPN
DRUGS IN JAPAN; ethical drugs. Text in Japanese. 1974. a. JPY 23,500 (effective 2001).
Related titles: CD-ROM ed.: Drugs in Japan D B. JPY 35,000 (effective 2000).
Published by: Japan Pharmaceutical Information Center/Nihon Iyaku Joho Senta, 3rd Fl Nagai-Kinenkan, 2-12-15 Shibuya, Shibuya-ku, Tokyo 150-0002, Japan. TEL 81-3-5466-1812, FAX 81-3-5466-1814.

344.042 USA
DRUGS IN LITIGATION: DAMAGE AWARDS INVOLVING PRESCRIPTION AND NONPRESCRIPTION DRUGS. Text in English. a., latest 1996. USD 80. **Description:** Summarizes hundreds of trial and appellate decisions involving drugs and medicines.
Published by: Lexis Law Publishing (Subsidiary of: Reed Elsevier plc), PO Box 7587, Charlottesville, VA 22906-7587. TEL 804-972-7600, 800-562-1197, FAX 804-562-1197, llp.customer.support@lexis-nexis.com, http://www.lexislawpublishing.com.

615.1 DEU ISSN 0012-6683
RS1 CODEN: DRMGAS
DRUGS MADE IN GERMANY. Text in English. 1958. 4/yr. DEM 50.85, EUR 26; DEM 58.67, EUR 30 print & online eds. combined (effective 2001). adv. bk.rev. charts, illus, pat, tr.lit. reprint service avail. from IRC,ISI. **Document type:** *Journal, Trade.* **Description:** Covers topics such as politics on health care and pharmaceutical issues, testing and approval of new drugs, legislation, marketing, and distribution.
Related titles: Online - full text ed.
Indexed: Agri.& Environ.Biotech.Abstr. (coverage dropped), Biol.Abstr., Chem.Abstr., Chem.Indus.Notes, Chem.Titles, Derwent Biotech.Abstr., Excerp.Med., I.P.A., Ind.Med. (coverage dropped), Ref.Zh.
—BLDSC (3629.900000), CASDDS, CINDOC, GNLM, Infotrieve, KNAW, Linda Hall. **CCC.**
Published by: Editio Cantor Verlag, Postfach 1255, Aulendorf 88322, Germany. TEL 49-7525-940135, FAX 49-7525-940180, info@ecv.de, http://www.ecv.de/drugshom.htm. Ed. Viktor Schramm. Adv. contact Holger Leupoldt. B&W page DEM 2,150; trim 192 x 270. Circ: 4,800 (paid and controlled).

615 619 ESP ISSN 0377-8282
RM1 CODEN: DRFUD4
DRUGS OF THE FUTURE. Text in English. 1976. m. USD 1,100 (effective 2000). adv. **Description:** Offers comprehensive drug monographs on new compounds, including their synthesis, pharmacological action, pharmacokinetics and metabolism, toxicity, and clinical studies.
Related titles: Online - full text ed.: (from Institute for Scientific Information).
Indexed: Biol.Abstr., Chem.Abstr., Curr.Cont., Excerp.Med., I.P.A., Inpharma, Pharm.&Out.News, Reac.
—CASDDS, CISTI, EMDOCS, GNLM, IDS, Infotrieve, KNAW. **CCC.**
Published by: Prous Science, PO Box 540, Barcelona 08080, Spain. TEL 34-93-4592220, FAX 34-93-4581535, service@prous.com. R&P Pat Leeson. Circ: 3,000.

615.1 ESP ISSN 0025-7656
CODEN: MDACAP
DRUGS OF TODAY/MEDICAMENTOS DE ACTUALIDAD. Text in English. 1965. m. USD 750 (effective 2000). adv. bk.rev. *Refereed.* **Description:** Provides physicians and other healthcare professionals with practical, up-to-date monographs on recently approved and launched drugs.
Related titles: Online - full text ed.: (from Institute for Scientific Information).
Indexed: Biol.Abstr., Chem.Abstr., Chem.Indus.Notes, Chem.Titles, Curr.Cont., Excerp.Med., I.P.A., Inpharma, Mass Spectr.Bull., Pharm.&Out.News, Reac., Rev.Med.& Vet.Mycol.
—CASDDS, CISTI, GNLM, IDS, Infotrieve, ingenta, KNAW. **CCC.**
Published by: Prous Science, PO Box 540, Barcelona 08080, Spain. TEL 34-93-4592220, FAX 34-93-4581535, service@prous.com. R&P Pat Leeson. Circ: 3,000.

615.1 GBR ISSN 1368-8529
DRUGS QUARTERLY. Text in English. 1997. q. GBP 37.50 domestic; GBP 45 foreign (effective 2000). **Document type:** *Academic/Scholarly.*
Indexed: I.P.A.
—BLDSC (3630.101500).
Published by: Pillar Publications Ltd., 45 Woodland Grove, Weybridge KT13 9EQ, United Kingdom. FAX 44-1932-868035, dq@bjhc.demon.co.uk. Ed. John Dunne. Pub. Hugh de Glanville.

619 CHE ISSN 0378-6501
CODEN: DECRDP
DRUGS UNDER EXPERIMENTAL AND CLINICAL RESEARCH. Short title: Drugs under Research. Text in English. 1977. bi-m. CHF 450 (effective 2002). reprint service avail. from PQC. *Refereed.* **Document type:** *Journal, Academic/Scholarly.* **Description:** Devoted to the study of compounds and molecules which may have possible therapeutic application. Covers animal and clinical pharmacology, medicinal chemistry, toxicology, teratology, mutagenesis, drug metabolism, pharmacokinetics, and clinical trials.
Related titles: Microform ed.: (from PQC); Online - full text ed.: (from Institute for Scientific Information).
Indexed: ASCA, Biol.Abstr., Chem.Abstr., Chem.Indus.Notes, Chem.Titles, Curr.Adv.Ecol.Sci., Curr.Cont. (coverage dropped), Derwent Biotech.Abstr., Excerp.Med., I.P.A., Ind.Med. (1977-), Inpharma, Int.Abstr.Biol.Sci., Neurosci.Cit.Ind., Nutr.Abstr., Pharm.&Out.News, Protozool.Abstr., Reac., Ref.Zh., Rev.Med.& Vet.Mycol., Sci.Cit.Ind. (coverage dropped).
—BLDSC (3629.820000), CASDDS, CISTI, EMDOCS, GNLM, IDS, ingenta, KNAW. **CCC.**
Published by: Bioscience Ediprint Inc., Rue Alexandre Gavard 16, Carouge 1227, Switzerland. TEL 41-22-3003383, FAX 41-22-3002489, TELEX 423355-BIOS-CH, bioscience.smey@gkb.com. Ed. A Bertelli.

615 RUS
DYABET. OBRAZ ZHIZNI. Text in Russian. q. USD 99.95 in United States.
Published by: Mezhdunarodnaya Programma Diabet, Chasovaya ul 20, Moscow 125315, Russian Federation. TEL 7-095-4900394, FAX 7-095-1521982. Ed. A S Ametov. **US dist. addr.:** East View Publications, 3020 Harbor Ln N, Minneapolis, MN 55447. TEL 612-550-0961.

DYABETIK. see *MEDICAL SCIENCES—Endocrinology*

DYABETOGRAFIYA. see *MEDICAL SCIENCES—Endocrinology*

615.1 ITA
E D I M E D. Text in Italian. a., latest 2001. EUR 108.46 (effective 2001). **Document type:** *Directory, Consumer.*
Formerly (until 2001): Notiziario Medico Farmaceutico (0029-439X)
Related titles: ♦ Supplement to: L' Informatore Farmaceutico. ISSN 0392-3010.
Published by: O E M F SpA, Via Filippo Palizzi, 88, PO Box 10434, Milan, MI 20157, Italy. TEL 39-02-332101, FAX 39-02-3551731, info@oemf.it, http://www.oemf.it. Ed. Dr. G Panagia. Adv. contact Delia Weissy. Circ: 6,500.

615 DEU ISSN 1381-4060
E H P*. (European Hospital Pharmacy) Text in German. 1995. q. membership. *Refereed.*
Indexed: I.P.A.
—BLDSC (3664.724000), GNLM.
Published by: (European Association of Hospital Pharmacists), Medicultura International B.V., c/o J. Kotwas, Universitaetsklinikum Steglitz Apotheke, Freie Universitaet Berlin, Hindenburgdamm 30, Berlin 12200, Germany.

615 GBR ISSN 1462-3129
E R A NEWS. (European Regulatory Affairs) Text in English. 1992. m. GBP 150 in Europe; GBP 155 in the Middle East; USD 300 in US & Canada; JPY 38,000 in Japan; GBP 175 rest of world (effective 2001). 16 p./no. 2 cols./p. back issues avail.; reprints avail. **Document type:** *Newsletter.* **Description:** Constitutes a regulatory affairs newsletter providing updates on European & national developments in the pharmaceutical, veterinary and medical device industry.
Formerly (until Jan. 1998): G P L C Update
Related titles: Online - full text ed.: (from Data-Star, The Dialog Corporation, S T N International).
Published by: P J B Publications Ltd., 18-20 Hill Rise, Richmond, Surrey TW10 6UA, United Kingdom. TEL 44-20-8948-3262, FAX 44-20-8332-8998, maria@pjbsubs.demon.co.uk, http://www.pjbpubs.com. Ed. Peter Rixon. Pub. Philip Brown. R&P Annette Watts TEL 44-20-8332-8961. Circ: 150 (paid). **Subscr. in N. America:** PharmaBooks, 1775 Broadway, Suite 511, New York, NY 10019. TEL 212-262-8230, FAX 212-262-8234.

615 840 DEU
E S - H W G - ENTSCHEIDUNGSSAMMLUNG HEILMITTELWERBEGESETZ. Text in German. base vol. plus irreg. updates. DEM 950. **Document type:** *Monographic series.*
Published by: P M I Verlag AG, August-Schanz-Str 8, Frankfurt Am Main 60433, Germany. TEL 49-69-548000-0, FAX 49-69-548000-77, pmiverlag@aol.com.

615.1 IND ISSN 0012-8872
CODEN: EAPHA6
THE EASTERN PHARMACIST. Text in English. 1958. m. USD 60 (effective 2000). adv. bk.rev. charts, illus, mkt, pat, tr.lit, tr.mk. *Refereed.* **Document type:** *Newspaper, Trade.*
Related titles: Online - full text ed.: (from Factiva).
Indexed: Bus.& Indus. (Sep.1994-), CBNB (1996-), Chem.Abstr., Chem.Indus.Notes, Chem.Titles, Curr.Adv.Ecol.Sci., I.P.A.
—BLDSC (3646.800000), CASDDS, CISTI, GNLM, KNAW.
Published by: Pamposh Publications, 507 Ashok Bhawan, 93 Nehru Place, New Delhi 110 019, India. TEL 91-11-6433315, FAX 91-11-6225885. Ed. Mohan C Bazaz. Adv. contact Kong Posh. Circ: 5,000 (paid).

ECONOMICS, MEDICINES, & HEALTH. see *BUSINESS AND ECONOMICS—Production Of Goods And Services*

615.1 EGY ISSN 0301-5068
RS1 CODEN: EJPSBZ
EGYPTIAN JOURNAL OF PHARMACEUTICAL SCIENCES. Text in English; Summaries in Arabic, English. 1960. 6/yr. USD 217 (effective 2000). charts, illus. reprint service avail. from IRC. **Document type:** *Academic/Scholarly.*
Former titles (until 1972): United Arab Republic Journal of Pharmaceutical Sciences (0301-5076); Journal of Pharmaceutical Sciences of the United Arab Republic (0022-3557)
Related titles: CD-ROM ed.; Online - full text ed.
Indexed: Biol.Abstr., Chem.Abstr., Chem.Indus.Notes, Chem.Titles, ExtraMED, Food Sci.& Tech.Abstr., Helminthol.Abstr., Hort.Abstr., I.P.A., Nutr.Abstr., Postharvest, Protozool.Abstr., Rev.Appl.Entomol., Rev.Med.& Vet.Mycol., Rev.Plant Path., Sugar Ind.Abstr.
—BLDSC (3664.410000), CASDDS, CISTI, GNLM, ingenta, Linda Hall.
Published by: (Research Department, Pharmaceutical Society of Egypt), National Information and Documentation Centre (NIDOC), Tahrir St., Dokki, Awqaf P.O., Cairo, Egypt. TEL 20-2-3371696. Ed. A A Abd El Rahman. Circ: 1,750.

615.9 RUS ISSN 0869-2092
RS1 CODEN: EKFAE9
EKSPERIMENTAL'NAYA I KLINICHESKAYA FARMAKOLOGIYA. Text in Russian; Summaries in English. 1938. bi-m. USD 100 in United States. adv. index. **Document type:** *Academic/Scholarly.* **Description:** Publishes articles devoted to the pharmacological study of medicinal preparations and of the effects produced by various poisons on animals and man.
Formerly (until 1992): Farmakologiya i Toksikologiya (0014-8318)
Related titles: ♦ Russian Translation: Russian Journal of Experimental and Clinical Pharmacology. ISSN 1026-3241.
Indexed: Agri.& Environ.Biotech.Abstr. (coverage dropped), Biol.Abstr., Chem.Abstr., Curr.Adv.Ecol.Sci., Curr.Cont. (coverage dropped), Dent.Ind., Derwent Biotech.Abstr., Excerp.Med., Helminthol.Abstr., INIS Atomind., I.P.A., Ind.Med. (coverage dropped), Ind.Sci.Rev., Nutr.Abstr., Psyclnfo, Psychol.Abstr. (1943-), Ref.Zh., Sci.Cit.Ind. (coverage dropped), e-psyche.
—BLDSC (0397.988500), CASDDS, CINDOC, CISTI, East View, EMDOCS, GNLM, Infotrieve, ingenta, Linda Hall. **CCC.**
Published by: Rossiiskaya Akademiya Meditsinskikh Nauk, Solyanka ul 14, Moscow 109801, Russian Federation. TEL 7-095-9172286. Ed. D A Kharkevich. Adv. contact V F Strizhova. Circ: 80,000. **Dist. by:** Mezhdunarodnaya Kniga, B Yakimanka 39, Moscow 117049, Russian Federation. TEL 7-095-2384967, FAX 7-095-2384634. **Co-sponsor:** Nauchnoe Obshchestvo Farmakologov.

615 USA ISSN 1061-6098
CODEN: EMPHFR
EMERGING PHARMACEUTICALS. Text in English. 1992. m. USD 467 in US & Canada; USD 487 elsewhere (effective 2001). tr.lit. back issues avail. **Document type:** *Newsletter.* **Description:** Focuses on the earliest stages of drug development - from discovery through preclinical trials and on small-molecule drugs. Audience: Presidents, researchers, executives of pharmaceutical and biotech companies.
Indexed: Chem.Abstr., Chem.Indus.Notes, Chem.Titles, Inpharma, Reac.
—CASDDS, Infotrieve. **CCC.**
Published by: C T B International Publishing Inc., PO Box 218, Maplewood, NJ 07040-0218. TEL 973-379-7749, FAX 973-379-1158, info@ctbintl.com, http://www.ctbintl.com. Eds. John Gever, Christopher Brogna. Pub. Oykue Brogna. R&P Christopher Brogna.

615.7 AUS ISSN 1034-8719
ENCAPSULATOR. Text in English. 1977. q. free per issue. back issues avail. *Refereed.* **Document type:** *Bulletin.*
Formerly (until 1989): Pharmacy Bulletin
Indexed: I.P.A.
Published by: Monash Medical Centre, Southern Health Care Network, Pharmacy Department, 246 Clayton Rd, Clayton, VIC 3168, Australia. TEL 61-3-95942596, FAX 61-3-95942595. Ed., Pub., R&P Ian Larmour. Circ: 1,500.

ENVIRONMENTAL TOXICOLOGY AND PHARMACOLOGY. see *ENVIRONMENTAL STUDIES—Toxicology And Environmental Safety*

EOS; rivista di immunologia ed immunofarmacologia. see *MEDICAL SCIENCES—Allergology And Immunology*

EPILEPSY RESEARCH. see *MEDICAL SCIENCES—Psychiatry And Neurology*

EPILEPSY RESEARCH SUPPLEMENTS. see *MEDICAL SCIENCES—Psychiatry And Neurology*

615.1 GRC ISSN 1011-6575
CODEN: EKFFE
EPITHEORESE KLINIKES FARMAKOLOGIAS KAI FARMAKOKINETIKAS (ELLENIKE EKDOSIS)/REVIEW OF CLINICAL PHARMACOLOGY AND PHARMACOKINETICS (ELLENIKE EKDOSIS). Text in Greek; Summaries in English. 1983. q. **Document type:** *Academic/Scholarly.*
Related titles: ♦ English ed.: Epitheorese Klinikes Farmakologias kai Farmakokinetikes (International Edition). ISSN 1011-6583; ♦ International ed.: Epitheorese Klinikes Farmakologias kai Farmakokinetikes (International Edition). ISSN 1011-6583.

P

Indexed: Excerp.Med.
—BLDSC (3794.274000), CASDDS, CISTI, EMDOCS, GNLM.
Published by: Pharmakon Press, 20 Daskalaki St, Athens 115 26, Greece. TEL 30-1-7778-101.

615.1 GRC ISSN 1011-6583 CODEN: EKIEE
EPITHEORESE KLINIKES FARMAKOLOGIAS KAI FARMAKOKINETIKES (INTERNATIONAL EDITION)/REVIEW OF CLINICAL PHARMACOLOGY AND PHARMACOKINETICS (INTERNATIONAL EDITION). Text in English. 1987. 3/yr. **Document type:** *Academic/Scholarly.*
Related titles: ♦ Greek ed.: Epitheorese Klinikes Farmakologias kai Farmakokinetikas (Ellenike Ekdosis). ISSN 1011-6575; ♦ International ed.: Epitheorese Klinikes Farmakologias kai Farmakokinetikas (Ellenike Ekdosis). ISSN 1011-6575.
Indexed: Chem.Abstr., Chem.Indus.Notes, Chem.Titles, Excerp.Med.
—BLDSC (7788.985000), CASDDS, EMDOCS, GNLM, KNAW.
Published by: Pharmakon Press, 20 Daskalaki St, Athens 115 26, Greece. TEL 30-1-7778-101.

615.321 635.7 ITA ISSN 1121-2896
L'ERBORISTA. Text in Italian. 1986. 8/yr. ITL 45,000; ITL 110,000 in Europe; ITL 160,000 elsewhere. adv.
Published by: Tecniche Nuove s.p.a., Via Ciro Menotti, 14, Milan, MI 20129, Italy. TEL 39-027570329, FAX 39-027570332, abbonamenti@tecnet.it; erborist@tecnet.it, http://www.tecnet.it/index1.html. adv.: B&W page ITL 1,960,000, color page ITL 3,136,000; trim 250 x 184. Circ: 5,043.

615 ITA
ESPRESSO FARMACEUTICO. Text in Italian. 1981. 10/yr. ITL 197,000; ITL 350,000 foreign.
Published by: Edizioni Effe s.r.l., Via Volta, 25, Corbetta, MI 20011, Italy. TEL 39-2-9770310, FAX 39-2-9772363. Ed. Mario Bernardi. Circ: 9,000.

615 CHE ISSN 1015-0919
ESSENTIAL DRUGS MONITOR. Text in English, French, Russian, Spanish, Chinese. 1986. s-a. free. **Document type:** *Bulletin, Trade.* **Description:** Contains regular features on national drug policies, rational drug use, supply, operational research and public education.
Related titles: Online - full text ed.
Indexed: CINAHL.
—BLDSC (3811.792510).
Published by: World Health Organization, Department of Essential Drugs & Medicines Policy, Geneva, 27 1211, Switzerland. FAX 41-22-7914167, darec@who.ch, http://www.who.int/medicines. Ed. D A Fresle. Circ: 200,000.

ESSENTIAL PSYCHOPHARMACOLOGY. see *MEDICAL SCIENCES—Psychiatry And Neurology*

ETHNOBOTANY. see *BIOLOGY—Botany*

615 614.4 USA ISSN 1056-179X
EUROPE DRUG & DEVICE REPORT. Text in English. 1991. bi-w., latest vol.12, 2002. USD 937 in North America; USD 962 elsewhere (effective Nov. 2001). Supplement avail.; back issues avail. **Document type:** *Newsletter.* **Description:** Reports on European rules and standards for the pharmaceutical and device and diagnostic products industries.
Related titles: E-mail ed.: (from Data-Star, The Dialog Corporation).
—Infotrieve. **CCC.**
Published by: Washington Business Information, Inc., 300 N Washington St, Ste 200, Falls Church, Arlington, VA 22046. TEL 703-538-7600, 703-538-7661, FAX 703 538-7676, ehinkle@fdanews.com, http://www.fdanews.com. Ed. Sara Lewis.

EUROPEAN AIDS DIRECTORY. see *MEDICAL SCIENCES—Communicable Diseases*

615.19 GBR ISSN 1369-0663
EUROPEAN BIOPHARMACEUTICAL REVIEW. Text in English. q.
—BLDSC (3829.489290).
Published by: Ballantyne Ross Ltd., 16 Hampden Gurney St, London W1H 5AL, United Kingdom. TEL 44-1717-245444, editor@balross.com, http://www.ballantyneross.com. Ed. Dr. Helen Abbott.

615 ITA ISSN 1122-2441
EUROPEAN BULLETIN OF DRUG RESEARCH. Text in English. 1994 (Jan., vol.3, no.1). 3/yr. ITL 120,000, USD 120. **Document type:** *Bulletin, Academic/Scholarly.* **Description:** Publishes original and innovative papers dealing with all aspects of drug research and development, such as medicinal chemistry, design and synthesis of new active substances, pharmacology and pharmacognosy, pharmaceutics and biopharmaceutics, and new drug-delivery systems.
—CISTI.
Published by: Europharma 2000 s.r.l., Via Ghibellina, 81, Florence, FI 50122, Italy. TEL 39-55-2478982, FAX 39-55-2478982.

615.1 DEU ISSN 0031-6970 CODEN: EJCPAS
EUROPEAN JOURNAL OF CLINICAL PHARMACOLOGY. Text in English. 1968. m. EUR 1,701.10 domestic; EUR 1,690.70 in Germany; EUR 167 newsstand/cover foreign (effective 2002). adv. bk.rev. illus. reprint service avail. from ISI. *Refereed.* **Document type:** *Journal, Academic/Scholarly.* **Description:** Publishes original papers, short communications, and letters to the editor on all aspects of clinical pharmacology and drug therapy in man. Focuses on clinical pharmacology and pharmacokinetics.
Related titles: Microform ed.: (from PQC); Online - full text ed.: ISSN 1432-1041 (from EBSCO Publishing, RoweCom Information Quest, Swets Blackwell, Springer LINK, Institute for Scientific Information).
Indexed: ASCA, Abstr.Inter.Med., Agri.& Environ.Biotech.Abstr. (coverage dropped), Biol.Abstr., C.I.S. Abstr., Chem.Abstr., Chem.Indus.Notes, Chem.Titles, Curr.Adv.Cancer Res., Curr.Adv.Ecol.Sci., Curr.Cont., Dairy Sci.Abstr., Dent.Ind., Derwent Biotech.Abstr., Excerp.Med., INIS Atomind., Ind.Med. (1970-), Ind.Sci.Rev., Inpharma, Int.Abstr.Biol.Sci., Int.Nurs.Ind., Kidney, Med.& Surg.Dermat., Neurosci.Cit.Ind., Nutr.Abstr., Pharm.&Out.News, Protozool.Abstr., Reac., Rev.Med.& Vet.Mycol., SSCI (coverage dropped), Sci.Cit.Ind., Sugar Ind.Abstr., THA.
—BLDSC (3829.728100), ADONIS, CASDDS, CISTI, GNLM, IDS, ingenta, KNAW, Linda Hall. **CCC.**
Published by: (European Association for Clinical Pharmacology and Therapeutics), Springer-Verlag (Subsidiary of: BertelsmannSpringer), Tiergartenstr 17, Heidelberg 69121, Germany. TEL 49-6221-345-0, FAX 49-6221-345229, subscriptions@springer.de, http://link.springer.de/link/service/journals/00228/index.htm, http://www.springer.de. Eds. L Offerhaus, R Dahlqvist. **Subscr. in N. America to:** Springer-Verlag New York Inc., PO Box 2485, Secaucus, NJ 07096-2485. TEL 212-460-1500, FAX 212-473-6272.

615.7 CHE ISSN 0378-7966
RM301 CODEN: EJDPD2
EUROPEAN JOURNAL OF DRUG METABOLISM AND PHARMACOKINETICS. Text in English, French. 1976. q. CHF 325, EUR 211.03 (effective 2002). *Refereed.* **Document type:** *Journal, Academic/Scholarly.*
Related titles: Online - full text ed.: (from Institute for Scientific Information).
Indexed: ASCA, Agri.& Environ.Biotech.Abstr. (coverage dropped), Biol.Abstr., Chem.Abstr., Chem.Indus.Notes, Chem.Titles, Curr.Adv.Ecol.Sci., Curr.Cont., Dent.Ind., Derwent Biotech.Abstr., Excerp.Med., I.P.A., Ind.Med. (coverage dropped), Ind.Sci.Rev., Inpharma, Int.Abstr.Biol.Sci., Mass Spectr.Bull., Nutr.Abstr., Pharm.&Out.News, Poult.Abstr., Protozool.Abstr., Reac., Rev.Appl.Entomol., Rev.Med.& Vet.Mycol., Sci.Cit.Ind.
—BLDSC (3829.728300), CASDDS, CISTI, EMDOCS, IDS, ingenta, KNAW. **CCC.**
Published by: Editions Medecine et Hygiene, Case Postale 456, Geneva, 4 1211, Switzerland. TEL 41-22-7029311, FAX 41-22-7029355, abonnements@medhyg.ch, http://www.medhyg.ch. Ed. A Benakis.

615 GBR ISSN 1352-4755
EUROPEAN JOURNAL OF HERBAL MEDICINE. Text in English. 1994. 3/yr. GBP 24.50 in British Isles to individuals; GBP 29.50 in the European Union to individuals; GBP 34.50 elsewhere to individuals; GBP 59.50 in British Isles to institutions; GBP 64.50 in the European Union to institutions; GBP 69.50 elsewhere to institutions (effective 2000). adv. bk.rev. *Refereed.* **Document type:** *Academic/Scholarly.* **Description:** Articles concerning theory, research and practice in herbal medicine.
Indexed: AMED.
—BLDSC (3829.729870).
Published by: National Institute of Medical Herbalists, 56 Longbrook St, Exeter EX4 6AH, United Kingdom. TEL 44-181-340-2900, FAX 44-181-341-7425, herbmed@dial.pipex.com. Ed., R&P Adrian McDermott. Adv. contact Christopher Menzies.

615 DEU ISSN 0939-9437
EUROPEAN JOURNAL OF HOSPITAL PHARMACY. Text in German. 1984. irreg. EUR 31.36 domestic; EUR 33.60 in Europe; EUR 42.60 elsewhere (effective 2002); EUR 7.70 newsstand/cover (effective (No. 2002). **Document type:** *Journal, Trade.*
Published by: Medpharm GmbH Scientific Publishers, Postfach 101061, Stuttgart 70009, Germany. TEL 49-711-25820, FAX 49-711-2582-290, service@medpharm.de, http://www.medpharm.de. Ed. Dr. Jochen Kotwas. Circ: 8,000.

EUROPEAN JOURNAL OF MEDICINAL CHEMISTRY. see *BIOLOGY—Biochemistry*

615.19 GBR ISSN 0964-4679
EUROPEAN JOURNAL OF PARENTERAL SCIENCES. Text in English. 1996. q. GBP 48 to individuals; GBP 96 to institutions (effective 2001). adv. bk.rev. index. back issues avail. *Refereed.* **Document type:** *Academic/Scholarly.* **Description:** Provides European forum for publishing original papers, editorials, and reviews on subjects that cover all aspects of the parenteral sciences, both practical and scientific.
Indexed: I.P.A.
—BLDSC (3829.733420). **CCC.**
Published by: (Parenteral Society), Euromed Communications Ltd., The Old Surgery, Liphook Rd, Haslemere, Surrey GU27 1NL, United Kingdom. TEL 44-1428-656665, FAX 44-1428-6t56643, info@euromed.uk.com, http://www.euromed.uk.com. Ed. Gerry Prout. Pub. Joe Ridge. Adv. contact Allan Andrews TEL 44-1621-851007. Circ: 2,500 (paid).

615.1 NLD ISSN 0928-0987
RM301.25 CODEN: EPSCED
EUROPEAN JOURNAL OF PHARMACEUTICAL SCIENCES. Text and summaries in English. 1993. m. EUR 719 in Europe to institutions; JPY 95,400 in Japan to institutions; USD 804 elsewhere to institutions (effective 2002). adv. index. *Refereed.* **Document type:** *Academic/Scholarly.* **Description:** Publishes original multidisciplinary research, short communications and reviews in the pharmaceutical sciences, from both academia and industry, including topics such as drug bioanalysis, medicinal chemistry and drug delivery, biomedical drug research and drug targeting, pharmacokinetics, pharmacodynamics, drug metabolism and toxicology, as well as pharmaceutical biotechnology.
Incorporates (1926-2000): Pharmaceutica Acta Helvetiae (0031-6865); Formed by the merger of (1977-1992): Acta Pharmaceutica Fennica (0356-3456); Which was formerly (1928-1976): Farmaseuttinen Aikakauslehti (0367-259X); (1989-1992): Acta Pharmaceutica Nordica (1100-1801); Which was formed by the merger of (1964-1988): Acta Pharmaceutica Suecica (0001-6675); (1983-1988): Norwegica Pharmaceutica Acta (0800-2606); Which was formerly (1939-1982): Norsk Farmaceutisk Selskap. Meddelelser (0029-1927); Which was formerly (until 1987): Archiv for Pharmaci og Chemi. Scientific Edition (0302-248X); (1926-1972): Dansk Tidsskrift for Farmaci (0011-6513)
Related titles: Microform ed.: (from PQC); Online - full text ed.: (from EBSCO Publishing, ingenta, Swets Blackwell, ScienceDirect, Institute for Scientific Information).
Indexed: ASCA, Agri.& Environ.Biotech.Abstr. (coverage dropped), Anal.Abstr., Biol.Abstr., Chem.Abstr., Chem.Indus.Notes, Chem.Titles, Curr.Adv.Ecol.Sci., Curr.Chem.React., Curr.Cont., Dairy Sci.Abstr., Derwent Biotech.Abstr., Eng.Ind., Excerp.Med. (1993-), Helminthol.Abstr., INIS Atomind., I.P.A., Ind.Chem., Ind.Med. (1993-), Ind.Sci.Rev., Inpharma, MOS, NPU, Pharm.&Out.News, Protozool.Abstr., RCI, Reac., Rev.Arom.& Med.Plants, Rev.Med.& Vet.Mycol., Sci.Cit.Ind.
—BLDSC (3829.733850), CASDDS, CINDOC, CISTI, Ei, EMDOCS, GNLM, IDS, Infotrieve, ingenta, KNAW, Linda Hall. **CCC.**
Published by: (European Federation for Pharmaceutical Sciences), Elsevier Science BV, PO Box 211, Amsterdam 1000 AE, Netherlands. TEL 31-20-485-3757, FAX 31-20-485-3432, TELEX 18582 ESPA NL, http://www.elsevier.com/locate/ejps. Eds. G Alderborn, P Artursson. **Subscr. in Australasia and the Far East to:** Elsevier Science (Singapore) Pte Ltd, No.1 Temasek Ave, 17-01 Millenia Tower, Singapore 039192, Singapore. TEL 65-434-3727, FAX 65-337-2230; **Subscr. in Japan to:** Elsevier Science Inc - Japan Regional Office, 9-15 Higashi-Azabu 1-chome, Minato-ku, Tokyo 106-0044, Japan. TEL 81-3-5561-5033, FAX 81-3-5561-5047; **Subscr. in the Americas to:** Elsevier Science, PO Box 945, New York, NY 10159-0945. TEL 212-633-3730, FAX 212-633-3680, usinfo-f@elsevier.com.

615 NLD ISSN 0939-6411
CODEN: EJPBEL
EUROPEAN JOURNAL OF PHARMACEUTICS AND BIOPHARMACEUTICS. Text in English, French, German. 1955. bi-m. EUR 483 in Europe to institutions; JPY 64,000 in Japan to institutions; USD 540 elsewhere to institutions (effective 2002). abstr. back issues avail. *Refereed.* **Document type:** *Academic/Scholarly.* **Description:** Provides a medium for publication of research from areas of pharmaceutical technology, drug delivery systems, controlled release systems, drug targeting, physical pharmacy, and pharmacodynamics and pharmacokinetics.
Formerly: Acta Pharmaceutica Technologica (0340-3157)
Related titles: Online - full text ed.: (from ingenta, Swets Blackwell, ScienceDirect, Institute for Scientific Information).
Indexed: ASCA, Agri.& Environ.Biotech.Abstr. (coverage dropped), BBCI, Chem.Abstr., Chem.Indus.Notes, Chem.Titles, Dairy Sci.Abstr., Derwent Biotech.Abstr., Excerp.Med., I.P.A., Ind.Med. (1991-), Protozool.Abstr., Rev.Med.& Vet.Mycol.
—BLDSC (3829.733900), CASDDS, CISTI, EMDOCS, GNLM, IDS, Infotrieve, ingenta, KNAW, Linda Hall. **CCC.**
Published by: (Arbeitsgemeinschaft fuer Pharmazeutische Verfahrenstechnik e.V. BRD), Elsevier Science BV, PO Box 211, Amsterdam 1000 AE, Netherlands. nlinfo-f@elsevier.nl, http://www.elsevier.com/locate/ejphabio. Ed. R Gurny. Circ: 2,000. **Subscr. in Australasia and the Far East to:** Elsevier Science (Singapore) Pte Ltd, No.1 Temasek Ave, 17-01 Millenia Tower, Singapore 039192, Singapore. TEL 65-434-3727; **Subscr. in Japan to:** Elsevier Science Inc - Japan Regional Office, 9-15 Higashi-Azabu 1-chome, Minato-ku, Tokyo 106-0044, Japan. TEL 81-3-5561-5033; **Subscr. in the Americas to:** Elsevier Science, PO Box 945, New York, NY 10159-0945. TEL 212-633-3730, FAX 212-633-3680.

615.1 NLD ISSN 0014-2999
RS1 CODEN: EJPHAZ
EUROPEAN JOURNAL OF PHARMACOLOGY; an international journal. Text in Dutch. 1967. 72/yr. EUR 7,512 in Europe to institutions; JPY 998,400 in Japan to institutions; USD 8,402 elsewhere to institutions (effective 2002). adv. charts, illus, abstr. back issues avail.; reprint service avail. from ISI. *Refereed.* **Document type:** *Journal, Academic/Scholarly.* **Description:** Publishes full length papers as well as short and rapid communications on the mechanisms of action of chemical substances affecting biological systems.
Incorporates (1989-1997): European Journal of Pharmacology. Molecular Pharmacology Section (0922-4106)
Related titles: Microform ed.: (from PQC); Online - full text ed.: (from EBSCO Publishing, ingenta, Swets Blackwell, ScienceDirect, Institute for Scientific Information).
Indexed: ASCA, Apic.Abstr., Aqua.Sci.& Fish.Abstr., BBCI, Biol.Abstr., Chem.Abstr., Chem.Indus.Notes, Chem.Titles, Curr.Adv.Ecol.Sci., Curr.Cont., Dairy Sci.Abstr., Dent.Ind., Derwent Biotech.Abstr., Environ.Sci.Poll.Mgmt., Excerp.Med., Helminthol.Abstr., INIS Atomind., Ind.Med. (1967-), Ind.Sci.Rev., Ind.Vet., Inpharma, Int.Abstr.Biol.Sci., Neurosci.Abstr. (coverage dropped), Neurosci.Cit.Ind., Nutr.Abstr., Pharm.&Out.News, Psychol.Abstr., Reac., Rev.Appl.Entomol., Rev.Arom.& Med.Plants, Rev.Med.& Vet.Mycol., SSCI (coverage dropped), Sci.Cit.Ind., THA, Vet.Bull., Wild.Rev.
—BLDSC (3829.734000), ADONIS, CASDDS, CISTI, GNLM, IDS, ingenta, KNAW, Linda Hall. **CCC.**
Published by: Elsevier Science BV, PO Box 211, Amsterdam 1000 AE, Netherlands. TEL 31-20-485-3757, FAX 31-20-485-3432, http://www.elsevier.com/locate/ejphar. Eds. D de Wied, J Bruinvels. **Subscr. in Australasia and the Far East to:** Elsevier Science (Singapore) Pte Ltd, No.1 Temasek Ave, 17-01 Millenia Tower, Singapore 039192, Singapore. TEL 65-434-3727, FAX 65-337-2230; **Subscr. in Japan to:** Elsevier Science Inc - Japan Regional Office, 9-15 Higashi-Azabu 1-chome, Minato-ku, Tokyo 106-0044, Japan. TEL 81-3-5561-5033, FAX 81-3-5561-5047; **Subscr. in the Americas to:** Elsevier Science, PO Box 945, New York, NY 10159-0945. TEL 212-633-3730, 888-437-4636, FAX 212-633-3680, usinfo-f@elsevier.com. **Dist. by:** Elsevier Science (Brazil).

EUROPEAN NEUROPSYCHOPHARMACOLOGY. see *MEDICAL SCIENCES—Psychiatry And Neurology*

615 GBR ISSN 1364-369X
EUROPEAN PHARMACEUTICAL CONTRACTOR. Text in English. 1996. q. free per issue. bk.rev. pat, stat, tr.lit. back issues avail. *Refereed.* **Document type:** *Directory, Trade.* **Description:** Covers contract research & development, clinical trials and outsourcing plus promotion of specific topics, Audience are decision makers in the pharmaceutical market, both contractor groups & pharmaceutical companies.
Related titles: Online - full text ed.
Published by: Ballantyne Ross Ltd., 16 Hampden Gurney St, London W1H 5AL, United Kingdom. TEL 44-1717-245444, FAX 44-1717-242632, clive@balross.com, http://www.balross.com. Ed. Graham Hughes. R&P Clive Baigent. adv.: color page GBP 2,750. Circ: 7,500 (controlled).

615 GBR
EUROPEAN PHARMACEUTICAL INTELLIGENCE BULLETIN. Abbreviated title: E P I B. Text in English. m. GBP 495 domestic; GBP 535 foreign (effective 2001). **Document type:** *Bulletin, Trade.* **Description:** Provides news, information and analysis on all aspects of the European pharmaceutical industry and healthcare reform.
Published by: SMi Publishing, 1 New Concordia Wharf, Mill St, London SE1 2BB, United Kingdom. TEL 44-207-827-6000, FAX 44-207-827-6001, epib@smipublishing.co.uk, ordering@smipublishing.co.uk, http://www.smipublishing.co.uk.

615 GBR ISSN 1360-8606
EUROPEAN PHARMACEUTICAL REVIEW; the quarterly review of pharmaceutical business and technology. Text in English. 1996. q. GBP 60 (effective 2001). adv. 100 p./no. *Refereed.* **Document type:** *Journal, Trade.* **Description:** Addresses the new technologies and developments in the European pharmaceutical industry.
—BLDSC (3829.776700).
Published by: Russell Publishing Ltd., 4 Bourlet Close, London W1W 7BJ, United Kingdom. TEL 44-20-7436-3642, FAX 44-20-7255-2223, 44-20-7436-3610, pharmaceutical@russellpublishing.com, admin@russellpublishing.com, http://www.russellpublishing.com/pages/pharmy/pharmy1.html. Ed. Ken Leiper. Pub. Ian Russell. R&P Vincent Vikentiom. Adv. contact Graeme Ringsell. color page GBP 4,477; trim 297 x 210. Circ: 220 (paid); 12,000 (controlled).

615.19 USA ISSN 0090-6654
EVALUATIONS OF DRUG INTERACTIONS. Text in English. 1973. base vol. plus bi-m. updates. USD 229; USD 89.95 renewals (effective 1999). adv. **Document type:** *Academic/Scholarly.* **Description:** Comprehensive reference source for prescription and OTC drug conflicts.
Related titles: Online - full text ed.
—CCC.
Published by: (American Pharmaceutical Association), First DataBank, Inc., Two Cityplace Dr., St. Louis, MO 63141. TEL 314-812-2552, 800-366-4737, FAX 314-812-2553, rick_zucchero@firstdatabank.com; mark_hogan@firstdatabank.com, http://www.firstdatabank.com. Eds. Fredric J Zucchero, Mark J Hogan. R&P Pat Bremerkamp. Adv. contact Christine D Schultz.

615 FRA ISSN 0755-8309
EVOLUTION PHARMACEUTIQUE. Text in French. m. FRF 120. adv.
Published by: Union Nationale des Grandes Pharmacies, 57 rue Spontini, Paris 75116, France. TEL 45-53-60-90. Ed. J Vigan. Circ: 4,500.

EXPERIMENTAL AND CLINICAL PSYCHOPHARMACOLOGY. see *PSYCHOLOGY*

EXPERIMENTAL AND TOXICOLOGIC PATHOLOGY. see *MEDICAL SCIENCES*

615 GBR
▼ **EXPERT OPINION ON DRUG SAFETY.** Text in English. forthcoming 2002 (April). q. GBP 425, USD 1,480 (effective 2002). abstr. Index. back issues avail.; reprints avail. *Refereed.* **Document type:** *Journal, Academic/Scholarly.* **Description:** Contains expert reviews on clinical tests and drug safety.
Related titles: Ed. forthcoming 2002.
Published by: Ashley Publications Ltd., Unitec House 3rd Fl, 2 Albert Place, Finchley Central, London N3 1QB, United Kingdom. TEL 44-20-8343-3883, FAX 44-20-8343-2313, jdrake@ashley-pub.com, http://www.ashley-pub.com. Ed. Joanne Heath. Pub. James Drake.

615.1 GBR ISSN 1472-8214
CODEN: EMDRFV
EXPERT OPINION ON EMERGING DRUGS. Text in English. 1996. s-a. GBP 470, USD 800 (effective 2002). abstr. 2 cols./p. back issues avail.; reprints avail. *Refereed.* **Document type:** *Journal, Academic/Scholarly, Corporate.* **Description:** Provides an expert assessment of the potential impact of the most promising areas of drug research on the current management of specific diseases. Profiles include background, existing treatments, medical need, compounds in development, scientific concepts, market size, development issues and evaluation.
Formerly (until June 2001): Emerging Drugs (1361-9195)
Related titles: Online - full content ed.: 1997. GBP 670, USD 1,040 (effective 2002).
Indexed: Derwent Biotech.Abstr.
Published by: Ashley Publications Ltd., Unitec House 3rd Fl, 2 Albert Place, Finchley Central, London N3 1QB, United Kingdom. TEL 44-20-8343-3883, FAX 44-20-8343-2313, jdrake@ashley-pub.com, http://www.ashley-pub.com. Ed. Katie Prickett. Pub. James Drake.

615 GBR ISSN 1472-8222
EXPERT OPINION ON EMERGING THERAPEUTIC TARGETS. Text in English. 1997. bi-m. GBP 975, USD 1,660 (effective 2002). abstr. 2 cols./p. back issues avail.; reprints avail. *Refereed.* **Document type:** *Journal, Academic/Scholarly, Corporate.* **Description:** Contains structured profiles of research projects for which the originators are seeking support from an industrial partner. Includes details of therapeutic target, mechanism of action, indications, advantages of approach, current research goals and type of collaborative research envisaged.
Formerly (until June 2001): Emerging Therapeutic Targets (1460-0412)
Related titles: Online - full content ed.: 1997. GBP 1,270, USD 2,160 (effective 2002).
Published by: Ashley Publications Ltd., Unitec House 3rd Fl, 2 Albert Place, Finchley Central, London N3 1QB, United Kingdom. TEL 44-20-8343-3883, FAX 44-20-8343-2313, jdrake@ashley-pub.com, http://www.ashley-pub.com. Ed. Henry Scowcroft. Pub. James Drake.

P

615.1 GBR ISSN 1354-3784
CODEN: CIDREE
EXPERT OPINION ON INVESTIGATIONAL DRUGS; authoritative analysis of R&D trends. Text in English. 1994. m. GBP 1,800, USD 3,060 (effective 2002). abstr. back issues avail. *Refereed.* **Document type:** *Journal, Academic/Scholarly, Corporate.* **Description:** Highlights important pharmacological and pharmaceutical developments; covers meetings and conferences; and reviews important worldwide developments.
Formerly (until 1994): Current Opinion in Investigational Drugs (0967-8298)
Related titles: Online - full text ed.: (from Institute for Scientific Information).
Indexed: Curr.Cont., Excerp.Med. (1994-), Ind.Med., Inpharma, Pharm.&Out.News, Reac.
—BLDSC (3500.775600), CASDDS, EMDOCS, GNLM, KNAW.
Published by: Ashley Publications Ltd., Unitec House 3rd Fl, 2 Albert Place, Finchley Central, London N3 1QB, United Kingdom. TEL 44-20-8343-3883, FAX 44-20-8343-2313, jdrake@ashley-pub.com, http://www.ashley-pub.com. Ed. Anja Johansen-Bibby. Pub. James Drake.

615 GBR ISSN 1465-6566
▼ **EXPERT OPINION ON PHARMACOTHERAPY.** Text in English. 1999. m. GBP 1,285, USD 2,185 (effective 2002). abstr. back issues avail. *Refereed.* **Document type:** *Journal, Academic/Scholarly.* **Description:** Contains drug evaluations and reviews.
Related titles: Online - full content ed.
Published by: Ashley Publications Ltd., Unitec House 3rd Fl, 2 Albert Place, Finchley Central, London N3 1QB, United Kingdom. TEL 44-20-8343-3883, FAX 44-20-8343-2313, jdrake@ashley-pub.com, http://www.ashley-pub.com. Ed. Jennifer Grey. Pub. James Drake.

615.1 GBR ISSN 1354-3776
CODEN: EOTPEG
EXPERT OPINION ON THERAPEUTIC PATENTS; authoritative analysis of patenting trends. Text in English. 1991. m. GBP 2,130, USD 3,620 (effective 2002). pat, abstr. back issues avail. *Refereed.* **Document type:** *Journal, Academic/Scholarly.* **Description:** Reviews and evaluates patents issued over the preceding six months, profiles companies and their patenting practices, selects the most significant patents issued each month.

Formerly (until Feb. 1994): Current Opinion on Therapeutic Patents (0962-2594)
Related titles: Online - full text ed.: (from Institute for Scientific Information).
Indexed: Curr.Cont., Excerp.Med. (1992-), Inpharma, Pharm.&Out.News, Reac.
—CASDDS, EMDOCS, GNLM.
Published by: Ashley Publications Ltd., Unitec House 3rd Fl, 2 Albert Place, Finchley Central, London N3 1QB, United Kingdom. TEL 44-20-8343-3883, FAX 44-20-8343-2313, jdrake@ashley-pub.com, http://www.ashley-pub.com. Ed. Katherine Fowler. Pub. James Drake.

615.1 616.992 GBR ISSN 1473-7140
▼ **EXPERT REVIEW OF ANTICANCER THERAPY**; an essential contribution to decision making in cancer care. Text in English. 2001. bi-m. GBP 680 domestic for print ed. only; USD 1,195 foreign for print ed. only; GBP 885 domestic for print & online eds. combined; USD 1,555 foreign for print & online eds. combined (effective 2002). bibl, abstr. back issues avail.; reprints avail. *Refereed.* **Document type:** *Journal, Academic/Scholarly.* **Description:** Provides expert appraisal and commentary on the major trends in cancer care and highlights the performance of new therapeutics and diagnostic approaches.
Related titles: Online - full content ed.
Published by: Future Drugs Ltd. (Subsidiary of: Ashley Publications Ltd.), 3rd floor, Unitec House, 2 Albert Pl, Finchley Central, London N3 1QB, United Kingdom. TEL 44-20-8349-2033, FAX 44-20-8343-2313, info@future-drugs.com, http://www.future-drugs.com. Ed. Phil Garner. Pub., R&P, Adv. contact David Hughes.

615.1 GBR ISSN 1473-7159
▼ **EXPERT REVIEW OF MOLECULAR DIAGNOSTICS**; new diagnostic technologies are set to revolutionise healthcare. Text in English. 2001. bi-m. GBP 680 domestic for print ed. only; USD 1,195 foreign for print ed. only; GBP 885 domestic for print & online eds. combined; USD 1,555 foreign for print & online eds. combined (effective 2002). abstr, bibl. back issues avail.; reprints avail. *Refereed.* **Document type:** *Journal, Academic/Scholarly.* **Description:** Provides a resource for commentary and debate that will help to shape decision-making in patient care.
Related titles: Online - full content ed.
Published by: Future Drugs Ltd. (Subsidiary of: Ashley Publications Ltd.), 3rd floor, Unitec House, 2 Albert Pl, Finchley Central, London N3 1QB, United Kingdom. TEL 44-20-8349-2033, FAX 44-20-8343-2313, info@future-drugs.com, http://www.future-drugs.com. Ed. Phil Garner. Pub., R&P, Adv. contact David Hughes.

615 616.8 GBR ISSN 1473-7175
▼ **EXPERT REVIEW OF NEUROTHERAPEUTICS**; a key contribution to decision making in the treatment of neurologic and neuropsychiatric disorders. Text in English. 2001. bi-m. GBP 680 domestic for print ed. only; USD 1,195 foreign for print ed. only; GBP 885 domestic for print & online eds. combined; USD 1,555 foreign for print & online eds. combined (effective 2002). abstr, bibl. back issues avail.; reprints avail. *Refereed.* **Document type:** *Journal, Academic/Scholarly.* **Description:** Provides expert appraisal and commentary on the major therapeutic and diagnostic advances in neurology and neuropsychiatry.
Related titles: Online - full content ed.
Published by: Future Drugs Ltd. (Subsidiary of: Ashley Publications Ltd.), 3rd floor, Unitec House, 2 Albert Pl, Finchley Central, London N3 1QB, United Kingdom. TEL 44-20-8349-2033, FAX 44-20-8343-2313, info@future-drugs.com, http://www.future-drugs.com. Ed. Phil Garner. Pub., R&P, Adv. contact David Hughes.

615 GBR ISSN 1473-7167
▼ **EXPERT REVIEW OF PHARMACOECONOMICS & OUTCOMES RESEARCH**; informing decision-making in the delivery of cost-effective healthcare. Text in English. 2001. bi-m. GBP 680 domestic for print ed. only; USD 1,195 foreign for print ed. only; GBP 885 domestic for print & online eds. combined; USD 1,555 foreign for print & online eds. combined (effective 2002). abstr, bibl. back issues avail.; reprints avail. *Refereed.* **Document type:** *Journal, Academic/Scholarly.* **Description:** Provides commentary and analysis on the growing relationship between economic factors and clinical prescribing decisions, providing a practical background to informed prescribing decisions and allocation of healthcare resources.
Related titles: Online - full content ed.
Published by: Future Drugs Ltd. (Subsidiary of: Ashley Publications Ltd.), 3rd floor, Unitec House, 2 Albert Pl, Finchley Central, London N3 1QB, United Kingdom. TEL 44-20-8349-2033, FAX 44-20-8343-2313, info@future-drugs.com, http://www.future-drugs.com. Ed. Phil Garner. Pub., R&P, Adv. contact David Hughes.

615 SWE ISSN 1400-6588
F A S S - LAEKEMEDEL I SVERIGE. Key Title: F A S S. Text in Swedish. 1966. a. SEK 669 (effective 2001). adv. **Document type:** *Catalog.*
Formerly (until 1995): F A S S - Farmacevtiska Specialiteter i Sverige (0430-1080)
Published by: LINFO - Laekemedelsinformation AB, Fack 17608, Stockholm 11892, Sweden. TEL 46-8-462-37-00, FAX 46-8-462-02-88. Ed. Anna Greta Hedstrand. R&P, Adv. contact Maia Sundberg TEL 46-8-462-37-74.

636.089 SWE ISSN 0347-1136
F A S S VET; laekemedel foer veterinaermedicinsk bruk. Text in Swedish. 1973. a. SEK 366 (effective 2001). adv. **Document type:** *Catalog.*
Published by: LINFO - Laekemedelsinformation AB, Fack 17608, Stockholm 11892, Sweden. TEL 46-8-462-37-00, FAX 46-8-462-02-88. Ed. Anna Greta Hedstrand. R&P, Adv. contact Maia Sundberg TEL 46-8-462-37-74.

F D A COMPLIANCE POLICY GUIDANCE. MANUAL. see *FOOD AND FOOD INDUSTRIES*

F D A CONSUMER. (Food and Drug Administration) see *CONSUMER EDUCATION AND PROTECTION*

F D A ENFORCEMENT MANUAL. (Food and Drug Administration) see *FOOD AND FOOD INDUSTRIES*

F D A ENFORCEMENT REPORT. (Food and Drug Administration) see *CRIMINOLOGY AND LAW ENFORCEMENT*

F D A INSPECTION OPERATIONS MANUAL. (Food and Drug Administration) see *FOOD AND FOOD INDUSTRIES*

615.1 USA ISSN 1063-8067
F D A MEDICAL BULLETIN. (Food and Drug Administration) Text in English. 1970. irreg. free. back issues avail. **Document type:** *Government.* **Description:** Reports on new drug approvals, adverse reactions, biological end-products and medical and radiological devices.
Formerly (until 1990): F D A Drug Bulletin (0361-4344)
Related titles: Online - full text ed.: (from Data-Star, The Dialog Corporation, Gale Group).
Indexed: Curr.Lit.Fam.Plan., Excerp.Med., I.P.A., Ind.Med. (coverage dropped), Ind.U.S.Gov.Per., Inpharma, MEDOC, Med.Care Rev., Reac., Telegen.
—GNLM.
Published by: U.S. Food and Drug Administration, Office of Public Affairs, 5600 Fishers Ln, Rockville, MD 20857. TEL 301-443-3220, http://www.fda.gov/medbull/contents.html. Ed. Eileen Parish. **Orders to:** National Technical Information Service, Government Research Center. FAX 703-321-8547.

615.1 USA ISSN 1069-5109
F D A NEWS; drugs, devices, cosmetics, and biologics. (Food and Drug Administration) Text in English. 1993. m. USD 245 for print or electronic eds.; USD 285 for print and electronic eds. (effective 2001). back issues avail.; reprints avail. **Document type:** *Newsletter.* **Description:** Acts as a digest of FDA and other regulatory activity in the area of drugs and cosmetics.
Related titles: E-mail ed.; Online - full content ed.
—CCC.
Published by: (Association of Food and Drug Officials), Sage Publications, Inc., 2111 W Hillcrest Dr, Thousand Oaks, CA 91320. Circ: 80 (paid).

F D A WEEK. (Food and Drug Administration) see *CONSUMER EDUCATION AND PROTECTION*

F D C CONTROL NEWSLETTER. (Food, Drug, and Cosmetics) see *FOOD AND FOOD INDUSTRIES*

F T BIOTECHNOLOGY & PHARMACEUTICAL COMPANIES DATABASE CD-ROM (YEARS). (Financial Times) see *BIOLOGY—Biotechnology*

615 GBR ISSN 1354-5299
FAR EAST FOCUS. Text in English. 1994. m. GBP 2,500 (effective 2001). adv. 2 cols./p. back issues avail. **Document type:** *Magazine, Trade.* **Description:** Data and analysis on Asian OTC markets.
Related titles: CD-ROM ed.; Online - full text ed.: (from LexisNexis).
Indexed: Bus.& Indus. (Apr.1994-).
Published by: Nicholas Hall & Company, 35 Alexandra St, Southend-on-Sea, Essex SS1 1BW, United Kingdom. TEL 44-1702-220200, FAX 44-1702-430787, fareastfocus@nicholashall.com, info@nicholashall.com. Ed. Mike Nash. R&P Nina Stimson. Adv. contact Scot Nisbet. B&W page GBP 750, color page GBP 1,200; trim 165 x 260.

615.19 660 AUT
FARBE AKTUELL PLUS. Text in German. m. **Document type:** *Trade.*
Formerly: Farbe Aktuell
Published by: Johann L. Bondi und Sohn, Industriestrasse 2, Perchtoldsdorf, N 2380, Austria. TEL 01-864921, FAX 01-86492144.

615.1 BGR
FARMA NEWS. Text in English, Bulgarian. q. USD 48 foreign (effective 2002). **Description:** Presents news on the field of pharmacology, clinical pharmacy, technology of medicine forms, analyses of medicines, herbalism.
Published by: Meditsinski Universitet - Sofia, Tsentur za Informatsiia po Meditsina/Medical University - Sofia, Medical Information Center, 1 Sv Georgi Sofiiski ul, Sofia 1431, Bulgaria. TEL 359-2-9522342, FAX 359-2-9522393, http://www.medun.acad.bg. **Dist. by:** Sofia Books, Ul Silivria 16, Sofia 1404, Bulgaria. TEL 359-2-9586257, sofiabooks@hotmail.com, http://www.sofiabooks.hit.bg.

615.1 DNK ISSN 0904-6542
FARMACEUTEN. Text in Danish; Summaries in English. 1890. w. DKK 675. adv. bk.rev. abstr, bibl, charts, illus, stat. index, cum.index.
Formerly (until 1989): Farmaceutisk Tidende (0367-1720)
Related titles: Online - full text ed.
Indexed: Chem.Abstr., I.P.A.
—GNLM.
Published by: Dansk Farmaceutforening/Danish Pharmacists' Association, Toldbodgade 36, Copenhagen K 1253, Denmark. Ed. Hans Otto Loldrup. Adv. contact Connie Faaborg Nielsen. page DKK 7,000; trim 175 x 260. Circ: 3,989.

615.1 SVK ISSN 0014-8172
CODEN: FAOBAS
FARMACEUTICKY OBZOR. Text in Czech, Slovak; Summaries in English, German, Russian. 1931. m. USD 90. adv. bk.rev. stat, abstr, charts, illus. index.
Related titles: Online - full text ed.
Indexed: Anal.Abstr., Biol.Abstr., Chem.Abstr., Chem.Indus.Notes, Chem.Titles, Excerp.Med., INIS Atomind., I.P.A.
—BLDSC (3881.850000), CASDDS, CISTI, GNLM, KNAW, Linda Hall.
Published by: Ministerstvo Zdravotnictva, Institut pre Dalsie Vzdelavanie Pracovnikov, Limbova 12, Bratislava 83339, Slovakia. Circ: 2,500. **Dist. by:** Slovart, Gottwaldovo nam 48, Bratislava 805 32, Czechoslovakia.

615 ESP ISSN 0213-7283
EL FARMACEUTICO; profesion y cultura. Text in Spanish. 1984. 19/yr. ESP 9,500 domestic; EUR 57.23 in Europe; USD 115 in United States (effective 2001). adv. bk.rev. **Document type:** *Academic/Scholarly, Trade.* **Description:** Addressed to all pharmacists, pharmaceutical industry, and pharmacy services in hospitals.
Indexed: I.P.A.
Published by: Ediciones Mayo S.A., Muntaner, 374-376 4o, Barcelona 08006, Spain. TEL 34-93-2090255, FAX 34-93-2020643, edmayo@app.es. Ed. Javier March. Pub. Josep Ma Ferrando. R&P Mercedes Mayoral. Adv. contact Jose Mayoral. Circ: 18,304.

615 ESP ISSN 0214-4697
EL FARMACEUTICO HOSPITALES. Text in Spanish. 1988. 10/yr. ESP 6,000 domestic; EUR 36.15 in Europe; USD 40 in United States (effective 2001). adv. **Document type:** *Academic/Scholarly, Trade.* **Description:** Contains interviews with prominent pharmacists, original articles about therapeutics and pharmacology, and reviews of international medical journals.
Indexed: I.P.A.
—GNLM.
Published by: Ediciones Mayo S.A., Muntaner, 374-376 4o, Barcelona 08006, Spain. TEL 34-93-2090090, FAX 34-93-2020643, edmayo@app.es. Ed. Josep M Ferrando. R&P Mercedes Mayoral. Adv. contact Jose Mayoral. Circ: 2,600.

615.1 BEL ISSN 0771-2367
FARMACEUTISCH TIJDSCHRIFT VOOR BELGIE. Text in Flemish. 1923. bi-m. **Document type:** *Journal, Trade.*

P

Formerly (until 1971): Pharmaceutisch Tijdschrift voor Belgie (0369-9714)
—Linda Hall.
Published by: Algemene Pharmaceutische Bond, Archimedesstraat 11, Brussels 1000, Belgium. TEL 32-2-2854200, FAX 32-2-2854285.

615.1 HRV ISSN 0014-8202
CODEN: FAGLAI
FARMACEUTSKI GLASNIK. Text in Croatian; Summaries in English. 1907. q. USD 100. adv. bk.rev. abstr, bibl, charts, illus, stat. index. *Refereed.* **Document type:** *Academic/Scholarly.*
Formerly (until 1944): Farmaceutski Vjesnik
Related titles: Online - full text ed.
Indexed: Agri.& Environ.Biotech.Abstr. (coverage dropped), Biol.Abstr., Chem.Abstr., Chem.Indus.Notes, Chem.Titles, Derwent Biotech.Abstr., Excerp.Med., I.P.A.
—BLDSC (3884.000000), CASDDS, CISTI, EMDOCS, KNAW.
Published by: Hrvatsko Farmaceutsko Drustvo/Croatian Pharmaceutical Society, Masarykova 2, Zagreb 10000, Croatia. TEL 385-1-427944, FAX 385-1-431301. Ed. Maja Jaksevac Miksa. Adv. contact Marina Carevic. Circ: 2,300.

615.1 SWE ISSN 0014-8210
FARMACEVTISK REVY. Text in Swedish. 1902. 8/yr. SEK 500 (effective 2001). adv. bk.rev. **Document type:** *Magazine, Trade.* **Description:** Promotes studies, scientific research and education, and fosters national and international solidarity between pharmacists.
Related titles: Audio cassette/tape ed.; Online - full text ed.
Indexed: Biol.Abstr., Chem.Abstr., I.P.A.
—GNLM, Linda Hall.
Published by: Sveriges Farmacevtfoerbund, Vasagatan 48, Box 3215, Stockholm 10364, Sweden. TEL 46-8-50799900, FAX 46-8-50799999, revyn@farmacevtforbundet.se, post@farmacevtforbundet.se, http://www.farmacevtforbundet.se. Ed., Pub. Aake Lindfors. adv.: B&W page SEK 11,600, color page SEK 18,200; trim 185 x 270. Circ: 7,700.

615.1 SVN ISSN 0014-8229
CODEN: FMVTAV
FARMACEVTSKI VESTNIK; strokovno glasilo slovenske farmacije. Text in Serbo-Croatian, Slovenian. 1950. q. USD 50. adv. bk.rev. charts, illus, tr.lit. index. reprint service avail. from PQC.
Related titles: Online - full text ed.
Indexed: Agri.& Environ.Biotech.Abstr. (coverage dropped), Biol.Abstr., Chem.Abstr., Chem.Indus.Notes, Chem.Titles, I.P.A.
—CASDDS, GNLM, Linda Hall.
Published by: Slovensko Farmacevtsko Drustvo, Masera Spasica 10, Box 311, Ljubljana 61001, Slovenia. TEL 061-221-078. Ed. Ales Krbavcic. Circ: 1,900.

615.1 DNK ISSN 0903-9198
CODEN: APCEAR
FARMACI. Text in Danish. 1844. m. DKK 600, USD 100; DKK 60, USD 10 newsstand/cover (effective 1997). bk.rev. abstr, charts, illus. index. back issues avail. **Document type:** *Academic/Scholarly, Trade.* **Description:** Features articles relating to Danish pharmacists, political and economic developments in the Danish pharmacy sector and abroad, Danish national health politics and scholarly articles relating to pharmacy.
Formerly: Archiv for Pharmaci og Chemi (0003-8938)
Related titles: Online - full text ed.
Indexed: Biol.Abstr., Chem.Abstr., INIS Atomind., I.P.A.
—CASDDS, CISTI, GNLM, Linda Hall.
Published by: Danmarks Apotekerforening/Danish Pharmaceutical Association, Bredgade 54, Copenhagen K 1260, Denmark. TEL 45-33-76-76-00, FAX 45-33-76-76-99, farmaci@daf.umi.dk, http://www.dpa.dk. Ed. Birger Lenvig. adv.: B&W page DKK 5,000, color page DKK 10,500. Circ: 2,400 (controlled).

615.1 ROM ISSN 0014-8237
CODEN: FRMBAZ
FARMACIA/PHARMACY. Text in Romanian; Summaries in English, French, German, Russian. 1953. 4/yr. USD 20. adv. bk.rev. abstr, charts.
Related titles: Online - full text ed.
Indexed: Abstr.Bulg.Sci.Med.Lit., Agri.& Environ.Biotech.Abstr. (coverage dropped), Chem.Abstr., Chem.Indus.Notes, Chem.Titles, Derwent Biotech.Abstr., Excerp.Med., I.P.A.
—BLDSC (3886.000000), CASDDS, CISTI, GNLM, Linda Hall.
Published by: Uniunea Societatilor de Stiinte Medicale din Rumania, Str. Progresului 8, Bucharest 70754, Romania. **Subscr. to:** ILEXIM, Str. 13 Decembrie 3, PO Box 136-137, Bucharest 70116, Romania.

615.1 PRT ISSN 0873-5301
FARMACIA DISTRIBUICAO. Text in Portuguese. 1991. m. PTE 8,640 domestic; PTE 15,552 foreign (effective 2001). adv. index. **Document type:** *Trade.* **Description:** Presents business news in the pharmacy and drugstore industry.
Published by: A J E Sociedade Editorial Lda., Rua Barao de Sabrosa, 165-A, Lisbon 1900, Portugal. TEL 351-21-8110100, FAX 351-21-8140044, aje@aje.pt, http://www.aje.pt. Ed. Carina Machado. Pub. A J Esteves. Adv. contact Paulo Silva. page PTE 330,000; trim 200 x 265. Circ: 6,000 (paid).

615 ITA ISSN 1121-1350
FARMACIA NATURALE. Key Title: Natom. Farmacia Naturale. Text in Italian. 1986. m. (9/yr.). ITL 70,000; ITL 140,000 in Europe; ITL 200,000 elsewhere. adv. **Description:** Covers phytotherapy, homeopathy and nutrition.
Former titles (until 1990): Natom (0394-8196); (until 1985): Naturopatia Omeopatia (0394-8188)
Published by: Tecniche Nuove s.p.a., Via Ciro Menotti, 14, Milan, MI 20129, Italy. TEL 39-027570321, FAX 39-027570332, abbonamenti@tecnet.it; farmacia@tecnet.it, http://www.tecnet.it/index1.html. Ed. Giorgio Albonetti. adv.: B&W page ITL 3,380,000, color page ITL 4,560,000; trim 250 x 184. Circ: 8,032.

615 ESP
FARMACIA PROFESIONAL✻. Text in Spanish. 11/yr.
Published by: Haymarket, S.A., Travesera Gracia 17-21, 5o 2o, Barcelona 08022, Spain. TEL 3-237-22-66, FAX 237-66-88. Ed. Enrique Medrano. Circ: 8,500.

615 ITA
FARMACIA REGIONE. Text in Italian. 10/yr.
Address: Via Emanuele Filiberto, 190, Rome, RM 00185, Italy. TEL 6-75-73-679, FAX 6-75-95-647. Circ: 16,000.

615.19 SWE ISSN 1102-8033
FARMACIFACKET. Text in Swedish. 1931. 10/yr. SEK 395 (effective 2001). adv. **Document type:** *Magazine, Trade.*
Former titles (until 1991): Apotekstjaenstemannen (0281-6040); (until 1983): Apoteksteknikern (0345-0945); (until 1956): Tekniska Apotekspersonalens Tidskrift; (until vol.4, 1932): Meddelande fraan Sveriges Tekniska Apotekspersonals Foerbundscentralstyrelse
Published by: Farmacifoerbundet, Vastmannagatan 66, Stockholm 11325, Sweden. TEL 46-8-31-64-10, FAX 46-8-34-08-08, farmaciforbundet@farmaciforbundet.se, http://www.farmacifacket.press.se, http://www.farmaciforbundet.se. Ed., Pub. Anita Wingaardh. adv.: B&W page SEK 8,500, color page SEK 16,000; trim 181 x 260. Circ: 7,000.

615.1 POL ISSN 0014-8261
CODEN: FAPOA4
FARMACJA POLSKA. Text in Polish, English, Russian. 1945. fortn. USD 180 (effective 1998). adv. bk.rev. charts, illus, tr.lit. index. back issues avail. **Description:** Devoted to scientific and social and professional problems of pharmacy.
Related titles: Online - full text ed.
Indexed: Agri.& Environ.Biotech.Abstr. (coverage dropped), Anal.Abstr., Chem.Abstr., Derwent Biotech.Abstr., Excerp.Med., INIS Atomind., I.P.A.
—BLDSC (3887.000000), CASDDS, CISTI, GNLM, Linda Hall.
Published by: Polskie Towarzystwo Farmaceutyczne/Polish Pharmaceutical Society, Ul Dluga 16, Warsaw 00238, Poland. TEL 48-22-8310241, FAX 48-22-8310243. Ed. Jerzy Lazowski. Circ: 4,000.

615.1 FRA ISSN 0014-827X
CODEN: FRMCE8
IL FARMACO. Text in English. 1945. m. EUR 80 in Europe to individuals; USD 89 elsewhere to individuals; EUR 431 in Europe to institutions; USD 350 elsewhere to institutions (effective 2002). adv. bk.rev. charts, illus, tr.lit. index. back issues avail. *Refereed.* **Document type:** *Academic/Scholarly.* **Description:** Publishes original scientific papers and articles on various aspects of medicinal chemistry and pharmaceutical sciences.
Related titles: Microfilm ed.: (from PMC); Online - full text ed.: (from ingenta, Swets Blackwell, ScienceDirect, Institute for Scientific Information).
Indexed: ASCA, Agri.& Environ.Biotech.Abstr. (coverage dropped), Anal.Abstr., Biol.Abstr., Biotech.& Bioeng.Abstr., Cal.Tiss.Abstr., Chem.Abstr., Chem.Cit.Ind., Chem.Indus.Notes, Chem.Infd., Chem.Titles, Curr.Adv.Ecol.Sci., Curr.Chem.React., Curr.Cont., Dairy Sci.Abstr., Derwent Biotech.Abstr., Environ.Sci.Poll.Mgmt., Excerp.Med., Food Sci.& Tech.Abstr., I.P.A., Ind.Chem., Ind.Med. (1989-), Ind.Sci.Rev., Inpharma, MOS, Mass Spectr.Bull., Microbiol.Abstr., NPU, Neurosci.Cit.Ind., Nutr.Abstr., Pharm.&Out.News, Protozool.Abstr., RCI, Reac., Ref.Zh., Rev.Med.& Vet.Mycol., Rev.Plant Path., Sci.Cit.Ind.
—BLDSC (3887.500000), CASDDS, CINDOC, GNLM, IDS, KNAW, Linda Hall.
Published by: (Societa Chimica Italiana ITA), Elsevier Paris, Editions Scientifiques et Medicales (Subsidiary of: Reed Elsevier plc. group), 23 rue Linois, Paris 75015, France. TEL 33-1-71724500, FAX 33-1-71724664, http://www.elsevier.fr. Ed. F Dall'Acqua. Circ: 1,500.

615 ITA ISSN 1126-4705
FARMACOECONOMIA NEWS. Text in Italian. 1997. q. ITL 20,000 (effective 2001). adv.
Published by: C I C Edizioni Internazionali s.r.l., Corso Trieste 42, Rome, RM 00198, Italy. TEL 39-06-8412673, FAX 39-06-8412688, info@gruppocic.it, 1160199510. Ed. A Koverech. adv.: B&W page XEU 1,601.02, color page XEU 2,014.18; 210 x 290.

615 BRA ISSN 1413-9626
FARMACOTERAPEUTICA. Text in Portuguese. 1996. q. free per issue. back issues avail. *Refereed.* **Document type:** *Bulletin.*
Related titles: Online - full text ed.
Published by: Conselho Federal de Farmacia, Centro Brasileiro de Informacoes sobre Medicamentos, SCRN 712-713, Bloco G, No. 30, Brasilia, DF 70760770, Brazil. TEL 55-61-3496552, FAX 55-61-3496553, cebrim@cff.org.br, http://www.cff.org.br. Circ: 5,000 (controlled).

P

615.19 ESP ISSN 0214-8935
FARMACOTERAPIA/JOURNAL OF PHARMACOLOGY. Text in Spanish. 1984. q. ESP 6,000 domestic; ESP 60 foreign (effective 2001). **Document type:** *Academic/Scholarly.*
—CISTI, Infotrieve. **CCC.**
Published by: Editores Medicos S.A., Gabriela Mistral, 2, Madrid 28035, Spain. TEL 34-91-3768140, FAX 34-91-3739907. Circ: 8,000.

615 UKR
FARMAKOLOHICHNYI VISNYK. Text in English, Russian, Ukrainian. 1996. bi-m. UAK 10 per issue domestic; USD 1.45 per issue foreign (effective 2001). adv. bk.rev. **Document type:** *Academic/Scholarly.*
Published by: Farmakolohichnyi Komitet Ministerstva Okhorony Zdorov'ya Ukrainy, Ul Grushevs'kogo 7, Kiev, Ukraine. TEL 380-44-2935439, FAX 380-44-2935439, journal@pharma.viaduk.net. Ed. Vladimir S Danilenko. **US dist. addr.:** East View Publications, 3020 Harbor Ln N, Minneapolis, MN 55447. TEL 612-550-0961.

615.1 BGR
FARMATSEVTICHEN MONITOR. Text in Bulgarian. q. USD 48 foreign (effective 2002). **Description:** Contains information surveys for pharmacologists.
Published by: Meditsinski Universitet - Sofia, Tsentur za Informatsiia po Meditsina/Medical University - Sofia, Medical Information Center, 1 Sv Georgi Sofiiski ul, Sofia 1431, Bulgaria. TEL 359-2-9522342, FAX 359-2-9522393, http://www.medun.acad.bg. **Dist. by:** Sofia Books, Ul Silivria 16, Sofia 1404, Bulgaria. TEL 359-2-9586257, sofiabooks@hotmail.com, http://www.sofiabooks.hit.bg.

615 RUS
FARMATSEVTICHESKII VESTNIK. Text in Russian. s-m. **Document type:** *Academic/Scholarly.*
Address: A-ya 1, Moscow 117420, Russian Federation. TEL 7-095-2031145, FAX 7-095-2031145. Ed. M V Zenin. **US dist. addr.:** East View Publications, 3020 Harbor Ln N, Minneapolis, MN 55447. TEL 612-550-0961.

615.1 UKR ISSN 0367-3057
RS1 CODEN: FRZKAP
FARMATSEVTYCHNYI ZHURNAL. Text in Ukrainian; Summaries in Russian. 1928-1942; resumed 1958. bi-m. USD 89. charts, illus. index. **Document type:** *Academic/Scholarly.*
Indexed: Agri.& Environ.Biotech.Abstr. (coverage dropped), Anal.Abstr., Apic.Abstr., Biol.Abstr., Chem.Abstr., Derwent Biotech.Abstr., Excerp.Med., INIS Atomind., I.P.A., Ind.Med. (coverage dropped).

—BLDSC (0389.100000), CASDDS, CISTI, East View, EMDOCS, GNLM, Infotrieve, KNAW, Linda Hall. **CCC.**
Published by: Vydavnytstvo Zdorov'ia, Kominterna ul 16, Kiev, Ukraine. TEL 380-44-2442892. Circ: 7,900. **Dist. by:** Mezhdunarodnaya Kniga, B Yakimanka 39, Moscow 117049, Russian Federation; **US dist. addr.:** East View Publications, 3020 Harbor Ln N, Minneapolis, MN 55447. TEL 612-550-0961.

615 BGR ISSN 0428-0296 CODEN: FMTYA2
FARMATSIA. Text and summaries in Bulgarian, English. 1951. q., latest vol.47, 2000. USD 48 foreign (effective 2002). adv. bk.rev. abstr. index. 48 p./no. back issues avail. *Refereed.* **Document type:** *Journal, Academic/Scholarly, Bibliography.* **Description:** Presents original articles and reviews of a range of pharmacy research topics.
Indexed: Abstr.Bulg.Sci.Med.Lit., Chem.Abstr., Excerp.Med., INIS Atomind., I.P.A., Ind.Med. (coverage dropped), Ref.Zh.
—CASDDS, CISTI, EMDOCS, GNLM.
Published by: Meditsinski Universitet - Sofia, Tsentur za Informatsiia po Meditsina/Medical University - Sofia, Medical Information Center, 1 Sv Georgi Sofiiski ul, Sofia 1431, Bulgaria. TEL 359-2-9522342, FAX 359-2-9522393, mutafov@sun.medun.acad.bg, http://www.medun.acad.bg. Ed. Ivan Assenov. R&P Dr. Christo Mutafov. Adv. contacts Dr. Christo Mutafov, St Nikolov TEL 359-2-9879874. B&W page USD 50, color page USD 125. Circ: 300. **Dist. by:** Sofia Books, Ul Silivria 16, Sofia 1404, Bulgaria. TEL 359-2-9586257, sofiabooks@hotmail.com, http://www.sofiabooks.hit.bg.

615.19 RUS ISSN 0367-3014 CODEN: FRMTAL
FARMATSIYA/PHARMACY. Text in Russian; Summaries in English. 1952. bi-m. RUR 300 domestic; USD 75 foreign (effective 1999). adv. bibl. *Refereed.* **Description:** Publishes actual pharmaceutical information, scientific articles, problem-oriented publications and reviews, latest achievements in pharmaceutical science and practice, materials on both domestic and foreign pharmaceutical companies. Regularly includes the columns: Branch Strategy, Investigation, Experiment, Current Events, History of Pharmacy, etc.. Also includes reviews, criticism, a discussion section, and news on conferences.
Indexed: Agri.& Environ.Biotech.Abstr. (coverage dropped), Anal.Abstr., Apic.Abstr., Biol.Abstr., Chem.Abstr., Chem.Indus.Notes, Chem.Titles, Curr.Cont. (coverage dropped), Derwent Biotech.Abstr., Excerp.Med., Hort.Abstr., I.P.A., Mass Spectr.Bull., Ref.Zh.
—BLDSC (0389.180000), CASDDS, CISTI, East View, EMDOCS, GNLM, Infotrieve. **CCC.**
Published by: Rossiiskii Tsentr Farmatsevticheskoi i Mediko-Tekhnicheskoi Informatsii, A-ya 195, Moscow 103051, Russian Federation. TEL 7-095-2115356, FAX 7-095-2115356, frmdin@dol.ru. Ed. S S Budarin. R&P Galina V Shashkova. Adv. contact Ludmila E Kononova. color page USD 1,200. Circ: 6,000. **Dist. by:** Mezhdunarodnaya Kniga, B Yakimanka 39, Moscow 117049, Russian Federation. TEL 7-095-2384967, FAX 7-095-2384634; **US dist. addr.:** Victor Kamkin Inc., 4956 Boiling Brook Pkwy, Rockville, MD 20852.

615.1 JPN ISSN 0014-8601 CODEN: FARUAW
FARUMASHIA. Text in Japanese. 1965. m. USD 120 to members (effective 2001). adv. bk.rev. abstr, bibl, charts, mkt, stat. index. 170 p./no. *Refereed.* **Document type:** *Journal, Academic/Scholarly.* **Description:** Covers all aspects of pharmaceutical sciences.
Indexed: Chem.Abstr., Chem.Indus.Notes, Chem.Titles, INIS Atomind., Mass Spectr.Bull.
—BLDSC (3896.500000), CASDDS, CISTI, Linda Hall. **CCC.**
Published by: Pharmaceutical Society of Japan/Nihon Yakugakkai, 2-12-15, Shibuya, Shibuya-ku, Tokyo 150-0002, Japan. TEL 81-3-3406-3321, FAX 81-3-3498-1835. Ed. Masakatsu Shbasaki. Circ: 22,000 (controlled).

615 ITA
FEDERFARMA NOTIZIE; organo d'informazione settimanale dei titolari di farmacia. Text in Italian. 1986. w. ITL 220,000, USD 150 to non-members. adv. bk.rev. back issues avail.
Formerly (until 1986): Farmacia Notizie
Published by: Editoriale Giornalidea s.r.l., Via Sebenico, 14, Milan, MI 20124, Italy. TEL 02-688875, FAX 02-6888780. Ed. Sossio Guarnaccia. Circ: 17,000.

FINANCIAL SURVEY. THE PHARMACEUTICAL INDUSTRY. see *BUSINESS AND ECONOMICS—Trade And Industrial Directories*

615 JPN
FINE D I WEEKLY. Text in Japanese. 1988. w.
Published by: Fukujin Co. Ltd., 23-5 Hatanaka 1-chome, Niiza-shi, Saitama-ken 352-0012, Japan.

FITOCIENCIA REVISTA. see *BIOLOGY—Botany*

FITOTERAPIA; journal for the study of medicinal plants - rivista di studi ed applicazioni delle piante medicinali. see *BIOLOGY—Botany*

615 658 USA
FLORIDA JOURNAL OF HEALTH-SYSTEM PHARMACY✱. Text in English. 198?. bi-m.
Formerly (until 1995): Florida Journal of Hospital Pharmacy (1074-0295)
Indexed: I.P.A.
Published by: Florida Society of Health-System Pharmacists, 2304 Killearn Center Blvd A, Tallahassee, FL 32308-3524. TEL 904-386-8855. Ed. Steve Glass.

615.1 USA ISSN 0897-4616
FLORIDA PHARMACY TODAY. Text in English. 1937. m. USD 36 to individuals; USD 5 newsstand/cover to individuals; USD 70 to institutions (effective 2000). adv. bk.rev. illus. *Refereed.* **Document type:** *Trade.*
Former titles: Florida Pharmacy Journal (0161-746X); Florida Pharmaceutical Journal (0015-4202); Florida Pharmacist
Indexed: AgeLine, I.P.A.
Published by: Florida Pharmacy Association, 3128 Crawfordville Hwy., Crawfordville, FL 32327. TEL 850-222-2400, FAX 850-561-6758. Ed., R&P Julia Hanway TEL 850-926-2405. Adv. contacts Julia Hanway TEL 850-926-2405, Paul Payne. B&W page USD 600, color page USD 1,100; trim 8 x 11. Circ: 3,200 (controlled).

615 GBR ISSN 1465-539X
FOCUS (GUILDFORD). Text in English. w. GBP 395; GBP 435 in the European Union; GBP 465 elsewhere. **Document type:** *Trade.*
Published by: Pharmafile Ltd., First House, Park St, Guildford, Surrey GU1 4XB, United Kingdom. TEL 44-1483-515300, FAX 44-1483-515301, s.benard@pharmafile.co.uk.

615 615.89 GBR ISSN 1465-3753
FOCUS ON ALTERNATIVE AND COMPLEMENTARY THERAPIES. Cover title: F A C T. Text in English. 1996. q. USD 105 in United States to individuals; GBP 65 elsewhere to individuals; USD 190 in United States to institutions; GBP 115 elsewhere to institutions (effective 2001). adv. bk.rev. back issues avail. *Refereed.* **Document type:** *Journal, Academic/Scholarly.* **Description:** Systematically considers both the mainstream medical and pharmaceutical literature along with complementary medicine related journals. The most importantant papers from all journals are then summarized and commented on in FACT.
Related titles: Online - full text ed.: (from RoweCom Information Quest).
Indexed: AMED.
—BLDSC (3964.203730).
Published by: Pharmaceutical Press (Subsidiary of: Euromed Communications Ltd.), 1 Lambeth High St, London SE1 7JN, United Kingdom. TEL 44-20-7735-9141, FAX 44-20-7735-5085, pharmpress@rpsgb.org.uk, http://www.pharmj.com. Ed. Edzard Ernst. Pub., R&P Charles Fry. Adv. contact Jack Richmond.

FOCUS ON PULMONARY PHARMACOLOGY AND TOXICOLOGY. see *ENVIRONMENTAL STUDIES—Toxicology And Environmental Safety*

615 CHE
FOLIA PHARMACEUTICA. Text in German. 9/yr.
Published by: Verlag Diethelm AG, Postfach 203, Pfaeffikon Sz 8808, Switzerland. TEL 01-7849693, FAX 01-7843503. Circ: 8,500.

615 JPN ISSN 0015-5691 CODEN: NYKZAU
FOLIA PHARMACOLOGICA JAPONICA/NIPPON YAKURIGAKU ZASSHI. Text in Japanese; Summaries in English. 1925. m. JPY 12,000 domestic (effective 2001 & 2002). adv. illus. index. reprint service avail. from PQC,ISI. *Refereed.* **Document type:** *Academic/Scholarly.*
Related titles: Microform ed.: (from PQC); Online - full text ed.: (from Institute for Scientific Information).
Indexed: Agri.& Environ.Biotech.Abstr. (coverage dropped), Biol.Abstr., Chem.Abstr., Curr.Adv.Ecol.Sci., Curr.Cont. (coverage dropped), Dairy Sci.Abstr., Dent.Ind., Derwent Biotech.Abstr., Excerp.Med., Helminthol.Abstr., INIS Atomind., Ind.Med. (1944-), Ind.Sci.Rev., Nutr.Abstr.
—BLDSC (3973.500000), CASDDS, CISTI, GNLM, IDS, KNAW, Linda Hall.
Published by: Japanese Pharmacological Society, Editorial Office/Nihon Yakuri Gakkai Henshuubu, Kantohya Bldg, Gokomachi-Ebisugawa, Nakagyo-ku, Kyoto-shi 604-0982, Japan. TEL 81-75-252-4641, FAX 81-75-252-4618, LDB00573@nifty.ne.jp, http://www.soc.nii.ac.jp/tjps/kyoto/fpj. Ed. Masamichi Satoh. Circ: 6,200.

615 664 GBR ISSN 0265-203X TX553.A3 CODEN: FACOEB
FOOD ADDITIVES AND CONTAMINANTS; analysis, surveillance, evaluation, control. Text in English. 1984. 12/yr. GBP 1,132, USD 1,869 to institutions (effective 2002). adv. bk.rev. illus. Index. back issues avail.; reprints avail. *Refereed.* **Document type:** *Journal, Trade.* **Description:** Contains original research and review articles relating to the detection, determination, occurrence, persistence, safety evaluation and control of naturally occurring and man-made additives and contaminants in the food chain.
Related titles: Online - full text ed.: ISSN 1464-5122 (from CatchWord Ltd., EBSCO Publishing, O C L C Online Computer Library Center, Inc., RoweCom Information Quest, Swets Blackwell, Institute for Scientific Information).
Indexed: AMED, ASCA, Abstr.Bull.Inst.Pap.Chem., Agricola, Agroforest.Abstr., Anal.Abstr., Aqua.Sci.& Fish.Abstr., Bibl.Agri., Biodet.Abstr., Chem.Abstr., Chem.Indus.Notes, Chem.Titles, Curr.Adv.Cancer Res., Curr.Adv.Ecol.Sci., Curr.Cont., Dairy Sci.Abstr., Environ.Abstr., Environ.Per.Bibl. (1991-), Environ.Sci.Poll.Mgmt., Excerp.Med., Field Crop Abstr., Food Sci.& Tech.Abstr., Forest Prod.Abstr., Forest.Abstr., Helminthol.Abstr., Hort.Abstr., INIS Atomind., Ind.Med. (1984-), Ind.Vet., Int.Packag.Abstr., METADEX, Maize Abstr., NRN, Nutr.Abstr., Packag.Sci.Tech., Pig News & Info., Plant Breed.Abstr., Pollut.Abstr., Postharvest, Potato Abstr., Poult.Abstr., Protozool.Abstr., RAPRA (1995-), Rev.Appl.Entomol., Rev.Med.& Vet.Mycol., Rev.Plant Path., Sci.Cit.Ind., Soyabean Abstr., Sugar Ind.Abstr., Triticale Abstr., Trop.Dis.Bull., Vet.Bull., Weed Abstr.
—BLDSC (3977.001000), CASDDS, CatchWord, CISTI, EMDOCS, GNLM, IDS, ingenta, Linda Hall. **CCC.**
Published by: Taylor & Francis Group, Taylor & Francis Ltd., 11 New Fetter Ln, London EC4P 4EE, United Kingdom. TEL 44-20-7583-9855, FAX 44-20-7842-2298, info@tandf.co.uk, http://www.tandf.co.uk/journals/tf/0265203X.html. Eds. J Gilbert, P M Scott. **Subscr. in N. America to:** Taylor & Francis Ltd., 325 Chestnut St, Suite 800, Philadelphia, PA 19016. TEL 800-354-1420, FAX 215-625-8914, info@taylorandfrancis.com.

FOOD AND DRUG ADMINISTRATION. REGULATORY MANUAL. see *LAW*

615 664 USA ISSN 1086-024X
FOOD & DRUG INSPECTION MONITOR. Text in English. 1996. m. USD 554 (effective 2001). 10 p./no. 2 cols./p. back issues avail.; reprints avail. **Document type:** *Newsletter, Trade.*
—CCC.
Published by: Washington Information Source, 6506 Old Stage Rd, Ste 100, Rockville, MD 20852-4326. TEL 301-770-5553. Ed., Pub., R&P Ken Reid.

FOOD AND DRUG LAW JOURNAL. see *LAW*

614 USA ISSN 0362-6466
FOOD AND DRUG LETTER. Text in English. 1976. bi-w. USD 1,095 in North America; USD 1,120 elsewhere (effective Nov. 2001). bk.rev. charts. 12 p./no. Supplement avail.; back issues avail. **Document type:** *Newsletter.* **Description:** Focuses on major regulatory issues of foods, drugs and cosmetics.
Incorporating: Nutrition Intelligence
Related titles: E-mail ed.: (from The Dialog Corporation).
—Infotrieve. **CCC.**
Published by: Washington Business Information, Inc., 300 N Washington St, Ste 200, Falls Church, Arlington, VA 22046. TEL 703-538-7600, 703-538-7660, FAX 703 538-7676, ehinkle@fdanews.com, http://www.fdanews.com. Ed. Phil Wallace.

FOOD & DRUG PACKAGING. see *PACKAGING*

FOOD, DRINKS & DRUGS INDUSTRY BULLETIN. see *LAW*

615 340 USA ISSN 0162-1122
FOOD DRUG COSMETIC LAW REPORTS (RX EDITION). Text in English. 1938. w. (50/yr.). USD 2,599 (effective 2001).
Related titles: CD-ROM ed.
—CCC.
Published by: C C H Incorporated, 2700 Lake Cook Rd., Riverwoods, IL 60015. TEL 847-267-7000, 800-449-9525, FAX 773-866-3895, http://www.cch.com. Pub. Catherine Wolfe.

615.1 USA ISSN 1082-801X
RA975.5.P5 CODEN: FORMF9
FORMULARY; a peer-reviewed drug management journal for managed care and hospital decision makers. Text in English. 1966. m., latest vol.36. USD 55 domestic; USD 80 in Canada & Mexico; USD 110 elsewhere; USD 6.50 newsstand/cover (effective 2001). adv. abstr, bibl, charts. index. 85 p./no. back issues avail.; reprints avail. *Refereed.* **Document type:** *Journal, Trade.* **Description:** Provides information on newly approved drugs, pharmaceutical comparisons for managing disease states, formulary management issues, rational prescribing approaches, and insights into effective formulary committee structure and function.
Former titles (until 1995): Hospital Formulary (0098-6909); (until 1975): Hospital Formulary Management (0018-5655)
Related titles: Microform ed.: (from PQC); Online - full text ed.: (from Northern Light Technology, Inc., ProQuest Information & Learning, LexisNexis, Institute for Scientific Information).
Indexed: ASCA, Agri.& Environ.Biotech.Abstr. (coverage dropped), Biol.Abstr., CINAHL, Chem.Abstr., Curr.Cont., Derwent Biotech.Abstr., Excerp.Med., Hosp.Lit.Ind., I.P.A., Inpharma, Pharm.&Out.News, Protozool.Abstr., Reac., Rev.Med.& Vet.Mycol., SSCI (coverage dropped).
—BLDSC (4008.805800), CASDDS, GNLM, IDS, ingenta, KNAW. **CCC.**
Published by: Advanstar Communications Inc., 7500 Old Oak Blvd, Cleveland, OH 44130. TEL 440-891-2689, FAX 440-891-2683, ksprague@advanstar.com; formul@en.com, http://www.formularyjournal.com, http://www.advanstar.com. Ed. David C Calabrese. Pub., R&P Steve Reichenstein TEL 732-225-9500. Circ: 46,000.

615.1 618.97 USA
FORMULARY GERIATRICS. Text in English. q.
Published by: Advanstar Communications Inc., 201 E Sandpointe Ave Ste 600, Santa Ana, CA 92707. TEL 440-891-2767, FAX 440-891-2683, http://www.advanstar.com.

615.1 CHE ISSN 0071-786X
RS122 CODEN: FAZMAE
FORTSCHRITTE DER ARZNEIMITTELFORSCHUNG/ PROGRES DES RECHERCHES PHARMACEUTIQUES/PROGRESS IN DRUG RESEARCH. Text in English. 1959. irreg. (1-2/yr.). price varies. **Document type:** *Monographic series, Academic/Scholarly.*
Related titles: Online - full text ed.
Indexed: Agri.& Environ.Biotech.Abstr. (coverage dropped), Biol.Abstr., Chem.Abstr., Chem.Indus.Notes, Chem.Titles, Derwent Biotech.Abstr., Excerp.Med., I.P.A., Ind.Med. (1968-).
—BLDSC (6868.200000), CASDDS, CINDOC, CISTI, GNLM, ingenta, KNAW, Linda Hall. **CCC.**
Published by: Birkhaeuser Verlag AG (Subsidiary of: BertelsmannSpringer), Klosterberg, Postfach 133, Basel 4010, Switzerland. TEL 41-61-2050707, FAX 41-61-2050792, orders@birkhauser.ch, http://www.birkhauser.ch. Ed. Ernst Jucker.

615 ZAF ISSN 1607-9620
FRONT SHOP. Text in English. 1994. m. ZAR 131.45 (effective 2001).
Published by: Primedia Publishing, 366 Pretoria Ave, Randburg, Transvaal 2194, South Africa. TEL 27-11-293-7400, FAX 27-11-787-5776, http://www.primemags.co.za.

615.1 660 USA
FRONTIERS IN BIOMEDICAL POLYMER APPLICATIONS. Text in English. irreg., latest vol.2, 1999. price varies. **Document type:** *Newsletter.*
Related titles: E-mail ed.; Online - full content ed.
—BLDSC.
Published by: C R C Press, LLC, 2000 Corporate Blvd, N W, Boca Raton, FL 33431. TEL 800-272-7737, FAX 561-994-0555, 800-374-3401, orders@crcpress.com, http://www.crcpress.com.

615.6 610.5 CHN
FUJIAN YIYAO ZAZHI/FUJIAN MEDICAL JOURNAL. Text in Chinese; Abstracts in English. 1979. bi-m. CNY 18 (effective 1999). adv. **Document type:** *Academic/Scholarly.* **Description:** Presents research results and developments in pharmacology and the medical sciences.
Published by: Fujiansheng Yixue Kexue Yanjiusuo/Fujian Institute of Medical Sciences, 7 Wusi Lu, Fuzhou, Fujian 350001, China. TEL 86-591-7516804, http://www.straitinto.com/publicat; http://netcity.fz.fi.cn. Ed., Pub. Chen Xin. Adv. contact Xin Chen. **Dist. overseas by:** Jiangsu Publications Import & Export Corp., 56 Gao Yun Ling, Nanjing, Jiangsu, China. **Co-sponsor:** Fujian Public Health Bureau - Fujiansheng Weisheng Ting.

615 JPN ISSN 0913-1736
CODEN: FDYKES
FUKUOKA DAIGAKU YAKUGAKU KIYO/FUKUOKA UNIVERSITY. PHARMACEUTICAL BULLETIN. Text in English, Japanese; Summaries in English. 1963. a.
Indexed: Chem.Abstr.
—BLDSC (6442.780000).
Published by: Fukuoka Daigaku, Sogo Kenkyusho/Fukuoka University, Central Research Institute, 19-1 Nanakuma 8-chome, Jonan-ku, Fukuoka-shi 814-0133, Japan. TEL 81-92-871-6631, FAX 81-92-866-2308.

615 JPN
FUKUOKA SOCIETY OF HOSPITAL PHARMACY. DRUG INFORMATION NEWS. Text in Japanese. 1965. q. membership.
Published by: Fukuokaken Byoin Yakuzaishikai, Kyushu Daigaku Igakubu Fuzoku Byoin Yakuzaibu, 1-1 Maidashi 3-chome, Higashi-ku, Fukuoka-shi 812-0054, Japan.

615 JPN ISSN 0288-724X
FUKUYAMA DAIGAKU YAKUGAKUBU KENKYU NENPO/FUKUYAMA UNIVERSITY. FACULTY OF PHARMACY & PHARMACEUTICAL SCIENCES. ANNUAL REPORT. Text in English, Japanese; Summaries in English. 1982. a.
Published by: Fukuyaka Daigaku, Yakugakubu, 985, Mikura, Higashimuracho, Fukuyama-shi, Hiroshimaken 729-02, Japan.

615.19 GBR ISSN 0767-3981
CODEN: FCPHEZ
FUNDAMENTAL AND CLINICAL PHARMACOLOGY. Text in English. 1970. bi-m., latest vol.16, 2002. GBP 100 in Europe to individuals; USD 159 in North America to individuals; GBP 110 elsewhere to individuals; GBP 345 in Europe to institutions; USD 548 in North America to institutions; GBP 380 elsewhere to institutions (effective 2002). adv. bk.rev. index. *Refereed.* **Document type:** *Academic/Scholarly.* **Description:** Publishes full-length articles and short communications in the entire field of pharmacology from molecular studies to clinical investigations.
Incorporates (in 1997): Archives Internationales de Pharmacodynamie et de Therapie (0003-9780); Which was formerly (until 1899): Archives Internationales de Pharmacodynamie (0301-4533); (until 1898): Archives de Pharmacodynamie (0770-1071)
Related titles: Microform ed.: (from PQC); Online - full text ed.: GBP 90 in Europe to individuals; USD 144 in North America to individuals; GBP 90 elsewhere to individuals; GBP 311 in Europe to institutions; USD 494 in North America to institutions; GBP 311 elsewhere to institutions (effective 2002) (from ingenta, Swets Blackwell, Institute for Scientific Information, RoweCom Information Quest).
Indexed: ASCA, Anim.Behav.Abstr., Aqua.Sci.& Fish.Abstr., Biol.Abstr., Chem.Abstr., Chem.Indus.Notes, Chem.Titles, Curr.Adv.Biochem., Curr.Chem.React., Curr.Cont., Derwent Biotech.Abstr., Excerp.Med., INIS Atomind., Ind.Chem., Ind.Med. (1987-), Inpharma, Int.Abstr.Biol.Sci., Neurosci.Abstr. (coverage dropped), Neurosci.Cit.Ind., Pharm.&Out.News, RCI, Reac., Rev.Med.& Vet.Mycol., Sci.Cit.Ind. (coverage dropped).
—BLDSC (4056.033000), ADONIS, CASDDS, CISTI, EMDOCS, GNLM, IDS, Infotrieve, ingenta, KNAW. **CCC.**
Published by: (Societe Francaise de Pharmacologie FRA), Blackwell Science Ltd., PO Box 88, Oxford OX2 0NE, United Kingdom. TEL 44-1865-206180, 44-1865-206002, FAX 44-1865-206219, jnl.orders@blacksci.co.uk, http://www.blackwell-science.com/~cgilib/jnlpage.asp?Journal=fcp&File=fcp, http://www.blackwellpublishing.com. Ed. Jean Francois Guidicelli.

615 340 JPN
G M P REGULATIONS OF JAPAN. Text in English, Japanese. irreg., latest 2001. price varies. **Description:** Covers G.M.P. provisions on drugs, sterile drug preparations, bulk pharmaceutical chemicals, medical devices, cosmetics and more.
Published by: (Japan. Ministry of Health and Welfare, Pharmaceutical Affairs Bureau, Inspection and Guidance Division), Yakuji Nippo Ltd., 1 Kanda-Izumi-cho, Chiyoda-ku, Tokyo 101-8648, Japan. TEL 81-3-3862-2141, FAX 81-3-5821-8757, shuppan@yakuji.co.jp, http://www.yakuji.co.jp/.

GAIKOKU BUNKEN DAIJESUTO. KAKU IGAKU/FOREIGN LITERATURE DIGEST. NUCLEAR MEDICINE. see *MEDICAL SCIENCES—Radiology And Nuclear Medicine*

615 JPN ISSN 0288-349X
GAKUJUTSU ZASSHI/KYOTO COLLEGE OF PHARMACY. SCIENTIFIC JOURNAL. Text in Japanese. 1968. a. **Document type:** *Academic/Scholarly.*
Published by: Kyoto Yakka Daigaku, Jichikai Gakujutsubu Shokubutsu Kenkyubu/Kyoto College of Pharmacy, 5 Misasagi-Nakauchi-cho, Yamashina-ku, Kyoto-shi 607-8414, Japan.

GASTROINTESTINAL HORMONES AND GASTRIC SECRETION. see *MEDICAL SCIENCES—Abstracting, Bibliographies, Statistics*

615 TUR ISSN 1015-9592
CODEN: GUEDE
GAZI UNIVERSITESI ECZACILIK FAKULTESI DERGISI. Text in Turkish. 1984. s-a. USD 100. Index. *Refereed.* **Document type:** *Academic/Scholarly, Abstract/Index.*
Indexed: Excerp.Med., I.P.A.
—BLDSC (3659.741500), CASDDS, EMDOCS, GNLM, KNAW.
Published by: Gazi Universitesi, Eczacilik Fakultesi/Gazi University, Faculty of Pharmacy, Etiler - Ankara 06330, Turkey. TEL 90-312-2227225, FAX 90-312-2235018. Ed. Dr. M. Fethi Sahin. Pub. Dr. Riza Ayhan.

615.19 DEU ISSN 0942-2951
GELBE LISTE PHARMINDEX. Text in German. 1971. q. DEM 107. adv. *Refereed.* **Document type:** *Directory.*
Formerly: Liste Pharmindex (0344-015X)
—GNLM.
Published by: Medi-Media (Subsidiary of: Medizinische Media Informations GmbH), Am Forsthaus Gravenbruch 9, Neu-Isenburg 63263, Germany. TEL 49-6102-5020, FAX 49-6102-53779, redaktion@medimedia.de, http://www.gelbe-liste.de. Ed. Marianne Kaemmer Reusch. Adv. contact Thomas Lang. B&W page DEM 14,100; trim 148 x 225. Circ: 43,000.

615 NLD ISSN 0304-4629
CODEN: GNMBA
GENEESMIDDELENBULLETIN. Text in Dutch. 1967. m., latest vol.35, 2001 (One volume per calendar year). NLG 80; free to qualified personnel. 10-year index. 12 p./no. 2 cols./p. back issues avail. *Refereed.* **Document type:** *Bulletin, Academic/Scholarly.*
Related titles: Online - full text ed.; ♦ Supplement to: Medisch Contact. ISSN 0025-8245.
Indexed: Excerp.Med.
—BLDSC (4096.468000), EMDOCS, GNLM, KNAW.
Published by: Stichting Geneesmiddelenbulletin, Lomanlaan 85, Utrecht 3526 XC, Netherlands. TEL 31-30-280-2660, http://www.geneesmiddelenbulletin.nl. Ed. Peter Admiraal. Circ: 46,750.

615.1 USA ISSN 0306-3623
RM1 CODEN: GEPHDP
GENERAL PHARMACOLOGY; the vascular system. Text in English. 1970. 12/yr. EUR 2,611 in Europe to institutions; JPY 346,800 in Japan to institutions; USD 2,920 elsewhere to institutions (effective 2002). adv. bk.rev. abstr, charts, illus, stat. index. back issues avail.; reprint service avail. from PQC. *Refereed.* **Document type:** *Journal, Academic/Scholarly.* **Description:** Covers all aspects of pharmacology.
Formerly: Comparative and General Pharmacology (0010-4035)
Related titles: Microfilm ed.: (from PQC); Online - full text ed.: (from ingenta, Swets Blackwell, ScienceDirect, Institute for Scientific Information).

P

Indexed: ASCA, Agri.& Environ.Biotech.Abstr. (coverage dropped), Agroforest.Abstr., Aqua.Sci.& Fish.Abstr., Biol.Abstr., Cal.Tiss.Abstr. (coverage dropped), Chem.Abstr., Chem.Indus.Notes, Chem.Titles, Curr.Adv.Biochem., Curr.Adv.Ecol.Sci., Curr.Cont., Dent.Ind., Derwent Biotech.Abstr., Excerp.Med., Forest Prod.Abstr., Helminthol.Abstr., Ind.Med. (1975-), Ind.Sci.Rev., Ind.Vet., Inpharma, Int.Abstr.Biol.Sci., Maize Abstr., Neurosci.Abstr., Neurosci.Cit.Ind., Nutr.Abstr., Pharm.&Out.News, Poult.Abstr., Protozool.Abstr., Reac., Ref.Zh., Rev.Appl.Entomol., Rev.Arom.& Med.Plants, Rev.Med.& Vet.Mycol., Sci.Cit.Ind., THA, Tox.Abstr. (coverage dropped), Triticale Abstr., Vet.Bull., Weed Abstr.
—BLDSC (4106.710000), ADONIS, CASDDS, CISTI, EMDOCS, GNLM, IDS, ingenta, KNAW, Linda Hall. **CCC.**
Published by: Elsevier Science, Box 945, New York, NY 10159-0945. TEL 212-989-5800, FAX 212-633-3990, usinfo-f@elsevier.com, http://www.elsevier.com/locate/genpharm. Eds. J Catravas, Mary Jane Ferraro. Circ: 1,000. **Subscr. in Australasia and the Far East to:** Elsevier Science (Singapore) Pte Ltd, No.1 Temasek Ave, 17-01 Millenia Tower, Singapore 039192, Singapore. TEL 65-434-3727, FAX 65-337-2230; **Subscr. in Japan to:** Elsevier Science Inc - Japan Regional Office, 9-15 Higashi-Azabu 1-chome, Minato-ku, Tokyo 106-0044, Japan. TEL 81-3-5561-5033; **Subscr. outside the Americas to:** Elsevier Science BV, PO Box 211, Amsterdam 1000 AE, Netherlands. TEL 31-20-485-3757.

615.1 332.6 USA ISSN 1076-884X
GENERIC LINE. Text in English. 1984. bi-w., latest vol.19, 2002. USD 495 in North America; USD 520 elsewhere (effective Nov. 2001). 8 p./no. back issues avail. **Document type:** *Newsletter.* **Description:** Aims at business leaders in the generic drug industry. Covers business, FDA and Congressional actions.
Related titles: E-mail ed.: (from Data-Star, The Dialog Corporation).
Published by: Washington Business Information, Inc., 300 N Washington St, Ste 200, Falls Church, Arlington, VA 22046. TEL 703-538-7600, 703-538-7660, FAX 703 538-7676, ddouglass@fdanews.com, http://www.fdanews.com. Ed. Robert Billings. Pub. David Swit.

615 USA ISSN 1061-2270
GENESIS REPORT - RX; business implications of technology innovation in pharmaceuticals. Text in English. 1991. bi-m. USD 1,195 domestic; USD 1,250 foreign (effective 2000). **Document type:** *Newsletter.*
Related titles: Online - full text ed.: (from Northern Light Technology, Inc., Gale Group).
—BLDSC (4111.842000).
Published by: Genesis Group Associates, Inc., 29 Park St, Montclair, NJ 07042. TEL 973-509-7735, FAX 973-509-7745, http://www.genesispov.com. Ed. James Kehoe.

615.1 USA
GEORGIA PHARMACIST QUARTERLY. Text in English. q. back issues avail. **Document type:** *Academic/Scholarly.*
Related titles: Online - full text ed.
Published by: University of Georgia, College of Pharmacy, Athens, GA 30602. TEL 706-542-5303, FAX 706-542-5269, robertson@rx.uga.edu, http://www.rx.uga.edu/publications/frames.html. Ed. Sheila Roberson.

615.1 DEU ISSN 0939-334X
GESCHICHTE DER PHARMAZIE. Text in German. 1948. q. EUR 17.76 domestic; EUR 18.40 in Europe; EUR 20.28 elsewhere; EUR 6 newsstand/cover (effective 2002); free with subscr. to Deutsche Apotheker Zeitung. bk.rev. illus. index. **Document type:** *Journal, Trade.*
Former titles: Beitraege zur Geschichte der Pharmazie (0341-0099); Zur Geschichte der Pharmazie (0044-5509)
Related titles: ♦ Supplement to: Deutsche Apotheker Zeitung. ISSN 0011-9857.
Indexed: Amer.Hist.& Life, Hist.Abstr. (1987-).
—BLDSC (4162.518000), GNLM.
Published by: (Internationale Gesellschaft fuer Geschichte der Pharmazie), Deutscher Apotheker Verlag, Postfach 101061, Stuttgart 70009, Germany. TEL 49-711-2582-0, FAX 49-711-2582290, daz@deutscher-apotheker-verlag.de, http://www.deutscher-apotheker-verlag.de. Ed. Wolf-Dieter Mueller-Jahncke.

615 JPN ISSN 0285-1458
GINKAI. Text in Japanese. 1964. m. JPY 500 per issue. adv. **Document type:** *Consumer.*
Published by: Senju Seiyaku K.K./Senju Pharmaceutical Co., Ltd., 5-8 Hirano-Machi 2-chome, Chuo-ku, Osaka-shi 541-0046, Japan. TEL 81-6-201-9612, FAX 81-6-203-7330. Ed., R&P, Adv. contact Nobuo Aonami.

615 JPN ISSN 0288-6537
GINSENG REVIEW. Text in Japanese; Summaries in English. 1983. a. **Document type:** *Proceedings.* **Description:** Contains medical and pharmacological research on panax ginseng.
Published by: Yakuyo Ninjin Kenkyukai/Medical Society for Red Ginseng Research, Nikkan Korai Ninjin K.K., 11-10 Motomachidori 3-chome, Chuo-ku, Kobe-shi, Hyogo-ken 650-0022, Japan. Ed. Akira Kumagai.

615.19 ITA ISSN 0393-8476
GIORNALE DEL FARMACISTA. Text in Italian. 1986. 18/yr. ITL 16,000 (effective 1999).
Published by: Masson S.p.A., Divisione Periodici, Via F.lli Bressan 2, Milan, MI 20126, Italy. TEL 39-2-270741, FAX 39-2-27074210. adv.: B&W page ITL 4,900,000, color page ITL 5,900,000; trim 285 x 212. Circ: 15,000.

GIORNALE DI NEUROPSICOFARMACOLOGIA. see *MEDICAL SCIENCES—Psychiatry And Neurology*

615 ITA ISSN 1120-3749
GIORNALE ITALIANO DI FARMACIA CLINICA; epidemiologia - informazione - ricerca. Text in Italian; Summaries in English. 1987. 4/yr. USD 107 (effective 2000). bk.rev. bibl. 64 p./no. **Document type:** *Journal, Academic/Scholarly.*
Indexed: Excerp.Med., I.P.A.
—BLDSC (4178.215500), EMDOCS, GNLM.
Published by: (Societa Italiana di Farmacia Ospedaliera), Il Pensiero Scientifico Editore s.r.l., Via Bradano, 3-C, Rome, RM 00199, Italy. TEL 39-06-862821, FAX 39-06-86282250, pensiero@pensiero.it, http://www.pensiero.it. Ed. Giovanna Scroccaro. Pub. Luca De Fiore. Circ: 2,500.

THE GIST. see *FOOD AND FOOD INDUSTRIES*

GLOBAL COSMETIC INDUSTRY. see *BEAUTY CULTURE—Perfumes And Cosmetics*

615.9 616.1 BRA ISSN 1414-0330
GLOSSARIUM CARDIOLOGIA. Text in Portuguese. 1993. a. BRL 40, USD 48.40 (effective 2000). adv. back issues avail. **Document type:** *Consumer, Trade.* **Description:** Provides dosing and administration information, along with indications and contraindications for heart medications.
Published by: Elea Ciencia Editorial Ltda., Rua Haddock Lobo, 86 Andar 6, Estacio, Rio De Janeiro, RJ 20260-132, Brazil. TEL 55-21-293-2112, FAX 55-21-293-7818, elea@openlink.com.br. Ed. Luiz Augusto Rodrigues. Adv. contact Alexandre Augusto Rodrigues. Circ: 6,000.

615.9 616.5 BRA ISSN 1414-0349
GLOSSARIUM DERMATOLOGIA. Text in Portuguese. 1995. a. BRL 40, USD 48.40 (effective 2000). adv. back issues avail. **Document type:** *Consumer, Trade.* **Description:** Compiles dosing and administration information, along with indications and contraindications for skin-treatment medications.
Published by: Elea Ciencia Editorial Ltda., Rua Haddock Lobo, 86 Andar 6, Estacio, Rio De Janeiro, RJ 20260-132, Brazil. TEL 55-21-293-2112, FAX 55-21-293-7818, elea@openlink.com.br. Ed. Luiz Augusto Rodrigues. Adv. contact Alexandre Augusto Rodrigues. Circ: 4,500.

615.9 616.99 BRA ISSN 1414-0284
GLOSSARIUM ONCOLOGIA. Text in Portuguese. 1995. a. BRL 40, USD 48 (effective 2000). adv. back issues avail. **Document type:** *Consumer, Trade.* **Description:** Supplies dosing and administration, along with indications and contraindications for cancer medications.
Published by: Elea Ciencia Editorial Ltda., Rua Haddock Lobo, 86 Andar 6, Estacio, Rio De Janeiro, RJ 20260-132, Brazil. TEL 55-21-293-2112, FAX 55-21-293-7818, elea@openlink.com.br. Ed. Luiz Augusto Rodrigues. Adv. contact Alexandre Augusto Rodrigues.

615 CHN ISSN 1000-8535
R97.7.C5
GUANGZHOU YIYAO/GUANGZHOU MEDICINE AND PHARMACOLOGY. Text in Chinese. 1970. bi-m. CNY 2 per issue. **Document type:** *Academic/Scholarly.*
Published by: Guangzhou Weisheng Ju/Guangzhou Health Bureau, No 484, Renmin Beilu, Guangzhou, Guangdong 510180, China. TEL 8853547. Ed. Yan Shufeng.

615.1 FRA ISSN 1155-1852
GUIDE NATIONAL DE PRESCRIPTION DES MEDICAMENTS✶. Abbreviated title: G N P. Text in French. 1987. a. FRF 370; FRF 390 foreign. **Description:** Provides product category information and selection, 8,000 ethical pharmaceuticals classified.
Published by: O.V.P. - Editions du Vidal, 33 av. de Wagram, Paris Cedex 17 75854, France. TEL 47-23-90-91, FAX 47-20-72-89, TELEX OVP 643 506 F. Circ: 10,000. **Dist. by:** EM-INTER, Allee de la Croix-Bossee, Cachan Cedex 94234, France. TEL 45-46-15-00.

615 USA ISSN 1098-0539
RM301.27
GUINEA PIG ZERO; a journal for human research subjects. Text in English. 1996. irreg. USD 15 domestic to individuals for 4 nos.; USD 20 in Canada & Mexico to individuals for 4 nos.; USD 24 out of North America to individuals for 4 nos.; USD 5 newsstand/cover domestic; USD 8 newsstand/cover in Canada (effective 2001). adv. bk.rev., film rev., play rev., tel.rev., video rev. illus, maps, tr.mk. back issues avail. *Refereed.* **Document type:** *Journal, Consumer, Trade.* **Description:** Serves as an occupational jobzine for people who are used as medical or pharmaceutical research subjects. Various sections are devoted to bioethics, historical facts, current news and research, evaluations of particular research facilities by volunteers, and true stories of guinea pig adventures.
Published by: Robert Helms, Ed. & Pub., PO Box 42531, Philadelphia, PA 19101. TEL 215-727-3582, gpzero@earthlink.net, gpzero@netaxs.com, http://www.guineapigzero.com, http://www.geocities.com/hotsprings/villa/2529/., http://hop.to/guineapigzero. R&P, Adv. contact Robert Helms. page USD 100; trim 5.5 x 8.5. Circ: 4,000.

615 CHN
GUOWAI YIXUE (YAOXUE FENCE)✶/FOREIGN MEDICAL SCIENCES (PHARMACY). Text in Chinese. bi-m. USD 17.40; USD 2.90 newsstand/cover (effective 2001).
Published by: (Junshi Yixue Kexueyuan, Duwu Yaowu Jianjiusuo/Military Academy of Medical Sciences, Institute of Poisonous and Medical Substances), China International Book Trading Corp/Zhongguo Guoji Tushu Maoyi Zonggongsi cibtc@mail.cibtc.com.cn, http://www.cibtc.com.cn. Ed. Zhang Qikai. **Dist. by:** 35, Chegongzhuang Xilu, Haidian District, Beijing 100044, China.

615.329 CHN ISSN 1001-8751
GUOWAI YIYAO (KANGSHENGSU FENCE)/WORLD NOTES ON ANTIBIOTICS. Text in Chinese. bi-m. USD 110 (effective 2000). **Document type:** *Academic/Scholarly.*
Published by: Sichuan Kangjunsu Gongye Yanjiusuo/Sichuan Industrial Institute of Antibiotics, 18, Shanbanqiao Lu, Chengdu, Sichuan 610051, China. TEL 86-28-4381243, FAX 86-28-4381243, cjap@mail.sc.cninfo.net.

615 CHN ISSN 1001-6856
GUOWAI YIYAO (ZHIWUYAO FENCE)/WORLD NOTES ON HERBAL MEDICINE. Text in Chinese. bi-m.
Published by: Guojia Yiyao Guanli-ju, Tianjin Yaowu Yanjiusuo, 308 Anshan Xidao, Tianjin 300193, China. TEL 711320. Ed. Liu Deyan.

615 659.1 USA
H M C NEWS✶. Text in English. 9/yr. membership only. **Document type:** *Trade.*
Formerly: P A Cer
Published by: H M C Council, Inc., 1525 Valley Center Pkwy, #150, Bethlehem, PA 18017-2279. Circ: 6,000.

615 JPN
H O P NYUSU/HOKKAIDO HOSPITAL PHARMACISTS' NEWSLETTER. Text in Japanese. 1991. s-a. **Document type:** *Newsletter.*
Published by: Hokkaido Byoin Yakuzaishikai, Hokkaido Daigaku Fuzoku Byoin Yakuzaibu, Nishi 5-chome, Kita 14-jo, Kita-ku, Sapporo-shi, Hokkaido 060, Japan.

H S R: HEALTH SUPPLEMENT RETAILER. see *NUTRITION AND DIETETICS*

615 SWE ISSN 1102-3899
HAELSOKURIREN; tidningen om haelsa och egenvaard. Text in Swedish. 1991. q.

P

Published by: Svenska Defence, Fack 812, Sundsvall 85123, Sweden.

615 SWE ISSN 0346-9751
HAESSLE INFORMATION. Text in Swedish. 1967. 10/yr. free per issue. charts, illus, stat. back issues avail. *Refereed.* **Description:** Provides a forum for doctors, hospitals and pharmacies for the exchange of medical information.
Published by: Haessle Laekemedel, Moelndal 43183, Sweden. TEL 46-31-776-3500, FAX 46-31-776-3501, info@hlakemedel.se.astra.com. Ed., R&P Marianne Hein. Circ: 18,500.

615.19 USA ISSN 0171-2004
CODEN: HEPHD2
HANDBOOK OF EXPERIMENTAL PHARMACOLOGY. Text in English. 1950. irreg., latest vol.120, 1996. price varies. reprint service avail. from ISI. **Document type:** *Academic/Scholarly.*
Indexed: Chem.Abstr., Chem.Indus.Notes, Chem.Titles.
—BLDSC (4250.460000), CASDDS, CISTI, ingenta. **CCC.**
Published by: Springer-Verlag, Journals (Subsidiary of: BertelsmannSpringer), 175 Fifth Ave, New York, NY 10010. TEL 212-460-1500, FAX 212-473-6272.

HANDBOOK OF NATURAL TOXINS. see *MEDICAL SCIENCES*

615 USA ISSN 0889-7816
RS250
HANDBOOK OF NON-PRESCRIPTION DRUGS. Text in English. 1967. irreg. **Document type:** *Monographic series.*
—CCC.
Published by: American Pharmaceutical Association, 2215 Constitution Ave, N W, Washington, DC 20037. TEL 202-628-4410.

615.9 USA
HANDBOOK ON INJECTABLE DRUGS. Text in English. 1976. base vol. plus biennial updates. USD 169.95 to non members; USD 139.95 to members (effective 2001). 1430 p./no. Supplement avail. **Document type:** *Academic/Scholarly.* **Description:** Comprehensive coverage of injectable drugs used in admixtures including investigational drugs. Monographs are cross-referenced and arranged according to non-proprietary name.
Related titles: CD-ROM ed.; Online - full text ed.: (from The Dialog Corporation).
Published by: American Society of Health-System Pharmacists, Product Development Office, 7272 Wisconsin Ave, Bethesda, MD 20814. TEL 301-657-3000, FAX 301-657-1251, 301-657-8857, pdiso@ashp.org, http://www.ashp.org. Ed. Lawrence A Trissel.

615.7 USA ISSN 1092-048X
HANSTEN AND HORN'S DRUG INTERACTIONS ANALYSIS AND MANAGEMENT*. Text in English. 1981. base vol. plus q. updates. USD 169 (effective 2000). adv. back issues avail. **Document type:** *Newsletter, Academic/Scholarly.* **Description:** Concise and authoritative guide to drug interactions. Includes a comprehensive index.
Supersedes: Drug Interactions and Updates; Former titles: Drug Interactions (Vancouver); (until vol.8, no.11, 1989): Drug Interactions Newsletter (0271-8707); Incorporates (in 1989): Drug Interactions (Philadelphia)
Indexed: I.P.A., Inpharma, Pharm.&Out.News, Reac.
—BLDSC (4262.337500), GNLM.
Published by: (Applied Therapeutics, Inc.), Facts and Comparisons, 111 W. Port Plaza, Ste. 300, St. Louis, MO 63146-3098. TEL 800-223-0554, FAX 314-878-5563. Eds. John R Horn, Philip D Hansten. R&P, Adv. contact Steven Naught.

615 CHN ISSN 1001-8131
HARBIN YIYAO/HARBIN MEDICINE. Text in Chinese. q.
Published by: Zhonghua Yixuehui (Harbin Fenhui)/Chinese Medical Association (Harbin Branch), 34, Xi 5 Daojie, Daoli-qu, Harbin, Heilongjiang 150010, China. TEL 413165. Ed. Zhao Zhongwu.

615 USA
HARPER HOSPITAL, PHARMACY & THERAPEUTICS NEWSLETTER. Text in English. 1970. bi-m. free per issue. **Document type:** *Newsletter.*
Former titles: Harper-Grace Hospitals, Pharmacy and Therapeutics Newsletter; Harper-Grace Hospital Drug Therapy Newsletter; Grace Hospital Drug Therapy Newsletter
Media: Duplicated (not offset).
Published by: Harper Hospital (Detroit), 3990 John, Detroit, MI 48201. TEL 313-745-2006, FAX 313-745-1793. Ed. Margo Farber. Circ: 500.

615 JPN ISSN 0914-9864
HATTATSU YAKURI YAKUBUTSU CHIRYO KENKYUKAI ZASSHI/JAPANESE JOURNAL OF DEVELOPMENTAL AND THERAPEUTIC PHARMACOLOGY. Text in Japanese; Summaries in English. 1988. a.
—BLDSC (4651.630000).
Published by: Hattatsu Yakuri Yakubutsu Chiryo Kenkyukai, Asahikawa Ika Daigaku Shonika, 3-11, 5-go, Nishikagura 4-sen, Asahikawa-shi, Hokkaido 078, Japan.

615 DEU
HAUSAPOTHEKE. Text in German. a. **Document type:** *Bulletin, Consumer.*
Published by: Otto Hoffmanns Verlag GmbH, Arnulfstr 10, Munich 80335, Germany. TEL 49-89-545845-0, FAX 49-89-54584520. adv.: B&W page DEM 32,500, color page DEM 44,200; trim 175 x 112. Circ: 1,850,000 (controlled).

615.1 USA ISSN 0073-1420
HAYES DRUGGIST DIRECTORY*. Text in English. 1912. a. USD 390.
Published by: Edward N. Hayes, Ed. & Pub., PO Box 3436, Mission Viejo, CA 92690-1436. TEL 714-756-9063, FAX 714-756-0921.

615.1 USA ISSN 1096-9160
HD9666.1
HEALTHCARE DISTRIBUTOR; the industry's multi-market information resource. Text in English. 1948. bi-m. USD 30; USD 5 newsstand/cover (effective 2001). adv. charts, illus, tr.lit, stat. back issues avail.; reprints avail. **Document type:** *Journal, Trade.* **Description:** Covers news as it affects the wholesale drug, chain drug industries, home-health care. Distributed nationwide as well as in Canada and abroad.
Formerly (until 1997): Wholesale Drugs Magazine (0743-3778)
Indexed: I.P.A.
Published by: E L F Publications, 5285 W Louisiana Ave, Ste 112, Lakewood, CO 80232-5976. TEL 303-975-0075, 800-922-8513, FAX 303-975-0132, elfedit@qwest.net, elfpub@qwest.net, http://www.elfpublications.com. Ed. Chuck Austin. Pubs. Judith D Lane, Ronald R Quam. Adv. contact Jerry Lester. B&W page USD 2,475; trim 10.88 x 8.38. Circ: 14,000 (controlled).

615.1 CHE ISSN 1422-9528
▼ **HEART DRUG.** Variant title: HeartDrug. Text in English. 2000. 6/yr. CHF 891, EUR 636.80 in Europe to institutions; CHF 908.40, USD 694 elsewhere to institutions (effective 2002). adv. **Document type:** *Journal, Academic/Scholarly.* **Description:** Provides a forum of high quality for researchers with a strong drive to achieve clinical results in the study of cardiovascular disorders.
Related titles: Online - full text ed.: ISSN 1424-0556. CHF 58, EUR 42, USD 45 to institutions with print edition (effective 2002) (from EBSCO Publishing, Swets Blackwell, RoweCom Information Quest).
—BLDSC (4275.327000).
Published by: S. Karger AG, Allschwilerstr 10, PO Box, Basel 4009, Switzerland. TEL 41-61-306-1111, FAX 41-61-306-1234, karger@karger.ch, http://www.online.karger.com/journals/hed, http://www.karger.com. Eds. D Atar, H Kusuoka, V L Serebruany. adv.: page USD 1,185.

615 CHN
HEBEI YIYAO/JOURNAL OF HEBEI MEDICINE. Text in Chinese. 1973. bi-m. **Document type:** *Academic/Scholarly.*
Published by: Hebei Yixue Kexueyuan/Hebei Academy of Medical Sciences, 62 Qingyuan Jie, Shijiazhuang, Hebei 050021, China. TEL 0311-612687. Ed. Wang Rongjie.

615 840 DEU
HEILMITTELWERBEGESETZ. Text in German. base vol. plus irreg. updates. DEM 250 per base vol.. **Document type:** *Monographic series.*
Published by: P M I Verlag AG, August-Schanz-Str 8, Frankfurt Am Main 60433, Germany. TEL 49-69-548000-0, FAX 49-69-548000-77, pmiverlag@aol.com.

HERBALGRAM; the journal of the American botanical council & the herb research foundation. see *BIOLOGY—Botany*

615.329 IND ISSN 0018-1935
RM265 CODEN: HINAAU
HINDUSTAN ANTIBIOTICS BULLETIN. Text in English. 1958. q. INR 200; USD 50 foreign (effective 2001). adv. bk.rev. bibl, charts, illus. index. 70 p./no. 2 cols./p. back issues avail. *Refereed.* **Document type:** *Bulletin.* **Description:** Features research articles and reviews on all aspects of microbial metabolites all over the world.
Indexed: Bio-Contr.News & Info., Biol.Abstr., Chem.Abstr., Chem.Indus.Notes, Chem.Titles, Excerp.Med., Ind.Med. (1958-), Indian Sci.Abstr., Rev.Appl.Entomol., Rev.Plant Path.
—BLDSC (4315.100000), CASDDS, CISTI, GNLM, KNAW, Linda Hall.
Published by: Hindustan Antibiotics Ltd., Editorial and Advertisement Office, Pimpri, Pune, Maharashtra 411 018, India. TEL 91-20-7476511, FAX 91-212-772327, hapune@pn3.vsnl.net.in, http://www.hindantibiotics.com. Ed., R&P, Adv. contact Dr. R K Nanda. Circ: 400.

615 JPN ISSN 0388-2616
CODEN: HBYNDA
HIROSHIMAKEN BYOIN YAKUZAISHIKAI GAKUJUTSU NENPO/HIROSHIMA SOCIETY OF HOSPITAL PHARMACISTS. ANNUAL RESEARCH REPORT. Text in Japanese. 1975. a. **Document type:** *Academic/Scholarly.*
Indexed: Chem.Abstr., Chem.Indus.Notes, Chem.Titles.
—CASDDS.
Published by: Hiroshimaken Byoin Yakuzaishikai, Daigaku Igakubu Byoin Yakuzaibu, 2-3 Kasumi 1-chome, Minami-ku, Hiroshima-shi 734-0037, Japan. Ed. Yoshida Minoru.

615 JPN ISSN 0389-4061
HIROSHIMAKEN HOSPITAL PHARMACISTS ASSOCIATION. DRUG INFORMATION NEWS. Text in Japanese. 1973. q. **Document type:** *Newsletter.*
Published by: Hiroshimaken Byoin Yakuzaishikai, Daigaku Igakubu Byoin Yakuzaibu, 2-3 Kasumi 1-chome, Minami-ku, Hiroshima-shi 734-0037, Japan. Ed. Masayoshi Okigawa.

HIV AND AIDS TREATMENTS DIRECTORY. see *MEDICAL SCIENCES—Communicable Diseases*

615 JPN ISSN 0917-0936
HOKKAIDO BYOIN YAKUZAISHIKAISHI/HOKKAIDO SOCIETY OF HOSPITAL PHARMACISTS. JOURNAL. Text in Japanese. 1960. s-a.
Published by: Hokkaido Byoin Yakuzaishikai, Hokkaido Daigaku Fuzoku Byoin Yakuzaibu, Nishi 5-chome, Kita 14-jo, Kita-ku, Sapporo-shi, Hokkaido 060, Japan.

615 JPN ISSN 0917-5245
HOKURIKU DAIGAKU YAKUGAKUBU SOYAKU KENKYU SHISETSU NENPO/HOKURIKU UNIVERSITY. RESEARCH LABORATORY FOR DEVELOPMENT OF MEDICINE. ANNUAL REPORT OF ACTIVITIES. Text in English, Japanese; Summaries in English. 1988. a.
Published by: Hokuriku Daigaku, Yakugakubu Soyaku Kenkyu Shisetsu, Ho-3, Kanakawamachi, Kanazawa-shi, Ishikawa-ken 920-1148, Japan.

HOME HEALTH PRODUCTS. see *MEDICAL SCIENCES*

615 JPN ISSN 0441-2559
CODEN: HYDKAK
HOSHI YAKKA DAIGAKU KIYO/HOSHI COLLEGE OF PHARMACY. ANNUAL REPORT. Text in English, Japanese; Summaries in English. 1951. a.
Indexed: Biol.Abstr., Chem.Abstr.
Published by: Hoshi Yakka Daigaku, 4-41 Ebara 2-chome, Shinagawa-ku, Tokyo 142-8501, Japan.

615 GBR ISSN 1352-7967
THE HOSPITAL PHARMACIST. Text in English. 1994. 10/yr. GBP 68 in United Kingdom; GBP 82 in the European Union; GBP 90 rest of world; GBP 7 newsstand/cover in United Kingdom (effective 2001); Free for members. adv. back issues avail. **Document type:** *Academic/Scholarly.* **Description:** Provides coverage of material devoted to hospital pharmacists.
Related titles: Online - full text ed.: (from RoweCom Information Quest).
Indexed: I.P.A.
—BLDSC (4333.206900).
Published by: (Euromed Communications Ltd.), Pharmaceutical Press (Subsidiary of: Euromed Communications Ltd.), 1 Lambeth High St, London SE1 7JN, United Kingdom. TEL 44-20-7735-9141, FAX 44-20-7735-5085, http://www.pharmj.com/Hospital/CurrentContents.html. Ed. Diane Langleben. Pub., R&P Charles Fry. Adv. contact Jack Richmond. Circ: 6,500.

P

615 USA ISSN 1052-3146
CODEN: HPRPEC

HOSPITAL PHARMACIST REPORT. Text in English. 1987. m. USD 39 domestic; USD 55 foreign; USD 10 newsstand/cover (effective 2001). adv. **Document type:** *Trade.* **Description:** Reports on clinical, professional, business, government and legal news and trends affecting hospital pharmacy management.
Related titles: Microform ed.: (from PQC).
Indexed: I.P.A.
—GNLM. **CCC.**
Published by: Medical Economics Co., Inc., 5 Paragon Dr, Montvale, NJ 07645-1742. TEL 201-358-7200. Ed. Valentine Cardinale. Circ: 30,000.

615.1 USA ISSN 0018-5787
CODEN: HOPHAZ

HOSPITAL PHARMACY. Text in English. 1966. m. USD 124.95 domestic to individuals; USD 184 foreign to individuals; USD 189.95 domestic to institutions; USD 208 foreign to institutions; USD 17 newsstand/cover (effective 2002). adv. illus. index. **Document type:** *Academic/Scholarly.*
Related titles: Microform ed.: (from PQC); Online - full text ed.: (from Ovid Technologies, Inc., Institute for Scientific Information).
Indexed: Abstr.Health Care Manage.Stud., Biol.Abstr., Excerp.Med., Hosp.Lit.Ind., I.P.A.
—BLDSC (4333.207200), GNLM, ingenta, KNAW, Linda Hall.
Published by: Lippincott Williams & Wilkins, 345 Hudson St, 16th Fl, New York, NY 10014-4502. TEL 212-840-7760, FAX 212-840-7813, http://www.lrpub.com. Ed. Neil M Davis. Pub. Nhora Cortes Comerer. R&P Kyle Booth. adv.: B&W page USD 2,980. Circ: 30,425.

615.9 610.73 USA ISSN 0739-957X

HOSPITAL PHARMACY DIRECTOR'S MONTHLY MANAGEMENT SERIES. Text in English. 1979. m. USD 50 (effective 2001). **Description:** Contains practical management information for pharmacy managers.
Published by: Rx-Data-Pac Service, 8907 Terwilliger s Tr, Cincinnati, OH 45249. TEL 513-489-0943, FAX 513-489-0943.

615.1 CAN

HOSPITAL PHARMACY IN ONTARIO✱. Text in English. 1964. q. membership. **Document type:** *Newsletter.*
Published by: Canadian Society of Hospital Pharmacists, Ontario Branch, 1145 Hunt Club Rd, Ste 350, Ottawa, ON K1V 0Y3, Canada. TEL 613-730-6228. Ed. Rosemarie Pavlakovic. Circ: 1,000.

615.19 658 USA ISSN 0739-9561

HOSPITAL PHARMACY SERVICE INSTANT UP-DATE. Text in English. 1978. m. USD 75 (effective 2001). back issues avail. **Description:** Contains current data with "its-a-fact" quizzes, to help meet JCAHO requirements for in-service staff. Includes photocopy rights.
Published by: Rx-Data-Pac Service, 8907 Terwilliger s Tr, Cincinnati, OH 45249. TEL 513-489-0943, FAX 513-489-0943. Ed. Dr. I H Goodman.

615 CHN ISSN 1006-0103
CODEN: HYZAE2

HUAXI YAOXUE ZAZHI/WEST CHINA JOURNAL OF PHARMACEUTICAL SCIENCES. Text in Chinese. 1985. q. CNY 3 newsstand/cover.
Indexed: Chem.Abstr., Chem.Indus.Notes, Chem.Titles, Mass Spectr.Bull.
—BLDSC (9298.863200), CASDDS.
Published by: Huaxi Yike Daxue/West China University of Medical Sciences, Yao Xueyuan, 17 Renmin Nanlu 3 Duan, Chengdu, Sichuan 610041, China. TEL 86-28-550-1400, FAX 86-28-558-7960.

HUAXI YIKE DAXUE XUEBAO/WEST CHINA UNIVERSITY OF MEDICAL SCIENCES. JOURNAL. see *MEDICAL SCIENCES*

HUMAN & EXPERIMENTAL TOXICOLOGY; an international journal. see *ENVIRONMENTAL STUDIES—Toxicology And Environmental Safety*

HUMAN PSYCHOPHARMACOLOGY: CLINICAL AND EXPERIMENTAL. see *MEDICAL SCIENCES—Psychiatry And Neurology*

HUMAN REPRODUCTION. see *MEDICAL SCIENCES—Obstetrics And Gynecology*

615 JPN ISSN 0916-7587

HYOGOKEN YAKUZAISHIKAISHI/HYOGO PHARMACEUTICAL SOCIETY. JOURNAL. Text in Japanese. 1951. m. JPY 300 per issue.
Published by: Hyogoken Yakuzaishikai, 45-3 Shimoyama-Tedori 6-chome, Chuo-ku, Kobe-shi, Hyogo-ken 650-0011, Japan.

615.1 JPN

I C H E5 HANDBOOK (YEAR). Text in English. a. USD 60 (effective 2001).
Related titles: Japanese ed.
Published by: Yakuji Nippo Ltd., 1 Kanda-Izumi-cho, Chiyoda-ku, Tokyo 101-8648, Japan. TEL 81-3-3862-2141, FAX 81-3-3866-8495, shuppan@yakuji.co.jp, http://www.yakuji.co.jp/.

615.1 IND

I D M A ANNUAL PUBLICATION. Text in English. 1963. a. INR 725 per issue. **Document type:** *Trade.*
Published by: Indian Drug Manufacturers' Association, 102 B Poonan Chambers, Dr. A.B. Rd., Worli, Mumbai, Maharashtra 400 018, India. TEL 91-22-494-4624, 91-22-497-4308, FAX 91-22-495-0723, idma@vsnl.com, http://www.idma-assn.org.

615.1 IND ISSN 0970-6054

I D M A BULLETIN. Text in English. 1970. w. INR 3,000 to non-members; INR 1,000 to members (effective 1999 & 2000); INR 25 newsstand/cover. **Document type:** *Bulletin, Trade.* **Description:** Discusses topics of interest to professionals in the Indian pharmaceutical manufacturing industry.
Indexed: INIS Atomind.
—BLDSC (4362.490500).
Published by: Indian Drug Manufacturers' Association, 102 B Poonan Chambers, Dr. A.B. Rd., Worli, Mumbai, Maharashtra 400 018, India. TEL 91-22-494-4624, 91-22-497-4308, FAX 91-22-495-0723, idma@vsnl.com, http://www.idma-assn.org.

615.19005 GBR ISSN 1369-7056

I DRUGS: THE INVESTIGATIONAL DRUGS JOURNAL. (Investigational) Variant title: 1 Drugs. Text in English. 1997. m. GBP 800, USD 1,300 to individuals; GBP 1,575, USD 2,600 to institutions (effective 2001 - 2002). **Document type:** *Journal, Academic/Scholarly, Trade.* **Description:** Presents information disclosed at scientific meetings as well as a selection of expert evaluations of investigational drugs and reviews highlighting important issues in drug research and analysis.
Published by: Current Drugs Ltd., 34-42 Cleveland St, Middlesex House, London W1P 6LB, United Kingdom. TEL 44-207-580-8393, FAX 44-207-580-5646, info@current-drugs.com, http://www.current-drugs.com. Ed. Tara Dyson. **Subscr. to:** Current Drugs Ltd., 400 Market St, Ste 700, Philadelphia, PA 19106. TEL 215-721-9700, FAX 215-721-9287.

615.1 NLD ISSN 1024-0268

I P S F NEWS BULLETIN. Text in English, French, German, Spanish. 1960. 3/yr., latest 2001. free to members. adv. charts, illus. index. 30 p./no. 2 cols./p. *Refereed.* **Document type:** *Bulletin, Trade, Newspaper-distributed.* **Description:** Contains articles, news, information and a calendar of worldwide pharmaceutical events of interest to pharmaceutical students.
Related titles: Online - full content ed.
Indexed: I.P.A.
Published by: International Pharmaceutical Students Federation, Andries Bickerweg 5, The Hague 2517 JP, Netherlands. TEL 31-70-3021992, FAX 31-70-3021999, ipsf@ipsf.org, http://www.ips.org, http://www.ipsf.org. adv.: page USD 700. Circ: 3,100 (controlled).

615 IRL ISSN 0332-2130

I P U REVIEW. Text in English. 1976. 11/yr. IEP 30 (effective 1998). adv. bk.rev. **Document type:** *Trade.* **Description:** Primary objectives are to reflect the authentic views of the pharmaceutical profession, to acquaint pharmacists of Union policy and information, and to ensure that developments in pharmacy are published and commented on as they occur.
Indexed: I.P.A.
Published by: Irish Pharmaceutical Union, 140 Grange Rd., Dublin 14, Ireland. TEL 01-4931801, FAX 01-4951082. Ed. David Butler. Adv. contact Michael Ryan. B&W page IEP 350, color page IEP 560; trim 297 x 210. Circ: 1,600.

I V S. (Index of Veterinary Specialists) see *VETERINARY SCIENCE*

I V S DESK REFERENCE. (Index of Veterinary Specialists) see *VETERINARY SCIENCE*

615 JPN ISSN 0285-1199

ICHIYAKU SOMOKU TSUSHIN. Text in Japanese. bi-m.
Published by: Daiichi Seiyaku Co. Ltd., 14-10 Nihonbashi 3-chome, Chuo-ku, Tokyo 103-0027, Japan.

615.1 USA ISSN 0019-1221

IDAHO PHARMACIST✱. Text in English. 1964. s-a. USD 15. adv. stat. **Document type:** *Newsletter.* **Description:** For registered pharmacists, pharmacies, hospitals, wholesale drug houses, colleges of pharmacy faculty members and students, drug travelers, nursing associations.
Indexed: I.P.A.
Published by: Idaho State Pharmacy Association, Inc., PO Box 140117, Boise, ID 83714-0117. TEL 208-376-2273, FAX 208-376-5814, condie@micron.net. Ed., R&P, Adv. contact Jo An Condie. page USD 275; trim 9.75 x 7.5. Circ: 500.

615 JPN ISSN 0389-3898
CODEN: IGYAEI

IGAKU TO YAKUGAKU/JOURNAL OF MEDICINE AND PHARMACEUTICAL SCIENCE. Text in Japanese. 1975. m. JPY 2,000 per issue.
Indexed: Chem.Abstr., Chem.Indus.Notes, Chem.Titles, Inpharma, Reac.
—CASDDS, GNLM.
Published by: Shizen Kagakusha Co. Ltd., 1-4 Iida-Bashi 2-chome, Chiyoda-ku, Tokyo 102-0072, Japan. TEL 81-3-3813-5401.

615.1 USA ISSN 0195-2099

ILLINOIS PHARMACIST. Text in English. 1977. bi-m. USD 36 (effective 2001). adv. tr.lit. back issues avail.; reprint service avail. from PQC. **Document type:** *Journal, Trade.*
Formerly: Illinois Journal of Pharmacy (0147-8222); Which was formed by the merger of (1963-1977): Illinois Pharmacist (0019-2163); (1904-1977): C R D A News (0007-9030)
Related titles: Microform ed.: (from PQC).
Indexed: I.P.A.
—Linda Hall. **CCC.**
Published by: Illinois Pharmacists Association, 204 W Cook St, Springfield, IL 62704-2526. TEL 217-522-7300, FAX 217-522-7349, ipha@ipha.org, http://www.ipha.org. Ed. Terri McEntaffer. Adv. contact Judith Ramsden. Circ: 42,024.

615 616.9 USA

IMMUNOFACTS VACCINES & IMMUNOLOGIC DRUGS. Text in English. 1993. base vol. plus s-a. updates. USD 125; USD 143.80 foreign (effective 1999). Supplement avail. **Description:** Provides information on all vaccines, toxoids, immune globulins, immunologic mediators and modulators, hypersensitivity agents and related non-immunologics.
Published by: Facts and Comparisons, 111 W. Port Plaza, Ste. 300, St. Louis, MO 63146-3098. TEL 800-223-0554, FAX 314-878-5563.

615 USA ISSN 0892-3973
CODEN: IITOEF

IMMUNOPHARMACOLOGY AND IMMUNOTOXICOLOGY. Text in English. 1979. q. USD 95 to individuals print and online eds.; USD 995 to institutions print only (effective 2002). adv. *Refereed.* **Document type:** *Academic/Scholarly.* **Description:** Offers readers an interdisciplinary approach to subjects integrating pharmacology and toxicology with immunology.
Former titles: Journal of Pharmacology and Immunotoxicology; Journal of Immunopharmacology (0163-0571)
Related titles: Microform ed.: (from RPI); Online - full content ed.; Online - full text ed.: (from Institute for Scientific Information, RoweCom Information Quest).
Indexed: AIDS & Cancer Res., ASCA, Agri.& Environ.Biotech.Abstr. (coverage dropped), Anim.Breed.Abstr., Aqua.Sci.& Fish.Abstr., Biol.Abstr., Biol.Dig., Chem.Abstr., Chem.Indus.Notes, Chem.Titles, Curr.Adv.Ecol.Sci., Curr.Cont., Derwent Biotech.Abstr., Environ.Sci.Poll.Mgmt., Excerp.Med., Helminthol.Abstr., INIS Atomind., Immun.Abstr., Ind.Med. (1987-), Ind.Sci.Rev., Ind.Vet., Inpharma, Int.Abstr.Biol.Sci., Microbiol.Abstr., Pharm.&Out.News, Pollut.Abstr., Poult.Abstr., Protozool.Abstr., Reac., Ref.Zh., Rev.Arom.& Med.Plants, Rev.Med.& Vet.Mycol., Risk Abstr., Saf.Sci.Abstr., Sci.Cit.Ind., Sugar Ind.Abstr., Tox.Abstr., Trop.Dis.Bull., Vet.Bull.
—BLDSC (4369.760200), CASDDS, CISTI, EMDOCS, GNLM, IDS, Infotrieve, ingenta, KNAW. **CCC.**
Published by: Marcel Dekker Inc., 270 Madison Ave, New York, NY 10016. TEL 212-696-9000, 800-228-1160, FAX 212-685-4540, http://www.dekker.com/servlet/product/productid/IPH. Ed. Michael A Chirigos. R&P Julia Mulligan. Adv. contact Diane Saulon. B&W page USD 800. Circ: 325.

615 GBR ISSN 0963-0759
THE INDEPENDENT COMMUNITY PHARMACIST. Text in English. 1990. m. GBP 45 (effective 2000). adv. bk.rev. **Document type:** *Trade.*
Published by: Independent Community Pharmacist, Plestor House, Farnham Rd, W Liss, Hants GU33 6JQ, United Kingdom. TEL 44-1703-894059, FAX 44-1703-895298. Ed. Richard Thomas. Pub. Paul Fenton. Adv. contact Ian Mogg. Circ: 10,500.

615.1 IND ISSN 0019-4360
INDIAN & EASTERN PHARMACY✱. Text in English. 1968. m. INR 40.
Published by: L. K. Pandeya Ed. & Pub., Block F, 105 C New Alipore, Kolkata, West Bengal 700 053, India.

615.1 IND ISSN 0019-462X
HD9672.I5 CODEN: INDRBA
INDIAN DRUGS. Text in English. 1963. 15/yr. INR 1,000, USD 300 (effective 2001). adv. bk.rev. charts, tr.lit. **Document type:** *Trade.*
Indexed: Anal.Abstr., Biol.Abstr., Chem.Abstr., Chem.Indus.Notes, Chem.Titles, Excerp.Med., INIS Atomind., I.P.A.
—BLDSC (4396.180000), CASDDS, GNLM, ingenta, KNAW.
Published by: (Indian Drug Manufacturers' Association), Scientific Publishers, 5-A New Pali Rd., P O Box 91, Jodhpur, Rajasthan 342 001, India. TEL 91-291-433323, FAX 91-291-512580, scienti@sancharnet.in, http://www.scientificpub.com. Circ: 6,000.

615.1 IND ISSN 0019-4638
CODEN: IDPIA6
INDIAN DRUGS AND PHARMACEUTICALS INDUSTRY. Text in English. 1966. bi-m. INR 20. adv. bk.rev. illus, stat.
—CASDDS.
Published by: Chary Publications, 14 Sidh Prasad, Ghatkopar Mahul Rd., Tilak Nagar, Mumbai, Maharashtra 400 089, India. Ed. S T Chary. Circ: 4,000.

615.1 IND ISSN 0019-526X
RA975.5.P5 CODEN: IJHPBU
INDIAN JOURNAL OF HOSPITAL PHARMACY. Text in English. 1965. bi-m. INR 400, USD 200 (effective 2000). adv. bk.rev. charts, illus, stat. index. *Refereed.* **Document type:** *Academic/Scholarly.* **Description:** Aims to develop advanced technology for the manufacture of several vital drugs ranging from antiasthmatics and cardiovascular medicines to antibacterials, antiarthritics, antiparasitics and medical aerosols.
Related titles: Online - full text ed.
Indexed: Biol.Abstr., Chem.Abstr., Chem.Indus.Notes, Chem.Titles, Excerp.Med., I.P.A.
—CASDDS, CISTI, GNLM, Linda Hall.
Published by: Indian Hospital Pharmacists' Association, R-566 New Rajinder Nagar, New Delhi 110 060, India. TEL 91-11-5754344. Ed. B D Miglani. Adv. contact A K Adhikari. page INR 1,000; 160 x 220. Circ: 5,000 (paid).

615.1 IND ISSN 0019-5464
RS119.I5 CODEN: IJPEB3
INDIAN JOURNAL OF PHARMACEUTICAL EDUCATION. Text in English. 1967. q. INR 1,000, USD 100 (effective 2001). adv. bk.rev. abstracted in international pharma abstract. 44 p./no. 2 cols./p. *Refereed.* **Document type:** *Journal, Academic/Scholarly.*
Related titles: CD-ROM ed.; Online - full content ed.
Indexed: Biol.Abstr., Chem.Abstr., I.P.A.
—BLDSC (4418.700000), CASDDS, CISTI.
Published by: Association of Pharmaceutical Teachers of India, c/o J.S.S. College of Pharmacy, S.S Nagara, Mysore, Karnataka 570 015, India. TEL 91-821-497583, FAX 91-821-495900, TELEX 833209 VVHC IN, jsspharma@mailcity.com, www.ijpc.org. Ed., Pub. B G Nagavi. Circ: 1,400.

615.1 IND ISSN 0250-474X
CODEN: IJSIDW
INDIAN JOURNAL OF PHARMACEUTICAL SCIENCES. Text in English. 1939. bi-m. INR 1,500, USD 100 (effective 2001). adv. bk.rev. reprint service avail. from PQC. *Refereed.* **Document type:** *Journal, Academic/Scholarly.*
Formerly (until 1978): Indian Journal of Pharmacy (0019-5472)
Related titles: CD-ROM ed.; Microfilm ed.: (from PQC); Online - full text ed.
Indexed: Agri.& Environ.Biotech.Abstr. (coverage dropped), Agroforest.Abstr., Anal.Abstr., Biol.Abstr., Chem.Abstr., Chem.Indus.Notes, Chem.Titles, Dairy Sci.Abstr., Derwent Biotech.Abstr., Excerp.Med., ExtraMED, Field Crop Abstr., Forest.Abstr., Helminthol.Abstr., Hort.Abstr., I.P.A., Ind.Vet., Mass Spectr.Bull., Nutr.Abstr., Plant Breed.Abstr., Plant Grow.Reg.Abstr., Postharvest, Protozool.Abstr., Ref.Zh., Rev.Arom.& Med.Plants, Rev.Med.& Vet.Mycol., Rev.Plant Path., Seed Abstr., Soils & Fert., Sugar Ind.Abstr.
—BLDSC (4418.750000), CASDDS, CISTI, EMDOCS, GNLM, ingenta, KNAW, Linda Hall.
Published by: Indian Pharmaceutical Association, Kalina Santacruz East, Mumbai, Maharashtra 400 098, India. TEL 91-22-612-2401, FAX 91-22-614-0480, ipacentr@bol.net.in, http://www.indianpharma.org. Ed. Rao V. S. V. Vadlamudi. adv.: page INR 900; trim 190 x 240. Circ: 1,200.

615 IND ISSN 0253-7613
CODEN: INJPD2
INDIAN JOURNAL OF PHARMACOLOGY. Text in English. 1969. bi-m. INR 2,000, USD 150 (effective 2000). adv. bk.rev. *Refereed.* **Document type:** *Academic/Scholarly.* **Description:** Contains original research articles, and reviews on pharmacology, clinical pharmacology, chemotherapy, ethnopharmacology and molecular biology related to drug action.
Related titles: CD-ROM ed.
Indexed: Biol.Abstr., Chem.Abstr., Chem.Indus.Notes, Chem.Titles, Curr.Adv.Ecol.Sci., Excerp.Med., ExtraMED, INIS Atomind., Nutr.Abstr., Rev.Arom.& Med.Plants, Rev.Med.& Vet.Mycol.
—BLDSC (4418.900000), CASDDS, CISTI, EMDOCS, GNLM, KNAW.
Published by: Indian Pharmacological Society, Department of Pharmacology, Jipmer, Pondicherry, Tamil Nadu 605 006, India. TEL 91-413-372380, FAX 91-413-372067, adithan@biogate.com, ijp@biogate.com, http://www.ijp-online.com. Ed., R&P, Adv. contact C Adithan TEL 91-413-371969. page USD 100. Circ: 1,750.

INDIAN JOURNAL OF PHYSIOLOGY AND PHARMACOLOGY. see *BIOLOGY—Physiology*

615.19 IND
INDIAN PHARMACEUTICAL DIRECTORY. Text in English. 1988. triennial. INR 750, USD 110 (effective 2000). adv. bk.rev. abstr, charts, illus. **Document type:** *Directory.*
Published by: Technical Press Publications, Eucharistic Congress Bldg. No.1, 5/1 Convent St, Colaba, Mumbai, Maharashtra 400 039, India. TEL 91-22-2021446, FAX 91-22-2871499. adv.: B&W page INR 1,750, color page INR 2,250; trim 18 x 23. Circ: 12,000.

615.1 IND ISSN 0073-6635
INDIAN PHARMACEUTICAL GUIDE. Text in English. 1963. a. USD 80 (effective 2000). adv. **Document type:** *Directory.* **Description:** Contains various information on drugs and pharmaceuticals produced in India for local consumption and exports.
Published by: Pamposh Publications, 507 Ashok Bhawan, 93 Nehru Place, New Delhi 110 019, India. TEL 91-11-6432797, FAX 91-11-6225885. Ed. Mohan C Bazaz. Adv. contact Kong Posh. Circ: 5,000.

615 USA ISSN 1083-4974
INDIANA PHARMACIST. Text in English. 1882. q. USD 15 (effective 2001). adv. **Document type:** *Magazine, Trade.* **Description:** Departments include pharmaceutical dynamics (new products, research developments carried as an extension service from the Purdue University School of Pharmacy and Pharmaceutical Sciences), biology, chemistry, pharmacy, including technical material from the Butler University College of Pharmacy.
Indexed: I.P.A.
Published by: Indiana Pharmacists Alliance, 729 N Pennsylvania St, Indianapolis, IN 46204-1171. TEL 317-634-4968, FAX 317-632-1219, http://www.indianapharmacists.org/. Ed. Larry Sage. adv.: B&W page USD 410. Circ: 1,700 (controlled).

615.19 ESP ISSN 0213-5574
INDUSTRIA FARMACEUTICA; investigacion y tecnologia. Text in Spanish. 1986. 6/yr. ESP 13,600, EUR 81.74 in Spain; ESP 18,000, EUR 108.18 in Europe; USD 160 elsewhere; ESP 8,200, EUR 49.28 in Spain to students; ESP 13,000, EUR 78.13 in Europe to students; USD 120 elsewhere to students (effective 2000). adv. bk.rev. illus. index. **Document type:** *Trade.*
Indexed: Ind.SST.
—CINDOC.
Published by: Editorial Alcion S.A., Medea, 4, Madrid 28037, Spain. TEL 34-91-4402920, FAX 34-91-4402931, alcion@tsai.es, http://www.tsai.es/pymes/alcion; http://www.alcion.es. Ed. Ramon R Madrid. Circ: 2,000.

615.1 GBR ISSN 1369-6831
THE INDUSTRIAL PHARMACIST; The Journal of the industrial Pharmacist Group of the Royal Pharmaceutical Society. Text in English. 1997. q. GBP 75 in United Kingdom to non-members; GBP 82 in Europe to non-members; GBP 87 elsewhere to non-members; GBP 25 in United Kingdom to members and qualified personnel; GBP 32 in Europe to members and qualified personnel; GBP 44 elsewhere to members and qualified personnel (effective 2001). adv. bk.rev. **Document type:** *Newsletter, Trade.* **Description:** Contains information on industry trends and products for industrial pharmacists.
Related titles: Online - full text ed.: (from RoweCom Information Quest).
Published by: Euromed Communications Ltd., The Old Surgery, Liphook Rd, Haslemere, Surrey GU27 1NL, United Kingdom. TEL 44-1428-656665, FAX 44-1428-656643, info@euromed.uk.com, http://www.euromed.uk.com/indpharm.htm. Ed. Joe Ridge.

615 BRA ISSN 0104-0219
INFARMA. Text in Portuguese. bi-m. free per issue. bk.rev. illus.
Formerly (until 1991): Brazil. Conselho Federal de Farmacia. Relatorio
Published by: Conselho Federal de Farmacia, SBS Quadra 01, Bloco K, Brasilia, DF 70093900, Brazil. TEL 061-224-68-49, FAX 061-224-68-25. Circ: 10,000 (controlled).

615 NLD ISSN 0923-9405
CODEN: IDTSEQ
INFLAMMATION AND DRUG THERAPY SERIES. Text in English. 1987. irreg., latest vol.5, 1992. price varies. *Refereed.* **Document type:** *Monographic series.*
Indexed: Chem.Abstr., Chem.Indus.Notes, Chem.Titles.
—CASDDS, KNAW.
Published by: Kluwer Academic Publishers Group (Subsidiary of: Wolters Kluwer N.V.), Spuiboulevard 50, PO Box 17, Dordrecht 3300 AA, Netherlands. FAX 31-78-639-2254, services@wkap.nl, http://www.wkap.nl. **Dist. by:** Journals Department, PO Box 322, Dordrecht 3300 AH, Netherlands. FAX 31-78-654-6474.

615 CHE ISSN 1023-3830
RM1 CODEN: INREFB
INFLAMMATION RESEARCH. Text in English. 1969. 14/yr. CHF 1,898, USD 1,357; CHF 164 newsstand/cover (effective 2002). index. *Refereed.* **Document type:** *Journal, Academic/Scholarly.* **Description:** Contains original research papers, short communications, reviews, commentaries, selected reviewed society proceedings and meeting reports on all aspects of inflammation and related fields.
Formerly (until 1995): Agents and Actions (0065-4299)
Related titles: Online - full text ed.: ISSN 1420-908X (from EBSCO Publishing, Swets Blackwell, Springer LINK, Institute for Scientific Information).
Indexed: AIDS & Cancer Res., ASCA, Agri.& Environ.Biotech.Abstr. (coverage dropped), Apic.Abstr., Biol.Abstr., Cal.Tiss.Abstr. (coverage dropped), Chem.Abstr., Chem.Indus.Notes, Chem.Titles, Curr.Adv.Biochem., Curr.Adv.Cancer Res., Curr.Adv.Ecol.Sci., Curr.Cont., Dairy Sci.Abstr., Dent.Ind., Derwent Biotech.Abstr., Environ.Sci.Poll.Mgmt., Excerp.Med., Helminthol.Abstr., Immun.Abstr., Ind.Med. (1995-), Ind.Sci.Rev., Inpharma, Int.Abstr.Biol.Sci., Neurosci.Cit.Ind., Nutr.Abstr., Pharm.&Out.News, Pollut.Abstr., Protozool.Abstr., Reac., Rev.Appl.Entomol., Rev.Med.& Vet.Mycol., Rev.Plant Path., Risk Abstr., Saf.Sci.Abstr., Sci.Cit.Ind., Tox.Abstr. (coverage dropped).
—BLDSC (4478.845300), ADONIS, CASDDS, CISTI, EMDOCS, GNLM, IDS, ingenta, KNAW, Linda Hall. **CCC.**
Published by: (European Histamine Research Society), Birkhaeuser Verlag AG (Subsidiary of: BertelsmannSpringer), Klosterberg, Postfach 133, Basel 4010, Switzerland. TEL 41-61-2050730, FAX 41-61-2050792, inflammation@birkhauser.ch, subscriptions@birkhauser.ch, http://www.birkhauser.ch/journals/1100/1100_tit.htm. Ed. M J Parnham. Circ: 900. **Dist. in N.America by:** Springer-Verlag, 333 Meadowlands Parkway, Secaucus, NJ 07094. TEL 800-777-4643, FAX 201-348-4505. **Co-sponsors:** European Workshop on Inflammation; American Inflammation Research Association; British Inflammation Research Association.

P

616.047 NLD ISSN 0925-4692
CODEN: IAOAES

INFLAMMOPHARMACOLOGY; experimental and clinical studies. Text in English. 1991. q. EUR 490, USD 568 includes online ed. (effective 2002). back issues avail.; reprint service avail. from SWZ. *Refereed.* **Document type:** *Journal, Academic/Scholarly.* **Description:** Publishes papers on all aspects of inflammation and its pharmacological control.
Related titles: Online - full content ed.: 2000 (from EBSCO Publishing, Swets Blackwell,PQC); Online - full text ed.: (from CatchWord Ltd.).
Indexed: Chem.Abstr., Chem.Indus.Notes, Chem.Titles, Excerp.Med. (1992-), Inpharma, Int.Abstr.Biol.Sci., Reac.
—BLDSC (4478.845700), CASDDS, CISTI, EMDOCS, GNLM, Infotrieve, KNAW. **CCC.**
Published by: V S P (Subsidiary of: Brill Academic Publishers), PO Box 346, Zeist 3700 AH, Netherlands. TEL 31-30-692-5790, FAX 31-30-693-2081, vsppub@compuserve.com, http://www.vsppub.com/journals/jn-Inf.html. Ed. K D Rainsford.

615 SWE ISSN 1101-7104

INFORMATION FRAAN LAEKEMEDELSVERKET. Text in Swedish. 1976. bi-m. free. **Document type:** *Bulletin, Trade.*
Formerly (until 1990): Information fraan Socialstyrelsens Laekemedelsavdeling (0347-5107)
Published by: Laekemedelsverket, Box 26, Uppsala 75103, Sweden. TEL 46-18-17-46-00, FAX 46-18-54-85-66, http://www.inpa.se, http://www.mpa.se. Ed. Gunnar Alvan. R&P Bjoern Beermann.

INFORMATION SOURCES IN CHEMISTRY. see *CHEMISTRY*

INFORMATIONS PHARMACEUTIQUES OMS. see *PUBLIC HEALTH AND SAFETY*

615 ITA ISSN 0392-3010

L'INFORMATORE FARMACEUTICO. Text in Italian. 1940. a. EUR 256.16 includes EDIMED (effective 2001). **Document type:** *Directory, Consumer.*
Former titles (until 1967): Informatore Farmacuetico Italiano (0443-1839); (until 1950): Informatore Farmaceutico (0073-7984)
Related titles: ♦ Supplement: E D I M E D.
—GNLM.
Published by: O E M F SpA, Via Filippo Palizzi, 88, PO Box 10434, Milan, MI 20157, Italy. TEL 39-02-332101, FAX 39-02-3551731, info@oemf.it, http://www.oemf.it. Ed. Dr. G Panagia. Adv. contact Delia Weissy. Circ: 11,000.

615 ITA ISSN 1121-1644

INFORMAZIONI SUI FARMACI. Text in Italian. 1977. bi-m. ITL 90,000 domestic to individuals; ITL 140,000 foreign to individuals; ITL 120,000 domestic to institutions; ITL 140,000 foreign to institutions (effective 1999). bk.rev. charts, stat. index. back issues avail. *Refereed.* **Document type:** *Bulletin.* **Description:** Contains information on individual drugs, selection of drugs, adverse drug reactions or interactions, drug treatment of diseases, patient information. Includes articles on selected topics.
Published by: Farmacie Comunali Riunite di Reggio Emilia, Servizio Informazione e Documentazione Scientifica, Via Doberdo, 9, Reggio Emilia, RE 42100, Italy. TEL 39-522-543450, FAX 39-522-550146, SIDS@fcr.re.it, http://www.fcr.re.it. Ed. Albano Del Favero. R&P Egidio Campari. Circ: 6,500.

INHALATION TOXICOLOGY. see *ENVIRONMENTAL STUDIES—Toxicology And Environmental Safety*

658 GBR ISSN 1369-8540

INSTITUTE OF PHARMACY MANAGEMENT INTERNATIONAL. INSTITUTE NEWS. Variant title: Institute of Pharmacy Management International. Institute News. Text in English. 1978. q., latest vol.23, 2001. GBP 40; GBP 10 newsstand/cover (effective 2001). bk.rev. back issues avail. **Document type:** *Newsletter, Academic/Scholarly.* **Description:** Covers management, finance and pharmacy practice.
Formerly: Journal of Management and Communication (0958-482X)
Published by: (Institute of Pharmacy Management International Ltd.), Communications International Group, 307 Linen Hall, 162-168 Regent St, London W1R 5TB, United Kingdom. TEL 44-20-7434-1530, FAX 44-20-7437-0915, grepharm@globalnet.co.uk, http://www.pharmweb.net/ipmi.net. Ed. Douglas Simpson. Circ: 1,000.

INTERKANTONALE KONTROLLSTELLE FUER HEILMITTEL. MONATSBERICHT/OFFICE INTERCANTONAL DE CONTROLE DE MEDICAMENTS. BULLETIN MENSUEL/UFFICIO INTERCANTONALE DI CONTROLLO DEI MEDICAMENTI. BOLLETTINO MENSILE. see *MEDICAL SCIENCES*

INTERNATIONAL CLINICAL PSYCHOPHARMACOLOGY. see *PSYCHOLOGY*

615 NLD ISSN 0074-3879

INTERNATIONAL CONGRESS OF PHARMACEUTICAL SCIENCES. PROCEEDINGS. Text in Dutch. a., latest vol.57, 1997. **Document type:** *Proceedings.* **Description:** Publishes papers on drug research presented at the International Congress of Pharmaceutical Sciences.
Published by: International Pharmaceutical Federation/Federation Internationale Pharmaceutique, PO Box 84200, The Hague 2508 AE, Netherlands. TEL 31-70-302-1970, FAX 31-70-302-1999, http://www.pharmweb.net/fip.html.

INTERNATIONAL DIRECTORY OF DRUGS AND PHARMACEUTICALS IMPORTERS. see *BUSINESS AND ECONOMICS—Trade And Industrial Directories*

615 USA

INTERNATIONAL DIRECTORY OF INVESTIGATORS IN PSYCHOPHARMACOLOGY✱. Text in English. 1973. irreg.
Published by: (Alcohol, Drug Abuse, and Mental Health Administration), U.S. Public Health Service, 5600 Fishers Ln, Rockville, MD 20857. TEL 301-496-4000. Ed. Alice A Leeds. Circ: 6,000. **Co-sponsor:** World Health Organization.

INTERNATIONAL DRUG THERAPY NEWSLETTER. see *MEDICAL SCIENCES—Psychiatry And Neurology*

615 616.97 GBR ISSN 1567-5769
CODEN: IJIMDS

▼ **INTERNATIONAL IMMUNOPHARMACOLOGY.** Text in English. 2001. m. EUR 1,674 in Europe to institutions; JPY 222,300 in Japan to institutions; USD 1,872 in Europe to institutions (effective 2002). adv. back issues avail.; reprint service avail. from PQC. *Refereed.* **Document type:** *Academic/Scholarly.* **Description:** Publishes contributions of clinical relevance which integrate pharmacology and immunology.
Formed by the merger of (1979-2001): International Journal of Immunopharmacology (0192-0561); (1978-2001): Immunopharmacology (0162-3109)
Related titles: Microfilm ed.: (from PQC); Online - full text ed.: (from ingenta, Swets Blackwell, ScienceDirect, Institute for Scientific Information).
Indexed: AIDS & Cancer Res., ASCA, Agri.& Environ.Biotech.Abstr. (coverage dropped), Biol.Abstr., Chem.Abstr., Chem.Indus.Notes, Chem.Titles, Curr.Adv.Ecol.Sci., Curr.Cont., Derwent Biotech.Abstr., Environ.Sci.Poll.Mgmt., Excerp.Med., Helminthol.Abstr., Immun.Abstr., Ind.Med. (1979-), Ind.Sci.Rev., Ind.Vet., Inpharma, Int.Abstr.Biol.Sci., Microbiol.Abstr., Nutr.Abstr., Pharm.&Out.News, Poult.Abstr., Protozool.Abstr., Reac., Ref.Zh., Rev.Appl.Entomol., Rev.Arom.& Med.Plants, Rev.Med.& Vet.Mycol., Sci.Cit.Ind., Vet.Bull., Weed Abstr.
—BLDSC (4541.038960), ADONIS, CASDDS, CISTI, GNLM, IDS, ingenta, KNAW. **CCC.**
Published by: Pergamon (Subsidiary of: Elsevier Science), The Boulevard, Langford Ln, East Park, Kidlington, Oxford OXB 1GB, United Kingdom. FAX 44-1865-843010, http://www.elsevier.com/locate/intimp. Ed. J Talmadge. Circ: 1,250. **Subscr. in Australasia and the Far East to:** Elsevier Science (Singapore) Pte Ltd, No.1 Temasek Ave, 17-01 Millenia Tower, Singapore 039192, Singapore. TEL 65-434-3727, FAX 65-337-2230; **Subscr. in the Americas to:** Elsevier Science, PO Box 945, New York, NY 10159-0945. TEL 212-633-3730, FAX 212-633-3680, usinfo-f@elsevier.com; **Subscr. to:** Elsevier Science BV, PO Box 211, Amsterdam 1000 AE, Netherlands. TEL 31-20-485-3757.

613.2 USA ISSN 0300-9831
QP771 CODEN: IVEBBN

INTERNATIONAL JOURNAL FOR VITAMIN AND NUTRITION RESEARCH. Text in English. 1930. q. USD 198 (effective 2000). adv. bk.rev. abstr, illus. Index. reprints avail. *Refereed.* **Document type:** *Journal, Academic/Scholarly.* **Description:** Provides a scientific international forum for work on the two vast and closely connected research fields of vitaminology and nutrition.
Former titles (until 1971): Internationale Zeitschrift fuer Vitaminforschung (0020-9406); Formerly: Zeitschrift fuer Vitaminforschung (0373-0239)
Related titles: Online - full text ed.: (from Institute for Scientific Information).
Indexed: ASCA, Agricola, Anim.Breed.Abstr., Biol.Abstr., Chem.Abstr., Chem.Indus.Notes, Chem.Titles, Curr.Adv.Ecol.Sci., Curr.Cont., Dairy Sci.Abstr., Derwent Biotech.Abstr., Environ.Sci.Poll.Mgmt., Excerp.Med., Food Sci.& Tech.Abstr., INIS Atomind., Ind.Med. (1971-), Ind.Sci.Rev., Ind.Vet., Inpharma, Int.Abstr.Biol.Sci., Maize Abstr., NRN, Nutr.Abstr., Pharm.&Out.News, Pig News & Info., Pollut.Abstr., Potato Abstr., Poult.Abstr., Reac., Rev.Med.& Vet.Mycol., Risk Abstr., Saf.Sci.Abstr., Sci.Cit.Ind., Soyabean Abstr., Sport Fish.Abstr., Sugar Ind.Abstr., Triticale Abstr., Trop.Dis.Bull., Trop.Oil Seeds Abstr., Vet.Bull., Wild.Rev.
—BLDSC (4542.698000), CASDDS, CINDOC, CISTI, EMDOCS, GNLM, IDS, ingenta, KNAW, Linda Hall. **CCC.**
Published by: Hogrefe & Huber Publishers, PO Box 2487, Kirkland, WA 98083. TEL 425-820-1500, FAX 425-823-8324, verlag@HansHuber.com, http://www.hhpub.com/journals. Ed. P Walter. Circ: 800.

615.1 DEU ISSN 0946-1965
RM1 CODEN: ICTHEK

INTERNATIONAL JOURNAL OF CLINICAL PHARMACOLOGY AND THERAPEUTICS. Text in English. 1967. m. DEM 380, EUR 194.29, USD 192 to individuals; USD 234 to institutions; DEM 40, EUR 20.45 newsstand/cover (effective 2001). adv. bibl, charts, illus, abstr. *Refereed.* **Document type:** *Journal, Academic/Scholarly.* **Description:** Presents articles and features on all aspects of clinical pharmacology including clinical trials, pharmacoepidemiology, pharmacodynamics, drug disposition and pharmacokinetics, quality assurance, pharmacogenetics, and biotechnological drugs such as cytokines and recombinant antibiotics.
Former titles (until 1994): International Journal of Clinical Pharmacology, Therapy and Toxicology (0174-4879); (until 1980): International Journal of Clinical Pharmacology and Biopharmacy (0340-0026); Internationale Zeitschrift fuer Klinische Pharmakologie, Therapie und Toxikologie (0020-9392)
Related titles: Online - full text ed.: (from Institute for Scientific Information).
Indexed: ASCA, Agri.& Environ.Biotech.Abstr. (coverage dropped), Biol.Abstr., Chem.Abstr., Chem.Indus.Notes, Chem.Titles, Compumath, Curr.Adv.Ecol.Sci., Curr.Cont., Curr.Ind.Stat., Dairy Sci.Abstr., Dent.Ind., Derwent Biotech.Abstr., Excerp.Med., Helminthol.Abstr., INIS Atomind., I.P.A., Ind.Med. (1994-), Ind.Sci.Rev., Inpharma, Int.Abstr.Biol.Sci., Pharm.&Out.News, Psychol.Abstr., Reac., Rev.Arom.& Med.Plants, Rev.Med.& Vet.Mycol., SSCI (coverage dropped), Sci.Cit.Ind., Sugar Ind.Abstr.
—BLDSC (4542.170700), CASDDS, CISTI, EMDOCS, GNLM, IDS, Infotrieve, ingenta, KNAW, Linda Hall. **CCC.**
Published by: Dustri-Verlag Dr. Karl Feistle, Bajuwarenring 4, Oberhaching 82041, Germany. TEL 49-89-613861-0, FAX 49-89-613-5412, info@dustri.de, http://www.dustri.de. Ed. B Woodcock. R&P Renate Lehmann. Adv. contact Joerg Feistle. Circ: 1,200.

615.19 CHE ISSN 0251-1649
CODEN: CPHRDE

INTERNATIONAL JOURNAL OF CLINICAL PHARMACOLOGY RESEARCH. Short title: Clinical Pharmacology Research. Text in English. 1981. q. CHF 400 (effective 2002). reprint service avail. from PQC. *Refereed.* **Document type:** *Journal, Academic/Scholarly.*
Related titles: Online - full text ed.: (from Institute for Scientific Information).
Indexed: ASCA, Chem.Abstr., Chem.Indus.Notes, Chem.Titles, Curr.Cont. (coverage dropped), Derwent Biotech.Abstr., Environ.Sci.Poll.Mgmt., Excerp.Med., Ind.Med. (1981-), Ind.Sci.Rev., Inpharma, Int.Abstr.Biol.Sci., Kidney, Neurosci.Cit.Ind., Pharm.&Out.News, Pollut.Abstr., Reac., Ref.Zh., Rev.Med.& Vet.Mycol., Saf.Sci.Abstr., Tox.Abstr.
—BLDSC (4542.170800), CASDDS, CISTI, EMDOCS, GNLM, IDS, Infotrieve, ingenta, KNAW. **CCC.**
Published by: Bioscience Ediprint Inc., Rue Alexandre Gavard 16, Carouge 1227, Switzerland. TEL 41-22-3003383, FAX 41-22-3002489, bioscience.smey@gkb.com. Ed. A Bertell.

INTERNATIONAL JOURNAL OF DRUG POLICY. see *DRUG ABUSE AND ALCOHOLISM*

INTERNATIONAL JOURNAL OF IMMUNOPATHOLOGY AND PHARMACOLOGY. see *MEDICAL SCIENCES—Allergology And Immunology*

P

615 658.8 GBR ISSN 1469-7025
▼ **INTERNATIONAL JOURNAL OF MEDICAL MARKETING**; facilitating excellence in device, diagnostic and pharmaceutical marketing. Text in English. 2000. q. GBP 100 in Europe to individuals in academics; USD 150 in North America to individuals in academics; GBP 105 rest of world to individuals in academics; GBP 200 in Europe to institutions; USD 300 in North America to institutions; GBP 195 rest of world to institutions (effective 2001). abstr. 96 p./no. 2 cols./p. back issues avail. *Refereed.* **Document type:** *Journal, Academic/Scholarly.* **Description:** Aims to facilitate excellence in medical marketing by providing a source of marketing expertise that is tailored specifically to pharmaceutical, medical device and diagnostic markets.
Related titles: Online - full text ed.
—BLDSC (4542.345620).
Published by: Henry Stewart Publications, Russell House, 28/30 Little St, London WC1A 2HN, United Kingdom. TEL 44-20-7404-3040, gweny@henrystewart.co.uk, http://www.henrystewart.co.uk/journals/ijmm/index.html, http://www.henrystewart.com. Ed. Brenda Rouse. R&P Paddy Walters TEL 44-20-7323-2916. Adv. contact Lorna Titley. **Subscr. addr. in N America:** Henry Stewart Publications, Subscriptions Office, PO Box 10812, Birmingham, AL 35202-1588. TEL 800-633-4931, FAX 205-955-1588, hsp@ebsco.com.

615.1 616.89 GBR ISSN 1461-1457
INTERNATIONAL JOURNAL OF NEURO-PSYCHOPHARMACOLOGY. Text in English. q. (plus one supplement). GBP 106 to individuals; USD 224 to institutions (effective 2002). adv. Supplement avail. *Refereed.* **Document type:** *Academic/Scholarly.* **Description:** Publishes original research in basic pharmacology, human psychopharmacological research, and related areas.
Related titles: Online - full text ed.: ISSN 1469-5111. 1998 (from EBSCO Publishing, O C L C Online Computer Library Center, Inc., RoweCom Information Quest, Swets Blackwell, Institute for Scientific Information).
Indexed: Curr.Cont., Focus on: Psychophar., e-psyche.
—BLDSC (4542.383000).
Published by: Cambridge University Press, Edinburgh Bldg, Shaftesbury Rd, Cambridge CB2 2RU, United Kingdom. FAX 44-1223-315052, information@cup.cam.ac.uk, information@cambridge.org, http://www.cup.org/journals/cupjnls.html. Ed. Bernard Lerer. R&P Linda Nicol. Adv. contact Rebecca Symons.

INTERNATIONAL JOURNAL OF NEUROPSYCHOPHARMACOLOGY. see *MEDICAL SCIENCES—Psychiatry And Neurology*

INTERNATIONAL JOURNAL OF ORIENTAL MEDICINE/GUOJI HANFANG YIYAO ZAZHI. see *ALTERNATIVE MEDICINE*

615 USA ISSN 1092-4221
INTERNATIONAL JOURNAL OF PHARMACEUTICAL COMPOUNDING. Text in English. 1997. bi-m. USD 95 domestic; USD 150 foreign (effective 2000). adv. cum. index: 1997-1999. back issues avail. *Refereed.* **Document type:** *Academic/Scholarly.* **Description:** Provides information about contemporary pharmaceutical compounding.
Related titles: Portuguese ed.
Indexed: CINAHL, I.P.A.
—BLDSC (4542.452930).
Published by: I.J.P.C., 122 N Bryant, Edmond, OK 73034-6301. TEL 405-330-0094, 800-757-4572, FAX 405-330-5622, lallen@ijpc.com, http:/www.ijpc.com. Ed. Loyd V Allen Jr. R&P Shelly Capps. Adv. contact Lauren Bernick. color page USD 4,100; trim 11 x 8.5. Circ: 10,000 (controlled). **Subscr. to:** PO Box 2849, Sugarland, TX 77487.

615 610 USA ISSN 1364-9027
CODEN: IJPMFV
INTERNATIONAL JOURNAL OF PHARMACEUTICAL MEDICINE. Text in English. 1985. bi-m. USD 222 domestic to individuals; USD 222 foreign to individuals; USD 540 per issue domestic to institutions; USD 540 per issue foreign to institutions; USD 80 newsstand/cover (effective 2002). bk.rev. back issues avail.; reprints avail. *Refereed.* **Document type:** *Academic/Scholarly.* **Description:** Assesses new and old methods used to test drugs for clinical use.
Formerly (until 1997): Pharmaceutical Medicine (London) (0265-0673)
Related titles: CD-ROM ed.; Microform ed.: (from PQC); Online - full text ed.: USD 702 domestic for academic site license; USD 702 foreign for academic site license; USD 783 domestic for corporate site license; USD 783 foreign for corporate site license (effective 2002) (from EBSCO Publishing).
Indexed: Aqua.Sci.& Fish.Abstr., Aquacult.Abstr., Derwent Biotech.Abstr., Excerp.Med., I.P.A., Inpharma, Int.Abstr.Biol.Sci., Pharm.&Out.News, Pollut.Abstr., Reac.
—BLDSC (4542.452950), ADONIS, CASDDS, CISTI, EMDOCS, GNLM, Infotrieve, KNAW. **CCC.**
Published by: Lippincott Williams & Wilkins (Philadelphia) (Subsidiary of: Wolters Kluwer N.V.), 530 Walnut St, Philadelphia, PA 19106-3621. TEL 215-521-8300, FAX 215-521-8902, http://www.Lww.com. Eds. N Snell, Robert Smith. Adv. contact Anthony Greford. Circ: 1,543. **Subscr. to:** PO Box 1600, Hagerstown, MD 21740-1600. TEL 800-777-2295, FAX 301-824-7390.

615 NLD ISSN 0378-5173
CODEN: IJPHDE
INTERNATIONAL JOURNAL OF PHARMACEUTICS. Text in English. 1978. 38/yr. EUR 422 in Europe to qualified personnel; JPY 57,000 in Japan to qualified personnel; USD 472 elsewhere to qualified personnel; EUR 5,679 in Europe to institutions; JPY 754,300 in Japan to institutions; USD 6,353 elsewhere to institutions (effective 2002). adv. abstr. back issues avail.; reprint service avail. from SWZ. *Refereed.* **Document type:** *Academic/Scholarly.* **Description:** Publishes research results dealing with all aspects of pharmaceutics including physical, chemical, analytical, biological and engineering studies related to drug delivery.
Related titles: Microform ed.: (from PQC); Online - full text ed.: (from EBSCO Publishing, ingenta, Swets Blackwell, ScienceDirect, Institute for Scientific Information).
Indexed: ASCA, Agri.& Environ.Biotech.Abstr. (coverage dropped), Aqua.Sci.& Fish.Abstr., Biodet.Abstr., Biol.Abstr., Chem.Abstr., Chem.Cit.Ind., Chem.Indus.Notes, Chem.Titles, Curr.Cont., Dairy Sci.Abstr., Derwent Biotech.Abstr., Environ.Sci.Poll.Mgmt., Excerp.Med., INIS Atomind., I.P.A., Ind.Med. (1978-), Ind.Sci.Rev., Inpharma, Mass Spectr.Bull., Mat.Sci.Cit.Ind. (coverage dropped), Pharm.&Out.News, Pollut.Abstr., Protozool.Abstr., Reac., Rev.Appl.Entomol., Rev.Med.& Vet.Mycol., Risk Abstr., Saf.Sci.Abstr., Sci.Cit.Ind., Sugar Ind.Abstr.
—BLDSC (4542.454000), ADONIS, CASDDS, CISTI, EMDOCS, GNLM, IDS, Infotrieve, ingenta, KNAW, Linda Hall. **CCC.**
Published by: Elsevier Science BV, PO Box 211, Amsterdam 1000 AE, Netherlands. TEL 31-20-485-2911, FAX 31-20-485-2457, http://www.elsevier.com/locate/ijpharm. Ed. A T Florence. **Subscr. in Australasia and the Far East to:** Elsevier Science (Singapore) Pte Ltd, No.1 Temasek Ave, 17-01 Millenia Tower, Singapore 039192, Singapore. TEL 65-434-3727, FAX 65-337-2230; **Subscr. in Japan to:** Elsevier Science Inc - Japan Regional Office, 9-15 Higashi-Azabu 1-chome, Minato-ku, Tokyo 106-0044, Japan. TEL 81-3-5561-5033; **Subscr. in the Americas to:** Elsevier Science, PO Box 945, New York, NY 10159-0945. TEL 212-633-3730, FAX 212-633-3680, usinfo-f@elsevier.com.

615 GBR ISSN 0961-7671
INTERNATIONAL JOURNAL OF PHARMACY PRACTICE. Text in English. 1991. q. GBP 115 in British Isles; GBP 125 in the European Union; GBP 130 rest of world; GBP 70 to members (effective 2001). adv. bk.rev. back issues avail. *Refereed.* **Document type:** *Academic/Scholarly.* **Description:** Publishes peer-reviewed papers describing research into all aspects of the practice of pharmacy and related fields.
Related titles: Online - full text ed.: (from RoweCom Information Quest).
Indexed: Excerp.Med. (1996-), I.P.A., Inpharma, Intl.Bibl.Soc.Sci., Pharm.&Out.News, Reac.
—BLDSC (4542.454300), CISTI, GNLM, Infotrieve, KNAW. **CCC.**
Published by: (Euromed Communications Ltd.), Pharmaceutical Press (Subsidiary of: Euromed Communications Ltd.), 1 Lambeth High St, London SE1 7JN, United Kingdom. TEL 44-20-7735-9141, FAX 44-20-7582-7327, http://www.pharmj.com/IJPP/IJPPIndex.html, http://www.pharmpress.com. Ed. Alison Blenkinsopp. Pub., R&P Charles Fry. Adv. contact Jack Richmond. Circ: 800.

INTERNATIONAL JOURNAL OF PSYCHOPATHOLOGY, PSYCHOPHARMACOLOGY, AND PSYCHOTHERAPY. see *PSYCHOLOGY*

INTERNATIONAL JOURNAL OF TOXICOLOGY. see *ENVIRONMENTAL STUDIES—Toxicology And Environmental Safety*

INTERNATIONAL MOCHIDA MEMORIAL SYMPOSIUM. see *MEDICAL SCIENCES*

615 USA ISSN 0257-3717
INTERNATIONAL NARCOTICS CONTROL BOARD. REPORT FOR (YEAR). Text in English. 1968. a. USD 18 (effective 1997). **Description:** Focuses on the operation of the international drug control system, with an analysis of the world drug situation.
Former titles: United Nations. International Narcotics Control Board. Annual Report; United Nations. Permanent Central Opium Board. Report of the Permanent Central Opium Board on Its Work; United Nations. Permanent Central Opium Board. Report to the Economic and Social Council on the Work of the Permanent Central Narcotics (Opium) Board (0082-8343)
Related titles: Microfiche ed.: (from CIS); French ed.: ISSN 0257-3725; Spanish ed.: ISSN 0257-3733.
Indexed: IIS.
Published by: (International Narcotics Control Board), United Nations Publications, Sales and Marketing Section, Room DC2 0853, New York, NY 10017. TEL 212-963-8302, 800-253-9646, FAX 212-963-3489, publications@un.org, http://www.un.org/publications.

615 FRA ISSN 1289-0146
INTERNATIONAL PHARMA NEWS. Text in English. 1998. 11/yr. EUR 990 (effective 2001). **Document type:** *Journal, Trade.* **Description:** Provides comprehensive international coverage of healthcare economics, company news, and regulatory and legislative developments.
Published by: Droit & Pharmacie, 12 rue de Lorraine, Levallois-Perret Cedex 92309, France. TEL 33-1-55-46-91-00, FAX 33-1-55-46-91-01, info@droit-et-pharmacie.fr, http://www.droit-et-pharmacie.fr. **Co-publisher:** Editio Cantor Verlag.

615.1 USA ISSN 0888-6393
INTERNATIONAL PHARMACEUTICAL REGULATORY MONITOR; a legal, medical & scientific information series for the pharmaceutical and biotech industry. Text in English. 1974. m. USD 595 domestic; CND 650 in Canada; USD 650 elsewhere (effective 2001). index. 50 p./no. back issues avail. **Document type:** *Newsletter.* **Description:** Contains international regulatory news affecting pharmaceutical manufacturers. Provides texts of official regulatory documents from around the world.
Supersedes in part (in 1993): International Drug and Device Regulatory Monitor (0888-6393); Which was formerly (until 1982): International Drug Regulatory Monitor (0198-7402)
—**CCC.**
Published by: Omniprint Inc., 9700 Philadelphia Ct, Lanham, MD 20706-4405. TEL 301-731-5202, 800-345-2611, FAX 301-731-5203, editor@omniprint.net. Ed. Joanne Eglovitch. Pub., R&P Michael Nagan.

615 NLD ISSN 1010-0423
CODEN: IPHJEN
INTERNATIONAL PHARMACY JOURNAL. Text in English; Summaries in French, German, Spanish. 1912. bi-m. NLG 200 to individuals; NLG 160 to students (effective 1999). adv. bk.rev. back issues avail. *Refereed.* **Document type:** *Academic/Scholarly.* **Description:** Publishes review and original articles on pharmacy practice, and up-to-date information on new drugs and drug reactions and interactions.
Former titles (until 1986): Pharmacy International (0167-3157); (until 1980): Journal Mondial de Pharmacie (0449-2099); Bulletin del la F I P
Related titles: Microform ed.
Indexed: AgeLine, Agri.& Environ.Biotech.Abstr. (coverage dropped), Biol.Abstr., Chem.Abstr., Curr.Adv.Ecol.Sci., Curr.Cont. (coverage dropped), Excerp.Med., Helminthol.Abstr., INIS Atomind., I.P.A., Inpharma, Pharm.&Out.News, Reac.
—CASDDS, CISTI, EMDOCS, GNLM, Infotrieve, KNAW. **CCC.**
Published by: International Pharmaceutical Federation/Federation Internationale Pharmaceutique, PO Box 84200, The Hague 2508 AE, Netherlands. TEL 31-70-302-1970, FAX 31-70-302-1999, k.moody@fip.nl, http://www.pharmweb.net/ftp.html. Ed. P Zethner Moller. Adv. contact K Moody. B&W page NLG 3,000, color page NLG 7,000; 269 x 185. Circ: 5,000.

INTERNATIONAL REINHARDSBRUNN SYMPOSIUM PROCEEDINGS. see *BIOLOGY—Botany*

615.1 DEU
CODEN: ISHPAO
INTERNATIONALE GESELLSCHAFT FUER GESCHICHTE DER PHARMAZIE. VEROEFFENTLICHUNGEN. NEUE FOLGE. Text in English, German. 1953; N.S.. irreg., latest vol.61, 1999. **Document type:** *Monographic series, Academic/Scholarly.*

P

—CASDDS, GNLM.
Published by: (Internationale Gesellschaft fuer Geschichte der Pharmazie), Wissenschaftliche Verlagsgesellschaft mbH, Postfach 101061, Stuttgart 70009, Germany. TEL 49-711-2582-0, FAX 49-711-2582-290, service@wissenschaftliche-verlagsgesellschaft.de, http://www.wissenschaftliche-verlagsgesellschaft.de. Eds. Frank Leimkugel, Wolf-Dieter Mueller-Jahncke.

615 USA ISSN 0167-6997
RC271.C5 CODEN: INNDDK
INVESTIGATIONAL NEW DRUGS; the journal of new anti-cancer agents. Text in English. 1983. q. USD 397, EUR 396 to institutions for print or online ed.; USD 476.40, EUR 475.20 to institutions for print & online eds. combined (effective 2002). adv. bk.rev. back issues avail.; reprint service avail. from SWZ,PQC. *Refereed.* **Document type:** *Journal, Academic/Scholarly.*
Related titles: Microform ed.: (from PQC); Online - full text ed.: (from EBSCO Publishing, O C L C Online Computer Library Center, Inc., RoweCom Information Quest, Swets Blackwell, Kluwer Online, Institute for Scientific Information).
Indexed: ASCA, Chem.Abstr., Chem.Indus.Notes, Chem.Titles, Curr.Cont., Derwent Biotech.Abstr., Excerp.Med., INIS Atomind., Ind.Med. (1983-), Ind.Sci.Rev., Inpharma, Int.Abstr.Biol.Sci., Pharm.&Out.News, Reac., Sci.Cit.Ind., Telegen.
—BLDSC (4559.885000), CASDDS, CISTI, GNLM, IDS, ingenta, KNAW. **CCC.**
Published by: Kluwer Academic Publishers Boston, 101 Philip Dr, Assinippi Park, Norwell, MA 02061. TEL 781-871-6600, FAX 781-871-9045, services@wkap.nl, http://www.wkap.nl/journalhome.htm/0167-6997. Ed. Eric K Rowinsky. R&P Rose Luongo TEL 781-871-6311. **Subscr. outside the Americas to:** Kluwer Academic Publishers Group, Journals Department, PO Box 322, Dordrecht 3300 AH, Netherlands. TEL 31-78-639-2392, FAX 31-78-654-6474; **Subscr. to:** Kluwer Academic - Plenum Publishers, 233 Spring St, New York, NY 10013-1578. TEL 212-620-8468, FAX 212-807-1047.

615 USA ISSN 0889-7735
IOWA PHARMACIST✶ . Text in English. m. adv.
Indexed: I.P.A.
Published by: Iowa Pharmacist Association, 8515 Douglas 16, Des Moines, IA 50322. Circ: 2,100.

615.1 IRL ISSN 0332-0707
IRISH PHARMACY JOURNAL. Text in English. 1923. m. IEP 35 (effective 2001). adv. bk.rev. illus, tr.lit. *Refereed.* **Document type:** *Journal, Consumer, Trade.*
Formerly (until 1972): Irish Chemist and Druggist (0021-1109)
Indexed: I.P.A.
—BLDSC (4574.640000).
Published by: (Pharmaceutical Society of Ireland), Irish Marine Press, 2 Lower Glenageary Rd., Dun Laoghaire, Dublin 4, Ireland. TEL 353-1-2846161, FAX 353-1-2846192, journal@pharmaceuticalsociety.ie, info@afloat.ie. Ed., R&P Val J Harte. Adv. contact Angela J Fealy TEL 353-1-2020374. B&W page IEP 650, color page IEP 850; trim 210 x 296. Circ: 2,300.

ISHI SHIKAISHI YAKUZAISHI CHOSA/SURVEY ON PHYSICIANS, DENTISTS AND PHARMACEUTISTS. see *MEDICAL SCIENCES*

615.1 ISR ISSN 0017-7865
ISRAEL PHARMACEUTICAL JOURNAL/ASSOCIATION PHARMACEUTIQUE D'ISRAEL. JOURNAL/HA-ROKEACH HA-IVRI. Text in English, French, Hebrew. 1941. 6/yr. adv. charts, illus.
Related titles: Online - full text ed.
Indexed: Biol.Abstr., Chem.Abstr., Excerp.Med., I.P.A.
Published by: Pharmaceutical Association of Israel, P O Box 566, Tel Aviv 65112, Israel. Eds. E Menczel, Z Tomer. Circ: 5,000.

ISTITUTO DI RICERCHE FARMACOLOGICHE MARIO NEGRI. ALUMNI NEWS. see *COLLEGE AND ALUMNI*

615 RUS ISSN 0137-026X
CODEN: INFKDZ
ITOGI NAUKI I TEKHNIKI. FARMAKOLOGIYA. KHIMIOTERAPEVTICHESKIE SREDSTVA. Text in Russian. irreg.
—CASDDS, Linda Hall.
Published by: Vserossiiskii Institut Nauchnoi i Tekhnicheskoi Informatsii (VINITI), Usievicha ul 20-a, Moscow 125315, Russian Federation. TEL 7-095-1526441, FAX 7-095-943-0060. **US dist. addr.:** East View Publications, 3020 Harbor Ln N, Minneapolis, MN 55447. TEL 612-550-0961.

615.1 JPN ISSN 0288-2906
IYAKU ANZENSEI KENKYUKAI KAIHO/JAPANESE SOCIETY FOR BIOPHARMACEUTICAL STATISTICS. BULLETIN. Text in English, Japanese. 1979. q. JPY 1,000 per issue.
Published by: (Iyaku Anzensei Kenkyukai/Japanese Society for Biopharmaceutical Statistics), Saientisutosha/Scientist Inc., 3-2 Kanda-Surugadai, Chiyoda-ku, Tokyo 101-0062, Japan.

615.1 JPN
IYAKU ANZENSEI KENKYUKAI TEIREIKAI SHIRYO/PROCEEDINGS OF REGULAR MEETINGS ON BIOPHARMACEUTICAL STATISTICS. Text in English, Japanese. q. **Document type:** *Proceedings.*
Published by: (Iyaku Anzensei Kenkyukai/Japanese Society for Biopharmaceutical Statistics), Saientisutosha/Scientist Inc., 3-2 Kanda-Surugadai, Chiyoda-ku, Tokyo 101-0062, Japan.

615 JPN ISSN 0287-4741
IYAKU JOURNAL/MEDICINE AND DRUG JOURNAL. Text in Japanese. 1965. m. JPY 35,385 (effective 2000). adv. **Document type:** *Academic/Scholarly.*
—BLDSC (5534.005700).
Published by: Iyaku Journal-sha/Medicine & Drug Journal Co., Ltd., 2-8 Hirano-Machi 3-chome, Chuo-ku, Osaka-shi 541-0046, Japan. TEL 81-6-6202-7280, FAX 81-6-6202-5295, iyakujor@skyblue.ocn.ne.jp, http://www.so-net.ne.jp/medipro/iyaku. Ed. Minoru Numata. R&P, Adv. contact Kiriko Numata.

615.19 JPN ISSN 1341-4607
IYAKU KANREN JOHO/J A P I C MONTHLY BULLETIN. Text in Japanese. 1973. m. JPY 100,000 to members (effective 2001). bk.rev. cum.index. **Document type:** *Bulletin.*
Former titles (until 1995): Nihon Iyaku Joho Senta. Joho (0915-163X); Japan Pharmaceutical Information Center. Information
Published by: Japan Pharmaceutical Information Center/Nihon Iyaku Joho Senta, 3rd Fl Nagai-Kinenkan, 2-12-15 Shibuya, Shibuya-ku, Tokyo 150-0002, Japan. TEL 81-3-5466-1812, FAX 81-3-5466-1814. Ed. H Miyake. Circ: 600.

615 JPN ISSN 0579-2762
IYAKU NO MON/GATEWAY TO MEDICINE. Text in Japanese. 1961. bi-m.
Published by: Torii Yakuhin K.K., 4-1 Nihonbashihoncho 3-chome, Chuo-ku, Tokyo 103-0023, Japan.

IYAKU TOKKYO SHOROKU/MEDICINE - PATENTS ABSTRACTS. see *PHARMACY AND PHARMACOLOGY—Abstracting, Bibliographies, Statistics*

615.9 JPN ISSN 1342-2049
IYAKUHIN FUKUSAYO BUNKEN JOHOSHU. YAKKOBETSU FUKUSAYO ICHIRAN-HEN/ADVERSE REACTIONS TO DRUGS INFORMATION COMPENDIUM FOR EXPERTS. PRODUCT - ADVERSE REACTION INFORMATION. Text in Japanese. 1975. s-a. JPY 50,000 includes Iyakuhin Fukusayo Bunken Johoshu. Shorokushu-Hen (effective 2001). **Document type:** *Academic/Scholarly.*
Supersedes in part (in 1995): Kokunai Iyakuhin Fukusayo Ichiran (0912-2133)
Published by: Japan Pharmaceutical Information Center/Nihon Iyaku Joho Senta, 3rd Fl Nagai-Kinenkan, 2-12-15 Shibuya, Shibuya-ku, Tokyo 150-0002, Japan. TEL 81-3-5466-1812, FAX 81-3-5466-1814. Ed. H Miyake. Circ: 3,000.

615 JPN ISSN 1342-2022
IYAKUHIN FUKUSAYO BUNKEN SOKUHO/MONTHLY REPORT ON ADVERSE REACTIONS TO DRUGS. Text in Japanese. 1986. m. JPY 19,800 (effective 2001).
Formerly (until 1993): Iyakuhin Fukusayo Bunken Geppo (0912-2141)
Published by: (Nihon Iyaku Joho Senta/Japan Pharmaceutical Information Center), Chuwa Insatsu K.K., 2-14 Irifune 2-chome, Chuo-ku, Tokyo 104-0042, Japan. TEL 03-3552-0426, FAX 03-3551-4604, soumu@chuwa-p.co.jp.

615 JPN ISSN 0286-6153
IYAKUHIN FUKUSAYO JOHO/INFORMATION ON SIDE EFFECTS OF DRUGS. Text in Japanese. 1977. irreg. JPY 3,800 per issue.
Published by: Yakuma Kohosha, 47-8-202 Koenji-Minami 3-chome, Suginami-ku, Tokyo 166-0003, Japan.

615 JPN
IYAKUHIN NO FUKUSAYO. ANNUAL REPORT/ADVERSE REACTIONS TO DRUGS. ANNUAL REPORT. Text in Japanese. 1990. a. JPY 7,560 (effective 1998). **Document type:** *Academic/Scholarly.*
Published by: Chugai Igakusha, 62 Yarai-cho, Shinjuku-ku, Tokyo 162-0805, Japan. R&P M Takahashi.

615 JPN ISSN 0911-9329
IYAKUHIN SEIZO SHISHIN. Text in Japanese. 1962. a.
Related titles: ♦ English ed.: Drug Approval and Licensing Procedures in Japan. ISSN 0289-9922.
Published by: (Society of Japanese Pharmacopoeia), Yakugyo Jiho Co. Ltd., 2-36 Kanda-Jinbo-cho, Chiyoda-ku, Tokyo 101-0051, Japan.

615.9 JPN ISSN 0385-5015
CODEN: ISSKEY
IYAKUHIN SOGO SAYO KENKYU/RESEARCH ON DRUG ACTIONS AND INTERACTIONS. Text in Japanese. 1975. s-a. JPY 3,000. bk.rev.
Indexed: Chem.Abstr., Chem.Indus.Notes, Chem.Titles.
—CASDDS.
Published by: Iyakuhin Sogo Sayo Kenkyukai/Research Society of Drug Actions and Interactions, Hirosaki Daigaku Igakubu Yakurigaku Kyoshitsu, 5 Zaifu-cho, Hirosaki-shi, Aomori-ken 036-8216, Japan. Circ: 1,200.

615 JPN ISSN 0918-3566
J P M A UPDATE. Text in English. 1991. s-a.
Published by: Japan Pharmaceutical Manufacturers Association/Nihon Seiyaku Kogyo Kyokai, 4-1 Nihonbashihoncho 3-chome, Chuo-ku, Tokyo 103-0023, Japan.

615.1029 JPN ISSN 1342-6826
JAPAN PHARMACEUTICAL REPORT. Text in Japanese. 1982. irreg., latest 1997. USD 850 (effective 1998). **Document type:** *Directory, Trade.* **Description:** Provides information on the pharmaceutical industry and pharmaceutical companies in Japan. Includes information on business operations, research and development, and products, as well as a directory.
Published by: Survey Japan, 16-603 Ichigaya-Hachiman-cho, Shinjuku-ku, Tokyo 162-0844, Japan. TEL 81-3-3235-3421, FAX 81-3-3235-3422.

615 JPN ISSN 0917-8678
JAPANESE ETHICAL PHARMACEUTICAL TARIFF. Text in English. 1984. biennial. JPY 21,000 per issue.
Published by: Pharmadata Publishing, 519-1, Minamicho, Marutamachi Agaru, Higashisanbongi Dori, Kamigyo-ku, Kyoto-shi 602, Japan.

JAPANESE JOURNAL OF ANTIBIOTICS. see *MEDICAL SCIENCES*

616.89 JPN ISSN 1340-7007
CODEN: NKRZE5
JAPANESE JOURNAL OF CHEMOTHERAPY. Text in English, Japanese. 1953. m. JPY 9,000; JPY 12,000 foreign (effective 2000). adv. abstr. index. *Refereed.* **Document type:** *Academic/Scholarly.*
Formerly (until 1994, vol.42): Nihon Kagaku Ryoho Gakkai Zasshi - Chemotherapy (0009-3165)
Related titles: Online - full text ed.: (from Institute for Scientific Information).
Indexed: Agri.& Environ.Biotech.Abstr. (coverage dropped), Biol.Abstr., Chem.Abstr., Curr.Adv.Ecol.Sci., Curr.Cont. (coverage dropped), Derwent Biotech.Abstr., Excerp.Med., INIS Atomind., I.P.A., Ind.Med. (coverage dropped), Ind.Sci.Rev., Inpharma, Pharm.&Out.News, Protozool.Abstr., Reac.
—BLDSC (4651.320000), CASDDS, CISTI, EMDOCS, GNLM, KNAW.
Published by: Nihon Kagaku Ryoho Gakkai/Japan Society of Chemotherapy, 2-20-8 Kami-Osaki, Shinagawa-ku, Tokyo 141-0021, Japan. TEL 81-3-3493-7129, FAX 81-3-5434-0843, karyo@jc4.so-net.ne.jp. Ed. Kohya Shiba. Circ: 4,000.

615.1 JPN ISSN 0021-5198
QP901 CODEN: JJPAAZ
THE JAPANESE JOURNAL OF PHARMACOLOGY. Text in English. 1951. m. JPY 20,000 domestic (effective 2001 & 2002); USD 250 foreign (effective 2001). illus. index. Supplement avail.; reprint service avail. from PQC,ISI. *Refereed.* **Document type:** *Academic/Scholarly.* **Description:** Publishes original research on the interactions between chemicals and biological systems.
Related titles: Microform ed.: (from PQC); Online - full text ed.: (from Institute for Scientific Information).

P

Indexed: ASCA, Agri.& Environ.Biotech.Abstr. (coverage dropped), Anim.Behav.Abstr. (coverage dropped), Aqua.Sci.& Fish.Abstr., Biol.Abstr., Chem.Abstr., Chem.Indus.Notes, Chem.Titles, Curr.Cont., Dent.Ind., Derwent Biotech.Abstr., Environ.Sci.Poll.Mgmt., Excerp.Med., Helminthol.Abstr., INIS Atomind., Ind.Med. (1951-), Ind.Sci.Rev., Ind.Vet., Inpharma, Int.Abstr.Biol.Sci., JTA, Neurosci.Abstr. (coverage dropped), Neurosci.Cit.Ind., Nutr.Abstr., P.A.I.S. (coverage dropped), Pharm.&Out.News, Pollut.Abstr., Protozool.Abstr., Psychol.Abstr., Reac., Rev.Arom.& Med.Plants, Rev.Med.& Vet.Mycol., Risk Abstr., Saf.Sci.Abstr., Sci.Cit.Ind., THA, Weed Abstr.
—BLDSC (4657.000000), CASDDS, CINDOC, CISTI, GNLM, IDS, ingenta, KNAW, Linda Hall. **CCC.**
Published by: Japanese Pharmacological Society, Editorial Office/Nihon Yakuri Gakkai Henshuubu, Kantohya Bldg, Gokomachi-Ebisugawa, Nakagyo-ku, Kyoto-shi 604-0982, Japan. TEL 81-75-252-4641, FAX 81-75-252-4618, LDB00573@nifty.ne.jp, http://wwwsoc.nacsis.ac.jp/tjps/fpj. Ed. Masamichi Satoh. Circ: 2,400.

JAPANESE JOURNAL OF TOXICOLOGY/CHUDOKU KENKYU. see *ENVIRONMENTAL STUDIES—Toxicology And Environmental Safety*

615 JPN
THE JAPANESE PHARMACOPOEIA. Text in Japanese, English. irreg., latest 2001, 14th Ed. JPY 53,000, USD 600 (effective 2001). **Document type:** *Government.* **Description:** Contains general notices, general rules for preparation, general tests, processes and apparatus, and monographs.
Formerly: Pharmacopoeia of Japan
Related titles: CD-ROM ed.: USD 12,000 (effective 2001); Supplement: The Japanese Pharmacopoeia. Supplement I. USD 85 (effective (No. 2001); The Japanese Pharmacopoeia. Supplement II. JPY 8,600, USD 100 (effective 2001).
Published by: (Society of Japanese Pharmacopoeia), Yakuji Nippo Ltd., 1 Kanda-Izumi-cho, Chiyoda-ku, Tokyo 101-8648, Japan. TEL 81-3-3862-2141, FAX 81-3-3866-8495, shuppan@yakuji.co.jp, http://www.yakuji.co.jp/.

615 JPN
JAPANESE PHARMACOPOEIAL FORUM. Variant title: J P Forum. Text in English, Japanese. 1992. q. USD 140.
—BLDSC (4660.250000).
Published by: Society of Japanese Pharmacopoeia, 2-12-15 Shibuya, Shibuya-ku, Tokyo 150-0002, Japan. TEL 81-3-3400-5634, FAX 81-3-3400-3158. **Subscr. to:** Yakuji Nippo Ltd., Kanda-Izumi-cho, Chiyoda-ku, Tokyo 101-0024, Japan. TEL 81-3-3862-2141, FAX 81-3-5821-8757.

615.19 JPN ISSN 0021-5201
JAPANESE WEEKLY ON PHARMACY AND CHEMISTRY✶ /YAKUGYO SHINBUN. Variant title: Weekly Drug News. Text in Japanese. 1946. w. JPY 3,000. adv. bk.rev. abstr, bibl, stat.
Formerly: Japanese Journal of Pharmacy and Chemistry
Indexed: Biol.Abstr., Chem.Abstr., I.P.A.
Address: 1-13-12 Kikawa-nishino-cho, Higoshi-yodogawa-ku, Osaka-shi, Japan. Ed. Y Taguchi. Circ: 20,000.

344.04233 JPN
JAPAN'S AND I C H GUIDELINES FOR NEW DRUG REGISTRATION (YEAR). Text in English. a. JPY 14,240 domestic; USD 160 elsewhere (effective 2001). **Document type:** *Government, Academic/Scholarly.*
Related titles: Supplement: JPY 7,350, USD 95 newsstand/cover (effective 2001).
Published by: Yakuji Nippo Ltd., 1 Kanda-Izumi-cho, Chiyoda-ku, Tokyo 101-8648, Japan. TEL 81-3-3862-2141, FAX 81-3-3866-8495, shuppan@yakuji.co.jp, http://www.yakuji.co.jp/.

JILIN ZHONGYIYAO/JILIN TRADITIONAL CHINESE MEDICINE. see *ALTERNATIVE MEDICINE*

615 USA
JOBWATCH. Text in English. 1997. m. USD 89 to non-members (effective 2001); free to members. adv. **Document type:** *Bulletin.* **Description:** Lists job and career opportunities in all areas of the pharmaceutical industry, including management, research, and informaton systems.
Published by: CenterWatch, Inc., 22 Thomson Pl, Bldg 36 Tl, Boston, MA 02210. TEL 617-856-5900, FAX 617-247-2535, jobwatch@centerwatch.com, http://www.centerwatch.com. Adv. contact Joan Kroll.

615 JPN ISSN 0913-5340
JOSAI DAIGAKU YAKUGAKUBU KENKYU GYOSEKISHU/JOSAI UNIVERSITY. PHARMACEUTICAL BULLETIN. Text in English, Japanese; Summaries in English. 1979. a.
Published by: Josai Daigaku, Yakugakubu/Josai University, Faculty of Pharmaceutical Science, 1-1 Keyakidai, Sakado-shi, Saitama-ken 350-0248, Japan.

615.19 FRA ISSN 0291-1981
CODEN: JPCLDE
JOURNAL DE PHARMACIE CLINIQUE; international journal of clinical pharmacy. Text in French. 1982. q. FRF 670 domestic to individuals; EUR 111 in Europe to individuals; FRF 770 elsewhere to individuals; FRF 1,120 domestic to institutions; EUR 180 in Europe to institutions; FRF 1,220 elsewhere to institutions; FRF 275 newsstand/cover (effective 2001). **Document type:** *Academic/Scholarly.* **Description:** Papers on all aspects of pharmaceutical sciences applied to human use.
Related titles: Online - full text ed.: FRF 670 to individuals; FRF 1,120 to institutions (effective 2001).
Indexed: Chem.Abstr., Chem.Indus.Notes, Chem.Titles, Derwent Biotech.Abstr., Excerp.Med., I.P.A., Inpharma, Reac.
—BLDSC (5032.050000), CASDDS, CISTI, EMDOCS, GNLM, Infotrieve, KNAW. **CCC.**
Published by: John Libbey Eurotext, 127 av. de la Republique, Montrouge 92120, France. TEL 33-01-46730660, FAX 33-01-40840999, marketing@jle.com, http://www.john-libbey-eurotext.fr/. Ed. Pierre A Sado. Circ: 1,300. **Subscr. to:** A T E I, 3 av. Pierre Kerautret, Romainville 92230, France. TEL 33-1-48408686, FAX 33-1-48400731, atei@club-internet.fr.

615 FRA ISSN 0047-2166
CODEN: JPBEAJ
JOURNAL DE PHARMACIE DE BELGIQUE. Text in French. 1919; N.S. 1945. 6/yr. FRF 851; FRF 880 foreign (effective 1997). adv. illus. Supplement avail.; reprint service avail. from ISI. **Document type:** *Academic/Scholarly.* **Description:** Contains original papers and reviews covering the entire field of pharmaceutical sciences: pharmacology, pharmakokinetics, pharmaceutical chemistry, galenics and phytotherapy.
Indexed: Agri.& Environ.Biotech.Abstr. (coverage dropped), Biol.Abstr., Chem.Abstr., Chem.Indus.Notes, Chem.Titles, Curr.Adv.Biochem., Derwent Biotech.Abstr., Excerp.Med., Hort.Abstr., I.P.A., Ind.Med. (1919-), Ind.Sci.Rev., Risk Abstr., Sci.Cit.Ind. (coverage dropped).
—BLDSC (5032.000000), CASDDS, CISTI, GNLM, Infotrieve, KNAW, Linda Hall. **CCC.**
Published by: (Association Pharmaceutique Belge BEL), Masson - Periodiques, 120 bd. St. Germain, Paris 75006, France. TEL 33-1-40466200, FAX 33-1-40466201. Eds. J Vervaeren, M Delfosse. **Subscr. to:** Societe de Periodiques Specialises, BP 22, Vineuil Cedex 41354, France. TEL 33-2-54504612, FAX 33-2-54504611.

615.1 DEU ISSN 1432-4334
JOURNAL FUER PHARMAKOLOGIE UND THERAPIE/JOURNAL OF PHARMACOLOGY AND THERAPY. Text in English, German. 1992. bi-m. DEM 120 (effective 2000). adv. **Document type:** *Journal, Academic/Scholarly.*
—BLDSC (5034.040000).
Published by: Verlag Perfusion GmbH, Regensburger Str 44-46, Nuernberg 90478, Germany. TEL 49-911-49108, FAX 49-911-493579. Ed. Brigitte Soellner. Adv. contact Sibylle Michna.

615.7 USA
CODEN: JGDTEF
JOURNAL OF AGING & PHARMACOTHERAPY. Text in English. 1987. q. USD 75 to individuals; USD 101 in Canada to individuals; USD 109 elsewhere to individuals; USD 125 to institutions; USD 169 in Canada to institutions; USD 181 elsewhere to institutions; USD 350 to libraries; USD 473 in Canada to libraries; USD 508 elsewhere to libraries (effective Aug. 2001). adv. bk.rev. reprint service avail. from HAW,ISI. *Refereed.* **Document type:** *Journal, Academic/Scholarly.* **Description:** Covers drug therapy and related issues in the geriatric population.
Formerly (until 1999): Journal of Geriatric Drug Therapy (8756-4629)
Related titles: Microfiche ed.: (from PQC); Microform ed.

Indexed: ASSIA, Abstr.Soc.Geront., AgeLine, Curr.Cont. (coverage dropped), Environ.Sci.Poll.Mgmt., Excerp.Med., Human Resour.Abstr., IMFL, Inpharma, Lang.& Lang.Behav.Abstr., Pharm.&Out.News, Pollut.Abstr., Psycinfo, Psychol.Abstr. (1986-), Reac., Ref.Zh., Risk Abstr., SOPODA, Saf.Sci.Abstr., Sage Fam.Stud.Abstr., Soc.Work Res.& Abstr., Sociol.Abstr., e-psyche.
—BLDSC (4995.073000), EMDOCS, GNLM, Haworth, ingenta, KNAW.
Published by: Haworth Press, Inc., 10 Alice St, Binghamton, NY 13904-1580. TEL 607-722-5857, 800-429-6784, FAX 607-722-6362, 800-895-0582, getinfo@haworthpressinc.com, http://www.haworthpress.com/journals/journallist.asp. Ed. Roy C. Parish. Pub. William Cohen. R&P Ruthann Heath TEL 607-723-5857 ext 316. Adv. contact Jackie Blakeslee TEL 607-722-5857 ext 346. B&W page USD 315, color page USD 550; trim 6 x 8.5. Circ: 400.

JOURNAL OF ANALYTICAL TOXICOLOGY. see *ENVIRONMENTAL STUDIES—Toxicology And Environmental Safety*

JOURNAL OF ANTIBIOTICS; an international journal devoted to research on bioactive microbial products. see *MEDICAL SCIENCES*

615 CHE ISSN 1029-2659
CODEN: JATHFI
JOURNAL OF APPLIED THERAPEUTIC RESEARCH. Text in English. 1997. 4/yr. EUR 294 to institutions; EUR 460 to corporations; USD 88 to individuals (effective 2001). **Document type:** *Journal, Academic/Scholarly.* **Description:** Focuses on the efficacy, safety and rational use of drugs following approval.
Formerly (until 1998): Journal of Applied Therapeutics (1072-1754)
Related titles: CD-ROM ed.; Online - full text ed.: (from EBSCO Publishing, RoweCom Information Quest).
Indexed: Derwent Biotech.Abstr., I.P.A., Inpharma, Pharm.&Out.News, Reac.
—BLDSC (4947.121000), CISTI.
Published by: Gordon and Breach - Harwood Academic (Subsidiary of: Taylor & Francis Group), PO Box 531, Lausanne 1000, Switzerland. TEL 41-21-6411280, FAX 41-21-6411281, luscombedk@cardiff.ac.uk, info@gbhap.com, http://www.gbhap.com. Ed. David K Luscombe. **Subscr. addr. in US:** International Publishers Direct, PO Box 32160, Newark, NJ 07102. FAX 215-750-6343.

JOURNAL OF APPLIED TOXICOLOGY. see *ENVIRONMENTAL STUDIES—Toxicology And Environmental Safety*

615.328 ISR ISSN 0792-6855
CODEN: RCBPEJ
JOURNAL OF BASIC AND CLINICAL PHYSIOLOGY AND PHARMACOLOGY. Text in English. 1980. q., latest vol.13. USD 300 (effective 2002). adv. bk.rev. illus. back issues avail. **Document type:** *Academic/Scholarly.*
Former titles (until 1987): Reviews in Clinical and Basic Pharmacology (0334-1534); (until 1985): Reviews in Pure and Applied Pharmacological Sciences (0197-2839)
Indexed: Biol.Abstr., Chem.Abstr., Chem.Indus.Notes, Chem.Titles, Curr.Adv.Ecol.Sci., Derwent Biotech.Abstr., Excerp.Med., I.P.A., Ind.Med. (1990-).
—BLDSC (4951.117000), CASDDS, CISTI, EMDOCS, GNLM, KNAW, Linda Hall.
Published by: (Israel Physiological and Pharmacological Society), Freund Publishing House, Ltd., P O Box 35010, Tel Aviv 61350, Israel. TEL 972-3-562-8540, FAX 972-3-562-8538, h_freund@netvision.net.il, http://www.angelfire.com/il/freund. Eds. M Horowitz, Y Oron.

615 616.1 USA ISSN 0160-2446
RM345 CODEN: JCPCDT
JOURNAL OF CARDIOVASCULAR PHARMACOLOGY. Text in English. 1979. m. USD 575 domestic to individuals for print & online eds.; USD 659 foreign to individuals for print & online eds.; USD 1,036 domestic to institutions for print & online eds.; USD 1,265 foreign to institutions for print & online eds.; USD 99 newsstand/cover (effective 2002). adv. bk.rev. index. back issues avail.; reprint service avail. from PQC. *Refereed.* **Document type:** *Academic/Scholarly.* **Description:** Publishes extensive reports on major new drugs affecting the heart and blood vessels.
Related titles: Online - full text ed.: USD 1,346.80 domestic academic site license; USD 1,575.80 foreign academic site license; USD 1,502.20 domestic corporate site license; USD 1,731.20 foreign corporate site license (effective 2002) (from Ovid Technologies, Inc., Institute for Scientific Information).

P

Indexed: ASCA, Agri.& Environ.Biotech.Abstr. (coverage dropped), Chem.Abstr., Chem.Indus.Notes, Chem.Titles, Curr.Cont., Derwent Biotech.Abstr., Environ.Sci.Poll.Mgmt., Excerp.Med., INIS Atomind., Ind.Med. (1979-), Ind.Sci.Rev., Inpharma, Int.Abstr.Biol.Sci., Kidney, Neurosci.Cit.Ind., Nutr.Abstr., Pharm.&Out.News, Pollut.Abstr., Reac., Risk Abstr., Saf.Sci.Abstr., Sci.Cit.Ind., THA.
—BLDSC (4954.868000), CASDDS, CISTI, IDS, ingenta, KNAW.
Published by: Lippincott Williams & Wilkins (Philadelphia) (Subsidiary of: Wolters Kluwer N.V.), 530 Walnut St, Philadelphia, PA 19106-3621. TEL 215-521-8300, FAX 215-521-8902, http://www.cardiovascularpharm.com/, http://www.Lww.com. Eds. Michael R Rosen, Paul M Vanhoutte. Pub. Shelley Johnson. R&P Margaret Becker. Adv. contact James Nagle. B&W page USD 760, color page USD 1,785. Circ: 961. **Subscr. to:** PO Box 1600, Hagerstown, MD 21740-1600. TEL 800-777-2295, FAX 301-824-7390.

615 616.1 USA ISSN 1074-2484
CODEN: JCPTFE
JOURNAL OF CARDIOVASCULAR PHARMACOLOGY AND THERAPEUTICS✱. Text in English. 1996. q. USD 139 domestic to individuals; USD 184 foreign to individuals; USD 196 domestic to institutions; USD 248 foreign to institutions; USD 65 domestic to students; USD 110 foreign to students; USD 63 per issue (effective 2000). **Document type:** *Academic/Scholarly.*
Indexed: Chem.Abstr., Chem.Indus.Notes, Chem.Titles, Ind.Med.
—BLDSC (4954.868500), CASDDS, CISTI, GNLM, Infotrieve, KNAW. **CCC.**
Published by: Churchill Livingstone (Subsidiary of: Harcourt Health Sciences), 15 E 26th St, Fl 15, New York, NY 10010-1505. TEL 212-206-5000, FAX 212-206-7808, http://www.churchillmed.com. Ed. Bramah N Singh. **Subscr. in the UK to:** Pearson Professional Ltd., Journals Subscription Department, Fourth Ave., PO Box 77, Harlow, Essex CM19 5AA, United Kingdom. TEL 44-1279-623924, 44-1279-629609.

P

JOURNAL OF CHEMOTHERAPY. see *MEDICAL SCIENCES—Oncology*

JOURNAL OF CHILD AND ADOLESCENT PSYCHOPHARMACOLOGY. see *MEDICAL SCIENCES—Psychiatry And Neurology*

615.19 CHN ISSN 1003-1057
CODEN: JCHSE4
JOURNAL OF CHINESE PHARMACEUTICAL SCIENCES. Text in English. 1992. q. USD 140 (effective 2000). adv. *Refereed.* **Document type:** *Academic/Scholarly.*
Description: Covers pharmaceutical sciences including medicinal chemistry, pharmacognosy and natural products, pharmaceutical analysis, pharmaceutics, pharmacology and antibiotics.
Indexed: Chem.Abstr., Chem.Indus.Notes, Chem.Titles.
—BLDSC (4958.128000), CASDDS, GNLM.
Published by: (Zhongguo Yaoxuehui/Chinese Pharmaceutical Association), Kexue Chubanshe/Science Press, 16 Donghuang Cheng Genbei Jie, Beijing 100717, China. Ed. Tonghui Zhou. R&P, Adv. contact Jianhui Wu. page USD 200. Circ: 1,000.

JOURNAL OF CLINICAL ONCOLOGY. see *MEDICAL SCIENCES—Oncology*

615.1 USA ISSN 0091-2700
CODEN: JCPCBR
JOURNAL OF CLINICAL PHARMACOLOGY. Text in English. 1960. m. USD 404 domestic; USD 491 foreign (effective 2002). adv. bk.rev. charts, illus. index. 112 p./no. back issues avail.; reprints avail. *Refereed.* **Document type:** *Journal, Academic/Scholarly.*
Description: Geared toward clinical pharmacologists and physicians concerned with and responsible for the appropriate selection, investigation and prescribing of drugs.
Former titles: Journal of Clinical Pharmacology and New Drugs (0021-9754); Journal of New Drugs (0096-0284)
Related titles: Microform ed.: (from PQC); Online - full text ed.: (from Ovid Technologies, Inc., EBSCO Publishing, O C L C Online Computer Library Center, Inc., RoweCom Information Quest, ingenta, Swets Blackwell, Institute for Scientific Information).
Indexed: ASCA, Agri.& Environ.Biotech.Abstr. (coverage dropped), Biol.Abstr., Chem.Abstr., Chem.Indus.Notes, Chem.Titles, Curr.Cont., Dairy Sci.Abstr., Dent.Ind., Derwent Biotech.Abstr., Environ.Sci.Poll.Mgmt., Excerp.Med. (1993-), INIS Atomind., I.P.A., Ind.Med. (1973-), Ind.Sci.Rev., Inpharma, Kidney, Mass Spectr.Bull., Med.& Surg.Dermat., Neurosci.Cit.Ind., Nutr.Abstr., Pharm.&Out.News, Psychol.Abstr., Reac., Rev.Med.& Vet.Mycol., SSCI (coverage dropped), Sci.Cit.Ind.
—BLDSC (4958.680000), CASDDS, CISTI, GNLM, IDS, Infotrieve, ingenta, KNAW, Linda Hall. **CCC.**
Published by: (American College of Clinical Pharmacology), Sage Publications, Inc., Sage Science Press, 2455 Teller Rd, Thousand Oaks, CA 91320. TEL 805-499-0721, FAX 805-499-0871, sagescience@sagepub.com, http://www.sagesciencepress.com. Ed. Dr. Deborah L Keefe. Pub. Susan Hanscom. R&P Peter Marino. Adv. contact Robert Vrooman. B&W page USD 770, color page USD 1,720; bleed 8.375 x 11. Circ: 1,706. **Overseas subscr. to:** Sage Publications Ltd., 6 Bonhill St, London EC2A 4PU, United Kingdom. TEL 44-20-7374-0645, FAX 44-20-7374-8741, info@sagepub.com.

615 GBR ISSN 0269-4727
CODEN: JCPTED
JOURNAL OF CLINICAL PHARMACY AND THERAPEUTICS. Text in English. 1976. bi-m., latest vol.27, 2002. GBP 455 in Europe; USD 722 in North America; GBP 501 elsewhere (effective 2002). adv. bk.rev. abstr, bibl. index. back issues avail.; reprint service avail. from ISI. *Refereed.* **Document type:** *Academic/Scholarly.* **Description:** Provides a forum for clinicians, pharmacists and other health-care professionals to explore and report on issues of common interest. Embraces all aspects of drug development and drug use.
Former titles: Journal of Clinical and Hospital Pharmacy (0143-3180); Journal of Clinical Pharmacy (0308-6593)
Related titles: Microform ed.: (from PQC); Online - full text ed.: ISSN 1365-2710. 1999. GBP 410 in Europe; USD 650 in North America; GBP 410 elsewhere (effective 2002) (from Ovid Technologies, Inc., EBSCO Publishing, O C L C Online Computer Library Center, Inc., RoweCom Information Quest, ingenta, Munksgaard & Blackwell Science's Synergy, Swets Blackwell, Institute for Scientific Information).
Indexed: ASCA, Agri.& Environ.Biotech.Abstr. (coverage dropped), Biol.Abstr., CINAHL, Chem.Abstr., Chem.Indus.Notes, Chem.Titles, Curr.Cont., Derwent Biotech.Abstr., Excerp.Med., I.P.A., Ind.Med. (1987-), Ind.Sci.Rev., Inpharma, Int.Nurs.Ind., Med.& Surg.Dermat., Pharm.&Out.News, Reac., Rev.Arom.& Med.Plants, Rev.Med.& Vet.Mycol., SSCI (coverage dropped), Sci.Cit.Ind., Trop.Dis.Bull.
—BLDSC (4958.685000), ADONIS, CASDDS, CISTI, EMDOCS, GNLM, IDS, Infotrieve, ingenta, KNAW. **CCC.**
Published by: Blackwell Science Ltd., PO Box 88, Oxford OX2 0NE, United Kingdom. TEL 44-1865-206180, 44-1865-206002, FAX 44-1865-206219, jnl.orders@blacksci.co.uk, http://www.blackwell-science.com/~cgilib/jnlpage.asp?Journal=jcpt&File=jcpt, http://www.blackwellpublishing.com. Eds. A Li Wan Po, M J Kendall. Pub. Elaine Stott. R&P Sophie Savage. Adv. contact Jenny Applin. Circ: 340.

615.19 USA ISSN 0271-0749
CODEN: JCPYDR
JOURNAL OF CLINICAL PSYCHOPHARMACOLOGY. Text in English. 1981. bi-m. USD 178 domestic to individuals for print & online eds.; USD 221 foreign to individuals for print & online eds; USD 350 domestic to institutions for print & online eds; USD 367 foreign to institutions for print & online eds; USD 56 newsstand/cover (effective 2002). adv. bk.rev. back issues avail. *Refereed.* **Document type:** *Academic/Scholarly.* **Description:** Publishes clinical papers for psychiatrists on antipsychotic, antianxiety, antidepressant medications and stimulants.
Related titles: CD-ROM ed.: (from Ovid Technologies, Inc.); Microform ed.: (from WWS); Online - full text ed.: USD 455 domestic academic site license; USD 472 foreign academic site license; USD 507.50 domestic corporate site license; USD 524.50 foreign corporate site license (effective 2002) (from Ovid Technologies, Inc., Institute for Scientific Information).
Indexed: A.D.& D., ASCA, Adol.Ment.Hlth.Abstr., Chem.Abstr., Chem.Indus.Notes, Chem.Titles, Chic.Per.Ind., Curr.Cont., Dairy Sci.Abstr., Dent.Ind., Derwent Biotech.Abstr., Excerp.Med., Focus on: Psychophar., Ind.Med. (1981-), Ind.Sci.Rev., Inpharma, Int.Nurs.Ind., Jrnl.Watch Psych., Neurosci.Cit.Ind., Pharm.&Out.News, PsycInfo, Psychol.Abstr. (1988-), Reac., Rev.Arom.& Med.Plants, Rev.Med.& Vet.Mycol., SSCI (coverage dropped), Sci.Cit.Ind., THA, e-psyche.
—BLDSC (4958.691000), CASDDS, CISTI, EMDOCS, GNLM, IDS, ingenta, KNAW.
Published by: Williams & Wilkins (Subsidiary of: Waverly International), 351 W Camden St, Baltimore, MD 21201-2436. TEL 410-528-4068, 800-222-3790, FAX 410-528-4452, Kmalamphy@wwilkins.com, http://www.wwilkins.com, http://www.Lww.com. Ed. Richard I Shader. Adv. contact Kathleen Malamphy. B&W page USD 825; trim 10.88 x 8.13. Circ: 8,431; 3,400 (paid); 5,031 (controlled).

615 GBR ISSN 1369-5207
JOURNAL OF CLINICAL RESEARCH. Text in English. 1997. irreg., latest vol.4 (Each paper is published within 21 days of acceptance.). Avail. with subscr. to Journal of Drug Assessment. adv. abstr. 2 cols./p. Supplement avail.; back issues avail.; reprints avail. *Refereed.* **Document type:** *Journal, Academic/Scholarly.*
Description: Specializes in the publication of studies determining the efficacy of new clinical interventions, from phase I through post-marketing investigations. It also encompasses studies from many therapeutic areas and reports the data in the form of RTC reports, specialists reviews and meetings summaries.
Formed by the merger of (1990-1997): British Journal of Clinical Research (0961-1053); (1991-1997): European Journal of Clinical Research (0961-3692)
Indexed: I.P.A.
Published by: Brookwood Medical Publications (Subsidiary of: P J B Publications Ltd.), 18-20 Hill Rise, Richmond, Surrey TW10 6UA, United Kingdom. TEL 44-20-8332-4600, FAX 44-20-8332-4610, maria@brookwd.demon.co.uk, http://www.pjbpubs.com/brookwood/. Ed., R&P Wendy Kimleer TEL 44-20-8332-4601. Pub. Dr. Philip J Brown. Adv. contact Jenefer Trevena TEL 44-20-8332-4605.

615.1 NLD ISSN 0168-3659
CODEN: JCREEC
JOURNAL OF CONTROLLED RELEASE. Text and summaries in English. 1984. 24/yr. EUR 2,400 in Europe to institutions; JPY 318,400 in Japan to institutions; USD 2,685 elsewhere to institutions (effective 2002). adv. bk.rev. abstr, bibl, illus, pat. index. back issues avail.; reprint service avail. from SWZ. *Refereed.* **Document type:** *Academic/Scholarly.*
Description: Publishes research and reviews on the science and technology of all types of controlled release of active agents, including applications in pharmacology, agricultural sciences, and relevant work in toxicology.
Related titles: Microform ed.: (from PQC); Online - full text ed.: (from ingenta, ScienceDirect, Swets Blackwell, Institute for Scientific Information).
Indexed: ASCA, AgBiotech, Anim.Breed.Abstr., Biotech.& Bioeng.Abstr., Chem.Abstr., Chem.Cit.Ind., Chem.Indus.Notes, Chem.Titles, Curr.Cont., Derwent Biotech.Abstr., Eng.Ind., Excerp.Med., I.P.A., Ind.Med. (1984-), Ind.Vet., Inpharma, Mat.Sci.Cit.Ind. (coverage dropped), Med.& Pharm.Biotech.Abstr., Pharm.&Out.News, Reac., Rev.Appl.Entomol., Rev.Arom.& Med.Plants, Rev.Med.& Vet.Mycol., Rev.Plant Path., Sci.Cit.Ind., Sugar Ind.Abstr., Vet.Bull., Weed Abstr.
—BLDSC (4965.260000), ADONIS, CASDDS, CISTI, Ei, GNLM, IDS, Infotrieve, KNAW, Linda Hall. **CCC.**
Published by: (Controlled Release Society), Elsevier Science BV, PO Box 211, Amsterdam 1000 AE, Netherlands. TEL 31-20-485-2911, FAX 31-20-485-2457, nlinfo-f@elsevier.nl, http://www.elsevier.nl/locate/jconrel. Eds. C G Pitt, W E Hennink. Circ: 700. **Subscr. in Australasia and the Far East to:** Elsevier Science (Singapore) Pte Ltd, No.1 Temasek Ave, 17-01 Millenia Tower, Singapore 039192, Singapore. TEL 65-434-3727, FAX 65-337-2230; **Subscr. in Japan to:** Elsevier Science Inc - Japan Regional Office, 9-15 Higashi-Azabu 1-chome, Minato-ku, Tokyo 106-0044, Japan; **Subscr. in the Americas to:** Elsevier Science, PO Box 945, New York, NY 10159-0945. TEL 212-633-3730, FAX 212-633-3680, usinfo-f@elsevier.com.

615.1 001.4 GBR ISSN 1369-9474
JOURNAL OF DRUG ASSESSMENT. Text in English. 1998. q. GBP 250 in Europe; USD 437 in US & Canada; JPY 62,500 in Japan; GBP 275 rest of world (effective 2001). adv. abstr. 2 cols./p. Supplement avail.; back issues avail.; reprints avail. *Refereed.* **Document type:** *Journal, Academic/Scholarly.* **Description:** Covers primary research on all aspects of drug development and clinical trials involving phases I-IV.
Indexed: Inpharma, Pharm.&Out.News, Reac.
—BLDSC (4970.525000), GNLM, KNAW.

Published by: Brookwood Medical Publications (Subsidiary of: P J B Publications Ltd.), 18-20 Hill Rise, Richmond, Surrey TW10 6UA, United Kingdom. TEL 44-20-8332-4600, FAX 44-20-8332-4610, maria@brookwd.demon.co.uk, http://www.pjbpubs.com/brookwood/. Ed., R&P Wendy Kimleer TEL 44-20-8332-4601. Pub. Dr. Philip J Brown. Adv. contact Jenefer Trevena TEL 44-20-8332-4605.

615.1 EGY ISSN 0085-2406
JOURNAL OF DRUG RESEARCH OF EGYPT. Cover title: Journal of Drug Research. Text in English; Summaries in Arabic, English. 1968. a. USD 12. bk.rev. illus. **Document type:** *Academic/Scholarly.*
Related titles: Online - full text ed.
Indexed: Anal.Abstr., Biol.Abstr., Chem.Abstr., Derwent Biotech.Abstr., Excerp.Med., Food Sci.& Tech.Abstr., I.P.A., Mass Spectr.Bull., Nutr.Abstr.
—BLDSC (4970.580000), GNLM.
Published by: National Organisation for Drug Control and Research, Drug Research and Control Center, 6, Abou-Hazem St., Pyramids Ave., P O Box 29, Cairo, Egypt.

615 CHE ISSN 1061-186X
RS199.5 CODEN: JDTAEH
JOURNAL OF DRUG TARGETING. Text in English. 1993. 6/yr. GBP 190, USD 231, EUR 254 to individuals; GBP 698, USD 918, EUR 932 to institutions; GBP 1,147, USD 1,504, EUR 1,528 to corporations (effective 2002). *Refereed.* **Document type:** *Journal, Academic/Scholarly.* **Description:** Publishes papers and reviews on all aspects of drug delivery and targeting, and the design and characterization of carrier systems, with an emphasis on 'in vivo' evaluation.
Related titles: CD-ROM ed.; Microform ed.; Online - full text ed.: (from EBSCO Publishing, RoweCom Information Quest, Institute for Scientific Information).
Indexed: ASCA, Curr.Cont., Derwent Biotech.Abstr., Excerp.Med. (1994-), I.P.A., Ind.Med. (1993-), Ind.Sci.Rev., Inpharma, Int.Abstr.Biol.Sci., Med.& Pharm.Biotech.Abstr., Reac., Sci.Cit.Ind.
—BLDSC (4970.582000), EMDOCS, GNLM, Infotrieve. **CCC.**
Published by: Gordon and Breach - Harwood Academic (Subsidiary of: Taylor & Francis Group), PO Box 531, Lausanne 1000, Switzerland. TEL 41-21-6411280, FAX 41-21-6411281, info@gbhap.com, http://www.gbhap.com/Drug_Targeting/. Eds. Ruth Duncan, Vincent Lee. **Subscr. addr. in US:** International Publishers Direct, PO Box 32160, Newark, NJ 07102. FAX 215-750-6343.

615.19 IRL ISSN 0378-8741
CODEN: JOETD7
JOURNAL OF ETHNOPHARMACOLOGY; an interdisciplinary journal devoted to bioscientific research on indigenous drugs. Text in English. 1979. 18/yr. EUR 1,574 in Europe to institutions; JPY 208,800 in Japan to institutions; USD 1,761 elsewhere to institutions (effective 2002). bk.rev. abstr. back issues avail.; reprint service avail. from SWZ. *Refereed.* **Document type:** *Academic/Scholarly, Abstract/Index.* **Description:** Publishes articles concerned with the observation and experimental investigation of the biological activities of plant and animal substances used in the traditional medicine of past and present cultures. Also provides abstracts of current literature screened from more than 100 journals.
Related titles: Microform ed.: (from PQC); Online - full text ed.: (from ingenta, ScienceDirect, Swets Blackwell, Institute for Scientific Information).
Indexed: AMED, ASCA, Abstr.Anthropol., Agricola, Agroforest.Abstr., Anthropol.Lit., Aqua.Sci.& Fish.Abstr., BBCI, Bibl.Agri., Biol.Abstr., Biotech.& Bioeng.Abstr., Chem.Abstr., Chem.Cit.Ind., Chem.Indus.Notes, Chem.Titles, Cott.& Trop.Fibr.Abstr., Curr.Cont., Dairy Sci.Abstr., Environ.Sci.Poll.Mgmt., Excerp.Med., Field Crop Abstr., Forest Prod.Abstr., Forest.Abstr., Helminthol.Abstr., Hort.Abstr., I.P.A., Ind.Med. (1979-), Ind.Sci.Rev., Ind.Vet., Inpharma, Int.Abstr.Biol.Sci., Microbiol.Abstr., Nutr.Abstr., Pharm.&Out.News, Plant Gen.Res.Abstr., Pollut.Abstr., Postharvest, Poult.Abstr., Protozool.Abstr., Reac., Rev.Appl.Entomol., Rev.Arom.& Med.Plants, Rev.Med.& Vet.Mycol., Rev.Plant Path., Risk Abstr., Rural Devel.Abstr., SSCI (coverage dropped), Saf.Sci.Abstr., Sci.Cit.Ind., Seed Abstr., Tox.Abstr., Trop.Dis.Bull., Trop.Oil Seeds Abstr., Vet.Bull., Weed Abstr., World Ag.Econ.& Rur.Soc.Abstr.
—BLDSC (4979.602400), CASDDS, CISTI, EMDOCS, GNLM, IDS, ingenta, KNAW. **CCC.**
Published by: Elsevier Science Ireland Ltd, Elsevier House, Brookvale Plaza, E. Park, Shannon, Co. Clare, Ireland. TEL 353-61-471944, FAX 353-61-472144, http://www.elsevier.com/locate/jethpharm. Eds. D D Soejarto, P J Houghton. **Subscr. in Australasia and the Far East to:** Elsevier Science (Singapore) Pte Ltd, No.1 Temasek Ave, 17-01 Millenia Tower, Singapore 039192, Singapore; **Subscr. in the Americas to:** Elsevier Science, PO Box 945, New York, NY 10159-0945. TEL 212-633-3730, FAX 212-633-3680, http://www.elsevier.com; **Subscr. to:** Elsevier Science BV, PO Box 211, Amsterdam 1000 AE, Netherlands. TEL 31-20-485-3757.

615.1 MLT ISSN 1023-3857
JOURNAL OF EUROMED PHARMACY. Text in English. 1994. irreg. MTL 5 per issue (effective 1998). *Refereed.* **Document type:** *Academic/Scholarly.* **Description:** Promotes pharmacy in the Mediterranean region. Includes research work by local and foreign pharmacy graduates and other papers relating to pharmacy.
Published by: University of Malta, Department of Pharmacy, Msida, Malta. TEL 56-343764, FAX 356-340427, http://www.cis.um.edu.mt/~phcy/euromed. Ed. Anthony Serracino Inglott. Pub. Bhabkar Sharma. Circ: 1,500.

615 KOR ISSN 1226-8453
SB295.G5 CODEN: KINHEK
JOURNAL OF GINSENG RESEARCH. Text in Korean. 1976. 3/yr. **Document type:** *Academic/Scholarly.* **Description:** Publishes research papers on original work, either experimental or theoretical, that advance our understanding of ginseng science, including questions on the cultivation, biology, chemistry, pharmacology and biochemistry of ginseng.
Formerly (until 1997): Korean Journal of Ginseng Science (1016-2615)
Indexed: Food Sci.& Tech.Abstr.
—BLDSC (4995.600000), CASDDS.
Published by: Korean Society of Ginseng, Seocho World Officetel Rm. 804, Seocho-dong Seocho-ku, Seoul 137070, Korea, S.. TEL 82-2-3473-8772, FAX 82-2-3474-2330.

JOURNAL OF HEALTH SCIENCE/EISEI KAGAKU. see *ENVIRONMENTAL STUDIES—Toxicology And Environmental Safety*

615.1 610 JPN ISSN 1341-321X
CODEN: JICHFN
JOURNAL OF INFECTION AND CHEMOTHERAPY. Text in English. 1995. q. (in 1 vol., 4 nos./vol.). JPY 18,000 domestic; USD 177 in North America; DEM 328 elsewhere; DEM 358, EUR 183.04 in Germany for print & online eds.; DEM 362.80, EUR 185.49 elsewhere for print & online eds. (effective 2001). *Refereed.* **Document type:** *Academic/Scholarly.* **Description:** Covers the combined area of infection and chemotherapy, including the pathogenesis, diagnosis, treatment and control of infectious diseases.
Related titles: Online - full text ed.: ISSN 1437-7780 (from EBSCO Publishing, RoweCom Information Quest, Swets Blackwell, Springer LINK).
Indexed: Chem.Abstr., Chem.Indus.Notes, Chem.Titles.
—BLDSC (5006.691000), CASDDS, CISTI, ingenta.
Published by: (Japan Society of Chemotherapy), Springer-Verlag Tokyo, Eastern Book Service, Inc. (Subsidiary of: BertelsmannSpringer), 3-13 Hongo 3-chome, Bunkyo-ku, Tokyo 113-0033, Japan. TEL 81-3-3812-0617, FAX 81-3-3812-4699, kyj04632@niftysrev.or.jp; 100466,2555@compuserve.com., http://link.springer-ny.com/link/service/journals/10156/index.htm, http://www.churchillmed.com. Ed. Kyoichi Totsuka. Circ: 1,500 (paid). **Subscr. in N. America to:** Springer-Verlag New York Inc., PO Box 2485, Secaucus, NJ 07096-2485. TEL 800-777-4643, 212-460-1526, FAX 201-348-4505, orders@springer-ny.com; **Subscr. in UK & Europe to:** Pearson Professional Ltd., Journals Subscription Department, Fourth Ave., PO Box 77, Harlow, Essex CM19 5AA, United Kingdom. TEL 44-1279-623924; **Subscr. to:** Eastern Book Service, Inc., 3-13 Hongo 3-chome, Bunkyo-ku, Tokyo 113-8480, Japan. TEL 81-3-3818-0861, FAX 81-3-3818-0864, orders@svt-ebs.co.jp; Springer-Verlag, c/o Gabriele Kubitza, Haberstrasse 7, Heidelberg 69126, Germany. TEL 49-6221-345242, FAX 49-6221-345229, http://link.springer.de, http://link.springer-ny.com.

615 616.9 USA ISSN 1068-7777
CODEN: JIDPFI
JOURNAL OF INFECTIOUS DISEASE PHARMACOTHERAPY; antimicrobial evaluation, development & clinical application. Text in English. 1995. q. USD 50 to individuals; USD 68 in Canada to individuals; USD 73 elsewhere to individuals; USD 85 to institutions; USD 115 in Canada to institutions; USD 123 elsewhere to institutions; USD 105 to libraries; USD 142 in Canada to libraries; USD 152 elsewhere to libraries (effective Aug. 2001). adv. bk.rev. back issues avail.; reprint service avail. from HAW. *Refereed.* **Document type:** *Journal, Academic/Scholarly, Trade.* **Description:** Focuses exclusively on infectious disease, pharmacotherapy and the surrounding issues which are important to pharmacists and other healthcare practitioners.
Formerly: Antimicrobial Evaluation, Development & Clinical Application
Related titles: Microfiche ed.: (from PQC); Microform ed.; Online - full text ed.
Indexed: Biol.Dig., Biotech.& Bioeng.Abstr., CINAHL, Environ.Sci.Poll.Mgmt., Excerp.Med. (1996-), I.P.A., Inpharma, Pharm.&Out.News, Pollut.Abstr., Reac., Ref.Zh., Virol.Abstr.
—BLDSC (5006.698000), EMDOCS, GNLM, Haworth, KNAW.
Published by: (Society of Infectious Disease Pharmacists), Haworth Press, Inc., Pharmaceutical Products Press, 10 Alice St, Binghamton, NY 13904-1580. TEL 607-722-5857, 800-429-6784, FAX 607-722-6362, 800-895-0582, getinfo@haworth.com, http://www.haworthpress.com/journallist.asp. Eds. David Nicolau, Michael Klepser. Pub. William Cohen. R&P Ruthann Heath TEL 607-723-5857 ext 316. Adv. contact Jackie Blakeslee TEL 607-722-5857 ext 346. B&W page USD 315, color page USD 550; trim 6 x 8.5. Circ: 225 (paid).

615 JPN ISSN 0389-1194
JOURNAL OF INTENSIVE CARE MEDICINE. Text in Japanese; Summaries in English, Japanese. 1977. m. JPY 2,000 per issue.
Indexed: INIS Atomind.
Published by: Igaku Tosho Shuppan Co. Ltd., 2-28-1 Tohgane Bldg, Hongo, Bunkyo-ku, Tokyo 113-0033, Japan.

615 USA ISSN 0194-5106
JOURNAL OF KANSAS PHARMACY. Text in English. 1964. q. USD 20; USD 8 newsstand/cover Journal of Kansas Pharmacy; USD 4 newsstand/cover Journal of Kansas Pharmacy Update Newsletter (effective 2000). adv. illus. stat. tr.lit. **Document type:** *Trade.* **Description:** Statewide pharmacy news; association news, reports, health-system pharmacy news; original articles; and president's editorials.
Indexed: I.P.A.
Published by: Kansas Pharmacists Association, 1020 SW Fairlawn Rd, Topeka, KS 66604. TEL 785-232-0439, FAX 785-232-3764, info@kansaspharmacy.org. Ed., R&P, Adv. contact Jenith Hoover TEL 785-232-0439. B&W page USD 500, color page USD 832; trim 11 x 8.5. Circ: 1,300 (controlled).

615.19 USA ISSN 0898-2104
RS201.L55 CODEN: JLREE7
JOURNAL OF LIPOSOME RESEARCH. Text in English. 1991. q. USD 95 to individuals print & online eds.; USD 895 to institutions print only (effective 2002). adv. *Refereed.* **Document type:** *Academic/Scholarly.* **Description:** Presents high quality liposome research. Subjects are broad, ranging from biophysical analysis of liposome membranes to clinical applications of liposome-encapsulated drugs.
Related titles: Microform ed.: (from RPI); Online - full text ed.: (from Institute for Scientific Information, RoweCom Information Quest).
Indexed: ASCA, Chem.Abstr., Chem.Titles, Curr.Cont., Derwent Biotech.Abstr., Inpharma, Int.Abstr.Biol.Sci., Med.& Pharm.Biotech.Abstr., Pharm.&Out.News, Reac., Ref.Zh., Telegen.
—BLDSC (5010.505000), CASDDS, CISTI, EMDOCS, GNLM, IDS, Infotrieve, KNAW. **CCC.**
Published by: Marcel Dekker Inc., 270 Madison Ave, New York, NY 10016. TEL 212-696-9000, 800-228-1160, FAX 212-685-4540, journals@dekker.com, http://www.dekker.com/servlet/product/productid/LPR. Ed. Andrew S Janoff. R&P Julia Mulligan. Adv. contact Diane Saulon. B&W page USD 800. Circ: 400.

JOURNAL OF MAINTENANCE IN THE ADDICTIONS; innovations in research, theory, & practice. see *DRUG ABUSE AND ALCOHOLISM*

P

615 368.382 USA ISSN 1083-4087
JOURNAL OF MANAGED CARE PHARMACY. Text in English. 1995. bi-m. USD 60; USD 80 foreign. *Refereed.* **Description:** Presents scholarly, peer-reviewed articles in the areas of managed care pharmacy practice, pharmacotherapy, research, education, economics, and other pertinent areas of pharmacy practice.
Indexed: I.P.A., Inpharma, Pharm.&Out.News, Reac.
—BLDSC (5011.080000).
Published by: Academy of Managed Care Pharmacy, 100 N Pitt St, 400, Alexandria, VA 22314-3134. TEL 703-683-8416, FAX 703-683-8417, ccampbell@mitchellpeterson.org, http://www.amcp.org. Ed. Craig Stern. Pub. Judith Cahill. R&P Tricia Rudis TEL 717-560-2001. Circ: 19,000.

615 USA ISSN 1534-9713
▼ **JOURNAL OF MANAGED PHARMACEUTICAL CARE.** Text in English. 2001 (Spr.). q. USD 48 domestic to individuals; USD 65 in Canada to individuals; USD 70 elsewhere to individuals; USD 90 domestic to institutions; USD 122 in Canada to institutions; USD 131 elsewhere to institutions; USD 200 domestic to libraries; USD 270 in Canada to libraries; USD 290 elsewhere to libraries (effective Aug. 2001). adv. *Refereed.* **Document type:** *Journal, Academic/Scholarly, Trade.* **Description:** Provides information and research related to managed pharmaceutical care and pharmacy practices around the world.
Published by: (Pharmaceutical Care Management Association), Haworth Press, Inc., 10 Alice St, Binghamton, NY 13904-1580. TEL 607-722-5857, 800-429-6784, FAX 607-722-6362, 800-895-0582, getinfo@haworthpressinc.com, http://www.haworthpress.com/journals/journallist.asp. Eds. Albert I Wertheimer, Jennifer Palcher. adv.: B&W page USD 315, color page USD 550; trim 6 x 8.5.

JOURNAL OF MEDICAL AND PHARMACEUTICAL MARKETING. see *BUSINESS AND ECONOMICS—Marketing And Purchasing*

615.19 610 USA ISSN 0022-2623
RS402 CODEN: JMCMAR
JOURNAL OF MEDICINAL CHEMISTRY. Text in English. 1958. bi-w. USD 1,419 in North America to institutions; USD 1,560 elsewhere to institutions; USD 1,703 in North America to institutions Print & online eds.; USD 1,844 elsewhere to institutions Print & online eds. (effective 2002); for additional pricing options for print and web editions contact inside sales specialist, Ms. Chako Dickinson, at 202-872-4063. adv. bk.rev. charts. index. back issues avail.; reprints avail. *Refereed.* **Document type:** *Journal, Academic/Scholarly.* **Description:** Focuses on the relationship of chemistry to biological activity. Provides valuable research findings and comprehensive book reviews on medicinal chemistry and related areas.
Formerly: Journal of Medicinal and Pharmaceutical Chemistry (0095-9065)
Related titles: Microfiche ed.: USD 1,419 in North America to institutions; USD 1,458 elsewhere to institutions (effective 2002); Microfilm ed.: USD 1,419 in North America to institutions; USD 1,439 elsewhere to institutions (effective 2002); Online - full text ed.: ISSN 1520-4804. USD 1,490 to institutions (effective 2002) (from EBSCO Publishing, Institute for Scientific Information).
Indexed: ASCA, Agri.& Environ.Biotech.Abstr. (coverage dropped), Aqua.Sci.& Fish.Abstr., BBCI, Biol.Abstr., Chem.Abstr., Chem.Cit.Ind., Chem.Indus.Notes, Chem.Titles, Curr.Adv.Biochem., Curr.Adv.Cancer Res., Curr.Adv.Ecol.Sci., Curr.Chem.React., Curr.Cont., Curr.Ind.Stat., Dairy Sci.Abstr., Dent.Ind., Derwent Biotech.Abstr., Environ.Sci.Poll.Mgmt., Excerp.Med., Genet.Abstr., Helminthol.Abstr., Hum.Gen.Abstr., INIS Atomind., Ind.Chem., Ind.Med. (1963-), Ind.Sci.Rev., Inpharma, MOS, Mass Spectr.Bull., Microbiol.Abstr., NPU, Neurosci.Abstr. (coverage dropped), Neurosci.Cit.Ind., Nuc.Acids Abstr., Nutr.Abstr., Pharm.&Out.News, Poult.Abstr., Protozool.Abstr., RCI, Reac., Rev.Appl.Entomol., Rev.Arom.& Med.Plants, Rev.Med.& Vet.Mycol., Rev.Plant Path., Sci.Cit.Ind., Sugar Ind.Abstr., Vet.Bull., Virol.Abstr. (coverage dropped).
—BLDSC (5017.200000), CASDDS, CINDOC, CISTI, EMDOCS, GNLM, IDS, ingenta, Linda Hall. **CCC.**
Published by: American Chemical Society, 1155 16th St, N W, Washington, DC 20036. TEL 202-332-5544, 800-333-9511, FAX 202-332-4559, service@acs.org, http://pubs.acs.org/jmc, http://www.acs.org. Ed. Dr. Philip S Portoghese. Circ: 4,425. **Subscr. to:** American Chemical Society, Member and Subscriber Services, PO Box 3337, Columbus, OH 43210. TEL 614-447-3674, FAX 614-447-3671.

616.01 GBR ISSN 0265-2048
RS201.C3 CODEN: JOMIEF
JOURNAL OF MICROENCAPSULATION. Text in English. 1984. bi-m. GBP 227, USD 374 to individuals; GBP 453, USD 750 to institutions (effective 2002). adv. *Refereed.* **Document type:** *Academic/Scholarly.* **Description:** Devoted to the preparation, properties and uses of individually encapsulated small particles. Its scope extends beyond microcapsules to all other small-particle dosage forms involving preparative manipulating.
Related titles: Online - full text ed.: ISSN 1464-5246 (from CatchWord Ltd., EBSCO Publishing, O C L C Online Computer Library Center, Inc., RoweCom Information Quest, Swets Blackwell, Institute for Scientific Information).
Indexed: ASCA, Chem.Abstr., Chem.Titles, Curr.Adv.Ecol.Sci., Curr.Cont., Derwent Biotech.Abstr., Food Sci.& Tech.Abstr., Ind.Med. (1984-), Ind.Sci.Rev., Inpharma, Intl.Polym.Sci.& Tech., Pharm.&Out.News, RAPRA (1988-), Reac., Sci.Cit.Ind., Sugar Ind.Abstr.
—BLDSC (5019.530000), CASDDS, CatchWord, CINDOC, CISTI, EMDOCS, GNLM, IDS, Infotrieve, KNAW. **CCC.**
Published by: Taylor & Francis Group, Taylor & Francis Ltd., 11 New Fetter Ln, London EC4P 4EE, United Kingdom. TEL 44-20-7583-9855, FAX 44-20-7842-2298, info@tandf.co.uk, http://www.tandf.co.uk. Ed. Tony L Whateley. **Subscr. in N. America to:** Taylor & Francis Ltd., 325 Chestnut St, Suite 800, Philadelphia, PA 19016. TEL 800-354-1420, FAX 215-625-8914, info@taylorandfrancis.com, http://www.taylorandfrancis.com/.

615 ZAF
JOURNAL OF MODERN PHARMACY; up-to-the-minute practical pharmacy. Cover title: Modern Pharmacy. Text in English. 1994. m. ZAR 333.68 foreign. adv. illus. **Document type:** *Trade.* **Description:** For pharmacists in community, hospital and health clinic pharmacies.
Published by: National Publishing (Pty) Ltd., PO Box 2271, Clareinch 7740, South Africa. TEL 27-21-611140, FAX 27-21-611389, accirc@natpub.co.za.

547.7 USA ISSN 0163-3864
QH1 CODEN: JNPRDF
JOURNAL OF NATURAL PRODUCTS. Text in English. 1938. m. USD 589 in North America to institutions; USD 630 elsewhere to institutions; USD 707 in North America to institutions Print & online eds.; USD 748 elsewhere to institutions Print & online eds. (effective 2002); for additional pricing options for print and web editions contact inside sales specialist, Ms. Chako Dickinson, at 202-872-4063. adv. bk.rev. charts, illus, stat. index. back issues avail. *Refereed.* **Document type:** *Journal, Academic/Scholarly.* **Description:** Covers natural products research - chemistry, biochemistry and biology of naturally occurring compounds.
Formerly (until vol.42, 1979): Lloydia (0024-5461)
Related titles: Online - full text ed.: ISSN 1520-6025. USD 618 to institutions (effective 2002) (from EBSCO Publishing, Institute for Scientific Information).
Indexed: AMED, ASCA, AgBiotech, Agri.& Environ.Biotech.Abstr. (coverage dropped), Agricola, Agroforest.Abstr., Anal.Abstr., Aqua.Sci.& Fish.Abstr., BBCI, Bibl.Agri., Bio-Contr.News & Info., Biol.& Agr.Ind. (Jan.1983-Mar.1989), Biol.Abstr., CEABA, Chem.Abstr., Chem.Cit.Ind., Chem.Infd., Chem.Titles, Chemorec.Abstr., Crop Physiol.Abstr., Curr.Adv.Biochem., Curr.Adv.Ecol.Sci., Curr.Biotech.Abstr., Curr.Chem.React., Curr.Cont., Deep Sea Res.& Oceanogr.Abstr., Derwent Biotech.Abstr., Entomol.Abstr., Environ.Sci.Poll.Mgmt., Excerp.Med., Field Crop Abstr., Food Sci.& Tech.Abstr., Forest Prod.Abstr., Forest.Abstr., Helminthol.Abstr., Herb.Abstr., Hort.Abstr., INIS Atomind., I.P.A., Ind.Chem., Ind.Med. (1979-), Ind.Sci.Rev., Ind.Vet., Inpharma, Int.Abstr.Biol.Sci., MOS, Maize Abstr., Mass Spectr.Bull., Med.& Pharm.Biotech.Abstr., Microbiol.Abstr., NPU, Nutr.Abstr., Ornam.Hort., Plant Breed.Abstr., Plant Grow.Reg.Abstr., Postharvest, Protozool.Abstr., RCI, Reac., Rev.Appl.Entomol., Rev.Arom.& Med.Plants, Rev.Med.& Vet.Mycol., Rev.Plant Path., Sci.Cit.Ind., Seed Abstr., So.Pac.Per.Ind., Soils & Fert., Soyabean Abstr., Vet.Bull., Weed Abstr., Zoo.Rec.
—BLDSC (5021.225000), CASDDS, CISTI, EMDOCS, GNLM, IDS, ingenta, Linda Hall. **CCC.**
Published by: American Society of Pharmacognosy, PO Box 12548, Glendale, AZ 85318. TEL 623-572-3500, FAX 623-572-3510, dslatk@arizona.midwestern.edu, http://pubs.acs.org/jnp, http://pubs.acs.org/journals/jnprdf/index.html. Ed. A Douglas Kinghorn. Circ: 2,300. **Co-sponsor:** American Chemical Society.

571.95 USA ISSN 1058-8108
CODEN: JNTOER
JOURNAL OF NATURAL TOXINS. Text in English. 1992. 4/yr. USD 160 in North America to individuals; USD 190 elsewhere to individuals; USD 280 in North America to institutions; USD 340 elsewhere to institutions (effective 2000). adv. bk.rev. back issues avail. *Refereed.* **Document type:** *Academic/Scholarly.* **Description:** Publishes original papers on all aspects of toxins, allergens and related compounds of natural origins.
Related titles: Online - full text ed.: (from Institute for Scientific Information).
Indexed: ASCA, Aqua.Sci.& Fish.Abstr., BBCI, Biol.Abstr., Chem.Abstr., Chem.Indus.Notes, Chem.Titles, Environ.Sci.Poll.Mgmt., Food Sci.& Tech.Abstr., Forest.Abstr., Ind.Med. (1992-), Ind.Vet., Int.Abstr.Biol.Sci., Mass Spectr.Bull., Microbiol.Abstr., Nutr.Abstr., Ocean.Abstr., Pollut.Abstr., Protozool.Abstr., Saf.Sci.Abstr., Sport Fish.Abstr., Trop.Dis.Bull., Vet.Bull., Weed Abstr., Wild.Rev., Zoo.Rec.
—BLDSC (5021.300200), CASDDS, CISTI, EMDOCS, GNLM, IDS, ingenta.
Published by: Alaken, Inc., 305 W. Magnolia St., PMB 196, Ft. Collins, CO 80521. TEL 970-223-5348, FAX 970-226-8655, info@alaken.com, http://www.alaken.com. Ed. Anthony T Tu. R&P Anthony Tu. Adv. contact Caroline Farley. Circ: 200.

615.1 USA ISSN 1089-4179
RM214 CODEN: JNFMFK
JOURNAL OF NUTRACEUTICALS, FUNCTIONAL & MEDICAL FOODS; innovations in research, practice, commercialization & policy. Text in English. q. USD 32 to individuals; USD 43 in Canada to individuals; USD 46 elsewhere to individuals; USD 60 to institutions; USD 81 in Canada to institutions; USD 87 elsewhere to institutions; USD 130 to libraries; USD 176 in Canada to libraries; USD 189 elsewhere to libraries (effective Aug. 2001). adv. back issues avail.; reprint service avail. from HAW. *Refereed.* **Document type:** *Journal, Academic/Scholarly.* **Description:** Offers a forum to explore the many product, business and policy issues that surround the technology allowing for the development of "superfoods.".
Related titles: Microform ed.
Indexed: AMED, Agricola, Aqua.Sci.& Fish.Abstr., Aquacult.Abstr., CINAHL, Dairy Sci.Abstr., Environ.Sci.Poll.Mgmt., Food Sci.& Tech.Abstr., Nutr.Abstr., Ref.Zh., Risk Abstr., Saf.Sci.Abstr., World Ag.Econ.& Rur.Soc.Abstr.
—BLDSC (5023.950000), Haworth.
Published by: Haworth Press, Inc., 10 Alice St, Binghamton, NY 13904-1580. TEL 607-722-5857, 800-429-6784, FAX 607-722-6362, 800-895-0582, getinfo@haworthpressinc.com, http://www.haworthpress.com/journals/journallist.asp. Eds. Nancy Maressa Childs, Robert Wildman. Pub. William Cohen. R&P Ruthann Heath TEL 607-723-5857 ext 316. Adv. contact Jackie Blakeslee TEL 607-722-5857 ext 346. B&W page USD 315, color page USD 550; trim 6 x 8.5.

JOURNAL OF OCULAR PHARMACOLOGY AND THERAPEUTICS. see *MEDICAL SCIENCES—Ophthalmology And Optometry*

615 616.99 USA ISSN 1078-1552
CODEN: JOPPFI
JOURNAL OF ONCOLOGY PHARMACY PRACTICE. Text in English. 1995. q. GBP 135 in Europe to individuals; USD 169 in North America to individuals; GBP 139 rest of world to individuals; GBP 332 in Europe to institutions; USD 375 in North America to institutions; GBP 339 rest of world to institutions; USD 55 in North America to members isopp; GBP 169 in developing nations; GBP 85 newsstand/cover in Europe; USD 99 newsstand/cover in North America; GBP 87 newsstand/cover rest of world (effective 2002). adv. abstr, bibl, charts, illus, stat. back issues avail.; reprints avail. *Refereed.* **Document type:** *Journal, Academic/Scholarly.* **Description:** Provides education and practice-related issues as well as original research, new therapies, patient management, and pharmacoeconomic evaluations for this emerging pharmacy specialty.
Related titles: Online - full text ed.: (from EBSCO Publishing, O C L C Online Computer Library Center, Inc., RoweCom Information Quest, ingenta, Swets Blackwell).
Indexed: Chem.Abstr., Chem.Indus.Notes, Chem.Titles, I.P.A.
—BLDSC (5026.314560), CASDDS, CISTI, GNLM, Infotrieve. **CCC.**

P

Published by: (International Society for Oncology Pharmacy Practitioners), Arnold Publishers (Subsidiary of: Hodder Headline plc.), 338 Euston Rd, London NW1 3BH, United Kingdom. TEL 44-20-7873-6337, FAX 44-20-7873-6325, arnoldjournals@hodder.co.uk, http://www.arnoldpublishers.com/journals/Journpages/10781552.htm, http://www.arnoldpublishers.com/journals/journtitles.htm. Eds. Barry R Goldspiel, Graham J Sewell, Jo-anne Brien.

615 362 GBR ISSN 1369-698X

JOURNAL OF OUTCOMES RESEARCH. Text in English. 1997. irreg., latest vol.5 (Each paper is published within 21 days of acceptance.). Avail. with subscr. to Journal of Drug Assessment. adv. abstr. index. 2 cols./p. Supplement avail.; back issues avail.; reprints avail. *Refereed.* **Document type:** *Journal, Academic/Scholarly.* **Description:** Covers quality of life aspects of drug development assessments.

Published by: Brookwood Medical Publications (Subsidiary of: P J B Publications Ltd.), 18-20 Hill Rise, Richmond, Surrey TW10 6UA, United Kingdom. TEL 44-20-8332-4600, FAX 44-20-8332-4610, maria@brookwd.demon.co.uk, http://www.pjbpubs.com/brookwood/. Ed., R&P Wendy Kimleer TEL 44-20-8332-4601. Pub. Dr. Philip J Brown. Adv. contact Jenefer Trevena TEL 44-20-8332-4605.

615 USA
RM319 CODEN: JPPSEX

JOURNAL OF PAIN & PALLIATIVE CARE PHARMACOTHERAPY; advances in acute, chronic and end of life symptom control. Text in English. 1993. q. USD 75 to individuals; USD 101 in Canada to individuals; USD 109 elsewhere to individuals; USD 175 to institutions; USD 236 in Canada to institutions; USD 254 elsewhere to institutions; USD 350 to libraries; USD 473 in Canada to libraries; USD 508 elsewhere to libraries (effective Aug. 2001). adv. bk.rev. reprint service avail. from HAW. *Refereed.* **Document type:** *Journal, Academic/Scholarly.*

Formerly (until 2002): Journal of Pharmaceutical Care in Pain & Symptom Control (1056-4950); Incorporates (in 2002): The Hospice Journal (0742-969X)

Related titles: Microfiche ed.: (from PQC); Microform ed.

Indexed: AMED, CINAHL, Excerp.Med. (1994-), I.P.A., Inpharma, Per.Islam. (1992-), Pharm.&Out.News, PsycInfo, Reac., Ref.Zh., e-psyche.

—BLDSC (5031.860000), EMDOCS, GNLM, Haworth, KNAW.

Published by: Haworth Press, Inc., 10 Alice St, Binghamton, NY 13904-1580. TEL 607-722-5857, 800-429-6784, FAX 607-722-6362, 800-895-0582, getinfo@haworthpressinc.com, http://www.haworthpressinc.com/journals/journallist.asp, http://www.haworthpress.com. Ed. Arthur Lipman. Pub. William Cohen. R&P Ruthann Heath TEL 607-723-5857 ext 316. Adv. contact Jackie Blakeslee TEL 607-722-5857 ext 346. B&W page USD 315, color page USD 550; trim 6 x 8.5.

615.19 NLD ISSN 0731-7085
CODEN: JPBADA

JOURNAL OF PHARMACEUTICAL AND BIOMEDICAL ANALYSIS. Text in English. 1983. 18/yr. EUR 2,109 in Europe to institutions; JPY 279,900 in Japan to institutions; USD 2,359 elsewhere to institutions (effective 2002). back issues avail. *Refereed.* **Document type:** *Academic/Scholarly.* **Description:** Publishes research reports and reviews on pharmaceutical and biomedical analysis.

Related titles: Microfilm ed.: (from PQC); Online - full text ed.: (from ingenta, ScienceDirect, Swets Blackwell, Institute for Scientific Information).

Indexed: ASCA, AgBiotech, Anal.Abstr., Anim.Breed.Abstr., BBCI, Chem.Abstr., Chem.Cit.Ind., Chem.Indus.Notes, Chem.Titles, Chromat.Abstr., Curr.Adv.Ecol.Sci., Curr.Cont., Curr.Ind.Stat., Dairy Sci.Abstr., Derwent Biotech.Abstr., Environ.Sci.Poll.Mgmt., Excerp.Med., Forest.Abstr., Helminthol.Abstr., Hort.Abstr., I.P.A., Ind.Med. (1983-), Ind.Sci.Rev., Ind.Vet., Inpharma, Int.Abstr.Biol.Sci., Mass Spectr.Bull., Nutr.Abstr., Pharm.&Out.News, Postharvest, Protozool.Abstr., Reac., Rev.Arom.& Med.Plants, Rev.Med.& Vet.Mycol., Sci.Cit.Ind., Tox.Abstr., Vet.Bull.

—BLDSC (5031.600000), ADONIS, CASDDS, CISTI, EMDOCS, GNLM, IDS, Infotrieve, KNAW. **CCC.**

Published by: Elsevier Science BV, PO Box 211, Amsterdam 1000 AE, Netherlands. TEL 31-20-485-2911, FAX 31-20-485-2457, nlinfo-f@elsevier.nl; usinfo-f@elsevier.com; forinfo-kyf04035@niftyserve.or.jp, http://www.elsevier.com/locate/jpba. Eds. Anthony Fell, Christopher M Riley. **Subscr. in Australasia and the Far East to:** Elsevier Science (Singapore) Pte Ltd, No.1 Temasek Ave, 17-01 Millenia Tower, Singapore 039192, Singapore. TEL 65-434-3727, FAX 65-337-2230; **Subscr. in Japan to:** Elsevier Science Inc - Japan Regional Office, 9-15 Higashi-Azabu 1-chome, Minato-ku, Tokyo 106-0044, Japan. TEL 81-3-5561-5033, FAX 81-3-5561-5047; **Subscr. in the Americas to:** Elsevier Science, PO Box 945, New York, NY 10159-0945. TEL 212-633-3730, FAX 212-633-3680, usinfo-f@elsevier.com.

615 610 NGA ISSN 0331-0604

JOURNAL OF PHARMACEUTICAL AND MEDICAL SCIENCES. Text in English. 1977. bi-m. USD 115.20. adv. illus.

Published by: Fred Atoki Publishing Co. Ltd., Plot 25 Kekere-Ekun St., Orile-Iganmu, PO Box 7313, Lagos, Nigeria. Ed. F O Atoki. Circ: 16,000.

615 USA

THE JOURNAL OF PHARMACEUTICAL CARE. Text in English. d. *Refereed.* **Document type:** *Academic/Scholarly.* **Description:** Serves as a resource to the academic and practice communities, and to enhance research and disseminate ideas pertaining to pharmaceutical care.

Media: Online - full text.

Published by: University of Louisiana at Monroe, 700 University Ave, Monroe, LA 71209. TEL 318-342-5272, pyhunter@alpha.nlu.edu, http://198.79.220.3/pharmacy/jpc/, http://www.ulm.edu. Ed. Dr. Tracy S Hunter.

615.19 658 USA ISSN 0883-7597
CODEN: JPMMEY

JOURNAL OF PHARMACEUTICAL MARKETING AND MANAGEMENT. Text in English. 1986. q. USD 60 to individuals; USD 81 in Canada to individuals; USD 87 elsewhere to individuals; USD 90 to institutions; USD 122 in Canada to institutions; USD 131 elsewhere to institutions; USD 275 to libraries; USD 371 in Canada to libraries; USD 399 elsewhere to libraries (effective Aug. 2001). adv. bk.rev. back issues avail.; reprint service avail. from HAW. *Refereed.* **Document type:** *Journal, Academic/Scholarly.* **Description:** Deals with solving problems of management and the marketing of pharmaceutical products and services.

Related titles: Microfiche ed.: (from PQC); Microform ed.; Online - full text ed.: (from Gale Group).

Indexed: Biostat., Human Resour.Abstr., I.P.A., Ind.Med. (coverage dropped), Mgmt.& Market.Abstr., P.A.I.S., Sage Fam.Stud.Abstr., Tr.& Indus.Ind.

—BLDSC (5031.880000), GNLM, Haworth, ingenta.

Published by: Haworth Press, Inc., 10 Alice St, Binghamton, NY 13904-1580. TEL 607-722-5857, 800-429-6784, FAX 607-722-6362, 800-895-0582, getinfo@haworthpressinc.com, http://www.haworthpress.com/journals/journallist.asp. Ed. Mickey C Smith. Pub. William Cohen. R&P Ruthann Heath TEL 607-723-5857 ext 316. Adv. contact Jackie Blakeslee TEL 607-722-5857 ext 346. B&W page USD 315, color page USD 550; trim 6 x 8.5.

615 GBR ISSN 0958-0581
CODEN: JPMDE7

JOURNAL OF PHARMACEUTICAL MEDICINE. Text in English. 1991. q. GBP 143 in Europe; GBP 157 elsewhere. adv. bk.rev. illus. index. back issues avail. *Refereed.* **Document type:** *Journal, Academic/Scholarly.*

Related titles: Microform ed.: (from PQC); Online - full text ed.: (from EBSCO Publishing).

Indexed: I.P.A., Ind.Vet., Pig News & Info., Vet.Bull.

—EMDOCS, GNLM, Infotrieve. **CCC.**

Published by: (Society of Pharmaceutical Medicine), Chapman & Hall Ltd. (Subsidiary of: International Thomson Publishing Group), Journals Department, Chapman & Hall, 2-6 Boundary Row, London SE1 8HN, United Kingdom. TEL 44-20-7865-0066, FAX 44-20-7522-9623, jhelp@chall.co.uk. Circ: 435. **Subscr. to:** international Publishing Services Ltd., Cheriton House, North Way, Walworth Industrial Estate, Andover, Hants SP10 5BE, United Kingdom. TEL 44-1264-342713, FAX 44-1264-342807.

615.1 JPN ISSN 0372-7629
CODEN: YAKUA2

JOURNAL OF PHARMACEUTICAL SCIENCE AND TECHNOLOGY/YAKUZAIGAKU. Text in English, Japanese; Summaries in English. 1940. q. JPY 5,356. **Document type:** *Academic/Scholarly.*

Formerly: Archives of Practical Pharmacy

Indexed: Biol.Abstr., Chem.Abstr., Chem.Indus.Notes, Chem.Titles, INIS Atomind., I.P.A.

—BLDSC (5031.890000), CASDDS, GNLM, Infotrieve, Linda Hall. **CCC.**

Published by: (Academy of Pharmaceutical Science and Technology), Business Center for Academic Societies Japan/Nihon Gakkai Jimu Senta, 5-16-9 Honkomagome, Bunkyo-ku, Tokyo 113-0021, Japan. TEL 81-3-5814-5811, FAX 81-3-5814-5822, TELEX 2722268 BCJSP J. Circ: 1,200.

615.1 USA ISSN 0022-3549
RS1 CODEN: JPMSAE

JOURNAL OF PHARMACEUTICAL SCIENCES. Text in English. 1961 (vol.50). a. USD 795 in United States; USD 795 in Canada & Mexico; USD 852 elsewhere; USD 835 combined subscription in United States for print and online eds.; USD 835 combined subscription in Canada & Mexico for print and online eds.; USD 892 combined subscription elsewhere for print and online eds. (effective 2002). adv. bk.rev. bibl, charts, illus. index. back issues avail. *Refereed.* **Document type:** *Academic/Scholarly.* **Description:** Primary research in pharmaceutical science; graduate level and above.

Related titles: Online - full text ed.: ISSN 1520-6017. USD 795 in United States; USD 795 in Canada & Mexico; USD 795 elsewhere (effective 2002) (from EBSCO Publishing, Wiley InterScience, Institute for Scientific Information).

Indexed: AIDS Abstr., ASCA, Agri.& Environ.Biotech.Abstr. (coverage dropped), Anal.Abstr., Biol.Abstr., Chem.Abstr., Chem.Cit.Ind., Chem.Indus.Notes, Chem.Infd., Chem.Titles, Chromat.Abstr., Compumath, Curr.Adv.Cancer Res., Curr.Adv.Ecol.Sci., Curr.Chem.React., Curr.Cont., Dairy Sci.Abstr., Dent.Ind., Derwent Biotech.Abstr., Environ.Sci.Poll.Mgmt., Excerp.Med., Helminthol.Abstr., Hort.Abstr., INIS Atomind., I.P.A., Ind.Chem., Ind.Med. (1961-), Ind.Sci.Rev., Inpharma, Mass Spectr.Bull., Mat.Sci.Cit.Ind. (coverage dropped), Nutr.Abstr., Pharm.&Out.News, Pollut.Abstr., Protozool.Abstr., RCI, Reac., Rev.Plant Path., Risk Abstr., Saf.Sci.Abstr., Sci.Cit.Ind., Sugar Ind.Abstr., Vet.Bull.

—BLDSC (5031.900000), CASDDS, CINDOC, CISTI, GNLM, IDS, ingenta, KNAW, Linda Hall. **CCC.**

Published by: (American Chemical Society), John Wiley & Sons, Inc., Journals (Subsidiary of: Wiley InterScience), 605 Third Ave, New York, NY 10158. TEL 212-850-6645, FAX 212-850-6021, subinfo@wiley.com, uscs-wis@wiley.com, http://www.wiley.com. Ed. William I Higuchi. Circ: 5,400. **Subscr. outside the Americas to:** John Wiley & Sons Ltd., Baffins Ln, Chichester, Sussex PO19 IUD, United Kingdom. TEL 44-1243-779777, FAX 44-1243-843232, cs-journals@wiley.co.uk.

615.19 USA ISSN 0896-6966
CODEN: JPHAE7

JOURNAL OF PHARMACOEPIDEMIOLOGY; innovations in pharmaceutical research and practice relating. Text in English. 1989. s-a. USD 75 to individuals; USD 101 in Canada to individuals; USD 109 elsewhere to individuals; USD 125 to institutions; USD 169 in Canada to institutions; USD 181 elsewhere to institutions; USD 175 to libraries; USD 236 in Canada to libraries; USD 254 elsewhere to libraries (effective Aug. 2001). adv. bk.rev. back issues avail.; reprint service avail. from HAW. *Refereed.* **Document type:** *Journal, Academic/Scholarly.* **Description:** Facilitates the dissemination and exchange of findings, assessments, and reports of research and practice dealing with the outcomes of drug treatment.

Related titles: Microform ed.: (from PQC).

Indexed: Biostat., Environ.Sci.Poll.Mgmt., Excerp.Med. (1993-), I.P.A., Inpharma, Pharm.&Out.News, Pollut.Abstr., Reac., Ref.Zh., Risk Abstr., Saf.Sci.Abstr.

—BLDSC (5032.500000), EMDOCS, GNLM, Haworth.

Published by: Haworth Press, Inc., 10 Alice St, Binghamton, NY 13904-1580. TEL 607-722-5857, 800-429-6784, FAX 607-722-6362, 800-895-0582, getinfo@haworthpressinc.com, http://www.haworthpress.com/journals/journallist.asp. Eds. Dennis Frate, Eugene Kolassa. Pub. William Cohen. R&P Ruthann Heath TEL 607-723-5857 ext 316. Adv. contact Jackie Blakeslee TEL 607-722-5857 ext 346. B&W page USD 315, color page USD 550; trim 6 x 8.5.

P

615 USA ISSN 1567-567X
RM1 CODEN: JPBPBJ

JOURNAL OF PHARMACOKINETICS AND PHARMACODYNAMICS. Text in English. 1973. bi-m. USD 645, EUR 644 to institutions for print or online ed.; USD 774, EUR 772.80 to institutions for print & online eds.combined (effective 2002). adv. index. back issues avail. *Refereed.* **Document type:** *Journal, Academic/Scholarly.* **Description:** Illustrates the importance of pharmacokinetic and biopharmaceutical applications in the understanding of drug action, design, therapy, and evaluation.
Formerly (until 2000): Journal of Pharmacokinetics and Biopharmaceutics (0090-466X)
Related titles: Microfilm ed.: (from PQC); Online - full text ed.: (from O C L C Online Computer Library Center, Inc., Swets Blackwell, Kluwer Online, Institute for Scientific Information, RoweCom Information Quest).
Indexed: ASCA, Agri.& Environ.Biotech.Abstr. (coverage dropped), BBCI, Biol.Abstr., Chem.Abstr., Chem.Indus.Notes, Chem.Titles, Compumath, Curr.Adv.Ecol.Sci., Curr.Cont., Derwent Biotech.Abstr., Excerp.Med., INIS Atomind., I.P.A., Ind.Med. (1973-), Ind.Sci.Rev., Inpharma, Int.Abstr.Biol.Sci., Pharm.&Out.News, Reac., Ref.Zh., SSCI (coverage dropped), Sci.Cit.Ind.
—BLDSC (5032.610000), ADONIS, CASDDS, CISTI, GNLM, IDS, KNAW, Linda Hall. **CCC.**
Published by: Kluwer Academic - Plenum Publishers (Subsidiary of: Wolters Kluwer N.V.), 233 Spring St, New York, NY 10013-1578. TEL 212-620-8000, 800-221-9369, FAX 212-463-0742, info@plenum.com, http://www.wkap.nl/journalhome.htm/1567-567X. Eds. Malcolm Rowland, Thomas M Ludden. R&P Rose Luongo TEL 781-871-6311. **Subscr. outside the Americas to:** Kluwer Academic Publishers Group, Journals Department, PO Box 322, Dordrecht 3300 AH, Netherlands. TEL 31-78-639-2392, FAX 31-78-654-6474.

P

JOURNAL OF PHARMACOLOGICAL AND TOXICOLOGICAL METHODS. see *ENVIRONMENTAL STUDIES—Toxicology And Environmental Safety*

615.1 USA ISSN 0022-3565
RS1 CODEN: JPETAB

JOURNAL OF PHARMACOLOGY AND EXPERIMENTAL THERAPEUTICS. Text in English. 1909. m. (4 vols./yr.). USD 235 domestic to individuals; USD 337 foreign to individuals; USD 540 domestic to institutions; USD 642 foreign to institutions (effective 2000); includes on-line ed.. adv. bibl, charts, illus. index. *Refereed.* **Document type:** *Academic/Scholarly.* **Description:** Documents interactions of chemicals with biological systems for pharmacologists, toxicologists and biochemists.
Related titles: Microfilm ed.: (from WWS); Online - full text ed.: ISSN 1521-0103. USD 176 domestic to individuals; USD 188 foreign to individuals; USD 432 domestic to institutions (effective 2000) (from HighWire Pr., EBSCO Publishing, Institute for Scientific Information).
Indexed: ASCA, Addic.Abstr., Agri.& Environ.Biotech.Abstr. (coverage dropped), Apic.Abstr., Aqua.Sci.& Fish.Abstr., BBCI, Biol.Abstr., Cal.Tiss.Abstr. (coverage dropped), Chem.Abstr., Chem.Indus.Notes, Chem.Titles, Curr.Adv.Ecol.Sci., Curr.Cont., Dairy Sci.Abstr., Dent.Ind., Derwent Biotech.Abstr., Environ.Sci.Poll.Mgmt., Excerp.Med., Helminthol.Abstr., INIS Atomind., I.P.A., Ind.Med. (1909-), Ind.Sci.Rev., Ind.Vet., Inpharma, Int.Abstr.Biol.Sci., Kidney, Mass Spectr.Bull., Med.& Surg.Dermat., Neurosci.Abstr. (coverage dropped), Neurosci.Cit.Ind., Nutr.Abstr., Pharm.&Out.News, Protozool.Abstr., PsycInfo, Psychol.Abstr. (1968-), Reac., Ref.Zh., Rev.Appl.Entomol., Rev.Arom.& Med.Plants, SSCI (coverage dropped), Sci.Cit.Ind., THA, Tox.Abstr. (coverage dropped), Vet.Bull., e-psyche.
—BLDSC (5033.000000), CASDDS, CINDOC, CISTI, GNLM, IDS, ingenta, KNAW, Linda Hall.
Published by: American Society for Pharmacology and Experimental Therapeutics (ASPET), 9650 Rockville Pike, Bethesda, MD 20814-3998. TEL 301-530-7024, FAX 301-571-5728, staff@dues.faseb.org, http://jpet.aspetjournals.org. Ed. S J Enna. R&P Richard Dodenhof TEL 301-571-5754. Adv. contact Frances Yates. B&W page USD 675; trim 10.88 x 8.38. Circ: 2,074; 2,034 (paid).

615 CAN ISSN 1482-1826

JOURNAL OF PHARMACY AND PHARMACEUTICAL SCIENCES. Text in English. 1998. q. free per issue. bk.rev. **Document type:** *Academic/Scholarly.* **Description:** Features original research articles, reviews, news and views on pharmaceutical sciences.
Media: Online - full text (from Institute for Scientific Information).
Indexed: Curr.Cont., Ind.Med. (1998-).
Published by: Canadian Society for Pharmaceutical Sciences, 3118 Dentistry/Pharmacy Centre, Univ of Alberta Campus, Edmonton, AB T6G 2N8, Canada. TEL 780-492-0950, FAX 780-492-0951, sandra.hutt@ualberta.ca, http://www.uablerta.ca/~csps. Ed. Fakhreddin Jamali.

615.1 GBR ISSN 0022-3573
CODEN: JPPMAB

JOURNAL OF PHARMACY AND PHARMACOLOGY. Text in English. 1949. m. GBP 520 in United Kingdom; GBP 540 in the European Union; USD 910 in United States; GBP 560 elsewhere (effective 2001). adv. bibl, charts, illus. index. back issues avail. *Refereed.* **Document type:** *Journal, Academic/Scholarly.* **Description:** Publishes original research papers and reviews articles about the development and evaluation of medicinal substances.
Incorporates (1995-2000): Pharmacy and Pharmacology Communications (1460-8081)
Related titles: Microfilm ed.; Online - full text ed.: (from ingenta, Institute for Scientific Information, RoweCom Information Quest).
Indexed: ASCA, Abstr.Hyg., Agri.& Environ.Biotech.Abstr. (coverage dropped), Agroforest.Abstr., Anal.Abstr., Apic.Abstr., Aqua.Sci.& Fish.Abstr., Biol.Abstr., Cal.Tiss.Abstr., Chem.Abstr., Chem.Cit.Ind., Chem.Indus.Notes, Chem.Titles, Curr.Adv.Ecol.Sci., Curr.Chem.React., Curr.Cont., Dairy Sci.Abstr., Dent.Ind., Derwent Biotech.Abstr., Environ.Sci.Poll.Mgmt., Excerp.Med., Forest Prod.Abstr., Helminthol.Abstr., INIS Atomind., I.P.A., Ind.Chem., Ind.Med. (1949-), Ind.Sci.Rev., Ind.Vet., Inpharma, Int.Abstr.Biol.Sci., Med.& Surg.Dermat., NPU, Neurosci.Abstr., Neurosci.Cit.Ind., Nutr.Abstr., Pharm.&Out.News, Pig News & Info., Pollut.Abstr., Protozool.Abstr., RCI, Reac., Ref.Zh., Rev.Appl.Entomol., Rev.Arom.& Med.Plants, Rev.Med.& Vet.Mycol., SSCI (coverage dropped), Sci.Cit.Ind., Sugar Ind.Abstr., THA, Trop.Dis.Bull., Vet.Bull.
—BLDSC (5034.000000), CASDDS, CINDOC, CISTI, GNLM, IDS, ingenta, KNAW, Linda Hall. **CCC.**
Published by: (Euromed Communications Ltd.), Pharmaceutical Press (Subsidiary of: Euromed Communications Ltd.), 1 Lambeth High St, London SE1 7JN, United Kingdom. TEL 44-20-7735-9141, FAX 44-20-7735-5085, http://www.pharmpress.com. Pub., R&P Charles Fry. Adv. contact Jack Richmond. Circ: 1,000. **Subscr. to:** PO Box 151, Wallingford, Oxford OX10 8QU, United Kingdom. TEL 44-1491-829272, FAX 44-1491-829292, rpsgb@cabi.org.

615 USA ISSN 0897-1900
RS1 CODEN: JPPREU

JOURNAL OF PHARMACY PRACTICE. Text in English. 1988. bi-m. USD 210 for print or electronic eds.; USD 240 for print and electronic eds. (effective 2001). back issues avail.; reprints avail. **Document type:** *Journal, Academic/Scholarly.* **Description:** Covers current information on new drugs, pharmocokinetics, drug administration, and adverse drug reactions. Also considers legal issues, economic concerns, and new problems rising from managed care.
Related titles: E-mail ed.; Online - full content ed.
Indexed: Excerp.Med. (1996-), I.P.A.
—BLDSC (5034.020000), GNLM, Infotrieve. **CCC.**
Published by: Sage Publications, Inc., 2111 W Hillcrest Dr, Thousand Oaks, CA 91320. Circ: 285 (paid).

615.071 USA ISSN 1044-0054
CODEN: JOPTET

JOURNAL OF PHARMACY TEACHING. Text in English. 1990. q. USD 60 to individuals; USD 81 in Canada to individuals; USD 87 elsewhere to individual members; USD 95 to institutions; USD 128 in Canada to institutions; USD 138 elsewhere to institutions; USD 105 to libraries; USD 142 in Canada to libraries; USD 152 elsewhere to libraries (effective Aug. 2001). adv. back issues avail.; reprint service avail. from HAW. *Refereed.* **Document type:** *Journal, Academic/Scholarly.* **Description:** Focuses on the communication of information with the goal of improved teaching in pharmacy.
Related titles: Microform ed.: (from PQC).
Indexed: Cont.Pg.Educ., ERA, I.P.A., Ref.Zh.
—BLDSC (5034.025000), GNLM, Haworth.
Published by: Haworth Press, Inc., 10 Alice St, Binghamton, NY 13904-1580. TEL 607-722-5857, 800-429-6784, FAX 607-722-6362, 800-895-0582, getinfo@haworthpressinc.com, http://www.haworthpress.com/journals/journallist.asp. Ed. Noel Wilkin. Pub. William Cohen. R&P Ruthann Heath TEL 607-723-5857 ext 316. Adv. contact Jackie Blakeslee TEL 607-722-5857 ext 346. B&W page USD 315, color page USD 550; trim 6 x 8.5.

615.329 USA ISSN 8755-1225
CODEN: JPTEEB

JOURNAL OF PHARMACY TECHNOLOGY. Text in English. 1985. bi-m. USD 49 to individuals; USD 130 to institutions; USD 30 to students; USD 10 newsstand/cover (effective 2001). adv. bk.rev., software rev. abstr, bibl, charts, illus. index. back issues avail.; reprints avail. *Refereed.* **Document type:** *Journal, Academic/Scholarly.* **Description:** Aimed at pharmacists and technicians. Covers therapeutic trends, current research and organizational, legal and educational activities. Includes information on new drugs and medical products and equipment.
Related titles: Microform ed.: (from PQC).
Indexed: Abstr.Health Care Manage.Stud., CINAHL, Chem.Abstr., Chem.Indus.Notes, Chem.Titles, Curr.Adv.Ecol.Sci., Excerp.Med., I.P.A., Inpharma, Pharm.&Out.News, Reac.
—BLDSC (5034.030000), CASDDS, CISTI, EMDOCS, GNLM.
Published by: Harvey Whitney Books Company, PO Box 42696, Cincinnati, OH 45242. TEL 513-793-3555, FAX 513-793-3600, customerserv@jpharmtechnol.com, http://www.jpharmtechnol.com. Ed., Pub. Harvey Whitney Jr. R&P, Adv. contact Greg J Johnson. Circ: 1,600.

JOURNAL OF PHYSIOLOGY AND PHARMACOLOGY. see *BIOLOGY—Physiology*

JOURNAL OF PLANAR CHROMATOGRAPHY - MODERN TLC (JPC). see *CHEMISTRY—Analytical Chemistry*

JOURNAL OF PSYCHOACTIVE DRUGS; a multidisciplinary forum. see *DRUG ABUSE AND ALCOHOLISM*

615.7 616.8 GBR ISSN 0269-8811
CODEN: JOPSEQ

JOURNAL OF PSYCHOPHARMACOLOGY. Text in English. 1987. q. GBP 59 to individuals; GBP 249 to institutions; GBP 16 newsstand/cover to individuals; GBP 63 newsstand/cover to institutions (effective 2002). adv. bk.rev. back issues avail.; reprint service avail. from PSC,SCH. *Refereed.* **Document type:** *Academic/Scholarly.* **Description:** Presents original research and review articles on both preclinical and clinical aspects of psychopharmacology.
Formerly: British Association for Psychopharmacology. Journal
Related titles: Online - full text ed.: (from EBSCO Publishing, O C L C Online Computer Library Center, Inc., RoweCom Information Quest, ingenta, Swets Blackwell, Institute for Scientific Information).
Indexed: ASCA, Addic.Abstr., Biol.Abstr., Chem.Abstr., Chem.Indus.Notes, Chem.Titles, Curr.Cont., Dairy Sci.Abstr., Derwent Biotech.Abstr., Excerp.Med., Focus on: Psychophar., Ind.Med. (1987-), Ind.Sci.Rev., Inpharma, Int.Abstr.Biol.Sci., Neurosci.Cit.Ind., Nutr.Abstr., Pharm.&Out.News, PsycInfo, Psychol.Abstr. (1987-), Reac., SSCI (coverage dropped), Sci.Cit.Ind., Viol.& Abuse Abstr., e-psyche.
—BLDSC (5043.450000), CASDDS, CISTI, EMDOCS, GNLM, Infotrieve, KNAW. **CCC.**
Published by: Sage Publications Ltd., 6 Bonhill St, London EC2A 4PU, United Kingdom. TEL 44-20-7374-0645, FAX 44-20-7374-8741, market@sagepub.co.uk, http://www.sagepub.co.uk. Eds. David Nutt, Martin Sarter. Adv. contact Jenny Kirby. page GBP 250; trim 230 x 175. Circ: 1,250.

615.19 330.9 USA ISSN 0896-6621
HD9666.1 CODEN: JRPEE5

JOURNAL OF RESEARCH IN PHARMACEUTICAL ECONOMICS. Text in English. 1989. q. USD 75 to individuals; USD 101 in Canada to individuals; USD 190 elsewhere to individuals; USD 150 to institutions; USD 203 in Canada to institutions; USD 218 elsewhere to institutions; USD 300 to libraries; USD 405 in Canada to libraries; USD 435 elsewhere to libraries (effective Aug. 2001). adv. bk.rev. back issues avail.; reprint service avail. from HAW. *Refereed.* **Document type:** *Journal, Academic/Scholarly.* **Description:** Deals with the analysis of economic questions and concerns related to the use of pharmaceutical products and services.
Related titles: Microfiche ed.: (from PQC); Microform ed.
Indexed: Excerp.Med. (1996-), I.P.A., Inpharma, J.of Econ.Lit., Pharm.&Out.News, Reac., Soc.Work Res.& Abstr.
—BLDSC (5052.026000), GNLM, Haworth.

Published by: Haworth Press, Inc., 10 Alice St, Binghamton, NY 13904-1580. TEL 607-722-5857, 800-429-6784, FAX 607-722-6362, 800-895-0582, getinfo@haworthpressinc.com, http://www.haworthpressinc.com, http://www.haworthpress.com. Ed. Mickey Smith. Pub. William Cohen. R&P Ruthann Heath TEL 607-723-5857 ext 316. Adv. contact Jackie Blakeslee TEL 607-722-5857 ext 346. B&W page USD 315, color page USD 550; trim 6 x 8.5.

615.9 500 610 IND ISSN 0253-7249 CODEN: JSRMDB
JOURNAL OF SCIENTIFIC RESEARCH IN PLANTS & MEDICINES. Text in English. 1981. s-a. INR 150 to individuals; INR 300 to institutions. bk.rev. back issues avail. **Document type:** *Trade.* **Description:** Covers the manufacturing of medicines and medicinal products from plants, herbs, and mineral rarely found on the higher altitudes of the Himalayan ranges.
Indexed: Biol.Abstr., Forest.Abstr., Hort.Abstr., Seed Abstr.
—CASDDS, CISTI.
Published by: Yogi Pharmacy Ltd. (Hardwar), Research & Publication Division, D-29-30 Industrial Area, Hardwar, Uttar Pradesh 249 401, India. TEL 91-133-420304, FAX 91-133-421111. Ed. C S Trivedi. Circ: 5,000.

615.19 SWE ISSN 0281-0662
JOURNAL OF SOCIAL AND ADMINISTRATIVE PHARMACY. Text in English. 1983. 6/yr. USD 140, EUR 150 (effective 2001). 40 p./no. back issues avail. *Refereed.* **Document type:** *Journal, Academic/Scholarly.*
Related titles: ♦ Supplement: Journal of Social and Administrative Pharmacy. Supplement. ISSN 0282-6607.
Indexed: IBZ, I.P.A., Lang.& Lang.Behav.Abstr., SOPODA, Sociol.Abstr.
—BLDSC (5064.714000), EMDOCS, GNLM, ingenta.
Published by: Swedish Pharmaceutical Press, Box 1136, Stockholm 11181, Sweden. TEL 46-8-723-50-00, 46-8-7235021, FAX 46-8-14-95-80, press@swepharm.se, http://www.swepharm.se/Forlag/Lakemedelsvarlden/aktuellt.html. Eds. G Nilsson, J Lars.

615.19 SWE ISSN 0282-6607
JOURNAL OF SOCIAL AND ADMINISTRATIVE PHARMACY. SUPPLEMENT. Text in English. 1984. irreg.
Related titles: ♦ Supplement to: Journal of Social and Administrative Pharmacy. ISSN 0281-0662.
Published by: Swedish Pharmaceutical Press, Box 1136, Stockholm 11181, Sweden. TEL 46-8-723-50-00, FAX 46-8-14-95-80, press@swepharm.se, http://www.swepharm.se/Forlag/Lakemedelsvarlden/aktuellt.html.

JOURNAL OF TOXICOLOGIC PATHOLOGY. see *ENVIRONMENTAL STUDIES—Toxicology And Environmental Safety*

JOURNAL OF TOXICOLOGICAL SCIENCES. see *ENVIRONMENTAL STUDIES—Toxicology And Environmental Safety*

JOURNAL OF TOXICOLOGY AND ENVIRONMENTAL HEALTH. PART A. see *ENVIRONMENTAL STUDIES—Toxicology And Environmental Safety*

JOURNAL OF TOXICOLOGY AND ENVIRONMENTAL HEALTH. PART B: CRITICAL REVIEWS. see *ENVIRONMENTAL STUDIES—Toxicology And Environmental Safety*

615 USA ISSN 0731-3810
RA1190 CODEN: JTCTDW
JOURNAL OF TOXICOLOGY. CLINICAL TOXICOLOGY. Text in English. 1963. 7/yr. USD 145 to individuals print & online eds.; USD 1,775 to institutions print only (effective 2002). adv. *Refereed.* **Document type:** *Academic/Scholarly.* **Description:** Correlates the various disciplines that deal directly with and contribute to the practical aspects of poisoning per se.
Supersedes (in 1981): Clinical Toxicology (0009-9309)
Related titles: Microform ed.: (from RPI); Online - full text ed.: (from Gale Group, EBSCO Publishing, O C L C Online Computer Library Center, Inc., RoweCom Information Quest, Swets Blackwell, Factiva, Institute for Scientific Information).
Indexed: AIM, ASCA, Abstr.Hyg., Agri.& Environ.Biotech.Abstr. (coverage dropped), Biol.Abstr., Biol.Dig., C.I.S. Abstr., Chem.Abstr., Chem.Indus.Notes, Chem.Titles, Curr.Adv.Ecol.Sci., Curr.Cont., Dairy Sci.Abstr., Dent.Ind., Derwent Biotech.Abstr., Energy Rev., Environ.Abstr., Environ.Per.Bibl. (1991-1994), Environ.Sci.Poll.Mgmt., Excerp.Med., INIS Atomind., I.P.A., Ind.Med. (1982-), Ind.Sci.Rev., Ind.Vet., Inpharma, Int.Abstr.Biol.Sci., Jrnl.Watch Emer.Med., Lab.Haz.Bull., Med.Abstr., NRN, Neurosci.Abstr., Nutr.Abstr., Pharm.&Out.News, Pig News & Info., Pollut.Abstr., Protozool.Abstr., Reac., Ref.Zh., Rev.Appl.Entomol., Rev.Arom.& Med.Plants, Rev.Med.& Vet.Mycol., Rev.Plant Path., Risk Abstr., Saf.Sci.Abstr., Sci.Cit.Ind., Sport Fish.Abstr., THA, Trop.Dis.Bull., Vet.Bull., Weed Abstr., Wild.Rev.
—BLDSC (5069.736000), CASDDS, CISTI, EMDOCS, GNLM, IDS, ingenta, KNAW, Linda Hall. **CCC.**
Published by: (American Academy of Clinical Toxicology), Marcel Dekker Inc., 270 Madison Ave, New York, NY 10016. TEL 212-696-9000, 800-228-1160, FAX 212-685-4540, http://www.dekker.com/servlet/product/productid/CLT. Ed. Carol R Angle. R&P Julia Mulligan. Adv. contact Diane Saulon. Circ: 1,500. **Co-sponsor:** European Association of Poison Centres and Clinical Toxicologists.

615.9 USA ISSN 0731-3829
RL803 CODEN: JTOTDO
JOURNAL OF TOXICOLOGY. CUTANEOUS AND OCULAR TOXICOLOGY. Text in English. 1982. q. USD 110 combined subscription to individuals for print & online eds.; USD 1,050 to institutions (effective 2002). *Refereed.* **Document type:** *Academic/Scholarly.* **Description:** Explores the phenomena of cutaneous and ocular irritation, sensitization, phototoxicity and photoallergenicity of cosmetics, etc. Contains in vitro and in vivo research as well as the clinical description, diagnosis, and treatment of such effects.
Related titles: Microform ed.: (from RPI); Online - full content ed.; Online - full text ed.: (from Institute for Scientific Information, RoweCom Information Quest).
Indexed: ASCA, Aqua.Sci.& Fish.Abstr., Biol.Abstr., Chem.Abstr., Chem.Indus.Notes, Chem.Titles, Curr.Adv.Ecol.Sci., Curr.Cont., Energy Rev., Environ.Abstr., Environ.Per.Bibl. (1982-), Environ.Sci.Poll.Mgmt., Excerp.Med., Ind.Sci.Rev., Inpharma, Int.Abstr.Biol.Sci., Lab.Haz.Bull., Pollut.Abstr., Reac., Ref.Zh., Saf.Sci.Abstr., Sci.Cit.Ind.
—BLDSC (5069.738500), CASDDS, CISTI, EMDOCS, GNLM, IDS, ingenta, KNAW. **CCC.**
Published by: Marcel Dekker Inc., 270 Madison Ave, New York, NY 10016. TEL 212-696-9000, 800-228-1160, FAX 212-685-4540, http://www.dekker.com/servlet/product/productid/CUS. Ed. Wallace Hayes. R&P Julia Mulligan. Adv. contact Diane Saulon. Circ: 425.

615.9 USA ISSN 0731-3837
RA1190 CODEN: JTTRD9
JOURNAL OF TOXICOLOGY. TOXIN REVIEWS. Text in English. 1982. q. USD 110 to individuals print & online eds.; USD 950 to institutions print only (effective 2002). *Refereed.* **Document type:** *Academic/Scholarly.* **Description:** Brings information on toxins (their characteristics, activities and mechanisms of action) from the full range of clinical and scientific disciplines in which toxins impinge.
Related titles: Microform ed.: (from RPI); Online - full text ed.: (from EBSCO Publishing, O C L C Online Computer Library Center, Inc., RoweCom Information Quest, Swets Blackwell, Institute for Scientific Information).
Indexed: ASCA, Aqua.Sci.& Fish.Abstr., Biol.Abstr., Chem.Abstr., Chem.Indus.Notes, Chem.Titles, Curr.Adv.Ecol.Sci., Curr.Cont., Dairy Sci.Abstr., Environ.Abstr., Environ.Sci.Poll.Mgmt., Excerp.Med., Ind.Sci.Rev., Inpharma, Maize Abstr., NRN, Nutr.Abstr., Pharm.&Out.News, Pig News & Info., Pollut.Abstr., Reac., Ref.Zh., Rev.Appl.Entomol., Rev.Med.& Vet.Mycol., Saf.Sci.Abstr., Sci.Cit.Ind., Sport Fish.Abstr., Wild.Rev., Zoo.Rec.
—BLDSC (5069.741000), CASDDS, CISTI, EMDOCS, GNLM, IDS, ingenta, KNAW. **CCC.**
Published by: Marcel Dekker Inc., 270 Madison Ave, New York, NY 10016. TEL 212-696-9000, 800-228-1160, FAX 212-685-4540, http://www.dekker.com/servlet/product/productid/TXR. Eds. A T Tu, W T Shier. R&P Julia Mulligan. Adv. contact Diane Saulon. Circ: 225.

615 JPN
CODEN: WIGAES
JOURNAL OF TRADITIONAL MEDICINES. Text in English, Japanese; Abstracts in English. 1967. 4/yr. JPY 10,000, USD 95. adv. back issues avail. *Refereed.* **Document type:** *Academic/Scholarly.* **Description:** Contains chemical, pharmaceutical, pharmacological and clinical studies on Sino-Japanese traditional medicines.
Former titles (until 1994): Medical and Pharmaceutical Society for Wakan-Yaku. Journal (0289-730X); (until 1984): Wakan-Yaku Shinpojumu (0388-7413)
Indexed: Nutr.Abstr., Rev.Arom.& Med.Plants.
—BLDSC (5069.755000), CASDDS.
Published by: (Medical and Pharmaceutical Society for Wakan-Yaku), Chuo Insatsu Co., 1-4-5 Shimo-Okui, Toyama-shi 930-0817, Japan. TEL 0764-32-6572. Ed. Hiroshi Watanabe. Circ: 1,300. **Subscr. to:** Toyama Medical & Pharmaceutical University, Research Institute for Wakan-Yaku, Toyama 930-01, Japan. TEL 81-764-34-2281, FAX 81-764-34-5056.

JOURNAL OF VENOMOUS ANIMALS AND TOXINS. see *BIOLOGY—Zoology*

615 636.089 GBR ISSN 0140-7783 CODEN: JVPTD9
JOURNAL OF VETERINARY PHARMACOLOGY AND THERAPEUTICS. Text in English. 1978. bi-m., latest vol.25, 2002. GBP 465 in Europe; USD 738 in North America; GBP 512 elsewhere (effective 2002). adv. bk.rev. bibl. back issues avail.; reprint service avail. from ISI. *Refereed.* **Document type:** *Academic/Scholarly.* **Description:** Devoted to the publication of scientific papers in the basic and clinical aspects of veterinary pharmacology and toxicology.
Related titles: Microform ed.: (from PQC); ♦ Online - full text ed.: Journal of Veterinary Pharmacology and Therapeutics Online. ISSN 1365-2885.
Indexed: ASCA, Agri.& Environ.Biotech.Abstr. (coverage dropped), Agricola, Chem.Abstr., Chem.Indus.Notes, Chem.Titles, Curr.Adv.Ecol.Sci., Curr.Cont., Dairy Sci.Abstr., Derwent Biotech.Abstr., Excerp.Med. (1992-), Focus on: Vet.Sci.& Med., Helminthol.Abstr., Ind.Med. (1978-), Ind.Sci.Rev., Ind.Vet., Nutr.Abstr., Pig News & Info., Postharvest, Poult.Abstr., Protozool.Abstr., Rev.Appl.Entomol., Rev.Med.& Vet.Mycol., Sci.Cit.Ind., Small Anim.Abstr., Sport Fish.Abstr., Triticale Abstr., Vet.Bull., Wild.Rev.
—BLDSC (5072.420000), ADONIS, CASDDS, CISTI, GNLM, IDS, Infotrieve, ingenta. **CCC.**
Published by: (Association for Veterinary Clinical Pharmacology & Therapeutics), Blackwell Science Ltd., PO Box 88, Oxford OX2 0NE, United Kingdom. TEL 44-1865-206180, 44-1865-206002, FAX 44-1865-206219, jnl.orders@blacksci.co.uk, http://www.blackwell-science.com/~cgilib/jnlpage.asp?Journal=jvpt&File=jvpt, http://www.blackwellpublishing.com. Eds. A Aronson, Q McKellar. Pub. Elaine Stott. R&P Sophie Savage. Adv. contact Jenny Applin. Circ: 445. **Co-sponsors:** American Academy of Veterinary Pharmacology and Therapeutics; European Association for Veterinary Pharmacology and Toxicology, American College of Veterinary Clinical Pharmacology.

615 636.089 GBR ISSN 1365-2885
▼ **JOURNAL OF VETERINARY PHARMACOLOGY AND THERAPEUTICS ONLINE.** Text in English. 1999. bi-m. GBP 419 in Europe; USD 665 in North America; GBP 419 elsewhere (effective 2002). *Refereed.* **Document type:** *Academic/Scholarly.*
Media: Online - full text (from EBSCO Publishing, ingenta, Munksgaard & Blackwell Science's Synergy, Swets Blackwell, Institute for Scientific Information, RoweCom Information Quest). **Related titles:** Microform ed.: (from PQC); ♦ Print ed.: Journal of Veterinary Pharmacology and Therapeutics. ISSN 0140-7783.
Published by: Blackwell Science Ltd., Osney Mead, Oxford OX2 0EL, United Kingdom. TEL 44-1685-206206, FAX 44-1685-721205, website@blacksci.com, journals.cs@blacksci.co.uk, http://www.blackwell-science.com.

615 SWE ISSN 1102-285X
JOURNALEN; aktuellt fraan Kabi Pharmacia AB. Text in Swedish. 1988. 10/yr.
Published by: Kabi Pharmacia AB, Stockholm 11287, Sweden.

KANAGAWA SEISHIN YAKURI/KANAGAWA JOURNAL OF PSYCHOPHARMACOLOGY. see *PSYCHOLOGY*

615 JPN ISSN 0285-4775 CODEN: KKBYDO
KANAGAWAKEN BYOIN YAKUZAISHIKAI KAISHI/KANAGAWA HOSPITAL PHARMACISTS ASSOCIATION. JOURNAL. Text in Japanese. 1968. 3/yr.
—CASDDS.
Published by: Kanagawaken Byoin Yakuzaishikai/Kanagawaken Hospital Pharmacists Association, Kitasato Byoin, 15-1 Kitaza-To 1-chome, Sagamihara-shi, Kanagawa-ken 228-0829, Japan.

P

615 JPN
KANPOYAKUHO/CHINESE DRUG NEWS. Text in Japanese. 1983. 3/yr.
Published by: Kinokuniya Kan'yakkyoku, 2-14 Sotokanda 1-chome, Chiyoda-ku, Tokyo 101-0021, Japan.

KAOHSIUNG JOURNAL OF MEDICAL SCIENCES. see *MEDICAL SCIENCES*

615.9 JPN ISSN 0287-2358
KAPUSERU/CAPSULE. Text in Japanese. 1982. irreg.
Published by: Nihon Seiyaku Kogyo Kyokai/Japan Pharmaceutical Manufacturers Association, 4-1 Nihonbashihoncho 3-chome, Chuo-ku, Tokyo 103-0023, Japan.

615 JPN ISSN 0289-4750
KATEIYAKU KENKYU/RESEARCH ON HOME MEDICINES. Text in Japanese. 1982. a.
Published by: Toyamaken Kateiyaku Kaihatsu Kenkyukai/Toyama Research Society for Home Medicine, 1-7 Shinsokawa, Toyama-shi 930-0006, Japan.

615 USA ISSN 0194-567X
THE KENTUCKY PHARMACIST. Text in English. 1878. m. USD 30. adv. bk.rev.
Indexed: I.P.A.
—Linda Hall.
Published by: Kentucky Pharmacists Association, Inc., 1228 U S 127 S, Frankfort, KY 40601. TEL 502-227-2303, FAX 502-227-2258. Ed. Robert L Barnett Jr. Circ: 1,800.

P

615 GBR
KEY NOTE MARKET REPORT: O T C PHARMACEUTICALS. (Over The Counter) Variant title: O T C Pharmaceuticals. Text in English. irreg., latest vol.8, 1997. GBP 355 (effective 1999). **Document type:** *Trade.*
Formerly: Key Note Report: O T C Pharmaceuticals (0956-8956)
Related titles: CD-ROM ed.; Online - full text ed.
Published by: Key Note Ltd., Field House, 72 Oldfield Rd, Hampton, Mddx TW12 2HQ, United Kingdom. TEL 44-20-8481-8750, FAX 44-20-8783-0049, http://www.keynote.co.uk.

615 GBR
KEY NOTE MARKET REPORT: PRESCRIBED PHARMACEUTICALS. Variant title: Prescribed Pharmaceuticals. Text in English. irreg., latest vol.12, 1997. GBP 265 (effective 1999). **Document type:** *Trade.*
Formerly: Key Note Report: Prescribed Pharmaceuticals (1352-7134)
Related titles: CD-ROM ed.; Online - full text ed.
Published by: Key Note Ltd., Field House, 72 Oldfield Rd, Hampton, Mddx TW12 2HQ, United Kingdom. TEL 44-20-8481-8750, FAX 44-20-8783-0049, http://www.keynote.co.uk.

615 GBR
KEY NOTE MARKET REPORT: RETAIL CHEMISTS & DRUG STORES. Variant title: Retail Chemists & Drug Stores. Text in English. 1993. irreg., latest vol.10, 1998. GBP 265 (effective 1999). **Document type:** *Trade.*
Formerly: Key Note Report: Retail Chemists and Drug Stores (1352-6979)
Related titles: CD-ROM ed.; Online - full text ed.
Published by: Key Note Ltd., Field House, 72 Oldfield Rd, Hampton, Mddx TW12 2HQ, United Kingdom. TEL 44-20-8481-8750, FAX 44-20-8783-0049, http://www.keynote.co.uk.

615 658.8 GBR
KEY NOTE MARKET REVIEW: U K PHARMACEUTICAL INDUSTRY. Variant title: U K Pharmaceutical Industry. Text in English. irreg., latest vol.2, 1995. GBP 465 (effective 1999). **Document type:** *Trade.*
Related titles: CD-ROM ed.; Online - full text ed.
Published by: Key Note Ltd., Field House, 72 Oldfield Rd, Hampton, Mddx TW12 2HQ, United Kingdom. TEL 44-20-8481-8750, FAX 44-20-8783-0049, http://www.keynote.co.uk.

615.1 RUS ISSN 0023-1134
RS402 CODEN: KHFZAN
KHIMIKO-FARMATSEVTICHESKII ZHURNAL. Text in Russian. 1967. m. USD 269.95. bk.rev., play rev. bibl, charts, illus. index. **Description:** Publishes articles on scientific-technical and production activities of chemo-pharmaceutic enterprises.
Related titles: Online - full text ed.; ♦ English Translation: Pharmaceutical Chemistry Journal. ISSN 0091-150X.
Indexed: Agri.& Environ.Biotech.Abstr. (coverage dropped), Anal.Abstr., Biol.Abstr., Chem.Abstr., Chem.Infd., Chem.Titles, Cott.& Trop.Fibr.Abstr., Curr.Adv.Ecol.Sci., Curr.Cont. (coverage dropped), Derwent Biotech.Abstr., Excerp.Med. (1993-), Helminthol.Abstr., Hort.Abstr., INIS Atomind., I.P.A., Ind.Chem. (coverage dropped), Ind.Sci.Rev., Plant Grow.Reg.Abstr., Ref.Zh., Soils & Fert., Sugar Ind.Abstr.
—BLDSC (0391.922000), CASDDS, CISTI, GNLM, Infotrieve, KNAW, Linda Hall. **CCC.**
Published by: (Tsentr Khimii i Lekarstvennykh Sredstv), Izdatel'stvo Folium, Dmitrovskoe shosse 58, Moscow 127474, Russian Federation. TEL 7-095-4825646, FAX 7-095-482-5590. Ed. R G Glushkov. **Dist. by:** Mezhdunarodnaya Kniga, B Yakimanka 39, Moscow 117049, Russian Federation. TEL 7-095-2384967, FAX 7-095-2384634; **US dist. addr.:** East View Publications, 3020 Harbor Ln N, Minneapolis, MN 55447. TEL 612-550-0961.

615.1 JPN ISSN 0023-1657
KINKI UNIVERSITY. BULLETIN OF PHARMACY/KINKI DAIGAKU YAKUGAKUBU KIYO. Text in Japanese. 1959. irreg.
Indexed: Biol.Abstr., Chem.Abstr., I.P.A.
Published by: Kinki University, Faculty of Pharmaceutical Sciences, 321 Kowakae, Higashiosaka-shi, Osaka-fu 577-0818, Japan. Ed. Shoji Takemura. Circ: 1,000.

615 JPN ISSN 0914-5079
KITASATO DAIGAKU DAIGAKUIN YAKUGAKU KENKYUKA RINSHO YAKUGAKU TOKURON KIYO/KITASATO UNIVERSITY. CLINICAL PHARMACY BULLETIN. Text in Japanese. 1982. a.
Published by: Kitasato Daigaku, Yakugakubu/Kitasato University, Faculty of Pharmacy, 9-1 Shirokane 5-chome, Minato-ku, Tokyo 108-0072, Japan.

615 RUS ISSN 0869-5490
KLINICHESKAYA FARMAKOLOGIYA I TERAPIYA. Text in Russian. q. USD 99.95 in United States.
Indexed: Ref.Zh.
—East View.
Published by: Klinika Terapii i Profzabolevenii, Ul Rossolimo 11-a, Moscow 119021, Russian Federation. TEL 7-095-2482544. **US dist. addr.:** East View Publications, 3020 Harbor Ln N, Minneapolis, MN 55447. TEL 612-550-0961.

615 SWE ISSN 0280-6185
KLINIK & TERAPI. Text in Swedish. 1965. 8/yr.
Former titles (until 1982): Astra-Nytt; (until 1970): Information fraan Astra Laekemedel AB
Published by: Astra Laekemedel AB, Soedertaelje 15185, Sweden.

615 DEU
KLINISCHE PHARMAKOLOGIE. Text in German. 1990. irreg., latest vol.18, 1999. **Document type:** *Academic/Scholarly.*
Indexed: Chem.Abstr., Chem.Indus.Notes, Chem.Titles.
—BLDSC (5099.464500).
Published by: W. Zuckschwerdt Verlag GmbH, Industriestr 1, Germering 82110, Germany. TEL 49-89-894349-0, FAX 49-89-89434950.

615 JPN ISSN 0911-9191
KOBE GAKUIN DAIGAKU YAKUGAKKAISHI/KOBE GAKUIN UNIVERSITY. PHARMACEUTICAL SOCIETY. ANNUAL BULLETIN. Text in English, Japanese. 1977. a. free per issue.
Indexed: Intl.Bibl.Soc.Sci.
Published by: Kobe Gakuin Daigaku, Yakugakubu/Kobe Gakuin University, Faculty of Pharmaceutical Science, 518, Arise, Ikawadanicho, Nishi-ku, Kobe-shi, Hyogo-ken 673, Japan. TEL 81-78-974-1551, FAX 81-78-974-5689, dean@pharm.kobegakuin.ac.jp.

615 JPN ISSN 0911-9183
KOBE GAKUIN DAIGAKU YAKUGAKUBU KIYO/KOBE GAKUIN UNIVERSITY. FACULTY OF PHARMACEUTICAL SCIENCES. MEMOIRS. Text in English, Japanese. 1978. every 5 yrs.
Published by: Kobe Gakuin Daigaku, Yakugakubu/Kobe Gakuin University, Faculty of Pharmaceutical Science, 518, Arise, Ikawadanicho, Nishi-ku, Kobe-shi, Hyogo-ken 673, Japan.

615 JPN ISSN 0915-1656
KOKUNAI IYAKUHIN TENPU BUNSHO JOHO/PACKAGE INSERT INFORMATION FOR DRUGS IN JAPAN. Text in Japanese. 1986. m. JPY 30,000 to non-members; JPY 20,000 to members.
Published by: Nihon Iyaku Joho Senta/Japan Pharmaceutical Information Center, Nagai Kinenkan, 12-15 Shibuya 2-chome, Shibuya-ku, Tokyo 150-0002, Japan. TEL 81-3-5466-1811. Ed. Kiyoshi Nagao. Pub. Hiroshi Miyake. Circ: 400.

615 JPN ISSN 0388-211X
KOKUSAI IYAKUHIN JOHO/INTERNATIONAL PHARMACEUTICAL INTELLIGENCE. Text in Japanese. 1972. 2/m. JPY 104,200.
Published by: Kokusai Shogyo Shuppan K.K./Kokusai Shogyo Publishing Corp., 14-5 Ginza 6-chome, Chuo-ku, Tokyo 104-0061, Japan.

615 JPN
KONNICHI NO CHIRYOYAKU/TODAY'S PHARMACY. Text in Japanese. 1977. a. JPY 4,200.
Published by: Nankodo Co. Ltd., 42-6 Hongo 3-chome, Bunkyo-ku, Tokyo 113-0033, Japan. TEL 81-3-3811-7239, FAX 81-3-3811-7230.

615.4 KOR ISSN 0253-3073
RS160 CODEN: SYHJAM
KOREAN JOURNAL OF PHARMACOGNOSY. Key Title: Sengyakhak-Hoeji (Sehur). Text in English, Korean; Summaries in English. 1970. q. USD 40. adv. bk.rev. back issues avail. **Document type:** *Academic/Scholarly.*
Indexed: AgBiotech, Chem.Abstr., Crop Physiol.Abstr., Excerp.Med., Food Sci.& Tech.Abstr., Forest Prod.Abstr., Forest.Abstr., Hort.Abstr., Nutr.Abstr., Plant Breed.Abstr., Plant Gen.Res.Abstr., Rev.Appl.Entomol., Rev.Arom.& Med.Plants, Rev.Med.& Vet.Mycol., Rev.Plant Path., Seed Abstr., Sugar Ind.Abstr.
—BLDSC (5113.572000), CASDDS, EMDOCS, GNLM, Linda Hall.
Published by: Korean Society of Pharmacognosy, c/o Natural Products Research Institute, Jongro-ku, 28 Yeongun dong, Seoul 110460, Korea, S.. TEL 82-2-740-8925, FAX 82-2-742-3323, sskang@plaza.snu.ac.kr. Ed. Jae Sue Choi. Circ: 800.

615 KOR ISSN 1226-4512
RM1 CODEN: TYCPAQ
KOREAN JOURNAL OF PHYSIOLOGY AND PHARMACOLOGY. Text and summaries in English. 1997. bi-m. USD 30 foreign to individuals; USD 50 foreign to institutions (effective 2000). back issues avail. *Refereed.* **Document type:** *Academic/Scholarly.* **Description:** Provides original research papers on physiological and pharmacological sciences.
Formed by the merger of (1965-1997): Korean Journal of Pharmacology - Daiham Yangrihag Jabji (0377-9459); (1967-1997): Korean Journal of Physiology - Daeham Saengri Haghoeji (0300-4015)
Related titles: Fax ed.; Online - full text ed.
Indexed: Biol.Abstr., Chem.Abstr., Chem.Indus.Notes, Chem.Titles, Excerp.Med.
—BLDSC (5113.573350), CASDDS, EMDOCS, GNLM, KNAW.
Published by: (Korean Society of Pharmacology), Eui-Hak Publishing and Printing Co., 448-13 Seokyo Dong, Mapo-Gu, Seoul 121210, Korea, S.. TEL 82-2-326-0370, FAX 82-2-326-0371, kosphar@kams.or.kr, kipp@netsgo.com, http://www.kosphar.or.kr. Ed. Soo Wan Chae. Pub. Jee-Chang Chang. Circ: 1,400. **Subscr. to:** Korean Society of Pharmacology, 443-13 euihak Bldg 2nd Fl, 448-13 Seokyo-dong Mapo-gu, Seoul 121-210, Korea, S. **Co-sponsor:** Korean Society of Physiology.

615 KOR ISSN 1225-5467
RM301.28
KOREAN SOCIETY FOR CLINICAL PHARMACOLOGY AND THERAPEUTICS. JOURNAL. Text in Korean. 1993. s-a. USD 30 (effective 1996). adv. *Refereed.* **Document type:** *Academic/Scholarly.* **Description:** Publishes articles dealing with the effects of drugs, including pharmacodynamics, clinical trials, pharmacoepidemiology, pharmacogenetics and other studies of drugs.
—BLDSC (4812.343900), EMDOCS.
Published by: Korean Society for Clinical Pharmacology and Therapeutics, c/o Seoul National University College of Medicine, Department of Neuropsychiatry, Chongno-gu, 28 Yongon dong, Seoul 110744, Korea, S.. TEL 740-8286, FAX 745-7996. Ed. Jung Sang Lee. Pub. Chung Kyoon Lee. Adv. contact Myoung Mook Lee.

615 JPN ISSN 0912-5027
KOSEI BUSSHITSU RYOHO/INDICATIONS IN ANTIBIOTIC THERAPY. Text in Japanese. 1985. s-a.
Published by: Sutandado Makkintaiya/Standard McIntyre, 3-7 Irifune 2-chome, Chuo-ku, Tokyo 104-0042, Japan.

615 DEU ISSN 0173-7597
CODEN: KRANDZ
KRANKENHAUSPHARMAZIE. Text in German; Summaries in English, German. 1950. m. EUR 155.76 domestic; EUR 170.88 elsewhere; EUR 17 newsstand/cover (effective 2002). **Document type:** *Journal, Trade.*
Formerly (until 1980): Krankenhaus-Apotheke (0075-7071)
Related titles: Online - full text ed.: (from Institute for Scientific Information).
Indexed: Agri.& Environ.Biotech.Abstr. (coverage dropped), Chem.Abstr., Derwent Biotech.Abstr., I.P.A., Inpharma, Reac.
—BLDSC (5118.146200), CASDDS, GNLM, IDS, Infotrieve, KNAW. **CCC.**
Published by: (Arbeitsgemeinschaft Deutscher Krankenhausapotheker), Deutscher Apotheker Verlag, Postfach 101061, Stuttgart 70009, Germany. TEL 49-711-2582-0, FAX 49-711-2582290, kph@deutscher-apotheker-verlag.de, service@deutscher-apotheker-verlag.de, http://www.deutscher-apotheker-verlag.de. Ed. Susanne Heinzl. Adv. contact Klaus Graef TEL 49-711-2582245.

615 JPN ISSN 0916-4758
KURAYA YAKUHO/KURAYA MEDICAL WEEKLY. Text in Japanese. 1986. w.
Published by: Kuraya Yakuhin K.K., Gakujutsubu, 24-7 Hongo 5-chome, Bunkyo-ku, Tokyo 113-0033, Japan.

615 JPN ISSN 0285-2713
KURINIKARU NYUSU/DAIICHI PURE CHEMICALS CO., LTD. CLINICAL NEWS. Text in Japanese. 1980. 3/yr.
Published by: Daiichi Kagaku Yakuhin K.K./Daiichi Pure Chemicals Co., Ltd., 13-5 Nihonbashi 3-chome, Chuo-ku, Tokyo 103-0027, Japan.

615 JPN
KUSURI HAKUBUTSUKAN DAYORI/NAITO MUSEUM. SEMI-ANNUAL REPORT. Text in Japanese. 1978. s-a. free per issue. adv. **Document type:** *Bulletin.*
Published by: Naito Kinen Kursuri Hakubutsukan/Naito Museum of Pharmaceutical Science and Industry, Hashima gun, Kawashima-cho, Gifu-ken 501-6195, Japan. TEL 81-58689-2101, FAX 81-58689-2197. Ed. Yasuo Miyake. Adv. contact Makiko Morita.

615 JPN ISSN 0452-9731
CODEN: KYDKAJ
KYORITSU YAKKA DAIGAKU KENKYU NENPO/KYORITSU COLLEGE OF PHARMACY. ANNUAL REPORT. Text in English, Japanese; Summaries in English. 1955. a.
Indexed: Chem.Abstr., Chem.Indus.Notes, Chem.Titles.
—BLDSC (1320.500000), CASDDS.
Published by: Kyoritsu Yakka Daigaku, 5-30 Shibakoen 1-chome, Minato-ku, Tokyo 105-0011, Japan.

615 JPN ISSN 0288-111X
KYOTOFU YAKUZAISHIKAI SHIKEN KENKYU SENTA NENPO/KYOTO PREFECTURAL PHARMACEUTICAL ASSOCIATION. ANNUAL REPORT OF THE LABORATORY. Text in Japanese. 1980. a.
Published by: Kyotofu Yakuzaishikai, Shiken Kenkyu Senta, Kyotofu Yakuzaishi Kaikan 563, Umebayashicho, Yamato Oji Higashi Iru 5 chome, Goji Dori, Higashiyama-ku, Kyoto-shi 605, Japan.

615 JPN ISSN 0368-7279
CODEN: KYYKBN
KYUSHU YAKUGAKKAI KAIHO/KYUSHU PHARMACEUTICAL SOCIETY. JOURNAL. Text in Japanese; Summaries in English. 1927. a.
Indexed: Chem.Abstr., Chem.Indus.Notes, Chem.Titles.
—BLDSC (5136.400000), CASDDS.
Published by: Kyushu Yamaguchi Yakugakkai, c/o Kyushu Daigaku Igakubu Fuzoku Byoin Yakuzaibu, 1-1 Maidashi 3-chome, Higashi-ku, Fukuoka-shi 812-0054, Japan.

615.1 DNK ISSN 0106-1275
LAEGEFORENINGENS MEDICINFORTEGNELSE. Text in Danish. 1963. biennial. DKK 400 (effective 2000).
Published by: Laegeforeningens Forlag, Esplanaden 8 A, Copenhagen K 1263, Denmark. TEL 45-35-44-85-00, FAX 45-35-44-81-99.

615.1 DNK ISSN 0105-287X
LAEGEMIDDELKATALOGET. Text in Danish. 1976. a. DKK 598; DKK 989 print & CD-ROM eds. (effective 1999). *Refereed.* **Document type:** *Catalog.*
Related titles: CD-ROM ed.: GBP 598 (effective 1999); ♦ Supplement: Laegemiddelkatalogets Prisliste. ISSN 0105-4600.
Address: Stroedamvej 50, Copenhagen Oe 2100, Denmark. TEL 45-39-27-44-88, FAX 45-39-27-59-10, lmk@dli.dk. Ed. Mogens Brandt Kristensen. R&P Aase Bak.

615.1 DNK ISSN 0105-4600
LAEGEMIDDELKATALOGETS PRISLISTE. Text in Danish. 1976. a.
Related titles: ♦ Supplement to: Laegemiddelkataloget. ISSN 0105-287X.
Published by: Laegemiddelkataloget, Stroedamvej 50, Copenhagen Oe 2100, Denmark. TEL 45-39-27-44-88, FAX 45-39-27-59-10, lmk@dli.dk.

615.5 SWE ISSN 0347-8343
LAEKEMEDELSBOKEN. Text in Swedish. 1977. biennial. SEK 300 (effective 2001). **Document type:** *Trade.*
Published by: Apoteket AB, Stockholm 13188, Sweden. TEL 46-8-466-10-00, FAX 46-8-466-15-15. Ed. Signe Bogentoft.

615.1 SWE
CODEN: SFTIAE
LAEKEMEDELSVAERLDEN. Text in Swedish. 1897. 10/yr. SEK 450; SEK 52 newsstand/cover (effective 2001). adv. bk.rev. illus, stat. 64 p./no. **Document type:** *Magazine, Trade.*
Formerly: Svensk Farmacevtisk Tidskrift (0039-6524)
Related titles: Microfilm ed.: (from PQC); Online - full text ed.
Indexed: Agri.& Environ.Biotech.Abstr. (coverage dropped), Biol.Abstr., Chem.Abstr., Excerp.Med., I.P.A., Ind.Med. (coverage dropped), PROMT.
—CASDDS, CISTI, Linda Hall.
Published by: (Apotekarsocieteten), Swedish Pharmaceutical Press, Box 1136, Stockholm 11181, Sweden. TEL 46-8-723-50-00, FAX 46-8-14-95-80, press@swepharm.se, http://www.lakemedelsvarlden.nu, http://www.swepharm.se. Ed. Fredrik Hed. Adv. contact Mats Lindkvist. B&W page SEK 12,000, color page SEK 20,000; trim 180 x 251. Circ: 11,200. **Affiliate:** Swedish Academy of Pharmaceutical Sciences.

LECTINS. see *BIOLOGY—Abstracting, Bibliographies, Statistics*

LEKARSKY OBZOR. see *MEDICAL SCIENCES*

615.1 FRA ISSN 0984-452X
LA LETTRE DU PHARMACOLOGUE. Text in French. 1987. m. FRF 460 domestic to individuals; FRF 580, USD 105 foreign to individuals; FRF 580 domestic to institutions; FRF 700, USD 127 foreign to institutions; FRF 290 domestic to students; USD 75 foreign to students (effective 2000). *Refereed.* **Document type:** *Academic/Scholarly.*
Related titles: ♦ Supplement: La Lettre du Pharmacologue. Supplement. ISSN 1245-4893.
—BLDSC (5185.215200), GNLM.
Published by: Edimark S.A., 62-64 rue Jean Jaures, Puteaux 92800, France. TEL 33-1-414-58000, FAX 33-1-41458025, contact@edimark.fr, http://www.edimark.fr. Ed. P Jaillon. Pub. Claudie Damour-Terrasson.

615.1 FRA ISSN 1245-4893
LA LETTRE DU PHARMACOLOGUE. SUPPLEMENT. Text in French. 1987. irreg. price varies. **Document type:** *Academic/Scholarly.*
Related titles: ♦ Supplement to: La Lettre du Pharmacologue. ISSN 0984-452X.
Published by: Edimark S.A., 62-64 rue Jean Jaures, Puteaux 92800, France. TEL 33-1-414-58000, FAX 33-1-41458025, contact@edimark.fr, http://www.edimark.fr. Ed. P Jaillon. Pub. C Damour Terrasson.

LIAONING ZHONGYI ZAZHI/LIAONING JOURNAL OF TRADITIONAL CHINESE MEDICINE. see *ALTERNATIVE MEDICINE*

▼ **LIFE SCIENCE LAW REVIEW.** see *LAW*

615 338 GBR ISSN 1470-4560
CODEN: PMREEC
LIFE SCIENCE TODAY. Text in English. bi-m. GBP 103 in United Kingdom; USD 232 in United States; GBP 133 elsewhere (effective 2000); GBP 38 newsstand/cover. adv. **Document type:** *Trade.* **Description:** Covers all aspects of pharmaceutical manufacturing, from raw materials to the packaged product, considering both management related topics and technological developments.
Formerly (until 2000): Pharmaceutical Manufacturing Review (0955-3894)
Related titles: Online - full text ed.: (from Gale Group, Northern Light Technology, Inc., Factiva).
Indexed: CBNB (1996-).
—BLDSC (5208.929980).
Published by: D M G World Media, Queensway House, 2 Queensway, Redhill, Surrey RH1 1QS, United Kingdom. TEL 44-1737-768611, FAX 44-1737-855477, http://www.dmgworldmedia.com/. Ed. Tom Mulligan TEL 44-1737-855080. Adv. contact Mark Harrington.

615 NLD ISSN 1381-3145
LIJFBLAD. Text in Dutch. 1995. m. adv. **Document type:** *Trade.* **Description:** Covers drug store products and educational matters for salespersons in drug stores and pharmacies.
Published by: Mediselect B.V., Postbus 63, Leusden 3830 AB, Netherlands. TEL 31-33-4229900, FAX 31-33-4229922, info@mediselect.nl. Ed. M Thewissen. Circ: 11,000 (controlled).

615 610.73 USA ISSN 1081-857X
RM301.12
LIPPINCOTT'S NURSING DRUG GUIDE. Variant title: Nursing Drug Guide. Text in English. 1996. irreg. **Document type:** *Trade.*
Published by: Lippincott Williams & Wilkins (Philadelphia) (Subsidiary of: Wolters Kluwer N.V.), 530 Walnut St, Philadelphia, PA 19106-3621. TEL 301-223-2300, 800-638-3030, FAX 301-223-2400, http://www.lww.com.

615 GBR
THE LOCUM. Text in English. bi-m.
Published by: Locum, The Old Fire Sta, 69 Albion St, Birmingham, Warks B1 3EA, United Kingdom. TEL 021-233-0233, FAX 021-233-0723. Circ: 3,500.

LOOKOUT - NONFOODS. see *BEAUTY CULTURE—Perfumes And Cosmetics*

615 USA ISSN 0192-3838
LOUISIANA PHARMACIST* . Text in English. 1943. bi-m. USD 20. adv. illus.
Indexed: I P A.
—Linda Hall.
Published by: Louisiana Pharmacists Association, PO Box 14446, Baton Rouge, LA 70898-4446. Ed. Linda Foreman. Circ: 2,000.

615.1 FRA ISSN 0024-7804
CODEN: LYPHAD
LYON PHARMACEUTIQUE. Text in French. 1929. 8/yr. FRF 800 (effective 1999). adv. charts, illus. back issues avail. *Refereed.* **Document type:** *Academic/Scholarly.* **Description:** Publishes scientific articles for students, pharmacists and hospital practitioners in the pharmacological and biological fields at the post-graduate level.
Related titles: Online - full text ed.: (from ingenta).
Indexed: Agri.& Environ.Biotech.Abstr. (coverage dropped), Biol.Abstr., Chem.Abstr., Chem.Indus.Notes, Chem.Titles, Derwent Biotech.Abstr., Excerp.Med. (1993-), INIS Atomind., I.P.A.
—CASDDS, GNLM, Infotrieve, KNAW, Linda Hall. **CCC.**
Published by: Association des Pharmaciens - Anciens Eleves - Amis de la Faculte de Pharmacie de Lyon, c/o Bernard Poggi, Sec Gen, Hotel Dieu de Lyon, Laboratoire de Biologie, 1 pl de l'Hopital, Lyon Cedex 4 69288, France. TEL 33-1-45589026, FAX 33-1-45589421, gilles.leboucher@chu-lyon.fr, http://www.univ-lyon1.fr/ispb/lyon-pharma. Ed. Gilles Legoucher. Circ: 2,500.

615 GBR
M C A BUSINESS PLAN. (Medicines Control Agency) Text in English. a. adv. **Document type:** *Government.*
Published by: Department of Health, Medicines Control Agency, Market Towers, 1 Nine Elms Ln, London SW8 5DA, United Kingdom. TEL 44-20-7273-0254, FAX 44-20-7273-0269. Ed. A Breckenridge. Adv. contact C Hepburn TEL 0-171-273-0954.

615 GBR
M C A EURODIRECT PUBLICATIONS. Text in English. 1993. m. GBP 300 (effective 2001). back issues avail. **Document type:** *Monographic series.*
Published by: Medicines Control Agency, 1 Nine Elms Ln, Rm 10-238, London SW8 5NQ, United Kingdom. FAX 44-20-7273-0353, 44-20-7273-0353, info@mca.gov.uk, http://www.mca.gov.uk. Circ: 160 (paid).

615.1 FIN ISSN 0024-8045
M D S. Text in Finnish; Summaries in English, Swedish. 1901. bi-m. FIM 150. adv. bk.rev. charts, illus, pat, stat, tr.lit.

P

Published by: Yliopiston Farmasiakunta r.y./University Pharmaceutical Association, Biokeskus 1 B, Viikinkaari 5, PLJ 6, Helsingin Yliopisto 00014, Finland. Ed. Liisa Rantanon. Circ: 1,000.

615 GBR ISSN 0957-9095
M I M S. (Monthly Index of Medical Specialties) Text in English. 1959. m. GBP 75 in United Kingdom; GBP 96 in Europe; GBP 176 in Australasia; GBP 161 elsewhere (effective 2001). adv. **Document type:** *Trade.*
—BLDSC (5775.410000), GNLM.
Published by: Haymarket Medical Ltd., 174 Hammersmith Rd, London W6 7JP, United Kingdom. TEL 44-20-8943-5000, 44-20-8606-7500, FAX 44-20-8606-7301, admin.mims@haynet.com, http://www.haymarketgroup.com. Ed. Ed Marritee TEL 44-20-8267-4870. Circ: 63,501.

615 GBR ISSN 0140-4415
M I M S AFRICA. Variant title: Monthly Index of Medical Specialities Africa. Text in English. 1961. bi-m. GBP 25 in United Kingdom; GBP 27.50 elsewhere (effective 2001). adv. 4 cols./p. **Document type:** *Directory, Trade, Abstract/Index.* **Description:** Lists prescription pharmaceuticals for medical practitioners.
Former titles (until 1976): African M I M S (0002-0079); Which incorporated: African Medical Practitioner
—CCC.
Published by: A.E. Morgan Publications Ltd., Stanley House, 9 West St, Epsom, Surrey KT18 7RL, United Kingdom. TEL 44-1372-741411, FAX 44-1372-744493. Pub. Terence Morgan. Adv. contact Geoff Donovan. color page GBP 1,370; 130 x 190. Circ: 8,300.

P

615.19 AUS ISSN 0725-4709
M I M S ANNUAL. Text in English. 1977. a. AUD 159 in New Zealand for 2000 ed.; AUD 169 to PNG, Asia & Pacific Region; AUD 189 to US & Middle East; AUD 201 elsewhere (effective 2000). adv. charts. **Document type:** *Directory.* **Description:** Full disclosure information on all pharmaceuticals available for prescription in Australia.
Related titles: CD-ROM ed.
Published by: M I M S Australia (Subsidiary of: Medimedia Australia), PO Box 3000, St Leonards, NSW 2065, Australia. TEL 02-99027700, FAX 02-99027701. Ed., R&P Amanda Caswell. Pub. Chris Wills. Adv. contact Sue McElroyy. Circ: 24,000.

615.19 AUS ISSN 1035-5723
M I M S BI-MONTHLY. Text in English. 1963. bi-m. AUD 193 in New Zealand; AUD 217 in PNG, Asia & Pacific Region; AUD 241 in US & Middle East; AUD 299 elsewhere (effective 2000). adv. **Description:** Therapeutically classified prescribing information on all products available for prescription in Australia.
Related titles: CD-ROM ed.
Published by: M I M S Australia (Subsidiary of: Medimedia Australia), PO Box 3000, St Leonards, NSW 2065, Australia. TEL 02-99027700, FAX 02-99027701. Ed., R&P Amanda Caswell. Pub. Chris Wills. Adv. contact Sue McElroy. Circ: 28,000.

615 GBR
M I M S CARIBBEAN. Variant title: Monthly Index of Medical Specialities Caribbean. Text in English. 1970. bi-m. GBP 23 domestic; GBP 24 foreign (effective 2002). adv. 4 cols./p. **Document type:** *Directory, Trade, Abstract/Index.* **Description:** Lists prescription drugs for medical practitioners.
Published by: A.E. Morgan Publications Ltd., Stanley House, 9 West St, Epsom, Surrey KT18 7RL, United Kingdom. TEL 44-1372-741411, FAX 44-1372-744493. Ed. Frances Wilson. Pub. Terence Morgan. Adv. contact Geoff Donovan. color page GBP 1,100; 130 x 190. Circ: 2,600.

615 ZAF ISSN 0076-8847
M I M S DESK REFERENCE. Text in English. 1965. a. ZAR 350 domestic; ZAR 516 in United States; ZAR 528 in Europe; ZAR 547 in Australia & New Zealand (effective 2000). adv. index. **Description:** Contains full product information on human medicines, tablet and capsule identification chart, and a reference section.
Formerly: M I M S Reference Manual
Published by: M I M S, Division of Times Media Limited, PO Box 2059, Pretoria 0001, South Africa. TEL 27-12-3485010, FAX 27-12-3617716. Ed. Jacques Snyman. Adv. contact Peter McGonigle. Circ: 6,800.

615 GBR ISSN 0302-4172
M I M S MIDDLE EAST. Variant title: Monthly Index of Medical Specialities Middle East. Text in English. 1971. bi-m. GBP 27.50 domestic; GBP 31 foreign (effective 2002). adv. 4 cols./p. **Document type:** *Directory, Trade, Abstract/Index.* **Description:** Lists prescription drugs for qualified medical practitioners.
Published by: A.E. Morgan Publications Ltd., Stanley House, 9 West St, Epsom, Surrey KT18 7RL, United Kingdom. TEL 44-1372-741411, FAX 44-1372-744493. Ed. Frances Wilson. Pub. Terence Morgan. Adv. contact Geoff Donovan. color page GBP 1,750; 130 x 190. Circ: 19,000.

615.19 AUS
M I M S - O T C. (Over the Counter) Text in English. 1998. a., latest 2000. AUD 40 per issue (effective 2000). adv. **Document type:** *Directory.* **Description:** Provides product information on non-prescription pharmaceutical and other healthcare products.
Published by: M I M S Australia (Subsidiary of: Medimedia Australia), PO Box 3000, St Leonards, NSW 2065, Australia. TEL 02-99027700, FAX 02-99027701. Pub. Chris Wills. R&P Amanda Caswell. Adv. contact Sue McElroy.

MAGNESIUM RESEARCH. see *MEDICAL SCIENCES*

615 GBR ISSN 1360-8738
MAIL. Text in English. 1973. bi-m. GBP 25 domestic; GBP 35 foreign (effective 2001). **Document type:** *Government.*
Published by: Medicines Control Agency, 1 Nine Elms Ln, Rm 10-238, London SW8 5NQ, United Kingdom. TEL 44-20-7273-0000, FAX 44-20-7273-0353, info@mca.gov.uk, http://www.mca.gov.uk. Circ: 4,000 (paid and controlled).

MAJOR PHARMACEUTICAL COMPANIES OF THE WORLD (YEAR). see *BUSINESS AND ECONOMICS—Trade And Industrial Directories*

362.1042580940 GBR ISSN 1366-9613
MANAGED CARE EUROPE. Text in English. 1997. m. **Document type:** *Bulletin, Trade.* **Description:** Analyzes developments in the pharmaceutical industry while providing insight into the European healthcare system.
Published by: SMi Publishing, 1 New Concordia Wharf, Mill St, London SE1 2BB, United Kingdom. TEL 44-207-827-6000, FAX 44-207-827-6001, ordering@smipublishing.co.uk, http:// www.smipublishing.co.uk.

615 USA ISSN 1075-2358
MANAGED PHARMACEUTICAL REPORT. Text in English. 1994. m. USD 425; USD 43 newsstand/cover (effective 2001). **Document type:** *Newsletter.* **Description:** Briefing service on managed pharmaceuticals that helps subscribers identify new business opportunities and keep costs down.
Published by: Aspen Publishers, Inc., 200 Orchard Ridge Dr, Ste 200, Gaithersburg, MD 20878. TEL 301-417-7500, 800-638-8437, FAX 301-695-7931, customer.service@aspenpubl.com, http:// www.aspenpub.com. Ed. Jane M Anderson. Pub. Marjorie Weiner. R&P Rossette Graham. **Dist. by:** Aspen Publishers Inc., Distribution Center, 7201 McKinney Circle, Frederick, MD 21701. TEL 301-698-7100, FAX 301-417-7550.

615 EGY ISSN 1110-1318
CODEN: MJPSEO
MANSOURA JOURNAL OF PHARMACEUTICAL SCIENCES/MAJALLAT AL-MANSURAH LIL-ULUM AL-SAYDALIYYAH. Text in Arabic, English. 1986. s-a. USD 80. *Refereed.* **Document type:** *Academic/Scholarly.*
Related titles: CD-ROM ed.
Indexed: Chem.Abstr., Chem.Indus.Notes, Chem.Titles, ExtraMED.
—BLDSC (5361.303000), CASDDS, GNLM.
Published by: University of Mansoura, Faculty of Pharmacy, University, P O Box 35516, Mansoura, Egypt.

615 ARG
MANUAL FARMACEUTICO. Text in Spanish. 1960. m. USD 240. adv.
Published by: Alfa Beta S A C I F Y S, Avda. Melian, 3136, Capital Federal, Buenos Aires 1430, Argentina. Ed. Juan Marrari. Circ: 15,000.

615 330.9 658.8 GBR
THE MARKET FOR O T C HEALTHCARE IN ASIA. (Over the Counter) Text in English. 1995. irreg. GBP 2,250; USD 4,500 in United States. charts, stat. **Document type:** *Trade.* **Description:** Asia specialists provide the expert analysis essential to understanding, participating and succeeding in this market.
Formerly: Market for O T C Healthcare in South East Asia
Published by: Euromonitor, 60-61 Britton St, London EC1M 5UX, United Kingdom. TEL 44-20-7251-8024, 800-577-3876, info@euromonitor.com, http://www.euromonitor.com.

615 330.9 658.8 GBR
THE MARKET FOR O T C HEALTHCARE IN CHINA AND HONG KONG. (Over the Counter) Text in English. 1996. irreg. GBP 1,495. charts, stat. **Document type:** *Trade.* **Description:** Contains market analyses of Hong Kong and China, including coverage by province. Attention given to retail networks and consumer attitudes. Product sectors include vitamins and dietary supplements, analgesics, cough and cold remedies, digestive remedies, medicated skincare, and traditional Chinese remedies.
Formerly: Market for O T C Healthcare in China
Published by: Euromonitor, 60-61 Britton St, London EC1M 5UX, United Kingdom. TEL 44-20-7251-8024, 800-577-3876, info@euromonitor.com, http://www.euromonitor.com.

615 330.9 658.8 GBR
THE MARKET FOR O T C HEALTHCARE IN EASTERN EUROPE. (Over the Counter) Text in English. irreg. GBP 1,950, USD 3,900 (effective 1999). charts, stat. **Description:** Contains market analysis, company profiles, and industry forecasts.
Published by: Euromonitor, 60-61 Britton St, London EC1M 5UX, United Kingdom. TEL 44-20-7251-8024, 800-577-3867, 800-577-3876, info@euromonitor.com, http://www.euromonitor.com. **for Asia-Pacific:** Euromonitor International (Asia) Pte Ltd., 40 Tras St, Singapore 078979, Singapore. TEL 65-429-0590, FAX 65-324-1867**; for the Americas:** Euromonitor International.

615 330.9 658.8 GBR
THE MARKET FOR O T C HEALTHCARE IN LATIN AMERICA. (Over the Counter) Text in English. 1996. irreg. GBP 1,950; USD 3,900 in United States. charts, stat. **Description:** Latin America specialists provide the analysis essential to understanding, participating and succeeding in this emerging market.
Published by: Euromonitor, 60-61 Britton St, London EC1M 5UX, United Kingdom. TEL 44-20-7251-8024, 800-577-3876, info@euromonitor.com, http://www.euromonitor.com.

615 338 658 GBR
▼ **THE MARKET FOR O T C HEALTHCARE IN WESTERN EUROPE.** (Over the Counter) Text in English. 1999. irreg. GBP 2,500; USD 5,000 in United States. **Document type:** *Trade.* **Description:** Provides essential data and analysis of the OTC industry in Western Europe.
Published by: Euromonitor, 60-61 Britton St, London EC1M 5UX, United Kingdom. TEL 44-20-7251-8024, info@euromonitor.com, http://www.euromonitor.com.

615.1 658 NLD ISSN 0929-8444
MARKETING RESULTS; vakblad voor verkopers van drogisterijartikelen. Text in Dutch. 1988. 20/yr. NLG 108.49 domestic; NLG 242 foreign (effective 2001). illus. **Document type:** *Journal, Trade.* **Description:** Covers the retail market for personal health care products.
Published by: Phoenix Publishers, De Haag 5, Houten 3993 AV, Netherlands. TEL 31-30-6342790, FAX 31-30-6342795, info@phoenixbu.ni. Eds. Linda Kattekamp, Loet Bergen. Pub. Leo Vogels. Adv. contact Paula Brinks.

615 GBR
MARTINDALE: THE COMPLETE DRUG REFERENCE. Text in English. 1883. triennial, latest vol.32, 32nd edition. GBP 235 per issue in United Kingdom; GBP 250 per issue elsewhere (effective 2001). adv. index. **Document type:** *Academic/Scholarly.* **Description:** Provides a concise summary of the properties, actions and uses of drugs and medicines for the practising pharmacists and medical practitioners.
Formerly (until 2001): Martindale: the Extra Pharmacopoeia (0263-5364); Incorporates: Squires Companion
Related titles: CD-ROM ed.; Online - full text ed.: (from Data-Star, The Dialog Corporation).

Published by: (Euromed Communications Ltd.), Pharmaceutical Press (Subsidiary of: Euromed Communications Ltd.), 1 Lambeth High St, London SE1 7JN, United Kingdom. TEL 44-20-7735-9141, FAX 44-20-7582-7327, pharmpress@rpsgb.org.uk, http://www.pharmpress.com. Eds. Kathleen Parfitt, Kathleen Parfitt. Pub. Charles Fry. R&Ps Charles Fry, Charles Fry. **Dist. in U.S. by:** Rittenhouse Book Distributors, 511 Feheley Drive, King of Prussia, PA 19406.

615.1 USA ISSN 0025-4347
MARYLAND PHARMACIST. Text in English. 1925. q. USD 30 (effective 2001). adv. bk.rev. charts, illus.
Indexed: Alt.Press Ind., Chem.Abstr., I.P.A.
—Linda Hall.
Published by: Maryland Pharmacists Association, 650 W Lombard St, Baltimore, MD 21201. TEL 410-727-0746, FAX 410-725-2253, mpha@erols.com, http://www.erols.com/mpha. Ed. Howard Schiff. R&P, Adv. contact Elsie Prince. page USD 350; trim 11 x 8.5. Circ: 1,100 (paid).

615.1 378 USA ISSN 0025-4789
MASSACHUSETTS COLLEGE OF PHARMACY. BULLETIN. Text in English. 1911. q. free per issue to qualified personnel. illus. **Document type:** *Bulletin.* **Description:** Contains organization news.
Published by: Massachusetts College of Pharmacy and Allied Health Sciences, 179 Longwood Ave, Boston, MA 02115. TEL 617-732-2850, FAX 617-732-2801. Ed. James J Larkin. Circ: 9,500 (controlled).

MATERIA MEDICA POLONA; the Polish journal of medicine and pharmacy. see *MEDICAL SCIENCES*

344.04233 615.35 USA ISSN 1097-5497
MEALEY'S LITIGATION REPORT: FEN-PHEN - REDUX. Text in English. 1997. m. USD 650; USD 710 foreign (effective 1999). adv. index. back issues avail. **Document type:** *Newsletter, Trade.* **Description:** Provides detailed coverage of the litigation surrounding fen-phen, Redux and other diet drugs.
Related titles: Diskette ed.; Online - full text ed.: (from West Group, LexisNexis).
Published by: Meadow Publications, Inc., 217 W Church Rd, PO Box 62090, King Of Prussia, PA 19406-0230. TEL 610-768-7800, 800-632-5397, FAX 610-768-0880, news@mealeys.com. Ed. Ed Sue Sutter. Pub., R&P Tom Hagy. Adv. contact Cathy Roach.

MED AD NEWS. see *BUSINESS AND ECONOMICS—Marketing And Purchasing*

615 GBR
MEDICAL DEVICE DEVELOPMENTS. Text in English. 1997. a. GBP 55. adv. **Document type:** *Journal, Trade.* **Description:** Contains technical articles and case histories on leading edge developments, new products and applications, drawing on the expertise of leading engineers and designers from around the globe.
Formerly: Medical Manufacturing International (1365-8786)
Published by: Sterling Publications Ltd. (Subsidiary of: Sterling Publishing Group Plc.), Brunel House, 55-57 North Wharf Rd, London W2 1LA, United Kingdom. TEL 44-20-7915-9660, FAX 44-20-7724-2089, mmi@sterlingpublications.com, info@sterlingpublications.com, http://www.sterlingpublications.com/publications/medicaldevice.html. Pub. Sarah Woddis. Circ: 10,000 (controlled).

615 USA ISSN 0025-732X
MEDICAL LETTER ON DRUGS AND THERAPEUTICS (ENGLISH EDITION); on drugs and therapeutics. Text in English. 1959. fortn. USD 55 (effective 2001). illus. index, cum.index every 5 yrs. back issues avail.; reprints avail. *Refereed.* **Document type:** *Newsletter.* **Description:** Provides critical evaluations of drugs for physicians and other members of the health professions.
Media: Diskette. **Related titles:** Online - full text ed.: (from ProQuest Information & Learning, Gale Group, Factiva, Institute for Scientific Information).
Indexed: AIM, ASCA, CINAHL, Curr.Cont. (coverage dropped), Dent.Ind., Diar.Dis.Res., Excerp.Med., FAMLI, Helminthol.Abstr., INIS Atomind., I.P.A., Ind.Med. (1959-), Ind.Sci.Rev., Inpharma, Pharm.&Out.News, Reac.
—BLDSC (5529.700000), GNLM, IDS, KNAW.
Published by: Medical Letter, Inc., 1000 Main St, New Rochelle, NY 10801. TEL 914-235-0500, 800-211-2769, FAX 914-576-3377, http://www.medletter.com. Ed. Dr. Mark Abramowicz. R&P Marianne Aschenbrenner. Circ: 150,000.

615 CHE ISSN 0253-8512
MEDICAL LETTER ON DRUGS AND THERAPEUTICS (FRENCH EDITION). Text in French. 1978. 26/yr. CHF 88, EUR 57.14 domestic; CHF 90, EUR 58.44 foreign (effective 2002). **Document type:** *Journal, Academic/Scholarly.*
Published by: Editions Medecine et Hygiene, Case Postale 456, Geneva, 4 1211, Switzerland. TEL 41-22-7029311, FAX 41-22-7029355, abonnements@medhyg.ch, http://www.medhyg.ch.

615 JPN ISSN 0910-6316
MEDICAL LETTER ON DRUGS AND THERAPEUTICS (JAPANESE EDITION). Text in Japanese. 1985. bi-w. JPY 20,000. **Document type:** *Newsletter.*
Published by: Fukumi Transpac Corp., 2-4-10 Kyodo Bldg, Iwamoto-cho 2-chome, Chiyoda-ku, Tokyo 101-0032, Japan. TEL 81-3-5687-2890, FAX 81-3-5687-2918, pharmisk@ask.ne.jp, http://www.ask.ne.jp/~pharmisk/. Ed., R&P Hiroyuki Kosuge. Pub. Junji Fukuoka. Circ: 3,000.

MEDICAL MALPRACTICE: PHARMACY LAW. see *LAW—Civil Law*

610 658.8 USA ISSN 0025-7354
HD9665.1 CODEN: MMKMBX
MEDICAL MARKETING & MEDIA. Short title: M M & M. Text in English. 1966. m. USD 96 domestic to individuals; USD 108 in Canada to individuals; USD 144 elsewhere to individuals; USD 108 domestic to institutions; USD 132 in Canada to institutions; USD 160 elsewhere to institutions (effective 2001). adv. bk.rev. charts, illus, stat. index. back issues avail.; reprints avail. **Document type:** *Trade.* **Description:** For the pharmaceutical, medical, marketing and advertising industry providing intra-industry communication and an information link with other industries and government.
Formerly: Pharmaceutical Marketing and Media
Related titles: Microfilm ed.: (from PQC); Online - full text ed.: (from Gale Group, ProQuest Information & Learning, Northern Light Technology, Inc., Factiva).
Indexed: ABI Inform. (Aug.1985-), BPIA, Bus.& Indus (Mar.1997-), I.P.A., PROMT.
—BLDSC (5529.950000), GNLM, Infotrieve. **CCC.**
Published by: C P S Communications, Inc., 7200 W Camino Real, Ste 215, PO Box 3011, Boca Raton, FL 33433. TEL 407-368-9301, FAX 407-368-7870, http://www.cpnet.com/Pubs/mmm.asp. Ed. David Gideon. Circ: 12,800 (controlled).

615.1 JPN ISSN 0025-7427
MEDICAL PHARMACY. Text in Japanese. 1967. bi-m. JPY 300 per issue. adv. index.
Indexed: Chem.Abstr.
Published by: Daiichi Seiyaku Co. Ltd., 14-10 Nihonbashi 3-chome, Chuo-ku, Tokyo 103-0027, Japan. Circ: 6,500.

615.1 610 CHE ISSN 1423-5765
▼ **MEDICAL PRESCRIPTION OF NARCOTICS.** Text in English. 1999. irreg., latest vol.2, 2000. CHF 60 in Europe; DEM 70 in Germany; USD 50 in United States (effective 2001). **Document type:** *Monographic series, Academic/Scholarly.* **Description:** Gives an account of the research reports of a Swiss study on prescription of narcotics to chronic heroin addicts.
—BLDSC (5531.190000).
Published by: S. Karger AG, Allschwilerstr 10, PO Box, Basel 4009, Switzerland. TEL 41-61-306-1111, FAX 41-61-306-1234, karger@karger.ch, http://www.karger.com/bookseries/MEPNA.

615 658.8 GBR
MEDICATED SKINCARE: THE INTERNATIONAL MARKET. Text in English. a. GBP 2,250. **Document type:** *Trade.* **Description:** Analyzes the market for nonprescription medicated skin care products for France, Germany, Italy, Spain, the U.K., the U.S., and Japan.
Related titles: Online - full text ed.: (from Data-Star, The Dialog Corporation).
Published by: Euromonitor, 60-61 Britton St, London EC1M 5UX, United Kingdom. TEL 44-20-7251-8024, info@euromonitor.com, http://www.euromonitor.com.

615.1 ESP ISSN 1134-248X
MEDICINA PALIATIVA. Text in Spanish; Abstracts in Spanish, English. 1994. bi-m. ESP 6,000 to individuals; ESP 10,000 to institutions. adv. abstr, bibl, illus, stat. back issues avail. *Refereed.* **Document type:** *Academic/Scholarly.*
—BLDSC (5533.637000).
Published by: (Sociedad Espanola de Cuidados Paliativos/Spanish Society of Palliative Medicine), Aran Ediciones S.A., Castello, 128 1o, Madrid 28006, Spain. TEL 34-91-782-0030, FAX 34-91-561-5787, edita@grupoaran.com, http://www.grupoaran.com. Ed. J Porta. Pub. Jose Jimenez. R&P Maria Dolores Linares TEL 34-1-7820035.

615.19 USA ISSN 0198-6325
RM300 CODEN: MRREDD
MEDICINAL RESEARCH REVIEWS. Text in English. 1981. bi-m. USD 1,230 in United States; USD 1,290 in Canada & Mexico; USD 1,341 elsewhere; USD 1,292 combined subscription in United States for print and online eds.; USD 1,352 combined subscription in Canada & Mexico for print and online eds.; USD 1,403 combined subscription elsewhere for print and online eds. (effective 2002). adv. back issues avail. *Refereed.* **Document type:** *Academic/Scholarly.* **Description:** Embraces all aspects of research addressing the study of disease and the consequent development of therapeutic agents.
Related titles: Microform ed.: (from PQC); Online - full text ed.: ISSN 1098-1128. 1996. USD 1,230 in United States; USD 1,230 in Canada & Mexico; USD 1,230 elsewhere (effective 2002) (from EBSCO Publishing, Wiley InterScience, Institute for Scientific Information).
Indexed: ASCA, Chem.Abstr., Chem.Infd., Chem.Titles, Curr.Adv.Biochem., Curr.Adv.Ecol.Sci., Curr.Cont., Derwent Biotech.Abstr., Ind.Med. (1981-), Ind.Sci.Rev., Inpharma, Int.Abstr.Biol.Sci., Pharm.&Out.News, Reac., Ref.Zh., SSCI (coverage dropped), Sci.Cit.Ind.
—BLDSC (5533.992000), CASDDS, CISTI, GNLM, IDS, Infotrieve, KNAW, Linda Hall. **CCC.**
Published by: John Wiley & Sons, Inc., Journals (Subsidiary of: Wiley InterScience), 605 Third Ave, New York, NY 10158. TEL 212-850-6645, FAX 212-850-6021, subinfo@wiley.com, uscs-wis@wiley.com, http://www.wiley.com. Ed. Lester Mitscher. adv.: B&W page GBP 640, color page GBP 1,515; trim 140 x 254. Circ: 550. **Subscr. outside the Americas to:** John Wiley & Sons Ltd., Baffins Ln, Chichester, Sussex PO19 IUD, United Kingdom. TEL 44-1243-779777, FAX 44-1243-843232, cs-journals@wiley.co.uk.

P

615 BGR ISSN 1311-5162
MEDICINSKI PREGLED. FARMA-NEWS. Text in Bulgarian; Summaries in Bulgarian, English. 1972. q., latest vol.30, 2001. BGL 14 domestic; USD 30 foreign (effective 2001 - 2002). adv. bk.rev. abstr, bibl. index. 48 p./no. back issues avail. *Refereed.* **Document type:** *Academic/Scholarly, Abstract/Index, Bibliography.* **Description:** Publishes original articles and abstracts on foreign publication on pharmacokinetics, pharmacotherapy, clinical pharmacology and pharmacy.
Former titles: Farma; Farmatsevtichen Pregled (0204-6008)
Published by: Meditsinski Universitet - Sofia, Tsentur za Informatsiia po Meditsina/Medical University - Sofia, Medical Information Center, 1 Sv Georgi Sofiiski ul, Sofia 1431, Bulgaria. TEL 359-2-9522342, FAX 359-2-9522393, mutafov@sun.medun.acad.bg, http://www.medun.acad.bg. Ed. E Minkov. R&P, Adv. contact Dr. Christo Mutafov. B&W page USD 50, color page USD 200; 12 x 18. Circ: 300.

615 DNK ISSN 0900-4858
MEDICINTAKST. Text in Danish. 1955. irreg. DKK 50.
Indexed: BHA.
Published by: Sundhedsstyrelsen, Amaliegade 13, PO Box 2020, Copenhagen K 1012, Denmark. **Dist. by:** Statens Informationstjeneste, PO Box 1103, Copenhagen K 1009, Denmark.

615 ZAF ISSN 1021-6987
MEDIFILE; drug information bulletin. Text in English. 1987. m. ZAR 60 (effective 1999). abstr, bibl. *Refereed.* **Document type:** *Bulletin.* **Description:** Provides the pharmacist with current, objective and accurate information on medicines.
Related titles: ♦ Supplement to: South African Pharmaceutical Journal. ISSN 0038-2558.
—BLDSC (5534.267380).
Published by: T P S Drug Information Centre, PO Box 31238, Braamfontein, Johannesburg 2017, South Africa. FAX 27-11-3393819. Ed. Geraldine Bartlett. Circ: 6,000.

615 RUS ISSN 0868-4898
MEDIKAL MARKET. Text in Russian. q.
Indexed: Ref.Zh.
—East View.
Address: Tsvetnoi bulv 30, etazh 3, Moscow 103051, Russian Federation. TEL 7-095-2002457, FAX 7-095-2002359. **US dist. addr.:** East View Publications, 3020 Harbor Ln N, Minneapolis, MN 55447. TEL 612-550-0961.

615 615.329 614.8 DEU ISSN 0171-3876
MEDIKAMENT & MEINUNG; Zeitschrift fuer Arzneimittel- und Gesundheitswesen. Text in German. 1978. m. free. adv. bk.rev. back issues avail. **Document type:** *Bulletin.*
—GNLM.
Published by: Bundesverband der Pharmazeutischen Industrie e.V., Karlstr 21, Frankfurt Am Main 60329, Germany. TEL 49-69-2556-1261, FAX 49-69-2556-1603, presse@bpi.de, http://www.bpi.de. Ed. Thomas Postina. Adv. contact Kerstin Freller. Circ: 30,000.

615.19 610 NGA ISSN 0331-4782
MEDIPHARM. Text in English. 1969. a. USD 130 (effective 2000). **Document type:** *Abstract/Index.* **Description:** Covers pharmaceutical specialties in Nigeria.
—GNLM.
Published by: Literamed Publications Nigeria Ltd, PMB 21068, Ikeja, Oregun Village, Lagos, Nigeria. TEL 234-64-962512, FAX 234-64-961037. Ed. L A Aladesuyi. Pub. O M Lawar Solarin. Circ: 10,000.

615.1 NLD ISSN 0168-7670
MEDISCH - FARMACEUTISCHE MEDELINGEN. Text in Dutch. 1963. m. NLG 106; BEF 2,000 in Belgium. **Document type:** *Academic/Scholarly.* **Description:** Reports on pharmaceutical research.
—KNAW.
Published by: Wegener Tijdschriften Groep BV (Subsidiary of: Wegener Arcade NV), Wildenborch 5, Postbus 1860, Diemen 1112 CD, Netherlands. TEL 31-20-660-3300, FAX 31-20-660-3303, info@wtg.wegener.nl, http://www.wegener.nl.

615 DEU ISSN 0939-6292
MEDIZIN OHNE NEBENWIRKUNGEN. Text in German. q. EUR 60.34 domestic; EUR 67.34 foreign; EUR 46.32 domestic to students; EUR 53.32 foreign to students; EUR 13.08 newsstand/cover (effective 2002). **Document type:** *Journal, Academic/Scholarly.*
—GNLM.
Published by: Urban und Vogel Medien und Medizin Verlagsgesellschaft mbH (Subsidiary of: BertelsmannSpringer), Neumarkter Str 43, Munich 81673, Germany. TEL 49-89-43721411, FAX 49-89-43721410, verlag@urban-vogel.de, http://www.medkomm.de. Ed. Dr. Monika Drelmann. Adv. contact Barbara Kanters. **Subscr. to:** Springer Auslieferungs Gesellschaft, Postfach 105160, Heidelberg 69041, Germany. TEL 49-6221-345244, FAX 49-6221-345244.

615.2 DEU ISSN 0934-9170
CODEN: MEKOEK
MEDIZINISCH-PHARMAKOLOGISCHES KOMPENDIUM. Text in German. 1985. irreg., latest vol.13, 2001. **Document type:** *Monographic series, Academic/Scholarly.*
Indexed: Biol.Abstr. (1988-).
Published by: Wissenschaftliche Verlagsgesellschaft mbH, Postfach 101061, Stuttgart 70009, Germany. TEL 49-711-2582-0, FAX 49-711-2582-290, service@wissenschaftliche-verlagsgesellschaft.de, http://www.wissenschaftliche-verlagsgesellschaft.de.

615 JPN ISSN 0543-3975
MEIJI YAKKA DAIGAKU KENKYU KIYO/MEIJI PHARMACEUTICAL UNIVERSITY. BULLETIN. Text in English, Japanese; Summaries in English. 1962. a.
Indexed: Chem.Abstr., INIS Atomind.
—BLDSC (2612.095500).
Published by: Meiji Yakka Daigaku/Meiji Pharmaceutical University, 2-522-1, Noshio, Kiyose, Tokyo 204-8588, Japan.

615 JPN ISSN 0911-9442
MEIJO DAIGAKU SENKOKA YAKUGAKU SENKO HOKOKUSHU. Text in Japanese. 1975. a.
Published by: Meijo Daigaku, Yakugakubu/Meijo University, Faculty of Pharmacy, 15 Yagotorayama-Tenpakucho, Tenpaku-ku, Nagoya-shi, Aichi-ken 468-0000, Japan.

MEINE GESUNDHEIT. see *TRAVEL AND TOURISM*

METAL-BASED DRUGS. see *CHEMISTRY—Analytical Chemistry*

615.19 ESP ISSN 0379-0355
CODEN: MFEPDX
METHODS AND FINDINGS IN EXPERIMENTAL AND CLINICAL PHARMACOLOGY. Text in English. 1979. 10/yr. USD 525 (effective 2000). adv. bk.rev. back issues avail. *Refereed.* **Document type:** *Academic/Scholarly.* **Description:** Forum for papers dealing with the methodology employed and the results obtained in the scientific assessment of drugs in animals and humans.
Related titles: Online - full text ed.: (from Institute for Scientific Information).
Indexed: ASCA, Agri.& Environ.Biotech.Abstr. (coverage dropped), Biol.Abstr., Chem.Abstr., Chem.Titles, Curr.Adv.Cancer Res., Curr.Adv.Ecol.Sci., Curr.Cont., Dent.Ind., Derwent Biotech.Abstr., Excerp.Med., Ind.Med. (1979-), Ind.Med.Esp., Ind.Sci.Rev., Inpharma, Int.Abstr.Biol.Sci., Neurosci.Cit.Ind., Pharm.&Out.News, Reac., Ref.Zh., Rev.Med.& Vet.Mycol., Sci.Cit.Ind.
—CASDDS, CISTI, EMDOCS, GNLM, IDS, ingenta, KNAW. **CCC.**
Published by: Prous Science, PO Box 540, Barcelona 08080, Spain. TEL 34-93-4592220, FAX 34-93-4581535, service@prous.com. R&P Pat Leeson. Circ: 3,000.

615.1 USA
▼ **METHODS IN PHARMACOLOGY AND TOXICOLOGY✱.** Text in English. forthcoming 2001. irreg. price varies. illus. back issues avail. *Refereed.* **Document type:** *Monographic series, Academic/Scholarly.* **Description:** Covers all aspects of pharmacology, including toxicology, physiology, and molecular and cell biology.
Published by: Humana Press Inc., 999 Riverview Dr, Ste 208, Totowa, NJ 07512. TEL 973-256-1699, FAX 973-256-8341, humana@humanapr.com, http://humanapress.com. Ed. Mannfred Hollinger. R&P Wendy A Warren.

METHODS IN TOXICOLOGY. see *ENVIRONMENTAL STUDIES—Toxicology And Environmental Safety*

615.7 NLD ISSN 0376-7396
RM302.5 CODEN: MSEFDQ
MEYLER'S SIDE EFFECTS OF DRUGS; the encyclopedia of adverse reactions. Text in English. 1956. irreg., latest vol.13, 1997. USD 316 (effective 1992). charts, illus. *Refereed.* **Document type:** *Trade.* **Description:** Lists the side effects of every type of prescription drug.
Formerly (until 1975): Side Effects of Drugs (0583-1881)
Related titles: CD-ROM ed.: (from SilverPlatter Information, Inc.); Online - full text ed.: (from Data-Star, The Dialog Corporation); ♦ Supplement: Side Effects of Drugs Annual. ISSN 0378-6080.
—BLDSC (5751.800000), CASDDS, Infotrieve, KNAW. **CCC.**
Published by: Elsevier Science BV, PO Box 211, Amsterdam 1000 AE, Netherlands. TEL 31-20-485-3757, 31-20-485-3911, FAX 31-20-485-3432, 31-20-485-3598, nlinfo-f@elsevier.nl, http://www.elsevier.nl. Ed. M N G Dukes. **Subscr. in Australasia and the Far East to:** Elsevier Science (Singapore) Pte Ltd, No.1 Temasek Ave, 17-01 Millenia Tower, Singapore 039192, Singapore. TEL 65-434-3727, FAX 65-337-2230, asiainfo@elsevier.com.sg; **Subscr. in Japan to:** Elsevier Science Inc - Japan Regional Office, 9-15 Higashi-Azabu 1-chome, Minato-ku, Tokyo 106-0044, Japan. TEL 81-3-5561-5033, FAX 81-3-5561-5047, info@elsevier.co.jp; **Subscr. in the Americas to:** Elsevier Science, PO Box 945, New York, NY 10159-0945. TEL 212-633-3730, 888-437-4636, FAX 212-633-3680, usinfo-f@elsevier.com, http://www.elsevier.com

615.1 USA ISSN 1081-6089
MICHIGAN PHARMACIST. Text in English. 1963. m. USD 40; USD 5 newsstand/cover (effective 2001). adv. bk.rev. charts, illus, stat. *Refereed.* **Document type:** *Trade.*
Formerly (until 1995): Journal Michigan Pharmacist (1045-6481)
Related titles: Microform ed.: (from PQC).
Indexed: I.P.A., Med.Care Rev., Mich.Mag.Ind.
Published by: Michigan Pharmacists Association, 815 N Washington Ave, Lansing, MI 48906. TEL 517-484-1466, FAX 517-484-4893, http://www.mipharm.com. Ed. Larry D Wagenknecht. R&P Jennifer Mou. Adv. contact Jennifer Pakkala. B&W page USD 630, color page USD 1,230; trim 11 x 8.5. Circ: 3,835 (controlled).

MICROBIAL DRUG RESISTANCE; mechanism, epidemiology, and disease. see *MEDICAL SCIENCES*

615.7 GBR ISSN 1461-1732
▼ **MICROSPHERES, MICROCAPSULES & LIPOSOMES.** Text in English. 1999. q. price varies. adv. abstr, bibl, charts, illus, pat, stat. back issues avail. *Refereed.* **Document type:** *Monographic series, Academic/Scholarly.* **Description:** Contains fundamental and state of the art information on microspheres, microcapsules and liposomes, their preparation, properties and applications in chemical and life sciences, medicine, biotechnology and related industries.
Media: E-mail. **Related titles:** Diskette ed.
Published by: Citus Books, 176 Franciscan Rd, London SW17 8HH, United Kingdom. TEL 44-207-639-3305, FAX 44-207-639-3305, 44-208-628-0940, books@citus.globalnet.co.uk. Ed., R&P, Adv. contact Reza Arshady.

616.97 JPN ISSN 0388-4783
MINOPHAGEN MEDICAL REVIEW. Text in Japanese. 1956. bi-m.
Indexed: Ref.Zh.
—BLDSC (5810.550000).
Published by: Minofagen Seiyaku Honpo/Minophagen Pharmaceutical Co., 10-22 Akasaka 8-chome, Minato-ku, Tokyo 107-0052, Japan.

615 JPN ISSN 0289-629X
MINOPHAGEN MEDICAL REVIEW. SUPPLEMENT. Text in Japanese. 1968. irreg.
Published by: Minofagen Seiyaku Honpo/Minophagen Pharmaceutical Co., 10-22 Akasaka 8-chome, Minato-ku, Tokyo 107-0052, Japan.

615.19 ISR
MIRKACHTON. Text in Hebrew. 1987. q.
Published by: Pharmaceutical Association of Israel, Pharmacies Branch, P O Box 566, Tel Aviv 65112, Israel. TEL 03-615085.

615.1 USA ISSN 0026-6663
MISSOURI PHARMACIST. Text in English. 1926. q. USD 30 (effective 1997). adv. bk.rev. **Description:** Includes news items, continuing education articles and professional articles of interest to Missouri pharmacists.
Indexed: I.P.A.
Published by: Missouri Pharmaceutical Association, 211 East Capitol Ave, Jefferson City, MO 65101. TEL 573-636-7522, FAX 573-636-7485. Ed., R&P Deedie K Bedosky. Circ: 1,200.

516.1 ISL ISSN 1021-0075
MIXTURA; blad lyfjafraedinema. Text in Icelandic. 1987. a. free per issue. adv. illus. back issues avail.
Published by: University of Iceland, Department of Pharmacy, Reykjavik 101, Iceland. TEL 354-569-4462, FAX 354-552-1331. Circ: 4,000.

615 JPN ISSN 0913-2147
MIYAGIKEN YAKUJI JOHO/MIYAGI PREFECTURE DRUG INFORMATION. Text in Japanese. 1982. s-a.
Published by: Miyagiken Hoken Kankyobu/Miyagi Prefectural Government, Healthy Environment Division, 8-1 Hon-cho 3-chome, Aoba-ku, Sendai-shi, Miyagi-ken 980-0014, Japan.

615 JPN ISSN 0917-6209
MIYAGIKEN YAKUJI JOHO YAKKYOKU YAKUTEN'YO/MIYAGI PREFECTURE DRUG INFORMATION FOR PHARMACY. Text in Japanese. 1990. a. free per issue. **Description:** Contains comprehensive drug information covering the pharmaceutical industry.
Published by: Miyagiken Hoken Fukushibu/Miyagi Prefectural Government, Pharmaceutical Affairs, 8-1 Hon-cho 3-chome, Aoba-ku, Sendai-shi, Miyagi-ken 980-0014, Japan. TEL 81-22-296-0911, FAX 81-22-296-0912. Ed. Suetugu Mue. Pub. Sei Saito. R&P Megumi Chida TEL 81-22-211-2652. Circ: 42,000.

615 610.73 USA ISSN 1044-0704
RS79
MODELL'S DRUGS IN CURRENT USE AND NEW DRUGS. Text in English. 1955. a., latest vol.47, 2001. USD 29.95 domestic; USD 33.80 foreign (effective 2001). adv. 360 p./no. back issues avail.; reprint service avail. from PQC. **Document type:** *Monographic series, Academic/Scholarly, Abstract/Index.* **Description:** Contains concise information on nearly 1,100 generic drugs, with 1,200 cross-references to their branded counterparts. Presents information on indications and contraindications, side effects, drug interactions, dosages and administration, and available preparations.
Formerly: Drugs in Current Use and New Drugs (0070-7392)
Related titles: Microform ed.: (from PQC).
—CISTI.
Published by: Springer Publishing Company, 536 Broadway, New York, NY 10012. TEL 212-431-4370, FAX 212-941-7842, springer@springerpub.com, http://www.springerjournals.com/store/page1396_6.html, http://www.springerpub.com. R&P Dorothy Kouwenberg. Circ: 1,200.

P

615.1 USA ISSN 1099-8209
MODERN DRUG DISCOVERY; chemical and biological perspectives. Text in English. m. USD 170 in North America to institutions; USD 239 elsewhere to institutions (effective 2002); for additional pricing options for print and web editions contact inside sales specialist, Ms. Chako Dickinson, at 202-872-4063. adv. back issues avail. **Document type:** *Magazine, Academic/Scholarly.* **Description:** Features articles on the newest areas in drugs and life sciences research. Coverage includes reporting on new technologies for finding drug candidates and targets and on current research fields of interest that include combinatorial chemistry, high-throughput screening, rational drug design, molecular modeling, bioinformatics and genomics.
Related titles: Online - full text ed.
Indexed: Biol.Dig.
—BLDSC (5886.197000), CISTI, Linda Hall.
Published by: American Chemical Society, Publications Marketing, 1155 16th St, N W, Washington, DC 20036. TEL 800-227-5558, FAX 202-872-6005, mdd@acs.org, http://pubs.acs.org/mdd, http://pubs.acs.org/journals/mdd/index.html/. Ed. James F Ryan. Circ: 40,000.

615.19 USA ISSN 0732-7218
RM301 CODEN: MMEPDE
MODERN METHODS IN PHARMACOLOGY. Text in English. 1982. irreg., latest vol.5, 1990. price varies. *Refereed.*
Indexed: Biol.Abstr., Chem.Abstr., Chem.Indus.Notes, Chem.Titles.
—CASDDS, CISTI.
Published by: John Wiley & Sons, Inc., Journals (Subsidiary of: Wiley InterScience), 605 Third Ave, New York, NY 10158. TEL 212-475-7700.

MODERN PROBLEMS OF PHARMACOPSYCHIATRY. see *MEDICAL SCIENCES—Psychiatry And Neurology*

615.7 USA
▼ **MOLECULAR INTERVENTIONS.** Text in English. 2001 (Apr.). bi-m. **Description:** Provides scientifically rigorous, cutting-edge reviews written for nonspecialists but sufficiently precise and detailed to command the attention and respect of experts in the field. It features articles on the interplay between science and society, interviews with leaders in pharmacology, information about relevant web sites, reviews of pharmacology and science in the media, and a comprehensive meetings calendar. All articles include creative and compelling graphics.
Related titles: Online - full text ed.
Published by: American Society for Pharmacology and Experimental Therapeutics (ASPET), 9650 Rockville Pike, Bethesda, MD 20814-3998. sack@stanford.edu, http://molinterv.aspetjournals.org, http://www.intl.molinterv.org.

616.4 USA ISSN 1076-1551
CODEN: MOMEF3
MOLECULAR MEDICINE. Text in English. 1995. m. USD 160 domestic to individuals; USD 575 domestic to institutions (effective 2002). adv. back issues avail. *Refereed.* **Document type:** *Journal, Academic/Scholarly.* **Description:** Focused on understanding the molecules that are key to the normal functioning of the body and those related to the fundamental mechanisms of disease.
Related titles: Online - full text ed.: ISSN 1528-3658. USD 446 domestic to institutions; USD 644 domestic to institutions with print ed (effective 2000) (from EBSCO Publishing, RoweCom Information Quest, Swets Blackwell, Institute for Scientific Information).
Indexed: BBCI, Chem.Abstr., Chem.Indus.Notes, Chem.Titles, Curr.Cont., Focus on: Mol.Med., Ind.Med. (1994-), Ind.Sci.Rev., Ind.Vet., Sci.Cit.Ind., Vet.Bull.
—BLDSC (5900.817920), ADONIS, CASDDS, GNLM, IDS, Infotrieve, KNAW. **CCC.**
Published by: (Molecular Medicine Society), Johns Hopkins University Press, Journals Publishing Division, 2715 N Charles St, Baltimore, MD 21218-4363. TEL 410-516-6900, FAX 410-516-6968, http://muse.jhu.edu/journals/molecular_medicine/, http://www.press.jhu.edu/press/journals. Ed. David Weatherall. adv.: page USD 450; trim 8.5 x 11. Circ: 500. **Co-publisher:** Picower Institute Press.

615.7 USA ISSN 0026-895X
QP901 CODEN: MOPMA3
MOLECULAR PHARMACOLOGY. Text in English. 1965. m. USD 147, USD 198 to individuals; USD 360, USD 410 to institutions (effective 2000); includes on-line ed.. adv. index. back issues avail. *Refereed.* **Document type:** *Academic/Scholarly.* **Description:** Covers research on drug action and selective toxicity at the molecular level, for pharmacologists and biochemists.
Related titles: Microfilm ed.: (from WWS); Online - full text ed.: ISSN 1521-0111. USD 118 to individuals; USD 288 to institutions (effective 2000) (from HighWire Pr., EBSCO Publishing, Institute for Scientific Information).
Indexed: ASCA, Agri.& Environ.Biotech.Abstr. (coverage dropped), Aqua.Sci.& Fish.Abstr., BBCI, Chem.Abstr., Chem.Cit.Ind., Chem.Indus.Notes, Chem.Titles, Curr.Adv.Biochem., Curr.Adv.Cancer Res., Curr.Adv.Ecol.Sci., Curr.Adv.Gen.& Molec.Biol., Curr.Cont., Dent.Ind., Derwent Biotech.Abstr., Excerp.Med., Genet.Abstr., Helminthol.Abstr., Hum.Gen.Abstr., INIS Atomind., Ind.Med. (1965-), Ind.Sci.Rev., Inpharma, Int.Abstr.Biol.Sci., Neurosci.Abstr. (coverage dropped), Neurosci.Cit.Ind., Nuc.Acids Abstr., Pharm.&Out.News, Protozool.Abstr., Reac., Rev.Appl.Entomol., Rev.Med.& Vet.Mycol., Sci.Cit.Ind., THA.
—BLDSC (5900.818000), CASDDS, CISTI, GNLM, IDS, ingenta, KNAW, Linda Hall.
Published by: American Society for Pharmacology and Experimental Therapeutics (ASPET), 9650 Rockville Pike, Bethesda, MD 20814-3998. TEL 301-530-7024, FAX 301-571-5728, staff@dues.faseb.org, http://www.molpharm.org. Ed. Joan Heller Brown. Adv. contact Frances Yates. Circ: 1,383; 1,318 (paid).

615.1 FRA ISSN 0026-9689
MONITEUR DES PHARMACIES ET DES LABORATOIRES. Text in French. 1946. w. FRF 890 domestic; FRF 926.50 foreign (effective 1999). adv. illus.
Published by: Groupe Liaisons S.A., 1 av. Edouard Belin, Rueil Malmaison Cedex 92856, France. TEL 33-1-43790630, FAX 33-1-43791775. Circ: 35,800.

615 FRA ISSN 0993-9199
MONITEUR HOSPITALIER. Text in French. 11/yr. FRF 350; FRF 585 foreign.
Published by: Groupe Liaisons S.A., 1 av. Edouard Belin, Rueil Malmaison Cedex 92856, France. TEL 33-1-43790630, FAX 33-1-43791775. Ed. Lawrence Flippone. Circ: 3,500.

615 ESP ISSN 0463-1536
MONITOR DE LA FARMACIA Y DE LA TERAPEUTICA. Text in Spanish. 1895. m. (11/yr.). ESP 3,000. adv. bk.rev. bibl.
Related titles: Cards ed.; Online - full text ed.
Indexed: Biol.Abstr., I.P.A.
Published by: Centros Farmaceuticos Nacional S.A., Julian Camarillo, 37, Madrid 28037, Spain. TEL 17754-43-84, FAX 1-754-56-59. Ed. Daniel Pacheco. Circ: 17,000.

610 USA ISSN 0883-0266
MONTHLY PRESCRIBING REFERENCE. Text in English. 1985. m. USD 79; USD 145 foreign (effective 1999). adv. back issues avail. **Document type:** *Monographic series.* **Description:** Provides up-to-date information to prescribing physicians including the latest Federal Drug Administration drug approvals.
Published by: Prescribing Reference, Inc., 170 Broadway, Ste 1612, New York, NY 10038. TEL 212-766-7200, FAX 212-732-2360. Ed. Jeanette Murphy. Pub., R&P Mark E Bugni. Circ: 124,226. **Subscr. to:** PO Box 412, Congers, NY 10920.

▼ **MULTINATIONAL PHARMACEUTICAL COMPANIES.** see *BUSINESS AND ECONOMICS—International Development And Assistance*

615.1 USA ISSN 8756-4483
N A B P NEWSLETTER. Text in English. 1971. 10/yr. USD 35 to non-members (effective 1999). abstr. charts, illus, stat. index. **Document type:** *Newsletter.*
Formerly: N A B P Quarterly (0027-5700)
Related titles: Online - full text ed.
Indexed: I.P.A.
Published by: National Association of Boards of Pharmacy, 700 Busse Hwy, Park Ridge, IL 60068-2402. TEL 847-698-6227. Eds. Carmen Catizone, Janice O Teplitz. Circ: 1,300 (controlled).

N A C D S ANNUAL REPORT. see *BUSINESS AND ECONOMICS—Management*

615.328 USA ISSN 1092-4272
N A C D S CHAIN PHARMACIST PRACTICE MEMO. Text in English. 1997. m. **Document type:** *Newsletter.* **Description:** Includes practice related information for the chain pharmacist.
Published by: National Association of Chain Drug Stores, PO Box 1417 D49, Alexandria, VA 22313-1417. TEL 703-549-3001, FAX 703-836-4869. Ed. Nancy J Olins.

615.328 USA ISSN 1079-1108
N A C D S FEDERAL REPORT. Text in English. q. membership. **Document type:** *Newsletter.*
Former titles: National Association of Chain Drug Stores. Legislative Newsletter; (until 1971): National Association of Chain Drug Stores. Legislative News Bulletin
Indexed: I.P.A.
Published by: National Association of Chain Drug Stores, PO Box 1417 D49, Alexandria, VA 22313-1417. TEL 703-549-3001, FAX 703-836-4869. Ed. David Lambert. Circ: 400.

N A C D S SOURCEBOOK. see *BUSINESS AND ECONOMICS—Management*

615 658 ZAF
N A P W NEWS* /N V F G NUUS. Text mainly in English; Text occasionally in Afrikaans. 1993. irreg. membership. **Document type:** *Newsletter.*
Published by: National Association of Pharmaceutical Wholesalers/Nasionale Vereniging van Farmaseutiese Groothandelaars, c/o SACOB, J C C House, Empire Rd, Milpark, Johannesburg, South Africa.

615.19 ITA ISSN 0393-3733
N C F. Text in Italian. 1970. m. (10/yr.). ITL 265,000; USD 270 foreign (effective 2000). adv. bk.rev. bibl. **Document type:** *Newspaper.* **Description:** Aims to present a global and current view of the technical and commercial evolution of this field.
Formerly (until 1983): Notiziario Chimico e Farmaceutico (0550-1156)
Indexed: I.P.A.
—BLDSC (6174.278000), CISTI, KNAW, Linda Hall.
Published by: Societa Editoriale Farmaceutica s.r.l., Via Ausonio, 12, Milan, MI 20123, Italy. TEL 02-89404545, FAX 02-89401168. Ed. M Rucci. Adv. contact Giancarlo Lubner. Circ: 6,000.

615.1 USA
HD9666.1
N C P A NEWSLETTER. Text in English. 1970. m. USD 50. **Document type:** *Newsletter.*
Formerly: N A R D Newsletter (0162-1602)
Published by: National Community Pharmacists Association, 205 Daingerfield Rd, Alexandria, VA 22314. TEL 703-683-8200, FAX 703-683-3619. Ed. Cary Boshamer. Circ: 15,350.

615.1029 USA ISSN 0890-6610
RS189
N D A PIPELINE. (New Drug Approval) Text in English. 1981. a. USD 1,295 (effective 2001). adv. back issues avail. **Document type:** *Trade.* **Description:** Contains a company-by-company compilation of Rx drug development activity in the U.S. throughout the past year - from new compounds in research to those that obtained FDA marketing approval.
Related titles: Online - full text ed.: (from Data-Star).
Published by: F-D-C Reports, Inc., 5550 Friendship Blvd, Ste One, Chevy Chase, MD 20815-7278. TEL 800-332-2181, FAX 301-664-7238, http://www.fdcreports.com. Ed. Cindy Frederick. R&P Laura Desimione. Adv. contact Michael Keville.

615 GBR
N P A SUPPLEMENT. Text in English. 1921. m. membership. index. **Document type:** *Newsletter.*
Formerly: N P U Supplement
Published by: National Pharmaceutical Association, 38-42 St Peters St, St. Albans, Herts, United Kingdom. TEL 44-1727-832161, FAX 44-1727-840858, npa@cix.co.uk, http://www.npa.co.uk. Ed. Veronica Wray. Circ: 10,500.

615 USA
N W D A EXECUTIVE NEWSLETTER. Text in English. 1913. m. USD 100 to non-members. **Document type:** *Newsletter.* **Description:** Covers services and programs of NWDA, news of membership and industry trends. Includes some statistics on sales and growth on monthly basis.
Published by: National Wholesale Druggists' Association, PO Box 2219, Reston, VA 22090. TEL 703-787-0000, FAX 703-787-6930. Ed. Lauren Asplen. Circ: 2,300 (controlled).

615.1 USA ISSN 0163-1586
N Y STATE PHARMACIST. Text in English. 1926. bi-m. USD 25 to non-members; USD 20 to members (effective 1999). adv. bk.rev. illus, mkt.
Formerly: New York State Pharmacist (0028-7660)
—Linda Hall.
Published by: Pharmacists Society of the State of New York, 201 Washington Avenue Ext, Albany, NY 12203-5221. TEL 518-869-6595. Ed. Anthony J Conte. Adv. contact Mary Prediger. Circ: 2,000.

P

615.1 POL ISSN 1426-0514
NACZELNA IZBA APTEKARSKA. BIULETYN. Text in Polish. q.
—BLDSC (2102.729000).
Published by: Naczelna Izba Aptekarska, ul. Dluga 16, Warszawa 00-238, Poland. TEL 48-22-7815102, FAX 48-227815102.

615.19 JPN ISSN 0369-5611 CODEN: NSDYAI
NAGOYA SHIRITSU DAIGAKU YAKUGAKUBU KENKYU NENPO/NAGOYA CITY UNIVERSITY. FACULTY OF PHARMACEUTICAL SCIENCE. ANNUAL REPORT. Text in English, Japanese. 1953. a. free per issue. bibl.
Indexed: Biol.Abstr., Chem.Abstr.
—CASDDS, KNAW, Linda Hall.
Published by: Nagoya Shiritsu Daigaku, Yakugakubu, 3-1 Tanabetori, Mizuho-ku, Nagoya-shi, Aichi-ken 467-0027, Japan. Circ: 400.

615 570 660 GBR ISSN 1360-3019
NAPRALERT ON CD-ROM. Text in English. 1998. s-a. GBP 4,000; GBP 3,000 renewals. **Description:** Comprehensive resource on the medicinal aspects of biological species. Covers marine and terrestrial organisms, their chemical constituents, biological and pharmacological activities, and their ethnomedical uses. Aimed at medicinal chemists and other drug researchers, pharmacologists and bioscientists with a related research interest.
Media: CD-ROM.
Published by: Chapman & Hall, Electronic Publishing Division, 2-6 Boundary Row, London E1 8HN, United Kingdom. TEL 44-20-7865-0066, FAX 44-20-7522-0101, cust.serv@chall.co.uk, http://epd.chapmanhall.com. **Dist. by:** Cheriton House, North Way, Andover, Hamps SP10 5BE, United Kingdom. TEL 44-1264-332424, FAX 44-1264-342787.

615 USA ISSN 0077-3263
NATIONAL ASSOCIATION OF BOARDS OF PHARMACY. PROCEEDINGS. Text in English. 1904. a. USD 15 (effective 1999). index. **Document type:** *Proceedings.*
Related titles: Online - full text ed.
Indexed: I.P.A.
Published by: National Association of Boards of Pharmacy, 700 Busse Hwy, Park Ridge, IL 60068-2402. TEL 847-698-6227. Ed. Carmen Catizone. Circ: 300.

NATIONAL ASSOCIATION OF CHAIN DRUG STORES. EXECUTIVE NEWSLETTER. see *BUSINESS AND ECONOMICS—Management*

615 USA
NATIONAL ASSOCIATION OF PHARMACEUTICAL MANUFACTURERS. NEWS BULLETIN*. Text in English. 1960. m. free per issue. **Document type:** *Newsletter, Bulletin.*
Published by: National Association of Pharmaceutical Manufacturers, 3279 Veterans Memorial Hwy no.D7, Ronkonkoma, NY 11779-7671. TEL 516-741-3699, FAX 516-741-3696, NAPMGenRX@aol.com. Ed. Robert S Milanese. Circ: 1,200.

615.1 USA ISSN 0027-9897
NATIONAL PHARMACEUTICAL ASSOCIATION. JOURNAL. Text in English. 1970 (vol.17). 3/yr. USD 25 to members. adv. **Document type:** *Academic/Scholarly.*
Related titles: Online - full text ed.
Indexed: I.P.A.
Published by: National Pharmaceutical Association, Inc., c/o Texas Southern University, College of Pharmacy, 3100 Cleburne, Houston, TX 77004. TEL 713-527-7164, FAX 713-639-1091. Ed. Dr. Henry Lewis III. Circ: 2,000.

615.1 JPN ISSN 1340-3443 CODEN: NMEDEO
NATURAL MEDICINES. Text in English, Japanese; Summaries in English. 1947. q. JPY 12,000. adv. bk.rev. charts, illus. cum.index.
Former titles (until 1994): Shoyakugaku Zasshi - Japanese Journal of Pharmacognosy (0037-4377); (until 1952): Yakuyo Shokubutsu to Shoyaku (0372-7831)
Indexed: Biol.Abstr., Chem.Abstr., Chem.Indus.Notes, Chem.Titles, Excerp.Med., Hort.Abstr., INIS Atomind., I.P.A., Rice Abstr., Seed Abstr.
—BLDSC (6040.735550), CASDDS, CISTI, EMDOCS, GNLM, Infotrieve, ingenta, KNAW, Linda Hall. **CCC.**
Published by: Japanese Society of Pharmacognosy/Nihon Shoyaku Gakkai, c/o Business Center for Academic Societies, 5-16-9 Honkomagome, Bunkyo-ku, Tokyo 113-0021, Japan. Ed. Hidezi Itokawa. Circ: 700.

615.535 613.286 USA ISSN 1089-4853
NATURAL PHARMACY. Text in English. 1996. 10/yr., latest vol.5, 2001. USD 89 domestic to individuals; USD 139 foreign to individuals; USD 139 domestic to institutions; USD 203 foreign to institutions (effective 2002). **Document type:** *Newspaper, Academic/Scholarly.* **Description:** Serves the business and professional needs of independent retail pharmacists who promote, sell and counsel clients on the responsible and successful use of vitamins, nutritional supplements, herbs, homeopathic preparations and other natural products.
Indexed: I.P.A.
Published by: Mary Ann Liebert, Inc. Publishers, 2 Madison Ave, Larchmont, NY 10538. TEL 914—834-3100, FAX 914-834-1388, info@liebertpub.com, www.liebertpub.com/nap, http://www.liebertpub.com.

615.4 KOR
NATURAL PRODUCT SCIENCES. Text in English. q. USD 30. **Document type:** *Academic/Scholarly.*
Indexed: Chem.Abstr., Chem.Indus.Notes, Chem.Titles, Forest Prod.Abstr., Nutr.Abstr., Ornam.Hort., Rev.Arom.& Med.Plants, Rev.Med.& Vet.Mycol., Seed Abstr., Sugar Ind.Abstr., Weed Abstr.
—BLDSC (6040.738200).
Published by: Korean Society of Pharmacognosy, c/o Natural Products Research Institute, Jongro-ku, 28 Yeongun dong, Seoul 110460, Korea, S.. TEL 82-2-740-8925, FAX 82-2-742-3323, sskang@plaza.snu.ac.kr.

NATURAL PRODUCTS NEWS. see *CHEMISTRY—Organic Chemistry*

NATURAL TOXINS. see *ENVIRONMENTAL STUDIES—Toxicology And Environmental Safety*

615.1 DEU ISSN 0028-1298 CODEN: NSAPCC
NAUNYN-SCHMIEDEBERG'S ARCHIVES OF PHARMACOLOGY. Text in German. 1873. m. EUR 1,575.90 domestic; EUR 1,556.70 in Germany; EUR 28 newsstand/cover foreign (effective 2002). adv. charts, illus. back issues avail.; reprint service avail. from ISI. *Refereed.* **Document type:** *Journal, Academic/Scholarly.* **Description:** Original papers, ranging from reports on the molecular effects of drugs within the cell to observations of their effects on the whole organism. Focuses on pharmacology and toxicology.
Formerly: Naunyn-Schmiedebergs Archiv fuer Pharmakologie und Experimentelle Pathologie
Related titles: Microform ed.: (from PQC,PMC); Online - full text ed.: ISSN 1432-1912 (from EBSCO Publishing, RoweCom Information Quest, Swets Blackwell, Springer LINK, Institute for Scientific Information).
Indexed: ASCA, Anim.Behav.Abstr. (coverage dropped), Aqua.Sci.& Fish.Abstr., Biol.Abstr., Chem.Abstr., Chem.Indus.Notes, Chem.Titles, Curr.Adv.Ecol.Sci., Curr.Chem.React., Curr.Cont., Dairy Sci.Abstr., Dent.Ind., Derwent Biotech.Abstr., Excerp.Med., INIS Atomind., Ind.Chem., Ind.Med. (1972-), Ind.Sci.Rev., Inpharma, Int.Abstr.Biol.Sci., Mass Spectr.Bull., Neurosci.Abstr. (coverage dropped), Neurosci.Cit.Ind., Pharm.&Out.News, RCI, Reac., Sci.Cit.Ind., THA.
—BLDSC (6060.200000), ADONIS, CASDDS, CINDOC, CISTI, GNLM, IDS, ingenta, Linda Hall. **CCC.**
Published by: (Deutsche Gesellschaft fuer experimentelle und klinische Pharmakologie und Toxikologie), Springer-Verlag (Subsidiary of: BertelsmannSpringer), Tiergartenstr 17, Heidelberg 69121, Germany. TEL 49-6221-345-0, FAX 49-6221-345229, subscriptions@springer.de, http://link.springer.de/link/service/journals/00210/index.htm, http://www.springer.de. Eds. K H Jakobs, M Goethert. **Subscr. in N. America to:** Springer-Verlag New York Inc., PO Box 2485, Secaucus, NJ 07096-2485. TEL 212-460-1500, FAX 212-473-6272.

615.1 USA ISSN 0028-1891
NEBRASKA MORTAR AND PESTLE. Text in English. 1937. m. USD 30 (effective 2001). adv. charts, illus. back issues avail. **Document type:** *Trade.* **Description:** Articles that relate to store operation, layout and management.
Indexed: I.P.A.
Published by: Nebraska Pharmacists Association, Inc., 6221 S 58th St, Ste A, Lincoln, NE 68516-3687. TEL 402-420-1500, FAX 402-420-1406, m&p@npharm.org, m+p@npharm.org. Ed., Adv. contact Darlene K Lowe. page USD 300; trim 8.5 x 11. Circ: 1,809 (paid).

615.1 378 ITA
NEGRI NEWS. Text in Italian. s-a. free per issue. **Document type:** *Newsletter.*
Media: Online - full text.
Published by: Istituto di Ricerche Farmacologiche Mario Negri, Via Eritrea, 62, Milan, MI 20157, Italy. TEL 39-2-390141, FAX 39-2-3546277, http://www.irfmn.mnegri.it/perp/nn/. Ed. Silvio Garattini.

NEPAL. DEPARTMENT OF MEDICINAL PLANTS. ANNUAL REPORT. see *BIOLOGY—Botany*

615 USA
NETSCI. Text in English. 1995. m. adv. bk.rev. *Refereed.* **Description:** Covers pharmaceutical R&D activities for scientists working in the pharmaceutical and biotech industries.
Media: Online - full text.
Published by: Network Science Corporation, 412 Carolina Blvd, Isle Of Palms, SC 29451. TEL 843-886-5008, FAX 843-886-5924, netsci@awod.com, http://www.netsci.org. Ed., R&P Allen B Richon. Adv. contact Merry Ambos.

615 DEU ISSN 0724-567X
NEUE ARZNEIMITTEL. Text in German. 1953. m. EUR 44.28 domestic; EUR 46.20 in Europe; EUR 51.84 elsewhere; EUR 4.50 newsstand/cover (effective 2002); free with subscr. to Deutsche Apotheker Zeitung. **Document type:** *Journal, Trade.*
Formerly: Neue Arzneimittel und Spezialitaeten (0548-2674)
Related titles: ♦ Supplement to: Deutsche Apotheker Zeitung. ISSN 0011-9857.
Indexed: Chem.Abstr., Excerp.Med.
—BLDSC (6077.237900), GNLM, Infotrieve. **CCC.**
Published by: Deutscher Apotheker Verlag, Postfach 101061, Stuttgart 70009, Germany. TEL 49-711-2582-0, FAX 49-711-2582290, daz@deutscher-apotheker-verlag.de, http://www.deutscher-apotheker-verlag.de. Ed. Bettina Hellwig.

615.1 GBR ISSN 0028-3908 RM315 CODEN: NEPHBW
NEUROPHARMACOLOGY. Text in English. 1962. 16/yr. EUR 357 in Europe to qualified personnel; JPY 47,400 in Japan to qualified personnel; USD 398 elsewhere to qualified personnel; EUR 2,618 in Europe to institutions; JPY 284,886 in Japan to institutions; USD 2,928 elsewhere to institutions (effective 2002). adv. bk.rev. bibl, charts, illus. index. back issues avail.; reprint service avail. from PQC. *Refereed.* **Document type:** *Academic/Scholarly.* **Description:** Furthers the understanding of the mechanisms of drug actions on the nervous system.
Formerly: International Journal of Neuropharmacology
Related titles: Microfilm ed.: (from PQC); Online - full text ed.: (from ingenta, ScienceDirect, Swets Blackwell, Institute for Scientific Information).
Indexed: ASCA, Agri.& Environ.Biotech.Abstr. (coverage dropped), Arts & Hum.Cit.Ind. (coverage dropped), BBCI, Biol.Abstr., Biotech.& Bioeng.Abstr., Chem.Abstr., Chem.Indus.Notes, Chem.Titles, Chemorec.Abstr., Curr.Adv.Ecol.Sci., Curr.Cont., Dent.Ind., Derwent Biotech.Abstr., Excerp.Med., Helminthol.Abstr., INIS Atomind., Ind.Med. (1970-), Ind.Sci.Rev., Inpharma, Int.Abstr.Biol.Sci., Int.Aerosp.Abstr., Neurosci.Abstr., Neurosci.Cit.Ind., Nutr.Abstr., Pharm.&Out.News, PsycInfo, Psychol.Abstr. (1970-), Reac., Rev.Appl.Entomol., Sci.Cit.Ind., THA, e-psyche.
—BLDSC (6081.517500), ADONIS, CASDDS, CISTI, GNLM, IDS, ingenta, KNAW, Linda Hall. **CCC.**
Published by: Pergamon (Subsidiary of: Elsevier Science), The Boulevard, Langford Ln, East Park, Kidlington, Oxford OXB 1GB, United Kingdom. FAX 44-1865-843010, http://www.elsevier.com/locate/neuropharm. Eds. Bridget L Craddock, G Collingridge. Circ: 1,500. **Subscr. in Australasia and the Far East to:** Elsevier Science (Singapore) Pte Ltd, No.1 Temasek Ave, 17-01 Millenia Tower, Singapore 039192, Singapore. TEL 65-434-3727, FAX 65-337-2230; **Subscr. in the Americas to:** Elsevier Science, PO Box 945, New York, NY 10159-0945. TEL 212-633-3730, FAX 212-633-3680, usinfo-f@elsevier.com; **Subscr. to:** Elsevier Science BV, PO Box 211, Amsterdam 1000 AE, Netherlands. TEL 31-20-485-3757.

NEUROPSYCHOBIOLOGY; international journal of experimental and clinical research in biological psychiatry, pharmacopsychiatry, biological psychology, pharmacopsychology and pharmacoelectroencephalography. see *MEDICAL SCIENCES—Psychiatry And Neurology*

NEUROPSYCHOPHARMACOLOGY. see *MEDICAL SCIENCES—Psychiatry And Neurology*

615.1 DEU
▼ **NEW DRUGS.** Text in English. 2001. bi-m. adv. **Document type:** *Magazine, Trade.* **Description:** Provides news and information of interest to international pharmaceutical research concerns.
Published by: Vogel Verlag und Druck GmbH & Co. KG, Max-Planck-Str 7-9, Wuerzburg 97064, Germany. TEL 49-931-4182518, FAX 49-931-4182750, http://www.vogel-medien.de.

615.1 NZL ISSN 0110-9510
NEW ETHICALS CATALOGUE; the basis of a system of independent drug information. Text in English. 1966. 2/yr. (plus m. updates). NZD 120 (effective 1999). adv.
Related titles: ♦ Supplement to: New Ethicals Journal. ISSN 1174-4502.
—GNLM, Infotrieve. **CCC.**
Published by: Adis International Limited, Mairangi Bay, Private Bag 65901, Auckland 1010, New Zealand. TEL 64-9-477-0700, FAX 64-9-477-0766, http://www.adis.com. Ed. Rhoda Saunders. Pub. Graeme Avery. R&P, Adv. contact Chris Lawson. Circ: 6,000.

615.1 NZL ISSN 1174-4502
CODEN: NEETEG
NEW ETHICALS JOURNAL. Text in English. 1998. m. NZD 135 (effective 1999). **Description:** Provides general practitioners and allied professionals with information on diagnosis, clinical management and practical drug treatment.
Formed by the merger of (1972-1998): New Zealand Patient Management (1172-630X); Which was formerly (until 1985): Patient Management (0110-4578); (1964-1998): New Ethicals (0111-0020); Which was formerly (until 1976): New Ethicals and Medical Progress (0548-4545); (until 1967): New Ethicals
Related titles: ♦ Supplement: New Ethicals Catalogue. ISSN 0110-9510.
Indexed: I.P.A., Ind.N.Z.Per., Inpharma, Pharm.&Out.News, Reac.
—BLDSC (6084.142000), GNLM.
Published by: Adis International Limited, Mairangi Bay, Private Bag 65901, Auckland 1010, New Zealand. TEL 64-9-477-0700, FAX 64-9-477-0766, http://www.adis.com. Ed. Kirsten Stone. Pub. Graeme Avery. R&P Jane Melville. Circ: 6,000.

615.1 USA ISSN 0028-5773
RS1
NEW JERSEY JOURNAL OF PHARMACY. Text in English. 1927. bi-m. USD 12; USD 55 foreign (effective 1999). adv. bk.rev. illus. reprint service avail. from PQC. *Refereed.* **Document type:** *Academic/Scholarly.* **Description:** Articles pertaining to the practice of pharmacy, both scientific and economic.
Related titles: Microform ed.: (from PQC).
Indexed: I.P.A.
—Linda Hall.
Published by: New Jersey Pharmacists Association, 3 Marlen Dr., Robbinsville, NJ 08691-1604. TEL 609-584-9063, FAX 609-586-8186, njpharm@aol.com, http://www.njpha.com. Ed., Adv. contact Patricia L Frasier. R&P Patricia L Frazier. Circ: 2,500.

615 GBR
NEW PRODUCT LAUNCH LETTER. Text in English. 1976. s-m. GBP 2,500. **Document type:** *Trade.*
Formerly (until 1990): New Product Card Index
Related titles: CD-ROM ed.; Online - full text ed.: (from Data-Star).
Published by: IMSWORLD Publications Ltd., 7 Harewood Ave, London NW1 6JB, United Kingdom. TEL 0171-393-5000, FAX 0171-393-5900.

615 USA ISSN 1080-1855
THE NEW YORK HEALTH SYSTEM PHARMACIST. Text in English. 1981. bi-m. membership. adv. **Document type:** *Academic/Scholarly.*
Former titles (until 1994): New York State Council of Hospital Pharmacists. Newsletter (1066-5617); (until 1992): New York State Journal of Pharmacy (0279-8778); Which supersedes (in 1981): New York State Council of Hospital Pharmacists. Newsletter (0199-6169)
Indexed: I.P.A.
Published by: New York State Council of Health System Pharmacists, 435 New Karner Rd, Albany, NY 12205-3833. Ed. Henry Cohen. Adv. contact Debra Feinberg. B&W page USD 700, color page USD 1,650; trim 7.5 x 10.

615.329 USA ISSN 0739-7062
NEW YORK STATE PHARMACIST - CENTURY II. Text in English. 1927. q. USD 25. adv.
Indexed: I.P.A.
Published by: Pharmacists Society of the State of New York, 201 Washington Avenue Ext, Albany, NY 12203-5221. TEL 518-869-6595. Ed. Anthony J Conte. Circ: 2,000.

NEW ZEALAND GAZETTE TRADE LISTS. REGISTER OF PHARMACIES. see *BUSINESS AND ECONOMICS—Trade And Industrial Directories*

615.1 NZL ISSN 0111-431X
NEW ZEALAND PHARMACY. Text in English. 1981. m. NZD 66. adv. bk.rev. **Document type:** *Trade.*
Formed by the merger of (1977-1981): Pharmacy Digest (0110-8832); (1910-1981): Pharmaceutical Journal of New Zealand (0031-6881)
Related titles: Online - full text ed.: (from Factiva).
Indexed: ABIX (Nov.1992-), Agri.& Environ.Biotech.Abstr. (coverage dropped), Biol.Abstr., Chem.Abstr., Curr.Adv.Ecol.Sci., I.P.A., Ind.N.Z.Per., Inpharma, Pharm.&Out.News, Protozool.Abstr., Reac.
—BLDSC (6096.495000), GNLM, Infotrieve. **CCC.**
Published by: (Pharmaceutical Society of New Zealand), Methode Media Ltd., PO Box 105 483, Auckland, New Zealand. TEL 64-9-3660404, FAX 64-9-3660402, methode@xtra.co.nz. Ed., Pub., R&P Lorraine Thomson. Adv. contact Carli Clark. B&W page NZD 1,550, color page NZD 1,950; trim 210 x 285. Circ: 3,200.

615.1 NLD ISSN 0927-0574
NIEUWE DROGIST. Text in Dutch. 1902. m. NLG 132.08 domestic; NLG 231.13 foreign (effective 2001). adv. bk.rev. illus. **Document type:** *Journal, Trade.* **Description:** Covers all aspects of the retail drug industry.
Formerly (until 1991): Drogist (0012-6330)
Indexed: Key to Econ.Sci.
Published by: Phoenix Publishers, De Haag 5, Houten 3993 AV, Netherlands. TEL 31-30-6342790, FAX 31-30-6342795, info@phoenixbu.ni. Ed. Linda Kattlekamp. Adv. contact Paula Brinks. Circ: 6,100 (paid and controlled).

615 JPN
NIKKEI DRUG INFORMATION. Text in Japanese. 1998. m. JPY 9,600. adv. **Document type:** *Consumer.* **Description:** Contains the latest information on pharmaceutical products provided by manufacturers. Includes information useful to pharmacists and drug store management.
Published by: Nikkei Business Publications Inc. (Subsidiary of: Nihon Keizai Shimbun, Inc.), 2-7-6 Hirakawa-cho, Chiyoda-ku, Tokyo 102-8622, Japan. TEL 81-3-5210-8311, FAX 81-3-5210-8530, info@nikkeibpnyc.com, info@nikkeibp-america.com, http://www.nikkeibp.com. Ed. Katsuniro Sekimoto. Pub. Hitoshi Sawai. Adv. contact Kenji Tameishi. B&W page JPY 440,000, color page JPY 640,000; trim 210 x 280. Circ: 40,589. **Dist. in America by:** Nikkei Business Publications America Inc., 575 Fifth Ave, 20th Fl, New York, NY 10017.

615 JPN ISSN 0914-0697
NIPPON BYOIN YAKUZAISHIKAI ZASSHI/JAPANESE SOCIETY OF HOSPITAL PHARMACISTS. JOURNAL. Text in Japanese. m. JPY 400 per issue.
Indexed: I.P.A.
—BLDSC (4809.452000).
Published by: Nihon Byoin Yakuzaishikai/Japanese Society of Hospital Pharmacists, 12-15-304 Shibuya 2-chome, Shibuya-ku, Tokyo 150-0002, Japan.

615.19 JPN
NIPPON KAYAKU. ANNUAL REPORT. Text in Japanese. a.
Published by: Nippon Kayaku Co., Fujimi Bldg, 11-2 Fujimi 1-chome, Chiyoda-ku, Tokyo 102-0071, Japan.

615 JPN
NIPPON KAYAKU SOGO KENKYUJO NENPO/NIPPON KAYAKU RESEARCH LABORATORIES. ANNUAL REPORT. Text in English, Japanese. 1984. a.
Published by: Nippon Kayaku K.K., Iryo Jigyo Honbu Sogo Kenkyujo/Nippon Kayaku Co., Ltd., Pharmaceuticals Group, Research Laboratories, 31-12 Shimo 3-chome, Kita-ku, Tokyo 115-0042, Japan.

615.328 CAN
NON-PRESCRIPTION DRUG REFERENCE FOR HEALTHCARE PROFESSIONALS. Text in English. quadrennial. CND 120 to non-members; CND 95 to members (effective 2000). **Document type:** *Directory.*
Former titles: Self-Medication; Canadian Self-Medication
Published by: Canadian Pharmacists Association, 1785 Alta Vista Dr, Ottawa, ON K1G 3Y6, Canada. TEL 613-523-7877, FAX 613-523-0445, cpha@cdnpharm.ca, http://www.cdnpharm.ca.

615 USA ISSN 1068-5316
NONPRESCRIPTION PHARMACEUTICALS AND NUTRITIONALS: THE TAN SHEET. Text in English. 1939. w. USD 970 domestic; USD 1,110 foreign (effective 2001). adv. charts, illus, stat, tr.lit. back issues avail.; reprints avail. **Document type:** *Newsletter, Trade.* **Description:** Provides in-depth coverage of nonprescription pharmaceuticals and dietary supplement-nutritionals.
Supersedes in part (in 1993): Prescription and O T C Pharmaceuticals: The Pink Sheet (0734-6514); Which was formerly (until 1982): F D C Reports. Ethical and O T C Pharmaceuticals (0272-913X)
Related titles: Online - full text ed.: (from Data-Star, The Dialog Corporation).
Indexed: P.N.I.
—Infotrieve. **CCC.**
Published by: F-D-C Reports, Inc., 5550 Friendship Blvd, Ste One, Chevy Chase, MD 20815-7278. TEL 800-332-2181, FAX 301-664-7238, http://www.fdcreports.com. Ed. Karl Uhlendorf. R&P Meghanne Malone. Adv. contact Richard Messmer.

615.1 NOR ISSN 0802-8400
NORGES APOTEKERFORENINGS TIDSSKRIFT. Text in Norwegian. 1893. 16/yr. NOK 400; NOK 450 foreign. adv. bk.rev. charts, illus. index. **Document type:** *Bulletin.*
Formerly (until 1985): NAT. Norges Apotekerforenings Tidsskrift (0332-8678)
Indexed: Biol.Abstr., Chem.Abstr., INIS Atomind., I.P.A.
Published by: Norges Apotekerforening, Generalsekretaeren, Postboks 5070, Majorstua, Oslo 0301, Norway. TEL 47-22-69-60-40, FAX 47-22-56-47-18. Ed. Ellen B Wickstrand. adv.: B&W page NOK 4,600, color page NOK 8,800; trim 210 x 297. Circ: 1,900.

P

615 610 382 POL ISSN 0209-3928
NOVOSTI FARMATSII I MEDITSINY/NEWS IN PHARMACOLOGY AND MEDICINE. Text in Russian; Summaries in English. 1967. q. adv. bk.rev. illus. **Description:** Covers all aspects of preparing, preserving, compounding and dispensing drugs.
Published by: (Osrodek Informacji Naukowej "Polfa"), AGPOL - Polexportpress, Ul Kierbedzia 4, Warsaw 00957, Poland. TEL 48-22-402391. Ed. Andrzej Werbeniec. Circ: 30,000.

615 636.08 POL ISSN 0860-3847
NOVOSTI VETERINARNOI FARMATSII I MEDITSINY. Text in Russian. 1985. q.
Formerly (until 1986): Polfa: Novosti Farmatsii i Veterinarnoi Meditsiny (0860-3154)
Published by: (Osrodek Informacji Naukowej "Polfa"), AGPOL - Polexportpress, Ul Kierbedzia 4, Warsaw 00957, Poland. TEL 48-22-402391, FAX 48-22-416061. Ed. Andrzej Werbeniec.

615 GBR ISSN 1358-6327
NUMARK NEWS. Text in English. 1973. bi-m. GBP 75. adv. **Document type:** *Trade.*
Formerly (until 1994): Numark Newsline
Published by: Numark Ltd., Numark House, 5-6 Fairway Ct, Business Park, Mercury Park, Amber Close, Tamworth, Staffs B77 4RP, United Kingdom. TEL 44-1827-69269, FAX 44-1827-62369. Ed. Val Pirie. Circ: 6,000 (controlled).

615 USA ISSN 1074-3871
NURSE PRACTITIONERS' PRESCRIBING REFERENCE. Text in English. 1994. q. USD 32 (effective 2000). *Refereed.* **Document type:** *Monographic series.*
Published by: Prescribing Reference, Inc., 170 Broadway, Ste 1612, New York, NY 10038. TEL 212-766-7200, FAX 212-732-2360. Ed. Jeanette Murphy. Pub., R&P Mark E Bugni. Adv. contact Scott Bugni.

NURSES' DRUG ALERT. see *MEDICAL SCIENCES—Nurses And Nursing*

NURSING (YEAR) DRUG HANDBOOK. see *MEDICAL SCIENCES—Nurses And Nursing*

615.1 GBR ISSN 1362-5411
NUTRACEUTICALS INTERNATIONAL. Text in English. 1996. m. GBP 399 (effective 2001). adv. back issues avail. **Document type:** *Newsletter, Trade.* **Description:** Contains legislation, product development, manufacturing technologies, company information, interviews, market data, marketing alliances, international conferences, worldwide news and views and forthcoming meetings. Aimed at executives in OTC pharmaceuticals, vitamin and health food manufactures, financial analysts and regulatory bodies.
Related titles: Online - full text ed.: (from Gale Group, Factiva).
Published by: Marketletter (Publications) Ltd., 54-55 Wilton Rd, London SW1V 1DE, United Kingdom. TEL 44-20-7828-7272, FAX 44-20-7828-0415, editorial@marketletter.com, http://www.marketletter.com. Ed., Pub. Barbara Obstoj. Adv. contact Robin Cardwell. B&W page GBP 595, color page GBP 1,365; trim 210 x 297. **Subscr. to:** Marketletter (Publications) Ltd, Connaught Housex, 65 Aldwych, PO Box 221, London WC2B 4EJ, United Kingdom.

615 330.9 GBR ISSN 1350-1097
O T C BULLETIN; the business newsletter for Europe's consumer healthcare industry. (Over the Counter) Text in English. 1993. 20/yr. GBP 445 in Europe First subscription; GBP 245 in Europe Subsequent subscriptions; GBP 475 elsewhere First subscription; GBP 275 elsewhere Subsequent subscriptions; GBP 25 newsstand/cover (effective 2002). adv. bk.rev., Website rev. 3 cols./p. back issues avail. **Document type:** *Newsletter, Trade.* **Description:** Contains news and information covering Europe's nonprescription medicine market.
—**CCC.**
Published by: O T C Publications Ltd., 54 Creynolds Ln, Shirley, Solihull, W Midlands B90 4ER, United Kingdom. TEL 44-121-733-8755, FAX 44-121-733-8744, infp@otc-bulletin.com, http://www.otc-bulletin.com. Ed., Pub. Deborah Wilkes. Adv. contact Val Davis. B&W page GBP 895, color page GBP 1,390; trim 297 x 210. Circ: 2,000 (paid).

338.476 GBR ISSN 1355-2449
O T C BUSINESS NEWS. Text in English. 1994. fortn. GBP 475, USD 775 (effective 2001). **Document type:** *Newsletter, Trade.*
Indexed: Bus.& Indus. (Jan.1996-).
Published by: Informa Global Pharmaceuticals & Healthcare (Subsidiary of: Financial Times Business.), Mortimer House, 37-41 Mortimer St, London W1N 7RJ, United Kingdom. TEL 44-1206-772113, FAX 44-20-7453-2386, enquiries@informa.com, http://www.informapharma.com/LS0184, http://www.informapharma,com. Ed. Sarah Walkley.

615 330.9 GBR
O T C HEALTHCARE: A WORLD SURVEY. (Over The Counter) Text in English. irreg., latest 1997. GBP 3,950, USD 7,900. **Document type:** *Trade.* **Description:** Looks at the latest trends and developments in the over-the-counter healthcare products market worldwide.
Published by: Euromonitor, 60-61 Britton St, London EC1M 5UX, United Kingdom. TEL 44-20-7251-8024, info@euromonitor.com, http://www.euromonitor.com.

615 GBR ISSN 1360-4619
O T C LATINA. (Over the Counter) Text in English. 1995. m. GBP 2,500 (effective 2001). 2 cols./p. back issues avail. **Document type:** *Magazine, Trade.* **Description:** Data and analysis on Latin American OTC markets.
Related titles: CD-ROM ed.
Indexed: Bus.& Indus. (Jul.1995-).
Published by: Nicholas Hall & Company, 35 Alexandra St, Southend-on-Sea, Essex SS1 1BW, United Kingdom. TEL 44-1702-220200, FAX 44-1702-430787, otclatina@nicholashall.com, info@nicholashall.com. Ed. Mark Doxey. R&P Nina Stimson. Adv. contact Scot Nisbet.

615 GBR ISSN 0956-2559
O T C NEWS AND MARKET REPORT. (Over the Counter) Text in English. 1988. m. GBP 1,150 (effective 2001). adv. back issues avail. **Document type:** *Magazine, Trade.* **Description:** Contains data and analysis on European OTC markets.
Related titles: CD-ROM ed.
Indexed: Bus.& Indus. (Jan.1994-).
Published by: Nicholas Hall & Company, 35 Alexandra St, Southend-on-Sea, Essex SS1 1BW, United Kingdom. TEL 44-1702-220200, FAX 44-1702-430787, otcnews@nicholashall.com, info@nicholashall.com. Ed., R&P Nina Stimson. Adv. contact Scot Nisbet. B&W page GBP 750, color page GBP 1,200.

615 GBR
O T C UPDATE. (Over The Counter) Text in English. 1990. m. GBP 2,500 (effective 2001). adv. 2 cols./p. back issues avail. **Document type:** *Magazine, Trade.* **Description:** Data and analysis on North American OTC markets.
Related titles: CD-ROM ed.
Indexed: Bus.& Indus. (Jan.1996-).
Published by: Nicholas Hall & Company, 35 Alexandra St, Southend-on-Sea, Essex SS1 1BW, United Kingdom. TEL 44-1702-220200, FAX 44-1702-430787, otcupdate@NicholasHall.com, info@nicholashall.com. Ed. Mike Nash. R&P Nina Stimson. Adv. contact Scot Nisbet. B&W page GBP 750, color page GBP 1,200; trim 165 x 260.

615.1 AUT ISSN 0029-8859
CODEN: OAZEAL
OESTERREICHISCHE APOTHEKER-ZEITUNG. Text in German. 1946. fortn. ATS 1,395.45 (effective 1998). adv. bk.rev. abstr. index. **Document type:** *Newspaper.* **Description:** Information and networking for Austrian pharmacists.
Indexed: Agri.& Environ.Biotech.Abstr. (coverage dropped), Chem.Abstr., INIS Atomind., I.P.A.
—CASDDS, CISTI, GNLM.
Published by: Oesterreichische Apotheker-Verlagsgesellschaft mbH, Spitalgasse 31, Vienna, W 1094, Austria. TEL 43-1-4023588, FAX 43-1-4085355. Ed. Gottfried Zimmermann. Circ: 4,500.

615 PRT ISSN 0872-962X
OFFARM. Text in Portuguese. 1993. m. (11/yr.). PTE 6,080. **Document type:** *Trade.*
Published by: Ferreira e Bento Lda., Rua D. Estefania 32-1o, Lisbon 1000, Portugal. TEL 351-1-791-2500, http://www.fbento.pt/FB/.

615 ESP ISSN 0212-047X
OFFARM* . Text in Spanish. 1982. 12/yr.
Published by: Haymarket, S.A., Travesera Gracia 17-21, 5o 2o, Barcelona 08022, Spain. TEL 3-237-22-66, FAX 3-237-66-88. Ed. Juan Mir Morato. Circ: 18,000.

615.1 USA ISSN 0030-1027
OHIO PHARMACIST. Text in English. 1952. m. USD 20. adv. illus. **Document type:** *Trade.*
Indexed: I.P.A.
Published by: Ohio Pharmacists Association, 6037 Frantz Rd, Ste 106, Dublin, OH 43017-3320. TEL 614-798-0037. Ed. Amy Bennett. Circ: 4,000.

ONKOLOGIYA. see *MEDICAL SCIENCES—Oncology*

615.19 AUS ISSN 1443-2285
ONLINE JOURNAL OF PHARMACOKINETICS. Text in English. 1996. bi-m. **Description:** Encourages submissions dealing with interactive pharmacokinetic profiles.
Media: Online - full text.
Published by: Pestsearch International Pty. Ltd., 173 Chatswood Rd, Daisy Hill, QLD 4127, Australia. http://www.uq.edu.au/~csvguerr/Pharkin.htm. Ed. D W A Bourne.

OPHTHALMIC DRUG FACTS. see *MEDICAL SCIENCES—Ophthalmology And Optometry*

615 CHE
OPTIPHARM. Text in French. m. **Document type:** *Magazine, Trade.* **Description:** Information for pharmacists and their assistants.
Published by: Editions Optima SA, Av de Chillon 90, Montreux 1820, Switzerland. TEL 41-21-9635161, FAX 41-21-9638679. Ed. Gerard Geiger. Circ: 10,344 (controlled).

615 PRT ISSN 0872-7554
ORDEM DOS FARMACEUTICOS. REVISTA. Text in Portuguese. 1994. bi-m. PTE 4,000 domestic; USD 24 foreign (effective 2001). adv. bk.rev. **Document type:** *Trade.* **Description:** Presents current information on the society's activities and short articles of interest to the average pharmacist.
Related titles: Online - full text ed.
Published by: Ordem dos Farmaceuticos, Rua da Sociedade Farmaceutica, 18, Lisbon, Lisboa 1169-075, Portugal. TEL 351-21-3191370, FAX 351-21-3191399, http://www.ordemfarmaceuticos.pt. Ed. Jose Aranda da Silv. R&P Ivana Silva. Adv. contact Antonio Viveiros. Circ: 8,500.

615 JPN ISSN 0387-480X
OSAKA UNIVERSITY. FACULTY OF PHARMACEUTICAL SCIENCES. MEMOIRS/OSAKA DAIGAKU YAKUGAKUBU KIYO. Text in English. 1970. a. free per issue. abstr. **Description:** Features the collection of abstracts of scientific papers published in the previous year by the faculty.
Published by: Osaka Daigaku, Yakugakubu/Osaka University, Faculty of Pharmaceutical Sciences, 1-6 Yamada-Oka, Suita-shi, Osaka-fu 565-0871, Japan. FAX 81-6-879-8154. Ed. Tadashi Mizoguchi. Circ: 300.

615.1 JPN ISSN 0030-669X
OTSUKA PHARMACEUTICAL FACTORY. JOURNAL/OTSUKA YAKUHO. Text in Japanese. 1950. 11/yr. JPY 2,000. illus.
Published by: Otsuka Pharmaceutical Factory/Otsuka Seiyaku Kojo, 115 Tateiwa-Muya-cho, Naruto-shi, Tokushima-ken 772-0000, Japan. Ed. M Ohsaka. Circ: 61,500.

615 JPN ISSN 0300-8533
CODEN: OYYAA2
OYO YAKURI/PHARMACOMETRICS. Text in English, Japanese. 1967. m. JPY 10,000, USD 120 (effective 2000). adv. bk.rev. index. back issues avail. *Refereed.* **Document type:** *Academic/Scholarly.* **Description:** Applied pharmacology, pharmacodynamics, pharmacokinetics and toxicity studies of new drugs.
Indexed: Chem.Abstr., Chem.Titles, Dairy Sci.Abstr., Excerp.Med., INIS Atomind., I.P.A., Inpharma, Pharm.&Out.News, Reac.
—BLDSC (6447.085000), CASDDS, CISTI, EMDOCS, GNLM, Infotrieve, KNAW. **CCC.**
Published by: Oyo Yakuri Kenkyukai/Japanese Society of Pharmacometrics, C.P.O. Box 180, Sendai 980-8691, Japan. TEL 81-22-267-3810, FAX 81-22-222-0515. Ed. Dr. Hikaru Ozawa. Adv. contact Oyo Yakuri Kenkyukai. Circ: 1,200.

615 USA ISSN 1052-1372
CODEN: PPTTEK
P & T; journal for formulary management. (Pharmacy & Therapeutic) Text in English. 1976. m. USD 87 in the Americas to institutions; USD 130 elsewhere to institutions (effective 2000). adv. *Refereed.* **Document type:** *Academic/Scholarly, Trade.*
Former titles (until Jul. 1990): Hospital Therapy (0160-9459); Drug Therapy (Hospital Edition); Drug Therapy Hospital
Related titles: Online - full text ed.
Indexed: Excerp.Med., I.P.A., Inpharma, Pharm.&Out.News, Reac.
—BLDSC (6327.163000), CISTI, EMDOCS, GNLM, Infotrieve, KNAW. **CCC.**
Published by: Quadrant HealthCom, 26 Main St, Ste A, Chatham, NJ 07928-2402. TEL 973-701-8900, FAX 973-701-8892. Ed. Debra Gitterman. Pub. Robert Morgan. Adv. contact Denise Andrade.

615.1 USA ISSN 1079-7440
CODEN: JPHTEU
P D A JOURNAL OF PHARMACEUTICAL SCIENCE AND TECHNOLOGY. Text in English. 1947. 6/yr. USD 195 (effective 2001). bk.rev. charts, illus. index. 80 p./no. back issues avail.; reprints avail. *Refereed.* **Document type:** *Journal, Academic/Scholarly.* **Description:** Technical articles in the field of pharmaceutical science and technology.
Former titles (until vol.48, no.5, 1994): Journal of Pharmaceutical Science and Technology (1076-397X); (until vol.48, no.1, 1994): Journal of Parenteral Science and Technology (0279-7976); (until 1981): Parenteral Drug Association. Journal (0161-1933); (until vol.32, 1978): Parenteral Drug Association. Bulletin (0048-2986).
Related titles: CD-ROM ed.; Online - full text ed.: (from Institute for Scientific Information); ♦ Supplement: P D A Technical Reports.
Indexed: ASCA, Agri.& Environ.Biotech.Abstr. (coverage dropped), Biol.Abstr., Chem.Abstr., Chem.Titles, Curr.Adv.Ecol.Sci., Derwent Biotech.Abstr., Excerp.Med., INIS Atomind., I.P.A., Ind.Med. (1994-), Mass Spectr.Bull., Sugar Ind.Abstr.
—BLDSC (6413.644300), CASDDS, CISTI, EMDOCS, GNLM, IDS, KNAW, Linda Hall.
Published by: P D A (Parenteral Drug Association), 7500 Old Georgetown Rd, Ste 620, Bethesda, MD 20814-6133. TEL 301-986-0293, FAX 301-986-0296, info@pda.org, http://www.pda.org. Ed. Dr. Lee E Kirsch. Pub. Edmund Fry. R&P Linda Williams. Adv. contact Nahid Kiani TEL 301-986-0293 ext 128. Circ: 10,500.

615.19 USA
P D A LETTER. Text in English. 1964. m. membership only. adv. 48 p./no. **Document type:** *Newsletter.* **Description:** Covers pharmaceutical science and technology news, PDA activities and events, member news, international regulatory updates and commentary, as well as services and publications of the PDA.
Published by: P D A (Parenteral Drug Association), 7500 Old Georgetown Rd, Ste 620, Bethesda, MD 20814-6133. TEL 301-986-0293, FAX 301-986-0296, info@pda.org, http://www.pda.org. Ed. Joe Bury. Pub. Edmund Fry. R&P Linda Williams. Adv. contact Nahid Kiani TEL 301-986-0293 ext 128. B&W page USD 1,650. Circ: 10,500.

615.19 USA
P D A TECHNICAL REPORTS. Text in English. 1978. irreg., latest vol.33. price varies. back issues avail. **Document type:** *Monographic series.*
Former titles: Parenteral Drug Association. Technical Report (0277-3406); (until 1981): Parenteral Drug Association. Technical Monograph (0196-3619)
Related titles: ♦ Supplement to: P D A Journal of Pharmaceutical Science and Technology. ISSN 1079-7440.
Indexed: I.P.A.
—KNAW.
Published by: P D A (Parenteral Drug Association), 7500 Old Georgetown Rd, Ste 620, Bethesda, MD 20814-6133. TEL 301-986-0293, FAX 301-986-0296, info@pda.org, http://www.pda.org. R&P Linda Williams.

615 DEU ISSN 0944-7032
CODEN: APKFA2
P K A AKTUELL; DAZ-Beilage fuer die Pharmazeutsich-kaufmaennische Angestellte. Text in German. 1952. bi-m. EUR 17.34 domestic; EUR 19.74 in Europe; EUR 21.30 elsewhere; EUR 3 newsstand/cover (effective 2002); free with subscr. to Deutsche Apotheker Zeitung. **Document type:** *Journal, Trade.* **Description:** Aimed at enlightening pharmaceutical assistants.
Former titles: Apothekenhelferin Heute (0939-3331); Apothekenhelferln (0570-4723)
Related titles: ♦ Supplement to: Deutsche Apotheker Zeitung. ISSN 0011-9857.
—CASDDS, GNLM.
Published by: Deutscher Apotheker Verlag, Postfach 101061, Stuttgart 70009, Germany. TEL 49-711-2582-0, FAX 49-711-2582290, daz@deutscher-apotheker-verlag.de, http://www.deutscher-apotheker-verlag.de. Ed. Klaus Feuerhelm.

615 DEU ISSN 0940-0508
P P I - PRO PHARMA INFORM; Informationsdienst und Presseschau fuer Fuehrungskraefte in Pharmaindustrie, Fachagenturen und Fachverlagen. Text in German. 20/yr. DEM 580. **Document type:** *Academic/Scholarly.*
Published by: P M I Verlag AG, August-Schanz-Str 8, Frankfurt Am Main 60433, Germany. TEL 49-69-548000-0, FAX 49-69-548000-77, pmiverlag@aol.com.

615.7 AUS ISSN 0156-0433
P S. (Postscript) Text in English. 1979. bi-m. AUD 30; AUD 45 foreign (effective 1999). back issues avail. **Document type:** *Trade.*
Published by: Australian Pharmaceutical Publishing Co. Ltd., 40 Burwood Rd, Hawthorn, VIC 3122, Australia. TEL 61-3-9810-9800, FAX 61-3-9819-1706, appco@hcn.net.au, http://www.aapco.com.au. Circ: 7,000.

615 DEU
P T A DIALOG. (Pharmazeutisch - Technische Assistentin) Text in German. 1987. q. DEM 20. back issues avail. **Document type:** *Academic/Scholarly.*
Published by: (Beiersdorf AG), Industrie-Contact GmbH, Bahrenfelder Marktplatz 7, Hamburg 22761, Germany. TEL 49-40-89966617, FAX 49-40-8902641, pr@ic-gruppe.com, http://www.ic-gruppe.com. Ed. Juergen Klimke.

615 DEU ISSN 0302-167X
CODEN: PTAHAF
P T A HEUTE; Zeitschrift der DAZ fuer die Pharmazeutisch-technische Assistentin. Text in German. 1954. m. EUR 42.60 domestic; EUR 31.20 to students; EUR 57.84 foreign; EUR 5 newsstand/cover (effective 2002). bk.rev. **Document type:** *Journal, Trade.*
Formerly: Apothekerpraktikant und Pharmazeutisch-Technische Assistent
Indexed: Chem.Abstr.
—CISTI, GNLM.
Published by: Deutscher Apotheker Verlag, Postfach 101061, Stuttgart 70009, Germany. TEL 49-711-2582-0, FAX 49-711-2582290, ptaheute@deutscher-apotheker-verlag.de, service@deutscher-apotheker-verlag.de, http://www.deutscher-apotheker-verlag.de. Ed. Reinhild Berger. Adv. contact Klaus Graef TEL 49-711-2582245. Circ: 54,700.

615 DEU ISSN 0722-1029
CODEN: PTAED9
DIE P T A IN DER APOTHEKE; Fachzeitschrift fuer pharmazeutisch-technische Assistenten. Text in German. m. DEM 117; DEM 94.80 to students (effective 2000). adv. **Document type:** *Journal, Trade.*
Former titles: P T A in der Praktischen Pharmazie; P T A in Apotheke und Industrie
Related titles: ♦ Supplement: P T A - Repetitorium. ISSN 0342-8397.
—CASDDS. **CCC.**
Published by: Umschau Zeitschriftenverlag Breidenstein GmbH, Stuttgarter Str 18-24, Frankfurt Am Main 60329, Germany. TEL 49-69-2600-670, FAX 49-69-2600-619. Ed. Julia Pflegel. Adv. contact Barbara Eckert. B&W page DEM 4,900, color page DEM 7,900; trim 176 x 247. Circ: 25,839.

615 DEU ISSN 0342-8397
P T A - REPETITORIUM. Text in German. 1972. m.
Related titles: ♦ Supplement to: Die P T A in der Apotheke. ISSN 0722-1029.
Published by: Umschau Zeitschriftenverlag Breidenstein GmbH, Stuttgarter Str 18-24, Frankfurt Am Main 60329, Germany. TEL 49-69-2600-621, FAX 49-69-2600-609.

615 DEU ISSN 0945-5566
CODEN: PZPREU
P Z PRISMA; Pharmazeutische Zeitung - Materialen zur Weiterbildung. Text in German. 1983. q. EUR 55.48; EUR 27.60 to students (effective 2002). adv. **Document type:** *Journal, Academic/Scholarly.*
Former titles (until 1994): P Z Wissenschaft (0935-5901); (until 1988): Pharmazeutische Zeitung. Scientific Edition (0724-6315)
Indexed: Biol.Abstr. (1990-), Chem.Abstr., Chem.Indus.Notes, Chem.Titles, I.P.A.
—BLDSC (7163.530500), CASDDS, EMDOCS, GNLM, KNAW. **CCC.**
Published by: (Bundesvereinigung Deutscher Apothekerverbaende), Govi Verlag Pharmazeutischer Verlag GmbH, Carl Mannich Str 26, Eschborn 65760, Germany. TEL 49-6196-928262, FAX 49-6196-928259, t.fast@govi.aponet.de. Adv. contact Hans Juergen Renn.

615 618.92 GBR ISSN 1463-0095
CODEN: PPDTF9
PAEDIATRIC AND PERINATAL DRUG THERAPY. Text in English. 1997. a. GBP 48 to individuals; GBP 53 foreign to individuals; GBP 100 to institutions; GBP 110 foreign to institutions (effective 2001 - 2002). adv. bk.rev. back issues avail. *Refereed.* **Document type:** *Academic/Scholarly.* **Description:** Features topical reviews of drug therapy in the fields of paediatrics and neonatology that are of clinical relevance, academic interest and educational value to health professionals.
Indexed: Derwent Biotech.Abstr.
—BLDSC (6333.399708).
Published by: Librapharm Ltd, Gemini House, 162 Craven Rd, Newbury, Berks RG14 5NR, United Kingdom. TEL 44-1635-522651, FAX 44-1635-36294, journals@librapharm.com, http://www.librapharm.com. Ed. Imti Choonara. Pub., R&P P.L. Dr. Clarke. Adv. contact P L Clarke. Circ: 350.

615 618.92 NZL ISSN 1174-5878
▼ **PAEDIATRIC DRUGS.** Text in English. 1999. q. USD 165 to individuals Print or Online ed.; USD 198 to individuals Print and Online combined eds.; USD 650 to institutions Print or Online ed.; USD 780 to institutions Print and Online combined eds. (effective 2001). back issues avail. **Description:** Offers practical advice and reviews on the safe and effective use of drugs in children.
Related titles: Online - full text ed.: (from Ovid Technologies, Inc., EBSCO Publishing, O C L C Online Computer Library Center, Inc., RoweCom Information Quest, ingenta, Swets Blackwell).
Indexed: Ind.Med., Inpharma, Pharm.&Out.News, Reac.
—BLDSC (6333.399732), ADONIS.
Published by: Adis International Limited, Mairangi Bay, Private Bag 65901, Auckland 1010, New Zealand. TEL 64-9-477-0700, FAX 64-9-477-0766, http://www.adis.com. Ed. Lynda Wiseman. **Americas subscr. to:** Adis International Inc., Attn: Subscription Dept, 860 Town Center Dr, Langhorne, PA 19047. TEL 877-872-2347.

615.19 PAK ISSN 1011-601X
CODEN: PJPSEN
PAKISTAN JOURNAL OF PHARMACEUTICAL SCIENCES. Text in English. s-a. PKR 150, USD 25. *Refereed.* **Document type:** *Academic/Scholarly.* **Description:** Publishes short research papers and reviews in pharmaceutical chemistry, pharmaceutics, pharmacognosy, pharmacology, and related studies in toxicology.
Related titles: CD-ROM ed.
Indexed: Chem.Abstr., Chem.Titles, ExtraMED, Food Sci.& Tech.Abstr.
—BLDSC (6341.690000), CASDDS, CISTI.
Address: University of Karachi, Faculty of Pharmacy, Karachi 75270, Pakistan. Ed. Dr. S Sabir Ali.

615 PAK ISSN 0255-7088
CODEN: PJPHEO
PAKISTAN JOURNAL OF PHARMACOLOGY. Text in English. 1983. s-a. USD 50. **Document type:** *Academic/Scholarly.*
Indexed: Chem.Abstr., Chem.Indus.Notes, Chem.Titles.
—CASDDS, CISTI.
Published by: University of Karachi, Department of Pharmacology, Karachi 75270, Pakistan. TEL 479001. Ed. S.I. Ahmad.

615 USA
PALMETTO PHARMACIST∗ **.** Text in English. m. USD 10. adv.
Indexed: I.P.A.
Published by: State Pharmaceutical Editorial Association, 204 W Cook St, Springfield, IL 62704. Ed. Sharon Fennell. Circ: 1,500.

P

615.19 USA
▼ **PART 11 COMPLIANCE REPORT.** Variant title: Part Eleven Compliance Report. Text in English. 2001. bi-w. USD 627 in North America; USD 652 elsewhere (effective Nov. 2001). 6 p./no. back issues avail. **Document type:** *Newsletter.*
Published by: Washington Business Information, Inc., 300 N Washington St, Ste 200, Falls Church, Arlington, VA 22046. TEL 703-538-7600, 703 538 7660, FAX 703-538-7676. Ed. Peter Riebling.

PARTICULATE SCIENCE AND TECHNOLOGY; an international journal. see *ENGINEERING—Chemical Engineering*

615.10272 GBR ISSN 1462-2394
PATENT FAST-ALERT. Text in English. 199?. w. USD 3,700, GBP 2,300 (effective 2002). **Document type:** *Trade.* **Description:** Provides a therapeutic patent monitoring service which includes clues to research trends and represents a vital competitive intelligence tool for research and development groups.
Formerly (until 1998): Investigational Drug Patent Fast-Alert (1357-7026)
Media: Online - full text (from EBSCO Publishing).
Published by: Current Drugs Ltd., 34-42 Cleveland St, Middlesex House, London W1P 6LB, United Kingdom. TEL 44-207-580-8393, FAX 44-207-580-5646, info@current-drugs.com, http://www.current-drugs.com. Ed. Tara Dyson. **Subscr. to:** Current Drugs Ltd., 400 Market St, Ste 700, Philadelphia, PA 19106. TEL 215-721-9700, FAX 215-721-9287.

615.9 USA
PATIENT DRUG FACTS. Text in English. 1989. q. USD 150; USD 172.50 foreign (effective 1999). **Description:** Drug information reference written in laymen's terms to aid health care professionals with the education and counseling of patients and drug therapy management.
Formerly: Professional's Guide to Patient Drug Facts
Related titles: Spanish ed.
Published by: Facts and Comparisons, 111 W. Port Plaza, Ste. 300, St. Louis, MO 63146-3098. TEL 800-223-0554, FAX 314-878-5563.

PEDIATRIC PHARMACOTHERAPY; a monthly review for health care professionals. see *MEDICAL SCIENCES—Pediatrics*

615.1 USA ISSN 0031-4633
PENNSYLVANIA PHARMACIST. Text in English. 1926. bi-m. (6 issues per year). USD 100 to non-members; USD 50 to members (effective 2000); includes Pharmacy News and Review. adv. bk.rev. illus, tr.lit. cum.index. 32 p./no. 3 cols./p. **Document type:** *Journal, Trade.* **Description:** Provides information on issues and concerns of interest to pharmacists.
Indexed: I.P.A.
—BLDSC (6421.748800), Linda Hall.

Published by: Pennsylvania Pharmacists Association, 508 N Third St, Harrisburg, PA 17101-1199. TEL 717-234-6151, FAX 717-236-1618, 717-236-1618, http://www.papharmacists.com. Ed. Carmen A Dicello. Adv. contact Judith A Kleinfelter. B&W page USD 800, color page USD 1,210; trim 11 x 8.5. Circ: 2,800.

615 658 GBR
PHARMA BUSINESS; the international magazine of pharmaceutical business and marketing. Text in English. 1995. 6/yr. USD 235 (effective 2002). **Document type:** *Trade.*
Related titles: Online - full content ed.
Indexed: Bus.& Indus. (Jul.1995-).
—BLDSC (6441.878000).
Published by: Euromoney Publications plc., Nestor House, Playhouse Yard, London EC4V 5EX, United Kingdom. TEL 44-20-7779-8935, FAX 44-20-7779-8541, http://www.euromoney.com. **Dist. in US by:** American Educational Systems, 173 W 81st St, New York, NY 10024. TEL 800-431-1579, aesbooks@aol.com.

615 DEU
PHARMA DATEN. Text in German. a. **Document type:** *Trade.*
Related titles: English ed.
Published by: Bundesverband der Pharmazeutischen Industrie e.V., Karlstr 21, Frankfurt Am Main 60329, Germany. TEL 49-69-2556-1261, FAX 49-69-2556-1603. Ed. Thomas Postina.

615 CHE ISSN 0378-7958
PHARMA-FLASH. Text in French. 1972. 6/yr. CHF 37, EUR 24.02 domestic; CHF 75, EUR 48.70 foreign (effective 2002). **Document type:** *Journal, Consumer.*
—**CCC.**
Published by: Editions Medecine et Hygiene, Case Postale 456, Geneva, 4 1211, Switzerland. TEL 41-22-7029311, FAX 41-22-7029355, abonnements@medhyg.ch, http://www.medhyg.ch.

615 CHE ISSN 0301-1348
CODEN: PHAID5
PHARMA INTERNATIONAL. Text in Multiple languages. 1973. bi-m. CHF 202; CHF 214 foreign (effective 2000). **Document type:** *Trade.*
Formed by the merger of (1968-1973): Pharma International. Deutsche Sprache Ausgabe (0340-2533); (19??-1973): Pharma International. English Edition (0301-1356); (19??-1973): Pharma International. Edition en Francais (0340-2630)
Indexed: Ref.Zh.
—BLDSC (6441.880000), CASDDS, CISTI, GNLM, Infotrieve. **CCC.**
Published by: Verlag Coating Thomas & Co., Bankgasse 8, St. Gallen 9001, Switzerland. TEL 41-71-2223239, FAX 41-71-2228761.

615 JPN ISSN 0285-4937
CODEN: PHAREX
PHARMA JAPAN; Japan drug industry news. Text in English. 1960. w. JPY 180,000. pat, stat. **Description:** Focuses on matters of importance in the Japanese pharmaceutical and medical industries.
Formerly (until 1975): Pharmaceutical Daily News
Related titles: Online - full text ed.: (from Northern Light Technology, Inc., LexisNexis).
Indexed: Bus.& Indus. (Dec.1994-), CBNB (1990-), CEABA, Chem.Abstr., Chem.Titles.
—BLDSC (6441.881000), CASDDS.
Published by: Yakugyo Jiho Co. Ltd., 2-36 Kanda-Jinbo-cho, Chiyoda-ku, Tokyo 101-0051, Japan. TEL 03-265-7751. **Dist. in N. America by:** F-D-C Reports, Inc., 5550 Friendship Blvd, Ste One, Chevy Chase, MD 20815-7278.

615 JPN
PHARMA JAPAN YEARBOOK. Text in English. a. JPY 9,000, USD 88. **Description:** Explains trends in Japanese pharmaceutical and medical fields.
Former titles: Japan Drug Industry Review; (until 1976): Handbook of the Japan Drug Industry
Published by: Yakugyo Jiho Co. Ltd., 2-36 Kanda-Jinbo-cho, Chiyoda-ku, Tokyo 101-0051, Japan. TEL 03-265-7751. **Dist. in N. America by:** F-D-C Reports, Inc., 5550 Friendship Blvd, Ste One, Chevy Chase, MD 20815-7278.

615 DEU ISSN 0948-7182
PHARMA KODEX. Text in German. a. DEM 56 (effective 2000). **Document type:** *Trade.*
Published by: Bundesverband der Pharmazeutischen Industrie e.V., Karlstr 21, Frankfurt Am Main 60329, Germany. TEL 49-69-2556-1261, FAX 49-69-2556-1603.

615 CHE ISSN 1010-5409
CODEN: PHKRFG
PHARMA KRITIK. Text in German. 1979. 20/yr. CHF 98, DEM 98, ATS 800; CHF 49, DEM 49, ATS 400 to students (effective 2000). *Refereed.* **Document type:** *Newsletter, Trade.*
—GNLM.
Published by: Infomed-Verlag, Bergliweg 17, Wil 9500, Switzerland. TEL 41-71-9100866, FAX 41-71-9100877, infomed@infomed.org, http://www.infomed.org/pharma-kritik/. Ed., Pub. Dr. Etzel Gysling. Circ: 5,500.

PHARMA-MARKETING JOURNAL. see *BUSINESS AND ECONOMICS—Marketing And Purchasing*

615 GBR ISSN 1355-8501
PHARMA MARKETLETTER. Text in English. 1974. 50/yr. GBP 525 (effective 2001). adv. index. back issues avail. **Document type:** *Journal, Trade.* **Description:** Aimed at executives in the pharmaceutcial industry, financial analysts and regulatory bodies. Contains worldwide markets, legislation and healthcare environmental matters, company news, start-ups, biotechnology, stock market commentaries, research and development, drug launches and sales progress.
Former titles (until 1994): Marketletter (0951-3175); I M S Pharmaceutical Marketletter (0140-4288); Which incorporates: I M S Monitor Report (0262-6756); Which was formerly: I M S Monitor Report: Europe (0140-4741)
Related titles: E-mail ed.; Online - full text ed.: (from Data-Star, Gale Group, Factiva).
Indexed: ABC, Bus.& Indus. (Oct.1994-), Inpharma, Pharm.&Out.News, Reac.
—BLDSC (6441.882000), Infotrieve. **CCC.**
Published by: Marketletter (Publications) Ltd., 54-55 Wilton Rd, London SW1V 1DE, United Kingdom. TEL 44-20-7828-7272, FAX 44-20-7828-0415, editorial@marketletter.com, http://www.marketletter.com. Ed. Joan Kairis. Pub. Barbara Obstoj. R&P, Adv. contact Robin Cardwell. B&W page GBP 900, color page GBP 1,760; trim 210 x 297. **Subscr. to:** Marketletter (Publications) Ltd, Connaught Housex, 65 Aldwych, PO Box 221, London WC2B 4EJ, United Kingdom.

615 JPN ISSN 0289-5803
CODEN: PMEDEC
PHARMA MEDICA. Text in Japanese. 1983. m. JPY 1,800 per issue (effective 1998).
Indexed: Chem.Abstr., Chem.Indus.Notes, Chem.Titles.
—BLDSC (6441.883000), CASDDS.
Published by: Medikaru Rebyusha/Medical Review Co., Ltd., 7-3 Hirano-Machi 1-chome, Chuo-ku, Osaka-shi 541-0046, Japan. TEL 81-6-223-1556, FAX 81-6-223-1414, medrev@osk2.3web.ne.jp.

615 GBR ISSN 1462-1428
PHARMA PATENT BULLETIN. Text in English. 1998. bi-m. GBP 295 (effective 2001). bk.rev. abstr, pat. back issues avail. *Refereed.* **Document type:** *Bulletin.* **Description:** Covers current comments and interpretation of patents and intellectual property issues in the pharmaceutical industry.
Published by: Marketletter (Publications) Ltd., 54-55 Wilton Rd, London SW1V 1DE, United Kingdom. TEL 44-20-7828-7272, FAX 44-20-7828-0415, editorial@marketletter.com, http://www.marketletter.com. Pub. Barbara Obstoj. Circ: 100 (paid).

344.0416 DEU ISSN 0172-6617
PHARMA RECHT. Text in German. 1979. m. DEM 510 (effective 1999). bk.rev. back issues avail. **Document type:** *Academic/Scholarly.* **Description:** Publishes current acts and court rulings concerning the production, distribution and marketing of pharmaceuticals, cosmetics, and dietary supplements.
—GNLM.
Published by: P M I Verlag AG, August-Schanz-Str 8, Frankfurt Am Main 60433, Germany. TEL 49-69-548000-0, FAX 49-69-548000-77, pmiverlag@aol.com. adv.: B&W page DEM 1,938; trim 280 x 210. Circ: 1,000 (paid).

615 NLD ISSN 0169-6882
PHARMA SELECTA. Text in Dutch, English; Summaries in English. 1985. bi-w. NLG 125, USD 110. adv. back issues avail. *Refereed.* **Document type:** *Newsletter, Trade.* **Description:** Provides pharmacotherapy and drug information for hospital and community pharmacists.
Related titles: Diskette ed.: NLG 200; Online - full text ed.: (from Institute for Scientific Information).
Published by: Stichting Pharma Selecta, Postbus 69, Buitenpost 9285 2W, Netherlands. TEL 31-597-646812, 31-511-542623, FAX 31-597-645174, 31-511-543660, pharma.selecta@pi.net. Circ: 2,800 (controlled).

615.014 DEU ISSN 0931-9700
PHARMA TECHNOLOGIE JOURNAL. Text in German. 1984. irreg. price varies. **Document type:** *Journal, Trade.* **Description:** Deals with special technological aspects of pharmaceutical processing.
—BLDSC (6441.887000).
Published by: (Concept Heidelberg), Editio Cantor Verlag, Postfach 1255, Aulendorf 88322, Germany. TEL 49-7525-940145, FAX 49-7525-940147, info@ecv.de, http://www.ecv.de.

615 AUT
PHARMA TIME; das unabhaengige Apothekerjournal. Text in German. 1984. m. ATS 300. adv. bk.rev. **Document type:** *Trade.*
Published by: Pharma Time Verlag, Klostergasse 16, Vienna, W 1180, Austria. TEL 0222-4703238, FAX 0222-470978430. Ed. Hans Jakesz. Circ: 8,000.

615.1 IND ISSN 0031-6849
CODEN: PHTIDW
PHARMA TIMES. Text in English. 1969. m. INR 6,000, USD 100 (effective 2001). adv. bk.rev. pat. *Refereed.* **Document type:** *Newsletter.*
Related titles: Online - full text ed.
Indexed: I.P.A.
—BLDSC (6441.890000), CASDDS, GNLM.
Published by: Indian Pharmaceutical Association, Kalina Santacruz East, Mumbai, Maharashtra 400 098, India. TEL 91-22-612-2401, FAX 91-22-614-0480, ipacentr@bol.net.in, http://www.indianpharma.org. Ed. K S Desai. adv.: B&W page INR 3,600, color page INR 6,000; trim 220 x 280. Circ: 8,000.

615.328 613.2 DEU ISSN 1434-8942
PHARMA UND FOOD; Hygiene - Produktion - Ausruestung. Text in German. 1998. 5/yr. DEM 100, DEM 105 (effective 2000). **Document type:** *Magazine, Academic/Scholarly.*
Published by: Huethig GmbH, Postfach 102869, Heidelberg 69018, Germany. TEL 49-6221-489-0, FAX 49-6221-489279, hvs_zeitschrift@huethig.de, http://www.huethig.de.

615.19 DEU ISSN 0933-0909
PHARMA UND WIR. Text in German. 1986. bi-m. DEM 13.48, EUR 6.60; DEM 2.15, EUR 1.10 newsstand/cover (effective 2001). **Document type:** *Bulletin, Catalog, Consumer.*
Published by: (Bundesverband der Pharmazeutischen Industrie e.V.), Werkschriften Verlag GmbH, Bachstr 14-16, Heidelberg 69121, Germany. TEL 49-6221-6446-0, FAX 49-6221-644640, info@haefner-verlag.de, http://www.haefner-verlag.de. R&P Dieter Neumann TEL 49-6221-64460. Circ: 5,200 (paid).

615.1 HRV ISSN 0031-6857
CODEN: PHAMBF
PHARMACA; casopis za farmakoterpiju. Text in Croatian; Summaries in English. 1963. q. USD 35 foreign (effective 1999). bk.rev. **Document type:** *Bulletin.*
Indexed: Biol.Abstr., Chem.Abstr., Chem.Titles, Excerp.Med.
—CASDDS, EMDOCS, GNLM, KNAW.
Published by: Udruga Zdravstva Zagreb/Association of Croatian Health Organizations, Savska cesta 41-VII, PO Box 878, Zagreb 10000, Croatia. TEL 385-1-6176100, FAX 385-1-213861, vrhovac@rebro.mef.hr. Ed. Bozidar Vrhovac. Circ: 3,500.

615 340 JPN
PHARMACEUTICAL ADMINISTRATION IN JAPAN. Text in English, Japanese. irreg., latest 10th Ed. JPY 16,800 domestic; USD 180 foreign (effective 2001). **Document type:** *Government.* **Description:** Gives a broad description of the Japanese Government's recent steps in the pharmaceutical administration.
Published by: (Japan. Ministry of Health and Welfare, Pharmaceutical Affairs Bureau), Yakuji Nippo Ltd., 1 Kanda-Izumi-cho, Chiyoda-ku, Tokyo 101-8648, Japan. TEL 81-3-3862-2141, FAX 81-3-3866-8495, shuppan@yakuji.co.jp, http://www.yakuji.co.jp/.

PHARMACEUTICAL & COSMETIC REVIEW; devoted to the manufacture & marketing of medicines, toiletries, soaps, detergents in South Africa. see *BEAUTY CULTURE—Perfumes And Cosmetics*

P

615 340 USA
KF8925.P4
PHARMACEUTICAL AND MEDICAL DEVICE LITIGATION BULLETIN. Text in English. 1998. m. USD 179 (effective 2001). index. back issues avail. *Refereed.* **Document type:** *Newsletter, Catalog.* **Description:** Source of news, updates, and medical and legal background on the Fen-Phen litigation explosion.
Formerly (until Dec. 2000): Fen-Phen Litigation Strategist (1099-9825)
Related titles: Online - full text ed.
Published by: American Lawyer Media, Inc., 345 Park Ave, S, 8th Fl, New York, NY 10010. TEL 212-545-6170, FAX 212-481-8161, http://www.ljx.com, http://www.americanlawyermedia.com. Ed. Julie Braun.

PHARMACEUTICAL & MEDICAL PACKAGING NEWS. see *PACKAGING*

615 USA ISSN 1086-2218
PHARMACEUTICAL APPROVALS MONTHLY. Text in English. 1996. m. USD 430 domestic; USD 480 foreign (effective 2001). adv. back issues avail.; reprints avail. **Document type:** *Trade.* **Description:** Provides an in-depth look at the process of FDA review and approval for drugs in the US.
Related titles: Online - full text ed.: (from Data-Star, The Dialog Corporation, LexisNexis).
Indexed: Inpharma, P.N.I., Pharm.&Out.News, Reac.
—CCC.
Published by: F-D-C Reports, Inc., 5550 Friendship Blvd, Ste One, Chevy Chase, MD 20815-7278. TEL 800-332-2181, FAX 301-664-7238, http://www.fdcreports.com. Ed. Melissa Carlson. R&P Laura Desimio. Adv. contact Michael Keville.

615 NLD ISSN 1388-0209
RS160 CODEN: PHBIFC
PHARMACEUTICAL BIOLOGY. Text in English. 1954; N.S. 1975. 6/yr., latest vol.39, 2001. NLG 830, USD 425 to individuals; NLG 1,502, USD 770 to institutions includes online ed (effective 2001). adv. bk.rev. charts, illus. Supplement avail.; reprint service avail. from SWZ. *Refereed.* **Document type:** *Journal, Academic/Scholarly.* **Description:** Covers all aspects of contemporary pharmacognosy, including the biological evaluation of natural products, and issues relating to the understanding of the efficacy or safety of natural product drugs.
Former titles (until 1998): International Journal of Pharmacognosy (0925-1618); Pharmacognosy; International Journal of Crude Drug Research (0167-7314); Quarterly Journal of Crude Drug Research (0033-5525)
Related titles: Microform ed.: N.S. (from SWZ); Online - full text ed.: N.S. (from EBSCO Publishing, O C L C Online Computer Library Center, Inc., RoweCom Information Quest, Swets Blackwell, Institute for Scientific Information).
Indexed: ASCA, Agri.& Environ.Biotech.Abstr. (coverage dropped), Agricola, Agroforest.Abstr., Aqua.Sci.& Fish.Abstr., BBCI, Bibl.Agri., Biol.Abstr., Chem.Abstr., Chem.Indus.Notes, Chem.Titles, Curr.Adv.Ecol.Sci., Derwent Biotech.Abstr., Environ.Sci.Poll.Mgmt., Excerp.Med., Forest Prod.Abstr., Forest.Abstr., Genet.Abstr. (coverage dropped), Helminthol.Abstr., Hort.Abstr., I.P.A., Ind.Vet., Int.Abstr.Biol.Sci., Med.& Pharm.Biotech.Abstr., Microbiol.Abstr., NPU, Nuc.Acids Abstr., Nutr.Abstr., Ocean.Abstr. (coverage dropped), Ornam.Hort., Plant Gen.Res.Abstr., Protozool.Abstr., Ref.Zh., Rev.Appl.Entomol., Rev.Arom.& Med.Plants, Rev.Med.& Vet.Mycol., Rev.Plant Path., Seed Abstr., Soils & Fert., Triticale Abstr., Trop.Dis.Bull.
—BLDSC (6442.767000), ADONIS, CASDDS, CISTI, EMDOCS, GNLM, IDS, Infotrieve, ingenta, Linda Hall. **CCC.**
Published by: Swets & Zeitlinger BV, PO Box 825, Lisse 2160 SZ, Netherlands. TEL 31-252-435111, FAX 31-252-415888, orders@swets.nl, http://www.swets.nl/sps/journals/pb.html. Ed. John M Pezzuto. R&P J van der Valk. Adv. contact Patrick Kliean. **Dist. in N. America by:** Swets & Zeitlinger, PO Box 582, Downingtown, PA 19335-998. TEL 800-477-9387, FAX 610-524-5366.

PHARMACEUTICAL BIOTECHNOLOGY. see *BIOLOGY—Biotechnology*

330 615 GBR ISSN 0956-0661
CODEN: PBNEEH
PHARMACEUTICAL BUSINESS NEWS; the executive newsletter for the pharmaceutical industry. Text in English. 1983. s-m. GBP 480 in United Kingdom; USD 890 in United States; GBP 525 elsewhere (effective 2001). adv. bk.rev. back issues avail. **Document type:** *Newsletter, Trade.* **Description:** Analyzes and forecasts the pharmaceutical market worldwide.
Incorporates (in 1997): Biotechnology Business News (0965-9595)
Related titles: Microform ed.: (from PQC); Online - full text ed.: (from Northern Light Technology, Inc., Gale Group, LexisNexis).
Indexed: Bus.& Indus. (Jan.1995-), CBNB (1995-), CEABA, Chem.Abstr., Chem.Indus.Notes, Chem.Titles.
—BLDSC (6443.245000), CASDDS.
Published by: Informa Global Pharmaceuticals & Healthcare (Subsidiary of: Financial Times Business.), Mortimer House, 37-41 Mortimer St, London W1N 7RJ, United Kingdom. TEL 44-1206-772113, FAX 44-20-7453-2386, enquiries@informa.com, http://www.informapharma.com/LS0191, http://www.informapharma,com. Ed. Alex Crawford.

615.19 USA ISSN 0091-150X
RS402 CODEN: PCJOAU
PHARMACEUTICAL CHEMISTRY JOURNAL. Text in English. 1967. m. EUR 2,269 to institutions for print or online ed.; EUR 2,722.80 to institutions print & online eds.combined (effective 2002). back issues avail. *Refereed.* **Document type:** *Academic/Scholarly.* **Description:** Reports scientific and technical research on the creation of new pharmaceuticals and on improvements in their manufacture.
Related titles: Microfilm ed.: (from PQC); Online - full text ed.: (from Swets Blackwell, Kluwer Online, RoweCom Information Quest); ♦ Translation of: Khimiko-farmatsevticheskii Zhurnal. ISSN 0023-1134.
Indexed: Biol.Abstr., Chem.Titles, Curr.Adv.Ecol.Sci., INIS Atomind., I.P.A., Int.Abstr.Biol.Sci.
—BLDSC (0416.770000), CISTI, GNLM, Infotrieve, ingenta. **CCC.**
Published by: (Tsentr Khimii i Lekarstvennykh Sredstv RUS), Kluwer Academic - Plenum Publishers (Subsidiary of: Wolters Kluwer N.V.), 233 Spring St, New York, NY 10013-1578. TEL 212-620-8468, FAX 212-463-0742, info@plenum.com; kluwer@wkap.com; services@wkap.nl, http://www.plenum.com. Ed. R G Glushkov.

615 330.9 GBR ISSN 1359-625X
PHARMACEUTICAL COMPANIES ANALYSIS. Text in English. 1995. m. GBP 895; GBP 1,075 cd-rom; GBP 1,075 combined (effective 2000). adv. **Document type:** *Directory.* **Description:** Reports the latest pharmaceutical business, product and company news.
Related titles: CD-ROM ed.: GBP 1,075; Online - full text ed.
Published by: Espicom Business Intelligence, Lincoln House, City Fields Business Park, City Fields Way, Tangmere, Chichester, W Sussex PO20 6FS, United Kingdom. TEL 44-1243-533322, FAX 44-1243-533418, sales_desk@espicom.com, http://www.espicom.com. Ed. Ros Smallman. R&P Nigel Chivers.

615 330 GBR
PHARMACEUTICAL COMPANY PROFILES. Text in English. 1991. m. GBP 10,900 for full set of 110. **Document type:** *Trade.*
Related titles: CD-ROM ed.; Online - full text ed.
Published by: IMSWORLD Publications Ltd., 7 Harewood Ave, London NW1 6JB, United Kingdom. TEL 0171-393-5000, FAX 0171-393-5900.

615.1 USA ISSN 1083-7450
CODEN: PDTEFS
PHARMACEUTICAL DEVELOPMENT AND TECHNOLOGY. Text in English. 1996. q. USD 110 to individuals print & online eds.; USD 495 to institutions print only (effective 2002). adv. bk.rev. back issues avail. *Refereed.* **Document type:** *Academic/Scholarly.* **Description:** Publishes articles exploring the research, design, development, manufacture and evaluation of traditional and novel drug delivery, with an emphasis on practical solutions and applications to theoretical and research-based problems.
Related titles: Online - full text ed.: (from EBSCO Publishing, O C L C Online Computer Library Center, Inc., RoweCom Information Quest, Swets Blackwell, Institute for Scientific Information).
Indexed: Aqua.Sci.& Fish.Abstr., Chem.Abstr., Chem.Titles, Environ.Sci.Poll.Mgmt., I.P.A., Ind.Med. (1996-), Med.& Pharm.Biotech.Abstr., Pollut.Abstr., Ref.Zh., Risk Abstr., Saf.Sci.Abstr.
—BLDSC (6443.625000), CASDDS, CISTI, Infotrieve. **CCC.**
Published by: (American Association of Pharmaceutical Scientists), Marcel Dekker Inc., 270 Madison Ave, New York, NY 10016. TEL 212-696-9000, 800-228-1160, FAX 212-685-4540, http://www.dekker.com/servlet/product/productid/PDT. Ed. Michael Akers. R&P Julia Mulligan. Adv. contact Anne Mullins. Circ: 1,500.

615.19 USA
PHARMACEUTICAL DIGEST** . Text in English. 1991. s-a. adv. **Description:** Contains listings of literature and catalog descriptions.
Published by: Centcom, Ltd., 676 E Swedesford Rd, no 202, Wayne, PA 19087-1612. Ed. Joan Moynihan. Circ: 30,391.

PHARMACEUTICAL ENGINEERING. see *ENGINEERING*

615 USA ISSN 0279-6570
RS1 CODEN: PHEXD2
PHARMACEUTICAL EXECUTIVE; for global business and marketing leaders. Text in English. 1981. m., latest vol.21. USD 64 in United States; USD 84 in Canada; USD 124 elsewhere; USD 7 newsstand/cover (effective 2001). adv. illus. back issues avail.; reprints avail. *Refereed.* **Document type:** *Magazine, Trade.* **Description:** Designed to meet the management and marketing needs of professionals in the pharmaceutical industry. Covers the latest marketing techniques, industry trends, sales, promotional strategies, and the legal and regulatory issues influencing product development and management.
Related titles: Online - full text ed.: (from Gale Group, ProQuest Information & Learning, Northern Light Technology, Inc., H. W. Wilson, Factiva); Supplement: e-Health.
Indexed: ABI Inform. (Sep.1994-), B.P.I. (Jan.1999-), BPIA, Bus.& Indus. (Nov.1996-), Curr.Pack.Abstr., I.P.A., Telegen.
—BLDSC (6443.680000). **CCC.**
Published by: Advanstar Communications Inc., 859 Willamette St, Eugene, OR 97401. TEL 541-343-1200, 800-346-0085 ext. 477, FAX 541-344-3514, tlarranaga@advanstar.com, http://www.pharmexec.com. Ed. Wayne Koberstein. Pub., R&P, Adv. contact Tom Larranaga. B&W page USD 3,835, color page USD 5,275; trim 8 x 10.75. Circ: 16,568 (paid and controlled). **Subscr. to:** 131 W First St, Duluth, MN 55802. TEL 888-527-7008.

615.19 USA ISSN 1531-2135
PHARMACEUTICAL FORMULATION & QUALITY; for product development and quality professionals. Text in English. 1996. bi-m. USD 160 foreign (effective 2001); free for qualified subscribers. adv. **Document type:** *Magazine, Trade.* **Description:** Covers the latest technologies, techniques and regulations affecting product development, formulation, quality assurance and quality control in the pharmaceutical industry.
Formerly: Pharmaceutical & Cosmetic Quality (1092-7522)
Published by: Carpe Diem Communications, Inc., 208 Floral Vale Blvd, Yardley, PA 19067. TEL 215-860-7800, FAX 215-860-7900, staff@carpediemcomm.com, http://www.pharmaquality.com/. Ed. Mark Devlin. adv.: B&W page USD 5,095, color page USD 6,445.

615 668.5 USA
PHARMACEUTICAL FORMULATION & QUALITY BUYERS' GUIDE. Text in English. a. **Document type:** *Directory, Trade.* **Description:** Lists products and services for the pharmaceutical and cosmetics industries.
Related titles: Online - full text ed.
Published by: Carpe Diem Communications, Inc., 208 Floral Vale Blvd, Yardley, PA 19067. TEL 215-860-7800, FAX 215-860-7900, staff@pharmaquality.com, staff@carpediemcomm.com, http://www.pharmaquality.com/buyguide.html.

615.1 GBR ISSN 0079-1393
RS61
PHARMACEUTICAL HISTORIAN. Text in English. 1967. q. GBP 4.60 domestic; GBP 5 foreign.
Indexed: I.P.A.
—BLDSC (6443.700000).
Published by: British Society for the History of Pharmacy, 36 York Pl, Edinburgh, Midlothian EH1 3HU, United Kingdom. TEL 44-131-556-4386. Ed. Dr. J G L Burnby.

338.616151 USA ISSN 1085-4185
PHARMACEUTICAL INDUSTRY GUIDE. Text in English. 1996. a. USD 49.95; USD 59.95 foreign (effective 1998). **Document type:** *Directory, Academic/Scholarly.* **Description:** Contains contact information for more than 400 top U.S. pharmaceutical companies including generics, biotechnology firms that specialize in therapeutics or vaccine development, and contract research organizations.
Published by: Institute for Biotechnology Information, c/o Mark Dibner, Pres., Box 14569, Research Triangle Park, NC 27709-4569. TEL 919-544-5111, FAX 919-544-5401, ibi@mindspring.com, http://www.bitechinfo.com.

P

615.1 GBR ISSN 0031-6873 CODEN: PHJOAV
PHARMACEUTICAL JOURNAL. Text in English. 1841. w. GBP 120 in British Isles; GBP 142 in the European Union; GBP 162 rest of world (effective 2001). adv. bk.rev. charts, tr.lit. index. back issues avail. **Document type:** *Journal, Academic/Scholarly.* **Description:** Provides comprehensive news coverage of all aspects of pharmacy in Great Britain and abroad.
Related titles: Microform ed.; Online - full text ed.: (from Institute for Scientific Information, RoweCom Information Quest); ♦ Supplement: The Pharmacy Assistant. ISSN 1365-0629.
Indexed: AMED, Abstr.Health Care Manage.Stud., Abstr.Hyg., Agri.& Environ.Biotech.Abstr. (coverage dropped), Biol.Abstr., Chem.Abstr., Curr.Adv.Cancer Res., Curr.Adv.Ecol.Sci., Dairy Sci.Abstr., Derwent Biotech.Abstr., Excerp.Med. (1994-), Helminthol.Abstr., High.Educ.Curr.Aware.Bull., I.P.A., Ind.Vet., Inpharma, LISA, Nutr.Abstr., Pharm.&Out.News, Protozool.Abstr., Reac., Rev.Arom.& Med.Plants, Rev.Med.& Vet.Mycol., Rural Recreat.Tour.Abstr., Sugar Ind.Abstr., Trop.Dis.Bull., Vet.Bull.
—BLDSC (6444.000000), CASDDS, CISTI, GNLM, IDS, Infotrieve, ingenta, KNAW, Linda Hall. **CCC.**
Published by: (Euromed Communications Ltd.), Pharmaceutical Press (Subsidiary of: Euromed Communications Ltd.), 1 Lambeth High St, London SE1 7JN, United Kingdom. TEL 44-20-7735-9141, FAX 44-20-7735-5085, http://www.pharmj.com. Ed. Olivia Timbs. Pub., R&P Charles Fry. Adv. contact Jack Richmond. Circ: 47,351.

615 ZWE
PHARMACEUTICAL JOURNAL OF ZIMBABWE. Variant title: Zimbabwe Pharmaceutical Journal. Text in English. bi-m. ZWD 250 to membership. adv. **Document type:** *Academic/Scholarly.*
Published by: Pharmaceutical Society of Zimbabwe, PO Box 1476, Harare, Zimbabwe. TEL 263-14-706967, FAX 263-14-706967. Ed. Rtee Mithal. adv.: B&W page ZWD 1,200. Circ: 350.

615 USA
PHARMACEUTICAL LABORATORY. Text in English. 1998. 9/yr. (plus annual directory). USD 42.95 domestic; USD 45.95 in Canada & Mexico; USD 64.95 elsewhere; USD 8 newsstand/cover domestic; USD 10 newsstand/cover foreign (effective 2001). adv. **Document type:** *Trade.* **Description:** For scientists, research and development personnel, and quality control and quality assurance staff at pharmaceutical manufacturers.
Published by: Cahners Business Information, New Product Information Unit (Subsidiary of: Reed Elsevier plc), 301 Gibraltar Dr, P O Box 650, Morris Plains, NJ 07950-0650. TEL 973-292-5100 ext.381, FAX 973-539-3476, wcurtis@cahners.com, http://www.pharmlab.com. Ed. Pamela Holland-Moritz TEL 973-292-5100 x259. Pub. Timothy J Canny. Circ: 22,000 (controlled).

615 USA
PHARMACEUTICAL: LATIN AMERICAN INDUSTRIAL REPORT★. (Avail. for each of 22 Latin American countries) Text in English. 1985. a. USD 435; per country report.
Published by: Aquino Productions, P O Box 15760, Stamford, CT 06901-0760. Ed. Andres C Aquino.

PHARMACEUTICAL LIBRARY BULLETIN/YAKUGAKU TOSHOKAN. see *LIBRARY AND INFORMATION SCIENCES*

PHARMACEUTICAL LITIGATION REPORTER; the national journal of record of pharmaceutical litigation. see *LAW—Civil Law*

PHARMACEUTICAL MANUFACTURERS OF JAPAN. see *BUSINESS AND ECONOMICS—Trade And Industrial Directories*

615 688.8 GBR ISSN 1463-1245
PHARMACEUTICAL MANUFACTURING & PACKING SOURCER. Text in English. 1998. q. GBP 62; GBP 70 foreign (effective 2000). adv. bk.rev. back issues avail. *Refereed.* **Document type:** *Trade.* **Description:** Targeted at senior decision makers in European pharmaceutical companies and their contract manufacturing and packaging partners. PMPS covers all aspects of pharmaceutical manufacturing from initial formulation development, drug delivery systems, pilot & bulk production through to packaging.
Related titles: E-mail ed.
Published by: (Technomark Consulting Services), Ballantyne Ross Ltd., 16 Hampden Gurney Rd, London W1H 5AL, United Kingdom. TEL 44-1717-245444, FAX 44-1717-242632, pmps@balross.com, http://www.ballentyneross.com. Ed. Dr. Patricia Lobo. Pub. Mike Goodwin. R&P Louise Mouzouris. adv.: page GBP 2,750. Circ: 500 (paid); 5,500 (controlled).

615 USA ISSN 0149-0885
HD9666.3
PHARMACEUTICAL MARKETERS DIRECTORY. Text in English. 1977. a. USD 175 (effective 1998). adv. **Document type:** *Directory.* **Description:** Covers the entire healthcare field including names, titles, addresses, phone, fax, e-mail and Internet addresses for over 1,500 pharmaceutical and healthcare manufacturers, 300 advertising agencies, over 800 healthcare journals, as well as alternative media. Includes suppliers to the health care industry.
Incorporates: Medical Products Marketers Directory
Published by: C P S Communications, Inc., Directories Division, 7200 W Camino Real, Ste 215, PO Box 3011, Boca Raton, FL 33433. TEL 561-368-9301, FAX 561-368-7870, pmd@cpsnet.com. Pub. Beverly Reynolds. Adv. contact Cathy Tracy. Circ: 2,500 (paid).

615 GBR ISSN 0969-3963
PHARMACEUTICAL MARKETING. Text in English. 1989. m. GBP 60 domestic; GBP 120 foreign (effective 2000). adv. **Document type:** *Trade.*
Related titles: ♦ Supplement: Pharmaceutical Marketing. Practical Guide Series. ISSN 0969-3971.
—BLDSC (6444.038000).
Published by: Pharmaceutical Marketing Limited, Vincent House, Vincent Ln, Dorking, Surrey RH4 3JD, United Kingdom. TEL 44-1306-740777, FAX 44-1306-741069, info@pharmark.co.uk. Ed. Andy Rice. Pub. Mark Savage. R&P Keith Shilson. Adv. contact Zoe Almeida. Circ: 7,800.

615 GBR ISSN 0969-3971
PHARMACEUTICAL MARKETING. PRACTICAL GUIDE SERIES. Text in English. 1992.
Related titles: ♦ Supplement to: Pharmaceutical Marketing. ISSN 0969-3963.
—BLDSC (6444.038100).
Published by: Pharmaceutical Marketing Limited, Vincent House, Vincent Ln, Dorking, Surrey RH4 3JD, United Kingdom. TEL 44-1306-740777, FAX 44-1306-741069. Ed. Andy Rice.

PHARMACEUTICAL MEDICINE (WORTHING); symposium proceedings. see *MEDICAL SCIENCES*

615.1 CHE ISSN 1071-894X CODEN: PHNEEP
PHARMACEUTICAL NEWS. Text in English. 6/yr. EUR 289 to institutions; EUR 449 to corporations; USD 47 to individuals (effective 2001). back issues avail. **Document type:** *Journal, Academic/Scholarly.*
—BLDSC (6444.063000), Infotrieve. **CCC.**
Published by: Gordon and Breach - Harwood Academic (Subsidiary of: Taylor & Francis Group), PO Box 531, Lausanne 1000, Switzerland. TEL 41-21-6411280, FAX 41-21-6411281, info@gbhap.com, http://www.gbhap.com/magazines/pharmanews. Ed. David J Triggle. **Subscr. addr. in US:** International Publishers Direct, PO Box 32160, Newark, NJ 07102. FAX 215-750-6343.

615.1 USA
PHARMACEUTICAL NEWS DAILY. Text in English. d. USD 239 domestic e-mail; USD 320 domestic fax; USD 360 in Canada; USD 405 in Western Europe; USD 575 in Eastern Europe; USD 734 in the Middle East; USD 750 in South & Central America; USD 790 in Asia; USD 793 in Africa (effective 2001). back issues avail. **Document type:** *Newsletter.* **Description:** Includes summaries of 8 to 12 business and product development stories.
Media: E-mail. **Related titles:** Fax ed.
Published by: C T B International Publishing Inc., PO Box 218, Maplewood, NJ 07040-0218. TEL 973-379-7749, FAX 973-379-1158, info@ctbintl.com, http://www.ctbintl.com.

615.19 USA ISSN 1049-9156 CODEN: PLPREY
PHARMACEUTICAL PROCESSING. Text in English. 1984. m. (plus buyers' guide). USD 69.95 domestic; USD 74.25 in Canada; USD 69.75 in Mexico; USD 94 elsewhere; USD 10 newsstand/cover domestic; USD 20 newsstand/cover foreign (effective 2001). adv. tr.lit. **Document type:** *Trade.* **Description:** Focuses on the processors and packagers of pharmaceuticals, biologicals, cosmetics and toiletry products.
Formerly: Pharmaceutical and Cosmetic Equipment (0895-2795)
Related titles: Online - full text ed.: (from Gale Group).
—**CCC.**
Published by: Cahners Business Information, New Product Information Unit (Subsidiary of: Reed Elsevier plc), 301 Gibraltar Dr, P O Box 650, Morris Plains, NJ 07950-0650. TEL 973-292-5100 x220, FAX 973-539-3476, bjramsey@cahners.com, http://www.pharmpro.com. Ed. Michael Auerbach TEL 973-292-5100 X273. Pub. Bud Ramsey. Circ: 31,000.

615 USA ISSN 0161-8415
PHARMACEUTICAL REPRESENTATIVE. Text in English. 1971. m. USD 37.95 domestic; USD 44.95 in Canada; USD 58.95 elsewhere; USD 4.95 newsstand/cover (effective 2001). bk.rev. abstr, charts, illus, stat, tr.lit. back issues avail. **Document type:** *Trade.* **Description:** Features new products, industry and research news, and market trends.
Formerly: Pharmaceutical Salesman (0048-3621)
Related titles: Microform ed.: (from PQC); Online - full text ed.: (from ProQuest Information & Learning).
—**CCC.**
Published by: McKnight Medical Communications (Subsidiary of: Medical Economics Publishing Co., Inc.), Two Northfield Plaza, Ste. 300, Northfield, IL 60093. TEL 847-441-3700, FAX 847-441-3701, pr@medec.com, www//medec.com/pr/. Ed. George Hardecky. Pub. Grett Havroth. Adv. contact Ronald Kamka. Circ: 47,000 (paid).

615.19 USA ISSN 0724-8741 CODEN: PHREEB
PHARMACEUTICAL RESEARCH. Text in English. 1983. m. NLG 2,178, EUR 988.50 to institutions for print or online ed.; NLG 2,613.60, EUR 1,186.20 to institutions print & online eds.combined (effective 2001). adv. bk.rev. back issues avail. *Refereed.* **Document type:** *Academic/Scholarly.* **Description:** Publishes innovative research, reports, and reviews of technological advances in the pharmaceutical and biomedical sciences.
Related titles: Microfilm ed.: (from PQC); Online - full content ed.: (from EBSCO Publishing, Swets Blackwell).
Indexed: ASCA, Chem.Abstr., Chem.Cit.Ind., Chem.Titles, Curr.Adv.Ecol.Sci., Curr.Cont., Excerp.Med., INIS Atomind., I.P.A., Ind.Med. (1984-), Ind.Sci.Rev., Inpharma, Mass Spectr.Bull., Mat.Sci.Cit.Ind. (coverage dropped), Neurosci.Cit.Ind., Pharm.&Out.News, Protozool.Abstr., Reac., Rev.Appl.Entomol., Rev.Arom.& Med.Plants, Rev.Med.& Vet.Mycol., Sci.Cit.Ind., Sugar Ind.Abstr.
—BLDSC (6444.080000), ADONIS, CASDDS, CatchWord, CISTI, EMDOCS, GNLM, IDS, Infotrieve, ingenta, KNAW, Linda Hall. **CCC.**
Published by: (University of Southern California, Department of Pharmaceutical Sciences, American Association of Pharmaceutical Scientists), Kluwer Academic - Plenum Publishers (Subsidiary of: Wolters Kluwer N.V.), 233 Spring St, New York, NY 10013-1578. TEL 212-620-8000, 800-221-9369, FAX 212-463-0742, TELEX 23-421139, info@plenum.com; kluwer@wkap.com; services@wkap.nl; vincent1@hsc.usc.edu, http://www.plenum.com; http://www.aaps.org. Ed. Vincent H L Lee.

615 KOR ISSN 0513-4242 CODEN: YAHOA3
PHARMACEUTICAL SOCIETY OF KOREA. JOURNAL/YAKHAK HOEJI. Text in Korean; Summaries in English. 1948. bi-m. USD 120 (effective 2000). adv. bk.rev. back issues avail. *Refereed.* **Document type:** *Academic/Scholarly.*
Indexed: Biol.Abstr., Chem.Abstr., Chem.Indus.Notes, Excerp.Med. (until 1993), INIS Atomind., I.P.A., Ind.Med. (coverage dropped).
—BLDSC (4840.050000), GNLM.
Published by: Pharmaceutical Society of Korea, 1489-3 Suhcho 3 dong, Suhcho-gu, Seoul 137073, Korea, S.. TEL 82-2-584-3257, FAX 82-2-521-1781, pskor@thrunet.com, pskor@chollian.net, http://www.psk.or.kr, http://www.apr.psk.or.kr, http://www.pharmbiomed.org. Ed. Uhtaek Oh. Pub. Chang Jong Kim. R&P, Adv. contact Young Choong Kim. Circ: 1,500.

615 330 USA ISSN 1090-4409
PHARMACEUTICAL STRATEGIC ALLIANCES; the drug and biotech alliances reference guide. Short title: P S A. Text in English. a. USD 2,100 domestic; USD 2,175 foreign (effective 2002). **Description:** Contains information on over 700 alliances and the companies that signed them. Tracks alliances signed by both public and private pharmaceutical and biotech companies worldwide.
Published by: Windhover Information, Inc., 10 Hoyt St, Norwalk, CT 06851 . TEL 203-838 4401, FAX 203-838 3214, custserv@windhoverinfo.com, http://www.windhoverinfo.com.

615 USA ISSN 0147-8087
RS1 CODEN: PTECDN
PHARMACEUTICAL TECHNOLOGY. Text in English. 1977. m., latest vol.25. USD 64 in United States; USD 84 in Canada; USD 124 elsewhere; USD 7 newsstand/cover (effective 2001). adv. abstr, charts, illus, pat, stat, tr.lit. cum.index. back issues avail. *Refereed.* **Document type:** *Magazine, Trade.* **Description:** Offers practical hands-on information about the manufacture of pharmaceutical products, focusing on applied technology.
Related titles: Online - full text ed.: (from Northern Light Technology, Inc., ProQuest Information & Learning, Gale Group).
Indexed: ABI Inform., Agri.& Environ.Biotech.Abstr. (coverage dropped), Bioeng.Abstr., Biotech.& Bioeng.Abstr., Bus.& Indus. (Nov.1996-), Chem.Abstr., Chem.Indus.Notes, Chem.Titles, Curr.Pack.Abstr., Derwent Biotech.Abstr., Eng.Ind., Excerp.Med., I.P.A., Telegen.
—BLDSC (6444.130000), CASDDS, CISTI, Ei, EMDOCS, GNLM, Infotrieve, ingenta, KNAW, Linda Hall. **CCC.**
Published by: Advanstar Communications Inc., 859 Willamette St, Eugene, OR 97401. TEL 541-343-1200, 800-346-0085 ext. 477, sschuber@advanstar.com, fulfill@superfill.com, http://www.pharma-connections.com/. Ed., R&P Stefan Schuber. Pub., Adv. contact Ralph Vitaro TEL 732-225-9500. Circ: 35,000.

615.1 HKG
PHARMACEUTICAL TECHNOLOGY ASIA. Text in English. s-a. GBP 30 in Asia & the Pacific; GBP 45 elsewhere; GBP 20 newsstand/cover (effective 2001); Free to qualified readers in Asia Pacific. **Document type:** *Academic/Scholarly.* **Description:** Contains peer-reviewed technical articles concerned with the practical aspects and regulatory issues involved in the manufacture and processing of pharmaceuticals and biopharmaceuticals.
Published by: Advanstar Asia Limited (Subsidiary of: Advanstar Communications Inc.), 2501-2, 25/F, Pacific Plaza, 401 Des Voeux Rd W, Hong Kong, Hong Kong. TEL 852-2589-1339, FAX 852-2559-2015, customer_service@telecomasia.net, http://www.telecomasia.net/, http://www.pharmaportal.com/.

615 GBR
CODEN: PTEUFB
PHARMACEUTICAL TECHNOLOGY EUROPE. Text in English. 1978; N.S. 1989. m., latest vol.13. GBP 85 in Europe; GBP 120 elsewhere; free to qualified personnel; GBP 20 newsstand/cover (effective 2001). adv. abstr, bibl, charts, illus, stat, tr.lit. reprints avail. *Refereed.* **Document type:** *Magazine, Trade.* **Description:** Targets the pharmaceutical industry in Europe; contains peer-reviewed technical articles on the manufacturing of pharmaceuticals and biopharmaceuticals.
Formerly (until 1994): Pharmaceutical Technology International (0164-6826)
Indexed: Bus.& Indus. (May 1997-), CEABA, Excerp.Med., I.P.A.
—BLDSC (6444.155000), CASDDS, GNLM. **CCC.**
Published by: Advanstar Communications, Lamb House, Church St, London CH1 4RN, United Kingdom. TEL 44-208-987-0900, FAX 44-208-987-0901, advanstar@advanstar.com, krobinson@advanstar.com, http://www.pharma-connections.com, http://www.pharmaportal.com. Ed. Kevin Robinson. Pub. Mike Clancy. Adv. contact Justin Longdon. B&W page GBP 2,745, color page GBP 3,655; trim 203 x 273. Circ: 18,086 (paid and controlled).

615 GBR ISSN 0963-6366
PHARMACEUTICAL TIMES. Text in English. 1988. 11/yr. GBP 60; GBP 94 foreign. adv. bk.rev. **Document type:** *Trade.*
Indexed: CBNB (1989-).
—BLDSC (6444.199000). **CCC.**
Address: 75 Sheen Ln, E Sheen, London SW14 8AD, United Kingdom. TEL 0181-878-8566, FAX 0181-876-8834. Ed., Pub. Geoff Frew. Adv. contact Annons Huset. Circ: 7,000.

PHARMACEUTICAL VENTURES. see *BUSINESS AND ECONOMICS—Investments*

615 GBR
PHARMACEUTICALS: A WORLD SURVEY. Text in English. irreg., latest 1997. GBP 3,950, USD 7,900. **Document type:** *Trade.* **Description:** Looks at the latest trends and developments in the pharmaceuticals industry and market worldwide.
Published by: Euromonitor, 60-61 Britton St, London EC1M 5UX, United Kingdom. TEL 44-20-7251-8024, info@euromonitor.com, http://www.euromonitor.com.

615.1029 GBR
PHARMACEUTICALS (YEAR): INTERNATIONAL YEARBOOK. Text in English. 1996. a. GBP 185, USD 296 (effective 1998). adv. **Document type:** *Directory.* **Description:** Contains detailed information on the top pharmaceutical companies worldwide. Includes company performance information, as well as an overview of the industry.
Published by: Financial Times Healthcare, Maple House, 149 Tottenham Ct Rd, London W1P 9LL, United Kingdom. TEL 44-207-896-2066, FAX 44-20-7896-2213, lizg@pearson-pro.com, http://www.fthealthcare.com. Ed. Olwen Glynn Owen. Adv. contact Liz Godden.

615.1 JPN ISSN 0016-5980
CODEN: YAKUD5
PHARMACEUTICALS MONTHLY/GEKKAN YAKUJI. Text in Japanese. 1959. m. JPY 1,200. adv. bk.rev. abstr. index. **Description:** Developments in medical treatment.
Related titles: Online - full text ed.
Indexed: Chem.Abstr., Chem.Indus.Notes, Chem.Titles, I.P.A.
—CASDDS.
Published by: (Pharmaceutical Research Association), Yakugyo Jiho Co. Ltd., 2-36 Kanda-Jinbo-cho, Chiyoda-ku, Tokyo 101-0051, Japan. Ed. Shozo Takeda. Circ: 14,400. **Subscr. to:** F-D-C Reports, Inc., 5550 Friendship Blvd, Ste One, Chevy Chase, MD 20815-7278.

615.1 NLD ISSN 1389-2827
▼ **PHARMACEUTICALS POLICY AND LAW.** Text in English. 1999. bi-m. (in 6 vols., 1 no./vol.). EUR 154, USD 137 to individuals (effective 2002). adv. back issues avail. *Refereed.* **Document type:** *Journal, Academic/Scholarly.* **Description:** Studies and evaluates the legal status of medicinal products in the EU, along with implications for markets in the US, Japan, and developing nations.
Related titles: Online - full text ed.: (from RoweCom Information Quest).
Published by: I O S Press, Nieuwe Hemweg 6B, Amsterdam 1013 BG, Netherlands. TEL 31-20-688-3355, FAX 31-20-620-3419, market@iospress.nl, http://www.iospress.nl. Ed. Jose Luis Valverde TEL 34-958-242326. R&P C Koolbergen TEL 31-20-638-2189. Adv. contact M Janmaat. **Subscr. to:** I O S Press, Inc, 5795-G Burke Centre Pkwy, Burke, VA 22015. TEL 703-323-5554, FAX 703-323-3668, iosbooks@iospress.com; Kinokuniya Company Ltd, Shinjuku 3-chome, Shinjuku-ku, Tokyo 160-0022, Japan. FAX 81-3-3439-1094, journal@kinokuniya.co.jp, http://www.kinokuniya.co.jp; Globe Publication Pvt. Ltd., C-62 Inderpuri, New Delhi 100 012, India. TEL 91-11-579-3211, 91-11-579-3212, FAX 91-11-579-8876, custserve@globepub.com, http://www.globepub.com.

615.19 BEL
PHARMACEUTISCH TIJDSCHRIFT. Text in Dutch. m. adv.
Address: 217 Av d'Huart, Kraainem 1950, Belgium. Circ: 3,200.

615.1 NLD ISSN 0031-6911
RS1.P53 CODEN: PHWEAW
PHARMACEUTISCH WEEKBLAD. Text in Dutch. 1864. w. NLG 270 (effective 2000). adv. bk.rev. abstr, charts, illus, mkt. index. *Refereed.* **Document type:** *Journal, Academic/Scholarly.* **Description:** Practice oriented journal aimed at improving the scientific and professional practice by community, hospital, industrial and other pharmacists.
Indexed: Agri.& Environ.Biotech.Abstr. (coverage dropped), Anal.Abstr., Biol.Abstr., Chem.Abstr., Chem.Titles, Crop Physiol.Abstr., Curr.Adv.Ecol.Sci., Derwent Biotech.Abstr., Excerp.Med., Forest Prod.Abstr., Hort.Abstr., INIS Atomind., I.P.A., Ind.Med. (coverage dropped), Key to Econ.Sci., Plant Grow.Reg.Abstr., Ref.Zh.
—BLDSC (6446.000000), CASDDS, CISTI, GNLM, KNAW, Linda Hall.
Published by: Koninklijke Nederlandse Maatschappij ter Bevordering der Pharmacie/Royal Netherlands Pharmaceutical Society, Alexanderstraat 11, The Hague 2514 JL, Netherlands. TEL 31-70-362-4111, FAX 31-70-346-4926, weekblad@knmp.nl, http://www.knmp.nl. Ed. Dr. F J Venema. Adv. contact Buro Weijer. Circ: 6,000 (paid); 7,000 (controlled).

615 ZAF
PHARMACIAE. Text in Afrikaans, English. 1985. q. illus. **Document type:** *Newsletter.*
Formerly (until 1993): South African Pharmacy Council. Report
Indexed: I.P.A.
Published by: Suid-Afrikaanse Aptekersraad/South African Pharmacy Council, Posbus 40040, Arcadia, Pretoria 0007, South Africa. TEL 27-12-211477, FAX 27-12-3261496, sapharmc@alpha.terranet.co.za. Ed. J S Du Toit. R&P Riana Steyn. Circ: 11,000.

615.1 FRA ISSN 0031-6938
PHARMACIEN DE FRANCE; organe d'informations scientifiques et professionnelles. Text in French. 1925. 20/yr. FRF 60.
Related titles: Online - full text ed.
Indexed: Biol.Abstr., Chem.Abstr., I.P.A.
Published by: Federation des Syndicats Pharmaceutiques de France, 13 rue Ballu, Paris 75009, France. TEL 42-81-15-96. Ed. Paul Duchein. Circ: 19,870.

615.8 658 FRA ISSN 0768-9179
PHARMACIEN HOSPITALIER. Text in French. 1966. q. FRF 285. adv.
Indexed: I.P.A.
—BLDSC (6446.155000).
Published by: Syndicat des Pharmaciens Gerants, 31 rue du Terrage, Paris 75010, France. TEL 42-06-23-25, FAX 42-09-09-10. Circ: 1,600.

615.1 FRA ISSN 0031-6954
PHARMACIEN RURAL* . Text in French. 1953. 5/yr. adv. bk.rev., rec.rev. charts, illus.
Related titles: Online - full text ed.: 1953.
Indexed: Chem.Abstr., I.P.A.
—CISTI.
Published by: Association de Pharmacie Rural, 24 rue de Vintimille, Paris 75009, France. TEL 48-74-64-26, FAX 45-26-13-37. Ed. Jean Calvet. Circ: 6,500.

615 658.8 GBR
PHARMACIES AND DRUGSTORES: A WORLD SURVEY. Text in English. irreg. GBP 3,950. **Document type:** *Trade.* **Description:** Analyzes the market for drugstores and pharmacies for France, Germany, Italy, Spain, the U.K., the U.S., and Japan.
Formerly: Pharmacies and Drugstores: The International Market
Related titles: Online - full text ed.: (from Data-Star, The Dialog Corporation).
Published by: Euromonitor, 60-61 Britton St, London EC1M 5UX, United Kingdom. TEL 44-20-7251-8024, info@euromonitor.com, http://www.euromonitor.com.

615.1 NLD
THE PHARMACIST. Text in Dutch. 1996. 4/yr. adv. **Document type:** *Trade.* **Description:** Covers continuing education, pharmacy business and management issues.
Published by: Mediselect B.V., Postbus 63, Leusden 3830 AB, Netherlands. TEL 31-33-4229900, FAX 31-33-4229922, info@mediselect.nl. Ed. M Fahey. Circ: (controlled).

615.1 CAN
PHARMACIST NEWS. Text in English. 14/yr. CND 38. adv. illus. **Document type:** *Newspaper, Trade.* **Description:** News about retail pharmacy and hospital and clinic-based pharmacists.
Formerly (until 1993): Drug Merchandising (0012-6586)
Related titles: Microfiche ed.: (from MML); Microform ed.: (from PQC,MML); Online - full text ed.; ♦ French ed.: L' Actualite Pharmaceutique. ISSN 1195-2857.
Indexed: Can.B.P.I., I.P.A.
Published by: Healthcare and Financial Publishing (Subsidiary of: Rogers Media Publishing Ltd), 777 Bay Street, 5th Fl, Toronto, ON M5W 1A7, Canada. TEL 416-596-5950. Ed. Polly Thompson. Circ: 16,600.

615 USA ISSN 0883-0371
PHARMACIST'S LETTER. Text in English. 1985. m. USD 85. index. back issues avail. *Refereed.* **Document type:** *Newsletter.* **Description:** Advises pharmacists on current drug therapy, including drug interactions, proper drug use, trends in therapy, new research findings, and new drugs.
Published by: Therapeutic Research Center, 2453 Grand Canal Blvd, Ste A, Box 8190, Stockton, CA 95208. TEL 209-472-2240, FAX 209-472-2249. R&P Jeff M Jellin.

615.1 NLD ISSN 0165-7208
CODEN: PHLIDQ
PHARMACOCHEMISTRY LIBRARY. Text in English. 1977. irreg., latest vol.30, 1998. price varies. back issues avail. *Refereed.* **Document type:** *Monographic series, Academic/Scholarly.* **Description:** Examines developments in the field of quantitative structure-activity relationships (QSARs).
Indexed: Chem.Abstr., Chem.Titles, Mass Spectr.Bull.
—BLDSC (6446.245000), CASDDS, CISTI, Infotrieve, KNAW. **CCC.**

P

Published by: Elsevier Science BV, PO Box 211, Amsterdam 1000 AE, Netherlands. TEL 31-20-485-3757, 31-20-485-3911, FAX 31-20-485-3432, 31-20-485-3598, nlinfo-f@elsevier.nl, http://www.elsevier.nl. **Subscr. in Australasia and the Far East to:** Elsevier Science (Singapore) Pte Ltd, No.1 Temasek Ave, 17-01 Millenia Tower, Singapore 039192, Singapore. TEL 65-434-3727, FAX 65-337-2230, asiainfo@elsevier.com.sg; **Subscr. in Japan to:** Elsevier Science Inc - Japan Regional Office, 9-15 Higashi-Azabu 1-chome, Minato-ku, Tokyo 106-0044, Japan. TEL 81-3-5561-5033, FAX 81-3-5561-5047, info@elsevier.co.jp; **Subscr. in the Americas to:** Elsevier Science, PO Box 945, New York, NY 10159-0945. TEL 212-633-3730, 888-437-4636, FAX 212-633-3680, usinfo-f@elsevier.com, http://www.elsevier.com

615 338 NZL ISSN 1170-7690
CODEN: PARMEK

PHARMACOECONOMICS. Text in English. 1992. m. USD 165 to individuals Print or Online ed.; USD 198 to individuals Print and Online combined eds.; USD 1,095 to institutions Print or Online ed.; USD 1,314 to institutions Print and Online combined eds. (effective 2001). back issues avail. *Refereed.* **Document type:** *Academic/Scholarly.* **Description:** Promotes the development and study of health economics as applied to rational drug therapy.

Related titles: Online - full text ed.: (from Ovid Technologies, Inc., EBSCO Publishing, O C L C Online Computer Library Center, Inc., RoweCom Information Quest, ingenta, Swets Blackwell, Institute for Scientific Information).

Indexed: ASCA, Chem.Abstr., Chem.Titles, Curr.Cont., Excerp.Med. (1995-), I.P.A., Inpharma, J.of Econ.Lit., Pharm.&Out.News, Reac., Rev.Med.& Vet.Mycol., Rural Devel.Abstr., SSCI (coverage dropped), Sci.Cit.Ind.

—BLDSC (6446.246500), ADONIS, CASDDS, CISTI, GNLM, IDS, Infotrieve, KNAW. **CCC.**

Published by: Adis International Limited, Mairangi Bay, Private Bag 65901, Auckland 1010, New Zealand. TEL 64-9-477-0700, FAX 64-9-477-0766, pecjournal@adis.co.nz, http://www.adis.com. Ed. Michelle Wilde. Pub. Paul Chrisp. R&P Will Charles. Circ: 1,200. **Subscr. in the Americas to:** Adis International Inc., Attn: Subscription Dept, 860 Town Center Dr, Langhorne, PA 19047. TEL 877-872-2347.

615 GBR ISSN 1053-8569
CODEN: PDSAEA

PHARMACOEPIDEMIOLOGY AND DRUG SAFETY. Text in English. 1992. 9/yr. USD 850 in United States; USD 850 in Canada & Mexico; USD 850 elsewhere; USD 893 combined subscription in United States for print and online eds.; USD 893 combined subscription in Canada & Mexico for print and online eds.; USD 893 combined subscription elsewhere for print and online eds. (effective 2002). adv. back issues avail.; reprint service avail. from SWZ. *Refereed.* **Document type:** *Academic/Scholarly.* **Description:** Provides an international forum for the communication and evaluation of data, methods and opinion in the emerging discipline of pharmacoepidemiology.

Incorporates (1986-1995): Post Marketing Surveillance (0269-2333)

Related titles: Microform ed.: (from PQC); Online - full text ed.: ISSN 1099-1557. 1997. USD 850 in United States; USD 850 in Canada & Mexico; USD 850 elsewhere (effective 2002) (from EBSCO Publishing, Wiley InterScience, Institute for Scientific Information).

Indexed: Chem.Abstr., Chem.Indus.Notes, Chem.Titles, Curr.Cont., Environ.Sci.Poll.Mgmt., Excerp.Med. (1992-), I.P.A., Inpharma, Int.Abstr.Biol.Sci., Pharm.&Out.News, Pollut.Abstr., Reac., Risk Abstr., Saf.Sci.Abstr., Sci.Cit.Ind., Stat.Theor.Meth.Abstr. (1996), Tox.Abstr.

—BLDSC (6446.248000), CASDDS, CISTI, EMDOCS, GNLM, IDS, Infotrieve, KNAW. **CCC.**

Published by: Wiley Europe Ltd., Baffins Ln, Chichester, W Sussex PO19 1UD, United Kingdom. TEL 44-1243-779777, FAX 44-1243-775878, customer@wiley.co.uk, http://www.wiley.co.uk. adv.: B&W page GBP 650, color page GBP 1,550; trim 200 x 260. Circ: 850. **Subscr. in the Americas to:** John Wiley & Sons, Inc., Journals, 605 Third Ave, New York, NY 10158. TEL 212-850-6021, 212-850-6645, subinfo@jwiley.com.

PHARMACOGENETICS. see *BIOLOGY—Genetics*

615 GBR ISSN 1462-2416

▼ **PHARMACOGENOMICS.** Text in English. 2000. q. GBP 595, USD 1,010 (effective 2002). abstr. back issues avail. *Refereed.* **Document type:** *Journal, Academic/Scholarly.* **Description:** Addresses major initiatives in genomics which are impacting on drug discovery and creating opportunities in molecular diagnostics.

Related titles: Online - full content ed.

—BLDSC (6446.249500).

Published by: Ashley Publications Ltd., Unitec House 3rd Fl, 2 Albert Place, Finchley Central, London N3 1QB, United Kingdom. TEL 44-20-8343-3883, FAX 44-20-8343-2313, jdrake@ashley-pub.com, http://www.ashley-pub.com. Ed. Henry Scowcroft. Pub. James Drake.

615 580 GBR

PHARMACOGNOSY, PHYTOCHEMISTRY, MEDICINAL PLANTS. Text in English. irreg. GBP 125, USD 197, EUR 200 per issue (effective 2001). stat, illus. **Description:** Contains more than 1300 literature references & the most recent statistics. Four dozen botanical families are classified alphabetically with over 350 plant species including plant monographs and numerous illustrations.

Published by: Intercept Ltd, PO Box 716, Andover, Hants SP10 1YG, United Kingdom. TEL 44-1264-334748, FAX 44-1264-334058, intercept@andover.co.uk, http://www.intercept.co.uk.

615.1 GBR ISSN 1043-6618
RS122 CODEN: PHMREP

PHARMACOLOGICAL RESEARCH. Text in English. 1969. m. GBP 550 to institutions (effective 2001). adv. reprint service avail. from SWZ. *Refereed.* **Document type:** *Academic/Scholarly.* **Description:** Presents papers on basic and applied pharmacological research in both animals and man for the specialist whose fields of study vary widely within the discipline of pharmacology.

Formerly: Pharmacological Research Communications (0031-6989)

Related titles: Online - full text ed.: (from EBSCO Publishing, O C L C Online Computer Library Center, Inc., RoweCom Information Quest, ingenta, Swets Blackwell, IDEAL Online Library, Institute for Scientific Information).

Indexed: ASCA, Biol.Abstr., Chem.Abstr., Chem.Titles, Curr.Adv.Biochem., Curr.Adv.Ecol.Sci., Curr.Cont., Dairy Sci.Abstr., Derwent Biotech.Abstr., Excerp.Med., Helminthol.Abstr., INIS Atomind., Ind.Med. (1989-), Ind.Sci.Rev., Ind.Vet., Inpharma, Int.Abstr.Biol.Sci., Neurosci.Cit.Ind., Nutr.Abstr., Pharm.&Out.News, Pig News & Info., Protozool.Abstr., Reac., Rev.Arom.& Med.Plants, Rev.Med.& Vet.Mycol., Risk Abstr., Sci.Cit.Ind., THA, Vet.Bull.

—BLDSC (6446.550000), ADONIS, CASDDS, CISTI, EMDOCS, GNLM, IDS, ingenta, KNAW, Linda Hall. **CCC.**

Published by: (Italian Pharmacological Society), Academic Press (Subsidiary of: Harcourt Publishers Ltd.), 24 Oval Rd, London NW1 7DX, United Kingdom. TEL 44-20-7267-4466, FAX 44-20-7482-2293, apsubs@acad.com, http://www.academicpress.com/pharmres; http://www.europe.idealibrary.com/. Ed. R Paoletti. R&P Catherine John. Adv. contact Nik Screen. **Subscr. to:** Harcourt Publishers Ltd., Foots Cray High St, Sidcup, Kent DA14 5HP, United Kingdom. TEL 44-20-8300-3322, FAX 44-20-8309-0807.

615.1 USA ISSN 0031-6997
RS1 CODEN: PAREAQ

PHARMACOLOGICAL REVIEWS. Text in English. 1951. q. USD 85 domestic to individuals; USD 112 foreign to individuals; USD 152 domestic to institutions; USD 180 foreign to institutions (effective 2000); includes online access. adv. bibl, charts. back issues avail. *Refereed.* **Document type:** *Academic/Scholarly.* **Description:** Contains review articles on topics of interest to pharmacologists, toxicologists and biochemists.

Related titles: Microfilm ed.: (from WWS); Online - full text ed.: ISSN 1521-0081. USD 68 to individuals; USD 122 to institutions (effective 1999) (from HighWire Pr., EBSCO Publishing, Institute for Scientific Information).

Indexed: ASCA, Agri.& Environ.Biotech.Abstr. (coverage dropped), Aqua.Sci.& Fish.Abstr., Chem.Abstr., Chem.Titles, Curr.Adv.Ecol.Sci., Curr.Cont., Dent.Ind., Derwent Biotech.Abstr., Diar.Dis.Res., Excerp.Med., INIS Atomind., I.P.A., Ind.Med. (1949-), Ind.Sci.Rev., Ind.Vet., Inpharma, Int.Abstr.Biol.Sci., Neurosci.Abstr., Nutr.Abstr., Pharm.&Out.News, Reac., SSCI (coverage dropped), Sci.Cit.Ind., THA, Vet.Bull.

—BLDSC (6447.000000), CASDDS, CINDOC, CISTI, GNLM, IDS, ingenta, KNAW, Linda Hall.

Published by: American Society for Pharmacology and Experimental Therapeutics (ASPET), 9650 Rockville Pike, Bethesda, MD 20814-3998. TEL 301-530-7024, FAX 301-530-5728, TELEX 87669, staff@dues.faseb.org, http://www.pharmrev.org/. Ed. David B Bylund. Adv. contact Christophe Valton. B&W page USD 630, color page USD 1,040; trim 10.88 x 8.38. Circ: 1,863.

615.1 USA ISSN 0031-7004
RM1 CODEN: PHMCAA

PHARMACOLOGIST. Text in English. 1959. q. USD 35 domestic to non-members; USD 50 foreign to non-members (effective 2000). abstr, charts, illus. index. back issues avail.; reprint service avail. from PQC. **Document type:** *Trade.*

Related titles: Microform ed.: (from PQC); Online - full text ed.

Indexed: Agri.& Environ.Biotech.Abstr. (coverage dropped), Biol.Abstr., Chem.Abstr., Derwent Biotech.Abstr., Excerp.Med., Inpharma, Pharm.&Out.News, Reac.

—BLDSC (6447.050000), CISTI, GNLM, ingenta, KNAW, Linda Hall.

Published by: American Society for Pharmacology and Experimental Therapeutics (ASPET), 9650 Rockville Pike, Bethesda, MD 20814-3998. wcline@aspet.org, http://www.faseb.org/aspet/tptocs.htm. Ed. William H Cline. Circ: 4,500.

615.1 CHE ISSN 0031-7012
RM1 CODEN: PHMGBN

PHARMACOLOGY; international journal of experimental and clinical pharmacology. Text in English. 1959. 8/yr. (in 2 vols.). CHF 2,226 in Europe to institutions; CHF 2,260.80 elsewhere to institutions; EUR 1,590.60 in Europe to institutions; USD 1,728 elsewhere to institutions (effective 2002). adv. abstr, bibl, charts, illus. index. back issues avail. *Refereed.* **Document type:** *Journal, Academic/Scholarly.* **Description:** Communicates basic and clinical research in general pharmacology and related fields. Covers biochemical pharmacology, molecular pharmacology, immunopharamacology, drug metabolism, pharmacogenetics, analytical toxicology, neuropsychopharmacology, pharmacokinetics, and clinical pharmacology.

Formerly: Medicina et Pharmacologia Experimentalis

Related titles: Microfilm ed.; Online - full text ed.: ISSN 1423-0313. 1999. CHF 174, EUR 126, USD 135 to institutions with print edition (effective 2002) (from EBSCO Publishing, O C L C Online Computer Library Center, Inc., RoweCom Information Quest, Swets Blackwell, Institute for Scientific Information).

Indexed: ASCA, Agri.& Environ.Biotech.Abstr. (coverage dropped), Aqua.Sci.& Fish.Abstr., Biol.Abstr., Chem.Abstr., Chem.Titles, Curr.Adv.Ecol.Sci., Curr.Cont., Dent.Ind., Derwent Biotech.Abstr., Environ.Sci.Poll.Mgmt., Excerp.Med., Helminthol.Abstr., Ind.Med. (1968-), Ind.Sci.Rev., Inpharma, Neurosci.Abstr., Neurosci.Cit.Ind., Nutr.Abstr., Pharm.&Out.News, Pollut.Abstr., Reac., Ref.Zh., Rev.Plant Path., Risk Abstr., Saf.Sci.Abstr., Sci.Cit.Ind., THA, Tox.Abstr.

—BLDSC (6447.060000), CASDDS, CISTI, GNLM, IDS, ingenta, KNAW, Linda Hall. **CCC.**

Published by: S. Karger AG, Allschwilerstr 10, PO Box, Basel 4009, Switzerland. TEL 41-61-306-1111, FAX 41-61-306-1234, karger@karger.ch, http://www.online.karger.com/journals/pha, http://www.karger.com. Eds. J Donnerer, M L Billingsley, T Watanabe. adv.: page USD 1,185. Circ: 1,150.

PHARMACOLOGY AND THE SKIN. see *MEDICAL SCIENCES—Dermatology And Venereology*

615.1 USA ISSN 0163-7258
RM1 CODEN: PHTHDT

PHARMACOLOGY AND THERAPEUTICS. Text in English. 1975. m. EUR 3,387 in Europe to institutions; JPY 449,600 in Japan to institutions; USD 3,787 elsewhere to institutions (effective 2002). adv. bk.rev. charts, illus, stat. index. reprints avail. *Refereed.* **Document type:** *Academic/Scholarly.* **Description:** Presents authoritative review articles covering recent developments in pharmacology, including chemotherapy, toxicology and clinical pharmacology.

Formed by the Jan. 1979 merger of: Pharmacology and Therapeutics. Part A. Chemotherapy, Toxicology and Metabolic Inhibitors (0362-5478); Pharmacology and Therapeutics. Part B. General and Systematic Pharmacology (0306-039X); Pharmacology and Therapeutics. Part C. Clinical Pharmacology and Therapeutics (0362-5486)

Related titles: Microfilm ed.: (from PQC); Online - full text ed.: (from ingenta, ScienceDirect, Swets Blackwell, Institute for Scientific Information).

Indexed: ASCA, Agri.& Environ.Biotech.Abstr. (coverage dropped), Biol.Abstr., Chem.Abstr., Chem.Cit.Ind., Chem.Indus.Notes, Chem.Titles, Curr.Adv.Biochem., Curr.Adv.Cancer Res., Curr.Adv.Ecol.Sci., Curr.Adv.Gen.& Molec.Biol., Curr.Cont., Dairy Sci.Abstr., Dent.Ind., Derwent Biotech.Abstr., Excerp.Med., Ind.Med. (1979-), Ind.Sci.Rev., Ind.Vet., Inpharma, Int.Abstr.Biol.Sci., Med.& Surg.Dermat., Neurosci.Abstr. (coverage dropped), Neurosci.Cit.Ind., Nutr.Abstr., Pharm.&Out.News, Reac., Rev.Med.& Vet.Mycol., SSCI (coverage dropped), Sci.Cit.Ind., THA.

—BLDSC (6447.061800), ADONIS, CASDDS, CISTI, GNLM, IDS, Infotrieve, ingenta, KNAW, Linda Hall. **CCC.**
Published by: (International Union of Pharmacology), Elsevier Science, 655 Ave of the Americas, New York, NY 10010. TEL 212-989-5800, FAX 212-633-3990, usinfo-f@elsevier.com, http://www.elsevier.nl/locate/pharmthera. Eds. Alan C Sartorelli, W C Bowman. **Subscr. in Australasia and the Far East to:** Elsevier Science (Singapore) Pte Ltd, No.1 Temasek Ave, 17-01 Millenia Tower, Singapore 039192, Singapore. TEL 65-434-3727, FAX 65-337-2230**; Subscr. in Japan to:** Elsevier Science Inc - Japan Regional Office, 9-15 Higashi-Azabu 1-chome, Minato-ku, Tokyo 106-0044, Japan. TEL 81-3-5561-5033, FAX 81-3-5561-5047**; Subscr. outside the Americas to:** Elsevier Science BV, PO Box 211, Amsterdam 1000 AE, Netherlands. TEL 31-20-485-3757, FAX 31-20-485-3432, nlinfo-f@elsevier.nl.

615.902 DNK ISSN 0901-9928
QP901 CODEN: PHTOEH
PHARMACOLOGY & TOXICOLOGY. Text in English. 1944. m. USD 372 in the Americas to institutions print & online eds. combined; GBP 258 elsewhere to institutions print & online eds. combined (effective 2002). bibl, charts, illus. index. reprint service avail. from ISI. *Refereed.* **Document type:** *Academic/Scholarly.*
Formerly: Acta Pharmacologica et Toxicologica (0001-6683)
Related titles: Microfilm ed.: (from PMC); ♦ Online - full text ed.: Pharmacology & Toxicology Online. ISSN 1600-0773; ♦ Supplement: Pharmacology & Toxicology. Supplementum. ISSN 0901-9936.
Indexed: ASCA, Agri.& Environ.Biotech.Abstr. (coverage dropped), Biol.Abstr., C.I.S. Abstr., Chem.Abstr., Curr.Adv.Cell & Devel.Biol., Curr.Adv.Ecol.Sci., Curr.Cont., Dairy Sci.Abstr., Dent.Ind., Derwent Biotech.Abstr., Excerp.Med., Helminthol.Abstr., INIS Atomind., I.P.A., Ind.Med. (1987-), Ind.Sci.Rev., Ind.Vet., Inpharma, Int.Abstr.Biol.Sci., Lab.Haz.Bull., NRN, Neurosci.Cit.Ind., Nutr.Abstr., Pharm.&Out.News, Psychol.Abstr., Reac., Rev.Med.& Vet.Mycol., SSCI (coverage dropped), Sci.Cit.Ind., Sel.Water Res.Abstr., THA, Trop.Dis.Bull., Vet.Bull., Weed Abstr.
—BLDSC (6447.070000), ADONIS, CASDDS, CINDOC, CISTI, EMDOCS, GNLM, IDS, ingenta, KNAW, Linda Hall. **CCC.**
Published by: (Nordic Pharmacological Society), Blackwell Munksgaard, Noerre Soegade 35, PO Box 2148, Copenhagen K 1016, Denmark. TEL 45-77-33-33-33, FAX 45-77-33-33-77, customerservice@munksgaard.dk, http://journals.munksgaard.dk/pharmtox, http://www.munksgaard.dk/journals/pharmacology/. Ed. Jens Schou. Adv. contact Eric Rozario TEL 45-77-33-33-01. Circ: 400.

615.902 DNK ISSN 1600-0773
PHARMACOLOGY & TOXICOLOGY ONLINE. Text in English. m. GBP 232 (effective 2002). *Refereed.* **Document type:** *Academic/Scholarly.*
Media: Online - full text (from Swets Blackwell, Ovid Technologies, Inc., Institute for Scientific Information). **Related titles:** Microfilm ed.: (from PMC); ♦ Print ed.: Pharmacology & Toxicology. ISSN 0901-9928.
Published by: Blackwell Munksgaard, Noerre Soegade 35, PO Box 2148, Copenhagen K 1016, Denmark. TEL 45-77-33-33-33, FAX 45-77-33-33-77, fsub@mail.munksgaard.dk, http://www.munksgaard.dk.

615.1 DNK ISSN 0901-9936
CODEN: PTSUEC
PHARMACOLOGY & TOXICOLOGY. SUPPLEMENTUM. Text in English. 1947. irreg. free with subscr. to Pharmacology & Toxicology. reprint service avail. from ISI. *Refereed.* **Document type:** *Academic/Scholarly.*
Formerly: Acta Pharmacologica et Toxicologica. Supplementum (0065-1508)
Related titles: Online - full text ed.: ISSN 1600-5570 (from Ovid Technologies, Inc.); ♦ Supplement to: Pharmacology & Toxicology. ISSN 0901-9928.
Indexed: Biol.Abstr., Chem.Abstr., Curr.Cont. (coverage dropped), Excerp.Med., INIS Atomind., Ind.Med. (coverage dropped), Int.Abstr.Biol.Sci., Nutr.Abstr., Ocean.Abstr. (coverage dropped).
—ADONIS, CASDDS, CISTI, EMDOCS, Infotrieve, KNAW, Linda Hall. **CCC.**
Published by: Blackwell Munksgaard, Noerre Soegade 35, PO Box 2148, Copenhagen K 1016, Denmark. TEL 45-77-33-33-33, FAX 45-77-33-33-77, customerservice@munksgaard.dk, http://www.munksgaard.dk/pharmtox. Ed. Jens Schou. Adv. contact Eric Rozario TEL 45-77-33-33-01.

615.1 USA ISSN 0091-3057
QP901 CODEN: PBBHAU
PHARMACOLOGY, BIOCHEMISTRY AND BEHAVIOR. Text in English. 1973. m. EUR 320 in Europe to individuals; JPY 42,600 in Japan to individuals; USD 359 elsewhere to individuals; EUR 2,950 in Europe to institutions; JPY 391,800 in Japan to institutions; USD 3,300 elsewhere to institutions (effective 2002). adv. illus. index. back issues avail.; reprint service avail. from PQC,ISI. *Refereed.* **Document type:** *Academic/Scholarly.* **Description:** Original reports of systematic studies in the areas of pharmacology, biochemistry, toxicology and behavior, in which the primary emphasis and theoretical context are behavioral.
Related titles: E-mail ed.; Microfilm ed.: (from PQC); Online - full text ed.: (from ingenta, ScienceDirect, Swets Blackwell, Institute for Scientific Information).
Indexed: ASCA, Addic.Abstr., Agri.& Environ.Biotech.Abstr. (coverage dropped), Anim.Behav.Abstr., Aqua.Sci.& Fish.Abstr., BBCI, Biol.Abstr., Chem.Abstr., Chem.Titles, Chemorec.Abstr., Curr.Adv.Ecol.Sci., Curr.Cont., Dairy Sci.Abstr., Dent.Ind., Derwent Biotech.Abstr., Environ.Sci.Poll.Mgmt., Excerp.Med., Focus on: Psychophar., INIS Atomind., Ind.Med. (1973-), Ind.Sci.Rev., Indian Psychol.Abstr., Inpharma, Int.Abstr.Biol.Sci., Neurosci.Abstr., Neurosci.Cit.Ind., Nutr.Abstr., Pharm.&Out.News, PsycInfo, Psychol.Abstr. (1973-), Reac., Rev.Appl.Entomol., Rev.Arom.& Med.Plants, Risk Abstr., SSCI (coverage dropped), Sci.Cit.Ind., Sport Fish.Abstr., Sugar Ind.Abstr., THA, Tox.Abstr., Wild.Rev., e-psyche.
—BLDSC (6447.078000), ADONIS, CASDDS, CISTI, GNLM, IDS, ingenta, KNAW. **CCC.**
Published by: Elsevier Science, 655 Ave of the Americas, New York, NY 10010. TEL 212-989-5800, FAX 212-633-3990, usinfo-f@elsevier.com, http://www.elsevier.nl/locate/pharmbiochembeh. Eds. George F Koob, Sandra E File. **Subscr. in Australasia and the Far East to:** Elsevier Science (Singapore) Pte Ltd, No.1 Temasek Ave, 17-01 Millenia Tower, Singapore 039192, Singapore. TEL 65-434-3727, FAX 65-337-2230**; Subscr. in Japan to:** Elsevier Science Inc - Japan Regional Office, 9-15 Higashi-Azabu 1-chome, Minato-ku, Tokyo 106-0044, Japan. TEL 81-3-5561-5033, FAX 81-3-5561 5047**; Subscr. outside the Americas to:** Elsevier Science BV, PO Box 211, Amsterdam 1000 AE, Netherlands. TEL 31-20-485-3757.

615 AUT ISSN 1437-6873
▼ **PHARMACOLOGY FAST.** Text in German. 1999. irreg. price varies. **Document type:** *Monographic series, Academic/Scholarly.*
Published by: Springer-Verlag Wien (Subsidiary of: BertelsmannSpringer), Sachsenplatz 4-6, PO Box 89, Vienna, W 1201, Austria. TEL 43-1-3302415-0, FAX 43-1-330242665, books@springer.at, http://www.springer.at. R&P Angela Foessl TEL 43-1-3302415517. **Dist. in N. America by:** Springer-Verlag, Journals. books@springer.at, http://www.springer-ny.com.

615 DEU
PHARMACOLOGY OF CEREBRAL ISCHEMIA. Text in German. 1994. biennial. EUR 126.80 per vol. (effective 2001). **Document type:** *Monographic series, Academic/Scholarly.*
Indexed: Neurosci.Cit.Ind.
—BLDSC (6447.078200).
Published by: Medpharm GmbH Scientific Publishers, Postfach 101061, Stuttgart 70009, Germany. TEL 49-711-25820, FAX 49-711-2582-290, service@medpharm.de, http://www.medpharm.de. Ed. Josef Krieglstein.

615 CHE ISSN 1028-8945
CODEN: PCMME9
PHARMACOLOGY REVIEWS AND COMMUNICATIONS. Text in English. 1992. 4/yr. GBP 89, USD 130, EUR 130 to individuals; GBP 377, USD 520, EUR 535 to institutions; GBP 562, USD 789, EUR 815 to corporations (effective 2002). **Document type:** *Academic/Scholarly.* **Description:** Publishes original short research reports on all aspects of basic and clinical pharmacology.
Formerly (until 1996): Pharmacology Communications (1060-4456)
Related titles: CD-ROM ed.; Microform ed.; Online - full text ed.: (from EBSCO Publishing, RoweCom Information Quest).
Indexed: Aqua.Sci.& Fish.Abstr., Environ.Sci.Poll.Mgmt., Excerp.Med. (1993-), Inpharma, Int.Abstr.Biol.Sci., Neurosci.Abstr., Pharm.&Out.News, Pollut.Abstr., Reac., Risk Abstr., Saf.Sci.Abstr.
—BLDSC (6447.083000), CISTI, EMDOCS, GNLM, Infotrieve. **CCC.**
Published by: Gordon and Breach - Harwood Academic (Subsidiary of: Taylor & Francis Group), PO Box 531, Lausanne 1000, Switzerland. http://www.gbhap.com/Pharmacology_Reviews_Communications/. Eds. Norman G Bowery, Robert R Ruffolo Jr. **Subscr. addr. in US:** International Publishers Direct, PO Box 32160, Newark, NJ 07102. FAX 215-750-6343.

615 USA ISSN 0363-4655
PHARMACOPEIAL FORUM. Text in English. 1975. bi-m. USD 310. **Document type:** *Directory.* **Description:** Presents proposed U.S.P. National Formulary revisions for public comment.
Indexed: ASCA, Curr.Cont. (coverage dropped), I.P.A., Sugar Ind.Abstr.
—BLDSC (6447.087400), GNLM, IDS.
Published by: United States Pharmacopeial Convention, Inc., 12601 Twinbrook Pkwy, Rockville, MD 20852. TEL 301-881-0666.

615 HKG
PHARMACOPOEIA OF THE PEOPLE'S REPUBLIC OF CHINA. Text in English. a.
Related titles: Chinese ed.
Published by: (China, People's Republic. Ministry of Public Health CHN), People's Medical Publishing House, 10 Tianxili Lu, Beijing, China. **Dist. by:** China Pharmaceutical Books Company, Rm. 1001-4 Champion Bldg, 287-291 Des Voeus Rd, Central, Hong Kong, Hong Kong.

PHARMACOPSYCHIATRY; clinical pharmacology, psychiatry, psychology, neurophysiology, neurobiology, gerontopsychiatry. see *MEDICAL SCIENCES—Psychiatry And Neurology*

PHARMACOPSYCHIATRY. SUPPLEMENT. see *MEDICAL SCIENCES—Psychiatry And Neurology*

615.19 USA ISSN 0277-0008
CODEN: PHPYDQ
PHARMACOTHERAPY; the journal of human pharmacology and drug therapy. Text in English. 1981. m. USD 65 domestic to individuals; USD 80 foreign to individuals; USD 95 domestic to institutions; USD 110 foreign to institutions; USD 45 domestic to students; USD 60 foreign to students (effective 2001). adv. bk.rev. charts, illus. index. 130 p./no. 2 cols./p. back issues avail.; reprint service avail. from PQC. *Refereed.* **Document type:** *Academic/Scholarly.* **Description:** Publishes original articles of interest to physicians, pharmacists, and other health professionals with major interests in drug therapy or clinical drug research.
Related titles: CD-ROM ed.; Microfilm ed.: (from PQC); Online - full content ed.; Online - full text ed.: (from Institute for Scientific Information, RoweCom Information Quest).
Indexed: ASCA, Biol.Abstr., Cal.Tiss.Abstr., Chem.Abstr., Curr.Cont., Dent.Ind., Derwent Biotech.Abstr., Environ.Sci.Poll.Mgmt., Excerp.Med., INIS Atomind., I.P.A., Ind.Med. (1981-), Ind.Sci.Rev., Inpharma, Int.Abstr.Biol.Sci., Int.Nurs.Ind., Kidney, Nutr.Abstr., Pharm.&Out.News, Pollut.Abstr., Protozool.Abstr., Reac., Ref.Zh., Rev.Arom.& Med.Plants, Rev.Med.& Vet.Mycol., Risk Abstr., SSCI (coverage dropped), Saf.Sci.Abstr., Sci.Cit.Ind., Sugar Ind.Abstr., THA, Tox.Abstr.
—BLDSC (6447.089000), CASDDS, CISTI, EMDOCS, GNLM, IDS, ingenta, KNAW. **CCC.**
Address: New England Medical Center, 806, 750 Washington St, Boston, MA 02111. TEL 617-636-5390, FAX 617-636-5318, PPIJournal@aol.com, http://accp.com. Ed. Richard T Scheife. R&P Wendy R Cramer. adv.: B&W page USD 1,300, color page USD 1,775. Circ: 7,000 (paid and free). **Dist. by:** I O S Press, Nieuwe Hemweg 6B, Amsterdam 1013 BG, Netherlands. TEL 31-20-688-3355, FAX 31-20-620-3419, market@iospress.nl, http://www.iospress.nl.

615.19 CAN ISSN 0834-065X
PHARMACTUEL; la revue de la pratique pharmaceutique en etablissement de sante au Quebec. Text in French. 1967. bi-m. CND 50 to non-members (effective 2000). adv. bk.rev., Website rev. abstr, charts, illus. index. back issues avail. *Refereed.* **Document type:** *Magazine, Academic/Scholarly, Abstract/Index.* **Description:** Presents articles regarding the pharmaceutical field, written by pharmacists, for members of the Association of Pharmacists of the Health Estabishments of Quebec (A. P. E. S.), subscribers and manufacturers.
Indexed: I.P.A.

P

Published by: Association des Pharmaciens des Etablissements de Sante du Quebec, 1470 Peel, Tour B, Bureau 900, Montreal, PQ H3A 1T1, Canada. TEL 514-286-0776, FAX 514-286-1081, lgermain@apesquebec.org, http://www.pharmactuel.com. Ed. Jude Goulet. R&P Lucie Germain. Adv. contact Clifford K Goodman. B&W page USD 1,000, color page USD 1,600; trim 10.88 x 8.13. Circ: 1,300 (controlled).

615 USA ISSN 1064-797X
RS122.5
PHARMACY CADENCE. Text in English. 1992. a. USD 17.95 (effective 2000). *Refereed.* **Description:** Overview of pharmacy for students and others new to the profession in the U.S. and Canada.
Published by: P E N S Pharmacy Editorial & News Services, Inc., PO Box 6565, Athens, GA 30604. TEL 706-613-0100, FAX 706-613-0200. Ed., Pub. L Michael Posey. Circ: 2,000 (paid).

615.1 CHE ISSN 1560-2214
▼ **PHARMACY EDUCATION.** Text in English. 2001. 4/yr. GBP 59, USD 90, EUR 99 to individuals; GBP 132, USD 200, EUR 220 to institutions; GBP 216, USD 328, EUR 360 to corporations (effective 2002). **Document type:** *Journal, Academic/Scholarly.* **Description:** Provides a forum for communication between academic teachers and practitioners, with an emphasis on new and established teaching and learning methods; new curriculum and syllabus directions; guidance on structuring courses and assessing achievement as well as the dissemination of new ideas.
Related titles: Online - full text ed.
Published by: Gordon and Breach - Harwood Academic (Subsidiary of: Taylor & Francis Group), PO Box 531, Lausanne 1000, Switzerland. TEL 41-21-6411280, FAX 41-21-6411281, info@gbhap.com, http://www.gbhap.com/Pharmacy_Education/. Ed. Ian Bates.

615.1 NLD
▼ **PHARMACY EDUCATION - A VISION OF THE FUTURE.** Text in English. 1999. a. **Document type:** *Academic/Scholarly.* **Description:** Provides a comprehensive and collaborative study by pharmacy students worldwide of essential developments in pharmacy education.
Formerly: Pharmacy Education
Related titles: Online - full content ed.
Published by: International Pharmaceutical Students Federation, Andries Bickerweg 5, The Hague 2517 JP, Netherlands. TEL 31-70-3021992, FAX 31-70-3021999, ipsf@ipsf.org, http://www.ipsf.org.

615.9 CAN
PHARMACY ELECTRONIC COMMUNICATIONS STANDARD. Text in English. biennial. CND 35 (effective 2000). **Document type:** *Trade.*
Former titles (until 1998): Pharmacy Claim Standard; Electronic Claim Standard
Published by: Canadian Pharmacists Association, 1785 Alta Vista Dr, Ottawa, ON K1G 3Y6, Canada. TEL 613-523-7877, FAX 613-523-0445, cpha@cdnpharm.ca, http://www.cdnpharm.ca.

615.19 AUS ISSN 1032-3279
PHARMACY GUILD OF AUSTRALIA. ANNUAL REPORT✱. Text in English. 1975. a.
Formerly: Pharmacy Guild of Australia. National Report
Published by: Pharmacy Guild of Australia, PO Box 2036, Canberra Mail Centre, ACT 2600, Australia. TEL 61-2-6270-1888, FAX 61-2-6270-1800, guild.nat@guild.org.au. Circ: 5,500.

615.19 AUS ISSN 0155-8595
PHARMACY GUILD OF AUSTRALIA. NATIONAL NEWSLETTER✱. Text in English. 1976. irreg. free per issue to members. back issues avail. **Document type:** *Newsletter.*
Published by: Pharmacy Guild of Australia, PO Box 2036, Canberra Mail Centre, ACT 2600, Australia. TEL 61-2-6270-1888, FAX 61-2-6270-1800, guild.nat@guild.org.au. Circ: 5,300.

615.9 610.73 614.8 USA ISSN 0739-9596
PHARMACY HEALTH-LINE. Text in English. 1982. m. USD 55 (effective 2001). back issues avail.
Published by: Rx-Data-Pac Service, 8907 Terwilliger s Tr, Cincinnati, OH 45249. TEL 513-489-0943, FAX 513-489-0943. Ed. Dr. I H Goodman.

615.1 USA ISSN 0031-7047
RS61 CODEN: PHHIB4
PHARMACY IN HISTORY. Text in English. 1959. q. USD 50 (effective 2000). adv. bk.rev. bibl, charts, illus. index every 3 yrs. reprint service avail. from PQC. **Document type:** *Academic/Scholarly.*
Related titles: Microfilm ed.: (from PQC); Online - full text ed.
Indexed: Amer.Hist.& Life, Hist.Abstr. (1972-), I.P.A.
—BLDSC (6447.350000), ingenta, Linda Hall.
Published by: American Institute of the History of Pharmacy, Pharmacy Bldg, Madison, WI 53706. TEL 608-262-5378. Ed. Gregory Higby. Circ: 1,200.

615.4 GBR ISSN 1358-1538
CODEN: HPPRE8
PHARMACY IN PRACTICE. Text in English. 1991. m. GBP 65 domestic; USD 120 foreign (effective 2000). **Document type:** *Academic/Scholarly.*
Formerly (until 1994): Hospital Pharmacy Practice (0962-9734)
Indexed: Derwent Biotech.Abstr., Excerp.Med. (1994-), I.P.A.
—BLDSC (6447.504000), EMDOCS, GNLM, KNAW.
Published by: Medicom Publishing, Churston House, Portsmouth Rd, Esher, Surrey KT10 9AD, United Kingdom. TEL 44-1372-471671, FAX 44-1372-471672. Ed. Elspeth Lee. Circ: 5,000.

615.19 340 USA ISSN 0149-1717
KF2915.P4
PHARMACY LAW DIGEST. Text in English. 1965. a. (plus s-a. updates). USD 100; USD 115 foreign (effective 1999). **Description:** Information on controlled substances, pharmacy inspection, civil liability, pertinent court cases, business and drug control law, with emphasis on federal law.
Published by: Facts and Comparisons, 111 W. Port Plaza, Ste. 300, St. Louis, MO 63146-3098. TEL 800-223-0554, FAX 314-878-5563.

615 GBR
PHARMACY MAGAZINE. Text in English. 1995. m. GBP 52; GBP 93 foreign (effective 2000). adv. **Document type:** *Trade.* **Description:** Provides trade information for pharmacists.
Published by: Communications International Group, 307 Linen Hall, 162-168 Regent St, London W1R 5TB, United Kingdom. TEL 44-20-7434-1530, FAX 44-20-7437-0915. R&P Anne Anstice. Adv. contact Simon Whiten. Circ: 19,468.

615.1 IND ISSN 0031-7063
PHARMACY NEWS✱. Text in English. 1962. m. INR 8. adv. bk.rev. illus, pat.
Incorporating: Modern Medical Practice
Related titles: Hindi ed.: 1962; Panjabi ed.: 1962; Urdu ed.: 1962.
Indexed: I.P.A.
Published by: (Punjab Pharmacists' Federation), Rajesh Publications, 1 Ansari Rd., Daryaganj, New Delhi 110 002, India. Ed. Dr. Kuldip Bhatia. Circ: 12,000 (controlled). **Co-sponsors:** All India Medical Practitioners' Association; All India Homeopathic League.

615 USA ISSN 8750-4790
PHARMACY NEWS AND REVIEW. Text in English. 6/yr. USD 100 to non-members; USD 50 to members (effective 2000). 8 p./no. **Document type:** *Newsletter, Trade.* **Description:** Covers current legal, administrative and medical issues affecting pharmacists.
Published by: Pennsylvania Pharmacists Association, 508 N Third St, Harrisburg, PA 17101-1199. TEL 717-234-6151, FAX 717-236-1618. Ed. Carmen Dicello.

615.1 GBR
PHARMACY ON-LINE; the international forum for pharmacy. Text in English. 1995. m. free per issue. bk.rev., software rev., video rev. illus. *Refereed.* **Document type:** *Journal, Academic/Scholarly.* **Description:** Covers pharmacy, pharmaceuticals and pharmacology.
Media: Online - full text.
Published by: Priory Lodge Education Ltd., 2 Cornflower Way, Moreton, Wirral CH46 1SV, United Kingdom. TEL 44-151-606-1796, FAX 44-151-606-1812, ben@priory.com, solutions@priory.com, http://www.priory.com/pharmol.htm. Ed. Dr. Ben Green. Circ: 40,000 (controlled).

615 CAN ISSN 1199-2131
PHARMACY POST; your news, business and otc market report. Text in English. 1993. m. CND 62.60 domestic; CND 95.50 foreign (effective 2001). adv. **Document type:** *Magazine, Trade.* **Description:** Complete resource for news, OTC drug information, and business management for Canada's 16,000 community pharmacists as well as 2,000 buyers and frontshop managers.
Indexed: CBCA Ref.
Published by: Rogers Media Publishing Ltd, 777 Bay St, 6th Fl, Toronto, ON M5W 1A7, Canada. TEL 416-596-5000, FAX 416-596-5881, http://www.pharmacyconnects.com. Ed. Karen Welds. Pub., Adv. contact Janet Smith. Circ: 12,636.

615.1 CAN ISSN 0829-2809
CODEN: PHRPEA
PHARMACY PRACTICE. Text in English. 1985. 12/yr. CND 62.60 domestic; CND 95.50 foreign (effective 2001). adv. **Document type:** *Magazine, Trade.* **Description:** Provides readers with information on the new and significant developments that affect the profession of pharmacy.
Indexed: I.P.A.
Published by: Rogers Media Publishing Ltd, 777 Bay St, 6th Fl, Toronto, ON M5W 1A7, Canada. TEL 416-596-5000, FAX 416-596-5881, http://www.pharmacyconnects.com, http://www.rogers.com. Ed. Anne Bokma. Pub., Adv. contact Janet Smith. B&W page CND 2,620. Circ: 20,100.

410 USA ISSN 1080-5737
PHARMACY PRACTICE MANAGEMENT QUARTERLY. Text in English. 1981. q. USD 134 domestic; USD 161 foreign (effective 2000). adv. **Document type:** *Academic/Scholarly.* **Description:** Provides detailed guidance to help pharmacists reduce pharmacy-related costs, improve patient care quality and outcomes, reduce risks, handle Joint Commission on Accreditation of Healthcare Organizations surveys (JCHAO), and manage more confidently.
Formerly (until 1995): Topics in Hospital Pharmacy Management (0271-1206)
Related titles: Microfiche ed.: (from PQC); Online - full text ed.: (from Ovid Technologies, Inc., ProQuest Information & Learning, Factiva).
Indexed: CINAHL, Hosp.Lit.Ind., I.P.A., Int.Nurs.Ind.
—BLDSC (6447.509000), CISTI, GNLM, Infotrieve, ingenta. **CCC.**
Published by: Aspen Publishers, Inc., 200 Orchard Ridge Dr, Ste 200, Gaithersburg, MD 20878. TEL 301-417-7500, 800-638-8437, FAX 301-695-7931, customer.service@aspenpubl.com, http://www.aspenpub.com. Ed. Andrew L Wilson. **Dist. by:** Aspen Publishers Inc., Distribution Center, 7201 McKinney Circle, Frederick, MD 21701. TEL 301-698-7100, FAX 301-417-7550.

615 USA ISSN 0886-988X
PHARMACY PRACTICE NEWS. Text in English. 1984. m. USD 60 domestic; USD 84 foreign (effective 2001); Free to qualified subscribers. adv. illus. **Document type:** *Trade.* **Description:** Provides health-system pharmacists with up-to-date information that improves their clinical practice, such as continuing education lessons, new FDA drug approvals and educational reviews.
Former titles (until 1985): Intravenous Therapy News (8750-3182); American Journal of Intravenous Therapy and Clinical Nutrition (0195-0282); American Journal of Intravenous Therapy (0161-3065); American Journal of I.V. Therapy (0095-4012)
Related titles: Online - full text ed.; Special ed.
Indexed: CINAHL, Excerp.Med., I.P.A.
—CISTI, GNLM. **CCC.**
Published by: McMahon Group, 545 W 45th St, 8th Fl, New York, NY 10036. TEL 212-957-5300, FAX 212-957-7230, dmacnamara@mcmahonmed.com, http://www.pharmacypracticenews.com/index.html, http://www.mcmahonmed.com. Ed. Damian McNamara. adv.: B&W page USD 4,200, color page USD 2,000. Circ: 24,577.

615 GBR
PHARMACY PRODUCTS REVIEW. Text in English. 1992. m. GBP 52; GBP 93 foreign (effective 2000). adv. **Document type:** *Trade.*
Published by: Communications International Group, 307 Linen Hall, 162-168 Regent St, London W1R 5TB, United Kingdom. TEL 44-20-7434-1530, FAX 44-20-7437-0915. Ed. Anne Anstice. Pub., Adv. contact Simon Whiten. Circ: 15,000 (controlled).

615 658 ZAF
PHARMACY RETAILER. Text in English. m. ZAR 60. adv. **Document type:** *Trade.*

Published by: Complete Publishing (Pty.) Ltd., PO Box 87745, Houghton, Johannesburg 2041, South Africa. TEL 27-11-7892112, FAX 27-11-789-5347. Ed. Roy Watson. Circ: 4,000.

615.19 AUS ISSN 0314-6316
PHARMACY REVIEW* . Text in English. 1976. q. AUD 40.
Description: Informs members about decisions relating to pharmacy in Australia.
Indexed: I.P.A.
Published by: Pharmacy Guild of Australia, PO Box 2036, Canberra Mail Centre, ACT 2600, Australia. TEL 61-2-6270-1888, FAX 61-2-6270-1800, guild.nat@guild.org.au. Ed. Wal Williams. Circ: 5,200.

615.1071 USA ISSN 0149-1113
RS110
PHARMACY SCHOOL ADMISSION REQUIREMENTS. Text in English. 1974. a. **Document type:** *Directory.*
Description: Informs students interested in getting into Pharmacy schools.
Published by: American Association of Colleges of Pharmacy, Office of Academic Affairs, 1426 Prince St, Alexandria, VA 22314-2815. FAX 703-836-8982.

615.1 USA ISSN 1098-1853
PHARMACY SOCIETY OF WISCONSIN. JOURNAL. Abbreviated title: J P S W. Text in English. 1930 (vol.40). bi-m. USD 60 to non-members (effective 2001); free to members. adv. back issues avail.
Document type: *Trade.*
Formerly (until 1997): Wisconsin Pharmacist (0043-6585)
Indexed: Chem.Abstr., I.P.A.
Published by: Pharmacy Society of Wisconsin, 701 Heartland Trail, Madison, WI 53717-1916. TEL 608-827-9200, FAX 608-827-9292. adv.: B&W page USD 440, color page USD 1,040. Circ: 2,200 (controlled).

615.10711 USA ISSN 0279-5272
PHARMACY STUDENT. Text in English. 1976 (vol.7). q. USD 25 to non-members (effective 2000).
Formerly (until vol.8, 1978): S A Ph A News
Indexed: I.P.A.
—CCC.
Published by: American Pharmaceutical Association, 2215 Constitution Ave, N W, Washington, DC 20037. TEL 202-628-4410. Ed. Rick Harding. Circ: 11,500.

615.1 USA ISSN 0003-0627
RS1
PHARMACY TIMES; practical information for today's pharmacist. Text in English. 1897. m. USD 43 domestic; USD 82 in Canada; USD 93 foreign; USD 22 domestic retired pharmacists (effective 2000). adv. bk.rev. abstr, illus. index. back issues avail.; reprints avail. **Document type:** *Magazine, Trade.* **Description:** Deals with pharmaceutical news, pharmacy economics and prescription practice.
Former titles (until 1969): American Professional Pharmacist (0096-0349); Practical Druggist; Spatula
Related titles: Microform ed.: (from PQC); Online - full text ed.
Indexed: AgeLine, Biol.Abstr., Chem.Abstr., I.P.A.
—CISTI, ingenta, Linda Hall.
Published by: Romaine Pierson Publishing Co. (Subsidiary of: Medical World Communications), 1065 Old Country Rd, Ste 213, Westbury, NY 11590-5628. TEL 516-997-0377, FAX 516-997-0344. Ed. Ann Latner. Pub. James Granato. Adv. contact Lara Fichera. Circ: 113,000.

615 USA ISSN 1042-0991
PHARMACY TODAY. Text in English. 1962. m. USD 50 (effective 2000). bibl, illus. **Description:** Reports on current news and opinions, including pharmacotherapeutic, legislative and socioeconomic news.
Former titles: Pharmacy Weekly; A-Ph-Armacy Weekly (0098-2814); A Ph A Newsletter (0567-4069)
Indexed: I.P.A.
—Infotrieve. **CCC.**
Published by: American Pharmaceutical Association, 2215 Constitution Ave, N W, Washington, DC 20037. TEL 202-628-4410, FAX 202-628-5425. Ed. Rick Harding. Circ: 40,000 (controlled).

615 GBR ISSN 0968-042X
PHARMACY TODAY. Text in English. 1986. 9/yr. adv.
Document type: *Magazine, Trade.* **Description:** Contains articles of interest to managers of independent pharmacies.
Related titles: Online - full text ed.: (from LexisNexis).

Published by: C M P Information (Subsidiary of: United Business Media), Sovereign House, Sovereign Way, Tonbridge, Kent TN9 1RW, United Kingdom. TEL 44-1732-377486, FAX 44-1732-353328, enquiries@cmpinformation.com, http://www.cmpinformation.com. Circ: 9,969 (controlled).

615.1 AUS ISSN 0031-7071
PHARMACY TRADE. Text in English. 1967. m. AUD 138.60 (effective 2001). adv. illus. **Document type:** *Trade.* **Description:** Provides independent news, health, marketing and business information about retail pharmacy.
Related titles: Online - full text ed.: (from Factiva).
Indexed: ABIX (Nov.1992-).
Published by: Reed Business Information Pty. Ltd. (Subsidiary of: Reed Elsevier plc), Locked Bag 2999, Chatswood, NSW 2067, Australia. matthew.eton@reedbusiness.com.au, http://www.reedbusiness.com.au/. Ed. Matthew Eton. Pub. Fadia Matouk. Adv. contact Bob Antic. Circ: 6,985.

615.1 USA
PHARMACY UPDATE. Text in English. bi-m. back issues avail. **Document type:** *Government.*
Related titles: Online - full text ed.
Published by: U.S. National Institutes of Health, Warren Grant Magnuson Clinical Center, Pharmacy Department, 10 Center Dr, Room iN257, Bethesda, MD 20892. TEL 301-496-4363, kcalis@nih.gov, http://www.cc.nih.gov/phar/updates/. Ed. Karim Anton Calis.

615 USA ISSN 1075-2552
PHARMACY WEEK. Text in English. 1992. w. free per issue to qualified personnel. adv. **Document type:** *Trade.* **Description:** For hospital and home health care pharmacists. Covers management and employment issues.
Related titles: Online - full text ed.
Address: 7 N Pinckney St, 200, Madison, WI 53703. TEL 608-251-1112, FAX 608-251-1155, info@pharmacyweek.com, pweek@pweek.com, http://www.pharmacyweek.com. R&P Ann Powers. Adv. contacts Rebecca Polk, Tracy Oswald. B&W page USD 2,500, color page USD 4,500; trim 11 x 8.5. Circ: 12,000 (controlled).

615 NLD ISSN 0928-1231
CODEN: PWSCED
PHARMACY WORLD AND SCIENCE; a journal devoted to rational drug use. Text in Dutch. 1979. bi-m. EUR 210 to institutions print & online eds.combined (effective 2002). adv. bk.rev. *Refereed.* **Document type:** *Academic/Scholarly.* **Description:** Provides a medium for the publication of articles within all fields of pharmaceutical sciences, with an emphasis on clinical pharmacy.
Formerly (until 1992): Pharmaceutisch Weekblad. Scientific Edition (0167-6555)
Related titles: Online - full content ed.: (from EBSCO Publishing, O C L C Online Computer Library Center, Inc., Swets Blackwell).
Indexed: ASCA, Chem.Abstr., Chem.Indus.Notes, Chem.Titles, Curr.Cont., Derwent Biotech.Abstr., Excerp.Med., INIS Atomind., I.P.A., Ind.Med. (1993-), Ind.Sci.Rev., Inpharma, Int.Nurs.Ind., Pharm.&Out.News, Protozool.Abstr., Reac., Rev.Med.& Vet.Mycol., SSCI (coverage dropped), Sci.Cit.Ind.
—BLDSC (6447.541000), CASDDS, CISTI, EMDOCS, GNLM, IDS, KNAW.
Published by: (Koninklijke Nederlandse Maatschappij ter Bevordering der Pharmacie/Royal Netherlands Pharmaceutical Society), Kluwer Academic Publishers Group (Subsidiary of: Wolters Kluwer N.V.), Spuiboulevard 50, PO Box 17, Dordrecht 3300 AA, Netherlands. FAX 31-78-639-2254, services@wkap.nl, http://www.wkap.nl/journalhome.htm/0928-1231. Ed. C W H Koks. **Dist. by:** Journals Department, PO Box 322, Dordrecht 3300 AH, Netherlands. TEL 781-871-6600, FAX 31-78-654-6474. **Co-sponsor:** European Society of Clinical Pharmacy.

615 GBR ISSN 1465-5403
▼ **PHARMAFOCUS.** Text in English. 1999. m. GBP 75 domestic; GBP 90 in the European Union; GBP 110 elsewhere; GBP 6.50 newsstand/cover. **Document type:** *Trade.*
Published by: Pharmafile Ltd., First House, Park St, Guildford, Surrey GU1 4XB, United Kingdom. TEL 44-1483-515300, FAX 44-1483-515301, s.benard@pharmafile.co.uk.

615 GRC ISSN 1105-4999
CODEN: PHMKE4
PHARMAKEFTIKI. Text in English, Greek. 1988. q. USD 80 to individuals; USD 100 to institutions. adv.
Document type: *Academic/Scholarly.*

Indexed: Chem.Abstr.
—CASDDS.
Published by: L & S Papathanasopoulou Ltd., 41 Stadiou St, Athens 105 59, Greece. TEL 30-1-3212533. Ed. P Macheras. R&P, Adv. contact Lida Papathanasopoulou.

615.1 DEU
RS1 CODEN: PHMRAL
PHARMARUNDSCHAU. Text in German. 1968. m. DEM 202, EUR 103.28 domestic; DEM 238, EUR 121.69 foreign (effective 2001). adv. bk.rev. **Document type:** *Journal, Trade.* **Description:** Contains pharmaceutical news and cover issues important to professional in the industy.
Formerly: Pharmazeutische Rundschau (0031-7128)
Indexed: Biol.Abstr., Excerp.Med.
—CISTI, Infotrieve. **CCC.**
Published by: P. Keppler Verlag GmbH und Co. KG, Industriestr 2, Heusenstamm 63150, Germany. TEL 49-6104-606-0, FAX 49-6104-606333, info@kepplermediengruppe.de, http://www.kepplermediengruppe.de. Ed. Silvia Schmidtke. Adv. contact Margitta Mueller. B&W page DEM 5,590; trim 185 x 263. Circ: 12,500.

615 GBR ISSN 1361-2018
RS51
PHARMASOURCE; dictionary of pharmacological agents plus the P D R Generics. Text in English. s-a. GBP 950; GBP 350 renewals. illus. **Description:** Contains complete contents of the Dictionary of Pharmacological Agents. Also includes full monographs on the top 2,000 drugs from the Physicians Desk Reference Generics which are hypertext-linked to each associated dictionary entry.
Formerly (until 1996): Dictionary of Drugs on CD-ROM
Media: CD-ROM.
Published by: Chapman & Hall, Electronic Publishing Division, Chapman & Hall, 2-6 Boundary Row, London SE1 8HN, United Kingdom. TEL 44-20-7865-0066, FAX 44-20-7522-0101, cust.serv@chall.co.uk, http://www.epd.chapmanhall.com. **Dist. by:** Cheriton House, North Way, Andover, Hamps SP10 5BE, United Kingdom. TEL 44-1264-332424, FAX 44-1264-332424.

615 USA
▼ **PHARMAVOICE.** Text in English. 2001. bi-m. adv.
Document type: *Magazine, Trade.* **Description:** Provides a forum for the views and opinions of pharmaceutical industry executives on key issues and trends.
Published by: PharmaLinx LLC, PO Box 327, Titusville, NJ 08650. TEL 609-730-0196, FAX 609-730-0197, http://www.pharmalinx.com/index.html. Ed. Taren Grom. Pub. Lisa Banket. adv.: B&W page USD 3,425, color page USD 4,825; trim 9.5 x 11.5. Circ: 10,000 (controlled).

615 DEU ISSN 0480-2624
DER PHARMAZEUTISCHE BETRIEB. Text in German, English. 1955. irreg. **Document type:** *Monographic series, Trade.*
Published by: Editio Cantor Verlag, Postfach 1255, Aulendorf 88322, Germany. TEL 49-7525-940145, FAX 49-7525-940147, info@ecv.de, http://www.ecv.de.

615.1 DEU ISSN 0031-711X
CODEN: PHINAN
DIE PHARMAZEUTISCHE INDUSTRIE. Text in English, German. 1939. m. DEM 318.80, EUR 163 domestic; DEM 377.48, EUR 193 foreign; DEM 367.70, EUR 188 domestic print & online eds.; DEM 415.81, EUR 212.60 foreign print & online eds. (effective 2001). adv. bk.rev. abstr, bibl, charts, illus, mkt, pat, tr.lit. index. reprint service avail. from IRC,ISI. *Refereed.* **Document type:** *Journal, Trade.* **Description:** Provides a forum for the pharmaceutical industry covering pharmaceutics, health care and social politics as well as public health affairs affecting the market members.
Related titles: Online - full text ed.: (from Institute for Scientific Information).
Indexed: ASCA, Agri.& Environ.Biotech.Abstr. (coverage dropped), Bus.& Indus. (Apr.1996-), CBNB (1997-), CEABA, Chem.Abstr., Chem.Titles, Derwent Biotech.Abstr., Excerp.Med., INIS Atomind., I.P.A., Int.Packag.Abstr., Key to Econ.Sci., PROMT, Ref.Zh., Sugar Ind.Abstr.
—BLDSC (6448.690000), CASDDS, CISTI, GNLM, IDS, Infotrieve, KNAW, Linda Hall. **CCC.**
Published by: Editio Cantor Verlag, Postfach 1255, Aulendorf 88322, Germany. TEL 49-7525-940135, FAX 49-7525-940180, info@ecv.de, http://www.ecv.de/phihome.htm. Ed. Viktor Schramm. Adv. contact Holger Leupoldt. B&W page DEM 2,638, color page DEM 4,621; trim 192 x 270. Circ: 4,000.

615.1 DEU ISSN 0031-7136 CODEN: PHZIAP
PHARMAZEUTISCHE ZEITUNG. Abbreviated title: P Z. Text in German. 1953. w. EUR 124.28 domestic; EUR 194.48 foreign (effective 2002). adv. bk.rev. bibl, charts, illus. index. **Document type:** *Newspaper, Trade.*
Formed by the merger of (1951-1953): Pharmazeutische Zeitung-Nachrichten (0369-9803); (1949-1953): Apotheker-Zeitung (0174-1675)
Indexed: Agri.& Environ.Biotech.Abstr. (coverage dropped), Chem.Abstr., Chem.Infd., Chem.Titles, Derwent Biotech.Abstr., Excerp.Med., INIS Atomind., I.P.A.
—BLDSC (6447.693000), CASDDS, CINDOC, CISTI, EMDOCS, GNLM, Infotrieve, KNAW, Linda Hall. **CCC.**
Published by: (Bundesvereinigung Deutscher Apothekerverbaende), Govi Verlag Pharmazeutischer Verlag GmbH, Carl Mannich Str 26, Eschborn 65760, Germany. TEL 49-6196-928271, FAX 49-6196-928294, t.fast@govi.aponet.de. Ed. Dr. Hartmut Morck. Circ: 36,500.

615.1 DEU ISSN 0031-7144
RS1 CODEN: PHARAT
DIE PHARMAZIE; an international journal of pharmaceutical sciences. Text in English, German. 1946. m. EUR 154.56 domestic; EUR 160.30 in the European Union; EUR 169.32 elsewhere (effective 2002). adv. bk.rev. abstr, bibl, charts, illus. index. *Refereed.* **Document type:** *Journal, Academic/Scholarly.*
Related titles: Online - full text ed.: (from Swets Blackwell, Institute for Scientific Information).
Indexed: ASCA, Agri.& Environ.Biotech.Abstr. (coverage dropped), Anal.Abstr., Biol.Abstr., CEABA, Chem.Abstr., Chem.Cit.Ind., Chem.Infd., Chem.Titles, Crop Physiol.Abstr., Curr.Adv.Ecol.Sci., Curr.Chem.React., Curr.Cont., Dairy Sci.Abstr., Dent.Ind., Derwent Biotech.Abstr., Excerp.Med., Field Crop Abstr., Forest.Abstr., Helminthol.Abstr., Herb.Abstr., Hort.Abstr., INIS Atomind., I.P.A., Ind.Chem., Ind.Med. (1946-), Ind.Sci.Rev., Ind.Vet., Inpharma, MOS, Mass Spectr.Bull., Mat.Sci.Cit.Ind. (coverage dropped), NPU, Nutr.Abstr., Pharm.&Out.News, Plant Breed.Abstr., Plant Grow.Reg.Abstr., Postharvest, Protozool.Abstr., RCI, Reac., Ref.Zh., Rev.Appl.Entomol., Rev.Arom.& Med.Plants, Rev.Med.& Vet.Mycol., Sci.Cit.Ind., Seed Abstr., Sugar Ind.Abstr., Weed Abstr.
—BLDSC (6448.000000), CASDDS, CINDOC, CISTI, GNLM, IDS, Infotrieve, KNAW, Linda Hall. **CCC.**
Published by: Govi Verlag Pharmazeutischer Verlag GmbH, Carl Mannich Str 26, Eschborn 65760, Germany. TEL 49-6196-928262, FAX 49-6196-928203, dingermann@em.uni-frankfurt.de, t.fast@govi.aponet.de. Eds. Dr. Peter Pflegel, Dr. Theodor Dingermann. Adv. contact Hans Juergen Renn. Circ: 800.

615.19 DEU ISSN 0369-979X CODEN: PHZHAM
PHARMAZIE HEUTE; Beilage der Deutschen Apotheker Zeitung zur Fortbildung. Text in German. 1971. irreg., latest vol.3. **Document type:** *Journal, Trade.*
Related titles: ♦ Supplement to: Deutsche Apotheker Zeitung. ISSN 0011-9857.
Indexed: Chem.Abstr., Chem.Indus.Notes, Chem.Titles.
—CASDDS, GNLM, Infotrieve. **CCC.**
Published by: Deutscher Apotheker Verlag, Postfach 101061, Stuttgart 70009, Germany. TEL 49-711-2582-0, FAX 49-711-2582290, ptaheute@deutscher-apotheker-verlag.de, daz@deutscher-apotheker-verlag.de, http://www.deutscher-apotheker-verlag.de. Ed. Ernst Mutschler.

615 DEU ISSN 0048-3664 CODEN: PHUZBI
PHARMAZIE IN UNSERER ZEIT. Text in German. 1972. bi-m. EUR 154 in Europe; CHF 239 in Switzerland & Liechtenstein; USD 176 elsewhere; EUR 162 combined subscription in Europe for print and online eds.; CHF 251 combined subscription in Switzerland & Liechtenstein, for print and online eds.; USD 185 combined subscription elsewhere for print and online eds. (effective 2002). adv. bk.rev. charts, illus. reprint service avail. from ISI. *Refereed.* **Document type:** *Journal, Academic/Scholarly.* **Description:** Presents review articles pertinent to all areas of drug research.
Related titles: Online - full text ed.: ISSN 1615-1003. EUR 154 in Europe; CHF 239 in Switzerland & Liechtenstein; USD 176 elsewhere (effective 2002) (from Wiley InterScience).
Indexed: Agri.& Environ.Biotech.Abstr. (coverage dropped), Biol.Abstr., Chem.Abstr., Chem.Titles, Derwent Biotech.Abstr., Excerp.Med., Ind.Med. (1972-).
—BLDSC (6448.600000), CASDDS, CISTI, GNLM, Infotrieve, KNAW, Linda Hall. **CCC.**
Published by: (Deutsche Pharmazeutische Gesellschaft), Wiley - V C H, Postfach 101161, Weinheim 69451, Germany. FAX 49-6201-606-117, subservice@wiley-vch.de, http://www.wiley-vch.de/home/pharmuz. Ed. P Pachaly. R&P Claudia Rutz. Adv. contact M Schaefer. Circ: 9,300. **Subscr. in the Americas to:** John Wiley & Sons, Inc., Journals. TEL 44-1243-779777, 212-850-6645, FAX 212-850-6021; **Subscr. outisde Germany, Austria & Switzerland to:** John Wiley & Sons Ltd., Baffins Ln, Chichester, Sussex PO19 IUD, United Kingdom. TEL 44-1243-779777, FAX 44-1243-843232.

615 AUT
PHARMIG INFO. Text in German. 10/yr. adv. **Document type:** *Magazine, Trade.*
Address: Zieglergasse 5, Vienna 1072, Austria. TEL 43-1-5232956, FAX 43-1-52329519, office@pharmig.at, http://www.pharmig.at. Ed. Ruth Mayrhofer. R&P, Adv. contact Karin Vallaszkovits. Circ: 4,000.

615.1 USA
▼ **PHARMSCI.** Text in English. 1999. m. free per issue. adv. back issues avail. **Description:** Covers all areas of the pharmaceutical sciences on scientific advances in drug discovery, development and therapy.
Media: Online - full text.
Published by: American Association of Pharmaceutical Scientists, 150 King St, 2nd Fl, Alexandria, VA 22314-2747. TEL 703-548-3000, FAX 703-684-7349, hemenway@aaos.org, http://www.pharmsci.org/journal/. Ed. Wolfgang Sade. Adv. contact Don Hemenway.

615 IND ISSN 0379-556X CODEN: PMSDBB
PHARMSTUDENT. Text in English. 1952. a. USD 8. adv.
Indexed: Chem.Abstr., I.P.A.
—CASDDS.
Published by: Pharmaceutical Society, c/o Department of Pharmaceutics, Banaras Hindu University, Varanasi, Uttar Pradesh 221 005, India. Ed. J K Pandit. Circ: 600.

615 USA ISSN 1056-5671 CODEN: PPOFEL
PHASE III DRUG PROFILES; international journal of pharmaceuticals in clinical trials. Text in English. 1991. 10/yr. price varies. index. back issues avail. **Document type:** *Monographic series.* **Description:** Provides comprehensive information on drugs waiting approval by the FDA. Reviews the pharmacology, adverse effects, pharmacokinetics, dosage and administration, latest clinical data and anticipated cost for each drug.
Indexed: Excerp.Med. (1993-).
—EMDOCS, GNLM.
Published by: BIOMEGA Corporation, 191, Waukegan, IL 60093-2743. TEL 847-446-5511, FAX 847-446-5572, biomega@biomega.com. Ed. Donald L Barbeau.

615.1 NLD
PHUTURE SUPPLEMENT. Text in English. 1998. 2/yr., latest 2001. illus. 1 cols./p. *Refereed.* **Document type:** *Journal, Academic/Scholarly.* **Description:** Contains review and research articles and information on relevant topics in pharmaceutical science.
Published by: International Pharmaceutical Students Federation, Andries Bickerweg 5, The Hague 2517 JP, Netherlands. TEL 31-70-3021992, FAX 31-70-3021999, ipsf@ipsf.org, http://www.ipsf.org.

615 USA ISSN 1074-388X
PHYSICIAN ASSISTANTS' PRESCRIBING REFERENCE. Text in English. 1994. q. USD 32 (effective 2000). *Refereed.* **Document type:** *Monographic series.*
Published by: Prescribing Reference, Inc., 170 Broadway, Ste 1612, New York, NY 10038. TEL 212-766-7200, FAX 212-732-2360. Ed. Jeanette Murphy. Pub., R&P Mark E Bugni. Adv. contact Scott Bugni.

PHYSICIANS' DESK REFERENCE FOR NONPRESCRIPTION DRUGS AND DIETARY SUPPLEMENTS. see *MEDICAL SCIENCES*

615 USA ISSN 1043-3953
RM301.12
PHYSICIAN'S DRUG HANDBOOK. Text in English. 1989. irreg., latest vol.7, 1997. USD 39.95.
Published by: Springhouse Corporation (Subsidiary of: Lippincott Williams & Wilkins (Philadelphia)), 1111 Bethlehem Tpk, Springhouse, PA 19477. TEL 215-646-8700, 800-346-7844, FAX 215-646-4508. Pub. Matt Cahill.

615.1058 USA
PHYSICIAN'S THERAPEUTICS & DRUG ALERT. Text in English. 1996. m. USD 119 domestic; USD 149 foreign; USD 20 newsstand/cover (effective 2001). **Document type:** *Newsletter.*
Published by: American Health Consultants (Subsidiary of: Medical Economics Co., Inc.), 3525 Piedmont Rd, N E, 6 Piedmont Center, Ste 400, Atlanta, GA 30305. TEL 404-262-5476, 404-262-7436, 800-688-2421, FAX 404-262-7837, 800-284-3291, custserv@ahcpub.com, http://www.ahcpub.com.

615.1 FRA ISSN 0031-8876 CODEN: PHPHA6
PHYTIATRIE-PHYTHOPHARMACIE. Text in French. 4/yr. FRF 80.
Indexed: Agri.& Environ.Biotech.Abstr. (coverage dropped), Chem.Abstr., Field Crop Abstr., Helminthol.Abstr., Herb.Abstr., Hort.Abstr., Rev.Appl.Entomol., Rev.Plant Path., Soils & Fert.
—CASDDS.
Published by: (Societe Francaise de Phytiatrie et de Phytopharmacie), C.N.R.A., Route de St. Cyr, Versailles 78-, France.

PICTORIAL DIRECTORY OF SPOKANE PHYSICIANS. see *MEDICAL SCIENCES*

615 USA
PILLS-A-GO-GO; journal of pills. Text in English. 1991. 6/yr. USD 12. adv. **Document type:** *Newsletter.* **Description:** Covers any issue having to do with pharmaceuticals, especially in pill form, including legal, medical, technical developments, news and essays on pill advertising and manufacture, lists of pills known to be taken by famous or notorious public figures.
Published by: Jim Hogshire, Ed. & Pub., 1202 E Pike St, Seattle, WA 98122. TEL 206-328-1586.

615.7 AUT ISSN 1608-5523
▼ **PLACEBO.** Text in English. 2000. q. USD 75 domestic; USD 115 foreign; USD 35 newsstand/cover (effective 2001). adv. back issues avail. *Refereed.* **Document type:** *Journal, Academic/Scholarly.* **Description:** Publishes articles, case reports, reviews, and letters that improve communication in the understanding of placebo research.
Related titles: Online - full text ed.
Published by: V I C E R Publishing, PO Box 14, Vienna A-1097, Austria. TEL 43-676-9568085, FAX 43-676-9568086, vicer@vicer.org, http://www.vicer.org. Ed., R&P Roland Hofbauer. adv.: B&W page USD 1,700, color page USD 2,200. Circ: 1,000 (paid and controlled).

615 DEU ISSN 0032-0943
RS164 CODEN: PLMEAA
PLANTA MEDICA; journal of medicinal plant research. Text in English. 1935. 8/yr. EUR 579.20 domestic to institutions; EUR 589.80 in Europe to institutions; EUR 605.80 elsewhere to institutions; EUR 58 newsstand/cover (effective 2002). adv. bk.rev. charts, illus, tr.lit. index. *Refereed.* **Document type:** *Journal, Academic/Scholarly.*
Related titles: Microfiche ed.; Online - full text ed.: ISSN 1439-0221 (from Institute for Scientific Information).
Indexed: AMED, ASCA, AgBiotech, Agri.& Environ.Biotech.Abstr. (coverage dropped), Agricola, Agroforest.Abstr., Apic.Abstr., BBCI, Bibl.Agri., Biol.Abstr., CEABA, Chem.Abstr., Chem.Cit.Ind., Chem.Indus.Notes, Chem.Titles, Crop Physiol.Abstr., Curr.Adv.Ecol.Sci., Curr.Biotech.Abstr., Curr.Cont., Derwent Biotech.Abstr., Excerp.Med., Field Crop Abstr., Food Sci.& Tech.Abstr., Forest Prod.Abstr., Forest.Abstr., Helminthol.Abstr., Herb.Abstr., Hort.Abstr., INIS Atomind., I.P.A., Ind.Med. (1953-), Ind.Sci.Rev., Ind.Vet., Int.Abstr.Biol.Sci., Mass Spectr.Bull., NPU, Nutr.Abstr., Ornam.Hort., Plant Breed.Abstr., Plant Grow.Reg.Abstr., Postharvest, Poult.Abstr., Protozool.Abstr., Rev.Appl.Entomol., Rev.Arom.& Med.Plants, Rev.Med.& Vet.Mycol., Rev.Plant Path., Sci.Cit.Ind., Seed Abstr., Soyabean Abstr., Sugar Ind.Abstr., Weed Abstr.
—BLDSC (6524.100000), ADONIS, CASDDS, CISTI, GNLM, IDS, ingenta, Linda Hall. **CCC.**
Published by: (Gesellschaft fuer Arzneipflanzenforschung), Georg Thieme Verlag, Ruedigerstr 14, Stuttgart 70469, Germany. TEL 49-711-8931-0, FAX 49-711-8931298, plantamedica@thieme.de, leser.service@thieme.de, http://www.thieme.de/plantamedica/index.html. Ed. Adolf Nahrstedt. R&P Alessandra Kreibaum. Circ: 1,200.

PODRAVKA; znanstveno-strucni casopis. see *AGRICULTURE*

615.1 POL ISSN 1230-6002
CODEN: PJPAE3
POLISH JOURNAL OF PHARMACOLOGY. Text and summaries in English. 1949. bi-m. USD 150 (effective 1998). bk.rev. charts, illus. index. *Refereed.* **Document type:** *Academic/Scholarly.* **Description:** Covers original experimental studies in the field of pharmacology in its broadest sense.
Former titles (until 1992): Polish Journal of Pharmacology and Pharmacy (0301-0244); (until 1973): Dissertationes Pharmaceuticae et Pharmacologicae (0012-3870)
Related titles: Online - full text ed.: (from Institute for Scientific Information).
Indexed: Agri.& Environ.Biotech.Abstr. (coverage dropped), Anal.Abstr., Aqua.Sci.& Fish.Abstr., BBCI, Biol.Abstr., Chem.Abstr., Chem.Titles, Curr.Adv.Ecol.Sci., Curr.Chem.React. (coverage dropped), Curr.Cont. (coverage dropped), Derwent Biotech.Abstr., Environ.Sci.Poll.Mgmt., Excerp.Med., Helminthol.Abstr., INIS Atomind., I.P.A., Ind.Chem. (coverage dropped), Ind.Med. (1993-), Int.Abstr.Biol.Sci., NPU, Pollut.Abstr., Ref.Zh., Risk Abstr., Saf.Sci.Abstr.
—BLDSC (6543.671450), CASDDS, CISTI, EMDOCS, GNLM, ingenta, KNAW, Linda Hall.
Published by: Polska Akademia Nauk, Instytut Farmakologii, Ul Smetna 12, Krakow 31343, Poland. TEL 48-12-6374022, FAX 48-12-6374500. Ed. Wladyslaw Lason. Circ: 725. **Dist. by:** Ars Polona, Krakowskie Przedmiescie 7, Warsaw, Poland.

615 FRA ISSN 0181-1169
PORPHYRE; revue professionnelle des preparatrices, preparateurs en pharmacie, collaborateurs de l'officine et candidats aux examens. Text in French. 1949. m. FRF 350; FRF 387 foreign. adv. bk.rev.
Published by: Groupe Liaisons S.A., 1 av. Edouard Belin, Rueil Malmaison Cedex 92856, France. TEL 33-1-41299935, FAX 33-1-41299705. Ed. Alain Rabelle. Adv. contact Frank Denis. Circ: 14,641.

615.1 JPN ISSN 0044-0035
PRACTICAL PHARMACY/YAKKYOKU. Variant title: Journal of Practical Pharmacy. Text in Japanese. 1950. m. JPY 28,980 (effective 2000). adv. **Document type:** *Academic/Scholarly.*
Indexed: Chem.Abstr., GeoRef, I.P.A.
—CISTI.
Published by: Nanzando Co. Ltd., 4-1-11 Yushima, Bunkyo-ku, Tokyo 113-0034, Japan. TEL 81-3-5689-7868, FAX 81-3-5689-7869, nanzando@magical.egg.or.jp, http://nanzando.com. Ed., Adv. contact Hisao Nakamura. Pub., R&P Hajime Suzuki. Circ: 15,500.

615 GBR ISSN 0959-6682
PRESCRIBER. Text in English. 1990. s-m. GBP 81 domestic; GBP 110 in Europe; GBP 130 elsewhere; GBP 7.75 newsstand/cover. adv. back issues avail. *Refereed.* **Document type:** *Trade.*
Indexed: Inpharma, Pharm.&Out.News, Reac.
—BLDSC (6609.700100).
Published by: A & M Publishing Ltd., Alexandra House, First Fl, 1-5 Alexandra Terr., Guildford, Surrey GU1 3DA, United Kingdom. TEL 44-1483-534888, FAX 44-1483-33316, ampublishing@am-publishing.co.uk. Ed., R&P Tim Dean. Pub. Marc Eisenstadt. Adv. contact Tony Norrington. Circ: 21,000.

615 USA ISSN 1073-7219
PRESCRIBER'S LETTER. Text in English. 1994. m. USD 88. index. back issues avail. *Refereed.* **Document type:** *Newsletter.* **Description:** Advises prescribing physicians on current drug therapy, including drug interactions, proper drug use, trends in therapy, new research findings, and new drugs.
Published by: Therapeutic Research Center, 2453 Grand Canal Blvd, Ste A, Box 8190, Stockton, CA 95208. TEL 209-472-2240, FAX 209-472-2249. Ed. Sandra Harley Counts. Pub., R&P Jeff M Jellin.

615 USA ISSN 1051-4171
PRESCRIBING REFERENCE FOR OBSTETRICIANS AND GYNECOLOGISTS. Text in English. 1991. s-a. USD 28 (effective 2000). *Refereed.* **Document type:** *Monographic series.*
Published by: Prescribing Reference, Inc., 170 Broadway, Ste 1612, New York, NY 10038. TEL 212-766-7200, FAX 212-732-2360. Ed. Jeanette Murphy. Pub., R&P Mark E Bugni. Adv. contact Scott Bugni.

615 USA ISSN 1051-3280
PRESCRIBING REFERENCE FOR PEDIATRICIANS. Text in English. 1990. s-a. USD 28 (effective 2000). *Refereed.* **Document type:** *Monographic series.*
Published by: Prescribing Reference, Inc., 170 Broadway, Ste 1612, New York, NY 10038. TEL 212-766-7200, FAX 212-732-2360. Ed. Jeanette Murphy. Pub., R&P Mark E Bugni. Adv. contact Scott Bugni.

615 USA ISSN 1068-5324
CODEN: FRPBEK
PRESCRIPTION PHARMACEUTICALS AND BIOTECHNOLOGY: THE PINK SHEET. Text in English. 1939. w. USD 1,200 domestic; USD 1,325 foreign (effective 2001). adv. charts, illus, stat, tr.lit. back issues avail.; reprints avail. **Document type:** *Trade.* **Description:** Provides in-depth news and analysis about developments affecting prescription medicines.
Supersedes in part (in 1993): Prescription and O T C Pharmaceuticals: The Pink Sheet (0734-6514); Which was formerly (until 1982): F D C Reports. Ethical and O T C Pharmaceuticals (0272-913X)
Related titles: Online - full text ed.: (from Data-Star, The Dialog Corporation).
Indexed: Inpharma, P.N.I., Pharm.&Out.News, Reac.
—CASDDS, Infotrieve. **CCC.**
Published by: F-D-C Reports, Inc., 5550 Friendship Blvd, Ste One, Chevy Chase, MD 20815-7278. TEL 800-332-2181, FAX 301-664-7238, http://www.fdcreports.com. Ed. Michael McCaughan. R&P Laura Desimio. Adv. contact Michael Keville.

615 FRA ISSN 1167-7422
CODEN: PRINFU
PRESCRIRE INTERNATIONAL. Text in English. 1992. bi-m. FRF 600, USD 85 to individuals; FRF 1,500, USD 210 to institutions; FRF 300, USD 45 to students (effective 2001). *Refereed.* **Document type:** *Bulletin.* **Description:** For health professionals concerned with therapeutics and medical evaluation.
Related titles: Online - full text ed.: (from Institute for Scientific Information); ♦ International ed.: La Revue Prescrire. ISSN 0247-7750.
Indexed: I.P.A., Inpharma, Pharm.&Out.News, Reac.
—BLDSC (6609.709200), EMDOCS, GNLM, IDS, Infotrieve. **CCC.**
Published by: Association Mieux Prescrire, B.P. 459, Paris Cedex 11 75527, France. TEL 33-1-49237265, FAX 33-1-48065237, international@prescrire.org. Ed. Christophe Kopp. R&P E Hoen. Circ: 500.

PREVENTION OF FOOD ADULTERATION CASES. see *LAW*

PREVISIONS GLISSANTES DETAILLEES EN PERSPECTIVES SECTORIELLES (VOL.22): PARACHIMIE. see *BUSINESS AND ECONOMICS—Economic Situation And Conditions*

615.1 NLD ISSN 1380-1775
PRIMA FARMA. Text in Dutch. 1994. m. (11/yr.). free per issue to qualified personnel. adv. **Document type:** *Trade.* **Description:** Provides pharmacists with drugstore and pharmacology news.
Published by: Elsevier Gezondheidszorg B.V., Tijdstroom (Subsidiary of: Reed Elsevier plc Group), Planetenbaan 1, Maarssen 3600 AK, Netherlands. TEL 31-346-577577, FAX 31-346-544287, http://www.tijdstroom.nl. **Subscr. to:** Elsevier Den Haag, Postbus 16500, The Hague 2500 BM, Netherlands. TEL 31-70-381-9900, FAX 31-70-333-8399.

615.7 USA ISSN 1061-0359
PRIMARY CARE MEDICINE DRUG ALERTS. Text in English. m., latest vol.22. USD 67 domestic; USD 83 in Canada; USD 91 elsewhere (effective 2001). index. 8 p./no. back issues avail. **Document type:** *Newsletter.* **Description:** Contains abstracts of journal articles regarding pharmacology and pharmacotherpy in a primary care setting.
Incorporates (1988-1991): Cardiovascular Drug Alerts (0897-3830); Incorporates: Women's Medicine Alerts; Formed by the Jan. 1992 merger of: Physicians Drug Alert; Drug Alerts for Internal Medicine
Published by: M.J. Powers & Co. Publishers, 65 Madison Ave Ste 220, Morristown, NJ 07960-6088. TEL 973-898-1200, FAX 973-898-1201, mjpcn@alertpubs.com, psych@alertpubs.com, http://www.alert[pubs.com, http://www.alertpubs.com. Ed. Trish Elliott. Pub. Michael Powers.

615 GBR ISSN 1469-1426
▼ **PRIMARY CARE PHARMACY.** Text in English. 1999. q. GBP 55 domestic to non-members; GBP 65 in the European Union to non-members; GBP 76 elsewhere to non-members; GBP 20 domestic to members; GBP 32 in the European Union to members; GBP 38 elsewhere to members (effective 2001). adv. back issues avail. **Document type:** *Magazine, Trade.* **Description:** Designed to give insight into the range of role models where pharmacists can provide input at different levels, from strategic planning to hands on service provision at patient level.
Related titles: Online - full text ed.: (from RoweCom Information Quest).
Published by: Pharmaceutical Press (Subsidiary of: Euromed Communications Ltd.), 1 Lambeth High St, London SE1 7JN, United Kingdom. TEL 44-20-7735-9141, FAX 44-20-7582-7327, primarycare@pharmj.org.uk, editor@pharmj.org.uk, http://www.pharmj.com. Ed. Sheena Macgregor. Adv. contact Jack Richmond. Circ: 4,240.

PROCHEM. see *ENGINEERING—Chemical Engineering*

PRODUCT ALERT. see *FOOD AND FOOD INDUSTRIES*

PRODUCT MANAGEMENT TODAY. see *BUSINESS AND ECONOMICS—Marketing And Purchasing*

344.04233 USA
PRODUCTS LIABILITY: PHARMACEUTICAL DRUG CASES. Text in English. 1988. irreg. USD 95 (effective 1995). Supplement avail. **Document type:** *Trade.*
Published by: Shepard's (Subsidiary of: Reed Elsevier plc), 555 Middle Creek Pkwy, Colorado Springs, CO 80921. TEL 800-743-7393, customer_service@shepards.com, http://www.shepards.com. Eds. Alexander E Slaughter, Donald E Vinson.

P

615.7 CHE ISSN 1011-0267
CODEN: PBCPET
PROGRESS IN BASIC AND CLINICAL PHARMACOLOGY. Text in English. 1988. irreg., latest vol.11. CHF 280 in Europe; DEM 335 in Germany; USD 240 in United States (effective 2001). *Refereed.* **Document type:** *Academic/Scholarly.* **Description:** Designed to promote a rational approach to drug treatment.
Related titles: Online - full text ed.: (from Institute for Scientific Information).
Indexed: Chem.Abstr., Chem.Indus.Notes, Chem.Titles.
—BLDSC (6865.955500), CASDDS, KNAW. **CCC.**
Published by: S. Karger AG, Allschwilerstr 10, PO Box, Basel 4009, Switzerland. TEL 41-61-306-1111, FAX 41-61-306-1234, karger@karger.ch, http://www.karger.com/bookseries/PRBCP.

615 CHE ISSN 0079-6085
CODEN: PBPHAW
PROGRESS IN BIOCHEMICAL PHARMACOLOGY. Text in English. 1965. irreg., latest vol.25. price varies. back issues avail.; reprint service avail. from ISI. *Refereed.* **Document type:** *Monographic series, Academic/Scholarly.* **Description:** Volumes in this series consider drugs as the therapeutic agents and curative measures for dealing with various conditions of human health.
Related titles: Online - full text ed.: (from Institute for Scientific Information).
Indexed: ASCA, BBCI, Biol.Abstr., Chem.Abstr., Chem.Titles, Curr.Cont. (coverage dropped), Ind.Med. (coverage dropped).
—BLDSC (6865.960000), CASDDS, CISTI, GNLM, Linda Hall. **CCC.**
Published by: S. Karger AG, Allschwilerstr 10, PO Box, Basel 4009, Switzerland. TEL 41-61-306-1111, FAX 41-61-306-1234, karger@karger.ch, http://www.karger.com/bookseries/PRBIP. Ed. R Paoletti. **Subscr. to:** S Karger Publishers Inc.

615 USA ISSN 0278-5846
RM315 CODEN: PNPPD7
PROGRESS IN NEURO-PSYCHOPHARMACOLOGY AND BIOLOGICAL PSYCHIATRY. Text in English. 1977. 8/yr. EUR 255 in Europe to individuals; JPY 33,800 in Japan to individuals; USD 285 elsewhere to individuals; EUR 1,366 in Europe to institutions; JPY 181,400 in Japan to institutions; USD 1,527 elsewhere to institutions (effective 2002). bk.rev. abstr. index. *Refereed.* **Document type:** *Academic/Scholarly.* **Description:** Aims to assure rapid publication of authoritative reviews and research papers dealing with experimental and clinical aspects of neuro-psychopharmacology and biological psychiatry.
Formerly: Progress in Neuro-Psychopharmacology (0364-7722)

Related titles: Microfilm ed.: (from PQC); Online - full text ed.: (from ingenta, Swets Blackwell, Institute for Scientific Information, ScienceDirect).
Indexed: ASCA, Biol.Abstr., Chem.Abstr., Chem.Titles, Curr.Adv.Ecol.Sci., Curr.Cont., Dent.Ind., Derwent Biotech.Abstr., Environ.Sci.Poll.Mgmt., Excerp.Med., Focus on: Psychophar., Ind.Med. (1982-), Ind.Sci.Rev., Indian Psychol.Abstr., Inpharma, Int.Abstr.Biol.Sci., Neurosci.Abstr., Neurosci.Cit.Ind., Pharm.&Out.News, PsycInfo, Psychol.Abstr. (1977-), Reac., Ref.Zh., Risk Abstr., SSCI (coverage dropped), Saf.Sci.Abstr., Sci.Cit.Ind., THA, e-psyche.
—BLDSC (6870.380000), ADONIS, CASDDS, CISTI, EMDOCS, GNLM, IDS, ingenta, KNAW. **CCC.**
Published by: Elsevier Science, PO Box 945, New York, NY 10159-0945. TEL 212-989-5800, FAX 212-633-3990, usinfo-f@elsevier.com, http://www.elsevier.com/locate/pnpbp. Ed. P Bedard. Circ: 1,000. **Subscr. in Australasia and the Far East to:** Elsevier Science (Singapore) Pte Ltd, No.1 Temasek Ave, 17-01 Millenia Tower, Singapore 039192, Singapore. TEL 65-434-3727, FAX 65-337-2230; **Subscr. in Japan to:** Elsevier Science Inc - Japan Regional Office, 9-15 Higashi-Azabu 1-chome, Minato-ku, Tokyo 106-0044, Japan. TEL 81-3-5561-5033; **Subscr. outside the Americas to:** Elsevier Science BV, PO Box 211, Amsterdam 1000 AE, Netherlands. TEL 31-20-485-3757.

PROTEASE INHIBITOR REFERENCE. see *BIOLOGY—Biochemistry*

615.9 CAN
PROVINCIAL DRUG BENEFIT PROGRAMS. Text in English. s-a. CND 275 to non-members; CND 220 to members. **Document type:** *Trade.*
Published by: Canadian Pharmacists Association, 1785 Alta Vista Dr, Ottawa, ON K1G 3Y6, Canada. TEL 613-523-7877, FAX 613-523-0445, cpha@cdnpharm.ca, http://www.cdnpharm.ca.

615 UKR
PROVIZOR. Text in Russian, Ukrainian. s-m. USD 225 in North America (effective 2000). adv. pat, charts, stat, illus, mkt. Index. back issues avail. **Document type:** *Journal, Academic/Scholarly.* **Description:** Covers different issues in pharmaceutical sciency and industry.
Related titles: Online - full content ed.
Published by: Megapolis, Pr-t Lenina 40, Khar'kov 61166, Ukraine. pro_adv@mega.kharkiv.com, http;//www.provizor.kharkov.ua. adv.: color page USD 2,250. **Dist. by:** East View Publications, 3020 Harbor Ln N, Minneapolis, MN 55447. TEL 763-550-0961, FAX 763-559-2931.

PSORIASIS RESOURCE. see *MEDICAL SCIENCES—Dermatology And Venereology*

615 USA ISSN 0894-4873
PSYCHIATRY DRUG ALERTS. Text in English. 1986. m. USD 67 domestic to individuals; USD 83 in Canada to individuals; USD 91 elsewhere to individuals (effective 2001). 8 p./no. **Document type:** *Newsletter.*
Indexed: e-psyche.
Published by: M.J. Powers & Co. Publishers, 65 Madison Ave Ste 220, Morristown, NJ 07960-6088. TEL 973-898-1200, FAX 973-898-1201, psych@alertpubs.com, http://www.alertpubs.com. Ed. Trish Elliott. Pub. Michael Powers.

615.1 DEU ISSN 0033-3158
RM315 CODEN: PSCHDL
PSYCHOPHARMACOLOGY. Text mainly in English. 1959. 24/yr. EUR 3,541.70 domestic; EUR 3,503.50 in Germany; EUR 172.50 newsstand/cover foreign (effective 2002). adv. charts, illus. back issues avail.; reprint service avail. from ISI. *Refereed.* **Document type:** *Journal, Academic/Scholarly.* **Description:** Original research into the effects of drugs on behavior.
Formerly (until vol.47, 1976): Psychopharmacologia
Related titles: Microform ed.: (from PQC); Online - full text ed.: ISSN 1432-2072 (from EBSCO Publishing, RoweCom Information Quest, Swets Blackwell, Springer LINK, Institute for Scientific Information).
Indexed: Addic.Abstr., Agri.& Environ.Biotech.Abstr. (coverage dropped), Anim.Behav.Abstr., Biol.Abstr., Biotech.& Bioeng.Abstr., Chem.Abstr., Chem.Titles, Chemorec.Abstr., Curr.Adv.Ecol.Sci., Curr.Cont., Derwent Biotech.Abstr., Excerp.Med., Focus on: Psychophar., Ind.Med. (1976-), Ind.Sci.Rev., Inpharma, Jrnl.Watch Psych., Neurosci.Abstr., Neurosci.Cit.Ind., Pharm.&Out.News, PsycInfo, Psychol.Abstr. (1965-), Reac., SSCI (coverage dropped), Sci.Cit.Ind., THA, e-psyche.
—BLDSC (6946.546500), ADONIS, CASDDS, CINDOC, CISTI, GNLM, IDS, ingenta, KNAW, Linda Hall. **CCC.**
Published by: Springer-Verlag (Subsidiary of: BertelsmannSpringer), Tiergartenstr 17, Heidelberg 69121, Germany. TEL 49-6221-345-0, FAX 49-6221-345229, subscriptions@springer.de, http://link.springer.de/link/service/journals/00213/index.htm, http://www.springer.de. Eds. J Gerlach, P J Cowen. **Subscr. in N. America to:** Springer-Verlag New York Inc., PO Box 2485, Secaucus, NJ 07096-2485. TEL 212-460-1500, FAX 212-473-6272.

615.1 150 USA ISSN 0048-5764
RM1 CODEN: PSYBB9
PSYCHOPHARMACOLOGY BULLETIN. Text in English. 1959. q. (plus special biennial no.). USD 21 domestic; USD 26.25 foreign; USD 16 newsstand/cover (effective 2000). cum.index: 1969-1975. back issues avail.; reprint service avail. from PQC. *Refereed.* **Document type:** *Bulletin, Government.* **Description:** Provides up-to-date and otherwise inaccessible information on ongoing psychopharmacological research and alerts readers to places and proceedings of national and international meetings.
Related titles: Microform ed.: (from PQC); Online - full text ed.: (from National Library of Medicine, ProQuest Information & Learning).
Indexed: ASCA, Addic.Abstr., AgeLine, Agri.& Environ.Biotech.Abstr. (coverage dropped), Biol.Abstr., Chem.Abstr., Chem.Indus.Notes, Chem.Titles, Curr.Adv.Ecol.Sci., Curr.Cont. (coverage dropped), Derwent Biotech.Abstr., Documentatieblad, Excerp.Med., Focus on: Psychophar. (coverage dropped), I.P.A., Ind.Med. (until 1999, dropped), Ind.Sci.Rev., Ind.U.S.Gov.Per., Indian Psychol.Abstr., Inpharma, Jrnl.Watch Psych., MEDOC, Neurosci.Cit.Ind., PsycInfo, Psychol.Abstr. (1990-), Reac., SSCI (coverage dropped), Sci.Cit.Ind. (coverage dropped), THA, e-psyche.
—CASDDS, CISTI, GNLM, IDS, ingenta, Linda Hall.
Published by: (Alcohol, Drug Abuse, and Mental Health Administration), U.S. Public Health Service, 5600 Fishers Ln, Rockville, MD 20857. TEL 301-496-4000. Circ: 3,500. **Subscr. to:** U.S. Government Printing Office, Superintendent of Documents.

615.1 USA
PSYCHOPHARMACOLOGY UPDATE. Text in English. 1990. m., latest vol.12, 2001. USD 167 domestic to individuals; USD 217 domestic to institutions; USD 227 in Canada to institutions; USD 237 elsewhere to institutions (effective 2001). 8 p./no. back issues avail.; reprints avail. *Refereed.* **Document type:** *Newsletter.* **Description:** Advises mental health professionals on treating behavioral disorders with pharmacological agents.
Related titles: E-mail ed.; Online - full text ed.: (from Gale Group, Factiva).
Indexed: e-psyche.
—CCC.
Published by: Manisses Communications Group, Inc., PO Box 9758, Providence, RI 02906-9758. TEL 401-831-6020, 800-333-7771, FAX 401-861-6370, manissescs@manisses.com, manissesCS@manisses.com, http://www.manisses.com. Ed. Stephen R Saklad. Pub. Betty R Lang. R&P Barbara Deekle.

615 DEU ISSN 0944-6877
PSYCHOPHARMAKOTHERAPIE; Rationale Pharmakotherapie psychischer Erkrankungen. Abbreviated title: P P T. Text in German. 1994. q. EUR 44.28 domestic; EUR 45.64 foreign; EUR 12 newsstand/cover (effective 2002). adv. *Refereed.* **Document type:** *Journal, Academic/Scholarly.*
Related titles: Online - full text ed.: (from Institute for Scientific Information).
Indexed: Excerp.Med., Focus on: Psychophar., Neurosci.Cit.Ind.
—BLDSC (6946.550600), GNLM, IDS, Infotrieve. **CCC.**
Published by: Wissenschaftliche Verlagsgesellschaft mbH, Postfach 101061, Stuttgart 70009, Germany. TEL 49-711-2582-0, FAX 49-711-2582-290, sheinzl@wissenschaftliche-verlagsgesellschaft.de, http://www.wissenschaftliche-verlagsgesellschaft.de. Ed. Susanne Heinzl. Adv. contact Klaus Graef TEL 49-711-2582245.

PULMONARY PHARMACOLOGY & THERAPEUTICS. see *MEDICAL SCIENCES—Respiratory Diseases*

615.1 USA ISSN 0033-4529
PURDUE PHARMACIST. Text in English. 1924. 3/yr. (Sep.-Jun.). free per issue. adv. cum.index: 1924-1935. **Description:** Alumni news from the Purdue University School of Pharmacy.
—Linda Hall.
Published by: Purdue University, School of Pharmacy, Lafayette, IN 47907. TEL 317-494-1363. Ed. Frank Murphy. Circ: 6,000.

615.1 PAK ISSN 0033-4790
Q I M P QUARTERLY. (Quick Index of Medical Preparations) Text in English. 1963. q. PKR 100, USD 25. adv.
Address: Salma Plaza, Mir Karam Ali Talpur Rd., Saddar, Karachi 0306, Pakistan. Ed. Dr. A H Qureshi. Circ: 4,000.

QUALITY ASSURANCE JOURNAL. see *MEDICAL SCIENCES*

615 USA ISSN 0163-2418
CODEN: QUCRB6
QUALITY CONTROL REPORTS: THE GOLD SHEET. Text in English. 1967. m. USD 485 domestic; USD 535 foreign (effective 2001). back issues avail.; reprints avail. **Document type:** *Trade.* **Description:** Focuses on important changes in the FDA's policies for regulating good manufacturing practices for pharmaceutical companies and their suppliers.
Related titles: Diskette ed.; Online - full text ed.: (from LexisNexis).
Indexed: P.N.I.
—Infotrieve. **CCC.**
Published by: F-D-C Reports, Inc., 5550 Friendship Blvd, Ste One, Chevy Chase, MD 20815-7278. TEL 800-332-2181, FAX 301-664-7238, http://www.fdcreports.com. Ed. William Paulson. R&P Laura Desimio.

615.19 DEU ISSN 0931-8771
RM301.42
QUANTITATIVE STRUCTURE-ACTIVITY RELATIONSHIPS. Abbreviated title: Q S A R. Text in English. 1982. bi-m. EUR 818 in Europe; CHF 1,378 in Switzerland & Liechtenstein; USD 1,078 elsewhere; EUR 859 combined subscription in Europe for print and online eds.; CHF 1,447 combined subscription in Switzerland & Liechtenstein, for print and online eds.; USD 1,132 combined subscription elsewhere for print and online eds. (effective 2002). adv. *Refereed.* **Document type:** *Journal, Academic/Scholarly.* **Description:** Interdisciplinary forum for contributions on molecular modelling, computer graphics and other computer-assisted methods helpful in the design and development of biologically active compounds as applied to medicinal, agricultural and environmental chemistry.
Formerly (until 1986): Quantitative Structure-Activity Relationships in Pharmacology, Chemistry and Biology (0722-3676)
Related titles: Online - full text ed.: ISSN 1521-3838. EUR 818 in Europe; CHF 1,378 in Switzerland & Liechtenstein; USD 1,078 elsewhere (effective 2002) (from EBSCO Publishing, Wiley InterScience, Institute for Scientific Information).
Indexed: ASCA, Chem.Abstr., Chem.Cit.Ind., Chem.Titles, Curr.Adv.Ecol.Sci., Curr.Cont., Derwent Biotech.Abstr., Ind.Sci.Rev., Inpharma, Int.Abstr.Biol.Sci., Reac., Rev.Appl.Entomol., Sci.Cit.Ind.
—BLDSC (7168.343000), CASDDS, CISTI, EMDOCS, GNLM, IDS, Infotrieve. **CCC.**
Published by: Wiley - V C H, Postfach 101161, Weinheim 69451, Germany. FAX 49-6201-606-117, subservice@wiley-vch.de, http://www.interscience.wiley.com. Eds. Ferenc Darvas, G Folkers, M Wiese. R&P Claudia Rutz. Circ: 930. **Subscr. in the Americas to:** John Wiley & Sons, Inc., Journals, 605 Third Ave, New York, NY 10158. TEL 44-1243-779777, 212-850-6645, FAX 212-850-6021; **Subscr. outside Germany, Austria & Switzerland to:** John Wiley & Sons Ltd., Baffins Ln, Chichester, Sussex PO19 IUD, United Kingdom. TEL 44-1243-779777, FAX 44-1243-843232.

615 FRA ISSN 0764-5104
QUOTIDIEN DU PHARMACIEN. Text in French. 1985. 100/yr. FRF 680 (effective 1999).
Published by: Societe d'Editions Scientifiques & Culturelles, 140 rue Jules Guesde, Levallois-Perret Cedex 92593, France. TEL 47307500, FAX 47307583. Ed. Jacques Gravier. Circ: 21,000.

615.1 USA
▼ **R A J EUROPE.** Text in English. 1999. m. GBP 1,050 in Europe; USD 2,192 in US & Canada; JPY 217,560 in Japan; GBP 1,190 rest of world (effective 2001); subscr. prices quoted for 1 user.. adv. **Document type:** *Trade.* **Description:** Provides the very latest documents to emerge from the regulatory authorities during the month prior to publication relating to human-use pharmaceuticals, veterinary medicinal products and medical devices.

Media: CD-ROM. **Related titles:** Diskette ed.
Published by: P J B Publications Ltd., Regulatory Affairs Journals Ltd., 18-20 Hill Rise, Richmond, Surrey TW10 6UA, United Kingdom. TEL 44-20-8948-3262, FAX 44-20-8332-8990, editors@raj.co.uk, info@pjbpubs.com, http://www.pjbpubs.co.uk/raj/europe/index.html, http://www.pjbpubs.com. Ed. Stewart Clarke. Adv. contact Sharon Clark.

615 GBR
R & D FOCUS. Text in English. 1978. w. GBP 3,670; includes Drug News and Meetings Diary. **Document type:** *Newsletter.*
Formerly: Drug License Opportunities
Related titles: CD-ROM ed.; Online - full text ed.: (from Data-Star, The Dialog Corporation).
Published by: IMSWORLD Publications Ltd., 7 Harewood Ave, London NW1 6JB, United Kingdom. TEL 0171-393-5000, FAX 0171-393-5900.

615.19 CHE ISSN 0748-6111
RADIOPHARMACY AND RADIOPHARMACOLOGY YEARBOOK SERIES. Text in English. 1985. irreg., latest vol.5. *Refereed.* **Document type:** *Monographic series.*
—GNLM.
Published by: Gordon and Breach - Harwood Academic (Subsidiary of: Taylor & Francis Group), PO Box 531, Lausanne 1000, Switzerland. Ed. P H Cox. **Subscr. addr. in US:** International Publishers Direct, PO Box 32160, Newark, NJ 07102. FAX 215-750-6343.

615.1 ESP ISSN 0034-0618
CODEN: ARAFAY
REAL ACADEMIA DE FARMACIA. ANALES. Text in English, French, Spanish; Summaries in English, French. 1932. q. ESP 6,500; ESP 8,500 foreign (effective 1998). bk.rev. bibl. index. back issues avail. *Refereed.* **Document type:** *Monographic series, Academic/Scholarly.*
Indexed: Biol.Abstr., Chem.Abstr., Chem.Indus.Notes, Chem.Titles, Curr.Adv.Ecol.Sci., Derwent Biotech.Abstr., Excerp.Med., GeoRef, I.P.A., Ind.Med. (coverage dropped), Ind.SST, Mass Spectr.Bull., Ref.Zh.
—BLDSC (0882.000000), CASDDS, CINDOC, CISTI, EMDOCS, GNLM, Infotrieve, KNAW. **CCC.**
Published by: Real Academia de Farmacia, Farmacia, 11, Madrid 28004, Spain. TEL 915-31-03-07, FAX 91-531-03-06. Ed. Antonio Portoles Alonso. Circ: 1,500.

615 GBR ISSN 0957-5545
CODEN: RACPD9
RECENT ADVANCES IN CLINICAL PHARMACOLOGY AND TOXICOLOGY. Text in English. irreg. **Document type:** *Monographic series, Academic/Scholarly.*
Formerly (until 1989): Recent Advances in Clinical Pharmacology (0143-8735)
—CASDDS, CISTI, GNLM.
Published by: Churchill Livingstone (Subsidiary of: Harcourt Publishers Ltd.), Robert Stevenson House, 1-3 Baxter's Pl, Leith Walk, Edinburgh, Midlothian EH1 3AF, United Kingdom. TEL 44-131-556-2424, FAX 44-131-459-1177, http://www.churchillmed.com. **US subscr. to:** Churchill Livingstone, 650 Ave of the Americas, New York, NY 10011. TEL 212-206-5000.

615 NLD ISSN 1381-3269
RECEPT MAGAZINE. Text in Dutch. 1994. m. (11/yr.). NLG 125, USD 110. bk.rev., software rev. illus. back issues avail.
Published by: Van Zuiden Communications B.V., Postbus 2122, Alphen aan den Rijn 2400 CC, Netherlands. TEL 31-172-476191, FAX 31-172-471882, 101617.2211@compuserve.com. Ed. J C F M Aghira. adv.: page NLG 3,600; trim 293 x 164. Circ: 8,000 (controlled).

615 NLD ISSN 0048-6914
RECEPTARIUS; maanduitgave van de bedrijfsgroep gezondheidszorg. Text in Dutch. 1907. m. NLG 60 (effective 1999). adv. bk.rev. back issues avail. **Document type:** *Trade.*
Published by: (Federatie Nederlandse Vakbeweging), F N V Bondgenoten, Postbus 9239, Amsterdam 1006 AE, Netherlands. TEL 31-3480-87752. Ed. Hilde Ter Doest. Circ: 4,000.

THE RECEPTORS. see *MEDICAL SCIENCES—Psychiatry And Neurology*

615 GBR ISSN 1351-0002
REDOX REPORT. Text in English. 1994. bi-m. GBP 126, USD 188 to individuals; GBP 292, USD 444 to institutions (effective 2002). bk.rev. back issues avail. *Refereed.* **Document type:** *Academic/Scholarly.* **Description:** Publishes reviews, research articles, hypotheses, debates, and correspondence on the role of free radicals, oxidative stress, activated oxygen, peroxidative, and redox processes, primarily in human biology and pathology.
Related titles: Online - full text ed.: (from Institute for Scientific Information).
Indexed: ASCA, BBCI, Chem.Abstr., Chem.Indus.Notes, Chem.Titles, Curr.Cont. (coverage dropped), Excerp.Med., Ind.Med. (1994-), Inpharma, Int.Abstr.Biol.Sci., Reac., Weed Abstr., Zoo.Rec.
—BLDSC (7331.315220).
Published by: Maney Publishing, Hudson Rd, Leeds, W Yorks LS9 7DL, United Kingdom. TEL 44-113-249-7481, FAX 44-113-248-6983, maney@maney.co.uk, http://www.maney.co.uk. Eds. J W Eaton, N H Hunt.

615 GBR ISSN 0960-7889
REGULATORY AFFAIRS JOURNAL. Abbreviated title: R A J. Text in English. 1990. m. GBP 890 in Europe for print ed. only; USD 1,635 in US & Canada for print ed. only; JPY 240,000 in Japan for print ed. only; GBP 960 rest of world for print ed. only; GBP 1,810 in Europe for CD-ROM & print eds.; USD 3,200 in US & Canada for CD-ROM & print eds.; JPY 548,000 in Japan for CD-ROM & print eds.; GBP 1,880 rest of world for CD-ROM & print eds. (effective 2001). adv. back issues avail.; reprints avail. *Refereed.* **Document type:** *Journal, Trade.* **Description:** Provides comprehensive coverage of licensing of pharmaceuticals for governments and the pharmaceutical industry worldwide.
Related titles: CD-ROM ed.
—BLDSC (7349.620000), GNLM.
Published by: P J B Publications Ltd., 18-20 Hill Rise, Richmond, Surrey TW10 6UA, United Kingdom. TEL 44-20-8948-3262, FAX 44-20-8332-8990, editors@raj.co.uk, info@pjbpubs.com, http://www.pjbpubs.com. Ed. Catherine Brunskill. Pub. Philip Brown. R&P Annette Watts TEL 44-20-8332-8961. Adv. contact Tom Jamison TEL 44-20-8332-8871. page GBP 600. **Subscr. addr. in N America:** Pharmabooks Ltd., 1775 Broadway, Ste 511, New York, NY 10019. TEL 212-262-8230, FAX 212-262-8234.

615 GBR ISSN 0969-4129
REGULATORY AFFAIRS JOURNAL. DEVICES. Abbreviated title: R A J Devices. Text in English. 1993. q. GBP 490 in Europe; USD 910 in US & Canada; JPY 133,000 in Japan; GBP 535 rest of world (effective 2001). back issues avail.; reprints avail. *Refereed.* **Document type:** *Trade.* **Description:** Provides comprehensive coverage of regulations affecting medical devices for governments and the medical device industry worldwide.
Related titles: CD-ROM ed.
—BLDSC (7349.620500).
Published by: P J B Publications Ltd., 18-20 Hill Rise, Richmond, Surrey TW10 6UA, United Kingdom. TEL 44-20-8948-3262, FAX 44-20-8332-8990, editors@raj.co.uk, info@pjbpubs.com, http://www.pjbpubs.com. Ed. Catherine Brunskill. Pub. Philip Brown. R&P Annette Watts TEL 44-20-8332-8961. Adv. contact Steve Day TEL 44-20-8332-8847. **Subscr. addr. in N America:** Pharmabooks Ltd., 1775 Broadway, Ste 511, New York, NY 10019. TEL 212-262-8230, FAX 212-262-8234.

615.1 GBR
REGULATORY AFFAIRS JOURNAL EUROPE. Abbreviated title: R A J Europe. Text in English. m. GBP 1,050 in Europe; USD 2,192 in US & Canada; JPY 217,560 in Japan; GBP 1,190 rest of world (effective 2001). reprints avail. **Description:** Provides a comprehensive archive of rules, regulations and guidelines that impact on the development, production, registration and sale of medicines in the EU - relating to human-use pharmaceuticals, veterinary medicinal products and medical devices.
Media: CD-ROM.
Published by: P J B Publications Ltd., 18-20 Hill Rise, Richmond, Surrey TW10 6UA, United Kingdom. TEL 44-20-8948-3262, FAX 44-20-8332-8990, info@pjbpubs.com, http://www.pjbpubs.com. Ed. Catherine Brunskill. Pub. Philip Brown. **Subscr. addr. in N America:** Pharmabooks Ltd., 1775 Broadway, Ste 511, New York, NY 10019. TEL 212-262-8230, FAX 212-262-8234.

REGULATORY TOXICOLOGY AND PHARMACOLOGY. see *ENVIRONMENTAL STUDIES—Toxicology And Environmental Safety*

REGULATORY WATCHDOG SERVICE. see *PUBLIC ADMINISTRATION*

RENIN, ANGIOTENSIN & KININS. see *BIOLOGY—Abstracting, Bibliographies, Statistics*

615.19 DEU ISSN 0179-8618
RESEARCH. Text in German. 1986. a. back issues avail. **Document type:** *Magazine, Academic/Scholarly.*
Related titles: ♦ Spanish ed.: Research. Spanish Edition. ISSN 1438-6747; English ed.: Research. English Edition. ISSN 0932-8394.
Published by: Bayer AG, Corporate Communications, Kaiser-Wilhelm-Allee, Leverkusen 51368, Germany. TEL 49-214-3058992, FAX 49-214-3071985, ute.bode.ub@bayer-ag.de, http://www.bayer.com. Ed. Ute Bode. Circ: 340,000.

615.19 157.6 616.8 USA ISSN 1080-8388
RC563 CODEN: RCAAE3
RESEARCH COMMUNICATIONS IN ALCOHOL & SUBSTANCES OF ABUSE. Text in English. 1980. q. USD 90; USD 105 foreign (effective 1998). adv. bk.rev. abstr. charts, illus. index. reprints avail. *Refereed.* **Document type:** *Academic/Scholarly.* **Description:** Focuses on clinical and human aspects of all abused substances: alcohol, drugs, and synthetic and natural substances.
Formerly (until 1994): Research Communications in Substances of Abuse (0193-0818)
Indexed: ASCA, Biol.Abstr., Chem.Abstr., Chem.Indus.Notes, Chem.Titles, Curr.Adv.Ecol.Sci., Curr.Cont. (coverage dropped), Excerp.Med., Int.Abstr.Biol.Sci., Sci.Cit.Ind. (coverage dropped).
—BLDSC (7736.400000), CASDDS, CISTI, GNLM, IDS, ingenta, KNAW. **CCC.**
Published by: P J D Publications Ltd, PO Box 966, Westbury, NY 11590. TEL 516-626-0650, FAX 516-626-5546. Ed. P D Wong.

RESEARCH COMMUNICATIONS IN MOLECULAR PATHOLOGY AND PHARMACOLOGY. see *MEDICAL SCIENCES*

615.19 DEU ISSN 1438-6747
RESEARCH. SPANISH EDITION. Text in Spanish. a. **Document type:** *Academic/Scholarly.*
Related titles: ♦ German ed.: Research. ISSN 0179-8618; English ed.: Research. English Edition. ISSN 0932-8394.
Published by: Bayer AG, Corporate Communications, Kaiser-Wilhelm-Allee, Leverkusen 51368, Germany. TEL 49-214-3058992, FAX 49-214-3071985, ute.bode.ub@bayer-ag.de, http://www.bayer.com.

615 USA ISSN 1061-6632
RESIDENTS' PRESCRIBING REFERENCE. Text in English. 1992. s-a. USD 28 (effective 2000). *Refereed.* **Document type:** *Monographic series.*
Published by: Prescribing Reference, Inc., 170 Broadway, Ste 1612, New York, NY 10038. TEL 212-766-7200, FAX 212-732-2360. Ed. Jeanette Murphy. Pub., R&P Mark E Bugni. Adv. contact Scott Bugni.

615 616.2 CHE
RESPIRATORY PHARMACOLOGY AND PHARMACOTHERAPY. Text in English. 1994. irreg. price varies. **Document type:** *Monographic series.*
Published by: Birkhaeuser Verlag AG (Subsidiary of: BertelsmannSpringer), Klosterberg, Postfach 133, Basel 4010, Switzerland. TEL 41-61-2050707, FAX 41-61-2050792, orders@birkhauser.ch, http://www.birkhauser.ch. Eds. D Raeburn, M Giembycz. **Dist. in N. America by:** Birkhauser, 333 Meadowlands Pkwy, Secaucus, NJ 07049-2491.

RESTORATIVE NEUROLOGY AND NEUROSCIENCE. see *MEDICAL SCIENCES—Psychiatry And Neurology*

615.1 658 AUS
RETAIL NEWS. Text in English. q. AUD 28; AUD 43 foreign (effective 1999). **Document type:** *Trade.*
Published by: Australian Pharmaceutical Publishing Co. Ltd., 40 Burwood Rd, Hawthorn, VIC 3122, Australia. TEL 61-3-9810-9800, FAX 61-3-9819-1706, appco@hcn.net.au, http://www.aapco.com.au.

615 AUS
RETAIL PHARMACY. Text in English. 1992. m. (except Jan.). AUD 50 domestic; AUD 60 foreign (effective 2000 - 2001). adv. **Description:** Provides general and industry news, and research material that relates to pharmacists and pharmaceutical industry. Includes case success stories of pharmacists and industry analyses.

P

Published by: Sterling Media, PO Box 6104, North Parramatta, NSW 2150, Australia. TEL 61-2-98901199, FAX 61-2-98907694. R&P John Allison. Adv. contact Jenifer Carter. page AUD 3,000. Circ: 7,124 (controlled).

615 USA
RETAIL PHARMACY MANAGEMENT NEWS. Text in English. m. USD 60 domestic; USD 70 foreign (effective 2001). **Document type:** *Trade.* **Description:** Covers front-end merchandising trends and clinical developments that have a direct impact on pharmacy operations.
Formerly: Retail Pharmacy News
Related titles: Online - full text ed.; Special ed.
Published by: McMahon Group, 545 W 45th St, 8th Fl, New York, NY 10036. TEL 212-957-5300, FAX 212-957-7230, dbron@mcmahonmed.com, http://www.retailpharmacynews.com/index.html, http://www.mcmahonmed.com. Ed. David Bronstein.

615.19 USA ISSN 1089-5302 CODEN: LRNSEP
REVIEW OF NATURAL PRODUCTS. Text in English. 1980. m. USD 159 (effective 2001). Supplement avail. **Document type:** *Trade.* **Description:** Provides referenced reviews of the history, chemistry, pharmacology and toxicity of natural products of medical, social and economic interest.
Formerly (until 1996): Lawrence Review of Natural Products (0734-4961)
Indexed: Biol.Abstr., I.P.A.
Published by: Facts and Comparisons, 111 W. Port Plaza, Ste. 300, St. Louis, MO 63146-3098. TEL 800-223-0554, FAX 314-878-5563.

615 GBR ISSN 0954-8602 CODEN: RCPHFW
REVIEWS IN CONTEMPORARY PHARMACOTHERAPY. Text in English. 1988. q. GBP 210 domestic; GBP 290, GBP 530 foreign (effective 2001). back issues avail. *Refereed.* **Document type:** *Academic/Scholarly.* **Description:** Presents an up-to-date and critical survey of the published work in important aspects of pharmacology.
Related titles: Online - full text ed.: (from Institute for Scientific Information).
Indexed: Curr.Cont., Inpharma, Pharm.&Out.News, Reac.
—BLDSC (7789.120000), CASDDS, GNLM, IDS, KNAW.
Published by: Marius Press, Marius Press, Over Kellet, PO Box 15, Carnforth, Lancs LA6 1HW, United Kingdom. TEL 44-1524-733027, FAX 44-1524-736659. Ed. S Johnson. R&P F N Johnson.

REVIEWS IN TOXICOLOGY. see *ENVIRONMENTAL STUDIES—Toxicology And Environmental Safety*

REVIEWS OF ENVIRONMENTAL CONTAMINATION AND TOXICOLOGY. see *ENVIRONMENTAL STUDIES—Toxicology And Environmental Safety*

REVIEWS OF PHYSIOLOGY, BIOCHEMISTRY AND PHARMACOLOGY. see *BIOLOGY—Physiology*

615.1 BRA ISSN 0370-372X CODEN: RBFAAH
REVISTA BRASILEIRA DE FARMACIA. Text in Portuguese; Summaries in English, Portuguese. 1920. q. USD 50. adv. charts, illus, stat. **Document type:** *Academic/Scholarly.* **Description:** Contains original papers in pharmacology and chemistry.
Former titles (until 1942): Associacao Brasileira de Farmaceuticos. Revista (0370-3126); (until 1937): Associacao Brasileira de Farmaceuticos. Boletim (0366-158X)
Indexed: Chem.Abstr., Chem.Titles, I.P.A., Rev.Arom.& Med.Plants.
—CASDDS, EMDOCS, GNLM.
Published by: (Associacao Brasileira de Farmaceuticos), Nuno Alvares Pereira Ed.& Pub., Rua dos Andradas, 96-Andar 10, Centro, Rio De Janeiro, RJ 20051-000, Brazil. FAX 55-21-2333672.

615.1 COL ISSN 0034-7418
RS402 CODEN: RCQFAQ
REVISTA COLOMBIANA DE CIENCIAS QUIMICO FARMACEUTICAS. Text in Spanish; Summaries in English. 1969. 2/yr. free per issue. illus. **Document type:** *Academic/Scholarly.*
Related titles: Online - full text ed.
Indexed: Biol.Abstr., Chem.Abstr., Chem.Indus.Notes, Chem.Titles, Excerp.Med., I.P.A.
—BLDSC (7851.401000), CASDDS.
Published by: Universidad Nacional de Colombia, Departamento de Farmacia, Apdo Aereo 14490, Bogota, Colombia. TEL 57-1-316-5045, rccqf@ciencias.ciencias.unal.edu.co. Ed. Jaime Rojas. Circ: 500.

615.1 CUB ISSN 0034-7515 CODEN: RCUFAC
REVISTA CUBANA DE FARMACIA. Text in Spanish; Summaries in English, Spanish. 1967. 3/yr. USD 34 in the Americas; USD 42 in Europe; USD 50 elsewhere. abstr, bibl, charts, illus. index. **Description:** Covers the fields of pharmacy, pharmacology and the drug industry.
Related titles: Online - full text ed.
Indexed: Chem.Abstr., Chem.Titles, Excerp.Med., Hort.Abstr., I.P.A., Ind.Med. (coverage dropped), Seed Abstr., Weed Abstr.
—CASDDS, CISTI, GNLM.
Published by: (Cuba. Ministerio de Salud Publica, Centro Nacional de Informacion de Ciencias Medicas), Editorial de Ciencias Medicas, O'Reilly No. 4, Habana, Cuba. TEL 809-62-8091. Ed. Ana Dolores del Campo. Circ: 1,300. **Co-sponsors:** Sociedad Cubana de Farmacia; Industria Medico-Farmaceutica de Cuba.

615.1 BRA ISSN 0101-3793 CODEN: RCIFDN
REVISTA DE CIENCIAS FARMACEUTICAS. Text in Portuguese. 1978. s-a. USD 30 (effective 2001); or exchange basis. charts, stat, abstr, bibl. back issues avail. *Refereed.* **Document type:** *Journal, Academic/Scholarly.* **Description:** Original articles, notes and technical reviews on clinical cases in all areas of pharmacology.
Formerly: Faculdade de Ciencias Farmaceuticas de Araraquara. Revista
Indexed: Anal.Abstr., Aqua.Sci.& Fish.Abstr., Biol.Abstr., Chem.Abstr., Chem.Indus.Notes, Chem.Titles, Environ.Sci.Poll.Mgmt., Excerp.Med., INIS Atomind., I.P.A., Protozool.Abstr., Ref.Zh.
—CASDDS, GNLM, KNAW.
Published by: Universidade Estadual Paulista, Ave. VICENTE FERREIRA, 1278, Centro, Caixa Postal 71, Marilia, SP 17515-901, Brazil. TEL 55-144-222504, FAX 55-144-222504, cgb@marilia.unesp.br. Ed. Luis Marcos da Fonseca. Circ: (controlled).

615.9 ESP ISSN 0212-7113 CODEN: REVTE9
REVISTA DE TOXICOLOGIA✱. Text in Spanish; Summaries in English. 1983. 3/yr. ESP 9,000 to non-members (effective 2001). adv. bk.rev. back issues avail. *Refereed.* **Document type:** *Journal, Academic/Scholarly.*
Indexed: Excerp.Med., Ind.SST, Int.Abstr.Biol.Sci.
—BLDSC (7873.150000), CASDDS, CINDOC, GNLM. **CCC.**
Published by: Asociacion Espanola de Toxicologia, c/o Centro de Ciencias Medioambientales, dpdo., Serrano, 115, Madrid 28006, Spain. TEL 34-91-7452500 ext 219, FAX 34-91-5640800, revista.toxicologia@coma.csic.es, http://www.tox.umh.es/aet/revista. Ed. Dr. Eduardo de la Pena de Torres. adv.: B&W page ESP 35,000, color page ESP 60,000. Circ: 800.

615.1 ARG ISSN 0034-9496 CODEN: RFABAN
REVISTA FARMACEUTICA. Text in Spanish. 1858. 12/yr. (in 6 double issues). USD 20. adv. bk.rev. bibl, charts, illus.
Related titles: Online - full text ed.
Indexed: Agri.& Environ.Biotech.Abstr. (coverage dropped), Biol.Abstr., Chem.Abstr., I.P.A., Ref.Zh.
—CASDDS, CISTI.
Published by: Academia Argentina de Farmacia y Bioquimica, Junin, 956, Capital Federal, Buenos Aires 1113, Argentina. Ed. Alfredo Jose Bandoni. Circ: 6,000.

615 MEX ISSN 1027-3956
REVISTA MEXICANA DE CIENCIAS FARMACEUTICAS. Text in Spanish, English. 1971. bi-m. free to members. **Document type:** *Journal, Magazine.*
—BLDSC (7866.240000).
Published by: Asociacion Farmaceutica Mexicana, A. C., Adolfo Prieto No. 1649-6to piso, Col. Del Valle, Mexico, D F 03100, Mexico. TEL 524-0993, 534-5397, FAX 534-5098, info@afmac.org.mx, http://www.afmac.org/. Ed. Emma D. Perez. Adv. contact Mario Trias TEL 669-1214. Circ: 3,500.

615 PRT ISSN 0484-811X CODEN: RPTFAU
REVISTA PORTUGUESA DE FARMACIA. Text in Portuguese; Summaries in English. 1951. q. PTE 7,500 domestic; USD 70 foreign (effective 2001). bk.rev. bibl, charts, stat. cum.index. back issues avail. **Document type:** *Academic/Scholarly.* **Description:** Presents original papers in pharmacy and pharmacology research.
Related titles: Online - full text ed.
Indexed: Agri.& Environ.Biotech.Abstr. (coverage dropped), Apic.Abstr., Biol.Abstr., Chem.Abstr., Chem.Indus.Notes, Chem.Titles, Food Sci.& Tech.Abstr., INIS Atomind., I.P.A., Mass Spectr.Bull., Sugar Ind.Abstr.
—BLDSC (7870.000000), CASDDS, CINDOC, CISTI, EMDOCS, GNLM, Linda Hall.
Published by: Ordem dos Farmaceuticos, Rua da Sociedade Farmaceutica, 18, Lisbon, Lisboa 1169-075, Portugal. TEL 351-21-3191370, FAX 351-21-3191399, dirnacional@ordemfarmaceuticos.pt, http://www.ordemfarmaceuticos.pt. Ed. Jose Aranda da Silv. R&P Ivana Silva. Circ: 1,500.

REVUE DE MEDECINES ET PHARMACOPEES AFRICAINES. see *MEDICAL SCIENCES*

615.1 FRA ISSN 0035-2349
REVUE D'HISTOIRE DE LA PHARMACIE. Text in French. 1913. q. FRF 540 (effective 2000). adv. bk.rev. abstr, illus, bibl. index, cum.index: 1913-1963, 1964-1983. **Document type:** *Academic/Scholarly, Bibliography.*
Indexed: I.P.A.
—GNLM.
Published by: Societe d'Histoire de la Pharmacie, 4 av. de l' Observatoire, Paris Cedex 6 75270, France. Ed. Thierry Lefebvre. Circ: 1,400.

615 610 FRA ISSN 0247-7750
LA REVUE PRESCRIRE. Text in French. 1980. m. (11/yr). FRF 1,200, EUR 182.94 to individuals; FRF 2,700, EUR 411.61 to institutions; FRF 600, EUR 91.47 to students (effective 2001). **Document type:** *Bulletin.*
Related titles: ♦ International ed. of: Prescrire International. ISSN 1167-7422.
—BLDSC (7943.440000).
Published by: Association Mieux Prescrire, 83 bd. Voltaire, Paris 75011, France. TEL 33-1-49237265, 33-1-49237280, FAX 33-1-48065237, revue@prescrire.org. Ed. Gilles Bardelay. Pub. Philippe Schilliger.

615.9 ITA ISSN 0390-6019 CODEN: RTSCDD
RIVISTA DI TOSSICOLOGIA SPERIMENTALE E CLINICA. Text in Italian. 1971. bi-m. ITL 66,000; ITL 132,000 foreign.
Formerly (until 1975): Rivista di Clinica Tossicologica (0390-6027)
Indexed: Biol.Abstr., Chem.Abstr., Chem.Indus.Notes, Chem.Titles, Excerp.Med.
—CASDDS, CISTI, GNLM.
Published by: (Centro Italiano Contro le Intossicazioni), Societa Editrice Universo, Via Giovanni Battista Morgagni, 1, Rome, RM 00161, Italy. Ed. Enrico Malizia.

615 DEU
ROTE LISTE. Text in German. 1935. a. DEM 119.31, EUR 61 (effective 2001). **Document type:** *Directory, Trade.* **Description:** Provides a comprehensive survey on drugs made in Germany from a pharmacological-therapeutic view as well as regarding the preparations, package sizes and prices.
Related titles: CD-ROM ed.: DEM 119.31, EUR 61 (effective 2001).
Published by: (Verbaende der Pharmazeutischen Industrie in Deutschland), Editio Cantor Verlag, Postfach 1255, Aulendorf 88322, Germany. TEL 49-7525-940145, FAX 49-7525-940147, info@ecv.de, http://www.ecv.de. Circ: 280,000.

615.9 RUS ISSN 1026-3241
RUSSIAN JOURNAL OF EXPERIMENTAL AND CLINICAL PHARMACOLOGY. Text in Russian. 1996. 4/yr. USD 248 domestic. index. **Document type:** *Academic/Scholarly.*
Related titles: ♦ Translation of: Eksperimental'naya i Klinicheskaya Farmakologiya. ISSN 0869-2092.
Published by: (Russian Academy of Medical Sciences), Izdatel'stvo Folium, Dmitrovskoe shosse 58, Moscow 127474, Russian Federation. TEL 7-095-482-5590, FAX 7-095-482-5590, jour@folium.msk.su, http://www.folium.ru/ecp/home.htm. Ed. D A Kharkevich. Circ: 80,000.

615 ZAF
S A PHARMACEUTICAL JOURNAL. Text in English. 1980. 10/yr. ZAR 75, USD 80 (effective 1995). adv. 64 p./no. 3 cols./p. back issues avail. *Refereed.* **Document type:** *Journal, Trade.* **Description:** Contains management and clinical articles written by South African specialists.
Formerly (until 2000): Pharmacy Management (1015-1362)
Indexed: I.P.A.
—BLDSC (6447.451000), GNLM.
Published by: Medpharm Publications, PO Box 786, Irene 0062, South Africa. TEL 27-12-664-5738, FAX 27-12-6646355, medpharm@iafrica.com, medpharm@shibbolet.co.za. Ed. Lorraine Osman. Pub., R&P Rene' F S Smulders. Adv. contact Sandy Barnarot. Circ: 6,500.

615 ZAF ISSN 1018-1474
S A RETAIL CHEMIST. Text in English; Text occasionally in Afrikaans. 1951. m. ZAR 91.20; ZAR 160 foreign (effective 1997). adv. bk.rev. illus. **Document type:** *Trade.* **Description:** Information of interest to all retail pharmacies in South Africa.
Formerly: South African Retail Chemist (0038-2639)
Indexed: I.P.A.
Published by: George Warman Publications (Pty.) Ltd., PO Box 704, Cape Town 8000, South Africa. TEL 27-21-24-5320, FAX 27-21-26-1332. Ed. Loren Kolevsohn. Circ: 4,100.

615 ITA ISSN 0081-0703
S.I.S.F. DOCUMENTI. Text in Italian. 1965. irreg. price varies. **Document type:** *Monographic series.*
Published by: Societa Italiana di Scienze Farmaceutiche, Viale Abruzzi, 32, Milan, MI 20131, Italy. TEL 39-02-29513303, FAX 39-02-29520179. Ed. Piero Sensi.

615.1 FRA ISSN 1157-1489
CODEN: STSSE5
S T P PHARMA SCIENCES. (Sciences Techniques Pratiques) Text in French; Summaries in English. 1953. 6/yr. FRF 900; FRF 950 foreign. bk.rev. charts, illus. index. *Refereed.*
Supersedes in part (in 1991): S T P Pharma (0758-6922); Former titles: Labo - Pharma Problems et Techniques (0458-5747); Labo-Pharma (0023-6470); Incorporating: Catalogue des Theses de Pharmacie Soutenues en France (0069-4665)
Related titles: Online - full text ed.: 1953 (from Institute for Scientific Information).
Indexed: ASCA, Agri.& Environ.Biotech.Abstr. (coverage dropped), Anal.Abstr., Chem.Abstr., Chem.Indus.Notes, Chem.Titles, Curr.Cont., Excerp.Med., INIS Atomind., I.P.A., Ind.Sci.Rev., Inpharma, Pharm.&Out.News, Reac., Ref.Zh., Rev.Med.& Vet.Mycol., Sci.Cit.Ind.
—BLDSC (8467.295000), CASDDS, CISTI, EMDOCS, GNLM, Infotrieve, KNAW, Linda Hall. **CCC.**
Published by: Editions de Sante, 49, rue Galilee, Paris 75116, France. TEL 1-40-701615, FAX 1-40-701614, editiondesante@editiondesante.com, http://www.editiondesante.fr. Ed. Dominique Dupont. Circ: 2,000.

615 JPN
SAIKIN NO SHINYAKU/NEW DRUGS IN JAPAN. Text in Japanese. 1950. a., latest vol.48. JPY 4,515 (effective 2001). adv. back issues avail. **Document type:** *Government.* **Description:** Description of old and new drugs marketed in Japan.
Published by: Yakuji Nippo Ltd., 1 Kanda-Izumi-cho, Chiyoda-ku, Tokyo 101-8648, Japan. TEL 81-3-3862-2141, FAX 81-3-3866-8495, shuppan@yakuji.co.jp, http://www.yakuji.co.jp/. Circ: 20,000.

615.19 JPN ISSN 1341-741X
CODEN: SKKNAJ
SANKYO RESEARCH LABORATORIES. ANNUAL REPORT. Text in English. 1946. a. free per issue. abstr. reprint service avail. from PQC. *Refereed.* **Document type:** *Corporate.*
Former titles (until 1991): Sankyo Kenkyusho Nempo (0080-6064); (until 1963): Takamine Kenkyujo Nenpo (0371-8670)
Indexed: Biol.Abstr., Chem.Abstr., INIS Atomind., Ref.Zh.
—BLDSC (1430.050000), CASDDS, KNAW.
Published by: Sankyo Co. Ltd., Research Institute/Sankyo K.K. Sogo Kenkyujo, 1-2-58 Hiro-Machi, Shinagawa-ku, Tokyo 140-0005, Japan. TEL 81-3-3492-3131, FAX 81-3-5436-7066, library@shina.sankyo.co.jp, http://www.sankyo.co.jp. Ed., R&P Tetsuo Hiraoka.

SASKATCHEWAN DRUG PLAN AND EXTENDED BENEFITS BRANCH. ANNUAL STATISTICAL REPORT. see *PHARMACY AND PHARMACOLOGY—Abstracting, Bibliographies, Statistics*

615.19 574.28 DEU
SCHERING ANNUAL REPORT (YEAR). Text in English. a. **Document type:** *Corporate.*
Related titles: German ed.
Published by: Schering AG, Corporate Communications, Muellerstr 178, Berlin 13342, Germany. TEL 49-30-4681111, FAX 49-30-46815896, TELEX 18203-0-SCH-D, http://www.schering.de.

615.1071 USA
SCHOOLS IN THE UNITED STATES AND CANADA OFFERING GRADUATE EDUCATION IN PHARMACOLOGY. Text in English. 1963. biennial. free. **Document type:** *Directory.*
Published by: American Society for Pharmacology and Experimental Therapeutics (ASPET), 9650 Rockville Pike, Bethesda, MD 20814-3998. Ed. Christine K Carrico.

615.1 CHE ISSN 1420-4932
CODEN: SAZTA8
SCHWEIZER APOTHEKERZEITUNG/GIORNALE SVIZZERO DI FARMACIA/JOURNAL SUISSE DE PHARMACIE. Text in German. 1863. s-m. CHF 170 domestic; CHF 200 foreign (effective 2000). adv. bk.rev. **Document type:** *Newspaper, Trade.*
Formerly (until 1994): Schweizerische Apotheker-Zeitung (0036-7508)
Indexed: Agri.& Environ.Biotech.Abstr. (coverage dropped), Biol.Abstr., Chem.Abstr., Excerp.Med., I.P.A.
—BLDSC (8108.900000), CASDDS, GNLM, KNAW, Linda Hall.
Published by: Schweizerischer Apothekerverein, Postfach, Bern-Liebefeld CH-3097, Switzerland. TEL 41-31-9785858, FAX 41-31-9785859, http://verlag.hanshuber.com. Ed. Markus Kamber. adv.: B&W page CHF 1,548, color page CHF 2,648; trim 297 x 210. Circ: 6,400.

615 CHE ISSN 0258-6983
SCHWEIZER HAUSAPOTHEKE. Text in German. 1930. 9/yr. CHF 18.75. adv. **Document type:** *Trade.*
Published by: Perpress Medien AG, Industriestr 5, Boesingen 3178, Switzerland. TEL 41-31-7409700, FAX 41-31-7409728. Ed. Silvia Felber. Adv. contact Christoph Tshang. B&W page CHF 13,770, color page CHF 16,799. Circ: 325,000.

615.1 AUT ISSN 0036-8709
CODEN: SCPHA4
SCIENTIA PHARMACEUTICA. Text in German. 1932. q. ATS 303 (effective 1998). adv. bk.rev. charts. index. **Document type:** *Academic/Scholarly.* **Description:** Covers all scientific aspects of pharmacy and related disciplines.
Related titles: Online - full text ed.
Indexed: Agri.& Environ.Biotech.Abstr. (coverage dropped), Anal.Abstr., Biol.Abstr., Chem.Abstr., Chem.Indus.Notes, Chem.Titles, Derwent Biotech.Abstr., Excerp.Med., I.P.A., MOS, Mass Spectr.Bull., NPU, Ref.Zh.
—BLDSC (8173.000000), CASDDS, CISTI, GNLM, KNAW, Linda Hall.
Published by: (Oesterreichische Apothekerkammer), Oesterreichische Apotheker-Verlagsgesellschaft mbH, Spitalgasse 31, Vienna, W 1094, Austria. TEL 43-1-4023588, FAX 43-1-4085355. Eds. Dr. Wilhelm Fleischhacker, Dr. Wolfgang Kubelka. Circ: 800.

615 GBR ISSN 1353-6303
SCRIP MAGAZINE. Text in English. 1992. m. GBP 130 in Europe; GBP 165 in the Middle East; USD 310 in US & Canada; JPY 48,000 in Japan; GBP 175 rest of world (effective 2001). adv. 4 cols./p. back issues avail.; reprints avail. **Document type:** *Magazine, Trade.* **Description:** An international magazine providing features, commentary, trends and analysis on the pharmaceutical industry.
Indexed: INIS Atomind., Inpharma, Pharm.&Out.News, Reac.
—BLDSC (8211.859355).
Published by: P J B Publications Ltd., 18-20 Hill Rise, Richmond, Surrey TW10 6UA, United Kingdom. TEL 44-20-8948-3262, FAX 44-20-8332-8990, info@pjbpubs.com, http://www.pjbpubs.com. Ed. Jenny Hone. Pub. Philip Brown. R&P Annette Watts TEL 44-20-8332-8961. Adv. contact Donna Lee TEL 44-20-8332-4616. Circ: 10,500 (paid). **Subscr. addr. in N America:** Pharmabooks Ltd., 1775 Broadway, Ste 511, New York, NY 10019. TEL 212-262-8230, FAX 212-262-8234.

615 GBR
THE SCRIP PHARMACEUTICAL COMPANIES FACT FILE. Text in English. 1994. a. (in 7 vols.). GBP 895, USD 1,880, JPY 215,000 per issue for printed edition 7 volumes; GBP 1,345, USD 2,825, JPY 323,000 combined subscription for print & CD-ROM (effective 2001); Print & CD-ROM combination includes 7 print volumes plus 4 quarterly CD-ROM editions.. abstr, charts, stat. back issues avail. *Refereed.* **Document type:** *Trade.* **Description:** Contains up-to-date profiles of over 1000 pharmaceutical & biotechnology companies worldwide. Includes details of joint ventures, biographies of major personnel, 12 month review of each company, licensing contacts and in-depth financial data.
Related titles: CD-ROM ed.: GBP 995, USD 1,995, JPY 239,000 (effective 2001 - 2002).
Published by: P J B Publications Ltd., 18-20 Hill Rise, Richmond, Surrey TW10 6UA, United Kingdom. TEL 44-20-8332-8964, FAX 44-20-8332-8992, custserv@repsinfo.demon.co.uk, http://www.pjbpubs.com, http://www.pjbpubs.com/scriprep/. Ed. Katherine Davies. R&P Annette Watts TEL 44-20-8332-8961.

615 GBR ISSN 0143-7690
CODEN: SCRIDK
SCRIP - WORLD PHARMACEUTICAL NEWS. Abbreviated title: Scrip. Text in English. 1972. 2/w. GBP 625 in United Kingdom; GBP 695 for rest of Europe; USD 1,305 in US & Canada; GBP 710 in the Middle East; JPY 216,000 in Japan; GBP 745 rest of world (effective 2001). adv. bk.rev. 2 cols./p. back issues avail.; reprints avail. **Document type:** *Newsletter.* **Description:** Covers company news, product developments politics, market data and regulatory affairs on the international pharmaceutical industry.
Related titles: Online - full text ed.: (from Data-Star, The Dialog Corporation, S T N International, Gale Group).
Indexed: ABC, Inpharma, P.N.I., Pharm.&Out.News, Reac.
—BLDSC (8211.859000), CASDDS, GNLM. **CCC.**
Published by: P J B Publications Ltd., 18-20 Hill Rise, Richmond, Surrey TW10 6UA, United Kingdom. TEL 44-20-8948-3262, FAX 44-20-8332-8990, info@pjbpubs.com, http://www.pjbpubs.com. Ed. John Davis. Pub. Philip Brown. R&P Annette Watts TEL 44-20-8332-8961. Adv. contact Peter Coltart TEL 44-20-8332-8802. Circ: 9,991 (paid). **Subscr. addr. in N America:** Pharmabooks Ltd., 1775 Broadway, Ste 511, New York, NY 10019. TEL 212-262-8230, FAX 212-262-8234.

P

615 GBR
▼ **SCRIP'S DRUG DELIVERY COMPANIES FACT FILE.** Text in English. 2001. a. GBP 750, USD 1,575, JPY 180,000 per issue (effective 2001). charts, pat. *Refereed.* **Document type:** *Trade.* **Description:** Drug delivery reference source containing details of over 100 drug delivery companies worldwide. Profiles include financial summaries, key information on proprietory drug delivery technologies, details of senior executives, and licensing contacts, patent information and R&D pipelines.
Published by: P J B Publications Ltd., 18-20 Hill Rise, Richmond, Surrey TW10 6UA, United Kingdom. TEL 44-20-8332-8964, FAX 44-20-8332-8992, custserv@repsinfo.demon.co.uk, http://www.pjbpubs.com, http://www.pjbpubs.com/scriprep/. Ed. Katherine Davies. R&P Annette Watts TEL 44-20-8332-8961.

615 GBR
SCRIP'S PHARMACEUTICAL COMPANY LEAGUE TABLES (YEAR). Text in English. 1982. a., latest 2001, 20th Edition. GBP 450 per issue in United Kingdom; USD 945, JPY 108,000 per issue elsewhere (effective 2001 - 2002). charts, stat. back issues avail. *Refereed.* **Document type:** *Yearbook, Trade.* **Description:** Guide to performance in the pharmaceutical marketplace. Containing the 200 top players in the pharmaceutical industry ranked in terms of sales, R&D, profitability, ROI, ROCE, EPS, geophysical sales, etc.
Published by: P J B Publications Ltd., 18-20 Hill Rise, Richmond, Surrey TW10 6UA, United Kingdom. TEL 44-20-8332-8964, FAX 44-20-8332-8992, paul@repsinfo.demon.co.uk, custserv@repsinfo.demon.co.uk, http://www.pjbpubs.com/scriprep/. Ed. Katherine Davies. R&P Annette Watts TEL 44-20-8332-8961.

615 GBR
SCRIP'S YEARBOOK (YEAR). Text in English. 1984. a., latest 17th Edition. GBP 450, USD 945, JPY 108,000 per issue (effective 2001). charts, mkt, stat, tr.lit. back issues avail. *Refereed.* **Document type:** *Yearbook, Trade.* **Description:** Contains company profiles, information on drugs in R&D, market data, background information and essential statistics on a wide range of diseases, and data on country markets.
Published by: P J B Publications Ltd., 18-20 Hill Rise, Richmond, Surrey TW10 6UA, United Kingdom. TEL 44-20-8332-8964, FAX 44-20-8332-8992, custserv@repsinfo.demon.co.uk, http://www.pjbpubs.com/scriprep/. Ed. Katherine Davies. R&P Annette Watts TEL 44-20-8332-8961.

615 USA
SCRIPTNEWS. Text in English. 1997. q. USD 525 per quarter for 1000 copies (effective 2001). **Document type:** *Newsletter, Consumer.* **Description:** Offers "relationship marketing" through newsletters for the community pharmacy.
Published by: Newsletters Ink, PO Box 2019, Lancaster, PA 17608-2019. TEL 717-393-1000, 800-379-5585, FAX 717-393-4702, http://www.newslettersink.com. Ed. Ann Mead Ash. Pub. Gregory A Gilson.

615 FIN ISSN 0049-0164
SEMINA. Text in Finnish; Summaries in Swedish. 1917. 17/yr. FIM 280 domestic; FIM 300 foreign (effective 2000). adv. bk.rev. **Document type:** *Newspaper.*
Indexed: Anim.Breed.Abstr., Chem.Abstr., Dairy Sci.Abstr., Food Sci.& Tech.Abstr., Forest.Abstr., Helminthol.Abstr., Hort.Abstr., Plant Grow.Reg.Abstr., Protozool.Abstr., Rev.Appl.Entomol., Rev.Plant Path., Seed Abstr., Sugar Ind.Abstr., Vet.Bull.
—BLDSC (8239.000000).
Published by: Suomen Farmasialiitto/Finish Pharmacists' Association, Iso Roobertinkatu 7 A, Helsinki 00120, Finland. TEL 385-9-696-22729, FAX 358-9-605112, marketta.harinen@tarmasialiitto.fi, www.tarmasialiitto.fi. Ed., Adv. contact Marketta Harinen. B&W page FIM 6,300, color page FIM 11,000. Circ: 7,500.

P

SEMINARS IN HEMATOLOGY. see *MEDICAL SCIENCES—Hematology*

SEMINARS IN ONCOLOGY NURSING. see *MEDICAL SCIENCES—Nurses And Nursing*

SHAANXI ZHONGYI XUEYUAN XUEBAO/SHAANXI INSTITUTE OF TRADITIONAL CHINESE MEDICINE. JOURNAL. see *MEDICAL SCIENCES*

SHANDONG YIYAO/SHANDONG MEDICAL JOURNAL. see *MEDICAL SCIENCES*

SHANGHAI ZHONGYIYAO ZAZHI/REVISTA DE MEDICINA TRADICIONAL CHINA DE SHANGHAI/REVUE DE MEDECINE TRADITIONNELLE CHINOISE/SHANGHAI JOURNAL OF TRADITIONAL CHINESE MEDICINE. see *ALTERNATIVE MEDICINE*

615 CHN ISSN 0253-9926
R97.7.C5 CODEN: SIYCDB
SHANXI YIYAO ZAZHI/SHANXI MEDICAL JOURNAL. Text in Chinese; Summaries in English. 1957. bi-m. CNY 3.50 newsstand/cover domestic; USD 3.50 newsstand/cover foreign (effective 2000). adv. abstr, bibl, charts, maps, stat. back issues avail. *Refereed.* **Document type:** *Academic/Scholarly.* **Description:** Offers reports, reviews, and columns, along with editorials, original articles, experimental studies, and clinical studies on quickening the blood and transforming stasis, diagnostic imaging, medical eletrophysiology, pharmaceutical reports, elementary knowledge forum, and clinical nursing cases reporting.
Related titles: CD-ROM ed.; Fax ed.
—CASDDS.
Published by: Chinese Medical Association - Shanxi Branch, 23 Donghuamen, Taiyuan, Shanxi 030013, China. TEL 86-351-3071551, FAX 86-351-3173607. Ed., R&P, Adv. contact Donghai Yuan TEL 86-351-3071551 ext 2153. Circ: 8,500 (paid); 200 (controlled). **Dist. by:** China International Book Trading Corp, 35 Chegongzhuang Xilu, Haidian District, Beijing 100044, China.

615 CHN ISSN 1006-2858
CODEN: SYXUE3
SHENYANG YAOKE DAXUE XUEBAO/SHENYANG PHARMACEUTICAL UNIVERSITY. JOURNAL. Text in Chinese. 1957. bi-m. USD 48 domestic; USD 60 foreign (effective 2001). adv. abstr. 80 p./no. *Refereed.* **Document type:** *Journal, Academic/Scholarly.* **Description:** Contains research reports on pharmaceutics, pharmaceutical analysis, pharmaceutical chemistry, pharmacology, traditional Chinese medicine and synthesis of drugs.
Formerly (until 1995): Shenyang Yaoxueyuan Xuebao/Shenyang College of Pharmacy. Journal (1000-1727)
Indexed: Chem.Abstr., Chem.Titles, Mass Spectr.Bull., Ref.Zh., Sugar Ind.Abstr.
—BLDSC (4874.937000), CASDDS, GNLM.
Published by: Shenyang Yaoke Daxue, Xuebao Bianjibu, 103 Wenhua Rd, Shenyang, Liaoning 110016, China. TEL 86-24-2384-3711, FAX 86-24-23994540, syyd@chinajournal.net.cn. Ed. Yao Xinsheng. R&P Gao Ming. Adv. contact Ren-yong Liu. page USD 1,200; trim 208 x 297. Circ: 2,200.

615.328 615.89 CHN ISSN 1004-0919
SHIZHEN GUOYAO YANJIU/SHIZHEN JOURNAL OF TRADITIONAL CHINESE MEDICINE RESEARCH. Text in Chinese; Abstracts in Chinese, English. 1990. bi-m. CNY 24; USD 24 foreign. adv. **Document type:** *Academic/Scholarly.* **Description:** Researches Li Shizhen, the reknowned ancient Chinese physician. Covers the pharmacology of traditional Chinese medicine and its clinical applications. Also examines the preparation of and recipes for traditional herbal medicines, along with modern medical research.
Published by: (Zhongguo Zhongyiyao Xuehui), Shizhen Guoyao Yanjiu Zazhishe, 169 Tianjin Lu, Huangshi, Hubei 435000, China. TEL 86-714-6225102, FAX 86-714-6225102. Ed. Xiao Peigen. Pub. Zhu Baohua. R&P, Adv. contact Baohua Zhu. page USD 4,000. Circ: 10,000 (paid); 3,000 (controlled). **Dist. overseas by:** China International Book Trading Corp, 35 Chegongzhuang Xilu, Haidian District, Beijing 100044, China.

615.1 340 DEU ISSN 0947-269X
SICHERHEITSVORSCHRIFTEN FUER MEDIZINPRODUKTE. Text in German. 1994. irreg. DEM 148 (effective 2000). **Document type:** *Monographic series, Trade.*
Published by: Erich Schmidt Verlag GmbH & Co. (Berlin), Genthiner Str 30G, Berlin 10785, Germany. TEL 49-30-250085-0, FAX 49-85-25008511, esv@esvmedien.de, http://www.erich-schmidt-verlag.de.

615.7 NLD ISSN 0378-6080
RM302.5 CODEN: SEDAD8
SIDE EFFECTS OF DRUGS ANNUAL; a yearly critical survey of the world's literature on adverse reactions to drugs. Text in Dutch. 1972. a., latest vol.23, 1999. NLG 400, EUR 181.51, USD 203 per vol.. *Refereed.* **Document type:** *Monographic series, Academic/Scholarly.*
Related titles: CD-ROM ed.: (from SilverPlatter Information, Inc.); Online - full text ed.: (from Data-Star, The Dialog Corporation); ♦ Supplement to: Meyler's Side Effects of Drugs. ISSN 0376-7396.
Indexed: Biol.Abstr., INIS Atomind.
—BLDSC (8271.735000), CASDDS, GNLM, KNAW. **CCC.**
Published by: Elsevier Science BV, PO Box 211, Amsterdam 1000 AE, Netherlands. TEL 31-20-485-3757, 31-20-485-3911, FAX 31-20-485-3432, 31-20-485-3598, nlinfo-f@elsevier.nl, http://www.elsevier.nl. Ed. J K Aronson. **Subscr. in Australasia and the Far East to:** Elsevier Science (Singapore) Pte Ltd, No.1 Temasek Ave, 17-01 Millenia Tower, Singapore 039192, Singapore. TEL 65-434-3727, FAX 65-337-2230, asiainfo@elsevier.com.sg; **Subscr. in Japan to:** Elsevier Science Inc - Japan Regional Office, 9-15 Higashi-Azabu 1-chome, Minato-ku, Tokyo 106-0044, Japan. TEL 81-3-5561-5033, FAX 81-3-5561-5047, info@elsevier.co.jp; **Subscr. in the Americas to:** Elsevier Science, PO Box 945, New York, NY 10159-0945. TEL 212-633-3730, 888-437-4636, FAX 212-633-3680, usinfo-f@elsevier.com, http://www.elsevier.com

615 SWE ISSN 0346-8453
SJUKHUSFARMACI. Text in Swedish. 1973. 4/yr. **Document type:** *Newspaper, Trade.*
Published by: Apoteket AB, Stockholm 13188, Sweden. TEL 46-8-466-10-00, FAX 46-8-466-15-15. Ed. Margareta Marcusson.

615.7 CHE ISSN 1422-2868
CODEN: SPAPFF
SKIN PHARMACOLOGY AND APPLIED SKIN PHYSIOLOGY. Text in English. 1988. bi-m. CHF 722 in Europe to institutions; CHF 739.40 elsewhere to institutions; EUR 515.80 in Europe to institutions; USD 564 elsewhere to institutions (effective 2002). adv. bk.rev. charts, illus. index. back issues avail. *Refereed.* **Document type:** *Journal, Academic/Scholarly.* **Description:** Includes articles on skin pharmacology, immunosuppressive topicals, and new strategies in the therapy of malignant melanoma and wound healing.
Formerly (until 1998): Skin Pharmacology (1011-0283); Which incorporates (1985-1990): Bioengineering and the Skin (0266-3082)
Related titles: Microform ed.: (from PQC); Online - full text ed.: ISSN 1422-2906. CHF 58, EUR 42, USD 45 to institutions with print edition (effective 2002) (from EBSCO Publishing, O C L C Online Computer Library Center, Inc., RoweCom Information Quest, Swets Blackwell, Institute for Scientific Information).
Indexed: ASCA, Chem.Abstr., Chem.Titles, Curr.Cont., Derwent Biotech.Abstr., Excerp.Med., Ind.Med. (1998-), Inpharma, Med.& Surg.Dermat., Pharm.&Out.News, Reac., Sci.Cit.Ind.
—BLDSC (8295.937000), CASDDS, CISTI, EMDOCS, GNLM, IDS, Infotrieve, KNAW. **CCC.**
Published by: (Skin Pharmacology Society), S. Karger AG, Allschwilerstr 10, PO Box, Basel 4009, Switzerland. TEL 41-61-306-1111, FAX 41-61-30161234, karger@karger.ch, http://www.online.karger.com/journals/sph, http://www.karger.com. Ed. H F Merk. adv.: page USD 1,195.

615.19 616.89 USA ISSN 1060-8427
SMART DRUG NEWS. Text in English. 1992. 10/yr. USD 44 domestic; USD 46 in Canada; USD 55 elsewhere; USD 6 newsstand/cover. bk.rev. illus. **Document type:** *Newsletter.* **Description:** Provides answers to questions related to drug research, particularly psychiatric pharmacology.
Indexed: e-psyche.
Published by: Cognitive Enhancement Research Institute, PO Box 4029, Menlo Park, CA 94026. TEL 415-321-CERI. Ed. Steven W Fowkes.

615.9 658 ESP ISSN 1130-8230
SOCIEDAD ESPANOLA DE FARMACIA HOSPITALARIA. BOLETIN INFORMATIVO. Cover title: Boletin Informativo - S E F H. Text in Spanish. q. ESP 4,000 to individuals; ESP 5,500 to institutions; USD 45 foreign (effective 2000). **Document type:** *Bulletin.*
Formerly (until 1989): Asociacion Espanola de Farmaceuticos de Hospitales. Boletin Informativo (1130-8222)
Indexed: BHA.
Published by: Sociedad Espanola de Farmacia Hospitalaria, General Orgaz, 23 1o A, Madrid 28020, Spain. TEL 34-1-5714487, FAX 34-1-5714586, sefh@sefh.es, http://www.sefh.es. Ed. Eduardo Echarri Arrieta. R&P Esteban Valverde Molina. Circ: 1,700.

615.1 ITA ISSN 0037-8798
CODEN: BSFOB3
SOCIETA ITALIANA DI FARMACIA OSPEDALIERA. BOLLETTINO. Text in Italian. 1955. bi-m. ITL 145,000 (effective 2000). adv. bk.rev. charts, illus, stat. 64 p./no. reprint service avail. from PQC. **Document type:** *Journal, Academic/Scholarly.*
Related titles: Microform ed.: (from PQC).
Indexed: Agri.& Environ.Biotech.Abstr. (coverage dropped), Biol.Abstr., Chem.Abstr., Derwent Biotech.Abstr., Excerp.Med., I.P.A.
—BLDSC (2231.200000), CASDDS, CISTI, GNLM.
Published by: (Societa Italiana di Farmacia Ospedaliera), Il Pensiero Scientifico Editore s.r.l., Via Bradano, 3-C, Rome, RM 00199, Italy. TEL 39-06-862821, FAX 39-06-86282250, pensiero@pensiero.it, http://www.pensiero.it. Pub. Luca De Fiore. Adv. contact Luciano De Fiore. Circ: 2,500.

615.1 FRA ISSN 0037-9093
CODEN: BSPBAD
SOCIETE DE PHARMACIE DE BORDEAUX. BULLETIN. Text in French. 1860. q. FRF 200. adv. bk.rev. abstr, charts. index. **Document type:** *Academic/Scholarly.*
Indexed: Agri.& Environ.Biotech.Abstr. (coverage dropped), Biol.Abstr., Chem.Abstr., Chem.Indus.Notes, Chem.Titles, Derwent Biotech.Abstr., GeoRef, I.P.A.
—BLDSC (2747.500000), CASDDS, GNLM.
Published by: Societe de Pharmacie de Bordeaux, c/o Faculte de Pharmacie, 3 place de la Victoire, Bordeaux Cedex 33076, France. Ed. Jean Cambar. Circ: 900.

615 FRA
SOCIETE DE PHARMACIE DE LILLE. BULLETIN. Text in French. 1946. q. FRF 160.

Indexed: Agri.& Environ.Biotech.Abstr. (coverage dropped), Biol.Abstr., Chem.Abstr., Excerp.Med., I.P.A., Nutr.Abstr.
Published by: (Societe de Pharmacie), Universite de Lille, 3 rue du Professeur Laguesse, Lille 59000, France.

615.1 FRA ISSN 0037-9131
CODEN: BPMSAS
SOCIETE DE PHARMACIE DE STRASBOURG. BULLETIN. Text in French. 1955. s-a. FRF 100. adv. bk.rev. charts, illus. cum.index: 1955-1964, 1965-1973, 1974-1978.
Indexed: Biol.Abstr., Chem.Abstr.
—CASDDS, GNLM.
Published by: Societe de Pharmacie de Strasbourg, Faculte de Pharmacie, B.P. 24, Illkirch Cedex 67401, France. Ed. Dr. Boymond. Circ: 600.

615 LKA
SRI LANKA PHARMACEUTICAL ASSOCIATION. QUARTERLY NEWSLETTER. Text in English. q. **Document type:** *Newsletter.*
Published by: Sri Lanka Pharmaceutical Association, c/o Dept. of Pharmacy, Faculty of Medicine, University of Sri Lanka, Colombo 8, Sri Lanka.

615.19 USA ISSN 1521-2467
STRATEGIC OUTSOURCING REPORT. Text in English. 1998. m., latest vol.4, 2002. USD 497 in North America; USD 512 elsewhere (effective Nov. 2001). 8 p./no. back issues avail. **Document type:** *Newsletter.*
Published by: Washington Business Information, Inc., 300 N Washington St, Ste 200, Falls Church, Arlington, VA 22046. TEL 703-538-7600, 703-538-7660, FAX 703 538-7676. Ed. Sean Oberle.

STREET PHARMACOLOGIST. see *DRUG ABUSE AND ALCOHOLISM*

615.1071 DEU ISSN 0721-8672
STUDENT UND PRAKTIKANT; Forum fuer die Pharmazeutische Ausbildung. Text in German. 1982. bi-m. adv. bk.rev. **Document type:** *Journal, Trade.*
Related titles: ♦ Supplement to: Deutsche Apotheker Zeitung. ISSN 0011-9857.
—BLDSC (8480.100000), GNLM.
Published by: Deutscher Apotheker Verlag, Postfach 101061, Stuttgart 70009, Germany. TEL 49-711-2582-0, FAX 49-711-2582291, daz@deutscher-apotheker-verlag.de, http://www.deutscher-apotheker-verlag.de. Ed. Wolfgang Caesar.

SUBSTANCE ABUSE REPORT; twice-monthly newsletter covering all aspects of drug abuse: its prevention, detection and treatment. see *DRUG ABUSE AND ALCOHOLISM*

615.9 340 USA ISSN 0098-714X
KF2915.P4
SURVEY OF PHARMACY LAW. Text in English. 1950. a. USD 20 (effective 1999). stat, charts.
Published by: National Association of Boards of Pharmacy, 700 Busse Hwy, Park Ridge, IL 60068-2402. TEL 847-698-6227. Ed. Carmen Catizone. Circ: 12,000.

615 CHE ISSN 0251-1673
SWISS PHARMA; Schweizerische Zeitschrift fuer die pharmazeutische industrie. Text in German, English. 1979. 10/yr. CHF 180 domestic; CHF 200 in Europe; CHF 340 elsewhere (effective 2001). adv. back issues avail. **Document type:** *Journal, Trade.* **Description:** Publishes original selected papers and interviews with top leaders in pharmaceutical production in Switzerland.
Indexed: I.P.A.
—CISTI, GNLM.
Published by: Verlag Dr. Felix Wuest AG, Kuesnachterstr 36, Postfach 161, Zumikon 8126, Switzerland. TEL 41-1-919-80-60, FAX 41-1-919-80-69. Ed., Pub., Adv. contact Dr. Felix Wuest. B&W page CHF 1,750, color page CHF 3,460; trim 185 x 265. Circ: 1,000 (paid).

610 CHE ISSN 0082-0504
SWITZERLAND. BUNDESAMT FUER SOZIALVERSICHERUNG. SPEZIALITAETENLISTE - LISTE DES SPECIALITES - ELENCO DELLE SPECIALITA. Text in French, German, Italian. 1955. a. CHF 34 (effective 2000). **Document type:** *Catalog, Government.* **Description:** List of drugs being reimbursed by Swiss sickness insurers.
Related titles: CD-ROM ed.
Published by: Bundesamt fuer Sozialversicherung, Effingerstr 20, Bern 3003, Switzerland. TEL 41-31-3229011, FAX 41-31-3227880, reinhard.kaempf@bsv.admin.ch, info@bsv.admin.ch, http://www.bsv.admin.ch. Ed. Reinhard Kampf. Circ: 24,000. **Dist. by:** Bundesamt fur Bauten und Logistik, Effingerstr 33, Bern 3003, Switzerland. TEL 41-31-3223908, FAX 41-31-9920023.

615 DEU ISSN 0936-3904
SYMBIOSE. Text in German. 1989. q. **Document type:** *Bulletin.*
—GNLM.
Published by: (Schaper und Bruemmer), Vereinigte Verlagsanstalten GmbH, Hoeherweg 278, Duesseldorf 40231, Germany. TEL 49-211-7357589, FAX 49-211-7357507, am@vva.de, http://www.vva.de. Circ: 50,000 (controlled).

615 AUS ISSN 1325-8559
T G A NEWS (ONLINE EDITION). Text in English. 3/yr.
Incorporates (1995-2001): Australian Therapeutic Device Bulletin (Online) (1325-8567)
Media: Online - full content. **Related titles:** ♦ Print ed.: T G A News (Print Edition).
Published by: Therapeutic Goods Administration, PO Box 100, Woden, ACT 2606, Australia. TEL 61-2-6232-8610, 61-2-6232-8444, FAX 61-2-6232-8222, tga-information-officer@health.gov.au, http://www.anzfa.gov.au/.

615 AUS
T G A NEWS (PRINT EDITION). Text in English. 1995. 3/yr. **Document type:** *Newsletter, Government.*
Incorporates (in 2001): Australian Therapeutic Device Bulletin (Print) (1031-8542); Which was formerly (until 1987): Therapeutic Device Bulletin (1030-1933)
Related titles: ♦ Online - full content ed.: T G A News (Online Edition). ISSN 1325-8559.
Published by: Therapeutic Goods Administration, PO Box 100, Woden, ACT 2606, Australia. TEL 61-2-6232-8610, 61-2-6232-8444, FAX 61-2-6232-8222, tga-information-officer@health.gov.au, http://www.anzfa.gov.au/.

615 USA ISSN 1096-9268
T P A SPEEDLETTER. Text in English. m. USD 15 (effective 1999). adv. bk.rev. back issues avail. **Document type:** *Newsletter.* **Description:** Covers items of interest to all areas of pharmacy practice, including industry news and mergers, pharmacy trends and professional announcements.
Published by: Texas Pharmacy Association, 1624 E Anderson Ln, Austin, TX 78752-1806. TEL 512-836-8350, 800-505-5463, FAX 512-836-0308, http://www.txpharmacy.com. Ed. Audra F Johnson. R&P, Adv. contact Lori S Alcala. Circ: 3,000 (paid).

TAKEDA RESEARCH LABORATORIES. JOURNAL. see *BIOLOGY*

615 613 DNK ISSN 0107-1181
TAL OG DATA, MEDICIN OG SUNDHEDSVAESEN/ FACTS, MEDICINE AND HEALTH CARE, DENMARK. Text in Danish, English. 1976. a. free per issue. illus.
Formerly: Tal og Data om Medicin
Published by: Foreningen af Danske Medicinfabrikker, Stroedamvej 50 A, Copenhagen Oe 2100, Denmark. TEL 45-39-27-00-88, FAX 45-32-27-00-50. Circ: 6,000.

TECHNOMARK REGISTER. CONTRACT PACKAGERS & MANUFACTURERS - EUROPE. see *BUSINESS AND ECONOMICS—Trade And Industrial Directories*

TECHNOMARK REGISTER. CONTRACT RESEARCH ORGANISATIONS - NORTH AMERICA. see *BUSINESS AND ECONOMICS—Trade And Industrial Directories*

TECHNOMARK REGISTER. EUROPEAN CONTRACT RESEARCH ORGANISATIONS. CLINICAL RESEARCH. see *BUSINESS AND ECONOMICS—Trade And Industrial Directories*

TECHNOMARK REGISTER. EUROPEAN CONTRACT RESEARCH ORGANISATIONS. TOXICOLOGY & ANALYSIS. see *BUSINESS AND ECONOMICS—Trade And Industrial Directories*

615 ITA
TEMA FARMACIA. Text in Italian. m. (except July & Aug.). adv.
Published by: U T E T SpA, Corso Raffaello 28, Turin 10125, Italy. TEL 39-2-29003555, FAX 39-2-6599049. Ed. Angelo Cambie. Adv. contact Corrado Trevisan. B&W page ITL 3,740,000, color page ITL 5,600,000; trim 246 x 185. Circ: 16,311.

615.19 USA ISSN 1047-0166
TENNESSEE PHARMACIST. Text in English. 1965. m. membership. adv. bk.rev. **Document type:** *Trade.*
Indexed: I.P.A.
Published by: Tennessee Pharmacists Association, 226 Capitol Blvd, Ste 810, Nashville, TN 37219. FAX 615-255-3528, tnpharm@aol.com. Ed. Baeteena Black. Adv. contact Marcia Williams. Circ: 2,500.

615 USA ISSN 0362-7926
CODEN: TXPDAE
TEXAS PHARMACY. Text in English. 1879. q. USD 30 to non-members (effective 2001). adv. bk.rev. index. *Refereed.* **Document type:** *Magazine, Trade.* **Description:** Contains news of interest to pharmacists and offers practice and management tips, trends in pharmacy, legislative issues coverage, profiles of outstanding practitioners, disease state information and new products information.
Indexed: I.P.A.
Published by: Texas Pharmacy Association, PO Box 14709, Austin, TX 78761-4709. http://www.txpharmacy.com. Ed. Audra F Johnson. Circ: 3,000 (paid and controlled).

615 USA ISSN 0163-4356
RM301.5 CODEN: TDMODV
THERAPEUTIC DRUG MONITORING. Text in English. 1979. bi-m., latest vol.23. USD 344 domestic to individuals; USD 404 foreign to individuals; USD 640 domestic to institutions; USD 690 foreign to institutions; USD 109 newsstand/cover (effective 2002). adv. bk.rev. illus. index. back issues avail.; reprint service avail. from PQC. *Refereed.* **Document type:** *Academic/Scholarly.*
Related titles: Online - full text ed.: USD 832 domestic academic site license; USD 882 foreign academic site license; USD 928 domestic corporate site license; USD 978 foreign corporate site license (2002) (from Ovid Technologies, Inc., Institute for Scientific Information).
Indexed: ASCA, Agri.& Environ.Biotech.Abstr. (coverage dropped), Anal.Abstr., Biol.Abstr., Chem.Abstr., Chem.Cit.Ind., Chem.Titles, Curr.Adv.Ecol.Sci., Curr.Cont., Dent.Ind., Derwent Biotech.Abstr., Excerp.Med., INIS Atomind., I.P.A., Ind.Med. (1979-), Inpharma, Int.Abstr.Biol.Sci., Kidney, Mass Spectr.Bull., Neurosci.Cit.Ind., Nutr.Abstr., Pharm.&Out.News, Protozool.Abstr., Reac., Rev.Med.& Vet.Mycol., Sci.Cit.Ind., THA.
—BLDSC (8814.643000), CASDDS, CISTI, GNLM, IDS, ingenta, KNAW.
Published by: Lippincott Williams & Wilkins (Philadelphia) (Subsidiary of: Wolters Kluwer N.V.), 530 Walnut St, Philadelphia, PA 19106-3621. TEL 215-521-8300, FAX 215-521-8902, www.drug-monitoring.com, http://www.lww.com. Eds. Dr. Folke Sjoeqvist, Steven J Soldin. Pub. Shelley Johnson. R&P Alice McElhinney. Adv. contact Ray Thibodeau. B&W page USD 850, color page USD 1,925; trim 11 x 8.25. Circ: 1,352. **Subscr. to:** PO Box 1600, Hagerstown, MD 21740-1600. TEL 800-777-2295, FAX 301-824-7390.

615 GBR
THERAPEUTIC DRUGS. SUPPLEMENT. Text in English. irreg., latest vol.2, 1994. adv. **Document type:** *Academic/Scholarly.*
Published by: Churchill Livingstone (Subsidiary of: Harcourt Publishers Ltd.), Robert Stevenson House, 1-3 Baxter's Pl, Leith Walk, Edinburgh, Midlothian EH1 3AF, United Kingdom. TEL 44-131-556-2424, FAX 44-131-459-1177, http://www.churchillmed.com. Ed. Colin Dollery. Adv. contact Kathy Crawford. **Subscr. to:** Harcourt Publishers Ltd., Foots Cray High St, Sidcup, Kent DA14 5HP, United Kingdom. TEL 44-20-8308-5700, FAX 44-20-8309-0807.

610.9 DNK ISSN 0082-4003
THERIACA; samlinger til farmaciens og medicinens historie. Text in Danish; Summaries in English. 1956. irreg., latest vol.31, 1998. price varies.
Published by: Dansk Farmacihistorisk Selskab/Danish Society of the History of Pharmacy, Institut for Samfundsfarmaci, Universitetsparken 2, Copenhagen O 2100, Denmark. Ed. Poul R Kruse.

615.1 USA
THIRD PARTY RX. Text in English. 1989. m. USD 50.
Published by: National Community Pharmacists Association, 205 Daingerfield Rd, Alexandria, VA 22314. TEL 703-683-8200, FAX 703-683-3619. Ed. Robert McCarthy. Circ: 3,000.

P

615 CHN ISSN 0253-9896
R97.7.C5 CODEN: TIYADG
TIANJIN YIYAO/TIANJIN PHARMACY. Text in Chinese. m.
Indexed: Chem.Abstr., Chem.Titles.
—BLDSC (8820.510000), CASDDS.
Published by: Tianjin Yixue Keji Qingbao Yanjiusuo/Tianjin Medical Science and Technology Information Institute, 131 Chengdu Dao, Heping-qu, Tianjin 300050, China. TEL 311705. Ed. Zhang Yingfu.

615 JPN ISSN 0285-368X
CODEN: TTQUDB
TOKYO TANABE QUARTERLY. Text in Japanese. 1967. q. free per issue. adv. bk.rev.
Indexed: Chem.Abstr.
—CASDDS.
Published by: Tokyo Tanabe Co. Ltd./Tokyo Tanabe K.K., 2-7-3 Nihonbashihoncho, Chuo-ku, Tokyo 103-0023, Japan. Circ: 20,000.

615 GBR ISSN 1470-5761
▼ **TOMORROW'S PHARMACIST.** Text in English. 1999. a. GBP 5 per issue in United Kingdom; GBP 7 per issue rest of world (effective 2001).
Published by: Euromed Communications Ltd., 1 Lambeth High St, London SE1 7JN, United Kingdom. TEL 44-20-7735-9141, editor@pharmj.org.uk, http://www.pharmj.com/about/tp.html, http://www.euromed.uk.com.

P

TOXIC EXPOSURE ADVISORY NEWSLETTER. see *ENVIRONMENTAL STUDIES—Toxicology And Environmental Safety*

TOXICOLOGICAL AND ENVIRONMENTAL CHEMISTRY. see *ENVIRONMENTAL STUDIES—Toxicology And Environmental Safety*

TOXICOLOGICAL SCIENCES. see *ENVIRONMENTAL STUDIES—Toxicology And Environmental Safety*

TOXICOLOGY; an international journal concerned with the effects of chemicals on living systems. see *ENVIRONMENTAL STUDIES—Toxicology And Environmental Safety*

TOXICOLOGY AND APPLIED PHARMACOLOGY; for those working in the fields of toxicology, pharmacology, biochemistry, nutrition, veterinary medicine. see *ENVIRONMENTAL STUDIES—Toxicology And Environmental Safety*

TOXICOLOGY AND INDUSTRIAL HEALTH; an international journal. see *ENVIRONMENTAL STUDIES—Toxicology And Environmental Safety*

TOXICOLOGY IN VITRO. see *ENVIRONMENTAL STUDIES—Toxicology And Environmental Safety*

TOXICOLOGY LETTERS; an international journal for the rapid publication of short reports on biochemical mechanisms of mammalian toxicity. see *ENVIRONMENTAL STUDIES—Toxicology And Environmental Safety*

TOXICOLOGY METHODS. see *ENVIRONMENTAL STUDIES—Toxicology And Environmental Safety*

615.9 GBR ISSN 0041-0101
QP631 CODEN: TOXIA6
TOXICON; an interdisciplinary journal on the toxins derived from animals, plants and microorganisms. Text in English, French, German, Spanish. 1962. m. EUR 1,644 in Europe to institutions; JPY 218,300 in Japan to institutions; USD 1,839 elsewhere to institutions (effective 2002). adv. bk.rev., software rev. abstr, charts, illus. index. back issues avail. *Refereed.* **Document type:** *Academic/Scholarly.* **Description:** Publishes original research on the chemical, pharmacological, zootoxicological and immunological properties of naturally occurring poisons, including clinical and therapeutic observations.
Related titles: Microfilm ed.: (from PQC); Online - full text ed.: (from ingenta, Swets Blackwell, Institute for Scientific Information, ScienceDirect).
Indexed: ASCA, Abstr.Hyg., Apic.Abstr., Aqua.Sci.& Fish.Abstr., Bibl.Agri., Bio-Contr.News & Info., Biol.Abstr., Chem.Abstr., Chem.Indus.Notes, Crop Physiol.Abstr., Curr.Adv.Biochem., Curr.Adv.Ecol.Sci., Curr.Cont., Dairy Sci.Abstr., Deep Sea Res.& Oceanogr.Abstr., Diar.Dis.Res., Entomol.Abstr., Environ.Sci.Poll.Mgmt., Excerp.Med., Field Crop Abstr., Forest Prod.Abstr., Forest.Abstr., Helminthol.Abstr., Herb.Abstr., Hort.Abstr., INIS Atomind., Ind.Med. (1962-), Ind.Sci.Rev., Ind.Vet., Inpharma, Int.Aerosp.Abstr., Maize Abstr., Mass Spectr.Bull., Microbiol.Abstr., Neurosci.Abstr. (coverage dropped), Neurosci.Cit.Ind., Nutr.Abstr., Ocean.Abstr., Pig News & Info., Pollut.Abstr., Postharvest, Poult.Abstr., Reac., Rev.Appl.Entomol., Rev.Arom.& Med.Plants, Rev.Med.& Vet.Mycol., Rev.Plant Path., Risk Abstr., Saf.Sci.Abstr., Sci.Cit.Ind., Sel.Water Res.Abstr., Small Anim.Abstr., Sport Fish.Abstr., Tox.Abstr., Trop.Dis.Bull., Vet.Bull., Weed Abstr., Wild.Rev., Zoo.Rec.
—BLDSC (8873.050000), ADONIS, CASDDS, CISTI, GNLM, IDS, ingenta, Linda Hall. **CCC.**
Published by: (International Society on Toxinology), Pergamon (Subsidiary of: Elsevier Science), The Boulevard, Langford Ln, East Park, Kidlington, Oxford OXB 1GB, United Kingdom. FAX 44-1865-843010, nlinfo-f@elsevier.nl; usinfo-f@elsevier.com; forinfo-kyf04035@niftyserve.or.jp, nlinfo-f@elsevier/nl; usinfo-f@elsevier.com; forinfo-kyf04035@niftyserve.or.jp, htt://www.elsevier.nl/inca/publications/store/2/5/9/. Eds. Alan Harvey, G E Russell, Gerhard G Habermehl. Circ: 1,000. **Subscr. in Australasia and the Far East to:** Elsevier Science (Singapore) Pte Ltd, No.1 Temasek Ave, 17-01 Millenia Tower, Singapore 039192, Singapore. TEL 65-434-3727, FAX 65-337-2230; **Subscr. in the Americas to:** Elsevier Science, PO Box 945, New York, NY 10159-0945. TEL 212-633-3730, FAX 212-633-3680, usinfo-f@elsevier.com; **Subscr. to:** Elsevier Science BV, PO Box 211, Amsterdam 1000 AE, Netherlands. TEL 31-20-485-3757, nlinfo-f@elsevier.nl.

TRANSMITTERS, RECEPTORS & SYNAPSES. see *PHARMACY AND PHARMACOLOGY—Abstracting, Bibliographies, Statistics*

TRANSPLANTATION PROCEEDINGS. see *MEDICAL SCIENCES—Surgery*

615.1 GBR ISSN 0165-6147
CODEN: TPHSDY
TRENDS IN PHARMACOLOGICAL SCIENCES. Text in English. 1979. m. GBP 92, EUR 115 in Europe to individuals; JPY 14,000 in Japan to individuals; USD 126 elsewhere to individuals; NLG 1,908, EUR 908 in Europe to institutions; JPY 125,900 in Japan to institutions; USD 1,015 elsewhere to institutions; GBP 47 in Europe to students; JPY 10,100 in Japan to students; USD 78 elsewhere to students; EUR 1,168.94 in Europe to institutions Print & online eds. combined; JPY 162,200 in Japan to institutions Print & online eds. combined; USD 1,308 elsewhere to institutions Print & online eds. combined; EUR 144 in Europe to qualified personnel; JPY 17,500 in Japan to qualified personnel; USD 157 elsewhere to qualified personnel (effective 2002). adv. bk.rev. bibl, illus, abstr. index. back issues avail.; reprint service avail. from SWZ. *Refereed.* **Document type:** *Academic/Scholarly.* **Description:** Covers the sciences of pharmacology and toxicology.
Related titles: Microform ed.: (from PQC); Online - full text ed.: (from ingenta, Gale Group, Swets Blackwell, Institute for Scientific Information, ScienceDirect).
Indexed: ASCA, Aqua.Sci.& Fish.Abstr., Biol.Abstr., Cal.Tiss.Abstr., Chem.Abstr., Chem.Indus.Notes, Chem.Titles, Curr.Adv.Biochem., Curr.Adv.Cancer Res., Curr.Adv.Ecol.Sci., Curr.Cont., Derwent Biotech.Abstr., Excerp.Med., I.P.A., Ind.Med. (1979-), Ind.Sci.Rev., Inpharma, Int.Abstr.Biol.Sci., Neurosci.Abstr., Neurosci.Cit.Ind., Nuc.Acids Abstr., Pharm.&Out.News, Protozool.Abstr., Reac., Rev.Arom.& Med.Plants, Rev.Med.& Vet.Mycol., Sci.Cit.Ind., Telegen.
—BLDSC (9049.675000), ADONIS, CASDDS, CISTI, GNLM, IDS, ingenta, KNAW. **CCC.**
Published by: Elsevier Science Ltd., Elsevier Trends Journals, 68 Hills Rd, Cambridge CB2 1LA, United Kingdom. TEL 44-1223-315961, FAX 44-1223-464430, tips@elsevier.co.uk, http://www.elsevier.nl/inca/publications/store/4/0/5/9/2/0/. Eds. A Smith, G MacKenzie, Sian Lewis. Adv. contact Thelma Reid. Circ: 4,000. **Subscr. in Australasia and the Far East to:** Elsevier Science (Singapore) Pte Ltd, No.1 Temasek Ave, 17-01 Millenia Tower, Singapore 039192, Singapore. TEL 65-434-3727, FAX 65-337-2230; **Subscr. in the Americas to:** Elsevier Science, PO Box 945, New York, NY 10159-0945. TEL 212-633-3730, FAX 212-633-3680, http://www.elsevier.com; **Subscr. to:** Elsevier Current Trends Subscriptions, PO Box 331, Haywards Heath, W Sussex RH16 3FG, United Kingdom. TEL 44-1444-475650, FAX 44-1444-445423. **Co-sponsors:** International Union of Pharmacology; International Union of Toxicology.

615 ITA
TUTTOSALUTE. Text in Italian. 4/yr. adv.
Related titles: German ed.
Published by: U T E T SpA, Corso Raffaello 28, Turin 10125, Italy. TEL 39-2-29003555, FAX 39-2-6599049. Ed. Romolo Saccomani. Adv. contact Corrado Trevisan. color page ITL 3,000,000; trim 245 x 180. Circ: 30,625.

U K AIDS DIRECTORY. see *MEDICAL SCIENCES—Communicable Diseases*

▼ **U N M C DISCOVER.** see *MEDICAL SCIENCES*

615 USA ISSN 0090-6816
RS55 CODEN: UUDNDB
U S A N AND THE U S P DICTIONARY OF DRUG NAMES. (United States Adopted Names and the United States Pharmacopeial Convention) Text in English. 1963. a. USD 105. **Description:** Lists more than 8,100 nonproprietary drug entries from the U.S., the U.K., and Japan.
—CASDDS, CISTI.
Published by: United States Pharmacopeial Convention, Inc., 12601 Twinbrook Pkwy, Rockville, MD 20852. TEL 301-881-0666.

615.1 USA ISSN 0077-4235
U.S. FOOD AND DRUG ADMINISTRATION. NATIONAL DRUG CODE DIRECTORY. Text in English. 1969. irreg. USD 76; includes supplements. **Document type:** *Directory, Government.*
Published by: U.S. Food and Drug Administration, Office of Public Affairs, 5600 Fishers Ln, Rockville, MD 20857. TEL 202-783-3054. **Orders to:** U.S. Government Printing Office, Superintendent of Documents. TEL 202-783-3238, FAX 202-783-2250.

615. USA ISSN 0730-1324
U S P - D I UPDATE. Text in English. 1980. m.
Incorporates (1980-1990): U S P - D I Review (1045-8301)
Related titles: ♦ Supplement to: U S P - D I, Volume 1. Drug Information for the Health Care Professional. ISSN 0740-4174; ♦ Supplement to: U S P - D I, Volume 2. Advice for the Patient. ISSN 0740-6916; ♦ Supplement to: U S P - D I, Volume 3. Approved Drug Products and Legal Requirements. ISSN 1045-8298.
Published by: United States Pharmacopeia, 12601 Twinbrook Pkwy, Rockville, MD 20852. TEL 800-227-8772, FAX 301-816-8148.

615 USA ISSN 0740-4174
RM300 CODEN: USPIE9
U S P - D I, VOLUME 1. DRUG INFORMATION FOR THE HEALTH CARE PROFESSIONAL. Text in English. 1980. a. (plus m. Update). USD 140; USD 158 in Canada; USD 179 elsewhere. **Document type:** *Trade.* **Description:** Contains information on both labeled and unlabeled U.S. and Canadian drug products, and selected therapeutic monographs for disease management.
Supersedes in part (in 1983): United States Pharmacopeia Dispensing Information (0276-5373)
Related titles: ♦ Supplement: U S P - D I Update. ISSN 0730-1324.
Published by: United States Pharmacopeia, 12601 Twinbrook Pkwy, Rockville, MD 20852. TEL 800-877-6733, FAX 802-864-7626, http://www.usp.org.

615 USA ISSN 0740-6916
RM300 CODEN: USPIE9
U S P - D I, VOLUME 2. ADVICE FOR THE PATIENT; drug information in lay language. Text in English. 1980. a. (plus m. Update). USD 80; USD 98 in Canada; USD 119 elsewhere; includes Update. **Document type:** *Trade.* **Description:** Contains information to educate and counsel patients on drug use, available dosage forms, side effects, and contraindications.
Supersedes in part (in 1983): United States Pharmacopeia Dispensing Information (0276-5373)
Related titles: Online - full text ed.: (from Gale Group); ♦ Supplement: U S P - D I Update. ISSN 0730-1324.
—GNLM.
Published by: United States Pharmacopeia, 12601 Twinbrook Pkwy, Rockville, MD 20852. TEL 800-877-7633, FAX 802-864-7626, http://www.usp.org.

615 340 USA ISSN 1045-8298
RS131.2
U S P - D I, VOLUME 3. APPROVED DRUG PRODUCTS AND LEGAL REQUIREMENTS. Text in English. 1989. a. USD 124; USD 142 in Canada; USD 163 elsewhere. **Document type:** *Trade.* **Description:** Contains important therapeutic equivalence information, as well as selected federal and state requirements that affect the prescribing and dispensing of prescription drugs and controlled substances.

Related titles: ♦ Supplement: U S P - D I Update. ISSN 0730-1324.
Published by: United States Pharmacopeia, 12601 Twinbrook Pkwy, Rockville, MD 20852. TEL 800-877-6733, FAX 802-864-7626, http://www.usp.org.

615 USA
U S P QUALITY REVIEW. (United States Pharmacopeia) Text in English. 1988. 10/yr. membership. **Document type:** *Academic/Scholarly.* **Description:** Presents information and advisories relating to the reported information gathered through the network.
Related titles: Online - full text ed.
Published by: U.S. Pharmacopoeial Practitioners' Reporting Network, 12601 Twinbrook Pky, Rockville, MD 20852. TEL 800-487-7776, http://www.usp.org. Ed., R&P Elizabeth Cowley TEL 301-816-8217.

615.105 USA ISSN 0148-4818
RS1
U S PHARMACIST. Text in English. 1976. m. USD 30. adv. index. back issues avail. *Refereed.* **Document type:** *Academic/Scholarly.*
Related titles: Online - full text ed.
Indexed: I.P.A.
—BLDSC (9124.762000), CISTI, GNLM, Infotrieve, ingenta, KNAW. **CCC.**
Published by: Jobson Publishing LLC, 100 Ave of Americas, New York, NY 10013-1678. TEL 212-274-7000, 800-747-1652, FAX 212-431-0500, uspharmacist@jobson.com, http://www.uspharmacist.com/. Eds. Angele D'Angelo, Joseph Cupolo. Adv. contact Frank Bennicasa. Circ: 103,000. **Subscr. to:** US Pharmacist, PO Box 7632, Riverton, NJ 08077-7632. TEL 609-764-2675.

615 DNK ISSN 0108-948X
RS67.D4
UNDERSOEGELSE OVER APOTEKERNES DRIFTSFORHOLD; regnskabsresultater fra apoteker. Text in Danish. 1944 (vol.9). a. DKK 75.
Published by: Sundhedsstyrelsen, Amaliegade 13, PO Box 2020, Copenhagen K 1012, Denmark. **Co-sponsor:** Apotekerfonden.

615.11 USA ISSN 0195-7996
RS141.2 CODEN: USPFDX
UNITED STATES PHARMACOPEIA - NATIONAL FORMULARY. Text in English. 1820. every 5 yrs. USD 450; includes annual supplement. **Description:** Compiles all the legally enforceable standards of strength, purity, packaging, labeling, and storage for drugs and excipients.
Formed by the 1980 merger of: National Formulary (0084-6414); United States Pharmacopeia; Which was formerly titled: Pharmacopeia of the United States of America (0079-1407)
—BLDSC (9100.172000), CASDDS, CISTI.
Published by: United States Pharmacopeia, 12601 Twinbrook Pkwy, Rockville, MD 20852. TEL 800-877-6733, FAX 802-864-7626, http://www.usp.org.

615.1 VEN ISSN 0041-8307
RM101 CODEN: RFFVA6
UNIVERSIDAD CENTRAL DE VENEZUELA. FACULTAD DE FARMACIA. REVISTA. Text in English, Spanish; Summaries in English. 1959. s-a. per issue exchange basis. bk.rev. abstr, bibl, charts, illus, stat. index. back issues avail. *Refereed.* **Document type:** *Academic/Scholarly.*
Related titles: Fax ed.
Indexed: Biol.Abstr., I.P.A.
—CASDDS, Linda Hall.
Published by: Universidad Central de Venezuela, Facultad de Farmacia, Apdo. 40109, Nueva Granada, Ciudad Universitaria, las Chaguaramos, Caracas, Venezuela. TEL 58-2-605-2731, FAX 58-2-605-2707, fcarrill@sagi.ucv.edu.ve. Ed. Fanny C Padilla. Pub. Miguel Garcia. Circ: 1,000.

615 ESP ISSN 0067-4176
UNIVERSIDAD DE BARCELONA. FACULTAD DE FARMACIA. MEMORIA✱ . Text in Spanish. biennial. Price varies.
Published by: Universidad de Barcelona, Facultad de Farmacia, Av. Jose Antonio 585, Barcelona, 7, Spain.

615 ESP ISSN 0214-1442
UNIVERSIDAD DE SEVILLA. SERIE: FARMACIA. Text in Spanish. 1983. irreg., latest vol.4.
Indexed: Ind.SST.
Published by: Universidad de Sevilla, Servicio de Publicaciones, Porvenir, 27, Sevilla 41013, Spain. TEL 34-5-4487446, FAX 34-5-4487443.

615.19 PER ISSN 0377-4708
RS1
UNIVERSIDAD NACIONAL MAYOR DE SAN MARCOS. FACULTAD DE FARMACIA Y BIOQUIMICA. REVISTA. Text in Spanish. 1939. s-a. charts, illus, stat. **Document type:** *Academic/Scholarly.*
Indexed: Biol.Abstr.
—CISTI.
Published by: Universidad Nacional Mayor de San Marcos, Facultad de Farmacia y Bioquimica, Apdo. 1760, Lima, Peru. Circ: 500.

615.19 BRA ISSN 0370-4726
RS1 CODEN: RFBUBI
UNIVERSIDADE DE SAO PAULO. REVISTA DE FARMACIA E BIOQUIMICA. Text in Portuguese. 1939. a. USD 40 to individuals; USD 45 to institutions. bk.rev. back issues avail. *Refereed.* **Document type:** *Academic/Scholarly.*
Formerly: Universidade de Sao Paulo. Faculdade de Farmacia e Bioquimica. Revista; Supersedes in part (in 1962): Universidade de Sao Paulo. Faculdade de Farmacia. Anais (0365-2181)
Related titles: Online - full text ed.
Indexed: Anal.Abstr., Chem.Abstr., Chem.Titles, Derwent Biotech.Abstr., Helminthol.Abstr., INIS Atomind., I.P.A., Mass Spectr.Bull., Nutr.Abstr., Rev.Med.& Vet.Mycol.
—CASDDS, CISTI, EMDOCS, GNLM, KNAW.
Published by: Universidade de Sao Paulo, Faculdade de Ciencias Farmaceuticas, Vl Leopoldina, Caixa Postal 66083, Sao Paulo, SP 05389-970, Brazil. TEL 55-11-8137251, FAX 55-11-2128194, bibcq@quim.iq.usp.br. Ed. Andrejus Korolkovas. Circ: 1,000.

615.329 547 BRA ISSN 0080-0228
UNIVERSIDADE FEDERAL DE PERNAMBUCO. INSTITUTO DE ANTIBIOTICOS. REVISTA. Text in Portuguese; Summaries in English, Portuguese. 1958. irreg., latest vol.23, 1986. per issue exchange basis. bibl, charts, illus. **Document type:** *Academic/Scholarly.*
Indexed: Chem.Abstr.
—GNLM.
Published by: Universidade Federal de Pernambuco, Departamento de Antibioticos, Recife, PERNAMBUCO, Brazil. TELEX 811267. Circ: 800.

615.1 BRA ISSN 0041-8846
UNIVERSIDADE FEDERAL DE SANTA MARIA. FACULDADE DE FARMACIA E BIOQUIMICA. REVISTA✱ . Text in Portuguese. s-a. charts, illus.
Published by: Universidade Federal de Santa Maria, Faculdade de Farmacie e Bioquimica, Caixa Postal 124, Santa Maria, R.G.S., Brazil.

615 ITA ISSN 0430-3210
UNIVERSITA DI FERRARA. ANNALI. SEZIONE 11: FARMACOLOGIA E TERAPIA. Text in Italian. 1953. 3/w.
Published by: (Universita di Ferrara), Casa Editrice Leo S. Olschki, Viuzzo Del Pozzetto, Florence, FI 50126, Italy. TEL 39-55-6530684, FAX 39-55-6530214.

615.1 SVK ISSN 0041-9087
UNIVERSITAS COMENIANA. ACTA FACULTATIS PHARMACEUTICAE. Text in English, German, Russian. 1958. irreg. per issue exchange basis. charts, illus. index.
Formerly: Acta Facultatis Pharmaceuticae Bohemoslovenicae
Indexed: Alloys Ind., Biol.Abstr., Chem.Abstr., I.P.A., Met.Abstr., Met.Abstr.Ind., Nonfer.Met.Alert, PCC Alert, Steels Alert.
Published by: Univerzita Komenskeho, Farmaceuticka Fakulta, Ustredna Kniznica, Odbojarov 10, Bratislava 83232, Slovakia. FAX 042-7060388. Ed. Milan Chalabala. Circ: 500.

615.1 USA
UNIVERSITY OF THE SCIENCES IN PHILADELPHIA BULLETIN. Text in English. 1865. q. free to alumni. illus. reprint service avail. from PQC. **Document type:** *Bulletin.* **Description:** Information pertaining to the University and its alumni.
Former title: Philadelphia College of Pharmacy and Science Bulletin (0031-725X)
Published by: University of the Sciences in Philadelphia, 600 S 43rd St, Philadelphia, PA 19104. TEL 215-596-8545, FAX 215-895-1177, h.gomon@usip.edu, http://www.usip.edu. Ed., R&P Harriet Gomon. Circ: 15,000 (controlled).

615 USA ISSN 8755-7142
RS1
UNLISTED DRUGS INDEX - GUIDE. Text in English. irreg., latest 1997 (every 2-3/yrs.). USD 680.
Published by: Pharmaco-Medical Documentation, Inc., 21 Green Village Rd, Madison, NJ 07940. TEL 973-822-9200, FAX 973-765-0722.

616.6 615 USA ISSN 1074-2921
VACCINE WEEKLY. Text in English. 1994. w. (43/yr.). USD 1,549 in North America; USD 1,649 elsewhere. **Document type:** *Newsletter.* **Description:** Brings together relevant news and breakthroughs from interrelated topics ranging from therapeutic vaccines for AIDS, cancer, and other diseases, efficacy and safety trials, FDA regulations and approvals, and prevention.
Related titles: Microform ed.: (from PQC); Online - full text ed.: (from Gale Group, Northern Light Technology, Inc., Factiva).
Indexed: Bus.& Indus. (Jan.1995-).
—CCC.
Published by: Charles W. Henderson, Ed. & Pub., PO Box 5528, Atlanta, GA 31107-0528. TEL 770-507-7777, FAX 770-507-7788, info@hendersonnet.atl.ga.us, http://www.newsfile.com.

615 USA
VALIDATION TIMES. Text in English. 1998. m. USD 699 (effective 2001). 20 p./no. back issues avail. **Document type:** *Newsletter.*
Formerly: Drug, Evaluation and Compliance Report; Validation Timer
Related titles: E-mail ed.; Online - full text ed.
Published by: Washington Information Source, 6506 Old Stage Rd, Ste 100, Rockville, MD 20852-4326. TEL 301-770-5553, http://www.fdainfo.com. Ed., Pub., R&P Ken Reid.

615.1 USA ISSN 1098-3015
CODEN: VIHLFM
VALUE IN HEALTH. Text in English. 1998. bi-m. USD 115 domestic to individuals; USD 130 in Canada & Mexico to individuals; USD 145 elsewhere to individuals; USD 200 domestic to institutions; USD 215 in Canada & Mexico to institutions; USD 230 elsewhere to institutions; USD 126.50 to individuals; USD 220 to institutions (effective 2001). adv. reprints avail. *Refereed.* **Document type:** *Academic/Scholarly.* **Description:** Evaluates medical technologies, including pharmaceutical, biologics, devices, procedures, and other medical interventions.
Related titles: Online - full text ed.: ISSN 1524-4733. USD 104 to individuals; USD 180 to institutions (effective 2001) (from EBSCO Publishing, O C L C Online Computer Library Center, Inc., RoweCom Information Quest, ingenta, Munksgaard & Blackwell Science's Synergy, Swets Blackwell).
Indexed: I.P.A., Inpharma, Pharm.&Out.News, Reac.
—BLDSC (9142.093500). **CCC.**
Published by: (International Society for Pharmacoeconomics and Outcomes Research), Blackwell Science Inc., Commerce Pl, 350 Main St, Malden, MA 02148-5018. TEL 781-388-8250, 800-759-6102, FAX 781-388-8255, journals@blacksci.com; isporjnl@hsc.usc.edu, http://www.blackwell-science.com. Ed. Joel W Hay. R&P Tracey Davies. Adv. contact Jenny Applin.

615.1 NOR ISSN 0042-3351
VENEFICUS; farmasistudentenes tidsskrift. Text in Norwegian. 1935. 6/yr. NOK 100, USD 6 domestic; NOK 125 foreign (effective 1999). adv. bk.rev. charts, illus. index. **Description:** Forum for pharmacy students' activities, with reviews of social events, articles on sports and scientific discussions.
Indexed: Chem.Abstr., I.P.A.
Published by: Studentforeningen Veneficus/Students Association Veneficus, Farmasoeytisk Institutt, Postboks 1068, Blindern, Oslo 0104, Norway. tidsskrift@farmasi.uio.no. Eds. Astrid H Fidjeland, Ragna H Stromman. Adv. contact Tone Brynn. page NOK 1,000. Circ: 600.

VETERINARY AND HUMAN TOXICOLOGY. see *ENVIRONMENTAL STUDIES—Toxicology And Environmental Safety*

615.1 USA ISSN 0042-6717
RS1
VIRGINIA PHARMACIST. Text in English. 1882. m. USD 50 domestic; USD 100 elsewhere (effective 2001). adv. bk.rev. charts, illus, mkt, pat, tr.lit. back issues avail. **Document type:** *Trade.* **Description:** Publishes articles of interest concerning the pharmaceutical industry for an audience of pharmacists and practitioners of related industries.
Indexed: I.P.A.
—Linda Hall.

P

Published by: Virginia Pharmaceutical Association, 5501 Patterson Ave, Ste 200, Richmond, VA 23226-2025. TEL 804-355-7941, FAX 804-285-4227, rphanow@erols.com. Ed. Rebecca P Snead. R&P Rebecca Snead TEL 804-285-4145. Adv. contact Peggy McLaughlin. Circ: 2,000 (paid).

615.1 COL ISSN 0121-4004
VITAE. Text in Spanish. 1991. s-a. COP 14,000 domestic; USD 10 foreign (effective 2000). back issues avail. **Document type:** *Academic/Scholarly.* **Description:** publishes original research in pharmaceutical chemistry, cosmetic and food sciences and technology.
Published by: Universidad de Antioquia, Facultad de Quimica Farmaceutica, Apartado Postal 1226, Medellin, Colombia. TEL 57-4-210-5475, FAX 57-4-210-5456, http://muiscas.udea.edu.co/~vitae/indice.html.

615.9 610.73 USA ISSN 0739-9588
VITAL SIGNS PHARMACY SERVICES NEWSLETTER. Text in English. 1978. m. USD 85 (effective 2001). back issues avail. **Document type:** *Newsletter.* **Description:** Hospital pharmacy-nursing newsletter with photocopy rights for facility. Helps meet JCAHO requirements for hospital staff continuing education.
Published by: Rx-Data-Pac Service, 8907 Terwilliger s Tr, Cincinnati, OH 45249. TEL 513-489-0943, FAX 513-489-0943. Ed. Dr. I H Goodman.

615.328 JPN ISSN 0006-386X
QP771 CODEN: BTMNA7
VITAMINS/BITAMIN. Text in Japanese; Summaries in English. 1948. m. USD 35.
Related titles: Online - full text ed.: (from Northern Light Technology, Inc.).
Indexed: Biol.Abstr., Chem.Abstr., Dairy Sci.Abstr., Excerp.Med., Food Sci.& Tech.Abstr., INIS Atomind., Jap.Per.Ind., Nutr.Abstr., Ref.Zh.
—BLDSC (9243.500000), CASDDS, CISTI, Infotrieve, Linda Hall. **CCC.**
Published by: Japan Vitamin Society/Nippon Bitamin Gakkai, Nippon Itaria Kyoto Kaikan, 3rd Fl, 4 Ushinomiya-cho, Yoshida, Sakyo-ku, Kyoto-shi 606, Japan. TEL 075-751-0314. Ed. Shyoichi Shimizu.

615.328 658.8 GBR
VITAMINS & DIETARY SUPPLEMENTS: THE INTERNATIONAL MARKET. Text in English. a. GBP 2,250, USD 4,500. **Document type:** *Trade.* **Description:** Analyzes the vitamin and dietary supplement market for France, Germany, Italy, Spain, the U.K., the U.S., and Japan.
Former titles: Slimming and Supplementary Nutrition: The International Market; Vitamins and Dietary Supplements: The International Market
Related titles: Online - full text ed.: (from Data-Star, The Dialog Corporation).
Published by: Euromonitor, 60-61 Britton St, London EC1M 5UX, United Kingdom. TEL 44-20-7251-8024, info@euromonitor.com, http://www.euromonitor.com.

615.328 612.405 USA ISSN 0083-6729
QP801.V5 CODEN: VIHOAQ
VITAMINS AND HORMONES: ADVANCES IN RESEARCH AND APPLICATIONS. Text in English. 1943. irreg., latest vol.54, 1998. index, cum.index: vols.1-5 (1943-1947), vols.6-10 (1948-1952), vols.11-15 (1953-1957). reprint service avail. from ISI. *Refereed.* **Document type:** *Academic/Scholarly.*
Related titles: Online - full text ed.: (from Institute for Scientific Information).
Indexed: ASCA, Agri.& Environ.Biotech.Abstr. (coverage dropped), Agricola, Anim.Breed.Abstr., BBCI, Biol.Abstr., Chem.Abstr., Curr.Adv.Ecol.Sci., Dairy Sci.Abstr., Derwent Biotech.Abstr., Excerp.Med., Ind.Med. (1943-), Ind.Sci.Rev., Nutr.Abstr., Sci.Cit.Ind., Vet.Bull.
—BLDSC (9244.000000), CASDDS, CISTI, GNLM, ingenta, Linda Hall. **CCC.**
Published by: Academic Press, Inc., Journal Division (Subsidiary of: Harcourt Brace & Company), 525 B St, Ste 1900, San Diego, CA 92101-4495. TEL 619-231-0926, FAX 619-699-6715. Eds. Donald B McCormick, G D Auerbach. **Subscr. to:** Order Dept., 6277 Sea Harbor Dr, 4th Fl, Orlando, FL 32887. TEL 800-321-5068.

615.328 DEU ISSN 0943-3163
VITAMINSPUR; Zeitschrift fuer Diaetetik, Ernaehrungsmedizin und angewandte Ernaehrungsberatung. Text in German; Summaries in English. 1986. 5/yr. EUR 75.40 domestic to institutions; EUR 81.90 in Europe to institutions; EUR 84.80 elsewhere to institutions; EUR 34.90 to students; EUR 16.90 newsstand/cover (effective 2002). adv. bk.rev., software rev., Website rev. abstr, bibl, charts, illus. back issues avail. *Refereed.* **Document type:** *Journal, Academic/Scholarly.*
Formerly (until 1992): Vitamine, Mineralstoffe, Spurenelemente in Medizin, Ernaehrung und Umwelt (0930-4827)
Indexed: Dairy Sci.Abstr., Nutr.Abstr.
—GNLM.
Published by: Hippokrates Verlag GmbH, Postfach 300504, Stuttgart 70445, Germany. TEL 49-711-8931-0, FAX 49-711-8931706, http://www.hippokrates.de. Ed. Hanno Kretschmer. Adv. contact Guenter Fecke TEL 49-711-8931714. Circ: 3,000 (paid).

615.9 USA ISSN 0507-2379
VOICE OF THE PHARMACIST. Text in English. 1946. q. USD 40. **Document type:** *Newsletter.*
Indexed: I.P.A.
Published by: American College of Apothecaries, PO Box 341266, Memphis, TN 38184. TEL 901-383-8119, FAX 901-383-8882. Ed. D C Huffman Jr. Circ: 1,000.

VOJENSKE ZDRAVOTNICKE LISTY. see *MEDICAL SCIENCES*

VOJNOSANITETSKI PREGLED/MILITARY MEDICAL AND PHARMACEUTICAL; casopis lekara i farmaceuta vojske Jugoslavije. see *MEDICAL SCIENCES*

VOPROSY BIOLOGICHESKOI, MEDITSINSKOI, I FARMATSEVTICHESKOI KHIMII/PROBLEMS OF BIOLOGICAL, MEDICAL AND PHARMACOLOGICAL. see *BIOLOGY*

W H O DRUG INFORMATION. see *PUBLIC HEALTH AND SAFETY*

615 JPN ISSN 0509-5832
WAKSMAN FOUNDATION OF JAPAN. REPORT. Text in English. 1962. a. per issue exchange basis.
—Linda Hall.
Published by: Waksman Foundation of Japan/Nihon Wakkusuman Zaidan, c/o Keio Daigaku Igakubu, 30-8 Daikyo-cho, Shinjuku-ku, Tokyo 160-0015, Japan.

WARNING LETTER BULLETIN. see *MEDICAL SCIENCES*

616 USA ISSN 0194-1291
KF3885.A15
WASHINGTON DRUG LETTER (WASHINGTON, 1979). Text in English. 1969. w., latest vol.34, 2002. USD 897 in North America; USD 947 elsewhere (effective Nov. 2001). bk.rev. 8 p./no. Supplement avail.; back issues avail. **Document type:** *Newsletter.* **Description:** Reports on regulation of the pharmaceutical and biotechnology industries by the FDA and Congress.
Former titles (until 1979): Washington Drug and Device Letter (0162-2994); Washington Drug Letter; Incorporates (in 1994): Pharmaceutical and Biotech Daily (1074-8636); Which was formed by the merger of (1993-1994): Pharmaceutical Daily (1071-5096); (1992-1994): Biotech Daily (1067-1196); Which superseded (1981-1992): Genetic Engineering Letter (0276-1882)
Related titles: E-mail ed.: (from The Dialog Corporation).
Indexed: P.N.I., Telegen.
—Infotrieve. **CCC.**
Published by: Washington Business Information, Inc., 300 N Washington St, Ste 200, Falls Church, Arlington, VA 22046. TEL 703-538-7661, FAX 703 538-7676, ehinkle@fdanews.com, http://www.fdanews.com. Ed. Elizabeth Tilley-Hinkle. Pub. David Swit.

615 USA ISSN 0745-7413
THE WASHINGTON PHARMACIST. Text in English. 1959. 4/yr. USD 24 domestic; USD 59 foreign; USD 6 newsstand/cover (effective 2000). adv. bk.rev. **Document type:** *Trade.* **Description:** Focuses on current issues and challenges of the profession. Appeals to a broad spectrum of pharmacy professionals with articles about new products.
Formerly: Washington - Alaska Pharmacist
Indexed: I.P.A.
Published by: Washington State Pharmacists Association, 1501 Taylor Ave, S W, Renton, WA 98055-3139. TEL 425-228-7171, FAX 425-277-3897, http://www.pharmcare.org. Ed. Rod Shafer. R&P Sheri Ray. Adv. contact Sheri L Ray. Circ: 2,000.

615.1 USA
THE WEEK ONLINE. Text in English. w. **Document type:** *Newsletter.* **Description:** Covers the drug war and the growing global reform movement, includes news from around the world and expert commentary from leading reform voices. Dedicated to raising awareness of the consequences of drug prohibition.
Media: Online - full text.
Published by: Drug Reform Coordination Network, 2000 P St, N W, 615, Washington, DC 20036. TEL 202-293-8340, FAX 202-293-8344, drcnet@drcnet.org, http://www.stopthedrugwar.org/. Ed. David Borden.

615.1 USA ISSN 0043-1893
CODEN: WPHRAR
WEEKLY PHARMACY REPORTS: THE GREEN SHEET. Text in English. 1951. w. USD 90 domestic; USD 140 foreign (effective 2001). back issues avail.; reprints avail. **Document type:** *Trade.* **Description:** News and information on the pharmacy profession and the pharmaceutical distribution system. Coverage of professional policy, pharmacy association activities, reimbursement issues, new drug introductions and pharmaceutical pricing and deals.
Related titles: Online - full text ed.
Indexed: P.N.I.
—**CCC.**
Published by: F-D-C Reports, Inc., 5550 Friendship Blvd, Ste One, Chevy Chase, MD 20815-7278. TEL 800-332-2181, FAX 301-664-7238, http://www.fdcreports.com. Ed. Scott Steinke. R&P Michael Keville.

WEHRMEDIZIN UND WEHRPHARMAZIE. see *MEDICAL SCIENCES*

615.19 DEU ISSN 0171-4449
WER UND WAS IN DER DEUTSCHEN PHARMAZEUTISCHEN - INDUSTRIE. Text in German. 1978. biennial. DEM 269 (effective 2000). **Document type:** *Directory, Trade.*
—GNLM.
Published by: B. Behr's Verlag GmbH, Averhoffstr 10, Hamburg 22085, Germany. TEL 49-40-2270080, FAX 49-40-2201091, behrs@behrs.de, http://www.behrs.de.

615.19 NGA ISSN 0303-691X
CODEN: WAJPAS
WEST AFRICAN JOURNAL OF PHARMACOLOGY AND DRUG RESEARCH. Text in English. 1974. biennial. USD 10.60 (effective 2000). *Refereed.* **Document type:** *Journal, Academic/Scholarly.*
Indexed: Biol.Abstr., Chem.Abstr., Excerp.Med. (until 1993), Ind.Med. (coverage dropped).
—CASDDS, GNLM.
Published by: (West African Society for Pharmacology), Literamed Publications Nigeria Ltd, PMB 21068, Ikeja, Oregun Village, Lagos, Nigeria. TEL 234-64-962512, FAX 234-64-961037. Pub. O M Lawal Solarin.

615.1 CAN ISSN 0043-3829
WESTERN HORIZONS; a quarterly magazine for Western Canadian pharmacists. Text in English. 1966. q. free per issue. adv. **Document type:** *Trade.*
Published by: National Drug & Chemical Co. of Canada Ltd., P O Box 758, Winnipeg, MB, Canada. TEL 204-774-4511. Ed. T H Glenwright. Circ: 3,200.

615.1 USA ISSN 0083-8969
CODEN: PWPSA8
WESTERN PHARMACOLOGY SOCIETY. PROCEEDINGS. Text in English. 1958. a. USD 35 (effective 2000). reprint service avail. from PQC. *Refereed.* **Document type:** *Proceedings, Academic/Scholarly.*
Related titles: Microform ed.: (from PQC).
Indexed: Anim.Behav.Abstr. (coverage dropped), Aqua.Sci.& Fish.Abstr., Biol.Abstr., Chem.Abstr., Chem.Indus.Notes, Chem.Titles, Curr.Adv.Ecol.Sci., Curr.Cont. (coverage dropped), Dairy Sci.Abstr., Excerp.Med., INIS Atomind., Ind.Med. (1958-), Neurosci.Abstr. (coverage dropped), Nutr.Abstr., Zoo.Rec.
—BLDSC (6834.200000), CASDDS, CISTI, GNLM, ingenta, KNAW, Linda Hall. **CCC.**
Published by: Western Pharmacology Society, Inc., University of Arizona, Department of Pharmacology, College of Medicine, Tucson, AZ 85724-5050. TEL 520-626-7843, FAX 520-626-6883, huxtable@u.arizona.edu. Ed. Dr. Ryan J Huxtable. Circ: 500 (paid).

615.1 USA
WHITE SHEET. Text in English. 1967. m. free to pharmacists. bk.rev.
Formerly (until 1977): Hospital Pharmacy (0018-5779)
Published by: Philips Roxane Laboratories, Inc., 330 Oak St, Columbus, OH 43216. TEL 614-228-5403. Ed. Richard E Surface. Circ: 25,000.

615 GBR ISSN 0140-4806
WORLD DRUG MARKET MANUAL. Text in English. 1975. a. GBP 5,100. **Document type:** *Trade.*
Related titles: CD-ROM ed.; Online - full text ed.

P

Published by: IMSWORLD Publications Ltd., 7 Harewood Ave, London NW1 6JB, United Kingdom. TEL 0171-393-5000, FAX 0171-393-5900, TELEX 8954520.

615 338 658 GBR
▼ **THE WORLD MARKET FOR O T C HEALTHCARE.** (Over the Counter) Text in English. 1999. irreg. GBP 4,750; USD 9,500 in United States. **Description:** Features global investigation into the worldwide OTC healthcare products industry. Includes in-depth sales, share and distribution analysis.
Published by: Euromonitor, 60-61 Britton St, London EC1M 5UX, United Kingdom. TEL 44-20-7251-8024, info@euromonitor.com, http://www.euromonitor.com.

615.7822 USA
WORLD OF DRUG INFORMATION. Text in English. q. back issues avail. **Document type:** *Newsletter.*
Related titles: Online - full text ed.
Published by: University of Iowa, College of Pharmacy, Iowa Drug Information Service, 100 Oakdale Campus, N330 OH, Iowa City, IA 52242-5000. TEL 319-335-4800, 800-525-4347, FAX 319-335-4440, idis@uiowa.edu, http://www.uiowa.edu/~idis/idisnews.htm. Ed., R&P Donna Brus. Circ: 2,500.

615 GBR CODEN: PMAIF8
WORLD PHARMACEUTICAL DEVELOPMENTS. Text in English. 198?. a. adv. **Document type:** *Journal, Trade.* **Description:** Covers the most important developments in the global pharmaceuticals industry.
Formerly: Pharmaceutical Manufacturing International (0951-9696)
—BLDSC (6444.036000), CASDDS, GNLM.
Published by: Sterling Publications Ltd. (Subsidiary of: Sterling Publishing Group Plc.), Brunel House, 55-57 North Wharf Rd, London W2 1LA, United Kingdom. TEL 44-20-7915-9660, FAX 44-20-7724-2089, wpd@sterlingpublications.com, info@sterlingpublications.com, http://www.worldpharmaceuticals.net, http://www.sterlingpublications.com. Pub. Sarah Woddis. Circ: 10,000 (controlled).

615.1029 USA ISSN 0276-2277
RM39
WORLD PHARMACEUTICAL DIRECTORY. Text in English. irreg., latest 1996 (every 2-3 yrs.). USD 640. **Document type:** *Directory.*
Published by: Pharmaco-Medical Documentation, Inc., 21 Green Village Rd, Madison, NJ 07940. TEL 973-822-9200, FAX 973-765-0722.

WORLDWIDE BIOTECH. see *BIOLOGY—Biotechnology*

XINZHONGYI/NEW JOURNAL OF TRADITIONAL CHINESE MEDICINE. see *ALTERNATIVE MEDICINE*

615.1 JPN ISSN 0913-0683
YAKKYOKU NO TOMO (TOKYO, 1975)/PHARMACY COMPANION. Text in Japanese. 1953. m. adv. charts, illus, tr.lit.
Formerly (until 1975): Yakkyoku no Tomo (Tokyo, 1953) (0044-0043)
Published by: Yamanouchi Pharmaceutical Co. Ltd./Yamanouchi Seiyaku K.K., 2-5 Nihonbashihoncho, Chuo-ku, Tokyo 103-0023, Japan. Circ: 20,000.

615.1 JPN ISSN 0031-6903 CODEN: YKKZAJ
YAKUGAKU ZASSHI/PHARMACEUTICAL JOURNAL. Variant title: Pharmaceutical Society of Japan. Journal. Text in English, Japanese; Abstracts and contents page in English. 1881. m. USD 90 to members (effective 2001). adv. tr.lit, tr.mk, bibl. index. 90 p./no. *Refereed.* **Document type:** *Bulletin, Academic/Scholarly.* **Description:** Covers all pharmaceutical sciences.
Related titles: Microform ed.: (from PMC); Online - full text ed.: (from Institute for Scientific Information).
Indexed: ASCA, Agri.& Environ.Biotech.Abstr. (coverage dropped), Anal.Abstr., Biol.Abstr., Chem.Abstr., Chem.Cit.Ind., Chem.Indus.Notes, Chem.Titles, Crop Physiol.Abstr., Curr.Adv.Biochem., Curr.Adv.Ecol.Sci., Curr.Chem.React., Curr.Cont., Dairy Sci.Abstr., Excerp.Med., Food Sci.& Tech.Abstr., Forest Prod.Abstr., Forest.Abstr., Helminthol.Abstr., Hort.Abstr., INIS Atomind., I.P.A., Ind.Chem., Ind.Med. (1881-), Ind.Sci.Rev., Inpharma, Mass Spectr.Bull., Nutr.Abstr., Pharm.&Out.News, RCI, Reac., Sci.Cit.Ind.
—BLDSC (4840.000000), CASDDS, CISTI, GNLM, IDS, Infotrieve, KNAW, Linda Hall. **CCC.**
Published by: Pharmaceutical Society of Japan/Nihon Yakugakkai, 2-12-15, Shibuya, Shibuya-ku, Tokyo 150-0002, Japan. TEL 81-3-3406-3321, FAX 81-3-3498-1835, ronb@pharm.or.jp, http://yakushi.or.jp. Ed. Mikio Yamazaki. Circ: 2,400.

615 KOR
YAKUP SHINMOON/PHARMACEUTICAL NEWS. Text in Korean. 1954. s-w. KRW 60,000. adv. bk.rev. **Document type:** *Newspaper.*
Address: 100-1, 2-ka, Cheongpa-Dong, Yongsan-Ku, Seoul 140, Korea, S.. TEL 82-2-3270-0114, FAX 02-3270-0159. Ed. Seung Joon Jin. Pub. Hahm Yong Hun. Adv. contact Ki Joo Ko.

615 JPN ISSN 0386-3603 CODEN: YACHDS
YAKURI TO CHIRYO/JAPANESE PHARMACOLOGY AND THERAPEUTICS. Text in Japanese; Summaries in English. 1973. m.
Related titles: Online - full text ed.: (from Institute for Scientific Information).
Indexed: Chem.Abstr., Chem.Indus.Notes, Excerp.Med., INIS Atomind., Inpharma, Reac.
—BLDSC (4660.200000), CASDDS, CISTI, EMDOCS, GNLM, KNAW.
Published by: Life Science Publishing Co. Ltd., 11-7 Nihonbashikobuna-cho, Chuo-ku, Tokyo 103-0024, Japan. TEL 3-3664-7750.

615 JPN ISSN 0910-5247
YAMAGUCHI UNIVERSITY. DRUG INFORMATION NEWS. Text in Japanese. 1966. q.
Published by: Yamaguchi Daigaku Igakubu, Fuzhoku Byoin D I Senta, 1144 Kogushi, Ube-shi, Yamaguchi-ken 755-0067, Japan.

615 CHN ISSN 0254-1793
RS189 CODEN: YFZADL
YAOWU FENXI ZAZHI/JOURNAL OF PHARMACEUTICAL ANALYSIS. Text in Chinese. 1981. bi-m. USD 25.20; USD 4.20 newsstand/cover (effective 2001). adv. *Refereed.* **Document type:** *Academic/Scholarly.*
Related titles: Online - full content ed.: (from WanFang Data Corp.).
Indexed: Anal.Abstr., Chem.Abstr., Chem.Indus.Notes, Chem.Titles, Excerp.Med. (1993-), Hort.Abstr., I.P.A., Mass Spectr.Bull., Rev.Plant Path.
—BLDSC (3180.473000), CASDDS, CISTI, EMDOCS, Linda Hall.
Published by: Zhongguo Yaoxuehui/Chinese Pharmaceutical Association, 2, Tianting Xili, Beijing 100050, China. TEL 86-1-67017755, ywfx@public.sti.ac.cn. **Dist. by:** China International Book Trading Corp, 35, Chegongzhuang Xilu, Haidian District, Beijing 100044, China. TEL 86-1-68413849, FAX 86-1-68412048, cibtc@mail.cibtc.com.cn, http://www.cibtc.com.cn.

615.19 CHN ISSN 0513-4870
RS1 CODEN: YHHPAL
YAOXUE XUEBAO/ACTA PHARMACEUTICA SINICA. Text in Chinese. 1953. m. USD 62.40 foreign; USD 19.20 newsstand/cover foreign; USD 8 newsstand/cover domestic (effective 2001).
Related titles: Online - full content ed.: (from WanFang Data Corp.).
Indexed: Abstr.Hyg., AgBiotech, Chem.Abstr., Chem.Indus.Notes, Chem.Titles, Crop Physiol.Abstr., Curr.Adv.Ecol.Sci., Curr.Cont. (coverage dropped), Field Crop Abstr., Forest Prod.Abstr., Forest.Abstr., Helminthol.Abstr., Hort.Abstr., I.P.A., Ind.Med. (1953-), Mass Spectr.Bull., Nutr.Abstr., Plant Breed.Abstr., Plant Gen.Res.Abstr., Poult.Abstr., Protozool.Abstr., Rev.Appl.Entomol., Rev.Arom.& Med.Plants, Rev.Med.& Vet.Mycol., Seed Abstr.
—BLDSC (0646.500000), CASDDS, CISTI, GNLM, KNAW, Linda Hall.
Published by: Zhonghua Yixuehui Zazhishe, 42 Dongsi Xidajie, Beijing 100710, China. TEL 86-1-63035116, FAX 86-1-63017757, yxxb@imm.ac.cn. Ed. Tong-Hui Zhou. **Dist. by:** China International Book Trading Corp, 35, Chegongzhuang Xilu, Haidian District, Beijing 100044, China. TEL 86-1-68413849, FAX 86-1-68412048, cibtc@mail.cibtc.com.cn, http://www.cibtc.com.cn.

615 CHN
YIYAO GONGCHENG SHEJI. Text in Chinese. bi-m.
Published by: Guojia Yiyao Guanli-ju, Shanghai Yiyao Sheji-yuan/State Administration of Pharmacy, Shanghai Pharmacy Design Academy, 1856 Nanjing Donglu, Shanghai 200040, China. TEL 2584840. Ed. Lu Zhendong.

YOKOHAMA MEDICAL JOURNAL. see *MEDICAL SCIENCES*

YUNNAN ZHONGYI ZAZHI/YUNNAN JOURNAL OF TRADITIONAL CHINESE MEDICINE. see *ALTERNATIVE MEDICINE*

615 EGY ISSN 1110-5089 CODEN: ZJPSEV
ZAGAZIG JOURNAL OF PHARMACEUTICAL SCIENCES. Text in Arabic, English. 1992. s-a. USD 150 (effective 1998). **Document type:** *Bulletin, Academic/Scholarly.*
Indexed: Chem.Indus.Notes, Chem.Titles.
—BLDSC (9425.516200), CASDDS.
Published by: Zagazig University, Faculty of Pharmacy, Zagazig, Egypt. TEL 20-55-323266, FAX 20-55-323266. Ed. Maher El Domiaty. R&P Abdelmonem Ateya.

615.1 DEU ISSN 1431-9292
ZEITSCHRIFT FUER ARZNEI- UND GEWUERZPFLANZEN. Text in German. 1997. q. DEM 208 (effective 2001). **Document type:** *Journal, Academic/Scholarly.*
Indexed: AMED, Food Sci.& Tech.Abstr., Hort.Abstr., Irr.& Drain.Abstr., Plant Breed.Abstr., Plant Gen.Res.Abstr., Postharvest, Rev.Appl.Entomol., Rev.Arom.& Med.Plants, Rev.Med.& Vet.Mycol., Rev.Plant Path., Seed Abstr., Soils & Fert., Weed Abstr., World Ag.Econ.& Rur.Soc.Abstr.
—BLDSC (9452.270000), GNLM.
Published by: Agrimedia GmbH, Spithal 4, Bergen-Dumme 29468, Germany. TEL 49-5845-9881-0, FAX 49-5845-988111, mail@agrimedia.com, http://www.agrimedia.com.

ZHEJIANG ZHONGYI XUEYUAN XUEBAO/ZHEJIANG COLLEGE OF TRADITIONAL CHINESE MEDICINE. JOURNAL. see *MEDICAL SCIENCES*

ZHEJIANG ZHONGYI ZAZHI/ZHEJIANG JOURNAL OF TRADITIONAL CHINESE MEDICINE. see *ALTERNATIVE MEDICINE*

615.328 615.89 CHN
ZHONG CAO YAO/CHINESE HERBAL MEDICINE. Text in Chinese. m. USD 0.80 per issue.
Indexed: Chem.Abstr.
Published by: China International Book Trading Corp/Zhongguo Guoji Tushu Maoyi Zonggongsi, 35 Chegongzhuang Xilu, Haidian District, Beijing 100044, China. TEL 86-1-68413849, FAX 86-1-68412048, cibtc@mail.cibtc.com.cn, http://www.cibtc.com.cn.

615 CHN ISSN 1001-1528
ZHONGCHENYAO/CHINESE TRADITIONAL PATENT MEDICINE. Text in Chinese; Abstracts occasionally in English. 1988. m. USD 62.40; USD 5.20 newsstand/cover (effective 2001). adv. bk.rev. *Refereed.* **Document type:** *Academic/Scholarly, Trade.* **Description:** Reports the recent research achievements in industry of Chinese patent medicine and introduces new products, dosage formulations, processes and new equipment used in this industry.
Published by: Guojia Yaoping Jiandu Guanli Ju, Nankai-qu, Anshan Xi Dao 308 Hao, Tianjin 300193, China. Circ: 10,000. **Dist. outside China by:** China International Book Trading Corp, 35, Chegongzhuang Xilu, Haidian District, Beijing 100044, China. TEL 86-1-68413849, FAX 86-1-68412048, cibtc@mail.cibtc.com.cn, http://www.cibtc.com.cn.

578.77 CHN ISSN 1002-3461
ZHONGGUO HAIYANG YAOWU ZAZHI/CHINESE JOURNAL OF MARINE DRUGS. Text in Chinese. 1982. bi-m. USD 23.40; CNY 7.50, USD 3.90 newsstand/cover (effective 2001). **Document type:** *Academic/Scholarly.*
Indexed: Aquacult.Abstr.
—BLDSC (3180.369500).
Published by: Zhongguo Yaoxuehui/Chinese Pharmaceutical Association, 2, Tianting Xili, Beijing 100050, China. TEL 86-532-2795937. Ed. Mei-Jun Guan.

615 CHN ISSN 1001-6821
ZHONGGUO LINCHUANG YAOLIXUE ZAZHI/CHINESE JOURNAL OF CLINICAL PHARMACOLOGY. Text in Chinese. 1981. bi-m. USD 22.20; CNY 7 newsstand/cover domestic; USD 3.70 newsstand/cover foreign (effective 2001). **Document type:** *Academic/Scholarly.*
Related titles: Online - full content ed.: (from WanFang Data Corp.).
—BLDSC (3180.303000).
Address: Haidian-qu, 38 Xueyuan Lu, Beijing 100083, China. TEL 86-1-62092540, FAX 86-1-62072817, lijt@cbm.imicams.ac.cn.

615 CHN ISSN 1005-1678
ZHONGGUO SHENGHUA YAOWU ZAZHI. Text in Chinese; Abstracts in English. 1992. bi-m. USD 25.20; USD 4.20 newsstand/cover (effective 2001). Index. 54 p./no. **Document type:** *Academic/Scholarly.*
Related titles: Online - full content ed.: (from WanFang Data Corp.).
—BLDSC (3180.295550).
Published by: (Nanjing Shenghua Zhiyao Yanjiusuo/Nanjing Institute of Biochemical Pharmaceutics, Zhongguo Shenghua Zhiyao Gongye Xiehui/Chinese Association of the Pharmaceutical Industry), Quanguo Shenghua Zhiyao Qingbao Zhongxinzhan/National Information Center of Biochemical Pharmaceutics, 18 Jiangdong Lu, Nanjing 210011, China. shyw@jloline.com. **Dist. outside of China by:** China International Book Trading Corp, 35 Chegongzhuang Xilu, Haidian District, Beijing 100044, China. TEL 86-10-68411769, FAX 86-10-68420340, bk@mail.cibtc.com.cn, http://www.cibtc.com.cn/.

615 CHN ISSN 1005-9903
ZHONGGUO SHIYAN FANGJIXUE ZAZHI/CHINESE JOURNAL OF EXPERIMENTAL TRADITIONAL MEDICAL FORMULAE. Text in Chinese. 1995. bi-m. USD 17.40; USD 2.90 newsstand/cover (effective 2001). **Document type:** *Academic/Scholarly.*
Published by: Zhongguo Zhongyi Yanjiuyuan, Zhongyi Yanjiusuo, 18 Bei Xincang, Beijing 100700, China. **Dist. by:** China International Book Trading Corp, 35, Chegongzhuang Xilu, Haidian District, Beijing 100044, China. TEL 86-1-68413849, FAX 86-1-68412048, cibtc@mail.cibtc.com.cn, http://www.cibtc.com.cn.

615 CHN ISSN 1007-7693
ZHONGGUO XIANDAI YINGYONG YAOXUE/CHINESE JOURNAL OF MODERN APPLIED PHARMACY. Text in Chinese. 1984. bi-m. USD 37.80; CNY 8, USD 6.30 newsstand/cover (effective 2001). **Document type:** *Abstract/Index.*
Related titles: Online - full content ed.: (from WanFang Data Corp.).
Published by: Zhongguo Yaoxuehui/Chinese Pharmaceutical Association, Muganshan Lu, 27, Wenbei Hang, Hangzhou, China. TEL 86-571-8843848, 86-571-8822697. Ed. Shu-Chun Liu. **Dist. by:** China International Book Trading Corp, 35, Chegongzhuang Xilu, Haidian District, Beijing 100044, China. TEL 86-1-68413849, FAX 86-1-68412048, cibtc@mail.cibtc.com.cn, http://www.cibtc.com.cn.

615 CHN ISSN 1007-7669
RM300 CODEN: XYLIEU
ZHONGGUO XINYAO YU LINCHUANG ZAZHI/CHINESE JOURNAL OF NEW DRUGS AND CLINICAL REMEDIES. Text in Chinese; Abstracts in English. 1982. m. (bi-m until 2002). USD 80 domestic; USD 180 foreign (effective 2002). adv. *Refereed.* **Document type:** *Academic/Scholarly.* **Description:** Covers the clinical research on new drugs (including new indications of old drugs), clinical trials, clinical verifications, pharmacology, adverse reactions, retional prescriptions, drug interactions, drug evaluation and other related news.
Formerly: Xinyao yu Linchuang - New Drugs and Clinical Remedies (1000-3843)
Related titles: Online - full content ed.
Indexed: Ref.Zh.
—BLDSC (3180.436600), CASDDS.
Published by: Shanghai Yaopin Jiandu Guanliju, Keji Qingbaosuo/Scientific and Technic Information Institute of Shanghai Municipal Drug Administration, No 50 Lane 532, Yuyuan Rd, Shanghai 200040, China. TEL 86-21-6252-5690, FAX 86-21-6252-5690, xyylc@21cn.com, cjndcr@citi2.net, http://chinainfo.gov.cn/periodical/zgxyylczz/. Ed. Guangsheng Ding. R&P Yao Song Yu. Adv. contact Yaosong Yu. page USD 2,000. Circ: 20,000. **Subscr. to:** China International Book Trading Corp, 35 Chegongzhuang Xilu, Haidian District, Beijing 100044, China. cibtc@mail.cibtc.com.cn, http://www.cibtc.com.cn. **Co-sponsor:** Zhongguo Yaoxuehui/Chinese Pharmaceutical Association.

615 CHN ISSN 1003-3734
ZHONGGUO XINYAO ZAZHI* /CHINESE NEW DRUGS JOURNAL. Text in Chinese. 1992. m. (10/yr.). USD 50.40; USD 4.20 newsstand/cover (effective 2001).
Related titles: Online - full content ed.: (from WanFang Data Corp.).
—GNLM.
Published by: China International Book Trading Corp/Zhongguo Guoji Tushu Maoyi Zonggongsi cibtc@mail.cibtc.com.cn, http://www.cibtc.com.cn. Ed. Yu Chuanlong. **Dist. by:** 35, Chegongzhuang Xilu, Haidian District, Beijing 100044, China.

615 CHN ISSN 1001-0408
ZHONGGUO YAOFANG/JOURNAL OF CHINA PHARMACY. Text in Chinese. 1990. bi-m. CNY 25.20. **Document type:** *Academic/Scholarly.*
Indexed: I.P.A.
—BLDSC (3180.217750).
Published by: Chongqing Weishengjuliju, Chongqing Yiyao Guanliju/Chongqing Bureau of Public Health, Chongqi Bureau of Drug Administration, 22 Meng Yung, Zhong Shan San Rd, Chongqing, China. TEL 023-63873050, FAX 023-63869472. Ed. Chen Congyuan. **Dist. by:** China International Book Trading Corp, 35 Chegongzhuang Xilu, Haidian District, Beijing 100044, China.

615 CHN ISSN 1000-5048
ZHONGGUO YAOKE DAXUE XUEBAO/CHINA PHARMACEUTICAL UNIVERSITY. JOURNAL. Text in Chinese. 1979. bi-m. USD 37.80; CNY 10, USD 6.30 newsstand/cover (effective 2001). **Document type:** *Academic/Scholarly.*
Related titles: Online - full content ed.: (from WanFang Data Corp.).
—BLDSC (4729.218950).
Published by: Zhongguo Yaoke Daxue/China Pharmaceutical University, Heping Qu, 92, Bei Er-Ma Lu, Chengyang 110001, China. Ed. Weiwei He. **Dist. by:** China International Book Trading Corp, 35, Chegongzhuang Xilu, Haidian District, Beijing 100044, China. TEL 86-1-68413849, FAX 86-1-68412048, cibtc@mail.cibtc.com.cn, http://www.cibtc.com.cn.

615.9 615.7 CHN ISSN 0253-9756
RM1 CODEN: CYLPDN
ZHONGGUO YAOLI XUEBAO. Text in Chinese. 1980. m. USD 245 (effective 2000). adv. reprint service avail. from ISI. *Refereed.* **Document type:** *Academic/Scholarly.* **Description:** Contains original articles on pharmacological and toxicological research, including the therapeutic effects, toxicities, metabolism, experimental uses and mechanisms of drugs, poisons, and biologically active substances.
Related titles: Online - full text ed.: (from Institute for Scientific Information); ♦ English ed.: Acta Pharmacologica Sinica.
Indexed: ASCA, Biol.Abstr., Chem.Abstr., Chem.Indus.Notes, Chem.Titles, Curr.Cont., Dairy Sci.Abstr., Derwent Biotech.Abstr., Excerp.Med., Helminthol.Abstr., Ind.Med. (coverage dropped), Inpharma, Neurosci.Cit.Ind., Nutr.Abstr., Reac., Rev.Appl.Entomol., Rev.Arom.& Med.Plants, SSCI (coverage dropped), Sci.Cit.Ind., Soyabean Abstr., Trop.Dis.Bull.
—BLDSC (0648.100000), CASDDS, CISTI, EMDOCS, GNLM, IDS, KNAW, Linda Hall.
Published by: (Chinese Society of Pharmacology), Kexue Chubanshe/Science Press, 16 Donghuang Cheng Genbei Jie, Beijing 100717, China. Circ: 10,000.

615 CHN ISSN 1001-1978
CODEN: ZYTOE
ZHONGGUO YAOLIXUE TONGBAO/CHINESE PHARMACOLOGICAL BULLETIN. Text in Chinese. 1985. bi-m. USD 15 newsstand/cover (effective 2000); USD 180 foreign. adv. bk.rev. *Refereed.* **Document type:** *Bulletin, Academic/Scholarly.* **Description:** Includes original articles, reviews, and new test methods.
Indexed: Chem.Abstr., Chem.Indus.Notes, Chem.Titles, Excerp.Med. (1993-), NPU, Ref.Zh.
—BLDSC (3181.046600), EMDOCS.
Published by: Zhongguo Yaoli Xuehui/Chinese Society of Pharmacology, c/o Anhui Medical University, 21 Meishen Lu, Hefei, Anhui 230032, China. TEL 86-551-363-7769, huanghs@mail.hf.ah.cn. Ed. Xu Shu Yun.

ZHONGGUO YAOLIXUE YU DULIXUE ZAZHI/CHINESE JOURNAL OF PHARMACOLOGY AND TOXICOLOGY. see *ENVIRONMENTAL STUDIES—Toxicology And Environmental Safety*

615 CHN ISSN 1002-7777
ZHONGGUO YAOSHI (BEIJING)/CHINESE PHARMACEUTICAL AFFAIRS. Text in Chinese. 1987. bi-m. CNY 48 domestic; USD 31.20 foreign; CNY 8 newsstand/cover domestic; USD 5.20 newsstand/cover foreign (effective 2001). **Document type:** *Academic/Scholarly.*
Related titles: Online - full content ed.: (from WanFang Data Corp.).
Published by: Zhongguo Yaopin Shengwu Zhipin Jiandingsuo, 2,Tiantan Xili, Beijing 100050, China. TEL 86-1-67033529. Ed. Guo-Wei Sang. **Dist. by:** China International Book Trading Corp, 35, Chegongzhuang Xilu, Haidian District, Beijing 100044, China. TEL 86-1-68413849, FAX 86-1-68412048, cibtc@mail.cibtc.com.cn, http://www.cibtc.com.cn.

615 CHN ISSN 1008-049X
ZHONGGUO YAOSHI (WUYI)/CHINA PHARMACIST. Text in Chinese. bi-m. USD 15; CNY 5, USD 2.50 newsstand/cover (effective 2001). **Document type:** *Academic/Scholarly.*
Related titles: Online - full content ed.: (from WanFang Data Corp.).
Published by: Yaowu Liuxingbingxue Zazhishe, 2, Lanling Lu, Wuyi, Hubei 430014, China. TEL 86-27-82835077, FAX 86-27-82778580, acjpe077@public.wh.hb.cn. Ed. Shi-Bin Zhu. **Dist. by:** China International Book Trading Corp, 35, Chegongzhuang Xilu, Haidian District, Beijing 100044, China. TEL 86-1-68413849, FAX 86-1-68412048, cibtc@mail.cibtc.com.cn, http://www.cibtc.com.cn.

615.19 CHN ISSN 1005-0108
CODEN: ZYHZEF
ZHONGGUO YAOWUHUAXUE ZAZHI/CHINESE JOURNAL OF MEDICINAL CHEMISTRY. Text in Chinese; Abstracts in English. 1990. bi-m. CNY 39 domestic; USD 40 foreign (effective 2001). adv. abstr. 64 p./no. back issues avail. **Document type:** *Journal, Academic/Scholarly.* **Description:** Contains original articles, research notes, and reviews relating to pharmaceutical chemistry.
Related titles: Online - full content ed.: (from WanFang Data Corp.).
—BLDSC (3180.428500), CASDDS.
Address: 103 Wenhua Rd, Shenyang, Liaoning 110016, China. TEL 86-24-23994540, FAX 86-24-23994540, zgyh@chinajournal.net.cn, http://www.zgyh.chinajournal.net.cn. Eds. Li-he Zhang, Shou-fang Zhang. Adv. contact Ren-yong Liu. page USD 300. Circ: 2,500. **Dist. by:** China International Book Trading Corp, 35 Chegongzhuang Xilu, Haidian District, Beijing 100044, China. cibtc@mail.cibtc.com.cn, http://www.cibtc.com.cn.

615.19 CHN ISSN 1001-2494
RS1 CODEN: ZYZAEU
ZHONGGUO YAOXUE ZAZHI/CHINESE PHARMACEUTICAL JOURNAL. Text in Chinese; Abstracts in English. m. CNY 5 per issue. **Document type:** *Academic/Scholarly.*
Formerly: Yaoxue Tongbao - Chinese Pharmaceutical Bulletin (0512-7343)
Related titles: CD-ROM ed.
Indexed: Anal.Abstr., Apic.Abstr., Aqua.Sci.& Fish.Abstr., Chem.Abstr., Chem.Indus.Notes, Chem.Titles, Eng.Ind., Environ.Sci.Poll.Mgmt., Excerp.Med. (1993-), ExtraMED, I.P.A., Mass Spectr.Bull., NPU, Pollut.Abstr., Risk Abstr., Saf.Sci.Abstr.
—BLDSC (3181.046000), CASDDS, EMDOCS, GNLM, Linda Hall.
Published by: Zhongguo Yaoxuehui/Chinese Pharmaceutical Association, 42 Dongsi Xidajie, Beijing 100710, China. TEL 86-1-5133311, FAX 86-1-8354609. **Dist. outside of China by:** China International Book Trading Corp, 35 Chegongzhuang Xilu, Haidian District, Beijing 100044, China.

615 CHN ISSN 1001-8255
CODEN: ZYGZEA
ZHONGGUO YIYAO GONGYE ZAZHI/JOURNAL OF CHINESE MEDICAL INDUSTRY. Text in Chinese. 1970. m. USD 50.40; USD 4.20 newsstand/cover (effective 2001). adv. bk.rev. **Document type:** *Academic/Scholarly.*
Formerly (until 1989): Yiyao Gongye/Pharmaceutical industry (0255-7223)
Indexed: Chem.Abstr., Chem.Indus.Notes, Chem.Titles, I.P.A., Mass Spectr.Bull.
—BLDSC (3180.473500), CASDDS, GNLM.
Published by: Shanghai Yiyao Gongye Yanjiuyuan/Shanghai Institute of Pharmaceutical Industry, 1320 Beijing Xilu, Shanghai 200040, China. TEL 86-21-6247-9808, FAX 86-21-6247-7965, sipind@public.sta.net.cn. Ed. Yixin Li. Pub. Houquan Shi. Adv. contact Peijun Shi. Circ: 8,000. **Dist. by:** China International Book Trading Corp, 35, Chegongzhuang Xilu, Haidian District, Beijing 100044, China. TEL 86-1-68413849, FAX 86-1-68412048, cibtc@mail.cibtc.com.cn, http://www.cibtc.com.cn.

P

615 CHN ISSN 1000-4971
R97.7.C5 CODEN: ZYIXEE
ZHONGGUO YIYAO XUEBAO/JOURNAL OF CHINESE PHARMACOLOGY. Text in Chinese. 1986. bi-m. USD 14.40; USD 2.40 newsstand/cover (effective 2001). 64 p./no. **Document type:** *Academic/Scholarly.*
Description: Covers the new developments and clinical applications of traditional Chinese medicine.
Published by: Zhongguo Zhongyiyao Xuehui, 18, Bei-Xincang, Dongzhimen, Beijing 100700, China. **Dist. overseas by:** China International Book Trading Corp, 35, Chegongzhuang Xilu, Haidian District, Beijing 100044, China. TEL 86-1-68413849, FAX 86-1-68412048, cibtc@mail.cibtc.com.cn, http://www.cibtc.com.cn. **Co-publisher:** Zhongguo Zhongyi Yanjiuyuan.

615 CHN ISSN 1001-5213
CODEN: ZYYAEP
ZHONGGUO YIYUAN YAOXUE ZAZHI/CHINESE JOURNAL OF HOSPITAL PHARMACY. Text in Chinese. 1981. m. USD 56.40; CNY 7.80, USD 4.70 newsstand/cover (effective 2001). **Document type:** *Academic/Scholarly.*
Related titles: Online - full content ed.: (from WanFang Data Corp.).
Indexed: Chem.Abstr., Chem.Indus.Notes, Chem.Titles, I.P.A.
—BLDSC (3180.352000), CASDDS.
Published by: Zhongguo Yaoxuehui (Hankou)/Chinese Pharmaceutical Association, Hankou Branch, 177 Shengli St, Hankou, Hubei 430014, China. TEL 86-27-82836596, pharmacy@public.wh.hb.cn. **Dist. overseas by:** China International Book Trading Corp, 35, Chegongzhuang Xilu, Haidian District, Beijing 100044, China. TEL 86-1-68413849, FAX 86-1-68412048, cibtc@mail.cibtc.com.cn, http://www.cibtc.com.cn.

615.328 615.89 CHN ISSN 1001-5302
CODEN: ZZZAE3
ZHONGGUO ZHONGYAO ZAZHI/CHINA JOURNAL OF CHINESE MATERIA MEDICA. Text in Chinese. 1955. m. USD 75.60 foreign; CNY 5 newsstand/cover domestic; USD 6.30 newsstand/cover foreign (effective 2001). bk.rev. 64 p./no. *Refereed.* **Document type:** *Academic/Scholarly.* **Description:** Contains researches on herbs, resources, production, and pharmacology of Chinese medicine.
Formerly (until 1989): Zhongyao Tongbao/Bulletin of Chinese Meteria Medica (0254-0029)
Related titles: Online - full content ed.: (from WanFang Data Corp.).
Indexed: Chem.Abstr., Chem.Indus.Notes, Chem.Titles, I.P.A., Ind.Med. (1989-), Mass Spectr.Bull.
—BLDSC (3180.180500), CASDDS, GNLM.
Published by: (Zhongguo Yaoxuehui/Chinese Pharmaceutical Association), Zhongguo Zhongyi Yanjiuyuan, Zhongyi Yanjiusuo, 18 Bei Xincang, Beijing 100700, China. TEL 86-1-64045830, FAX 86-1-64045830. **Dist. overseas by:** China International Book Trading Corp, 35, Chegongzhuang Xilu, Haidian District, Beijing 100044, China. TEL 86-1-68413849, FAX 86-1-68412048, cibtc@mail.cibtc.com.cn, http://www.cibtc.com.cn.

ZHONGHUA FENGSHIBINGXUE ZAZHI/CHINESE JOURNAL OF RHEUMATOLOGY. see *MEDICAL SCIENCES—Rheumatology*

615 CHN ISSN 1003-9783
ZHONGYAO XINYAO YU LINGCHUANG YAOLI/TRADITIONAL CHINESE DRUG RESEARCH & CLINICAL PHARMACOLOGY. Text in Chinese. 1990. bi-m. USD 22.20; CNY 7, USD 3.70 newsstand/cover (effective 2001). **Document type:** *Academic/Scholarly.*
Description: Covers the latest development in traditional Chinese drug research and clinical pharmacology in China.
Related titles: Online - full content ed.: (from WanFang Data Corp.).
Published by: Guangzhou Zhongyiyao Daxue/Guangzhou University of Traditional Chinese Medicine, 12, Jichang Lu, Guangzhou, Guangdong 510405, China. TEL 86-20-86552367, 86-20-86591233 ext 2483, zyxylc@publiclguangzhou.gd.cn. Ed. Ou Ming. **Dist. overseas by:** China International Book Trading Corp, 35, Chegongzhuang Xilu, Haidian District, Beijing 100044, China. TEL 86-1-68413849, FAX 86-1-68412048, cibtc@mail.cibtc.com.cn, http://www.cibtc.com.cn.

615 CHN ISSN 1001-859X
ZHONGYAO YAOLI YU LINCHUANG/PHARMACOLOGY AND CLINICS OF CHINESE MATERIA MEDICA. Text in Chinese. 1985. bi-m. USD 20. **Document type:** *Bulletin, Academic/Scholarly.*
—BLDSC (6447.060750).
Published by: Sichuan Sheng Zhongyao Yanjiusuo/Sichuan Institute of Chinese Materia Medica, Chongqingshi Nan'an, Huangjiaoya, Sichuan 630065, China. TEL 481615.

ZHONGYI ZAZHI. see *ALTERNATIVE MEDICINE*

615 DEU ISSN 0177-6290
ZULASSUNGEN UND REGISTRIERUNGEN VON ARZNEIMITTELN. Short title: Z R v A. Text in German. irreg. **Document type:** *Monographic series.*
Published by: P M I Verlag AG, August-Schanz-Str 8, Frankfurt Am Main 60433, Germany. TEL 49-69-548000-0, FAX 49-69-548000-77, pmiverlag@aol.com.

PHARMACY AND PHARMACOLOGY—Abstracting, Bibliographies, Statistics

016.6151 USA ISSN 0065-8111
RS355
AMERICAN DRUG INDEX. Text in English. 1950. a. USD 49.95 domestic; USD 57.40 foreign (effective 1999). **Document type:** *Abstract/Index.* **Description:** Lists over 20,000 drug entries in dictionary style with cross-indexing of brands, generic and chemical names.
Related titles: CD-ROM ed.: USD 79.95 domestic; USD 91.90 foreign (effective 1999).
Indexed: Inpharma, Reac.
—GNLM.
Published by: Facts and Comparisons, 111 W. Port Plaza, Ste. 300, St. Louis, MO 63146-3098. TEL 800-223-0554, FAX 314-878-5563. Ed. Norman F Billups.

615 USA ISSN 0898-4654
AMERICAN STATISTICAL ASSOCIATION. BIOPHARMACEUTICAL SECTION. PROCEEDINGS. Text in English. a. price varies. **Document type:** *Proceedings.*
Indexed: Curr.Ind.Stat.
—BLDSC (6661.250000), Linda Hall.
Published by: American Statistical Association, 1429 Duke St, Alexandria, VA 22314-3415. TEL 703-684-1221, FAX 703-684-2036.

ATRIAL NATRIURETIC FACTORS. see *MEDICAL SCIENCES—Abstracting, Bibliographies, Statistics*

615.19 USA ISSN 1051-3957
CODEN: CBUPEA
C A S BIOTECH UPDATES. SLOW-RELEASE PHARMACEUTICALS. Text in English. 1991. s-w. USD 270 (effective 2001). **Document type:** *Abstract/Index.*
Description: Covers slow-release pharmaceutical dosage forms, including controlled- and sustained-release systems; newer dosage forms such as osmotic-release devices, transdermal systems, polymer conjugates, and other materials giving regulated drug release rates.
Published by: Chemical Abstracts Service (Subsidiary of: American Chemical Society), 2540 Olentangy River Rd, Box 3012, Columbus, OH 43210-0012. TEL 614-447-3600, 800-753-4227, FAX 614-447-3751.

016.615 USA ISSN 1051-3884
CODEN: CAAOE2
C A SELECTS. ALKOXYLATED OLEOCHEMICALS. Text in English. 1990. s-w. USD 275 (effective 2001). **Document type:** *Abstract/Index.* **Description:** Covers analysis, preparation, properties, reactions, and uses of ethoxylated and - or propoxylated alcohols.
Published by: Chemical Abstracts Service (Subsidiary of: American Chemical Society), 2540 Olentangy River Rd, Box 3012, Columbus, OH 43210-0012. TEL 614-447-3600, 800-753-4227, FAX 614-447-3751.

C A SELECTS. ANTIARRHYTHMICS. see *MEDICAL SCIENCES—Abstracting, Bibliographies, Statistics*

350 USA ISSN 0148-2459
CODEN: CSBADM
C A SELECTS. BETA-LACTAM ANTIBIOTICS. Text in English. s-w. USD 275 (effective 2001). **Document type:** *Abstract/Index.* **Description:** Covers synthesis, biosynthesis, chemical reactivity, antimicrobial activity, pharmacodynamics, metabolism, toxicology, analysis, and formulation.
Published by: Chemical Abstracts Service (Subsidiary of: American Chemical Society), 2540 Olentangy River Rd, Box 3012, Columbus, OH 43210-0012. TEL 614-447-3600, 800-753-4227, FAX 614-447-3751.

016.572516 USA ISSN 1051-3906
CODEN: CASBEJ
C A SELECTS. CALCIUM CHANNEL BLOCKERS. Text in English. 1990. s-w. USD 275 (effective 2001). **Document type:** *Abstract/Index.* **Description:** Covers agents that act as calcium antagonists; biochemical and pharmacological effects, mechanisms of action, synthesis, physicochemical properties, modeling, QSAR, and structure-activity studies.
Published by: Chemical Abstracts Service (Subsidiary of: American Chemical Society), 2540 Olentangy River Rd, Box 3012, Columbus, OH 43210-0012. TEL 614-447-3600, 800-753-4227, FAX 614-447-3751.

016.615 USA ISSN 1045-8530
CODEN: CSDTEM
C A SELECTS. DRUG ANALYSIS BIOLOGICAL FLUIDS & TISSUES. Text in English. s-w. USD 275 (effective 2001). **Document type:** *Abstract/Index.* **Description:** Covers newly developed methods (gas chromatography, HPLC, mass spectrometry, immunoassay) for the analysis of drugs in biological fluids (blood, urine, saliva) and tissues (liver, lungs, kidneys).
Published by: Chemical Abstracts Service (Subsidiary of: American Chemical Society), 2540 Olentangy River Rd, Box 3012, Columbus, OH 43210-0012. TEL 614-447-3600, 800-753-4227, FAX 614-447-3751.

615.9 USA ISSN 0162-7775
CODEN: CSDTDL
C A SELECTS. DRUG & COSMETIC TOXICITY. Text in English. s-w. USD 275 (effective 2001). **Document type:** *Abstract/Index.* **Description:** Covers toxic manifestations of drugs, cosmetics, and ingredients of drug and cosmetic preparations, e.g., mutagenicity, teratogenicity, carcinogenicity, allergic potential; health hazards, side effects, and safety of drugs.
Published by: Chemical Abstracts Service (Subsidiary of: American Chemical Society), 2540 Olentangy River Rd, Box 3012, Columbus, OH 43210-0012. TEL 614-447-3600, 800-753-4227, FAX 614-447-3751.

615.19 USA ISSN 1047-8205
CODEN: CSDIEN
C A SELECTS. DRUG INTERACTIONS. Text in English. 1987. s-w. USD 275 (effective 2001). **Document type:** *Abstract/Index.* **Description:** Covers adverse, metabolic, and physicochemical drug interactions. Includes drug-drug, food-drug, and drug-alcohol interactions.
Formerly (until 1989): BIOSIS CAS Selects: Drug Interactions
Published by: Chemical Abstracts Service (Subsidiary of: American Chemical Society), 2540 Olentangy River Rd, Box 3012, Columbus, OH 43210-0012. TEL 614-447-3600, 800-753-4227, FAX 614-447-3751.

C A SELECTS. FOOD, DRUGS, & COSMETICS - LEGISLATIVE & REGULATORY ASPECTS. see *FOOD AND FOOD INDUSTRIES—Abstracting, Bibliographies, Statistics*

615 USA ISSN 0895-5875
CODEN: CSNAEF
C A SELECTS. NEW ANTIBIOTICS. Text in English. 1988. s-w. USD 275 (effective 2001). **Document type:** *Abstract/Index.* **Description:** Covers production, isolation, characterization, structure determination, and antimicrobial activity of antibiotics, both natural and synthetic.
Published by: Chemical Abstracts Service (Subsidiary of: American Chemical Society), 2540 Olentangy River Rd, Box 3012, Columbus, OH 43210-0012. TEL 614-447-3600, 800-753-4227, FAX 614-447-3751.

615.19 USA ISSN 0890-1910
CODEN: CAPCE7
C A SELECTS. PHARMACEUTICAL CHEMISTRY (JOURNALS). Text in English. 1987. s-w. USD 275 (effective 2001). **Document type:** *Abstract/Index.*
Description: Covers all aspects of pharmaceutical chemistry: drug standards, pharmacopeia, formulations, prosthetic materials, surgical goods, and properties of pharmaceuticals.
Published by: Chemical Abstracts Service (Subsidiary of: American Chemical Society), 2540 Olentangy River Rd, Box 3012, Columbus, OH 43210-0012. TEL 614-447-3600, 800-753-4227, FAX 614-447-3751.

615.19 USA ISSN 0890-1929
CODEN: CPCPEI
C A SELECTS. PHARMACEUTICAL CHEMISTRY (PATENTS). Text in English. 1987. s-w. USD 275 (effective 2001). **Document type:** *Abstract/Index.*
Description: Covers formulations, prosthetic materials, and surgical goods.

P

Published by: Chemical Abstracts Service (Subsidiary of: American Chemical Society), 2540 Olentangy River Rd, Box 3012, Columbus, OH 43210-0012. TEL 614-447-3600, 800-753-4227, FAX 614-447-3751.

350 USA ISSN 1084-2349
CODEN: CSDFFF

C A SELECTS PLUS. DRUG DELIVERY SYSTEMS & DOSAGE FORMS. Text in English. 1989. s-w. USD 275 (effective 2001). **Document type:** *Abstract/Index.* **Description:** Covers pharmaceutical dosage forms, such as tablets, capsules, ointments; newer delivery systems and forms such as controlled-release devices, transdermal systems, ocular inserts. osmotic devices, antibody conjugates. and liposomes; properties, formulation bioavailability, and pharmacokinetic studies of drugs from the delivery systems and dosage forms.
Formerly: C A Selects. Drug Delivery Systems and Dosage Forms (1040-7162)
Published by: Chemical Abstracts Service (Subsidiary of: American Chemical Society), 2540 Olentangy River Rd, Box 3012, Columbus, OH 43210-0012. TEL 614-447-3600, 800-753-4227, FAX 614-447-3751.

615.19 USA
CODEN: CPPAFS

C A SELECTS PLUS. PHARMACEUTICAL ANALYSIS. Text in English. 1987. s-w. USD 260 to non-members; USD 80 to members (effective 1999). **Document type:** *Abstract/Index.* **Description:** Covers analysis of drugs in pure form or in pharmaceutical preparations.
Formerly: C A Selects. Pharmaceutical Analysis (0890-1902)
Published by: Chemical Abstracts Service (Subsidiary of: American Chemical Society), 2540 Olentangy River Rd, Box 3012, Columbus, OH 43210-0012. TEL 614-447-3600, 800-753-4227, FAX 614-447-3751.

P

C A SELECTS. STEROIDS (CHEMICAL ASPECTS). see *CHEMISTRY—Abstracting, Bibliographies, Statistics*

016.6157 616.1 GBR ISSN 0263-7243

CARDIOVASCULAR PHARMACOLOGY. Text in English. s-m. GBP 120 for print or e-mail eds. (effective 2001). adv. back issues avail. **Document type:** *Abstract/Index.* **Description:** Current awareness service for researchers in clinical and life sciences. Covers anti-hypertensives, calcium channel blockers, vasoconstrictors, and vasodilators.
Related titles: E-mail ed.; Online - full text ed.: GBP 108 (effective 2001).
—GNLM. **CCC.**
Published by: S U B I S (Subsidiary of: Sheffield Academic Press Ltd), Mansion House, 19 Kingfield Rd, Sheffield, S Yorks S11 9AS, United Kingdom. TEL 44-114-255-4433, FAX 44-114-255-4626, subis@sheffac.demon.co.uk, http://www.shef-ac-press.co.uk/subis. Ed. S Huntridge. Adv. contact C Evans.

016.615 USA ISSN 0069-4770

CLIN-ALERT. Text in English. 1962. 24/yr. USD 155 for print or electronic eds.; USD 175 for print and electronic eds. (effective 2001). q. cum.index. back issues avail.; reprints avail. **Document type:** *Newsletter, Abstract/Index.* **Description:** Reference summaries of and conclusions about prescription drug reactions-interactions.
Related titles: E-mail ed.; Online - full content ed.
—Infotrieve. **CCC.**
Published by: Sage Publications, Inc., 2111 W Hillcrest Dr, Thousand Oaks, CA 91320. Circ: 620 (paid).

615 JPN ISSN 0385-6747

CONTENTS. Text in Japanese. 1971. w. JPY 100,000 (effective 2001). **Document type:** *Bibliography.* **Description:** Lists titles of medical and pharmaceutical journals.
Published by: Japan Pharmaceutical Information Center/Nihon Iyaku Joho Senta, 3rd Fl Nagai-Kinenkan, 2-12-15 Shibuya, Shibuya-ku, Tokyo 150-0002, Japan. TEL 81-3-5466-1812, FAX 81-3-5466-18184. Ed. H Miyake. Circ: 900.

016.615105 GBR ISSN 1354-5337
CODEN: CMPHE4

CURRENT MEDICAL LITERATURE. INTERNATIONAL HOSPITAL PHARMACY. Text in English. 1990. q. GBP 25, USD 40 to individuals; GBP 75, USD 120 to institutions (effective 1999). back issues avail. **Document type:** *Abstract/Index.*
Formerly (until 1994): Current Medical Literature. Hospital Pharmacy (0958-9384)
—CCC.
Published by: (Royal Society of Medicine), Current Medical Literature Ltd., 40-42 Osnaburgh St, London NW1 3ND, United Kingdom. TEL 44-20-7465-8377, FAX 44-20-7465-8380, enquiries@curmedlit.com. **Dist. by:** Cassis Publishing Ltd., Realpage House, Abingdon Science Park, Barton Ln., Abingdon, Oxon OX13 3NB, United Kingdom. TEL 44-1235-537352, FAX 44-1235-537353.

DRUG FILE UPDATE; a current awareness index to publications on drugs and doping in sport. see *SPORTS AND GAMES—Abstracting, Bibliographies, Statistics*

016.61519 GBR ISSN 0952-0317

DRUG TARGETING. Text in English. 1988. s-m. GBP 120 fpr print or e-mail eds. (effective 2001). adv. bk.rev. back issues avail. **Document type:** *Abstract/Index.* **Description:** Current awareness service for researchers in clinical and life sciences.
Related titles: E-mail ed.; Online - full text ed.: GBP 108 (effective 2001).
—Infotrieve. **CCC.**
Published by: S U B I S (Subsidiary of: Sheffield Academic Press Ltd), Mansion House, 19 Kingfield Rd, Sheffield, S Yorks S11 9AS, United Kingdom. TEL 44-114-255-4433, FAX 44-114-255-4626, subis@sheffac.demon.co.uk, http://www.shef-ac-press.co.uk/subis. Ed. S Huntridge. Adv. contact C Evans.

016.6151 NLD ISSN 0927-2798

EXCERPTA MEDICA. SECTION 30: CLINICAL AND EXPERIMENTAL PHARMACOLOGY. Text in English. 1948. 32/yr. EUR 4,525 in Europe to institutions; JPY 599,896 in Japan to institutions; USD 5,062 elsewhere to institutions (effective 2002). adv. abstr. index, cum.index. **Document type:** *Abstract/Index, Academic/Scholarly.* **Description:** Provides a comprehensive current-awareness service of clinical and academic articles covering all aspects of experimental and clinical pharmacology, including pharmacokinetics, pharmacodynamics, methodology, mathematical models, and experimental studies on human organs, tissues, and cells and on the mechanisms of action of exogenous substances.
Formerly (until 1992): Excerpta Medica. Section 30: Pharmacology (0167-9643); Supersedes: Excerpta Medica. Section 30: Pharmacology and Toxicology (0014-4347)
Related titles: CD-ROM ed.: (from SilverPlatter Information, Inc.); Online - full text ed.: (from DIMDI, Data-Star, The Dialog Corporation, JICST).
—GNLM, Infotrieve, Linda Hall. **CCC.**
Published by: Excerpta Medica Medical Communications BV (Subsidiary of: Reed Elsevier plc), Rooseveltweg 15, Almere-Stad 1314 SJ, Netherlands. TEL 31-36-538-5600, FAX 31-36-538-5650, http://www.elsevier.nl/locate/clinexppharm, http://www.excerptamedica.com. **Subscr. in Australasia and the Far East to:** Elsevier Science (Singapore) Pte Ltd, No.1 Temasek Ave, 17-01 Millenia Tower, Singapore 039192, Singapore. TEL 65-434-3727, FAX 65-337-2230, asiainfo@elsevier.com.sg; **Subscr. in Japan to:** Elsevier Science Inc - Japan Regional Office, 9-15 Higashi-Azabu 1-chome, Minato-ku, Tokyo 106-0044, Japan. TEL 81-3-5561-5033, FAX 81-3-5561-5047, info@elsevier.co.jp; **Subscr. in the Americas to:** Elsevier Science, PO Box 945, New York, NY 10159-0945. TEL 212-633-3730, 888-437-4636, FAX 212-633-3680, usinfo-f@elsevier.com, http://www.elsevier.com. **Dist. by:** Elsevier Science (Brazil).; Elsevier Science BV, PO Box 211, Amsterdam 1000 AE, Netherlands. TEL 31-20-485-3757, FAX 31-20-485-3432, nlinfo-f@elsevier.nl, http://www.elsevier.nl.

016.615 NLD ISSN 0167-9090
CODEN: ADRTA

EXCERPTA MEDICA. SECTION 38: ADVERSE REACTIONS TITLES. Text in English. 1966. m. EUR 10,730 in Europe to institutions; JPY 1,422,623 in Japan to institutions; USD 12,004 elsewhere to institutions (effective 2002). adv. index, cum.index. **Document type:** *Abstract/Index, Academic/Scholarly.* **Description:** Offers a comprehensive awareness service for articles and other academic and professional writings dealing with pharmacological adverse reactions.
Formerly (until 1966): Adverse Reactions Titles (0001-8848)
Related titles: CD-ROM ed.: (from SilverPlatter Information, Inc.); Online - full text ed.: (from DIMDI, Data-Star, The Dialog Corporation, JICST).
—Infotrieve. **CCC.**
Published by: Excerpta Medica Medical Communications BV (Subsidiary of: Reed Elsevier plc), Rooseveltweg 15, Almere-Stad 1314 SJ, Netherlands. TEL 31-36-538-5600, FAX 31-36-538-5650, http://www.elsevier.nl/located/advreactions, http://www.excerptamedica.com. **Subscr. in Australasia and the Far East to:** Elsevier Science (Singapore) Pte Ltd, No.1 Temasek Ave, 17-01 Millenia Tower, Singapore 039192, Singapore. TEL 65-434-3727, FAX 65-337-2230; **Subscr. in Japan to:** Elsevier Science Inc - Japan Regional Office, 9-15 Higashi-Azabu 1-chome, Minato-ku, Tokyo 106-0044, Japan. TEL 81-3-5561-5033, FAX 81-3-5561-5047; **Subscr. in the Americas to:** Elsevier Science, PO Box 945, New York, NY 10159-0945. TEL 212-633-3730, 888-437-4636, FAX 212-633-3680, usinfo-f@elsevier.com, http://www.elsevier.com. **Dist. by:** Elsevier Science (Brazil).; Elsevier Science BV, PO Box 211, Amsterdam 1000 AE, Netherlands. TEL 31-20-485-3757, FAX 31-20-485-3432.

EXCERPTA MEDICA. SECTION 52: TOXICOLOGY. see *ENVIRONMENTAL STUDIES—Abstracting, Bibliographies, Statistics*

016.615 USA

FOCUS ON: PSYCHOPHARMACOLOGY. Text in English. m. USD 345 (effective 1998). **Document type:** *Abstract/Index.* **Description:** Covers more than 1,100 source items per issue regarding the clinical and experimental studies of psychotropic drugs in humans and animals.
Media: Diskette.
Published by: Institute for Scientific Information, 3501 Market St., Philadelphia, PA 19104. TEL 215-386-0100, 800-336-4474, FAX 215-386-2911, webmaster@isinet.com, http://www.isinet.com. **Dist. in Europe by:** ISI Europe, Brunel Science Park, Kingston Ln, Uxbridge, Mddx UB8 3PQ, United Kingdom. TEL 44-1895-270016, FAX 44-1895-256710.

615 FRA

FRANCE. SERVICE D'ETUDE DES STRATEGIES ET DES STATISTIQUES INDUSTRIELLES. RESULTATS MENSUELS DES ENQUETES DE BRANCHE. INDUSTRIE PHARMACEUTIQUE. Text in French. m. FRF 260; FRF 310 foreign (effective 1991). stat. **Description:** Follows developments in the pharmaceutical industry through the performance of selected indicators.
Published by: Service d'Etude des Strategies et des Statistiques Industrielles (SESSI), 85 bd. du Montparnasse, Paris Cedex 6 75270, France. TEL 45-56-42-34, FAX 45-56-40-71.

615.19 AUS ISSN 0155-9885

GUILD DIGEST (YEAR)* . Key Title: Pharmacy Guild Digest. Text in English. 1974. a. AUD 100. index. back issues avail. **Description:** Compares interfirm survey statistics on financial performance of pharmacies and some detail of drug usage and cost.
Former titles: Community Pharmacy in Australia; Guild Digest
Published by: Pharmacy Guild of Australia, PO Box 2036, Canberra Mail Centre, ACT 2600, Australia. TEL 61-2-6270-1888, FAX 61-2-6270-1800, guild.nat@guild.org.au. Ed. Vasken Demirian. Circ: 5,500.

016.61519 GBR ISSN 0261-4707

HIGH PERFORMANCE LIQUID CHROMATOGRAPHY. Text in English. 1982. s-m. (diskette m.). GBP 115 (effective 1999). adv. **Document type:** *Abstract/Index.* **Description:** Current awareness service for researchers focusing on pharmacological substances.
Related titles: Diskette ed.: USD 120 (effective 1999); E-mail ed.: USD 115 (effective 1999); Online - full text ed.: USD 100 (effective 1999).
—CCC.
Published by: S U B I S (Subsidiary of: Sheffield Academic Press Ltd), Mansion House, 19 Kingfield Rd, Sheffield, S Yorks S11 9AS, United Kingdom. TEL 44-114-255-4433, FAX 44-114-255-4626, subis@sheffac.demon.co.uk, http://www.shef-ac-press.co.uk/subis. Ed. S Huntridge. Adv. contact C Evans.

615.19 IND

INDIAN CHEMICALS AND PHARMACEUTICALS STATISTICS. Text in English. 1967. a. free per issue. stat. **Document type:** *Academic/Scholarly.*
Published by: Ministry of Chemicals and Fertilizers, Economics and Statistics Division, New Delhi, India. Circ: (controlled).

016.6151 NZL ISSN 1173-8324
INPHARMA WEEKLY; rapid alerts to news on drugs and drug therapy. Text in English. 1975. w. USD 2,745 Print or Online ed.; USD 3,294 Print and Online combined eds. (effective 2001). back issues avail. **Document type:** *Abstract/Index.* **Description:** Provides brief evaluated summaries of all important pharmacological and therapeutic news from the world biomedical literature and from international meetings.
Formerly: Inpharma (0156-2703)
Related titles: CD-ROM ed.: (from SilverPlatter Information, Inc.); Online - full text ed.: (from Data-Star, The Dialog Corporation, EBSCO Publishing, ingenta, Swets Blackwell, Institute for Scientific Information).
Indexed: Pharm.&Out.News, Reac.
—BLDSC (4515.936000), IDS. **CCC.**
Published by: Adis International Limited, Mairangi Bay, Private Bag 65901, Auckland 1010, New Zealand. TEL 64-9-477-0700, FAX 64-9-477-0766, will.charles@adis.co.nz, http://www.adis.com; http://biomednet.com/library/jinp. Ed. Teresa Szabo. Pub. Paul Chrisp. R&P Knight Ridder. Circ: 900. **Americas subscr. to:** Adis International Inc., Attn: Subscription Dept, 860 Town Center Dr, Langhorne, PA 19047. TEL 877-872-2347.

614 USA
INTERNATIONAL NARCOTICS CONTROL BOARD. PSYCHOTROPIC SUBSTANCES; assessments of medical and scientific requirements for substances in schedules II, III and IV. Requirements of import authorization for substances in schedules III and IV. Text in English, French, Spanish. 1977. a. USD 42 (effective 1997). **Document type:** *Academic/Scholarly.*
Former titles: International Narcotics Control Board. Statistics on Psychotropic Substances for (Year); International Narcotics Control Board. Statistics on Psychotropic Substances Furnished by Governments in Accordance with the Convention of 1971 on Psychotropic Substances (0253-9403)
Related titles: Microfiche ed.: (from CIS).
Indexed: IIS.
Published by: (International Narcotics Control Board), United Nations Publications, Sales and Marketing Section, Room DC2 0853, New York, NY 10017. TEL 212-963-8302, 800-253-9646, FAX 212-963-3489, publications@un.org, http://www.un.org/publications.

615 016 USA ISSN 0020-8264
RS1 CODEN: IPMAAH
INTERNATIONAL PHARMACEUTICAL ABSTRACTS; key to the world's literature of pharmacy. Text in English. 1964. s-m. USD 565 domestic to non-members; USD 595 foreign to non-members (effective 2001). index. back issues avail.; reprint service avail. from PQC. **Document type:** *Academic/Scholarly, Abstract/Index.* **Description:** Covers approximately 600 worldwide pharmaceutical, cosmetics, medical and health care publications.
Related titles: CD-ROM ed.: (from The Dialog Corporation, SilverPlatter Information, Inc.); Microform ed.: (from PQC); Online - full text ed.: (from DIMDI, Data-Star, The Dialog Corporation, National Library of Medicine, EBSCO Publishing).
—BLDSC (4544.924000), GNLM, Linda Hall. **CCC.**
Published by: American Society of Health-System Pharmacists, 7272 Wisconsin Ave, Bethesda, MD 20814. TEL 301-657-3000, FAX 301-657-1251, 301-657-8857, ipa@ashp.org, pdiso@ashp.org, http://www.ashp.org. Ed. Victoria Ferretti-Aceto. Circ: 2,000.

615 JPN
IYAKU TOKKYO SHOROKU/MEDICINE - PATENTS ABSTRACTS. Text in Japanese. 1972. s-m. JPY 300,000.
Published by: Aiaru Shuppan K.K./Information Retrieval Publishing Co., Ltd., 50-101 Wada 3-chome, Suginami-ku, Tokyo 166-0012, Japan. TEL 81-3-5377-1841, FAX 81-3-5377-1861.

016.615 JPN ISSN 1342-2030
IYAKUHIN FUKUSAYO BUNKEN JOHOSHU. SHOROKUSHU-HEN/ADVERSE REACTION TO DRUGS INFORMATION COMPENDIUM FOR EXPERTS. ABSTRACTS. Text in Japanese. 1975. s-a. JPY 50,000 includes Iyakuhin Fukusayo Bunken Johoshu. Yakkobeetsu Fukusayo Ichiran-hen (effective 2000).
Supersedes in part (in 1995): Kokunai Iyakuhin Fukusayo Ichiran
Published by: Japan Pharmaceutical Information Center/Nihon Iyaku Joho Senta, 3rd Fl Nagai-Kinenkan, 2-12-15 Shibuya, Shibuya-ku, Tokyo 150-0002, Japan. TEL 81-3-5466-1812, FAX 81-3-5466-1814.

615 310 USA ISSN 1054-3406
RS57 CODEN: JBSTEL
JOURNAL OF BIOPHARMACEUTICAL STATISTICS. Text in English. 1991. q. USD 85 to individuals print & online eds.; USD 795 to institutions print only (effective 2002). adv. *Refereed.* **Document type:** *Academic/Scholarly.* **Description:** Applications of statistics in biopharmaceutical research and development and expositions of statistical methodology with applicability to such work.
Related titles: Online - full text ed.: (from EBSCO Publishing, O C L C Online Computer Library Center, Inc., RoweCom Information Quest, Swets Blackwell).
Indexed: Curr.Cont. (1991-, dropped), Curr.Ind.Stat., Excerp.Med. (1994-), Ind.Med. (1991-), Ref.Zh., Stat.Theor.Meth.Abstr. (1991-), Zent.Math.
—BLDSC (4953.910000), CISTI, EMDOCS, GNLM, Infotrieve, KNAW. **CCC.**
Published by: Marcel Dekker Inc., 270 Madison Ave, New York, NY 10016. TEL 212-696-9000, 800-228-1160, FAX 212-685-4540, http://www.dekker.com/servlet/product/productid/BIP. Ed. A Lawrence Gould. R&P Julia Mulligan. Adv. contact Diane Saulon. B&W page USD 800. Circ: 550.

L M S ALERT. PAIN CONTROL. (Literature Monitoring and Evaluation Service) see *MEDICAL SCIENCES—Abstracting, Bibliographies, Statistics*

016.6151 NZL ISSN 1172-1545
L M S ALERT. PHARMACOECONOMICS. (Literature Monitoring and Evaluation Service) Text in English. 1993. m. charts. *Refereed.* **Document type:** *Abstract/Index.*
Related titles: CD-ROM ed.; Online - full text ed.
Published by: Adis International Limited, Mairangi Bay, Private Bag 65901, Auckland 1010, New Zealand. TEL 64-9-477-0700, FAX 64-9-477-0784, pauline.mcwilliams@adis.com, http://www.adis.com. Eds. Laura Hunt, Pauline McWilliams. Pub. Christopher J Mellor.

615.19 ISR
M E D I C. (Monthly Ethical Drug Index Complication) Text in English. 1971. 6/yr. USD 65. adv.
Published by: Shirol Publications Ltd., P O Box 2066, Herzlia, Israel. FAX 972-9-507604. Ed. S H Bergman. Circ: 7,000.

M I M S MEDICAL SPECIALITIES. (Monthly Index of Medical Specialties) see *MEDICAL SCIENCES—Abstracting, Bibliographies, Statistics*

MEDICAL & PHARMACEUTICAL BIOTECHNOLOGY ABSTRACTS. see *MEDICAL SCIENCES—Abstracting, Bibliographies, Statistics*

615 JPN
MEDICAL COMPANIES GUIDE TO JAPAN. Text in English. 1987. irreg. JPY 23,447. **Document type:** *Directory.* **Description:** Lists pharmaceutical companies and those dealing with diagnostic agents and medical apparatuses with up-to-date information including company name, address, turnover, features, and main products.
Formerly (until 1992): Japan Medical and Pharmaceutical Directory
Published by: Chemical Daily Co. Ltd., International Affairs, 3-16-8 Nihonbashihama-cho, Chuo-ku, Tokyo 103-0007, Japan. TEL 81-3-3663-7932, FAX 81-3-3663-7275, chemnews@tky.threewebnet.or.jp, http://www.chemnews-japan.com/.

MEDITSINSKI PREGLED. KLINIKA I PREDKLINIKA. see *MEDICAL SCIENCES—Abstracting, Bibliographies, Statistics*

615 USA ISSN 0076-6518
MERCK INDEX: AN ENCYCLOPEDIA OF CHEMICALS AND DRUGS. Text in English. 1889. irreg., latest vol.12, 1996. USD 45 (effective 2000). **Document type:** *Monographic series.*
Related titles: Online - full text ed.: (from CISTI, The Dialog Corporation, S T N International, Telesystemes-Questel).
Published by: Merck Publishing Group, 126 E Lincoln Ave, PO Box 2000, Rahway, NJ 07065. TEL 732-594-4600, FAX 732-388-9778. Ed. Susan Budavari.

300 614.35 AUT ISSN 1013-3453
HV5800
NARCOTIC DRUGS: ESTIMATED WORLD REQUIREMENTS FOR (YEAR). Text in English, French, Spanish. 1989. a. USD 38 (effective 1997).
Formed by the 1989 merger of: United Nations. International Narcotics Control Board. Statistics on Narcotics Drugs for (Year) (1014-8817); Which was formerly: United Nations. International Narcotics Control Board. Statistics on Narcotic Drugs Furnished by Governments in Accordance with the International Treaties; United Nations. International Narcotics Control Board. Comparative Statement of Estimates and Statistics on Narcotic Drugs for (Year) (0255-9374); Which was formerly: United Nations. International Narcotics Control Board. Comparative Statement of Estimates and Statistics on Narcotics Drugs Furnished by Governments in Accordance with the International Treaties; Estimated World Requirements of Narcotic Drugs (0082-8335); United Nations. International Narcotics Control Board. Statistics on Narcotic Drugs Furnished by Governments in Accordance with the International Treaties; Which was formerly (until 1984): United Nations. International Narcotics Control Board. Statistics on Narcotic Drugs Furnished by Governments in Accordance with the International Treaties and Maximum Level of Opium Stocks (0566-7658)
Related titles: Microfiche ed.: (from CIS).
Indexed: IIS, Russ.Acad.Sci.Bibl.
Published by: (International Narcotics Control Board USA, Vienna International Center), United Nations Publications, Sales and Marketing Section, Room DC2 0853, New York, NY 10017. TEL 212-963-9302, 800-253-9646, FAX 212-963-3489, publications@un.org, http://www.un.org/publications.

016.615 JPN ISSN 0915-1621
NIHON IYAKU BUNKEN SHOROKUSHU/JAPAN PHARMACEUTICAL ABSTRACTS. Text in Japanese. 1972. bi-m. JPY 300,000 to members (effective 2001). **Document type:** *Abstract/Index.*
Published by: Japan Pharmaceutical Information Center/Nihon Iyaku Joho Senta, 3rd Fl Nagai-Kinenkan, 2-12-15 Shibuya, Shibuya-ku, Tokyo 150-0002, Japan. TEL 81-3-5466-1811, FAX 81-3-5466-1814. Circ: 1,100 (controlled).

615.19 USA
P M A STATISTICAL FACTBOOK; pharmaceuticals, in-vivo diagnostic. Text in English. a. USD 21.50. charts, stat.
Formerly: Prescription Drug Industry Fact Book
Indexed: SRI.
Published by: Pharmaceutical Manufacturers Association, 1100 15th St, N W, Washington, DC 20005. TEL 202-835-3400, FAX 202-835-3595. Circ: 1,500.

615 USA ISSN 1043-5905
RS356
PHARMACEUTICAL ACTIVITIES INDEX - DIRECTORY. Text in English. irreg., latest 1993 (every 3-4/yrs.). USD 570. **Document type:** *Directory.*
Published by: Pharmaco-Medical Documentation, Inc., 21 Green Village Rd, Madison, NJ 07940. TEL 973-822-9200, FAX 973-765-0722.

615 USA
PHARMACEUTICAL MANUFACTURERS ASSOCIATION. ANNUAL SURVEY REPORT. Text in English. a. free per issue. stat. **Description:** Provides annual and historical statistical information on pharmaceutical industry sales and research.
Indexed: SRI.
Published by: Pharmaceutical Manufacturers Association, 110 15th St, N W, Washington, DC 20005. TEL 202-835-3400, FAX 202-835-3595.

016.615 NZL ISSN 1173-5503
PHARMACOECONOMICS AND OUTCOMES NEWS; rapid alerts to world pharmacoeconomic news, views and practical application. Text in English. 1994. w. USD 1,095 Print or Online ed.; USD 1,314 Print and Online combined eds. (effective 2001). back issues avail. **Document type:** *Academic/Scholarly.* **Description:** Provides brief, evaluated summaries of current pharmacoeconomic and outcomes research from the world biomedical literature.
Formerly: PharmacoResources (1172-8299)
Related titles: CD-ROM ed.: (from SilverPlatter Information, Inc.); Online - full text ed.: (from Data-Star, The Dialog Corporation, EBSCO Publishing, ingenta, Swets Blackwell, Institute for Scientific Information).
Indexed: Inpharma, Reac.
—Infotrieve. **CCC.**
Published by: Adis International Limited, Mairangi Bay, Private Bag 65901, Auckland 1010, New Zealand. TEL 64-9-477-0700, FAX 64-9-477-0766, pecnews@adis.co.nz, http://www.adis.com; http://biomednet.com/library/jpon. Ed. Amanda Cameron. Pub. Paul Chrisp. R&P Will Charles. Circ: 600. **Americas subscr. to:** Adis International Inc., Attn: Subscription Dept, 860 Town Center Dr, Langhorne, PA 19047. TEL 877-872-2347.

P

PHILIPPINES INDEX OF MEDICAL SPECIALITIES. see *MEDICAL SCIENCES—Abstracting, Bibliographies, Statistics*

016.615 NZL ISSN 0114-9954
REACTIONS WEEKLY; rapid alerts to adverse drug experience. Text in English. 1979. w. USD 1,095 Print or Online ed.; USD 1,314 Print and Online combined eds. (effective 2001). bk.rev. q. cum.index. back issues avail. **Document type:** *Abstract/Index.* **Description:** Rapid alerts to adverse drug experiences reported in international medical journals.
Formerly (until 1990): Reactions (0157-7271)
Related titles: CD-ROM ed.: (from SilverPlatter Information, Inc.); Online - full text ed.: (from Data-Star, The Dialog Corporation, EBSCO Publishing, ingenta, Swets Blackwell, Institute for Scientific Information).
Indexed: Inpharma, Pharm.&Out.News.
—CISTI. **CCC.**
Published by: Adis International Limited, Mairangi Bay, Private Bag 65901, Auckland 1010, New Zealand. TEL 64-9-477-0700, FAX 64-9-477-0766, will.charles@adis.co.nz, http://www.adis.com; http://biomednet.com/library/jrea. Ed. Rosie Stather. Pub. Paul Chrisp. R&P Will Charles. Circ: 700. **US subscr. to:** Adis International Inc., Subscriptions Dept, Ste F 10, 940 Town Center Dr, Langhorne, PA 19047. TEL 877-872-2347, 877-234-7329.

016.615 RUS ISSN 0202-5132
REFERATIVNYI ZHURNAL. FARMAKOLOGIYA EFFEKTORNYKH SISTEM. KHIMIOTERAPEVTICHESKIE SREDSTVA. Text in Russian. 1958. m. USD 351. **Document type:** *Abstract/Index.*
—East View.
Published by: Vserossiiskii Institut Nauchnoi i Tekhnicheskoi Informatsii (VINITI), Usievicha ul 20-a, Moscow 125315, Russian Federation. TEL 7-095-1526441, FAX 7-095-943-0060. **Dist. by:** Mezhdunarodnaya Kniga, B Yakimanka 39, Moscow 117049, Russian Federation. TEL 7-095-2384967, FAX 7-095-2384634; **US dist. addr.:** East View Publications, 3020 Harbor Ln N, Minneapolis, MN 55447. TEL 612-550-0961.

615 RUS ISSN 0134-580X
REFERATIVNYI ZHURNAL. FARMAKOLOGIYA OBSHCHAYA. FARMAKOLOGIYA NERVNOI SISTEMY. Text in Russian. 1958. m. USD 251. **Document type:** *Abstract/Index.*
Published by: Vserossiiskii Institut Nauchnoi i Tekhnicheskoi Informatsii (VINITI), Usievicha ul 20-a, Moscow 125315, Russian Federation. TEL 7-095-1526441. **Dist. by:** Mezhdunarodnaya Kniga, B Yakimanka 39, Moscow 117049, Russian Federation. TEL 7-095-2384967, FAX 7-095-2384634; **US dist. addr.:** East View Publications, 3020 Harbor Ln N, Minneapolis, MN 55447. TEL 612-550-0961.

016.615 RUS ISSN 0869-4109
REFERATIVNYI ZHURNAL. FARMAKOLOGIYA: TOKSIKOLOGIYA. Text in Russian. m. USD 1,995 in United States. **Document type:** *Abstract/Index.*
—BLDSC (0142.160000), East View.
Published by: Vserossiiskii Institut Nauchnoi i Tekhnicheskoi Informatsii (VINITI), Usievicha ul 20-a, Moscow 125315, Russian Federation. TEL 7-095-1526441, FAX 7-095-943-0060. **US dist. addr.:** East View Publications, 3020 Harbor Ln N, Minneapolis, MN 55447. TEL 612-550-0961.

016.615 RUS ISSN 0202-9162
REFERATIVNYI ZHURNAL. KLINICHESKAYA FARMAKOLOGIYA. Text in Russian. 1979. m. USD 399. **Document type:** *Abstract/Index.*
Published by: Vserossiiskii Institut Nauchnoi i Tekhnicheskoi Informatsii (VINITI), Usievicha ul 20-a, Moscow 125315, Russian Federation. TEL 7-095-1526441. **Dist. by:** Mezhdunarodnaya Kniga, B Yakimanka 39, Moscow 117049, Russian Federation. TEL 7-095-2384967, FAX 7-095-2384634; **US dist. addr.:** East View Publications, 3020 Harbor Ln N, Minneapolis, MN 55447. TEL 612-559-2931, 612-550-0961.

016.6159 RUS ISSN 0202-9219
RA1190 CODEN: RZTODS
REFERATIVNYI ZHURNAL. TOKSIKOLOGIYA. Text in Russian. 1958. m. USD 288. **Document type:** *Abstract/Index.*
Indexed: Chem.Abstr.
—CASDDS, East View.
Published by: Vserossiiskii Institut Nauchnoi i Tekhnicheskoi Informatsii (VINITI), Usievicha ul 20-a, Moscow 125315, Russian Federation. TEL 7-095-1526441, FAX 7-095-943-0060. **Dist. by:** Mezhdunarodnaya Kniga, B Yakimanka 39, Moscow 117049, Russian Federation. TEL 7-095-2384967, FAX 7-095-2384634; **US dist. addr.:** East View Publications, 3020 Harbor Ln N, Minneapolis, MN 55447. TEL 612-550-0961.

615.1021 CAN ISSN 1487-198X
HD7103.5.C2
SASKATCHEWAN DRUG PLAN AND EXTENDED BENEFITS BRANCH. ANNUAL STATISTICAL REPORT. Text in English. 1976. a. **Document type:** *Government.*
Former titles (1991-1996): Saskatchewan Health. Prescription Drug Services Branch. Annual Statistical Report (1187-8991); (1989-1990): Saskatchewan Health. Statistical Supplement to the Annual Report (1182-218X); (1976-1988): Saskatchewan. Prescription Drug Plan. Annual Report (0707-0152)
Published by: Saskatchewan Health, Prescription Drug Services Branch, 3475 Albert St, Regina, SK S4S 6X6, Canada. TEL 306-787-3317, FAX 306-787-8679. Circ: 700.

615.9 016 RUS ISSN 0233-6588
SIGNAL'NAYA INFORMATSIYA. TOKSIKOLOGIYA LEKARSTVENNAYA. Text in Russian. m. **Document type:** *Abstract/Index.*
Formerly: Signal'naya Informatsiya. Toksikologiya (0202-8514)
Published by: Vserossiiskii Institut Nauchnoi i Tekhnicheskoi Informatsii (VINITI), Usievicha ul 20-a, Moscow 125315, Russian Federation. TEL 7-095-1526441. **Dist. by:** Mezhdunarodnaya Kniga, B Yakimanka 39, Moscow 117049, Russian Federation. TEL 7-095-2384967, FAX 7-095-2384634.

016.6151 GBR ISSN 0143-4241
TRANSMITTERS, RECEPTORS & SYNAPSES. Text in English. 1980. s-m. GBP 120 for print ed. or e-mail (effective 2001). adv. **Document type:** *Abstract/Index.* **Description:** Current awareness service for researchers. Covers synapses, neuromuscular junction, transmitters and neuromodulators.
Related titles: E-mail ed.; Online - full text ed.: GBP 108 to individuals (effective 2001).
—CCC.
Published by: S U B I S (Subsidiary of: Sheffield Academic Press Ltd), Mansion House, 19 Kingfield Rd, Sheffield, S Yorks S11 9AS, United Kingdom. TEL 44-114-255-4433, FAX 44-114-255-4626, subis@sheffac.demon.co.uk, http://www.shef-ac-press.co.uk/subis. Ed. S Huntridge. Adv. contact C Evans.

PHARMACY AND PHARMACOLOGY—Computer Applications

610.285 USA
COMPUTERTALK; for contemporary pharmacy management. Text in English. 1981. bi-m. USD 50 domestic; USD 75 foreign (effective 2001). adv. back issues avail. **Document type:** *Magazine, Trade.* **Description:** Offers practical advice to familiarize pharmacists with computers and computer applications. Short articles cover a broad range of topics.
Formerly: ComputerTalk for the Pharmacist (0736-3893)
Indexed: I.P.A.
—ingenta.
Published by: ComputerTalk Associates, Inc., 492 Norristown Rd, 160, Blue Bell, PA 19422-2355. TEL 610-825-7686, FAX 610-825-7641, maggie@computertalk.com, http://www.computertalk.com. Ed. Margaret L Lockwood. Pub., Adv. contact William A Lockwood Jr. B&W page USD 4,820, color page USD 6,115; trim 10.75 x 8. Circ: 36,000.

610.285 USA
COMPUTERTALK PHARMACY SYSTEMS BUYERS GUIDE. Text in English. 1982. a. USD 25 (effective 2001). adv. 85 p./no. **Document type:** *Magazine, Trade.* **Description:** A guide to available computer systems and services designed for pharmacy use. Information contained within product profiles written by vendors. Articles cover a range of topics on computers and applications.
Formerly: ComputerTalk Directory of Pharmacy Systems (0736-3877)
Published by: ComputerTalk Associates, Inc., 492 Norristown Rd, 160, Blue Bell, PA 19422-2355. TEL 610-825-7686, FAX 610-825-7641, maggie@computertalk.com, http://www.computertalk.com. Ed. Margaret L Lockwood. Pub., Adv. contact William A Lockwood Jr. B&W page USD 4,900, color page USD 5,500; trim 8 x 10.75. Circ: 38,000.

PHILATELY

see also HOBBIES

769.56 610.9 USA ISSN 0048-9255
SCALPEL AND TONGS; medical philately. Text in English. 1955. bi-m. USD 15 domestic to membership; USD 18 foreign to membership (effective 1999). adv. bk.rev. **Document type:** *Academic/Scholarly.* **Description:** Deals with all aspects of philately related to medicine and allied subjects, such as nursing and blood transfusion. Covers the history of medicine as well.
Related titles: Microform ed.: (from PQC).
Published by: American Topical Association, Inc., Medical Subjects Unit, c/o Ranes Chakravorty, Ed, 5049 Cherokee Hills Dr, Salem, VA 24153-5848. TEL 540-380-2362, FAX 540-224-1961, rcc9u@virginia.edu. Ed., Pub., R&P, Adv. contact Ranes C Chakravorty. Circ: 400 (paid).

PHILOSOPHY

see also RELIGIONS AND THEOLOGY

174.957 USA
ADVANCES IN BIOETHICS. Text in English.
—BLDSC (0699.960000).
Published by: Jai Press, Incorporated (Subsidiary of: Elsevier Science), 100 Prospect St., Stamford, CT 06904-0811. Eds. Edwards E Bittar, Rem B Edwards.

100 150.19 ITA ISSN 1120-9364
ATQUE; materiali tra filosofia e psicoterapia. Text in Italian. 1990. s-a. ITL 35,000 to individuals. **Description:** Covers relational studies between philosophy and psychotherapy.
Indexed: e-psyche.
Published by: Moretti e Vitalli Editori, Via Betty Ambiveri 15, Bergamo, BG 24126, Italy. TEL 39-35-321588, FAX 39-35-321647. Ed. Paolo Francesco Pieri.

174.957 GBR ISSN 0269-9702
QH332
BIOETHICS. Text in English. q. GBP 269 to institutions in UK & Europe (effective 2001); USD 506 to institutions; GBP 351 elsewhere to institutions (effective 2002). bk.rev. illus. reprint service avail. from SWZ. *Refereed.* **Document type:** *Academic/Scholarly.*
Related titles: Online - full text ed.: (from EBSCO Publishing, O C L C Online Computer Library Center, Inc., RoweCom Information Quest, ingenta, Gale Group, Swets Blackwell, Institute for Scientific Information).
Indexed: ASCA, ASSIA, Arts & Hum.Cit.Ind. (coverage dropped), Curr.Cont., Fam.Ind., Gen.Sci.Ind. (Jul.1997-), IBZ, Ind.Philos., Intl.Bibl.Soc.Sci., Lang.& Lang.Behav.Abstr., Phil.Ind., Rel.Ind.One, Rel.Ind.Two, Russ.Acad.Sci.Bibl., SOPODA, SSCI, Soc.Sci.Ind. (Jul.1999-), Soc.Serv.Abstr., Sociol.Abstr., Stud.Wom.Abstr.
—BLDSC (2072.119500), CISTI, GNLM, IDS, Infotrieve, ingenta. **CCC.**
Published by: Blackwell Publishers Ltd., 108 Cowley Rd, Oxford OX4 1JF, United Kingdom. TEL 44-1865-791100, FAX 44-1865-791347, jnlinfo@blackwellpublishers.co.uk, http://www.blacksci.co.uk/. Eds. Ruth Chadwick, Udo Schuklenk.

BIOETHICS FORUM. see *HUMANITIES: COMPREHENSIVE WORKS*

174.95 AUS ISSN 1037-6410
BIOETHICS OUTLOOK. Text in English. 1990. q. AUD 48 domestic to individuals; AUD 63 foreign to individuals; AUD 65 domestic to institutions; AUD 78 foreign to institutions; AUD 20 domestic to students; AUD 35 foreign to students (effective 2000). bk.rev. back issues avail. **Document type:** *Newsletter.* **Description:** Contains articles on current issues in bioethics (euthanasia, informed consent, resource allocation).
—BLDSC (2072.121800).

P

Published by: Plunkett Centre for Ethics, St. Vincents Hospital, Darlinghurst, NSW 2010, Australia. TEL 61-2-93612869, FAX 61-2-93610975, plunkett@plunkett.edu.au. Ed., R&P Bernadette Tobin. Circ: 400.

BIOETHICS YEARBOOK. see *RELIGIONS AND THEOLOGY*

BIOMEDICAL ETHICS REVIEWS. see *MEDICAL SCIENCES*

BLAUWE WEGWIJZER. see *SOCIOLOGY*

BODYWORK SERIES. see *NEW AGE PUBLICATIONS*

BREATH SERIES; a progression of pranayama practices. see *NEW AGE PUBLICATIONS*

150 616.8 NLD ISSN 0924-0314
BRILL'S STUDIES IN EPISTEMOLOGY, PSYCHOLOGY AND PSYCHIATRY. Text in Dutch. 1989. irreg., latest vol.3, 1993. price varies. back issues avail. *Refereed.* **Document type:** *Monographic series.*
Indexed: e-psyche.
Published by: Brill Academic Publishers, PO Box 9000, Leiden 2300 PA, Netherlands. TEL 31-71-535-3500, FAX 31-71-531-7532, cs@brill.nl. R&P Elizabeth Venekamp.

BULLETIN OF MEDICAL ETHICS. see *MEDICAL SCIENCES*

CHRISTIAN BIOETHICS; non-ecumenical studies in medical morality. see *MEDICAL SCIENCES*

CLINICAL MEDICAL ETHICS. see *MEDICAL SCIENCES*

▼ **COGNITION, TECHNOLOGY AND WORK.** see *PSYCHOLOGY*

170 FRA ISSN 1260-8599
COMITE CONSULTATIF NATIONAL D'ETHIQUE POUR LES SCIENCES DE LA VIE ET DE LA SANTE. LES CAHIERS. Text in French. 1985. q. FRF 200 domestic; FRF 250 foreign (effective 2000). bk.rev. *Refereed.* **Document type:** *Bulletin.*
Former titles (until 1993): Comite Consultatif National d'Ethique pour les Sciences de la Vie et de la Sante. Lettre (1169-1476); (until 1991): Comite Consultatif National d'Ethique pour les Sciences de la Vie et de la Sante. Lettre d'Information (0296-4074)
Related titles: Microfiche ed.
Published by: Comite Consultatif National d'Ethique pour les Sciences de la Vie et de la Sante, 71 rue Saint Dominique, Paris 75007, France. TEL 33-01-44424852, FAX 33-01-44424848, contact@ccne-ethique.org, http://www.ccne-ethique.org, http://www.comite-ethique.fr. Pub. Didier Sicard. R&P Anne Bernard. Circ: 1,000 (paid). **Subscr. to:** Biomedition, 18 rue Camille Desmoulins, Levallois Perret 92300, France. TEL 33-1-41340260.

COMMENTS & CRITICISMS. see *PSYCHOLOGY*

D W D NEWSLETTER. see *GERONTOLOGY AND GERIATRICS*

100 IND ISSN 0011-6734
B1
DARSHANA INTERNATIONAL; an international quarterly of philosophy, psychology, sociology, psychical research, religion and mysticism. Text in English. 1961. q. INR 200, USD 40. adv. bk.rev. charts, illus. index. **Document type:** *Academic/Scholarly.*
Indexed: Bibl.Asian Stud. (1975-1991), Curr.Cont. (coverage dropped), Phil.Ind., e-psyche.
Published by: Darashna International, Moradabad 244 001, India. TEL 91-591-314370, FAX 91-591-320678. Ed. J P Atreya. Adv. contact J.P. Atreya. Circ: 500.

128 155.937 178 USA
▼ **DEATH & DYING SOURCEBOOK.** Text in English. 1999. irreg., latest 1999. USD 78 per issue (effective 2001). charts, bibl. Index. **Document type:** *Consumer.* **Description:** Basic information for the layperson about end-of-life care and related ethical and legal issues.
Published by: Omnigraphics, Inc., 615 Griswold St, Detroit, MI 48226. TEL 313-961-1340, 800-234-1340, FAX 313-961-1383, 800-875-1340, info@omnigraphics.com, http://www.omnigraphics.com/cgi-bin/loadpage.cgi?user_id=29079&file=0-7808-0230-6.html. Ed. Annemarie S Muth.

DICTIONNAIRE PERMANENT: BIOETHIQUE ET BIOTECHNOLOGIES. see *BIOLOGY—Biotechnology*

ETHICS, LAW, AND AGING REVIEW. see *GERONTOLOGY AND GERIATRICS*

170 610 DEU ISSN 0935-7335
ETHIK IN DER MEDIZIN. Text in German. 1989. q. EUR 111.90 domestic; EUR 109.50 in Germany; EUR 30.80 newsstand/cover foreign (effective 2001). *Refereed.* **Document type:** *Journal, Academic/Scholarly.* **Description:** Discusses ethical issues encountered in clinical medicine, research and development, and psychology.
Related titles: Microform ed.: (from PQC); Online - full text ed.: ISSN 1437-1618 (from EBSCO Publishing, RoweCom Information Quest, Swets Blackwell, Springer LINK).
—GNLM, Infotrieve. **CCC.**
Published by: (Akademie fuer Ethik in der Medizin), Springer-Verlag (Subsidiary of: BertelsmannSpringer), Tiergartenstr 17, Heidelberg 69121, Germany. TEL 49-6221-345-0, FAX 49-6221-345229, subscriptions@springer.de, http://link.springer.de/link/service/journals/00481/index.htm, http://www.springer.de. Eds. D Birnbacher, K Gahl. **Subscr. in N. America to:** Springer-Verlag New York Inc., PO Box 2485, Secaucus, NJ 07096-2485. TEL 212-460-1500, FAX 212-473-6272.

EUBIOS JOURNAL OF ASIAN AND INTERNATIONAL BIOETHICS. see *BIOLOGY*

EUROPEAN STUDIES IN PHILOSOPHY OF MEDICINE. see *MEDICAL SCIENCES*

EVOLUTION AND COGNITION. see *PSYCHOLOGY*

FILOZOFSKI FAKULTET - ZADAR. RAZDIO FILOZOFIJE, PSIHOLOGIJE, SOCIOLOGIJE I PEDAGOGIJE. RADOVI. see *EDUCATION*

GENETHICS NEWS. see *BIOLOGY—Biotechnology*

GLOBAL BIOETHICS. see *BIOLOGY*

H E C FORUM; an interprofessional journal on healthcare institutions' ethical and legal issues. (HealthCare Ethics Committee) see *HEALTH FACILITIES AND ADMINISTRATION*

HASTINGS CENTER REPORT. see *MEDICAL SCIENCES*

HAWLIYAT KULLIYAT AL-A'DAAB/ANNALS OF THE FACULTY OF ARTS. see *HUMANITIES: COMPREHENSIVE WORKS*

HISTORY AND PHILOSOPHY OF THE LIFE SCIENCES. see *BIOLOGY*

HOSPITAL ETHICS. see *HEALTH FACILITIES AND ADMINISTRATION*

HUMAN REPRODUCTION AND GENETIC ETHICS; an international journal. see *BIOLOGY*

HUMANES LEBEN - HUMANES STERBEN. see *MEDICAL SCIENCES*

628 GBR
IAN RAMSEY CENTRE. PUBLICATIONS. Text in English. 1989 (no.2). irreg. **Document type:** *Academic/Scholarly.* **Description:** Studies ethical problems arising from scientific and medical research and practice; examines the underlying philosophical and theological issues. Reviews religious beliefs in relation to the sciences.
Published by: Ian Ramsey Centre, Theology Faculty Centre, 41 St Giles, Oxford, Oxon OX1 3LW, United Kingdom. TEL 44-1865-270792, FAX 44-1865-270792, ian-ramsey-centre@theology.oxford.ac.uk. **Co-sponsor:** University of Wales, College of Cardiff, Centre for Applied Statistics.

THE INTERBEHAVIORIST; a quarterly newsletter of interbehavioral psychology. see *PSYCHOLOGY*

INTERNATIONAL JOURNAL OF CHILDREN'S SPIRITUALITY. see *PSYCHOLOGY*

INTERNATIONAL JOURNAL OF TRANSPERSONAL STUDIES. see *PSYCHOLOGY*

JOURNAL FOR THE THEORY OF SOCIAL BEHAVIOUR. see *PSYCHOLOGY*

JOURNAL OF BIBLICAL ETHICS IN MEDICINE. see *MEDICAL SCIENCES*

JOURNAL OF CONSCIOUSNESS STUDIES; controversies in science & the humanities. see *PSYCHOLOGY*

JOURNAL OF MEDICAL ETHICS. see *MEDICAL SCIENCES*

JOURNAL OF MEDICAL HUMANITIES. see *MEDICAL SCIENCES*

THE JOURNAL OF MEDICINE AND PHILOSOPHY; a forum for bioethics and philosophy of medicine. see *MEDICAL SCIENCES*

JOURNAL OF MIND AND BEHAVIOR. see *PSYCHOLOGY*

▼ **JOURNAL OF MUNDANE BEHAVIOR.** see *SOCIOLOGY*

155.937 128 USA ISSN 0891-4494
BF789.D4 CODEN: JNDAE7
JOURNAL OF NEAR-DEATH STUDIES. Text in English. 1981. q. USD 398, EUR 397 to institutions for print or online ed.; USD 490.80, EUR 476.40 to institutions for print & online eds.combined (effective 2002). adv. bk.rev. illus. reprint service avail. from PQC. *Refereed.* **Document type:** *Journal, Academic/Scholarly.* **Description:** Publishes articles on the empirical effects and theoretical implications of near-death experiences.
Formerly (until 1986): Anabiosis: The Journal for Near-Death Studies (0743-6238)
Related titles: Online - full text ed.: (from EBSCO Publishing, O C L C Online Computer Library Center, Inc., Swets Blackwell, Kluwer Online, RoweCom Information Quest).
Indexed: AMED, Abstr.Anthropol., IBR, IBZ, IMFL, Ind.Philos., PsycInfo, Psychol.Abstr. (1981-), Soc.Work Res.& Abstr., e-psyche.
—BLDSC (5021.392000), GNLM, Infotrieve, ingenta. **CCC.**
Published by: (International Association for Near-Death Studies), Kluwer Academic - Plenum Publishers (Subsidiary of: Wolters Kluwer N.V.), 233 Spring St, New York, NY 10013-1578. TEL 212-620-8000, 800-221-9369, FAX 212-463-0742, info@plenum.com, http://www.wkap.nl/journalhome.htm/0891-4494. Ed. Dr. Bruce Greyson. **Subscr. outside the Americas to:** Kluwer Academic Publishers Group, Journals Department, PO Box 322, Dordrecht 3300 AH, Netherlands. TEL 31-78-639-2392, FAX 31-78-654-6474.

JOURNAL OF PSYCHOLOGY AND JUDAISM. see *RELIGIONS AND THEOLOGY—Judaic*

JOURNAL OF THEORETICAL & PHILOSOPHICAL PSYCHOLOGY. see *PSYCHOLOGY*

KENNEDY INSTITUTE OF ETHICS. JOURNAL. see *MEDICAL SCIENCES*

KENNEDY INSTITUTE OF ETHICS. SCOPE NOTE. see *MEDICAL SCIENCES*

LAST RIGHTS. see *MEDICAL SCIENCES*

153.6 170 USA
LIES PEOPLE TELL; welcome to the truth about lies. Text in English. 1997. w. **Description:** Reports on lies people all over the world tell themselves and others everyday.
Media: Online - full text.
Indexed: e-psyche.
Published by: Rise and Shine Press webs@liespeopletell, http://www.liespeopletell.com. Ed., Pub. Chris Riseley.

LOVING BROTHERHOOD NEWSLETTER; a journal for personal and planetary transformation. see *HOMOSEXUALITY*

MACROBIOTICS TODAY. see *NUTRITION AND DIETETICS*

MEDICAL ETHICS ADVISOR. see *MEDICAL SCIENCES*

▼ **MEDICAL HUMANITIES.** see *MEDICAL SCIENCES*

MEDICINE, HEALTH CARE AND PHILOSOPHY. see *MEDICAL SCIENCES*

MEDIZIN UND ETHIK. see *MEDICAL SCIENCES*

P

100 DEU
MEDIZIN UND PHILOSOPHIE; Beitraege aus der Forschung. Abbreviated title: M Ph. Text in German. 1995. irreg., latest vol.5, 2000. price varies. **Document type:** *Monographic series, Academic/Scholarly.* **Description:** Contains current topics involving the relationships between medicine and philosophy.
Published by: Friedrich Frommann Verlag Guenther Holzboog, Koenig-Karl-Str 27, Stuttgart 70372, Germany. TEL 49-711-9559690, FAX 49-711-9559691, vertrieb@frommann-holzboog.de, http://www.frommann-holzboog.de.

174.95 344 AUS ISSN 1321-2753
MONASH BIOETHICS REVIEW. Text in English. 1981. q. AUD 45 to individuals; AUD 65 to institutions. **Document type:** *Academic/Scholarly.* **Description:** Presents the study of the ethical, social and legal problems arising out of medical and biomedical research.
—BLDSC (5901.591450), ingenta, KNAW.
Published by: Monash University, Centre for Human Bioethics, Clayton, VIC 3168, Australia. TEL 61-3-9905-4278, FAX 61-3-9905-3279, john.mckie@arts.monash.edu.au. Ed. Udo Schukleuk. Circ: 1,000.

THE NOETIC JOURNAL; an international forum on the cosmology of consciousness. see *PHYSICS*

▼ **NURSING PHILOSOPHY**; an international journal for healthcare professionals. see *MEDICAL SCIENCES—Nurses And Nursing*

P

170 610.78 USA
OF VALUE✱. Text in English. 1969. q. membership. **Document type:** *Newsletter.*
Formerly: Society for Health and Human Values. Bulletin
Published by: Society for Health & Human Values, 4700 W Lake Ave, Glenview, IL 60025-1468. TEL 703-556-9222, FAX 703-556-8729. Circ: 800.

ON COURSE; inspiration for the inner journey. see *NEW AGE PUBLICATIONS*

THE PARK RIDGE CENTER. BULLETIN. see *MEDICAL SCIENCES*

PHILOSOPHICAL PSYCHOLOGY. see *PSYCHOLOGY*

100 610 NLD ISSN 0376-7418
CODEN: PHIMDN
PHILOSOPHY AND MEDICINE. Text in English. 1975. irreg., latest vol.47, 1994. price varies. *Refereed.* **Document type:** *Monographic series.*
Indexed: Biol.Abstr.
—BLDSC (6464.580000), CISTI, Infotrieve, KNAW. **CCC.**
Published by: Kluwer Academic Publishers Group (Subsidiary of: Wolters Kluwer N.V.), Spuiboulevard 50, PO Box 17, Dordrecht 3300 AA, Netherlands. FAX 31-78-639-2254, services@wkap.nl, http://www.wkap.nl. Eds. H Tristam Engelhardt Jr., Stuart F Spicker. **Dist. by:** Journals Department, PO Box 322, Dordrecht 3300 AH, Netherlands. FAX 31-78-654-6474.

616.89001 USA ISSN 1071-6076
RC437.5
PHILOSOPHY, PSYCHIATRY & PSYCHOLOGY. Text in English. 1994. q. USD 85 to individuals; USD 158 to institutions (effective 2002). bk.rev. illus. back issues avail.; reprints avail. *Refereed.* **Document type:** *Academic/Scholarly.* **Description:** Focuses on the overlap among three fields, making clinical material and theory more accessible to philosophers.
Related titles: Online - full text ed.: Philosophy, Psychiatry, and Psychology Online. ISSN 1086-3303. 1996. USD 132.30 to institutions (effective 2001) (from Project MUSE, EBSCO Publishing, O C L C Online Computer Library Center, Inc., RoweCom Information Quest, Swets Blackwell).
Indexed: Phil.Ind., PsycInfo, Psychol.Abstr., e-psyche.
—BLDSC (6464.980000), GNLM, Infotrieve, ingenta. **CCC.**
Published by: Johns Hopkins University Press, Journals Publishing Division, 2715 N Charles St, Baltimore, MD 21218-4363. TEL 800-548-1784, FAX 410-516-6968, jlorder@jhupress.jhu.edu, http://www.press.jhu.edu/press/journals/ppp/. Eds. John Sadler, K W M Fulford. Adv. contact Anastasia Scherr. Circ: 592. **Co-sponsors:** Association for the Advancement of Philosophy and Psychiatry; Royal College of Psychiatrists Philosophy Group, Royal Institute of Philosophy.

215 610 509 USA
PITTSBURGH SERIES IN PHILOSOPHY & HISTORY OF SCIENCE. Text in English. 1982. irreg., latest vol.14, 1992. price varies. back issues avail. *Refereed.* **Document type:** *Monographic series.* **Description:** Examines philosophical issues in the history of medical and physical sciences.
Published by: University of California Press, Journals Division, 2000 Center St, Ste 303, Berkeley, CA 94704-1223. TEL 510-642-4247, FAX 510-643-7127. **Orders to:** California-Princeton Fulfillment Services, Princeton, NJ 08618. TEL 800-777-4726, FAX 800-999-1958.

PROEFDIERVRIJ. see *ANIMAL WELFARE*

128 NLD ISSN 1381-2866
RELEVANT. Text in Dutch. 1975. q. NLG 30 (effective 2000). bk.rev. **Document type:** *Consumer.* **Description:** Discusses issues concerning euthanasia and the right to die for persons with terminal illnesses and their families.
Former titles (until 1994): Euthanasie (0921-2396); N V V E Kwartaalblad (0921-240X)
Related titles: Audio cassette/tape ed.
Published by: Nederlandse Vereniging voor Vrijwillige Euthanasie/Dutch Voluntary Euthanasia Society, Postbus 75331, Amsterdam 1070 AH, Netherlands. TEL 31-20-620-0690, FAX 31-20-420-7216, euthanasie@nvve.nl, http://www.nvve.nl.

THE RESHAPING OF PSYCHOANALYSIS; from Sigmund Freud to Ernest Becker. see *PSYCHOLOGY*

REVIEW OF EXISTENTIAL PSYCHOLOGY AND PSYCHIATRY. see *PSYCHOLOGY*

RIVISTA DI PSICOLOGIA DELL'ARTE. see *ART*

SELF & SOCIETY; European journal of humanistic psychology. see *PSYCHOLOGY*

153 BEL
SEMIOTIC AND COGNITIVE STUDIES. Text in English, Italian. 1995. irreg., latest vol.7, 2000. price varies. back issues avail. **Document type:** *Monographic series.* **Description:** Publishes interdisciplinary studies in the fields of cognitive sciences, psychology, psycholinguistics, the philosophy of mind, and artificial intelligence.
Indexed: e-psyche.
—BLDSC.
Published by: (University of San Marino, International Center for Semiotic and Cognitive Studies), N.V. Brepols, Steenweg op Tielen 68, Turnhout 2300, Belgium. FAX 32-14-42-89-19, publishers@brepols.com. Eds. Patrizia Violi, Umberto Eco.

142.7 616.89 GBR ISSN 0958-0476
SOCIETY FOR EXISTENTIAL ANALYSIS. JOURNAL. Text in English. 1989. s-a. GBP 20 in Europe to individuals; GBP 26 rest of world to individuals; GBP 30 in Europe to institutions; GBP 36 rest of world to institutions (effective 2000). adv. bk.rev. 200 p./no. back issues avail. *Refereed.* **Document type:** *Journal, Academic/Scholarly.* **Description:** Presents papers relating to the analysis of existence from philosophical and psychological-psychotherapeutic perspectives.
Indexed: e-psyche.
—BLDSC (4887.220000).
Published by: Society for Existential Analysis, BM Existential, London WC1N 3XX, United Kingdom. TEL 44-171-254-2707, FAX 44-171-538-0050, exist@cwcom.net, http://www.existential.mcmail.com/. Eds. John Heaton TEL 44-0207-487-7555, Simon Du Plock. Adv. contact D Scoular TEL 44-0207-538-0500. Circ: 500 (paid).

SPRINGER SERIES ON ETHICS, LAW, AND AGING. see *GERONTOLOGY AND GERIATRICS*

STUDIES IN COGNITIVE SYSTEMS. see *PSYCHOLOGY*

STUDIES IN LINGUISTICS AND PHILOSOPHY. see *PSYCHOLOGY*

SUBTLE ENERGIES AND ENERGY MEDICINE; an interdisciplinary journal of energetic and informational interactions. see *PHYSICS*

TAKING SIDES: CLASHING VIEWS ON CONTROVERSIAL BIOETHICAL ISSUES. see *MEDICAL SCIENCES*

TAROT NETWORK NEWS. see *NEW AGE PUBLICATIONS*

THEOLOGY AND MEDICINE. see *RELIGIONS AND THEOLOGY*

THEORETICAL MEDICINE AND BIOETHICS; philosophy of medical research and practice. see *MEDICAL SCIENCES*

100 SWE ISSN 0040-5825
B1 CODEN: THRAA5
THEORIA; a Swedish journal of philosophy. Text in English. 1935. 3/yr. SEK 150, USD 35 (effective 1998). adv. bk.rev. bibl. **Document type:** *Academic/Scholarly.*
Indexed: Bibl.Engl.Lang.& Lit., Curr.Cont. (coverage dropped), IBR, IBZ, Ind.Philos., Lang.& Lang.Behav.Abstr., Math.R., P C I, Phil.Ind., Psychol.Abstr., RILM, Russ.Acad.Sci.Bibl., SOPODA, SSCI (coverage dropped), Sociol.Abstr., e-psyche.
—ingenta.
Published by: Thales, c/o Theoria Filosofiska Institutionen, Kungshuset, Lund 22222, Sweden. FAX 46-46-222-44-24, theoria@fil.lu.se. Ed. Wlodek Rabinowicz. R&P, Adv. contact Jonas Josefsson.

174.2 610.9 360 GBR
THERAPEUTIC COMMUNITIES. Text in English. 1998. irreg., latest vol.8, 2001. back issues avail. *Refereed.* **Document type:** *Monographic series, Academic/Scholarly.* **Description:** Features Therapeutic Community movement, which holds a multidisciplinary view of health based on ideas of collective responsibility, citizenship and empowerment. Its principles are applicable in a wide variety of settings, as the series reflects.
Published by: Jessica Kingsley Publishers, 116 Pentonville Rd, London N1 9JB, United Kingdom. TEL 44-207-833-2307, post@jkp.com, http://www.jkp.com. Eds. Jan Lees, Rex Haigh. **Dist. by:** Plymbridge Distributors Ltd, Plymbridge House, Estover Rd, Plymouth, Devon PL6 7PY, United Kingdom. TEL 44-1752-202300, FAX 44-1752-202330.

THINKING & REASONING. see *PSYCHOLOGY*

TIJDSCHRIFT VOOR GENEESKUNDE EN ETHIEK. see *MEDICAL SCIENCES*

150 NLD ISSN 0167-7411
B1
TOPOI; an international review of philosophy. Text in English. 1982. s-a. EUR 294 to institutions for print or online ed.; EUR 352.80 to institutions print & online eds.combined (effective 2002). adv. bk.rev. index. back issues avail.; reprint service avail. from SWZ. *Refereed.* **Document type:** *Academic/Scholarly.* **Description:** Publishes articles, reviews and discussions of philosophy and the history of philosophy.
Related titles: Microform ed.: (from PQC); Online - full text ed.: (from EBSCO Publishing, O C L C Online Computer Library Center, Inc., RoweCom Information Quest, Swets Blackwell, Kluwer Online, Institute for Scientific Information).
Indexed: ASCA, Arts & Hum.Cit.Ind., Curr.Cont., Math.R., Phil.Ind., SSCI (coverage dropped), e-psyche.
—BLDSC (8867.499800), IDS, ingenta. **CCC.**
Published by: Kluwer Academic Publishers Group (Subsidiary of: Wolters Kluwer N.V.), Spuiboulevard 50, PO Box 17, Dordrecht 3300 AA, Netherlands. FAX 31-78-639-2254, services@wkap.nl, http://www.wkap.nl/journalhome.htm/0167-7411. Ed. Ermanno Bencivenga. **Dist. by:** Journals Department, PO Box 322, Dordrecht 3300 AH, Netherlands. TEL 781-871-6600, FAX 31-78-654-6474.

100 ESP
UNIVERSIDAD DE SEVILLA. SERIE FILOSOFIA Y PSICOLOGIA. Text in Spanish. 1990. irreg. back issues avail. **Document type:** *Academic/Scholarly.*
Published by: Universidad de Sevilla, Servicio de Publicaciones, Porvenir, 27, Sevilla 41013, Spain. TEL 34-95-448-7446, FAX 34-95-448-7443.

179 174.95 AUS ISSN 1321-0599
V.E. BULLETIN. (Voluntary Euthanasia) Text in English. 1984. 3/yr. AUD 14 domestic; AUD 18 foreign (effective 2001). bk.rev. **Document type:** *Newsletter.* **Description:** Promotes a change to the law so that in appropriate circumstances and with defined safeguards a medically assisted or induced death is allowed as an option of last resort in medical practice.
Published by: South Australian Voluntary Euthanasia Society, PO Box 2151, Kent Town, SA 5071, Australia. TEL 61-8-83793421, FAX 61-8-82652287, raym@adam.com.au, http://www.on.net/clients/saves/. Ed. Julia Anaf.

179 GBR ISSN 1467-2200
V E NEWS; the campaign journal of the Voluntary Euthanasia Society. Text in English. 1978. 3/yr. GBP 15 to membership (effective 2000). bk.rev. back issues avail. **Document type:** *Newsletter.* **Description:** Brings news and articles on the right to self-determination in dying.
Former titles (until 1998): V E S Newsletter (1360-161X); Exit; Exit News; Right to Die
Published by: Voluntary Euthanasia Society, 13 Prince Of Wales Terr, London W8 5PG, United Kingdom. TEL 44-171-937-7770, FAX 44-171-376-2648, info@ves.org.uk, http://www.ves.org.uk. Ed., R&P Jenni Burt. Circ: 18,500 (paid).

VS; quaderni di studi semiotici. see *LINGUISTICS*

100 CHN ISSN 1002-0772
YIXUE YU ZHEXUE/MEDICINE AND PHILOSOPHY. Text in Chinese. 1980. m. USD 34.80; CNY 5.50, USD 2.90 newsstand/cover (effective 2001). **Document type:** *Academic/Scholarly.*
Related titles: Online - full content ed.: (from WanFang Data Corp.).
Published by: Zhongguo Ziran Bianzhengfa Yanjiuhui, 3, Nanshi Jie Bingyin Hang, Dalian 116013, China. TEL 86-411-2496559, Yizhe@dalian-gov.net, yizhe@yizhe.net, http://www.Yizhe.net. Ed. Zhi-Zheng Du. **Dist. by:** China International Book Trading Corp, 35, Chegongzhuang Xilu, Haidian District, Beijing 100044, China. TEL 86-1-68413849, FAX 86-1-68412048, cibtc@mail.cibtc.com.cn, http://www.cibtc.com.cn. **Co-sponsor:** Zhongguo Ziran Bianzhengfa Yanjiuhui.

YOGA AND HEALTH. see *PHYSICAL FITNESS AND HYGIENE*

181.45 294.54 IND ISSN 0970-1737
YOGA AND TOTAL HEALTH. Text in English. 1933. m. INR 150, USD 25; INR 15 newsstand/cover (effective 2001). adv. bk.rev. abstr, bibl, charts, illus. 28 p./no. back issues avail. *Refereed.* **Document type:** *Magazine, Academic/Scholarly.* **Description:** Contains articles on Yoga education therapy, Yoga philosophy and techniques, as well as research on cardiac, respiratory, diabetes, orthopaedic problems.
Formerly: Yoga Institute. Journal (0044-0493)
Indexed: Russ.Acad.Sci.Bibl.
Published by: Yoga Institute, Santa Cruz East, Mumbai, Maharashtra 400 055, India. TEL 91-22-6110506, yoga@vsnl.net, FAX http://www.yogainstitute.org. Ed., Pub. Jayadeva Yogendra. R&P A N Desai. Circ: 2,000 (paid).

YOGA INTERNATIONAL. see *NEW AGE PUBLICATIONS*

ZEITSCHRIFT FUER MEDIZINISCHE ETHIK. see *MEDICAL SCIENCES*

ZHONG WAI YI XUE ZHE ZUE/CHINESE AND INTERNATIONAL PHILOSOPHY OF MEDICINE. see *MEDICAL SCIENCES*

PHILOSOPHY—Abstracting, Bibliographies, Statistics

NEW TITLES IN BIOETHICS. see *MEDICAL SCIENCES—Abstracting, Bibliographies, Statistics*

PHOTOGRAPHY

see also MOTION PICTURES

770 IND
INDIAN JOURNAL OF MEDICAL PHOTOGRAPHY. Text in English. 1965. q. INR 6.
Published by: Biological Photographic Association, Indian Chapter, 10-D Medical Enclave, Patiala, Punjab, India.

614.19 USA
JOURNAL OF EVIDENCE PHOTOGRAPHY. Variant title: E P I C Journal. Text in English. 1968. s-a. adv. reprint service avail. from PQC. **Document type:** *Trade.* **Description:** Features articles advancing knowledge in the field of forensic photography.
Related titles: Microform ed.: (from PQC).
Published by: Evidence Photographers International Council, 600 Main St, Honesdale, PA 18431. TEL 570-253-5450, FAX 570-253-5011, http://www.epic-photo.org. Ed. William Amptman. R&P, Adv. contact Robert F Jennings. page USD 250. Circ: 2,500.

TAUCHEN; internationales Unterwasser-Magazin. see *SPORTS AND GAMES*

PHYSICAL CHEMISTRY

see CHEMISTRY—Physical Chemistry

PHYSICAL FITNESS AND HYGIENE

see also MEDICAL SCIENCES; NUTRITION AND DIETETICS; PUBLIC HEALTH AND SAFETY; SPORTS AND GAMES

A B C NEWSLETTER. see *MEDICAL SCIENCES—Hematology*

613.0711 USA ISSN 0002-7952
A C H A ACTION. Text in English. 1970. 4/yr. membership. adv. **Document type:** *Newsletter.* **Description:** Covers current issues in college health for those interested in student health services.
Formerly: A C H Action; Supersedes: American College Health Association. Newsletter
Published by: American College Health Association, PO Box 28937, Baltimore, MD 21240-8937. TEL 410-859-1500, FAX 410-859-1510. Ed. Rebecca Kerins. Pub. Charley Hartman. Adv. contact Susan Ainsworth. Circ: 4,300.

A C H P E R HEALTHY LIFESTYLES JOURNAL. see *EDUCATION*

613.7 USA ISSN 1091-5397
A C S M'S HEALTH & FITNESS JOURNAL. Variant title: American College of Sports Medicine Health and Fitness Journal. Health & Fitness Journal. Text in English. 1997. bi-m. USD 40 domestic; USD 50 foreign; USD 9 (effective 2002). **Document type:** *Journal.* **Description:** Promotes and distributes accurate, unbiased, and authoritative information on health and fitness.
Related titles: Online - full text ed.: (from Institute for Scientific Information).
Indexed: Focus on: Sports Sci.& Med.
—BLDSC (0578.950700).
Published by: (American College of Sports Medicine), Lippincott Williams & Wilkins (Philadelphia) (Subsidiary of: Wolters Kluwer N.V.), 530 Walnut St, Philadelphia, PA 19106-3621. TEL 215-521-8300, FAX 215-521-8902, custserv@lww.com, http://acsm-healthfitness.org, http://www.lww.com/. Ed. Lawrence A Golding. **Subscr. addr.:** Lippincott Williams & Wilkins, Order Dept, 16522 Hunters Green Pkwy, Hagerstown, MD 21740. TEL 301-714-2334, FAX 301-824-7390. **Affiliates:** Lippincott Williams & Wilkins Asia; Lippincott Williams & Wilkins Pty, Ltd.; Lippincott Williams & Wilkins, Ltd.

A S H SMOKING AND HEALTH REVIEW. see *LAW*

613.7 330 USA ISSN 1067-1714
A W H P ACTION. Text in English. 1975. q. free for members. adv. **Document type:** *Newsletter.*
Formerly: A F B Action (0891-7450)
Media: Online - full text.
Indexed: Sportsearch (1983-).
Published by: Association for Worksite Health Promotion, 60 Revere Dr, Ste 500, Northbrook, IL 60062-1577. TEL 847-480-9574, FAX 847-480-9282, http://www.awhp.org. Ed. Patricia Sullivan. Pub. Greg Schultz. R&P, Adv. contact Rick Koepke. Circ: 3,000 (controlled).

363.8 GBR ISSN 1364-3959
A - Z OF CALORIES. Text in English. 1996. q. GBP 1.99 newsstand/cover. **Document type:** *Consumer.* **Description:** Contains information about calories and how to count them, as well as low-calorie food selection advice.
Published by: Octavo Publications Ltd., Tolland, Lydeard St Lawrence, Taunton TA4 3PS, United Kingdom. TEL 44-1984-623014, FAX 44-1984-623901. Ed. Gertrud Pertl. **Dist. by:** Marketforce, 247 Tottenham Ct Rd, London W1P 0AU, United Kingdom. TEL 44-171-261-5199, FAX 44-171-261-7341.

613.7 AUS ISSN 1321-1609
ACTIVE AND HEALTHY; the ACHPER magazine for physical educators, health educators and fitness leaders. Text in English. q. AUD 39.60 domestic; AUD 55 foreign (effective 2001). adv. back issues avail. **Document type:** *Consumer.* **Description:** Aims to improve the health and life-styles of Australians by the dissemination of classroom ideas, teaching strategies and trends for fitness, health and physical education.
Formed by the 1994 merger of: Physical Education Teacher Newsletter; Health and Fitness Newsletter (0814-754X); Health Education and Lifestyle Promotion Newsletter; Which was formerly (until 1991): Health Education and Lifestyle Project Newsletter
Published by: Australian Council for Health Physical Education and Recreation Inc., PO Box 304, Hindmarsh, SA 5007, Australia. TEL 61-8-8340-3388, FAX 61-8-8340-3399, membership@achper.org.au, http://www.achper.org.au/. Adv. contact Lyndall Bryden.

ADAPTED PHYSICAL ACTIVITY QUARTERLY. see *EDUCATION—Special Education And Rehabilitation*

ADIPOSITAS. see *NUTRITION AND DIETETICS*

330 613 USA ISSN 0731-2199
RA410.A1
ADVANCES IN HEALTH ECONOMICS AND HEALTH SERVICES RESEARCH. Text in English. 1979. irreg., latest vol.16. USD 73.25. *Refereed.* **Document type:** *Monographic series.*
Formerly (until 1981): Research in Health Economics (0197-0690)
Indexed: Abstr.Health Care Manage.Stud., Inpharma, Reac. —BLDSC (0709.008000), GNLM, Infotrieve, ingenta. **CCC.**
Published by: J A I Press Inc., 100 Prospect St, Box 811, Stamford, CT 06904-0811. TEL 203-323-9606, FAX 203-357-8446, jai@jaipress.com. Eds. Louis F Rossiter, Richard M Scheffler.

613 USA ISSN 0896-1255
ADVANCES IN HEALTH EDUCATION AND PROMOTION. Text in English. 1986. irreg. **Document type:** *Monographic series.*
Published by: Taylor & Francis Ltd. (Subsidiary of: Taylor & Francis Group), 325 Chestnut St, Suite 800, Philadelphia, PA 19016. info@taylorandfrancis.com, http://www.taylorandfrancis.com/. **Subscr. addr. in Europe:** Taylor & Francis Group, Journals Customer Service, Rankine Rd, Basingstoke, Hants RG24 8PR, United Kingdom. TEL 44-1256-813000, FAX 44-1256-479438, enquiry@tanf.co.uk, http://www.tandf.co.uk/journals.

ADVANCES IN HEALTH EDUCATION: CURRENT RESEARCH. see *EDUCATION—Teaching Methods And Curriculum*

613.7 USA ISSN 0888-9287
RJ133
ADVANCES IN MOTOR DEVELOPMENT RESEARCH. Text in English. 1987. a. USD 37.50. bk.rev. index. back issues avail. *Refereed.* **Description:** Original research and review in the study of motor development.
—CISTI, GNLM.
Published by: A M S Press, Inc., 56 E 13th St, New York, NY 10003. TEL 212-777-4700, FAX 212-995-5413. Eds. James H Humphrey, Jane E Clark.

613.7 USA
AEROBIC BEAT. Text in English. 1984. bi-m. USD 25. adv. bk.rev., music rev. **Document type:** *Newsletter.* **Description:** Designed to help in the location of the latest and most appropriate music for aerobic workouts, jogging, step training and other fitness activities done with music.
Address: 7985 Santa Monica Blvd, Ste 109, Los Angeles, CA 90046-5186. TEL 310-659-2503, FAX 213-655-5223. Eds. Ken Alan, Randy Sills.

AGEING AND ERGONOMICS SERIES. see *OCCUPATIONAL HEALTH AND SAFETY*

AIDS EDUCATION AND PREVENTION; an interdisciplinary journal. (Acquired Immune Deficiency Syndrome) see *PUBLIC HEALTH AND SAFETY*

613.7 AUT
AKTIV; Magazin fuer Gesundheit, Ernaehrung und Schoenheit. Text in German. bi-m. adv. **Document type:** *Consumer.*
Published by: Oesterreichischer Wirtschaftsverlag GmbH, Nikolsdorfer Gasse 7-11, Vienna, W 1051, Austria. TEL 43-1-54664, FAX 43-1-54663360, office@oewv.at, http://www.oewv.at. Ed. Wolfgang Friedrich. Adv. contact Christine Fasching. B&W page ATS 36,400, color page ATS 45,000; trim 252 x 185. Circ: 77,000 (paid).

613.7 USA
THE AKWA LETTER. Text in English. 1986. bi-m. USD 48 to members. adv. **Document type:** *Newsletter.*
Published by: Aquatic Exercise Association, Inc., PO Box 1609, Nokomis, FL 34274-1609. TEL 941-486-8600, FAX 941-486-8820, aea@ix.netcom.com. Ed. Julie See. R&P Tracy Fryer. Adv. contact Kim Huff. Circ: 6,000.

P

613.2 CAN ISSN 0228-586X
CODEN: ACOLEL
ALIVE; Canadian journal of health and nutrition. Text in English. 1975. 12/yr. CND 34, USD 40 domestic; CND 54 foreign (effective 2000). adv. bk.rev. *Refereed.* **Document type:** *Consumer.* **Description:** Covers nutrition and alternative health information, issues and therapies.
Indexed: INIS Atomind., Mid.East: Abstr.& Ind.
—CCC.
Published by: Canadian Health Reform Products Ltd., 7436 Fraser Park Dr, Burnaby, BC V5J 5B9, Canada. TEL 604-435-1919, FAX 604-435-4888. Ed., Pub., R&P, Adv. contact Siegfried Gursche. Circ: 230,000. **Subscr. to:** P O Box 80055, Burnaby, BC V5J 3X5, Canada.

613.7 USA ISSN 0893-5238
CODEN: AAFIEL
AMERICAN FITNESS. Text in English. 1983. bi-m. USD 27 (effective 2000). adv. bk.rev. **Document type:** *Trade.* **Description:** Provides news and information concerning health and fitness.
Supersedes (in 1987): Aerobics and Fitness (0749-8942); Formerly (until 1984): Aerobics and Fitness Association of America. Journal
Related titles: Microform ed.: (from PQC); Online - full text ed.: (from Gale Group, The Dialog Corporation, ProQuest Information & Learning, Northern Light Technology, Inc., Factiva).
Indexed: Phys.Ed.Ind., Sportsearch (1987-).
—BLDSC (0815.220000).
Published by: Aerobics and Fitness Association of America, 15250 Ventura Blvd, Sherman Oaks, CA 91403. TEL 818-905-0040. Ed. Peg Jordan, R.N. Pub. Roscoe Fawcett. R&P Peg Jordan Jordan, R N. Adv. contact Cindy Schofield. Circ: 30,000.

613.7 USA ISSN 1523-3359
RA773 CODEN: AMHEEZ
AMERICAN HEALTH; smart ways women stay well . Abbreviated title: A H. Cover title: Health. Text in English. 1982. 10/yr. USD 18.97 domestic; USD 27.97 foreign; USD 1.95 newsstand/cover. adv. bk.rev. illus. reprints avail. **Document type:** *Consumer.* **Description:** Research-based consumer magazine on health, fitness, medicine and nutrition.
Former titles (until 1999): American Health for Women (1092-1656); (until 1996): American Health (0730-7004)
Indexed: AgeLine, Alloys Ind. (1980-1981), Amer.Bibl.Slavic & E.Eur.Stud., CHNI, CINAHL, Consum.Ind. (1989-), Gen.Sci.Ind. (Dec.1996-Dec.1998), Hlth.Ind., Met.Abstr. (1980-1981), Met.Abstr.Ind. (1980-1981), NRN, Nonfer.Met.Alert (1980-1981), PCC Alert (1980-1981), Phys.Ed.Ind., R.G. (1988-Oct.1999), R.G.Abstr. (1988-Oct.1999), Steels Alert (1980-1981).
—GNLM, ingenta.
Published by: R D Publications, Inc, 260 Madison Ave, New York, NY 10016. TEL 212-366-8900, FAX 212-627-3833, http://www.americanhealth.com. Ed. Freddi Greenberg. Pub. Margery Gladstone. Adv. contact Robyn Borok. B&W page USD 34,980, color page USD 43,100; trim 10.5 x 7.88. Circ: 926,430 (paid). **Subscr. to:** PO Box 3017, Harlan, IA 51537.

613.7 USA ISSN 1087-3244
RA421
AMERICAN JOURNAL OF HEALTH BEHAVIOR. Text in English. 1977. bi-m. USD 78 to individuals; USD 90 in Canada & Mexico to individuals; USD 110 elsewhere to individuals; USD 124 to institutions; USD 136 in Canada & Mexico to institutions; USD 156 elsewhere to institutions (effective 2000). adv. bk.rev. illus. index. back issues avail.; reprints avail. *Refereed.* **Document type:** *Academic/Scholarly.* **Description:** Seeks to provide a comprehensive understanding of the relationships among personal behavior, social structure and health, and to disseminate knowledge of major behavioral science principles and strategies to assist in designing and implementing programs to prevent disease and promote health.
Formerly (until 1996): Health Values (0147-0353)
Related titles: Microform ed.: (from PQC); Online - full text ed.: (from Institute for Scientific Information).
Indexed: ASCA, ASSIA, AgeLine, CHNI, C.I.J.E., CINAHL, Crim.Just.Abstr., Curr.Cont., Educ.Admin.Abstr., Environ.Sci.Poll.Mgmt., Fam.Ind., Lang.& Lang.Behav.Abstr., NRN, Ocean.Abstr., Phys.Ed.Ind., Pollut.Abstr., PsycInfo, Psychol.Abstr. (1990-), Risk Abstr., SOPODA, SSCI, Saf.Sci.Abstr., Sage Fam.Stud.Abstr., Soc.Serv.Abstr., Sociol.Abstr., e-psyche.
—BLDSC (0824.700000), CISTI, GNLM, IDS, ingenta. **CCC.**
Published by: P N G Publications, PO Box 4593, Star City, WV 26504-4593. TEL 304-293-4699, FAX 304-293-4693, pglover@wvu.edu, http://www.ajhb.org. Ed., Pub. Elbert D Glover. R&P, Adv. contact Penny N Glover. Circ: 2,000 (paid).

AMERICAN JOURNAL OF HEALTH PROMOTION. see *PUBLIC HEALTH AND SAFETY*

613 DEU ISSN 0402-270X
AMPHORA. Text in German. 1955. m. adv. **Document type:** *Magazine, Consumer.*
Published by: Gebr. Storck GmbH, Bebelstr 102, Oberhausen 46049, Germany. TEL 49-208-848020, FAX 49-208-8480242. adv.: page DEM 42,000. Circ: 1,653,990 (controlled).

613 USA ISSN 0278-4653
RA773
ANNUAL EDITIONS: HEALTH. Text in English. 1975. a. USD 12.25. illus. *Refereed.* **Document type:** *Academic/Scholarly.*
Former titles (1980-1981): Readings in Health (0730-8930); Annual Editions: Readings in Health (0360-9766)
Published by: Dushkin - McGraw-Hill, Sluice Dock, Guilford, CT 06437-9989. TEL 203-453-4351, FAX 203-453-6000. Ed. Rick Yarian. Pub. Ian Nielsen. R&P Cheryl Greenleaf.

ANNUAL EDITIONS: NUTRITION. see *NUTRITION AND DIETETICS*

ANTROPO-EKOLOGIIA. see *ENVIRONMENTAL STUDIES*

613.7 AUT
APA-JOURNAL. GESUNDHEIT. Variant title: A P A - Journal. Gesundheit. Text in German. w. ATS 480 per month (effective 2000). **Document type:** *Journal, Trade.*
Published by: Austria Presse Agentur (APA), Gunoldstrasse 14, Vienna, W 1199, Austria. TEL 43-1-360605555, FAX 43-1-360605199, journale@apa.at, http://www.apa.at.

613 IND ISSN 0003-6498
APKA SWASTHYA. Text in Hindi. 1953. m. INR 361.
Published by: Indian Medical Association, I.M.A. House, Indraprastha Marg, New Delhi 110 002, India. Circ: 3,500. **Subscr. to:** Apka Swasthya, I.M.A. Building, C. 7-31 Chet Ganj, Varanasi, Uttar Pradesh 1, India.

613 DEU
APOTHEKE; Ratgeber fuer Ihre Gesundheit. Text in German. m. adv. **Document type:** *Magazine, Consumer.*
Published by: Gebr. Storck GmbH, Bebelstr 102, Oberhausen 46049, Germany. TEL 49-208-848020, FAX 49-208-8480242. adv.: page DEM 42,000. Circ: 1,653,990 (controlled).

613 DEU
APOTHEKEN-MAGAZIN FUER SENIOREN & DIABETIKER. Text in German. bi-m. adv. **Document type:** *Magazine, Consumer.*
Published by: Gebr. Storck GmbH, Bebelstr 102, Oberhausen 46049, Germany. TEL 49-208-848020, FAX 49-208-8480242. adv.: page DEM 5,800. Circ: 105,500 (controlled).

613.7 610 DEU ISSN 0402-7108
APOTHEKEN UMSCHAU; das Gesundheits-Magazin. Text in German. 1957. m. **Document type:** *Consumer.*
Published by: Wort und Bild Verlag Konradshoehe GmbH, Konradshoehe, Baierbrunn 82065, Germany. TEL 49-89-74433-0, FAX 49-89-74433150, http://www.wortundbild.de. Ed. Dr. Gudrun Starringer.

613.7 RUS
ARGUMENTY I FAKTY. ZDOROV'E. Text in Russian. w. USD 145 in United States.
Related titles: ♦ Supplement to: Argumenty i Fakty. ISSN 0204-0476.
Published by: Redaktsiya Argumenty i Fakty, Myasnitskaya ul 42, Moscow 101000, Russian Federation. TEL 7-095-9281294, zdorovie@aif.ru. Ed. V Romanenko. **US dist. addr.:** East View Publications, 3020 Harbor Ln N, Minneapolis, MN 55447. TEL 612-550-0961.

613.7 USA
ARIZONA HEALTH ECONOMICS. Text in English. q. **Document type:** *Newsletter.* **Description:** Provides analysis of costs and usage of health care in Arizona.
Published by: Arizona State University, Center for Business Research, College of Business, Box 874406, Tempe, AZ 85287-4406. TEL 602-965-3961, FAX 602-965-5458, asubr@asuvm.inre.asu.edu. **Co-sponsor:** Blue Cross Blue Shield of Arizona.

613.7 610 IND ISSN 0253-682X
CODEN: AROGD8
AROGYA; a journal of health sciences. Text in English. 1975. s-a. free per issue. adv. bk.rev.
Indexed: Chem.Abstr., Food Sci.& Tech.Abstr., INIS Atomind., Rev.Med.& Vet.Mycol.
—CASDDS, CISTI, GNLM.
Published by: Kasturba Medical College Trust Manipal, Department of Clinical Biochemistry, c/o Arogyal, Ed., Manipal 576 119, India. TEL 20060. Ed. Sudhakar S Nayak. Circ: 1,000 (controlled).

613.7 TWN ISSN 1015-1990
ASIAN JOURNAL OF PHYSICAL EDUCATION. Text in Chinese. 1978. q.
Indexed: Sportsearch (1978-).
Address: No3, Ln 153, Sec 2, Cahng An East Rd, Taipei, Taiwan.

613 616.8 AUS ISSN 1329-6884
AUSTRALIAN COUNCIL ON SMOKING AND HEALTH NEWSLETTER. Text in English. 1984. irreg. back issues avail. **Document type:** *Newsletter.*
Formerly (until 1997): Smoking or Health (1032-8416)
Media: Online - full content. **Related titles:** Online - full text ed.
Published by: Australian Council on Smoking and Health, PO Box 327, Subiaco, W.A. 6008, Australia. TEL 61-8-9388-3342, FAX 61-8-9382-4611, library@acosh.org, http://www.acosh.org. Ed. Peter Markham. Circ: 2,000.

AUSTRALIAN SURF LIFESAVER. see *SPORTS AND GAMES—Outdoor Life*

AUSTRALIAN SWIMMING AND FITNESS. see *SPORTS AND GAMES*

613.7 CAN ISSN 1201-6144
AVANTE. Text in English, French. 1995. 3/yr. CND 65 domestic to individuals; CND 83 foreign to individuals; CND 100 domestic to institutions; CND 118 foreign to institutions. adv. *Refereed.* **Document type:** *Academic/Scholarly.* **Description:** Designed to stimulate and communicate Canadian research and critical thought on issues pertaining to health, physical education and recreation.
—BLDSC (1837.119520).
Published by: Canadian Association for Health, Physical Education, Recreation and Dance, Place R Tait McKenzie, 1600 James Naismith Dr, Gloucester, ON K1B 5N4, Canada. TEL 613-748-5622, FAX 613-748-5737, agrantha@rtm.activeliving.ca. Adv. contact Andrea Grantham. Circ: 600.

363.8 GBR ISSN 0956-5345
BE SLIM. Text in English. 1989. q. GBP 1.60 newsstand/cover. **Document type:** *Consumer.* **Description:** Offers advice and guidance on how to lose weight in a smart and healthy manner.
Published by: Octavo Publications Ltd., Tolland, Lydeard St Lawrence, Taunton TA4 3PS, United Kingdom. TEL 44-1984-623014, FAX 44-1984-623901. **Dist. by:** MarketForce UK Ltd, 247 Tottenham Court Rd, London, Middx W1T 7AU, United Kingdom. TEL 44-207-261-5199, FAX 44-207-261-7341.

613.7 USA
BEAUTY HANDBOOK. Text in English. 1982. q. USD 0.99 newsstand/cover (effective 2000). adv. illus. **Document type:** *Consumer.* **Description:** Enables men and women to improve their own and their families' health and fitness through improving nutrition, reducing stress, and generally engaging in healthful lifestyles.
Formerly: Health Handbook
Published by: Compendium Systems Corp., 346 N. Main, Port Chester, NY 10573. TEL 914-935-1000, FAX 914-935-1063. Pub. John McAuliffe. adv.: B&W page USD 18,000, color page USD 35,000. Circ: 2,800,000.

613.7 610 USA
BETTER HEALTH. Text in English. 1979. bi-m.
Published by: Better Health Magazine, 1450 Chapel St, New Haven, CT 06511-4440. TEL 203-789-3972, FAX 203-789-4053. Ed. Cynthia Wolfe Boynton. Adv. contact Meredith Long. Circ: 500,000.

613.7 USA
BEYOND P E* . (Physical Education) Text in English. 1991. bi-m. USD 18. adv. back issues avail. **Document type:** *Consumer.* **Description:** Covers topics in bodybuilding, fitness and health for the urban man and woman, including aerobics, yoga, nutrition, massage and healing.
Formerly (until 1993): New York Bodies

P

Address: 209 E 59th St, Apt 4F, New York, NY 10022-1412. TEL 212-779-0294, FAX 212-779-1526. Ed. Ronald L Dobrin. Circ: 80,000 (controlled).

613.7 DEU ISSN 0949-4642
BIO MAGAZIN. Text in German. 1984. bi-m. DEM 42; DEM 48 foreign (effective 1999). adv. bk.rev. back issues avail. **Document type:** *Consumer.* **Description:** Contains information on achieving health through natural means and procedures.
Formerly: Bio Spezial Magazin
Published by: Bio Ritter GmbH, Monatshauserstr 8, Tutzing 82327, Germany. TEL 49-8158-8021, FAX 49-8158-7142, bioritter@aol.com, http://www.magazin-bio.de. Ed., R&P Monica Ritter. Adv. contact Edith Vonhafenbraedl. Circ: 60,000.

613 DEU ISSN 0006-3487
BIONOMICA. Text in German. 1950. bi-m. DEM 20. adv. bk.rev. **Document type:** *Bulletin.*
Published by: (Bionomica-Gemeinschaft e.V.), Bionomica Verlag, Duesseldorfer Str 9-11, Mannheim 68219, Germany. TEL 49-621-895061, FAX 49-621-814962. Ed. Ewald Koenemann.

BODY BULLETIN NEWSLETTER. see *OCCUPATIONAL HEALTH AND SAFETY*

613.7 USA ISSN 1092-0129
BOTTOM LINE - HEALTH. Text in English. 1987. m. USD 29.95 (effective 2000). **Document type:** *Newsletter, Consumer.* **Description:** Offers consumers valuable expert insider tips on all aspects of personal health and fitness.
Formerly (until 1997): Health Confidential (0894-4172)
Indexed: CINAHL.
—BLDSC (2264.025500).
Published by: Boardroom, Inc, 55 Railroad Ave, PO Box 2614, Greenwich, CT 06936-2614. TEL 203-625-5900, FAX 203-861-7057, editors@boardroom.com, http://www.boardroom.com. R&P Bradley Smith TEL 203-861-7443. Circ: 30,000. **Subscr. to:** PO Box 53408, Boulder, CO 80322-3408. TEL 800-289-0409, FAX 303-604-7455, blhealth@boardroom.com, http://www.blp.net/subscription.html.

613.7 DEU
BURDA AKTIV UND GESUND. Text in German. 1953. m. adv. back issues avail. **Document type:** *Magazine, Consumer.*
Formerly: Burda International (0937-356X)
Indexed: Russ.Acad.Sci.Bibl.
Published by: Verlag Aenne Burda, Am Kestendamm 2, Offenburg 77652, Germany. TEL 49-781-8402, FAX 49-781-843291, TELEX 752804-BUMOD-D. Ed. Susanne Walsleben. Pub. Aenne Burda. Adv. contact Corinna Lohrenz. color page DEM 13,800. Circ: 150,000.

613.7 USA
▼ **BURN.** Text in English. 1999. bi-m. USD 19.97; USD 4.95 newsstand/cover; CND 5.95 newsstand/cover in Canada (effective 1999). **Document type:** *Consumer.* **Description:** Deals with fitness issues for men from 18 to 28.
Published by: Celebrity Style Inc., 230 W 41st St, Ste 1500, New York, NY 10036. TEL 212-840-0309, FAX 212-840-3911, burnmail@aol.com, http://www.mediafinder.com. **Dist. by:** Kable Distribution Service, 641 Lexington Ave, New York, NY 10022. TEL 212-705-4600, FAX 212-705-4666.

613.7 ZMB
BWINO: HEALTH CARE NEWS. Text in English. 1981. bi-m. free per issue. **Document type:** *Newsletter, Government.*
Published by: Ministry of Health, Health Education Unit, PO Box 30205, Lusaka, Zambia. Circ: 6,000.

C P H A HEALTH DIGEST. see *PUBLIC HEALTH AND SAFETY*

613.7 CAN ISSN 1187-0818
CANADIAN INTRAMURAL RECREATION ASSOCIATION. BULLETIN; the voice of intramurals in Canada. Text in English, French. 1977. bi-m. CND 45 (effective 1997). adv. bk.rev. abstr. illus. **Document type:** *Bulletin, Catalog, Newsletter.* **Description:** Contains ideas, information and hands-on practical and user-friendly information on intramurals for practitioners and participants.
Published by: Canadian Intramural Recreation Association/Association Canadienne de Loisirs Intramuros, 1600 James Naismith Dr, Ste 809, Gloucester, ON K1B 5N4, Canada. TEL 613-748-5639, FAX 613-748-5737, cira@rtm.activeliving.ca, http://www.activeliving.ca. Ed., R&P, Adv. contact Rick Turnbull. Circ: 1,500.

CANADIAN JOURNAL OF DIABETES CARE. see *MEDICAL SCIENCES—Endocrinology*

616.1 USA ISSN 0194-2557
CARDIAC ALERT. Text in English. 1979. m. USD 39. index.
—CCC.
Published by: Phillips Publishing, Inc., Consumer Publishing, 7811 Montrose Rd, Potomac, MD 20854. TEL 301-340-2100, FAX 301-424-7034. Ed. Dr. Jorge C Rios.

CHEMECOLOGY; covering health, safety and the environment. see *ENVIRONMENTAL STUDIES*

CHINESE ACADEMIC JOURNAL. MEDICINE & HYGIENE. see *MEDICAL SCIENCES*

613.7 640.73 AUS ISSN 1324-8065
CHOICE HEALTH READER. Text in English. 1995. 10/yr. AUD 55 domestic to individuals; AUD 33 foreign to individuals; AUD 62 domestic to institutions; AUD 84 foreign to institutions (effective 2001). **Document type:** *Magazine, Consumer.* **Description:** Contains information about the latest developments in health, fitness and medical research for consumers.
Published by: Australian Consumers' Association, 57 Carrington Rd, Marrickville, NSW 2204, Australia. TEL 61-2-9577-3333, FAX 61-2-9577-3377, ausconsumer@choice.com.au, http://www.choice.com.au. Eds. Dr. Garry Egger, Dr. Norman Swan. Circ: 4,000.

CLINICAL JOURNAL OF SPORT MEDICINE. see *MEDICAL SCIENCES—Sports Medicine*

CLINICAL KINESIOLOGY. see *MEDICAL SCIENCES—Physical Medicine And Rehabilitation*

613.7 USA ISSN 0747-8283
CLUB INDUSTRY. Text in English. 1984. m. USD 68. adv. tr.lit. back issues avail. **Document type:** *Trade.* **Description:** Educates club owners, operators, general managers and directors on the latest market trends and recent product releases relating to health clubs and gyms.
Related titles: Online - full text ed.: (from H. W. Wilson, Gale Group).
Indexed: B.P.I. (Jan.1999-), Lod.Restr.& Tour.Ind.
—ingenta.
Published by: Primedia Business Magazines & Media, Inc. (Atlanta), 6151 Powers Ferry Rd, N W, Atlanta, GA 30339-2941. TEL 770-955-2500, FAX 770-955-0400, http://industryclick.com/magazine.asp?magazineid=123&siteid=18, http://www.primediabusiness.com/. Ed. Jerry Janda. Pub. Barry Lecerf. adv.: B&W page USD 5,150, color page USD 6,600. Circ: 30,000. **Subscr. to:** Primedia Business Magazines & Media, Inc., PO Box 12914, Overland Park, KS 66282-2914. TEL 800-441-0294, FAX 913-967-1903.

613.7 616.12 FRA ISSN 0335-5306
COEUR ET SANTE. Text in French. 1974. bi-m. FRF 100. adv. **Document type:** *Newspaper.*
Published by: (Federation Francaise de Cardiologie), Edicardio, 50 rue du Rocher, Paris 75008, France. TEL 44-90-83-67, FAX 42-93-38-97. Ed. Guy Malherbe. Pub. Armand Schaller.

613 ITA ISSN 1124-1705
COME STAI; mensile della salute per la famiglia. Text in Italian. 1995. m. ITL 35,000 domestic; USD 19.26 in United States; ITL 35,000 newsstand/cover. adv. illus. **Document type:** *Consumer.* **Description:** Provides health and fitness tips and articles for the whole family.
Published by: World Servizi Editoriali s.r.l. (Subsidiary of: Casa Editrice Universo S.p.A.), Via Cusani, 4, Milan, MI 20121, Italy. TEL 39-02-723311, FAX 39-02-8051119. Ed. Monica Sori. R&P Elisabetta Savoca TEL 39-2-72331435. Adv. contact Rodolfo Milosa. color page ITL 9,375,000; trim 277 x 218. Circ: 124,003 (paid).

COMPLEMENTARY CARE JOURNAL. see *SOCIOLOGY*

CONDITION; Ratgebermagazin fuer Lauf- und Ausdauersport. see *SPORTS AND GAMES*

613.7 155.937 USA
CONNECTICUT HOSPICE NEWSLETTER; making today count. Text in English. 1979. s-a. free per issue. **Description:** Provides information related to timely medical issues as they impact hospice care; includes features about hospice services.
Indexed: e-psyche.
Published by: Connecticut Hospice Inc., 61 Burban Dr, Branford, CT 06405. TEL 203-481-6231, FAX 203-483-9539. Circ: 50,000.

CONNELLY REPORT. see *NUTRITION AND DIETETICS*

613 GBR
CONSULTANT. Text in English. q. free per issue. adv.
Indexed: Bus.Ind., Hospit.Ind., Tr.& Indus.Ind.
Published by: Hospital Consultants and Specialists Association, No. One Kingsclere Rd, Overton, Basingstoke, Hants RG25 3JP, United Kingdom. TEL 0265-771777, FAX 0265-770999. Circ: 7,000.

613.7 USA ISSN 1058-0832
CODEN: CREHEI
CONSUMER REPORTS ON HEALTH. Text in English. 1989. m. USD 24; USD 30 foreign (effective 1997). illus. Index. reprints avail. **Document type:** *Consumer.* **Description:** Provides current information in making wise decisions concerning family health care services and products.
Formerly: Consumer Reports Health Letter (1044-3193)
Related titles: Online - full text ed.: (from Gale Group, The Dialog Corporation, LexisNexis, Factiva); ♦ Supplement to: Consumer Reports. ISSN 0010-7174.
Indexed: Biol.Dig., CINAHL.
—BLDSC (3424.551000).
Published by: Consumers Union of the United States, Inc., 101 Truman Ave, Yonkers, NY 10703-1057. TEL 914-378-2000, FAX 914-378-2919. Ed. Ronni Sandroff. Pub. James D Davis. Circ: 360,000. **Subscr. to:** PO Box 56356, Boulder, CO 80322-6356.

P

613.7 JPN
CONTEMPORARY HEALTH DIGEST. Text in Japanese. 1986. a.
Published by: Snow Brand Milk Products Co. Ltd., Health & Nutrition Institute/Yukijirushi Nyugyo K.K. Kenko Seikatsu Kenkyujo, 13 Honshio-cho, Shinjuku-ku, Tokyo 160-0003, Japan.

613.7 790.1 ESP
CORRICOLARI; el corredor y su mundo. Text in Spanish. m. ESP 6,000; ESP 500 newsstand/cover (effective 2001). adv. illus. back issues avail. **Document type:** *Magazine, Consumer.* **Description:** Covers the world of racing: marathons, race courses, athletics, nutrition, and the physiology of sport.
Published by: Grupo Arthax, Paseo Marques de Monistrol, 7-20, Madrid 28011, Spain. TEL 34-91-5268080, FAX 34-91-5261012, airelibre@airelibre.com, grupoarthax@airelibre.com, http://www.airelibre.com. Pub., R&P Paloma Fernandez. Adv. contact Pilar Fernandez. B&W page ESP 230,000, color page ESP 300,000; trim 270 x 250. Circ: 35,000.

613 790.1 ESP
CURATE REGENERATE. Text in Spanish. 12/yr.
Address: Cuatro Caminos 27 y Jaime Cancer 33, Barcelona 080222, Spain. TEL 85-23-65-10.

613.7 USA
CURRENT AWARENESS IN HEALTH EDUCATION. Text in English. m. USD 24.
Related titles: Online - full text ed.
Published by: U.S. Bureau of Health Education, Department of Health and Human Services, Washington, DC 20201. TEL 202-655-4000. **Subscr. to:** Supt. of Documents, Govt Printing Office, Washington, DC 20402.

CURRENT HEALTH 1; the beginning guide to health education. see *EDUCATION—Teaching Methods And Curriculum*

CURRENT HEALTH 2; the continuing guide to health education. see *EDUCATION—Teaching Methods And Curriculum*

613.7 CHN ISSN 1002-574X
DAZHONG JIANKANG/ORDINARY PEOPLE'S HEALTH. Text in Chinese. 1985. m.
Published by: Jiankang Baoshe, 11 Shuangsi, Jiu Gulou Dajie, Beijing 100009, China. TEL 4015114. Ed. Li Zhimin.

613 DEU ISSN 0343-3838
DER DEUTSCHE BADEBETRIEB. Short title: D D B. Text in German. 1909. m. DEM 115. **Document type:** *Trade.*
Formerly: Kurbad; Which incorporated: Bad
Published by: (Verband Deutscher Badebetriebe e.V.), Ebert Verlag GmbH, Blankenseer Str 6-8, Luebeck 23562, Germany. TEL 49-451-501011, FAX 49-4509-2241. Ed. Hans Juergen Ebert. Circ: 14,400.

DIABETES DIALOGUE. see *MEDICAL SCIENCES—Endocrinology*

613.7 USA
DIET & FITNESS MAGAZINE. Text in English. 1989. q. USD 5.99 per issue (effective 2000). adv. **Document type:** *Consumer.* **Description:** For adults interested in health, nutrition, weight loss, and healthy living.
Formerly: Diet and Health Magazine (1048-8391); Incorporates: Diet and Health Series
Published by: Lifetime Periodicals, Inc., 2131 Hollywood Blvd, Hollywood, FL 33020. TEL 954-925-5242, FAX 954-925-5244, FELLPUB@aol.com, http://www.lifetimebooks.com. Ed. Callie Rucker. Pub. Donald Lessne. Adv. contact Berbara Newman. Circ: 65,000.

DIET & NUTRITION SOURCEBOOK. see *NUTRITION AND DIETETICS*

613.7 610 ITA
DIMENSIONE SALUTE. Text in Italian. m. ITL 35,000.
Published by: Valentini Editore s.r.l., Via Fabio Filzi, 19, Milan, MI 20124, Italy. TEL 02-6696471. Ed. Aldo Quinto Lazzari.

P

613.7 AUS ISSN 1039-3145
DIRECTION; a journal on the Alexander Technique. Text in English. 1984. irreg. AUD 35 in Australia & New Zealand; GBP 22 in Europe; USD 39 elsewhere (effective 2002). adv. back issues avail. **Document type:** *Trade.* **Description:** For teachers of the Alexander Technique. Each issue explores an application of the work.
Published by: Chance Media Pty Ltd, PO Box 770, Spit Junction, NSW 2088, Australia. TEL 61-2-9960-7728, FAX 61-2-9960-7729, help@DirectionJournal.com; direction_journal@compuserve.com, info@directionjournal.com, http://www.directionjournal.com. Ed., Pub. Jeremy Chance. Adv. contact Nick Chance. **Dist. in UK & Europe by:** The Old Schoolhouse, Ide Hill Sevenoaks, Kent TN14 6JT, United Kingdom. TEL 44-1732-750062, 800-344-4224, FAX 44-1732-75-0662, uk@directionjournal.com.

613.714 ESP ISSN 0212-2308
DOJO. Text in Spanish. 1976. m. ESP 3,500; ESP 350 newsstand/cover (effective 1999). bibl, illus. back issues avail. *Refereed.* **Document type:** *Consumer.* **Description:** Covers martial arts: training, philosophy, nutrition, and masters.
Formerly (until 1981): Budo (0212-2294)
Published by: Ediciones A.M. S.L., Ferraz, 11, Madrid 28008, Spain. TEL 34-91-5401880, FAX 34-91-5415055, edijardin@arrakis.es. Pub., R&P Mariano Alonso. adv.: color page ESP 160,000. Circ: 90,000.

362.1 GBR ISSN 1368-891X
DR. VERNON COLEMAN'S HEALTH LETTER. Text in English. 1996. m. GBP 44.95 domestic; GBP 49.95, USD 79.95 foreign (effective 2000 - 2001). bk.rev. back issues avail. **Document type:** *Newsletter.* **Description:** Covers a wide range of medical, psychological, and social welfare issues.
Related titles: E-mail ed.
Address: Publishing House, Trinity Pl, Barnstaple, Devon EX32 9HJ, United Kingdom. TEL 44-1271-328892, FAX 44-1271-328768, mail@vernoncoleman.com, http://www.vernoncoleman.com. Ed. Dr. Vernon Coleman. Pub., R&P Sue Ward. Circ: 2,500 (paid).

613.7 USA
EHEALTH. Text in English. q. **Document type:** *Newsletter, Consumer.* **Description:** Contains articles and features on health and wellness.
Related titles: ♦ Online - full content ed.: eHealth.com.
Published by: McMurry Publishing, 1010 E Missouri Ave, Phoenix, AZ 85014-2601. TEL 602-395-5850, 888-626-8779, FAX 602-395-5853, info@mcmurry.com, http://www.mcmurry.com.

613.7 USA
EHEALTH.COM. Text in English. q. **Document type:** *Consumer.*
Media: Online - full content. **Related titles:** ♦ Print ed.: eHealth.
Published by: McMurry Publishing, 1010 E Missouri Ave, Phoenix, AZ 85014-2601. TEL 602-395-5850, 888-626-8779, FAX 602-395-5853, info@mcmurry.com, http://www.ehealth.com, http://www.mcmurry.com.

▼ **EMPLOYER HEALTH REGISTER.** see *OCCUPATIONAL HEALTH AND SAFETY*

368.382 BEL ISSN 0013-6964
EN MARCHE; journal bimensuel d'information pour les beneficiaires des soins de sante. Text in French. 1948. s-m. BEF 600. adv. bk.rev. charts, illus, stat. **Description:** Discusses various aspects of health and relevant fields, such as insurance.
Published by: Alliance Nationale des Mutualites Chretiennes, Rue de la Loi 121, Brussels 1040, Belgium. TEL 32-2-2374627, FAX 32-2-2373300. Ed. Christian van Rompeal. Circ: 460,000.

▼ **ENERGY FOR WOMEN**; how to energize your life. see *WOMEN'S HEALTH*

ENVIRONMENTAL HEALTH MONTHLY. see *ENVIRONMENTAL STUDIES*

DIE ERSATZKASSE. see *SOCIAL SERVICES AND WELFARE*

613.7 MNG
ERUUL MEND/HEALTH. Text in Mongol. 1959. q. MNT 160.
Published by: Ministry of Health, Ulan Bator, Mongolia. TEL 976-1-321307, FAX 976-1-321278, TELEX 247 MINHE MH. Ed. T Ochirkhuu. Circ: 25,000.

ESPRIT LIBRE. see *PSYCHOLOGY*

613.7 IND
EXECUTIVE HEALTH AND PHYSICAL FITNESS REPORT. Text in English. w. INR 715, USD 85 (effective 1999). **Document type:** *Newsletter.* **Description:** Reports on health and physical fitness.
Published by: International Press Cutting Service, PO Box 121, Allahabad, Uttar Pradesh 211 001, India. TEL 91-532-622392.

614 USA
EXECUTIVE HEALTH'S GOOD HEALTH REPORT. Text in English. 1963. m. (plus 1 bonus issue). USD 34; USD 40 in Canada & Mexico; USD 58 elsewhere. adv. bk.rev. index. back issues avail.; reprint service avail. from PQC. **Document type:** *Newsletter.* **Description:** Disseminates information on health issues, along with regular features, including nutrition and exercise.
Former titles (until June 1991): Executive Health Report (0882-2131); Executive Health
Related titles: Microfiche ed.: (from PQC); Microfilm ed.: (from PQC); Online - full text ed.: (from Gale Group, Factiva).
Indexed: Consum.Ind., Hlth.Ind., Sportsearch.
—CISTI.
Published by: Executive Health, 383 Route 46 W, Fairfield, NJ 07004-2402. TEL 201-227-5599. Ed. Deborah Hauss. Pub. Daniel Glassman. Adv. contact Gene L Goldborg. Circ: 15,000.

EXERCISE & HEALTH; the complete fitness guide for men. see *MEN'S HEALTH*

613.7 USA ISSN 0882-4657
EXERCISE FOR MEN ONLY. Text in English. 1985. bi-m. USD 35.15; USD 40.95 foreign; USD 4.95 newsstand/cover foreign; GBP 2.75 newsstand/cover in United Kingdom (effective 2001). bk.rev. illus. reprints avail. **Document type:** *Consumer.*
Published by: Chelo Publishing Inc., Empire State Bldg, 50 Fifth Ave, New York, NY 10118. TEL 212-947-4322, FAX 212-563-4774. Ed., Pub., R&P Cheh N Low. Adv. contact Robert B Rose. **UK dist. addr.:** Seymour, 86 Newman St, London W1P 3EX, United Kingdom. TEL 44-20-7396-8000, FAX 44-20-7396-8002.

613.7 USA ISSN 0748-3155
QP301
EXERCISE PHYSIOLOGY: CURRENT SELECTED RESEARCH. Text in English. 1985. a. USD 45. index. back issues avail. **Description:** Research articles on various topics of exercise science and sports medicine.
—CISTI, GNLM.
Published by: A M S Press, Inc., 56 E 13th St, New York, NY 10003. TEL 212-777-4700, FAX 212-995-5413. Eds. Charles O Dotson, James H Humphrey.

EXERCISE STANDARDS AND MALPRACTICE REPORTER. see *LAW*

613.7 USA ISSN 0895-2906
EXTENDED CARE PRODUCT NEWS. Text in English. 1987. bi-m. free. adv. **Document type:** *Magazine, Trade.*
Published by: H M P Communications, LLC, 950 W Valley Rd, Ste 2800, Wayne, PA 19087. TEL 610-688-8220, FAX 610-688-8050, pnorris@voicenet.com, http://www.extendedcarenews.com. Ed., R&P Elizabeth Klumpp. Pub. Peter Norris. Adv. contact Tom Gillespie. B&W page USD 4,365, color page USD 5,665. Circ: 50,011.

▼ **F H M BIONIC**; we can rebuild you. (For Him Magazine) see *MEN'S HEALTH*

613.7 USA ISSN 0899-9562
FAMILY PRACTICE ALERT. Text in English. 1988-1990; resumed 1997. m. USD 189; USD 219 foreign (effective 1998). **Document type:** *Newsletter.*
Related titles: Audio cassette/tape ed.; Online - full text ed.: (from Northern Light Technology, Inc.).
Published by: American Health Consultants (Subsidiary of: Medical Economics Co., Inc.), 3525 Piedmont Rd, N E, 6 Piedmont Center, Ste 400, Atlanta, GA 30305. TEL 404-262-5476, custserv@ahcpub.com, http://www.ahcpub.com.

FIBROUS MATERIALS IN THE ENVIRONMENT. see *ENVIRONMENTAL STUDIES—Toxicology And Environmental Safety*

FIRST YEAR OF LIFE; a guide to your baby's growth and development month by month. see *CHILDREN AND YOUTH—About*

613.7 ITA ISSN 1125-6737
FIT FOR FUN. Text in Italian. 1997. m. ITL 4,000 newsstand/cover. adv. illus. **Document type:** *Consumer.* **Description:** Offers young, active, sports and fitness-minded readers articles and information on ways to keep fit as part of a fun lifestyle.
Published by: R C S Periodici S.p.A. (Subsidiary of: R C S, Rizzoli - Corriere della Sera), Via Angelo Rizzoli, 2, Milan, MI 20132, Italy. TEL 39-02-2584-3647, FAX 39-02-2584-3903, fitforfun.pub@agora.stm.it, info@periodici.rcs.it, http://www.rcs.it/inforcs/uk/strutt/periodic/testate/fit/scheda.htm, http://www.rcs.it/periodici. Ed. Paolo Bonnani. Adv. contact Flavio Biondi. Circ: 174,435 (paid). **Dist. in UK by:** Seymour, 86 Newman St, London W1P 3EX, United Kingdom. TEL 44-20-7396-8000, FAX 44-207-396-8002.

FIT PREGNANCY. see *MEDICAL SCIENCES—Obstetrics And Gynecology*

▼ **FIT PREGNANCY EN ESPANOL.** see *MEDICAL SCIENCES—Obstetrics And Gynecology*

613.7 DEU
FIT UND FUENFZIG. Text in German. 6/yr. adv. **Document type:** *Magazine, Consumer.* **Description:** Provides health and fitness tips and advice for those over 50 years of age.
Published by: Marken-Verlag GmbH, Hugo-Junkers-Str 20, Cologne 50739, Germany. TEL 49-221-957427-0, FAX 49-221-95742777, marken-info@markenverlag.de, http://www.markenverlag.de. adv.: B&W page DEM 4,190, color page DEM 6,700. Circ: 98,000 (paid and controlled).

613.082 USA ISSN 1060-9237
GV482
FITNESS; mind - body - spirit for women. Text in English. 1983. m. (10/yr.). USD 19.98; USD 2.99 newsstand/cover domestic; GBP 2.25 newsstand/cover in United Kingdom; CND 3.95 newsstand/cover in Canada (effective 2000). adv. illus. reprints avail. **Document type:** *Consumer.* **Description:** Covers beauty and fashion, health, fitness and wellness for women.
Formerly (until 1992): Family Circle's Fitness Now
Published by: Gruner + Jahr U.S.A. Publishing (Subsidiary of: Gruner und Jahr AG & Co.), 375 Lexington Ave, New York, NY 10017-5514. TEL 212-499-2000, FAX 212-499-1586. Ed. Emily Listfield. Pub. Diane Newman. adv.: B&W page USD 51,092, color page USD 65,254; trim 10.5 x 7.94. Circ: 1,050,000 (paid). **Dist. in UK by:** Seymour, 86 Newman St, London W1P 3EX, United Kingdom. TEL 44-20-7396-8000, FAX 44-207-396-8002.

613.7 790.1 ITA ISSN 1121-2586
FITNESS. Text in Italian. m. ITL 54,000; ITL 7,000, EUR 3.62 newsstand/cover (effective 1999). **Document type:** *Consumer.* **Description:** Contains general-interest articles on health and fitness, sports such as hang gliding, bicycling, and surfing, as well as exercise techniques.
Published by: Gruppo Editoriale Futura, Via XXV Aprile, 39, Bresso, MI 20091, Italy. TEL 39-02-66526257, FAX 39-02-66526243, fitness@futura-ge.com. Ed. Paolo Reina. **Subscr. to:** Gruppo Editoriale Futura S.p.A., Casella Postale 88, Bresso, MI 20091, Italy. TEL 39-02-66526213, FAX 39-02-66526300. **Dist. by:** SO. DI. P., Via Bettola 18, Cinisello Balsamo, MI 20092, Italy. TEL 39-02-660301.

613.7 CAN ISSN 0820-6163
FITNESS BULLETIN. Text in English. 1978. m. USD 30 (effective 1995 & 1996). bk.rev. back issues avail. **Document type:** *Newsletter.* **Description:** Contains health and fitness news, and instructive articles for subscribers and institute members.
Formerly (until 1982): Fitness Institute Bulletin (0826-4341)
Published by: Fitness Institute, 2235 Sheppard Ave., E, Atria 11, PO Box 63, Willowdale, ON M2J 5B5, Canada. Ed. David Steen. Circ: 4,000.

613.7 658 USA ISSN 0882-0481
FITNESS MANAGEMENT. Text in English. m. USD 24 (effective 1999). adv. back issues avail. **Document type:** *Trade.* **Description:** Presents scientific and professional health fitness and management information in non-technical language to owners, managers and pro shop buyers of commerical community and corporate physical fitness centers.
Indexed: Sportsearch (1991-).
—BLDSC (3948.229200), ingenta.
Published by: Leisure Publications, Inc., 4160 Wilshire Blvd, Los Angeles, CA 90010. TEL 323-964-4800, FAX 323-964-4837, fitmgt@earthlink.net, http://www.fitnessworld.com. Ed. Ronale Tucker. Pubs. David Levy, Ed Pitts. R&P Ed Pitts. Adv. contact David Levy. B&W page USD 3,985, color page USD 4,960. Circ: 25,000.

613.7 USA
FITNESS NEWS. Text in English. fortn. free per issue. **Document type:** *Newsletter.*
Media: Online - full text.
Published by: E G W Publishing Co., 1041 Shary Circle, Concord, CA 94518. TEL 925-671-9852, FAX 510-671-0692, hstevens@egw.com, http://www.naturalland.com/efv/efnc.htm.

613.7 RUS
FIZICHESKAYA KUL'TURA: OBRAZOVANIE, TRENIROVKA, VOSPITANIE. Text in Russian. q. USD 75 in United States. **Document type:** *Abstract/Index.*
Published by: Rossiiskia Akademiya Fizicheskoi Kul'tury, Sirenevyi bulv 4, Moscow 105122, Russian Federation. TEL 7-095-1663734, FAX 7-095-1663774. Ed. V V Kuzin. **US dist. addr.:** East View Publications, 3020 Harbor Ln N, Minneapolis, MN 55447. TEL 612-550-0961.

613.7 RUS ISSN 0130-5581
FIZICHESKAYA KUL'TURA V SHKOLE. Text in Russian. bi-m. USD 49 foreign (effective 2000). **Document type:** *Academic/Scholarly.*
—East View.
Published by: Izdatel'stvo Shkola Press, Rustaveli ul 10-3, Moscow 127254, Russian Federation. TEL 7-095-2198380, FAX 7-095-2195289. Ed. A V Komarov. **US dist. addr.:** East View Publications, 3020 Harbor Ln N, Minneapolis, MN 55447. TEL 612-550-0961.

613.7 RUS
FIZICHESKOE OBRAZOVANIE V VUZAKH. Text in Russian. q. USD 149 in United States. **Document type:** *Academic/Scholarly.*
Indexed: Ref.Zh.
Published by: Moskovskoe Fizicheskoe Obshchestvo, Leninskii pr-t 53, Moscow 117924, Russian Federation. TEL 7-095-1326651, FAX 7-095-1357995. Ed. O N Krokhin. **US dist. addr.:** East View Publications, 3020 Harbor Ln N, Minneapolis, MN 55447. TEL 612-550-0961.

613 BGR ISSN 0861-6485
CODEN: KUFIAT
FIZIKALNA, KURORTNA I REKHABILITATSIONNA MEDITSINA/JOURNAL OF PHYSICAL, HEALTH RESORT AND REHABILITATION MEDICINE. Text in Bulgarian; Summaries in English, Russian. q. BGL 10; USD 44 foreign (effective 2002). **Document type:** *Journal.*
Formerly (until 1992): Kurortologija i Fizioterapija (0368-7066)
Indexed: Abstr.Bulg.Sci.Med.Lit., Excerp.Med. (until 1993, 1996-), INIS Atomind.
—CASDDS, CISTI, EMDOCS.
Published by: (Bulgaria. Ministerstvo na Narodnoto Zdrave), Izdatelstvo Meditsina i Fizkultura, 11 Pl Slaveikov, Sofia 1080, Bulgaria. Ed. St Bankov. Circ: 850. **Distr. by:** Hemus, 6 Rouski blvd, Sofia 1000, Bulgaria. **Co-sponsor:** Nauchno Druzhestvo po Kurortologija, Fizioterapija i Rehabilitacija.

613.7 GBR ISSN 0955-1212
FLEX. Text in English. 1986. m. USD 29.97 domestic; USD 46.97 foreign; USD 4.99 newsstand/cover (effective 2001). illus. **Document type:** *Magazine, Consumer.*
Related titles: Online - full text ed.: (from America Online, Inc.).
Published by: Weider Publishing, 10 Windsor Ct, Clarence Dr, Harrogate, N Yorks HG1 2PE, United Kingdom. TEL 44-1423-504516, FAX 44-1423-523294, ukpub@weider.demon.co.uk, http://www.flexonline.com. **Dist. by:** Comag, Tavistock Works, Tavistock Rd, W Drayton, Middx UB7 7QX, United Kingdom. TEL 44-1895-433600, FAX 44-189-543-3606.

613.7 USA
▼ **FLEX: MR. OLYMPIA PREVIEW.** Text in English. 2001 (Oct.). a. USD 5.99 newsstand/cover; USD 6.99 newsstand/cover in Canada (effective 2001). **Document type:** *Magazine, Consumer.* **Description:** Covers all aspects of the Mr. Olympia bodybuilding competition.
Published by: Weider Publications, 21100 Erwin St, Woodland Hills, CA 91367. TEL 818-884-6800, 800-998-0731, FAX 818-716-5626.

FOCUS ON FEDERAL EMPLOYEE HEALTH AND ASSISTANCE PROGRAMS. see *OCCUPATIONAL HEALTH AND SAFETY*

FODOR'S HEALTHY ESCAPES. see *TRAVEL AND TOURISM*

FRONTIERS OF HEALTH SERVICES MANAGEMENT. see *HEALTH FACILITIES AND ADMINISTRATION*

613.7 CHE ISSN 1422-0970
FUER UNS VITA SANA; Magazin fuer Dialog und Gesundheit. Text in German. 1997. 10/yr. CHF 49.50; CHF 65 in Europe; CHF 82 elsewhere; CHF 5.80 newsstand/cover (effective 2000). adv. **Document type:** *Magazine, Consumer.* **Description:** Contains information, tips and products on healthy lifestyles.
Formed by the merger of (1975-1997): Vita Sana Magazin (1421-4334); (1978-1997): Fuer Uns (1422-111X)
Published by: Vita Sana Verlag AG, Postfach 468, Breganzona 6932, Switzerland. TEL 41-91-9681110, FAX 41-91-9667183, fu-vsm@alicom.ch. Adv. contact Markus Mettler. Circ: 102,500 (controlled).

613.7 POL ISSN 1232-1907
GAZETA O ZDROWIU I URODZIE. Text in Polish. 1993. irreg.
Related titles: ♦ Supplement to: Gazeta Wyborcza. ISSN 0860-908X.
Published by: Agora S.A., Ul Czerska 8-10, Warsaw 00732, Poland. TEL 48-22-6994301, FAX 48-22-6994603, http://www.gazeta.pl.

613 FRA ISSN 0995-6301
GAZETTE OFFICIELLE DU THERMALISME✱ . Text in French. 1988. bi-m. FRF 250.
Published by: Office des Nouvelles Internationales, Agence de Presse, 16 rue de l'Estrapade, Paris 75005, France. TEL 59-30-03-28. Ed. Nicole Belval. **Co-sponsor:** Federation Thermale et Climatique Francaise.

GENEESKUNDE EN SPORT. see *MEDICAL SCIENCES—Sports Medicine*

GESICHERTES LEBEN. see *SOCIAL SERVICES AND WELFARE*

613 DEU ISSN 0016-9234
GESUND LEBEN. Text in German. 1952. 12/yr. DEM 34.30; DEM 53.40 foreign (effective 2000). adv. charts, illus. **Document type:** *Bulletin.*
—CCC.
Published by: Verlag M. und H. Schaper GmbH, Borsigstr 5, Alfeld 31061, Germany. TEL 49-5181-8009-0, FAX 49-5181-8009-33, info@schaper-verlag.de, http://www.schaper-verlag.de. Ed. A Peter. Circ: 60,000.

613 DEU ISSN 0016-9250
GESUNDES LEBEN✱ ; Medizinalpolitische Rundschau, Zeitschrift fuer natuerliche Lebensordnung. Text in German. 1924. m. adv. bk.rev. tr.lit.
Indexed: AMED.
—BLDSC (4163.900000), GNLM.
Published by: Praxiswissen und Fachfortbildungs Gesellschaft mbH, Kraillingerstr 12, Stockdorf 82131, Germany. Circ: 5,000.

613 DEU ISSN 0016-9269
GESUNDHEIT (BADEN-BADEN). Text in German. 1949. bi-m. DEM 6 (effective 1999). adv. bk.rev. illus. **Document type:** *Magazine, Consumer.*
Former titles: Gesundheit in Betrieb und Familie; Gesundheit
Related titles: Microform ed.: (from PQC).
Published by: Agis Verlag GmbH, Ooser Luisenstr 23, Baden-Baden 76532, Germany. TEL 49-7221-95750, FAX 49-7221-66810, info@agis-verlag.de, http://www.agis-verlag.de. Ed. Karin Grochowiak. Adv. contact Wolfgang Jacob. Circ: 2,700,000.

613.7 610 DEU
GESUNDHEIT (BAIERBRUNN). Text in German. m. adv. **Document type:** *Consumer.*
Formerly: Gesundheit in Wort und Bild
Published by: Wort und Bild Verlag Konradshoehe GmbH, Konradshoehe, Baierbrunn 82065, Germany. TEL 49-89-74433-0, FAX 49-89-74433150, http://www.wortundbild.de. Adv. contact Wolfgang Smeilus.

GESUNDHEIT IN DER EINEN WELT; Nachrichten aus der Aerzlichen Mission. see *RELIGIONS AND THEOLOGY*

613.7 CHE ISSN 1423-5536
GESUNDHEIT-SPRECHSTUNDE. Text in German. 1998. fortn. adv. **Document type:** *Magazine, Consumer.* **Description:** Presents articles and information on leading and maintaining a healthy and active lifestyle.
Published by: Ringier AG, Dufourstr 47, Zuerich 8008, Switzerland. TEL 41-1-2596483, FAX 41-1-2596996, ges@ringier.ch, info@ringier.ch, http://www.gesundheit-sprechstunde.ch, http://www.ringier.ch. Ed. Emil Mahnig. adv.: B&W page CHF 9,020, color page CHF 11,000. Circ: 68,899 (paid).

614 RUS ISSN 0016-9900
CODEN: GISAAA
GIGIENA I SANITARIYA/HYGIENE AND SANITATION. Text in Russian; Summaries in English. 1922. bi-m. USD 185 foreign (effective 2000). adv. bk.rev., Website rev. bibl. index. reprints avail. **Document type:** *Journal, Academic/Scholarly.* **Description:** Publishes papers on all the branches of hygienic science and sanitary practice.
Indexed: Abstr.Hyg., Anal.Abstr., Biol.Abstr., C.I.S. Abstr., Chem.Abstr., Chem.Indus.Notes, Chem.Titles, Dairy Sci.Abstr., Dent.Ind., Field Crop Abstr., Food Sci.& Tech.Abstr., INIS Atomind., Ind.Med. (1936-), Ind.Vet., Int.Aerosp.Abstr., Irr.& Drain.Abstr., Nutr.Abstr., Packag.Sci.Tech., Pig News & Info., Plant Grow.Reg.Abstr., Pollut.Abstr., Potato Abstr., Poult.Abstr., Protozool.Abstr., Ref.Zh., Rev.Appl.Entomol., Soils & Fert., Soyabean Abstr., Trop.Dis.Bull., Vet.Bull., W.R.C.Inf., Weed Abstr., World Bibl.Soc.Sec.
—BLDSC (0048.000000), CASDDS, CISTI, East View, GNLM, Infotrieve, Linda Hall. **CCC.**
Published by: Izdatel'stvo Meditsina, Petroverigskii per 6-8, Moscow 101000, Russian Federation. TEL 7-095-9248785, 7-095-928-86-48, FAX 7-095-9211355, 7-095-9286003, http://www.medit.ru. Ed. G I Rumyantsev. Pub. A M Stochik. R&P V Sinitsina. Adv. contact O A Fadeeva TEL 7-095-923-51-40. Circ: 2,500. **Dist. by:** Mezhdunarodnaya Kniga, B Yakimanka 39, Moscow 117049, Russian Federation. TEL 7-095-2384967, FAX 7-095-2384634; **US dist. addr.:** East View Publications, 3020 Harbor Ln N, Minneapolis, MN 55447. TEL 612-550-0961.

GLOBAL HEALTH DIRECTORY. see *MEDICAL SCIENCES*

614.8 GBR ISSN 1365-7070
GOOD HEALTH; look good - feel great - be healthy. Text in English. 1997. bi-m. GBP 2.30 newsstand/cover (effective 2001). adv. **Document type:** *Magazine, Consumer.* **Description:** Covers natural therapies, healthy eating, nutritional information, and exercise for the whole family.

P

Published by: Attic Futura Ltd., 16-18 Berners St, London W1P 3DD, United Kingdom. TEL 44-20-7664-6400, FAX 44-20-7323-1854, goodhealth@atticfutura.co.uk, viviencotterill@atticfutura.co.uk, http://www.good-health.co.uk, http://www.atticfutura.co.uk. Ed. Christina Neal. Pub. Bridget Marrison. Adv. contact Caroline Brookes. B&W page GBP 2,100, color page USD 3,200; trim 213 x 300. Circ: 50,000 (paid). **Dist. by:** Comag, Tavistock Works, Tavistock Rd, W Drayton, Middx UB7 7QX, United Kingdom. TEL 44-1895-444055, FAX 44-1895-433602.

613.7 USA
GOOD HEALTH MAGAZINE. Text in English. q. back issues avail. **Document type:** *Magazine, Consumer.* **Description:** Covers the latest in health issues for central Texas.
Related titles: Online - full text ed.: Good Health Magazine.
Published by: Seton Healthcare Network, 1201 W 38th St, Austin, TX 78705. TEL 512-324-1980, FAX 512-324-1972, ggranberry@seton.org, http://www.goodhealth.com, http://www.seton.net.

613.7 AUS
GOOD MEDICINE. Text in English. m. AUD 52; AUD 5.40 newsstand/cover (effective 2001). adv. **Document type:** *Magazine, Consumer.* **Description:** Covers the latest news and views in traditional/alternative medicine, emotional health, beauty, nutrition, weight management, body image and fitness.
Published by: Good Medicine Magazine, 54 Park St, Sydney, NSW 2000, Australia. TEL 61-02-92828426, http://lifestyle.ninemsn.com.au/goodmedicine/. Ed. Jennifer Gilbert.

GREAT BODY. see *NUTRITION AND DIETETICS*

613.25 USA
GREG LANDRY'S FITNESS NEWSLETTER. Text in English. w. free per issue. **Document type:** *Newsletter, Consumer.* **Description:** Provides information and motivation for individuals interested in a healthy, permanent approach to weight loss and fitness.
Formerly: All about Weight Loss, Health, and Fitness
Media: E-mail.
Published by: Greg Landry, Ed. & Pub., 2805 Newkirk Ave, Wilmington, NC 28412. greg@landry.com, http://www.landry.com.

613.7 CHN
GUOWAI YIXUE (WEISHENGXUE FENCE)/FOREIGN MEDICAL SCIENCES (HYGIENICS). Text in Chinese. bi-m. USD 17.40; USD 2.90 newsstand/cover (effective 2001). **Document type:** *Academic/Scholarly.*
Published by: China International Book Trading Corp/Zhongguo Guoji Tushu Maoyi Zonggongsi cibtc@mail.cibtc.com.cn, http://www.cibtc.com.cn. **Dist. by:** 35, Chegongzhuang Xilu, Haidian District, Beijing 100044, China.

613.7 305.31 USA
▼ **GYM**; for the physical man. Text in English. 1999. bi-m. USD 19.97; USD 4.95 newsstand/cover; GBP 2.95 newsstand/cover in United Kingdom. adv. illus. **Document type:** *Consumer.* **Description:** Covers topics on fitness for men.
Published by: Celebrity Style Inc., 230 W 41st St, Ste 1500, New York, NY 10036. TEL 212-252-0698, FAX 212-686-9098, gymmagmail@aol.com.

614 USA
H E F NEWS. Text in English. 1977. q. USD 15. **Document type:** *Newsletter.* **Description:** Provides information and perspectives on health behavior and lifestyle, written in layperson language.
Published by: Health Education Foundation, Inc., 2600 Virginia Ave, N W, Ste 502, Washington, DC 20037. TEL 202-338-3501. Ed. Marion Donovan Chafetz. Circ: 900.

613.7 USA
H E - XTRA. Text in English. 5/yr. USD 100 to members (effective 1998). adv. **Document type:** *Newsletter.* **Description:** Seeks to advance health by encouraging, supporting, and assisting health professionals concerned with health promotion through education and other systematic strategies.
Published by: American Association for Health Education, 1900 Association Dr, Reston, VA 20191-1599. TEL 703-476-3437, FAX 703-476-6638, aahe@aahperd.org. Ed., R&P, Adv. contact Linda M Moore.

HAELSOKURIREN; tidningen om haelsa och egenvaard. see *PHARMACY AND PHARMACOLOGY*

613.7 HTI
HAITI SANTE. Text in French. 1980. q. USD 7.
Published by: Centre d'Hygiene Familiale, 10, 1ere Impasse Lavand, BP 430, Port-au-Prince, Haiti. Ed. Ary Bordes. Circ: 4,000.

HANDBOOK OF PSYCHOLOGY AND HEALTH SERIES. see *PSYCHOLOGY*

051 USA ISSN 1052-1577
RC81.A1 CODEN: HHLEET
HARVARD HEALTH LETTER; a publication for the general readership, designed to provide accurate and timely health information. Text in English. 1975. m. USD 28 domestic; USD 40 in Canada; USD 47 elsewhere (effective 2000). illus. index. back issues avail.; reprints avail. *Refereed.* **Document type:** *Newsletter, Consumer, Academic/Scholarly, Trade.* **Description:** Interprets timely health information for the general reader in layman's terms.
Formerly: Harvard Medical School Health Letter (0161-7486)
Related titles: Online - full text ed.: (from Gale Group, Northern Light Technology, Inc., Factiva).
Indexed: Biol.Dig., CHNI, CINAHL, Consum.Ind. (1989-), Hlth.Ind., Mag.Ind., R.G., Ref.Zh., Sportsearch, WMB. —BLDSC (4267.127000), CASDDS, GNLM.
Published by: (Harvard Medical School), Harvard Health Publications Group (Subsidiary of: Harvard Medical School), 164 Longwood Ave, Boston, MA 02115. TEL 617-432-1485, FAX 617-432-1506, jrudin@warren.med.edu, hhp@hms.harvard.edu, http://www.health.harvard.edu/newsletters/hltext.html. Eds. Peter Wehrein, Dr. Thomas H Lee. Circ: 300,000 (paid). **Subscr. to:** PO Box 420099, Palm Coasat, FL 32142-0099. TEL 800-829-9045.

613 IND ISSN 0017-8861
HEALTH; devoted to healthful living. Text in English. 1923. m. INR 60; INR 480 foreign (effective 1999). reprint service avail. from PQC. **Document type:** *Trade.*
Published by: Professional Publications Ltd., Satya Sai Nagar, P O Box 2, Madurai, Tamil Nadu 625 003, India. TEL 0452-673701, FAX 0452-674602. Pub. R Lakshmipathy. adv.: B&W page INR 2,000, color page INR 3,000; trim 125 x 200. Circ: 11,872.

613.7 344 USA ISSN 0897-3598
KF3821.A15
HEALTH ADVOCATE. Text in English. 1971. 4/yr. USD 85 (effective 2000). bk.rev. **Document type:** *Newsletter.* **Description:** Covers legal aspects of current health care issues, including Medicaid, managed care, access to health care, and more.
Former titles (until 1982): N H E L P Health Advocate (0272-7102); (until 1980): Health Law Newsletter (0160-7227)
Indexed: Med.Care Rev.
Published by: National Health Law Program, 2639 S La Cienega Blvd, Los Angeles, CA 90034. TEL 310-204-6010, FAX 310-204-0891, nhelp@healthlaw.org, http://www.healthlaw.org. Ed. Laurence Lavin. R&P, Adv. contact Brendan McTaggart TEL 202-289-7661. Circ: 1,700.

613.7 GBR ISSN 0957-5928
HEALTH AND FITNESS; all you need for life!. Text in English. 1984. m. GBP 27.60 domestic; GBP 37.70 in Europe; GBP 65 elsewhere; GBP 2.30 newsstand/cover (effective 1999). adv. illus. back issues avail. **Document type:** *Consumer.* **Description:** Informs readers of the many ways in which to maintain one's health and fitness through exercise, good nutrition, and a healthy lifestyle.
Formerly (until 1989): Fitness
—BLDSC (4274.811500).
Published by: Nexus Media Ltd., Nexus House, Azalea Dr, Swanley, Kent BR8 8HU, United Kingdom. TEL 44-1322-660070, FAX 44-1322-667633, http://www.fitpro.com. Ed. Mary Comber. Adv. contact Vanessa Spiers. Circ: 49,000. **Subscr. to:** Tower House, Lathkill St, Tower House, Sovereign Park, Market Harborough, Leics LE16 9EF, United Kingdom. TEL 44-1858-435344, FAX 44-1858-434958. **Dist. by:** Comag, Tavistock Works, Tavistock Rd, W Drayton, Middx UB7 7QX, United Kingdom. TEL 44-1895-444055, FAX 44-1895-433602.

613.7 USA ISSN 1048-8405
HEALTH & FITNESS MAGAZINE FOR HEALTHY, SOUND LIVING. Short title: H F. Text in English. 1989. q. USD 5.99 newsstand/cover (effective 2000). adv. **Document type:** *Consumer.* **Description:** Probes current health and fitness issues for all ages.
Incorporates: Health Series
Published by: Lifetime Periodicals, Inc., 2131 Hollywood Blvd, Hollywood, FL 33020. TEL 954-925-5242, FAX 954-925-5244, FELLPUB@aol.com, http://www.lifetimebooks.com. Ed. Callie Ruckner. Pub. Donald Lessne. Adv. contact Barbara Newman. Circ: 30,000.

613 GBR ISSN 0265-2021
HEALTH AND HEALING. Text in English. 1982. 3/yr. GBP 5 (effective 2000). bk.rev. **Document type:** *Newsletter.* **Description:** To serve Christians who care and heal, to share ideas and information, and to explore the churches' theological and spiritual role in health and healing.
Published by: Churches' Council for Health and Healing, St Luke's Hospital, 12 Fitzroy Square, London W1P 5HQ, United Kingdom. TEL 44-171-486-9644. Ed. Stephens Maisons. Circ: 3,000.

613 USA
HEALTH & HEALING. Text in English. 1991. m. USD 39.95 (effective 1992). Supplement avail. **Document type:** *Newsletter.*
Published by: Phillips Publishing, Inc., Consumer Publishing, 7811 Montrose Rd, Potomac, MD 20854. TEL 800-777-5005, FAX 301-424-7034. Ed. Dr. Julian Whitaker.

613.7 ZAF
HEALTH & HYGIENE. Text in English. ZAR 85.50 (effective 2000). adv. **Document type:** *Trade.*
Published by: Malnor (Pty) Ltd., Private Bag X20, Auckland Park, Johannesburg 2006, South Africa. TEL 27-11-7263081, FAX 27-11-7263017, malnor@iafrica.com. Ed. Cornelia Fick. R&P Ken Nortje. adv.: B&W page ZAR 4,445, color page ZAR 5,495; trim 210 x 297.

HEALTH AND PHYSICAL EDUCATION/HOKEN TAIIKU KYOSHITSU. see *EDUCATION*

613.7 USA
▼ **HEALTH CARE INTERNET RESOURCES.** Text in English. 1999. q. USD 295; includes CD-ROM. **Document type:** *Bulletin.*
Related titles: CD-ROM ed.; Online - full text ed.: USD 195.
Published by: Nova Science Publishers, Inc., 227 Main St, Ste 100, Huntington, NY 11743-6907. TEL 516-499-3103, FAX 516-499-3146, novascience@earthlink.net, http://nexusworld.com/nova.

362.1 USA
HEALTH CARE JOURNAL. Text in English. irreg. adv. back issues avail.
Related titles: Online - full text ed.
Published by: American City Business Journals, Inc. (Charlotte), 120 W Morehead St, Ste 400, Charlotte, NC 28202. TEL 800-486-3289, webmaster@amcity.com, http://www.amcity.com/journals/health_care.

HEALTH CARE ON THE INTERNET; a journal for medical professionals, consumers & librarians. see *COMPUTERS—Internet*

HEALTH CARE STRATEGIC MANAGEMENT; the newsletter for hospital strategists. see *HEALTH FACILITIES AND ADMINISTRATION*

HEALTH COUNTER NEWS. see *NUTRITION AND DIETETICS*

HEALTH DIET & NUTRITION. see *NUTRITION AND DIETETICS*

362.1 USA
▼ **HEALTH E-ZINE.** Text in English. 1999. w. free per issue. back issues avail. **Document type:** *Newsletter.* **Description:** Provides summaries of health related issues.
Media: Online - full text.
Published by: Alt Health, c/o Vitamin Discount Connection, 645 Kolter Dr, Ste 2, Indiana, PA 15701. TEL 724-349-6828, FAX 724-349-3711, bvdries@vitamindiscount.com, http://www.alt-health.com/signup.html. Ed. Bruce Dires.

613 GBR ISSN 0965-4283
RA440.3.G7
HEALTH EDUCATION. Text in English. 1996. bi-m. USD 1,289 in North America; EUR 1,429 in Europe; AUD 1,629 in Australasia; GBP 839 in the UK & rest of the world (effective 2002). adv. reprint service avail. from SCH,PSC. **Document type:** *Academic/Scholarly.*

Related titles: Online - full text ed.: (from EBSCO Publishing, O C L C Online Computer Library Center, Inc., RoweCom Information Quest, ingenta, Swets Blackwell).
Indexed: Emrld.Intell.
—BLDSC (4274.968700), Infotrieve. **CCC.**
Published by: Emerald, 60-62 Toller Ln, Bradford, W Yorks BD8 9BY, United Kingdom. TEL 44-1274-777700, FAX 44-1274-785200, info@emeraldinsight.com, http://www.emeraldinsight.com/he.htm, http://www.mcb.co.uk/, http://www.emeraldinsight.com/journals/. Ed. Dr. Katherine Weare TEL 44-23-8059-3707. Adv. contact Jeremy Wright.

HEALTH EDUCATION JOURNAL. see *PUBLIC HEALTH AND SAFETY*

HEALTH EFFECTS OF OZONE AND NITROGEN OXIDES IN AN INTEGRATED ASSESSMENT OF AIR POLLUTION. see *ENVIRONMENTAL STUDIES—Pollution*

HEALTH LAW DIGEST. see *LAW*

HEALTH LAW JOURNAL. see *LAW*

HEALTH MASTER. see *PSYCHOLOGY*

613.7 USA
HEALTH MEASURES. Text in English. 12/yr. USD 50; USD 70 foreign (effective 1999).
Related titles: Online - full text ed.
Published by: Miller Freeman, Inc. (Subsidiary of: United Newspapers), 600 Harrison St, San Francisco, CA 94107. TEL 415-905-2200, FAX 415-905-2233, jpaine@mfi.com, http://www.healthmeasure.com/.

630 CAN ISSN 1188-9500
HEALTH NATURALLY. Text in English. 1992. 6/yr. CND 21; CND 30 in United States; CND 36 elsewhere. adv. bk.rev. **Document type:** *Consumer.* **Description:** Features natural health products, books, services and therapies. Stresses the positive aspects of natural alternatives.
Indexed: Can.Per.Ind. (Dec.1995-).
Published by: Health Naturally Publications Inc., 74 James St, Parry Sound, ON P2A 1T8, Canada. TEL 705-746-7839, FAX 705-746-7893. Ed. Lorrie Imbert. Pub. Bonnie Rowland. R&P Gloria Marshall. Adv. contact Jean Embury. B&W page CND 2,125, color page CND 2,500; trim 10.88 x 8.13. Circ: 40,000.

HEALTH NEWS. see *NUTRITION AND DIETETICS*

HEALTH PHYSICS; the radiation protection journal. see *MEDICAL SCIENCES*

613 USA ISSN 1059-938X
RA773
HEALTH (SAN FRANCISCO). Text in English. 1992. 9/yr. USD 19.97 domestic; USD 27.97 in Canada; USD 31.97 elsewhere; USD 2.99 newsstand/cover foreign (effective 2000). adv. bk.rev. charts, illus, stat. reprint service avail. from PQC. **Document type:** *Consumer.* **Description:** Features a wide range of articles on how to maintain good health, including nutrition and physical fitness.
Formed by the merger of (1990-1992): In Health (1047-0549); (1969-1991): Health (New York) (0279-3547); Which was formerly (1969-1981): Family Health (0014-7249); Which incorporated (1950-1976): Today's Health (0040-8514)
Related titles: Microform ed.: (from PQC); Online - full text ed.: (from ProQuest Information & Learning, Gale Group, Factiva).
Indexed: Acad.Ind., AgeLine, Biol.Abstr., Biol.Dig., CHNI, CINAHL, Can.Per.Ind., Consum.Ind. (1990-), Curr.Lit.Fam.Plan., Gen.Sci.Ind. (Jun.1992-), GeoRef, Hlth.Ind., Mag.Ind., PMR, Phys.Ed.Ind., R.G. (Jan.1991-), R.G.Abstr. (Jan.1983-Dec.1991, Feb.1992-), Sportsearch, TOM.
—CISTI, ingenta, Linda Hall.
Published by: Time Inc. Health (Subsidiary of: Time Warner, Inc.), 2 Embarcadero Center, Ste 600, San Francisco, CA 94111. TEL 415-248-2700, FAX 415-248-2779. Ed. Barbara Paulsen. Pub. Mary Morgan. adv.: B&W page USD 50,700, color page USD 59,900; trim 10.75 x 8. Circ: 1,084,535 (paid). **Subscr. to:** PO Box 56892, Boulder, CO 80322-6892.

HEALTH SCIENCE; living in harmony with nature. see *NUTRITION AND DIETETICS*

HEALTH, SOCIETY AND CULTURE. see *SOCIOLOGY*

613.7 GBR
HEALTH TODAY MAGAZINE. Text in English. 1993. bi-m. adv. **Document type:** *Consumer.*
Published by: Media Partners CPR, Northern Rock House, 20 Market Pl, Guisborough, Cleveland TS14 6HF, United Kingdom. TEL 44-1287-639111, FAX 44-1287-637201. Ed. Sarah Hovington. Adv. contact Kay Chapman. Circ: 120,000.

613 GBR
HEALTH WHICH?. Text in English. 1983. bi-m. bk.rev. cum.index. **Document type:** *Consumer.* **Description:** Independent food and health magazine for the lay person. Features and information on self-care and on major illnesses, health promotion and provisions in Britain; independent testing of health products and services, and information on nutrition.
Former titles (until 1995): Which? Way to Health (0957-1728); (until 1988): Self Health (0265-5497)
Related titles: Online - full text ed.
Indexed: Brit.Nur.Ind., Food Sci.& Tech.Abstr.
—BLDSC (4275.247512).
Published by: (Consumers' Association Ltd.), Which? Ltd., 2 Marylebone Rd, London NW1 4DF, United Kingdom. TEL 44-20-7830-6000, FAX 44-20-7830-7664, health@which.co.uk, http://www.which.net. Ed. Charlotte Gann. R&P Joanna McHale. Circ: 71,000 (paid). **Subscr. to:** Consumers' Association Ltd., PO Box 44, Hertford SG14 1SH, United Kingdom. TEL 44-1992-822803.

613.7 USA ISSN 0741-9368
HEALTHCARE MARKETING REPORT. Text in English. m.
Related titles: Online - full text ed.: (from Gale Group, Factiva).
Published by: H M R Publications Group, PO Box 76002, Atlanta, GA 30358-1002. TEL 404-457-6105, FAX 404-457-0049. Ed. Beverly Seitz. Circ: 1,900.

613.7 USA
HEALTHCARE NEW ORLEANS. Text in English. m. **Document type:** *Trade.* **Description:** Contains articles of interest to local healthcare professionals.
Published by: CityBusiness - New Orleans Publishing Group, 111 Veterans Blvd, Rm 1810, Metairie, LA 70005. TEL 504-834-9292, FAX 504-837-2258. Ed. Brian Ettinger. Circ: 25,000 (controlled).

613 USA
HEALTHCARE U S A*. Text in English. m. **Document type:** *Consumer.*
Published by: Sport Tech Labs, 2434 N Greenview Ave, Chicago, IL 60614-2013. TEL 312-929-7398, FAX 312-929-5733. adv.: B&W page USD 3,950, color page USD 4,950.

362.1 USA
▼ **HEALTHOLOGY.** Text in English. 1999. m. **Description:** Includes news that communicates health information between health care professionals and the public.
Media: Online - full text.
Published by: Healthology, LLC, 1333 Broadway, Ste 500, New York, NY 10018. TEL 212-431-5100, Info@healthology.com, http://healthology.com/. Ed. Steven Haimowitz.

HEALTHSMART MAGAZINE. see *GERONTOLOGY AND GERIATRICS*

613.7 USA ISSN 1051-8770
RC81.A1
HEALTHWISE HANDBOOK. Text in English. 1976. irreg.
Published by: Doubleday & Company, Inc., 501 Franklin Ave, Garden City, NY 11530.

HEALTHY & NATURAL JOURNAL. see *ALTERNATIVE MEDICINE*

HEALTHY EATING. see *NUTRITION AND DIETETICS*

HEALTHY KIDS. see *CHILDREN AND YOUTH—About*

613.7 NZL ISSN 1170-6058
HEALTHY OPTIONS. Text in English. 1984. m. NZD 42; NZD 4.95 newsstand/cover (effective 2001). bk.rev. tr.lit. 88 p./no. back issues avail. **Document type:** *Consumer.* **Description:** Provides information on New Zealand's natural health and environmental issues.
Published by: Healthy Options Ltd., 100 Grage Rd, PO Box 13209, Tauranga, New Zealand. editorial@healthyoptions.co.nz, http://www.healthyoptions.co.nz. Ed., Pub. Janice-Ann Priest. Adv. contact Alan Morton TEL 64-7-5700560 ext 201. Circ: 18,000. **Dist. by:** Gordon & Gotch. TEL 64-9-625-3000, FAX 64-9-625-3001.

613.7 USA
HEALTHY TIMES (NORTH BERGEN). Text in English. bi-m.
Published by: Vitamin Shoppe, 4700 Westside Ave, North Bergen, NJ 07047. TEL 800-223-1216, FAX 201-866-9513. Ed. Helen Howard.

613.7 USA ISSN 1092-1974
RA776.5
HEART & SOUL. Text in English. 1993. 10/yr. USD 16.97 domestic (effective 2000); USD 2.95 newsstand/cover; CND 3.50 newsstand/cover in Canada; GBP 2.25 newsstand/cover in United Kingdom. adv. bk.rev., music rev. illus. reprints avail. **Document type:** *Magazine, Consumer.* **Description:** Covers health, beauty and fitness for African-American women.
Formerly (until 199?): Rodale's Heart and Soul (1072-7345)
Related titles: Online - full text ed.: (from Northern Light Technology, Inc.).
Indexed: Gend.Watch, Ind.Per.Blacks.
—ingenta. **CCC.**
Published by: (B E T), Vanguarde Media, Inc, 315 Park Ave S, 11th fl, New York, NY 10010. TEL 646-654-4200, FAX 646-654-4260, http://www.heartandsoul.comde.com, http://www.vanguarde.com. Ed. Corynne L. Corbett. Circ: 200,000. **Subscr. to:** B E T, PO Box 7412, Red Oak, IA 51591. **Dist. in UK by:** MarketForce (UK), 247 Tottenham Court Rd, London W1P 0AU, United Kingdom. TEL 44-20-7261-1599, FAX 44-20-7261-7341.

613.7 USA
THE HEARTH BEAT. Text in English. m. free per issue. bk.rev. **Description:** Deals with heart health and fitness.
Media: Online - full text.
Published by: Hearth Beat siva@dencats.org, http://www.dencats.org/heart/nl/nl.html. Ed. Mani Rajan.

HELAN MEDICAL MAGAZINE. see *MEDICAL SCIENCES*

613 DNK ISSN 0018-0149
HELSE; familiens laegemagasin. Text in Danish. 1955. m. DKK 228 (effective 2000). adv. **Document type:** *Magazine, Consumer.*
Published by: (Almindelige Danske Laegeforening/Danish Medical Association), Helse - Familiens Laegemagasin, Oestbanegade 55, Copenhagen Oe 2100, Denmark. TEL 45-35-25-05-25, FAX 45-35-26-87-60, helse@helse.dk, http://www.helse.dk. Ed. Leif Hansgaard. Adv. contact Bjarne Hedegaard. B&W page DKK 35,055, color page DKK 49,020; trim 185 x 252. Circ: 300,000 (paid and controlled).

613.2 GBR ISSN 0018-0696
HERE'S HEALTH; a monthly guide to health, nutrition, natural food and natural therapy. Text in English. 1956. m. GBP 19.98; GBP 2.30 newsstand/cover (effective 1999). adv. bk.rev. illus. back issues avail. **Document type:** *Consumer.* **Description:** Covers all aspects of natural health including nutrition and alternative medicine.
Incorporates: Health for All (0017-8985)
Indexed: AMED.
—BLDSC (4300.025000), Infotrieve. **CCC.**
Published by: Emap Elan Ltd. (Subsidiary of: Emap Consumer Magazines Ltd.), Endeavour House, 189 Shaftesbury Ave, London WC2H 8JG, United Kingdom. TEL 44-20-7208-3209, FAX 44-20-7208-3583, http://www.emap.com. Ed. Elaine Griffiths. **Subscr. to:** Tower Publishing Services Ltd., Tower House, Sovereign Park, Lathkill St, Market Harborough, Leics LE16 9EF, United Kingdom. TEL 44-1858-435339, FAX 44-1858-432164. **Dist. by:** Frontline Ltd., Unit 6, Stockwell Centre, Stephenson Way, Crawley, W Sussex RH10 1TN, United Kingdom. TEL 44-1293-415000, FAX 44-1293-415009.

HIMAN CHIRYO KENKYUKAI KOENSHU/JAPANESE SOCIETY FOR OBESITY THERAPY. PROCEEDINGS. see *NUTRITION AND DIETETICS*

613 JPN ISSN 0018-3342
HOKEN NO KAGAKU/HEALTH CARE. Text in Japanese. 1959. m. JPY 10,200. index.
Published by: (Health Science Research Association/Hoken Kagaku Kenkyukai), Kyorin Shoin, 4-2-1 Yushima, Bunkyo-ku, Tokyo 113-0034, Japan. Ed. Fusao Akiyama. Circ: 710.

301.16 613.7 USA ISSN 0891-3374
HOPE HEALTH LETTER. Text in English. 1978. m. USD 19.80; USD 42 foreign (effective 1999). illus. **Document type:** *Newsletter.* **Description:** Covers many subjects on health including smoking, exercise, family matters, substance abuse, stress management, diet, self-care, health-care, cost-containment. Written for all levels.
Formerly (until 1986): Hope Newsletter
Published by: (Hope Heart Institute), International Health Awareness Center Inc., 350 E Michigan Ave, Ste 301, Kalamazoo, MI 49007-3851. TEL 616-343-0770, FAX 616-343-6260, hopeinfo@aol.com, http://www.hithope.com. Ed. Carol P Garzona.

613.7 616.1 USA
HORIZONS (LIVINGSTON). Text in English. q. free per issue. illus. *Refereed.* **Description:** Offers cancer patients and their families advice on the treatment and prevention of cancer. Provides news of the Cancer Center and related departments at Saint Barnabas Medical Center, along with sponsored programs.
Published by: Saint Barnabas Medical Center, Cancer Center, Dept of Public Relations, 95 Old Short Hills Rd, Livingston, NJ 07039. http://www.saintbarnabas.com. Ed. Lydia T Dorsky.

HUMAN MOVEMENT SCIENCE; journal devoted to pure and applied research on human movement. see *MEDICAL SCIENCES*

HUMAN SEXUALITY SUPPLEMENT. see *EDUCATION—Teaching Methods And Curriculum*

613 CZE ISSN 1210-7840
RA421 CODEN: HGIEE7
HYGIENA; casopis pro ochranu a podporu zdravi. Text in Czech, Slovak; Summaries in Czech, English. 1955. q. EUR 64, USD 84 (effective 2001). adv. bk.rev. bibl, charts, illus. index. *Refereed.*
Formerly (until 1994): Ceskoslovenska Hygiena (0009-0573)
Indexed: Abstr.Hyg., Biol.Abstr., C.I.S. Abstr., Cadscan, Chem.Abstr., Chem.Indus.Notes, Chem.Titles, Dairy Sci.Abstr., Dent.Ind., Ergon.Abstr., Excerp.Med., Food Sci.& Tech.Abstr., INIS Atomind., Lead Abstr., Protozool.Abstr., Rev.Med.& Vet.Mycol., Trop.Dis.Bull., Zincscan.
—BLDSC (4352.236200), CASDDS, CISTI, EMDOCS, GNLM, Infotrieve. **CCC.**
Published by: (Ceska Lekarska Spolecnost J.E. Purkyne/Czech Medical Association), Nakladatelske Stredisko C L S J.E. Purkyne, Sokolska 31, Prague 12026, Czech Republic. TEL 42-2-24911420, FAX 42-2-24911420, nts@iol.cz, http://www.clsjep.cz, http://www.medical.cz. Ed. J Lener. adv.: B&W page CZK 19,900, color page CZK 31,000; 197 x 136. Circ: 600. **Dist. by:** Abont s.r.o., Chlumova 17, Prague, 3 130 00, Czech Republic; **Dist. in Western Countries by:** Kubon & Sagner, Hesstr 39-41, Munich 80798, Germany.

613.7 USA
I C H P E R - S D CONGRESS PROCEEDINGS. Text in English. 1958. biennial. price varies. **Document type:** *Proceedings.* **Description:** Covers physical fitness.
Former titles: I C H P E R Congress Proceedings; I C H P E R Congress Reports (0074-4417)
Indexed: Sportsearch.
Published by: International Council on Health, Physical Education, Recreation, Sport and Dance, 1900 Association Dr, Reston, VA 20191. TEL 703-476-3462, FAX 703-476-9527.

613.7 USA
I D E A FITNESS EDGE. Text in English. 1998. 5/yr. membership.
Published by: (International Dance-Exercise Association), I D E A Health & Fitness Inc., 6190 Cornerstone Court E, Ste 204, San Diego, CA 92121. TEL 619-535-8979, FAX 619-535-8234, member@ideafit.com, http://www.ideafit.com.

613.7 USA
I D E A FITNESS MANAGER. Text in English. 5/yr. membership. **Document type:** *Newsletter, Trade.*
Published by: (International Dance-Exercise Association), I D E A Health & Fitness Inc., 190 Cornerstone Ct, Ste 204, San Diego, CA 92121-3773. TEL 619-535-8979, 800-999-4332, FAX 619-535-8234, member@ideafit.com, http://www.ideafit.com, http://www.idea.fit.com. Circ: 3,600 (paid).

613.7 USA ISSN 1073-7952
I D E A FITNESS MANAGER NEWSLETTER. Text in English. 5/yr. membership. **Document type:** *Newsletter.* **Description:** Offers fitness business owners, program directors and managers information needed to build business, support staff and be effective administrators.
Published by: I D E A Health & Fitness Inc., 6190 Cornerstone Court E, Ste 204, San Diego, CA 92121. TEL 619-535-8979, 800-999-4332. Ed. Patricia Ryan. Pub. Peter Davis. Circ: 5,000.

613.7 USA ISSN 1096-8156
RA781.15
I D E A HEALTH & FITNESS SOURCE. Text in English. 1984. 10/yr. membership. adv. bk.rev. index. back issues avail. *Refereed.* **Document type:** *Trade.* **Description:** Covers exercise science, research and teaching skills, motivation and communication skills, programming, nutrition and weight loss, business operations and marketing, and association news for exercise instructors, personal trainers and business operators.
Former titles (until 1998): I D E A Today; (until 1988): Dance Exercise Today (0882-1399)
Related titles: Online - full text ed.: (from Gale Group).
Indexed: Phys.Ed.Ind., Sportsearch (1988-).
—BLDSC (4362.371650).
Published by: I D E A Health & Fitness Inc., 6190 Cornerstone Court E, Ste 204, San Diego, CA 92121. TEL 619-535-8979, 800-999-4332, http://www.ideafit.com, http://www.idea.fit.com. Ed. Diane Lofshult. Pub. Peter Davis. R&P Michelle Zamora. adv.: B&W page USD 1,778, color page USD 2,850; trim 11 x 8.25. Circ: 23,000.

613.7 USA ISSN 1068-087X
I D E A PERSONAL TRAINER. Text in English. 1990. 10/yr. membership. **Document type:** *Trade.* **Description:** Enables trainers to operate successful businesses, plan prudent exercise programs and motivate clients to pursue a healthy lifestyle.
Published by: (International Dance Exercise Association), I D E A Health & Fitness Inc., 6190 Cornerstone Court E, Ste 204, San Diego, CA 92121. TEL 619-535-8979, 800-999-4332, FAX 619-535-8234, member@ideafit.com, http://www.ideafit.com, http://www.idea.fit.com. Ed. Patricia Ryan. Pub. Peter Davis. adv.: B&W page USD 1,115, color page USD 1,795; trim 11.25 x 8.5. Circ: 10,000.

I E H REPORT ON FACTORS AFFECTING THE ABSORPTION OF TOXIC METALS FROM THE DIET. see *ENVIRONMENTAL STUDIES—Toxicology And Environmental Safety*

I E H REPORT ON HEALTH EFFECTS OF WASTE COMBUSTION PRODUCTS. see *ENVIRONMENTAL STUDIES—Pollution*

I E H REPORT ON PERINATEL DEVELOPMENTAL NEUROTOXCITY. see *ENVIRONMENTAL STUDIES—Toxicology And Environmental Safety*

613 ITA ISSN 0019-1655
CODEN: IGMPAX
IGIENE MODERNA; rivista di igiene, microbiologia, epidemiologia. Text in English, Italian, Spanish. 1908. m. ITL 150,000, USD 180 (effective 1994). adv. bk.rev. abstr, charts, illus. index. **Description:** Covers the Italian Society of Hygiene, Preventive Medicine and Public Health; includes microbiology and epidemiology.
Indexed: Abstr.Hyg., AgBiotech, Aqua.Sci.& Fish.Abstr., Aquacult.Abstr., Biol.Abstr., C.I.S. Abstr., Chem.Abstr., Curr.Adv.Ecol.Sci., Dairy Sci.Abstr., Environ.Sci.Poll.Mgmt., Excerp.Med., Food Sci.& Tech.Abstr., Helminthol.Abstr., Hort.Abstr., Ind.Med. (coverage dropped), Ind.Vet., Microbiol.Abstr., Nutr.Abstr., Pollut.Abstr., Postharvest, Poult.Abstr., Protozool.Abstr., Rev.Appl.Entomol., Rev.Med.& Vet.Mycol., Rev.Plant Path., Risk Abstr., Saf.Sci.Abstr., Soils & Fert., Trop.Dis.Bull., Vet.Bull., Weed Abstr.
—BLDSC (4363.440000), CASDDS, CISTI, GNLM, KNAW.
Published by: European Journal of Epidemiology Publishers S.r.l., Pratti, Via Riccardo Zandonai, 11, Rome, RM 00194, Italy. TEL 06-36309593, FAX 06-3290343, TELEX 611330 UCATRO. Ed. Dr. Giovanni Fadda. Adv. contact Cristina Delmonte.

INSTITUTUL DE SUBINGINERI ORADEA. LUCRARI STIINTIFICE: SERIA EDUCATIE FIZICA SI SPORT. see *SPORTS AND GAMES*

613.7 USA ISSN 1091-2193
GV201
INTERNATIONAL COUNCIL FOR HEALTH, PHYSICAL EDUCATION, RECREATION, SPORT AND DANCE. JOURNAL. Text in English, Spanish, German, French, Arabic. q. USD 35 (effective 2001). adv. **Document type:** *Academic/Scholarly.* **Description:** Contains articles, research papers, worldwide developments in the professional areas of sport, dance and physical fitness.
Formerly: International Council for Health, Physical Education and Recreation. Journal (1046-3380)
Indexed: C.I.J.E., Sportsearch (1988-).
—BLDSC (4802.218000), ingenta.
Published by: International Council for Health, Physical Education and Recreation, Sport and Dance, 1900 Association Dr, Reston, VA 20191. TEL 703-476-3462, FAX 703-476-9527, ichper@aahperd.org, http://www.ichpersd.org/. Ed. Julian U Stein.

613.7071 GBR ISSN 1463-5240
INTERNATIONAL JOURNAL OF HEALTH PROMOTION AND EDUCATION. Text in English. 1962. q. GBP 25 to non-members (effective 2001). adv. bk.rev., film rev. index. *Refereed.* **Document type:** *Academic/Scholarly.* **Description:** Serves as a platform for new ideas and practical research, publishing research articles for a wide range of health and teaching professionals.
Former titles (until 1998): International Journal of Health Education (1368-1222); (until 1997): Institute of Health Education. Journal (0307-3289)
Indexed: Abstr.Hyg., Addic.Abstr., Brit.Nur.Ind., Cont.Pg.Educ., Curr.Adv.Ecol.Sci., Nutr.Abstr., Trop.Dis.Bull.
—BLDSC (4542.277700), GNLM.
Published by: Institute of Health Promotion and Education, University Dental Hospital, Higher Cambridge St, Manchester M15 6FH, United Kingdom. TEL 44-161-275-6610, FAX 44-161-275-6610. Ed., R&P Anthony S Blinkhorn. Circ: 1,000 (paid).

INTERNATIONAL JOURNAL OF OBESITY. see *NUTRITION AND DIETETICS*

ISOKINETICS AND EXERCISE SCIENCE. see *MEDICAL SCIENCES—Sports Medicine*

613 JPN ISSN 0021-5082
CODEN: NEZAAQ
JAPANESE JOURNAL OF HYGIENE/NIHON EISEIGAKU ZASSHI. Text in English, Japanese; Abstracts in English. 1946. bi-m. JPY 4,500; JPY 6,500 foreign. adv. **Document type:** *Academic/Scholarly.*
Indexed: Art.Hosp.& Tour., C.I.S. Abstr., Excerp.Med., Food Sci.& Tech.Abstr., Helminthol.Abstr., INIS Atomind., Ind.Med. (1946-), Int.Nurs.Ind., Nutr.Abstr.
—BLDSC (4655.300000), CASDDS, CISTI, GNLM, Infotrieve, ingenta. **CCC.**
Published by: Japanese Society for Hygiene/Nihon Eisei Gakkai, c/o Dept of Hygiene and Preventive Medicine, Faculty of Medicine, University of, 7-3-1 Hongo, Bunkyo-ku, Tokyo 113-0033, Japan. FAX 81-3-5684-2297. Ed. K Morimoto. Circ: 2,700.

610 613.7 JPN ISSN 0039-906X
JAPANESE JOURNAL OF PHYSICAL FITNESS AND SPORTS MEDICINE. Text in English, Japanese. 1950. bi-m. JPY 12,000 (effective 1998). adv. *Refereed.* **Document type:** *Academic/Scholarly.*
Formerly: Japanese Journal of Physical Fitness
Related titles: Online - full text ed.: (from Institute for Scientific Information).
Indexed: ASCA, Excerp.Med., Focus on: Sports Sci.& Med., Nutr.Abstr.
—BLDSC (4657.420000).
Published by: Japanese Society of Physical Fitness and Sports Medicine, Business Center for Academic Societies Japan, 5-16-9 Honkomagome, Bunkyo-ku, Tokyo 113-0021, Japan. TEL 81-3-5814-5811. Ed. Masahisa Usami. Circ: 4,800.

JEWISH VEGETARIAN. see *NUTRITION AND DIETETICS*

613.7 CHN ISSN 1002-297X
JIANKANG* /HEALTH MAGAZINE. Text in Chinese. 1980. m. USD 19.20; USD 1.60 newsstand/cover (effective 2001). adv. **Document type:** *Government.* **Description:** Covers general medical and disease prevention knowledge.
Published by: (Beijing Jiankang Jiaoyusuo/Beijing Municipal Institute of Health Education), China International Book Trading Corp/Zhongguo Guoji Tushu Maoyi Zonggongsi cibtc@mail.cibtc.com.cn, http://www.cibtc.com.cn. Ed. Chen Shianshan. Circ: 100,000. **Dist. by:** 35, Chegongzhuang Xilu, Haidian District, Beijing 100044, China. **Co-sponsor:** Beijing Municipal Health Bureau.

613.2 CHN
JIANKANG BAO/HEALTH NEWS. Text in Chinese. 6/w. CNY 70.56. **Document type:** *Newspaper, Consumer.*
Indexed: Int.Nurs.Ind.
Published by: China Books & Periodicals, Inc, 2929 24th St, San Francisco, CA 94110. **Dist. by:** China International Book Trading Corp, 35, Chegongzhuang Xilu, Haidian District, Beijing 100044, China. TEL 86-1-68413849, FAX 86-1-68412048, cibtc@mail.cibtc.com.cn, http://www.cibtc.com.cn; TEL 415-282-0994, 415-282-2994.

613.7 CHN ISSN 1003-000X
JIANKANG GUWEN/GUIDE TO GOOD HEALTH. Text in Chinese. 1980. bi-m. USD 26.40; USD 2.20 newsstand/cover (effective 2001). **Document type:** *Consumer.*
Published by: Renmin Tiyu Chubanshe/People's Sports Publishing House, 8 Tiyuguan Lu, Chongwen-qu, Beijing 100061, China. TEL 86-1-6714-2466, FAX 86-1-6711-6129. Ed. Pei Jiarong. **Dist. by:** China International Book Trading Corp, 35, Chegongzhuang Xilu, Haidian District, Beijing 100044, China. TEL 86-1-68413849, FAX 86-1-68412048, cibtc@mail.cibtc.com.cn, http://www.cibtc.com.cn.

613.7 CHN ISSN 1005-4596
JIANKANG SHIJIE/HEALTH WORLD. Text in Chinese. m. **Document type:** *Academic/Scholarly.*
Related titles: Online - full content ed.: (from WanFang Data Corp.).
Published by: Zhonghua Yixuehui Zazhishe, 42 Dongsi Xidajie, Beijing 100710, China. TEL 86-1-65221632, cmajk@public.sti.ac.cn. Ed. Jing-He Lang. **Dist. by:** China International Book Trading Corp, 35, Chegongzhuang Xilu, Haidian District, Beijing 100044, China. TEL 86-1-68413849, FAX 86-1-68412048, cibtc@mail.cibtc.com.cn, http://www.cibtc.com.cn.

613.7 CHN
JIANKANG TIANDI/HEALTH WORLD. Text in Chinese. bi-m.
Published by: Hebei Fangyi Zhan/Hebei Epidemic Prevention Station, 18 Hongqi Lu, Baoding, Hebei 071000, China. TEL 24911. Ed. Zhang Furui.

613.7 CHN ISSN 1002-8714
JIANKANG ZHI YOU/FRIEND OF HEALTH. Text in Chinese. 1985. bi-m.
Published by: Xin Tiyu Zazhishe, 8 Tiyuguan Lu, Beijing 100061, China. TEL 757161. Ed. Cao Yan.

613.7 CHN
JIANKANG ZHINAN (ZHONG LAO NAN)/GUIDE TO HEALTH. Text in Chinese. 1988. bi-m. USD 24; CNY 4, USD 2 newsstand/cover (effective 2001).
Related titles: Online - full content ed.: (from WanFang Data Corp.).
Published by: Quanguo Laoganbu Jiankang Zhidao Weiyuanhui/National Health Committee for Senior Officials, c/o Beijing Yike Daxue, Shenghua-lou 212-shi, Beijing 100083, China. TEL 86-1-62091682. Ed. Jun-Bo Zhi. **Dist. by:** China International Book Trading Corp, 35, Chegongzhuang Xilu, Haidian District, Beijing 100044, China. TEL 86-1-68413849, FAX 86-1-68412048, cibtc@mail.cibtc.com.cn, http://www.cibtc.com.cn.

613.7 CHN ISSN 1000-9701
JIEFANGJUN JIANKANG/P L A HEALTH. Text in Chinese. 1987. bi-m. USD 10.20; USD 17 newsstand/cover (effective 2001). **Document type:** *Academic/Scholarly.*
Published by: China International Book Trading Corp/Zhongguo Guoji Tushu Maoyi Zonggongsi cibtc@mail.cibtc.com.cn, http://www.cibtc.com.cn. **Dist. by:** 35, Chegongzhuang Xilu, Haidian District, Beijing 100044, China.

JOGGING - LA GRANDE CORSA. see *SPORTS AND GAMES*

JOURNAL OF AGING AND PHYSICAL ACTIVITY. see *GERONTOLOGY AND GERIATRICS*

613.7 USA ISSN 0744-8481
RA564.5
JOURNAL OF AMERICAN COLLEGE HEALTH. Text in English. 1952. bi-m., latest vol.50, 2001. USD 66 domestic to individuals; USD 81 foreign to individuals; USD 117 domestic to institutions; USD 132 foreign to institutions; USD 19.50 newsstand/cover (effective 2001 - 2002). adv. bk.rev. charts, illus. index. back issues avail.; reprints avail. *Refereed.* **Document type:** *Academic/Scholarly.* **Description:** It covers developments and research in this broad field, including administration, clinical and preventive medicine, environmental health and safety, nursing diagnosis, pharmacy, and sports medicine.
Formerly (until 1982): American College Health Association. Journal (0002-7944); Incorporates: American College Health Association. Proceedings
Related titles: CD-ROM ed.: (from ProQuest Information & Learning); Microform ed.; Online - full text ed.: (from Northern Light Technology, Inc., H. W. Wilson, ProQuest Information & Learning, Gale Group, LexisNexis, Institute for Scientific Information).
Indexed: ASCA, ASSIA, Biol.Abstr., C.I.J.E., CINAHL, C.I.S. Abstr., CWI, Chem.Abstr., Curr.Cont., Curr.Lit.Fam.Plan., Educ.Ind. (Oct.1982-), Environ.Sci.Poll.Mgmt., Excerp.Med., High.Educ.Abstr., Hosp.Lit.Ind., IBZ, Ind.Med. (1982-), Int.Nurs.Ind., Phys.Ed.Ind., Pollut.Abstr., PsycInfo, Psychol.Abstr. (1971-), Risk Abstr., SSCI, Saf.Sci.Abstr., THA, e-psyche.
—BLDSC (4927.231000), CISTI, EMDOCS, GNLM, IDS, Infotrieve, ingenta, KNAW. **CCC.**
Published by: (American College Health Association), Heldref Publications, 1319 Eighteenth St, N W, Washington, DC 20036-1802. TEL 202-296-6267, 800-365-9753, FAX 202-293-6130, jach@heldref.org; orders@allenpress.com, http://www.heldref.org; http://www.allenpress.com. Ed. Martha Wedemen. Adv. contact Grant Williams. Circ: 650. **Subscr. to:** Allen Press Inc., PO Box 1897, Lawrence, KS 66044-8897. **Co-sponsor:** Helen Dwight Reid Educational Foundation.

JOURNAL OF BIOENERGETICS AND BIOMEMBRANES. see *BIOLOGY—Biochemistry*

613 610 USA ISSN 1044-2790
JOURNAL OF HEALTH & HEALING. Text in English. 1975. q. USD 10 domestic; USD 13 foreign (effective 2000). adv. charts, illus. index. back issues avail. **Document type:** *Academic/Scholarly.*
Published by: Wildwood Lifestyle Center & Hospital, PO Box 129, Wildwood, GA 30757-0129. TEL 404-820-1493, FAX 706-820-1474, journalhh@yahoo.com, http://www.tagnet.org/wildwood/. Ed. Dr. Marjorie Baldwin. Circ: 10,000.

613.7 200 USA ISSN 0885-4726
BV4335
JOURNAL OF HEALTH CARE CHAPLAINCY. Text in English. 1987. s-a. USD 50 to individuals; USD 68 in Canada to individuals; USD 73 elsewhere to individuals; USD 95 to institutions; USD 128 in Canada to institutions; USD 138 elsewhere to institutions; USD 150 to libraries; USD 203 in Canada to libraries; USD 218 elsewhere to libraries (effective Aug. 2001). adv. bk.rev. back issues avail.; reprint service avail. from HAW. *Refereed.* **Document type:** *Journal, Academic/Scholarly.* **Description:** Promotes both foundational and applied interdisciplinary research related to chaplaincy as practiced in community hospitals, medical centers, nursing homes, and other health care institutions.
Related titles: Microfiche ed.: (from PQC); Microform ed.; Online - full text ed.: free with subscr. to the print ed.
Indexed: Abstr.Soc.Geront., AgeLine, Curr.Cont. (coverage dropped), IMFL, Ind.Med. (coverage dropped), Int.Nurs.Ind., Per.Islam. (1990-), Rel.& Theol.Abstr., Rel.Ind.One, Rel.Ind.Two.
—GNLM, Haworth.
Published by: Haworth Press, Inc., 10 Alice St, Binghamton, NY 13904-1580. TEL 607-722-5857, 800-429-6784, FAX 607-722-6362, 800-895-0582, getinfo@haworthpressinc.com, http://www.haworthpress.com/journals/journallist.asp. Ed. Larry Vandecreek. Pub. William Cohen. R&P Ruthann Heath TEL 607-723-5857 ext 316. Adv. contact Jackie Blakeslee TEL 607-722-5857 ext 346. B&W page USD 315, color page USD 550; trim 6 x 8.5. Circ: 575.

JOURNAL OF HEALTH SCIENCE. see *NUTRITION AND DIETETICS*

613.907 155.3 USA ISSN 0161-4576
HQ1 CODEN: JSETE2
JOURNAL OF SEX EDUCATION AND THERAPY. Text in English. 1975-1995; resumed 1997. q. USD 40 to individuals; USD 60 foreign to individuals; USD 75 to institutions; USD 95 foreign to institutions (effective 1999). adv. bk.rev., video rev. charts, illus, stat. reprint service avail. from PQC. *Refereed.* **Document type:** *Academic/Scholarly.* **Description:** Publishes selected research on sex education as well as sex counseling and therapy.
Indexed: ASCA, Abstr.Anthropol., Abstr.Crim.& Pen., Child Devel.Abstr., Commun.Abstr., Cont.Pg.Educ., Curr.Cont. (coverage dropped), Curr.Lit.Fam.Plan., ERA, Fam.Ind., IBZ, Ind.Philos., Lang.& Lang.Behav.Abstr., Mid.East: Abstr.& Ind., Mult.Ed.Abstr., PsycInfo, Psychol.Abstr. (1985-), SOPODA, Sage Fam.Stud.Abstr., Soc.Serv.Abstr., Soc.Work Res.& Abstr., Sociol.Abstr., Stud.Wom.Abstr., e-psyche.
—BLDSC (5064.019000), IDS, Infotrieve, ingenta. **CCC.**
Published by: American Association of Sex Educators, Counselors and Therapists, 103 Ave S, Ste 2 A, Box 238, Mount Vernon, IA 52314-0238. TEL 319-895-8407, FAX 319-895-6203, aasect@worldnet.att.net, http://www.aasect.org. Ed. S Michael Plaut. Pub. Robert Matloff. Adv. contact Marian Robinson. Circ: 2,700.

THE JOURNAL OF SPORTS MEDICINE AND PHYSICAL FITNESS. see *MEDICAL SCIENCES—Sports Medicine*

JOURNAL OF STRENGTH AND CONDITIONING RESEARCH; the research journal of the National Strength and Conditioning Association. see *MEDICAL SCIENCES—Sports Medicine*

613.7 USA
JOURNEY TO HEALTH. Text in English. bi-m. **Document type:** *Newsletter.* **Description:** Provides information, tips and motivation for a healthier lifestyle. Covers exercise, diet, vegetarianism, preventative health, voluntary simplicity and more.
Media: Online - full text.
Address: cherylstkf@earthlink.net, http://home.earthlink.net/cherylstkf/webdocs/index.html.

796 613.7 FIN ISSN 0782-4971
JUOKSIJA. Text in Finnish. 1971. m. FIM 297, EUR 50 domestic; FIM 380, EUR 60 in Europe; FIM 430, EUR 70 elsewhere (effective 2002). adv. bk.rev. 96 p./no. 3 cols./p. **Document type:** *Consumer.* **Description:** Devoted to running, cross-country skiing, and physical fitness.
Published by: Kustannusyhtio Juoksija Oy, Olympic Stadium, B 10, Helsinki 00250, Finland. TEL 358-9-4342040, FAX 358-9-434-20444, juoksija-lehti@stadion.fi. Ed. Ari Paunonen. Pub., R&P Tapio Pekola. Adv. contact Ilkka Kalermo. B&W page FIM 6,500, color page FIM 9,900; trim 30 x 21. Circ: 13,000.

613.7 CHN
KANGLI SHIJIE/HEALTH AND HAPPINESS. Text in Chinese. bi-m. USD 14.40; USD 2.40 newsstand/cover (effective 2001). **Document type:** *Academic/Scholarly.*
Published by: China International Book Trading Corp/Zhongguo Guoji Tushu Maoyi Zonggongsi cibtc@mail.cibtc.com.cn, http://www.cibtc.com.cn. **Dist. by:** 35, Chegongzhuang Xilu, Haidian District, Beijing 100044, China.

613.7 AUT
KNEIPP ZEITSCHRIFT; das oesterreichische Gesundheitsmagazin. Text in German. 10/yr. adv. **Document type:** *Magazine, Consumer.*
Published by: Oesterreichischer Kneippbund, Kunigundenweg 10, Leoben, St 8700, Austria. TEL 43-3842-21718, FAX 43-3842-2171819. Adv. contact Helma Urschler. B&W page ATS 29,400, color page ATS 37,300; 266 x 190. Circ: 62,000 (controlled).

613.7 DEU ISSN 0323-4916
KOERPERERZIEHUNG; Fachzeitschrift fuer Sportlehrerinnen und Sportlehrer. Text in German. 1951. 6/yr. DEM 103.60; DEM 74 to students; DEM 16.20 newsstand/cover (effective 2000). **Document type:** *Journal, Academic/Scholarly.*
Indexed: IBR, IBZ.
Published by: Paedagogischer Zeitschriftenverlag, Postfach 269, Berlin 10107, Germany. TEL 49-30-20183592, FAX 49-30-20183593, http://cthulhu.hsd.de/pzv. Ed. Wolfgang Hartisch. Adv. contact Constanze Richter. Circ: 2,800. **Subscr. to:** CVK Cornelsen Verlagskontor, Postfach 100271, Bielefeld 33502, Germany. TEL 49-521-9719-0.

P

613 FIN ISSN 0787-9385
KOTILAAKARI. Text in Finnish. 1889. m. FIM 349 (effective 2001). adv. illus. **Document type:** *Magazine, Consumer.* **Description:** Features diverse, challenging contents and a holistic approach to health.
Incorporates: Terveys (0040-3911); Former titles (until 1978): T H Kotilaakari (0355-1903); Terveydenhoitolehti (0040-3903)
Published by: Yhtyneet Kuvalehdet Oy/United Magazines Ltd., Maistraatinportti 1, Helsinki 00015, Finland. TEL 358-9-156-6273, 358-9-15661, FAX 358-9-156-6505, 358-9-145650. Ed. Vuokko Jaervilehto. adv.: B&W page FIM 13,500, color page FIM 19,800; trim 280 x 217. Circ: 54,703.

613.7 USA ISSN 0024-1288
TX341
LET'S LIVE; America's foremost health & preventive medicine magazine. Text in English. 1933. m. USD 15.95; USD 3.95 newsstand/cover (effective 2000). adv. bk.rev. *Refereed.* **Document type:** *Magazine, Consumer.* **Description:** Publishes articles on holistic and alternative medicine, homeopathy and naturopathy, sports nutrition and fitness.
Related titles: Online - full text ed.: (from Gale Group, Factiva).
Indexed: Hlth.Ind., Plant Sci.
Published by: Franklin Publications (Subsidiary of: Basic Media Group), 320 N Larchmont Blvd, 3rd Fl, Box 74908, Los Angeles, CA 90004. TEL 310-479-4545, FAX 310-479-8663, letslive@earthlink.net, b-salamon@letslivemag.com, http://www.letsliveonline.com. Ed., R&P Beth Salmon. Pub. Lee Kelley. Adv. contact Karen Dion. B&W page USD 17,600, color page USD 23,500; trim 10.5 x 8. Circ: 1,400,000.

LIFE EXTENSION; the ultimate source for new health and medical findings from around the world. see *ALTERNATIVE MEDICINE*

LIFELINES (TORONTO); the voice of Toronto's vegetarian community. see *NUTRITION AND DIETETICS*

613 USA
LIVEWELL★ . Text in English. 1988. m. USD 2.50 per issue. adv. **Description:** Focuses on heart attacks, cancer, lung disease, and strokes; discusses prevention and aftercare.
Address: 4353 E 119th Way, Denver, CO 80233-1738. TEL 303-292-3343. Ed. Pam Avery. Circ: 150,000.

613.2 SWE ISSN 0346-6280
MAA BRA; specialtidningen foer kropp & sjael. Text in Swedish. 1976. 12/yr. SEK 389 (effective 2001). adv. 4 cols./p. **Document type:** *Magazine, Consumer.* **Description:** Presents articles and features on how to lead a healthy life without sacrificing pleasure.
Published by: Aller Specialtidningar AB, Landskronavaegen 25A, Helsingborg 25185, Sweden. TEL 46-42-17-35-00, FAX 46-42-17-35-99. Ed., Pub. Inger Ridstroem. Adv. contact Aake Borgstroem. B&W page SEK 37,500, color page SEK 43,000; trim 190 x 265. Circ: 111,900 (paid).

362.1 USA
▼ **MANAGED CARE INSIDER ENEWS.** Text in English. 1999. m. free. back issues avail. **Document type:** *Newsletter.* **Description:** Designed for health care providers and professionals in the health care industry.
Media: Online - full text.
Published by: Scheur Managed Group, Inc., 255 Washington St, Ste 100, Newton, MA 02458-1611. TEL 617-969-7500, insider@scheur.com, http://www.scheur.com/ITechnology/webpage/Ezine.nsf/subscriber?openform.

MARKETING HEALTH SERVICES. see *BUSINESS AND ECONOMICS—Marketing And Purchasing*

615.82 USA
MASSAGE AND BODYWORK. Text in English. 1988. 6/yr. USD 26 in US & Canada; USD 60 elsewhere; GBP 4.95 newsstand/cover domestic; CND 5.95 newsstand/cover in Canada (effective 2001). adv. bk.rev., music rev., video rev. tr.lit. 168 p./no. back issues avail. **Document type:** *Magazine, Consumer, Trade.* **Description:** For an International audience of massage, bodywork, somatic and esthetic therapy professionals. The latest research, historical perspectives massage techniques, business information, professional trends and a variety of regularly featured columns keep the audience in touch with their work, their clients and their health.
Former titles (until 1997): Massage and Bodywork Quarterly (1066-9337); Associated Bodywork and Massage Professionals News (1053-458X)
Related titles: Diskette ed.
Published by: Associated Bodywork and Massage Professionals, 1271 Sugarbush Dr, Evergreen, CO 80439-9766. TEL 303-674-8478, 800-458-2267, FAX 303-674-0859, expectmore@abmp.com, http://www.abmp.com. Ed., R&P Karrie Mowen. Adv. contact Kris Centeno. B&W page USD 1,125, color page USD 1,625; trim 10.88 x 8.25. Circ: 110,000 (paid and controlled). **Dist. by:** IPD, 3360 Industrial Rd, Harrisburg, PA 17110.

613.7 USA ISSN 1091-367X
GV436 CODEN: MPESFC
MEASUREMENT IN PHYSICAL EDUCATION AND EXERCISE SCIENCE. Text in English. 1997. q. USD 50 in US & Canada to individuals; USD 80 elsewhere to individuals; USD 295 in US & Canada to institutions; USD 325 elsewhere to institutions (effective 2002). adv. **Document type:** *Journal, Academic/Scholarly.* **Description:** Covers research, test development, and evaluation of theoretical and methodological issues in measurement and statistics as they apply to physical education and exercise science.
Related titles: Online - full text ed.: ISSN 1532-7841. USD 45 to individuals; USD 265.50 to institutions (effective 2002) (from CatchWord Ltd., EBSCO Publishing, O C L C Online Computer Library Center, Inc., RoweCom Information Quest, Swets Blackwell).
Indexed: Rural Recreat.Tour.Abstr.
—BLDSC (5413.567300), CatchWord. **CCC.**
Published by: (American Association for Active Lifestyles and Fitness), Lawrence Erlbaum Associates, Inc., 10 Industrial Ave, Mahwah, NJ 07430-2262. TEL 201-760-3735, 800-926-6579, FAX 201-236-0072, journals@erlbaum.com, http://www.erlbaum.com/Journals/journals/MPEE/mpee.htm. Eds. Barbara E Jensen, William J Considine. adv.: page USD 300; trim 5 x 8.

MEDECINE DU SPORT. see *MEDICAL SCIENCES—Sports Medicine*

MEDECINE ET HYGIENE. see *MEDICAL SCIENCES*

MEDICAL AND HEALTH ANNUAL. see *MEDICAL SCIENCES*

613 USA ISSN 0749-9973
R118.4.U6
MEDICAL & HEALTH INFORMATION DIRECTORY. Text in English. 1978. triennial, latest vol.10. USD 590 3 vol. set (effective 1999). **Description:** Guide to medical and health information in the U.S.
Published by: Gale Group (Subsidiary of: The Thomson Corporation), 27500 Drake Rd, Farmington Hills, MI 48331-3535. TEL 248-699-4253, 800-877-4253, FAX 248-699-8061, galeord@gale.com, http://www.gale.com. Ed. Bridgett Travers.

613.7 USA
MEDICAL UPDATE; a Saturday Evening Post monthly medical newsletter. Text in English. 1976. m. USD 15. **Document type:** *Newsletter.* **Description:** Covers all areas of health, nutrition and fitness.
Related titles: Online - full text ed.: (from Gale Group).
Indexed: CHNI, CINAHL, Hlth.Ind.
—BLDSC (5532.085500).
Published by: American Foundation for Preventive Medicine, 1102 Stadium Dr, PO Box 2166, Indianapolis, IN 46202. FAX 317-637-0126. Ed. Edwin W Brown. Pub. Dr. Cory Servaas. R&P Jack Grambling. Circ: 21,000.

613 DEU ISSN 0179-0404
MEDIZIN HEUTE; die gesunden Seiten des Lebens. Text in German. 1950. m. DEM 38.40, EUR 19.63; DEM 27 to students; DEM 57.60 foreign; DEM 4.10, EUR 2.10 newsstand/cover (effective 2000). adv. bk.rev. illus. **Document type:** *Magazine, Trade.*
Published by: Deutscher Aerzte-Verlag GmbH, Dieselstr 2, Cologne 50859, Germany. TEL 49-2234-7011-0, FAX 49-2234-7011515, http://www.medizinheute.com, http://www.aerzteverlag.de. Ed. Johann Friedrich Jeurink. Adv. contact Renate Peters. B&W page DEM 9,880, color page DEM 16,280. Circ: 160,000 (paid).

MEDIZINI. see *CHILDREN AND YOUTH—For*

MELPOMENE JOURNAL; a journal for women's health research. see *WOMEN'S HEALTH*

613.7 USA ISSN 1043-8475
MEMPHIS HEALTH CARE NEWS. Text in English. fortn. **Document type:** *Trade.*
—CCC.
Published by: Mid-South Communications, Inc., 88 Union, Rm 200, Memphis, TN 38103-5100. TEL 901-526-2007, FAX 901-526-5240. Ed. Deborah Dubois. Circ: 12,601.

MEN'S FITNESS; when performance counts. see *MEN'S HEALTH*

613 USA ISSN 0164-1336
RA440.A1
MICHIGAN HEALTH EDUCATOR. Text in English. 1976. bi-m. USD 7.50. adv. bk.rev. index. back issues avail.
Published by: Michigan Health Educator Company, 2843 Hilton Rd, Ferndale, MI 48220. Ed. E Dewey Little. Circ: 10,200.

613.7 ITA
MISSIONE SALUTE; Bimestrale di cultura e salute sul mondo della sanita. Text in Italian. 1988. bi-m. ITL 40,000 domestic; ITL 60,000 foreign (effective 2002). adv. 84 p./no.
Published by: Provincia Lombardo Veneta dei Camilliani d'Italia, Via Francesco Nava, 31, Milan, MI 20159, Italy. TEL 39-02-69516156, FAX 39-02-69516157, missionesalute.camillians@interbusiness.it, http://www.camilliani.org. Ed. P Domenico Fantin. adv.: B&W page ITL 2,500,000, color page ITL 3,500,000. Circ: 20,000.

613 USA
MONTROSE HEALTH E-LETTER★ . Text in English. w. bk.rev. back issues avail. **Document type:** *Newsletter.* **Description:** Provides timely information and articles for health conscious adults.
Media: Online - full text.
Published by: Montrose Integrated Research, PO Box 292193, Temple Terrace, FL 33687-2193. TEL 813-899-1938, editor@montrose-research.com, http://www.montrose-research.com/newsletter.htm/. Ed. Robert T Wallen.

MOTHERING; the magazine of natural family living. see *WOMEN'S HEALTH*

613.7 GBR ISSN 0955-1387
MUSCLE AND FITNESS. Text in English. 1988. m. GBP 26.97; GBP 2.95 newsstand/cover (effective 1999). illus. **Document type:** *Consumer.* **Description:** Offers persons engaged or interested in body building features and tips on general training, nutrition, and fitness.
Published by: Weider Publishing, 10 Windsor Ct, Clarence Dr, Harrogate, N Yorks HG1 2PE, United Kingdom. TEL 44-1423-504516, FAX 44-1423-523294, ukpub@weider.demon.co.uk. **Subscr. to:** Tower Publishing Services Ltd., Tower House, Sovereign Park, Lathkill St, Market Harborough, Leics LE16 9EF, United Kingdom. TEL 44-1858-435346, FAX 44-1858-434958. **Dist. by:** Comag, Tavistock Works, Tavistock Rd, W Drayton, Middx UB7 7QX, United Kingdom. TEL 44-1895-444055, FAX 44-189-543-3606.

613.7 USA
▼ **MUSCLE & FITNESS HERS.** Text in English. 2000. m. USD 17.97 domestic; USD 29.97 foreign; USD 3.99 newsstand/cover per academic year (effective 2001). adv. **Document type:** *Magazine, Consumer.* **Description:** Provides tips, advice and instruction for women who want more out of fitness.
Related titles: Online - full text ed.: (from America Online, Inc.).
Published by: Weider Publications, 21100 Erwin St, Woodland Hills, CA 91367. http://www.muscleandfitnesshers.com/. adv.: color page USD 10,000; trim 8 x 10.5.

613.7 USA
▼ **MUSCLE & FITNESS MILITARY.** Text in English. 2001 (Sep.). a. USD 5.99 newsstand/cover; USD 6.99 newsstand/cover in Canada (effective 2001). **Document type:** *Magazine, Consumer.* **Description:** Contains articles and information on exercise routines and nutrition strategies used by all branches of the U.S. military.
Published by: Weider Publications, 21100 Erwin St, Woodland Hills, CA 91367. TEL 818-884-6800, 800-998-0731, FAX 818-716-5626.

613 796.41 USA
MUSCULAR DEVELOPMENT. Cover title: Muscular Development Magazine. Text in English. 1964. m. USD 35.88; USD 55 foreign; USD 4.99 newsstand/cover; GBP 2.75 newsstand/cover in United Kingdom; CND 5.99 newsstand/cover in Canada (effective 1999). adv. charts, illus, tr.lit. **Document type:** *Consumer.* **Description:** Offers comprehensive coverage of bodybuilding, sports nutrition, muscular development and strength training.

Former titles (until 1999): All Natural Muscular Development; (until 1997): Muscular Development Fitness and Health; Muscular Development (0047-8415)
Indexed: Phys.Ed.Ind., Sportsearch.
—ingenta.
Published by: Advanced Research Press, Inc., 150 Motor Pkwy, Ste 210, Hauppauge, NY 11788. TEL 516-467-3140, FAX 516-467-2973, allnat.md@aol.com, http://www.musculardevelopment.com, http://www.advancedresearchpress.com/. Ed. Alan Paul. Pub. Steve Blechman. R&P Roy Ulin. Adv. contact Angela Frizalone. Circ: 125,000 (paid). **Dist. in UK by:** Seymour, 86 Newman St, London W1P 3EX, United Kingdom. TEL 44-20-7396-8000, FAX 44-20-7396-8002.

613.7 USA
NATIONAL STRENGTH & CONDITIONING ASSOCIATION BULLETIN. Text in English. bi-m. membership. bk.rev. back issues avail. **Document type:** *Bulletin, Newsletter.* **Description:** Keeps readers informed about the latest products, current industry events, and upcoming conferences.
Related titles: Online - full text ed.
Indexed: Sportsearch (1986-).
Published by: (National Strength & Conditioning Association), Allen Press Inc., PO Box 1897, Lawrence, KS 66044-8897. nsca@iex.net, http://www.nsca-lift.org, http://www.nsca-lift.org/. Ed. Lori Marker. Adv. contact Kris Clark. Circ: 16,000.

613.7 USA
NATURAL BEAUTY & HEALTH. Variant title: Magical Blend's Natural Beauty & Health. Text in English. 2/yr. USD 3.99 newsstand/cover (effective 2001). **Document type:** *Magazine, Consumer.* **Description:** Focuses on today's hottest wellness trends as well as advice on healthy eating, great workouts, travel and much more.
Published by: M B Media, 133 1/2 Broadway, Chico, CA 95928. TEL 530-893-9037, FAX 530-893-9076, magical@magicalblend.com, http://www.nbhonline.com, http://www.magicalblend.com. **Dist. by:** International Publishers Direct, 674 Via de la Valle, Ste 200, Solana Beach, CA 92075. TEL 619-481-5928, FAX 619-259-7580.

613.7 USA ISSN 1071-555X
NATURAL BODYBUILDING AND FITNESS. Text in English. 1988. q. USD 12.90 (effective 1998). adv. **Document type:** *Consumer.*
Formerly (until 1993): Natural Physique (1044-6583)
Published by: Chelo Publishing Inc., Empire State Bldg, 50 Fifth Ave, New York, NY 10118. TEL 212-947-4322, FAX 212-563-4774. Ed., R&P Cheh N Low. Adv. contact Robert B Rose.

613.7 GBR
NATURAL CHOICE MAGAZINE. Text in English. 1993. bi-m. adv. **Document type:** *Consumer.*
Published by: Media Partners CPR, Northern Rock House, 20 Market Pl, Guisborough, Cleveland TS14 6HF, United Kingdom. TEL 44-1287-639111, FAX 44-1287-637201. Ed. Heather Welford. Adv. contact Susan Calvert. Circ: 150,000 (controlled).

790.1 GBR ISSN 1369-9385
NATURAL DEVELOPMENT. Text in English. 1997. m. GBP 2.50 newsstand/cover. adv. **Document type:** *Consumer.* **Description:** Contains recommendations and tips on how to train naturally and successfully.
Published by: Fitness Publications Ltd., 53 Lichfield Rd, Aston, Birmingham B6 5RW, United Kingdom. TEL 44-121-327-7525, FAX 44-121-327-0847, natural@fit-pubs.demon.co.uk. Ed., Pub. David McInerney. Adv. contact Jay Roe. **Dist. by:** M M C Ltd., Octagon House, White Hart Meadows, Ripley, Woking, Surrey GU23 6HR, United Kingdom. TEL 44-1483-211222, FAX 44-1483-224541.

NATURAL HEALTH. see *NUTRITION AND DIETETICS*

NATURAL HEALTH. see *ALTERNATIVE MEDICINE*

NATURAL HEALTH. see *ALTERNATIVE MEDICINE*

▼ **NATURAL HEALTH HOLLYWOOD.** see *ALTERNATIVE MEDICINE*

613 AUS
NATURAL HEALTH REVIEW. Text in English. 1998. bi-m. AUD 52.80 (effective 2001). adv. **Document type:** *Trade.*
Published by: Publishing Services (Australia) Pty. Ltd., 244 St Pauls Terrace, Fortitude Valley, Brisbane, QLD 4000, Australia. TEL 61-7-3854-1286, FAX 61-7-3252-4829, nhr@pubserv.com.au, http://www.nhr.com.au. adv.: B&W page AUD 3,440, color page AUD 4,920; trim 275 x 205. Circ: 10,866.

613.7 612.3 USA
NATURAL LAND NEWS. Text in English. w. free per issue. **Document type:** *Newsletter.* **Description:** Latest information on a wide range of natural living topics.
Media: Online - full text.
Published by: E G W Publishing Co., 1041 Shary Circle, Concord, CA 94518. TEL 925-671-9852, FAX 510-671-0692, hstevens@egw.com, http://www.naturalland.com/news.htm. Ed. Andrew Ligon.

613.7 USA
NATURAL MUSCLE MAGAZINE. Text in English. m. USD 19.95 (effective 1998). **Document type:** *Consumer.* **Description:** Information on all aspects of natural bodybuilding, training, weightlifting, and supplements.
Address: totalh@aol.com; natmuslmag@aol.com, http://www.naturalmuscle.net. Pub. Debbie Baigrie.

NATURAL REMEDIES. see *ALTERNATIVE MEDICINE*

613.194 ITA ISSN 0392-4173
NATURISMO; rivista naturista e umanitaria. Text in Italian. 1972. s-a. free per issue. bk.rev. **Description:** Covers gymnosophy, the philosophy of nudism, and nature and the unconscious being.
Published by: Unione Naturisti Italiani, Via Claudio Luigi Berthollet, 10, Turin, TO 10125, Italy. Ed. Gianfranco Ribolzi. Circ: 1,500.

NEBRASKA JOURNAL. see *EDUCATION*

613.7 ALB
NENA DHE FEMIJA. Text in Albanian. 3/yr.
Published by: Ministria e Shendetesise/Ministry of Health, Tirana, Albania. TELEX 4205.

613.7 USA
NEW BODY DIET AND EXERCISE. Text in English. 5/yr.
Published by: G C R Publishing Group, Inc., 1700 Broadway, 34th Fl, New York, NY 10019. TEL 212-541-7100, FAX 212-245-1241. Pub. Jason Goodman.

NEW LIFE; for those who are changing. see *NEW AGE PUBLICATIONS*

613.7 USA
NEW LIVING. Text in English. 1991. m. USD 12.95 (effective 2000). adv. bk.rev. **Document type:** *Newspaper.*
Published by: Christine Lynn Harvey, Ed. & Pub., PO Box 1519, Stony Brook, NY 11790. TEL 516-751-8819, FAX 516-751-8910, http://www.newliving.com. Ed., Pub., R&P Christine Lynn Harvey. Adv. contact Bill Stevens. B&W page USD 1,295. Circ: 100,000.

NEW OHIO JOURNAL. see *ENVIRONMENTAL STUDIES*

613.7 003.4 USA ISSN 1468-9928
▼ **THE NEW REVIEW OF HEALTH INFORMATICS.** Text in English. 2000. a. GBP 70, USD 130 per vol. (effective 2001). **Document type:** *Journal.* **Description:** Features a number of current issues and activities, and covers a wide range of issues, problems and techniques, Electronic Health Records, Patient Administration Systems online drug prescribing, hospital information management systems and more. Members of the Editorial Board come from medicine, nursing, medical science, IT and computing, health education and training, and health informatics.
Published by: Taylor Graham Publishing, 48 Regent St, Cambridge CB2 1FD, United Kingdom. http://www.taylorgraham.com/journals/nrhi.html. Ed. Michael Brittain.

613.2 IND ISSN 0029-070X
NISARG ANE AROGYA. Text in Gujarati. 1966. m. INR 3. adv. bk.rev.
Published by: S.A. Pandit, Ed. & Pub., Arya Kanya Gurukul, Rajwadi, Porbandar, Gujarat, India. Circ: 600.

613.7 USA ISSN 1081-8928
NORTHWEST HEALTH. Text in English. 1958. q. USD 12 (effective 2001). bk.rev. **Document type:** *Consumer.* **Description:** Covers health and fitness life-styles for western Washington State.
Formerly: View (Seattle) (0504-264X)
Related titles: Online - full text ed.
Published by: Group Health Cooperative, 521 Wall St, Seattle, WA 98121. TEL 206-448-5999, FAX 206-448-4010, nwhealth@ghc.org, http://www.ghc.org. Ed. Pat Bailey. Pub. Clarice Hutchison. Circ: 300,000 (controlled).

NURSING SPECTRUM - FLORIDA EDITION. see *MEDICAL SCIENCES—Nurses And Nursing*

NUTRIDATE. see *NUTRITION AND DIETETICS*

NUTRITION AND HEALTH. see *NUTRITION AND DIETETICS*

▼ **OBESITY.** see *MEDICAL SCIENCES*

OBESITY MATTERS. see *NUTRITION AND DIETETICS*

OBESITY RESEARCH. see *MEDICAL SCIENCES*

▼ **OBESITY REVIEWS.** see *NUTRITION AND DIETETICS*

▼ **OBESITY REVIEWS ONLINE.** see *NUTRITION AND DIETETICS*

OCCUPATIONAL HEALTH; a journal for the occupational health team. see *MEDICAL SCIENCES—Nurses And Nursing*

OESTERREICHISCHES JUGENDROTKREUZ. ARBEITSBLAETTER. see *SOCIAL SERVICES AND WELFARE*

OLYMPIAN'S NEWS. see *SPORTS AND GAMES*

OLYMPIC HEALTH NEWS (EDITION FRANCAISE). see *MEDICAL SCIENCES—Sports Medicine*

ONTARIO WRESTLER MAGAZINE. see *SPORTS AND GAMES*

613.7 ITA ISSN 1121-3264
OPTIMA SALUTE. Text in Italian. 1990. m. (10/yr.). ITL 25,000. **Document type:** *Consumer.*
Published by: Editoriale Optima s.r.l., Largo Augusto, 8, Milan, MI 20122, Italy. TEL 39-2-76017397, FAX 39-2-76014959. Ed. Giacomo Casarotto. adv.: B&W page ITL 9,450,000, color page ITL 14,000,000. Circ: 245,000.

ORTOPEDICI E SANITARI. see *MEDICAL SCIENCES—Orthopedics And Traumatology*

362.6 USA ISSN 1078-5035
OVER 50 AND FIT; life before 50 is the warm-up. Text in English. 1995. m. USD 29. bk.rev. back issues avail. **Document type:** *Newsletter.* **Description:** Covers health and fitness topics for older adults, including medical, dietary and exercise related questions.
Published by: Newsletter Publishers Association, 1202 E Pike St, Ste 740, Seattle, WA 98122-9917. TEL 800-527-6240, FAX 506-527-6651, fiftyfit@aol.com. Ed. Karissa D Collins. Pub. Alan A Cooper.

PELIZZA'S POSITIVE PRINCIPLES FOR BETTER LIVING. see *PSYCHOLOGY*

613.7 612.3 USA
PERSONAL CARE NEWS. Text in English. fortn. free per issue. **Document type:** *Newsletter.*
Media: Online - full text.
Published by: E G W Publishing Co., 1041 Shary Circle, Concord, CA 94518. TEL 925-671-9852, FAX 510-671-0692, hstevens@egw.com, http://www.naturalland.com/pcv/pcnc.htm.

613.7 USA ISSN 0738-7857
PERSONAL FITNESS. Text in English. 1983. m. USD 67 (effective 2001). bk.rev. abstr, charts, illus. back issues avail.
Published by: (Personal Fitness Consultants), Cromwell - Sloan Publishing Company, 63 Vine Rd, Stamford, CT 06905-2012. TEL 203-323-4810. Ed. Paul Sloan. Circ: 32,000.

613.7 USA ISSN 1520-8397
PHYSICAL. Text in English. 1998. m. USD 15.98 (effective 2000). adv. **Document type:** *Magazine, Consumer.* **Description:** Provides information and motivation for high-energy activities and sports nutrition.

P

Published by: Franklin Publications (Subsidiary of: Basic Media Group), 320 N Larchmont Blvd, 3rd Fl, Box 74908, Los Angeles, CA 90004. TEL 323-469-3901, 800-388-1979, FAX 323-469-9597, http://www.physicalmag.com.

▼ **PHYSICAL & MENTAL ISSUES IN AGING SOURCEBOOK.** see *MEDICAL SCIENCES*

615.8 DEU ISSN 0031-9392
PHYSIOTHERAPIE. Text in German. 1909. m. DEM 115 (effective 1996). adv. bk.rev. charts. index. **Document type:** *Bulletin.*
Formerly: Fachblatt der Physikalischen Therapie
—GNLM.
Published by: (Verband Deutscher Badebetriebe e.V.), Ebert Verlag GmbH, Blankenseer Str 6-8, Luebeck 23562, Germany. TEL 49-451-501011, FAX 49-4509-2241. Ed. Hans Juergen Ebert. Circ: 9,500.

613 GBR ISSN 1356-3963
POSITIVE HEALTH; integrated medicine for the 21st century. Text in English. 1994. m. GBP 36; GBP 3.50 newsstand/cover; GBP 75 foreign (effective 2000). adv. bk.rev. back issues avail. **Document type:** *Magazine, Consumer, Academic/Scholarly, Trade.* **Description:** Features news and articles on alternative healing, including such methods as nutrition, massage, acupressure techniques, aromatheraphy.
Related titles: CD-ROM ed.; Online - full text ed.
Indexed: CINAHL.
Published by: Positive Health Publications Ltd., 1 Queen Sq, Bristol BS1 4JQ, United Kingdom. TEL 44-117-983-8851, FAX 44-117-908-0097, admin@positivehealth.com, http://www.positivehealth.com. Ed., R&P Dr. Sandra Goodman. Adv. contact Mike Howell. color page GBP 800. **Dist. by:** Diamond Magazine Distribution Ltd., Unit 7, Rother Ironworks, Fishmarket Rd, Rye, E Sussex TN31 7LR, United Kingdom. TEL 44-1797-225229, FAX 44-1797-225657.

P

613 USA ISSN 0032-8006
RA421 CODEN: PRVEAT
PREVENTION; the magazine for better health. Text in English. 1950. m. USD 15.94 domestic; CND 23.97 in Canada; USD 1.99 newsstand/cover (effective 2001). adv. bk.rev. illus. index. reprint service avail. from PQC. **Document type:** *Magazine, Consumer.* **Description:** Reports on new developments in nutrition, preventive medicine, fitness, natural living and drugless therapies. Emphasis is on practicality and self-improvement.
Related titles: Microform ed.: (from PQC); Online - full text ed.: (from ProQuest Information & Learning, Gale Group); ♦ Esperanto ed.: Prevention en Espanol. ISSN 1529-370X.
Indexed: CHNI, Can.Per.Ind. (Jun.1999-), Environ.Per.Bibl., Gen.Sci.Ind. (Jun.1992-), Hlth.Ind., Jun.High Mag.Abstr., Mag.Ind., PMR, R.G. (Jan.1984-), R.G.Abstr. (Jan.1984-).
—GNLM, IDS, ingenta, Linda Hall.
Published by: Rodale, 33 E Minor St, Emmaus, PA 18098. TEL 610-967-5171, FAX 610-967-7725, 212-297-1531, TELEX 847338, prevention@rodalepress.com, customer_service@rodale.com, http://www.prevention.com. Ed. Anne Alexander. Pub. Barb Newton. adv.: B&W page USD 74,360, color page USD 86,790; trim 7.44 x 5.25. Circ: 3,000,000. **Subscr. to:** PO Box 7319, Red Oak, IA 51591-7319.

613.7 USA
PREVENTION WEIGHT LOSS. Text in English. a. adv. **Document type:** *Consumer.*
Published by: Rodale, 33 E Minor St, Emmaus, PA 18098. TEL 610-967-5171, FAX 610-967-7725.

PRIME TIMES MAGAZINE (MADISON). see *CONSUMER EDUCATION AND PROTECTION*

613.7 RUS
PROFILAKTIKA ZABOLEVANII I UKREPLENIE ZDOROVIA/DISEASES PREVENTION AND HEALTH PROMOTION. Text in Russian. 1997. bi-m. RUR 216 for 6 mos. to individuals; RUR 450 for 6 mos. to institutions (effective 2002).
Published by: Media Sfera, Dmitrovskoe shosse 46, korp 2, etazh 4, P.O. Box 54, Moscow 127238, Russian Federation. TEL 7-095-4824329, FAX 7-095-4824312, mediashp@mediasphera.ru.

PROGRESS IN OBESITY RESEARCH (YEAR). see *MEDICAL SCIENCES*

PROMOTION & EDUCATION; international journal of health promotion and education. see *PUBLIC HEALTH AND SAFETY*

PSYCHOLOGY AND SOCIOLOGY OF SPORT: CURRENT SELECTED RESEARCH. see *PSYCHOLOGY*

▼ **PSYCHOLOGY OF SPORT & EXERCISE.** see *PSYCHOLOGY*

PUERTO RICO. DEPARTMENT OF HEALTH. BOLETIN ESTADISTICO. see *PUBLIC HEALTH AND SAFETY—Abstracting, Bibliographies, Statistics*

PUERTO RICO. DEPARTMENT OF HEALTH. INFORME ESTADISTICO DE FACILIDADES DE SALUD. see *HEALTH FACILITIES AND ADMINISTRATION*

613.7 CHE ISSN 1424-6082
PULS-DOSSIER. Text in German. 1996. irreg. CHF 28 newsstand/cover. **Document type:** *Consumer.*
Published by: K I Media GmbH, Hottingerstr 12, Postfach 75, Zurich 8024, Switzerland. TEL 41-1-2661717, FAX 41-1-2661700, redaktion@puls-tip.ch, http://www.puls-tip.ch/pulstip/PDossier/PDos.html, http://www.ki-media.ch. Adv. contact Yvonne Mueller.

613.7 CHE ISSN 1424-6090
PULS-TIP. Text in German. 1994. 11/yr. CHF 24; CHF 2.90 newsstand/cover (effective 2000). adv. **Document type:** *Magazine, Consumer.* **Description:** Contains articles and features on maintaining a healthy lifestyle.
Published by: K I Media GmbH, Hottingerstr 12, Postfach 75, Zurich 8024, Switzerland. TEL 41-1-2661717, FAX 41-1-2661700, redaktion@puls-tip.ch, http://www.puls-tip.ch, http://www.ki-media.ch. Ed. Tobias Frey. Adv. contact Yvonne Mueller. B&W page CHF 7,995, color page CHF 10,800; trim 209 x 287. Circ: 140,763 (paid).

PUNJAB MEDICAL JOURNAL. see *MEDICAL SCIENCES*

613.7 CHN ISSN 1000-825X
QIGONG. Text in Chinese. m. **Document type:** *Academic/Scholarly.*
Published by: Zhejiang-sheng Zhongyiyao Yanjiuyuan/Zhejiang Academy of Traditional Chinese Medicine, Tianmushan Lu 26 Hao, Hangzhou, Zhejiang 310007, China. TEL 86-571-8842882, FAX 86-571-8845196. Ed. Shen Hancheng.

613.7 CHN
QINGCHUN YU JIANKANG/YOUTH AND HEALTH. Text in Chinese. 1985. m. CNY 7.20.
Published by: (Shanghai Shi Weisheng Jiaoyu-guan/Shanghai Health Education Institute), Qingchun yu Jiankang Zazhishe, 394 Zhoushan Lu, Shanghai 200082, China. TEL 5460177. Ed. Hu Jinhua. Circ: 200,000.

QINGSHAONIAN YU JIANKANG/YOUTH AND HEALTH. see *CHILDREN AND YOUTH—About*

613.85 USA
QUIT SMOKING REPORT EZINE. Text in English. 1998. bi-m. back issues avail. **Document type:** *Newsletter.* **Description:** Contains quit smoking tips, encouragement, success stories from other smokers, questions, pleas for help, plus information about products on how to quit smoking.
Media: Online - full text.
Published by: Quit Smoking Company, 3675 Glennvale Court, Cummings, GA 30041. TEL 770-346-9222, FAX 770-475-5007, info@quitsmoking.com, http://www.quitsmoking.com/ezine/index.htm.

RADIANCE ONLINE; the magazine for large women. see *WOMEN'S INTERESTS*

613 DEU ISSN 1438-2865
RATGEBER AUS IHRER APOTHEKE. Text in German. 1922. s-m. free. adv. bk.rev. illus. **Document type:** *Magazine, Consumer.*
Former titles (until 1999): Ratgeber aus der Apotheke (0722-9062); (until 1972): Ratgeber fuer Kranke und Gesunde (0033-9997)
Published by: Gebr. Storck GmbH, Bebelstr 102, Oberhausen 46049, Germany. TEL 49-208-848020, FAX 49-208-8480242. Ed. Wilhelm Doe. adv.: page DEM 42,000. Circ: 1,653,990 (paid and free).

613 NPL
RE PRODUCTIONS. Text in English. irreg. back issues avail. **Document type:** *Newsletter.* **Description:** Dedicated to disseminating work by scholars, activists, and organizations exploring discourses of reproductive health and rights in South Asia.
Media: Online - full text.
Published by: Joshi /Sushma, Ed., PO Box 140, Kathmandu, Nepal. http://www.hsph.harvard.edu/Organizations/healthnet/SAsia/frontpage.html. Ed. Joshi Shusma.

RECRUITMENT DIRECTIONS. see *OCCUPATIONS AND CAREERS*

613.7 610 USA
REMEDY MAGAZINE; prescriptions for a healthy life. Text in English. 1992. bi-m.
Published by: Remedy, Inc., 120 Post Rd W, Westport, CT 06880. Ed. Shari Miller Sims. Circ: 2,200,000.

613.7 USA ISSN 0270-1367
GV201 CODEN: RQESD4
RESEARCH QUARTERLY FOR EXERCISE AND SPORT. Text in English. 1930. q. USD 175 in US & Canada to institutions; USD 42 newsstand/cover (effective 2001). adv. bibl, charts, illus. index, cum.index every 10 yrs.: 1930-1969 (in 4 vols.). reprint service avail. from PQC,SCH,PSC,ISI. *Refereed.* **Document type:** *Academic/Scholarly.* **Description:** Includes research articles in the art and science of human movement that lead to the development of theory or the application of new techniques.
Formerly (until 1980): American Alliance for Health, Physical Education and Recreation. Research Quarterly (0034-5377)
Related titles: Microform ed.: (from PMC); ISSN 0364-9857 (from PQC); Online - full text ed.: (from Gale Group, ProQuest Information & Learning, Factiva, Institute for Scientific Information).
Indexed: AMED, ASCA, AgeLine, Arts & Hum.Cit.Ind. (coverage dropped), Biol.Abstr., C.I.J.E., Curr.Cont., Educ.Ind. (Jun.1983-), Ergon.Abstr., Excerp.Med., Focus on: Sports Sci.& Med., IBZ, Ind.Med. (1980-), Inpharma, NRN, Pharm.&Out.News, Phys.Ed.Ind., Psychol.Abstr., Reac., Russ.Acad.Sci.Bibl., SSCI, Sportsearch (1980-).
—BLDSC (7759.172000), GNLM, ingenta, KNAW.
Published by: American Alliance for Health, Physical Education, Recreation, and Dance, 1900 Association Dr, Reston, VA 20191-1599. TEL 703-476-3484, 800-213-7193, FAX 703-476-9527, info@aahperd.org, http://www.aahperd.org/aahperd/publications-qes.html. Eds. Amy Maurer, T Gilmore Reeve. Circ: 8,000.

REVISTA CUBANA DE HIGIENE Y EPIDEMIOLOGIA. see *PUBLIC HEALTH AND SAFETY*

REVISTA DE EDUCACAO FISICA. see *EDUCATION—Teaching Methods And Curriculum*

613 610 ROM ISSN 1220-1146
RA523.R8 CODEN: IGIBA5
REVISTA DE IGIENA, BACTERIOLOGIE, VIRUSOLOGIE, PARAZITOLOGIE, PNEUMOFTIZIOLOGIE. IGIENA. Text in Romanian; Summaries in English, French, German, Russian. 1952. 4/yr. USD 20. adv. bk.rev. abstr, bibl, charts, illus.
Indexed: Biol.Abstr., Chem.Abstr., Nutr.Abstr.
—CISTI.
Published by: Uniunea Societatilor de Stiinte Medicale din Rumania, Str. Progresului 8, Bucharest 70754, Romania. **Subscr. to:** ILEXIM, Str. 13 Decembrie 3, PO Box 136-137, Bucharest 70116, Romania.

613 ITA ISSN 0035-6921
RA421 CODEN: RIIGAV
RIVISTA ITALIANA D'IGIENE. Text in Italian; Summaries in English, Italian. 1965 (vol.25). bi-m. ITL 100,000; ITL 120,000 foreign (effective 1996). adv. bibl, charts, illus, stat. index. **Document type:** *Academic/Scholarly.*
Indexed: Abstr.Hyg., Biol.Abstr., Chem.Abstr., Chem.Titles, Excerp.Med., INIS Atomind., Nutr.Abstr., Ref.Zh., Trop.Dis.Bull.
—CASDDS, CISTI, GNLM.
Published by: Nistri-Lischi Editori, Via Ventiquattro Maggio, 28, Pisa, PI 56123, Italy. TEL 39-50-563371, FAX 39-50-562726. Ed. Giuseppe Armani. Adv. contact Giuseppe Caroli.

ROBERT WOOD JOHNSON FOUNDATION. ANNUAL REPORT. see *MEDICAL SCIENCES*

RODALE'S FITNESS SWIMMER; technique - nutrition - workouts. see *SPORTS AND GAMES*

613.7 GBR ISSN 1360-497X
ROSEMARY CONLEY DIET & FITNESS. Text in English. 1996. bi-m. GBP 1.90 newsstand/cover. **Document type:** *Consumer.* **Description:** Promotes health and well-being through special exercise and diet plans and examples. Includes special interest stories, celebrity interviews, entertainment articles, and fashion spreads.

Published by: Quorn House Publishing Ltd., Quorn House, Meeting St, Quorn, Leics LE12 8EX, United Kingdom. TEL 44-1509-620444, FAX 44-1509-620555. Circ: 161,007 (paid). **Dist. by:** Comag, Tavistock Works, Tavistock Rd, W Drayton, Middx UB7 7QX, United Kingdom. TEL 44-1895-444055, FAX 44-1895-433602.

ROYAL SOCIETY FOR THE PROMOTION OF HEALTH. JOURNAL. see *SOCIAL SERVICES AND WELFARE*

613.2 USA ISSN 0898-5162
RUNNING & FITNEWS. Text in English. 1983. m. USD 25 to members; USD 40 to libraries (effective 2001). bk.rev. charts, illus. index. back issues avail.; reprints avail. *Refereed.* **Document type:** *Newsletter.* **Description:** Dedicated to helping runners and recreational athletes get the most from their exercise program by providing information on exercise, nutrition, training, sports medicine, injury prevention and long-term health.
Former titles (until 1984): Running and Fitness; Jogger (0164-694X)
Indexed: CINAHL, Sportsearch (1984-).
Published by: American Running Association, 4405 East West Hwy, Ste 405, Bethesda, MD 20814. TEL 301-913-9517, FAX 301-913-9520, run@americanrunning.org, http:// www.americanrunning.org. Ed. Carol Newman. R&P Susan Kalish. Circ: 15,000 (paid); 20,000 (controlled).

S T A P S; Review STAPS & bulletin de Liaison. (Sciences et Techniques des Activites Physiques et Sportives) see *MEDICAL SCIENCES—Sports Medicine*

613.7 305.86 USA ISSN 1527-0440
LA SALUD HISPANA; previniendo enfermedades. Text in English, Spanish. 1994. bi-m. USD 12.99; USD 1.95 newsstand/cover (effective 2001). adv. *Refereed.* **Document type:** *Magazine, Consumer.* **Description:** Promotes good health and disease prevention among people in the Spanish-speaking community.
Published by: La Salud Hispana, Inc., 225 Broadway, Ste 3009, New York, NY 10007. TEL 212-791-7177, 888-887-2583, FAX 201-568-9023, editor@lasaludhispana.com, http:// www.lasaludhispana.com. Ed., Pub. Dr. Rodrigo Cardenas. Adv. contact Alberto Colagreco. B&W page USD 4,124, color page USD 5,500; trim 8.125 x 10.812. Circ: 35,000 (paid); 65,000 (controlled).

▼ **SALUTE NATURALE**; la nuova via del vivere bene. see *ALTERNATIVE MEDICINE*

613.7 FRA ISSN 0397-0329
SANTE MAGAZINE. Text in French. 1976. m. FRF 165; FRF 18 newsstand/cover (effective 2000). adv. **Document type:** *Magazine, Consumer.* **Description:** Offers short articles and advice on every day health issues.
Address: 110 rue Marius-Aufan, BP 318, Levallois-Perret Cedex 92304, France. TEL 33-1-41494149, FAX 33-1-40890430, direction@santemagazine.fr, http://www.santemagazine.fr. Ed. Christine Vilet. Pub. Andre Giovanni. adv.: B&W page FRF 101,500, color page FRF 132,000; trim 205 x 280. Circ: 418,555.

SATURDAY EVENING POST. see *GENERAL INTEREST PERIODICALS—United States*

SCHLANK UND FIT. see *NUTRITION AND DIETETICS*

SCRIPPS CLINIC PERSONAL HEALTH LETTER. see *MEDICAL SCIENCES*

614.8 USA ISSN 1068-1930
SEARCH FOR HEALTH. Text in English. m.
Published by: U.S. National Institutes of Health, News Branch, Bldg 31, Rm 28 10, Bethesda, MD 20892. TEL 301-496-2535. Ed. Helen Ou.

SEX & HEALTH. see *MEN'S HEALTH*

SHANDONG TIYU XUEYUAN XUEBAO/SHANDONG PHYSICAL EDUCATION INSTITUTE. JOURNAL. see *EDUCATION—Teaching Methods And Curriculum*

SHAPE. see *WOMEN'S HEALTH*

SHAPE. see *WOMEN'S HEALTH*

▼ **SHAPE SOUTH AFRICA.** see *WOMEN'S HEALTH*

613.7 362.41 GBR
SHAPING UP. Text in English. m. GBP 18 (effective 2000). **Document type:** *Consumer.* **Description:** Gives information about health and fitness, with health news, product reviews, articles on alternative therapies, and tips on keeping in shape.
Media: Braille. **Related titles:** Diskette ed.
Published by: Royal National Institute for the Blind, 224 Great Portland St, London W1N 6AA, United Kingdom. FAX 44-1733-371555, webmaster @rnib.org.uk, cservices@rnib.org.uk, webmaster@rnib.org.uk, http://www.rnib.org.uk. **Subscr. to:** RNIB Customer Services, PO Box 173, Peterborough, Cambs PE2 6WS, United Kingdom. TEL 44-1733-370777.

613.972 JPN ISSN 0037-4113
SHONI HOKEN KENKYU/JOURNAL OF CHILD HEALTH. Text in Japanese. 1933. bi-m. bk.rev. stat. index.
Published by: Nihon Shoni Hoken Kenkyukai/Japanese Society of Child Health, 1-12 Kata-Machi, Shinjuku-ku, Tokyo 160-0001, Japan.

SIMPLY BETTER. see *LIFESTYLE*

613.2 AUS
▼ **SIMPLYLITE**; low-fat food - no-fuss fitness. Text in English. 2001. q. AUD 4.95 newsstand/cover (effective 2002). adv. **Document type:** *Magazine, Consumer.* **Description:** Devoted to delicious low-fat recipes along with health and fitness advice.
Published by: A C P Publishing Pty. Ltd., 54-58 Park St, Sydney, NSW 1028, Australia. TEL 61-2-9282-8000, FAX 61-2-9267-4361, info@acp.com.au, http://www.acp.com.au. Ed. Sue Wannan. Adv. contact Patricia Connolly. Circ: 33,384 (paid and controlled).

613.7 USA ISSN 1058-2940
SLIM & FIT DIET & EXERCISE. Text in English. 1989. q. USD 3.99 newsstand/cover; CND 4.95 newsstand/cover in Canada; GBP 2.50 newsstand/cover in United Kingdom. **Document type:** *Consumer.* **Description:** features articles on exercise, diets, exercise machines, and nutrition.
Published by: Harris Publications, Inc., 1115 Broadway, New York, NY 10010. TEL 212-807-7100.

SLIMMER. see *NUTRITION AND DIETETICS*

SLIMMING. see *NUTRITION AND DIETETICS*

613 USA
SMOKING AND HEALTH NEWSLETTER* . Text in English. 1965. q. free per issue.
Media: Duplicated (not offset).
Published by: National Interagency Council on Smoking and Health, 7320 Greenville Ave, Dallas, TX 75231. TEL 214-750-5359. Ed. Robert E Wallace. Circ: 10,000.

613.7 USA ISSN 1088-7482
SO YOUNG!; dedicated to a youthful body, mind and spirit. Text in English. 1996. bi-m. USD 35 in US & Canada (effective 2001). adv. bk.rev., music rev. illus. 12 p./no. back issues avail. **Document type:** *Newsletter, Consumer.* **Description:** Informs on holistic self-help, cutting-edge, and anti-aging information. Covers all aspects of anti-aging: beauty, diet, nutrition, hormone replacement therapy, exercise, and medical breakthroughs.
Published by: Anti-Aging Press, Inc., PO Box 141489, Coral Gables, FL 33114. TEL 305-662-3928, FAX 305-661-4123, julia2@gate.net. Ed., R&P Julia M Busch. Circ: 500 (paid); 500 (controlled).

613 USA ISSN 0147-5231
SOMATICS; magazine - journal of the mind - body arts and sciences. Text in English. 1976. s-a. USD 20 domestic to individuals; USD 27 in Canada & Mexico to individuals; USD 33 elsewhere to individuals; USD 25 domestic to institutions (effective 2001). adv. bk.rev. back issues avail. **Description:** Publishes articles for professionals and laypersons in the mind and body field. Covers issues relating to holistic health care, fitness, movement, dance, psychology and philosophy.
Indexed: Psychol.Abstr., Sociol.Abstr., e-psyche.
—GNLM.
Published by: Novato Institute for Somatic Research and Training, 1516 Grant Avenue, Ste 212, Novato, CA 94945. TEL 415-892-0617, http://www.somaticsed.com. Ed. Eleanor Criswell Hanna TEL 415-897-0336. Circ: 1,300.

613.7 DEU ISSN 1437-1057
SPA; das Wellness Magazin. Text in German. q. DEM 4 newsstand/cover (effective 2000). adv. **Document type:** *Magazine, Consumer.* **Description:** Covers all aspects of producing and maintaining good health through nutrition, exercise and well-being.
Published by: AMIGO Verlag GmbH und Co KG, Postfach 1409, Roesrath 51495, Germany. TEL 49-2205-911240, FAX 49-2205-911241, spa.news@amigo-verlag.de, http://www.spa-magazin.de. Ed. Ingo Loehmer.

613.7 910.09 USA
SPA FINDER. Text in English. 1987. q. USD 17.95; USD 5.95 newsstand/cover (effective 2001). adv. maps. **Document type:** *Magazine, Consumer.* **Description:** Contains information on the world's great spas and fitness resorts for health, fitness and beauty enthusiasts.
Published by: Spa Finders - Travel Arrangements Ltd., 91 Fifth Ave, New York, NY 10003-3039. TEL 212-924-6800, FAX 212-924-7240, allspas@spafinders.com, http://www.spafinders.com. Ed. Frank Van Patten. Pubs. Frank Van Patten, Jed Horowitz. Adv. contact Jed Horowitz. B&W page USD 9,500, color page USD 9,900; trim 10.75 x 8.5. Circ: 150,000.

613.7 362.41 GBR
SPECTRUM (PETERBOROUGH). Text in English. m. **Document type:** *Consumer.* **Description:** Tackles fitness and diet, along with other subjects concerning the well-being of individuals with visual impairments.
Media: Braille. **Related titles:** Diskette ed.
Published by: Royal National Institute for the Blind, PO Box 173, Peterborough, Cambs PE2 6WX, United Kingdom. TEL 44-1733-3707777, FAX 44-1733-238-541, http://www.rnib.org.uk.

P

613.7 DEU ISSN 0171-6298
SPIRIDON LAUFMAGAZIN. Text in German. 1975. m. DEM 75. adv. bk.rev. illus. index. back issues avail. **Document type:** *Consumer.*
Published by: Spiridon Verlags GmbH, Dorfstr 18 a, Erkrath 40699, Germany. TEL 49-211-726364, FAX 49-211-786823. Ed., Pub. Manfred Steffny. Adv. contact Christian Stanetzek. Circ: 17,000.

SPIRITUALITY & HEALTH; the soul body connection. see *ALTERNATIVE MEDICINE*

SPLASH! (COLORADO SPRINGS). see *SPORTS AND GAMES*

SPORT & MEDICINA. see *MEDICAL SCIENCES—Sports Medicine*

SPORTS MEDICINE ALERT; the clinician's practical guide to diagnosis, treatment, rehabilitation and prevention of injury and disease. see *MEDICAL SCIENCES—Sports Medicine*

SPORTS MEDICINE BULLETIN. see *MEDICAL SCIENCES—Sports Medicine*

613.17 USA
ST. PATRICK HOSPITAL MESSENGER. Text in English. 1979. m. free per issue. back issues avail. **Document type:** *Newsletter.* **Description:** Health issues forum for consumers.
Published by: St. Patrick Hospital, 500 W Broadway, Box 4587, Missoula, MT 59806. TEL 406-543-7271, FAX 406-543-6836. Ed. Joann Hoven. Circ: 6,000.

613.7 USA ISSN 1524-1602
GV514
STRENGTH AND CONDITIONING JOURNAL. Abbreviated title: S & C. Text in English. 1979. bi-m. USD 90 domestic to institutions; USD 98 foreign to institutions (effective 2001). adv. bk.rev. charts, illus, stat. Index. back issues avail.; reprints avail. *Refereed.* **Document type:** *Academic/Scholarly.* **Description:** Focuses on resistance training, conditioning, sports science and medicine and current issues in strength and conditioning.
Former titles (until 1999): Strength and Conditioning (1073-6840); (until 1994): N S C A Journal (1073-2721); (until 1992): National Strength and Conditioning Journal (0744-0049); (until 1981): National Strength Coaches Association Journal (0199-610X)
Related titles: Online - full text ed.: (from Institute for Scientific Information).
Indexed: ASCA, CINAHL, Focus on: Sports Sci.& Med., IBZ, Phys.Ed.Ind., Sportsearch (1981-).
—BLDSC, IDS, ingenta. **CCC.**

Published by: (National Strength and Conditioning Association), Allen Press Inc., PO Box 1897, Lawrence, KS 66044-8897. TEL 785-843-1235, 800-627-0932, FAX 785-843-1274, 785-843-1853, nsca@allenpress.com, nsca@ncsa-lift.org, http://www.nsca-lift.org, http://www.nsca-lift.org/. Ed. Jeff Chandler. Pub. Theresa Pickel. R&P Harvey Newton. Adv. contact Kris Clark. B&W page USD 900, color page USD 600; trim 11 x 8.5. Circ: 17,420 (paid).

613.7 POL ISSN 0867-1079
STUDIES IN PHYSICAL CULTURE AND TOURISM. Text in English. 1990. a. PLZ 60 domestic; USD 20 foreign (effective 2000). bk.rev. back issues avail. **Document type:** *Academic/Scholarly.* **Description:** Generally contains works on humanistic subjects connected with physical education, sports and tourism and is aimed at physical education teachers and specialists in the area of physical culture or qualified sports.
Published by: Akademia Wychowania Fizycznego w Poznaniu/University School of Physical Education in Poznan, Ul Krolowej Jadwigi 27-39, Poznan 61871, Poland. TEL 48-61-8355202, FAX 48-61-8330087. Ed. Wojciech Liponski. R&P Michal Bronikowski. Circ: 120 (paid); 80 (controlled).

612.044 790.072 ZAF ISSN 0379-9069
SUID-AFRIKAANSE TYDSKRIF VIR NAVORSING IN SPORT, LIGGAAMLIKE OPVOEDKUNDE EN ONTSPANNING/SOUTH AFRICAN JOURNAL FOR RESEARCH IN SPORT, PHYSICAL EDUCATION AND RECREATION. Text in Afrikaans, English; Summaries in English. 1978. s-a. ZAR 40 (effective 1993). bk.rev. back issues avail. **Document type:** *Academic/Scholarly.* **Description:** Aimed at scientists involved in the areas of physical fitness, sport, sports medicine, movement education and recreation.
Indexed: Ind.S.A.Per., Sport Fish.Abstr., Sportsearch (1980-).
—BLDSC (8053.668500).
Published by: Southern African Federation for Movement and Leisure Sciences, PO Box 13206, Clubview 0014, South Africa. TEL 27-12-6633290, FAX 27-12-6633294. Ed. B C Andrews. Circ: 600.

SWIMMING POOLS TODAY. see *SPORTS AND GAMES—Outdoor Life*

613.7 USA
SYRACUSE HEALTH & FITNESS✶. Text in English. m.
Address: Syracuse, NY 13206-1103. TEL 315-635-3921. Ed. Dave Grieves.

613.7 USA ISSN 0889-0846
T A H P E R D JOURNAL. Text in English. 1954. 3/yr. USD 39 to individuals; USD 50 to institutions (effective 2000). adv. *Refereed.* **Document type:** *Academic/Scholarly.*
Indexed: Sportsearch (1983-).
Published by: Texas Association for Health, Physical Education, Recreation and Dance, 6300 La Calma Dr, 100, Austin, TX 78752. TEL 512-459-1299, FAX 512-459-1290, http://www.tahperd.sfasu.org, http://www.tahperd.org. Ed., R&P Quentin A Christian. Adv. contact Lee James. Circ: 5,000.

613.7 DEU
▼ **T Z GESUNDHEITSM@GAZIN.** (TagesZeitung) Text in German. 2000. fortn. adv. **Document type:** *Magazine, Consumer.* **Description:** Contains information and advice on better health and how to lead a more active lifestyle.
Published by: Gesundheitsmedien GmbH & Co. KG, Herriotstr 3, Frankfurt Am Main 60528, Germany. TEL 49-69-95633-0, FAX 49-69-95633333, info@gesundheitsmedien.de, http://www.gesundheitsmedien.de. Ed. Klaus Rehnig. Pub. Karl Dieter Greese. Adv. contact Natalie Groppler. B&W page DEM 106,333, color page DEM 159,500; trim 230 x 290. Circ: 5,531,167 (controlled).

613.85 FRA
TABAC ET SANTE; tabagisme. Text in French. 1970. q. FRF 50. adv. bk.rev.
Published by: (Comite National Contre le Tabagisme), Nouvelles Editions Touristiques et Artistiques, 19 rue Bergere, Paris 75009, France. Ed. J P Lejard. Circ: 3,000.

TAI CHI & ALTERNATIVE HEALTH. see *ORIENTAL STUDIES*

TAL OG DATA, MEDICIN OG SUNDHEDSVAESEN/ FACTS, MEDICINE AND HEALTH CARE, DENMARK. see *PHARMACY AND PHARMACOLOGY*

613.7 USA ISSN 0890-1597
TENNESSEE JOURNAL OF HEALTH, PHYSICAL EDUCATION, RECREATION AND DANCE. Text in English. 196?. s-a.
Indexed: Phys.Ed.Ind., Sportsearch.
Published by: Tennessee Association of Health, Physical Education, Recreation and Dance, Peabody College of Vanderbilt University, Box 513, Nashville, TN 37203.

613.7 ITA
TERME EUROPA; mensile di turismo, salute, bellezza e vacanze - benessere. Text in Italian. 1991. m. (10/yr.). ITL 40,000; ITL 70,000 foreign. adv. back issues avail. **Document type:** *Consumer.* **Description:** Deals with spas, health and tourism, with medical information about hydrological and spa treatments.
Published by: Gestione Periodici Riuniti, Residenza Mestieri Milano Due, Segrate, MI 20090, Italy. TEL 39-2-26413274, FAX 39-2-26413409. Ed. Giorgio Pozzani. R&P Franco Bomprezzi. Adv. contact Marco Zulberti. B&W page ITL 3,200,000, color page ITL 5,300,000; trim 275 x 210. Circ: 73,000.

TIYU KEYAN/SPORTS SCIENCE RESEARCH. see *MEDICAL SCIENCES—Sports Medicine*

613.7 USA
TO YOUR GOOD HEALTH; a health care newsletter. Text in English. 1993. q. free per issue. adv. illus. **Document type:** *Newspaper.* **Description:** Covers general health care information.
Published by: Larry Fox Associates, Inc., PO Box 918, Dennis, MA 02638. TEL 508-790-2761, FAX 508-771-3745, lFox@ma.ultranet.com, http://www.capecod.com/goodhealth. Ed., Pub., R&P Larry Fox. Adv. contact Jane Cushman. page USD 4,200; trim 170 x 110. Circ: 120,000. **Co-sponsor:** Cape Cod Healthcare, Inc.

613.7 USA
▼ **TODAY'S HEALTH AND WELLNESS.** Text in English. 2000. bi-m. USD 20 (effective 2001). adv. 80 p./no. back issues avail. **Document type:** *Consumer.* **Description:** Provides information for men & women who take an active role in maximizing the quality of life for themselves and family, featuring special report pull-out section.
Published by: North American Media Group, Inc., 12301 Whitewater Dr, Ste 260, Minnetonka, MN 55343. TEL 952-936-9333, FAX 952-936-9169, http://www.healthandwellnessclub.com/. Ed. Claire Lewis. Pub., Adv. contact Lee Sarles. color page USD 6,250. Circ: 125,000 (paid).

TOKYO JIKEIKAI IKA DAIGAKU TAIRYOKU IGAKU KENKYUSHITSU NENPO/JIKEI UNIVERSITY. SCHOOL OF MEDICINE. ANNUAL REPORT OF LABORATORY SPORTS MEDICINE. see *MEDICAL SCIENCES—Sports Medicine*

613.7 ITA
TOP SALUTE. Text in Italian. 1993. m. (10/yr.). ITL 40,000; ITL 100,000 foreign. adv. **Document type:** *Consumer.*
Published by: Alberto Peruzzo Editore s.r.l., Via Marelli, 165, Sesto San Giovanni, MI 20099, Italy. TEL 39-2-242021. Ed. Nadia Gelmi. adv.: B&W page ITL 6,000,000, color page ITL 7,000,000.

613.7 NLD ISSN 1381-1770
TOP SANTE. Text in Dutch. 1994. m. adv. illus. back issues avail. **Document type:** *Magazine, Consumer.* **Description:** Offers health and fitness tips.
Published by: V N U Tijdschriften B.V., Postbus 1900, Hoofddorp 2130 JH, Netherlands. TEL 31-23-556-6770, FAX 31-23-556-6771, ServiceTeam@tijdschriften.vnu.com, www.vnu.nl/vnu/organisatie/t373.html, http://www.vnu.nl.

613.2 USA
TOPS NEWS. Text in English. 1949. m. membership. back issues avail. *Refereed.* **Document type:** *Newspaper.* **Description:** News and features about weight-control and nutrition. Covers activities of the organization.
Published by: Tops Club Inc., 4575 S Fifth St, Box 070360, Milwaukee, WI 53207-0360. TEL 414-482-4620, http://www.tops.org. Ed., R&P Kathleen Davis. Circ: 303,692.

613.7 615.53 USA
TOUCH FOR HEALTH. Text in English. 1982. q. USD 20. adv. bk.rev. **Document type:** *Newsletter.* **Description:** Offers commentary and news concerning holistic health promotion, wellness, healing, kinesiology, acupressure, subtle energies, world views and beliefs.
Published by: Touch for Health Education, Inc., 6162 La Gloria Dr, Malibu, CA 90265-3105. TEL 310-589-5269. Ed. John F Thie. R&P John Thie. Circ: 2,000.

613.7 DEU
TRIATHLON MAGAZIN. Text in German. 1985. 4/yr. DEM 27 (effective 1999). adv. bk.rev. index. back issues avail. **Document type:** *Consumer.*
Published by: Spiridon Verlags GmbH, Dorfstr 18 a, Erkrath 40699, Germany. TEL 49-211-726364, FAX 49-211-786823. Ed., Pub. Manfred Steffny. Adv. contact Christian Stanetzek. Circ: 4,000.

613 COL
UNIVERSIDAD DE ANTIOQUIA. FACULTAD NACIONAL DE SALUD PUBLICA. REVISTA. Text in Spanish. 1983. s-a. USD 9 (effective 2000). back issues avail. **Document type:** *Academic/Scholarly.*
Published by: Universidad de Antioquia, Facultad Nacional de Salud Publica, Apartado Postal 51922, Medellin, Colombia. TEL 57-4-510-6870, FAX 57-4-511-2506, lbermu@guajiros.udea.edu.co, revfnsp@caribe.udea.edu.co.

613.7 USA ISSN 0748-9234
RA773 CODEN: UCWLE9
UNIVERSITY OF CALIFORNIA, BERKELEY. WELLNESS LETTER; the newsletter of nutrition, fitness, and stress management. Text in English. 1984. m. USD 28 domestic; CND 36 in Canada; USD 39 elsewhere (effective 2000). illus. back issues avail.; reprints avail. **Document type:** *Newsletter.* **Description:** Provides information for physicians, nutritionists, and other professionals in the health care field; focuses on staying well rather than coping with illness.
Related titles: Online - full text ed.: (from Gale Group).
Indexed: Biol.Dig., CINAHL, Consum.Ind. (1989-1996), Hlth.Ind.
—BLDSC (9104.436000). **CCC.**
Published by: (School of Public Health, University of California at Berkeley), Health Letter Associates, PO Box 412, Prince St Sta, New York, NY 10012-0007. TEL 510-642-8061, 800-829-9170, FAX 212-505-5462, http://www.wellnessletter.com/. Pub. Rodney M Friedman. Circ: 500,000 (paid). **Subscr. to:** PO Box 420148, Palm Coast, FL 32142.

613.7 USA ISSN 0739-4217
THE UNIVERSITY OF TEXAS LIFETIME HEALTH LETTER; useful news about health, fitness, nutrition, and mental well-being. Text in English. 1989. m. USD 24. *Refereed.* **Document type:** *Newsletter.* **Description:** Contains articles on health habits people can practice to improve the quality of their physical and mental lives.
Formerly (until 1989): Health Letter
Indexed: CHNI, CINAHL.
Published by: University of Texas, Houston Health Science Center, 7000 Fannin St, Houston, TX 77030. TEL 713-792-4265, FAX 713-794-4738, sdeaner@uthouston.edu, http://www.uth.tmc.edu/uth-orgs/pub-affairs/lifetime.html. Ed. Linda Barth. Pub., R&P Susan Deaner. Circ: 65,000. **Subscr. to:** PO Box 420342, Palm Coast, FL 32142-0342.

613.7 790.1 USA ISSN 0739-4586
V A H P E R D JOURNAL. Text in English. 1978. s-a. USD 25 (effective 1998). adv. back issues avail. **Document type:** *Academic/Scholarly.*
Indexed: Sportsearch (1979-).
Published by: Virginia Association for Health, Physical Education and Dance, c/o Dr Robert Davis, 12 Westmoreland St, Richmond, VA 23226. TEL 804-355-6955, FAX 804-355-6955, vahperd@erols.com. Ed., R&P Dr. G.B. Darden. Adv. contact G B Darden. Circ: 1,000.

▼ **V O I C E**; victory over incontinence/continence education. see *PUBLIC HEALTH AND SAFETY*

VEGETARIAN VOICE. see *NUTRITION AND DIETETICS*

613.2 USA ISSN 0749-3509
R773
VIBRANT LIFE; abundant living for you and your family. Text in English. 1904. bi-m. USD 16.95 (effective 2001). adv. bk.rev. abstr. charts, illus. index. reprint service avail. from PQC. **Document type:** *Magazine, Consumer.*
Former titles: Your Life and Health (0279-2680); Life and Health (0024-3035)
Related titles: Online - full text ed.: (from Gale Group, Northern Light Technology, Inc., ProQuest Information & Learning, Factiva).
Indexed: CCR, CHNI, CINAHL, Hlth.Ind.

P

Published by: Review and Herald Publishing Association, 55 W Oak Ridge Dr, Hagerstown, MD 21740. TEL 301-393-3000, vibrantlife@rhpa.org, http://vibrantlife.com, http://www.rhpa.org. Ed. Larry Becker. Adv. contact Melynie Tooley TEL 301-393-3165. Circ: 50,000.

613.2 FRA ISSN 0042-5524
VIE ET SANTE; le mensuel du mieux-etre. Text in French. 1890. m. FRF 288; FRF 29 newsstand/cover (effective 1997). adv. bk.rev.
Related titles: CD-ROM ed.
Indexed: ExtraMED, Pt.de Rep. (1979-).
—GNLM.
Published by: Editions Vie et Sante, 60 av. Emile Zola, BP 59, Dammarie-les-Lys Cedex 77192, France. TEL 33-1-64393826, FAX 33-1-64870066. Ed. Jean Claude Roeland. Pub. Aldo Monet. Circ: 31,447 (controlled).

613.7 USA ISSN 0886-6554
VIM & VIGOR; America's family health magazine. Text in English. 1985. q. USD 7. adv. bk.rev. tr.lit. back issues avail. **Document type:** *Consumer.* **Description:** Directed to health-conscious people who are interested in a variety of health issues including diagnosis, treatment, diet, fitness, and exercise.
Published by: McMurry Publishing, 1010 E Missouri Ave, Phoenix, AZ 85014-2601. FAX 602-395-5853. Ed. Jennifer Dack Woolson. Pub. Fred Petronsky. Adv. contact Greg Ottersbach. Circ: 1,000,000 (controlled).

VISIONARY. see *MEDICAL SCIENCES—Ophthalmology And Optometry*

613 GRC ISSN 1108-6033
VITA. Text in Greek. 1997. m. adv. **Document type:** *Magazine, Consumer.* **Description:** Aims to inform and educate on vital health-related issues, healthy lifestyles, and physical fitness options.
Published by: Lambrakis Press SA, Panepistimiou 18, Athens 106 72, Greece. TEL 30-1-3686-452, FAX 30-1-3686-445, dolinfo@dol.gr, http://www.dol.gr. Circ: 44,714 (paid).

613 ITA ISSN 0042-7268
VITA E SALUTE; rivista mensile di medicina preventiva. Text in Italian. 1952. m. ITL 55,000 (effective 1998). bk.rev. charts, illus. index.
Published by: Edizioni A.D.V., Via Chiantigiana, 30, Falciani, Impruneta, FI 50023, Italy. TEL 39-55-2326291. Ed. Ennio Battista. adv.: color page ITL 7,000,000. Circ: 40,000.

613 DEU ISSN 0507-1747
VITAL; wellcome to wellness. Text in German. 1969. m. DEM 48; DEM 4 newsstand/cover; GBP 2.75 newsstand/cover in United Kingdom (effective 2000). adv. **Document type:** *Magazine, Consumer.*
Formerly: Vital Gesundheit, Freizeit, Lebensfreude
Published by: Jahreszeiten Verlag GmbH, Possmoorweg 5, Hamburg 22301, Germany. TEL 49-40-2717-0, FAX 49-40-27172059, redaktion@vital-online.de, http://www.jalag.de/zundz/vital/index.html. Ed. Angela Oelckers. Pub. Thomas Ganske. Adv. contact Monika Krieger. B&W page DEM 17,920, color page DEM 25,010; trim 193 x 257. Circ: 320,000 (paid). **Dist. in UK by:** Seymour, 86 Newman St, London W1P 3EX, United Kingdom. TEL 44-20-7396-8000, FAX 44-20-7396-8002.

613.7 USA
VITALIDA AHORA. Text in Spanish. q. **Document type:** *Newsletter, Consumer.* **Description:** Covers health and wellness items of interest to Spanish-speaking communities.
Published by: McMurry Publishing, 1010 E Missouri Ave, Phoenix, AZ 85014-2601. TEL 602-395-5850, 888-626-8779, FAX 602-395-5853, info@mcmurry.com, http://www.mcmurry.com.

613 USA ISSN 1074-5831
VITALITY. Text in English. 1986. m. USD 13.90 (effective 2001). adv. bk.rev. 28 p./no. **Document type:** *Magazine, Consumer.* **Description:** Features health diet, fitness, parenting, and personal productivity.
Published by: Vitality Magazine, 9400 N. Central Expy., Ste.1202, Dallas, TX 75231-5027. TEL 214-691-5572, FAX 214-691-8156, http://www.vitality.com. Ed. Barbara Floria. Pub., R&P Sue Quate TEL 214-691-5572. adv.: B&W page USD 13,560, color page USD 16,950. Circ: 565,000 (controlled).

VITALITY. see *NUTRITION AND DIETETICS*

613.7 ITA
VIVA. Text in Italian. 1985. bi-m. ITL 35,000. **Document type:** *Consumer.*
Published by: Valentini Editore s.r.l., Via Fabio Filzi, 41, Milan, MI 20124, Italy. TEL 39-2-66804467, FAX 39-2-6887740, TELEX 330299 VALEDI I. Ed. Pietro Paolo Valentini. adv.: B&W page ITL 1,700,000, color page ITL 3,500,000. Circ: 24,000.

613.7 646.7 ITA
VIVER SANI E BELLI; settimanale di salute e belleza. Text in Italian. 1992. w. ITL 95,000 domestic; USD 52.20 in United States; ITL 2,000 newsstand/cover. adv. illus. **Document type:** *Consumer.* **Description:** Offers women advice on enhancing and maintaining their health and beauty.
Published by: D.E. Didieffe s.r.l. (Subsidiary of: Casa Editrice Universo S.p.A.), Via Cusani, 4, Milan, MI 20121, Italy. TEL 39-2-723311, FAX 39-2-861328, viversaniebelli@iol.it. Ed. Silvia Huen. R&P Elisabetta Savoca TEL 39-2-72331435. Adv. contact Rodolfo Milosa. color page ITL 215,000,000. Circ: 227,831.

613 ESP
VIVIR CON SALUD; la revista decana del naturismo espanol. Key Title: Vivir. Text in Spanish. 1953. 5/yr. ESP 4,200, USD 50 (effective 2001). bk.rev. bibl, illus, tr.mk. index. 56 p./no. back issues avail. **Document type:** *Consumer.*
Formerly: Vivir (0042-7578)
Published by: (Centro de Estudios Naturistas), Ediciones CEDEL, Mallorca, 257, Barcelona 08008, Spain. TEL 34-3-4877349, FAX 34-3-4873145, cen@federacioaccap.org, http://www.perso.wanadoo.es/cden. Ed. Jose Avila. Pub. Gabriel Alomar. Circ: 5,000.

613.7 FIN ISSN 0780-1122
VOI HYVIN. Text in Finnish. 1986. 6/yr. FIM 300 in Europe; FIM 324 elsewhere (effective 2001). **Document type:** *Consumer.* **Description:** Provides information on healthy living to modern, well educated people.
Published by: A-Lehdet Oy, Hitsaajankatu 10-3, Helsinki 00081, Finland. TEL 358-9-75961, FAX 358-9-786341, a-tilaus@a-lehdet.fi, http://www.a-lehdet.fi. Ed. Arja Sihvola. Circ: 64,780 (controlled).

613 DEU ISSN 0042-8493
VOLKSGESUNDHEIT✶ ; Monatszeitschrift fuer gesundes Leben und naturgemaesse Heilverfahren. Text in German. 1924. m. DEM 32. adv. abstr, illus.
—GNLM.
Published by: Helfer-Verlag, Postfach 1645, Bad Homburg 61286, Germany. Ed. Emil Schwabe.

613.7 USA ISSN 1042-2102
GV199
WALKING MAGAZINE; the magazine of smart health and fitness. Text in English. 1986. 7/yr. USD 11.95 domestic; USD 23.95 foreign; USD 2.99 newsstand/cover (effective 2000). adv. bk.rev. illus. reprints avail. **Document type:** *Magazine, Consumer.* **Description:** Contains information for recreational and fitness walkers. Focuses on health, fitness, nutrition, travel, and equipment.
—CCC.
Published by: (Reader's Digest Association, Inc), R D Publications Inc. (Subsidiary of: Reader's Digest Association), 28 W 23rd St, New York, NY 10010. TEL 212-366-8600, 800-345-6563, FAX 212-366-8899, letters@walking.com, http://www.walkingmag.com. Pub. Charles S McNiff. adv.: B&W page USD 22,580, color page USD 28,190; trim 10.5 x 7.88. Circ: 629,000 (paid). **Subscr. to:** Reader's Digest Association, Inc, Reader's Digest Walking, PO Box 420 235, Palm Coast, FL 32142. TEL 800-829-5585.

WEIGHT LOSS NEWS. see *NUTRITION AND DIETETICS*

WEIGHT WATCHERS MAGAZINE. see *NUTRITION AND DIETETICS*

613.7 USA
WEIGHTLIFTING U S A. Text in English. 1983. q. USD 20 domestic; USD 30 foreign (effective 2000). adv. bk.rev. back issues avail. **Document type:** *Newsletter.* **Description:** Covers USA weightlifting, coaching, health and fitness, sports medicine, and local, national, and international competition results.
Published by: U S A Weightlifting Federation, One Olympic Plaza, Colorado Springs, CO 80909-5764. TEL 719-578-4508, FAX 719-578-4741, usaw@usaw.org, http://www.usaw.org. Ed., Adv. contact James J Fox. R&P Laurie Lopez. Circ: 3,300.

613.7 CHN ISSN 1000-8020
WEISHENG YANJIU/JOURNAL OF HYGIENE RESEARCH. Text in Chinese. 1972. bi-m. USD 20.40; USD 3.40 newsstand/cover (effective 2001). **Document type:** *Academic/Scholarly.*
Indexed: Ind.Med.
—BLDSC (5004.200000).
Published by: China International Book Trading Corp/Zhongguo Guoji Tushu Maoyi Zonggongsi cibtc@mail.cibtc.com.cn, http://www.cibtc.com.cn. **Dist. by:** 35, Chegongzhuang Xilu, Haidian District, Beijing 100044, China.

613.7 AUS ISSN 1328-7540
WELLBEING MAGAZINE; personal and planetary healing. Text in English. 1984. q. AUD 48; AUD 12 newsstand/cover; GBP 5 newsstand/cover in United Kingdom (effective 2000). adv. bk.rev. back issues avail. **Document type:** *Consumer.*
Formerly: Australian Well Being (0812-8227)
Indexed: WMB.
—CCC.
Published by: Wellspring Publishers Pty Ltd., 317 Pacific Hwy, Private Bag 2102, North Sydney, NSW 2060, Australia. TEL 61-2-99227800, FAX 61-2-99661638, wellbeing@wellbeing.com.au, http://www.wellbeing.com.au. Ed., R&P Terry Robson. Pub. Barbara McGregor. Adv. contact Katinka Robertson. Circ: 35,000.

▼ **WELLFIT.** see *WOMEN'S HEALTH*

WHOLE LIFE TIMES. see *NEW AGE PUBLICATIONS*

WORLD BOOK HEALTH AND MEDICAL ANNUAL. see *ENCYCLOPEDIAS AND GENERAL ALMANACS*

613.7 CAN
Y M C A WEEKLY NEWS. (Young Men's Christian Association) Text in English. w.
Published by: Vancouver Downtown Young Men's Christian Association, 955 Burrard St, Vancouver, BC V6Z 1Y2, Canada. TEL 604-681-0221. Ed. Terry Connolly. Circ: 1,000.

613.2 GBR ISSN 0953-2161
YOGA AND HEALTH. Text in English. 1975. m. GBP 22; GBP 26 foreign; GBP 2.30 newsstand/cover (effective 1999). adv. bk.rev. back issues avail. **Document type:** *Consumer.* **Description:** European's leading independent yoga magazine. Also contains features on health issues, complementary therapies and healthy nutrition suggestions.
Formerly (until 1988): Yoga Today (0308-3349)
Published by: Yoga Today Ltd., 21 Caburn Crescent, Lewes, E Sussex BN7 1NR, United Kingdom. TEL 44-480-5656, FAX 44-480-5656, fotodirect@mistral.co.uk. Ed. Jane Sill. Adv. contact P Barnes. Circ: 15,000. **Dist. by:** Diamond Magazine Distribution Ltd., Unit 7 Rother Ironworks, Fishmarket Rd, Rye TN31 7LR, United Kingdom. TEL 44-1797-225229, FAX 44-1797-225657.

YOGA AND TOTAL HEALTH. see *PHILOSOPHY*

613.7 DEU ISSN 1430-3345
YOGA UND GANZHEITLICHE GESUNDHEIT. Text in German. 1996. q. DEM 30 in Europe; DEM 60 elsewhere (effective 2001). charts, illus. 24 p./no. 2 cols./p. back issues avail. **Document type:** *Newsletter, Consumer.* **Description:** Covers the technical, psychological, philosophical, medical, scientific, and emotional aspects of yoga.
Published by: Hella Naura Verlag, Gerckensplatz 18, Hamburg 22339, Germany. TEL 49-40464997, hnaura@t-online.de, http://www.ganzheitlicher-yoga.de. Ed. Hella Naura. Circ: 300.

YOUR GREATEST GUIDE TO CALORIES. see *NUTRITION AND DIETETICS*

613.7 USA ISSN 0889-4329
YOUR HEALTH (BOCA RATON). Text in English. 1963. bi-w. USD 19.77; USD 2.25 newsstand/cover (effective 1997). bk.rev., software rev., video rev. back issues avail. **Document type:** *Consumer.* **Description:** Presents health issues, diet news, alternative therapies and medical breakthroughs.
Former titles: Your Health and Medical Bulletin (0745-4627); Medical Bulletin (0273-5342)
Published by: American Media, 5401 N W Broken Sound Blvd, Boca Raton, FL 33487. TEL 561-997-7733, FAX 561-997-9210. Ed. Susan Gregg. Pub. Donald McLachlan. Adv. contact Len Seminara. Circ: 50,000 (paid).

P

613.7 USA
YOUR HEALTH DAILY. Text in English. 1997. d.
Document type: *Magazine, Consumer.*
Media: Online - full content.
Published by: New York Times Company, 100 Ave. of the Americas, New York, NY 10013. http://www.yourhealthdaily.com.

613 057.87 SVK ISSN 0044-1953
ZDRAVIE✶ ; fit, krasa, pohoda. Text in Slovak. m. SKK 240; SKK 512 foreign (effective 1999). adv. bk.rev. illus.
Description: Covers beauty culture, birth control, health aids, medical sciences, men's health, psychology, rational nutrition, and healthy lifestyles.
Formerly: Zdravie Ludu
Published by: Spolocnost 7 Plus s.r.o., Ruzova dolina 27, Bratislava 82506, Slovakia. TEL 421-7-53413970, pluska@internet.sk. Ed. Katarina Chlapikova. R&P Stefan Simak. Adv. contact Juran Pucher. page SKK 65,000. Circ: 48,000. **Dist. by:** ABOPRESS, Radlinskeho 27, Bratislava 81107, Slovakia.

ZDROWIE, URODA I ZYCIE. see *BEAUTY CULTURE*

ZEST; the health and beauty magazine. see *WOMEN'S INTERESTS*

613.7 CHN
ZHONG LAO NIAN BAOJIAN. Text in Chinese. bi-m.
Published by: Zhongri Youhao Yiyuan, Yinghuayuan Dongjie, Beijing 100029, China. TEL 86-1-6420-6649. Ed. Ma Xiuye.

613.7 CHN ISSN 1001-2001
ZHONGGUO KANGFU/CHINESE JOURNAL OF REHABILITATION. Text in Chinese. 1986. q. USD 11.60; USD 2.90 newsstand/cover (effective 2001).
Document type: *Academic/Scholarly.*
Published by: China International Book Trading Corp/Zhongguo Guoji Tushu Maoyi Zonggongsi cibtc@mail.cibtc.com.cn, http://www.cibtc.com.cn. **Dist. by:** 35, Chegongzhuang Xilu, Haidian District, Beijing 100044, China.

ZHONGGUO QIGONG KEXUE/CHINA QIGONG SCIENCE. see *ALTERNATIVE MEDICINE*

613.7 CHN ISSN 1000-4610
ZHONGHUA QIGONG/CHINESE BREATH EXERCISE. Text in Chinese. 1982. q. USD 22.80; USD 3.90 newsstand/cover (effective 2001). **Document type:** *Academic/Scholarly.*
Related titles: Online - full content ed.: (from WanFang Data Corp.).
Published by: Zhongguo Zhongyiyao Xuehui, 18, Bei-Xincang, Dongzhimen, Beijing 100700, China. **Dist. by:** China International Book Trading Corp, 35, Chegongzhuang Xilu, Haidian District, Beijing 100044, China. TEL 86-1-68413849, FAX 86-1-68412048, cibtc@mail.cibtc.com.cn, http://www.cibtc.com.cn.
Co-publisher: Zhongguo Zhongyi Yanjiuyuan.

613.7 CHN ISSN 0529-5548
R97.7.C5
ZHONGJI YIKAN. Text in Chinese. m. USD 2.70.
Document type: *Academic/Scholarly.*
Published by: Renmin Weisheng Chubanshe, 10 Tiantan Xili, Beijing 100050, China. TEL 7015802. Ed. Liu Yiqing. Circ: 110,000.

ZORG & WELZIJN; opiniemagazine voor de sector zorg en welzijn. see *SOCIAL SERVICES AND WELFARE*

PHYSICAL FITNESS AND HYGIENE—Abstracting, Bibliographies, Statistics

613.7021 AUS
AUSTRALIA. BUREAU OF STATISTICS. OCCASIONAL PAPER: CIGARETTE SMOKING AMONG INDIGENOUS AUSTRALIANS. Text in English. 1995. irreg., latest 1994. AUD 15 (effective 2001). **Document type:** *Government, Academic/Scholarly, Trade.*
Published by: Australian Bureau of Statistics, PO Box 10, Belconnen, ACT 2616, Australia. TEL 61-2-6252-5249, FAX 61-2-6252-6778, http://www.abs.gov.au.

613.7021 AUS
AUSTRALIA. BUREAU OF STATISTICS. OCCASIONAL PAPER: OVERWEIGHT AND OBESITY, INDIGENOUS AUSTRALIANS. Text in English. 1998. irreg. AUD 19.50 (effective 2001). **Document type:** *Government, Academic/Scholarly, Trade.*
Published by: Australian Bureau of Statistics, PO Box 10, Belconnen, ACT 2616, Australia. TEL 61-2-6252-5249, FAX 61-2-6252-6778, http://www.abs.gov.au.

613.7021 AUS
AUSTRALIA. BUREAU OF STATISTICS. OCCASIONAL PAPER: SELF-ASSESSED HEALTH STATUS, INDIGENOUS AUSTRALIANS. Text in English. 1994. irreg. AUD 18.50 (effective 2001). **Document type:** *Government, Academic/Scholarly.*
Published by: Australian Bureau of Statistics, PO Box 10, Belconnen, ACT 2616, Australia. TEL 61-2-6252-5249, FAX 61-2-6252-6778, http://www.abs.gov.au.

613.7021 AUS ISSN 1441-2004
AUSTRALIA. BUREAU OF STATISTICS. THE HEALTH AND WELFARE OF AUSTRALIA'S ABORIGINAL AND TORRES STRAIT ISLANDER PEOPLES. Text in English. 1997. biennial. AUD 46 (effective 2001).
Document type: *Government.*
Published by: Australian Bureau of Statistics, PO Box 10, Belconnen, ACT 2616, Australia. TEL 61-2-6252-5249, FAX 61-2-6252-6778, http://www.abs.gov.au.
Co-sponsor: Australian Institute of Health and Welfare.

016 613.85 USA ISSN 0067-7361
RA1242.T6
BIBLIOGRAPHY ON SMOKING AND HEALTH. Text in English. 1967. a. free per issue. index. **Document type:** *Bibliography, Government.* **Description:** Lists articles pertaining to the prevention and cessation of tobacco use and the protection of nonsmokers.
Supersedes (in 1989): Smoking and Health Bulletin (0081-0363); Which was formerly: Smoking and Health Bibliographical Bulletin
Related titles: Microfiche ed.: (from CIS).
Indexed: Amer.Stat.Ind. (1979-), MEDOC.
—GNLM.
Published by: U.S. Centers for Disease Control, National Center for Chronic Disease Prevention and Health Promotion, Office on Smoking and Health, 4770 Buford Hwy, NE, MS K 50, Atlanta, GA 30341-3724. TEL 404-488-5705, 800-CDC-1311, FAX 404-488-5939. Circ: (controlled). **Orders to:** U.S. Government Printing Office, Superintendent of Documents.

BRITISH JOURNAL OF PHYSICAL EDUCATION. RESEARCH SUPPLEMENT. see *EDUCATION—Teaching Methods And Curriculum*

613.7 CAN ISSN 1201-2319
CANADIAN ASSOCIATION FOR HEALTH, PHYSICAL EDUCATION, RECREATION AND DANCE. JOURNAL. Short title: C A H P E R D Journal. Text in English, French. 1933. 4/yr. CND 65 domestic to individuals; CND 118 foreign to individuals; CND 100 domestic to institutions; CND 118 foreign to institutions (effective 1999). adv. bk.rev. illus. **Document type:** *Academic/Scholarly.*
Former titles: Canadian Association for Health, Physical Education and Recreation. Journal (0834-1915); C A H P E R Journal (0226-5478)
Media: Duplicated (not offset). **Related titles:** Microfilm ed.: (from MML).
Indexed: Can.B.P.I., Can.Educ.Ind., Can.Per.Ind. (Jan.1988-), Sportsearch (1952-).
—BLDSC (4722.320000), GNLM, Infotrieve, ingenta. **CCC.**
Published by: Canadian Association for Health, Physical Education, Recreation and Dance, Place R Tait McKenzie, 1600 James Naismith Dr, Gloucester, ON K1B 5N4, Canada. TEL 613-748-5622, FAX 613-748-5737. Ed. Andrea Grantham. Circ: 2,200.

FITNESS IN AMERICA. see *SPORTS AND GAMES—Abstracting, Bibliographies, Statistics*

HAWAII. DEPARTMENT OF HEALTH. RESEARCH AND STATISTICS OFFICE. R & S REPORT. see *POPULATION STUDIES—Abstracting, Bibliographies, Statistics*

613.7 790 USA ISSN 1526-1956
Z6121
HEALTH, PHYSICAL EDUCATION AND RECREATION, EXERCISE AND SPORT SCIENCES MICROFORM PUBLICATIONS BULLETIN; a subject and author index of dissertations and theses including abstracts. Text in English. 1949. a. USD 1,210 (effective 2001). abstr. cum.index: 1949-1999. back issues avail. **Document type:** *Bulletin, Abstract/Index, Academic/Scholarly.* **Description:** Serves as an index to a collection of microfiches representing dissertations and theses in the area of physical education, sport and exercise science, health, dance and recreational studies.
Former titles (until 1992): Health, Physical Education and Recreation Microform Publications Bulletin (0090-5119); (until 1972): Health, Physical Education, and Recreation Microcard Bulletin (0017-906X); (until 1964): Health and Physical Education Microcard Bulletin (0732-4804); (until 1955): Health and Physical Education Microcards (0732-4790)
Related titles: Microfiche ed.
Published by: (International Institute for Sport & Human Performance), Microform Publications of Human Movement Studies, 1243 University of Oregon, Eugene, OR 97403-1243. TEL 541-346-4117, FAX 541-346-0935, hheiny@oregon.uoregon.edu, http://www.uoregon.edu/~micropub/. Ed. Henriette Heiny.

MEDICAL ABSTRACTS NEWSLETTER; your direct pipeline to the latest breakthroughs in health care. see *MEDICAL SCIENCES—Abstracting, Bibliographies, Statistics*

613 016 USA
N T I S ALERTS: HEALTH CARE. Text in English. 1987. s-m. USD 210 in North America; USD 275 elsewhere (effective 1999). index. back issues avail. **Document type:** *Newsletter, Bibliography, Government.*
Description: Reports on methodology, health services, facilities utilization and health needs. Also covers health care assessment quality assurance, forecasting and measurement methods and legislation and regulations.
Former titles: Abstract Newsletter: Health Care; Abstract Newsletter: Health Planning and Health Services Research; Weekly Abstract Newsletter: Health Planning and Health Services Research; Weekly Government Abstracts. Health Planning and Health Services Research (0199-9974); Weekly Government Abstracts. Health Planning (0017-9086)
Related titles: Microform ed.: (from NTI).
—GNLM.
Published by: U.S. National Technical Information Service, 5285 Port Royal Rd, Springfield, VA 22161. TEL 703-605-6000, 800-363-2068, FAX 703-605-6900, orders@ntis.fedworld.gov; subscriptions@ntis.fedworld.gov, http://www.ntis.gov/alerts.htm.

613 011 USA ISSN 0161-603X
HV5825
U.S. NATIONAL INSTITUTE ON DRUG ABUSE. STATISTICAL SERIES D. DATA FROM THE CLIENT ORIENTED DATA ACQUISITION PROCESS. QUARTERLY REPORT. PROVISIONAL DATA. Text in English. 1973-1979; resumed 1982. q. charts, stat.
Formerly: U.S. National Institute on Drug Abuse. Statistical Series D. Client Oriented Data Acquisition Process. Quarterly Report (0145-1065)
Indexed: Amer.Stat.Ind.
Published by: U.S. National Institute on Drug Abuse, 5600 Fishers Ln, Rm 111, Rockville, MD 20857. TEL 301-443-6637.

613.7 CHN ISSN 1002-3674
ZHONGGUO WEISHENG TONGJI/CHINESE JOURNAL OF HEALTH STATISTICS. Text in Chinese. 1984. bi-m. CNY 34.80 domestic; USD 16.80 foreign; CNY 5.80 newsstand/cover domestic; USD 2.80 newsstand/cover foreign (effective 2001). **Document type:** *Academic/Scholarly.*
Related titles: Online - full content ed.: (from WanFang Data Corp.).
Published by: Zhongguo Yike Daxue/Chinese University of Medical Sciences, 92 Er-ma Lu, Hepin Qu Bei, Chenyang 110001, China. Ed. Yude Chen. **Dist. by:** China International Book Trading Corp, 35, Chegongzhuang Xilu, Haidian District, Beijing 100044, China. TEL 86-1-68413849, FAX 86-1-68412048, cibtc@mail.cibtc.com.cn, http://www.cibtc.com.cn.

613.7 CHN ISSN 1001-134X
ZHONGGUO YIXUE WENZHAI (WEISHENGXUE)/ CHINESE MEDICAL DIGEST (HYGIENICS). Text in Chinese. 1984. bi-m. USD 17.40; USD 2.90 newsstand/cover (effective 2001). **Document type:** *Abstract/Index.*
Published by: Zhongguo Yufang Yixue Kexueyuan/Chinese Academy of Preventive Medicine, 27 Nanwei Rd, Beijing 100050, China. TEL 86-1-4377008. **Dist. by:** China International Book Trading Corp, 35, Chegongzhuang Xilu, Haidian District, Beijing 100044, China. TEL 86-1-68413849, FAX 86-1-68412048, cibtc@mail.cibtc.com.cn, http://www.cibtc.com.cn.

PHYSICAL MEDICINE AND REHABILITATION

see MEDICAL SCIENCES—Physical Medicine And Rehabilitation

PHYSICALLY IMPAIRED

see HANDICAPPED—Physically Impaired

PHYSICS

see also PHYSICS—Electricity; PHYSICS—Heat; PHYSICS—Mechanics; PHYSICS—Nuclear Physics; PHYSICS—Optics; PHYSICS—Sound

A C O NEWSLETTER. see *MEDICAL SCIENCES—Psychiatry And Neurology*

ADVANCES IN COLLOID AND INTERFACE SCIENCE. see *CHEMISTRY—Physical Chemistry*

AUSTRALASIAN PHYSICAL & ENGINEERING SCIENCES IN MEDICINE. see *MEDICAL SCIENCES—Experimental Medicine, Laboratory Technique*

CHEMICAL SOCIETY OF JAPAN. SYMPOSIUM ON PHYSICAL AND CHEMICAL ASPECTS OF ULTRASOUND. PROCEEDINGS/ONPA NO BUSSEI TO KAGAKU TORONKAI KOEN RONBUNSHU. see *CHEMISTRY*

530 510 540 610 FIN ISSN 0788-5717
Q60 CODEN: CPMCET
COMMENTATIONES PHYSICO-MATHEMATICAE ET CHEMICO-MEDICAE. Text in English. 1923. irreg. price varies. charts, illus. index. **Document type:** *Academic/Scholarly.*
Formerly: Commentationes Physico-Mathematicae (0069-6609)
Indexed: Chem.Abstr., Curr.Cont. (coverage dropped), Curr.Ind.Stat., Deep Sea Res.& Oceanogr.Abstr., GeoRef, INIS Atomind., INSPEC (pre-1969-), Ind.Sci.Rev., Phys.Ber., Sci.Cit.Ind. (coverage dropped), Zent.Math.
—AskIEEE, CASDDS, CISTI, Linda Hall.
Published by: Societas Scientiarum Fennica/Finnish Society of Sciences and Letters, Sofiankatu 5, Helsinki 00170, Finland. TEL 358-9-633-005, FAX 358-9-661-065. Circ: 600.

CONCEPTS IN MAGNETIC RESONANCE; an educational quarterly. see *MEDICAL SCIENCES—Radiology And Nuclear Medicine*

ELECTROMAGNETIC FIELD LITIGATION REPORTER. see *ENERGY—Electrical Energy*

ELEKTRONENMIKROSKOPIE. see *BIOLOGY—Microscopy*

FORMA. see *BIOLOGY*

539.735 NLD
HANDBOOK ON SYNCHROTRON RADIATION. Text in English. 1983. irreg., latest vol.4, 1991. price varies. back issues avail. *Refereed.* **Document type:** *Monographic series, Academic/Scholarly.* **Description:** Discusses applications of synchrotron radiation in various areas of physics and chemistry and examines properties of sources, elements of instrumentation, and applications to biological and medical research.
Published by: Elsevier Science BV, PO Box 211, Amsterdam 1000 AE, Netherlands. TEL 31-20-485-3757, 31-20-485-3911, FAX 31-20-485-3432, 31-20-485-3598, nlinfo-f@elsevier.nl; usinfo-f@elsevier.com; forinfo-kyf04035@niftyserve.or.jp, http://www.elsevier.nl/. Eds. D E Eastman, Y Farge. **Subscr. in Australasia and the Far East to:** Elsevier Science (Singapore) Pte Ltd, No.1 Temasek Ave, 17-01 Millenia Tower, Singapore 039192, Singapore. TEL 65-434-3727, FAX 65-337-2230, asiainfo@elsevier.com.sg; **Subscr. in Japan to:** Elsevier Science Inc - Japan Regional Office, 9-15 Higashi-Azabu 1-chome, Minato-ku, Tokyo 106-0044, Japan. TEL 81-3-5561-5033, FAX 81-3-5561-5047, info@elsevier.co.jp; **Subscr. in the Americas to:** Elsevier Science, PO Box 945, New York, NY 10159-0945. TEL 212-633-3730, 888-437-4636, FAX 212-633-3680, usinfo-f@elsevier.com, http://www.elsevier.com

INSTITUTE OF PHYSICS AND ENGINEERING IN MEDICINE. REPORT. see *MEDICAL SCIENCES—Radiology And Nuclear Medicine*

INTERNATIONAL JOURNAL OF RADIATION BIOLOGY. see *MEDICAL SCIENCES—Oncology*

J A M P NEWS. see *MEDICAL SCIENCES*

JIKI KYOMEI IGAKKAI PUROGURAMU/SOCIETY OF MAGNETIC RESONANCE IN MEDICINE. PROCEEDINGS OF ANNUAL CONFERENCE. see *MEDICAL SCIENCES—Radiology And Nuclear Medicine*

JIKI KYOMEI TO IGAKU/MAGNETIC RESONANCE IN MEDICINE. see *MEDICAL SCIENCES—Radiology And Nuclear Medicine*

JOURNAL OF ORGONOMY. see *MEDICAL SCIENCES—Psychiatry And Neurology*

MAGNETIC RESONANCE IN MEDICINE. see *MEDICAL SCIENCES—Radiology And Nuclear Medicine*

MEDICAL PHYSICS. see *MEDICAL SCIENCES*

MEDICAL SCIENCE SERIES. see *MEDICAL SCIENCES*

530 571 100 150 USA ISSN 1094-0359
THE NOETIC JOURNAL; an international forum on the cosmology of consciousness. Text in English. 1997. q. USD 34 to individuals; USD 52 to institutions (effective 2000). adv. abstr, bibl, charts, illus. back issues avail. *Refereed.* **Document type:** *Journal, Proceedings, Academic/Scholarly.*
Related titles: CD-ROM ed.; Online - full text ed.
Published by: (The International Noetic University), The Noetic Press, 120 Village Sq, #49, Orinda, CA 94567-2502. TEL 510-832-6059, noeticj@mindspring.com, http://www.mindspring.com/~noeticj/. Ed., Pub., R&P Dr. Richard L Amoroso. adv.: B&W page USD 485, color page USD 1,750. Circ: 4,500 (paid and controlled).

ORGONOMIC FUNCTIONALISM; a journal devoted to the work of Wilhelm Reich. see *MEDICAL SCIENCES—Psychiatry And Neurology*

PHYSICA MEDICA. see *MEDICAL SCIENCES*

PHYSIOLOGICAL MEASUREMENT. see *MEDICAL SCIENCES*

RAUM UND ZEIT; die neue Dimension der Wissenschaft. see *MEDICAL SCIENCES*

530 USA
RESONANCE (SUMTERVILLE). Text in English; Summaries in English, French, Georgian, German, Urdu. 1985. s-a. USD 10 domestic; USD 13 in Canada & Mexico; USD 15 elsewhere. bk.rev. abstr, bibl, charts, illus, pat, tr.lit. index. back issues avail. **Document type:** *Newsletter.* **Description:** Tracks the interaction between electric and magnetic fields and living organisms.
Published by: (Bioelectromagnetics Special Interest Group (BEM SIG), American Mensa Ltd.), Judy Wall, Ed. & Pub., C R 535, Sumterville, FL 33585. TEL 352-793-8748. Circ: 150 (paid).

530 GBR
SCOPE (YORK). Text in English. 1951. q. membership. adv. bk.rev.
Formerly: H P A Bulletin (Hospital Physicists Association)
Published by: Institute of Physics and Engineering in Medicine., PO Box 303, York YO1 2WR, United Kingdom. TEL 44-1904-610821, FAX 44-1904-612279, office@ipem.org.uk. Ed. Patrick Hill. Circ: 1,500.

615.89 110 USA ISSN 1099-6591
WMLC 93/3448
SUBTLE ENERGIES AND ENERGY MEDICINE; an interdisciplinary journal of energetic and informational interactions. Text in English. 1990. 3/yr. USD 50 domestic; USD 68 foreign. bk.rev. abstr, charts, illus, stat. back issues avail. *Refereed.* **Document type:** *Journal, Academic/Scholarly.* **Description:** Concerns the study of subtle energies and energy medicine, self-regulation and alternative therapies.
Formerly (until 1996): Subtle Engergies (1084-2209)
—BLDSC (8503.537000).
Published by: International Society for the Study of Subtle Energies and Energy Medicine, 11005 Ralston Rd Ste 100D, Arvada, CO 80004. TEL 303-425-4625, FAX 303-425-4685, TELEX 159294488, issseem@compuserve.com, http://www.issseem.org. Ed. Steven L Fahrion. R&P Christa Hankins. Circ: 1,200.

TRANSYLVANIA UNIVERSITY OF BRASOV. BULLETIN. SERIES B; mathematics, economical sciences, philology, medicine, physics, chemistry, sports. see *MATHEMATICS*

ULTRASONIC IMAGING; an international journal. see *MEDICAL SCIENCES—Radiology And Nuclear Medicine*

PHYSICS—Abstracting, Bibliographies, Statistics

016.5397 GBR ISSN 1464-1437
RA569 CODEN: AHPAES
RADIATION PROTECTION ABSTRACTS. Text in English. 1974. q. GBP 101 domestic; USD 186 foreign (effective 2002). adv. abstr. 72 p./no. back issues avail. **Document type:** *Journal, Abstract/Index.* **Description:** Covers all aspects of radiation protection.
Formerly (until 1999): Applied Health Physics Abstracts and Notes (0305-7615)
—GNLM.
Published by: Nuclear Technology Publishing, PO Box 7, Ashford, Kent TN23 1JW, United Kingdom. TEL 44-1233-641683, FAX 44-1233-610021, subscriptions@ntp.org.uk, http://www.ntp.org.uk/rpa/rpaind.html. Ed. E P Goldfinch. Adv. contact L Richmond. Circ: 500.

PHYSICS—Electricity

EXTRACTS FROM EUROPEAN PATENT SPECIFICATIONS. PART 2. ELECTRICITY, PHYSICS, PRECISION ENGINEERING, OPTICS AND ACOUSTICS. see *PATENTS, TRADEMARKS AND COPYRIGHTS*

537 USA
INTERNATIONAL TESLA SOCIETY. BULLETIN* . Text in English. m. USD 39 domestic to individual members; USD 44 in Canada & Mexico to individual members; USD 64 elsewhere to individual members; includes Tesla: a journal of modern science. **Document type:** *Newsletter.* **Description:** Keeps members up-to-date on news of the society, news of chapters, and events or items of interest.
Published by: International Tesla Society, Inc., PO Box 5636, Colorado Springs, CO 80931. TEL 719-475-0918, FAX 719-475-0582. Ed. David Hanson.

PHYSICS—Heat

CRYOGAS INTERNATIONAL; the source of timely and relevant information for the industrial gas and cryogenics industries. see *ENGINEERING—Mechanical Engineering*

JOURNAL OF FLOW VISUALIZATION AND IMAGE PROCESSING. see *ENGINEERING—Mechanical Engineering*

PHYSICS—Mechanics

BIOMEKHANIKA/BIOMECHANICS. see *BIOLOGY—Biophysics*

JOURNAL OF FLOW VISUALIZATION AND IMAGE PROCESSING. see *ENGINEERING—Mechanical Engineering*

PHYSICS—Nuclear Physics

539 616 GBR ISSN 0969-8043
QC770 CODEN: ARISEF
APPLIED RADIATION AND ISOTOPES. Text in English. 1956. m. EUR 301 in Europe to qualified personnel; JPY 40,000 in Japan to qualified personnel; USD 336 elsewhere to qualified personnel; EUR 1,987 in Europe to institutions; JPY 264,000 in Japan to institutions; USD 2,224 elsewhere to institutions (effective 2002). adv. bk.rev. charts, illus. index. back issues avail.; reprint service avail. from PQC. *Refereed.* **Document type:** *Academic/Scholarly.* **Description:** Publishes papers relating to the production, measurement and application of radionuclides and radiation in all branches of science and technology.

Incorporates (1987-1995): Nuclear Geophysics (0969-8086); Which was formerly (until 1993): International Journal of Radiation Applications and Instrumentation. Part E: Nuclear Geophysics (0886-0130); Former titles (until 1993): International Journal of Radiation Applications and Instrumentation. Part A: Applied Radiation and Isotopes (0883-2889); (until 1985): International Journal of Applied Radiation and Isotopes (0020-708X)
Related titles: Microfilm ed.: (from PQC); Online - full text ed.: (from ingenta, Swets Blackwell, ScienceDirect, Institute for Scientific Information).
Indexed: AESIS, ASCA, Agri.& Environ.Biotech.Abstr. (coverage dropped), Anal.Abstr., Aqua.Sci.& Fish.Abstr., Bioeng.Abstr., Biol.Abstr., Biwk.Pap.Rad.Chem.& Photochem., Chem.Abstr., Chem.Cit.Ind., Chem.Indus.Notes, Chem.Titles, Comput.& Info.Sys., Curr.Adv.Ecol.Sci., Curr.Cont., Dairy Sci.Abstr., Deep Sea Res.& Oceanogr.Abstr., Derwent Biotech.Abstr., Energy Info.Abstr., Eng.Ind., Environ.Abstr., Environ.Sci.Poll.Mgmt., Excerp.Med., Food Sci.& Tech.Abstr., Geo.Abstr.H.G., GeoRef, Geol.Abstr., INIS Atomind., INSPEC (pre-1969-), Ind.Med. (1993-), Ind.Sci.Rev., Ind.Vet., Int.Abstr.Biol.Sci., MOS, Maize Abstr., Mass Spectr.Bull., Mat.Sci.Cit.Ind. (coverage dropped), NPU, Nutr.Abstr., Ocean.Abstr. (coverage dropped), Petrol.Abstr. (coverage dropped), Pollut.Abstr., RCI, Rev.Med.& Vet.Mycol., SSCI (coverage dropped), Saf.Sci.Abstr., Sci.Cit.Ind., Sel.Water Res.Abstr., Soils & Fert., Soyabean Abstr., Tox.Abstr., Triticale Abstr., Vet.Bull.
—BLDSC (1576.565000), ADONIS, AskIEEE, CASDDS, CISTI, Ei, EMDOCS, GNLM, IDS, Infotrieve, ingenta, Linda Hall. **CCC.**
Published by: Elsevier Science Ltd., Pergamon, PO Box 800, Kidlington, Oxon 0X5 1DX, United Kingdom. TEL 44-1865-843000, FAX 44-1865-843010, nlinfo-f@elsevier.nl; usinfo-f@elsevier.com; forinfo-kyf04035@niftyserve.or.jp, http://www.elsevier.com/locate/apradiso, http://www.elsevier.nl/ . Eds. D M Taylor, P M Coursey. adv.: B&W page USD 550, color page USD 1,350. Circ: 2,000. **Subscr. in Australasia and the Far East to:** Elsevier Science (Singapore) Pte Ltd, No.1 Temasek Ave, 17-01 Millenia Tower, Singapore 039192, Singapore. TEL 65-434-3727, FAX 65-337-2230; **Subscr. in the Americas to:** Elsevier Science, PO Box 945, New York, NY 10159-0945. TEL 212-633-3730, FAX 212-633-3680, usinfo-f@elsevier.com, http://www.elsevier.com; **Subscr. to:** Elsevier Science BV, PO Box 211, Amsterdam 1000 AE, Netherlands. TEL 31-20-485-3757, FAX 31-20-485-3432, nlinfo-f@elsevier.nl, http://www.elsevier.nl.

C Y R I C ANNUAL REPORT. (Cyclotron Radioisotope Center) see *MEDICAL SCIENCES—Radiology And Nuclear Medicine*

EGYPTIAN JOURNAL OF RADIATION SCIENCES & APPLICATIONS. see *MEDICAL SCIENCES—Radiology And Nuclear Medicine*

539.7 363.7 362.1 610 GBR ISSN 1473-6691
▼ **JOURNAL OF THE I C R U.** Text in English. 2001. 3/yr. (Frequency will change to semi-annually in 2002). GBP 139 domestic; USD 236 foreign (effective 2002). adv. bk.rev. 250 p./no. 2 cols./p. *Refereed.* **Document type:** *Journal, Academic/Scholarly.*
Published by: (International Commission on Radiation Units & Measurements (ICRU)), Nuclear Technology Publishing, PO Box 7, Ashford, Kent TN23 1JW, United Kingdom. TEL 44-1233-641683, FAX 44-1233-610021, subscriptions@ntp.org.uk, http://www.ntp.org.uk. Ed. Mitio Inokuti. R&P E P Goldfinch. Adv. contact L Richmond. Circ: 1,000.

543.0877 GBR ISSN 1352-8661
CODEN: MRBMEQ
MAGNETIC RESONANCE MATERIALS IN PHYSICS, BIOLOGY AND MEDICINE. Short title: M A G M A. Text in English. 1993. bi-m. EUR 389 in Europe to institutions; JPY 51,600 in Japan to institutions; USD 435 elsewhere to institutions (effective 2002). adv. bk.rev. back issues avail.; reprints avail. *Refereed.* **Document type:** *Academic/Scholarly.* **Description:** Presents the latest research, development, and application of techniques in magnetic resonance imaging and spectroscopy.
Formerly (until 1995): Magma (0968-5243); Which was previously announced as: Magma Magnetic Resonance Materials
Related titles: Online - full text ed.: (from ingenta, ScienceDirect, Swets Blackwell).
Indexed: ASCA, Chem.Abstr., Chem.Indus.Notes, Chem.Titles, Excerp.Med. (1994-), INSPEC (Mar.1993-Mar.1994, Jul.1994-Dec.1997, Aug.1998-), Ind.Med. (1993-), Int.Abstr.Biol.Sci.
—BLDSC (5334.854000), AskIEEE, CASDDS, CISTI, GNLM, IDS, Infotrieve. **CCC.**
Published by: (European Society for Magnetic Resonance in Medicine and Biology), Pergamon (Subsidiary of: Elsevier Science), The Boulevard, Langford Ln, East Park, Kidlington, Oxford OXB 1GB, United Kingdom. FAX 44-1865-843010, nlinfo-f@elsevier.nl; usinfo-f@elsevier.com; forinfo-kyf04035@niftyserve.or.jp, nlinfo-f@elsevier/nl; usinfo-f@elsevier.com; forinfo-kyf04035@niftyserve.or.jp, http://www.elsevier.com/locate/magma. Eds. Axel Haase, Dieter Matthaei. **Subscr. in Australasia and the Far East to:** Elsevier Science (Singapore) Pte Ltd, No.1 Temasek Ave, 17-01 Millenia Tower, Singapore 039192, Singapore. TEL 65-434-3727, FAX 65-337-2230; **Subscr. in the Americas to:** Elsevier Science, PO Box 945, New York, NY 10159-0945. TEL 212-633-3730, FAX 212-633-3680, usinfo-f@elsevier.com; **Subscr. to:** Elsevier Science BV, PO Box 211, Amsterdam 1000 AE, Netherlands. TEL 31-20-485-3757, FAX 31-20-485-3432, nlinfo-f@elsevier.nl.

539.7 USA
N R C T L D DIRECT RADIATION MONITORING NETWORK. Text in English. q. USD 23 (effective 2001). **Document type:** *Government.* **Description:** Presents the radiation levels measured in the vicinity of NRC licensed facility sites throughout the country.
Published by: U.S. Nuclear Regulatory Commission, 1 White Flint North Bldg, 11555 Rockville Pike, Rockville, MD 20852-2738. http://www.nrc.gov/NRC/NUREGS/ABSTRACTS/index.html. **Subscr. to:** U.S. Government Printing Office, Superintendent of Documents, PO Box 371954, Pittsburgh, PA 15250-7954. TEL 202-512-1800, FAX 202-512-2250, orders@gpo.gov, http://www.access.gpo.gov.

NUCLEAR MEDICINE AND BIOLOGY. see *MEDICAL SCIENCES—Radiology And Nuclear Medicine*

PROGRESS IN NUCLEAR MAGNETIC RESONANCE SPECTROSCOPY. see *CHEMISTRY—Analytical Chemistry*

R S O MAGAZINE. (Radiation Safety Officer) see *OCCUPATIONAL HEALTH AND SAFETY*

363.7 GBR ISSN 0144-8420
R905 CODEN: RPDODE
RADIATION PROTECTION DOSIMETRY. Text in English. 1981. 20/yr. (in 5 vols.). GBP 853 domestic; USD 1,710 foreign (effective 2002). adv. bk.rev. 96 p./no. 2 cols./p. back issues avail. *Refereed.* **Document type:** *Journal, Academic/Scholarly.* **Description:** Provides international coverage of biological aspects, physical concepts, external and internal dosimetry and monitoring, environmental and work place monitoring, as well as dosimetry monitoring related to the protection of patients.
Related titles: Online - full text ed.: (from Institute for Scientific Information).
Indexed: ASCA, Aqua.Sci.& Fish.Abstr., Chem.Abstr., Chem.Indus.Notes, Chem.Titles, Curr.Cont. (coverage dropped), Energy Ind., Energy Info.Abstr., Environ.Abstr., Environ.Sci.Poll.Mgmt., IBR, INIS Atomind., INSPEC (1981-), Lab.Haz.Bull., Mat.Sci.Cit.Ind. (coverage dropped), Pollut.Abstr., Ref.Zh., Risk Abstr., Saf.Sci.Abstr., Sci.Cit.Ind., Sel.Water Res.Abstr., Tox.Abstr.
—BLDSC (7227.993000), AskIEEE, CASDDS, CISTI, GNLM, IDS, Linda Hall.
Published by: Nuclear Technology Publishing, PO Box 7, Ashford, Kent TN23 1JW, United Kingdom. TEL 44-1233-641683, FAX 44-1233-610021, subscriptions@ntp.org.uk, http://www.ntp.org.uk/rpd/rpdind.html. Ed. J C McDonald. R&P E P Goldfinch. Adv. contact L Richmond. Circ: 750.

RADIATION PROTECTION MANAGEMENT; the journal of applied health physics. see *OCCUPATIONAL HEALTH AND SAFETY*

PHYSICS—Optics

535 617.7 658.8 GBR ISSN 1470-7152
BUSINESS RATIO. THE OPTICAL INDUSTRY. Text in English. 1980. a. GBP 275 (effective 2001). charts, stat. **Document type:** *Trade.*
Former titles (until 2000): Business Ratio Plus: Optical Industry (1354-8735); (until 1994): Business Ratio Report. Optical Industry (0261-9172)
Published by: The Prospect Shop Ltd., Field House, 72 Oldfield Rd, Hampton, Middx TW12 2HQ, United Kingdom. TEL 44-20-8461-8730, 44-20-8481-8720, FAX 44-20-8783-1940, info@theprospectshop.co.uk.

535 610.284 USA ISSN 1083-3668
R857.O6 CODEN: JBOPFO
JOURNAL OF BIOMEDICAL OPTICS. Text in English. 1996. q. USD 225 in North America to non-members; USD 245 elsewhere to non-members; USD 50 in North America to members (effective 2001). adv. illus. *Refereed.* **Document type:** *Academic/Scholarly.* **Description:** Applications of modern optics technology to biomedical research.
Related titles: CD-ROM ed.; Online - full text ed.: USD 25 to members (effective 2001) (from EBSCO Publishing, Institute for Scientific Information).
Indexed: C.P.I., Chem.Abstr., Chem.Indus.Notes, Chem.Titles, Curr.Cont., Eng.Ind., INSPEC (pre-1969-), Ind.Med., Inpharma, Pharm.&Out.News, Reac., SPINweb, Sci.Cit.Ind.
—BLDSC (4953.760000), AskIEEE, CASDDS, CISTI, GNLM, IDS, Infotrieve. **CCC.**
Published by: International Society for Optical Engineering (SPIE), 1000 20th St, PO Box 10, Bellingham, WA 98227-0010. TEL 360-676-3290, FAX 360-647-1445, journal@spie.org, http://www.spie.org/web/journals. Ed. Bruce J Tromberg. R&P Eric Pepper. Adv. contact Michele Hurst. **Co-sponsor:** International Biomedical Optics Society.

535 NLD ISSN 0022-2313
QC476.4 CODEN: JLUMA8
JOURNAL OF LUMINESCENCE; an interdisciplinary journal of research on excited state processes in condensed matter. Text in English, French, German; Summaries in English. 1970. 20/yr. EUR 2,012 in Europe to institutions; JPY 267,000 in Japan to institutions; USD 2,251 elsewhere to institutions (effective 2002). adv. bk.rev. bibl, charts, illus. index, cum.index. back issues avail. *Refereed.* **Document type:** *Academic/Scholarly.* **Description:** Provides a means of communication between scientists in different disciplines who share a common interest in the electronic excited state of molecular, ionic and covalent system, whether crystalline, amorphous, or liquid.
Related titles: Microform ed.: (from PQC); Online - full text ed.: (from ingenta, ScienceDirect, Swets Blackwell, Institute for Scientific Information).
Indexed: ASCA, Biol.Abstr., Biwk.Pap.Rad.Chem.& Photochem., Cadscan, Chem.Abstr., Chem.Cit.Ind., Chem.Indus.Notes, Chem.Titles, Curr.Cont., Electron.& Communic.Abstr.J., Eng.Ind., Environ.Eng.Abstr., Environ.Sci.Poll.Mgmt., GeoRef, INIS Atomind., INSPEC (Apr.1970-), Ind.Sci.Rev., Lead Abstr., Mass Spectr.Bull., Mat.Sci.Cit.Ind. (coverage dropped), Phys.Ber., Ref.Zh., Sci.Cit.Ind., Solid St.Abstr., Zincscan.
—BLDSC (5010.650000), AskIEEE, CASDDS, CISTI, Ei, IDS, ingenta, Linda Hall. **CCC.**
Published by: North-Holland (Subsidiary of: Elsevier Science BV), PO Box 211, Amsterdam 1000 AE, Netherlands. TEL 31-20-485-3911, FAX 31-20-485-3598, nlinfo-f@elsevier.nl, http://www.elsevier.com/locate/jlumin, http://www.elsevier.nl. Ed. R S Meltzer. **Subscr. in Australasia and the Far East to:** Elsevier Science (Singapore) Pte Ltd, No.1 Temasek Ave, 17-01 Millenia Tower, Singapore 039192, Singapore. TEL 65-434-3727, FAX 65-337-2230, asiainfo@elsevier.com.sg; **Subscr. in Japan to:** Elsevier Science Inc - Japan Regional Office, 9-15 Higashi-Azabu 1-chome, Minato-ku, Tokyo 106-0044, Japan. TEL 81-3-5561-5033, FAX 81-3-5561-5047, info@elsevier.co.jp; **Subscr. in the Americas to:** Elsevier Science, PO Box 945, New York, NY 10159-0945. TEL 212-633-3730, FAX 212-633-3680, usinfo-f@elsevier.com.

535.3 621.36 NLD ISSN 0921-8564
LASER HANDBOOK. Text in English. 1972. irreg., latest vol.6, 1990. price varies. charts, stat. back issues avail. *Refereed.* **Document type:** *Monographic series, Academic/Scholarly.* **Description:** Reports investigations into applications of lasers in applied and theoretical physics research.
Published by: Elsevier Science BV, PO Box 211, Amsterdam 1000 AE, Netherlands. TEL 31-20-485-3911, FAX 31-20-485-3432, 31-20-485-3598, nlinfo-f@elsevier.nl; usinfo-f@elsevier.com; forinfo-kyf04035@niftyserve.or.jp, http://www.elsevier.nl/. **Subscr. in Australasia and the Far East to:** Elsevier Science (Singapore) Pte Ltd, No.1 Temasek Ave, 17-01 Millenia Tower, Singapore 039192, Singapore. TEL 65-434-3727, FAX 65-337-2230, asiainfo@elsevier.com.sg; **Subscr. in Japan to:** Elsevier Science Inc - Japan Regional Office, 9-15 Higashi-Azabu 1-chome, Minato-ku, Tokyo 106-0044, Japan. TEL 81-3-5561-5033, FAX 81-3-5561-5047, info@elsevier.co.jp; **Subscr. in the Americas to:** Elsevier Science, PO Box 945, New York, NY 10159-0945. TEL 212-633-3730, 888-437-4636, FAX 212-633-3680, usinfo-f@elsevier.com, http://www.elsevier.com

LASERS IN MEDICAL SCIENCE. see *MEDICAL SCIENCES*

LASERS IN SURGERY AND MEDICINE. see *MEDICAL SCIENCES—Surgery*

535 570 CHE ISSN 0886-0467 CODEN: LLSCES
LASERS IN THE LIFE SCIENCES. Text in English. 1986. q. EUR 610, USD 671 to institutions; EUR 952, USD 1,047 to corporations; USD 171 to individuals (effective 2001). *Refereed.* **Document type:** *Journal, Academic/Scholarly.*
Related titles: Microform ed.
Indexed: Aqua.Sci.& Fish.Abstr., Environ.Sci.Poll.Mgmt., INSPEC (1986-1999, dropped), Pollut.Abstr., Risk Abstr., Saf.Sci.Abstr.
—BLDSC (5156.680500), AskIEEE, CISTI, EMDOCS, GNLM, ingenta. **CCC.**
Published by: Gordon and Breach - Harwood Academic (Subsidiary of: Taylor & Francis Group), PO Box 531, Lausanne 1000, Switzerland. TEL 41-21-6411280, FAX 41-21-6411281, info@gbhap.com, http://www.gbhap.com. Ed. V S Letokhov. **Subscr. addr. in US:** International Publishers Direct, PO Box 32160, Newark, NJ 07102. FAX 215-750-6343.

535.58 610 USA
MEDICAL LASER INSIGHT. Text in English. m. USD 300; USD 345 foreign (effective 1999). **Description:** Focuses on market analysis, industry news, technology assessment and identifying new business opportunities.
Indexed: Bus.& Indus. (Feb.1997-).
Published by: Biomedical Market Newsletter, Inc., 3237 Idaho Pl, Costa Mesa, CA 92626-2207. TEL 714-434-9500, 800-875-8181, FAX 714-434-9755. Ed. Michael Moretti. Pub. David G Anast.

535.58 610 USA
MEDICAL LASER REPORT. Text in English. 1986. 12/yr. USD 365 Print or e-mail; USD 465 Print & e-mail (effective 2001). Supplement avail. **Description:** Features news and reports about trends and developments in the medical laser business. Includes information on new technologies, market opportunities, product trends, and relevant FDA decisions.
Formerly: Medical Laser Industrial Report
Related titles: Fax ed.: USD 475 (effective 2001).
Published by: PennWell Publishing Co. (Nashua), 98 Spit Brook Rd, Nashua, NH 03062. TEL 603-891-0123, 847-559-7501, 800-331-4463, FAX 603-891-0574, http://www.pennwell.com. Ed. David Kales. Circ: 700.

MICROSCOPY SOCIETY OF SOUTHERN AFRICA. PROCEEDINGS/MIKROSKOPIEVERENIGING VAN SUIDELIKE AFRIKA. VERRIGTINGS. see *BIOLOGY—Microscopy*

535 JPN ISSN 0913-5510
MYU. Text in Japanese. 1987. s-a. **Document type:** *Academic/Scholarly.*
Published by: Meisei Daigaku, Kobunkaino Bunseki Denshi Kenbikyo Senta/Meisei University, High Resolution Analytical Electron Microscopy Research Center, 1-1 Hodokubo 2-chome, Hino-shi, Tokyo-to 191-0042, Japan.

OPHTHALMIC AND PHYSIOLOGICAL OPTICS. see *MEDICAL SCIENCES—Ophthalmology And Optometry*

OPTOMAGAZINE. see *MEDICAL SCIENCES—Ophthalmology And Optometry*

L'OROPTERO; rivista di scienze della visione. see *MEDICAL SCIENCES—Ophthalmology And Optometry*

SCANNING MICROSCOPY; an international journal of scanning electron microscopy, related techniques, and applications. see *BIOLOGY—Microscopy*

ZHONGGUO JIGUANG YIXUE ZAZHI/CHINESE JOURNAL OF LASER MEDICINE & SURGERY. see *MEDICAL SCIENCES*

PHYSICS—Sound

see also SOUND RECORDING AND REPRODUCTION

CLINICS IN DIAGNOSTIC ULTRASOUND. see *MEDICAL SCIENCES—Radiology And Nuclear Medicine*

534 IND ISSN 0256-4637
JOURNAL OF PURE AND APPLIED ULTRASONICS. Text in English. 1979. q. USD 100 (effective 2000). adv. bk.rev. index. back issues avail. *Refereed.* **Document type:** *Academic/Scholarly.*
Indexed: INIS Atomind., INSPEC (Jan.1984-).
—BLDSC (5043.682000), AskIEEE.
Published by: (Ultrasonics Society of India), Scientific Publishers, 5-A New Pali Rd., P O Box 91, Jodhpur, Rajasthan 342 001, India. TEL 91-291-433323, FAX 91-291-512580, scienti@sancharnet.in, http://www.scientificpub.com. Ed. Dr. Ashok Kumar. R&P, Adv. contact Dr. Y Kumar. Circ: 300.

JOURNAL OF ULTRASOUND IN MEDICINE. see *MEDICAL SCIENCES—Radiology And Nuclear Medicine*

ULTRASOUND IN MEDICINE & BIOLOGY. see *BIOLOGY*

534 DEU ISSN 1435-4691 CODEN: AUKADP
ZEITSCHRIFT FUER AUDIOLOGIE/AUDIOLOGICAL ACOUSTICS. Text in English, German. 1962. 4/yr. EUR 39 domestic; EUR 44.50 foreign (effective 2002). adv. bk.rev. bibl, charts, illus. index. **Document type:** *Magazine, Academic/Scholarly, Trade.*
Former titles (until 1998): Audiologische Akustik (0172-8261); Zeitschrift fuer Hoergeraete Akustik (0044-2860)
Indexed: Acoust.Abstr., Excerp.Med., INSPEC (Sep.1982-), NBA, Ref.Zh.
—BLDSC (9453.251500), AskIEEE, GNLM, Infotrieve, Linda Hall. **CCC.**
Published by: Median-Verlag von Killisch-Horn GmbH, Hauptstr 64, Heidelberg 69117, Germany. TEL 49-6221-90509-0, FAX 49-6221-9050920, median-verlag@t-online.de, http://www.median-verlag.de. Circ: 2,300.

534 DEU ISSN 0174-1098
TD891
ZEITSCHRIFT FUER LAERMBEKAEMPFUNG. Text in German. 1954. bi m. EUR 174.50 (effective 2002). adv. bk.rev. abstr, charts, illus, tr.lit. back issues avail.; reprint service avail. from ISI. **Document type:** *Magazine, Academic/Scholarly.* **Description:** Publishes papers on all aspects of noise control.
Formerly: Kampf dem Laerm (0022-8249)
Related titles: Microform ed.: (from PQC); Online - full text ed.: (from EBSCO Publishing, RoweCom Information Quest).
Indexed: Acoust.Abstr., Dok.Str., Excerp.Med.
—BLDSC (9468.750000), CISTI, GNLM, Infotrieve. **CCC.**
Published by: (Deutscher Arbeitsring fuer Laermbekaempfung e.V.), Springer V D I Verlag, Heinrichstr 24, Duesseldorf 40239, Germany. TEL 49-211-6103-0, FAX 49-211-6103414, anzeigen@technikwissen.de, info@technikwissen.de, http://www.technikwissen.de. Ed. E Zimmermann. Adv. contact Karin Assig TEL 49-211-6103312. B&W page XEU 1,404; trim 185 x 270. Circ: 2,000.

PHYSIOLOGY

see BIOLOGY—Physiology

PLASTICS

see also CHEMISTRY—Physical Chemistry; ENGINEERING—Chemical Engineering

BIOMEDICAL MATERIALS; an international newsletter. see *MEDICAL SCIENCES*

▼ **FOCUS ON POLYVINYL CHLORIDE.** see *CHEMISTRY—Organic Chemistry*

▼ **MICROSPHERES, MICROCAPSULES & LIPOSOMES.** see *PHARMACY AND PHARMACOLOGY*

668.4 614 USA ISSN 1065-1896
REGULATORY UPDATE; government legislation and regulations related to plastics industry. Text in English. 1983. m. USD 95 domestic; USD 105 foreign (effective 2000). back issues avail. **Document type:** *Newsletter, Trade.* **Description:** Covers regulatory (Federal Register) and legislative updates in public health and safety and environmental developments affecting the plastics industry.
Related titles: Diskette ed.; Online - full text ed.: USD 49.95 (effective 2000).
Published by: Lewis B. Weisfeld, Ed. & Pub., 1 Franklin Town Blvd, Ste 1204, Philadelphia, PA 19103. TEL 215-567-7235, FAX 215-567-7235, Lweisfeld@aol.com@aol.com, http://www.regup.plastics.com/. Ed., Pub., R&P Lewis B Weisfeld.

POETRY

see LITERATURE—Poetry

POLITICAL SCIENCE

see also LITERARY AND POLITICAL REVIEWS; POLITICAL SCIENCE—Civil Rights; POLITICAL SCIENCE—International Relations; PUBLIC ADMINISTRATION

320.3 USA ISSN 0010-4140
JA3
COMPARATIVE POLITICAL STUDIES. Text in English. 1968. 10/yr. USD 83, GBP 85 to individuals; USD 495, GBP 407 to institutions; USD 20 newsstand/cover to individuals; USD 60 newsstand/cover to institutions (effective 2002). adv. bk.rev. bibl, charts, stat, illus. index. back issues avail.; reprints avail. *Refereed.* **Document type:** *Academic/Scholarly.* **Description:** Publishes theoretical and empirical research articles by scholars engaged in comparative, cross-national studies.
Related titles: Microform ed.: (from PQC); Online - full text ed.: (from EBSCO Publishing, O C L C Online Computer Library Center, Inc., RoweCom Information Quest, ProQuest Information & Learning, Gale Group, ingenta, Swets Blackwell, Institute for Scientific Information).
Indexed: A.B.C.Pol.Sci., ASCA, ASSIA, Abstr.Crim.& Pen., Amer.Bibl.Slavic & E.Eur.Stud., Arts & Hum.Cit.Ind. (coverage dropped), Bibl.Asian Stud. (1971-1991), Commun.Abstr., Curr.Cont., Curr.Ind.Stat., Hist.Abstr. (1969-1998, dropped), IBR, Int.Polit.Sci.Abstr., Intl.Bibl.Soc.Sci., Mid.East: Abstr.& Ind., P C I, P.A.I.S., Peace Res.Abstr., Per.Islam. (1991-), Polit.Sci.Abstr., Pub.Admin.Abstr., Rural Recreat.Tour.Abstr., Russ.Acad.Sci.Bibl., SSCI, Sage Pub.Admin.Abstr., Soc.Sci.Ind. (Jan.1983-), Soc.Serv.Abstr., Sociol.Abstr., Sociol.Educ.Abstr., Stud.Wom.Abstr., World Ag.Econ.& Rur.Soc.Abstr.
—BLDSC (3363.795000), IDS, ingenta. **CCC.**
Published by: Sage Publications, Inc., 2455 Teller Rd, Thousand Oaks, CA 91320. TEL 805-499-0721, FAX 805-499-0871, info@sagepub.com, http://www.sagepub.co.uk/journals/details/j0193.html, http://www.sagepub.com. Ed. James A Caporaso. R&P Tanya Udin. Adv. contact DeAnna Vega Hammersley. Circ: 1,650. **Overseas subscr. to:** Sage Publications Ltd., 6 Bonhill St, London EC2A 4PU, United Kingdom; Sage Publications India Pvt. Ltd., 4215, New Delhi 110 048, India.

320 USA
FOOD FIRST NEWS & VIEWS. Text in English. 1978. 4/yr. USD 35; USD 40 foreign (effective 2001). bk.rev. 4 p./no. 2 cols./p. back issues avail.; reprints avail. **Document type:** *Newsletter, Corporate.* **Description:** Provides alternative analysis of the root causes of hunger and environmental degredation. Issues include foreign aid, organic farming, structural adjustment impact on the poor, alternatives to the Third World development, and more.
Formerly: Food First News (0749-9825)
Published by: Institute for Food & Development Policy, 398 60th St, Oakland, CA 94618-1212. TEL 510-654-4400, FAX 510-654-4551, foodfirst@foodfirst.org, http://www.foodfirst.org. Ed. Sal Glynn. Pub. Peter Rosset. R&P Martha Fernandez TEL 510-654-4400. Circ: 9,000.

FREE ASSOCIATIONS; psychoanalysis, groups, politics, culture. see *PSYCHOLOGY*

L'HOMME LIBRE; fils de la terre. see *PSYCHOLOGY*

JOURNAL OF HEALTH POLITICS, POLICY AND LAW. see *MEDICAL SCIENCES*

THE LEADERSHIP QUARTERLY; an international journal of political, social and behavioral science. see *BUSINESS AND ECONOMICS—Management*

P

320 USA ISSN 0887-378X
RA418.3.U6 CODEN: MIQUES
THE MILBANK QUARTERLY; a journal of public health and health care policy . Text in English. 1923. q. GBP 98 to institutions in UK & Europe; USD 119 to institutions in the Americas & Caribbean; GBP 98 elsewhere to institutions (effective 2002). adv. charts, illus, stat. Index. back issues avail.; reprint service avail. from PSC,SCH. *Refereed.* **Document type:** *Journal, Academic/Scholarly.* **Description:** Contains scholarly articles on research and policy analysis in health care focusing on economic, social, demographic, ethical and philosophical aspects.
Former titles (until 1985): Health and Society (0160-1997); (until 1973): Milbank Memorial Fund Quarterly (0026-3745); (until 1934): Milbank Memorial Fund Quarterly Bulletin (0276-5187)
Related titles: Microfiche ed.; Microform ed.: (from PQC); Online - full text ed.: (from Gale Group, Ovid Technologies, Inc., Northern Light Technology, Inc., EBSCO Publishing, O C L C Online Computer Library Center, Inc., RoweCom Information Quest, ingenta, Swets Blackwell, Institute for Scientific Information).
Indexed: ASCA, ASSIA, Abstr.Health Care Manage.Stud., Abstr.Hyg., Abstr.Soc.Geront., Acad.Ind., AgeLine, Aqua.Sci.& Fish.Abstr., Arts & Hum.Cit.Ind. (coverage dropped), B.P.I. (Mar.1986-Sep.1988), BPIA, Bibl.Asian Stud. (1970), Biol.Abstr., Chem.Abstr., Curr.Cont., Curr.Lit.Fam.Plan., Fam.Ind., Fut.Surv., Hlth.Ind., Hosp.Lit.Ind., Human Resour.Abstr., Ind.Med. (1986-), Intl.Bibl.Soc.Sci., Lang.& Lang.Behav.Abstr., Med.Care Rev., Mid.East: Abstr.& Ind., Nutr.Abstr., P.A.I.S., PsycInfo, Psychol.Abstr. (1988-), Risk Abstr., SOPODA, SSCI, Sage Fam.Stud.Abstr., Sage Pub.Admin.Abstr., Sci.Cit.Ind., Soc.Sci.Ind. (Mar.1987-), Soc.Serv.Abstr., Soc.Work Res.& Abstr., Sociol.Abstr., THA, Tr.& Indus.Ind., e-psyche.
—BLDSC (5766.040000), CISTI, GNLM, IDS, ingenta, KNAW. **CCC.**
Published by: (Milbank Memorial Fund), Blackwell Publishers, 350 Main St, Malden, MA 02148. TEL 781-388-8200, 800-835-6770, FAX 781-388-8232, subscript@blackwellpub.com, http://www.blackwellpub.com, http://www.blackwellpublishers.co.uk/journals/diph. Ed. Dr. Paul D Cleary. R&P Gretchen Voter TEL 781-388-0423. Adv. contact Anne Marie Sheehy TEL 781-388-0427. Circ: 3,000.

320 USA ISSN 0162-895X
JA74.5 CODEN: POPSEO
POLITICAL PSYCHOLOGY. Text in English. 1979. q. GBP 426 to institutions in UK & Europe; USD 538 to institutions in the Americas & Caribbean; GBP 426 elsewhere to institutions (effective 2002). adv. bk.rev. illus. back issues avail.; reprints avail. *Refereed.* **Document type:** *Journal, Academic/Scholarly.* **Description:** Interdisciplinary journal dedicated to the analysis of the inter-relationships between psychological and political processes.
Related titles: Microfilm ed.: (from PQC); Online - full text ed.: (from EBSCO Publishing, O C L C Online Computer Library Center, Inc., RoweCom Information Quest, ingenta, Swets Blackwell, Institute for Scientific Information).
Indexed: ASCA, ASSIA, Amer.Bibl.Slavic & E.Eur.Stud., Arts & Hum.Cit.Ind. (coverage dropped), Curr.Cont., Environ.Sci.Poll.Mgmt., Indian Psychol.Abstr., Int.Polit.Sci.Abstr., Intl.Bibl.Soc.Sci., Peace Res.Abstr., Polit.Sci.Abstr., PsycInfo, Psychol.Abstr. (1980-), Risk Abstr., Russ.Acad.Sci.Bibl., SSCI, Saf.Sci.Abstr., e-psyche.
—BLDSC (6543.888500), IDS, Infotrieve, ingenta. **CCC.**
Published by: (International Society of Political Psychology), Blackwell Publishers, 350 Main St, Malden, MA 02148. TEL 781-388-8200, 800-835-6770, FAX 781-388-8232, subscript@blackwellpub.com, http://www.blackwellpublishers.co.uk/journals/diph. Eds. Eugene Borgida, John L Sullivan, Wendy Rahn. R&P Gretchen Voter TEL 781-388-0423. Adv. contact Anne Marie Sheehy TEL 781-388-0427.

320 USA ISSN 0730-9384
JA80
POLITICS AND THE LIFE SCIENCES. Text in English. 1982. s-a. GBP 59, USD 97 worldwide to institutions; GBP 48, USD 80 in developing nations; GBP 29, USD 49 per issue (effective 2001). adv. bk.rev. bibl, charts, illus. back issues avail. *Refereed.* **Document type:** *Academic/Scholarly.* **Description:** Provides a forum for scholars interested in both the methods and the findings of research in the life sciences that relates to the study of politics and public policy.
Related titles: Online - full content ed.: ISSN 1471-5457 (from Gale Group); Online - full text ed.: (from CatchWord Ltd., Factiva, Institute for Scientific Information, H. W. Wilson).
Indexed: A.B.C.Pol.Sci., ASCA, AgeLine, Arts & Hum.Cit.Ind. (coverage dropped), Biol.Abstr., Biol.Dig., CLOSS, Crim.Just.Abstr., Curr.Cont., Fam.Ind., Int.Polit.Sci.Abstr., Intl.Bibl.Soc.Sci., Lang.& Lang.Behav.Abstr., Per.Islam. (1991-), Polit.Sci.Abstr., SOPODA, SSCI, Soc.Sci.Ind. (Jan.1994-), Soc.Serv.Abstr., Sociol.Abstr.
—BLDSC (6543.941850), CatchWord, CISTI, IDS, ingenta. **CCC.**
Published by: Association for Politics and the Life Sciences, c/o Gary Johnson, Ed., Lake Superior State University, Saulte Sainte Marie, MI 49783-1699. page@scipol.demon.co.uk, http://www.scipol.demon.co.uk. Circ: 750 (paid). **Dist by:** Turpin Distribution Services Ltd., Blackhorse Rd, Letchworth, Herts SG6 1HN, United Kingdom. TEL 44-1462-488900, FAX 44-1462-483011.

PSYCHOLOGY, PUBLIC POLICY, AND LAW. see *PSYCHOLOGY*

REGULATORY WATCHDOG SERVICE. see *PUBLIC ADMINISTRATION*

RESEARCH IN ORGANIZATIONAL BEHAVIOR. see *PSYCHOLOGY*

SATYA; magazine of vegetarianism, environmentalism, and animal advocacy. see *NUTRITION AND DIETETICS*

SCIENCE AS CULTURE. see *SCIENCES: COMPREHENSIVE WORKS*

SYNTHESIS - REGENERATION: A MAGAZINE OF GREEN SOCIAL THOUGHT. see *ENVIRONMENTAL STUDIES*

POLITICAL SCIENCE—Civil Rights

BRAILLE MONITOR (INKPRINT EDITION). see *HANDICAPPED—Visually Impaired*

323.4 AUS
C C H R NEWSLETTER. Text in English. 1972. irreg., latest 1985, Nov. AUD 12, USD 15. back issues avail.
Published by: Citizens Committee on Human Rights, 24 Waymouth St, Adelaide, SA 5000, Australia. Ed. Colin Harris. Circ: 350.

EVERYONE'S BACKYARD. see *ENVIRONMENTAL STUDIES—Waste Management*

GAY AND LESBIAN MEDICAL ASSOCIATION. JOURNAL. see *MEDICAL SCIENCES*

GRAUER PANTHER. see *GERONTOLOGY AND GERIATRICS*

HEALTH AND HUMAN RIGHTS; an international journal. see *PUBLIC HEALTH AND SAFETY*

HIV POLICY WATCH. see *PUBLIC HEALTH AND SAFETY*

INTERNATIONAL JOURNAL OF GROUP TENSIONS; an interdisciplinary quarterly of behavioral sciences devoted to the study of conflict and violence in human relationships. see *PSYCHOLOGY*

INTERNATIONAL JOURNAL OF SEXUALITY AND GENDER STUDIES. see *HOMOSEXUALITY*

MIND FREEDOM JOURNAL; human rights in mental health. see *MEDICAL SCIENCES—Psychiatry And Neurology*

N A A F A NEWSLETTER. see *NUTRITION AND DIETETICS*

323.40715 USA
NETWORK NEWS (SHERMAN). Text in English. 1966. s-a. USD 35 to membership (effective 2000). back issues avail. **Document type:** *Newsletter.*
Formerly: Newsletter for Soulmates
Published by: Center for Nonviolent Communication, PO Box 2662, Sherman, TX 75091-2662. TEL 903-893-3886, FAX 903-893-2935, cnvc@compuserve.com, http://www.cnvc.org. Ed. Rita Herzog. Circ: 25,000. **Co-publisher:** Center for Nonviolent Communication.

323.4 SWE
OESTERSJOEJUDISKT FORUM. Text in Swedish. 1973. irreg. (4-6/yr.). membership. charts. *Refereed.* **Document type:** *Newsletter.*
Former titles (until 1997): Judarna i f.d. Sovjet (1104-4950); (until vol.5, 1991): Judarna i Sovjet
Indexed: Inform.Sci.Abstr.
Published by: Baltic Jewish Forum, Fack 5053, Stockholm 10242, Sweden. TEL 46-8-664-53-38, FAX 46-8-664-05-91. Ed., R&P Barbro Sollbe. Circ: 2,600 (controlled).

323.4 USA ISSN 1054-1675
JC571
P H R RECORD. Text in English. 1986. q. USD 40; USD 75 to physicians. bk.rev. **Document type:** *Newsletter.*
Related titles: Microform ed.
Published by: Physicians for Human Rights, 100 Boylston St, Ste 702, Boston, MA 02116-4610. TEL 617-695-0041, FAX 617-695-0307, phrusa@phrusa.org, http://www.phrusa.org. Eds. Barbara Ayotte, Susannah Sirkin. R&P Barbara Ayotte. Circ: 5,000 (controlled).

PRO-LIFE ACTION NEWS. see *BIRTH CONTROL*

RAGGED EDGE. see *HANDICAPPED—Visually Impaired*

REPORT ON DISABILITY PROGRAMS. see *SOCIAL SERVICES AND WELFARE*

SAGE SERIES ON VIOLENCE AGAINST WOMEN. see *SOCIOLOGY*

SCHIEDSAMTSZEITUNG. see *LAW*

323.4 330.968 ZAF ISSN 1023-5310
T R A C NEWSLETTER. (Transvaal Rural Action Committee) Text in English. 1983. irreg. (1-4/yr.). ZAR 2.50 per issue. illus. **Document type:** *Newsletter.* **Description:** Examines issues in civil rights in agricultural and mining contexts. Also explores environmental issues in these areas.
Published by: T R A C, PO Box 62535, Marshalltown, Johannesburg 2107, South Africa. TEL 27-11-833-1060, FAX 27-11-834-8385, trac@wn.apc.org, http://www.oneworld.org/trac. R&P Stuart Marr. Circ: 500.

VIOLENCE AGAINST WOMEN; an international and interdisciplinary journal. see *SOCIOLOGY*

THE WEEK ONLINE. see *PHARMACY AND PHARMACOLOGY*

POLITICAL SCIENCE—International Relations

see also LAW—International Law

FOOD FIRST NEWS & VIEWS. see *POLITICAL SCIENCE*

INTERNATIONAL MINDS. see *PSYCHOLOGY*

MEDICINE, CONFLICT AND SURVIVAL; international medical concerns on global security issues. see *MEDICAL SCIENCES*

P S R MONITOR. see *PUBLIC HEALTH AND SAFETY*

P S R REPORTS. see *PUBLIC HEALTH AND SAFETY*

PSYCHOLOGISTS FOR SOCIAL RESPONSIBILITY. NEWSLETTER. see *PSYCHOLOGY*

POLLUTION

see ENVIRONMENTAL STUDIES—Pollution

POPULATION STUDIES

see also BIRTH CONTROL

BELGIUM. INSTITUT NATIONAL DE STATISTIQUE. STATISTIQUES DES CAUSES DE DECES. see *POPULATION STUDIES—Abstracting, Bibliographies, Statistics*

BELGIUM. NATIONAAL INSTITUUT VOOR DE STATISTIEK. STATISTIEK VAN DOODSOORZAKEN. see *POPULATION STUDIES—Abstracting, Bibliographies, Statistics*

BOGEON SAHOE YEONGU/HEALTH AND SOCIAL WELFARE REVIEW. see *SOCIAL SERVICES AND WELFARE*

P

BOLETIN CHILENO DE PARASITOLOGIA. see *BIOLOGY—Microbiology*

BULLETIN ON AGEING. see *GERONTOLOGY AND GERIATRICS*

362 FRA ISSN 0007-9995
RA18
CAHIERS DE SOCIOLOGIE ET DE DEMOGRAPHIE MEDICALES. Text in French. 1961. q. FRF 420, EUR 64 domestic (effective 2000); FRF 440, EUR 67 foreign (effective 1999). bk.rev. charts, stat. index. 1 cols./p. back issues avail. **Document type:** *Journal, Proceedings.*
Indexed: Abstr.Hyg., Biol.Abstr., Excerp.Med., Ind.Med. (1961-), Trop.Dis.Bull.
—BLDSC (2952.240000), GNLM.
Published by: Centre de Sociologie et Demographie Medicales, 168A ne de Grenelle, Paris 75007, France. TEL 33-1-45557377, FAX 33-1-45558794, csdm.fic@wanadoo.fr.

CELEBRATE LIFE (STAFFORD). see *BIRTH CONTROL*

325 363.96 612.6 BEL
CHOICES; sexual and reproductive health and rights in Europe. Text in English. 1972. a., latest vol.28, 2000. free per issue. bk.rev. cum.index: 1972-1976, 1977-1990. back issues avail. **Document type:** *Journal, Academic/Scholarly.*
Formerly (until 1995): Planned Parenthood in Europe (1017-8538)
Related titles: Online - full content ed.
Indexed: CWI, Curr.Lit.Fam.Plan.
Published by: International Planned Parenthood, European Network, I P P F European Network, 146 Rue Royale, Brussels 1000, Belgium. TEL 32-2500950, FAX 32-2500969, info@ippfen.org, http://www.ippf.org/regional/europe. Ed. Evert Ketting. R&P Nicoletta Confalone. Circ: 2,000.

CHRONIC DISEASES NOTES & REPORTS. see *PUBLIC HEALTH AND SAFETY*

EUGENICS SPECIAL INTEREST GROUP BULLETIN. see *BIOLOGY—Genetics*

GEORGIA VITAL STATISTICS REPORT. see *POPULATION STUDIES—Abstracting, Bibliographies, Statistics*

304.6 610 GBR ISSN 0072-6400
GREAT BRITAIN. STUDIES ON MEDICAL AND POPULATION SUBJECTS. Text in English. 1948. irreg. price varies. reprint service avail. from PQC. **Document type:** *Government.*
—BLDSC (8491.101000), CISTI.
Published by: (Great Britain. Office for National Statistics), Stationery Office, 51 Nine Elms Ln, London SW8 5DA, United Kingdom. TEL 44-20-7873-0011, FAX 44-20-7873-8247.

HEALTH INFORMATION FOR INTERNATIONAL TRAVEL. see *PUBLIC HEALTH AND SAFETY*

304.6 GBR ISSN 1465-1645
HEALTH STATISTICS QUARTERLY. Text in English. q. GBP 75; GBP 20 newsstand/cover. stat. **Document type:** *Academic/Scholarly.* **Description:** Contains commentary on the latest findings, topical articles on relevant subjects illustrated with colour charts and diagrams, regularly updated statistical tables and graphs, showing trends and the latest quarterly information: on deaths, childhood mortality, cancer survival, abortions, congenital anomalies, morbidity etc.
—BLDSC (4275.201500).
Published by: Office for National Statistics, 1 Drummond Gate, London SW1V 2QQ, United Kingdom. TEL 44-20-7533-6262. Eds. David Pearce, Karen Dunnell.

304.6 BEL ISSN 0771-2022
HB848
I U S S P NEWSLETTER/U I E S P BULLETIN DE LIAISON. Text in English, French. 3/yr. USD 10 per issue. charts, stat. back issues avail.
Published by: International Union for the Scientific Study of Population, Rue des Augustins 34, Liege 4000, Belgium. FAX 32-4-2223847. Circ: 2,000.

304.6 BEL ISSN 0253-4010
I U S S P PAPERS/U I E S P DOCUMENTS DE L'UNION. Text in English. 1974. irreg. price varies. bibl, charts, illus, stat. back issues avail.
Published by: International Union for the Scientific Study of Population, Rue des Augustins 34, Liege 4000, Belgium. FAX 32-4-2223847.

INDIAN HEALTH TRENDS AND SERVICES. see *PUBLIC HEALTH AND SAFETY*

304.6 BEL ISSN 0074-9338
INTERNATIONAL POPULATION CONFERENCE. PROCEEDINGS. Text in English. quadrennial. price varies. **Document type:** *Proceedings.*
Related titles: French ed.: Congres International de la Population. Proceedings. ISSN 0254-5217.
Indexed: Popul.Ind.
Published by: International Union for the Scientific Study of Population, Rue des Augustins 34, Liege 4000, Belgium. FAX 32-4-2223847, TELEX 42648 POPUN.

325 613.9 USA ISSN 0887-0241
JOHNS HOPKINS UNIVERSITY. POPULATION INFORMATION PROGRAM. POPULATION REPORTS. ENGLISH EDITION. Text in English. 1973. 4/yr. free per issue to qualified personnel. bibl, charts, illus, stat. back issues avail.; reprints avail. **Document type:** *Monographic series.*
Formerly: George Washington University. Population Information Program. Population Reports
Indexed: Popul.Ind.
Published by: Johns Hopkins University, Population Information Program, 111 Market Pl, Baltimore, MD 21202-4012. TEL 410-659-6300, TELEX 240430, PopRepts@welchlink.welch.jhu.edu, http://www.juccp.org. Ed. Bryant Robey. Circ: 81,000.

325 613.9 USA ISSN 0887-025X
JOHNS HOPKINS UNIVERSITY. POPULATION INFORMATION PROGRAM. POPULATION REPORTS. FRENCH EDITION. Text in English. 1973. 4/yr. free per issue to qualified personnel. bibl, charts, illus, stat. back issues avail. **Document type:** *Monographic series.*
Formerly: George Washington University. Population Information Program. Population Reports
Indexed: Popul.Ind.
Published by: Johns Hopkins University, Population Information Program, 111 Market Pl, Baltimore, MD 21202-4012. TEL 410-659-6300, PopRepts@welchlink.welch.jhu.edu, http://www.juccp.org. Ed. Bryant Robey. R&P Merridy Gottleib. Circ: 11,000.

325 613.9 USA ISSN 0887-0276
JOHNS HOPKINS UNIVERSITY. POPULATION INFORMATION PROGRAM. POPULATION REPORTS. PORTUGUESE EDITION. Text in English. 1973. 4/yr. free per issue to qualified personnel. bibl, charts, illus, stat. back issues avail. **Document type:** *Monographic series.*
Formerly: George Washington University. Population Information Program. Population Reports
Indexed: Popul.Ind.
Published by: Johns Hopkins University, Population Information Program, 111 Market Pl, Baltimore, MD 21202-4012. TEL 410-659-6300, PopRepts@welchlink.welch.jhu.edu, PoPrepts@jhuccp.org, http://www.charm.net/~nccp, http://www.jhuccp.org. Ed. Stephen Goldstein. Circ: 14,000.

325 613.9 USA ISSN 0887-0268
JOHNS HOPKINS UNIVERSITY. POPULATION INFORMATION PROGRAM. POPULATION REPORTS. SPANISH EDITION. Text in English. 1973. 4/yr. free per issue to qualified personnel. bibl, charts, illus, stat. back issues avail. **Document type:** *Monographic series.*
Formerly: George Washington University. Population Information Program. Population Reports
Indexed: Popul.Ind.
Published by: Johns Hopkins University, Population Information Program, 111 Market Pl, Baltimore, MD 21202-4012. TEL 410-659-6300, PopRepts@welchlink.welch.jhu.edu, http://www.juccp.org. Ed. Stephen Goldstein. Circ: 40,000.

JOURNAL OF HEALTH & POPULATION IN DEVELOPING COUNTRIES. see *PUBLIC HEALTH AND SAFETY*

301.32 MYS ISSN 0126-8104
MALAYSIA. NATIONAL POPULATION AND FAMILY DEVELOPMENT BOARD. BULLETIN KELUARGA. Text in English. 1969. q. free per issue. abstr, stat. **Document type:** *Government.* **Description:** Discusses family development, population and family planning.
Published by: National Population and Family Development Board, Jalan Raja Laut, PO Box 10416, Kuala Lumpur 50712, Malaysia. TEL 2937555, TELEX POPMAL MA 31911. Ed. Raj Abdul Karim.

MORBIDITY AND MORTALITY WEEKLY REPORT. see *PUBLIC HEALTH AND SAFETY*

304.64 USA ISSN 0085-428X
RA407.4.N8
NORTH CAROLINA COMMUNICABLE DISEASE MORBIDITY STATISTICS. Text in English. 1918. a., latest 1988. free per issue. stat. **Document type:** *Government.*
Published by: Department of Environment, Health and Natural Resources, Division of Epidemiology, PO Box 27687, Raleigh, NC 27611-7687. TEL 919-733-3419, FAX 919-733-0490. Circ: 600.

304.63 USA
NORTH CAROLINA REPORTED PREGNANCIES. Text in English. a. free per issue. **Document type:** *Government.*
Supersedes: North Carolina Reported Abortions (0098-3217)
Published by: Department of Health and Human Services, State Center for Health Statistics, PO Box 29538, Raleigh, NC 27626-0538. TEL 919-733-4728.

304.6 614 USA
OKLAHOMA. DEPARTMENT OF HEALTH. MONTHLY VITAL STATISTICS REPORT. Text in English. 1974. m. **Document type:** *Government.*
Published by: Department of Health, N E Tenth and Stonewall, Box 53551, Oklahoma City, OK 73105. TEL 405-271-5600. Circ: 400.

PASSAGES (WASHINGTON, D.C.). see *CHILDREN AND YOUTH—About*

PLANNED PARENTHOOD TODAY; news from the most trusted advocate for reproductive choice. see *BIRTH CONTROL*

POPULATION AND ENVIRONMENT. see *PSYCHOLOGY*

304.6 613.9 CHN ISSN 1005-4235
RENKOUXUE YU JIHUA SHENGYU/DEMOGRAPHY AND FAMILY PLANNING. Text in Chinese. 1980. bi-m. USD 27 (effective 2001). 120 p./no. **Description:** Covers the history and present situation of Chinese and world population studies. Also covers Chinese birth control policies.
Formerly (until 1993): Renkouxue (1001-3458)
Indexed: Russ.Acad.Sci.Bibl.
Published by: Zhongguo Renmin Daxue Shubao Zilio Zhongxin/Renmin University's Social Science Information Center, PO Box 1122, Beijing 100007, China. TEL 86-10-64015080, FAX 86-10-64030674, cmktg@public3.bta.net.cn, http://www.confucius.cn.net. **Dist. in US by:** China Publications Service, PO Box 49614, Chicago, IL 60649. TEL 312-288-3291, FAX 312-288-8570.

REPRODUCTIONS. see *BIOLOGY*

304.6 325 DOM
RESUMENES SOBRE POBLACION DOMINICANA. Text in Spanish. 1984. s-a. USD 9.
Published by: Asociacion Dominicana pro Bienestar de la Familia, Socorro Sanchez No. 64 Zona 1, Apdo Postal 1053, Santo Domingo, Dominican Republic. **Affiliate:** International Planned Parenthood Federation. **Co-sponsor:** Federacion Internacional de Planificacion de la Familia.

306.85 USA ISSN 0039-3665
HQ763 CODEN: SFPLA3
STUDIES IN FAMILY PLANNING. Text in English. 1963. q. USD 32 (effective 2001). bk.rev. charts, abstr, illus. index. back issues avail.; reprint service avail. from PQC. *Refereed.* **Document type:** *Academic/Scholarly.* **Description:** Publishes articles concerned with all aspects of reproductive health, fertility regulation and family planning programs, and their relation to health and development in both developed and developing countries.
Incorporates: Current Publications in Family Planning (0011-3867)
Related titles: Microform ed.: (from NRP,PQC); Online - full text ed.: (from Gale Group, JSTOR (Web-based Journal Archive), Northern Light Technology, Inc., Factiva, Institute for Scientific Information).

P

Indexed: ASCA, ASSIA, Abstr.Hyg., Adol.Ment.Hlth.Abstr., Amer.Bibl.Slavic & E.Eur.Stud., Arts & Hum.Cit.Ind. (coverage dropped), Bibl.Asian Stud. (1971-1998), Biol.Abstr., CINAHL, CWI, Curr.Cont., Curr.Lit.Fam.Plan., Ekist.Ind., Environ.Abstr., Environ.Ind., Excerp.Med., Fam.Ind., Geo.Abstr.H.G., Geo.Abstr.P.G., IBZ, IDA, IMFL, I.P.A., Ind.Med. (1963-), Intl.Bibl.Soc.Sci., Lang.& Lang.Behav.Abstr., Mid.East: Abstr.& Ind., Mult.Ed.Abstr., Nutr.Abstr., P C I, P.A.I.S., Peace Res.Abstr., Popul.Ind., Rural Devel.Abstr., Rural Ext.Educ.& Tr.Abstr., Rural Recreat.Tour.Abstr., SOPODA, SSCI, Sage Fam.Stud.Abstr., So.Pac.Per.Ind., Soc.Serv.Abstr., Sociol.Abstr., Sp.Ed.Needs Abstr., Stud.Wom.Abstr., Trop.Dis.Bull., Viol.& Abuse Abstr., World Ag.Econ.& Rur.Soc.Abstr. —BLDSC (8490.545000), GNLM, IDS, ingenta, KNAW.
Published by: Population Council, 1 Dag Hammarskjold Plaza, New York, NY 10017. TEL 212-339-0500, FAX 212-755-6052, jstor-info@umich.edu, http://www.jstor.org/fcgi-bin/jstor/listjournal.fcg/. Ed. Julie Reich. R&P Julie Sitney. Circ: 6,000 (paid and free).

304.6 PRY
TEMAS DE POBLACION. Text in Spanish. 1968. bi-m. free per issue or exchange basis. bk.rev.
Formerly: Temas Medicos
Published by: Centro Paraguayo de Estudios de Poblacion, Edif. El Dorado piso 8, Manduvira y O'Leary, Asuncion, Paraguay. TEL 447334. Ed. Helio Vera. Circ: 3,500.

THEORETICAL POPULATION BIOLOGY; an international journal. see *BIOLOGY*

U.S. CENTERS FOR DISEASE CONTROL. MORBIDITY AND MORTALITY WEEKLY REPORT. RECOMMENDATIONS AND REPORT. see *PUBLIC HEALTH AND SAFETY*

304.6 USA ISSN 0199-0071
THE Z P G REPORTER. Text in English. 1970. q. USD 25 (effective 2000); donation. adv. bk.rev. charts, stat. back issues avail. **Document type:** *Consumer.* **Description:** Contains articles and special features on a range of population-related social, economic and environmental issues.
Formerly: Z P G National Reporter (0049-8718)
Related titles: Online - full text ed.
Indexed: Curr.Lit.Fam.Plan., Environ.Abstr. —CIS.
Published by: Zero Population Growth, Inc., 1400 16th St, N W, Ste 320, Washington, DC 20036. TEL 202-332-2200, 800-767-1956, FAX 202-332-2302, info@zpg.org, http://www.zpg.org. Ed. Lee Polamsky. Circ: 60,000.

POPULATION STUDIES—Abstracting, Bibliographies, Statistics

011 FRA ISSN 1261-0674
50 TITRES SUR... Text in French. 1995. irreg.
Related titles: ♦ Supplement to: Choisir. ISSN 1261-0666.
Published by: Centre National de Documentation Pedagogique, 29 rue d'Ulm, Paris Cedex 5 75230, France. TEL 33-1-46349000, FAX 33-1-46345544. Ed. Bernard Piens.

BELGIUM. INSTITUT NATIONAL DE STATISTIQUE. ACCIDENTS DE LA CIRCULATION SUR LA VOIE PUBLIQUE AVEC TUES ET BLESSES. see *PUBLIC HEALTH AND SAFETY—Abstracting, Bibliographies, Statistics*

304.64 BEL ISSN 1370-1770
BELGIUM. INSTITUT NATIONAL DE STATISTIQUE. STATISTIQUES DES CAUSES DE DECES. Text in French. 1976. a. BEF 430 per vol. foreign (effective 2000). charts. back issues avail. **Document type:** *Government.* **Description:** Analyzes statistical data reflecting the current state and trends in the causes of death in Belgium.
Related titles: ♦ Dutch ed.: Belgium. Nationaal Instituut voor de Statistiek. Statistiek van Doodsoorzaken. ISSN 1370-1789.
Published by: Institut National de Statistique/Nationaal Instituut voor de Statistiek (Subsidiary of: Ministere des Affaires Economiques), Rue de Louvain 44, Brussels 1000, Belgium. TEL 32-2-548-6211, FAX 32-2-5486367, http://www.statbel.gfov.be.

304.6021 BEL ISSN 1370-1789
BELGIUM. NATIONAAL INSTITUUT VOOR DE STATISTIEK. STATISTIEK VAN DOODSOORZAKEN. Text in Dutch. 1976. a. BEF 430 per vol. foreign (effective 2000). charts. **Document type:** *Government.* **Description:** Analyzes statistical data reflecting the current state and trends in the causes of death in Belgium.
Related titles: ♦ French ed.: Belgium. Institut National de Statistique. Statistiques des Causes de Deces. ISSN 1370-1770.
Published by: Institut National de Statistique/Nationaal Instituut voor de Statistiek (Subsidiary of: Ministere des Affaires Economiques), Rue de Louvain 44, Brussels 1000, Belgium. TEL 32-2-548-6211, FAX 32-2-548-6367, http://www.statbel.fgov.be.

BELGIUM. NATIONAAL INSTITUUT VOOR DE STATISTIEK. VERKEERSONGEVALLEN OP DE OPENBARE WEG MET DODEN OF GEWONDEN. see *PUBLIC HEALTH AND SAFETY—Abstracting, Bibliographies, Statistics*

304.6 ITA ISSN 1121-0958
RA407.5.I8
CAUSE DI MORTE. Text in Italian. 1989. a. ITL 41,000. **Document type:** *Government.* **Description:** Presents data relevant to the causes of death and infant mortality.
Published by: Istituto Nazionale di Statistica (I.S.T.A.T.), Via Cesare Balbo, 16, Rome, RM 00184, Italy. FAX 39-6-46735198.

330.9 312 GHA
DEMOGRAPHIC AND HEALTH SURVEY (YEAR). Text in English. irreg., latest 1993. USD 10. **Document type:** *Government.*
Published by: Statistical Service, Information Section, PO Box 1098, Accra, Ghana. TEL 233-21-663758, FAX 233-21-667069.

614 363.12509489 DNK ISSN 0070-3516
HE5614.5.D4
DENMARK. DANMARKS STATISTIK. FAERDSELSUHELD. Text in Danish; Notes in English. 1930. a. DKK 164.80 (effective 2000). **Document type:** *Government.*
Indexed: Russ.Acad.Sci.Bibl.
Published by: Danmarks Statistik, Sejroegade 11, Copenhagen Oe 2100, Denmark. TEL 45-39-17-39-17, FAX 45-31-18-48-01.

304.6 DNK ISSN 0108-5646
HB1441
DOEDSAARSAGERNE/CAUSES OF DEATH IN DENMARK. Text in Danish, English. 1980. a. DKK 75. **Document type:** *Government.*
Formerly: Doedsaarsagerne i Kongeriget Danmark
Published by: Sundhedsstyrelsen, Amaliegade 13, PO Box 2020, Copenhagen K 1012, Denmark. **Orders to:** Statens Informationstjeneste, PO Box 1103, Copenhagen K 1009, Denmark.

304.644897 FIN ISSN 0787-0132
FINLAND. TILASTOKESKUS. KUOLEMANSYYT/ FINLAND. STATISTICS FINLAND. CAUSES OF DEATH IN FINLAND/FINLAND. STATISTIKCENTRALEN. DOEDSORSAKER. Text in English, Finnish, Swedish. 1939. a. FIM 155, EUR 26.07 (effective 2001). **Document type:** *Government.*
Formerly (until 1988): Sluomen Virallinen Tilasto. 6 B, Kuolemansyyt (0355-2144)
Published by: Tilastokeskus/Statistics Finland, Tyopajakatu 13, Statistics Finland, Helsinki 00022, Finland. TEL 358-9-17341, FAX 358-9-1734-2750.

304.6 USA
GEORGIA VITAL STATISTICS REPORT. Text in English. 1947. a. price varies. **Document type:** *Government.* **Description:** Disseminates selected information by race and age on births, deaths, marriages, divorces, abortions and projected populations for the calendar year.
Former titles (until 1983): Georgia Vital Statistics Data Book; Georgia Vital and Health Statistics (0362-0662); Georgia Vital Morbidity Statistics (0072-1379)
Indexed: SRI.
Published by: Department of Human Resources, Division of Public Health, 2 Peachtree St, S W, Ste 3 522, Atlanta, GA 30303-3186. TEL 404-657-6300, gdphinfo@ph.dhr.state.ga.us, http://www.ph.dhr.state.ga.us. R&P Wilma Barshaw. Circ: 650 (controlled).

304.6 USA ISSN 0093-3481
HB3525.H3
HAWAII. DEPARTMENT OF HEALTH. RESEARCH AND STATISTICS OFFICE. R & S REPORT. Key Title: R & S Report (Honolulu). Text in English. 1973. irreg. free per issue. stat. **Document type:** *Government.*
Published by: Department of Health, PO Box 3378, Honolulu, HI 96801. TEL 808-586-4600, FAX 808-586-4606, byhori@pixi.com, http://www.hawaii.gov/health, http://www.hawaii.gov/healthstatistics.

304.6 ITA
ITALY. ISTITUTO NAZIONALE DI STATISTICA. NASCITE E DECESSI. Text in Italian. 1988. a. ITL 52,500.
Supersedes in part: Statistiche Demografiche. Tomo 2. Parte Prima
Published by: Istituto Nazionale di Statistica (I.S.T.A.T.), Via Cesare Balbo, 16, Rome, RM 00184, Italy. FAX 39-6-46735198.

304.6 USA
MISSOURI MONTHLY VITAL STATISTICS. Text in English. 1967. m. free per issue. charts, stat. **Document type:** *Government.* **Description:** Contains vital statistics data and short analytical article concerning public health issues.
Published by: Department of Health, Center for Health Information Management & Epidemiology, PO Box 570, Jefferson City, MO 65102. TEL 314-751-6272. Ed. Garland Land. Circ: 800.

304.6 USA
HA203
NATIONAL VITAL STATISTICS REPORTS. Text in English. 1952. m. free per issue. Supplement avail.; reprint service avail. from CIS. *Refereed.* **Document type:** *Government.*
Formerly (until Aug. 1998): U.S. National Center for Health Statistics. Monthly Vital Statistics Report (0364-0396)
Related titles: Microfiche ed.: (from CIS).
Indexed: Abstr.Health Care Manage.Stud., Abstr.Hyg., Amer.Stat.Ind. (1972-), Curr.Lit.Fam.Plan., Ind.Med. (coverage dropped), MEDOC, Nutr.Abstr., PROMT, Popul.Ind., Rehabil.Lit., Sage Race Rel.Abstr., Trop.Dis.Bull. —GNLM.
Published by: U.S. National Center for Health Statistics, Data Dissemination Branch, 6525 Belcrest Rd, Hyattsville, MD 20782. TEL 301-458-4636, nchsquery@cdc.gov, http://www.cdc.gov/nchs/.

NEW ZEALAND HEALTH INFORMATION SERVICE. SELECTED MORBIDITY FOR PUBLICLY FUNDED HOSPITALS. see *HEALTH FACILITIES AND ADMINISTRATION—Abstracting, Bibliographies, Statistics*

NEW ZEALAND. STATISTICS NEW ZEALAND. HOUSEHOLD HEALTH SURVEY. see *PUBLIC HEALTH AND SAFETY—Abstracting, Bibliographies, Statistics*

304.6 USA ISSN 0078-1371
NORTH CAROLINA VITAL STATISTICS. Text in English. 1916. a. free per issue. **Document type:** *Government.*
Indexed: SRI.
Published by: Department of Health and Human Services, State Center for Health Statistics, PO Box 29538, Raleigh, NC 27626-0538. TEL 919-733-4728.

U.S. NATIONAL CENTER FOR HEALTH STATISTICS. CATALOG OF PUBLICATIONS. see *PUBLIC HEALTH AND SAFETY—Abstracting, Bibliographies, Statistics*

U.S. NATIONAL CENTER FOR HEALTH STATISTICS. VITAL AND HEALTH STATISTICS. SERIES 1. PROGRAMS AND COLLECTION PROCEDURES. see *PUBLIC HEALTH AND SAFETY—Abstracting, Bibliographies, Statistics*

U.S. NATIONAL CENTER FOR HEALTH STATISTICS. VITAL AND HEALTH STATISTICS. SERIES 10. DATA FROM THE HEALTH INTERVIEW SURVEY. see *PUBLIC HEALTH AND SAFETY—Abstracting, Bibliographies, Statistics*

U.S. NATIONAL CENTER FOR HEALTH STATISTICS. VITAL AND HEALTH STATISTICS. SERIES 11. DATA FROM THE HEALTH AND NUTRITION EXAMINATION SURVEY. see *PUBLIC HEALTH AND SAFETY—Abstracting, Bibliographies, Statistics*

U.S. NATIONAL CENTER FOR HEALTH STATISTICS. VITAL AND HEALTH STATISTICS. SERIES 14. DATA ON HEALTH RESOURCES. see *PUBLIC HEALTH AND SAFETY—Abstracting, Bibliographies, Statistics*

U.S. NATIONAL CENTER FOR HEALTH STATISTICS. VITAL AND HEALTH STATISTICS. SERIES 2. DATA EVALUATION AND METHODS RESEARCH. see *PUBLIC HEALTH AND SAFETY—Abstracting, Bibliographies, Statistics*

U.S. NATIONAL CENTER FOR HEALTH STATISTICS. VITAL AND HEALTH STATISTICS. SERIES 20. DATA ON MORTALITY. see *PUBLIC HEALTH AND SAFETY—Abstracting, Bibliographies, Statistics*

U.S. NATIONAL CENTER FOR HEALTH STATISTICS. VITAL AND HEALTH STATISTICS. SERIES 21. DATA ON NATALITY, MARRIAGE, AND DIVORCE. see *PUBLIC HEALTH AND SAFETY—Abstracting, Bibliographies, Statistics*

U.S. NATIONAL CENTER FOR HEALTH STATISTICS. VITAL AND HEALTH STATISTICS. SERIES 23. DATA FROM THE NATIONAL SURVEY OF FAMILY GROWTH. see *PUBLIC HEALTH AND SAFETY—Abstracting, Bibliographies, Statistics*

U.S. NATIONAL CENTER FOR HEALTH STATISTICS. VITAL AND HEALTH STATISTICS. SERIES 24. COMPILATIONS OF DATA ON NATALITY, MORTALITY, DIVORCE, AND INDUCED TERMINATIONS OF PREGNANCY. see *PUBLIC HEALTH AND SAFETY—Abstracting, Bibliographies, Statistics*

U.S. NATIONAL CENTER FOR HEALTH STATISTICS. VITAL AND HEALTH STATISTICS. SERIES 3. ANALYTICAL STUDIES. see *PUBLIC HEALTH AND SAFETY—Abstracting, Bibliographies, Statistics*

U.S. NATIONAL CENTER FOR HEALTH STATISTICS. VITAL AND HEALTH STATISTICS. SERIES 4. DOCUMENTS AND COMMITTEE REPORT. see *PUBLIC HEALTH AND SAFETY—Abstracting, Bibliographies, Statistics*

U.S. NATIONAL CENTER FOR HEALTH STATISTICS. VITAL AND HEALTH STATISTICS. SERIES 5. COMPARATIVE INTERNATIONAL VITAL AND HEALTH STATISTICS REPORTS. see *PUBLIC HEALTH AND SAFETY—Abstracting, Bibliographies, Statistics*

U.S. NATIONAL CENTER FOR HEALTH STATISTICS. VITAL AND HEALTH STATISTICS. SERIES 6. COGNITION AND SURVEY MEASUREMENT. see *PSYCHOLOGY—Abstracting, Bibliographies, Statistics*

VITAL STATISTICS OF THE UNITED STATES. see *PUBLIC HEALTH AND SAFETY—Abstracting, Bibliographies, Statistics*

POSTAL AFFAIRS

see *COMMUNICATIONS—Postal Affairs*

POULTRY AND LIVESTOCK

see *AGRICULTURE—Poultry And Livestock*

PRODUCTION OF GOODS AND SERVICES

see *BUSINESS AND ECONOMICS—Production Of Goods And Services*

PROTESTANTISM

see *RELIGIONS AND THEOLOGY—Protestant*

PSYCHIATRY AND NEUROLOGY

see *MEDICAL SCIENCES—Psychiatry And Neurology*

PSYCHOLOGY

see also *MEDICAL SCIENCES—Psychiatry And Neurology*

155 USA
A B A NEWSLETTER (KALAMAZOO). Text in English. 1977. q. USD 30 to non-members. adv. bk.rev. **Document type:** *Newsletter.* **Description:** Covers association activities, news and conference announcements.
Published by: Association for Behavior Analysis, Western Michigan University, Kalamazoo, MI 49008-5052. TEL 616-387-8341, FAX 616-387-8354. Ed. Matthew Miller. Circ: 2,300.

152.4 USA
A D A A REPORTER. Text in English. 1990. q. USD 30 (effective 1999). adv. bk.rev. **Document type:** *Newsletter.* **Description:** Includes scientific, research and clinical articles, self-helps information, and association news items.
Indexed: e-psyche.
Published by: Anxiety Disorders Association of America, 11900 Parklawn Dr, Ste 100, Rockville, MD 20852-2624. TEL 301-231-9350, FAX 301-231-7392, anxdis@adaa, http://www.adaa.org. Ed., R&P David Rapoport. Adv. contact Michelle Alonso. Circ: 6,000.

A D A M H A NEWS. (Alcohol, Drug Abuse, and Mental Health Administration) see *DRUG ABUSE AND ALCOHOLISM*

A E C A RESEARCH IN PRACTICE. see *CHILDREN AND YOUTH—About*

A E P APPOINTMENTS BROADSHEET. see *OCCUPATIONS AND CAREERS*

370.15 USA ISSN 1041-956X
A H A F JOURNAL. Text in English. 1967. bi-m. USD 50 (effective Jan. 2001). adv. bk.rev. charts, illus. back issues avail. *Refereed.* **Document type:** *Journal, Academic/Scholarly, Bibliography.* **Description:** Covers educational material pertaining to graphology and questioned documents. Includes international graphological "hand-holding" exchange with analysts around the world.
Formerly (until 1985): A H A F News
Indexed: e-psyche.
Published by: American Handwriting Analysis Foundation, PO Box 6210, San Jose, CA 95150. TEL 804-979-2848. Ed., R&P, Adv. contact Jeanette Farmer. B&W page USD 100. Circ: 300.

158 USA
A H P PERSPECTIVE. Text in English. 1962. bi-m. members only. adv. bk.rev. back issues avail. *Refereed.* **Document type:** *Newsletter, Directory, Academic/Scholarly, Trade.* **Description:** Aimed at international community of people with diverse talents and interests who are dedicated to building a more humane world.
Formerly: A H P Newsletter
Related titles: Online - full text ed.
Indexed: e-psyche.
Published by: Association for Humanistic Psychology, 45 Franklin St, Ste 315, San Francisco, CA 94102. TEL 415-435-1604, FAX 415-435-2815, erickson.editorial@att.net, http://ahpweb.org/pub/perspective/menu.html. Ed., R&P, Adv. contact Kathleen E Erickson. Circ: 5,500 (paid).

A M S STUDIES IN MODERN SOCIETY. see *PUBLIC HEALTH AND SAFETY*

155.4 610 USA
A N A D: WORKING TOGETHER. Text in English. 1979. q. USD 25 to members. bk.rev. **Document type:** *Newsletter.* **Description:** Discusses issues and challenges facing persons suffering from eating disorders and related afflictions.
Indexed: e-psyche.
Published by: National Association of Anorexia Nervosa and Associated Disorders, PO Box 7, Highland, IL 60035. TEL 847-831-3438, FAX 847-433-4632. Circ: 15,000.

A N R E D. see *MEDICAL SCIENCES—Psychiatry And Neurology*

150 USA
A P A RESEARCH PSYCHOLOGY FUNDING BULLETIN. Text in English. irreg. back issues avail. **Document type:** *Bulletin.* **Description:** Includes news and announcements of conferences and special events of interest to research psychologists.
Media: Online - full text.
Published by: American Psychological Association, 750 First St., N.E., Washington, DC 20002-4242. TEL 202-336-6000, FAX 202-336-5953, science@apa.org, http://www.apa.org/science/bulletin.html.

152 IND
A P R C JOURNAL OF EXPERIMENTAL PSYCHOLOGY. Text in English. 1978. 2/yr. USD 181.75. reprint service avail. from ISI. **Document type:** *Academic/Scholarly.*
Indexed: e-psyche.
Published by: Agra Psychological Research Cell, Tiwari Kothi, Belanganj, Agra, Uttar Pradesh 282 004, India. Ed. Govind Tiwari.

150 USA ISSN 1050-4672
A P S OBSERVER. Text in English. 1988. bi-m. USD 35 domestic to individuals; USD 50 foreign to individuals; USD 50 domestic to institutions; USD 65 foreign to institutions. adv. illus. reprints avail. **Document type:** *Newsletter, Trade.* **Description:** Covers the Society activities and news on political and research issues of importance to scientific psychologists.
Indexed: e-psyche.
Published by: American Psychological Society, 1010 Vermont Ave, NW, Ste 1100, Washington, DC 20005-4907. TEL 202-783-2077, FAX 202-783-2083, aps@aps.washington.dc.us, ewr@aps.washington.dc.us, http://www.hanover.edu./psych/APS/aps.html. Ed. Elizabeth Ruksznis. Pub. Alan Kraut. R&P K Lee Herring. Adv. contact Kristen Bourke. B&W page USD 1,450; trim 11 x 8.5. Circ: 15,030.

301.1 150 VEN ISSN 1011-6281
A V E P S O FASCICULO. Text in Spanish. 1983. a. VEB 45, USD 6. back issues avail.
Indexed: Psychol.Abstr., e-psyche.
Published by: Asociacion Venezolana de Psicologia Social, Los Chaguaramos, Apdo 47101, Caracas, DF 1040, Venezuela. TEL 6624751; 619811-30, Ext. 2643, 3043. Ed. Beatriz Rodriguez. Circ: 500.

150 DNK ISSN 0906-6659
AARHUS UNIVERSITET. PSYKOLOGISK SKRIFTSERIE. Text in Danish; Summaries in English. 1976. irreg. price varies. *Refereed.* **Document type:** *Monographic series.*
Former titles (until 1990): Aarhus Universitet. Psykologisk Skriftserie Aarhus (0900-8527); (until 1979): Psychological Reports Aarhus (0105-2861)
Indexed: Psychol.Abstr., e-psyche.
Published by: Aarhus Universitet, Psykologisk Institut, Aarhus C 8000, Denmark. TEL 45-89-42-49-00, FAX 45-89-42-49-01, aske@psy.aau.dk. Ed., R&P Ask Elklit.

ABHIGYAN; the journal of foundation for organization research and education. see *SOCIAL SCIENCES: COMPREHENSIVE WORKS*

150 USA
ACADEMIC PRESS SERIES IN COGNITION AND PERCEPTION. Text in English. 1973. irreg., latest 1988. reprint service avail. from ISI. *Refereed.* **Document type:** *Monographic series.*
Indexed: e-psyche.
Published by: Academic Press, Inc., Journal Division (Subsidiary of: Harcourt Brace & Company), 525 B St, Ste 1900, San Diego, CA 92101-4495. TEL 619-231-0926, FAX 619-699-6715. Eds. Edward C Carterette, Morton P Friedman. **Subscr. to:** Order Dept., 6277 Sea Harbor Dr, 4th Fl, Orlando, FL 32887. TEL 800-321-5068.

150 USA ISSN 0192-1088
RC500
ACADEMY FORUM. Text in English. 1956. s-a. USD 20 in North America; USD 30 elsewhere (effective 2000). adv. bk.rev. *Refereed.* **Document type:** *Academic/Scholarly.* **Description:** Provides an opportunity for members to present their views on issues pertaining to practice, social conflict and change, literary criticism, the arts, and the state of the world.
Formerly (until 1977): Academy (0197-5781)
Indexed: e-psyche.
Published by: American Academy of Psychoanalysis, 47 E 19th St, 6th Fl, New York, NY 10003-1323. TEL 212-475-7980, FAX 212-425-8101, aapny@aol.com. Ed., R&P, Adv. contact Jane Simon. Circ: 1,000.

150.195 ARG ISSN 0329-9147
BF175.4.C84
ACHERONTA; revista de psicoanalisis y cultura. Text in Spanish. 1995. irreg. adv. bk.rev. **Description:** Includes articles on psychology and psychoanalisis, including Freud theory.
Media: Online - full text.

P

Address: Coronel Diaz 1785 - 1C, Buenos Aires 1425, Argentina. acheronta@psiconet.com, http://www.acheronta.org/, http://www.psiconet.com/acheronta/. Ed. Michel Sauval.

ACTA ETHOLOGICA. see *BIOLOGY—Zoology*

ACTA ETHOLOGICA ONLINE. see *BIOLOGY*

ACTA MEDICA ROMANA. see *MEDICAL SCIENCES*

ACTA PAEDOLOGICA; an international journal of child development. see *CHILDREN AND YOUTH—About*

150 NLD ISSN 0001-6918
BF1 CODEN: APSOAZ
ACTA PSYCHOLOGICA; international journal of psychonomics. Text in English. 1941. 9/yr. EUR 294 in Europe to individuals; JPY 39,000 in Japan to individuals; USD 329 elsewhere to individuals; EUR 732 in Europe to institutions; JPY 97,200 in Japan to institutions; USD 818 elsewhere to institutions (effective 2002). adv. bk.rev. bibl, illus. index. back issues avail.; reprint service avail. from PSC,SCH. *Refereed.* **Document type:** *Journal, Academic/Scholarly.* **Description:** Publishes original papers reporting on experimental studies, as well as theoretical and review articles, in human experimental psychology.
Related titles: Microform ed.: (from PQC); Online - full text ed.: (from ingenta, Swets Blackwell, ScienceDirect, Institute for Scientific Information).
Indexed: ASCA, ASSIA, Addic.Abstr., AgeLine, Bibl.Ind., Biol.Abstr., Commun.Abstr., Curr.Cont., Environ.Sci.Poll.Mgmt., Ergon.Abstr., Ind.Med. (1935-), Lang.& Lang.Behav.Abstr., Mid.East: Abstr.& Ind., Neurosci.Cit.Ind., Pollut.Abstr., PsycInfo, Psychol.Abstr. (1950-), Res.High.Educ.Abstr., Risk Abstr., Russ.Acad.Sci.Bibl., SOPODA, SSCI, Saf.Sci.Abstr., Sociol.Abstr., Stud.Wom.Abstr., e-psyche.
—BLDSC (0661.490000), CISTI, IDS, ingenta, KNAW. **CCC.**
Published by: North-Holland (Subsidiary of: Elsevier Science BV), PO Box 211, Amsterdam 1000 AE, Netherlands. TEL 31-20-485-3911, FAX 31-20-485-3598, nlinfo-f@elsevier.nl, http://www.elsevier.com/locate/actpsy, http://www.elsevier.nl. Ed. M. W. van der Molen. **Subscr. in Australasia and the Far East to:** Elsevier Science (Singapore) Pte Ltd, No.1 Temasek Ave, 17-01 Millenia Tower, Singapore 039192, Singapore. TEL 65-434-3727, FAX 65-337-2230, asiainfo@elsevier.com.sg; **Subscr. in Japan to:** Elsevier Science Inc - Japan Regional Office, 9-15 Higashi-Azabu 1-chome, Minato-ku, Tokyo 106-0044, Japan. TEL 81-3-5561-5033, FAX 81-3-5561-5047, info@elsevier.co.jp; **Subscr. in the Americas to:** Elsevier Science, PO Box 945, New York, NY 10159-0945. TEL 212-633-3730, 888-437-4636, FAX 212-633-3680, usinfo-f@elsevier.com, http://www.elsevier.com. **Dist. by:** Elsevier Science (Brazil).

P

152 FIN ISSN 0515-3115
ACTA PSYCHOLOGICA FENNICA. Text in Finnish. 1951. irreg. (1-2/yr.). FIM 100 (effective 1998). **Document type:** *Academic/Scholarly.*
Indexed: e-psyche.
Published by: Finnish Psychological Society, Sofiankatu 16 A, Helsinki 00170, Finland. TEL 358-9-278-21-22. Ed. Marja Vauras. Circ: 700.

150 POL
L51
ACTA UNIVERSITATIS LODZIENSIS: FOLIA PSYCHOLOGICA. Text in German, Polish; Summaries in English, German. 1955-1974; N.S. 1980; N.S. 1995. irreg. charts. **Document type:** *Academic/Scholarly.* **Description:** Contains articles from the fields of psychology, as well as proceeding of scientific conferences organized by Department of Pedagogics and Psychology in the University of Lodz.
Supersedes in part (in 1995): Acta Universitatis Lodziensis: Folia Padagogica et Psychologica (0208-6093); Which superseded in part: Uniwersytet Lodzki. Zeszyty Naukowe. Seria 1: Nauki Humanistyczno-Spoleczne (0076-0358)
Indexed: e-psyche.
—KNAW.
Published by: (Uniwersytet Lodzki, Wydzial Pedagogiki i Psychologii), Wydawnictwo Uniwersytetu Lodzkiego, Ul. Jaracza 34, Lodz, Poland. TEL 48-42-331671.

150 POL ISSN 0137-110X
ACTA UNIVERSITATIS WRATISLAVIENSIS. PRACE PSYCHOLOGICZNE. Text in Polish. 1972. irreg. price varies. **Document type:** *Academic/Scholarly.*
Indexed: Russ.Acad.Sci.Bibl., e-psyche.
—KNAW.
Published by: (Uniwersytet Wroclawski/Polish Chemical Society), Wydawnictwo Uniwersytetu Wroclawskiego Spolka z o.o., Pl Uniwersytecki 9-13, Wroclaw 50137, Poland. TEL 48-71-441006, FAX 48-71-402735. Ed. Maria Stras Romanowska. Circ: 300.

ADOLESCENCE (SAN DIEGO); an international quarterly devoted to the physiological, psychological, psychiatric, sociological, and educational aspects of the second decade of human life. see *CHILDREN AND YOUTH—About*

ADOLESCENT PSYCHIATRY; annals of the American Society for Adolescent Psychiatry. see *MEDICAL SCIENCES—Psychiatry And Neurology*

150 JPN ISSN 0918-1490
ADORERIAN/ADLERIAN. Text in Japanese. 1984. 3/yr. JPY 5,000. adv. *Refereed.* **Document type:** *Academic/Scholarly.* **Description:** Covers the theories and practices of adlerian or individual psychology.
Indexed: e-psyche.
Published by: Nihon Adora Shinri Gakkai/Japanese Society of Adlerian Psychology, 5-12-15-301 Nishinaka-Jima, Yodogawa-ku, Osaka-shi 532-0011, Japan. TEL 81-6-6306-4699, FAX 81-6-1306-0160. Ed., R&P, Adv. contact Samuel M Kamata.

155.4 USA ISSN 1524-6817
▼ **ADULTSPAN.** Text in English. 1999. 2/yr. USD 25 to individuals; USD 52 to institutions (effective 2001). adv. abstr, bibl. 64 p./no. back issues avail. *Refereed.* **Document type:** *Journal, Academic/Scholarly.* **Description:** Covers development through youth, middle age, and older adulthood.
Related titles: Microfilm ed.
Published by: (Association for Adult Development and Ageing), American Counseling Association, 5999 Stevenson Ave, Alexandria, VA 22304-3300. TEL 703-823-9800, FAX 703-823-0252, http://www.counseling.org. Ed. Catherine B Roland. R&P Cynthia Peay TEL 703-823-9800 x 249. Adv. contact Kathy Maguire TEL 703-823-9800 ext 207. Circ: 1,500.

150 USA
ADVANCED PSYCHOLOGY TEXTS. Text in English. irreg., latest vol.2, 1995. **Document type:** *Academic/Scholarly.*
Indexed: e-psyche.
—BLDSC (0696.923000).
Published by: Sage Publications, Inc., Books, 2455 Teller Rd, Thousand Oaks, CA 91320. TEL 805-499-0721, FAX 805-499-0871, order@sagepub.com. Ed. Ronald Kellogg.

155 USA
BF712
ADVANCES IN APPLIED DEVELOPMENTAL PSYCHOLOGY. Text in English. 1985. a. price varies. **Document type:** *Academic/Scholarly.*
Former titles: Annual Advances in Applied Developmental Psychology (1042-2463); (until 1987): Advances in Applied Developmental Psychology (0748-8572)
Indexed: Psychol.Abstr., e-psyche.
—BLDSC (0698.940000). **CCC.**
Published by: Ablex Publishing Corporation (Subsidiary of: Greenwood Publishing Group Inc.), 88 Post Rd W, Westport, CT 06881. TEL 203-323-9606, FAX 203-357-8446. Ed. Irving Siegel.

155 591 USA ISSN 0099-6246
CODEN: ADBBBW
ADVANCES IN BEHAVIORAL BIOLOGY. Text in English. 1971. irreg., latest vol.49, 1999. price varies. back issues avail. *Refereed.* **Document type:** *Monographic series.*
Indexed: Chem.Abstr., Chem.Indus.Notes, Chem.Titles, e-psyche.
—BLDSC (0699.910000), CASDDS, CISTI, GNLM, Infotrieve, ingenta, KNAW. **CCC.**
Published by: Kluwer Academic - Plenum Publishers (Subsidiary of: Wolters Kluwer N.V.), 233 Spring St, New York, NY 10013-1578. TEL 212-620-8000, 800-221-9369, FAX 212-463-0742, info@plenum.com, http://www.plenum.com.

152.8 330.9 USA ISSN 0890-0159
HB1
ADVANCES IN BEHAVIORAL ECONOMICS. Text in English. 1987. irreg., latest vol.3, 1996. USD 73.25. **Document type:** *Academic/Scholarly.*
Indexed: e-psyche.
—BLDSC (0699.911200).
Published by: Ablex Publishing Corporation (Subsidiary of: Greenwood Publishing Group Inc.), 88 Post Rd W, Westport, CT 06881. TEL 302-661-7602, FAX 203-661-0792. Eds. John Kagel, Leonard Green.

155 618.92 USA ISSN 0065-2407
BF721 CODEN: ADCDA8
ADVANCES IN CHILD DEVELOPMENT AND BEHAVIOR. Text in English. 1963. irreg., latest vol.26, 1996. index. reprint service avail. from ISI. *Refereed.* **Document type:** *Monographic series.*
Related titles: Online - full text ed.: (from Institute for Scientific Information).
Indexed: ASCA, Biol.Abstr., Ind.Med. (1963-), SSCI, e-psyche.
—BLDSC (0703.800000), CISTI, GNLM, ingenta. **CCC.**
Published by: Academic Press, Inc., Journal Division (Subsidiary of: Harcourt Brace & Company), 525 B St, Ste 1900, San Diego, CA 92101-4495. TEL 619-231-0926, FAX 619-699-6715. Eds. Charles C Spiegel, L P Lipsitt. **Subscr. to:** Order Dept., 6277 Sea Harbor Dr, 4th Fl, Orlando, FL 32887. TEL 800-321-5068.

150 616.8 USA ISSN 0940-8606
ADVANCES IN CHILD NEUROPSYCHOLOGY. Text in English. irreg., latest vol.3, 1995. **Document type:** *Monographic series, Academic/Scholarly.*
Indexed: e-psyche.
Published by: Springer-Verlag, Journals (Subsidiary of: BertelsmannSpringer), 175 Fifth Ave, New York, NY 10010. TEL 212-460-1500, FAX 212-473-6272. Eds. Michael Tramontana, Stephen Hooper.

ADVANCES IN CLINICAL NEUROPSYCHOLOGY. see *MEDICAL SCIENCES—Psychiatry And Neurology*

ADVANCES IN COGNITION AND EDUCATIONAL PRACTICE. see *EDUCATION*

150 USA
ADVANCES IN COMPARATIVE PSYCHOLOGY. Text in English. 1991. irreg. price varies. **Document type:** *Monographic series.*
Indexed: e-psyche.
Published by: Praeger Publishers (Subsidiary of: Greenwood Publishing Group Inc.), 88 Post Rd W, Box 5007, Westport, CT 06881-5007. TEL 203-226-3571, FAX 203-222-1502.

152 NLD ISSN 1381-589X
ADVANCES IN CONSCIOUSNESS RESEARCH. Text in English. 1995. irreg., latest vol.21, 2000. price varies. back issues avail. *Refereed.* **Document type:** *Monographic series, Academic/Scholarly.* **Description:** Provides a forum for scholars from various scientific disciplines and fields of knowledge relating to all aspects of consciousness, including cognitive psychology, linguistics, brain science, and philosophy.
Indexed: MLA Intl.Bibl., e-psyche.
—BLDSC (0704.135000).
Published by: John Benjamins Publishing Co., PO Box 36224, Amsterdam 1020 ME, Netherlands. TEL 31-20-630-4747, FAX 31-20-673-9773, http://www.benjamins.nl/jbp/index.html, http://www.benjamins.com. Eds. Gordon G Globus, Maxim I Stamenov. **In N America:** John Benjamins Publishing Co., PO Box 27519, Philadelphia, PA 19118-0519. TEL 215-836-1200, FAX 215-836-1204.

ADVANCES IN EXPERIMENTAL SOCIAL PSYCHOLOGY. see *SOCIOLOGY*

ADVANCES IN HEALTH EDUCATION: CURRENT RESEARCH. see *EDUCATION—Teaching Methods And Curriculum*

332.1 NLD ISSN 0921-2647
TA166
ADVANCES IN HUMAN FACTORS - ERGONOMICS. Text in Dutch. 1984. irreg., latest 1997, vol 21 A&B. price varies. *Refereed.* **Document type:** *Monographic series, Proceedings, Academic/Scholarly.* **Description:** Reports on research and development in the specialty field of ergonomics.
Indexed: Eng.Ind., e-psyche.
—BLDSC (0709.067000), CISTI, Ei, Infotrieve. **CCC.**

Published by: Elsevier Science BV, PO Box 211, Amsterdam 1000 AE, Netherlands. TEL 31-20-485-3757, 31-20-485-3911, FAX 31-20-485-3432, 31-20-485-3598, nlinfo-f@elsevier.nl; usinfo-f@elsevier.com; forinfo-kyf04035@niftyserve.or.jp, http://www.elsevier.nl/. Ed. Gavriel Salvendy. **Subscr. in Australasia and the Far East to:** Elsevier Science (Singapore) Pte Ltd, No.1 Temasek Ave, 17-01 Millenia Tower, Singapore 039192, Singapore. TEL 65-434-3727, FAX 65-337-2230, asiainfo@elsevier.com.sg; **Subscr. in Japan to:** Elsevier Science Inc - Japan Regional Office, 9-15 Higashi-Azabu 1-chome, Minato-ku, Tokyo 106-0044, Japan. TEL 81-3-5561-5033, FAX 81-3-5561-5047, info@elsevier.co.jp; **Subscr. in the Americas to:** Elsevier Science, PO Box 945, New York, NY 10159-0945. TEL 212-633-3730, 888-437-4636, FAX 212-633-3680, usinfo-f@elsevier.com, http://www.elsevier.com

ADVANCES IN INFANCY RESEARCH. see *MEDICAL SCIENCES—Pediatrics*

ADVANCES IN LEARNING AND BEHAVIORAL DISABILITIES. see *EDUCATION—Special Education And Rehabilitation*

614.58 USA ISSN 0749-7423
BF501
ADVANCES IN MOTIVATION AND ACHIEVEMENT. Text in English. 1984. a. USD 78.50 to institutions.
Indexed: e-psyche.
—BLDSC (0709.453000), ingenta. **CCC.**
Published by: J A I Press Inc., 100 Prospect St, Box 811, Stamford, CT 06904-0811. TEL 203-323-9606, FAX 203-357-8446. Ed. Martin L Maehr.

150 NLD ISSN 0166-4115
CODEN: ADPSEK
ADVANCES IN PSYCHOLOGY. Text in Dutch. 1980. irreg., latest vol.129, 1999. price varies. *Refereed.* **Document type:** *Monographic series, Academic/Scholarly.* **Description:** Reports on developments and research in clinical and applied psychology.
Indexed: e-psyche.
—BLDSC (0711.065000), CISTI. **CCC.**
Published by: Elsevier Science BV, PO Box 211, Amsterdam 1000 AE, Netherlands. TEL 31-20-485-3757, 31-20-485-3911, FAX 31-20-485-3432, 31-20-485-3598, nlinfo-f@elsevier.nl; usinfo-f@elsevier.com; forinfo-kyf04035@niftyserve.or.jp, http://www.elsevier.nl/. Ed. G E Stelmach. **Subscr. in Australasia and the Far East to:** Elsevier Science (Singapore) Pte Ltd, No.1 Temasek Ave, 17-01 Millenia Tower, Singapore 039192, Singapore. TEL 65-434-3727, FAX 65-337-2230, asiainfo@elsevier.com.sg; **Subscr. in Japan to:** Elsevier Science Inc - Japan Regional Office, 9-15 Higashi-Azabu 1-chome, Minato-ku, Tokyo 106-0044, Japan. TEL 81-3-5561-5033, FAX 81-3-5561-5047, info@elsevier.co.jp; **Subscr. in the Americas to:** Elsevier Science, PO Box 945, New York, NY 10159-0945. TEL 212-633-3730, 888-437-4636, FAX 212-633-3680, usinfo-f@elsevier.com, http://www.elsevier.com

155.937 362 USA ISSN 0196-1934
BD444
ADVANCES IN THANATOLOGY✱ . Text in English. q. USD 66.50. adv. back issues avail. **Description:** Articles cover life threatening disease, dying, death, bereavement, hospice care, and widowhood.
Formerly: Journal of Thanatology (0047-2832)
Related titles: Microform ed.: (from PQC).
Indexed: IBR, e-psyche.
—BLDSC (0711.605000), GNLM.
Published by: Foundation of Thanatology, Foundation Book & Periodical Division, 630 W 168th St, New York, NY 10032. TEL 212-928-2066. Ed. David Peretz.

150 USA ISSN 0065-3454
QL750 CODEN: ADSBBF
ADVANCES IN THE STUDY OF BEHAVIOR. Text in English. 1965. irreg., latest vol.27, 1998. index. reprint service avail. from ISI. *Refereed.*
Related titles: Online - full text ed.: (from Institute for Scientific Information).
Indexed: ASCA, Agricola, Biol.Abstr., Curr.Adv.Ecol.Sci., Dairy Sci.Abstr., Ind.Sci.Rev., P C I, SSCI (coverage dropped), Sci.Cit.Ind., Sport Fish.Abstr., Zoo.Rec., e-psyche.
—BLDSC (0711.590000), CASDDS, CISTI. **CCC.**
Published by: Academic Press, Inc., Journal Division (Subsidiary of: Harcourt Brace & Company), 525 B St, Ste 1900, San Diego, CA 92101-4495. TEL 619-231-0926, FAX 619-699-6715. **Subscr. to:** Order Dept., 6277 Sea Harbor Dr, 4th Fl, Orlando, FL 32887. TEL 800-321-5068.

616.89 USA
THE ADVOCATE (ALEXANDRIA). Text in English. 1976. bi-m. USD 25 to non-members (effective 2000). adv. bk.rev. **Document type:** *Newsletter.* **Description:** Covers professional issues, legal issues, licensure and certification, third-party payment, consumer concerns.
Related titles: Microform ed.
Indexed: L.R.I., e-psyche.
Published by: American Mental Health Counselors Association, 801 N Fairfax St, Ste 304, Alexandria, VA 22314. TEL 800-326-2642, FAX 703-548-4775, http://www.amhca.org. Ed. Bill Wheeler. Pub., Adv. contact Erin Liposky. Circ: 5,500.

ADVOCATE (BETHESDA). see *EDUCATION—Special Education And Rehabilitation*

AFTERLOSS; the monthly newsletter to comfort and care for those who mourn. see *MEDICAL SCIENCES—Psychiatry And Neurology*

616.89 GBR ISSN 1359-1789
RC569.5.A34 CODEN: AVBEFZ
AGGRESSION AND VIOLENT BEHAVIOR; a review journal. Text in English. 1996. bi-m. EUR 82 in Europe to qualified personnel; JPY 10,800 in Japan to qualified personnel; USD 90 elsewhere to qualified personnel; EUR 404 in Europe to institutions; JPY 53,600 in Japan to institutions; USD 452 elsewhere to institutions (effective 2002). adv. back issues avail. *Refereed.* **Document type:** *Academic/Scholarly.* **Description:** Provides multidisciplinary forum for publication of review articles and summary reports of innovative and ongoing clinical research programs relating to the field of aggression and violent behavior.
Related titles: Online - full text ed.: (from ingenta, Swets Blackwell, ScienceDirect, Institute for Scientific Information).
Indexed: AgeLine, Crim.Just.Abstr., Curr.Cont., Indian Psychol.Abstr., PsycInfo, SSCI, e-psyche.
—BLDSC (0736.284200), IDS, ingenta. **CCC.**
Published by: Pergamon (Subsidiary of: Elsevier Science), The Boulevard, Langford Ln, East Park, Kidlington, Oxford OXB 1GB, United Kingdom. FAX 44-1865-843010, http://www.elsevier.com/locate/aggviobeh. Eds. M Hersen, V B van Hasselt. **Subscr. in Australasia and the Far East to:** Elsevier Science (Singapore) Pte Ltd, No.1 Temasek Ave, 17-01 Millenia Tower, Singapore 039192, Singapore. TEL 65-434-3727, FAX 65-337-2230; **Subscr. in the Americas to:** Elsevier Science, PO Box 945, New York, NY 10159-0945. TEL 212-633-3730, FAX 212-633-3680; **Subscr. to:** Elsevier Science BV. TEL 31-20-485-3757, FAX 31-20-485-3432.

350 USA ISSN 0096-140X
BF575.A3 CODEN: AGBEDU
AGGRESSIVE BEHAVIOR; a multidisciplinary journal devoted to the experimental and observational analysis of conflict in humans and animals. Text in English. 1975. bi-m. USD 1,450 in United States; USD 1,510 in Canada & Mexico; USD 1,561 elsewhere; USD 1,523 combined subscription in United States for print and online eds.; USD 1,583 combined subscription in Canada & Mexico for print and online eds.; USD 1,634 combined subscription elsewhere for print and online eds. (effective 2002). adv. bk.rev. bibl, charts, illus, abstr. index. back issues avail.; reprint service avail. from ISI. *Refereed.* **Document type:** *Academic/Scholarly.* **Description:** Devoted to the empirical and theoretical analysis of conflict and the scientific understanding of agression in humans and animals.
Related titles: Microform ed.: (from PQC); Online - full text ed.: ISSN 1098-2337. 1996. USD 1,450 in United States; USD 1,450 in Canada & Mexico; USD 1,450 elsewhere (effective 2002) (from EBSCO Publishing, Gale Group, Wiley InterScience, Institute for Scientific Information).
Indexed: ASCA, Adol.Ment.Hlth.Abstr., AgeLine, Anim.Behav.Abstr., Aqua.Sci.& Fish.Abstr., Biol.Abstr., Chem.Abstr., Chem.Indus.Notes, Chem.Titles, Commun.Abstr., Crim.Just.Abstr., Curr.Adv.Ecol.Sci., Curr.Cont., Environ.Sci.Poll.Mgmt., Excerp.Med., Fam.Ind., Ind.Sci.Rev., Ind.Vet., Inpharma, Mid.East: Abstr.& Ind., Neurosci.Cit.Ind., Peace Res.Abstr., Pig News & Info., PsycInfo, Psychol.Abstr. (1974-), Reac., Ref.Zh., Risk Abstr., SSCI, Saf.Sci.Abstr., Sci.Cit.Ind., Sport Fish.Abstr., Vet.Bull., Wild.Rev., Zoo.Rec., e-psyche.
—BLDSC (0736.285000), CASDDS, CISTI, EMDOCS, GNLM, IDS, ingenta. **CCC.**
Published by: (International Society for Research on Agression), John Wiley & Sons, Inc., Journals (Subsidiary of: Wiley InterScience), 605 Third Ave, New York, NY 10158. TEL 212-850-6645, FAX 212-850-6021, uscs-wis@wiley.com, http://www.interscience.wiley.com/jpages/0096-140 X, http://www.wiley.com. Ed. Ronald Baenninger. adv.: B&W page GBP 640, color page GBP 1,515; trim 178 x 254. Circ: 550. **Subscr. outside the Americas to:** John Wiley & Sons Ltd., Baffins Ln, Chichester, Sussex PO19 IUD, United Kingdom. TEL 44-1243-779777, FAX 44-1243-843232, cs-journals@wiley.co.uk, http://www.wiley.co.uk.

AGING & MENTAL HEALTH. see *GERONTOLOGY AND GERIATRICS*

AIDS & BEHAVIOR. see *MEDICAL SCIENCES—Allergology And Immunology*

AIDS PREVENTION AND MENTAL HEALTH. see *MEDICAL SCIENCES—Communicable Diseases*

AIIKU TSUSHIN/LETTERS OF HUMAN GROWTH. see *EDUCATION*

ALABAMA COUNSELING ASSOCIATION. JOURNAL. see *OCCUPATIONS AND CAREERS*

AMERICAN ACADEMY OF PSYCHIATRY AND THE LAW. NEWSLETTER. see *LAW*

150.19 USA ISSN 0090-3604
RC500 CODEN: JAAPCC
AMERICAN ACADEMY OF PSYCHOANALYSIS. JOURNAL. Text in English. 1973. q. USD 50 domestic to individuals; USD 75 foreign to individuals; USD 185 domestic to institutions; USD 210 foreign to institutions (effective 2000). adv. bk.rev. index. back issues avail.; reprint service avail. from PQC,PSC,SCH,ISI. *Refereed.* **Document type:** *Academic/Scholarly.*
Related titles: Microform ed.; Online - full text ed.: (from ProQuest Information & Learning, CatchWord Ltd., RoweCom Information Quest).
Indexed: Adol.Ment.Hlth.Abstr., AgeLine, Biol.Abstr., Curr.Cont. (coverage dropped), Environ.Sci.Poll.Mgmt., Excerp.Med., Ind.Med. (1973-), Indian Psychol.Abstr., Int.Nurs.Ind., PSI, Pollut.Abstr., PsycInfo, Psychoanal.Abstr., Psychol.Abstr. (1973-), Psychol.R.G., Risk Abstr., SSCI (coverage dropped), Saf.Sci.Abstr., Soc.Work Res.& Abstr., e-psyche.
—BLDSC (4683.735000), CISTI, GNLM, ingenta, KNAW. **CCC.**
Published by: (American Academy of Psychoanalysis), Guilford Publications, Inc., 72 Spring St, 4th Fl, New York, NY 10012. TEL 212-431-9800, FAX 212-966-6708, info@guilford.com. Ed. Jules Bemporad. Pub. Robert Matloff. R&P Kathy Kuehl. Adv. contact Susan Pavliscak. Circ: 1,500.

362.28 USA
AMERICAN ASSOCIATION OF SUICIDOLOGY. PROCEEDINGS OF THE ANNUAL MEETING. Text in English. 1975 (8th). a. price varies. back issues avail. **Document type:** *Proceedings.*
Indexed: e-psyche.
Published by: American Association of Suicidology, 4201 Connecticut Ave, Ste 408, Washington, DC 20008-1158. TEL 202-237-2280. Ed. Dr. David Lester. Circ: 1,000.

614.58 614.58 USA ISSN 0895-8009
CODEN: MAMREB
AMERICAN ASSOCIATION ON MENTAL RETARDATION. MONOGRAPHS. Text in English. 1973. irreg. price varies. **Document type:** *Monographic series, Academic/Scholarly.*
Formerly (until 1987): American Association on Mental Deficiency. Monographs (0730-7128)
Indexed: e-psyche.
Published by: American Association on Mental Retardation, 444 N Capitol St, Washington, DC 20001-1512. TEL 202-387-1968, 800-424-3688, FAX 202-387-2193. Ed. David Braddock. Pub. M Doreen Croser. R&P Stephen Stidinger.

AMERICAN BEHAVIORAL SCIENTIST. see *SOCIAL SCIENCES: COMPREHENSIVE WORKS*

306.85 USA
AMERICAN FAMILY THERAPY ACADEMY NEWSLETTER. Text in English. 1980. 3/yr. USD 24 (effective 2000). adv. bk.rev. back issues avail. *Refereed.* **Document type:** *Newsletter.*
Formerly: American Family Therapy Association Newsletter
Indexed: e-psyche.

P

Published by: American Family Therapy Academy, Inc., PMB 273, 2020 Pennsylvania Ave, NW, Washington, DC 20006. TEL 202-994-2776, FAX 202-994-2775, afta@afta.org. Ed. Volker Thomas. R&P Barbro Miles. Adv. contact Silas Flashman. Circ: 1,000.

616.89 USA ISSN 0742-3187
AMERICAN GROUP PSYCHOTHERAPY MONOGRAPH SERIES. Text in English. 1984. irreg., latest vol.7. price varies. *Refereed.* **Document type:** *Monographic series.*
Indexed: e-psyche.
Published by: International Universities Press, Inc., 59 Boston Post Rd, Box 1524, Madison, CT 06443-1524. TEL 203-245-4000, FAX 203-245-0775, http://www.iup.com. Ed. Dr. Howard Kibel.

AMERICAN IMAGO; studies in psychoanalysis and culture. see *MEDICAL SCIENCES—Psychiatry And Neurology*

AMERICAN INDIAN AND ALASKA NATIVE MENTAL HEALTH RESEARCH. see *NATIVE AMERICAN STUDIES*

AMERICAN INSTITUTE OF GERONTOLOGY AND HUMAN DEVELOPMENT. BROOKDALE INSTITUTE OF GERONTOLOGY AND HUMAN DEVELOPMENT. RESEARCH REPORTS. see *GERONTOLOGY AND GERIATRICS*

AMERICAN JOURNAL OF COMMUNITY PSYCHOLOGY. see *SOCIOLOGY*

AMERICAN JOURNAL OF DANCE THERAPY. see *DANCE*

306.85 USA ISSN 0192-6187
RC488.5 CODEN: IJFPDM
AMERICAN JOURNAL OF FAMILY THERAPY. Text in English. 1973. 5/yr. GBP 52, USD 85 to individuals; GBP 106, USD 175 to institutions (effective 2002). adv. bk.rev. illus. index. reprint service avail. from PQC,PSC,SCH. *Refereed.* **Document type:** *Academic/Scholarly.* **Description:** Provides an interdisciplinary forum for innovation, theory, research and clinical practice in family therapy.
Former titles (until 1979): International Journal of Family Counseling (0147-1775); (until 1976): Journal of Family Counseling (0093-3171)
Related titles: Microform ed.: 1973 (from PQC); Online - full text ed.: ISSN 1521-0383. 1973 (from CatchWord Ltd., Northern Light Technology, Inc., EBSCO Publishing, O C L C Online Computer Library Center, Inc., RoweCom Information Quest, ProQuest Information & Learning, Gale Group, Swets Blackwell, Institute for Scientific Information).
Indexed: ASCA, Adol.Ment.Hlth.Abstr., AgeLine, C.I.J.E., Curr.Cont., ERA, Fam.Ind., IMFL, L.R.I., Lang.& Lang.Behav.Abstr., Mid.East: Abstr.& Ind., Mult.Ed.Abstr., P C I, PsycInfo, Psychol.Abstr. (1973-), SOPODA, SSCI, Sage Fam.Stud.Abstr., Soc.Sci.Ind. (Mar.1987-), Soc.Serv.Abstr., Soc.Work Res.& Abstr., Sociol.Abstr., Sp.Ed.Needs Abstr., e-psyche.
—BLDSC (0824.620000), CatchWord, GNLM, IDS, ingenta. **CCC.**
Published by: Brunner - Routledge (Subsidiary of: Taylor & Francis Group), 325 Chestnut St, Ste 800, Philadelphia, PA 19106. TEL 215-625-8900, FAX 215-625-8900, info@taylorandfrancis.com, http://www.tandf.co.uk/. Circ: 2,000. **Subscr. to:** Taylor & Francis Group, Journals Customer Service, Rankine Rd, Basingstoke, Hants RG24 8PR, United Kingdom. TEL 44-1256-813000, FAX 44-1256-479438, enquiry@tanf.co.uk, http://www.tandf.co.uk/journals.

301.1 340 USA ISSN 0733-1290
K1
AMERICAN JOURNAL OF FORENSIC PSYCHOLOGY; interfacing issues of psychology and law. Text in English. 1983. q., latest vol.20, 2002. USD 75 in US & Canada; USD 100 elsewhere (effective 2002). bk.rev. 90 p./no. 1 cols./p. back issues avail.; reprint service avail. from WSH. *Refereed.* **Document type:** *Journal, Academic/Scholarly.* **Description:** For psychologists used as expert witnesses in civil and criminal court cases.
Related titles: Microfiche ed.: (from WSH); Microfilm ed.: (from PMC,WSH).
Indexed: Crim.Just.Abstr., Excerp.Med. (1996-), PsycInfo, Psychol.Abstr., e-psyche.
—BLDSC (0824.645000).
Published by: American College of Forensic Psychology, PO Box 5870, Balboa Island, CA 92662. TEL 949-673-7773, FAX 949-673-7710, psychlaw@sover.net, http://www.forensicpsychology.org/journal/journalpg.html. Ed. Debbie Miller. Pub. Edward Miller. Circ: 500.

616.89 USA ISSN 0002-9432
RA790.A1 CODEN: AJORAG
AMERICAN JOURNAL OF ORTHOPSYCHIATRY. Text in English. 1930. q. USD 70 per vol. domestic to individuals; USD 90 per vol. domestic to institutions; USD 80 per vol. foreign to individuals; USD 100 per vol. foreign to institutions (effective 2001); free to members. adv. bibl, charts, illus. index, cum.index. reprint service avail. from PQC,PSC,SCH. *Refereed.* **Document type:** *Academic/Scholarly.*
Related titles: Microform ed.: (from PQC); Online - full text ed.: (from Gale Group, Factiva, Institute for Scientific Information).
Indexed: ASCA, ASSIA, Abstr.Crim.& Pen., Acad.Ind., Adol.Ment.Hlth.Abstr., AgeLine, Bibl.Dev.Med.& Child Neur., Bibl.Ind., Biol.Abstr., Bk.Rev.Dig. (Jan.1983-Mar.1986), CINAHL, Chem.Abstr., Child Devel.Abstr., Crim.Just.Abstr., Curr.Adv.Ecol.Sci., Curr.Cont., Curr.Lit.Fam.Plan., ERA, Educ.Ind. (coverage dropped), Environ.Sci.Poll.Mgmt., Except.Child Educ.Abstr., Excerp.Med., Fam.Ind., Hosp.Lit.Ind., IMFL, INIS Atomind., Ind.Med. (1930-), Ind.Sci.Rev., Inpharma, Int.Nurs.Ind., Intl.Bibl.Soc.Sci., Lang.& Lang.Behav.Abstr., Ment.Retard.Abstr., Mult.Ed.Abstr., Nutr.Abstr., Pharm.&Out.News, Pollut.Abstr., PsycInfo, Psychol.Abstr. (1930-), Psycscan C.P., Psycscan D.P., Reac., Risk Abstr., SOPODA, SSCI, Saf.Sci.Abstr., Sage Fam.Stud.Abstr., Sage Race Rel.Abstr., Sci.Cit.Ind., Soc.Sci.Ind. (Jul.1982-), Soc.Serv.Abstr., Soc.Work Res.& Abstr., Sociol.Abstr., Sociol.Educ.Abstr., Sp.Ed.Needs Abstr., Stud.Wom.Abstr., THA, e-psyche.
—BLDSC (0829.250000), CISTI, EMDOCS, GNLM, IDS, ingenta, KNAW. **CCC.**
Published by: American Orthopsychiatric Association, Inc., 330 Seventh Ave, 18th Fl, New York, NY 10001. TEL 212-564-5930, FAX 212-564-6180, amerortho@aol.com., http://www.amerortho.org/ajo.htm. Ed. Carlos E. Sluzki. R&P Robert Keizer. Adv. contact Joan Adler. Circ: 13,000. **Subscr. to:** 49 Sheridan Ave, Albany, NY 12201-1413.

291.61 USA ISSN 1094-6098
BV4012.2
AMERICAN JOURNAL OF PASTORAL COUNSELING. Text in English. 1952. q. USD 45 to individuals; USD 61 in Canada to individuals; USD 65 elsewhere to individuals; USD 75 to institutions; USD 101 in Canada to institutions; USD 109 elsewhere to institutions; USD 95 to libraries; USD 128 in Canada to libraries; USD 138 elsewhere to libraries (effective (No. 2001). adv. bk.rev. back issues avail.; reprint service avail. from HAW,PQC,ISI. *Refereed.* **Document type:** *Journal, Academic/Scholarly.* **Description:** Aimed at therapists and researchers who are interested in the role and dynamic of religion in the healing process of psychotherapy.
Former titles: Journal of Religion in Psychotherapy (1045-5876); (until 1990): Journal of Pastoral Psychotherapy (0886-5477)
Related titles: Microform ed.: (from PQC).
Indexed: CCR, CERDIC, Curr.Cont. (coverage dropped), G.Soc.Sci.& Rel.Per.Lit., IBZ, Ind.Philos., Past.Care & Couns.Abstr., Psychol.Abstr., Ref.Zh., Rel.& Theol.Abstr. (1987-), Rel.Ind.One, SSCI (coverage dropped), Soc.Work Res.& Abstr., e-psyche.
—BLDSC (0829.550000), GNLM, Haworth.
Published by: Haworth Press, Inc., 10 Alice St, Binghamton, NY 13904-1580. TEL 607-722-5857, 800-429-6784, FAX 607-722-6362, 800-895-0582, getinfo@haworthpressinc.com, http://www.haworthpress.com/journals/journallist.asp. Ed. Richard Dayringer. Pub. William Cohen. R&P Ruthann Heath TEL 607-723-5857 ext 316. Adv. contact Jackie Blakeslee TEL 607-722-5857 ext 346. B&W page USD 315, color page USD 550; trim 6 x 8.5. Circ: 825.

AMERICAN JOURNAL OF PRIMATOLOGY. see *BIOLOGY—Zoology*

616.891 USA ISSN 0002-9548
RC321 CODEN: AJPYA8
AMERICAN JOURNAL OF PSYCHOANALYSIS. Text in English. 1941. q. USD 360, EUR 359 to institutions for print or online ed.; USD 59, EUR 59 to individuals for print or online ed.; USD 432, EUR 430.80 to institutions for print & online eds. combined (effective 2002). adv. bk.rev. bibl. index, cum.index: 1941-1965. reprint service avail. from PQC,PSC,SCH. *Refereed.* **Document type:** *Journal, Academic/Scholarly.* **Description:** Intended to communicate modern concepts of psychoanalytic theory and practice, plus related investigations in allied fields.
Related titles: Microform ed.: (from PQC); Online - full text ed.: (from Northern Light Technology, Inc., EBSCO Publishing, O C L C Online Computer Library Center, Inc., RoweCom Information Quest, ProQuest Information & Learning, Gale Group, Swets Blackwell, Kluwer Online, Factiva).
Indexed: AgeLine, Biol.Abstr., Chem.Abstr., Chicago Psychoanal.Lit.Ind., Curr.Cont. (coverage dropped), Educ.Ind. (coverage dropped), Excerp.Med., IBR, IBZ, IMFL, Ind.Med. (1941-), Ind.Philos., MLA Intl.Bibl., Mid.East: Abstr.& Ind., P C I, PsycInfo, Psychoanal.Abstr., Psychol.Abstr. (1928-), SSCI (coverage dropped), Soc.Sci.Ind. (Mar.1987-), Soc.Work Res.& Abstr., e-psyche.
—BLDSC (0835.300000), CISTI, EMDOCS, GNLM, ingenta. **CCC.**
Published by: (Association for the Advancement of Psychoanalysis), Kluwer Academic - Plenum Publishers (Subsidiary of: Wolters Kluwer N.V.), 233 Spring St, New York, NY 10013-1578. TEL 212-620-8000, 800-221-9369, FAX 212-463-0742, services@wkap.nl, info@plenum.com, http://www.wkap.nl/journalhome.htm/0002-9548. Eds. Douglas H Ingram, Giselle P Galdi. **Subscr. outside the Americas to:** Kluwer Academic Publishers Group, Journals Department, PO Box 322, Dordrecht 3300 AH, Netherlands. TEL 31-78-639-2392, FAX 31-78-654-6474.

150 USA ISSN 0002-9556
BF1 CODEN: AJPCAA
AMERICAN JOURNAL OF PSYCHOLOGY. Text in English. 1887. q. USD 58 to individuals; USD 125 to institutions (effective 2001). adv. bk.rev. bibl, charts, stat, illus. index, cum.index every 25 vols. back issues avail.; reprint service avail. from PSC,PQC,SCH. *Refereed.* **Document type:** *Academic/Scholarly.* **Description:** Explores the basic science of the mind, publishing reports of original research in experimental psychology, theoretical presentations, combined theoretical and experimental analyses, historical commentaries, and obituaries of prominent psychologists.
Related titles: Microform ed.: (from MIM,PQC,PMC); Online - full text ed.: (from Gale Group, Northern Light Technology, Inc., ProQuest Information & Learning, Factiva, Institute for Scientific Information).
Indexed: ASCA, ASSIA, Abstr.Anthropol., Acad.Ind., Adol.Ment.Hlth.Abstr., AgeLine, Arts & Hum.Cit.Ind. (coverage dropped), Biol.Abstr., Bk.Rev.Ind. (1980-), C.I.S. Abstr., Chem.Abstr., Child.Bk.Rev.Ind. (1980-), Commun.Abstr., Curr.Cont., Ergon.Abstr., Gen.Sci.Ind. (Jun.1992-), IBR, IBZ, INIS Atomind., Ind.Med. (1887-), Ind.Per.Art.Relat.Law, Ind.Philos., Lang.& Lang.Behav.Abstr., Mid.East: Abstr.& Ind., Mult.Ed.Abstr., P C I, Pers.Lit., PsycInfo, Psychol.Abstr. (1925-), Ref.Zh., Russ.Acad.Sci.Bibl., SSCI, Soc.Sci.Ind. (Sep.1982-), Soc.Serv.Abstr., Sociol.Abstr., e-psyche.
—BLDSC (0835.500000), CISTI, IDS, ingenta. **CCC.**
Published by: (University of Illinois at Urbana-Champaign), University of Illinois Press, 1325 S Oak St, Champaign, IL 61820. TEL 217-244-0950, FAX 217-244-8082, http://www.press.uillinois.edu/journals/main.html. Ed. Don Dulany. Adv. contact Clydette Wantland TEL 217-244-6496. B&W page USD 300. Circ: 2,200 (paid).

AMERICAN POLYGRAPH ASSOCIATION NEWSLETTER. see *CRIMINOLOGY AND LAW ENFORCEMENT*

370.15 USA ISSN 1052-7958
RC500
AMERICAN PSYCHOANALYST. Text in English. 1967. q., latest vol.35, 2001. USD 29.50 in US & Canada to individuals; USD 49.50 elsewhere to individuals; USD 63 in US & Canada to institutions; USD 83 elsewhere to institutions; USD 8.50 newsstand/cover in US & Canada; USD 11.50 newsstand/cover elsewhere (effective 2001). adv. back issues avail. **Document type:** *Newsletter.* **Description:** Features information of the association, essays on the history of psychoanalysis in America, and interviews with leading analysts.
Formerly: American Psychoanalytic Association. Newsletter
Indexed: e-psyche.
Published by: (American Psychoanalytic Association), Analytic Press, Inc. (Subsidiary of: Lawrence Erlbaum Associates, Inc.), 101 West St, Hillsdale, NJ 07642. TEL 201-358-9477, FAX 201-358-4700, TAP@analyticpress.com, http://www.analyticpress.com/newsletter.html. Ed. Prudence Leib. R&P, Adv. contact Joan Riegel. page USD 850; trim 7.25 x 9.75. Circ: 4,000. **Subscr. to:** Journals, 810 E 10th St, PO Box 1897, Lawrence, KS 66044-8897. TEL 785-843-1274, 800-627-0629, FAX 785-843-1274. **Dist. by:** Eurospan University Press Group.

616.891 USA ISSN 0003-0651
BF173.A2 CODEN: JAPOAE
AMERICAN PSYCHOANALYTIC ASSOCIATION. JOURNAL. Variant title: J A P A. Text in English. 1953. q., latest vol.49. USD 120 in US & Canada to individuals; USD 155 elsewhere to individuals; USD 225 in US & Canada to institutions; USD 260 elsewhere to institutions; USD 35 newsstand/cover in US & Canada; USD 45 newsstand/cover elsewhere (effective 2001). adv. bk.rev. abstr, bibl, charts, illus. index, cum.index: vols.1-22, vols.23-33. Supplement avail.; back issues avail.; reprint service avail. from PSC,SCH. *Refereed.* **Document type:** *Academic/Scholarly.* **Description:** Covers articles in clinical and theoretical applied psychoanalytic studies.
Related titles: CD-ROM ed.; Online - full text ed.: (from Institute for Scientific Information).
Indexed: ASCA, ASSIA, Adol.Ment.Hlth.Abstr., AgeLine, BHA, Biol.Abstr., Curr.Cont., Excerp.Med., Fam.Ind., IBZ, Ind.Med. (1953-), Ind.Philos., Lang.& Lang.Behav.Abstr., Mid.East: Abstr.& Ind., PsycInfo, Psychoanal.Abstr., Psychol.Abstr. (1953-), SOPODA, SSCI, Sociol.Abstr., e-psyche.
—BLDSC (4692.070000), CISTI, GNLM, IDS, ingenta. **CCC.**
Published by: (American Psychoanalytic Association), Analytic Press, Inc. (Subsidiary of: Lawrence Erlbaum Associates, Inc.), 101 West St, Hillsdale, NJ 07642. TEL 201-358-9477, FAX 201-358-4700, TAP@analyticpress.com, http://www.analyticpress.com/japa.html. Ed. Arnold D Richards. R&P, Adv. contact Joan Riegel. page USD 630; trim 5 x 8. Circ: 6,500.

150 USA ISSN 0065-9843
AMERICAN PSYCHOANALYTIC ASSOCIATION. JOURNAL. MONOGRAPH. Text in English. 1953. irreg. *Refereed.* **Document type:** *Monographic series, Academic/Scholarly.*
Indexed: Biol.Abstr., SSCI (coverage dropped).
Published by: (American Psychoanalytic Association), International Universities Press, Inc., 59 Boston Post Rd, Box 1524, Madison, CT 06443-1524. TEL 203-245-4000, FAX 203-245-0775, http://www.iup.com.

150.19 USA
AMERICAN PSYCHOANALYTIC ASSOCIATION. WORKSHOP SERIES. Text in English. 1985. irreg., latest vol.8. price varies. *Refereed.*
Indexed: e-psyche.
—BLDSC.
Published by: (American Psychoanalytic Association), International Universities Press, Inc., 59 Boston Post Rd, Box 1524, Madison, CT 06443-1524. TEL 203-245-4000, FAX 203-245-0775, http://www.iup.com. Ed. Scott Dowling.

AMERICAN PSYCHOLOGICAL ASSOCIATION. DIRECTORY. see *BIOGRAPHY*

150 USA ISSN 0003-066X
BF1 CODEN: AMPSAB
AMERICAN PSYCHOLOGIST. Text in English. 1946. m. USD 198 domestic to non-members; USD 238 foreign to non-members; USD 12 to members; USD 424 domestic to institutions; USD 512 foreign to institutions (effective 2001). adv. illus. index. back issues avail.; reprint service avail. from PSC,SCH. *Refereed.* **Document type:** *Academic/Scholarly.* **Description:** Publishes empirical, theoretical and practical articles.
Related titles: Microform ed.: (from PQC,PMC); Online - full text ed.: (from Gale Group, Factiva, Institute for Scientific Information).
Indexed: ASCA, ASSIA, Acad.Ind., Addic.Abstr., Adol.Ment.Hlth.Abstr., AgeLine, Amer.Bibl.Slavic & E.Eur.Stud., Arts & Hum.Cit.Ind. (coverage dropped), Biol.Abstr., CERDIC, C.I.J.E., Chem.Abstr., Child Devel.Abstr., Commun.Abstr., Crim.Just.Abstr., Curr.Adv.Ecol.Sci., Curr.Cont., Curr.Ind.Stat., ERA, Environ.Sci.Poll.Mgmt., Fam.Ind., Fut.Surv., IBR, IBZ, Ind.Med. (1946-), Ind.Per.Art.Relat.Law, Ind.Philos., Indian Psychol.Abstr., Int.Nurs.Ind., Intl.Bibl.Soc.Sci., L.R.I., Lang.& Lang.Behav.Abstr., M.L.A., MLA Intl.Bibl., Mid.East: Abstr.& Ind., Mult.Ed.Abstr., P C I, PSI, Peace Res.Abstr., Pers.Lit., Pollut.Abstr., PsycInfo, Psychol.Abstr. (1946-), Rel.Ind.One, Rel.Ind.Two, Res.High.Educ.Abstr., Risk Abstr., Russ.Acad.Sci.Bibl., SSCI, Saf.Sci.Abstr., Sage Fam.Stud.Abstr., Sage Pub.Admin.Abstr., Sage Race Rel.Abstr., Soc.Sci.Ind. (Dec.1982-), Soc.Serv.Abstr., Soc.Work Res.& Abstr., Sociol.Abstr., Sp.Ed.Needs Abstr., Stud.Wom.Abstr., THA, Tech.Educ.Abstr., e-psyche.
—BLDSC (0853.400000), CISTI, GNLM, IDS, ingenta. **CCC.**
Published by: American Psychological Association, 750 First St., N.E., Washington, DC 20002-4242. TEL 202-336-5600, 800-374-2721, FAX 202-336-5568, subscriptions@apa.org, http://www.apa.org/journals/amp.html. Eds. Ed Diener, Raymond D Fowler. Circ: 102,000.

362.29 USA ISSN 0740-0454
AMERICAN UNIVERSITY STUDIES. SERIES 8. PSYCHOLOGY. Text in English. 1983. irreg. price varies. *Refereed.* **Document type:** *Monographic series, Academic/Scholarly.* **Description:** Explores theoretical, practical, and clinical issues in psychology.
Indexed: e-psyche.
Published by: Peter Lang Publishing, Inc., 275 Seventh Ave, 28th Fl, New York, NY 10001. TEL 212-647-7706, 800-770-5264, FAX 212-475-7707, customerservice@plang.com, http://www.peterlang.com. Ed., Pub. Christopher Myers. R&P Stephanie Archer. Adv. contact Patricia Mulrane.

AMSTERDAM STUDIES IN THE THEORY AND HISTORY OF LINGUISTIC SCIENCE. SERIES 2: CLASSICS IN PSYCHOLINGUISTICS. see *LINGUISTICS*

370.15 ESP ISSN 0212-9728
ANALES DE PSICOLOGIA. Text in English, Spanish. 1955. s-a. ESP 3,000 (effective 2001). back issues avail. *Refereed.* **Document type:** *Academic/Scholarly.* **Description:** Publishes theoretical, empirical and methodological papers covering all aspects related to basic and applied scientific psychology.
Supersedes in part (in 1984): Universidad de Murcia. Anales. Filosofia y Letras (0463-9863)
Indexed: PsycInfo, e-psyche.
—CINDOC, KNAW.
Published by: Universidad de Murcia, Servicio de Publicaciones, C Actor Isidoro Maiquez 9, Murcia 30007, Spain. TEL 34-68-363207, FAX 34-68-363414, vgm@um.es, http://www.um.es/spumweb. Ed. Agustin Romero Medina. Circ: 155.

158 PRT ISSN 0870-8231
RC500
ANALISE PSICOLOGICA. Text in Portuguese. 1977. q. USD 77 in Europe; USD 87 elsewhere. adv. bk.rev. **Document type:** *Academic/Scholarly.*
Indexed: PsycInfo, Psychol.Abstr. (1992-), e-psyche.
Published by: Instituto Superior de Psicologia Aplicada, Rua Jardim do Tabaco, 44, Lisbon 1100, Portugal. TEL 351-1-8863184, FAX 351-1-8860954. Ed. Frederico Pereira. Adv. contact Jorge Senos.

150.19 808.8 USA
ANALYTICAL PSYCHOLOGY CLUB OF NEW YORK. BULLETIN. Text in English. 1938. 8/yr. membership. bk.rev., film rev. **Description:** Covers club business, programs and brief accounts of talks.
Indexed: e-psyche.
Published by: Analytical Psychology Club of New York, 28 E 39th St, New York, NY 10016. TEL 212-697-7877. Circ: 300.

616.89 DEU ISSN 0945-6740
ANALYTISCHE KINDER- UND JUGENDLICHEN-PSYCHOTHERAPIE. Text in German. 1970. q. EUR 49 domestic; EUR 52 foreign (effective 2001). bk.rev. **Document type:** *Newsletter, Academic/Scholarly.*
Former titles (until 1994): Beitraege zur Analytischen Kinder- und Jugendlichenpsychotherapie (0942-069X); (until 1992): Kind und Umwelt (0721-1791); (until 1980): Beitraege zur Analytischen Kinder- und Jugendlichenpsychotherapie (0343-2777)
Indexed: IBR, IBZ, Ind.Philos., e-psyche.
—GNLM.
Published by: Brandes und Apsel Verlag GmbH, Scheidswaldstr 33, Frankfurt Am Main 60385, Germany. TEL 49-69-95730186, FAX 49-69-95730187, brandes-apsel@t-online.de, http://www.brandes-apsel-verlag.de.

150 CHE ISSN 0301-3006
RC500 CODEN: ANAPC4
ANALYTISCHE PSYCHOLOGIE. Text in German; Summaries in English, German. 1970. q. CHF 213, EUR 152.20 in Europe to institutions; CHF 224.60, USD 169 overseas to institutions (effective 2002). adv. bk.rev. bibl. back issues avail. *Refereed.* **Document type:** *Journal, Academic/Scholarly.*
Supersedes: Zeitschrift fuer Analytische Psychologie und ihre Grenzgebiete (0049-8580)
Related titles: Microform ed.: (from PQC); Online - full text ed.: ISSN 1421-9689. CHF 58, EUR 42, USD 45 (effective 2002) (from EBSCO Publishing, O C L C Online Computer Library Center, Inc., RoweCom Information Quest, Swets Blackwell).
Indexed: ASCA, Arts & Hum.Cit.Ind. (coverage dropped), Biol.Abstr., Curr.Cont. (coverage dropped), P C I, PsycInfo, Psychoanal.Abstr., Psychol.Abstr. (1974-), SSCI, e-psyche.
—BLDSC (0897.170000), CISTI, GNLM, IDS, Infotrieve, KNAW. **CCC.**
Published by: S. Karger AG, Allschwilerstr 10, PO Box, Basel 4009, Switzerland. TEL 41-61-306-1111, FAX 41-61-306-1234, karger@karger.ch, http://www.online.karger.com/journals/aps, http://www.karger.com. Eds. H Dieckmann, V Kast. adv.: page USD 1,195. Circ: 1,700.

150 410 USA ISSN 0895-366X
ANCHOR POINT MAGAZINE; the practical journal of NLP. Text in English. 1987. m. USD 39 domestic; USD 49 in Canada; USD 59 elsewhere (effective 2000). adv. bk.rev. charts, illus. back issues avail. **Document type:** *Trade.*
Indexed: e-psyche.
Published by: Anchor Point Productions, Inc., 259 S 500 E, Salt Lake City, UT 84102-2017. TEL 801-534-1022, 800-544-6480, FAX 801-532-2113, info@nlpanchorpoint.com, http://www.nlpanchorpoint.com. Ed. Terry Fieland. Adv. contact Anita Sholiton. Circ: 1,300 (paid).

301.1 150 IDN ISSN 0126-1215
ANDA; majalah psikologi populer. Text in Indonesian. irreg.
Indexed: e-psyche.
Published by: Yayasan Bina Psikologi, c/o Mulyono & Associates, Gedung Pant Trisula, Jalan Menteng Raya 35, Box 3216, Jakarta, Indonesia.

150 USA
ANDROS DIGEST✱ . Text in English. 1982. 17/yr. USD 39.
Indexed: e-psyche.
Published by: PeopleScience, Inc., 20 Pine Valley Ln, Jamesburg, NJ 08831-2705. Ed. Fred Streit.

150.19 FRA ISSN 0294-653X
L'ANE; le magazine freudien. Text in French. 1980. 4/yr. FRF 280 domestic; FRF 320 foreign; FRF 80 newsstand/cover (effective 1999). bk.rev. **Description:** Covers art, literature and social sciences with a psychoanalysis influence.
Indexed: e-psyche.
Published by: Ane, 74 rue d'Assas, Paris 75006, France. TEL 33-1-45485672, judithm@easynet.fr. Ed. Judith Miller. Pub. Dominique Kalfon. **Subscr. to:** 31 rue de Navarin, Paris 75009, France.

150 001.3 ITA
ANIMA. Text in Italian. 1988. a. ITL 60,000 for 2 yrs. domestic to individuals; USD 60 for 2 yrs. foreign to individuals; ITL 100,000 for 2 yrs. domestic to institutions; USD 100 for 2 yrs. foreign to institutions. **Description:** Multidisciplinary forum featuring readings on archetypical psychology, religion, art and humanities.
Indexed: e-psyche.
Published by: Moretti e Vitalli Editori, Via Betty Ambiveri 15, Bergamo, BG 24126, Italy. TEL 39-35-321588, FAX 39-35-321647. Ed. Francesco Donfrancesco. Circ: 450.

ANIMAL BEHAVIOUR. see *BIOLOGY—Zoology*

155 DEU ISSN 1435-9448
ANIMAL COGNITION. Text in English. 1998. 4/yr. EUR 283 domestic; EUR 279.60 in Germany; EUR 80.70 newsstand/cover foreign (effective 2002). *Refereed.* **Document type:** *Journal, Academic/Scholarly.* **Description:** Aims to establish the course of the evolution of intelligence, of the mechanisms, functions and adaptive value of basic and complex cognitive abilities, and of the evolution of intelligent behavior and intelligent systems from invertebrates to humans.
Related titles: Online - full text ed.: ISSN 1435-9456 (from EBSCO Publishing, RoweCom Information Quest, Swets Blackwell).
Indexed: Zoo.Rec., e-psyche.
—BLDSC (0903.180000).
Published by: Springer-Verlag (Subsidiary of: BertelsmannSpringer), Tiergartenstr 17, Heidelberg 69121, Germany. TEL 49-6221-345-0, FAX 49-6221-345229, subscriptions@springer.de, http://link.springer.de/link/service/journals/10071/index.htm, http://www.springer.de. **Subscr. in N. America to:** Springer-Verlag New York Inc., PO Box 2485, Secaucus, NJ 07096-2485. TEL 212-460-1500, FAX 212-473-6272.

P

591.5 USA ISSN 0090-4996
CODEN: ALBVAB
ANIMAL LEARNING & BEHAVIOR. Text in English. 1973. q. USD 118 in United States; USD 127 foreign (effective 2001). adv. illus. back issues avail.; reprint service avail. from PQC,SCH,PSC. *Refereed.* **Document type:** *Academic/Scholarly.* **Description:** Includes articles on animal learning, motivation, emotion, and comparative behavior.
Related titles: Microform ed.: (from NRP,PQC); Online - full text ed.: (from CatchWord Ltd., Gale Group, Factiva, Institute for Scientific Information).
Indexed: ASCA, Agricola, Anim.Behav.Abstr., Aqua.Sci.& Fish.Abstr., Biol.Abstr., Curr.Adv.Ecol.Sci., Curr.Cont., Entomol.Abstr., Excerp.Med., Gen.Sci.Ind. (Aug.1984-), Ind.Sci.Rev., Inpharma, Int.Abstr.Biol.Sci., Neurosci.Abstr., Neurosci.Cit.Ind., Nutr.Abstr., PsycInfo, Psychol.Abstr. (1973-), Psycscan B.A.& T., Reac., Rev.Med.& Vet.Mycol., Risk Abstr., SSCI, Sci.Cit.Ind., Sport Fish.Abstr., Wild.Rev., Zoo.Rec., e-psyche.
—BLDSC (0905.002000), CISTI, IDS, ingenta. **CCC.**
Published by: Psychonomic Society, Inc., 1710 Fortview Rd, Austin, TX 78704. TEL 512-462-2442, FAX 512-462-1101, jbellquist@psychonomic.org, http://www.sig.net/~psysoc/home.htm, http://www.psychonomic.org. Ed. Ralph R Miller. R&P Cinnamon Nemec. Adv. contact Robert Samford. page USD 140; trim 10.75 x 8. Circ: 1,220.

616.8 FRA ISSN 0003-4487
CODEN: AMPYAT
ANNALES MEDICO-PSYCHOLOGIQUES. Text in French. 1843. 10/yr. EUR 175 in Europe to individuals; USD 213 elsewhere to individuals; EUR 293 in Europe to institutions; USD 347 elsewhere to institutions (effective 2002). bk.rev. abstr, illus. index. reprint service avail. from ISI. *Refereed.* **Document type:** *Academic/Scholarly.* **Description:** Deals with topical matters such as the training of psychologists, the relation between psychiatry and neurology, the development of psychotherapy.
Related titles: Online - full text ed.: (from Institute for Scientific Information).
Indexed: ASCA, Agri.& Environ.Biotech.Abstr. (coverage dropped), Biol.Abstr., C.I.S. Abstr., Curr.Cont., Derwent Biotech.Abstr., Excerp.Med., INIS Atomind., Ind.Med. (coverage dropped), Inpharma, Neurosci.Cit.Ind., Pharm.&Out.News, PsycInfo, Psychol.Abstr. (1927-), Reac., SSCI (coverage dropped), e-psyche.
—BLDSC (0984.150000), CISTI, EMDOCS, GNLM, IDS, Infotrieve, KNAW. **CCC.**
Published by: (Societe Medico-Psychologique), Elsevier France, Editions Scientifiques et Medicales (Subsidiary of: Reed Elsevier plc), 23 rue Linois, Paris 75015, France. Ed. J-F Allilaire. Circ: 2,000. **Subscr. to:** Societe de Periodiques Specialises, BP 22, Vineuil Cedex 41354, France. TEL 33-2-54504612, FAX 33-2-54504611.

ANNALES UNIVERSITATIS MARIAE CURIE-SKLODOWSKA. SECTIO J. PAEDAGOGIA - PSYCHOLOGIA. see *EDUCATION*

150 FRA ISSN 0003-5033
BF2
L'ANNEE PSYCHOLOGIQUE. Text in French; Summaries in English, French. 1884. q. EUR 75 domestic to individuals; EUR 84 foreign to individuals (effective 2002). bk.rev. charts. index. reprint service avail. from PSC,SCH. *Refereed.* **Document type:** *Academic/Scholarly.* **Description:** Presents original research, critical reviews, bibliographic analyses.
Related titles: Microform ed.; Online - full text ed.: (from Institute for Scientific Information).
Indexed: Curr.Cont., Ind.Med. (coverage dropped), Lang.& Lang.Behav.Abstr., Neurosci.Cit.Ind., P C I, PsycInfo, Psychol.Abstr. (1925-), Russ.Acad.Sci.Bibl., SOPODA, SSCI, Sociol.Abstr., e-psyche.
—BLDSC (1049.250000), IDS, Infotrieve. **CCC.**
Published by: Presses Universitaires de France, Departement des Revues, 6 av. Reille, Paris 75685 Cedex 14, France. TEL 33-1-60873030, FAX 33-1-60792045, revues@puf.com. Ed. J Segui. Circ: 1,500.

616.89 USA
ANNUAL EDITIONS: ABNORMAL PSYCHOLOGY. Text in English. 1996. a. USD 12.25. illus. **Document type:** *Academic/Scholarly.*
Indexed: e-psyche.
Published by: Dushkin - McGraw-Hill, Sluice Dock, Guilford, CT 06437-9989. TEL 203-453-4351, FAX 203-453-6000. Ed. Joseph J Palladino.

155.6 USA
ANNUAL EDITIONS: ADOLESCENT PSYCHOLOGY. Text in English. 1997. a. USD 12.25. illus. **Document type:** *Academic/Scholarly.*
Published by: Dushkin - McGraw-Hill, Sluice Dock, Guilford, CT 06437-9989. TEL 203-453-4351, FAX 203-453-6000. Eds. Anita M Meehan, Eileen Astor Stetson.

150 USA
ANNUAL EDITIONS: BIOPSYCHOLOGY. Text in English. 1995. a. USD 12.25. illus. **Document type:** *Academic/Scholarly.*
Indexed: e-psyche.
Published by: Dushkin - McGraw-Hill, Sluice Dock, Guilford, CT 06437-9989. TEL 203-453-4351, FAX 203-453-6000. Ed. Boyce M Jubilan.

ANNUAL EDITIONS: CHILD GROWTH & DEVELOPMENT. see *MEDICAL SCIENCES—Pediatrics*

302 USA
ANNUAL EDITIONS: DYING, DEATH, AND BEREAVEMENT. Text in English. 1993. a. USD 12.25. illus. **Document type:** *Academic/Scholarly.*
Indexed: e-psyche.
Published by: Dushkin - McGraw-Hill, Sluice Dock, Guilford, CT 06437-9989. TEL 203-453-4351, FAX 203-453-6000. Pub. Ian Nielsen. R&P Cheryl Greenleaf.

ANNUAL EDITIONS: EDUCATIONAL PSYCHOLOGY. see *EDUCATION*

ANNUAL EDITIONS: HUMAN SEXUALITY. see *BIOLOGY*

158.105 USA ISSN 0198-912X
BF698.A1
ANNUAL EDITIONS: PERSONAL GROWTH AND BEHAVIOR. Text in English. 1975. a. USD 12.25. illus. index. back issues avail. *Refereed.* **Document type:** *Academic/Scholarly.*
Formerly: Annual Editions: Readings in Personality and Adjustment (0361-3836)
Indexed: e-psyche.
Published by: Dushkin - McGraw-Hill, Sluice Dock, Guilford, CT 06437-9989. TEL 203-453-4351, FAX 203-453-6000. Ed. Karen G Duffy. Pub. Ian Nielsen. R&P Cheryl Greenleaf.

150 USA ISSN 0272-3794
BF149
ANNUAL EDITIONS: PSYCHOLOGY. Text in English. 1971. a. USD 12.25. illus. *Refereed.* **Document type:** *Academic/Scholarly.*
Formerly: Annual Editions: Readings in Psychology (0197-0542)
Indexed: e-psyche.
Published by: Dushkin - McGraw-Hill, Sluice Dock, Guilford, CT 06437-9989. TEL 203-453-4351, FAX 203-453-6000. Ed. Karen G Duffy. Pub. Ian Nielsen. R&P Cheryl Greenleaf.

302 USA
ANNUAL EDITIONS: SOCIAL PSYCHOLOGY. Text in English. 1997. a. USD 12.25. illus. **Document type:** *Academic/Scholarly.*
Indexed: e-psyche.
Published by: Dushkin - McGraw-Hill, Sluice Dock, Guilford, CT 06437-9989. TEL 203-453-4351, FAX 203-453-6000. Ed. Mark Davis.

150 USA ISSN 0092-5055
RC500 CODEN: APSACT
ANNUAL OF PSYCHOANALYSIS. Text in English. 1973. a., latest 28. price varies. **Document type:** *Academic/Scholarly.*
Indexed: AgeLine, Biol.Abstr., PsycInfo, Psychoanal.Abstr., Psychol.Abstr. (1973-), e-psyche.
—BLDSC (1092.900000), CISTI, GNLM, Infotrieve, ingenta. **CCC.**
Published by: (Chicago Institute for Psychoanalysis), Analytic Press, Inc. (Subsidiary of: Lawrence Erlbaum Associates, Inc.), 101 West St, Hillsdale, NJ 07642. TEL 201-358-9477, TAP@analyticpress.com, http://www.analyticpress.com/books/300-3.html. Ed. Jerome A Winer. **Dist. addr. in Africa:** Overseas Publications, P O Box 12292, Centrahil 6006, South Africa; **Dist. addr. in Australia, New Zealand & Papua New Guinea:** DAInformation Services, 648 Whitehouse Rd, Mitcham, VIC 3132, Australia. TEL 61-3-9210-7788, FAX 61-3-9210-7724; **Dist. addr. in India, Bangladesh & Sri Lanka:** VivaBooks Private Ltd, 4325/2 Ansari Rd, Darya Ganj, New Delhi 11002, India. TEL 91-11-327-9280, FAX 91-11-326-7224; **Dist. addr. in the UK, Europe & the Middle East:** Eurospan University Press Group, Order Dept, 3 Henrietta St, London WC2E 8LU, United Kingdom. TEL 44-20-7240-0856, FAX 44-20-7379-0609, http://www.eurospan.co.uk.

150 USA ISSN 0066-4308
BF30 CODEN: ARPSAC
ANNUAL REVIEW OF PSYCHOLOGY. Text in English. 1950. a. USD 60 domestic to individuals; USD 65 foreign to individuals; USD 130 domestic to institutions print ed.; USD 135 foreign to institutions print ed.; USD 130 domestic to institutions online ed.; USD 130 foreign to institutions online ed.; USD 145 domestic to institutions print & online eds.; USD 150 foreign to institutions print & online eds. (effective 2001). adv. bibl, charts, illus. index, cum.index. back issues avail.; reprint service avail. from PSC,SCH. *Refereed.* **Document type:** *Academic/Scholarly.* **Description:** Synthesizes and filters primary research to identify the principal contributions in the field of psychology.
Related titles: CD-ROM ed.: (from Ovid Technologies, Inc.); Microfilm ed.: (from PQC); Online - full text ed.: (from Gale Group, HighWire Pr., Ovid Technologies, Inc., Northern Light Technology, Inc., EBSCO Publishing, H. W. Wilson, Factiva, Institute for Scientific Information).
Indexed: ASCA, Adol.Ment.Hlth.Abstr., AgeLine, Bibl.Asian Stud. (1990), Biol.Abstr., Chem.Abstr., Child Devel.Abstr., Crim.Just.Abstr., Curr.Adv.Ecol.Sci., Curr.Cont., DSH Abstr., Environ.Sci.Poll.Mgmt., Excerp.Med., IBR, IBZ, INIS Atomind., Ind.Med. (1950-), Ind.Philos., Ind.Sci.Rev., Inpharma, Intl.Bibl.Soc.Sci., Lang.& Lang.Behav.Abstr., Media Rev.Dig., P C I, Pharm.&Out.News, Pollut.Abstr., PsycInfo, Psychol.Abstr. (1950-), Psycscan D.P., Reac., Risk Abstr., Russ.Acad.Sci.Bibl., SOPODA, SSCI, Saf.Sci.Abstr., Sci.Cit.Ind., Soc.Sci.Ind. (Jan.1983-), Soc.Serv.Abstr., Sociol.Abstr., e-psyche.
—BLDSC (1528.400000), CASDDS, GNLM, IDS, ingenta. **CCC.**
Published by: Annual Reviews Inc., 4139 El Camino Way, Box 10139, Palo Alto, CA 94303-0139. TEL 650-493-4400, 800-523-8635, FAX 650-424-0910, service@annurev.org; orders@allenpress.com, http://www.biomedical.annualreviews.org. Ed. Susan T. Fiske. R&P, Adv. contact Swati Aneja TEL 650-843-6634. **Subscr.to:** Allen Press Inc., PO Box 1897, Lawrence, KS 66044-8897.

306.7 USA ISSN 1053-2528
HQ60 CODEN: ARXREJ
ANNUAL REVIEW OF SEX RESEARCH. Text in English. 1990. a., latest vol.11. USD 56 domestic to individuals; USD 66 foreign to individuals; USD 92 domestic to institutions; USD 103 foreign to institutions (effective 2001). charts, illus, stat. back issues avail. **Document type:** *Journal, Academic/Scholarly.* **Description:** Publishes 7-10 chapters that integrate multidisciplinary research and provide up-to-date summaries of knowledge on selected human sexological issues.
Related titles: Online - full text ed.: (from Northern Light Technology, Inc., H. W. Wilson, ProQuest Information & Learning, Gale Group).
Indexed: ASSIA, Abstr.Anthropol., Biol.Abstr., Child Devel.Abstr., Crim.Just.Abstr., Curr.Lit.Fam.Plan., IBZ, IMFL, Ind.Med. (1990-), Ind.Per.Art.Relat.Law, Ind.Philos., Lang.& Lang.Behav.Abstr., PsycInfo, Psychol.Abstr. (1990-), SOPODA, Sage Fam.Stud.Abstr., Soc.Sci.Ind. (Jan.1999-), Soc.Serv.Abstr., Soc.Work Res.& Abstr., Sociol.Abstr., Stud.Wom.Abstr., Viol.& Abuse Abstr., e-psyche.
—BLDSC (1528.830000), GNLM, ingenta. **CCC.**
Published by: Society for the Scientific Study of Sexuality, PO Box 416, Allentown, PA 18105. TEL 610-530-2483, FAX 610-530-2485, thesociety@inetmail.att.net, http://www.sexscience.org. Ed. Julia C Heiman. Circ: 500.

ANTHROPOLOGY OF CONSCIOUSNESS. see *ANTHROPOLOGY*

150 ESP ISSN 0066-5126
ANUARIO DE PSICOLOGIA. Text in Spanish, English, French; Summaries in English, French, Spanish. 1969. q. USD 63 in Europe; USD 73 in the Americas (effective 2001). bk.rev. back issues avail.
Indexed: PsycInfo, Psychol.Abstr. (1962-), e-psyche.
—BLDSC (1565.132000), CINDOC. **CCC.**
Published by: (Universidad de Barcelona, Facultad de Psicologia), Ediciones Paidos Iberoamerica, S.A., Mariano Cubi 92, Barcelona 08021, Spain. TEL 34-93-2419250, FAX 34-93-2022954, paidos@paidos.com, http://www.ub.es/psicolog/anuari/anuari1.html. Ed. Miguel Siguan. Adv. contact Maria Jose Quevedo. Circ: 1,000. **Dist. by:** Editorial Fontalba S.A., Valencia, 359 6o 1a, Barcelona 08009, Spain. TEL 93-458-5508, FAX 93-458-6602

150 340 ESP ISSN 1133-0740
ANUARIO DE PSICOLOGIA JURIDICA. Text in Spanish. 1991. a. **Document type:** *Academic/Scholarly.*
Indexed: e-psyche.
—CINDOC.
Published by: Colegio Oficial de Psicologos de Madrid, Cuesta de San Vicente, 4 6o, Madrid 28008, Spain. TEL 34-91-541-7009, FAX 34-91-547-2284, dmadrid@correo.cop.es, http://www.cop.es/publicaciones/juridica/. Ed. Victor Sancha.

ANXIETY DISORDERS FOUNDATION OF AUSTRALIA. NEWSLETTER. see *MEDICAL SCIENCES—Psychiatry And Neurology*

152.46 CHE ISSN 1061-5806
BF575.A6 CODEN: AXSCEP
ANXIETY, STRESS AND COPING. Text in English. 1988. 4/yr. GBP 106, USD 128, EUR 141 to individuals; GBP 413, USD 530, EUR 550 to institutions; GBP 673, USD 868, EUR 899 to corporations (effective 2002). illus. reprint service avail. from SCH,PSC. *Refereed.* **Document type:** *Journal, Academic/Scholarly.* **Description:** Emphasizes research reports, theoretical papers, and interpretive reviews or meta-analysis of the literature.
Formerly: Anxiety Research (0891-7779)
Related titles: Microform ed.; Online - full text ed.: (from Institute for Scientific Information).
Indexed: ASCA, Curr.Cont., ERA, Environ.Sci.Poll.Mgmt., Fam.Ind., Indian Psychol.Abstr., Lang.& Lang.Behav.Abstr., Mult.Ed.Abstr., Neurosci.Cit.Ind., Pollut.Abstr., PsycInfo, Psychol.Abstr. (1988-), Risk Abstr., SOPODA, SSCI, Saf.Sci.Abstr., Soc.Serv.Abstr., Sociol.Abstr., Sp.Ed.Needs Abstr., Stud.Wom.Abstr., e-psyche.
—GNLM, ingenta. **CCC.**
Published by: Gordon and Breach - Harwood Academic (Subsidiary of: Taylor & Francis Group), PO Box 531, Lausanne 1000, Switzerland. TEL 41-21-6411280, FAX 41-21-6411281, info@gbhap.com, http://www.gbhap.com/journals/356/356-top.htm. Eds. Reinhard Pekrun, S E Hobfoll. **Subscr. addr. in US:** International Publishers Direct, PO Box 32160, Newark, NJ 07102. FAX 215-750-6343.

150.19 GBR ISSN 0962-1849
RC467
APPLIED AND PREVENTIVE PSYCHOLOGY. Text in English. 1992. q. GBP 92, USD 152 to institutions (effective 2001). adv. back issues avail. *Refereed.* **Document type:** *Academic/Scholarly.* **Description:** Focuses on the scientific, epidemiological, or public health approach to psychological problems.
Related titles: Online - full text ed.: (from Institute for Scientific Information).
Indexed: ASCA, Crim.Just.Abstr., Curr.Cont., Fam.Ind., IMFL, PsycInfo, Psychol.Abstr. (1974-), SSCI, THA, e-psyche.
—BLDSC (1571.442000), GNLM, IDS, ingenta. **CCC.**
Published by: (American Association of Applied and Preventive Psychology), Cambridge University Press, Edinburgh Bldg, Shaftesbury Rd, Cambridge CB2 2RU, United Kingdom. FAX 44-1223-315052, TELEX 851917256, information@cup.cam.ac.uk, information@cambridge.org, http://www.cup.org/journals/CUPJNLS.html. Ed. David Smith. R&P Linda Nicol. Adv. contact Rebecca Symons.

APPLIED ANIMAL BEHAVIOUR SCIENCE; an international scientific journal reporting on the application of ethology to animals used by man. see *BIOLOGY—Zoology*

150 GBR ISSN 1068-8595
H96 CODEN: ABSREI
APPLIED BEHAVIORAL SCIENCE REVIEW. Text in English. 1993. s-a. USD 95 domestic to individuals; USD 115 foreign to individuals; USD 195 domestic to institutions; USD 215 foreign to institutions. back issues avail. **Document type:** *Academic/Scholarly.*
Related titles: Microform ed.: (from PQC); Online - full text ed.: (from ingenta, ScienceDirect).
Indexed: Lang.& Lang.Behav.Abstr., SOPODA, Soc.Serv.Abstr., Sociol.Abstr., e-psyche.
—**CCC.**
Published by: Elsevier Press Ltd., The Boulevard, Langford Ln, Kidlington, Oxfords OX5 1GB, United Kingdom. TEL 44-1865-843000, FAX 44-1865-843010, http://www.elsevier.com. Ed. David W Britt.

370.15 150 GBR ISSN 0888-4080
BF311 CODEN: ACPSED
APPLIED COGNITIVE PSYCHOLOGY. Text in English. 1987. 7/yr. USD 925 in United States; USD 925 in Canada & Mexico; USD 925 elsewhere; USD 972 combined subscription in United States for print and online eds.; USD 972 combined subscription in Canada & Mexico for print and online eds.; USD 972 combined subscription elsewhere for print and online eds. (effective 2002). adv. bk.rev. charts, illus. index. back issues avail.; reprint service avail. from SWZ,PQC. *Refereed.* **Document type:** *Academic/Scholarly.* **Description:** Reviews and reports papers dealing with psychological analyses of problems of memory, learning, thinking, language, and consciousness as they are reflected in the real world.
Formerly (until 1987): Human Learning (0277-6707)
Related titles: Microform ed.: (from PQC); Online - full text ed.: ISSN 1099-0720. 1996. USD 925 in United States; USD 925 in Canada & Mexico; USD 925 elsewhere (effective 2002) (from EBSCO Publishing, Wiley InterScience, Institute for Scientific Information).
Indexed: ASCA, ASSIA, Abstr.Hum.Comp.Inter., AgeLine, Cont.Pg.Educ., Crim.Just.Abstr., Curr.Cont., ERA, Educ.Tech.Abstr., Ergon.Abstr., Fam.Ind., IBR, IBZ, Ind.Philos., Lang.& Lang.Behav.Abstr., PsycInfo, Ref.Zh., Russ.Acad.Sci.Bibl., SOPODA, SSCI, Sociol.Abstr., e-psyche.
—BLDSC (1571.936500), CISTI, IDS, ingenta. **CCC.**
Published by: (Society for Applied Research in Memory and Cognition), Wiley Europe Ltd., Baffins Ln, Chichester, W Sussex PO19 1UD, United Kingdom. TEL 44-1243-779777, FAX 44-1243-775878, cs-journals@wiley.co.uk, customer@wiley.co.uk, http://www.interscience.wiley.com/jpages/0888-4080/, http://www.wiley.co.uk. Ed. Louis Nirenberg. adv.: B&W page GBP 650, color page GBP 1,550; trim 165 x 248. Circ: 575. **Subscr. in the US to:** John Wiley & Sons, Inc., Journals, 605 Third Ave, New York, NY 10158. TEL 212-820-6021, 212-850-6645, subinfo@jiley.com.

301 USA ISSN 1088-8691
CODEN: ADSCFM
APPLIED DEVELOPMENTAL SCIENCE. Text in English. 1997. q. USD 45 in US & Canada to individuals; USD 75 elsewhere to individuals; USD 260 in US & Canada to institutions; USD 290 elsewhere to institutions (effective 2002). adv. **Document type:** *Journal, Academic/Scholarly.* **Description:** Synthesis of research and application that reflect the view that individual and family functioning is a combined and interactive product of biology, and the physical and social environments that continuously evolve and change over time.
Related titles: Online - full text ed.: ISSN 1532-480X. USD 40.50 to individuals; USD 234 to institutions (effective 2002) (from CatchWord Ltd., EBSCO Publishing, O C L C Online Computer Library Center, Inc., RoweCom Information Quest, Swets Blackwell).
Indexed: Child Devel.Abstr., PsycInfo, Sociol.Abstr., e-psyche.
—BLDSC (1571.946000), CatchWord, Infotrieve, ingenta. **CCC.**
Published by: Lawrence Erlbaum Associates, Inc., 10 Industrial Ave, Mahwah, NJ 07430-2262. TEL 201-760-3735, 800-926-6579, FAX 201-236-0072, journals@erlbaum.com, http://www.erlbaum.com/Journals/journals/ADS/ads.htm. Eds. Celia B Fisher, Richard M Lerner. adv.: page USD 275; trim 7 x 10.

APPLIED ERGONOMICS; human factors in technology and society. see *ENGINEERING*

150 658.3 USA ISSN 1055-9094
APPLIED H.R.M. RESEARCH. (Human Resources Management) Text in English. 1990-1996; resumed 1997. s-a. USD 40 to individuals; USD 70 to institutions (effective 2000). adv. back issues avail. *Refereed.* **Document type:** *Academic/Scholarly.* **Description:** Publishes scientific articles of interest to professionals in human resource management and industrial psychology, as well as personnel specialists and industrial psychologists.
Indexed: PsycInfo, e-psyche.
Published by: Society of I-O Graduates, Department of Psychology, Radford University, Radford, VA 24142. TEL 540-831-5513. Ed., Pub., R&P, Adv. contact Michael G Aamodt.

APPLIED NEUROPSYCHOLOGY. see *MEDICAL SCIENCES—Psychiatry And Neurology*

APPLIED PSYCHOLINGUISTICS; psychological studies of language processes. see *LINGUISTICS*

APPLIED PSYCHOLINGUISTICS AND COMMUNICATION DISORDERS. see *LINGUISTICS*

150 USA ISSN 0146-6216
BF39
APPLIED PSYCHOLOGICAL MEASUREMENT. Text in English. 1976. q. USD 55 to individuals; USD 325 to institutions; USD 20 newsstand/cover to individuals; USD 75 newsstand/cover to institutions (effective 2002). adv. bk.rev. illus. Index. back issues avail.; reprints avail. *Refereed.* **Document type:** *Academic/Scholarly.* **Description:** Presents empirical research on the application of techniques of psychological measurement to substantive problems in all areas of psychology and related disciplines.
Related titles: Microfiche ed.: (from PQC); Online - full text ed.: (from EBSCO Publishing, O C L C Online Computer Library Center, Inc., RoweCom Information Quest, ProQuest Information & Learning, ingenta, Swets Blackwell, Institute for Scientific Information).
Indexed: ASCA, Biol.Abstr., C.I.J.E., Child Devel.Abstr., Curr.Cont., IBZ, Ind.Philos., PsycInfo, Psychol.Abstr. (1977-), Psycscan A.P., Russ.Acad.Sci.Bibl., SSCI, e-psyche.
—BLDSC (1576.550000), IDS, ingenta. **CCC.**
Published by: (Applied Psychological Measurement, Inc.), Sage Publications, Inc., 2455 Teller Rd, Thousand Oaks, CA 91320. TEL 805-449-0721, FAX 805-499-0871, info@sagepub.com, http://www.sagepub.com. Ed. David J Weiss. Pub. Sara Miller McCune. R&P Tanya Udin. Adv. contact DeAnna Vega Hammersley. Circ: 975 (paid). **Overseas subscr. to:** Sage Publications Ltd., 6 Bonhill St, London EC2A 4PU, United Kingdom; Sage Publications India Pvt. Ltd., 4215, New Delhi 110 048, India.

150 USA
APPLIED PSYCHOLOGY. Text in English. irreg. **Document type:** *Monographic series.*
Published by: Lawrence Erlbaum Associates, Inc., 10 Industrial Ave, Mahwah, NJ 07430-2262. TEL 201-236-9500, 800-926-6579, FAX 201-236-0072, jamsel@erlbaum.com, http://www.erlbaum.com. Ed. Edwin Fleishman.

158 GBR ISSN 0269-994X
BF636.A1 CODEN: ADPYE4
APPLIED PSYCHOLOGY; an international review. Text in English; Abstracts in French. 1951. q. GBP 295 to institutions in UK & Europe; USD 453 to institutions in the Americas & Caribbean; GBP 295 elsewhere to institutions non-members (effective 2002). back issues avail. *Refereed.* **Document type:** *Journal, Academic/Scholarly.* **Description:** Serves as a forum for the scholarly exchange of research findings and professional standards and promotes awareness of important professional issues.
Formerly: International Review of Applied Psychology
Related titles: Online - full text ed.: ISSN 1464-0597 (from CatchWord Ltd., EBSCO Publishing, O C L C Online Computer Library Center, Inc., RoweCom Information Quest, ingenta, Swets Blackwell, Institute for Scientific Information).
Indexed: ASCA, ASSIA, Adol.Ment.Hlth.Abstr., Bibl.Asian Stud. (1970), Cont.Pg.Manage., Curr.Cont., ERA, Environ.Sci.Poll.Mgmt., Ergon.Abstr., Indian Psychol.Abstr., Lang.& Lang.Behav.Abstr., Mult.Ed.Abstr., Pollut.Abstr., PsycInfo, Psychol.Abstr. (1968-), Psycscan A.P., Risk Abstr., SOPODA, SSCI, Saf.Sci.Abstr., Soc.Serv.Abstr., Sociol.Abstr., Stud.Wom.Abstr.
—BLDSC (1576.555000), CatchWord (psych), CISTI, IDS, Infotrieve. **CCC.**

P

Published by: (International Association of Applied Psychology, Technion - Israel Institute of Technology, William Davidson Faculty of Industrial Engineering and Management ISR), Blackwell Publishers Ltd., 108 Cowley Rd, Oxford OX4 1JF, United Kingdom. TEL 44-1865-791100, FAX 44-1865-791347, jnlinfo@blackwellpublishers.co.uk, http://www.blackwellpulishers.co.uk. Ed. Prof. Miriam Erez TEL 972-4829-4444. Circ: 2,000. **Subscr. in N. America to:** Taylor & Francis Ltd.. FAX 215—269-0363.

613 USA ISSN 1090-0586
BF319.5.B5 CODEN: APSBFZ
APPLIED PSYCHOPHYSIOLOGY AND BIOFEEDBACK. Text in English. 1975. q. USD 484, EUR 483 to institutions for print or online ed.; USD 580.80, EUR 579.60 to institutions for print & online eds. (effective 2002). adv. bk.rev. illus. Index. back issues avail.; reprints avail. *Refereed.* **Document type:** *Academic/Scholarly.* **Description:** Emphasizes empirical research, basic and applied, in the theory, practice, and evaluation of applied psychophysiology and biofeedback.
Formerly (until 1997): Biofeedback and Self Regulation (0363-3586)
Related titles: Microfilm ed.: (from PQC); Online - full text ed.: (from EBSCO Publishing, O C L C Online Computer Library Center, Inc., Swets Blackwell, Kluwer Online, Institute for Scientific Information, RoweCom Information Quest).
Indexed: AMED, ASCA, Adol.Ment.Hlth.Abstr., AgeLine, Biol.Abstr., Curr.Adv.Ecol.Sci., Curr.Cont., Dent.Ind., ERA, Excerp.Med., INSPEC (Mar.1979-Dec.1996, Mar.1997-), Ind.Med. (1997-), Indian Psychol.Abstr., PsycInfo, Psychol.Abstr. (1977-), Psycscan B.A.& T., Ref.Zh., SSCI, Sp.Ed.Needs Abstr., e-psyche.
—BLDSC (1576.562000), AskIEEE, CISTI, GNLM, IDS, Infotrieve, ingenta, KNAW. **CCC.**
Published by: Kluwer Academic - Plenum Publishers (Subsidiary of: Wolters Kluwer N.V.), 233 Spring St, New York, NY 10013-1578. TEL 212-620-8000, 800-221-9369, FAX 212-463-0742, info@plenum.com, http://www.wkap.nl/journalhome.htm/1090-0586. Ed. F Andrasik. R&P Rose Luongo TEL 781-871-6311. **Subscr. outside the Americas:** Kluwer Academic Publishers Group, Journals Department, PO Box 322, Dordrecht 3300 AH, Netherlands. TEL 31-78-639-2392, FAX 31-78-654-6474.

150 ESP ISSN 0213-3334
APUNTES DE PSICOLOGIA. Text in Spanish. 1982. 3/yr. ESP 2,200; ESP 3,000 in the European Union and Latin America; ESP 4,000 elsewhere. back issues avail. *Refereed.* **Document type:** *Academic/Scholarly.*
Formerly (until 1983): Colegio Oficial de Psicologos, Delegacion de Andalucia Occidental. Boletin Informativo (0213-3342)
Indexed: PsycInfo, e-psyche.
—CINDOC.
Published by: Colegio Oficial de Psicologos. Andalucia Occidental, C. Carlos de Capeda 2, 2a Planta, Sevilla 41005, Spain. TEL 34-95-446-3076, FAX 34-95-465-9237, dsevilla@correo.cop.es, http://www.cop.es/publicaciones/apuntes/. Ed. Francisco Fernandez Serra.

302 DEU
ARBEITEN ZUR SOZIALWISSENSCHAFTLICHEN PSYCHOLOGIE. Text in German. 1972. irreg. price varies. **Document type:** *Monographic series, Academic/Scholarly.*
Published by: Aschendorffsche Verlagsbuchhandlung, Soester Str 13, Muenster 48155, Germany. TEL 49-251-690-0, FAX 49-251-690143, buchverlag@aschendorff.de, http://www.aschendorff.de/buch. R&P Dirk F Passmann. Adv. contact Petra Landsknecht.

616.89 DEU
ARBEITSHEFTE GRUPPENANALYSE. Text in German. s-a. **Document type:** *Academic/Scholarly.*
Indexed: e-psyche.
Published by: (Foerderverein Gruppentherapie e.V.), Votum Verlag GmbH, Grevener Str 89-91, Muenster 48159, Germany. TEL 49-251-26514-0, FAX 49-251-2651420, info@votum-verlag.de, http://www.votum-verlag.de.

150.19 DEU ISSN 0721-9628
ARBEITSHEFTE KINDERPSYCHOANALYSE. Text in German. 1982. a. DEM 22. bk.rev. back issues avail. **Document type:** *Journal, Academic/Scholarly.* **Description:** Contains articles on psychoanalysis discussing theoretical questions, case studies, and child psychoanalytical work in institutions.
Indexed: e-psyche.
Published by: Gesamthochschule Kassel, Wissenschaftliches Zentrum II, Gottschalkstr 26, Kassel 34127, Germany. TEL 49-561-8042807, FAX 49-561-8042811, wz2@hrz.uni-kassel.de, http://www.uni-kassel.de/wz2/publikationen/arbeitshefte/index.htm. Ed. Hilde Kipp. Circ: 700.

150 ITA
ARCADIA. Text in Italian. 1994. irreg., latest vol.5, 1998. price varies. **Document type:** *Monographic series.*
Indexed: e-psyche.
Published by: Liguori Editore srl, Via Posillipo, 394, Naples, NA 80123, Italy. TEL 39-81-7206111, FAX 39-81-7206244, http://www.liguori.it. Pub. Guido Liguori. Adv. contact Maria Liguori.

301.1 150 GBR ISSN 0260-4523
ARCHITECTURAL PSYCHOLOGY NEWSLETTER. Text in English. 1969. 4/yr. GBP 8. **Document type:** *Newsletter.* **Description:** Research concerned with the interrelationship between people and their physical surroundings.
Indexed: e-psyche.
—CISTI.
Published by: Architectural Psychology Research Unit, Kingston Polytechnic, Knights Park, Kingston Upon Thames, Surrey KT1 2QJ, United Kingdom. TEL 44-181-549-6151.

ARCHITECTURE & BEHAVIOUR/ARCHITECTURE ET COMPORTEMENT. see *ARCHITECTURE*

ARCHIV FUER RELIGIONSPSYCHOLOGIE. see *RELIGIONS AND THEOLOGY*

150 CHE ISSN 0003-9640
BF2
ARCHIVES DE PSYCHOLOGIE. Text in English, French. 1901. q. CHF 90, EUR 58.44 to individuals; CHF 160, EUR 103.89 to institutions (effective 2002). bk.rev. charts. cum.index irreg. back issues avail. **Document type:** *Journal, Academic/Scholarly.*
Indexed: IBR, IBZ, Ind.Philos., P C I, PsycInfo, Psychol.Abstr. (1959-), Ref.Zh., e-psyche.
—BLDSC (1640.450000), Infotrieve, ingenta. **CCC.**
Published by: (Universite de Geneve/University of Geneva, Faculte de Psychologie et des Sciences de l'Education BEL, Section de Psychologie), Editions Medecine et Hygiene, Case Postale 456, Geneva, 4 1211, Switzerland. TEL 41-22-7029311, FAX 41-22-7029355, abonnements@medhyg.ch, http://www.medhyg.ch. Circ: 600.

ARCHIVES OF CLINICAL NEUROPSYCHOLOGY. see *MEDICAL SCIENCES—Psychiatry And Neurology*

▼ **ARCHIVES OF PSYCHIATRY AND PSYCHOTHERAPY.** see *MEDICAL SCIENCES—Psychiatry And Neurology*

ARCHIVES OF WOMEN'S MENTAL HEALTH. see *WOMEN'S HEALTH*

306.7 MEX ISSN 1405-1923
ARCHIVOS HISPANOAMERICANOS DE SEXOLOGIA. Text in Spanish. 1995. s-a. MXP 80, USD 35 (effective 2000). adv. bk.rev. back issues avail.; reprints avail. *Refereed.* **Document type:** *Academic/Scholarly.* **Description:** Designed for educators, psychologists, physicians, social scientists and professionals interested in sex education and sexology. Presents research papers in sexuality, gender issues, rehabilitation and education of the disabled, sex education, therapy and social aspects of sex.
Indexed: e-psyche.
Published by: Instituto Mexicano de Sexologia, TEPIC 86, Col Roma, Mexico City, DF 06760, Mexico. TEL 52-5-5642850, http://www.imesex.edu.mx/. Ed. Dr. Juan Luis Alvarez-Gayou Jurgenson. R&P Juan Luis Alvarez Gayou Jurgenson. Adv. contact Cristina Torices. Circ: 500. **Co-sponsors:** Facultad de Psicologia; Universidad Pedagogica Nacional; Sociedad Mexicana de Psicologia.

AROMA-CHOLOGY REVIEW. see *BEAUTY CULTURE—Perfumes And Cosmetics*

ARQUIVOS DE SAUDE MENTAL DO ESTADO DE SAO PAULO. see *MEDICAL SCIENCES—Psychiatry And Neurology*

ARQUIVOS DE SAUDE MENTAL DO ESTADO DE SAO PAULO. SUPLEMENTO. see *MEDICAL SCIENCES—Psychiatry And Neurology*

616.89 GBR ISSN 0197-4556
RC489.A7 CODEN: APCYAJ
THE ARTS IN PSYCHOTHERAPY; an international journal. Text in English. 1973. 5/yr. EUR 99 in Europe to individuals; JPY 13,200 in Japan to individuals; USD 112 elsewhere to individuals; EUR 509 in Europe to institutions; JPY 67,500 in Japan to institutions; USD 570 elsewhere to institutions (effective 2002). adv. bk.rev. reprint service avail. from PQC,ISI. *Refereed.* **Document type:** *Academic/Scholarly.* **Description:** Innovative research in artistic inquiry and expression and its use in the treatment of mental disorders.
Formerly (until 1980): Art Psychotherapy (0090-9092)
Related titles: Microfilm ed.: (from PQC); Online - full text ed.: (from ingenta, Swets Blackwell, ScienceDirect, Institute for Scientific Information).
Indexed: AMED, ASCA, AgeLine, Artbibl.Mod., Arts & Hum.Cit.Ind. (coverage dropped), Biol.Abstr., Curr.Cont., Except.Child Educ.Abstr., Excerp.Med., Fam.Ind., PsycInfo, Psychol.Abstr. (1973-), SSCI, e-psyche.
—BLDSC (1736.825000), GNLM, IDS, Infotrieve, ingenta, KNAW. **CCC.**
Published by: Pergamon (Subsidiary of: Elsevier Science), The Boulevard, Langford Ln, East Park, Kidlington, Oxford OXB 1GB, United Kingdom. FAX 44-1865-843010, nlinfo-f@elsevier/nl; usinfo-f@elsevier.com; forinfo-kyf04035@niftyserve.or.jp, http://www.artspsycho, http://www.elsevier.nl/. Eds. H Smeijsters, I Dosamantes. **Subscr. in Australasia and the Far East to:** Elsevier Science (Singapore) Pte Ltd, No.1 Temasek Ave, 17-01 Millenia Tower, Singapore 039192, Singapore. TEL 65-434-3727, FAX 65-337-2230; **Subscr. in the Americas to:** Elsevier Science, PO Box 945, New York, NY 10159-0945. TEL 212-633-3730, FAX 212-633-3680, usinfo-f@elsevier.com, http://www.elsevier.com; **Subscr. to:** Elsevier Science BV, PO Box 211, Amsterdam 1000 AE, Netherlands. TEL 31-20-485-3757, FAX 31-20-485-3432, nlinfo-f@elsevier.nl, http://www.elsevier.nl.

ASIAN JOURNAL OF PSYCHOLOGY AND EDUCATION. see *EDUCATION*

302 GBR ISSN 1367-2223
HM1001
ASIAN JOURNAL OF SOCIAL PSYCHOLOGY. Text in English. 1998. 3/yr. GBP 168 to institutions in UK & Europe; USD 274 to institutions in the Americas & Caribbean; GBP 168 elsewhere to institutions (effective 2002). bk.rev. **Document type:** *Academic/Scholarly.* **Description:** Aims to stimulate research and encourage academic exchanges for the advancement of social psychology in Asia. Publishes both theoretical and empirical papers.
Related titles: Online - full text ed.: (from EBSCO Publishing, O C L C Online Computer Library Center, Inc., RoweCom Information Quest, ingenta, Swets Blackwell).
Indexed: PsycInfo, Soc.Serv.Abstr., Sociol.Abstr., e-psyche.
—BLDSC (1742.576000). **CCC.**
Published by: Blackwell Publishers Ltd., 108 Cowley Rd, Oxford OX4 1JF, United Kingdom. TEL 44-1865-791100, FAX 44-1865-791347, jnlinfo@blackwellpublishers.co.uk, http://www.blackwellpublishers.co.uk. Ed. Kwok Leung.

301.1 150 VEN
ASOCIACION VENEZOLANA DE PSICOLOGIA SOCIAL. REVISTA. Text in Spanish. 1978. q. USD 25 to individuals; USD 30 to institutions. adv. bk.rev. back issues avail. **Document type:** *Academic/Scholarly.* **Description:** Features theoretical and methodological papers and information about social psychology in Latin America.
Formerly (until 1994): Asociacion Venezolana de Psicologia Social. Boletin (1011-6273)
Indexed: e-psyche.
Published by: Asociacion Venezolana de Psicologia Social, Los Chaguaramos, Apdo 47101, Caracas, DF 1040, Venezuela. TEL 619811-30 Ext. 2643. Ed. Leoncio Barrios. Circ: 500.

616.8 USA ISSN 1073-1911
BF176
ASSESSMENT. Text in English. 1993. q. USD 50 domestic to individuals; USD 60 foreign to individuals; USD 150 domestic to institutions; USD 180 foreign to institutions (effective 2000). abstr. back issues avail. *Refereed.* **Document type:** *Academic/Scholarly.* **Description:** Publishes articles derived from psychometric research, clinical comparisons or theoretical formulations and literature reviews that fall within the broad domain of clinical and applied assessment.
Related titles: Online - full text ed.: (from ProQuest Information & Learning, Institute for Scientific Information).

Indexed: AgeLine, C.I.J.E., Crim.Just.Abstr., Curr.Cont., Ind.Med. (1994-), PsycInfo, Psycscan C.P., SSCI, e-psyche.
—BLDSC (1746.636200), GNLM, IDS, ingenta.
Published by: Psychological Assessment Resources, Inc., 16204 N Florida Ave, Lutz, FL 33549. TEL 813-968-3003, FAX 813-968-2598, http://www.parinc.com. Ed. Robert P Archer. R&P Brenda Vanantwerp. Adv. contact Daphne Lambright.

150 610 USA
BF319.5.B5
ASSOCIATION FOR APPLIED PSYCHOPHYSIOLOGY AND BIOFEEDBACK. PROCEEDINGS OF THE ANNUAL MEETING. Text in English. 1972. a. USD 30 to non-members; USD 15 to members (effective 1999). abstr, illus. **Document type:** *Proceedings, Abstract/Index.*
Formerly: Biofeedback Society of America. Proceedings of the Annual Meeting (0094-0895)
Media: Online - full content.
Indexed: e-psyche.
—BLDSC (6841.323200).
Published by: Association for Applied Psychophysiology and Biofeedback, 10200 W 44th Ave, Ste 304, Wheat Ridge, CO 80033-2840. TEL 303-422-8436, FAX 303-422-8894, aapb@resourcenter.com, http://www.aapb.org. Ed. Michael Thompson. R&P, Adv. contact Michael P Thompson. Circ: 2,000.

ASSOCIATION FOR CHILD PSYCHOANALYSIS. NEWSLETTER. see *CHILDREN AND YOUTH—About*

155.937 USA
ASSOCIATION FOR DEATH EDUCATION & COUNSELING. FORUM NEWSLETTER. Text in English. 6/yr. USD 115 to individuals; USD 230 to institutions (effective 1999). adv. bk.rev. **Document type:** *Newsletter.*
Indexed: e-psyche.
Published by: Association for Death Education & Counseling, 342 North Main St, West, Hartford, CT 06117-2507. TEL 860-586-7503, FAX 860-586-7550, adecofice@aol.com, http://www.adec.org. R&P Nickie Meeles. Adv. contact Nickie Meeks. Circ: 2,000.

370.15 USA ISSN 1054-0792
ASSOCIATION FOR PAST-LIFE RESEARCH AND THERAPIES. NEWSLETTER. Variant title: A P R T Newsletter. Text in English. 1980. a. USD 10 (effective 1998). adv. bk.rev. **Document type:** *Newsletter.* **Description:** Articles by past-life regression therapists and researchers; includes case histories and techniques, alternative therapies.
Indexed: e-psyche.
Published by: Association for Past-Life Research and Therapies, Inc., PO Box 20151 0151, Riverside, CA 92516. TEL 909-784-1570, pastlife@empirenet.com. Ed. Terry Nash. Circ: 800.

616.891 USA ISSN 0004-542X
RC500
ASSOCIATION FOR PSYCHOANALYTIC MEDICINE. BULLETIN. Text in English. 1961. s-a. USD 20 (effective 1999). bk.rev. cum.index: 1961-1967. **Document type:** *Academic/Scholarly.*
Indexed: e-psyche.
—CISTI.
Published by: Association for Psychoanalytic Medicine, 252 W 85 St, New York, NY 10024. TEL 212-595-7441. Ed. Dr. David Stein. Circ: 1,500 (controlled).

155.4 USA
ASSOCIATION FOR THE STUDY OF PLAY NEWSLETTER. Text in English. 1974. 3/yr. USD 15. back issues avail. **Document type:** *Newsletter.* **Description:** Covers social science and humanistic study of play behavior.
Indexed: e-psyche.
Published by: Association for the Study of Play, PO Box 6375, Georgetown, TX 78626. Ed. Dan Hilliard. Circ: 200. **Subscr. to:** c/o E.P. Jonnsen, Dept of Educational Psychology, University of Kansas, Lawrence, KS 66945-2338.

158 ITA
ASSOCIAZIONE ITALIANA STUDI DI MUSICOTERAPIA. BOLLETTINO. Text in Italian. 1982. s-a. ITL 15,000 (effective 2000). **Document type:** *Bulletin.*
Published by: Associazione Italiana Studi di Musicoterapia, Via Brignole De Ferrari, 6-2, Genoa, GE 16125, Italy. TEL 39-10-2512393.

ATQUE; materiali tra filosofia e psicoterapia. see *PHILOSOPHY*

155 GBR ISSN 1461-6734
▼ **ATTACHMENT AND HUMAN DEVELOPMENT.** Text in English. 1999. 3/yr. GBP 53, USD 87 to individuals; GBP 189, USD 312 to institutions (effective 2002). bk.rev. back issues avail. *Refereed.* **Document type:** *Academic/Scholarly.* **Description:** Provides a new forum for research, case studies and debate for clinicians and academics concerned with the development of social and emotional relationships across the lifespan.
Related titles: Online - full content ed.: ISSN 1469-2988 (from EBSCO Publishing, O C L C Online Computer Library Center, Inc., Swets Blackwell); Online - full text ed.: (from CatchWord Ltd., RoweCom Information Quest).
Indexed: e-psyche.
—BLDSC (1772.775300), CatchWord.
Published by: (International Attachment Network), Routledge (Subsidiary of: Taylor & Francis Group), 11 New Fetter Ln, London EC4P 4EE, United Kingdom. TEL 44-20-7583-9855, FAX 44-20-7842-2298, info@routledge.co.uk, http://www.tandf.co.uk/journals. Eds. Howard Stehle, Jude Cassidy. **Subscr. in US & Canada to:** Routledge, Taylor & Francis Ltd, 29 W 35th St, New York, NY 10001-2299. TEL 212-216-7800; **Subscr. to:** Subscriptions, PO Box 362, Abingdon, Oxon OX14 3WB, United Kingdom. TEL 44-1235-401060, FAX 44-1235-401075.

152 USA ISSN 1047-0387
BF321
ATTENTION AND PERFORMANCE. Text in English. irreg. *Refereed.* **Document type:** *Monographic series.*
Related titles: Online - full text ed.: (from Institute for Scientific Information).
Indexed: ASCA, Neurosci.Cit.Ind., SSCI, e-psyche.
—BLDSC (1772.810000), IDS.
Published by: Lawrence Erlbaum Associates, Inc., 10 Industrial Ave, Mahwah, NJ 07430-2262. TEL 201-236-9500, FAX 201-236-0072, jamsel@erlbaum.com, http://www.erlbaum.com.

ATTI DELLO PSICODRAMMA. see *THEATER*

155.2 ITA ISSN 0394-3747
ATTUALITA GRAFOLOGICA; Trimestrale dell'associazione grafologica italiana. Text in Italian. 1981. q. ITL 30,000 (effective 2000). bk.rev. bibl. 48 p./no. 2 cols./p. *Refereed.* **Document type:** *Bulletin, Academic/Scholarly, Bibliography.* **Description:** Contains news about graphology and psychology initiatives.
Indexed: e-psyche.
Published by: Associazione Grafologica Italiana, Casella Postale 178, Scale San Francesco, 8, Ancona, AN 60121, Italy. TEL 39-071-206100, FAX 39-071-206100, info@a-g-i.it, http://www.a-g-i.it. Ed. Pacifico Cristofanelli. Pub. Iride Conficoni. Circ: 1,400 (paid).

616.89 AUS
AUSTRALASIAN JOURNAL OF PSYCHOTHERAPY. Text in English. 1982. s-a. AUD 55 domestic to individuals; AUD 65 in New Zealand to individuals; AUD 80 elsewhere to individuals; AUD 77 to institutions (effective 2001). adv. bk.rev. back issues avail. *Refereed.* **Document type:** *Academic/Scholarly.* **Description:** A journal of clinical and general interest for practitioners and others.
Formerly: Australian Journal of Psychotherapy (0728-6155)
Indexed: PsycInfo, e-psyche.
—GNLM.
Published by: Psychoanalytic Psychotherapy Association of Australia, Ste 303, 89 High St, Kew, VIC 3101, Australia. dmeadows@netspace.net.au. Ed., R&P Don Meadows TEL 61-3-94890115. Adv. contact Peter Fullerton. Circ: 400 (paid and controlled).

AUSTRALIAN AND NEW ZEALAND JOURNAL OF FAMILY THERAPY; innovative and contextual approaches to human problems. see *SOCIOLOGY*

150 AUS ISSN 1037-2911
AUSTRALIAN JOURNAL OF GUIDANCE & COUNSELLING. Text in English. 1990. a. AUD 25. **Document type:** *Academic/Scholarly.*
Indexed: Aus.Educ.Ind.
—BLDSC (1808.375000).
Published by: Australian Guidance & Counselling Association Ltd., 12 Croydon Rd, Surrey Hills, VIC 3127, Australia. TEL 03-98362952. Ed. Dr. Ivan Watson. Circ: 1,200.

150 331 AUS ISSN 1440-4567
AUSTRALIAN JOURNAL OF MANAGEMENT AND ORGANISATIONAL BEHAVIOUR. Text in English. 1998. s-a. back issues avail. *Refereed.* **Description:** Aims to act as a learning aid for students of the university and be a forum whereby practitioners and academics can share their knowledge, experiences and ideas.
Media: Online - full text.
Published by: University of Southern Queensland, Department of Human Resource Management and Employment Relations, Toowoomba, QLD 4350, Australia. hrm@usq.edu.au, http://www.usq.edu.au/faculty/business/dept_hrm/HRMJournal/. Eds. Cec Pedersen, Tesera Marchant.

150 AUS ISSN 0004-9530
BF1 CODEN: ASJPAE
AUSTRALIAN JOURNAL OF PSYCHOLOGY. Text in English. 1949. 3/yr. AUD 89 domestic to individuals; AUD 90 foreign to individual members; AUD 100 domestic to institutions; AUD 110 foreign to institutions (effective 2001). bk.rev. abstr, bibl, charts, illus. index. cum.index approx. every 10 yrs. back issues avail.; reprint service avail. from PSC,SCH. *Refereed.* **Document type:** *Academic/Scholarly.* **Description:** Presents articles and book reviews on any topic with a central reference to psychology and an emphasis on academic or archival functions.
Related titles: Online - full text ed.: (from Institute for Scientific Information).
Indexed: ASCA, ASSIA, Addic.Abstr., Adol.Ment.Hlth.Abstr., AgeLine, Arts & Hum.Cit.Ind. (coverage dropped), Aus.Educ.Ind., Aus.P.A.I.S., Biol.Abstr., Child Devel.Abstr., Curr.Cont., DSH Abstr., Ergon.Abstr., Fam.Ind., IBR, Ind.Philos., Lang.& Lang.Behav.Abstr., Mid.East: Abstr.& Ind., Neurosci.Cit.Ind., P C I, PsycInfo, Psychol.Abstr. (1949-), Res.High.Educ.Abstr., Risk Abstr., Russ.Acad.Sci.Bibl., SOPODA, SSCI, Soc.Serv.Abstr., Sociol.Abstr., Stud.Wom.Abstr., WMB, e-psyche.
—BLDSC (1811.300000), ingenta.
Published by: Australian Psychological Society, 1 Grattan Street,, Carlton, VIC 3053, Australia. TEL 61-3-86623300, FAX 61-3-96636177, http://www.psychsociety.com.au/. Ed. Christina Lee. Circ: 4,000.

AUSTRALIAN PARAPSYCHOLOGICAL REVIEW. see *PARAPSYCHOLOGY AND OCCULTISM*

150 AUS ISSN 0005-0067
CODEN: AUPCBK
AUSTRALIAN PSYCHOLOGIST. Text in English. 1966. 3/yr. AUD 61 to individuals; AUD 72 to institutions. adv. bk.rev. abstr, charts, illus. index. *Refereed.* **Document type:** *Academic/Scholarly.* **Description:** Publishes articles of relevance to professional and applied psychology, and generally to Australian psychologists.
Related titles: Online - full text ed.: (from Institute for Scientific Information).
Indexed: ASCA, ASSIA, AgeLine, Arts & Hum.Cit.Ind. (coverage dropped), Aus.Educ.Ind., Aus.P.A.I.S., Biol.Abstr., Child Devel.Abstr., Crim.Just.Abstr., Curr.Cont., Fam.Ind., Ind.Philos., Indian Psychol.Abstr., Lang.& Lang.Behav.Abstr., P C I, PsycInfo, Psychol.Abstr. (1966-), Res.High.Educ.Abstr., SOPODA, SSCI, Sociol.Abstr., e-psyche.
—BLDSC (1818.350000), CISTI, ingenta, KNAW. **CCC.**
Published by: Australian Psychological Society, c/o Dr. Christina Lee, Department of Psychology, University of Newcastle, Newcastle, NSW 2308, Australia. Adv. contact Joanne Linzner. Circ: 10,500. **Subscr. to:** PO Box 126, Carlton South, VIC 3053, Australia. TEL 61-3-9663-6166, FAX 61-3-9663-6177.

AUTISM; the international journal of research and practice. see *MEDICAL SCIENCES—Psychiatry And Neurology*

AUTISM RESEARCH REVIEW INTERNATIONAL. see *MEDICAL SCIENCES—Psychiatry And Neurology*

152 COL ISSN 0120-3797
AVANCES EN PSICOLOGIA CLINICA LATINOAMERICANA. Text in Spanish. 1982. a. USD 7 to individuals; USD 14 to institutions (effective 2000 & 2001). adv. bk.rev. bibl, illus, stat. **Document type:** *Academic/Scholarly.* **Description:** Articles on all areas of psychology as a science and as a profession.
Indexed: Biol.Abstr., Curr.Cont. (coverage dropped), IBZ, Ind.Philos., PsycInfo, Psychol.Abstr. (1982-), e-psyche.
—BLDSC (1837.110500). **CCC.**
Published by: Foundation for the Advancement of Psychology, PO Box 92621, Bogota, CUND, Colombia. TEL 57-1-256-7527. Ed. Ruben Ardila. Circ: 2,500.

P

150 JPN ISSN 0386-1856
BAIOFIDOBAKKU KENKYU/JAPANESE JOURNAL OF BIOFEEDBACK RESEARCH. Text in English, Japanese. 1973. 2/yr. JPY 1,000.
Indexed: PsycInfo, Psychol.Abstr. (1990-), e-psyche.
Published by: Nihon Baiofidobakku Gakkai/Society of Japanese Biofeedback Research, Jochi Daigaku Bungakubu Shinrigaku Kenkyushitsu, 7 Kioi-cho, Chiyoda-ku, Tokyo 102-0094, Japan.

370.15 USA
BANFF INTERNATIONAL BEHAVIORAL SCIENCES SERIES. Text in English. irreg.
—BLDSC (1861.598700).
Published by: Sage Publications, Inc., 2455 Teller Rd, Thousand Oaks, CA 91320. TEL 805-499-0871, FAX 805-706-0871, http://www.sagepub.com. Ed. Jim Nageotte.

150 BGD ISSN 1022-7466
BANGLADESH JOURNAL OF PSYCHOLOGY. Text in English. 1968. a. USD 10. reprints avail. **Document type:** *Academic/Scholarly.* **Description:** Contains research and review articles on all branches of psychology.
Indexed: PsycInfo, e-psyche.
Published by: Bangladesh Psychological Association, Dept. of Psychology, University of Dhaka, Dhaka 1000, Bangladesh. TEL 88-2-864553. Ed. A Khaleque. Circ: 400.

301.1 150 USA ISSN 0197-3533
HM251 CODEN: BASPEG
BASIC AND APPLIED SOCIAL PSYCHOLOGY. Text in English. 1980. q. USD 65 in US & Canada to individuals; USD 95 elsewhere to individuals; USD 450 in US & Canada to institutions; USD 480 elsewhere to institutions (effective 2002). adv. bk.rev. abstr, bibl, charts, illus, stat. *Refereed.* **Document type:** *Journal, Academic/Scholarly.* **Description:** Presents material relevant to basic and applied research in all areas of social psychology in order to bring relevant social psychological studies from other specialties and disciplines to the attention of social psychologists.
Related titles: Online - full text ed.: ISSN 1532-4834. USD 58.50 to individuals; USD 405 to institutions (effective 2002) (from CatchWord Ltd., EBSCO Publishing, O C L C Online Computer Library Center, Inc., RoweCom Information Quest, Swets Blackwell, Institute for Scientific Information).
Indexed: ASCA, ASSIA, AgeLine, Curr.Cont., Fam.Ind., IBZ, Ind.Philos., PsycInfo, Psychol.Abstr. (1980-), Psycscan A.P., SSCI, Soc.Serv.Abstr., Sociol.Abstr., e-psyche.
—BLDSC (1863.913300), CatchWord. **CCC.**
Published by: Lawrence Erlbaum Associates, Inc., 10 Industrial Ave, Mahwah, NJ 07430-2262. TEL 201-760-3735, 800-926-6579, FAX 201-236-0072, journals@erlbaum.com, http://www.erlbaum.com/Journals/journals/BASP/basp.htm. Ed. Michael J Strube. adv.: page USD 275; trim 7 x 10. Circ: 1,000.

158 USA
BE YOUR OWN THERAPIST NEWSLETTER. Text in English. bi-m. free per issue. **Document type:** *Newsletter.* **Description:** Self-help psychology newsletter featuring tips and suggestions for changing your life.
Media: Online - full text.
Indexed: e-psyche.
Address: thayerw@aol.com, http://members.aol.com/purplepara. Ed. Thayer White.

150 USA ISSN 0738-6729
BF199
THE BEHAVIOR ANALYST. Text in English. 1978. s-a. USD 35 to individuals; USD 50 foreign to individuals; USD 85 to institutions; USD 95 foreign to institutions; USD 15 to students; USD 23 foreign to students. adv. bk.rev. cum.index. back issues avail. *Refereed.* **Document type:** *Academic/Scholarly.* **Description:** Devoted to trend issues, policies, and developments in behavior analysis.
Related titles: Audio cassette/tape ed.; Online - full text ed.: (from Institute for Scientific Information).
Indexed: ASCA, Behav.Abstr., Curr.Cont., PsycInfo, Psychol.Abstr. (1982-), Psycscan B.A.& T., SSCI, e-psyche.
—BLDSC (1876.652500), IDS, ingenta.
Published by: Association for Behavior Analysis, 213 West Hall, Western Michigan University, Kalamazoo, MI 49008-5052. TEL 616-387-8341, FAX 616-387-8354. Ed. Phill Chase. Adv. contact Tim Castanon. Circ: 2,900.

150 USA ISSN 1053-8348
BF199 CODEN: BEPHE5
BEHAVIOR AND PHILOSOPHY. Text in English. 1972. 1/yr. USD 60 domestic to individuals; USD 70 foreign to individuals (effective 1999). adv. bk.rev. illus. 100 p./no. reprint service avail. from PSC,SCH. *Refereed.* **Document type:** *Journal, Academic/Scholarly.* **Description:** Publishes the philosophical reflections of psychologists and the psychological ruminations of philosophers in papers that are both scientifically sound and philosophically significant.
Formerly (until vol.12, no.2, 1982): Behaviorism (0090-4155)
Related titles: Online - full text ed.: (from Institute for Scientific Information).
Indexed: ASCA, Adol.Ment.Hlth.Abstr., Biol.Abstr., Curr.Cont., Excerp.Med., IBR, IBZ, Mid.East: Abstr.& Ind., P C I, Phil.Ind., PsycInfo, Psychol.Abstr. (1972-), Psycscan B.A.& T., Ref.Zh., Rel.Ind.One, Rel.Ind.Two, SSCI, e-psyche.
—IDS, ingenta.
Published by: Behaviorists For Social Responsibility, 336 Baker Ave, Concord, MA 01742-2107. TEL 978-369-2227, FAX 978-369-8584, center@behavior.org, http://www.behavior.org/journals_B&P/BandP_index.cfm. Ed. J E R Staddon. R&P Betsy Constantine. Circ: 600. **Subscr. to:** Boyd Printing, 49 Sheridan Ave, Albany, NY 12210.

302 USA ISSN 1064-9506
BF199
BEHAVIOR AND SOCIAL ISSUES. Text in English. 1978. 2/yr. USD 35 to individuals; USD 60 to institutions. adv. bk.rev. illus. 100 p./no. 1 cols./p. back issues avail. *Refereed.* **Document type:** *Journal, Academic/Scholarly.* **Description:** Publishes scholarly articles that advance the analysis of human social behavior, particularly with application to understanding existing social problems.
Former titles (until 1990): Behavior Analysis and Social Action (1065-1047); (until 1986): Behaviorists for Social Action Journal (0739-5051)
Related titles: Online - full text ed.: (from ProQuest Information & Learning).
Indexed: PsycInfo, Psychol.Abstr. (1991-), Psycscan B.A.& T., e-psyche.
Published by: Behaviorists For Social Responsibility TEL 978-369-2227, FAX 978-369-8584, bfsr@bfsr.org, center@behavior.org, http://www.bfsr.org, http://www.behavior.org. Ed. Dwight Harshbarger. R&P Betsy Constantine. Circ: 400. **Subscr. to:** Boyd Printing, 49 Sheridan Ave, Albany, NY 12210.

150 USA ISSN 0145-4455
BF637.B4
BEHAVIOR MODIFICATION. Text in English. 1977. 5/yr. USD 80 to individuals; USD 395 to institutions; USD 25 newsstand/cover to individuals; USD 80 newsstand/cover to institutions (effective 2002). adv. bk.rev. illus. index. back issues avail.; reprint service avail. from PSC,SCH. *Refereed.* **Document type:** *Academic/Scholarly.* **Description:** Describes assessment and modification techniques for problems in psychiatric, clinical, educational, and rehabilitational settings.
Related titles: Online - full text ed.: (from EBSCO Publishing, O C L C Online Computer Library Center, Inc., RoweCom Information Quest, ProQuest Information & Learning, ingenta, Swets Blackwell, Institute for Scientific Information).
Indexed: ASCA, Adol.Ment.Hlth.Abstr., AgeLine, C.I.J.E., Curr.Cont., Educ.Ind. (Jul.1992-Jun.1997), Except.Child Educ.Abstr., Excerp.Med., Fam.Ind., Human Resour.Abstr., Ind.Med. (1977-), Int.Nurs.Ind., PsycInfo, Psychol.Abstr. (1977-), Psychol.R.G., Psycscan B.A.& T., SSCI, Sage Fam.Stud.Abstr., Sage Race Rel.Abstr., Sage Urb.Stud.Abstr., Soc.Sci.Ind. (coverage dropped), Soc.Serv.Abstr., Sociol.Abstr., Viol.& Abuse Abstr., e-psyche.
—BLDSC (1876.720000), EMDOCS, GNLM, IDS, ingenta. **CCC.**
Published by: Sage Publications, Inc., 2455 Teller Rd, Thousand Oaks, CA 91320. TEL 805-499-0721, FAX 805-499-0871, libraries@sagepub.com., libaries@sagepub.com, http://www.sagepub.co.uk/, http://www.sagepub.com. Eds. Alan S Bellack, Michel Hersen. Pub. Sara Miller McCune. R&P Tanya Udin. Adv. contact DeAnna Vega Hammersley. Circ: 1,500. **Overseas subscr. to:** Sage Publications Ltd., 6 Bonhill St, London EC2A 4PU, United Kingdom; Sage Publications India Pvt. Ltd., 4215, New Delhi 110 048, India.

572 USA ISSN 0743-3808
BF180 CODEN: BRMCEW
BEHAVIOR RESEARCH METHODS, INSTRUMENTS, AND COMPUTERS; a journal of the Psychonomic Society . Text in English. 1968. q. USD 68 domestic to individuals; USD 77 foreign to individuals; USD 151 domestic to institutions; USD 160 foreign to institutions (effective 2001); USD 160 domestic to institutions; USD 170 foreign to institutions (effective 2002). adv. bk.rev. illus. Index. back issues avail.; reprint service avail. from PQC. *Refereed.* **Document type:** *Academic/Scholarly.* **Description:** Contains articles in the areas of methods, techniques and instrumentation of research in experimental psychology.
Formerly (until 1984): Behavior Research Methods and Instrumentation (0005-7878)
Related titles: Microform ed.: (from NRP,PQC); Online - full text ed.: (from CatchWord Ltd., Institute for Scientific Information).
Indexed: ASCA, Anim.Behav.Abstr., Biol.Abstr., Compumath, Curr.Adv.Ecol.Sci., Curr.Cont., Curr.Ind.Stat., Ergon.Abstr., IBR, INSPEC (Jan.1973-Jan.1985, Apr.1985-), Ind.Med. (1984-), Ind.Philos., Lang.& Lang.Behav.Abstr., Mid.East: Abstr.& Ind., PsycInfo, Psychol.Abstr. (1968-), Russ.Acad.Sci.Bibl., SOPODA, SSCI, Sociol.Abstr., Sport Fish.Abstr., Wild.Rev., Zoo.Rec., e-psyche.
—BLDSC (1876.832000), AskIEEE, CISTI, IDS, ingenta. **CCC.**
Published by: Psychonomic Society, Inc., 1710 Fortview Rd, Austin, TX 78704. TEL 512-462-2442, FAX 512-462-1101, jbellquist@psychonomic.org, http://www.psychonomic.org. Ed. Jonathan Vaughn. R&P Cinnamon Nemec. Adv. contact Robert Samford. page USD 110; trim 10.75 x 8. Circ: 1,150.

301.1 USA ISSN 0278-8403
THE BEHAVIOR THERAPIST. Text in English. 1978. 10/yr. USD 38 domestic; USD 48 in Canada & Mexico; USD 65 elsewhere (effective 2001). adv. bk.rev., software rev. back issues avail. **Document type:** *Academic/Scholarly.* **Description:** Aims to be a vehicle of communication among behavioral scientists, educators, practitioners, admini strators, students and job seekers.
Formerly: Association for Advancement of Behavior Therapy. Newsletter
Indexed: Psychol.Abstr., Yrbk.Assoc.Educ.& Rehab.Blind, e-psyche.
—BLDSC (1876.900000), ingenta. **CCC.**
Published by: Association for Advancement of Behavior Therapy, 305 Seventh Ave, Ste 16A, New York, NY 10001. TEL 212-647-1890, FAX 212-647-1865, http://www.aabt.org. Ed. George Ronan. Pub. David Teisler. R&P Felicia Robinson. Adv. contact Stephanie Schwartz. B&W page USD 400. Circ: 4,500.

150 USA ISSN 0005-7894
RC489.B4 CODEN: BHVTAK
BEHAVIOR THERAPY. Text in English. 1970. 4/yr. USD 75 domestic to individuals; USD 150 domestic to institutions; USD 163 in Canada & Mexico; USD 183 elsewhere (effective 2001). adv. illus. Index. back issues avail.; reprint service avail. from PSC,SCH. *Refereed.* **Document type:** *Academic/Scholarly.* **Description:** Interdisciplinary journal which presents treatment research covering theory, methodology, clinical and ethical issues.
Related titles: Online - full text ed.: (from Gale Group, Factiva, Institute for Scientific Information).
Indexed: ASCA, Addic.Abstr., Adol.Ment.Hlth.Abstr., AgeLine, Behav.Med.Abstr., Biol.Abstr., Crim.Just.Abstr., Curr.Cont., Curr.Ind.Stat., Except.Child Educ.Abstr., Excerp.Med., Fam.Ind., Jrnl.Watch Psych., Mid.East: Abstr.& Ind., Mult.Ed.Abstr., P C I, PsycInfo, Psychol.Abstr. (1970-), Psycscan B.A.& T., Psycscan C.P., SSCI, Soc.Sci.Ind. (Jan.1994-), Sp.Ed.Needs Abstr., Stud.Wom.Abstr., THA, e-psyche.
—BLDSC (1876.930000), EMDOCS, GNLM, IDS, ingenta, KNAW. **CCC.**
Published by: Association for Advancement of Behavior Therapy, 305 Seventh Ave, Ste 16A, New York, NY 10001. publication@aabt.org. Ed. David A. F. Haaga. Pub. David Teisler. R&P Teresa Wimmer. Adv. contact Stephanie Schwartz. B&W page USD 275. Circ: 3,500.

150 574 616.8 GBR ISSN 0140-525X
QP360 CODEN: BBSCDH
BEHAVIORAL AND BRAIN SCIENCES; an international journal of current research and theory with open peer commentary. Text in English. 1978. bi-m. GBP 160 to individuals; USD 470 to institutions (effective 2002). adv. bk.rev. charts, illus. index. back issues avail.; reprint service avail. from SWZ,PSC,SCH. *Refereed.* **Document type:** *Academic/Scholarly.* **Description:** Covers psychology, neuroscience, behavioral biology, and cognitive science.

Related titles: Microform ed.: (from PQC); Online - full text ed.: (from EBSCO Publishing, O C L C Online Computer Library Center, Inc., RoweCom Information Quest, Gale Group, Swets Blackwell, Factiva, Institute for Scientific Information).
Indexed: ASCA, Anim.Behav.Abstr., Art.Int.Abstr., Arts & Hum.Cit.Ind. (coverage dropped), Biol.Abstr., Curr.Adv.Ecol.Sci., Curr.Cont., Excerp.Med., IBR, IBZ, INSPEC (Mar.1987-), Ind.Med. (1978-), Ind.Philos., Ind.Sci.Rev., Inpharma, Int.Abstr.Biol.Sci., Intl.Bibl.Soc.Sci., Lang.& Lang.Behav.Abstr., Neurosci.Abstr., Neurosci.Cit.Ind., P C I, Pharm.&Out.News, PsycInfo, Psychol.Abstr. (1978-), Psycscan B.A.& T., Reac., Russ.Acad.Sci.Bibl., SOPODA, SSCI, Sci.Cit.Ind., Soc.Serv.Abstr., Sociol.Abstr., Sport Fish.Abstr., THA, Telegen, e-psyche.
—BLDSC (1877.293000), AskIEEE, CISTI, GNLM, IDS, ingenta. **CCC.**
Published by: Cambridge University Press, Edinburgh Bldg, Shaftesbury Rd, Cambridge CB2 2RU, United Kingdom. FAX 44-1223-315052, information@cambridge.org, http://cogsci.ecs.soton.ac.uk/~harnad/bbs.html. Ed. Stevan Harnad. R&P Linda Nicol. Adv. contact Rebecca Symons.

150 616.8 USA ISSN 1534-5823
▼ **BEHAVIORAL & COGNITIVE NEUROSCIENCE REVIEWS.** Text in English. 2002 (Jan). q. USD 94, GBP 65 to individuals; USD 911, GBP 628 to institutions; USD 26, GBP 17 newsstand/cover to individuals; USD 251, GBP 158 newsstand/cover to institutions (effective (2002). reprints avail. *Refereed.* **Document type:** *Journal, Academic/Scholarly.* **Description:** Focuses on brain mechanisms and how they give rise to behavioral functions in humans and animals.
Related titles: Online - full text ed.: forthcoming 2002 (Online version of print journal, record 355107, to begin publication March 2002.).
Published by: Sage Publications, Inc., Sage Science Press, 2455 Teller Rd, Thousand Oaks, CA 91320. TEL 805-499-0721, FAX 805-499-0871, info@sagepub.com, http://www.sagepub.com. Ed. Joesph E Steinmetz. Pub. Susan Hanscom. R&P Peter Marino. Adv. contact Robert Vrooman.

BEHAVIORAL ECOLOGY AND SOCIOBIOLOGY. see *ENVIRONMENTAL STUDIES*

BEHAVIORAL EDUCATOR. see *EDUCATION—Teaching Methods And Curriculum*

BEHAVIORAL HEALTH ACCREDITATION & ACCOUNTABILITY ALERT; outcomes best practices performance measures reimbursements coding. see *MEDICAL SCIENCES—Psychiatry And Neurology*

158 362.2 USA ISSN 1063-8490
BEHAVIORAL HEALTHCARE TOMORROW. Text in English. 1992. bi-m., latest vol.10, 2001. USD 74 domestic to individuals; USD 117 domestic to institutions; USD 127 in Canada to institutions; USD 147 elsewhere to institutions; USD 15 newsstand/cover (effective 2001). bk.rev., software rev., video rev. back issues avail.; reprints avail. *Refereed.* **Document type:** *Magazine, Trade.* **Description:** Addresses issues in mental-health care practice and theory, particularly in the context of the continuing trend toward managed health.
Related titles: Online - full text ed.: (from Institute for Scientific Information).
Indexed: Curr.Cont., Int.Nurs.Ind., Ref.Zh., SSCI, e-psyche.
—BLDSC (1877.480000), IDS.
Published by: (Institute for Behavioral Healthcare), Manisses Communications Group, Inc., PO Box 9758, Providence, RI 02906-9758. TEL 401-831-6020, 800-333-7771, FAX 401-861-6370, manissesCS@manisses.com, http://www.manisses.com. Ed. Gary A Enos. Pub. Fraser A Lang. R&P Barbara Deekle. Adv. contact Paul Newman. Circ: 3,500 (paid); 18,500 (controlled).

616.8 USA ISSN 0896-4289
RB152 CODEN: BEMEEF
BEHAVIORAL MEDICINE; investigations of environmental influences on health and behavior. Text in English. 1975. q., latest vol.28, 2002. USD 63 domestic to individuals; USD 76 foreign to individuals; USD 118 domestic to institutions; USD 131 foreign to institutions; USD 29.50 newsstand/cover (effective 2001 - 2002). adv. bk.rev. charts, stat. index. back issues avail.; reprint service avail. from PSC,SCH. *Refereed.* **Document type:** *Academic/Scholarly.* **Description:** Interdisciplinary journal for physicians, psychologists, nurses, educators, and all who are concerned with behavioral and social influences on mental and physical health.
Formerly: Journal of Human Stress (0097-840X)
Related titles: CD-ROM ed.: (from ProQuest Information & Learning); Microfilm ed.; Online - full text ed.: (from Ovid Technologies, Inc., Northern Light Technology, Inc., ProQuest Information & Learning, Gale Group, LexisNexis, Institute for Scientific Information).
Indexed: ASCA, ASSIA, Abstr.Anthropol., Adol.Ment.Hlth.Abstr., AgeLine, Behav.Med.Abstr., Biol.Abstr., Curr.Cont., Excerp.Med., INIS Atomind., Ind.Med. (1988-), Ind.Philos., Int.Nurs.Ind., Mid.East: Abstr.& Ind., PsycInfo, Psychol.Abstr. (1975-), Psycscan A.P., Russ.Acad.Sci.Bibl., SSCI, e-psyche.
—BLDSC (1877.560000), EMDOCS, GNLM, IDS, ingenta. **CCC.**
Published by: (Helen Dwight Reid Educational Foundation), Heldref Publications, 1319 Eighteenth St, N W, Washington, DC 20036-1802. TEL 202-296-6267, 800-365-9753, FAX 202-293-6130, bmed@heldref.org, http://www.heldref.org/. Ed. Martha Wedeman. Adv. contact Grant Williams. Circ: 1,000. **Subscr. to:** Allen Press Inc., PO Box 1897, Lawrence, KS 66044-8897.

156 616.8 USA ISSN 0735-7044
BF1 CODEN: BENEDJ
BEHAVIORAL NEUROSCIENCE. Text in English. 1947. bi-m. USD 199 domestic to non-members; USD 219 foreign to non-members; USD 114 domestic to members; USD 126 foreign to members; USD 473 domestic to institutions; USD 517 foreign to institutions (effective 2001). adv. charts, illus. index. reprint service avail. from PSC,SCH. *Refereed.* **Document type:** *Academic/Scholarly.* **Description:** Covers research in the broad field of the biological bases of behavior; includes occasional reviews and theoretical articles that make original contributions to the field.
Supersedes in part (in 1983): Journal of Comparative and Physiological Psychology (0021-9940)
Related titles: Microform ed.: (from PQC,PMC); Online - full text ed.: (from Gale Group, Factiva, Institute for Scientific Information).
Indexed: ASCA, Abstr.Anthropol., Agricola, Anim.Behav.Abstr., Anim.Breed.Abstr., Aqua.Sci.& Fish.Abstr., Biol.& Agr.Ind. (Feb.1983-), Biol.Abstr., Chem.Abstr., Chemorec.Abstr., Curr.Adv.Ecol.Sci., Curr.Cont., Dairy Sci.Abstr., Dent.Ind., Excerp.Med., INIS Atomind., Ind.Med. (1983-), Ind.Sci.Rev., Inpharma, NRN, Neurosci.Abstr., Neurosci.Cit.Ind., Nutr.Abstr., P C I, Pharm.&Out.News, Poult.Abstr., PsycInfo, Psychol.Abstr. (1983-), Reac., Russ.Acad.Sci.Bibl., SSCI (coverage dropped), Sci.Cit.Ind., Soc.Sci.Ind. (Feb.1983-), Sport Fish.Abstr., THA, Wild.Rev., Zoo.Rec., e-psyche.
—BLDSC (1877.610000), CASDDS, CISTI, EMDOCS, GNLM, IDS, ingenta, KNAW. **CCC.**
Published by: American Psychological Association, 750 First St., N.E., Washington, DC 20002-4242. TEL 202-336-5600, 800-374-2721, FAX 202-336-5568, subscriptions@apa.org, http://www.apa.org/journals/bne.html. Eds. Ed Diener, Michela Gallagher. Circ: 1,700.

BEHAVIORAL RESEARCH IN ACCOUNTING. see *BUSINESS AND ECONOMICS—Accounting*

150 340 GBR ISSN 0735-3936
K2 CODEN: BSLADR
BEHAVIORAL SCIENCES AND THE LAW. Text in English. 1983. 6/yr. USD 715 in United States; USD 715 in Canada & Mexico; USD 715 elsewhere; USD 751 combined subscription in United States for print and online eds.; USD 751 combined subscription in Canada & Mexico for print and online eds.; USD 751 combined subscription elsewhere for print and online eds. (effective 2002). adv. reprint service avail. from SWZ,WSH. *Refereed.* **Document type:** *Academic/Scholarly.* **Description:** Provides current and comprehensive information in focused topics at the interface of the law and behavioral sciences.
Related titles: Microform ed.: (from PQC); Online - full text ed.: ISSN 1099-0798. USD 715 in United States; USD 715 in Canada & Mexico; USD 715 elsewhere (effective 2002) (from EBSCO Publishing, Gale Group, Wiley InterScience, Institute for Scientific Information).
Indexed: ASCA, ASSIA, AgeLine, C.L.I., Crim.Just.Abstr., Curr.Cont., ERA, Excerp.Med., Ind.Med. (1983-), Int.Nurs.Ind., L.R.I. (Jan.1984-), Lang.& Lang.Behav.Abstr., Leg.Per. (Sep.1993-), PsycInfo, Psychol.Abstr. (1983-), Rel.Ind.One, Rel.Ind.Two, SOPODA, SSCI, Soc.Serv.Abstr., Sociol.Abstr., Stud.Wom.Abstr., e-psyche.
—BLDSC (1877.905000), EMDOCS, GNLM, IDS, Infotrieve, ingenta. **CCC.**
Published by: Wiley Europe Ltd., Baffins Ln, Chichester, W Sussex PO19 1UD, United Kingdom. TEL 44-1243-779777, FAX 44-1243-775878, cs-journals@wiley.co.uk, customer@wiley.co.uk, http://www.interscience.wiley.com/japges/0735-3936/, http://www.wiley.co.uk. adv.: B&W page GBP 650, color page GBP 1,550; trim 165 x 248. Circ: 1,000. **Subscr. in the Americas to:** John Wiley & Sons, Inc., Journals, 605 Third Ave, New York, NY 10158. TEL 212-850-6021, 212-850-6645, subinfo@jwiley.com.

154.6 USA
▼ **BEHAVIORAL SLEEP MEDICINE.** Text in English. forthcoming 2003. **Document type:** *Journal, Academic/Scholarly.* **Description:** Addresses behavioral dimensions of normal and abnormal sleep mechanisms and the prevention, assessment, and treatment of sleep disorders and associated behavioral and emotional problems.
Published by: Lawrence Erlbaum Associates, Inc., 10 Industrial Ave, Mahwah, NJ 07430-2262. TEL 201-760-3735, 800-926-6579, FAX 201-236-0072, journals@erlbaum.com, http://www.erlbaum.com/Journals/journals/BSM/bsm.htm. Ed. Kenneth L Lichstein.

155.9 304 USA ISSN 1047-8663
BF199
BEHAVIOROLOGY. Text in English. 1993. a. USD 25 to individual members; USD 40 to institutions (effective 1999). adv. back issues avail. *Refereed.* **Document type:** *Academic/Scholarly.* **Description:** Features papers that contribute to the experimental analysis of functional relations between environment and behavior.
Indexed: e-psyche.
Published by: (Department of Psychology, Lafayette College), The International Society for Behaviorology, Robert W. Allen, Dept of Psychology, Lafayette College, Easton, PA 18042. TEL 610-330-5291, FAX 610-330-5349, allanr@lafayette.edu; orders@allenpress.com, http://www.allenpress.com. Ed., R&P Robert W Allan. **Subscr. to:** Allen Press Inc., PO Box 1897, Lawrence, KS 66044-8897.

BEHAVIOUR; an international journal of behaviourial biology. see *BIOLOGY—Zoology*

301.1 150 GBR ISSN 0144-929X
QA75.5 CODEN: BEITD5
BEHAVIOUR AND INFORMATION TECHNOLOGY; an international journal on the human aspects of computing. Text in English. 1982. bi-m. GBP 160, USD 264 to individuals; GBP 395, USD 652 to institutions (effective 2002). adv. bk.rev. illus. Index. back issues avail.; reprint service avail. from SCH,PSC. *Refereed.* **Document type:** *Academic/Scholarly.* **Description:** Covers all aspects of human-computer interaction.
Related titles: Online - full text ed.: ISSN 1362-3001 (from CatchWord Ltd., EBSCO Publishing, O C L C Online Computer Library Center, Inc., RoweCom Information Quest, Swets Blackwell, Institute for Scientific Information).
Indexed: ASCA, ASSIA, Abstr.Hum.Comp.Inter., Abstr.Soc.Geront., AgeLine, Art.Hosp.& Tour., Commun.Abstr., Compumath, Comput.Abstr., Comput.Lit.Ind., Cont.Pg.Educ., Curr.Cont., ERA, Educ.Admin.Abstr., Eng.Ind., Ergon.Abstr., Human Resour.Abstr., INSPEC (Jan.1983-), LISA, PsycInfo, Psychol.Abstr. (1982-), Robomat., SSCI, e-psyche.
—BLDSC (1876.660000), AskIEEE, CASDDS, CatchWord, CISTI, Ei, IDS. **CCC.**
Published by: Taylor & Francis Group, Taylor & Francis Ltd., 11 New Fetter Ln, London EC4P 4EE, United Kingdom. TEL 44-20-7583-9855, FAX 44-20-7842-2298, info@tandf.co.uk, http://www.tandf.co.uk. Ed. T F M Stewart. **Subscr. in N. America to:** Taylor & Francis Ltd., 325 Chestnut St, Suite 800, Philadelphia, PA 19016. TEL 800-354-1420, FAX 215-625-8914, info@taylorandfrancis.com, http://www.taylorandfrancis.com/.

150 AUS ISSN 0813-4839
RC489.B4 CODEN: BHCAE8
BEHAVIOUR CHANGE. Text in English. 1984. q. AUD 42 domestic to individuals; AUD 55 in New Zealand to individuals; AUD 75 elsewhere to individuals; AUD 80 domestic to institutions; AUD 92 in New Zealand to institutions; AUD 105 elsewhere to institutions (effective 2000). back issues avail. *Refereed.* **Document type:** *Academic/Scholarly.* **Description:** Publishes research involving the application of behavioural and cognitive-behavioural principles and techniques to the assessment and treatment of health, social, organizational, community and educational problems.
Related titles: Online - full text ed.: (from Institute for Scientific Information).

P

Indexed: ASCA, Curr.Cont., Excerp.Med., Lang.& Lang.Behav.Abstr., PsycInfo, Psychol.Abstr. (1984-), Psycscan B.A.& T., SOPODA, SSCI, Sociol.Abstr., Sp.Ed.Needs Abstr., e-psyche.
—BLDSC (1876.679000), EMDOCS, GNLM, IDS, Infotrieve, ingenta, KNAW. **CCC.**
Published by: (Australian Association for Cognitive and Behaviour Therapy), Australian Academic Press Pty. Ltd., 32 Jeays St, Bowen Hills, QLD 4006, Australia. TEL 61-7-32571176, FAX 61-7-32525908, australianacademicpress@compuserve.com, http://www.australianacademicpress.com.au. Ed. Alan M Hudson.

150 GBR ISSN 0005-7967
RC321 CODEN: BRTHAA
BEHAVIOUR RESEARCH AND THERAPY; an international multi-disciplinary journal. Text in English. 1963. m. EUR 1,186 in Europe to institutions; JPY 157,500 in Japan to institutions; USD 1,326 elsewhere to institutions; EUR 278 in Europe to qualified personnel; JPY 37,000 in Japan to qualified personnel; USD 312 elsewhere to qualified personnel (effective 2002). adv. bk.rev. charts, illus. index. back issues avail.; reprint service avail. from SCH,PSC. *Refereed.* **Document type:** *Academic/Scholarly.* **Description:** Focuses on the application of existing modern learning theory to psychiatric and social problems, relating learning to maladaptive behavior.
Incorporates (1978-1995): Advances in Behaviour Research and Therapy (0146-6402); (1979-1992): Behavioral Assessment (0191-5401)
Related titles: Microfiche ed.: (from MIM); Microfilm ed.: (from PQC); Online - full text ed.: (from ingenta, Gale Group, Swets Blackwell, ScienceDirect, Factiva, Institute for Scientific Information).
Indexed: ASCA, ASSIA, Abstr.Crim.& Pen., Addic.Abstr., Adol.Ment.Hlth.Abstr., AgeLine, Aqua.Sci.& Fish.Abstr., Behav.Med.Abstr., Bibl.Dev.Med.& Child Neur., Biol.Abstr., CINAHL, Child Devel.Abstr., Curr.Adv.Ecol.Sci., Curr.Cont., Dent.Ind., Environ.Sci.Poll.Mgmt., Excerp.Med., Fam.Ind., High.Educ.Abstr., IBR, Ind.Med. (1963-), Ind.Philos., Ind.Sci.Rev., Int.Abstr.Biol.Sci., Lang.& Lang.Behav.Abstr., M.L.A., MLA Intl.Bibl. (coverage dropped), PsycInfo, Psychol.Abstr. (1963-), Psycscan B.A.& T., Psycscan C.P., SOPODA, SSCI, Soc.Sci.Ind. (Jan.1987-), Soc.Work Res.& Abstr., Sociol.Abstr., THA, e-psyche.
—BLDSC (1876.810000), CISTI, EMDOCS, GNLM, IDS, ingenta, KNAW. **CCC.**
Published by: Elsevier Science Ltd., Pergamon, PO Box 800, Kidlington, Oxon 0X5 1DX, United Kingdom. TEL 44-1865-843000, FAX 44-1865-843010, nlinfo-f@elsevier.nl; usinfo-f@elsevier.com; forinfo-kyf04035@niftyserve.or.jp, http://www.elsevier.com/locate/brat, http://www.elsevier.nl/. Ed. S Rachman. Circ: 4,300. **Subscr. in Australasia and the Far East to:** Elsevier Science (Singapore) Pte Ltd, No.1 Temasek Ave, 17-01 Millenia Tower, Singapore 039192, Singapore. TEL 65-434-3727, FAX 65-337-2230; **Subscr. in the Americas to:** Elsevier Science, PO Box 945, New York, NY 10159-0945. TEL 212-633-3730, FAX 212-633-3680, usinfo-f@elsevier.com, http://www.elsevier.com; **Subscr. to:** Elsevier Science BV, PO Box 211, Amsterdam 1000 AE, Netherlands. TEL 31-20-485-3757, nlinfo-f@elsevier.nl, http://www.elsevier.nl.

150 GBR ISSN 1352-4658
RC489.B4
BEHAVIOURAL AND COGNITIVE PSYCHOTHERAPY. Text in English. 1972. q. GBP 78 to individuals; USD 188 to institutions (effective 2002). adv. bk.rev. **Document type:** *Academic/Scholarly.* **Description:** Multidisciplinary original research, of an experimental or clinical nature, that contributes to the theory, practice, and evaluation of behavior therapy.
Former titles (until 1993): Behavioural Psychotherapy (0141-3473); (until 1978): B A B P Bulletin
Related titles: Online - full text ed.: (from EBSCO Publishing, O C L C Online Computer Library Center, Inc., RoweCom Information Quest, Swets Blackwell).
Indexed: AMED, ASSIA, Addic.Abstr., PsycInfo, Psychol.Abstr. (1981-), Psycscan B.A.& T., SSCI (coverage dropped), Sp.Ed.Needs Abstr., e-psyche.
—BLDSC (1877.293500), EMDOCS, GNLM, IDS, KNAW. **CCC.**
Published by: (British Association for Behavioural and Cognitive Psychotherapy), Cambridge University Press, Edinburgh Bldg, Shaftesbury Rd, Cambridge CB2 2RU, United Kingdom. FAX 44-1223-315052, information@cup.cam.ac.uk, information@cambridge.org, http://www.cup.org/journals/CUPJNLS.html. Ed. Paul Salkovskis. Pub. Penelope Head. Circ: 2,000.

BEHAVIOURAL PHARMACOLOGY. see *PHARMACY AND PHARMACOLOGY*

150 GBR ISSN 0953-7074
BEHAVIOURAL PSYCHOTHERAPIST. Text in English. 1981. 3/yr. GBP 15 to non-members. adv. bk.rev. **Document type:** *Newsletter.* **Description:** Gives news of the association's events and allows for the exchange of information among members.
Formerly: British Association for Behavioural Psychotherapy. Newsletter (0262-3110)
Indexed: e-psyche.
Published by: British Association for Behavioural and Cognitive Psychotherapy, c/o Harrow Psychological Health Services, Northwick Park Hospital, Watford Rd, Harrow, Mddx HA1 3UJ, United Kingdom. TEL 44-181-8692326, FAX 44-181-8692317. Ed., R&P John Rose. Circ: 2,000. **Subscr. to:** Howard Lomas, 23 Partridge Dr, Accrington, Lancs BB5 2RL, United Kingdom.

150 DEU ISSN 0722-8902
BEITRAEGE ZUR INDIVIDUALPSYCHOLOGIE. Text in German. 1978. irreg., latest vol.25, 1999. price varies. **Document type:** *Monographic series, Academic/Scholarly.*
Indexed: e-psyche.
Published by: Ernst Reinhardt Verlag, Kemnatenstr 46, Munich 80639, Germany. TEL 49-89-1780160, FAX 49-89-17801630.

155.4 DEU ISSN 0340-0123
BEITRAEGE ZUR PSYCHODIAGNOSTIK DES KINDES. Text in German. 1973. irreg., latest vol.7, 1984. price varies. **Document type:** *Monographic series.*
Indexed: e-psyche.
Published by: Ernst Reinhardt Verlag, Kemnatenstr 46, Munich 80639, Germany. TEL 49-89-1780160, FAX 49-89-17801630. Eds. G Biermann, M Kos.

302 DEU ISSN 0173-0967
BEITRAEGE ZUR PSYCHOLOGIE UND SOZIOLOGIE DES KRANKEN MENSCHEN. Text in German. 1974. irreg., latest vol.6, 1986. price varies. **Document type:** *Monographic series.*
Indexed: e-psyche.
Published by: Ernst Reinhardt Verlag, Kemnatenstr 46, Munich 80639, Germany. TEL 49-89-1780160, FAX 49-89-17801630. Eds. G Biermann, J von Troschke.

614.58 USA
THE BELL. Text in English. 1980-1993; N.S. 1995. m. USD 36. adv. bk.rev. back issues avail. **Document type:** *Newsletter.* **Description:** Provides information on issues relating to mental health, including research in psychology and psychiatry, the effects of managed mental health care, prevention efforts, legislation and public education.
Supersedes (in 1995): Focus (Alexandria)
Indexed: Diver.Y.World.
Published by: National Mental Health Association, 1021 Prince St, Alexandria, VA 22314-2971. TEL 703-684-7722, FAX 703-684-5968, http://www.nmha.org. Ed. Sandy Alexander. Adv. contact Tonya McCreary. Circ: 2,500.

155.4 DEU ISSN 1439-5916
▼ **BERATUNG AKTUELL**; Zeitschrift fuer Theorie und Praxis der Beratung. Text in German; Summaries in English. 2000. 4/yr. DEM 49; DEM 39.50 to students; DEM 15 newsstand/cover (effective 2000). adv. **Document type:** *Magazine, Academic/Scholarly.* **Description:** Provides information on various types of psychological counseling.
Related titles: ♦ Online - full text ed.: Beratung Aktuell (Internet). ISSN 1437-3181.
Published by: Junfermann Verlag, Imadstr 40, Paderborn 33102, Germany. TEL 49-5251-13440, FAX 49-5251-134444, ju@junfermann.de, http://www.junfermann.de, http://www.beratung-aktuell.de. Ed. Dr. Rudolf Sanders. Adv. contact Ruth Frerker.

155.4 DEU ISSN 1437-3181
▼ **BERATUNG AKTUELL (INTERNET).** Text in German; Summaries in English. 1999. 4/yr. **Document type:** *Academic/Scholarly.*
Media: Online - full text. **Related titles:** ♦ Print ed.: Beratung Aktuell. ISSN 1439-5916.
Published by: Junfermann Verlag, Imadstr 40, Paderborn 33102, Germany. TEL 49-5251-13440, FAX 49-5251-134444, ju@junfermann.de, http://www.beratung-aktuell.de.

BEREAVEMENT CARE; an international journal for those who help bereaved people. see *SOCIAL SERVICES AND WELFARE*

150 610 USA ISSN 1081-5937
BIOFEEDBACK (WHEAT RIDGE). Text in English. a. **Document type:** *Bulletin.*
Related titles: Online - full content ed.
Indexed: e-psyche.
Published by: Association for Applied Psychophysiology and Biofeedback, 10200 W 44th Ave, Ste 304, Wheat Ridge, CO 80033-2840. TEL 303-422-8436, FAX 303-422-8894. Ed. Francine Butler. R&P Michael P Thompson.

570 NLD ISSN 0301-0511
QP360 CODEN: BLPYAX
BIOLOGICAL PSYCHOLOGY. Text in Dutch. 1974. 9/yr. EUR 1,025 in Europe to institutions; JPY 136,200 in Japan to institutions; USD 1,147 elsewhere to institutions (effective 2002). adv. bk.rev. charts. index. back issues avail.; reprint service avail. from ISI. *Refereed.* **Document type:** *Academic/Scholarly.* **Description:** Publishes original scientific papers on the biological aspects of psychological states and processes.
Related titles: Microform ed.: (from PQC); Online - full text ed.: (from ingenta, Swets Blackwell, ScienceDirect, Institute for Scientific Information).
Indexed: ASCA, AgeLine, Behav.Med.Abstr., Chem.Abstr., Commun.Abstr., Curr.Adv.Ecol.Sci., Curr.Cont., Curr.Ind.Stat., Dent.Ind., Excerp.Med., IBZ, Ind.Med. (1973-), Ind.Philos., Int.Abstr.Biol.Sci., Neurosci.Cit.Ind., PsycInfo, Psychol.Abstr. (1973-), SSCI, Sci.Cit.Ind., e-psyche.
—BLDSC (2077.560000), CASDDS, CISTI, EMDOCS, GNLM, IDS, ingenta. **CCC.**
Published by: North-Holland (Subsidiary of: Elsevier Science BV), PO Box 211, Amsterdam 1000 AE, Netherlands. TEL 31-20-485-3911, FAX 31-20-485-3598, http://www.elsevier.com/locate/biopsycho. Ed. R Simons. Circ: 375. **Subscr. in Australasia and the Far East to:** Elsevier Science (Singapore) Pte Ltd, No.1 Temasek Ave, 17-01 Millenia Tower, Singapore 039192, Singapore. TEL 65-434-3727, FAX 65-337-2230; **Subscr. in Japan to:** Elsevier Science Inc - Japan Regional Office, 9-15 Higashi-Azabu 1-chome, Minato-ku, Tokyo 106-0044, Japan. TEL 81-3-5561-5033, FAX 81-3-5561-5047; **Subscr. in the Americas to:** Elsevier Science, PO Box 945, New York, NY 10159-0945. TEL 212-633-3730, FAX 212-633-3680.

BIRD BEHAVIOR; an international and interdisciplinary multimedia journal. see *BIOLOGY—Ornithology*

150 618 USA ISSN 0734-3124
RG658
BIRTH PSYCHOLOGY BULLETIN. Text in English. 1979. s-a. USD 9 (effective 2001). bk.rev. back issues avail. **Document type:** *Bulletin, Academic/Scholarly.* **Description:** Clinical, theoretical, and empirical articles on the psychological impact of pregnancy, birth, and the neonatal period.
Indexed: C.I.J.E. (coverage dropped), Psychol.Abstr., e-psyche.
Published by: Association for Birth Psychology, 444 E 82nd St, New York, NY 10028. TEL 212-988-6617. Ed., R&P Leslie Feher. Circ: 500.

BLEIKT OG BLATT. see *SOCIOLOGY*

BODYWORK SERIES. see *NEW AGE PUBLICATIONS*

270.15 CUB ISSN 0253-5742
BOLETIN DE PSICOLOGIA. Text in Spanish. 1971. s-a. free per issue. adv. *Refereed.* **Description:** Covers health, clinical, child, and adolescent psychology, and related areas.
Indexed: PsycInfo, Psychol.Abstr., e-psyche.
—CINDOC.
Published by: Ministerio de Salud Publica, Hospital Psiquiatrico de la Habana, Avenida de Independencia No. 26520, Mazorra (Havana), Cuba. TEL 5683-2465. Ed. Dr. Noemi Perez. Circ: 6,000 (paid).

158 ITA ISSN 0006-6761
BOLLETTINO DI PSICOLOGIA APPLICATA. Text in Italian. 1954. 3/yr. ITL 70,000 domestic to individuals; ITL 100,000 foreign to individuals; ITL 100,000 domestic to institutions; ITL 130,000 foreign to institutions (effective 2000). adv. bk.rev. bibl, charts. reprint service avail. from PQC. *Refereed.* **Document type:** *Bulletin.* **Description:** Covers all topics concerning applied psychology in clinical, educational and work fields.
Related titles: Microform ed.: (from PQC).

P

Indexed: Biol.Abstr., Lang.& Lang.Behav.Abstr., PsycInfo, Psychol.Abstr. (1956-), SOPODA, SSCI (coverage dropped), Sociol.Abstr., e-psyche.
—BLDSC (2240.700000).
Published by: Organizzazioni Speciali, Via Fra' Paolo Sarpi, 7-A, Florence, FI 50136, Italy. TEL 39-55-672580, FAX 39-55-669446, o.s.@iol.it. Ed. Saulo Sirigatti. Pub. Jacopo Tarantino. R&P, Adv. contact Silvia Delgrosso. Circ: 1,000.

150 USA ISSN 0278-2626
QP376
BRAIN AND COGNITION; journal of clinical, experimental, and theoretical research. Text in English. 1982. 9/yr. USD 775 in US & Canada to institutions; USD 825 elsewhere to institutions (effective 2001). adv. back issues avail. *Refereed.* **Document type:** *Academic/Scholarly.* **Description:** Presents clinical case histories, original research papers, reviews, notes, and commentaries on neuropsychology.
Related titles: Online - full text ed.: (from EBSCO Publishing, O C L C Online Computer Library Center, Inc., RoweCom Information Quest, ingenta, Swets Blackwell, IDEAL Online Library, Institute for Scientific Information).
Indexed: ASCA, Abstr.Anthropol., AgeLine, CINAHL, Child Devel.Abstr., Curr.Adv.Ecol.Sci., Curr.Cont., Fam.Ind., INIS Atomind., Ind.Med. (1982-), Ind.Sci.Rev., Inpharma, Int.Abstr.Biol.Sci., Lang.& Lang.Behav.Abstr., Neuropsych.Abstr., Neurosci.Abstr. (coverage dropped), Neurosci.Cit.Ind., Pharm.&Out.News, PsycInfo, Psychol.Abstr. (1982-), Reac., Russ.Acad.Sci.Bibl., SOPODA, SSCI, Sci.Cit.Ind., Sociol.Abstr., e-psyche.
—BLDSC (2268.032000), ADONIS, CISTI, EMDOCS, GNLM, IDS, ingenta, KNAW. **CCC.**
Published by: Academic Press, Inc., Journal Division (Subsidiary of: Harcourt Brace & Company), 525 B St, Ste 1900, San Diego, CA 92101-4495. TEL 619-230-1840, FAX 619-699-6800, apsubs@acad.com, http://www.academicpress.com/b&c. Ed. Harry A Whitaker.

150 410 USA ISSN 0093-934X
RC423.A1
BRAIN AND LANGUAGE. Text in English. 1974. 12/yr. USD 950 in US & Canada to institutions; USD 1,025 elsewhere to institutions (effective 2001). back issues avail. *Refereed.* **Document type:** *Academic/Scholarly.* **Description:** Original theoretical, clinical, and experimental papers on human language and communication: speech, hearing, reading, writing, and higher language functions, as they relate to brain structure and function.
Related titles: Online - full text ed.: (from EBSCO Publishing, O C L C Online Computer Library Center, Inc., RoweCom Information Quest, ingenta, Swets Blackwell, IDEAL Online Library, Institute for Scientific Information).
Indexed: AMED, ASCA, Abstr.Anthropol., AgeLine, Arts & Hum.Cit.Ind. (coverage dropped), Bibl.Dev.Med.& Child Neur., Bibl.Ling., CINAHL, Curr.Adv.Ecol.Sci., Curr.Cont., Dent.Ind., Excerp.Med., INIS Atomind., Ind.Med. (1974-), Ind.Sci.Rev., Indian Psychol.Abstr., Inpharma, Int.Abstr.Biol.Sci., Jrnl.Watch Neuro., Lang.& Lang.Behav.Abstr. (1974-), Ling.Abstr., M.L.A., MLA Intl.Bibl., Neuropsych.Abstr., Neurosci.Abstr. (coverage dropped), Neurosci.Cit.Ind., Pharm.&Out.News, PsycInfo, Psychol.Abstr. (1974-), Reac., Russ.Acad.Sci.Bibl., SOPODA, SSCI, Sci.Cit.Ind., Sociol.Abstr., e-psyche.
—BLDSC (2268.040000), ADONIS, CISTI, EMDOCS, GNLM, IDS, ingenta. **CCC.**
Published by: Academic Press, Inc., Journal Division (Subsidiary of: Harcourt Brace & Company), 525 B St, Ste 1900, San Diego, CA 92101-4495. TEL 619-230-1840, FAX 619-699-6800, apsubs@acad.com, http://www.academicpress.com/b&l. Ed. Harry A Whitaker.

BRAIN - MIND; bulletin of breakthroughs. see *MEDICAL SCIENCES—Psychiatry And Neurology*

362.2 616.89 GBR ISSN 1363-898X
BREAKTHROUGH; international mental health journal. Text in English. 1996. q. GBP 34 in Europe to individuals; GBP 40 elsewhere to individuals; GBP 52 in Europe to institutions; GBP 59 elsewhere to institutions. **Document type:** *Academic/Scholarly.* **Description:** Covers a wide range of mental health issues throughout the world. Previous topics have included: multicultural mental health issues in Australia; mental health in Romania; dissident psychiatry in Ukraine; mental health advocacy in the UK; psychosis in Hong Kong; and mental health rights in Latvia.
Indexed: e-psyche.
Published by: British Association of Social Workers, 16 Kent St, Birmingham, Warks B5 6RD, United Kingdom. TEL 44-121-622-3911, FAX 44-121-622-4860.
Co-sponsor: Anglia Polytechnic University.

BREATH SERIES; a progression of pranayama practices. see *NEW AGE PUBLICATIONS*

616.89 GBR ISSN 0954-0350
BRITISH ASSOCIATION OF PSYCHOTHERAPISTS. JOURNAL. Text in English. 1968. s-a. USD 49 in North America to individuals; GBP 27 rest of world to individuals; USD 99 in North America to institutions; GBP 55 rest of world to institutions (effective 2001). adv. bk.rev. **Document type:** *Academic/Scholarly.* **Description:** Covers topics related to Freudian or Jungian psycho-dynamic psychotherapy.
Formerly: British Association of Psychotherapists. Bulletin (0268-6643)
Indexed: e-psyche.
—BLDSC (4712.930000).
Published by: (British Association of Psychotherapists), Whurr Publishers Ltd., 19b Compton Terr, London N1 2UN, United Kingdom. TEL 44-20-7359-5979, FAX 44-20-7226-5290, info@whurr.co.uk, http://www.whurrjournals.co.uk/, http://www.whurr.co.uk. Eds. Arna Davis, Mary Adams. Circ: 700. **Subscr. in N America to:** Whurr Publishers Ltd., PO Box 1897, Lawrence, KS 66044-8897. TEL 913-843-1221, FAX 913-843-1274, am&m@allenpress.com. **Subscr. to:** Turpin Distribution Services Ltd., Blackhorse Rd, Letchworth, Herts SG6 1HN, United Kingdom. TEL 44-1462-488900, FAX 44-1462-483011, custservturpin@turpinltd.com.

301.1 150 GBR ISSN 0144-6657
BF1 CODEN: BJCPDW
BRITISH JOURNAL OF CLINICAL PSYCHOLOGY. Text in English. 1962. q., latest vol.40. GBP 145 in the European Union to institutions; USD 268 rest of world to institutions; GBP 45 newsstand/cover in the European Union; USD 84 newsstand/cover rest of world (effective 2001). adv. bk.rev. charts, illus, abstr. index. back issues avail.; reprint service avail. from SWZ,ISI. *Refereed.* **Document type:** *Academic/Scholarly.* **Description:** Aims to reflect the broad role of clinical psychologists and include descriptive studies as well as studies of the aetiology, assessment and amelioration of disorders of all kinds, in all settings, and among all age groups.
Supersedes in part (in 1981): British Journal of Social and Clinical Psychology (0007-1293)
Related titles: Microform ed.: (from PQC,SWZ); Online - full text ed.: free with print (from CatchWord Ltd., Northern Light Technology, Inc., EBSCO Publishing, ProQuest Information & Learning, Swets Blackwell, Institute for Scientific Information).
Indexed: AMED, ASCA, ASSIA, Abstr.Crim.& Pen., Addic.Abstr., Adol.Ment.Hlth.Abstr., AgeLine, Behav.Med.Abstr., Bibl.Dev.Med.& Child Neur., Biol.Abstr., Brit.Nur.Ind., CINAHL, Curr.Adv.Ecol.Sci., Curr.Cont., Dent.Ind., ERA, Environ.Sci.Poll.Mgmt., Excerp.Med., Fam.Ind., IMFL, Ind.Med. (1981-), Ind.Philos., Int.Nurs.Ind., Intl.Bibl.Soc.Sci., Lang.& Lang.Behav.Abstr., Mult.Ed.Abstr., Neurosci.Cit.Ind., Pollut.Abstr., PsycInfo, Psychol.Abstr. (1981-), Psycscan C.P., Ref.Zh., Risk Abstr., SOPODA, SSCI, Saf.Sci.Abstr., Soc.Serv.Abstr., Sociol.Abstr., Sociol.Educ.Abstr., THA, e-psyche.
—BLDSC (2307.230000), CISTI, GNLM, IDS, ingenta, KNAW. **CCC.**
Published by: The British Psychological Society, St Andrews House, 48 Princess Rd E, Leicester LE1 7DR, United Kingdom. TEL 44-116-252-9580, FAX 44-116-254-8824, journals@bps.org.uk, http://www.bps.org.uk/publications/jCP_1.cfm. Eds. Brendan Bradley, Karin Mogg. R&P, Adv. contact J Neason TEL 44-116-252-9580. page GBP 288; 135 x 210. Circ: 2,900. **Subscr. to:** Turpin Distribution Services Ltd., Blackhorse Rd, Letchworth, Herts SG6 1HN, United Kingdom. TEL 44-1462-488900, FAX 44-1462-483011.

THE BRITISH JOURNAL OF CRIMINOLOGY; delinquency and deviant social behaviour. see *CRIMINOLOGY AND LAW ENFORCEMENT*

BRITISH JOURNAL OF DEVELOPMENTAL DISABILITIES. see *EDUCATION—Special Education And Rehabilitation*

155 GBR ISSN 0261-510X
BF712
BRITISH JOURNAL OF DEVELOPMENTAL PSYCHOLOGY. Text in English. 1983. q., latest vol.19. GBP 140 in the European Union to institutions; USD 260 rest of world to institutions; GBP 44 newsstand/cover in the European Union; USD 82 newsstand/cover rest of world (effective 2001). adv. bk.rev. charts, illus, abstr. index. 160 p./no. back issues avail.; reprint service avail. from SWZ,ISI. *Refereed.* **Document type:** *Journal, Academic/Scholarly.* **Description:** Publishes empirical, conceptual, and review articles on all aspects of development.
Related titles: Magnetic Tape ed.; Microfiche ed.; Microform ed.: (from PQC,SWZ); Online - full text ed.: 1999. free with print (from CatchWord Ltd., Northern Light Technology, Inc., EBSCO Publishing, ProQuest Information & Learning, Swets Blackwell, Institute for Scientific Information).
Indexed: ASCA, ASSIA, AgeLine, Arts & Hum.Cit.Ind. (coverage dropped), Bibl.Dev.Med.& Child Neur., Br.Educ.Ind., Brit.Nur.Ind., Child Devel.Abstr., Curr.Cont., IBR, IBZ, IMFL, Ind.Philos., Lang.& Lang.Behav.Abstr., PsycInfo, Psychol.Abstr. (1983-), Psycscan D.P., Ref.Zh., SOPODA, SSCI, Soc.Serv.Abstr., Sociol.Abstr., Yrbk.Assoc.Educ.& Rehab.Blind, e-psyche.
—BLDSC (2307.480000), CISTI, IDS, ingenta. **CCC.**
Published by: The British Psychological Society, St Andrews House, 48 Princess Rd E, Leicester LE1 7DR, United Kingdom. TEL 44-116-252-9580, FAX 44-116-254-8824, journals@bps.org.uk. Ed. Gavin Bremner. R&P, Adv. contact J Neason TEL 44-116-252-9580. page GBP 214; 135 x 210. Circ: 1,800. **Subscr. to:** Turpin Distribution Services Ltd., Blackhorse Rd, Letchworth, Herts SG6 1HN, United Kingdom. TEL 44-1462-488900, FAX 44-1462-483011.

370.15 GBR ISSN 0007-0998
LB1051.A2 CODEN: BJESAE
BRITISH JOURNAL OF EDUCATIONAL PSYCHOLOGY. Text in English. 1931. q., latest vol.71. GBP 94 in the European Union to institutions; USD 173 rest of world to institutions; GBP 28 newsstand/cover in the European Union; USD 50 newsstand/cover rest of world (effective 2001). adv. bk.rev. bibl, charts, illus, abstr. index. 144 p./no. back issues avail.; reprint service avail. from SWZ,PSC,SCH. *Refereed.* **Document type:** *Journal, Academic/Scholarly.* **Description:** Focuses on psychological research that makes a significant contribution to the understanding and practice of education. Includes empirical and theoretical studies, action research as well as psychometric and statistical methods.
Related titles: Magnetic Tape ed.; Microfiche ed.; Microform ed.: (from SWZ); Online - full text ed.: 1999. free with print (from CatchWord Ltd., Northern Light Technology, Inc., EBSCO Publishing, ProQuest Information & Learning, Swets Blackwell, Institute for Scientific Information).
Indexed: ASCA, ASSIA, Adol.Ment.Hlth.Abstr., AgeLine, Arts & Hum.Cit.Ind. (coverage dropped), Bibl.Dev.Med.& Child Neur., Biol.Abstr., Br.Educ.Ind., C.I.J.E. (coverage dropped), Child Devel.Abstr., Child.Lit.Abstr., Cont.Pg.Educ., Curr.Cont., Curr.Ind.Stat., ERA, Educ.Ind. (Jun.1983-), Educ.Tech.Abstr., High.Educ.Abstr., High.Educ.Curr.Aware.Bull., IBR, IBZ, Ind.Med. (1931-), Ind.Philos., Lang.& Lang.Behav.Abstr., Lang.Teach.& Ling.Abstr., P C I, PsycInfo, Psychol.Abstr. (1931-), Res.High.Educ.Abstr., Russ.Acad.Sci.Bibl., SOMA, SOPODA, SSCI, Sociol.Abstr., Sociol.Educ.Abstr., Stud.Wom.Abstr., Tech.Educ.Abstr., e-psyche.
—BLDSC (2307.650000), IDS, ingenta. **CCC.**
Published by: The British Psychological Society, St Andrews House, 48 Princess Rd E, Leicester LE1 7DR, United Kingdom. TEL 44-116-252-9580, FAX 44-116-254-8824, journals@bps.org.uk, http://www.bps.org.uk/publications/jEP_1.cfm. Ed. P Tomlinson. R&P, Adv. contact J Neason TEL 44-116-252-9580. page GBP 288. Circ: 2,500. **Subscr. to:** Turpin Distribution Services Ltd., Blackhorse Rd, Letchworth, Herts SG6 1HN, United Kingdom. TEL 44-1462-488900, FAX 44-1462-483011.

BRITISH JOURNAL OF GUIDANCE AND COUNSELLING. see *OCCUPATIONS AND CAREERS*

P

616.8 GBR ISSN 1359-107X
R726.7 CODEN: BJHPFP
BRITISH JOURNAL OF HEALTH PSYCHOLOGY. Text in English. 1996. q., latest vol.6. GBP 120 in the European Union to institutions; USD 223 rest of world to institutions; GBP 36 newsstand/cover in the European Union; USD 68 newsstand/cover rest of world (effective 2001). adv. bk.rev. bibl, charts, illus, abstr. index. 104 p./no. back issues avail.; reprint service avail. from SWZ. *Refereed.* **Document type:** *Journal, Academic/Scholarly.* **Description:** Covers all areas of psychological factors relating to health and illness across the life span, including experimental and clinical research on aetiology and the management of acute and chronic illness, responses to ill health, screening and medical procedures, research on health behaviour, and psychological aspects of prevention.
Related titles: Magnetic Tape ed.; Microfiche ed.; Online - full text ed.: 1999. free with print (from CatchWord Ltd., EBSCO Publishing, Swets Blackwell, Institute for Scientific Information).
Indexed: ASSIA, Addic.Abstr., AgeLine, Curr.Cont., ERA, IBZ, Ind.Philos., Lang.& Lang.Behav.Abstr., PsycInfo, Ref.Zh., SOPODA, SSCI, Sociol.Abstr., THA, e-psyche.
—BLDSC (2309.080000), IDS, Infotrieve, ingenta, KNAW. **CCC.**
Published by: The British Psychological Society, St Andrews House, 48 Princess Rd E, Leicester LE1 7DR, United Kingdom. TEL 44-116-252-9580, FAX 44-116-254-8824, journals@bps.org.uk, http://www.bps.org.uk/publications/jHH_1.cfm. Eds. A Steptoe, J Wardle. R&P, Adv. contact J Neason TEL 44-116-252-9580. page GBP 288; trim 135 x 210. Circ: 2,100. **Subscr. to:** Turpin Distribution Services Ltd., Blackhorse Rd, Letchworth, Herts SG6 1HN, United Kingdom. TEL 44-1462-488900, FAX 44-1462-483011.

P

152.8 GBR ISSN 0007-1102
BF1
BRITISH JOURNAL OF MATHEMATICAL AND STATISTICAL PSYCHOLOGY. Text in English. 1948. s-a., latest vol.54. GBP 128 in the European Union to institutions; USD 242 rest of world to institutions; GBP 78 newsstand/cover in the European Union; GBP 146 newsstand/cover rest of world (effective 2001). adv. bk.rev. charts, illus. index. reprint service avail. from SWZ,PSC,SCH,ISI. *Refereed.* **Document type:** *Academic/Scholarly.* **Description:** Contains papers on all aspects of quantitative psychology, including mathematical psychology, statistics, psychometrics, psychophysics, and relevant areas of mathematics, computing and computer software.
Related titles: Magnetic Tape ed.; Microfiche ed.; Microform ed.: (from PQC,SWZ); Online - full text ed.: 1999. free with print (from CatchWord Ltd., EBSCO Publishing, ProQuest Information & Learning, Swets Blackwell, Institute for Scientific Information).
Indexed: ASCA, C.C.M.J., Compumath, Comput.Abstr., Curr.Cont. (1993-), Curr.Ind.Stat., IBR, IBZ, Ind.Med. (1965-), Ind.Philos., J.Cont.Quant.Meth., Mark.Res.Abstr. (1965-1991), Math.R., PsycInfo, Psychol.Abstr. (1953-), Psycscan A.P., Ref.Zh., Russ.Acad.Sci.Bibl., SSCI, Stat.Theor.Meth.Abstr. (1993-), Trop.Dis.Bull., Zent.Math., e-psyche.
—BLDSC (2311.300000), CISTI, GNLM, IDS, ingenta. **CCC.**
Published by: The British Psychological Society, St Andrews House, 48 Princess Rd E, Leicester LE1 7DR, United Kingdom. TEL 44-116-254-9568, FAX 44-116-247-0787, journals@bps.org.uk, http://www.bps.org.uk/publications/jMS_1.cfm. Ed. Pat Lovie. R&P, Adv. contact J Neason TEL 44-116-252-9580. page GBP 165. Circ: 700. **Subscr. to:** Turpin Distribution Services Ltd., Blackhorse Rd, Letchworth, Herts SG6 1HN, United Kingdom. TEL 44-1462-488900, FAX 44-1462-483011.

616.89 150 GBR ISSN 0007-1129
RC321 CODEN: BJMPAB
BRITISH JOURNAL OF MEDICAL PSYCHOLOGY. Text in English. 1920. q., latest vol.74. GBP 144 in the European Union to institutions; USD 268 rest of world to institutions; GBP 45 newsstand/cover in the European Union; USD 84 newsstand/cover rest of world (effective 2001). adv. bk.rev. charts, illus, abstr. index. 144 p./no. reprint service avail. from SWZ,PSC,SCH,ISI. *Refereed.* **Document type:** *Journal, Academic/Scholarly.* **Description:** Contains original theory and research from psychodynamic and interpersonal psychology. Emphasizes research from these fields with a bearing upon vulnerability to, adjustment to and recovery from both medical and psychological disorders.
Related titles: Magnetic Tape ed.; Microfiche ed.; Microform ed.: (from PQC,SWZ); Online - full text ed.: 1999. free with print (from CatchWord Ltd., Northern Light Technology, Inc., EBSCO Publishing, ProQuest Information & Learning, Swets Blackwell, Institute for Scientific Information).
Indexed: AMED, ASCA, Addic.Abstr., Adol.Ment.Hlth.Abstr., AgeLine, Arts & Hum.Cit.Ind. (coverage dropped), Behav.Med.Abstr., Bibl.Dev.Med.& Child Neur., Biol.Abstr., CINAHL, Chem.Abstr., Curr.Adv.Ecol.Sci., Curr.Cont., Dent.Ind., Environ.Sci.Poll.Mgmt., Excerp.Med., Fam.Ind., IBR, IMFL, Ind.Med. (1923-), Ind.Philos., Ind.Sci.Rev., Inpharma, Int.Nurs.Ind., Lang.& Lang.Behav.Abstr., Mid.East: Abstr.& Ind., Nutr.Abstr., Pharm.&Out.News, Pollut.Abstr., PsycInfo, Psychol.Abstr. (1926-), Reac., Ref.Zh., Risk Abstr., SOPODA, SSCI, Saf.Sci.Abstr., Sci.Cit.Ind., Sociol.Abstr., THA, e-psyche.
—BLDSC (2311.850000), CISTI, GNLM, IDS, ingenta, KNAW. **CCC.**
Published by: The British Psychological Society, St Andrews House, 48 Princess Rd E, Leicester LE1 7DR, United Kingdom. TEL 44-116-252-9580, FAX 44-116-254-8824, journals@bps.org.uk, http://www.bps.org/uk/publications/jHP_1.cfm. Ed. P Richardson. R&P, Adv. contact J Neason TEL 44-116-252-9580. page GBP 256; 135 x 210. Circ: 2,100. **Subscr. to:** Turpin Distribution Services Ltd., Blackhorse Rd, Letchworth, Herts SG6 1HN, United Kingdom. TEL 44-1462-488900, FAX 44-1462-483011.

616.89 GBR ISSN 0309-7757
CODEN: BJPSD4
BRITISH JOURNAL OF PROJECTIVE PSYCHOLOGY. Text in English. 1955. a. GBP 20. adv. bk.rev. back issues avail. **Document type:** *Academic/Scholarly.* **Description:** Devoted to projective approaches and research in psychology.
Formerly: British Journal of Projective Psychology and Personality Study
Indexed: PsycInfo, Psychol.Abstr. (1968-), e-psyche.
—Infotrieve, ingenta. **CCC.**
Published by: British Society for Projective Psychology, Department of Psychology, Parkhead Hospital, 81 Salamanca St, Glasgow G31 5ES, United Kingdom. TEL 041-554-7951, FAX 041-551-8318. Ed. Zahid Mahmood. Circ: 200.

150 GBR ISSN 0007-1269
BF1 CODEN: BJSGAE
BRITISH JOURNAL OF PSYCHOLOGY. Text in English. 1904. q., latest vol.92. GBP 196 in the European Union to institutions; USD 367 rest of world to institutions; GBP 58 newsstand/cover in the European Union; USD 108 newsstand/cover rest of world (effective 2001). adv. bk.rev. bibl, charts, illus, abstr. index. 144 p./no. back issues avail.; reprint service avail. from SWZ,PSC,SCH,ISI. *Refereed.* **Document type:** *Journal, Academic/Scholarly.* **Description:** Publishes reports of empirical studies, critical reviews, and theoretical contributions geared towards academic and research workers in experimental, cognitive and general psychology.
Related titles: Magnetic Tape ed.; Microfiche ed.; Microform ed.: (from PQC); Online - full text ed.: (from ProQuest Information & Learning, CatchWord Ltd., Gale Group, Northern Light Technology, Inc., EBSCO Publishing, H. W. Wilson, Swets Blackwell, Factiva, Institute for Scientific Information).
Indexed: ASCA, ASSIA, Abstr.Crim.& Pen., Adol.Ment.Hlth.Abstr., AgeLine, Arts & Hum.Cit.Ind. (coverage dropped), Bibl.Dev.Med.& Child Neur., Biol.Abstr., Br.Educ.Ind., Br.Hum.Ind., Brit.Nur.Ind., C.I.J.E. (coverage dropped), Commun.Abstr., Crim.Just.Abstr., Curr.Adv.Ecol.Sci., Curr.Cont., Curr.Ind.Stat., ERA, Environ.Sci.Poll.Mgmt., Ergon.Abstr., IBR, IBZ, IMFL, INSPEC (coverage dropped), Ind.Med. (1904-), Ind.Philos., Intl.Bibl.Soc.Sci., L.R.I., Lang.& Lang.Behav.Abstr., M.L.A., MLA Intl.Bibl., Mid.East: Abstr.& Ind., Neurosci.Cit.Ind., P C I, Pollut.Abstr., PsycInfo, Psychol.Abstr. (1926-), Ref.Zh., Res.High.Educ.Abstr., Risk Abstr., Russ.Acad.Sci.Bibl., SOPODA, SSCI, Saf.Sci.Abstr., So.Pac.Per.Ind., Soc.Sci.Ind. (Feb.1982-), Soc.Serv.Abstr., Sociol.Abstr., THA, Tech.Educ.Abstr., WMB, e-psyche.
—BLDSC (2321.000000), CISTI, IDS, ingenta. **CCC.**
Published by: The British Psychological Society, St Andrews House, 48 Princess Rd E, Leicester LE1 7DR, United Kingdom. TEL 44-116-252-9580, FAX 44-116-254-8824, http://www.bps.org.uk. Ed. Geoffrey Underwood. R&P, Adv. contact J Neason TEL 44-116-252-9580. page GBP 288; 135 x 210. Circ: 3,100. **Subscr. to:** Turpin Distribution Services Ltd., Blackhorse Rd, Letchworth, Herts SG6 1HN, United Kingdom. TEL 44-1462-488900, FAX 44-1462-483011.

301.1 150 GBR ISSN 0144-6665
BF1 CODEN: BJSPDA
BRITISH JOURNAL OF SOCIAL PSYCHOLOGY. Text in English. 1962. q., latest vol.40. GBP 140 in the European Union to institutions; USD 258 rest of world to institutions; GBP 42 newsstand/cover in the European Union; USD 78 newsstand/cover rest of world (effective 2001). adv. bk.rev. charts, illus, abstr. index. 160 p./no. back issues avail.; reprint service avail. from SWZ,SCH,PSC,ISI. *Refereed.* **Document type:** *Journal, Academic/Scholarly.* **Description:** Describes applications of social psychology. Includes research, review and methodological papers in addition to empirical papers of theoretical significance.
Supersedes in part (in 1981): British Journal of Social and Clinical Psychology (0007-1293)
Related titles: Magnetic Tape ed.; Microfiche ed.; Microform ed.: (from PQC); Online - full text ed.: 1999. free with print (from CatchWord Ltd., Northern Light Technology, Inc., EBSCO Publishing, ProQuest Information & Learning, Swets Blackwell, Institute for Scientific Information).
Indexed: ASCA, ASSIA, Abstr.Crim.& Pen., Addic.Abstr., Adol.Ment.Hlth.Abstr., Bibl.Dev.Med.& Child Neur., Biol.Abstr., Br.Hum.Ind., Brit.Nur.Ind., Commun.Abstr., Crim.Just.Abstr., Curr.Adv.Ecol.Sci., Curr.Cont., Curr.Ind.Stat., ERA, Environ.Sci.Poll.Mgmt., Excerp.Med., Fam.Ind., High.Educ.Curr.Aware.Bull., IBR, IMFL, Ind.Med. (1981-), Ind.Philos., Intl.Bibl.Soc.Sci., Lang.& Lang.Behav.Abstr., Mark.Res.Abstr. (1981-), Mid.East: Abstr.& Ind., Pollut.Abstr., PsycInfo, Psychol.Abstr. (1981-), Res.High.Educ.Abstr., Risk Abstr., Russ.Acad.Sci.Bibl., SOPODA, SSCI, Saf.Sci.Abstr., Soc.Serv.Abstr., Sociol.Abstr., Sociol.Educ.Abstr., Stud.Wom.Abstr., THA, e-psyche.
—BLDSC (2324.784000), CISTI, GNLM, IDS, ingenta. **CCC.**
Published by: The British Psychological Society, St Andrews House, 48 Princess Rd E, Leicester LE1 7DR, United Kingdom. TEL 44-116-252-9580, FAX 44-116-254-8824, journals@bps.org.uk. Eds. Margaret Wetherell, Stephen Reicher. R&P, Adv. contact J Neason TEL 44-116-252-9580. page GBP 256; 135 x 210. Circ: 2,000. **Subscr. to:** Turpin Distribution Services Ltd., Blackhorse Rd, Letchworth, Herts SG6 1HN, United Kingdom. TEL 44-1462-488900, FAX 44-1462-483011.

BRITISH JOURNAL OF SPECIAL EDUCATION; a journal of the National Association for Special Educational Needs. see *EDUCATION—Special Education And Rehabilitation*

150 GBR ISSN 0309-7773
BF11
BRITISH PSYCHOLOGICAL SOCIETY. ANNUAL REPORT. Text in English. a. free per issue. **Document type:** *Corporate.*
Indexed: e-psyche.
—BLDSC (1127.250000).
Published by: The British Psychological Society, St Andrews House, 48 Princess Rd E, Leicester LE1 7DR, United Kingdom. TEL 44-116-254-9568, FAX 44-116-247-0787, mail@bps.org.uk. Circ: 23,000.

BRITISH SOCIETY FOR MUSIC THERAPY. BULLETIN. see *MUSIC*

BROWN UNIVERSITY CHILD AND ADOLESCENT BEHAVIOR LETTER; monthly reports on the problems of children and adolescents growing up. see *CHILDREN AND YOUTH—About*

616.89 USA ISSN 1053-4474
CODEN: BIPSEW
BRUNNER - MAZEL INTEGRATIVE PSYCHOTHERAPY SERIES✶. Text in English. 1987. irreg. **Document type:** *Monographic series.*
Indexed: e-psyche.
Published by: Brunner - Routledge (Subsidiary of: Taylor & Francis Group), 325 Chestnut St, Ste 800, Philadelphia, PA 19106. TEL 215-269-0400, FAX 215-269-0363, postmaster@bmpub.com.

BRUNNER - MAZEL PSYCHOSOCIAL STRESS SERIES. see *MEDICAL SCIENCES—Hematology*

150 JPN ISSN 0288-3538
BUKKYO DAIGAKU SHINRIGAKU KENKYUJO KIYO/JOURNAL OF PSYCHOLOGY. Text in Japanese. 1983. a.
Related titles: Online - full text ed.
Indexed: Soc.Sci.Ind. (coverage dropped), e-psyche.

Published by: Bukkyo Daigaku, Shinrigaku Kenkyujo/Bukkyo University, Research Institute for Psychology, Murasakino-Kitahananobo-cho, Kita-ku, Kyoto-shi 603-8301, Japan.

150 BGR
BULGARSKO SPISANIE PO PSIKHOLOGIA. Text in Bulgarian. q. USD 36 foreign (effective 2002). **Document type:** *Journal, Academic/Scholarly.* **Description:** Presents theoretical and experimental material in all fields of psychology and related sciences.
Published by: Druzhestvo na Psycholosite v Bulgaria/Bulgarian Psychological Society, 14 Lulin Planina St, Sofia 1606, Bulgaria. TEL 359-2-541295. **Dist. by:** Sofia Books, Ul Silivria 16, Sofia 1404, Bulgaria. TEL 359-2-9586257, sofiabooks@hotmail.com, http://www.sofiabooks.hit.bg.

150 FRA ISSN 0007-4403
BULLETIN DE PSYCHOLOGIE. Text in French. 1947. q. FRF 530 to individuals; FRF 750 to institutions (effective 2000). adv. bk.rev. abstr, bibl, charts. back issues avail.; reprint service avail. from PSC,SCH. **Document type:** *Academic/Scholarly.*
Formerly (until 1951): Universite de Paris. Groupe d'Etudes de Psychologie. Bulletin (0242-5432)
Indexed: IBR, Psychol.Abstr. (1962-), e-psyche.
—BLDSC (2884.450000).
Published by: Universite de Paris, 17 rue de la Sorbonne, Paris 75005, France. TEL 33-1-46989941, petard@claranet.fr. Ed. Marcel Turbiaux. Pub. Jean Pierre Petard. Adv. contact J P Petard. Circ: 700.

375 USA
BUROS DESK REFERENCE. Text in English. 1994. irreg. **Document type:** *Academic/Scholarly.* **Description:** Contains descriptions and candidly critical reviews of commercially available tests in specific areas. Editions available include School Psychology and Substance Abuse.
Indexed: e-psyche.
Published by: Buros Institute of Mental Measurements, 135 Bancroft Hall, University of Nebraska Lincoln, Lincoln, NE 68588-0348. TEL 402-472-6203, FAX 402-472-6207, bimm@unlinfo.unl.edu, http://www.unl.edu/buros. Eds. James C Impara, Linda L Murphy. **Dist by:** University of Nebraska Press, 233 N 8th St, Lincoln, NE 68588-0255. TEL 800-755-1105, FAX 402-4726214.

371.3 USA
BUROS - NEBRASKA SERIES ON MEASUREMENT AND TESTING. Text in English. 1982. irreg. **Document type:** *Academic/Scholarly.* **Description:** Each publication in the series focuses on an individual issue within the assessment field.
Indexed: e-psyche.
Published by: Buros Institute of Mental Measurements, 135 Bancroft Hall, University of Nebraska Lincoln, Lincoln, NE 68588-0348. TEL 402-472-6203, FAX 402-472-6207, bimm@unlinfo.unl.edu, http://www.unl.edu/buios. Ed. Linda L Murphy.

370.15 150 USA ISSN 1052-3103
C A C D JOURNAL. Text in English. 1989 (vol.9). a. USD 8 (effective 1998). adv. charts, stat. **Document type:** *Monographic series, Academic/Scholarly.* **Description:** Presents articles in the field of counseling and guidance for professionals.
Indexed: e-psyche.
Published by: California Association for Counseling and Development, 2555 E Chapman Ave, Ste 201, Fullerton, CA 92631-3617. TEL 714-871-6460, FAX 714-871-5132. Ed. Dr. Patricia Wickwire. R&P Richard Hoover. Adv. contact Sharon Barth. Circ: 3,000.

C A P S REPORT NEWSLETTER; fellowship, personal news, membership, convention. see *RELIGIONS AND THEOLOGY*

150 BRA
CADERNOS DE PSICOLOGIA APLICADA* . Text in Portuguese. s-a. bibl.
Indexed: Psychol.Abstr., e-psyche.
Published by: Centro de Orientacao e Selecao Psicoterapia, Rua Jacinto Gomes, 540, Santana, Porto Alegre, RGS 90040-270, Brazil.

155.5 FRA ISSN 1295-7364
CAHIERS ALFRED BINET; education, psychologie et sciences de l'enfance. Text in French. 1900. q. EUR 30 domestic; EUR 38.50 foreign (effective 2001).
Published by: Editions Eres, 11 rue des Alouettes, Ramonville Saint-Agne 31520, France. TEL 33-05-61751576, FAX 33-05-61735289, eres@editions-eres.com. Ed. Guy Avanzini.

616.89156 BEL ISSN 0241-5453
CAHIERS CRITIQUES DE THERAPIE FAMILIALE ET DE PRATIQUES DE RESEAUX. Text in French. s-a. BEF 1,965 domestic; BEF 2,295 in the European Union; BEF 2,342 in Europe; BEF 2,625 elsewhere; BEF 1,075 newsstand/cover (effective 2000 - 2001). bk.rev. abstr. 200 p./no. back issues avail. *Refereed.* **Document type:** *Monographic series, Academic/Scholarly.* **Description:** Covers issues relating to family psychotherapy, group therapy, and short-term therapy.
Indexed: IBZ, Ind.Philos., e-psyche.
Published by: De Boeck Universite (Subsidiary of: De Boeck et Larcier S.A.), Rue des Minimes 39, Brussels 1000, Belgium. TEL 32-2-5480711, FAX 32-2-5139009, http://www.deboeck.be. Ed. Mony Elkaim. **Subscr. to:** Acces S.P.R.L., Fond Jean Paques 4, Louvain-la-Neuve 1348, Belgium. TEL 32-10-482570, FAX 32-10-482519, acces+@deboeck.be.

616.89 BEL ISSN 1370-074X
CAHIERS DE PSYCHOLOGIE CLINIQUE; une revue interdisciplinaire en psychologie clinique et psychotherapie. Text in French. 1994. s-a. BEF 2,090 domestic; BEF 2,420 in the European Union; BEF 2,467 in Europe; BEF 2,750 elsewhere; BEF 1,075 newsstand/cover (effective 2000 - 2001). bk.rev. 230 p./no. *Refereed.* **Document type:** *Monographic series, Academic/Scholarly.* **Description:** Takes a multidisciplinary approach to the study of clinical psychology and psychotherapy.
Indexed: IBZ, e-psyche.
Published by: De Boeck Universite (Subsidiary of: De Boeck et Larcier S.A.), Rue des Minimes 39, Brussels 1000, Belgium. TEL 2-32-10482570, FAX 2-32-10-482650, http://www.deboeck.be. Eds. Alex Lefebvre, Philippe Van Meerbeeck. **Subscr. to:** Acces S.P.R.L., Fond Jean Paques 4, Louvain-la-Neuve 1348, Belgium. TEL 32-10-482570, FAX 32-10-482519, acces+@deboeck.be.

150 FRA ISSN 0249-9185
CAHIERS DE PSYCHOLOGIE COGNITIVE/CURRENT PSYCHOLOGY OF COGNITION. Abbreviated title: C P C. Text in French. 1962. bi-m. FRF 816.80 (effective 2000). *Refereed.* **Description:** Features papers emphasizing experimental work, and target articles focusing on significant and controversial contributions. Also includes theoretical, review, advance and integrative empirical articles.
Formerly (until 1980): Cahiers de Psychologie (0373-8965)
Related titles: Online - full text ed.: (from Institute for Scientific Information).
Indexed: Curr.Cont., Lang.& Lang.Behav.Abstr., Neurosci.Cit.Ind., PsycInfo, Psychol.Abstr. (1981-), Ref.Zh., SOPODA, SSCI, Sociol.Abstr., e-psyche.
—BLDSC (3501.620000), IDS. **CCC.**
Published by: Association pour la Diffusion des Recherches en Sciences Cognitives de Langue Francaise, CNRS - CRNC, 31 chemin Joseph Aiguier, Marseille Cedex 20 13402, France. TEL 33-4-91164279, FAX 33-4-91714938, cpc@lnf.cnrs-mrs.fr. Ed. Bruno Poucet. R&P Francoise Joubaud.

301.1 150 BEL ISSN 0777-0707
CAHIERS INTERNATIONAUX DE PSYCHOLOGIE SOCIALE. Text in French; Summaries in English, French, Spanish. 1989. q. BEF 3,320 domestic; BEF 3,770 in the European Union; BEF 3,870 in Europe; BEF 4,120 elsewhere; BEF 950 newsstand/cover (effective 2000 - 2001). bk.rev. 128 p./no. *Refereed.* **Document type:** *Monographic series, Academic/Scholarly.* **Description:** Discusses various aspects of social psychology.
Indexed: IBZ, Ind.Philos., PsycInfo, Psychol.Abstr. (1989-), Soc.Serv.Abstr., Sociol.Abstr., e-psyche.
Published by: De Boeck Universite (Subsidiary of: De Boeck et Larcier S.A.), Rue des Minimes 39, Brussels 1000, Belgium. TEL 2-32-10482570, FAX 2-32-10-482650, dbu@deboeck.be, http://www.deboeck.be. Ed. Pierre de Visscher. **Subscr. to:** Acces S.P.R.L., Fond Jean Paques 4, Louvain-la-Neuve 1348, Belgium. TEL 32-10-482500, FAX 32-10-482519.

150.19 FRA ISSN 0980-5508
CAHIERS POUR LA RECHERCHE FREUDIENNE. Text in French. 1986. irreg., latest 1989. price varies. **Document type:** *Academic/Scholarly.*
Indexed: e-psyche.
Published by: (Universite de Paris X - Nanterre, Centre de Recherches et d'Etudes Freudiennes), Publidix, 200 av. de la Republique, Nanterre Cedex 92001, France. TEL 33-1-40977590, FAX 33-1-40975698, publidix@u-paris10.fr.

614.58 USA ISSN 1062-8193
RC488.5
CALIFORNIA THERAPIST. Text in English. 1989. bi-m. USD 36 to non-members (effective 2001). bk.rev. charts, illus, stat, tr.lit. **Document type:** *Trade.* **Description:** For and about CA licensed marriage, family and child therapists.
Indexed: e-psyche.
Published by: California Association of Marriage and Family Therapists, 7901 Raytheon Rd, San Diego, CA 92111-1606. TEL 858-292-2638, FAX 858-292-2666, http://www.camft.org. Ed. Mary Riemersma. R&P, Adv. contact Lori Greenberg. Circ: 25,200 (paid and free).

150.1953 CAN
THE CANADIAN JOURNAL OF ADLERIAN PSYCHOLOGY. Text in English. 1991. s-a. CND 35; USD 30 foreign. bk.rev. bibl, charts, illus, stat. back issues avail. *Refereed.* **Document type:** *Academic/Scholarly.* **Description:** Provides theoretical and practical information for practicing therapists and counselors who use Adlerian psychology.
Related titles: E-mail ed.; Fax ed.; Online - full text ed.
Indexed: e-psyche.
Published by: Adlerian Psychology Association of British Columbia, No 401-1195 W Broadway, Vancouver, BC V6H 3X5, Canada. TEL 604-874-4614, FAX 604-874-4634, cjap@adler.bc.ca, http://www.adler.bc.ca. Ed., R&P Steven Slavik. Circ: 500 (paid).

370.15 CAN ISSN 0008-400X
BF1 CODEN: CJBSAA
CANADIAN JOURNAL OF BEHAVIOURAL SCIENCE/REVUE CANADIENNE DES SCIENCES DU COMPORTEMENT. Text in English, French. 1969. q. CND 45 domestic to individuals; USD 45 foreign to individuals; CND 85 domestic to institutions; USD 85 foreign to institutions (effective 2000). adv. bk.rev. charts, tr.lit. index. back issues avail.; reprint service avail. from PSC,SCH. *Refereed.* **Description:** Covers abnormal, behavioral, community, counselling, educational, environmental, developmental, health, industrial-organizational, clinical neuropsychological, personality, psychometrics, and social.
Related titles: Microfiche ed.: (from MML); Microform ed.: (from PQC,MML); Online - full text ed.: (from ProQuest Information & Learning, LexisNexis, Institute for Scientific Information).
Indexed: ASCA, Adol.Ment.Hlth.Abstr., AgeLine, Biol.Abstr., CBCA Ref., Can.B.P.I., Can.Per.Ind. (Apr.1989-), Can.Wom.Per.Ind., Curr.Adv.Ecol.Sci., Curr.Cont., ERA, Excerp.Med., Ind.Philos., Ind.Sci.Rev., Lang.& Lang.Behav.Abstr., Mid.East: Abstr.& Ind., Mult.Ed.Abstr., PsycInfo, Psychol.Abstr. (1969-), SOPODA, SSCI, Sage Race Rel.Abstr., Sci.Cit.Ind. (coverage dropped), Soc.Serv.Abstr., Sociol.Abstr., Sp.Ed.Needs Abstr., e-psyche.
—BLDSC (3028.700000), CISTI, IDS, ingenta. **CCC.**
Published by: Canadian Psychological Association, 151 Slater St, Ste 205, Ottawa, ON K1P 5H3, Canada. TEL 613-237-2144, FAX 613-237-1674, warren_eaton@umanitoba.ca, cpapubs@cpa.ca, http://www.cpa.ca. Ed. Warren Eaton. R&P Ivan Parisien. Adv. contact Mary Franklin. Circ: 3,800.

150 301.1 CAN ISSN 0713-3936
CANADIAN JOURNAL OF COMMUNITY MENTAL HEALTH/REVUE CANADIENNE DE SANTE MENTALE COMMUNAUTAIRE. Text in English, French. 1982. 2/yr. CND 25 domestic to individuals; USD 30 in United States to individuals; USD 35 elsewhere to individuals; CND 55 domestic to institutions; USD 60 in United States to institutions; USD 65 elsewhere to institutions; CND 20 to students; CND 25 newsstand/cover; USD 27.50 newsstand/cover in United States; USD 30 newsstand/cover elsewhere (effective 2002). index. **Document type:** *Academic/Scholarly.* **Description:** Devoted to the sharing of information and valid knowledge about phenomena pertinent to the mental well-being of Canadians and their communities.
Indexed: CINAHL, Child Devel.Abstr., P.A.I.S., PsycInfo, Psychol.Abstr. (1983-), Sage Fam.Stud.Abstr., Soc.Work Res.& Abstr., Viol.& Abuse Abstr., e-psyche.
—BLDSC (3031.046000), EMDOCS, GNLM, Infotrieve, KNAW. **CCC.**
Published by: (Canadian Periodical for Community Studies Inc.), Wilfrid Laurier University Press, 75 University Ave W, Waterloo, ON N2L 3C5, Canada. TEL 519-884-1970, FAX 519-725-1399, press@wlu.ca, http://www.wlupress.wlu.ca. Ed. Eli Teram.

158 CAN ISSN 0828-3893
CANADIAN JOURNAL OF COUNSELLING/REVUE CANADIENNE DE COUNSELING. Text in English, French. 1966. q. CND 50 domestic to non-members; CND 61.35 in United States to non-members; CND 66.70 elsewhere to non-members (effective 2001). adv. bk.rev. index. back issues avail.; reprint service avail. from PQC. *Refereed.* **Document type:** *Journal, Academic/Scholarly.* **Description:** Publishes current research and reports with relevance to psychological counselling practitioners.
Formerly: Canadian Counsellor (0008-333X)
Related titles: Microfiche ed.: (from MML); Microform ed.: 1967 (from PQC,MML).
Indexed: C.I.J.E., Can.Educ.Ind., High.Educ.Abstr., PsycInfo, Psychol.Abstr. (1972-), Res.High.Educ.Abstr., Sage Race Rel.Abstr., Sp.Ed.Needs Abstr., Tech.Educ.Abstr., e-psyche.
—BLDSC (3031.122000), ingenta. **CCC.**
Published by: Canadian Counselling Association/ Association Canadienne de Counseling, 116 Albert St, Ste 702, Ottawa, ON K1P 5G3, Canada. TEL 613-237-1099, 877-765-5565, FAX 613-237-9786, http://cjc-rcc.icaap.org/index-e.html, http://www.ccacc.ca. Ed. Max R Uhlemann. adv.: page CND 375; 6 x 9. Circ: 2,000 (paid).

150 CAN ISSN 1196-1961
BF1
CANADIAN JOURNAL OF EXPERIMENTAL PSYCHOLOGY/REVUE CANADIENNE DE PSYCHOLOGIE EXPERIMENTALE. Text in English, French. 1947. q. CND 45 domestic to individuals; USD 45 foreign to individuals; CND 85 domestic to institutions; USD 85 foreign to institutions (effective 2000). adv. bibl, charts, illus. index, cum.index: 1947-1961. reprint service avail. from PQC,SCH,PSC. *Refereed.* **Document type:** *Academic/Scholarly.* **Description:** Publishes original research papers that advance understanding of the broad field of general experimental psychology. This includes, but is not restricted to, cognition, perception, sensorimotor processes, memory, learning, language, decision making, development, and neuroscience.
Former titles (until 1993): Canadian Journal of Psychology (0008-4255); (until 1947): Canadian Psychology Association. Bulletin (0382-8654)
Related titles: Microfiche ed.: (from MML); Microform ed.: (from PQC,MML); Online - full text ed.: (from Northern Light Technology, Inc., ProQuest Information & Learning, Gale Group, LexisNexis, Factiva, Institute for Scientific Information).
Indexed: ASCA, ASSIA, Adol.Ment.Hlth.Abstr., AgeLine, Arts & Hum.Cit.Ind. (coverage dropped), Biol.Abstr., CBCA Ref., Can.B.P.I., Can.Per.Ind. (Mar.1993-), Child Devel.Abstr., Curr.Adv.Ecol.Sci., Curr.Cont., Ergon.Abstr., Ind.Med. (1993-), Ind.Philos., Lang.& Lang.Behav.Abstr., Mult.Ed.Abstr., Neurosci.Cit.Ind., P C I, PsycInfo, Psychol.Abstr. (1947-), Pt.de Rep., Russ.Acad.Sci.Bibl., SOPODA, SSCI, Soc.Sci.Ind. (Nov.1982-Dec.1992), Sociol.Abstr., Sp.Ed.Needs Abstr., Yrbk.Assoc.Educ.& Rehab.Blind, e-psyche.
—BLDSC (3031.410000), CISTI, GNLM, IDS, Infotrieve, ingenta. **CCC.**
Published by: Canadian Psychological Association, 151 Slater St, Ste 205, Ottawa, ON K1P 5H3, Canada. TEL 613-237-2144, FAX 613-237-1674, m_singer@umanitoba.ca. Ed. Murray Singer. R&P Ivan Parisien. Adv. contact Mary Franklin. Circ: 2,000.

155.3 616.6 CAN ISSN 1188-4517
CODEN: CJHSEA
CANADIAN JOURNAL OF HUMAN SEXUALITY. Text in English. 1986. q. CND 45 in Canada to individuals; CND 50 in United States to individuals; CND 70 elsewhere to individuals; CND 65 in Canada to institutions; CND 70 in United States to institutions; CND 90 elsewhere to institutions; CND 30 in Canada to students; CND 35 in United States to students; CND 55 elsewhere to students (effective 2001). bk.rev. reprints avail. *Refereed.* **Document type:** *Academic/Scholarly.* **Description:** Includes scholarly articles, research papers, reviews, conference announcements and special theme issue.
Formerly (until 1992): S I E C C A N Journal (0844-3718)
Related titles: Online - full text ed.: (from ProQuest Information & Learning, Gale Group, LexisNexis).
Indexed: ASSIA, CBCA Ref., CINAHL, Can.B.P.I., Can.Educ.Ind., Can.Per.Ind. (Mar.1995-), Child Devel.Abstr., Cont.Pg.Educ., Curr.Lit.Fam.Plan., ERA, Educ.Admin.Abstr., Environ.Sci.Poll.Mgmt., Excerp.Med. (1996-), Intl.Bibl.S.S.Soc.Cult.Anthro., Intl.Bibl.Soc.Sci., Lang.& Lang.Behav.Abstr., Mult.Ed.Abstr., Pollut.Abstr., PsycInfo, Psychol.Abstr., Ref.Zh., Res.High.Educ.Abstr., SOPODA, Sage Fam.Stud.Abstr., Soc.Serv.Abstr., Sociol.Abstr., Sociol.Educ.Abstr., Sp.Ed.Needs Abstr., Stud.Wom.Abstr., Viol.& Abuse Abstr., e-psyche.
—BLDSC (3031.710000), EMDOCS, GNLM, Infotrieve, ingenta. **CCC.**
Published by: Sex Information and Education Council of Canada, 850 Coxwell Ave, York, ON M4C 5R1, Canada. TEL 416-466-5304, FAX 416-778-0785, sieccan@web.net, http://www.sieccan.org. Ed. F Michael Barrett. R&P, Adv. contact Alex McKay. Circ: 1,000.

CANADIAN JOURNAL OF MUSIC THERAPY/REVUE CANADIENNE DE MUSICOTHERAPIE. see *MUSIC*

CANADIAN JOURNAL OF SCHOOL PSYCHOLOGY. see *EDUCATION*

150 CAN ISSN 0068-9211
CANADIAN MENTAL HEALTH ASSOCIATION. ANNUAL REPORT/ASSOCIATION CANADIENNE POUR LA SANTE MENTALE. RAPPORT ANNUEL. Text in English. 1926. a. free per issue. **Document type:** *Corporate.*
Indexed: Curr.Cont. (coverage dropped), e-psyche.
Published by: Canadian Mental Health Association, 2160 Yonge St, Toronto, ON M4S 2Z3, Canada. TEL 416-484-7750.

150 CAN ISSN 0708-5591
BF1 CODEN: CPSGD2
CANADIAN PSYCHOLOGY. Text in English, French. 1959. q. CND 85 to individuals; CND 45 foreign to individuals; CND 45 to institutions; CND 85 foreign to institutions (effective 1999). adv. bk.rev. illus. Index. back issues avail.; reprint service avail. from PSC,SCH. *Refereed.* **Document type:** *Academic/Scholarly.* **Description:** Publishes generelist articles in areas of theory, research, and practice that are potentially of interest to a broad cross-section of psychologists.
Former titles: Canadian Psychological Review (0318-2096); Canadian Psychologist
Related titles: Microfiche ed.: (from MML); Microform ed.; Online - full text ed.: (from ProQuest Information & Learning, Institute for Scientific Information).
Indexed: ASCA, ASSIA, AgeLine, Arts & Hum.Cit.Ind. (coverage dropped), Biol.Abstr., CBCA Ref., Can.B.P.I., Can.Per.Ind. (Jan.1988-), Can.Wom.Per.Ind., Curr.Cont., Ind.Philos., Lang.& Lang.Behav.Abstr., Mid.East: Abstr.& Ind., PsycInfo, Psychol.Abstr. (1960-), SOPODA, SSCI, Sage Race Rel.Abstr., Soc.Serv.Abstr., Sociol.Abstr., e-psyche.
—BLDSC (3044.105000), CISTI, IDS, ingenta. **CCC.**
Published by: Canadian Psychological Association, 151 Slater St, Ste 205, Ottawa, ON K1P 5H3, Canada. TEL 613-237-2144, FAX 613-237-1674, catano@husky1.stmarys.ca, http://www.cpa.ca/ Psynopsis/scholar.html. Ed. Dr. Victor Catano. R&P Ivan Parisien. Adv. contact Mary Franklin. Circ: 4,600.

THE CAREER DEVELOPMENT QUARTERLY. see *OCCUPATIONS AND CAREERS*

CARIBBEAN JOURNAL OF CRIMINOLOGY & SOCIAL PSYCHOLOGY. see *CRIMINOLOGY AND LAW ENFORCEMENT*

155.937 618 USA
CARING NOTES; a professional newsletter by S H A R E. Text in English. 1995. q. USD 35 (effective 2000). bk.rev., video rev., Website rev. **Document type:** *Newsletter.* **Description:** For SHARE group facilitators and other caregivers, reaching out to the bereaved experiencing a pregnancy loss, stillbirth or neonatal death. Offers professional articles on clinical and psychological aspects of perinatal loss.
Indexed: e-psyche.
Published by: S H A R E Pregnancy & Infant Loss Support National Office, St Joseph Health, 300 First Capitol Dr, Center, MO 63301. TEL 636-947-6164, 800-821-6819, FAX 314-947-7486, share@nationalshareoffice.com, http:// www.nationalshareoffice.com. Eds. Catherine A Lammert, Jane Borman. Circ: 150.

150.19 155.4 USA
CARNEGIE-MELLON SYMPOSIA ON COGNITION SERIES. Variant title: Carnegie Symposium on Cognition. Text in English. 1974. irreg., latest vol.23, 1992. **Document type:** *Monographic series.*
Indexed: Curr.Cont. (coverage dropped), Psychol.Abstr., e-psyche.
Published by: Lawrence Erlbaum Associates, Inc., 10 Industrial Ave, Mahwah, NJ 07430-2262. TEL 201-236-9500, FAX 201-236-0072, jamsel@erlbaum.com, http://www.erlbaum.com. Ed. David Klahr.

616.89 AUS ISSN 1321-9324
CASE STUDIES; in brief and family therapy. Text in English. 1986. s-a. AUD 25 to individuals; AUD 36 to institutions. **Description:** Designed to provide practical examples and information for working therapists.
Formerly (until vol.8, 1994): Family Therapy Case Studies (0818-3538)
Indexed: e-psyche.
Published by: (Eastwood Family Therapy Centre), Michael Durrant & Assoc. Pty. Ltd., PO Box 630, Epping, NSW 2121, Australia. TEL 61-2-8682799, FAX 61-2-8768943. Ed. Michael Durrant.

150 USA
CENTENNIAL PSYCHOLOGY SERIES. Text in English. 1982. irreg. price varies. **Document type:** *Monographic series.*
Indexed: e-psyche.
Published by: Praeger Publishers (Subsidiary of: Greenwood Publishing Group Inc.), 88 Post Rd W, Box 5007, Westport, CT 06881-5007. TEL 203-226-3571, FAX 203-222-1502.

616.89 ITA ISSN 0392-3398
CENTRO RICERCHE BIOPSICHICHE. Text in Italian; Summaries in English. 1957. irreg. free per issue. bk.rev. **Document type:** *Bulletin, Academic/Scholarly.*
Indexed: Psychol.Abstr., e-psyche.
Address: Via Dante, 60, Padua, PD 35139, Italy. TEL 39-49-657996. Ed. Giorgio Foresti. Circ: 600.

150 CZE ISSN 1211-216X
CESKA AKADEMIE VED. PSYCHOLOGICKY USTAV. BULLETIN. Text in Czech. 1995. irreg. **Document type:** *Academic/Scholarly.* **Description:** Covers the research of members of the Prague branch of the institute.
Published by: Ceska Akademie Ved, Psychologicky Ustav, Husova 4, Prague, 1 110 00, Czech Republic. TEL 42-2-24220979, FAX 42-2-2314436, http://www.lib.cas.cz/knav/journals/ Bulletin_Psychologickeho_ustavu.htm.

150 CZE ISSN 0009-062X
BF8.C9 CODEN: CEPSBC
CESKOSLOVENSKA PSYCHOLOGIE/CZECHOSLOVAK PSYCHOLOGY. Text mainly in Czech, Slovak; Text occasionally in English, German, Russian; Summaries in English. 1957. bi-m. DEM 141. adv. bk.rev. charts, illus, stat. index. *Refereed.* **Description:** Covers all fields of psychology, theoretical and applied. Includes basic research into general and social psychology, survey studies which have been given preference and reports on important conferences and institutes.
Related titles: Online - full text ed.: (from Institute for Scientific Information).
Indexed: ASCA, Arts & Hum.Cit.Ind. (coverage dropped), Bibl.Ling., Biol.Abstr., C.I.S. Abstr., Child Devel.Abstr., Curr.Cont., Ergon.Abstr., Neurosci.Cit.Ind., PsycInfo, Psychol.Abstr. (1957-), Russ.Acad.Sci.Bibl., SSCI, e-psyche.
—BLDSC (3122.500000).
Published by: Ceska Akademie Ved, Psychologicky Ustav, Husova 4, Prague, 1 110 00, Czech Republic. TEL 42-2-24220979, FAX 42-2-2314436, http://www.lib.cas.cz/knav/journals/ Bulletin_Psychologickeho_ustavu.htm. Ed. Miluse Sedlakova. Circ: 2,800. **Dist. in Western countries by:** Kubon & Sagner, Postfach 24, Munich 34 8000, Germany.

150 POL ISSN 1427-695X
CHARAKTERY; magazyn psychologiczny dla kazdego. Text in Polish. 1997. m. PLZ 4 newsstand/cover (effective 2000). adv. dance rev., music rev., play rev., tel.rev., video rev. bibl, illus. back issues avail. **Description:** Offers practical knowledge indispensable in professional, social and family life.
Published by: Wydawnictwo Naukowe P W Nowe, Ul Miodowa 10, Warsaw 00251, Poland. TEL 48-22-6954270, FAX 48-22-6954272, http://www.pwn.com.pl. Pub., R&P Bogdan Bialek. Adv. contact Beata Michalak. color page PLZ 4,800; trim 210 x 297. Circ: 40,000.

CHEIRON NEWSLETTER. see *SOCIAL SCIENCES: COMPREHENSIVE WORKS*

CHICOREL INDEX SERIES. see *BIBLIOGRAPHIES*

CHILD; the essential guide for parents. see *CHILDREN AND YOUTH—About*

CHILD ABUSE REVIEW. see *SOCIAL SERVICES AND WELFARE*

P

CHILD AND ADOLESCENT SOCIAL WORK JOURNAL. see *SOCIOLOGY*

155.4 157 USA ISSN 0731-7107
RJ504
CHILD & FAMILY BEHAVIOR THERAPY. Text in English. 1978. q. USD 65 to individuals; USD 88 in Canada to individuals; USD 94 elsewhere to individuals; USD 250 to institutions; USD 338 in Canada to institutions; USD 363 elsewhere to institutions; USD 500 to libraries; USD 675 in Canada to libraries; USD 725 elsewhere to libraries (effective Aug. 2001). adv. bk.rev., film rev. bibl, charts, stat, illus. back issues avail.; reprint service avail. from HAW. *Refereed.* **Document type:** *Journal, Academic/Scholarly.* **Description:** Offers an interdisciplinary journal devoted to research and clinical applications in behavior therapy with children and adolescents, as well as the enhancement of parenting.
Formerly (until 1982): Child Behavior Therapy (0162-1416)
Related titles: Microfiche ed.: (from PQC); Microform ed.; Online - full text ed.: (from Institute for Scientific Information).
Indexed: ASCA, Abstr.Crim.& Pen., Addic.Abstr., Adol.Ment.Hlth.Abstr., Behav.Abstr., C.I.J.E., Child Devel.Abstr., Crim.Just.Abstr., Curr.Cont., ERA, Educ.Ind. (coverage dropped), Environ.Sci.Poll.Mgmt., Except.Child Educ.Abstr., Fam.Ind., IMFL, Lang.& Lang.Behav.Abstr., Mult.Ed.Abstr., Peace Res.Abstr., PsycInfo, Psychol.Abstr. (1979-), Psycscan B.A.& T., Rehabil.Lit., Risk Abstr., SOPODA, SSCI, Saf.Sci.Abstr., Sage Fam.Stud.Abstr., Soc.Serv.Abstr., Soc.Work Res.& Abstr., Sociol.Abstr., Sociol.Educ.Abstr., Sp.Ed.Needs Abstr., Stud.Wom.Abstr., Viol.& Abuse Abstr., e-psyche.
—BLDSC (3172.915100), GNLM, Haworth, IDS, ingenta.
Published by: Haworth Press, Inc., 10 Alice St, Binghamton, NY 13904-1580. TEL 607-722-5857, 800-429-6784, FAX 607-722-6362, 800-895-0582, getinfo@haworthpressinc.com, http://www.haworthpress.com/journals/journallist.asp. Ed. Cyril M Franks. Pub. William Cohen. R&P Ruthann Heath TEL 607-723-5857 ext 316. Adv. contact Jackie Blakeslee TEL 607-722-5857 ext 346. B&W page USD 315, color page USD 550; trim 6 x 8.5. Circ: 750.

CHILD AND YOUTH CARE FORUM; an independent journal of day and residential child and youth care practice. see *CHILDREN AND YOUTH—About*

CHILD ASSESSMENT NEWS. see *CHILDREN AND YOUTH—About*

CHILD BEHAVIOR AND DEVELOPMENT. see *MEDICAL SCIENCES—Pediatrics*

CHILD DEVELOPMENT. see *CHILDREN AND YOUTH—About*

CHILD MALTREATMENT. see *CHILDREN AND YOUTH—About*

155.4 GBR ISSN 1360-6417
RJ499.A1
CHILD PSYCHOLOGY AND PSYCHIATRY REVIEW. Text in English. 1996. q. GBP 70, USD 112 to institutions (effective 2001). adv. bk.rev., software rev. *Refereed.* **Document type:** *Academic/Scholarly.* **Description:** Provides a forum for the exchange of clinical experience, ideas and research. Aims to foster good clinical practice.
Supersedes in part (in 1996): A C P P Review and Newsletter (1354-5329); Which was formerly (until 1993): Association for Child Psychology and Psychiatry. Newsletter. (0265-4520); (until 1983): Association for Child Psychology and Psychiatry. News
Related titles: Online - full text ed.: (from EBSCO Publishing, O C L C Online Computer Library Center, Inc., RoweCom Information Quest, Swets Blackwell).
Indexed: PsycInfo, e-psyche.
—BLDSC (3172.945540). **CCC.**
Published by: Cambridge University Press, Edinburgh Bldg, Shaftesbury Rd, Cambridge CB2 2RU, United Kingdom. FAX 44-1223-315052, information@cup.cam.ac.uk, information@cambridge.org, http://www.cup.org/journals/CUPJNLS.html. Eds. Linda Dowdney, Orlee Udwin, Stephen Scott. R&P Linda Nicol. Adv. contact Rebecca Symons.

CHILD STUDY JOURNAL. see *EDUCATION*

155.4 GBR
CHILDREN'S ENVIRONMENTS; theory, research, policy and applications. Text in English. 1984. q. GBP 35 to individuals; GBP 99 in the European Union to institutions; USD 169 in North America to institutions; USD 109 elsewhere to institutions (effective 1999). adv. bk.rev. bibl. reprints avail. *Refereed.* **Document type:** *Academic/Scholarly.* **Description:** Serves as both a forum among child environment research scholars and a bridge to practice and policy in environmental design, planning, and education for children.
Former titles (until vol.9, 1992): Children's Environments Quarterly (0886-0505); (until 1984): Childhood City Quarterly (0738-1484); Childhood City Newsletter
Indexed: Child Devel.Abstr., Fam.Ind., PsycInfo, Psychol.Abstr. (1986-), e-psyche.
—ingenta. **CCC.**
Published by: (Center for Human Environments USA), Chapman & Hall, Journals Department (Subsidiary of: International Thomson Publishing Group), Chapman & Hall, 2-6 Boundary Row, London SE1 8HN, United Kingdom. TEL 44-20-7865-0066, FAX 44-20-7522-9623, TELEX 290164 CHAPMA G, jhelp@chall.co.uk, http://www.chaphall.com/chaphall/journals.html. Ed. Roger A Hart. Circ: 500. **Subscr. to:** 400 Market St, Philadelphia, PA 19106. **Dist. by:** International Thompson Publishing Services Ltd., Cheriton House, North Way, Walworth Industrial Estate, Andover, Hants SP10 5BE, United Kingdom. TEL 44-1264-342713, FAX 44-1264-642807.

155 616 614 USA
CHILDREN'S MENTAL HEALTH SERVICES. Text in English. irreg., latest vol.2, 1996. bibl. **Description:** Covers the mental health system for children and adolescents.
Indexed: e-psyche.
—BLDSC (3172.992040).
Published by: Sage Publications, Inc., 2455 Teller Rd, Thousand Oaks, CA 91320. TEL 805-499-0721, FAX 805-499-0871, libraries@sagepub.com, libraries@sagepub.com., http://www.sagepub.com. Eds. Carol T Nixon, Craig Anne Heflinger. **Subscr. to:** Sage Publications Ltd., 6 Bonhill St, London EC2A 4PU, United Kingdom; Sage Publications India Pvt. Ltd., 32-m Market, Greater Kailash-I, New Delhi 110 048, India.

150 130 TWN ISSN 1013-9656
CHINESE JOURNAL OF PSYCHOLOGY. Text in Chinese, English; Abstracts in Chinese, English. 1958. s-a. USD 40 (effective 1996). adv. back issues avail. *Refereed.* **Document type:** *Academic/Scholarly.*
Formerly: Acta Psychologica Taiwanica (0065-1613)
Indexed: ASCA, Bibl.Asian Stud. (1971-1972), Biol.Abstr., Curr.Cont. (coverage dropped), PsycInfo, Psychol.Abstr. (1990-), SSCI (coverage dropped), e-psyche.
Published by: Chinese Psychological Association, c/o Department of Psychology, National Taiwan University, Taipei 10764, Taiwan. FAX 886-2-3629909, chhsu@ccms.ntu.edu.tw. Ed. Chia Hung Hsu. R&P Chia Huang Hsu. Circ: 500.

CHOWANNA. see *EDUCATION*

150 ESP ISSN 1135-5956
CIENCIA PSICOLOGICA. Text in Spanish. 1995. s-a. bibl. **Document type:** *Academic/Scholarly.* **Description:** Publishes scientific articles from the world of psychology and related sciences.
Indexed: e-psyche.
—CINDOC.
Published by: Colegio Oficial de Psicologos, Delegacion de Extremadura, Apdo. de Correos 1, Badajoz 06080, Spain. TEL 34-924-317660, FAX 34-924-312015, recisico@ba.unex.es, http://www.cop.es/publicaciones/cpsicolo.

CLASSIFICATION LITERATURE AUTOMATED SEARCH SERVICE. see *MATHEMATICS*

150.19 ESP ISSN 0210-0657
RC475
CLINICA Y ANALISIS GRUPAL; revista de psicoterapia, psicoanalisis y grupo. Text in Spanish; Summaries in English, French. 1976. 3/yr. ESP 7,000 domestic; USD 100 in Europe; USD 120 elsewhere (effective 2000). adv. bk.rev. index. back issues avail. **Document type:** *Academic/Scholarly.*
Indexed: PsycInfo, Psychol.Abstr. (1984-), e-psyche.
—CINDOC.
Published by: Imago Clinica Psicoanalitica, Oquendo, 14 B, Madrid 28006, Spain. TEL 34-91-411-2020, FAX 34-91-745-2630, isanfeliu@nexo.es. Ed. Isabel Sanfeliu. Adv. contact Nicolas Caparros. Circ: 1,500.

158 ESP ISSN 1130-5274
CLINICA Y SALUD; revista de psicologia clinica y salud. Text in Spanish. 1990. q. adv. abstr, bibl. back issues avail. **Document type:** *Academic/Scholarly.* **Description:** Includes articles and tips on psychology and general health for clinical psychologists to incorporate into their practices.
Indexed: PsycInfo, e-psyche.
—CINDOC.
Published by: Colegio Oficial de Psicologos de Madrid, Cuesta de San Vicente, 4 6o, Madrid 28008, Spain. TEL 34-91-541-8504, FAX 34-91-559-0303, dmadrid2@correo.cop.es, http://www.cop.es/publicaciones/clinica. Ed. Alejandro Avila Espada.

▼ **CLINICAL CASE STUDIES.** see *MEDICAL SCIENCES—Psychiatry And Neurology*

155 USA ISSN 1096-4037
RJ503.3 CODEN: CCFPFB
CLINICAL CHILD AND FAMILY PSYCHOLOGY REVIEW. Text in English. 1998. q. USD 45 in the Americas to individuals for print or online ed.; EUR 45 elsewhere to individuals for print or online ed.; USD 180 in the Americas to institutions for print or online ed.; EUR 179 elsewhere to institutions for print or online ed.; USD 216 in the Americas to institutions for print & online eds. combined; EUR 214.80 elsewhere to institutions for print & online eds. combined (effective 2002). *Refereed.* **Document type:** *Journal, Academic/Scholarly.* **Description:** Covers behavioral issues concerning infants, children, adolescents, and families. Publishes research, review articles, position papers, and conceptual and theoretical articles that explore the psychological treatment of these special populations.
Related titles: Online - full text ed.: (from EBSCO Publishing, O C L C Online Computer Library Center, Inc., Swets Blackwell, Kluwer Online, RoweCom Information Quest).
Indexed: Ind.Med., PsycInfo, e-psyche.
—BLDSC (3286.268350), Infotrieve, ingenta. **CCC.**
Published by: Kluwer Academic - Plenum Publishers (Subsidiary of: Wolters Kluwer N.V.), 233 Spring St, New York, NY 10013-1578. TEL 212-620-8000, 800-221-9369, FAX 212-463-0742, services@wkap.nl, info@plenum.com, http://www.wkap.nl/journalhome.htm/1096-4037. Eds. Ronald J Prinz, Thomas H Ollendick. R&P Rose Luongo TEL 781-871-6311. **Subscr. outside the Americas to:** Kluwer Academic Publishers Group, Journals Department, PO Box 322, Dordrecht 3300 AH, Netherlands. TEL 31-78-639-2392, FAX 31-78-654-6474.

CLINICAL CHILD PSYCHOLOGY & PSYCHIATRY. see *CHILDREN AND YOUTH—About*

616.89 USA ISSN 0009-9244
BF1
THE CLINICAL PSYCHOLOGIST. Text in English. 1946. q. USD 30 in United States to institutions; USD 35 in Canada to institutions; USD 40 elsewhere to institutions (effective 2000). adv. *Refereed.* **Document type:** *Bulletin.*
Indexed: Psychol.Abstr., Psycscan C.P., Rehabil.Lit., e-psyche.
—BLDSC (3286.343000), CISTI.
Published by: American Psychological Association, Division of Clinical Psychology, PO Box 1082, Niwot, CO 80544-1082. TEL 303-652-3126. Ed. Paul D Rokke. R&P, Adv. contact Lynn Peterson. Circ: 6,250.

616.86 GBR ISSN 1473-8279
CODEN: CPFOFV
CLINICAL PSYCHOLOGY. Text in English. 1986. m. GBP 30 to individuals; GBP 60 to institutions. reprint service avail. from ISI. *Refereed.*
Formerly (until May 2001): Clinical Psychology Forum (0269-0144)
Indexed: e-psyche.
—BLDSC (3286.344000).
Published by: The British Psychological Society, St Andrews House, 48 Princess Rd E, Leicester LE1 7DR, United Kingdom. TEL 44-116-254-9568, FAX 44-116-247-0787, ezbp001@ulcc.ac.uk. Ed. Craig Wewyes.

P

616.89 USA ISSN 0969-5893
RC467

CLINICAL PSYCHOLOGY; science and practice. Text in English. 1994. q. GBP 60, USD 95 to individuals; GBP 175, USD 280 to institutions (effective Feb. 2002). adv. bk.rev. illus. Index. back issues avail.; reprints avail. *Refereed.* **Document type:** *Journal, Academic/Scholarly.* **Description:** Publishes topical reviews of research, theory and application, including assessment, intervention, service delivery, and professional issues.

Related titles: Online - full text ed.: ISSN 1468-2850. GBP 157, USD 252 to institutions Online only (effective Feb. 2002) (from EBSCO Publishing, O C L C Online Computer Library Center, Inc., RoweCom Information Quest, HighWire Pr., ingenta, Swets Blackwell, Institute for Scientific Information).

Indexed: ASCA, AgeLine, Curr.Cont., PsycInfo, Psycscan C.P., SSCI, e-psyche.

—BLDSC (3286.343400), IDS, Infotrieve. **CCC.**

Published by: (American Psychological Association), Oxford University Press, Academic Division, Great Clarendon St, Oxford OX2 6DP, United Kingdom. TEL 44-1865-267907, FAX 44-1865-267835, jnl.info@oup.co.uk, http://www.oup.co.uk/journals. Ed. D H Barlow. Pub. Erich Staib. adv.: B&W page GBP 700, B&W page USD 1,260; 165 x 215. Circ: 6,000. **Subscr outside N. Americas to:** Journals Marketing, Great Clarendon St, Oxford OX2 6DP, United Kingdom.

616.89 GBR ISSN 1063-3995
CODEN: CPPSEO

CLINICAL PSYCHOLOGY & PSYCHOTHERAPY; an international journal of theory and practice. Text in English. 1993. 5/yr. USD 520 in United States; USD 520 in Canada & Mexico; USD 520 elsewhere; USD 546 combined subscription in United States for print and online eds.; USD 546 combined subscription in Canada & Mexico for print and online eds.; USD 546 combined subscription elsewhere for print and online eds. (effective 2002). adv. back issues avail.; reprint service avail. from SWZ,PSC,SCH. *Refereed.* **Document type:** *Academic/Scholarly.* **Description:** Presents papers on various presentations within clinical psychology and psychotherapy, with special emphasis on theoretical papers outlining innovations within existing approaches.

Related titles: Microform ed.: (from PQC); Online - full text ed.: ISSN 1099-0879. 1997. USD 520 in United States; USD 520 in Canada & Mexico; USD 520 elsewhere (effective 2002) (from EBSCO Publishing, Wiley InterScience, Institute for Scientific Information).

Indexed: ASCA, AgeLine, Curr.Cont., Fam.Ind., SSCI, e-psyche.

—BLDSC (3286.343500), GNLM, IDS, Infotrieve. **CCC.**

Published by: Wiley Europe Ltd., Baffins Ln, Chichester, W Sussex PO19 1UD, United Kingdom. TEL 44-1243-779777, FAX 44-1243-775878, customer@wiley.co.uk, http://www.interscience.wiley.com/jpages/1063-3995/, http://www.wiley.co.uk. adv.: B&W page GBP 650, color page GBP 1,550; trim 200 x 260. Circ: 500. **Subscr. to:** John Wiley & Sons, Inc., Journals, 605 Third Ave, New York, NY 10158. TEL 212-850-6021, 212-850-6645, subinfo@jwiley.com.

616.89 GBR ISSN 0272-7358
RC467 CODEN: CPSRDZ

CLINICAL PSYCHOLOGY REVIEW. Text in English. 1981. 8/yr. EUR 197 in Europe to individuals; JPY 26,100 in Japan to individuals; USD 221 elsewhere to individuals; EUR 880 in Europe to institutions; JPY 116,800 in Japan to institutions; USD 984 elsewhere to institutions (effective 2002). adv. bk.rev. illus. back issues avail.; reprint service avail. from PSC,SCH. *Refereed.* **Document type:** *Academic/Scholarly.* **Description:** Publishes original research and reviews on topics germane to clinical psychology, including psychopathology, psychotherapy, community mental health, behavioral medicine and child development.

Related titles: Microfilm ed.: (from PQC); Online - full text ed.: (from ingenta, Swets Blackwell, ScienceDirect, Institute for Scientific Information).

Indexed: Abstr.Crim.& Pen., AgeLine, Crim.Just.Abstr., Curr.Cont., Dok.Arbeitsmed., Excerp.Med., Fam.Ind., Ind.Med. (1981-), PsycInfo, Psychol.Abstr. (1981-), Psycscan C.P., SSCI, e-psyche.

—BLDSC (3286.345500), EMDOCS, GNLM, IDS, ingenta, KNAW. **CCC.**

Published by: Pergamon (Subsidiary of: Elsevier Science), The Boulevard, Langford Ln, East Park, Kidlington, Oxford OXB 1GB, United Kingdom. FAX 44-1865-843010, http://www.elsevier.com/locate/clinpsychrev. Eds. Alan S Bellack, Michel Hersen. adv.: B&W page USD 550, color page USD 1,350. **Subscr. in Australasia and the Far East to:** Elsevier Science (Singapore) Pte Ltd, No.1 Temasek Ave, 17-01 Millenia Tower, Singapore 039192, Singapore. TEL 65-434-3727, FAX 65-337-2230; **Subscr. in the Americas to:** Elsevier Science, PO Box 945, New York, NY 10159-0945. TEL 212-633-3730, FAX 212-633-3680, usinfo-f@elsevier.com, http://www.elsevier.com; **Subscr. to:** Elsevier Science BV, PO Box 211, Amsterdam 1000 AE, Netherlands. TEL 31-20-485-3757, FAX 31-20-485-3432, nlinfo-f@elsevier.nl, http://www.elsevier.nl.

CLINICAL SOCIOLOGY: RESEARCH AND PRACTICE. see *SOCIAL SCIENCES: COMPREHENSIVE WORKS*

152 USA ISSN 8756-3207

CLINICIAN'S RESEARCH DIGEST; Briefings in Behavioral Science. Text in English. 1983. m. USD 87 domestic to non-members; USD 127 foreign to non-members; USD 48 domestic to members; USD 66 foreign to members; USD 131 domestic to institutions; USD 219 foreign to institutions (effective 2001). adv. *Refereed.* **Document type:** *Newsletter.* **Description:** Highlights current information on clinical research and professional practice in a concise manner.

Indexed: e-psyche.

Published by: American Psychological Association, 750 First St., N.E., Washington, DC 20002-4242. TEL 202-336-5600, 800-374-2721, FAX 202-336-5568, subscriptions@apa.org, http://www.apa.org/journals/crd.html. Ed. Jane Goodman-Delahunty. Circ: 5,200.

150 USA

CLINICIAN'S TOOLBOX. Text in English. irreg. **Document type:** *Monographic series.* **Description:** Consists of ready-to-use books, manuals and computer programs designed for working practitioners.

Indexed: e-psyche.

Published by: Guilford Publications, Inc., 72 Spring St, New York, NY 10012. TEL 212-431-9800, 800-365-7006, FAX 212-966-6708, info@guilford.com, http://www.guilford.com. Ed. Edward L Zuckerman.

616.89 FRA ISSN 1281-6124

CLINIQUE PSYCHANALITIQUE ET PSYCHO-PATHOLOGIE. Text in French. 1988. a. adv. 200 p./no. **Document type:** *Academic/Scholarly.* **Description:** Studies practical observations, clinical interventions.

Formerly: Annales des Cliniques Psychologiques (0992-5481)

Indexed: e-psyche.

Published by: (Laboratoire de Cliniques Psychologiques), Presses Universitaires de Rennes, Campus Rennes 2 - La Harpe, 2 rue du Doyen D. Leroy, Rennes Cedex 35044, France. TEL 33-2-99141401, FAX 33-2-99141407. Eds. Francois Sauvagnat, Laurent Ottavi. Adv. contact Jerome Besin.

COGNITIO; Kognitions- und neurowissenschaftliche Beitraege zur natuerlichen Sprachverarbeitung. see *LINGUISTICS*

153.4 NLD ISSN 0010-0277
BF311 CODEN: CGTNAU

COGNITION; international journal of cognitive psychology. Text in English; Summaries in French. 1972. m. EUR 192 in Europe to qualified personnel; JPY 25,600 in Japan to qualified personnel; USD 215 elsewhere to qualified personnel; EUR 1,070 in Europe to institutions; JPY 142,000 in Japan to institutions; USD 1,196 elsewhere to institutions (effective 2002). adv. bibl. charts, illus. index. back issues avail.; reprint service avail. from SWZ,PSC,SCH. *Refereed.* **Document type:** *Journal, Academic/Scholarly.* **Description:** Publishes theoretical and experimental papers covering all aspects of the study of the mind. Includes research papers in the fields of psychology, linguistics, neuroscience, ethology, philosophy and epistemology.

Related titles: Microform ed.: (from PQC); Online - full text ed.: (from ingenta, Swets Blackwell, ScienceDirect, Institute for Scientific Information).

Indexed: A.I.Abstr., AMED, Adol.Ment.Hlth.Abstr., Arts & Hum.Cit.Ind. (coverage dropped), Bibl.Ling., Biol.Abstr., CAD CAM Abstr., C.I.J.E., Child Devel.Abstr., Cont.Pg.Educ., Curr.Cont., Eng.Ind., IBR, Ind.Med. (1972-), Intl.Bibl.Soc.Sci., Lang.& Lang.Behav.Abstr., Lang.Teach.& Ling.Abstr., Ling.Abstr., M.L.A., MLA Intl.Bibl., Neurosci.Abstr. (coverage dropped), Phil.Ind., PsycInfo, Psychol.Abstr. (1972-), Russ.Acad.Sci.Bibl., SOPODA, SSCI, Sci.Cit.Ind. (coverage dropped), Sociol.Abstr., e-psyche.

—BLDSC (3292.870000), IDS, ingenta. **CCC.**

Published by: Elsevier Science BV, PO Box 211, Amsterdam 1000 AE, Netherlands. TEL 31-20-485-3757, FAX 31-20-485-3432, TELEX 18582 ESPA NL, nlinfo-f@elsevier.nl, http://www.elsevier.com/locate/cognit, http://www.elsevier.nl. Eds. Jacques Mehler, Thomas G Bever. **Subscr. in Australasia and the Far East to:** Elsevier Science (Singapore) Pte Ltd, No.1 Temasek Ave, 17-01 Millenia Tower, Singapore 039192, Singapore. TEL 65-434-3727, FAX 65-337-2230, asiainfo@elsevier.com.sg; **Subscr. in Japan to:** Elsevier Science Inc - Japan Regional Office, 9-15 Higashi-Azabu 1-chome, Minato-ku, Tokyo 106-0044, Japan. TEL 81-3-5561-5033, FAX 81-3-5561-5047, info@elsevier.co.jp; **Subscr. in the Americas to:** Elsevier Science, PO Box 945, New York, NY 10159-0945. TEL 212-633-3730, 888-437-4636, FAX 212-633-3680, usinfo-f@elsevier.com, http://www.elsevier.com. **Dist. by:** Elsevier Science (Brazil).

301.1 150 USA ISSN 0269-9931
BF309 CODEN: COEMEC

COGNITION AND EMOTION. Text in English. 1987. bi-m. GBP 140, USD 232 to individuals; GBP 369, USD 608 to institutions (effective 2002). adv. bk.rev. back issues avail. *Refereed.* **Document type:** *Academic/Scholarly.* **Description:** Explores the interrelationship of cognition and emotion.

Related titles: Online - full text ed.: ISSN 1464-0600 (from CatchWord Ltd., EBSCO Publishing, O C L C Online Computer Library Center, Inc., RoweCom Information Quest, Swets Blackwell, Institute for Scientific Information).

Indexed: ASCA, ASSIA, Arts & Hum.Cit.Ind. (coverage dropped), Curr.Cont., ERA, Fam.Ind., Lang.& Lang.Behav.Abstr., PsycInfo, Psychol.Abstr. (1987-), Russ.Acad.Sci.Bibl., SOPODA, SSCI, Soc.Serv.Abstr., Sociol.Abstr., Stud.Wom.Abstr., e-psyche.

—BLDSC (3292.871500), CatchWord, GNLM, IDS, ingenta. **CCC.**

Published by: Psychology Press (Subsidiary of: Taylor & Francis Ltd.), 325 Chestnut St, Ste 800, Philadelphia, PA 19106. TEL 215-625-8900, FAX 215-625-2940, info@taylorandfrancis.com, http://www.journals.tandf.co.uk/journals/pp/0269931.html, http://www.psypress.com/. Ed. Craig Smith. Circ: 1,000. **Subscr. addr. outside N America:** Psychology Press, Journals Customer Service, Taylor & Francis Group, Rankine Rd, Basingstoke, Hants RG24 8PR, United Kingdom. TEL 44-1256-813002, FAX 44-1256-479438, enquiry@tandf.co.uk.

370.152 USA ISSN 0737-0008
LB1060

COGNITION AND INSTRUCTION. Text in English. 1984. q. USD 45 in US & Canada to individuals; USD 75 elsewhere to individuals; USD 365 in US & Canada to institutions; USD 395 elsewhere to institutions (effective 2002). adv. *Refereed.* **Document type:** *Journal, Academic/Scholarly.* **Description:** Interdisciplinary journal devoted to cognitive investigations of instruction and learning.

Related titles: Online - full text ed.: ISSN 1532-690X. USD 40.50 to individuals; USD 328.50 to institutions (effective 2002) (from CatchWord Ltd., EBSCO Publishing, O C L C Online Computer Library Center, Inc., RoweCom Information Quest, Swets Blackwell, Institute for Scientific Information).

Indexed: ASCA, Abstr.Hum.Comp.Inter., Arts & Hum.Cit.Ind. (coverage dropped), C.I.J.E., Chic.Per.Ind., Child Devel.Abstr., Cont.Pg.Educ., Curr.Cont., ERA, Educ.Ind. (Jul.1992-), Educ.Tech.Abstr., Lang.& Lang.Behav.Abstr., PsycInfo, Psychol.Abstr. (1985-), SOPODA, SSCI, Sociol.Abstr., Sp.Ed.Needs Abstr., Tech.Educ.Abstr., e-psyche.

—BLDSC (3292.872000), CatchWord, Infotrieve, ingenta. **CCC.**

Published by: Lawrence Erlbaum Associates, Inc., 10 Industrial Ave, Mahwah, NJ 07430-2262. TEL 201-760-3735, 800-926-6579, FAX 201-236-0072, journals@erlbaum.com, http://www.erlbaum.com/Journals/journals/CI/ci.htm. Eds. Deborah McCutchen, Ralph Putnam. adv.: page USD 450; trim 5 x 8.

COGNITION AND LANGUAGE; a series in psycholinguistics. see *LINGUISTICS*

153.4 GBR ISSN 1435-5558

▼ **COGNITION, TECHNOLOGY AND WORK.** Text in English. 1999. q. EUR 191, EUR 188.70; EUR 54 newsstand/cover (effective 2002). **Document type:** *Academic/Scholarly.* **Description:** An international journal for the analysis, design and use of joint cognitive systems.

Related titles: Online - full text ed.: ISSN 1435-5566 (from EBSCO Publishing, RoweCom Information Quest, Swets Blackwell, Springer LINK).

Indexed: Ergon.Abstr., INSPEC (1999-), e-psyche.
—BLDSC (3292.872650).
Published by: Springer-Verlag London Ltd. (Subsidiary of: BertelsmannSpringer), Sweetapple House, Catteshall Rd, Godalming, Surrey GU7 3DJ, United Kingdom. TEL 44-1483-418800, FAX 44-1483-415144, alex@svl.co.uk, http://link.springer.de. Eds. Erik Hollnagel, Pietro Cacciabue.

150 ESP ISSN 0214-3550
COGNITIVA. Text in English, Spanish. 1988. s-a. ESP 3,200 per issue (effective 1999). adv. *Refereed.* **Document type:** *Academic/Scholarly.* **Description:** Publishes original empirical and theoretical contributions concerning human cognitive processes.
Related titles: Online - full text ed.: (from CatchWord Ltd.).
Indexed: PsycInfo, Psychol.Abstr., e-psyche.
—CINDOC.
Published by: Fundacion Infancia y Aprendizaje, Ctra. de Canillas 138, 16C, Madrid 28043, Spain. TEL 34-91-388-3874, FAX 34-91-300-3527. Ed. Manuel de Vega. Circ: 1,100.

152.05 USA ISSN 1530-7026
QP360 CODEN: PSYBEC
COGNITIVE, AFFECTIVE, & BEHAVIORAL NEUROSCIENCE. Text in English. 1973. q. USD 104 to individuals; USD 112 foreign to individuals; USD 98.80 to institutions; USD 106.80 foreign to institutions (effective 1999 - 2000). adv. illus. back issues avail.; reprint service avail. from PQC,PSC,SCH. *Refereed.* **Document type:** *Journal, Academic/Scholarly.* **Description:** Publishes original research articles and reviews in the disciplines of cognitive neuroscience and affective neuroscience. Focuses on behavior and brain processes in humans, both normal subjects and patients with brain injury.
Former titles (until 2001): Psychobiology (0889-6313); (until 1987): Physiological Psychology (0090-5046)
Related titles: Microform ed.: (from NRP,PQC); Online - full content ed.: ISSN 1531-135X; Online - full text ed.: (from CatchWord Ltd., Institute for Scientific Information).
Indexed: ASCA, Biol.Abstr., Chem.Abstr., Chem.Titles, Curr.Adv.Ecol.Sci., Curr.Cont., Dairy Sci.Abstr., Ergon.Abstr., Excerp.Med., IBR, IBZ, Ind.Philos., Ind.Sci.Rev., Inpharma, Int.Abstr.Biol.Sci., Neurosci.Abstr. (coverage dropped), Neurosci.Cit.Ind., Nutr.Abstr., PsycInfo, Psychol.Abstr. (1973-), Reac., Russ.Acad.Sci.Bibl., SSCI, Sci.Cit.Ind., e-psyche.
—BLDSC (6946.276530), CASDDS, CISTI, EMDOCS, GNLM, IDS, Infotrieve, KNAW. **CCC.**
Published by: Psychonomic Society, Inc., 1710 Fortview Rd, Austin, TX 78704. TEL 512-462-2442, FAX 512-462-1101, psysoc@sig.net, jbellquist@psychonomic.org, http://www.sig.net/~psysoc/home.htm, http://www.psychonomic.org. Ed. John Jonides. R&P Cinnamon Nemec. Adv. contact Robert Sanford. page USD 105; trim 10.75 x 8. Circ: 1,120.

158 USA ISSN 1077-7229
RC489.B4 CODEN: CBPRFQ
COGNITIVE AND BEHAVIORAL PRACTICE. Text in English. 1994. q. USD 145 domestic (effective 2001); USD 163 in Canada & Mexico; USD 183 elsewhere (2001). adv. *Refereed.* **Document type:** *Academic/Scholarly.* **Description:** Interdisciplinary journal that presents treatment techniques that have been empirically validated. Covers behavior therapy and cognitive therapy.
Related titles: Online - full text ed.: (from Institute for Scientific Information).
Indexed: ASCA, AgeLine, Curr.Cont., Excerp.Med. (1996-), PsycInfo, SSCI, e-psyche.
—BLDSC (3292.872900), EMDOCS, Infotrieve. **CCC.**
Published by: Association for Advancement of Behavior Therapy, 305 Seventh Ave, Ste 16A, New York, NY 10001. TEL 212-647-1890, FAX 212-647-1865. Ed. Anne Marie Albano. Pub. David Teisler. R&P Teresa Wimmer. Adv. contact Stephanie Schwartz. B&W page USD 275.

THE COGNITIVE BEHAVIOURAL SOCIAL WORK REVIEW. see *SOCIAL SERVICES AND WELFARE*

370.15 150 GBR ISSN 0885-2014
BF1 CODEN: CODEFI
COGNITIVE DEVELOPMENT. Text in English. 1986. q. EUR 103 in Europe to individuals; JPY 13,600 in Japan to individuals; USD 115 elsewhere to individuals; EUR 246 in Europe to institutions; JPY 32,600 in Japan to institutions; USD 275 elsewhere to institutions (effective 2002). adv. bk.rev. illus. index. back issues avail.; reprint service avail. from PSC,SCH,ISI. *Refereed.* **Document type:** *Academic/Scholarly.* **Description:** Examines the development of perception, memory, language, concepts, thinking, problem solving, metacognition, and social cognition.
Related titles: Online - full text ed.: (from ingenta, Swets Blackwell, ScienceDirect, Institute for Scientific Information).
Indexed: ASCA, C.I.J.E., Child Devel.Abstr., Curr.Cont., Indian Psychol.Abstr., Lang.& Lang.Behav.Abstr., PsycInfo, Psychol.Abstr. (1983-), Russ.Acad.Sci.Bibl., SOPODA, SSCI, Sociol.Abstr., e-psyche.
—BLDSC (3292.876600), ingenta. **CCC.**
Published by: Elsevier Science, The Boulevard, Langford Ln, Kidlington, Oxon OX5 1GB, United Kingdom. TEL 44-1865-843000, FAX 44-1865-843010, nlinfo-f@elsevier.nl; usinfo-f@elsevier.com; forinfo-ky04035@niftyserve.or.jp, http://www.elsevier.com/locate/cogdev, http://www.elsevier.com/locate/cogdedv. Ed. Peter Bryant. Circ: 500. **Subscr. in Australasia and the Far East to:** Elsevier Science (Singapore) Pte Ltd, No.1 Temasek Ave, 17-01 Millenia Tower, Singapore 039192, Singapore. TEL 65-434-3727, FAX 65-337-2230; **Subscr. in the Americas to:** Elsevier Science, PO Box 945, New York, NY 10159-0945. TEL 212-633-3730, FAX 212-633-3680; **Subscr. to:** Elsevier Science BV, PO Box 211, Amsterdam 1000 AE, Netherlands. TEL 31-20-485-3757, FAX 31-20-485-3432, nlinfo-f@elsevier.nl.

COGNITIVE LINGUISTICS. see *LINGUISTICS*

COGNITIVE LINGUISTICS RESEARCH. see *LINGUISTICS*

616.89 GBR ISSN 1354-6805
QP360
COGNITIVE NEUROPSYCHIATRY. Text in English. 1996. q. USD 118, GBP 71 to individuals; USD 242, GBP 147 to institutions (effective 2002). adv. **Document type:** *Academic/Scholarly.* **Description:** Promotes the study of cognitive processes underlying psychological and behavioral abnormalities, including psychotic symptoms, with and without organic brain disease.
Related titles: Online - full text ed.: ISSN 1464-0619 (from CatchWord Ltd., EBSCO Publishing, O C L C Online Computer Library Center, Inc., RoweCom Information Quest, Swets Blackwell).
Indexed: e-psyche.
—BLDSC (3292.878800), CatchWord, GNLM.
Published by: Psychology Press (Subsidiary of: Taylor & Francis Group), 27 Church Rd, Hove, E Sussex BN3 2FA, United Kingdom. TEL 44-1273-207411, FAX 44-1273-205612, information@psypress.co.uk, http://www.journals.tandf.co.uk/journals/pp/13546805.html, http://www.psypress.co.uk. Eds. Anthony S David, Peter W Halligan. R&P Zoe Peden TEL 44-20-7842-2363. Adv. contact Claire Buckminster. **Subscr. addr. in N America:** Psychology Press, Journals Customer Service, Taylor & Francis Group, 325 Chestnut St, Philadelphia, PA 19106. TEL 800-354-1420, FAX 215-625-8914, info@taylorandfrancis.com, http://www.psypress.com.

153.4 USA ISSN 0010-0285
BF309 CODEN: CGPSBQ
COGNITIVE PSYCHOLOGY. Text in English. 1970. 8/yr. USD 475 in US & Canada to institutions; USD 520 elsewhere to institutions (effective 2001). adv. abstr, bibl, charts, stat, illus. back issues avail.; reprint service avail. from SWZ,PSC,SCH. *Refereed.* **Document type:** *Academic/Scholarly.* **Description:** Concerned with advances in the study of memory, language processing, perception, problem solving, and thinking. Presents original empirical, theoretical, and tutorial papers, methodological articles, and critical reviews.
Related titles: Online - full text ed.: (from EBSCO Publishing, O C L C Online Computer Library Center, Inc., RoweCom Information Quest, ingenta, Gale Group, Swets Blackwell, IDEAL Online Library, Factiva, Institute for Scientific Information).
Indexed: ASCA, Adol.Ment.Hlth.Abstr., C.I.J.E., Child Devel.Abstr., Commun.Abstr., Curr.Cont., Educ.Ind. (Jul.1992-), Ergon.Abstr., IBZ, INSPEC (Jul.1971-Oct.1986, dropped), Ind.Med. (1970-), Ind.Philos., Lang.& Lang.Behav.Abstr., M.L.A., MLA Intl.Bibl., Mid.East: Abstr.& Ind., Neurosci.Cit.Ind., PsycInfo, Psychol.Abstr. (1970-), Psycscan D.P., Russ.Acad.Sci.Bibl., SOPODA, SSCI, Soc.Sci.Ind. (Oct.1982-), Sociol.Abstr., e-psyche.
—BLDSC (3292.880000), IDS, ingenta. **CCC.**
Published by: Academic Press, Inc., Journal Division (Subsidiary of: Harcourt Brace & Company), 525 B St, Ste 1900, San Diego, CA 92101-4495. TEL 619-230-1840, FAX 619-699-6800, apsubs@acad.com, http://www.academicpress.com/cogpsych. Ed. Keith Holyoak.

020 410 GBR ISSN 0364-0213
BF311 CODEN: COGSD5
COGNITIVE SCIENCE; a multidisciplinary journal of artificial intelligence, linguistics, neuroscience, philosophy and psychology. Text in English. 1977. bi-m. EUR 125 in Europe to individuals; JPY 16,500 in Japan to individuals; USD 140 elsewhere to individuals; EUR 299 in Europe to institutions; JPY 39,700 in Japan to institutions; USD 335 elsewhere to institutions (effective 2002). adv. illus. index. back issues avail.; reprint service avail. from ISI. *Refereed.* **Document type:** *Academic/Scholarly.* **Description:** Publishes articles on such topics as knowledge representation, inference, memory process, learning, problem solving, planning, perception, natural language understanding, connectionism, brain theory, motor control, intentional systems, and other areas of multidisciplinary concern.
Related titles: Online - full text ed.: (from ingenta, Gale Group, Swets Blackwell, ScienceDirect, Institute for Scientific Information).
Indexed: A.I.Abstr., ASCA, Abstr.Anthropol., Abstr.Hum.Comp.Inter., Art.Int.Abstr., Bibl.Ling., CAD CAM Abstr., C.I.J.E. (coverage dropped), Compumath, Curr.Cont., Ergon.Abstr., Excerp.Med., INSPEC (Jan.1987-), Ind.Philos., Intl.Bibl.Soc.Sci., Lang.& Lang.Behav.Abstr., M.L.A., MLA Intl.Bibl., PsycInfo, Psychol.Abstr. (1977-), Russ.Acad.Sci.Bibl., SOPODA, SSCI, Sociol.Abstr., e-psyche.
—BLDSC (3292.885000), AskIEEE, CISTI, ingenta. **CCC.**
Published by: Elsevier Science, The Boulevard, Langford Ln, Kidlington, Oxon OX5 1GB, United Kingdom. TEL 44-1865-843000, FAX 44-1865-843010, http://www.elsevier.com/locate/cogsci. Circ: 2,400.

153 FRA ISSN 1466-6553
▼ **COGNITIVE SCIENCE QUARTERLY.** Text in English. 2000. q. EUR 50 in Europe to individuals; EUR 70 elsewhere to individuals; EUR 180 in Europe to institutions; EUR 195 elsewhere to institutions (effective 2000).
—BLDSC (3292.885300).
Published by: (University of Freiburg DEU), Hermes Science Publications, 8, quai du Marche-Neuf, Paris 75004, France. FAX 33-1-53101521, hermes@iway.fr, http://www.iig.uni-freiburg.de/cognition/csq, http://www.hermes-science.com. Ed. Gerhard Strube.

301.1 USA ISSN 0732-1295
COGNITIVE SCIENCE SERIES (CAMBRIDGE). Text in English. irreg., latest vol.9, 1989. price varies. adv. *Refereed.* **Document type:** *Monographic series.*
Indexed: e-psyche.
Published by: Harvard University Press, 79 Garden St, Cambridge, MA 02138. TEL 617-495-2600, FAX 617-495-5898, http://www.hup.harvard.edu. R&P Mindy Koyanis TEL 617-495-2619. Adv. contact Denise Waddington.

150 USA
COGNITIVE SCIENCE SERIES: TECHNICAL MONOGRAPHS AND EDITED COLLECTIONS. Text in English. 1981. irreg., latest vol.13, 1991. USD 99.95. bibl, charts, illus. *Refereed.* **Document type:** *Monographic series.*
Indexed: Curr.Cont. (coverage dropped), Psychol.Abstr., e-psyche.
Published by: Lawrence Erlbaum Associates, Inc., 10 Industrial Ave, Mahwah, NJ 07430-2262. TEL 201-236-9500, FAX 201-236-0072, journals@erlbaum, http://www.erlbaum.com. Ed. Andrew Ortony.

153 USA
BF311
COGNITIVE SCIENCE SOCIETY. ANNUAL CONFERENCE. PROCEEDINGS. Text in English. 1986. a. adv. **Document type:** *Proceedings.*
Formerly: Cognitive Science Society. Annual Conference. Program (1047-1316)
Indexed: e-psyche.
—BLDSC (6840.278010).
Published by: Lawrence Erlbaum Associates, Inc., 10 Industrial Ave, Mahwah, NJ 07430-2262. TEL 201-236-9500, FAX 201-236-0072, journals@erlbaum.com, http://www.erlbaum.com. Adv. contact Sharon Levy.

P

153 NLD ISSN 0256-663X
COGNITIVE SYSTEMS. Text in Dutch. 1985. irreg. (4 nos./vol.), latest vol.5, 1997. NLG 140. bk.rev. back issues avail. **Document type:** *Academic/Scholarly.*
Indexed: Psychol.Abstr., e-psyche.
—BLDSC (3292.892500).
Published by: European Society for the Study of Cognitive Systems, c/o Dept for Psychology, University of Groningen, PO Box 72, Groningen 9700 AB, Netherlands. FAX 31-50-3636304. Ed. G J Dalenoort. Circ: 60.

150 USA ISSN 0147-5916
BF311 CODEN: CTHRD8
COGNITIVE THERAPY AND RESEARCH. Text in English. 1977. bi-m. USD 80 in the Americas to individuals for print or online ed.; EUR 80 elsewhere to individuals for print or online ed.; USD 699 in the Americas to institutions for print or online ed.; EUR 698 elsewhere to institutions for print or online ed.; USD 838.80 in the Americas to institutions for print & online eds. combined; EUR 837.60 elsewhere to institutions for print & online eds. combined (effective 2002). adv. illus. Index. back issues avail.; reprints avail. *Refereed.* **Document type:** *Journal, Academic/Scholarly.* **Description:** Examines the role of cognitive processes in human adaptation and adjustment, drawing from the divergent fields of cognitive psychology, philosophy of science, and behavioral psychotherapy.
Related titles: Microfilm ed.: (from PQC); Online - full text ed.: (from CatchWord Ltd., EBSCO Publishing, O C L C Online Computer Library Center, Inc., RoweCom Information Quest, Swets Blackwell, Kluwer Online, Institute for Scientific Information).
Indexed: ASCA, Addic.Abstr., Adol.Ment.Hlth.Abstr., AgeLine, Behav.Abstr., Biol.Abstr., Curr.Cont., ERA, Excerp.Med., IMFL, Jrnl.Watch Psych., Mult.Ed.Abstr., PsycInfo, Psychol.Abstr. (1977-), Psycscan C.P., Ref.Zh., SSCI, Sp.Ed.Needs Abstr., e-psyche.
—BLDSC (3292.895000), CatchWord, CISTI, GNLM, IDS, ingenta. **CCC.**
Published by: Kluwer Academic - Plenum Publishers (Subsidiary of: Wolters Kluwer N.V.), 233 Spring St, New York, NY 10013-1578. TEL 212-620-8000, 800-221-9369, FAX 212-463-0742, services@wkap.nl, info@plenum.com, http://www.wkap.nl/journalhome.htm/0147-5916. Ed. Rick E Ingram. R&P Rose Luongo TEL 781-871-6311. **Subscr. outside the Americas to:** Kluwer Academic Publishers Group, Journals Department, PO Box 322, Dordrecht 3300 AH, Netherlands. TEL 31-78-639-2392, FAX 31-78-654-6474.

P

150 ESP
COLEGIO OFICIAL DE PSICOLOGOS DE MADRID. MONOGRAFIA. Text in Spanish. 1995. irreg. ESP 2,500 per issue to non-members; ESP 1,500 per issue to members. back issues avail. **Document type:** *Monographic series.*
Related titles: Online - full text ed.
Indexed: e-psyche.
Published by: Colegio Oficial de Psicologos de Madrid, Cuesta de San Vicente, 4 6o, Madrid 28008, Spain. TEL 34-91-541-7009, FAX 34-91-547-2284, dmadrid@correo.cop.es, http://www.cop.es/publicaciones/monografia/.

150 ESP ISSN 0213-5973
COLEXIO OFICIAL DE PSICOLOGOS DE GALICIA. CADERNOS DE PSICOLXIA. Key Title: Cadernos de Psicolxia. Text in Spanish. 1986. 3/yr. *Refereed.* **Document type:** *Academic/Scholarly.*
Indexed: e-psyche.
—CINDOC.
Published by: Colexio Oficial de Psicologos de Galicia, Rua Espineira, 10 Bajo, Santiago De Compostela 15706, Spain. dgalicia@correo.cop.es, http://www.cop.es/delegaci/cadernos.html. Ed. Elixio Domarco Alvarez.

COLLECTION ORIENTATIONS. see *EDUCATION*

156 FRA ISSN 0993-7536
COLLECTION PSYCHOLOGIE✱. Text in French. irreg. price varies.
Indexed: e-psyche.
Published by: Editions Scientifiques et Psychologiques, c/o Office de Justification de la Diffusion Controle (O J D), 40 Bd. Malesherbes, Paris 75008, France. TEL 46-45-38-12, FAX 40-95-73-32. Ed. T Ego.

152 790.1 FRA
COLLECTION PSYCHOLOGIE ET PEDAGOGIE DU SPORT✱. Text in French. irreg. price varies.
Indexed: e-psyche.
Published by: Editions Scientifiques et Psychologiques, c/o Office de Justification de la Diffusion Controle (O J D), 40 Bd. Malesherbes, Paris 75008, France. TEL 46-45-38-12, FAX 40-95-73-32. Ed. A Vom Hofe.

158.7 FRA ISSN 0981-7727
COLLECTION PSYCHOLOGIE ET PEDAGOGIE DU TRAVAIL✱. Text in French. 1986. irreg. price varies.
Indexed: e-psyche.
Published by: Editions Scientifiques et Psychologiques, c/o Office de Justification de la Diffusion Controle (O J D), 40 Bd. Malesherbes, Paris 75008, France. TEL 46-45-38-12, FAX 40-95-73-32, TELEX 270 105 F. Ed. B Gillet.

156 FRA ISSN 1242-5028
COLLECTION TESTS PSYCHOLOGIQUES✱. Text in French. 1992. irreg. price varies.
Indexed: e-psyche.
Published by: Editions Scientifiques et Psychologiques, c/o Office de Justification de la Diffusion Controle (O J D), 40 Bd. Malesherbes, Paris 75008, France. TEL 46-45-38-12, FAX 40-95-73-32, TELEX 270 104 F. Ed. R Simonnet.

150 CAN
COLLEGE OF PSYCHOLOGISTS OF ONTARIO. BULLETIN. Text in English. 1973. q. CND 15 (effective 1999). index. back issues avail. **Document type:** *Bulletin.* **Description:** Covers professional affairs, discipline, licensing, training and public policy.
Formerly: Ontario Board of Examiners in Psychology. Bulletin
Indexed: e-psyche.
Published by: College of Psychologists of Ontario, 1246 Yonge St, Ste 201, Toronto, ON M4T 1W5, Canada. TEL 416-961-8817, 800-489-8388, FAX 416-961-2635, cpo@cpo.on.ca, http://www.cpo.on.ca. Ed., R&P Dr. Rich Morris. Circ: 2,400 (controlled).

156 109 USA ISSN 0267-9469
COMMENTS & CRITICISMS. Text in English. 1983. irreg. bk.rev. **Document type:** *Academic/Scholarly.*
Indexed: e-psyche.
Published by: Prytaneum Press, 1015 Bryan, Amarillo, TX 79102. TEL 806-372-7888, prytaneumpress@juno.com. Ed. Don D Davis. Circ: 500.

616.89 200 USA ISSN 0885-8500
COMMON BOUNDARY; exploring spirituality, psychotherapy, and creativity. Text in English. 1980. bi-m. USD 24.95; USD 35 foreign (effective 1999). adv. bk.rev. back issues avail. **Document type:** *Consumer.* **Description:** Publishes articles, news, and research for people interested in the relationship of psychology, spirituality and creativity.
Related titles: Microform ed.: (from PQC).
Indexed: Rel.Ind.One, Rel.Ind.Two, e-psyche.
—ingenta.
Published by: Common Boundary, Inc., 4304 East-West Hwy, Bethesda, MD 20814. TEL 301-652-9495, FAX 301-652-0579, connect@commonboundary.org, http://www.commonboundary.org. Ed. Anne A Simpkinson. Pub. Charles Simpkinson. R&P Anne Simpkinson. Adv. contact Geoff Goldstein. B&W page USD 1,240. Circ: 20,000 (paid).

301.1 USA
COMMON GROUND HAWAII✱. Text in English. 4/yr. USD 4. adv.
Indexed: e-psyche.
Address: 750 Amana St, Ste 301, Honolulu, HI 96814-5002. TEL 808-239-7190.

COMMON GROUND (SAN ANSELMO); resources for personal transformation. see *NEW AGE PUBLICATIONS*

370 USA ISSN 0164-775X
COMMUNIQUE (BETHESDA). Text in English. 8/yr. USD 30. adv. bk.rev. **Document type:** *Newsletter.* **Description:** Publishes practical professional articles to help school psychologists. Also includes research, job listings, convention information, organizational news, and legislative updates.
Indexed: e-psyche.
Published by: National Association of School Psychologists, 4340 East West Hwy, Ste 402, Bethesda, MD 20814-4411. TEL 301-657-0270, FAX 301-657-3127, nasp8455@aol.com. Ed. Paul Mendez. Circ: 19,000 (paid).

COMMUNITY MENTAL HEALTH JOURNAL. see *SOCIAL SERVICES AND WELFARE*

COMMUNITY PSYCHIATRY JOURNAL. see *MEDICAL SCIENCES—Psychiatry And Neurology*

370.15 150 ISR
COMMUNITY STRESS PREVENTION. Text in English. 1985. a., latest no.4, 1999. ILS 35 domestic; USD 8 foreign (effective 2001). bk.rev. Index. back issues avail. *Refereed.* **Document type:** *Bulletin, Academic/Scholarly.* **Description:** Covers the work and activities of the Centre.
Formerly: School Psychology Emergency Centre. Newsletter
Indexed: e-psyche.
Published by: Community Stress Prevention Centre Tel Hai College, P O Box 797, Kiryat Shmona 11012, Israel. TEL 972-4-6900891, FAX 972-4-6950740, cspc@isdn.net.il, http://ispc.telhai.ac.il. Eds. Mooli Lahad, Ofra Ayalon. R&P Alan Cohen. Circ: 100.

COMPREHENSIVE PSYCHIATRY. see *MEDICAL SCIENCES—Psychiatry And Neurology*

616.89 CHE ISSN 0275-7222
RC475
COMPREHENSIVE PSYCHOTHERAPY. Text in English. 1980. irreg., latest vol.3, 1984. *Refereed.* **Document type:** *Monographic series.*
Indexed: e-psyche.
—GNLM.
Published by: Gordon and Breach - Harwood Academic (Subsidiary of: Taylor & Francis Group), PO Box 531, Lausanne 1000, Switzerland. Ed. P Olsen. **Subscr. addr. in US:** International Publishers Direct, PO Box 32160, Newark, NJ 07102. FAX 215-750-6343.

COMPUTERS IN HUMAN BEHAVIOR. see *SOCIOLOGY—Computer Applications*

301.1 150 ITA ISSN 0392-7504
BF1
COMUNICAZIONI SCIENTIFICHE DI PSICOLOGIA GENERALE. Text in Italian. 1976. s-a. ITL 66,000 to individuals; ITL 80,000 to institutions.
Formerly (until 1981): Communicazioni Scientifiche della Cattedra di Psicologia Generale IV (0392-7555)
Indexed: Ind.Philos., e-psyche.
Published by: Edizioni Scientifiche Italiane S.p.A., Via Chiatamone, 7, Naples, NA 80121, Italy. TEL 39-81-7645443, FAX 39-81-7646477, esi@dial.it, http://www.dial.it. Ed. Marta Olivetti Belardinelli.

150 USA
CONFESS✱. Text in English. 1996. d. **Description:** Covers embarrassment, guilt, and catharsis.
Media: Online - full text.
Indexed: e-psyche.
Address: 24425 Wax Orchard Rd SW, Vashon, WA 98070-7514. bluesnow@halcyon.com, http://www.fess-up.com. Ed. John Anderson.

347.73 302 USA ISSN 1536-5581
KF9084.A15
CONFLICT RESOLUTION QUARTERLY. Text in English. 1983. q. USD 160 in United States; USD 200 in Canada; USD 234 elsewhere (effective 2002). bk.rev., software rev., video rev. back issues avail.; reprint service avail. from WSH. *Refereed.* **Document type:** *Journal, Academic/Scholarly.* **Description:** Covers the latest developments in the theory and practice of mediation, dispute resolution and conflict resolution.
Formerly (until 2002): Mediation Quarterly (0739-4098)
Related titles: Microfiche ed.: (from PQC); Online - full text ed.: (from O C L C Online Computer Library Center, Inc.).
Indexed: Amer.Bibl.Slavic & E.Eur.Stud., Crim.Just.Abstr., Fam.Ind., Human Resour.Abstr., IMFL, Ind.Per.Art.Relat.Law, Intl.Bibl.Soc.Sci., Lang.& Lang.Behav.Abstr., PsycInfo, Psychol.Abstr. (1983-), SOPODA, Sage Fam.Stud.Abstr., Sage Urb.Stud.Abstr., Soc.Serv.Abstr., Sociol.Abstr., e-psyche.
—BLDSC (5525.380000), ingenta.
Published by: (Association for Conflict Resolution), Jossey-Bass Inc., Publishers (Subsidiary of: John Wiley & Sons, Inc., Journals), 350 Sansome St, San Francisco, CA 94104-1342. TEL 415-433-1740, 888-378-2537, FAX 800-605-2665, 415-433-0499, jbsubs@jbp.com, http://www.josseybass.com. Ed. Tricia S Jones. Pub. Sue Lewis. Circ: 4,000 (paid).

150.9 FRA ISSN 0245-8829
CONFLUENTS PSYCHANALYTIQUES. Text in French. 1980. irreg.
Indexed: e-psyche.
Published by: Societe d'Edition les Belles Lettres, 95 bd. Raspail, Paris 75006, France. TEL 1-45485826, FAX 1-45485860.

CONNECTICUT HOSPICE NEWSLETTER; making today count. see *PHYSICAL FITNESS AND HYGIENE*

302 FRA ISSN 0337-3126
CONNEXIONS. Text in French. 1972. s-a. EUR 46 domestic; EUR 52 foreign (effective 2001).
Former titles (until 199?): Connexions Psychosociologie Sciences Humaines; Connexions - Psychologie - Sciences Humaines
Related titles: Online - full text ed.: (from Northern Light Technology, Inc.).
Indexed: Int.Lab.Doc., Psychol.Abstr., Russ.Acad.Sci.Bibl., e-psyche.
Published by: (Association pour la Recherche et Intervention Psychosociologiques), Editions Eres, 11 rue des Alouettes, Ramonville Saint-Agne 31520, France. TEL 33-5-61751576, FAX 33-5-61735289, eres@editions-eres.com. Ed. Jean Claude Rouchy. **Subscr. to:** Service abonnements, BP16, Fenouillet Cedex 31151, France.

153.4 USA ISSN 1053-8100
BF309 CODEN: COCOF9
CONSCIOUSNESS AND COGNITION; an international journal. Text in English. 1992. q. USD 320 in US & Canada to institutions; USD 425 elsewhere to institutions (effective 2001). bk.rev. back issues avail. *Refereed.* **Document type:** *Academic/Scholarly.* **Description:** Provides a forum for a natural-science approach to the issues of consciousness, voluntary control, and self. Features two types of articles: empirical research (in the form of regular articles and short reports) and theoretical articles.
Related titles: Online - full text ed.: (from EBSCO Publishing, O C L C Online Computer Library Center, Inc., RoweCom Information Quest, ingenta, Swets Blackwell, IDEAL Online Library, Institute for Scientific Information).
Indexed: ASCA, AgeLine, Arts & Hum.Cit.Ind. (coverage dropped), Chem.Abstr., Curr.Cont., Ind.Med. (1992-), Lang.& Lang.Behav.Abstr., PsycInfo, Psychol.Abstr. (1992-), SOPODA, SSCI, Sociol.Abstr., e-psyche.
—BLDSC (3417.864800), ADONIS, GNLM, IDS, ingenta. **CCC.**
Published by: Academic Press, Inc., Journal Division (Subsidiary of: Harcourt Brace & Company), 525 B St, Ste 1900, San Diego, CA 92101-4495. TEL 619-230-1840, FAX 619-699-6800, apsubs@acad.com, http://www.academicpress.concog. Eds. Bernard Baars, William Banks.

152.4 NLD ISSN 1566-5836
▼ **CONSCIOUSNESS & EMOTION.** Text in English. 2000. s-a., latest vol.2, 2001. EUR 150 (effective 2002). back issues avail. *Refereed.* **Document type:** *Journal, Academic/Scholarly.* **Description:** Presents thoughtful analysis of the implications of both empirical and experiential (eg, clinical psychological) approaches to emotion.
Related titles: Online - full content ed.: 2000. included with institutional subscr (from ingenta).
—BLDSC (3417.864900).
Published by: John Benjamins Publishing Co., PO Box 36224, Amsterdam 1020 ME, Netherlands. TEL 31-20-630-4747, FAX 31-20-673-9773, subscriptions@benjamins.nl, http://www.benjamins.nl/jbp/journals/C&e_info.html, http://www.benjamins.com. Eds. Natika Newton, Ralph D Ellis.

152 USA ISSN 0146-5457
QP411
CONSCIOUSNESS AND SELF-REGULATION: ADVANCES IN RESEARCH AND THEORY. Text in English. 1976. irreg., latest vol.4, 1986. price varies. *Refereed.* **Document type:** *Monographic series.*
Formerly: Consciousness and Self-Regulation: Advances in Research
Indexed: e-psyche.
Published by: Kluwer Academic - Plenum Publishers (Subsidiary of: Wolters Kluwer N.V.), 233 Spring St, New York, NY 10013-1578. TEL 212-620-8000, 800-221-9369, FAX 212-463-0742, info@plenum.com, http://www.plenum.com. Eds. David Shapiro, Gary Schwartz.

800 700 USA ISSN 1052-8164
NX165
CONSTRUCTIVE CRITICISM; a journal of construct psychology and the arts. Text in English. 1991. s-a. USD 25; USD 30 foreign. film rev., play rev. bibl. back issues avail. **Description:** Covers the application of construct psychology to the arts.
Indexed: e-psyche.
Published by: Constructive Publishing, Inc., PO Box 162, Gambier, OH 43022. TEL 614-393-2834. Ed. Cintra Whitehead.

150.19 USA ISSN 1061-4087
BF637.C56
CONSULTING PSYCHOLOGY JOURNAL: PRACTICE AND RESEARCH. Text in English. 1992. q. USD 60 domestic to non-members; USD 75 foreign to non-members; USD 32 domestic to members; USD 42 foreign to members; USD 102 domestic to institutions; USD 134 foreign to institutions (effective 2001). adv. illus. reprints avail. *Refereed.* **Document type:** *Academic/Scholarly.* **Description:** Publishes articles that provide knowledge and ideas in the field of consultation to the community of psychologists and others interested in consultation.
Indexed: PsycInfo, Psychol.Abstr. (1992-), Russ.Acad.Sci.Bibl., e-psyche.
—BLDSC (3424.011000).
Published by: American Psychological Association, 750 First St., N.E., Washington, DC 20002-4242. TEL 202-336-5600, 800-374-3721, FAX 202-336-5568, subscriptions@apa.org, http://www.apa.org/journals/cpb.html. Ed. Richard Diedrich. adv.: B&W page USD 175; trim 9.25 x 6.88. Circ: 1,100. **Co-publisher:** Educational Publishing Foundation.

CONTEMPORARY EDUCATIONAL PSYCHOLOGY. see *EDUCATION*

CONTEMPORARY ERGONOMICS. see *ENGINEERING*

306.85 USA ISSN 0892-2764
RC488.5
CONTEMPORARY FAMILY THERAPY; an international journal. Text in English. 1979. q. USD 523, EUR 522 to institutions for print or online ed.; USD 627.60, EUR 626.40 to institutions for print & online eds.combined (effective 2002). adv. bk.rev. reprint service avail. from PQC,PSC,SCH,ISI. *Refereed.* **Document type:** *Journal, Academic/Scholarly.* **Description:** Presents the latest theory, research, and practice with an emphasis on examination of the family within the socioeconomic matrix of which it is an integral part.
Formerly (until 1986): International Journal of Family Therapy (0148-8384)
Related titles: Online - full text ed.: (from EBSCO Publishing, O C L C Online Computer Library Center, Inc., RoweCom Information Quest, Swets Blackwell, Kluwer Online, Institute for Scientific Information).
Indexed: ASCA, ASSIA, Abstr.Soc.Geront., Adol.Ment.Hlth.Abstr., AgeLine, Amer.Bibl.Slavic & E.Eur.Stud., Biol.Abstr., C.I.J.E. (coverage dropped), Curr.Cont., ERA, Fam.Ind., IBR, IBZ, IMFL, Ind.Philos., Mult.Ed.Abstr., Past.Care & Couns.Abstr., PsycInfo, Psychol.Abstr. (1979-), Rel.Ind.One, Rel.Ind.Two, SSCI, Sage Fam.Stud.Abstr., Soc.Work Res.& Abstr., Sp.Ed.Needs Abstr., Stud.Wom.Abstr., Viol.& Abuse Abstr., e-psyche.
—BLDSC (3425.181810), GNLM, IDS, ingenta. **CCC.**
Published by: Kluwer Academic - Plenum Publishers (Subsidiary of: Wolters Kluwer N.V.), 233 Spring St, New York, NY 10013-1578. TEL 212-620-8000, 800-221-9369, FAX 212-463-0742, services@wkap.nl, info@plenum.com, http://www.wkap.nl/journalhome.htm/0892-2764. Ed. William C Nichols. **Subscr. outside the Americas:** Kluwer Academic Publishers Group, Journals Department, PO Box 322, Dordrecht 3300 AH, Netherlands. TEL 31-78-639-2392, FAX 31-78-654-6474.

CONTEMPORARY HYPNOSIS. see *MEDICAL SCIENCES—Hypnosis*

616.89 USA ISSN 0010-7530
RC500 CODEN: CPPSBL
CONTEMPORARY PSYCHOANALYSIS. Text in English. 1964. q. USD 59.50 domestic to individuals; USD 71.50 foreign to individuals; USD 89 domestic to institutions; USD 101 foreign to institutions (effective 2000). bk.rev. index. back issues avail. *Refereed.* **Document type:** *Academic/Scholarly.* **Description:** Presents a scholarly approach to the contemporary psychoanalytic scene. Covers a wide range of subjects, from schizophrenia and the neuroses, to group processes and community psychiatry, from a clinical perspective.
Related titles: Online - full text ed.: (from Institute for Scientific Information).
Indexed: ASCA, Arts & Hum.Cit.Ind. (coverage dropped), Biol.Abstr., Curr.Cont., Fam.Ind., IBZ, Ind.Philos., Lang.& Lang.Behav.Abstr., Mid.East: Abstr.& Ind., PsycInfo, Psychoanal.Abstr., Psychol.Abstr. (1968-), Ref.Zh., SOPODA, SSCI, Soc.Work Res.& Abstr., Sociol.Abstr., e-psyche.
—BLDSC (3425.230000), GNLM, IDS, ingenta, KNAW. **CCC.**
Published by: William Alanson White Psychoanalytic Institute, 20 W 74th St, New York, NY 10023. TEL 212-873-0725, FAX 212-362-6967. Ed. Jay Greenberg. R&P Fred Antonoff. Circ: 1,650.

155 USA
BF1
CONTEMPORARY PSYCHOLOGY: A P A REVIEW OF BOOKS; a journal of reviews. Text in English. 1956. bi-m. USD 125 domestic to non-members; USD 145 foreign to non-members; USD 50 domestic to members; USD 62 foreign to members; USD 306 domestic to institutions; USD 350 foreign to institutions (effective 2001). adv. bk.rev., film rev. illus. index. reprint service avail. from PSC,SCH. *Refereed.* **Document type:** *Academic/Scholarly.* **Description:** Publishes articles dealing with new concepts, trends and issues in every arena of psychology.
Formerly: Contemporary Psychology (0010-7549)
Related titles: Microform ed.; Online - full text ed.: (from Institute for Scientific Information).
Indexed: ASCA, Adol.Ment.Hlth.Abstr., Arts & Hum.Cit.Ind. (coverage dropped), Biol.Abstr., Bk.Rev.Ind. (1975-), Chic.Per.Ind., Child.Bk.Rev.Ind. (1975-), Curr.Cont., Curr.Ind.Stat., IBR, Neurosci.Cit.Ind., P C I, Risk Abstr., Russ.Acad.Sci.Bibl., SSCI.
—BLDSC (3425.250000), IDS. **CCC.**
Published by: American Psychological Association, 750 First St., N.E., Washington, DC 20002-4242. TEL 202-336-5600, 800-374-2721, FAX 202-336-5568, http://www.apa.org/journals/cnt.html. Eds. Ed Diener, Robert J Sternberg. Circ: 2,900.

150 GBR
CONTEMPORARY PSYCHOLOGY SERIES. Text in English. irreg., latest vol.10, 1994. **Document type:** *Monographic series.*
Indexed: Curr.Cont. (coverage dropped), e-psyche.
Published by: Taylor & Francis Group, Taylor & Francis Ltd., 11 New Fetter Ln, London EC4P 4EE, United Kingdom. TEL 44-20-7583-9855, FAX 44-20-7842-2298, info@tandf.co.uk, http://www.tandf.co.uk. **Subscr. in N America to:** Taylor & Francis Ltd., 325 Chestnut St, Suite 800, Philadelphia, PA 19016. TEL 800-354-1420, FAX 215-625-8914, info@taylorandfrancis.com, http://www.taylorandfrancis.com/.

306.7 USA ISSN 1094-5725
CONTEMPORARY SEXUALITY; the international resource for educators, researchers and therapists. Text in English. 1967. m. USD 42 domestic to individuals; USD 72 foreign to individuals; USD 65 domestic to institutions; USD 95 foreign to institutions. adv. charts, illus, stat. **Document type:** *Newsletter.* **Description:** Publishes research, news and information of interest to sex educators, researchers, and therapists in addition to news and announcements of the association.
Indexed: e-psyche.
—**CCC.**
Published by: American Association of Sex Educators, Counselors and Therapists, PO Box 238, Mt. Vernon, IA 52314-0238. TEL 319-895-8407, FAX 319-895-6203, mawlula@indigo.ie. Ed. Ann Williams. Adv. contact Mary Ann Williams. Circ: 2,100.

301.1 150 USA ISSN 1041-3030
HM251
CONTEMPORARY SOCIAL PSYCHOLOGY. Text in English. 1974. q. USD 22 (effective 1999 & 2000). adv. index. back issues avail. *Refereed.* **Document type:** *Academic/Scholarly.* **Description:** Covers all aspects of social psychology.
Indexed: e-psyche.
—BLDSC (3425.302750).
Published by: Society for the Advancement of Social Psychology, Department of Psychology, Mercer University, 1400 Coleman Ave, Macon, GA 31207-0001. TEL 912-752-2972, FAX 912-752-2956. Ed., Pub., Adv. contact Francis C Dane. R&P Frances C Dane. Circ: 450.

150 USA
CONTEMPORARY TOPICS IN VOCATIONAL PSYCHOLOGY. Text in English. irreg. **Document type:** *Monographic series.*
Indexed: e-psyche.
Published by: Lawrence Erlbaum Associates, Inc., 10 Industrial Ave, Mahwah, NJ 07430-2262. TEL 201-236-9500, 800-926-6579, FAX 201-236-0072, orders@erlbaum.com, http://www.erlbaum.com. Eds. Samuel Osipow, W Bruce Walsh.

616.89 GBR ISSN 0969-1936
CONTEXT (CANTERBURY); a magazine of family therapy and systemic practice. Text in English. 1989. bi-m. GBP 15 (effective 2001). adv. bk.rev., film rev., play rev. index. back issues avail. **Document type:** *Magazine, Consumer.* **Description:** Covers the study and psychotherapeutic treatment of families.
Indexed: e-psyche.

P

Published by: A F T Publishing, 47 St Augustines Rd, Canterbury, Kent CT1 1XR, United Kingdom. TEL 44-1227-452155, FAX 44-1227-786322, august@cathcity.demon.co.uk. Ed. John Hills. Adv. contact Kate Hills. Circ: 1,600. **Subscr. to:** Chris Frederick, 12 Mabledon Close, Heald Green, Cheadle, Ches SK8 3DB, United Kingdom. TEL 44-161-4939012.

616.89 BRA

CONTRIBUICOES EM PSICOLOGIA, PSIQUIATRIA E PSICANALISE. Text in Portuguese. irreg. **Document type:** *Monographic series.*

Indexed: e-psyche.

Published by: Editora Campus Ltda. (Subsidiary of: Elsevier Science (Brazil)), Rua Sete se Setembro 111-16 andar, Centro, Rio De Janeiro, RJ 20159-900, Brazil. TEL 021-222-5340, FAX 021-252-2904.

150 USA ISSN 0736-2714

CONTRIBUTIONS IN PSYCHOLOGY. Text in English. 1983. irreg. price varies. bibl. index.

Indexed: e-psyche.

—BLDSC (3461.153000).

Published by: Greenwood Press, Inc. (Subsidiary of: Greenwood Publishing Group Inc.), 88 Post Rd W, Box 5007, Westport, CT 06881. TEL 203-226-3571, FAX 203-226-1502.

155.4 USA

CONTRIBUTIONS TO RESIDENTIAL TREATMENT. Text in English. 1957. a. USD 20 (effective 1998). back issues avail. **Document type:** *Proceedings.*

Indexed: e-psyche.

Published by: American Association of Children's Residential Centers, 440 First St N W, 3rd Fl, Washington, DC 20001-2028. TEL 202-628-1816, FAX 202-638-4004. Circ: 200.

COUNSELING AND VALUES. see *RELIGIONS AND THEOLOGY—Roman Catholic*

158.3 USA ISSN 0011-0000
BF637.C6 CODEN: CPSYB

THE COUNSELING PSYCHOLOGIST. Text in English. 1973. bi-m. USD 75 to individuals; USD 395 to institutions; USD 20 newsstand/cover to individuals; USD 70 newsstand/cover to institutions (effective 2002). adv. illus. back issues avail.; reprint service avail. from PQC,PSC,SCH. *Refereed.* **Document type:** *Academic/Scholarly.* **Description:** Presents timely coverage, especially in new or developing areas of practice and research, of topics of immediate interest to counseling psychologists.

Related titles: Microform ed.: (from PQC); Online - full text ed.: (from ProQuest Information & Learning, Gale Group, ingenta, Institute for Scientific Information).

Indexed: ASCA, ASSIA, Adol.Ment.Hlth.Abstr., AgeLine, Amer.Bibl.Slavic & E.Eur.Stud., C.I.J.E., Child Devel.Abstr., Crim.Just.Abstr., Curr.Cont., Educ.Admin.Abstr., Educ.Ind. (coverage dropped), Environ.Sci.Poll.Mgmt., Fam.Ind., High.Educ.Abstr., Human Resour.Abstr., IMFL, Mid.East: Abstr.& Ind., P C I, Pollut.Abstr., PsycInfo, Psychol.Abstr. (1969-), Risk Abstr., Russ.Acad.Sci.Bibl., SSCI, Saf.Sci.Abstr., Sage Race Rel.Abstr., Soc.Sci.Ind. (Dec.1982-), Viol.& Abuse Abstr., e-psyche.

—BLDSC (3481.330000), IDS, ingenta. **CCC.**

Published by: (Division 17, American Psychological Association), Sage Publications, Inc., 2455 Teller Rd, Thousand Oaks, CA 91320. TEL 805-499-0721, FAX 805-499-0871, info@sagepub.com, http://www.sagepub.com. Ed. Paul Heppner. Pub. Sara Miller McCune. R&P Tanya Udin. Adv. contact DeAnna Vega Hammersley. Circ: 5,400. **Overseas subscr. to:** Sage Publications Ltd., 6 Bonhill St, London EC2A 4PU, United Kingdom; Sage Publications India Pvt. Ltd., 4215, New Delhi 110 048, India.

371.42 USA ISSN 1078-8719

COUNSELING TODAY. Text in English. 1958. m. USD 76 (effective 2001). adv. bk.rev., film rev. 48 p./no. back issues avail.; reprint service avail. from PQC. **Document type:** *Newspaper, Academic/Scholarly.*

Formerly (until 1994): Guidepost (0017-5323)

Related titles: Online - full text ed.

Indexed: e-psyche.

—CCC.

Published by: American Counseling Association, 5999 Stevenson Ave, Alexandria, VA 22304-3300. TEL 703-823-9800, FAX 703-823-0252, http://www.counseling.org. Ed. Shawn Schmitt. Adv. contact Kathy Maguire TEL 703-823-9800 ext 207. Circ: 54,000.

616.89 GBR ISSN 0264-9977

COUNSELLING; the monthly professional journal for counsellors. Text in English. 1981. m. GBP 60 domestic; GBP 70 foreign; GBP 8 newsstand/cover (effective 2000). adv. bk.rev. index. back issues avail. *Refereed.* **Document type:** *Newsletter, Academic/Scholarly, Abstract/Index.* **Description:** Directed to those interested in working in counselling and psychotherapy and to members of related professions, including nursing and teaching.

Related titles: Diskette ed.

Indexed: Br.Educ.Ind., Brit.Nur.Ind., e-psyche.

Published by: British Association for Counseling, 1 Regent Pl, Rugby, Warks CV21 2PJ, United Kingdom. TEL 44-1788-550899, FAX 44-1788-562189, bac@bac.co.uk, http://www.counselling.co.uk. Adv. contact Nicholas Temple-Smith. page GBP 529; trim. Circ: 19,200.

150 616.8 GBR ISSN 0951-5070
CODEN: CPQUEZ

COUNSELLING PSYCHOLOGY QUARTERLY. Text in English. 1988. q. GBP 117, USD 197 to individuals; GBP 413, USD 711 to institutions (effective 2002). adv. bk.rev. *Refereed.* **Document type:** *Academic/Scholarly.*

Related titles: Microfiche ed.; Online - full content ed.: ISSN 1469-3674 (from EBSCO Publishing, O C L C Online Computer Library Center, Inc., ProQuest Information & Learning, Swets Blackwell); Online - full text ed.: (from CatchWord Ltd., RoweCom Information Quest).

Indexed: ASSIA, Addic.Abstr., CINAHL, Crim.Just.Abstr., ERA, Human Resour.Abstr., Lang.& Lang.Behav.Abstr., Mult.Ed.Abstr., PsycInfo, Psychol.Abstr. (1988-), SOPODA, Sage Fam.Stud.Abstr., Sociol.Abstr., Sp.Ed.Needs Abstr., Stud.Wom.Abstr., Viol.& Abuse Abstr., e-psyche.

—BLDSC (3481.338300), CatchWord, EMDOCS, GNLM, ingenta. **CCC.**

Published by: Carfax Publishing Limited (Subsidiary of: Taylor & Francis Group), PO Box 25, Abingdon, Oxon OX14 3UE, United Kingdom. TEL 44-1235-401000, FAX 44-1235-401550, enquiries@carfax.co.uk, enquiry@tandf.co.uk, http://www.carfax.co.uk. Ed. W J Alladin.

616.89 USA ISSN 1047-7314

COUNSELOR; the magazine for addiction professionals. Variant title: Counselor Magazine. Text in English. 1986. bi-m., latest vol.2, no.4, 2001. USD 26 domestic; USD 34 in Canada; USD 43 elsewhere (effective 2001). adv. bk.rev. 80 p./no. back issues avail. **Document type:** *Magazine, Trade.* **Description:** Features articles about mental health counseling, addictions treatment and prevention. Covers the clinical, social and political aspects of addictions.

Former titles (until Oct. 2000): Professional Counselor (1086-3397); (until 1995): Professional Counselor Magazine (1042-7570); N A A D A C Counselor

Indexed: e-psyche.

—ingenta. **CCC.**

Published by: Health Communications, Inc., 3201 S.W. 15th St., Deerfield, FL 33442-8190. TEL 954-360-0909, FAX 954-360-0034, info@counselormagazine.com, http://www.counselormagazine.com/. Ed. Ria Romano. Pub. Peter Vegso. R&P Fred Courtright TEL 908-537-7559. Adv. contact Neca Logan TEL 800-851-9100 ext 236. B&W page USD 2,285; trim 8.375 x 11.125. Circ: 30,000.

COUNSELOR EDUCATION AND SUPERVISION. see *EDUCATION*

COUNTRY LIVING'S HEALTHY LIVING; the magazine that refreshes body, mind, and soul. see *ALTERNATIVE MEDICINE*

CREATIVITY IN ACTION. see *EDUCATION*

301.1 150 USA ISSN 1040-0419

CREATIVITY RESEARCH JOURNAL. Text in English. 1988. q. USD 55 in US & Canada to individuals; USD 85 elsewhere to individuals; USD 300 in US & Canada to institutions; USD 330 elsewhere to institutions (effective 2002). adv. abstr. bibl. back issues avail.; reprint service avail. from SCH,PSC. *Refereed.* **Document type:** *Journal, Academic/Scholarly.* **Description:** Publishes scholarly research capturing the full range of approaches to the study of creativity: aesthetic, behavioral, clinical, cognitive, cross-cultural, developmental, educational, genetic, organizational, psychoanalytic, and psychometric.

Related titles: Online - full text ed.: ISSN 1532-6934. USD 49.50 to individuals; USD 270 to institutions (effective 2002) (from CatchWord Ltd., O C L C Online Computer Library Center, Inc., RoweCom Information Quest, Swets Blackwell, Institute for Scientific Information).

Indexed: ASCA, Arts & Hum.Cit.Ind. (coverage dropped), Curr.Cont., Except.Child Educ.Abstr., PsycInfo, Psychol.Abstr. (1988-), SSCI, e-psyche.

—BLDSC (3487.252000), CatchWord, ingenta. **CCC.**

Published by: Lawrence Erlbaum Associates, Inc., 10 Industrial Ave, Mahwah, NJ 07430-2262. TEL 201-760-3735, 800-926-6579, FAX 201-236-0072, journals@erlbaum.com, http://www.erlbaum.com/Journals/journals/CRJ/crj.htm. Ed. Mark Runco. adv.: page USD 425; trim 7 x 10. Circ: 400.

CRIMINAL JUSTICE & BEHAVIOR. see *CRIMINOLOGY AND LAW ENFORCEMENT*

150 CHE ISSN 1064-5136
RC480.6 CODEN: CITTEW

CRISIS INTERVENTION AND TIME-LIMITED TREATMENT. Text in English. 1994. 3/yr. GBP 53, USD 64, EUR 70 to individuals; GBP 164, USD 190, EUR 190 to institutions; GBP 232, USD 274, EUR 281 to corporations (effective 2002). *Refereed.* **Document type:** *Academic/Scholarly.* **Description:** Focuses on the latest clinical innovations and research of those working in crisis intervention settings.

Related titles: Microform ed.; Online - full text ed.: (from Institute for Scientific Information).

Indexed: ASCA, ASSIA, Crim.Just.Abstr., Curr.Cont., Fam.Ind., P.A.I.S., PsycInfo, SSCI, Sage Urb.Stud.Abstr., Viol.& Abuse Abstr., e-psyche.

—BLDSC (3487.383500), Infotrieve. **CCC.**

Published by: Gordon and Breach - Harwood Academic (Subsidiary of: Taylor & Francis Group), PO Box 531, Lausanne 1000, Switzerland. Ed. Albert R Roberts. **Subscr. addr. in US:** International Publishers Direct, PO Box 32160, Newark, NJ 07102. FAX 215-750-6343.

362.28 USA ISSN 0227-5910
HV6549

CRISIS (KIRKLAND); the journal of crisis intervention and suicide prevention. Text in English. 1980. q. USD 54 (effective 2001). adv. bk.rev. back issues avail. *Refereed.* **Document type:** *Journal, Academic/Scholarly.* **Description:** Articles on the research and clinical aspects of how to prevent suicides, and how to intervene in severe emotional crises.

Indexed: AgeLine, Crim.Just.Abstr., Hist.Abstr. (1969-1988, dropped), Ind.Med. (1980-), Ind.Philos., Indian Psychol.Abstr., P C I, PsycInfo, Psychol.Abstr. (1980-), Soc.Sci.Ind. (coverage dropped).

—BLDSC (3487.382350), GNLM, ingenta. **CCC.**

Published by: (International Association for Suicide Prevention), Hogrefe & Huber Publishers, PO Box 2487, Kirkland, WA 98083. TEL 425-820-1500, FAX 425-823-8324, hh@hhpub.com, http://www.hhpub.com/journals. Ed. A J F M Kerkhof. Adv. contact Iris Pruegl.

618.92 USA

CRITICAL ISSUES IN DEVELOPMENTAL & BEHAVIORAL PEDIATRICS. Text in English. 1987. irreg., latest vol.3. price varies. back issues avail. *Refereed.* **Document type:** *Monographic series.*

Formerly: Developmental and Behavioral Pediatrics: Selected Topics

Indexed: e-psyche.

Published by: Kluwer Academic - Plenum Publishers (Subsidiary of: Wolters Kluwer N.V.), 233 Spring St, New York, NY 10013-1578. TEL 212-620-8000, 800-221-9369, FAX 212-463-0742, info@plenum.com, http://www.plenum.com. Ed. Martin Gottlieb.

150.19 GBR ISSN 1471-4167

▼ **CRITICAL PSYCHOLOGY.** Text in English. 2000 (Oct). 3/yr. GBP 40, USD 65 to individuals; GBP 120, USD 190 to institutions; GBP 15, USD 24 newsstand/cover to individuals; GBP 45, USD 60 newsstand/cover to institutions (effective 2001). adv. bk.rev. 192 p./no. back issues avail. *Refereed.* **Document type:** *Journal, Academic/Scholarly.* **Description:** Provides a forum for new research in the rapidly expanding field of critical psychology, including such topics as feminist psychology, the anti-psychiatry movement, and black socio-political thought.

—BLDSC (3487.459350).

Published by: Lawrence & Wishart Ltd, 99a Wallis Rd, London E9 5LN, United Kingdom. TEL 44-20-8533-2506, FAX 44-20-8533-7369, mailroom@l-w-bks.demon.co.uk, lw@l-w-bks.demon.co.uk, http://www.l-w-bks.co.uk/crit-psych/cp-discussion.html, http://www.l-w-bks.co.uk/index.html. Ed. Valerie Walkerdine. R&P Vanna Derosas. adv.: page GBP 200; trim 105 x 175.

P

156 572 USA ISSN 0710-068X
CROSS-CULTURAL PSYCHOLOGY BULLETIN. Text in English. 1967. q. USD 20 to membership (effective 2000). adv. bk.rev. abstr, bibl. back issues avail. **Document type:** *Newsletter, Academic/Scholarly.* **Description:** Presents a forum to present and discussissues relevant to cross-cultural psychology and to the IACCP.
Former titles: Cross-Cultural Psychology Newsletter; (until vol.15, 1981): International Association for Cross-Cultural Psychology. Newsletter
Indexed: Child Devel.Abstr., e-psyche.
—BLDSC (3488.810000).
Published by: International Association for Cross-Cultural Psychology, c/o Ted Singelis, Treas, Dept of Psychology, California State University, Chico, CA 95929-0234. TEL 916-898-5363, FAX 916-898-4740, tsingelis@oavax.csuchico.edu, http://www.fit.edu/CampusLife/clubs-org/iaccp/bulletin/main.html. Ed. William K Gabrenya Jr. R&P Theodore M Singelis TEL 530-898-4009. Circ: 850.

CROSS-CULTURAL RESEARCH; the journal of comparative social science. see *SOCIAL SCIENCES: COMPREHENSIVE WORKS*

306.4 USA
CROSS-CULTURAL RESEARCH AND METHODOLOGY SERIES. Text in English. 1977. irreg. price varies. adv. back issues avail. **Document type:** *Monographic series, Academic/Scholarly.*
Former titles: Cross-Cultural Research Methods; Sage Series in Cross-Cultural Research and Methodology; Cross-Cultural Research and Methodology Series
Indexed: e-psyche.
Published by: Sage Publications, Inc., Books, 2455 Teller Rd, Thousand Oaks, CA 91320. TEL 805-499-0721, FAX 805-499-0871, libraries@sagepub.com, http://www.sagepub.com. Eds. John W Berry, Walter J Lonner. Adv. contact Margaret Travers. **Overseas subscr. to:** Sage Publications Ltd., 6 Bonhill St, London EC2A 4PU, United Kingdom; Sage Publications India Pvt. Ltd., 4215, New Delhi 110 048, India.

150 USA ISSN 0272-1678
CROSSCURRENTS IN CONTEMPORARY PSYCHOLOGY. Text in English. irreg. **Document type:** *Monographic series.*
Indexed: e-psyche.
Published by: Lawrence Erlbaum Associates, Inc., 10 Industrial Ave, Mahwah, NJ 07430-2262. TEL 201-236-9500, 800-926-6579, FAX 201-236-0072, orders@erlbaum.com, http://www.erlbaum.com. Ed. Marc Bornstein.

150 COL ISSN 0120-4653
CUADERNOS DE PSICOLOGIA. Text in Spanish. 1976. 2/yr. USD 10. adv. bk.rev. **Document type:** *Academic/Scholarly.*
Indexed: Psychol.Abstr., e-psyche.
Published by: Universidad del Valle, Departamento de Psicologia, Apartado Aereo 25360, Cali, VALLE, Colombia. FAX 57-23-392311. Ed. Sonia Meluk. Circ: 1,000.

155.4 USA
CULTURAL CONTEXT OF INFANCY. Text in English. 1989. irreg., latest vol.2, 1991. USD 78.50; price varies. **Document type:** *Academic/Scholarly.*
Indexed: e-psyche.
Published by: Ablex Publishing Corporation (Subsidiary of: Greenwood Publishing Group Inc.), 88 Post Rd W, Westport, CT 06881. TEL 203-323-9606, FAX 203-357-8446, http://www.jal.com. Ed. J Kevin Nugent.

CULTURAL DIVERSITY & ETHNIC MINORITY PSYCHOLOGY. see *SOCIOLOGY*

306 GBR ISSN 1354-067X
BF1 CODEN: CUPSFQ
CULTURE & PSYCHOLOGY. Text in English. 1995. q. GBP 41 to individuals; GBP 215 to institutions; GBP 11 newsstand/cover to individuals; GBP 55 newsstand/cover to institutions (effective 2002). adv. *Refereed.* **Document type:** *Academic/Scholarly.* **Description:** Addresses the centrality of culture to our understanding of human behaviour, identity, intersubjective experiences, emotions, development and language.
Related titles: Online - full text ed.: (from EBSCO Publishing, O C L C Online Computer Library Center, Inc., RoweCom Information Quest, ingenta, Swets Blackwell, Institute for Scientific Information).
Indexed: ASSIA, Curr.Cont., IBZ, Ind.Philos., Indian Psychol.Abstr., Lang.& Lang.Behav.Abstr., PsycInfo, SOPODA, SSCI, Soc.Serv.Abstr., Sociol.Abstr., Sociol.Educ.Abstr., e-psyche.
—BLDSC (3491.668740), IDS, Infotrieve, ingenta. **CCC.**
Published by: Sage Publications Ltd., 6 Bonhill St, London EC2A 4PU, United Kingdom. TEL 44-20-7374-0645, FAX 44-20-7374-8741, market@sagepub.co.uk, http://www.sagepub.co.uk. Ed. Jaan Valsiner. Adv. contact Jenny Kirby. page GBP 195.

CURRENT CONTENTS: SOCIAL & BEHAVIORAL SCIENCES. see *PSYCHOLOGY—Abstracting, Bibliographies, Statistics*

150.19 USA ISSN 0963-7214
BF1 CODEN: CDPSE8
CURRENT DIRECTIONS IN PSYCHOLOGICAL SCIENCE. Text in English. 1992. bi-m. GBP 225 to institutions in UK& Europe; USD 263 to institutions in the Americas & Caribbean; GBP 225 elsewhere to institutions (effective 2002). adv. illus. back issues avail.; reprint service avail. from PSC,SCH. *Refereed.* **Document type:** *Journal, Academic/Scholarly.* **Description:** Contains concise reviews of important trends and controversies in psychology.
Related titles: Online - full text ed.: (from EBSCO Publishing, O C L C Online Computer Library Center, Inc., RoweCom Information Quest, ingenta, Swets Blackwell, Institute for Scientific Information).
Indexed: ASCA, AgeLine, Child Devel.Abstr., Curr.Cont., Ergon.Abstr., Fam.Ind., PsycInfo, Psychol.Abstr. (1992-), SSCI, e-psyche.
—BLDSC (3496.357000), IDS, ingenta. **CCC.**
Published by: (American Psychological Society), Blackwell Publishers, 350 Main St, Malden, MA 02148. TEL 781-388-8200, 800-835-6770, FAX 781-388-8232, subscript@blackwellpub.com, http://www.blackwellpublishers.co.uk/journals/diph. Ed. Alan E Kazdin. R&P Gretchen Voter TEL 781-388-0423. Adv. contact Anne Marie Sheehy TEL 781-388-0427.

616.89 USA
CODEN: CIPPEY
CURRENT ISSUES IN PSYCHOANALYTIC PRACTICE. MONOGRAPHS✱ . Text in English. 1984. irreg. price varies. back issues avail. **Document type:** *Monographic series, Academic/Scholarly.*
Formerly: Current Issues in Psychoanalytic Practice. Journal (0737-7851)
Indexed: Excerp.Med., Psychol.Abstr., e-psyche.
—BLDSC (3499.075500), GNLM.
Published by: Brunner - Routledge (Subsidiary of: Taylor & Francis Group), 325 Chestnut St, Ste 800, Philadelphia, PA 19106. TEL 215-269-0400, FAX 215-269-0363, postmaster@bmp.com, info@taylorandfrancis.com. Ed. Herbert S Strean.

150 USA
CURRENT PSYCHOLOGY (HENDERSONVILLE). Text in English. 1979. m. USD 25.
Related titles: Microform ed.: (from PQC).
Indexed: Curr.Cont. (coverage dropped), Psychol.Abstr., SSCI (coverage dropped), e-psyche.
Published by: Psychological Press, PO Box 309, Hendersonville, TN 37075.

150 BEL ISSN 1376-2095
CURRENT PSYCHOLOGY LETTERS: BEHAVIOR, BRAIN AND COGNITION. Text in English. 3/yr. BEF 2,765 domestic; BEF 3,215 in the European Union; BEF 3,315 in Europe; BEF 3,565 elsewhere; BEF 1,230 newsstand/cover (effective 2001). bk.rev. abstr. 128 p./no. *Refereed.* **Document type:** *Monographic series, Academic/Scholarly.*
Published by: De Boeck Universite (Subsidiary of: De Boeck et Larcier S.A.), Rue des Minimes 39, Brussels 1000, Belgium. TEL 2-32-10482570, FAX 2-32-10-482650, http://www.deboeck.be. Eds. Jacques Vauclair, Jean-Paul Caverni. **Subscr. to:** Acces S.P.R.L., Fond Jean Paques 4, Louvain-la-Neuve 1348, Belgium. acces+@deboeck.be.

150 USA ISSN 1046-1310
BF1
CURRENT PSYCHOLOGY (NEW BRUNSWICK); developmental - learning - personality - social. Text in English. 1981. q. USD 80 to individuals; USD 196 to institutions (effective 2001). adv. *Refereed.* **Document type:** *Academic/Scholarly.* **Description:** Provides an international forum for the rapid dissemination of new psychological information. Includes significant empirical contributions from all areas of psychology.
Former titles: Current Psychological Research and Reviews (0737-8262); Current Psychological Research; Current Psychological Reviews
Related titles: Online - full text ed.: (from CatchWord Ltd., EBSCO Publishing, Gale Group, Institute for Scientific Information).
Indexed: Amer.Bibl.Slavic & E.Eur.Stud., Crim.Just.Abstr., Curr.Cont., HRIS, IMFL, Ind.Philos., Lang.& Lang.Behav.Abstr., PsycInfo, Psychol.Abstr. (1981-), SOPODA, SSCI, Sage Fam.Stud.Abstr., Soc.Sci.Ind. (coverage dropped), Soc.Serv.Abstr., Sociol.Abstr., e-psyche.
—BLDSC (3501.601000), CatchWord, IDS, ingenta. **CCC.**
Published by: Transaction Publishers, 35 Berrue Circle, Rutgers University, Piscataway, NJ 08854-8042. TEL 732-445-2280, FAX 732-445-3138, http://www.transactionpub.com. Eds. Nathaniel Pallone, Noel P Sheehy. Pub. Mary Curtis. R&P Marlena Davidian TEL 732-445-2280 ext 100. Adv. contact Alicja Garbie. page USD 300; 5.125 x 7.625. Circ: 500. **Subscr. address in US:** Transaction Distribution Center, 390 Campus Dr, Somerset, NJ 08873. TEL 732-748-0300, FAX 732-748-1886; **Subscr. in Europe and Israel to:** Swets & Zeitlinger bv, Heereweg 347, Lisse 2161 CA, Netherlands. TEL 31-2521-35111, 31-2521-15888.

302 USA ISSN 1088-7423
HM251
CURRENT RESEARCH IN SOCIAL PSYCHOLOGY. Text in English. 1995. irreg. free per issue. illus. back issues avail.; reprints avail. *Refereed.* **Document type:** *Monographic series, Academic/Scholarly.* **Description:** Covers a variety of topics in social psychology.
Media: Online - full text.
Indexed: e-psyche.
Published by: University of Iowa, Department of Sociology, Center for the Study of Group Processes, Iowa City, IA 52242-1401. http://www.uiowa.edu/~grpproc/crisp/crisp.html. Ed. Michael J Lovaglia.

152.4 GBR
CURRENT REVIEW OF MOOD DISORDERS. Text in English. 1997. q. **Document type:** *Academic/Scholarly.*
Indexed: e-psyche.
Published by: Current Science Ltd, Middlesex House, 34-42 Cleveland St, London W1P 6LB, United Kingdom. FAX 44-20-7636-6911.

150 USA ISSN 1092-2067
CURRENT THINKING AND RESEARCH IN BRIEF THERAPY. Text in English. a. **Description:** Provides access to a wide range of theoretical ideas, clinical cases, and empirically based research related to solution-focused strategic, and narrative brief therapies.
—BLDSC (3504.840000).
Published by: Taylor & Francis Ltd. (Subsidiary of: Taylor & Francis Group), 325 Chestnut St, Suite 800, Philadelphia, PA 19016. TEL 215-625-8900, FAX 215-625-2940, info@taylorandfrancis.com, http://www.taylorandfrancis.com/. **Subscr. addr. in Europe:** Taylor & Francis Group, Journals Customer Service, Rankine Rd, Basingstoke, Hants RG24 8PR, United Kingdom. TEL 44-1256-813000, FAX 44-1256-479438, enquiry@tanf.co.uk, http://www.tandf.co.uk/journals.

150 USA ISSN 8755-0040
BF431
CURRENT TOPICS IN HUMAN INTELLIGENCE. Text in English. 1985. a., latest 1996. USD 78.50. **Document type:** *Academic/Scholarly.* **Description:** Focuses on selected topics in human intelligence of interest to researchers in the filed. Designed to provide forum for extensive discussion of issues from multiple points of view.
Indexed: Psychol.Abstr., e-psyche.
—BLDSC (3504.883950). **CCC.**
Published by: Ablex Publishing Corporation (Subsidiary of: Greenwood Publishing Group Inc.), 88 Post Rd W, Westport, CT 06881. TEL 203-323-9606, FAX 203-357-8446. Ed. Douglas K Detterman.

CZLOWIEK I SPOLECZENSTWO. see *EDUCATION*

616.89 DEU ISSN 0935-2066
D G I P - INTERN. Text in German. 1982. q. DEM 160 to membership (effective 2001). adv. bk.rev. **Document type:** *Newsletter, Academic/Scholarly.*
Indexed: e-psyche.
Published by: Deutsche Gesellschaft fuer Individualpsychologie e.V., Marktstr 12, Gotha 99867, Germany. TEL 49-3621-29691, FAX 49-3621-29691, dgip-gotha@t-online.de, http://www.dgip.de. Ed., Adv. contact Horst Groener. Circ: 1,800.

D W D NEWSLETTER. see *GERONTOLOGY AND GERIATRICS*

DARSHANA INTERNATIONAL; an international quarterly of philosophy, psychology, sociology, psychical research, religion and mysticism. see *PHILOSOPHY*

▼ **DEATH & DYING SOURCEBOOK.** see *PHILOSOPHY*

P

302 USA ISSN 0748-1187
BF789.D4 CODEN: DESTEA

DEATH STUDIES; education - counseling - care - law - ethics. Text in English. 1977. 10/yr. GBP 102, USD 169 to individuals; GBP 271, USD 447 to institutions (effective 2002). adv. bk.rev. abstr, bibl, charts, illus. index. back issues avail.; reprint service avail. from PQC,SCH,PSC. *Refereed.* **Document type:** *Academic/Scholarly.* **Description:** Provides an international and interdisciplinary forum in the field of death studies. Refereed papers cover education, counseling, bioethics, and psychosocial research.

Formerly (until 1985): Death Education (0145-7624)

Related titles: Microform ed.: (from PQC); Online - full text ed.: ISSN 1091-7683 (from CatchWord Ltd., EBSCO Publishing, O C L C Online Computer Library Center, Inc., RoweCom Information Quest, ProQuest Information & Learning, Gale Group, Swets Blackwell, Institute for Scientific Information).

Indexed: AMED, ASCA, Abstr.Soc.Geront., AgeLine, CERDIC, C.I.J.E. (coverage dropped), CINAHL, Cont.Pg.Educ., Curr.Cont., ERA, Excerp.Med., Fam.Ind., L.R.I., Lang.& Lang.Behav.Abstr., Mult.Ed.Abstr., P C I, Past.Care & Couns.Abstr., Per.Islam. (1991-), PsycInfo, Psychol.Abstr. (1977-), Rel.Ind.One, Rel.Ind.Two, Res.High.Educ.Abstr., Risk Abstr., SOMA, SOPODA, SSCI, Sage Fam.Stud.Abstr., Soc.Sci.Ind. (Jan.1987-), Soc.Serv.Abstr., Soc.Work Res.& Abstr., Sociol.Abstr., Sp.Ed.Needs Abstr., Stud.Wom.Abstr., Viol.& Abuse Abstr., WMB, e-psyche.

—BLDSC (3535.960460), CatchWord, EMDOCS, GNLM, IDS, Infotrieve, ingenta, KNAW. **CCC.**

Published by: Taylor & Francis Ltd. (Subsidiary of: Taylor & Francis Group), 325 Chestnut St, Suite 800, Philadelphia, PA 19016. TEL 215-625-8900, FAX 215-625-2940, beverley.acreman@tandf.co.uk, info@taylorandfrancis.com, http://www.tandf.co.uk/journals/default.html. Ed. Robert A Neimeyer. Circ: 800. **Subscr. addr. in Europe:** Taylor & Francis Group, Journals Customer Service, Rankine Rd, Basingstoke, Hants RG24 8PR, United Kingdom. TEL 44-1256-813000, FAX 44-1256-479438, enquiry@tanf.co.uk, http://www.tandf.co.uk/journals.

155.904 616.8 USA ISSN 1091-4269
RC531 CODEN: DEANF5

DEPRESSION AND ANXIETY. Text in English. 1997. 8/yr. USD 425 in United States; USD 505 in Canada & Mexico; USD 573 elsewhere; USD 447 combined subscription in United States for print and online eds.; USD 527 combined subscription in Canada & Mexico for print and online eds.; USD 595 combined subscription elsewhere for print and online eds. (effective 2002). *Refereed.* **Document type:** *Academic/Scholarly.* **Description:** Publishes reports of novel research on the etiology, pathophysiology, epidemiology, nosology, symptomatology, and treatment of mood and anxiety disorders.

Formed by the merger of (1993-1997): Depression (1062-6417); (1994-1997): Anxiety (1070-9797)

Related titles: Online - full text ed.: ISSN 1520-6394. USD 425 in United States; USD 425 in Canada & Mexico; USD 425 elsewhere (effective 2002) (from EBSCO Publishing, Wiley InterScience, Institute for Scientific Information).

Indexed: AgeLine, Curr.Cont., Ind.Med. (1997-), Inpharma, Jrnl.Watch Psych., Pharm.&Out.News, Reac., Ref.Zh., SSCI, Sci.Cit.Ind., e-psyche.

—BLDSC (3554.590040), CISTI, GNLM, IDS, Infotrieve, KNAW. **CCC.**

Published by: John Wiley & Sons, Inc., Journals (Subsidiary of: Wiley InterScience), 605 Third Ave, New York, NY 10158. TEL 212-850-6645, FAX 212-850-6021, subinfo@jwiley.com, uscs-wis@wiley.com, http://www.wiley.com. Eds. Charles Nemeroff, Thomas Uhde. **Subscr. to:** John Wiley & Sons Ltd., Baffins Ln, Chichester, Sussex PO19 IUD, United Kingdom. TEL 44-1243-779777, FAX 44-1243-843232, cs-journals@wiley.co.uk, http://www.wiley.co.uk. **Dist. in UK by:** John Wiley & Sons Ltd.

DEPRESSION: DISEASE STATE MANAGEMENT RESOURCE. see *MEDICAL SCIENCES—Psychiatry And Neurology*

616.89 USA ISSN 0893-8636

DEPRESSIVE ILLNESS SERIES. Text in English. 1988. irreg., latest vol.4. **Document type:** *Monographic series.*

Indexed: e-psyche.

—CCC.

Published by: Kluwer Academic - Human Sciences Press (Subsidiary of: Wolters Kluwer N.V.), 233 Spring St, New York, NY 10013-1578. TEL 212-620-8000, FAX 212-463-0742.

▼ **DERMATOLOGY AND PSYCHOSOMATICS/ DERMATOLOGIE UND PSYCHOSOMATIK.** see *MEDICAL SCIENCES—Dermatology And Venereology*

150 GBR ISSN 0954-5794
RC454.4

DEVELOPMENT AND PSYCHOPATHOLOGY. Text in English. 1989. q. GBP 85 to individuals; USD 220 to institutions (effective 2002). adv. back issues avail.; reprint service avail. from SWZ. *Refereed.* **Document type:** *Academic/Scholarly.* **Description:** Devoted to the publication of original empirical, theoretical and review papers that address the interrelationship of normal and pathological development in adults and children.

Related titles: Online - full text ed.: (from EBSCO Publishing, O C L C Online Computer Library Center, Inc., RoweCom Information Quest, Swets Blackwell, Institute for Scientific Information).

Indexed: AMED, ASCA, Curr.Cont., Fam.Ind., IMFL, Ind.Med. (1989-), Int.Nurs.Ind., P C I, PsycInfo, Psychol.Abstr. (1989-), SSCI, e-psyche.

—BLDSC (3578.855000), GNLM, IDS, ingenta. **CCC.**

Published by: Cambridge University Press, The Edinburgh Building, Shaftesbury Rd, Cambridge CB2 2RU, United Kingdom. TEL 44-1223-312393, FAX 44-1223-315052, information@cup.cam.ac.uk; journals_subscriptions@cup.org, http://www.cup.cam.ac.uk, http://www.uk.cambridge.org/journals/pmu. Eds. Barry Nurcombe, Dante Cicchetti. R&P Linda Nicol. Adv. contact Rebecca Symons.

616.89 USA

DEVELOPMENTAL APPROACHES TO PSYCHOPATHOLOGY. Text in English. irreg. **Document type:** *Monographic series.* **Description:** Addresses common psychiatric disorders in children and adolescents from a developmental perspective.

Indexed: e-psyche.

Published by: Guilford Publications, Inc., 72 Spring St, New York, NY 10012. TEL 212-431-9800, 800-365-7006, FAX 212-966-6708, info@guilford.com, http://www.guilford.com. Ed. Hans Steiner.

155 613.62 USA

DEVELOPMENTAL DISABILITIES SPECIAL INTEREST SECTION QUARTERLY. Text in English. 1989 (vol.12, no.2). q. USD 20 (effective 1999). **Document type:** *Newsletter.*

Former titles (until 199?): Developmental Disabilities Special Interest Section Newsletter (0279-4098); American Occupational Therapy Association. Developmental Disabilities Specialty Section. Newsletter (0194-6390)

Published by: American Occupational Therapy Association, Inc., 4720 Montgomery Lane, Bethesda, MD 20814-3425. TEL 301-652-2682, FAX 301-652-7711.

370.15 USA ISSN 8756-5641
WMLC 93/1384 CODEN: DENEE8

DEVELOPMENTAL NEUROPSYCHOLOGY; an international journal of life-span issues in neuropsychology. Text in English. 1985. bi-m. USD 100 in US & Canada to individuals; USD 145 elsewhere to individuals; USD 750 in US & Canada to institutions; USD 795 elsewhere to institutions (effective 2002). adv. back issues avail. *Refereed.* **Document type:** *Journal, Academic/Scholarly.* **Description:** Covers issues concerning the structure and function of both the developing and the aging brain.

Related titles: Online - full text ed.: ISSN 1532-6942. USD 90 to individuals; USD 675.50 to institutions (effective 2002) (from CatchWord Ltd., EBSCO Publishing, O C L C Online Computer Library Center, Inc., RoweCom Information Quest, Swets Blackwell, Institute for Scientific Information).

Indexed: ASCA, AgeLine, Child Devel.Abstr., Curr.Cont., Environ.Sci.Poll.Mgmt., Ind.Med. (1985-), Neurosci.Abstr., Neurosci.Cit.Ind., PsycInfo, Psychol.Abstr. (1985-), Risk Abstr., SSCI, Saf.Sci.Abstr., e-psyche.

—BLDSC (3579.057300), CatchWord, GNLM, Infotrieve, ingenta. **CCC.**

Published by: Lawrence Erlbaum Associates, Inc., 10 Industrial Ave, Mahwah, NJ 07430-2262. TEL 201-760-3735, 800-926-6579, FAX 201-236-0072, journals@erlbaum.com, http://www.erlbaum.com/Journals/journals/DN/dn.htm. Ed. Dennis L Molfese. adv.: page USD 400; trim 5 x 8. Circ: 750.

DEVELOPMENTAL PSYCHOBIOLOGY. see *BIOLOGY*

155 USA ISSN 0012-1649
BF699 CODEN: DEVPA9

DEVELOPMENTAL PSYCHOLOGY. Text in English. 1969. bi-m. USD 174 domestic to non-members; USD 194 foreign to non-members; USD 87 domestic to members; USD 99 foreign to members; USD 404 domestic to institutions; USD 448 foreign to institutions (effective 2001). adv. bibl, charts, stat, illus. back issues avail.; reprint service avail. from PSC,PQC,SCH. *Refereed.* **Document type:** *Academic/Scholarly.* **Description:** Empirical contributions that advance knowledge and theory about human psychological growth and development from infancy to old age.

Related titles: Microform ed.: (from PQC); Online - full text ed.: (from Gale Group, Factiva, Institute for Scientific Information).

Indexed: ASCA, ASSIA, Abstr.Crim.& Pen., Adol.Ment.Hlth.Abstr., AgeLine, Arts & Hum.Cit.Ind. (coverage dropped), Bibl.Dev.Med.& Child Neur., Bibl.Ling., Biol.Abstr., C.I.J.E., Chic.Per.Ind., Child Devel.Abstr., Commun.Abstr., Crim.Just.Abstr., Curr.Adv.Ecol.Sci., Curr.Cont., ERA, Educ.Ind. (Jul.1992-), Energy Ind., Energy Info.Abstr., Fam.Ind., IBZ, Ind.Med. (1969-), Ind.Philos., M.L.A., MLA Intl.Bibl., Mid.East: Abstr.& Ind., Mult.Ed.Abstr., P C I, PsycInfo, Psychol.Abstr. (1969-), Psycscan D.P., Russ.Acad.Sci.Bibl., SSCI, Soc.Sci.Ind. (Sep.1982-), Soc.Work Res.& Abstr., Sp.Ed.Needs Abstr., Stud.Wom.Abstr., e-psyche.

—BLDSC (3579.059000), CISTI, IDS, ingenta. **CCC.**

Published by: American Psychological Association, 750 First St., N.E., Washington, DC 20002-4242. TEL 202-336-5600, 800-374-2721, FAX 202-336-5568, subscriptions@apa.org, http://www.apa.org/journals/dev.html. Ed. Jane Goodman-Delahunty. Circ: 5,000.

150 USA ISSN 0273-2297
BF721

DEVELOPMENTAL REVIEW; perspectives in behavior and cognition. Text in English. 1981. q. USD 300 to institutions (effective 2001). adv. illus. index. back issues avail.; reprint service avail. from SWZ. *Refereed.* **Document type:** *Academic/Scholarly.* **Description:** Provides child and developmental, child clinical, and educational psychologists with articles that reflect current thinking and covers scientific developments.

Related titles: Online - full text ed.: (from EBSCO Publishing, O C L C Online Computer Library Center, Inc., RoweCom Information Quest, ingenta, Swets Blackwell, IDEAL Online Library, Institute for Scientific Information).

Indexed: ASCA, AgeLine, C.I.J.E., Child Devel.Abstr., Curr.Cont., Fam.Ind., IBZ, Ind.Philos., Lang.& Lang.Behav.Abstr., PsycInfo, Psychol.Abstr. (1981-), Psycscan D.P., Russ.Acad.Sci.Bibl., SOPODA, SSCI, Sociol.Abstr., e-psyche.

—BLDSC (3579.059780), IDS, ingenta. **CCC.**

Published by: Academic Press, Inc., Journal Division (Subsidiary of: Harcourt Brace & Company), 525 B St, Ste 1900, San Diego, CA 92101-4495. TEL 619-230-1840, FAX 619-699-6800, eb@acad.com, http://www.academicpress.com/dr. Ed. C J Brainerd.

155 GBR ISSN 1363-755X
BF712

DEVELOPMENTAL SCIENCE. Text in English. 1998. q. BPS 220 to institutions in UK & Europe; USD 317 Sat. to institutions in the Americas & Caribbean; GBP 220 elsewhere to institutions (effective 2002). **Document type:** *Academic/Scholarly.* **Description:** Aims to represent contemporary scientific developmental psychology both in the presentation of theory and in reporting new data.

Related titles: Online - full text ed.: (from EBSCO Publishing, O C L C Online Computer Library Center, Inc., RoweCom Information Quest, ingenta, Swets Blackwell, Institute for Scientific Information).

Indexed: Zoo.Rec., e-psyche.

—BLDSC (3579.059785). **CCC.**

Published by: Blackwell Publishers Ltd., 108 Cowley Rd, Oxford OX4 1JF, United Kingdom. TEL 44-1865-791100, FAX 44-1865-791347, jnlinfo@blackwellpublishers.co.uk, http://www.blackwellpublishers.co.uk. Ed. George Butterworth.

DEVIANCE ET SOCIETE. see *SOCIOLOGY*

DEVIANT BEHAVIOR. see *SOCIOLOGY*

DEVON COUNTY COUNCIL. SPECIAL EDUCATIONAL NEEDS SERIES. see *EDUCATION—Special Education And Rehabilitation*

DI CYAN BULLETIN. see *MEDICAL SCIENCES—Psychiatry And Neurology*

P

155.28 DEU ISSN 0012-1924
CODEN: DGNSAQ
DIAGNOSTICA; Zeitschrift fuer Psychologische Diagnostik und Differentielle Psychologie, zugleich Informationsorgan ueber psychologische Tests und Untersuchungsmethoden. Text in German; Summaries in English. 1955. q. DEM 108 (effective 2001). adv. bk.rev. bibl, charts. reprint service avail. from PSC,SCH. *Refereed.* **Document type:** *Journal, Academic/Scholarly.*
Related titles: Microfiche ed.: (from PQC); Online - full text ed.: (from Institute for Scientific Information).
Indexed: ASCA, Biol.Abstr., Curr.Cont., Ger.J.Psych., IBR, IBZ, Ind.Philos., PsycInfo, Psychol.Abstr. (1964-), Ref.Zh., SSCI.
—BLDSC (3579.670000), CISTI, GNLM, IDS.
Published by: Hogrefe Verlag GmbH und Co. KG, Rohnsweg 25, Goettingen 37085, Germany. TEL 49-551-496090, FAX 49-551-4960988, verlag@hogrefe.de, http://www.hogrefe.de. Ed. D Leutner. Circ: 1,200.

DIAGNOSTIQUE. see *EDUCATION—Special Education And Rehabilitation*

150 USA
DIALOGUES IN CONTEMPORARY PSYCHOLOGY SERIES. Text in English. 1981. irreg. price varies. **Document type:** *Monographic series.*
Indexed: e-psyche.
Published by: Praeger Publishers (Subsidiary of: Greenwood Publishing Group Inc.), 88 Post Rd W, Box 5007, Westport, CT 06881-5007. TEL 203-226-3571, FAX 203-222-1502.

DIMENSIONS (RIMROCK). see *PARAPSYCHOLOGY AND OCCULTISM*

301.1 USA
DIPLOMATE✶ **.** Text in English. 1981. s-a. membership. bk.rev. **Document type:** *Newsletter.* **Description:** Contains news for members.
Indexed: e-psyche.
Published by: American Board of Professional Psychology, 514 E Capitol Ave, Jefferson City, MO 65101-3008. TEL 573-875-1267, FAX 573-443-1199. Ed. Robert W Goldberg. Circ: 3,000 (controlled).

616.89 USA ISSN 1062-0788
DIRECTIONS IN MENTAL HEALTH COUNSELING. Text in English. 1991. q., latest vol.11, 2001. USD 165; USD 195 foreign (effective 2001). index. back issues avail.; reprints avail. *Refereed.* **Document type:** *Journal, Academic/Scholarly.* **Description:** Presents developments in mental health counseling. Approved by various boards for continuing education credits.
Indexed: e-psyche.
Published by: Hatherleigh Company Ltd., 5-22 46th Ave, Ste 200, Long Island City, NY 11101-5215. TEL 212-832-1584, 800-367-2550, FAX 212-832-1502, info@hatherleigh.com. Eds. Gerald Corey, Jane E Myers.

DIRECTORY FOR EXCEPTIONAL CHILDREN; a listing of educational and training facilities. see *EDUCATION—Special Education And Rehabilitation*

362.28 USA
DIRECTORY OF SUICIDE PREVENTION AND CRISIS INTERVENTION CENTERS. Text in English. a. USD 15 (effective 2000). **Document type:** *Directory.*
Indexed: e-psyche.
Published by: American Association of Suicidology, 4201 Connecticut Ave, Ste 408, Washington, DC 20008-1158. TEL 202-237-2280.

156 FRA ISSN 0766-5350
DIRES. Text in French. 2/yr. FRF 80; FRF 50 newsstand/cover; FRF 85.30 foreign (effective 1997). bk.rev. **Description:** Presents poetical and analytical research.
Indexed: MLA Intl.Bibl., e-psyche.
Published by: Universite Montpellier III (Universite Paul Valery), Centre d'Etudes Freudiennes de Montpellier, B.P. 5043, Montpellier Cedex 1 34032, France. TEL 33-467-142406 609, FAX 33-467-142332, serpub@alor.univ.montp3.fr.

150.19 COL
DISCERNIMIENTO. Text and summaries in Spanish, English. 1998. irreg., latest vol.5, 1999. free. back issues avail. **Description:** Examines possiblities and potentials in the field of psychology, along with the directions in which it can go.
Media: Online - full content.
Published by: Universidad del Norte, Division de Humanidades, Programa de Psicologia, Bolque D, 3er piso, Baranquilla, Colombia. http://www.uninorte.edu.co/publicacion/discernimiento, http://www.uninorte.edu.co/division/humanidades.

302 GBR ISSN 0957-9265
P302 CODEN: DISOEN
DISCOURSE & SOCIETY; an international journal for the study of discourse and communication in their social, political and cultural contexts. Text in English. 1990. q. GBP 41 to individuals; GBP 267 to institutions; GBP 8 newsstand/cover to individuals; GBP 46 newsstand/cover to institutions (effective 2002). adv. *Refereed.* **Document type:** *Academic/Scholarly.* **Description:** Explores the relevance of discourse analysis to the social sciences, with a particular focus on the political implications of discourse and communication.
Related titles: Online - full text ed.: (from EBSCO Publishing, O C L C Online Computer Library Center, Inc., RoweCom Information Quest, Gale Group, ingenta, Swets Blackwell, Institute for Scientific Information).
Indexed: ASCA, ASSIA, Arts & Hum.Cit.Ind. (coverage dropped), Bibl.Ling., Commun.Abstr., Curr.Cont., Educ.Admin.Abstr., Film Lit.Ind., Human Resour.Abstr., IBR, IBZ, Int.Bibl.Soc.Sci., Int.Polit.Sci.Abstr., Intl.Bibl.Soc.Sci., Lang.& Lang.Behav.Abstr., Ling.Abstr., M.L.A., MLA Intl.Bibl., Peace Res.Abstr., Res.High.Educ.Abstr., SOPODA, SSCI, Sage Fam.Stud.Abstr., Sage Pub.Admin.Abstr., Sage Urb.Stud.Abstr., Soc.Serv.Abstr., Sociol.Abstr., Stud.Wom.Abstr., Viol.& Abuse Abstr., e-psyche.
—BLDSC (3595.810000), ingenta. **CCC.**
Published by: Sage Publications Ltd., 6 Bonhill St, London EC2A 4PU, United Kingdom. TEL 44-20-7374-0645, FAX 44-20-7374-8741, market@sagepub.co.uk, http://www.sagepub.co.uk. Ed. Teun A van Dijk. Adv. contact Jenny Kirby. page GBP 195.

▼ **DISCOURSE STUDIES**; an interdisciplinary journal for the study of text and talk. see *LINGUISTICS*

150 USA
DISTINGUISHED CONTRIBUTIONS IN PSYCHOLOGY. Text in English. irreg. **Document type:** *Monographic series.* **Description:** Offers research in developmental, social and personality psychology.
Indexed: e-psyche.
Published by: Guilford Publications, Inc., 72 Spring St, New York, NY 10012. TEL 212-431-9800, 800-365-7006, FAX 212-966-6708, info@guilford.com, http://www.guilford.com. Eds. E Tory Higgins, Kurt W Fischer.

DIVAN. see *LITERARY AND POLITICAL REVIEWS*

DOCTOR - PATIENT STUDIES. see *MEDICAL SCIENCES*

616.891 FRA ISSN 0012-477X
DOCUMENTS ET DEBATS. Text in French. 1970. irreg. (4-5/yr.). membership. bk.rev. abstr, bibl. **Document type:** *Bulletin.* **Description:** Explores psychoanalytic techniques.
Media: Duplicated (not offset).
Indexed: e-psyche.
Published by: Association Psychoanalytique de France, 24 place Dauphine, Paris 75001, France. Circ: 200.

▼ **DOMESTIC VIOLENCE AND CHILD ABUSE SOURCEBOOK.** see *CRIMINOLOGY AND LAW ENFORCEMENT*

155.3 236 367 USA
DOMINANT NEWSLETTER. Text in English. 1975. 10/yr. USD 20. adv. bk.rev. back issues avail.
Indexed: e-psyche.
Published by: Skye Publishing, PO Box 324, Riverside, IL 60546. Ed. Jonathan Lee. Circ: 300.

150 JPN ISSN 0389-312X
DOSHISHA SHINRI/DOSHISHA PSYCHOLOGICAL REVIEW. Text in Japanese. a.
Indexed: e-psyche.
Published by: Doshisha Daigaku, Bungakubu/Doshisha University, Faculty of Letters, Department of Psychology, Shinrigaku Kenkyushitsu, 601, Genbucho, Karasuma Higashi Iru, Imadegawa Dori, Kamigyo-ku, Kyoto-shi 602, Japan.

DOWN SYNDROME: RESEARCH AND PRACTICE. see *MEDICAL SCIENCES—Psychiatry And Neurology*

DREAM NETWORK; a quarterly journal exploring dreams and myth. see *NEW AGE PUBLICATIONS*

DREAM SWITCHBOARD. see *EDUCATION*

152 USA
DREAM TIME✶ **.** Text in English. 1984. q. membership. bk.rev. abstr, bibl, charts, illus. back issues avail. *Refereed.* **Document type:** *Magazine, Academic/Scholarly.* **Description:** International, multidisciplinary, basic and applied dream research.
Formerly: A S D Newsletter
Indexed: e-psyche.
Published by: Association for the Study of Dreams, PO Box 1592, Merced, CA 95341. asdreams@aol.com, http://www.outreach.org/gmcc/asd. Ed., R&P, Adv. contact Alan Seigel TEL 510-652-4185. Circ: 1,000.

158 DNK
DRIFT (VANLOESE); tidsskrift for psykoanalyse. Text in Danish. 3/yr. DKK 240; DKK 90 newsstand/cover (effective 2001). **Document type:** *Academic/Scholarly.*
Published by: Tommy Thambour & Rene Rasmussen, Eds. & Pubs., Rebildvej 14, Vanloese 2720, Denmark. TEL 45-38-88-50-86. Eds. Rene Rasmussen, Tommy Thambour.

150 USA
DYNAMICAL PSYCHOLOGY. Text in English. 1993. irreg. *Refereed.*
Formerly (until 1995): PsychoScience
Media: Online - full text.
Address: http://goertzel.org/dynapsyc/dynacon.html. Ed. Ben Goertzel.

E A P DIGEST. (Employee Assistance Programs) see *DRUG ABUSE AND ALCOHOLISM*

▼ **EARLY CHILDHOOD RESEARCH & PRACTICE.** see *EDUCATION*

155.4 USA
EARLY CHILDHOOD UPDATE. Text in English. 1996. s-a. free. back issues avail. **Document type:** *Newsletter, Government.* **Description:** Discusses topics of interest to persons involved in teaching young children in preschool, kindergarden, and the primary elementary grades.
Indexed: e-psyche.
Published by: (U.S. Department of Education), National Institute on Early Childhood Development and Education, Early Childhood Research Working Group, 555 New Jersey Ave, N W, Washington, DC 20208. TEL 202-219-1935, FAX 202-273-4768, eci@inet.ed.gov, http://www.ed.gov/offices/OERI/EDI.

EARLY EDUCATION AND DEVELOPMENT. see *EDUCATION*

EATING AND WEIGHT DISORDERS; Studies on Anorexia, Bulimia and Obesity. see *MEDICAL SCIENCES—Psychiatry And Neurology*

150 NLD ISSN 1471-0153
▼ **EATING BEHAVIORS.** Text in English. 2000. q. NLG 277, NLG 125.70 in Europe to individuals; JPY 17,400 in Japan to individuals; USD 146 elsewhere to individuals; NLG 646, EUR 293.14 in Europe to institutions; JPY 40,700 in Japan to institutions; USD 338 elsewhere to institutions; USD 1,196 to institutions with Addictive Behaviors (effective 2001).
Related titles: Online - full text ed.: (from ingenta, ScienceDirect).
—BLDSC (3646.939080).
Published by: Elsevier Science BV, Sara Burgerhartstraat 25, Amsterdam 1055 KV, Netherlands. TEL 31-20-485-2911, FAX 31-20-485-2457, nlinfo-f@elsevier.nl, http://www.elsevier.com/locate/eatbeh, http://www.elsevier.nl.

616.89 USA ISSN 1064-0266
RC552.E18
EATING DISORDERS; the journal of treatment and prevention. Text in English. 1992. q. GBP 47, USD 78 to individuals; GBP 104, USD 172 to institutions (effective 2002). back issues avail. *Refereed.* **Document type:** *Academic/Scholarly.* **Description:** Provides a wide range of practical and informative viewpoints for professionals involved in the treatment of and education in eating disorders.
Related titles: Online - full text ed.: 1992 (from CatchWord Ltd.).
Indexed: PsycInfo, e-psyche.
—BLDSC (3646.939100), KNAW.
Published by: Brunner - Routledge (Subsidiary of: Taylor & Francis Group), 325 Chestnut St, Ste 800, Philadelphia, PA 19106. TEL 215-269-0400, FAX 215-269-0363, postmaster@bmpub.com. Ed. Leigh Cohn.

P

158 ITA ISSN 0394-1310
ECOLOGIA DELLA MENTE. Text in Italian; Summaries in English, Spanish. 1986. s-a. USD 73 (effective 2000). adv. **Document type:** *Academic/Scholarly.*
Indexed: PsycInfo, e-psyche.
Published by: (Centro Studi di Terapia Familiare e Relazionale), Il Pensiero Scientifico Editore s.r.l., Via Bradano, 3-C, Rome, RM 00199, Italy. TEL 39-06-862821, FAX 39-06-86282250, pensiero@pensiero.it, http://www.pensiero.it. Ed. Luigi Cancrini. Adv. contact Luciano De Fiore. Circ: 2,000.

370.1 USA ISSN 1040-7413
BF353 CODEN: ECPSEN
ECOLOGICAL PSYCHOLOGY. Text in English. 1989. q. USD 55 in US & Canada to individuals; USD 85 elsewhere to individuals; USD 395 in US & Canada to institutions; USD 420 elsewhere to institutions (effective 2002). adv. *Refereed.* **Document type:** *Journal, Academic/Scholarly.* **Description:** Presents empirical, theoretical, and methodological papers in the form of research reports, target articles and commentary.
Related titles: Online - full text ed.: ISSN 1532-6969. USD 49.50 to individuals; USD 355.50 to institutions (effective 2002) (from CatchWord Ltd., EBSCO Publishing, O C L C Online Computer Library Center, Inc., RoweCom Information Quest, Swets Blackwell, Institute for Scientific Information).
Indexed: ASCA, Curr.Cont., Ergon.Abstr., PsycInfo, Psychol.Abstr. (1989-), SSCI, e-psyche.
—BLDSC (3649.050000), CatchWord, Infotrieve, ingenta. **CCC.**
Published by: (International Society for Ecological Psychology), Lawrence Erlbaum Associates, Inc., 10 Industrial Ave, Mahwah, NJ 07430-2262. TEL 201-760-3735, 800-926-6579, FAX 201-236-0072, journals@erlbaum.com, http://www.erlbaum.com/Journals/journals/ECO/eco.htm. Ed. William Mace. adv.: page USD 275; trim 5 x 8.

EDUCATION AND PSYCHOLOGY OF THE GIFTED SERIES. see *EDUCATION—Special Education And Rehabilitation*

EDUCATION AND PSYCHOLOGY REVIEW. see *EDUCATION*

370.15 150 155.4 GBR
EDUCATIONAL & CHILD PSYCHOLOGY. Text in English. 1984. q. GBP 40 domestic; GBP 60 foreign (effective 1999). back issues avail. *Refereed.* **Document type:** *Academic/Scholarly.* **Description:** Deals with the research and professional practice of educational and child psychology.
Formerly: British Psychology Society. Division of Educational and Child Psychology. Papers (0267-1611)
Indexed: Br.Educ.Ind., Cont.Pg.Educ., ERA, Mult.Ed.Abstr., PsycInfo, Psychol.Abstr. (1985-), Sp.Ed.Needs Abstr., e-psyche.
—BLDSC (3661.363300). **CCC.**
Published by: The British Psychological Society, Division of Educational and Child Psychology, St Andrews House, 48 Princess Rd E, Leicester LE1 7DR, United Kingdom. Ed. Peter Graves. Circ: 1,000.

EDUCATIONAL AND PSYCHOLOGICAL INTERACTIONS. see *EDUCATION*

155.28 370.15 USA ISSN 0013-1644
BF1 CODEN: EPMEAJ
EDUCATIONAL AND PSYCHOLOGICAL MEASUREMENT; devoted to the development and application of measures of individual differences. Text in English. 1941. bi-m. USD 95 to individuals; USD 395 to institutions; USD 25 newsstand/cover to individuals; USD 75 newsstand/cover to institutions (effective 2002). adv. bk.rev. bibl, charts. index. back issues avail.; reprint service avail. from PQC,PSC,SCH. *Refereed.* **Document type:** *Academic/Scholarly.* **Description:** Discusses problems in the field of measuring individual differences and reports research on the development and use of tests and measurements in education.
Related titles: Microform ed.: (from PQC); Online - full text ed.: (from EBSCO Publishing, H. W. Wilson, O C L C Online Computer Library Center, Inc., RoweCom Information Quest, ProQuest Information & Learning, Gale Group, ingenta, Swets Blackwell, Institute for Scientific Information).
Indexed: ASCA, Abstr.Anthropol., Acad.Ind., Adol.Ment.Hlth.Abstr., C.I.J.E., CINAHL, Chem.Abstr., Compumath, Cont.Pg.Educ., Curr.Cont., Curr.Ind.Stat., Educ.Admin.Abstr., Educ.Ind. (Jun.1983-), Except.Child Educ.Abstr., Fam.Ind., High.Educ.Abstr., High.Educ.Curr.Aware.Bull., IBR, IBZ, Ind.Philos., Mark.Res.Abstr. (1963-), Mid.East: Abstr.& Ind., Mult.Ed.Abstr., P C I, Pers.Lit., PsycInfo, Psychol.Abstr. (1941-), Psycscan A.P., Res.High.Educ.Abstr., SSCI, Soc.Sci.Ind. (Jan.1994-), Sp.Ed.Needs Abstr., e-psyche.
—BLDSC (3661.366000), IDS, ingenta. **CCC.**
Published by: Sage Publications, Inc., 2455 Teller Rd, Thousand Oaks, CA 91320. TEL 805-499-0721, FAX 805-499-0871, info@sagepub.com, http://www.sagepub.com. Eds. Bruce Thompson, Michael E Roloff. Pub. Sara Miller McCune. R&P Tanya Udin. Adv. contact DeAnna Vega Hammersley. Circ: 2,700 (paid). **Overseas subscr. to:** Sage Publications Ltd., 6 Bonhill St, London EC2A 4PU, United Kingdom; Sage Publications India Pvt. Ltd., 4215, New Delhi 110 048, India.

370.15 USA ISSN 0046-1520
LB1051 CODEN: EDPSDT
EDUCATIONAL PSYCHOLOGIST. Text in English. 1963. q. USD 50 in US & Canada to individuals; USD 80 elsewhere to individuals; USD 370 in US & Canada to institutions; USD 400 elsewhere to institutions (effective 2002). adv. illus. index. reprint service avail. from PQC. *Refereed.* **Document type:** *Journal, Academic/Scholarly.* **Description:** Provides detailed explorations of new educational concepts and accepted educational practices.
Related titles: Microform ed.: (from PQC); Online - full text ed.: ISSN 1532-6985. USD 45 to individuals; USD 333 to institutions (effective 2002) (from CatchWord Ltd., EBSCO Publishing, O C L C Online Computer Library Center, Inc., RoweCom Information Quest, Swets Blackwell, Institute for Scientific Information).
Indexed: ASCA, Cont.Pg.Educ., Curr.Cont., Curr.Ind.Stat., ERA, Educ.Ind. (Apr.1983-), Mult.Ed.Abstr., PsycInfo, Psychol.Abstr. (1973-), SSCI, Sociol.Educ.Abstr., Sp.Ed.Needs Abstr., Tech.Educ.Abstr., e-psyche.
—BLDSC (3661.530000), CatchWord, ingenta. **CCC.**
Published by: (Division of Educational Psychology, American Psychological Association), Lawrence Erlbaum Associates, Inc., 10 Industrial Ave, Mahwah, NJ 07430-2262. TEL 201-760-3735, 800-926-6579, FAX 201-236-0072, journals@erlbaum.com, http://www.erlbaum.com/Journals/journals/EP/ep.htm. Eds. Lyn Corno, Philip H Winne. adv.: page USD 425; trim 7 x 10. Circ: 3,700.

EDUCATIONAL PSYCHOLOGY; an international journal of experimental educational psychology. see *EDUCATION*

EDUCATIONAL PSYCHOLOGY IN PRACTICE. see *EDUCATION*

EDUCATIONAL PSYCHOLOGY REVIEW. see *EDUCATION*

158 RUS ISSN 0321-2173
EKSPERIMENTAL'NAYA I PRIKLADNAYA PSIKHOLOGIYA. Text in Russian. 1968. irreg.
Indexed: e-psyche.
Published by: Sankt-Peterburgskii Universitet, Universitetskaya nab 7-9, St Petersburg 199034, Russian Federation. Circ: 5,150.

150 RUS
EKSPERIMENTAL'NOE ISSLEDOVANIE LICHNOSTI I TEMPERAMENTA. Text in Russian. irreg. illus.
Indexed: e-psyche.
Published by: Permskii Gosudarstvennyi Pedagogicheskii Institut, Perm, Russian Federation. Ed. Bronislaw Aleksandrovich Vyatkin.

154.6 USA ISSN 1089-4284
ELECTRIC DREAMS. Text in English. 1994. m. USD 200. **Document type:** *Newsletter.* **Description:** Publishes dreams, comments on dreams, articles on dream sharing and dreamwork, as well as news on public dream related events both on- and off-line.
Related titles: Online - full text ed.
Indexed: e-psyche.
Published by: Dream Gate, 4644 Geary Blvd PMB 171, San Francisco, CA 94118. TEL 415-221-3239, ed@dreamgate.com, http://www.dreamgate.com/electric-dreams. Ed. Richard Catlett Wilkerson.

616.89 CAN ISSN 1492-1103
THE ELECTRONIC JOURNAL OF COMMUNICATIVE PSYCHOANALYSIS; an independent multilingual international publication. Text in English. 1998. q. abstr. back issues avail. *Refereed.* **Document type:** *Academic/Scholarly.* **Description:** Promotes free scholarly discussion of ideas in psychoanalysis, psychotherapy, psychology, and psychiatry.
Media: Online - full text.
Indexed: e-psyche.
Published by: Electronic Journal of Communicative Psychoanalysis, Office 301, 1055 W Broadway, Vancouver, BC V6H 1E2, Canada. FAX 604-261-3931, editor.ejcp@mortimer.com, http://www.mortimer.com/psychoanalysiscom/. Ed. V A Bonac.

THE ELEMENTARY SCHOOL JOURNAL. see *EDUCATION*

150 USA ISSN 1528-3542
▼ **EMOTION.** Text in English. 2001 (Spring). q. USD 70 domestic to non-members; USD 85 foreign to non-members; USD 35 domestic to members; USD 45 foreign to members; USD 150 domestic to institutions; USD 182 foreign to institutions; USD 19 domestic to students; USD 29 foreign to students (effective 2001). **Document type:** *Academic/Scholarly.* **Description:** Publishes articles that advance knowledge and theory about all aspects of emotional processes, including reports of substantial empirical studies, scholarly reviews, and major theoretical articles.
Published by: American Psychological Association, 750 First St., N.E., Washington, DC 20002-4242. TEL 202-336-5600, FAX 202-336-5568, subscriptions@apa.org, http://www.apa.org/journals/emo.html. Eds. Jane Goodman-Delahunty, Klaus R Scherer.

152.4 USA
EMOTIONS AND SOCIAL BEHAVIOR. Text in English. irreg. **Document type:** *Monographic series.* **Description:** Explores complex human emotions.
Indexed: e-psyche.
Published by: Guilford Publications, Inc., 72 Spring St, New York, NY 10012. TEL 212-431-9800, 800-365-7006, FAX 212-966-6708, info@guilford.com, http://www.guilford.com. Ed. Peter Salovey.

EMPLOYEE ASSISTANCE REPORT; supporting EAP and HR professionals. see *BUSINESS AND ECONOMICS—Personnel Management*

EMPLOYEE TESTING & THE LAW; reporting legal, technical, and business developments in employee testing. see *BUSINESS AND ECONOMICS—Personnel Management*

616.89 USA
ENCOUNTERER. Text in English. 1971. irreg. USD 5.
Indexed: e-psyche.
Published by: Golden Gate Foundation for Group Treatment, PO Box 1141, Vallejo, CA 94590. Ed. Dr. F H Ernst.

150.19 USA
ENCOUNTERING JUNG. Text in English. 1995. irreg., latest vol.7, 1999. price varies; not for sale in the Commonwealth. back issues avail. **Document type:** *Monographic series, Academic/Scholarly.* **Description:** Examines the life and work of Carl Gustav Jung and his contributions to psychoanalytic psychology.
Published by: Princeton University Press, 41 William St, Princeton, NJ 08540. TEL 609-258-4900, FAX 609-258-6305, http://pup.princeton.edu. **in Canada:** University Press Group; **in continental Europe & Africa:** John Wiley & Sons Ltd.

370.15 USA
ENCYCLOPEDIC DICTIONARY OF PSYCHOLOGY. Text in English. irreg., latest vol.3, 1985. USD 14.95. illus.
Published by: Dushkin - McGraw-Hill, Sluice Dock, Guilford, CT 06437-9989. TEL 203-453-4351, FAX 203-453-6000. Ed. Terry F Pettijohn. Pub. Jeffrey Hahn. R&P Cheryl Greenleaf.

150 CHE ISSN 0938-3522
ENERGIE UND CHARAKTER✶. Text in German. 1990. s-a. CHF 60 (effective 2000). adv. bk.rev. index. back issues avail. *Refereed.* **Document type:** *Magazine, Academic/Scholarly.*
Indexed: e-psyche.
Address: Benzenrueti 6, Heiden 9410, Switzerland. TEL 41-71-8916855, FAX 41-71-8915855, biosynthesis@bluewin.ch. Ed. David Boadella. Circ: 1,000 (controlled).

150 USA ISSN 1050-5326
RC489.B5
ENERGY & CONSCIOUSNESS; international journal of core energetics. Text in English. 1991. s-a. USD 25 domestic; USD 45 foreign (effective 2000). adv. bk.rev. back issues avail. **Document type:** *Academic/Scholarly.* **Description:** Articles are theoretical and clinical, focussing on the theory and practice of Core Energetic psychotherapy. Research reports and literature reviews are included.
Indexed: e-psyche.
Published by: Institute of Core Energetics, 115 E 92nd St, #2A, New York, NY 10010. TEL 212-987-4969, FAX 914-427-0264, jacarleton@aol.com. Ed. Dr. Jacqueline Carleton. R&P, Adv. contact Joan Groom TEL 908-276-5867. Circ: 500.

ENFANCE; psychologie, pedagogie, neuro-psychiatrie, sociologie. see *CHILDREN AND YOUTH—About*

ENFANCE & PSY. see *CHILDREN AND YOUTH—About*

158 MEX ISSN 0185-1594
ENSENANZA E INVESTIGACION EN PSICOLOGIA. Text in Spanish. 1975. a. MXP 290, USD 25. adv. bk.rev. abstr, bibl. index. reprint service avail. from PQC. **Document type:** *Academic/Scholarly.*
Related titles: Microfilm ed.: (from PQC).
Indexed: Biol.Abstr., Psychol.Abstr., e-psyche.
Published by: Consejo Nacional para la Ensenanza e Investigacion en Psicologia, c/o Universidad Iberoamericana, Mexico, PROL PASEO DE LA REFORMA 880, Lomas de Santa Fe, Ciudad De Mexico, DF 01219, Mexico. Ed. Dr. Juan Lafarga. Circ: 1,000.

150 ARG
ENTREDICHOS. Text in Spanish. 1983. m.
Address: La Rioja, 718, Capital Federal, Buenos Aires 1221, Argentina.

ENVIRONMENT AND BEHAVIOR. see *SOCIOLOGY*

EOS; revista Argentina de arte y psicoanalisis. see *ART*

152.4 CAN
EQUILIBRIUM (TORONTO). Text in English. bi-m. **Document type:** *Newsletter.*
Indexed: e-psyche.
Published by: Mood Disorders Association of Metropolitan Toronto, 40 Orchard View Blvd, Ste 222, Toronto, ON M4R 1B9, Canada. TEL 416-486-8046, FAX 416-486-8127. Ed. Eric Jonasson.

EQUINE BEHAVIOUR. see *SPORTS AND GAMES—Horses And Horsemanship*

ERGONOMIA; prodotti, lavoro, ricerca. see *ENGINEERING*

ERGONOMICS; an international journal of research and practice in human factors and ergonomics. see *ENGINEERING*

ERGONOMICS IN DESIGN; the magazine of human factors applications. see *ENGINEERING*

THE ERGONOMIST. see *ENGINEERING*

150 USA
ESALEN CATALOG. Text in English. 1961. 3/yr. USD 15. **Document type:** *Catalog.*
Published by: Esalen Institute, Big Sur, CA 93920. TEL 408-667-3000, FAX 408-667-2724. Ed. Margaret Livingston. Circ: 25,000.

150 FRA ISSN 1270-7864
ESPRIT LIBRE. Text in French. 1958; N.S. 1996. q. FRF 20; FRF 30 foreign (effective 2001). **Description:** How-to style journal helps the reader get free from obstinate opinions, prejudices, fixed convictions, social conditioning and political and religious phantasms.
Media: Duplicated (not offset).
Indexed: e-psyche.
Published by: Georges Krassovsky, Ed. & Pub., B.P. 164, Paris Cedex 14 75664, France. Circ: 1,000.

150 USA ISSN 0959-4779
ESSAYS IN COGNITIVE PSYCHOLOGY. Text in English. 1988. irreg. **Document type:** *Monographic series.*
Indexed: e-psyche.
Published by: Lawrence Erlbaum Associates, Inc., 10 Industrial Ave, Mahwah, NJ 07430-2262. TEL 201-236-9500, 800-926-6579, FAX 201-236-0072, orders@erlbaum.com, http://www.erlbaum.com.

150 USA ISSN 0959-3977
ESSAYS IN DEVELOPMENTAL PSYCHOLOGY. Text in English. 1990. irreg. **Document type:** *Monographic series.*
Indexed: e-psyche.
Published by: Lawrence Erlbaum Associates, Inc., 10 Industrial Ave, Mahwah, NJ 07430-2262. TEL 201-236-9500, 800-926-6579, FAX 201-236-0072, orders@erlbaum.com, http://www.erlbaum.com.

150 USA
ESSENTIALS OF ADOLESCENCE* . Text in English. 1975. m. (11/yr.). USD 25. back issues avail.
Formerly: Essence of Adolescence
Indexed: e-psyche.
Published by: PeopleScience, Inc., 20 Pine Valley Ln, Jamesburg, NJ 08831-2705. Ed. Fred Streit. Circ: 2,200.

150 ESP ISSN 0210-9395
BF5
ESTUDIOS DE PSICOLOGIA. Text in Spanish. 1980. s-a. ESP 3,200 per issue foreign. adv. *Refereed.* **Document type:** *Academic/Scholarly.* **Description:** Publishes empirical research, theoretical essays and bibliographic reviews in the field of current general psychology.
Related titles: Online - full text ed.: (from CatchWord Ltd.).
Indexed: PsycInfo, e-psyche.
—CINDOC.
Published by: Fundacion Infancia y Aprendizaje, Cr Canillas, 138, 2o 16C, Madrid 28043, Spain. TEL 34-91-388-3874, FAX 34-91-300-3527. Ed. Angel Riviere. Circ: 1,100.

150 BRA ISSN 0103-166X
ESTUDOS DE PSICOLOGIA. Text in Portuguese; Summaries in Portuguese. 1983. every 4 mos. BRL 10 domestic; USD 5 foreign (effective 1999). bk.rev. back issues avail. *Refereed.* **Document type:** *Magazine, Academic/Scholarly.* **Description:** Provides current research and scientific communications for students and professionals in the fields of psychology and psychiatry.
Related titles: E-mail ed.; Fax ed.; Online - full text ed.
Published by: Pontificia Universidade Catolica de Campinas, Departamento de Pos-Graduacao em Psicologia, Rua Waldemar Cesar da Silveira, 105 Swift, Campinas, SP 13045-270, Brazil. TEL 55-19-2307180, FAX 55-19-2307180, vraposo@mpc.comu.br, http://www.epub.org.br/epsico. Ed., R&P Vera Lucia Adami Raposo do Amaral.

301.1 150 ITA ISSN 0392-0658
RJ131
ETA EVOLUTIVA; rivista di scienze dello sviluppo. Text in Italian; Summaries in English. 1978. 3/yr. ITL 75,000 domestic; ITL 85,000 foreign (effective 2001). back issues avail. **Document type:** *Academic/Scholarly.* **Description:** Contains theoretical work and experimental research on the evolutive age, covering several areas of interest: psychology, sociology, pedagogy, genetics, and psychoanalysis.
Indexed: Ind.Philos., PsycInfo, Psychol.Abstr. (1979-), e-psyche.
Published by: Giunti Gruppo Editoriale S.p.A., Via Bolognese, 165, Florence, FI 50139, Italy. TEL 39-55-5062236, FAX 39-55-5062397, promoper@giunti.it, http://www.giunti.it. Circ: 1,300.

370.15 150 USA ISSN 1050-8422
BJ1725
ETHICS & BEHAVIOR. Text in English. 1991. q. USD 35 in US & Canada to individuals; USD 65 elsewhere to individuals; USD 390 in US & Canada to institutions; USD 420 elsewhere to institutions (effective 2002). adv. bk.rev. illus. reprints avail. *Refereed.* **Document type:** *Journal, Academic/Scholarly.* **Description:** Publishes articles on an array of topics pertaining to various moral issues and conduct.
Related titles: Online - full text ed.: ISSN 1532-7019. USD 31.50 to individuals; USD 351 to institutions (effective 2002) (from CatchWord Ltd., EBSCO Publishing, O C L C Online Computer Library Center, Inc., RoweCom Information Quest, Swets Blackwell, Institute for Scientific Information).
Indexed: ASCA, ASSIA, Curr.Cont., Environ.Sci.Poll.Mgmt., Fam.Ind., P.A.I.S., Phil.Ind., PsycInfo, Psychol.Abstr. (1991-), Risk Abstr., SSCI, Saf.Sci.Abstr., Soc.Serv.Abstr., Sociol.Abstr., e-psyche.
—CatchWord, ingenta. **CCC.**
Published by: Lawrence Erlbaum Associates, Inc., 10 Industrial Ave, Mahwah, NJ 07430-2262. TEL 201-760-3735, 800-926-6579, FAX 201-236-0072, journals@erlbaum.com, http://www.erlbaum.com/Journals/journals/EB/eb.htm. Ed. Gerald P Koocher. adv.: page USD 375; trim 5 x 8.

155.82 DEU ISSN 0937-4523
ETHNOPSYCHOANALYSE. Text in German. 1990. biennial, latest vol.6, 2001. EUR 19.90 per vol. (effective 2001). bk.rev. **Document type:** *Monographic series, Academic/Scholarly.*
Indexed: IBR, IBZ, Ind.Philos., e-psyche.
Published by: Brandes und Apsel Verlag GmbH, Scheidswaldstr 33, Frankfurt Am Main 60385, Germany. TEL 49-69-95730186, FAX 49-69-95730187, brandes-apsel@t-online.de, http://www.brandes-apsel-verlag.de.

150 DEU ISSN 0940-9882
ETHNOPSYCHOLOGISCHE MITTEILUNGEN. Text in German; Summaries in English, German. 1992. s-a. DEM 40. bk.rev. **Document type:** *Academic/Scholarly.*
Indexed: e-psyche.
Published by: Universitaet Koblenz-Landau, Fachbereich Psychologie, Im Fort 7, Landau In Der Pfalz 76829, Germany. TEL 49-6341-280249, FAX 49-6341-280101. Ed. Renaud van Quekelberghe. Circ: 140.

ETHOLOGY. see *BIOLOGY—Zoology*

ETHOLOGY ONLINE. see *BIOLOGY—Zoology*

ETOLOGIA. see *BIOLOGY—Zoology*

616.89 BEL
ETUDES PSYCHANALYTIQUES. Text in French. 1970. s-a. BEF 1,965; BEF 2,295 in the European Union; BEF 2,625 elsewhere (effective 2000). **Document type:** *Academic/Scholarly.* **Description:** Covers psychoanalytic techniques involving the waking dream state.
Formerly (until 1999): Etudes Psychotherapiques (1372-8210)
Indexed: Biol.Abstr., IBZ, Psychoanal.Abstr., Psychol.Abstr., e-psyche.
—BLDSC (3821.620000).
Published by: Groupe International du Reve-Eveille en Psychanalyse, 18 rue Bertholet, Paris 75005, France.

616.8526 301.1 GBR ISSN 1072-4133
RC552.E18 CODEN: EEDRE8
EUROPEAN EATING DISORDERS REVIEW. Text in English. 1986. 5/yr. USD 335 in United States; USD 335 in Canada & Mexico; USD 335 elsewhere; USD 352 combined subscription in United States for print and online eds.; USD 352 combined subscription in Canada & Mexico for print and online eds.; USD 352 combined subscription elsewhere for print and online eds. (effective 2002). adv. bk.rev. back issues avail.; reprint service avail. from SWZ. *Refereed.* **Document type:** *Academic/Scholarly.* **Description:** Covers all aspects of bulimia and anorexia nervosa for the complete range of professionals who deal with patients suffering from these eating disorders.
Former titles (until 1994): Eating Disorders Review (1067-1633); (until 1993): British Review of Bulimia and Anorexia Nervosa (0950-3005)
Related titles: Microform ed.: (from PQC); Online - full text ed.: ISSN 1099-0976. USD 335 in United States; USD 335 in Canada & Mexico; USD 335 elsewhere (effective 2002) (from EBSCO Publishing, ingenta, Wiley InterScience, Institute for Scientific Information).
Indexed: ASCA, Curr.Cont., Excerp.Med., Nutr.Abstr., PsycInfo, Psychol.Abstr., SSCI, e-psyche.
—BLDSC (3829.693600), CISTI, EMDOCS, GNLM, IDS, Infotrieve. **CCC.**
Published by: (Eating Disorders Association), Wiley Europe Ltd., Baffins Ln, Chichester, W Sussex PO19 1UD, United Kingdom. TEL 44-1243-779777, FAX 44-1243-775878, customer@wiley.co.uk, http://www.wiley.co.uk. adv.: B&W page GBP 650, color page GBP 1,550; trim 165 x 248. Circ: 750. **Subscr. in the Americas to:** John Wiley & Sons, Inc., Journals, 605 Third Ave, New York, NY 10158. TEL 212-850-6021, 212-850-6645, subinfo@jwiley.com.

155 GBR ISSN 0954-1446
BF309 CODEN: EJCPEW
EUROPEAN JOURNAL OF COGNITIVE PSYCHOLOGY. Text in English. 1989. q. GBP 131, USD 216 to individuals; GBP 262, USD 432 to institutions (effective 2002). adv. *Refereed.* **Document type:** *Academic/Scholarly.* **Description:** Focuses on articles of either a theoretical or a review nature to provide an integrated rather than empirical approach.
Formerly: European Cognitive Psychology
Related titles: Online - full text ed.: ISSN 1464-0635 (from CatchWord Ltd., EBSCO Publishing, O C L C Online Computer Library Center, Inc., RoweCom Information Quest, Swets Blackwell, Institute for Scientific Information).
Indexed: ASCA, AgeLine, Bibl.Ling., Curr.Cont., Ergon.Abstr., Lang.& Lang.Behav.Abstr., PsycInfo, Psychol.Abstr. (1989-), SOPODA, SSCI, Sociol.Abstr., e-psyche.
—BLDSC (3829.728150), CatchWord, GNLM, IDS, Infotrieve, ingenta. **CCC.**
Published by: (European Society for Cognitive Psychology), Psychology Press (Subsidiary of: Taylor & Francis Group), 27 Church Rd, Hove, E Sussex BN3 2FA, United Kingdom. TEL 44-1273-207411, FAX 44-1273-205612, information@psypress.co.uk, http://www.journals.tandf.co.uk/, http://www.psypress.co.uk. Ed. Phillip Smith. R&P Zoe Peden TEL 44-20-7842-2363. Adv. contact Claire Buckminster. **Subscr. addr. in N America:** Psychology Press, Journals Customer Service, Taylor & Francis Group, 325 Chestnut St, Philadelphia, PA 19106. TEL 800-354-1420, FAX 215-625-8914, info@taylorandfrancis.com, http://www.psypress.com.

P

156 GBR ISSN 0890-2070
BF698.A1
EUROPEAN JOURNAL OF PERSONALITY. Text in English; Summaries in English, French, German. 1987. bi-m. USD 895 in United States; USD 895 in Canada & Mexico; USD 895 elsewhere; USD 940 combined subscription in United States for print and online eds.; USD 940 combined subscription in Canada & Mexico for print and online eds.; USD 940 combined subscription elsewhere for print and online eds. (effective 2002). adv. bk.rev. back issues avail.; reprint service avail. from SWZ. *Refereed.* **Document type:** *Academic/Scholarly.* **Description:** Reflects all areas of current research in personality psychology with emphasis on human individuality.
Related titles: Microform ed.: (from PQC); Online - full text ed.: ISSN 1099-0984. USD 895 in United States; USD 895 in Canada & Mexico; USD 895 elsewhere (effective 2002) (from EBSCO Publishing, ingenta, Wiley InterScience, Institute for Scientific Information).
Indexed: ASCA, ASSIA, AgeLine, Curr.Cont., ERA, Lang.& Lang.Behav.Abstr., Mult.Ed.Abstr., PsycInfo, Psychol.Abstr. (1987-), Ref.Zh., SOPODA, SSCI, Sociol.Abstr., e-psyche.
—BLDSC (3829.733800), IDS, ingenta. **CCC.**
Published by: (European Association of Personality Psychology), Wiley Europe Ltd., Baffins Ln, Chichester, W Sussex PO19 1UD, United Kingdom. TEL 44-1243-779777, FAX 44-1243-775878, customer@wiley.co.uk, http://www.wiley.co.uk. adv.: B&W page GBP 650, color page GBP 1,550; trim 165 x 248. Circ: 500. **Subscr. in the Americas to:** John Wiley & Sons, Inc., Journals, 605 Third Ave, New York, NY 10158. TEL 212-850-6021, 212-850-6645, subinfo@jwiley.com.

152 USA ISSN 1015-5759
EUROPEAN JOURNAL OF PSYCHOLOGICAL ASSESSMENT. Text in English. 3/yr. USD 74 to individuals; USD 139 to institutions (effective 2001). bk.rev. abstr. back issues avail. *Refereed.* **Document type:** *Journal, Academic/Scholarly.* **Description:** Presents articles which provide seminal information on both theoretical and applied developments in the field of psychological testing.
Related titles: Online - full text ed.: (from Institute for Scientific Information).
Indexed: ASCA, Curr.Cont., IBZ, PsycInfo, Psychol.Abstr. (1985-), SSCI, e-psyche.
—BLDSC (3829.737800), IDS, Infotrieve. **CCC.**
Published by: (European Association of Psychological Assessment), Hogrefe & Huber Publishers, PO Box 2487, Kirkland, WA 98083. TEL 425-820-1500, FAX 425-823-8324, hh@hhpub.com, http://www.hhpub.com/journals. Eds. R Fernandez-Ballesteros, R Steyer. Adv. contact Iris Pruegl.

EUROPEAN JOURNAL OF PSYCHOLOGY OF EDUCATION. see *EDUCATION*

302 GBR ISSN 0046-2772
HM251 CODEN: EJSPA6
EUROPEAN JOURNAL OF SOCIAL PSYCHOLOGY. Text in English. 1971. 8/yr. USD 895 in United States; USD 895 in Canada & Mexico; USD 895 elsewhere; USD 940 combined subscription in United States for print and online eds.; USD 940 combined subscription in Canada & Mexico for print and online eds.; USD 940 combined subscription elsewhere for print and online eds. (effective 2002). adv. charts. back issues avail.; reprint service avail. from SWZ,PQC,ISI. *Refereed.* **Document type:** *Academic/Scholarly.* **Description:** Promotes communication among social psychology researchers in Europe and provides a bridge between European and other research traditions.
Related titles: Microform ed.: (from PQC); Online - full text ed.: ISSN 1099-0992. USD 895 in United States; USD 895 in Canada & Mexico; USD 895 elsewhere (effective 2002) (from EBSCO Publishing, Wiley InterScience, Institute for Scientific Information).
Indexed: ASCA, ASSIA, Adol.Ment.Hlth.Abstr., Commun.Abstr., Curr.Cont., ERA, Excerp.Med., IBZ, Ind.Philos., Intl.Bibl.Soc.Sci., Lang.& Lang.Behav.Abstr., Mid.East: Abstr.& Ind., Mult.Ed.Abstr., PsycInfo, Psychol.Abstr. (1971-), Ref.Zh., SOPODA, SSCI, Soc.Serv.Abstr., Sociol.Abstr., Sociol.Educ.Abstr., Sp.Ed.Needs Abstr., Stud.Wom.Abstr., e-psyche.
—BLDSC (3829.739000), IDS, ingenta. **CCC.**
Published by: Wiley Europe Ltd., Baffins Ln, Chichester, W Sussex PO19 1UD, United Kingdom. TEL 44-1243-779777, FAX 44-1243-775878, customer@wiley.co.uk, http://www.wiley.co.uk. adv.: B&W page GBP 650, color page GBP 1,550; trim 165 x 248. Circ: 1,650. **Subscr. to:** John Wiley & Sons, Inc., Journals, 605 Third Ave, New York, NY 10158. TEL 212-850-6021, 212-850-6645, subinfo@jwiley.com.

158.7 GBR ISSN 1359-432X
CODEN: EWOPED
EUROPEAN JOURNAL OF WORK AND ORGANIZATIONAL PSYCHOLOGY. Text in English. 1991. q. GBP 109, USD 179 to individuals; GBP 236, USD 390 to institutions (effective 2002). adv. bk.rev. **Document type:** *Academic/Scholarly.* **Description:** Provides a bridge between academies which enlarge the knowledge base of work psychology and practitioners who apply this knowledge to clients and organizations.
Formerly: European Work and Organizational Psychologist (0960-2003)
Related titles: Online - full text ed.: ISSN 1464-0643 (from CatchWord Ltd., EBSCO Publishing, O C L C Online Computer Library Center, Inc., RoweCom Information Quest, Swets Blackwell).
Indexed: Ergon.Abstr., Lang.& Lang.Behav.Abstr., SOPODA, Soc.Serv.Abstr., Sociol.Abstr., e-psyche.
—BLDSC (3829.747370), CatchWord, Infotrieve. **CCC.**
Published by: (International Association of Applied Psychology), Psychology Press (Subsidiary of: Taylor & Francis Group), 27 Church Rd, Hove, E Sussex BN3 2FA, United Kingdom. TEL 44-1273-207411, FAX 44-1273-205612, information@psypress.co.uk, http://www.psypress.co.uk. Ed. Dr. Fred R H Zijlstra. R&P Zoe Peden TEL 44-20-7842-2363. Adv. contact Claire Buckminster. **Subscr. addr. in N America:** Psychology Press, Journals Customer Service, Taylor & Francis Group, 325 Chestnut St, Philadelphia, PA 19106. TEL 800-354-1420, FAX 215-625-8914, info@taylorandfrancis.com, http://www.psypress.com.

301.15 USA ISSN 0892-7286
EUROPEAN MONOGRAPHS IN SOCIAL PSYCHOLOGY. Text in English. 1971. irreg., latest vol.35, 1985. reprint service avail. from ISI. **Document type:** *Monographic series.*
Indexed: Psychol.Abstr., e-psyche.
Published by: (European Association of Experimental Social Psychology), Academic Press, Inc., Journal Division (Subsidiary of: Harcourt Brace & Company), 525 B St, Ste 1900, San Diego, CA 92101-4495. TEL 619-231-0926, FAX 619-699-6715. Ed. H Tajfel. **Subscr. to:** Order Dept., 6277 Sea Harbor Dr, 4th Fl, Orlando, FL 32887. TEL 800-321-5068.

150 USA ISSN 1016-9040
BF1 CODEN: EUPSFE
EUROPEAN PSYCHOLOGIST. Text in English. 1977. q. USD 49 to non-members; USD 39 to members; USD 89 to institutions (effective 2001). adv. bk.rev. abstr, tr.lit, illus. back issues avail.; reprint service avail. from SCH,PSC. *Refereed.* **Document type:** *Journal, Academic/Scholarly.*
Formerly (until 1995): German Journal of Psychology (0705-5870)
Indexed: ASSIA, IBZ, Ind.Philos., PsycInfo, Soc.Serv.Abstr., Sociol.Abstr., e-psyche.
—BLDSC (3829.842730), ingenta.
Published by: (European Federation of Professional Psychology Associations), Hogrefe & Huber Publishers, PO Box 2487, Kirkland, WA 98083. TEL 425-820-1500, FAX 425-823-8324, hh@hhpub.com, http://www.hhpub.com/catalogue/EP.html, http://www.hhpub.com/journals. Ed. Kurt Pawlik. Adv. contact Iris Pruegl.

150 790.1 DEU ISSN 1433-1462
EUROPEAN YEARBOOK OF SPORT PSYCHOLOGY. Text in English. 1997. a. DEM 46 (effective 2000). **Document type:** *Academic/Scholarly.*
Indexed: e-psyche.
—BLDSC (3830.371755).
Published by: (European Federation of Sport Psychology), Academia Verlag GmbH, Postfach 1663, Sankt Augustin 53734, Germany. TEL 49-2241-34521-0, FAX 49-2241-345316, kontakt@academia-verlag.de, http://www.raps.com/academia.

EVIDENCE - BASED MENTAL HEALTH. see *MEDICAL SCIENCES—Psychiatry And Neurology*

155 AUT ISSN 0938-2623
EVOLUTION AND COGNITION. Text in English. 1991. s-a. ATS 500 (effective 2001). 100 p./no. back issues avail. *Refereed.* **Document type:** *Journal, Academic/Scholarly.* **Description:** Interdisciplinary forum devoted to all aspects of cognition, at both the animal and human level.
Related titles: Microfilm ed.: (from PQC).
Indexed: Zoo.Rec., e-psyche.
—BLDSC (3834.210000), CISTI, Infotrieve. **CCC.**
Published by: Konrad-Lorenz-Institut fuer Evolutions- und Kognitionsforschung, Adolf-Lorenz-Gasse 2, Altenberg A-3422, Austria. TEL 43-2242-323900, FAX 43-2242-323904, sec@kla.univie.ac.at, http://www.kli.ac.at. Eds. Manfred Wimmer, Rupert Riedl.

EVOLVING WOMAN; A Woman's Guide to Wholeness. see *WOMEN'S INTERESTS*

EXCEPTIONAL CHILDREN. see *EDUCATION—Special Education And Rehabilitation*

EXISTENZANALYSE. see *MEDICAL SCIENCES—Psychiatry And Neurology*

612.67 USA ISSN 0361-073X
QP86 CODEN: EAGRDS
EXPERIMENTAL AGING RESEARCH. Text in English. 1975. q. GBP 50, USD 82 to individuals; GBP 204, USD 336 to institutions (effective 2002). adv. bk.rev. illus. index. back issues avail.; reprint service avail. from PQC. *Refereed.* **Document type:** *Academic/Scholarly.* **Description:** Takes a multidisciplinary, scientific approach in dealing with all areas of scientific inquiry, human and animal, involving aging and the elderly.
Related titles: Microform ed.: (from PQC); Online - full text ed.: ISSN 1096-4657 (from CatchWord Ltd., EBSCO Publishing, O C L C Online Computer Library Center, Inc., RoweCom Information Quest, Swets Blackwell, Institute for Scientific Information).
Indexed: ASCA, Abstr.Soc.Geront., AgeLine, Behav.Med.Abstr., Biol.Abstr., CINAHL, Chem.Abstr., Curr.Cont., Curr.Ind.Stat., Ergon.Abstr., Excerp.Med., Fam.Ind., Helminthol.Abstr., INIS Atomind., Ind.Med. (1975-), Ind.Sci.Rev., Inpharma, Int.Abstr.Biol.Sci., NRN, Pharm.&Out.News, PsycInfo, Psychol.Abstr. (1975-), Reac., SSCI (coverage dropped), Sci.Cit.Ind., e-psyche.
—BLDSC (3838.570000), CASDDS, CatchWord, CISTI, EMDOCS, GNLM, IDS, ingenta, KNAW. **CCC.**
Published by: Taylor & Francis Ltd. (Subsidiary of: Taylor & Francis Group), 325 Chestnut St, Suite 800, Philadelphia, PA 19016. TEL 215-625-8900, FAX 215-625-2940, info@taylorandfrancis.com, http://www.taylorandfrancis.com/. Ed. Jeffrey W Elias. Circ: 1,500. **Subscr. addr. in Europe:** Taylor & Francis Group, Journals Customer Service, Rankine Rd, Basingstoke, Hants RG24 8PR, United Kingdom. TEL 44-1256-813000, FAX 44-1256-479438, enquiry@tanf.co.uk, http://www.tandf.co.uk/journals.

150 615 USA ISSN 1064-1297
RM315 CODEN: ECLPES
EXPERIMENTAL AND CLINICAL PSYCHOPHARMACOLOGY. Text in English. 1993. q. USD 92 domestic to non-members; USD 107 foreign to non-members; USD 46 domestic to members; USD 56 foreign to members; USD 184 domestic to institutions; USD 216 foreign to institutions (2001). adv. back issues avail. *Refereed.* **Document type:** *Academic/Scholarly.* **Description:** Advances research and development of theory in psychopharmacology.
Related titles: Online - full text ed.: (from Institute for Scientific Information).
Indexed: Addic.Abstr., Chem.Abstr., Chem.Indus.Notes, Chem.Titles, Excerp.Med. (1995-), Focus on: Psychophar., Ind.Med. (1993-), PsycInfo, Psychol.Abstr. (1993-), Psycscan B.A.& T., SSCI, e-psyche.
—BLDSC (3838.654000), CISTI, GNLM, IDS, ingenta, KNAW. **CCC.**
Published by: American Psychological Association, 750 First St., N.E., Washington, DC 20002-4242. TEL 202-336-5600, 800-374-2721, FAX 202-336-5568, subscriptions@apa.org; orders@allenpress.com, http://www.apa.org/journals/pha.html; http://www.apa.org/journals/pha.html, http://www.apa.org/journals/pha.html; http://www.allenpress.com. Ed. Patricia Sutker. Circ: 1,100. **Subscr. to:** Allen Press Inc., PO Box 1897, Lawrence, KS 66044-8897.

150 USA ISSN 1092-0803
BF11
EYE ON PSI CHI. Text in English. 1934. q. USD 10 (effective 2000).
Formerly (until 1996): Psi Chi Newsletter (0033-2569)
Indexed: e-psyche.
Published by: Psi Chi National Office, PO Box 709, Chattanooga, TN 37401-0709. TEL 423-756-2044, FAX 423-265-1529. Ed., R&P Kay Wilson. Circ: 27,000.

153.1 347.91 USA ISSN 1069-0484
F M S FOUNDATION NEWSLETTER* . (False Memory Syndrome) Text in English. 1992. 6/yr. USD 30 domestic; USD 35 in Canada; USD 40 elsewhere; USD 15 domestic to students; USD 20 foreign to students (effective 2000). bk.rev. bibl. **Document type:** *Newsletter.* **Description:** Reviews news events, including legal cases involving persons with recovered or repressed memories.
Indexed: Pollut.Abstr.
Published by: False Memory Syndrome Foundation, PO Box34580, Philadelphia, PA 19101-4580. TEL 215-387-1865, FAX 215-387-1917, pjf@saul.cis.upenn.edu, http://www.FMSLonline.org; www.MemoryandReality.org. Ed. Pamela Freyd. Circ: 4,000 (paid).

FALLING LEAF. see *MILITARY*

306.85 DEU ISSN 0342-2747
CODEN: FDYNF4
FAMILIENDYNAMIK; interdisziplinaere Zeitschrift fuer systemorientierte Praxis und Forschung. Text in German. 1976. q. DEM 115, EUR 58.80; DEM 87, EUR 44.48 to students (effective 2000). adv. **Document type:** *Magazine, Academic/Scholarly.*
Indexed: IBR, IBZ, Ind.Philos., e-psyche.
—GNLM. **CCC.**
Published by: Verlag Klett-Cotta, Rotebuehlstr 77, Stuttgart 70178, Germany. TEL 49-711-66721648, FAX 49-711-66722032. Eds. Arnold Retzer, Fritz Simon. Adv. contact Thomas Kleffner. B&W page DEM 1,100; trim 113 x 180. Circ: 3,800.

FAMILIENMAGAZIN. see *CHILDREN AND YOUTH—About*

150 306.8 USA ISSN 1066-4807
RC488.5
THE FAMILY JOURNAL; counseling and therapy for couples and families. Text in English. 1993. q. USD 60 to individuals; USD 140 to institutions; USD 20 newsstand/cover to individuals; USD 50 newsstand/cover to institutions (effective 2002). **Description:** Emphasizes practical information based on the most up-to-date research and therapies on marriage and family counseling.
Related titles: Online - full text ed.: (from EBSCO Publishing, O C L C Online Computer Library Center, Inc., RoweCom Information Quest, ProQuest Information & Learning, ingenta, Swets Blackwell).
Indexed: C.I.J.E., Human Resour.Abstr., PsycInfo, Soc.Serv.Abstr., Sociol.Abstr., e-psyche.
—BLDSC (3865.564279). **CCC.**
Published by: (International Association of Marriage and Family Counselors), Sage Publications, Inc., 2455 Teller Rd, Thousand Oaks, CA 91320. TEL 805-499-0721, FAX 805-499-0871, info@sagepub.com, http://www.sagepub.com. Ed. Jon Carlson. R&P Tanya Udin. Adv. contact DeAnna Vega Hammersley. Circ: 7,000. **Overseas subscr. to:** Sage Publications Ltd., 6 Bonhill St, London EC2A 4PU, United Kingdom. TEL 44-20-7374-0645, FAX 44-20-7374-8741; Sage Publications India Pvt. Ltd., 4215, New Delhi 110 048, India. TEL 91-11-641-9884, FAX 91-11-647-2426.

306.85 USA ISSN 0014-7370
RC488.5.A1 CODEN: FAPRA
FAMILY PROCESS. Text in English. 1962. q. USD 47 domestic to individuals; USD 124 domestic to individuals Print with CD-ROM; USD 59 foreign to individuals; USD 134 foreign to individuals Print with CD-ROM; USD 97 domestic to institutions; USD 251 domestic to institutions Print with CD-ROM; USD 109 foreign to institutions; USD 262 foreign to institutions Print with CD-ROM; USD 24 domestic to students; USD 36 foreign to students (effective 2000). adv. bk.rev. abstr, bibl, charts, illus. index. 128 p./no. back issues avail.; reprint service avail. from SWZ,PQC,PSC,SCH. *Refereed.* **Document type:** *Journal, Academic/Scholarly.* **Description:** Covers family mental health and psychotherapy.
Related titles: CD-ROM ed.: USD 99 to individuals; USD 199 to institutions (effective 2000) (from ProQuest Information & Learning); Online - full text ed.: (from ProQuest Information & Learning, Gale Group, Institute for Scientific Information).
Indexed: ASCA, ASSIA, Adol.Ment.Hlth.Abstr., AgeLine, CINAHL, Commun.Abstr., Crim.Just.Abstr., Curr.Cont., Excerp.Med., Fam.Ind., IBR, IBZ, IMFL, Ind.Med. (1962-), Ind.Philos., Int.Nurs.Ind., Lang.& Lang.Behav.Abstr., Mid.East: Abstr.& Ind., Mult.Ed.Abstr., Past.Care & Couns.Abstr., PsycInfo, Psychol.Abstr. (1962-), Ref.Zh., Russ.Acad.Sci.Bibl., SOPODA, SSCI, Sage Fam.Stud.Abstr., Sage Race Rel.Abstr., Soc.Serv.Abstr., Soc.Work Res.& Abstr., Sociol.Abstr., Stud.Wom.Abstr., Viol.& Abuse Abstr., e-psyche.
—BLDSC (3865.576000), GNLM, IDS, Infotrieve, ingenta. **CCC.**
Published by: Family Process, Inc., PO Box 23980, Rochester, NY 14692-3980. TEL 716-482-7390, FAX 716-482-2902, info@familyprocess.org, http://www.familyprocess.org. Ed. Carol Anderson. Pub., R&P, Adv. contact William Steger TEL 716-482-7390. Circ: 3,800 (paid).

306.85 USA ISSN 0277-6464
FAMILY THERAPY NEWS. Text in English. 1969. bi-m. USD 20 to individuals; USD 35 to institutions. reprint service avail. from PQC. **Document type:** *Newsletter.*
Formerly: American Association for Marriage and Family Therapy Newsletter
Indexed: e-psyche.
—CCC.
Published by: American Association for Marriage and Family Therapy, 1133 15th St, N W, Ste 300, Washington, DC 20005. Ed. Jennifer Daw. adv.: B&W page USD 1,400. Circ: 21,000.

150 TWN
▼ **FEICHANG XILIE XINLI CEYAN.** Text in English. 2000. m. TWD 88 newsstand/cover (effective 2001). **Document type:** *Magazine, Consumer.* **Description:** Contains monthly psychological and personality tests on love, stress,.
Published by: Jianduan Chuban Qufen Youxian Gongsi/Sharp Point Publishing Ltd., Inc., 231 Xindiansi, Fuyu-Lu 43-Hao 8-Lou, Taipei, Taiwan. TEL 886-2-2218-1582, FAX 886-2-2218-1583, janey@spp.com.tw, http://www.spp.com.tw/.

150 305.4 GBR ISSN 0959-3535
HQ1206 CODEN: FEPSFF
FEMINISM & PSYCHOLOGY; an international journal. Text in English. 1991. q. GBP 41 to individuals; GBP 219 to institutions; GBP 11 newsstand/cover to individuals; GBP 56 newsstand/cover to institutions (effective 2002). adv. bk.rev. illus. reprints avail. *Refereed.* **Document type:** *Journal, Academic/Scholarly.* **Description:** Fosters the development of feminist theory and practice in psychology and represents the concerns of women in a wide range of contexts across the academic-applied 'divide'.
Related titles: Online - full text ed.: (from EBSCO Publishing, O C L C Online Computer Library Center, Inc., RoweCom Information Quest, ingenta, Swets Blackwell, Institute for Scientific Information).
Indexed: ASCA, ASSIA, AgeLine, Arts & Hum.Cit.Ind. (coverage dropped), Curr.Cont., ERA, Fam.Ind., Fem.Per. (1991-), IBR, IBZ, Ind.Philos., Intl.Bibl.Soc.Sci., Lang.& Lang.Behav.Abstr., Mult.Ed.Abstr., PsycInfo, Psychol.Abstr. (1991-), SOPODA, SSCI, Sage Fam.Stud.Abstr., Soc.Serv.Abstr., Sociol.Abstr., Stud.Wom.Abstr., Wom.Stud.Abstr., e-psyche.
—BLDSC (3905.195980), Infotrieve, ingenta. **CCC.**
Published by: Sage Publications Ltd., 6 Bonhill St, London EC2A 4PU, United Kingdom. TEL 44-20-7374-0645, FAX 44-20-7374-8741, order@sagepub.com, market@sagepub.co.uk, http://www.sagepub.co.uk/journals/details/j0191.html. Ed. Sue Wilkinson. Adv. contact Jenny Kirby. page GBP 220; trim 185 x 114. Circ: 1,000.

150 BEL
FIGURES OF THE UNCONSCIOUS. Text in Multiple languages. 1998. irreg. price varies. **Document type:** *Academic/Scholarly.*
Published by: Leuven University Press, Blijde Inkomststraat 5, Leuven 3000, Belgium. TEL 32-16-325345, FAX 32-16-325352, university.press@upers.kuleuven.ac.be, http://www.lup.be.

FILOZOFSKI FAKULTET - ZADAR. RAZDIO FILOZOFIJE, PSIHOLOGIJE, SOCIOLOGIJE I PEDAGOGIJE. RADOVI. see *EDUCATION*

FOCUS GROUP KIT. see *TECHNOLOGY: COMPREHENSIVE WORKS*

301.1 150 ITA ISSN 0393-5418
FOGLI DI INFORMAZIONE. Text in Italian; Summaries in English. 1972. m. ITL 100,000, USD 30 (effective 2000).
Indexed: e-psyche.
Published by: Associazione Centro di Documentazione, Casella Postale 347, Via Orafi, 29, Pistoia, PT 51100, Italy. TEL 39-573-977353, FAX 39-573-977353, cdocumen@tin.it, giorlima@tin.it.

FORENSISCHE PSYCHIATRIE UND PSYCHOTHERAPIE. see *MEDICAL SCIENCES—Psychiatry And Neurology*

616.89 FRA ISSN 0769-184X
FORTUNA. Text in French. 1986. s-a. FRF 80; FRF 40 newsstand/cover (effective 2000). bk.rev.
Indexed: e-psyche.
Published by: Universite Montpellier III (Universite Paul Valery), Groupe d'Etudes Szondiennes de Montpellier, Montpellier Cedex 5 34199, France. TEL 33-4-67142516, FAX 33-4-67142152. Ed. Anne Gayral. Circ: 300.

150.19 DEU ISSN 0178-7667
FORUM DER PSYCHOANALYSE; Zeitschrift fuer klinische Theorie und Praxis. Text in German. 1985. q. EUR 245.55 domestic; EUR 228.65 in Germany (effective 2002). back issues avail.; reprint service avail. from ISI. *Refereed.* **Document type:** *Journal, Academic/Scholarly.* **Description:** Journal for the clinical theory and practice of psychoanalysis.
Related titles: Microform ed.: (from PQC); Online - full text ed.: ISSN 1437-0751 (from EBSCO Publishing, RoweCom Information Quest, Swets Blackwell, Springer LINK, Institute for Scientific Information).
Indexed: ASCA, Curr.Cont., Excerp.Med., PsycInfo, Psychoanal.Abstr., Psychol.Abstr. (1993-), SSCI, e-psyche.
—BLDSC (4024.098000), GNLM, IDS. **CCC.**
Published by: Springer-Verlag (Subsidiary of: BertelsmannSpringer), Tiergartenstr 17, Heidelberg 69121, Germany. TEL 49-6221-345-0, FAX 49-6221-345229, subscriptions@springer.de, http://link.springer.de/link/service/journals/00451/index.htm, http://www.springer.de. **Subscr. in N. America to:** Springer-Verlag New York Inc., PO Box 2485, Secaucus, NJ 07096-2485. TEL 212-460-1500, FAX 212-473-6272.

156 DEU ISSN 0720-0447
BF3
FORUM KRITISCHE PSYCHOLOGIE. Text in German. 1978. s-a. DEM 34; DEM 28 to students (effective 1999). back issues avail. **Document type:** *Academic/Scholarly.*
Indexed: e-psyche.
Published by: Argument-Verlag GmbH, Eppendorfer Weg 95A, Hamburg 20259, Germany. TEL 49-40-401800-0, FAX 49-40-40180020. Ed. Klaus Holzkamp.

155.937 USA ISSN 0160-7081
FOUNDATION OF THANATOLOGY. ARCHIVES. Text in English. q. USD 72. back issues avail. **Description:** Contains abstracts of conference proceedings on aging, dying, death, bereavement, and grief.
Related titles: Microform ed.: (from PQC).
Indexed: AgeLine, e-psyche.
—GNLM.
Published by: Foundation of Thanatology, Foundation Book & Periodical Division, 630 W 168th St, New York, NY 10032. TEL 212-928-2066, FAX 914-793-0813, rhalporn@pipeline.com. Ed. Austin H Kutscher.

616.89 GBR ISSN 0267-0887
BF173.A2
FREE ASSOCIATIONS; psychoanalysis, groups, politics, culture. Text in English. 1984. q. GBP 30 domestic to individuals; GBP 35 foreign to individuals; GBP 70 domestic to institutions; GBP 80 foreign to institutions. adv. bk.rev. abstr, bibl. index. back issues avail.; reprint service avail. from PQC. **Document type:** *Academic/Scholarly.* **Description:** Covers from clinical to cultural studies on psychodynamic approaches to human nature, culture and society.
Related titles: Microform ed.: (from PQC); Online - full text ed.
Indexed: ASSIA, Alt.Press Ind., Chicago Psychoanal.Lit.Ind., IBR, IBZ, Ind.Philos., Lang.& Lang.Behav.Abstr., Left Ind. (1985-), P C I, PsycInfo, Psychoanal.Abstr., Psychol.Abstr. (1993-), SOPODA, Sociol.Abstr., e-psyche.
—CCC.
Published by: Process Press, 26 Freegrove Rd, London N7 9RQ, United Kingdom. TEL 44-20-7609-1597, FAX 44-20-7609-4837, pp@rmy1.demon.co.uk, http://www.human-nature.com/free-associations/index.html, http://www.human-nature.com/process-press/index.html. Ed. Robert M Young. Circ: 2,000. **Subscr. to:** World Wide Subscription Service Ltd., Unit 4, Gibbs Reed Farm, Ticehurst, E Sussex TN5 7HE, United Kingdom. **Co-publisher:** Guilford Publications, Inc.

P

155.937 CAN ISSN 1180-3479
CODEN: FRONFI
FRONTIERES; les vivants et les morts. Text in English. 1988. 3/yr. CND 27 domestic to individuals; CND 35 foreign to individuals; CND 40 domestic to institutions; CND 50 foreign to institutions. adv. bk.rev., film rev. bibl, illus, stat. back issues avail. **Description:** Discusses death and grieving for professionals and volunteers in the health services.
Indexed: Pt.de Rep., Soc.Serv.Abstr., Sociol.Abstr., e-psyche.
Published by: Universite du Quebec a Montreal, Service des Publications, Succ Centre Ville, C P 8888, Montreal, PQ H3C 3P8, Canada. TEL 514-987-8537, FAX 514-987-0307, frontier@er.uqam.ca. Ed. Giuseppe Samona. Circ: 1,500 (controlled).

150 JPN ISSN 0917-8163
FUKUSHIMA SHINRIGAKU ZASSHI/FUKUSHIMA JOURNAL OF PSYCHOLOGY. Text in Japanese. 1990. a. **Document type:** *Academic/Scholarly.*
Indexed: e-psyche.
Published by: Fukushima Shinri Gakkai/Fukushima Psychological Association, c/o Fukushima Daigaku Kyoikugakubu, Kyoiku Shinrigaku Kyoshitsu, 2 Sugumichi, Asakawa, Matsukawamachi, Fukushima-shi, Fukushima-ken 960-12, Japan. TEL 81-245-48-5151, FAX 81-245-48-3181, kfukuda@post.ipc.fukushima-u.ac.jp.

155.937 USA
G E I NEWSLETTER✱ . Text in English. 1979. q. USD 5. bk.rev. **Document type:** *Newsletter.*
Indexed: e-psyche.
Published by: Grief Education Institute, 3540 S Poplar St, Ste 202, Denver, CO 80237-1362. Ed. Carole Rawland. Circ: 2,000.

P

301.1 150 510 USA ISSN 0899-8256
QA269 CODEN: GEBEEF
GAMES AND ECONOMIC BEHAVIOR. Text in English. 1989. 8/yr. USD 545 in US & Canada to institutions; USD 600 elsewhere to institutions (effective 2001). adv. illus. Index. back issues avail.; reprints avail. *Refereed.* **Document type:** *Academic/Scholarly.* **Description:** Deals with game-theoretic modeling in the social, biological and mathematical sciences. Addresses the beliefs in the importance of interchange of game-theoretic ideas leading to a mathematical science of games and economic behavior.
Related titles: Online - full text ed.: (from EBSCO Publishing, O C L C Online Computer Library Center, Inc., RoweCom Information Quest, ingenta, Swets Blackwell, IDEAL Online Library, Institute for Scientific Information).
Indexed: ASCA, Arts & Hum.Cit.Ind. (coverage dropped), C.C.M.J., Curr.Cont., Environ.Sci.Poll.Mgmt., INSPEC (Mar.1990-), Intl.Bibl.Soc.Sci., J.of Econ.Lit., Risk Abstr., Russ.Acad.Sci.Bibl., SSCI, Saf.Sci.Abstr., Zent.Math., e-psyche.
—BLDSC (4069.168000), AskIEEE, IDS, ingenta. **CCC.**
Published by: Academic Press, Inc., Journal Division (Subsidiary of: Harcourt Brace & Company), 525 B St, Ste 1900, San Diego, CA 92101-4495. TEL 619-230-1840, FAX 619-699-6800, apsubs@acad.com, http://www.academicpress.com/games. Ed. Ehud Kalai.

150 NLD ISSN 0921-5360
BF8.D8 CODEN: GEGEE6
GEDRAG & GEZONDHEID; het wetenschappelijke tijdschrift voor psychologie en gezondheid. Text in Dutch, English. 1952. bi-m. NLG 195 foreign; free to qualified personnel. adv. bk.rev. bibl, charts, illus. index. **Document type:** *Trade.* **Description:** Offers advice to professionals in all areas of caring for persons with both physical and mental disorders.
Supersedes (in 1986): Gedrag (0377-7308); Which was formed by the 1973 merger of: Hypothese (0018-8352); Nijmeegs Tijdschrift voor Psychologie (0029-0475); Which was formerly (until 1969): Gawein (0016-5271)
Indexed: Biol.Abstr., Curr.Cont. (coverage dropped), IBR, PsycInfo, Psychol.Abstr. (1973-), Risk Abstr., SSCI (coverage dropped), e-psyche.
—BLDSC (4095.760900), KNAW.
Published by: Elsevier Gezondheidszorg B.V., Tijdstroom (Subsidiary of: Reed Elsevier plc Group), Planetenbaan 1, Maarssen 3600 AK, Netherlands. TEL 31-346-577577, FAX 31-346-554287, http://www.tijdstroom.nl. Ed. G J J Calis. Circ: 450 (controlled). **Subscr. to:** Elsevier Den Haag, Postbus 16500, The Hague 2500 BM, Netherlands. TEL 31-70-381-9900, FAX 31-70-333-8399.

615.8 NLD ISSN 0167-7454
GEDRAGSTHERAPIE. Text in Dutch. 1982. q. NLG 90. adv. **Document type:** *Academic/Scholarly.*
Indexed: PsycInfo, e-psyche.
—BLDSC (4095.761600), KNAW.
Published by: (Stichting Tijdschrift voor Gedragstherapie), Bohn Stafleu van Loghum B.V. (Subsidiary of: Wolters Kluwer N.V.), Postbus 246, Houten 3990 GA, Netherlands. TEL 31-3403-95711, FAX 31-3403-50903. Circ: 2,300.

GEISTIGE BEHINDERUNG; Fachzeitschrift der Lebenshilfe fuer geistig Behinderte. see *EDUCATION—Special Education And Rehabilitation*

150.19 616.9 USA ISSN 1091-6318
GENDER & PSYCHOANALYSIS; an interdisciplinary journal. Text in English. 1996. q. USD 53 domestic to individuals; USD 72 foreign to individuals; USD 94 domestic to institutions; USD 102 foreign to institutions (effective 2002). adv. bk.rev. charts, illus. back issues avail. *Refereed.* **Document type:** *Journal, Academic/Scholarly.* **Description:** Devoted to provide a lively intellectual forum linking and critiquing diverse psychoanalytic views of gender, taking a multidisciplinary approach.
Indexed: Alt.Press Ind., CINAHL, Fem.Per. (1997-), Lang.& Lang.Behav.Abstr., PsycInfo, SOPODA, Soc.Serv.Abstr., Sociol.Abstr., e-psyche.
Published by: International Universities Press, Incorporated, 59 Boston Post Rd., P.O. Box 1524, Madison, CT 06443-1524. Ed. Dr. Margaret Emery. adv.: page USD 360; 4.25 x 7.

121.3 USA ISSN 0740-9583
BF712
GENETIC EPISTEMOLOGIST. Text in English. 1971. q. USD 70 to members; USD 30 to students. adv. bk.rev. *Refereed.* **Document type:** *Newsletter.* **Description:** Interdisciplinary study of human knowledge and its development.
Indexed: e-psyche.
—BLDSC (4111.849000).
Published by: Jean Piaget Society, Department of Psychology, Franklin and Arshall College, Box 3003, Lancaster, PA 17604. Ed. Ed Reed. Circ: 550 (paid). **Subscr. to:** Wm. M. Gray, Treas, Jean Piaget Society, Dept of Educational Psychology, University of Toledo, Toledo, OH 43606-3390. TEL 419-530-2481.

156 155 USA ISSN 8756-7547
LB1101 CODEN: GSGMEQ
GENETIC, SOCIAL, AND GENERAL PSYCHOLOGY MONOGRAPHS. Text in English. 1926. q., latest vol.128, 2002. USD 136 domestic; USD 149 foreign; USD 34 newsstand/cover (effective 2001 - 2002). bibl, charts. s-a. index. back issues avail.; reprint service avail. from SWZ,PQC,PSC,SCH. *Refereed.* **Document type:** *Academic/Scholarly.*
Formerly: Genetic Psychology Monographs (0016-6677)
Related titles: CD-ROM ed.: (from ProQuest Information & Learning); Online - full text ed.: (from ProQuest Information & Learning, Gale Group, Institute for Scientific Information).
Indexed: ASCA, AgeLine, Biol.Abstr., Chic.Per.Ind., Child Devel.Abstr., Curr.Adv.Ecol.Sci., Curr.Cont., DSH Abstr., ERA, Except.Child Educ.Abstr., Fam.Ind., IBR, IBZ, INIS Atomind., Ind.Med. (1985-), Ind.Philos., Indian Psychol.Abstr., Lang.& Lang.Behav.Abstr., Mult.Ed.Abstr., PsycInfo, Psychol.Abstr. (1926-), Psycscan D.P., Ref.Zh., Risk Abstr., Russ.Acad.Sci.Bibl., SOPODA, SSCI, Sage Race Rel.Abstr., Soc.Serv.Abstr., Soc.Work Res.& Abstr., Sociol.Abstr., Stud.Wom.Abstr., e-psyche.
—BLDSC (4111.916000), CISTI, GNLM, IDS, Infotrieve, ingenta. **CCC.**
Published by: (Helen Dwight Reid Educational Foundation), Heldref Publications, 1319 Eighteenth St, N W, Washington, DC 20036-1802. TEL 202-296-6267, FAX 202-296-5149, http://www.heldref.org. Ed. Doris Chalfin. Circ: 500.

GESELLSCHAFT FUER LOGOTHERAPIE UND EXISTENZANALYSE. TAGUNGSBERICHTE. see *MEDICAL SCIENCES—Psychiatry And Neurology*

150 ARE ISSN 1091-1766
GESTALT!. Text in English. 1997. irreg. back issues avail. **Document type:** *Journal, Academic/Scholarly.*
Media: Online - full content.
Published by: Gestalt Global Corporation http://www.g-g.org/gej/index.html, http://www.g-g.org/gestalt-global/index.html.

150 616.89 USA ISSN 0190-0412
BF203
GESTALT JOURNAL. Text in English. 1978. s-a. USD 35 domestic to individuals; USD 45 foreign to individuals; USD 50 domestic to institutions; USD 60 foreign to institutions (effective 1999). bk.rev. back issues avail. **Document type:** *Academic/Scholarly.* **Description:** Features articles and reviews relating to the theory and practice of Gestalt therapy.
Indexed: PsycInfo, Psychol.Abstr. (1978-), e-psyche.
—BLDSC (4163.350000), ingenta. **CCC.**
Published by: Center for Gestalt Development, Inc., PO Box 990, Highland, NY 12528-0990. TEL 914-691-7192, tgjournal@gestalt.org, http://www.gestalt.org. Ed., Pub., R&P Joe Wysong. Circ: 2,500.

616.89 USA ISSN 1084-8657
GESTALT REVIEW. Text in English. 1997. 3/yr. USD 49.50 in US & Canada to individuals; USD 69.50 elsewhere to individuals; USD 155 in US & Canada to institutions; USD 175 elsewhere to institutions; USD 15 per issue in US & Canada; USD 21 per issue elsewhere (effective 2001). adv. back issues avail. *Refereed.* **Document type:** *Academic/Scholarly.* **Description:** Concentrates on the Gestalt approach to clinical, family, group and organizational topics.
Related titles: Online - full content ed.; Online - full text ed.: (from CatchWord Ltd.).
Indexed: e-psyche.
—BLDSC (4163.380000), CatchWord. **CCC.**
Published by: The Gestalt International Study Center, PO Box 515, South Wellfleet, MA 02663. TEL 508-349-7900, FAX 508-349-7908, gestaltrev@aol.com, office@gisc.org, GestaltStudyIntl@aol.com, http://www.gisc.org/gestaltreview/index.html. Ed. Joseph Melnick. adv.: page USD 265; trim 5 x 8.

150.19 AUT ISSN 0170-057X
BF203
GESTALT THEORY; an international multidisciplinary journal. Text in English, German. 1979. q. adv. bk.rev. **Document type:** *Journal, Academic/Scholarly.*
Indexed: Ger.J.Psych., IBZ, Ind.Philos., PsycInfo, Psychol.Abstr. (1979-), e-psyche.
—BLDSC (4163.400000). **CCC.**
Published by: (Society for Gestalt Theory and Its Applications (GTA) DEU), Buchhandlung Krammer, Camillo-Sitte-Gasse 20, Vienna 1150, Austria. TEL 43-1-9852119, FAX 43-1-985211915, buchhandlung_krammer@aon.at, http://www.psycho.uni-osnabrueck.de/fach/gta/. Eds. G Stemberger, H.-J Walter, J Kriz. Circ: 550.

GIFU SHISHUNKI KENKYU/GIFU SOCIETY OF ADOLESCENTOLOGY. JOURNAL. see *CHILDREN AND YOUTH—About*

▼ **GIORNALE ITALIANO DI PSICO-ONCOLOGIA.** see *MEDICAL SCIENCES—Oncology*

150.5 ITA ISSN 0390-5349
BF1
GIORNALE ITALIANO DI PSICOLOGIA/ITALIAN JOURNAL OF PSYCHOLOGY. Text in Italian. 1974. q. ITL 124,000 to individuals; ITL 180,000 foreign to individuals; ITL 178,000 to institutions; ITL 220,000 foreign to institutions (effective 2000). adv. index. back issues avail. **Document type:** *Academic/Scholarly.*
Indexed: Child Devel.Abstr., Ind.Philos., Lang.& Lang.Behav.Abstr., PsycInfo, Psychol.Abstr. (1981-), Ref.Zh., SOPODA, Sociol.Abstr., e-psyche.
—BLDSC (4178.243000).
Published by: Societa Editrice Il Mulino, Strada Maggiore, 37, Bologna, BO 40125, Italy. TEL 39-51-256011, FAX 39-51-256034, diffusione@mulino.it, http://www.mulino.it/. Ed. C A Umilta. Adv. contact M Luisa Vezzali. Circ: 1,300.

150 ITA ISSN 0391-2515
BF84
GIORNALE STORICO DI PSICOLOGIA DINAMICA. Text in Italian. 1977. s-a. ITL 30,000; price varies. adv. **Document type:** *Monographic series.*
Indexed: PsycInfo, Psychoanal.Abstr., Psychol.Abstr. (1981-), e-psyche.
Published by: Liguori Editore srl, Via Posillipo, 394, Naples, NA 80123, Italy. TEL 39-81-7206111, FAX 39-81-7206244, http://www.liguorieditore.com/. Ed. Aldo Carotenuto. Pub. Guido Liguori. Adv. contact Maria Liguori.

150 016 SWE ISSN 0301-0996
CODEN: GPSRDB
GOETEBORG PSYCHOLOGICAL REPORTS. Text in English. 1971. irreg. (5-8/yr.). SEK 25, USD 7.50 per issue (effective 2001). **Document type:** *Academic/Scholarly.*

Indexed: Curr.Ind.Stat., Psychol.Abstr., e-psyche.
Published by: Goeteborgs Universitet, Department of Psychology, P O Box 500, Goeteborg 40530, Sweden. TEL 46-31-773-1668, FAX 46-31-773-4628, eve.gunne@psy.gu.se. Ed. Anders Biel. Circ: 400.

GOING BONKERS; a magazine for our times. see *NEW AGE PUBLICATIONS*

150 CHE ISSN 0172-3421
GORGO. Text in German. 1979. 2/yr. CHF 47. adv. bk.rev. illus. **Document type:** *Academic/Scholarly.*
Indexed: e-psyche.
—CCC.
Published by: Edition I K M AG, Rauchackerstr 31, Oberengstringen 8102, Switzerland. TEL 41-1-7502920, FAX 41-1-7502943. Ed. Allan Guggenbuehl. Adv. contact Monika Menne. page CHF 400. **Subscr. to:** Buch Service Basel, Postfach, Basel 4002, Switzerland. TEL 41-61-2729470.

GORILLA. see *BIOLOGY—Zoology*

150.71 USA
BF77
GRADUATE STUDY IN PSYCHOLOGY. Text in English. 1969. a. USD 21.95 to non-members; USD 19.95 to members (effective 1999). adv. **Document type:** *Directory.*
Former titles (until 1991): Graduate Study in Psychology and Associated Fields (0742-7220); (until 1983): Graduate Study in Psychology (0072-5277)
Indexed: Psychol.Abstr., e-psyche.
Published by: American Psychological Association, 211 E 70th St, New York, NY 10021. TEL 202-336-1003, FAX 202-336-5633. Ed. Ed Diener. Circ: 15,000.

155.282 GBR
GRAPHOLOGY DIGEST. Text in English. 1994. m. GBP 15, EUR 10, USD 10 (effective 2001). Website rev. 4 p./no. 1 cols./p. **Document type:** *Newsletter, Academic/Scholarly.* **Description:** Includes graphology related news with a bias to British and European graphology.
Media: E-mail.
Published by: NR Bradley, 91 Hawksley Ave, Chesterfield, Derbyshire S40 4JT, United Kingdom. bradlen@graphology.ws, http://www.leylines.com/titles.htm#digest, http://www.graphology.ws. Ed. Nigel Bradley.

616.8 GBR ISSN 0533-3164
GROUP ANALYSIS; journal of group-analytic psychotherapy. Text in English. 1967. q. GBP 48 to individuals; GBP 197 to institutions; GBP 13 newsstand/cover to individuals; GBP 50 newsstand/cover to institutions (effective 2002). adv. bk.rev. *Refereed.* **Document type:** *Academic/Scholarly.* **Description:** Centered upon the theory, practice and experience of analytic group psychotherapy, using an integrative approach based on the view that we are all primarily group beings.
Formerly: Group Analysis: International Panel and Correspondence (0533-3164)
Related titles: Online - full text ed.: (from EBSCO Publishing, O C L C Online Computer Library Center, Inc., RoweCom Information Quest, ingenta, Swets Blackwell).
Indexed: ASSIA, ERA, Excerp.Med., Human Resour.Abstr., IBR, IBZ, Ind.Philos., Lang.& Lang.Behav.Abstr., Mult.Ed.Abstr., PsycInfo, Psychol.Abstr. (1990-), SOPODA, Soc.Serv.Abstr., Sociol.Abstr., Sp.Ed.Needs Abstr., Stud.Wom.Abstr., e-psyche.
—BLDSC (4220.170000), EMDOCS, GNLM, ingenta. **CCC.**
Published by: Sage Publications Ltd., 6 Bonhill St, London EC2A 4PU, United Kingdom. TEL 44-20-7374-0645, FAX 44-20-7374-8741, market@sagepub.co.uk, http://www.sagepub.co.uk. Ed. Malcolm Pines. Adv. contact Jenny Kirby. page GBP 220; trim 170 x 100. Circ: 1,250.

GROUP & ORGANIZATION MANAGEMENT; an international journal. see *EDUCATION*

616.89 USA
GROUP CIRCLE. Text in English. q. **Document type:** *Newsletter.*
Formerly: A G P A Newsletter
Indexed: e-psyche.
Published by: American Group Psychotherapy Association, 25 E 21st St, 6th Fl, New York, NY 10010. TEL 212-477-2677, FAX 212-979-6627. Ed. Harold S Bernard. Circ: 4,000 (controlled).

152 USA ISSN 1089-2699
HM131 CODEN: GRDYF7
GROUP DYNAMICS; theory, research, and practice. Variant title: Group Dynamics: Theory, Research and Practice. Text in English. 1997. q. USD 48 domestic to non-members; USD 63 foreign to non-members; USD 36 domestic to members; USD 46 foreign to members; USD 108 domestic to institutions; USD 140 foreign to institutions (effective 2001). adv. back issues avail. *Refereed.* **Document type:** *Journal, Academic/Scholarly.* **Description:** Covers empirical analyses dealing with topics that extend our knowledge of groups. Revitalizes the link between the scientific study of group dynamics and the application of that scientific understanding in applied settings.
Related titles: Online - full text ed.
Indexed: PsycInfo, e-psyche.
—BLDSC (4220.174600). **CCC.**
Published by: American Psychological Association, 750 First St., N.E., Washington, DC 20002-4242. TEL 202-336-5560, 800-374-2721, FAX 202-336-5633, subscriptions@apa.org, http://www.apa.org/journals/gdn.html. Ed. Donelson Forsyth. Circ: 1,000 (paid).

616.89 USA ISSN 0362-4021
RC488.A1 CODEN: GROUDE
GROUP (NEW YORK); journal of the Eastern Group Psychotherapy Society. Text in English. 1977. q. USD 213, EUR 212 to institutions for print or online ed.; USD 255.60, EUR 255.60 to institutions for print & online eds. combined (effective 2002). bk.rev. index. reprint service avail. from PQC,PSC,SCH,ISI. *Refereed.* **Document type:** *Journal, Academic/Scholarly.* **Description:** Publishes advances, theoretical and clinical contributions, and research in dynamic group psychotherapy.
Related titles: Microform ed.: (from PQC); Online - full text ed.: (from EBSCO Publishing, O C L C Online Computer Library Center, Inc., Swets Blackwell, Kluwer Online, Institute for Scientific Information, RoweCom Information Quest).
Indexed: AgeLine, Biol.Abstr., Curr.Cont., Excerp.Med., IMFL, PsycInfo, Psychol.Abstr. (1982-), SSCI, e-psyche. GNLM, IDS, ingenta.
Published by: (Eastern Group Psychotherapy Society), Kluwer Academic - Plenum Publishers (Subsidiary of: Wolters Kluwer N.V.), 233 Spring St, New York, NY 10013-1578. TEL 212-620-8000, 800-221-9369, FAX 212-463-0742, info@plenum.com, http://www.wkap.nl/journalhome.htm/0362-4021. Ed. Jeffrey L Kleinberg. Circ: 1,200. **Subscr. outside the Americas to:** Kluwer Academic Publishers Group, Journals Department, PO Box 322, Dordrecht 3300 AH, Netherlands. TEL 31-78-639-2392, FAX 31-78-654-6474.

GROUPWORK. see *SOCIAL SERVICES AND WELFARE*

616.89 DEU ISSN 0939-4273
GRUPPENANALYSE; Zeitschrift fuer gruppenanalytische Psychotherapie, Beratung und Supervision. Text in German; Summaries in English, German. 1991. 2/yr. DEM 42.40 (effective 2001 & 2002). adv. bk.rev. back issues avail. **Document type:** *Magazine, Academic/Scholarly.*
Indexed: e-psyche.
Published by: (Institut fuer Gruppenanalyse Heidelberg e.V.), Mattes Verlag GmbH, Postfach 103866, Heidelberg 69028, Germany. TEL 49-6221-459321, FAX 49-6221-459322, journals@mattes.de. adv.: B&W page DEM 300; trim 160 x 240.

302 DEU
CODEN: GRUPDT
GRUPPENDYNAMIK UND ORGANISATIONSBERATUNG; Zeitschrift fuer angewandte Sozialpsychologie. Text in German. 1970. q. EUR 50 domestic; EUR 53.50 foreign; EUR 38.75 domestic to students; EUR 42.25 foreign to students; EUR 12.50 newsstand/cover (effective 2002). adv. bk.rev. back issues avail.; reprint service avail. from PSC,SCH. *Refereed.* **Document type:** *Journal, Academic/Scholarly.*
Formerly: Gruppendynamik (0046-6514)
Related titles: Online - full text ed.: (from Institute for Scientific Information).
Indexed: ASCA, Arts & Hum.Cit.Ind. (coverage dropped), Curr.Cont., Ger.J.Psych., IBR, IBZ, Ind.Philos., PsycInfo, Psychol.Abstr. (1970-), Ref.Zh., SSCI, e-psyche.
—BLDSC (4223.459000), IDS. **CCC.**
Published by: Verlag Leske und Budrich GmbH, Postfach 300551, Leverkusen 51334, Germany. TEL 49-2171-4907-0, FAX 49-2171-4907-11, leske-budrich@t-online.de, http://www.leske-budrich.de. adv.: page DEM 1,050; 125 x 190. Circ: 1,000 (paid).

150 DEU ISSN 0085-1302
GRUPPENPSYCHOTHERAPIE UND GRUPPENDYNAMIK. BEIHEFTE. Text in German. 1972. irreg., latest vol.22, 1986. DEM 49 per issue. **Document type:** *Monographic series, Academic/Scholarly.*
Indexed: Curr.Cont. (coverage dropped), Excerp.Med., e-psyche.
Published by: Vandenhoeck und Ruprecht, Robert-Bosch-Breite 6, Goettingen 37079, Germany. TEL 49-551-6959-0, FAX 49-551-695917. Ed. Dr. Annelise Heigl Evers. Circ: 1,900.

306.85 USA
GUILFORD FAMILY THERAPY SERIES. Text in English. irreg. (approx. biennial). **Document type:** *Monographic series, Academic/Scholarly.* **Description:** Equips therapists and social workers with theoretical and clinical texts on family development and family therapy. The influences of ethnicity, therapist behavior, life transitions, social changes, personal authority, intervention and resistance on families are examined.
Indexed: e-psyche.
Published by: Guilford Publications, Inc., 72 Spring St, New York, NY 10012. TEL 212-431-9800, 800-365-7006, FAX 212-966-6708, info@guilford.com. Ed. Seymour Weingarten. Pub. Robert Matloff. R&P David Mitchell. Adv. contact Christine Luberto.

370.15 150 USA
GUILFORD SCHOOL PRACTITIONER SERIES. Text in English. irreg. (approx. 3-4/yr.). **Document type:** *Monographic series.* **Description:** Provides focused, readable, and prescriptive accounts of techniques for changing children's behavior.
Indexed: e-psyche.
Published by: Guilford Publications, Inc., 72 Spring St, New York, NY 10012. TEL 212-431-9800, 800-365-7006, FAX 212-966-6708, info@guilford.com, http://www.guilford.com. Ed. Seymour Weingarten. Pub. Robert Matloff. R&P David Mitchell. Adv. contact Christine Luberto.

302 USA
GUILFORD SERIES ON SOCIAL AND EMOTIONAL DEVELOPMENT. Text in English. irreg. **Document type:** *Monographic series.*
Indexed: e-psyche.
Published by: Guilford Publications, Inc., 72 Spring St, New York, NY 10012. TEL 212-431-9800, 800-365-7006, FAX 212-966-6708, info@guilford.com, http://www.guilford.com. Eds. Claire Kopp, Steven Asher.

155.4 613.7 USA ISSN 0899-3122
CODEN: HPHEAR
HANDBOOK OF PSYCHOLOGY AND HEALTH SERIES. Text in English. 1982. irreg., latest vol.5, 1987. USD 49.95. back issues avail. *Refereed.* **Document type:** *Monographic series.*
Indexed: Curr.Cont. (coverage dropped), Psychol.Abstr., e-psyche.
Published by: Lawrence Erlbaum Associates, Inc., 10 Industrial Ave, Mahwah, NJ 07430-2262. TEL 201-236-9500, FAX 201-236-0072, jamsel@erlbaum.com, http://www.erlbaum.com. Eds. Andrew Baum, Jerome E Singer.

THE HARVARD MENTAL HEALTH LETTER. see *MEDICAL SCIENCES—Psychiatry And Neurology*

150 GBR ISSN 0266-4771
BF173
HARVEST; journal for Jungian studies. Text in English. 1954. s-a., latest vol.47, 2001. GBP 20, USD 30 (effective 2001). adv. bk.rev. 200 p./no. 1 cols./p. back issues avail. *Refereed.* **Document type:** *Journal, Academic/Scholarly.* **Description:** Promotes a specific genre of Jungian writing which makes use of personal experience in a reflexive style in order to develop theoretical and clinical insights.
Published by: Karnac Books, 6 Pembroke Buildwos, London NW 10, United Kingdom. TEL 44-20-89694454, FAX 44-20-89695585, apc@pipemedia.co.uk, shop@karnacbooks.com, jungclub-london.org.uk, http://www.karnacbooks.com. Ed. Renos Papadopoulos. adv.: B&W page GBP 100. Circ: 500. **U.S. dist. by:** Other Books, 224 West 20th Street, New York 1, NY 10011. TEL 860-874-3428, 860-974-3195.

155 JPN ISSN 0915-9029
HATTATSU SHINRIGAKU KENKYU/JAPANESE JOURNAL OF DEVELOPMENTAL PSYCHOLOGY. Text in Japanese; Summaries in English. 1990. s-a.
Indexed: PsycInfo, Psychol.Abstr. (1990-), e-psyche.
—BLDSC (4651.650000).

P

Published by: Nihon Hattasu Shinri Gakkai/Japan Society of Developmental Psychology, Shirayuri Joshi Daigaku Jido Bunka Gakka, 1-25 Midorigaoka, Chofu-shi, Tokyo-to 182-0001, Japan. FAX 03-3326-9417.

HAWLIYAT KULLIYAT AL-A'DAAB/ANNALS OF THE FACULTY OF ARTS. see *HUMANITIES: COMPREHENSIVE WORKS*

301.1 150 613.7 USA
HEALTH MASTER. Text in English. 1983. s-a. USD 1 (effective 2000). adv. bk.rev. back issues avail. **Document type:** *Catalog, Newsletter.* **Description:** Health & wellness improvement through biofeedback, stress management, relaxation, communications skills, diet, exercise and more.
Former titles: Stress Master; Gentle Places and Quiet Spaces
Indexed: e-psyche.
Published by: Conscious Living Foundation, Inc., PO Box 9, Drain, OR 97435. TEL 503-836-2358, FAX 503-836-2930, info@cliving.org, http://www.cliving.org. Ed. Dr. Tim Lowenstein. Circ: 80,000.

150 USA ISSN 0278-6133
R726.5
HEALTH PSYCHOLOGY. Text in English. 1982. bi-m. USD 81 domestic to non-members; USD 101 foreign to non-members; USD 50 domestic to members; USD 62 foreign to members; USD 224 domestic to institutions; USD 268 foreign to institutions (effective 2001). adv. bk.rev. abstr, bibl, charts, illus, stat. reprint service avail. from PSC,SCH. *Refereed.* **Document type:** *Academic/Scholarly.* **Description:** Publishes empirical studies that promote the understanding of scientific relationships between behavioral principles and physical health and illness.
Related titles: Online - full text ed.: (from Gale Group, Institute for Scientific Information).
Indexed: AIDS Abstr., ASSIA, Abstr.Anthropol., Addic.Abstr., AgeLine, Behav.Med.Abstr., Curr.Cont., Environ.Sci.Poll.Mgmt., Fam.Ind., Food Sci.& Tech.Abstr., INIS Atomind., Ind.Med. (1982-), Int.Nurs.Ind., NRN, Pollut.Abstr., PsycInfo, Psychol.Abstr. (1982-), Risk Abstr., Russ.Acad.Sci.Bibl., SSCI, Saf.Sci.Abstr., Soc.Sci.Ind. (Jul.1999-), Soc.Work Res.& Abstr., THA, e-psyche.
—BLDSC (4275.105200), GNLM, IDS, ingenta. **CCC.**
Published by: American Psychological Association, Division of Health Psychology, 750 First St., N.E., Washington, DC 20002-4242. TEL 202-336-5600, 800-336-2721, FAX 202-336-5568, subscriptions@apa.org, www.apa.org/journals/hea.html. Ed. Arthur A Stone. Circ: 7,700.

HEALTHY MINDS. see *CHILDREN AND YOUTH—About*

150 CAN ISSN 0085-1493
HERE AND NOW; a brief of news from the IPR. Text and summaries in French. 1969. irreg. free per issue. adv. bk.rev. **Document type:** *Bulletin.*
Indexed: e-psyche.
Published by: Institute of Psychological Research, Inc., 34 Fleury St W, Montreal, PQ H3L 1S9, Canada. TEL 514-382-3000, FAX 514-382-3007. Ed. Marie Paule Chevrier. Circ: 2,000 (controlled).

155 JPN
HERUSU SAIKOROJISUTO/HEALTH PSYCHOLOGIST. Text in Japanese. q.
Indexed: e-psyche.
Published by: Nihon Kenko Shinri Gakkai/Japanese Association of Health Psychology, Waseda Daigaku Bungakubu Oda Kenkyushitsu, 24-1, Toyama 1-chome, Shinjuku-ku, Tokyo 162, Japan.

155 610 JPN ISSN 0917-6934
HIROSHIMA SHUDO DAIGAKU RINSHO SHINRIGAKU KENKYU/HIROSHIMA SHUDO UNIVERSITY. BULLETIN OF CLINICAL PSYCHOLOGY. Text in Japanese; Summaries in English. 1991. a. JPY 2,500. adv. bk.rev. *Refereed.* **Document type:** *Bulletin.*
Indexed: e-psyche.
Published by: Hiroshima Shudo Daigaku, Shinrigaku Kyoshitsu/Hiroshima Shudo University, Department of Psychology, 1717, Otsuka, Numatacho, Asaminami-ku, Hiroshima-shi 731-31, Japan. TEL 81-82-830-1139, FAX 81-82-848-6633. Adv. contact Mamoru Asada.

150 301.1 USA ISSN 0739-9863
RC451.5.H57 CODEN: HJBSEZ
HISPANIC JOURNAL OF BEHAVIORAL SCIENCES. Text in English, Spanish. 1979. q. USD 345 domestic; GBP 249 UK, Europe, Middle East & Africa; USD 361 elsewhere (effective 2002). adv. bk.rev., film rev. illus. index. back issues avail.; reprint service avail. from PQC,PSC,SCH. *Refereed.* **Document type:** *Academic/Scholarly.* **Description:** Contains empirical articles, case study reports, and scholarly notes of theoretical or methodological interest pertaining to Hispanics. Focuses on the fields of anthropology, linguistics, psychology, public health, and sociology.
Related titles: Microfilm ed.: (from PQC); Online - full text ed.: (from EBSCO Publishing, O C L C Online Computer Library Center, Inc., RoweCom Information Quest, ProQuest Information & Learning, Gale Group, ingenta, Swets Blackwell, Institute for Scientific Information).
Indexed: ASCA, Abstr.Soc.Geront., AgeLine, C.I.J.E., Chic.Per.Ind. (1979-), Crim.Just.Abstr., Curr.Cont., Educ.Admin.Abstr., Fam.Ind., High.Educ.Abstr., Hisp.Amer.Per.Ind. (1989-), IMFL, Lang.& Lang.Behav.Abstr., Mult.Ed.Abstr., PsycInfo, Psychol.Abstr. (1979-), SOPODA, SSCI, Sage Fam.Stud.Abstr., Sage Race Rel.Abstr., Soc.Sci.Ind. (Jan.1994-), Soc.Serv.Abstr., Sociol.Abstr., Sp.Ed.Needs Abstr., Viol.& Abuse Abstr., e-psyche.
—BLDSC (4315.772700), IDS, Infotrieve, ingenta. **CCC.**
Published by: Sage Publications, Inc., 2455 Teller Rd, Thousand Oaks, CA 91320. TEL 805-499-0721, FAX 805-706-0871, 805-499-0871, libraries@sagepub.com., info@sagepub.com, http://www.sagepub.com. Ed. Dr. Amado M Padilla. Pub. Sara Miller McCune. R&P Tanya Udin. Adv. contact DeAnna Vega Hammersley. Circ: 1,200. **Overseas subscr. to:** Sage Publications Ltd., 6 Bonhill St, London EC2A 4PU, United Kingdom. TEL 44-20-7374-0645, FAX 44-20-7374-8741, subscription@sagepub.co.uk, http://www.sagepub.co.uk; Sage Publications India Pvt. Ltd., 4215, New Delhi 110 048, India. TEL 91-11-641-9884, FAX 91-11-647-2426.

152 USA ISSN 1093-4510
HISTORY OF PSYCHOLOGY. Text in English. 1998. q. USD 40 domestic to non-members; USD 55 foreign to non-members; USD 34 domestic to members; USD 44 foreign to members; USD 82 domestic to institutions; USD 114 foreign to institutions (effective 2001). adv. illus. reprints avail. *Refereed.* **Document type:** *Journal, Academic/Scholarly.* **Description:** Addresses all aspects of psychology's past and its interrelationship with the many contexts within which it has emerged and has been practiced.
Indexed: Amer.Hist.& Life, Hist.Abstr., PsycInfo, e-psyche.
—BLDSC (4318.409500), Infotrieve. **CCC.**
Published by: American Psychological Association, 750 First St., N.E., Washington, DC 20002-4242. TEL 202-336-5500, 800-374-2721, FAX 202-336-5568, subscriptions@apa.org, http://www.apa.org/journals/hop.html. Ed. Michael M Sokal. Pub. Susan Knapp. R&P Karen Thomas. Circ: 860.

150 FRA ISSN 0018-4314
L'HOMME LIBRE; fils de la terre. Text in French. 1960. q. FRF 50; FRF 64 foreign (effective 1997). bk.rev. bibl.
Indexed: e-psyche.
Published by: Cercle d'Etudes Psychologiques, BP 205, St Etienne Cedex 1 42005, France. Ed. Marcel Renoulet.

HUMAN COGNITIVE PROCESSING. see *LINGUISTICS—Computer Applications*

153.6 USA ISSN 0360-3989
P91.3
HUMAN COMMUNICATION RESEARCH. Text in English. 1974. q. GBP 55, USD 75 to individuals includes free online access; GBP 180, USD 280 to institutions includes free online access (effective 2002). adv. bk.rev. abstr, illus. back issues avail.; reprint service avail. from PQC,SCH,PSC. *Refereed.* **Document type:** *Journal, Academic/Scholarly.* **Description:** Publishes important research and reports that contribute to the expanding body of knowledge about human communication.
Related titles: Microform ed.: (from PQC); Online - full text ed.: ISSN 1468-2885 (from ProQuest Information & Learning, Gale Group, Institute for Scientific Information).
Indexed: ASCA, Abstr.Anthropol., Abstr.Soc.Geront., AgeLine, Arts & Hum.Cit.Ind. (coverage dropped), C.I.J.E., Commun.Abstr., Curr.Cont., Film Lit.Ind., IJCS (1974-), IMFL, L.R.I., Lang.& Lang.Behav.Abstr., Mid.East: Abstr.& Ind., Mult.Ed.Abstr., Peace Res.Abstr., PsycInfo, Psychol.Abstr. (1975-), SOMA, SOPODA, SSCI, Sage Fam.Stud.Abstr., Sage Pub.Admin.Abstr., Soc.Sci.Ind. (Jan.1994-), Soc.Serv.Abstr., Sociol.Abstr., Viol.& Abuse Abstr., e-psyche.
—BLDSC (4336.043000), IDS. **CCC.**
Published by: (International Communication Association GBR), Oxford University Press, Academic Division, Great Clarendon St, Oxford OX2 6DP, United Kingdom. TEL 44-1865-267907, FAX 44-1865-267835, jnlorders@oup-usa.org, jnl.info@oup.co.uk, http://www3.oup.co.uk/humcom/, http://www.oup.co.uk/journals. Ed. Edward Fink. Pub. Erich Staib. Adv. contact Helen Pearson TEL 44-1235-201904. page GBP 220, page USD 365. Circ: 4,400. **Subscr. outside N. America to:** Journals Marketing, Great Clarendon St, Oxford OX2 6DP, United Kingdom.

HUMAN - COMPUTER INTERACTION (MAHWAH); a journal of theoretical, empirical, and methodological issues of user psychology and of system design. see *COMPUTERS*

305.8 USA
HUMAN ETHOLOGY BULLETIN. Text in English. 1974. q. USD 25; USD 25 foreign (effective 1999). adv. bk.rev. back issues avail. *Refereed.* **Document type:** *Academic/Scholarly.* **Description:** Publishes essays, brief research reports, listings of current literature, announcements.
Formerly: Human Ethology Newsletter (0739-2036)
Indexed: Intl.Bibl.Soc.Sci., e-psyche.
Published by: International Society for Human Ethology, University of Maine, Department of Psychology, Orono, ME 04469. TEL 207-581-2044, FAX 207-581-6128, peterlaf@maine.edu;barbara.fuller@uchsc.edu, http://evolution.humb.univie.ac.at. Ed., R&P Peter Lafreniere. Circ: 400 (paid). **Dist.by:** Dr. Barbara F. Fuller, School of Nursing, Univ of Colorado, 4200E N Ave, Boulder, CO 80220. TEL 303-315-8929, FAX 303-315-5666.

HUMAN EVOLUTION, BEHAVIOR, AND INTELLIGENCE. see *BIOLOGY—Genetics*

HUMAN FACTORS. see *ENGINEERING*

HUMAN FACTORS AND ERGONOMICS IN MANUFACTURING. see *ENGINEERING—Industrial Engineering*

HUMAN FACTORS AND ERGONOMICS SOCIETY ANNUAL MEETING. PROCEEDINGS. see *ENGINEERING*

HUMAN FACTORS AND ERGONOMICS SOCIETY BULLETIN. see *ENGINEERING*

HUMAN FACTORS IN INFORMATION TECHNOLOGY. see *COMPUTERS—Information Science And Information Theory*

616.89 GBR ISSN 1473-4850
HUMAN GIVENS; radical psychology today. Text in English. 1993. q. GBP 30 domestic (effective 2001); GBP 35 foreign (effective 2000). bk.rev. 52 p./no. back issues avail. *Refereed.* **Document type:** *Journal, Academic/Scholarly.* **Description:** Discusses psychology, human development, and medical and economic topics relating to the work of complementary and orthodox health care workers.
Former titles (until April 2001): The New Therapist (1467-5676); (until 2000): Therapist (1350-4614)
—BLDSC (6088.870780).
Published by: (European Therapy Studies Institute), Human Givens Publishing Ltd., The Barn, Church Farm, Chalvington, N. Hailsham, E Sussex BN27 3TD, United Kingdom. TEL 44-1323-811662, FAX 44-1323-811486, editor@humangivens.com, info@humangivens.com, thhp://www.humangivens.com. Eds. Denise Winn TEL 44-20-84505646, Ivan Tyrrell. Circ: 1,500 (paid).

HUMAN MOVEMENT SCIENCE; journal devoted to pure and applied research on human movement. see *MEDICAL SCIENCES*

HUMAN NATURE; an interdisciplinary biosocial perspective. see *SOCIAL SCIENCES: COMPREHENSIVE WORKS*

152 USA ISSN 0895-9285
BF636.A1
HUMAN PERFORMANCE. Text in English. 1988. q. USD 60 in US & Canada to individuals; USD 90 elsewhere to individuals; USD 380 in US & Canada to institutions; USD 410 elsewhere to institutions (effective 2002). adv. *Refereed.* **Document type:** *Journal, Academic/Scholarly.* **Description:** Provides information for behavioral scientists interested in the factors that motivate and influence excellence in human behavior. Publishes research and theory that investigates the nature of goal-directed human activity.

Related titles: Online - full text ed.: ISSN 1532-7043. USD 54 to individuals; USD 342 to institutions (effective 2002) (from CatchWord Ltd., EBSCO Publishing, O C L C Online Computer Library Center, Inc., RoweCom Information Quest, Swets Blackwell, Institute for Scientific Information).
Indexed: ASCA, Curr.Cont., Environ.Sci.Poll.Mgmt., Ergon.Abstr., Pollut.Abstr., PsycInfo, Psychol.Abstr. (1988-), Risk Abstr., SSCI, Saf.Sci.Abstr., e-psyche.
—BLDSC (4336.265000), CatchWord, Infotrieve, ingenta. **CCC.**
Published by: Lawrence Erlbaum Associates, Inc., 10 Industrial Ave, Mahwah, NJ 07430-2262. TEL 201-760-3735, 800-926-6579, FAX 201-236-0072, journals@erlbaum.com, http://www.erlbaum.com/Journals/journals/HP/hp.htm. Ed. James Farr. adv.: page USD 275; trim 5 x 8.

158.2 302 GBR
HUMAN RELATIONS, AUTHORITY AND JUSTICE; experiences and critiques. Text in English. irreg. back issues avail. **Document type:** *Academic/Scholarly.* **Description:** Focuses on bringing psychoanalytic and related psychodynamic approaches to bear on group, institutional, cultural and political processes.
Media: Online - full text.
Indexed: e-psyche.
Published by: Human Nature Trust, 26 Freegrove Rd, London N7 9RQ, United Kingdom. TEL 44-20-7607-8306, FAX 44-20-7609-4837, robert@rmy1.demon.co.uk; ttbb@sf.cit.bg, http://www.human-nature.com/hraj/home.html, http://www.human-nature.com/HRAJ/home.html. Eds. Robert M Young, Toma Tomov.

302.3 USA ISSN 0885-1174
BF575.S75
HUMAN STRESS: CURRENT SELECTED RESEARCH. Text in English. 1986. a. USD 37.50. bk.rev. index. back issues avail. **Description:** Articles on biological and behavioral problems related to stress.
Formerly: Human Stress Current Advances in Research
Indexed: e-psyche.
—BLDSC (4336.466800).
Published by: A M S Press, Inc., 56 E 13th St, New York, NY 10003. TEL 212-777-4700, FAX 212-995-5413. Ed. James H Humphrey.

150 GBR ISSN 0960-9830
HUMAN SYSTEMS; the journal of systemic consultation and management. Text in English. 1990. q. GBP 30 domestic to individuals; GBP 37.70 in Europe to individuals; GBP 40 elsewhere to individuals; GBP 40 domestic to institutions; GBP 48 in Europe to institutions; GBP 54 elsewhere to institutions. adv. bk.rev., software rev., video rev. *Refereed.* **Document type:** *Academic/Scholarly.* **Description:** Creates a forum for exchanging and developing ideas and practices, investigates and discusses emerging concepts applicable to clinical and organizational practice, and provides a specialist field that includes research and theoretical papers focusing on systematic and constructionist ideas.
Indexed: e-psyche.
—BLDSC (4336.467500).
Published by: University of Leeds, Department of Psychology, Leeds Family Therapy & Research Centre, Leeds, W Yorks LS2 9JT, United Kingdom. TEL 44-113-2335728, FAX 44-113-2335700, peters@psychology.leeds.ac.uk. Eds. Peter Stratton, Philippa Seligman. Adv. contact Peter Lang. Circ: 750 (paid). **Subscr. to:** K C C International, 2 Wyvil Ct, Trenchold St, London SW8 2TG, United Kingdom. TEL 44-20-7720-7301, FAX 44-20-7720-7302. **Co-sponsor:** Kensington Consultation Centre.

150 USA ISSN 0887-3267
THE HUMANISTIC PSYCHOLOGIST. Text in English. 1973. 3/yr. USD 20 domestic to individuals; USD 24 foreign to individuals; USD 40 domestic to institutions; USD 44 foreign to institutions (effective 2000). adv. bk.rev. back issues avail. *Refereed.* **Document type:** *Academic/Scholarly.* **Description:** Publishes contributions that advance the field of humanistic psychology, broadly defined.
Indexed: PsycInfo, Psychol.Abstr. (1986-), e-psyche.
—BLDSC (4336.530800). **CCC.**
Published by: American Psychological Association, Division of Humanistic Psychology, Psychology Dept, University of West Georgia, Carrollton, GA 30118-2130. TEL 770-836-4578, FAX 770-836-6791, aanstoos@westga.edu, http://www.westga.edu/~thp. Ed., R&P Christopher M Anastoos. Adv. contact Greg Kuschwara. Circ: 1,200 (paid).

HUMOR; international journal of humor research. see *SOCIOLOGY*

152.4 362.2 USA
HYGEIA; an online journal for pregnancy and neonatal loss. Text in English. 1995. m. (plus d. updates). free. *Refereed.* **Document type:** *Consumer.* **Description:** Shares information about support groups, resources and references. Provides updates of relevant medical news, reviews, and multidiscipline insights into the nature of pregnancy, perinatal and neonatal loss.
Media: Online - full text.
Indexed: GeoRef, e-psyche.
Address: PO Box 3943, Amity Sta, New Haven, CT 06525. berman@hygeia.org, http://hygeia.org. Ed., Pub., R&P Dr. Michael R Berman.

HYPNOTHERAPY TODAY. see *MEDICAL SCIENCES—Hypnosis*

150 NGA ISSN 1117-1421
I F E PSYCHOLOGIA; psychology in Africa. Text in English. 1993. s-a. NGN 500, USD 40 (effective 2001). adv. bk.rev. abstr, bibl, charts, maps, stat, tr.lit. back issues avail. *Refereed.* **Document type:** *Journal, Academic/Scholarly.* **Description:** Deals with psychology and science.
Related titles: CD-ROM ed.: A P A. 1993; Online - full text ed.: Africa Online, INASP London. 1999.
Indexed: PsycInfo, e-psyche.
—BLDSC (4363.282195).
Published by: (Psychologia Ltd GHA), I F E Centre for Psychological Studies, PO Box 1548, Ile Ife, Osun State, Nigeria. solowu@oauife.edu.ng. Ed. A A Olowu. Adv. contact Samson Akinyele. page USD 100. Circ: 1,000.

I P O ANNUAL PROGRESS REPORT. (Instituut voor Perceptie Onderzoek) see *LINGUISTICS*

I S P T JOURNAL OF RESEARCH IN EDUCATIONAL & PSYCHOLOGICAL TESTING & MEASUREMENT. see *EDUCATION*

152.8 IND
I S P T QUARTERLY BULLETIN. Text in English. q. INR 50, USD 50. **Description:** Provides information regarding Institute members, news, awards, honors and its publication.
Indexed: e-psyche.
Published by: Institute for Studies in Psychological Testing, 101 Doon, Jakhan, Rajpur Rd., Dehra Dun, Uttar Pradesh 248 001, India.

616.89 USA
I S S D NEWS. Text in English. 1983. bi-m. USD 120 to members (effective 2001). back issues avail. **Document type:** *Newsletter.* **Description:** Focuses on recent news from other organizations of interest to members, news for US and international affiliates, and current issues concerning the field of multiple personality and dissociative states.
Formerly: I S S M P and D News (1075-7783)
Indexed: e-psyche.
Published by: International Society for the Study of Dissociation, 60 Revere Dr, Ste 500, Northbrook, IL 60062. TEL 847-480-0899, FAX 847-480-9282, cmcomstock@worldnet.att.net. Ed., R&P Christine Comstock TEL 440-845-9011. Circ: 1,500 (paid).

614.58 ITA ISSN 0019-1647
IGIENE MENTALE. Text in Italian. 1957. q. ITL 10,000. adv. bk.rev. abstr, charts, illus, stat. index, cum.index.
Indexed: Excerp.Med., e-psyche.
Published by: Lega Italiana di Igiene e Profilassi Mentale, Ospedale Psichiatrico Provinciale di Trapani, Trapani, TP 91100, Italy. Circ: 250.

370.15 150 USA ISSN 1041-8377
IMAGERY TODAY. Text in English. 1983. s-a. USD 10 (effective 2000).
Indexed: e-psyche.
Published by: (International Imagery Association), Brandon House, Inc., PO Box 240, Bronx, NY 10471. Circ: 14,941.

133 152 USA ISSN 0276-2366
BF311
IMAGINATION, COGNITION AND PERSONALITY. Text in English. q. USD 58 to individuals; USD 218 to institutions (effective 2001). adv. bk.rev. back issues avail.; reprints avail. *Refereed.* **Document type:** *Journal, Academic/Scholarly.* **Description:** Authoritative articles examine the diverse uses of imagery, fantasy, consciousness in psychotherapy, behavior modification, and related areas of study.
Supersedes (in 1981): Journal of Altered States of Consciousness (0094-5498); Which was formerly (until 1973): International Journal of Altered States of Consciousness
Indexed: Abstr.Anthropol., Biol.Abstr., Excerp.Med., IBR, IBZ, Ind.Philos., PsycInfo, Psychol.Abstr. (1981-), Russ.Acad.Sci.Bibl., Stud.Wom.Abstr., e-psyche.
—BLDSC (4368.996200), ingenta. **CCC.**
Published by: Baywood Publishing Co., Inc., 26 Austin Ave, Box 337, Amityville, NY 11701. TEL 631-691-1270, 800-638-7819, FAX 631-691-1770, info@baywood.com, baywood@baywood.com, http://baywood.com/search/PreviewJournal.asp?qsRecord=4, http://www.baywood.com. Eds. Jerome Singer, Kenneth Pope. R&P Julie Krempa. Adv. contact Joi Tamber-Brooks.

IMAGO; revista de psicoanalisis, psiquiatria y psicologia. see *MEDICAL SCIENCES—Psychiatry And Neurology*

IMPACT (AUSTIN). see *MEDICAL SCIENCES—Psychiatry And Neurology*

IN THE FAMILY; the magazine for lesbians, gays, bisexuals and their relations. see *HOMOSEXUALITY*

150 ITA ISSN 0391-3198
INCONSCIO E CULTURA. Text in Italian. 1978. irreg., latest vol.21, 1999, numbers not consecutive. price varies. adv. **Document type:** *Monographic series.*
Indexed: e-psyche.
Published by: Liguori Editore srl, Via Posillipo, 394, Naples, NA 80123, Italy. TEL 39-81-7206111, FAX 39-81-7206244, http://www.liguori.it. Ed. Aldo Carotenuto. Pub. Guido Liguori. Adv. contact Maria Liguori.

P

158 IND ISSN 0019-4247
BF636.A1
INDIAN ACADEMY OF APPLIED PSYCHOLOGY. JOURNAL. Text in English. 1974 (vol.17). 2/yr. INR 50, USD 10 to individuals; INR 150, USD 25 to institutions. charts, stat. index. **Document type:** *Academic/Scholarly.*
Indexed: Indian Psychol.Abstr., PsycInfo, Psychol.Abstr. (1964-), e-psyche.
—BLDSC (4761.900000).
Published by: Indian Academy of Applied Psychology, University of Madras, Department of Psychology, Chennai, Tamil Nadu 600 005, India. Ed. Habib Ahmed. Adv. contact V Natarajan.

158 IND ISSN 0019-5073
BF636.A1 CODEN: IJAPBI
INDIAN JOURNAL OF APPLIED PSYCHOLOGY. Text in English. 1964. s-a. USD 50. adv. bk.rev. charts. index. reprint service avail. from PQC.
Related titles: Microfilm ed.: (from PQC).
Indexed: Bibl.Asian Stud. (1971-1990), Biol.Abstr., Indian Psychol.Abstr., Psychol.Abstr., Sp.Ed.Needs Abstr., e-psyche.
—BLDSC (4410.300000), ingenta.
Published by: University of Madras, Department of Psychology, c/o Director, Publications Division, Chennai, Tamil Nadu 600 005, India. TEL 91-44-568778, FAX 91-44-566693, TELEX 416376 ONOMIN. Ed. P Anantha Krishnan. Circ: 200.

152 IND ISSN 0303-2582
RC467
INDIAN JOURNAL OF CLINICAL PSYCHOLOGY. Text in English. 1974. s-a. INR 200, USD 50 (effective 1999). adv. bk.rev. abstr, bibl. index. **Document type:** *Academic/Scholarly.*
Indexed: Indian Psychol.Abstr., Lang.& Lang.Behav.Abstr., PsycInfo, Psychol.Abstr. (1974-), Psychol.R.G., Sociol.Abstr., e-psyche.
—BLDSC (4410.750000), CISTI.
Published by: Indian Association of Clinical Psychologists, C-135A Dayanand Marg, Tilak Nagar, Jaipur, Rajasthan 302 004, India. TEL 91-0141-621477, FAX 91-0141-652784. Ed. S Nathawat. R&P, Adv. contact S. Nathawat. B&W page INR 1,000, color page INR 3,000. Circ: 700.

150 IND ISSN 0970-3748
INDIAN JOURNAL OF CURRENT PSYCHOLOGICAL RESEARCH. Text in English. 1986. s-a. INR 100, USD 32 to individuals; INR 125, USD 40 to institutions. adv. bk.rev. **Description:** Publishes empirical and critical review articles in the field of psychology.
Indexed: Psychol.Abstr. (1986-), e-psyche.
Published by: National Psychological Corporation, Bhargava Bhavan, 4-230 Kacheri Ghat, Agra, Uttar Pradesh 282 004, India. TEL 65780. Ed. S N Rai.

370.15 150 IND ISSN 0046-9009
INDIAN JOURNAL OF PSYCHOMETRY AND EDUCATION. Text in English. 1970. s-a. INR 100, USD 10. adv. bk.rev. bibl, charts.
Indexed: Indian Psychol.Abstr., Lang.& Lang.Behav.Abstr., PsycInfo, Psychol.Abstr. (1970-), e-psyche.
—BLDSC (4420.321000).
Published by: Indian Psychometric and Educational Research Association, University of Patna, Dept. of Education, Patna, Bihar 800 004, India. Ed. R P Singh. Circ: 500. **Dist. by:** Nandini Enterprises, 23-451 Wazirpura, Agra, Uttar Pradesh 282 003, India.

156 IND ISSN 0019-6215
BF1
INDIAN PSYCHOLOGICAL REVIEW. Text in English. 1964. q. (plus 1 special. issue). USD 445 (effective 2000). adv. bk.rev. reprint service avail. from ISI. **Document type:** *Academic/Scholarly.*
Indexed: Bibl.Asian Stud. (1976-1991), Psychol.Abstr., e-psyche.
—BLDSC (4428.200000), ingenta.
Published by: Agra Psychological Research Cell, Tiwari Kothi, Belanganj, Agra, Uttar Pradesh 282 004, India. TEL 91-562-362964. Eds. Dr. Jay Prakash, S Jalota.

INFANCIA Y APRENDIZAJE/JOURNAL FOR THE STUDY OF EDUCATION AND DEVELOPMENT. see *EDUCATION*

155.4 GBR ISSN 1522-7227
HQ771 CODEN: EDPAEA
INFANT AND CHILD DEVELOPMENT. Text in English. 1992. q. USD 405 in United States; USD 405 in Canada & Mexico; USD 405 elsewhere; USD 426 combined subscription in United States for print and online eds.; USD 426 combined subscription in Canada & Mexico for print and online eds.; USD 426 combined subscription elsewhere for print and online eds. (effective 2002). adv. back issues avail.; reprint service avail. from SWZ. *Refereed.* **Document type:** *Academic/Scholarly.* **Description:** Publishes theoretical, empirical and methodological papers covering all aspects of psychological development during infancy and early childhood.
Formerly (until 1999): Early Development and Parenting (1057-3593)
Related titles: Microform ed.: (from PQC); Online - full text ed.: ISSN 1522-7219. USD 405 in United States; USD 405 in Canada & Mexico; USD 405 elsewhere (effective 2002) (from EBSCO Publishing, Wiley InterScience, Institute for Scientific Information).
Indexed: ASSIA, Curr.Cont., Fam.Ind., PsycInfo, SSCI, e-psyche.
—BLDSC (4478.257000), GNLM, IDS. **CCC.**
Published by: Wiley Europe Ltd., Baffins Ln, Chichester, W Sussex PO19 1UD, United Kingdom. TEL 44-1243-779777, FAX 44-1243-775878, customer@wiley.co.uk, http://www.wiley.co.uk. adv.: B&W page GBP 650, color page GBP 1,550; trim 200 x 260. Circ: 400. **Subscr. to:** John Wiley & Sons, Inc., Journals, 605 Third Ave, New York, NY 10158. TEL 212-850-6021, 212-850-6645, subinfo@jwiley.com.

618.92 GBR ISSN 0163-6383
BF719 CODEN: IBDEDP
INFANT BEHAVIOR AND DEVELOPMENT; an international & interdisciplinary journal. Text in English. 1978. q. EUR 103 in Europe to individuals; JPY 13,600 in Japan to individuals; USD 115 elsewhere to individuals; EUR 300 in Europe to institutions; JPY 39,900 in Japan to institutions; USD 337 elsewhere to institutions (effective 2002). bk.rev. index. back issues avail.; reprint service avail. from PSC,SCH,ISI. *Refereed.* **Document type:** *Academic/Scholarly.* **Description:** Presents original, empirical and theoretical studies directed toward the understanding of infancy. Each study is methodologically complete with a documented replicability of results.
Related titles: Online - full text ed.: (from ingenta, Swets Blackwell, ScienceDirect, Institute for Scientific Information).
Indexed: ASCA, Bibl.Dev.Med.& Child Neur., Biol.Abstr., Chicago Psychoanal.Lit.Ind., Child Devel.Abstr., Curr.Cont., ERA, Excerp.Med., Fam.Ind., IBR, IBZ, Ind.Philos., Lang.& Lang.Behav.Abstr., M.L.A., MLA Intl.Bibl., Mult.Ed.Abstr., PsycInfo, Psychol.Abstr. (1979-), Psycscan D.P., SOPODA, SSCI, Sociol.Abstr., Sp.Ed.Needs Abstr., e-psyche.
—BLDSC (4478.270000), GNLM, ingenta. **CCC.**
Published by: (International Society for Infant Studies.), Elsevier Science, The Boulevard, Langford Ln, Kidlington, Oxon OX5 1GB, United Kingdom. TEL 44-1865-843000, FAX 44-1865-843010, http://www.elsevier.com/locate/inbede. Eds. G Savelsbergh, L Lipsitt. Circ: 1,500.

INFANT MENTAL HEALTH JOURNAL. see *MEDICAL SCIENCES—Pediatrics*

INFANZIA. see *CHILDREN AND YOUTH—About*

155.4 157 ITA
INFANZIA PSICOANALISI E ISTITUZIONI. Text in Italian. 1981. irreg., latest vol.9, 1997. price varies. adv. **Document type:** *Monographic series.*
Indexed: e-psyche.
Published by: Liguori Editore srl, Via Posillipo, 394, Naples, NA 80123, Italy. TEL 39-81-7206111, FAX 39-81-7206244, http://www.liguori.it. Ed. Bianca Iaccarino. Pub. Guido Liguori. Adv. contact Maria Liguori.

302.2 USA ISSN 0740-5502
P87
INFORMATION AND BEHAVIOR. Text in English. 1985. a. USD 54.95 (effective 2001). back issues avail. **Document type:** *Academic/Scholarly.* **Description:** Examines the forms, technologies, organization, and use of information, and how they affect human behavior. Coverage includes the effect of new technology on office and home life, regulation and control of information, and the economics of information.
Indexed: Int.Polit.Sci.Abstr., e-psyche.
—BLDSC (4481.758500). **CCC.**
Published by: Transaction Publishers, 35 Berrue Circle, Rutgers University, Piscataway, NJ 08854-8042. TEL 732-445-2280, FAX 732-445-3138, trans@transactionpub.com, http://www.transactionpub.com. Ed. Brent D Ruben. Pub. Mary Curtis. R&P Marlena Davidian TEL 732-445-2280 ext 100. Adv. contact Alicja Garbie. Circ: 4,000. **Subscr. to:** Transaction Distribution Center, 390 Campus Dr, Somerset, NJ 08873. TEL 732-748-0300, FAX 732-748-1886.

INFORMATIONSBULLETINEN; tidskrift foer livskvalitet. see *SOCIAL SCIENCES: COMPREHENSIVE WORKS*

150 ZAF ISSN 1022-0798
INNOVANT. Text in Afrikaans, English. 1993. 3/yr. ZAR 15, USD 2.50 (effective 1999). adv. *Refereed.* **Document type:** *Academic/Scholarly.*
Indexed: e-psyche.
Published by: Sentrum vir Mensilike Ontwikkeling in Psigososiele Konteks - SEMKO/Centre for Human Advancement in Psychosocial Context, Department of Psychology, University of Pretoria, Lynnwood Rd., Brooklyn, Pretoria 0181, South Africa. TEL 27-12-4203430, FAX 27-12-4202404, fieddijk@libarts.up.ac.za, http://www.up.ac.za/academic/psychol/cemco/cemco.html. Ed., Adv. contact Carina Fiedeldey-Van Dijk. R&P Carina Fiedeldey Van Dijk. Circ: 400.

616.890 150 USA
RC467.7
INSIDER'S GUIDE TO GRADUATE PROGRAMS IN CLINICAL AND COUNSELING PSYCHOLOGY (YEARS). Text in English. 1990. biennial. USD 21.95 (effective 2000). charts, stat. **Description:** Outlines strategies for getting into graduate school in psychology and gives an inside look at all to the programs available in the US and Canada.
Formerly: Insider's Guide to Graduate Programs in Clinical Psychology (1061-7132)
Indexed: e-psyche.
Published by: Guilford Publications, Inc., 72 Spring St, New York, NY 10012. TEL 212-431-9800, 800-365-7006, FAX 212-966-6708, info@guilford.com, http://www.guilford.com. Ed. Seymour Weingarten. Pub. Robert Matloff. R&P David Mitchell. Adv. contact Christine Luberto.

INSIGHT-PSICOTERAPIA. see *MEDICAL SCIENCES—Psychiatry And Neurology*

616.89 CAN ISSN 0832-7475
INSTITUT DE RECHERCHES PSYCHOLOGIQUES. BULLETIN. Key Title: Bulletin I R P. Text in French. 1986. irreg. price varies. **Document type:** *Bulletin.*
Published by: Institut de Recherches Psychologiques, 34 Fleury St W, Montreal, PQ H3L 1S9, Canada. TEL 514-382-3000, FAX 514-382-3007. Eds. Malko von Osten, Marie-Paule Chevrier.

150 GBR ISSN 0073-9561
INSTITUTE OF PSYCHOPHYSICAL RESEARCH. PROCEEDINGS. Text in English. 1968. irreg. GBP 30 per vol.. back issues avail. **Document type:** *Proceedings, Monographic series.*
Published by: Institute of Psychophysical Research, 118 Banbury Rd, Oxford OX2 6JU, United Kingdom. TEL 44-1865-58787, FAX 44-1865-58064. Circ: 2,500. **Dist. in the U.S. by:** State Mutual Book & Periodical Service Ltd., 521 Fifth Ave, New York, NY 10017.

INSTITUTUL DE SUBINGINERI ORADEA. LUCRARI STIINTIFICE: SERIA PEDAGOGIE, PSIHOLOGIE, METODICA. see *EDUCATION*

150 658.3 GBR ISSN 1461-5320
INTAND NEWSLETTER; the newsletter of the international network for transactional analysis, neuro-linguistic programming. Text in English. 1993. q. GBP 12; GBP 18 foreign (effective 2002). bk.rev. illus. back issues avail. **Document type:** *Newsletter, Magazine.* **Description:** Contains theory, techniques for consultants, educators & trainers applying developmental and organizational transactional analysis, neuro-linguistic programming and similar.
Published by: Sherwood Publishing, 7 Oxhey Rd, Watford, Herts WD1 4QF, United Kingdom. TEL 44-1923-224737, FAX 44-1923-210648, instand@adinternational.com. Ed., Pub. Julie Hay. Circ: 76. **Co-sponsor:** A D International.

INTEGRAL'NOE ISSLEDOVANIE INDIVIDUAL'NOSTI. see *EDUCATION*

INTEGRATIVE PHYSIOLOGICAL AND BEHAVIORAL SCIENCE. see *MEDICAL SCIENCES—Psychiatry And Neurology*

155.4 DEU ISSN 0342-6831
INTEGRATIVE THERAPIE; Zeitschrift fuer vergleichende Psychotherapie und Methodenintegration. Text in German; Summaries in English. 1975. q. DEM 70; DEM 55 to students (effective 2000). adv. bk.rev. index. **Document type:** *Magazine, Academic/Scholarly.*
Indexed: IBR, IBZ, Ind.Philos., e-psyche.
—GNLM.
Published by: (Fritz Perls Institut), Junfermann Verlag, Imadstr 40, Paderborn 33102, Germany. TEL 49-5251-13440, FAX 49-5251-134444, ju@junfermann.de. Ed. Hilarion Petzold. Circ: 2,500.

370.15 150 GBR ISSN 0160-2896
BF431 CODEN: NTLLDT
INTELLIGENCE (KIDLINGTON); a multidisciplinary journal. Text in English. 1977. 6/yr. EUR 138 in Europe to individuals; JPY 18,300 in Japan to individuals; USD 154 elsewhere to individuals; EUR 333 in Europe to institutions; JPY 44,200 in Japan to institutions; USD 372 elsewhere to institutions (effective 2002). bk.rev. index. back issues avail.; reprint service avail. from PSC,SCH,ISI. *Refereed.* **Document type:** *Academic/Scholarly.* **Description:** Publishes original research and theoretical studies and review papers that substantially contribute to the understanding of intelligence. Includes papers in psychometrics, test and measurement, and other empirical and theoretical studies in intelligence and mental retardation.
Related titles: Online - full text ed.: (from ingenta, Gale Group, ScienceDirect, Factiva, Institute for Scientific Information).
Indexed: A.I.Abstr., ASSIA, Biol.Abstr., C.I.J.E., Child Devel.Abstr., Cont.Pg.Educ., Curr.Cont., Ind.Philos., Lang.& Lang.Behav.Abstr., PsycInfo, Psychol.Abstr. (1977-), Russ.Acad.Sci.Bibl., SOPODA, SSCI, Sociol.Abstr.
—BLDSC (4531.826500), CISTI, ingenta. **CCC.**
Published by: Elsevier Science, The Boulevard, Langford Ln, Kidlington, Oxon OX5 1GB, United Kingdom. TEL 44-1865-843000, FAX 44-1865-843010, http://www.elsevier.com/locate/intell. Ed. Douglas K Detterman. Circ: 650.

150.19 ITA
INTERAZIONI; clinica e ricerca psicoanalitica su individuo-coppia-famiglia. Text in Italian. s-a. ITL 50,000; ITL 85,000 foreign (effective 1993).
Indexed: PsycInfo, e-psyche.
Published by: (Istituto di Psicoterapia Psicoanalitica della Famiglia), Franco Angeli Editore, Viale Monza, 106, Milan, MI 20127, Italy. Ed. Anna M Nicolo.

370.15 150 100 USA ISSN 8755-612X
THE INTERBEHAVIORIST; a quarterly newsletter of interbehavioral psychology. Text in English. ceased; resumed 1970. q. USD 13 domestic to individuals; USD 15 foreign to individuals; USD 20 to institutions. adv. bk.rev. back issues avail. **Document type:** *Newsletter.* **Description:** Includes news, information, discussions, comments and brief articles pertaining to interbehavioral psychology. Provides a contextualistic, integrated-field approach to the natural science of behavior.
Indexed: e-psyche.

Published by: Context Press, c/o Dr Linda Hayes, Ed, Dept of Psychology 296, University of Nevada, Reno, NV 89557-0062. TEL 702-784-4998, FAX 702-784-1126. R&P Linda Hayes. Circ: 125.

150 300 ARG ISSN 0325-8203
BF5
INTERDISCIPLINARIA; revista de psicologia y ciencias afines/journal of psychology and related sciences. Text in English, Spanish. 1980. s-a. USD 30 domestic to individuals; USD 42 foreign to individuals; USD 40 domestic to institutions; USD 47 foreign to institutions (effective 1999). bk.rev. **Document type:** *Monographic series, Academic/Scholarly.*
Indexed: PsycInfo, Psychol.Abstr. (1983-), e-psyche.
—BLDSC (4533.356240).
Published by: (National Research Council of Argentina), Centro Interamericano de Investigaciones Psicologicas y Ciencias Afines, Tte. Gral. Juan D. Peron 2158, Buenos Aires 1040, Argentina. TEL 54-1-953-1477, FAX 54-1-953-3541, ciipme@ssdnet.com.ar. Eds. Horacio J A Rimoldi, Maria Cristina Richaud. Circ: 600.

155 ARG ISSN 0326-1913
INTERDISCIPLINARIA MONOGRAPHS. Text in Spanish, English. 1982. irreg. price varies. **Document type:** *Monographic series, Academic/Scholarly.* **Description:** Covers the study of some perceptual and personality correlations of problem-solving solutions.
Published by: (National Research Council of Argentina), Centro Interamericano de Investigaciones Psicologicas y Ciencias Afines, Tte. Gral. Juan D. Peron 2158, Buenos Aires 1040, Argentina. TEL 54-114-9531477, FAX 54-114-9533541, ciipme@ssdnet.com.ar. Eds. Horacio J A Rimoldi, Maria Cristina Richaud. Circ: 500.

INTERFACES: LINGUISTICS, PSYCHOLOGY AND HEALTH THERAPEUTICS; an international journal of research, notes and commentary. see *LINGUISTICS*

150 NLD
INTERNATIONAL ASSOCIATION FOR CROSS-CULTURAL PSYCHOLOGY. INTERNATIONAL CONFERENCE. SELECTED PAPERS. Text in English. irreg., latest vol.13, 1999. NLG 155, NLG 84 per vol. Vol 13 (effective 2000). back issues avail. **Document type:** *Proceedings, Academic/Scholarly.* **Description:** Examines psychological issues pertaining to all aspects of cultural identity.
Indexed: e-psyche.
Published by: (International Association for Cross-Cultural Psychology USA), Swets & Zeitlinger BV, PO Box 825, Lisse 2160 SZ, Netherlands. TEL 31-252-435111, FAX 31-252-415888, pub@swets.nl, orders@swets.nl, http://www.szp.swets.nl/sps/books/psych.html, http://www.swets.nl. **Dist. in N. America by:** Swets & Zeitlinger, PO Box 582, Downingtown, PA 19335-998. TEL 800-477-9387, FAX 610-524-5366.

572 IND ISSN 0020-613X
H1
INTERNATIONAL BEHAVIOURAL SCIENTIST. Text in English. 1969. q. INR 25, USD 6.50. adv. bk.rev. abstr, bibl, charts, illus. reprint service avail. from PQC.
Related titles: Microfilm ed.: (from PQC).
Indexed: Curr.Cont. (coverage dropped), Int.Polit.Sci.Abstr., Lang.& Lang.Behav.Abstr., Sociol.Abstr., e-psyche.
Published by: Sadhna Prakashan, Rastogi St., Subhash Bazar, Meerut, Uttar Pradesh 2, India. Ed. D P Rastogi. Circ: 500.

150 USA ISSN 1094-6039
INTERNATIONAL BULLETIN OF POLITICAL PSYCHOLOGY. Text in English. 1996 (Nov.). w.
Media: Online - full text.
Published by: Embry-Riddle Aeronautical University, Humanities and Social Science Department, 3200 Willow Creek Rd, Prescott, AZ 86301. FAX 520-708-6988, http://www.pr.erau.edu/~security/index.html, http://coas.pr.erau.edu/index.html. Ed. Richard W Bloom.

615.78 USA ISSN 0268-1315
CODEN: ICLPE4
INTERNATIONAL CLINICAL PSYCHOPHARMACOLOGY. Text in English. 1986. bi-m. USD 289 domestic to individuals; USD 289 foreign to individuals; USD 785 per issue domestic to institutions; USD 785 per issue foreign to institutions; USD 119 newsstand/cover (effective 2002). adv. index. back issues avail. *Refereed.* **Document type:** *Academic/Scholarly.* **Description:** Bridges the gap between research and clinical practice in psychopharmacology.
Related titles: CD-ROM ed.; Online - full text ed.: USD 1,020.50 domestic academic site license; USD 1,020.50 foreign academic site license; USD 1,138.25 domestic corporate site license; USD 1,138.25 foreign corporate site license (2002) (from EBSCO Publishing, Institute for Scientific Information).
Indexed: ASCA, Curr.Cont., Derwent Biotech.Abstr., Excerp.Med. (1993-), Focus on: Psychophar., Ind.Med. (1986-), Ind.Sci.Rev., Inpharma, Int.Abstr.Biol.Sci., Int.Nurs.Ind., Neurosci.Cit.Ind., Pharm.&Out.News, PsycInfo, Psychol.Abstr. (1986-), Reac., SSCI (coverage dropped), Sci.Cit.Ind., e-psyche.
—BLDSC (4538.674500), ADONIS, CISTI, EMDOCS, GNLM, IDS, ingenta, KNAW.
Published by: Lippincott Williams & Wilkins (Philadelphia) (Subsidiary of: Wolters Kluwer N.V.), 530 Walnut St, Philadelphia, PA 19106-3621. TEL 215-521-8300, FAX 215-521-8902, http://www.Lww.com. Eds. Martin B Keller, Dr. Stuart Montgomery. Adv. contact Gemma Heiser. Circ: 1,000. **Subscr. to:** PO Box 1600, Hagerstown, MD 21740-1600. TEL 800-777-2295, FAX 301-824-7390.

INTERNATIONAL CONFERENCE ON ENGINEERING PSYCHOLOGY AND COGNITIVE ERGONOMICS. see *ENGINEERING*

150 CHE ISSN 0074-3364
INTERNATIONAL CONGRESS FOR ANALYTICAL PSYCHOLOGY. PROCEEDINGS. Text in English. 1983. triennial, latest 1998, 14th, Florence. illus, bibl. Index. back issues avail. **Document type:** *Proceedings, Academic/Scholarly.*
Indexed: e-psyche.
Published by: (International Association for Analytical Psychology), Daimon Verlag AG, Hauptstr 85, Einsiedeln 8840, Switzerland. TEL 41-55-4122266, FAX 41-55-4122231, daimon@compuserve.com, http://www.daimon.ch. Eds. Mary Ann Mattoon, Robert Hinshaw. R&P Heidy Fassler.

150 GBR ISSN 0085-2112
INTERNATIONAL CONGRESS OF PSYCHOLOGY. PROCEEDINGS. (Published by host national organization: Great Britain, 1969; Japan, 1972; France, 1976; German Democratic Republic, 1980; Mexico, 1984) Text in English. quadrennial, latest 1996, 26th, Canada. *Refereed.* **Document type:** *Proceedings, Academic/Scholarly.*
Indexed: e-psyche.
Published by: (International Union of Psychological Science DEU), Psychology Press (Subsidiary of: Taylor & Francis Group), 27 Church Rd, Hove, E Sussex BN3 2FA, United Kingdom. TEL 44-1273-207411, FAX 44-1273-205612, information@psypress.co.uk, http://www.psypress.co.uk.

616.89 NOR ISSN 0803-706X
BF173.A2 CODEN: IFOPE6
INTERNATIONAL FORUM OF PSYCHOANALYSIS. Text in English. 1992. q. GBP 59, USD 98 to individuals; GBP 105, USD 173 to institutions (effective 2002). adv. **Document type:** *Academic/Scholarly.* **Description:** Promotes articles demonstrating clinical experience and interest in revising or expanding psychoanalytic theory.
Related titles: Online - full text ed.: (from EBSCO Publishing, O C L C Online Computer Library Center, Inc., RoweCom Information Quest, CatchWord Ltd., ingenta, Swets Blackwell).
Indexed: Excerp.Med. (1994-), PsycInfo, Psychoanal.Abstr., Psychol.Abstr. (1981-), e-psyche.
—BLDSC (4540.345505), EMDOCS, GNLM, Infotrieve. **CCC.**
Published by: (International Federation of Psychoanalytic Societies (IFPS)), Taylor & Francis AS (Subsidiary of: Taylor & Francis Group), Cort Adelersgt. 17, Solli, PO Box 2562, Oslo 0202, Norway. TEL 47-22-12-98-80, FAX 47-22-12-98-90, journals@tandf.no, http://www.tandf.co.uk/tfas. Ed. Jan Steensen.

THE INTERNATIONAL JOURNAL FOR THE PSYCHOLOGY OF RELIGION. see *RELIGIONS AND THEOLOGY*

150.19 USA ISSN 1096-7680
RC488.A1
THE INTERNATIONAL JOURNAL OF ACTION METHODS; psychodrama, skill training and role playing. Text in English. 1947. q., latest vol.55, 2002. USD 57 domestic to individuals; USD 69 foreign to individuals; USD 95 domestic to institutions; USD 107 foreign to institutions; USD 23.75 (effective 2001 - 2002). adv. bk.rev. reprint service avail. from PSC,SCH. *Refereed.* **Document type:** *Academic/Scholarly.* **Description:** Articles on the application of action methods to psychotherapy, consulting, and education.
Former titles (until 1997): Journal of Group Psychotherapy, Psychodrama and Sociometry (0731-1273); (until 1982): Group Psychotherapy, Psychodrama and Sociometry (0146-6178); Handbook of International Sociometry (0160-4635); (until 1975): Group Psychotherapy and Psychodrama (0096-0586); Group Psychotherapy (0017-4734); Sociometry - A Journal of Interpersonal Relations
Related titles: CD-ROM ed.: (from ProQuest Information & Learning); Microform ed.; Online - full text ed.: (from ProQuest Information & Learning, ingenta, Gale Group).
Indexed: ASSIA, Curr.Cont. (coverage dropped), IBZ, Ind.Philos., Lang.& Lang.Behav.Abstr., PsycInfo, Psychol.Abstr. (1950-), Ref.Zh., SOPODA, SSCI (coverage dropped), Sociol.Abstr., e-psyche.
—BLDSC (4541.532000), GNLM, ingenta. **CCC.**
Published by: (American Society of Group Psychotherapy and Psychodrama), Heldref Publications, 1319 Eighteenth St, N W, Washington, DC 20036-1802. TEL 202-296-6267, FAX 202-296-5149, http://www.heldref.org. Ed. Helen Kress. Adv. contact Grant Williams. Circ: 400. **Co-sponsor:** Helen Dwight Reid Educational Foundation.

INTERNATIONAL JOURNAL OF ADOLESCENCE AND YOUTH. see *CHILDREN AND YOUTH—About*

THE INTERNATIONAL JOURNAL OF AVIATION PSYCHOLOGY. see *TRANSPORTATION—Air Transport*

155 GBR ISSN 0165-0254
BF712 CODEN: IJBDDY
INTERNATIONAL JOURNAL OF BEHAVIORAL DEVELOPMENT. Text in English. 1978. bi-m. GBP 117, USD 193 to individuals; GBP 470, USD 775 to institutions (effective 2002). adv. bk.rev. *Refereed.* **Document type:** *Academic/Scholarly.* **Description:** Promotes the discovery and application of knowledge about developmental processes at all stages of the lifespan, from infancy through old age.
Related titles: Microform ed.: (from PQC); Online - full text ed.: ISSN 1464-0651 (from CatchWord Ltd., EBSCO Publishing, O C L C Online Computer Library Center, Inc., RoweCom Information Quest, Swets Blackwell, Institute for Scientific Information).
Indexed: ASCA, ASSIA, AgeLine, Arts & Hum.Cit.Ind. (coverage dropped), Biol.Abstr., C.I.J.E. (coverage dropped), CINAHL, Chic.Per.Ind., Child Devel.Abstr., Crim.Just.Abstr., Curr.Cont., ERA, Fam.Ind., IBZ, IMFL, Ind.Philos., Indian Psychol.Abstr., Lang.& Lang.Behav.Abstr., Mult.Ed.Abstr., PSI, PsycInfo, Psychol.Abstr. (1978-), Psycscan D.P., Russ.Acad.Sci.Bibl., SOPODA, SSCI, Soc.Serv.Abstr., Sociol.Abstr., Sp.Ed.Needs Abstr., Stud.Wom.Abstr., e-psyche.
—BLDSC (4542.128000), CatchWord, IDS, ingenta. **CCC.**
Published by: (International Society for the Study of Behavioral Development), Psychology Press (Subsidiary of: Taylor & Francis Group), 27 Church Rd, Hove, E Sussex BN3 2FA, United Kingdom. TEL 44-1273-207411, FAX 44-1273-205612, information@psypress.co.uk, http://www.psypress.co.uk. Ed. Rainer Silbereisen. R&P Zoe Peden TEL 44-20-7842-2363. Adv. contact Claire Buckminster. **Subscr. addr. in N America:** Psychology Press, Journals Customer Service, Taylor & Francis Group, 325 Chestnut St, Philadelphia, PA 19106. TEL 800-354-1420, FAX 215-625-8914, info@taylorandfrancis.com, http://www.psypress.com.

302 USA ISSN 1070-5503
R726.5
INTERNATIONAL JOURNAL OF BEHAVIORAL MEDICINE. Text in English. 1994. q. USD 50 in Canada & Mexico to individuals; USD 80 elsewhere to individuals; USD 310 in US & Canada to institutions; USD 340 elsewhere to institutions (effective 2002). adv. *Refereed.* **Document type:** *Journal, Academic/Scholarly.* **Description:** Devoted to furthering an understanding of scientific relations between sociocultural, psychosocial, and behavioral principles on the one hand and biological processes, physical health, and illness on the other.
Related titles: Online - full text ed.: ISSN 1532-7558. USD 45 to individuals; USD 279 to institutions (effective 2002) (from CatchWord Ltd., EBSCO Publishing, O C L C Online Computer Library Center, Inc., RoweCom Information Quest, Swets Blackwell, Institute for Scientific Information).
Indexed: ASCA, AgeLine, Curr.Cont., Environ.Sci.Poll.Mgmt., Indian Psychol.Abstr., Pollut.Abstr., PsycInfo, Risk Abstr., SSCI, Saf.Sci.Abstr., e-psyche.
—BLDSC (4542.128700), CatchWord, Infotrieve. **CCC.**

P

Published by: (International Society of Behavioral Medicine), Lawrence Erlbaum Associates, Inc., 10 Industrial Ave, Mahwah, NJ 07430-2262. TEL 201-760-3735, 800-926-6579, FAX 201-236-0072, journals@erlbaum.com, http://www.erlbaum.com/Journals/journals/IJBM/ijbm.htm. Ed. Ulf Lundberg TEL 46-8-167-847. adv.: page USD 400; trim 5 x 8.

300 150 IND ISSN 0971-3190
INTERNATIONAL JOURNAL OF BEHAVIOURAL SCIENCES. Text in English. 1981. 2/yr. INR 300 domestic; USD 150 foreign (effective 2000). adv. bk.rev. **Document type:** *Academic/Scholarly.*
Published by: Scientific Publishers, 5-A New Pali Rd., P O Box 91, Jodhpur, Rajasthan 342 001, India. TEL 91-291-433323, FAX 91-291-512580, scienti@sancharnet.in, http://www.scientificpub.com. adv.: B&W page USD 100, color page USD 500; trim 9.5 x 6.25.

INTERNATIONAL JOURNAL OF BIOSOCIAL AND MEDICAL RESEARCH; bridging the gap between the natural and social sciences to better understand human behavior. see *NUTRITION AND DIETETICS*

155.25 GBR ISSN 1364-436X
INTERNATIONAL JOURNAL OF CHILDREN'S SPIRITUALITY. Text in English. 1966. 3/yr. GBP 36, USD 59 to individuals; GBP 147, USD 242 to institutions (effective 2002). **Document type:** *Academic/Scholarly.* **Description:** Aims to provide an international and multicultural forum for persons involved in research and development of children's and young people's spirituality. Includes an examination of the nature and possible expressions of spirituality, the philosophical and practical foundations for morality, and their relationships in a rapidly changing world.
Related titles: Online - full text ed.: ISSN 1469-8455 (from CatchWord Ltd., EBSCO Publishing, Swets Blackwell, RoweCom Information Quest).
Indexed: Br.Educ.Ind., Cont.Pg.Educ., ERA, Rel.& Theol.Abstr., e-psyche.
—CatchWord. **CCC.**
Published by: Carfax Publishing Limited (Subsidiary of: Taylor & Francis Group), c/o Sue Dommett, PO Box 25, Abingdon, Oxford OX14 3UE, United Kingdom. TEL 44-1235-401000, FAX 44-1235-041550, enquiries@carfax.co.uk, enquiries@carfax.co.uk/, http://www.carfax.co.uk. Eds. Clive Erricker, Jane Erricker.

150 004 NLD ISSN 1569-2167
▼ **INTERNATIONAL JOURNAL OF COGNITION & TECHNOLOGY**; co-existence, convergence and co-evolution. Text in English. 2002. s-a. EUR 175 (effective 2002). 400 p./no. **Document type:** *Journal.* **Description:** Brings theoretical and empirical studies that examine the co-evolution of technology and its users. Its concern is human cognitive adaptation to computer technology.
Related titles: Online - full text ed.
Published by: (Cognitive Technology Society USA), John Benjamins Publishing Co., PO Box 36224, Amsterdam 1020 ME, Netherlands. TEL 31-20-630-4747, FAX 31-20-673-9773, http://www.benjamins.com. Eds. Barbara Gorayska, Jacob Mey.

153.1 USA ISSN 1088-6362
TA166
INTERNATIONAL JOURNAL OF COGNITIVE ERGONOMICS. Text in English. 1997. q. USD 50 in Canada & Mexico to individuals; USD 80 elsewhere to individuals; USD 270 in Canada & Mexico to institutions; USD 300 elsewhere to institutions (effective 2001). adv. **Document type:** *Journal, Academic/Scholarly.* **Description:** Publishes articles in cognitive ergonomics as it relates to the analysis, design, and operation of cognitive activities.
Related titles: Online - full text ed.: ISSN 1532-7566. USD 45 to individuals; USD 243 to institutions (effective 2001) (from CatchWord Ltd., EBSCO Publishing, O C L C Online Computer Library Center, Inc., RoweCom Information Quest, Swets Blackwell).
Indexed: Environ.Sci.Poll.Mgmt., Ergon.Abstr., Pollut.Abstr., PsycInfo, Risk Abstr., Saf.Sci.Abstr., e-psyche.
—BLDSC (4542.172270), CatchWord, CISTI, Infotrieve. **CCC.**
Published by: Lawrence Erlbaum Associates, Inc., 10 Industrial Ave, Mahwah, NJ 07430-2262. TEL 201-760-3735, 800-926-6579, FAX 201-236-0072, journals@erlbaum.com, http://www.erlbaum.com/Journals/journals/IJCE/ijce.htm. Eds. Gavriel Salvendy, Michael J Smith. adv.: page USD 275; trim 6 x 9.

THE INTERNATIONAL JOURNAL OF COMMUNICATIVE PSYCHOANALYSIS & PSYCHOTHERAPY. see *MEDICAL SCIENCES—Psychiatry And Neurology*

150 USA
▼ **INTERNATIONAL JOURNAL OF COMPARATIVE PSYCHOANALYSIS.** Text in English. forthcoming 2002. q. USD 48 domestic to individuals; USD 65 foreign to individuals; USD 85 domestic to institutions; USD 114 foreign to institutions (effective 2002). **Document type:** *Journal, Academic/Scholarly.*
Published by: International Universities Press, Inc., 59 Boston Post Rd, Box 1524, Madison, CT 06443-1524. TEL 203-245-4000, FAX 203-245-0775, office@iup.com, http://www.iup.com.

156 USA ISSN 0889-3667
BF671 CODEN: IJCPE8
INTERNATIONAL JOURNAL OF COMPARATIVE PSYCHOLOGY* . Text in English. 1987. q. USD 95 in United States to institutions; USD 110 elsewhere to institutions (effective 2001). adv. back issues avail.; reprint service avail. from PQC. *Refereed.* **Document type:** *Academic/Scholarly.* **Description:** Explores how the study of the development and evolution of behavior elucidates behavior, and investigates relationship of scientific research and theory to fundamental concepts about the evolutionary history and nature of humanity.
Indexed: Ind.Philos., Indian Psychol.Abstr., PsycInfo, Psychol.Abstr. (1987-), Russ.Acad.Sci.Bibl., Soc.Work Res.& Abstr., e-psyche.
—ingenta. **CCC.**
Published by: International Society for Comparative Psychology, Department of Psychology, Texas Christian University, Box 298920, Fort Worth, TX 76129. TEL 785-843-1235, FAX 785-843-1274, iscp@allenpress.com, http://rana.uqam.ca/iscp/IJCP.htm, http://www.psy.tcu.edu/psy/iscp/iscp.html. Ed. Nancy K Innis. R&P David Byrd Stadler. **Subscr. to:** Allen Press Inc., PO Box 1897, Lawrence, KS 66044-8897.

INTERNATIONAL JOURNAL OF EATING DISORDERS. see *NUTRITION AND DIETETICS*

616.8 USA ISSN 0020-7284
RC488 CODEN: IJGPAO
INTERNATIONAL JOURNAL OF GROUP PSYCHOTHERAPY. Text in English. 1951. q. USD 75 domestic to individuals; USD 87 foreign to individuals; USD 230 domestic to institutions; USD 222 foreign to institutions (effective 2000). adv. bk.rev. abstr, bibl, charts, stat, illus. index. back issues avail.; reprint service avail. from PQC,PSC,SCH,ISI. *Refereed.* **Document type:** *Academic/Scholarly.* **Description:** Devoted to reporting and interpreting the research and practice of group psychotherapy.
Related titles: Online - full text ed.: (from Northern Light Technology, Inc., ProQuest Information & Learning, CatchWord Ltd., Institute for Scientific Information, RoweCom Information Quest).
Indexed: ASCA, ASSIA, Adol.Ment.Hlth.Abstr., AgeLine, Biol.Abstr., Crim.Just.Abstr., Curr.Cont., Excerp.Med., Fam.Ind., Ind.Med. (1951-), Int.Nurs.Ind., Lang.& Lang.Behav.Abstr., PsycInfo, Psychol.Abstr. (1951-), SOPODA, SSCI, Soc.Sci.Ind. (Jul.1999-), Soc.Serv.Abstr., Soc.Work Res.& Abstr., Sociol.Abstr., e-psyche.
—BLDSC (4542.270000), CISTI, GNLM, IDS, ingenta, KNAW. **CCC.**
Published by: (American Group Psychotherapy Association), Guilford Publications, Inc., 72 Spring St, 4th Fl, New York, NY 10012. TEL 212-431-9800, 800-365-7006, FAX 212-966-6708, info@guilford.com. Ed. Dr. William Piper. Pub. Robert Matloff. R&P Kathy Kuehl. Adv. contact Susan Pavliscak. Circ: 5,400.

301 USA ISSN 0047-0732
HN1 CODEN: IJGTB3
INTERNATIONAL JOURNAL OF GROUP TENSIONS; an interdisciplinary quarterly of behavioral sciences devoted to the study of conflict and violence in human relationships. Text in English. 1971. q. USD 371, EUR 370 to institutions for print or online ed.; USD 445.20, EUR 444 to institutions for print & online eds. combined (effective 2002). adv. bk.rev. bibl. index. reprint service avail. from PQC,PSC,SCH. *Refereed.* **Document type:** *Journal, Academic/Scholarly.* **Description:** Publishes research findings and theoretical analysis pertaining to bias, prejudice, discrimination, hostility, and violence - and methods of resolving these conflicts.
Related titles: Microform ed.: (from PQC); Online - full text ed.: (from EBSCO Publishing, O C L C Online Computer Library Center, Inc., Swets Blackwell, Kluwer Online, RoweCom Information Quest).
Indexed: AgeLine, Amer.Bibl.Slavic & E.Eur.Stud., Int.Polit.Sci.Abstr., Lang.& Lang.Behav.Abstr., Mid.East: Abstr.& Ind., Peace Res.Abstr., Polit.Sci.Abstr., Psychol.Abstr., Russ.Acad.Sci.Bibl., SOPODA, SSCI (coverage dropped), Soc.Serv.Abstr., Sociol.Abstr., e-psyche.
—BLDSC (4542.272000), Infotrieve, ingenta. **CCC.**
Published by: (International Organization for the Study of Group Tensions), Kluwer Academic - Plenum Publishers (Subsidiary of: Wolters Kluwer N.V.), 233 Spring St, New York, NY 10013-1578. TEL 212-620-8000, 800-221-9369, FAX 212-463-0742, info@plenum.com, http://www.wkap.nl/journalhome.htm/0047-0732. Ed. Uwe P Gielen. **Subscr. outside the Americas to:** Kluwer Academic Publishers Group, Journals Department, PO Box 322, Dordrecht 3300 AH, Netherlands. TEL 31-78-639-2392, FAX 31-78-654-6474.

614.58 362.2 USA ISSN 0020-7411
RA790.A1 CODEN: IJMHBV
INTERNATIONAL JOURNAL OF MENTAL HEALTH. Text in English. 1972. q. USD 125 domestic to individuals; USD 181 foreign to individuals; USD 711 domestic to institutions; USD 790 foreign to institutions (effective 2001). adv. bk.rev. back issues avail. *Refereed.* **Document type:** *Academic/Scholarly.* **Description:** Presents in-depth articles on research, clinical practice, and the organization and delivery of mental health services. Covers both industrial and developing nations.
Related titles: Online - full text ed.: (from H. W. Wilson, Gale Group).
Indexed: ASCA, ASSIA, Adol.Ment.Hlth.Abstr., AgeLine, Amer.Bibl.Slavic & E.Eur.Stud., Arts & Hum.Cit.Ind. (coverage dropped), Biol.Abstr., Child Devel.Abstr., Curr.Cont. (coverage dropped), Excerp.Med., Fam.Ind., Mid.East: Abstr.& Ind., PsycInfo, Psychol.Abstr. (1972-), SSCI, Soc.Sci.Ind. (Jan.1999-), Stud.Wom.Abstr., e-psyche.
—BLDSC (4542.352000), CISTI, GNLM, IDS, ingenta, KNAW. **CCC.**
Published by: (World Association for Psychosocial Rehabilitation), M.E. Sharpe, Inc., 80 Business Park Dr, Armonk, NY 10504. TEL 914-273-1800, 800-541-6563, FAX 914-273-2106, custserv@mesharpe.com, http://www.mesharpe.com. Ed. Martin Gittelman. Adv. contact Barbara Ladd. page USD 300; trim 8 x 5.

INTERNATIONAL JOURNAL OF NEURO-PSYCHOPHARMACOLOGY. see *PHARMACY AND PHARMACOLOGY*

150 AUS ISSN 1440-5377
INTERNATIONAL JOURNAL OF ORGANISATIONAL BEHAVIOUR. Text in English. 1998. s-a.
Media: Online - full text.
Published by: University of Southern Queensland, Department of Human Resource Management and Employment Relations, Toowoomba, QLD 4350, Australia. hrm@usq.edu.au, http://www.usq.edu.au/faculty/business/dept_hrm/HRMJournal/IJOBHome.htm.

INTERNATIONAL JOURNAL OF PSYCHIATRY IN MEDICINE; an international journal of medical psychology and psychiatry in the general hospital. see *MEDICAL SCIENCES—Psychiatry And Neurology*

150.19 GBR ISSN 0020-7578
BF173.A2 CODEN: IJPSAA
THE INTERNATIONAL JOURNAL OF PSYCHO-ANALYSIS. Text in English; Summaries in French, German, Spanish. 1920. bi-m. USD 196 in US & Canada to individuals; GBP 122 elsewhere to individuals; USD 386 in US & Canada to institutions; GBP 191 in the European Union to institutions; GBP 235 elsewhere to institutions (effective 2001). adv. bk.rev. illus. index. back issues avail.; reprint service avail. from PSC,SCH. *Refereed.* **Document type:** *Proceedings, Academic/Scholarly.*
Incorporates (in 1992): International Psycho-Analytical Association. Bulletin (0306-2643)
Related titles: Online - full text ed.: (from CatchWord Ltd., EBSCO Publishing, Swets Blackwell, Institute for Scientific Information).
Indexed: ASCA, AgeLine, Arts & Hum.Cit.Ind. (coverage dropped), Biol.Abstr., Curr.Cont., Excerp.Med., Fam.Ind., IBR, IBZ, Ind.Med. (1920-), Ind.Philos., Intl.Bibl.Soc.Sci., Lang.& Lang.Behav.Abstr., Mid.East: Abstr.& Ind., Mult.Ed.Abstr., P C I, Psychoanal.Abstr., Psychol.Abstr. (1929-), Russ.Acad.Sci.Bibl., SOPODA, SSCI, Sociol.Abstr.
—BLDSC (4542.498000), GNLM, IDS, ingenta, KNAW. **CCC.**
Published by: Institute of Psychoanalysis, 112A Shirland Rd., London W9 2EQ, United Kingdom. TEL 44-20-7563 5000, FAX 44-20-7563 5001, 10066.2236@compuserve.com, subs@ijpa.org, http://www.ijpa.org. Ed. Glen Gabbard. Adv. contact Sophie Leighton TEL 44-20-7563-5013. Circ: 7,200.

INTERNATIONAL JOURNAL OF PSYCHOLINGUISTICS. see *LINGUISTICS*

P

150 USA ISSN 0020-7594
BF1 CODEN: IJPSBB
INTERNATIONAL JOURNAL OF PSYCHOLOGY/ JOURNAL INTERNATIONAL DE PSYCHOLOGIE. Text in English, French. 1966. bi-m. GBP 69, USD 113 to individuals; GBP 294, USD 485 to institutions (effective 2002). adv. bk.rev. abstr, charts, illus, stat. reprint service avail. from SWZ,PSC,SCH,ISI. *Refereed.* **Document type:** *Academic/Scholarly.*
Related titles: Microform ed.; Online - full text ed.: ISSN 1464-066X (from CatchWord Ltd., EBSCO Publishing, O C L C Online Computer Library Center, Inc., RoweCom Information Quest, Swets Blackwell, Institute for Scientific Information).
Indexed: ASCA, ASSIA, Adol.Ment.Hlth.Abstr., AgeLine, Arts & Hum.Cit.Ind. (coverage dropped), Bibl.Asian Stud. (1969-1970), Biol.Abstr., Curr.Cont., ERA, Ergon.Abstr., Fam.Ind., Ind.Philos., Indian Psychol.Abstr., Lang.& Lang.Behav.Abstr., Mid.East: Abstr.& Ind., PsycInfo, Psychol.Abstr. (1966-), Russ.Acad.Sci.Bibl., SOPODA, SSCI, Soc.Serv.Abstr., Sociol.Abstr., Stud.Wom.Abstr., Tech.Educ.Abstr., e-psyche.
—BLDSC (4542.506000), CatchWord, IDS, ingenta. **CCC.**
Published by: (International Union of Psychological Science GBR), Psychology Press (Subsidiary of: Taylor & Francis Ltd.), 325 Chestnut St, Ste 800, Philadelphia, PA 19106. TEL 215-625-8900, FAX 215-625-2940, info@taylorandfrancis.com, http://www.psypress.com/. Ed. Francois Y Dore. Circ: 1,500. **Subscr. addr. in N America:** Journals Customer Service, Taylor & Francis Group, 325 Chestnut St, Philadelphia, PA 19106. TEL 800-354-1420, FAX 215-625-8914, info@taylorandfrancis.com; **Subscr. addr. outside N America:** Psychology Press, Journals Customer Service, Taylor & Francis Group, Rankine Rd, Basingstoke, Hants RG24 8PR, United Kingdom. TEL 44-1256-813002, FAX 44-1256-479438, enquiry@tandf.co.uk, http://www.psypress.co.uk.

150 616.891 615.1 USA ISSN 1088-6710
INTERNATIONAL JOURNAL OF PSYCHOPATHOLOGY, PSYCHOPHARMACOLOGY, AND PSYCHOTHERAPY. Text in English. 1996. irreg. free per issue. bk.rev., software rev., video rev. illus. reprints avail. *Refereed.* **Document type:** *Academic/Scholarly.* **Description:** Publishes review papers, research reports, case reports, comments and letters to the editor.
Media: Online - full text.
Indexed: e-psyche.
Published by: PsyCom.Net, 1346 Lexington Ave, New York, NY 10128. psydoc@psycom.net, http://www.psycom.net/ijppp.html. Ed. Ivan Goldberg.

150 NLD ISSN 0167-8760
CODEN: IJPSEE
INTERNATIONAL JOURNAL OF PSYCHOPHYSIOLOGY. Text in English. 1983. 12/yr., latest vol.39. EUR 1,745 in Europe to institutions; JPY 231,600 in Japan to institutions; USD 1,951 elsewhere to institutions (effective 2002). adv. bk.rev. back issues avail. *Refereed.* **Document type:** *Academic/Scholarly.* **Description:** Covers all aspects of psychophysiology. Aims to integrate the neurosciences and psychological sciences.
Related titles: Microform ed.: (from PQC); Online - full text ed.: (from ingenta, Swets Blackwell, ScienceDirect, Institute for Scientific Information).
Indexed: ASCA, AgeLine, Curr.Cont., Excerp.Med., IBZ, Ind.Med. (1983-), Ind.Philos., Ind.Sci.Rev., Inpharma, Int.Abstr.Biol.Sci., Neurosci.Abstr., Neurosci.Cit.Ind., Pharm.&Out.News, PsycInfo, Psychol.Abstr. (1983-), Reac., SSCI, Sci.Cit.Ind., e-psyche.
—BLDSC (4542.506500), CISTI, GNLM, IDS, ingenta, KNAW. **CCC.**
Published by: (International Organization of Psychophysiology), Elsevier Science BV, PO Box 211, Amsterdam 1000 AE, Netherlands. TEL 31-20-485-2911, FAX 31-20-485-2457, nlinfo-f@elsevier.nl; usinfo-f@elsevier.com; forinfo-kyf04035@niftyserve.or.jp, http://www.elsevier.com/locate/ijpsycho. Eds. John H Gruzelier, John L Andreassi. Circ: 750. **Subscr. in Australasia and the Far East to:** Elsevier Science (Singapore) Pte Ltd, No.1 Temasek Ave, 17-01 Millenia Tower, Singapore 039192, Singapore. TEL 65-434-3727, FAX 65-337-2230; **Subscr. in Japan to:** Elsevier Science Inc - Japan Regional Office, 9-15 Higashi-Azabu 1-chome, Minato-ku, Tokyo 106-0044, Japan. TEL 81-3-5561-5033; **Subscr. in the Americas to:** Elsevier Science, PO Box 945, New York, NY 10159-0945. TEL 212-633-3730, FAX 212-633-3680, usinfo-f@elsevier.com.

616.89 USA
INTERNATIONAL JOURNAL OF REALITY THERAPY. Text in English. 1981. s-a. USD 10. back issues avail. *Refereed.*
Formerly (until 1997): Journal of Reality Therapy (0743-0493)
Indexed: PsycInfo, e-psyche.
—BLDSC (4542.525300), ingenta.
Published by: Northeastern University, 203 Lake Hall, Boston, MA 02115. TEL 617-373-2470, FAX 617-373-8892. Ed. Larry Litwack. **Co-sponsor:** William Glaser Institute.

INTERNATIONAL JOURNAL OF REHABILITATION AND HEALTH. see *HANDICAPPED*

THE INTERNATIONAL JOURNAL OF SELF-HELP AND SELF-CARE. see *NEW AGE PUBLICATIONS*

INTERNATIONAL JOURNAL OF SEXUALITY AND GENDER STUDIES. see *HOMOSEXUALITY*

INTERNATIONAL JOURNAL OF SPORT PSYCHOLOGY. see *MEDICAL SCIENCES—Sports Medicine*

▼ **INTERNATIONAL JOURNAL OF TESTING.** see *EDUCATION*

150.5 200 AUS ISSN 1321-0122
INTERNATIONAL JOURNAL OF TRANSPERSONAL STUDIES. Text in English. 1982. s-a. AUD 50 to individuals; AUD 75 to institutions. bk.rev. back issues avail. *Refereed.* **Document type:** *Academic/Scholarly.* **Description:** Discusses holism from multidisciplinary perspective.
Formerly: Australian Journal of Transpersonal Psychology (0725-0061)
Indexed: e-psyche.
—ingenta.
Published by: Bolda-Lok Publishing and Educational Enterprises, PO Box 5513, Stafford Heights, QLD 4053, Australia. TEL 61-7-33592547, FAX 61-7-33592547, e.neill@gut.edu.au. Ed. E M Neill.

150 GBR
INTERNATIONAL LIBRARY OF GROUP ANALYSIS. Text in English. 1998. irreg., latest vol.14, 2001. back issues avail. *Refereed.* **Document type:** *Monographic series, Academic/Scholarly.* **Description:** Aims to represent innovative work in group psychotherapy, particularly but not exclusively group analysis.
Published by: Jessica Kingsley Publishers, 116 Pentonville Rd, London N1 9JB, United Kingdom. FAX 44-20-7837-2917, post@jkp.com, http://www.jkp.com. Ed. Malcolm Pines. **Dist. by:** Plymbridge Distributors Ltd, Plymbridge House, Estover Rd, Plymouth, Devon PL6 7PY, United Kingdom. TEL 44-1752-202300, FAX 44-1752-202330.

327 GBR ISSN 0957-1299
INTERNATIONAL MINDS. Text in English. 1989. s-a. GBP 24 in Europe to members; GBP 32 elsewhere to members; GBP 12 in Europe to students; GBP 16 elsewhere to students (effective 1999). adv. bk.rev. **Document type:** *Academic/Scholarly.* **Description:** Features speeches, reports and debates.
Indexed: Intl.Bibl.Soc.Sci., e-psyche.
Published by: Hugo Publications, 19 Hugh St, London SW1V 1QJ, United Kingdom. TEL 44-20-7255-1007, FAX 44-20-7976-6567. Pub. George Bull. R&P, Adv. contact Jennie West. Circ: 300 (paid and controlled).

155.4 GBR ISSN 0965-2531
GV1201
INTERNATIONAL PLAY JOURNAL. Text in English; Summaries in French, Spanish. 1993. 3/yr. GBP 79 in the European Union to institutions; USD 135 in North America to institutions; GBP 85 elsewhere to institutions. adv. reprints avail. *Refereed.* **Document type:** *Academic/Scholarly.* **Description:** Publishes research papers and practice-based articles on all aspects of play.
Related titles: Online - full text ed.
Indexed: ERA, Lang.& Lang.Behav.Abstr., Mult.Ed.Abstr., SOPODA, Sociol.Abstr., e-psyche.
—BLDSC (4542.470250). **CCC.**
Published by: Chapman & Hall, Journals Department (Subsidiary of: International Thomson Publishing Group), Chapman & Hall, 2-6 Boundary Row, London SE1 8HN, United Kingdom. TEL 44-20-7865-0066, FAX 44-20-7522-9623, jhelp@chall.co.uk, http://www.chaphall.com/chaphall/journals.html. Ed. Bob Hughes. **Dist. by:** International Thompson Publishing Services Ltd., Cheriton House, North Way, Walworth Industrial Estate, Andover, Hants SP10 5BE, United Kingdom. TEL 44-1264-342713, FAX 44-1264-342807.

150 GBR ISSN 1564-0361
INTERNATIONAL PSYCHOANALYSIS. Text in English. 1992. s-a. USD 10 per issue worldwide (effective 2000). **Document type:** *Newsletter.* **Description:** Contains information on aspects of professional psychoanalytic life, and administrative news for members of the IPA.
Related titles: Online - full text ed.: ISSN 1564-0051.
Indexed: e-psyche.
Published by: International Psychoanalytical Association, Broomhills, Woodside Ln, London N12 8UD, United Kingdom. FAX 44-20-8445-4729, janice@ipa.org.uk, http://www.ipa.org.uk. Ed. Dr. Alex Holder. R&P Janice Ahmed TEL 44-20-8446-8324. Circ: 10,000.

150 USA ISSN 0047-116X
BF1
INTERNATIONAL PSYCHOLOGIST. Text in English. 1959. q. USD 28 to individuals; USD 48 to institutions. adv. bk.rev. abstr. back issues avail. **Document type:** *Academic/Scholarly.*
Indexed: e-psyche.
Published by: International Council of Psychologists, Inc., c/o John M Davis, Secy Gen, Dept of Psychology, Southwest Texas State Univ, San Marcos, TX 78666-4616. FAX 512-245-3153. Ed. Pittu Laungani. Circ: 1,700.

INTERNATIONAL REGISTRY OF ORGANIZATION DEVELOPMENT PROFESSIONALS AND ORGANIZATION DEVELOPMENT HANDBOOK. see *BUSINESS AND ECONOMICS—Personnel Management*

150 GBR
INTERNATIONAL REVIEW OF HEALTH PSYCHOLOGY. Text in English. 1992. irreg. USD 368.95 (effective 1999). **Document type:** *Academic/Scholarly.* **Description:** Provides a series of annual of volumes offering and useful overview of the field. Review-type chapters by international contributors cover general concepts and methodology, health behavior and promotion, illness conduct and health care, and practical and professional issues.
Indexed: e-psyche.
Published by: Wiley Europe Ltd., Baffins Ln, Chichester, W Sussex PO19 1UD, United Kingdom. TEL 44-1243-779777, FAX 44-1243-843232, cs-journals@wiley.co.uk, http://www.wiley.co.uk. **Subscr. in the Americas to:** John Wiley & Sons, Inc., Journals, 605 Third Ave, New York, NY 10158. TEL 212-850-6645, FAX 212-850-6021, http://www.wiley.co.uk.

158.7 GBR ISSN 0886-1528
HF5548.7
INTERNATIONAL REVIEW OF INDUSTRIAL AND ORGANIZATIONAL PSYCHOLOGY. Text in English. 1986. a. USD 140 in United States; USD 140 in Canada & Mexico; USD 140 elsewhere (effective 2002). adv. back issues avail. *Refereed.* **Document type:** *Academic/Scholarly.* **Description:** Provides reviews in the field of industrial and organizational psychology.
Related titles: Microform ed.: (from PQC).
Indexed: e-psyche.
—BLDSC (4547.325000), Infotrieve. **CCC.**
Published by: Wiley Europe Ltd., Baffins Ln, Chichester, W Sussex PO19 1UD, United Kingdom. TEL 44-1243-779777, FAX 44-1243-775878, info-assets@wiley.co.uk, customer@wiley.co.uk, http://www.wiley.co.uk. adv.: B&W page GBP 595, color page GBP 1,495; trim 153 x 229. Circ: 700. **Subscr. in the Americas to:** John Wiley & Sons, Inc., Journals, 605 Third Ave, New York, NY 10158. TEL 212-850-6021, 212-850-6645, subinfo@jwiley.com.

156 GBR ISSN 1058-4994
BF531
INTERNATIONAL REVIEW OF STUDIES ON EMOTION. Text in English. 1991. biennial. **Document type:** *Academic/Scholarly.*
Indexed: e-psyche.
—GNLM.
Published by: Wiley Europe Ltd., Baffins Ln, Chichester, W Sussex PO19 1UD, United Kingdom. TEL 44-1243-779777, FAX 44-1243-843232, cs-journals@wiley.co.uk, http://www.wiley.co.uk.

INTERNATIONAL SERIES IN THE PSYCHOLOGY OF RELIGIONS. see *RELIGIONS AND THEOLOGY*

P

302 AUT ISSN 0254-928X
INTERNATIONALE ZEITSCHRIFT FUER SOZIALPSYCHOLOGIE UND GRUPPENDYNAMIK; in Wirtschaft und Gesellschaft. Text in German, English. 1975. q. ATS 380 domestic; DEM 69 foreign; ATS 120 newsstand/cover. 48 p./no. **Document type:** *Journal, Academic/Scholarly.* **Description:** Contains articles and research involving social psychology and group dynamics.
Indexed: IBZ, Ind.Philos.
Published by: Psychologische Gesellschaft fuer Persoenlichkeits und Organisationsentwicklung, Fraungrubergasse 4-5-13, Vienna 1120, Austria. TEL 43-663-9140514, FAX 43-1-9854653. Ed., R&P Dr. Rudolf Zucha.

INTERNATIONALES SYMPOSIUM GEGEN DROGEN IN DER SCHWEIZ. see *DRUG ABUSE AND ALCOHOLISM*

150 302 ESP ISSN 1132-0559
INTERVENCION PSICOSOCIAL. Text in Spanish. 1992. 3/yr. ESP 4,200, USD 60 to non-members; USD 2,900 to members. back issues avail. **Document type:** *Academic/Scholarly.*
Indexed: e-psyche.
—CINDOC.
Published by: Colegio Oficial de Psicologos de Madrid, Cuesta de San Vicente, 4 6o, Madrid 28008, Spain. TEL 34-91-541-7009, FAX 34-91-547-2284, dmadrid@correo.cop.es, http://www.cop.es/publicaciones/psicosocial/.

INTERVENTION IN SCHOOL AND CLINIC. see *EDUCATION—Special Education And Rehabilitation*

IRISH JOURNAL OF PSYCHOLOGICAL MEDICINE. see *MEDICAL SCIENCES—Psychiatry And Neurology*

150 GBR ISSN 0303-3910
CODEN: IRJPAR
IRISH JOURNAL OF PSYCHOLOGY. Text in English. 1971. q. USD 80, IEP 48. adv. bk.rev. bibl, charts. *Refereed.* **Document type:** *Academic/Scholarly.*
Indexed: ASCA, AgeLine, Biol.Abstr., Br.Educ.Ind., Curr.Cont., Fam.Ind., IMFL, Lang.& Lang.Behav.Abstr., PsycInfo, Psychol.Abstr. (1971-), SOPODA, SSCI, Soc.Serv.Abstr., Sociol.Abstr., e-psyche.
—BLDSC (4572.200000), CISTI, IDS, ingenta.
Published by: Psychological Society of Ireland, c/o Queen's University, School of Psychology, Belfast, Co Antrim, N Ireland BT7 1NN, United Kingdom. TEL 44-1232-245133, FAX 44-1232-664144, c.mc.guinness@qub.ac.uk. Eds. Carol McGuinness, Kenneth Brown. Circ: 1,200.

616.89 156 ISR ISSN 0334-6080
BF8.H4
ISRAEL QUARTERLY OF PSYCHOLOGY. Text in Hebrew. irreg. (1-2/yr.). membership. adv. bk.rev. **Document type:** *Academic/Scholarly.*
Indexed: Ind.Heb.Per. (1984-1987), e-psyche.
Published by: Histadrut Hapsikologim B'yisrael/Israel Psychological Association, Frishman 74, Tel Aviv 65456, Israel. FAX 972-3-5230763. Circ: 3,000.

364 345 GBR ISSN 1468-4756
ISSUES IN FORENSIC PSYCHOLOGY. Text in English. 1981. irreg., latest vol.28, 1996. GBP 2.50 per issue. back issues avail. *Refereed.* **Document type:** *Monographic series.* **Description:** Conveys recent research and debate in the fields of criminology and legal psychology to an academic readership.
Formerly (until 1999): Issues in Criminological and Legal Psychology (0266-6863)
Indexed: Crim.Just.Abstr., PsycInfo, Psychol.Abstr. (1981-), e-psyche.
—BLDSC (4584.244500). **CCC.**
Published by: The British Psychological Society, Division of Forensic Psychology, St Andrews House, 48 Princess Rd E, Leicester LE1 7DR, United Kingdom. TEL 44-116-254-9568, FAX 44-116-247-0787, bps1@uk.ac.le, http://www.bps.org.uk/index.cfm. Eds. Geoffrey Stephenson, Noel Clark. Circ: 250.

ISSUES IN MENTAL HEALTH NURSING. see *MEDICAL SCIENCES—Nurses And Nursing*

616.89 USA
ISSUES IN THE PRACTICE OF PSYCHOLOGY. Text in English. 1996. irreg., latest 2000. **Document type:** *Monographic series.* **Description:** Examines professional matters within the mental health services.
Indexed: e-psyche.
Published by: Kluwer Academic - Plenum Publishers (Subsidiary of: Wolters Kluwer N.V.), 233 Spring St, New York, NY 10013-1578. TEL 212-620-8000, 800-221-9369, FAX 212-463-0742, info@plenum.com, http://www.plenum.com. Ed. George Stricker.

J A S C T NEWSLETTER. see *MEDICAL SCIENCES*

150 DEU ISSN 0075-2363
JAHRBUCH DER PSYCHOANALYSE; Beitraege zur Theorie, Praxis und Geschichte. Text in German. 1960. 2/yr. EUR 50 (effective 2002). adv. back issues avail.; reprint service avail. from SCH,PSC. *Refereed.* **Document type:** *Journal, Academic/Scholarly.* **Description:** Consists of theoretical, clinical and historical contributions, mainly by psychoanalysts.
Indexed: IBR, Ind.Philos., P C I, PsycInfo, Psychoanal.Abstr., Psychol.Abstr. (1981-).
—BLDSC (4632.050000), GNLM.
Published by: Friedrich Frommann Verlag Guenther Holzboog, Koenig-Karl-Str 27, Stuttgart 70372, Germany. TEL 49-711-9559690, FAX 49-711-9559691, vertrieb@frommann-holzboog.de, http://www.frommann-holzboog.de. Eds. Claudia Frank, Helmut Hinz, Ludger Hermanns. Adv. contact Sybille Wittmann. page DEM 580; 107 x 157. Circ: 700.

JAHRBUCH DER PSYCHOONKOLOGIE. see *MEDICAL SCIENCES—Oncology*

301.1 DEU ISSN 0938-183X
JAHRBUCH FUER PSYCHOANALYTISCHE PAEDAGOGIK. Text in German. 1989. a. DEM 38 (effective 2000). **Document type:** *Academic/Scholarly.*
Indexed: Ind.Philos., e-psyche.
Published by: Psychosozial Verlag, Friedrichstr 35, Giessen 35392, Germany. TEL 49-641-77819, FAX 49-641-77742, psychosozial-verlag@t-online.de.

150 DEU ISSN 0939-5806
GR880
JAHRBUCH FUER TRANSKULTURELLE MEDIZIN UND PSYCHOTHERAPIE/YEARBOOK OF CROSS-CULTURAL MEDICINE AND PSYCHOTHERAPY. Text in English, German. 1990. a. EUR 34 (effective 2001 & 2002). back issues avail. **Document type:** *Yearbook, Academic/Scholarly.* **Description:** Contains research on all aspects of ethnic and alternative healing methods.
Indexed: IBZ, e-psyche.
—GNLM.
Published by: (Internationales Institut fuer Kulturvergleichende Therapieforschung), V W B - Verlag fuer Wissenschaft und Bildung, Zossener Str 55, Berlin 10961, Germany. TEL 49-30-2510415, FAX 49-30-2511136, 100615.1565@compuserve.com, http://www.vwb-verlag.com.

JAPANESE BULLETIN OF ARTS THERAPY. see *ART*

364.3 JPN ISSN 0017-7547
JAPANESE JOURNAL OF CRIMINAL PSYCHOLOGY/HANZAI SHINRIGAKU KENKYU. Text in Japanese; Summaries in English. 1963. 3/yr. JPY 2,400, USD 30. **Document type:** *Academic/Scholarly.*
Indexed: PsycInfo, Psychol.Abstr. (1969-), e-psyche.
Published by: Japanese Association of Criminal Psychology, 2-11-7 Hikawadai, Nerima-ku, Tokyo 179-0084, Japan. TEL 03-3559-5084. Ed. Kosuke Tsubouchi. Circ: 1,200.

370.15 150 JPN ISSN 0021-5015
CODEN: JJEPAP
JAPANESE JOURNAL OF EDUCATIONAL PSYCHOLOGY. Text in Japanese; Contents page in English. 1953. q. JPY 16,000 (effective 2000). adv. bk.rev. charts. *Refereed.* **Document type:** *Academic/Scholarly.*
Related titles: Online - full text ed.: (from Institute for Scientific Information).
Indexed: ASCA, Bibl.Asian Stud. (1969), Child Devel.Abstr., Curr.Cont., PsycInfo, Psychol.Abstr. (1956-), SSCI, e-psyche.
—BLDSC (4651.750000), IDS.
Published by: Japanese Association of Educational Psychology/Nihon Kyoiku Shinri Gakkai, 5-26-5-701 Hongo, Bunkyo-ku, Tokyo 113-0033, Japan. Ed. Kanae Miura. Circ: (controlled).

618.89 JPN ISSN 0389-3723
JAPANESE JOURNAL OF PSYCHOPATHOLOGY/RINSHO SEISHIN BYORI. Text in Japanese. 1980. s-a.
Indexed: e-psyche.
Published by: Seiwa Shoten Co. Ltd., 2-5 Kami-Takai-Do 1-chome, Suginami-ku, Tokyo 168-0074, Japan. TEL 03-304-3822.

150 JPN ISSN 0021-5368
BF76.5 CODEN: JPREAV
JAPANESE PSYCHOLOGICAL RESEARCH. Text in English. 1954. q. GBP 92 to institutions in UK & Europe; USD 132 to institutions in the Americas & Caribbean; GBP 92 elsewhere to institutions (effective 2002). abstr, charts, illus. index. back issues avail. *Refereed.* **Document type:** *Journal, Academic/Scholarly.* **Description:** International in focus, the journal's analysis of problem-oriented research contributes significantly to all fields of psychology. Containing original articles, together with news and notes, are intended to raise awareness of psychological research in Japan amongst psychologists worldwide.
Related titles: Online - full text ed.: 1954 (from EBSCO Publishing, O C L C Online Computer Library Center, Inc., RoweCom Information Quest, ingenta, Swets Blackwell, Institute for Scientific Information).
Indexed: ASCA, Arts & Hum.Cit.Ind. (coverage dropped), Bibl.Asian Stud. (1970-1998), Biol.Abstr., Curr.Cont., Curr.Ind.Stat., Ergon.Abstr., Lang.& Lang.Behav.Abstr., PsycInfo, Psychol.Abstr. (1954-), Ref.Zh., Russ.Acad.Sci.Bibl., SOPODA, SSCI, Sociol.Abstr., e-psyche.
—BLDSC (4661.100000), CISTI, IDS, ingenta. **CCC.**
Published by: (Japanese Psychological Association), Blackwell Publishers Ltd., 108 Cowley Rd, Oxford OX4 1JF, United Kingdom. TEL 44-1965-791100, FAX 44-1865-791347, jnlinfo@blackwellpublishers.co.uk, http://www.blackwellpublishers.co.uk, http://www.blackwellpulishers.co.uk. Ed. Sotohiro Kojima. Circ: 6,300. **Dist. by:** Business Center for Academic Societies Japan. TEL 81-3-5814-5811.

158 USA ISSN 0193-3922
BF637.C6
JOURNAL FOR SPECIALISTS IN GROUP WORK. Text in English. 1978. q. USD 140 domestic; GBP 108 UK, Europe, Middle East & Africa; USD 156 elsewhere (effective 2002). bk.rev. reprint service avail. from PQC,PSC,SCH. **Document type:** *Academic/Scholarly.* **Description:** Includes empirical research, history of group work, work with groups, theoretical discussions and current group literature reviews.
Formerly: Together (Washington, 1975) (0161-0333)
Related titles: Microfiche ed.; Online - full text ed.: (from ProQuest Information & Learning, ingenta).
Indexed: C.I.J.E., High.Educ.Abstr., Human Resour.Abstr., IBZ, Lang.& Lang.Behav.Abstr., PsycInfo, Psychol.Abstr. (1979-), SOPODA, Soc.Serv.Abstr., Soc.Work Res.& Abstr., Sociol.Abstr., Sp.Ed.Needs Abstr., e-psyche.
—BLDSC (5066.138000), ingenta. **CCC.**
Published by: (Association for Specialists in Group Work, American Counseling Association), Sage Publications, Inc., 2455 Teller Rd, Thousand Oaks, CA 91320. TEL 805-499-0721, FAX 805-499-0871, info@sagepub.com, http://www.sagepub.com. Ed. Janice Delucia Waack. Circ: 6,000.

302 USA ISSN 1088-0763
BF175.4.C84
JOURNAL FOR THE PSYCHOANALYSIS OF CULTURE & SOCIETY. Text in English. 1996. s-a., latest vol.6, 2001. USD 30 domestic to individuals; USD 42.10 in Canada to individuals; USD 40 elsewhere to individuals; USD 40 domestic to institutions; USD 52.80 in Canada to institutions; USD 50 elsewhere to institutions (effective 2001). bk.rev. illus. back issues avail. **Document type:** *Journal, Academic/Scholarly.* **Description:** Publishes works that employ psychoanalytic theories, concepts to address the psychological roots or consequences of social and cultural phenomena in such a way as to promote beneficial social change.
Indexed: MLA Intl.Bibl., PsycInfo, e-psyche.
—BLDSC (5043.264000).
Published by: (Association for the Psychoanalysis of Culture and Society, Kent State University, Department of English), Ohio State University Press, 1070 Carmack Rd, Columbus, OH 43210. TEL 614-292-6930, FAX 614-292-2065, moffet.8@osu.edu, http://www.ohiostatepress.org. Ed. Mark Bracher. R&P, Adv. contact Ava Stinnett. Circ: 400 (paid).

155 300 GBR ISSN 0021-8308
HM132
JOURNAL FOR THE THEORY OF SOCIAL BEHAVIOUR. Text in English. 1971. q. GBP 201 to institutions in UK & Europe; USD 308 to institutions in the Americas & Caribbean; GBP 241 elsewhere to institutions (effective 2002). adv. reprint service avail. from SWZ,PQC,PSC,SCH. *Refereed.* **Document type:** *Academic/Scholarly.*
Related titles: Online - full text ed.: (from EBSCO Publishing, O C L C Online Computer Library Center, Inc., RoweCom Information Quest, ingenta, Swets Blackwell, Institute for Scientific Information).

P

Indexed: ASCA, ASSIA, Adol.Ment.Hlth.Abstr., Curr.Cont., ERA, IBR, Int.Polit.Sci.Abstr., Intl.Bibl.Soc.Sci., Lang.& Lang.Behav.Abstr., Mid.East: Abstr.& Ind., Mult.Ed.Abstr., Phil.Ind., PsycInfo, Psychol.Abstr. (1971-), Res.High.Educ.Abstr., SOPODA, SSCI, Sage Race Rel.Abstr., Soc.Serv.Abstr., Sociol.Abstr., Sociol.Educ.Abstr., e-psyche.
—BLDSC (5069.076000), IDS, Infotrieve, ingenta. **CCC.**
Published by: Blackwell Publishers Ltd., 108 Cowley Rd, Oxford OX4 1JF, United Kingdom. TEL 44-1865-791100, FAX 44-1865-791347, jnlinfo@blackwellpublishers.co.uk, http://www.blackwellpublishers.co.uk. Ed. Charles W Smith TEL 718-997-2840. Circ: 800.

150 DEU ISSN 0942-2285
JOURNAL FUER PSYCHOLOGIE; Theorie - Forschung - Praxis. Text in German. 1992. q. DEM 98. **Document type:** *Academic/Scholarly.*
Indexed: e-psyche.
Published by: (Neue Gesellschaft fuer Psychologie), Roland Asanger Verlag GmbH, Rohrbacher Str 18, Heidelberg 69115, Germany. TEL 49-6221-183104, FAX 49-6221-160415. Ed. Roland Asanger.

155.4 USA ISSN 0091-0627
RJ499.A1 CODEN: JABCAA
JOURNAL OF ABNORMAL CHILD PSYCHOLOGY. Text in English. 1973. bi-m. USD 671, EUR 670 to institutions for print or online ed.; USD 100, EUR 100 to individuals for print or online ed.; USD 805.20, EUR 804 to institutions for print & online eds. combined (effective 2002). adv. bibl, charts, illus. back issues avail.; reprint service avail. from PSC,SCH. *Refereed.* **Document type:** *Journal, Academic/Scholarly.* **Description:** Brings together scientists and practicing professionals from a wide range of disciplines to focus on child and adolescent psychopathology.
Related titles: Microfilm ed.: (from PQC); Online - full text ed.: (from Northern Light Technology, Inc., EBSCO Publishing, O C L C Online Computer Library Center, Inc., RoweCom Information Quest, ProQuest Information & Learning, Gale Group, Swets Blackwell, Kluwer Online, Factiva, Institute for Scientific Information).
Indexed: AMED, ASCA, ASSIA, Abstr.Crim.& Pen., Adol.Ment.Hlth.Abstr., Behav.Med.Abstr., Bibl.Dev.Med.& Child Neur., Biol.Abstr., C.I.J.E. (coverage dropped), Child Devel.Abstr., Crim.Just.Abstr., Curr.Cont., Except.Child Educ.Abstr., Excerp.Med., Fam.Ind., IBR, IBZ, IMFL, Ind.Med. (1973-), Ind.Philos., Mid.East: Abstr.& Ind., Mult.Ed.Abstr., P C I, PsycInfo, Psychol.Abstr. (1977-), Psycscan D.P., Ref.Zh., SSCI, Soc.Sci.Ind. (Mar.1987-), Sp.Ed.Needs Abstr., e-psyche.
—BLDSC (4918.820000), CISTI, GNLM, IDS, ingenta. **CCC.**
Published by: Kluwer Academic - Plenum Publishers (Subsidiary of: Wolters Kluwer N.V.), 233 Spring St, New York, NY 10013-1578. TEL 212-620-8000, 800-221-9369, FAX 212-463-0742, info@plenum.com, http://www.wkap.nl/journalhome.htm/0091-0627. Ed. Susan B Campbell. R&P Rose Luongo TEL 781-871-6311. **Subscr. outside the Americas to:** Kluwer Academic Publishers Group, Journals Department, PO Box 322, Dordrecht 3300 AH, Netherlands. TEL 31-78-639-2392, FAX 31-78-654-6474.

616.89 USA ISSN 0021-843X
RC321 CODEN: JAPCAC
JOURNAL OF ABNORMAL PSYCHOLOGY. Text in English. 1906. q. USD 107 domestic to non-members; USD 122 foreign to non-members; USD 53 domestic to members; USD 63 foreign to members; USD 238 domestic to institutions; USD 270 foreign to institutions (effective 2001). adv. charts, illus. index. back issues avail.; reprint service avail. from PSC,PQC,SCH. *Refereed.* **Document type:** *Academic/Scholarly.* **Description:** Provides articles on basic research and theory in the broad field of abnormal behavior.
Supersedes in part (in 1965): Journal of Abnormal and Social Psychology (0096-851X)
Related titles: Microform ed.: (from PQC,PMC); Online - full text ed.: (from Gale Group, Factiva, Institute for Scientific Information).
Indexed: AMED, ASCA, ASSIA, Abstr.Crim.& Pen., Abstr.Health Care Manage.Stud., Acad.Ind., Addic.Abstr., AgeLine, Behav.Med.Abstr., Biol.Abstr., Biol.Dig., Chic.Per.Ind., Crim.Just.Abstr., Curr.Cont., Curr.Ind.Stat., Dok.Arbeitsmed., ERA, Except.Child Educ.Abstr., Excerp.Med., Fam.Ind., Hlth.Ind., Ind.Med. (1965-), Jrnl.Watch Psych., M.L.A., MLA Intl.Bibl., Mid.East: Abstr.& Ind., Neurosci.Cit.Ind., P C I, PsycInfo, Psychol.Abstr. (1925-), Psycscan C.P., Russ.Acad.Sci.Bibl., SSCI, Sage Fam.Stud.Abstr., Soc.Sci.Ind. (Oct.1982-), Soc.Work Res.& Abstr., Sp.Ed.Needs Abstr., Stud.Wom.Abstr., e-psyche.
—BLDSC (4918.840000), CISTI, IDS, ingenta. **CCC.**
Published by: American Psychological Association, 750 First St., N.E., Washington, DC 20002-4242. TEL 202-336-5600, 800-374-2721, FAX 202-336-5568, subscriptions@apa.org, http://www.apa.org/journals/abn.html. Ed. Timothy B Baker. Circ: 6,700.

364 USA ISSN 1055-3835
HV9275
JOURNAL OF ADDICTIONS & OFFENDER COUNSELING. Text in English. 1980. s-a. USD 30 domestic to institutions; USD 42 foreign to institutions (effective 2001). adv. abstr, bibl, illus. 48 p./no. back issues avail.; reprint service avail. from PQC. *Refereed.* **Document type:** *Journal, Academic/Scholarly.* **Description:** Covers sexual crime, drug and alcohol abuse and prison overcrowding.
Formerly (until 1990): Journal of Offender Counseling (0275-8598)
Related titles: Microform ed.: (from PQC); Online - full text ed.: (from Northern Light Technology, Inc., ProQuest Information & Learning, H. W. Wilson).
Indexed: C.I.J.E., Crim.Just.Abstr., Educ.Ind. (Jan.2001-), PsycInfo, Psychol.Abstr. (1990-), Soc.Work Res.& Abstr., e-psyche.
—ingenta. **CCC.**
Published by: (International Association of Addictions and Offender Counselors), American Counseling Association, 5999 Stevenson Ave, Alexandria, VA 22304-3300. TEL 703-823-9800, FAX 703-823-0252, http://www.counseling.org, http://www.ncda.org. Ed. Virginia A Kelly. R&P Cynthia Peay TEL 703-823-9800 x 249. Adv. contact Kathy Maguire TEL 703-823-9800 ext 207. Circ: 2,200.

JOURNAL OF ADOLESCENCE. see *CHILDREN AND YOUTH—About*

155.5 USA ISSN 0743-5584
HQ796
JOURNAL OF ADOLESCENT RESEARCH. Text in English. 1986. bi-m. USD 70 to individuals; USD 350 to institutions; USD 20 newsstand/cover to individuals; USD 65 newsstand/cover to institutions (effective 2002). adv. back issues avail.; reprints avail. *Refereed.* **Document type:** *Academic/Scholarly.* **Description:** Takes an interdisciplinary perspective in providing professionals and practitioners with current and relevant information on many aspects of individuals 10-20 years old.
Related titles: Microform ed.; Online - full text ed.: (from EBSCO Publishing, O C L C Online Computer Library Center, Inc., RoweCom Information Quest, ProQuest Information & Learning, ingenta, Swets Blackwell, Institute for Scientific Information).
Indexed: ASCA, Bibl.Agri., C.I.J.E., Chic.Per.Ind., Child Devel.Abstr., Crim.Just.Abstr., Curr.Cont., Educ.Admin.Abstr., Educ.Ind. (coverage dropped), Environ.Sci.Poll.Mgmt., Fam.Ind., IMFL, Lang.& Lang.Behav.Abstr., Pollut.Abstr., PsycInfo, Psychol.Abstr. (1986-), Risk Abstr., SOPODA, SSCI, Saf.Sci.Abstr., Sage Fam.Stud.Abstr., Soc.Serv.Abstr., Soc.Work Res.& Abstr., Sociol.Abstr., THA, Viol.& Abuse Abstr., e-psyche.
—BLDSC (4918.943500), GNLM, IDS. **CCC.**
Published by: Sage Publications, Inc., 2455 Teller Rd, Thousand Oaks, CA 91320. TEL 805-499-0721, FAX 805-499-0871, info@sagepub.com, http://www.sagepub.com. Ed. Gerald R Adams. R&P Tanya Udin. Adv. contact DeAnna Vega Hammersley. Circ: 1,000. **Overseas subscr. to:** Sage Publications Ltd., 6 Bonhill St, London EC2A 4PU, United Kingdom. TEL 44-20-7374-0645, FAX 44-20-7374-8741, subscription@sagepub.co.uk, http://www.sagepub.co.uk; Sage Publications India Pvt. Ltd., 4215, New Delhi 110 048, India. TEL 91-11-641-9884, FAX 91-11-647-2426.

155.6 USA ISSN 1068-0667
HQ799.95 CODEN: JADEEU
JOURNAL OF ADULT DEVELOPMENT. Text in English. 1994. q. USD 292, EUR 291 to institutions for print or online ed.; USD 50, EUR 50 to individuals for print or online ed.; USD 350.40, EUR 349.20 to institutions for print & online eds. combined (effective 2002). *Refereed.* **Document type:** *Journal, Academic/Scholarly.* **Description:** Publishes broad studies of the positive aspects of adult development, pure cognition or reasoning from an interdisciplinary approach, and appreciations of a range of developmental theories and methodologies for understanding adults across the life span.
Related titles: Microfilm ed.: (from PQC); Online - full text ed.: (from EBSCO Publishing, O C L C Online Computer Library Center, Inc., Swets Blackwell, Kluwer Online, Institute for Scientific Information, RoweCom Information Quest).
Indexed: ASCA, Abstr.Soc.Geront., AgeLine, Curr.Cont., Fam.Ind., PsycInfo, SSCI, e-psyche.
—BLDSC (4918.943600), IDS, Infotrieve, ingenta. **CCC.**
Published by: (Society for Research in Adult Development), Kluwer Academic - Plenum Publishers (Subsidiary of: Wolters Kluwer N.V.), 233 Spring St, New York, NY 10013-1578. TEL 212-620-8000, 800-221-9369, FAX 212-463-0742, info@plenum.com, http://www.wkap.nl/journalhome.htm/1068-0667. Ed. Jack Demick. R&P Rose Luongo TEL 781-871-6311. **Subscr. outside the Americas to:** Kluwer Academic Publishers Group, Journals Department, PO Box 322, Dordrecht 3300 AH, Netherlands. TEL 31-78-639-2392, FAX 31-78-654-6474.

150 USA ISSN 1092-6771
RC569.5.V55 CODEN: JAMTFJ
JOURNAL OF AGGRESSION, MALTREATMENT & TRAUMA. Text in English. s-a. USD 60 to individuals; USD 81 in Canada to individuals; USD 87 elsewhere to individuals; USD 200 to institutions; USD 270 in Canada to institutions; USD 290 elsewhere to institutions; USD 300 to libraries; USD 405 in Canada to libraries; USD 435 elsewhere to libraries (effective Aug. 2001). adv. back issues avail.; reprint service avail. from HAW. **Document type:** *Journal, Academic/Scholarly.*
Indexed: Crim.Just.Abstr., Environ.Sci.Poll.Mgmt., IBZ, Ind.Philos., Ref.Zh., Risk Abstr., Saf.Sci.Abstr., Sage Urb.Stud.Abstr., Soc.Serv.Abstr., Sociol.Abstr., e-psyche.
—BLDSC (4919.997810), Haworth, ingenta.
Published by: Haworth Press, Inc., 10 Alice St, Binghamton, NY 13904-1580. TEL 607-722-5857, 800-429-6784, FAX 607-722-6362, 800-895-0582, getinfo@haworthpressinc.com, http://www.haworthpress.com/journals/journallist.asp. Ed. Robert Geffner. Pub. William Cohen. R&P Ruthann Heath TEL 607-723-5857 ext 316. Adv. contact Jackie Blakeslee TEL 607-722-5857 ext 346. B&W page USD 315, color page USD 550; trim 6 x 8.5.

JOURNAL OF AGING & IDENTITY. see *GERONTOLOGY AND GERIATRICS*

616.89 GBR ISSN 0021-8774
BF173.A2 CODEN: JANPA7
JOURNAL OF ANALYTICAL PSYCHOLOGY. Text in English. 1955. q. GBP 155 to institutions in UK & Europe; USD 223 to institutions in the Americas & Caribbean; GBP 155 elsewhere to institutions (effective 2002). adv. bk.rev. bibl. index. *Refereed.* **Document type:** *Academic/Scholarly.*
Related titles: Microfilm ed.; Online - full text ed.: (from EBSCO Publishing, O C L C Online Computer Library Center, Inc., RoweCom Information Quest, ingenta, Swets Blackwell, Institute for Scientific Information).
Indexed: ASCA, ASSIA, Arts & Hum.Cit.Ind. (coverage dropped), Biol.Abstr., Curr.Cont., Excerp.Med., IBR, IBZ, Ind.Med. (1955-), Ind.Philos., Mid.East: Abstr.& Ind., PsycInfo, Psychoanal.Abstr., Psychol.Abstr. (1955-), Rel.Ind.One, Rel.Ind.Two, Russ.Acad.Sci.Bibl., SSCI, Yrbk.Assoc.Educ.& Rehab.Blind, e-psyche.
—BLDSC (4928.500000), CISTI, GNLM, IDS, ingenta. **CCC.**
Published by: Blackwell Publishers Ltd., 108 Cowley Rd, Oxford OX4 1JF, United Kingdom. TEL 44-1865-791100, FAX 44-1865-791347, jnlinfo@blackwellpublishers.co.uk, http://www.blackwellpublishers.co.uk. Eds. Barbara Wharton TEL 44-20-7794-3640, Coline Covington TEL 44-20-7607-5078, Joseph Cambray. adv.: page GBP 200; trim 190 x 115. Circ: 1,800.

616.85 152.4 GBR ISSN 0887-6185
RC531 CODEN: JADIE8
JOURNAL OF ANXIETY DISORDERS. Text in English. 1987. bi-m. EUR 114 in Europe to individuals; JPY 15,100 in Japan to individuals; USD 127 elsewhere to individuals; EUR 487 in Europe to institutions; JPY 64,700 in Japan to institutions; USD 544 elsewhere to institutions (effective 2002). illus. index. back issues avail.; reprint service avail. from PSC,SCH. *Refereed.* **Document type:** *Journal, Academic/Scholarly.* **Description:** Publishes interdisciplinary research dealing with all aspects of anxiety disorders for all age groups (child, adolescent, adult and geriatric), including assessment, diagnosis, psychosocial and pharmacological treatment, epidemiology and prevention.
Related titles: Microfilm ed.: (from PQC); Online - full text ed.: (from ingenta, Swets Blackwell, ScienceDirect, Institute for Scientific Information).
Indexed: ASCA, AgeLine, Curr.Cont., Environ.Sci.Poll.Mgmt., Excerp.Med., Ind.Med. (1987-), Inpharma, Pollut.Abstr., PsycInfo, Psychol.Abstr. (1987-), Reac., Risk Abstr., SSCI, Saf.Sci.Abstr., e-psyche.
—BLDSC (4939.300000), CISTI, EMDOCS, GNLM, IDS, ingenta, KNAW. **CCC.**

P

Published by: Pergamon (Subsidiary of: Elsevier Science), The Boulevard, Langford Ln, East Park, Kidlington, Oxford OXB 1GB, United Kingdom. FAX 44-1865-843010, http://www.elsevier.com/locate/janxdis. Ed. Michel Hersen. Circ: 1,500. **Subscr. in Australasia and the Far East to:** Elsevier Science (Singapore) Pte Ltd, No.1 Temasek Ave, 17-01 Millenia Tower, Singapore 039192, Singapore. TEL 65-434-3727, FAX 65-337-2230; **Subscr. in the Americas to:** Elsevier Science, PO Box 945, New York, NY 10159-0945. TEL 212-633-3730, FAX 212-633-3680, usinfo-f@elsevier.com; **Subscr. to:** Elsevier Science BV, PO Box 211, Amsterdam 1000 AE, Netherlands. TEL 31-20-485-3757, nlinfo-f@elsevier.nl, http://www.elsevier.nl.

JOURNAL OF APPLIED ANIMAL WELFARE SCIENCE. see *ANIMAL WELFARE*

155 USA ISSN 0021-8855
BF636.A1 CODEN: JOABAW
JOURNAL OF APPLIED BEHAVIOR ANALYSIS. Text in English. 1968. q. USD 28 to individuals; USD 72 to institutions; USD 14 to students (effective 2000). adv. bk.rev. charts, illus. index. back issues avail.; reprint service avail. from PSC,SCH. *Refereed.* **Description:** Publishes experimental research about applications of the experimental analysis of behavior to problems of social importance.
Related titles: Microfilm ed.; Online - full text ed.: (from H. W. Wilson, Gale Group, Factiva, Institute for Scientific Information).
Indexed: ABI Inform. (Win.1973-Fall 1974), AMED, ASCA, ASSIA, Adol.Ment.Hlth.Abstr., AgeLine, Biol.Abstr., C.I.J.E., Child Devel.Abstr., Commun.Abstr., Cont.Pg.Manage., Curr.Cont., Curr.Ind.Stat., Except.Child Educ.Abstr., INIS Atomind., Ind.Med. (1968-), Int.Nurs.Ind., Mid.East: Abstr.& Ind., PsycInfo, Psychol.Abstr. (1968-), Psycscan A.P., Psycscan B.A.& T., SSCI, Soc.Sci.Ind. (Mar.1982-), Yrbk.Assoc.Educ.& Rehab.Blind, e-psyche.
—BLDSC (4940.450000), GNLM, IDS, ingenta.
Published by: Society for the Experimental Analysis of Behavior, Inc. (Lawrence), c/o Department of Human Development, University of Kansas, Lawrence, KS 66045. TEL 785-843-0008, http://sage.und.nodak.edu/org/jBAT/jbatinfo.html. Ed. Charles F Mace. Circ: 4,000 (paid).

150.1943 USA ISSN 0021-8863
H1 CODEN: JABHAP
JOURNAL OF APPLIED BEHAVIORAL SCIENCE. Text in English. 1965. q. USD 78, GBP 65 to individuals; USD 390, GBP 280 to institutions; USD 25 newsstand/cover to individuals; USD 90 newsstand/cover to institutions (effective 2002). adv. bk.rev. abstr, charts, illus. index. back issues avail.; reprint service avail. from PSC,SCH. *Refereed.* **Document type:** *Academic/Scholarly.* **Description:** Reports the latest interdisciplinary research on behavioral science and its applications to social policy, organization development, and community activity.
Related titles: Online - full text ed.: (from ProQuest Information & Learning, Gale Group, ingenta, Swets Blackwell).
Indexed: A.B.C.Pol.Sci., ABI Inform. (Jul.1971-), ASSIA, AgeLine, Amer.Bibl.Slavic & E.Eur.Stud., BPIA, Cont.Pg.Manage., Curr.Cont. (coverage dropped), Curr.Ind.Stat., ERA, Educ.Admin.Abstr., Ergon.Abstr., Human Resour.Abstr., Int.Polit.Sci.Abstr., Lang.& Lang.Behav.Abstr., Manage.Cont., Mult.Ed.Abstr., Pers.Lit., PsycInfo, Psychol.Abstr. (1965-), Psycscan A.P., Russ.Acad.Sci.Bibl., SCIMP, SOPODA, SSCI (coverage dropped), Sage Fam.Stud.Abstr., Sage Pub.Admin.Abstr., Soc.Sci.Ind. (Sep.1982-), Soc.Serv.Abstr., Soc.Work Res.& Abstr., Sociol.Abstr., Stud.Wom.Abstr., Tech.Educ.Abstr., e-psyche.
—BLDSC (4940.500000), CISTI, ingenta. **CCC.**
Published by: Sage Publications, Inc., 2455 Teller Rd, Thousand Oaks, CA 91320. TEL 805-499-0721, 800-818-7243, FAX 805-706-0871, 800-583-2665, info@sagepub.com, http://www.sagepub.com.uk/journals/details/j0059.html. Ed. Clayton Alderfer. R&P Tanya Udin. Adv. contact DeAnna Vega Hammersley. Circ: 2,800. **Overseas subscr. to:** Sage Publications Ltd., 6 Bonhill St, London EC2A 4PU, United Kingdom; Sage Publications India Pvt. Ltd., 4215, New Delhi 110 048, India. **Co-sponsor:** N T L Institute for Applied Behavioral Science.

150 USA ISSN 1071-2089
R726.7
JOURNAL OF APPLIED BIOBEHAVIORAL RESEARCH. Text in English. 1993. s-a. USD 50; USD 55 foreign (effective 1998). abstr, bibl, charts. index. *Refereed.* **Document type:** *Academic/Scholarly.*
Related titles: Online - full text ed.: (from Institute for Scientific Information).
Indexed: Curr.Cont., PsycInfo, SSCI, e-psyche.
Published by: Bellwether Publishing, Ltd., 8640 Guilford Rd, Ste 200, Columbia, MD 21046. TEL 410-290-3870, FAX 410-290-8726, bellpub@bellpub.com, http://www.bellpub.com. Ed. Andrew Baum.

155 GBR ISSN 0193-3973
BF636.A1
JOURNAL OF APPLIED DEVELOPMENTAL PSYCHOLOGY; an international lifespan journal. Text in English. 1980. bi-m. EUR 121 in Europe to individuals; JPY 16,000 in Japan to individuals; USD 135 elsewhere to individuals; EUR 299 in Europe to institutions; JPY 39,700 in Japan to institutions; USD 336 elsewhere to institutions (effective 2002). back issues avail.; reprint service avail. from PSC,SCH,ISI. *Refereed.* **Document type:** *Academic/Scholarly.* **Description:** Covers study of change in humans over time, bridging the gap between research in developmental psychology and its application.
Related titles: Online - full text ed.: (from ingenta, Swets Blackwell, ScienceDirect, Institute for Scientific Information).
Indexed: ASCA, Biol.Abstr., Child Devel.Abstr., Curr.Cont., Fam.Ind., Ind.Philos., Lang.& Lang.Behav.Abstr., PsycInfo, Psychol.Abstr. (1980-), Psycscan D.P., SOPODA, SSCI, Sociol.Abstr., e-psyche.
—BLDSC (4942.450000), CISTI, ingenta. **CCC.**
Published by: Elsevier Science, Langford Ln, Kidlington, Oxon OX5 1GB, United Kingdom. TEL 44-1865-843000, FAX 44-1865-843010, http://www.elsevier.com/locate/jappdp. Eds. Irving E Sigel, Radney Cocking. Circ: 500.

150 301 300 AUS ISSN 1442-0872
JOURNAL OF APPLIED HEALTH BEHAVIOUR. Text in English. 1995. s-a. AUD 40 (effective 2001). back issues avail. *Refereed.* **Document type:** *Academic/Scholarly.* **Description:** Examines the empirical research into health related behavior and the teachings into health related behaviours.
Formerly (until 1998): Journal of Applied Social Behaviour (1325-782X)
Published by: University of Sydney, School of Behavioural and Community Health, PO Box 170, Lidcombe, NSW 2141, Australia. TEL 61-2-93519587, FAX 61-2-93519540, http://www.cchs.usyd.edu.au/bach/. Ed., R&P Dr. C J Lennings. Pub. Dr. Ross Menzies. Circ: 30.

302 USA ISSN 1521-1401
BF173.A2 CODEN: JPSSFF
▼ **JOURNAL OF APPLIED PSYCHOANALYTIC STUDIES.** Text in English. 1999. q. USD 45, EUR 45 to individuals for print or online ed.; USD 202, EUR 201 to institutions for print or online ed.; USD 242.40, EUR 241.20 to institutions for print & online eds. combined (effective 2002). adv. bk.rev. back issues avail.; reprints avail. *Refereed.* **Document type:** *Journal, Academic/Scholarly.* **Description:** Discusses all aspects of psychoanalysis, not only from a psychological context but also from the perspectives of sociology, anthropology, criminal justice, education, political science, and history.
Related titles: Online - full text ed.: (from EBSCO Publishing, O C L C Online Computer Library Center, Inc., RoweCom Information Quest, Swets Blackwell, Kluwer Online).
Indexed: Intl.Bibl.Soc.Sci.
—BLDSC (4946.800000).
Published by: Kluwer Academic - Plenum Publishers (Subsidiary of: Wolters Kluwer N.V.), 233 Spring St, New York, NY 10013-1578. TEL 212-620-8000, 800-221-9369, FAX 212-463-0742, info@plenum.com, http://www.wkap.nl/journalhome.htm/1521-1401. Eds. Nadia Ramzy, Stuart W Twemlow. **Subscr. outside the Americas to:** Kluwer Academic Publishers Group, Journals Department, PO Box 322, Dordrecht 3300 AH, Netherlands. TEL 31-78-639-2392, FAX 31-78-654-6474.

158 USA ISSN 0021-9010
BF1 CODEN: JAPGBP
JOURNAL OF APPLIED PSYCHOLOGY. Text in English. 1917. bi-m. USD 153 domestic to non-members; USD 173 foreign to non-members; USD 76 domestic to members; USD 88 foreign to members; USD 362 domestic to institutions; USD 406 foreign to institutions (effective 2001). adv. bibl, charts, illus. index. reprint service avail. from PSC,PQC,SCH. *Refereed.* **Document type:** *Academic/Scholarly.* **Description:** Research on applications of psychology in work settings such as industry, correction systems, government, and educational institutions.
Related titles: Microform ed.: (from PQC,PMC); Online - full text ed.: (from Gale Group, Institute for Scientific Information).
Indexed: ABI Inform. (Oct.1971-), ASCA, ASSIA, Abstr.Crim.& Pen., Acad.Ind., Adol.Ment.Hlth.Abstr., AgeLine, BPIA, Biol.Abstr., CINAHL, Commun.Abstr., Comput.Abstr., Cont.Pg.Manage., Crim.Just.Abstr., Curr.Cont., Curr.Ind.Stat., Dok.Arbeitsmed., ERA, Educ.Admin.Abstr., Educ.Ind. (coverage dropped), Ergon.Abstr., Excerp.Med., Fam.Ind., Hlth.Ind., IBZ, Ind.Med. (1917-), Ind.Philos., Int.Aerosp.Abstr., Int.Lab.Doc., Int.Nurs.Ind., Intl.Bibl.Soc.Sci., Mid.East: Abstr.& Ind., Mult.Ed.Abstr., P C I, Pers.Lit., PsycInfo, Psychol.Abstr. (1926-), Psycscan A.P., Res.High.Educ.Abstr., Risk Abstr., Russ.Acad.Sci.Bibl., SCIMP, SOMA, SSCI, Sage Race Rel.Abstr., Soc.Sci.Ind. (Oct.1982-), Sp.Ed.Needs Abstr., Stud.Wom.Abstr., e-psyche.
—BLDSC (4947.000000), CISTI, GNLM, IDS, ingenta. **CCC.**
Published by: American Psychological Association, 750 First St., N.E., Washington, DC 20002-4242. TEL 202-336-5600, 800-374-2721, FAX 202-336-5568, subscriptions@apa.org, http://www.apa.org/journals/apl.html. Ed. Kevin R Murphy. Circ: 5,100.

158 USA ISSN 0021-9029
HM251 CODEN: JASPBX
JOURNAL OF APPLIED SOCIAL PSYCHOLOGY. Text in English. 1971. 12/yr. USD 679 in North America; USD 699 elsewhere (effective 1999 - 2000). abstr, charts, illus, stat. index. back issues avail.; reprint service avail. from PSC,SCH. *Refereed.* **Document type:** *Academic/Scholarly.*
Related titles: Online - full text ed.: (from Gale Group, Institute for Scientific Information).
Indexed: ASCA, ASSIA, Abstr.Crim.& Pen., AgeLine, Chic.Per.Ind., Crim.Just.Abstr., Curr.Cont., Curr.Lit.Fam.Plan., ERA, Environ.Sci.Poll.Mgmt., Excerp.Med., Fam.Ind., Food Sci.& Tech.Abstr., High.Educ.Abstr., IBZ, Ind.Philos., Indian Psychol.Abstr., Intl.Bibl.Soc.Sci., L.R.I., Mid.East: Abstr.& Ind., Mult.Ed.Abstr., P C I, PsycInfo, Psychol.Abstr. (1971-), Psycscan A.P., Risk Abstr., Russ.Acad.Sci.Bibl., SSCI, Saf.Sci.Abstr., Sage Race Rel.Abstr., Soc.Sci.Ind. (May 1981-), Sociol.Educ.Abstr., Sp.Ed.Needs Abstr., Sportsearch, Stud.Wom.Abstr., e-psyche.
—BLDSC (4947.080000), IDS, ingenta. **CCC.**
Published by: V.H. Winston & Son, Inc., c/o Bellwether Publishing, Ltd, 8640 Guilford Rd, Ste 200, Columbia, MD 21046. TEL 410-290-3870, FAX 410-290-8726, bellpub@bellpub.com, http://www.bellpub.com. Ed. Andrew Baum. Circ: 1,100.

JOURNAL OF APPLIED SPORT PSYCHOLOGY. see *MEDICAL SCIENCES—Sports Medicine*

JOURNAL OF AUTISM AND DEVELOPMENTAL DISORDERS. see *EDUCATION—Special Education And Rehabilitation*

THE JOURNAL OF BEHAVIOR THERAPY AND EXPERIMENTAL PSYCHIATRY; an interdisciplinary journal. see *MEDICAL SCIENCES—Psychiatry And Neurology*

JOURNAL OF BEHAVIORAL EDUCATION. see *EDUCATION*

JOURNAL OF BEHAVIORAL HEALTH SERVICES AND RESEARCH. see *PUBLIC HEALTH AND SAFETY*

JOURNAL OF BEHAVIORAL MEDICINE. see *MEDICAL SCIENCES—Psychiatry And Neurology*

JOURNAL OF BIBLICAL COUNSELING. see *RELIGIONS AND THEOLOGY*

155.84 USA ISSN 0095-7984
E185.625 CODEN: JBPSE3
JOURNAL OF BLACK PSYCHOLOGY. Text in English. 1974. q. USD 320 domestic; GBP 232; USD 336 elsewhere (effective 2002). adv. bk.rev. illus. back issues avail.; reprint service avail. from PQC. *Refereed.* **Document type:** *Academic/Scholarly.* **Description:** Publishes scholarly contributions within the field of psychology on the experience of Black and other minority populations from an Afrocentrist perspective in such issues as cognition, personality, social behavior, child development, education, and clinical application.
Related titles: Microform ed.: (from PQC); Online - full text ed.: (from ProQuest Information & Learning, Gale Group, ingenta).

P

Indexed: ASSIA, Abstr.Anthropol., Adol.Ment.Hlth.Abstr., C.I.J.E., Crim.Just.Abstr., Environ.Sci.Poll.Mgmt., High.Educ.Abstr., Human Resour.Abstr., IMFL, Ind.Per.Blacks, Intl.Bibl.Soc.Sci., Lang.& Lang.Behav.Abstr., PsycInfo, Psychol.Abstr. (1974-), Risk Abstr., SOPODA, Saf.Sci.Abstr., Sage Race Rel.Abstr., Soc.Sci.Ind. (Jan.1994-), Soc.Serv.Abstr., Sociol.Abstr., e-psyche.
—BLDSC (4954.180000), ingenta. **CCC.**
Published by: (Association of Black Psychologists), Sage Publications, Inc., 2455 Teller Rd, Thousand Oaks, CA 91320. TEL 805-499-0721, FAX 805-499-0871, libraries@sagepub.com., info@sagepub.com, http://sagepub.co.uk/journals/usdetails/. Ed. Dr. Ann Kathleen Burlew. Pub. Sara Miller McCune. R&P Tanya Udin. Adv. contact DeAnna Vega Hammersley. Circ: 2,600. **Overseas subscr. to:** Sage Publications Ltd., 6 Bonhill St, London EC2A 4PU, United Kingdom.

158.7 330 USA ISSN 0889-3268
JOURNAL OF BUSINESS & PSYCHOLOGY. Text in English. 1986. q. USD 74, EUR 74 to individuals for print or online ed.; USD 507, EUR 506 to institutions for print or online ed.; USD 608.40, EUR 607.20 to institutions for print & online eds.combined (effective 2002). adv. reprint service avail. from PQC,PSC,SCH. *Refereed.* **Document type:** *Journal, Academic/Scholarly.* **Description:** Highlights empirical research, case studies, and literature reviews dealing with psychological programs implemented in business settings.
Related titles: Online - full text ed.: (from EBSCO Publishing, O C L C Online Computer Library Center, Inc., Swets Blackwell, Kluwer Online, Institute for Scientific Information, RoweCom Information Quest).
Indexed: ASCA, B.P.I. (00/1989-), Curr.Cont., Educ.Admin.Abstr., Fam.Ind., Human Resour.Abstr., Ind.Philos., Peace Res.Abstr., PsycInfo, Psychol.Abstr. (1986-), Russ.Acad.Sci.Bibl., SSCI, Stud.Wom.Abstr., Tech.Educ.Abstr., e-psyche.
—BLDSC (4954.661070), IDS, Infotrieve, ingenta. **CCC.**
Published by: (Business Psychology Research Institute), Kluwer Academic - Plenum Publishers (Subsidiary of: Wolters Kluwer N.V.), 233 Spring St, New York, NY 10013-1578. TEL 212-620-8000, 800-221-9369, FAX 212-463-0742, info@plenum.com, http://www.wkap.nl/journalhome.htm/0889-3268. Ed. John W Jones. **Subscr. outside the Americas:** Kluwer Academic Publishers Group, Journals Department, PO Box 322, Dordrecht 3300 AH, Netherlands. TEL 31-78-639-2392, FAX 31-78-654-6474.

150 658.3 USA ISSN 1069-0727
HF5381.A1 CODEN: JOAAEX
JOURNAL OF CAREER ASSESSMENT. Text in English. 1993. q. USD 40 domestic to individuals; USD 48 foreign to individuals; USD 120 domestic to institutions; USD 140 foreign to institutions (effective 2000). adv. abstr. index. back issues avail. *Refereed.* **Document type:** *Academic/Scholarly.* **Description:** Focuses on the process and techniques by which counselors and others gain understanding of the individual faced with the necessity of making informed career decisions.
Related titles: Online - full text ed.: (from Northern Light Technology, Inc., ProQuest Information & Learning, Institute for Scientific Information).
Indexed: ASCA, C.I.J.E., Curr.Cont., PsycInfo, SSCI, e-psyche.
—BLDSC (4954.874000), IDS, ingenta.
Published by: Psychological Assessment Resources, Inc., 16204 N Florida Ave, Lutz, FL 33549. TEL 813-968-3003, FAX 813-968-2598, http://www.parinc.com. Ed. Robert P Archer. R&P Brenda Vanantwerp. Adv. contact Daphne Lambright.

150 USA ISSN 1062-1024
RJ499.A1 CODEN: JCFSES
JOURNAL OF CHILD AND FAMILY STUDIES. Text in English. 1992. q. USD 71, EUR 71 to individuals for print or online ed.; USD 273, EUR 272 to institutions for print or online ed.; USD 327.60, EUR 326.40 combined subscription to institutions for print & online eds. (effective 2002). adv. bk.rev. *Refereed.* **Document type:** *Journal, Academic/Scholarly.* **Description:** Publishes original papers on basic and applied research, program evaluation, service delivery and policy issues. Studies the emotional disorders in children and adolescents and their effect on the family unit.
Related titles: Online - full text ed.: (from EBSCO Publishing, O C L C Online Computer Library Center, Inc., Gale Group, Swets Blackwell, Kluwer Online, Factiva, RoweCom Information Quest).
Indexed: ASSIA, Crim.Just.Abstr., Environ.Sci.Poll.Mgmt., Fam.Ind., Intl.Bibl.Soc.Sci., Lang.& Lang.Behav.Abstr., PsycInfo, Psychol.Abstr. (1992-), Risk Abstr., SOPODA, Saf.Sci.Abstr., Sage Fam.Stud.Abstr., Sage Race Rel.Abstr., Soc.Sci.Ind. (Jan.1994-), Soc.Serv.Abstr., Soc.Work Res.& Abstr., Sociol.Abstr., e-psyche.
—BLDSC (4957.426000), Infotrieve, ingenta. **CCC.**
Published by: Kluwer Academic - Plenum Publishers (Subsidiary of: Wolters Kluwer N.V.), 233 Spring St, New York, NY 10013-1578. TEL 212-620-8000, 800-221-9369, FAX 212-463-0742, info@plenum.com, http://kapis1.wkap.nl/journalhome.htm/1062-1024, http://www.wkap.nl. Ed. Nirbhay N Singh. Adv. contact Daniel S Lipner. **Subscr. outside the Americas to:** Kluwer Academic Publishers Group, Journals Department, PO Box 322, Dordrecht 3300 AH, Netherlands. TEL 31-78-639-2392, FAX 31-78-654-6474.

JOURNAL OF CHILD LANGUAGE. see *CHILDREN AND YOUTH—About*

155.4 GBR ISSN 0021-9630
RJ499.A1 CODEN: JPPDAI
JOURNAL OF CHILD PSYCHOLOGY & PSYCHIATRY & ALLIED DISCIPLINES. Text in English. 1960. 8/yr. GBP 264 to institutions in UK & Europe; USD 388 to institutions in the Americas & Caribbean; GBP 264 elsewhere to institutions (effective 2002). adv. bk.rev. charts, illus. index. back issues avail.; reprint service avail. from PQC,PSC,SCH. *Refereed.* **Document type:** *Academic/Scholarly.* **Description:** Primarily concerned with child and adolescent psychology and psychiatry, including experimental and developmental studies and especially developmental psychopathology.
Related titles: Microform ed.: (from PQC); Online - full text ed.: (from EBSCO Publishing, O C L C Online Computer Library Center, Inc., RoweCom Information Quest, ingenta, Gale Group, Swets Blackwell, Factiva, Institute for Scientific Information).
Indexed: AMED, ASCA, ASSIA, Abstr.Crim.& Pen., Adol.Ment.Hlth.Abstr., AgeLine, Bibl.Dev.Med.& Child Neur., Biol.Abstr., Br.Educ.Ind., Brit.Nur.Ind., C.I.J.E. (coverage dropped), CINAHL, Child Devel.Abstr., Crim.Just.Abstr., Curr.Cont., Educ.Ind. (Jul.1983-), Environ.Sci.Poll.Mgmt., Except.Child Educ.Abstr., Excerp.Med., Fam.Ind., Ind.Med. (1960-), Indian Psychol.Abstr., Int.Nurs.Ind., Lang.& Lang.Behav.Abstr., Mid.East: Abstr.& Ind., Mult.Ed.Abstr., Neurosci.Cit.Ind., Nutr.Abstr., Pollut.Abstr., PsycInfo, Psychol.Abstr. (1960-), Psycscan D.P., Risk Abstr., SOPODA, SSCI, Saf.Sci.Abstr., Soc.Sci.Ind. (Jan.1994-), Soc.Serv.Abstr., Sociol.Abstr., Sp.Ed.Needs Abstr., e-psyche.
—BLDSC (4957.800000), CISTI, GNLM, IDS, ingenta, KNAW. **CCC.**
Published by: (Association of Child Psychology and Psychiatry), Cambridge University Press, Edinburgh Bldg, Shaftesbury Rd, Cambridge CB2 2RU, United Kingdom. FAX 44-1223-315052, information@cambridge.org, http://www.cup.org. Eds. Dorothy Bishop, Eric Taylor, Francesca Happe, Frank C. Verhulst, Jim Stevenson. R&P Linda Nicol. Adv. contact Rebecca Symons. Circ: 4,700.

155.4 616.89 GBR ISSN 0075-417X
JOURNAL OF CHILD PSYCHOTHERAPY. Text in English. 1963. 3/yr. GBP 52, USD 81 to individuals; GBP 153, USD 250 to institutions (effective 2002). adv. bk.rev. reprints avail. **Document type:** *Academic/Scholarly.* **Description:** Contains articles on theory, technique, and the practice of psychoanalytic psychotherapy with children, young people, and their families.
Related titles: Online - full text ed.: ISSN 1469-9370 (from CatchWord Ltd., EBSCO Publishing, O C L C Online Computer Library Center, Inc., RoweCom Information Quest, Swets Blackwell).
Indexed: ASSIA, Biol.Dig., Br.Educ.Ind., Child Devel.Abstr., Excerp.Med. (1996-), Mid.East: Abstr.& Ind., PsycInfo, Psychol.Abstr. (1977-), Soc.Work Res.& Abstr., e-psyche.
—BLDSC (4957.900000), CatchWord, EMDOCS, GNLM, ingenta.
Published by: (Association of Child Psychotherapists), Routledge (Subsidiary of: Taylor & Francis Group), 11 New Fetter Ln, London EC4P 4EE, United Kingdom. TEL 44-207-842-2001, FAX 44-20-7842-2298, journals@routledge.com, http://www.routledge.com/routledge/journal/journals.html. Eds. Judith Edwards, Monica Lanyado. R&P Sally Sweet. adv.: page GBP 150; trim 190 x 115. Circ: 2,000. **Subscr. to:** Subscriptions, PO Box 362, Abingdon, Oxon OX14 3WB, United Kingdom. TEL 44-1235-401060, FAX 44-1235-401075.

JOURNAL OF CLASSIFICATION. see *MATHEMATICS*

616.89 USA ISSN 1532-3285
▼ **JOURNAL OF CLINICAL ACTIVITIES, ASSIGNMENTS & HANDOUTS IN PSYCHOTHERAPY PRACTICE;** innovations in resources for treatment & intervention. Text in English. 2001 (Spr.). q. USD 38 domestic to individuals; USD 51 in Canada to individuals; USD 55 elsewhere to individuals; USD 65 domestic to institutions; USD 88 in Canada to institutions; USD 94 elsewhere to institutions; USD 90 domestic to libraries; USD 122 in Canada to libraries; USD 131 elsewhere to libraries (effective Aug. 2001). adv. back issues avail.; reprints avail. *Refereed.* **Document type:** *Journal, Academic/Scholarly.* **Description:** Contains articles and features reflecting up-to-the-minute developments in eclectic, problem-solving and task-oriented psychotherapy practice.
Related titles: Online - full text ed.: free with subscr. to the print ed.
Published by: Haworth Press, Inc., 10 Alice St, Binghamton, NY 13904-1580. TEL 607-722-5857, 800-429-6784, FAX 607-722-6362, 800-895-0582, getinfo@haworthpressinc.com, http://www.haworthpress.com/journals/journallist.asp. Ed. Lorna Hecker. Pub. William Cohen. R&P Ruthann Heath TEL 607-723-5857 ext 316. Adv. contact Jackie Blakeslee TEL 607-722-5857 ext 346. B&W page USD 315, color page USD 550; trim 6 x 8.5.

155.4 USA ISSN 1537-4416
BF721 CODEN: JCCPD3
JOURNAL OF CLINICAL CHILD AND ADOLESCENT PSYCHOLOGY. Text in English. 1972. q. USD 55 in US & Canada to individuals; USD 85 elsewhere to individuals; USD 435 in US & Canada to institutions; USD 465 elsewhere to institutions (effective 2002). adv. bk.rev. illus. Index. reprint service avail. from PQC. *Refereed.* **Document type:** *Journal, Academic/Scholarly.* **Description:** Features the research and viewpoints of child advocates in all disciplines.
Formerly (until 2001): Journal of Clinical Child Psychology (0047-228X)
Related titles: Microform ed.; Online - full text ed.: ISSN 1532-7639. USD 49.50 to individuals; USD 391.50 to institutions (effective 2002) (from CatchWord Ltd., EBSCO Publishing, O C L C Online Computer Library Center, Inc., RoweCom Information Quest, Gale Group, Swets Blackwell, Factiva, Institute for Scientific Information).
Indexed: ASCA, ASSIA, Abstr.Crim.& Pen., Bibl.Dev.Med.& Child Neur., Child Devel.Abstr., Crim.Just.Abstr., Curr.Cont., Environ.Sci.Poll.Mgmt., Except.Child Educ.Abstr., Fam.Ind., IMFL, Ind.Med. (1971-), Mid.East: Abstr.& Ind., Neurosci.Cit.Ind., Pollut.Abstr., PsycInfo, Psychol.Abstr. (1972-), Psycscan C.P., Psycscan D.P., Risk Abstr., SSCI, Saf.Sci.Abstr., Soc.Sci.Ind. (Mar.1987-), e-psyche.
—BLDSC (4958.384000), CatchWord, CISTI, GNLM, ingenta. **CCC.**
Published by: (Clinical Child Psychology, American Psychological Association), Lawrence Erlbaum Associates, Inc., 10 Industrial Ave, Mahwah, NJ 07430-2262. TEL 201-760-3735, 800-926-6579, FAX 201-236-0072, journals@erlbaum.com, http://www.erlbaum.com/Journals/journals/JCCP/jccp.htm. Ed. Wendy K Silverman. adv.: page USD 475; trim 7 x 10. Circ: 1,700.

JOURNAL OF CLINICAL GEROPSYCHOLOGY. see *GERONTOLOGY AND GERIATRICS*

616.891 USA ISSN 1076-044X
CODEN: JCIPEY
JOURNAL OF CLINICAL PSYCHOANALYSIS. Text in English. 1992. q. USD 71 domestic to individuals; USD 106 foreign to individuals; USD 106 domestic to institutions; USD 127 foreign to institutions (effective 2002). adv. bk.rev. back issues avail. *Refereed.* **Document type:** *Journal, Academic/Scholarly.* **Description:** Explains, in jargon-free language, what actually happens in an analysis.
Indexed: ASSIA, Excerp.Med. (1994-), PsycInfo, Psychoanal.Abstr., Psychol.Abstr. (1992-), e-psyche.
—BLDSC (4958.689000), GNLM.
Published by: International Universities Press, Incorporated, 59 Boston Post Rd., P.O. Box 1524, Madison, CT 06443-1524. adv.: page USD 580; 4.25 x 7.

P

616.891 USA ISSN 0021-9762
RC475
JOURNAL OF CLINICAL PSYCHOLOGY. Text in English. 1945. 8/yr. USD 460 in United States; USD 544 in Canada & Mexico; USD 544 elsewhere; USD 483 combined subscription in United States for print and online eds.; USD 567 combined subscription in Canada & Mexico for print and online eds.; USD 567 combined subscription elsewhere for print and online eds. (effective 2002). adv. bk.rev. charts. index. back issues avail.; reprint service avail. from PSC,SCH. *Refereed.* **Document type:** *Academic/Scholarly.* **Description:** Includes research studies, articles on contemporary professional issues, and single case research. Covers psycopathology, psychodiagnostics, and the psychotherapeutic process, as well as psychotherapy effectiveness research, psychological assessment and treatment matching, and clinical outcomes.
Incorporates (1995-1998): In Session: Psychotherapy in Practice (1077-2413)
Related titles: Microform ed.: (from PQC); Online - full text ed.: ISSN 1097-4679. 1996. USD 460 in United States; USD 460 in Canada & Mexico; USD 460 elsewhere (effective 2002) (from EBSCO Publishing, Gale Group, Wiley InterScience, Factiva, Institute for Scientific Information).
Indexed: ASCA, ASSIA, Abstr.Crim.& Pen., Abstr.Health Care Manage.Stud., Addic.Abstr., Adol.Ment.Hlth.Abstr., AgeLine, Biol.Abstr., C.I.J.E. (coverage dropped), CINAHL, Chem.Abstr., Chic.Per.Ind., Commun.Abstr., Crim.Just.Abstr., Curr.Cont., Curr.Ind.Stat., Dent.Ind., Environ.Sci.Poll.Mgmt., Excerp.Med., Fam.Ind., Hosp.Lit.Ind., Human Resour.Abstr., IMFL, Ind.Med. (1945-), Ind.Sci.Rev., Indian Psychol.Abstr., Int.Nurs.Ind., Lang.& Lang.Behav.Abstr., Mid.East: Abstr.& Ind., Neurosci.Cit.Ind., Nutr.Abstr., Pollut.Abstr., PsycInfo, Psychol.Abstr. (1945-), Psycscan C.P., Ref.Zh., Rel.Ind.One, Rel.Ind.Two, Risk Abstr., SOPODA, SSCI, Saf.Sci.Abstr., Sage Fam.Stud.Abstr., Sci.Cit.Ind. (coverage dropped), Soc.Sci.Ind. (Jul.1982-), Soc.Work Res.& Abstr., Sociol.Abstr., THA, e-psyche.
—BLDSC (4958.690000), CISTI, GNLM, IDS, ingenta, KNAW. **CCC.**
Published by: John Wiley & Sons, Inc., Journals (Subsidiary of: Wiley InterScience), 605 Third Ave, New York, NY 10158. TEL 212-850-6645, FAX 212-850-6021, subinfo@wiley.com, uscs-wis@wiley.com, http://www.wiley.com. Eds. Kenneth I Howard, Larry E Beutler. adv.: B&W page GBP 640, color page GBP 1,515; trim 172 x 254. Circ: 2,529. **Subscr. outside the Americas to:** John Wiley & Sons Ltd., Baffins Ln, Chichester, Sussex PO19 IUD, United Kingdom. TEL 44-1243-779777, FAX 44-1243-843232, cs-journals@wiley.co.uk, http://www.wiley.co.uk.

616.89 USA ISSN 1068-9583
CODEN: JLPSE5
JOURNAL OF CLINICAL PSYCHOLOGY IN MEDICAL SETTINGS. Text in English. 1994. q. USD 292, EUR 291 to institutions for print or online ed.; USD 350.40, EUR 349.20 to institutions for print & online eds.combined (effective 2002). adv. bk.rev. back issues avail. *Refereed.* **Document type:** *Journal, Academic/Scholarly.* **Description:** Explores theoretical and applied research in clinical science, clinical practice and service delivery, education and professional issues.
Related titles: Microfilm ed.: (from PQC); Online - full text ed.: (from EBSCO Publishing, O C L C Online Computer Library Center, Inc., RoweCom Information Quest, Swets Blackwell, Kluwer Online, Institute for Scientific Information).
Indexed: ASCA, AgeLine, Curr.Cont., Fam.Ind., Lang.& Lang.Behav.Abstr., PsycInfo, SOPODA, SSCI, Sociol.Abstr., e-psyche.
—BLDSC (4958.690550), CISTI, GNLM, IDS, Infotrieve, ingenta, KNAW. **CCC.**
Published by: (Evanston Hospital, Department of Psychiatry), Kluwer Academic - Plenum Publishers (Subsidiary of: Wolters Kluwer N.V.), 233 Spring St, New York, NY 10013-1578. TEL 212-620-8000, 800-221-9369, FAX 212-463-0742, info@plenum.com, http://www.wkap.nl/journalhome.htm/1068-9583. Ed. Ronald H Rozensky. R&P Rose Luongo TEL 781-871-6311. **Subscr. outside the Americas to:** Kluwer Academic Publishers Group, Journals Department, PO Box 322, Dordrecht 3300 AH, Netherlands. TEL 31-78-639-2392, FAX 31-78-654-6474.

153.4 NLD ISSN 1567-7095
▼ **JOURNAL OF COGNITION AND CULTURE.** Text in English. 2001. 4/yr. EUR 63, USD 73 to individuals; EUR 148.50, USD 172 to institutions (effective 2002). **Document type:** *Journal, Academic/Scholarly.* **Description:** Provides an interdisciplinary forum for exploring the mental foundations of culture and the culture foundations of mental life.
Related titles: Online - full text ed.: (from CatchWord Ltd.).
Published by: Brill Academic Publishers, PO Box 9000, Leiden 2300 PA, Netherlands. TEL 31-71-535-3500, FAX 31-71-531-7532, cs@brill.nl, http://www.brill.nl. Eds. E T Lawson, Justin Barrett, Pascal Boyer.

155 USA ISSN 1524-8372
▼ **JOURNAL OF COGNITION AND DEVELOPMENT.** Text in English. 2000. q. USD 60 in US & Canada to individuals; USD 90 elsewhere to individuals; USD 220 in US & Canada to institutions; USD 250 elsewhere to institutions (effective 2002). adv. bk.rev. *Refereed.* **Document type:** *Journal, Academic/Scholarly.* **Description:** Provides articles and empirical reports covering the area of cognitive development. Features theoretical essays and reviews of new and significant books.
Related titles: Online - full text ed.: ISSN 1532-7647. USD 45 to individuals (effective 2n2002); USD 198 to institutions (effective 2002) (from CatchWord Ltd., EBSCO Publishing, O C L C Online Computer Library Center, Inc., RoweCom Information Quest, Swets Blackwell).
—BLDSC (4958.798100), CatchWord.
Published by: (Cognitive Development Society), Lawrence Erlbaum Associates, Inc., 10 Industrial Ave, Mahwah, NJ 07430-2262. TEL 201-760-3735, 800-926-6579, FAX 201-236-0072, journals@erlbaum.com, http://www.erlbaum.com/Journals/journals/JCD/jcd.htm. Ed. Philip David Zelazo TEL 416-978-3904. adv.: page USD 375; trim 5 x 8.

JOURNAL OF COGNITIVE EDUCATION. see *EDUCATION*

150 USA ISSN 1527-3946
▼ **JOURNAL OF COGNITIVE LIBERTIES.** Text in English. 2000. 3/yr. USD 40 domestic to individuals; USD 50 foreign to individuals; USD 65 domestic to institutions; USD 80 foreign to institutions (effective 2001). back issues avail. **Document type:** *Journal, Academic/Scholarly.* **Description:** Designed to express thoughts about the importance of cognitive freedom.
Published by: Alchemind Society, Box 73481, Davis, CA 95617-3481. TEL 1-888-950-6463, info@alchemind.org, http://www.alchemind.org/jcl/jclabout.htm. Ed. Sharon O'Toole-Dubois.

JOURNAL OF COGNITIVE NEUROSCIENCE. see *MEDICAL SCIENCES—Psychiatry And Neurology*

616.89 USA ISSN 0889-8391
JOURNAL OF COGNITIVE PSYCHOTHERAPY; an international quarterly. Text in English. 1987. q., latest vol.15, 2001, Spring. USD 56 in United States to individuals; USD 94 for 2 yrs. in United States to individuals; USD 65 foreign to individuals; USD 111 for 2 yrs. foreign to individuals; USD 123 in United States to institutions; USD 209 for 2 yrs. in United States to institutions; USD 141 foreign to institutions; USD 240 for 2 yrs. foreign to institutions (effective 2001). adv. bk.rev., software rev., video rev., Website rev. abstr, bibl. 70 p./no. back issues avail.; reprints avail. *Refereed.* **Document type:** *Academic/Scholarly.* **Description:** Devoted to the advancement of the clinical practice of cognitive psychotherapy in its broadest sense. Merges theory, research and practice to provide an international forum investigating clinical implications of theoretical developments and research findings.
Indexed: AgeLine, Excerp.Med., Lang.& Lang.Behav.Abstr., PsycInfo, Psychol.Abstr. (1987-), SOPODA, Sociol.Abstr., e-psyche.
—BLDSC (4958.799200), EMDOCS, GNLM, Infotrieve, ingenta. **CCC.**
Published by: (International Association of Cognitive Psychotherapy), Springer Publishing Company, 536 Broadway, New York, NY 10012. TEL 212-431-4370, FAX 212-941-7842, springer@springerpub.com, http://www.springerpub.com. Ed. Robert L Leahy. Pub. Ursula Springer. R&P Dorothy Kouwenberg. Adv. contact Bob Friel. B&W page USD 300; 4.5 x 7.5.

155 USA ISSN 1389-0417
▼ **JOURNAL OF COGNITIVE SYSTEMS RESEARCH.** Text in English. 1999. irreg. free per issue. adv. bk.rev. *Refereed.* **Document type:** *Academic/Scholarly.* **Description:** Explores new approaches in studying cognitive processes in human and computer contexts from the perspectives of multiple disciplines.
Related titles: Online - full text ed.: (from ScienceDirect).
Indexed: e-psyche.
—BLDSC (3292.893000).
Published by: University of Missouri at Columbia, Department of Computer Engineering and Computer Science, 201 Engineering Building West, Columbia, MO 65211. TEL 573-884-7662, FAX 573-882-8318, rsun@cecs.missouri.edu, http://www.cecs.missouri.edu. Ed. Ron Sun. R&P, Adv. contact Wilma Wezenbeek.

378.17 USA ISSN 0897-5264
LB2343
JOURNAL OF COLLEGE STUDENT DEVELOPMENT. Text in English. 1959. bi-m. USD 45 in North America; USD 55 elsewhere. adv. bk.rev. abstr, illus. index. reprint service avail. from PQC,SCH,PSC. *Refereed.* **Document type:** *Academic/Scholarly.* **Description:** In-depth coverage of topics such as student psychosocial and cognitive development, needs of special student populations and career planning.
Formerly (until 1987): Journal of College Student Personnel (0021-9789)
Related titles: Microform ed.: (from PQC); Online - full text ed.: (from ProQuest Information & Learning, Institute for Scientific Information).
Indexed: ASCA, AgeLine, C.I.J.E., Chic.Per.Ind., Cont.Pg.Educ., Curr.Cont., ERA, Educ.Admin.Abstr., Educ.Ind. (Mar.1983-Nov.1987), Fam.Ind., High.Educ.Abstr., Mult.Ed.Abstr., PSI, PsycInfo, Psychol.Abstr. (1965-), SSCI, Soc.Work Res.& Abstr., Sp.Ed.Needs Abstr., Tech.Educ.Abstr., e-psyche.
—BLDSC (4958.816000), ingenta.
Published by: American College Personnel Association, One Dupont Circle, N W, Ste 300, Washington, DC 20036-1110. TEL 202-835-2272, FAX 202-296-3286, info@acpa.nche.edu, http://www.acpa.nche.edu/pubs/public.htm. Ed. Gregory Blimling. R&P John Salzman. Circ: 8,000 (paid).

616.8914 378.3 USA ISSN 8756-8225
RC451.4.S7
JOURNAL OF COLLEGE STUDENT PSYCHOTHERAPY. Text in English. 1986. q. USD 60 to individuals; USD 81 in Canada to individuals; USD 87 elsewhere to individuals; USD 95 to institutions; USD 128 in Canada to institutions; USD 138 elsewhere to institutions; USD 400 to libraries; USD 540 in Canada to libraries; USD 580 elsewhere to libraries (effective Aug. 2001). adv. bk.rev. back issues avail.; reprint service avail. from HAW. *Refereed.* **Document type:** *Journal, Academic/Scholarly.* **Description:** Enhances the lives of college and university students by stimulating high-quality practice theory, and research in mental and personal development.
Related titles: Microfiche ed.: (from PQC); Microform ed.
Indexed: ASSIA, C.I.J.E. (coverage dropped), Cont.Pg.Educ., ERA, Educ.Admin.Abstr., High.Educ.Abstr., IMFL, Lang.& Lang.Behav.Abstr., Mult.Ed.Abstr., PsycInfo, Psychol.Abstr. (1986-), SOPODA, Sage Fam.Stud.Abstr., Sage Pub.Admin.Abstr., Soc.Serv.Abstr., Soc.Work Res.& Abstr., Sociol.Abstr., Sociol.Educ.Abstr., Sp.Ed.Needs Abstr., Stud.Wom.Abstr., Tech.Educ.Abstr., e-psyche.
—BLDSC (4958.830000), GNLM, Haworth, ingenta.
Published by: Haworth Press, Inc., 10 Alice St, Binghamton, NY 13904-1580. TEL 607-722-5857, 800-429-6784, FAX 607-722-6362, 800-895-0582, getinfo@haworthpressinc.com, http://www.haworthpress.com/journals/journallist.asp. Ed. Leighton C Whitaker. Pub. William Cohen. R&P Ruthann Heath TEL 607-723-5857 ext 316. Adv. contact Jackie Blakeslee TEL 607-722-5857 ext 346. B&W page USD 315, color page USD 550; trim 6 x 8.5. Circ: 630.

617.8 USA ISSN 0021-9924
RC423.A1 CODEN: JCDIAI
JOURNAL OF COMMUNICATION DISORDERS. Text in English. 1968. bi-m. EUR 209 in Europe to individuals; JPY 27,800 in Japan to individuals; USD 234 elsewhere to individuals; EUR 562 in Europe to institutions; JPY 74,600 in Japan to institutions; USD 629 elsewhere to institutions (effective 2002). adv. bk.rev. charts, illus. reprint service avail. from SWZ,PSC,SCH. *Refereed.* **Document type:** *Journal, Academic/Scholarly.* **Description:** Provides up-to-date information on clinical and research advances in a wide range of hearing and speech disorders.
Incorporates (1991-1994): Clinics in Communication Disorders (1054-8505)
Related titles: Microform ed.: (from PQC); Online - full text ed.: (from ingenta, ScienceDirect, Swets Blackwell, Institute for Scientific Information).
Indexed: AMED, ASCA, ASSIA, AgeLine, Bibl.Dev.Med.& Child Neur., Biol.Abstr., C.I.J.E., CINAHL, Curr.Cont., DSH Abstr., Dent.Ind., Except.Child Educ.Abstr., Excerp.Med., Fam.Ind., INIS Atomind., Ind.Med. (1967-), Lang.& Lang.Behav.Abstr. (1977-), Mid.East: Abstr.& Ind., PsycInfo, Psychol.Abstr. (1967-), Rehabil.Lit., SOPODA, SSCI, Sociol.Abstr., Yrbk.Assoc.Educ.& Rehab.Blind, e-psyche.
—BLDSC (4961.600000), GNLM, IDS, Infotrieve, ingenta. **CCC.**

Published by: Elsevier Science, PO Box 945, New York, NY 10159-0945. TEL 212-633-3730, FAX 212-633-3680, TELEX 420643 AEP UI, usinfo-f@elsevier.com, http://www.elsevier.nl/locate/jcomdis, http://www.elsevier.com. Eds. A L Holland, Theodore J Glattke. **Subscr. in Australasia and the Far East to:** Elsevier Science (Singapore) Pte Ltd, No.1 Temasek Ave, 17-01 Millenia Tower, Singapore 039192, Singapore. TEL 65-434-3727, FAX 65-337-2230, asiainfo@elsevier.com.sg; **Subscr. in Japan to:** Elsevier Science Inc - Japan Regional Office, 9-15 Higashi-Azabu 1-chome, Minato-ku, Tokyo 106-0044, Japan. TEL 81-3-5561-5033, FAX 81-3-5561-5047, info@elsevier.co.jp. **Subscr. outside the Americas to:** Elsevier Science BV, PO Box 211, Amsterdam 1000 AE, Netherlands. TEL 31-20-485-3757, FAX 31-20-485-3432, nlinfo-f@elsevier.nl.; **Dist. by:** Elsevier Science (Brazil).

302 150 GBR ISSN 1052-9284
HM251 CODEN: JLCPEX

JOURNAL OF COMMUNITY AND APPLIED SOCIAL PSYCHOLOGY. Text in English. 1986. bi-m. USD 630 in United States; USD 630 in Canada & Mexico; USD 630 elsewhere; USD 662 combined subscription in United States for print and online eds.; USD 662 combined subscription in Canada & Mexico for print and online eds.; USD 662 combined subscription elsewhere for print and online eds. (effective 2002). adv. back issues avail.; reprint service avail. from SWZ. *Refereed.* **Document type:** *Academic/Scholarly.* **Description:** Fosters international communication among those concerned with the social psychological analysis and critical understanding of community issues and problems and to develop this understanding in the context of proposals for intervention and social policy.

Formerly (until 1990): Social Behaviour (0885-6249)

Related titles: Microform ed.: (from PQC); Online - full text ed.: ISSN 1099-1298. 1996. USD 630 in United States; USD 630 in Canada & Mexico; USD 630 elsewhere (effective 2002) (from EBSCO Publishing, Wiley InterScience, Institute for Scientific Information).

Indexed: ASCA, ASSIA, AgeLine, Crim.Just.Abstr., Curr.Cont., ERA, Fam.Ind., IBZ, Ind.Philos., Intl.Bibl.Soc.Sci., Lang.& Lang.Behav.Abstr., Mult.Ed.Abstr., PsycInfo, Psychol.Abstr. (1987-), Russ.Acad.Sci.Bibl., SOPODA, SSCI, Soc.Serv.Abstr., Sociol.Abstr., Stud.Wom.Abstr., e-psyche.

—BLDSC (4961.693000), IDS, ingenta. **CCC.**

Published by: Wiley Europe Ltd., Baffins Ln, Chichester, W Sussex PO19 1UD, United Kingdom. TEL 44-1243-779777, FAX 44-1243-775878, customer@wiley.co.uk, http://www.wiley.co.uk. adv.: B&W page GBP 650, color page GBP 1,550; trim 165 x 248. Circ: 400. **Subscr. in the Americas to:** John Wiley & Sons, Inc., Journals, 605 Third Ave, New York, NY 10158. TEL 212-850-6021, 212-850-6645, subinfo@jwiley.com.

302 USA ISSN 0090-4392
RC467 CODEN: JCPSD9

JOURNAL OF COMMUNITY PSYCHOLOGY. Text in English. 1973. bi-m. USD 360 in United States; USD 408 in Canada & Mexico; USD 408 elsewhere; USD 378 combined subscription in United States for print and online eds.; USD 426 combined subscription in Canada & Mexico for print and online eds.; USD 426 combined subscription elsewhere for print and online eds. (effective 2002). adv. index. back issues avail.; reprint service avail. from PSC,SCH. *Refereed.* **Document type:** *Academic/Scholarly.* **Description:** Devoted to research, evaluation, assessment, and intervention, and review articles that deal with human behavior in community settings. For psychologists, psychiatrists, social workers, counselors and mental health professionals.

Related titles: Microform ed.: (from PQC); Online - full text ed.: ISSN 1520-6629. 1996. USD 360 in United States; USD 360 in Canada & Mexico; USD 360 elsewhere (effective 2002) (from EBSCO Publishing, Wiley InterScience, Institute for Scientific Information).

Indexed: ASCA, Adol.Ment.Hlth.Abstr., AgeLine, Chic.Per.Ind., Commun.Abstr., Crim.Just.Abstr., Curr.Cont., Fam.Ind., IMFL, INIS Atomind., Lang.& Lang.Behav.Abstr., Mid.East: Abstr.& Ind., PSI, PsycInfo, Psychol.Abstr. (1973-), SSCI, Sage Pub.Admin.Abstr., Sage Race Rel.Abstr., THA, e-psyche.

—BLDSC (4961.750000), IDS, ingenta. **CCC.**

Published by: John Wiley & Sons, Inc., Journals (Subsidiary of: Wiley InterScience), 605 Third Ave, New York, NY 10158. TEL 212-850-6645, FAX 212-850-6021, subinfo@wiley.com, uscs-wis@wiley.com, http://www.wiley.com. Ed. Dr. Raymond P Lorion. adv.: B&W page GBP 640, color page GBP 1,515; trim 172 x 254. Circ: 820. **Subscr. outside the Americas to:** John Wiley & Sons Ltd., Baffins Ln, Chichester, Sussex PO19 IUD, United Kingdom. TEL 44-1243-779777, FAX 44-1243-843232, cs-journals@wiley.co.uk, http://www.wiley.co.uk.

156 USA ISSN 0735-7036
BF1 CODEN: JCOPDT

JOURNAL OF COMPARATIVE PSYCHOLOGY. Text in English. 1947. q. USD 61 domestic to non-members; USD 76 foreign to non-members; USD 31 domestic to members; USD 41 foreign to members; USD 144 domestic to institutions; USD 176 foreign to institutions (effective 2001). adv. charts, illus. index. reprint service avail. from PQC,PSC,SCH. *Refereed.* **Document type:** *Academic/Scholarly.* **Description:** Laboratory and field studies of the behavioral patterns of various species as they relate to evolution, development, ecology, control and functional significance.

Supersedes in part (in 1983): Journal of Comparative and Physiological Psychology (0021-9940)

Related titles: Microform ed.: (from PQC); Online - full text ed.: (from Gale Group, Factiva, Institute for Scientific Information).

Indexed: ASCA, Abstr.Anthropol., Adol.Ment.Hlth.Abstr., Anim.Breed.Abstr., Biol.& Agr.Ind. (Mar.1983-), Biol.Abstr., Chem.Abstr., Curr.Cont., Ecol.Abstr., INIS Atomind., Ind.Med. (1983-), Ind.Sci.Rev., Inpharma, Neurosci.Cit.Ind., P C I, PsycInfo, Psychol.Abstr. (1926-), Reac., Russ.Acad.Sci.Bibl., SSCI, Sci.Cit.Ind., Soc.Sci.Ind. (Mar.1983-), Zoo.Rec., e-psyche.

—BLDSC (4963.300000), CASDDS, CISTI, GNLM, IDS, ingenta. **CCC.**

Published by: American Psychological Association, 750 First St., N.E., Washington, DC 20002-4242. TEL 202-336-5600, 800-374-2721, FAX 202-336-5568, subscriptions@apa.org, http://www.apa.org/journals/com.html. Eds. Ed Diener, Meredith J West. Circ: 1,400.

153 500 GBR ISSN 1355-8250
BF309

JOURNAL OF CONSCIOUSNESS STUDIES; controversies in science & the humanities. Text in English. 1994. m. GBP 62, USD 96 to individuals (effective 2001 & 2002); GBP 146, USD 226 to institutions (effective 2001); GBP 160.50, USD 248.50 to institutions; GBP 9.50, USD 14.50 newsstand/cover to individuals; USD 22, USD 35 newsstand/cover to institutions (effective 2002). adv. bk.rev. back issues avail. *Refereed.* **Document type:** *Academic/Scholarly.* **Description:** Publishes original scholarship and reviews in the new field of consciousness research, integrating developments in the sciences and humanities.

Related titles: Online - full text ed.: (from Institute for Scientific Information).

Indexed: Arts & Hum.Cit.Ind., Curr.Cont., PsycInfo, SSCI, e-psyche.

—BLDSC (4965.160000), Infotrieve, ingenta. **CCC.**

Published by: Imprint Academic, PO Box 1, Thorverton, Devon EXS 5YX, United Kingdom. TEL 44-1392-841600, FAX 44-1392-841478, sandra@imprint.co.uk, http://www.imprint.co.uk. Ed. Joseph Goguen. Pub. Keith Sutherland. R&P Sandra Good. Adv. contact Anthony Freeman. page GBP 250, page USD 400. Circ: 2,500 (paid).

155 USA ISSN 1072-0537
BF698.9.P47 CODEN: JCPYES

JOURNAL OF CONSTRUCTIVIST PSYCHOLOGY. Text in English. 1988. q. GBP 87, USD 143 to individuals; GBP 182, USD 300 to institutions (effective 2002). reprint service avail. from PQC. *Refereed.* **Document type:** *Academic/Scholarly.* **Description:** Presents empirical research, conceptual analyses, critical reviews, case studies on personal construct theory and related approaches to psychology.

Formerly (until 1994): International Journal of Personal Construct Psychology (0893-603X)

Related titles: Microform ed.: (from PQC); Online - full text ed.: ISSN 1521-0650 (from CatchWord Ltd., EBSCO Publishing, O C L C Online Computer Library Center, Inc., RoweCom Information Quest, Swets Blackwell, Institute for Scientific Information).

Indexed: ASCA, Curr.Cont., PsycInfo, Psychol.Abstr. (1988-), SSCI, e-psyche.

—BLDSC (4965.194000), CatchWord, IDS, Infotrieve. **CCC.**

Published by: Taylor & Francis Ltd. (Subsidiary of: Taylor & Francis Group), 325 Chestnut St, Suite 800, Philadelphia, PA 19016. TEL 215-625-8900, FAX 215-625-2940, info@taylorandfrancis.com, http://www.taylorandfrancis.com/. Eds. Greg J Neimeyer, Robert A Neimeyer. **Subscr. addr. in Europe:** Taylor & Francis Group, Journals Customer Service, Rankine Rd, Basingstoke, Hants RG24 8PR, United Kingdom. TEL 44-1256-813000, FAX 44-1256-479438, enquiry@tanf.co.uk, http://www.tandf.co.uk/journals.

158.3 USA ISSN 0022-006X
BF1 CODEN: JCLPBC

JOURNAL OF CONSULTING AND CLINICAL PSYCHOLOGY. Text in English. 1937. bi-m. USD 183 domestic to non-members; USD 203 foreign to non-members; USD 92 domestic to members; USD 104 foreign to members; USD 408 domestic to institutions; USD 452 foreign to institutions (effective 2001). adv. bibl, charts, illus. index. reprint service avail. from PSC,PQC,SCH. *Refereed.* **Document type:** *Academic/Scholarly.* **Description:** Research on techniques of diagnosis and treatment in disordered behavior as well as studies of populations of clinical interest.

Formerly (until 1967): Journal of Consulting Psychology (0095-8891)

Related titles: Microform ed.: (from PQC,PMC); Online - full text ed.: (from Gale Group, Factiva, Institute for Scientific Information).

Indexed: AMED, ASCA, ASSIA, Abstr.Crim.& Pen., Acad.Ind., Addic.Abstr., Adol.Ment.Hlth.Abstr., AgeLine, Behav.Med.Abstr., Biol.Abstr., C.I.J.E. (coverage dropped), Commun.Abstr., Crim.Just.Abstr., Curr.Cont., Curr.Ind.Stat., Dok.Arbeitsmed., Except.Child Educ.Abstr., Excerp.Med., Fam.Ind., Hlth.Ind., IBR, INIS Atomind., Ind.Med. (1968-), Jrnl.Watch Psych., Mid.East: Abstr.& Ind., Mult.Ed.Abstr., P C I, Peace Res.Abstr., PsycInfo, Psychol.Abstr. (1937-), Psycscan C.P., Risk Abstr., Russ.Acad.Sci.Bibl., SSCI, Sage Fam.Stud.Abstr., Soc.Sci.Ind. (Aug.1982-), Soc.Work Res.& Abstr., Sp.Ed.Needs Abstr., THA, Viol.& Abuse Abstr., e-psyche.

—BLDSC (4965.195000), CISTI, GNLM, IDS, ingenta, KNAW. **CCC.**

Published by: American Psychological Association, 750 First St., N.E., Washington, DC 20002-4242. TEL 202-336-5600, 800-374-2721, FAX 202-336-5568, subscriptions@apa.org, http://www.apa.org/journals/ccp.html. Ed. Philip C Kendall. Circ: 7,800.

JOURNAL OF CONSUMER PSYCHOLOGY. see *ADVERTISING AND PUBLIC RELATIONS*

JOURNAL OF CONSUMER SATISFACTION, DISSATISFACTION AND COMPLAINING BEHAVIOR. see *BUSINESS AND ECONOMICS—Marketing And Purchasing*

JOURNAL OF CONTEMPLATIVE PSYCHOTHERAPY. see *MEDICAL SCIENCES—Psychiatry And Neurology*

616.89 USA ISSN 0022-0116
RC475 CODEN: JCPTBA

JOURNAL OF CONTEMPORARY PSYCHOTHERAPY. Text in English. 1970. q. USD 441, EUR 441 to institutions for print or online ed.; USD 529.20, EUR 529.20 to institutions for print & online eds.combined (effective 2002). adv. bk.rev. bibl, charts. reprint service avail. from PQC,PSC,SCH,ISI. *Refereed.* **Document type:** *Journal, Academic/Scholarly.* **Description:** Presents progressive research and clinical papers covering advances in psychotherapeutic concepts and methodology. Offers an eclectic approach to the promotion of emotional health and maturity.

Related titles: Microfilm ed.: (from PQC); Online - full text ed.: (from EBSCO Publishing, O C L C Online Computer Library Center, Inc., Swets Blackwell, Kluwer Online, RoweCom Information Quest).

Indexed: Excerp.Med., IMFL, Mid.East: Abstr.& Ind., PsycInfo, Psychol.Abstr. (1968-), Ref.Zh., Rehabil.Lit., SSCI (coverage dropped), Soc.Work Res.& Abstr., e-psyche.

—BLDSC (4965.240000), CISTI, GNLM, ingenta. **CCC.**

Published by: Kluwer Academic - Plenum Publishers (Subsidiary of: Wolters Kluwer N.V.), 233 Spring St, New York, NY 10013-1578. TEL 212-620-8000, 800-221-9369, FAX 212-463-0742, info@plenum.com, http://www.wkap.nl/journalhome.htm/0022-0116. Ed. Ira Moses. **Subscr. outside the Americas to:** Kluwer Academic Publishers Group, Journals Department, PO Box 322, Dordrecht 3300 AH, Netherlands. TEL 31-78-639-2392, FAX 31-78-654-6474.

371.4 USA ISSN 0748-9633
HF5381.A1
JOURNAL OF COUNSELING & DEVELOPMENT. Text in English. 1922. q. USD 138 to institutions (effective 2001). adv. abstr, bibl, illus. index. 128 p./no. back issues avail.; reprint service avail. from PSC,SCH,PQC. *Refereed.* **Document type:** *Journal, Academic/Scholarly.* **Description:** Publishes archival materials and contains authoritative in-depth articles on professional and scientific issues, research of interest to practitioners, and new techniques or practices.
Formerly (until 1984): Personnel and Guidance Journal (0031-5737)
Related titles: CD-ROM ed.; Microform ed.: (from PQC); Online - full text ed.: (from Factiva, Institute for Scientific Information, H. W. Wilson); Cumulative ed.: 1999. USD 295 to non-members; USD 195 to members; USD 495 for multiple user license (effective 2001) (from ProQuest Information & Learning, Northern Light Technology, Inc., Gale Group).
Indexed: ABI Inform. (Oct.1971-Jun.1975), ASSIA, Acad.Ind., AgeLine, Bk.Rev.Ind. (1965-1984, 1986-1987), C.I.J.E., Chic.Per.Ind., Child.Bk.Rev.Ind. (1965-1984, 1986-1987), Curr.Cont., Educ.Admin.Abstr., Educ.Ind. (Oct.1982-Jun.1984), Except.Child Educ.Abstr., High.Educ.Abstr., Hlth.Ind., Human Resour.Abstr., Mag.Ind., Mult.Ed.Abstr., P C I, Past.Care & Couns.Abstr., Psycinfo, Psychol.Abstr. (1952-), Psycscan A.P., Rehabil.Lit., Rel.Ind.One, Rel.Ind.Two, Res.High.Educ.Abstr., Risk Abstr., Russ.Acad.Sci.Bibl., SOMA, SSCI, Sage Fam.Stud.Abstr., Sage Pub.Admin.Abstr., Soc.Sci.Ind. (Jul.1999-), Soc.Work Res.& Abstr., Sp.Ed.Needs Abstr., Work Rel.Abstr., e-psyche.
—BLDSC (4965.445000), IDS, ingenta. **CCC.**
Published by: American Counseling Association, 5999 Stevenson Ave, Alexandria, VA 22304-3300. TEL 703-823-9800, FAX 703-823-0252, http://www.counseling.org, http://www.ncda.org. Ed. Earl Ginter. Pub. Carolyn Baker. R&P Cynthia Peay TEL 703-823-9800 x 249. Adv. contact Kathy Maguire TEL 703-823-9800 ext 207. Circ: 55,000 (paid).

150 371.4 USA ISSN 0022-0167
BF637.C6
JOURNAL OF COUNSELING PSYCHOLOGY. Text in English. 1954. q. USD 76 domestic to non-members; USD 91 foreign to non-members; USD 38 domestic to members; USD 48 foreign to members; USD 170 domestic to institutions; USD 202 foreign to institutions (effective 2001). adv. bk.rev. bibl, charts, illus. index. reprint service avail. from PQC,PSC,SCH. *Refereed.* **Document type:** *Academic/Scholarly.* **Description:** Empirical studies about counseling processes and interventions, theoretical articles about counseling, and studies dealing with evaluation of counseling applications and programs.
Related titles: Microform ed.: (from PQC); Online - full text ed.: (from Gale Group, Factiva, Institute for Scientific Information).
Indexed: ABI Inform. (May 1971-Jul.1975), ASCA, ASSIA, Abstr.Crim.& Pen., Addic.Abstr., Adol.Ment.Hlth.Abstr., AgeLine, Bk.Rev.Ind. (1965-1979), C.I.J.E., Chic.Per.Ind., Child Devel.Abstr., Child.Bk.Rev.Ind. (1965-1979), Crim.Just.Abstr., Curr.Cont., ERA, Educ.Ind. (Jul.1983-), Fam.Ind., High.Educ.Abstr., Ind.Philos., Mid.East: Abstr.& Ind., Mult.Ed.Abstr., Psycinfo, Psychol.Abstr. (1954-), Psycscan C.P., Rehabil.Lit., Res.High.Educ.Abstr., Russ.Acad.Sci.Bibl., SSCI, Sage Fam.Stud.Abstr., Sage Race Rel.Abstr., Soc.Sci.Ind. (Sep.1982-), Soc.Work Res.& Abstr., Sp.Ed.Needs Abstr., Stud.Wom.Abstr., Tech.Educ.Abstr., e-psyche.
—BLDSC (4965.450000), IDS, ingenta. **CCC.**
Published by: American Psychological Association, 750 First St., N.E., Washington, DC 20002-4242. TEL 202-336-5600, 800-374-2721, FAX 202-336-5568, subscriptions@apa.org, http://www.apa.org/journals/cou.html. Ed. Jo-Ida Hansen. Circ: 8,900.

616.89 USA ISSN 1533-2691
RC488.5 CODEN: JCTHEV
▼ **JOURNAL OF COUPLE & RELATIONSHIP THERAPY.** Text in English. 2001 (Spr.). q. USD 60 domestic to individuals; USD 81 in Canada to individuals; USD 87 elsewhere to individuals; USD 95 domestic to institutions; USD 128 in Canada to institutions; USD 138 elsewhere to institutions; USD 250 domestic to libraries; USD 338 in Canada to libraries; USD 363 elsewhere to libraries (effective Aug. 2001). adv. bk.rev. reprint service avail. from HAW. *Refereed.* **Document type:** *Journal, Academic/Scholarly.* **Description:** Deals with the study of human bonding and intimacy for couples, therapists, marriage, family and clinical practitioners.
Formerly (until 2001): Journal of Couples Therapy (0897-4446)
Related titles: Microfiche ed.: (from PQC); Microform ed.
Indexed: Crim.Just.Abstr., Fam.Ind., IMFL, Lang.& Lang.Behav.Abstr., Ref.Zh., SOPODA, Sage Fam.Stud.Abstr., Soc.Serv.Abstr., Soc.Work Res.& Abstr., Sociol.Abstr., Stud.Wom.Abstr., e-psyche.
—GNLM, Haworth, ingenta.
Published by: Haworth Press, Inc., 10 Alice St, Binghamton, NY 13904-1580. TEL 607-722-5857, 800-429-6784, FAX 607-722-6362, 800-895-0582, getinfo@haworthpressinc.com, http://www.haworthpress.com/journals/journallist.asp. Ed. Joseph L. Wetchler. Pub. William Cohen. R&P Ruthann Heath TEL 607-723-5857 ext 316. Adv. contact Jackie Blakeslee TEL 607-722-5857 ext 346. B&W page USD 315, color page USD 550; trim 6 x 8.5.

THE JOURNAL OF CREATIVE BEHAVIOR. see *EDUCATION*

155 USA ISSN 1088-0755
JOURNAL OF CREDIBILITY ASSESSMENT AND WITNESS PSYCHOLOGY. Text in English. 1997. bi-m.?. **Document type:** *Academic/Scholarly.* **Description:** Features original empirical, review, and theoretical work in all areas of the scientific study of credibility assessment and witness psychology.
Media: Online - full text.
Indexed: e-psyche.
Address: honts@truth.idbsu.edu, http://truth.idbsu.edu/jcaawp/.

155.8 USA ISSN 0022-0221
BF728 CODEN: JCPGB5
JOURNAL OF CROSS-CULTURAL PSYCHOLOGY. Text in English. 1970. bi-m. USD 80 to individuals; USD 410 to institutions; USD 20 newsstand/cover to individuals; USD 70 newsstand/cover to institutions (effective 2002). adv. bk.rev. charts, illus. cum.index. back issues avail.; reprint service avail. from PQC,PSC,SCH. *Refereed.* **Document type:** *Journal, Academic/Scholarly.* **Description:** Presents behavioral and social research concentrating on psychological phenomena as differentially conditioned by culture, focusing on individual members of cultural groups.
Related titles: Microfilm ed.: (from PQC); Online - full text ed.: (from EBSCO Publishing, ProQuest Information & Learning, Gale Group, ingenta, Swets Blackwell, Institute for Scientific Information, RoweCom Information Quest).
Indexed: ASCA, ASSIA, Abstr.Anthropol., Abstr.Crim.& Pen., Adol.Ment.Hlth.Abstr., AgeLine, Amer.Bibl.Slavic & E.Eur.Stud., Arts & Hum.Cit.Ind. (coverage dropped), Bibl.Asian Stud. (1970-1991), C.I.J.E., Chic.Per.Ind., Child Devel.Abstr., Commun.Abstr., Curr.Cont., Fam.Ind., Human Resour.Abstr., IBZ, Ind.Philos., Indian Psychol.Abstr., Lang.& Lang.Behav.Abstr., Mid.East: Abstr.& Ind., Mult.Ed.Abstr., Peace Res.Abstr., Psycinfo, Psychol.Abstr. (1970-), Psychol.R.G., SOPODA, SSCI, Sage Fam.Stud.Abstr., Soc.Sci.Ind. (Jan.1994-), Soc.Serv.Abstr., Sociol.Abstr., Stud.Wom.Abstr., Viol.& Abuse Abstr., e-psyche.
—BLDSC (4965.670000), IDS. **CCC.**
Published by: (International Association for Cross-Cultural Psychology), Sage Publications, Inc., 2455 Teller Rd, Thousand Oaks, CA 91320. TEL 805-499-0721, FAX 805-499-0871, info@sagepub.com, http://www.fit.edu/CampusLife/clubs-org/iaccp/JCCP/jccp.html, http://www.sagepub.com. Ed. Fons Van de Vijver. Pub. Sara Miller McCune. R&P Tanya Udin. Adv. contact DeAnna Vega Hammersley. Circ: 2,000. **Overseas subscr. to:** Sage Publications Ltd., 6 Bonhill St, London EC2A 4PU, United Kingdom; Sage Publications India Pvt. Ltd., 4215, New Delhi 110 048, India. **Co-sponsor:** Western Washington University, Center for Cross-Cultural Research.

JOURNAL OF DEVELOPMENTAL AND BEHAVIORAL PEDIATRICS. see *MEDICAL SCIENCES—Pediatrics*

150 USA ISSN 1533-2802
▼ **JOURNAL OF DIAGNOSIS & ASSESSMENT IN MENTAL HEALTH.** Text in English. 2002. q. USD 48 to individuals; USD 65 in Canada to individuals; USD 70 elsewhere to individuals; USD 65 to institutions; USD 88 in Canada to institutions; USD 94 elsewhere to institutions; USD 75 to libraries; USD 101 in Canada to libraries; USD 109 elsewhere to libraries (effective Aug. 2001). adv. **Document type:** *Journal, Academic/Scholarly.* **Description:** Designed to meet the needs of both clinical social workers relatively new to diagnosis and assessment as well as the seasoned practitioner and diagnostician.
Published by: Haworth Press, Inc., 10 Alice St, Binghamton, NY 13904-1580. TEL 607-722-5857, 800-429-6784, FAX 607-722-6362, 800-895-0582, getinfo@haworthpressinc.com, http://www.haworthpress.com/journals/journallist.asp. Ed. Carlton E Munson. Pub. William Cohen. R&P Ruthann Heath TEL 607-723-5857 ext 316. Adv. contact Jackie Blakeslee TEL 607-722-5857 ext 346. B&W page USD 315, color page USD 550; trim 6 x 8.5.

JOURNAL OF EARLY ADOLESCENCE. see *CHILDREN AND YOUTH—About*

THE JOURNAL OF ECONOMIC PSYCHOLOGY. see *BUSINESS AND ECONOMICS—Marketing And Purchasing*

JOURNAL OF EDUCATION AND PSYCHOLOGY. see *EDUCATION*

JOURNAL OF EDUCATIONAL AND PSYCHOLOGICAL CONSULTATION. see *EDUCATION*

JOURNAL OF EDUCATIONAL PSYCHOLOGY. see *EDUCATION*

152.4 158.2 USA ISSN 1092-6798
RC569.5.P75 CODEN: JEABFZ
JOURNAL OF EMOTIONAL ABUSE; interventions, research & theories of psychological maltreatment, trauma & nonphysical aggression. Text in English. 1998. q. USD 45 to individuals; USD 61 in Canada to individuals; USD 65 elsewhere to individuals; USD 85 to institutions; USD 115 in Canada to institutions; USD 123 elsewhere to institutions; USD 95 to libraries; USD 128 in Canada to libraries; USD 138 elsewhere to libraries (effective Aug. 2001). adv. back issues avail.; reprint service avail. from HAW. **Document type:** *Journal, Academic/Scholarly.* **Description:** Focuses on nonphysical aggression, intimidation and harassment in the family, in the school, and in the workplace.
Related titles: Microform ed.
Indexed: Child Devel.Abstr., Environ.Sci.Poll.Mgmt., IBZ, Pollut.Abstr., Ref.Zh., Risk Abstr., Saf.Sci.Abstr., Soc.Serv.Abstr., Soc.Work Res.& Abstr., Sociol.Abstr., Stud.Wom.Abstr., e-psyche.
—BLDSC (4977.460000), Haworth.
Published by: Haworth Press, Inc., 10 Alice St, Binghamton, NY 13904-1580. TEL 607-722-5857, 800-429-6784, FAX 607-722-6362, 800-895-0582, getinfo@haworthpressinc.com, http://www.haworthpress.com/journals/journallist.asp. Eds. Marti Loring, Robert A Geffner. Pub. William Cohen. R&P Ruthann Heath TEL 607-723-5857 ext 316. Adv. contact Jackie Blakeslee TEL 607-722-5857 ext 346. B&W page USD 315, color page USD 550; trim 6 x 8.5.

371.42 USA ISSN 0022-0787
HF5382.5.U5 CODEN: JECODE
JOURNAL OF EMPLOYMENT COUNSELING. Text in English. 1965. q. USD 40 to non-members (effective 2001). adv. bk.rev. illus, abstr, bibl. index. 64 p./no. back issues avail.; reprint service avail. from PQC. *Refereed.* **Document type:** *Journal, Academic/Scholarly.* **Description:** Focuses on trends in organizational behavior and state-of-the-art personnel practices.
Related titles: Microform ed.: (from PQC); Online - full text ed.: (from Northern Light Technology, Inc., ProQuest Information & Learning, Institute for Scientific Information, H. W. Wilson).
Indexed: ASCA, ASSIA, AgeLine, BPIA, C.I.J.E., Curr.Cont., ERA, Educ.Ind. (Dec.2000-), Fam.Ind., High.Educ.Abstr., Int.Lab.Doc., Psycinfo, Psychol.Abstr. (1969-), SSCI, Sage Fam.Stud.Abstr., Soc.Work Res.& Abstr., e-psyche.
—BLDSC (4977.700000), IDS, ingenta. **CCC.**
Published by: (National Employment Counselors Association), American Counseling Association, 5999 Stevenson Ave, Alexandria, VA 22304-3300. TEL 703-823-9800, FAX 703-823-0252, http://www.geocities.com/Athens/Acropolis/6491/neca.html, http://www.ncda.org. Ed. Norman E Amundson. R&P Cynthia Peay TEL 703-823-9800 x 249. Adv. contact Kathy Maguire TEL 703-823-9800 ext 207. Circ: 1,700.

150 GBR ISSN 0272-4944
BF353 CODEN: JEPSEO
JOURNAL OF ENVIRONMENTAL PSYCHOLOGY. Text in English. 1980. q. GBP 160 to institutions (effective 2001). adv. bk.rev. illus. reprint service avail. from SWZ. *Refereed.* **Document type:** *Academic/Scholarly.* **Description:** Publishes international research contributions in a broad range of disciplines relating to the study of the transactions and interrelationships between people and their sociophysical surroundings (including man-made and natural environments), as well as relevant applications to the social and biological sciences and the environmental professions.
Related titles: Online - full text ed.: (from EBSCO Publishing, O C L C Online Computer Library Center, Inc., RoweCom Information Quest, ingenta, Swets Blackwell, IDEAL Online Library, Institute for Scientific Information).
Indexed: ASCA, ASSIA, AgeLine, Art.Hosp.& Tour., Br.Tech.Ind., Crim.Just.Abstr., Curr.Cont., Environ.Sci.Poll.Mgmt., Ergon.Abstr., Ind.Philos., Indian Psychol.Abstr., Pollut.Abstr., PsycInfo, Psychol.Abstr. (1981-), Psycscan A.P., Risk Abstr., Russ.Acad.Sci.Bibl., SSCI, Sage Fam.Stud.Abstr., Sage Urb.Stud.Abstr., e-psyche.
—BLDSC (4979.389000), CISTI, IDS, ingenta. **CCC.**
Published by: Academic Press (Subsidiary of: Harcourt Publishers Ltd.), 24 Oval Rd, London NW1 7DX, United Kingdom. TEL 44-20-7267-4466, FAX 44-20-7482-2293, apsubs@acad.com, http://www.academicpress.com/jcp; http://www.europe.idealibrary.com/. Ed. David V Canter. R&P Catherine John. Adv. contact Nik Screen. **Subscr. to:** Harcourt Publishers Ltd., Foots Cray High St, Sidcup, Kent DA14 5HP, United Kingdom. TEL 44-20-8300-3322, FAX 44-20-8309-0807.

150 USA ISSN 0737-4828
PN56.P93
JOURNAL OF EVOLUTIONARY PSYCHOLOGY. Text in English. 1979. s-a. USD 12 domestic; USD 14 foreign (effective 2000). film rev., play rev. 130 p./no. *Refereed.* **Document type:** *Academic/Scholarly.* **Description:** Presents psychological interpretation of literature, art, film and poetry.
Related titles: CD-ROM ed.
Indexed: M.L.A., MLA Intl.Bibl., e-psyche.
—BLDSC (4979.643000).
Published by: Institute for Evolutionary Psychology, 4625 Fifth Ave, Apt 605, Pittsburgh, PA 15213-3644. TEL 412-621-7057. Ed. Paul Neumarkt. Circ: 200.

158 CAN ISSN 1496-9955
JOURNAL OF EXCELLENCE. Text in English. 1998. s-a. CND 44.95 domestic to individuals; USD 34.95 foreign to individuals; CND 149.99 domestic to institutions; USD 99.99 foreign to institutions (effective 2001). abstr, bibl, charts, stat. back issues avail. *Refereed.* **Document type:** *Journal, Consumer.* **Description:** Devoted to nurturing excellence in all human endeavors including sport, performing arts, education, the work place, health and quality living. The goal is education for better people, better performers and a better world.
Related titles: Online - full content ed.
Published by: (International Society for Mental Training and Excellence USA), Zone of Excellence, PO Box 1807, Chelsea, PQ J9B 1A1, Canada. http://www.%20zoneofexcellence.com/Journal.html. Ed. Louise Zitzelsberger. Pub. Terry Orlick. Circ: 382 (paid); 50 (free).

155.4 152 USA ISSN 0022-0965
BF721 CODEN: JECPAE
JOURNAL OF EXPERIMENTAL CHILD PSYCHOLOGY. Text in English. 1964. m. USD 1,000 in US & Canada to institutions; USD 1,000 elsewhere to institutions (effective 2001). adv. charts, illus. index. back issues avail.; reprint service avail. from PSC,SCH. *Refereed.* **Document type:** *Academic/Scholarly.* **Description:** Covers all aspects of the behavior of children.
Related titles: Online - full text ed.: (from EBSCO Publishing, O C L C Online Computer Library Center, Inc., RoweCom Information Quest, ingenta, Gale Group, Swets Blackwell, IDEAL Online Library, Factiva, Institute for Scientific Information).
Indexed: ASCA, ASSIA, Adol.Ment.Hlth.Abstr., Bibl.Dev.Med.& Child Neur., Biol.Abstr., C.I.J.E., Child Devel.Abstr., Curr.Cont., Curr.Ind.Stat., Educ.Ind. (coverage dropped), Fam.Ind., IBZ, Ind.Med. (1964-), Ind.Philos., MLA Intl.Bibl., Mid.East: Abstr.& Ind., PsycInfo, Psychol.Abstr. (1964-), Psycscan D.P., Russ.Acad.Sci.Bibl., SSCI, Sci.Cit.Ind. (coverage dropped), Soc.Sci.Ind. (Apr.1982-), e-psyche.
—BLDSC (4981.300000), CISTI, GNLM, IDS, ingenta. **CCC.**
Published by: Academic Press, Inc., Journal Division (Subsidiary of: Harcourt Brace & Company), 525 B St, Ste 1900, San Diego, CA 92101-4495. TEL 619-230-1840, FAX 619-699-6800, apsubs@acad.com, http://www.academicpress.com/jecp. Ed. Lynn S Liben.

152 USA ISSN 0097-7403
BF1
JOURNAL OF EXPERIMENTAL PSYCHOLOGY: ANIMAL BEHAVIOR PROCESSES; Animal Behavior Processes. Short title: J E P: A B P. Text in English. 1916. q. USD 76 domestic to non-members; USD 91 foreign to non-members; USD 38 domestic to members; USD 48 foreign to members; USD 170 domestic to institutions; USD 202 foreign to institutions (effective 2001). adv. illus. Index. reprint service avail. from PQC,PSC,SCH. *Refereed.* **Document type:** *Academic/Scholarly.* **Description:** Experimental studies on the basic mechanisms of perception, learning, motivation and performance, especially in nonhuman animals.
Supersedes in part (in 1975): Journal of Experimental Psychology (0022-1015)
Related titles: Microform ed.: (from PQC); Online - full text ed.: (from Gale Group, Institute for Scientific Information).
Indexed: ASCA, Anim.Behav.Abstr., Aqua.Sci.& Fish.Abstr., Biol.Abstr., Child Devel.Abstr., Curr.Cont., IBR, IBZ, Ind.Med. (1975-), Ind.Philos., Ind.Sci.Rev., Inpharma, Neurosci.Abstr., Neurosci.Cit.Ind., PsycInfo, Psychol.Abstr. (1975-), Psycscan B.A.& T., Reac., Russ.Acad.Sci.Bibl., SSCI, Sci.Cit.Ind., Soc.Sci.Ind. (Oct.1982-), Sport Fish.Abstr., Wild.Rev., Zoo.Rec., e-psyche.
—BLDSC (4982.501000), CISTI, IDS, ingenta. **CCC.**
Published by: American Psychological Association, 750 First St., N.E., Washington, DC 20002-4242. TEL 202-336-5600, 800-374-2721, FAX 202-336-5568, subscriptions@apa.org, http://www.apa.org/journals/xan.html. Ed. Mark E Bouton. Circ: 2,000.

152 USA ISSN 1076-898X
BF180
JOURNAL OF EXPERIMENTAL PSYCHOLOGY: APPLIED. Text in English. 1995. q. USD 61 domestic to non-members; USD 76 foreign to non-members; USD 31 domestic to members; USD 41 foreign to members; USD 136 domestic to institutions; USD 168 foreign to institutions (effective 2001). adv. *Refereed.* **Document type:** *Academic/Scholarly.* **Description:** Publishes empirical investigations in experimental psychology that bridge practically oriented problems and psychological theory, focusing on the testing of models of cognitive processing or behavior in applied settings.
Related titles: Online - full text ed.: (from Institute for Scientific Information).
Indexed: ASCA, AgeLine, Curr.Cont., Ergon.Abstr., IBZ, Ind.Med., Ind.Philos., PsycInfo, Psycscan A.P., SSCI, e-psyche.
—BLDSC (4982.501100), IDS, Infotrieve. **CCC.**
Published by: American Psychological Association, 750 First St., N.E., Washington, DC 20002-4242. TEL 202-336-5500, 800-374-2721, FAX 202-336-5568, subscriptions@apa.org, http://www.apa.org/journals/xap.html. Ed. Raymond S Nickerson. Circ: 1,500.

152 USA ISSN 0096-3445
BF1
JOURNAL OF EXPERIMENTAL PSYCHOLOGY: GENERAL. Short title: J E P: GEN. Text in English. 1916. q. USD 61 domestic to non-members; USD 76 foreign to non-members; USD 31 domestic to members; USD 41 foreign to members; USD 144 domestic to institutions; USD 176 foreign to institutions (effective 2001). adv. charts, illus, stat. index. back issues avail.; reprint service avail. from PSC,PQC,SCH. *Refereed.* **Document type:** *Academic/Scholarly.* **Description:** Presents reports of interest to all experimental psychologists.
Supersedes in part (in 1975): Journal of Experimental Psychology (0022-1015)
Related titles: Microform ed.: (from PQC); Online - full text ed.: (from Gale Group, Factiva, Institute for Scientific Information).
Indexed: ASCA, AgeLine, Biol.Abstr., Child Devel.Abstr., Curr.Cont., Curr.Ind.Stat., Ergon.Abstr., Fam.Ind., IBZ, Ind.Med. (1975-), Ind.Philos., Mid.East: Abstr.& Ind., P C I, PsycInfo, Psychol.Abstr. (1926-), Risk Abstr., Russ.Acad.Sci.Bibl., SSCI, Soc.Sci.Ind. (Dec.1982-), Yrbk.Assoc.Educ.& Rehab.Blind, e-psyche.
—BLDSC (4982.503000), CISTI, GNLM, IDS, Infotrieve, ingenta. **CCC.**
Published by: American Psychological Association, 750 First St., N.E., Washington, DC 20002-4242. TEL 202-336-5600, 800-374-2721, FAX 202-336-5568, subscriptions@apa.org, http://www.apa.org/journals/xge.html. Ed. Nora S Newcombe. Circ: 3,100.

152.05 USA ISSN 0096-1523
BF1
JOURNAL OF EXPERIMENTAL PSYCHOLOGY: HUMAN PERCEPTION AND PERFORMANCE. Short title: J E P: H P P. Text in English. 1916. bi-m. USD 244 domestic to non-members; USD 264 foreign to non-members; USD 122 domestic to members; USD 134 foreign to members; USD 509 domestic to institutions; USD 553 foreign to institutions (effective 2001). adv. reprint service avail. from PQC,PSC,SCH. *Refereed.* **Document type:** *Academic/Scholarly.* **Description:** Covers current research in perception, formulation, control of action, and related cognitive processes, articles include research on all sensory modalities, all types of motor behavior, empirical studies of human action, machine and animal research, as well as theoretical notes and commentaries. Areas covered include visual attention, word perception, musical context effects, perceptual integration, taste, and tacticle discrimination.
Supersedes in part (in 1975): Journal of Experimental Psychology (0022-1015)
Related titles: Microform ed.: (from PQC); Online - full text ed.: (from Gale Group, Factiva, Institute for Scientific Information).
Indexed: AMED, ASCA, ASSIA, Biol.Abstr., C.I.J.E. (coverage dropped), Child Devel.Abstr., Commun.Abstr., Compumath, Curr.Cont., Dent.Ind., Ergon.Abstr., Ind.Med. (1975-), Ind.Philos., Lang.& Lang.Behav.Abstr., MLA Intl.Bibl., Neurosci.Cit.Ind., PsycInfo, Psychol.Abstr. (1975-), Russ.Acad.Sci.Bibl., SOPODA, SSCI, Soc.Sci.Ind. (Feb.1982-), Sociol.Abstr., e-psyche.
—BLDSC (4982.507000), CISTI, GNLM, IDS, ingenta. **CCC.**
Published by: American Psychological Association, 750 First St., N.E., Washington, DC 20002-4242. TEL 202-336-5600, 800-374-2721, FAX 202-336-5568, subscriptions@apa.org, http://www.apa.org/journals/xhp.html. Ed. David Rosenbaum. Circ: 2,500.

152 USA ISSN 0278-7393
BF1
JOURNAL OF EXPERIMENTAL PSYCHOLOGY: LEARNING, MEMORY, AND COGNITION. Short title: J E P: L M C. Text in English. 1916. bi-m. USD 244 domestic to non-members; USD 264 foreign to non-members; USD 122 domestic to members; USD 134 foreign to members; USD 509 domestic to institutions; USD 553 foreign to institutions (effective 2001). adv. reprint service avail. from PQC,PSC,SCH. *Refereed.* **Document type:** *Academic/Scholarly.* **Description:** Experimental studies on fundamental encoding, transfer, memory, and cognitive processes in human behavior.
Formerly (until Jan. 1982): Journal of Experimental Psychology: Human Learning and Memory (0096-1515); Which supersedes in part (in 1975): Journal of Experimental Psychology (0022-1015)
Related titles: Microform ed.: (from PQC); Online - full text ed.: (from Gale Group, Factiva, Institute for Scientific Information).
Indexed: ASCA, AgeLine, Arts & Hum.Cit.Ind. (coverage dropped), Biol.Abstr., C.I.J.E. (coverage dropped), Child Devel.Abstr., Curr.Cont., Ergon.Abstr., Ind.Med. (1982-), Ind.Philos., Lang.& Lang.Behav.Abstr., MLA Intl.Bibl., Neurosci.Cit.Ind., P C I, PsycInfo, Psychol.Abstr. (1975-), SOPODA, SSCI, Soc.Sci.Ind. (Nov.1982-), Sociol.Abstr., e-psyche.
—BLDSC (4982.509000), CISTI, GNLM, IDS, Infotrieve, ingenta. **CCC.**
Published by: American Psychological Association, 750 First St., N.E., Washington, DC 20002-4242. TEL 202-336-5600, 800-374-2721, FAX 202-336-5568, subscriptions@apa.org, http://www.apa.org/journals/xlm.html. Ed. Thomas O Nelson. Circ: 2,900.

302 USA ISSN 0022-1031
HM251 CODEN: JESPAQ
JOURNAL OF EXPERIMENTAL SOCIAL PSYCHOLOGY. Text in English. 1965. bi-m. USD 550 in US & Canada to institutions; USD 575 elsewhere to institutions (effective 2001). adv. illus. back issues avail.; reprint service avail. from PSC,SCH. *Refereed.* **Document type:** *Academic/Scholarly.* **Description:** Publishes original research and theory on human social behavior and related phenomena.
Related titles: Online - full text ed.: (from EBSCO Publishing, O C L C Online Computer Library Center, Inc., RoweCom Information Quest, ingenta, Gale Group, Swets Blackwell, IDEAL Online Library, Factiva, Institute for Scientific Information).
Indexed: ASCA, ASSIA, Abstr.Crim.& Pen., Arts & Hum.Cit.Ind. (coverage dropped), Biol.Abstr., Commun.Abstr., Crim.Just.Abstr., Curr.Cont., IBZ, Ind.Philos., Intl.Bibl.Soc.Sci., L.R.I., Mid.East: Abstr.& Ind., P C I, PsycInfo, Psychol.Abstr. (1965-), Rel.Ind.One, Rel.Ind.Two, Russ.Acad.Sci.Bibl., SSCI, Soc.Sci.Ind. (Sep.1982-), e-psyche.

P

—BLDSC (4982.700000), IDS, ingenta. **CCC.**
Published by: Academic Press, Inc., Journal Division (Subsidiary of: Harcourt Brace & Company), 525 B St, Ste 1900, San Diego, CA 92101-4495. TEL 619-230-1840, FAX 619-699-6800, apsubs@acad.com, http://www.academicpress.com/jesp. Ed. Russell H. Fazio.

150 USA ISSN 1058-0476
HQ1 CODEN: JFEIEE
JOURNAL OF FAMILY AND ECONOMIC ISSUES. Text in English. 1978. q. USD 431, EUR 430 to institutions for print or online ed.; USD 517.20, EUR 516 to institutions for print & online eds.combined (effective 2002). adv. bk.rev., film rev. bibl, charts, stat, illus. index. back issues avail.; reprint service avail. from PQC. *Refereed.* **Document type:** *Journal, Academic/Scholarly.* **Description:** Covers family consumer behavior, household division of labor and productivity, the relationship between economic and noneconomic decisions, and interrelationships between work and family life.
Former titles (until 1991): Lifestyles: Family and Economic Issues (0882-3391); Alternative Lifestyles (0161-570X)
Related titles: Online - full text ed.: (from EBSCO Publishing, O C L C Online Computer Library Center, Inc., Swets Blackwell, Kluwer Online, RoweCom Information Quest).
Indexed: AgeLine, Community Ment.Health Rev., Curr.Cont. (coverage dropped), Educ.Ind. (coverage dropped), Except.Child Educ.Abstr., Fam.Ind., IMFL, Lang.& Lang.Behav.Abstr., Mid.East: Abstr.& Ind., PsycInfo, Psychol.Abstr. (1980-), Russ.Acad.Sci.Bibl., SOPODA, SSCI (coverage dropped), Sage Fam.Stud.Abstr., Soc.Serv.Abstr., Soc.Work Res.& Abstr., Sociol.Abstr., e-psyche.
—BLDSC (4983.645000), ingenta. **CCC.**
Published by: Kluwer Academic - Plenum Publishers (Subsidiary of: Wolters Kluwer N.V.), 233 Spring St, New York, NY 10013-1578. TEL 212-620-8000, 800-221-9369, FAX 212-463-0742, info@plenum.com, http://www.wkap.nl/journalhome.htm/1058-0476. Eds. Barbara R Rowe, Gong Soog Hong. **Subscr. outside the Americas to:** Kluwer Academic Publishers Group, Journals Department, PO Box 322, Dordrecht 3300 AH, Netherlands. TEL 31-78-639-2392, FAX 31-78-654-6474.

155 USA ISSN 0893-3200
JOURNAL OF FAMILY PSYCHOLOGY. Text in English. 1987. q. USD 92 domestic to non-members; USD 107 foreign to non-members; USD 46 domestic to members; USD 56 foreign to members; USD 146 domestic to institutions; USD 178 foreign to institutions (effective 2001). adv. illus. Index. reprints avail. *Refereed.* **Document type:** *Academic/Scholarly.* **Description:** Delivers a variety of perspectives on the study of family systems, emphasizing empirical research on a wide range of family-related topics.
Related titles: Online - full text ed.: (from Gale Group, Factiva, Institute for Scientific Information).
Indexed: ASCA, ASSIA, Addic.Abstr., Crim.Just.Abstr., Curr.Cont., ERA, Educ.Ind., Fam.Ind., IMFL, Ind.Med. (1987-), Lang.& Lang.Behav.Abstr., Mult.Ed.Abstr., PsycInfo, Psychol.Abstr. (1987-), Russ.Acad.Sci.Bibl., SOPODA, SSCI, Soc.Sci.Ind. (Jan.1994-), Soc.Serv.Abstr., Soc.Work Res.& Abstr., Sociol.Abstr., Sp.Ed.Needs Abstr., Stud.Wom.Abstr., e-psyche.
—BLDSC (4983.733000), IDS, ingenta. **CCC.**
Published by: American Psychological Association, Division of Family Psychology, 750 First St., N.E., Washington, DC 20002-4242. TEL 202-336-5600, FAX 202-336-5568, subscriptions@apa.org, http://www.apa.org/journals/fam.html. Ed. Ross D Parke. Circ: 4,800.

616.89 USA ISSN 0897-5353
RC488.5 CODEN: JFAPEF
JOURNAL OF FAMILY PSYCHOTHERAPY; the official journal of the International Family Therapy Association. Text in English. 1985. q. USD 65 to individuals; USD 88 in Canada to individuals; USD 94 elsewhere to individuals; USD 125 to institutions; USD 169 in Canada to institutions; USD 181 elsewhere to institutions; USD 335 to libraries; USD 452 in Canada to libraries; USD 486 elsewhere to libraries (effective Aug. 2001). adv. bk.rev. back issues avail.; reprint service avail. from HAW. *Refereed.* **Document type:** *Journal, Academic/Scholarly.* **Description:** Provides an exchange for clinicians across the disciplines to share solutions to difficult family problems. Offers detailed clinical case studies, descriptions of successful treatment programs, innovative strategies in clinical practice.
Formerly (until 1988): Journal of Psychotherapy and the Family (0742-9703)
Related titles: Microfiche ed.: (from PQC); Microform ed.; Online - full text ed.: free with subscr. to the print ed.
Indexed: Biol.Dig., Curr.Cont. (coverage dropped), DNP, ERA, Environ.Sci.Poll.Mgmt., Excerp.Med., Fam.Ind., IMFL, Ind.Med. (coverage dropped), Ind.Per.Art.Relat.Law, Lang.& Lang.Behav.Abstr., Mult.Ed.Abstr., Past.Care & Couns.Abstr., PsycInfo, Psychol.Abstr. (1985-), Ref.Zh., Risk Abstr., Russ.Acad.Sci.Bibl., SOPODA, Saf.Sci.Abstr., Sage Fam.Stud.Abstr., Soc.Serv.Abstr., Soc.Work Res.& Abstr., Sociol.Abstr., Sp.Ed.Needs Abstr., Stud.Wom.Abstr., Viol.& Abuse Abstr., e-psyche.
—BLDSC (4983.735000), EMDOCS, GNLM, Haworth, ingenta.
Published by: (International Family Therapy Association), Haworth Press, Inc., 10 Alice St, Binghamton, NY 13904-1580. TEL 607-722-5857, 800-429-6784, FAX 607-722-6362, 800-895-0582, getinfo@haworthpressinc.com, http://www.haworthpress.com/journals/journallist.asp. Ed. Terry S Trepper. Pub. William Cohen. R&P Ruthann Heath TEL 607-723-5857 ext 316. Adv. contact Jackie Blakeslee TEL 607-722-5857 ext 346. B&W page USD 315, color page USD 550; trim 6 x 8.5. Circ: 1,275.

JOURNAL OF FAMILY STUDIES. see *MATRIMONY*

JOURNAL OF FAMILY THERAPY. see *MEDICAL SCIENCES—Psychiatry And Neurology*

JOURNAL OF FAMILY VIOLENCE. see *CRIMINOLOGY AND LAW ENFORCEMENT*

JOURNAL OF FEMINIST FAMILY THERAPY; an international forum. see *WOMEN'S STUDIES*

302 USA ISSN 0094-730X
RC423.A1 CODEN: JFDID8
JOURNAL OF FLUENCY DISORDERS. Text in English. 1974. q. EUR 176 in Europe to individuals; JPY 23,400 in Japan to individuals; USD 198 elsewhere to individuals; EUR 429 in Europe to institutions; JPY 57,000 in Japan to institutions; USD 479 elsewhere to institutions (effective 2002). adv. bk.rev. back issues avail. *Refereed.* **Document type:** *Academic/Scholarly.* **Description:** Provides comprehensive coverage of clinical, experimental, and theoretical aspects of stuttering, including the latest remediation techniques.
Related titles: Microform ed.: (from PQC); Online - full text ed.: (from ingenta, ScienceDirect, Swets Blackwell, Institute for Scientific Information).
Indexed: AMED, ASCA, AgeLine, Biol.Abstr., CINAHL, Curr.Cont., DSH Abstr., ERA, Excerp.Med., Fam.Ind., Lang.& Lang.Behav.Abstr. (1978-), PsycInfo, Psychol.Abstr. (1981-), Rehabil.Lit., SOPODA, SSCI, Sociol.Abstr., Sp.Ed.Needs Abstr., e-psyche.
—BLDSC (4984.450000), CISTI, GNLM, IDS, Infotrieve, ingenta. **CCC.**
Published by: Elsevier Science, 655 Ave of the Americas, New York, NY 10010. TEL 212-989-5800, FAX 212-633-3990, usinfo-f@elsevier.com, http://www.elsevier.com/locate/jfludis. Eds. J van Borsel, R F Curlee. **Subscr. in Australasia and the Far East to:** Elsevier Science (Singapore) Pte Ltd, No.1 Temasek Ave, 17-01 Millenia Tower, Singapore 039192, Singapore. TEL 65-434-3727, FAX 65-337-2230; **Subscr. in Japan to:** Elsevier Science Inc - Japan Regional Office, 9-15 Higashi-Azabu 1-chome, Minato-ku, Tokyo 106-0044, Japan. TEL 81-3-5561-5033; **Subscr. outside the Americas to:** Elsevier Science BV, PO Box 211, Amsterdam 1000 AE, Netherlands. TEL 31-20-485-3757.

150 345 USA
▼ **JOURNAL OF FORENSIC PSYCHOLOGY PRACTICE.** Text in English. 2001 (Spr.). q. USD 60 to individuals; USD 81 in Canada to individuals; USD 87 elsewhere to individuals; USD 95 to institutions; USD 128 in Canada to institutions; USD 138 elsewhere to institutions; USD 150 to libraries; USD 203 in Canada to libraries; USD 218 elsewhere to libraries (effective Aug. 2001). adv. bk.rev. *Refereed.* **Document type:** *Journal, Academic/Scholarly.* **Description:** Presents new programs and techniques, analyzes existing policies and programs in their social context, and evaluates specific institutions and forensic procedures.
—BLDSC (4984.599100), Haworth.
Published by: Haworth Press, Inc., 10 Alice St, Binghamton, NY 13904-1580. TEL 607-722-5857, 800-429-6784, FAX 607-722-6362, 800-895-0582, getinfo@haworthpressinc.com, http://www.haworthpress.com/journals/journallist.asp. Ed. Bruce A Arrigo. Pub. William Cohen. R&P Ruth Ann Heath. Adv. contact Jackie Blakeslee TEL 607-722-5857 ext 346. B&W page USD 315, color page USD 550; trim 6 x 8.5.

626.8583406 USA ISSN 0891-7140
RC558 CODEN: JGLPE9
JOURNAL OF GAY & LESBIAN PSYCHOTHERAPY. Text in English. 1988. q. USD 50 domestic to individuals; USD 68 in Canada to individuals; USD 73 elsewhere to individuals; USD 85 domestic to institutions; USD 115 in Canada to institutions; USD 123 elsewhere to institutions; USD 110 domestic to libraries; USD 149 in Canada to libraries; USD 160 elsewhere to libraries (effective Aug. 2001). adv. bk.rev. illus. reprint service avail. from HAW,ISI. *Refereed.* **Document type:** *Journal, Academic/Scholarly.* **Description:** Provides a multidisciplinary professional forum for issues relating to the use of psychotherapy for gay, lesbian and bisexual clients. Goal is to facilitate the quality of life for gays and foster effective therapy for those who require support.
Related titles: Microfiche ed.: (from PQC); Microfilm ed.; Microform ed.; Online - full text ed.: (from Gale Group).
Indexed: Abstr.Anthropol., CWI, Environ.Sci.Poll.Mgmt., Fam.Ind., Gend.Watch, IMFL, Lang.& Lang.Behav.Abstr., Psychol.Abstr. (1989-), Risk Abstr., SOPODA, Soc.Serv.Abstr., Soc.Work Res.& Abstr., Sociol.Abstr., e-psyche.
—BLDSC (4987.640000), GNLM, Haworth, ingenta.
Published by: Haworth Press, Inc., 10 Alice St, Binghamton, NY 13904-1580. TEL 607-722-5857, 800-429-6784, FAX 607-722-6362, 800-895-0582, getinfo@haworthpressinc.com, http://www.haworthpress.com/journals/journallist.asp. Ed. Dr. Jack Drescher. Pub. William Cohen. R&P Ruthann Heath TEL 607-723-5857 ext 316. Adv. contact Jackie Blakeslee TEL 607-722-5857 ext 346. B&W page USD 315, color page USD 550; trim 6 x 8.5. Circ: 1,600.

150 USA ISSN 0022-1309
BF1 CODEN: JGPSAY
THE JOURNAL OF GENERAL PSYCHOLOGY; experimental, physiological, and comparative psychology. Text in English. 1927. q., latest vol.129, 2002. USD 135 domestic; USD 148 foreign; USD 33.75 newsstand/cover (effective 2001 - 2002). bibl, charts. index. back issues avail.; reprint service avail. from SWZ,PSC,SCH. *Refereed.* **Document type:** *Academic/Scholarly.*
Related titles: CD-ROM ed.: (from ProQuest Information & Learning); Microform ed.; Online - full text ed.: (from ProQuest Information & Learning, Gale Group, Northern Light Technology, Inc., H. W. Wilson, Factiva, Institute for Scientific Information).
Indexed: ASCA, ASSIA, Abstr.Crim.& Pen., AgeLine, Biol.& Agr.Ind. (coverage dropped), Biol.Abstr., C.I.J.E. (coverage dropped), Chem.Abstr., Child Devel.Abstr., Commun.Abstr., Curr.Adv.Ecol.Sci., Curr.Cont., Curr.Ind.Stat., Curr.Ref.Fish Res., Dent.Ind., Ergon.Abstr., Except.Child Educ.Abstr., IBR, IBZ, Ind.Med. (1928-), Ind.Philos., Indian Psychol.Abstr., Lang.& Lang.Behav.Abstr., P C I, PsycInfo, Psychol.Abstr. (1928-), Ref.Zh., Russ.Acad.Sci.Bibl., SOPODA, SSCI, Soc.Sci.Ind. (Jul.1982-), Soc.Serv.Abstr., Soc.Work Res.& Abstr., Sociol.Abstr., e-psyche.
—BLDSC (4989.200000), CISTI, GNLM, IDS, ingenta. **CCC.**
Published by: (Helen Dwight Reid Educational Foundation), Heldref Publications, 1319 Eighteenth St, N W, Washington, DC 20036-1802. TEL 202-296-6267, FAX 202-296-5149, http://www.heldref.org. Ed. Elisa Subin. Pub. Douglas Kirkpatrick. Adv. contact Ali Mayhew. Circ: 1,143.

150 USA ISSN 1059-7700
RB155.7 CODEN: JGCOET
JOURNAL OF GENETIC COUNSELING. Text in English. 1992. bi-m. USD 376, EUR 376 to institutions for print or online ed.; USD 451.20, EUR 451.20 to institutions for print & online eds.combined (effective 2002). adv. abstr. *Refereed.* **Document type:** *Journal, Academic/Scholarly.* **Description:** Covers psychosocial issues, educational and counseling techniques, legislation and regulations affecting genetic counseling, and other issues related to providing counseling services.
Related titles: Online - full text ed.: (from EBSCO Publishing, O C L C Online Computer Library Center, Inc., RoweCom Information Quest, Swets Blackwell, Kluwer Online).
Indexed: CINAHL, Fam.Ind., IMFL, Lang.& Lang.Behav.Abstr., PsycInfo, Psychol.Abstr. (1992-), SOPODA, Sage Fam.Stud.Abstr., Soc.Work Res.& Abstr., Sociol.Abstr., e-psyche.
—BLDSC (4989.700000), GNLM, Infotrieve, ingenta, KNAW. **CCC.**

Published by: (National Society of Genetic Counselors, Inc.), Kluwer Academic - Plenum Publishers (Subsidiary of: Wolters Kluwer N.V.), 233 Spring St, New York, NY 10013-1578. TEL 212-620-8000, 800-221-9369, FAX 212-463-0742, info@plenum.com, http://www.wkap.nl/journalhome.htm/1059-7700. Ed. Allyn McConkie-Rosell. **Subscr. outside the Americas to:** Kluwer Academic Publishers Group, Journals Department, PO Box 322, Dordrecht 3300 AH, Netherlands. TEL 31-78-639-2392, FAX 31-78-654-6474.

THE JOURNAL OF GENETIC PSYCHOLOGY; developmental and clinical psychology. see *BIOLOGY—Genetics*

130 USA ISSN 0022-1449
JOURNAL OF GRAPHOANALYSIS. Text in English. 1929. m. USD 90. bk.rev. abstr, bibl, charts, illus, tr.lit. **Document type:** *Academic/Scholarly.*
Indexed: e-psyche.
Published by: International Graphoanalysis Society, 111 N Canal St, Chicago, IL 60606. TEL 312-930-9446, FAX 312-930-5903, headquarters@igas.com, http://www.igas.com. Ed. William Harms. Pub. Kathleen Kusta. Circ: 35,000.

158 NLD ISSN 1389-4978
▼ **JOURNAL OF HAPPINESS STUDIES**; an interdisciplinary forum on subjective well-being. Text in English. 2000 (Mar). q. EUR 273, USD 274 to institutions for print or online ed.; EUR 327.60, USD 328.80 to institutions for print & online eds.combined (effective 2001). bk.rev. reprints avail. *Refereed.* **Document type:** *Journal, Academic/Scholarly.* **Description:** Explores the psychological and sociological conditions leading to individual happiness and overall well-being.
Related titles: Online - full text ed.: (from EBSCO Publishing, Swets Blackwell, Kluwer Online).
—BLDSC (4996.623800).
Published by: (International Society for Quality of Life Studies), Kluwer Academic Publishers Group (Subsidiary of: Wolters Kluwer N.V.), Spuiboulevard 50, PO Box 17, Dordrecht 3300 AA, Netherlands. TEL 31-78-639-2392, FAX 31-78-654-2254, services@wkap.nl, http://www.wkap.nl/journalhome.htm/1389-4978. Eds. Alex C Michalos, Ed Diener, Ruut Veenhoven. Pub. Sabine Wesseldijk. **Subscr. in the Americas to:** Kluwer Academic - Plenum Publishers, 233 Spring St, New York, NY 10013-1578. TEL 212-620-8468, FAX 212-807-1047; **Subscr. to:** Journals Department, PO Box 322, Dordrecht 3300 AH, Netherlands. TEL 31-78-639-2392, FAX 31-78-654-6474.

616.8 GBR ISSN 1359-1053
R726.7 CODEN: JHPSFC
JOURNAL OF HEALTH PSYCHOLOGY; an interdisciplinary, international journal. Text in English. 1996. bi-m. GBP 39 to individuals; GBP 279 to institutions; GBP 8 newsstand/cover to individuals; GBP 48 newsstand/cover to institutions (effective 2002). adv. bk.rev. *Refereed.* **Document type:** *Academic/Scholarly.* **Description:** Provides an international forum for the best research in health psychology from around the world.
Related titles: Online - full text ed.: (from EBSCO Publishing, O C L C Online Computer Library Center, Inc., RoweCom Information Quest, ingenta, Swets Blackwell, Institute for Scientific Information).
Indexed: ASSIA, Curr.Cont., Excerp.Med., Lang.& Lang.Behav.Abstr., PsycInfo, SOPODA, SSCI, Soc.Serv.Abstr., Sociol.Abstr., e-psyche.
—BLDSC (4996.870100). **CCC.**
Published by: Sage Publications Ltd., 6 Bonhill St, London EC2A 4PU, United Kingdom. TEL 44-20-7374-0645, FAX 44-20-7374-8741, market@sagepub.co.uk, http://www.sagepub.co.uk. Ed. David Marks. Adv. contact Jenny Kirby. page GBP 220; trim 200 x 135. Circ: 900.

152.4 610 GBR ISSN 0306-7297
QP303 CODEN: JHMSDT
JOURNAL OF HUMAN MOVEMENT STUDIES. Text in English. 1975. m. GBP 355; GBP 475 in the European Union; GBP 875 in the Americas. bk.rev. cum.index. *Refereed.* **Document type:** *Academic/Scholarly.*
Related titles: Online - full text ed.: (from Institute for Scientific Information).
Indexed: AMED, ASCA, AgeLine, Biol.Abstr., Curr.Cont. (coverage dropped), Ergon.Abstr., Excerp.Med., Focus on: Sports Sci.& Med., Lang.& Lang.Behav.Abstr., Phys.Ed.Ind., SSCI (coverage dropped), Sportsearch (1975-), e-psyche.
—BLDSC (5003.418000), CISTI, GNLM, IDS, ingenta, KNAW. **CCC.**

Published by: Teviot Scientific Publications Ltd., 82 Great King St, Edinburgh EH3 6QU, United Kingdom. TEL 44-131-220-8209, FAX 44-131-226-5435. Ed. W J Irvine.

371.42 USA ISSN 0735-6846
LB1715
JOURNAL OF HUMANISTIC COUNSELING, EDUCATION AND DEVELOPMENT. Text in English. 1962. 2/yr. USD 37 domestic to institutions; USD 49 foreign to institutions (effective 2001). adv. abstr, bibl, illus. 128 p./no. back issues avail.; reprint service avail. from PQC. *Refereed.* **Document type:** *Academic/Scholarly.* **Description:** Addresses issues and concerns affecting counselors and educators committed to developing humanistic education practices in schools.
Former titles (until July 1999): Journal of Humanistic Education and Development (0735-6846); (until 1982): Humanistic Educator (0362-9783); (until 1975): Student Personnel Association for Teacher Education. Journal (0036-1836)
Related titles: Microform ed.: (from PQC); Online - full text ed.: (from H. W. Wilson).
Indexed: C.I.J.E., Cont.Pg.Educ., ERA, Educ.Ind. (Jul.1997-Jun.1999), Fam.Ind., High.Educ.Abstr., Mult.Ed.Abstr., Psychol.Abstr., Soc.Work Res.& Abstr., Sociol.Educ.Abstr., Sp.Ed.Needs Abstr., Stud.Wom.Abstr., e-psyche.
—BLDSC (5003.443500), ingenta. **CCC.**
Published by: (Association for Humanistic Counseling, Education and Development), American Counseling Association, 5999 Stevenson Ave, Alexandria, VA 22304-3300. TEL 703-823-9800, FAX 703-823-0252, http://www.counseling.org. Ed. Roger D Herring. R&P Cynthia Peay TEL 703-823-9800 x 249. Adv. contact Kathy Maguire TEL 703-823-9800 ext 207. Circ: 1,500.

150 170 USA ISSN 0022-1678
BF1
JOURNAL OF HUMANISTIC PSYCHOLOGY. Text in English. 1961. q. USD 65 to individuals; USD 345 to institutions; USD 25 newsstand/cover to individuals; USD 90 newsstand/cover to institutions (effective 2002). adv. bk.rev. stat, illus. index, cum.index: 1961-1979. back issues avail.; reprint service avail. from PQC,PSC,SCH. *Refereed.* **Document type:** *Academic/Scholarly.* **Description:** Provides an interdisciplinary forum for contributions and controversies in humanistic psychology as applied to personal growth, interpersonal encounters, social problems, and philosophical issues.
Related titles: Microfilm ed.: (from PQC); Online - full text ed.: (from EBSCO Publishing, O C L C Online Computer Library Center, Inc., RoweCom Information Quest, ProQuest Information & Learning, Gale Group, ingenta, Swets Blackwell, Institute for Scientific Information).
Indexed: ASCA, ASSIA, AgeLine, Amer.Bibl.Slavic & E.Eur.Stud., Arts & Hum.Cit.Ind. (coverage dropped), C.I.J.E. (coverage dropped), Commun.Abstr., Curr.Cont., Human Resour.Abstr., IMFL, Lang.& Lang.Behav.Abstr., Mid.East: Abstr.& Ind., Mult.Ed.Abstr., Per.Islam. (1996-), PsycInfo, Psychol.Abstr. (1961-), Rel.Ind.One, Rel.Ind.Two, Russ.Acad.Sci.Bibl., SOPODA, SSCI, Soc.Sci.Ind. (Jan.1994-Sep.1998), Sociol.Abstr., Sociol.Educ.Abstr., e-psyche.
—BLDSC (5003.450000), IDS, Infotrieve, ingenta. **CCC.**
Published by: (Association for Humanistic Psychology), Sage Publications, Inc., 2455 Teller Rd, Thousand Oaks, CA 91320. TEL 805-499-0721, FAX 805-499-0871, info@sagepub.com, http://www.sagepub.com. Ed. Thomas C Greening. Pub. Sara Miller McCune. R&P Tanya Udin. Adv. contact DeAnna Vega Hammersley. Circ: 3,000. **Overseas subscr. to:** Sage Publications Ltd., 6 Bonhill St, London EC2A 4PU, United Kingdom; Sage Publications India Pvt. Ltd., 4215, New Delhi 110 048, India.

302 USA ISSN 1529-4129
JOURNAL OF IMAGO RELATIONSHIP THERAPY. Text in English. 1996. s-a. USD 97 worldwide (effective 2002). adv. bk.rev. **Document type:** *Journal, Academic/Scholarly.* **Description:** Presents research and case studies concerning the use of imago therapy, pioneered by Dr. Harville Hendrix.
Indexed: ASSIA, Lang.& Lang.Behav.Abstr., PsycInfo, SOPODA, Sociol.Abstr., e-psyche.
Published by: (Institute for Imago Relationship Therapy), International Universities Press, Incorporated, 59 Boston Post Rd., P.O. Box 1524, Madison, CT 06443-1524. adv.: page USD 375; 4.25 x 7.

301.1 150 IND ISSN 0379-3885
BF1
JOURNAL OF INDIAN PSYCHOLOGY. Text in English. 1977. s-a. USD 6 to individuals; USD 9 to institutions. **Document type:** *Academic/Scholarly.*

Formerly: Indian Psychology
Indexed: Bibl.Asian Stud. (1986-1991), Indian Psychol.Abstr., PsycInfo, Psychol.Abstr. (1978-), e-psyche.
—BLDSC (5005.330000), ingenta.
Published by: (Andhra University, Department of Psychology & Parapsychology), Andhra University Press and Publications, Waltair, Visakhapatnam, Andhra Pradesh 530 003, India.

150 USA
BF1
JOURNAL OF INDIVIDUAL PSYCHOLOGY; the journal of Adlerian research, theory & practice. Text in English. 1982. q. USD 42 domestic to individuals; USD 54 in Canada & Mexico to individuals; USD 64 rest of world to individuals; USD 77 domestic to institutions; USD 89 in Canada & Mexico to institutions; USD 99 per issue rest of world to institutions (effective 2001 - 2002); USD 17 per issue domestic to individuals; USD 19.50 per issue in Canada & Mexico to individuals; USD 22 per issue rest of world to individuals; USD 26 per issue domestic to institutions; USD 28.50 per issue in Canada & Mexico to institutions; USD 31 per issue rest of world to institutions (effective 2001). adv. bk.rev. bibl, charts, stat. index. back issues avail.; reprint service avail. from PSC,PQC,SCH. **Document type:** *Academic/Scholarly.* **Description:** Presents current scholarly and professional research dealing with all aspects of the theories founded by Alfred Adler.
Formerly (until 1997): Individual Psychology (0277-7010); Which was formed by the merger of (1963-1982): Individual Psychologist (0019-7149); (1957-1982): Journal of Individual Psychology (0022-1805); Which was formerly (until 1956): American Journal of Individual Psychology (0091-7788); Individual Psychology Bulletin; Individual Psychology News
Indexed: ASCA, Abstr.Anthropol., Adol.Ment.Hlth.Abstr., AgeLine, Arts & Hum.Cit.Ind. (coverage dropped), Biol.Abstr., Curr.Cont. (coverage dropped), Curr.Lit.Fam.Plan., Fam.Ind., IMFL, Ind.Med. (coverage dropped), Ind.Philos., Lang.& Lang.Behav.Abstr., Mid.East: Abstr.& Ind., P C I, PsycInfo, Psychoanal.Abstr., Psychol.Abstr. (1982-), Res.High.Educ.Abstr., SOPODA, SSCI (coverage dropped), Soc.Work Res.& Abstr., Sociol.Abstr., e-psyche.
—BLDSC (5005.350000), GNLM, IDS, Infotrieve, ingenta. **CCC.**
Published by: (North American Society of Adlerian Psychology), University of Texas Press, Journals Division, PO Box 7819, Austin, TX 78713. TEL 512-471-4531, FAX 512-232-7178, journals@uts.cc.utexas.edu, http://www.utexas.edu. Eds. Roy Kern, William Curlette. R&P Stacey Salling TEL 512-232-7621. Adv. contact Leah Dixon TEL 512-232-7618. Circ: 1,900.

JOURNAL OF INSTRUCTIONAL PSYCHOLOGY. see *EDUCATION*

JOURNAL OF INTERPERSONAL VIOLENCE; concerned with the study and treatment of victims and perpetrators of physical and sexual violence. see *CRIMINOLOGY AND LAW ENFORCEMENT*

JOURNAL OF INVITATIONAL THEORY AND PRACTICE. see *EDUCATION*

302 USA ISSN 0261-927X
P40
JOURNAL OF LANGUAGE AND SOCIAL PSYCHOLOGY. Text in English. 1982. q. USD 75 to individuals; USD 365 to institutions; USD 25 newsstand/cover to individuals; USD 95 newsstand/cover to institutions (effective 2002). adv. bk.rev. index. back issues avail.; reprints avail. *Refereed.* **Document type:** *Academic/Scholarly.* **Description:** Explores the social dimensions of language and the linguistic implications of social life.
Related titles: Online - full text ed.: (from EBSCO Publishing, O C L C Online Computer Library Center, Inc., RoweCom Information Quest, ProQuest Information & Learning, ingenta, Swets Blackwell, Institute for Scientific Information).
Indexed: ASCA, AgeLine, Bibl.Ling., Commun.Abstr., Curr.Cont., IBR, IBZ, Ind.Philos., Intl.Bibl.Soc.Sci., Lang.& Lang.Behav.Abstr. (1985-), Lang.Teach.& Ling.Abstr., Ling.Abstr., MLA Intl.Bibl., Peace Res.Abstr., PsycInfo, Psychol.Abstr. (1983-), Ref.Zh., Russ.Acad.Sci.Bibl., SOPODA, SSCI, Sage Fam.Stud.Abstr., Soc.Serv.Abstr., Sociol.Abstr., Viol.& Abuse Abstr., e-psyche.
—BLDSC (5010.096000), IDS, ingenta. **CCC.**

P

Published by: (Multilingual Matters Ltd. GBR), Sage Publications, Inc., 2455 Teller Rd, Thousand Oaks, CA 91320. TEL 805-499-0721, FAX 805-499-0871, info@sagepub.com, http://www.sagepub.com. Eds. Howard Giles, James Bradac. R&P Tanya Udin. Adv. contact DeAnna Vega Hammersley. Circ: 500. **Overseas subscr. to:** Sage Publications Ltd., 6 Bonhill St, London EC2A 4PU, United Kingdom. TEL 44-20-7374-0645, FAX 44-20-7374-8741, subscription@sagepub.co.uk, http://www.sagepub.co.uk; Sage Publications India Pvt. Ltd., 4215, New Delhi 110 048, India. TEL 91-11-641-9884, FAX 91-11-647-2426.

JOURNAL OF LEARNING DISABILITIES. see *EDUCATION—Special Education And Rehabilitation*

JOURNAL OF LESBIAN STUDIES. see *HOMOSEXUALITY*

150 USA ISSN 1532-5024
BF575.D35 CODEN: JPILFC

JOURNAL OF LOSS & TRAUMA. Text in English. 1996. q. GBP 46, USD 76 to individuals; GBP 131, USD 216 to institutions (effective 2002). *Refereed.* **Document type:** *Academic/Scholarly.* **Description:** Forum on personal losses relating to family, health and aging issues, and interpersonal losses surrounding such areas as marriage and divorce.
Formerly (until 2001): Journal of Personal & Interpersonal Loss (1081-1443)
Related titles: Online - full text ed.: (from CatchWord Ltd., Institute for Scientific Information).
Indexed: AgeLine, C.I.J.E., Curr.Cont., SSCI, e-psyche.
—BLDSC (5030.820000), IDS, Infotrieve. **CCC.**
Published by: Taylor & Francis Ltd. (Subsidiary of: Taylor & Francis Group), 325 Chestnut St, Suite 800, Philadelphia, PA 19016. TEL 215-625-8900, FAX 215-625-2940, info@taylorandfrancis.com, http://www.taylorandfrancis.com/. **Subscr. addr. in Europe:** Taylor & Francis Group, Journals Customer Service, Rankine Rd, Basingstoke, Hants RG24 8PR, United Kingdom. TEL 44-1256-813000, FAX 44-1256-479438, enquiry@tanf.co.uk, http://www.tandf.co.uk/journals.

P

JOURNAL OF MANAGERIAL PSYCHOLOGY. see *BUSINESS AND ECONOMICS—Management*

306.43 USA ISSN 0194-472X
HQ1

JOURNAL OF MARITAL AND FAMILY THERAPY. Text in English. 1975. q. USD 45 to individuals; USD 75 to institutions. adv. bk.rev. illus. Index. reprint service avail. from PQC,PSC,SCH. *Refereed.* **Document type:** *Academic/Scholarly.*
Formerly (until 1979): Journal of Marriage and Family Counseling (0094-5102)
Related titles: Microform ed.: (from PQC); Online - full text ed.: (from ProQuest Information & Learning, H. W. Wilson, Gale Group, Factiva, Institute for Scientific Information).
Indexed: ASCA, Abstr.Soc.Geront., Addic.Abstr., Adol.Ment.Hlth.Abstr., AgeLine, Biol.Abstr., CERDIC, C.I.J.E., Curr.Cont., Excerp.Med., Fam.Ind., IMFL, Ind.Med. (1979-), Int.Nurs.Ind., Lang.& Lang.Behav.Abstr., Past.Care & Couns.Abstr., PsycInfo, Psychol.Abstr. (1975-), Russ.Acad.Sci.Bibl., SOPODA, SSCI, Sage Fam.Stud.Abstr., Soc.Sci.Ind. (Apr.1987-), Soc.Serv.Abstr., Soc.Work Res.& Abstr., Sociol.Abstr., Stud.Wom.Abstr., Viol.& Abuse Abstr., e-psyche.
—BLDSC (5012.060000), IDS, Infotrieve, ingenta, KNAW. **CCC.**
Published by: American Association for Marriage and Family Therapy, 1133 15th St, N W, Ste 300, Washington, DC 20005. http://www.aamft.org/index.htm. Ed. Douglas Sprenkle. Circ: 20,000.

150 USA ISSN 0022-2496
BF1 CODEN: JMTPAJ

JOURNAL OF MATHEMATICAL PSYCHOLOGY. Text in English. 1964. bi-m. USD 695 in US & Canada to institutions; USD 850 elsewhere to institutions (effective 2001). adv. bk.rev. bibl, charts, illus. Index. back issues avail.; reprint service avail. from PSC,SCH. *Refereed.* **Document type:** *Academic/Scholarly.* **Description:** Presents theoretical and empirical research in all areas of mathematical psychology.
Related titles: Online - full text ed.: (from EBSCO Publishing, O C L C Online Computer Library Center, Inc., RoweCom Information Quest, ingenta, Swets Blackwell, IDEAL Online Library, Institute for Scientific Information).
Indexed: ASCA, Biol.Abstr., C.C.M.J., Child Devel.Abstr., Compumath, Curr.Cont., Curr.Ind.Stat., IBZ, INIS Atomind., INSPEC (Mar.1992-), Ind.Philos., J.Cont.Quant.Meth., Math.R., PsycInfo, Psychol.Abstr. (1964-), Russ.Acad.Sci.Bibl., SSCI, Zent.Math., e-psyche.
—BLDSC (5012.420000), AskIEEE, CISTI, IDS, ingenta. **CCC.**
Published by: (Society for Mathematical Psychology), Academic Press, Inc., Journal Division (Subsidiary of: Harcourt Brace & Company), 525 B St, Ste 1900, San Diego, CA 92101-4495. TEL 619-230-1840, FAX 619-699-6800, apsubs@acad.com, http://www.academicpress.com/jmp. Ed. Richard Schweikert.

JOURNAL OF MEMORY AND LANGUAGE. see *LINGUISTICS*

JOURNAL OF MENTAL HEALTH AND AGING. see *GERONTOLOGY AND GERIATRICS*

362.2 USA ISSN 1040-2861
BF637.C6

JOURNAL OF MENTAL HEALTH COUNSELING. Text in English. 1979. q. USD 131 domestic to individuals; USD 143 foreign to individuals (effective 2000). abstr, charts. reprint service avail. from PSC,SCH. **Document type:** *Academic/Scholarly.* **Description:** Disseminates pertinent theory, therapeutic applications, and research related to mental health counseling.
Formerly (until 1987): A M H C A Journal (0193-1830)
Related titles: Online - full text ed.: (from Northern Light Technology, Inc., ProQuest Information & Learning).
Indexed: AgeLine, C.I.J.E., Environ.Sci.Poll.Mgmt., High.Educ.Abstr., Pollut.Abstr., PsycInfo, Psychol.Abstr. (1983-), Risk Abstr., Saf.Sci.Abstr., Soc.Work Res.& Abstr., e-psyche.
—BLDSC (5017.687000), GNLM, ingenta. **CCC.**
Published by: American Mental Health Counselors Association, 801 N Fairfax St, Ste 304, Alexandria, VA 22314. TEL 205-995-1567, 800-326-2642, FAX 205-995-1588, kkelly@purdue.edu, http://www.amhca.org. Ed. Kevin Kelly. Circ: 13,500.

150 USA ISSN 0364-5541
BF367

JOURNAL OF MENTAL IMAGERY. Text in English. 1977. 4/yr. USD 40 to individuals; USD 80 to institutions (effective 2000). adv. bk.rev. charts. back issues avail.
Indexed: Curr.Cont. (coverage dropped), IBR, Ind.Philos., PsycInfo, Psychol.Abstr. (1977-), Russ.Acad.Sci.Bibl., Soc.Sci.Ind. (coverage dropped), e-psyche.
—BLDSC (5017.690000), ingenta.
Published by: (International Imagery Association), Brandon House, Inc., PO Box 240, Bronx, NY 10471. Ed. Dr. Akhter Ahsen.

150 121 USA ISSN 0271-0137
BF1

JOURNAL OF MIND AND BEHAVIOR. Text in English. 1980. q., latest vol.22, 2001 (One volume per year; four issues per volume). USD 46 to individuals; USD 111 to institutions; USD 32 to students (effective 2001). adv. bk.rev. abstr, charts, illus, stat, bibl. index in issue #4. 160 p./no. 1 cols./p. back issues avail.; reprints avail. *Refereed.* **Document type:** *Journal, Academic/Scholarly.* **Description:** Publishes articles pertaining to mind and body epistemology in the social sciences, theory of consciousness and ideation, and historical investigations of science and issues pertaining to the ethical study of cognition, self-awareness and higher functions of consciousness in animals.
Related titles: Online - full text ed.: (from Institute for Scientific Information).
Indexed: ASCA, Curr.Cont., Excerp.Med. (1996-), INSPEC (Sum.1991-), Ind.Philos., Lang.& Lang.Behav.Abstr., Per.Islam. (1992-), Phil.Ind., PsycInfo, Psychol.Abstr. (1981-), SOPODA, SSCI, Soc.Serv.Abstr., Soc.Work Res.& Abstr., Sociol.Abstr., e-psyche.
—BLDSC (5020.140000), AskIEEE, IDS, ingenta.
Published by: Institute of Mind & Behavior, PO Box 522, Village Sta, New York, NY 10014. TEL 212-595-4853, www.kramer.ume.maine.edu/~jmb/, http://kramer.ume.maine.edu/~jmb/. Ed. Dr. Raymond C Russ. R&P, Adv. contact Richard Schenkman TEL 212-595-4853. Circ: 1,190 (controlled).

152.3 USA ISSN 0022-2895
QP303 CODEN: JMTBAB

JOURNAL OF MOTOR BEHAVIOR. Short title: J M B. Text in English. 1969. q., latest vol.34, 2002. USD 77 domestic to individuals; USD 95 foreign to individuals; USD 155 domestic to institutions; USD 173 foreign to institutions; USD 38.75 newsstand/cover (effective 2001 - 2002). adv. abstr, bibl, charts, illus. back issues avail.; reprints avail. *Refereed.* **Document type:** *Academic/Scholarly.* **Description:** Devoted to an understanding of the basic processes and mechanisma underlying motor control, learning and development.
Related titles: CD-ROM ed.: (from ProQuest Information & Learning); Microform ed.; Online - full text ed.: (from Northern Light Technology, Inc., ProQuest Information & Learning, Gale Group, Institute for Scientific Information).
Indexed: AMED, ASCA, AgeLine, Biol.Abstr., Child Devel.Abstr., Curr.Cont., ERA, Ergon.Abstr., Excerp.Med., Focus on: Sports Sci.& Med., Ind.Med., Ind.Philos., Lang.& Lang.Behav.Abstr., Neurosci.Cit.Ind., Phys.Ed.Ind., PsycInfo, Psychol.Abstr. (1970-), Ref.Zh., Russ.Acad.Sci.Bibl., SSCI, Sci.Cit.Ind., Sp.Ed.Needs Abstr., Sportsearch (1974-), e-psyche.
—BLDSC (5021.050000), CISTI, IDS, Infotrieve, ingenta. **CCC.**
Published by: (Helen Dwight Reid Educational Foundation), Heldref Publications, 1319 Eighteenth St, N W, Washington, DC 20036-1802. TEL 202-296-6267, 800-365-9753, FAX 202-293-6130, jmb@heldref.org, http://www.heldref.org; http://www.allenpress.com. Ed. Betty Adelman. Circ: 1,100. **Subscr. to:** Allen Press Inc., PO Box 1897, Lawrence, KS 66044-8897.

371.9 USA ISSN 0883-8534
LC3701

JOURNAL OF MULTICULTURAL COUNSELING AND DEVELOPMENT. Text in English. 1972. q. USD 60 (effective 2001). adv. illus, abstr, bibl. 64 p./no. back issues avail.; reprint service avail. from PQC,PSC,SCH. *Refereed.* **Document type:** *Journal, Academic/Scholarly.* **Description:** Issues include state-of-the-art multicultural counseling research and reports on applications of the latest theoretical ideas and concepts.
Formerly (until 1985): Journal of Non-White Concerns in Personnel and Guidance (0090-5461)
Related titles: Microform ed.: (from PQC); Online - full text ed.: (from H. W. Wilson, ProQuest Information & Learning, Institute for Scientific Information).
Indexed: ASCA, C.I.J.E., Chic.Per.Ind., Curr.Cont., Educ.Ind. (Oct.1983-Apr.1985), High.Educ.Abstr., Ind.Per.Blacks, PsycInfo, Psychol.Abstr. (1973-), SSCI, Sage Race Rel.Abstr., Soc.Work Res.& Abstr., e-psyche.
—BLDSC (5021.058000), IDS, ingenta. **CCC.**
Published by: (Association for Multicultural Counseling and Development), American Counseling Association, 5999 Stevenson Ave, Alexandria, VA 22304-3300. TEL 703-823-9800, FAX 703-823-0252, http://www.counseling.org. Ed. Donald B Pope Davis. R&P Cynthia Peay TEL 703-823-9800 x 249. Adv. contact Kathy Maguire TEL 703-823-9800 ext 207. Circ: 3,200.

▼ **JOURNAL OF MUNDANE BEHAVIOR.** see *SOCIOLOGY*

JOURNAL OF NEAR-DEATH STUDIES. see *PHILOSOPHY*

301.3 150 USA ISSN 0191-5886
BF353 CODEN: JNVBDV

JOURNAL OF NONVERBAL BEHAVIOR. Text in English. 1976. q. USD 507, EUR 506 to institutions for print or online ed.; USD 608.40, EUR 607.20 to institutions for print & online eds.combined (effective 2002). adv. illus. reprint service avail. from PQC,ISI. *Refereed.* **Document type:** *Journal, Academic/Scholarly.* **Description:** Presents theoretical and empirical research on nonverbal communications, including paralanguage, proxemics, facial expressions, eye contact, face-to-face interaction, and nonverbal emotive expression.
Formerly (until 1979): Environmental Psychology and Nonverbal Behavior (0361-3496)
Related titles: Microform ed.: (from PQC); Online - full text ed.: (from EBSCO Publishing, O C L C Online Computer Library Center, Inc., ProQuest Information & Learning, Gale Group, Swets Blackwell, Kluwer Online, Factiva, Institute for Scientific Information, RoweCom Information Quest).
Indexed: ASCA, AgeLine, Biol.Abstr., C.I.J.E. (coverage dropped), Child Devel.Abstr., Commun.Abstr., Crim.Just.Abstr., Curr.Adv.Ecol.Sci., Curr.Cont., ERA, Educ.Admin.Abstr., Fam.Ind., Human Resour.Abstr., IBR, IMFL, Lang.& Lang.Behav.Abstr., M.L.A., MLA Intl.Bibl., Mult.Ed.Abstr., P C I, Peace Res.Abstr., PsycInfo, Psychol.Abstr. (1976-), Psychol.R.G., SOPODA, SSCI, Saf.Sci.Abstr., Sage Fam.Stud.Abstr., Soc.Sci.Ind. (Mar.1987-), Soc.Serv.Abstr., Soc.Work Res.& Abstr., Sociol.Abstr., Sp.Ed.Needs Abstr., Stud.Wom.Abstr., Viol.& Abuse Abstr., e-psyche.
—BLDSC (5022.843000), CISTI, IDS, ingenta. **CCC.**

Published by: Kluwer Academic - Plenum Publishers (Subsidiary of: Wolters Kluwer N.V.), 233 Spring St, New York, NY 10013-1578. TEL 212-620-8000, 800-221-9369, FAX 212-463-0742, info@plenum.com, http://www.wkap.nl/journalhome.htm/0191-5886. Ed. Ronald E Riggio. **Subscr. outside the Americas to:** Kluwer Academic Publishers Group, Journals Department, PO Box 322, Dordrecht 3300 AH, Netherlands. TEL 31-78-639-2392, FAX 31-78-654-6474.

158 GBR ISSN 0963-1798
HF5548.8 CODEN: JOCCEF
JOURNAL OF OCCUPATIONAL AND ORGANIZATIONAL PSYCHOLOGY. Text in English. 1922. q., latest vol.74. GBP 132 in the European Union to institutions; USD 244 rest of world to institutions; GBP 40 newsstand/cover in the European Union; USD 75 newsstand/cover rest of world (effective 2001). adv. bk.rev. charts, illus, abstr. index. 128 p./no. back issues avail.; reprint service avail. from SWZ,SCH,PSC,ISI. *Refereed.* **Document type:** *Journal, Academic/Scholarly.* **Description:** Examines industrial and organizational psychology. Describes, and interprets new research about people at work.
Former titles: Journal of Occupational Psychology (0305-8107); Occupational Psychology (0029-7976)
Related titles: Magnetic Tape ed.; Microfiche ed.; Microform ed.; Online - full text ed.: 1999. free with print (from CatchWord Ltd., Gale Group, EBSCO Publishing, ProQuest Information & Learning, Swets Blackwell, Factiva, Institute for Scientific Information).
Indexed: ABI Inform. (Jan.1978-), ASCA, ASSIA, Account.& Data Proc.Abstr., AgeLine, BMT, BPIA, Biol.Abstr., Br.Educ.Ind., Br.Hum.Ind., Brit.Nur.Ind., Bus.Ind., C.I.S. Abstr., Cont.Pg.Manage., Curr.Cont., Curr.Ind.Stat., ERA, Emerald, Environ.Sci.Poll.Mgmt., Ergon.Abstr., Hlth.Ind., IBR, IBZ, INSPEC (1983-Dec.1991, Mar.1992-), Ind.Med. (coverage dropped), Ind.Philos., Int.Lab.Doc., Intl.Bibl.Soc.Sci., Lang.& Lang.Behav.Abstr., Manage.Cont., Mult.Ed.Abstr., Noise Pollut.Publ.Abstr., P C I, Pers.Lit., Pollut.Abstr., PsycInfo, Psychol.Abstr. (1975-), Psycscan A.P., Res.High.Educ.Abstr., Risk Abstr., Russ.Acad.Sci.Bibl., SCIMP, SOPODA, SSCI, Saf.Sci.Abstr., Soc.Serv.Abstr., Sociol.Abstr., Sp.Ed.Needs Abstr., Stud.Wom.Abstr., Tech.Educ.Abstr., Tr.& Indus.Ind., e-psyche.
—BLDSC (5026.082000), AskIEEE, IDS, ingenta. **CCC.**
Published by: The British Psychological Society, St Andrews House, 48 Princess Rd E, Leicester LE1 7DR, United Kingdom. TEL 44-116-252-9580, FAX 44-116-254-8824, journals@bps.org.uk, http://www.bps.org.uk/publications/journals.cfm. Ed. Henk Thierry. R&P, Adv. contact J Neason TEL 44-116-252-9580. page GBP 288; 135 x 210. Circ: 3,100. **Subscr. to:** Turpin Distribution Services Ltd., Blackhorse Rd, Letchworth, Herts SG6 1HN, United Kingdom. TEL 44-1462-488900, FAX 44-1462-483011.

JOURNAL OF OFFENDER REHABILITATION; a multidisciplinary journal of innovation in research, services, and programs in corrections and criminal justice. see *CRIMINOLOGY AND LAW ENFORCEMENT*

150 USA ISSN 0160-8061
HD58.7 CODEN: JOBMF7
JOURNAL OF ORGANIZATIONAL BEHAVIOR MANAGEMENT. Text in English. 1977. s-a. USD 75 to individuals; USD 101 in Canada to individuals; USD 109 elsewhere to individuals; USD 200 to institutions; USD 270 in Canada to institutions; USD 290 elsewhere to institutions; USD 400 to libraries; USD 540 in Canada to libraries; USD 580 elsewhere to libraries (effective Aug. 2001). adv. bk.rev. illus. back issues avail.; reprint service avail. from HAW. *Refereed.* **Document type:** *Journal, Academic/Scholarly.* **Description:** Deals with behavior management in organizations; provides systematic and effective approaches to behavior management.
Related titles: Microfiche ed.: (from PQC); Microform ed.; Online - full text ed.: (from ProQuest Information & Learning, Gale Group, Factiva, Institute for Scientific Information).
Indexed: ABI Inform. (Spr.1981-), ASCA, Abstr.Health Care Manage.Stud., BPIA, Behav.Abstr., Bus.Educ.Ind., Bus.Ind., Curr.Cont., Educ.Admin.Abstr., Environ.Sci.Poll.Mgmt., Ergon.Abstr., Human Resour.Abstr., IBZ, Lang.& Lang.Behav.Abstr., Manage.Cont., Mgmt.& Market.Abstr., Oper.Res.Manage.Sci., Pers.Lit., Pers.Manage.Abstr., Pollut.Abstr., PsycInfo, Psychol.Abstr. (1978-), Psycscan A.P., Psycscan B.A.& T., Qual.Contr.Appl.Stat., Risk Abstr., SOPODA, SSCI, Saf.Sci.Abstr., Sage Pub.Admin.Abstr., Sociol.Abstr., Tr.& Dev.Alert, Tr.& Indus.Ind., e-psyche.
—BLDSC (5027.068000), Haworth, IDS, ingenta.

Published by: Haworth Press, Inc., 10 Alice St, Binghamton, NY 13904-1580. TEL 607-722-5857, 800-429-6784, FAX 607-722-6362, 800-895-0582, getinfo@haworthpressinc.com, http://www.haworthpress.com/journals/journallist.asp. Ed. Thomas C Mawhinney. Pub. William Cohen. R&P Ruthann Heath TEL 607-723-5857 ext 316. Adv. contact Jackie Blakeslee TEL 607-722-5857 ext 346. B&W page USD 315, color page USD 550; trim 6 x 8.5. Circ: 1,050.

302 GBR ISSN 0894-3796
HD6951 CODEN: JORBEJ
JOURNAL OF ORGANIZATIONAL BEHAVIOUR. Text in English. 1979. 10/yr. USD 1,295 in United States; USD 1,295 in Canada & Mexico; USD 1,295 elsewhere; USD 1,360 combined subscription in United States for print and online eds.; USD 1,360 combined subscription in Canada & Mexico for print and online eds.; USD 1,360 combined subscription elsewhere for print and online eds. (effective 2002). adv. illus. back issues avail.; reprint service avail. from SWZ,PQC,ISI. *Refereed.* **Document type:** *Academic/Scholarly.* **Description:** Aims to report and review the growing research in the industry-organizational behavior fields, and in all topics associated with occupational-organizational behavior.
Formerly (until 1988): Journal of Occupational Behaviour (0142-2774)
Related titles: Microform ed.: (from PQC); Online - full text ed.: ISSN 1099-1379. USD 1,295 in United States; USD 1,295 in Canada & Mexico; USD 1,295 elsewhere (effective 2002) (from EBSCO Publishing, Gale Group, Wiley InterScience, Factiva, Institute for Scientific Information).
Indexed: ABI Inform. (Jan.1988-), ASCA, ASSIA, AgeLine, BPIA, Bus.Ind., Commun.Abstr., Cont.Pg.Manage., Crim.Just.Abstr., Curr.Cont., ERA, Emerald, Environ.Sci.Poll.Mgmt., Ergon.Abstr., Fam.Ind., Human Resour.Abstr., IBR, IBZ, Ind.Philos., Int.Lab.Doc., Lang.& Lang.Behav.Abstr., Mult.Ed.Abstr., Noise Pollut.Publ.Abstr., Peace Res.Abstr., PsycInfo, Psychol.Abstr. (1982-), Psycscan A.P., Risk Abstr., Russ.Acad.Sci.Bibl., SCIMP (1982-), SOPODA, SSCI, Saf.Sci.Abstr., Sage Fam.Stud.Abstr., Sociol.Abstr., Stud.Wom.Abstr., Tr.& Indus.Ind., Viol.& Abuse Abstr., e-psyche.
—BLDSC (5027.066000), IDS, ingenta. **CCC.**
Published by: Wiley Europe Ltd., Baffins Ln, Chichester, W Sussex PO19 1UD, United Kingdom. TEL 44-1243-779777, FAX 44-1243-775878, customer@wiley.co.uk, http://www.wiley.co.uk. adv.: B&W page GBP 650, color page GBP 1,550; trim 200 x 260. **Subscr. in the Americas to:** John Wiley & Sons, Inc., Journals, 605 Third Ave, New York, NY 10158. TEL 212-850-6021, 212-850-6645, subinfo@jwiley.com.

JOURNAL OF OUTCOME MEASUREMENT; dedicated to health, education, and social science. (JOM) see *EDUCATION*

JOURNAL OF PARAPSYCHOLOGY; a scientific quarterly dealing with extrasensory perception, the psychokinetic effect and related topics. see *PARAPSYCHOLOGY AND OCCULTISM*

THE JOURNAL OF PASTORAL CARE. see *RELIGIONS AND THEOLOGY*

155.4 USA ISSN 0146-8693
RJ503.3 CODEN: JPPSDW
JOURNAL OF PEDIATRIC PSYCHOLOGY. Text in English. 1976. 8/yr. GBP 65, USD 92 to individuals; GBP 255, USD 375 to institutions; GBP 25, USD 36 to students (effective 2002). bk.rev. illus. Index. back issues avail.; reprints avail. *Refereed.* **Document type:** *Academic/Scholarly.* **Description:** Emphasis in on the dissemination of original research relating broadly to the multidimensional functioning and development of children, adolescents and families or issues related to pediatric health and illness.
Formerly: Pediatric Psychology
Related titles: Microfilm ed.: (from PQC); Online - full text ed.: ISSN 1465-735X. USD 229, GBP 337 to institutions Online only (effective 2002) (from HighWire Pr., EBSCO Publishing, O C L C Online Computer Library Center, Inc., RoweCom Information Quest, ingenta, Swets Blackwell, Institute for Scientific Information).
Indexed: ASCA, Behav.Med.Abstr., Bibl.Dev.Med.& Child Neur., Biol.Abstr., CINAHL, Child Devel.Abstr., Curr.Cont., ERA, Environ.Sci.Poll.Mgmt., Excerp.Med., Fam.Ind., IMFL, Ind.Med. (1976-), Int.Nurs.Ind., Lang.& Lang.Behav.Abstr., Pollut.Abstr., PsycInfo, Psychol.Abstr. (1975-), Psycscan D.P., Risk Abstr., SOPODA, SSCI, Saf.Sci.Abstr., Sage Fam.Stud.Abstr., Soc.Work Res.& Abstr., Sociol.Abstr., Sp.Ed.Needs Abstr., e-psyche.

—BLDSC (5030.260000), CISTI, GNLM, IDS, ingenta, KNAW. **CCC.**
Published by: (Society of Pediatric Psychology GBR), Oxford University Press, Academic Division, Great Clarendon St, Oxford OX2 6DP, United Kingdom. TEL 44-1865-267907, FAX 44-1865-267835, jnl.info@oup.co.uk, http://www.oup.co.uk/jpepsy/, http://www.oup.co.uk/journals. Ed. Anne Ekazak Barnett. Pub. Janet Fox. Circ: 2,000.

155.2 USA ISSN 0022-3506
CODEN: JOPEAE
JOURNAL OF PERSONALITY. Text in English. 1932. bi-m. GBP 386 to institutions in UK & Europe; USD 461 to institutions in the Americas & Caribbeans; GBP 386 elsewhere to institutions (effective 2002). adv. bibl, charts, illus. index. reprint service avail. from PSC,SCH. *Refereed.* **Document type:** *Journal, Academic/Scholarly.* **Description:** Publishes studies in the fields of personality and behavior dynamics that focus on personality development and individual differences in the cognitive affective and interpersonal domains. Reflects and stimulates growth in new theoritical and methodological approaches.
Related titles: Online - full text ed.: (from EBSCO Publishing, O C L C Online Computer Library Center, Inc., RoweCom Information Quest, ingenta, Gale Group, Swets Blackwell, Factiva, Institute for Scientific Information).
Indexed: ASCA, ASSIA, Acad.Ind., Adol.Ment.Hlth.Abstr., AgeLine, Arts & Hum.Cit.Ind. (coverage dropped), Biol.Abstr., Commun.Abstr., Curr.Cont., Educ.Ind. (coverage dropped), Fam.Ind., IBR, IBZ, Ind.Med. (1945-), Ind.Philos., Intl.Bibl.Soc.Sci., Lang.& Lang.Behav.Abstr., Mid.East: Abstr.& Ind., P C I, Past.Care & Couns.Abstr., PsycInfo, Psychol.Abstr. (1945-), Risk Abstr., Russ.Acad.Sci.Bibl., SOPODA, SSCI, Sage Fam.Stud.Abstr., Soc.Sci.Ind. (Sep.1982-), Soc.Serv.Abstr., Sociol.Abstr., Stud.Wom.Abstr., e-psyche.
—BLDSC (5030.900000), GNLM, IDS, ingenta. **CCC.**
Published by: Blackwell Publishers, 350 Main St, Malden, MA 02148. TEL 781-388-8200, 800-835-6770, FAX 781-388-8232, subscript@blackwellpub.com, http://www.blackwellpublishers.co.uk/journals/diph. Ed. Howard Tennen. R&P Gretchen Voter TEL 781-388-0423. Adv. contact Anne Marie Sheehy TEL 781-388-0427. Circ: 2,000.

152 158.3 IND ISSN 0970-1206
JOURNAL OF PERSONALITY AND CLINICAL STUDIES. Text in English. bi-m. **Document type:** *Academic/Scholarly.*
Indexed: Indian Psychol.Abstr., PsycInfo, Psychol.Abstr. (1985-), e-psyche.
—BLDSC (5030.900500).
Published by: (Association of Clinical Psychologists), Habib Ahmad, c/o Samar Offset Printers, 1788 Kalan Mahal Daryaganj, New Delhi 110 002, India.

155.2 USA ISSN 0022-3514
HM251 CODEN: JPSPB2
JOURNAL OF PERSONALITY AND SOCIAL PSYCHOLOGY. Text in English. 1925. m. USD 340 domestic to non-members; USD 380 foreign to non-members; USD 170 domestic to members; USD 188 foreign to members; USD 863 domestic to institutions; USD 951 foreign to institutions (effective 2001). adv. charts, stat, illus. index. reprint service avail. from PQC,PSC,SCH. *Refereed.* **Document type:** *Academic/Scholarly.* **Description:** Covers research in three major areas: attitudes and social cognition; interpersonal relations and group processes; and personality processes and individual differences.
Supersedes in part (in 1965): Journal of Abnormal and Social Psychology (0096-851X)
Related titles: Microform ed.: (from PQC); Online - full text ed.: (from Gale Group, Factiva, Institute for Scientific Information).
Indexed: ASCA, ASSIA, Acad.Ind., Addic.Abstr., Adol.Ment.Hlth.Abstr., AgeLine, Amer.Bibl.Slavic & E.Eur.Stud., Arts & Hum.Cit.Ind. (coverage dropped), Bibl.Asian Stud. (1970-1971), Biol.Abstr., C.I.J.E. (coverage dropped), Chic.Per.Ind., Child Devel.Abstr., Commun.Abstr., Crim.Just.Abstr., Curr.Cont., Curr.Ind.Stat., ERA, Educ.Admin.Abstr., Fam.Ind., High.Educ.Abstr., IBZ, INIS Atomind., Ind.Med. (1965-), Ind.Philos., Int.Nurs.Ind., Int.Polit.Sci.Abstr., Intl.Bibl.Soc.Sci., Lang.& Lang.Behav.Abstr., M.L.A., MLA Intl.Bibl., Mark.Res.Abstr. (1965-), Mid.East: Abstr.& Ind., Mult.Ed.Abstr., P C I, PSI, PsycInfo, Psychol.Abstr. (1965-), Psycscan D.P., Rel.Ind.One, Rel.Ind.Two, Russ.Acad.Sci.Bibl., SOPODA, SSCI, Sage Fam.Stud.Abstr., Sage Urb.Stud.Abstr., Soc.Sci.Ind. (Jun.1982-), Soc.Serv.Abstr., Soc.Work Res.& Abstr., Sociol.Abstr., Sp.Ed.Needs Abstr., Sportsearch, Stud.Wom.Abstr., e-psyche.
—BLDSC (5030.901000), GNLM, IDS, ingenta. **CCC.**

P

Published by: American Psychological Association, 750 First St., N.E., Washington, DC 20002-4242. TEL 202-336-5600, 800-374-2721, FAX 202-336-5568, subscriptions@apa.org, http://www.apa.org/journals/psp.html. Eds. Arie W Kruglanski, Chester A Insko, Ed Diener. Circ: 5,100.

155.2 USA ISSN 0022-3891
BF698.4
JOURNAL OF PERSONALITY ASSESSMENT. Text in English. 1970 (vol.34). bi-m. (in 2 vols.). USD 85 in US & Canada to individuals; USD 130 elsewhere to individuals; USD 395 in US & Canada to institutions; USD 440 elsewhere to institutions (effective 2002). adv. bk.rev. abstr, bibl, charts, illus. index. reprint service avail. from PSC,SCH,PQC. *Refereed.* **Document type:** *Journal, Academic/Scholarly.* **Description:** Presents commentaries, case reports, and research studies dealing with the application of methods of personality assessment.
Formerly: Journal of Projective Techniques and Personality Assessment
Related titles: Microform ed.: (from PQC); Online - full text ed.: ISSN 1532-7752. USD 76.50 to individuals; USD 355.50 to institutions (effective 2002) (from CatchWord Ltd., EBSCO Publishing, O C L C Online Computer Library Center, Inc., RoweCom Information Quest, Swets Blackwell, Institute for Scientific Information).
Indexed: ASCA, ASSIA, Adol.Ment.Hlth.Abstr., AgeLine, Biol.Abstr., C.I.S. Abstr., Child Devel.Abstr., Curr.Cont., Environ.Sci.Poll.Mgmt., Except.Child Educ.Abstr., Excerp.Med., Fam.Ind., Ind.Med. (1971-), Indian Psychol.Abstr., Int.Nurs.Ind., Lang.& Lang.Behav.Abstr., Mid.East: Abstr.& Ind., P C I, Pollut.Abstr., PsycInfo, Psychol.Abstr. (1971-), Psycscan C.P., Risk Abstr., Russ.Acad.Sci.Bibl., SSCI, Saf.Sci.Abstr., e-psyche.
—BLDSC (5030.950000), CatchWord, EMDOCS, GNLM, ingenta. **CCC.**
Published by: (Society for Personality Assessment), Lawrence Erlbaum Associates, Inc., 10 Industrial Ave, Mahwah, NJ 07430-2262. TEL 201-760-3735, 800-926-6579, FAX 201-236-0072, journals@erlbaum.com, http://www.erlbaum.com/Journals/journals/JPA/jpa.htm. Ed. Bill N Kinder. adv.: page USD 600; trim 5 x 8. Circ: 2,700.

370.15 USA ISSN 0885-579X
RC554
JOURNAL OF PERSONALITY DISORDERS. Text in English. 1986. q. USD 50 domestic to individuals; USD 75 foreign to individuals; USD 172 domestic to institutions; USD 197 foreign to institutions (effective 2000). adv. bk.rev. index. reprint service avail. from PQC,ISI. *Refereed.* **Document type:** *Academic/Scholarly.* **Description:** Presents new research, and clinical techniques for assessing, diagnosing and treating personality disorders.
Related titles: Online - full text ed.: (from Northern Light Technology, Inc., ProQuest Information & Learning, CatchWord Ltd., Institute for Scientific Information, RoweCom Information Quest).
Indexed: ASCA, Biol.Abstr., Curr.Cont., Excerp.Med., Fam.Ind., IBZ, Ind.Med. (1987-), Lang.& Lang.Behav.Abstr., PsycInfo, Psychol.Abstr. (1987-), SOPODA, SSCI, Soc.Work Res.& Abstr., Sociol.Abstr., e-psyche.
—BLDSC (5030.955000), EMDOCS, GNLM, IDS, ingenta, KNAW. **CCC.**
Published by: (International Society for the Study of Personality Disorders), Guilford Publications, Inc., 72 Spring St, 4th Fl, New York, NY 10012. TEL 212-431-9800, 800-365-7006, FAX 212-966-6708, info@guilford.com. Ed. W John Livesley. Pub. Robert Matloff. R&P Kathy Kuehl. Adv. contact Susan Pavliscak. Circ: 1,300.

150 USA ISSN 0047-2662
BF204.5 CODEN: JPHPAE
JOURNAL OF PHENOMENOLOGICAL PSYCHOLOGY. Text in English. 1970. s-a. EUR 72, USD 84 includes online ed. (effective 2002). adv. bk.rev. index. back issues avail. *Refereed.* **Document type:** *Journal, Academic/Scholarly.* **Description:** Publishes articles that advance the discipline of psychology from a phenomenological perspective as understood by scholars who work within the continental sense of phenomenology.
Related titles: Microform ed.: (from PQC); Online - full text ed.: (from Northern Light Technology, Inc., ProQuest Information & Learning, CatchWord Ltd.).
Indexed: ASCA, Arts & Hum.Cit.Ind. (coverage dropped), Curr.Cont. (coverage dropped), IBR, IBZ, PsycInfo, Psychol.Abstr. (1970-), Russ.Acad.Sci.Bibl., SSCI (coverage dropped), e-psyche.
—BLDSC (5034.100000), IDS, ingenta. **CCC.**

Published by: Brill Academic Publishers, Inc., 112 Water St, Ste 400, Boston, MA 02109. TEL 617-263-2323, 877-999-7575, FAX 617-263-2324, cs@brillusa.com. Ed. Frederick J Wertz. Pub., R&P Lynne Moser. Adv. contact Katy Stenhouse. B&W page USD 150; trim 9 x 6. Circ: 200.

JOURNAL OF POETRY THERAPY; the interdisciplinary journal of practice, theory, research, and education. see *LITERATURE—Poetry*

JOURNAL OF POLICE AND CRIMINAL PSYCHOLOGY. see *CRIMINOLOGY AND LAW ENFORCEMENT*

JOURNAL OF POLYMORPHOUS PERVERSITY. see *LITERARY AND POLITICAL REVIEWS*

150 USA ISSN 1098-3007
▼ **JOURNAL OF POSITIVE BEHAVIOR INTERVENTIONS.** Text in English. 1999. 4/yr., latest vol.3. USD 43 in North America to individuals; USD 71 elsewhere to individuals; USD 109 in North America to institutions; USD 138 elsewhere to institutions (effective 2002). **Document type:** *Journal, Academic/Scholarly.* **Description:** Provides a forum for researchers, professionals, families, and policymakers concerned with the behavior of individuals with developmental and behavioral disabilities.
Related titles: Online - full text ed.: (from ProQuest Information & Learning, CatchWord Ltd.).
—BLDSC (5041.147700).
Published by: Pro-Ed Inc., 8700 Shoal Creek Blvd, Austin, TX 78757-6897. TEL 512-451-3246, proed1@aol.com, http://www.proedinc.com. Eds. Glen Dunlap, Robert L Koegel. Pub. Donald D Hammill. R&P Barbara Rivera TEL 512-451-3246 ext 653.

JOURNAL OF PRENATAL & PERINATAL PSYCHOLOGY & HEALTH. see *MEDICAL SCIENCES—Obstetrics And Gynecology*

613 USA ISSN 0278-095X
RA790.A1 CODEN: JPPRDT
THE JOURNAL OF PRIMARY PREVENTION. Text in English. 1980. q. USD 540, EUR 538 to institutions for print or online ed.; USD 648, EUR 645.60 to institutions for print & online eds.combined (effective 2002). adv. bk.rev. reprint service avail. from PQC,ISI. *Refereed.* **Document type:** *Journal, Academic/Scholarly.* **Description:** Presents theoretical, empirical, and methodological research on preventative intervention in human services, and discusses innovative programs and concepts.
Formerly (until 1981): Journal of Prevention (0163-514X)
Related titles: Online - full text ed.: (from EBSCO Publishing, O C L C Online Computer Library Center, Inc., Swets Blackwell, Kluwer Online, RoweCom Information Quest).
Indexed: Adol.Ment.Hlth.Abstr., Biol.Abstr., Crim.Just.Abstr., Excerp.Med., IBZ, IMFL, Lang.& Lang.Behav.Abstr., PsycInfo, Psychol.Abstr. (1980-), SOPODA, Soc.Serv.Abstr., Sociol.Abstr., e-psyche.
—BLDSC (5042.370000), EMDOCS, GNLM, Infotrieve, ingenta, KNAW. **CCC.**
Published by: (Vermont Conference on Primary Prevention of Psychopathology), Kluwer Academic - Plenum Publishers (Subsidiary of: Wolters Kluwer N.V.), 233 Spring St, New York, NY 10013-1578. TEL 212-620-8000, 800-221-9369, FAX 212-463-0742, info@plenum.com, http://www.wkap.nl/journalhome.htm/0278-095X. Ed. Martin Bloom. **Subscr. outside the Americas to:** Kluwer Academic Publishers Group, Journals Department, PO Box 322, Dordrecht 3300 AH, Netherlands. TEL 31-78-639-2392, FAX 31-78-654-6474.

JOURNAL OF PSYCHOACTIVE DRUGS; a multidisciplinary forum. see *DRUG ABUSE AND ALCOHOLISM*

JOURNAL OF PSYCHOEDUCATIONAL ASSESSMENT. see *EDUCATION*

900 150 USA ISSN 0145-3378
HQ768 CODEN: JOPSDP
JOURNAL OF PSYCHOHISTORY. Text in English. 1973. q. USD 54 to individuals; USD 129 to institutions (effective 2001). adv. bk.rev. illus. reprint service avail. from PQC,PSC,SCH. *Refereed.* **Document type:** *Academic/Scholarly.* **Description:** Contains research in the psychological study of history.
Incorporates (1978-1988): Journal of Psychoanalytic Anthropology (0278-2944); Formerly (until 1976): History of Childhood Quarterly (0091-4266)
Related titles: Microfilm ed.: (from PQC); Online - full text ed.: (from Institute for Scientific Information).
Indexed: ASCA, Amer.Hist.& Life, Anthropol.Lit., Arts & Hum.Cit.Ind. (coverage dropped), BHA, Bibl.Asian Stud. (1974), Child Devel.Abstr., Child.Lit.Abstr., Curr.Cont., Curr.Lit.Fam.Plan., Hist.Abstr. (1973-), IMFL, Lang.& Lang.Behav.Abstr., Mid.East: Abstr.& Ind., Polit.Sci.Abstr., PsycInfo, Psychoanal.Abstr., Psychol.Abstr. (1973-), Ref.Zh., Rel.Ind.One, Rel.Ind.Two, SOPODA, SSCI, Sociol.Abstr., Viol.& Abuse Abstr., e-psyche.
—BLDSC (5043.280000), IDS, Infotrieve, ingenta. **CCC.**
Published by: Association for Psychohistory, Inc., 140 Riverside Dr, New York, NY 10024-2605. TEL 212-799-2294, FAX 212-799-2294, psychhst@tiac.net. Ed., Pub., R&P, Adv. contact Lloyd de Mause. Circ: 6,000 (paid).

JOURNAL OF PSYCHOLINGUISTIC RESEARCH. see *LINGUISTICS*

150 USA
JOURNAL OF PSYCHOLOGICAL PRACTICE. Variant title: Journal of the Northamerican Association of Masters in Psyhcology. Text in English. q.
Indexed: e-psyche.
—BLDSC (5043.304000).
Published by: Cleveland State University, Psychology Department, Euclid at East 24th St, Cleveland, OH 44115. TEL 216-687-2525, FAX 216-687-9294. Ed. Steve Slane.

150 IND ISSN 0022-3972
BF1 CODEN: JPSRB8
JOURNAL OF PSYCHOLOGICAL RESEARCHES. Text in English. 1957. 3/yr. USD 75. adv. bk.rev. charts. index. reprint service avail. from PQC. **Document type:** *Academic/Scholarly.*
Related titles: Microform ed.: (from PQC).
Indexed: Bibl.Asian Stud. (1969-1984), Biol.Abstr., Indian Psychol.Abstr., Psychol.Abstr., e-psyche.
—BLDSC (5043.310000), ingenta.
Published by: Madras Psychology Society, University of Madras, Department of Psychology, Chennai, Tamil Nadu 600 005, India. TEL 91-44-568778, FAX 91-44-566693, TELEX 416376 ONOMIN. Ed. K V Kaliappan. Circ: 400.

150 USA ISSN 0895-8750
JOURNAL OF PSYCHOLOGICAL TYPE. Text in English. 1977. 4/yr. USD 88 domestic; USD 99 foreign (effective 2000). adv. back issues avail.; reprint service avail. from PSC,SCH. *Refereed.* **Document type:** *Academic/Scholarly.* **Description:** Publishes research, theoretical discussions and applications of psychological type and the Myers-Briggs Type Indicator.
Formerly (until vol.7): Research in Psychological Type
Indexed: PsycInfo, Psychol.Abstr. (1991-), e-psyche.
—BLDSC (5043.321000), ingenta.
Published by: (Association for Psychological Type), Dr. Thomas G. Carskadon, Ed. & Pub., c/o Department of Psychology, Mississippi State Univ, Box 6161, Mississippi State, MS 39762. TEL 662-325-7655, FAX 662-325-7212, tomcar@ra.msstate.edu. R&P, Adv. contact Dr. Thomas G Carskadon. Circ: 5,500 (paid).

150 USA ISSN 0733-4273
BR110
JOURNAL OF PSYCHOLOGY AND CHRISTIANITY. Text in English. 1982. q. USD 65 to libraries (effective 2002). adv. bk.rev. back issues avail.; reprint service avail. from PQC,PSC,SCH. *Refereed.* **Document type:** *Academic/Scholarly.* **Description:** Investigation of theoretical and applied issues in the relationship of Christianity and the psychological and pastorial professions.
Supersedes (1974-1981): Christian Association for Psychological Studies. Bulletin; Incorporates: Christian Association for Psychological Studies. Proceedings (0092-072X)
Related titles: Microfilm ed.: (from PQC).
Indexed: A.S.& T.Ind. (coverage dropped), Chr.Per.Ind., Educ.Ind. (coverage dropped), Fam.Ind., G.Soc.Sci.& Rel.Per.Lit., IBZ, Ind.Philos., PSI, PsycInfo, Psychol.Abstr. (1982-), R.G. (coverage dropped), Rel.& Theol.Abstr. (1986-), Rel.Ind.One, Rel.Ind.Two, Soc.Sci.Ind. (coverage dropped), e-psyche.
—BLDSC (5043.405000), ingenta.
Published by: Christian Association for Psychological Studies, Inc., PO Box 310400, New Braunfels, TX 78131-0400. TEL 830-629-2277, FAX 830-629-2342, capsintl@compuvision.net. Ed. Peter C Hill. Adv. contact Brian Eck. Circ: 2,400 (paid).

150 332 USA ISSN 1520-8834
▼ **JOURNAL OF PSYCHOLOGY AND FINANCIAL MARKETS.** Text in English. 2000. q. USD 75 in US & Canada to individuals; USD 105 elsewhere to individuals; USD 220 in US & Canada to institutions; USD 250 elsewhere to institutions (effective 2002). adv. back issues avail. **Document type:** *Journal, Academic/Scholarly.* **Description:** Addresses the implications of current research on individual and group emotion, cognition, and action related to individual behavior in the context of financial markets, on the part of both persons in the field and investors.
Related titles: Online - full content ed.: ISSN 1532-7760. USD 67.50 to individuals; USD 198 to institutions (effective 2002) (from EBSCO Publishing, O C L C Online Computer Library Center, Inc., Swets Blackwell); Online - full text ed.: (from CatchWord Ltd., RoweCom Information Quest).
Indexed: e-psyche.
—BLDSC (5043.406000), CatchWord. **CCC.**
Published by: (Institute of Psychology and Markets), Lawrence Erlbaum Associates, Inc., 10 Industrial Ave, Mahwah, NJ 07430-2262. TEL 201-760-3735, 800-926-6579, FAX 201-236-0072, journals@erlbaum.com, http://www.erlbaum.com/Journals/journals/JPFM/jpfm.htm. Ed. Gunduz Caganalp. adv.: page USD 275; trim 7 x 10.

155.3 USA ISSN 0890-7064
BF692 CODEN: JPSXET
JOURNAL OF PSYCHOLOGY & HUMAN SEXUALITY. Text in English. 1988. q. USD 75 to individuals; USD 101 in Canada to individuals; USD 109 elsewhere to individuals; USD 240 to institutions; USD 324 in Canada to institutions; USD 348 elsewhere to institutions; USD 360 to libraries; USD 486 in Canada to libraries (effective Aug. 2001); USD 522 elsewhere to libraries (effective Apr. 2001). adv. bk.rev. back issues avail.; reprint service avail. from HAW. *Refereed.* **Document type:** *Journal, Academic/Scholarly.* **Description:** Publishes original articles and reviews about human sexuality.
Related titles: Microform ed.: (from PQC).
Indexed: Abstr.Anthropol., Biol.Dig., Environ.Sci.Poll.Mgmt., Gend.Watch, High.Educ.Abstr., IBZ, IMFL, Ind.Philos., Indian Psychol.Abstr., Lang.& Lang.Behav.Abstr., Per.Islam. (1988-), PsycInfo, Psychol.Abstr. (1988-), Ref.Zh., Risk Abstr., SOPODA, Saf.Sci.Abstr., Sage Fam.Stud.Abstr., Soc.Serv.Abstr., Soc.Work Res.& Abstr., Sociol.Abstr., Stud.Wom.Abstr., Viol.& Abuse Abstr., e-psyche.
—BLDSC (5043.408000), GNLM, Haworth, ingenta.
Published by: Haworth Press, Inc., 10 Alice St, Binghamton, NY 13904-1580. TEL 607-722-5857, 800-429-6784, FAX 607-722-6362, 800-895-0582, getinfo@haworthpressinc.com, http://www.haworthpress.com/journals/journallist.asp. Ed. Eli Coleman. Pub. William Cohen. R&P Ruthann Heath TEL 607-723-5857 ext 316. Adv. contact Jackie Blakeslee TEL 607-722-5857 ext 346. B&W page USD 315, color page USD 550; trim 6 x 8.5. Circ: 560.

JOURNAL OF PSYCHOLOGY AND JUDAISM. see *RELIGIONS AND THEOLOGY—Judaic*

150 200 USA ISSN 0091-6471
BF1 CODEN: JPSTDG
JOURNAL OF PSYCHOLOGY AND THEOLOGY; an evangelical forum for the integration of psychology and theology. Text in English. 1973. q. USD 40 domestic; USD 42 foreign surface mail; USD 52 foreign airmail (effective 2001). adv. bk.rev. bibl. charts, illus. index, cum index. back issues avail.; reprint service avail. from PQC. *Refereed.* **Document type:** *Journal, Academic/Scholarly.* **Description:** Communicates recent scholarly thinking on the interrelationships of psychological and theological concepts and considers the application of these concepts to a variety of professional settings.
Related titles: CD-ROM ed.; Microfilm ed.: (from PQC); Online - full text ed.: (from The Dialog Corporation, ProQuest Information & Learning, Institute for Scientific Information).
Indexed: ASCA, AgeLine, Arts & Hum.Cit.Ind., CCR, CERDIC, Chic.Per.Ind., Chr.Per.Ind., Curr.Cont., G.Soc.Sci.& Rel.Per.Lit., IBR, IBZ, IMFL, Ind.Philos., Old Test.Abstr., Past.Care & Couns.Abstr., PsycInfo, Psychol.Abstr. (1973-), Psychol.R.G., Rel.& Theol.Abstr. (1973-), Rel.Ind.One, Rel.Ind.Two, SSCI, e-psyche.
—BLDSC (5043.420000), IDS.
Published by: Biola University, Rosemead School of Psychology, 13800 Biola Ave, La Mirada, CA 90639-0001. TEL 562-903-4727, FAX 562-906-4500, journal_editorial@peter.biola.edu, journal_subscriptions@peter.biola.edu, http://www.biola.edu/admin/jpt, http://www.rosemead.edu. Ed., R&P Patricia L Pike TEL 562-903-4867. Adv. contact Tora Massey. Circ: 1,700.

150 DEU ISSN 1433-0237
JOURNAL OF PSYCHOLOGY IN AFRICA. Text in English. 1988. 2/yr. DEM 36 per issue to individuals; DEM 59 per issue to institutions (effective 2000). **Document type:** *Academic/Scholarly.* **Description:** Forum for dissemination and utilization of psychological research in Africa and related regions.
Indexed: PsycInfo, Soc.Serv.Abstr., Sociol.Abstr., e-psyche.
Published by: I K O - Verlag fuer Interkulturelle Kommunikation, Postfach 900421, Frankfurt Am Main 60444, Germany. TEL 49-69-784808, FAX 49-69-7896575, ikoverlag@t-online.de, http://www.iko-verlag.de.

150 HKG ISSN 1563-3403
JOURNAL OF PSYCHOLOGY IN CHINESE SOCIETIES. Text in English. 1978. s-a. USD 180, USD 24 to individuals; HKD 310, USD 40 to institutions (effective 2001). bk.rev. 155 p./no. *Refereed.* **Document type:** *Journal, Academic/Scholarly.* **Description:** Aims to create a new and integrative forum for discussions and exchanges of research and information across disciplinary and national boundaries by focusing on both differences and similarities in approaches to researching Chinese psychology and empirical data relevant to psychological issues within Chinese societies, including but not limited to social, cognitive, developmental, physiological, and clinical studies.
Formerly (until Feb. 2000): Hong Kong Psychological Society. Bulletin (0379-4490)
—BLDSC (5043.422000).
Published by: (Hong Kong Psychological Society Ltd.), Chinese University Press, Sha Tin, New Territories, Hong Kong. TEL 852-2609-6508, FAX 852-2603-7355, cup@cuhk.edu.hk, http://www.chineseupress.com/. Eds. Leung Y.K. Freedom, Tardif Twila. R&P, Adv. contact Angelina Wong TEL 852-26096500.

150 USA
BF1
JOURNAL OF PSYCHOLOGY: INTERDISCIPLINARY & APPLIED; the general field of psychology. Text in English. 1936. bi-m., latest vol.136, 2002. USD 155 domestic; USD 170 foreign; USD 38.75 (effective 2001 - 2002). adv. bibl. index. back issues avail.; reprint service avail. from SWZ,SCH,PSC. *Refereed.* **Document type:** *Academic/Scholarly.* **Description:** Publishes a variety of research and theoretical articles in the field of psychology, with an emphasis on articles that integrate divergent data and theories, explore new avenues for thinking and research, or present outrageous criticisms of the present status of the behavioral disciplines.
Formerly: Journal of Psychology (0022-3980)
Related titles: Online - full text ed.: (from Gale Group, H. W. Wilson, ProQuest Information & Learning, Factiva, Institute for Scientific Information).
Indexed: Acad.Ind., Addic.Abstr., AgeLine, Arts & Hum.Cit.Ind. (coverage dropped), Biol.Abstr., CERDIC, C.I.J.E. (coverage dropped), Chem.Abstr., Chic.Per.Ind., Child Devel.Abstr., Commun.Abstr., Crim.Just.Abstr., Curr.Cont., DSH Abstr., Environ.Sci.Poll.Mgmt., Ergon.Abstr., Except.Child Educ.Abstr., Fam.Ind., Ind.Med. (1935-), Ind.Philos., Indian Psychol.Abstr., Int.Polit.Sci.Abstr., Intl.Bibl.Soc.Sci., Lang.& Lang.Behav.Abstr., Mid.East: Abstr.& Ind., Mult.Ed.Abstr., P C I, PsycInfo, Psychol.Abstr. (1935-), Ref.Zh., Rel.Ind.One, Rel.Ind.Two, Risk Abstr., Russ.Acad.Sci.Bibl., SOPODA, SSCI, Saf.Sci.Abstr., Sage Race Rel.Abstr., Soc.Sci.Ind. (Jan.1987-), Soc.Serv.Abstr., Soc.Work Res.& Abstr., Sociol.Abstr., Stud.Wom.Abstr., e-psyche.
—BLDSC (5043.400000), CISTI, GNLM, IDS, ingenta. **CCC.**
Published by: (Helen Dwight Reid Educational Foundation), Heldref Publications, 1319 Eighteenth St, N W, Washington, DC 20036-1802. TEL 202-296-6267, 800-365-9753, FAX 202-293-6130, jrl@heldref.org, http://www.heldref.org. Ed. Doris Chalfin. Circ: 1,420. **Subscr. to:** Allen Press Inc., PO Box 1897, Lawrence, KS 66044-8897.

150 USA ISSN 0882-2689
BF698.4 CODEN: JPBAEB
JOURNAL OF PSYCHOPATHOLOGY AND BEHAVIORAL ASSESSMENT. Text in English. 1979. q. USD 506, EUR 505 to institutions for print or online ed.; USD 607.20, EUR 606 to institutions for print & online eds.combined (effective 2002). adv. back issues avail.; reprint service avail. from PSC,SCH. *Refereed.* **Document type:** *Journal, Academic/Scholarly.*
Formerly (until 1986): Journal of Behavioral Assessment (0164-0305)
Related titles: Microfilm ed.: (from PQC); Online - full text ed.: (from EBSCO Publishing, O C L C Online Computer Library Center, Inc., Swets Blackwell, Kluwer Online, Institute for Scientific Information, RoweCom Information Quest).
Indexed: ASCA, Adol.Ment.Hlth.Abstr., Biol.Abstr., Curr.Cont., ERA, Excerp.Med., Fam.Ind., IMFL, Mult.Ed.Abstr., PsycInfo, Psychol.Abstr. (1979-), Psycscan B.A.& T., Ref.Zh., Russ.Acad.Sci.Bibl., SSCI, Soc.Work Res.& Abstr., Sp.Ed.Needs Abstr., e-psyche.
—BLDSC (5043.430000), CISTI, EMDOCS, GNLM, IDS, ingenta, KNAW. **CCC.**
Published by: Kluwer Academic - Plenum Publishers (Subsidiary of: Wolters Kluwer N.V.) http://www.wkap.nl/journalhome.htm/0882-2689. Eds. Henry E Adams, Patricia B Sutker. **Subscr. outside the Americas to:** Kluwer Academic Publishers Group, Journals Department, PO Box 322, Dordrecht 3300 AH, Netherlands. TEL 31-78-639-2392, FAX 31-78-654-6474.

JOURNAL OF PSYCHOPHARMACOLOGY. see *PHARMACY AND PHARMACOLOGY*

616.8 USA ISSN 0269-8803
JOURNAL OF PSYCHOPHYSIOLOGY. Text in English. 1987. q. USD 149 (effective 2001). adv. bk.rev. back issues avail. *Refereed.* **Document type:** *Journal, Academic/Scholarly.* **Description:** Outlet for original research in all areas employing psychophysiological techniques.
Related titles: Online - full text ed.: (from Institute for Scientific Information).
Indexed: ASCA, Addic.Abstr., Excerp.Med., IBR, IBZ, Ind.Philos., Int.Abstr.Biol.Sci., Neurosci.Cit.Ind., PsycInfo, Psychol.Abstr. (1987-), SSCI, e-psyche.
—BLDSC (5043.465000), EMDOCS, GNLM, IDS, ingenta, KNAW. **CCC.**
Published by: Hogrefe & Huber Publishers, PO Box 2487, Kirkland, WA 98083. TEL 425-820-1500, FAX 425-823-8324, hh@hhpub.com, http://www.hhpub.com/journals. Ed. G Barrett. Adv. contact Iris Pruegl.

158 USA ISSN 0894-9085
RC489.R3 CODEN: JRCTFK
JOURNAL OF RATIONAL - EMOTIVE AND COGNITIVE - BEHAVIOR THERAPY. Text in English. 1983. q. USD 480, EUR 479 to institutions for print or online ed.; USD 576, EUR 574.80 to institutions for print & online eds.combined (effective 2002). adv. bk.rev. illus. reprint service avail. from PQC. *Refereed.* **Document type:** *Journal, Academic/Scholarly.* **Description:** Provides a forum for the stimulation and maintenance of rational-emotive therapy and other forms of cognitive-behavior therapy.
Formerly (until 1987): Journal of Rational-Emotive Therapy (0748-1985); Supersedes (1966-1983): Rational Living (0034-0049)
Related titles: Microform ed.: (from PQC); Online - full text ed.: (from EBSCO Publishing, O C L C Online Computer Library Center, Inc., RoweCom Information Quest, Swets Blackwell, Kluwer Online).
Indexed: Adol.Ment.Hlth.Abstr., IBR, IBZ, Ind.Philos., Lang.& Lang.Behav.Abstr., PsycInfo, Psychol.Abstr. (1966-), Psycscan B.A.& T., e-psyche.
—BLDSC (5046.800000), ingenta. **CCC.**
Published by: (Institute for Rational-Emotive Therapy), Kluwer Academic - Plenum Publishers (Subsidiary of: Wolters Kluwer N.V.), 233 Spring St, New York, NY 10013-1578. TEL 212-620-8000, 800-221-9369, FAX 212-463-0742, info@plenum.com, http://www.wkap.nl/journalhome.htm/0894-9085. Ed. Michael E Bernard. **Subscr. outside the Americas to:** Kluwer Academic Publishers Group, Journals Department, PO Box 322, Dordrecht 3300 AH, Netherlands. TEL 31-78-639-2392, FAX 31-78-654-6474.

370.1 USA ISSN 1054-0830
RC489.R43
JOURNAL OF REGRESSION THERAPY. Text in English. 1986. a. USD 18 (effective 1998). bk.rev. *Refereed.* **Document type:** *Academic/Scholarly.* **Description:** Compilation of articles submitted by professionals in the field of Regression Therapy. Includes case histories, therapeutic principles and techniques, and research.
Indexed: e-psyche.
Published by: Association for Past-Life Research and Therapies, Inc., PO Box 20151 0151, Riverside, CA 92516. TEL 909-784-1570, FAX 909-789-8440, pastlife@empirenet.com. Ed. Thelma Freedman. Circ: 1,200.

155.3 155.4 GBR ISSN 0264-6838
CODEN: JRIPE3
JOURNAL OF REPRODUCTIVE AND INFANT PSYCHOLOGY. Abbreviated title: J R I P. Text in English. 1983. q. GBP 74, USD 123 to individuals; GBP 242, USD 401 to institutions (effective 2002). bk.rev. *Refereed.* **Document type:** *Academic/Scholarly.* **Description:** Reports and reviews research on the psychological, behavioral, medical and social aspects of reproduction, birth and infancy.

P

Related titles: Online - full text ed.: ISSN 1469-672X (from CatchWord Ltd., EBSCO Publishing, O C L C Online Computer Library Center, Inc., ProQuest Information & Learning, Swets Blackwell, Institute for Scientific Information, RoweCom Information Quest).

Indexed: ASSIA, Brit.Nur.Ind., Curr.Cont., IBZ, Ind.Philos., Lang.& Lang.Behav.Abstr., Mult.Ed.Abstr., PsycInfo, Psychol.Abstr. (1983-), SOPODA, SSCI, Sociol.Abstr., Stud.Wom.Abstr., e-psyche.

—BLDSC (5049.620000), CatchWord, GNLM, Infotrieve. **CCC.**

Published by: (Society for Reproductive and Infant Psychology), Carfax Publishing Limited (Subsidiary of: Taylor & Francis Group), PO Box 25, Abingdon, Oxon OX14 3UE, United Kingdom. TEL 44-1235-401000, FAX 44-1235-401550, enquiries@carfax.co.uk, enquiry@tandf.co.uk, http://www.carfax.co.uk. Eds. Ken Gannon, Suzanne Zeedayk.

152 USA ISSN 0092-6566
BF1 CODEN: JRPRA6

JOURNAL OF RESEARCH IN PERSONALITY. Text in English. 1965. q. USD 400 in US & Canada to institutions; USD 475 elsewhere to institutions (effective 2001). adv. charts. back issues avail.; reprint service avail. from PSC,SCH. *Refereed.* **Document type:** *Academic/Scholarly.* **Description:** Examines issues in the field of personality and in related fields basic to the understanding of personality.

Formerly: Journal of Experimental Research in Personality (0022-1023)

Related titles: Online - full text ed.: (from EBSCO Publishing, O C L C Online Computer Library Center, Inc., RoweCom Information Quest, ingenta, Swets Blackwell, IDEAL Online Library, Institute for Scientific Information).

Indexed: ASCA, ASSIA, Adol.Ment.Hlth.Abstr., AgeLine, Biol.Abstr., Commun.Abstr., Crim.Just.Abstr., Curr.Adv.Ecol.Sci., Curr.Cont., Excerp.Med., IBZ, Ind.Philos., Mid.East: Abstr.& Ind., PsycInfo, Psychol.Abstr. (1971-), Russ.Acad.Sci.Bibl., SSCI, Soc.Work Res.& Abstr., e-psyche.

—BLDSC (5052.025000), GNLM, IDS, Infotrieve, ingenta. **CCC.**

Published by: Academic Press, Inc., Journal Division (Subsidiary of: Harcourt Brace & Company), 525 B St, Ste 1900, San Diego, CA 92101-4495. TEL 619-230-1840, FAX 619-699-6800, apsubs@acad.com, http://www.academicpress.com/jrp. Ed. David Funder.

JOURNAL OF RESEARCH ON ADOLESCENCE. see *CHILDREN AND YOUTH—About*

JOURNAL OF RISK AND UNCERTAINTY. see *BUSINESS AND ECONOMICS—Economic Systems And Theories, Economic History*

150 USA ISSN 1061-0405
BF1

JOURNAL OF RUSSIAN AND EAST EUROPEAN PSYCHOLOGY; a journal of translations. Text in English. 1962. bi-m. USD 125 domestic to individuals; USD 198 foreign to individuals; USD 890 domestic to institutions; USD 998 foreign to institutions (effective 2001). adv. charts. illus. index. back issues avail.; reprint service avail. from SCH,PSC. *Refereed.* **Document type:** *Journal, Academic/Scholarly.* **Description:** Contains original submissions and selected translations from the Russian and East European tradition in psychology. Offers insights into the history and development of the field, contains innovations in method or theory, and covers areas of special research of interest to Western scholars.

Formerly: Soviet Psychology (0038-5751)

Indexed: Adol.Ment.Hlth.Abstr., Biol.Abstr., P.A.I.S., PsycInfo, Psychol.Abstr. (1979-), Russ.Acad.Sci.Bibl., e-psyche.

—BLDSC (5052.128950), CISTI, GNLM, Infotrieve, ingenta. **CCC.**

Published by: M.E. Sharpe, Inc., 80 Business Park Dr, Armonk, NY 10504. TEL 914-273-1800, 800-541-6563, FAX 914-273-2106, custserv@mesharpe.com, http://www.mesharpe.com/rpo_main.html. Ed. Michael Cole. Adv. contact Barbara Ladd. page USD 300; 8 x 5.

370.15 GBR ISSN 0022-4405
LB3013.6 CODEN: JSCPAA

JOURNAL OF SCHOOL PSYCHOLOGY. Text in English. 1963. bi-m. EUR 62 in Europe to individuals; JPY 8,200 in Japan to individuals; USD 68 elsewhere to individuals; EUR 294 in Europe to institutions; JPY 39,000 in Japan to institutions; USD 329 elsewhere to institutions (effective 2002). adv. bk.rev. abstr, bibl, illus. index. back issues avail.; reprint service avail. from PQC,PSC,SCH,ISI. *Refereed.* **Document type:** *Academic/Scholarly.* **Description:** Publishes original articles on research and practice relevant to the development of school psychology as both a scientific and an applied specialty.

Related titles: Microfilm ed.: (from PQC); Online - full text ed.: (from ingenta, ScienceDirect, Swets Blackwell, Institute for Scientific Information).

Indexed: ASCA, Adol.Ment.Hlth.Abstr., C.I.J.E., Cont.Pg.Educ., Curr.Cont., Curr.Ind.Stat., ERA, Educ.Ind. (Jan.1983-), Except.Child Educ.Abstr., Fam.Ind., Lang.& Lang.Behav.Abstr., Mult.Ed.Abstr., PsycInfo, Psychol.Abstr. (1963-), SOMA, SOPODA, SSCI, Sociol.Abstr., Sp.Ed.Needs Abstr., e-psyche.

—IDS, ingenta. **CCC.**

Published by: Elsevier Science Ltd., Pergamon, PO Box 800, Kidlington, Oxon 0X5 1DX, United Kingdom. TEL 44-1865-843000, FAX 44-1865-843010, http://www.elsevier.com/locate/jschpsyc. Eds. B Morris, Robert C Pianta. Circ: 2,000. **Subscr. in Australasia and the Far East to:** Elsevier Science (Singapore) Pte Ltd, No.1 Temasek Ave, 17-01 Millenia Tower, Singapore 039192, Singapore. TEL 65-434-3727, FAX 65-337-2230; **Subscr. in the Americas to:** Elsevier Science, PO Box 945, New York, NY 10159-0945. TEL 212-633-3730, FAX 212-633-3680, usinfo-f@elsevier.com; **Subscr. to:** Elsevier Science BV, PO Box 211, Amsterdam 1000 AE, Netherlands. TEL 31-20-485-3757.

155.3 GBR ISSN 0092-623X
RC556 CODEN: JSMTB

JOURNAL OF SEX & MARITAL THERAPY. Text in English. 1974. 5/yr. GBP 59, USD 98 to individuals; GBP 135, USD 222 to institutions (effective 2002). adv. bk.rev. illus. index. reprint service avail. from PQC,PSC,SCH,ISI. *Refereed.* **Document type:** *Journal, Academic/Scholarly.* **Description:** Provides a contemporary forum on new clinical techniques, conceptualizations and research in sex and marital therapy.

Related titles: Microform ed.: 1974 (from PQC); Online - full text ed.: ISSN 1521-0715. 1974 (from CatchWord Ltd., EBSCO Publishing, O C L C Online Computer Library Center, Inc., RoweCom Information Quest, Swets Blackwell, Institute for Scientific Information).

Indexed: ASCA, Abstr.Soc.Geront., Adol.Ment.Hlth.Abstr., AgeLine, Behav.Med.Abstr., Biol.Abstr., Curr.Cont., Excerp.Med., Fam.Ind., Ind.Med. (1974-), Indian Psychol.Abstr., Lang.& Lang.Behav.Abstr., Mid.East: Abstr.& Ind., Mult.Ed.Abstr., PsycInfo, Psychol.Abstr. (1974-), Russ.Acad.Sci.Bibl., SOPODA, SSCI, Sage Fam.Stud.Abstr., Sage Race Rel.Abstr., Sociol.Abstr., Stud.Wom.Abstr., Viol.& Abuse Abstr., e-psyche.

—BLDSC (5064.017000), CatchWord, GNLM, IDS, ingenta, KNAW.

Published by: Brunner - Routledge (Subsidiary of: Taylor & Francis Group), 27 Church Rd, Hove, E Sussex BN3 2FA, United Kingdom. TEL 44-1273-207411, FAX 44-1273-205612, information@brunner-routledge.co.uk, http://www.brunner-routledge.co.uk/. Eds. Clifford J Sager, R Taylor Segraves. Circ: 2,000. **Subscr. to:** Taylor & Francis Group, Journals Customer Service, Rankine Rd, Basingstoke, Hants RG24 8PR, United Kingdom. TEL 44-1256-813000, FAX 44-1256-479438, enquiry@tanf.co.uk. **Dist. addr. in US:** Taylor & Francis Inc, c/o Taylor & Francis Group, Customer Services, 7625 Empire Dr, Florence, KY 41024. TEL 800-634-7064, FAX 800-248-4724, cserv@routledge-ny.com. **Affiliate:** Brunner - Routledge.

JOURNAL OF SEX EDUCATION AND THERAPY. see *PHYSICAL FITNESS AND HYGIENE*

306.7 USA ISSN 0022-4499
HQ5 CODEN: JSXRAJ

JOURNAL OF SEX RESEARCH. Text in English. 1965. q., latest vol.38, no.1. USD 99 domestic to individuals; USD 126 foreign to individuals; USD 158 domestic to institutions; USD 168 foreign to institutions (effective 2001). adv. bk.rev. charts, illus, stat. back issues avail.; reprint service avail. from SWZ,PQC,PSC,SCH. *Refereed.* **Document type:** *Journal, Academic/Scholarly.* **Description:** Publishes selected research on issues in human sexuality.

Related titles: Microfilm ed.: (from PQC); Online - full text ed.: (from ProQuest Information & Learning, Northern Light Technology, Inc., H. W. Wilson, Gale Group, Factiva, Institute for Scientific Information).

Indexed: ASCA, ASSIA, Abstr.Anthropol., Adol.Ment.Hlth.Abstr., AgeLine, Arts & Hum.Cit.Ind. (coverage dropped), Behav.Med.Abstr., Bibl.Asian Stud. (1972-1991), Chic.Per.Ind., Child Devel.Abstr., Commun.Abstr., Crim.Just.Abstr., Curr.Cont., Curr.Lit.Fam.Plan., Excerp.Med., Fam.Ind., IBZ, IMFL, Ind.Per.Art.Relat.Law, Ind.Philos., Indian Psychol.Abstr., Lang.& Lang.Behav.Abstr., Mid.East: Abstr.& Ind., Mult.Ed.Abstr., PsycInfo, Psychol.Abstr. (1967-), Ref.Zh., SOPODA, SSCI, Sage Fam.Stud.Abstr., Soc.Sci.Ind. (Feb.1987-), Soc.Serv.Abstr., Soc.Work Res.& Abstr., Sociol.Abstr., Stud.Wom.Abstr., Viol.& Abuse Abstr., e-psyche.

—BLDSC (5064.020000), CISTI, GNLM, Infotrieve, ingenta. **CCC.**

Published by: Society for the Scientific Study of Sexuality, PO Box 416, Allentown, PA 18105. TEL 610-530-2483, FAX 610-530-2485, thesociety@inetmail.att.net, http://www.sexscience.org. Ed. John D DeLamater. Circ: 1,750.

364.153 GBR ISSN 1355-2600
CODEN: JSAGFC

JOURNAL OF SEXUAL AGGRESSION. Text in English. 1994. s-a. GBP 47.50 domestic; USD 80 in North America; GBP 55 elsewhere (effective 2000). bk.rev. **Document type:** *Academic/Scholarly.*

Indexed: ASSIA, Crim.Just.Abstr., ERA, IBZ, Ind.Philos., Lang.& Lang.Behav.Abstr., SOPODA, Sage Fam.Stud.Abstr., Soc.Serv.Abstr., Sociol.Abstr., Sp.Ed.Needs Abstr., Stud.Wom.Abstr., Viol.& Abuse Abstr., e-psyche.

—BLDSC (5064.040000), Infotrieve. **CCC.**

Published by: (National Association for the Development of Work with Sex Offenders), Whiting & Birch Ltd., PO Box 872, London SE23 3HL, United Kingdom. TEL 44-20-8244-2421, FAX 44-20-8244-2448, savpub@dircon.co.uk.

JOURNAL OF SLEEP RESEARCH. see *MEDICAL SCIENCES*

▼ **JOURNAL OF SLEEP RESEARCH ONLINE.** see *MEDICAL SCIENCES*

JOURNAL OF SLEEP RESEARCH. SUPPLEMENT. see *MEDICAL SCIENCES*

301.1 USA ISSN 0736-7236
RC467 CODEN: JSCPFF

JOURNAL OF SOCIAL AND CLINICAL PSYCHOLOGY. Text in English. 1983. q. USD 50 domestic to individuals; USD 72 foreign to individuals; USD 175 domestic to institutions; USD 197 foreign to institutions (effective 2000). adv. bk.rev. index. back issues avail.; reprint service avail. from PQC,ISI. *Refereed.* **Document type:** *Academic/Scholarly.* **Description:** Covers theory, research and practice in the growing interface of social and clinical psychology.

Related titles: Online - full text ed.: (from ProQuest Information & Learning, CatchWord Ltd., Institute for Scientific Information, RoweCom Information Quest).

Indexed: ASCA, ASSIA, AgeLine, Curr.Cont., Fam.Ind., IBZ, Ind.Philos., Intl.Bibl.Soc.Sci., Lang.& Lang.Behav.Abstr., Mult.Ed.Abstr., PsycInfo, Psychol.Abstr. (1983-), SOPODA, SSCI, Soc.Serv.Abstr., Soc.Work Res.& Abstr., Sociol.Abstr., Sp.Ed.Needs Abstr., Stud.Wom.Abstr., Viol.& Abuse Abstr., e-psyche.

—BLDSC (5064.718000), GNLM, IDS, ingenta. **CCC.**

Published by: Guilford Publications, Inc., 72 Spring St, 4th Fl, New York, NY 10012. TEL 212-431-9800, 800-365-7006, FAX 212-966-6708. Ed. C R Snyder. Pub. Robert Matloff. R&P Kathy Kuehl. Adv. contact Susan Pavliscak. Circ: 700.

150 574 GBR ISSN 1061-7361
GN365.9 CODEN: JSESEX

JOURNAL OF SOCIAL AND EVOLUTIONARY SYSTEMS. Text in English. 1978. q. NLG 646, EUR 293.14 in Europe to institutions; JPY 43,300 in Japan to institutions; USD 328 elsewhere to institutions; NLG 286, EUR 129.78 in Europe to individuals; JPY 19,200 in Japan to individuals; USD 145 elsewhere to individuals; USD 80 newsstand/cover (effective 2001). adv. bk.rev. bibl. back issues avail. *Refereed.* **Document type:** *Academic/Scholarly.* **Description:** Concerned with the unity, analogy, and relationships, theoretical and practical, between biological dynamics and mechanisms such as evolution, natural selection, and individual development.

Supersedes (in 1991): Journal of Social and Biological Structures (0140-1750)

Related titles: Microform ed.: (from PQC); Online - full text ed.: (from ingenta).

P

Indexed: ASCA, Amer.Bibl.Slavic & E.Eur.Stud., Arts & Hum.Cit.Ind. (coverage dropped), Bibl.Ling., Curr.Cont. (coverage dropped), Fam.Ind., IBR, Intl.Bibl.Soc.Sci., Lang.& Lang.Behav.Abstr., Phil.Ind., Psychol.Abstr., SOPODA, SSCI (coverage dropped), Soc.Serv.Abstr., Sociol.Abstr., e-psyche.
—BLDSC (5064.735000), GNLM, ingenta. **CCC.**
Published by: Elsevier Science, The Boulevard, Langford Ln, Kidlington, Oxon OX5 1GB, United Kingdom. TEL 44-1865-843000, FAX 44-1865-843010, usinfo-f@elsevier.com, http://www.elsevier.com/locate/jsevsy. Ed. Paul Levinson.

150 GBR ISSN 0265-4075
HM132 CODEN: JSRLE9
JOURNAL OF SOCIAL AND PERSONAL RELATIONSHIPS. Text in English. 1984. bi-m. GBP 58 to individuals; GBP 325 to institutions; GBP 11 newsstand/cover to individuals; GBP 55 newsstand/cover to institutions (effective 2002). adv. bk.rev. *Refereed.* **Document type:** *Academic/Scholarly.* **Description:** Multidisciplinary examination of personal relationships, drawing on materials from the fields of social, clinical and developmental psychology, communications, and sociology.
Related titles: Online - full content ed.: (from EBSCO Publishing, O C L C Online Computer Library Center, Inc., ingenta, Swets Blackwell); Online - full text ed.: (from Institute for Scientific Information, RoweCom Information Quest).
Indexed: ASCA, ASSIA, AgeLine, Commun.Abstr., Curr.Cont., ERA, Fam.Ind., Human Resour.Abstr., IBZ, Ind.Philos., Lang.& Lang.Behav.Abstr., PsycInfo, Psychol.Abstr. (1988-), Russ.Acad.Sci.Bibl., SOPODA, SSCI, Sage Fam.Stud.Abstr., Soc.Serv.Abstr., Sociol.Abstr., Sociol.Educ.Abstr., Stud.Wom.Abstr., Viol.& Abuse Abstr., e-psyche.
—BLDSC (5064.740000), ingenta. **CCC.**
Published by: Sage Publications Ltd., 6 Bonhill St, London EC2A 4PU, United Kingdom. TEL 44-20-7374-0645, FAX 44-20-7374-8741, market@sagepub.co.uk, http://www.sagepub.co.uk. Ed. Mark Fine. Adv. contact Jenny Kirby. page GBP 195; trim 190 x 114. Circ: 1,400.

155.205 302 USA ISSN 0886-1641
BF698.A1 CODEN: JSBPE9
JOURNAL OF SOCIAL BEHAVIOR AND PERSONALITY. Text in English. 1986. q. USD 30 domestic to individuals; USD 70 domestic to libraries; USD 78 foreign to libraries. back issues avail. *Refereed.* **Document type:** *Trade.* **Description:** Studies psychology, sociology, speech, management and other social sciences from an academic approach.
Related titles: Online - full text ed.: (from Institute for Scientific Information).
Indexed: ASCA, AgeLine, Chic.Per.Ind., Commun.Abstr., Crim.Just.Abstr., Curr.Cont., Fam.Ind., IBZ, Ind.Philos., Lang.& Lang.Behav.Abstr., Peace Res.Abstr., PsycInfo, Psychol.Abstr. (1986-), SOPODA, SSCI, Soc.Serv.Abstr., Sociol.Abstr., e-psyche.
—BLDSC (5064.751500), IDS, ingenta. **CCC.**
Published by: Select Press, PO Box 37, Corte Madera, CA 94976-0037. TEL 415-924-1612, FAX 415-924-7179. Ed., R&P Rick Crandall.

JOURNAL OF SOCIAL DISTRESS AND THE HOMELESS. see *SOCIAL SERVICES AND WELFARE*

302 USA ISSN 0022-4537
HN51 CODEN: JSISAF
JOURNAL OF SOCIAL ISSUES. Text in English. 1944. q. GBP 292 to institutions in UK& Europe; USD 379 to institutions in the Americas & Caribbean; GBP 292 elsewhere to institutions (effective 2002); Subscr. includes online journal, Analyses of Social Issues and Public Policy.. adv. abstr, bibl, charts, illus. index, cum.index. reprints avail. *Refereed.* **Document type:** *Journal, Academic/Scholarly.*
Related titles: Microfilm ed.: (from PQC,PMC); Online - full content ed.: (from EBSCO Publishing, O C L C Online Computer Library Center, Inc., ingenta, Gale Group, Swets Blackwell); Online - full text ed.: (from Institute for Scientific Information, RoweCom Information Quest).
Indexed: A.B.C.Pol.Sci., ASCA, ASSIA, Abstr.Anthropol., Abstr.Crim.& Pen., Acad.Ind., AgeLine, Bibl.Asian Stud. (1971-1990), Bus.Ind., C.I.J.E. (coverage dropped), Chic.Per.Ind., Commun.Abstr., Crim.Just.Abstr., Curr.Cont., Curr.Lit.Fam.Plan., Educ.Admin.Abstr., Environ.Sci.Poll.Mgmt., Fam.Ind., Geo.Abstr.H.G., Geo.Abstr.P.G., Hist.Abstr. (1971-1992, dropped), IBR, IDA, IMFL, Ind.Philos., Int.Polit.Sci.Abstr., Intl.Bibl.Soc.Sci., L.R.I., Lang.& Lang.Behav.Abstr., Mark.Res.Abstr. (1963-), Mid.East: Abstr.& Ind., Mult.Ed.Abstr., P C I, P.A.I.S., Peace Res.Abstr., Polit.Sci.Abstr., PsycInfo, Psychol.Abstr. (1945-), Psycscan A.P., Rel.Ind.One, Rel.Ind.Two, Risk Abstr., Russ.Acad.Sci.Bibl., SOPODA, SSCI, Saf.Sci.Abstr., Sage Fam.Stud.Abstr., Sage Race Rel.Abstr., Sage Urb.Stud.Abstr., Soc.Sci.Ind. (Sep.1982-), Soc.Work Res.& Abstr., Sociol.Abstr., Sp.Ed.Needs Abstr., Stud.Wom.Abstr., THA, e-psyche.
—BLDSC (5064.755000), IDS, ingenta. **CCC.**
Published by: (Society for the Psychological Study of Social Issues), Blackwell Publishers, 350 Main St, Malden, MA 02148. TEL 781-388-8200, 800-835-6770, FAX 781-388-8232, subscript@blackwellpub.com, http://www.blackwellpublishers.co.uk/asp/journal.asp?ref=0022-4537, http://www.blackwellpublishers.co.uk/journals/diph. Eds. Irene Hanson Frieze, Phyllis Katz. R&P Gretchen Voter TEL 781-388-0423. Adv. contact Anne Marie Sheehy TEL 781-388-0427.

301.1 150 USA ISSN 0022-4545
HM251.A1 CODEN: JSPSAG
THE JOURNAL OF SOCIAL PSYCHOLOGY. Text in English. 1929. bi-m., latest vol.142, 2002. USD 155 domestic; USD 170 foreign; USD 26 newsstand/cover (effective 2001 - 2002). adv. bibl, charts, illus. index. back issues avail.; reprint service avail. from SWZ,PSC,SCH. *Refereed.* **Document type:** *Academic/Scholarly.* **Description:** Publishes experimental, empirical and field studies of groups, cultural effects, cross-national problems, and language and ethnicity.
Related titles: Microfilm ed.: (from PQC); Online - full text ed.: (from Gale Group, ProQuest Information & Learning, Northern Light Technology, Inc., H. W. Wilson, LexisNexis, Factiva, Institute for Scientific Information).
Indexed: ASCA, ASSIA, Abstr.Crim.& Pen., Addic.Abstr., Adol.Ment.Hlth.Abstr., AgeLine, Arts & Hum.Cit.Ind. (coverage dropped), Bibl.Asian Stud. (1970-1971), Biol.Abstr., C.I.J.E., CWI, Chic.Per.Ind., Child Devel.Abstr., Commun.Abstr., Crim.Just.Abstr., Curr.Cont., DSH Abstr., Except.Child Educ.Abstr., Excerp.Med., Fam.Ind., High.Educ.Abstr., IBR, INIS Atomind., Ind.Med. (1930-), Indian Psychol.Abstr., Int.Nurs.Ind., Int.Polit.Sci.Abstr., Intl.Bibl.Soc.Sci., L.R.I., Lang.& Lang.Behav.Abstr., Mid.East: Abstr.& Ind., Mult.Ed.Abstr., P C I, PSI, Peace Res.Abstr., Pers.Lit., PsycInfo, Psychol.Abstr. (1929-), Res.High.Educ.Abstr., Russ.Acad.Sci.Bibl., SOMA, SOPODA, SSCI, Sage Race Rel.Abstr., Sage Urb.Stud.Abstr., Soc.Sci.Ind. (Aug.1982-), Soc.Serv.Abstr., Soc.Work Res.& Abstr., Sociol.Abstr., Stud.Wom.Abstr., Tech.Educ.Abstr., e-psyche.
—BLDSC (5064.800000), IDS, ingenta. **CCC.**
Published by: (Helen Dwight Reid Educational Foundation), Heldref Publications, 1319 Eighteenth St, N W, Washington, DC 20036-1802. TEL 202-296-6267, 800-365-9753, FAX 202-293-6130, soc@heldref.org, http://www.heldref.org. Ed. Elisa Subin. Circ: 1,700. **Subscr. to:** Allen Press Inc., PO Box 1897, Lawrence, KS 66044-8897.

150 USA ISSN 0895-2779
GV706.4
JOURNAL OF SPORT AND EXERCISE PSYCHOLOGY. Short title: J S E P. Text in English. 1979. q. USD 45 to individuals; USD 135 to institutions (effective 2001). adv. bk.rev. bibl, charts, illus, stat. index. back issues avail.; reprint service avail. from PSC,SCH. *Refereed.* **Document type:** *Academic/Scholarly.* **Description:** Multidisciplinary journal designed to stimulate and communicate research and theory. Examines the influence of psychological variables on sport performance and the influence of sport participation on psychological phenomena.
Formerly: Journal of Sport Psychology (0163-433X)
Related titles: Online - full text ed.: (from Gale Group, Factiva, Institute for Scientific Information).
Indexed: AMED, ASCA, Biol.Abstr., Child Devel.Abstr., Curr.Cont., Educ.Ind. (Jan.1983-Dec.1987), Environ.Sci.Poll.Mgmt., Ergon.Abstr., Focus on: Sports Sci.& Med., IBZ, Ind.Philos., Phys.Ed.Ind., Pollut.Abstr., PsycInfo, Psychol.Abstr. (1979-), Risk Abstr., Rural Recreat.Tour.Abstr., SSCI, Saf.Sci.Abstr., Soc.Sci.Ind. (Jul.1999-), Sportsearch (1988-), e-psyche.
—BLDSC (5066.183500), IDS, Infotrieve, ingenta. **CCC.**
Published by: Human Kinetics Publishers, Inc., PO Box 5076, Champaign, IL 61825-5076. TEL 217-351-5076, FAX 217-351-2674, http://www.humankinetics.com. Ed. Steven Petruzzello. Pub. Rainer Martens. R&P Cheri Banks TEL 217-351-5076 ext 2275. Adv. contact Patty Rodriguiz. Circ: 1,299 (paid).

JOURNAL OF SPORT BEHAVIOR. see *SPORTS AND GAMES*

370.15 CHE ISSN 1027-1015
L11
JOURNAL OF STRUCTURAL LEARNING AND INTELLIGENT SYSTEMS. Text in French. 1968. 4/yr. USD 485 to institutions; USD 757 to corporations (effective 1999). adv. index. back issues avail.; reprint service avail. from SCH,PSC. *Refereed.* **Document type:** *Academic/Scholarly.* **Description:** Includes structural process theories, design methodologies and research in artificial intelligence, cognitive and cognitive developmental psychology, individual differences measurement, mathematics, language and other subject matter learning and instructional systems.
Formerly (until 1997): Journal of Structural Learning (0022-4774)
Related titles: CD-ROM ed.; Microform ed.; Online - full text ed.: (from EBSCO Publishing).
Indexed: Cont.Pg.Educ., Curr.Cont. (coverage dropped), ERA, Educ.Tech.Abstr., IBZ, Intl.Bibl.Soc.Sci., PsycInfo, Psychol.Abstr. (1971-), SSCI (coverage dropped), Stud.Wom.Abstr., Tech.Educ.Abstr., Zent.Math., e-psyche.
—BLDSC (5066.880100), ingenta. **CCC.**
Published by: (International Study Group for Mathematics Learning), Gordon and Breach - Harwood Academic (Subsidiary of: Taylor & Francis Group), PO Box 531, Lausanne 1000, Switzerland. http://www.gbhap.com/Structural_Learning_Intelligent_Systems/; http://biomednet.com/library/165. Ed. Joseph M Scandura. **Subscr. addr. in US:** International Publishers Direct, PO Box 32160, Newark, NJ 07102. FAX 215-750-6343. **Co-sponsor:** Structural Learning Society.

616.89 USA ISSN 1195-4396
JOURNAL OF SYSTEMIC THERAPIES. Text in English. 1981. q. USD 36 domestic to individuals; USD 46 foreign to individuals; USD 105 domestic to institutions; USD 115 foreign to institutions (effective 2000). adv. bk.rev. back issues avail. **Document type:** *Academic/Scholarly.* **Description:** Presents provocative ideas and methods that work with families, individuals and groups. Explores brief therapies, solution-focused models, narrative therapies, constructionism and therapeutic conversations.
Formerly: Journal of Strategic and Systematic Therapies (0711-5075)
Related titles: Online - full text ed.: (from CatchWord Ltd., RoweCom Information Quest).
Indexed: Fam.Ind., PsycInfo, Psychol.Abstr. (1983-), e-psyche.
—BLDSC (5068.064000), GNLM, Infotrieve, ingenta. **CCC.**
Published by: Guilford Publications, Inc., 72 Spring St, New York, NY 10012. TEL 212-431-9800, 800-365-7006, FAX 212-966-6708, info@guilford.com. Ed. Don Efron. Pub. Robert Matloff. R&P Kathy Kuehl. Adv. contact Susan Pavliscak. Circ: 1,200.

371.42 USA
▼ **JOURNAL OF TECHNOLOGY IN COUNSELING.** Text in English. 1999. 3/yr. *Refereed.* **Document type:** *Academic/Scholarly.* **Description:** Publishes articles related to the use of technology in training, teaching, and practice of professional counseling.
Media: Online - full text.
Published by: Columbus State University, Department of Counseling and Educational Leadership, 4225 University Ave, Jordan Hall, Columbus, GA 31907. TEL 706-568-2222, FAX 706-569-3134, http://jtc.colstate.edu/. Eds. Marty Jencius, Michael L Baltimore.

152 USA ISSN 0022-5002
BF1 CODEN: JEABAU
JOURNAL OF THE EXPERIMENTAL ANALYSIS OF BEHAVIOR. Abbreviated title: J E A B. Text in English. 1958. bi-m. USD 28 domestic to individuals; USD 38 foreign to individuals; USD 127 domestic to institutions; USD 137 foreign to institutions (effective 2000). adv. bk.rev. bibl, charts. index, cum.index: vols.1-20; 21-40; 41-60. back issues avail.; reprint service avail. from PSC,SCH. *Refereed.* **Document type:** *Academic/Scholarly.* **Description:** Presents original experiments relevant to the behavior of individual organisms.
Related titles: Microfilm ed.: (from PMC); Online - full text ed.: (from Gale Group, Factiva, Institute for Scientific Information).

P

Indexed: ASCA, ASSIA, AgeLine, Anim.Behav.Abstr., Aqua.Sci.& Fish.Abstr., Biol.Abstr., Chem.Abstr., Curr.Cont., Excerp.Med., IBR, IBZ, INIS Atomind., Ind.Med. (1958-), Ind.Philos., Inpharma, Mid.East: Abstr.& Ind., PsycInfo, Psychol.Abstr. (1958-), Psychol.R.G., Psycscan B.A.& T., Reac., Russ.Acad.Sci.Bibl., SSCI, Sci.Cit.Ind., Soc.Sci.Ind. (Sep.1982-), e-psyche.
—BLDSC (4979.700000), CASDDS, CISTI, GNLM, IDS, ingenta.
Published by: Society for the Experimental Analysis of Behavior, Inc., c/o Psychology Department, Indiana University, Bloomington, IN 47405. TEL 812-339-4718, jeab@indiana.edu, http://www.envmed.rochester.edu/wwwrap/behavior/jeabjaba.htm. Ed. Kennon A Lattal. R&P, Adv. contact Devonia Stein. Circ: 2,000.

JOURNAL OF THE HISTORY OF SEXUALITY. see *SOCIOLOGY*

150 USA ISSN 0022-5061
BF1 CODEN: JHBSA5
JOURNAL OF THE HISTORY OF THE BEHAVIORAL SCIENCES. Text in English. 1965. q. USD 240 in United States; USD 268 in Canada & Mexico; USD 268 elsewhere; USD 252 combined subscription in United States for print and online eds.; USD 280 combined subscription in Canada & Mexico for print and online eds.; USD 280 combined subscription elsewhere for print and online eds. (effective 2002). adv. bk.rev. illus. index. back issues avail.; reprint service avail. from PQC,PSC,SCH. *Refereed.* **Document type:** *Academic/Scholarly.*
Related titles: Microform ed.: (from PQC); Online - full text ed.: ISSN 1520-6696. 1996. USD 240 in United States; USD 240 in Canada & Mexico; USD 240 elsewhere (effective 2002) (from EBSCO Publishing, Wiley InterScience, Institute for Scientific Information).
Indexed: ASCA, ASSIA, Abstr.Anthropol., Amer.Bibl.Slavic & E.Eur.Stud., Amer.Hist.& Life, Arts & Hum.Cit.Ind. (coverage dropped), Chic.Per.Ind., Curr.Cont., Hist.Abstr. (1970-95, 1997-), Ind.Med. (1965-), Intl.Bibl.Soc.Sci., Lang.& Lang.Behav.Abstr., Mid.East: Abstr.& Ind., PsycInfo, Psychol.Abstr. (1965-), Psychol.R.G., Ref.Zh., Russ.Acad.Sci.Bibl., SOPODA, SSCI, Sociol.Abstr., e-psyche.
—BLDSC (5000.600000), GNLM, IDS, Infotrieve, ingenta. **CCC.**
Published by: John Wiley & Sons, Inc., Journals (Subsidiary of: Wiley InterScience), 605 Third Ave, New York, NY 10158. TEL 212-850-6645, FAX 212-850-6021, uscs-wis@wiley.com, http://www.wiley.com. Ed. Raymond E Fancher. adv.: B&W page GBP 640, color page GBP 1,515; trim 172 x 254. Circ: 800. **Subscr. outside the Americas to:** John Wiley & Sons Ltd., Baffins Ln, Chichester, Sussex PO19 IUD, United Kingdom. TEL 44-1243-779777, FAX 44-1243-843232, cs-journals@wiley.co.uk, http://www.wiley.co.uk.

P

JOURNAL OF THE LEARNING SCIENCES; a journal of ideas and their applications. see *EDUCATION*

JOURNAL OF THE PSYCHOLOGY OF RELIGION. see *RELIGIONS AND THEOLOGY*

150 100 USA
JOURNAL OF THEORETICAL & PHILOSOPHICAL PSYCHOLOGY. Text in English. s-a. **Description:** Encourages and facilities informed exploration and discussion of psychological theories and issues in both their scientific and philosophical dimensions and interrelationships.
—BLDSC (5069.074750).
Published by: American Psychological Association, Division 14, Administrative Office, 750 First St., N E, Washington, DC 2002-4242. TEL 202-336-6013, FAX 202-218-3599, kcooke@apa.org, http://www.cas.utulsa.edu. Ed. Daniel Robinson.

▼ **JOURNAL OF THREAT ASSESSMENT.** see *MEDICAL SCIENCES—Forensic Sciences*

158 USA ISSN 0022-524X
BF1 CODEN: JTPSAN
JOURNAL OF TRANSPERSONAL PSYCHOLOGY. Text in English. 1969. s-a. USD 29 domestic to individuals; USD 48 foreign to individuals; USD 45, USD 56 domestic to institutions; USD 12 newsstand/cover domestic; USD 16 newsstand/cover foreign (effective 2002). bk.rev. back issues avail.; reprint service avail. from PSC,SCH. **Document type:** *Journal, Academic/Scholarly.* **Description:** Focuses on psychological and spiritual states, experiences, practices and concepts.
Related titles: Microform ed.: (from PQC).
Indexed: AgeLine, Curr.Cont. (coverage dropped), Ind.Philos., PsycInfo, Psychol.Abstr. (1969-), Psychol.R.G., Rel.Ind.One, Rel.Ind.Two, Russ.Acad.Sci.Bibl., SSCI (coverage dropped), Soc.Sci.Ind. (coverage dropped), e-psyche.
—BLDSC (5069.870000), IDS, ingenta.
Published by: (Association for Transpersonal Psychology), InnoVision Communications, 169 Saxony Rd, Ste 104, Encinitas, CA 92024. TEL 760-633-3910, FAX 760-633-3918, 866-828-2962, info@invcom.com, http://www.atpweb.org/journal/journal.html. Ed. Kaisa Puhakka. Circ: 3,000.

616.852 USA ISSN 1529-9732
▼ **JOURNAL OF TRAUMA AND DISSOCIATION**; the official journal of the International Society for the Study of Dissociation. Text in English. 1999. q. USD 60 to individuals; USD 81 in Canada to individuals; USD 87 elsewhere to individuals; USD 95 to institutions; USD 128 in Canada to institutions; USD 138 elsewhere to institutions; USD 135 to libraries; USD 182 in Canada to libraries; USD 196 elsewhere to libraries (effective Aug. 2001). adv. **Document type:** *Journal, Academic/Scholarly.* **Description:** Provides scientific literature in dissociation, dissociative disorders, psychological trauma, and aspects of memory associated with trauma and dissociation.
Published by: (International Society for the Study of Dissociation), Haworth Press, Inc., 10 Alice St, Binghamton, NY 13904-1580. TEL 607-722-5857, FAX 607-722-6362, 800-895-0582, getinfo@haworthpressinc.com, http://www.haworthpress.com/journals/journallist.asp. Pub. William Cohen. R&P Ruthann Heath TEL 607-723-5857 ext 316. Adv. contact Jackie Blakeslee TEL 607-722-5857 ext 346. B&W page USD 315, color page USD 550; trim 6 x 8.5.

150 USA
▼ **JOURNAL OF TRAUMA PRACTICE.** Text in English. 2002 (Spr.). q. USD 48 domestic to individuals; USD 65 in Canada to individuals; USD 70 elsewhere to individuals; USD 75 domestic to institutions; USD 101 in Canada to institutions; USD 109 elsewhere to institutions; USD 110 domestic to libraries; USD 149 in Canada to libraries; USD 160 elsewhere to libraries (effective Aug. 2001). **Document type:** *Journal, Academic/Scholarly.* **Description:** Covers the latest developments in trauma scholarship.
Published by: Haworth Press, Inc., 10 Alice St, Binghamton, NY 13904-1580. TEL 607-722-5857, 800-429-6784, FAX 607-722-6362, 800-895-0582, getinfo@haworthpressinc.com, http://www.haworthpress.com/journals/journallist.asp. Eds. Jan Faust, Steven N. Gold. R&P Ruthann Heath TEL 607-723-5857 ext 316. Adv. contact Jackie Blakeslee TEL 607-722-5857 ext 346.

370.15 150 USA ISSN 0894-9867
RC552.P67 CODEN: JTSTEB
JOURNAL OF TRAUMATIC STRESS. Text in English. 1988. q. USD 461, EUR 460 to institutions for print or online ed.; USD 553.20, EUR 552 to institutions for print & online eds.combined (effective 2002). adv. bk.rev. back issues avail.; reprint service avail. from PSC,SCH. *Refereed.* **Document type:** *Journal, Academic/Scholarly.* **Description:** Examines the biopsychosocial aspects of trauma through theoretical formulations, research, treatment, prevention, education and training, and legal and policy concerns.
Related titles: Microfilm ed.: (from PQC); Online - full text ed.: (from EBSCO Publishing, O C L C Online Computer Library Center, Inc., RoweCom Information Quest, Swets Blackwell, Kluwer Online, Institute for Scientific Information).
Indexed: ASCA, AgeLine, Crim.Just.Abstr., Curr.Cont., Environ.Sci.Poll.Mgmt., Excerp.Med. (1995-), Fam.Ind., IMFL, Ind.Med. (1988-), Int.Nurs.Ind., Lang.& Lang.Behav.Abstr., Pollut.Abstr., PsycInfo, Psychol.Abstr. (1988-), Risk Abstr., SOPODA, SSCI, Saf.Sci.Abstr., Soc.Serv.Abstr., Sociol.Abstr., e-psyche.
—BLDSC (5070.520000), CISTI, GNLM, IDS, ingenta, KNAW. **CCC.**
Published by: (International Society for Traumatic Stress Studies), Kluwer Academic - Plenum Publishers (Subsidiary of: Wolters Kluwer N.V.), 233 Spring St, New York, NY 10013-1578. TEL 212-620-8000, 800-221-9369, FAX 212-463-0742, info@plenum.com, http://www.wkap.nl; http://www.wkap.nl/journalhome.htm/0894-9867. Ed. Dean G Kilpatrick. R&P Rose Luongo TEL 781-871-6311. **Subscr. to:** Kluwer Academic Publishers Group, Journals Department, PO Box 322, Dordrecht 3300 AH, Netherlands. TEL 31-78-639-2392, FAX 31-78-654-6474.

158 USA ISSN 0001-8791
HF5381.A1 CODEN: JVBHA2
JOURNAL OF VOCATIONAL BEHAVIOR. Text in English. 1971. bi-m. USD 675 in US & Canada to institutions; USD 750 elsewhere to institutions (effective 2001). adv. illus. index. back issues avail.; reprints avail. *Refereed.* **Document type:** *Academic/Scholarly.* **Description:** Publishes empirical and theoretical articles that expand knowledge of vocational behavior and career development across the life span.
Related titles: Online - full text ed.: (from EBSCO Publishing, O C L C Online Computer Library Center, Inc., RoweCom Information Quest, ingenta, Swets Blackwell, IDEAL Online Library, Institute for Scientific Information).
Indexed: ASCA, ASSIA, AgeLine, C.I.J.E., CINAHL, Chic.Per.Ind., Curr.Cont., Curr.Ind.Stat., Fam.Ind., High.Educ.Abstr., Lang.& Lang.Behav.Abstr., Mid.East: Abstr.& Ind., Pers.Lit., PsycInfo, Psychol.Abstr. (1971-), Psycscan A.P., Russ.Acad.Sci.Bibl., SOPODA, SSCI, Soc.Serv.Abstr., Sociol.Abstr., Stud.Wom.Abstr., e-psyche.
—BLDSC (5072.510000), IDS, ingenta. **CCC.**
Published by: Academic Press, Inc., Journal Division (Subsidiary of: Harcourt Brace & Company), 525 B St, Ste 1900, San Diego, CA 92101-4495. TEL 619-230-1840, FAX 619-699-6800, apsubs@acad.com, http://www.academicpress.com/jvb. Ed. Mark L Savickas.

JOURNAL OF YOUTH AND ADOLESCENCE; a multidisciplinary research publication. see *CHILDREN AND YOUTH—About*

JOURNAL OF YOUTH STUDIES. see *CHILDREN AND YOUTH—About*

JOURNALS OF GERONTOLOGY. SERIES B: PSYCHOLOGICAL SCIENCES & SOCIAL SCIENCES. see *GERONTOLOGY AND GERIATRICS*

155 301.1 MYS ISSN 0127-8029
BF8.M35
JURNAL PSIKOLOGI MALAYSIA. Text in English, Malay. 1972. a. USD 15. **Description:** Discusses various fields of psychology such as social, developmental, physiological, industrial, counseling, and others particularly relevant to Malaysia.
Indexed: e-psyche.
—ingenta.
Published by: Penerbit Universiti Kebangsaan Malaysia, Ukm Bangi, Selangor 43600, Malaysia.

JYVASKYLA STUDIES IN EDUCATION, PSYCHOLOGY AND SOCIAL RESEARCH. see *EDUCATION*

616.8 615.7 JPN ISSN 0918-0354
KANAGAWA SEISHIN YAKURI* /KANAGAWA JOURNAL OF PSYCHOPHARMACOLOGY. Text in Japanese. 1988. a.
Indexed: e-psyche.
Published by: Kanagawa Seishin Yakuri Konwakai/Kanagawa Society of Psychopharmacology, c/o Japanese Pharmacological Society, 2-4-16 Yayoi, Bunkyo-ku, Tokyo 113-0032, Japan.

153.4 GBR ISSN 0952-1194
KEELE COGNITION SEMINARS. Text in English. 1987. biennial. price varies. **Document type:** *Proceedings.*
Indexed: e-psyche.
Published by: Oxford University Press, Oxford Journals, Walton St, Oxford OX2 6DP, United Kingdom. TEL 44-1865-56767, FAX 44-1865-56646, jnlorders@oup.co.uk, jnl.orders@oup.co.uk, http://www.oup.co.uk. **Orders in N. America to:** Oxford University Press, Journals. TEL 919-677-0977, FAX 919-677-1714, http://www.oup.co.uk.

DAS KIND. see *CHILDREN AND YOUTH—About*

616.89 DEU ISSN 0942-6051
CODEN: KINDF9
KINDERANALYSE. Text in German. 1992. q. DEM 120, EUR 61.36; DEM 110, EUR 56.24 to students (effective 2000). adv. **Document type:** *Magazine, Academic/Scholarly.*
Indexed: IBZ, Ind.Philos., PsycInfo, Psychoanal.Abstr., e-psyche.
—GNLM.
Published by: Verlag Klett-Cotta, Rotebuehlstr 77, Stuttgart 70178, Germany. TEL 49-711-66721648, FAX 49-711-66722032. Ed. Jochen Stork. Adv. contact Thomas Kleffner. B&W page DEM 950; trim 113 x 180. Circ: 1,700.

616.89 JPN ISSN 0910-6529
KODO RYOHO KENKYU/JAPANESE JOURNAL OF BEHAVIOR THERAPY. Text in English, Japanese; Summaries in English. 1974. s-a. JPY 3,260. adv. bk.rev. index. back issues avail. *Refereed.* **Document type:** *Academic/Scholarly.* **Description:** Covers experimental and clinical research in behavior therapy.
Indexed: PsycInfo, Psychol.Abstr. (1984-), Psycscan B.A.& T., e-psyche.
—BLDSC (4651.010000).
Published by: Nihon Kodo Ryoho Gakkai/Japanese Association of Behavior Therapy, c/o Masahiko Sugiyama Sec-Gen, Institute of Special Education, University of Tsukuba, 1-1-1 Tenno-Dai, Tsukuba-shi, Ibaraki-ken 305-0006, Japan. TEL 81-298-53-6719, FAX 81-298-53-6719. Ed., R&P, Adv. contact Yuji Sakano. Circ: 1,200.

150 DEU ISSN 0949-1821
GN502
KOELNER BEITRAEGE ZUR ETHNOPSYCHOLOGIE UND TRANSKULTURELLEN PSYCHOLOGIE. Text in German. 1995. irreg., latest vol.3, 1997. DEM 55 (effective 2000). **Document type:** *Academic/Scholarly.*
Indexed: Anthropol.Lit., e-psyche.
Published by: Holos Verlag, Ermekeilstr 15, Bonn 53113, Germany. FAX 49-228-212435. Ed. Hannes Stubbe. Circ: 300 (paid).

KOELNER ZEITSCHRIFT FUER SOZIOLOGIE UND SOZIALPSYCHOLOGIE. see *SOCIOLOGY*

370.15 150 DNK ISSN 0906-6225
KOGNITION OG PAEDAGOGIK. Text in Danish. 1991. q. DKK 225 in the European Union to individuals; DKK 180 elsewhere to individuals; DKK 345 in the European Union to institutions; DKK 276 elsewhere to institutions; DKK 80 per issue in the European Union; DKK 64 per issue elsewhere (effective 2002). bk.rev. 80 p./no. **Document type:** *Journal, Academic/Scholarly.*
Published by: (Center for Kognitiv Forskning og Paedagogik, Aarhus Universitet), Dansk Psykologisk Forlag/Danish Psychological Publishers, Stockholmsgade 29, Copenhagen Oe 2100, Denmark. TEL 45-35-38-16-55, FAX 45-35-38-16-65, dk-psych@dpf.dk, http://www.dpf.dk. Ed. Kjeld Fredens.

156 DEU ISSN 0938-7986
BF309 CODEN: KOGNEB
KOGNITIONSWISSENSCHAFT. Text in German. 1990. q. DEM 396.40 domestic; DEM 400 foreign (effective 2001). *Refereed.* **Document type:** *Journal, Academic/Scholarly.* **Description:** Contains scientific papers on all aspects of cognition and related fields.
Related titles: Microform ed.: (from PQC); Online - full text ed.: ISSN 1432-1483 (from EBSCO Publishing, RoweCom Information Quest, Swets Blackwell, Springer LINK).
Indexed: IBZ, Ind.Philos., Lang.& Lang.Behav.Abstr., SOPODA, Sociol.Abstr., e-psyche.
—CCC.
Published by: (Gesellschaft fuer Kognitionswissenschaft), Springer-Verlag (Subsidiary of: BertelsmannSpringer), Tiergartenstr 17, Heidelberg 69121, Germany. TEL 49-6221-345-0, FAX 49-6221-345229, subscriptions@springer.de, http://link.springer.de/link/service/journals/00197/index.htm, http://www.springer.de. Ed. G Weber. **Subscr. in N. America to:** Springer-Verlag New York Inc., PO Box 2485, Secaucus, NJ 07096-2485. TEL 212-460-1500, FAX 212-473-6272.

616.89 ITA
KOINOS - GRUPPO E FUNZIONE ANALITICA. Text in Italian. s-a. ITL 60,000 domestic to individuals; USD 70 foreign to individuals; ITL 70,000 domestic to institutions; USD 90 foreign to institutions.
Indexed: e-psyche.
Published by: (Gruppo de Pollaiolo, Centro Ricerche), Edizioni Borla s.r.l., Via Delle Fornaci, 50, Rome, RM 00165, Italy. TEL 39-6-39376728, FAX 39-6-39376620.

616.8 JPN ISSN 0023-2807
KOKORO TO SHAKAI/MIND AND SOCIETY. Text in Japanese. 1969. q. JPY 1,500, USD 5.
Indexed: e-psyche.
—BLDSC (5775.552000).
Published by: Nihon Seishin Eiseikai/Japan Mental Health Society, 91 Benten-cho, Shinjuku-ku, Tokyo 162-0851, Japan. Ed. Dr. Haruo Akimoto.

150 DEU ISSN 0720-1079
KONTEXT; Zeitschrift fuer Familientherapie. Text in German. 1979. s-a. DEM 49; DEM 39 to students (effective 2000). **Document type:** *Journal, Academic/Scholarly.*
Indexed: IBZ, Ind.Philos., e-psyche.
—GNLM.
Published by: (Deutsche Arbeitsgemeinschaft fuer Familientherapie e.V.), Vandenhoeck und Ruprecht, Robert-Bosch-Breite 6, Goettingen 37079, Germany. TEL 49-551-6959-0, FAX 49-551-695917.

616.89 DEU ISSN 0937-289X
KRANKENHAUSPSYCHIATRIE. Text in German. 1990. q. EUR 123.80 domestic to institutions; EUR 124.80 in Europe to institutions; EUR 128.80 elsewhere to institutions; EUR 36 newsstand/cover (effective 2002). adv. reprint service avail. from IRC. **Document type:** *Journal, Academic/Scholarly.*
Related titles: Online - full text ed.: ISSN 1439-3816.
Indexed: PsycInfo, e-psyche.
—GNLM.
Published by: Georg Thieme Verlag, Ruedigerstr 14, Stuttgart 70469, Germany. TEL 49-711-8931-0, FAX 49-711-8931133, kunden.service@thieme.de, http://www.thieme.de.

616.89 NLD ISSN 0167-238X
KWARTAALSCHRIFT VOOR DIRECTIEVE THERAPIE EN HYPNOSE. Text in Dutch. q. NLG 115 to individuals; NLG 165 to institutions; NLG 85 to students. adv. bk.rev. **Document type:** *Trade.*
Indexed: e-psyche.
—GNLM.
Published by: Bohn Stafleu van Loghum B.V. (Subsidiary of: Wolters Kluwer N.V.), Postbus 246, Houten 3990 GA, Netherlands. TEL 31-3403-95711, FAX 31-3403-50903. Circ: 2,000.

KYOIKU SHINRIGAKU NENPO/ANNUAL REPORT OF EDUCATIONAL PSYCHOLOGY IN JAPAN. see *EDUCATION*

616.89 JPN ISSN 0285-4562
KYUSHU DAIGAKU SHINRI RINSHO KENKYU/KYUSHU UNIVERSITY. PSYCHOLOGICAL CLINIC. ARCHIVES. Text in Japanese. 1982. a. for sale only to clinician. **Document type:** *Academic/Scholarly.*
Indexed: e-psyche.
Published by: Kyushu Daigaku, Kyoikugakubu, Shinri Kyoiku Sodanshitsu, 19-1 Hakozaki 6-chome, Higashi-ku, Fukuoka-shi 812-8581, Japan. TEL 81-92-642-3144, FAX 81-92-646-4330. Ed. Seiichi Tajima.

THE L D READER. (Learning Disabilities) see *EDUCATION—Special Education And Rehabilitation*

150.195 USA
LACANIAN STUDIES*. Text in English. 1987. s-a. USD 30 to individuals; USD 40 to institutions. bk.rev. *Refereed.* **Document type:** *Academic/Scholarly.* **Description:** Dedicated to the study of Jacques Lacan's oral teaching as presented in the seminars (1953-81) and the Ecrits (1966).
Former titles (until 1997): Askew; Newsletter of the Freudian Field (0894-1750)
Indexed: e-psyche.
Published by: (Foundation Freudian Field), Ellie Ragland, Ed. & Pub., 502 W Rockcreek Dr, Columbia, MO 65203-1664. TEL 573-884-6212, FAX 314-882-5785. Circ: 200 (paid).

LANGUAGE AND COGNITIVE PROCESSES. see *LINGUISTICS*

LATERALITY. see *MEDICAL SCIENCES—Psychiatry And Neurology*

808.87 USA ISSN 0731-1788
LAUGHING MATTERS. Text in English. 1981. q. USD 15. bk.rev. illus. cum.index. back issues avail.
Indexed: e-psyche.
Published by: Saratoga Institute, Humor Project, 480 Broadway, 210, Saratoga Springs, NY 12866-2230. TEL 518-587-8770, mail@humorproject.com, http://www.humorproject.com. Ed. Dr. Joel Goodman. Circ: 10,000.

LAW AND HUMAN BEHAVIOR. see *LAW*

LAW AND PSYCHOLOGY REVIEW. see *LAW*

THE LEADERSHIP QUARTERLY; an international journal of political, social and behavioral science. see *BUSINESS AND ECONOMICS—Management*

LEARNING AND INDIVIDUAL DIFFERENCES; a multidisciplinary journal in education. see *EDUCATION*

LEARNING AND INSTRUCTION. see *EDUCATION*

LEARNING AND MOTIVATION. see *EDUCATION*

▼ **LEARNING DISABILITY PRACTICE.** see *EDUCATION—Special Education And Rehabilitation*

LEBENDIGE SEELSORGE; Zeitschrift fuer alle Fragen der Seelsorge. see *RELIGIONS AND THEOLOGY—Protestant*

152.335 USA
LEFTHANDER. Text in English. 1975. bi-m. USD 15; USD 33 foreign. adv. bk.rev. back issues avail. **Description:** Publishes interviews with left-handed celebrities, research on left-handedness, superstitions and facts about left-handedness and parenting skills; includes catalog product section.
Former titles: Lefthander Magazine; Lefty Magazine
Indexed: e-psyche.
Published by: Lefthanders International, 3600 N E Sardov Bldg 2, Box 8249, Topeka, KS 66608. TEL 913-234-2177. Ed. Kim Kipers. Adv. contact Carol Riddle. Circ: 25,000.

158 364 614.19 GBR ISSN 1355-3259
K12 CODEN: LCPSFX
LEGAL AND CRIMINOLOGICAL PSYCHOLOGY. Text in English. 1996. s-a., latest vol.6. GBP 70 in the European Union to institutions; USD 128 rest of world to institutions; GBP 38 newsstand/cover in the European Union; USD 72 newsstand/cover rest of world (effective 2001). adv. bk.rev. abstr. 128 p./no. back issues avail.; reprint service avail. from SWZ. *Refereed.* **Document type:** *Journal, Academic/Scholarly.* **Description:** Covers theoretical, empirical and review studies in the field as broadly defined. Topics include new legislation, victimology, theories of delinquency, public attitudes, mental health and the law, policing and crime detection.
Related titles: Magnetic Tape ed.; Microfiche ed.; Online - full text ed.: 1999. free with print (from CatchWord Ltd., EBSCO Publishing, Swets Blackwell).
Indexed: ASSIA, Crim.Just.Abstr., IBZ, Ind.Philos., PsycInfo, Soc.Serv.Abstr., Sociol.Abstr., e-psyche.
—BLDSC (5181.312110). **CCC.**
Published by: The British Psychological Society, St Andrews House, 48 Princess Rd E, Leicester LE1 7DR, United Kingdom. TEL 44-116-252-9580, FAX 44-116-254-8824, journals@bps.org.uk, http://www.bps.org.uk/publications/journals.cfm. Ed. Ron Blackburn. R&P, Adv. contact J Neason TEL 44-116-252-9580. page GBP 165; 135 x 210. Circ: 1,200. **Subscr. to:** Turpin Distribution Services Ltd., Blackhorse Rd, Letchworth, Herts SG6 1HN, United Kingdom. TEL 44-1462-488900, FAX 44-1462-483011.

LEISURE SCIENCES; an interdisciplinary journal. see *LEISURE AND RECREATION*

LESBIAN AND GAY COUNSELLING NEWS. see *HOMOSEXUALITY*

301.1 150 GBR ISSN 0267-7172
LIBERTARIAN ALLIANCE. PSYCHOLOGICAL NOTES. Text in English. 1985. irreg. GBP 15, USD 30 (effective 1999). **Document type:** *Monographic series.*
Indexed: e-psyche.
Published by: Libertarian Alliance, 25 Chapter Chambers, Esterbrooke St, London SW1P 4NN, United Kingdom. TEL 44-20-7821-5502, FAX 44-20-7834-2031, liberty@capital.demon.co.uk, http://www.digiweb.com/igeldard/la. Pub. Chris Tame.

LIES PEOPLE TELL; welcome to the truth about lies. see *PHILOSOPHY*

A LIFE IN THE DAY; work and daytime opportunities for people who use mental health services. see *SOCIAL SERVICES AND WELFARE*

LINGDALE PAPERS. see *RELIGIONS AND THEOLOGY*

LITERATURE AND PSYCHOLOGY; a quarterly journal of literary criticism as informed by depth psychology. see *LITERATURE*

150.19 ITA
L'OMBRA; tracce e percorsi a partire da Jung. Text in Italian. 1996. s-a. ITL 25,000. **Description:** Covers studies in psychoanalysis since Jung.
Indexed: e-psyche.
Published by: Moretti e Vitalli Editori, Via Betty Ambiveri 15, Bergamo, BG 24126, Italy. TEL 39-35-321588, FAX 39-35-321647. Ed. Fulvio Salza.

LONGITUDINAL RESEARCH IN THE SOCIAL AND BEHAVIORAL SCIENCES; an interdisciplinary series. see *SOCIAL SCIENCES: COMPREHENSIVE WORKS*

370.15 150 USA ISSN 8756-4610
R726.5
LOSS, GRIEF & CARE; a journal of professional practice. Text in English. 1986. q. USD 75 domestic to individuals; USD 101 in Canada to individuals; USD 109 elsewhere to individuals; USD 125 domestic to institutions; USD 169 in Canada to institutions; USD 181 elsewhere to institutions; USD 185 domestic to libraries; USD 250 in Canada to libraries; USD 268 elsewhere to libraries (effective 2001). adv. bk.rev. illus. reprint service avail. from HAW. *Refereed.* **Document type:** *Journal, Academic/Scholarly.* **Description:** Explores the critical issues of psychosocial care for chronically, critically, and terminally ill patients and their family members.
Related titles: Microfiche ed.: (from PQC); Microform ed.
Indexed: AMED, ASSIA, CINAHL, IBZ, IMFL, Ind.Philos., Int.Polit.Sci.Abstr., LISA, Lang.& Lang.Behav.Abstr., Past.Care & Couns.Abstr., Psychol.Abstr., Ref.Zh., SOPODA, Soc.Serv.Abstr., Soc.Work Res.& Abstr., Sociol.Abstr., e-psyche.
—BLDSC (5294.735000), GNLM, Haworth, ingenta.
Published by: Haworth Press, Inc., 10 Alice St, Binghamton, NY 13904-1580. TEL 607-722-5857, 800-429-6784, FAX 607-722-6362, 800-895-0582, getinfo@haworthpressinc.com, http://www.haworthpress.com/journals/journallist.asp. Ed. Austin H Kutscher. Pub. William Cohen. R&P Ruthann Heath TEL 607-723-5857 ext 316. Adv. contact Jackie Blakeslee TEL 607-722-5857 ext 346. B&W page USD 315, color page USD 550; trim 6 x 8.5. Circ: 385.

LOVING BROTHERHOOD NEWSLETTER; a journal for personal and planetary transformation. see *HOMOSEXUALITY*

LUND STUDIES IN PSYCHOLOGY OF RELIGION. see *RELIGIONS AND THEOLOGY*

150 DEU ISSN 0933-3347
BF173.A2
LUZIFER-AMOR; Zeitschrift zur Geschichte der Psychoanalyse. Text in German. 1988. s-a. DEM 60 (effective 2000). adv. bk.rev. back issues avail. **Document type:** *Magazine, Academic/Scholarly.*
Indexed: IBR, Ind.Philos., PsycInfo, Psychoanal.Abstr., e-psyche.
—GNLM.
Published by: Edition Diskord, Schwarzlocherstr 104-b, Tuebingen 72070, Germany. TEL 49-7071-40102, FAX 49-7071-44710, ed.diskord@t-online.de, http://www.edition-diskord.de. Ed. Ludger Hermanns. R&P Gerd Kimmerle. Circ: 800.

150 HUN ISSN 0025-0279
BF8.H8
MAGYAR PSZICHOLOGIAI SZEMLE/HUNGARIAN PSYCHOLOGICAL REVIEW. Text in Hungarian; Summaries in English, Russian. 1928. q. USD 76 (effective 2002). adv. bk.rev. abstr. illus. index. 150 p./no. back issues avail. **Document type:** *Journal, Academic/Scholarly.* **Description:** Latest Hungarian and occasional foreign results in fields of general and evolutionary, medical, pedagogical, social psychology, psychology of art, and criminal psychology research..
Related titles: Online - full text ed.
Indexed: C.I.S. Abstr., Curr.Cont. (coverage dropped), Lang.& Lang.Behav.Abstr., PsycInfo, Psychol.Abstr. (1934-), Russ.Acad.Sci.Bibl., SOPODA, Sociol.Abstr., e-psyche.
Published by: (Magyar Tudomanyos Akademia), Akademiai Kiado Rt., PO Box 245, Budapest 1519, Hungary. TEL 36-1-4648233, FAX 36-1-4648297, http://www.akkrt.hu. Ed. Csaba Pleh. **Co-sponsor:** Magyar Pszichologiai Tarsasag.

150 301 574 IND ISSN 0025-1615
MANAB MON; a journal depicting the modern trends in psychology, biology, and sociology. Text in English. 1972. q. INR 8, USD 1. adv. bk.rev.
Indexed: e-psyche.
Published by: Pavlov Institute, 132-1A Bidhan Sarani, Kolkata, West Bengal 700 004, India. Ed. Dr. D N Ganguly. Circ: 1,000.

MANAGEMENT KINDEROPVANG. see *CHILDREN AND YOUTH—About*

MANKIND QUARTERLY; an international quarterly journal dealing with both physical and cultural anthropology including related subjects such as psychology, demography, genetics, linguistics and mythology. see *ANTHROPOLOGY*

150 CZE ISSN 1211-3522
MASARYKOVA UNIVERZITA. FILOZOFICKA FAKULTA. SBORNIK PRACI. P: RADA PSYCHOLOGICKA. ANNALES PSYCHOLOGICI. Text in Czech; Summaries in Multiple languages. 1996. a. price varies. bk.rev. **Document type:** *Academic/Scholarly.* **Description:** Covers all aspects of psychology.
Supersedes in part (in 1996): Masarykova Univerzita. Filozoficka Fakulta. Sbornik Praci. I: Rada Pedagogicko - Psychologicka; Which was formerly: Univerzita J.E. Purkyne. Filozoficka Fakulta. Sbornik Praci. I: Rada Pedagogicko - Psychologicka (0068-2705)
Indexed: IBR, Lang.& Lang.Behav.Abstr., Psychol.Abstr., SOPODA, Sociol.Abstr., e-psyche.
Published by: Masarykova Univerzita, Filozoficka Fakulta, A Novaka 1, Brno 66088, Czech Republic. TEL 420-5-41121102, FAX 420-5-41121406, exchange@phil.muni.cz. Ed. Milos Stedron TEL 420-5-41121337.

150 658 USA
MASSACHUSETTS PSYCHOLOGIST. Text in English. 1993. m. Free to qualified subscribers. adv. back issues avail. **Document type:** *Magazine, Trade.* **Description:** Targets business and marketplace issues that affect clinical practices.
Related titles: Online - full content ed.
Address: P O Box 812068, Wellesley, MA 02482-0013. TEL 781-237-9909, feedback@masspsy.com, http://www.masspsy.com. Pub. Denise M. Yocum.

MATERIALIEN AUS DER BILDUNGSFORSCHUNG. see *EDUCATION*

152 510 GBR ISSN 1354-6791
QA11.A1 CODEN: MTCIFY
MATHEMATICAL COGNITION. Text in English. 1995. s-a. GBP 48, USD 80 to institutions. adv. back issues avail. **Document type:** *Academic/Scholarly.* **Description:** Aims to provide a forum for explorations of how human beings understand mathematics and acquire mathematical concepts.
Related titles: Online - full text ed.: ISSN 1464-0724 (from CatchWord Ltd., EBSCO Publishing, O C L C Online Computer Library Center, Inc., RoweCom Information Quest, Swets Blackwell).
Indexed: C.I.J.E., e-psyche.
—BLDSC (5401.920000), CatchWord. **CCC.**
Published by: Psychology Press (Subsidiary of: Taylor & Francis Group), 27 Church Rd, Hove, E Sussex BN3 2FA, United Kingdom. TEL 44-1273-207411, FAX 44-1273-205612, information@psypress.co.uk, http://www.psypress.co.uk. Ed. Brian Butterworth. R&P Zoe Peden TEL 44-20-7842-2363. Adv. contact Claire Buckminster. **Subscr. addr. outside N America:** Journals Customer Service, Taylor & Francis Group, Rankine Rd, Basingstoke, Hants RG24 8PR, United Kingdom. TEL 44-1256-813002, FAX 44-1256-479438, enquiry@tandf.co.uk; **subscr. addr. in N America:** Psychology Press, Journals Customer Service, Taylor & Francis Group, 325 Chestnut St, Philadelphia, PA 19106. TEL 800-354-1420, FAX 215-625-8914, info@taylorandfrancis.com, http://www.psypress.com.

▼ **MATHEMATICAL THINKING AND LEARNING**; an international journal. see *MATHEMATICS*

616.89 DNK ISSN 0109-646X
MATRIX; nordisk tidsskrift for psykoterapi. Text in Danish; Abstracts in English. 1984. q. DKK 335 in the European Union to individuals; DKK 268 elsewhere to individuals; DKK 553 in the European Union to institutions; DKK 442 elsewhere to institutions; DKK 100 per issue in the European Union; DKK 80 per issue elsewhere (effective 2002). bk.rev. 80 p./no. **Document type:** *Journal, Academic/Scholarly.*
Indexed: e-psyche.
Published by: Dansk Psykologisk Forlag/Danish Psychological Publishers, Stockholmsgade 29, Copenhagen Oe 2100, Denmark. TEL 45-35-38-16-55, FAX 45-35-38-16-65, dk-psych@dpf.dk, http://www.dpf.dk. Ed. Soeren Aagaard.

MEASUREMENT AND EVALUATION IN COUNSELING AND DEVELOPMENT. see *EDUCATION*

302.23 USA ISSN 1521-3269
▼ **MEDIA PSYCHOLOGY.** Text in English. 1999. q. USD 55 in US & Canada to individuals; USD 85 elsewhere to individuals; USD 250 in US & Canada to institutions; USD 280 elsewhere to institutions (effective 2002). adv. *Refereed.* **Document type:** *Journal, Academic/Scholarly.* **Description:** Publishes theoretical and empirical research in the area where the fields of psychology and media communication intersect.
Related titles: Online - full text ed.: ISSN 1532-785X. USD 49.50 to individuals; USD 225 to institutions (effective 2002) (from CatchWord Ltd., EBSCO Publishing, O C L C Online Computer Library Center, Inc., RoweCom Information Quest, Swets Blackwell, Institute for Scientific Information).
Indexed: Arts & Hum.Cit.Ind., Curr.Cont., SSCI, e-psyche.
—BLDSC (5525.258750), CatchWord. **CCC.**
Published by: Lawrence Erlbaum Associates, Inc., 10 Industrial Ave, Mahwah, NJ 07430-2262. TEL 201-760-3735, 800-926-6579, FAX 201-236-0072, journals@erlbaum.com, http://www.erlbaum.com/Journals/journals/MEP/mep.htm, http://www.erlbaum.com/journal.html. Eds. David Roskos-Ewoldsen, Jennings Bryant. adv.: page USD 275; trim 5 x 8.

MEDICAL HYPNOANALYSIS JOURNAL. see *MEDICAL SCIENCES—Hypnosis*

MEDICINA, PSICHE E ADOLESCENZA/MEDICINE, MIND AND ADOLESCENCE; semestrale di psicologia medica e di filosofia della medicina - semi-annual journal of philosophy of medicine, medical psychology and adolescentology. see *MEDICAL SCIENCES—Psychiatry And Neurology*

302 DEU ISSN 0936-7780
P96.P75
MEDIENPSYCHOLOGIE; Zeitschrift fuer Individual- und Massenkommunikation. Text in German, English. 1989. q. EUR 69.39, EUR 70.56 (effective 2001). adv. bk.rev. index. back issues avail. **Document type:** *Journal, Academic/Scholarly.*
Indexed: IBZ, Ind.Philos., PsycInfo, Psychol.Abstr. (1992-), e-psyche.
—BLDSC (5534.258000).
Published by: Hogrefe Verlag GmbH und Co. KG, Rohnsweg 25, Goettingen 37085, Germany. TEL 49-551-50688-0, FAX 49-551-5068824, verlag@hogrefe.de, http://www.hogrefe.de/zmp/. Eds. Corinna Kastner, Sabine Trepte. Circ: 500.

MEGAMOT; behavioural sciences journal. see *SOCIOLOGY*

152 GBR ISSN 0965-8211
BF371 CODEN: MEMOFV
MEMORY. Text in English. 1993. bi-m. GBP 114, USD 188 to individuals; GBP 230, USD 379 to institutions (effective 2002). adv. *Refereed.* **Document type:** *Academic/Scholarly.* **Description:** Covers high-quality research in all areas of memory, including experimental studies and developmental, educational, neuropsychological, clinical, and social research on memory.
Related titles: Online - full text ed.: ISSN 1464-0686 (from CatchWord Ltd., EBSCO Publishing, O C L C Online Computer Library Center, Inc., RoweCom Information Quest, Swets Blackwell, Institute for Scientific Information).
Indexed: AMED, ASCA, AgeLine, Curr.Cont., Ergon.Abstr., Ind.Med. (1993-), Lang.& Lang.Behav.Abstr., PsycInfo, SOPODA, SSCI, Sociol.Abstr., e-psyche.
—BLDSC (5678.000000), CatchWord, IDS, Infotrieve. **CCC.**
Published by: Psychology Press (Subsidiary of: Taylor & Francis Group), 27 Church Rd, Hove, E Sussex BN3 2FA, United Kingdom. TEL 44-1273-207411, FAX 44-1273-205612, information@psypress.co.uk, http://www.psypress.co.uk. Eds. Martin A Conway, Susan E Gathercole. R&P Zoe Peden TEL 44-20-7842-2363. Adv. contact Claire Buckminster. Circ: 250. **Subscr. addr. in N America:** Psychology Press, Journals Customer Service, Taylor & Francis Group, 325 Chestnut St, Philadelphia, PA 19106. TEL 800-354-1420, FAX 215-625-8914, info@taylorandfrancis.com, http://www.psypress.com; **Subscr. addr. outside of N America:** Journals Customer Service, Taylor & Francis Group, Rankine Rd, Basingstoke, Hants RG24 8PR, United Kingdom. TEL 44-1256-813002, FAX 44-1256-479438, enquiry@tandf.co.uk.

152 USA ISSN 0090-502X
BF371 CODEN: MYCGAO
MEMORY AND COGNITION. Text in English. 1973. 8/yr. USD 181 in United States; USD 197 foreign (effective 2001). adv. bibl. illus. back issues avail.; reprint service avail. from PQC,PSC,SCH. *Refereed.* **Document type:** *Academic/Scholarly.* **Description:** Covers human memory, learning, conceptual processes, psycholinguistics, and problem solving, along with reports of work in computer simulation and experimental social psychology.
Related titles: Microform ed.: (from NRP,PQC); Online - full text ed.: (from CatchWord Ltd., Gale Group, Factiva, Institute for Scientific Information).

Indexed: ASCA, AgeLine, Arts & Hum.Cit.Ind. (coverage dropped), Biol.Abstr., CINAHL, Child Devel.Abstr., Commun.Abstr., Curr.Adv.Ecol.Sci., Curr.Cont., Ergon.Abstr., Excerp.Med., IBR, Ind.Med. (1973-), Ind.Philos., Lang.& Lang.Behav.Abstr., M.L.A., MLA Intl.Bibl., Mid.East: Abstr.& Ind., Mult.Ed.Abstr., Neurosci.Abstr. (coverage dropped), Neurosci.Cit.Ind., Psychol.Abstr. (1973-), Russ.Acad.Sci.Bibl., SOPODA, SSCI, Soc.Sci.Ind. (Jan.1987-), Sociol.Abstr., e-psyche. —BLDSC (5678.300000), GNLM, IDS, ingenta. **CCC.**
Published by: Psychonomic Society, Inc., 1710 Fortview Rd, Austin, TX 78704. TEL 512-462-2442, FAX 512-462-1101, jbellquist@psychonomic.org, http://www.sig.net/~psysoc.home.htm, http://www.psychonomic.org. Ed. Morton A Gernsbacher. R&P Cinnamon Nemec. Adv. contact Robert Samford. page USD 165; trim 10.75 x 8. Circ: 2,400.

MENNINGER CLINIC. BULLETIN; a journal for the mental health professions. see *MEDICAL SCIENCES—Psychiatry And Neurology*

MENNINGER PERSPECTIVE. see *MEDICAL SCIENCES—Psychiatry And Neurology*

MENTAL CAPACITY: MEDICAL AND LEGAL ASPECTS OF THE AGING. see *GERONTOLOGY AND GERIATRICS*

614.58 790.1 USA
THE MENTAL EDGE. Text in English. q. USD 15. **Document type:** *Newsletter.* **Description:** Covers specific procedures to enhance sports performance and discusses how top athletes use mental training to boost their athletic skills.
Published by: Mental Edge, 18607 Ventura Blvd, Ste 310, Tarzana, CA 91356. TEL 818-344-4464, Compuserve 76473,546. Ed. J P Erickson.

MENTAL HEALTH CARE. see *MEDICAL SCIENCES—Psychiatry And Neurology*

616.89 USA
MENTAL HEALTH DISORDERS SOURCEBOOK. Text in English. 1995. irreg., latest 1999, 2nd edition. USD 78 per issue (effective 2001). charts. Index. **Document type:** *Consumer.* **Description:** Basic information about schizophrenia, depression, bipolar disorder, panic disorder, obsessive-compulsive disorder, phobias and other anxiety disorders, paranoia and other personality disorders, eating disorders, and sleep disorders, along with Information about treatment and therapies.
Published by: Omnigraphics, Inc., 615 Griswold St, Detroit, MI 48226. TEL 313-961-1340, 800-234-1340, FAX 313-961-1383, 800-875-1340, info@omnigraphics.com, jjts@sprynet.com, http://www.omnigraphics.com. Ed. Karen Bellenir.

155.4 362.7 616.8 USA
MENTAL HEALTH IN CHILDREN. Text in English. 1975. irreg. USD 69.95. back issues avail. **Document type:** *Academic/Scholarly.* **Description:** Articles for professionals in the area of child mental health.
Indexed: e-psyche.
Published by: P J D Publications Ltd, PO Box 966, Westbury, NY 11590. TEL 516-626-0650, FAX 516-626-5546. Ed. Dr. D V Siva Sankar. Pub. Barbara Sankar.

MENTAL HEALTH LAW BULLETIN. see *LAW—Civil Law*

MENTAL HEALTH LAW NEWS. see *LAW—Civil Law*

MENTAL HEALTH LAW REPORTER. see *LAW—Civil Law*

150 USA
MENTAL HEALTH LIBRARY SERIES. Text in English. irreg., latest vol.3, 1994. **Document type:** *Monographic series, Academic/Scholarly.*
Indexed: e-psyche.
—BLDSC (235658).
Published by: International Universities Press, Inc., 59 Boston Post Rd, Box 1524, Madison, CT 06443-1524. TEL 203-245-4000, FAX 203-245-0775, http://www.iup.com. Ed. Dr. George H Pollock.

MENTAL HEALTH MATTERS. see *MEDICAL SCIENCES—Psychiatry And Neurology*

616.89 CAN ISSN 1196-5304
MENTAL HEALTH MATTERS. Text in English, French. q. **Document type:** *Newsletter.* **Description:** Audience consists of members of the association, people who have had mental illness, mental health professionals, and family members.
Formerly: National - Canadian Mental Health Association National Office (1196-0337)
Published by: Canadian Mental Health Association, 2160 Yonge St, Toronto, ON M4S 2Z3, Canada. TEL 416-484-7750, FAX 416-484-4617. Ed. Nancy MacMillan. Circ: 1,500 (controlled).

616.89 GBR ISSN 0963-0201
MENTAL HEALTH MATTERS. Text in English. 1962. q. membership. bk.rev. **Document type:** *Newsletter.*
Former titles (until 1991): Beacon House Bulletin (0144-2368); Northern Ireland Association for Mental Health. Newsletter; Beacon House News
Published by: Northern Ireland Association for Mental Health, 80 University St, Belfast, N Ireland BT7 1HE, United Kingdom. FAX 0232-234940. Ed. Margery Magee. Circ: 1,500 (controlled).

155.82 GBR ISSN 1367-4676
MENTAL HEALTH, RELIGION & CULTURE. Text in English. 1998. 3/yr. GBP 52, USD 86 to individuals; GBP 128, USD 211 to institutions (effective 2002). **Document type:** *Academic/Scholarly.* **Description:** Publishes empirically-based work exploring the relationships between mental health and aspects of religion and culture, and discussing conceptual and philosophical aspects.
Related titles: Online - full content ed.: ISSN 1469-9737 (from EBSCO Publishing, O C L C Online Computer Library Center, Inc., Swets Blackwell); Online - full text ed.: (from CatchWord Ltd., RoweCom Information Quest).
Indexed: PsycInfo, Soc.Serv.Abstr., Sociol.Abstr., e-psyche. —CatchWord. **CCC.**
Published by: Carfax Publishing Limited (Subsidiary of: Taylor & Francis Group), PO Box 25, Abingdon, Oxon OX14 3UE, United Kingdom. TEL 44-1235-401000, FAX 44-1235-401550, enquiries@carfax.co.uk, enquiry@tandf.co.uk, http://www.carfax.co.uk. Eds. Kate Miriam Loewenthal, Simon Dein.

MENTAL HEALTH REPORT. see *SOCIAL SERVICES AND WELFARE*

614.58 GBR
MENTAL HEALTH RESEARCH REVIEW. Text in English. 1994. m. free per issue (2001). **Document type:** *Journal, Academic/Scholarly.* **Description:** Presents mental health care research carried out by the PSSRU and the Centre for the Economics of Mental Health (CEMH).
Indexed: e-psyche.
—BLDSC (5678.584700).
Published by: P S S R U, University of Kent at Canterbury, Canterbury, Kent CT2 7NF, United Kingdom. TEL 44-1227-764000, FAX 44-1227-764327, pssru@ukc.ac.uk, http://www.ukc.ac.uk/pssru. Eds. David McDaid, Paul McCrone. **Co-publisher:** C E M H.

THE MENTAL HEALTH REVIEW. see *MEDICAL SCIENCES—Psychiatry And Neurology*

MENTAL HEALTH REVIEW TRIBUNALS FOR ENGLAND AND WALES. ANNUAL REPORT. see *PUBLIC HEALTH AND SAFETY*

150 USA ISSN 1522-3434
CODEN: MHSRFN
▼ **MENTAL HEALTH SERVICES RESEARCH.** Text in English. 1999. q. EUR 230 to institutions for print or online ed.; EUR 276 to institutions print & online eds.combined (effective 2002). *Refereed.* **Document type:** *Academic/Scholarly.* **Description:** Focuses on how the need for services can be conceptualized and measured, how services are utilized, the fit between service needs and utilization, service quality and service cost, how consumer outcomes can be conceptualized and measured, and how measures pertaining to services are associated with consumer outcomes.
Related titles: Online - full text ed.: (from EBSCO Publishing, O C L C Online Computer Library Center, Inc., RoweCom Information Quest, Swets Blackwell, Kluwer Online).
Indexed: e-psyche.
—BLDSC (5678.585735). **CCC.**
Published by: (Vanderbilt University Institute for Public Policy Studies), Kluwer Academic - Plenum Publishers (Subsidiary of: Wolters Kluwer N.V.), 233 Spring St, New York, NY 10013-1578. TEL 212-620-8000, 800-221-9369, FAX 212-463-0742, services@wkap.nl, http://www.wkap.nl; http://www.wkap.nl/journalhome.htm/1522-3434. Ed. Leonard Bickman. R&P Rose Luongo TEL 781-871-6311.

370.15 613.62 USA
MENTAL HEALTH SPECIAL INTEREST SECTION QUARTERLY. Text in English. 1989 (vol.12, no.4). q. USD 20 (effective 1999). **Document type:** *Newsletter.*
Former titles (until 199?): Mental Health Special Interest Section Newsletter (0279-4136); American Occupational Therapy Association. Mental Health Specialty Section. Newsletter (0194-6382)
Indexed: e-psyche.
Published by: American Occupational Therapy Association, Inc., 4720 Montgomery Lane, Bethesda, MD 20814-3425. TEL 301-652-2682, FAX 301-652-7711.

362.2 301.1 USA ISSN 1058-1103
MENTAL HEALTH WEEKLY; news for policy and program decision-makers. Text in English. 48/yr., latest vol.11, 2001 (48/yr.). USD 499 domestic to individuals; USD 647 domestic to institutions; USD 657 in Canada to institutions; USD 667 elsewhere to institutions (effective 2001). 8 p./no. back issues avail.; reprints avail. **Document type:** *Newsletter.* **Description:** Covers the latest news and analysis of public policy, business trends and treatment issues affecting mental health administrators in the public, private and nonprofit sectors.
Incorporates (in 1991): Addiction Program Management (0897-4934); (1970-1991): Behavior Today (0005-7924); Which incorporates: Sexuality Today (0148-883X); Marriage and Divorce Today (0148-8821)
Related titles: E-mail ed.; Online - full text ed.: (from Gale Group).
Indexed: Except.Child Educ.Abstr., Pers.Lit., Soc.Work Res.& Abstr., e-psyche.
—Infotrieve. **CCC.**
Published by: Manisses Communications Group, Inc., PO Box 9758, Providence, RI 02906-9758. TEL 401-861-6020, 800-333-7771, FAX 401-861-6370, manissesCS@manisses.com, http://www.manisses.com. Ed. Gary A Enos. R&P Barbara Deekle.

P

153.93 371.26 USA ISSN 0076-6461
Z5814.P8
MENTAL MEASUREMENTS YEARBOOK. Text in English. 1938. biennial. price varies. *Refereed.* **Document type:** *Directory.* **Description:** Contains descriptions and candidly critical reviews of commercially available test instruments. Reviews done by professionals in the assessment, measurement or subject area.
Indexed: e-psyche.
—BLDSC (5678.605000).
Published by: Buros Institute of Mental Measurements, 135 Bancroft Hall, University of Nebraska Lincoln, Lincoln, NE 68588-0348. TEL 402-472-6203, FAX 402-472-6207, bimm@unlinfo.unl.edu, http://www.unl.edu. Eds. Barbara S Plake, James C Impara. **Dist. by:** University of Nebraska Press, 233 N 8th St, Lincoln, NE 68588-0255. TEL 800-755-1105, FAX 402-4726214.

MENTALITIES/MENTALITES; an interdisciplinary journal. see *HISTORY*

301.1 150 ITA
MENTE E SOCIETA. Text in Italian. 1985. irreg., latest vol.13, 1999. price varies. adv. **Document type:** *Monographic series.*
Indexed: e-psyche.
Published by: Liguori Editore srl, Via Posillipo, 394, Naples, NA 80123, Italy. TEL 39-81-7206111, FAX 39-81-7206244, http://www.liguori.it. Ed. Guglielmo Bellelli. Pub. Guido Liguori. Adv. contact Maria Liguori.

MERIDIAN; Zeitschrift fuer Kosmobiologie, Astrologie und angewandte Psychologie. see *NEW AGE PUBLICATIONS*

150 301 USA ISSN 0272-930X
HQ1 CODEN: MPQUA5
MERRILL - PALMER QUARTERLY. Text in English. 1954. q. USD 50 to individuals; USD 98 to institutions; USD 28 to students (effective 2000). adv. bk.rev. charts, illus. index. reprint service avail. from SCH,PSC. *Refereed.* **Document type:** *Academic/Scholarly.* **Description:** Publishes theoretical and empirical papers in the areas of human development and family-child relationships.
Former titles (until 1960): Merrill - Palmer Quarterly of Behavior and Development (0026-0150); (until 1958): Merrill - Palmer Quarterly (0272-9679)
Related titles: Microform ed.: (from PQC); Online - full text ed.: (from H. W. Wilson, ProQuest Information & Learning, Gale Group, Swets Blackwell, Institute for Scientific Information, RoweCom Information Quest).

Indexed: ASCA, Adol.Ment.Hlth.Abstr., AgeLine, Arts & Hum.Cit.Ind. (coverage dropped), Bibl.Dev.Med.& Child Neur., Biol.Abstr., C.I.J.E., Child Devel.Abstr., Curr.Cont., DSH Abstr., ERA, Educ.Ind. (Jul.1982-), Except.Child Educ.Abstr., Fam.Ind., Human Resour.Abstr., IBR, IBZ, IMFL, Ind.Philos., Lang.& Lang.Behav.Abstr., Mid.East: Abstr.& Ind., Mult.Ed.Abstr., PSI, PsycInfo, Psychol.Abstr. (1954-), Psycscan D.P., SOPODA, SSCI, Sage Fam.Stud.Abstr., Soc.Serv.Abstr., Soc.Work Res.& Abstr., Sociol.Abstr., Sociol.Educ.Abstr., Sp.Ed.Needs Abstr., Stud.Wom.Abstr., Viol.& Abuse Abstr., e-psyche.
—BLDSC (5682.280000), IDS, Infotrieve, ingenta. **CCC.**
Published by: (Merrill - Palmer Institute), Wayne State University Press, The Leonard N. Simons Bldg, 4809 Woodward Ave, Detroit, MI 48201-1309. TEL 313-577-6120, 313-577-6119, FAX 313-577-6131, ac3707@wayne.edu, http://www.press.uchicago.edu/cgi-bin/hfx.cgi/66/wayne_state/mpq.ctl. Ed. Carolyn Shantz. R&P Mary Garcia TEL 313-577-6257. Adv. contact Alison Reeves. Circ: 1,290.

METAPHOR AND SYMBOL. see *LINGUISTICS*

METHODOLOGIA; pensiero linguaggio modelli - thought language models. see *LINGUISTICS*

150 DEU
METHODS OF PSYCHOLOGICAL RESEARCH. Variant title: M P R - Online. Text in English. 1996. irreg., latest vol.6, no.3, 2001. **Document type:** *Journal, Academic/Scholarly.*
Media: Online - full content.
Published by: German Psychology Society http://www.mpr-online.de/.

P

150.72 ESP
▼ **METODOLOGIA DE LAS CIENCIAS DEL COMPORTAMIENTO.** Text in Spanish. 1999. s-a.?. **Document type:** *Journal, Academic/Scholarly.* **Description:** Covers behavioral research methodology.
—CINDOC.
Published by: Asociacion Espanola de Metodologia de las Ciencias del Comportamiento, c/o Dept. de Psicologia Basica y Metodologia, Univ. de Murcia, Campus de Espinardo, Apdo. 4021, Murcia 30080, Spain.

MILITAERPSYKOLOGISKE MEDDELELSER. see *MILITARY*

355 USA ISSN 0899-5605
U22.3
MILITARY PSYCHOLOGY. Text in English. 1989. q. USD 55 in US & Canada to individuals; USD 85 elsewhere to individuals; USD 375 in US & Canada to institutions; USD 405 elsewhere to institutions (effective 2002). adv. *Refereed.* **Document type:** *Journal, Academic/Scholarly.* **Description:** Presents behavioral science research papers having military applications in clinical and health psychology, cognition and training, human factors, manpower and personnel, social and organizational systems, and testing and measurement.
Related titles: Online - full text ed.: ISSN 1532-7876. USD 49.50 to individuals; USD 337.50 to institutions (effective 2002) (from CatchWord Ltd., EBSCO Publishing, O C L C Online Computer Library Center, Inc., RoweCom Information Quest, Swets Blackwell, Institute for Scientific Information).
Indexed: ASCA, Compumath, Curr.Cont., Eng.Ind., Environ.Sci.Poll.Mgmt., Ergon.Abstr., Fam.Ind., Pollut.Abstr., PsycInfo, Psychol.Abstr. (1989-), Risk Abstr., SSCI, Saf.Sci.Abstr., e-psyche.
—BLDSC (5768.167000), CatchWord, Ei, Infotrieve, ingenta. **CCC.**
Published by: (Division 19, American Psychological Association), Lawrence Erlbaum Associates, Inc., 10 Industrial Ave, Mahwah, NJ 07430-2262. TEL 201-760-3735, 800-926-6579, FAX 201-236-0072, journals@erlbaum.com, http://www.erlbaum.com/Journals/journals/MP/mp.htm. Ed. Martin F Wiskoff. adv.: page USD 325; trim 5 x 8.

MIMESIS (BAURU); revista da area de ciencias humanas. see *SOCIAL SCIENCES: COMPREHENSIVE WORKS*

150.19 300 USA ISSN 1071-6866
MIND & HUMAN INTERACTION. Text in English. 1989. q. USD 63 domestic to individuals; USD 69 foreign to individuals; USD 99 domestic to institutions; USD 107 foreign to institutions (effective 2002). adv. **Document type:** *Journal, Academic/Scholarly.* **Description:** Seeks to open windows between psychoanalysis and politics, history, sociology, anthropology and other social sciences disciplines.
Published by: (University of Virginia, School of Medicine, Center for the Study of Mind and Human Interaction), International Universities Press, Incorporated, 59 Boston Post Rd., P.O. Box 1524, Madison, CT 06443-1524. adv.: page USD 360; 5 x 8.5.

363.7 USA
MIND MATTERS REVIEW. Text in English. 1988. q. USD 15; USD 20 foreign (effective 1999). adv. bk.rev. back issues avail. **Description:** Forum for discussion on the politics of mind, encompassing politics of religion, psychiatry, science, ideology.
Indexed: e-psyche.
Published by: Carrie L. Drake, Ed. & Pub., 2040 Polk St, Box 234, San Francisco, CA 94109. R&P Carrie L Drake. Adv. contact Carrie Drake. Circ: 1,000.

150 ITA
MINOTAURO; problemi e ricerche di psicologia del profondo. Text in Italian. 1974. s-a. ITL 25,000, USD 20 (effective 2000). adv. bk.rev. bibl. index. *Refereed.* **Document type:** *Academic/Scholarly.* **Description:** Covers analytical psychology (C.G. Jung) for students, psychoanalysts and psychotherapists.
Indexed: e-psyche.
Published by: Gruppo Autonomo di Psicologia Analitica, Via Della Consulta, 50, Rome, RM 00184, Italy. TEL 39-6-4885304, FAX 39-6-36303643. Ed. Francesco Paolo Ranzato. adv.: page ITL 500,000. Circ: 800 (paid).

616.89 DEU ISSN 0342-3174
MITEINANDER LEBEN LERNEN; Zeitschrift fuer Tiefenpsychologie, Persoenlichkeitsbildung und Kulturforschung. Text in German. bi-m. DEM 28. **Document type:** *Academic/Scholarly.*
Formerly (until 1976): Leben Lernen (0341-8286)
Indexed: e-psyche.
Published by: Institut fuer Tiefenpsychologie, Eichenallee 6, Berlin 14050, Germany. TEL 030-3023034. Ed. Josef Rattner.

150 USA ISSN 0361-5227
RC500
MODERN PSYCHOANALYSIS. Text in English. 1976. s-a. USD 48 domestic to individuals; USD 48 foreign to individuals; USD 48 domestic to institutions; USD 59 foreign to institutions (effective 2002). adv. bk.rev. index. reprint service avail. from PSC,SCH. *Refereed.* **Document type:** *Academic/Scholarly.* **Description:** Dedicated to extending the theory and practice of psychoanalysis to the full range of emotional disorders.
Indexed: CINAHL, Chicago Psychoanal.Lit.Ind., IBR, IBZ, Ind.Philos., Mid.East: Abstr.& Ind., PsycInfo, Psychoanal.Abstr., Psychol.Abstr. (1976-), e-psyche.
—BLDSC (5894.420000), CISTI, ingenta.
Published by: (Center for Modern Psychoanalytic Studies), International Universities Press, Inc., 59 Boston Post Rd, Box 1524, Madison, CT 06443-1524. TEL 203-245-4000, FAX 203-245-0775, office@iup.com, http://www.iup.com. Pub. Sara Sheftel. R&P Carol Brod. adv.: page USD 580; 4.25 x 7. Circ: 1,000 (paid).

150 USA ISSN 1529-4978
BF1
MONITOR ON PSYCHOLOGY. Text in English. 1970. m. USD 45 domestic to non-members; USD 85 foreign to non-members; USD 75 domestic to institutions; USD 163 foreign to institutions (effective 2001). adv. charts, illus, tr.lit. back issues avail.; reprints avail. *Refereed.* **Document type:** *Newspaper.* **Description:** Reports on the science, practice, and social responsibility activities of psychology, including latest legislative developments affecting mental health, education, and research support.
Formerly: A P A Monitor (0001-2114); Incorporates: American Psychological Association. Employment Bulletin
Related titles: Microform ed.: (from PQC); Online - full text ed.
—BLDSC (5908.960250).
Published by: American Psychological Association, 750 First St., N.E., Washington, DC 20002-4242. TEL 202-336-5500, 800-374-2721, FAX 202-336-5568, letters.monitor@apa.org, http://www.apa.org/monitor/. Eds. Ed Diener, Sara Martin. adv.: B&W page USD 5,145, color page USD 6,345. Circ: 116,000.

573.8 612.8 CHE ISSN 0749-1190
CODEN: MPSYEV
MONOGRAPHS IN PSYCHOBIOLOGY. Text in English. 1985. irreg., latest vol.6, 1989. price varies. *Refereed.* **Document type:** *Monographic series.*
Indexed: e-psyche.
Published by: Gordon and Breach - Harwood Academic (Subsidiary of: Taylor & Francis Group), PO Box 531, Lausanne 1000, Switzerland. Ed. S A Corson. **Subscr. addr. in US:** International Publishers Direct, PO Box 32160, Newark, NJ 07102. FAX 215-750-6343.

155.6 RUS ISSN 0137-0936
MOSKOVSKII GOSUDARSTVENNYI UNIVERSITET. VESTNIK. SERIYA 14: PSIKHOLOGIYA. Text in Russian. q. USD 85 in United States.
Indexed: PsycInfo, Ref.Zh., Russ.Acad.Sci.Bibl., e-psyche.
—BLDSC (0032.697100), East View.
Published by: (Moskovskii Gosudarstvennyi Universitet), Izdatel'stvo Moskovskogo Gosudarstvennogo Universiteta, B Nikitskaya 5-7, Moscow 103009, Russian Federation. TEL 7-095-2033128. **US dist. addr.:** East View Publications, 3020 Harbor Ln N, Minneapolis, MN 55447. TEL 612-550-0961.

150 USA ISSN 0146-7239
BF683 CODEN: MOEMDJ
MOTIVATION AND EMOTION. Text in English. 1977. q. EUR 489 to institutions for print or online ed. (effective 2002); NLG 1,174.80 to institutions Print & Online eds.combined (effective 2001); EUR 586.80 to institutions Print & Online eds.combined (effective 2002). adv. back issues avail. *Refereed.* **Document type:** *Academic/Scholarly.* **Description:** Publishes theoretical papers and original research reports of either a basic or applied nature from any area of psychology or other behavioral science.
Related titles: Microfilm ed.: (from PQC); Online - full text ed.: (from EBSCO Publishing, O C L C Online Computer Library Center, Inc., Swets Blackwell, Kluwer Online, Institute for Scientific Information, RoweCom Information Quest).
Indexed: ASCA, Arts & Hum.Cit.Ind. (coverage dropped), Biol.Abstr., Child Devel.Abstr., Curr.Cont., IBZ, Ind.Philos., PsycInfo, Psychol.Abstr. (1977-), Ref.Zh., Rel.Ind.One, Rel.Ind.Two, SSCI, e-psyche.
—BLDSC (5969.060000), CISTI, IDS, ingenta. **CCC.**
Published by: Kluwer Academic - Plenum Publishers (Subsidiary of: Wolters Kluwer N.V.), 233 Spring St, New York, NY 10013-1578. TEL 212-620-8000, 800-221-9369, FAX 212-463-0742, services@wkap.nl, http://www.wkap.nl/journalhome.htm/0146-7239. Ed. Alice M Isen.

155.4 DEU
MULTIMIND - N L P AKTUELL. Text in German. 1992. bi-m. DEM 94 (effective 2000). adv. bk.rev. index. back issues avail. **Document type:** *Magazine, Academic/Scholarly.*
Indexed: e-psyche.
Published by: Junfermann Verlag, Imadstr 40, Paderborn 33102, Germany. TEL 49-5251-13440, FAX 49-5251-134444, ju@junfermann.de. Adv. contact Ruth Frerker. B&W page DEM 1,850, color page DEM 4,070; trim 265 x 184.

▼ **MULTIPLE INTELLIGENCES NEWSLETTER.** see *EDUCATION—Teaching Methods And Curriculum*

152 USA ISSN 0027-3171
BF39 CODEN: MVBRAV
MULTIVARIATE BEHAVIORAL RESEARCH. Text in English. 1966. q. USD 50 in US & Canada to individuals; USD 80 elsewhere to individuals; USD 380 in US & Canada to institutions; USD 410 elsewhere to institutions (effective 2002). adv. index. back issues avail.; reprint service avail. from PSC,SCH. *Refereed.* **Document type:** *Journal, Academic/Scholarly.* **Description:** Reports results of behavioral research employing multivariate methods.
Related titles: Microform ed.: (from PQC); Online - full text ed.: ISSN 1532-7906. USD 45 to individuals; USD 342 to institutions (effective 2002) (from CatchWord Ltd., EBSCO Publishing, O C L C Online Computer Library Center, Inc., RoweCom Information Quest, Swets Blackwell, Institute for Scientific Information).
Indexed: ASCA, AgeLine, Biol.Abstr., Biostat., C.I.J.E., Commun.Abstr., Compumath, Curr.Cont., Curr.Ind.Stat., Fam.Ind., IBZ, Ind.Philos., J.Cont.Quant.Meth., Lang.& Lang.Behav.Abstr., Mid.East: Abstr.& Ind., PsycInfo, Psychol.Abstr. (1966-), Psycscan A.P., SOPODA, SSCI, Sci.Cit.Ind. (coverage dropped), Sociol.Abstr., e-psyche.
—BLDSC (5983.300000), CatchWord, ingenta. **CCC.**
Published by: Lawrence Erlbaum Associates, Inc., 10 Industrial Ave, Mahwah, NJ 07430-2262. TEL 201-760-3735, 800-926-6579, FAX 201-236-0072, journals@erlbaum.com, http://www.erlbaum.com/Journals/journals/MBR/mbr.htm. Ed. Roger E Millsap. adv.: page USD 350; trim 5 x 8. Circ: 905.

616.89 USA ISSN 0147-3964
BF698.A1 CODEN: MCREDA
MULTIVARIATE EXPERIMENTAL CLINICAL RESEARCH; a journal for basic behavioral research into personality dynamics and clinical psychology. Text in English. 1973. irreg. USD 29 to individuals; USD 35 foreign to individuals; USD 50 to institutions; USD 56 foreign to institutions (effective 1999). adv. bk.rev. **Document type:** *Academic/Scholarly.* **Description:** Outlet for clinical and personality researches using sophisticated, multivariate experimental methods. Both manipulative and non-manipulative research is accepted.
Formerly: Journal of Multivariate Experimental Personality and Clinical Psychology (0149-9688)
Media: Duplicated (not offset).
Indexed: Biol.Abstr., Curr.Cont. (coverage dropped), Curr.Ind.Stat., Excerp.Med., IMFL, PsycInfo, Psychol.Abstr., Psycscan C.P., SSCI (coverage dropped), Sci.Cit.Ind. (coverage dropped), e-psyche.
—CISTI, GNLM, ingenta, KNAW.
Published by: Psychology Press (Subsidiary of: Taylor & Francis Ltd.), c/o Dr Charles Burdsal, Ed, Wichita State University, Dept of Psychology, 1845 Fairmount, Wichita, KS 67260-0034. TEL 316-978-3170, burdsal@wsuhub.uc.twsu.edu. Ed. Charles Burdsal. Circ: 200.

MUSIC THERAPY PERSPECTIVES. see *MUSIC*

MUSIKPSYCHOLOGIE. see *MUSIC*

616.89 DEU ISSN 0172-5505
ML3920
MUSIKTHERAPEUTISCHE UMSCHAU. Text in German; Summaries in English. 4/yr. DEM 109; DEM 81 to students (effective 2000). **Document type:** *Journal, Academic/Scholarly.* **Description:** Publication containing studies in music oriented therapy, and its application in medicine, psychotherapy, and psychology.
Indexed: Dok.Arbeitsmed., Excerp.Med., IBZ, Ind.Philos., Int.Ind.Mus.Per., Music Ind., Psychol.Abstr., RILM, e-psyche.
—GNLM, Infotrieve. **CCC.**
Published by: Vandenhoeck und Ruprecht, Robert-Bosch-Breite 6, Goettingen 37079, Germany. TEL 49-551-6959-26, FAX 49-551-695917. Ed. V Bernius.

300 NLD ISSN 0258-123X
CODEN: NADSDD
N A T O ADVANCED SCIENCE INSTITUTES SERIES D: BEHAVIOURAL AND SOCIAL SCIENCES. Text in English. 1974. irreg., latest vol.82, 1995. *Refereed.* **Document type:** *Monographic series.*
Formerly: N A T O Advanced Study Institutes Series D: Behavioural and Social Sciences
Related titles: Online - full text ed.: (from European Space Agency).
Indexed: Math.R., Zoo.Rec., e-psyche.
—CASDDS, CISTI, Infotrieve. **CCC.**
Published by: (Scientific Affairs Division BEL, North Atlantic Treaty Organization BEL), Kluwer Academic Publishers Group (Subsidiary of: Wolters Kluwer N.V.), Spuiboulevard 50, PO Box 17, Dordrecht 3300 AA, Netherlands. FAX 31-78-639-2254, services@wkap.nl, http://www.wkap.nl. **Dist. by:** Journals Department, PO Box 322, Dordrecht 3300 AH, Netherlands. FAX 31-78-654-6474.

370.15 150 USA ISSN 1067-1161
NATIONAL CHARACTER LABORATORY NEWSLETTER. Text in English. 1971. q. USD 5 (effective 2000). bk.rev. abstr, bibl, stat. **Document type:** *Newsletter.* **Description:** Reports research results on character, and encourages and coordinates further research.
Indexed: e-psyche.
Published by: National Character Laboratory, 4635 Leeds Ave, El Paso, TX 79903. TEL 915-562-5046. Ed. A J Stuart Jr. Circ: 150.

150.19 USA ISSN 0077-5339
NATIONAL PSYCHOLOGICAL ASSOCIATION FOR PSYCHOANALYSIS. BULLETIN. Text in English. 1950. biennial. **Document type:** *Bulletin.*
Indexed: e-psyche.
Published by: National Psychological Association for Psychoanalysis, Inc., 150 W 13th St, New York, NY 10011. TEL 212-924-7440. Circ: 7,000.

150.19 USA
NATIONAL PSYCHOLOGICAL ASSOCIATION FOR PSYCHOANALYSIS. NEWS AND REVIEWS. Text in English. 1970. 3/yr. USD 10. **Document type:** *Newsletter.*
Indexed: e-psyche.
Published by: National Psychological Association for Psychoanalysis, Inc., 150 W 13th St, New York, NY 10011. TEL 212-924-7440, FAX 212-989-7543. Ed. Harvey A Kaplan. Circ: 1,000.

NATIONAL REGISTER OF PROFESSIONAL HYPNOTHERAPISTS. see *MEDICAL SCIENCES—Hypnosis*

153.1534 USA ISSN 0146-7875
BF683 CODEN: NSMPB3
NEBRASKA SYMPOSIUM ON MOTIVATION (PUBLICATION). Text in English. 1953. a., latest vol.47, 2000. USD 50 (effective 2001). index, cum.index. back issues avail. **Document type:** *Monographic series, Academic/Scholarly.* **Description:** Includes timely paper topics for the Nebraska Symposium which deal with all aspects of motivation.
Formerly: Current Theory and Research in Motivation (0070-2099)
Related titles: Online - full text ed.: (from Institute for Scientific Information).
Indexed: ASCA, Ind.Med. (1954-), Psychol.Abstr., SSCI, e-psyche.
—BLDSC (6068.380000), IDS, ingenta.
Published by: (Department of Psychology, University of Nebraska), University of Nebraska Press, 233 N 8th St, Lincoln, NE 68588-0255. TEL 402-472-3581, FAX 402-472-6214. Eds. Alan C Kamil, Daniel W Leger, Jeffrey A French. R&P Elaine Maruhn.

150 616.89 NLD ISSN 0028-2235
BF8.N2
NEDERLANDS TIJDSCHRIFT VOOR DE PSYCHOLOGIE EN HAAR GRENSGEBIEDEN. Text in Dutch. 1934. bi-m. NLG 152.50. **Document type:** *Academic/Scholarly.*
Indexed: PsycInfo, e-psyche.
—BLDSC (6072.200000), GNLM, KNAW.
Published by: Bohn Stafleu van Loghum B.V. (Subsidiary of: Wolters Kluwer N.V.), Postbus 246, Houten 3990 GA, Netherlands. TEL 31-3403-95712, FAX 31-3403-50903. Ed. Dr. J van Heerden.

NEODIDAGMATA. see *EDUCATION—Teaching Methods And Curriculum*

▼ **NEURO-PSYCHOANALYSIS**; an interdisciplinary journal for psychoanalysis and the neurosciences. see *MEDICAL SCIENCES—Psychiatry And Neurology*

NEUROBIOLOGY OF LEARNING AND MEMORY. see *MEDICAL SCIENCES—Psychiatry And Neurology*

NEUROPSYCHOLOGICAL REHABILITATION; an international journal. see *MEDICAL SCIENCES—Psychiatry And Neurology*

NEUROPSYCHOLOGY. see *MEDICAL SCIENCES—Psychiatry And Neurology*

NEUROPSYCHOLOGY AND COGNITION. see *MEDICAL SCIENCES—Psychiatry And Neurology*

616.8 NLD ISSN 1380-3395
CODEN: JCENE8
NEUROPSYCHOLOGY, DEVELOPMENT AND COGNITION. SECTION A: JOURNAL OF CLINICAL AND EXPERIMENTAL NEUROPSYCHOLOGY. Cover title: Journal of Clinical and Experimental Neuropsychology. Text in English. 1979. bi-m., latest vol.23, 2001. NLG 631, USD 351 to individuals; NLG 1,393, USD 714 to institutions includes online ed; NLG 2,755, USD 1,413 to institutions includes sections B, C, D (effective 2001). adv. bk.rev. abstr, illus. Index. back issues avail.; reprint service avail. from SWZ. *Refereed.* **Document type:** *Journal, Academic/Scholarly.* **Description:** Publishes original empirical research comprising methodological and theoretical papers, critical reviews, and case studies.
Supersedes (in 1994): Journal of Clinical and Experimental Neuropsychology (0168-8634); Which was formerly: Journal of Clinical Neuropsychology (0165-0475)
Related titles: Online - full text ed.: (from EBSCO Publishing, O C L C Online Computer Library Center, Inc., RoweCom Information Quest, Swets Blackwell, Institute for Scientific Information).
Indexed: ASCA, AgeLine, Behav.Med.Abstr., Biol.Abstr., Child Devel.Abstr., Curr.Cont., Except.Child Educ.Abstr., Excerp.Med., Fam.Ind., Ind.Med. (1985-), Ind.Sci.Rev., Inpharma, Lang.& Lang.Behav.Abstr., Neuropsych.Abstr., Neurosci.Cit.Ind., Pharm.&Out.News, PsycInfo, Psychol.Abstr. (1979-), Psycscan C.P., Reac., SOPODA, SSCI, Sci.Cit.Ind., Sociol.Abstr., THA, e-psyche.
—BLDSC (4958.375000), ADONIS, CISTI, GNLM, IDS, ingenta. **CCC.**
Published by: Swets & Zeitlinger BV, PO Box 825, Lisse 2160 SZ, Netherlands. TEL 31-252-435111, FAX 31-252-415888, orders@swets.nl, http://www.swets.nl/sps/journals/neuro.html. Ed. Wilfred G van Gorp. R&P J van der Valk. Adv. contact Patrick Kliean. **Dist. in N. America by:** Swets & Zeitlinger, PO Box 582, Downingtown, PA 19335-998. TEL 800-477-9387, FAX 610-524-5366.

618.97 NLD ISSN 1382-5585
CODEN: AGCOEW
NEUROPSYCHOLOGY, DEVELOPMENT AND COGNITION. SECTION B: AGING, NEUROPSYCHOLOGY AND COGNITION; a journal on normal and dysfunctional development. Cover title: Aging, Neuropsychology and Cognition. Text in English. 1994. q. NLG 199, USD 111 to individuals; NLG 544, USD 278 to institutions includes online ed; NLG 2,755, USD 1,413 to institutions includes sections A, C, D (effective 2001). adv. abstr. back issues avail.; reprint service avail. from SWZ. *Refereed.* **Document type:** *Journal, Academic/Scholarly.* **Description:** Publishes research in normal and dysfunctional aspects of cognitive development in adulthood and aging, integrating theory, method and research findings in the fields of cognitive gerontology and neuropsychology.
Formerly (until 1996): Aging and Cognition (0928-9917)
Related titles: Online - full text ed.: (from EBSCO Publishing, O C L C Online Computer Library Center, Inc., RoweCom Information Quest, Swets Blackwell, Institute for Scientific Information).
Indexed: ASCA, AgeLine, Curr.Cont., Excerp.Med. (1995-), Lang.& Lang.Behav.Abstr., PsycInfo, SOPODA, SSCI, Sociol.Abstr., e-psyche.
—BLDSC (0736.364400), ADONIS, CISTI, EMDOCS, IDS, ingenta. **CCC.**
Published by: Swets & Zeitlinger BV, PO Box 825, Lisse 2160 SZ, Netherlands. TEL 31-252-435111, FAX 31-252-415888, orders@swets.nl, http://www.swets.nl/sps/. Eds. David F Hultsch, Linas A Bieftuskas. R&P J van der Valk. Adv. contact Patrick Kliean. **Dist. in N. America by:** Swets & Zeitlinger, PO Box 582, Downingtown, PA 19335-998. TEL 800-477-9387, FAX 610-524-5366.

P

616.8 155.4 NLD ISSN 0929-7049
CODEN: CHNEFJ
NEUROPSYCHOLOGY, DEVELOPMENT, AND COGNITION. SECTION C: CHILD NEUROPSYCHOLOGY; a journal on normal and abnormal development in childhood and adolescence. Cover title: Child Neuropsychology. Text and summaries in English. 1995. q. NLG 190, USD 105 to individuals; NLG 520, USD 267 to institutions includes online ed; NLG 2,755, USD 1,413 to institutions includes sections A, B, D (effective 2001). adv. bk.rev. abstr. index. back issues avail. *Refereed.* **Document type:** *Journal, Academic/Scholarly.* **Description:** Publishes research on the neuropsychological dimension of development in childhood and adolescence, and promotes the integration of theories, methods and research findings in child and developmental neuropsychology.
Related titles: Microfilm ed.: (from SWZ); Online - full text ed.: (from EBSCO Publishing, O C L C Online Computer Library Center, Inc., RoweCom Information Quest, Swets Blackwell, Institute for Scientific Information).
Indexed: Excerp.Med. (1996-), Ind.Med., Lang.& Lang.Behav.Abstr., Neurosci.Cit.Ind., PsycInfo, SOPODA, Sociol.Abstr., e-psyche.
—BLDSC (3172.944795), ADONIS, CISTI, EMDOCS, IDS, Infotrieve. **CCC.**
Published by: Swets & Zeitlinger BV, PO Box 825, Lisse 2160 SZ, Netherlands. TEL 31-252-435111, FAX 31-252-415888, orders@swets.nl, http://www.swets.nl/sps/journals/child.html. Ed. Robert F Asarnow. R&P J van der Valk. Adv. contact Patrick Kliean. Circ: 750 (paid). **Dist. in N. America by:** Swets & Zeitlinger, PO Box 582, Downingtown, PA 19335-998. TEL 800-477-9387, FAX 610-524-5366.

616.8 NLD ISSN 1385-4046
CODEN: CLNEEC
NEUROPSYCHOLOGY, DEVELOPMENT AND COGNITION. SECTION D: THE CLINICAL NEUROPSYCHOLOGIST. Cover title: Clinical Neuropsychologist. Text in English. 1987. q. NLG 259, USD 144 to individuals; NLG 606, USD 310 to institutions includes online ed; NLG 2,755, USD 1,413 to institutions includes sections A, B, C (effective 2001). adv. Supplement avail.; back issues avail.; reprint service avail. from SWZ. *Refereed.* **Document type:** *Journal, Academic/Scholarly.* **Description:** Covers all matters relevant to the practicing clincical neuropsychologist.
Supersedes: Clinical Neuropsychologist (0920-1637)

Related titles: Online - full text ed.: (from EBSCO Publishing, O C L C Online Computer Library Center, Inc., RoweCom Information Quest, Swets Blackwell, Institute for Scientific Information).
Indexed: ASCA, AgeLine, Child Devel.Abstr., Curr.Cont., Except.Child Educ.Abstr., Excerp.Med., Ind.Med. (1987-), Lang.& Lang.Behav.Abstr., Neuropsych.Abstr., Neurosci.Cit.Ind., PsycInfo, Psychol.Abstr. (1987-), SOPODA, SSCI, Sociol.Abstr., e-psyche.
—BLDSC (3286.310680), ADONIS, CISTI, GNLM, IDS, Infotrieve, ingenta, KNAW. **CCC.**
Published by: Swets & Zeitlinger BV, PO Box 825, Lisse 2160 SZ, Netherlands. TEL 31-252-435111, FAX 31-252-415888, orders@swets.nl, http://www.swets.nl/sps/journals/tcn.html. Eds. Byron P Rourke, Kenneth M Adams. R&P J van der Valk. Adv. contact Patrick Kliean. Circ: 3,000. **Dist in N. America by:** Swets & Zeitlinger, PO Box 582, Downingtown, PA 19335-998. TEL 800-477-9387, FAX 610-524-5366.

NEUROPSYCHOLOGY REVIEW. see *MEDICAL SCIENCES—Psychiatry And Neurology*

NEW BABYLON: STUDIES IN THE SOCIAL SCIENCES. see *SOCIAL SCIENCES: COMPREHENSIVE WORKS*

210 USA
NEW CRUCIBLE; a magazine about man and his environment. Variant title: Crucible. Text in English. 1964. irreg. USD 24. adv. bk.rev. **Document type:** *Consumer.* **Description:** Deals with the total human environment including all ecological factors impacting upon man such as political, psychological, religious, and physical.
Incorporates: Naturalist (8756-3592); Former titles: Crucible and Scientific Atheist (8756-1247); Scientific Atheist
Indexed: Environ.Sci.Poll.Mgmt., e-psyche.
Published by: De Young Press, RR 1 Box 76, Stark, KS 66775-9802. Ed. Garry De Young. R&P Mary De Young. Adv. contact Gary De Young. Circ: 2,500.

155.4 USA ISSN 1520-3247
BF721 CODEN: NDCDDI
NEW DIRECTIONS FOR CHILD AND ADOLESCENT DEVELOPMENT. Text in English. 1978. q. USD 144 in United States; USD 184 in Canada; USD 218 elsewhere; USD 152 combined subscription in United States for print and online eds.; USD 192 combined subscription in Canada for print and online eds.; USD 226 combined subscription elsewhere for print and online eds. (effective 2002). bibl. Index. back issues avail.; reprint service avail. from PQC. **Document type:** *Journal, Academic/Scholarly.* **Description:** Covers the latest findings in developmental psychology; addresses children's cognitive, social, moral, and emotional growth.
Formerly (until 1998): New Directions for Child Development (0195-2269)
Related titles: Microfiche ed.: (from PQC); Online - full text ed.: ISSN 1534-8687. USD 144 in United States; USD 144 in Canada; USD 144 elsewhere (effective 2002) (from O C L C Online Computer Library Center, Inc.).
Indexed: Biol.Abstr., C.I.J.E., Child Devel.Abstr., Educ.Ind. (coverage dropped), Ind.Med. (1998-), Lang.& Lang.Behav.Abstr., Psychol.Abstr., SOPODA, Sociol.Abstr., e-psyche.
—BLDSC (6083.323000), GNLM, ingenta.
Published by: Jossey-Bass Inc., Publishers (Subsidiary of: John Wiley & Sons, Inc., Journals), 350 Sansome St, San Francisco, CA 94104-1342. TEL 415-433-1740, 888-378-2537, FAX 800-605-2665, 415-433-0499, jbsubs@jbp.com, http://www.josseybass.com. Ed. William Damon. Pub. Sue Lewis. Circ: 425.

158 USA
NEW HARVEST NEWSLETTER. Text in English. bi-m. free per issue. **Document type:** *Newsletter.* **Description:** Provides assistance with abuse recovery, stress management, chemical dependency, crisis intervention, communication skills, and trauma recovery.
Media: Online - full text.
Indexed: e-psyche.
Published by: Personal Development Center Associates, 6345 Balboa Blvd, Ste 212, Encino, CA 91316. TEL 818-503-2144, FAX 818-776-0312, pdca@pdcaonline.com, http://www.pdcaonline.com/. Ed. Karen Kenney.

150 GBR ISSN 0732-118X
BF1
NEW IDEAS IN PSYCHOLOGY; international journal of innovative theory in psychology. Text in English. 1983. 3/yr. EUR 138 in Europe to qualified personnel; JPY 18,400 in Japan to qualified personnel; USD 155 elsewhere to qualified personnel; EUR 471 in Europe to institutions; JPY 62,500 in Japan to institutions; USD 526 elsewhere to institutions (effective 2002). adv. back issues avail. *Refereed.* **Document type:** *Academic/Scholarly.* **Description:** Acts as a forum for theorizers striving to integrate the fragmented ideas and theories currently found in theoretical psychology.
Related titles: Microfilm ed.: (from PQC); Online - full text ed.: (from ingenta, ScienceDirect, Swets Blackwell, Institute for Scientific Information).
Indexed: ASCA, Arts & Hum.Cit.Ind. (coverage dropped), Curr.Adv.Ecol.Sci., Curr.Cont., P C I, PsycInfo, Psychol.Abstr. (1983-), Russ.Acad.Sci.Bibl., SSCI, e-psyche.
—BLDSC (6084.249500), IDS, Infotrieve, ingenta. **CCC.**
Published by: Pergamon (Subsidiary of: Elsevier Science), The Boulevard, Langford Ln, East Park, Kidlington, Oxford OXB 1GB, United Kingdom. FAX 44-1865-843010, nlinfo-f@elsevier.nl; usinfo-f@elsevier.com; forinfo-kyf04053@niftyserve.or.jp, http://www.elsevier.com/locate/newideapsych. Ed. Richard Kitchener. adv.: B&W page USD 550, color page USD 1,350. **Subscr. in Australasia and the Far East to:** Elsevier Science (Singapore) Pte Ltd, No.1 Temasek Ave, 17-01 Millenia Tower, Singapore 039192, Singapore. TEL 65-434-3727, FAX 65-337-2230; **Subscr. in the Americas to:** Elsevier Science, PO Box 945, New York, NY 10159-0945. TEL 212-633-3730, FAX 212-633-3680; **Subscr. to:** Elsevier Science BV, PO Box 211, Amsterdam 1000 AE, Netherlands. TEL 31-20-485-3757, FAX 31-20-485-3432.

150 USA ISSN 0077-9008
BF173.A2
NEW YORK PSYCHOANALYTIC INSTITUTE. KRIS STUDY GROUP. MONOGRAPHS. Text in English. 1965. irreg., latest vol.7, 1984. price varies. *Refereed.* **Document type:** *Monographic series.*
Indexed: Biol.Abstr., e-psyche.
Published by: (New York Psychoanalytic Institute, Kris Study Group), International Universities Press, Inc., 59 Boston Post Rd, Box 1524, Madison, CT 06443-1524. TEL 203-245-4000, FAX 203-245-0775, http://www.iup.com. Ed. Dr. Edward Joseph.

150 USA ISSN 0028-7687
NEW YORK STATE PSYCHOLOGIST✶. Text in English. 1948. m. USD 20. adv. bk.rev. charts, illus, stat, tr.lit. back issues avail.
Indexed: Psychol.Abstr., e-psyche.
Published by: Foundation of New York State Psychological Association, Inc., Executive Park E, Albany, NY 12203. TEL 212-787-6487, FAX 914-683-5223. Ed. Laurence S Baker. Circ: 4,000.

150 NZL ISSN 0112-109X
CODEN: NZJPF7
NEW ZEALAND JOURNAL OF PSYCHOLOGY. Text in English. 1972. s-a. (Jun. & Dec.). NZD 40 (effective 2001). adv. bk.rev. 48 p./no. back issues avail. *Refereed.* **Document type:** *Journal, Academic/Scholarly.*
Formerly (until 1983): New Zealand Psychologist
Related titles: Online - full text ed.: (from Northern Light Technology, Inc., ProQuest Information & Learning, Gale Group, Institute for Scientific Information).
Indexed: ASCA, AgeLine, Curr.Cont., Fam.Ind., Ind.N.Z.Per., Lang.& Lang.Behav.Abstr., PsycInfo, Psychol.Abstr. (1972-), Risk Abstr., SOPODA, SSCI, Soc.Serv.Abstr., Sociol.Abstr., e-psyche.
—BLDSC (6094.655000), IDS, Infotrieve. **CCC.**
Published by: New Zealand Psychological Society, c/o Business Manager, PO Box 4092, Wellington, New Zealand. TEL 64-4-8015414, FAX 64-4-8015366, office@psychology.org.nz, linden@psychology.org.nz. Ed. Michael P O'Driscoll TEL 64-7-8562889. R&P, Adv. contact Linden Williams. B&W page NZD 200; trim 265 x 175. Circ: 700 (controlled).

362.28 USA
NEWSLINK (WASHINGTON). Text in English. q. membership. **Description:** Provides suicide prevention information.
Indexed: e-psyche.
Published by: American Association of Suicidology, 4201 Connecticut Ave, Ste 408, Washington, DC 20008-1158. TEL 202-237-2280. Circ: 1,500.

616.89 JPN
NIHON KODO RYOHO GAKKAI NYUZU RETA/JAPANESE ASSOCIATION OF BEHAVIOR THERAPY. NEWSLETTER. Text in Japanese. s-a. **Document type:** *Newsletter.*
Indexed: e-psyche.
Published by: Nihon Kodo Ryoho Gakkai/Japanese Association of Behavior Therapy, c/o Masahiko Sugiyama Sec-Gen, Institute of Special Education, University of Tsukuba, 1-1-1 Tenno-Dai, Tsukuba-shi, Ibaraki-ken 305-0006, Japan. TEL 81-298-53-6719, FAX 81-298-53-6719.

NINTH STREET CENTER JOURNAL. see *HOMOSEXUALITY*

616.89 617 JPN ISSN 0917-950X
NO SHINKEI GEKA JANARU/JAPANESE JOURNAL OF NEUROSURGERY. Text in Japanese; Summaries in English, Japanese. 1992. q. JPY 2,039 (effective 1999). adv. **Document type:** *Academic/Scholarly.*
Indexed: Excerp.Med. (1994-), INIS Atomind., e-psyche.
—BLDSC (4656.643000), EMDOCS, GNLM.
Published by: Nihon No Shinkei Geka Konguresu/Japanese Congress of Neurological Surgeons, 2-1-1 Hongo, Bunkyo-ku, Tokyo 113-0033, Japan. Ed. Masao Matsutani. Pub., Adv. contact Miwa Shoten.

THE NOETIC JOURNAL; an international forum on the cosmology of consciousness. see *PHYSICS*

153 AUS ISSN 1324-6038
NOETICA; a cognitive science forum. Text in English. 1995. irreg.
Media: Online - full text.
Published by: (Australian Cognitive Science Society), University of Queensland, School of Psychology, Brisbane, QLD 4072, Australia. TEL 61-7-3365-6230, noetica@psy.uq.edu.au, http://www2.psy.uq.edu.au/CogPsych/Noetica/. Ed. Simon Dennis.

003.75 300 USA ISSN 1090-0578
BF1 CODEN: NDPSFS
NONLINEAR DYNAMICS, PSYCHOLOGY, AND LIFE SCIENCES. Text in English. 1997. q. EUR 185 to institutions for print or online ed.; EUR 222 to institutions print & online eds.combined (effective 2002). adv. bk.rev. *Refereed.* **Document type:** *Academic/Scholarly.* **Description:** Publishes applications of nonlinear dynamics research to problems in the psychological, life and social sciences.
Related titles: Online - full text ed.: (from EBSCO Publishing, O C L C Online Computer Library Center, Inc., RoweCom Information Quest, Swets Blackwell, Kluwer Online).
Indexed: PsycInfo, e-psyche.
—BLDSC (6117.316720), ingenta.
Published by: (Society for Chaos Theory in Psychology & Life Sciences), Kluwer Academic - Plenum Publishers (Subsidiary of: Wolters Kluwer N.V.), 233 Spring St, New York, NY 10013-1578. TEL 212-620-8000, 800-221-9369, FAX 212-463-0742, info@plenum.com; kluwer@wkap.com; services@wkap.nl, http://www.plenum.com. Ed. Stephen J Guastello.

150 DNK ISSN 0029-1463
BF8.D3 CODEN: NOPSAW
NORDISK PSYKOLOGI. Text mainly in Danish, Norwegian, Swedish; Text occasionally in English; Summaries in English. 1949. q. DKK 600 in the European Union; DKK 160 per issue in the European Union; DKK 480 elsewhere; DKK 128 per issue elsewhere (effective 2002). adv. bk.rev. bibl, charts, illus, stat. index. 80 p./no. back issues avail. *Refereed.* **Document type:** *Journal, Academic/Scholarly.*
Related titles: Online - full text ed.: (from Institute for Scientific Information).
Indexed: ASCA, Biol.Abstr., Chem.Abstr., Lang.& Lang.Behav.Abstr., PsycInfo, Psychol.Abstr. (1949-), Russ.Acad.Sci.Bibl., SOPODA, SSCI, Soc.Serv.Abstr., Sociol.Abstr., e-psyche.
—IDS. **CCC.**
Published by: Dansk Psykologisk Forlag/Danish Psychological Publishers, Stockholmsgade 29, Copenhagen Oe 2100, Denmark. TEL 45-35-38-16-55, FAX 45-35-38-16-65, dk-psych@dpf.dk. Ed. Peter Elsass. Circ: 1,500.

NORDISK TIDSSKRIFT FOR SPESIALPEDAGOGIKK. see *EDUCATION—Special Education And Rehabilitation*

158 370.15 306.43 USA ISSN 1527-7143
▼ **NORTH AMERICAN JOURNAL OF PSYCHOLOGY.** Text in English. 1999. 3/yr. USD 30 domestic to individuals; USD 37 in Canada to individuals; USD 38 elsewhere to individuals; USD 65 domestic to institutions; USD 73 foreign to institutions (effective 2001). bk.rev. abstr. back issues avail. *Refereed.* **Document type:** *Journal, Academic/Scholarly.* **Description:** Publishes original studies in a wide variety of areas of psychology, as well as education and sociology. Includes interviews with renowned psychologists and reviews, with an editorial bias favoring topics of broad concern to social scientists.
Address: 240 Harbor Dr, Winter Garden, FL 34787. TEL 407-877-8364, FAX 407-877-8364, najp@mpinet.net, http://najp.8m.com. Ed., Pub., R&P Dr. Lynn McCutcheon. Circ: 200 (paid); 300 (controlled).

150.1953 USA ISSN 0889-9428
NORTH AMERICAN SOCIETY OF ADLERIAN PSYCHOLOGY. NEWSLETTER. Text in English. 1967. bi-m. USD 20 to non-members (effective 2000). bk.rev. **Document type:** *Newsletter.* **Description:** Contains information on news and activities of the Society. Covers recent conventions in the field.
Indexed: e-psyche.
Published by: North American Society of Adlerian Psychology, 65 E Wacker Pl, Ste 1710, Chicago, IL 60601-7298. TEL 312-629-8801, FAX 312-629-8859, nasap@msn.com, http://www.alfredadler.com. Ed., R&P Jerianne Garber. Circ: 1,000.

NUTRITION HEALTH REVIEW; The Consumer's Medical Journal. see *NUTRITION AND DIETETICS*

150 USA
O P A NEWSGRAM. Text in English. 1959. 10/yr. USD 35 to non-members (effective 2000). adv. bk.rev. **Document type:** *Newsletter.*
Former titles: Oregon Psychology; Oregon Psychological Association. Newsletter (0471-9336)
Indexed: e-psyche.
Published by: Oregon Psychological Association, 147 S E 102nd Ave, Portland, OR 97216-2703. Ed. Rodger Bufford. Adv. contact Rod Harriman. Circ: 700 (controlled).

ODENSE UNIVERSITY STUDIES IN PSYCHIATRY AND MEDICAL PSYCHOLOGY. see *MEDICAL SCIENCES—Psychiatry And Neurology*

OKEE. see *MEDICAL SCIENCES—Psychiatry And Neurology*

614.58 USA
OKLAHOMA. DEPARTMENT OF MENTAL HEALTH AND SUBSTANCE ABUSE SERVICES. ANNUAL REPORT. Text in English. a. free per issue. **Document type:** *Government.*
Former titles: Oklahoma. Department of Mental Health. Annual Report; Mental Health Care in Oklahoma. Annual Report
Indexed: e-psyche.
Published by: Department of Mental Health, Biometrics Division, P O Box 53277, Oklahoma City, OK 73105. TEL 405-522-3908, FAX 405-522-3650. Ed. Rosemary Brown. Circ: 1,000.

155.937 USA ISSN 0030-2228
BF789.D4 CODEN: OMGABX
OMEGA: JOURNAL OF DEATH AND DYING. Text in English. 1969. 8/yr. (in 2 vols., 4 nos./vol.). USD 76 to individuals; USD 298 to institutions (effective 2001). adv. bk.rev. abstr, bibl, charts, illus. back issues avail.; reprints avail. *Refereed.* **Document type:** *Journal, Academic/Scholarly.* **Description:** Guide for clinicians, social workers, and health professionals dealing with problems in crisis management, such as terminal illness, fatal accidents, catastrophes, suicide and bereavement.
Related titles: Online - full text ed.: (from Gale Group, Factiva, Institute for Scientific Information).
Indexed: AMED, ASCA, ASSIA, Abstr.Anthropol., Abstr.Soc.Geront., AgeLine, Arts & Hum.Cit.Ind. (coverage dropped), Biol.Abstr., C.I.J.E. (coverage dropped), CINAHL, Compumath, Crim.Just.Abstr., Curr.Cont., Excerp.Med. (until 1992), IBR, IBZ, Ind.Philos., Lang.& Lang.Behav.Abstr., P C I, PsycInfo, Psychol.Abstr. (1970-), Ref.Zh., Rel.Ind.One, Rel.Ind.Two, SOPODA, SSCI, Soc.Sci.Ind. (Jan.1982-), Soc.Serv.Abstr., Sociol.Abstr., e-psyche.
—BLDSC (6256.425000), GNLM, IDS, ingenta. **CCC.**
Published by: Baywood Publishing Co., Inc., 26 Austin Ave, Box 337, Amityville, NY 11701. TEL 631-691-1270, FAX 631-691-1770, info@baywood.com, baywood@baywood.com, http://baywood.com/search/PreviewJournal.asp?qsRecord=22, http://www.baywood.com. Ed. Kenneth Doka. R&P Julie Krempa. Adv. contact Joi Tamber-Brooks.

ON COURSE; inspiration for the inner journey. see *NEW AGE PUBLICATIONS*

▼ **ON FERTILE GROUND.** see *MEDICAL SCIENCES—Obstetrics And Gynecology*

150 CAN ISSN 0030-3054
RC467
ONTARIO PSYCHOLOGIST. Text in English. 1969. q. CND 60. bk.rev. bibl, charts, illus, stat. reprint service avail. from PQC. **Document type:** *Newsletter.*
Related titles: Microfiche ed.: (from MML); Microform ed.: (from PQC,MML).
Indexed: Psychol.Abstr., e-psyche.
—Infotrieve. **CCC.**
Published by: Ontario Psychological Association, 730 Yonge St, Ste 221, Toronto, ON M4Y 2B7, Canada. TEL 416-961-5552, FAX 416-961-5516, ont@hookup.net. Ed. Dr. D Rudzinski. R&P Ruth Berman. adv.: B&W page USD 750; trim 9.94 x 7.5. Circ: 1,400.

ORGANISATIONSBERATUNG, SUPERVISION, COACHING. see *BUSINESS AND ECONOMICS—Personnel Management*

150 USA
ORGANIZATIONAL AND OCCUPATIONAL PSYCHOLOGY. Text in English. 1979. irreg., latest vol.18, 1987. reprint service avail. from ISI. **Document type:** *Monographic series.*
Indexed: e-psyche.
Published by: Academic Press, Inc., Journal Division (Subsidiary of: Harcourt Brace & Company), 525 B St, Ste 1900, San Diego, CA 92101-4495. TEL 619-231-0926, FAX 619-699-6715. Ed. P Warr. **Subscr. to:** Order Dept., 6277 Sea Harbor Dr, 4th Fl, Orlando, FL 32887. TEL 800-321-5068.

ORGANIZATIONAL BEHAVIOR AND HUMAN DECISION PROCESSES; a journal of fundamental research and theory in applied psychology. see *BUSINESS AND ECONOMICS—Management*

158.3 FRA ISSN 0249-6739
ORIENTATION SCOLAIRE ET PROFESSIONNELLE. Text in French. 1972. q. FRF 280 domestic; FRF 350 foreign (effective 2000). adv. bk.rev. abstr, bibl, charts, stat. index. back issues avail. *Refereed.* **Document type:** *Academic/Scholarly.*
Formerly (until 1972): B I N O P Bulletin (0005-3147)
Indexed: PsycInfo, Psychol.Abstr. (1972-), Ref.Zh., Russ.Acad.Sci.Bibl., e-psyche.
—BLDSC (6291.213000).
Published by: Institut National d'Etude du Travail et d'Orientation Professionnelle, 41 rue Gay Lussac, Paris 75005, France. TEL 33-1-44107877, FAX 33-1-44107911, peylet@cnam.fr. Ed. Serge Blanchard. Pub. Jean Guichard. Adv. contact Renee Delblond. Circ: 2,000. **Co-sponsor:** Institut National des Arts et Metiers.

OUR GIFTED CHILDREN. see *CHILDREN AND YOUTH—About*

150 USA
P S C P TIMES✶. Text in English. 1971. irreg. (6-8/yr.). USD 5.
Indexed: e-psyche.
Published by: Philadelphia Society of Clinical Psychologists, Cedarbrook Hill Apts, E Mall Bld 1, Wyncote, PA 19095-2601. Eds. Frank A Melone, Lita L Schwartz. Circ: 200.

155.3 NLD ISSN 0167-4749
PAEDO ALERT NEWS MAGAZINE. Short title: P A N Magazine. Text in Dutch. 1979. 5/yr. NLG 40, USD 20. adv. bk.rev. illus.
Indexed: e-psyche.
Published by: Spartacus International Ltd., Postbus 3496, Amsterdam 1001 AG, Netherlands. Ed. Roger Hunt. Circ: 4,000.

PAIDIKA; the journal of paedophilia. see *SOCIOLOGY*

150 PAK ISSN 1019-438X
PAKISTAN JOURNAL OF CLINICAL PSYCHOLOGY; clinical psychology. Text in English. 1992. s-a. PKR 150, USD 34 (effective 2001). back issues avail. *Refereed.* **Document type:** *Academic/Scholarly.* **Description:** Publishes experimental, clinical and theoretical articles, social surveys, comments and special reviews of clinical issues in psychology.
Related titles: CD-ROM ed.
Indexed: ExtraMED, e-psyche.
Published by: University of Karachi, Institute of Clinical Psychology, Gulistan-e-Jauhar, 118, Block 20 Abul Asar Hafeez Jalindhri Rd, Karachi 75290, Pakistan. TEL 92-021-8113584, PJPICP@hotline.com, pjpicp@hotline.com. Ed. Farrukh Z Ahmad. Circ: 500.

150 PAK ISSN 0030-9869
BF1
PAKISTAN JOURNAL OF PSYCHOLOGY; psychology. Text in English. 1965-1976 (Dec.); resumed 1979. 2/yr. USD 34, PKR 150 (effective 2001). adv. bk.rev. charts. back issues avail. *Refereed.* **Document type:** *Journal, Academic/Scholarly.* **Description:** Publishes theoretical and research articles covering a wide range of issues in psychology.
Related titles: CD-ROM ed.
Indexed: Bibl.Asian Stud. (1975-1990), ExtraMED, Psychol.Abstr., e-psyche.
Published by: University of Karachi, Institute of Clinical Psychology, Gulistan-e-Jauhar, 118, Block 20 Abul Asar Hafeez Jalindhri Rd, Karachi 75290, Pakistan. TEL 92-021-8113584, pjpicp@hotline.com, icpuok@usa.net. Ed., R&P Farrukh Z Ahmad. Circ: 500.

PALLIATIVE CARE INDEX. see *MEDICAL SCIENCES—Abstracting, Bibliographies, Statistics*

PALO ALTO REVIEW; journal of ideas. see *EDUCATION*

158 615.89 USA
THE PANIC RELIEF NEWS. Text in English. 1994. irreg. (approx. 4/yr.). USD 12; USD 16 foreign (effective 1996). adv. illus. **Document type:** *Newsletter.* **Description:** Informs persons suffering from panic disorders and offers support from a holistic health perspective, often from personal experience. Seeks to inspire people to take control of their lives and regain or improve self-esteem.
Indexed: e-psyche.
Published by: Panic Relief, Inc., 981 Shephard Ave, North Brunswick, NJ 08902-2252. TEL 908-937-4832, slepian@eclipse.net. Ed., Pub. Don Slepian.

150 ESP ISSN 0214-7823
PAPELES DEL PSICOLOGO. Text in Spanish. 198?. bi-m. *Refereed.* **Document type:** *Academic/Scholarly.*
Formerly (until 1989): Colegio Oficial de Psicologos. Delegacion de Madrid. Papeles del Colegio (0211-7851)
Indexed: e-psyche.
—CINDOC.
Published by: Colegio Oficial de Psicologos. Espana, Secretaria Estatal, Claudio Coello, 46, 2o Dcha., Madrid 28001, Spain. TEL 34-91-435-5212, FAX 34-91-577-9172, secop@correo.cop.es, http://www.cop.es/publicaciones/papeles/. Pub. Juan Carlos Duro Martinez.

150 200 USA ISSN 0031-2789
BV4012
PASTORAL PSYCHOLOGY. Text in English. 1952. bi-m. EUR 566 to institutions for print or online ed.; EUR 679.20 to institutions print & online eds.combined (effective 2002). adv. bk.rev., film rev. reprint service avail. from PQC,PSC,SCH,ISI. *Refereed.* **Document type:** *Academic/Scholarly.* **Description:** Examines pastoral counseling, and brings psychological and behavioral science into relation and dialogue with the work of the ministry.
Related titles: Microfilm ed.: (from PQC); Online - full text ed.: (from O C L C Online Computer Library Center, Inc., Swets Blackwell, Kluwer Online, RoweCom Information Quest).
Indexed: CCR, G.Soc.Sci.& Rel.Per.Lit., IBR, IBZ, Ind.Philos., PsycInfo, Psychol.Abstr. (1982-), Rel.& Theol.Abstr. (1969-), Rel.Ind.One, Rel.Ind.Two, e-psyche.
—BLDSC (6409.300000), ingenta. **CCC.**
Published by: (Princeton Theological Seminary), Kluwer Academic - Plenum Publishers (Subsidiary of: Wolters Kluwer N.V.), 233 Spring St, New York, NY 10013-1578. TEL 212-620-8000, 800-221-9369, FAX 212-463-0742, info@plenum.com; kluwer@wkap.com; services@wkap.nl, http://www.plenum.com. Ed. Lewis R Rambo.

P

301.1 USA
PATHWAYS (BETHESDA); DC resources. Text in English. 1978. 4/yr. USD 10. adv. bk.rev.
Published by: Pathways, 4931 St. Elmo Ave, Bethesda, MD 20814. TEL 301-656-3127, FAX 301-656-3023, pathwaysmag@earthlink.net, http://www.pathwaysmag.com. Ed. Lou de Sabla. Circ: 40,000.

150 USA ISSN 1078-1919
JX1901
PEACE AND CONFLICT; journal of peace psychology. Text in English. 1995. q. USD 40 in US & Canada to individuals; USD 70 elsewhere to individuals; USD 275 in US & Canada to institutions; USD 305 elsewhere to institutions (effective 2002). adv. bk.rev. illus. Index. reprints avail. *Refereed.* **Document type:** *Journal, Academic/Scholarly.* **Description:** Reflects the essential reality of human consciousness and social and societal relations.
Related titles: Online - full text ed.: ISSN 1532-7949. USD 36 to individuals; USD 247.50 to institutions (effective 2002) (from CatchWord Ltd., EBSCO Publishing, O C L C Online Computer Library Center, Inc., RoweCom Information Quest, Swets Blackwell).
Indexed: Environ.Sci.Poll.Mgmt., Int.Polit.Sci.Abstr., Intl.Bibl.Soc.Sci., P.A.I.S., Peace Res.Abstr., PsycInfo, e-psyche.
—BLDSC (6413.759000), CatchWord. **CCC.**
Published by: (Division of Peace Psychology, American Psychological Association), Lawrence Erlbaum Associates, Inc., 10 Industrial Ave, Mahwah, NJ 07430-2262. TEL 201-760-3735, 800-926-6579, FAX 201-236-0072, journals@erlbaum.com, http://www.erlbaum.com/Journals/journals/PAC/pac.htm. Ed. Richard Wagner. adv.: page USD 300; trim 5 x 8.

P

370.5 155.4 SWE ISSN 0346-5004
PEDAGOGISK-PSYKOLOGISKA PROBLEM. Text in Swedish. 1964. irreg. back issues avail. **Document type:** *Journal, Academic/Scholarly.*
Indexed: Psychol.Abstr., e-psyche.
Published by: Malmoe University, Department of Education, Fack 23501, Malmo 20045, Sweden. FAX 46-40-325-210.

PEER COUNSELLOR JOURNAL. see *SOCIAL SERVICES AND WELFARE*

150 613.7 USA ISSN 1070-6674
PELIZZA'S POSITIVE PRINCIPLES FOR BETTER LIVING. Text in English. 1993. q. USD 29.95 for 3 yrs. (effective 2001). adv. bk.rev. **Document type:** *Newsletter.* **Description:** Provides information and tips to maximize personal and professional productivity.
Indexed: e-psyche.
Published by: Pelizza & Associates, PO Box 225, North Chatham, NY 12132. TEL 518-766-4849, FAX 518-766-4849, john@pelizza.com, http://www.pelizza.com. Ed. Phillip Niles. Pub. John Pelizza. R&P, Adv. contact Bonnie Pelizza. Circ: 3,000 (paid).

150 617.7 GBR ISSN 0301-0066
BF311 CODEN: PCTNBA
PERCEPTION. Text in English. 1972. m., latest vol.30, no.12, 2001. USD 697; USD 69 newsstand/cover (effective 2001). adv. bk.rev. index. back issues avail.; reprints avail. *Refereed.* **Document type:** *Journal, Academic/Scholarly.* **Description:** Reports experimental results and theoretical ideas in the fields of animal, human and machine perception, and artificial intelligence.
Related titles: CD-ROM ed.; Online - full text ed.: (from Institute for Scientific Information).
Indexed: ASSIA, Abstr.Hum.Comp.Inter., Arts & Hum.Cit.Ind. (coverage dropped), Can.Per.Ind. (Jan.1988-), Commun.Abstr., Curr.Cont., Dent.Ind., Excerp.Med., Ind.Med. (1972-), Ind.Philos., Mid.East: Abstr.& Ind., Neurosci.Cit.Ind., P C I, Photo.Abstr., PsycInfo, Psychol.Abstr. (1972-), SSCI, e-psyche.
—BLDSC (6423.150000), CISTI, GNLM, ingenta.
Published by: Pion Ltd., 207 Brondesbury Park, London NW2 5JN, United Kingdom. TEL 44-20-8459-0066, FAX 44-20-8451-6454, sales@pion.co.uk, http:www.perceptionweb.com, http://www.pion.co.uk/perception, http://www.perceptionweb.com. Ed. R L Gregory. Pub. Adam Gelbtuch. R&P, Adv. contact Diana Harrop TEL 44-20-8459-0069. page USD 280; trim 132 x 230.

152 USA ISSN 0191-2518
PERCEPTION AND PERCEPTUAL DEVELOPMENT. Text in English. 1978. irreg. **Document type:** *Monographic series.*
Indexed: e-psyche.
Published by: Kluwer Academic - Plenum Publishers (Subsidiary of: Wolters Kluwer N.V.), 233 Spring St, New York, NY 10013-1578. TEL 212-620-8000, 800-221-9369, FAX 212-463-0742, info@plenum.com, http://www.plenum.com.

152 USA ISSN 0031-5117
BF233 CODEN: PEPSBJ
PERCEPTION & PSYCHOPHYSICS. Text in English. 1966. 8/yr. USD 216 domestic; USD 232 foreign (effective 2001). adv. charts, illus. index. back issues avail.; reprint service avail. from PQC,PSC,SCH. *Refereed.* **Document type:** *Academic/Scholarly.* **Description:** Contains articles that deal with sensory processes, perception and psychophysics. Some theoretical and evaluative reviews are published.
Related titles: Microform ed.: (from NRP,PQC); Online - full text ed.: (from CatchWord Ltd., Institute for Scientific Information).
Indexed: ASCA, AgeLine, Arts & Hum.Cit.Ind. (coverage dropped), Biol.Abstr., Commun.Abstr., Compumath, Curr.Adv.Ecol.Sci., Curr.Cont., Curr.Ind.Stat., Dent.Ind., Ergon.Abstr., Excerp.Med., IBR, Ind.Med. (1966-), Ind.Philos., Int.Aerosp.Abstr., Lang.& Lang.Behav.Abstr., M.L.A., MLA Intl.Bibl., Neurosci.Cit.Ind., PsycInfo, Psychol.Abstr. (1966-), RILM, SOPODA, SSCI, Sci.Cit.Ind. (coverage dropped), Sociol.Abstr., Sp.Ed.Needs Abstr., e-psyche.
—BLDSC (6423.200000), CISTI, GNLM, IDS, ingenta. **CCC.**
Published by: Psychonomic Society, Inc., 1710 Fortview Rd, Austin, TX 78704. TEL 512-462-2442, FAX 512-462-1101, jbellquist@psychonomic.org, http://www.sig.net/~psysoc/home.htm, http://www.psychonomic.org. Ed. Neil Macmillan. R&P Cinnamon Nemec. Adv. contact Robert Sanford. page USD 145; trim 10.75 x 8. Circ: 1,800.

152 USA ISSN 0031-5125
BF311 CODEN: PMOSAZ
PERCEPTUAL AND MOTOR SKILLS. Text in English. 1949. bi-m., latest 2001, Jun. (2 vols./yr.). USD 320 (effective 2001). bk.rev. bibl, charts, illus, abstr, stat. index. 352 p./no. back issues avail.; reprint service avail. from PSC,SCH. *Refereed.* **Document type:** *Journal, Academic/Scholarly.* **Description:** Encourages scientific originality and creativity. Includes experimental or theoretical articles dealing with perception or motor skills, especially as affected by experience.
Related titles: Microform ed.; Online - full text ed.: (from Factiva, Institute for Scientific Information).
Indexed: AMED, ASCA, Abstr.Anthropol., AgeLine, Arts & Hum.Cit.Ind. (coverage dropped), Bibl.Dev.Med.& Child Neur., Biol.Abstr., C.I.J.E. (coverage dropped), CINAHL, Chic.Per.Ind., Child Devel.Abstr., Commun.Abstr., Curr.Cont., Curr.Ind.Stat., DSH Abstr., Dent.Ind., Ergon.Abstr., Except.Child Educ.Abstr., Excerp.Med., Fam.Ind., HRIS, High.Educ.Abstr., IBZ, INIS Atomind., Ind.Med. (1955-), Ind.Philos., Indian Psychol.Abstr., Int.Nurs.Ind., Lang.& Lang.Behav.Abstr., M.L.A., MLA Intl.Bibl., Neurosci.Cit.Ind., Nutr.Abstr., Phys.Ed.Ind., PsycInfo, Psychol.Abstr. (1952-), RILM, Risk Abstr., Russ.Acad.Sci.Bibl., SOPODA, SSCI, Sci.Cit.Ind. (coverage dropped), Soc.Sci.Ind. (Aug.1982-), Sociol.Abstr., Sp.Ed.Needs Abstr., Sportsearch (1974-), Stud.Wom.Abstr.
—BLDSC (6423.300000), GNLM, ingenta, Linda Hall.
Published by: Dr. C.H. Ammons, Ed. & Pub., PO Box 9229, Missoula, MT 59807. TEL 406-728-1710. R&P C H Ammons TEL 406-728-1702. Circ: 2,000.
Co-publisher: Behavioral Engineering Assoc.

150 GBR ISSN 0191-8869
BF698.A1 CODEN: PEIDD9
PERSONALITY AND INDIVIDUAL DIFFERENCES; an international journal of research into the structure and development of personality and the causation of individual differences. Text in English. 1980. 16/yr. EUR 1,576 in Europe to institutions; JPY 209,200 in Japan to institutions; USD 1,763 elsewhere to institutions (effective 2002). adv. back issues avail.; reprints avail. *Refereed.* **Document type:** *Academic/Scholarly.* **Description:** Publishes experimental, theoretical and review articles that aim to integrate the major factors of personality with empirical paradigms from experimental, physiological, animal, clinical, educational, criminological or industrial psychology.
Related titles: Microform ed.: (from PQC,PMC); Online - full text ed.: (from ingenta, ScienceDirect, Swets Blackwell, Institute for Scientific Information).
Indexed: ASCA, ASSIA, Addic.Abstr., AgeLine, Amer.Bibl.Slavic & E.Eur.Stud., Arts & Hum.Cit.Ind. (coverage dropped), Biol.Abstr., Br.Educ.Ind., Crim.Just.Abstr., Curr.Cont., Fam.Ind., Indian Psychol.Abstr., Neurosci.Cit.Ind., PSI, PsycInfo, Psychol.Abstr., Russ.Acad.Sci.Bibl., SSCI, e-psyche.
—BLDSC (6428.010500), GNLM, IDS, ingenta. **CCC.**
Published by: (International Society for the Study of Individual Differences), Pergamon (Subsidiary of: Elsevier Science), The Boulevard, Langford Ln, East Park, Kidlington, Oxford OXB 1GB, United Kingdom. FAX 44-1865-843010, http://www.elsevier.com/locate/paid. Eds. G H Gudjonsson, H J Eysenck. Circ: 1,500. **Subscr. in Australasia and the Far East to:** Elsevier Science (Singapore) Pte Ltd, No.1 Temasek Ave, 17-01 Millenia Tower, Singapore 039192, Singapore. TEL 65-434-3727, FAX 65-337-2230; **Subscr. in the Americas to:** Elsevier Science, PO Box 945, New York, NY 10159-0945. TEL 212-633-3730, FAX 212-633-3680; **Subscr. to:** Elsevier Science BV, PO Box 211, Amsterdam 1000 AE, Netherlands. TEL 31-20-485-3757, FAX 31-20-485-3432.

150 USA
PERSONALITY AND PSYCHOPATHOLOGY. Text in English. irreg. **Document type:** *Monographic series.*
Indexed: e-psyche.
Published by: Guilford Publications, Inc., 72 Spring St, New York, NY 10012. TEL 212-431-9800, 800-365-7006, FAX 212-966-6708, info@guilford.com, http://www.guilford.com. Eds. Theodore Millon, W John Livesley.

150 USA ISSN 0146-1672
BF698.A1
PERSONALITY AND SOCIAL PSYCHOLOGY BULLETIN. Text in English. 1975. m. USD 150 to individuals; USD 735 to institutions; USD 20 newsstand/cover to individuals; USD 70 newsstand/cover to institutions (effective 2002). adv. illus. back issues avail.; reprint service avail. from PQC,PSC,SCH. *Refereed.* **Document type:** *Bulletin.* **Description:** Publishes theoretical articles and empirical reports of research in all areas of personality and social psychology.
Formerly: American Psychological Association. Division of Personality and Social Psychology. Proceedings
Related titles: Microform ed.: (from PQC); Online - full text ed.: (from ProQuest Information & Learning, Gale Group, ingenta, Institute for Scientific Information, RoweCom Information Quest).
Indexed: ASCA, ASSIA, Adol.Ment.Hlth.Abstr., AgeLine, C.I.J.E. (coverage dropped), Commun.Abstr., Curr.Cont., Curr.Ind.Stat., ERA, Environ.Sci.Poll.Mgmt., Fam.Ind., IBZ, IMFL, Ind.Philos., Mult.Ed.Abstr., PSI, PsycInfo, Psychol.Abstr. (1974-), Risk Abstr., Russ.Acad.Sci.Bibl., SSCI, Saf.Sci.Abstr., Sage Fam.Stud.Abstr., Sage Race Rel.Abstr., Sage Urb.Stud.Abstr., Soc.Sci.Ind. (Sep.1982-), Soc.Serv.Abstr., Sociol.Abstr., Stud.Wom.Abstr., Viol.& Abuse Abstr., e-psyche.
—BLDSC (6428.011500), IDS, ingenta. **CCC.**
Published by: (Society for Personality and Social Psychology), Sage Publications, Inc., 2455 Teller Rd, Thousand Oaks, CA 91320. TEL 805-499-0721, FAX 805-499-0871, info@sagepub.com, http://www.sagepub.com. Ed. Jerry Suls. Pub. Sara Miller McCune. R&P Tanya Udin. Adv. contact DeAnna Vega Hammersley. Circ: 4,200. **Overseas subscr. to:** Sage Publications Ltd., 6 Bonhill St, London EC2A 4PU, United Kingdom; Sage Publications India Pvt. Ltd., 4215, New Delhi 110 048, India.

155.28 302 USA ISSN 1088-8683
BF698.A1 CODEN: PSPRFG
PERSONALITY AND SOCIAL PSYCHOLOGY REVIEW. Text in English. 1997. q. USD 55 in US & Canada to individuals; USD 85 elsewhere to individuals; USD 285 in US & Canada to institutions; USD 315 elsewhere to institutions (effective 2002). adv. **Document type:** *Journal, Academic/Scholarly.* **Description:** Publishes theory-based reviews and offers integrative theoretical formulations in personality and social psychology.
Related titles: Online - full text ed.: USD 49.50 to individuals; USD 256.50 to institutions (effective 2002) (from CatchWord Ltd., EBSCO Publishing, O C L C Online Computer Library Center, Inc., RoweCom Information Quest, Swets Blackwell, Institute for Scientific Information).
Indexed: Curr.Cont., Lang.& Lang.Behav.Abstr., PsycInfo, SOPODA, SSCI, Soc.Serv.Abstr., Sociol.Abstr., e-psyche.
—BLDSC (6428.011530), CatchWord, ingenta. **CCC.**
Published by: (Society for Personality and Social Psychology), Lawrence Erlbaum Associates, Inc., 10 Industrial Ave, Mahwah, NJ 07430-2262. TEL 201-760-3735, 800-926-6579, FAX 201-236-0072, journals@erlbaum.com, http://www.erlbaum.com/Journals/journals/PSPR/pspr.htm. Ed. Elliot R Smith. adv.: page USD 450; trim 7 x 10.

150 NLD
PERSONALITY PSYCHOLOGY IN EUROPE. Text in Dutch. irreg., latest vol.6, 1998. **Document type:** *Monographic series.*
Indexed: e-psyche.

Published by: Tilburg University Press, Postbus 90153, Tilburg 5000 LE, Netherlands. TEL 31-13-466-2909, FAX 31-13-466-3288.

150 USA ISSN 0079-0931
CODEN: PEPSDL
PERSONALITY, PSYCHOPATHOLOGY AND PSYCHOTHERAPY; a series of texts, monographs and treatises. Text in English. 1967. irreg., latest 1993. reprint service avail. from ISI. *Refereed.* **Document type:** *Monographic series.*
Formerly: Personality and Psychopathology
Indexed: Chem.Abstr., e-psyche.
—CASDDS. **CCC.**
Published by: Academic Press, Inc., Journal Division (Subsidiary of: Harcourt Brace & Company), 525 B St, Ste 1900, San Diego, CA 92101-4495. TEL 619-231-0926, FAX 619-699-6715. Eds. David T Lykken, Philip C Kendall. **Subscr. to:** Order Dept., 6277 Sea Harbor Dr, 4th Fl, Orlando, FL 32887. TEL 800-321-5068.

156 IND ISSN 0970-8111
PERSONALITY STUDY AND GROUP BEHAVIOUR. Text in English. 1981. a. INR 30 to individuals; INR 40 to institutions (effective 1999). **Document type:** *Academic/Scholarly.* **Description:** Examines research reports and other related scholarly endeavors which have a theoretical, empirical orientation.
Indexed: Psychol.Abstr., e-psyche.
Published by: Guru Nanak Dev University, Publication Office, Press & Publications Dept., Amritsar, Punjab 143 005, India. TEL 91-183-258837, FAX 91-183-258820, TELEX 384 274 GNDU IN. Ed. Satvir Singh. Pub. Jagjit Singh Walia. Circ: 250.

158 USA ISSN 0031-5826
HF5549.A2 CODEN: PPSYAQ
PERSONNEL PSYCHOLOGY. Text in English. 1948. q. USD 70 domestic; USD 79.50 foreign (effective 2002 - 2003). adv. bk.rev. charts, illus. index. 280 p./no. back issues avail.; reprint service avail. from PSC,SCH. *Refereed.* **Document type:** *Journal, Academic/Scholarly.* **Description:** Research articles on industrial psychology, employees and the workplace.
Related titles: Microform ed.: (from PQC); Online - full text ed.: (from ProQuest Information & Learning, Gale Group, Northern Light Technology, Inc., H. W. Wilson, Factiva, Institute for Scientific Information).
Indexed: ABI Inform. (Fall 1971-), ASCA, AgeLine, B.P.I. (Jan.1982-), BPIA, Bk.Rev.Ind. (1980-), Bus.Ind., C.I.J.E. (coverage dropped), Child.Bk.Rev.Ind. (1980-), Commun.Abstr., Cont.Pg.Manage., Curr.Cont., Educ.Admin.Abstr., Emerald, Environ.Sci.Poll.Mgmt., Fam.Ind., Manage.Cont., P C I, Pers.Lit., Pers.Manage.Abstr., Pollut.Abstr., PsycInfo, Psychol.Abstr. (1949-), Psycscan A.P., Risk Abstr., Russ.Acad.Sci.Bibl., SCIMP, SSCI, Saf.Sci.Abstr., Tr.& Dev.Alert, Work Rel.Abstr., e-psyche.
—BLDSC (6428.095000), CISTI, IDS, ingenta. **CCC.**
Published by: Personnel Psychology, Inc., 520 Ordway Ave, Bowling Green, OH 43402-2756. TEL 419-352-1562, FAX 419-352-2645, ppsych@personnelpsychology.com, http://www.personnelpsychology.com/. Ed. John R Hollenbeck. Pub. Milton D Hakel. R&P, Adv. contact Lee Hakel. Circ: 2,800.

301.1 150 COL ISSN 0120-3878
BF5
PERSPECTIVAS EN PSICOLOGIA. Text in Spanish. 1982. a. COP 400, USD 6. bk.rev.
Related titles: English ed.
Indexed: Psychol.Abstr., e-psyche.
Published by: Fundacion Universidad de Manizales, Facultad de Psicologia, Apartado Aereo 868, Manizales, CAL, Colombia. Circ: 1,000.

PERSPECTIVES IN LAW AND PSYCHOLOGY. see *LAW*

PERSPECTIVES IN PSYCHOLOGICAL RESEARCHES. see *EDUCATION*

616.89 CHE ISSN 0735-4037
PERSPECTIVES IN PSYCHOTHERAPY. Text in English. 1983. irreg., latest vol.2. *Refereed.* **Document type:** *Monographic series.*
Indexed: e-psyche.
Published by: Gordon and Breach - Harwood Academic (Subsidiary of: Taylor & Francis Group), PO Box 531, Lausanne 1000, Switzerland. Ed. P Olsen. **Subscr. addr. in US:** International Publishers Direct, PO Box 32160, Newark, NJ 07102. FAX 215-750-6343.

306.88 USA ISSN 0733-6217
PERSPECTIVES ON DEATH AND DYING SERIES. Text in English. 1980. irreg., latest vol.5. **Document type:** *Monographic series.*
Indexed: e-psyche.
Published by: Baywood Publishing Co., Inc., 26 Austin Ave, Box 337, Amityville, NY 11701. TEL 631-691-1270, 800-638-7819, FAX 631-691-1770, baywood@baywood.com, http://baywood.com. Eds. Kenneth Doka, Stuart Cohen. R&P Julie Krempa. Adv. contacts Marcie Cohen, Valerie Ford.

PHARMACOLOGY, BIOCHEMISTRY AND BEHAVIOR. see *PHARMACY AND PHARMACOLOGY*

616.89 PHL
PHILIPPINE JOURNAL OF COUNSELING PSYCHOLOGY. Text in English. 1987. a. PHP 30, USD 3.20. adv. bk.rev. **Document type:** *Academic/Scholarly.* **Description:** Publishes original contributions on counseling in different populations. Emphasizes empirical studies on counseling techniques and intervention strategies; the development and validation of assessment instruments; group treatment programs; and counselor education and supervision. Also accepts reviews, concept papers, and research notes.
Indexed: e-psyche.
Published by: (De La Salle University, Department of Psychology, Guidance and Counseling), De La Salle University Press, 2401 Taft Ave, Manila, Philippines. TEL 2-59-48-32, FAX 632-521-9094. Circ: 300. **Co-sponsor:** Philippine Association for Counselor Education, Research & Supervision (PACERS).

150 PHL
PHILIPPINE JOURNAL OF PSYCHOLOGY. Text in English. 1968. s-a. PHP 40, USD 5. adv. charts, illus.
Indexed: Bibl.Asian Stud. (1974-1998), Ind.Phil.Per., Psychol.Abstr., e-psyche.
Published by: Psychological Association of the Philippines, Philippine Social Science Council (PSSC) Bldg, Commonwealth Ave, Diliman, Quezon City, Philippines. Ed. Allen L Tan. Circ: 175.

156 GBR ISSN 0951-5089
PHILOSOPHICAL PSYCHOLOGY. Text in English. 1988. q. GBP 124, USD 207 to individuals; GBP 375, USD 622 to institutions (effective 2002). abstr. back issues avail.; reprint service avail. from PSC,SCH. *Refereed.* **Document type:** *Academic/Scholarly.* **Description:** Deals with the application of philosophical psychology to the cognitive and brain sciences, and to areas of applied psychology. Of interest to advanced students in philosophy, psychology, computer science, linguistics and the neurosciences.
Related titles: Online - full text ed.: ISSN 1465-394X (from CatchWord Ltd., Northern Light Technology, Inc., EBSCO Publishing, O C L C Online Computer Library Center, Inc., RoweCom Information Quest, ProQuest Information & Learning, Swets Blackwell, Institute for Scientific Information).
Indexed: ASCA, Arts & Hum.Cit.Ind. (coverage dropped), Curr.Cont., Lang.& Lang.Behav.Abstr., P C I, Phil.Ind., PsycInfo, Psychol.Abstr. (1988-), Russ.Acad.Sci.Bibl., SOPODA, SSCI, Sociol.Abstr., e-psyche.
—BLDSC (6462.260000), CatchWord, IDS, Infotrieve, ingenta. **CCC.**
Published by: Carfax Publishing Limited (Subsidiary of: Taylor & Francis Group), PO Box 25, Abingdon, Oxon OX14 3UE, United Kingdom. TEL 44-1235-401000, FAX 44-1235-401550, enquiries@carfax.co.uk, enquiry@tandf.co.uk, http://www.carfax.co.uk. Eds. Bill Bechtel, John Rust.

PHILOSOPHY, PSYCHIATRY & PSYCHOLOGY. see *PHILOSOPHY*

150.19 ITA ISSN 0390-3206
PICCOLO HANS. Text in Italian. 1974. a. ITL 40,000 to individuals; ITL 60,000 foreign to individuals; ITL 100,000 to institutions. Supplement avail. **Description:** Essays in psychoanalysis, art and literature.
Indexed: e-psyche.
Published by: Moretti e Vitalli Editori, Via Betty Ambiveri 15, Bergamo, BG 24126, Italy. Ed. Sergio Finzi. Circ: 4,000.

PLENUM SERIES IN REHABILITATION AND HEALTH. see *MEDICAL SCIENCES—Physical Medicine And Rehabilitation*

153.9 USA
▼ **PLENUM SERIES ON HUMAN EXCEPTIONALITY.** Text in English. 1999. irreg. price varies. **Document type:** *Monographic series.* **Description:** Goes beyond the traditional academic and cognitive domains to explore the psychological, social, cultural, educational, and legal aspects of human exceptionality.
Published by: Kluwer Academic - Plenum Publishers (Subsidiary of: Wolters Kluwer N.V.), 233 Spring St, New York, NY 10013-1578. TEL 212-620-8000, FAX 212-463-0742, info@plenum.com; kluwer@wkap.com; orderdept@kluwer.nl, http://www.plenum.com. Eds. Donald H Saklolfske, Moshe Zeidner. **Orders to:** Order Dept., 101 Philip Dr, Norwell, MA 02061. TEL 781-871-6000, FAX 781-681-9045.

150 POL ISSN 0079-2993
BF1 CODEN: PPBUDY
POLISH PSYCHOLOGICAL BULLETIN. Text in English. 1970. q. USD 40. bibl. **Document type:** *Bulletin.*
Indexed: Bibl.Ling., Curr.Cont. (coverage dropped), IBZ, PsycInfo, Psychol.Abstr. (1970-), Russ.Acad.Sci.Bibl., SSCI (coverage dropped), Sage Fam.Stud.Abstr., Sp.Ed.Needs Abstr., e-psyche.
—BLDSC (6543.723000), ingenta.
Published by: Polska Akademia Nauk, Komitet Nauk Psychologicznych, Ul Stawki 5-7, pok. 316, Warsaw 00183, Poland. Ed. Dariusz Dolinski. R&P Zofia Oleszkiewicz Zsurzs. Circ: 350. **Dist. by:** Ars Polona, Krakowskie Przedmiescie 7, Warsaw, Poland.

POLITICAL PSYCHOLOGY. see *POLITICAL SCIENCE*

POLYGRAPH. see *CRIMINOLOGY AND LAW ENFORCEMENT*

150 CHN
POPULAR PSYCHOLOGY/DAZHONG XINLIXUE. Text in Chinese. bi-m.
Indexed: e-psyche.
Published by: Huadong Shifan Daxue/East China Normal University, Department of Physics, Jiaoyu Kexue Xueyuan, 3663 Zhongshan Beilu, Shanghai, 4 200062, China. TEL 2518532, http://http://www.ecnu.edu.cn/english/ecnu.htm. **Co-sponsor:** Shanghai Society of Psychology.

158 USA ISSN 0199-0039
HB848 CODEN: PENVDK
POPULATION AND ENVIRONMENT. Text in English. 1978. bi-m. EUR 566 to institutions for print or online ed. (effective 2002); NLG 1,372.80 to institutions print & online eds.combined (effective 2001); EUR 679.20 to institutions print & online eds.combined (effective 2002). adv. bk.rev. charts, illus. index. reprint service avail. from PQC,ISI. *Refereed.* **Document type:** *Academic/Scholarly.* **Description:** Explores relationships between population and societal, cultural, and physical environments. Covers demographic variables linked to lifestyle, law, health, business, economics, and international relations.
Former titles (until vol.4, 1981): Journal of Population (0146-1052); Population (New York)
Related titles: Microfilm ed.: (from PQC); Online - full text ed.: (from O C L C Online Computer Library Center, Inc., Gale Group, Swets Blackwell, Kluwer Online, Factiva, Institute for Scientific Information, RoweCom Information Quest).
Indexed: ASCA, Abstr.Hyg., AgeLine, Aqua.Sci.& Fish.Abstr., Biol.Abstr., C.I.J.E. (coverage dropped), Curr.Adv.Ecol.Sci., Curr.Cont., Curr.Lit.Fam.Plan., Environ.Abstr., Environ.Per.Bibl. (1989-), Environ.Sci.Poll.Mgmt., Excerp.Med., Fam.Ind., G.Soc.Sci.& Rel.Per.Lit., High.Educ.Abstr., IBR, IBZ, Intl.Bibl.Soc.Sci., Lang.& Lang.Behav.Abstr., P.A.I.S., Peace Res.Abstr., Pollut.Abstr., Popul.Ind., PsycInfo, Psychol.Abstr. (1978-), Psycscan A.P., Risk Abstr., SOPODA, SSCI, Saf.Sci.Abstr., Sage Urb.Stud.Abstr., Soc.Serv.Abstr., Soc.Work Res.& Abstr., Sociol.Abstr., e-psyche.
—BLDSC (6552.022000), CISTI, IDS, Infotrieve, ingenta. **CCC.**
Published by: (California State University, Long Beach, Department of Psychology, American Psychological Association, Division of Population and Environmental Psychology), Kluwer Academic - Plenum Publishers (Subsidiary of: Wolters Kluwer N.V.), 233 Spring St, New York, NY 10013-1578. TEL 212-620-8000, 800-221-9369, FAX 212-463-0742, info@plenum.com; kluwer@wkap.com; services@wkap.nl, http://www.plenum.com. Ed. Kevin MacDonald.

P

150 USA
PRACTICING PROFESSIONAL SERIES. Text in English. irreg. (approx. 2/yr.). **Document type:** *Monographic series, Academic/Scholarly.* **Description:** Devoted to communicating practical information about counseling and psychotherapy. Serves as an accessible and understandable source for practical knowledge about specific issues.
Indexed: e-psyche.
Published by: Guilford Publications, Inc., 72 Spring St, New York, NY 10012. TEL 212-431-9800, 800-365-7006, FAX 212-966-6708, info@guilford.com, http://www.guilford.com. Ed. Seymour Weingarten. Pub. Robert Matloff. R&P David Mitchell. Adv. contact Christine Luberto.

150 ITA ISSN 1120-9380
PRATICA ANALITICA; saggi di psicologia junghiana. Text in Italian. 1977. s-a. ITL 35,000 domestic to individuals; USD 35 foreign to individuals; ITL 100,000 domestic to institutions; USD 80 foreign to institutions. **Document type:** *Monographic series.*
Indexed: e-psyche.
Published by: Moretti e Vitalli Editori, Via Betty Ambiveri 15, Bergamo, BG 24126, Italy. TEL 39-35-321588, FAX 39-35-321647. Ed. Salvatore Zingale.

PRAXIS DER KINDERPSYCHOLOGIE UND KINDERPSYCHIATRIE. see *MEDICAL SCIENCES—Psychiatry And Neurology*

150 616.89 DEU ISSN 0085-5073
PRAXIS DER KINDERPSYCHOLOGIE UND KINDERPSYCHIATRIE. BEIHEFTE. Text in German. 1958. irreg., latest vol.29, 1989. price varies. **Document type:** *Monographic series.*
Indexed: Curr.Cont. (coverage dropped), Ind.Med. (1958-), Lang.& Lang.Behav.Abstr., Psychol.Abstr., SSCI (coverage dropped), e-psyche.
Published by: Vandenhoeck und Ruprecht, Robert-Bosch-Breite 6, Goettingen 37079, Germany. TEL 49-551-6959-0, FAX 49-551-695917. Ed. Annemarie Duehrssen.

PRAXIS SPIEL UND GRUPPE. see *EDUCATION*

150 DEU ISSN 0941-7192
PRAXISREPORT PSYCHOLOGISCHE THERAPIEN UND PSYCHOTHERAPIEN. Text in German; Summaries in English, German. 1993. s-a. DEM 28 to individuals; DEM 44 to institutions. bk.rev. index. back issues avail. *Refereed.* **Document type:** *Academic/Scholarly.*
Indexed: e-psyche.
Published by: Psychomedia Verlags GmbH, Postfach 465, Berlin 12214, Germany. TEL 49-30-4927200, FAX 49-30-7749176. Ed. L. Gawe. R&P L Gawe. Circ: 500 (controlled).

PREVENTION & TREATMENT. see *MEDICAL SCIENCES—Psychiatry And Neurology*

PREVENTION IN PRACTICE LIBRARY. see *MEDICAL SCIENCES*

150 USA ISSN 0164-5056
PRIMAL INSTITUTE NEWSLETTER. Text in English. 1978. q. USD 11 domestic; USD 15 foreign (effective 2000). bk.rev. index. back issues avail. **Document type:** *Newsletter.* **Description:** Contains personal narratives and experiences of patients and therapists involved with primal therapy. Also discusses scientific, medical and psychological discoveries relating to primal therapy.
Supersedes (1973-1978): Journal of Primal Therapy (0091-9772)
Indexed: e-psyche.
—CISTI, GNLM.
Published by: Primal Institute, 10379 W Pico Blvd, Los Angeles, CA 90064-2608. TEL 310-785-9456, FAX 310-785-9481, janov@primalinstitute.com. Ed., R&P Vivian Janov. Circ: 1,600.

PRIMATES; journal of primatology. see *BIOLOGY—Zoology*

306.85 DEU ISSN 0175-2960
PRO FAMILIA MAGAZIN; die Zeitschrift fuer Sexualpaedagogik, Sexualberatung und Familienplanung. Text in German. 1971. q. DEM 39 (effective 2000). adv. bk.rev. back issues avail. **Document type:** *Consumer.*
Formerly (until 1983): Sexualpaedagogik und Familienplanung (0721-1228); Which was formed by the merger of (1969-1981): Sexualpaedagogik (0344-5380); Which was formerly (until 1977): Medien und Sexual Paedagogik (0343-0189); (until 1973): Sexual Paedagogik (0343-0421); (1971-1981): Pro Familia Informationen (0721-1198)
Related titles: Online - full text ed.
Indexed: IBZ, e-psyche.
—GNLM.
Published by: (Pro Familia - Deutsche Gesellschaft fuer Familienplanung, Sexualpaedagogik und Sexualberatung), Psychosozial Verlag, Friedrichstr 35, Giessen 35392, Germany. TEL 49-641-77819, FAX 49-641-77742, psychosozial-verlag@t-online.de. R&P Andrea Stroh. Circ: 7,500 (paid).

370.15 150 USA ISSN 0731-2326
PROBLEM BEHAVIOR MANAGEMENT; educator's resource service. Text in English. 1982. base vol. plus s-a. updates (2nd ed., 1992).
Indexed: e-psyche.
Published by: Aspen Publishers, Inc., 200 Orchard Ridge Dr, Ste 200, Gaithersburg, MD 20878. TEL 301-417-7500, FAX 301-417-7550.

158.7 USA ISSN 0277-4178
PROBLEMS OF INDUSTRIAL PSYCHIATRIC MEDICINE SERIES. Text in English. irreg., latest vol.11, 1985. prices varies. reprint service avail. from PQC. *Refereed.* **Document type:** *Monographic series.*
Indexed: e-psyche.
Published by: Kluwer Academic - Human Sciences Press (Subsidiary of: Wolters Kluwer N.V.), 233 Spring St, New York, NY 10013-1578. TEL 212-620-8000, FAX 212-463-0742. Ed. Sherman N Keiffer.

150 USA ISSN 0735-7028
RC467
PROFESSIONAL PSYCHOLOGY: RESEARCH AND PRACTICE. Text in English. 1969. bi-m. USD 92 domestic to non-members; USD 112 foreign to non-members; USD 46 domestic to members; USD 58 foreign to members; USD 216 domestic to institutions; USD 260 foreign to institutions (effective 2001). adv. illus. index. back issues avail.; reprint service avail. from PQC,PSC,SCH. *Refereed.* **Document type:** *Academic/Scholarly.* **Description:** Articles on techniques and practices used in the application of psychology, including applications of research, standards of practice, interprofessional relations, delivery of services, and training.
Formerly (until 1982): Professional Psychology (0033-0175)
Related titles: Microform ed.: (from PQC); Online - full text ed.: (from Gale Group, Factiva, Institute for Scientific Information).
Indexed: ASCA, Abstr.Health Care Manage.Stud., Adol.Ment.Hlth.Abstr., AgeLine, Chic.Per.Ind., Crim.Just.Abstr., Curr.Cont., Fam.Ind., Mid.East: Abstr.& Ind., PsycInfo, Psychol.Abstr. (1969-), Psycscan C.P., Rel.Ind.One, Rel.Ind.Two, Russ.Acad.Sci.Bibl., SSCI, Sage Fam.Stud.Abstr., Soc.Sci.Ind. (Jan.1994-), e-psyche.
—BLDSC (6864.211000), IDS, ingenta. **CCC.**
Published by: American Psychological Association, 750 First St., N.E., Washington, DC 20002-4242. TEL 202-336-5600, 800-374-2721, FAX 202-336-5568, subscriptions@apa.org, http://www.apa.org/journals/pro.html, http://www.apa.org/journals/pro/html. Ed. Mary Beth Kenkel. Circ: 7,800.

PROFESSIONAL SCHOOL COUNSELING. see *EDUCATION*

131 USA ISSN 0363-0951
QP351 CODEN: PPPPDL
PROGRESS IN PSYCHOBIOLOGY AND PHYSIOLOGICAL PSYCHOLOGY. Text in English. 1967. irreg., latest vol.17, 1998. reprint service avail. from ISI. *Refereed.* **Document type:** *Monographic series.*
Former titles: Psychobiology and Physiological Psychology; (until vol.6): Progress in Physiological Psychology (0079-6670)
Related titles: Online - full text ed.: (from Institute for Scientific Information).
Indexed: ASCA, Curr.Adv.Ecol.Sci., IBZ, Ind.Philos., Ind.Sci.Rev., Neurosci.Cit.Ind., SSCI (coverage dropped), Sci.Cit.Ind., e-psyche.
—CASDDS, CISTI, GNLM, ingenta. **CCC.**
Published by: Academic Press, Inc., Journal Division (Subsidiary of: Harcourt Brace & Company), 525 B St, Ste 1900, San Diego, CA 92101-4495. TEL 619-231-0926, FAX 619-699-6715. Ed. Alan N Epstein. **Subscr. to:** Order Dept., 6277 Sea Harbor Dr, 4th Fl, Orlando, FL 32887. TEL 800-321-5068.

616.89 USA ISSN 0893-5483
BF697
PROGRESS IN SELF PSYCHOLOGY; conversations in self psychology. Text in English. 1985. a., latest vol.17. USD 47.50 per vol. (effective 2000). bibl. back issues avail.; reprints avail. *Refereed.* **Document type:** *Academic/Scholarly.* **Description:** Presents new concepts and controversies in the field of self psychology.
Indexed: e-psyche.
—BLDSC (6924.539000), Infotrieve. **CCC.**
Published by: Analytic Press, Inc. (Subsidiary of: Lawrence Erlbaum Associates, Inc.), 101 West St, Hillsdale, NJ 07642. TEL 201-358-9477, FAX 201-358-4700, tapbooks@analyticpress.com, TAP@analyticpress.com, http://www.analyticpress.com/books/346-1.html. Ed. Arnold Goldberg. Pub. Lawrence Erlbaum. R&P, Adv. contact John Riegel. **Orders in the Americas, Caribbean, China & the Far East to:** Journals, 810 E 10th St, PO Box 1897, Lawrence, KS 66044-8897. **Dist. addr. in Africa:** Overseas Publications, P O Box 12292, Centrahil 6006, South Africa.; **Dist. addr. in Australia, New Zealand & Papua New Guinea:** DAInformation Services, 648 Whitehouse Rd, Mitcham, VIC 3132, Australia. TEL 61-3-9210-7788, FAX 61-3-9210-7724.; **Dist. addr. in Inda, Bangladesh & Sri Lanka:** VivaBooks Private Ltd, 4325/2 Ansari Rd, Darya Ganj, New Delhi 11002, India. TEL 91-11-327-9280, FAX 91-11-326-7224.; **Dist. addr. in the UK, Europe & the Middle East:** Eurospan University Press Group, Order Dept, 3 Henrietta St, London WC2E 8LU, United Kingdom. TEL 44-20-7240-0856, FAX 44-20-7379-0609, http://www.eurospan.co.uk.

155.4 USA
PROGRESS NOTES. Text in English. 1976. 3/yr. membership. adv.
Formerly: Society of Pediatric Psychology. Newsletter
Indexed: I.P.A., e-psyche.
Published by: Society of Pediatric Psychology, Ferkauf Graduate School of Psychology, Yeshiva University, Mazer Hall, 1300 Morris Park Ave, Bronx, NY 10461. TEL 212-430-4201, FAX 212-430-3252. Ed. Lawrence J Siegel. Circ: 1,000. **Subscr. to:** Debra Bendelt Estroff, 887 Praderia Circle, Fremont, CA 94539.

150 POL ISSN 0048-5675
BF26 CODEN: PRZPBF
PRZEGLAD PSYCHOLOGICZNY/PSYCHOLOGICAL REVIEW. Text in Polish; Summaries in English, Russian. 1952. q. USD 54. bk.rev. index. reprint service avail. from PQC,PSC.
Related titles: Microform ed.: (from PQC).
Indexed: Acad.Ind., C.I.J.E. (coverage dropped), Compumath, Curr.Adv.Ecol.Sci., IBR, Lang.& Lang.Behav.Abstr., PsycInfo, Psychol.Abstr. (1952-), Russ.Acad.Sci.Bibl., e-psyche.
Published by: Polskie Towarzystwo Psychologiczne, Ul Stawki 5-7, Warsaw 00183, Poland. Ed. R Stachowski. Circ: 2,200. **Dist. by:** Ars Polona, Krakowskie Przedmiescie 7, Warsaw, Poland.

150 BRA ISSN 1413-0556
PSICANALISE E UNIVERSIDADE/PSYCHOANALYSIS AND UNIVERSITY. Text in Portuguese. 1993. s-a. back issues avail. *Refereed.* **Document type:** *Academic/Scholarly.*
Published by: (Pontificia Universidade Catolica de Sao Paulo), Nucleo de Estudos e Pesquisas em Psicanalise, Rua Monte Alegre, 984, Perdizes, Sao Paulo, SP 05014-001, Brazil. TEL 55-11-38628213, FAX 55-11-36708501, psiclin@exatas.pucsp.br. Ed. Maria Lucia Vieira Violante. Circ: 500.

616.89 ITA
PSICHE; rivista di cultura psicoanalitica. Text in Italian. s-a. ITL 60,000 domestic to individuals; USD 90 foreign to individuals; ITL 80,000 domestic to institutions; USD 110 foreign to institutions.
Indexed: e-psyche.
Published by: Edizioni Borla s.r.l., Via Delle Fornaci, 50, Rome, RM 00165, Italy. TEL 39-6-39376728, FAX 39-6-39376620.

150 ITA
PSICHIATRIA E PSICOTERAPIA. Text in Italian. 1994. irreg., latest vol.3, 1997. price varies. **Document type:** *Monographic series.*
Indexed: e-psyche.
Published by: Liguori Editore srl, Via Posillipo, 394, Naples, NA 80123, Italy. TEL 39-81-7206111, FAX 39-81-7206244, http://www.liguori.it. Ed. Nicola Lalli. Pub. Guido Liguori. Adv. contact Maria Liguori.

PSICHIATRIA E PSICOTERAPIA ANALITICA/ANALYTIC PSYCHOTHERAPY AND PSYCHOPATHOLOGY. see *MEDICAL SCIENCES—Psychiatry And Neurology*

158 ITA ISSN 1125-4963
PSICOANALISI. Text in Italian. 1997. s-a. USD 73 (effective 2000). bk.rev. illus. index. 128 p./no. **Document type:** *Journal, Academic/Scholarly.*
Indexed: e-psyche.
Published by: (Associazione Italiana di Psicoanalisi), Il Pensiero Scientifico Editore s.r.l., Via Bradano, 3-C, Rome, RM 00199, Italy. TEL 39-06-862821, FAX 39-06-86282250, pensiero@pensiero.it, http://www.pensiero.it. Ed. Jacqueline Amati Mehler. Pub. Luca De Fiore. Circ: 600.

158 ITA
PSICOANALISI E METODO; materiali per il piacere della psicoanalisi. Text in Italian. 1983. s-a. ITL 50,000 domestic to individuals; USD 60 foreign to individuals; ITL 60,000 domestic to institutions; USD 70 foreign to institutions. bk.rev. back issues avail. **Document type:** *Monographic series, Proceedings.*
Formerly: Materiali per il Piacere della Psicoanalisi (0394-8102)
Indexed: e-psyche.
Published by: (Associazione Materiali per il Piacere della Psicoanalisi), Edizioni Borla s.r.l., Via Delle Fornaci, 50, Rome, RM 00165, Italy. TEL 39-6-39376728, FAX 39-6-39676620. Ed. Giuseppe Maffei.

616.89 VEN ISSN 0798-4308
PSICOLOGIA. Text in Spanish. 1974. s-a. USD 40. *Refereed.* **Description:** Covers general, scholarly, clinical, educational, industrial, and social psychology.
Indexed: e-psyche.
Published by: (Universidad Central de Venezuela, Escuela de Psicologia), Fondo Editorial Tropykos, Calle El Escorial, Edif. Luxor 7 Fl., Las Acacias, Caracas, Venezuela. TEL 2-6930565, FAX 2-6624926. Eds. Aristides Medina Rubio, Armando Gil Navarro. **Subscr. to:** UCV, Escuela de Psicologia, Avda. Los Ilustres, Caracas, Venezuela. TEL 6052917.

158 ITA
PSICOLOGIA CLINICA DELLO SVILUPPO. Text in Italian. 1997. 3/yr. ITL 78,000 to individuals; ITL 150,000 foreign to individuals; ITL 108,000 to institutions; ITL 195,000 foreign to institutions (effective 2000). **Document type:** *Academic/Scholarly.*
Indexed: e-psyche.
Published by: Societa Editrice Il Mulino, Strada Maggiore, 37, Bologna, BO 40125, Italy. TEL 39-51-256011, FAX 39-51-256034, diffusione@mulino.it, http://www.mulino.it.

150 ESP ISSN 1132-9483
PSICOLOGIA CONDUCTUAL/BEHAVIORAL PSYCHOLOGY; revista internacional de psicologia clinica y de la salud. Text in Spanish; Summaries in Spanish, English. 1993. 3/yr. EUR 36; EUR 50 foreign (effective for 2 yrs. 2001 & 2002); EUR 13 newsstand/cover. adv. bk.rev. abstr. back issues avail. *Refereed.* **Document type:** *Journal, Academic/Scholarly.* **Description:** Directed to psychologists, psychiatrists, social workers and others interested in clinical and/or health psychology from an empirical standpoint, mainly cognitive, behavioral or cognitive-behavioral.
—BLDSC (6945.850000), CINDOC.
Published by: Fundacion VECA, Asociacion Psicologia Iberoamericana de Clinica y Salud, Apartado de Correos 1245, Granada 18080, Spain. TEL 34-902-117486, FAX 34-902-117486, apicsa@attglobal.net, http://www.apicsa.com. Ed. Dr. Vicente E Caballo. Circ: 1,000.

150 ITA ISSN 0390-346X
PSICOLOGIA CONTEMPORANEA. Text in Italian. 1974. bi-m. ITL 28,000 domestic; ITL 39,000 foreign (effective 2001). adv.
Indexed: Ind.Philos., PsycInfo, e-psyche.
Published by: Giunti Gruppo Editoriale S.p.A., Via Bolognese, 165, Florence, FI 50139, Italy. TEL 39-55-5062236, FAX 39-55-5062397, periodici@giunti.it, http://www.giunti.it. Ed. Massimo Casini. adv.: B&W page ITL 3,750,000, color page ITL 6,000,000.

150.19 COL ISSN 0123-417X
PSICOLOGIA DESDE EL CARIBE. Text in Spanish. 1985. s-a. COP 10,000 domestic; COP 6,000 per issue domestic. *Refereed.* **Document type:** *Journal, Academic/Scholarly.* **Description:** Showcases academic scholarship and research in psychology of interest to professors and students in the field conducted in northern Colombia.
Published by: Universidad del Norte, Division de Humanidades, Programa de Psicologia, Bolque D, 3er piso, Baranquilla, Colombia. http://www.uninorte.edu.co/publicacion/discernimiento/ppal/index.html, http://www.uninorte.edu.co/division/humanidades. Ed. Kary Cabrera.

158.7 ITA ISSN 0048-5691
PSICOLOGIA E LAVORO. Text in Italian. 1968. q. ITL 70,000, EUR 36.15 domestic; ITL 80,000, EUR 41.32 foreign (effective 2001). back issues avail. **Document type:** *Academic/Scholarly.* **Description:** Focuses on psycology in workplace settings through research and opinion articles.
Indexed: Psychol.Abstr., e-psyche.
Published by: Patron Editore, Via Badini, 12, Quarto Inferiore, Bologna, BO 40127, Italy. TEL 39-51-767003, FAX 39-51-768252, patroned@tin.it, http://www.patroneditore.com. Ed. Enzo Spaltro.

PSICOLOGIA E SCUOLA; giornale italiano di psicologia dell'educazione e pedagogia sperimentale. see *EDUCATION*

150 BRA
PSICOLOGIA EM REVISTA. Text in Portuguese. s-a. **Document type:** *Journal, Academic/Scholarly.*
Formerly (until 1999): Cadernos de Psicologia (0104-4370)
Published by: Pontificia Universidade Catolica de Minas Gerais, Av Dom Jose Gaspar, 500, C Eucaristico, Belo Horizonte, MG 30535-610, Brazil. TEL 55-31-33194271, FAX 55-31-33194129, proex@pucminas.br, http://www.pucminas.br.

150 MEX ISSN 1405-0943
PSICOLOGIA IBEROAMERICANA. Text in Spanish. 1988; N.S. 1993. q. USD 40 (effective 2000). bibl, illus. **Document type:** *Academic/Scholarly.* **Description:** Presents contributions in the research, teaching, and profession of psychology.
Formerly (until 1993): Universidad Iberoamericana. Departamento de Psicologia. Revista
Indexed: e-psyche.
Published by: Universidad Iberoamericana, Departamento de Psicologia, Prol Paseo de la Reforma 880, Col Lomas de Santa Fe, Mexico City, DF 01210, Mexico. TEL 52-5-2674046, FAX 52-2-2674289, antonio.tena@uia.mx. Ed. Antonio Tena. Circ: 1,000.

150 ITA ISSN 0393-1064
PSICOLOGIA ITALIANA. Text in Italian. 1979. 3/yr. ITL 72,000; ITL 82,000 foreign (effective 2000). **Document type:** *Academic/Scholarly.* **Description:** Explores all branches of psychological science and the many forms it can assume in society. Includes news, opinion, and discussion.
Indexed: e-psyche.
Published by: (Associazione Italiana di Psicologia), Patron Editore, Via Badini, 12, Quarto Inferiore, Bologna, BO 40127, Italy. TEL 39-51-767003, FAX 39-51-768252. Ed. Enzo Spaltro.

150 BRA ISSN 0102-7972
PSICOLOGIA: REFLEXAO E CRITICA. Text in Portuguese. 1986. s-a., latest vol.12, no.3, 1999. BRL 75 domestic; USD 50 foreign; BRL 40 newsstand/cover domestic; USD 25 newsstand/cover foreign (effective 2000). bk.rev. back issues avail. **Document type:** *Academic/Scholarly.* **Description:** Provides research reports, theoritical studies, article reviews, and other information pertaining to the field of psychology.
Related titles: Online - full text ed.: (from SciELO).
Indexed: PsycInfo, e-psyche.
Published by: Universidade Federal do Rio Grande do Sul, Curso de Pos-Graduacao em Psicologia, Rua Ramiro Barcelos, 2600 Sala 110, Porto Alegre, RGS 90035-003, Brazil. TEL 55-51-316-5246, FAX 55-51-330-4797, revista@psico.ufrgs.br, http://www.scielo.br/prc. Eds. Cleonice Bosa, Silivia Helena Koller. R&P Silivia Helena Koller.

150 BRA
PSICOLOGIA REVISTA. Text in Portuguese; Summaries in English, Portuguese. 1995. s-a. BRL 12, USD 10. adv. bk.rev. abstr, bibl, illus, stat. *Refereed.* **Document type:** *Academic/Scholarly.* **Description:** Deals with broad subjects in the area of psychology and discusses new challenges.
Published by: (Pontificia Universidade Catolica da Sao Paulo, Faculdade de Psicologia), Editora da Pontificia Universidade Catolica de Sao Paulo, R. Ministro Godoi 1213, Sao Paulo, Sao Paulo 05014-001, Brazil. TEL 55-11-38733359, FAX 55-11-2626003, educ@pucsp.br. Ed. Ana Bahia Bock.

370.15 150 BRA ISSN 0102-3772
BF5
PSICOLOGIA: TEORIA E PESQUISA/PSYCHOLOGY: THEORY AND RESEARCH. Text in Portuguese; Summaries in English, Portuguese. 1985. q. BRL 48, USD 48 domestic to individuals; BRL 75, USD 75 foreign to institutions; BRL 42, USD 42 to students (effective 2001). bk.rev. back issues avail. *Refereed.* **Document type:** *Academic/Scholarly.* **Description:** Publishes research reports, theoretical studies, reports of professional experience, critical reviews, and technical notes related to psychology.
Related titles: Online - full text ed.
Indexed: INIS Atomind., PsycInfo, Psychol.Abstr. (1985-), e-psyche.
Published by: Universidade de Brasilia, Instituto de Psicologia, Campus Universitario, Brasilia, DF 70910900, Brazil. TEL 55-61-2746455, FAX 55-61-2736378, revptp@unb.br, http://www.unb.br/ip/ip.htm. Ed. Norberto Abreu E Silva Neto. Adv. contact Claudio Vaz Torres. Circ: 1,000.

150 BRA ISSN 0103-6564
PSICOLOGIA U S P. Text in Portuguese. 1990. s-a. back issues avail.
Related titles: Online - full text ed.: (from SciELO).
Published by: Universidade do Sao Paulo, Instituto de Psicologia, Ave. Prof. Lucio Martins Rodrigues, Trav.4, 399 Bl. 23, Cidade Universitaria, Sao Paulo, SP 05508-900, Brazil. TEL 55-11-8184452, FAX 55-11-8184462, revpsico@edu.usp.br, http://www.scielo.br.

152 ESP ISSN 0211-2159
PSICOLOGICA; journal of methodology and experimental psychology. Text mainly in Spanish; Text occasionally in English. 1980. s-a. ESP 3,000 domestic to individuals; USD 20 foreign to individuals; ESP 6,000 domestic to institutions; USD 36 foreign to institutions (effective 2000). adv. bk.rev. abstr, bibl. back issues avail. *Refereed.* **Document type:** *Academic/Scholarly.* **Description:** Includes articles on experimental psychology as well as the methodological and statistical aspects of psychology.
Related titles: Online - full text ed.
Indexed: PsycInfo, e-psyche.
—CINDOC.
Published by: Universitat de Valencia, Departamento de Metodologia, Psicobiologia e Psicologia Social, Avda Blasco Ibanez, 21, Valencia 46010, Spain. TEL 39-6-3864420 ext. 6264, FAX 39-6-3864668, algarabe@uv.es, http://www.uv.es.psicologica/. Ed., R&P Salvador Algarabel.

P

150 ESP ISSN 0214-9915
PSICOTHEMA: REVISTA DE PSICOLOGIA. Text in English, Spanish. 1989. q. ESP 6,000, USD 45 (effective 2001). adv. bk.rev., software rev. stat. back issues avail.; reprints avail. *Refereed.* **Document type:** *Academic/Scholarly.*
Related titles: Online - full text ed.: (from Institute for Scientific Information).
Indexed: ASCA, Curr.Cont., PsycInfo, Psychol.Abstr. (1993-), SSCI, e-psyche.
—BLDSC (6945.865500), CINDOC, IDS.
Published by: Colegio Oficial de Psicologos Asturias, Idelfonso Sanchez del Rio, 4, 1-B, Oviedo 33001, Spain. TEL 34-98-528-5778, FAX 34-98-528-1374, dasturias@correo.cop.es, http://www.cop.es/publicaciones/psicothema/. Ed. Jose Muniz Fernandez. Pub., Adv. contact Jose R Hermida. R&P Jorge Arias. Circ: 2,000.

150 ROM ISSN 1220-689X
PSIHOLOGIA. Text in Romanian. 1991. bi-m. ROL 17,000; USD 10 foreign. adv. bk.rev. back issues avail. **Document type:** *Academic/Scholarly.*
Indexed: e-psyche.
Published by: Stiinta & Tehnica S.A., Piata Presei Libere 1, Bucharest 79781, Romania. TEL 40-1-6175833, FAX 40-1-2228494. Ed. Alexandrian Chelcea. Pub., Adv. contact Ioan Albescu. R&P Iaon Albescu. B&W page USD 300; trim 270 x 135. Circ: 20,000.

158 RUS
PSIKHOLOGICHESKIE ISSLEDOVANIYA. Text in Russian. 1976 (no.6). irreg. **Document type:** *Academic/Scholarly.*
Indexed: e-psyche.
Published by: (Moskovskii Gosudarstvennyi Universitet), Izdatel'stvo Moskovskogo Gosudarstvennogo Universiteta, B Nikitskaya 5-7, Moscow 103009, Russian Federation. TEL 7-095-2295091. Circ: 5,500.

100 RUS ISSN 0205-9592
PSIKHOLOGICHESKII ZHURNAL. Text in Russian. 1980. bi-m. *Refereed.*

Related titles: Online - full text ed.: (from Institute for Scientific Information).
Indexed: Curr.Cont., Ref.Zh., Russ.Acad.Sci.Bibl., SSCI, e-psyche.
—BLDSC (0134.678000).
Published by: (Russian Academy of Sciences), Izdatel'stvo Nauka, Profsoyuznaya ul 90, Moscow 117864, Russian Federation. TEL 7-095-2340584.

150 BGR ISSN 0204-644X
PSIKHOLOGIIA✱ . Text in Bulgarian. 1973. q. BGL 1.60.
Indexed: Psychol.Abstr., Russ.Acad.Sci.Bibl., e-psyche.
Published by: Druzhestvo na Psikholozite, c/o Kathedre of Psychology, Sofia University, 15 Rouski blvd, Sofia, Bulgaria. Ed. S Ganovski. Circ: 500. **Dist. by:** Hemus, 6 Rouski blvd, Sofia 1000, Bulgaria.

158.7 RUS
PSIKHOLOGIYA V BIZNESE. Text in Russian. s-a. USD 55 in United States.
Published by: Biznes Shkola Intel-Sintez, Profsoyuznaya ul 3, ofis 620, Moscow 117036, Russian Federation. TEL 7-095-1299212, FAX 7-095-1246809. Ed. N A Litvintseva. **US dist. addr.:** East View Publications, 3020 Harbor Ln N, Minneapolis, MN 55447. TEL 612-550-0961.

PSIQUIS; revista de psiquiatria, psicologia y psicosomatica. see *MEDICAL SCIENCES—Psychiatry And Neurology*

158 NLD ISSN 1385-7630
PSY; tijdschrift over de geestelijke gezondheidszorg. Text in Dutch. 1997. m. **Document type:** *Academic/Scholarly.*
Formed by the merger of (1995-1996): Mentaal (1382-3000); (1993-1996): Gazet (1382-3620); Which superseded (1973-1993): G G Z Nieuwsbrief (0929-3663); (1992-1996): Buitengewoon (1381-2599); Which superseded (1987-1992): Nederlandse Vereniging van Beschermede Woonvormen (N V B W). Nieuwsbrief; (1993-1996): Addictum (0929-7375); Which was formed by the merger of (1989-1993): Cadans (1380-7900); (1985-1993): JoJo Info Bulletin (1380-7943); (1990-1993): Kommissie Gezamenlijk Overlag Drugshulpverlenigsinstellingen (K G O D). Nieuwsbrief (1381-0049)
Indexed: e-psyche.
Published by: G G Z Nederland, Postbus 8305, Utrecht 3503 RH, Netherlands. TEL 31-30-2874020, FAX 31-30-2874021, psy@ggznederland.nl.

PSYCH DISCOURSE. see *EDUCATION*

150 ITA
PSYCHE; rassegna di psicoterapia umanistico-esistenziale, di psicoterapia autogena e psicoterapie brevi. Text in Italian. 1981; N.S. 1993. 3/yr. ITL 70,000.
Published by: C I S S P A T, Piazza De Gasperi, 41, Padua, PD 35100, Italy. TEL 049-650861. Ed. Marilla Malugani.

150.19 DEU ISSN 0033-2623
BF173.A2 CODEN: PSYEDK
PSYCHE; Zeitschrift fuer Psychoanalyse und ihre Anwendungen. Text in German. 1947. 11/yr. DEM 190, EUR 97.15; DEM 150, EUR 76.69 to students (effective 2000). adv. bk.rev. abstr, bibl, charts. index. reprint service avail. from PSC,SCH. *Refereed.* **Document type:** *Magazine, Academic/Scholarly.*
Related titles: Online - full text ed.: (from Institute for Scientific Information).
Indexed: ASCA, Arts & Hum.Cit.Ind. (coverage dropped), Curr.Cont., Excerp.Med., Ger.J.Psych., IBR, IBZ, INIS Atomind., Ind.Med. (coverage dropped), Ind.Philos., PsycInfo, Psychoanal.Abstr., Psychol.Abstr. (1947-), Russ.Acad.Sci.Bibl., SSCI.
—BLDSC (6946.115000), CISTI, GNLM, IDS. **CCC.**
Published by: Verlag Klett-Cotta, Rotebuehlstr 77, Stuttgart 70178, Germany. TEL 49-711-66721648, FAX 49-711-66722032. Ed. Werner Bohleber. Adv. contact Thomas Kleffner. B&W page DEM 1,500; trim 113 x 180. Circ: 7,000.

513 USA
PSYCHE (GREENVILLE, ONLINE EDITION); an interdisciplinary journal of research on consciousness. Text in English. 1994. irreg. free. *Refereed.* **Document type:** *Academic/Scholarly.* **Description:** Dedicated to supporting the interdisciplinary exploration of the nature of consciousness and its relation to the brain.
Media: Online - full text.
Published by: Association for the Scientific Study of Consciousness, Caltech, Div of Biology, 139-74, Pasadena, CA 91125. http://psyche.cs.monash.edu.au, http://psyche.cs.monash.edu.au/.

PSYCHIATRIC & PSYCHOLOGICAL EVIDENCE. see *LAW*

PSYCHIATRIC REHABILITATION JOURNAL. see *MEDICAL SCIENCES—Psychiatry And Neurology*

PSYCHIATRY PSYCHOLOGY AND LAW. see *MEDICAL SCIENCES—Psychiatry And Neurology*

150 616.8 USA ISSN 1366-9869
PSYCHNEWS INTERNATIONAL. Text in English. 1994. m. (10/yr.). free per issue. illus. back issues avail.; reprints avail. **Document type:** *Academic/Scholarly.* **Description:** Covers the issues in psychology, psychiatry and the social sciences.
Formerly (until 1996): InterPsych Newsletter (1355-2562)
Media: Online - full text.
Indexed: e-psyche.
Published by: Mental Health Net - C M H C Systems fu03c2dj@zedat.FU-Berlin.de, http://www.mhnet.org/pni/. Ed. Sunkyo Kwon.

616.89 ZAF ISSN 1023-0548
PSYCHO-ANALYTIC PSYCHOTHERAPY IN SOUTH AFRICA. Text in English. 1992. 2/yr., latest vol.9, no.2, 2001. ZAR 80 domestic to individuals; USD 15 foreign to individuals; ZAR 100 domestic to institutions; USD 20 foreign to institutions (effective 2001). adv. bk.rev. back issues avail. *Refereed.* **Document type:** *Journal, Academic/Scholarly.* **Description:** Publishes articles of interest to psychotherapists working psycho-analytically in South Africa.
Indexed: PsycInfo, Psychoanal.Abstr., e-psyche.
—BLDSC (6946.269760).
Address: PO Box 16115, Vlaeberg, Cape Town 8018, South Africa. TEL 27-21-4232550, FAX 27-21-4232550, http://www.psa.za.org. Ed. Trevor Lubbe.

PSYCHO-LINGUA; a biannual research journal devoted to communicative behavior. see *LINGUISTICS*

PSYCHO-ONCOLOGY; journal of the psychological, social and behavioral dimensions of cancer. see *MEDICAL SCIENCES—Oncology*

616.89 NLD ISSN 0924-6290
PSYCHOANALYSE EN CULTUUR/PSYCHOANALYSIS AND CULTURE. Text in Dutch, English. 1990. irreg., latest vol.10, 2000. price varies. illus. back issues avail. *Refereed.* **Document type:** *Monographic series, Academic/Scholarly.* **Description:** Examines the interaction of psychoanalysis and culture.
Indexed: e-psyche.
Published by: Rodopi, Tijnmuiden 7, Amsterdam 1046 AK, Netherlands. TEL 31-20-611-4821, FAX 31-20-447-2979, F.van.der.Zee@Rodopi.nl, orders-queries@Rodopi.nl, http://www.rodopi.nl. Ed. Walter Schonau. **Dist. by:** Nordeal; Rodopi (USA), One Rockefeller Plaza, Ste. 1420, New York, NY 10020. TEL 212-265-6360, 800-225-3998, FAX 212-265-6402.

PSYCHOANALYSIS AND HISTORY. see *HISTORY*

616.891 USA ISSN 1057-5723
PSYCHOANALYSIS AND PSYCHOTHERAPY. Text in English. 1983. s-a. USD 52 domestic to individuals; USD 64 foreign to individuals; USD 52 domestic to institutions; USD 105 foreign to institutions (effective 2002). adv. bk.rev. index. **Document type:** *Journal, Academic/Scholarly.* **Description:** Represents contemporary thinking, application and recent advances in the art and techniques of dynamic psychotherapy and psychoanalysis.
Formerly (until 1989): Dynamic Psychotherapy (0736-508X)
Indexed: PsycInfo, Psychoanal.Abstr., Psychol.Abstr., e-psyche.
—BLDSC (6946.265300), GNLM, ingenta.
Published by: (Postgraduate Center for Mental Health), International Universities Press, Incorporated, 59 Boston Post Rd., P.O. Box 1524, Madison, CT 06443-1524. adv.: page USD 360; 4.25 x 7. Circ: 1,000.

616.89 USA ISSN 1044-2103
BF173.A2
PSYCHOANALYTIC BOOKS; a quarterly journal of reviews. Text in English. 1990. q. USD 55 domestic to individuals; USD 65 foreign to individuals; USD 95 domestic to institutions; USD 105 foreign to institutions (effective 1999). adv. bk.rev. index. back issues avail. **Document type:** *Academic/Scholarly.* **Description:** Reviews of books in psychoanalysis including Freudian studies, history of psychoanalysis, psychobiography, psychohistory, and psychoanalytic study of literature and the arts.
Indexed: e-psyche.
Published by: Psychoanalytic Books, Inc., 211 E 70th St, New York, NY 10021. TEL 212-628-8792, FAX 212-628-8453, psabooks@datagram.com. Ed. Dr. Joseph Reppen. R&P Victoria Schwartz. Adv. contact Francesca Reppen. B&W page USD 250. Circ: 1,000 (paid).

150.19 616.891 USA
PSYCHOANALYTIC CROSSCURRENTS. Text in English. 1985. irreg. price varies. **Document type:** *Monographic series.*
Indexed: e-psyche.
Published by: New York University Press, 70 Washington Square So, New York, NY 10012. TEL 212-998-2575, 800-996-3833, FAX 212-995-3833. Ed. Leo Goldberger. R&P Susan Conn.

616.89 USA ISSN 1048-1885
RC500
PSYCHOANALYTIC DIALOGUES; a journal of relational perspectives. Text in English. 1991. bi-m. USD 75 in US & Canada to individuals; USD 105 elsewhere to individuals; USD 230 in US & Canada to institutions; USD 260 elsewhere to institutions; USD 15 per issue in US & Canada; USD 21 per issue elsewhere (effective 2001). adv. back issues avail. *Refereed.* **Document type:** *Academic/Scholarly.* **Description:** Psychoanalytic contributions on interpersonal psychoanalysis, object relations theory, self psychology, infant research and child development.
Related titles: Online - full content ed.; Online - full text ed.: (from CatchWord Ltd., Institute for Scientific Information).
Indexed: Curr.Cont., IBR, Ind.Philos., PsycInfo, Psychoanal.Abstr., Psychol.Abstr. (1991-), SSCI, e-psyche.
—BLDSC (6946.267000), CatchWord, Infotrieve. **CCC.**
Published by: Analytic Press, Inc. (Subsidiary of: Lawrence Erlbaum Associates, Inc.), 365 Broadway, Hillsdale, NJ 07642. TEL 201-666-4110, FAX 201-358-0621, TAPJournals@analyticpress.com, TAP@analyticpress.com, http://www.analyticpress.com/psychoanalytic_dialogues.html. Eds. Jody Messler Davies, Neil Altman. adv.: page USD 410; trim 5 x 8. Circ: 2,500. **Subscr. to:** Journals, 810 E 10th St, PO Box 1897, Lawrence, KS 66044-8897.

150 USA ISSN 0735-1690
RC500
PSYCHOANALYTIC INQUIRY; a topical journal for mental health professionals. Text in English. 1980. 5/yr. USD 79.50 in US & Canada to individuals; USD 109.50 elsewhere to individuals; USD 295 domestic to institutions; USD 325 foreign to institutions (effective 2002). adv. back issues avail. *Refereed.* **Document type:** *Academic/Scholarly.* **Description:** Each issue dedicated to a specific topic in psychoanalysis, psychotherapy, infant research or child development.
Related titles: Online - full content ed.; Online - full text ed.: (from CatchWord Ltd., Institute for Scientific Information).
Indexed: ASCA, Curr.Cont., IBR, IBZ, Ind.Philos., PsycInfo, Psychoanal.Abstr., Psychol.Abstr. (1983-), SSCI, e-psyche.
—BLDSC (6946.269000), CatchWord, GNLM, IDS. **CCC.**
Published by: Analytic Press, Inc. (Subsidiary of: Lawrence Erlbaum Associates, Inc.), 365 Broadway, Hillsdale, NJ 07642. TEL 201-666-4110, FAX 201-358-0621, TAPJournals@analyticpress.com, TAP@analyticpress.com, http://www.analyticpress.com/psychoanalytic_inquiry.html. Ed. Joseph D Lichtenberg. adv.: page USD 375; trim 5 x 8. Circ: 1,500. **Subscr. to:** Journals, 810 E 10th St, PO Box 1897, Lawrence, KS 66044-8897. **Dist. by:** Lawrence Erlbaum Associates, Inc., 10 Industrial Ave, Mahwah, NJ 07430-2262.

150 616.8 USA ISSN 0736-9735
BF173.A2
PSYCHOANALYTIC PSYCHOLOGY; Journal of the Division of Psychoanalysis, American Psychological Association. Text in English. 1984. q. USD 60 domestic to non-members; USD 75 foreign to non-members; USD 45 domestic to members; USD 55 foreign to members; USD 255 domestic to institutions; USD 287 foreign to institutions (effective 2001). adv. bk.rev. abstr, bibl. 600 p./no. 1 cols./p. reprint service avail. from PSC,SCH. *Refereed.* **Document type:** *Academic/Scholarly.* **Description:** Forum for the study of psychoanalytic issues in psychology and psychological issues in psychoanalysis.
Related titles: Online - full text ed.: (from Institute for Scientific Information).
Indexed: ASCA, Curr.Cont., PsycInfo, Psychoanal.Abstr., Psychol.Abstr. (1984-), SSCI, e-psyche.
—BLDSC (6946.269600), EMDOCS, GNLM, Infotrieve, ingenta, KNAW. **CCC.**

P

Published by: American Psychological Association, Division of Psychoanalytic Psychology, 211 E 70th St, New York, NY 10021. TEL 212-628-8792, 202-336-5600, 800-374-3721, FAX 212-628-8453, 202-336-5568, subscriptions@apa.org, www.apa.org/journals.pap.html, http://www.apa.org/journals/pap.html, http://www.apa.org/. Ed. Dr. Joseph Reppen. adv.: B&W page USD 175; trim 10 x 7. Circ: 3,300 (paid).

616.890 GBR ISSN 0266-8734
PSYCHOANALYTIC PSYCHOTHERAPY. Text in English. 1984. 3/yr. GBP 40, USD 66 to individuals; GBP 72, USD 119 to institutions; GBP 13.50 to members (effective 2002). *Refereed.* **Document type:** *Journal, Academic/Scholarly.* **Description:** Promotes standards of excellence and to act as a vehicle for the exchange of views and the dissemination of research throughout the public sphere.
Related titles: Online - full content ed.; Online - full text ed.: (from CatchWord Ltd.).
Published by: (Association for Psychoanalytic Psychotherapy in the National Health Service), Routledge (Subsidiary of: Taylor & Francis Group), 11 New Fetter Ln, London EC4P 4EE, United Kingdom. TEL 44-20-7583-9855, FAX 44-20-7842-2298, info@routledge.co.uk, http://www.tandf.co.uk/journals/routledge/02668734.html, http://www.routledge.com. Ed. Marilyn Lawrence.

616.89 USA ISSN 0033-2828
BF173.A2 CODEN: PSQAAX
PSYCHOANALYTIC QUARTERLY. Text in English. 1932. q. USD 92.50 domestic; USD 107.50 foreign (effective 2001). bk.rev. abstr, bibl. index, cum.index: vols.1-35, 36-45, 46-55. reprint service avail. from PSC,SCH. *Refereed.* **Document type:** *Journal, Academic/Scholarly.* **Description:** Original contributions in the field of theoretical, clinical, and applied psychoanalysis. Departments include book reviews, abstracts, notes.
Related titles: Online - full text ed.: (from Institute for Scientific Information).
Indexed: ASCA, AgeLine, Amer.Bibl.Slavic & E.Eur.Stud., Arts & Hum.Cit.Ind. (coverage dropped), Chicago Psychoanal.Lit.Ind., Curr.Cont., Documentatieblad, Ind.Med. (1932-), Indian Psychol.Abstr., Lang.& Lang.Behav.Abstr., Mid.East: Abstr.& Ind., PsycInfo, Psychoanal.Abstr., Psychol.Abstr. (1932-), Ref.Zh., Rel.Ind.One, Rel.Ind.Two, Russ.Acad.Sci.Bibl., SOPODA, SSCI, Soc.Work Res.& Abstr., Sociol.Abstr., e-psyche.
—BLDSC (6946.270000), CISTI, EMDOCS, GNLM, IDS, ingenta.
Published by: (Psychoanalytic Quarterly, Inc), Other Press, LLC, 377 W. 11th St., Ste. 2-D, New York, NY 10014. TEL 212-414-0747, FAX 212-255-5736. Ed. Dr. Owen Renik. Pub. Michael Moskowitz. Circ: 3,300 (paid).

150 616.89 USA ISSN 0033-2836
BF1 CODEN: PSREAG
THE PSYCHOANALYTIC REVIEW. Text in English. 1913. bi-m. USD 55 domestic to individuals; USD 85 foreign to individuals; USD 235 domestic to institutions; USD 265 foreign to institutions (effective 2000). adv. bk.rev., film rev., play rev. bibl. index. back issues avail.; reprint service avail. from PSC,SCH,ISI. *Refereed.* **Document type:** *Journal, Academic/Scholarly.* **Description:** Covers contemporary psychoanalytical theory and practice, and psychoanalytical themes in art, film and literature.
Incorporates (1952-19??): Psychoanalysis
Related titles: Microform ed.: (from PQC); Online - full text ed.: (from Northern Light Technology, Inc., ProQuest Information & Learning, CatchWord Ltd., RoweCom Information Quest).
Indexed: ASSIA, Abstr.Anthropol., Abstr.Crim.& Pen., Abstr.Engl.Stud., AgeLine, Amer.Bibl.Slavic & E.Eur.Stud., Arts & Hum.Cit.Ind. (coverage dropped), Biol.Abstr., Curr.Cont. (coverage dropped), Excerp.Med., Film Lit.Ind. (1985-), IBR, IBZ, IMFL, Ind.Med. (1963-), Ind.Philos., Lang.& Lang.Behav.Abstr., MLA Intl.Bibl., Mid.East: Abstr.& Ind., P C I, PsycInfo, Psychoanal.Abstr., Psychol.Abstr. (1926-), Ref.Zh., Rel.Ind.One, Rel.Ind.Two, Russ.Acad.Sci.Bibl., SOPODA, SSCI (coverage dropped), Sci.Cit.Ind. (coverage dropped), Soc.Work Res.& Abstr., Sociol.Abstr., Yrbk.Assoc.Educ.& Rehab.Blind, e-psyche.
—BLDSC (6946.273000), GNLM, IDS, ingenta. **CCC.**
Published by: (National Psychological Association for Psychoanalysis, Inc.), Guilford Publications, Inc., 72 Spring St, 4th Fl, New York, NY 10012. TEL 212-431-9800, 800-365-7006, FAX 212-966-6708, info@guilford.com. Ed. Martin Schulman. Pub. Robert Matloff. R&P Kathy Kuehl. Adv. contact Susan Pavliscak. Circ: 1,600.

PSYCHOANALYTIC SOCIAL WORK. see *SOCIAL SERVICES AND WELFARE*

150 GBR ISSN 1460-8952
▼ **PSYCHOANALYTIC STUDIES.** Text in English. 1999. q. GBP 52, USD 86 to individuals; GBP 198, USD 328 to institutions (effective 2001). *Refereed.* **Description:** Devoted to the academic, scholarly discussion of all aspects of psychoanalysis, including its history, its institutions, and its application to a wide range of disciplines.
Related titles: Online - full text ed.: ISSN 1470-1049 (from CatchWord Ltd., EBSCO Publishing, O C L C Online Computer Library Center, Inc., RoweCom Information Quest, Swets Blackwell).
Indexed: e-psyche.
—BLDSC (6946.274500), CatchWord.
Published by: Carfax Publishing Limited (Subsidiary of: Taylor & Francis Group), PO Box 25, Abingdon, Oxon OX14 3UE, United Kingdom. TEL 44-1235-401000, FAX 44-1235-401550, enquiries@carfax.co.uk, enquiry@tandf.co.uk, http://www.carfax.co.uk. Ed. Geraldine Shipton.

155.4 USA ISSN 0079-7308
BF721 CODEN: PYACAZ
PSYCHOANALYTIC STUDY OF THE CHILD. Text in English. 1945. a. price varies. reprint service avail. from PSC,SCH.
Related titles: Online - full text ed.: (from Institute for Scientific Information).
Indexed: ASCA, Biol.Abstr., Educ.Ind. (Jan.1983-Dec.1991), Excerp.Med., Ind.Med. (1945-), P C I, PsycInfo, Psychoanal.Abstr., Psychol.Abstr. (1945-), SSCI, Yrbk.Assoc.Educ.& Rehab.Blind, e-psyche.
—BLDSC (6946.275000), CISTI, GNLM, ingenta, KNAW.
Published by: Yale University Press, PO Box 209040, New Haven, CT 06520. TEL 203-432-0940, FAX 616-592-2618, chla@mlc.lib.mi.us, http://www.yale.edu. Ed. Dr. Albert J Solnit.

PSYCHOANALYTISCHE BLAETTER ZU KLINIK, FORSCHUNG, ZEITGESCHEHEN. see *MEDICAL SCIENCES—Psychiatry And Neurology*

150 JPN ISSN 0033-2852
BF1 CODEN: PYLGAY
PSYCHOLOGIA/PUSHIKOROGIA; an international journal of psychology in the Orient. Text in English. 1957. q. JPY 8,000 domestic to individuals; JPY 7,000 foreign to individuals; JPY 11,000 domestic to institutions; JPY 10,000 foreign to institutions (effective 2001). adv. bk.rev. index. 75 p./no. back issues avail.; reprint service avail. from PSC,SCH. *Refereed.* **Document type:** *Journal, Academic/Scholarly.* **Description:** Publishes symposia, general surveys, reviews, brief reports, notes and discussions, as well as representative original works in very broad field of psychology.
Related titles: Online - full text ed.: (from Institute for Scientific Information).
Indexed: ASCA, Arts & Hum.Cit.Ind. (coverage dropped), Bibl.Asian Stud. (1969-1991), Curr.Cont., Documentatieblad, IBR, Indian Psychol.Abstr., Lang.& Lang.Behav.Abstr., Mid.East: Abstr.& Ind., P C I, PsycInfo, Psychol.Abstr. (1957-), Russ.Acad.Sci.Bibl., SOPODA, SSCI, Sociol.Abstr., e-psyche.
—BLDSC (6946.278000), CISTI, IDS, ingenta.
Published by: Psychologia Society/Pushikorogia-kai, Dept of Cognitive Psychology in Education, Graduate School of Education, Kyoto University, Yoshida-Honmachi, Sakyo-ku, Kyoto 606-8501, Japan. psysoc@www.educ.kyoto-u.ac.jp, http://www.educ.kyoto-u.ac.jp/cogpsy/psycholoeng/psycholo.htm. Ed. Masuo Koyasu. Circ: 900.

370.15 SVK ISSN 0555-5574
PSYCHOLOGIA A PATOPSYCHOLOGIA DIETATA. Text in Slovak, Czech; Summaries in English, German. 1966. q. USD 65 (effective 2001 - 2002). bk.rev. *Refereed.* **Document type:** *Journal, Academic/Scholarly.*
Indexed: Bibl.Ling., PsycInfo, Psychol.Abstr. (1966-), e-psyche.
—BLDSC (6946.279000).
Published by: (Vyskumny Ustav Detskej Psychologie a Patopsychologie/Research Institue for Child Psychology and Pathopsychology), Slovak Academic Press Ltd., Nam Slobody 6, PO Box 57, Bratislava 81005, Slovakia. http://www.elis.sk. Ed. Vladimir Dockal. Circ: 800.

150 BEL ISSN 0033-2879
BF30 CODEN: PBELAN
PSYCHOLOGICA BELGICA. Text and summaries in English. 1954. q. BEF 1,500 (effective 2000). adv. abstr. cum.index. Supplement avail.; back issues avail. *Refereed.* **Document type:** *Academic/Scholarly.*
Related titles: Online - full text ed.: (from Institute for Scientific Information).
Indexed: ASCA, Biol.Abstr., C.I.S. Abstr., Compumath, Curr.Cont., PsycInfo, Psychol.Abstr. (1961-), Ref.Zh., SSCI, e-psyche.
—BLDSC (6946.287000), IDS.
Published by: Societe Belge de Psychologie/Belgische Vereniging voor Psychologie, Tiensestraat 102, Leuven 3000, Belgium. TEL 32-16-326013, FAX 32-16-326118, betty.vandenbaviere@psy.kuleuven.ac.be, http://www.ulb.ac.be/bps/docs/pubs/psybel.html. Ed., R&P, Adv. contact Axel Cleeremans. Circ: 450.

152 USA ISSN 1040-3590
CODEN: PYASEJ
PSYCHOLOGICAL ASSESSMENT. Text in English. 1989. q. USD 92 domestic to non-members; USD 107 foreign to non-members; USD 46 domestic to members; USD 56 foreign to members; USD 204 domestic to institutions; USD 236 foreign to institutions (effective 2001). adv. illus. reprints avail. *Refereed.* **Document type:** *Academic/Scholarly.* **Description:** Original empirical articles concerning clinical assessment and evaluations.
Related titles: Online - full text ed.: (from Gale Group, Factiva, Institute for Scientific Information).
Indexed: ASCA, AgeLine, C.I.J.E., Curr.Cont., Ergon.Abstr., Excerp.Med. (1995-), Fam.Ind., Ind.Med. (1989-), PsycInfo, Psychol.Abstr. (1989-), Psycscan C.P., Russ.Acad.Sci.Bibl., SSCI, Soc.Sci.Ind. (Jan.1994-), e-psyche.
—BLDSC (6946.293500), CISTI, EMDOCS, GNLM, IDS, ingenta. **CCC.**
Published by: American Psychological Association, 750 First St., N.E., Washington, DC 20002-4242. TEL 202-336-5600, 800-374-2721, FAX 202-336-5568, subscriptions@apa.org, http://www.apa.org/journals/pas.html. Ed. Stephen N Haynes. Circ: 5,700.

P

150 ZAF
PSYCHOLOGICAL ASSOCIATION OF SOUTH AFRICA. PROCEEDINGS. Text in Afrikaans, English. 1962. a. free per issue. **Document type:** *Proceedings.*
Formerly: Psychological Institute of the Republic of South Africa. Proceedings
Indexed: e-psyche.
Published by: Psychological Association of South Africa, PO Box 74119, Lynnwood Ridge, Pretoria 0040, South Africa. TEL 27-12-326-1981.

150 USA ISSN 0033-2909
BF1 CODEN: PSBUAI
PSYCHOLOGICAL BULLETIN. Text in English. 1904. bi-m. USD 153 domestic to non-members; USD 173 foreign to non-members; USD 76 domestic to members; USD 88 foreign to members; USD 340 domestic to institutions; USD 384 foreign to institutions (effective 2001). adv. charts, illus. index. reprint service avail. from PSC,PQC,SCH. *Refereed.* **Document type:** *Academic/Scholarly.* **Description:** Comprehensive and integrative reviews and interpretations of critical substantive and methodological issues and practical problems from all the areas of psychology.
Related titles: Microform ed.: (from PQC,PMC); Online - full text ed.: (from Gale Group, Factiva, Institute for Scientific Information).
Indexed: ABI Inform., ASCA, ASSIA, Abstr.Crim.& Pen., Acad.Ind., Addic.Abstr., Adol.Ment.Hlth.Abstr., AgeLine, Arts & Hum.Cit.Ind. (coverage dropped), Biol.Abstr., C.I.J.E. (coverage dropped), Child Devel.Abstr., Compumath, Crim.Just.Abstr., Curr.Adv.Ecol.Sci., Curr.Cont., Curr.Ind.Stat., ERA, Educ.Admin.Abstr., Ergon.Abstr., Fam.Ind., IBR, IBZ, INIS Atomind., Ind.Med. (1904-), Ind.Philos., Ind.Sci.Rev., Inpharma, Intl.Bibl.Soc.Sci., M.L.A., MLA Intl.Bibl., Mark.Res.Abstr. (1963-), Mid.East: Abstr.& Ind., Neurosci.Cit.Ind., Nutr.Abstr., P C I, Pharm.&Out.News, PsycInfo, Psychol.Abstr. (1926-), Psycscan A.P., Psycscan C.P., Psycscan D.P., Reac., Russ.Acad.Sci.Bibl., SOMA, SSCI, Sci.Cit.Ind., Soc.Sci.Ind. (Nov.1982-), Soc.Work Res.& Abstr., Sp.Ed.Needs Abstr., Stud.Wom.Abstr., e-psyche.
—BLDSC (6946.300000), GNLM, IDS, ingenta. **CCC.**
Published by: American Psychological Association, 750 First St., N.E., Washington, DC 20002-4242. TEL 202-336-5500, 800-374-2721, FAX 202-336-5568, subscriptions@apa.org, http://www.apa.org/journals/bul.html. Eds. Ed Diener, Nancy Eisenberg. Circ: 5,800.

370.15 150 USA ISSN 1047-840X
BF1 CODEN: PINQEY
PSYCHOLOGICAL INQUIRY; an international journal of peer commentary and review. Text in English. 1990. q. USD 50 in US & Canada to individuals; USD 80 elsewhere to individuals; USD 455 in US & Canada to institutions; USD 485 elsewhere to institutions (effective 2002). adv. bk.rev. illus. reprints avail. *Refereed.* **Document type:** *Journal, Academic/Scholarly.* **Description:** Publishes theoretical and issue-oriented articles in the areas of personality, social, developmental, health, and clinical psychology.
Related titles: Online - full text ed.: ISSN 1532-7965. USD 45 to individuals; USD 409.50 to institutions (effective 2002) (from CatchWord Ltd., EBSCO Publishing, O C L C Online Computer Library Center, Inc., RoweCom Information Quest, Swets Blackwell, Institute for Scientific Information).
Indexed: ASCA, Curr.Cont., Lang.& Lang.Behav.Abstr., PsycInfo, Psychol.Abstr. (1990-), SOPODA, SSCI, Soc.Serv.Abstr., Sociol.Abstr., e-psyche.
—BLDSC (6946.380000), CatchWord, Infotrieve, ingenta. **CCC.**
Published by: Lawrence Erlbaum Associates, Inc., 10 Industrial Ave, Mahwah, NJ 07430-2262. TEL 201-760-3735, 800-926-6579, FAX 201-236-0072, journals@erlbaum.com, http://www.erlbaum.com/Journals/journals/PI/pi.htm. Eds. Constantine Sedikides, Roy F Baumeister. adv.: page USD 375; trim 7 x 10.

616.89 GBR ISSN 0264-1801
PSYCHOLOGICAL MEDICINE. MONOGRAPH SUPPLEMENT. Text in English. 1982. irreg. **Document type:** *Academic/Scholarly.*
Related titles: ♦ Supplement to: Psychological Medicine. ISSN 0033-2917.
Indexed: e-psyche.
—CISTI, ingenta. **CCC.**
Published by: Cambridge University Press, Edinburgh Bldg, Shaftesbury Rd, Cambridge CB2 2RU, United Kingdom. FAX 44-1223-315052, information@cup.cam.ac.uk, information@cambridge.org, http://www.cup.cam.ac.uk, http://www.uk.cambridge.org/journals/pmu. R&P Linda Nicol.

150 USA ISSN 1082-989X
PSYCHOLOGICAL METHODS. Text in English. 1996. q. USD 60 domestic to non-members; USD 75 foreign to non-members; USD 34 domestic to members; USD 44 foreign to members; USD 149 domestic to institutions; USD 181 foreign to institutions (effective 2001). adv. illus. Index. reprints avail. *Refereed.* **Document type:** *Journal, Academic/Scholarly.* **Description:** Devoted to the development and dissemination of methods for collecting, analyzing, understanding and interpreting psychological data.
Related titles: Online - full text ed.: (from Institute for Scientific Information).
Indexed: ASSIA, Curr.Cont., Ergon.Abstr., Ind.Med., PsycInfo, SSCI, e-psyche.
—BLDSC (6946.485000), IDS, Infotrieve, ingenta. **CCC.**
Published by: American Psychological Association, 750 First St., N.E., Washington, DC 20002-4242. TEL 202-336-5600, 800-374-2721, FAX 202-336-5568, subscriptions@apa.org, http://www.apa.org/journals/met.html. Ed. Stephen G West. Circ: 5,100.

150 USA ISSN 0033-2925
BF173.A2
PSYCHOLOGICAL PERSPECTIVES; a Jungian review. Text in English. 1970. s-a. USD 32; USD 37 foreign (effective 2001). adv. bk.rev., film rev. index. back issues avail.; reprint service avail. from PQC. **Document type:** *Academic/Scholarly.* **Description:** Features articles, interviews, poetry, and fiction. Explores themes and issues of personal, cultural, and global interest from a unique perspective which integrates archetypal and leading edge thinking in the arts and sciences.
Related titles: Microform ed.: (from PQC).
Indexed: Psychol.Abstr., Ref.Zh., e-psyche.
—BLDSC (6946.510000), ingenta. **CCC.**
Published by: C.G. Jung Institute of Los Angeles, 10349 W Pico Blvd, Los Angeles, CA 90064-2608. TEL 310-556-1193, FAX 310-556-2290, http://www.junginla.org/psychological_perspectives.htm. Eds. Gilda Frantz, Margaret Johnson. Circ: 1,300 (paid).

PSYCHOLOGICAL PERSPECTIVES ON LESBIAN AND GAY ISSUES. see *HOMOSEXUALITY*

150 152 USA ISSN 0033-2933
BF1 CODEN: PYRCAI
THE PSYCHOLOGICAL RECORD; a quarterly journal in theoretical and experimental psychology. Text in English. 1937. q. USD 45 to individuals; USD 55 foreign to individuals; USD 95 to institutions; USD 105 foreign to institutions; USD 25 to students; USD 30 foreign to students (effective 1999). adv. bk.rev. index. back issues avail.; reprint service avail. from PQC,PSC,SCH,ISI. *Refereed.* **Document type:** *Academic/Scholarly.*
Related titles: Microform ed.: (from PQC); Online - full text ed.: (from Gale Group, ProQuest Information & Learning, Northern Light Technology, Inc., H. W. Wilson, Factiva, Institute for Scientific Information).
Indexed: ASCA, ASSIA, Abstr.Crim.& Pen., Adol.Ment.Hlth.Abstr., AgeLine, Amer.Bibl.Slavic & E.Eur.Stud., Bibl.Asian Stud. (1971), Biol.Abstr., Child Devel.Abstr., Crim.Just.Abstr., Curr.Adv.Ecol.Sci., Curr.Cont., High.Educ.Abstr., IBR, IBZ, INIS Atomind., Ind.Med. (coverage dropped), Ind.Philos., Lang.& Lang.Behav.Abstr., Mid.East: Abstr.& Ind., Nutr.Abstr., PsycInfo, Psychol.Abstr. (1937-), Psycscan B.A.& T., Ref.Zh., SOPODA, SSCI, Sci.Cit.Ind. (coverage dropped), Soc.Sci.Ind. (Apr.1982-), Sociol.Abstr., e-psyche.
—BLDSC (6946.520000), IDS, Infotrieve, ingenta. **CCC.**
Published by: Psychological Record, Kenyon College, Gambier, OH 43022-9623. TEL 740-427-5377, FAX 740-427-5390, psychrecord@kenyon.edu. Ed. Charles E Rice. R&P Charles Rice. Circ: 1,500.

150 USA ISSN 0033-2941
BF21 CODEN: PYRTAZ
PSYCHOLOGICAL REPORTS. Text in English. 1955. bi-m. (2 vols./yr.). USD 365 in United States (effective 2001). bk.rev. charts, illus, stat, abstr, bibl. index. 352 p./no. back issues avail.; reprint service avail. from PSC,SCH. *Refereed.* **Document type:** *Journal, Academic/Scholarly.* **Description:** Publishes experimental, theoretical, and speculative articles in the field of general psychology.
Related titles: Microfilm ed.; Online - full text ed.: (from Institute for Scientific Information).
Indexed: ASCA, Abstr.Crim.& Pen., Adol.Ment.Hlth.Abstr., AgeLine, Amer.Bibl.Slavic & E.Eur.Stud., Arts & Hum.Cit.Ind. (coverage dropped), Biol.Abstr., CERDIC, CINAHL, Chic.Per.Ind., Child Devel.Abstr., Commun.Abstr., Crim.Just.Abstr., Curr.Cont., Curr.Ind.Stat., Curr.Lit.Fam.Plan., Dent.Ind., Documentatieblad, Ergon.Abstr., Excerp.Med., Fam.Ind., High.Educ.Abstr., IBR, IBZ, IMFL, INIS Atomind., Ind.Med. (1955-), Ind.Philos., Indian Psychol.Abstr., Int.Nurs.Ind., L.R.I., Lang.& Lang.Behav.Abstr., Mid.East: Abstr.& Ind., Mult.Ed.Abstr., PSI, PsycInfo, Psychol.Abstr. (1955-), Rel.Ind.One, Rel.Ind.Two, Res.High.Educ.Abstr., Risk Abstr., Russ.Acad.Sci.Bibl., SSCI, Sage Fam.Stud.Abstr., Sci.Cit.Ind. (coverage dropped), Soc.Sci.Ind. (Oct.1982-), Stud.Wom.Abstr., THA, e-psyche.
—BLDSC (6946.525000), GNLM, ingenta, KNAW, Linda Hall.
Published by: Dr. C.H. Ammons, Ed. & Pub., PO Box 9229, Missoula, MT 59807. TEL 406-728-1702. Eds. Bruce Ammons, Douglas Ammons, S.A. Isbell. R&P C H Ammons TEL 406-728-1702. Circ: 1,800.
Co-publisher: Behavioral Engineering Assoc.

150 DEU ISSN 0340-0727
BF3 CODEN: PSREDJ
PSYCHOLOGICAL RESEARCH; an international journal of perception, attention, memory and action. Text in English. 1921. s-a. EUR 614.40 domestic; EUR 610.60 in Germany; EUR 172.50 newsstand/cover foreign (effective 2002). cum.index: vols.1-36. reprint service avail. from ISI. *Refereed.* **Document type:** *Journal, Academic/Scholarly.* **Description:** Publishes articles that contribute to a basic understanding of human perception, attention, memory and action. Emphasizes the theoretical implications of the research reported.
Supersedes: Psychologische Forschung
Related titles: Microform ed.: (from PQC); Online - full text ed.: (from EBSCO Publishing, RoweCom Information Quest, Swets Blackwell, Springer LINK, Institute for Scientific Information).
Indexed: ASCA, AgeLine, Biol.Abstr., Compumath, Curr.Cont., IBZ, Ind.Med. (1974-), Ind.Philos., Mid.East: Abstr.& Ind., Neurosci.Cit.Ind., P C I, PsycInfo, Psychol.Abstr. (1973-), Russ.Acad.Sci.Bibl., SSCI, e-psyche.
—BLDSC (6946.527000), CISTI, IDS, ingenta. **CCC.**
Published by: Springer-Verlag (Subsidiary of: BertelsmannSpringer), Tiergartenstr 17, Heidelberg 69121, Germany. TEL 49-6221-345-0, FAX 49-6221-345229, subscriptions@springer.de, http://link.springer.de/link/service/journals/00426/index.htm, http://www.springer.de. Ed. J Engelkamp. **Subscr. in N. America to:** Springer-Verlag New York Inc., PO Box 2485, Secaucus, NJ 07096-2485. TEL 212-460-1500, FAX 212-473-6272.

150 SWE ISSN 0555-5620
BF21.A1 CODEN: PRBUDE
PSYCHOLOGICAL RESEARCH BULLETIN. Text in English. 1961. irreg. (approx. 6/yr.). free per issue to qualified personnel. bibl, charts. cum.index. *Refereed.* **Document type:** *Academic/Scholarly.* **Description:** Empirical psychological studies, frequently concerned with personality.
Indexed: Psychol.Abstr., e-psyche.
—BLDSC (6946.528000), ingenta.
Published by: Lund University, Department of Psychology, Paradisgatan 5 P, Lund 22350, Sweden. TEL 46-46-2228770, FAX 46-46-2224209, postmaster@psykol.lu.se, http://www.psykol.lu.se. Ed. Bert Westerlundh. Circ: 450.

150 IND ISSN 0970-6097
BF76.5
PSYCHOLOGICAL RESEARCH JOURNAL. Text in English. 1977. s-a. INR 50, USD 20. adv. bk.rev. index. **Document type:** *Academic/Scholarly.*
Indexed: Documentatieblad, G.Indian Per.Lit., Indian Psychol.Abstr., Psychol.Abstr., e-psyche.
Published by: Psychological Research Academy, Ste.9, 37 Syed Amir Ali Ave., Kolkata, West Bengal 700 019, India.

150 USA ISSN 0033-295X
BF1 CODEN: PSRVAX
PSYCHOLOGICAL REVIEW. Text in English. 1894. q. USD 115 domestic to non-members; USD 130 foreign to non-members; USD 57 domestic to members; USD 67 foreign to members; USD 264 domestic to institutions; USD 296 foreign to institutions (effective 2001). adv. bibl, charts, illus. index. reprint service avail. from PSC,SCH. *Refereed.* **Document type:** *Academic/Scholarly.* **Description:** Includes articles that make theoretical contributions to all areas of scientific psychology.
Related titles: Microform ed.: (from PQC,PMC); Online - full text ed.: (from Gale Group, Factiva, Institute for Scientific Information).
Indexed: ASSIA, Acad.Ind., Addic.Abstr., AgeLine, Biol.Abstr., C.I.J.E., Child Devel.Abstr., Compumath, Cont.Pg.Manage., Curr.Adv.Ecol.Sci., Curr.Cont., Curr.Lit.Fam.Plan., Environ.Sci.Poll.Mgmt., Ergon.Abstr., IBR, IBZ, INIS Atomind., Ind.Med. (1894-), Ind.Philos., Ind.Sci.Rev., Inpharma, Intl.Bibl.Soc.Sci., Lang.& Lang.Behav.Abstr., M.L.A., MLA Intl.Bibl., Mid.East: Abstr.& Ind., Neurosci.Cit.Ind., P C I, Pollut.Abstr., PsycInfo, Psychol.Abstr. (1924-), Psycscan D.P., Reac., Risk Abstr., Russ.Acad.Sci.Bibl., SSCI, Saf.Sci.Abstr., Sci.Cit.Ind., Soc.Sci.Ind. (Nov.1982-), Soc.Work Res.& Abstr., Sp.Ed.Needs Abstr., Stud.Wom.Abstr., Work Rel.Abstr., Yrbk.Assoc.Educ.& Rehab.Blind, e-psyche.
—BLDSC (6946.530000), CISTI, GNLM, IDS, ingenta. **CCC.**
Published by: American Psychological Association, 750 First St., N.E., Washington, DC 20002-4242. TEL 202-336-5600, FAX 202-336-5568, http://www.apa.org/journals/rev.html. Ed. Walter Mischel. Circ: 5,100.

150.19 USA ISSN 0956-7976
BF1 CODEN: PSYSET
PSYCHOLOGICAL SCIENCE. Text in English. 1990. bi-m. GBP 294 to institutions in UK & Europe; USD 356 to institutions in the Americas & Caribbean; GBP 294 elsewhere to institutions (effective 2002). adv. bk.rev. illus. back issues avail.; reprint service avail. from PSC,SCH. *Refereed.* **Document type:** *Journal, Academic/Scholarly, Trade.* **Description:** Provides a forum for research, theory and application in psychology and the closely related behavioral, cognitive, neural and social sciences.
Related titles: Online - full content ed.: (from EBSCO Publishing, O C L C Online Computer Library Center, Inc., ingenta, Gale Group, Swets Blackwell); Online - full text ed.: (from Factiva, Institute for Scientific Information, RoweCom Information Quest); Supplement: Psychological Science in the Public Interest.
Indexed: ASCA, AgeLine, Arts & Hum.Cit.Ind. (coverage dropped), Curr.Cont., Ergon.Abstr., Fam.Ind., High.Educ.Abstr., Ind.Med. (1990-), Lang.& Lang.Behav.Abstr., Neurosci.Cit.Ind., Peace Res.Abstr., Per.Islam. (1990-), PsycInfo, Psychol.Abstr. (1990-), Russ.Acad.Sci.Bibl., SOPODA, SSCI, Soc.Sci.Ind. (Jan.1994-), Soc.Serv.Abstr., Soc.Work Res.& Abstr., Sociol.Abstr., e-psyche.

—BLDSC (6946.530300), IDS, Infotrieve, ingenta. **CCC.**
Published by: (American Psychological Society), Blackwell Publishers, 350 Main St, Malden, MA 02148. TEL 781-388-8200, 800-835-6770, FAX 781-388-8232, subscript@blackwellpub.com, http://www.blackwellpublishers.co.uk/journals/PSCI, http://www.blackwellpublishers.co.uk/journals/diph. Ed. Sam Glucksberg. R&P Gretchen Voter TEL 781-388-0423. Adv. contact Anne Marie Sheehy TEL 781-388-0427.

150 USA ISSN 1040-404X
PSYCHOLOGICAL SCIENCE AGENDA. Text in English. 1988. bi-m. free. back issues avail. **Document type:** *Newsletter.* **Description:** Discusses current news in the field of psychological science (research), and what is happening at the American Psychological Association's Science Directorate.
Related titles: Online - full text ed.
Indexed: e-psyche.
—CCC.
Published by: American Psychological Association, Science Directorate, 211 E 70th St, New York, NY 10021. TEL 202-336-6000, FAX 202-336-5953, science@apa,org, science@apa.org, http://www.apa.org/psa/psacover.html. Ed. David Rosenbaum. Circ: 25,000.

150 IND ISSN 0033-2968
BF1
PSYCHOLOGICAL STUDIES. Text in English. 1956. 3/yr. INR 240, USD 30 (effective 1999). adv. bk.rev. charts, illus, stat. index. reprint service avail. from ISI. *Refereed.* **Document type:** *Academic/Scholarly.*
Indexed: Bibl.Asian Stud. (1971-1991), Documentatieblad, Indian Psychol.Abstr., PsycInfo, Psychol.Abstr. (1956-), SSCI (coverage dropped), Sci.Cit.Ind. (coverage dropped), e-psyche.
—BLDSC (6946.531100), ingenta.
Address: 623, Bogadi Extension, Stage 2, Mysore, Karnataka 570 006, India. Ed., R&P, Adv. contact M.A. Faroqi. Pub. M A Faroqi. Circ: 500.

150 NLD ISSN 0167-6598
PSYCHOLOGIE. Text in Dutch. 1982. m. (11/yr.). NLG 85 (effective 1995). back issues avail. **Document type:** *Consumer.* **Description:** Covers current psychological knowledge for an educated lay readership.
Indexed: e-psyche.
Published by: Weekbladpers B.V., Postbus 1050, Amsterdam 1000 BB, Netherlands. TEL 31-20-5518711, FAX 31-20-6251288. Ed. Rita Kohnstamm. Pub. H Verwoort. **Dist. in N. America by:** Swets & Zeitlinger, 440 Creamery Way, Ste A, Exton, PA 19341. TEL 800-447-9387.

150 FRA ISSN 1265-5449
PSYCHOLOGIE CLINIQUE ET PROJECTIVE. Text in French. 1952. s-a.
Former titles (until 1993): Societe Francaise du Rorschach et des Methodes Projectives. Bulletin (0373-6261); (until 1962): Groupement Francais du Rorschach. Bulletin (1148-828X)
Indexed: Ind.Philos., PsycInfo, e-psyche.
Published by: Dunod, 5 rue Laromiguiere, Paris 75005, France. TEL 33-1-40466200, FAX 33-1-40466201, gauthier.villars@mail.sgip.fr, http://www.gauthier-villars.fr. **Subscr. to:** Societe de Periodiques Specialises, BP 22, Vineuil Cedex 41354, France. TEL 33-2-54504612, FAX 33-2-54504611.

150 NLD ISSN 0168-9223
PSYCHOLOGIE EN MAATSCHAPPIJ. Text in Dutch. 1976. q. NLG 95 to individuals; NLG 129.95 to institutions. adv. bk.rev. index. back issues avail. *Refereed.* **Document type:** *Academic/Scholarly.* **Description:** Publishes scholarly studies of psychology and society.
Indexed: e-psyche.
—KNAW.
Published by: Elsevier Gezondheidszorg B.V., Tijdstroom (Subsidiary of: Reed Elsevier plc Group), Planetenbaan 1, Maarssen 3600 AK, Netherlands. TEL 31-346-577577, FAX 31-346-554287, http://www.tijdstroom; http://www.socsci.kun.nl/psy/cultuur/users/theo/p&m/. adv.: B&W page NLG 500. **Subscr. to:** Elsevier Den Haag, Postbus 16500, The Hague 2500 BM, Netherlands. TEL 31-70-381-9900, FAX 31-70-333-8399.

PSYCHOLOGIE & EDUCATION. see *EDUCATION*

152.8 FRA ISSN 0296-8770
PSYCHOLOGIE ET PSYCHOMETRIE* . Text in French. s-a. FRF 110.
Indexed: e-psyche.
Published by: Editions Scientifiques et Psychologiques, c/o Office de Justification de la Diffusion Controle (O J D), 40 Bd. Malesherbes, Paris 75008, France. TEL 46-45-38-12, FAX 40-95-73-32. Eds. Francis Van Dam, Pierre Favreau.

150 FRA ISSN 0033-2984
BF2 CODEN: PSFRAT
PSYCHOLOGIE FRANCAISE. Text in French. 1956. q. FRF 480, EUR 73.18 domestic to individuals; FRF 540, EUR 82.32 foreign to individuals; FRF 240 domestic to students (effective 2000). bibl, charts, illus. index. reprint service avail. from SWZ. **Description:** Publishes reviews of original investigations, articles covering theoretical reflection regarding the practice of psychology.
Indexed: Biol.Abstr., IBZ, Ind.Philos., Lang.& Lang.Behav.Abstr., PsycInfo, Psychol.Abstr. (1956-), Russ.Acad.Sci.Bibl., SSCI (coverage dropped), e-psyche.
—BLDSC (6946.532200), Infotrieve. **CCC.**
Published by: (Societe Francaise de Psychologie), Dunod, 5 rue Laromiguiere, Paris 75005, France. TEL 33-1-40466200, FAX 33-1-40466201, TELEX 634 916 F. Ed. R Ghiglione. Circ: 2,800. **Subscr. to:** Presses Universitaires de Grenoble, B.P. 47, Grenoble Cedex 9 38040, France. TEL 33-4-76825980, FAX 33-4-76827835.

150 DEU ISSN 0340-1677
PSYCHOLOGIE HEUTE. Text in German. 1974. m. DEM 108; DEM 10 newsstand/cover (effective 2000). adv. bk.rev. bibl, charts, illus, stat. index. **Document type:** *Journal, Academic/Scholarly.* **Description:** Covers the behavioral sciences.
Indexed: Excerp.Med., INIS Atomind., Ind.Philos., Russ.Acad.Sci.Bibl., e-psyche.
—BLDSC (6946.532240). **CCC.**
Published by: Verlag Julius Beltz GmbH, Werderstr. 10, Weinheim 69469, Germany. TEL 49-6201-60070, FAX 49-6201-6007382. Ed., R&P Heiko Ernst. Adv. contact Brigitte Bell. B&W page DEM 6,583, color page DEM 11,307. Circ: 85,000.

301.1 150 CAN ISSN 0714-3494
PSYCHOLOGIE PREVENTIVE. Text in English. 1982. s-a. CND 16 domestic to individuals; CND 20 foreign to individuals; CND 12 domestic to institutions; CND 25 foreign to institutions (effective 2000). adv. bk.rev. index. back issues avail. **Document type:** *Consumer.* **Description:** Covers problems of family, youth, education and health.
Indexed: Pt.de Rep. (1987-), e-psyche.
Published by: Societe de Recherche en Orientation Humaine Inc., 2120 E Rue Sherbrooke, Bur 212, Montreal, PQ H2K 1C3, Canada. TEL 514-523-5677, FAX 514-523-9999, frederike.d@sympatico.ca. Ed. Yves Brissette. Pub., R&P Moncef Guitouni. Circ: 1,000.

150 DEU ISSN 0170-0537
PSYCHOLOGIE UND GESELLSCHAFTSKRITIK. Text in German. 1977. q. DEM 65 (effective 1998). adv. bk.rev. index. back issues avail. **Document type:** *Academic/Scholarly.* **Description:** Critique of mainstream psychology in theory and practice; social foundation of psychology.
Indexed: IBZ, Ind.Philos., e-psyche.
Published by: (Initiative Kritischer Psychologinnen und Psychologen e.V.), Mabuse Verlag GmbH, Kasseler Str 1A, Frankfurt Am Main 60486, Germany. TEL 49-69-97074071, FAX 49-69-704152, mabuse@oeko-net.de, http://www.oeko-net.de/mabuse/. Ed. Siegfried Grubitzsch. Adv. contact Wolrad Bode. page DEM 780; trim 170 x 110. Circ: 2,750.

150 DEU ISSN 0079-7405
PSYCHOLOGIE UND PERSON. Text in German. 1961. irreg., latest vol.26, 1990. price varies. **Document type:** *Monographic series.*
Indexed: e-psyche.
Published by: Ernst Reinhardt Verlag, Kemnatenstr 46, Munich 80639, Germany. TEL 49-89-1780160, FAX 49-89-17801630.

150 790.1 DEU ISSN 0945-6031
PSYCHOLOGIE UND SPORT. Text in German. q. EUR 30; EUR 25 to students; EUR 9 newsstand/cover (effective 2002). **Document type:** *Journal, Academic/Scholarly.*
Indexed: e-psyche.
Published by: (Arbeitsgemeinschaft fuer Sportpsychologie), Verlag Karl Hofmann, Postfach 1360, Schorndorf 73603, Germany. TEL 49-7181-402127, FAX 49-7181-402111, info@hofmann-verlag.de, http://www.hofmann-verlag.de.

158 CZE ISSN 0033-300X
HF5548.8 CODEN: PSVPB2
PSYCHOLOGIE V EKONOMICKE PRAXI/APPLIED INDUSTRIAL PSYCHOLOGY; casopis pro pomoc hospodarske praxi. Text in Czech, Slovak; Summaries in English, German. 1966. s-a. CZK 30, USD 13 (effective 1999). bk.rev. abstr, bibl, charts, illus, stat. index. **Document type:** *Academic/Scholarly.*
Related titles: Microform ed.
Indexed: C.I.S. Abstr., Ergon.Abstr., Psychol.Abstr., Russ.Acad.Sci.Bibl., e-psyche.
Published by: (Univerzita Karlova, Filozoficka Fakulta), Vydavatelstvi Karolinum, Ovocny trh 5, Prague 116 36, Czech Republic. FAX 42-2-24212041, edice@cuni.cz; kat.psychologie@ruk.cuni.cz. Eds. Jiri Hoskovec, Jiri Stikar. Circ: 500. **Subscr. to:** Knihovna Katedry Psychologie FF UK, Celetna 20, Prague 11636, Czech Republic. TEL 42-2-24491406, FAX 42-2-24812166.

150 DEU ISSN 0941-3049
PSYCHOLOGIE VERSTEHEN; das Erleben und Verhalten der Lebewesen. Text in German, English. 1992. s-a. DEM 18 (effective 2001). adv. bk.rev. **Document type:** *Journal, Academic/Scholarly.*
Indexed: e-psyche.
Published by: Verlag Ursula Guss, Am Hexenteich 17, Borgentreich 34434, Germany. TEL 49-5643-8344, FAX 49-5643-948688. Ed. Kurt Guss.

054.1 FRA
PSYCHOLOGIES; Mieux vivre sane. Text in French. 1970. m. (11/yr.). FRF 220; FRF 25 newsstand/cover (effective 1999). adv. bk.rev. illus. index.
Formerly (until 1983): Psychologie (0032-1583)
Indexed: Curr.Cont. (coverage dropped), Pt.de Rep. (1979-), SSCI (coverage dropped), e-psyche.
Published by: Loft International, B.P. 703, Sainte Genevieve Cedex 60732, France. TEL 33-3-44034414, PSYCHOLOGIES@Wanadoo.fr. Ed. Jean Louis Servan Schreiber. Circ: 93,000. **Subscr. to:** Florence Raudon, 1 rue Lord Byron, Paris 75008, France. TEL 33-1-44958933, FAX 33-1-45636144.

150 DEU ISSN 0033-3018
BF3
PSYCHOLOGISCHE BEITRAEGE; Vierteljahresschrift fuer alle Gebiete der Psychologie. Text in English, German; Summaries in English, French, German. 1953. q. DEM 121 (effective 2001). adv. bk.rev. abstr, bibl, charts. index, cum.index every 10 yrs. reprint service avail. from PSC,SCH. *Refereed.* **Document type:** *Journal, Academic/Scholarly.* **Description:** Publishes original articles on all aspects and discplines of psychology.
Related titles: Online - full text ed.: (from ProQuest Information & Learning).
Indexed: BHA, Biol.Abstr., Curr.Cont. (coverage dropped), Curr.Ind.Stat., Ergon.Abstr., Ger.J.Psych., IBR, IBZ, Ind.Philos., Lang.& Lang.Behav.Abstr., P C I, PsycInfo, Psychol.Abstr. (1953-), Ref.Zh., SOPODA, SSCI (coverage dropped), Sociol.Abstr., e-psyche.
Published by: (Deutsche Gesellschaft fuer Psychologie), Pabst Science Publishers, Am Eichengrund 28, Lengerich 49525, Germany. TEL 35-5484-308, FAX 35-5484-550, pabst.publishers@t-online.de, http://www.pabst-publishers.de/psybeit/.

150 DEU ISSN 0033-3042
BF3
PSYCHOLOGISCHE RUNDSCHAU; Offizielles Orgen des Deutschen Gesellschaft fuer Psychologie zugleich Informationsorgan des Berufsverbandes Deutscher Psychologinnen und Psychologen. Text in German; Summaries in English. 1949. q. DEM 74 to individuals; DEM 138 to institutions (effective 2001). adv. bk.rev. abstr, charts. index. reprint service avail. from PSC,SCH. *Refereed.* **Document type:** *Journal, Academic/Scholarly.*
Related titles: Online - full text ed.: (from Institute for Scientific Information).
Indexed: ASCA, Child Devel.Abstr., Curr.Cont., IBR, IBZ, INIS Atomind., Ind.Philos., MLA Intl.Bibl., PsycInfo, Psychol.Abstr. (1929-), Ref.Zh., Russ.Acad.Sci.Bibl., SSCI, e-psyche.
—IDS.
Published by: (Deutsche Gesellschaft fuer Psychologie), Hogrefe Verlag GmbH und Co. KG, Rohnsweg 25, Goettingen 37085, Germany. TEL 49-551-496090, FAX 49-551-4960988, verlag@hogrefe.de, http://www.hogrefe.de. Ed. J Lukas. Circ: 6,200.
Co-sponsor: Berufsverband Deutscher Psychologinnen und Psychologen e.V.

150 GBR ISSN 0952-8229
THE PSYCHOLOGIST. Text in English. 1988. m. GBP 66 domestic to non-members; GBP 75 foreign to non-members (effective 2001). adv. bk.rev., software rev. abstr. reprint service avail. from SWZ,PQC,SCH,PSC,ISI. *Refereed.* **Document type:** *Academic/Scholarly.* **Description:** Contains articles on issues and events of general psychological interest, society news, regular columns on the media, computer and software news.
Formerly (until 1988): British Psychological Society. Bulletin (0007-1692)
Related titles: Microform ed.: (from PQC); Online - full text ed.: (from Northern Light Technology, Inc., ProQuest Information & Learning, Institute for Scientific Information).
Indexed: AMED, ASCA, AgeLine, Br.Hum.Ind., Curr.Adv.Ecol.Sci., Curr.Cont., Ergon.Abstr., Fam.Ind., PsycInfo, Psychol.Abstr., Ref.Zh., SSCI, e-psyche.
—BLDSC (6946.534680), IDS, Infotrieve, ingenta. **CCC.**
Published by: The British Psychological Society, St Andrews House, 48 Princess Rd E, Leicester LE1 7DR, United Kingdom. FAX 44-116-254-8824, psychologist@bps.org.uk, http://www.bps.org.uk. Ed. Jon Sutton. R&P P Dillon-Hooper TEL 44-116-254-9568. Adv. contact Nisha Gohel TEL 44-116-252-9552. B&W page GBP 650; trim 187 x 256. Circ: 30,000.

150 USA
PSYCHOLOGISTS FOR SOCIAL RESPONSIBILITY. NEWSLETTER. Text in English. 1982. q. USD 40 to members. **Document type:** *Newsletter.* **Description:** Networking newsletter for professional psychologists, students of psychology, and others interested in conflict resolution and prevention of war.
Indexed: e-psyche.
Published by: Psychologists for Social Responsibility, 2607 Connecticut Ave, N W, Washington, DC 20008. TEL 202-745-7084. Ed. Anne Anderson.

PSYCHOLOGY AND AGING. see *GERONTOLOGY AND GERIATRICS*

150 IND ISSN 0971-3336
PSYCHOLOGY AND DEVELOPING SOCIETIES. Text in English. 1989. biennial. INR 325 to individuals; INR 620 to institutions; USD 14 SAARC to individuals; USD 24 SAARC to institutions; INR 185 newsstand/cover to individuals; INR 355 newsstand/cover to institutions; USD 10 newsstand/cover SAARC to individuals; USD 14 newsstand/cover SAARC to institutions (effective 2002). adv. bk.rev. abstr. back issues avail.; reprints avail. *Refereed.* **Document type:** *Journal, Academic/Scholarly.* **Description:** Provides an international forum for psychologists concerned with problems of developing societies. Publishes theoretical, empirical, and review papers that further our understanding of the problems of these societies.
Indexed: Documentatieblad, IMFL, Indian Psychol.Abstr., Intl.Bibl.Soc.Sci., Lang.& Lang.Behav.Abstr., Per.Islam. (1992-), PsycInfo, Psychol.Abstr. (1989-), SOPODA, Soc.Serv.Abstr., Sociol.Abstr., e-psyche.
—BLDSC (6946.535321).
Published by: (University of Allahabad, Center for Advanced Study in Psychology), Sage Publications India Pvt. Ltd., M-32 Market, Greater Kailash-1, PO Box 4215, New Delhi 110 024, India. TEL 91-11-6419884, 91-11-6444958, FAX 91-11-6472426, sageindia@sagepub.com, http://indiasage.com/jdisp.asp?id=09713336. Ed. R C Tripathi. Pub. Tejeshwar Singh. Adv. contact Sunanda Ghosh. page USD 75. Circ: 500. **Affiliates:** Sage Publications Ltd.; Sage Publications, Inc.

370.15 USA
BF1 CODEN: PYCHBR
PSYCHOLOGY & EDUCATION; an interdisciplinary journal. Text in English. 1964. q. USD 22; USD 26.50 foreign (effective 1999). adv. bk.rev. reprint service avail. from PQC,PSC,SCH. *Refereed.* **Document type:** *Journal, Academic/Scholarly.* **Description:** Devoted to the basic research, theory and techniques in the general field of psychology.
Formerly (until vol.38, 2001): Psychology (0033-3077)
Related titles: Microform ed.: (from PQC); Online - full text ed.: (from Institute for Scientific Information).
Indexed: ASCA, AgeLine, Arts & Hum.Cit.Ind. (coverage dropped), Biol.Abstr., C.I.J.E. (coverage dropped), Commun.Abstr., Curr.Cont., High.Educ.Abstr., Int.Polit.Sci.Abstr., Lang.& Lang.Behav.Abstr., PsycInfo, Psychol.Abstr. (1965-), Rel.Ind.One, Rel.Ind.Two, SSCI, e-psyche.
—BLDSC (6946.535200), IDS, ingenta, KNAW, Linda Hall.
Published by: Institute for Leadership and Organization Effectiveness, 1409 Mt Ayr, Bowling Green, KY 42101. TEL 502-745-2343, 270-842-3436, FAX 502-842-0432, 270-842-0432. Eds. Cash J Kowalski TEL 803-536-7133, Dr. Joel Snell, Joseph Cangemi. R&P, Adv. contact Cash J Kowalski TEL 803-536-7133. Circ: 1,100.

155 CHE ISSN 0887-0446
R726.7 CODEN: PSHEE4
PSYCHOLOGY & HEALTH; an international journal. Text in English. 1987. bi-m. GBP 79, USD 96, EUR 106 to individuals; GBP 534, USD 702, EUR 711 to institutions; GBP 1,068, USD 1,278, EUR 1,424 to corporations (effective 2002). adv. illus. reprint service avail. from PSC,SCH. *Refereed.* **Document type:** *Journal, Academic/Scholarly.* **Description:** Health psychology forum dealing with the psychological and social factors in the etiology and outcome of physical illnesses. Promotes physical well-being through health education, prevention and behavior change.
Related titles: Microform ed.; Online - full text ed.: (from Institute for Scientific Information).
Indexed: ASCA, AgeLine, Behav.Med.Abstr., CINAHL, Curr.Cont., ERA, Fam.Ind., Mult.Ed.Abstr., PsycInfo, Psychol.Abstr. (1987-), SSCI, Stud.Wom.Abstr., e-psyche.
—BLDSC (6946.535325), GNLM, ingenta. **CCC.**
Published by: Gordon and Breach - Harwood Academic (Subsidiary of: Taylor & Francis Group), PO Box 531, Lausanne 1000, Switzerland. TEL 41-21-6411280, FAX 41-21-6411281, info@gbhap.com, http://www.gbhap-us.com/journals/340/340-top.htm, http://www.gbhap.com. Ed. Paul Norman. **Subscr. addr. in US:** International Publishers Direct, PO Box 32160, Newark, NJ 07102. FAX 215-750-6343.

616.89 GBR
PSYCHOLOGY AND HEALTH SERIES. Text in English. a. GBP 79 to individuals (effective 2002); price varies. index. back issues avail. **Document type:** *Monographic series.*
Indexed: e-psyche.
Published by: Chapman & Hall Ltd. (Subsidiary of: International Thomson Publishing Group), Journals Department, Chapman & Hall, 2-6 Boundary Row, London SE1 8HN, United Kingdom. TEL 44-20-7865-0066, FAX 44-20-7522-9623, jhelp@chall.co.uk. Ed. Donald Marcer. **Dist. by:** International Thompson Publishing Services Ltd., Cheriton House, North Way, Walworth Industrial Estate, Andover, Hants SP10 5BE, United Kingdom. TEL 44-1264-342713, FAX 44-1264-342807.

301.1 150 USA ISSN 0742-6046
HF5415.34 CODEN: PSMAFI
PSYCHOLOGY & MARKETING. Text in English. 1984. 8/yr. USD 925 in United States; USD 1,045 in Canada & Mexico; USD 1,147 elsewhere; USD 972 combined subscription in United States for print and online eds.; USD 1,092 combined subscription in Canada & Mexico for print and online eds.; USD 1,194 combined subscription elsewhere for print and online eds. (effective 2002). adv. illus. Index. back issues avail.; reprint service avail. from PSC,SCH. *Refereed.* **Document type:** *Academic/Scholarly.* **Description:** Promotes an understanding of the nature and operation of psychological principles, as applied to strategies in the marketing industry.
Related titles: Microform ed.: (from PQC); Online - full text ed.: ISSN 1520-6793. 1996. USD 925 in United States; USD 925 in Canada & Mexico; USD 925 elsewhere (effective 2002) (from EBSCO Publishing, Wiley InterScience, Factiva, Institute for Scientific Information).
Indexed: ABI Inform., ASCA, Abstr.Soc.Geront., AgeLine, B.P.I. (Jun.1905-), Commun.Abstr., Crim.Just.Abstr., Curr.Cont., Fam.Ind., PsycInfo, Psychol.Abstr. (1988-), SSCI, Viol.& Abuse Abstr., e-psyche.
—BLDSC (6946.535340), IDS, ingenta. **CCC.**
Published by: John Wiley & Sons, Inc., Journals (Subsidiary of: Wiley InterScience), 605 Third Ave, New York, NY 10158. TEL 212-850-6645, FAX 212-850-6021, subinfo@wiley.com, uscs-wis@wiley.com, http://www.wiley.com. Ed. Dr. Ronald J Cohen. Adv. contact Roberta Frederick. B&W page GBP 640, color page GBP 1,515; trim 153 x 229. Circ: 800. **Subscr. outside the Americas to:** John Wiley & Sons Ltd., Baffins Ln, Chichester, Sussex PO19 IUD, United Kingdom. TEL 44-1243-779777, FAX 44-1243-843232, cs-journals@wiley.co.uk.

302 USA ISSN 0885-7423
GV706
PSYCHOLOGY AND SOCIOLOGY OF SPORT: CURRENT SELECTED RESEARCH. Text in English. 1986. a. USD 37.50. index. back issues avail. **Description:** Research on contemporary problems of interest to behavioral scientists in the area of sport.
Indexed: e-psyche.
—BLDSC (6946.535430).
Published by: A M S Press, Inc., 56 E 13th St, New York, NY 10003. TEL 212-777-4700, FAX 212-995-5413. Eds. James H Humphrey, Lee Vander Velden.

616.89 ZAF
PSYCHOLOGY BULLETIN. Text in English. 1990. s-a. *Refereed.* **Document type:** *Academic/Scholarly.*
Formerly (until vol.3, no.1, 1993): Psychology Quarterly
Indexed: e-psyche.
Published by: (Department of Psychology, University of the Western Cape), Psychology Resource Centre, Private Bag X17, Bellville 7535, South Africa. TEL 27-21-959-2283, FAX 27-21-959-3515. Eds. Ashley van Niekerk, Norman Duncan. Circ: 1,000 (controlled).

345 CHE ISSN 1068-316X
CODEN: PCLAE2
PSYCHOLOGY, CRIME AND LAW. Text in English. 1994. 4/yr. GBP 68, USD 82, EUR 90 to individuals; GBP 159, USD 205, EUR 213 to institutions; GBP 268, USD 335, EUR 356 to corporations (effective 2002). back issues avail. *Refereed.* **Document type:** *Journal, Academic/Scholarly.* **Description:** Aims to promote the study and application of psychological approaches to crime, criminal and civil law, and the influence of law on behavior.
Related titles: Online - full text ed.: (from Institute for Scientific Information).
Indexed: ASCA, Crim.Just.Abstr., Curr.Cont., PsycInfo, SSCI, e-psyche.
—BLDSC (6946.535550), IDS, Infotrieve, ingenta. **CCC.**
Published by: Gordon and Breach - Harwood Academic (Subsidiary of: Taylor & Francis Group), PO Box 531, Lausanne 1000, Switzerland. TEL 41-21-6411280, FAX 41-21-6411281, info@gbhap.com, http://www.gbhap.com/journals/394/394-top.htm. Ed. Clive E Hollin. **Subscr. addr. in US:** International Publishers Direct, PO Box 32160, Newark, NJ 07102. FAX 215-750-6343.

152.4 GBR ISSN 1461-6661
▼ **PSYCHOLOGY, EVOLUTION AND GENDER.** Text in English. 1999. 3/yr. GBP 52, USD 85 to individuals; GBP 216, USD 358 to institutions (effective 2002). adv. bk.rev. back issues avail. *Refereed.* **Document type:** *Academic/Scholarly.* **Description:** Examines the psychology of gender-specific behaviors, including gender roles, gender differences and gender relations.
Related titles: Online - full text ed.: ISSN 1470-1073 (from CatchWord Ltd., EBSCO Publishing, RoweCom Information Quest, Swets Blackwell).
Indexed: e-psyche.
—BLDSC (6946.535586), CatchWord.
Published by: Routledge (Subsidiary of: Taylor & Francis Group), 11 New Fetter Ln, London EC4P 4EE, United Kingdom. TEL 44-207-842-2001, journals@routledge.com, http://journals.routledge.com/. Eds. David Buss, Paula Nicolson. R&P Sally Sweet. **Subscr. in US & Canada to:** Routledge, Taylor & Francis Ltd, 29 W 35th St, New York, NY 10001-2299. TEL 212-216-7800; **Subscr. to:** Subscriptions, PO Box 362, Abingdon, Oxon OX14 3WB, United Kingdom. TEL 44-1235-401060, FAX 44-1235-401075.

616.89 GBR ISSN 1354-8506
R726.5 CODEN: PHMEFL
PSYCHOLOGY, HEALTH & MEDICINE. Text in English. 1996. q. GBP 71, USD 117 to individuals; GBP 259, USD 425 to institutions (effective 2002). *Refereed.* **Document type:** *Academic/Scholarly.* **Description:** Provides a forum to report on issues of psychology and health in practice.
Related titles: Online - full text ed.: ISSN 1465-3966 (from CatchWord Ltd., EBSCO Publishing, O C L C Online Computer Library Center, Inc., RoweCom Information Quest, ProQuest Information & Learning, Swets Blackwell).
Indexed: ASSIA, CINAHL, Environ.Sci.Poll.Mgmt., Lang.& Lang.Behav.Abstr., Pollut.Abstr., PsycInfo, Risk Abstr., SOPODA, Saf.Sci.Abstr., Soc.Serv.Abstr., Sociol.Abstr., e-psyche.
—BLDSC (6946.535588), CatchWord, Infotrieve. **CCC.**
Published by: Carfax Publishing Limited (Subsidiary of: Taylor & Francis Group), PO Box 25, Abingdon, Oxon OX14 3UE, United Kingdom. TEL 44-1235-401000, FAX 44-1235-401550, enquiries@carfax.co.uk, enquiry@tandf.co.uk, http://www.carfax.co.uk/phm-ad.htm. Ed. Dr. Lorraine Sherr. Pub. Michael Gallico.

P

150 ESP ISSN 1137-9685
PSYCHOLOGY IN SPAIN. Text in English. 1998. a. USD 15 to individuals; USD 25 to institutions. **Document type:** *Academic/Scholarly.* **Description:** Disseminates selected articles published in Colegio Oficial de Psicologos (COP - Spanish Psychological Association) journals.
Indexed: e-psyche.
—CINDOC.
Published by: Colegio Oficial de Psicologos. Espana, Secretaria Estatal, Claudio Coello, 46, 2o Dcha., Madrid 28001, Spain. TEL 34-91-435-5212, FAX 34-91-577-9172, psyspain@correo.cop.es, http://www.cop.es/publicaciones/psyspain/. Ed. Jose Ramon Fernandez Hermida.

370.15 USA ISSN 0033-3085
LB1101
PSYCHOLOGY IN THE SCHOOLS. Text in English. 1964. q. USD 325 in United States; USD 367 in Canada & Mexico; USD 367 elsewhere; USD 342 combined subscription in United States for print and online eds.; USD 384 combined subscription in Canada & Mexico for print and online eds.; USD 384 combined subscription elsewhere for print and online eds. (effective 2002). adv. bk.rev. bibl, illus, abstr. index. back issues avail.; reprint service avail. from PSC,SCH. *Refereed.* **Document type:** *Journal, Academic/Scholarly.* **Description:** Provides information devoted to research, opintion, and practice.
Related titles: Microform ed.: (from PQC); Online - full text ed.: ISSN 1520-6807. USD 325 in United States; USD 325 in Canada & Mexico; USD 325 elsewhere (effective 2002) (from EBSCO Publishing, Wiley InterScience, Institute for Scientific Information).
Indexed: ASCA, Adol.Ment.Hlth.Abstr., AgeLine, C.I.J.E., Cont.Pg.Educ., Curr.Cont., ERA, Educ.Ind. (Jul.1983-), Except.Child Educ.Abstr., Fam.Ind., IBR, IBZ, IMFL, Ind.Philos., Lang.& Lang.Behav.Abstr., Mult.Ed.Abstr., PsycInfo, Psychol.Abstr. (1965-), SOMA, SOPODA, SSCI, Sociol.Abstr., Sp.Ed.Needs Abstr., Tech.Educ.Abstr., e-psyche.
—BLDSC (6946.536400), IDS, Infotrieve, ingenta. **CCC.**
Published by: John Wiley & Sons, Inc., Journals (Subsidiary of: Wiley InterScience), 605 Third Ave, New York, NY 10158. TEL 212-850-6645, FAX 212-850-6021, uscs-wis@wiley.com, http://www.wiley.com. Ed. Dr. Gerald B Fuller. adv.: B&W page GBP 640, color page GBP 1,515; trim 172 x 254. Circ: 1,700. **Subscr. outside the Americas to:** John Wiley & Sons Ltd., Baffins Ln, Chichester, Sussex PO19 IUD, United Kingdom. TEL 44-1243-779777, FAX 44-1243-843232, cs-journals@wiley.co.uk.

PSYCHOLOGY OF ADDICTIVE BEHAVIORS. see *DRUG ABUSE AND ALCOHOLISM*

THE PSYCHOLOGY OF EDUCATION REVIEW. see *EDUCATION*

152.5 USA ISSN 0079-7421
BF683 CODEN: PYLMAI
PSYCHOLOGY OF LEARNING AND MOTIVATION: ADVANCES IN RESEARCH AND THEORY. Text in English. 1967. irreg., latest vol.38, 1998. reprint service avail. from SCH,PSC,ISI. **Document type:** *Monographic series.*
Related titles: Online - full text ed.: (from Institute for Scientific Information).
Indexed: ASCA, Educ.Ind. (Jun.1983-), IBZ, Ind.Philos., SSCI, e-psyche.
—BLDSC (6946.535700), ingenta. **CCC.**
Published by: Academic Press, Inc., Journal Division (Subsidiary of: Harcourt Brace & Company), 525 B St, Ste 1900, San Diego, CA 92101-4495. TEL 619-231-0926, FAX 619-699-6715. Ed. K W Spence. **Subscr. to:** Order Dept., 6277 Sea Harbor Dr, 4th Fl, Orlando, FL 32887. TEL 800-321-5068.

155 USA ISSN 1524-9220
▼ **PSYCHOLOGY OF MEN & MASCULINITY.** Text in English. 2000. s-a. USD 56 domestic to non-members; USD 63.50 foreign to non-members; USD 36 domestic to members; USD 41 foreign to members; USD 140 domestic to institutions; USD 156 foreign to institutions (effective 2001). **Description:** Devoted to the dissemination of research, theory and clinical scholarship that advances the discipline of the psychology of men and masculinity.
—BLDSC (6946.535760).
Published by: American Psychological Association, 750 First St., N.E., Washington, DC 20002-4242. TEL 800-374-2721, 202-336-5600, FAX 202-336-5568, subscriptions@apa.org, http://www.apa.org/journals/men.html. Ed. David Lisak.

PSYCHOLOGY OF MUSIC. see *MUSIC*

150 613.71 NLD ISSN 1469-0292
▼ **PSYCHOLOGY OF SPORT & EXERCISE.** Text in English. 2000. q. EUR 128 in Europe to individuals; JPY 16,900 in Japan to individuals; USD 143 elsewhere to individuals; EUR 254 in Europe to institutions; JPY 33,700 in Japan to institutions; USD 284 elsewhere to institutions (effective 2002). back issues avail. *Refereed.* **Document type:** *Journal, Academic/Scholarly.* **Description:** Provides an international forum for scholarly reports in the psychology of sport and exercise.
Related titles: Online - full text ed.: (from ingenta, ScienceDirect).
—BLDSC (6946.536590).
Published by: (European Federation of Sport Psychology DEU), Elsevier Science BV, Sara Burgerhartstraat 25, Amsterdam 1055 KV, Netherlands. TEL 31-20-485-2911, FAX 31-20-485-2457, nlinfo-f@elsevier.nl, http://www.elsevier.com/locate/psychsport, http://www.elsevier.nl. Ed. S Biddle.

150 347.052 USA
THE PSYCHOLOGY OF THE AMERICAN JURY. Text in English. 1987. base vol. plus a. updates. USD 55. Supplement avail. **Description:** Discusses problems faced by lawyers in jury trials and offers practical solutions.
Indexed: e-psyche.
Published by: Lexis Law Publishing (Subsidiary of: Reed Elsevier plc), PO Box 7587, Charlottesville, VA 22906-7587. TEL 804-972-7600, 800-562-1197, FAX 804-972-7666, llp.customer.support@lexis-nexis.com, http://www.lexislawpublishing.com. Ed. Jeffrey T Frederick.

155 305.4 GBR ISSN 0361-6843
HQ1206 CODEN: PWOQDY
PSYCHOLOGY OF WOMEN QUARTERLY. Text in English. 1976. q. GBP 135 to institutions in UK & Europe; USD 200 to institutions in the Americas & Caribbean; GBP 135 elsewhere to institutions (effective 2002). adv. bk.rev. illus. Index. back issues avail.; reprint service avail. from SWZ,SCH,PSC. *Refereed.* **Document type:** *Academic/Scholarly.* **Description:** Publishes current and important findings in the field of psychology of women and gender.
Related titles: Microform ed.: (from PQC); Online - full text ed.: (from Gale Group, Factiva, Institute for Scientific Information, RoweCom Information Quest).
Indexed: ASCA, ASSIA, Abstr.Anthropol., Adol.Ment.Hlth.Abstr., AgeLine, Amer.Bibl.Slavic & E.Eur.Stud., C.I.J.E., Child Devel.Abstr., Crim.Just.Abstr., Curr.Cont., Curr.Lit.Fam.Plan., ERA, Environ.Sci.Poll.Mgmt., Fam.Ind., Fem.Per. (1982-), High.Educ.Abstr., Human Resour.Abstr., IMFL, Ind.Philos., Intl.Bibl.Soc.Sci., Lang.& Lang.Behav.Abstr., Mult.Ed.Abstr., P C I, Pollut.Abstr., PsycInfo, Psychol.Abstr. (1976-), Res.High.Educ.Abstr., Risk Abstr., SOPODA, SSCI, Saf.Sci.Abstr., Sage Pub.Admin.Abstr., Sage Race Rel.Abstr., Sage Urb.Stud.Abstr., Soc.Sci.Ind. (Dec.1982-), Soc.Serv.Abstr., Soc.Work Res.& Abstr., Sociol.Abstr., Sp.Ed.Needs Abstr., Stud.Wom.Abstr., Wom.Stud.Abstr. (1976-), Wom.Stud.Ind., e-psyche.
—BLDSC (6946.538000), IDS, ingenta. **CCC.**
Published by: (Division 35, American Psychological Association USA), Cambridge University Press, Edinburgh Bldg, Shaftesbury Rd, Cambridge CB2 2RU, United Kingdom. FAX 44-1223-315052, information@cambridge.org, http://www.uk.cambridge.org/journals/pmu. Ed. Jacquelyn W White. R&P Linda Nicol. Adv. contact Rebecca Symons.

150 GBR ISSN 1466-3724
PSYCHOLOGY OF WOMEN SECTION REVIEW. Text in English. 1988. s-a.
Formerly (until 1998): British Psychological Society. Psychology of Women Section. Newsletter (1362-6345)
—BLDSC (6946.538500).
Published by: The British Psychological Society, St Andrews House, 48 Princess Rd E, Leicester LE1 7DR, United Kingdom. TEL 44-116-254-9568, FAX 44-116-247-0787, psychologist@bps.org.uk, http://www.bps.org.uk/publications/journals.cfm.

150 USA ISSN 1076-8971
K16
PSYCHOLOGY, PUBLIC POLICY, AND LAW. Text in English. 1995. q. USD 61 domestic to non-members; USD 76 foreign to non-members; USD 31 domestic to members; USD 41 foreign to members; USD 136 domestic to institutions; USD 168 foreign to institutions (effective 2001). adv. illus. reprints avail. *Refereed.* **Document type:** *Academic/Scholarly.* **Description:** Links psychological science with policy and law. Evaluates the contributions of psychology to policy and law issues, assesses policy alternatives, and articulates research needs in psychology that address policy and legal issues.
Related titles: Online - full text ed.: (from LexisNexis, Institute for Scientific Information).
Indexed: ASCA, Crim.Just.Abstr., Curr.Cont., PsycInfo, SSCI, e-psyche.
—BLDSC (6946.536170), IDS, ingenta. **CCC.**
Published by: American Psychological Association, 750 First St., N.E., Washington, DC 20002-4242. TEL 202-336-5600, 800-374-2721, FAX 202-336-5568, subscriptions@apa.org, http://www.apa.org/journals/law.html. Ed. Jane Goodman-Delahunty. Circ: 2,300.

150 PAK ISSN 0033-3093
PSYCHOLOGY QUARTERLY. Text in English. 1964. q. PKR 30, USD 15. bk.rev. charts, stat.
Formerly: Journal of Psychology
Indexed: CINAHL, Psychol.Abstr., e-psyche.
Published by: Government College, Psychology Department, Lahore, Pakistan. Ed. Syed Azhar Ali Rizvi. Circ: 300.

150 GBR ISSN 0960-2925
PSYCHOLOGY RESEARCH. Text in English. q. GBP 5. adv. bk.rev. **Document type:** *Academic/Scholarly.*
Formerly (until 1990): Psychology Research on Placement
Indexed: e-psyche.
Address: Salomons Centre, Southborough, Broomhill Rd, Tunbridge Wells, Kent TN3 0TG, United Kingdom. TEL 44-1892-515152, FAX 44-1892-539102. Adv. contact Jenny Miah.

150 GBR ISSN 1354-1129
PSYCHOLOGY REVIEW. Text in English. 1994. 4/yr. GBP 18.95 in United Kingdom; GBP 26 in Europe; GBP 31 elsewhere (effective Sep. 2001). adv. **Document type:** *Academic/Scholarly.*
Indexed: e-psyche.
—BLDSC (6946.536350), Infotrieve. **CCC.**
Published by: Philip Allan Updates, Market Pl, Deddington, Banbury, Oxon OX15 0SE, United Kingdom. TEL 44-1869-338652, FAX 44-1869-338803, sales@philipallan.co.uk, http://www.philipallan.co.uk. Ed. Patrick Fox. R&P Ceri Jenkins.

150 USA ISSN 0033-3107
BF1 CODEN: PSTOAM
PSYCHOLOGY TODAY. Text in English. 1967-1989 (Dec.); resumed 1991. bi-m. USD 18 domestic; USD 26 in Canada; USD 30 elsewhere; USD 3.50 newsstand/cover domestic; CND 3 newsstand/cover in Canada; GBP 2.75 newsstand/cover in United Kingdom (effective 2000). adv. bk.rev. bibl, charts, illus, stat. index. reprint service avail. from PSC,SCH. *Refereed.* **Document type:** *Consumer.* **Description:** Explores the emotional, physical and spiritual aspects of daily life.
Related titles: CD-ROM ed.: (from ProQuest Information & Learning); Microfiche ed.: (from NBI); Online - full text ed.: (from ProQuest Information & Learning, The Dialog Corporation, Gale Group, Northern Light Technology, Inc., H. W. Wilson, Factiva).
Indexed: ABI Inform., ASSIA, Acad.Ind., AgeLine, Biol.Dig., Bk.Rev.Dig. (Jan.1983-Oct.1989), Bk.Rev.Ind. (1973-), CBCA Ref., CCR, Can.B.P.I., Can.Per.Ind. (Jan.1988-), Child.Bk.Rev.Ind. (1973-), Crim.Just.Abstr., Curr.Cont. (coverage dropped), Curr.Lit.Fam.Plan., Except.Child Educ.Abstr., Excerp.Med., Film Lit.Ind. (1983-), Fut.Surv., G.Soc.Sci.& Rel.Per.Lit., High.Educ.Curr.Aware.Bull., Hlth.Ind., Ind.Per.Art.Relat.Law, L.R.I., Mag.Ind., Mid.East: Abstr.& Ind., Music Ind., P C I, PMR, Peace Res.Abstr., Pers.Lit., R.G. (Jan.1983-), R.G.Abstr. (Jan.1983-), Rel.Ind.One, Rel.Ind.Two, Russ.Acad.Sci.Bibl., SSCI (coverage dropped), Soc.Sci.Ind. (Oct.1982-), Sportsearch, TOM, WMB, e-psyche.
—BLDSC (6946.537000), CISTI, ingenta.
Published by: Sussex Publishers Inc., 49 E 21st St, 11th Fl, New York, NY 10010. TEL 212-260-7210, FAX 212-260-7445. Ed. Robert Epstein. Circ: 350,000. **Dist. in UK by:** Comag, Tavistock Works, Tavistock Rd, W Drayton, Middx UB7 7QX, United Kingdom. TEL 44-1895-433600, FAX 44-189-543-3606.

P

150 NLD ISSN 0033-3115
DE PSYCHOLOOG. Text in Dutch. 1966. m. NLG 105 to individuals; NLG 195 to institutions (effective 2000). adv. bk.rev. abstr, bibl. index, cum.index. **Document type:** *Academic/Scholarly.*
Indexed: PsycInfo, Psychol.Abstr. (1972-), e-psyche.
—BLDSC (6946.539300), KNAW.
Published by: (Nederlands Instituut van Psychologen/Netherlands Psychological Association), Van Gorcum en Co. B.V., PO Box 43, Assen 9400 AA, Netherlands. TEL 31-592-379555, FAX 31-592-379552, assen@vgorcum.nl, http://www.vgorcum.nl. Circ: 11,000.

616.89 DEU ISSN 0935-2937
PSYCHOMED. Text in German. 1989. q. DEM 99; DEM 120.50 foreign; DEM 79.20 to students (effective 2000). **Document type:** *Academic/Scholarly.*
Indexed: Ind.Philos., e-psyche.
—GNLM.
Published by: Ernst Reinhardt Verlag, Kemnatenstr 46, Munich 80639, Germany. TEL 49-89-1780160, FAX 49-89-17801630.

150 CAN ISSN 0033-3123
BF1
PSYCHOMETRIKA; a journal devoted to the development of psychology as a quantitative rational science. Text in English. 1936. q. USD 100. adv. bk.rev. abstr, bibl, charts, illus. index. reprint service avail. from PQC,PSC,SCH. *Refereed.* **Document type:** *Academic/Scholarly.*
Related titles: Microform ed.: (from PQC); Online - full text ed.: (from Institute for Scientific Information).
Indexed: ASCA, Biol.Abstr., C.C.M.J., C.I.J.E., Child Devel.Abstr., Commun.Abstr., Compumath, Curr.Cont. (1984-), Curr.Ind.Stat., Ergon.Abstr., IBR, IBZ, Ind.Philos., J.Cont.Quant.Meth., Math.R., Mid.East: Abstr.& Ind., P C I, PsycInfo, Psychol.Abstr. (1936-), Psycscan A.P., Russ.Acad.Sci.Bibl., SSCI, Stat.Theor.Meth.Abstr. (1984-), Zent.Math., e-psyche.
—BLDSC (6946.540000), CISTI, GNLM, IDS, ingenta. **CCC.**
Published by: Psychometric Society, c/o Ontario Institute for Studies in Education, 252 Bloor St W, Toronto, ON M5S 1V6, Canada. http://www.psychometrika.org. Ed. Ulf Bockenholt. Adv. contact Cynthia Null. Circ: 2,200. **Subscr. to:** Dr. Ralph DeAyala, University of Maryland, Dept of Measurement, Statistics and Evaluation, 1230 Benjamin Bldg, College Park, MD 20742-1115.

P

PSYCHOMUSICOLOGY; a journal of research in music cognition. see *MUSIC*

150 USA ISSN 1069-9384
BF1 CODEN: PBUREN
PSYCHONOMIC BULLETIN & REVIEW. Text in English. 1973; N.S. 1994. q. USD 130 in United States; USD 139 rest of world (effective 2001). adv. illus. Index. back issues avail.; reprint service avail. from PQC,PSC,SCH. *Refereed.* **Document type:** *Bulletin, Academic/Scholarly.* **Description:** Publishes theoretical and review articles on topics in all areas of experimental psychology.
Formerly (until 1994): Psychonomic Society. Bulletin (0090-5054)
Related titles: Microform ed.: N.S. (from NRP,PQC); Online - full text ed.: (from CatchWord Ltd., Institute for Scientific Information).
Indexed: ASCA, AgeLine, Biol.Abstr., Curr.Adv.Ecol.Sci., Curr.Cont., Curr.Ind.Stat., Ergon.Abstr., High.Educ.Abstr., IBZ, IMFL, Ind.Med. (1994-), Ind.Philos., Lang.& Lang.Behav.Abstr., M.L.A., MLA Intl.Bibl., Mid.East: Abstr.& Ind., PsycInfo, Psychol.Abstr., SOPODA, SSCI, Sociol.Abstr., Sport Fish.Abstr., e-psyche.
—BLDSC (6946.540550), CASDDS, GNLM, IDS, ingenta. **CCC.**
Published by: Psychonomic Society, Inc., 1710 Fortview Rd, Austin, TX 78704. TEL 512-462-2442, FAX 512-462-1101, psysoc@sig.net, jbellquist@psychonomic.org, http://www.psychonomic.org. Ed. John T Wixted. R&P Cinnamon Nemec. Adv. contact Robert Sanford. page USD 190; trim 10.75 x 8. Circ: 2,200.

158 AUT ISSN 1434-1883
PSYCHOPRAXIS; Zeitschrift fuer praktische Psychiatrie und Grenzgebiete. Text in German. 1998. bi-m. EUR 47.70 domestic; EUR 45.10 in Germany; EUR 8 newsstand/cover foreign (effective 2002). back issues avail. **Document type:** *Journal, Academic/Scholarly.*
Related titles: Online - full text ed.: (from Springer LINK).
Indexed: e-psyche.
Published by: Springer-Verlag Wien (Subsidiary of: BertelsmannSpringer), Sachsenplatz 4-6, PO Box 89, Vienna, W 1201, Austria. TEL 43-1-3302415-0, FAX 43-1-330242665, journals@springer.at, http://www.springer.at/psychopraxis. Eds. Hans Zapotoczky, Walter Poeldinger. R&P Angela Foessl TEL 43-1-3302415517. Adv. contact Michael Katzenberger TEL 43-1-3302415220. **Subscr. in N. America to:** Springer-Verlag, Journals. TEL 212-460-1500, FAX 212-473-6272, orders@springer-ny.com.

301.1 150 CHE ISSN 1013-5987
PSYCHOSCOPE. Text in French, German. 1980. 10/yr. CHF 72; CHF 43 to students. adv. bk.rev. **Document type:** *Bulletin.*
Formerly: Schweizer Psychologen. Bulletin
Indexed: e-psyche.
Published by: Foederation der Schweizer Psychologen (FSP), Administration Psychoscope, Choisystr 11, Bern, 14 3000, Switzerland. TEL 41-31-3820856, FAX 41-31-3820857. Ed. Beatrice Thelen. Circ: 4,400.

301.1 150 DEU ISSN 0171-3434
PSYCHOSOZIAL; Zeitschrift fuer Analyse, Praevention und Therapie psychosozialer Konflikte und Krankheiten. Text in German. 1978. q. DEM 98; DEM 49 to students (effective 2000). adv. bk.rev. **Document type:** *Academic/Scholarly.*
Indexed: e-psyche.
—GNLM.
Published by: Psychosozial Verlag, Friedrichstr 35, Giessen 35392, Germany. TEL 49-641-77819, FAX 49-641-77742, psychosozial-verlag@t-online.de. Ed. Hans-Juergen Wirth. Pub. Hans Juergen Wirth. R&P Stephan Vogel. Circ: 4,500.

PSYCHOTERAPIA. see *MEDICAL SCIENCES—Psychiatry And Neurology*

PSYCHOTHERAPEUT. see *MEDICAL SCIENCES—Psychiatry And Neurology*

616.89 DEU ISSN 0946-3453
DIE PSYCHOTHERAPEUTIN. Text in German. 1994. s-a. DEM 45 (effective 1999). **Document type:** *Academic/Scholarly.*
Indexed: e-psyche.
—GNLM.
Published by: Psychiatrie Verlag GmbH, Thomas-Mann-Str 49A, Bonn 53111, Germany. TEL 49-228-72534-0, FAX 49-228-7253420. Ed. Dr. Ulrike Hoffmann Richter.

616.89 AUT ISSN 0943-1950
CODEN: PSFOEO
PSYCHOTHERAPIE FORUM. Text in German. 1993. q. EUR 57.50 domestic; EUR 55.80 in Germany; EUR 15 newsstand/cover foreign (effective 2002). back issues avail. **Document type:** *Journal, Academic/Scholarly.*
Related titles: Online - full text ed.: (from Springer LINK).
Indexed: IBZ, Ind.Philos., e-psyche.
—GNLM.
Published by: Springer-Verlag Wien (Subsidiary of: BertelsmannSpringer), Sachsenplatz 4-6, PO Box 89, Vienna, W 1201, Austria. TEL 43-1-3302415-0, FAX 43-1-330242665, journals@springer.at, http://www.springer.at/psychotherapie. R&P Angela Foessl TEL 43-1-3302415517. Adv. contact Michael Katzenberger TEL 43-1-3302415220. **Subscr. in N. America to:** Springer-Verlag, Journals, 175 Fifth Ave, New York, NY 10010. TEL 212-460-1500, FAX 212-473-6272, orders@springer-ny.com, http://www.springer-ny.com.

616.89 CHE ISSN 0251-737X
CODEN: PSYTEW
PSYCHOTHERAPIES. Text in French. 1981. 3/yr. CHF 100, EUR 64.93 to individuals; CHF 160, EUR 103.89 to institutions (effective 2002). adv. bk.rev. reprint service avail. from PQC. **Document type:** *Journal, Academic/Scholarly.*
Indexed: Int.Nurs.Ind., e-psyche.
—BLDSC (6946.558400), EMDOCS, GNLM. **CCC.**
Published by: Editions Medecine et Hygiene, Case Postale 456, Geneva, 4 1211, Switzerland. TEL 41-22-7029311, FAX 41-22-7029355, abonnements@medhyg.ch, http://www.medhyg.ch. Circ: 900.

616.89 USA ISSN 0033-3204
RC475 CODEN: PSYOAD
PSYCHOTHERAPY. Variant title: Psychotherapy: Theory, Research, Practice Training. Text in English. 1963. q. USD 75 domestic to individuals; USD 90 foreign to individuals; USD 95 domestic to institutions; USD 105 foreign to institutions; USD 35 domestic to students; USD 50 foreign to students (effective 2000). adv. bk.rev. charts. index. reprint service avail. from PQC,PSC,SCH,ISI. *Refereed.* **Document type:** *Academic/Scholarly.* **Description:** Offers a wide variety of articles relevant to the field of psychotherapy, both theoretical contributions and research studies.
Related titles: Online - full text ed.: (from Institute for Scientific Information).
Indexed: ASCA, Adol.Ment.Hlth.Abstr., AgeLine, Arts & Hum.Cit.Ind. (coverage dropped), Biol.Abstr., Chem.Abstr., Chem.Indus.Notes, Crim.Just.Abstr., Curr.Cont., Excerp.Med., PsycInfo, Psychol.Abstr. (1963-), Psycscan C.P., SSCI, e-psyche.
—BLDSC (6946.558530), GNLM, IDS, ingenta, KNAW.
Published by: American Psychological Association, Division of Psychotherapy, 1390 S. Dixie Hwy. Ste. 2222, Coral Gables, FL 33146-2946. TEL 305-669-6757, FAX 305-669-3289. Ed. Wade H Silverman. Pub. C L Hutson. R&P, Adv. contact Jane Sinagub. page USD 350; trim 254 x 170. Circ: 6,900.

616.89 USA ISSN 0164-078X
PSYCHOTHERAPY DIGEST. Text in English. 1976. bi-m. USD 15. bk.rev. back issues avail.
Indexed: e-psyche.
Address: PO Box 1167, Del Mar, CA 92014. Ed. Victor Kops. Circ: 1,000.

616.89156 USA ISSN 1535-573X
RC488.5
PSYCHOTHERAPY NETWORKER. Text in English. 1982. bi-m. USD 24 domestic; USD 30 foreign (effective 2001 & 2002). adv. bk.rev. illus. back issues avail.; reprints avail. **Document type:** *Newsletter, Trade.* **Description:** Professional journal for social workers, psychologists, therapists and educators.
Formerly (until Mar. 2001): Family Therapy Networker (0739-0882)
Indexed: Alt.Press Ind., Soc.Work Res.& Abstr., e-psyche.
—BLDSC, ingenta.
Published by: Family Therapy Network, Inc., 7705 13th St, N W, Washington, DC 20012. TEL 202-829-2452, FAX 202-726-7983, info@psychnetworker.org, http://www.familytherapynetworker.com. Ed. Richard Simon. R&P Brett Topping TEL 202-291-4259. Adv. contact Karen Sundquist. B&W page USD 1,775, color page USD 2,375. Circ: 65,000. **Subscr. to:** 8528 Bradford Rd, Silver Spring, MD 20901. TEL 800-464-6607.

616.89 USA ISSN 0738-6176
CODEN: PSPAEW
THE PSYCHOTHERAPY PATIENT; a quarterly journal of attribute-focused practice. Text in English. 1984. s-a. USD 50 to individuals; USD 68 in Canada to individuals; USD 73 elsewhere to individuals; USD 125 to institutions; USD 169 in Canada to institutions; USD 181 elsewhere to institutions; USD 225 to libraries; USD 304 in Canada to libraries; USD 326 elsewhere to libraries (effective Aug. 2001). adv. bk.rev. back issues avail.; reprint service avail. from HAW. *Refereed.* **Document type:** *Journal, Academic/Scholarly.* **Description:** Devotes each issue to diagnostic, behavioral, and phenomenological groupings.
Related titles: Microfiche ed.: (from PQC); Microform ed.
Indexed: IMFL, Psychol.Abstr., Soc.Work Res.& Abstr., e-psyche.
—BLDSC (6946.559300), GNLM, Haworth, ingenta.
Published by: Haworth Press, Inc., 10 Alice St, Binghamton, NY 13904-1580. TEL 607-722-5857, 800-429-6784, FAX 607-722-6362, 800-895-0582, getinfo@haworthpressinc.com, http://www.haworthpress.com/journals/journallist.asp. Ed. E Mark Stern. Pub. William Cohen. R&P Ruthann Heath TEL 607-723-5857 ext 316. Adv. contact Jackie Blakeslee TEL 607-722-5857 ext 346. B&W page USD 315, color page USD 550; trim 6 x 8.5. Circ: 250.

370.15 616.8 USA
PSYCHOTHERAPY, RECOVERY AND PERSONAL GROWTH UPDATE. Text in English. 1987. m. USD 67 (effective 2001). bk.rev. abstr, charts, illus. back issues avail.
Formerly: Understanding People
Indexed: e-psyche.
Published by: Cromwell - Sloan Publishing Company, 63 Vine Rd, Stamford, CT 06905-2012. TEL 203-323-4810. Ed. Paul Sloan. Circ: 6,400.

616.89 USA ISSN 1050-3307
RC475
PSYCHOTHERAPY RESEARCH. Text in English. 1991. q. GBP 60, USD 80 to individuals; GBP 99, USD 135 to institutions; GBP 32, USD 40 to students (effective Mar. 2002). adv. back issues avail. *Refereed.* **Document type:** *Journal, Academic/Scholarly.* **Description:** Seeks to encourage the development of the field of psychotherapy research, foster the utilization of research findings in training, practice and policy formation, and enhance the scientific quality and social relevance of psychotherapy.
Related titles: Online - full text ed.: ISSN 1468-4381. GBP 89, USD 121 to institutions online only (effective Mar. 2002) (from HighWire Pr., Northern Light Technology, Inc., ProQuest Information & Learning, Swets Blackwell, Institute for Scientific Information, RoweCom Information Quest).
Indexed: ASCA, Curr.Cont., PsycInfo, Psychol.Abstr. (1991-), Ref.Zh., SSCI, e-psyche.
—BLDSC (6946.559430), GNLM, IDS, Infotrieve. **CCC.**
Published by: (Society for Psychotherapy Research), Oxford University Press, Academic Division, Great Clarendon St, Oxford OX2 6DP, United Kingdom. TEL 44-1865-267907, FAX 44-1865-267835, jnlorders@oup-usa.org, jnl.info@oup.co.uk, http://ptr.oupjournals.org/, http://www.oup.co.uk/journals. Pub. J Fox. adv.: page GBP 230, page USD 420. Circ: 1,260. **Subscr. outside N. America to:** Journals Marketing, Great Clarendon St, Oxford OX2 6DP, United Kingdom.

150 BEL ISSN 1245-2092
PSYCHOTROPES (PARIS); revue internationale des toxicomanies. Text in French. q. BEF 2,460 domestic; BEF 2,910 in the European Union; BEF 3,010 in Europe; BEF 3,260 elsewhere; BEF 980 newsstand/cover (effective 2000 - 2001). bk.rev. abstr, bibl. 128 p./no. *Refereed.* **Document type:** *Monographic series, Academic/Scholarly.*
Indexed: IBZ, e-psyche.
—BLDSC (6946.559532).
Published by: De Boeck Universite (Subsidiary of: De Boeck et Larcier S.A.), Rue des Minimes 39, Brussels 1000, Belgium. TEL 2-32-10482570, FAX 2-32-10-482650, http://www.deboeck.be. **Subscr. to:** Acces S.P.R.L., Fond Jean Paques 4, Louvain-la-Neuve 1348, Belgium. TEL 32-10-482500, FAX 32-10-482519.

150 GBR ISSN 1055-0143
PSYCOLOQUY; a refereed journal of peer commentary in psychology, neuroscience and cognitive science. Text in English. 1990. irreg. free. bk.rev. illus. Index. reprints avail. *Refereed.* **Document type:** *Academic/Scholarly.*
Media: Online - full text.
Indexed: PsycInfo, e-psyche.
Address: c/o Cognitive Sciences Centre, Dept. of Electronics & Computer Science,, Univ. of Southampton, Zepler Bldg, Highfield, Southampton SO17 1BJ, United Kingdom. psyc@pucc.princeton.edu, http://www.cogsci.soton.ac.uk/cgi/psyc/newpsy, http://www.cogsci.soton.ac.uk/~harnad/psyc.html. Ed., R&P Stevan Harnad.

PSYCSCAN: CLINICAL PSYCHOLOGY. see *PSYCHOLOGY—Abstracting, Bibliographies, Statistics*

150 DNK ISSN 0107-1211
PSYKE & LOGOS. Text in Danish; Abstracts in English. 1980. 2/yr. DKK 295 in the European Union; DKK 215 per issue in the European Union; DKK 236 elsewhere; DKK 172 per issue elsewhere (effective 2002). bk.rev. 400 p./no. back issues avail. **Document type:** *Journal, Academic/Scholarly.*
Indexed: PsycInfo, Psychol.Abstr. (1981-), e-psyche.
—BLDSC (6946.559790).
Published by: Dansk Psykologisk Forlag/Danish Psychological Publishers, Stockholmsgade 29, Copenhagen Oe 2100, Denmark. TEL 45-35-38-16-55, FAX 45-35-38-16-65, dk-psych@dpf.dk, http://www.dpf.dk. Ed. Benny Karpatschof. Circ: 600.

616.89 362.2 SWE ISSN 0033-3212
PSYKISK HAELSA/MENTAL HEALTH. Text in Swedish. 1960. q. SEK 260 to members (effective 1999). bk.rev. **Document type:** *Academic/Scholarly.*
Indexed: Psychol.Abstr., e-psyche.
—CISTI.
Published by: Svenska Foereningen foer Psykisk Haelsa/Swedish Association for Mental Health, Saltmaetargatan 5 2, Fack 3445, Stockholm 10369, Sweden. TEL 46-8-34-70-65, FAX 46-8-32-88-75, info@sfph.se, http://www.sfph.se. Ed. Eggert Nielsen. Circ: 6,000.

150 DNK ISSN 0900-5625
PSYKOLOGISK FORSKNINGSRAPPORT. Text in Danish; Summaries in English. 1983. irreg. free per issue.
Formerly (until 1984): Psykologisk Laboratorium. Forskningsrapport (0107-3060)
Indexed: e-psyche.
Published by: University of Copenhagen, Department of Psychology, Njalsgade 94, Copenhagen S 2300, Denmark. Ed. Benny Karpauschof. Circ: 200.

370.15 150 DNK ISSN 0906-219X
PSYKOLOGISK PAEDAGOGISK RAADGIVNING/ JOURNAL OF SCHOOL PSYCHOLOGY; tidsskrift for paedagogisk psykologi og raadgivning. Text in Danish. 1964. bi-m. DKK 330 in the European Union; DKK 264 elsewhere; DKK 80 per issue in the European Union; DKK 64 per issue elsewhere (effective 2002). adv. bk.rev. abstr, bibl. index. 80 p./no. Supplement avail.; back issues avail. **Document type:** *Journal, Academic/Scholarly.*
Formerly (until 1991): Skolepsykologi (0037-6493)
Indexed: C.I.J.E. (coverage dropped), Fam.Ind., PsycInfo, Psychol.Abstr. (1968-), SSCI (coverage dropped), Soc.Work Res.& Abstr., e-psyche.
Published by: Dansk Psykologisk Forlag/Danish Psychological Publishers, Stockholmsgade 29, Copenhagen Oe 2100, Denmark. TEL 45-35-38-16-55, FAX 45-35-38-16-65, palle.johansen@skolekom.dk; dk-psych@dpf.dk, http://www.dpf.dk. Ed. Palle Johansen. Circ: 1,400.

150 DNK ISSN 0906-2483
PSYKOLOGISK SET. Text in Danish. 1982. q. DKK 255 in the European Union; DKK 80 per issue in the European Union; DKK 264 elsewhere; DKK 64 per issue elsewhere (effective 2002). bk.rev. illus. **Document type:** *Journal, Academic/Scholarly.*
Formerly (until 1990): Psykologi (0107-8755)
Indexed: Psychol.Abstr., e-psyche.
—BLDSC.
Published by: Dansk Psykologisk Forlag/Danish Psychological Publishers, Stockholmsgade 29, Copenhagen Oe 2100, Denmark. TEL 45-35-38-16-55, FAX 45-35-38-16-65, http://www.dpf.dk/ defPSYKSET.htm. Ed. Charlotte Mathiassen.

150 SWE ISSN 0280-9702
PSYKOLOGTIDNINGEN. Text in Swedish. 1954. 21/yr. SEK 520 (effective 2001). adv. bk.rev. charts, illus. **Document type:** *Magazine, Trade.*
Formerly (until 1983): Psykolognytt/Psychologist News (0033-3220)
Published by: Sveriges Psykologfoerbund/Swedish Psychological Association, Box 3287, Stockholm 10365, Sweden. TEL 46-8-567-06-450, FAX 46-8-567-06-490, rr@psykologforbundet.se, http:// www.psykologforbundet.se/psykologforbundet1.html. Ed., Pub. Eva Brita Jaernefors. Adv. contact Rosa Maria Risberg. B&W page SEK 12,880, color page SEK 18,400; trim 185 x 269. Circ: 4,000.

150 HUN ISSN 0079-7456
BF636.A1
PSZICHOLOGIA A GYAKORLATBAN/PSYCHOLOGY IN THE PRACTICE. Text in Hungarian. 1963. irreg., latest vol.50, 1997. price varies. back issues avail. **Document type:** *Academic/Scholarly.*
Indexed: e-psyche.
Published by: Akademiai Kiado Rt., PO Box 245, Budapest 1519, Hungary. TEL 36-1-4648233, FAX 36-1-4648297, pp@akkert.hu, http://www.akkrt.hu.

150 HUN ISSN 0079-7464
PSZICHOLOGIAI TANULMANYOK/PSYCHOLOGICAL STUDIES. Text in Hungarian; Summaries in English, German. 1958. irreg., latest vol.18, 2000. price varies. back issues avail. **Document type:** *Academic/Scholarly.*
Indexed: Psychol.Abstr., Russ.Acad.Sci.Bibl., e-psyche.
Published by: Akademiai Kiado Rt., PO Box 245, Budapest 1519, Hungary. TEL 36-1-4648233, FAX 36-1-4648297, pp@akkrt.hu, http://www.akkrt.hu.

150 USA
PUBLICATIONS FOR THE ADVANCEMENT OF THEORY AND HISTORY IN PSYCHOLOGY*. Text in English. 1980. irreg. price varies. **Document type:** *Academic/Scholarly.*
Indexed: e-psyche.
Published by: Ablex Publishing Corporation (Subsidiary of: Greenwood Publishing Group Inc.), 88 Post Rd W, Westport, CT 06881. TEL 203-661-7602, FAX 203-661-0792. Ed. David Bakan.

PULSE OF THE PLANET. see *ENVIRONMENTAL STUDIES*

616.89 ITA ISSN 0390-0320
QUADRANGOLO. Text in Italian. 1974. q. ITL 45,000.
Indexed: e-psyche.
Published by: (Centro Studi Psicologici "Lo Spazio"), Bulzoni Editore, Via Dei Liburni, 14, Rome, RM 00185, Italy. Ed. Emiliana Mazzonis. **Co-sponsor:** Societa Italiana di Psicoterapia di Gruppo.

150 USA ISSN 0033-5010
BF173.A2
QUADRANT. Text in English. 1967. s-a. USD 32 to individuals; USD 32 to institutions; USD 39.95 foreign (effective 2000). adv. bk.rev. charts, illus. reprint service avail. from PSC,SCH. **Document type:** *Academic/Scholarly.*
Formerly: Journal of Contemporary Jungian Thought
Related titles: Online - full text ed.: (from Gale Group).
Indexed: M.L.A., Psychoanal.Abstr., Psychol.Abstr. (1985-), e-psyche.
—ingenta.
Published by: C.G. Jung Foundation for Analytical Psychology, Inc., 28 E 39th St, New York, NY 10016. TEL 212-697-6430, FAX 201-953-3989, TELEX 135-393. Ed. V Walter Odajnyk. R&P Janet Careswell. Adv. contact Arnold Devera. B&W page USD 350. Circ: 2,000 (controlled).

QUALE SCUOLA?; periodico di educazione per una scuola diversa. see *EDUCATION*

QUALITY OF LIFE NEWSLETTER. see *MEDICAL SCIENCES*

152 GBR ISSN 0272-4987
QP351 CODEN: QJEADQ
QUARTERLY JOURNAL OF EXPERIMENTAL PSYCHOLOGY. SECTION A: HUMAN EXPERIMENTAL PSYCHOLOGY. Text in English. 1948. q. GBP 51, USD 113 to individuals; GBP 259, USD 528 to institutions (effective 2002). adv. bk.rev. bibl, charts. index. reprint service avail. from PSC,SCH. *Refereed.* **Document type:** *Academic/Scholarly.* **Description:** Presents original papers in all branches of human experimental psychology without limitation.
Supersedes in part (in 1981): Quarterly Journal of Experimental Psychology (0033-555X)
Related titles: Online - full text ed.: ISSN 1464-0740 (from CatchWord Ltd., EBSCO Publishing, O C L C Online Computer Library Center, Inc., RoweCom Information Quest, Gale Group, Swets Blackwell, Institute for Scientific Information).
Indexed: ASCA, ASSIA, AgeLine, Arts & Hum.Cit.Ind. (coverage dropped), Biol.Abstr., Br.Educ.Ind., Curr.Adv.Cell & Devel.Biol., Curr.Cont., Dent.Ind., Ergon.Abstr., IBZ, Ind.Med. (1981-), Ind.Philos., Lang.& Lang.Behav.Abstr., Mid.East: Abstr.& Ind., Neurosci.Cit.Ind., P C I, PsycInfo, Psychol.Abstr. (1981-), Russ.Acad.Sci.Bibl., SOPODA, SSCI, Soc.Sci.Ind. (Jul.1999-), Sociol.Abstr., e-psyche.
—BLDSC (7190.100000), CatchWord, CISTI, GNLM, IDS, ingenta. **CCC.**
Published by: (Experimental Psychology Society), Psychology Press (Subsidiary of: Taylor & Francis Group), 27 Church Rd, Hove, E Sussex BN3 2FA, United Kingdom. TEL 44-1273-207411, FAX 44-1273-205612, information@psypress.co.uk, http://www.psypress.co.uk. Ed. Dianne Berry. R&P Zoe Peden TEL 44-20-7842-2363. Adv. contact Claire Buckminster. Circ: 1,600. **Subscr. addr. in N America:** Psychology Press, Journals Customer Service, Taylor & Francis Group, 325 Chestnut St, Philadelphia, PA 19106. TEL 800-354-1420, FAX 215-625-8914, info@taylorandfrancis.com, http://www.psypress.com; **Subscr. addr. outside N America:** Journals Customer Service, Taylor & Francis Group, Rankine Rd, Basingstoke, Hants RG24 8PR, United Kingdom. TEL 44-1256-813002, FAX 44-1256-479438, enquiry@tandf.co.uk.

152 GBR ISSN 0272-4995
QP351 CODEN: QJEBDT
QUARTERLY JOURNAL OF EXPERIMENTAL PSYCHOLOGY. SECTION B: COMPARATIVE AND PHYSIOLOGICAL PSYCHOLOGY. Text in English; Abstracts in French, Spanish. 1981. q. GBP 29, USD 64 to individuals; GBP 104, USD 215 to institutions (effective 2002). adv. bk.rev. index. reprint service avail. from SCH,PSC. *Refereed.* **Document type:** *Academic/Scholarly.* **Description:** Features articles on any topic within the field of animal psychology, not only on such traditional topics as conditioning, learning and motivation, but also on any aspect of animal behavior, comparative psychology, and ethology.
Supersedes in part (in 1981): Quarterly Journal of Experimental Psychology (0033-555X)

P

Related titles: Online - full text ed.: ISSN 1464-1321 (from CatchWord Ltd., EBSCO Publishing, O C L C Online Computer Library Center, Inc., RoweCom Information Quest, Swets Blackwell, Institute for Scientific Information).
Indexed: ASCA, ASSIA, AgeLine, Anim.Behav.Abstr., Arts & Hum.Cit.Ind. (coverage dropped), Biol.Abstr., Curr.Adv.Cell & Devel.Biol., Curr.Cont., Dent.Ind., Ergon.Abstr., IBZ, Ind.Med. (1981-), Ind.Philos., Inpharma, Neurosci.Cit.Ind., P C I, PsycInfo, Psychol.Abstr. (1981-), Psycscan B.A.& T., Reac., Russ.Acad.Sci.Bibl., SSCI, Sci.Cit.Ind., e-psyche.
—BLDSC (7190.200000), CatchWord, CISTI, GNLM, IDS, ingenta. **CCC.**
Published by: (Experimental Psychology Society), Psychology Press (Subsidiary of: Taylor & Francis Group), 27 Church Rd, Hove, E Sussex BN3 2FA, United Kingdom. TEL 44-1273-207411, FAX 44-1273-205612, information@psypress.co.uk, http://www.psypress.co.uk. Ed. John Pearce. R&P Zoe Peden TEL 44-20-7842-2363. Adv. contact Claire Buckminster. **Subscr. addr. in N America:** Psychology Press, Journals Customer Service, Taylor & Francis Group, 325 Chestnut St, Philadelphia, PA 19106. TEL 800-354-1420, FAX 215-625-8914, info@taylorandfrancis.com, http://www.psypress.com; **Subscr. addr. outside N America:** Journals Customer Service, Taylor & Francis Group, Rankine Rd, Basingstoke, Hants RG24 8PR, United Kingdom. TEL 44-1256-813002, FAX 44-1256-479438, enquiry@tandf.co.uk.

RAAKPUNT. see *MEDICAL SCIENCES—Psychiatry And Neurology*

301.1 150 ITA
RASSEGNA DI PSICOLOGIA. Text in Italian. 1984; N.S.. 3/yr. ITL 45,000; ITL 70,000 foreign (effective 1993).
Indexed: IBZ, PsycInfo, e-psyche.
Published by: (Universita di Roma La Sapienza, Dipartimenti di Psicologia e Psicologia dei Processi di Sviluppo e Socializzazione), Franco Angeli Editore, Viale Monza, 106, Milan, MI 20127, Italy. TEL 02-28-27-651. Eds. C Pontecorvo Pipermo, P Bonaiuto.

READING AND WRITING; an interdisciplinary journal. see *LINGUISTICS*

READING PSYCHOLOGY; an international quarterly. see *EDUCATION*

READINGS; a journal of reviews and commentary in mental health. see *MEDICAL SCIENCES—Psychiatry And Neurology*

REALITY CHANGE; the global Seth journal. see *NEW AGE PUBLICATIONS*

614.58 616.8 340 DEU ISSN 0724-2247
RECHT & PSYCHIATRIE. Text in German. 1983. q. DEM 70; DEM 78 foreign (effective 1999). back issues avail. **Document type:** *Academic/Scholarly.* **Description:** Examines law and psychiatry.
Indexed: Crim.Just.Abstr., IBZ, PsycInfo, Psychol.Abstr. (1987-), e-psyche.
—GNLM.
Published by: Psychiatrie Verlag GmbH, Thomas-Mann-Str 49A, Bonn 53111, Germany. TEL 49-228-72534-0, FAX 49-228-7253420. Ed. Ingeborg Rakete. Circ: 900.

155.4 USA ISSN 1089-5701
HV741 CODEN: RCYOFU
RECLAIMING CHILDREN AND YOUTH; the journal of emotional and behavioral problems. Text in English. 1992. q. USD 39 domestic to individuals; USD 64 foreign to individuals (effective 2001); USD 95 domestic to institutions; USD 120 foreign to institutions (effective 2001). adv. *Refereed.* **Document type:** *Journal, Academic/Scholarly.* **Description:** Interdisciplinary journal networking practitioners and policy leaders from diverse backgrounds who serve children and youth in conflict with self, family, school and community. Articles blend research with practical wisdom and a holistic perspective.
Formerly (until 1995): Journal of Emotional and Behavioral Problems (1064-7023)
Related titles: Microform ed.: (from PQC); Online - full text ed.: (from ProQuest Information & Learning).
Indexed: C.I.J.E., Educ.Ind., Except.Child Educ.Abstr., Lang.& Lang.Behav.Abstr., SOPODA, Soc.Serv.Abstr., Sociol.Abstr., e-psyche.
—BLDSC (7309.659000), ingenta. **CCC.**
Address: PO Box 57, Lennox, SD 57039. TEL 605-647-2532, 888-647-2532, FAX 605-647-5212, courage@reclaiming.com, http://www.reclaiming.com/journal/. Eds. Larry K Brendtro, Nicholas J Long. Circ: 3,500 (paid). **Subscr. to:** Compassion Publications, Ltd., Circulation Department, 3315 N 124th St, Ste J, Brookfield, WI 53005. TEL 262-317-3493, 800-285-7910.

RECOVERY TODAY; the newsmagazine for today's recovering community. see *DRUG ABUSE AND ALCOHOLISM*

REFLECTIONS: NARRATIVES OF PROFESSIONAL HELPING. see *EDUCATION—Special Education And Rehabilitation*

155.916 USA ISSN 0090-5550
RM930.A1
REHABILITATION PSYCHOLOGY. Text in English. 1954. q. USD 45 domestic to non-members; USD 60 foreign to non-members; USD 32 domestic to members; USD 42 foreign to members; USD 92 domestic to institutions; USD 124 foreign to institutions (effective 2001). adv. bk.rev., film rev. charts, illus. back issues avail.; reprints avail. *Refereed.* **Document type:** *Academic/Scholarly.* **Description:** Takes an interdisciplinary approach in addressing psychosocial and behavioral aspects of rehabilitation; covers topics that relate to the experience of chronic illness and disability throughout the lifespan.
Formerly (until 1971): Psychological Aspects of Disability (0091-178X)
Related titles: Online - full text ed.: (from Institute for Scientific Information).
Indexed: AMED, ASCA, AgeLine, Behav.Med.Abstr., CINAHL, Curr.Cont., Excerp.Med., IMFL, PsycInfo, Psychol.Abstr. (1972-), Rehabil.Lit., SSCI, Yrbk.Assoc.Educ.& Rehab.Blind, e-psyche.
—BLDSC (7350.290000), GNLM, IDS, ingenta, KNAW. **CCC.**
Published by: American Psychological Association, Division of Rehabilitation Psychology, 750 First St., N.E., Washington, DC 20002-4242. TEL 202-336-5600, 800-374-2721, FAX 202-336-5568, http://www.apa.org/journals/rep.html. Ed. Bruce M Caplan. adv.: B&W page USD 175; trim 10 x 7. Circ: 1,700 (paid). **Subscr. to:** Allen Press Inc., PO Box 1897, Lawrence, KS 66044-8897.

302 URY ISSN 0797-9754
BF5
RELACIONES. Text in Spanish. 1984. m. USD 60 (effective 2001). adv. bk.rev. *Refereed.* **Document type:** *Academic/Scholarly.* **Description:** Devoted to human sciences.
Published by: Editorial Periodica S.R.L., Avda. Luis A. de Herrera, 1042, Ap. 708, Montevideo 11300, Uruguay. TEL 598-2-6221108, FAX 598-2-6221108, relacion@adinet.com.uy, http://chasque.apc.org/relacion. Ed. Saul Paciuk. Adv. contact Rosa Verdier. Circ: 4,000.

616.89 DEU ISSN 0344-9602
REPORT PSYCHOLOGIE. Text in German. 1974. 10/yr. DEM 105 domestic; DEM 140 foreign (effective 2001). adv. bk.rev. *Refereed.* **Document type:** *Newsletter, Academic/Scholarly.*
Indexed: IBZ, e-psyche.
—GNLM.
Published by: Deutscher Psychologen Verlag GmbH, Heilsbachstr 22, Bonn 53123, Germany. TEL 49-228-9873118, FAX 49-228-9873170, dpv@bdp-verband.org, http://www.bdp-verband.org. Ed., Pub., R&P, Adv. contact Petra Walkenbach TEL 49-228-98731-18. page DEM 2,200; trim 169 x 232. Circ: 18,500 (paid).

155.3 USA
REPRESENTATIONS BOOKS SERIES. Text in English. 1987. irreg., latest vol.7, 1996. price varies. back issues avail. **Document type:** *Monographic series.* **Description:** Examines sexuality throughout Western history.
Indexed: e-psyche.
Published by: University of California Press, Journals Division, 2000 Center St, Ste 303, Berkeley, CA 94704-1223. TEL 510-642-7127, FAX 510-643-7127. **Orders to:** California-Princeton Fulfillment Services, Princeton, NJ 08618. TEL 800-777-4726, FAX 800-999-1958.

302 USA ISSN 0034-4907
HM251 CODEN: RRSPD4
REPRESENTATIVE RESEARCH IN SOCIAL PSYCHOLOGY. Text in English. 1970. a. USD 8 to individuals; USD 10 in Canada & Mexico to individuals; USD 12 elsewhere to individuals; USD 15 to institutions; USD 17 in Canada & Mexico to institutions; USD 19 elsewhere to institutions (effective 1999 - 2000). bk.rev. *Refereed.* **Document type:** *Academic/Scholarly.* **Description:** Covers methodologically sound research in basic and applied social psychology including null findings and replication studies.
Related titles: Microform ed.: (from PMC).
Indexed: Adol.Ment.Hlth.Abstr., Curr.Cont. (coverage dropped), Curr.Ind.Stat., Fam.Ind., PsycInfo, Psychol.Abstr., Russ.Acad.Sci.Bibl., SSCI (coverage dropped), e-psyche.
—BLDSC (7692.000000), ingenta.
Published by: University of North Carolina at Chapel Hill, Department of Psychology, Social Psychology Graduate Students, Davie Hall, Campus Box 3270, Chapel Hill, NC 27599-3270. TEL 919-962-7636, FAX 919-962-2537, rrsp@email.unc.edu. Ed. Brad Pinter. R&P Jody Davis. Circ: 300.

150 616.8 362.7 USA ISSN 1087-0695
BF1 CODEN: RCBPFK
RESEARCH COMMUNICATIONS IN BEHAVIORAL PSYCHOLOGY AND PSYCHIATRY; including behavioral and neurosciences. Text in English. 1976. q. USD 90; USD 105 foreign (effective 1998). adv. bk.rev. abstr, charts, illus. index. reprint service avail. from ISI. *Refereed.* **Description:** Information of value to experimental psychologists, psychiatrists, behavioral scientists, psychopharmacologists and basic and clinical scientists.
Formerly (until 1995): Research Communications in Psychology, Psychiatry and Behavior (0362-2428)
Indexed: Biol.Abstr., Chem.Abstr., Curr.Adv.Ecol.Sci., Curr.Cont. (coverage dropped), Curr.Lit.Fam.Plan., Excerp.Med., PsycInfo, Psychol.Abstr. (1976-), e-psyche.
—BLDSC (7736.450000), CASDDS, CISTI, EMDOCS, GNLM, Infotrieve, ingenta, KNAW. **CCC.**
Published by: P J D Publications Ltd, PO Box 966, Westbury, NY 11590. TEL 516-626-0650, FAX 516-626-5546.

RESEARCH IN COMMUNITY AND MENTAL HEALTH; an annual compilation of research. see *PUBLIC HEALTH AND SAFETY*

302 USA ISSN 0191-3085
HD28
RESEARCH IN ORGANIZATIONAL BEHAVIOR. Text in English. 1979. irreg., latest vol.20, 1998. USD 78.50. *Refereed.* **Document type:** *Monographic series.*
Related titles: Online - full text ed.: (from Institute for Scientific Information).
Indexed: ASCA, Int.Lab.Doc., Int.Polit.Sci.Abstr., Psychol.Abstr., SSCI, e-psyche.
—BLDSC (7750.600000), CISTI, ingenta. **CCC.**
Published by: J A I Press Inc., 100 Prospect St, Box 811, Stamford, CT 06904-0811. TEL 203-323-9606, FAX 203-357-8446, jai@jaipress.com. Eds. Barry M Staw, L L Cummings.

RESEARCH ON SOCIAL WORK PRACTICE. see *SOCIOLOGY*

150.19 100 USA ISSN 1059-3551
THE RESHAPING OF PSYCHOANALYSIS; from Sigmund Freud to Ernest Becker. Text in English. irreg. price varies. **Document type:** *Monographic series, Academic/Scholarly.* **Description:** Studies of Freud and neo-Freudians such as Ernest Becker, concerned with the reshaping and revitalization of psychoanalysis.
Indexed: e-psyche.
Published by: Peter Lang Publishing, Inc., 275 Seventh Ave, 28th Fl, New York, NY 10001. TEL 212-647-7706, 800-770-5264, FAX 212-475-7707, customerservice@plang.com, http://www.peterlang.com. Ed. Barry R Arnold. Pub. Christopher Myers. R&P Stephanie Archer. Adv. contact Patricia Mulrane.

155.4 USA
RESIDENTIAL TREATMENT NEWS. Text in English. 1986. bi-m. USD 50 (effective 1998). **Document type:** *Newsletter.*
Formerly: A A C R C Newsletter
Indexed: e-psyche.
Published by: American Association of Children's Residential Centers, 440 First St N W, 3rd Fl, Washington, DC 20001-2028. TEL 202-628-1816, FAX 202-638-4004. Circ: 350.

150 616.8 100 800 USA ISSN 0361-1531
RC321 CODEN: REXPB4
REVIEW OF EXISTENTIAL PSYCHOLOGY AND PSYCHIATRY. Text in English. 1961. 3/yr. USD 98, USD 116 (effective 2001). adv. bk.rev. cum. index. back issues avail.; reprint service avail. from PSC,SCH. *Refereed.* **Document type:** *Journal, Academic/Scholarly.* **Description:** Applies existential and phenomenological approaches to the study of problems in human existence.
Former titles (until 1971): Human Inquiries (0363-2326); (until 1969): Review of Existential Psychology and Psychiatry (0034-656X)
Indexed: Curr.Cont. (coverage dropped), IBR, IBZ, Ind.Philos., Phil.Ind., Psychol.Abstr., e-psyche.
—Infotrieve, ingenta. **CCC.**
Address: PO Box 15680, Seattle, WA 98115. TEL 206-367-5764, FAX 206-365-3036. Ed., Pub., R&P, Adv. contact Keith Hoeller. B&W page USD 295; trim 6 x 9. Circ: 300.

152 USA ISSN 1089-2680
BF1.R48
REVIEW OF GENERAL PSYCHOLOGY. Text in English. 1997. q. USD 60 domestic to non-members; USD 75 foreign to non-members; USD 29 domestic to members; USD 39 foreign to members; USD 110 domestic to institutions; USD 142 foreign to institutions (effective 2001). adv. 100 p./no. 1 cols./p. back issues avail.; reprints avail. *Refereed.* **Description:** Includes innovative theoretical, conceptual, and methodological articles that cross-cut the traditional subdisciplines of psychology.
Indexed: PsycInfo, e-psyche.
—BLDSC (7790.741000). **CCC.**
Published by: American Psychological Association, 750 First St., N.E., Washington, DC 20002-4242. TEL 202-336-5600, 800-374-2721, FAX 202-336-5568, subscriptions@apa.org, www.apa.org/journals/gpr.html. Ed. Peter Salovey. Circ: 2,500 (paid); 2,500 (paid and controlled).

150 HRV ISSN 1330-6812
BF8.S4 CODEN: RPSHDY
REVIEW OF PSYCHOLOGY. Text in Croatian. 1971. s-a. HRK 70 to individuals; DEM 30 foreign to individuals; HRK 96 to institutions; DEM 76 foreign to institutions (effective 1999). adv. bk.rev. **Document type:** *Academic/Scholarly.* **Description:** Publishes original scientific papers, theoretical contributions and critical surveys of research in all fields of psychology and related disciplines, as well as relevant professional papers and news.
Formerly (until 1991): Revija za Psihologiju (0352-1605)
Indexed: PsycInfo, Psychol.Abstr., e-psyche.
Published by: Drustvo Psihologa S R Hrvatske/Croatian Psychologica, Salajeva 3, Zagreb, Croatia. TEL 385-1-41613155, FAX 385-1-41513834. Ed. Vladimir Kolesaric. Circ: 1,000.

REVISTA ARGENTINA DE PSICOPEDAGOGIA. see *EDUCATION*

150 COL ISSN 0121-5469
BF5
REVISTA COLOMBIANA DE PSICOLOGIA. Text in Spanish; Summaries in English, French, Spanish. 1956. irreg. per issue exchange basis. adv. bk.rev. abstr, bibl, illus. **Document type:** *Academic/Scholarly.* **Description:** Includes original papers and clinical case work on psychology.
Formerly: Revista de Psicologia (0120-2901)
Indexed: e-psyche.
Published by: Universidad Nacional de Colombia, Departamento de Psicologia, Apdo Aereo 14490, Bogota DC, Colombia. TEL 57-1-3681565, FAX 57-1-2225285, revcopis@usc.usc.unal.edu.co, revcopis@usc.unal.edu.co. Ed. Luis Bernardo Lopez Caicedo. Circ: 1,000.

301.1 150 CUB ISSN 0257-4322
REVISTA CUBANA DE PSICOLOGIA. Text in Spanish; Summaries in English, Spanish. 3/yr. USD 17 in North America; USD 18 in South America; USD 22 elsewhere.
Indexed: Russ.Acad.Sci.Bibl., e-psyche.
—KNAW.
Published by: Universidade de La Habana, Calle I No. 302, Entre 15 y 17, Havana 4, Cuba. TEL 32-5556-60. **Dist. by:** Ediciones Cubanas, Obispo No. 527, Apdo. 605, Havana, Cuba.

150 ESP
▼ **REVISTA DE METODOLOGIA DE LAS CIENCIAS DE COMPORTAMIENTO.** Text in Spanish. 1999.
Published by: Espanola de Metodologia de las Ciencias del Comportamiento, Departamento de Psiclogia Basica y Metodologia, Universidad de Murcia - Campus de Espinardo, Apartado 4021, Murcia 30080, Spain. TEL 34-968-363477, FAX 34-968-364115, fulmarin@fcu.um.es. Ed. Fulgencio Marin.

616.89 BRA ISSN 0102-4205
REVISTA DE PSICANALISE INTEGRAL✶ . Text in Portuguese. 1978. a. USD 4. adv. **Document type:** *Academic/Scholarly.*
Formerly: Analytical Trilogy
Indexed: e-psyche.
Published by: (Sociedad Internacional de Trilogia Analitica/International Society of Analytical Trilogy), Proton Editora Ltda., Av Reboucas, 3819, Pinheiros, Sao Paulo, SP 05401-450, Brazil. Ed. Marc Andre R Keppe. Circ: 1,500.

616.89 ARG ISSN 0034-8740
RC321
REVISTA DE PSICOANALISIS. Text in Spanish; Summaries in English, French. 1943. 6/yr. USD 80. bk.rev. abstr. index.
Media: Duplicated (not offset).
Indexed: Excerp.Med., IBR, PsycInfo, Psychoanal.Abstr., Psychol.Abstr. (1934-), e-psyche.
—BLDSC (7870.130000).
Published by: Asociacion Psicoanalitica Argentina, Pena Rodriguez, 1674, Capital Federal, Buenos Aires 1021, Argentina. Circ: 2,000.

150 PER ISSN 0254-9247
REVISTA DE PSICOLOGIA. Text in Spanish. 1983. s-a. USD 28. adv. *Refereed.* **Document type:** *Academic/Scholarly.*
Indexed: PsycInfo, e-psyche.
Published by: Pontificia Universidad Catolica del Peru, Departamento de Humanidades, Fondo Editorial, Apdo. 1761, Lima 100, Peru. TEL 51-14-626390, FAX 51-14-611785, editorial@pucp.edu.pe, http://www.pucp.edu.pe. Ed. Cecilia Thorne. Circ: 1,000.

155.4 370.15 ESP
REVISTA DE PSICOLOGIA EDUCATIVA; revista de los psicologos de la educacion. Text in Spanish. irreg. (1-2/yr.). back issues avail. **Document type:** *Academic/Scholarly.*
Related titles: Online - full text ed.
Indexed: e-psyche.
Published by: Colegio Oficial de Psicologos de Madrid, Cuesta de San Vicente, 4 6o, Madrid 28008, Spain. TEL 34-91-541-7009, FAX 34-91-547-2284, dmadrid@correo.es, http://www.cop.es/publicaciones/educativa/. Ed. Adolfo Fernandez Barroso.

150 ESP ISSN 0373-2002
REVISTA DE PSICOLOGIA GENERAL Y APLICADA. Text in Spanish; Summaries in English, Spanish. 1946. q., latest vol.54. ESP 6,000 domestic to individuals; ESP 9,800 domestic to institutions; ESP 12,000 foreign (effective 2001). bk.rev. bibl, charts. *Refereed.* **Document type:** *Journal, Academic/Scholarly.* **Description:** Reviews clinical and applied psychology.
Related titles: Online - full text ed.: IberPsicologia. 1996.
Indexed: Curr.Ind.Stat., Lang.& Lang.Behav.Abstr., PsycInfo, SOPODA, Sociol.Abstr., e-psyche.
—CINDOC, Infotrieve. **CCC.**
Published by: Federacion Espanola de Asociaciones de Psicologia, Seminario de Psicologia Basica, Facultad de Filosofia, Edif. A, Desp. 41, Universidad Complutense, Madrid 28040, Spain. http://fs-morente.filos.ucm.es/publicaciones/. Ed. Helio Carpintero. Pub. Jose Pascual.

150 ESP ISSN 0213-4748
REVISTA DE PSICOLOGIA SOCIAL. Text in Spanish. 1986. s-a. ESP 3,200 per issue foreign. adv. *Refereed.* **Document type:** *Academic/Scholarly.* **Description:** Publishes articles on empirical and theoretical research concerning the study of behavior from a theoretical perspective.
Related titles: Online - full text ed.: (from CatchWord Ltd.).
Indexed: PsycInfo, Psychol.Abstr. (1988-), e-psyche.
—CINDOC.
Published by: Fundacion Infancia y Aprendizaje, Ctra. de Canillas 138, 16C, Madrid 28043, Spain. TEL 34-91-388-3874, FAX 34-91-300-3527. Circ: 1,100.

150 ROM ISSN 0034-8759
BF8.R7
REVISTA DE PSIHOLOGIE. Text in Romanian. 1955. q. bk.rev. index. **Document type:** *Academic/Scholarly.*
Indexed: Biol.Abstr., C.I.S. Abstr., Child Devel.Abstr., Ergon.Abstr., Lang.& Lang.Behav.Abstr., Nutr.Abstr., PsycInfo, Psychol.Abstr. (1961-), Russ.Acad.Sci.Bibl., e-psyche.
—KNAW.
Published by: (Institutul de Psihologie, Academia Romana), Editura Academiei Romane, Calea 13 Septembrie 13, Bucharest 76117, Romania. Ed. Constantin Voicu. Circ: 1,400. **Dist. by:** Rodipet S.A.. TEL 401-618-5103, FAX 401-222-6407.

150 ESP ISSN 1137-8492
BF1
REVISTA ELECTRONICA DE PSICOLOGIA. Variant title: Psicologia.Com. Text in Spanish. 1997. q. free per issue to qualified personnel. back issues avail. **Document type:** *Academic/Scholarly.* **Description:** Publishes papers on pscyhology research.
Media: Online - full text.
Published by: Internet y Salud, Apdo. de Correos 20018, Palma De Marrorca, Baleares 07080, Spain. TEL 34-971-282839, FAX 34-971-220503, info@psiquiatria.com, http://www.psiquiatria.com/psicologia.

150 COL ISSN 0120-0534
BF5 CODEN: RLPSBM
REVISTA LATINOAMERICANA DE PSICOLOGIA. Text in Spanish. 1969. 3/yr. USD 25 to individuals; USD 35 to institutions (effective 2000 & 2001). adv. bk.rev. abstr, bibl, illus, stat. index. **Document type:** *Academic/Scholarly.* **Description:** International journal of all areas of psychology.
Related titles: Online - full text ed.: (from Institute for Scientific Information).
Indexed: ASCA, Arts & Hum.Cit.Ind. (coverage dropped), Biol.Abstr., Curr.Cont., IBR, IBZ, Ind.Philos., PsycInfo, Psychol.Abstr. (1969-), SSCI, e-psyche.
—BLDSC (7863.513000), Infotrieve. **CCC.**
Published by: Foundation for the Advancement of Psychology, PO Box 92621, Bogota, CUND, Colombia. TEL 57-1-256-7527. Ed. Ruben Ardila. Circ: 2,500.

P

150 MEX ISSN 0185-4534
REVISTA MEXICANA DE ANALISIS DE LA CONDUCTA/MEXICAN JOURNAL OF BEHAVIOR ANALYSIS. Text in English, Spanish. 1975. 3/yr. USD 20 to individuals; USD 25 in Europe to individuals; USD 35 to institutions; USD 40 in Europe to institutions. adv. bk.rev. bibl, charts, illus, stat. index. back issues avail. **Description:** Presents original research in behavior analysis and technical notes on diverse subjects of interest to behavioral scientists.
Indexed: Adol.Ment.Hlth.Abstr., Curr.Cont. (coverage dropped), Curr.Ind.Stat., PsycInfo, Psychol.Abstr., Psycscan B.A.& T., e-psyche.
Published by: (Mexican Society of Behavior Analysis), Editorial Trillas, Apdo. Postal 21-182, Mexico City, DF 04000, Mexico. TEL 5 547632. Ed., Adv. contact Florente Lopez. Circ: 1,000.

150 MEX ISSN 0185-6073
REVISTA MEXICANA DE PSICOLOGIA/MEXICAN JOURNAL OF PSYCHOLOGY. Text in English, Spanish; Summaries in English, Spanish. 1984. s-a. USD 20 domestic; USD 40 foreign (effective 2000); USD 10 newsstand/cover. adv. back issues avail.; reprints avail. *Refereed.* **Document type:** *Journal, Academic/Scholarly.* **Description:** Publishes original articles representing different theoretical and methodological approaches as well as contributions from different applied fields of psychology.
Related titles: Online - full text ed.: (from Institute for Scientific Information).
Indexed: ASCA, Curr.Cont., PsycInfo, SSCI, e-psyche.
—BLDSC (7866.402000), IDS.
Published by: Sociedad Mexicana de Psicologia, Indiana No. 260, Despacho 608, Mexico City, DF 03710, Mexico. TEL 52-5-5989566, FAX 52-5-6234046, prado@servidor.unam.mx, http://www.psicologia.org.mx/. Ed. Dr. Roberto A Prado Alcala. adv.: page USD 150. Circ: 500 (paid).

150.19 PRT
REVISTA PORTUGUESA DE PSICANALISE✶ . Text in Portuguese. 1985. irreg., latest vol.16, 1997. PTE 2,400 domestic (effective 1999); PTE 4,500 in Europe; PTE 5,500 elsewhere.
Indexed: PsycInfo, Psychoanal.Abstr., e-psyche.
Published by: (Sociedade Portuguesa de Psicanalise), Edicoes Afrontamento, Lda., Rua de Costa Cabral, 859, Apdo. 52009, Porto Codex 4201, Portugal. TEL 351-22-5074220, FAX 351-22-5074229. Eds. Carlos Amaral Dias, Jaime Milheiro.

150 URY ISSN 0797-4876
REVISTA URUGUAYA DE PSICOLOGIA. Text in Spanish. 1978. s-a. USD 10; (or exchange basis). bk.rev.
Indexed: PsycInfo, Psychol.Abstr. (1977-), e-psyche.
Published by: (Asociacion de Psicologos Universitarios del Uruguay), Editorial Imago s.r.l., Treinta Y Tres, 1324, Montevideo 11007, Uruguay. Ed. Ricardo Landeira.

REVUE CANADIENNE DE PSYCHO-EDUCATION. see *EDUCATION*

REVUE DE NEUROPSYCHOLOGIE. see *MEDICAL SCIENCES—Psychiatry And Neurology*

150 FRA ISSN 0297-1194
REVUE DE PSYCHOTHERAPIE PSYCHANALYTIQUE DE GROUPE. Text in French. 1985. s-a. FRF 290 domestic; FRF 330 foreign (effective 2000). **Document type:** *Academic/Scholarly.* **Description:** Contains reviews concerning groups dealing with psychoanalytic psychotherapy.
Published by: Editions Eres, 11 rue des Alouettes, Ramonville Saint-Agne 31520, France. TEL 33-5-61751576, FAX 33-5-61735289, eres@editions-eres.com. Eds. Jacqueline Falguiere, Jean Claude Rouchy. **Subscr. to:** Service abonnements, BP16, Fenouillet Cedex 31151, France.

158 NLD
BF636.A1
REVUE EUROPEENE DE PSYCHOLOGIE APPLIQUEE/EUROPEAN REVIEW OF APPLIED PSYCHOLOGY. Text in English, French. 1951. q. USD 110 (effective 2000). adv. bk.rev. bibl, charts, illus. index. *Refereed.* **Document type:** *Academic/Scholarly.* **Description:** Devoted to European developments in applied psychology.
Formerly (until 1991): Revue de Psychologie Appliquee (0035-1709)
Related titles: Online - full text ed.
Indexed: ASCA, AgeLine, Child Devel.Abstr., Curr.Cont. (coverage dropped), Ergon.Abstr., Excerp.Med., INSPEC (coverage dropped), PsycInfo, Psychol.Abstr. (1950-), SSCI (coverage dropped), e-psyche.
—BLDSC (3829.942000), Infotrieve. **CCC.**
Published by: (Centre de Psychologie Appliquee), Swets & Zeitlinger BV, PO Box 825, Lisse 2160 SZ, Netherlands. TEL 31-252-435111, FAX 31-252-415888, orders@swets.nl, http://www.swets.nl. R&P J van der Valk. Adv. contact Patrick Kliean. **Dist. in N. America by:** Swets & Zeitlinger, PO Box 582, Downingtown, PA 19335-998. TEL 800-477-9387, FAX 610-524-5366.

616.89 FRA ISSN 0035-2942
BF173.A2
REVUE FRANCAISE DE PSYCHANALYSE. Text in French. 1927. q. FRF 710 domestic to individuals; FRF 850 foreign to individuals (effective 2000 & 2001). adv. abstr, bibl, charts. index. reprint service avail. from PSC,SCH. *Refereed.* **Description:** Covers all aspects of psychoanalysis.
Related titles: Supplement: Congres de Psychanalyse des Langues Romanes. Rapports.
Indexed: ASCA, Arts & Hum.Cit.Ind. (coverage dropped), BHA, Excerp.Med., IBR, Ind.Med. (coverage dropped), P C I, PsycInfo, Psychoanal.Abstr., Psychol.Abstr. (1928-), Russ.Acad.Sci.Bibl., SSCI (coverage dropped), e-psyche.
—BLDSC (7904.280000), GNLM, IDS, Infotrieve. **CCC.**
Published by: (Societe Psychanalytique de Paris), Presses Universitaires de France, Departement des Revues, 6 av. Reille, Paris 75685 Cedex 14, France. TEL 33-1-60873030, FAX 33-1-60792045, revues@puf.com. Ed. Powe Denis.

301.1 150 FRA ISSN 0992-986X
CODEN: RIPSE4
REVUE INTERNATIONALE DE PSYCHOLOGIE SOCIALE/INTERNATIONAL REVIEW OF SOCIAL PSYCHOLOGY. Text in English, French. 1976. s-a. FRF 250 domestic to individuals; FRF 300 foreign to individuals; FRF 380 to institutions (effective 2000). **Description:** Publishes critical overviews, theoretical notes, and empirical research from all areas of social psychologie.
Formerly (until 1988): Psychologie et Education (0151-2137)
Indexed: Psychol.Abstr., e-psyche.
—BLDSC (7925.260000), Infotrieve. **CCC.**
Published by: Presses Universitaires de Grenoble, B.P. 47, Grenoble Cedex 9 38040, France. FAX 33-4-76827835.

301.1 150 ROM ISSN 1220-5419
BF1
REVUE ROUMAINE DE PSYCHOLOGIE. Text in English, French, German, Russian, Spanish. 1964. s-a. bk.rev. charts.
Formerly (until 1990): Revue Roumaine des Sciences Sociales. Serie de Psychologie (0035-3892)
Indexed: Child Devel.Abstr., Ergon.Abstr., Psychol.Abstr. (1964-), Russ.Acad.Sci.Bibl., e-psyche.
—BLDSC (7946.502000), KNAW.
Published by: (Academia Romana), Editura Academiei Romane, Calea 13 Septembrie 13, Bucharest 76117, Romania. Ed. P Groza. Circ: 750. **Dist. by:** Rodipet S.A.. TEL 401-618-5103, FAX 401-222-6407.

REVUE ZAIROISE DE PSYCHOLOGIE ET DE PEDAGOGIE. see *EDUCATION*

616.89 ITA ISSN 0391-996X
RICERCHE DI PSICOLOGIA. Text in Italian; Summaries in English, Italian. 1968. q. ITL 95,000; ITL 130,000 foreign (effective 1993). adv. bk.rev.
Formerly (until 1972): Annali di Psicologia
Indexed: Anim.Behav.Abstr. (coverage dropped), Ind.Philos., PsycInfo, Psychol.Abstr. (1979-), e-psyche.
—BLDSC.
Published by: (Universita degli Studi di Milano, Istituto di Psicologia), Franco Angeli Editore, Viale Monza, 106, Milan, MI 20127, Italy. TEL 02-28-27-651. Ed. Marcello Cesa Bianchi.

155.4 ITA ISSN 1121-9602
RICHARD E PIGGLE. Text in Italian. 1993. 3/yr. USD 89 (effective 2000). adv. 128 p./no. **Document type:** *Journal.*
Indexed: PsycInfo, Psychoanal.Abstr., e-psyche.
Published by: (Associazione Italiana di Psicoterapia Psicoanalitica Infantile), Il Pensiero Scientifico Editore s.r.l., Via Bradano, 3-C, Rome, RM 00199, Italy. TEL 39-06-862821, FAX 39-06-86282250, pensiero@pensiero.it, http://www.pensiero.it. Eds. Giuliana Micana, Luisa Carbone Tirelli, Vincenzo Bonaminio. Pub. Luca De Fiore. Circ: 600.

155.937 USA
RIGHT-TO-DIE NEWSLETTER. Text in English. 1980. biennial. bk.rev., tel.rev., Website rev. 8 p./no. 2 cols./p. back issues avail. **Document type:** *Journal, Internal.*
Formerly: Right to Die Societies Newsletter
Media: Online - full content. **Related titles:** Online - full text ed.
Published by: World Federation of Right to Die Societies, 24829 Norris Lane, Junction City, OR 97448. TEL 541-998-1873, 541-998-1873, derkhumphry@starband.net, http://www.worldrtd.ort, http://www.efn.org/~ergo/right.news.html. Ed. Derek Humphry. Circ: 200 (controlled).

158 ITA
RISORSA UOMO. Text in Italian. 1993. 3/yr. ITL 48,000; ITL 70,000 foreign (effective 1993).
Indexed: e-psyche.
Published by: Franco Angeli Editore, Viale Monza, 106, Milan, MI 20127, Italy. TEL 02-28-27-651. Ed. V Majer.

616.89 CHE ISSN 1019-1976
RISS* ; Zeitschrift fuer Psychoanalyse. Text in German. 1986. 3/yr. CHF 30.
Indexed: e-psyche.
Address: Minervastr 13, Zuerich 8032, Switzerland. Circ: 300.

616.89 ITA ISSN 0035-6492
RIVISTA DI PSICOANALISI/ITALIAN PSYCHOANALYTICAL SOCIETY. JOURNAL. Text in Italian. 1955. q. ITL 100,000, USD 114; ITL 120,000 domestic to institutions; USD 130 foreign to institutions. bk.rev. bibl, charts. index. reprint service avail. from ISI. **Description:** Covers research and study in the field of psychoanalysis.
Related titles: English ed.
Indexed: Ind.Philos., Psychol.Abstr., e-psyche.
—GNLM.
Published by: (Societa Psicoanalitica Italiana), Edizioni Borla s.r.l., Via Delle Fornaci, 50, Rome, RM 00165, Italy. TEL 39-6-39376728, FAX 39-6-39376620. Ed. Antonio Valdina. Circ: 1,500.

150.19 ITA ISSN 0392-9787
RIVISTA DI PSICOLOGIA ANALITICA. Text in Italian. 1970. s-a. ITL 50,000. bk.rev. **Document type:** *Academic/Scholarly.* **Description:** Covers research and study in the field of analytical psychology.
Indexed: e-psyche.
Published by: Casa Editrice Astrolabio, Via Gallonio 8, Rome, RM 00161, Italy. TEL 4270177, FAX 06-429590. Ed. A Carotenuto. Circ: 1,500.

RIVISTA DI PSICOLOGIA DELL'ARTE. see *ART*

616.89 ITA
RIVISTA ITALIANA DI ANALISI TRANSAZIONALE E METODOLOGIE PSICOTERAPEUTICHE. Text in Italian; Summaries in English. 1981. s-a. ITL 50,000; ITL 70,000 foreign (effective 1998). bk.rev. bibl. index. back issues avail. *Refereed.* **Document type:** *Academic/Scholarly.* **Description:** Presents theoretical research on transactional analysis as a philosophy and scientific theory. Reports on its application in psychiatry, medicine, in schools and in the training of adults.
Indexed: e-psyche.
Published by: Societa Italiana di Metodologie Psicoterapeutiche e Analisi Transazionale, Via Filippo Nicolai, 70, Rome, RM 00136, Italy. TEL 39-6-35344043, FAX 39-6-35402495. Ed. Maria Teresa Romanini. Circ: 1,000 (paid).

152 USA ISSN 1056-6511
ROCHESTER SYMPOSIUM ON DEVELOPMENTAL PSYCHOPATHOLOGY. Text in English. ceased; resumed 1989. a. **Document type:** *Proceedings.*
Indexed: e-psyche.
—BLDSC (8001.320000). **CCC.**
Published by: University of Rochester Press, c/o Susan Dykstra Poel, Box 41026, Rochester, NY 14604-4126. TEL 716-275-0419, FAX 716-271-8778, urpress@uhura.cc.rochester.edu, http://www.boydell.co.uk.

159.9 USA ISSN 1192-5604
RORSCHACHIANA; yearbook of the international rorschach society. Text in English. 1945. a. USD 38. **Document type:** *Journal, Academic/Scholarly.* **Description:** Provides updates on current uses of the Rorschach instrument in various countries and highlights recent results of research and theory.
Published by: (International Rorschach Society FRA), Hogrefe & Huber Publishers, PO Box 2487, Kirkland, WA 98083. TEL 425-820-1500, FAX 425-823-8324, http://www.hhpub.com/journals. Ed. Anne Andronikof-Sanglade.

150 GBR
ROUTLEDGE PROGRESS IN PSYCHOLOGY. Text in English. irreg. **Document type:** *Monographic series, Academic/Scholarly.*
Indexed: e-psyche.
—BLDSC.
Published by: Routledge (Subsidiary of: Taylor & Francis Group), 11 New Fetter Ln, London EC4P 4EE, United Kingdom. TEL 44-20-7583-9855, FAX 44-20-7842-2298, info.journals@routledge.com, http://www.routledge.com/routledge/journal/journals.html. Ed. Pertti Saariluoma.

150 ITA
RUOLO TERAPEUTICO; la formazione psicologica e la pratica professionale degli operatori sociosanitari. Text in Italian. 1972. 3/yr.
Indexed: IBZ, e-psyche.
Address: Via Giovanni Milani, 12, Milan, MI 20133, Italy. TEL 39-2-70636457. Circ: 800 (paid).

158 USA
RUTGERS SERIES ON SELF AND SOCIAL IDENTITY. Text in English. 1997. irreg., latest vol.2. price varies. back issues avail. **Document type:** *Monographic series, Proceedings, Academic/Scholarly.* **Description:** Examines issues in psychology relating to social identity and self-perception.
—BLDSC.
Published by: (Rutgers University, Department of Psychology), Oxford University Press Inc., 198 Madison Ave, New York, NY 10016. TEL 212-726-6000, http://www.oup-usa.org/catalogs/general/series/Rutgers_Series_on_Self_and_Social_Identity.html. Eds. Richard D Ashmore, Richard J Contrada.

616.89 USA
S C I PSYCHOSOCIAL PROCESS. (Spinal Cord Injury) Text in English. 1988. q. free per issue. bk.rev. charts, illus. *Refereed.* **Document type:** *Academic/Scholarly.* **Description:** For psychologists and social workers caring for spinal cord injured persons.
Indexed: CINAHL, Soc.Work Res.& Abstr., e-psyche.
—BLDSC.
Published by: Eastern Paralyzed Veterans Association, 75-20 Astoria Blvd., Jackson Heights, NY 11370-1177. TEL 718-803-3782, FAX 718-803-0414, info@EPVA.org. Ed. Jason Mask. Circ: 1,200.

S R C D NEWSLETTER. see *CHILDREN AND YOUTH—About*

155 USA
SAGE SERIES ON INDIVIDUAL DIFFERENCES AND DEVELOPMENT. Text in English. irreg., latest vol.6, 1994. price varies. adv. back issues avail. **Document type:** *Monographic series.* **Description:** Provides a forum for a new wave of research that focuses on individual differences in behavioral development.
Indexed: e-psyche.
Published by: Sage Publications, Inc., Books, 2455 Teller Rd, Thousand Oaks, CA 91320. TEL 805-499-0721, FAX 805-499-0871, libraries@sagepub.com, http://www.sagepub.com. Ed. Robert Plomin. Adv. contact Margaret Travers. **Overseas subscr. to:** Sage Publications Ltd., 6 Bonhill St, London EC2A 4PU, United Kingdom; Sage Publications India Pvt. Ltd., 4215, New Delhi 110 048, India.

SAMENWERKINGSVERBAND JEUGDHULPVERLENING UTRECHT. NIEUWSBRIEF. see *CHILDREN AND YOUTH—About*

150 IND ISSN 0971-3492
SAMIKSA. Text in English. 1947. a., latest vol.52. USD 40 (effective 1999). bk.rev. back issues avail. **Document type:** *Academic/Scholarly.* **Description:** Presents scientific discussion of various aspects of psychoanalysis and related subjects.
Indexed: Documentatieblad, Excerp.Med., Indian Psychol.Abstr., Psychol.Abstr., e-psyche.
Published by: Indian Psychoanalytical Society, 14 Parsibagan Ln., Kolkata, West Bengal 700 009, India. TEL 91-33-3508788. Ed. Hironmoy Ghosal. adv.: B&W page USD 20, color page USD 30. Circ: 400. **Affiliate:** International Psychoanalytical Association.

150 CAN ISSN 0383-6320
CODEN: SMQUEK
SANTE MENTALE AU QUEBEC. Text in French; Summaries in English, French. 1976. s-a. CND 31.06, FRF 150 to individuals; CND 42.56, FRF 200 to institutions; CND 24.16, FRF 140 to students (effective 2000). *Refereed.* **Document type:** *Academic/Scholarly.* **Description:** Publishes articles on experimental research and social innovation. Aims to fulfill the needs in development of scientific, academic and clinical knowledge.
Indexed: CINAHL, Int.Nurs.Ind., Intl.Bibl.Soc.Sci., Lang.& Lang.Behav.Abstr., Pt.de Rep. (1982-), SOPODA, Sage Race Rel.Abstr., Soc.Serv.Abstr., Soc.Work Res.& Abstr., Sociol.Abstr., e-psyche.
—BLDSC (8075.341000), GNLM, KNAW.
Published by: Revue Sante Mentale au Quebec, Succ Place d Armes, C P 548, Montreal, PQ H2Y 3H3, Canada. TEL 514-523-0607, FAX 514-523-0797, rsmq@cam.org, http://www.cam.org/~rsmq/. Ed. Suzanne Cloutier. Circ: 1,200.

150 SWE ISSN 0346-8100
SCANDINAVIAN JOURNAL OF BEHAVIOR THERAPY. SUPPLEMENTUM. Text in English. 1976. irreg.
Related titles: ♦ Supplement to: Scandinavian Journal of Behaviour Therapy. ISSN 0284-5717.
Published by: Scandinavian University Press (Subsidiary of: Taylor & Francis Ltd.), Postboks 2959, Toeyen, Oslo 0608, Norway. TEL 47-22-575400, FAX 47-22-57-53-53.

150 NOR ISSN 0284-5717
CODEN: NTBEDQ
SCANDINAVIAN JOURNAL OF BEHAVIOUR THERAPY/NORDISK TIDSKRIFT FOER BETEENDETERAPI. Text in English, Multiple languages. 1971. 4/yr. GBP 36, USD 60 to individuals; GBP 60, USD 99 to institutions (effective 2002). adv. bk.rev. charts, illus. back issues avail. **Document type:** *Academic/Scholarly.* **Description:** Devoted to the application of the behavioural and cognitive sciences to clinical psychology and psychotherapy.
Former titles (until vol.3, 1984): Nordisk Tidskrift foer Beteendeterapi; (until 1957): Beteendeterapi
Related titles: Online - full text ed.: (from EBSCO Publishing, O C L C Online Computer Library Center, Inc., RoweCom Information Quest, CatchWord Ltd., ingenta, Swets Blackwell); ♦ Supplement: Scandinavian Journal of Behavior Therapy. Supplementum. ISSN 0346-8100.
Indexed: AMED, Behav.Med.Abstr., ERA, PsycInfo, Psychol.Abstr. (1975-), Psycscan B.A.& T., Sp.Ed.Needs Abstr., e-psyche.
—BLDSC (8087.490000), GNLM.
Published by: (Swedish Association for Behaviour Therapy), Taylor & Francis AS (Subsidiary of: Taylor & Francis Group), Cort Adelersgt. 17, Solli, PO Box 2562, Oslo 0202, Norway. TEL 47-22-12-98-80, FAX 47-22-12-98-90, journals@tandf.no, http://www.tandf.co.uk/tfas. Ed. Gerhard Andersson. Circ: 1,000.

150 GBR ISSN 0036-5564
BF1 CODEN: SJPYA2
SCANDINAVIAN JOURNAL OF PSYCHOLOGY. Text in English. 1960. q. GBP 231 to institutions in UK & Europe; USD 360 to institutions in the Americas & Caribbean; GBP 250 elsewhere to institutions (effective 2002). bibl, charts, illus. index, cum.index every 5 yrs. *Refereed.* **Document type:** *Academic/Scholarly.* **Description:** Devoted to original scientific contributions from all fields of psychology.
Related titles: Online - full text ed.: (from EBSCO Publishing, O C L C Online Computer Library Center, Inc., RoweCom Information Quest, ingenta, Swets Blackwell, Institute for Scientific Information).
Indexed: ASCA, ASSIA, Addic.Abstr., Adol.Ment.Hlth.Abstr., AgeLine, Behav.Abstr., Biol.Abstr., Child Devel.Abstr., Curr.Cont., Curr.Ind.Stat., Dent.Ind., Environ.Sci.Poll.Mgmt., Ergon.Abstr., Fam.Ind., IMFL, Ind.Med. (1960-), Lang.& Lang.Behav.Abstr., Mid.East: Abstr.& Ind., Mult.Ed.Abstr., PsycInfo, Psychol.Abstr. (1960-), Risk Abstr., Russ.Acad.Sci.Bibl., SOPODA, SSCI, Saf.Sci.Abstr., Soc.Serv.Abstr., Sociol.Abstr., THA, e-psyche.
—BLDSC (8087.520000), CISTI, GNLM, IDS, ingenta. **CCC.**
Published by: (Psychological Associations of Denmark, Finland, Norway and Sweden), Blackwell Publishers Ltd., 108 Cowley Rd, Oxford OX4 1JF, United Kingdom. TEL 44-1865-791100, FAX 44-1865-791347, jnlinfo@blackwellpublishers.co.uk, http://www.blackwellpublishers.co.uk. Ed. Kenneth Hugdahl TEL 47-55-586-277. Circ: 1,400.

SCHOOL PSYCHOLOGY INTERNATIONAL. see *EDUCATION—Teaching Methods And Curriculum*

370.15 USA ISSN 1045-3830
LB1027.55 CODEN: SPSQE5
SCHOOL PSYCHOLOGY QUARTERLY. Text in English. 1960. q. USD 50 domestic to individuals; USD 62 foreign to individuals; USD 165 domestic to institutions; USD 167 foreign to institutions (effective 2000). adv. bk.rev. illus. index. reprint service avail. from PQC. *Refereed.* **Description:** Focuses on the scientific understanding of school psychology; covers new concepts in enhancing life experiences of children, families and schools.
Formerly: Professional School Psychology (0079-5933)
Related titles: Online - full text ed.: (from Northern Light Technology, Inc., ProQuest Information & Learning, CatchWord Ltd., Institute for Scientific Information, RoweCom Information Quest).
Indexed: ASCA, C.I.J.E., Cont.Pg.Educ., Curr.Cont., Fam.Ind., Lang.& Lang.Behav.Abstr., PsycInfo, Psychol.Abstr. (1986-), SOPODA, SSCI, Sociol.Abstr., e-psyche.
—BLDSC (8092.926500), IDS, ingenta. **CCC.**
Published by: (Division of School Psychology, American Psychological Association), Guilford Publications, Inc., 72 Spring St, 4th Fl, New York, NY 10012. TEL 212-431-9800, 800-365-7006, FAX 212-966-6708, info@guilford.com. Ed. Terry Gutkin. R&P Kathy Kuehl. Adv. contact Susan Pavliscak. Circ: 2,700.

370.15 USA ISSN 0279-6015
LB1051
SCHOOL PSYCHOLOGY REVIEW. Text in English. 1972. q. USD 50 to individuals; USD 55 in Canada to individuals; USD 75 elsewhere to individuals; USD 80 to institutions; USD 85 in Canada to institutions; USD 105 elsewhere to institutions. adv. bk.rev. abstr, bibl, charts, stat, illus. back issues avail.; reprint service avail. from PQC,PSC,SCH. *Refereed.* **Document type:** *Academic/Scholarly.* **Description:** Covers research, training, and practice in school psychology.
Formerly (until 1979): School Psychology Digest (0160-5569)
Related titles: Microform ed.: (from PQC); Online - full text ed.: (from Northern Light Technology, Inc., H. W. Wilson, ProQuest Information & Learning, Institute for Scientific Information).
Indexed: ASCA, C.I.J.E., Cont.Pg.Educ., Curr.Cont., Educ.Ind. (Apr.1983-), PsycInfo, Psychol.Abstr. (1972-), SSCI, Sage Race Rel.Abstr., e-psyche.
—BLDSC (8092.926600), IDS, ingenta.
Published by: National Association of School Psychologists, 4340 East West Hwy, Ste 402, Bethesda, MD 20814-4411. TEL 301-657-0270, FAX 301-657-3127, nasp8455@aol.com. Ed. Susan M Sheridan. Circ: 19,000 (paid).

150 CHE ISSN 1421-0185
SCHWEIZERISCHE ZEITSCHRIFT FUER PSYCHOLOGIE/REVUE SUISSE DE PSYCHOLOGIE/SWISS JOURNAL OF PSYCHOLOGY. Text in French, German; Abstracts in English, German. 1942. 4/yr. DEM 96 domestic; DEM 110 foreign (effective 2001). adv. bk.rev. abstr, bibl, charts. 48 p./no. *Refereed.* **Document type:** *Journal, Academic/Scholarly.*
Related titles: Online - full text ed.: (from Institute for Scientific Information).
Indexed: ASCA, Arts & Hum.Cit.Ind. (coverage dropped), Biol.Abstr., Curr.Cont., Fam.Ind., Ger.J.Psych., PsycInfo, Psychol.Abstr. (1973-), Risk Abstr., Russ.Acad.Sci.Bibl., SSCI, e-psyche.
—BLDSC (8576.760500), IDS.
Published by: (Societe Suisse de Psychologie), Hans Huber AG, Laengassstr 76, Bern, 9 3000, Switzerland. TEL 41-31-3004500, FAX 41-31-3004591, zeitschriften@hanshuber.com, http://www.hanshuber.com. Eds. Dr Gabriel Mugny, Dr M Oswald. Adv. contact Rene Waelchli. B&W page CHF 930, color page CHF 2,070; trim 170 x 250. Circ: 950.

150 USA
SCIENCE AND PRACTICE OF NEUROPSYCHOLOGY. Text in English. irreg. **Document type:** *Monographic series.* **Description:** Focuses on the connections of scientific foundations and clinical practice.
Indexed: e-psyche.
Published by: Guilford Publications, Inc., 72 Spring St, New York, NY 10012. TEL 212-431-9800, 800-365-7006, FAX 212-966-6708, info@guilford.com, http://www.guilford.com. Ed. Robert A Bornstein.

P

150 CAN ISSN 0841-7741
SCIENCE ET COMPORTEMENT; revue internationale et multidisciplinaire. Text in French; Summaries in English, French. 1970-1994; resumed. 3/yr. CND 60 domestic to individuals; CND 75 foreign to individuals; CND 35 domestic to students; CND 45 foreign to students (effective 1999). adv. bk.rev. *Refereed.* **Description:** Covers psychology, special education and rehabilitation and psychiatry.
Formerly: Revue de Modification du Comportement (0383-056X)
Indexed: PsycInfo, Psychol.Abstr. (1979-), Psycscan B.A.& T., Pt.de Rep. (1983-), e-psyche.
—BLDSC (8142.917000).
Published by: Association Scientifique pour la Modification du Comportement, 309 rue Godin, Repentigny, PQ J6A 5Z8, Canada. TEL 514-253-8200, FAX 514-585-9935. Ed., Adv. contact Michel Roberge. Circ: 300.

616.8 USA ISSN 0164-7393
SCRIPT. Text in English. 9/yr. membership. **Document type:** *Newsletter.*
Indexed: e-psyche.
Published by: International Transactional Analysis Association, 436 14th St, Ste 1301, Oakland, CA 94612-2710. TEL 510-625-7720, FAX 510-625-7725, itaa@itaa-net.org, http://www.itaa-net.org. Ed., R&P Robin Fryer.

155.2 ITA ISSN 0391-4224
SCRITTURA (URBINO); rivista di problemi grafologici. Text in Italian. 1971. q. ITL 45,000 (effective 2001). bk.rev. index. 100 p./no. **Document type:** *Magazine.*
Indexed: e-psyche.
Published by: Istituto Grafologico G. Moretti, Piazza San Francesco, 7, Urbino, PS 61029, Italy. info@grafologia.it, http://www.grafologia.it. Ed. Pacifico Cristofanelli. Circ: 1,300.

150 ITA ISSN 1122-3065
SCUOLA JUNGHIANA. ANNALI. Text in Italian. 1991. a., latest vol.4, 1994. ITL 30,000; USD 30 foreign. **Document type:** *Consumer.* **Description:** Aims at people interested in psychology and in C.G. Jung.
Related titles: Online - full text ed.
Indexed: e-psyche.
Published by: (Scuola Junghiana), Scriptorium, Via Pietro Giannone, 9, Milan, MI 20154, Italy. http://www.formazione.it. Ed., R&P Maurilio Orbecchi TEL 39-02-3491778.

616.89 DEU ISSN 1615-343X
▼ **SELBSTPSYCHOLOGIE/SELF PSYCHOLOGY**; europaeische Zeitschrift fuer psychoanalytische Therapie und Forschung. Text in German, English. 2000. q. EUR 49 domestic; EUR 52 foreign (effective 2001). **Document type:** *Magazine, Academic/Scholarly.* **Description:** Contains articles on various aspects of psychoanalytical therapy and research.

Published by: Brandes und Apsel Verlag GmbH, Scheidswaldstr 33, Frankfurt Am Main 60385, Germany. TEL 49-69-95730186, FAX 49-69-95730187, brandes-apsel@t-online.de, http://www.brandes-apsel-verlag.de.

SELECTION AND DEVELOPMENT REVIEW. see *BUSINESS AND ECONOMICS—Management*

152 USA ISSN 1529-8868
▼ **SELF AND IDENTITY.** Text in English. forthcoming 2002. q. GBP 52, USD 78 to individuals; GBP 153, USD 229 to institutions (effective 2002). **Document type:** *Journal.* **Description:** Devoted to the study of social and psychological processes, such as, cognition, motivation, emotion, and interpersonal behavior, that involve the human capacity for self-awareness, self-representation, and self-regulation.
Related titles: Online - full text ed.: forthcoming (from CatchWord Ltd.).
Published by: Psychology Press (Subsidiary of: Taylor & Francis Ltd.), 325 Chestnut St, Ste 800, Philadelphia, PA 19106. TEL 215-625-8900, FAX 215-625-2940, info@taylorandfrancis.com, http://www.psypress.com/. Ed. Mark Leary. **Subscr. addr. in N America:** Journals Customer Service, Taylor & Francis Group, 325 Chestnut St, Philadelphia, PA 19106. TEL 800-354-1420, FAX 215-625-8914**; Subscr. addr. outside N America:** Psychology Press, Journals Customer Service, Taylor & Francis Group, Rankine Rd, Basingstoke, Hants RG24 8PR, United Kingdom. TEL 44-1256-813002, FAX 44-1256-479438, enquiry@tandf.co.uk, http://www.psypress.co.uk.

301.1 150 GBR ISSN 0306-0497
SELF & SOCIETY; European journal of humanistic psychology. Text in English. 1973. bi-m. GBP 10. adv. bk.rev. **Description:** Discusses human potential and research work in psychology and sociology: promotes a holistic view of life and the importance of the individual.
Indexed: Russ.Acad.Sci.Bibl., e-psyche.
—BLDSC (8235.350000).
Published by: (Association for Humanistic Psychology in Britain), Gale Centre Publications, Whitakers Way, Loughton, Essex IG10 1SQ, United Kingdom. TEL 081-508-9344, FAX 081-508-1240. Ed. David Jones. Circ: 1,200.

SELF-HELP AND PSYCHOLOGY MAGAZINE. see *SOCIAL SERVICES AND WELFARE*

THE SELF-HELP SOURCEBOOK; your guide to community and online support group. see *SOCIAL SERVICES AND WELFARE*

616.072 CAN ISSN 1198-7340
SEMINARS IN HEADACHE MANAGEMENT. Text in English. 1996. q. USD 65 in US & Canada to individuals; USD 90 elsewhere to individuals; USD 95 in US & Canada to institutions; USD 125 elsewhere to institutions. back issues avail. **Document type:** *Academic/Scholarly.* **Description:** Covers clinical and research issues in the management of all types of headaches.
Related titles: Online - full text ed.: (from Northern Light Technology, Inc., ProQuest Information & Learning).
Indexed: e-psyche.
—CISTI, KNAW.
Published by: B.C. Decker Inc., 20 Hughson St S, LCD 1, P O Box 620, Hamilton, ON L8N 3K7, Canada. TEL 905-522-7017, 800-568-7281, FAX 905-522-7839, info@bcdecker.com, http://www.bcdecker.com. Eds. Alan M Rapoport, Fred O Sheftell.

SEMIOTIC AND COGNITIVE STUDIES. see *PHILOSOPHY*

150.18 USA ISSN 0894-4520
QP431
SENSORY SYSTEMS. Text in English. 1987. q. USD 920 domestic to institutions; USD 1,075 foreign to institutions (effective 2000). bibl, illus. index. back issues avail. *Refereed.* **Document type:** *Academic/Scholarly.* **Description:** Disseminates important research and theoretical papers in the fields of neuroscience, physiology, biochemistry, bioengineering, biophysics, psychology, and general medicine.
Related titles: Microfilm ed.: (from PQC); Online - full text ed.; Translation of: Sensornye Sistemy. ISSN 0235-0092. 1987.
Indexed: Aqua.Sci.& Fish.Abstr., Chemorec.Abstr., Environ.Sci.Poll.Mgmt., Pollut.Abstr., PsycInfo, Psychol.Abstr. (1987-), e-psyche.
—CISTI, GNLM, Infotrieve, ingenta. **CCC.**
Published by: (Rossiiskaya Akademiya Nauk/Russian Academy of Sciences RUS), Kluwer Academic - Plenum Publishers (Subsidiary of: Wolters Kluwer N.V.), 233 Spring St, New York, NY 10013-1578. TEL 212-620-8468, 800-221-9369, FAX 212-463-0742, info@plenum.com; kluwer@wkap.com; services@wkap.nl, http://www.plenum.com. Ed. M A Ostrovskii.

155.670711 USA ISSN 0275-3510
SERIES IN DEATH EDUCATION, AGING, AND HEALTH CARE. Variant title: Death Education Series. Text in English. 1979. irreg., latest 1991 (unnumbered). price varies. bibl, charts, illus. index. back issues avail.; reprint service avail. from PQC. *Refereed.* **Document type:** *Monographic series.*
Indexed: e-psyche.
—**CCC.**
Published by: Taylor & Francis Ltd. (Subsidiary of: Taylor & Francis Group), 325 Chestnut St, Suite 800, Philadelphia, PA 19016. TEL 215-625-8900, FAX 215-625-2940, info@taylorandfrancis.com, http://www.taylorandfrancis.com/. **Subscr. addr. in Europe:** Taylor & Francis Group, Journals Customer Service, Rankine Rd, Basingstoke, Hants RG24 8PR, United Kingdom. TEL 44-1256-813000, FAX 44-1256-479438, enquiry@tanf.co.uk, http://www.tandf.co.uk/journals.

THE SERIES ON SOCIAL EMOTIONAL LEARNING. see *EDUCATION*

150.19 ITA ISSN 1124-3899
SETTING. Text in Italian. 1990. s-a. ITL 40,000 to individuals; ITL 80,000 to institutions. **Description:** Publishes studies of the association covering the field of psychoanalysis.
Indexed: e-psyche.
Published by: (Associazione di Studi Psicoanalitici), Moretti e Vitalli Editori, Via Betty Ambiveri 15, Bergamo, BG 24126, Italy. TEL 39-35-321588, FAX 39-35-321647. Ed. Ciro Elia.

306.7 USA ISSN 0360-0025
HQ768 CODEN: SROLDH
SEX ROLES. Text in English. 1975. s-m. EUR 977 to institutions for print or online ed.; USD 979 to institutions for pirnt or online ed.; EUR 1,172.40 to institutions Print & Online eds.combined (effective 2002). adv. bk.rev. bibl, charts, illus. Index. back issues avail.; reprint service avail. from PSC,SCH. *Refereed.* **Document type:** *Academic/Scholarly.* **Description:** Publishes original research, theory, and reviews concerned with the underlying processes and consequences of gender role socialization, perceptions, and attitudes.
Related titles: Microfilm ed.: (from PQC); Online - full text ed.: (from CatchWord Ltd., Gale Group, EBSCO Publishing, O C L C Online Computer Library Center, Inc., RoweCom Information Quest, ProQuest Information & Learning, Swets Blackwell, Kluwer Online, Factiva, Institute for Scientific Information).
Indexed: ASCA, ASSIA, Abstr.Anthropol., Adol.Ment.Hlth.Abstr., AgeLine, Amer.Bibl.Slavic & E.Eur.Stud., Anthropol.Lit. (coverage dropped), Arts & Hum.Cit.Ind. (coverage dropped), C.I.J.E., Child Devel.Abstr., Commun.Abstr., Compumath, Crim.Just.Abstr., Curr.Cont., ERA, Excerp.Med., Fam.Ind., Fem.Per. (1982-), High.Educ.Abstr., IBR, IMFL, Ind.Philos., Lang.& Lang.Behav.Abstr., Mid.East: Abstr.& Ind., Mult.Ed.Abstr., PsycInfo, Psychol.Abstr. (1978-), Ref.Zh., Res.High.Educ.Abstr., Risk Abstr., Russ.Acad.Sci.Bibl., SOMA, SOPODA, SSCI, Sage Fam.Stud.Abstr., Soc.Sci.Ind. (Sep.1982-), Soc.Serv.Abstr., Soc.Work Res.& Abstr., Sociol.Abstr., Sociol.Educ.Abstr., Sp.Ed.Needs Abstr., Stud.Wom.Abstr., Wom.Stud.Abstr. (1975-), e-psyche.
—BLDSC (8254.457000), CatchWord, GNLM, IDS, Infotrieve, ingenta. **CCC.**
Published by: Kluwer Academic - Plenum Publishers (Subsidiary of: Wolters Kluwer N.V.), 233 Spring St, New York, NY 10013-1578. TEL 212-620-8000, 800-221-9369, FAX 212-463-0742, http://www.wkap.nl/journalhome.htm/0360-0025. Ed. Sue Rosenberg Zalk. R&P Rose Luongo TEL 781-871-6311.

306.7 USA ISSN 1079-0632
RC560.S47 CODEN: SAJTEY
SEXUAL ABUSE; a journal of research and treatment. Text in English. 1988. q. EUR 296 to institutions for print or online ed.; EUR 355.20 to institutions print & online eds.combined (effective 2002). adv. illus. back issues avail. *Refereed.* **Document type:** *Academic/Scholarly.* **Description:** Publishes clinical and theoretical material relating to the field of sexual abuse. Addresses causes, treatment and consequences for both perpetrators and victims.
Formerly (until 1995): Annals of Sex Research (0843-4611)
Related titles: Online - full text ed.: (from EBSCO Publishing, O C L C Online Computer Library Center, Inc., RoweCom Information Quest, Swets Blackwell, Kluwer Online).
Indexed: Crim.Just.Abstr., Curr.Cont. (coverage dropped), Ind.Med. (1995-), PsycInfo, Psychol.Abstr. (1988-), Soc.Serv.Abstr., Sociol.Abstr., e-psyche.
—BLDSC (8254.482000), GNLM, Infotrieve, ingenta. **CCC.**
Published by: (Association for the Treatment of Sexual Abusers), Kluwer Academic - Plenum Publishers (Subsidiary of: Wolters Kluwer N.V.), 233 Spring St, New York, NY 10013-1578. TEL 212-620-8000, 800-221-9369, FAX 212-463-0742, services@wkap.nl, http://www.wkap.nl/journalhome.htm/1079-0632. Ed. Judith V. Becker. R&P Rose Luongo TEL 781-871-6311.

616.89 USA ISSN 1072-0162
RC560.S43
SEXUAL ADDICTION & COMPULSIVITY; the journal of treatment and prevention. Text in English. 1994. q. GBP 39, USD 70 to individuals; GBP 105, USD 174 to institutions (effective 2002). bk.rev. index. **Document type:** *Academic/Scholarly.* **Description:** Deals with topics pertaining to the growing disorder of sexual addiction and compulsivity.
Related titles: Online - full text ed.: 1994 (from CatchWord Ltd.).
Indexed: Crim.Just.Abstr., ERA, PsycInfo, e-psyche.
—BLDSC (8254.482500).
Published by: (National Council on Sexual Addiction and Compulsivity), Brunner - Routledge (Subsidiary of: Taylor & Francis Group), 325 Chestnut St, Ste 800, Philadelphia, PA 19106. TEL 215-269-0400, FAX 215-269-0363, postmaster@bmpub.com. Ed. Patrick J Carnes. Circ: 1,000.

155.3 610 GBR ISSN 1468-1994
SEXUAL AND RELATIONSHIP THERAPY. Text in English. 1986. q. GBP 130, USD 214 to individuals; GBP 390, USD 647 to institutions (effective 2002). adv. bk.rev. illus, stat. index, cum.index. back issues avail.; reprints avail. *Refereed.* **Document type:** *Academic/Scholarly.*
Formerly (until vol.15): Sexual and Marital Therapy (0267-4653)
Related titles: Microfiche ed.; Online - full content ed.: ISSN 1468-1749 (from EBSCO Publishing, O C L C Online Computer Library Center, Inc., ProQuest Information & Learning, Swets Blackwell); Online - full text ed.: (from CatchWord Ltd., RoweCom Information Quest).
Indexed: ASSIA, Bibl.Asian Stud. (1998), CINAHL, Curr.Adv.Ecol.Sci., ERA, Lang.& Lang.Behav.Abstr., Mult.Ed.Abstr., PsycInfo, Psychol.Abstr. (1986-), SOPODA, Sage Fam.Stud.Abstr., Soc.Serv.Abstr., Sociol.Abstr., Sp.Ed.Needs Abstr., Stud.Wom.Abstr., Viol.& Abuse Abstr., e-psyche.
—BLDSC (8254.483150), CatchWord, EMDOCS, GNLM, Infotrieve, ingenta. **CCC.**
Published by: (Association of Sexual and Marital Therapists), Carfax Publishing Limited (Subsidiary of: Taylor & Francis Group), PO Box 25, Abingdon, Oxon OX14 3UE, United Kingdom. TEL 44-1235-401000, FAX 44-1235-401550, enquiries@carfax.co.uk, enquiry@tandf.co.uk, http://www.carfax.co.uk. Eds. A J Riley, P d'Ardenne.

306.7 USA ISSN 1094-5717
SEXUAL SCIENCE. Text in English. q. USD 20 (effective 1997). charts, illus, stat. **Document type:** *Newsletter.* **Description:** Includes announcements and news of the society, as well as news and current information of interest to sex researchers, therapists, educators, and clinicians.
Formerly (until 1996): Society Newsletter
Indexed: e-psyche.
—**CCC.**
Published by: Society for the Scientific Study of Sexuality, PO Box 416, Allentown, PA 18105. TEL 610-530-2483, FAX 610-530-2485, thesociety@worldnet.att.net, thesociety@inetmail.att.net, http://www.sexscience.org. Ed. Erica C Neuman. Circ: 1,200.

306.7 GBR ISSN 1363-4607
HQ21
SEXUALITIES; studies in culture and society. Text in English. 1998. q. GBP 40 to individuals; GBP 191 to institutions; GBP 11 newsstand/cover to individuals; GBP 49 newsstand/cover to institutions (effective 2002). adv. bk.rev. illus. Index. back issues avail.; reprints avail. *Refereed.* **Document type:** *Journal, Academic/Scholarly.* **Description:** Publishes work of an analytical and ethnographic nature which describes, analyzes, theorizes and provides a critique on the changing nature of the social organization of human sexual experience in the late modern world.

Related titles: Online - full text ed.: (from EBSCO Publishing, O C L C Online Computer Library Center, Inc., RoweCom Information Quest, ingenta, Swets Blackwell).
Indexed: IBZ, Ind.Philos., Soc.Serv.Abstr., Sociol.Abstr., Stud.Wom.Abstr., Viol.& Abuse Abstr., e-psyche.
—BLDSC (8254.485170). **CCC.**
Published by: Sage Publications Ltd., 6 Bonhill St, London EC2A 4PU, United Kingdom. TEL 44-20-7374-0645, FAX 44-20-7374-8741, market@sagepub.co.uk, http://www.sagepub.co.uk. Ed. Ken Plummer. Adv. contact Jenny Kirby. page GBP 195; 114 x 185. Circ: 1,200.

155.937 618 USA
SHARING (ST. CHARLES); the official newsletter of S H A R E. Text in English. 1978. bi-m. USD 20 donation (effective 2001). bk.rev., film rev., video rev., Website rev. bibl. reprints avail. **Document type:** *Newsletter.* **Description:** Provides guidance in bereavement following the death of a baby through miscarriage, stillbirth or newborn death. Includes writing from parents and information on support groups.
Formerly: S H A R E Newsletter
Indexed: e-psyche.
Published by: S H A R E Pregnancy & Infant Loss Support National Office, St Joseph Health, 300 First Capitol Dr, Center, MO 63301. TEL 636-947-6164, 800-821-6819, share@nationalshareoffice.com, http://www.nationalshareoffice.com. Ed. Sue Friedeck. R&P Catherine Lammert. Circ: 4,500.

150 JPN ISSN 0386-1058
BF8.J3 CODEN: SHHYDJ
SHINRIGAKU HYORON/JAPANESE PSYCHOLOGICAL REVIEW. Text in Japanese; Abstracts occasionally in English. 1957. q. JPY 6,500 to individuals; JPY 12,000 to institutions (effective 1999). illus. *Refereed.* **Description:** Contains review articles on experimental psychology.
Indexed: PsycInfo, Psychol.Abstr. (1969-), e-psyche.
—BLDSC (4661.150000).
Published by: Kyoto University, Graduate School of Letters/Kyoto Daigaku Bungakubu Shinrigaku Kyoshitsu, Department of Psychology, Yoshidahon-Machi, Sakyo-ku, Kyoto-shi 606-8317, Japan. FAX 81-75-753-2835, hyouron@kupsy.kyoto-u.ac.jp, http://www.kupsy.kyoto-u.ac.jp/jpn/hyoron. Ed. Naoyuki Osaka. Circ: 2,500 (controlled).

150 JPN ISSN 0021-5236
BF8.J3 CODEN: SHKEA5
SHINRIGAKU KENKYU/JAPANESE JOURNAL OF PSYCHOLOGY. Text in Japanese; Summaries in English. 1926. bi-m. USD 193. adv. abstr, charts, illus. index. *Refereed.* **Document type:** *Journal, Academic/Scholarly.*
Indexed: ASCA, Arts & Hum.Cit.Ind. (coverage dropped), Biol.Abstr., Curr.Cont., Ind.Med. (1926-), Int.Nurs.Ind., Lang.& Lang.Behav.Abstr., PsycInfo, Psychol.Abstr. (1929-), Ref.Zh., Russ.Acad.Sci.Bibl., SOPODA, SSCI, Soc.Serv.Abstr., Sociol.Abstr., e-psyche.
—BLDSC (4658.300000), GNLM, IDS, ingenta.
Published by: Japanese Psychological Association, 5-23-13-7f Hongo, Bunkyo-ku, Tokyo 113-0033, Japan. TEL 81-3-3814-3953, FAX 81-3-3814-3954. Circ: 8,000. **Dist. by:** Business Center for Academic Societies Japan. TEL 81-3-5814-5811, FAX 81-3-5814-5822.

SIKSHA. see *EDUCATION*

SINISTRALIAN. see *CLUBS*

616.89 NOR ISSN 0049-0563
SINNETS HELSE. Text in Norwegian. 1920. 8/yr. NOK 145. adv. bk.rev. bibl.
Indexed: e-psyche.
—CCC.
Published by: Mental Barnehjelp, Arbins Gate 1, Oslo 0253, Norway. Ed. Kirsten Weidemann Ycharff. Circ: 12,000.

154.6 USA ISSN 1531-3034
▼ **SLEEP REVIEW**; the journal for sleep specialists. Text in English. 2000. q. Free to qualified subscribers. adv. **Document type:** *Journal, Trade.* **Description:** Publishes information on the clinical as well as the business management side of sleep medicine.
Related titles: Online - full content ed.
Published by: Curant Communications, Inc. (Subsidiary of: Medical World Communications), 6701 Center Drive W #450, Los Angeles, CA 90045-1556. TEL 310-642-4400, FAX 310-641-0831, http://www.sleepreviewmag.com. Eds. Paige Smith, Tony Ramos. Pub. Tony Ramos. adv.: color page USD 4,125.

302 USA ISSN 1046-4964
HM133 CODEN: SGREE3
SMALL GROUP RESEARCH; an international journal of theory, investigation and application. Text in English. 1970. bi-m. USD 85 to individuals; USD 375 to institutions; USD 20 newsstand/cover to individuals; USD 70 newsstand/cover to institutions (effective 2002). adv. bk.rev. charts, abstr. index. back issues avail.; reprint service avail. from PQC,PSC,SCH. *Refereed.* **Document type:** *Academic/Scholarly.* **Description:** Addresses three vital areas of study: the psychology of small groups, communication within small groups, and the organizational behavior of small groups. Brings together research that probes all aspects of small group functioning, including processes, dynamics, outcomes, and relationship to environment.
Formerly: Small Group Behavior (0090-5526); Incorporates: International Journal of Small Group Research (8756-0275); Comparative Group Studies (0010-4108)
Related titles: Microform ed.: (from PQC); Online - full text ed.: (from EBSCO Publishing, O C L C Online Computer Library Center, Inc., RoweCom Information Quest, ProQuest Information & Learning, ingenta, Swets Blackwell, Institute for Scientific Information).
Indexed: ASCA, ASSIA, Adol.Ment.Hlth.Abstr., AgeLine, C.I.J.E. (coverage dropped), Commun.Abstr., Curr.Cont., ERA, Educ.Admin.Abstr., Educ.Tech.Abstr., Human Resour.Abstr., Lang.& Lang.Behav.Abstr., Mid.East: Abstr.& Ind., PsycInfo, Psychol.Abstr. (1970-), Russ.Acad.Sci.Bibl., SOPODA, SSCI, Sage Fam.Stud.Abstr., Sage Pub.Admin.Abstr., Sage Urb.Stud.Abstr., Soc.Serv.Abstr., Soc.Work Res.& Abstr., Sociol.Abstr., Tech.Educ.Abstr., e-psyche.
—BLDSC (8309.995000), IDS, ingenta. **CCC.**
Published by: Sage Publications, Inc., 2455 Teller Rd, Thousand Oaks, CA 91320. TEL 805-499-0721, 800-818-7243, FAX 805-499-0871, info@sagepub.com, http://www.sagepub.com. Eds. Charles Garvin, Richard Brian Polley. Pub. Sara Miller McCune. R&P Tanya Udin. Adv. contact DeAnna Vega Hammersley. page USD 225. Circ: 800 (paid). **Overseas subscr. to:** Sage Publications Ltd., 6 Bonhill St, London EC2A 4PU, United Kingdom; Sage Publications India Pvt. Ltd., 4215, New Delhi 110 048, India.

SMITH COLLEGE STUDIES IN SOCIAL WORK. see *SOCIAL SERVICES AND WELFARE*

340 USA ISSN 0272-765X
K23
SOCIAL ACTION AND THE LAW. Text in English. 1973. 4/yr. USD 20 to individuals; USD 30 to institutions. adv. bk.rev.
Related titles: Microfiche ed.; Online - full text ed.: (from Gale Group).
Indexed: C.I.J.E. (coverage dropped), C.L.I., L.R.I. (Jan.1981-), Lang.& Lang.Behav.Abstr., Psychol.Abstr., Sociol.Abstr., e-psyche.
Address: c/o Robert Buckhout, Pub, Brooklyn College, Center for Responsive Psychology, Brooklyn, NY 11210. TEL 718-780-5960. Ed. Frank J Sotolongo. Circ: 1,000.

302 NZL ISSN 0301-2212
HM1 CODEN: SBHPAF
SOCIAL BEHAVIOR AND PERSONALITY; an international journal. Text in English. 1973. every 6 wks. USD 480 (effective 2002). adv. bibl, illus, mkt, stat. 104 p./no. back issues avail.; reprint service avail. from ISI. *Refereed.* **Document type:** *Journal, Academic/Scholarly.* **Description:** Publishes papers on all aspects of social psychology, developmental psychology, and personality.
Incorporates (1984-1991): Psychology and Human Development (1011-5021); (1978-1990): Third Force Psychology
Related titles: CD-ROM ed.; Microform ed.: (from PQC); Online - full text ed.: (from ProQuest Information & Learning, Institute for Scientific Information).
Indexed: ASCA, ASSIA, Abstr.Crim.& Pen., Addic.Abstr., AgeLine, Bibl.Asian Stud. (1998), Biol.Abstr., C.I.J.E. (coverage dropped), Child Devel.Abstr., Curr.Cont., Fam.Ind., High.Educ.Abstr., IBZ, IMFL, Ind.Med. (coverage dropped), Ind.Philos., Lang.& Lang.Behav.Abstr., PsycInfo, Psychol.Abstr. (1973-), SOPODA, SSCI, Soc.Serv.Abstr., Sociol.Abstr., Sportsearch, e-psyche.
—BLDSC (8318.054500), IDS, ingenta. **CCC.**
Published by: Society for Personality Research (Inc.), 30 Summerhill Dr., PO Box 1539, Palmerston North 5331, New Zealand. TEL 64-6-355-5736, FAX 64-6-355-5424, stewart@sbp-journal.com, http://www.sbp-journal.com. Ed., R&P, Adv. contact Robert A.C. Stewart. Pub. Robert A C Stewart. Circ: 1,600.

155 USA ISSN 0278-016X
BF311
SOCIAL COGNITION; a journal of social, personality and developmental psychology. Text in English. 1982. q. USD 80 domestic to individuals; USD 105 foreign to individuals; USD 265 domestic to institutions; USD 290 foreign to institutions (effective 2001). adv. bk.rev. abstr. index. back issues avail.; reprint service avail. from PQC. *Refereed.* **Document type:** *Academic/Scholarly.* **Description:** Examines the role of cognitive process in the study of personality, development and social behavior.
Related titles: Online - full text ed.: (from Northern Light Technology, Inc., ProQuest Information & Learning, Gale Group, CatchWord Ltd., Factiva, Institute for Scientific Information, RoweCom Information Quest).
Indexed: ASCA, Biol.Abstr., Curr.Cont., ERA, IBZ, IMFL, Ind.Philos., Intl.Bibl.Soc.Sci., Lang.& Lang.Behav.Abstr., Mult.Ed.Abstr., PsycInfo, Psychol.Abstr. (1982-), Russ.Acad.Sci.Bibl., SOPODA, SSCI, Sage Race Rel.Abstr., Soc.Serv.Abstr., Sociol.Abstr., Sociol.Educ.Abstr., Sp.Ed.Needs Abstr., Stud.Wom.Abstr., e-psyche.
—BLDSC (8318.073000), IDS, Infotrieve, ingenta. **CCC.**
Published by: Guilford Publications, Inc., 72 Spring St, 4th Fl, New York, NY 10012. TEL 212-431-9800, 800-365-7006, FAX 212-966-6708, info@guilford.com, http://www.guilford.com/. Ed. Donal Carlston. Pub. Robert Matloff. R&P Kathy Kuehl. Adv. contact Susan Pavliscak. Circ: 760.

302 USA
HM251
SOCIAL PSYCHOLOGICAL APPLICATIONS TO SOCIAL ISSUES. Text in English. irreg., latest vol.4, 1998. *Refereed.* **Document type:** *Monographic series.*
Formerly (until 1988): Applied Social Psychology Annual (0196-4151)
Indexed: Psychol.Abstr., e-psyche.
—BLDSC. **CCC.**
Published by: (Society for the Psychological Study of Social Issues), Kluwer Academic - Plenum Publishers (Subsidiary of: Wolters Kluwer N.V.), 233 Spring St, New York, NY 10013-1578. TEL 212-620-8000, 800-221-9369, FAX 212-463-0742, info@plenum.com, http://www.plenum.com.

SOCIAL PSYCHOLOGY OF EDUCATION; an international journal. see *EDUCATION*

SOCIAL PSYCHOLOGY QUARTERLY. see *SOCIOLOGY*

SOCIAL SERVICE JOBS. see *OCCUPATIONS AND CAREERS*

302 USA
SOCIAL WORK PRACTICE WITH CHILDREN AND FAMILIES. Text in English. irreg. **Document type:** *Monographic series.* **Description:** Features detailed discussions of assessment, intervention, and professional and value issues.
Indexed: e-psyche.
Published by: Guilford Publications, Inc., 72 Spring St, New York, NY 10012. TEL 212-431-9800, 800-365-7006, FAX 212-966-6708, info@guilford.com, http://www.guilford.com. Ed. Nancy Boyd Webb.

SOCIETY & ANIMALS; social scientific studies of the human experience of other animals. see *ANIMAL WELFARE*

SOCIETY FOR COMPANION ANIMAL STUDIES. JOURNAL. see *ANIMAL WELFARE*

SOCIETY FOR EXISTENTIAL ANALYSIS. JOURNAL. see *PHILOSOPHY*

SOCIETY FOR RESEARCH IN CHILD DEVELOPMENT. MONOGRAPHS. see *CHILDREN AND YOUTH—About*

SOCIOLOGUS; Zeitschrift fuer empirische Ethnosoziologie und Ethnopsychologie. see *SOCIOLOGY*

370.15 USA
SOLVING PROBLEMS IN THE TEACHING OF LITERACY. Text in English. irreg. **Document type:** *Monographic series.* **Description:** Links research with the daily practice of educators and professionals responsible for staff development.
Indexed: e-psyche.
Published by: Guilford Publications, Inc., 72 Spring St, New York, NY 10012. TEL 212-431-9800, 800-365-7006, FAX 212-966-6708, info@guilford.com, http://www.guilford.com. Ed. Cathy Collins Block.

SOMATICS; magazine - journal of the mind - body arts and sciences. see *PHYSICAL FITNESS AND HYGIENE*

P

SOMNOLOGIE/SOMNOLOGY; Zeitschrift fuer Schlafforschung und Schlafmedizin. see *MEDICAL SCIENCES*

SOTSIONIKA, MENTOLOGIYA I PSIKHOLOGIYA LICHNOSTI/SOCIONICS, MENTOLOGY AND PERSONALITY PSYCHOLOGY. see *SOCIOLOGY*

SOUTH AFRICAN JOURNAL OF MUSIC THERAPY/SUID-AFRIKAANSE TYDSKRIF VIR MUSIEKTERAPIE. see *MUSIC*

150 ZAF ISSN 0081-2463
BF1 CODEN: SAJPDL
SOUTH AFRICAN JOURNAL OF PSYCHOLOGY/SUID-AFRIKAANSE TYDSKRIF VIR SIELKUNDE. Text and summaries in English. 1970. q. ZAR 212 domestic to institutions; USD 88 foreign to institutions (effective 2000). adv. bk.rev. bibl, charts, illus, stat. *Refereed.* **Document type:** *Journal, Academic/Scholarly.* **Description:** Publishes empirical research, theoretical and methodological papers, review articles and short communications in the field of psychology.
Incorporates (in July 1983): Psychologia Africana (0079-7332); (in Jan. 1979): South African Psychologist; Which was formerly: Journal of Behavioural Science (0075-4145)
Related titles: Online - full text ed.: (from Institute for Scientific Information).
Indexed: ASCA, Arts & Hum.Cit.Ind. (coverage dropped), Biol.Abstr., CINAHL, Curr.Cont., ERA, Ergon.Abstr., IBR, IBZ, Ind.Philos., Ind.S.A.Per., Indian Psychol.Abstr., Mult.Ed.Abstr., PsycInfo, Psychol.Abstr. (1970-), Russ.Acad.Sci.Bibl., SSCI, Sociol.Educ.Abstr., Sp.Ed.Needs Abstr., Stud.Wom.Abstr., e-psyche.
—BLDSC (8339.750000), IDS.
Published by: (Psychological Society of South Africa), South African Bureau for Scientific Publications, PO Box 11663, Pretoria, Hatfield 0028, South Africa. TEL 27-12-4202016, FAX 27-12-320-7803, bspman@icon.co.za, african.zoology@up.ac.za, http://www.safest.org.za/bsp, http://www.up.ac.za/academic/acadorgs/zssa/. Ed., Adv. contact L J Nicholas. Circ: 1,500.

P

150 BGD ISSN 1025-773X
SOUTH ASIAN JOURNAL OF PSYCHOLOGY. Text in English. 1996. s-a. USD 50 (effective 2000). **Document type:** *Academic/Scholarly.* **Description:** Publishes articles in all branches of psychology.
Indexed: e-psyche.
Published by: South Asian Association of Psychologists, c/o Dept. of Psychology, University of Dhaka, Dhaka 110007, Bangladesh. TEL 880-2-864553, FAX 880-2-865583. Ed. Arun K Sen. R&P, Adv. contact Muhammad R Ali TEL 880-2-883240.

150 NZL ISSN 1329-2617
SOUTH PACIFIC JOURNAL OF PSYCHOLOGY. Text in English; Summaries in English, Spanish. 1984. s-a. USD 50 (effective 2001). adv. bk.rev. *Refereed.* **Document type:** *Academic/Scholarly.* **Description:** Focuses on the human factor and its role in national and international development within the South Pacific Region. Includes quantitative and qualitative methods; long and short papers; papers interfacing psychology and technology; cultural, cross-cultural, inter-cultural issues; international and domestic aid; and community development.
Indexed: e-psyche.
Published by: Massey University, School of Psychology, North Shore Mail Centre, Private Bag 102 904, Auckland, New Zealand. TEL 64-9-443-9799, s.c.carry@massey.ac.nz, http://spjp.massey.ac.nz/. Ed., Pub., R&P, Adv. contact Carr Stuart. Circ: 2,245.
Co-sponsor: University of Papua New Guinea.

301.1 616.8 360 DEU ISSN 0171-4538
SOZIALPSYCHIATRISCHE INFORMATIONEN. Text in German. 1971. q. DEM 54; DEM 62 foreign (effective 1999). adv. back issues avail. **Document type:** *Academic/Scholarly.* **Description:** A journal for people working in psychiatry: psychiatrists, doctors, social workers and nurses.
Indexed: e-psyche.
—GNLM.
Published by: Psychiatrie Verlag GmbH, Thomas-Mann-Str 49A, Bonn 53111, Germany. TEL 49-228-72534-0, FAX 49-228-7253420. Ed. Dr. Haselbeck. Circ: 2,000.

150 ESP
THE SPANISH JOURNAL OF PSYCHOLOGY. Text in Spanish. 1997. s-a. ESP 1,200, USD 15 (effective 2001). **Document type:** *Academic/Scholarly.* **Description:** Aims to disseminate empirical research and methodological proposals in different areas of specialization within psychology.
Indexed: e-psyche.
—CINDOC.
Published by: Universidad Complutense de Madrid, Facultad de Psicologia, Servicio de Publicaciones, C. Isaac Peral s/n, Madrid 28040, Spain. TEL 34-1-3946934, FAX 34-1-3946978, psyjour@sis.ucm.es, http://www.ucm.es/info/extensio/publicaciones/sepindex.htm. Ed. Juan Fernandez.

150 NLD ISSN 1387-5868
▼ **SPATIAL COGNITION AND COMPUTATION.** Text in Dutch. 1999. q. EUR 221.50 to institutions for print or online ed.; EUR 266.40 to institutions print & online eds.combined (effective 2002). back issues avail. **Description:** Aims to concentrate the presentation of research into spatial cognition and computation, and to explicitly encourage an interdisciplinary dialogue.
Related titles: Online - full text ed.: (from EBSCO Publishing, O C L C Online Computer Library Center, Inc., RoweCom Information Quest, Swets Blackwell, Kluwer Online).
Indexed: INSPEC (1999-), e-psyche.
—BLDSC (8361.785150). **CCC.**
Published by: Wolters Kluwer N.V., Kluwer Academic Publishers Group, Postbus 17, Dordrecht 3300 AA, Netherlands. TEL 31-78-639-2392, FAX 31-78-939-2254, servides@wkap.nl, http://www.wkap.nl/journalhome.htm/1387-5868. **Dist. by:** Kluwer Academic Publishers Group, Journals Department, PO Box 322, Dordrecht 3300 AH, Netherlands. TEL 781-871-6600, FAX 31-78-639-2254, 31-78-654-6474.

SPATIAL VISION. see *MATHEMATICS—Computer Applications*

LO SPECCHIO DI PSICHE. see *MEDICAL SCIENCES—Psychiatry And Neurology*

SPECIAL INSIGHT. see *RELIGIONS AND THEOLOGY*

SPECIAL SERVICES IN THE SCHOOLS. see *EDUCATION—Special Education And Rehabilitation*

150.19 790.1 USA ISSN 0888-4781
GV706.4 CODEN: SPPSEU
THE SPORT PSYCHOLOGIST. Short title: T S P. Text in English. 1987. q. USD 45 to individuals; USD 135 to institutions; USD 30 to students (effective 2001). adv. bk.rev. bibl, charts, illus. back issues avail.; reprint service avail. from PSC,SCH. *Refereed.* **Document type:** *Academic/Scholarly.* **Description:** Designed for educational and clinical sport psychologists. Focuses on applied research and practical application of results in providing psychological services to coaches and athletes.
Related titles: Online - full text ed.: (from Institute for Scientific Information).
Indexed: ASCA, Curr.Cont., Focus on: Sports Sci.& Med., IBZ, Ind.Philos., Lang.& Lang.Behav.Abstr., Phys.Ed.Ind., PsycInfo, Psychol.Abstr. (1987-), Rural Recreat.Tour.Abstr., SOPODA, SSCI, Sociol.Abstr., Sportsearch (1987-), e-psyche.
—IDS, ingenta. **CCC.**
Published by: (International Society of Sport Psychology), Human Kinetics Publishers, Inc., PO Box 5076, Champaign, IL 61825-5076. TEL 217-351-5076, 800-747-4457, FAX 217-351-2674, http://www.humankinetics.com. Ed. Vikky Krane. Pub. Rainer Martens. R&P Cheri Banks TEL 217-351-5076 ext 2275. Adv. contact Patty Rodriguiz. Circ: 1,250 (paid).

150 CHE ISSN 0253-4533
P37
SPRACHE & KOGNITION; Zeitschrift fuer Sprach- und Kognitionspsychologie und ihre Grenzgebiete. Text in German; Summaries in English, German. 1982. q. CHF 112 to individuals; CHF 156 to institutions (effective 2001). adv. bk.rev. index. 48 p./no. *Refereed.* **Document type:** *Journal, Academic/Scholarly.*
Related titles: Online - full text ed.: (from Institute for Scientific Information).
Indexed: ASCA, Curr.Cont., Ger.J.Psych., Lang.& Lang.Behav.Abstr., MLA Intl.Bibl., P C I, PsycInfo, Psychol.Abstr. (1982-), SOPODA, SSCI, Sociol.Abstr., e-psyche.
—BLDSC (8419.869250), IDS, Infotrieve. **CCC.**
Published by: Hans Huber AG, Laengassstr 76, Bern, 9 3000, Switzerland. TEL 41-31-3004500, FAX 41-31-3004591, zeitschriften@hanshuber.com, http://www.hanshuber.com. Ed. Werner Deutsch. Adv. contact Rene Waelchli. B&W page DEM 1,140, color page DEM 2,540; trim 170 x 250. Circ: 300.

150 USA ISSN 0362-0522
BF173.A2 CODEN: SAATDM
SPRING JOURNAL; a journal of archetype and culture. Text in English. 1941. s-a. USD 24 to individuals; USD 17.50 newsstand/cover to individuals; USD 35 to institutions. adv. bk.rev. back issues avail.; reprint service avail. from PSC,SCH. *Refereed.* **Document type:** *Academic/Scholarly, Trade.* **Description:** Contains seminal articles on archetypal psychology that examine culture from an archetypal point of view. As the oldest journal on Jungian psychology, examines critically Jung's ideas in the light of post-Jungian developments.
Indexed: PMR, Psychol.Abstr., e-psyche.
—ingenta.
Address: PO Box 583, Putnam, CT 06260. TEL 203-974-3428, FAX 203-974-3195. Ed. Charles Boer. Pub. Jay Livernois. R&P Christopher Ludwig TEL 860-974-3428. Adv. contact Jessica Reiner. Circ: 3,000.

SPRINGER SERIES: FOCUS ON MEN. see *MEN'S HEALTH*

SPRINGER SERIES: FOCUS ON WOMEN. see *WOMEN'S HEALTH*

158 616.8 USA ISSN 0278-6729
SPRINGER SERIES ON BEHAVIOR THERAPY AND BEHAVIORAL MEDICINE. Text in English. 1976. irreg., latest vol.30, 1997. price varies. **Document type:** *Monographic series.* **Description:** Focuses on psychological and psychiatric treatment from a behaviorist perspective.
Formerly (until 1980): Springer Series in Behavior Modification (0272-9636)
Indexed: e-psyche.
Published by: Springer Publishing Company, 536 Broadway, New York, NY 10012. TEL 212-431-4370, FAX 212-941-7842, springer@springerpub.com, http://www.springerpub.com. Ed. Cyril M Franks. R&P Dorothy Kouwenberg.

616.89 USA
SPRINGER SERIES ON COMPARATIVE TREATMENTS FOR PSYCHOLOGICAL DISORDERS. Text in English. irreg. **Document type:** *Monographic series, Academic/Scholarly.* **Description:** Compares and integrates theoretical models that address common clinical concerns of therapists.
Published by: Springer Publishing Company, 536 Broadway, New York, NY 10012. TEL 212-431-4370, 877-687-7476, FAX 212-941-7842, springer@springerpub.com, http://www.springerjournals.com/store/SSCTP.html, http://www.springerpub.com. Ed. Arthur Freeman.

155.937 USA ISSN 0271-1192
SPRINGER SERIES ON DEATH AND SUICIDE. Variant title: Thanatos, the Springer Series on Death and Suicide. Text in English. 1979. irreg., latest vol.14, 1997. price varies. **Document type:** *Monographic series.* **Description:** Approaches topics on death and suicide from a psychological perspective.
Indexed: e-psyche.
Published by: Springer Publishing Company, 536 Broadway, New York, NY 10012. TEL 212-431-4370, FAX 212-941-7842, springer@springerpub.com, http://www.springerpub.com. Ed. Dr. Robert J Kastenbaum. R&P Dorothy Kouwenberg.

STATE PLAN FOR DEVELOPMENTAL DISABILITIES. see *SOCIAL SERVICES AND WELFARE*

150 SWE ISSN 0345-0139
CODEN: RPUSB7
STOCKHOLMS UNIVERSITET. PSYKOLOGISKA INSTITUTIONEN. REPORT SERIES. Text in English. 1954. irreg. (approx. 20/yr.). USD 25. index.
Indexed: Psychol.Abstr., e-psyche.
Published by: Stockholms Universitet, Psykologiska Institutionen, Stockholm 10691, Sweden. FAX 468-159342. Circ: 500.

150 USA ISSN 1053-2161
BF575.S75
STRESS AND EMOTION. Text in English. 1975. irreg., latest vol.16, 1996. price varies. bibl, charts, illus. index. back issues avail.; reprint service avail. from PQC. *Refereed.* **Document type:** *Monographic series, Academic/Scholarly.* **Description:** Aimed at educators, students, researchers, and professionals in the social, behavioral, and medical sciences.
Formerly (until no.14, 1991): Stress and Anxiety (0364-1112)
Indexed: Psychol.Abstr., e-psyche.
—BLDSC (8474.128650), Infotrieve, KNAW. **CCC.**

Published by: Taylor & Francis Ltd. (Subsidiary of: Taylor & Francis Group), 325 Chestnut St, Suite 800, Philadelphia, PA 19016. TEL 215-625-8900, FAX 215-625-2940, info@taylorandfrancis.com, http://www.taylorandfrancis.com/. **Subscr. addr. in Europe:** Taylor & Francis Group, Journals Customer Service, Rankine Rd, Basingstoke, Hants RG24 8PR, United Kingdom. TEL 44-1256-813000, FAX 44-1256-479438, enquiry@tanf.co.uk, http://www.tandf.co.uk/journals.

617.1 155.9042 FRA
▼ **STRESS & TRAUMA**; revue francophone du Stress et du Trauma. Text in French; Summaries in English, French. 2000. q. EUR 69 in Europe to individuals; EUR 85 elsewhere to individuals; EUR 49 in Europe to students; EUR 90 in Europe to institutions; EUR 110 elsewhere to institutions; EUR 23 newsstand/cover (effective 2002). **Description:** Features articles on stress and psychotraumatology. Includes clinics, therapeutics, work on the field, epidemiology and pathogeny.
Indexed: e-psyche.
Published by: Princeps Editions, 64 av. du General de Gaulle, Issy-les-Moulineaux 92130, France. TEL 33-01-46382414, FAX 33-01-40957215.

STRESS MANAGEMENT FOR LAW ENFORCEMENT; behind the shield: combating trauma. see *CRIMINOLOGY AND LAW ENFORCEMENT*

362.2 SWE ISSN 0280-2783
STRESSFORSKNINGSRAPPORTER. Text in English, Swedish. 1967. irreg., latest vol.231, 1991. SEK 125 (effective 1998). index. back issues avail. *Refereed.* **Document type:** *Monographic series.* **Description:** Aims to study the influence of psychosocial risk situations on the one hand and man's emotional, behavioural and physiological reactions on the other, as well as their relation to mental and somatic morbidity and mortality.
Related titles: Online - full text ed.
Indexed: e-psyche.
—BLDSC (8474.141000).
Published by: Karolinska Institutet, Institutionen foer Klinisk Neurovetenskap, Sektionen foer Stressforskning, Fack 230, Stockholm 17177, Sweden. TEL 46-08-7286400, FAX 46-08-344143, http://www.ki.se/ipm/. Ed. Toeres Theorell.

302 USA ISSN 1070-5511
QA278
STRUCTURAL EQUATION MODELING; a multidisciplinary journal. Text in English. 1994. q. USD 45 in US & Canada to individuals; USD 75 elsewhere to individuals; USD 420 in US & Canada to institutions; USD 450 elsewhere to institutions (effective 2002). adv. bk.rev. **Document type:** *Journal, Academic/Scholarly.* **Description:** Covers all academic disciplines with an interest in structural equation modeling, including psychology, sociology, educational research, political science, economics and management.
Related titles: Online - full text ed.: ISSN 1532-8007. USD 40.50 to individuals (effective 2001 & 2002); USD 378 to institutions (effective 2002) (from CatchWord Ltd., EBSCO Publishing, O C L C Online Computer Library Center, Inc., RoweCom Information Quest, Swets Blackwell).
Indexed: C.I.J.E., Curr.Ind.Stat., PsycInfo, e-psyche.
—BLDSC (8477.210000), CatchWord. **CCC.**
Published by: Lawrence Erlbaum Associates, Inc., 10 Industrial Ave, Mahwah, NJ 07430-2262. TEL 201-760-3735, 800-926-6579, FAX 201-236-0072, journals@erlbaum.com, http://www.erlbaum.com/Journals/journals/SEM/sem.htm. Ed. George A Marcoulides. adv.: page USD 725; trim 5 x 8.

STUDI DI PSICOLOGIA DELL'EDUCAZIONE. see *EDUCATION*

150 BEL
STUDIA PSYCHOLOGICA. Text in Multiple languages. 1954. irreg. price varies. **Document type:** *Academic/Scholarly.*
Published by: Leuven University Press, Blijde Inkomststraat 5, Leuven 3000, Belgium. TEL 32-16-325345, FAX 32-16-325352, university.press@upers.kuleuven.ac.be, http://www.lup.be.

150 SVK ISSN 0039-3320
CODEN: STPSAK
STUDIA PSYCHOLOGICA; journal for basic research in psychological sciences. Text in English; Summaries in Czech, Slovak, English. 1958. 5/yr. USD 135 (effective 2002). adv. bk.rev. charts, illus. index. *Refereed.* **Document type:** *Academic/Scholarly.* **Description:** Publishes original experimental and theoretical studies about results of investigations carried out in Slovakia and abroad in the field of basic psychological research.
Related titles: Online - full text ed.: (from Institute for Scientific Information).
Indexed: ASCA, AgeLine, Arts & Hum.Cit.Ind. (coverage dropped), Biol.Abstr., Child Devel.Abstr., Curr.Cont., Fam.Ind., Lang.& Lang.Behav.Abstr., PsycInfo, Psychol.Abstr. (1960-), Russ.Acad.Sci.Bibl., SOPODA, SSCI, Soc.Serv.Abstr., Sociol.Abstr., e-psyche.
—BLDSC (8483.202000), IDS.
Published by: (Slovak Academy of Sciences, Institute of Experimental Psychology), Slovak Academic Press Ltd., Nam Slobody 6, PO Box 57, Bratislava 81005, Slovakia. expspro@savba.savba.sk, http://www.elis.sk. Ed. Dr. Damian Kovac. R&P M Skultety. Adv. contact M. Skultety. Circ: 1,300. **Dist. by:** Mezhdunarodnaya Kniga, B Yakimanka 39, Moscow 117049, Russian Federation. TEL 7-095-2384967, FAX 7-095-2384634.

STUDIA PSYCHOLOGICA ET PAEDAGOGICA; series altera. see *EDUCATION*

150 SWE ISSN 0586-8858
STUDIA PSYCHOLOGICA UPSALIENSIA. Text in Multiple languages. 1969. irreg. price varies. **Document type:** *Monographic series, Academic/Scholarly.*
Published by: (Uppsala Universitet), Acta Universitatis Upsaliensis (Subsidiary of: Uppsala University), PO Box 256, Uppsala 75105, Sweden. **Dist. by:** Almqvist & Wiksell International.

150 POL ISSN 0081-685X
CODEN: SPSLBL
STUDIA PSYCHOLOGICZNE. Text in Polish; Summaries in English, Polish. 1956. s-a. PLZ 10 domestic; USD 18 foreign (effective 2000 & 2001). *Refereed.* **Document type:** *Academic/Scholarly.* **Description:** Works concerning historical and experimental psychology, theoretical and methodological problems, social perception, personal communication.
Indexed: Ind.Philos., Lang.& Lang.Behav.Abstr., PsycInfo, Psychol.Abstr. (1970-), Russ.Acad.Sci.Bibl., e-psyche.
Published by: Polska Akademia Nauk, Instytut Psychologii, Ul Podlesna 61, Warsaw 01673, Poland. TEL 48-22-8340907, FAX 48-22-8340907, jacekj@atos.psychpan.waw.pl. Ed. Magdalena Marszal-Wisniewska. Pub. Jacek Jarymowicz.

STUDIA UNIVERSITATIS "BABES-BOLYAI". PSYCHOLOGIA - PAEDAGOGIA. see *EDUCATION*

STUDIEN UND BERICHTE. see *EDUCATION*

155.4 DEU ISSN 0255-6715
STUDIEN ZUR KINDERPSYCHOANALYSE. JAHRBUCH. Text in German. 1981. a. DEM 35.10 (effective 2000). adv. *Refereed.* **Document type:** *Academic/Scholarly.* **Description:** Examines questions and problems concerning theories and techniques within child psychoanalysis.
Indexed: e-psyche.
—GNLM.
Published by: (Oesterreichische Studiengesellschaft fuer Kinderpsychoanalyse), Vandenhoeck und Ruprecht, Robert-Bosch-Breite 6, Goettingen 37079, Germany. TEL 49-551-6959-0, FAX 49-551-695917, vandenhoek@aol.com, info@vandenhoeck-ruprecht.de, http://www.vandenhoeck-ruprecht.de. Pub. Bernd Rachel. R&P Gerlinde Eggeling. Adv. contact Anja Kuetemeyer. Circ: 450.

153.4 121 NLD ISSN 0924-0780
STUDIES IN COGNITIVE SYSTEMS. Text in English. 1988. irreg., latest vol.15, 1993. price varies. **Document type:** *Monographic series.*
Indexed: Zent.Math., e-psyche.
Published by: Kluwer Academic Publishers Group (Subsidiary of: Wolters Kluwer N.V.), Spuiboulevard 50, PO Box 17, Dordrecht 3300 AA, Netherlands. FAX 31-78-639-2254, services@wkap.nl, http://www.wkap.nl. **Dist. by:** Journals Department, PO Box 322, Dordrecht 3300 AH, Netherlands. FAX 31-78-654-6474.

STUDIES IN EATING DISORDERS: AN INTERNATIONAL SERIES. see *MEDICAL SCIENCES—Psychiatry And Neurology*

STUDIES IN EDUCATION AND PSYCHOLOGY. see *EDUCATION*

150 401 NLD ISSN 0924-4662
STUDIES IN LINGUISTICS AND PHILOSOPHY. Text in Dutch. 1978. irreg., latest vol.50, 1993. price varies. reprint service avail. from PSC. *Refereed.* **Document type:** *Monographic series.*
Formerly (until 1989): Synthese Language Library
Indexed: Bibl.Ling., C.C.M.J., MLA Intl.Bibl. (coverage dropped), Math.R., Russ.Acad.Sci.Bibl., Zent.Math., e-psyche.
—BLDSC (8491.028000).
Published by: Kluwer Academic Publishers Group (Subsidiary of: Wolters Kluwer N.V.), Spuiboulevard 50, PO Box 17, Dordrecht 3300 AA, Netherlands. FAX 31-78-639-2254, services@wkap.nl, http://www.wkap.nl. **Dist. by:** Journals Department, PO Box 322, Dordrecht 3300 AH, Netherlands. FAX 31-78-654-6474.

STUDIES IN THE PSYCHOLOGY OF RELIGION. see *RELIGIONS AND THEOLOGY*

158 IRL
THE SUCCESS EXPRESS JOURNAL. Text in English. 1995. w. **Description:** Contains articles on personal improvement, motivation and success.
Media: Online - full text.
Indexed: e-psyche.
Published by: Life - Press Communications, PO Box 1062, Grand Cayman, Ireland. kaizen@success.ie, http://www.success.ie. Ed. Eric Edmeades.

150.19 USA
SUGGESTION QUARTERLY. Text in English. 1962. q. membership only. bk.rev. **Document type:** *Bulletin, Academic/Scholarly.*
Indexed: e-psyche.
Published by: Association to Advance Ethical Hypnosis, c/o Nell R Orndorf, M A, 2675 Oakwood Dr, Cuyahoga Falls, OH 44221. Circ: 1,200.

362.28 USA ISSN 0363-0234
RC569 CODEN: SLBEDP
SUICIDE AND LIFE-THREATENING BEHAVIOR; the official journal of the American Association of Suicidology . Text in English. 1970. q. USD 60 domestic to individuals; USD 85 foreign to individuals; USD 239 domestic to institutions; USD 264 foreign to institutions (effective 2001). adv. bk.rev. abstr. bibl, illus. index. back issues avail.; reprint service avail. from PQC,PSC,SCH,ISI. *Refereed.* **Document type:** *Academic/Scholarly.* **Description:** Biological, statistical, psychological and sociological approaches to the full range of suicide issues.
Former titles: Suicide (0360-1390); Life Threatening Behavior (0047-4592)
Related titles: Microform ed.: (from PQC); Online - full text ed.: (from ProQuest Information & Learning, Gale Group, CatchWord Ltd., Factiva, Institute for Scientific Information, RoweCom Information Quest).
Indexed: ASCA, Abstr.Anthropol., Abstr.Crim.& Pen., Abstr.Soc.Geront., Adol.Ment.Hlth.Abstr., AgeLine, Biol.Abstr., CERDIC, C.I.J.E., Commun.Abstr., Community Ment.Health Rev., Crim.Just.Abstr., Curr.Cont., Excerp.Med., Fam.Ind., Human Resour.Abstr., Ind.Med. (1976-), Int.Nurs.Ind., Lang.& Lang.Behav.Abstr., P C I, Peace Res.Abstr., PsycInfo, Psychol.Abstr. (1971-), SOPODA, SSCI, Sage Fam.Stud.Abstr., Sage Urb.Stud.Abstr., Soc.Sci.Ind. (Mar.1987-), Soc.Serv.Abstr., Sociol.Abstr., Viol.& Abuse Abstr., e-psyche.
—BLDSC (8514.141000), EMDOCS, GNLM, IDS, Infotrieve, ingenta. **CCC.**
Published by: (American Association of Suicidology), Guilford Publications, Inc., 72 Spring St, 4th Fl, New York, NY 10012. TEL 212-431-9800, 800-365-7006, FAX 212-966-6708, info@guilford.com, http://www.guilford.com/cartscript.cgi?page=periodicals/jnsl.htm&cart_id=668979.21709. Ed. Morton Silverman. Pub. Robert Matloff. R&P Kathy Kuehl. Adv. contact Susan Pavliscak. Circ: 2,000.

SVEUCILISTE U ZAGREBU. FILOZOFSKI FAKULTET. INSTITUT ZA PEDAGOGIJSKA ISTRAZIVANJA. ZBORNIK RADOVA. see *EDUCATION*

150 USA
SWISS MONOGRAPHS IN PSYCHOLOGY. Text in English. irreg., latest vol.4. **Document type:** *Monographic series, Academic/Scholarly.*
Indexed: e-psyche.
—BLDSC.
Published by: (Swiss Psychological Society), Hogrefe & Huber Publishers, PO Box 2487, Kirkland, WA 98083. TEL 425-820-1500, FAX 425-823-8324.

P

616.89 DEU ISSN 0724-7923
BF173.A2
SYSTEM UBW; Zeitschrift fuer klassische Psychoanalyse. Text in German; Summaries in English, French. 1983. irreg. DEM 52 for 4 nos. (effective 2001). bk.rev. 100 p./no. back issues avail. **Document type:** *Magazine, Academic/Scholarly.* **Description:** Scientific periodical for psychoanalysis in the tradition of Sigmund Freud.
Indexed: IBZ, Russ.Acad.Sci.Bibl., e-psyche.
—GNLM.
Published by: Ahriman Verlag GmbH, Postfach 6569, Freiburg Im Breisgau 79041, Germany. TEL 49-761-502303, FAX 49-761-502247, ahriman@t-online.de, http://www.ahriman.com. Eds. Fritz Erik Hoevels, Peter Priskil. **Dist. by:** Thanilo Verlag und Vertriebs GmbH, Postfach 710, Freiburg Im Breisgau 79007, Germany. TEL 49-761-502303, FAX 49-761-502247, thanilo@t-online.de.

150 CHE ISSN 0891-4451
SYSTEMS RESEARCH IN PHYSIOLOGY. Text in English. 1982. irreg., latest vol.4, 1990. *Refereed.* **Document type:** *Monographic series.*
Indexed: e-psyche.
—CISTI.
Published by: Gordon and Breach - Harwood Academic (Subsidiary of: Taylor & Francis Group), PO Box 531, Lausanne 1000, Switzerland. Ed. K V Sudakov. **Subscr. addr. in US:** International Publishers Direct, PO Box 32160, Newark, NJ 07102. FAX 215-750-6343.

150 USA
TAKING SIDES: CLASHING VIEWS ON CONTROVERSIAL ISSUES IN HUMAN SEXUALITY. Text in English. irreg., latest vol.6, 1997. USD 13. illus. **Document type:** *Academic/Scholarly.*
Indexed: e-psyche.
Published by: Dushkin - McGraw-Hill, Sluice Dock, Guilford, CT 06437-9989. TEL 203-453-4351, FAX 203-453-6000. Ed. Robert T Francoeur. Pub. David Dean. R&P Cheryl Greenleaf.

150 USA
TAKING SIDES: CLASHING VIEWS ON CONTROVERSIAL MORAL ISSUES. Text in English. irreg., latest vol.6, 1997. USD 13. illus. **Document type:** *Academic/Scholarly.*
Published by: Dushkin - McGraw-Hill, Sluice Dock, Guilford, CT 06437-9989. TEL 203-453-4351, FAX 203-453-6000. Ed. Stephen Satris. Pub. David Dean. R&P Cheryl Greenleaf.

150 USA
TAKING SIDES: CLASHING VIEWS ON CONTROVERSIAL PSYCHOLOGICAL ISSUES. Text in English. irreg., latest vol.10, 1997. USD 13. illus. **Document type:** *Academic/Scholarly.*
Indexed: e-psyche.
Published by: Dushkin - McGraw-Hill, Sluice Dock, Guilford, CT 06437-9989. TEL 203-453-4351, FAX 203-453-6000. Eds. Brent Slife, Joseph Rubinstein. Pub. David Dean. R&P Cheryl Greenleaf.

TAROT NETWORK NEWS. see *NEW AGE PUBLICATIONS*

150.71 USA ISSN 0098-6283
BF77
TEACHING OF PSYCHOLOGY. Text in English. 1974. q. USD 35 in US & Canada to individuals; USD 65 elsewhere to individuals; USD 275 in US & Canada to institutions; USD 305 elsewhere to institutions (effective 2002). adv. bk.rev., film rev. bibl, charts, illus. index. back issues avail.; reprint service avail. from PQC,PSC,SCH. *Refereed.* **Document type:** *Journal, Academic/Scholarly.* **Description:** Provides information to improving the learning-teaching process at all educational levels: from secondary through college and graduate school, to continuing education.
Related titles: Microform ed.: (from PQC); Online - full text ed.: ISSN 1532-8023. USD 31.50 to individuals; USD 247.50 to institutions (effective 2002) (from CatchWord Ltd., EBSCO Publishing, O C L C Online Computer Library Center, Inc., RoweCom Information Quest, Swets Blackwell, Institute for Scientific Information).
Indexed: ASCA, AgeLine, Amer.Bibl.Slavic & E.Eur.Stud., C.I.J.E., Cont.Pg.Educ., Curr.Cont., ERA, Educ.Ind. (Oct.1983-), Educ.Tech.Abstr., Mult.Ed.Abstr., PsycInfo, Psychol.Abstr. (1974-), Psychol.R.G., SSCI, Tech.Educ.Abstr., e-psyche.
—BLDSC (8614.330000), CatchWord, Infotrieve, ingenta. **CCC.**

Published by: (Division Two, American Psychological Association), Lawrence Erlbaum Associates, Inc., 10 Industrial Ave, Mahwah, NJ 07430-2262. TEL 201-760-3735, 800-926-6579, FAX 201-236-0072, journals@erlbaum.com, http://www.erlbaum.com/Journals/journals/TOP/top.htm. Ed. Randolph A Smith. adv.: page USD 450; trim 7 x 10. Circ: 3,200.

150 158.7 CAN
TELL-A-TYPE. Text in English. q. membership. **Document type:** *Newsletter.*
Published by: Ontario Association for the Application of Personality Type, 116 Viceroy Rd, Unit B1, Concord, ON L4K 2M2, Canada. TEL 905-760-1339, FAX 905-760-0113, dhughes@career-lifeskills.

TERAPIA FAMILIARE. see *LAW—Family And Matrimonial Law*

TESTIMONI; quindicinale di informazione e aggiornamento per istituti di vita consacrata. see *RELIGIONS AND THEOLOGY*

371.3 USA ISSN 0361-025X
Z5814.E9
TESTS IN PRINT. Text in English. 1961. quinquennial, latest vol.5, 1999. price varies. bibl. cum.index. back issues avail. **Document type:** *Academic/Scholarly.* **Description:** A reference listing over 4,000 test instruments that are commercially available in English. Includes description of tests, intended population, scores available, current pricing, and publisher name and address.
Indexed: e-psyche.
Published by: Buros Institute of Mental Measurements, 135 Bancroft Hall, University of Nebraska Lincoln, Lincoln, NE 68588-0348. TEL 402-472-6203, FAX 402-472-6207, bimm@unlinfo.unl.edu, http://www.unl.edu/buros. Ed. Linda L Murphy. **Dist. by:** University of Nebraska Press, 233 N 8th St, Lincoln, NE 68588-0255. TEL 800-755-1105, FAX 402-4726214.

THANATOLOGY ABSTRACTS. see *PSYCHOLOGY—Abstracting, Bibliographies, Statistics*

155.937 USA
THANATOLOGY LIBRARIAN; news of books on death, bereavement, loss & grief. Text in English. 1979. s-a. USD 15. bk.rev. back issues avail.
Indexed: e-psyche.
Published by: Center for Thanatology Research and Education Inc., 391 Atlantic Ave, Brooklyn, NY 11217-1701. TEL 718-858-3026. Ed. Roberta Halporn. Circ: 4,000.

156 DEU ISSN 0934-5272
HM291
THEMENZENTRIERTE INTERAKTION. Text and summaries in English, German. 1987. s-a. DEM 32 (effective 2001). adv. bk.rev. back issues avail. **Document type:** *Magazine, Academic/Scholarly.*
Indexed: e-psyche.
Published by: Matthias Gruenewald Verlag GmbH, Max-Hufschmidt-Str 4A, Mainz 55130, Germany. TEL 49-6131-9286-0, FAX 49-6131-928626, mail@gruenewaldverlag.de, http://www.engagementbuch.de. Ed. Josef Wagner. Adv. contact Antje Weber TEL 49-6131-928613. B&W page DEM 1,050; trim 150 x 200. Circ: 2,800 (paid).

THEORIA; a Swedish journal of philosophy. see *PHILOSOPHY*

370.15 150 GBR ISSN 0959-3543
BF1 CODEN: THPSEJ
THEORY & PSYCHOLOGY. Text in English. 1990. bi-m. GBP 44 to individuals; GBP 299 to institutions; GBP 8 newsstand/cover to individuals; GBP 51 newsstand/cover to institutions (effective 2002). adv. bk.rev. *Refereed.* **Document type:** *Academic/Scholarly.* **Description:** Fosters theoretical dialogue and innovation within psychology, focusing on the emergent themes at the center of contemporary psychological debate.
Related titles: Online - full text ed.: (from EBSCO Publishing, O C L C Online Computer Library Center, Inc., RoweCom Information Quest, ingenta, Swets Blackwell, Institute for Scientific Information).
Indexed: ASCA, Arts & Hum.Cit.Ind. (coverage dropped), Curr.Cont., Fam.Ind., Human Resour.Abstr., IBZ, Ind.Philos., Lang.& Lang.Behav.Abstr., PsycInfo, Psychol.Abstr. (1991-), Russ.Acad.Sci.Bibl., SOPODA, SSCI, Sage Fam.Stud.Abstr., Soc.Serv.Abstr., Sociol.Abstr., Stud.Wom.Abstr., Viol.& Abuse Abstr., e-psyche.
—BLDSC (8814.628600), IDS, Infotrieve, ingenta. **CCC.**

Published by: Sage Publications Ltd., 6 Bonhill St, London EC2A 4PU, United Kingdom. TEL 44-20-7374-0645, FAX 44-20-7374-8741, market@sagepub.co.uk, http://www.sagepub.co.uk. Ed. Henderikus J Stam. Adv. contact Jenny Kirby. page GBP 195.

150 USA ISSN 1061-4362
THERAPISTS REPORT. Text in English. 1985. q. USD 49 (effective 2000). adv. back issues avail. **Document type:** *Newsletter.* **Description:** Disseminates information to behavioral therapists on what is new in the behavioral sciences.
Indexed: e-psyche.
Published by: American Association of Behavioral Therapists, PO Box 1737, Ormond Beach, FL 32175-1735. Ed., Pub., R&P, Adv. contact Dan J Allen. Circ: 1,000.

150 100 GBR ISSN 1354-6783
BF441 CODEN: THREFM
THINKING & REASONING. Text in English. 1995. q. GBP 73, USD 120 to individuals; GBP 149, USD 245 to institutions (effective 2002). adv. **Document type:** *Academic/Scholarly.* **Description:** Dedicated to the understanding of human thought processes, particularly reasoning. The primary focus is on psychological studies of thinking.
Related titles: Online - full text ed.: ISSN 1464-0708 (from CatchWord Ltd., EBSCO Publishing, O C L C Online Computer Library Center, Inc., RoweCom Information Quest, Swets Blackwell).
Indexed: Ergon.Abstr., INSPEC (1995-), Lang.& Lang.Behav.Abstr., PsycInfo, SOPODA, Sociol.Abstr., e-psyche.
—BLDSC (8820.134600), AskIEEE, CatchWord.
Published by: Psychology Press (Subsidiary of: Taylor & Francis Group), 27 Church Rd, Hove, E Sussex BN3 2FA, United Kingdom. TEL 44-1273-207411, FAX 44-1273-205612, information@psypress.co.uk, http://www.psypress.co.uk. Ed. Jonathan Evans. **Subscr. addr. in N America:** Psychology Press, Journals Customer Service, Taylor & Francis Group, 325 Chestnut St, Philadelphia, PA 19106. TEL 800-354-1420, FAX 215-625-8914, info@taylorandfrancis.com, http://www.psypress.com; **Subscr. addr. outside N America:** Journals Customer Service, Taylor & Francis Group, Rankine Rd, Basingstoke, Hants RG24 8PR, United Kingdom. TEL 44-1256-813002, FAX 44-1256-479438, enquiry@tandf.co.uk.

158 616.89 NLD ISSN 1380-7161
TIJDSCHRIFT VOOR CLIENTGERICHTE PSYCHOTHERAPIE. Text in Dutch. 1984. q. **Document type:** *Academic/Scholarly.* **Description:** Examines client-directed psychotherapy.
Former titles (until 1994): V R T - Periodiek (0165-9014); (until 1989): Vereniging voor Rogeriaanse Therapie. Mededelingenblad (0923-9189)
Published by: (Vereniging voor Clientgerichte Psychotherapie te Utrecht), Elsevier Gezondheidszorg B.V., Tijdstroom (Subsidiary of: Reed Elsevier plc Group), Planetenbaan 1, Maarssen 3600 AK, Netherlands. TEL 31-346-577577, FAX 31-346-554287, http://www.tijdstroom.nl. **Subscr. to:** Elsevier Den Haag, Postbus 16500, The Hague 2500 BM, Netherlands. TEL 31-70-381-9900, FAX 31-70-333-8399. **Co-sponsor:** Vlaamse Vereniging voor Clientgerichte Psychotherapie te Leuven, BE.

615.85 NLD ISSN 0169-6912
TIJDSCHRIFT VOOR CREATIEVE THERAPIE. Text in Dutch; Summaries in English. 1965. q. NLG 85 domestic to individuals; NLG 100 foreign to individuals; NLG 125 domestic to institutions; NLG 140 foreign to institutions (effective 2000). adv. bk.rev. **Document type:** *Journal, Trade.* **Description:** Publishes articles on the practice and methods of art, drama, dance, music, and horticulture therapies.
Formed by the 1982 merger of: Nederlandse Vereniging voor Kreatieve Therapie. Documentatieblad; Stichting voor Muziektherapie. Documentatieblad
Indexed: e-psyche.
Published by: Nederlandse Vereniging voor Creatieve Therapie, Fivelingo 253, Utrecht 3524 BN, Netherlands. TEL 31-30-280-0432, FAX 31-30-289-3086, nvkt@casema.net. Ed. Willemijn van Welzen. adv.: B&W page NLG 600. Circ: 1,425.

TIROLER SCHULE. see *EDUCATION*

150 USA
TODAY (BUFFALO). Text in English. m. free per issue. **Document type:** *Newspaper, Consumer.*
Indexed: e-psyche.

P

Published by: Mental Health Association of Erie County, 999 Delaware Ave, Buffalo, NY 14209. TEL 716-886-1242. Ed., R&P Sandra Majewski. Circ: 3,000.

150.19 370.15 371.3 USA ISSN 1098-9277
TODAY'S SCHOOL PSYCHOLOGIST. Text in English. 1997. m. USD 130 (effective 1999). **Document type:** *Newsletter.* **Description:** In-depth guide to a school psychologist's job, offering practical strategies and tips for handling day to day tasks and responsibilities, encouraging change, and improving professional standing and performance.
—CCC.
Published by: L R P Publications, 747 Dresher Rd, Box 980, Horsham, PA 19044. TEL 800-341-7874, FAX 215-784-9639, custserve@lrp.com, http://www.lrp.com. Pub. Kenneth F Kahn.

150 JPN ISSN 0040-8743
BF1 CODEN: TPSFAD
TOHOKU PSYCHOLOGICA FOLIA. Text in English, French, German. 1933. a. per issue exchange basis. charts, illus. index. *Refereed.* **Document type:** *Academic/Scholarly.* **Description:** Contains full paper and short research notes, technical or instrument notes, and letters on the study of psychology.
Indexed: Biol.Abstr., Child Devel.Abstr., Curr.Cont. (coverage dropped), Lang.& Lang.Behav.Abstr., PsycInfo, Psychol.Abstr. (1933-), SOPODA, Sociol.Abstr., e-psyche.
—BLDSC (8862.350000).
Published by: Tohoku Daigaku, Bungakubu Shinrigaku Kyoshitsu/Tohoku University, Faculty of Arts and Letters, Department of Psychology, Kawauchi, Aoba-ku, Sendai-shi, Miyagi-ken 980-0862, Japan. TEL 81-22-217-6048, FAX 81-22-217-3703, ohbuchi@sal.tohoku.ac.jp, http://www.sal.tohoku.ac.jp/psychology/folia/folia.htm. Ed. Hideshi Ohashi. Circ: 525.

302 ARG
TOPIA REVISTA; psicoanalisis, sociedad y cultura. Text in Spanish. 1991. 3/yr. ARS 23; USD 25 foreign. adv. bk.rev. **Document type:** *Newsletter.*
Indexed: e-psyche.
Address: Juan Maria Gutierrez, 3809 3o A, Capital Federal, Buenos Aires 1425, Argentina. TEL 54-114-8025434, FAX 54-114-9430968, tp@topia.psico.net. Eds. Alejandro Vainer, Enrique Carpintero.

TOPIQUE - REVUE FREUDIENNE. see *MEDICAL SCIENCES—Psychiatry And Neurology*

TOPOI; an international review of philosophy. see *PHILOSOPHY*

TOTAL HEALTH; for longevity. see *NUTRITION AND DIETETICS*

616.89 361.06 GBR
TRAINING IN COUNSELLING & PSYCHOTHERAPY. Text in English. 1984. a., latest 2000, 16th Ed. **Document type:** *Directory.*
—BLDSC.
Published by: British Association for Counseling, 1 Regent Pl, Rugby, Warks CV21 2PJ, United Kingdom. TEL 44-1788-578328.

616.8 370 USA ISSN 0362-1537
RC489.T7
TRANSACTIONAL ANALYSIS JOURNAL. Text in English. 1962. q. USD 50. adv. bk.rev. abstr, charts. index. back issues avail.; reprint service avail. from PSC,SCH.
Formerly: Transactional Analysis Bulletin (0041-1051)
Related titles: Microform ed.: (from PQC).
Indexed: ASCA, AgeLine, Curr.Cont. (coverage dropped), Indian Psychol.Abstr., PsycInfo, Psychol.Abstr. (1974-), SSCI (coverage dropped), e-psyche.
—BLDSC (9020.564000), GNLM, ingenta.
Published by: International Transactional Analysis Association, 436 14th St, Ste 1301, Oakland, CA 94612-2710. TEL 510-625-7720, FAX 510-625-7725, itaa@itaa-net.org, http://www.itaa-net.org. Ed., R&P, Adv. contact Robin Fryer. Circ: 2,500.

155.34 USA
TRANSGENDER TAPESTRY; the journal for persons interested in crossdressing & transsexualism. Text in English. 1978. q. USD 40; USD 55 foreign (effective 1997). adv. bk.rev. illus. back issues avail.; reprints avail. **Document type:** *Consumer.* **Description:** Provides a forum for people in the community on gender and related matters.
Formerly: T V - T S Tapestry (0884-9749)
Indexed: e-psyche.
Published by: International Foundation for Gender Education, Inc., PO Box 229, Waltham, MA 02254. TEL 617-899-2212, FAX 617-899-5703, IFGE@World.STD.COM, http://www.ifge.org. Ed. Jean Marie Stine. R&P Alison Laing. Adv. contact Yvonne Cook Riley. Circ: 10,000 (paid).

301 DEU
TRANSKULTURELLE PSYCHOFORUM. Text in German. 1997. irreg., latest vol.2, 1997. **Document type:** *Monographic series, Academic/Scholarly.*
Indexed: e-psyche.
Published by: V W B - Verlag fuer Wissenschaft und Bildung, Zossener Str 55, Berlin 10961, Germany. TEL 49-30-2510415, FAX 49-30-2510412, 100615.1565@compuserve.com, http://www.vwb-verlag.com. Eds. Judith Schuler, Thomas Heise.

TRANSNATIONAL NETWORK FOR THE STUDY OF PHYSICAL, PSYCHOLOGICAL & SPIRITUAL WELL-BEING. NEWSLETTER. see *RELIGIONS AND THEOLOGY*

▼ **TRANSPORTATION HUMAN FACTORS.** see *TRANSPORTATION*

320.82 FRA ISSN 0041-1868
T58.A2 CODEN: TRHUAH
LE TRAVAIL HUMAIN. Text in French; Text occasionally in English. 1937. q. EUR 63 domestic; EUR 77 foreign (effective 2002). bk.rev. charts, illus. index. reprint service avail. from PSC,SCH. *Refereed.* **Description:** Covers ergonomics, organization of work, personnel recruitment, and occupational health and safety.
Related titles: Online - full text ed.: (from Institute for Scientific Information).
Indexed: ASCA, Biol.Abstr., C.I.S. Abstr., Chem.Abstr., Child Devel.Abstr., Compumath, Curr.Cont., Curr.Ind.Stat., Ergon.Abstr., Excerp.Med., Ind.Philos., Int.Lab.Doc., P.A.I.S., PsycInfo, Psychol.Abstr. (1933-), Ref.Zh., Russ.Acad.Sci.Bibl., SSCI, e-psyche.
—BLDSC (9027.300000), CISTI, IDS. **CCC.**
Published by: Presses Universitaires de France, Departement des Revues, 6 av. Reille, Paris 75685 Cedex 14, France. TEL 33-1-60873030, FAX 33-1-60792045, revues@puf.com. Ed. J M Hoe. Circ: 1,500.

155.3 USA ISSN 1052-3995
RC569.5.C55
TREATING ABUSE TODAY; trauma, treatment and trends. Text in English. 1991. 6/yr. USD 49 domestic to individuals; USD 59 in Canada & Mexico to individuals; USD 69 elsewhere to individuals; USD 72 domestic to institutions; USD 82 in Canada & Mexico to institutions; USD 92 elsewhere to institutions; USD 29 domestic to students; USD 39 in Canada & Mexico to students; USD 49 elsewhere to students; USD 7.95 newsstand/cover. adv. bk.rev. back issues avail. **Document type:** *Academic/Scholarly.* **Description:** Contains timely information, contemporary issues and expert guidance regarding the treatment and recovery of survivors of sexual abuse.
Former titles (until 1998): Trauma: An Interdisciplinary Magazine of Abuse Survivorship and Therapy; (until 1996): Treating Abuse Today (1052-3995)
—BLDSC (9046.830000).
Published by: Survivors And Victims Empowered (SAVE), PO Box 3030, Lancaster, PA 17604-3030. TEL 717-291-1940, FAX 717-291-5977, TreatAbuse@aol.com, TAT@s-a-v-e.org, http://www.idealist.com/tat, http://www.geocities.com/treatingabusetoday. Ed. Christina M DiCola. Pub. Phil Sheldon. Adv. contact Anna Machan. Circ: 4,000 (paid).

158 USA
TREATMENT. Text in English. irreg. membership. *Refereed.* **Document type:** *Academic/Scholarly.* **Description:** Publishes major empirical research on the outcome of psychological and biologically oriented therapy and their combination for the alleviation of mental illness.
Media: Online - full text.
Indexed: e-psyche.
Published by: American Psychological Association, 211 E 70th St, New York, NY 10021. TEL 202-336-5560, 800-374-3721, FAX 202-336-5568, admin@apa.org, http://journals.apa.org/treatment/. **Co-sponsor:** American Psychiatric Association.

150 USA
TREATMENT MANUALS FOR PRACTITIONERS. Text in English. irreg. (approx. 1/yr.). **Document type:** *Monographic series, Academic/Scholarly.* **Description:** Presents results of successful treatment programs for specific psychological disorders. Each manual targets problems and illustrates step-by-step treatment protocols.
Indexed: e-psyche.
Published by: Guilford Publications, Inc., 72 Spring St, New York, NY 10012. TEL 212-431-9800, 800-365-7006, FAX 212-966-6708, info@guilford.com. Ed. Seymour Weingarten. Pub. Robert Matloff. R&P David Mitchell. Adv. contact Christine Luberto.

153 GBR ISSN 1364-6613
QP360.5 CODEN: TCSCFK
TRENDS IN COGNITIVE SCIENCES. Text in English. 1997. m. GBP 92, EUR 115 in Europe to individuals; JPY 14,000 in Japan to individuals; USD 126 elsewhere to individuals; EUR 9,081 in Europe to institutions; JPY 125,900 in Japan to institutions; USD 1,015 elsewhere to institutions; GBP 47 in Europe to students (effective 2002); JPY 10,100 in Japan to students (effective 2001); USD 78 elsewhere to students; USD 1,308 to institutions Print & online eds. combined; EUR 144 in Europe to qualified personnel; JPY 17,500 to qualified personnel; USD 157 elsewhere to qualified personnel (effective 2002). adv. bk.rev., software rev. illus. back issues avail.; reprints avail. *Refereed.* **Document type:** *Academic/Scholarly.* **Description:** Explores all the cognitive sciences, bringing together such diverse disciplines as psychology, psychiatry, the neurosciences, artificial intelligence, philosophy, and anthropology.
Related titles: Online - full text ed.: (from ingenta, Swets Blackwell, Institute for Scientific Information, ScienceDirect).
Indexed: Curr.Cont., Eng.Ind., Ergon.Abstr., Excerp.Med., Int.Abstr.Biol.Sci., SSCI, Sci.Cit.Ind. (coverage dropped), Soc.Sci.Ind. (coverage dropped), e-psyche.
—BLDSC (9049.559000), IDS. **CCC.**
Published by: Elsevier Science Ltd., Elsevier Trends Journals, Elsevier Trends Journals, 86 Hills Rd, Cambridge CB2 1LA, United Kingdom. TEL 44-1223-615961, FAX 44-1223-464430, tics@elsevier.co.uk, http://www.elsevier.nl/inca/publications/store/6/0/0/3/5/6/. Eds. J Ogilvie, Peter Collins. Adv. contact Thelma Reid. **Subscr. in Australasia and the Far East to:** Elsevier Science (Singapore) Pte Ltd, No.1 Temasek Ave, 17-01 Millenia Tower, Singapore 039192, Singapore. TEL 65-434-3727, FAX 65-337-2230; **Subscr. in the Americas to:** Elsevier Science, PO Box 945, New York, NY 10159-0945. TEL 212-633-3730, FAX 212-633-3680, http://www.elsevier.com; **Subscr. to:** Elsevier Current Trends Subscriptions, PO Box 331, Haywards Heath, W Sussex RH16 3FG, United Kingdom. TEL 44-1444-475650, FAX 44-1444-445423.

150 347 USA
TRIAL PSYCHOLOGY; communication and persuasion in the courtroom. Text in English. 1987. base vol. plus a. updates. USD 95. **Description:** Shows how to win over the jury, from in-depth juror assessment and coordinating the proper appearance of clients and counsel, to voir dire and shadow juries.
Indexed: e-psyche.
Published by: Lexis Law Publishing (Subsidiary of: Reed Elsevier plc), PO Box 7587, Charlottesville, VA 22906-7587. TEL 804-972-7600, 800-562-1197, FAX 804-972-7666, llp.customer.support@lexis-nexis.com, http://www.lexislawpublishing.com. Ed. Margaret C Roberts.

616.89 DEU
TRIERER PSYCHOLOGISCHE BERICHTE. Text and summaries in English, German. 1974. irreg. free per issue. cum.index: 1974-1998. *Refereed.* **Document type:** *Academic/Scholarly.*
Indexed: e-psyche.
Published by: Universitaet Trier, Fachgebiet Psychologie, Universitaetsring 8, Trier 54286, Germany. TEL 49-651-201-2970, FAX 49-651-201-2971, graeser@uni-trier.de, http://www.psychologie.uni-trier.de:8000/. Eds. Horst Graeser, Reinhold Scheller. Circ: 100.

150 TUR ISSN 1300-4433
TURK PSIKOLOJI DERGISI/TURKISH JOURNAL OF PSYCHOLOGY. Text in Multiple languages. 1978. s-a. *Refereed.* **Document type:** *Journal, Academic/Scholarly.*
Related titles: Online - full text ed.: (from Institute for Scientific Information).
Indexed: Curr.Cont., SSCI.
Published by: Turk Psikologlar Dernegi/Turkish Psychologists Association, PK 117, Ankara 06662, Turkey.

150 FIN ISSN 0356-8741
TURUN YLIOPISTO. PSYKOLOGIAN TUTKIMUKSIA. Short title: Psykologian Tutkimuksia. Text in Finnish. 1976. irreg. price varies. **Document type:** *Academic/Scholarly.*
Indexed: e-psyche.

P

Published by: Turun Yliopisto, Psykologian Laitos/University of Turku, Department of Psychology, Turku 20500, Finland. TEL 358-2-333-5430, FAX 358-2-333-5060. Ed. P Niemi. Circ: 500.

150.19 USA ISSN 8756-4963
CODEN: TYREE4
TYPE REPORTER; a monthly publication on psychological type. Text in English. 1984. 8/yr. USD 16 (effective 1999). bk.rev. charts, illus. back issues avail. **Document type:** *Newsletter.*
Indexed: e-psyche.
Published by: Type Reporter, Inc., 11314 Chapel Rd, Fairfax, VA 22039-1523. TEL 703-823-3730. Ed. Susan Scanlon. Circ: 3,000.

301.1 150 ZAF ISSN 0256-8896
U N I S A PSYCHOLOGIA. Text in English. 1974. s-a. ZAR 20, USD 5 (effective 2001). adv. bk.rev. back issues avail. *Refereed.* **Document type:** *Journal, Academic/Scholarly.* **Description:** Includes scientific articles and synopses of psychology's sub-disciplines from students and lecturers.
Indexed: Ind.S.A.Per., e-psyche.
Published by: (University of South Africa), Unisa Press, Periodicals, PO Box 392, Pretoria 0003, South Africa. TEL 27-12-429-3081, FAX 27-12-429-3221, unisa-press@unisa.ac.za, http://www.unisa.ac.za/press. Ed., Adv. contact Henning Viljoen. B&W page ZAR 400. Circ: 16,000.

▼ **UNDERSTANDING STATISTICS**; statistical issues in psychology, education, and the social sciences. see *STATISTICS*

155.9042 616.8 GBR ISSN 1353-2723
UNDERSTANDING STRESS, ANXIETY AND DEPRESSION. Text in English. 1994. bi-m. **Document type:** *Academic/Scholarly.*
Indexed: e-psyche.
Published by: N C N Publishing, 8 Bovingdon Rd, London SW6 2AP, United Kingdom. TEL 44-20-7371-7674, FAX 44-20-7371-9790. Ed. Richard Hornsby.

UNHAPPY. see *LITERATURE*

UNIVERSIDAD DE SEVILLA. SERIE FILOSOFIA Y PSICOLOGIA. see *PHILOSOPHY*

150 FIN ISSN 0359-0216
UNIVERSITY OF TURKU. PSYCHOLOGICAL RESEARCH REPORTS. Key Title: Psychological Research Reports. Text in English. 1963. irreg. price varies. **Document type:** *Academic/Scholarly.*
Supersedes (in 1981): Turun Yliopisto. Psykologian Laitos. Reports (0356-8733)
Indexed: e-psyche.
Published by: Turun Yliopisto, Psykologian Laitos/University of Turku, Department of Psychology, Turku 20500, Finland. TEL 358-2-333-5430, FAX 358-2-333-5060. Ed. P Niemi. Circ: 500.

150 SVK ISSN 0083-419X
BF26 CODEN: PSYAD8
UNIVERZITA KOMENSKEHO. FILOZOFICKA FAKULTA. ZBORNIK: PSYCHOLOGICA. Text in Slovak; Summaries in English, German, Russian. 1961. irreg. per issue exchange basis. **Document type:** *Academic/Scholarly.* **Description:** Covers all aspects of psychology.
Indexed: Psychol.Abstr., Russ.Acad.Sci.Bibl., e-psyche.
Published by: Univerzita Komenskeho, Filozoficka Fakulta, c/o Ustredna Kniznica Filozofickej Fakulty, Gondova 2, Bratislava 81801, Slovakia. Circ: 400.

UNIWERSYTET IM. ADAMA MICKIEWICZA. PSYCHOLOGIA-PEDAGOGIKA. see *EDUCATION*

158.7 POL ISSN 1428-8664
UNIWERSYTET SLASKI W KATOWICACH. PRACE NAUKOWE. PSYCHOLOGIA. BADANIA I APLIKACJE. Text in Polish; Summaries in English, Russian. 1980. irreg. price varies. *Refereed.* **Document type:** *Academic/Scholarly.* **Description:** Provides social psychological studies of human behaviour at work, especially on interpersonal relations, trust, injustice, leadership, and resistance to change. Also covers attitudes to work and stress.
Formerly (until 1997): Uniwersytet Slaski w Katowicach. Prace Naukowe. Psychologiczne Problemy Funkncjonowania Czlowieka w Sytuacji Pracy (0208-5569)
Indexed: Russ.Acad.Sci.Bibl., e-psyche.
Published by: (Uniwersytet Slaski w Katowicach), Wydawnictwa Szkolne i Pedagogiczne, Ul Bankowa 12 B, Katowice 40007, Poland. TEL 48-32-596915, FAX 48-32-599-605, wydawus@us.edu.pl, http://www.us.edu.pl/uniwersytet/jednostki/ogolne. R&P Barbara Woznica. **Dist. by:** CHZ Ars Polona, Biblioteka PAN w Warszawie, PO Box 1001, Warsaw 00950, Poland.

UOMINI E IDEE. see *LITERATURE*

153.4 GBR
VANCOUVER STUDIES IN COGNITIVE SCIENCE. Text in English. irreg. price varies. **Document type:** *Proceedings.*
Indexed: e-psyche.
—BLDSC.
Published by: (Simon Fraser University), Oxford University Press, Oxford Journals, Walton St, Oxford OX2 6DP, United Kingdom. TEL 44-1865-56767, FAX 44-1865-56646, jnlorders@oup.co.uk, jnl.orders@oup.co.uk, http://www.oup.co.uk. **Orders in N. America to:** Oxford University Press, Journals. TEL 919-677-0977, FAX 919-677-1714, http://www.oup.co.uk.

616.89 DEU ISSN 0721-7234
VERHALTENSTHERAPIE UND PSYCHOSOZIALE PRAXIS. Text in German; Summaries in English. 1976. q. DEM 60; DEM 20 newsstand/cover (effective 2000). adv. bk.rev. abstr. bibl. back issues avail. **Document type:** *Academic/Scholarly.* **Description:** Focuses on behavior therapy (associated with the German Association of Behavior Therapy) and aims at an audience of psychologists, social workers and public health employees.
Indexed: e-psyche.
—GNLM.
Published by: (Deutsche Gesellschaft fuer Verhaltenstherapie), D G V T - Verlag, Hechinger Str 203, Tuebingen 72072, Germany. TEL 49-7071-792850, FAX 49-7071-792851. Ed. Otmar Koschar. R&P Cathrin Steppuhn. adv.: B&W page DEM 1,320; trim 155 x 185. Circ: 6,000.

VICTIMOLOGY; an international journal. see *CRIMINOLOGY AND LAW ENFORCEMENT*

VIERTELJAHRESSCHRIFT FUER HEILPAEDAGOGIK UND IHRE NACHBARGEBIETE. see *EDUCATION—Special Education And Rehabilitation*

VIOLENCE AND VICTIMS. see *SOCIOLOGY*

150 USA
VISIONS (SAN FRANCISCO). Text in English. 1987. s-a. free per issue. adv. tr.lit. **Document type:** *Newsletter.* **Description:** Covers the following areas of psychology: clinical, organizational, forensic, health, cross-cultural, and multicultural. Intended for CSPP alumni as well as outside audiences.
Indexed: e-psyche.
Published by: California School of Professional Psychology, 2728 Hyde St No. 100, San Francisco, CA 94109. TEL 415-346-4500, FAX 415-931-8322, mginsberg@cspp.edu, http://www.cspp.edu. Ed., R&P, Adv. contact Meryl Ginsberg. Circ: 8,000 (controlled).

152 USA ISSN 1064-5578
VISITOR STUDIES; theory, research, and practice. Text in English. 1988. a. **Document type:** *Proceedings, Academic/Scholarly.* **Description:** Contains selected conference papers.
Indexed: e-psyche.
—BLDSC (9240.973800).
Published by: Visitor Studies Association, PO Box 1111, Jacksonville, AL 36265. TEL 205-782-5640. Ed. Stephen C Bitgood.

150 GBR ISSN 1350-6285
BF241 CODEN: VICOF6
VISUAL COGNITION. Text in English. 1994. 8/yr. GBP 129, USD 213 to individuals; GBP 299, USD 493 to institutions (effective 2002). adv. *Refereed.* **Document type:** *Academic/Scholarly.* **Description:** Publishes research papers on all aspects of visual cognition, including studies of visual object and face recognition, texture and surface perception, perceptual organization, visual attention, visual memory, and more.
Related titles: Online - full text ed.: ISSN 1464-0716 (from CatchWord Ltd., EBSCO Publishing, O C L C Online Computer Library Center, Inc., RoweCom Information Quest, Swets Blackwell, Institute for Scientific Information).
Indexed: Curr.Cont., Ergon.Abstr., INSPEC (Mar.1995-), Lang.& Lang.Behav.Abstr., PsycInfo, SOPODA, SSCI, Sociol.Abstr., e-psyche.
—BLDSC (9241.234000), AskIEEE, CatchWord, IDS, Infotrieve. **CCC.**
Published by: Psychology Press (Subsidiary of: Taylor & Francis Group), 27 Church Rd, Hove, E Sussex BN3 2FA, United Kingdom. TEL 44-1273-207411, FAX 44-1273-205612, information@psypress.co.uk, http://www.psypress.co.uk. Ed. Glyn W Humphreys. R&P Zoe Peden TEL 44-20-7842-2363. Adv. contact Claire Buckminster. **Subscr. addr. in N America:** Psychology Press, Journals Customer Service, Taylor & Francis Group, 325 Chestnut St, Philadelphia, PA 19106. TEL 800-354-1420, FAX 215-625-8914, info@taylorandfrancis.com, http://www.psypress.com; **Subscr. addr. outside N America:** Journals Customer Service, Taylor & Francis Group, Rankine Rd, Basingstoke, Hants RG24 8PR, United Kingdom. TEL 44-1256-813002, FAX 44-1256-479438, enquiry@tandf.co.uk.

VITA DELL'INFANZIA. see *EDUCATION*

616.89 USA ISSN 0042-8272
RC475
VOICES (NEW BERN)✶ ; the art and science of psychotherapy. Text in English. 1965. q. USD 40 domestic to individuals; USD 55 foreign to individuals; USD 80 domestic to institutions; USD 95 foreign to institutions. adv. bk.rev. illus. cum.index. reprint service avail. from PQC. *Refereed.* **Document type:** *Academic/Scholarly.*
Related titles: Audio cassette/tape ed.: 1965; Microform ed.: 1965 (from PQC).
Indexed: Psychol.R.G., e-psyche.
—BLDSC (9251.465000), GNLM, ingenta.
Published by: American Academy of Psychotherapists, PO Box 1611, New Bern, NC 28563-1611. TEL 404-299-6336, FAX 404-299-0206. Ed. Monique Savlin. Circ: 1,500.

150 RUS ISSN 0042-8841
BF8.R8 CODEN: VOPSAI
VOPROSY PSIKHOLOGII. Text in Russian; Summaries in English. 1955. bi-m. *Refereed.*
Related titles: Online - full text ed.: (from Institute for Scientific Information).
Indexed: ASCA, Arts & Hum.Cit.Ind. (coverage dropped), Biol.Abstr., Child Devel.Abstr., Curr.Cont., INIS Atomind., Int.Aerosp.Abstr., Lang.& Lang.Behav.Abstr., PsycInfo, Psychol.Abstr. (1955-), Ref.Zh., Russ.Acad.Sci.Bibl., SOPODA, SSCI, Sociol.Abstr., e-psyche.
—BLDSC (0044.130000), East View, IDS. **CCC.**
Published by: (Rossiiskaya Akademiya Obrazovaniya), Voprosy Psikhologii, Mokhovaya ul 9-V, Moscow 103009, Russian Federation. TEL 7-095-2029609, FAX 7-095-2029609. Ed., R&P E.V. Shchedrina. Pub. E V Shchedrina. **Dist. by:** Mezhdunarodnaya Kniga, B Yakimanka 39, Moscow 117049, Russian Federation. TEL 7-095-2384967, FAX 7-095-2384634; **Dist. in U.S. by:** Victor Kamkin Inc., 4956 Boiling Brook Pkwy, Rockville, MD 20852.

VS; quaderni di studi semiotici. see *LINGUISTICS*

VYCHOVAVATEL. see *EDUCATION*

616.8 USA ISSN 0083-8977
W P S PROFESSIONAL HANDBOOK SERIES. Text in English. 1965. irreg. price varies. adv. *Refereed.* **Document type:** *Monographic series.* **Description:** Serves as handbooks for psychological assessment.
Indexed: e-psyche.
Published by: Western Psychological Services, 12031 Wilshire Blvd, Los Angeles, CA 90025. TEL 310-478-2061, 800-648-8857, FAX 310-478-7838, weinberg@wpspublish.com. Ed. Scott Colby. Pub. Sarah Manson. R&P Susan Weinberg. Adv. contact Susan Madden.

WASHINGTON COUNSELETTER. see *OCCUPATIONS AND CAREERS*

155.937 USA
WE NEED NOT WALK ALONE. Text in English. 1998. q. USD 20 (effective 2001). **Document type:** *Magazine, Consumer.* **Description:** Focuses on grief-related issues and features poetry and original articles by bereaved parents, siblings, grandparents, and professionals.
Formed by the merger of (1993-1998): S T A G E S Sibling Newsletter; We Need Not Walk Alone Newsletter; Which was formerly: Compassionate Friends National Newsletter; Compassionate Friends Newsletter
Indexed: e-psyche.

P

Published by: Compassionate Friends, Inc., Box 3696, Oak Brook, Oak Brook, IL 60522-3696. TEL 630-990-0010, 877-969-0010, FAX 630-990-0246, http://www.compassionatefriends.org/index.html. Ed. Wayne Loder. R&P Terry Eubanks.

WELFARE WORLD. see *SOCIAL SERVICES AND WELFARE*

301 AUT ISSN 0257-3601
WERKBLATT; Zeitschrift fuer Psychoanalyse und Gesellschaftskritik. Text in German. 1984. 2/yr. ATS 315 domestic; ATS 385 foreign (effective 2001). 128 p./no. **Document type:** *Journal, Academic/Scholarly.*
Indexed: e-psyche.
Address: Platzl 2/III, Salzburg, A, Sa 5020, Austria. FAX 43-662-650011, maetzler@salsburg.co.at, maetzler@alpin.or.at, http://home.subnetac.at/werkblatt, http://hhobel.phl.univie.ac.at/werkblatt.

WEST BENGAL. BUREAU OF EDUCATIONAL AND PSYCHOLOGICAL RESEARCH. see *EDUCATION*

616.58 USA
WILLIAM ALANSON WHITE PSYCHOANALYTIC INSTITUTE. RECORD. Text in English. 1966. 3/yr. membership. bk.rev. illus. **Document type:** *Newsletter.*
Formerly (until 1994): W A W Newsletter (0042-9511)
Indexed: e-psyche.
Published by: William Alanson White Psychoanalytic Institute, 20 W 74th St, New York, NY 10023. TEL 212-873-0725, FAX 212-362-6967. Ed. James Garofallou. Circ: 2,500.

WINGSPAN (LA JOLLA); journal of the male spirit. see *MEN'S STUDIES*

158.7 DEU ISSN 1615-7729
WIRTSCHAFTSPSYCHOLOGIE. Text in German. 1993. q. EUR 45, USD 40 (effective 2001). *Refereed.* **Document type:** *Journal, Academic/Scholarly.*
Formerly (until 1999): Arbeit Betrieb Organisation Aktuell (0945-6201)
Published by: Pabst Science Publishers, Am Eichengrund 28, Lengerich 49525, Germany. TEL 49-5484-308, FAX 49-5484-550, pabst.publishers@t-online.de, http://www.wirtschafts-psychologie.net/, http://www.pabst-publishers.de. Ed. Dr. Eckhard Gros. Adv. contact Birgit Heiter. Circ: 3,900 (paid and controlled).

158 305.4 USA ISSN 0270-3149
RC451.4.W6 CODEN: WOTHDJ
WOMEN & THERAPY; a feminist quarterly. Text in English. 1982. q. USD 60 to individuals; USD 81 in Canada to individuals; USD 87 elsewhere to individuals; USD 180 to institutions; USD 243 in Canada to institutions; USD 261 elsewhere to institutions; USD 335 to libraries; USD 452 in Canada to libraries; USD 486 elsewhere to libraries (effective Aug. 2001). adv. bk.rev. illus. back issues avail.; reprint service avail. from HAW. *Refereed.* **Document type:** *Journal, Academic/Scholarly.* **Description:** Explores the multidimensional relationship between women and therapy, with a feminist orientation. Publishes descriptive, theoretical, clinical, and empirical perspectives on the topic and the therapeutic process.
Formerly: Women - Counseling Therapy and Mental Health Services
Related titles: Microfiche ed.: (from PQC); Microform ed.; Online - full text ed.; (from LexisNexis, Northern Light Technology, Inc., ProQuest Information & Learning, Gale Group, Factiva, Institute for Scientific Information).
Indexed: ASCA, AgeLine, Alt.Press Ind., Amer.Bibl.Slavic & E.Eur.Stud., Biol.Abstr., CWI, Curr.Cont., Fam.Ind., Fem.Per. (1982-), Gend.Watch, High.Educ.Abstr., IBZ, IMFL, Ind.Philos., Mult.Ed.Abstr., PsycInfo, SSCI, Sage Fam.Stud.Abstr., Soc.Serv.Abstr., Soc.Work Res.& Abstr., Sociol.Abstr., Stud.Wom.Abstr., Viol.& Abuse Abstr., Wom.Stud.Abstr. (1982-), Wom.Stud.Ind., e-psyche.
—BLDSC (9343.276000), GNLM, Haworth, IDS, ingenta.
Published by: Haworth Press, Inc., 10 Alice St, Binghamton, NY 13904-1580. TEL 607-722-5857, 800-429-6784, FAX 607-722-6362, 800-895-0582, getinfo@haworthpressinc.com, http://bubl.ac.uk/journals/soc/wat/, http://www.haworthpress.com. Eds. Doris Howard, Ellyn Kaschak. Pub. William Cohen. R&P Ruthann Heath TEL 607-723-5857 ext 316. Adv. contact Jackie Blakeslee TEL 607-722-5857 ext 346. B&W page USD 315, color page USD 550; trim 6 x 8.5. Circ: 750.

WOMEN'S MENTAL HEALTH & DEVELOPMENT. see *WOMEN'S HEALTH*

158.7 GBR ISSN 0267-8373
HF5548.85
WORK AND STRESS. Text in English. 1987. q. GBP 94, USD 156 to individuals; GBP 189, USD 312 to institutions (effective 2002). adv. back issues avail. *Refereed.* **Document type:** *Academic/Scholarly.* **Description:** Features academic papers relating to stress, health and safety, and associated areas and scholarly articles of concern to the policy-makers, managers and trades unionists who have to deal with such issues.
Related titles: Online - full text ed.: ISSN 1464-5335 (from CatchWord Ltd., EBSCO Publishing, O C L C Online Computer Library Center, Inc., RoweCom Information Quest, Swets Blackwell, Institute for Scientific Information).
Indexed: ASCA, ASSIA, AgeLine, Behav.Med.Abstr., CINAHL, Cont.Pg.Manage., Crim.Just.Abstr., Curr.Cont., Environ.Sci.Poll.Mgmt., Ergon.Abstr., Fam.Ind., Lang.& Lang.Behav.Abstr., Pollut.Abstr., PsycInfo, Psychol.Abstr. (1987-), Risk Abstr., SOPODA, SSCI, Saf.Sci.Abstr., Soc.Serv.Abstr., Sociol.Abstr., e-psyche.
—BLDSC (9348.102000), CatchWord, CISTI, EMDOCS, GNLM, IDS, Infotrieve, ingenta. **CCC.**
Published by: Taylor & Francis Group, Taylor & Francis Ltd., Journals Customer Service, Rankine Rd, Basingstoke, Hants RG24 8PR, United Kingdom. Ed. Tom Cox TEL 44-1158-466623. **Subscr. in N. America to:** Taylor & Francis Ltd., 325 Chestnut St, Suite 800, Philadelphia, PA 19016. TEL 800-354-1420, FAX 215-625-8914, info@taylorandfrancis.com, http://www.taylorandfrancis.com/.

616.89 614.582 USA
WORLD FEDERATION FOR MENTAL HEALTH. ANNUAL REPORT. Text in English. 1984. a. USD 35 to membership; USD 15 to membership low income countries (effective 2000). **Document type:** *Proceedings, Corporate.* **Description:** Reviews the organization's international activities of the past year.
Indexed: e-psyche.
Published by: World Federation for Mental Health, 1021 Prince St, Alexandria, VA 22314-2971. TEL 703-838-7543, FAX 703-519-7648, wfmh@erols.com, http://www.wfmh.org. Ed. Dr. Eugene B Brody. Circ: 3,000 (controlled).

616.89 614.582 USA
WORLD FEDERATION FOR MENTAL HEALTH. NEWSLETTER. Text in English. 1948. q. USD 35 to membership; USD 15 to membership low income countries (effective 2000). bibl. **Document type:** *Newsletter.* **Description:** Provides members with information on the federation's activities at the United Nations, the World Health Organization, and around the world. Comments on mental health issues and contains a calendar of events.
Indexed: e-psyche.
Published by: World Federation for Mental Health, 1021 Prince St, Alexandria, VA 22314-2971. TEL 703-838-7543, FAX 703-519-7648, wfmh@erols.com, http://www.wfmh.org. Ed. Dr. Eugene B Brody. Circ: 4,000.

150 USA ISSN 1078-8468
WORLD PSYCHOLOGY. Text in English. 1995. q. USD 45 to individuals; USD 120 to institutions. *Refereed.* **Document type:** *Academic/Scholarly.* **Description:** Presents international trends and a global perspective on psychology.
Indexed: e-psyche.
Published by: International Council of Psychologists, Inc., c/o John M Davis, Secy Gen, Dept of Psychology, Southwest Texas State Univ, San Marcos, TX 78666-4616. FAX 512-245-3153. Ed. Uwe P Gielen.

150 USA
WRITE-UP. Text in English. 1972. bi-m. USD 40 (effective 2001). bk.rev. back issues avail. **Document type:** *Newsletter, Academic/Scholarly.* **Description:** Discusses topics of interest pertaining to the study of handwriting.
Formerly: National Society for Graphology Newsletter
Indexed: e-psyche.
Published by: National Society for Graphology, 250 W 57th St, Rm 2017, New York, NY 10107. TEL 212-265-1148, FAX 212-307-5671. Ed. Carole F. Schuler. R&Ps Janice Klein, Louise Erpelding. Circ: 300.

510.71 POL
WYZSZA SZKOLA PEDAGOGICZNA IM. KOMISJI EDUKACJI NARODOWEJ W KRAKOWIE. ROCZNIK NAUKOWO-DYDAKTYCZNY. PRACE PSYCHOLOGICZNE. Text in Polish. 1963. irreg., latest vol.2, 1988. price varies.
Indexed: e-psyche.
Published by: (Wyzsza Szkola Pedagogiczna im. Komisji Edukacji Narodowej w Krakowie), Wydawnictwo Naukowe W S P, Ul Karmelicka 41, Krakow 31128, Poland. TEL 33-78-20. **Co-sponsor:** Ministerstwo Edukacji Narodowej.

150 CHN ISSN 1000-6648
BF8.C5
XINLI KEXUE TONGXUN* /INFORMATION ON PSYCHOLOGICAL SCIENCES. Text in Chinese. 1965. bi-m.
Indexed: PsycInfo, Psychol.Abstr. (1984-), e-psyche.
Published by: Zhongguo Xinli Xuehui, Huadong Shifan Daxue, 3663 Zhongshan Beilu, Shanghai 200062, China. TEL 2577577. **Dist. in US by:** China Books & Periodicals, Inc, 2929 24th St, San Francisco, CA 94110. TEL 415-282-2994.

155 CHN ISSN 0439-755X
PN1991
XINLI XUEBAO/ACTA PSYCHOLOGICA SINICA. Text in Chinese; Summaries in English. 1956. q. USD 80 (effective 2000). adv. *Refereed.* **Document type:** *Academic/Scholarly.* **Description:** Covers the basic theories of psychology, general, medical, physiological, child, and educational psychology. Also covers the history of psychology, and contains evaluations of academic studies and information on current academic activities.
Indexed: PsycInfo, Psychol.Abstr., Russ.Acad.Sci.Bibl., e-psyche.
Published by: Kexue Chubanshe/Science Press, 16 Donghuang Cheng Genbei Jie, Beijing 100717, China. Circ: 32,000.

150 CHN ISSN 1001-2532
XINLIXUE/PSYCHOLOGY. Text in Chinese. 1978. m. USD 50.40 (effective 2001). 96 p./no. **Description:** Contains reprints of articles on psychology and related fields.
Indexed: e-psyche.
Published by: Zhongguo Renmin Daxue Shubao Zilio Zhongxin/Renmin University's Social Science Information Center, PO Box 1122, Beijing 100007, China. TEL 86-10-64015080, FAX 86-10-64030674, cmktg@public3.bta.net.cn, http://www.confucius.cn.net. **Dist. in US by:** China Publications Service, PO Box 49614, Chicago, IL 60649. TEL 312-288-3291, FAX 312-288-8570.

YOGA INTERNATIONAL. see *NEW AGE PUBLICATIONS*

155.4 CHN ISSN 1006-3595
YOU'ER ZHILI SHIJIE/INFANTS' INTELLIGENCE WORLD. Text in Chinese. 1986. s-m. (m. before 2002). CNY 91.20 domestic; CNY 3.80 newsstand/cover (effective 2002). adv. Index. back issues avail. *Refereed.* **Document type:** *Consumer.*
Media: Large Type (14 pt.).
Indexed: e-psyche.
Published by: Zhejiang Shaonian Ertong Chubanshe/Zhejiang Juvenile and Children's Publishing House, No.347 Tiyuchang Rd, Hangzhou, Zhjiang Province 310006, China. TEL 86-571-85102968, FAX 86-571-85176984, zjsrs@mail.hz.zj.cn, http://www.ses.zjcb.com. Eds. Mingjun Chen, Wen Chen. Pub. Chunyue Chen. R&P Ying Wu TEL 86-571-5102968. Adv. contact Mingjun Chen. color page CNY 20,000; trim 187 x 216. Circ: 450,000. **Dist. by:** China International Book Trading Corp, 35 Chegongzhuang Xilu, Haidian District, Beijing 100044, China. TEL 86-10-68411769, FAX 86-10-68420340, bk@mail.cibtc.com.cn, http://www.cibtc.com.cn/.

616.89 PAK
ZEHAN. Text in Urdu. 1978. q. PKR 12, USD 1.50. adv. bk.rev.
Indexed: e-psyche.
Published by: Psychope, G P O Box 1964, Lahore, Pakistan. Ed. Dr. Syed Azhar Ali Rizvi. Circ: 500.

150 158 DEU ISSN 0932-4089
ZEITSCHRIFT FUER ARBEITS- UND ORGANISATIONSPSYCHOLOGIE. Short title: A & O. Text in German. 1956. q. DEM 148 (effective 2001). adv. bk.rev. bibl. charts. *Refereed.* **Document type:** *Journal, Academic/Scholarly.*
Former titles (until 1987): Psychologie und Praxis; Psychologie und Praxis Arbeits- und Organisationspsychologie; Psychologie und Praxis (0033-2992)
Related titles: Online - full text ed.: (from Institute for Scientific Information).
Indexed: ASCA, Bibl.Asian Stud. (1971), C.I.S. Abstr., Curr.Cont., Documentatieblad, Dok.Arbeitsmed., Ger.J.Psych., IBR, IBZ, Ind.Philos., Indian Psychol.Abstr., PsycInfo, Psychol.Abstr. (1959-), Ref.Zh., SSCI, e-psyche.

P

—IDS, Infotrieve. **CCC.**
Published by: Hogrefe Verlag GmbH und Co. KG, Rohnsweg 25, Goettingen 37085, Germany. TEL 49-551-496090, FAX 49-551-4960988, verlag@hogrefe.de, http://www.hogrefe.de. Ed. Uwe Kleinbeck. Circ: 2,000.

152 CHE ISSN 0170-1789
ZEITSCHRIFT FUER DIFFERENTIELLE UND DIAGNOSTISCHE PSYCHOLOGIE. Text in German; Summaries in English. 1980. q. CHF 132 (effective 2001). adv. 80 p./no. **Document type:** *Journal, Academic/Scholarly.*
Indexed: IBZ, Ind.Philos., PsycInfo, Psychol.Abstr. (1980-), e-psyche.
—BLDSC (9457.686000), GNLM, Infotrieve. **CCC.**
Published by: Hans Huber AG, Laengassstr 76, Bern, 9 3000, Switzerland. TEL 41-31-3004500, FAX 41-31-3004591, zeitschriften@hanshuber.com, http://www.hanshuber.com. Ed. Dr H Haecker. Adv. contact Rene Waelchli. B&W page DEM 1,100, color page DEM 2,450; trim 216 x 283. Circ: 350.

370.15 150 DEU ISSN 0049-8637
L31 CODEN: ZEPPBI
ZEITSCHRIFT FUER ENTWICKLUNGSPSYCHOLOGIE UND PAEDAGOGISCHE PSYCHOLOGIE. Text in German; Summaries in English. 1969. q. DEM 108 (effective 2001). adv. bk.rev. abstr, bibl. *Refereed.* **Document type:** *Journal, Academic/Scholarly.*
Related titles: Online - full text ed.: (from Institute for Scientific Information).
Indexed: ASCA, Child Devel.Abstr., Curr.Cont., Ger.J.Psych., IBR, IBZ, Ind.Philos., PsycInfo, Psychol.Abstr. (1969-), Ref.Zh., SSCI, e-psyche.
—BLDSC (9458.600000), IDS.
Published by: Hogrefe Verlag GmbH und Co. KG, Rohnsweg 25, Goettingen 37085, Germany. TEL 49-551-496090, FAX 49-551-4960988, verlag@hogrefe.de, http://www.hogrefe.de. Ed. Gisela Trommsdorff. Circ: 2,400.

152 DEU ISSN 0949-3964
BF3
ZEITSCHRIFT FUER EXPERIMENTELLE PSYCHOLOGIE. Text in German; Summaries in English, German. 1953. q. DEM 178 (effective 2001). adv. bk.rev. bibl, charts, illus. *Refereed.* **Document type:** *Journal, Academic/Scholarly.*
Formerly: Zeitschrift fuer Experimentelle und Angewandte Psychologie (0044-2712)
Related titles: Online - full text ed.: (from Institute for Scientific Information).
Indexed: ASCA, Compumath, Curr.Cont., Curr.Ind.Stat., Excerp.Med., Ger.J.Psych., IBR, IBZ, Ind.Med. (1995-), Ind.Philos., Lang.& Lang.Behav.Abstr., PsycInfo, Psychol.Abstr. (1953-), Russ.Acad.Sci.Bibl., SOPODA, SSCI, Sociol.Abstr., e-psyche.
—CISTI, GNLM, IDS, Infotrieve. **CCC.**
Published by: Hogrefe Verlag GmbH und Co. KG, Rohnsweg 25, Goettingen 37085, Germany. TEL 49-551-496090, FAX 49-551-4960988, verlag@hogrefe.de, http://www.hogrefe.de. Ed. Karl Christoph Klauer. Circ: 800.

150 DEU ISSN 0943-8149
ZEITSCHRIFT FUER GESUNDHEITSPSYCHOLOGIE. Text in German. 1993. q. DEM 108 to individuals; DEM 198 to institutions (effective 2001). adv. bk.rev. abstr, bibl, illus. **Document type:** *Journal, Academic/Scholarly.*
Indexed: IBR, IBZ, Ind.Philos., e-psyche.
—GNLM.
Published by: Hogrefe Verlag GmbH und Co. KG, Rohnsweg 25, Goettingen 37085, Germany. TEL 49-551-496090, FAX 49-551-4960988, verlag@hogrefe.de, http://www.hogrefe.de. Ed. M Jerusalem. Circ: 2,000.

150 DEU ISSN 0342-393X
ZEITSCHRIFT FUER INDIVIDUALPSYCHOLOGIE. Text in German. 1976. q. DEM 99; DEM 79.20 to students (effective 2000). adv. bk.rev. reprint service avail. from PQC,ISI. **Document type:** *Journal, Academic/Scholarly.*
Indexed: IBR, IBZ, Ind.Philos., PsycInfo, Psychoanal.Abstr., Psychol.Abstr. (1984-), Ref.Zh., e-psyche.
—GNLM. **CCC.**
Published by: Ernst Reinhardt Verlag, Kemnatenstr 46, Munich 80639, Germany. TEL 49-89-1780160, FAX 49-89-17801630. Circ: 2,800.

ZEITSCHRIFT FUER KLINISCHE PSYCHOLOGIE, PSYCHOPATHOLOGIE UND PSYCHOTHERAPIE. see *MEDICAL SCIENCES—Psychiatry And Neurology*

616.89 DEU ISSN 1616-3443
ZEITSCHRIFT FUER KLINISCHE PSYCHOLOGIE UND PSYCHOTHERAPIE - FORSCHUNG UND PRAXIS. Text in German; Summaries in English. 1972. q. DEM 128 (effective 2001). adv. bk.rev. **Document type:** *Journal, Academic/Scholarly.*
Formerly (until 2000): Zeitschrift fuer Klinische Psychologie - Forschung und Praxis (0084-5345)
Related titles: Online - full text ed.: (from Institute for Scientific Information).
Indexed: ASCA, Curr.Cont., Excerp.Med., Ger.J.Psych., IBR, IBZ, Ind.Philos., PsycInfo, Psychol.Abstr. (1972-), Ref.Zh., SSCI, e-psyche.
—BLDSC (9467.775000), GNLM, IDS, KNAW.
Published by: Hogrefe Verlag GmbH und Co. KG, Rohnsweg 25, Goettingen 37085, Germany. TEL 49-551-496090, FAX 49-551-4960988, verlag@hogrefe.de, http://www.hogrefe.de. Ed. Martin Hautzinger. Circ: 3,600.

150 DEU ISSN 0940-5569
ZEITSCHRIFT FUER MEDIZINISCHE PSYCHOLOGIE. Text in German. 1992. q. EUR 60 to individuals; EUR 105 to institutions (effective 2001). adv. bk.rev. 48 p./no. 3 cols./p. back issues avail. *Refereed.* **Document type:** *Magazine, Academic/Scholarly.*
Indexed: IBZ, Ind.Philos., e-psyche.
—GNLM.
Published by: Akademische Verlagsgesellschaft Aka GmbH, Neue Promenade 6, Berlin 10178, Germany. TEL 49-30-24729840, FAX 49-30-24729840. Ed. Dr. H D Basler. Pub. Dr. Ekkehard Hundt.

150 CHE ISSN 1016-264X
ZEITSCHRIFT FUER NEUROPSYCHOLOGIE. Text in German; Summaries in English. 1990. 4/yr. CHF 136 to individuals; CHF 205 to institutions (effective 2001). adv. bk.rev., Website rev. 96 p./no. **Document type:** *Academic/Scholarly.*
Indexed: PsycInfo, e-psyche.
—GNLM.
Published by: Hans Huber AG, Laengassstr 76, Bern, 9 3000, Switzerland. TEL 41-31-3004500, FAX 41-31-3004591, zeitschriften@hanshuber.com, http://www.hanshuber.com. Ed. Dr. Siegfried Gaugel. Adv. contact Rene Waelchli. B&W page DEM 1,140, color page DEM 2,540; trim 216 x 283. Circ: 1,500.

370.15 CHE ISSN 1010-0652
LB1051 CODEN: ZPPSE5
ZEITSCHRIFT FUER PAEDAGOGISCHE PSYCHOLOGIE. Text in English, German. 1987. q. CHF 136 to individuals; CHF 205 to institutions (effective 2001). adv. bk.rev. back issues avail. *Refereed.* **Document type:** *Journal, Academic/Scholarly.*
Related titles: Online - full text ed.: (from Institute for Scientific Information).
Indexed: ASCA, Cont.Pg.Educ., Curr.Cont., ERA, Educ.Tech.Abstr., IBR, Ind.Philos., Lang.& Lang.Behav.Abstr., P C I, PsycInfo, Psychol.Abstr. (1987-), SOPODA, SSCI, Soc.Serv.Abstr., Sociol.Abstr., Sociol.Educ.Abstr., Sp.Ed.Needs Abstr., Tech.Educ.Abstr., e-psyche.
—BLDSC (9475.803000), IDS.
Published by: Hans Huber AG, Laengassstr 76, Bern, 9 3000, Switzerland. TEL 41-31-3004500, FAX 41-31-3004591, zeitschriften@hanshuber.com, http://www.hanshuber.com. Ed. Andreas Knapp. Adv. contact Rene Waelchli. color page DEM 2,540; trim 170 x 250. Circ: 500.

150 DEU ISSN 0044-3409
QP351
ZEITSCHRIFT FUER PSYCHOLOGIE; mit Zeitschrift fuer angewandte Psychologie. Text in German. 1792. q. DEM 194 to institutions (effective 2000). adv. bk.rev. bibl, charts, illus. index. reprint service avail. from SWZ,PSC,SCH. *Refereed.* **Document type:** *Academic/Scholarly.* **Description:** Publishes papers on experimental and theoretical psychology.
Formed by the merger of: Zeitschrift fuer Angewandte Psychologie und Charakterkunde (0323-8296); Zeitschrift fuer Psychologie (0323-8342); Which was formerly (until 1940): Zeitschrift fuer Psychologie und Physiologie des Sinnesorgane. 1. Abteilung. Zeitschrift fuer Psychologie (0233-2353)
Related titles: Online - full text ed.: (from Institute for Scientific Information).
Indexed: ASCA, Arts & Hum.Cit.Ind. (coverage dropped), Biol.Abstr., Curr.Cont., Curr.Ind.Stat., Ger.J.Psych., IBR, IBZ, Ind.Med. (coverage dropped), Ind.Philos., Lang.& Lang.Behav.Abstr., P C I, PsycInfo, Psychol.Abstr. (1929-), Ref.Zh., Russ.Acad.Sci.Bibl., SOPODA, SSCI, Sociol.Abstr., e-psyche.
—BLDSC (9485.100000), CISTI, IDS, Infotrieve. **CCC.**

Published by: Johann Ambrosius Barth Verlag in Medizinverlage Heidelberg GmbH & Co. KG, Ruedigerstr 14, Stuttgart 70469, Germany. TEL 49-6221-489251, FAX 49-711-8931422, zpsych@huethig.de, http://www.huethig.de, http://www.thieme.de. Ed. F Klix. Adv. contact Petra Schoene. B&W page DEM 700; trim 240 x 167. Circ: 800.

ZEITSCHRIFT FUER PSYCHOSOMATISCHE MEDIZIN UND PSYCHOANALYSE. MONOGRAPHIEN. see *MEDICAL SCIENCES—Psychiatry And Neurology*

137.7 AUT ISSN 1607-5579
ZEITSCHRIFT FUER SCHRIFTPSYCHOLOGIE UND SCHRIFTVERGLEICHUNG. Text in German. 1925. q. EUR 40 (effective 2002). adv. bk.rev. charts. cum.index every 2 yrs. **Document type:** *Journal, Academic/Scholarly.*
Former titles (until 2000): Zeitschrift fuer Menschenkunde. Zentralblatt fuer Schriftpsychologie und Schriftvergleichung (0379-4458); Zeitschrift fuer Menschenkunde und Zentralblatt fuer Graphologie, Ausdruckswissenschaft und Charakterkunde (0044-3085); Zeitschrift fuer Menschenkunde und Zentralblatt fuer Graphologie
Indexed: IBR, IBZ, Ind.Philos., e-psyche.
Published by: Wilhelm Braumueller Universitaets-Verlagsbuchhandlung GmbH, Servitengasse 5, Vienna, W 1092, Austria. TEL 43-1-3191159, FAX 43-1-3102805, office@braumueller.at, http://www.braumueller.at. Ed. Angelika Seibt. Adv. contact Susanne Mondl. Circ: 1,000.

ZEITSCHRIFT FUER SEXUALFORSCHUNG. see *MEDICAL SCIENCES*

302 CHE ISSN 0044-3514
ZEITSCHRIFT FUER SOZIALPSYCHOLOGIE. Text in German; Summaries in English. 1970. q. CHF 136 to individuals; CHF 205 to institutions (effective 2001). adv. bk.rev. abstr, bibl. reprint service avail. from SCH,PSC. *Refereed.* **Document type:** *Journal, Academic/Scholarly.*
Related titles: Online - full text ed.: (from Institute for Scientific Information).
Indexed: ASCA, Can.Rev.Comp.Lit., Curr.Cont., Ger.J.Psych., IBR, IBZ, Lang.& Lang.Behav.Abstr., PsycInfo, Psychol.Abstr. (1970-), Russ.Acad.Sci.Bibl., SOPODA, SSCI, Soc.Serv.Abstr., Sociol.Abstr., e-psyche.
—BLDSC (9486.380000), IDS.
Published by: Hans Huber AG, Laengassstr 76, Bern, 9 3000, Switzerland. TEL 41-31-3004500, FAX 41-31-3004591, zeitschriften@hanshuber.com, http://www.hanshuber.com. Adv. contact Rene Waelchli. color page DEM 2,540; trim 170 x 250. Circ: 350.

616.89 DEU ISSN 0723-9505
ZEITSCHRIFT FUER SYSTEMISCHE THERAPIE. Text in German. q. DEM 64 in Europe; DEM 72 elsewhere (effective 1999). **Document type:** *Academic/Scholarly.*
Indexed: IBR, IBZ, Ind.Philos., e-psyche.
—GNLM.
Published by: Verlag Modernes Lernen - Dortmund, Hohe Str 39, Dortmund 44139, Germany. TEL 49-231-128048, FAX 49-231-128009. Ed. Klaus Deissler. Circ: 2,100.

616.89 DEU ISSN 0176-9855
ZEITSCHRIFT FUER TRANSAKTIONSANALYSE IN THEORIE UND PRAXIS. Text in German; Summaries in English. 1984. q. DEM 60 (effective 2000). index. back issues avail. **Document type:** *Magazine, Academic/Scholarly.*
Indexed: e-psyche.
Published by: (Deutsche Gesellschaft fuer Transaktions-Analyse e.V.), Junfermann Verlag, Imadstr 40, Paderborn 33102, Germany. TEL 49-5251-13440, FAX 49-5251-134444, ju@junfermann.de.

150 CHN ISSN 1000-6729
ZHONGGUO XINLI WEISHENG ZAZHI/CHINESE MENTAL HEALTH JOURNAL. Text in Chinese; Abstracts in English. 1987. m. (bi-m. until 2002). USD 96; USD 8 newsstand/cover (effective until 2003). adv. *Refereed.* **Document type:** *Journal, Academic/Scholarly.* **Description:** Publishes postgraduate dissertations, research articles, and clinical practices in the fields of medicine, psychology, pedagogy and sociology, focusing on mental health issues.
Related titles: Online - full text ed.: (from The Dialog Corporation, WanFang Data Corp.).
Indexed: PsycInfo, Psychol.Abstr. (1992-), e-psyche.
—BLDSC (3181.015100).

P

Published by: Zhongguo Xinli Weisheng Xiehui/Chinese Mental Health Association, Beijing Daxue, Jingshen Weisheng Yanjiusuo, 51, Huayuan Bei Lu, Beijing 100083, China. xlwsh@public.fhnet.cn.net. Ed. Ruicong Peng. adv.: page USD 800. Circ: 15,000 (paid). **Dist. by:** China International Book Trading Corp, 35, Chegongzhuang Xilu, Haidian District, Beijing 100044, China. TEL 86-1-68413849, FAX 86-1-68412048, cibtc@mail.cibtc.com.cn, http://www.cibtc.com.cn.

150 DEU ISSN 0724-3766
ZWISCHENSCHRITTE; Beitraege zu einer morphologischen Psychologie. Text in German. 1982. s-a. price varies. adv. bk.rev., film rev., play rev. bibl, illus. back issues avail. **Document type:** *Academic/Scholarly.*
Indexed: IBR, Ind.Philos., e-psyche.
Published by: (Arbeitskreis Morphologische Psychologie e.V.), Bouvier Verlag Herbert Grundmann, Am Hof 28, Bonn 53113, Germany. TEL 49-228-7290184, FAX 49-228-7290179, verlag@books.de. Adv. contact Signe Krichel. Circ: 1,500.

PSYCHOLOGY—Abstracting, Bibliographies, Statistics

310 150 JPN ISSN 0385-7417
BF76.5
BEHAVIORMETRIKA. Text mainly in English. 1974. s-a. USD 40 (effective 2001). 88 p./no. back issues avail. *Refereed.* **Document type:** *Academic/Scholarly.*
Indexed: Curr.Cont. (1988-, dropped), Curr.Ind.Stat., J.Cont.Quant.Meth., Lang.& Lang.Behav.Abstr., PsycInfo, Psychol.Abstr. (1983-), SOPODA, Sociol.Abstr., Stat.Theor.Meth.Abstr. (1988-), e-psyche.
—BLDSC (1878.070000), ingenta.
Published by: Nihon Kodo Keiryo Gakkai/Behaviormetric Society of Japan, 6-7 Minami-Azabu 4-chome, Minato-ku, Tokyo 106-0047, Japan. FAX 81-3-5421-8707, yoshino@ism.ac.jp. Ed. Yutaka Kanou.

016 150 ARG ISSN 0523-1698
BIBLIOGRAFIA ARGENTINA DE PSICOLOGIA✱ . Text in Spanish. irreg., latest 1970, nos. 5-6. **Document type:** *Government.*
Published by: Ministerio de Cultura y Educacion, Direccion de Bibliotecos, Pizzurno, 900, Capital Federal, Buenos Aires 1020, Argentina.

150 011 USA ISSN 0360-277X
Z7203
BIBLIOGRAPHIC GUIDE TO PSYCHOLOGY. Text in Multiple languages. a. USD 295. **Document type:** *Bibliography, Abstract/Index.* **Description:** Lists all aspects of psychology catalogued during the past year by the Research Libraries of the N Y P L; includes additional entries from LC MARC tapes.
Formerly: Psychology Book Guide
Published by: G.K. Hall & Co., Macmillan Library Reference, Box 159, Thorndike, ME 04986. TEL 212-654-8452, 800-223-6121, FAX 207-948-2863, http://www.mir.com/thorndike, http://www.mlr.com/thorndike. **Subscr. to:** Simon & Schuster, Library Reference Order Processing, 200 Old Tappan Rd., Old Tappan, NJ 07675. TEL 800-223-2336.

016.3011 DEU ISSN 1436-2104
Z7203
BIBLIOGRAPHIE PSYCHOLOGISCHER LITERATUR AUS DEN DEUTSCHSPRACHIGEN LAENDERN. Text in German. 1972. a. DEM 348 (effective 2001). back issues avail. **Document type:** *Bibliography.* **Description:** Lists sources in the German-language psychological literature.
Formerly (until 1996): Bibliographie der Deutschsprachigen Psychologischen Literatur (0303-5999)
—GNLM.
Published by: (Universitaet Trier, Zentralstelle fuer Psychologische Information und Dokumentation), Vittorio Klostermann, Frauenlobstr 22, Frankfurt Am Main 60487, Germany. TEL 49-69-970816-0, FAX 49-69-708038, verlag@klostermann.de, http://www.klostermann.de.

150 USA ISSN 0742-681X
BIBLIOGRAPHIES AND INDEXES IN PSYCHOLOGY. Text in English. 1984. irreg. price varies.
Indexed: e-psyche.
Published by: Greenwood Press, Inc. (Subsidiary of: Greenwood Publishing Group Inc.), 88 Post Rd W, Box 5007, Westport, CT 06881. TEL 203-226-3571, FAX 203-226-1502.

011.15 ESP
COLEGIO OFICIAL DE PSICOLOGOS DE MADRID. DOCUMENTACION PSICOLOGICA. Text in Spanish. bi-m. ESP 2,900 to non-members; ESP 1,900 to members. abstr, bibl. **Document type:** *Bibliography.* **Description:** Informs readers and reviews Spanish and foreign books and serials received at the library of the Colegio Oficial de Psicologos de Madrid.
Indexed: e-psyche.
Published by: Colegio Oficial de Psicologos de Madrid, Cuesta de San Vicente, 4 6o, Madrid 28008, Spain. TEL 34-91-541-7009, FAX 34-91-541-2284, dmadrid@correo.cop.es, http://www.cop.es/publicaciones/documenta/documen.htm. Ed. Cristina Sanchez Martin.

016.5 ESP
COLEGIO OFICIAL DE PSICOLOGOS DE MADRID. SELECCIONES DE PRENSA. Text in Spanish. m. ESP 8,900 to members; ESP 6,900 to non-members. **Document type:** *Abstract/Index.* **Description:** Summarizes the most noteworthy articles on psychology from more than 90 daily and 35 weekly newspapers and at least 195 magazines and journals.
Indexed: e-psyche.
Published by: Colegio Oficial de Psicologos de Madrid, Cuesta de San Vicente, 4 6o, Madrid 28008, Spain. TEL 34-91-541-7009, FAX 34-91-547-2284, http://www.cop.es/publicaciones/selecciones/prensa.htm. Ed. Javier Martinez.

016.15 USA ISSN 0092-6361
CURRENT CONTENTS: SOCIAL & BEHAVIORAL SCIENCES. Short title: C C: S & B S. Text in English. 1969. w. USD 730. Index. **Document type:** *Academic/Scholarly, Bibliography.* **Description:** Tables of contents of the world's leading publications covering social and behavioral sciences.
Formerly: C C B S E (Current Contents, Behavioral, Social and Educational Sciences) (0011-3387)
Related titles: CD-ROM ed.: (from Institute for Scientific Information); Diskette ed.; Magnetic Tape ed.; Online - full text ed.: (from The Dialog Corporation).
Indexed: AgeLine, Popul.Ind., Russ.Acad.Sci.Bibl.
—BLDSC (3496.209500).
Published by: Institute for Scientific Information, 3501 Market St., Philadelphia, PA 19104. TEL 215-386-0100, FAX 215-386-2911.

016.15 USA
E-PSYCHE. Text in English. 1998. w. **Document type:** *Abstract/Index.* **Description:** Covers the field of psychology and related disciplines for professionals, students and the general public.
Media: Online - full text (from CSA, EBSCO Publishing).
Published by: e-psyche, LLC, 2425 Ridgecrest Dr. S.E., Ste. 149, Albuquerque, NM 87108. TEL 505-262-7607, FAX 505-262-7043, contact@e-psyche.net, http://www.e-psyche.net.

ERGONOMICS ABSTRACTS. see *ENGINEERING—Abstracting, Bibliographies, Statistics*

HUMAN SEXUALITY. see *MEDICAL SCIENCES—Abstracting, Bibliographies, Statistics*

016.15 IND ISSN 0971-524X
INDIAN PSYCHOLOGICAL ABSTRACTS AND REVIEWS. Text in English; Summaries in English. 1972. biennial. INR 270 to individuals India, Nepal & Bhutan; USD 13 SAARC to individuals Pakistan, Bangladesh, Sri Lanka & Maldives; USD 23 SAARC to institutions; INR 545 to institutions; INR 155 newsstand/cover to individuals; INR 315 newsstand/cover to institutions; USD 9 newsstand/cover SAARC to individuals; USD 13 newsstand/cover SAARC to institutions (effective 2002). adv. bk.rev. abstr. back issues avail. *Refereed.* **Document type:** *Journal, Academic/Scholarly, Abstract/Index.* **Description:** The journal disseminates relevant research based information in the form of abstracts and review articles on contemporary issues in phychology and related disciplines in India.
Formerly (until 1994): Indian Psychological Abstracts (0250-9679)
Indexed: Intl.Bibl.Soc.Sci., Russ.Acad.Sci.Bibl., e-psyche.
Published by: Indian Council of Social Science Research, PO Box 10528, Aruna Asaf Ali Marg, New Delhi 110067, India. TEL 91-11-6179832, FAX 91-11-6179836, info@icssr.org, http://indiasage.com/jdisp.asp?id=0971524X, www.icssr.org. Ed. B N Puhan. Pub. Tejeshwar Singh. Adv. contact Sunanda Ghosh. page USD 75. Circ: 500. **Subscr. to:** Sage Publications India Pvt. Ltd., M-32 Market, Greater Kailash-1, PO Box 4215, New Delhi 110 024, India. TEL 91-11-6419884, 91-11-6444958, FAX 91-11-6472426, sageindia@sagepub.com, http://indiasage.com/. **Affiliates:** Sage Publications, Inc.; Sage Publications Ltd. **Co-sponsor:** Indian Psychological Association.

150 016 614 USA ISSN 1085-2352
RA421
JOURNAL OF PREVENTION AND INTERVENTION IN THE COMMUNITY. Text in English. 1976. s-a. USD 75 to individuals; USD 101 in Canada to individuals; USD 109 elsewhere to individuals; USD 175 to institutions; USD 236 in Canada to institutions; USD 254 elsewhere to institutions; USD 250 to libraries; USD 338 in Canada to libraries; USD 363 elsewhere to libraries (effective Aug. 2001). adv. bk.rev. abstr, bibl, illus. cum.index. back issues avail.; reprint service avail. from HAW. *Refereed.* **Document type:** *Journal, Academic/Scholarly, Abstract/Index.* **Description:** Deals with the application of the philosophy of prevention in mental health and other human services.
Former titles (until 1996): Prevention in Human Services (0270-3114); (until 1981): Community Mental Health Review (0363-1605)
Related titles: Microfiche ed.: (from PQC); Microform ed.
Indexed: Child Devel.Abstr., IBZ, PsycInfo, Ref.Zh., Sage Urb.Stud.Abstr., Soc.Serv.Abstr., Soc.Work Res.& Abstr., Sociol.Abstr., Viol.& Abuse Abstr., e-psyche.
—BLDSC (5042.227300), EMDOCS, GNLM, Haworth, ingenta.
Published by: Haworth Press, Inc., 10 Alice St, Binghamton, NY 13904-1580. TEL 607-722-5857, 800-429-6784, FAX 607-722-6362, 800-895-0582, getinfo@haworthpressinc.com, http://www.haworthpress.com/journals/journallist.asp. Ed. Joseph Ferrari. Pub. William Cohen. R&P Ruthann Heath TEL 607-723-5857 ext 316. Adv. contact Jackie Blakeslee TEL 607-722-5857 ext 346. B&W page USD 315, color page USD 550; trim 6 x 8.5. Circ: 300.

150 ITA
LETTERA; percorsi bibliografici in psichiatria. Text in Italian. 1986. s-a. ITL 45,000. back issues avail. **Document type:** *Newsletter, Bibliography.* **Description:** Contains reviews on topics about psychiatry and bibliographic selection. Informs professionals on current literature.
Indexed: e-psyche.
Published by: Istituto di Ricerche Farmacologiche Mario Negri, Via Eritrea, 62, Milan, MI 20157, Italy. TEL 39-2-390141, FAX 39-2-3546277, http://www.irfmn.mnegri.it/perp/it, http://www.marionegri.it. Ed. Lucilla Frattura. Circ: 400.

MENTAL HEALTH STATISTICAL NOTES. see *SOCIAL SERVICES AND WELFARE—Abstracting, Bibliographies, Statistics*

150 GBR ISSN 1350-4126
HM132 CODEN: PRRLEY
PERSONAL RELATIONSHIPS. Text in English. 1994. q. GBP 172 to institutions in UK & Europe; USD 215 to institutions in the Americas & Caribbean; GBP 172 elsewhere to institutions (effective 2002). adv. back issues avail. *Refereed.* **Document type:** *Academic/Scholarly.* **Description:** Promotes scholarship in personal relationships through a broad range of disciplines, including psychology, psychiatry, communication studies, sociology, anthropology, and family studies.
Related titles: Online - full text ed.: (from Institute for Scientific Information).
Indexed: ASCA, AgeLine, Curr.Cont., Fam.Ind., IMFL, Lang.& Lang.Behav.Abstr., PsycInfo, SOPODA, SSCI, Soc.Serv.Abstr., Sociol.Abstr., e-psyche.
—BLDSC (6427.885200), IDS, Infotrieve, ingenta. **CCC.**
Published by: (International Society for the Study of Personal Relationships), Cambridge University Press, Edinburgh Bldg, Shaftesbury Rd, Cambridge CB2 2RU, United Kingdom. information@cup.cam.ac.uk, http://www.cup.cam.ac.uk. Eds. Anita Vangelisti, Deborah A. Kashy, Garth Fletcher, Jeffry A Simpson, Leigh A. Leslie, Steven Beach. R&P Linda Nicol. Adv. contact Rebecca Symons.

P

016.15 ESP
PSICODOC. Text in Spanish. 1997. a. ESP 29,000 to non-members; ESP 11,600 to members. **Document type:** *Abstract/Index.* **Description:** Compiles some 27,000 bibliographic references from more than 200 Spanish-language scholarly and trade publications and the proceedings of 100 congresses.
Media: CD-ROM.
Indexed: e-psyche.
Published by: Colegio Oficial de Psicologos de Madrid, Cuesta de San Vicente, 4 6o, Madrid 28008, Spain. TEL 34-91-541-9998, FAX 34-91-547-2284, http://www.cop.es/delegaci/madrid/cd-rom/psicodoc.html.

150.19 011 USA ISSN 1066-9884
PSYCHOANALYTIC ABSTRACTS. Text in English. 1985. q. USD 59 domestic to non-members; USD 74 foreign to non-members; USD 39 domestic to members; USD 49 foreign to members; USD 116 domestic to institutions; USD 148 foreign to institutions (effective 2001). adv. **Document type:** *Abstract/Index.* **Description:** Produced in collaboration with APA Division 39 (Psychoanalysis). Covers international literature in the field of psychoanalysis, including advances in psychoanalytic theory, therapy and interpretation, as well as the history of psychoanalysis.
Former titles: PsycSCAN: Psychoanalysis (0889-5236); Psychoanalysis Abstracts
Published by: American Psychological Association, 750 First St., N.E., Washington, DC 20002-4242. TEL 202-336-5600, 800-374-2721, FAX 202-336-5568, subscriptions@apa.org, www.apa.org/psycinfo/products/scan-analysis.html, http://www.apa.org/journals/psy.html. Circ: 4,100.

016.15 150 USA ISSN 0033-2887
BF1
PSYCHOLOGICAL ABSTRACTS. Text in English. 1927. m. USD 1,139 domestic to non-members and institutions; USD 1,217 foreign to non-members and institutions; USD 799 domestic to members; USD 877 foreign to members (effective 2001). adv. illus. cum.index. reprint service avail. from PSC,PQC,SCH. **Document type:** *Abstract/Index.* **Description:** Contains summaries (abstracts, bibliographic information, and indexing) of English-language journal articles, technical reports, book chapters, and books in the field of psychology.
Related titles: CD-ROM ed.: ClinPsyc (from Ovid Technologies, Inc., SilverPlatter Information, Inc.); Microform ed.: (from PQC,PMC); ♦ Online - full text ed.: PsycINFO; Print ed.: PsycFirst (from NISC).
Indexed: Ergon.Abstr., Russ.Acad.Sci.Bibl.
—BLDSC (6946.290000), Linda Hall.
Published by: American Psychological Association, 750 First St., N.E., Washington, DC 20002-4242. TEL 202-336-5600, 800-374-2721, FAX 202-336-5568, subscriptions@apa.org, http://www.apa.org/psycinfo/products/psycabs.html. Circ: 1,600.

152 USA ISSN 0272-0582
PSYCHOLOGICAL CINEMA REGISTER; films and video in the behavioral sciences. Abbreviated title: P C R. Text in English. 1944. a. **Document type:** *Catalog.*
Indexed: e-psyche.
Published by: Pennsylvania State University, Audio-Visual Services, University Park, PA 16802. TEL 800-826-0132, FAX 814-863-2574. Circ: 9,000.

016.15 USA
PSYCINFO. Text in English. m. **Document type:** *Abstract/Index.* **Description:** Offers comprehensive coverage of topics in, and applications of, behavior and psychology.
Media: Online - full text (from NISC, DIMDI, Data-Star, The Dialog Corporation, Questel Orbit Inc., EBSCO Publishing). **Related titles:** CD-ROM ed.: ClinPsyc (from Ovid Technologies, Inc., SilverPlatter Information, Inc.); Microform ed.: (from PQC,PMC); ♦ Print ed.: Psychological Abstracts. ISSN 0033-2887; PsycFirst (from NISC).
Published by: American Psychological Association, 211 E 70th St, New York, NY 10021. TEL 202-336-5500, 800-374-2722, sales@nisc.com, http://www.nisc.com.

370.15 USA
PSYCINFO NEWS. Text in English. 1981. q. free. **Document type:** *Newsletter.* **Description:** Contains search tips and news about forthcoming and existing PsycINFO products.
Related titles: Online - full text ed.
—BLDSC.
Published by: American Psychological Association, PsycINFO User Services, 211 E 70th St, New York, NY 10021. TEL 212-628-8792, 800-374-2722, FAX 212-628-8453, psycinfo@apa.org, http://www.apa.org/psychifo/pin, http://www.apa.org/psycinfo/pin. R&P William C Hayward. Circ: 11,500.

150 USA ISSN 0271-7506
BF636.A1
PSYCSCAN: APPLIED PSYCHOLOGY. Text in English. 1981. q. USD 49 domestic to non-members; USD 64 foreign to non-members; USD 29 domestic to members; USD 39 foreign to members; USD 84 domestic to institutions; USD 116 foreign to institutions (effective 2001). adv. reprint service avail. from PSC,SCH. **Document type:** *Abstract/Index.* **Description:** Abstracts from a cluster of subscriber-selected journals in general area of applied psychology.
Published by: American Psychological Association, 750 First St., N.E., Washington, DC 20002-4242. TEL 202-336-5600, 800-374-2721, FAX 202-336-5568, subscriptions@apa.org, http://www.apa.org/psycinfo/products/scan-applied.html, http://www.apa.org/journals/psa.html. Circ: 2,200.

158 USA ISSN 1078-3946
PSYCSCAN: BEHAVIOR ANALYSIS AND THERAPY. Text in English. 1995. q. USD 49 domestic to non-members; USD 64 foreign to non-members; USD 29 domestic to members; USD 39 foreign to members; USD 84 domestic to institutions; USD 116 foreign to institutions (effective 2001). **Document type:** *Academic/Scholarly.* **Description:** Lists abstracts from subscriber selected journals in basic and applied research in behavioral psychology and related topics.
Published by: American Psychological Association, 750 First St., N.E., Washington, DC 20002-4242. TEL 202-336-5600, 800-374-2721, FAX 202-336-5568, subscriptions@apa.org, http://www.apa.org/psycinfo/products/scan-bat.html, http://www.apa.org/journals/psb.html. Circ: 1,600.

016.61686 USA ISSN 0197-1484
RC467
PSYCSCAN: CLINICAL PSYCHOLOGY. Text in English. 1980. q. USD 49 domestic to non-members; USD 64 foreign to non-members; USD 29 domestic to members; USD 39 foreign to members; USD 84 domestic to institutions; USD 116 foreign to institutions (effective 2001). adv. back issues avail. **Document type:** *Abstract/Index.* **Description:** Abstracts from subscriber-selected journals of interest to clinical psychologists.
Published by: American Psychological Association, 750 First St., N.E., Washington, DC 20002-4242. TEL 202-336-5600, 800-374-2721, FAX 202-336-5568, subscriptions@apa.org, http://www.apa.org/psycinfo/products/scan-clin.html, http://www.apa.org/journals/psc.html. Circ: 5,300.

150 USA ISSN 0197-1492
PSYCSCAN: DEVELOPMENTAL PSYCHOLOGY. Text in English. 1980. q. USD 49 domestic to non-members; USD 64 foreign to non-members; USD 29 domestic to members; USD 39 foreign to members; USD 84 domestic to institutions; USD 116 foreign to institutions (effective 2001). adv. **Document type:** *Abstract/Index.* **Description:** Abstracts from subscriber-selected journals of interest to developmental psychologists.
Published by: American Psychological Association, 750 First St., N.E., Washington, DC 20002-4242. TEL 202-336-5600, 800-374-2721, FAX 202-336-5568, subscriptions@apa.org, http://www.apa.org/psycinfo/products/scan-dev.html, http://www.apa.org/journals/psd.html. Circ: 2,600.

016.15 RUS ISSN 0869-4133
REFERATIVNYI ZHURNAL. PSIKHOLOGIYA. Text in Russian. 1990. m. USD 545 in United States. **Document type:** *Abstract/Index.*
—BLDSC (0142.108000), East View.
Published by: Vserossiiskii Institut Nauchnoi i Tekhnicheskoi Informatsii (VINITI), Usievicha ul 20-a, Moscow 125315, Russian Federation. TEL 7-095-1526441, FAX 7-095-943-0060. **US dist. addr.:** East View Publications, 3020 Harbor Ln N, Minneapolis, MN 55447. TEL 612-550-0961.

150 DEU
TESTZENTRALE TESTKATALOG. Text in German. a. DEM 10 newsstand/cover (effective 2001). **Document type:** *Catalog, Academic/Scholarly.* **Description:** Contains information on a wide variety of diagnostic tests available to psychologists.
Related titles: CD-ROM ed.: DEM 49.80 (effective 2000).
Indexed: e-psyche.
Published by: (Testzentrale), Hogrefe Verlag GmbH und Co. KG, Rohnsweg 25, Goettingen 37085, Germany. TEL 49-551-50688-0, FAX 49-551-5068824, testzentrale@hogrefe.de, verlag@hogrefe.de, http://www.hogrefe.de. Circ: 110,000 (paid).

155.937 USA ISSN 0196-0121
HQ1073
THANATOLOGY ABSTRACTS✶ . Text in English. biennial. USD 20 per issue. adv. back issues avail. **Document type:** *Abstract/Index.* **Description:** Covers articles from 120 magazines.
Formerly: Funeral Service Abstracts
—GNLM.
Published by: Foundation of Thanatology, Foundation Book & Periodical Division, 630 W 168th St, New York, NY 10032. TEL 212-928-2066. Ed. Dr. Otto Margolis.

153.021 USA
U.S. NATIONAL CENTER FOR HEALTH STATISTICS. VITAL AND HEALTH STATISTICS. SERIES 6. COGNITION AND SURVEY MEASUREMENT. Text in English. 1989. irreg., latest vol.8. price varies. **Document type:** *Monographic series, Government.* **Description:** Comprises research from the National Laboratory for Collaborative Research in Cognition and Survey Measurement, using methods of cognitive science to design, evaluate, and test survey instruments.
Indexed: Excerp.Med.
Published by: U.S. National Center for Health Statistics, Data Dissemination Branch, 6525 Belcrest Rd, Hyattsville, MD 20782. TEL 301-458-4636, http://www.cdc.gov/nchs/. **Orders to:** U.S. Government Printing Office, Superintendent of Documents.

PUBLIC ADMINISTRATION

see also HOUSING AND URBAN PLANNING; POLITICAL SCIENCE; PUBLIC ADMINISTRATION—Municipal Government; SOCIAL SERVICES AND WELFARE

ANDERSON'S OHIO E P A ON CD-ROM. see *ENVIRONMENTAL STUDIES—Toxicology And Environmental Safety*

CAMBRIDGESHIRE COUNTY COUNCIL. ROAD SAFETY PLAN (YEAR). see *TRANSPORTATION—Roads And Traffic*

351.71 CAN ISSN 0045-4893
CANADIAN GOVERNMENT PROGRAMS AND SERVICES. Text in English. bi-m. CND 490. index. **Document type:** *Trade.* **Description:** Authoritative guide to federal government organizations, programs and services, government relations. Information on all departments: their structure, key personnel with addresses and phone numbers, jurisdictions, responsibilities, budgets, etc.
Related titles: Online - full text ed.: (from LexisNexis).
Indexed: CBCA Bus. (1996-).
Published by: C C H Canadian Ltd., 90 Sheppard Ave E, Ste 300, North York, ON M2N 6X1, Canada. TEL 416-224-2248, 800-268-4522, FAX 416-224-2243, http://camelot.ca.cch.com.

353.6 USA ISSN 1052-6552
COMMUNITY HEALTH FUNDING REPORT. Text in English. 1990. s-m. USD 329 domestic (effective 2001). 18 p./no. back issues avail. **Document type:** *Newsletter.* **Description:** Reviews of public and private health grant opportunities, including reports on eligibility requirements, funding levels and deadlines.
Incorporates (1988-1993): Public Assistance Funding Report (1056-7100); Which is formerly (until 1991): Public Assistance Success (1050-3447); Which incorporates (1988-1991): Helping the Homeless (1050-3439)
Published by: (Community Development Services, Inc.), C D Publications, 8204 Fenton St, Silver Spring, MD 20910-2889. TEL 301-588-6380, FAX 301-588-6385, chf@cdpublications.com, cdpubs@clark.net. Ed. David Adler. Pub. Mike Gerecht.

353.6 USA
DRUGS, HEALTH, AND SOCIAL POLICY SERIES. Text in English. 1996. q. price varies. back issues avail. **Document type:** *Monographic series.* **Description:** Provides students and professionals in the fields of substance abuse, AIDS, public health, and criminal justice access to current research and policy.
—BLDSC (3629.855000).
Published by: Sage Publications, Inc., Books, 2455 Teller Rd, Thousand Oaks, CA 91320. TEL 605-499-0721, order@sagepub.com, http://www.sagepub.com. Ed. James A Inciardi. **Overseas orders to:** Sage Publications Ltd., 6 Bonhill St, London EC2A 4PU, United Kingdom; Sage Publications India Pvt. Ltd., 32-m Market, Greater Kailash-I, New Delhi 110 048, India.

353.6 FRA
RA440.87.F8
FRANCE. MINISTERE DES AFFAIRES SOCIALES DE LA SANTE ET DE LA VILLE. BULLETIN OFFICIEL. Text in French. w. FRF 512; FRF 669 foreign. **Document type:** *Bulletin.*
Former titles: France. Ministere des Affaires Sociales et de l'Integration. Bulletin Officiel; France. Ministere des Affaires Sociales et de la Solidarite Nationale. Secretariat d'Etat Charge de la Sante. Bulletin Officiel (0758-1998)
Related titles: Microfiche ed.
Published by: Ministere des Affaires Sociales de la Sante et de la Ville, 1 place de Fontenoy, Paris Cedex 7 75350, France. FAX 40-56-60-00. **Subscr. to:** Direction des Journaux Officiels, 26 rue Desaix, Paris Cedex 15 75727, France.

353.6 GBR
GUIDE TO HEALTH SERVICES OF THE WORLD. Text in English. irreg., latest vol.2, 1994. GBP 16. charts, stat. **Document type:** *Academic/Scholarly.* **Description:** Provides an overview of the health services in more than 60 nations, along with health and hospital statistics.
Published by: International Hospital Federation, 4 Abbots Pl, London NW6 4NP, United Kingdom. TEL 44-207-372-7181, FAX 44-207-328-7433. Ed. Dr. Errol Pickering. R&P Carl Richmond.

GULF WAR REVIEW; information for veterans who served in Desert Shield - Desert Storm. see *ENVIRONMENTAL STUDIES—Toxicology And Environmental Safety*

352.73 USA ISSN 0194-2352
HEALTH GRANTS & CONTRACTS WEEKLY; selected federal project opportunities. Text in English. 1978. 50/yr. USD 435 to individuals; USD 10 newsstand/cover (effective 2002). **Document type:** *Newsletter.* **Description:** Alerts health researchers, administrators and fundseekers to the latest funding announcements for federal health grants and contracts. Includes facts on scope of work, eligibility, amount of funds, application deadline and contact officers.
Related titles: Online - full text ed.: (from NewsNet).
—Infotrieve. **CCC.**
Published by: Aspen Publishers Inc, 200 Orchard Ridge Dr, Gaithersburg, MD 20878. TEL 301-417-7500, 800-638-8437, FAX 301-417-7550, customer.service@aspenpubl.com, http://www.aspenpub.com. Pub. Marjorie Weiner. R&P Rossette Graham. **Dist. by:** Aspen Publishers Inc., Distribution Center, 7201 McKinney Circle, Frederick, MD 21701. TEL 301-698-7100, FAX 301-417-7550.

321.023 362.1 USA
HEALTH POLICY MONITOR. Text in English. q. USD 30 (effective 2001). **Document type:** *Journal, Government.* **Description:** Addresses late-breaking and significant issues affecting health reform efforts in the states.
Published by: Council of State Governments, 2760 Research Park Dr, Box 11910, Lexington, KY 40578-1910. TEL 606-244-8000, 800-800-1910, FAX 606-244-8001, info@csg.org, http://www.csg.com/.

JAPAN'S AND I C H GUIDELINES FOR NEW DRUG REGISTRATION (YEAR). see *PHARMACY AND PHARMACOLOGY*

▼ **JOURNAL OF HEALTH MANAGEMENT.** see *MEDICAL SCIENCES*

353.690973 USA ISSN 0270-6768
NATIONAL INTELLIGENCE REPORT; the biweekly on Medicare policy for laboratories, blood banks & physician services. Text in English. 1979. fortn. USD 264 domestic to individuals; USD 289 foreign to individuals (effective 2000); includes the Washington Insider's Focus, special Alerts, periodic supplements, and semi-annual subject index.. adv. charts. back issues avail. **Document type:** *Newsletter.* **Description:** Covers third-party payment and billing news, C.L.I.A. developments, system fraud and abuse. Aimed at laboratory and hospital administrators, attorneys, physicians, and blood bank directors.
Published by: Washington G-2 Reports, 1111 14th St, N W, Ste 500, Washington, DC 20005. TEL 202-789-1034, 800-LAB-REGS, FAX 202-289-4062, washg2@aol.com, http://www.nashg2.com. Ed. Jim Curren. Pub. Dennis W Weissman. Adv. contact Paulette A Washington. Circ: 2,000.

NEW ZEALAND. LAND TRANSPORT SAFETY AUTHORITY. RULES. see *TRANSPORTATION*

351 USA ISSN 0883-3648
K14
NOTRE DAME JOURNAL OF LAW, ETHICS & PUBLIC POLICY. Text in English. 1984. s-a. USD 20 (effective 1999). adv. reprint service avail. from WSH. **Document type:** *Academic/Scholarly.* **Description:** Applies normative and ethical concerns to public policy and legal issues.
Related titles: Microfiche ed.: (from WSH); Microform ed.: (from WSH); Online - full text ed.: (from LexisNexis, H. W. Wilson, Gale Group).
Indexed: C.L.I., L.R.I. (Sep.1984-), Lang.& Lang.Behav.Abstr., Leg.Per. (Sep.1987-), P.A.I.S., Phil.Ind., Rel.Ind.One, Rel.Ind.Two, SOPODA, Soc.Serv.Abstr., Sociol.Abstr.
—BLDSC (6175.405000), ingenta.
Published by: University of Notre Dame, Thomas J. White Center on Law and Government, Notre Dame Law School, Rm 341, Notre Dame, IN 46556. TEL 219-631-5913, FAX 219-631-6371. Ed., R&P, Adv. contact Todd Barker TEL 219-631-488. Circ: 1,000.

OCCUPATIONAL HEALTH & SAFETY LEGISLATION SERVICE. see *OCCUPATIONAL HEALTH AND SAFETY*

PESTICIDES MONITOR; a monthly listing of UK approvals and other announcements on pesticides. see *ENVIRONMENTAL STUDIES—Toxicology And Environmental Safety*

POLITICS AND THE LIFE SCIENCES. see *POLITICAL SCIENCE*

351 USA
PUBLIC ADMINISTRATION AND PUBLIC POLICY. Text in English. 1978. irreg., latest vol.73, 1999. adv. **Document type:** *Monographic series.*
Indexed: Intl.Bibl.Soc.Sci., Russ.Acad.Sci.Bibl.
—BLDSC.
Published by: Marcel Dekker, Inc., Attn: Eridania Perrez, 270 Madison Ave, New York, NY 10016-0602. TEL 212-696-9000, 800-228-1160, FAX 212-685-4540, marketing@dekker.com, http://www.dekker.com. Pub. Russell Dekker. R&P Julia Mulligan. Adv. contact Eridania Perez.

PUBLIC ASSISTANCE & WELFARE TRENDS - STATE CAPITALS. see *LAW*

PUBLIC HEALTH - STATE CAPITALS. see *LAW*

PUBLIC SAFETY AND JUSTICE POLICIES - STATE CAPITALS. see *LAW*

352.63 NZL ISSN 0110-6945
PUBLIC SERVICE ASSOCIATION JOURNAL. Short title: P S A Journal. Text in English. 1913. 10/yr. free per issue to members. adv. bk.rev., rec.rev. **Document type:** *Newspaper.* **Description:** Covers economic and social issues, international trade union news, personality profiles, health and safety, and PSA news.
Published by: New Zealand Public Service Association, Private Bag, Wellington, New Zealand. TEL 64-4-4942000, FAX 64-4-4942019. Ed. Pat Martin.

REGULATORY AFFAIRS FOCUS. see *MEDICAL SCIENCES*

352.88 USA ISSN 0275-0902
REGULATORY WATCHDOG SERVICE. Text in English. 1975. w. USD 289 in North America (effective Nov. 2001). bk.rev. index. back issues avail. **Document type:** *Newsletter.* **Description:** Reports on government documents available from Congress, FDA, and other federal agencies. Focuses on pharmaceuticals.
Former titles: Regulatory Safety Watchdog Service; Product Safety Watchdog Service (0146-4639)
—CCC.
Published by: Washington Business Information, Inc., 300 N Washington St, Ste 200, Falls Church, Arlington, VA 22046. TEL 703-538-7600, 703-538-7662, FAX 703 538-7676, mwright@fdanews.com, http://www.fdanews.com. Ed. Michelle Wright.

SAIGAI NO JITTAI TO SHOBO NO GENKYO/ANNUAL REPORT OF FIRE AND DISASTER PREVENTION. see *FIRE PREVENTION*

U.S. DEFENSE LOGISTICS AGENCY. D O D HAZARDOUS MATERIALS INFORMATION SYSTEM: HAZARDOUS ITEM LISTING. see *PUBLIC HEALTH AND SAFETY*

U.S. NUCLEAR REGULATORY COMMISSION. RULES AND REGULATIONS FOR MEDICAL LICENSEES. see *MEDICAL SCIENCES—Radiology And Nuclear Medicine*

PUBLIC ADMINISTRATION—Abstracting, Bibliographies, Statistics

AGENT ORANGE REVIEW; for veterans who served in Vietnam. see *ENVIRONMENTAL STUDIES—Toxicology And Environmental Safety*

EXCERPTA MEDICA. SECTION 36: HEALTH POLICY, ECONOMICS AND MANAGEMENT. see *HEALTH FACILITIES AND ADMINISTRATION—Abstracting, Bibliographies, Statistics*

PUBLIC ADMINISTRATION—Municipal Government

see also HOUSING AND URBAN PLANNING; SOCIAL SERVICES AND WELFARE

352.14 DEU
AMTSBLATT DES KREISES WESEL; Amtliches Verkuendungsblatt. Text in German. 1975. w. **Document type:** *Bulletin.*
Published by: Kreiseigene Druckerei, Reeser Landstr 31, Wesel 46483, Germany. TEL 49-281-2070. Circ: 1,000.

352.14 GBR
AUDIT COMMISSION. HEALTH INFORMATION BULLETIN. Text in English. 1993. bi-m. USD 55 (effective 1999). **Document type:** *Bulletin, Government.*
Supersedes (in 1999): Audit Commission. Health and Personal Social Services. Bulletin (1353-2979)
—BLDSC (4274.827000).
Published by: Audit Commission for Local Authorities and the National Health Service in England and Wales, 1 Vincent Sq, London SW1P 2PN, United Kingdom. TEL 44-20-7828-1212, http://www.audit-commission.gov.uk. **Dist. by:** Bookpoint, 39 Milton Park, Milton, Abingdon, Oxon OX14 4TD, United Kingdom. TEL 44-1235-400400, FAX 44-20-7400454.

332.1 GBR
AUDIT COMMISSION. LOCAL GOVERNMENT INFORMATION BULLETIN. Text in English. 1993. bi-m. GBP 55 (effective 1999). **Document type:** *Monographic series, Government.*
Supersedes (in 1999): Audit Commission. Local Government Bulletin (1353-2987)
—BLDSC (5290.012800).
Published by: Audit Commission for Local Authorities and the National Health Service in England and Wales, 1 Vincent Sq, London SW1P 2PN, United Kingdom. TEL 44-207- 8281212, FAX 44-20-7630-0182, http:/www.audit-commission.gov.uk, http://www.audit-commission.gov.uk. **Dist. by:** Bookpoint, 39 Milton Park, Milton, Abingdon, Oxon OX14 4TD, United Kingdom. TEL 44-1235-400400, FAX 44-1235-400454.

AUDIT COMMISSION. LOCAL GOVERNMENT REPORTS. see *BUSINESS AND ECONOMICS—Banking And Finance*

AUDIT COMMISSION. REPORTS. see *BUSINESS AND ECONOMICS—Banking And Finance*

HIV PREVENTION AND SERVICES TECHNICAL ASSISTANCE REPORTS. (Human Immunodeficiency Virus) see *PUBLIC HEALTH AND SAFETY*

HIV PREVENTION CASE STUDY SERIES. (Human Immunodeficiency Virus) see *PUBLIC HEALTH AND SAFETY*

LANDSTINGSVAERLDEN. see *MEDICAL SCIENCES*

LOCAL HEALTH OFFICERS NEWS. see *PUBLIC HEALTH AND SAFETY*

352 360 614.4 330 RUS
LOSINKA. Text in Russian. 1990. s-m. free per issue. adv. play rev., music rev. bibl. *Refereed.* **Document type:** *Newspaper, Government.* **Description:** Provides information about work of Moscow municipal governments (7 municipal districts), pension foundation, social and welfare protection, public health and safety, new medical methods, current events.
Related titles: Diskette ed.

P

Published by: (Moscow. Severo-Vostochnoi Administrativnoi Okrug Moskvy), Losinka, Letchika Babushkina ul 1, Moscow 129344, Russian Federation. Ed. Valentina Kutlovskaya. Pub. Valentina Kutlovsakaya. Adv. contact Marina Volnaya. page RUR 10,000, page USD 400. Circ: 15,000 (controlled).

PUBLIC FINANCE, TAXATION

see BUSINESS AND ECONOMICS—Public Finance, Taxation

PUBLIC HEALTH AND SAFETY

see also BIRTH CONTROL; DRUG ABUSE AND ALCOHOLISM; ENVIRONMENTAL STUDIES; FIRE PREVENTION; FUNERALS; HEALTH FACILITIES AND ADMINISTRATION; MEDICAL SCIENCES; OCCUPATIONAL HEALTH AND SAFETY

9-1-1 MAGAZINE. see *COMMUNICATIONS*

A A M A EXECUTIVE. see *MEDICAL SCIENCES*

A C P M NEWS. see *MEDICAL SCIENCES*

A H A GUIDE TO THE HEALTH CARE FIELD. see *HEALTH FACILITIES AND ADMINISTRATION—Abstracting, Bibliographies, Statistics*

A H C A NOTES. see *SOCIAL SERVICES AND WELFARE*

614.8 360 USA ISSN 0275-8407
A M S STUDIES IN MODERN SOCIETY. Text in English. 1972. irreg., latest vol.24, 1994. price varies. back issues avail. **Description:** Monographs, reference works and bibliographies on contemporary social issues.
Indexed: e-psyche.
Published by: A M S Press, Inc., 56 E 13th St, New York, NY 10003. TEL 212-777-4700, FAX 212-995-5413.

A Q I S BULLETIN. see *AGRICULTURE*

A S D A NEWS. see *MEDICAL SCIENCES—Psychiatry And Neurology*

A S D W A UPDATE. see *WATER RESOURCES*

362.1 USA ISSN 1085-2174
A W H P'S WORKSITE HEALTH. Text in English. q. USD 60 (effective 2001). adv. **Description:** Covers news in the field of worksite health promotion.
Published by: Association for Worksite Health Promotion, 60 Revere Dr, Ste 500, Northbrook, IL 60062-1577. TEL 847-480-9574, FAX 847-480-9282, http://www.awhp.org. Ed. Patricia Sullivan. adv.: B&W page USD 1,075, color page USD 1,775. Circ: 3,250 (paid and controlled).

614.8 AUS ISSN 1037-3403
ABORIGINAL AND ISLANDER HEALTH WORKER JOURNAL; a national resource journal for Aboriginal and Islander community education workers. Text in English. 1977. bi-m. AUD 30 to individuals; AUD 35 to institutions; AUD 40 foreign (effective 1999). adv. back issues avail. **Document type:** *Bulletin.*
Former titles: Aboriginal and Islander Health Worker; Aboriginal Health Worker (0155-0357)
—ingenta.
Published by: (Australia. Human Services and Health Department), Aboriginal and Islander Health Worker, PO Box 502, Matraville, NSW 2036, Australia. TEL 61-2-9311-2593, FAX 61-2-9311-2814. Ed., R&P Donnaleen Campbell. Adv. contact Donna Daly. B&W page USD 800. Circ: 11,000.

614.8 GBR ISSN 0001-4575
HV675.A1 CODEN: AAPVB5
ACCIDENT ANALYSIS & PREVENTION. Text in English. 1969. bi-m. EUR 273 in Europe to qualified personnel; JPY 36,200 in Japan to qualified personnel; USD 305 elsewhere to qualified personnel; EUR 1,070 in Europe to institutions; JPY 142,000 in Japan to institutions; USD 1,196 elsewhere to institutions (effective 2002). adv. bk.rev. charts, illus. Index. back issues avail.; reprints avail. *Refereed.* **Document type:** *Academic/Scholarly.* **Description:** Provides wide coverage of the general areas relating to accidental injury and damage, including the pre-injury and immediate post-injury phases.
Related titles: Microform ed.: (from PQC); Online - full text ed.: (from ingenta, Swets Blackwell, ScienceDirect, Institute for Scientific Information).
Indexed: ASCA, Abstr.Crim.& Pen., AgeLine, Aqua.Sci.& Fish.Abstr., Bioeng.Abstr., Biol.Abstr., C.I.S. Abstr., Comput.& Info.Sys., Crim.Just.Abstr., Curr.Cont., Curr.Ind.Stat., Eng.Ind., Environ.Sci.Poll.Mgmt., Ergon.Abstr., Excerp.Med., HRIS, IBR, INIS Atomind., ISMEC, Ind.Med. (1969-), Int.Abstr.Oper.Res., Int.Nurs.Ind., Intl.Civil Eng.Abstr., Pollut.Abstr., Psyclnfo, Psychol.Abstr. (1969-), Psycscan A.P., Risk Abstr., Russ.Acad.Sci.Bibl., SSCI, Saf.Sci.Abstr., Soft.Abstr.Eng., e-psyche.
—BLDSC (0573.130000), CISTI, Ei, GNLM, IDS, Infotrieve, Linda Hall. **CCC.**
Published by: Pergamon (Subsidiary of: Elsevier Science), The Boulevard, Langford Ln, East Park, Kidlington, Oxford OXB 1GB, United Kingdom. FAX 44-1865-843010, nlinfo-f@elsevier/nl; usinfo-f@elsevier.com; forinfo-kyf04035@niftyserve.or.jp, http://www.elsevier.nl/locate/aap. Ed. Frank A Haight. **Subscr. in Australasia and the Far East to:** Elsevier Science (Singapore) Pte Ltd, No.1 Temasek Ave, 17-01 Millenia Tower, Singapore 039192, Singapore. TEL 65-434-3727, FAX 65-337-2230; **Subscr. in the Americas to:** Elsevier Science, PO Box 945, New York, NY 10159-0945. TEL 212-633-3730, FAX 212-633-3680, usinfo-f@elsevier.com; **Subscr. to:** Elsevier Science BV, PO Box 211, Amsterdam 1000 AE, Netherlands. TEL 31-20-485-3757, FAX 31-20-485-3432, nlinfo-f@elsevier.nl.

614.8 USA ISSN 0148-6039
HA217
ACCIDENT FACTS. Text in English. a. USD 37.95 (effective 2001). **Description:** Compendium of statistical information relating to accidents.
Related titles: Microfiche ed.: (from CIS).
Indexed: SRI.
—Linda Hall.
Published by: National Safety Council, Statistics Department, 1121 Spring Lake Dr, Itasca, IL 60143. TEL 708-775-2281. Ed. Alan F Hoskin.

ACTA HYDROCHIMICA ET HYDROBIOLOGICA; journal for water and wastewater research. see *WATER RESOURCES*

ADMINISTRATION AND POLICY IN MENTAL HEALTH. see *MEDICAL SCIENCES*

ADVANCED RESCUE TECHNOLOGY. see *MEDICAL SCIENCES—Orthopedics And Traumatology*

614 551.5 NLD
ADVANCES IN NATURAL AND TECHNOLOGICAL HAZARDS RESEARCH. Text in Dutch. 1993. irreg., latest vol.5, 1995. back issues avail. *Refereed.* **Document type:** *Proceedings.*
Indexed: GeoRef, Meteor.& Geoastrophys.Abstr.
—BLDSC.
Published by: Kluwer Academic Publishers Group (Subsidiary of: Wolters Kluwer N.V.), Spuiboulevard 50, PO Box 17, Dordrecht 3300 AA, Netherlands. FAX 31-78-639-2254, services@wkap.nl, http://www.wkap.nl. Ed. Mohammed I El Sabh. **Dist. by:** Journals Department, PO Box 322, Dordrecht 3300 AH, Netherlands. FAX 31-78-654-6474.

ADVANCES IN THANATOLOGY. see *PSYCHOLOGY*

AFRICA MEDICINE AND HEALTH. see *MEDICAL SCIENCES*

AIDS & HEALTH NEWS. see *MEDICAL SCIENCES—Communicable Diseases*

AIDS & PUBLIC POLICY JOURNAL. (Acquired Immune Deficiency Syndrome) see *MEDICAL SCIENCES—Communicable Diseases*

AIDS & T B WEEKLY ARTICLE SUMMARIES. (Tuberculosis) see *MEDICAL SCIENCES—Abstracting, Bibliographies, Statistics*

AIDS BULLETIN. see *MEDICAL SCIENCES—Communicable Diseases*

362.1 USA ISSN 0899-9546
RA644.A25 CODEN: AEPREO
AIDS EDUCATION AND PREVENTION; an interdisciplinary journal. (Acquired Immune Deficiency Syndrome) Text in English. 1989. bi-m. USD 50 domestic to individuals; USD 80 foreign to individuals; USD 160 domestic to institutions; USD 190 foreign to institutions (effective 2000). adv. reprint service avail. from PQC. *Refereed.* **Document type:** *Academic/Scholarly.* **Description:** Provides information on prevention of AIDS geared towards all professionals: epidemiologists, physicians, health educators, psychologists, social workers, counselors and legislators.
Related titles: Online - full text ed.: (from ProQuest Information & Learning, CatchWord Ltd., Institute for Scientific Information, RoweCom Information Quest).
Indexed: AIDS & Cancer Res., AIDS Abstr., ASCA, Abstr.Hyg., Addic.Abstr., AgeLine, CINAHL, Chic.Per.Ind., Curr.Cont., Educ.Ind. (Jul.1997-), Environ.Sci.Poll.Mgmt., Fam.Ind., Ind.Med. (1989-), Lang.& Lang.Behav.Abstr., Microbiol.Abstr., Pollut.Abstr., Psyclnfo, Psychol.Abstr. (1989-), Risk Abstr., SOPODA, SSCI, Saf.Sci.Abstr., Sage Race Rel.Abstr., Soc.Serv.Abstr., Soc.Work Res.& Abstr., Sociol.Abstr., THA, Trop.Dis.Bull., Virol.Abstr., e-psyche.
—BLDSC (0773.083360), EMDOCS, GNLM, IDS, ingenta, KNAW. **CCC.**
Published by: Guilford Publications, Inc., 72 Spring St, 4th Fl, New York, NY 10012. TEL 212-431-9800, 800-365-7006, FAX 212-966-6708, info@guilford.com. Ed. Dr. Francisco Sy. Pub. Robert Matloff. R&P Kathy Kuehl. Adv. contact Susan Pavliscak. Circ: 1,700.

AIDS INFORMATION EXCHANGE. (Acquired Immune Deficiency Syndrome) see *MEDICAL SCIENCES—Communicable Diseases*

614 616.9 GBR ISSN 1356-9880
THE AIDS LEADER; covering business, economic policy and employment implications of AIDS & HIV. Text in English. 1992. bi-m. GBP 145, USD 240 (effective 2000). bk.rev. back issues avail. **Document type:** *Newsletter.* **Description:** Aims to promote high standards in corporate and organizational responses to HIV and Aids by encouraging behaviours which avoid infections and do not discriminate against people with (or thought to have) HIV or any chronic life-shortening condition.
Formerly: Digest of Organisational Responses to AIDS and HIV (0965-5840)
—BLDSC (0773.083486).
Published by: Healthworks Ltd., 30-38 Dock St, Leeds LS10 1JF, United Kingdom. TEL 44-1-113-242-6624, FAX 44-113-242-7782, insafe@modus-op.demon.co.uk, aidslead@modus-op.demon.co.uk, http://www.modus-op.demon.co.uk, http://www.healthworks.co.uk. Ed., Pub. Adam Christie. R&P Chris Aspinall. Circ: 500 (paid).

AIDS LITERATURE & LAW REVIEW. see *MEDICAL SCIENCES—Abstracting, Bibliographies, Statistics*

AIDS POLICY AND LAW. (Acquired Immune Deficiency Syndrome) see *LAW*

AIDS THERAPIES. see *MEDICAL SCIENCES—Communicable Diseases*

AIDS WEEKLY PLUS. see *MEDICAL SCIENCES—Communicable Diseases*

614 DEU ISSN 0172-2131
AKADEMIE FUER OEFFENTLICHES GESUNDHEITSWESEN. SCHRIFTENREIHE. Text in German. 1973. irreg. price varies. **Document type:** *Monographic series, Academic/Scholarly, Government.*
Formerly: Akademie fuer Staatsmedizin, Duesseldorf. Jahrbuch (0065-5392)
Published by: Akademie fuer Oeffentliches Gesundheitswesen, Auf'm Hennekamp 70, Duesseldorf 40225, Germany.

613 USA ISSN 0145-6857
ALABAMA'S HEALTH. Text in English. 1967. m. free. bk.rev. **Document type:** *Newsletter, Government.* **Description:** Describes events and topics of interest to public health professionals.
Published by: Alabama Department of Public Health, 0201 Monroe St, Montgomery, AL 36130-3017. TEL 334-206-5510, FAX 334-206-5534, http://www.alapubhealth.org. Ed., R&P Arrol Sheehan. Pub. Dr. Jim McVay. Circ: 1,200 (controlled).

ALERT; maandblad voor rampenbestrijding en crisisbeheersing. see *CIVIL DEFENSE*

362.1 ITA ISSN 1122-4991
AMBIENTE ENERGIA LAVORO. Text in Italian. 1992. m. ITL 150,000; ITL 300,000 foreign (effective 1999). **Document type:** *Trade.* **Description:** Covers public health and safety, health law, and personnel management.
Published by: De Lillo Editore s.r.l., Via Mecenate, 76,3, Milan, MI 20138, Italy. TEL 39-2-58013112, FAX 39-2-58012450. Ed. Pietro de Lillo. Circ: 8,500.

AMBIENTE RISORSE SALUTE; scienza, tecnica e cultura per uno sviluppo di qualita. see *ENVIRONMENTAL STUDIES*

AMERICAN HEALTH CARE ASSOCIATION. PROVIDER. see *SOCIAL SERVICES AND WELFARE*

614 USA
AMERICAN HEALTH LINE. Text in English. d. **Document type:** *Newsletter.*
Media: Online - full text. **Related titles:** E-mail ed.; Fax ed.
Indexed: NRN.
Published by: National Journal Grmoup, Inc., 3129 Mount Vernon Ave, Alexandria, VA 22305. TEL 800-717-3245, FAX 202-672-5700, ahl@advisory.com, http://www.ahl.com. Ed. Patricia Miller. Pubs. Doug Bailey, Roger Craver.

613.2 USA ISSN 0890-1171
CODEN: AJHPED
AMERICAN JOURNAL OF HEALTH PROMOTION. Short title: A J H P. Text in English. 1986. bi-m. USD 99.95 domestic to individuals; USD 108.95 in Canada & Mexico to individuals; USD 117.95 elsewhere to individuals; USD 119.95 domestic to institutions; USD 128.95 in Canada & Mexico to institutions; USD 137.95 elsewhere to institutions (effective 2001); Health Promotion: Global Perspectives - included. adv. bk.rev., film rev. abstr, charts, stat, illus. back issues avail.; reprints avail. *Refereed.* **Document type:** *Academic/Scholarly.* **Description:** Covers the science and art of helping people change their lifestyle to move toward a state of optimal health.
Related titles: Online - full text ed.: (from Institute for Scientific Information).
Indexed: ABI Inform. (coverage dropped), ASCA, ASSIA, Access, AgeLine, C.I.J.E., CINAHL, Curr.Cont., Environ.Sci.Poll.Mgmt., Excerp.Med., Fam.Ind., Human Resour.Abstr., Lang.& Lang.Behav.Abstr., NRN, PSI, Pollut.Abstr., PsycInfo, Psychol.Abstr. (1986-), Risk Abstr., SOPODA, SSCI, Saf.Sci.Abstr., Sage Fam.Stud.Abstr., Soc.Serv.Abstr., Sociol.Abstr., e-psyche.
—BLDSC (0824.760000), EMDOCS, GNLM, ingenta, KNAW.
Address: P O Box 15847, N. Hollywood, CA 91615-1584. TEL 800-783-9913, FAX 818-985-0687, http://www.healthpromotion.com, http:// www.healthpromotionjournal.com. adv.: B&W page USD 1,125, color page USD 2,030; trim 11 x 8.5. Circ: 4,567. **Subscr.to:** Allen Press Inc.

AMERICAN JOURNAL OF PREVENTIVE MEDICINE. see *MEDICAL SCIENCES*

614 USA ISSN 0090-0036
RA421 CODEN: AJHEAA
AMERICAN JOURNAL OF PUBLIC HEALTH. Text in English. 1911. m. USD 165 domestic to individuals; USD 255 foreign to individuals; USD 200 domestic to institutions; USD 265 foreign to institutions (effective 2001). adv. charts, illus. index. back issues avail.; reprints avail. *Refereed.* **Document type:** *Journal, Academic/Scholarly.* **Description:** Contains reports of original research, demonstrations, evaluations, and other articles covering current aspects of public health.
Supersedes in part (in 1971): American Journal of Public Health and the Nation's Health (0002-9572); Which was formed by the 1927 merger of: American Journal of Public Health (0271-4353); Nation's Health (1076-0704)
Related titles: CD-ROM ed.: (from Ovid Technologies, Inc.); Microform ed.: (from PQC,PMC); Online - full text ed.: (from ProQuest Information & Learning, Ovid Technologies, Inc., Northern Light Technology, Inc., H. W. Wilson, Gale Group, Factiva, Institute for Scientific Information).
Indexed: ABI Inform. (Mar.1975-Feb.1977), AIDS Abstr., AIM, ASCA, ASSIA, Abstr.Anthropol., Abstr.Health Care Manage.Stud., Abstr.Hyg., Abstr.Soc.Geront., Acad.Ind., Addic.Abstr., AgeLine, Amer.Bibl.Slavic & E.Eur.Stud., Arts & Hum.Cit.Ind. (coverage dropped), Behav.Med.Abstr., Bibl.Agri., Bibl.Dev.Med.& Child Neur., Biol.Abstr., Biol.Dig., C.I.J.E. (coverage dropped), CINAHL, C.I.S. Abstr., Chem.Abstr., Chic.Per.Ind., Crim.Just.Abstr., Curr.Adv.Cancer Res., Curr.Adv.Ecol.Sci., Curr.Cont., Curr.Ind.Stat., Curr.Lit.Fam.Plan., Curr.Tit.Dent., Dairy Sci.Abstr., Deep Sea Res.& Oceanogr.Abstr., Dent.Abstr., Dent.Ind., Diar.Dis.Res., Dok.Arbeitsmed., Environ.Abstr., Environ.Per.Bibl. (1972-1994), Environ.Sci.Poll.Mgmt., Excerp.Med., Fam.Ind., Food Sci.& Tech.Abstr., Gen.Sci.Ind. (Sep.1983-), HRIS, Helminthol.Abstr., Hlth.Ind., Hosp.Lit.Ind., Human Resour.Abstr., INIS Atomind., I.P.A., Ind.Med. (1971-), Ind.Sci.Rev., Ind.Vet., Inpharma, Int.Nurs.Ind., Irr.& Drain.Abstr., Jrnl.Watch Wom.Hlth., Kidney, MEDSOC, Med.& Surg.Dermat., Med.Care Rev., Mult.Ed.Abstr., NRN, Nutr.Abstr., Ocean.Abstr. (coverage dropped), P C I, Pharm.&Out.News, Phys.Ed.Ind., Pollut.Abstr., Popul.Ind., Protozool.Abstr., PsycInfo, Psychol.Abstr. (1991-), Reac., Res.High.Educ.Abstr., Rev.Appl.Entomol., Rev.Med.& Vet.Mycol., Risk Abstr., Rural Recreat.Tour.Abstr., SRI, SSCI, Saf.Sci.Abstr., Sage Fam.Stud.Abstr., Sage Race Rel.Abstr., Sci.Cit.Ind., Sel.Water Res.Abstr., Small Anim.Abstr., Soc.Sci.Ind. (Oct.1982-), Soc.Work Res.& Abstr., Sp.Ed.Needs Abstr., Stud.Wom.Abstr., THA, Tech.Educ.Abstr., Trop.Dis.Bull., Vet.Bull., Virol.Abstr. (coverage dropped), W.R.C.Inf., Weed Abstr., World Ag.Econ.& Rur.Soc.Abstr., e-psyche.
—BLDSC (0835.900000), CASDDS, CIS, CISTI, EMDOCS, GNLM, IDS, Infotrieve, ingenta, KNAW, Linda Hall. **CCC.**
Published by: American Public Health Association, 1015 15th St, N W, Washington, DC 20005. TEL 202-789-5674, 202-777-2462, FAX 202-789-5661, 202-777-2532, ajph-feedback@forsythe.stanford.edu, http://www.ajph.org, http://www.apha.org. Ed. Dr. Michael Ibrahim. Circ: 35,000. **Subscr. to:** APHA, Subscription Dept 5037, Washington, DC 20061-5037.

614 USA ISSN 0273-4737
AMERICAN SOCIETY OF SAFETY ENGINEERS. SOCIETY UPDATE. Text in English. 1974. m. included in association membership. **Document type:** *Newsletter.* **Description:** ASSE members in the news; chapter and division highlights; society activities and new programs.
Published by: American Society of Safety Engineers, 1800 E Oakton St, Des Plaines, IL 60018-2187. TEL 847-768-3433, FAX 847-296-3769. Ed. Tina Ellingsen. Circ: 30,000.

AMERICAN SOCIETY OF SANITARY ENGINEERING. YEAR BOOK. see *HEATING, PLUMBING AND REFRIGERATION*

614.85 USA
AMERISURE SAFETY NEWS. Text in English. 1921. q. free to policyholders. adv. back issues avail. **Document type:** *Newsletter.* **Description:** Provides safety tips for use in the home, on the road and at the workplace.
Former titles: Michigan Mutual Safety News; Amerisure Companies Safety News; Shopman
Published by: Amerisure Insurance, 26777 Halstead, Farmington, MI 48331. TEL 278-615-9000. Ed., Adv. contact Jeff Marzolf. Circ: 7,000. **Co-sponsor:** Amerisure Companies.

AMTSBLATT DES KREISES WESEL; Amtliches Verkuendungsblatt. see *PUBLIC ADMINISTRATION—Municipal Government*

362.1 ESP ISSN 1137-6627
R71 CODEN: ASSNFO
ANALES DEL SISTEMA SANITARIO DE NAVARRA. Text in Spanish. 1959-1984; resumed 1997. 3/yr. ESP 3,000 (effective 1999). **Document type:** *Government.*
Supersedes (1959-1984): Instituto Medico Beneficencia. Anales
Related titles: ♦ Supplement: Anales del Sistema Sanitario de Navarra. Suplemento. ISSN 1137-814X.
—CINDOC.
Published by: (Departamento de Salud), Gobierno de Navarra, Fondo de Publicaciones, Navas de Tolosa, 21, Pamplona, Navarra 31002, Spain.

362.1 ESP ISSN 1137-814X
ANALES DEL SISTEMA SANITARIO DE NAVARRA. SUPLEMENTO. Text in Spanish. 1997. 3/yr.
Related titles: ♦ Supplement to: Anales del Sistema Sanitario de Navarra. ISSN 1137-6627.
Published by: Gobierno de Navarra, Fondo de Publicaciones, Navas de Tolosa, 21, Pamplona, Navarra 31002, Spain. TEL 34-48-427123, FAX 34-48-427123.

614 ITA ISSN 0021-3071
CODEN: ADSAAB
ANNALI DELLA SANITA PUBBLICA. Text in Italian. 1970 (vol.23). m. ITL 52,000. bk.rev.
Indexed: Biol.Abstr., Chem.Abstr., Helminthol.Abstr., INIS Atomind., Trop.Dis.Bull.
—CASDDS, GNLM.
Published by: Ministero della Sanita, Piazzale dell' Industria, Rome, RM, Italy. Ed. Dr. Fausto Federici. Circ: 3,000.

613 ITA ISSN 1120-9135
CODEN: NAIMAH
ANNALI DI IGIENE, MEDICINA PREVENTIVA E DI COMUNITA. Text in Italian; Summaries in English. 1895. bi-m. ITL 60,000; ITL 120,000 foreign. adv. bk.rev. illus. index.
Former titles (until 1989): Nuovi Annali di Igiene e Microbiologia (0029-6287); (until 1950): Annali d'Igiene (0365-4842); (until 1916): Annali d'Igiene Sperimentale (0365-3161)
Indexed: Abstr.Hyg., Biol.Abstr., C.I.S. Abstr., Chem.Abstr., Dairy Sci.Abstr., Dent.Ind., INIS Atomind., Ind.Med. (1989-), Ind.Vet., Ref.Zh., Trop.Dis.Bull., Vet.Bull.
—BLDSC (1014.180000), CASDDS, CISTI, GNLM.
Published by: (Istituto di Igiene Giuseppe Sanarelli), Societa Editrice Universo, Via Giovanni Battista Morgagni, 1, Rome, RM 00161, Italy. Ed. G M Fara. Circ: 3,000.

614 USA ISSN 1047-2797
RA648.5 CODEN: ANNPE3
ANNALS OF EPIDEMIOLOGY. Text in English. 1990. 8/yr. EUR 212 in Europe to individuals; JPY 28,200 in Japan to individuals; USD 238 elsewhere to individuals; EUR 406 in Europe to institutions; JPY 53,800 in Japan to institutions; USD 454 elsewhere to institutions (effective 2002). adv. back issues avail. *Refereed.* **Document type:** *Academic/Scholarly.* **Description:** Provides reports of original research in epidemiology of chronic and acute diseases of interest to clinical and public-health researchers.
Related titles: Microform ed.: (from PQC); Online - full text ed.: (from ingenta, Swets Blackwell, ScienceDirect, Institute for Scientific Information).
Indexed: Abstr.Hyg., Aqua.Sci.& Fish.Abstr., CINAHL, Cal.Tiss.Abstr., Curr.Cont., Curr.Ind.Stat., Diar.Dis.Res., Environ.Sci.Poll.Mgmt., Excerp.Med. (1992-), Ind.Med. (1990-), Inpharma, Int.Abstr.Biol.Sci., Med.& Surg.Dermat., NRN, Nutr.Abstr., Pharm.&Out.News, Pollut.Abstr., Protozool.Abstr., Reac., Risk Abstr., Rural Recreat.Tour.Abstr., Saf.Sci.Abstr., Sci.Cit.Ind., THA, Trop.Dis.Bull., Wild.Rev.
—BLDSC (1040.470000), CISTI, EMDOCS, GNLM, IDS, Infotrieve, ingenta, KNAW. **CCC.**
Published by: (American College of Epidemiology), Elsevier Science, PO Box 945, New York, NY 10159-0945. TEL 212-989-5800, FAX 212-633-3990, usinfo-f@elsevier.com, http://www.elsevier.com/locate/ annepidem. Eds. Dr. A Franks, Dr. R Rothenberg. adv.: B&W page USD 855, color page USD 1,175. **Subscr. in Australasia and the Far East to:** Elsevier Science (Singapore) Pte Ltd, No.1 Temasek Ave, 17-01 Millenia Tower, Singapore 039192, Singapore. TEL 65-434-3727, FAX 65-337-2230; **Subscr. in Japan to:** Elsevier Science Inc - Japan Regional Office, 9-15 Higashi-Azabu 1-chome, Minato-ku, Tokyo 106-0044, Japan. TEL 81-3-5561-5033, FAX 81-3-5561-5047; **Subscr. outside the Americas to:** Elsevier Science BV, PO Box 211, Amsterdam 1000 AE, Netherlands. TEL 31-20-485-3757, FAX 31-20-485-3432, nlinfo-f@elsevier.nl.

628 USA
ANNUAL CONFERENCE ON ACTIVATED SLUDGE PROCESS CONTROL. PROCEEDINGS. Text in English. 1981. a. **Document type:** *Proceedings.*
Published by: Arthur Technology, Inc., PO Box 1236, Fond Du Lac, WI 54935-6836. Ed. Robert M Arthur.

614 USA ISSN 0163-7525
RA421 CODEN: AREHDT
ANNUAL REVIEW OF PUBLIC HEALTH. Text in English. 1980. a. USD 64 domestic to individuals; USD 69 foreign to individuals; USD 128 domestic to institutions; USD 138 foreign to institutions (effective 1999). adv. bibl, charts. index, cum.index. back issues avail.; reprints avail. *Refereed.* **Document type:** *Academic/Scholarly.* **Description:** Synthesizes and filters primary research to identify the principal contributions in the field of public health.

P

Related titles: Microfilm ed.: (from PQC); Online - full text ed.: (from HighWire Pr., EBSCO Publishing, Institute for Scientific Information).
Indexed: ASCA, Abstr.Health Care Manage.Stud., Abstr.Hyg., Adol.Ment.Hlth.Abstr., AgeLine, CINAHL, Crim.Just.Abstr., Curr.Cont., Curr.Ind.Stat., Deep Sea Res.& Oceanogr.Abstr., Dok.Arbeitsmed., Environ.Sci.Poll.Mgmt., INIS Atomind., Ind.Med. (1980-), Inpharma, Intl.Bibl.Soc.Sci., Microbiol.Abstr., Pollut.Abstr., Reac., Rev.Appl.Entomol., Risk Abstr., SSCI, Saf.Sci.Abstr., Sci.Cit.Ind., THA.
—BLDSC (1528.450000), ADONIS, CASDDS, CISTI, EMDOCS, GNLM, IDS, ingenta, KNAW. **CCC.**
Published by: Annual Reviews Inc., 4139 El Camino Way, Box 10139, Palo Alto, CA 94303-0139. TEL 650-493-4400, 800-523-8635, FAX 650-424-0910, service@annurev.org; orders@allenpress.com, http://www.annualreviews.org. Ed. Samuel Gubins. R&P, Adv. contact Swati Aneja TEL 650-843-6634.
Subscr.to: Allen Press Inc., PO Box 1897, Lawrence, KS 66044-8897.

ANNUAL REVIEW OF WOMEN'S HEALTH. see *WOMEN'S HEALTH*

362.1 CHN ISSN 1002-3631
ANQUAN/SAFETY. Text in Chinese. 1980. bi-m. CNY 6 per issue domestic (effective 2000). back issues avail. **Document type:** *Academic/Scholarly.*
Related titles: Online - full content ed.: (from WanFang Data Corp.).
Published by: Beijingshi Laodong Baohu Kexue Yanjiusuo, 55 Taoranting Lu, Beijing 100054, China. TEL 86-1-63524191. Ed. Kaili Zhang.

APA-JOURNAL. GESUNDHEIT. see *PHYSICAL FITNESS AND HYGIENE*

APPLIED OCCUPATIONAL & ENVIRONMENTAL HYGIENE. see *OCCUPATIONAL HEALTH AND SAFETY*

362.1 DEU ISSN 0948-0935
ARBEIT UND GESUNDHEIT. SONDERAUSGABE VERKEHR. Text in German. 197?. a. DEM 1.03. **Document type:** *Magazine, Trade.*
Formerly (until 1994): Blickpunkt Arbeitssicherheit. Sondernummer (0930-9101)
Published by: Universum Verlagsanstalt GmbH KG, Taunusstr 54, Wiesbaden 65183, Germany. TEL 49-611-9030-0, FAX 49-611-9030382, uv@universum.de, http://www.universum.de.

613.62 DEU ISSN 0944-6052
RC963 CODEN: ASOUEO
ARBEITSMEDIZIN, SOZIALMEDIZIN, UMWELTMEDIZIN; Zeitschrift fuer Praxis, Klinik, Forschung, Begutachtung. Text in German. 1965. m. DEM 291.60; DEM 302.40 foreign (effective 2000). adv. bk.rev. abstr, charts, illus. index. **Document type:** *Magazine, Academic/Scholarly.*
Former titles (until 1993): Arbeitsmedizin, Sozialmedizin, Praeventivmedizin (0300-581X); Arbeitsmedizin, Sozialmedizin, Arbeitshygiene (0003-7753)
Related titles: ♦ Supplement: Arbeitsmedizin, Sozialmedizin, Umweltmedizin. Supplement. ISSN 0944-6419.
Indexed: Abstr.Hyg., Biol.Abstr., C.I.S. Abstr., CSNB, Curr.Cont. (coverage dropped), Excerp.Med., INIS Atomind., Lab.Haz.Bull., Nutr.Abstr., Trop.Dis.Bull.
—BLDSC (1587.402750), CISTI, EMDOCS, GNLM, KNAW.
Published by: (Deutsche Gesellschaft fuer Arbeitsmedizin), Gentner Verlag Stuttgart, Forststr 131, Stuttgart 70193, Germany. TEL 49-711-63672-0, FAX 49-711-63672-11. Eds. Dr. Georg Zerlett, Dr. Gerhard Triebig. R&P Gernot Keuchen. Adv. contact Corinna Zepter. Circ: 3,587.
Co-sponsor: Oesterreichische Gesellschaft fuer Arbeitsmedizin.

613.62 DEU ISSN 0944-6419
CODEN: AUMSE
ARBEITSMEDIZIN, SOZIALMEDIZIN, UMWELTMEDIZIN. SUPPLEMENT. Text in German. 1966. irreg. **Document type:** *Academic/Scholarly.*
Former titles: Arbeitsmedizin, Sozialmedizin, Praeventivmedizin. Sonderheft (0720-0013); Arbeitsmedizin, Sozialmedizin, Arbeitshygiene. Sonderheft (0570-5878)
Related titles: ♦ Supplement to: Arbeitsmedizin, Sozialmedizin, Umweltmedizin. ISSN 0944-6052.
Indexed: Excerp.Med. (1995-).
—BLDSC (1587.402755), EMDOCS, KNAW.
Published by: (Deutsche Gesellschaft fuer Arbeitsmedizin), Gentner Verlag Stuttgart, Forststr 131, Stuttgart 70193, Germany. TEL 49-711-63672-0, FAX 49-711-63672-11. Ed. Dr. Georg Zerlett. R&P Gernot Keuchen. Adv. contact Corinna Zepter.

362.1 616 BEL ISSN 0778-7367
CODEN: ABMHAM
ARCHIVES BELGES DE SANTE PUBLIQUE. Key Title: Archives of Public Health. Text and summaries in English, Flemish, French. 1938. bi-m. BEF 1,500, USD 40. bk.rev. abstr, bibl, charts. index. *Refereed.* **Document type:** *Government, Academic/Scholarly.*
Former titles (until 1990): Archives Belges de Medecine Sociale, Hygiene, Medecine du Travail et Medecine (0003-9578); (until 1947): Archives Belges de Medicine Sociale et d'Hygiene (0365-4648); (until 1938): Revue de Pathologie et de Physiologie du Travail (0771-6192); (until 1931): Revue de Medecine et de Chirurgie des Accidents de Travail et des Maladies Professionnelles (0771-1301)
Indexed: Abstr.Hyg., Biol.Abstr., C.I.S. Abstr., Chem.Abstr., Dairy Sci.Abstr., Excerp.Med., Food Sci.& Tech.Abstr., INIS Atomind., Ind.Med. (coverage dropped), Nutr.Abstr., Protozool.Abstr., Trop.Dis.Bull.
—BLDSC (1640.530000), CASDDS, CISTI, GNLM, KNAW.
Published by: Archives de Medecine Sociale et d'Hygiene, Cite Administrative de l'Etat, Quartier Esplanade 6, Brussels 1010, Belgium. TEL 32-2-642-5233, FAX 32-2-642-5610, andre.stroobant@ihe.be. Ed. Andre Stroobant. Circ: 600.

353.9 USA ISSN 0362-1421
RA21
ARIZONA. DEPARTMENT OF HEALTH SERVICES. ANNUAL REPORT. Key Title: Annual Report of the Arizona Department of Health Services. Text in English. 1974. a. free per issue. illus. **Document type:** *Government.*
Published by: Department of Health Services, 1740 W Adams St, Phoenix,, AZ 85007. TEL 602-542-1001, FAX 602-542-1062. Ed. Brad Christensen. Circ: 500 (controlled).

614 360 USA
ARIZONA MEDICINE. Text in English. 1990. bi-m. USD 100. adv. cum.index. **Document type:** *Newspaper.*
Published by: Arizona Medical Association, 810 W Bethany Home Rd, Phoenix, AZ 85013. TEL 602-246-8901, FAX 602-242-6283, http://www.surgeon.org/contacts/listings/ama2.htm. Ed. Marshall B Block. Adv. contact Mariam Paulson. Circ: 4,300.

ARIZONA RADIATION REGULATORY AGENCY. ANNUAL REPORT. see *ENERGY—Nuclear Energy*

ARZT IN NIEDEROESTERREICH. see *MEDICAL SCIENCES*

362.296 613.85 343 AUS ISSN 0816-4347
ASHES TO DUST. Text in English. 1983-1985; resumed 1999 (Jan.-Jun; vol.16, no.1-2). s-a. AUD 30 to membership (effective 2000). charts, stat. 20 p./no. 1 cols./p. back issues avail. **Document type:** *Newsletter.* **Description:** Provides information for members of Canberra A S H Incorporated, a voluntary organization dedicated to a tobacco free world. Complimentary copies are send to kindred organizations in Australia and abroad, librarians and politicians.
Published by: Canberra A S H Incorporated, POB 280, Dickson, ACT 2602, Australia. TEL 61-6257-3853, FAX 61-6247-1022, ashroot@interact.net.au. Ed., Pub. Geraldine Spencer. Circ: 200.

614 362.1 USA
ASIAN AMERICAN AND PACIFIC ISLANDER JOURNAL OF HEALTH. Text in English. 1993. s-a. USD 64 (effective 1999). bk.rev. abstr, illus. **Document type:** *Academic/Scholarly.*
Published by: Asian American and Pacific Islander Health Promotion, 5525 Corey Swirl Dr, Dublin, OH 43017-3057. Ed. Moon S Chen Jr. R&P Moon Chen TEL 614-766-5219. Adv. contact Catherina Chen.

ASIAN ENVIRONMENT; journal of environmental science and technology for balanced development. see *ENVIRONMENTAL STUDIES*

614 362.2 USA
ASSOCIATION OF BEHAVIORAL HEALTH MANAGEMENT NEWSLETTER. Text in English. 1963. bi-m. membership. adv. bk.rev. **Document type:** *Newsletter.*
Formerly: Association of Mental Health Administrators. Newsletter (1055-260X)
Published by: Association of Behavioral Health Management, 60 Revere Dr, Ste 500, Northbrook, IL 60062. TEL 847-480-9626. Ed. Angelo Artemakis. Circ: 1,300 (controlled).

614 AUS ISSN 1032-6138
RA371
AUSTRALIA. BUREAU OF STATISTICS. AUSTRALIA'S HEALTH. Text in English. 1988. biennial, latest 2000. AUD 44 (effective 2001). **Document type:** *Bulletin, Government.* **Description:** Provides current information on all aspects of health and health services in Australia.
Published by: (Australia. Australian Institute of Health and Welfare), Australian Bureau of Statistics, PO Box 10, Belconnen, ACT 2616, Australia. TEL 61-2-6252-5249, FAX 61-2-6252-6778, http://www.abs.gov.au.

362.1 AUS
AUSTRALIA. DEPARTMENT OF THE TREASURY. ADVISORY PANEL ON THE MARKETING OF INFANT FORMULA. ANNUAL REPORT. Text in English. a. charts, stat. back issues avail. **Document type:** *Government.* **Description:** Reports on the efforts of the Australian Government to enforce the World Health Organization International Code of Marketing of Breast-Milk Substitutes.
Related titles: Online - full text ed.
Published by: (Australia. Department of the Treasury, Australia. Advisory Panel on the Marketing of Infant Formula. Annual Report), AusInfo, GPO Box 1920, Canberra Mc, ACT 2610, Australia. TEL 61-2-6295-4512, FAX 61-2-6295-4455, http://www.treasury.gov.au; http://www.ausinfo.gov.au.
Orders to: AusInfo Mail Order Sales, GPO Box 84, Canberra, ACT 2601, Australia. FAX 61-2-6295-4888.

616.9 AUS ISSN 1326-0200
HV88 CODEN: AZPHF6
AUSTRALIAN AND NEW ZEALAND JOURNAL OF PUBLIC HEALTH. Text in English. 1977. bi-m. AUD 182 to individuals; AUD 268 to institutions (effective 2001). adv. bk.rev. 112 p./no. reprint service avail. from PQC. *Refereed.* **Document type:** *Journal, Academic/Scholarly.* **Description:** Publishes research reports, reviews and letters on epidemiology, health policy, health services and health promotion.
Former titles: Australian Journal of Public Health (1035-7319); (until Dec. 1990): Community Health Studies (0149-2047)
Related titles: Microfilm ed.: (from PQC); Online - full text ed.: (from ProQuest Information & Learning, Gale Group, Factiva, Institute for Scientific Information).
Indexed: ABI Inform. (Mar.1993-), ASCA, AgeLine, Aus.P.A.I.S., CINAHL, Curr.Cont., Dent.Ind., Excerp.Med., Fam.Ind., IMFL, Ind.Med. (1996-), Ind.N.Z.Per., Int.Nurs.Ind., NRN, Risk Abstr., SSCI, Soc.Sci.Ind. (coverage dropped), THA.
—BLDSC (1796.894000), EMDOCS, GNLM, IDS, ingenta, KNAW. **CCC.**
Published by: Public Health Association of Australia, PO Box 319, Curtin, ACT 2605, Australia. TEL 61-2-62852373, FAX 61-2-62825438, phaa@phaa.net.au, http://www.phaa.net.au. Eds. Jeanne Daly, Judith Lumley. R&P Julie Woollacott. adv.: page AUD 902; 18.5 x 26. Circ: 2,500.

362.1 AUS
AUSTRALIAN DEPARTMENT OF HEALTH & AGED CARE. ANNUAL REPORT. Text in English. a., latest 1998. **Document type:** *Government.*
Related titles: Online - full content ed.
Published by: Australian Prescriber, GPO Box 9848, Canberra City, ACT 2601, Australia. TEL 61-2-6289-1555, 61-2-6289-7777, 800-020-103, FAX 61-2-6281-6946, webmaster@health.gov.au.

362.1 AUS
AUSTRALIAN DEPARTMENT OF HEALTH & AGED CARE. BUDGET PAPERS. Text in English. a., latest 1999. back issues avail. **Document type:** *Government.*
Related titles: Online - full content ed.
Published by: Australian Prescriber, GPO Box 9848, Canberra City, ACT 2601, Australia. TEL 61-2-6289-1555, 61-2-6289-7777, 800-020-103, FAX 61-2-6281-6946, webmaster@health.gov.au, http://www.health.gov.au.

632.1 AUS
AUSTRALIAN DEPARTMENT OF HEALTH & AGED CARE. CHIEF MEDICAL OFFICER'S REPORT. Text in English. irreg., latest 1997. **Document type:** *Government.*
Published by: Australian Prescriber, GPO Box 9848, Canberra City, ACT 2601, Australia. TEL 61-2-6289-1555, 61-2-6289-7777, 800-020-103, FAX 61-2-6281-6946, webmaster@health.gov.au, http://www.health.gov.au.

632.1 AUS
AUSTRALIAN DEPARTMENT OF HEALTH & AGED CARE. CORPORATE PLAN. Text in English. a., latest 1998. back issues avail. **Document type:** *Government.*

Related titles: Online - full content ed.
Published by: Australian Prescriber, GPO Box 9848, Canberra City, ACT 2601, Australia. TEL 61-2-6289-1555, 61-2-6289-7777, 800-020-103, FAX 61-2-6281-6946, webmaster@health.gov.au, http://www.health.gov.au.

362.1 AUS
AUSTRALIAN DEPARTMENT OF HEALTH & AGED CARE. HEALTH AND AGED CARE OCCASIONAL PAPERS NEW SERIES. Text in English. ; N.S. (no.6). irreg. **Document type:** *Government.*
Formerly: Australian Department of Health & Aged Care. Health and Aged Care Occasional Papers Series
Published by: Australian Prescriber, GPO Box 9848, Canberra City, ACT 2601, Australia. TEL 61-2-6289-1555, 61-2-6289-7777, 800-020-103, FAX 61-2-6281-6946, webmaster@health.gov.au, http://www.health.gov.au.

632.1 AUS
AUSTRALIAN DEPARTMENT OF HEALTH & AGED CARE. HEALTH FINANCING SERIES OCCASIONAL PAPERS. Text in English. irreg. **Document type:** *Government.*
Related titles: Online - full content ed.
Published by: Australian Prescriber, GPO Box 9848, Canberra City, ACT 2601, Australia. TEL 61-2-6289-1555, 61-2-6289-7777, 800-020-103, FAX 61-2-6281-6946, webmaster@health.gov.au, http://www.health.gov.au.

AUSTRALIAN DOCTOR. see *MEDICAL SCIENCES*

AUSTRALIAN FLUORIDATION NEWS. AQUA-PURA. see *WATER RESOURCES*

613 AUS ISSN 1445-7253
AUSTRALIAN INDIGENOUS HEALTH BULLETIN. Text in English. 1997. q. bk.rev. **Document type:** *Journal, Academic/Scholarly.*
Formerly (until Jul. 2001): Aboriginal and Torres Strait Islander Health Bulletin (1329-3362)
Media: Online - full content.
Published by: (Aboriginal and Torres Strait Islander Studies Unit), Australian Indigenous Health Info Net, c/o School of Nursing and Public Health, Edith Cowan University, 100 Joondalup Dr, Joondalup, W.A. 6027, Australia. TEL 61-8-9400-5104, FAX 61-8-9400-5449, healthinfonet@ecu.edu.au, http://www.healthinfonet.ecu.edu.au/html/html-bulletin/bulletin_home.htm. Ed. Sean Ulm.

THE AUSTRALIAN JOURNAL OF EMERGENCY MANAGEMENT. see *CIVIL DEFENSE*

362.1042505 AUS ISSN 1038-5282
CODEN: AJRHF6
AUSTRALIAN JOURNAL OF RURAL HEALTH. Text in English. 1983. bi-m. AUD 160 domestic to individuals; AUD 145 in New Zealand to individuals; USD 248 elsewhere to individuals; AUD 369 domestic to institutions; AUD 335 in New Zealand to institutions; USD 459 elsewhere to institutions; AUD 176 combined subscription domestic to individuals for print & online eds.; AUD 160 combined subscription in New Zealand to individuals for print & online eds.; USD 273 combined subscription elsewhere to individuals for print & online eds.; AUD 406 combined subscription domestic to institutions for print & online eds.; AUD 369 combined subscription in New Zealand to institutions for print & online eds.; USD 505 combined subscription elsewhere to institutions for print & online eds. (effective 2001). adv. **Document type:** *Academic/Scholarly.* **Description:** Reports on all aspects of rural health from a variety of health and related disciplines.
Related titles: Online - full text ed.: ISSN 1440-1584. AUD 144 domestic to individuals; AUD 131 in New Zealand to individuals; USD 224 elsewhere to individuals; AUD 333 domestic to institutions; AUD 302 in New Zealand to institutions; USD 414 elsewhere to institutions (effective 2001) (from EBSCO Publishing, O C L C Online Computer Library Center, Inc., RoweCom Information Quest, ingenta, Munksgaard & Blackwell Science's Synergy, Swets Blackwell).
Indexed: ASSIA, Aus.P.A.I.S. (Coverage Dropped), CINAHL, Dairy Sci.Abstr., Environ.Sci.Poll.Mgmt., Int.Nurs.Ind., Lang.& Lang.Behav.Abstr., Ling.Abstr., Nutr.Abstr., Pollut.Abstr., Risk Abstr., SOPODA, Saf.Sci.Abstr., Soc.Serv.Abstr., Sociol.Abstr.
—BLDSC (1811.870000), Infotrieve, ingenta. **CCC.**
Published by: (National Rural Health Alliance), Blackwell Science Asia Pty Ltd, PO Box 378, Carlton South, VIC 3053, Australia. TEL 61-3-9347-0300, FAX 61-3-9347-5001, info@blacksci-asia.com.au; hegney@usq.edu.au, http://www.blacksci.co.uk. Ed. Desley Hegney. Adv. contact Kathryn O'Brien. B&W page AUD 1,012, color page AUD 2,057; trim 210 x 275.

AUSTRALIAN MEDICINE. see *MEDICAL SCIENCES*

AUSTRALIAN PRESCRIBER. see *PHARMACY AND PHARMACOLOGY*

362.1 AUS
AUSTRALIAN RECALLS AND CANCELLATIONS. Text in English. 11/yr. AUD 75.90 domestic; AUD 79 foreign (effective 2001). back issues avail. **Document type:** *Government.*
Published by: Therapeutic Goods Administration, PO Box 100, Woden, ACT 2606, Australia. TEL 61-2-6232-8610, 61-2-6232-8444, FAX 61-2-6232-8222, tga-information-officer@health.gov.au, http://www.anzfa.gov.au/.

614 AUS ISSN 0067-2165
AUSTRALIAN STUDIES IN HEALTH SERVICE ADMINISTRATION. Text in English. 1968. irreg., latest vol.80, 1996. price varies. **Document type:** *Monographic series.*
Published by: University of New South Wales, School of Health Services Management, Sydney, NSW 2052, Australia. FAX 61-2-9385-1036. R&P Sam Sheridan. Circ: 300.

AUSTRALIAN SURF LIFESAVER. see *SPORTS AND GAMES—Outdoor Life*

B E L L E NEWSLETTER. (Biological Effects of Low Level Exposures) see *ENVIRONMENTAL STUDIES—Toxicology And Environmental Safety*

614.5 USA
B M F T RISIKO- UND SICHERHEITSFORSCHUNG. Text in English. 1982. irreg., latest 1986. price varies. **Document type:** *Monographic series.*
Indexed: Chem.Abstr.
Published by: (Bundesministerium fuer Forschung und Technologie DEU), Springer-Verlag, Journals (Subsidiary of: BertelsmannSpringer), 175 Fifth Ave, New York, NY 10010. TEL 212-460-1500, FAX 212-473-6272.

614 USA ISSN 1068-1213
KF3605.A15
B N A'S HEALTH CARE POLICY REPORT. Text in English. 1993. 50/yr. USD 977 (effective 2001). s-a. index. 40 p./no. back issues avail. **Description:** Covers federal, state and private sector efforts to reform and manage the U.S. health care system.
Related titles: Online - full text ed.: ISSN 1521-5369 (from Bureau of National Affairs, Inc., (BNA), The).
—**CCC.**
Published by: The Bureau of National Affairs, Inc., 1231 25th St, N W, Washington, DC 20037. TEL 202-452-4200, 800-372-1033, 800-452-7773, FAX 202-822-8092, customercare@bna.com, bnaplus@bna.com, http://www.bna.com/. Ed. Paul Albergo. Pub. Gregory McCaffery.

B T - L M & S. (Building Technology - Land Management & Safety) see *BUILDING AND CONSTRUCTION*

BAD TOELZ AKTUELL; Informationen und Veranstaltungen. see *TRAVEL AND TOURISM*

610 BRB
BARBADOS. MINISTRY OF HEALTH. CHIEF MEDICAL OFFICER. ANNUAL REPORT. Text in English. 1972. a. free per issue. charts, illus, stat. **Document type:** *Government.*
Former titles: Barbados. Ministry of Health and Community Services. Chief Medical Officer. Annual Report; Barbados. Ministry of Health and Welfare. Chief Medical Officer. Annual Report
Published by: Ministry of Health, Bridgetown, Barbados. FAX 246-426-5570. Circ: 300.

BEZPECNOST A HYGIENA PRACE/SAFETY AND HYGIENE OF WORK. see *LABOR UNIONS*

363.7 POL ISSN 0867-4752
BEZPIECZENSTWO JADROWE I OCHRONA RADIOLOGICZNA. Text in Polish. 1989. q.
Indexed: INIS Atomind.
Published by: (Panstwowy Dozor Bezpieczenstwa Jadrowego i Ochrony Radiologicznej), Panstwowa Agencja Atomistyki, Ul Krucza 36, Warsaw 00525, Poland. TEL 48-22-298593, FAX 48-22-290164. Ed. Leszek Mlynarczyk.

362.1 460 USA
BILINGUAL HANDBOOK FOR PUBLIC SAFETY PROFESSIONALS; a concise guide to fit into any memo book, pocket, briefcase. Text in English, Spanish. 1994. irreg. USD 23.95 includes audio cassette (effective 2000). **Document type:** *Trade.* **Description:** Provides the means to communicate critical information on Spanish-speaking subjects in a variety of situations.
Published by: Gould Publications, Inc., 1333 N US Hwy 17 92, Longwood, FL 32750-3724. TEL 407-695-9500, 800-717-7917, FAX 407-695-2906, info@gouldlaw.com, http://www.gouldlaw.com.

614 CHE ISSN 0006-4629
BLAUES KREUZ. Text in German. 1896. 10/yr. CHF 32 (effective 1999). bk.rev. illus. **Document type:** *Newsletter.*
Published by: (Blue Cross of Switzerland), Blaukreuz Verlag, Lindenrain 5 A, Bern 3001, Switzerland. TEL 41-31-3005866, FAX 41-31-3005869. Circ: 3,700.

628 VEN ISSN 0798-037X
BOLETIN DE SALUD PUBLICA. Text in Spanish. 1941. a. charts, illus. **Document type:** *Government.*
Supersedes: Venezuela. Consejo de Salud Publica. Boletin
Published by: Ministerio de Sanidad y Asistencia Social, Direccion de Salud Publica, c/o Oficina de Publicaciones Biblioteca y Archivo,, Centro Simon Bolivar, Torre Sur 5o, Caracas, DF 1010, Venezuela. **Co-sponsor:** Venezuela. Oficina de los Servicios Regionales de Salud.

P

BOLETIN DE VIGILANCIA EPIDEMIOLOGICA DE LA RABIA PARA LAS AMERICAS. see *VETERINARY SCIENCE*

614 MEX
BOLETIN EPIDEMIOLOGICO. Text in Spanish. 1973. a. free per issue. stat.
Formerly: Boletin Epidemiologico Anual
Published by: Instituto Mexicano del Seguro Social, Subdireccion General Medica, Jefatura de Servicios de Medicina Preventiva, Apdo. Postal 12976, Mexico City, DF 03001, Mexico. Circ: 2,000.

614 USA
BORDER EPIDEMIOLOGICAL BULLETIN/BOLETIN EPIDEMIOLOGICO FRONTERIZO. Text in English, Spanish. 1975. bi-m. **Document type:** *Bulletin.* **Description:** Covers U.S.-Mexico border public health and epidemiology issues.
Published by: Pan American Health Organization, El Paso Field Office, 6006 N Mesa, Ste 600, El Paso, TX 79912. TEL 915-581-6645, FAX 915-833-4768, epi@usmeha.org, http://www.epfo.org. Ed. Dr. Joaquin Salcedo.

BOTSWANA. CENTRAL STATISTICS OFFICE. HEALTH STATISTICS REPORT. see *MEDICAL SCIENCES—Abstracting, Bibliographies, Statistics*

616.9 BWA ISSN 0258-8846
BOTSWANA. MINISTRY OF HEALTH. EPIDEMIOLOGICAL BULLETIN. Key Title: Botswana Epidemiological Bulletin. Text in English. 1982. q. **Document type:** *Academic/Scholarly, Government.*
Published by: Ministry of Health, Epidemiological Unit, Private Bag 0038, Gaborone, Botswana. TEL 267-352000. **Subscr. to:** Government Printer, Private Bag 0081, Gaborone, Botswana. TEL 267-353202, FAX 267-312001, http://www.gov.bw.

614 BWA ISSN 0253-5629
RA352.B6
BOTSWANA. MINISTRY OF HEALTH. REPORT. Text in English. a. **Document type:** *Government.*
Former titles (until 1974): Botswana. Department of Health. Report (0377-3949); (until 1963): Bechuanaland Protectorate. Director of Medical Services. Medical and Sanitary Report for (Year) (0258-4530); (until 1961): Bechuanaland Protectorate. Director of Medical Services. Annual Medical and Sanitary Report for (Year) (0258-4549)
Published by: Ministry of Health, Epidemiological Unit, Private Bag 0038, Gaborone, Botswana. TEL 267-352000.

BREAKTHROUGH; international mental health journal. see *PSYCHOLOGY*

BRIEFINGS ON HOSPITAL SAFETY; the newsletter for hospital safety committees. see *HEALTH FACILITIES AND ADMINISTRATION*

614.8 CAN ISSN 0706-4810
RA185.B7
BRITISH COLUMBIA. MINISTRY OF HEALTH. ANNUAL REPORT. Text in English. 1975. a. free per issue. **Document type:** *Government.*
Formerly: British Columbia. Department of Health. Annual Report (0701-5372)
—CISTI.
Published by: Ministry of Health, 1515 Blanshard St, 7th Fl, Victoria, BC V8W 3C8, Canada. TEL 604-387-2323. Circ: 4,000.

BULLETIN OF EPIDEMIOLOGICAL SURVEILLANCE OF RABIES FOR THE AMERICAS. see *VETERINARY SCIENCE*

614 DEU ISSN 1436-9990
BUNDESGESUNDHEITSBLATT - GESUNDHEITSFORSCHUNG - GESUNDHEITSSCHUTZ. Text in German. 1958. m. EUR 121.49 domestic; EUR 105.99 in Germany; EUR 9.20 newsstand/cover foreign (effective 2002). adv. bk.rev. bibl, charts, stat. index. *Refereed.* **Document type:** *Bulletin, Academic/Scholarly.* **Description:** Covers all aspects of public health care services and programs.
Formerly: Bundesgesundheitsblatt (0007-5914)
Related titles: ♦ Online - full content ed.: Bundesgesundheitsblatt - Gesundheitsforschung - Gesundheitsschutz Online. ISSN 1437-1588; Online - full text ed.: (from Springer LINK, RoweCom Information Quest).
Indexed: Biol.Abstr., C.I.S. Abstr., Dairy Sci.Abstr., Dok.Arbeitsmed., Excerp.Med., Food Sci.& Tech.Abstr., INIS Atomind., Ind.Vet., Int.Packag.Abstr., Nonwov.Abstr., Nutr.Abstr., Packag.Sci.Tech., Paper & Bd.Abstr., Sugar Ind.Abstr., Vet.Bull.
—BLDSC (2930.200000), GNLM, Infotrieve. **CCC.**
Published by: (Germany. Robert-Koch-Institut), Springer-Verlag (Subsidiary of: BertelsmannSpringer), Tiergartenstr 17, Heidelberg 69121, Germany. TEL 49-6221-345-0, FAX 49-6221-345229, subscriptions@springer.de, http://link.springer.de/link/service/journals/00103/index.htm, http://www.springer.de. Circ: 2,300. **Co-sponsors:** Bundesinstitut fuer Gesundheitlichen Verbraucherschutz und Veterinaermedizin; Bundesinstitut fuer Arzneimittel und Medizinprodukte; Institut fuer Wasser-, Boden- und Lufthygiene des Umweltbundesamtes.

614 DEU ISSN 1437-1588
BUNDESGESUNDHEITSBLATT - GESUNDHEITSFORSCHUNG - GESUNDHEITSSCHUTZ ONLINE. Text in German. m. **Document type:** *Academic/Scholarly.*
Media: Online - full content (from EBSCO Publishing, Swets Blackwell). **Related titles:** Online - full text ed.: (from Springer LINK, RoweCom Information Quest); ♦ Print ed.: Bundesgesundheitsblatt - Gesundheitsforschung - Gesundheitsschutz. ISSN 1436-9990.
Published by: Springer-Verlag (Subsidiary of: BertelsmannSpringer), Tiergartenstr 17, Heidelberg 69121, Germany. TEL 49-6221-345-0, FAX 49-6221-345229, subscriptions@springer.de, http://link.springer.de/link/service/journals/00103/index.htm, http://www.springer.de.

344.04 GBR
BUTTERWORTHS FOOD LAW. Text in English. 1990. irreg., latest 2000, 2nd ed. GBP 50 per vol. (effective 2000). **Document type:** *Trade.* **Description:** Explains UK legislation affecting food safety and standards.
Published by: Butterworths Tolley (Subsidiary of: Reed Elsevier plc), Halsbury House, 35 Chancery Ln, London WC2A 1EL, United Kingdom. TEL 44-20-7400-2500, FAX 44-20-7400-2842, TELEX DX Chancery Lane 1023, http://www.butterworths.co.uk. Ed. Barry Atwood.

614.4 USA ISSN 1077-8373
RA644.6
C D P FILE. (Chronic Disease Prevention) Variant title: C D P File on CD-ROM. (In 6 parts: Health Promotion and Education; AIDS School Health Education; Cancer Prevention and Control; a combination of the first 3 parts; Chronic Disease Prevention Directory; State Profile.) Text in English. 1991. q. USD 83 (effective 2001). back issues avail. **Document type:** *Directory, Government, Abstract/Index.* **Description:** Contains 8 databases: health promotion and education, AIDS school health education, cancer prevention and control, a combination of the first 3 databases, chronic disease prevention directory, and a State profile. The databases include: abstracts of information from a variety of published and unpublished documents; information on Federal, State, and local government programs; and key contacts in health promotion and disease prevention.
Media: CD-ROM.
Published by: U.S. Centers for Disease Control, National Center for Chronic Disease Prevention and Health Promotion, 4770 Buford Hwy, NE, MS K 50, Atlanta, GA 30341-3724. TEL 404-488-5705, FAX 404-488-5739. **Orders to:** U.S. Government Printing Office, Superintendent of Documents, PO Box 371954, Pittsburgh, PA 15250-7954. TEL 202-512-1800, FAX 202-512-2250, orders@gpo.gov, http://www.access.gpo.gov.

C D R SUPPLEMENT. (Communicable Disease Report) see *MEDICAL SCIENCES—Communicable Diseases*

C D R WEEKLY. (Communicable Disease Report) see *MEDICAL SCIENCES—Communicable Diseases*

C H R I A NEWS. see *BUSINESS AND ECONOMICS—International Development And Assistance*

614 GBR ISSN 0964-7902
C H S S OCCASIONAL PAPER. Text in English. irreg., latest vol.4. **Document type:** *Monographic series.*
Published by: Centre for Health Services Studies, University of Warwick, Warwick Business School, Coventry, W Mids CV4 7AL, United Kingdom. TEL 44-1203-523985.

C O N C A W E REVIEW. see *ENVIRONMENTAL STUDIES*

614 USA ISSN 0272-9148
C O T H SURVEY OF HOUSE STAFF STIPENDS, BENEFITS, AND FUNDING. Text in English. 1969. a. USD 35 (effective 1999). **Document type:** *Corporate.*
Former titles (until 1979): C O T H Survey of House Staff Policy and Related Information (0272-9156); C O T H Survey of House Staff Policy and Related Issues (0164-1573); (until 1974): C O T H Survey of House Staff Policy (0093-7045)
Published by: (Council of Teaching Hospitals), Association of American Medical Colleges, 2450 N St N W, Washington, DC 20037-1126. TEL 202-828-0497.

613.7 CAN ISSN 0703-5624
C P H A HEALTH DIGEST. Text in English. 1977. q. free per issue to members. **Document type:** *Newsletter.*
Related titles: French ed.: A C S P Selection Sante.
Published by: Canadian Public Health Association, 1565 Carling Ave, Ste 400, Ottawa, ON K1Z 8R1, Canada. TEL 613-725-3769, FAX 613-725-9826. Ed. Gerald Dafoe. Circ: 3,000.

C S P DIRECTORY AND INTERNATIONAL REGISTRY OF CERTIFIED SAFETY PROFESSIONALS. see *OCCUPATIONAL HEALTH AND SAFETY*

614 BRA ISSN 0102-311X
RA421 CODEN: CSAQEW
CADERNOS DE SAUDE PUBLICA/REPORTS IN PUBLIC HEALTH. Text in Portuguese, Spanish, English. 1980. bi-m. BRL 65 domestic to individuals; USD 120 foreign to individuals; BRL 150 domestic to institutions; USD 200 foreign to institutions (effective 2001 - 2002). adv. bk.rev. back issues avail. *Refereed.* **Document type:** *Academic/Scholarly.* **Description:** Publishes original research reports and reviews on all aspects of public health, international health, preventive medicine, epidemiology, public health services, health policy and planning, and social sciences in health (including antropology, sociology, and psychology).
Formed by the 1985 merger of: Cadernos de Saude Publica. Serie Ensaio (0101-2231); Cadernos de Saude Publica. Serie Pesquisa (0101-5729); Cadernos de Saude Publica. Serie Documento (0102-3128)
Related titles: Online - full text ed.
Indexed: Abstr.Hyg., AgBiotech, Anim.Breed.Abstr., Dairy Sci.Abstr., Helminthol.Abstr., Ind.Med. (1985-), Ind.Vet., Lang.& Lang.Behav.Abstr., Nutr.Abstr., Protozool.Abstr., Rev.Appl.Entomol., Rev.Med.& Vet.Mycol., Rural Devel.Abstr., SOPODA, Soc.Serv.Abstr., Sociol.Abstr., Trop.Dis.Bull., Vet.Bull., World Ag.Econ.& Rur.Soc.Abstr.
—BLDSC (2947.170850), GNLM.
Published by: Escola Nacional de Saude Publica, Rua Leopoldo Bulhoes, 1480, Terreo, Bonsucesso, Rio De Janeiro, RJ 21041-210, Brazil. TEL 55-21-2598-2511, FAX 55-21-2598-2737, cadernos@ensp.fiocruz.br. Eds. Carlos E A Coimbra Jr., Luis David Castiel. Adv. contact Delfina Araujo TEL 55-11-2552-4114. Circ: 1,200 (paid); 300 (controlled).

CAHIERS DE SOCIOLOGIE ET DE DEMOGRAPHIE MEDICALES. see *POPULATION STUDIES*

CAHIERS D'ETUDES ET DE RECHERCHES FRANCOPHONES. SANTE. see *MEDICAL SCIENCES*

CALIFORNIA FIRE SERVICE. see *FIRE PREVENTION*

614 USA
CALIFORNIA WORKPLACE MONITOR. Text in English. 1993. bi-w. USD 317 (effective 2001). back issues avail. **Description:** Features comprehensive coverage of laws, regulations and litigation affecting California's health care industry.
Former titles: California Health Law Monitor; B N A California Health Care Reporter (1070-5414)
Published by: M. Lee Smith Publishers LLC, 5201 Virginia Way, PO Box 5094, Brentwoood, TN 37024-5094. TEL 615-373-7517, FAX 615-373-5183. Ed. Barrett McBride.

CAMBRIDGESHIRE COUNTY COUNCIL. ROAD SAFETY PLAN (YEAR). see *TRANSPORTATION—Roads And Traffic*

614 610 CAN ISSN 1188-4169
CODEN: CDWSE9
CANADA COMMUNICABLE DISEASE REPORT/RELEVE DES MALADIES TRANSMISSIBLES AU CANADA. Text in English, French. 1975. bi-m. CND 80 domestic; USD 105 foreign (effective 2000). charts, illus, stat. index. Supplement avail. **Document type:** *Newsletter, Government.*
Former titles (until 1992): Canada Diseases Weekly Report (0382-232X); Epidemiological Bulletin (0425-1474)
Indexed: Abstr.Hyg., Biodet.Abstr., Curr.Adv.Ecol.Sci., Dairy Sci.Abstr., Ind.Med. (1992-), Protozool.Abstr., Rev.Appl.Entomol., Rev.Med.& Vet.Mycol., Rev.Plant Path.
—BLDSC (3016.417400), CISTI, GNLM, Infotrieve. **CCC.**
Published by: Department of National Health and Welfare, Laboratory Centre for Disease Control, Tunney s Pasture, P L 0602C2, Ottawa, ON K1A 0L2, Canada. TEL 613-957-1788, FAX 613-952-7009, http://www.hc-sc.gc.ca/hpb/lcdc. Ed., R&P Eleanor Paulson. Circ: 2,500.

CANADIAN HEALTH FACILITIES LAW GUIDE. see *LAW*

CANADIAN JOURNAL OF COMMUNITY MENTAL HEALTH/REVUE CANADIENNE DE SANTE MENTALE COMMUNAUTAIRE. see *PSYCHOLOGY*

614 CAN ISSN 0008-4263
CODEN: CJPEA4
CANADIAN JOURNAL OF PUBLIC HEALTH/REVUE CANADIENNE DE SANTE PUBLIQUE. Text in English. 1910. bi-m. CND 86 domestic (effective 1999); USD 105 in United States; USD 135 elsewhere. adv. bk.rev. charts, illus. Index. reprint service avail. from PQC. *Refereed.* **Description:** Covers all aspects of public health, preventive medicine, health promotion, and public policy related to health.
Related titles: Microform ed.: (from PQC,PMC); Online - full text ed.: (from Northern Light Technology, Inc., ProQuest Information & Learning, Institute for Scientific Information).
Indexed: ASCA, Abstr.Anthropol., Abstr.Hyg., AgeLine, Aqua.Sci.& Fish.Abstr., Bibl.Dev.Med.& Child Neur., Bio-Contr.News & Info., Biol.Abstr., Biol.Dig., CBCA Ref., CINAHL, Can.B.P.I., Chem.Abstr., Curr.Cont., Dairy Sci.Abstr., Dent.Ind., Dok.Arbeitsmed., Environ.Sci.Poll.Mgmt., Excerp.Med., Fam.Ind., Food Sci.& Tech.Abstr., INIS Atomind., Ind.Med. (1943-), Ind.Vet., Int.Nurs.Ind., Med.Care Rev., NRN, Nutr.Abstr., Ocean.Abstr. (coverage dropped), Pig News & Info., Pollut.Abstr., Protozool.Abstr., Rev.Appl.Entomol., Rev.Med.& Vet.Mycol., Rev.Plant Path., Risk Abstr., SSCI, Saf.Sci.Abstr., Sel.Water Res.Abstr., Small Anim.Abstr., Sportsearch (1977-), THA, Triticale Abstr., Trop.Dis.Bull., Vet.Bull., W.R.C.Inf.

—BLDSC (3035.000000), CISTI, EMDOCS, GNLM, IDS, ingenta, KNAW, Linda Hall. **CCC.**
Published by: Canadian Public Health Association, 1565 Carling Ave, Ste 400, Ottawa, ON K1Z 8R1, Canada. TEL 613-725-3769, FAX 613-725-9826. Ed. Gerald Dafoe. Adv. contact Karen Craven. Circ: 3,000.

CANADIAN MENTAL HEALTH ASSOCIATION. ANNUAL REPORT/ASSOCIATION CANADIENNE POUR LA SANTE MENTALE. RAPPORT ANNUEL. see *PSYCHOLOGY*

CANADIAN NURSE/L'INFIRMIERE CANADIENNE. see *MEDICAL SCIENCES—Nurses And Nursing*

362.1 USA ISSN 1083-7183
CAPITATION MANAGEMENT REPORT. Text in English. 1997. m. USD 299; USD 309 in Canada & Mexico; USD 319 elsewhere. **Document type:** *Newsletter.*
Published by: National Health Information, LLC, PO Box 15429, Atlanta, GA 30333. TEL 404-607-9500. Ed. Marie Powers. Pub. David Schwartz.

362.1 USA ISSN 1090-1574
CAPITATION RATES AND DATA. Text in English. 1996. m. USD 359; USD 369 in Canada & Mexico; USD 379 elsewhere. stat. **Document type:** *Trade.*
Published by: National Health Information, LLC, PO Box 15429, Atlanta, GA 30333. TEL 404-607-9500.

362.1 614.8 GBR
CARE ON THE ROAD. Text in English. 1972. bi-m. GBP 14.12 to non-members; GBP 12 to members; GBP 16.59 foreign to members (effective 2000). adv. bk.rev. illus, stat. **Description:** Covers road safety, relating to drivers, motorcyclists, cyclists and pedestrians.
Supersedes: Safety News (0036-2522)
Indexed: HRIS.
Published by: Royal Society for the Prevention of Accidents, Edgbaston Park, 353 Bristol Rd, Edgbaston, Birmingham, Worcs B5 7ST, United Kingdom. TEL 44-121-248-2000, FAX 44-121-248-2001, help@rospa.com.uk, http://www.rospa.com.uk. Ed. Janice Cave. Circ: 30,000.

614 360 GBR ISSN 1355-0454
CARE PLAN. Text in English. 1995. q. GBP 18 to individuals; GBP 35 to institutions. adv. **Document type:** *Trade.* **Description:** Contains detailed information relating to individual care planning and care management for professionals working in health and social services.
—BLDSC (3051.588000).
Published by: Anglia Polytechnic University, Faculty of Health and Social Work, 84 Dowanhill Rd, London SE6 1SY, United Kingdom. Ed., Pub. Derek Heptinstall. Circ: 1,000.

614 362.1 GBR ISSN 1462-8120
CARIBBEAN HEALTH. Text in English. 1998. bi-m. GBP 54 in Europe; USD 132 in United States; GBP 79 elsewhere (effective 2002). adv. bk.rev. **Description:** Contains review articles, news and letters for healthcare professionals in the Caribbean.
Published by: F S G MediMedia Ltd., Vine House, The Barn, Fair Green, Reach, Cambridge CB5 0JD, United Kingdom. TEL 44-1638-743633, FAX 44-1638-743998, info@fsg.co.uk, http://www.fsg.co.uk. Ed. Paul Chinnock. Pub. Bryan Pearson. Adv. contact Stuart Marritt. Circ: 4,500.

614.88 GBR ISSN 0008-7580
CASUALTY SIMULATION; to simulate realism in first aid, nursing and rescue training. Text in English. 1946. 4/yr. free worldwide to members (effective 2000); GBP 15 worldwide for accociate members (effective 2001). adv. bk.rev. charts, illus. index, cum.index. 28 p./no. back issues avail. *Refereed.* **Document type:** *Bulletin, Newsletter.* **Description:** Aims to simulate realism in first aid, nursing and rescue training.
—BLDSC.
Published by: Casualties Union, PO Box 1942, London E17 6YU, United Kingdom. TEL 08700-780590, hq@casualtiesunion.org.uk. Eds. D Maceachran, Susan Rawlings. Pub., Adv. contact P A Tupman. Circ: 1,500 (controlled).

614.49 CZE ISSN 1210-7778
RA421 CODEN: CEJHEK
CENTRAL EUROPEAN JOURNAL OF PUBLIC HEALTH. Text and summaries in English. 1956. q. EUR 128, USD 172 (effective 2001). adv. bk.rev. bibl, charts, illus. index. *Refereed.* **Document type:** *Academic/Scholarly.* **Description:** Presents research papers on public health, health problems of the population and different population groups.
Formerly (until 1993): Journal of Hygiene, Epidemiology, Microbiology and Immunology (0022-1732)
Indexed: Abstr.Hyg., Agri.& Environ.Biotech.Abstr. (coverage dropped), Agri.Eng.Abstr., Biol.Abstr., C.I.S. Abstr., Chem.Abstr., Chem.Indus.Notes, Chem.Titles, Curr.Adv.Ecol.Sci., Curr.Cont. (coverage dropped), Dairy Sci.Abstr., Derwent Biotech.Abstr., Environ.Sci.Poll.Mgmt., Excerp.Med., Food Sci.& Tech.Abstr., Forest Prod.Abstr., Helminthol.Abstr., INIS Atomind., Ind.Med. (1993-), Ind.Vet., Nutr.Abstr., Pollut.Abstr., Poult.Abstr., Protozool.Abstr., Rev.Appl.Entomol., Rev.Plant Path., Saf.Sci.Abstr., Soils & Fert., Trop.Dis.Bull., Vet.Bull.
—BLDSC (3106.138200), CASDDS, CISTI, EMDOCS, GNLM, Infotrieve, ingenta, Linda Hall. **CCC.**
Published by: (Statni Zdravotni Ustavy), Nakladatelske Stredisko C L S J.E. Purkyne, Sokolska 31, Prague 12026, Czech Republic. TEL 420-2-24911420, FAX 420-2-24911420, nts@iol.cz, http://www.clsjep.cz, http://www.medical.cz. Ed. Dr. B Tichacek. adv.: B&W page CZK 17,700, color page CZK 26,600; 260 x 176. Circ: 1,000. **Dist. by:** Abont s.r.o., Chlumova 17, Prague, 3 130 00, Czech Republic; **Dist. in Western countries by:** Kubon & Sagner, Hesstr 39-41, Munich 80798, Germany.

614 BRA ISSN 0009-0131
SF793
CENTRO PAN-AMERICANO DE FEBRE AFTOSA. BOLETIN. Text in Portuguese. 1963. q. free per issue. **Description:** Covers foot and mouth disease.
Formerly: Centro Pan-Americano de Febre Aftosa. Cuadernos
Indexed: Biol.Abstr., Ind.Vet., Vet.Bull.
—BLDSC (2162.050000), CISTI.
Published by: World Health Organization, Centro Pan Americano de Febre Aftosa, Pan American Health Organization, Centro, Caixa Postal 589 Z 000, Rio De Janeiro, RJ 20001-970, Brazil. Circ: 1,500.

CERAM ENVIRONMENT BULLETIN. see *ENVIRONMENTAL STUDIES*

CEYLON JOURNAL OF MEDICAL SCIENCE. see *MEDICAL SCIENCES*

THE CHALLENGE. see *MEDICAL SCIENCES—Respiratory Diseases*

CHARTERED INSTITUTE OF PUBLIC FINANCE AND ACCOUNTANCY. ENVIRONMENTAL HEALTH STATISTICS. ACTUALS. see *PUBLIC HEALTH AND SAFETY—Abstracting, Bibliographies, Statistics*

CHARTERED INSTITUTION OF WATER AND ENVIRONMENTAL MANAGEMENT. JOURNAL. see *WATER RESOURCES*

CHEMICAL REGULATION REPORTER: HAZARDOUS MATERIALS TRANSPORTATION. see *TRANSPORTATION*

CHILD ABUSE PREVENTION; national child protection clearing house newsletter. see *SOCIAL SERVICES AND WELFARE*

CHILDREN'S HEALTH & SAFETY. see *CHILDREN AND YOUTH—About*

CHILDREN'S MENTAL HEALTH SERVICES. see *PSYCHOLOGY*

614.427 USA ISSN 1041-5513
CHRONIC DISEASES NOTES & REPORTS. Text in English. 1988. irreg. **Document type:** *Government.*
Related titles: ♦ Supplement to: Morbidity and Mortality Weekly Report. ISSN 0149-2195.
Published by: U.S. Department of Health and Human Services, Centers for Disease Control (MS: A28), Epidemiology Program Office, 1600 Clifton Rd, NE, Atlanta, GA 30333. TEL 800-843-6356. Ed. John W Ward. **Subscr. to:** U.S. Government Printing Office, Superintendent of Documents.

CLEVELAND FOUNDATION. ANNUAL REPORT. see *SOCIAL SERVICES AND WELFARE*

CLUB NEWS; caring for the carers. see *LEISURE AND RECREATION*

COLLETTIVITA - CONVIVENZE. see *HEALTH FACILITIES AND ADMINISTRATION*

COMBUSTION SCIENCE AND TECHNOLOGY. see *CHEMISTRY—Physical Chemistry*

COMMON SENSE ABOUT AIDS. see *MEDICAL SCIENCES—Communicable Diseases*

▼ **COMMUNITY CARE REVIEW NEWSLETTER.** see *SOCIAL SERVICES AND WELFARE*

COMMUNITY DENTISTRY AND ORAL EPIDEMIOLOGY. see *MEDICAL SCIENCES—Dentistry*

COMMUNITY DENTISTRY AND ORAL EPIDEMIOLOGY ONLINE. see *MEDICAL SCIENCES—Dentistry*

362.1 GBR
COMMUNITY HEALTH UK ACTION; journal of community health UK. Text in English. 1983. q. GBP 20 to individuals; GBP 80 to libraries; GBP 50 to institutions statutory; GBP 4 newsstand/cover (effective 2001). adv. bk.rev. **Document type:** *Journal.* **Description:** Aims to promote local community health initiatives and to publicize their work.
Formerly (until 199?): Community Health Action (1360-6115); Which was formed by the 1983 merger of: London Health News; Community Health Initiatives Resource Unit. Newsletter
—BLDSC (3363.629700).
Published by: Community Health UK, Freshford, PO Box 2977, Bath BA2 7YR, United Kingdom. TEL 44-1225-723779, FAX 44-1225-722024, mail@chuk.org, http://www.chuk.org. Ed. Terry Drummond. R&P Linda Benn. Circ: 450 (paid).

614.8 USA
COMPLIANCE PROGRAM GUIDANCE MANUALS. Text in English. irreg. USD 425 in North America; USD 850 elsewhere. **Document type:** *Government.* **Description:** Provides the latest information on and helps maintain program plans and instructions directed to F.D.A. field operations. These plans and instructions are surveillance or compliance-oriented and provide the needed direction from headquarters offices and bureaus in accomplishing F.D.A. regulatory obligations.
Published by: U.S. Food and Drug Administration, Office of Public Affairs, 5600 Fishers Ln, Rockville, MD 20857. TEL 301-443-3220. **Orders to:** National Technical Information Service, Government Research Center. FAX 703-321-8547.

CONCERN NEWS. see *SOCIAL SERVICES AND WELFARE*

614.8 388.3 ESP
CONCIENCIA VIAL. Text in Spanish. 12/yr.
Address: Boters, 10 intra Sr de Thorson, Barcelona 08002, Spain. TEL 3-207-19-73. Ed. Fernando Rubio Mila.

628 USA ISSN 0069-8474
TD5
CONFERENCE OF STATE SANITARY ENGINEERS. REPORT OF PROCEEDINGS. Text in English. 1920. a. **Document type:** *Proceedings.*
Published by: U.S. Public Health Service, Department of Health and Human Services, Washington, DC 20201. TEL 202-245-6761.

CONSUMER PRODUCT SAFETY REVIEW. see *CONSUMER EDUCATION AND PROTECTION*

363 USA ISSN 1040-4376
CONTEMPORARY ISSUES IN RISK ANALYSIS. Text in English. 1986. irreg., latest vol.5, 1991. price varies. back issues avail. *Refereed.* **Document type:** *Proceedings.*
—KNAW.
Published by: (Society for Risk Analysis), Kluwer Academic - Plenum Publishers (Subsidiary of: Wolters Kluwer N.V.), 233 Spring St, New York, NY 10013-1578. TEL 212-620-8000, 800-221-9369, FAX 212-463-0742, info@plenum.com, http://www.plenum.com.

CONTRACEPTIVE EDUCATION BULLETIN. see *BIRTH CONTROL*

614 ITA
CORRIERE A V I S. Text in Italian. 1956. s-a. free per issue. adv. **Description:** Includes news and articles on medical subjects related to blood transfusions.
Published by: Associazione Volontari Italiani del Sangue (Turin), Via Pietro Baiardi, 5, Turin, TO 10126, Italy. TEL 011-658095, FAX 011-678831. Eds. Piero Onida, Sandro Fisso. Circ: 45,000.

P

362.1 GBR ISSN 0958-1596
CRITICAL PUBLIC HEALTH. Text in English. 1979. q. GBP 62, USD 102 to individuals; GBP 179, USD 295 to institutions (effective 2002). **Document type:** *Academic/Scholarly.* **Description:** Provides a multidisciplinary forum for those researching and developing public health practice. Addresses social and cultural implications of changes.
Formerly (until 1990): Radical Community Medicine (0265-0851)
Related titles: Online - full content ed.: ISSN 1469-3682 (from EBSCO Publishing, O C L C Online Computer Library Center, Inc., Swets Blackwell); Online - full text ed.: (from CatchWord Ltd., RoweCom Information Quest).
Indexed: Soc.Serv.Abstr., Sociol.Abstr.
—BLDSC (3487.459500), CatchWord, GNLM. **CCC.**
Published by: Carfax Publishing Limited (Subsidiary of: Taylor & Francis Group), PO Box 25, Abingdon, Oxon OX14 3UE, United Kingdom. TEL 44-1235-401000, FAX 44-1235-401550, enquiries@carfax.co, http://www.carfax.co.uk. Ed. Robin Bunton.

614 610 CUB ISSN 1013-2821
CUADERNOS DE HISTORIA DE LA SALUD PUBLICA. Text in Spanish. 1952. a. USD 10 in the Americas; USD 12 elsewhere.
Indexed: Biol.Abstr.
Published by: (Cuba. Ministerio de Salud Publica, Centro Nacional de Informacion de Ciencias Medicas, Cuba. Oficina del Historiador de Salud Publica), Editorial de Ciencias Medicas, O'Reilly No. 4, Habana, Cuba. TEL 62-8091, FAX 338187. Ed. Jose Antonio Fidalgo. Circ: 1,300.

614 362.1 GBR ISSN 1076-7762
RA421
CURRENT ISSUES IN PUBLIC HEALTH. Text in English. 1995. bi-m. GBP 45, USD 65 to individuals; GBP 90, USD 129 to institutions. adv. back issues avail. **Document type:** *Academic/Scholarly.* **Description:** Serves as a forum for timely topics of interest to the public health practitioner.
Related titles: Online - full text ed.
Indexed: Environ.Sci.Poll.Mgmt., Microbiol.Abstr., Pollut.Abstr., Saf.Sci.Abstr., Virol.Abstr. (coverage dropped).
Published by: Rapid Science Publishers, 2-6 Boundary Row, London SE1 8HN, United Kingdom. TEL 44-207-865-0198, FAX 44-207-410-6600, rapid@rapidcom.co.uk, http://www.chapmanhall.com/ci/default.html. Ed. Jonathan Mann.

614.3 GBR
CURRENT PROBLEMS IN PHARMACOVIGILANCE. Text in English. 1975. q. *Refereed.* **Document type:** *Government.*
Indexed: Inpharma, Pharm.&Out.News, Reac.
—BLDSC (3501.398000).
Published by: Department of Health, Medicines Control Agency, Market Towers, 1 Nine Elms Ln, London SW8 5DA, United Kingdom. TEL 44-20-7273-0254, FAX 44-20-7273-0269. Ed. A Breckenridge. R&P C Hepburn TEL 0-171-273-0954. **Co-sponsor:** Committee on Safety of Medicines.

CURRENT RESEARCH IN FAMILY & COMMUNITY SCIENCES. see *HOME ECONOMICS*

614.8 USA ISSN 1522-0389
D E S ACTION VOICE✶; a focus on diethylstilbestrol exposure. (Diethylstilbestrol) Text in English. 1979. q. USD 35 (effective 2000). bk.rev. abstr. back issues avail. **Document type:** *Newsletter.* **Description:** Covers the latest medical and legal information for D E S mothers, daughters and sons.
Published by: D E S Action USA, 610 16th St #301, Oakland, CA 94612-1229. TEL 510-465-4011, FAX 510-465-4815, desact.well.com, http://www.desaction.org. Ed., R&P Pat Cody. Circ: 3,000 (paid).

DAIRY, FOOD AND ENVIRONMENTAL SANITATION; a publication for food safety professionals. see *FOOD AND FOOD INDUSTRIES*

362.1 USA
DATA STRATEGIES AND BENCHMARKS. Text in English. 1997. m. USD 299; USD 309 in Canada & Mexico; USD 319 elsewhere. **Document type:** *Trade.*
Indexed: Int.Nurs.Ind.
Published by: National Health Information, LLC, PO Box 15429, Atlanta, GA 30333. TEL 404-607-9500. Ed. Marie Powers Terry Redman. Pubs. David Schwartz, Terry Redman.

614 PER
DE LA MANO CON LA SALUD. Text in Spanish. 1995. irreg. price varies. **Document type:** *Monographic series.*
Published by: Centro de Estudios Regionales Andinos "Bartolome de Las Casas", Apdo Postal 140087, Lince, Lima 14, Peru. TEL 51-14-429992, FAX 51-14-427894, cbcimpta@apu.cbc.org.pe. Pub. Andres Chirinos Rivera.

DENMARK. DANMARKS STATISTIK. FAERDSELSUHELD. see *POPULATION STUDIES—Abstracting, Bibliographies, Statistics*

362.1 AUS
DEPARTMENT OF HUMAN SERVICES, VICTORIA. ANNUAL REPORT (YEAR). Text in English. a. **Document type:** *Government.*
Related titles: Online - full content ed.
Published by: Department of Human Services, 555 Collins St, Melbourne, VIC 3000, Australia. TEL 61-3-9616-7777, 61-3-9637-4684, http://www.dhs.vic.gov.au/.

362 NLD ISSN 0927-4987
DEVELOPMENTS IN HEALTH ECONOMICS AND PUBLIC POLICY. Text in English. 1992. irreg., latest vol.2, 1992. price varies. back issues avail. **Document type:** *Monographic series.*
—BLDSC (3579.075100).
Published by: Kluwer Academic Publishers Group (Subsidiary of: Wolters Kluwer N.V.), Spuiboulevard 50, PO Box 17, Dordrecht 3300 AA, Netherlands. FAX 31-78-639-2254, services@wkap.nl, http://www.wkap.nl. **Dist. by:** Journals Department, PO Box 322, Dordrecht 3300 AH, Netherlands. FAX 31-78-654-6474.

614 ITA ISSN 0012-2653
CODEN: DISOAJ
DIFESA SOCIALE. Text in Italian; Summaries in English, Italian. 1922. bi-m. free per issue. bk.rev. abstr. index. **Document type:** *Government.* **Description:** Provides a forum to cover the social issues of medicine. Includes articles on the socialization of people with handicaps, pollution issues, drug addiction and alcoholism, and the elderly.
Indexed: Biol.Abstr., C.I.S. Abstr., Excerp.Med., Psychol.Abstr.
—BLDSC (3584.000000), CISTI.
Published by: Istituto Italiano di Medicina Sociale, Via Pasquale Stanislao Mancini, 28, Rome, RM 00196, Italy. TEL 06-3200641. Ed. Giovanni Maria Pirone. Circ: 4,500.

613 USA
DIRECTORY OF PREVENTIVE CARE RESOURCES. Text in English. 1997. a. USD 89. **Description:** Lists resources for planning, implementing, and evaluating preventive care programs.
Published by: Aspen Publishers, Inc., 200 Orchard Ridge Dr, Ste 200, Gaithersburg, MD 20878. TEL 800-638-8437, FAX 301-417-7550, http://www.aspenpub.com.

DIRITTO SANITARIO MODERNO. see *HEALTH FACILITIES AND ADMINISTRATION*

614 USA ISSN 0251-4486
HV553
DISASTER PREPAREDNESS AND MITIGATION IN THE AMERICAS; news and information for the international disaster community. Text in English. q. **Document type:** *Newsletter.*
Indexed: Environ.Abstr.
Published by: Pan American Health Organization (Subsidiary of: World Health Organization), PO Box 465, Hanover, PA 17331. TEL 202-974-3525, FAX 202-775-4578, disaster@paho.org, http://www.paho.org/english/disaster.htm. Circ: 26,000.

614.84 JPN ISSN 0006-7873
DISASTER PREVENTION/BOSAI. Text in Japanese. 1947. bi-m. JPY 780. adv.
Indexed: Abstr.J.Earthq.Eng.
Published by: Tokyo Consolidated Fire Prevention Association/Tokyo Rengo Boka Kyokai, c/o Tokyo Shobo-cho, 3-5, Otemachi Ichome, Chiyoda-ku, Tokyo 100, Japan. Ed. Bunkichi Sawaguri. Circ: 12,000.

614 GBR ISSN 0965-3562
HV551.2 CODEN: DPMAEY
DISASTER PREVENTION AND MANAGEMENT. Text in English. 1992. 5/yr. USD 3,559 in North America; EUR 3,809 in Europe; AUD 5,399 in Australasia; GBP 2,239 in the UK & rest of the world (effective 2002). reprint service avail. from SWZ. **Document type:** *Academic/Scholarly.*
Related titles: Online - full text ed.: (from EBSCO Publishing, O C L C Online Computer Library Center, Inc., RoweCom Information Quest, ingenta, Swets Blackwell).
Indexed: Aqua.Sci.& Fish.Abstr., Emerald, Emrld.Intell., Environ.Sci.Poll.Mgmt., Geo.Abstr.P.G., Lang.& Lang.Behav.Abstr., Pollut.Abstr., Ref.Zh., Risk Abstr., Rural Devel.Abstr., SOPODA, Saf.Sci.Abstr., Sel.Water Res.Abstr., Sociol.Abstr.
—BLDSC (3595.462000). **CCC.**
Published by: Emerald, 60-62 Toller Ln, Bradford, W Yorks BD8 9BY, United Kingdom. TEL 44-1274-777700, FAX 44-1274-785200, info@emeraldinsight.com, http://www.emeraldinsight.com/dpm.htm, http://www.mcb.co.uk/, http://www.emeraldinsight.com/journals/.

362.1 USA ISSN 1531-5681
DISEASE MANAGEMENT ADVISOR. Text in English. m. USD 359 domestic; USD 369 in North America; USD 379 elsewhere (effective 2000). back issues avail.
Former titles (until July 2000): Healthcare Demand and Disease Management (1094-2521); (until 1997): Healthcare Demand Management (1083-7191)
Indexed: Int.Nurs.Ind.
—BLDSC (3598.083500).
Published by: National Health Information, LLC, PO Box 15429, Atlanta, GA 30333. TEL 404-607-9500, nhi@nhionline.net, http://www.nhionline.net. Ed. Terry Hartnett. Pub. David Schwartz.

DISEASE MANAGEMENT AND CLINICAL OUTCOMES. see *MEDICAL SCIENCES*

628 ITA
DISINFESTAZIONE. Text in Italian. 1984. bi-m. ITL 100,000. adv. **Description:** Concerned with pest control.
Published by: MO.ED.CO. s.r.l., Via Paolo da Cannobio, 9, Milan, MI 20122, Italy. TEL 39-02-878577, FAX 39-02-89010728. Circ: 5,000.

DIZHEN KANAN ANQUAN. see *EARTH SCIENCES—Geology*

614 USA
DOCTOM'S ONLINE SELF-CARE JOURNAL. Text in English. 1996. irreg.
Media: Online - full content.
Published by: Harvard Medical School, Center for Clinical Computing, Boston, MA 02115. http://www.healthy.net/selfcare. Ed. Tom Ferguson.

614 HRV ISSN 1331-2499
DOKTOR U KUCI. Text in Croatian. 1998. m. **Document type:** *Magazine, Consumer.*
Published by: Arena d.d., Slavonska Avenija 4, Zagreb 10000, Croatia. TEL 385-1-6166666, FAX 385-1-6162065, doktor@eph.hr. Ed. Mladen Gerovac.

362.1 CHN
DONGFANG JIAN. Text in Chinese. m. **Document type:** *Consumer.*
Published by: China International Book Trading Corp/Zhongguo Guoji Tushu Maoyi Zonggongsi cibtc@mail.cibtc.com.cn, http://www.cibtc.com.cn. **Dist. by:** 35, Chegongzhuang Xilu, Haidian District, Beijing 100044, China.

DRINKING WATER & BACKFLOW PREVENTION. see *ENGINEERING—Civil Engineering*

DRUG G M P REPORT. (Good Manufacturing Practices) see *PHARMACY AND PHARMACOLOGY*

DRUGLINK. see *PHARMACY AND PHARMACOLOGY*

614.8 USA
DRUGS AND BIOLOGY GUIDANCE MANUAL. Text in English. irreg. USD 135 in North America; USD 270 elsewhere. **Document type:** *Government.* **Description:** Provides the latest information on and helps maintain program plans and instructions directed to F.D.A. field operations. These plans and instructions are surveillance or compliance oriented and provide the needed direction from headquarters offices and bureaus in accomplishing F.D.A. regulatory obligations.
Published by: U.S. Food and Drug Administration, Office of Public Affairs, 5600 Fishers Ln, Rockville, MD 20857. TEL 301-443-3220. **Orders to:** National Technical Information Service, Government Research Center. FAX 703-321-8547.

DRUGS AND DEVICE RECALL BULLETIN. see *PHARMACY AND PHARMACOLOGY*

P

DRUGS, HEALTH, AND SOCIAL POLICY SERIES. see *PUBLIC ADMINISTRATION*

DU & JOBBET; arbetsmiljoetidningen. see *OCCUPATIONAL HEALTH AND SAFETY*

E H P SUPPLEMENTS. (Environmental Health Perspectives) see *ENVIRONMENTAL STUDIES*

628.5 USA
E M A NEWS. Text in English. q. USD 150 to members. adv. **Document type:** *Newsletter.*
Published by: Environmental Management Association, 1721 Pheasant Lane, Jeffersonville, PA 19403-3333. TEL 610-539-8588, FAX 610-539-9999, emapress@aol.com, http://www.emantional.org. R&P Barry M Dressler. Adv. contact Slobodan Djurdjevic.

E M F HEALTH & SAFETY DIGEST. (Electric and Magnetic Field) see *OCCUPATIONAL HEALTH AND SAFETY*

362.1 DEU ISSN 0949-8567
E U INFORMATIONSBRIEF GESUNDHEIT. (European Union) Text in German. 1994. bi-m. DEM 126; DEM 152 foreign (effective 2000). **Document type:** *Newsletter.* **Description:** Provides current and background information on European policies in the fields of health issues and consumer protection.
Published by: Europa-Kontakt e.V., Postfach 580139, Berlin 10411, Germany. TEL 49-30-42851570, FAX 49-30-4250353, http://www.europa-kontakt.de.

614 EGY ISSN 1020-3397
EASTERN MEDITERRANEAN HEALTH JOURNAL/REVUE DE SANTE DE LA MEDITERRANEE ORIENTALE. Text in English. 1995. s-a. USD 24; USD 5 newsstand/cover (effective 2000). **Description:** It is a forum for the presentation and promotion of new policies and initiatives in health services and for the exchange of ideas, concepts, epidemiological data, research findings and other information, with special reference to the Eastern Mediterranean Region.
Indexed: Abstr.Hyg., Dairy Sci.Abstr., IIS, Ind.Med., Ind.Vet., Irr.& Drain.Abstr., Nutr.Abstr., Protozool.Abstr., Rev.Med.& Vet.Mycol., Rural Devel.Abstr., Soils & Fert., Trop.Dis.Bull.
—BLDSC (3646.669520).
Published by: World Health Organization, Regional Office for the Eastern Mediterranean, P O Box 1517, Alexandria 21563, Egypt. TEL 20-3-4830090, FAX 20-3-4838916, TELEX 54028 WHO UN, khayat@who.sci.eg. Ed. Haytham Khayat.

ECONOMICS, MEDICINES, & HEALTH. see *BUSINESS AND ECONOMICS—Production Of Goods And Services*

ECOTOXICOLOGY AND ENVIRONMENTAL SAFETY. see *ENVIRONMENTAL STUDIES—Toxicology And Environmental Safety*

628 ESP
EDUCACION SANITARIA. Text in Spanish. 1983. irreg., latest vol.3, 1986. price varies.
Published by: (Universidad de Navarra, Facultad de Medicina), Ediciones Universidad de Navarra S.A., Apartado 396, Pamplona, Navarra 31080, Spain. TEL 94 825 6850.

EDUCATION SANITAIRE ET NUTRITIONNELLE D'AFRIQUE CENTRALE. see *NUTRITION AND DIETETICS*

614 HUN ISSN 0073-4012
EGESZSEGNEVELES SZAKKONYVTARA. Text in Hungarian. 1967. irreg. price varies.
Published by: Medicina Kiado, Beloiannisz utca 8, Budapest 1054, Hungary.

614 EGY ISSN 0013-2446
CODEN: JEGPAY
EGYPTIAN PUBLIC HEALTH ASSOCIATION JOURNAL. Text in Arabic. 1970 (vol.45). 6/yr. USD 18.
Indexed: Biol.Abstr., Chem.Abstr., Excerp.Med., Ind.Med. (1926-).
—CASDDS, CISTI, GNLM.
Published by: Egyptian Public Health Association, Shousha Bldg., Block A, Apt. 116, 31 Sharia 26 July, Cairo, Egypt. Ed. Dr. S El Kholy. Circ: 750.

614 JPN
RA421 CODEN: ESKHA5
EISEI KENKYUJO HOKOKU/NATIONAL INSTITUTE OF HEALTH SCIENCES. BULLETIN. Text in Japanese; Summaries in English. 1886. a. free per issue. adv. **Document type:** *Bulletin, Academic/Scholarly.* **Description:** Disseminates research activities of NIHS.
Formerly: Eisei Shinkenjo Hokoku (0077-4715)
Indexed: Biol.Abstr., Chem.Abstr., Dairy Sci.Abstr., Excerp.Med., Field Crop Abstr., Food Sci.& Tech.Abstr., Hort.Abstr., INIS Atomind., Ind.Med. (coverage dropped), Rev.Med.& Vet.Mycol., Rev.Plant Path., Triticale Abstr., Trop.Dis.Bull.
—BLDSC (2640.170000), CASDDS, GNLM, KNAW.
Published by: National Institute of Health Sciences, 1-18-1 Kami-Yoga, Setagaya-ku, Tokyo 158-0098, Japan. TEL 81-3-3700-1141, FAX 81-3-3700-7592, kaminuma@nihs.go.jp, http://www.nihs.go.jp/index.html. Ed. Tadao Terao. Adv. contact Tsugutika Kaminuma. Circ: 1,000.

614 USA ISSN 1086-2897
ELECTRICAL SENSITIVITY NEWS. Text in English. ceased; resumed 1996. bi-m. USD 20 domestic; USD 35 foreign (effective 2000). bk.rev. back issues avail. **Document type:** *Newsletter.* **Description:** Covers the latest environmental illness, electrical sensitivity from electromagnetic fields.
Published by: Weldon Publishing, PO Box 4146, Prescott, AZ 86302. http://www.northlink.com/~1grant. Ed. Lucinda Grant.

614.8 614.86 USA ISSN 0747-816X
T55.3.H3
EMERGENCY RESPONSE GUIDEBOOK. Text in English. a. **Description:** Provides information for police and fire personnel on steps to be taken in the first critical minutes after a hazardous materials transportation accident.
Published by: U.S. Department of Transportation, Materials Transportation Bureau, Washington, DC 20590.

362.1969 616.9 USA ISSN 1080-6059
EMERGING INFECTIOUS DISEASES (ONLINE EDITION). Text in English. 6/yr. **Document type:** *Academic/Scholarly.*
Media: Online - full text (from H. W. Wilson, Gale Group, Institute for Scientific Information). **Related titles:** ♦ Print ed.: Emerging Infectious Diseases (Print Edition). ISSN 1080-6040; Chinese Translation; French Translation; Esperanto Translation: Enfermedades Infecciosas Emergentes.
Published by: U.S. National Center for Infectious Diseases, 1600 Clifton Rd, Mailstop D61, Atlanta, GA 30333.

362.1969 616.9 USA ISSN 1080-6040
RA648.5 CODEN: EIDIFA
EMERGING INFECTIOUS DISEASES (PRINT EDITION). Text in English. 1995. 6/yr. free per issue. bk.rev. illus. reprints avail. *Refereed.* **Document type:** *Academic/Scholarly, Government.* **Description:** Reports on emerging infectious diseases worldwide, including reviews and analyses, epidemiologic and laboratory issues, and prevention strategies.
Related titles: ♦ Online - full text ed.: Emerging Infectious Diseases (Online Edition). ISSN 1080-6059.
Indexed: ASCA, Abstr.Hyg., Curr.Cont., Derwent Biotech.Abstr., Environ.Sci.Poll.Mgmt., Gen.Sci.Ind. (Jul.1997-), Ind.Med. (1995-), Ind.Vet., Inpharma, Jrnl.Watch Inf.Dis., Pig News & Info., Pollut.Abstr., Poult.Abstr., Protozool.Abstr., Reac., Rev.Appl.Entomol., Rev.Med.& Vet.Mycol., Risk Abstr., Rural Recreat.Tour.Abstr., Saf.Sci.Abstr., Sci.Cit.Ind., Sel.Water Res.Abstr., Trop.Dis.Bull., Vet.Bull., Wild.Rev., Zoo.Rec.
—BLDSC (3733.426050), CASDDS, IDS, ingenta.
Published by: U.S. National Center for Infectious Diseases, 1600 Clifton Rd, Mailstop D61, Atlanta, GA 30333. TEL 404-371-5329, FAX 404-371-5449, eideditor@cdc.gov; orders@allenpress.com, http://www.cdc.gov/eid; http://www.allenpress.com. Ed. Joseph E McDade. Circ: 23,500. **Subscr. to:** Allen Press Inc., PO Box 1897, Lawrence, KS 66044-8897. **Affiliate:** Centers for Disease Control and Prevention.

ENVIRONMENT & ASSESSMENT. see *ENVIRONMENTAL STUDIES*

ENVIRONMENT AND SAFETY BRIEFING. see *ENVIRONMENTAL STUDIES*

615.9 GBR ISSN 0964-5322
ENVIRONMENT INFORMATION BULLETIN. Abbreviated title: E I B. Text in English. 1991. m. (10/yr.). GBP 99; GBP 115 foreign. index. **Document type:** *Trade.*
Related titles: ♦ Supplement to: Health, Safety and Environment Bulletin. ISSN 1353-1638.
Indexed: CSNB.
—BLDSC (3791.251000).
Published by: Eclipse Group Ltd., Industrial Relations Services, 18 Highbury Park, London N5 2AB, United Kingdom. TEL 44-20-7354-5858, FAX 44-207-226-8618, rose.riddell@ireclipse.co.uk, http://www.irseclipse.co.uk. Ed. Rosemary Riddell. Pub. Andrew Brode.

ENVIRONMENT INTERNATIONAL; a journal of environmental science, risk & health. see *ENVIRONMENTAL STUDIES*

ENVIRONMENTAL COMPLIANCE & LITIGATION STRATEGY. see *LAW*

616.98 GBR ISSN 0013-9270
ENVIRONMENTAL HEALTH. Abbreviated title: E H. Text in English. 1895. m. GBP 82 Includes Environmental Health News; GBP 100 foreign Includes Environmental Health News (effective 1999). adv. bk.rev. bibl, charts, illus, stat, tr.lit. index. reprint service avail. from PQC. **Document type:** *Trade.* **Description:** Includes articles about food hygiene, health and safety, housing, pest control, pollution, waste management, and noise pollution.
Formerly: Public Health Inspector
Related titles: Microform ed.: (from PQC).
Indexed: ASSIA, Abstr.Hyg., Art.Hosp.& Tour., Biol.Abstr., C.I.S. Abstr., Curr.Adv.Ecol.Sci., Dairy Sci.Abstr., Diar.Dis.Res., Environ.Abstr., Environ.Per.Bibl., Excerp.Med., Food Sci.& Tech.Abstr., Helminthol.Abstr., Ind.Vet., Lab.Haz.Bull., Ocean.Abstr. (coverage dropped), Pollut.Abstr., Poult.Abstr., RICS, Rev.Appl.Entomol., Risk Abstr., Sport Fish.Abstr., Trop.Dis.Bull., WasteInfo, Wild.Rev.
—CISTI, ingenta, Linda Hall.
Published by: Chartered Institute of Environmental Health, Publishing and Communications Division, Chadwick Court, 15 Hatfields, London SE1 8DJ, United Kingdom. TEL 44-20-7928-6006, FAX 44-20-7827-5866, m.randall@chgl.com, http://www.cieh.org.uk. Ed. Claire Brown. R&P Nicola Rose. Adv. contact Paul Prior. B&W page GBP 600, color page GBP 1,050; trim 190 x 270. Circ: 11,725.

614 614.85 GBR ISSN 0964-914X
ENVIRONMENTAL HEALTH BRIEFING. Text in English. 1989. w. GBP 675. bk.rev. **Document type:** *Bulletin, Abstract/Index.* **Description:** Provides concise summaries of newly published U.K. and E.C. legislation, reports, and important information concerning environmental control, health, safety, housing, and food safety.
Related titles: CD-ROM ed.; Diskette ed.; Ed.
Published by: Barbour Index, New Lodge, Drift Rd, Winkfield, Windsor, Berks SL4 4RQ, United Kingdom. TEL 44-1344-884121, FAX 44-1344-884112. Ed. D Denton.

ENVIRONMENTAL HEALTH CRITERIA. see *ENVIRONMENTAL STUDIES*

614 GBR ISSN 0969-9856
ENVIRONMENTAL HEALTH NEWS. Short title: E H N. Text in English. 1986. w. GBP 82 domestic; GBP 100 foreign; includes EH: Environmental Health. **Document type:** *Trade.* **Description:** Reports on what has happened in that particular week in the world of environmental health.
Published by: Chartered Institute of Environmental Health, Publishing and Communications Division, Chadwick Court, 15 Hatfields, London SE1 8DJ, United Kingdom. TEL 44-20-7928-6006, FAX 44-20-7827-5866, m.randall@chgl.com, http://www.cieh.org.uk. Ed. B Randall. Circ: 10,700.

ENVIRONMENTAL HEALTH PERSPECTIVES. see *ENVIRONMENTAL STUDIES*

ENVIRONMENTAL HEALTH PERSPECTIVES SUPPLEMENT. see *ENVIRONMENTAL STUDIES*

616.98 GBR
ENVIRONMENTAL HEALTH REPORT (YEAR). Text in English. a. GBP 8.50. **Document type:** *Trade.* **Description:** Looks at the work of local authority environmental health departments in England and Wales. The report is based on information provided on a voluntary basis by local authorities in response to a questionnaire.
Published by: Chartered Institute of Environmental Health, Publishing and Communications Division, Chadwick Court, 15 Hatfields, London SE1 8DJ, United Kingdom. TEL 44-20-7928-6006, FAX 44-20-7827-5866, m.randall@chgl.com, http://www.cieh.org.uk.

P

363.72 CAN ISSN 0319-6771
ENVIRONMENTAL HEALTH REVIEW. Text in English. 1956. q. CND 30 domestic; CND 38 in United States; CND 45 overseas (effective 2002). adv. bk.rev. *Refereed.* **Document type:** *Journal, Academic/Scholarly.*
Indexed: Biol.Dig.
—CISTI, GNLM.
Published by: D2 C3 Enterprises, White Rock Pastal Outlet, P O Box 75264, White Rock, BC V4B 5L4, Canada. FAX 604-543-0904, dlosito@cnx.net. Ed., Pub., R&P Domenic Losito TEL 604-543-0999. Adv. contact Debra Losito. Circ: 1,500.

ENVIRONMENTAL MANAGEMENT NEWS. see *ENVIRONMENTAL STUDIES*

ENVIRONMENTAL RADIATION SURVEILLANCE IN WASHINGTON STATE. ANNUAL REPORT. see *ENVIRONMENTAL STUDIES*

ENVIRONMENTAL REGULATORY ADVISOR. see *ENVIRONMENTAL STUDIES—Waste Management*

ENVIRONMENTAL TOXICOLOGY AND CHEMISTRY. see *ENVIRONMENTAL STUDIES—Toxicology And Environmental Safety*

628 USA
EPI-GRAM. Text in English. m. **Document type:** *Government.*
Published by: Department of Human Services, Division of Disease Control, State House, Sta 11, Augusta, ME 04333. FAX 207-289-4172. Ed. Dr. Kathleen F Gensheiner.

614.4 616.8 ITA ISSN 1121-189X
EPIDEMIOLOGIA E PSICHIATRIA SOCIALE. Text in Italian. 1992. 4/yr. USD 107 (effective 2000). adv. 80 p./no. **Document type:** *Journal.*
Indexed: Excerp.Med. (1996-), Ind.Med. (1992-), Lang.& Lang.Behav.Abstr., Ref.Zh., SOPODA, Sociol.Abstr., e-psyche.
—BLDSC (3793.537000).
Published by: Il Pensiero Scientifico Editore s.r.l., Via Bradano, 3-C, Rome, RM 00199, Italy. TEL 39-06-862821, FAX 39-06-86282250, pensiero@pensiero.it, http://www.pensiero.it. Ed. Michele Tansella. Pub. Luca De Fiore. R&P Andrea De Fiore. Adv. contact Luciano De Fiore. Circ: 800.

EPIDEMIOLOGICAL BULLETIN. see *MEDICAL SCIENCES*

614.4 USA ISSN 1044-3983
RA648.5 CODEN: EPIDEY
EPIDEMIOLOGY. Text in English. 1990. bi-m. USD 181 domestic to individuals for print & online eds.; USD 235 foreign to individuals for print & online eds.; USD 360 domestic to institutions for print & online eds.; USD 377 foreign to institutions for print & online eds. (effective 2002); USD 58 newsstand/cover. adv. *Refereed.* **Document type:** *Trade, Academic/Scholarly.* **Description:** Targets epidemiologists, public health investigators, and other practicing health professionals interested in scientific discussion on principles and methods in data analysis.
Related titles: Online - full text ed.: USD 468 domestic academic site license; USD 485 foreign academic site license; USD 522 domestic corporate site license; USD 539 foreign corporate site license (effective 2002) (from Ovid Technologies, Inc., Institute for Scientific Information).
Indexed: ASCA, Abstr.Hyg., Aqua.Sci.& Fish.Abstr., CSNB, Crim.Just.Abstr., Curr.Cont., Curr.Ind.Stat., Environ.Sci.Poll.Mgmt., Fam.Ind., INIS Atomind., Ind.Med. (1990-), Inpharma, Int.Abstr.Biol.Sci., Int.Nurs.Ind., Jrnl.Watch Wom.Hlth., METADEX, NRN, Nutr.Abstr., Pharm.&Out.News, Pollut.Abstr., Reac., Rev.Med.& Vet.Mycol., Risk Abstr., SSCI (coverage dropped), Saf.Sci.Abstr., Sage Race Rel.Abstr., Sci.Cit.Ind., THA, Tox.Abstr., Trop.Dis.Bull.
—BLDSC (3793.574000), CISTI, EMDOCS, GNLM, IDS, ingenta, KNAW.
Published by: (Epidemiology Resources Inc.), Williams & Wilkins (Subsidiary of: Waverly International), 351 W Camden St, Baltimore, MD 21201-2436. TEL 410-528-4068, FAX 410-222-3790, cbrooks@wwilkins.com, http://www.wwilkins.com, http://www.Lww.com. Ed. Kenneth J Rothman. Adv. contact Carol Brooks. B&W page USD 495; trim 10.88 x 8.13. Circ: 1,747 (controlled); 1,251 (paid).

ERUUL MEND/HEALTH. see *PHYSICAL FITNESS AND HYGIENE*

614 362.1 ETH ISSN 1021-6790
THE ETHIOPIAN JOURNAL OF HEALTH DEVELOPMENT. Text in English. 1984. 3/yr. ETB 60 domestic; USD 75 foreign (effective 2001). bk.rev. *Refereed.* **Document type:** *Academic/Scholarly.* **Description:** Publishes analytical, descriptive, and methodological papers as well as original research on public health problems, management of health services, health care needs, and socio-economic and political factors related to health and development.
Indexed: Abstr.Anthropol., Agroforest.Abstr., INIS Atomind., Rev.Arom.& Med.Plants.
—BLDSC (3814.782000), GNLM.
Published by: Ethiopian Public Health Association, Tikur Anbessa Hospital, PO Box 32812, Addis Ababa, Ethiopia. TEL 251-1-513628, FAX 251-1-514870, rhr.aau@telecom.net.et, http://www.cih.uib.no/journals/EJHD. Ed. Yemane Berhane. R&P Yemane Berane. Adv. contact Simon Tekle Haimanot. Circ: 1,000. **Co-sponsor:** Addis Ababa University.

616.009 305.8 GBR ISSN 1355-7858
CODEN: ETHEFR
ETHNICITY AND HEALTH. Text in English. 1996. 4/yr. GBP 81, USD 133 to individuals; GBP 222, USD 367 to institutions (effective 2002). **Document type:** *Academic/Scholarly.*
Related titles: Online - full text ed.: ISSN 1465-3419 (from CatchWord Ltd., EBSCO Publishing, O C L C Online Computer Library Center, Inc., RoweCom Information Quest, ProQuest Information & Learning, Swets Blackwell, Institute for Scientific Information).
Indexed: ASSIA, CINAHL, Curr.Cont., Environ.Sci.Poll.Mgmt., Geo.Abstr.H.G., Ind.Med. (1996-), Lang.& Lang.Behav.Abstr., Nutr.Abstr., Pollut.Abstr., PsycInfo, Risk Abstr., SOPODA, SSCI, Saf.Sci.Abstr., Soc.Serv.Abstr., Sociol.Abstr., Trop.Dis.Bull., e-psyche.
—BLDSC (3814.840700), CatchWord, Infotrieve, KNAW. **CCC.**
Published by: Carfax Publishing Limited (Subsidiary of: Taylor & Francis Group), PO Box 25, Abingdon, Oxon OX14 3UE, United Kingdom. TEL 44-1235-401000, FAX 44-1235-401550, enquiries@carfax.co.uk, enquiry@tandf.co.uk, http://www.carfax.co.uk.

614 300 GBR
EUROHEALTH. Text in English. 195?. q. **Document type:** *Academic/Scholarly.* **Description:** Acts as a vehicle for scientists, policy-makers and experts to express their views on health policy issues and therefore contribute to a constructive debate on public health policy in Europe.
Indexed: Abstr.Hyg., Trop.Dis.Bull.
—BLDSC (3829.268610).
Published by: London School of Economics, Houghton St, London WC2 2AE, United Kingdom. TEL 44-20-7955-7540, FAX 44-20-7955-6803, d.nicolaou@lse.ac.uk. **Co-sponsor:** European Health Policy Research Network.

EUROPE DRUG & DEVICE REPORT. see *PHARMACY AND PHARMACOLOGY*

EUROPEAN JOURNAL OF EPIDEMIOLOGY. see *MEDICAL SCIENCES*

EUROPEAN JOURNAL OF HEALTH LAW. see *MEDICAL SCIENCES*

614 GBR ISSN 1101-1262
RA483 CODEN: EJPHF6
EUROPEAN JOURNAL OF PUBLIC HEALTH. Text in English. 1991. q. GBP 99, USD 160 to individuals; GBP 150, USD 245 to institutions (effective Mar. 2002). adv. bk.rev. back issues avail. *Refereed.* **Document type:** *Journal, Academic/Scholarly.* **Description:** Provides a forum for the discussion and debate of current public health issues in the European region.
Related titles: Online - full text ed.: ISSN 1464-360X. GBP 135, USD 220 to institutions Online only (effective Mar. 2002) (from EBSCO Publishing, ingenta, Swets Blackwell, Institute for Scientific Information, RoweCom Information Quest).
Indexed: Abstr.Hyg., Addic.Abstr., AgeLine, CINAHL, Curr.Cont., Inpharma, Lang.& Lang.Behav.Abstr., Nutr.Abstr., Pharm.&Out.News, Reac., SOPODA, SSCI, Sci.Cit.Ind., Soc.Serv.Abstr., Sociol.Abstr., Trop.Dis.Bull.
—BLDSC (3829.738030), CISTI, GNLM, IDS, Infotrieve, KNAW. **CCC.**
Published by: (Stichting Journals for Public Health and Science NLD), Oxford University Press, Academic Division, Great Clarendon St, Oxford OX2 6DP, United Kingdom. TEL 44-1865-267907, FAX 44-1865-267835, jnl.info@oup.co.uk, http://www3.oup.co.uk/eurpub/, http://www.oup.co.uk/journals. Eds. Carlo La Vecchina, Johan Mackenbach, Martin McKee. Pub. Mandy Sketch. R&P Fionna Willis. adv.: page GBP 410, page USD 740. Circ: 9,300. **U.S. subscr. to:** Oxford University Press, Journals, 2001 Evans Rd, Cary, NC 27513. TEL 800-852-7323, FAX 919-677-0977, jnlorders@oup-usa.org; **Subscr. to:** Journals Marketing, Great Clarendon St, Oxford OX2 6DP, United Kingdom.

362.1 GBR
EUROPEAN SAFETY NEWSLETTER. Abbreviated title: E S N. Text in English. 1993. 6/yr. GBP 75 (effective 1998). adv. bk.rev., video rev. **Document type:** *Newsletter.*
Address: PO Box 4, Haslemere, Surrey GU27 3XX, United Kingdom. TEL 44-1428-724911, FAX 44-1428-724911. Ed. John Manos. Circ: 1,500 (paid).

EVIDENCE - BASED CARDIOVASCULAR MEDICINE. see *MEDICAL SCIENCES—Cardiovascular Diseases*

614 362 GBR ISSN 1462-9410
EVIDENCE - BASED HEALTHCARE; a scientific approach to health policy. Text in English. 1997. q. GBP 70 to individuals; GBP 185 to institutions (effective 2002). adv. *Refereed.* **Document type:** *Journal, Academic/Scholarly.* **Description:** Provides health managers and policy makers with the best evidence available about the financing, organization and management of healthcare in the form of summaries from authorative journals in the field.
Formerly (until 1998): Evidence - Based Health Policy and Management (1363-4038)
Related titles: Online - full text ed.: (from IDEAL Online Library, Ovid Technologies, Inc.).
—BLDSC (3831.036670).
Published by: Churchill Livingstone (Subsidiary of: Harcourt Publishers Ltd.), Robert Stevenson House, 1-3 Baxter's Pl, Leith Walk, Edinburgh, Midlothian EH1 3AF, United Kingdom. TEL 44-131-556-2424, FAX 44-131-459-1177, http://www.harcourt-international.com/journals/ebhc. Ed. Dr. Anna Donald. R&P Greg Davies. **Subscr. to:** Harcourt Publishers Ltd., Foots Cray High St, Sidcup, Kent DA14 5HP, United Kingdom. TEL 44-20-8308-5700, FAX 44-20-8309-0807.

EVIDENCE - BASED OBSTETRICS & GYNAECOLOGY. see *MEDICAL SCIENCES—Obstetrics And Gynecology*

363.78 USA
EXECUTIVE REPORTS. Cover title: Pest Control Executive Reports. Text in English. 1991. m., latest vol.11. USD 69 domestic; USD 72 in Canada & Mexico; USD 80 elsewhere (effective 2001). bk.rev. charts, illus, stat, tr.lit. annual index. 6 p./no. back issues avail. **Document type:** *Newsletter, Trade.* **Description:** Provides management information relating to pest control, for owners, managers and supervisors of pest control businesses.
Published by: Pinto & Associates, Inc., 29839 Oak Rd, Mechanicsville, MD 20659. TEL 301-884-3020, FAX 301-884-4068. Ed., R&P Sandra Kraft. Pub. Lawrence J Pinto. Circ: 350 (paid).

EYE TO EYE. see *MEDICAL SCIENCES—Ophthalmology And Optometry*

614.8 IND
F R C H NEWSLETTER. Text in English, Hindi. 1986. bi-m. USD 4 newsstand/cover (effective 1999). bk.rev. **Document type:** *Newsletter.* **Description:** Carries articles related to community health with emphasis on holistic health care.
Published by: Foundation for Research in Community Health, 3 & 4 Trimiti B Apts., Aundh, 85 Anand Park, Pune, Maharashtra 411 007, India. TEL 91-22-4938601. Ed. Vaijayanti Aphale. Circ: 1,000.

FACT SHEET ON THE NETHERLANDS. see *SOCIAL SERVICES AND WELFARE*

FACTS AND ADVICE FOR AIRLINE PASSENGERS. see *TRANSPORTATION—Air Transport*

610 USA ISSN 0160-6379
RA421
FAMILY AND COMMUNITY HEALTH; the journal of health promotion and maintenance. Text in English. 1978. q. USD 172 to individuals; USD 52 newsstand/cover (effective 2002). bk.rev. illus. reprint service avail. from PQC. *Refereed.* **Document type:** *Journal.* **Description:** Presents creative, multidisciplinary perspectives and approaches for effective public health programs.
Related titles: Microform ed.: (from PQC); Online - full text ed.: (from Ovid Technologies, Inc., ProQuest Information & Learning, Gale Group, Institute for Scientific Information).
Indexed: ASCA, Abstr.Hyg., AgeLine, CINAHL, Crim.Just.Abstr., Curr.Cont., Environ.Sci.Poll.Mgmt., FAMLI, Fam.Ind., IMFL, Lang.& Lang.Behav.Abstr., NRN, Nurs.Abstr., Pollut.Abstr., PsycInfo, Psychol.Abstr. (1982-), Risk Abstr., SOPODA, SSCI, Saf.Sci.Abstr., Soc.Serv.Abstr., Sociol.Abstr., e-psyche.
—BLDSC (3865.558000), GNLM, IDS, Infotrieve, ingenta. **CCC.**
Published by: Aspen Publishers, Inc., 200 Orchard Ridge Dr, Ste 200, Gaithersburg, MD 20878. TEL 301-417-7500, 800-638-8437, FAX 301-417-7550, customer.service@aspenpubl.com, http://www.aspenpub.com. Ed. Jeanette Lancaster. Circ: 1,900 (paid). **Dist. by:** Aspen Publishers Inc., Distribution Center, 7201 McKinney Circle, Frederick, MD 21701. TEL 301-698-7100, FAX 301-417-7550.

362.1 AUS
FAMILY AND NEIGHBOURHOOD SERVICES EXTRA. Text in English. 1998 (Dec.). **Document type:** *Newsletter, Government.*
Media: Online - full content.
Published by: Community Care Division (Subsidiary of: Department of Human Services), Level 13, 555 Collin St, Melbourne, VIC 3000, Australia. TEL 61-3-9616-7121, michael.aughton@dhs.vic.gov.au.

614.42 CAN ISSN 0830-0305
FAMILY HEALTH. Text in English. 1985. bi-m. CND 13.75, USD 13.75 domestic; CND 13.75 foreign (effective 1997). adv. **Description:** Informs and increases health consciousness of Albertans through professional information.
Related titles: Online - full text ed.: (from LexisNexis).
Indexed: AgeLine, CBCA Ref., Can.Per.Ind. (Mar.1995-).
Address: P O Box 2421, Edmonton, AB T5J 2S6, Canada.

614.8 USA ISSN 0749-310X
TX150
FAMILY SAFETY & HEALTH. Text in English. 1961. q. USD 16.75 to members; USD 21.25 to non-members (effective 2001). adv. illus. reprint service avail. from PQC. **Document type:** *Consumer.* **Description:** Dedicated to preventing off-the-job injuries and to promoting health and fitness through consumer education.
Formerly (until 1984): Family Safety (0014-7397)
Related titles: Microform ed.: (from PQC); Online - full text ed.
—ingenta.
Published by: National Safety Council, 1121 Spring Lake Dr, Itasca, IL 60143. TEL 630-285-1121, 800-621-7619, FAX 630-285-1315, http://www.nsc.org/pubs/fsh/. Ed. Laura Coyne. Pubs. John H Kennedy, Suzanne Powills. adv.: page USD 24,225. Circ: 550,000.

FEDERAL MOTOR CARRIER SAFETY ADMINISTRATION REGISTER; a daily summary of motor carrier applications and of decisions and notices. see *TRANSPORTATION—Automobiles*

614 USA ISSN 1070-9029
FEDERAL PHYSICIAN. Text in English. 1979. bi-m. USD 37.50 (effective 2000). adv. back issues avail. **Document type:** *Newsletter.* **Description:** Covers changes in federal physician pay and benefits, updates on changes affecting federal employees, news of federal health programs.
Published by: Federal Physicians Association, PO Box 45150, Washington, DC 20026. TEL 703-455-5947, FAX 703-455-8282. Ed. Dennis W Boyd. Adv. contact Nick Cordovana. Circ: 1,000 (controlled).

FEDERAL VETERINARIAN. see *VETERINARY SCIENCE*

FIRE FOCUS. see *FIRE PREVENTION*

614 JPN ISSN 0917-3625
FIRUMU BADJI NYUSU/FILM BADGE NEWS. Text in Japanese. 1985. m. JPY 400 per issue. adv.
Published by: Chiyoda Hoan Yohin K.K./Chiyoda Safety Appliance Co., Ltd., 3-40-11 Hongo, Bunkyo-ku, Tokyo 113-0033, Japan. Ed. Michihiko Watanabe. Adv. contact Tadashi Matsutani.

FLIGHT SAFETY BULLETIN. see *AERONAUTICS AND SPACE FLIGHT*

FLYING SAFETY. see *AERONAUTICS AND SPACE FLIGHT*

614 PHL ISSN 0046-4317
FOCUS ON MENTAL HEALTH. Text in English, Tagalog. 1951. q. USD 3.60 to individuals; USD 37 to institutions (effective 2000). charts, illus, stat. **Document type:** *Newsletter.* **Description:** Covers public health and safety, community mental health, psychology and psychiatry, social work and social development.
Indexed: Ind.Phil.Per.
Published by: Philippine Mental Health Association, 18 East Ave, PO Box 1040, Quezon City CPO, Quezon City Mm 1100, Philippines. Ed. Regina G. De Jesus. Circ: 1,500.

614 CAN ISSN 0015-5195
FOCUS: SOCIAL AND PREVENTIVE MEDICINE. Text in English. 1964. 4/yr. CND 20 (effective 1999). adv. bk.rev. illus. *Refereed.* **Document type:** *Newsletter.*
Published by: Community Health Services Association, 455 2nd Ave N, Saskatoon, SK S7K 2C2, Canada. TEL 306-652-0300, FAX 306-664-4120, ad136@sfn.saskatoon.sk.ca. Ed., R&P Ingrid Larson. Adv. contact Ingrid Larsen. Circ: 5,300.

FOEDEVARENYT. see *FOOD AND FOOD INDUSTRIES*

614.8 USA
FOOD AND COSMETICS GUIDANCE MANUAL. Text in English. irreg. USD 140 in North America; USD 280 elsewhere. **Document type:** *Government.* **Description:** Provides the latest information on and helps maintain surveillance or compliance-oriented program plans and instructions directed to F.D.A. field operations, providing needed direction from headquarter offices and bureaus in accomplishing the F.D.A. regulatory obligations.
Published by: U.S. Food and Drug Administration, Office of Public Affairs, 5600 Fishers Ln, Rockville, MD 20857. TEL 301-443-3220. **Orders to:** National Technical Information Service, Government Research Center. FAX 703-321-8547.

362.1 GBR
FOOD FORUM. Text in English. q. GBP 88; GBP 108 foreign (effective 1999). **Document type:** *Bulletin, Trade.* **Description:** Provides current information to persons responsible for food safety.
Indexed: Food Sci.& Tech.Abstr.
Published by: Chartered Institute of Environmental Health, Publishing and Communications Division, Chadwick Court, 15 Hatfields, London SE1 8DJ, United Kingdom. TEL 44-20-7928-6006, FAX 44-20-7827-5866, m.randall@chgl.com, http://www.cieh.org.uk.

613.2 JPN ISSN 0015-6426
RA601 CODEN: SKEZAP
FOOD HYGIENIC SOCIETY OF JAPAN. JOURNAL/SHOKUHIN EISEIGAKU ZASSHI. Text in English, Japanese. 1960. bi-m. USD 72 to individuals; USD 180 to institutions. adv. bk.rev. abstr, charts, illus. index. *Refereed.* **Document type:** *Academic/Scholarly.*
Related titles: Online - full text ed.: (from Institute for Scientific Information).
Indexed: AESIS, Abstr.Hyg., AgBiotech, Anal.Abstr., Apic.Abstr., Aqua.Sci.& Fish.Abstr., Biol.Abstr., Chem.Abstr., Chem.Indus.Notes, Chem.Titles, Curr.Adv.Ecol.Sci., Curr.Cont., Dairy Sci.Abstr., Environ.Sci.Poll.Mgmt., Excerp.Med., Field Crop Abstr., Food Sci.& Tech.Abstr., Forest Prod.Abstr., Hort.Abstr., INIS Atomind., Ind.Med., Ind.Vet., Maize Abstr., Mass Spectr.Bull., Nutr.Abstr., Plant Breed.Abstr., Plant Grow.Reg.Abstr., Pollut.Abstr., Postharvest, Potato Abstr., Poult.Abstr., Protozool.Abstr., Rev.Appl.Entomol., Rev.Arom.& Med.Plants, Rev.Med.& Vet.Mycol., Rev.Plant Path., Rice Abstr., Risk Abstr., Saf.Sci.Abstr., Seed Abstr., Soyabean Abstr., Sugar Ind.Abstr., Triticale Abstr., Trop.Dis.Bull., Vet.Bull., Weed Abstr.
—BLDSC (4754.400000), CASDDS, CISTI, GNLM, IDS.
Published by: Food Hygienic Society of Japan/Nihon Shokuhin Eisei Gakkai, 2-6-1 Jingu-Mae, Shibuya-ku, Tokyo 150-0001, Japan. FAX 03-3470-2933.

613 USA ISSN 0884-0806
CODEN: FPREEP
FOOD PROTECTION REPORT. Text in English. 1985. m. (11/yr.). USD 149 (effective Oct. 2001). bk.rev. back issues avail.; reprints avail. **Document type:** *Newsletter.* **Description:** Includes information on food safety news, concerns, and techniques for members of the food industry, the government, and academia.
—BLDSC (3981.865100).
Published by: Pike & Fischer, Inc. (Subsidiary of: The Bureau of National Affairs, Inc.), 1010 Wayne Ave, Ste. 1400, Silver Springs, MD 20910-5600. TEL 301-562-1530, 800-255-8131, FAX 301-562-1521, pike@pf.com, http://www.pf.com. Ed. Ellen Morton. Pub., R&P U. Joseph Hecker.

363.19 GBR ISSN 0968-1647
FOOD SAFETY CONCERNS BULLETIN. Text in English. 1991. m. EUR 210 (effective 2002). **Document type:** *Trade.* **Description:** Contains compilation of articles on food safety issues as reported in the UK daily press. The Bulletin highlights topical issues, and subjects of continuing concern, both in the UK and worldwide.
Published by: Leatherhead Food R.A., Randalls Rd, Leatherhead, Surrey KT22 7RY, United Kingdom. TEL 44-1372-376761, FAX 44-1372-386228, hbennett@lfra.co.uk, http://www.lfra.co.uk. Ed. Richard Lawley.

▼ **FOOD SAFETY SOURCEBOOK.** see *FOOD AND FOOD INDUSTRIES*

614 FRA ISSN 0245-7466
FRANCE. MINISTERE CHARGE DE LA SANTE. BULLETIN EPIDEMIOLOGIQUE HEBDOMADAIRE. Abbreviated title: B E H. Text in French. w. FRF 280; FRF 380 in Europe; FRF 600 elsewhere. **Description:** For the practitioner; provides practical information, covers new diseases and recommendations for travelers.
Former titles: France. Ministere des la Sante et de la Famille. Bulletin Hebdomdaire d'Information Epidemiologique (0245-7474); France. Ministere des Affaires Sociales et de la Solidarite Nationale. Bulletin Epidemiologique; France. Ministere de la Sante et de la Famille. Bulletin Epidemiologique; France. Ministere de la Sante et de la Famille. Bulletin Epidemiologique
Indexed: Abstr.Hyg., Dairy Sci.Abstr., Helminthol.Abstr., Ind.Vet., Nutr.Abstr., Protozool.Abstr., Rev.Appl.Entomol., Rev.Med.& Vet.Mycol., Trop.Dis.Bull., Vet.Bull.
—BLDSC (2853.440000).
Published by: (France. Ministere Charge de la Sante), Imprimerie Nationale, 25 rue de la Convention, Paris Cedex 15 75732, France. TEL 33-1-40157000, FAX 33-1-40157230. Circ: 650.

P

614 FRA
FRANCE. MINISTERE DE LA SANTE ET DE LA SECURITE SOCIALE. BULLETIN OFFICIEL. Text in French. w. FRF 110.
Published by: Ministere de la Sante et de la Securite Sociale, 8 av. de Segur, Paris 75700, France.

614 FRA
FRANCE. MINISTERE DE LA SANTE ET DE LA SECURITE SOCIALE. NOTES D'INFORMATION. Text in French. 1969. irreg., latest vol.145, 1980. free per issue.
Former titles: France. Ministere de la Sante. Note d'Information (0071-8882); (until 1969): France. Ministere des Affaires Sociales. Information Actualites
Published by: Ministere de la Sante et de la Securite Sociale, 8 av. de Segur, Paris 75700, France.

FRANCE. MINISTERE DE LA SOLIDARITE, DE LA SANTE ET DE LA PROTECTION SOCIALE. BULLETIN OFFICIEL. see *BIBLIOGRAPHIES*

614 FRA ISSN 0755-3374
RA407.5.F7
FRANCE. MINISTERE DE L'EMPLOI ET DE LA SOLIDARITE. ANNUAIRE DES STATISTIQUES SANITAIRES ET SOCIALES. Text in French. 1971. a., latest 1998. FRF 320 newsstand/cover. **Document type:** *Government.*
Supersedes: France. Ministere de la Sante et de la Securite Sociale. Tableaux Statistiques "Sante et Securite Sociale"; France. Ministere de la Sante. Tableaux Sante et Securite Sociale; France. Ministere de la Sante Publique et de la Securite Sociale. Annuaire Statistique de la Sante et de l'Action Sociale (0071-8866)
Published by: (France. Ministere des Affaires Sociales et de la Solidarite Nationale, Ministere Charge de l 'Emploi, France. Ministere de l'Emploi et de la Solidarite), Documentation Francaise, 29-31 quai Voltaire, Paris Cedex 7 75344, France. FAX 33-1-40157230, libparis@ladocfrancaise.gouv.fr.

FRANCE. MINISTERE DES AFFAIRES SOCIALES DE LA SANTE ET DE LA VILLE. BULLETIN OFFICIEL. see *PUBLIC ADMINISTRATION*

614.86 CHE
FREIE FAHRT/ROUTE LIBRE. Text in French, German. 1923. m. CHF 10. adv. illus. **Document type:** *Bulletin.*
Former titles: Strasse und Nuechternheit (0039-2170); Abstinenter Rad- und Motorfahrer
Published by: Schweizerischer Abstinenten-Verkehrsverband/Association Suisse des Conducteurs Abstinents, Zentralsekretariat, Langwiesstr 22, Zuerich 8050, Switzerland. TEL 01-3115880. Ed. Peter Ritschard Inaunen. Circ: 2,000.

362.1 USA
FUNDING WATCH. Text in English. 1990. m. free in state. **Document type:** *Newsletter, Government.* **Description:** Reports on public health-related funding to organizations in Texas.
Formerly (until July 1996): HIV Funding Watch
Published by: Texas Department of Health, Funding Information Center, 1100 W 49th St, Austin, TX 78756-3199. TEL 512-458-7684, FAX 512-458-7683, fundctr@tdh.state.tx.us, http://www.tdh.state.tx.us. Ed. Darlene Murray. Circ: (controlled).

362.1 NLD
FUTURE HEALTH SCENARIOS. Text in English. 1987. irreg., latest vol.23, 1994. price varies. back issues avail. **Document type:** *Proceedings.* **Description:** Publishes studies on changes and projections in health care and health technology.
Published by: (Scenario Commission on Future Health Care Technology), Kluwer Academic Publishers Group (Subsidiary of: Wolters Kluwer N.V.), Spuiboulevard 50, PO Box 17, Dordrecht 3300 AA, Netherlands. FAX 31-78-639-2254, services@wkap.nl, http://www.wkap.nl. **Dist. by:** Journals Department, PO Box 322, Dordrecht 3300 AH, Netherlands. FAX 31-78-654-6474.

P

THE FUTURE OF CHILDREN. see *CHILDREN AND YOUTH—About*

363.7 DEU ISSN 0932-6200
CODEN: GHBUEG
G I - GESUNDHEITS INGENIEUR; Haustechnik - Bauphysik - Umwelttechnik. Text in German. 1877. bi-m. DEM 296 domestic; DEM 302 foreign (effective 2001). adv. bk.rev. abstr, bibl, charts, illus, pat. index. **Document type:** *Journal, Trade.*
Former titles (until 1985): Haustechnik, Bauphysik, Umwelttechnik (0172-8199); Gesundheits-Ingenieur (0016-9277)
Indexed: Biol.Abstr., Chem.Abstr., Eng.Ind., Excerp.Med., INIS Atomind., Ind.Med. (coverage dropped), Int.Build.Serv.Abstr., W.R.C.Inf.
—CASDDS, CISTI, GNLM, Infotrieve, Linda Hall. **CCC.**
Published by: Oldenbourg Wissenschaftsverlag GmbH, Rosenheimer Str 145, Munich 81571, Germany. TEL 49-89-45051339, FAX 49-89-45051333, vertrieb-zs@verlag.oldenbourg.de, http://www.oldenbourg.de. Circ: 4,000.

610 ESP ISSN 0213-9111
GACETA SANITARIA. Text in Spanish; Summaries in English. 1982. bi-m. ESP 10,800 to individuals; ESP 18,000 to institutions; ESP 8,640 to students (effective 2001). adv. bk.rev. bibl, charts. back issues avail.; reprints avail. *Refereed.* **Document type:** *Academic/Scholarly.*
Former titles (until 1986): Gaseta Sanitaria de Barcelona (0212-0542); (1888-1910): Gaceta Sanitaria de Barcelona (0212-2030)
Related titles: Online - full text ed.: 1996.
Indexed: Abstr.Hyg., Ind.Med. (1987-), Ind.Med.Esp., Int.Nurs.Ind.
—BLDSC (4066.169000), CINDOC, GNLM, Infotrieve. **CCC.**
Published by: (Sociedad Espanola de Salud Publica y Administracion Sanitaria), Ediciones Doyma S.A., Traversa de Gracia, 17-21, Barcelona 08021, Spain. TEL 34-93-200-0711, gs@doyma.es, doyma@doyma.es, http://www.doyma.es/gs. Ed. Antoni Plasencia. R&P Monica Barnes. Adv. contact Jose Antonio Hernandez. B&W page ESP 10,300, color page ESP 124,000; 280 x 210. Circ: 3,000.

614 GBR
GATESHEAD AND SOUTH TYNESIDE HEALTH AUTHORITY. DIRECTOR OF PUBLIC HEALTH. ANNUAL REPORT. Text in English. a. **Document type:** *Government.*
Former titles: South of Tyne Health Commission. Director of Public Health. Annual Report; South Tyneside Health Authority. Director of Public Health. Annual Report
—BLDSC (1230.356000).
Published by: Gateshead and South Tyneside Health Authority, Director of Public Health, Horsley Hill Rd, S. Shields, Tyne & Wear NE33 3BN, United Kingdom. TEL 44-191-401-4500, FAX 44-191-401-4520. R&P Rajan Madhok.

DE GEHEEL-ONTHOUDER. see *DRUG ABUSE AND ALCOHOLISM*

GENETIC RESOURCE. see *BIOLOGY—Genetics*

613 AUT
GESUNDE STADT. Text in German. q. adv. **Document type:** *Magazine, Consumer.*
Published by: D und R Verlagsgesellschaft mbH, Leberstr 122, Vienna 1110, Austria. TEL 43-1-740770, FAX 43-1-74077841, office@d-r.at. Ed. Uschi Korda. Adv. contact Michael Scharnagl. B&W page XEU 2,180.19, color page XEU 2,906.91; trim 210 x 297. Circ: 20,000 (controlled).

614 DEU ISSN 0948-3438
GESUNDHEITSPOLITIK. Text in German. 1995. bi-m. DEM 250 (effective 1999). **Document type:** *Academic/Scholarly.*
—GNLM.
Published by: P M I Verlag AG, August-Schanz-Str 8, Frankfurt Am Main 60433, Germany. TEL 49-69-548000-0, FAX 49-69-548000-77, pmiverlag@aol.com.

614 CHE ISSN 1420-5947
GESUNDHEITSPOLITISCHE INFORMATIONEN/ POLITIQUE DE LA SANTE: INFORMATIONS. Short title: G P I. Text in Multiple languages. 1977. 4/yr. USD 60 (effective 2001). bk.rev., Website rev. abstr, bibl, charts, stat. 46 p./no. **Document type:** *Newsletter, Consumer.* **Description:** Examines health policies, health economics, medical sociology, patients' legal and human rights as well as related economic topics.
Published by: Schweizerische Gesellschaft fuer Gesundheitspolitik/Societe Suisse pour la Politique de la Sante (Swiss Society for Health Policy), Haldenweg 10 A, Muri B. Bern 3074, Switzerland. TEL 41-31-9526655, FAX 41-31-952-6800, info@sggp.ch. Ed. Gerhard Kocher. Circ: 2,200.

614 DEU ISSN 0941-3790
CODEN: GHWNFX
DAS GESUNDHEITSWESEN; Sozialmedizin, Gesundheits-System-Forschung, Public Health, Education, Oeffentlicher Gesundheitsdienst, Medizinischer Dienst. Text in German. 1939. 12/yr. EUR 196.40 domestic to institutions; EUR 207.20 in Europe to institutions; EUR 216.80 elsewhere to institutions; EUR 19 newsstand/cover (effective 2002). adv. bk.rev. abstr, charts, illus. index. reprint service avail. from PQC. *Refereed.* **Document type:** *Journal, Academic/Scholarly.*
Former titles (until 1992): Oeffentliche Gesundheitswesen (0029-8573); Oeffentliche Gesundheitsdienst
Related titles: Microform ed.: (from PQC); Online - full text ed.: ISSN 1439-4421 (from Institute for Scientific Information).
Indexed: Abstr.Hyg., C.I.S. Abstr., Curr.Cont., Food Sci.& Tech.Abstr., Helminthol.Abstr., INIS Atomind., Ind.Med. (1992-), Ind.Vet., Int.Nurs.Ind., Nutr.Abstr., Protozool.Abstr., Rev.Appl.Entomol., SSCI, Sci.Cit.Ind. (coverage dropped), Soils & Fert., Trop.Dis.Bull., Vet.Bull.
—BLDSC (4165.078500), CISTI, GNLM, IDS, Infotrieve, KNAW. **CCC.**
Published by: (Bundesverband der Aerzte des Oeffentlichen Gesundheitsdienstes e.V.), Georg Thieme Verlag, Ruedigerstr 14, Stuttgart 70469, Germany. TEL 49-711-8931-0, FAX 49-711-8931298, kunden.service@thieme.de, http://www.thieme.de/gesu. Ed. J Gostomzyk. R&P Peter Eich. adv.: page DEM 2,300; 175 x 250. Circ: 1,800. **Co-sponsors:** Berufsverband der Sozialversicherungsaerzte Deutschlands e.V.; Deutsche Gesellschaft fuer Sozialmedizin und Praevention; Deutsche Gesellschaft fuer Public Health e.V.; Gesellschaft fuer Medizinische Ausbildung e.V.

353.6 NLD ISSN 1389-5702
▼ **GLOBAL CHANGE & HUMAN HEALTH.** Text in English. 2000. s-a. EUR 407, USD 408 to institutions for print or online ed.; EUR 488.40, USD 489.60 to institutions for print & online eds combined (effective 2001). **Document type:** *Journal, Academic/Scholarly.* **Description:** Covers the health impact of various social, economic, technological and environmental global changes.
Related titles: Online - full text ed.: (from Swets Blackwell, Kluwer Online, RoweCom Information Quest).
—BLDSC (4195.358320).
Published by: Kluwer Academic Publishers Group (Subsidiary of: Wolters Kluwer N.V.), Spuiboulevard 50, PO Box 17, Dordrecht 3300 AA, Netherlands. TEL 31-78-639-2392, FAX 31-78-654-2254, services@wkap.nl, http://www.wkap.nl/journalhome.htm/1389-5702. Eds. Jonathan Patz, Pim Martens, Tony McMichael. **Subscr. in the Americas to:** Kluwer Academic - Plenum Publishers, 233 Spring St, New York, NY 10013-1578. TEL 212-620-8468, FAX 212-807-1047; **Subscr. to:** Journals Department, PO Box 322, Dordrecht 3300 AH, Netherlands. TEL 31-78-639-2392, FAX 31-78-654-6474.

628 642.9 VGB ISSN 1461-765X
GLOBAL HEALTH (ASIAN EDITION). Text in English. 1980. m. adv. illus. **Document type:** *Journal, Trade.*
Formerly (until 1996): Far East Health (0143-0645)
Related titles: ♦ Regional ed.: Global Health (Middle East Edition). ISSN 1367-353X.
Indexed: ASSIA.
Published by: P D S Ltd, Cutlass House, Wickham Quay, Tortola, Virgin Isl., UK. Pub. Brian Wilkie. Circ: 5,875.

614 VGB ISSN 1367-353X
GLOBAL HEALTH (MIDDLE EAST EDITION). Text in English. 1977. m. adv. illus. **Document type:** *Trade.* **Description:** Publishes clinical and experimental articles on health issues worldwide.
Former titles (until 1996): Middle East Health (0263-1016); Which incorporated (in 1986): Middle East Dentistry; Formerly (until 1981): Middle East Health Supply and Services (0309-2003)
Related titles: ♦ Regional ed.: Global Health (Asian Edition). ISSN 1461-765X.
—CISTI.
Published by: P D S Ltd, Cutlass House, Wickham Quay, Tortola, Virgin Isl., UK. claremed@dircon.co.uk. Pub. Brian Wilkie. Circ: 60,000.

GOOD PRACTICE SERIES. see *SOCIAL SERVICES AND WELFARE*

GREAT BRITAIN. DEPARTMENT OF EDUCATION AND SCIENCE. SAFETY IN EDUCATION. see *EDUCATION—School Organization And Administration*

614 GBR ISSN 0072-6087
RA241
GREAT BRITAIN. DEPARTMENT OF HEALTH. ON THE STATE OF THE PUBLIC HEALTH. Key Title: On the State of the Public Health. Text in English. 1921. a. price varies. reprint service avail. from PQC. **Document type:** *Government.*
Formerly: Great Britain. Department of Health and Social Security. On the State of the Public Health
—CISTI. **CCC.**
Published by: (Great Britain. Department of Health), Stationery Office, 51 Nine Elms Ln, London SW8 5DA, United Kingdom. TEL 44-20-7873-0011, FAX 44-20-7873-8247, book.orders@theso.co.uk, http://www.national-publishing.co.uk.

614 GBR
GREAT BRITAIN. DEPARTMENT OF HEALTH. WELSH OFFICE AND SCOTTISH OFFICE. BACKGROUND PAPER. Text in English. irreg. **Document type:** *Monographic series, Government.*
Published by: Scottish Office, Home and Health Department, Scottish Office, St Andrews House, Regent Rd, Edinburgh EH1 3DG, United Kingdom.

362.1 363.11 GBR ISSN 1363-0695
GREAT BRITAIN. HEALTH & SAFETY EXECUTIVE. TECHNOLOGY AND HEALTH SCIENCES DIVISION. SPECIALIST INSPECTOR REPORTS. Text in English. irreg. back issues avail. **Document type:** *Monographic series, Government.* **Description:** Examines issues in public and occupational health and safety.
Formerly (until 1992): Great Britain. Health & Safety Executive. Technology Division. Specialist Inspector Reports (0963-3472)
Published by: Health and Safety Executive, Rose Ct, 2 Southwark Bridge, London SE1 9HS, United Kingdom. public.enquiries@hse.gov.uk, http://www.hse.gov.uk.

614.3 GBR
GREAT BRITAIN. MEDICINES ACT 1968 ADVISORY BODIES. ANNUAL REPORT. Text in English. 1971. a., latest 1998. GBP 8. **Document type:** *Government.* **Description:** Contains the reports of the Medicines Commission, the Committee on Safety of Medicines, the Veterinary Products Committee, the British Pharmacopoeia Commission, and the Advisory Board on the Registration of Homeopathic Products.

Former titles: Great Britain. Medicines Commission. Annual Report.; Great Britain. Committee on Safety of Medicines. Report
Published by: Department of Health, Medicines Control Agency, Market Towers, 1 Nine Elms Ln, London SW8 5DA, United Kingdom. TEL 44-20-7273-0648, FAX 44-20-7273-0020. Ed. Sue Jones. R&P Juliet Male TEL 44-171-273-0677. Circ: 600.

628 ITA
GUIDA MONACI. ANNUARIO DELLA SANITA. Text in Italian. 1952. a. ITL 340,000 (effective 1999). adv. index. **Document type:** *Directory.* **Description:** Directory of all Italian public health organizations and bodies, medical products and equipment manufacturers.
Formerly: Guida Monaci. Annuario Sanitario Italiano; Guida Monaci. Annuario Sanitario (0390-9263); (until 1974): Rome Sanitaria
Published by: Guida Monaci S.p.A., Via Salaria, 1319, Rome, RM 00138, Italy. TEL 39-6-3331333, FAX 39-6-3335555, guida.monaci@italybygm.it, http://www.italybygm.it. adv.: B&W page ITL 11,500,000; trim 260 x 186.

613.69 USA
GUIDE TO DELEGATE PREPARATION. MODEL U.N. SURVIVAL KIT. Text in English. 1989. a. USD 15. **Document type:** *Academic/Scholarly.*
Indexed: Appl.Mech.Rev.
Published by: United Nations Association of the USA, 801 Second Ave, New York, NY 10017-4706. TEL 212-907-1300, FAX 212-682-9185, unahq@unausa.org. Ed. Fernando A Flores. R&P Susan Woolfson.

GUILDER. see *HANDICAPPED—Hearing Impaired*

THE GUTTMACHER REPORT ON PUBLIC POLICY. see *BIRTH CONTROL*

614 PHL
H E A P JOURNAL. Text in English. 1961. q. PHP 2, USD 1.25. bk.rev.
Formerly: School Health Bulletin (0048-9417)
Published by: Philippine Normal College, Community-School Health Education Center, Taft Ave, Manila 2801, Philippines. Ed. Carmen F del Rosario. Circ: 100.

HANDGUN CONTROL. SEMI-ANNUAL PROGRESS REPORT. see *LAW*

628 DEU
HARTMANNBUND IN BADEN - WUERTTEMBERG. Text in German. 1949. q. **Document type:** *Journal, Trade.*
Published by: Hartmannbund - Verband der Aerzte Deutschlands e.V., Godesberger Allee 54, Bonn 53175, Germany. TEL 49-228-8104-0, FAX 49-228-8104155, hb-info@hartmannbund.de, http://www.hartmannbund.de.

616.98 USA
HARVARD MEDICAL SCHOOL. CENTER FOR HEALTH AND THE GLOBAL ENVIRONMENT. NEWSLETTER. Text in English. q. **Document type:** *Newsletter.* **Description:** Covers current research, news reports, events and debates concerning human health and the global environmental change.
Media: Online - full text.
Address: 164 Longwood Ave, Boston, MA 02115. chge@warren.med.harvard.edu, http://www.med.harvard.edu/chge/newstoc.html.

614 IND ISSN 0017-8241
RA312.H37
HARYANA HEALTH JOURNAL. Text in English. 1970. q. free per issue. charts, illus. **Description:** Presents information about developments in medical and health services, oriented to health care professionals.
Published by: State Health Education Bureau, Directorate of Health Services, 36 Madhaya Marg, Sector 7C, Chandigarh, Haryana, India. Ed. G G Saxena. Circ: (controlled).

HAWAII. DEPARTMENT OF HEALTH. MENTAL HEALTH SERVICES FOR CHILDREN AND YOUTH; children's MH services branch. see *SOCIAL SERVICES AND WELFARE*

614 USA ISSN 1053-9662
HAWAII HEALTH MESSENGER. Text in English. 1941. q. free per issue. charts, illus. **Document type:** *Newsletter.*
Published by: Department of Health, Communication Office, PO Box 3378, Honolulu, HI 96801. TEL 808-586-4442, FAX 808-586-4444. Ed. Barbara Hastings. Circ: 5,500 (controlled).

614 AUS ISSN 1320-0593
HAZARD. Text in English. 1988. q. *Refereed.* **Document type:** *Bulletin.* **Description:** Disseminates information about injuries and their prevention.
Published by: Victorian Injury Surveillance and Applied Research System, Accident Research Centre, Monash University, PO Box 70A, Clayton, VIC 3800, Australia. TEL 61-3-9905-1805, FAX 61-3-9905-1809, visar.enquire@general.monash.edu.au, http://www.general.monash.edu.au/muarc/visar/Haz.htm. R&P Karen Ashby.

614.8 USA ISSN 0743-8826
TA169.7
HAZARD PREVENTION∗ . Text in English. 1965. q. USD 45 to non-members. adv. bk.rev. back issues avail. **Description:** Technical information and news of topical interest to those associated with the practice of system and product safety.
Related titles: Microfiche ed.: 1965.
Indexed: Aqua.Sci.& Fish.Abstr., Environ.Sci.Poll.Mgmt., Pollut.Abstr., Risk Abstr., Saf.Sci.Abstr.
—CISTI.
Published by: System Safety Society, Inc., 30363 Hicks Rd, Spotsylvania, VA 22553-5525. TEL 703-444-6520. Ed. Sonya Kaiser. Circ: 1,700.

HAZARD TECHNOLOGY. see *CIVIL DEFENSE*

363.17 USA ISSN 0889-3454
HAZARDOUS MATERIALS NEWSLETTER. Text in English. 1980. bi-m. USD 47 in North America; USD 55 elsewhere (effective 2001). adv. bk.rev. abstr, bibl, tr.lit. 12 p./no. back issues avail. **Document type:** *Newsletter.* **Description:** Addresses leak, fire, spill control for incident commanders and experienced responders. Covers incident causes, prevention, remedial action, chemical and biological agents.
Published by: Hazardous Materials Publishing, 89 Silver Circle, PO Box 204, Barre, VT 05641. TEL 802-479-2307, haznews@aol.com. Ed., R&P John R Cashman TEL 888-433-5366. Adv. contact Maralyn Nolan TEL 888-433-5366. Circ: 467 (paid and free).

363.73 USA ISSN 1076-8920
HAZARDOUS SUBSTANCES & PUBLIC HEALTH. Text in English. 1990. q. free per issue. adv. bk.rev. illus. reprints avail. **Document type:** *Newsletter, Government.* **Description:** Aims to increase awareness and educate environmental and public health professionals and others about the effect of hazardous substances on health; how to prevent exposure to hazardous substances; and how to more effectively communicate hazardous substances and environmental health information.
Indexed: CINAHL, Environ.Abstr., Ind.Hyg.Dig.
—BLDSC (4274.451300).
Published by: U.S. Department of Health and Human Services, Agency for Toxic Substances and Disease Registry, 1600 Clifton Rd, N E, Mail Stop E 33, Atlanta, GA 30333. TEL 404-639-5017, FAX 404-639-0560, GBM7@cdc.gov, http://atsdr1.atsdr.cdc.gov:8080/HEC?hsphhome.html. Ed., R&P, Adv. contact Georgia Moore. Circ: 10,000.

HAZARDOUS WASTE CONSULTANT. see *ENVIRONMENTAL STUDIES—Waste Management*

HAZARDOUS WASTE REGULATORY ANALYSIS SERVICE. see *ENVIRONMENTAL STUDIES—Waste Management*

HAZARDS MAGAZINE. see *OCCUPATIONAL HEALTH AND SAFETY*

614 GBR ISSN 1363-4593
RA418
HEALTH; an interdisciplinary journal for the social study of health, illness and medicine. Text in English. 1997. q. GBP 39 to individuals; GBP 195 to institutions; GBP 11 newsstand/cover to individuals; GBP 50 newsstand/cover to institutions (effective 2002). adv. bk.rev. back issues avail. *Refereed.* **Document type:** *Academic/Scholarly.* **Description:** Focuses on the changing place of health matters in modern society.
Related titles: Online - full text ed.: (from EBSCO Publishing, O C L C Online Computer Library Center, Inc., RoweCom Information Quest, ingenta, Swets Blackwell).
Indexed: Brit.Nur.Ind., Soc.Serv.Abstr., Sociol.Abstr.
—BLDSC (4274.694140).
Published by: Sage Publications Ltd., 6 Bonhill St, London EC2A 4PU, United Kingdom. TEL 44-20-7374-0645, FAX 44-20-7374-8741, market@sagepub.co.uk, http://www.sagepub.co.uk. Ed. Alan Radley. Adv. contact Jenny Kirby. page GBP 220; trim 189 x 114. Circ: 850.

614 JOR
HEALTH/SIHHAH. Text in Arabic. 1966. m.
Published by: Ministry of Health, P O Box 86, Amman, Jordan. Ed. Dr. Ahmad Al Nabulsi.

368.382 USA ISSN 0278-2715
RA410.A1
HEALTH AFFAIRS; the policy journal of the health sphere. Text in English. 1981. bi-m. USD 85 domestic to individuals; USD 140 out of North America to individuals; USD 139 domestic to institutions; USD 175 out of North America to institutions (effective 1999). bk.rev. back issues avail.; reprint service avail. from PQC. *Refereed.* **Document type:** *Academic/Scholarly.* **Description:** A health care policy and managed care journal that addresses health care system change from the perspectives of all its players, through data, analysis, policy proposals, and commentary.
Related titles: Microform ed.: (from PQC); Online - full text ed.: (from ProQuest Information & Learning, Northern Light Technology, Inc., LexisNexis, O C L C Online Computer Library Center, Inc., CatchWord Ltd., Factiva, Institute for Scientific Information).
Indexed: ABI Inform. (Spr.1987-), ASCA, Abstr.Health Care Manage.Stud., AgeLine, BPIA, Biostat., Brit.Nur.Ind., Crim.Just.Abstr., Curr.Cont., Excerp.Med., Hosp.Lit.Ind., I.P.A., Ind.Med. (1981-), Int.Nurs.Ind., Int.Polit.Sci.Abstr., Manage.Cont., P.A.I.S., PSI, Ref.Zh., SSCI, Sci.Cit.Ind.
—BLDSC (4274.710000), CISTI, EMDOCS, GNLM, IDS, ingenta, KNAW. **CCC.**
Published by: Project Hope, 7500 Old Georgetown Rd, 600, Bethesda, MD 20814-6133. TEL 301-656-7401, FAX 301-654-2845, healthaffair@projhope.org; orders@allenpress.com, http://www.projhope.org/HA/; http://www.allenpress.com. Ed. John K Iglehart. R&P Judie Tucker. Circ: 8,000 (paid). **Subscr. to:** Allen Press Inc., PO Box 1897, Lawrence, KS 66044-8897. **Dist. by:** P O Box 148, Congers, NY 10920.

614 GBR
HEALTH & HOUSING INSIGHT. Text in English. q. GBP 65; GBP 72 foreign. **Document type:** *Bulletin, Trade.* **Description:** Places the legal aspects of housing issues under the spotlight, interpreting the law and its effect on housing professionals.
Published by: Chartered Institute of Environmental Health, Publishing and Communications Division, Chadwick Court, 15 Hatfields, London SE1 8DJ, United Kingdom. TEL 44-20-7928-6006, FAX 44-20-7827-5866, m.randall@chgl.com, http://www.cieh.org.uk.

362.1 USA ISSN 1079-0969
RA394 CODEN: HHRIF4
HEALTH AND HUMAN RIGHTS; an international journal. Text in English; Summaries in English, French, Spanish. 1995. 2/yr. USD 28 domestic to individuals; USD 34 in Canada to individuals; USD 36 elsewhere to individuals; USD 60 domestic to institutions; USD 66 in Canada to institutions; USD 68 elsewhere to institutions; USD 15 newsstand/cover (effective 2000). bk.rev. bibl. back issues avail. *Refereed.* **Document type:** *Journal, Academic/Scholarly.* **Description:** Examines the impacts of health policies, programs, and practices on human rights and the effects of human rights violations on public health.
Indexed: ASSIA, Geo.Abstr.H.G., IDA, Ind.Med. (1994-), Intl.Bibl.Soc.Sci., Lang.& Lang.Behav.Abstr., P.A.I.S., Per.Islam. (1994-), SOPODA, Soc.Serv.Abstr., Sociol.Abstr.
—BLDSC (4274.814900).
Published by: Harvard School for Public Health, Francois-Xavier Bagnoud Center for Health and Human Rights, 651 Huntington Ave, 7th fl, Boston, MA 02115. TEL 617-432-0656, FAX 617-432-4310, fxbcenter@igc.org, http://www.hri.ca/partners/fxbcenter; http://www.harvard.edu. Ed. Sofia Gruskin. R&P Laura Horton TEL 617-432-4311. Circ: 449 (paid); 619 (controlled). **Subscr. to:** 651 Huntington Ave., 7th fl., Boston, MA 02115. TEL 617-432-4611. **Co-sponsor:** Association Francois-Xavier Bagnoud.

614 GBR ISSN 0140-2986
RA421 CODEN: HEHYDD
HEALTH AND HYGIENE. Text in English. 1977. q. GBP 48 in Europe; GBP 53 elsewhere (effective 2000). adv. bk.rev. back issues avail. *Refereed.* **Document type:** *Academic/Scholarly.* **Description:** Contains information on environmental health, health education, food hygiene and medical and social issues the food industry, as well as the teaching, nursing and medical professions. Also includes legislation updates and sample answers to RIPHH exam questions.
Related titles: Online - full text ed.: (from ProQuest Information & Learning).
Indexed: Abstr.Hyg., Curr.Adv.Ecol.Sci., Excerp.Med., Ind.Vet., Trop.Dis.Bull.
—BLDSC (4274.815000), GNLM.

P

Published by: Royal Institute of Public Health and Hygiene, 28 Portland Pl, London W1N 4DE, United Kingdom. TEL 44-207-580-2731, FAX 44-207-580-6157, health.hygiene@riphh.org.uk. Ed. Dr. Rosalind Stanwell Smith. R&P A C Lagden. Circ: 2,600.

HEALTH AND MEDICINE MUSEUMS NEWSLETTER. see *MUSEUMS AND ART GALLERIES*

614 GBR
HEALTH AND PERSONAL SOCIAL SERVICES STATISTICS. Text in English. a. GBP 16.50. reprint service avail. from PQC. **Document type:** *Government.*
Formerly: Digest of Health Statistics for England and Wales (0070-4849)
Related titles: Microfiche ed.: (from CHL).
—BLDSC (4274.828000).
Published by: Stationery Office, 51 Nine Elms Ln, London SW8 5DA, United Kingdom. TEL 44-20-7873-0011, FAX 44-20-7873-8247, book.orders@theso.co.uk, http://www.national-publishing.co.uk.

HEALTH & PLACE; an international journal. see *GEOGRAPHY*

614 GBR
HEALTH & SAFETY BULLETIN. Text in English. q. GBP 90; GBP 100 foreign. **Document type:** *Bulletin, Trade.* **Description:** Aimed at enforcement professionals. Provides a forum for sharing sensitive health and safety information, news of liaisons, details of prosecutions, and updates on the newest regulations.
Indexed: Mgmt.& Market.Abstr.
Published by: Chartered Institute of Environmental Health, Publishing and Communications Division, Chadwick Court, 15 Hatfields, London SE1 8DJ, United Kingdom. TEL 44-20-7928-6006, FAX 44-20-7827-5866, m.randall@chgl.com, http://www.cieh.org.uk.

HEALTH & SAFETY MARKETGUIDE. see *BUSINESS AND ECONOMICS—Trade And Industrial Directories*

628 621.3 GBR ISSN 0142-5021
HEALTH & SAFETY NEWSLINE; for the engineering industry (UK). Text in English. 1968. bi-m. GBP 45 (effective 2000). bk.rev., film rev. **Document type:** *Newsletter, Trade.* **Description:** Keeps company management abreast of occupational health, safety and environmental developments in the UK.
Formerly (until 1984): Industrial Health and Safety
Published by: Engineering Employers' Federation, Broadway House, Tothill St, London SW1H 9NQ, United Kingdom. TEL 44-207-222-7777, FAX 44-20-7976-8056. Ed. Steve Walters. Circ: 8,000 (controlled).

362.1 341 NLD
HEALTH AND SAFETY REGULATIONS; international and national laws. Text in English. base vol. plus a. updates. Supplement avail. **Description:** Considers health and safety regulations in an international setting. Covers the EU, US, Japan and other major trading nations.
Published by: Kluwer Law International (Subsidiary of: Wolters Kluwer N.V.), Laan van Meerdervoort 70, PO Box 85889, The Hague 2508 CN, Netherlands. TEL 31-70-308-1500, FAX 31-70-308-1515, services@wkap.nl, http://www.wkap.nl. Ed. Kenneth S Kilimnik. **Dist. by:** Libresso Distribution Centre, PO Box 23, Deventer 7400 GA, Netherlands. TEL 31-570-633155, FAX 31-570-633834.

HEALTH AND SAFETY SCIENCE ABSTRACTS. see *PUBLIC HEALTH AND SAFETY—Abstracting, Bibliographies, Statistics*

362.1 363.1 GBR
HEALTH & SAFETY SPECIFIERS; health, safety and environmental safety. Text in English. 1974. 6/yr. GBP 24 (effective 2000). adv. bk.rev. **Document type:** *Trade.*
Former titles: Health and Safety Specifications; Caution Magazine
Published by: Specifiers Journals Ltd, 32 Portland St, Cheltenham, Glos GL52 2PB, United Kingdom. TEL 44-1242-236336, FAX 44-1242-222331. Ed. Debbie Preece. R&P David Constantine. Adv. contact Peter Hebblethwaite. Circ: 14,433.

614 GBR ISSN 0966-0410
HV1 CODEN: HSCCEL
HEALTH AND SOCIAL CARE IN THE COMMUNITY. Text in English. 1993. bi-m., latest vol.10, 2002. GBP 66 in Europe to individuals; USD 106 in North America to individuals; GBP 73 elsewhere to individuals; GBP 299 in Europe to institutions; USD 474 in North America to institutions; GBP 329 elsewhere to institutions (effective 2002). adv. bk.rev. bibl. index. back issues avail. *Refereed.* **Document type:** *Academic/Scholarly.* **Description:** Publishes original papers that reflect the broad range of practical and theoretical issues underpinning the provision of care in the community.
Related titles: Microform ed.: (from PQC); ♦ Online - full text ed.: Health and Social Care in the Community Online. ISSN 1365-2524.
Indexed: AMED, ASCA, ASSIA, AgeLine, Brit.Nur.Ind., CINAHL, Curr.Cont., Fam.Ind., SSCI, Soc.Serv.Abstr., Sociol.Abstr.
—BLDSC (4274.874000), GNLM, IDS, Infotrieve. **CCC.**
Published by: Blackwell Science Ltd., PO Box 88, Oxford OX2 0NE, United Kingdom. TEL 44-1865-206180, 44-1865-206002, FAX 44-1865-206219, jnl.orders@blacksci.co.uk, http://www.blackwell-science.com/products/journals/hscc.htm, http://www.blackwellpublishing.com. Ed. Karen A Luker. Pub. Elaine Stott. R&P Sophie Savage. Adv. contact Jenny Applin. Circ: 425.

614 GBR ISSN 1365-2524
▼ **HEALTH AND SOCIAL CARE IN THE COMMUNITY ONLINE.** Text in English. 1999. bi-m. GBP 60 in Europe to individuals; USD 96 in North America to individuals; GBP 60 elsewhere to individuals; GBP 270 in Europe to institutions; USD 427 in North America to institutions; GBP 270 elsewhere to institutions (effective 2002). *Refereed.* **Document type:** *Academic/Scholarly.*
Media: Online - full text (from EBSCO Publishing, Munksgaard & Blackwell Science's Synergy, O C L C Online Computer Library Center, Inc., RoweCom Information Quest, ingenta, Swets Blackwell, Institute for Scientific Information). **Related titles:** Microform ed.: (from PQC); ♦ Print ed.: Health and Social Care in the Community. ISSN 0966-0410.
Published by: Blackwell Science Ltd., Osney Mead, Oxford OX2 0EL, United Kingdom. TEL 44-1685-206206, FAX 44-1685-721205, website@blacksci.com, journals.cs@blacksci.co.uk, http://www.blackwell-science.com.

614 360 CAN ISSN 1184-650X
HEALTH AND SOCIAL SERVICE WORKFORCE IN ALBERTA. Text in English. 1979. a. back issues avail. **Description:** Contains data and information on the health and social services of employers and self-employed professionals.
Former titles (until 1990): Health and Social Service Personnel Working in Alberta (1184-6496); (until 1986): Survey of Health and Social Service Personnel Working in Alberta (1184-6488); (until 1984): Survey of Employers of Health and Social Service Personnel in Alberta (1184-647X); (until 1981): Survey of the Major Employers of Health and Social Service Personnel (1184-6461); (until 1980): Semi-Annual Surveys of the Major Employers of Health and Social Service Personnel (0225-9834)
Published by: Health and Social Service Disciplines Committee, Kensington Place, 5th Fl, 10011 109th St, Edmonton, AB T5J 3S8, Canada. TEL 403-427-2655.

HEALTH & SOCIAL WORK. see *SOCIAL SERVICES AND WELFARE*

362.1 USA ISSN 1088-4653
HEALTH CARE COST REENGINEERING REPORT. Variant title: Cost Reengineering Report. Text in English. 1996. m. USD 279; USD 289 in Canada & Mexico; USD 299 elsewhere. **Document type:** *Trade.*
Indexed: Int.Nurs.Ind.
Published by: National Health Information, LLC, PO Box 15429, Atlanta, GA 30333. TEL 404-607-9500.

614 USA
HEALTH CARE FACILITIES GUIDE. Text in English. 1994. m. USD 599 (effective 1999). back issues avail. **Document type:** *Newsletter.*
Formerly: B N A's Health Care Facilities Guide
Published by: Opus Communications, PO Box 1168, Marblehead, MA 01945. TEL 781-639-1872, 800-650-6787, FAX 800-639-8511, customer_service@opuscomm.com, http://www.opuscomm.com. Ed. Randy Kubetin.

338.43 362.1 USA ISSN 1057-9389
HEALTH CARE FINANCING REVIEW. SUPPLEMENT. Text in English. 1979. a. USD 26 (effective 2001). back issues avail.; reprint service avail. from CIS. **Document type:** *Government.*
Related titles: Microfiche ed.: (from CIS); Microform ed.: (from PQC); ♦ Supplement to: Health Care Financing Review. ISSN 0195-8631.
Indexed: ABI Inform. (coverage dropped), Abstr.Health Care Manage.Stud., Abstr.Soc.Geront., AgeLine, Amer.Stat.Ind. (1979-), Excerp.Med., Hosp.Lit.Ind., Ind.U.S.Gov.Per., MEDOC, Med.Care Rev., PROMT, Soc.Work Res.& Abstr., World Bibl.Soc.Sec.
Published by: U.S. Health Care Financing Administration (Subsidiary of: U.S. Department of Health and Human Services), 7500 Security Blvd, Baltimore, MD 21244. TEL 410-786-6572, FAX 410-786-5768. Ed. Linda F Wolf. **Subscr. to:** U.S. Government Printing Office, Superintendent of Documents, PO Box 371954, Pittsburgh, PA 15250-7954. TEL 202-512-1800, FAX 202-512-2250, orders@gpo.gov, http://www.access.gpo.gov.

614.8 USA ISSN 1041-0236
R118 CODEN: HECOER
HEALTH COMMUNICATION. Text in English. 1989. q. USD 45 in US & Canada to individuals; USD 75 elsewhere to individuals; USD 365 in US & Canada to institutions; USD 395 elsewhere to institutions (effective 2002). adv. bk.rev. *Refereed.* **Document type:** *Journal, Academic/Scholarly.* **Description:** Features articles from scholars in communication, psychology, medicine, nursing and allied health fields.
Related titles: Online - full text ed.: ISSN 1532-7027. USD 40.50 to individuals; USD 328.50 to institutions (effective 2002) (from CatchWord Ltd., EBSCO Publishing, O C L C Online Computer Library Center, Inc., RoweCom Information Quest, Swets Blackwell, Institute for Scientific Information).
Indexed: ASCA, ASSIA, Abstr.Soc.Geront., AgeLine, Brit.Nur.Ind., Commun.Abstr., Curr.Cont., Educ.Admin.Abstr., Environ.Sci.Poll.Mgmt., Ind.Med. (1989-), Lang.& Lang.Behav.Abstr., NRN, Pollut.Abstr., PsycInfo, Psychol.Abstr. (1989-), Risk Abstr., SOPODA, SSCI, Saf.Sci.Abstr., Soc.Serv.Abstr., Sociol.Abstr., Viol.& Abuse Abstr., e-psyche.
—BLDSC (4274.953900), CatchWord, GNLM, Infotrieve, ingenta. **CCC.**
Published by: Lawrence Erlbaum Associates, Inc., 10 Industrial Ave, Mahwah, NJ 07430-2262. TEL 201-760-3735, 800-926-6579, FAX 201-236-0072, journals@erlbaum.com, http://www.erlbaum.com/Journals/journals/HC/hc.htm. Ed. Teresa L Thompson. adv.: page USD 400; trim 5 x 8.

614 GBR
HEALTH ECHO. Text in English. 1988. q. free per issue. adv. **Document type:** *Newspaper.*
Published by: Lincolnshire Publishing Ltd., Brayford Wharf East, Lincoln LN5 7AT, United Kingdom. TEL 44-1522-525252, FAX 44-1522-521600. Ed. Cliff Smith. Adv. contact Lorraine Wadsley. Circ: 40,000.

HEALTH ECONOMICS. see *MEDICAL SCIENCES*

610 USA ISSN 1090-1981
RA440.A1 CODEN: HEDBFS
HEALTH EDUCATION & BEHAVIOR. Text in English. 1957-1978; resumed 1980. bi-m. USD 95 to individuals; USD 550 to institutions; USD 25 newsstand/cover to individuals; USD 100 newsstand/cover to institutions (effective 2002). adv. bk.rev. illus. Index. Supplement avail.; back issues avail.; reprint service avail. from PQC. *Refereed.* **Document type:** *Academic/Scholarly.* **Description:** Discusses the promotion of public health by elevating the quality of health education, improving medical practice, and stimulating research.
Formerly (until vol.24, 1997): Health Education Quarterly (0195-8402); Which superseded (in 1980): Health Education Monographs (0073-1455)
Related titles: Microform ed.: (from PQC); Online - full text ed.: (from ProQuest Information & Learning, ingenta, Institute for Scientific Information).
Indexed: ASCA, ASSIA, AgeLine, C.I.J.E. (coverage dropped), CINAHL, Cont.Pg.Educ., Crim.Just.Abstr., Curr.Cont., Educ.Ind. (Jun.1992-Dec.1996), Environ.Sci.Poll.Mgmt., Excerp.Med., Fam.Ind., INIS Atomind., Ind.Med. (1997-), Int.Nurs.Ind., Lang.& Lang.Behav.Abstr., NRN, Phys.Ed.Ind., Pollut.Abstr., PsycInfo, Psychol.Abstr. (1970-), Risk Abstr., SOPODA, SSCI, Saf.Sci.Abstr., Sage Fam.Stud.Abstr., Sage Race Rel.Abstr., Soc.Serv.Abstr., Soc.Work Res.& Abstr., Sociol.Abstr., THA, Viol.& Abuse Abstr., e-psyche.
—BLDSC (4274.977000), CISTI, GNLM, IDS, ingenta. **CCC.**

P

Published by: (Society for Public Health Education), Sage Publications, Inc., 2455 Teller Rd, Thousand Oaks, CA 91320. TEL 805-499-0721, FAX 805-499-0871, libraries@sagepub.com., info@sagepub.com, http://www.sagepub.com. Ed. Mark Zimmerman. R&P Tanya Udin. Adv. contact DeAnna Vega Hammersley. Circ: 2,200. **Subscr. outside the Americas to:** Sage Publications Ltd., 6 Bonhill St, London EC2A 4PU, United Kingdom; Sage Publications India Pvt. Ltd., PO Box 4125, New Delhi 110 048, India.

362.1 GBR ISSN 0017-8969
RA421
HEALTH EDUCATION JOURNAL. Text in English. 1943. q. GBP 37 in Europe to individuals; USD 79 in United States to individuals; GBP 42 elsewhere to individuals; GBP 65 in Europe to institutions; USD 125 in United States to institutions; GBP 71 elsewhere to institutions (effective 2002). adv. bk.rev. index. reprint service avail. from PQC. *Refereed.* **Document type:** *Journal, Academic/Scholarly.*
Related titles: Microform ed.: (from PQC); Online - full text ed.: (from Gale Group).
Indexed: ASSIA, Abstr.Hyg., Addic.Abstr., Bibl.Agri., Br.Educ.Ind., Brit.Nur.Ind., CINAHL, Cont.Pg.Educ., Curr.Adv.Ecol.Sci., Diar.Dis.Res., ERA, Educ.Tech.Abstr., Environ.Sci.Poll.Mgmt., Excerp.Med., Nutr.Abstr., Res.High.Educ.Abstr., Risk Abstr., SSCI (coverage dropped), Saf.Sci.Abstr., Stud.Wom.Abstr., Tech.Educ.Abstr., Trop.Dis.Bull., World Ag.Econ.& Rur.Soc.Abstr.
—BLDSC (4275.000000), CISTI, GNLM, ingenta.
Published by: (Health Education Authority), Royal Society of Medicine Press Ltd, 1 Wimpole St, London W1M 8AE, United Kingdom. TEL 44-20-7290-2921, FAX 44-20-7290-2929, rsmjournals@rsm.ac.uk, http://www.roysocmed.ac.uk/pub/hej.htm. Ed. Anthony Blinkhorn. Circ: 3,000.

614.8 USA ISSN 0193-5232
HEALTH EDUCATION REPORTS. Text in English. 24/yr. USD 198. **Document type:** *Newsletter.* **Description:** Covers health promotion and disease prevention. Reports on policy and legislation, reviews literature and meetings.
Published by: Feistritzer Publications, 4401 A Connecticut Ave, N W, Ste 212, Washington, DC 20088. TEL 202-362-3444, FAX 202-362-3493. Ed. Lawrence O'Rourke. Pub. David T Chester.

362.1 USA
HEALTH EDUCATOR. Text in English. 1969. s-a. USD 20 domestic; USD 35 foreign (effective 2000); USD 6 newsstand/cover. adv. bk.rev. bibl, charts, illus. back issues avail. *Refereed.* **Document type:** *Journal, Academic/Scholarly.* **Description:** Publishes articles and research of interest to students in the national health education honor society. Includes health education research, service and teaching reports for all ages in all settings.
Indexed: C.I.J.E.
Published by: Eta Sigma Gamma, 2000 University Ave, Muncie, IN 47306. TEL 765-285-2258, FAX 765-285-3210, etasigmagam@bsuvc.bsu.edu, http://www.cast.ilstu.edu/temple/esq.htm. Ed., Pub., R&P, Adv. contact Judith K Luebke TEL 507-389-5938. B&W page USD 200. Circ: 4,500 (paid).

614 GBR ISSN 1369-6513
HEALTH EXPECTATIONS. Text in English. 1998. q., latest vol.5, 2002. GBP 88 in Europe to individuals; USD 140 in North America to individuals; GBP 97 elsewhere to individuals; GBP 249 in Europe to institutions; USD 395 in North America to institutions; GBP 274 elsewhere to institutions (effective 2002). adv. *Refereed.* **Document type:** *Academic/Scholarly.* **Description:** Aims to promote critical thinking and informed debate about all aspects of public participation in health care and health policy.
Related titles: Online - full text ed.: ISSN 1369-7625. USD 321 in North America to institutions; USD 126 in North America to individuals; GBP 189 elsewhere to institutions; GBP 72 elsewhere to individuals (effective 2001) (from EBSCO Publishing, O C L C Online Computer Library Center, Inc., RoweCom Information Quest, ingenta, Munksgaard & Blackwell Science's Synergy, Swets Blackwell).
Indexed: CINAHL.
—BLDSC (4275.015545).
Published by: Blackwell Science Ltd., PO Box 88, Oxford OX2 0NE, United Kingdom. TEL 44-1865-206180, 44-1865-206002, FAX 44-1865-206219, jnl.orders@blacksci.co.uk, http://www.blackwell-science.com/~cgilib/jnlpage.asp?Journal=hex&File=hex, http://www.blackwellpublishing.com. Ed. Angela Coulter. Pub. Elaine Stott. R&P Sophie Savage. Adv. contact Jenny Applin.

HEALTH FACILITIES DIRECTORY. see *SOCIAL SERVICES AND WELFARE*

613 USA ISSN 0749-4742
RA395.A3
HEALTH FREEDOM NEWS. Text in English. 1955. bi-m. USD 36 to individuals; USD 48 in Canada to individuals (effective 1999). adv. bk.rev. charts, illus, stat. back issues avail. **Document type:** *Consumer.* **Description:** Covers educational, legislative and legal topics related to health.
Former titles (until 1982): Public Scrutiny (0743-5053); National Health Federation. Bulletin (0027-9420)
—CISTI, GNLM.
Published by: National Health Federation, 212 W Foothill Blvd, Monrovia, CA 91016. TEL 818-357-2181, FAX 818-303-0642. Ed. James F Scheer. Circ: 6,000 (paid). **Subscr. to:** PO Box 688, Monrovia, CA 91016.

HEALTH GRANTS & CONTRACTS WEEKLY; selected federal project opportunities. see *PUBLIC ADMINISTRATION*

614.427 USA ISSN 0095-3539
RA783.5
HEALTH INFORMATION FOR INTERNATIONAL TRAVEL. Text in English. 1974. a. USD 20 (effective 1999). **Document type:** *Government.* **Description:** Provides current information on vaccination, prophylaxis, and country entry requirements; U.S. Public Health Service recommendations; geographical distribution of potential health hazards; and how to avoid health problems while visiting foreign countries.
Related titles: ♦ Supplement to: Morbidity and Mortality Weekly Report. ISSN 0149-2195.
—GNLM.
Published by: U.S. Department of Health and Human Services, Centers for Disease Control (MS: CO8), Epidemiology Program Office, 1600 Clifton Rd N E, Atlanta, GA 30333. TEL 800-843-6356. **Subscr. to:** U.S. Government Printing Office, Superintendent of Documents.

614 610 340 USA ISSN 0549-804X
HEALTH LAW BULLETIN. Text in English. 1958. irreg. bibl. **Document type:** *Bulletin.* **Description:** Each issue deals with a current legal issue in the health care field. Reports the results of recent litigation and the effects of newly enacted legislation.
Published by: University of North Carolina at Chapel Hill, Institute of Government, CB#3330 Knapp Bldg, Chapel Hill, NC 27599-3330. TEL 919-966-4119, FAX 919-962-2707, http://ncinfo.iog.unc.edu/. Eds. Anne M Dellinger, Jeffrey C Koeze. R&P Katrina W Hunt. Circ: 500 (controlled).

HEALTH LETTER (WASHINGTON). see *MEDICAL SCIENCES*

614 USA ISSN 0735-9683
HEALTH MARKETING QUARTERLY. Text in English. 1978. q. USD 75 to individuals; USD 101 in Canada to individuals; USD 109 elsewhere to individuals; USD 125 to institutions; USD 169 in Canada to institutions; USD 181 elsewhere to institutions; USD 500 to libraries; USD 675 in Canada to libraries; USD 725 elsewhere to libraries (effective Aug. 2001). adv. bk.rev. abstr, bibl. back issues avail.; reprint service avail. from HAW. *Refereed.* **Document type:** *Journal, Academic/Scholarly.* **Description:** Each issue is devoted to a select health service, and serves as a basic resource for marketing the selected service. Covers group practice marketing, mental health marketing, and long-term care marketing.
Former titles (until 1984): Topics in Strategic Planning for Health Care (0731-714X); Topics in Health Care; Health and Medical Care Services Review (0160-7618)
Related titles: Microfiche ed.: (from PQC); Microform ed.; Online - full text ed.: (from ProQuest Information & Learning, Gale Group).
Indexed: ABI Inform. (Win.1984-), Abstr.Health Care Manage.Stud., Abstr.Soc.Geront., AgeLine, Aqua.Sci.& Fish.Abstr., Chicago Psychoanal.Lit.Ind., Commun.Abstr., Environ.Sci.Poll.Mgmt., Excerp.Med., Hosp.Abstr., Hosp.Lit.Ind., IBZ, J.of Econ.Lit., Lang.& Lang.Behav.Abstr., Med.Care Rev., Mgmt.& Market.Abstr., Pollut.Abstr., Psychol.Abstr., Risk Abstr., SOPODA, Saf.Sci.Abstr., Soc.Work Res.& Abstr., Sociol.Abstr.
—BLDSC (4275.052850), GNLM, Haworth, ingenta.
Published by: Haworth Press, Inc., 10 Alice St, Binghamton, NY 13904-1580. TEL 607-722-5857, 800-429-6784, FAX 607-722-6362, 800-895-0582, getinfo@haworthpressinc.com, http://www.haworthpress.com/journals/journallist.asp. Eds. David Paul, Earl Honeycutt. Pub. William Cohen. R&P Ruthann Heath TEL 607-723-5857 ext 316. Adv. contact Jackie Blackeslee. B&W page USD 315, color page USD 550; trim 6 x 8.5. Circ: 610.

613 USA
HEALTH - P A C BULLETIN*. Text in English. 1968. q. USD 35 to individuals; USD 45 to institutions. adv. bk.rev. charts, illus, stat, tr.lit. index. back issues avail. **Document type:** *Bulletin.* **Description:** Analysis and commentary on health care and health policy advocating decent, accessible health care for all.
Supersedes (in 1987): Health and Medicine; Formerly: Health-Pac (0017-9051)
Related titles: Microform ed.: 1968 (from PQC).
Indexed: Alt.Press Ind., Med.Care Rev., P.A.I.S.
—GNLM, Infotrieve, ingenta. **CCC.**
Published by: Health Policy Advisory Center, 237 Thompson St, New York, NY 10012-1017. TEL 212-614-1660, FAX 212-614-1665. Ed. Ellen Bilofsky. Circ: 1,100.

614 370 IRL ISSN 0168-8510
HEALTH POLICY. Text in English. 1979. m. EUR 173 in Europe to individuals; JPY 22,800 in Japan to individuals; USD 193 elsewhere to individuals; EUR 1,237 in Europe to institutions; JPY 164,400 in Japan to institutions; USD 1,384 elsewhere to institutions (effective 2002). Supplement avail.; back issues avail.; reprint service avail. from SWZ,ISI. *Refereed.* **Document type:** *Academic/Scholarly.* **Description:** Forum for discussion of health policy issues among health policy researchers, legislators, decision makers and other professionals.
Incorporates (in 1986): Effective Health Care (0167-871X); Formerly (until 1984): Health Policy and Education (0165-2281)
Related titles: Online - full text ed.: (from ingenta, Swets Blackwell, ScienceDirect, Institute for Scientific Information).
Indexed: ASCA, ASSIA, Abstr.Anthropol., Abstr.Health Care Manage.Stud., Adol.Ment.Hlth.Abstr., AgeLine, Arts & Hum.Cit.Ind. (coverage dropped), B.P.I. (Jul.1995-May 1999), Cont.Pg.Educ., Curr.Cont., Environ.Sci.Poll.Mgmt., Excerp.Med., Hosp.Abstr., Hosp.Lit.Ind., Inpharma, Int.Nurs.Ind., Intl.Bibl.Soc.Sci., P.A.I.S., Reac., Risk Abstr., SSCI, Sci.Cit.Ind. (coverage dropped), THA.
—BLDSC (4275.102700), CISTI, GNLM, IDS, Infotrieve, ingenta. **CCC.**
Published by: (European Health Policy Forum), Elsevier Science Ireland Ltd, Elsevier House, Brookvale Plaza, E. Park, Shannon, Co. Clare, Ireland. TEL 353-61-471944, FAX 353-61-472144, http://www.elsevier.com/locate/healthpol. Eds. K Kesteloot, M Defever. **Subscr. in Australasia and the Far East to:** Elsevier Science (Singapore) Pte Ltd, No.1 Temasek Ave, 17-01 Millenia Tower, Singapore 039192, Singapore. TEL 65-434-3727; **Subscr. in the Americas to:** Elsevier Science, PO Box 945, New York, NY 10159-0945. TEL 212-633-3730, FAX 212-633-3680, usinfo-f@elsevier.com**; Subscr. to:** Elsevier Science BV, PO Box 211, Amsterdam 1000 AE, Netherlands. TEL 31-20-485-3757.

614 GBR ISSN 0268-1080
RA441.5
HEALTH POLICY AND PLANNING; a journal on health in development. Text in English. 1986. q. GBP 75, USD 130 to individuals; GBP 175, USD 310 to institutions; GBP 88, USD 155 in developing nations to institutions (effective (No. 2002). adv. bk.rev. back issues avail. *Refereed.* **Document type:** *Journal, Academic/Scholarly.* **Description:** Covers issues in health policy, planning, management and evaluation in the developing world.
Related titles: Online - full text ed.: ISSN 1460-2245. GBP 155, USD 280 to institutions Online only; GBP 50, USD 88 in developing nations to institutions Online only (effective Mar. 2002) (from HighWire Pr., EBSCO Publishing, O C L C Online Computer Library Center, Inc., RoweCom Information Quest, ingenta, Swets Blackwell, Institute for Scientific Information).

P

Indexed: ASCA, ASSIA, Abstr.Hyg., AgeLine, Brit.Nur.Ind., Curr.Adv.Ecol.Sci., Curr.Cont., Dairy Sci.Abstr., Diar.Dis.Res., ERA, Environ.Sci.Poll.Mgmt., Excerp.Med., Fam.Ind., Helminthol.Abstr., IDA, Intl.Bibl.Soc.Sci., Lang.& Lang.Behav.Abstr., Nutr.Abstr., P C I, P.A.I.S., Pollut.Abstr., Protozool.Abstr., Refug.Abstr., Rev.Appl.Entomol., Rev.Med.& Vet.Mycol., Risk Abstr., Rural Devel.Abstr., SOPODA, SSCI, Saf.Sci.Abstr., Sel.Water Res.Abstr., Soc.Serv.Abstr., Sociol.Abstr., Stud.Wom.Abstr., Trop.Dis.Bull., World Ag.Econ.& Rur.Soc.Abstr.
—BLDSC (4275.103300), EMDOCS, GNLM, IDS, ingenta. **CCC.**
Published by: (London School of Hygiene and Tropical Medicine), Oxford University Press, Academic Division, Great Clarendon St, Oxford OX2 6DP, United Kingdom. TEL 44-1865-267907, FAX 44-1865-267835, jnl.info@oup.co.uk, http://www.heapol.oupjournals.org, http://www.oup.co.uk/journals. Eds. Anne Mills, R Brugha. Pub. Mandy Sketch. R&P Fiona Willis. adv.: B&W page GBP 260, B&W page USD 470; trim 210 x 150. Circ: 1,000. **Subscr. to:** Journals Marketing, Great Clarendon St, Oxford OX2 6DP, United Kingdom. **Affiliate:** Oxford University Press, Journals.

HEALTH POLICY MONITOR. see *PUBLIC ADMINISTRATION*

614 USA ISSN 0732-7439
HEALTH POLICY WEEK. Text in English. 1971. w. USD 395. **Document type:** *Newsletter.* **Description:** Offers an inside look at federal and state government actions affecting the financing and delivery of health care services.
—**CCC.**
Published by: United Communications Group, 1300 Rockville Pike, Ste 1100, Rockville, MD 20852-3030. TEL 301-816-8950, FAX 301-816-8945. Ed. Burt Schorr.

614 GBR ISSN 0957-4824
RA427.8 CODEN: HPINET
HEALTH PROMOTION INTERNATIONAL. Text in English. 1986. q. GBP 90, USD 160 to individuals; GBP 185, USD 310 to institutions (effective Mar. 2002). adv. bk.rev. back issues avail. *Refereed.* **Document type:** *Journal, Academic/Scholarly.* **Description:** Presents original articles, major reviews, and an editorial concerned with major health promotion themes.
Formerly (until 1989): Health Promotion (0268-1099)
Related titles: Online - full text ed.: ISSN 1460-2245. 1986. GBP 165, USD 280 to institutions Online only (effective Mar. 2002) (from HighWire Pr., EBSCO Publishing, O C L C Online Computer Library Center, Inc., RoweCom Information Quest, Swets Blackwell, Institute for Scientific Information).
Indexed: ASCA, ASSIA, AgeLine, Brit.Nur.Ind., CINAHL, Curr.Cont., ERA, Excerp.Med., Fam.Ind., Hosp.Abstr., Lang.& Lang.Behav.Abstr., Media Rev.Dig., PsycInfo, Psychol.Abstr. (1993-), SOPODA, SSCI, Soc.Serv.Abstr., Sociol.Abstr., Tech.Educ.Abstr., e-psyche.
—BLDSC (4275.105183), EMDOCS, GNLM, IDS, Infotrieve, ingenta, KNAW. **CCC.**
Published by: Oxford University Press, Academic Division, Great Clarendon St, Oxford OX2 6DP, United Kingdom. TEL 44-1865-267907, FAX 44-1865-267835, jnl.info@oup.co.uk, http://heapro.oupjournals.org/, http://www.oup.co.uk/journals. Ed. John Catford. Pub. Mandy Sketch. R&P Fiona Willis. adv.: page GBP 260, page USD 470. Circ: 1,000. **U.S. subscr. to:** Oxford University Press, Journals, 2001 Evans Rd, Cary, NC 27513. TEL 919-677-0977, 800-852-7323, FAX 919-677-1714, jnlorders@oup-usa.org; **Subscr. to:** Journals Marketing, Great Clarendon St, Oxford OX2 6DP, United Kingdom.

614 AUS ISSN 1036-1073
HEALTH PROMOTION JOURNAL OF AUSTRALIA. Text in English. 1991. 3/yr. AUD 165 to individuals; AUD 362.50 to institutions (effective 2001). **Description:** Aims to facilitate communication between researchers, practitioners, and policymakers involved in health promotion activities.
Related titles: Online - full text ed.
—BLDSC (4275.105184).
Published by: Australian Health Promotion Association, PO Box 4, Maroochydore, QLD 4558, Australia. TEL 61-3-9345-3200, FAX 61-3-9345-3222, http://vhpax.vichealth.vic.gov.au/hpja/. Ed. Rob Moodie.

613 614 610 USA ISSN 1524-8399
▼ **HEALTH PROMOTION PRACTICE.** Text in English. 2000. q. USD 100 to individuals; USD 300 to institutions; USD 20 newsstand/cover to individuals; USD 70 newsstand/cover to institutions (effective 2002). adv. back issues avail. *Refereed.* **Description:** Publishes authoritative, peer-reviwed articles devoted to the practical application of health promotion and education. Focus on critical and strategic information for professionals engaged in the practice of developing, implementing and evaluating health promotion and disease prevention programs.
Related titles: Online - full text ed.: (from EBSCO Publishing, O C L C Online Computer Library Center, Inc., RoweCom Information Quest, ingenta, Swets Blackwell).
—BLDSC (4275.105187).
Published by: (Society for Public Health Education), Sage Publications, Inc., 2455 Teller Rd, Thousand Oaks, CA 91320. TEL 805-499-9821, FAX 805-499-0721, http://www.sagepub.com. Ed. Randy Schwartz.

HEALTH PSYCHOLOGY. see *PSYCHOLOGY*

614.4 NZL ISSN 1170-4195
HEALTH RESEARCH COUNCIL OF NEW ZEALAND NEWSLETTER. Text in English. 1991. q. free. **Document type:** *Newsletter.*
Published by: Health Research Council of New Zealand, P.O. Box 5541, Auckland, 1, New Zealand. TEL 64-9-3798227, FAX 64-9-3779988, info@hrc.govt.nz, http://www.hrc.govt.nz. Ed., Pub. Jenny Rankine. Circ: 2,000.

362.1 300 GBR ISSN 1369-8575
▼ **HEALTH, RISK & SOCIETY.** Text in English. 1999. 3/yr. GBP 50, USD 71 to individuals; GBP 161, USD 266 to institutions (effective 2002). *Refereed.* **Document type:** *Academic/Scholarly.* **Description:** Aims to understand the social processes which influence the ways in which risks are taken, communicated, assessed and managed in relationship to health and health care.
Related titles: Online - full text ed.: ISSN 1469-8331 (from CatchWord Ltd., EBSCO Publishing, O C L C Online Computer Library Center, Inc., RoweCom Information Quest, Swets Blackwell, Institute for Scientific Information).
Indexed: Addic.Abstr., Curr.Cont., Environ.Sci.Poll.Mgmt., Ergon.Abstr., Pollut.Abstr., Risk Abstr., SSCI, Saf.Sci.Abstr.
—BLDSC (4275.106444), CatchWord.
Published by: Carfax Publishing Limited (Subsidiary of: Taylor & Francis Group), PO Box 25, Abingdon, Oxon OX14 3UE, United Kingdom. TEL 44-1235-401000, FAX 44-1235-401550, enquiries@carfax.co.uk, enquiry@tandf.co.uk, http://www.carfax.co.uk. Ed. Andy Alaszewski.

HEALTH, SAFETY AND ENVIRONMENT BULLETIN. see *ENVIRONMENTAL STUDIES—Toxicology And Environmental Safety*

362.1 AUS
HEALTH SERVICES ACT SURVIVAL KITS - COMMUNITY HEALTH CENTRES KIT. Text in English. irreg., latest 1994, Jan. price varies. **Document type:** *Government.*
Published by: Law Press (Victoria), 52-58 Chetwynd St, West Melbourne, VIC 3003, Australia. TEL 61-3-93208686, FAX 61-3-93208699.

▼ **HEALTH SERVICES AND OUTCOMES RESEARCH METHODOLOGY**; an international journal devoted to quantitative methods for the study of utilization, quality, cost and outcomes of health. see *MEDICAL SCIENCES*

HEALTH SERVICES MANAGEMENT RESEARCH. see *MEDICAL SCIENCES*

HEALTH SERVICES RESEARCH. see *HEALTH FACILITIES AND ADMINISTRATION*

362.1 AUS
HEALTH STREAM NEWSLETTER. Text in English. 1996. q. free per issue. **Document type:** *Newsletter.* **Description:** Includes conference reports, news items and information about the center on water quality and public health.
Media: Online - full text.
Published by: University of South Australia, School of Chemical Technology, C R C for Water Quality and Treatment, The Levels Campus, Mawson Lakes, SA, SA 5108, Australia. TEL 91-8-8302-3068, FAX 61-3-9276-6576, martha.sinclair@med.monash.edu.au, http://www.med.monash.edu.au/epidemiology/crc/crcpubs/. Ed. Martha Sinclair.

658 658 USA ISSN 0361-0195
HEALTH SYSTEMS MANAGEMENT* . Text in English. 1974. irreg., latest vol.18, 1985.
Published by: S P Medical & Scientific Books, Inc. (Subsidiary of: Spectrum Publications, Inc.), c/o Fisher, 200 Park Ave S, New York, NY 10003-1503. Ed. Dr. Samuel Levey.

HEALTH TRENDS. see *MEDICAL SCIENCES*

614 USA
HEALTH WATCH (WASHINGTON D C). Text in English. 1996. m.
Media: Online - full content.
Published by: Health Care Financing Administration, 200 Independence Ave S W, Washington, DC 20201. http://www.hcfa.gov/news/newsltrs/newsltrs.htm.

614 360 CAN ISSN 1195-7506
RA410.9.C2
HEALTH WORKFORCE IN ALBERTA. ANNUAL REPORT. Text in English. 1977. a. free per issue. **Document type:** *Government.* **Description:** Contains the results of the annual survey of health employers in Alberta concerning the number of personnel employed, their status, vacancy and turnover rates, and recruitment difficulties.
Formerly (until 1993): Alberta. Health and Social Services Disciplines Committee. Annual Report (0707-1434)
Published by: Alberta Health, Practitioner Services Division, 10025 Jasper Ave, 16th Fl, Edmonton, AB T5J 2N3, Canada. TEL 403-427-3276, FAX 403-422-2880. Ed. D Chesley. Circ: 500.

614 USA
HEALTHCARE 1500. Text in English. 1991. a. USD 295 (effective 2000). **Document type:** *Directory.* **Description:** Profiles influential federal and state health policy makers, advisors, lobbyists and health industry leaders, with addresses and telephone numbers. Also includes a review of healthcare budgets at the state level.
Former titles: HealthCare 1000; (until 1992): HealthCare 500
Published by: Thompson Financial / I M G Media, Healthcare Information Center (Subsidiary of: Thompson Publishing Group), 11 Penn Plaza, 17th Fl, New York, NY 10001-2006. TEL 212-967-7000. Ed. Beth Rosenthal.

HEALTHCARE ADVERTISING REVIEW; creative forum for the people who plan and create healthcare advertising programs. see *ADVERTISING AND PUBLIC RELATIONS*

363 USA ISSN 1523-7575
HEALTHCARE LIFE SAFETY COMPLIANCE. Text in English. 1995. m. USD 197 print or online ed.; USD 246 print & online eds. (effective 2001).
Formerly (until Jan. 1999): Healthcare Fire Protection (1083-9747)
Related titles: Online - full text ed.
Published by: Opus Communications, PO Box 1168, Marblehead, MA 01945. TEL 800-650-6787, FAX 781-639-7857, http://www.opuscomm.com.

368.382 GBR ISSN 1354-2915
HEALTHCARE TODAY; journal for NHS boards. Text in English. 1992. m. GBP 48; USD 100 in United States. adv. charts, illus, stat, tr.lit. **Document type:** *Trade.* **Description:** Covers a variety of health policy issues, including management of National Health Service trusts, government spending on health, along with national and local budgets, and studies of new practices such as collaborative care and telemedicine. Also discusses clinical risk management and problems such as clinical negligence claims. Intended for the board of directors of NHS organisations, such as health authorities and NHS trusts.
Published by: (National Health Service Confederation), Enterprise Events Ltd., Beech House, 840 Brighton Rd, Purley, Surrey CR8 2BH, United Kingdom. TEL 44-20-8763-2727, FAX 44-20-8763-2914, hct@entevents.co.uk. Ed. Dan Jellinek. Pub. John Neame. Adv. contact Martyn L James. color page GBP 1,700; 240 x 330.

HEALTHFACTS. see *MEDICAL SCIENCES*

610 USA ISSN 0736-7929
HEALTHLINE✱; helping keep well people well. Text in English. 1981. m. USD 24 domestic; USD 36 foreign (effective 2000). bk.rev. illus. cum.index. back issues avail.; reprints avail. **Document type:** *Magazine, Consumer.* **Description:** Offers current information on health and wellness, written in nontechnical language by healthcare professionals and medical journalists.
Related titles: Online - full text ed.: (from Gale Group).
Indexed: AgeLine, CHNI, CINAHL, Consum.Ind. (1990-).
—BLDSC (4275.247978).
Published by: Healthline Publishers Inc., 702 Marshall St, Ste 611, Redwood City, CA 94063-1827. TEL 650-780-0546, 800-325-4177, FAX 650-780-0547, health@healthline.com, http://www.healthline.com. Ed. Paul Insel. R&P Linda Lydon. Adv. contact Sue London. Circ: 11,000.

362.1 614.4 GBR ISSN 0969-336X
HEALTHLINES. Text in English. 1993. 10/yr. GBP 30 (effective 1999). bk.rev. **Document type:** *Trade.* **Description:** Discusses various aspects of health promotion and provides updates on research, publications, and events.
Related titles: Supplement: Healthlines Plus. ISSN 0969-3378.
Indexed: Brit.Nur.Ind.
Published by: Health Education Authority, Trevelyan House, 30 Great Peter St, London SW1P 2HW, United Kingdom. TEL 44-20-7413-1920, http://www.hea.org.uk. Ed. Sue Jelley. Circ: 3,000.

613 USA ISSN 1043-2779
S605.5
HEALTHY HARVEST. Text in English. 1985. biennial.
Published by: (National Institute for Science, Law, and Public Policy), Potomac Valley Press, 1424 16th St N W, Ste 105, Washington, DC 20036.

▼ **HEALTHY TRAVELER.** see *TRAVEL AND TOURISM*

614 USA
HEARTWEB✱. Text in English. 1995. irreg. *Refereed.*
Media: Online - full content.
Indexed: Curr.Cont.
Published by: Amadeus Multimedia Technologies, Ltd., One Bridge St Ste 93, Irvington, NY 10533. http://www.heartweb.org. Ed. Seymour Furman.

361 NOR
HELSENYTT FOR ALLE; et popuaervitenskaplig medisinsk tidsskrift. Text in Norwegian. 1910. bi-m. NOK 160. adv. **Document type:** *Newspaper, Consumer.* **Description:** Deals with medical issues in easy lay terms. Each issue has a main theme which is dealt with thoroughly.
Former titles (until 1970): Helsenytt (0018-0157); (until 1963): Nasjonalforeningen mot Tuberkulosen for Folkehelsen (0333-287X)
—**CCC.**
Published by: Nasjonalforeningen for Folkehelsen, Postboks 7139, Majorstua, Oslo 0307, Norway. Ed. Terje Fugelli. Adv. contact Henrik Sandberg.

614 BGR ISSN 0018-8247
CODEN: KHZDAN
HIGIENA I ZDRAVEOPAZVANE. Text in Bulgarian; Summaries in English, Russian. 1958. q. adv. bk.rev. abstr, charts, illus, stat. index. **Document type:** *Academic/Scholarly.*
Indexed: Abstr.Bulg.Sci.Med.Lit., Biol.Abstr., Chem.Abstr., Excerp.Med. (until 1993, 1996-), INIS Atomind., Nutr.Abstr.
—CASDDS, CISTI, EMDOCS.
Published by: (Bulgaria. Ministerstvo na Narodnoto Zdrave), Izdatelstvo Meditsina i Fizkultura, 11 Pl Slaveikov, Sofia 1080, Bulgaria. Ed. E Efremov. Circ: 1,402. **Co-sponsor:** Nauchno Druzhestvo po Higiena i Organizacia na Zdraveopazvaneto.

362.196 323.4 USA
HIV POLICY WATCH. Text in English. m.
Published by: San Francisco AIDS Foundation, PO Box 426182, San Francisco, CA 94142-6182. TEL 415-487-8060, 800-833-0159, FAX 415-487-8069, beta@sfaf.org, http://www.sfaf.org.

614 USA
HIV PREVENTION AND SERVICES TECHNICAL ASSISTANCE REPORTS. (Human Immunodeficiency Virus) Text in English. irreg. free per issue. **Document type:** *Monographic series.*
Published by: U.S. Conference of Mayors, Office of Public Affairs, 1620 Eye St, N W, Washington, DC 20006. TEL 202-293-7330, FAX 202-293-2352. Ed. J Thomas Cochran.

614 USA
HIV PREVENTION CASE STUDY SERIES. (Human Immunodeficiency Virus) Text in English. irreg. USD 5 per issue. **Document type:** *Monographic series.*
Published by: U.S. Conference of Mayors, Office of Public Affairs, 1620 Eye St, N W, Washington, DC 20006. TEL 202-293-7330.

HOPE HEALTH LETTER. see *PHYSICAL FITNESS AND HYGIENE*

614 USA
HOPE NEWS. Text in English. 1963. 2/yr. free per issue. adv. **Document type:** *Newsletter.*
Published by: People-to-People Health Foundation, Inc., Project Hope Health Sciences Education Center, Millwood, VA 22646. TEL 540-837-2100, FAX 540-837-1813, lpetrosi@projhope.org, http://www.projhope.org. Ed. Laura Petrosian. R&P, Adv. contact Mary Stine. Circ: 100,000.

HUANJING YU JIANKANG ZAZHI/JOURNAL OF ENVIRONMENT AND HEALTH. see *ENVIRONMENTAL STUDIES*

362.1 610.9 SWE
▼ **HYGIEA INTERNATIONALIS.** Text in English. 1999. irreg. Free access. back issues avail. *Refereed.* **Document type:** *Academic/Scholarly.* **Description:** Promotes, in the broadest sense, the study of the history of collective efforts for the improvement of the health of populations from antiquity to modernity with particular emphasis on the interdisciplinary analysis of the interaction between ideas on public health, organizations created to carry out these ideas, their implementation, and their social and demographic consequences.
Media: Online - full content.
Published by: International Network for the History of Public Health, Department of Health and Society, Linkoeping University, Linkoeping 581 83, Sweden. TEL 46-13-282309, FAX 46-13-282995, jasun@tema.liu.se, http://www.tema.liu.se/inhph/journal/. Eds. Jan Sundin, Marie C Nelson.

HYGIENES. see *HEALTH FACILITIES AND ADMINISTRATION*

628 614.8 FIN ISSN 1236-3081
HYVA TERVEYS. Text in Finnish. 1985. 9/yr. FIM 261 (effective 1997). **Document type:** *Consumer.* **Description:** Results of research in health care and medical research.
Formerly (until 1993): Terveys 2000 (0782-3789)
Published by: Helsinki Media Magazines, PL 100, Helsinki Media 00040, Finland. TEL 358-9-1201, FAX 358-9-120-5456. Ed. Jali Ruuskanen. adv.: B&W page FIM 9,420, color page FIM 12,900; 248 x 194. Circ: 53,000 (paid).

614 621.48 AUT ISSN 1020-525X
HD7269.A6 CODEN: SSAEAW
I A E A SAFETY STANDARDS SERIES. Text in English, French, Russian, Spanish, Arabic, Chinese. 1960. irreg. price varies. **Document type:** *Monographic series, Trade.*
Former titles (until 1996): International Atomic Energy Agency. Safety Series (1022-5420); I A E A Safety Series (0074-1892)
Related titles: CD-ROM ed.
Indexed: Biol.Abstr., GeoRef, I.M.M.Abstr., Pollut.Abstr.
—BLDSC, CISTI, Linda Hall.
Published by: (International Labour Office CHE), International Atomic Energy Agency/Agence Internationale de l'Energie Atomique, Division of Conference and Document Services, Wagramer Str 5, Postfach 100, Vienna, W 1400, Austria. TEL 43-1-2600-0, FAX 43-1-2600-29302, sales.publications@iaea.org, http://www.iaea.org.

614.8 USA ISSN 1063-9918
I A E M BULLETIN. (International Association of Emergency Managers) Text in English. 1983. m. USD 115 (effective 2001). adv. **Document type:** *Bulletin.*
Formerly: N C C E M's Official Monthly Newsletter; N C C E M Bulletin
Published by: International Association of Emergency Managers, 111 Park Pl, Falls Church, VA 22046-4513. TEL 703-538-1795, FAX 703-241-5603, IAEM@aol.com, http://www.iaem.com. Ed. Karen Thompson. Circ: 1,800.

613 USA ISSN 1093-1376
I C H F NEWSLETTER. Text in English. 1997. q. **Document type:** *Newsletter.*
Published by: International Council for Health Freedom, 5580 La Jolla Blvd, B429, La Jolla, CA 92037. TEL 619-483-8569, FAX 619-581-6640. Ed. Michael L Culbert.

I E & S NEWS. see *ENVIRONMENTAL STUDIES*

I E H ASSESSMENT INDOOR AIR QUALITY IN THE HOME: CARBON MONOXIDE. see *ENVIRONMENTAL STUDIES—Pollution*

▼ **I E H REPORT ON APPROACHES TO PREDICTING TOXICITY FROM OCCUPATIONAL EXPOSURE TO DUSTS.** see *ENVIRONMENTAL STUDIES—Toxicology And Environmental Safety*

▼ **I E H REPORT ON U K BLOOD LEAD SURVEYS.** see *ENVIRONMENTAL STUDIES—Toxicology And Environmental Safety*

I E H SPECIAL REPORT ON ORGANOPHOSPHORUS ESTERS; an evaluation of chronic neurotoxic effects. see *CHEMISTRY—Organic Chemistry*

I E Q STRATEGIES; a guide to the practical control of indoor air problems. (Indoor Environmental Quality) see *ENVIRONMENTAL STUDIES—Pollution*

362.1 GBR ISSN 1366-8331
I H S M HEALTH & SOCIAL SERVICES YEARBOOK. Text in English. 1996. a. GBP 120, USD 192. **Document type:** *Trade.* **Description:** Provides information about the NHS and related government organisations as well as independent hospitals and health services.
Incorporates: Burdett's Hospitals and Charities; Formerly (until 1995): Health Services Year Book
Related titles: CD-ROM ed.: I H S M Health and Social Services Database CD-ROM. GBP 250.
—BLDSC (4363.586350).
Published by: (Institute of Health Services Management), Financial Times Healthcare, Maple House, 149 Tottenham Ct Rd, London W1P 9LL, United Kingdom. TEL 44-207-896-2066, FAX 44-20-7896-2213, lizg@pearson-pro.com, http://www.fthealthcare.com. Ed. Guy Howland.

614 USA ISSN 1054-7053
I S S A TODAY. Text in English. 1975. m. USD 75 (effective 2000). adv. back issues avail. **Document type:** *Trade.*
Published by: International Sanitary Supply Association, Inc., 7373 N, Lincoln, IL 60712. TEL 847-982-0800, FAX 847-982-0995, info@issa.com, http://www.issa.com. Ed. Lisa Veeck. R&P Bill Balek. Adv. contact Charlie Walden. Circ: 4,600 (controlled).

I Z A. (Illustrierte Zeitschrift fuer Arbeitssicherheit) see *OCCUPATIONAL HEALTH AND SAFETY*

ICHIEFS ON SCENE. see *FIRE PREVENTION*

IDAHO. DEPARTMENT OF HEALTH AND WELFARE. RESEARCH AND STATISTICS SECTION. QUARTERLY WELFARE STATISTICAL BULLETIN. see *SOCIAL SERVICES AND WELFARE—Abstracting, Bibliographies, Statistics*

IDAHO. DEPARTMENT OF HEALTH AND WELFARE. VITAL STATISTICS (YEAR). see *PUBLIC HEALTH AND SAFETY—Abstracting, Bibliographies, Statistics*

362.1 ESP
I+G OGASUN LAGUNTZAK/AYUDAS I+D EN SALUD. Text in Spanish, Basque; Summaries in Spanish, Basque. 1988. a. free per issue (effective 2000). **Document type:** *Magazine, Government.*
Published by: Eusko Jaurlaritzaren Argitalpen-Zerbitzu Nagusia/Servicio Central de Publicaciones del Gobierno Vasco, Donostia-San Sebastian, 1, Vitoria-gasteiz, Alava 01010, Spain. TEL 34-945-018561, FAX 34-945-018709, hac-sabd@ej-gv.es, http://www.ej-gv.net/publicaciones.

614 ITA ISSN 0019-1639
CODEN: ISPRA2
IGIENE E SANITA PUBBLICA. Text in Italian; Summaries in English, French, German, Italian. 1945. bi-m. ITL 125,000; ITL 160,000 foreign (effective 1997). adv. bk.rev. charts, illus. index. **Document type:** *Academic/Scholarly.*
Related titles: Microform ed.: (from PQC).
Indexed: Abstr.Hyg., Biol.Abstr., Chem.Abstr., Curr.Adv.Ecol.Sci., Dairy Sci.Abstr., Excerp.Med., Helminthol.Abstr., INIS Atomind., Nutr.Abstr., Protozool.Abstr., Trop.Dis.Bull.
—CASDDS, Linda Hall. **CCC.**

P

Published by: Nebo Sas Editore, Piazza Monteleone Di Spoleto, 8, Rome, RM 00191, Italy. TEL 39-6-70300693, FAX 39-6-70303122. Ed. Augusto Pana. Pub., Adv. contact Giuseppe Cananzi. Circ: 2,000.

IGIENE MENTALE. see *PSYCHOLOGY*

614 USA
IN SIGHT. Text in English. 1978. s-a. free per issue.
Document type: *Newspaper.*
Formerly (until 1987): H K I Report
Published by: Helen Keller Worldwide, 352 Park Ave S, 12th Fl, New York, NY 10010. TEL 212-532-0544, FAX 212-943-1220, info@hki.org, http://www.hki.org. Ed. James E Ryan. R&P Louis Lo Re. Circ: 3,000.

613 310 USA ISSN 0885-9914
RA448.5.I5
INDIAN HEALTH TRENDS AND SERVICES. Text in English. 1969. irreg. free per issue. stat.
Published by: U.S. Public Health Service, Resources and Services Administration, 5600 Fishers Ln, Rockville, MD 20857. TEL 202-545-6700. Circ: 15,000. **Orders to:** Supt. of Documents, Govt Printing Office, Washington, DC 20402.

363.72 IND ISSN 0367-827X
RA565.A1 CODEN: IJEHBP
INDIAN JOURNAL OF ENVIRONMENTAL HEALTH. Text in English. 1959. q. adv. bk.rev. bibl, charts, illus, tr.lit.
Formerly: Environmental Health (0013-9289)
Indexed: Aqua.Sci.& Fish.Abstr., Biol.Abstr., CSNB, Chem.Abstr., Chem.Indus.Notes, Chem.Titles, Curr.Leather Lit., Environ.Per.Bibl., Environ.Sci.Poll.Mgmt., Excerp.Med., INIS Atomind., Ind.Med., Microbiol.Abstr., Ocean.Abstr. (coverage dropped), Pollut.Abstr., Sel.Water Res.Abstr., Soils & Fert., W.R.C.Inf.
—BLDSC (4412.100000), CASDDS, CISTI, GNLM, ingenta, Linda Hall.
Published by: National Environmental Engineering Research Institute, Documentation and Library Services, Nehru Marg, Nagpur, Maharashtra 440 020, India. Ed. S B Dabadghao. Circ: 1,200. **Affiliate:** Council of Scientific and Industrial Research.

614 IND ISSN 0019-557X
RA421 CODEN: IPBHAH
INDIAN JOURNAL OF PUBLIC HEALTH. Text in English. 1956. q. INR 100, USD 30. adv. bk.rev. abstr, charts, illus, stat. index.
Indexed: Abstr.Hyg., Biol.Abstr., Chem.Abstr., Dairy Sci.Abstr., Diar.Dis.Res., Food Sci.& Tech.Abstr., Helminthol.Abstr., Ind.Med. (1957-), Ind.Vet., Int.Nurs.Ind., Nutr.Abstr., Protozool.Abstr., Small Anim.Abstr., Vet.Bull.
—BLDSC (4420.400000), CISTI, GNLM.
Published by: Indian Public Health Association, 110 Chittaranjan Ave., Kolkata, West Bengal 700 073, India. Ed. A K Chakraborty. Circ: 2,500.

THE INDIAN PRACTITIONER; a monthly journal of medicine, surgery & public health. see *MEDICAL SCIENCES*

614 IDN ISSN 0216-3527
INDONESIAN JOURNAL OF PUBLIC HEALTH/MAJALAH KESEHATAN MASYARAKAT INDONESIA. Text and summaries in English, Indonesian. 1969. m. IDR 3,500 per issue. adv. bk.rev. charts, illus, stat.
Former titles: Indonesian Public Health Association. Journal; Indonesian Journal of Public Health
Published by: Indonesian Public Health Association/Ikatan Ahli Kesehatan Masyarakat Indonesia, Pegangsaan Timur 16, Jakarta, Indonesia. Ed. Azrul Azwar. Circ: 10,000.

613.5 697 DNK ISSN 0905-6947
TD883.1 CODEN: INAIE5
INDOOR AIR; international journal of indoor air quality and climate. Text in English. 1991. q. USD 257 in the Americas to institutions print & online eds. combined; GBP 178 elsewhere to institutions print & online eds. combined (effective 2002). adv. charts, illus. reprints avail. *Refereed.* **Document type:** *Academic/Scholarly.*
Related titles: ♦ Online - full text ed.: Indoor Air Online. ISSN 1600-0668; ♦ Supplement: Indoor Air. Supplement. ISSN 0908-5920.
Indexed: ASCA, Chem.Abstr., Chem.Indus.Notes, Chem.Titles, Curr.Cont., INIS Atomind., Ind.Med. (1991-), Int.Build.Serv.Abstr., Sci.Cit.Ind.
—BLDSC (4438.046530), CASDDS, CISTI, IDS, Infotrieve. **CCC.**
Published by: (International Society of Indoor Air Quality and Climate), Blackwell Munksgaard, Noerre Soegade 35, PO Box 2148, Copenhagen K 1016, Denmark. TEL 45-77-33-33-33, FAX 45-77-33-33-77, fsub@munksgaard.dk, http://journals.munksgaard.dk/indoorair, http://www.munksgaard.dk. Ed. Jan Sundell. Adv. contact Eric Rozario TEL 45-77-33-33-01. Circ: 1,200.

613.5 DNK ISSN 1600-0668
INDOOR AIR ONLINE. Text in English. q. DKK 160 (effective 2002). **Document type:** *Academic/Scholarly.*
Media: Online - full text (from EBSCO Publishing, ingenta, Swets Blackwell, Institute for Scientific Information).
Related titles: ♦ Print ed.: Indoor Air. ISSN 0905-6947.
Published by: Blackwell Munksgaard, Noerre Soegade 35, PO Box 2148, Copenhagen K 1016, Denmark. TEL 45-77-33-33-33, FAX 45-77-33-33-77, fsub@mail.munksgaard.dk, http://journals.munksgaard.dk/indoorair, http://www.munksgaard.dk.

613.5 DNK ISSN 0908-5920
INDOOR AIR. SUPPLEMENT. Text in English. 1993. irreg.
Related titles: ♦ Supplement to: Indoor Air. ISSN 0905-6947.
Published by: Blackwell Munksgaard, Noerre Soegade 35, PO Box 2148, Copenhagen K 1016, Denmark. TEL 45-77-33-33-33, FAX 45-7733-3333, http://www.munksgaard.dk/indoorair. Ed. Jan Sundell. Adv. contact Eric Rozario TEL 45-77-33-33-01.

▼ **INDOOR ENVIRONMENT CONNECTIONS**; the newspaper for the iaq marketplace. (indoor air quality) see *ENVIRONMENTAL STUDIES*

362.1 GBR ISSN 1461-085X
INFECTION SAFETY. Text in English. 1998. m. GBP 99 domestic; USD 145 foreign; GBP 9.50 newsstand/cover (effective 2000). **Description:** Covers biological agents and information sources from a safety perspective, including news of infection outbreaks worldwide, blood safety, precautions for travelers, occupational safety and health developments, new products, resources and educational opportunities.
Published by: Modus Operandi, PO Box HP346, Leeds LS6 1UL, United Kingdom. TEL 44-113-294-1212, http://www.modus-op.demon.co.uk. Ed., Pub. Adam Christie.

614.8 CHE ISSN 1011-5706
INFORMATIONS PHARMACEUTIQUES OMS. Text in French. 1987. q.
Related titles: ♦ English ed.: W H O Drug Information. ISSN 1010-9609.
Published by: World Health Organization, Marketing and Dissemination, Geneva, 27 1211, Switzerland. TEL 41-22-791-2476, FAX 41-22-791-4875.

INFORMAZIONE INNOVATIVA; agenzia quindicinale di documentazione internazionale servizio di informazione innovativa scientifica tecnologica legislativa per la produzione, l'ambiente, la sanita. see *ENVIRONMENTAL STUDIES*

362.1 ESP ISSN 1134-914X
INFORME DE SALUD PUBLICA. Text in Spanish; Summaries in Spanish. 1992. a. free per issue (effective 2000).
Published by: Eusko Jaurlaritzaren Argitalpen-Zerbitzu Nagusia/Servicio Central de Publicaciones del Gobierno Vasco, Donostia-San Sebastian, 1, Vitoria-gasteiz, Alava 01010, Spain. TEL 34-945-018561, FAX 34-945-018709, hac-sabd@ej-gv.es, http://www.ej-gv.net/publicaciones.

628 ITA ISSN 0394-5871
CODEN: IGEABH
INGEGNERIA AMBIENTALE. Key Title: I A Ingegneria Ambientale. Text in Italian; Summaries in English, Italian. 1972. 9/yr. ITL 165,000 domestic; ITL 265,000 foreign (effective 2000). adv. bk.rev. Index. 70 p./no.
Formerly (until 1986): Ingegneria Ambientale Inquinamento e Depurazione (0302-7775)
Indexed: Chem.Abstr., Chem.Indus.Notes, Chem.Titles, Environ.Sci.Poll.Mgmt., INIS Atomind., Pollut.Abstr., Saf.Sci.Abstr.
—BLDSC (4500.650000), CASDDS, CISTI.
Published by: (Centro di Ingegneria per la Protezione dell'Ambiente), C I P A s.a.s, Via Palladio, 26, Milan, MI 20135, Italy. TEL 39-02-58301528, FAX 39-02-58301550, cipami@tin.it. adv.: B&W page ITL 1,650,000, color page ITL 2,100,000; trim 210 x 297. Circ: 1,300.

628 ITA
INGEGNERIA AMBIENTALE QUADERNI. Text in Italian; Summaries in English, Italian. 1984. 2/yr. ITL 80,000.
Document type: *Monographic series.*
Formerly: Ingegneria Ambientale Inquinamento e Depurazione Quaderni
Indexed: Chem.Abstr., Pollut.Abstr.
Published by: (Centro di Ingegneria per la Protezione dell'Ambiente), C I P A s.a.s, Via Palladio, 26, Milan, MI 20135, Italy. TEL 39-02-58301528, FAX 39-02-58301550, cipami@tin.it.

628 ITA
INGEGNERIA SANITARIA AMBIENTALE; rivista tecnica bimestrale. Text in Italian. 1952; N.S. 1989. bi-m. ITL 110,000 (effective 1996). bk.rev. abstr, bibl, charts, illus.
Formerly (until 1990): Ingegneria Sanitaria (0020-0980)
Indexed: Chem.Abstr., INIS Atomind.
—Linda Hall.
Published by: (Associazione Nazionale di Ingegneria Sanitaria), Maggioli Editore, Divisione Periodici, Rimini, FO 47037, Italy. TEL 39-541-626777, FAX 39-0541-622020. Ed. Luigi Mendia. adv.: B&W page ITL 1,600,000, color page ITL 2,500,000; trim 270 x 160. Circ: 3,800.

628 BRA ISSN 0446-2424
TD4
INGENIERIA SANITARIA. Text in English, French, Portuguese, Spanish. 1946. q. USD 16 (effective 2000). adv. bk.rev.
Indexed: Pollut.Abstr., Repindex.
—CISTI.
Published by: Interamerican Association of Sanitary and Environmental Engineering, Rua Nicolau Gagliardi, 354, Sao Paulo, SP 05429, Brazil. TEL 011-212-4080, FAX 011-814-2441, TELEX 11-81453. Eds. Osvaldo Rey, Luiz Augusto de Lima Pontes. Circ: 8,000.

INJURY PREVENTION AND SAFETY PROMOTION. see *CONSUMER EDUCATION AND PROTECTION*

INSIDE INFORMATION. see *HEALTH FACILITIES AND ADMINISTRATION*

INSPECTOR. see *OCCUPATIONAL HEALTH AND SAFETY*

614 610 FRA ISSN 0755-4168
INSTITUT NATIONAL DE LA SANTE ET DE LA RECHERCHE MEDICALE. ACTUALITES. Key Title: INSERM Actualites. Text in French. 1950. m. free per issue. stat.
Former titles: Institut National de la Sante et de la Recherche Medicale. Bulletin d'Information; Institut National de la Sante et de la Recherche Medicale. Bulletin (0015-9603)
Indexed: INIS Atomind.
Published by: Institut National de la Sante et de la Recherche Medicale, 101 rue de Tolbiac, Paris Cedex 13 75654, France. TEL 33-1-44236000, FAX 33-1-44236099. Circ: 1,400.

614 JPN
INSTITUTE OF PUBLIC HEALTH. ANNUAL REPORT/KOKURITSU KOSHU EISEI-IN NENPO. Text in Japanese. 1948. a.
—BLDSC.
Published by: National Institute of Public Health, 4-6-1 Shirokanedai, Minato-ku, Tokyo 108-0071, Japan. Ed. Dr. Hidesuke Kobayashi.

INSTITUTION OF ENGINEERS (INDIA). ENVIRONMENTAL ENGINEERING DIVISION. JOURNAL. see *ENVIRONMENTAL STUDIES*

616.988 PRT ISSN 0303-7762
CODEN: AIHTDH
INSTITUTO DE HIGIENE E MEDICINA TROPICAL. ANAIS. Text and summaries in English, French, Portuguese. 1943. irreg., latest vol.10, 1984. PTE 1,500 (effective 2001). bk.rev. **Document type:** *Trade.*
Formerly: Lisbon. Escola Nacional de Saude de Medicina Tropical. Anais (0075-9767)
Indexed: Abstr.Hyg., Aqua.Sci.& Fish.Abstr., Aquacult.Abstr., Biol.Abstr., Environ.Sci.Poll.Mgmt., Excerp.Med., Helminthol.Abstr., Ind.Med. (coverage dropped), Ind.Vet., Rev.Appl.Entomol., Trop.Dis.Bull., Vet.Bull.
—CISTI, GNLM.
Published by: Instituto de Higiene e Medicina Tropical, Servico de Documentacao e Informacao Cientifica, Rua Junqueira, 96, Lisboa 1300-344, Portugal. TEL 351-1-3652600, FAX 351-1-3632105, biblio@ihmt.unl.pt, http://www.ihmt.unl.pt. Ed. Dr. Filomena Exposto. Circ: 1,000.

P

613 CHL ISSN 0716-1387
RA465 CODEN: BICHDZ
INSTITUTO DE SALUD PUBLICA DE CHILE. BOLETIN. Text in Spanish; Summaries in English. 1942. 2/yr. USD 6. adv. bk.rev. bibl, charts, illus.
Formerly: Instituto Bacteriologico de Chile. Boletin (0374-6224)
Indexed: Biol.Abstr., Chem.Abstr., Ind.Med. (coverage dropped), Trop.Dis.Bull.
—CASDDS.
Published by: Instituto de Salud Publica de Chile, Casillo 48, Marathon, 1000, Santiago, Chile. Eds. J Hernan Lobos R, Julio Garcia M. Circ: 628.

614 MEX
INSTITUTO MEXICANO DEL SEGURO SOCIAL. BOLETIN ESTADISTICO. Text in Spanish. 1972. a. free per issue.
Published by: Instituto Mexicano del Seguro Social, Subdireccion General Medica, Jefatura de Servicios de Medicina Preventiva, Apdo. Postal 12976, Mexico City, DF 03001, Mexico. Circ: 2,000.

614 MEX
INSTITUTO MEXICANO DEL SEGURO SOCIAL. BOLETIN SOBRE MORBILIDAD HOSPITALARIA. Text in Spanish. 1982. a. free per issue.
Published by: Instituto Mexicano del Seguro Social, Subdireccion General Medica, Jefatura de Servicios de Medicina Preventiva, Apdo. Postal 12976, Mexico City, DF 03001, Mexico. Circ: 2,000.

614 MEX
INSTITUTO MEXICANO DEL SEGURO SOCIAL. BOLETIN SOBRE MORTALIDAD. Text in Spanish. 1977. a. free per issue.
Published by: Instituto Mexicano del Seguro Social, Subdireccion General Medica, Jefatura de Servicios de Medicina Preventiva, Apdo. Postal 12976, Mexico City, DF 03001, Mexico. Circ: 2,000.

614 MEX
INSTITUTO MEXICANO DEL SEGURO SOCIAL. BOLETIN SOBRE MOTIVOS DE CONSULTA. Text in Spanish. 1980. a. free per issue.
Published by: Instituto Mexicano del Seguro Social, Subdireccion General Medica, Jefatura de Servicios de Medicina Preventiva, Apdo. Postal 12976, Mexico City, DF 03001, Mexico. Circ: 2,000.

614.86 USA ISSN 0018-988X
HE5614
INSURANCE INSTITUTE FOR HIGHWAY SAFETY. STATUS REPORT. Text in English. 1961. m. free per issue. index. reprint service avail. from PQC. **Document type:** *Newsletter, Consumer.*
Formerly: I I H S Report
Related titles: Microform ed.: (from PQC).
Indexed: Consum.Ind. (1990-).
Published by: Insurance Institute for Highway Safety, 1005 North Glebe Rd, Arlington, VA 22201. TEL 703-247-1500. Eds. Anne Fleming, Kim Stewart. Circ: 17,000.

INTERFACE (BETHESDA). see *COMPUTERS*

362.1 USA
INTERNATIONAL CLASSIFICATION OF DISEASES. CLINICAL MODIFICATION: CODING MANUAL. Short title: I C D - 9 - C M: Coding Manual. Text in English. 1978. base vol. plus irreg. updates. USD 25; USD 31.25 foreign. **Document type:** *Government.* **Description:** Presents guidelines that provide general assistance in coding and reporting medical conditions.
Published by: U.S. Public Health Service, 5600 Fishers Ln, Rockville, MD 20857. **Subscr. to:** National Technical Information Service, Government Research Center. FAX 703-321-8547. **Co-sponsor:** U.S. Department of Health and Human Services. Health Care Financing Administration.

INTERNATIONAL DIRECTORY OF SAFETY, SECURITY AND FIRE FIGHTING EQUIPMENT IMPORTERS. see *BUSINESS AND ECONOMICS—Trade And Industrial Directories*

INTERNATIONAL FOOD SAFETY NEWS. see *FOOD AND FOOD INDUSTRIES*

INTERNATIONAL JOURNAL OF CIRCUMPOLAR HEALTH. see *MEDICAL SCIENCES*

INTERNATIONAL JOURNAL OF EPIDEMIOLOGY. see *MEDICAL SCIENCES*

362 368.384 USA ISSN 1389-6563
▼ **INTERNATIONAL JOURNAL OF HEALTH CARE FINANCE AND ECONOMICS.** Text in English. 2001. q. USD 295, EUR 295 to institutions for print or online ed.; USD 354, EUR 354 combined subscription to institutions for print & online eds. (effective 2002). **Document type:** *Journal, Academic/Scholarly.*
Related titles: Online - full text ed.: (from Kluwer Online).
Published by: Kluwer Academic Publishers Boston, 101 Philip Dr, Assinippi Park, Norwell, MA 02061. TEL 781-871-6600, FAX 781-871-9045, services@wkap.nl, http://www.wkap.nl/journalhome.htm/1389-6563. Eds. Mark Pauly, Peter Zweifel. **Subscr. outside the Americas to:** Kluwer Academic Publishers Group, Journals Department, PO Box 322, Dordrecht 3300 AH, Netherlands. TEL 31-78-639-2392, FAX 31-78-654-6474; **Subscr. to:** Kluwer Academic - Plenum Publishers, 233 Spring St, New York, NY 10013-1578. TEL 212-620-8468, FAX 212-807-1047.

614 USA ISSN 0020-7314
RA421 CODEN: IJUSC3
INTERNATIONAL JOURNAL OF HEALTH SERVICES. Text in English. 1970. q. USD 56 to individuals; USD 218 to institutions (effective 2001). adv. bk.rev. abstr, illus. back issues avail.; reprints avail. *Refereed.* **Document type:** *Journal, Academic/Scholarly.* **Description:** Contains current and authoritative information on the development of the health care industry worldwide.
Related titles: Online - full text ed.: (from Institute for Scientific Information).
Indexed: ASCA, ASSIA, Abstr.Anthropol., Abstr.Health Care Manage.Stud., Abstr.Hyg., AgeLine, Alt.Press Ind., Amer.Bibl.Slavic & E.Eur.Stud., Biol.Abstr., CINAHL, C.I.S. Abstr., Crim.Just.Abstr., Curr.Cont., Diar.Dis.Res., ERA, Environ.Sci.Poll.Mgmt., Excerp.Med., Fam.Ind., Geo.Abstr.H.G., Hosp.Abstr., Hosp.Lit.Ind., IBZ, IDA, IMFL, INIS Atomind., I.P.A., Ind.Med. (1971-), Ind.Vet., Intl.Bibl.Soc.Sci., Lang.& Lang.Behav.Abstr., Med.Care Rev., Mid.East: Abstr.& Ind., Mult.Ed.Abstr., P.A.I.S., Polit.Sci.Abstr., Pollut.Abstr., Ref.Zh., Risk Abstr., Rural Devel.Abstr., SOPODA, SSCI, Saf.Sci.Abstr., Sage Race Rel.Abstr., Soc.Serv.Abstr., Sociol.Abstr., Sp.Ed.Needs Abstr., Stud.Wom.Abstr., Trop.Dis.Bull., Weed Abstr.
—BLDSC (4542.278000), CISTI, GNLM, IDS, ingenta, KNAW. **CCC.**
Published by: Baywood Publishing Co., Inc., 26 Austin Ave, Box 337, Amityville, NY 11701. TEL 631-691-1270, 800-638-7819, FAX 631-691-1770, info@baywood.com, baywood@baywood.com, http://baywood.com/search/PreviewJournal.asp?qsRecord=6. Ed. Vicente Navarro. R&P Julie Krempa. Adv. contact Joi Tamber-Brooks.

614.44 610 DEU ISSN 1438-4639
QR46 CODEN: ZHUMEO
INTERNATIONAL JOURNAL OF HYGIENE AND ENVIRONMENTAL HEALTH. Text in English; Summaries in English, German. 1883. 6/yr. EUR 3,370 to individuals; EUR 411 to institutions; GBP 117 to individuals; GBP 286 to institutions (effective 2002). *Refereed.* **Document type:** *Journal, Academic/Scholarly.* **Description:** Covers the entire field of human activity influencing health, regarding both the private and public health services.
Former titles: Zentralblatt fuer Hygiene und Umweltmedizin (0934-8859); Which incorporated (1955-1991): Zeitschrift fuer die Gesamte Hygiene und Ihre Grenzgebiete (0049-8610); (until 1989): Zentralblatt fuer Bakteriologie, Mikrogiologie und Hygiene. Serie B, Umwelthygiene, Krankenhaushygiene, Arbeitshygiene, Praventive Medizin (0932-6073); (until 1985): Zentralblatt fuer Bakteriologie, Mikrobiologie und Hygiene.1 Abt. Originale B, Hygiene (0174-3015); (until 1980): Zentralblatt fuer Bakteriologie. 1 Abt. Originale B, Hygiene, Krankenhaushygiene, Betriebshygiene, Praventive Medizin (0172-5602); (until 1979): Zentralblatt fuer Bakteriologie, Parasitenkunde, Infektionskrankheiten und Hygiene. 1. Abteilung. Originale. Reihe B, Hygiene, Praventive Medizin (0300-9661); (until 1971): Archiv fuer Hygiene und Bakteriologie (0003-9144); (until 1929): Archiv fuer Hygiene (0365-2955)
Related titles: Microfilm ed.: (from VCI,PMC); Online - full text ed.; (from Institute for Scientific Information).
Indexed: ASCA, Abstr.Hyg., Arts & Hum.Cit.Ind. (coverage dropped), Biol.Abstr., Chem.Indus.Notes, Chem.Titles, Curr.Cont., Dairy Sci.Abstr., Dent.Ind., Derwent Biotech.Abstr., Environ.Sci.Poll.Mgmt., Excerp.Med., Food Sci.& Tech.Abstr., INIS Atomind., Ind.Med. (2000-), Ind.Vet., Inpharma, Nutr.Abstr., Pollut.Abstr., Protozool.Abstr., Reac., Rev.Appl.Entomol., Rev.Med.& Vet.Mycol., SSCI (coverage dropped), Sci.Cit.Ind., Soils & Fert., Vet.Bull.
—BLDSC (4542.292000), CASDDS, CISTI, GNLM, IDS, Infotrieve. **CCC.**
Published by: Urban & Fischer Verlag, Loebdergraben 14A, Jena 07743, Germany. TEL 49-3641-626444, FAX 49-3641-626421, info@urbanfischer.de, http://www.urbanfischer.de. Eds. Dr. Hillel Koren, Dr. Michael Wilhem. R&P Martin Huber TEL 49-3641-626430.

INTERNATIONAL JOURNAL OF INFECTIOUS DISEASES. see *MEDICAL SCIENCES—Communicable Diseases*

INTERNATIONAL JOURNAL OF MASS EMERGENCIES AND DISASTERS. see *SOCIAL SERVICES AND WELFARE*

INTERNATIONAL JOURNAL OF MENTAL HEALTH. see *PSYCHOLOGY*

362.1 616.8 GBR ISSN 1462-3730
▼ **THE INTERNATIONAL JOURNAL OF MENTAL HEALTH PROMOTION**; promoting mental health, preventing mental disorders. Text in English. 1999. q. GBP 45 to individuals; GBP 135 to institutions. bk.rev. back issues avail. *Refereed.* **Document type:** *Bulletin, Academic/Scholarly.* **Description:** Coordinates the dissemination of new research to persons involved in policy making and promoting mental health.
—BLDSC (4542.352050).
Published by: (Clifford Beers Foundation), Pavilian Publishing Ltd., 8 St George's Pl, Brighton, E Essex BN1 4GB, United Kingdom. TEL 44-1273-623222, FAX 44-1273-625526, pavpub@pavilion.co.uk, http://www.pavpub.com. Ed. Michael Murray.

INTERNATIONAL JOURNAL OF OCCUPATIONAL MEDICINE AND ENVIRONMENTAL HEALTH. see *OCCUPATIONAL HEALTH AND SAFETY*

INTERNATIONAL JOURNAL OF PEST MANAGEMENT. see *AGRICULTURE—Crop Production And Soil*

▼ **INTERNATIONAL JOURNAL OF RADIATION MEDICINE/MEZHDUNARODNYI ZHURNAL RADIATSIONNOI MEDITSINYICINE.** see *MEDICAL SCIENCES—Radiology And Nuclear Medicine*

INTERNATIONAL JOURNAL OF TOXICOLOGY. see *ENVIRONMENTAL STUDIES—Toxicology And Environmental Safety*

INTERNATIONAL NARCOTICS CONTROL BOARD. REPORT FOR (YEAR). see *PHARMACY AND PHARMACOLOGY*

613 USA ISSN 0272-684X
RA440.A1
INTERNATIONAL QUARTERLY OF COMMUNITY HEALTH EDUCATION. Text in English. 1981. q. USD 56 to individuals; USD 218 to institutions (effective 2001). adv. bk.rev. abstr, illus. back issues avail.; reprints avail. *Refereed.* **Document type:** *Journal, Academic/Scholarly.* **Description:** Focuses on the systematic application of social science and health education theory and methodology to public health problems. Applies consumer-directed approaches to control preventive and curative health services.
Indexed: Abstr.Anthropol., Anthropol.Lit. (coverage dropped), Bibl.Asian Stud. (1996-1997), CINAHL, Cont.Pg.Educ., Curr.Lit.Fam.Plan., ERA, Lang.& Lang.Behav.Abstr., Mult.Ed.Abstr., NRN, PsycInfo, Psychol.Abstr. (1993-), Rural Devel.Abstr., SOPODA, Soc.Serv.Abstr., Sociol.Abstr., Sociol.Educ.Abstr., Tech.Educ.Abstr., e-psyche.
—BLDSC (4545.510000), CISTI, ingenta. **CCC.**
Published by: Baywood Publishing Co., Inc., 26 Austin Ave, Box 337, Amityville, NY 11701. TEL 631-691-1270, 800-638-7819, FAX 631-691-1770, info@baywood.com, baywood@baywood.com, http://baywood.com/search/PreviewJournal.asp?qsRecord=8. Ed. Dr. George P Cernada. R&P Julie Krempa. Adv. contact Joi Tamber-Brooks.

614.8 USA
INTERNATIONAL SYSTEM SAFETY CONFERENCE. PROCEEDINGS* . Text in English. 1971. biennial. USD 75. back issues avail. **Document type:** *Proceedings.* **Description:** Technical papers on system and product safety.
Published by: System Safety Society, Inc., 30363 Hicks Rd, Spotsylvania, VA 22553-5525. Circ: 550.

P

613.68 CHE ISSN 1020-0169
RA638
INTERNATIONAL TRAVEL AND HEALTH: VACCINATION REQUIREMENTS AND HEALTH ADVICE. Text in English. a. USD 15.30 (effective 1999). **Description:** Serves to alert physicians, health authorities and airline and shipping companies to changes in required and recommended vaccinations for travellers to every country in the world.
Former titles: Vaccination Certificate Requirements and Health Advice for International Travel (0257-912X); Vaccination Certificate Requirements for International Travel and Health Advice to Travellers (0254-296X); Vaccination Certificate Requirements for International Travel (0512-3011)
Related titles: French ed.: Voyages Internationaux et Sante. Vaccinations Exigees et Conseils d'Hygiene; German ed.
Indexed: Abstr.Hyg., Protozool.Abstr., Trop.Dis.Bull. —GNLM.
Published by: World Health Organization, Marketing and Dissemination, Geneva, 27 1211, Switzerland. TEL 41-22-791-2476, FAX 41-22-791-4857, publications@who.ch, http://www.who.int. Circ: 15,000.

INTERNATIONAL UNION AGAINST TUBERCULOSIS AND LUNG DISEASE. CONFERENCE PROCEEDINGS. see *MEDICAL SCIENCES—Respiratory Diseases*

362.1 USA
▼ **THE INTERNET JOURNAL OF HEALTH.** Text in English. 2000. s-a. free per issue. adv. bk.rev. back issues avail. *Refereed.* **Document type:** *Academic/Scholarly.* **Description:** Provides information from the field of general health, disease prevention, fitness and nutrition; contains original articles, reviews, case reports, streaming slide shows, streaming videos, letters to the editor, press releases, and meeting information.
Media: Online - full content.
Published by: Internet Scientific Publications, L.L.C., 23 Rippling Creek Dr, Sugar Land, TX 77479. TEL 281-240-1533, FAX 281-240-1533, http://www.ispub.com/. R&P, Adv. contact Hope Morrow TEL 832-754-0335.

613 AUS ISSN 1328-7443
RA427.8
INTERNET JOURNAL OF HEALTH PROMOTION. Text in English. 1995. irreg. *Refereed.* **Description:** Dedicated to public health and health care awareness issues.
Media: Online - full text.
Published by: Monash University, Department of Medicine, 246 Clayton Rd, Clayton, VIC 3168, Australia. TEL 61-3-9550-5523, FAX 61-3-9550-5524, Bridge.Hsu-Hage@med.monash.edu.au, http://www.monash.edu.au/health/IJHP. Ed. Dr. Bridget Hsu Hage.

362.1 DNK ISSN 1437-9619
▼ **INTERNET JOURNAL OF PUBLIC HEALTH EDUCATION.** Text in English. 1999. irreg. back issues avail. **Document type:** *Journal, Academic/Scholarly.* **Description:** Purses the systematic development and evaluation of public health and health sciences education and training.
Media: Online - full content.
Published by: University of Bielefeld, Faculty of Health Sciences, POB 100131, Bielefeld 33501, Denmark. http://www.ensp.fr/aspher/i-jphe/. Eds. Eliot Pearlman, Susanne Jordan, Thomas Kugel.

614 360 CAN
RA410.9.C2
INVENTORY OF HEALTH WORKFORCE IN ALBERTA. Text in English. 1978. a. free per issue. back issues avail. **Document type:** *Government.* **Description:** Contains the results of the annual survey of professional associations in Alberta concerning information and statistical data on the number of personnel registered with each association.
Former titles (until 1992): Inventory of Health & Social Service Personnel (0848-7332); Health and Social Service Manpower in Alberta (0714-1904)
Published by: Alberta Health, Practitioner Services Division, 10025 Jasper Ave, 16th Fl, Edmonton, AB T5J 2N3, Canada. TEL 403-427-3276, FAX 403-422-2880. Ed. D Chesley. Circ: 500.

614 IRN ISSN 0304-4556
CODEN: IJPHCD
IRANIAN JOURNAL OF PUBLIC HEALTH/MAJALLE-YE BEHDASHT-E IRAN. Text and summaries in English, Persian, Modern. 1972. q. IRR 1,000, USD 25. illus. index. **Document type:** *Academic/Scholarly.*
Related titles: CD-ROM ed.
Indexed: Abstr.Hyg., Biol.Abstr., Chem.Abstr., Dairy Sci.Abstr., Entomol.Abstr. (coverage dropped), Excerp.Med. (until 19??), ExtraMED, Helminthol.Abstr., INIS Atomind., Ind.Vet., Nutr.Abstr., Protozool.Abstr., Rev.Appl.Entomol., Rev.Med.& Vet.Mycol., Trop.Dis.Bull. —CASDDS, GNLM.
Published by: Iranian Public Health Association, University of Teheran, Teheran, Iran. Ed. D Farhud. Circ: 2,000.

363.179 615.902 IRL
IRELAND. DEPARTMENT OF AGRICULTURE AND FOOD. PESTICIDE RESIDUES IN FOOD. Text in English. a. **Document type:** *Government.*
Published by: Department of Agriculture and Food/An Roinn Talmhaiochta agus Bia, Agriculture House, Kildare St, Dublin, Dublin 2, Ireland. TEL 353-1-607-2000, information@daff.irlgov.ie, http://www.irlgov.ie/daff, http://www.irlgov.ie/daff/.

614 ISR
ISRAEL. MINISTRY OF HEALTH. DIVISION OF EPIDEMIOLOGY. INFECTIOUS DISEASES SURVEILLANCE. Text in English. s-a. **Document type:** *Government.*
Published by: Ministry of Health, Division of Epidemiology, 107 Hebron Rd, Jerusalem 91000, Israel.

614 ISR
ISRAEL. MINISTRY OF HEALTH. DIVISION OF EPIDEMIOLOGY. WEEKLY EPIDEMIOLOGICAL RECORD. Text in English. w. **Document type:** *Government.*
Published by: Ministry of Health, Division of Epidemiology, 107 Hebron Rd, Jerusalem 91000, Israel.

ISSUES IN CHILD ABUSE PREVENTION. see *SOCIAL SERVICES AND WELFARE*

ISSUES IN LAW AND MEDICINE. see *MEDICAL SCIENCES*

610 636.089 ITA ISSN 0021-2571
R61 CODEN: AISSAW
ISTITUTO SUPERIORE DI SANITA. ANNALI. Text and summaries in English, Italian. 1965. q., latest vol.37, 2001. ITL 110,000 domestic; ITL 130,000 foreign (effective 2001). adv. bk.rev. abstr, bibl, illus, charts, maps, stat. index, cum.index. back issues avail. *Refereed.* **Document type:** *Journal, Academic/Scholarly.* **Description:** Original articles, monographs, reviews and technical notes on health issues in many areas of public health.
Formerly: Istituto Superiore di Sanita. Rendiconti
Related titles: Online - full text ed.
Indexed: Abstr.Hyg., Biol.Abstr., CEABA, Chem.Abstr., Chem.Indus.Notes, Chem.Titles, Dairy Sci.Abstr., Excerp.Med., Food Sci.& Tech.Abstr., INIS Atomind., INSPEC (pre-1969-1970, 1980-), Ind.Med. (1965-), Ind.Vet., Nutr.Abstr., Protozool.Abstr., Ref.Zh., Rev.Appl.Entomol., Rev.Med.& Vet.Mycol., Soils & Fert., Triticale Abstr., Trop.Dis.Bull., Vet.Bull., Zoo.Rec. —BLDSC (1008.045000), AskIEEE, CASDDS, CINDOC, CISTI, GNLM, IDS, ingenta, KNAW, Linda Hall.
Published by: Istituto Superiore di Sanita, Viale Regina Elena 299, Rome, RM 00161, Italy. TEL 39-06-49901, FAX 39-06-49902253, pubblicazioni@iss.it, http://www.iss.it/publicazioni/annali.htm, http://www.iss.it/pubblicazioni. Ed. Enrico Alleva. Circ: 1,000. **Subscr. to:** Istituto Poligrafico e Zecca dello Stato, Funzione Editoria - Settore Abbonamenti, Piazza Verdi 10, Rome, RM 00198, Italy. TEL 39-06-85081.

610 ITA ISSN 0394-9303
ISTITUTO SUPERIORE DI SANITA. NOTIZIARIO. Text in Italian; Abstracts in English. 1988. m., latest vol.14, 2001. free to qualified personnel. Website rev. bibl, charts, illus, stat, abstr, maps. cum.index: 1988-1994. 24 p./no. back issues avail. **Document type:** *Newsletter, Academic/Scholarly.* **Description:** Presents activities of the institute, which is the scientific and technical body of the Italian national health service.
Related titles: Online - full text ed.; Supplement: Strumenti di Riferimento.
Published by: Istituto Superiore di Sanita, Viale Regina Elena 299, Rome, RM 00161, Italy. TEL 39-06-49901, FAX 39-06-49902253, notiziario@iss.it, http://www.iss.it/notiziario. Ed. Paola De Castro. Circ: 5,000 (controlled).

J D C - BROOKDALE INSTITUTE OF GERONTOLOGY AND HUMAN DEVELOPMENT. ANNUAL REPORT. see *GERONTOLOGY AND GERIATRICS*

J D C - BROOKDALE INSTITUTE OF GERONTOLOGY AND HUMAN DEVELOPMENT. RESEARCH SERIES. see *GERONTOLOGY AND GERIATRICS*

614 BGD ISSN 1012-8697
J O P S O M. (Journal of Preventive and Social Medicine) Text in Bengali. 1982. s-a. BDT 150 to individuals; BDT 200 to institutions. adv. back issues avail.
Indexed: Diar.Dis.Res.
Published by: National Institute of Preventive and Social Medicine, Mohakhali, Dhaka 1212, Bangladesh. Ed. M Mobarak Ali. Circ: 500.

JAHRBUCH KRITISCHE MEDIZIN. see *MEDICAL SCIENCES*

362.1 JPN
CODEN: GHKKEV
JAPAN. GIFU PREFECTURAL INSTITUTE OF HEALTH AND ENVIRONMENTAL SCIENCES. REPORT. Text in Japanese. 1972. a. **Document type:** *Government.*
Former titles (until 1996): Japan. Gifu Prefectural Health and Environment Research Center. Report (1340-2676); (until 1993): Japan. Gifu Prefectural Institute of Public Health. Report (0385-1575)
—BLDSC, CASDDS.
Published by: Gifu Prefectural Institute of Health and Environmental Sciences, 4-6-3 Noisshiki, Gifu-shi 500-8226, Japan. TEL 81-58-246-1101, FAX 81-58-246-1104.

628.2 JPN ISSN 0021-4639
TD511 CODEN: GSKSAQ
JAPAN SEWAGE WORKS ASSOCIATION. JOURNAL/GESUIDO KYOKAISHI. Text in Japanese. 1964. m. JPY 1,000 newsstand/cover. adv. bibl, charts, illus, mkt, tr.lit. index. **Document type:** *Academic/Scholarly.*
Indexed: Chem.Abstr., INIS Atomind., Mass Spectr.Bull. —BLDSC (4805.900000), CISTI.
Published by: Japan Sewage Works Association/Nihon Gesuido Kyokai, 6-2 Ote-Machi 2-chome, Chiyoda-ku, Tokyo 100-0004, Japan. TEL 81-3-5200-0816, FAX 81-3-5200-0847. Ed. Shogo Saito. Pub. Tsugio Furusawa. Adv. contact Yasuhiko Tanaka. Circ: 12,000.

362.1 CHN
JIANKANG WENZHAI BAO/DIGEST OF HEALTH NEWSPAPER. Text in Chinese. w. CNY 16.20. **Document type:** *Newspaper.*
Published by: China International Book Trading Corp/Zhongguo Guoji Tushu Maoyi Zonggongsi cibtc@mail.cibtc.com.cn, http://www.cibtc.com.cn. **Dist. by:** 35, Chegongzhuang Xilu, Haidian District, Beijing 100044, China.

614.8 USA ISSN 0277-8327
JOINT COMMISSION PERSPECTIVES. Text in English. 1952. bi-m. USD 80; USD 90 foreign. cum.index: 1983-1986. back issues avail. **Description:** Informs readers of new and revised Joint Commission standards, scoring guidelines, new and revised policies and procedures; covers the organization's quality improvement initiatives.
Formerly: J C A H Perspectives
Related titles: Online - full text ed.
Indexed: I.P.A., Int.Nurs.Ind.
—BLDSC (4672.252490).
Published by: (Joint Commission on Accreditation of Healthcare Organizations), Mosby Year, Inc. (Subsidiary of: Harcourt General, Inc.), Mosby, MO 63146-3318. TEL 800-453-4351, FAX 314-432-1380. Ed. Ruth Carol. Circ: 22,718.

614 USA ISSN 0449-122X
TX537
JOINT F A O - W H O CODEX ALIMENTARIUS COMMISSION. REPORT OF THE SESSION. Text in English. 1963. irreg., latest 1999, 23rd, Geneva, Switzerland. USD 12 (effective 2000). **Document type:** *Government.*
Related titles: French ed.; Spanish ed.
—BLDSC.
Published by: Food and Agriculture Organization of the United Nations, c/o Bernan Associates, 4611 F Assembly Dr, Lanham, MD 20706-4391. TEL 301-459-7666, FAX 301-459-0056.

JOURNAL: NEWS OF THE BLOOD PROGRAMME IN CANADA. see *MEDICAL SCIENCES—Hematology*

JOURNAL OF AGRICULTURAL SAFETY AND HEALTH. see *AGRICULTURE*

P

614 USA ISSN 0090-7421
R690
JOURNAL OF ALLIED HEALTH. Text in English. 1972. q., latest vol.30, 2001. USD 75 domestic; USD 92 foreign; USD 25 newsstand/cover domestic; USD 30 newsstand/cover foreign (effective 2001). adv. bk.rev. abstr. back issues avail.; reprint service avail. from PQC. *Refereed.* **Document type:** *Journal, Academic/Scholarly.* **Description:** Publishes scholarly papers, reports and findings related to research and development in allied health education, practice, history and current trends.
Related titles: Microform ed.: (from PQC,MIM).
Indexed: AMED, AgeLine, Biol.Abstr., C.I.J.E. (coverage dropped), CINAHL, Dent.Ind., Ind.Med. (1972-), Int.Nurs.Ind.
—BLDSC (4927.150000), CISTI, GNLM, ingenta.
Published by: (Association of Schools of Allied Health Professions), Hanley & Belfus, Inc., 210 S 13th St, Philadelphia, PA 19107. TEL 215-546-7293, FAX 215-790-9330. Ed. Dr. Kevin J Lyons. Adv. contact Diane Sherel. B&W page USD 640; 11 x 8.5. Circ: 2,000 (paid). **Subscr. to:** Publications Coordinator, Association of Schools of Allied Health Professions, 1730 M St, N W, Ste 500, Washington, DC 20036.

614.8 360 USA ISSN 1094-3412
JOURNAL OF BEHAVIORAL HEALTH SERVICES AND RESEARCH. Text in English. 1972. q. USD 69 to individuals; USD 21 newsstand/cover (effective 2002). adv. bk.rev. charts, illus, stat, abstr. index. back issues avail.; reprints avail. *Refereed.* **Document type:** *Journal, Academic/Scholarly.* **Description:** Publishes original research on the organization, financing, delivery and outcomes of mental health services and substance abuse treatment services.
Formerly (until 1997): Journal of Mental Health Administration (0092-8623)
Related titles: Microfilm ed.: (from PQC); Online - full text ed.: (from ProQuest Information & Learning, Institute for Scientific Information).
Indexed: ABI Inform. (Sum.1991-), ASSIA, AgeLine, Biostat., Crim.Just.Abstr., Curr.Cont., Excerp.Med. (1993-), Fam.Ind., Hosp.Lit.Ind., Human Resour.Abstr., Ind.Med. (1998-), Int.Nurs.Ind., Lang.& Lang.Behav.Abstr., P.A.I.S., PsycInfo, Psychol.Abstr. (1986-), SOPODA, SSCI, Sage Fam.Stud.Abstr., Sage Pub.Admin.Abstr., Soc.Serv.Abstr., Soc.Work Res.& Abstr., Sociol.Abstr., Viol.& Abuse Abstr., e-psyche.
—BLDSC (4951.261000), GNLM, IDS, ingenta. **CCC.**
Published by: (Association of Behavioral Healthcare Management), Aspen Publishers Inc, 200 Orchard Ridge Dr, Gaithersburg, MD 20878. TEL 301-417-7500, 800-234-1660, FAX 301-695-7931, customer.service@aspenpubl.com, http://www.aspenpub.com/. Ed. Bruce Levin. Circ: 2,000.

614 USA ISSN 1093-0019
RA446.5.M49
JOURNAL OF BORDER HEALTH* /REVISTA DE SALUD FRONTERIZA. Text in English, Spanish. 1984. q. USD 75 to individuals; USD 500 to institutions. *Refereed.* **Document type:** *Academic/Scholarly.* **Description:** Covers U.S.-Mexico border public health and environmental issues.
Formerly (until 1996): Border Health (1086-4512)
Indexed: Chic.Per.Ind., IIS.
Published by: (United States - Mexico Border Health Association), El Paso Field Office, 6006 N Mesa, Ste 600, El Paso, TX 79912. TEL 915-581-6645, FAX 915-833-4768, uph@usmbha.org. Ed. Dr. Guilleraio Mendoza. Circ: 800.

THE JOURNAL OF CLINICAL EPIDEMIOLOGY; including pharmacoepidemiology reports; devoted to the problems and management of chronic illness in all age groups. see *MEDICAL SCIENCES*

JOURNAL OF COMMUNITY HEALTH; the publication for health promotion and disease prevention. see *MEDICAL SCIENCES*

JOURNAL OF CRASH PREVENTION AND INJURY CONTROL. see *ENGINEERING—Mechanical Engineering*

JOURNAL OF ENVIRONMENTAL HEALTH. see *ENVIRONMENTAL STUDIES*

JOURNAL OF ENVIRONMENTAL PATHOLOGY, TOXICOLOGY AND ONCOLOGY. see *ENVIRONMENTAL STUDIES—Toxicology And Environmental Safety*

JOURNAL OF ENVIRONMENTAL SCIENCE AND HEALTH. PART A: TOXIC HAZARDOUS SUBSTANCES AND ENVIRONMENTAL ENGINEERING. see *ENVIRONMENTAL STUDIES—Toxicology And Environmental Safety*

JOURNAL OF ENVIRONMENTAL SCIENCE AND HEALTH. PART B: PESTICIDES, FOOD CONTAMINANTS, AND AGRICULTURAL WASTES. see *ENVIRONMENTAL STUDIES*

614.4 570 GBR ISSN 1359-5229
JOURNAL OF EPIDEMIOLOGY AND BIOSTATISTICS. Text in English. 1996. 6/yr. GBP 140, USD 240 to individuals; GBP 265, USD 440 to institutions (effective 2002).
Related titles: Online - full text ed.: (from ingenta, CatchWord Ltd.).
Indexed: Abstr.Hyg., Ind.Med. (1996-), Ind.Vet., Pig News & Info., Vet.Bull.
—GNLM.
Published by: Isis Medical Media Ltd. (Subsidiary of: Martin Dunitz Ltd.), The Livery House, 7-9 Pratt St, London NW1 0AE, United Kingdom. TEL 44-20-7482-2202, FAX 44-20-7267-0159, http://www.dunitz.co.uk, info@dunitz.co.uk, http://www.dunitz.co.uk/.

JOURNAL OF EPIDEMIOLOGY & COMMUNITY HEALTH. see *MEDICAL SCIENCES*

JOURNAL OF FOOD PROTECTION. see *FOOD AND FOOD INDUSTRIES*

JOURNAL OF HEALTH AND HUMAN SERVICES ADMINISTRATION. see *HEALTH FACILITIES AND ADMINISTRATION*

613 USA ISSN 1095-8940
JOURNAL OF HEALTH & POPULATION IN DEVELOPING COUNTRIES. Text in English. 1997. s-a. USD 15 to individuals; USD 30 to institutions (effective 2000). **Document type:** *Academic/Scholarly.*
—BLDSC (4996.715000).
Published by: University of North Carolina at Chapel Hill, Department of Health Policy and Administration, 1107 McGavran-Greenberg Bldg, Pittsboro St, Chapel Hill, NC 27599. TEL 919-966-1938, FAX 919-966-6961, hpjournal@unc.edu. Ed. Sagar C Jain.

JOURNAL OF HEALTH & SOCIAL POLICY. see *SOCIAL SERVICES AND WELFARE*

614 NLD ISSN 0167-6296
JOURNAL OF HEALTH ECONOMICS. Text in English. 1982. bi-m. EUR 81 in Europe to individuals; JPY 10,700 in Japan to individuals; USD 85 elsewhere to individuals; EUR 823 in Europe to institutions; JPY 109,300 in Japan to institutions; USD 921 elsewhere to institutions (effective 2002). adv. bk.rev. illus. back issues avail.; reprint service avail. from SWZ. *Refereed.* **Document type:** *Academic/Scholarly.* **Description:** Publishes articles related to the economics of health and medical care.
Related titles: Microform ed.: (from PQC); Online - full text ed.: (from EBSCO Publishing, ingenta, Gale Group, ScienceDirect, Swets Blackwell, Factiva, Institute for Scientific Information).
Indexed: ABI Inform. (Dec.1984-), ASCA, ASSIA, Abstr.Health Care Manage.Stud., Abstr.Hyg., Abstr.Soc.Geront., AgeLine, C.R.E.J., Curr.Cont., Environ.Sci.Poll.Mgmt., Excerp.Med., Geo.Abstr.H.G., Human Resour.Abstr., IDA, Inpharma, Int.Nurs.Ind., Intl.Bibl.Soc.Sci., J.of Econ.Lit., Med.Care Rev., P.A.I.S., Peace Res.Abstr., Pollut.Abstr., Reac., Risk Abstr., Russ.Acad.Sci.Bibl., SSCI, Saf.Sci.Abstr., Sage Fam.Stud.Abstr., Sage Pub.Admin.Abstr., Sci.Cit.Ind.
—BLDSC (4996.750000), CISTI, GNLM, IDS, ingenta. **CCC.**
Published by: North-Holland (Subsidiary of: Elsevier Science BV), PO Box 211, Amsterdam 1000 AE, Netherlands. TEL 31-20-485-3911, FAX 31-20-485-3598, http://www.elsevier.com/locate/jhealeco. Eds. A J Culyer, Joseph P Newhouse. **Subscr. in Australasia and the Far East to:** Elsevier Science (Singapore) Pte Ltd, No.1 Temasek Ave, 17-01 Millenia Tower, Singapore 039192, Singapore. TEL 65-434-3727, FAX 65-337-2230**; Subscr. in Japan to:** Elsevier Science Inc - Japan Regional Office, 9-15 Higashi-Azabu 1-chome, Minato-ku, Tokyo 106-0044, Japan. TEL 81-3-5561-5033**; Subscr. in the Americas to:** Elsevier Science, PO Box 945, New York, NY 10159-0945. TEL 212-633-3730, FAX 212-633-3680, usinfo-f@elsevier.com.

JOURNAL OF HEALTH SCIENCE/EISEI KAGAKU. see *ENVIRONMENTAL STUDIES—Toxicology And Environmental Safety*

JOURNAL OF HEALTH SERVICES RESEARCH & POLICY. see *MEDICAL SCIENCES*

JOURNAL OF HEPATOLOGY, GASTROENTEROLOGY, INFECTIOUS DISEASES. see *MEDICAL SCIENCES—Communicable Diseases*

JOURNAL OF HIV - AIDS PREVENTION & EDUCATION FOR ADOLESCENTS & CHILDREN. see *MEDICAL SCIENCES—Communicable Diseases*

▼ **JOURNAL OF HUMAN FACTORS AND AEROSPACE SAFETY.** see *AERONAUTICS AND SPACE FLIGHT*

JOURNAL OF PESTICIDE REFORM. see *ENVIRONMENTAL STUDIES—Pollution*

JOURNAL OF PHARMACOEPIDEMIOLOGY; innovations in pharmaceutical research and practice relating. see *PHARMACY AND PHARMACOLOGY*

JOURNAL OF PUBLIC HEALTH DENTISTRY. see *MEDICAL SCIENCES—Dentistry*

368.382 USA ISSN 1078-4659
RA395.A3
JOURNAL OF PUBLIC HEALTH MANAGEMENT AND PRACTICE. Text in English. 1995. bi-m. USD 172 to individuals; USD 34 newsstand/cover (effective 2002). adv. reprints avail. *Refereed.* **Document type:** *Journal, Academic/Scholarly.* **Description:** Addresses public health administration and profiles local programs and initiatives.
Related titles: Microform ed.: (from PQC); Online - full text ed.: (from ProQuest Information & Learning).
Indexed: CINAHL.
—BLDSC (5043.553000), ingenta.
Published by: Aspen Publishers, Inc., 200 Orchard Ridge Dr, Ste 200, Gaithersburg, MD 20878. TEL 301-417-7500, 800-638-8437, FAX 301-417-7550, customer.service@aspenpubl.com, http://www.aspenpub.com. Ed. Dr. Lloyd Novick. Pub. Michael B Brown. Adv. contact Frances S Ray. **Dist. by:** Aspen Publishers Inc., Distribution Center, 7201 McKinney Circle, Frederick, MD 21701. TEL 301-698-7100, FAX 301-417-7550.

JOURNAL OF PUBLIC HEALTH MEDICINE. see *SOCIAL SERVICES AND WELFARE*

362.1 USA ISSN 0197-5897
RA421 CODEN: JPPODK
JOURNAL OF PUBLIC HEALTH POLICY. Text in English. 1980. q. USD 130 (effective 2001). adv. bk.rev. back issues avail. *Refereed.* **Document type:** *Academic/Scholarly.* **Description:** Publishes contributions advancing the discussion of public health policy issues in the US and on an international level.
Related titles: Online - full text ed.: (from Institute for Scientific Information).
Indexed: ASCA, Abstr.Health Care Manage.Stud., AgeLine, Curr.Cont., Diar.Dis.Res., Dok.Arbeitsmed., Environ.Abstr., Environ.Per.Bibl. (1991-), Environ.Sci.Poll.Mgmt., Excerp.Med., Fam.Ind., Ind.Med. (1980-), Lang.& Lang.Behav.Abstr., NRN, P.A.I.S., Pollut.Abstr., Ref.Zh., Risk Abstr., Rural Devel.Abstr., SSCI, Saf.Sci.Abstr., Sage Race Rel.Abstr., Soc.Serv.Abstr., Sociol.Abstr., THA.
—BLDSC (5043.570000), CIS, CISTI, GNLM, IDS, ingenta, KNAW.
Published by: Journal of Public Health Policy, Inc., 208 Meadowood Dr, South Burlington, VT 05403. TEL 802-658-0136, FAX 802-862-4011, jphpterris@aol.com, http://members.aol.com/jphpterris/jphp.htm. Ed. Dr. Milton Terris. Circ: 1,800.

THE JOURNAL OF RURAL HEALTH. see *MEDICAL SCIENCES*

613 USA ISSN 0022-4391
LB3401 CODEN: JSHEA2
JOURNAL OF SCHOOL HEALTH. Text in English. 1930. m. (Aug.-May). USD 95 domestic to individuals; USD 115 foreign to individuals; USD 120 domestic to institutions; USD 140 foreign to institutions (effective 2001). adv. bk.rev. abstr, bibl, charts, stat. index, cum.index every 10 yrs. reprint service avail. from PQC. *Refereed.* **Document type:** *Academic/Scholarly.*
Formerly: School Physicians Bulletin
Related titles: Microform ed.: (from PQC); Online - full text ed.: (from Gale Group, ProQuest Information & Learning, Northern Light Technology, Inc., H. W. Wilson, Factiva, Institute for Scientific Information).

P

Indexed: ASCA, Acad.Ind., Adol.Ment.Hlth.Abstr., AgeLine, Biog.Ind., Biol.Abstr., C.I.J.E., CINAHL, Cont.Pg.Educ., Crim.Just.Abstr., Curr.Cont., Curr.Lit.Fam.Plan., Dent.Ind., Diar.Dis.Res., Educ.Ind. (May 1983-), Educ.Tech.Abstr., Environ.Sci.Poll.Mgmt., Except.Child Educ.Abstr., Fam.Ind., Hlth.Ind., IMFL, Ind.Med. (1937-), Int.Nurs.Ind., Media Rev.Dig. (Jan.1989-Dec.1991), Mult.Ed.Abstr., NRN, Nurs.Abstr., Phys.Ed.Ind., Pollut.Abstr., Psychol.Abstr., Res.High.Educ.Abstr., Risk Abstr., SOMA, SSCI, Saf.Sci.Abstr., Sp.Ed.Needs Abstr., Sportsearch (1976-), Stud.Wom.Abstr., THA, Tech.Educ.Abstr., WMB.
—BLDSC (5052.650000), GNLM, IDS, ingenta, KNAW.
Published by: American School Health Association, PO Box 708, Kent, OH 44240. TEL 216-678-1601, FAX 216-678-4526. Ed. R Morgan Pigg Jr. R&P Thomas Reed. Adv. contact Rick Gabler. Circ: 10,000.

▼ **JOURNAL OF THE I C R U.** see *PHYSICS—Nuclear Physics*

JOURNAL OF TOXICOLOGY AND ENVIRONMENTAL HEALTH. PART A. see *ENVIRONMENTAL STUDIES—Toxicology And Environmental Safety*

JOURNAL OF TOXICOLOGY AND ENVIRONMENTAL HEALTH. PART B: CRITICAL REVIEWS. see *ENVIRONMENTAL STUDIES—Toxicology And Environmental Safety*

JOURNAL OF TOXICOLOGY. CLINICAL TOXICOLOGY. see *PHARMACY AND PHARMACOLOGY*

JOURNAL OF TRAFFIC SAFETY EDUCATION. see *TRANSPORTATION—Automobiles*

JUGENDROTKREUZ. see *CHILDREN AND YOUTH—For*

KEEPING THE TRUST. see *SOCIAL SERVICES AND WELFARE*

616.9 KEN ISSN 0140-5071
KENYA. MINISTRY OF HEALTH. HEALTH INFORMATION BULLETIN. Text in English. 1977. q. free per issue. **Document type:** *Bulletin, Government.*
Published by: Ministry of Health, Division of Communicable Diseases Control and Epidemiology, PO Box 20781, Nairobi, Kenya. Circ: 500.

KIDSAFE. see *CHILDREN AND YOUTH—About*

362.1 DEU ISSN 1438-5066
▼ **KINDER, KINDER**; sicher - gesund. Text in German. 1999. q. DEM 14 (effective 2001). **Document type:** *Magazine, Trade.*
Published by: Universum Verlagsanstalt GmbH KG, Taunusstr 54, Wiesbaden 65183, Germany. TEL 49-611-9030-0, FAX 49-611-9030382, redaktion.kk@universum.de, uv@universum.de, http://www.universum.de/univ/arbeit_gesundheit/index_kk_main.html. Circ: 44,000 (paid).

KOKORO TO SHAKAI/MIND AND SOCIETY. see *PSYCHOLOGY*

614.8 JPN
KOKUTETSU CHUO HOKEN KANRIJOHO; health control. Text and summaries in English, Japanese. 1955. a. free per issue. back issues avail.
Published by: Japanese National Railways, Central Health Institute, 2-1 Yoyogi, Shibuya-ku, Tokyo 151-0053, Japan. Circ: 1,000.

614 DEU ISSN 0943-4100
KONTENRAHMEN FUER DIE TRAEGER DER GESETZLICHEN KRANKENVERSICHERUNG, KONTENRAHMEN FUER DIE TRAEGER DER SOZIALEN PFLEGEVERSICHERUNG UND DEN AUSGLEICHSFONDS. Text in German. 1981. irreg. DEM 96 (effective 2000). **Document type:** *Bulletin, Trade.*
Published by: Erich Schmidt Verlag GmbH & Co. (Berlin), Genthiner Str 30G, Berlin 10785, Germany. TEL 49-30-250085-0, FAX 49-30-25008521, vertrieb@esvmedien.de, http://www.erich-schmidt-verlag.de.

614 KOR ISSN 0023-401X
RA421 CODEN: KOPOAL
KOREAN JOURNAL OF PUBLIC HEALTH/BO KUN HAK NON ZIP. Key Title: Gonjun Bogen Jabji. Text in English, Korean. 1964. s-a. free per issue. **Description:** Contains research articles on public health and population.
Indexed: Biol.Abstr.
Published by: Seoul National University, School of Public Health, 28 Yunkun-dong, Chongro-ku, Seoul, Korea, S.. TEL 02-762-9101. Ed. Moonshik Zong. Circ: 1,000.

628 JPN ISSN 0368-5187
KOSHU EISEI/JOURNAL OF PUBLIC HEALTH PRACTICE. Text in Japanese. 1946. m. JPY 25,200.
Indexed: INIS Atomind., Ref.Zh.
Published by: Igaku-Shoin Ltd., 5-24-3 Hongo, Bunkyo-ku, Tokyo 113-0033, Japan. TEL 81-3-3817-5718. Ed. Kozo Tatara. Circ: 3,500.

614 DEU ISSN 0936-076X
KRANKENVERSICHERUNG DER RENTNER. Text in German. 1982. irreg. DEM 88 (effective 2000). **Document type:** *Bulletin.*
Published by: Erich Schmidt Verlag GmbH & Co. (Berlin), Genthiner Str 30G, Berlin 10785, Germany. TEL 49-30-250085-0, FAX 49-30-25008521, vertrieb@esvmedien.de, http://www.erich-schmidt-verlag.de.

614 697 JPN ISSN 0386-4081
TH6014
KUKI CHOWA EISEI KOGAKU/HEATING, AIR-CONDITIONING AND SANITARY ENGINEERING. Text in Japanese; Summaries in English, Japanese. 1917. m. USD 218.
Indexed: INIS Atomind.
—CISTI, Linda Hall.
Published by: Kuki Chowa Eisei Kogakkai/Society of Heating, Air-Conditioning and Sanitary Engineering of Japan, 8-1 Kitashinjuku 1-chome, Shinjuku-ku, Tokyo 160-0000, Japan. **Dist by:** International Marketing Corp., I.P.O. Box 5056, Tokyo 100-30, Japan. TEL 81-3-3661-7458, FAX 81-3-3667-9646.

614 ISR
KUPAT-HOLIM. INFORMATION SERIES AND SPECIAL STUDIES AND SURVEYS ON MEDICAL MANPOWER SOCIOLOGY AND MEDICAL ECONOMICS. Text in English. 1962. q. bk.rev. stat. **Document type:** *Academic/Scholarly.*
Former titles: Kupat Holim. Information Series: Special Studies on Medical Manpower and Sociology; Kupat-Holim. Information Series: Special Studies and Surveys on Medical Sociology and Health Economics; (until 1973): Kupat-Holim. Information Series. "Meida" on Medical Sociology and Health
Media: Duplicated (not offset).
Published by: (Kupat-Holim Health Insurance Institution, Research Department), Kupat Holim Center, P O Box 16250, Tel Aviv, Israel. TEL 972-3-6923532, FAX 972-3-433474. Ed. Dr. Nelu Shavitt. Circ: 150.

614 ISR ISSN 0301-4843
CODEN: SFYBAI
KUPAT-HOLIM YEARBOOK. Text in English. 1971. a. free per issue.
Related titles: Hebrew ed.
Indexed: Biol.Abstr., Chem.Abstr.
—CASDDS.
Published by: Kupat Holim Health Insurance Institution, 101 Arlosoroff St., P O Box 16250, Tel Aviv, Israel.

614 JPN ISSN 0454-7675
TA495 CODEN: DPKBAN
KYOTO UNIVERSITY. DISASTER PREVENTION RESEARCH INSTITUTE. BULLETIN/KYOTO DAIGAKU BOSAI KENKYUJO KIYO. Text in English. 1951. q. per issue exchange basis. **Document type:** *Bulletin.*
Indexed: GeoRef, J.of Ferroc., Meteor.& Geoastrophys.Abstr.
—CISTI, ingenta, Linda Hall.
Published by: Kyoto University, Disaster Prevention Research Institute/Kyoto Daigaku Bosai Kenkyujo, Gokasho, Uji-shi, Kyoto-Fu 611-0011, Japan. Circ: 650.

614 300 GBR
L S E HEALTH DISCUSSION PAPER. Text in English. irreg., latest vol.2, 1995. **Document type:** *Monographic series.*
—BLDSC (5300.408500).
Published by: London School of Economics and Political Science, Houghton St., London WC2A 2AE, United Kingdom. TEL 44-20-7955-7540, FAX 44-20-7955-7546.

LABORATORY INFORMATION BULLETIN. see *MEDICAL SCIENCES—Experimental Medicine, Laboratory Technique*

628 USA ISSN 1079-784X
LABORATORY SAFETY & ENVIRONMENTAL MANAGEMENT. Text in English. 1993. bi-m. USD 250. **Document type:** *Academic/Scholarly.*
Indexed: CSNB, Lab.Haz.Bull.
—BLDSC (5141.595700).
Published by: Target Group, 1907 W Burbank Blvd, 2nd Fl, Burbank, CA 91506. TEL 818-842-4777, FAX 818-842-0578. Eds. Cynthia L Salisbury, Frank J Priznar. Pub. Don Meeker.

▼ **LAMY HYGIENE ET SECURITE.** see *LAW*

614.83 USA ISSN 0277-9196
LAURISTON S. TAYLOR LECTURE SERIES. Text in English. 1977. a. USD 25 (effective 1999). back issues avail. **Document type:** *Monographic series.*
—CISTI, Linda Hall.
Published by: National Council on Radiation Protection and Measurements, 7910 Woodmont Ave, Ste 800, Bethesda, MD 20814. TEL 301-657-2652. Ed. William M Beckner. R&P Eric K Kearsley.

363.7384 AUS ISSN 1324-6011
LEAD ACTION NEWS. Text in English. 1993. q. AUD 30 to individuals; AUD 120 to institutions. adv. bk.rev. bibl, charts, illus, maps, stat. back issues avail. **Document type:** *Newsletter.* **Description:** Aims to eliminate childhood lead poisoning in Australia by the year 2002 and to protect the environment from lead.
Published by: Lead Group Incorporated, PO Box 161, Summer Hill, NSW 2130, Australia. TEL 61-2-97160014, FAX 61-2-97169005, leadnet@peg.apc. Ed., Pub., R&P, Adv. contact Elizabeth O'Brien. Circ: 500.

614 CHE
LEBEN UND GESUNDHEIT; monatlicher Ratgeber zur Foerderung einer naturgemaessen Lebensweise. Text in German. 1929. m. CHF 59 (effective 2000). adv. bk.rev. index. back issues avail. **Document type:** *Magazine, Consumer.*
Published by: Advent Verlag, Wylerhalde, Krattigen 3704, Switzerland. TEL 41-33-6541065, FAX 41-33-6544431, adventverlag@swissonline.ch. Ed., Adv. contact Gunther Klenk. B&W page CHF 1,623, color page CHF 2,751. Circ: 15,000.

614 LBR
LIBERIA. MINISTRY OF HEALTH AND SOCIAL WELFARE. ANNUAL REPORT*. Text in English. a., latest 1975.
Published by: Ministry of Health and Social Welfare, Monrovia, Liberia.

614.8 CAN ISSN 0714-5896
LIVING SAFETY. Text in English. 1983. q. CND 9.95 (effective 2000). **Document type:** *Consumer.*
Published by: Canada Safety Council, 1020 Thomas Spratt Pl, Ottawa, ON K1G 5L5, Canada. TEL 613-739-1535, FAX 613-739-1566. Ed. Jack A Smith. R&P Carole Deavey. Circ: 25,000.

614 USA
LOCAL HEALTH OFFICERS NEWS. Text in English. bi-m. USD 35. **Document type:** *Newsletter.* **Description:** Offers mayors and municipal health officials updates on policy, legislation, meetings, and other items of interest.
Published by: U.S. Conference of Mayors, Office of Public Affairs, 1620 Eye St, N W, Washington, DC 20006. TEL 202-293-7330.

LOSINKA. see *PUBLIC ADMINISTRATION—Municipal Government*

614.86 USA ISSN 0741-4439
LOUISIANA. DEPARTMENT OF PUBLIC SAFETY. SUMMARY OF MOTOR VEHICLE TRAFFIC ACCIDENTS. KENNER. Text in English. 1971. s-a. free per issue. charts, stat. **Document type:** *Government.*
Supersedes in part: Louisiana. Department of Public Safety. Summary of Motor Vehicle Accident Reports
Related titles: Microfiche ed.: (from CIS); Microfilm ed.
Indexed: SRI.
Published by: Department of Public Safety, Traffic Records Unit, PO Box 66614, Baton Rouge, LA 70896. TEL 504-925-6348. Circ: 350.

614.86 388.41 USA ISSN 0741-434X
LOUISIANA. DEPARTMENT OF PUBLIC SAFETY. SUMMARY OF MOTOR VEHICLE TRAFFIC ACCIDENTS. RURAL. Text in English. 1981. s-a. free per issue. **Document type:** *Government.*
Supersedes in part: Louisiana Department of Public Safety. Summary of Motor Vehicle Accident Reports
Indexed: SRI.
Published by: Department of Public Safety, Traffic Records Unit, PO Box 66614, Baton Rouge, LA 70896. TEL 504-925-6348.

614.86 388.41 USA ISSN 0741-4382
LOUISIANA. DEPARTMENT OF PUBLIC SAFETY. SUMMARY OF MOTOR VEHICLE TRAFFIC ACCIDENTS. SHREVEPORT. Text in English. s-a. free per issue. **Document type:** *Government.*
Supersedes in part: Louisiana. Department of Public Safety. Summary of Motor Vehicle Accident Reports
Indexed: SRI.
Published by: Department of Public Safety, Traffic Records Unit, PO Box 66614, Baton Rouge, LA 70896. TEL 504-925-6348.

614.86 388.41 USA ISSN 0741-4358
LOUISIANA. DEPARTMENT OF PUBLIC SAFETY. SUMMARY OF MOTOR VEHICLE TRAFFIC ACCIDENTS. STATEWIDE. Text in English. s-a. free per issue. **Document type:** *Government.*
Supersedes in part: Louisiana. Department of Public Safety. Summary Motor Vehicle Accident Reports
Published by: Department of Public Safety, Traffic Records Unit, PO Box 666614, Baton Rouge, LA 70896. TEL 504-925-6348.

362.1 ZMB
LUSAKA. MEDICAL OFFICER OF HEALTH. ANNUAL REPORT. Text in English. 1966. a. free per issue. stat.
Published by: Health and Welfare Department, Medical Officer of Health, Public Health Department, PO Box 789, Lusaka, Zambia. Circ: 300.

M E - TIDNINGEN. see *BUILDING AND CONSTRUCTION*

352.3 USA
M F D REGISTER. (Milwaukee Fire Department) Text in English. 1961. m. USD 10. **Description:** News, articles, and announcements on issues of interest to the Milwaukee Fire Department, its retirees and affiliated organizations.
Indexed: Ref.Zh.
Published by: Milwaukee Fire Department Athletic Association, 711 W Wells St, Milwaukee, WI 53233. TEL 414-276-5656. Ed. Carl W Klitzke. Circ: (controlled).

M I O S H A NEWS. (Michigan Occupational Safety and Health Act) see *OCCUPATIONAL HEALTH AND SAFETY*

MAINTAINING SAFE SCHOOLS - SCHOOL VIOLENCE ALERT. see *EDUCATION—School Organization And Administration*

361.3068 360 GBR ISSN 1360-936X
MANAGEMENT ISSUES IN SOCIAL CARE. Text in English. 1994. q. free per issue. bk.rev. **Document type:** *Bulletin.* **Description:** Discusses management theory, good practice, welfare issues, and examples of innovation.
—BLDSC (5359.041800).
Published by: O L M Consulting, Howard House Commercial Centre, Howard St., North Shields NE3 1AR, United Kingdom. TEL 44-191-296-5333, FAX 1344-884495, gill@olmconsulting.co.uk. Ed. Gill Smith TEL 01344- 882806. Circ: 750.

MASS CYCLIST. see *SPORTS AND GAMES—Bicycles And Motorcycles*

MATERNAL AND CHILD HEALTH JOURNAL. see *MEDICAL SCIENCES—Obstetrics And Gynecology*

614 MUS
MAURITIUS. MINISTRY OF HEALTH. REPORT. Text in English. irreg., latest 1988. price varies. **Document type:** *Government.*
Published by: Government Printing Office, Elizabeth II Ave, Port Louis, Mauritius. TEL 230-2345330, FAX 230-2345322. **Subscr. to:** La Tour Koenig, Pointe-aux-sables, Mauritius.

MEAT AND POULTRY INSPECTION REGULATIONS; meat inspection, poultry inspection, rabbit inspection, voluntary inspection and certificate service of meat and poultry, humane slaughter of livestock. see *AGRICULTURE—Poultry And Livestock*

MEDECINS DES HOPITAUX PUBLICS. see *MEDICAL SCIENCES*

614.8 USA
MEDICAL AND RADIOLOGICAL DEVICES GUIDANCE MANUAL. Text in English. irreg. USD 140 in North America; USD 280 elsewhere. **Document type:** *Government.* **Description:** Provides the latest information on and helps maintain program plans and instructions directed to F.D.A. field operations. These plans and instructions are surveillance or compliance oriented and provide the needed direction from headquarters offices and bureaus in accomplishing F.D.A. regulatory obligations.
Published by: U.S. Food and Drug Administration, Office of Public Affairs, 5600 Fishers Ln, Rockville, MD 20857. TEL 301-443-3220. **Orders to:** National Technical Information Service, Government Research Center. FAX 703-321-8547.

MEDICAL CARE. see *MEDICAL SCIENCES*

614.8 619 USA
MEDICAL DEVICE ESTABLISHMENT REGISTRATION MASTER FILE. Text in English. q. USD 360 in North America; USD 720 elsewhere. **Document type:** *Government.* **Description:** Contains information required to be submitted by owner-operators of medical device establishments in accordance with Section 510 of the Federal Food, Drug, and Cosmetics Act.
Media: Magnetic Tape.
Published by: U.S. Food and Drug Administration, Office of Public Affairs, 5600 Fishers Ln, Rockville, MD 20857. TEL 301-443-3220. **Subscr. to:** National Technical Information Service, Government Research Center. TEL 703-487-4630, FAX 703-321-8547.

614.8 619 USA
MEDICAL DEVICE PROBLEMS REPORT FROM THE D E N: REPORTS FROM MEDICAL DEVICE USERS. (Device Experience Network) Text in English. m. USD 225 in North America; USD 450 elsewhere. **Document type:** *Government.* **Description:** Reports are arranged by specific medical specialty such as anaesthesia, cardiovascular or by general health areas. Each report is divided into six parts: accession number, date of report, product name, manufacturer name, serial number, and report narrative.
Published by: U.S. Food and Drug Administration, Office of Public Affairs, 5600 Fishers Ln, Rockville, MD 20857. TEL 301-443-3220. **Subscr. to:** National Technical Information Service, Government Research Center. TEL 703-487-4630, FAX 703-321-8547.

614.8 619 USA
MEDICAL DEVICE REPORTING FROM THE D E N: REPORTS FROM MEDICAL DEVICE MANUFACTURERS. (Device Experience Network) Text in English. m. USD 450 in North America; USD 900 elsewhere. **Document type:** *Government.* **Description:** Arranged by specific medical specialty such as anaesthesia, cardio-vascular or general health areas such as general hospital. Each report is divided into six parts: accession number, date of report, product name, manufacturer name, serial number, and report narrative.
Published by: U.S. Food and Drug Administration, Office of Public Affairs, 5600 Fishers Ln, Rockville, MD 20857. TEL 301-443-3220. **Subscr. to:** National Technical Information Service, Government Research Center. TEL 703-487-4630, FAX 703-321-8547.

MEDICARE. PART A. INTERMEDIARY MANUAL. PART 3. CLAIMS PROCESS. see *INSURANCE*

MEDICARE. PART B. CARRIER MANUAL. PART 3. CLAIMS PROCESS. see *INSURANCE*

614 658 BGR ISSN 1311-6770
MEDITSINSKI PREGLED. PRAKTICHESKA MEDITSINA. Text in Bulgarian; Summaries in Bulgarian, English. 1970. q., latest vol.32, 2001. BGL 14 domestic; USD 35 foreign (effective 2002). bk.rev. abstr, bibl. index. 48 p./no. back issues avail.; reprints avail. *Refereed.* **Document type:** *Journal, Academic/Scholarly, Abstract/Index, Bibliography.* **Description:** Provides information about advances in Bulgarian medical science and practice, and methods adopted in management and administration of health care services.
Formerly: Iz Opita na Zdravnite Zavedeniia (0323-9233)
Indexed: Abstr.Bulg.Sci.Med.Lit.
Published by: Meditsinski Universitet - Sofia, Tsentur za Informatsiia po Meditsina/Medical University - Sofia, Medical Information Center, 1 Sv Georgi Sofiiski ul, Sofia 1431, Bulgaria. TEL 359-2-9522342, FAX 359-2-9522393, mutafov@sun.medun.acad.bg, http://www.medun.acad.bg. Ed. S Stoinov. R&P, Adv. contact Dr. Christo Mutafov. Circ: 200. **Dist. by:** Sofia Books, Ul Silivria 16, Sofia 1404, Bulgaria. TEL 359-2-9586257, sofiabooks@hotmail.com, http://www.sofiabooks.hit.bg.

MENSEN OP STRAAT. see *TRANSPORTATION—Roads And Traffic*

614 USA
MENTAL HEALTH DIRECTORY. Text in English. 1971. quinquennial. USD 35. **Document type:** *Directory, Government.*
Published by: U.S. Center for Mental Health Services, Substance Abuse and Mental Health Services Administration, 5600 Fishers Ln, Rockville, MD 20857. TEL 301-443-2792. Ed. Mary Anne Sonnenschein. **Subscr. to:** U.S. Government Printing Office, Superintendent of Documents.

MENTAL HEALTH MATTERS. see *PSYCHOLOGY*

614 150 GBR
MENTAL HEALTH REVIEW TRIBUNALS FOR ENGLAND AND WALES. ANNUAL REPORT. Text in English. a. **Document type:** *Government.*
Formed by the 1994 merger of: Mental Health Review Tribunal for England. Annual Report (Year); Mental Health Review Tribunal for Wales. Annual Report for (Year)
Indexed: e-psyche.
—BLDSC (5678.585300).
Published by: Department of Health, SD2, Rm 804, Hannibal House, Elephant and Castle, London SE1 6TE, United Kingdom. TEL 44-171-972-2193.

614 AUT ISSN 0026-010X
MERKUR MAGAZIN FUER VOLKSGESUNDHEIT. Text in German. 1958. q. free per issue. adv. charts, illus, mkt, stat.
Indexed: CINAHL.
Published by: Merkur Wechselseitige Versicherungsanstalt, Neutorgasse 57, Graz, St 8010, Austria. Circ: 200,000.

614.8 USA ISSN 0275-6595
CODEN: MIWNE3
MICROWAVE NEWS; a report on non-ionizing radiation. Text in English. 1981. bi-m. USD 325 domestic; USD 350 foreign (effective 2001). adv. bk.rev. back issues avail.; reprints avail. **Document type:** *Newsletter.* **Description:** Health and safety issues related to electromagnetic fields and radiation with emphasis on power lines, cell phones, radar, radio and TV transmitters, appliances, etc.
—BLDSC (5761.220800), CASDDS. **CCC.**
Address: PO Box 1799, Grand Central Sta, New York, NY 10163-1799. TEL 212-517-2800, FAX 212-734-0316, mwn@pobox.com, http://www.microwavenews.com. Ed., Pub., R&P Louis Slesin. Adv. contact Lesli Rice.

MIELENTERVEYS/MENTAL HEALTH. see *MEDICAL SCIENCES—Psychiatry And Neurology*

THE MILBANK QUARTERLY; a journal of public health and health care policy . see *POLITICAL SCIENCE*

MISSOURI. DIVISION OF HIGHWAY SAFETY (YEAR). HIGHWAY SAFETY PLAN. see *TRANSPORTATION—Roads And Traffic*

MITIGATION AND ADAPTATION STRATEGIES FOR GLOBAL CHANGE; an international journal devoted to scientific, engineering, socio-economic and policy responses to environmental change. see *ENVIRONMENTAL STUDIES*

614 JPN ISSN 0917-3331
CODEN: MEKNEH
MIYAZAKIKEN EISEI KANKYO KENKYUJO NENPO/MIYAZAKI PREFECTURAL INSTITUTE FOR PUBLIC HEALTH AND ENVIRONMENT. ANNUAL REPORT. Text in Japanese; Summaries in English. 1991. a.
Formed by the merger of: Miyazakiken Kogai Senta Nenpo; Miyazakiken Eisei Kenkyujoho
—BLDSC (1355.370000), CASDDS.
Published by: Miyazakiken Eisei Kankyo Kenkyujo, 3-2 Gakuenkibanadai-Nishi 2-chome, Miyazaki-shi 889-2155, Japan. TEL 0985-58-0930, FAX 0985-58-1410.

THE MOBILITY FORUM; journal of the Air Mobility Command. see *MILITARY*

614.8 DEU ISSN 0544-7119
MODERNE UNFALLVERHUETUNG. Text in German. 1956. a. DEM 40. adv. bk.rev. back issues avail. **Document type:** *Trade.*
Indexed: INIS Atomind.
—GNLM.

P

Published by: Vulkan Verlag GmbH, Postfach 103962, Essen 45039, Germany. TEL 49-201-8200214, FAX 49-201-8200240. Circ: 3,500.

MONASH UNIVERSITY ACCIDENT RESEARCH CENTRE. CONSULTANTS' REPORTS SERIES. see *TRANSPORTATION—Roads And Traffic*

MONASH UNIVERSITY ACCIDENT RESEARCH CENTRE. MINOR REPORTS SERIES. see *TRANSPORTATION—Roads And Traffic*

MONASH UNIVERSITY ACCIDENT RESEARCH CENTRE. OTHER REPORTS SERIES. see *TRANSPORTATION—Roads And Traffic*

MONATSBERICHT ANGEZEIGTER FLUGUNFAELLE. see *TRANSPORTATION—Air Transport*

614.4 570 GBR ISSN 0740-0845 CODEN: MEBIEP
MONOGRAPHS IN EPIDEMIOLOGY AND BIOSTATISTICS. Text in English. 1981. irreg. price varies. *Refereed.* **Document type:** *Monographic series.*
—BLDSC (5915.431000), KNAW. **CCC.**
Published by: Oxford University Press, Oxford Journals, Walton St, Oxford OX2 6DP, United Kingdom. TEL 44-1865-56767, FAX 44-1865-566646, jnlorders@oup.co.uk, jnl.orders@oup.co.uk, http://www.oup.co.uk. **Orders in N. America to:** Oxford University Press, Journals. TEL 919-677-0977, FAX 919-677-1714, http://www.oup.co.uk.

MONTHLY PRESCRIBING REFERENCE. see *PHARMACY AND PHARMACOLOGY*

614.4273 USA ISSN 0149-2195
RA407.3
MORBIDITY AND MORTALITY WEEKLY REPORT. Variant title: M M W R. Text in English. 1951. w. USD 255 (effective 2001). illus, stat. Index. back issues avail.; reprint service avail. from CIS. *Refereed.* **Document type:** *Bulletin, Government.* **Description:** Provides an account of communicable diseases, ranging from AIDS to malaria, on a state, regional, and national basis.
Formerly (until 1976): U.S. National Communicable Disease Center. Morbidity and Mortality (0091-0031); Formerly: U.S. Centers for Disease Control, Morbidity and Mortality Weekly Report
Related titles: Microfiche ed.: (from CIS); Microform ed.: (from PQC); Online - full text ed.: (from Gale Group, NewsNet, EBSCO Publishing, ProQuest Information & Learning, LexisNexis, Factiva); ♦ Supplement: Health Information for International Travel. ISSN 0095-3539; ♦ Chronic Diseases Notes & Reports. ISSN 1041-5513.
Indexed: AIDS Abstr., Abstr.Hyg., Agri.Eng.Abstr., Amer.Stat.Ind. (1973-), CINAHL, CWI, Chic.Per.Ind., Crim.Just.Abstr., Curr.Lit.Fam.Plan., Curr.Tit.Dent., Diar.Dis.Res., Environ.Abstr., Environ.Sci.Poll.Mgmt., Food Sci.& Tech.Abstr., Hlth.Ind., I.P.A., Ind.Med. (1976-), Ind.Vet., Inpharma, Int.Nurs.Ind., Jrnl.Watch, Jrnl.Watch Emer.Med., Jrnl.Watch Inf.Dis., Jrnl.Watch Wom.Hlth., MEDOC, Med.& Surg.Dermat., NRN, Nutr.Abstr., Pharm.&Out.News, Pollut.Abstr., Poult.Abstr., Protozool.Abstr., Reac., Rev.Appl.Entomol., Rev.Med.& Vet.Mycol., Rural Devel.Abstr., Rural Recreat.Tour.Abstr., Saf.Sci.Abstr., Sage Race Rel.Abstr., THA, Triticale Abstr., Trop.Dis.Bull., Vet.Bull.
—BLDSC (5966.650000), CISTI, GNLM, IDS, KNAW.
Published by: U.S. Department of Health and Human Services, Centers for Disease Control (MS: CO8), Epidemiology Program Office, 1600 Clifton Rd N E, Atlanta, GA 30333. TEL 404-639-3636, FAX 404-639-4198, mmwrq@cdc.gov, http://www.cdc.gov/epo/mmwr/mmwr.html. Ed. Dr. John W Ward. Circ: 30,000 (paid); 20,000 (controlled). **Subscr. to:** U.S. Government Printing Office, Superintendent of Documents, PO Box 371954, Pittsburgh, PA 15250-7954. TEL 202-512-1800, FAX 202-512-2250, orders@gpo.gov, http://www.access.gpo.gov.

614 URY
MORBILIDAD. Text in Spanish. irreg. stat.
Published by: Ministerio de Salud Publica, Departamento de Estadistica, Montevideo, Uruguay.

614 GBR ISSN 1357-6275
HQ1073 CODEN: MORTF5
MORTALITY. Text in English. 1996. 3/yr. GBP 53, USD 87 to individuals; GBP 172, USD 283 to institutions (effective 2002). **Document type:** *Academic/Scholarly.*
Related titles: Online - full content ed.: ISSN 1469-9885 (from EBSCO Publishing, O C L C Online Computer Library Center, Inc., ProQuest Information & Learning, Swets Blackwell); Online - full text ed.: (from CatchWord Ltd., RoweCom Information Quest).
Indexed: ASSIA, Br.Hum.Ind., CINAHL, Lang.& Lang.Behav.Abstr., Mult.Ed.Abstr., PsycInfo, SOPODA, Soc.Serv.Abstr., Sociol.Abstr.
—BLDSC (5967.451500), CatchWord, Infotrieve, ingenta. **CCC.**
Published by: Carfax Publishing Limited (Subsidiary of: Taylor & Francis Group), PO Box 25, Abingdon, Oxon OX14 3UE, United Kingdom. TEL 44-1235-401000, FAX 44-1235-401550, enquiries@carfax.co.uk, enquiry@tandf.co.uk, http://www.carfax.co.uk.

614.862 388.41 USA ISSN 0191-488X
TL242
MOTOR VEHICLE SAFETY; a report on activities under the National Traffic and Motor Vehicle Safety Act of 1966. Text in English. 1966. a. **Document type:** *Government.*
Published by: U.S. National Highway Traffic Safety Administration, 400 Seventh St, N W, Washington, DC 20590. **Co-sponsor:** Prepared with: U.S. Federal Highway Administration.

628 DEU ISSN 0027-2957 CODEN: MUABD8
MUELL UND ABFALL; Fachzeitschrift fuer Behandlung und Beseitigung von Abfaellen. Text in German. 1969. m. DEM 223.20; DEM 175.20 to students; DEM 21 newsstand/cover (effective 2001). adv. bk.rev. **Document type:** *Newspaper, Trade.* **Description:** Emphasis is on sanitary engineering.
Indexed: Chem.Abstr., Chem.Indus.Notes, Chem.Titles, GeoRef, IBR, IBZ, INIS Atomind., Repindex, WasteInfo.
—BLDSC (5982.650000), CASDDS, Infotrieve, Linda Hall. **CCC.**
Published by: Erich Schmidt Verlag GmbH & Co. (Berlin), Genthiner Str 30G, Berlin 10785, Germany. TEL 49-30-250085-0, FAX 49-30-25008521, esv@esvmedien.de, http://www.erich-schmidt-verlag.de. Ed. M Ferber.

MUNAZZAMAT AL-SIHHAH AL-'ALAMIYYAH. SILSILAT AL-TAQARIR AL-FANNIYYAH. see *MEDICAL SCIENCES*

N A C A NEWS. see *PETS*

614.84 GBR
N A F O MAGAZINE. Text in English. 1975. q. membership.
Published by: National Association of Fire Officers, Hayes Court, W. Common Rd, Keston, Bromley, Kent BR2 7AU, United Kingdom. Circ: 5,000.

614 USA
N A H S E'S RESUME✶. Text in English. 1972. q. USD 5. adv. bk.rev. stat. back issues avail.
Published by: National Association of Health Services Executives, 8630 Fenton St, Ste 328, Silver Spring, MD 20910-3803. Circ: 1,500.

THE N A WAY MAGAZINE. (Narcotics Anonymous) see *DRUG ABUSE AND ALCOHOLISM*

N B S GAZETTE. see *MEDICAL SCIENCES—Nurses And Nursing*

614.8 USA ISSN 0890-3417
N C A H F NEWSLETTER; quality in the health marketplace. (National Council Against Health Fraud) Text in English. 1977. bi-m., latest vol.24, 2001. USD 15; USD 18 to libraries. bk.rev. index. 4 p./no. 3 cols./p. back issues avail. **Document type:** *Newsletter.* **Description:** Focuses on health misinformation, fraud and quackery as public health problems. Contains summaries (with commentary) of current medical findings, reports on controversial health practices and other consumer health issues.
Formerly (until 2001): N C R H I Newsletter (National Council for Reliable Health Information, Inc.
Related titles: Microform ed.: (from PQC); Online - full text ed.: (from Gale Group).
Indexed: CHNI, Hlth.Ind.
Published by: National Council Against Health Fraud, Inc., PO Box 1276, Loma Linda, CA 92354. TEL 978-532-9383, FAX 978-532-9450, http://www.primenet.com/~ncahf/. Ed. John M London. R&P Dr. Robert S Baratz. Circ: 2,000 (paid).

614.83 USA
N C R P COMMENTARY. Text in English. 1980. irreg., latest vol.15, 1998. price varies.
Published by: National Council on Radiation Protection and Measurements, 7910 Woodmont Ave, Ste 800, Bethesda, MD 20814. TEL 301-657-2652. Ed. William M Beckner.

614.8 355.23 USA ISSN 0083-209X CODEN: NCRDBG
N C R P REPORT. Text in English. 1931. irreg., latest vol.129, 1999. price varies.
Indexed: Biol.Abstr., Energy Info.Abstr., Environ.Abstr., Excerp.Med., GeoRef, INIS Atomind., Ref.Zh.
—BLDSC (6067.817100), CISTI, KNAW, Linda Hall.
Published by: National Council on Radiation Protection and Measurements, 7910 Woodmont Ave, Ste 800, Bethesda, MD 20814. TEL 301-657-2652. Ed. William M Beckner.

614.83 USA
N C R P SYMPOSIUM PROCEEDINGS. Text in English. 1982. irreg., latest vol.3, 1997. USD 30. **Document type:** *Proceedings.*
Published by: National Council on Radiation Protection and Measurements, 7910 Woodmont Ave, Ste 800, Bethesda, MD 20814. TEL 301-657-2652. Ed. W Roger Ney.

N E C N P NEWSLETTER. see *ENERGY*

362.1 GBR
N H S CONFEDERATION. BEST PRACTICE PAPERS. Text in English. 1997. irreg. GBP 22 to non-members; GBP 15 to members (effective 2000). back issues avail. **Document type:** *Academic/Scholarly, Government.* **Description:** Analyzes major problems that the NHS faces, with emphasis on models of best practice.
Published by: (Great Britain. National Health Service, Great Britain. Publications Department), N H S Confederation Trading Company Ltd., Birmingham Research Park, Vincent Dr, Birmingham, Worcs B15 2SQ, United Kingdom. TEL 44-121-471-4444, FAX 44-121-471-1120, http://www.nhsconfed.net.

362.1 GBR
N H S CONFEDERATION. RESEARCH PAPERS. Text in English. 1989. irreg. price varies. back issues avail. **Document type:** *Monographic series, Academic/Scholarly, Government.* **Description:** Publishes research projects commissioned or undertaken by the NHS Confederation.
Published by: (Great Britain. National Health Service, Great Britain. Publications Department), N H S Confederation Trading Company Ltd., Birmingham Research Park, Vincent Dr, Birmingham, Worcs B15 2SQ, United Kingdom. TEL 44-121-471-4444, FAX 44-121-414-1120, http://www.nhsconfed.net.

362.1 GBR ISSN 0953-8623
THE N H S HANDBOOK (YEAR). Text in English. 198?. a. GBP 45 domestic to non-members; GBP 56.95 foreign to non-members; GBP 41.95 domestic to members; GBP 53.95 foreign to members (effective 2000). **Document type:** *Government.* **Description:** Describes the NHS structure and organization, including the year's changes.
Published by: (Great Britain. National Health Service, Great Britain. Publications Department), N H S Confederation Trading Company Ltd., Birmingham Research Park, Vincent Dr, Birmingham, Worcs B15 2SQ, United Kingdom. TEL 44-121-471-4444, FAX 44-121-414-1120, http://www.nhsconfed.net. Ed. Peter Merry.

614 GBR
N H S HEALTH ADVISORY SERVICE. ANNUAL REPORT OF THE DIRECTOR. (National Health Service) Text in English. a. GBP 14.95. **Document type:** *Government, Corporate.*
Formerly: N H S Health Advisory Service. Annual Report
Published by: National Health Service, Health Advisory Service, Sutherland House, 29-37 Brighton Rd, Sutton, Surrey, United Kingdom. **Subscr. to:** H.M.S.O., Publications Centre, PO Box 276, London SW8 5DT, United Kingdom. TEL 44- 207-873-9090, FAX 44-20-7873-8200.

614 GBR ISSN 1359-4443
N H S MAGAZINE. (National Health Service) Text in English. 1995. q. **Document type:** *Bulletin.*
—BLDSC (6109.523700).
Published by: National Health Service, External Communications Unit, Quarry House, Quarry Hill, Leeds LS2 7UE, United Kingdom. TEL 44-113-254-5610. Ed. Stan Abbott. Pub. Peter Addison. Adv. contact John Wheelhouse.

614 GBR ISSN 1354-2362
N H S NEWS. (National Health Service) Text in English. m. adv. **Document type:** *Bulletin.*
Formerly (until 1994): N H S Management Executive News (0963-5688)

Published by: National Health Service, External Communications Unit, Quarry House, Quarry Hill, Leeds LS2 7UE, United Kingdom. TEL 44-113-254-5610. Ed. Geoff Wilson. Adv. contact John Wheelhouse.

N R C T L D DIRECT RADIATION MONITORING NETWORK. see *PHYSICS—Nuclear Physics*

362.1 USA
N R H A ENEWS. Text in English. 1978. m. USD 75 (effective 2001). **Description:** Information on rural health issues, policy and projects.
Former titles: Rural Health F Y I (1083-6829); (until 1995): Rural Health Care
Indexed: CINAHL.
—CCC.
Published by: National Rural Health Association, 1 W Armour Blvd, Ste 203, Kansas City, MO 64111. TEL 816-756-3140, FAX 816-756-3144, pubs@nrharural.org, http://www.NRHArural.org. Ed. Tammy Houck Talbott. R&P Gregory Rieger. Circ: 3,900 (controlled).

362.1 AUS ISSN 1034-7674
N S W PUBLIC HEALTH BULLETIN. (New South Wales) Text in English. 1990. m. stat. cum.index: 1990-2000. 24 p./no. back issues avail. *Refereed.* **Document type:** *Bulletin, Government.* **Description:** Serves as an information vehicle for the whole public health community in New South Wales. Provides its readers with population health data as a means to motivate effective public health action.
Related titles: Online - full text ed.
Published by: Health Department, Locked Mail Bag 961, North Sydney, NSW 2059, Australia. TEL 61-2-9391-9241, FAX 61-2-9391-9232, phbulletin@doh.health.nsw.gov.au, http://www.health.nsw.gov.au/public-health/phb/phb.html. Ed. Dr. Lynne Madden. R&P Dr. Michael Giffin. Circ: 7,000.

614.40715 JPN ISSN 0287-9549
NARA JOSHI DAIGAKU HOKEN KANRI SENTA NENPO/NARA WOMEN'S UNIVERSITY. HEALTH ADMINISTRATION CENTER. ARCHIVES OF HEALTH CARE. Text in Japanese; Contents page in English. 1978. a. charts. **Document type:** *Academic/Scholarly.*
Formerly (until 1983): Nara Joshi Daigaku Hoken Kanri Senta Kiyo (0286-505X)
Published by: Nara Joshi Daigaku, Hoken Kanri Senta/Nara Women's University, Health Administration Center, Kita-Uoyahigashi-Machi, Nara-shi 630-8285, Japan. Ed. Kimihiro Yamamoto. Circ: 500.

614.8 IND
NATIONAL CONFERENCE ON SAFETY. PROCEEDINGS. Text in English. 1970. a. INR 10. charts. **Document type:** *Proceedings.*
Published by: National Safety Council, Central Labour Institute Bldg., Sion, Mumbai, Maharashtra 400 022, India. Ed. A A Krishnan. Circ: 2,000.

614.83 355.23 USA ISSN 0195-7740
CODEN: PNRME9
NATIONAL COUNCIL ON RADIATION PROTECTION AND MEASUREMENTS. PROCEEDINGS OF THE ANNUAL MEETING. Text in English. 1979 (15th). a. price varies. **Document type:** *Proceedings.*
Indexed: GeoRef.
—CASDDS, Linda Hall.
Published by: National Council on Radiation Protection and Measurements, 7910 Woodmont Ave, Ste 800, Bethesda, MD 20814. TEL 301-657-2652.

NATIONAL DIRECTORY OF SAFETY CONSULTANTS. see *ENGINEERING*

614 JPN
RA421 CODEN: KEKHA7
NATIONAL INSTITUTE OF PUBLIC HEALTH. JOURNAL. Text in English, Japanese. 1952. q. free per issue or exchange basis. abstr, bibl, charts, illus. index. **Document type:** *Bulletin.*
Former titles: Koshu Eisei Kenkyu - Institute of Public Health. Bulletin (0916-6823); (until 1990): Koshu Eiseiin Kenkyu Hokoku - Institute of Public Health. Bulletin (0020-3106)
Indexed: Abstr.Hyg., Biol.Abstr., Chem.Abstr., Excerp.Med., INIS Atomind., Ind.Vet., Ref.Zh., Rev.Appl.Entomol., Rural Devel.Abstr., Soils & Fert., Trop.Dis.Bull., Vet.Bull., Weed Abstr.
—CASDDS, GNLM.
Published by: National Institute of Public Health, 4-6-1 Shirokanedai, Minato-ku, Tokyo 108-0071, Japan. Ed. Dr. Toshiro Tango. Circ: 1,200.

362.5 USA
NATIONAL PEDICULOSIS ASSOCIATION. PROGRESS. Text in English. 1984. q. USD 60 (effective 1992). film rev. bibl, illus. back issues avail. **Document type:** *Newsletter.* **Description:** Newsletter reporting on health and prevention issues concerning head lice in young children.
Published by: National Pediculosis Association, PO Box 610189, Newton, MA 02161. TEL 617-449-6487, FAX 617-449-8129, linda@headlice.org, http://www.headlice.org. Eds. Deborah L Altschuler, Linda Menditto. R&P Linda Menditto.

614.8 ZAF ISSN 0028-0097
NATIONAL SAFETY/NASIONALE VEILIGHEID; and occupational hygiene - en Beroepshigiene. Text mainly in English; Text occasionally in Afrikaans. 1938. bi-m. ZAR 25; ZAR 35 foreign (effective 1995). adv. bk.rev. illus, stat, tr.lit. **Document type:** *Trade.* **Description:** Aims to prevent accidents by promoting an awareness of accident situations as they exist in day-to-day living among members of the community.
Indexed: C.I.S. Abstr., Environ.Sci.Poll.Mgmt., INIS Atomind., Pollut.Abstr., Saf.Sci.Abstr.
Published by: Safety First Association, 7 Pitcairn Rd, Blairgowrie, Johannesburg 2194, South Africa. TEL 27-11-7827698. Ed. Debbie Myer. Circ: 3,200 (controlled). **Subscr. to:** PO Box 400, Pinegowrie, Transvaal 2123, South Africa.

614 USA ISSN 0028-0496
RA421
THE NATION'S HEALTH. Text in English. 1911. 11/yr. USD 40 domestic; USD 58 foreign (effective 2001). adv. bk.rev. charts, illus. reprint service avail. from PQC. **Document type:** *Newspaper, Trade.* **Description:** Covers public health policy, including legislative and other federal action.
Supersedes in part (in 1971): American Journal of Public Health and the Nation's Health (0002-9572); Which was formed by the 1927 merger of: American Journal of Public Health (0271-4353); Nation's Health (1076-0709)
Related titles: Microform ed.: (from PQC); Online - full text ed.: (from Northern Light Technology, Inc., ProQuest Information & Learning, Gale Group, Factiva).
Indexed: Biol.Dig., Curr.Adv.Ecol.Sci., Hlth.Ind., Med.Care Rev., Rehabil.Lit., Telegen.
—CISTI, Infotrieve, Linda Hall. **CCC.**
Published by: American Public Health Association, 1015 15th St, N W, Washington, DC 20005. TEL 202-789-5674, FAX 202-789-5661, http://www.apha.org/journal/nation/tnhhome.htm. Ed. Kathryn Foxhall. Circ: 35,000. **Subscr. to:** APHA, Subscription Dept 5037, Washington, DC 20061-5037.

NATURAL HAZARDS REVIEW. see *ENVIRONMENTAL STUDIES*

614.88 NLD ISSN 0925-6040
NEDERLANDS TIJDSCHRIFT VOOR E H B O EN REDDINGWEZEN. Text in Dutch. 1912. 6/yr. NLG 35 (effective 1995). bk.rev. bibl, charts, illus.
Formerly: Reddingwezen (0034-2114)
Published by: (Koninklijke Nationale Bond voor Reddingwezen en Eerste Hulp bij Ongelukken "Het Oranje Kruis"), S M D Educatieve Uitgevers, PO Box 63, Leiden 2300 AB, Netherlands. FAX 31-71-323340. adv.: B&W page NLG 645. Circ: 5,700.

NEEDLE TIPS AND THE HEPATITIS B COALITION NEWS. see *MEDICAL SCIENCES—Allergology And Immunology*

614 CAN ISSN 0838-3693
RA450.N5
NEW BRUNSWICK. DEPARTMENT OF HEALTH AND COMMUNITY SERVICES. ANNUAL REPORT. Text in English, French. 1918. a. free per issue. stat. **Document type:** *Government.*
Formerly: New Brunswick. Department of Health. Annual Report
Published by: Department of Health and Community Services, P O Box 5100, Fredericton, NB E3B 5G8, Canada. TEL 506-453-2536, FAX 506-444-4697, http://www.gov.nb.ca/hcs. Ed. Gerald Weseen. Circ: 700.

614 344.032 USA
NEW HAMPSHIRE STATUTES PERTAINING TO HEALTH AND HUMAN SERVICES. Text in English. a. USD 40. index.
Published by: Lexis Law Publishing (Subsidiary of: Reed Elsevier plc), PO Box 7587, Charlottesville, VA 22906-7587. TEL 804-972-7566, 800-562-1197, FAX 800-643-1280, llp.customer.support@lexis-nexis.com, http://www.lexislawpublishing.com. Ed. George Harley.

610 USA ISSN 0885-842X
R15
NEW JERSEY MEDICINE; health care in the Garden State. Text in English. 1904. m. USD 55 domestic (effective 2001); USD 70 foreign (effective 1999). adv. bk.rev. abstr, bibl, charts, illus. index. *Refereed.* **Document type:** *Trade.* **Description:** Publishes health policy, N.J. legislative articles and health care system news.
Formerly (until 1985): Medical Society of New Jersey. Journal (0025-7524)
Related titles: Microfilm ed.: (from PQC).
Indexed: Excerp.Med., INIS Atomind., Ind.Med. (1985-), Int.Nurs.Ind.
—BLDSC (6084.310900), GNLM, KNAW.
Published by: Medical Society of New Jersey, 2 Princess Rd, Lawrenceville, NJ 08648. TEL 609-896-1766, FAX 609-896-1368. Ed. Dr. Paul J Hirsch. adv.: B&W page USD 750, color page USD 1,350. Circ: 10,000 (paid and controlled).

NEW JERSEY STATE FIRE CODE. see *FIRE PREVENTION*

NEW SOLUTIONS; a journal of environmental and occupational health policy. see *OCCUPATIONAL HEALTH AND SAFETY*

614 USA ISSN 1077-1344
NEW YORK HEALTH LAW UPDATE. Text in English. 1994. m. USD 177 (effective 2001). **Document type:** *Newsletter.* **Description:** Reports state-specific new public health laws that affect companies in New York.
Formerly: New York Health Law Alert (1073-0443)
Related titles: Online - full text ed.: (from LexisNexis).
Published by: (DeForest & Duer), M. Lee Smith Publishers LLC, 5201 Virginia Way, PO Box 5094, Brentwoood, TN 37024-5094. TEL 615-373-7517, 800-274-6774, FAX 615-373-5183. Pub. M Lee Smith.

P

614 USA
NEW YORK (STATE). HEALTH PLANNING COMMISSION. ADMINISTRATIVE PROGRAM FOR HEALTH PLANNING AND DEVELOPMENT. Text in English. a.
Published by: Health Planning Commission, Empire State Plaza, Tower Bldg Rm 1683, Albany, NY 12237.

614 310 NZL
NEW ZEALAND. HEALTH STATISTICAL SERVICES. CLIENT SERVICES NEWSLETTER. Text in English. m. **Document type:** *Newsletter.*
Published by: Health Statistical Services, P.O. Box 5013, Wellington, New Zealand. TEL 04-496-2049, FAX 04-496-2050.

NEW ZEALAND. LAND TRANSPORT SAFETY AUTHORITY. RULES. see *TRANSPORTATION*

614 616.9 NZL ISSN 1173-0250
NEW ZEALAND PUBLIC HEALTH REPORT. Text in English. 1994. 11/yr. NZD 50 (effective 2001). abstr, charts, stat. 8 p./no. back issues avail. *Refereed.* **Document type:** *Bulletin, Academic/Scholarly.* **Description:** Contains surveillance, outbreak and research reports.
Formerly (until 1994): Communicable disease New Zealand Weekly (1171-8064); Which superseded in part (in 1992): C A B Current Awareness bulletin (1171-722X)
Indexed: CINAHL, Ind.N.Z.Per.
—BLDSC (6096.835000).
Published by: Institute of Environmental Science & Research, P.O. Box 50 348, Porirua 6215, New Zealand. TEL 64-4-2370149, FAX 64-4-2372370, craig.thornley@esr.cri.nz, http://www.esr.cri.nz. Ed. C Thornley. Circ: 4,700.

NEW ZEALAND. STATISTICS NEW ZEALAND. PUBLIC HEALTH FINANCIAL STATISTICS. see *BUSINESS AND ECONOMICS—Public Finance, Taxation*

▼ **NICOTINE & TOBACCO RESEARCH.** see *TOBACCO*

614 JPN ISSN 0546-1766
CODEN: NKEZA4
NIHON KOSHU EISEI ZASSHI/JAPANESE JOURNAL OF PUBLIC HEALTH. Text in Japanese; Summaries in English, Japanese. 1954. m. JPY 1,000 per issue. adv.
Indexed: Chem.Abstr., INIS Atomind., Ind.Med. (1954-), Int.Nurs.Ind., Jap.Per.Ind.
—BLDSC (4658.400000), CASDDS, CISTI, GNLM, ingenta.
Published by: Nihon Koshu Eisei Gakkai/Japanese Society of Public Health, 29-8 Shinjuku 1-chome, Shinjuku-ku, Tokyo 160-0022, Japan. TEL 03-3352-4281, FAX 03-3352-4605.

NIPPON NOYAKU GAKKAISHI. see *ENGINEERING—Chemical Engineering*

615.952 AUS
NON-SMOKERS' UPDATE. Text in English. 1978. q. AUD 40 to individual members (effective 2001). adv. bk.rev. back issues avail. **Document type:** *Newsletter.* **Description:** Covers politics and health effects of tobacco, concentrating on Australia.
Formerly (until 1994): Clean Air Clarion (0155-2899)
Published by: Non-Smokers' Movement of Australia Inc., 4 Goulburn St, PO Box 6 TRADES HALL, Sydney, NSW 2000, Australia. TEL 61-2-92646243, FAX 61-2-92674393, nsma@nlc.net.au, http://www.nsma.org.au. Ed., R&P Brian McBride. Circ: 2,500.

NORSK V V S. see *HEATING, PLUMBING AND REFRIGERATION*

NORWAY. DIREKTORATET FOR BRANN OG EKSPLOSJONSVERN. AARSBERETNING. see *FIRE PREVENTION*

NUCLEAR LEMONS; an assessment of America's worst commercial nuclear reactors. see *ENERGY—Nuclear Energy*

NUCLEAR PLANT JOURNAL. see *ENERGY—Nuclear Energy*

NUCLEUS (CAMBRIDGE). see *ENERGY*

614 GBR
NUFFIELD INSTITUTE FOR HEALTH. WORKING PAPERS. Text in English. irreg. **Document type:** *Academic/Scholarly.*
Published by: University of Leeds, Nuffield Institute for Health, Nuffield Institute For Health, 71-75 Clarendon Rd, Leeds LS2 9PL, United Kingdom. TEL 0532-459034.

NURSING & POLICY FORUM. see *MEDICAL SCIENCES—Nurses And Nursing*

THE O E M REPORT. (Occupational and Environmental Medicine) see *OCCUPATIONAL HEALTH AND SAFETY*

362.1 AUS
O H S DIRECTORY. (Occupational Health & Safety) Text in English. a. AUD 185 (effective 1999). **Document type:** *Directory.* **Description:** Provides key contacts for all areas of occupational health and safety: government departments, occupational health consultants, authorities and courts, licensed insurers and claim agents, associations, training courses, equipment and computer systems.
Published by: Newsletter Information Services, PO Box 693, Manly, NSW 2095, Australia. TEL 61-2-9977-7500, FAX 61-2-9977-3310, customer.support@newsinfo.com.au, http://www.newsinfo.com.au. Ed. Anna Lockwood.

O S H A AND SAFETY MEETINGS HANDBOOK. (Occupational Safety and Health Administration) see *OCCUPATIONAL HEALTH AND SAFETY*

O S H A REGULATIONS, DOCUMENTS, AND TECHNICAL INFORMATION ON CD-ROM. see *OCCUPATIONAL HEALTH AND SAFETY*

614.8 USA ISSN 0146-3632
OCCUPATIONAL SAFETY AND HEALTH SERIES (NEW YORK). Text in English. 1976. irreg., latest vol.27, 1996. price varies. adv. *Refereed.* **Document type:** *Monographic series.*
—BLDSC (6231.150000), CISTI, Infotrieve. **CCC.**
Published by: Marcel Dekker, Inc., Attn: Eridania Perrez, 270 Madison Ave, New York, NY 10016-0602. TEL 212-696-9000, 800-228-1160, FAX 212-658-4540, marketing@dekker.com, http://www.dekker.com. Pub. Russell Dekker. R&P Julia Mulligan. Adv. contact Eridania Perez.

OKLAHOMA. DEPARTMENT OF HEALTH. MONTHLY VITAL STATISTICS REPORT. see *POPULATION STUDIES*

614.8 BEL ISSN 0771-2588
OPERATIE VEILIGHEID. Text in Dutch. 1964. m. (10/yr.). BEF 880 (effective 1994). adv. bk.rev. illus.
Related titles: ♦ French ed.: Objectif Prevention. ISSN 0771-2634.
Published by: Nationale Vereniging tot Voorkoming van Arbeidsongevallen (NVVA), Gachardstraat 88, Bus 4, Brussels 1050, Belgium. TEL 32-2-6480337, FAX 32-2-6486867. Ed. B Schoenmaekers. Circ: 27,000.

OPHTHALMIC EPIDEMIOLOGY. see *MEDICAL SCIENCES—Ophthalmology And Optometry*

614 USA
OREGON HEALTH. Text in English. 1998. 3/yr. free per issue. illus.
Published by: Oregon Health Sciences University, 3181 S W Sam Jackson Park Rd, Portland, OR 97201. TEL 503-494-8231, FAX 503-494-8246. Eds. Marlys Levin Pierson, Todd Schwartz. Circ: 5,600.

ORGANISATION MONDIALE DE LA SANTE. SERIE DE RAPPORTS TECHNIQUES. see *MEDICAL SCIENCES*

ORGANISATIONS CONCERNED WITH HEALTH AND SAFETY INFORMATION. see *BUSINESS AND ECONOMICS—Trade And Industrial Directories*

ORGANIZACION MUNDIAL DE LA SALUD. SERIE DE INFORMES TECNICOS. see *MEDICAL SCIENCES*

613.9 USA ISSN 0737-3732
OUTLOOK (SEATTLE); reproductive health. Text in English. 1983. q. USD 40 (effective 1999 - 2000). back issues avail. **Document type:** *Academic/Scholarly.*
Related titles: Chinese ed.; Indonesian ed.; Portuguese ed.; Russian ed.; Spanish ed.
Indexed: I.P.A., P.A.I.S.
Published by: Program for Appropriate Technology in Health, 4 Nickerson St, Seattle, WA 98109. TEL 206-285-3500, FAX 206-285-6619, TELEX 4740049 PATH UI, outlook@path.org, http://www.path.org/outlook.index.htm. Ed. Jacqueline Sherris. R&P Michele Burns. Circ: 5,000.

OVERVIEW (OLYMPIA). see *SOCIAL SERVICES AND WELFARE*

327.1747 USA
P S R MONITOR. Text in English. 1984. q. membership. **Document type:** *Monographic series.* **Description:** Covers health dangers of nuclear arms testing and social and environmental costs of nuclear arms race. Recommends legislative action.
Published by: Physicians for Social Responsibility, 1101 14th St, N W, Ste 700, Washington, DC 20005-5601. TEL 202-898-0150. Ed. Meg Duskin. Circ: 5,000.

614.8 USA ISSN 0894-6264
P S R REPORTS. Text in English. 1979. 4/yr. membership. adv. bk.rev. **Document type:** *Newsletter.* **Description:** Articles on the health and environmental impact of nuclear war, the nuclear arms race and military spending.
Formerly: P S R Newsletter
Published by: Physicians for Social Responsibility, 1101 14th St, N W, Ste 700, Washington, DC 20005-5601. TEL 202-898-0150. Ed. Meg Duskin. Circ: 25,000.

P S S R U BULLETIN. see *SOCIAL SERVICES AND WELFARE*

PACIFIC DIET ADVISORY LEAFLET. see *NUTRITION AND DIETETICS*

614 PAK ISSN 0030-9834
PAKISTAN JOURNAL OF HEALTH. Text in English. 1951. biennial. complementary. adv. bk.rev. charts, illus, stat. **Document type:** *Academic/Scholarly.*
Related titles: CD-ROM ed.
Indexed: Biol.Abstr., Chem.Abstr., ExtraMED.
Published by: College of Community Medicine, 6 Birdwood Rd., Lahore, Pakistan. TEL 92-42-7583945, FAX 92-42-7586395, jphpk@yahoo.com. Ed. Dr. Ilyas Ahmed Faridi. Circ: 1,000 (paid).

362.1 614 USA
PAN AMERICAN HEALTH ORGANIZATION. SCIENTIFIC AND TECHNICAL PUBLICATION. Text in English. 1953. irreg.
Formerly: Pan American Health Organization. Scientific Publication (0555-8913)
Related titles: Spanish ed.
Indexed: Abstr.Hyg., Trop.Dis.Bull.
Published by: Pan American Health Organization (PAHO), 525 23rd St., NW, Washington, DC 20037.

614 USA ISSN 1020-4989
RA442 CODEN: RPSPFQ
PAN AMERICAN JOURNAL OF PUBLIC HEALTH/REVISTA PANAMERICANA DE SALUD PUBLICA. Text in English, Spanish, Portuguese. 1997. m. USD 87 in US & Canada; USD 50 in Latin America & the Caribbean (effective 2002). adv. bk.rev. abstr, bibl, illus. index. 80 p./no. back issues avail. *Refereed.* **Document type:** *Journal, Academic/Scholarly.* **Description:** Provides a vehicle for disseminating information to public health personnel and researchers throughout the Americas.
Formed by the merger of (1967-1997): Pan American Health Organization. Bulletin (0085-4638); (1922-1997): Oficina Sanitaria Panamericana. Boletin (0030-0632)
Related titles: Microfiche ed.: (from CIS); Online - full text ed.: (from Ovid Technologies, Inc., CatchWord Ltd.).
Indexed: Abstr.Hyg., Aqua.Sci.& Fish.Abstr., Bio-Contr.News & Info., Biodet.Abstr., Biol.Abstr., CINAHL, Chem.Abstr., Curr.Adv.Ecol.Sci., Dairy Sci.Abstr., Dent.Ind., Ecol.Abstr., Environ.Abstr., Environ.Sci.Poll.Mgmt., Excerp.Med. (1996-), Food Sci.& Tech.Abstr., Geo.Abstr.H.G., Helminthol.Abstr., IDA, IIS, INIS Atomind., I.P.A., Ind.Med. (1997-), Ind.Vet., Microbiol.Abstr., Nutr.Abstr., Pig News & Info., Pollut.Abstr., Popul.Ind., Protozool.Abstr., Repindex, Rev.Appl.Entomol., Rev.Med.& Vet.Mycol., Risk Abstr., Rural Devel.Abstr., Saf.Sci.Abstr., Soc.Serv.Abstr., Sociol.Abstr., Trop.Dis.Bull., Vet.Bull., World Bibl.Soc.Sec.
—BLDSC (6356.445000), CISTI, EMDOCS, GNLM, Infotrieve, ingenta, KNAW, Linda Hall. **CCC.**
Published by: Pan American Health Organization (Subsidiary of: World Health Organization), 525 23rd St, N W, Washington, DC 20037. TEL 202-974-3877, FAX 202-338-0869, publiper@paho.org. Ed. Maria Luisa Clark. Adv. contact Evelin Rodriguez. Circ: 9,000.

614.4 POL ISSN 0035-7715
CODEN: RPZHAW
PANSTWOWY ZAKLAD HIGIENY. ROCZNIKI. Short title: Roczniki P Z H. Text in Polish; Summaries in English. 1950. q. USD 150 foreign (effective 2002). bk.rev. abstr, charts, illus, stat. index. **Document type:** *Academic/Scholarly.* **Description:** Covers hygiene, toxicology, food sciences, environment.
Indexed: AgroLibrex, Anim.Breed.Abstr., Bio-Contr.News & Info., Biol.Abstr., Biotech.& Bioeng.Abstr., Chem.Abstr., Dairy Sci.Abstr., Dent.Ind., Excerp.Med., Field Crop Abstr., Food Sci.& Tech.Abstr., Hort.Abstr., INIS Atomind., Ind.Med. (1950-), Nutr.Abstr., Plant Breed.Abstr., Postharvest, Potato Abstr., Rev.Appl.Entomol., Rev.Med.& Vet.Mycol., Rev.Plant Path., Rural Recreat.Tour.Abstr., Tox.Abstr.
—CASDDS, CISTI, GNLM, KNAW.
Published by: Panstwowy Zaklad Higieny/National Institute of Hygiene, Ul Chocimska 24, Warsaw 00791, Poland. TEL 48-22-6461538, FAX 48-22-8497484, TELEX 816712, http://www.pzh.gov.pl/biblioteka/roczniki/index.htm. Ed. Kazimiera Cwiek Ludwicka. **Dist. by:** Ars Polona, Krakowskie Przedmiescie 7, Warsaw, Poland. TEL 48-22-8261201.

614 IRL ISSN 0738-3991
R727.3
PATIENT EDUCATION AND COUNSELING; an interdisciplinary journal for patient education researchers and managers. Text in English. 1979. 9/yr. EUR 927.13 in Europe to individuals; JPY 12,000 in Japan to individuals; USD 102 elsewhere to individuals; EUR 773 in Europe to institutions; JPY 102,600 in Japan to institutions; USD 865 elsewhere to institutions (effective 2002). back issues avail.; reprints avail. *Refereed.* **Document type:** *Academic/Scholarly.* **Description:** For patient education researchers, managers, clinicians, and others involved in patient education and counseling services and administration.
Formerly (until 1983): Patient Counselling and Health (0190-2040); Incorporates (in 1986): Patient Education Reports; Which was formerly titled: Patient Education Newsletter
Related titles: Online - full text ed.: (from ingenta, ScienceDirect, Swets Blackwell, Institute for Scientific Information).
Indexed: ASCA, Abstr.Health Care Manage.Stud., AgeLine, Behav.Med.Abstr., C.I.J.E., CINAHL, Cont.Pg.Educ., Curr.Cont., Educ.Tech.Abstr., Excerp.Med., FAMLI, Fam.Ind., Helminthol.Abstr., Hosp.Lit.Ind., I.P.A., Ind.Med. (coverage dropped), Inpharma, Int.Nurs.Ind., NRN, Nutr.Abstr., Pharm.&Out.News, PsycInfo, Psychol.Abstr. (1985-), Reac., Rel.Ind.One, Rel.Ind.Two, Res.High.Educ.Abstr., SSCI, e-psyche.
—BLDSC (6412.864600), CISTI, EMDOCS, GNLM, IDS, ingenta, KNAW. **CCC.**

Published by: Elsevier Science Ireland Ltd, Elsevier House, Brookvale Plaza, E. Park, Shannon, Co. Clare, Ireland. TEL 353-61-471944, FAX 353-61-472144, http://www.elsevier.nl/locate/pateducou. Eds. A Visser, C Herbert, J Hall, L W Green. R&P Annette Moloney. **Subscr. in Australasia and the Far East to:** Elsevier Science (Singapore) Pte Ltd, No.1 Temasek Ave, 17-01 Millenia Tower, Singapore 039192, Singapore. TEL 65-434-3727, FAX 65-337-2230; **Subscr. in the Americas to:** Elsevier Science, PO Box 945, New York, NY 10159-0945. TEL 212-633-3730, FAX 212-633-3680, usinfo-f@elsevier.com; **Subscr. to:** Elsevier Science BV, PO Box 211, Amsterdam 1000 AE, Netherlands. TEL 31-20-485-3757.

614 635 USA ISSN 1067-4276
PEOPLE PLANT CONNECTION. Text in English. 1973. m. USD 3 per issue to non-members (effective 2000). **Document type:** *Newsletter.* **Description:** Designed to further the aims of A.H.T.A. by reviewing and communicating developments in the field of horticultural therapy. Aimed at medical professionals and interested individuals.
Published by: American Horticultural Therapy Association, 909 York St, Denver, CO 80206-3751. TEL 303-331-3862, FAX 303-331-0095, ahta@ahta.org, http://www.ahta.org. R&P Steven H Davis. Circ: 1,000.

628 ESP ISSN 0188-0012
PERSPECTIVAS EN SALUD PUBLICA. Text in English, Spanish. 1987. irreg. **Document type:** *Monographic series.*
Published by: Instituto Nacional de Salud Publica, Secretaria de Salud, Av. Universidad, 665, Planta Baja, Col. Santa Maria Ahuacatitlad, Cuernavaca, MORELOS 62508, Mexico. TEL 13-17-89, FAX 13-88-90. Circ: 2,000.

PERU. POLICIA NACIONAL. REVISTA DE LA SANIDAD. see *MEDICAL SCIENCES*

614.8 628.96 USA
PESTICIDE ANALYTICAL MANUAL. Text in English. irreg. USD 274; USD 548 foreign. **Document type:** *Government.*
—BLDSC (6428.358000).
Published by: U.S. Food and Drug Administration, Office of Public Affairs, 5600 Fishers Ln, Rockville, MD 20857. TEL 301-443-3220. **Subscr. to:** National Technical Information Service, Government Research Center. FAX 703-321-8547.

614 615.902 363.179 USA ISSN 0587-5943
PESTICIDE RESIDUES IN FOOD. Text in English. 1966. 3/yr. price varies. **Document type:** *Monographic series.*
Formerly: Codex Committee on Pesticide Residues. Report on the Meeting
Indexed: Rev.Plant Path.
Published by: Food and Agriculture Organization of the United Nations, c/o Bernan Associates, 4611 F Assembly Dr, Lanham, MD 20706-4391. TEL 301-459-7666, FAX 301-459-0056.

PFLEGE- UND KRANKENHAUSRECHT. see *LAW—Civil Law*

362.1 DEU ISSN 1439-7420
▼ **PFLEGEMAGAZIN**; Zeitschrift fuer den gesamten Pflegebereich. Text in German. 2000. bi-m. EUR 35.50 domestic; EUR 40.50 foreign (effective 2001). adv. bk.rev. illus. back issues avail. *Refereed.* **Document type:** *Magazine, Academic/Scholarly.* **Description:** Covers all aspects of the health care industry.
Published by: Juventa Verlag GmbH, Ehretstr 3, Weinheim 69469, Germany. TEL 49-6201-90200, FAX 49-6201-902013, juventa@juventa.de, http://www.juventa.de. Ed. Juliane Falk. adv.: B&W page DEM 1,300; 140 x 202.

362.1 DEU ISSN 0937-0277
PFLEGEN AMBULANT; das Magazin fuer Pflege - Organisation - Betriebsfuehrung. Text in German. 1990. bi-m. DEM 59.40, EUR 30.37 domestic; DEM 72, EUR 36.81 foreign; DEM 12, EUR 6.14 newsstand/cover (effective 2001). **Document type:** *Journal, Academic/Scholarly, Trade.* **Description:** Contains information and advice on various types of home and hospice care.
Published by: Bibliomed - Medizinische Verlagsgesellschaft mbH, Postfach 1150, Melsungen 34201, Germany. TEL 49-5661-7344-0, FAX 49-5661-8360, info@bibliomed.de, http://www.bibliomed.de.

614 DEU
PHARMA BRIEF. Text in German. 1981. 10/yr. EUR 15 domestic; EUR 28 foreign (effective 2001). bk.rev. back issues avail. **Document type:** *Newsletter, Consumer, Trade.* **Description:** Provides information on drug policy, rational use and prescribing of drugs in Germany and developing nations, and the marketing practices of German pharmaceutical manufacturers in developing countries.
Published by: B U K O Pharma-Kampagne, August-Bebel-Str 62, Bielefeld 33602, Germany. TEL 49-521-60550, FAX 49-521-63789, 100270.272@compuserve.com, http://www.bukopharma.de. Ed. Joerg Schaaber. Circ: 2,000.

PHARMACY HEALTH-LINE. see *PHARMACY AND PHARMACOLOGY*

PHYSICIANS' MEDICARE GUIDE. see *INSURANCE*

362.1 DEU ISSN 0930-7796
PLUSPUNKT; Sicherheit und Gesundheit in der Schule. Text in German. 1972. q. DEM 14 (effective 2001). **Document type:** *Magazine, Trade.*
Formerly (until 1976): Gib Acht Spezial (0930-780X)
Published by: Universum Verlagsanstalt GmbH KG, Taunusstr 54, Wiesbaden 65183, Germany. TEL 49-611-9030-0, FAX 49-611-9030382, uv@universum.de, http://www.universum.de. Circ: 71,000 (paid).

540 362.1 POL ISSN 1231-868X
PODSTAWY I METODY OCENY SRODOWISKA PRACY/PRINCIPLES AND METHODS OF ASSESSING THE WORKING ENVIRONMENT. Text in Polish; Summaries in English, Polish. 1985. q. PLZ 72; PLZ 18 newsstand/cover (effective 2001). charts, illus. index. back issues avail. *Refereed.* **Document type:** *Bulletin.* **Description:** Contains complete documentation on the harmful effects of definite chemical and physical agents on the human organism, together with the justification of MAC and MAI for these agents, adopted in Poland, and methods for their determination in the working environment. Helps to assess the hazards in the working environment and to establish appropriate medical prevention.
Published by: Centralny Instytut Ochrony Pracy/Central Institute for Labour Protection, Ul Czerniakowska 16, Warsaw 00701, Poland. TEL 48-22-6233698, FAX 48-22-6233693, oinip@ciop.pl. Ed. Danuta Koradecka. Circ: 500 (paid).

POLITECHNIKA WROCLAWSKA. INSTYTUT INZYNIERII OCHRONY SRODOWISKA. PRACE NAUKOWE. MONOGRAFIE. see *ENVIRONMENTAL STUDIES*

362.1 ITA ISSN 1590-069X
▼ **POLITICHE SANITARIE**; economia organizzazione e valutazione dei servizi sanitari. Text in Italian; Summaries in English. 2000. bi-m., latest vol.1, 2000. ITL 190,000, USD 150 (effective 2000). adv. bk.rev. 56 p./no. back issues avail. *Refereed.* **Document type:** *Journal, Academic/Scholarly.*
Published by: Il Pensiero Scientifico Editore s.r.l., Via Bradano, 3-C, Rome, RM 00199, Italy. TEL 39-06-862821, FAX 39-06-86282250, politiche@pensiero.it, http://www.pensiero.it. Ed. Gilberto Muraro. Pub. Francesco De Fiore. Adv. contact Luciano De Fiore. B&W page XEU 1,033, color page XEU 1,549; 21 x 28. Circ: 700 (paid).

POLSKA AKADEMIA NAUK. KOMITET GOSPODARKI WODNEJ. PRACE I STUDIA. see *WATER RESOURCES*

362.1 USA
POST-ACUTE PAYMENT REPORT. Text in English. 1997. m. USD 259; USD 269 in Canada & Mexico; USD 279 elsewhere. **Document type:** *Newsletter.*
Incorporates (in May 1999): Post-Acute Data Report; Which was formerly: Managed Home Care (1083-7205)
Published by: National Health Information, LLC, PO Box 15429, Atlanta, GA 30333. TEL 404-607-9500. Eds. Caralyn Davis, Melinda Young. Pubs. Cheli Brown, David Schwartz. **Subscr. to:** PO Box 670505, Marietta, GA 30066-9702.

POZ; health, hope & HIV. see *MEDICAL SCIENCES—Communicable Diseases*

PRAKTIKAN. see *MEDICAL SCIENCES—Dentistry*

PRATIQUE; newsletter of the disinfected mail study circle. see *COMMUNICATIONS—Postal Affairs*

614.8 ESP ISSN 0034-8732
PREVENCION (SAN SEBASTIAN). Text in Spanish. 1962. q. membership. adv. bk.rev.
Formerly (until 1975): Revista de Prevencion (1132-3140)
Indexed: C.I.S. Abstr.
—CCC.
Published by: Asociacion para la Prevencion de Accidentes, Echaide, 4 Piso 2, San Sebastian-donostia, Guipuzcoa 20005, Spain. TEL 43-42-56-45, FAX 43-42-91-32. Ed. Ramon Zamanillo Tellitu. Circ: 6,326.

614.44 610 GBR ISSN 0300-2659
RA421
PREVENT* ; the journal for all who would prevent disease. Text in English. 1973. bi-m. GBP 5. bibl, illus.
—CISTI, GNLM.
Published by: Fitzken Publishers, 3 Alma Sq, London NW8 6QD, United Kingdom. Ed. Dr. J McMurdoch.

371 USA
RE1
PREVENT BLINDNESS AMERICA. ANNUAL REPORT. Text in English. a. **Document type:** *Corporate.*
Former titles: National Society to Prevent Blindness. Annual Report (0270-4234); National Society for the Prevention of Blindness. Report
Published by: Prevent Blindness America, 500 E Remington Rd, Schaumburg, IL 60173. TEL 847-843-2020, FAX 847-843-8458. Ed. Jody Kenyon. R&P Joan Boyes.

362.41 USA
PREVENT BLINDNESS NEWS. Text in English. 1951. 3/yr. USD 10 to members (effective 2000). illus. **Document type:** *Newsletter.*
Former titles: National Society to Prevent Blindness. Member News; Insight (Schaumburg); Prevent Blindness News (0032-8014); Incorporates: Wise Owl News (0043-6755)
Published by: Prevent Blindness America, 500 E Remington Rd, Schaumburg, IL 60173. TEL 847-843-2020, FAX 847-843-8458. Ed., R&P Jody Kenyon. Circ: 25,000.

614.8 FRA ISSN 0032-8030
PREVENTION ROUTIERE DANS L'ENTREPRISE* . Text in French. 1970 (vol.18). bi-m. FRF 105. adv. charts, illus.
Address: 32 rue Alexandre Dumas, Paris Cedex 11 75543, France. TEL 43-67-03-62, FAX 43-67-28-43. Ed. Monique Anquetil. Circ: 52,000.

PREVENTIVE MEDICINE; an international journal devoted to practice and theory. see *MEDICAL SCIENCES*

PREVOYANCE. see *OCCUPATIONAL HEALTH AND SAFETY*

362.1 614 ZAF
PRIMARY HEALTH CARE NEWS. Text in English. 1993. bi-m. **Document type:** *Government.*
Published by: Department of Health, Private Bag X54348, Durban, KwaZulu-Natal 4000, South Africa.

354 614 CAN
PRINCE EDWARD ISLAND. DEPARTMENT OF HEALTH AND SOCIAL SERVICES. ANNUAL REPORT. Text in English. a. **Document type:** *Government.*
Formerly: Prince Edward Island. Department of Health. Annual Report (0317-4530)
—CISTI.
Published by: Department of Health and Social Services, P O Box 2000, Charlottetown, PE C1A 7N8, Canada. TEL 902-368-4900, FAX 902-368-4969. Circ: 500.

614 USA ISSN 1522-645X
PRIORITIES FOR HEALTH. Text in English. 1979. q. USD 25. adv. reprints avail. **Document type:** *Consumer.* **Description:** Consumer education magazine concerned with issues related to food nutrition, chemicals, pharmaceuticals, lifestyles, the environment and health.
Former titles (until 1999): Priorities for Long Life and Good Health (1089-3490); (until 1979): A C S H News and Views (0737-8637)
Related titles: Online - full text ed.
Indexed: AgeLine, CHNI, CINAHL, NRN, e-psyche.
—BLDSC (6615.527000).
Published by: American Council on Science and Health, 1995 Broadway, 2nd Fl, New York, NY 10023-5560. TEL 212-362-7044, FAX 212-362-4919, acsh@acsh.org, http://www.prioritiesforhealth.com. Ed. Jack Rasso. Pub. Dr. Elizabeth Whelan. R&P Mary Ellen Kelly. Adv. contact Adam Lieberman. Circ: 7,000.

P

614 RUS
PROBLEMY SOTSIALNOI GIGIENY, ZDRAVOOKHRANENIYA, I ISTORII MEDITSINY/PROBLEMS OF SOCIAL HYGIENE, HEALTH SERVICE AND HISTORY OF MEDICINE. Text in Russian; Summaries in English. 1942. bi-m. USD 186 foreign (effective 2000). adv. bk.rev. abstr, bibl, charts, illus, stat. index. **Document type:** *Journal, Academic/Scholarly.* **Description:** Discusses theoretical problems of social hygiene and public health organization, the main trends in the development of health protection, scientific bases of planning, prognosticating and management in public health service.
Former titles: Problemy Sotsialnoi Gigieny, i Istoriya Meditsiny (0869-866X); Sovetskoe Zdravookhranenie (0038-5239)
Indexed: Abstr.Hyg., Biol.Abstr., C.I.S. Abstr., Chem.Abstr., Curr.Dig.Sov.Press, Dent.Ind., INIS Atomind., Ind.Med. (1994-), Int.Nurs.Ind., Ref.Zh., Russ.Acad.Sci.Bibl., Trop.Dis.Bull., World Bibl.Soc.Sec.
—BLDSC (0133.774330), CISTI, East View, GNLM.
Published by: Izdatel'stvo Meditsina, Petroverigskii per 6-8, Moscow 101000, Russian Federation. TEL 7-095-9248785, 7-095-928-86-48, FAX 7-095-9211355, meditsina@iname.com, http://www.medit.ru. Ed. O P Shchepin. Pub. A M Stochik. R&P T Scheglova. Adv. contact O A Fadeeva TEL 7-095-923-51-40. Circ: 500. **Dist. by:** Mezhdunarodnaya Kniga, B Yakimanka 39, Moscow 117049, Russian Federation. TEL 7-095-2384967, FAX 7-095-2384634.

643 USA ISSN 0092-7732
KF3945.A73
PRODUCT SAFETY & LIABILITY REPORTER; a weekly review of consumer safety developments. Text in English. 1973. w. USD 1,493 (effective 2001). index. back issues avail. **Description:** Notification and reference service providing coverage of current administrative, legislative, judicial, and industry developments relating to product safety and product liability.
Related titles: Online - full text ed.: ISSN 1522-5259 (from Bureau of National Affairs, Inc., (BNA), The).
—CCC.
Published by: The Bureau of National Affairs, Inc., 1231 25th St, N W, Washington, DC 20037. TEL 202-452-4200, 800-372-1033, 800-452-7773, FAX 202-822-8092, customercare@bna.com, bnaplus@bna.com, http://www.bna.com/. Pub. Gregory McCaffery.

600 USA ISSN 0098-7530
PRODUCT SAFETY LETTER. Text in English. 1972. w., latest vol.31, 2002. USD 997 in North America; USD 1,047 elsewhere (effective Nov. 2001). bk.rev. charts. index. 4 p./no. Supplement avail.; back issues avail. **Document type:** *Newsletter.* **Description:** Contains information for executives concerned with government regulation of consumer products.
—CCC.
Published by: Washington Business Information, Inc., 300 N Washington St, Ste 200, Falls Church, Arlington, VA 22046. TEL 703-538-7600, 703-538-7661, FAX 703 538-7676, ehinkle@fdanews.com, http://www.fdanews.com. Ed. Joan Murphy.

362.1 GBR
PROFESSIONAL ADVICE AND SUPPORT PROGRAMMES (YEARS). Text in English. biennial.
Formerly (until 1995): Professional Advice and Support Programmes in the Community (Other than Maternity) (Years)
—BLDSC.
Published by: Department of Health, Statistics Division 2B, Room 430B, Skipton House, 80 London Rd, London SE1 6LH, United Kingdom. TEL 44-171-972-5540.

362.1 GBR
PROFESSIONAL PEST CONTROLLER. Text in English. 1992. 3/yr. free per issue. adv. bk.rev. charts, illus, tr.lit. back issues avail. **Document type:** *Trade.* **Description:** Aims to provide readers with an unbiased, high quality and professional magazine relevant to the pest control industry.
Published by: British Pest Control Association, 3 St James Court, Friar Gate, Derby DE1 1BT, United Kingdom. TEL 44-1332-294288, FAX 44-1332-295904, enquiry@bpca.org.uk, http://www.bpca.org.uk. Ed. Frances McKim TEL 44-1509-233219. adv.: page GBP 800; trim 185 x 260. Circ: 4,000 (controlled).

628 USA
PROFESSIONAL SANITARIAN. Text in English. irreg. (1-2/yr.).
Published by: National Society of Professional Sanitarians, 1224 Hoffman Dr, Jefferson City, MO 65101.

900 USA
PROGRESS (COLUMBUS). Text in English. 1984. 5/yr. free per issue to qualified personnel. charts, illus.
Published by: Department of Health, PO Box 118, Columbus, OH 43216. TEL 614-462-8562. Circ: 3,000.

362.1 GBR ISSN 1368-6445
PROMOTING HEALTH; the journal of health promotion for Northern Ireland. Text in English. 1997. q. *Refereed.* **Document type:** *Bulletin.*
—BLDSC (6925.161200).
Published by: Health Promotion Agency for Northern Ireland, 18 Ormeau Ave, Belfast, Co Antrim BT2 8HS, United Kingdom. FAX 44-1232-311711, http://www.healthpromotionagency.org.uk. Ed. Rachel Kelly. R&P Fionuala Boyd TEL 44-1232-311611. Circ: 5,000.

600 FRA ISSN 1025-3823
RA427.8
PROMOTION & EDUCATION; international journal of health promotion and education. Text in English, French, Spanish. 1958. q., latest vol.8. FRF 200, USD 35 in Africa; FRF 200, USD 35 in Latin America (effective 2001). adv. bibl, charts, illus, stat. biennial index. 48 p./no. back issues avail.; reprint service avail. from PQC. *Refereed.* **Document type:** *Journal.* **Description:** Presents theoretical research and practical papers on experiences, opinions and research leading to applications for health promotion and health education internationally.
Former titles: Hygie (0751-7149); (until 1982): International Journal of Health Education (0020-7306)
Related titles: Microfilm ed.: (from PQC); Online - full text ed.: (from ProQuest Information & Learning).
Indexed: Adol.Ment.Hlth.Abstr., Biol.Abstr., Br.Educ.Ind., C.I.S. Abstr., Cont.Pg.Educ., Curr.Cont. (coverage dropped), Excerp.Med., FAMLI, Ind.Med. (1993-), NRN, SSCI (coverage dropped), Trop.Dis.Bull.
—BLDSC (6925.172000), GNLM, ingenta, Linda Hall.
Published by: Union Internationale de Promotion de la Sante et d'Education pour la Sante/International Union for Health Promotion and Education, 2 rue Auguste Comte, Vanves 92170, France. TEL 33-1-46450059, FAX 33-1-46450045, iuhpecj@worldnet.fr, http://www.iuhpe.org. R&P, Adv. contact Catherine Jones. B&W page USD 11,500; 210 x 297. Circ: 4,000.

PROSPETTIVE SOCIALI E SANITARIE. see *SOCIAL SERVICES AND WELFARE*

614.49 POL ISSN 0033-2100
PRZEGLAD EPIDEMIOLOGICZNY. Text in Polish; Summaries in English. 1947. q. USD 120 foreign (effective 2002). adv. bk.rev. abstr, charts, illus. index, cum.index. **Document type:** *Academic/Scholarly.* **Description:** Discusses epidemiology, bacteriology, parasitology, pathology and clinical aspects of infectious diseases.
Indexed: Abstr.Hyg., Biol.Abstr., Chem.Abstr., Dent.Ind., Dok.Arbeitsmed., Excerp.Med., Forest Prod.Abstr., Forest.Abstr., Helminthol.Abstr., INIS Atomind., Ind.Med. (1947-), Ind.Vet., Protozool.Abstr., Rev.Appl.Entomol., Rev.Med.& Vet.Mycol., Rev.Plant Path., Trop.Dis.Bull., Weed Abstr.
—BLDSC (6940.100000), CISTI, GNLM.
Published by: Panstwowy Zaklad Higieny/National Institute of Hygiene, Ul Chocimska 24, Warsaw 00791, Poland. TEL 48-22-6464487, FAX 48-22-8497484, pzh@med.stat.waw.pl, azielinski@pzh.gov.pl. Ed., R&P Andrzej Zielinski. Circ: 750. **Dist. by:** Ars Polona, Krakowskie Przedmiescie 7, Warsaw, Poland. TEL 48-22-8261201. **Co-sponsor:** Polskie Towarzystwo Epidemiologow i Lekarzy Chorob Zakaznych - Polish Association of Epidemiologists and Infectionists.

PUBLIC ASSISTANCE & WELFARE TRENDS - STATE CAPITALS. see *LAW*

614 UGA
PUBLIC HEALTH AND HYGIENE*. Text in English. 1972 (vol.4). a. adv. bibl, illus.
Published by: Public Health Inspectors' Association, PO Box 46, Kampala, Uganda. Ed. Wazarwahi Bwengye.

PUBLIC HEALTH (BASINGSTOKE). see *MEDICAL SCIENCES*

362.1 GBR ISSN 1367-2509
PUBLIC HEALTH FORUM. Text in English. 1997. q.
—BLDSC (6964.170000).
Published by: King's Fund, 11-13 Cavendish Sq, London W1M 0AN, United Kingdom. TEL 44-171-307-2586, FAX 44-171-307-2801.

362.1 USA
PUBLIC HEALTH G I S NEWS AND INFORMATION. (Geographic Information Systems) Text in English. bi-m. **Document type:** *Newsletter.* **Description:** Provides timely information on a wide range of geographic information systems (GIS) topics, including assistance with applications of GIS technology, progressional meetings and conferences, and public health GIS literature.
Media: Online - full text.
Published by: National Center for Health Statistics, Centers for Disease Control and Prevention, Office of Research and Methodology, Rm 915, 6225 Belcrest Rd, Hyattsville, MD 20782. TEL 301-436-7904, cmc2@cdc.gov, http://atsdr1.atsdr.cdc.gov:8080/hec/hsph71-2.html#gis. Ed. Charles M Croner.

PUBLIC HEALTH LABORATORY SERVICE BOARD. REPORT. see *MEDICAL SCIENCES—Communicable Diseases*

362.1 614 GBR
PUBLIC HEALTH (LONDON). Text in English. 1888. bi-m. GBP 157 in Europe; GBP 167 elsewhere; GBP 168 in Europe print & online; GBP 181 elsewhere print & online (effective 2000). bk.rev. *Refereed.* **Document type:** *Academic/Scholarly.* **Description:** An international coverage of preventative medicine, epidemiology, and social and community medicine. Includes research papers on child health, communicable disease control, health service provision and management and other topics.
Related titles: Online - full text ed.: GBP 153 (effective 2000).
Indexed: Int.Abstr.Biol.Sci.
Published by: Nature Publishing Group Specialist Journals (Subsidiary of: Holtzbrink Publishers), Houndmills, Basingstoke, Hants RG21 6XS, United Kingdom. TEL 44-1256-329242, FAX 44-1256-328339, public.health@riphh.org.uk, subscriptions@nature.com, http://www.naturepublishing.com, http://www.nature.com. Ed. Dr. Richard Slack.

614 GBR ISSN 1465-1505
▼ **PUBLIC HEALTH MEDICINE.** Text in English. 1999. q. GBP 60 domestic to individuals; GBP 90 foreign to individuals; GBP 90 domestic to institutions; GBP 120 foreign to institutions (effective 2000). *Refereed.* **Document type:** *Academic/Scholarly.* **Description:** Provides articles on epidemiology, care groups, needs assessment, health service evaluation, clinical effectiveness and good practice, achieving change, public health around the world and a wide range of other public health topics.
Indexed: Protozool.Abstr., Trop.Dis.Bull.
Published by: Rila Publications Ltd., 73 Newman St, London W1A 4PG, United Kingdom. TEL 44-20-7631-1299, FAX 44-20-7580-7166, http://www.rila.co.uk. Eds. Jennifer Bennett, Salman Rawaf.

614 USA ISSN 0079-7596
PUBLIC HEALTH MONOGRAPH*. Text in English. 1951 (no.3). irreg.
Continues: Public Health Technical Monograph
Indexed: Biol.Abstr., Ind.Med. (coverage dropped).
—CISTI, GNLM.
Published by: U.S. Public Health Service, Dept of Health Education and Welfare, Bethesda, MD 20014. TEL 301-444-6656.

PUBLIC HEALTH NURSING. see *MEDICAL SCIENCES—Nurses And Nursing*

PUBLIC HEALTH NUTRITION. see *NUTRITION AND DIETETICS*

614 USA ISSN 0090-2918
RA11 CODEN: HSRPAT
PUBLIC HEALTH REPORTS; the public health journal that you want to read. Text in English. 1878. bi-m. GBP 40, USD 50 to individuals; GBP 65, USD 85 to institutions (effective Feb. 2002). adv. bk.rev. bibl, charts, illus, stat, abstr. index. back issues avail.; reprint service avail. from CIS,PQC. *Refereed.* **Document type:** *Journal, Government, Academic/Scholarly.* **Description:** Covers research, policy, and commentary on public health issues.
Former titles (until 1974): Health Services Reports; (until 1972): H S M H A Health Reports; (until 1970): Public Health Reports (0033-3549)

Related titles: Microfiche ed.: (from CIS); Microform ed.: (from PQC,PMC); Online - full text ed.: ISSN 1468-2877. GBP 58, USD 76 to institutions online only (effective Feb. 2002) (from ProQuest Information & Learning, Gale Group, LexisNexis, HighWire Pr., Northern Light Technology, Inc., EBSCO Publishing, H. W. Wilson, ingenta, Swets Blackwell, Factiva, Institute for Scientific Information, RoweCom Information Quest).
Indexed: AIDS Abstr., AIM, ASCA, Abstr.Health Care Manage.Stud., Abstr.Hyg., Acad.Ind., AgeLine, Agri.& Environ.Biotech.Abstr. (coverage dropped), Agricola, Amer.Bibl.Slavic & E.Eur.Stud., Amer.Stat.Ind. (1972-), Aqua.Sci.& Fish.Abstr., Bibl.Dev.Med.& Child Neur., CINAHL, Chem.Abstr., Chic.Per.Ind., Crim.Just.Abstr., Curr.Adv.Ecol.Sci., Curr.Cont., Dent.Abstr., Derwent Biotech.Abstr., Diar.Dis.Res., Dok.Arbeitsmed., Eng.Ind., Environ.Sci.Poll.Mgmt., Excerp.Med., Fam.Ind., Gen.Sci.Ind. (Jul.1984-), Helminthol.Abstr., Hlth.Ind., Hosp.Lit.Ind., INIS Atomind., I.P.A., Ind.Hyg.Dig., Ind.Med. (1974-), Ind.Sci.Rev., Ind.U.S.Gov.Per., Inpharma, Int.Nurs.Ind., Mid.East: Abstr.& Ind., NRN, Nutr.Abstr., P.A.I.S., Pharm.&Out.News, Pollut.Abstr., Popul.Ind., Protozool.Abstr., Reac., Ref.Zh., Rev.Appl.Entomol., Rev.Med.& Vet.Mycol., Risk Abstr., Russ.Acad.Sci.Bibl., SSCI, Saf.Sci.Abstr., Sage Race Rel.Abstr., Sci.Cit.Ind., Sel.Water Res.Abstr., Soc.Sci.Ind. (Nov.1982-), Soc.Work Res.& Abstr., THA, Trop.Dis.Bull., W.R.C.Inf.
—BLDSC (6965.000000), CISTI, GNLM, IDS, ingenta, KNAW.
Published by: (Association of Schools of Public Health), Oxford University Press, Academic Division, Great Clarendon St, Oxford OX2 6DP, United Kingdom. TEL 44-1865-267907, FAX 44-1865-267835, jnl.info@oup.co.uk, http://phr.oupjournals.org, http://www.oup.co.uk/journals. Pub. J Fox. adv.: page GBP 536, page USD 965. Circ: 8,000. **Subscr. outside N. America to:** Journals Marketing, Great Clarendon St, Oxford OX2 6DP, United Kingdom.

614 ISR ISSN 0301-0422
CODEN: PBHRAM
PUBLIC HEALTH REVIEWS; an international quarterly. Text in English. 1972. q. USD 150 (effective 1999). adv. bk.rev. abstr, bibl. index, cum.index. *Refereed.* **Document type:** *Academic/Scholarly.* **Description:** Presents reviews and critical evaluations of topics in public health, including epidemiology, environmental and occupational health. Publishes concise reports of research, surveys, long-term studies, and trends in morbidity and mortality. Also publishes proceedings and abstracts of conferences.
Indexed: Biol.Abstr., CINAHL, Curr.Adv.Ecol.Sci., Curr.Cont. (coverage dropped), Energy Ind., Energy Info.Abstr., Excerp.Med., Food Sci.& Tech.Abstr., Hosp.Lit.Ind., Ind.Med. (1972-), NRN, SSCI (coverage dropped), Virol.Abstr.
—BLDSC (6966.300000), CISTI, EMDOCS, GNLM, IDS, ingenta.
Published by: Technosdar Ltd., P O Box 31684, Tel Aviv 61316, Israel. TEL 972-3-5607418, FAX 972-3-5604932, TELEX 341667 RMYM. Ed. Sigmund Geller. R&P, Adv. contact Abraham Weiss.

PUBLIC HEALTH - STATE CAPITALS. see *LAW*

363.1 USA ISSN 0001-2165
PUBLIC SAFETY COMMUNICATIONS. Key Title: A P C O Bulletin. Text in English. 1935. m. membership. adv. bk.rev. back issues avail. **Document type:** *Trade.* **Description:** For persons who operate, maintain, install, design and manufacture the emergency communications systems used to answer the public's calls for police, fire and EMS services.
Published by: Association of Public-Safety Communications Officials International, Inc., 2040 S Ridgewood Ave, Daytona Beach, FL 32119-8437. TEL 904-322-2500, FAX 904-322-2501, bulletin@apcointl.org, http://www.apcointl.org. Ed., R&P Cindy Lorow. Adv. contact Terry D Diehl. B&W page USD 1,540, color page USD 2,610; trim 10.13 x 7.75. Circ: 13,000 (controlled).

362.1 USA ISSN 1084-9483
PUBLIC SECTOR CONTRACTING REPORT. Text in English. 1995. m. USD 299; USD 309 in Canada & Mexico; USD 319 elsewhere. **Document type:** *Trade.*
Indexed: Int.Nurs.Ind.
Published by: National Health Information, LLC, PO Box 15429, Atlanta, GA 30333. TEL 404-607-9500.

628 ITA ISSN 0393-1072
PULIZIA INDUSTRIALE E SANIFICAZIONE. Text in Italian. 1968. m. ITL 100,000. adv.
Published by: MO.ED.CO. s.r.l., Via Paolo Da Cannobio, 9, Milan, MI 20122, Italy. TEL 02-878577, FAX 02-89040728. Circ: 5,500.

QUADERNI DI COOPERAZIONE SANITARIA/CAHIERS DE COOPERATION MEDICALE/HEALTH COOPERATION PAPERS. see *MEDICAL SCIENCES—Communicable Diseases*

QUALITY OF LIFE NEWSLETTER. see *MEDICAL SCIENCES*

362.1 GBR
QUESTION AND ANSWER BRIEFING. Short title: Q and A Briefing. Text in English. irreg., latest vol.6, 1997. **Document type:** *Bulletin.*
Published by: West Sussex Health Authority, West Sussex Health Authority, 1 The Causeway, Goring-By-Sea, Durrington, Worthing BN12 6BT, United Kingdom. TEL 44-1903-708400, FAX 44-1903-700981.

R F L. (Rundschau Fleischhygiene und Lebensmittelueberwachung) see *FOOD AND FOOD INDUSTRIES*

R S O MAGAZINE. (Radiation Safety Officer) see *OCCUPATIONAL HEALTH AND SAFETY*

R T E C S. (Registry of Toxic Effects of Chemical Substances) see *ENVIRONMENTAL STUDIES—Toxicology And Environmental Safety*

614.8 IND ISSN 0972-0464
RADIATION PROTECTION AND ENVIRONMENT. Text in English. 1997. q. INR 50 to individuals; INR 100 to institutions; USD 25 to individuals; USD 50 to institutions (effective 2000). adv.
Formerly: Bulletin of Radiation Protection (0253-6897)
Indexed: Eng.Ind., INIS Atomind.
—BLDSC (7227.991700).
Published by: Indian Association for Radiation Protection, Radiation Safety Systems Division, Bhabha Atomic Research Centre, Trombay, Mumbai 400 085, India. TEL 91-22-5505050, FAX 91-22-5505150, ucm@magnum.barct1.ernet.in. adv.: page USD 3,500.

RADIATION PROTECTION DOSIMETRY. see *PHYSICS—Nuclear Physics*

RADIATION PROTECTION MANAGEMENT; the journal of applied health physics. see *OCCUPATIONAL HEALTH AND SAFETY*

363.7289 NZL ISSN 0113-4795
RADIATION PROTECTION NEWS AND NOTES. Text in English. 1988. q. NZD 28.12; NZD 50 foreign. bk.rev. charts, illus. back issues avail. **Document type:** *Academic/Scholarly.* **Description:** Covers items of interest in radiation protection, nationally and internationally.
Indexed: INIS Atomind.
Published by: (Singapore. Ministry of Health SGP), National Radiation Laboratory, P.O. Box 25-099, Christchurch, New Zealand. TEL 64-3-366-5059, FAX 64-3-366-1156, ursula@nrl.moh.govt.nz. Ed. A C McEwan.

LA RADIOACTIVITE DES PRINCIPALES SOURCES D'EAU MINERALE EN BELGIQUE. see *WATER RESOURCES*

362.1 ITA ISSN 1120-1762
RAGIUSAN; rassegna giuridica della sanita. Text in Italian. 1984. m. ITL 950,000, EUR 490.63. adv. bk.rev. back issues avail.
Published by: Sipis s.r.l., Viale Parioli, 77, Rome, RM 00197, Italy. TEL 39-6-8073368, FAX 39-6-8085817, sipis@tin.it. Ed. Luigi D'Elia. Pub., R&P, Adv. contact Anna Gemma Gonzales. page ITL 2,000,000.

RAUMPLANUNG UND UMWELTSCHUTZ IM KANTON ZURICH. see *HOUSING AND URBAN PLANNING*

614 MDG
RAVINTSARA. Text in French; Summaries in English, French. 2/yr. MGF 54, USD 9.
Published by: Centre d'Information et de Documentation Scientifique et Technique, BP 6224, Antananarivo 101, Madagascar. TEL 33288.

RE PRODUCTIONS. see *PHYSICAL FITNESS AND HYGIENE*

▼ **REAL HEALTHCARE.** see *HEALTH FACILITIES AND ADMINISTRATION*

RECYCLING MAGAZIN; Fachblatt des gesamten Handels mit Alt- und Abfallstoffen. see *TECHNOLOGY: COMPREHENSIVE WORKS*

614 COL
REGISTRO DE ORGANISMOS DE SALUD. Text in Spanish. 1976. a.
Published by: Departamento Administrativo Nacional de Estadistica, Banco Nacional de Datos, Centro Administrativo Nacional, Avda. Eldorado, Apdo. Aereo 80043, Bogota, DE, Colombia.

REGULATORY UPDATE; government legislation and regulations related to plastics industry. see *PLASTICS*

362.1 CHN
RENMIN GONGAN BAO/PEOPLE'S PUBLIC SECURITY REVIEW. Text in Chinese. 6/w. CNY 106.08. **Document type:** *Newspaper, Government.*
Published by: China International Book Trading Corp/Zhongguo Guoji Tushu Maoyi Zonggongsi cibtc@mail.cibtc.com.cn, http://www.cibtc.com.cn. **Dist. by:** 35, Chegongzhuang Xilu, Haidian District, Beijing 100044, China.

RENT I DANMARK. see *BUSINESS AND ECONOMICS—Management*

616 551.48 JPN
REPORTS OF INVESTIGATIONS ABOUT LAKE BIWA. Text in English. 1984. irreg.
Published by: Shiga Prefectural Institute of Public Health and Environmental Science/Shiga Kenritsu Eisei Kankyo Senta, 13-45 Goten-Hama, Otsu-shi, Shiga-ken 520-0834, Japan.

616.89 150 USA ISSN 0192-0812
RA790.A1
RESEARCH IN COMMUNITY AND MENTAL HEALTH; an annual compilation of research. Text in English. 1979. irreg., latest vol.9, 1998. USD 73.25. **Document type:** *Monographic series.*
Indexed: Chic.Per.Ind., Lang.& Lang.Behav.Abstr., Psychol.Abstr., SOPODA, Soc.Serv.Abstr., Sociol.Abstr., e-psyche.
—BLDSC (7736.700000), GNLM. **CCC.**
Published by: J A I Press Inc., 100 Prospect St, Box 811, Stamford, CT 06904-0811. TEL 203-323-9606, FAX 203-357-8446, jai@jaipress.com. Ed. Joseph Morrissey.

RESEARCH IN THE SOCIOLOGY OF HEALTH CARE. see *MEDICAL SCIENCES*

363.7 RUS
RET - INFO. Text in Russian. 1992. q. RUR 60,000. bk.rev. back issues avail. **Document type:** *Bulletin.* **Description:** Covers hygienic and epidemiologic control in urban and rural territories.
Published by: Nauchno-kommercheskaya Firma "Ret", Nizhnemaslovka ul 14-69, Moscow, Russian Federation. TEL 7-095-9454034, FAX 7-095-9456349. Ed. Valentin Rylnikov. adv.: page USD 300. Circ: 1,000.

REVIEWS ON ENVIRONMENTAL HEALTH. see *ENVIRONMENTAL STUDIES*

614 BRA ISSN 0100-0233
RA464.B33
REVISTA BAIANA DE SAUDE PUBLICA. Text in Portuguese; Summaries in English. 1974. q. per issue exchange basis. bibl, charts, stat.
Indexed: Abstr.Hyg.
—CISTI, KNAW.
Published by: Secretaria da Saude do Estado da Bahia, Centro Administrativo da Bahia, 4 a, Av. Plataforma 06, Cab, Caixa Postal 631, Salvador, BA 41745-000, Brazil. TEL 55-71-3704273, TELEX 7136. Circ: 1,000.

371.71 BRA ISSN 1413-3415
REVISTA BRASILEIRA DE SAUDE ESCOLAR/ BRAZILIAN JOURNAL OF SCHOOL HEALTH. Text in Portuguese. 199?. a. *Refereed.*
—BLDSC (7845.730000).
Published by: Associacao Brasileira de Saude Escolar, Prof. Rubiao Meira 61, Praca 02, Ciudade Universitaria, Sao Paulo, SP 05508-900, Brazil. Ed. Paschoal Luiz Tambucci.

614.4 CUB ISSN 0253-1151
CODEN: RCHEDF
REVISTA CUBANA DE HIGIENE Y EPIDEMIOLOGIA. Text in Spanish; Summaries in English, French, Spanish. 1963. s-a. USD 36 in the Americas; USD 44 in Europe; USD 52 elsewhere. abstr, bibl, charts, illus. index.
Formerly: Boletin de Higiene y Epidemiologia (0006-629X)
Related titles: Online - full text ed.
Indexed: Abstr.Hyg., Biol.Abstr., Chem.Abstr., Chem.Titles, Dairy Sci.Abstr., Excerp.Med., INIS Atomind., Ind.Med. (coverage dropped), Repindex, Trop.Dis.Bull.
—CASDDS, CISTI.

P

Published by: Ministerio de Salud Publica, Centro Nacional de Informacion de Ciencias Medicas, O'Reilly No. 4, Havana, Cuba. TEL 809-62-8091. Ed. Haydee Alfonso. Circ: 1,400. **Co-sponsors:** Instituto Nacional de Higiene, Epidemiologia y Microbiologia; Sociedad Cubana de Higiene y Epidemiologia.

614 CUB ISSN 0864-3466
RA456.C7
REVISTA CUBANA DE SALUD PUBLICA. Text in Spanish; Summaries in English, Spanish. 1975. 3/yr. USD 30 in the Americas; USD 38 in Europe; USD 46 elsewhere. bibl, charts, illus. index. **Description:** Covers the field of social medicine and organization and administration of the Cuban health system.
Formerly: Revista Cubana de Administracion de Salud (0252-1903)
Related titles: Online - full text ed.
Indexed: Abstr.Hyg., Curr.Adv.Ecol.Sci., Curr.Ind.Stat., IBR, Ind.Med. (coverage dropped), Lang.& Lang.Behav.Abstr., Popul.Ind., SOPODA, Sociol.Abstr.
Published by: (Cuba. Ministerio de Salud Publica, Centro Nacional de Informacion de Ciencias Medicas), Editorial de Ciencias Medicas, O'Reilly No. 4, Habana, Cuba. TEL 809-62-8091. Ed. Maria Julia Zamorano. Circ: 1,500. **Co-sponsor:** Sociedad Cubana de Administracion de Salud.

614 BRA ISSN 0034-8910
RA421 CODEN: RSPUB9
REVISTA DE SAUDE PUBLICA. Text in English, Portuguese, Spanish; Summaries in English, Portuguese. 1967. bi-m. BRL 34, USD 48 to individuals; BRL 38, USD 48 to institutions (effective 2000). bk.rev. bibl, charts, illus. index. back issues avail. *Refereed.* **Document type:** *Academic/Scholarly.* **Description:** Reflects scientific advances in the public health field through original research prepared by specialists, both domestic and foreign.
Supersedes: Universidade de Sao Paulo. Faculdade de Higiene e Saude Publica. Archivos
Related titles: Online - full text ed.: (from SciELO, Institute for Scientific Information).
Indexed: ASCA, Abstr.Hyg., Aqua.Sci.& Fish.Abstr., Biol.Abstr., C.I.S. Abstr., Curr.Cont., Dairy Sci.Abstr., Dent.Ind., Entomol.Abstr., Environ.Sci.Poll.Mgmt., Excerp.Med., Helminthol.Abstr., INIS Atomind., Ind.Med. (1967-), Ind.Vet., Microbiol.Abstr., Nutr.Abstr., Postharvest, Protozool.Abstr., Ref.Zh., Rev.Appl.Entomol., Rev.Med.& Vet.Mycol., Rice Abstr., Risk Abstr., Rural Devel.Abstr., Rural Recreat.Tour.Abstr., SSCI, Saf.Sci.Abstr., Sel.Water Res.Abstr., Soyabean Abstr., Sugar Ind.Abstr., Trop.Dis.Bull., Vet.Bull., Virol.Abstr. (coverage dropped), Wild.Rev., World Ag.Econ.& Rur.Soc.Abstr., Zoo.Rec.
—BLDSC (7870.635000), CASDDS, GNLM, IDS, KNAW.
Published by: Universidade de Sao Paulo, Faculdade de Saude Publica, Av. Dr. Arnaldo 715, Sao Paulo, SP 01246-904, Brazil. TEL 55-11-2809163, revsp@org.usp.br, http://www.scielo.br/. Ed. Dr. Oswaldo Paulo Forattini. Circ: 1,500.

614 ESP ISSN 1135-5727
REVISTA ESPANOLA DE SALUD PUBLICA. Text in Spanish; Summaries in English. 1926. 6/yr. bk.rev. abstr, bibl, charts, illus. **Document type:** *Bulletin.* **Description:** Includes original papers on public health, sanitation and epidemiology.
Formerly (until 1995): Revista de Sanidad e Higiene Publica (0034-8899)
Related titles: Online - full text ed.
Indexed: Abstr.Hyg., Biol.Abstr., Chem.Abstr., Dairy Sci.Abstr., Helminthol.Abstr., Ind.Med. (1995-), Ind.Med.Esp., Ind.SST, Ind.Vet., Int.Nurs.Ind., Nutr.Abstr., Poult.Abstr., Protozool.Abstr., Rev.Appl.Entomol., Trop.Dis.Bull.
—BLDSC (7854.315000), CINDOC, CISTI, EMDOCS, GNLM, Infotrieve. **CCC.**
Published by: Ministerio de Sanidad y Consumo, Paseo del Prado 18-20, Madrid 28071, Spain. TEL 34-91-5964176, FAX 34-91-5964195, resp@msc.es, http://www.msc.es/revistas/resp/home.htm. Ed. Cristina Perez Andres. Circ: 5,000.

614 MOZ ISSN 0254-5705
REVISTA MEDICA DE MOCAMBIQUE. Text in Portuguese. 1982. 4/yr. USD 60. adv. back issues avail. *Refereed.* **Document type:** *Academic/Scholarly.*
Related titles: CD-ROM ed.
Indexed: ExtraMED.
—GNLM.
Published by: Ministerio da Saude, Instituto Nacional de Saude, Universidade Eduardo Mondlane, Faculdade de Medicina, C.P. 264, Maputo, Mozambique. TEL 258-1-431103, FAX 258-1-431103, mdgedge@malarins.uem.mz. Eds. Dr. Joao Schwalbach, Martinho Dgedge. Circ: 1,500.

614 VEN ISSN 0035-0583
RA421
REVISTA VENEZOLANA DE SANIDAD Y ASISTENCIA SOCIAL. Text in Spanish; Summaries in Multiple languages. 1936. q. free per issue. charts, illus, stat. index.
Indexed: Biol.Abstr., Chem.Abstr., Ind.Med. (coverage dropped), Nutr.Abstr., P.A.I.S., Rev.Appl.Entomol.
—CISTI, GNLM.
Published by: Ministerio de Sanidad y Asistencia Social, c/o Oficina de Publicaciones Biblioteca y Archivo,, Centro Simon Bolivar, Torre Sur 5o, Caracas, DF 1010, Venezuela. Ed. Manuel Boet. Circ: 3,000.

614 FRA ISSN 0398-7620
CODEN: RESPDF
REVUE D'EPIDEMIOLOGIE ET DE SANTE PUBLIQUE. Text in French; Summaries in English. 1953. 6/yr. FRF 1,249; FRF 1,487 foreign (effective 2000). bk.rev. illus. index. reprint service avail. from ISI. *Refereed.* **Document type:** *Academic/Scholarly.* **Description:** Publishes work on contagious diseases, together with research on cardiovascular disease, cancer, suicide, and other topics that affect public health.
Former titles (until 1976): Revue d'Epidemiologie, Medecine Sociale et Sante Publique (0035-2438); Revue d'Hygiene et de Medecine Sociale
Related titles: Microform ed.: (from PQC); Online - full text ed.: (from Institute for Scientific Information, RoweCom Information Quest).
Indexed: ASCA, Abstr.Hyg., Anim.Breed.Abstr., Aqua.Sci.& Fish.Abstr., Bibl.Dev.Med.& Child Neur., Biol.Abstr., C.I.S. Abstr., Curr.Adv.Ecol.Sci., Curr.Cont., Dairy Sci.Abstr., Environ.Sci.Poll.Mgmt., Excerp.Med., Helminthol.Abstr., INIS Atomind., Ind.Med. (1976-), Ind.Vet., Inpharma, Int.Nurs.Ind., Med.Care Rev., Microbiol.Abstr., Nutr.Abstr., Pharm.&Out.News, Pollut.Abstr., Protozool.Abstr., Reac., Rev.Appl.Entomol., Risk Abstr., Rural Devel.Abstr., SSCI (coverage dropped), Saf.Sci.Abstr., Trop.Dis.Bull., Vet.Bull.
—BLDSC (7900.109000), CISTI, EMDOCS, GNLM, IDS, Infotrieve, KNAW. **CCC.**
Published by: Masson - Periodiques, 120 bd. St. Germain, Paris 75006, France. TEL 33-1-40466200, FAX 33-1-40466201. Ed. Ducimetiere. Circ: 1,300. **Subscr. to:** Societe de Periodiques Specialises, BP 22, Vineuil Cedex 41354, France. TEL 33-2-54504612, FAX 33-2-54504611.

REVUE MEDICALE RWANDAISE. see *MEDICAL SCIENCES*

614 USA ISSN 1073-8673
K22
RISK: HEALTH, SAFETY & ENVIRONMENT. Text in English. 1990. q. USD 35 to individuals; USD 60 to institutions; USD 70 foreign to institutions. adv. bk.rev. reprint service avail. from WSH. *Refereed.* **Document type:** *Academic/Scholarly.* **Description:** Explores public and private efforts to manage science and technology for net reduction in the probability, severity and aversive quality of health, safety and environmental impacts.
Formerly (until Jan. 1994): Risk, Issues in Health and Safety (1047-0484)
Related titles: Diskette ed.; Online - full text ed.: (from West Group, H. W. Wilson, Gale Group).
Indexed: Aqua.Sci.& Fish.Abstr., Energy Abstr., Environ.Abstr., Environ.Per.Bibl. (1990-), Environ.Sci.Poll.Mgmt., L.R.I. (Jan.1990-Sep.1993, Jan.1994-), Leg.Per. (Jul.1992-Sep.1993), P.A.I.S., Pollut.Abstr., Risk Abstr., Saf.Sci.Abstr.
—BLDSC (7972.576000), CIS, ingenta.
Published by: Franklin Pierce Law Center, 2 White St, Concord, NH 03301. TEL 603-228-1541, FAX 603-224-3342, risk@fplc.edu; cruh@fplc.edu, http://www.flpc.edu/tfield/PRORISK.htm. Ed., R&P Thomas G Field Jr. Adv. contact Carol Ruh. Circ: 315 (paid). **Co-sponsor:** Risk Assessment and Policy Association.

614.8 ITA ISSN 0035-6891
RIVISTA ITALIANA DI PREVIDENZA SOCIALE. Text in Italian. 1948. bi-m.
Address: Via Nicola Marchese, 20, Rome, RM 00141, Italy. Ed. U Chiapelli.

ROUTE. see *TRANSPORTATION—Automobiles*

614.8 GBR ISSN 0968-7726
THE ROYAL LIFE SAVING SOCIETY U.K. LIFEGUARD. Text in English. 1965. q. membership. adv. bk.rev. **Document type:** *Trade.* **Description:** Provides up-to-date news, information and advise to those interested in life saving, lifeguarding and life support.
Former titles: Royal Life Saving Society U.K. Lifesaver U.K.; Royal Life Saving Society - U.K. Quarterly Journal (0048-8704)
Indexed: Sportsearch.
Published by: Royal Life Saving Society UK, River House, High St, Broom, Alcester, Warks B50 4HN, United Kingdom. TEL 44-1789-773994, FAX 44-1789-773995, lifesavers@rlss.org.uk. Ed. Lynn Patey. R&P, Adv. contact Sandra Caldwell. Circ: 15,000.

ROYAL SOCIETY FOR THE PROMOTION OF HEALTH. JOURNAL. see *SOCIAL SERVICES AND WELFARE*

614 RWA
RWANDA. MINISTERE DE LA SANTE PUBLIQUE. RAPPORT ANNUEL. Text in French. a.
Published by: Ministere de la Sante Publique, BP 84, Kigali, Rwanda. Circ: 200.

S A H O NEWS. see *HEALTH FACILITIES AND ADMINISTRATION*

614 CAN ISSN 1195-907X
S.A.R. NEWS. Text in English. 1988. q. CND 16. back issues avail. **Description:** Contains land search, rescue articles with sharing information.
Published by: Search and Rescue Society of British Columbia, P O Box 187, Victoria, BC V8W 2M6, Canada. TEL 604-384-6696, FAX 604-383-6849. Ed. Mike Doyle. Adv. contact Dave Houseman. B&W page USD 815, color page USD 1,223. Circ: 3,500.

S B Z - SANITAER, HEIZUNGS- UND KLIMATECHNIK. see *HEATING, PLUMBING AND REFRIGERATION*

614 AUT
S - GESUENDER LEBEN. Text in German. 6/yr. **Document type:** *Consumer.*
Formerly: S Kontakt
Published by: S P V Printmedien GmbH, Talgasse 15, Markt Piesting, N 2753, Austria. TEL 43-1-71170271, FAX 43-1-71170310. Ed. Ingeborg Plaschka. Circ: 80,000.

614 SWE ISSN 0346-8445
S P R I INFORMERAR. Text in Swedish. 1968. 10/yr. free per issue. **Document type:** *Bulletin.*
Published by: Haelso och Sjukvaardens Utvecklingsinstitut/Swedish Institute for Health Services Development, Fack 70487, Stockholm 10726, Sweden. TEL 08-702-4600, FAX 08-702-4799.

614 SWE ISSN 0586-1691
S P R I RAPPORT. Text in Swedish. 1968. irreg. price varies. **Document type:** *Monographic series.*
Indexed: Abstr.Health Care Manage.Stud., Russ.Acad.Sci.Bibl.
Published by: Haelso och Sjukvaardens Utvecklingsinstitut/Swedish Institute for Health Services Development, Fack 70487, Stockholm 10726, Sweden. TEL 08-702-4600, FAX 08-702-4799.

362.1 613.62 614.85 NZL ISSN 0113-9533
SAFEGUARD (AUCKLAND); the magazine for better safety and health at the workplace. Text in English. 1992. bi-m. NZD 59 (effective 2001). adv. bk.rev., video rev. illus, stat, tr.lit. 74 p./no. back issues avail. **Document type:** *Magazine, Trade.* **Description:** Presents articles on working environments and safety issues.
Related titles: ♦ Supplement: Safeguard - Buyers Guide. ISSN 1172-9872.
Indexed: Ind.N.Z.Per.
Published by: Safeguard Publications Ltd., P.O. Box 34-355, Birkenhead, Auckland, New Zealand. TEL 64-9-418-2502, FAX 64-9-418-2089, cwshop@nznet.gen.nz, http://www.safeguard.co.nz. Ed. Peter Bateman TEL editor@safeguard.co.nz. Pub. Terry Barnett. Adv. contact Angela M J Kilikolly. B&W page NZD 1,370, color page NZD 1,920. Circ: 7,000 (paid).

362.1 613.62 614.85 NZL ISSN 1172-9872
SAFEGUARD - BUYERS GUIDE. Text in English. 1994. a. adv. 128 p./no. back issues avail. **Document type:** *Directory, Trade.* **Description:** Covers health, safety products and services directory.
Related titles: Online - full content ed.; ♦ Supplement to: Safeguard (Auckland). ISSN 0113-9533.
Published by: Safeguard Publications Ltd., P.O. Box 34-355, Birkenhead, Auckland, New Zealand. TEL 64-9-418-2502, FAX 64-9-418-2089, cwshop@nznet.gen.nz, http://www.safeguard.co.nz. Ed. Peter Bateman TEL editor@safeguard.co.nz. Adv. contact Angela M J Kilikolly.

SAFETY AND HEALTH; the international safety, health and environmental magazine. see *OCCUPATIONAL HEALTH AND SAFETY*

P

614.8 GBR ISSN 0958-479X CODEN: SAFPDZ
THE SAFETY & HEALTH PRACTITIONER. Text in English. m. GBP 59 (effective 2000). bk.rev. *Refereed.* **Document type:** *Magazine, Trade.*
Formerly: Safety Practitioner (0265-4792); Which superseded: Safety Surveyor and Protection
Related titles: Microform ed.: (from PQC); Online - full text ed.: (from ProQuest Information & Learning).
Indexed: ABI Inform. (Jan.1993-), AESIS, Art.Hosp.& Tour., Br.Ceram.Abstr., C.I.S. Abstr., CSNB, Eng.Ind., Ergon.Abstr., INIS Atomind., Ind.Vet., Lab.Haz.Bull., Mgmt.& Market.Abstr., Ref.Zh., World Surf.Coat.
—BLDSC (8065.716000), CISTI, GNLM.
Published by: C M P Information (Subsidiary of: United Business Media), 17-21 Shenley Rd, Borehamwood, Herts WD6 1RT, United Kingdom. TEL 44-20-8207-5599, FAX 44-20-8207-2598, shpeditor@cmpinformation.com, http://www.safetymags.com/, http://www.cmpinformation.com. Ed. J Balian. R&P A Edwards. Adv. contact D Bishop. Circ: 27,155.

614 GBR
SAFETY AND RESCUE. Text in English. 1959. m. GBP 1, USD 7. adv. bk.rev.
Indexed: C.I.S. Abstr.
Published by: British Safety Council, 70 Chancellors Rd, London W6 9RS, United Kingdom. TEL 44-20-8741-1231, FAX 44-20-8741-4555, 1bsc1@mail.britishsafetycouncil.co.uk, mail@britsafe.org, http://www.britishsafetycouncil.co.uk, http://www.britsafe.org/. Circ: 75,000.

SAFETY BRIEF. see *ENGINEERING—Mechanical Engineering*

614.8 350.78 USA ISSN 0036-245X
SAFETY BRIEFS. Text in English. 1938. 4/yr. free per issue. bk.rev. charts, stat.
Published by: New Jersey State Safety Council, 6 Commerce Dr, Cranford, NJ 07016-3597. TEL 201-272-7712, FAX 201-276-6622. Ed. Carolann Dillon. Circ: 19,000.

614.862 CAN ISSN 0048-8968
SAFETY CANADA. Text in English. 1957. q. free per issue. bk.rev. **Document type:** *Newsletter, Consumer.*
Formerly: Highway Safety News
Related titles: French ed.: Prevention au Canada.
Indexed: HRIS.
Published by: Canada Safety Council, 1020 Thomas Spratt Pl, Ottawa, ON K1G 5L5, Canada. TEL 613-739-1535, FAX 613-739-1566, csc@safety-council.org, http://www.safety-council.org. Ed. Ethel Archard. Circ: 400 (controlled).

614 GBR ISSN 0459-2034
SAFETY EDUCATION. Text in English. 1966. 3/yr. GBP 10.29 to non-members; GBP 8.75 to members (effective 2000). adv. bk.rev. **Document type:** *Academic/Scholarly.* **Description:** News items, reviews, informational articles, case studies, and technical advice on instruction to children and young adults in the adoption of safety practices.
Indexed: Br.Educ.Ind.
—BLDSC (8065.750000).
Published by: Royal Society for the Prevention of Accidents, Edgbaston Park, 353 Bristol Rd, Edgbaston, Birmingham, Worcs B5 7ST, United Kingdom. TEL 44-121-248-2000, FAX 44-121-248-2001, help@rospa.com.uk, http://www.rospa.com.uk. Ed. Carole Wale. Circ: 5,000.

SAFETY FOCUS NEWSLETTER. see *OCCUPATIONAL HEALTH AND SAFETY*

SAFETY MEETING REPROS. see *OCCUPATIONAL HEALTH AND SAFETY*

SAFETY SCIENCE. see *OCCUPATIONAL HEALTH AND SAFETY*

363.1 AUS ISSN 1443-8844
SAFETY SCIENCE MONITOR. Text in English. 1997. irreg. back issues avail. *Refereed.* **Document type:** *Journal, Academic/Scholarly.* **Description:** Provides a forum for debate, reviews and communications between academics and professionals in the fields of safety.
Media: Online - full text.
Published by: I P S O Australia, PO Box 516, Mt Eliza, VIC 3930, Australia. http://www.ipso.asn.au/index.htm. Ed. Tore J Larsson.

628 JPN
SAITAMA-KEN EISEI TOKEI NENPO/ANNUAL REPORT OF PUBLIC HEALTH, SAITAMA PREFECTURE. Text in Japanese. 1950. a. free per issue.
Published by: Saitama-ken, Eisei-bu/Saitama Prefecture, Bureau of Public Health, 15-1 Takasago 3-chome, Urawa-shi, Saitama-ken 336-0000, Japan.

614 MEX ISSN 0036-3634
SALUD PUBLICA DE MEXICO/PUBLIC HEALTH OF MEXICO. Text in Spanish; Summaries in English, Spanish. 1959. bi-m. MXP 180 domestic; USD 55 in Latin America; USD 77 elsewhere; MXP 150 domestic to students; MXP 40 newsstand/cover domestic; USD 12 newsstand/cover in Latin America; USD 15 newsstand/cover elsewhere (effective 2000). adv. bk.rev. bibl. reprints avail. *Refereed.* **Document type:** *Journal, Academic/Scholarly.* **Description:** Publishes results of public health research.
Incorporates (in 1977): Investigacion en Salud Publica
Related titles: CD-ROM ed.; Online - full text ed.: Salud Publica de Mexico Online. ISSN 1606-7916 (from DIMDI, Data-Star, The Dialog Corporation, SciELO, Institute for Scientific Information).
Indexed: ASCA, Abstr.Hyg. (1992-), Artemisa, Biol.Abstr., C.I.S. Abstr., Curr.Cont. (1993-), Dairy Sci.Abstr., Excerp.Med., Helminthol.Abstr., Ind.Med. (1959-), Int.Nurs.Ind., Nutr.Abstr., P.A.I.S., Protozool.Abstr., Rev.Appl.Entomol., Rev.Arom.& Med.Plants, Rev.Med.& Vet.Mycol., Rural Devel.Abstr., Rural Recreat.Tour.Abstr., SSCI (1993-), Trop.Dis.Bull., World Ag.Econ.& Rur.Soc.Abstr.
—BLDSC (8071.800000), CISTI, GNLM, IDS.
Published by: Instituto Nacional de Salud Publica, Secretaria de Salud, Av. Universidad, 665, Planta Baja, Col. Santa Maria Ahuacatitlad, Cuernavaca, MORELOS 62508, Mexico. TEL 91-73-175745 ext 2281, 91-73-110111 ext 3055, FAX 91-73-175745, eoropeza@insp3.insp.mx, http://www.insp.mx/salud. Ed., Pub., R&P Carlos Oropeza-Abundez. Adv. contact Monica Fuentes-Ramirez. Circ: 4,000.

614 362.1 COL ISSN 0120-5552
SALUD UNINORTE. Text in Spanish. 1986. s-a. **Document type:** *Journal, Academic/Scholarly.* **Description:** Discusses topics and research in all areas of public health and epidemiology.
Published by: Universidad del Norte, Division de Ciencias de la Salud, Comite Editorial, Barranquilla, Colombia. http://www.uninorte.edu.co/publicacion/salud/ppal.htm, http://www.uninorte.edu.co/division/salud. Ed. Carlo Vinicio Caballero.

614.8 ROM ISSN 1222-7633
SANATATEA. Text in Romanian. 1952. m.
Published by: Societatea Nationala de Cruce Rosie a Romania, Str. Biserica Amzei 29, Bucharest, Romania. Ed. Gheorghe M George. Circ: 140,000.

628 ITA ISSN 0393-4101
SANITA PUBBLICA; rivista mensile amministrativa per gli operatori della sanita. Text in Italian. 1981. m. (10/yr.). ITL 148,000 to individuals; ITL 245,000 to institutions. adv. **Description:** Provides information on public health for both doctors and health administrators.
Published by: Maggioli Editore, Casella Postale 290, Viale Vespucci, 12-n, Rimini, FO 47037, Italy. TEL 39-541-625777, FAX 39-0541-622020. Ed. Fabio Roversi Monaco. adv.: B&W page ITL 1,450,000, color page ITL 2,300,000; trim 195 x 115.

SANITAER UND HEIZUNGS REPORT. see *HEATING, PLUMBING AND REFRIGERATION*

628 USA ISSN 0036-4436
HD9999.S383
SANITARY MAINTENANCE; the journal of the sanitary supply industry. Text in English. 1943. m. USD 55 (effective 2000). adv. illus, tr.lit. index. reprint service avail. from PQC. **Document type:** *Trade.* **Description:** Serves the needs of distribution executives in the sanitary supply industry by covering market trends, product news, application methods, and management.
Related titles: Microfilm ed.: (from PQC); Online - full text ed.: (from Northern Light Technology, Inc., ProQuest Information & Learning).
—Linda Hall.
Published by: Trade Press Publishing Corp., 2100 W Florist Ave, PO Box 694, Milwaukee, WI 53209. TEL 414-228-7701, FAX 414-228-1134. Ed. Matt Schlag Mendenhall. Pub., Adv. contact Rob Geissler. R&P Tim Rowe TEL 414-228-7701 ext 515. Circ: 16,000.

614 DZA
SANTE. Text in French. 1956. bi-m.
Indexed: Pt.de Rep.
Published by: Federation Nationale de la Sante, Maison du Peuple, Place du 1 Mai, Algiers, Algeria.

362.1 CAN ISSN 1203-3669
SANTE ET SERVICES SOCIAUX AU QUEBEC. Text in English. biennial. CND 52.95 (effective 2000). **Document type:** *Directory.* **Description:** Contains listings of hospitals, health center, health associations, pharmaceutical companies, unions, research centers and pharmaceutical centers in Quebec.
Published by: Quebec dans le Monde, C P 8503, Sainte Foy, PQ G1V 4N5, Canada. TEL 418-659-5540, FAX 418-659-4143.

614 FRA ISSN 0995-3914 CODEN: SPBQA
SANTE PUBLIQUE. Text in French. 1978. bi-m. FRF 390 to members; FRF 490 to non-members. adv. bk.rev. **Document type:** *Academic/Scholarly.*
Formed by the 1988 merger of: Revue Francaise de la Sante Publique (0182-8819); Ecole Nationale de la Sante Publique. Cahiers (0984-9289)
Indexed: Excerp.Med. (1993-), Ind.Med. (1988-), Int.Nurs.Ind.
—BLDSC (8075.350100), CISTI, EMDOCS, GNLM.
Published by: Societe Francaise de Sante Publique, 2, av. du Doyen J. Parisot, B.P. 7, Vandoeuvre-les-Nancy Cedex 54501, France. TEL 33-3-83448747, FAX 33-3-83443776, sfsp@cmp.u-nancy.fr. Ed. Denis Zmirou. R&P Daniel Oberle. Adv. contact Therese Doucet.

610 BRA ISSN 0104-1290
SAUDE E SOCIEDADE. Text in Portuguese. 1991. s-a. USD 20 or exchange basis (effective 2000). **Document type:** *Academic/Scholarly.* **Description:** Provides articles and notes on public health.
Published by: Universidade de Sao Paulo, Faculdade de Saude Publica, Av. Dr. Arnaldo 715, Sao Paulo, SP 01246-904, Brazil. TEL 55-11-853-5411, saudesoc@edu.usp.br, bibfsp@org.usp.br. Eds. Augusta Thereza de Alvarenga, Jose da Rocha Carvalheiro.
Co-sponsor: Associacao Paulista de Saude Publica.

600 FRA ISSN 0294-0337 CODEN: SSSAEC
SCIENCES SOCIALES ET SANTE. Text in French. q. FRF 550 domestic to individuals; EUR 93 in Europe to individuals; FRF 640 elsewhere to individuals; FRF 980 domestic to institutions; EUR 159 in Europe to institutions; FRF 1,070 elsewhere to institutions; FRF 350 domestic to students; EUR 63 in Europe to students; FRF 450 elsewhere to students; FRF 220 newsstand/cover (effective 2001). *Refereed.* **Document type:** *Academic/Scholarly.* **Description:** Serves as an information exchange between all health care fields.
Related titles: Online - full text ed.: (from Institute for Scientific Information).
Indexed: ASCA, Curr.Cont., Lang.& Lang.Behav.Abstr., P.A.I.S., SOPODA, SSCI, Soc.Serv.Abstr., Sociol.Abstr.
—GNLM, IDS.
Published by: John Libbey Eurotext, 127 av. de la Republique, Montrouge 92120, France. TEL 33-01-46730660, FAX 33-01-40840999, marketing@jle.com, http://www.john-libbey-eurotext.fr/. Ed. Doris Bonnet. **Subscr. to:** A T E I, 3 av. Pierre Kerautret, Romainville 92230, France. TEL 33-1-48408686, FAX 33-1-48400731, atei@club-internet.fr.

353.6 USA
▼ **SCIPOLICY**; the journal of science & health policy. Text in English. 2000. s-a. USD 20; USD 25 to qualified personnel; USD 10 newsstand/cover; USD 15 newsstand/cover to qualified personnel (effective 2000). back issues avail. *Refereed.* **Document type:** *Academic/Scholarly.*
Related titles: Online - full text ed.
—CCC.
Published by: Sacks Research, PO Box 504, Haverford, PA 19041. TEL 610-658-2332, mail@scipolicy.net, http://www.scipolicy.net. Ed., Pub. Stephen Milese Sacks.

SECURITY SPECIFIER. see *CRIMINOLOGY AND LAW ENFORCEMENT—Security*

SEGURIDAD SOCIAL. see *SOCIAL SERVICES AND WELFARE*

SEIKATSU TO KANKYO/LIFE AND ENVIRONMENT. see *ENVIRONMENTAL STUDIES*

P

614 JPN ISSN 0916-7226
CODEN: SEKEEM
SENDAI-SHI EISEI KENKYUJOHO/SENDAI MUNICIPAL INSTITUTE OF PUBLIC HEALTH. Text in Japanese. 1966. a. **Document type:** *Academic/Scholarly.*
Formerly (until 1988): Sendai-shi Eisei Shikenjoho (0387-9771)
—BLDSC (7604.578460). **CCC.**
Published by: Sendai Municipal Institute of Public Health/Sendai-shi Eisei Kenkyujo, 2-5-10 Oroshimachi-Higashi, Wakabayashi-ku, Sendai-shi, Miyagi-ken 984-0002, Japan. TEL 81-22-236-7722, FAX 81-22-236-8601.

362.1 USA
SENIOR CARE MANAGEMENT. Text in English. 1998. m. USD 289; USD 299 in Canada & Mexico; USD 309 elsewhere. **Document type:** *Trade.*
Published by: National Health Information, LLC, PO Box 15429, Atlanta, GA 30333. TEL 404-607-9500. Eds. Dorothy Brooks, Kim McCormick. Pub. Terry Redman.

SEXUAL HEALTH EXCHANGE. see *MEDICAL SCIENCES—Communicable Diseases*

614.4 USA
SHEDDING LIGHT ON LEGISLATION. Text in English. irreg. **Document type:** *Newsletter.*
Published by: National Health Federation, 212 W Foothill Blvd, Monrovia, CA 91016. TEL 626-357-2181, FAX 626-303-0642. R&P Patrick von Mauck.

613 ALB
SHENDETI✱ . Text in Albanian. bi-m. USD 6.16.
Published by: Ministere de la Sante Publique, Tirana, Albania.

SICHERHEIT ZUERST. see *TRANSPORTATION—Railroads*

614.8 HRV ISSN 0350-6886
SIGURNOST/SAFETY. Text in Croatian; Abstracts and contents page in English. 1959. 4/yr. USD 100 (effective 2001). adv. bk.rev. charts, illus. index, cum.index. *Refereed.* **Document type:** *Journal.* **Description:** Covers safety issues in the work organization and living environment.
Formerly (until 1972): Sigurnost u Pogonu (0037-508X)
Indexed: C.I.S. Abstr., Environ.Sci.Poll.Mgmt., Fluidex, Pollut.Abstr., Saf.Sci.Abstr., Sel.Water Res.Abstr., Water Resour.Abstr., World Text.Abstr.
—BLDSC (8276.480000).
Published by: Zavod za Istrazivanje i Razvoj Sigurnosti/Institute of Safety Research and Development, Ul Grada Vukovara 68, Zagreb 10000, Croatia. TEL 385-1-6111334, FAX 385-1-6119812, zirs@zg.tel.hr, http://www.mzt.hr. Ed. Kresimir Telebec. Adv. contact Ljubica Dunaj Mutak. Circ: 1,000; 1,000 (paid). **Co-sponsor:** Ministarstvo Znanosti i Tehnologije Republike Hrvatske.

SINNETS HELSE. see *PSYCHOLOGY*

SOCIAL WORK IN HEALTH CARE; the journal of health care work. see *SOCIAL SERVICES AND WELFARE*

SOCIAL WORK LEADER. see *SOCIAL SERVICES AND WELFARE*

614 GBR ISSN 0037-8119
SOCIALISM AND HEALTH. Text in English. 1960. bi-m. GBP 18 to members. bk.rev. back issues avail. **Document type:** *Newsletter.*
Published by: Socialist Health Association, 16 Charles Sq, London N1 6HP, United Kingdom. TEL 44-171-490-0057. Ed., R&P John Biggs. Circ: 1,500 (paid).

613 NGA ISSN 0037-9905
SOCIETY OF HEALTH OF NIGERIA. JOURNAL✱ . Text in English. 1966. q. USD 7. adv.
Published by: Nigeria Medical Council, Plot PC 13, Victoria Island, 25 Ahmed Onidudo St, PMB 12611, Lagos, Nigeria.

SOUTHEAST ASIAN JOURNAL OF TROPICAL MEDICINE AND PUBLIC HEALTH. see *MEDICAL SCIENCES—Communicable Diseases*

614 CHE
SOZIALE MEDIZIN. Text in German. 1974. 6/yr. CHF 65; CHF 70 foreign (effective 1996). adv. bk.rev. **Document type:** *Bulletin.*
Published by: Schweizerische Gesellschaft fuer ein Soziales Gesundheitswesen, Postfach, Basel 4007, Switzerland. TEL 41-61-6911332. Ed. Ruedi Spoendlin. Adv. contact Fritz Wilechi. Circ: 2,500.

SOZIALGESETZBUCH: PFLEGEVERSICHERUNG. see *LAW—Civil Law*

363.1 USA
SPEAKING OF SAFETY. Text in English. 3/yr. USD 20 domestic; USD 25 in Canada & Mexico; USD 30 foreign (effective 2000). **Document type:** *Newsletter.*
Published by: Laboratory Safety Institute, 192 Worcester Rd, Natick, MA 01760. TEL 508-647-1900, FAX 508-647-0062, labsafe@aol.com, http://www.labsafety.org. Ed. Patricia Hamn. Circ: 2,000 (paid).

614 USA
STATE HEALTH NOTES. Text in English. 1979. bi-w. USD 277 to private sector; USD 197 to government, non-profit & universities (effective 2000). charts, stat. back issues avail. **Document type:** *Newsletter.* **Description:** Identifies and analyzes important health-related trends and innovations within state government.
Published by: Forum For State Health Policy Leadership, 444 N Capitol St, N W, Ste 515, Washington, DC 20001. TEL 202-624-3574, FAX 202-737-1069, ihpp@ncsl.org, http://www.ncsl.org/ihpp. Ed., R&P Linda Demkovich. Circ: 2,000.

614 SWE ISSN 0085-6738
STATUS. Text in Swedish. 1938. 8/yr. SEK 75 (effective 1999). adv. bk.rev.
Published by: Riksfoerbundet foer Hjaert- och Lungsjuka/Swedish Heart and Lung Association, Fack 9090, Stockholm 10272, Sweden. TEL 46-8-556-06-200, FAX 46-8-668-23-85. Circ: 32,000.

354.489 DNK ISSN 0905-0035
RA257
STATUS OG VISIONER - SUNDHEDSSTYRELSEN. Text in Danish. 1978. a. free per issue.
Formerly (until 1988): Sundhedsstyrelsen. Aarsberetning (0105-5151)
Published by: Sundhedsstyrelsen, Amaliegade 13, PO Box 2020, Copenhagen K 1012, Denmark.

614.85 GBR ISSN 1354-2249
STAYING ALIVE; staying alive with water & leisure. Text in English. 1968. q. GBP 17.65 to non-members (effective 2000); GBP 15 to members; GBP 20.74 foreign to members (effective 1999). bk.rev. charts, illus, stat. **Document type:** *Bulletin, Consumer.* **Description:** Discusses issues relating to safety in and around the home.
Former titles (until 1994): Care in the Home (0300-5909); Home Safety Journal (0018-4136)
Indexed: ASSIA.
—BLDSC (8459.501500).
Published by: Royal Society for the Prevention of Accidents, Edgbaston Park, 353 Bristol Rd, Edgbaston, Birmingham, Worcs B5 7ST, United Kingdom. TEL 44-121-248-2000, FAX 44-121-248-2001, help@rospa.com.uk, http://www.rospa.com.uk. Ed., Pub., R&P Janice Cave. Circ: 2,000 (paid).

614.48 AUS ISSN 0725-7066
STERILIZATION IN AUSTRALIA. Text in English. 1981. q. AUD 45 (effective 1998 & 1999). adv. back issues avail. **Document type:** *Trade.* **Description:** Covers infection control, cleaning, disinfection, sterilization, new technologies in sterilization.
—ingenta.
Published by: Sterilizing Research and Advisory Council of Australia (N.S.W.) Inc., GPO Box 4834, Sydney, NSW 2001, Australia. TEL 61-2-8453835. Ed., Adv. contact Rosslyn Fowler. B&W page AUD 300. Circ: 500.

363.7 NOR ISSN 0804-4910
STRAALEVERNRAPPORT/N R P A REPORT. Variant title: Norwegian Radiation Protection Authority Report. Text in Multiple languages. 1979. irreg. NOK 100 per issue (effective 2001). **Document type:** *Monographic series, Government.*
Former titles (until 1994): Statens Straalevern. Rapport (0804-2098); (until 1993): S I S Rapport (0800-4137)
Related titles: Online - full text ed.
Indexed: Aqua.Sci.& Fish.Abstr.
—BLDSC (8470.450000).
Published by: Statens Straalevern/Norwegian Radiation Protection Authority, Postboks 55, Oesteraas 1332, Norway. TEL 47-67-16-25-00, FAX 47-67-14-74-07, http://www.nrpa.no.

STRAHLENTELEX MIT ELEKTROSMOG-REPORT; unabhaengiger Informationsdienst zu Radioaktivitaet, Strahlung und Gesundheit. see *ENVIRONMENTAL STUDIES—Toxicology And Environmental Safety*

STUDIES ON CURRENT HEALTH PROBLEMS. see *MEDICAL SCIENCES*

STUDIES ON EMERGENCIES AND DISASTER RELIEF. see *CIVIL DEFENSE*

614 IND ISSN 0586-1179
SWASTH HIND. Text in English. 1957. m. INR 6, USD 5. adv. bk.rev. charts, illus, stat. index.
Published by: Ministry of Health and Family Welfare, Central Health Education Bureau, Kotla Rd., New Delhi 110 002, India. TEL 3315032. Ed. M L Mehta. Circ: 8,500.

SWIMMING POOLS TODAY. see *SPORTS AND GAMES—Outdoor Life*

614.8 USA
SYSTEM SAFETY SOCIETY. DIRECTORY OF CONSULTANTS✱ . Text in English. a. USD 50; to non-members; members $10. **Document type:** *Directory.* **Description:** Lists consultants in system and product safety.
Published by: System Safety Society, Inc., 30363 Hicks Rd, Spotsylvania, VA 22553-5525. TEL 703-444-6520. Circ: 1,100.

T B MONITOR. (Tuberculosis) see *MEDICAL SCIENCES—Respiratory Diseases*

T B SOURCEBOOK. (Tuberculosis) see *MEDICAL SCIENCES—Respiratory Diseases*

614 USA
TAKING SIDES: CLASHING VIEWS ON CONTROVERSIAL ISSUES IN HEALTH AND SOCIETY. Text in English. 1993. irreg., latest vol.3, 1997. USD 13. illus. **Document type:** *Academic/Scholarly.*
Published by: Dushkin - McGraw-Hill, Sluice Dock, Guilford, CT 06437-9989. TEL 203-453-4351, FAX 203-453-4351. Ed. Eileen Daniel. Pub. David Dean. R&P Cheryl Greenleaf.

363.72 USA ISSN 0883-8828
TECHLETTER; for pest control technicians. Text in English. 1985. bi-w., latest vol.17. USD 49 domestic; USD 57 in Canada & Mexico; USD 70 elsewhere (effective 2001). bk.rev. illus, tr.lit. annual index. 4 p./no. back issues avail. **Document type:** *Newsletter, Trade.* **Description:** Training information for exterminators.
Published by: Pinto & Associates, Inc., 29839 Oak Rd, Mechanicsville, MD 20659. TEL 301-884-3020, FAX 301-884-4068. Ed., R&P Sandra Kraft. Pub. Lawrence J Pinto. Circ: 1,000 (paid).

614 ITA ISSN 0392-8144
TECNICA SANITARIA E MEDICINA DI COMUNITA. Text in Italian. 1963. bi-m. ITL 60,000, USD 45. adv. bk.rev. abstr, bibl, charts, illus, stat. index.
Formerly (until 1976): Tecnica Sanitaria (0040-1897)
Indexed: Food Sci.& Tech.Abstr.
Published by: (Associazione Nazionale Ufficiali Sanitari Medici Igienisti), Tecnisan s.r.l., Via Giardini, 818, Modena, MO 41100, Italy. TEL 39-59-343785. Ed. Ferruccio Vivoli. Circ: 1,000.

TEMAS DE POBLACION. see *POPULATION STUDIES*

614 BEL ISSN 1370-0650
TEST SANTE. Text in French. 1994. 6/yr. BEF 1,188; BEF 1,392 foreign. **Document type:** *Consumer.*
Related titles: Dutch ed.: Test Gezondheid. ISSN 1370-0847.
Published by: Association des Consommateurs/ Verbruikersunie, Rue de Hollande 13, Brussels 1060, Belgium. TEL 32-2-5423211, FAX 32-2-5423250.

614 USA
TEXAS. DEPARTMENT OF HEALTH. ANNUAL REPORT. Text in English. 1987. irreg., latest 1995. free per issue. **Document type:** *Government.*
Formerly: Texas. Department of Health Resources. Biennial Report (0163-1667)
Published by: Department of Health, 1100 W 49th St, Austin, TX 78756. TEL 512-458-7761, FAX 512-458-7476, http://www.tdh.state.tx.us.

TEXAS WATER UTILITIES JOURNAL. see *WATER RESOURCES*

344 NLD ISSN 0165-0874
CODEN: TGEZD
TIJDSCHRIFT VOOR GEZONDHEIDSRECHT. Text in Dutch. 1977. bi-m.
Indexed: ELLIS, Excerp.Med. (until 1992).
—KNAW.
Published by: Samsom H.D. Tjeenk Willink B.V. (Subsidiary of: Wolters Kluwer N.V.), Postbus 316, Alphen aan den Rijn 2400 AH, Netherlands. TEL 31-1720-66822, FAX 31-1720-66639. Circ: 1,200 (paid).

TIJDSCHRIFT VOOR SOCIALE GEZONDHEIDSZORG; gezondheid & samenleving. see *MEDICAL SCIENCES*

TOKYO TORITSU EISEI KENKYUJO KENKYU NENPO/TOKYO METROPOLITAN RESEARCH LABORATORY OF PUBLIC HEALTH. ANNUAL REPORT. see *MEDICAL SCIENCES*

614 TON ISSN 0082-4895
TONGA. MINISTER OF HEALTH. REPORT. Text in English. 1951. a. USD 25.
Published by: Government Printer, Nuku'alofa, Tonga. Circ: 660.

TOXIC EXPOSURE ADVISORY NEWSLETTER. see *ENVIRONMENTAL STUDIES—Toxicology And Environmental Safety*

604.7 USA
TOXIC TORTS; litigation of hazardous substance cases. Text in English. 1984. irreg., latest 2nd. USD 190. **Document type:** *Trade.* **Description:** Covers the specific hows, whys and wherefores for successfully handling chemical and hazardous waste litigation.
Published by: Shepard's (Subsidiary of: Reed Elsevier plc), 555 Middle Creek Pkwy, Colorado Springs, CO 80921. TEL 800-743-7393, customer_service@shepards.com, http://www.shepards.com. Ed. G Z Nothstein.

TOYAMA-KEN EISEI TOKEI NENPO/TOYAMA PREFECTURE. ANNUAL REPORT OF PUBLIC HEALTH. see *PUBLIC HEALTH AND SAFETY—Abstracting, Bibliographies, Statistics*

614.8 380.5 USA ISSN 8756-4408
TRANSPORTATION SAFETY RECOMMENDATIONS. Text in English. irreg. (approx. 12/yr.). price varies. **Document type:** *Government.* **Description:** Provides reports on the board's safety oversight and accident information prevention activities and information on important transportation problems, issues, and other activities.
Published by: (U.S. Department of Transportation, National Transportation Safety Board, Bureau of Safety Programs), U.S. National Technical Information Service, 5825 Port Royal Rd, Springfield, VA 22161. TEL 703-605-6000, 800-553-6847, FAX 703-605-6880, orders@ntis.fedworld.gov, http://www.ntis.gov.

614.8 USA
TRANSPORTATION SAFETY SPECIAL REPORTS. Text in English. irreg. (approx. 5/yr.). price varies. **Document type:** *Government.* **Description:** Includes safety studies and reports, accident investigation reports, as well as highway and railroad accident reports.
Published by: (U.S. Department of Transportation, National Transportation Safety Board, Bureau of Accident Investigation), U.S. National Technical Information Service, 5825 Port Royal Rd, Springfield, VA 22161. TEL 703-605-6000, 800-553-6847, FAX 703-650-6860, orders@ntis.fedworld.gov, http://www.ntis.gov.

353.6 610 USA ISSN 1524-8380
TRAUMA, VIOLENCE & ABUSE; a review journal. Text in English. q. USD 65 to individuals; USD 215 to institutions; USD 25 newsstand/cover to individuals; USD 45 newsstand/cover to institutions (effective 2002). **Description:** Devoted to organizing, synthesizing and expanding knowledge on all forms of trauma, violence and abuse. Didicated to professionals and advanced students in clinical training who work in all forms of trauma, violence and abuse and is intended to compile knowledge that impacts practice, policy and research.
Related titles: Online - full text ed.: (from EBSCO Publishing, O C L C Online Computer Library Center, Inc., RoweCom Information Quest, ingenta, Swets Blackwell).
Indexed: Crim.Just.Abstr., Sage Fam.Stud.Abstr., Viol.& Abuse Abstr.
—BLDSC (9026.857330).
Published by: Sage Publications, Inc., 2455 Teller Rd, Thousand Oaks, CA 91320. TEL 805-499-9821, FAX 805-499-0721, http://www.sagepub.com. Ed. Jon R Conte.

614 USA
TRENDS (WASHINGTON, 1969). Text in English. 1969. m. USD 55 domestic; USD 70 foreign (effective 2000). adv. bk.rev. **Document type:** *Newsletter.*
Formerly: Allied Health Trends
Published by: Association of Schools of Allied Health Professions, 1730 M St, N W, 500, Washington, DC 20036-4505. TEL 202-293-4848, FAX 202-293-4852, asahp2@asahp.org, http://www.asahp.org. Ed., Pub., R&P, Adv. contact Thomas W Elwood. B&W page USD 350. Circ: 800.

TRIODYNE SAFETY BULLETIN. see *OCCUPATIONAL HEALTH AND SAFETY*

616.988 GBR ISSN 1360-2276
RC960 CODEN: TMIHFL
TROPICAL MEDICINE & INTERNATIONAL HEALTH. Text in English. 1996. m., latest vol.7, 2002. GBP 58 in Europe to individuals; USD 100 in North America to individuals; GBP 63 elsewhere to individuals; GBP 440 in Europe to institutions; USD 710.50 in North America to institutions; GBP 447 elsewhere to institutions (effective 2002). adv. bk.rev. back issues avail.; reprint service avail. from SWZ. *Refereed.* **Document type:** *Academic/Scholarly.* **Description:** Covers all aspects of tropical medicine.
Formed by the merger of (1898-1996): Journal of Tropical Medicine and Hygiene (0022-5304); (1948-1996): Tropical and Geographical Medicine (0041-3232); Which incorporated (1926-1991): Acta Leidensia (0065-1362); (1985-1996): Tropical Medicine and Parasitology (0177-2392); (1972-1996): Societe Belge de Medecine Tropicale. Annales (0772-4128); Which was formerly titled (until 1972): Annales des Societes Belges de Medecine Tropicale, de Parasitologie et de Mycologie (0037-9638); (until 1971): Annales des Societes Belges de Medecine Tropicale, de Parasitologie et de Mycologie Humaine et Animale (0373-2487); (1920-1964): Societe Belge de Medecine Tropicale. Annales (0365-6527); Tropical Medicine and Parasitology was formerly titled (until 1985): Tropenmedizin und Parasitologie (0303-4208); (1950-1974): Zeitschrift fuer Tropenmedizin und Parasitologie (0044-359X)
Related titles: Microform ed.: (from PQC); Online - full text ed.: Tropical Medicine & International Health Online. ISSN 1365-3156. 1999. GBP 52.50 in Europe to individuals; USD 90 in North America to individuals; GBP 52.50 elsewhere to individuals; GBP 396 in Europe to institutions; USD 639.45 in North America to institutions; GBP 396 elsewhere to institutions (effective 2002) (from Ovid Technologies, Inc., EBSCO Publishing, O C L C Online Computer Library Center, Inc., RoweCom Information Quest, ingenta, Munksgaard & Blackwell Science's Synergy, Swets Blackwell, Institute for Scientific Information).
Indexed: ASCA, Abstr.Hyg., Abstr.Rural Dev.Trop., Agri.& Environ.Biotech.Abstr. (coverage dropped), Agroforest.Abstr., Aqua.Sci.& Fish.Abstr., Bibl.Asian Stud. (1975-1978), Biol.Abstr., Chem.Abstr., Chem.Indus.Notes, Chem.Titles, Curr.Adv.Ecol.Sci., Curr.Cont., Dairy Sci.Abstr., Dent.Ind., Derwent Biotech.Abstr., Diar.Dis.Res., Dok.Arbeitsmed., E.I., Ecol.Abstr., Environ.Sci.Poll.Mgmt., Excerp.Med., Geo.Abstr.H.G., Geo.Abstr.P.G., Helminthol.Abstr., Ind.Med. (1996-), Ind.Sci.Rev., Ind.Vet., Inpharma, Int.Abstr.Biol.Sci., Int.Nurs.Ind., Maize Abstr., Med.& Surg.Dermat., Nutr.Abstr., Pharm.&Out.News, Pig News & Info., Pollut.Abstr., Protozool.Abstr., Reac., Rev.Appl.Entomol., Rev.Arom.& Med.Plants, Rev.Med.& Vet.Mycol., Rev.Plant Path., Rural Devel.Abstr., SSCI (coverage dropped), Sci.Cit.Ind., Sel.Water Res.Abstr., So.Pac.Per.Ind., Sport Fish.Abstr., THA, Trop.Dis.Bull., Vet.Bull., Zoo.Rec.
—BLDSC (9056.402000), ADONIS, CASDDS, CISTI, EMDOCS, GNLM, IDS, ingenta, KNAW. **CCC.**
Published by: Blackwell Science Ltd., Osney Mead, Oxford OX2 0EL, United Kingdom. TEL 44-1865-206206, FAX 44-1865-721205, journals.cs@blacksci.co.uk, http://www.blackwell-science.com. Ed. D Bradley. Pub. Elizabeth Whelan. R&P Sophie Savage. Adv. contact Jenny Applin. Circ: 1,890. **Co-sponsors:** Bernhard Nacht Institut, Hamburg; Foundation Tropical and Geographical Medicine, Amsterdam; Belgian Institute of Tropical Medicine, Antwerp; London School of Hygiene & Tropical Medicine.

TUBERCULOSIS & AIRBORNE DISEASE WEEKLY. see *MEDICAL SCIENCES—Communicable Diseases*

U C S F MAGAZINE. see *MEDICAL SCIENCES*

U.S. CENTERS FOR DISEASE CONTROL. ABORTION SURVEILLANCE. ANNUAL SUMMARY. see *BIRTH CONTROL*

U.S. CENTERS FOR DISEASE CONTROL. DIPHTHERIA SURVEILLANCE REPORT. see *MEDICAL SCIENCES—Communicable Diseases*

615.9 USA ISSN 0098-6623
RC143
U.S. CENTERS FOR DISEASE CONTROL. FOODBORNE & WATERBORNE DISEASE OUTBREAKS. ANNUAL SUMMARY. Key Title: Foodborne & Waterborne Disease Outbreaks. Annual Summary. Text in English. a. **Document type:** *Government.*
Formerly: U.S. Centers for Disease Control. Foodborne Outbreaks. Annual Summary.
Published by: U.S. Centers for Disease Control, 1600 Clifton Rd, Atlanta, GA 30333. TEL 404-639-3311.

U.S. CENTERS FOR DISEASE CONTROL. LEPROSY SURVEILLANCE REPORT. see *MEDICAL SCIENCES—Communicable Diseases*

U.S. CENTERS FOR DISEASE CONTROL. MALARIA SURVEILLANCE REPORT. see *MEDICAL SCIENCES—Communicable Diseases*

304.6 USA ISSN 1057-5987
RA407.A1
U.S. CENTERS FOR DISEASE CONTROL. MORBIDITY AND MORTALITY WEEKLY REPORT. RECOMMENDATIONS AND REPORT. Key Title: Morbidity and Mortality Weekly Report. Recommendations and Report. Text in English. 1989. irreg.
Indexed: Lab.Haz.Bull.
—CISTI.
Published by: U.S. Department of Health and Human Services, Centers for Disease Control (MS: A28), Epidemiology Program Office, 1600 Clifton Rd, NE, Atlanta, GA 30333. TEL 800-843-6356. **Orders to:** Supt. of Documents, Govt Printing Office, Washington, DC 20402.

P

614 USA
U.S. CENTERS FOR DISEASE CONTROL. SALMONELLA SURVEILLANCE. ANNUAL SUMMARY. Text in English. 1962. a. free per issue. charts, stat. **Document type:** *Government.*
Published by: U.S. Centers for Disease Control, Bureau of Epidemiology. Bacterial Disease Division, 1600 Clifton Rd, Atlanta, GA 30333. TEL 404-639-3311. Circ: 3,000.

355.4 USA
U.S. DEFENSE LOGISTICS AGENCY. D O D HAZARDOUS MATERIALS INFORMATION SYSTEM: HAZARDOUS ITEM LISTING* . Text in English. irreg. (base. vol. plus updates). USD 155; USD 193.75 foreign (effective 1994). **Document type:** *Government.* **Description:** Provides data elements for items included in the Department of Defense Materials Information System, primarily for Defense officials to use to comply with the regulatory controls established for hazardous materials.
Media: Microfiche.
Published by: U.S. Defense Logistics Agency, 8725 John J Kingman Rd, Ste 2533, Fort Belvoir, VA 22060-6221. TEL 703-545-6700. **Subscr. to:** U.S. Government Printing Office, Superintendent of Documents.

U.S. DEPARTMENT OF AGRICULTURE. FOOD SAFETY AND INSPECTION SERVICE. MEAT AND POULTRY INSPECTION DIRECTORY. see *FOOD AND FOOD INDUSTRIES*

U.S. HEALTH CARE FINANCING ADMINISTRATION. MEDICARE COVERAGE ISSUES MANUAL. see *INSURANCE*

U.S. HEALTH CARE FINANCING ADMINISTRATION. MEDICARE HOME HEALTH AGENCY MANUAL. see *INSURANCE*

U.S. HEALTH CARE FINANCING ADMINISTRATION. MEDICARE HOSPITAL MANUAL. see *INSURANCE*

U.S. HEALTH CARE FINANCING ADMINISTRATION. MEDICARE PROVIDER REIMBURSEMENT MANUAL. see *INSURANCE*

U.S. HEALTH CARE FINANCING ADMINISTRATION. MEDICARE SKILLED NURSING FACILITY MANUAL. see *INSURANCE*

362 USA
U.S. NATIONAL CENTER FOR HEALTH STATISTICS. VITAL AND HEALTH STATISTICS. SERIES 13. DATA ON HEALTH RESOURCES UTILIZATION. Text in English. 1966. irreg., latest vol.140. price varies. **Document type:** *Government.*
Incorporates: U.S. National Center for Health Care Statistics. Vital and Health Statistics. Series 12. Data from the Institutional Population Surveys (0083-1964); Formerly: U.S. National Center for Health Care Statistics. Vital and Health Statistics. Series 13. Data from the Hospital Discharge Survey (0083-2006)
Indexed: Excerp.Med., Ind.Med. (1966-).
Published by: U.S. National Center for Health Statistics, Data Dissemination Branch, 6525 Belcrest Rd, Hyattsville, MD 20782. TEL 301-458-4636, http://www.cdc.gov/nchs/. **Orders to:** U.S. Government Printing Office, Superintendent of Documents.

U Z MAGAZINE. (Universitaire Ziekenhuis) see *HEALTH FACILITIES AND ADMINISTRATION*

628 AUT ISSN 0049-5131
UMWELTSCHUTZ. Text in German. 1963. 10/yr. ATS 680 domestic; ATS 830 foreign (effective 2000). adv. bk.rev. illus. **Document type:** *Bulletin, Trade.*
Indexed: Biol.Abstr., Ref.Zh.
Published by: Bohmann Druck und Verlag GmbH & Co. KG, Leberstrasse 122, Vienna, W 1110, Austria. TEL 43-1-74095-0, FAX 43-1-74095-183, umweltschutz.zv@bohmann.co.at, http://www.umweltschutz.co.at. Ed. Leopold Lukschanderl. Adv. contact Josef Brodacz. B&W page ATS 42,000, color page ATS 56,000; trim 185 x 250. Circ: 14,000.

UNIT COSTS OF HEALTH & SOCIAL CARE. see *SOCIAL SERVICES AND WELFARE*

614 ARE
UNITED ARAB EMIRATES. WIZARAT AL-SIHHAH. IDARAT AL-TIBB AL-WAQA'I. AL-TAQRIR AL-SANAWI/UNITED ARAB EMIRATES. MINISTRY OF HEALTH. PREVENTIVE MEDICINE DEPARTMENT. ANNUAL REPORT. Text in Arabic, English. 1981. a. stat. **Description:** Comprehensive review of the department's activities, including communicable disease control, health education, maternal and children's health services.
Published by: Wizarat al-Sihhah, Idarat al-Tibb al-Waqa'i/Ministry of Health, Preventive Medicine Department, PO Box 344, Abu Dhabi, United Arab Emirates. TEL 333485. Circ: 1,000 (controlled).

614 USA
UNITED STATES - MEXICO BORDER HEALTH ASSOCIATION. NEWS - NOTICIAS. Text in English. 1976. q. USD 75 to individuals; USD 500 to institutions; includes all organization publications. **Description:** Reports on the activities of the association and its membership.
Published by: United States - Mexico Border Health Association, 5400 Suncrest Dr, no.C6, El Paso, TX 79912-5615. TEL 915-581-6645, FAX 915-833-4768, officer@usmbha.org, http://www.usmbha.org. Ed. Dr. Gerardo De Cosio. Circ: 800.

THE UNIVERSAL HEALTHCARE ALMANAC. see *STATISTICS*

628 GTM
UNIVERSIDAD DE SAN CARLOS. FACULTAD DE INGENIERIA. ESCUELA REGIONAL DE INGENIERIA SANITARIA. CARTA PERIODICA. Text in Spanish. 1966. irreg. bibl, charts, illus.
Formerly: Brujula
Published by: Universidad de San Carlos de Guatemala, Escuela Regional de Ingenieria Sanitaria, Ciudad Universitaria, zona 12, Edificio de Rectoria, Of 307, Guatemala City, Guatemala. Ed. Arturo Acajabon Mendoza.

UNIVERSIDAD INDUSTRIAL DE SANTANDER. REVISTA - SALUD. see *MEDICAL SCIENCES*

363.119378 GBR ISSN 1361-4266
UNIVERSITIES SAFETY ASSOCIATION. DIGEST. Text in English. s-a. **Document type:** *Bulletin.*
Formerly (until 1995): Universities Safety Association. Safety Digest (0951-3299)
Published by: Universities Safety Association, Kingston University, Millennium House, 21 Eden St, Kingston Upon Thames, Surrey KT1 1BL, United Kingdom. Ed. Martin Larmour.

UNIVERSITY OF OCCUPATIONAL AND ENVIRONMENTAL HEALTH. JOURNAL. see *OCCUPATIONAL HEALTH AND SAFETY*

UNSCHEDULED EVENTS; research committee on disasters newsletter. see *SOCIOLOGY*

393.1 AUT ISSN 0042-0581
UNTERNEHMER; Magazin fuer Fuehrungskraefte der Wirtschaftskammern. Text in German. 1960. m. adv. **Document type:** *Trade.*
Published by: (Bundeskammer der Gewerblichen Wirtschaft), Oesterreichischer Wirtschaftsverlag GmbH, Nikolsdorfer Gasse 7-11, Vienna, W 1051, Austria. TEL 43-1-54664, FAX 43-1-54664360, office@oewv.at, http://www.oewv.at. Ed. Ernst Hofbauer. Adv. contact Hildegard Ribarich. B&W page ATS 17,400, color page ATS 35,800; trim 240 x 185. Circ: 14,333.

614 ZAF
URBAN HEALTH AND DEVELOPMENT BULLETIN. Text in English. 1989. q. free per issue. **Document type:** *Newsletter, Bulletin.* **Description:** Contains information about urbanization and related health matters of interest to community health groups and organizations involved in urban policy formulation.
Formerly (until 1998): Urbanisation and Health Newsletter
Indexed: Ind.S.A.Per.
Published by: Medical Research Council, National Urbanisation and Health Research Programme, PO Box 19070, Tygerberg 7505, South Africa. TEL 27-21-938-0417, FAX 27-21-938-0342, http://www.mrc.ac.za/urbanheal/newsletter.htm. Ed. Dr. John Seager. R&P Pam Cerff. Circ: 800.

V F D B: ZEITSCHRIFT FUER FORSCHUNG UND TECHNIK IM BRANDSCHUTZ. see *ENGINEERING—Chemical Engineering*

613 305.21 613.7 052 AUS
▼ **V O I C E**; victory over incontinence/continence education. Text in English. 1999. q. free per issue. adv. bk.rev. 16 p./no. 7 cols./p. **Document type:** *Newspaper.* **Description:** Increases awareness and knowledge of incontinence problems and treatment. For parents of bedwetters, aged persons and prostate sufferers.
Published by: (Continence Foundation of Australia), The Victorian Senior, PO Box 1899, Geelong, VIC 3220, Australia. TEL 03-5221-9051, FAX 03-5221-9052, info@contfound.org.au, http://www.contfound.org.au/voice/voice.html. adv.: B&W page AUD 2,750, color page AUD 3,500.

VACCINE WEEKLY. see *PHARMACY AND PHARMACOLOGY*

VERKEHRSPSYCHOLOGISCHER INFORMATIONSDIENST. see *TRANSPORTATION—Roads And Traffic*

614.8 USA
VETERINARY MEDICINE GUIDANCE MANUAL. Text in English. irreg. USD 80 in North America; USD 160 elsewhere. **Document type:** *Government.* **Description:** Provides the latest information on and helps maintain surveillance of compliance-oriented plans and instructions directed to F.D.A. field operations, providing the needed direction from headquarters offices and bureaus in accomplishing F.D.A. regulatory obligations.
Published by: U.S. Food and Drug Administration, Office of Public Affairs, 5600 Fishers Ln, Rockville, MD 20857. TEL 301-443-3220. **Orders to:** U.S. National Technical Information Service, 5285 Port Royal Rd, Springfield, VA 22161. TEL 703-487-4650.

614.8 USA ISSN 0199-1345
VIRGINIA'S HEALTH. Text in English. 1970. bi-m. free per issue.
Published by: Department of Health, Office of Health Education and Information, PO Box 2448, Ste 245, Richmond, VA 23218. TEL 804-786-3552, FAX 804-371-6152. Ed. Dudley Olsson. Circ: 6,000.

355 USA
VITAL SIGNS (CAMBRIDGE). Text in English. 1988. 2/yr. USD 25 domestic; USD 35 foreign (effective 2000). bk.rev., film rev. charts, illus. back issues avail. *Refereed.* **Document type:** *Newsletter.* **Description:** Unites an international federation of 80 physicians' organizations worldwide practicing global social responsibility.
Related titles: Online - full text ed.
Published by: International Physicians for the Prevention of Nuclear War, 727 Massachusetts Ave, Cambridge, MA 02139-3323. TEL 617-868-5050, FAX 617-868-2560, ippnwbos@ippnw.org, http://www.ippnw.org. Ed., R&P Lynn Martin. Circ: 30,000.

628 RUS ISSN 0321-4044
CODEN: VSTEAO
VODOSNABZHENIE I SANITARNAYA TEKHNIKA. Text in Russian. 1913. m. USD 149. bk.rev. bibl. index.
Indexed: C.I.S. Abstr., Chem.Abstr., Chem.Indus.Notes, Chem.Titles, GeoRef, Int.Build.Serv.Abstr., Pollut.Abstr., Ref.Zh.
—BLDSC (0041.000000), CASDDS, CISTI, East View, Infotrieve, Linda Hall. **CCC.**
Published by: Stroiizdat, Komsomol'skii pr-t 42, Moscow 119826, Russian Federation. TEL 7-095-9782737, FAX 7-095-2459780, http://www.vstmag.ru. Ed. V N Shvetsov. Circ: 17,000. **Dist. by:** Mezhdunarodnaya Kniga, B Yakimanka 39, Moscow 117049, Russian Federation; **US dist. addr.:** East View Publications, 3020 Harbor Ln N, Minneapolis, MN 55447. TEL 612-550-0961.

▼ **VOEDINGSMIDDELENPRAKTIJK.** see *FOOD AND FOOD INDUSTRIES*

614 DEU ISSN 0934-8794
VORDRUCKE FUER DIE KASSENAERZTLICHE UND VERTRAGSAERZTLICHE VERSORGUNG. Text in German. 1978. irreg. DEM 89.80 (effective 2000). **Document type:** *Bulletin, Trade.*
Published by: Erich Schmidt Verlag GmbH & Co. (Berlin), Genthiner Str 30G, Berlin 10785, Germany. TEL 49-30-250085-0, FAX 49-30-25008521, vertrieb@esvmedien.de, http://www.erich-schmidt-verlag.de.

VSEMIRNAYA ORGANIZATSIYA ZDRAVOOKHRANENIYA. SERIYA TEKHNICHESKIKH DOKLADOV. see *MEDICAL SCIENCES*

614.8 CHE ISSN 1010-9609
RS189 CODEN: WDINE8
W H O DRUG INFORMATION. Text in English. q. CHF 75 (effective 2001). **Document type:** *Academic/Scholarly.* **Description:** Communicates medicinal drug information that is either developed and issued by WHO or transmitted to WHO by research and regulatory agencies throughout the world.
Related titles: Online - full text ed.: (from ProQuest Information & Learning, Gale Group, Factiva); ♦ French ed.: Informations Pharmaceutiques OMS. ISSN 1011-5706.
Indexed: CINAHL, Helminthol.Abstr., I.P.A., Ind.Vet., Inpharma, Pharm.&Out.News, Protozool.Abstr., Reac.
—BLDSC (9311.903000), CASDDS, EMDOCS, GNLM, ingenta.
Published by: World Health Organization, Marketing and Dissemination, Geneva, 27 1211, Switzerland. TEL 41-22-791-2476, FAX 41-22-791-4875, publications@who.ch, http://www.who.int. Circ: 1,848.

W H O TECHNICAL REPORT SERIES. see *MEDICAL SCIENCES*

W N Y F. (With New York Firefighters) see *FIRE PREVENTION*

614 IDN
WARTA DINAS KESEHATAN. Text in Indonesian. m. illus.
Formerly: Warta Kesehatan (0377-6549)
Published by: Dinas Kesehatan, Jl. Kesehatan 10, Jakarta, Indonesia.

WARY CANARY; a news network for allergics, "sensitive birds," & environmental health advocates. see *ENVIRONMENTAL STUDIES*

WASHINGTON (STATE). DEPARTMENT OF SOCIAL AND HEALTH SERVICES. INCOME MAINTENANCE, COMMUNITY SOCIAL SERVICES AND MEDICAL ASSISTANCE. see *SOCIAL SERVICES AND WELFARE*

WATER QUALITY NEWS. see *WATER RESOURCES*

WATER SEWAGE AND EFFLUENT. see *WATER RESOURCES*

P

614 CHE ISSN 0049-8114
RA651
WEEKLY EPIDEMIOLOGICAL RECORD. Text in English, French. 1925. w. CHF 230 (effective 2001). bibl, charts, illus, stat. index. back issues avail. **Document type:** *Trade.* **Description:** Provides an essential instrument for the collation and dissemination of data, including global number of AIDS cases, useful in disease surveillance and control on a global level.
Related titles: Microfiche ed.: (from CIS); Online - full text ed.: (from Northern Light Technology, Inc., ProQuest Information & Learning).
Indexed: AIDS Abstr., Abstr.Hyg., CINAHL, Diar.Dis.Res., Excerp.Med., Helminthol.Abstr., IIS, Ind.Med. (1970-), Ind.Vet., Int.Nurs.Ind., Irr.& Drain.Abstr., Nutr.Abstr., Protozool.Abstr., Rev.Appl.Entomol., Rev.Med.& Vet.Mycol., Trop.Dis.Bull.
—BLDSC (9284.780000), CISTI, GNLM, Linda Hall.
Published by: World Health Organization, Marketing and Dissemination, Geneva, 27 1211, Switzerland. TEL 41-22-791-2476, FAX 41-22-791-4857, publications@who.ch; wer@who.ch, http://www.who.int/wer/wer_home.html. Circ: 7,000.

610 USA ISSN 1085-7125
WELLNESS PROGRAM MANAGEMENT ADVISOR. Text in English. 1996. 12/yr. USD 237 (effective 2000). index. back issues avail. **Document type:** *Newsletter.* **Description:** Designed to help professionals manage their organizations' health promotion and wellness programs more effectively by demonstrating return on investment, incentive and disincentive programs, overcoming barriers to success, industry trends, and in-depth profiles of wellness programs around the country.
—CCC.
Published by: American Business Publishing, 1913 Atlantic Ave, Ste F4, Manasquan, NJ 08736. TEL 732-292-1100, FAX 732-292-1111, info@wellnessjunction.com, http://www.wellnessjunction.com. Ed. Jennifer L DeFalco. Pub. Robert K Jenkins.

614.8 658 GBR
WHO'S WHO IN THE EMERGENCY & RESCUE SERVICES (YEAR). Text in English. 1988. a. GBP 27.50 domestic; GBP 29 foreign (effective 1999). **Document type:** *Directory.*
Published by: Lincoln Publications, 28 Centre Point House, St Giles High St, London WC2H 8LW, United Kingdom. TEL 44-207-240-5562, FAX 44-207-497-2811. Ed. James Hardwick.

628 DEU ISSN 0342-5967
WOHNMEDIZIN. Text in German. 1962. bi-m. DEM 55 (effective 2001). bk.rev. back issues avail. **Document type:** *Journal, Academic/Scholarly.*
—GNLM.
Published by: Deutsche Gesellschaft fuer Hygiene und Umweltmedizin, c/o Dr. K. Fiedler, Institut fuer Hygiene, Fuerstengraben 23, Jena 07743, Germany. TEL 49-3641-937900, FAX 49-3641-937902.

614 658.3 USA ISSN 1053-492X
WORKSITE WELLNESS WORKS* . Text in English. 1986. m. membership. bk.rev. back issues avail. **Document type:** *Newsletter.* **Description:** Provides a forum for corporate health promotion and wellness programs, cost-benefits of health promotion programs, information from the Wellness Council National Network, and the names of the healthiest companies in the U.S.
Published by: Wellness Councils of America, 9802 Nicholas St, Ste 315, Omaha, NE 68114-2106. TEL 402-572-3590, FAX 402-572-3594, welcoa@welcoa.org. Ed., R&P Sandra Wendel. Circ: 3,000.

363.348 NLD ISSN 0929-0850
WORLD DISASTERS REPORT. Text in English. 1993. a. price varies.
Related titles: Arabic ed.; French ed.; Spanish ed.
—BLDSC (9354.235000).
Published by: (International Federation of Red Cross and Red Crescent Societies), Martinus Nijhoff Publishers, Human Rights and International Law (Subsidiary of: Kluwer Academic Publishers Group), Postbus 163, Dordrecht 3300 AD, Netherlands. TEL 31-78-334911, FAX 31-78-334254. **Dist. by:** Kluwer Academic Publishers Group, Journals Department, PO Box 322, Dordrecht 3300 AH, Netherlands. TEL 31-78-524400, FAX 31-78-524474.

WORLD FEDERATION FOR MENTAL HEALTH. ANNUAL REPORT. see *PSYCHOLOGY*

WORLD FEDERATION FOR MENTAL HEALTH. NEWSLETTER. see *PSYCHOLOGY*

614 CHE ISSN 0301-0740
RA8
WORLD HEALTH ORGANIZATION. HANDBOOK OF RESOLUTIONS AND DECISIONS OF THE WORLD HEALTH ASSEMBLY AND THE EXECUTIVE BOARD. Text in English. 1948. biennial.
Related titles: Arabic ed.: Munazzamat al-Sihhiyyah al-'Alamiyyah. Dalil Qararat Jam'iyyah al-Sihhiyyah wal-Majlis al-Tanfidhi. ISSN 1010-0202; Chinese ed.: Shijie Weisheng Dahui Ji Zhixing Weiyuanui Jueyi e Jueding Shouce. ISSN 1010-0245; French ed.: Recueil des Resolutions et Decisions de l'Assemblee Mondiale de la Sante et du Conseil Executif. ISSN 1010-0229; Russian ed.: Vsemirnaya Assambleya Zdravookhraneniya i Ispolnitel'nogo Komiteta. Sbornik Rezolyutsii i Reshenii. ISSN 1010-0237; Spanish ed.: Asamblea Mundial de la Salud y del Consejo Ejecutivo. Manual de Resoluciones y Decisiones. ISSN 1010-0210.
Published by: World Health Organization, Marketing and Dissemination, Geneva, 27 1211, Switzerland. TEL 41-22-791-2476, FAX 41-22-791-4857, publications@who.ch, http://www.who.int. Circ: 8,000.

614 EGY
WORLD HEALTH ORGANIZATION. REGIONAL OFFICE FOR THE EASTERN MEDITERRANEAN. ANNUAL REPORT OF THE REGIONAL DIRECTOR. Text in Arabic, English. 1950. a. free per issue to qualified personnel. **Document type:** *Corporate.*
Former titles (until 1989): World Health Organization. Regional Office for the Eastern Mediterranean. Biennial Report of Regional Director; (until 1979): World Health Organization. Regional Office for the Eastern Mediterranean. Annual Report of the Regional Director (0512-3089)
Related titles: Microfiche ed.: (from CIS); Abridged ed.
Indexed: IIS.
—GNLM.
Published by: World Health Organization, Regional Office for the Eastern Mediterranean, P O Box 1517, Alexandria 21563, Egypt. FAX 20-3-4838916, TELEX 54028 WHO UN, http://www.who.sci.eg/rd/index.htm. Eds. Christopher Zielinski, Haytham Khayat. Circ: 3,000.

614 CHE ISSN 1020-3311
RA8
THE WORLD HEALTH REPORT. Text in English. 1948. a. USD 13.50 (effective 1999). **Description:** Reports on important diseases and assesses the impact of knowledge and technology on controlling them. Suggests needed actions and estimates their cost.
Formerly (until 1995): World Health Organization. Work of W H O (0509-2558)
Related titles: Microfiche ed.: (from CIS); Online - full text ed.: ISSN 1564-0809; French ed.: ISSN 1020-332X.
Indexed: CWI, Helminthol.Abstr., IIS, Russ.Acad.Sci.Bibl., Trop.Dis.Bull.
—BLDSC (9356.048000), GNLM.
Published by: World Health Organization, Marketing and Dissemination, Geneva, 27 1211, Switzerland. TEL 41-22-791-2476, FAX 41-22-791-4857, publications@who.ch, http://www.who.int. Circ: 8,000.

WORLDWATCH READER. see *ENVIRONMENTAL STUDIES*

353.9 614 USA
WYOMING. DEPARTMENT OF HEALTH. ANNUAL REPORT. Text in English. 1975. a. **Document type:** *Government.*
Formerly: Wyoming. Department of Health and Social Services. Annual Report (0098-6984)
Published by: Department of Health, 117 Hathaway Bldg, Cheyenne, WY 82002. TEL 307-777-7656, FAX 307-777-7439. Ed. Marcia Benedict. Circ: 500.

628 JPN ISSN 0915-0498
CODEN: YEKHET
YAMAGUCHIKEN EISEI KOGAI KENKYU SENTA GYOSEKI HOKOKU. Text in Japanese; Contents page in English. 1958. a. per issue exchange basis. charts, bibl. **Description:** Contains original papers, technical reports and investigation articles on public health. Includes analyses of chemical constituents and pollutants in regional rivers and lakes, reservoirs, and wastewater, as well as investigations of atmospheric concentrations of chlorofluorocarbons and hazardous air pollutants in specific cities.
Supersedes (in 1988): Yamaguchiken Eisei Kenkyujo Gyoseki Hokoku (0513-4757)
—CASDDS.
Published by: Yamaguchiken Eisei Kogai Kenkyu Senta/Yamaguchi Prefectural Research Institute of Health, 5-67 Aoi 2-chome, Yamaguchi-shi 753-0821, Japan. TEL 81-839-22-7630, FAX 81-839-22-7632.

628 333.91 USA
YEARS AHEAD. Text in English. 1982. q. USD 10.
Published by: Pure Water of New England, 103 Union St, Watertown, MA 02172. TEL 617-924-0959. Ed. Patrick E Mertens. Circ: 10,000.

628 JPN ISSN 0912-2826
YOKOHAMA CITY INSTITUTE OF HEALTH. ANNUAL REPORT. Text in Japanese; Summaries in English. 1962. a.
Published by: Yokohama City Institute of Health, 2-17 Takigashira 1-chome, Isogo-ku, Yokohama-shi, Kanagawa-ken 235-0000, Japan. Circ: 300.

YOKOHAMA MEDICAL JOURNAL. see *MEDICAL SCIENCES*

614 USA
YOUR HEALTH TODAY. Text in English. 1997. d.
Media: Online - full content.
Published by: Jobson Publishing LLC, 100 Ave of Americas, New York, NY 10013-1678. http://www.yourhealthtoday.com.

614 RUS ISSN 0044-1945
CODEN: ZDRVA4
ZDOROV'E. Text in Russian. 1955. m. RUR 390 for 6 mos. (effective 2000). adv. bk.rev. bibl. index. back issues avail. *Refereed.* **Document type:** *Magazine, Consumer.* **Description:** Focuses on healthy living and includes features on nutrition, beauty, travel, preventive medicine, new medical technologies, drug use, child care. Also includes reports from medical institutes.
Related titles: CD-ROM ed.; Diskette ed.; Fax ed.
Indexed: Chem.Abstr.
—East View.
Published by: Izdatel'stvo Zdorov'e, Bumazhnyi pr 14, Moscow 101454, Russian Federation. TEL 7-095-2505828, FAX 7-095-2573251, zdorovie@zdorovie.fipc.ru, red@zdorovie.ad.ru, http://zdorovie.ad.ru. Ed. T Efimova. R&P T. Efimova TEL 7-05-2121403. adv.: color page USD 6,000. Circ: 185,000 (paid and controlled). **Dist. by:** Mezhdunarodnaya Kniga, B Yakimanka 39, Moscow 117049, Russian Federation. TEL 7-095-2384967, FAX 7-095-2385634; **US dist. addr.:** East View Publications, 3020 Harbor Ln N, Minneapolis, MN 55447. TEL 612-550-0961.

362.1 RUS
ZDOROV'E NASELENIYA I SREDA OBITANIYA. Text in Russian. m. USD 179.95 in United States.
Indexed: Ref.Zh.
Published by: Gosudarstvennogo Komiteta Sanitarno Epidemiologicheskogo Nadzora, Vadkovskii per 18-20, Moscow 103055, Russian Federation. TEL 7-095-9732671. **US dist. addr.:** East View Publications, 3020 Harbor Ln N, Minneapolis, MN 55447. TEL 612-550-0961.

362.1 RUS
ZDRAVOOKHRANENIE. Text in Russian. m. USD 199 in United States.
Indexed: Ref.Zh.
Published by: Mezhdunarodnyi Tsentr Finansovo-Ekonomicheskogo Razvitiya, Ul Komdiva Orlova 2-37, korp 3, Moscow 126106, Russian Federation. TEL 7-095-2825123, FAX 7-095-2157680. **US dist. addr.:** East View Publications, 3020 Harbor Ln N, Minneapolis, MN 55447. TEL 612-550-0961.

614 BLR
CODEN: ZDBEA9
ZDRAVOOKHRANENIE. Text in Russian. 1924-19??; resumed 1955. m. BYB 120,000; USD 149 foreign (effective 1999). adv. bk.rev. charts, illus, stat. index. back issues avail. *Refereed.* **Document type:** *Academic/Scholarly.*
Former titles: Zdravookhranenie Belarusi; (until 1995): Zdravookhranenie Belorussii (0044-1961); (until 1941): Meditsinsky Zhurnal B.S.S.R.; (until 1938): Belorusskaya Meditsinskaya Mysl
Related titles: Fax ed.
Indexed: Biol.Abstr., Chem.Abstr., INIS Atomind., Russ.Acad.Sci.Bibl.
—CASDDS, GNLM.
Published by: Ministerstvo Zdravookhraneniya/Ministry of Public Health, Vul Fabritsyusa 28, Minsk 220001, Belarus. TEL 7-172-2262167. Ed. V Ulashchik. Pub. M Podgainy. R&P V. Ulashchik TEL 7-172-2221682. Adv. contact Myshkovskaya. B&W page USD 250, color page USD 450. Circ: 11,000. **US dist. addr.:** East View Publications, 3020 Harbor Ln N, Minneapolis, MN 55447. TEL 612-550-0961.

P

362.1 RUS ISSN 0869-6306
ZDRAVOOKHRANENIE BASHKORTOSTANA. Text in Russian; Abstracts in English. bi-m. USD 40 to individuals; USD 56 to institutions (effective 2000). adv. bk.rev. *Refereed.* **Description:** Includes articles on health service, public health, theoretical medicine, and clinical medicine.
Indexed: Ref.Zh.
Address: Ul Lenina 3, Ufa 450000, Russian Federation. TEL 7-3472-227350, FAX 7-3472-223751, bsmu@anrb.ru, http://www.bsmu.amb.ru. Ed. S V Shagarova. Adv. contact N V Akhmetova. **US dist. addr.:** East View Publications, 3020 Harbor Ln N, Minneapolis, MN 55447. TEL 612-550-0961.

362.1 KAZ
ZDRAVOOKHRANENIE KAZAKHSTANA. Text in Russian. m. USD 149 in United States.
Indexed: Russ.Acad.Sci.Bibl.
Address: Ul Kunaeva 86, Almaty 480100, Kazakstan. TEL 3272-616294. **US dist. addr.:** East View Publications, 3020 Harbor Ln N, Minneapolis, MN 55447. TEL 612-550-0961.

570 RUS ISSN 0044-197X
ZDRAVOOKHRANENIE ROSSIISKOI FEDERATSII/ PUBLIC HEALTHCARE OF THE RUSSIAN FEDERATION. Text in Russian; Contents page in English. 1957. bi-m. USD 94 foreign (effective 2000). **Document type:** *Academic/Scholarly.* **Description:** Publishes scientific and practical materials on the health status of the population and on the development of public health services in autonomous republics, territories, regions and districts of the RSFSR.
Indexed: Biol.Abstr., INIS Atomind., Ind.Med. (coverage dropped), Int.Aerosp.Abstr., Ref.Zh., Russ.Acad.Sci.Bibl.
—CISTI, East View, GNLM.
Published by: Izdatel'stvo Meditsina, Petroverigskii per 6-8, Moscow 101000, Russian Federation. TEL 7-095-9246740, FAX 7-095-9211355, meditsina@iname.com, http://www.medit.ru. Ed. A I Potapov. Pub. A M Stochik. R&P T Kurushina. Adv. contact O A Fadeeva TEL 7-095-923-51-40. Circ: 3,800. **Dist. by:** Mezhdunarodnaya Kniga, B Yakimanka 39, Moscow 117049, Russian Federation. TEL 7-095-2384967, FAX 7-095-2384634.

362.1 TKM ISSN 0513-8736
CODEN: ZDTUAB
ZDRAVOOKHRANENIE TURKMENISTANA. Text in Russian. bi-m.
Indexed: INIS Atomind., Russ.Acad.Sci.Bibl.
—CASDDS, GNLM.
Published by: Ministry of Public Health, Ul Kerbabaeva 39-57, Ashgabat 744004, Turkmenistan. TEL 993-12-391621. **US dist. addr.:** East View Publications, 3020 Harbor Ln N, Minneapolis, MN 55447. TEL 612-550-0961.

614 CZE ISSN 0044-1996
ZDRAVOTNICKE NOVINY; tydenik pracovniku ve zdravotnictvi. Text in Czech. 1955. w. CZK 650; CZK 12.50 newsstand/cover. adv. **Document type:** *Magazine, Consumer.*
Published by: Strategie Praha s.r.o., Drtinova 8, Prague, 5 150 00, Czech Republic. TEL 420-2-57323578, FAX 420-2-57018362, strategie.praha@istrategie.cz, http://www.zdn.cz, http://www.istrategie.cz. Ed. Jiri Matous. adv.: page CZK 79,000; trim 277 x 428. Circ: 35,000. **Subscr. to:** Artia, Ve Smeckach 30, Prague, 1 111 27, Czechoslovakia.

614 SVK ISSN 1335-4477
ZDRAVOTNICKE NOVINY. Text in Slovak. 1996. w. adv. **Document type:** *Magazine, Trade.*
Published by: Strategie na Slovensku s.r.o., Tehelna 16, Bratislava 83103, Slovakia. TEL 421-7-44373376, FAX 421-7-44373356.

614 POL ISSN 0044-2011
RA421
ZDROWIE PUBLICZNE. Text in Polish. 1885. m. USD 150. bk.rev. abstr, charts, illus, stat. index. **Description:** Deals with social medicine, health care organization and health policy.
Indexed: Biol.Abstr., Excerp.Med., Ind.Med. (coverage dropped).
—GNLM.
Published by: Ministerstwo Zdrowia i Opieki Spolecznej/Ministry of Health and Social Welfare, Ul Miodowa 15, Warsaw 00923, Poland. TEL 48-22-312144, FAX 48-22-6359245. Circ: 2,377. **Dist. by:** Ars Polona, Krakowskie Przedmiescie 7, Warsaw, Poland.

614 DEU ISSN 0943-1853
ZEITSCHRIFT FUER GESUNDHEITSWISSENSCHAFTEN/ JOURNAL OF PUBLIC HEALTH. Text in English, German. 1993. q. EUR 63.20 domestic; EUR 69.50 foreign (effective 2001). adv. bk.rev. **Document type:** *Magazine, Academic/Scholarly.*
Indexed: Crim.Just.Abstr.
—EMDOCS, GNLM.
Published by: Juventa Verlag GmbH, Ehretstr 3, Weinheim 69469, Germany. TEL 49-6201-90200, FAX 49-6201-902013, juventa@juventa.de, http://www.juventa.de. Ed. Nora Merker. Circ: 700 (paid).

ZEITSCHRIFT FUER LAERMBEKAEMPFUNG. see *PHYSICS—Sound*

614 CHN ISSN 1004-1257
ZHIYE YU JIANKANG✱ /OCCUPATION AND HEALTH. Text in Chinese. 1985. bi-m. USD 44.40; USD 3.70 newsstand/cover (effective 2001). *Refereed.* **Document type:** *Academic/Scholarly.* **Description:** Popular science magazine for medical workers and safety-control technicians in industrial companies.
Published by: (Tianjin Shi Laodong Weisheng Zhiyebing Yanjiusuo/Tianjin Institute of Industrial Hygiene and Occupational Diseases), China International Book Trading Corp/Zhongguo Guoji Tushu Maoyi Zonggongsi cibtc@mail.cibtc.com.cn, http://www.cibtc.com.cn. Ed. Zhang Yinde. Circ: 100,000 (controlled). **Dist. by:** 35, Chegongzhuang Xilu, Haidian District, Beijing 100044, China.

362.1 CHN ISSN 1005-2720
ZHONGGUO BAOJIAN/CHINESE HEALTH CARE. Text in Chinese. 1993. m. USD 62.40; USD 2.20 newsstand/cover (effective 2001). 48 p./no.
Published by: (Zhongguo Yiliao Baojian Guoji Jiaoliu Cujinhui), Zhongguo Baojian Zazhishe, Zuojiazhuang 1 Xiao Nei, No. 4 Zuojiazhuang Houjie, Chaoyang-qu, Beijing 100028, China. TEL 86-1-4615875. Ed. Xiao Jianzhong. **Dist. overseas by:** China International Book Trading Corp, 35, Chegongzhuang Xilu, Haidian District, Beijing 100044, China. TEL 86-1-68413849, FAX 86-1-68412048, cibtc@mail.cibtc.com.cn, http://www.cibtc.com.cn.

614 CHN ISSN 1001-0580
ZHONGGUO GONGGONG WEISHENG/CHINA'S PUBLIC HEALTH. Text in Chinese. 1985. m. USD 19.20. adv.
Published by: Zhonghua Yufang Yixuehui (Shenyang)/China Preventive Medical Society (Shenyang), Jixian Jie, Heping-qu, Shenyang, Liaoning 110005, China. TEL 363643. Ed. Dai Zhicheng. Adv. contact Xiying Li. B&W page USD 300, color page USD 500. Circ: 10,000. **Dist. overseas by:** China International Book Trading Corp, 35 Chegongzhuang Xilu, Haidian District, Beijing 100044, China. TEL 8413063.

614 CHN ISSN 1001-0572
CODEN: ZGWXEQ
ZHONGGUO GONGGONG WEISHENG XUEBAO/CHINESE JOURNAL OF PUBLIC HEALTH. Text in Chinese. 1982. bi-m. USD 12. adv.
Indexed: Chem.Abstr., Chem.Indus.Notes, Chem.Titles, Environ.Sci.Poll.Mgmt., Microbiol.Abstr., Pollut.Abstr., Risk Abstr., Saf.Sci.Abstr.
—CASDDS.
Published by: Zhonghua Yufang Yixuehui (Shenyang)/China Preventive Medical Society (Shenyang), Jixian Jie, Heping-qu, Shenyang, Liaoning 110005, China. TEL 363643. Ed. Kan Xuegui. Adv. contact Xiying Li. B&W page USD 300, color page USD 500. Circ: 3,000. **Dist. overseas by:** China International Book Trading Corp, 35 Chegongzhuang Xilu, Haidian District, Beijing 100044, China. TEL 8413063.

ZHONGGUO JISHENGCHONG YU JISHENGCHONGBING ZAZHI/CHINESE JOURNAL OF PARASITOLOGY AND PARASITIC DISEASES. see *MEDICAL SCIENCES—Communicable Diseases*

ZHONGGUO JISHENGCHONGBING FANGZHI ZAZHI/CHINESE JOURNAL OF PARASITIC DISEASE CONTROL. see *MEDICAL SCIENCES—Communicable Diseases*

ZIVOT I ZDRAVIJE; obitelski casopis za proucavanje i promicanje prirodnih zdravstvenih nacela. see *MEDICAL SCIENCES*

PUBLIC HEALTH AND SAFETY— Abstracting, Bibliographies, Statistics

310 USA
ADVANCES IN RISK ANALYSIS. Text in English. 1983. irreg., latest vol.9, 1991. back issues avail. *Refereed.* **Document type:** *Monographic series.*
Published by: (Society for Risk Analysis), Kluwer Academic - Plenum Publishers (Subsidiary of: Wolters Kluwer N.V.), 233 Spring St, New York, NY 10013-1578. TEL 212-620-8000, 800-221-9369, FAX 212-463-0742, info@plenum.com, http://www.plenum.com.

AIDS & T B WEEKLY ABSTRACTS FROM CONFERENCE PROCEEDINGS. (Tuberculosis) see *MEDICAL SCIENCES—Abstracting, Bibliographies, Statistics*

614 318 ARG
ARGENTINA. MINISTERIO DE SALUD Y ACCION SOCIAL. PROGRAMA NACIONAL DE ESTADISTICAS DE SALUD. BOLETIN. (Subseries avail.: 2: Evaluacion de Datos, 3: Conclusiones y Recomendaciones de Congresos, 4: Estadisticas Hospitalarias; 5: Estadisticas Vitales; 8: Analisis de Datos; 9: Material de Ensenanza; 10: Encuesta a Poblacion) Text in Spanish. 1976 (no.6). irreg., latest vol.73, 1995. **Document type:** *Monographic series, Government.*
Formerly: Argentina. Secretaria de Estado de Salud Publica. Programa Nacional de Estadisticas de Salud. Boletin
Published by: Ministerio de Salud y Accion Social, Direccion de Estadisticas de Salud, Of. 606, Avda. 9 De Julio, 1925 Piso 6, Capital Federal, Buenos Aires 1332, Argentina.

362.1021 AUS
AUSTRALIA. BUREAU OF STATISTICS. AUSTRALIAN HEALTH TRENDS. Text in English. 1995. irreg., latest 2000. AUD 21.50 (effective 2001). **Document type:** *Government.*
Published by: Australian Bureau of Statistics, PO Box 10, Belconnen, ACT 2616, Australia. TEL 61-2-6252-5249, FAX 61-2-6252-6778, http://www.abs.gov.au. **Co-sponsor:** Australian Institute of Health and Welfare.

362.1021 AUS
AUSTRALIA. BUREAU OF STATISTICS. HEALTH IN AUSTRALIA - WHAT YOU SHOULD KNOW. Text in English. 1995. irreg. AUD 14.95 (effective 1998). **Document type:** *Government.*
Published by: Australian Bureau of Statistics, PO Box 10, Belconnen, ACT 2616, Australia. TEL 61-2-6252-5249, FAX 61-2-6252-6778, http://www.abs.gov.au. **Co-sponsor:** Australian Institute of Health and Welfare.

362.1021 AUS
AUSTRALIA. BUREAU OF STATISTICS. NATIONAL HEALTH INFORMATION MODEL. Text in English. 1995. irreg. AUD 25 (effective 1998). **Document type:** *Government.*
Published by: Australian Bureau of Statistics, PO Box 10, Belconnen, ACT 2616, Australia. TEL 61-2-6252-5249, FAX 61-2-6252-6778, http://www.abs.gov.au.

362.1021 AUS
AUSTRALIA. BUREAU OF STATISTICS. NATIONAL HEALTH SURVEY: ABORIGINAL AND TORRES STRAIT ISLANDER RESULTS, AUSTRALIA. Text in English. 1995. irreg. AUD 21 (effective 2001).
Published by: Australian Bureau of Statistics, PO Box 10, Belconnen, ACT 2616, Australia. TEL 61-2-6252-5249, FAX 61-2-6252-6778, http://www.abs.gov.au.

362.1021 AUS
AUSTRALIA. BUREAU OF STATISTICS. NATIONAL HEALTH SURVEY: HEALTH RISK FACTORS, AUSTRALIA. Text in English. 1998. irreg. AUD 16.50 (effective 1998). **Document type:** *Government.*
Published by: Australian Bureau of Statistics, PO Box 10, Belconnen, ACT 2616, Australia. TEL 61-2-6252-5249, FAX 61-2-6252-6778, http://www.abs.gov.au.

362.1021 AUS
AUSTRALIA. BUREAU OF STATISTICS. NATIONAL HEALTH SURVEY: SUMMARY OF RESULTS. Text in English. 1990. irreg., latest 1995. AUD 23 (effective 2001). **Document type:** *Government.*
Published by: Australian Bureau of Statistics, PO Box 10, Belconnen, ACT 2616, Australia. TEL 61-2-6252-5249, FAX 61-2-6252-6778, http://www.abs.gov.au.

362.1021 AUS
AUSTRALIA. BUREAU OF STATISTICS. NATIONAL HEALTH SURVEY: SUMMARY RESULTS, AUSTRALIAN STATES AND TERRITORIES. Text in English. 1995. irreg. AUD 21 (effective 2001). **Document type:** *Government.*
Published by: Australian Bureau of Statistics, PO Box 10, Belconnen, ACT 2616, Australia. TEL 61-2-6252-5249, FAX 61-2-6252-6778, http://www.abs.gov.au.

362.1021 AUS
AUSTRALIA. BUREAU OF STATISTICS. NATIONAL HEALTH SURVEY: USERS' GUIDE. Text in English. 1990. irreg., latest 1995. AUD 20 (effective 2000). **Document type:** *Government.*
Published by: Australian Bureau of Statistics, PO Box 10, Belconnen, ACT 2616, Australia. TEL 61-2-6252-5249, FAX 61-2-6252-6778, http://www.abs.gov.au.

362.1021 AUS
AUSTRALIA. BUREAU OF STATISTICS. NORTHERN TERRITORY OFFICE. NATIONAL HEALTH SURVEY: DARWIN-PALMERSTON AND ALICE SPRINGS. Text in English. 1995. irreg., latest 1995. AUD 18 (effective 2001). **Document type:** *Government.*
Published by: Australian Bureau of Statistics, Northern Territory Office, 5th Fl., 81 Smith St, Darwin, N.T. 0800, Australia. TEL 61-8-8943-2110, FAX 61-8-8981-1218, http://www.abs.gov.au.

362.1021 305.4021 AUS
AUSTRALIA. BUREAU OF STATISTICS. WOMEN'S SAFETY SURVEY, UNIT RECORD FILE, AUSTRALIA. Text in English. 1996. irreg. AUD 8,000 (effective 2001). **Document type:** *Government.*
Media: Diskette.
Published by: Australian Bureau of Statistics, PO Box 10, Belconnen, ACT 2616, Australia. TEL 61-2-6252-5249, FAX 61-2-6252-6778, http://www.abs.gov.au.

614.86021 BEL ISSN 0770-237X
HE5614.5.B4
BELGIUM. INSTITUT NATIONAL DE STATISTIQUE. ACCIDENTS DE LA CIRCULATION SUR LA VOIE PUBLIQUE AVEC TUES ET BLESSES. Key Title: Accidents de la Circulation sur la Voie Publique avec Tues et Blesses. Text in French. 1954. a. EUR 10 per issue; EUR 41 (effective 2001). charts. back issues avail. **Document type:** *Government.* **Description:** Provides a statistical overview of deaths and injuries in traffic accidents on public highways.
Former titles (until 1973): Belgium. Institut National de Statistique. Statistique des Accidents de la Circulation sur la Voie Publique (0067-5504); (until 1962): Belgium. Institut National de Statistique. Statistique des Accidents de Roulage (0067-5512)
Related titles: ♦ Dutch ed.: Belgium. Nationaal Instituut voor de Statistiek. Verkeersongevallen op de Openbare Weg met Doden of Gewonden. ISSN 0771-0577.
Published by: Institut National de Statistique/Nationaal Instituut voor de Statistiek (Subsidiary of: Ministere des Affaires Economiques), Rue de Louvain 44, Brussels 1000, Belgium. TEL 32-2-548-6211, FAX 32-2-548-6367, http://www.statbel.fgov.be.

310 BEL
BELGIUM. MINISTERE DES AFFAIRES SOCIALES DE LA SANTE PUBLIQUE ET DE L'ENVIRONNEMENT. ADMINISTRATION DES SOINS DE SANTE. ANNUAIRE STATISTIQUE DES HOPITAUX/BELGIUM. MINISTERIE VAN VOLKSGEZONDHEID EN LEEFMILIEU. BESTUUR VOOR DE VERZORGINGSINSTELLINGEN. STATISTISCH JAARBOEK VAN DE ZIEKENHUIZEN. (In 8 parts: Liste d'Adresses; Rapport Annuel; Activite dans les Hopitaux; Origine des Patients; Duree de Sejour Detaille; Activite des Medecins Hopitaliers; Personnel des Hopitaux; List d'Adresses des M R S) Text in Dutch, French. 1962. a. free per issue. **Document type:** *Government.*
Former titles: Belgium. Ministere de la Sante Publique et de la Famille. Annuaire Statistique des Hopitaux; Belgium. Ministere de la Sante et de la Famille. Premiers et Principaux Resultats Statistiques de l'Enquete dans les Etablissements de Soins
Published by: Ministere des Affaires Sociales de la Sante Publique et de l'Environnement, Administration des Soins de Sante/Ministerie van Volksgezondheid en Leefmilieu, Bestuursafdeling voor de Verzorgingsinstellingen, Studiedienst, Cite Administrative de l'Etat, Quartier Vesale 502, Brussels 1010, Belgium. TEL 32-2-210-45-11. Circ: 1,500.

614.86021 BEL ISSN 0771-0577
BELGIUM. NATIONAAL INSTITUUT VOOR DE STATISTIEK. VERKEERSONGEVALLEN OP DE OPENBARE WEG MET DODEN OF GEWONDEN. Key Title: Verkeersongevallen op de Openbare Weg met Doden of Gewonden. Text in Dutch. 1954. a. BEF 190 domestic; BEF 400 foreign (effective 2000). charts. **Document type:** *Government.* **Description:** Provides a statistical overview of deaths and injuries in traffic accidents on public highways.
Formerly (until 1973): Belgium. Nationaal Instituut voor de Statistiek. Statistiek van de Verkeersongevallen op de Openbare Weg (0522-7593)
Related titles: ♦ French ed.: Belgium. Institut National de Statistique. Accidents de la Circulation sur la Voie Publique avec Tues et Blesses. ISSN 0770-237X.
Published by: Institut National de Statistique/Nationaal Instituut voor de Statistiek (Subsidiary of: Ministere des Affaires Economiques), Rue de Louvain 44, Brussels 1000, Belgium. TEL 32-2-548-6211, FAX 32-2-548-6367, http://www.statbel.fgov.be.

304.6 CAN ISSN 1188-1437
BRITISH COLUMBIA. DIVISION OF VITAL STATISTICS AGENCY. QUARTERLY DIGEST. Text in English. 1991. q. free per issue. **Document type:** *Government.* **Description:** Presents current statistical data for selected health status indicators on a regional basis, and discusses public health issues affecting British Columbia.
Published by: Ministry of Health Services, B.C. Vital Statistics Agency, 818 Fort St, Victoria, BC V8W 1H8, Canada. TEL 250-952-2558, FAX 250-952-2594, http://www.vs.gov.bc.ca/stats/quarter/index.html. Ed. Julie M Macdonald.

614 616.99 USA
CANCER INCIDENCE AND MORTALITY MICHIGAN. Text in English. 1985. a. free per issue. **Document type:** *Government.* **Description:** Statistical tables, graphs and text containing data on cancer incidence and mortality for Michigan resident population.
Published by: Department of Community Health, Division for Vital Records and Health Statistics, 3423 N Martin Luther King Jr Blvd, Box 30619, Lansing, MI 48909. TEL 517-335-8705, FAX 517-335-8711, spivak@state.mi.us, http://www.mdch.state.mi.us.

614 GBR ISSN 0957-4956
RA630.G73
CHARTERED INSTITUTE OF PUBLIC FINANCE AND ACCOUNTANCY. CEMETERIES STATISTICS. ACTUALS. Text in English. 1982. a. GBP 55. back issues avail.
Supersedes in part (in 1989): Chartered Institute of Public Finance and Accountancy. Cemeteries and Crematoria Statistics. Actuals (0263-2969); Which was formed by the merger of (1956-1982): Chartered Institute of Public Finance and Accountancy. Crematoria Statistics. Actuals (0534-2104); (1979-1982): Chartered Institute of Public Finance and Accountancy. Cemeteries Statistics. Actuals (0260-9959)
Published by: Chartered Institute of Public Finance and Accountancy, Statistical Information Service, 3 Robert St, London WC2N 6RL, United Kingdom. TEL 44-20-7543-5800, FAX 44-20-7543-5700, http://www.cipfa.org.uk.

614 GBR ISSN 0956-1439
RA630.G73
CHARTERED INSTITUTE OF PUBLIC FINANCE AND ACCOUNTANCY. CREMATORIA STATISTICS. ACTUALS. Text in English. 1982. a. GBP 55. back issues avail.
Supersedes in part (in 1989): Chartered Institute of Public Finance and Accountancy. Cemeteries and Crematoria Statistics. Actuals (0263-2969); Which was formed by the merger of (1956-1982): Chartered Institute of Public Finance and Accountancy. Crematoria Statistics. Actuals (0534-2104); (1979-1982): Chartered Institute of Public Finance and Accountancy. Cemeteries Statistics. Actuals (0260-9959)
Published by: Chartered Institute of Public Finance and Accountancy, Statistical Information Service, 3 Robert St, London WC2N 6RL, United Kingdom. TEL 44-20-7543-5800, FAX 44-20-7543-5700, http://www.cipfa.org.uk.

614.8 GBR ISSN 0266-9552
RA566.5.G7
CHARTERED INSTITUTE OF PUBLIC FINANCE AND ACCOUNTANCY. ENVIRONMENTAL HEALTH STATISTICS. ACTUALS. Text in English. 1984. a. GBP 80.
Published by: Chartered Institute of Public Finance and Accountancy, Statistical Information Service, 3 Robert St, London WC2N 6RL, United Kingdom. TEL 44-20-7543-5800, FAX 44-20-7543-5700, http://www.cipfa.org.uk.

614 CHL
CHILE. INSTITUTO NACIONAL DE ESTADISTICAS. ESTADISTICAS DE SALUD. RECURSOS Y ATENCIONES. Text in Spanish. 1965. a. CLP 1,450 domestic; USD 9.50 in United States; USD 10.20 elsewhere (effective 1999).
Published by: Instituto Nacional de Estadisticas, Casilla 498, Correo 3, Ave. Bulnes, 418, Santiago, Chile. TEL 56-2-6991441, FAX 56-2-6712169.

614 CYP
CYPRUS. MINISTRY OF HEALTH. ANNUAL REPORT. Text in Greek. 1920. a. charts, stat. **Document type:** *Government.*
Supersedes (in 1991): Cyprus. Ministry of Health. Department of Medical and Public Health Services. Annual Report; And the reports of the other departments: Psychiatric Services, Dental Services, General State Laboratory, and Pharmaceutical Services
Published by: Ministry of Health, Nicosia, Cyprus. FAX 357-2-303498, TELEX 5734. Ed. Dr. G Malliotis. Circ: 200.

E C M T STATISTICAL REPORT ON ROAD ACCIDENTS. see *TRANSPORTATION—Abstracting, Bibliographies, Statistics*

610 JPN
EISEI TOKEI KARA MITA AICHI-KEN NO SUGATA. Text in Japanese. 1985. a.
Published by: Aichi-ken Eiseibu Somu-Ka, 1-2, 3-chome, Sannomaru, Naka-ku, Nagoya-shi, Japan. Circ: 200.

016.614 NLD ISSN 0924-5723
CODEN: EMPHA
EXCERPTA MEDICA. SECTION 17: PUBLIC HEALTH, SOCIAL MEDICINE AND EPIDEMIOLOGY. Text in English. 1955. s-m. EUR 3,030 in Europe to institutions; JPY 401,657 in Japan to institutions; USD 3,389 elsewhere to institutions (effective 2002). adv. index, cum.index. back issues avail. **Document type:** *Abstract/Index, Academic/Scholarly.* **Description:** Provides a comprehensive current-awareness service of trade and scholarly articles covering all facets of public health and social medicine, and includes health planning and education, epidemiology and prevention of communicable disease, public health aspects of risk populations, food and nutrition and environmental radiation, medical ethics, the influence of lifestyle on health, and the epidemiological aspects of water supply and purification.
Formerly: Excerpta Medica. Section 17: Public Health, Social Medicine and Hygiene (0014-4215)
Related titles: CD-ROM ed.: (from SilverPlatter Information, Inc.); Online - full text ed.: (from DIMDI, Data-Star, The Dialog Corporation, JICST).
—GNLM, Infotrieve. **CCC.**
Published by: Excerpta Medica Medical Communications BV (Subsidiary of: Reed Elsevier plc), Rooseveltweg 15, Almere-Stad 1314 SJ, Netherlands. TEL 31-36-538-5600, FAX 31-36-538-5650, http://www.elsevier.com/locate/phsme, http://www.excerptamedica.com. **Subscr. in Australasia and the Far East to:** Elsevier Science (Singapore) Pte Ltd, No.1 Temasek Ave, 17-01 Millenia Tower, Singapore 039192, Singapore. TEL 65-434-3727, FAX 65-337-2230; **Subscr. in Japan to:** Elsevier Science Inc - Japan Regional Office, 9-15 Higashi-Azabu 1-chome, Minato-ku, Tokyo 106-0044, Japan. TEL 81-3-5561-5033, FAX 81-3-5561-5047; **Subscr. in the Americas to:** Elsevier Science, PO Box 945, New York, NY 10159-0945. TEL 212-633-3730, 888-437-4636, FAX 212-633-3680, usinfo-f@elsevier.com, http://www.elsevier.com. **Dist. by:** Elsevier Science (Brazil).; Elsevier Science BV, PO Box 211, Amsterdam 1000 AE, Netherlands. TEL 31-20-485-3757, FAX 31-20-485-3432.

EXCERPTA MEDICA. SECTION 35: OCCUPATIONAL HEALTH AND INDUSTRIAL MEDICINE. see *MEDICAL SCIENCES—Abstracting, Bibliographies, Statistics*

614 CHE ISSN 0250-8664
EZHEGODNIK MIROVOI SANITARNOI STATISTIKI. Text in Russian. 1962. a.
Related titles: ♦ English ed.: World Health Statistics Annual. ISSN 0250-3794.
Published by: World Health Organization, Marketing and Dissemination, Geneva, 27 1211, Switzerland.

P

FINLAND. TILASTOKESKUS. ELINOLOT. see *SOCIAL SERVICES AND WELFARE—Abstracting, Bibliographies, Statistics*

362.1021 FIN ISSN 0784-8412
FINLAND. TILASTOKESKUS. TERVEYS. Text in Finnish. irreg. FIM 220 (effective 2000). stat. **Document type:** *Government.*
Published by: Tilastokeskus/Statistics Finland, Tyopajakatu 13, Statistics Finland, Helsinki 00022, Finland. TEL 358-9-17341.

614 312 DEU ISSN 0072-1840
GERMANY. STATISTISCHES BUNDESAMT. FACHSERIE 12, GESUNDHEITSWESEN, REIHE 1: AUSGEWAEHLTE ZAHLEN FUER DAS GESUNDHEITSWESEN. Text in German. 1959. a. DEM 17.10. **Document type:** *Government.*
Published by: Statistisches Bundesamt, Gustav-Stresemann-Ring 11, Wiesbaden 65180, Germany. TEL 49-611-75-1, FAX 49-611-724000, http://www.statistik-bund.de.

GREECE. NATIONAL STATISTICAL SERVICE. SOCIAL WELFARE AND HEALTH STATISTICS. see *SOCIAL SERVICES AND WELFARE—Abstracting, Bibliographies, Statistics*

016 363.11 USA ISSN 0892-9351
HD7260
HEALTH AND SAFETY SCIENCE ABSTRACTS. Text in English. 1973. q. USD 1,085 for print & online eds. combined (effective 2002). bk.rev. index, cum.index. back issues avail.; reprints avail. **Document type:** *Abstract/Index.* **Description:** Abstracts journal on public health, occupational safety, and industrial hygiene.
Former titles: Safety Science Abstracts Journal (0160-1342); Safety Science Abstracts (0092-542X)
Related titles: Online - full text ed.: USD 815 (effective 2002) (from NISC, Questel Orbit Inc., EBSCO Publishing, S T N International, CSA).
—GNLM, Linda Hall.
Published by: (Institute of Safety and Systems Management), Cambridge Scientific Abstracts, 7200 Wisconsin Ave., Suite 601, Bethesda, MD 20814. TEL 301-961-6798, FAX 301-961-6799, journals@csa.com, http://www.csa.com/journals. Ed. Evelyn Beck. Pub. Ted Caris.

362.10973 USA ISSN 1065-1403
RA407.3
HEALTH CARE STATE RANKINGS; health care in the 50 United States. Text in English. 1993. a. USD 54.95 (effective 2002). 540 p./no. **Description:** Provides detailed, comparative statistical information on health care and health care finance in more than 500 categories for each of the 50 states.
—GNLM.
Published by: Morgan Quitno Corporation, PO Box 1656, Lawrence, KS 66044. TEL 785-841-3534, 800-457-0742, FAX 785-841-3568, http://www.morganquitno.com. Ed. Kathleen O'Leary Morgan.

HEALTH STATISTICS WALES. see *SOCIAL SERVICES AND WELFARE—Abstracting, Bibliographies, Statistics*

362.1021 USA ISSN 0362-9279
HA331
IDAHO. DEPARTMENT OF HEALTH AND WELFARE. VITAL STATISTICS (YEAR). Key Title: Annual Summary of Vital Statistics (Boise). Cover title: Vital Statistics, Idaho. Text in English. 1946. a. USD 8 (effective 2000). illus, stat. **Document type:** *Government.* **Description:** Covers statistics of Idaho. Includes population census, natality, mortality, marriages and divorces, induced abortions and more.
Related titles: Microfiche ed.: (from CIS).
Indexed: SRI.
Published by: Department of Health and Welfare, Center for Vital Statistics and Health Policy, 450 W State, 1st Fl, PO Box 83720, Boise, ID 83720-0036. TEL 208-334-5992, FAX 208-332-7261, http://www2.state.id.us/dhw/hwgd_www/health/vs/stats1998.htm. Ed. Janet Wick. Circ: 800.

ILLINOIS. DEPARTMENT OF HUMAN SERVICES. DIVISION OF DISABILITY AND BEHAVIORAL HEALTH SERVICES. ILLINOIS STATISTICS. see *SOCIAL SERVICES AND WELFARE—Abstracting, Bibliographies, Statistics*

614 600 USA
INDEX AND ABSTRACTS OF A P I HEALTH-RELATED RESEARCH (YEARS). Text in English. 1978. irreg., latest vol.13, 1995. free per issue. **Document type:** *Abstract/Index.*
Former titles: American Petroleum Institute. Health and Environmental Sciences Department. Report and Other Publications, Index and Abstracts (1058-675X); American Petroleum Institute. Health and Environmental Sciences Department. Research Reports; American Petroleum Institute. Medicine and Biological Science Department. Medical Research Reports; American Petroleum Institute. Committee of Medicine and Environmental Health. Medical Research Reports
Indexed: API Catal., API Hlth.& Environ., API Oil., API Pet.Ref., API Pet.Subst., API Transport.
Published by: American Petroleum Institute, Publications Section, 1220 L St, N W, Washington, DC 20005. TEL 202-682-8378, http://www.api.org.

614 USA ISSN 1077-1212
HN51
INDEX OF SOCIAL HEALTH. Text in English. a.
Published by: Fordham Institute for Innovation in Social Policy, Fordham Graduate Center, Tarrytown, NY 10591.

INTERNATIONAL NARCOTICS CONTROL BOARD. PSYCHOTROPIC SUBSTANCES; assessments of medical and scientific requirements for substances in schedules II, III and IV. Requirements of import authorization for substances in schedules III and IV. see *PHARMACY AND PHARMACOLOGY—Abstracting, Bibliographies, Statistics*

368.384 ITA ISSN 0075-188X
ITALY. ISTITUTO NAZIONALE DI STATISTICA. STATISTICA DEGLI INCIDENTI STRADALI. Text in Italian. 1953. a. ITL 30,000 (effective 1998). **Document type:** *Government.*
Published by: Istituto Nazionale di Statistica (I.S.T.A.T.), Via Cesare Balbo, 16, Rome, RM 00184, Italy. FAX 39-6-46735198.

614 ITA ISSN 1121-1008
RA407.5.I8
ITALY. ISTITUTO NAZIONALE DI STATISTICA. STATISTICHE DELLA SANITA. Text in Italian. 1958. a. ITL 40,000 (effective 1998). **Document type:** *Government.*
Former titles (until 1989): Italy. Istituto Centrale di Statistica. Statistiche Sanitarie (1121-0990); (until 1985): Italy. Istituto Centrale di Statistica. Annuario di Statistiche Sanitarie (0075-1758)
Published by: Istituto Nazionale di Statistica (I.S.T.A.T.), Via Cesare Balbo, 16, Rome, RM 00184, Italy. FAX 39-6-46735198. Circ: 1,150.

628 360 JPN ISSN 0911-8403
HV411
JAPAN. MINISTRY OF HEALTH AND WELFARE. STATISTICS AND INFORMATION DEPARTMENT. HANDBOOK OF HEALTH AND WELFARE STATISTICS. Key Title: Kosei Tokei Yoran. Text in Japanese. 1969. a. JPY 2,940. **Document type:** *Government.*
Related titles: English ed.: Health and Welfare Statistics in Japan.
Published by: Ministry of Health and Welfare, Statistics and Information Department/Koseisho Daijin Kanbo Tokei Johobu, 1-2-3 Kasumigaseki, Chiyoda-ku, Tokyo 100-0013, Japan. TEL 91-3-3503-1711, FAX 91-3-3595-1607. **Subscr. to:** Health & Welfare Statistics Association, 5-13-14 Roppongi, Minato-ku, Tokyo 106-0032, Japan. TEL 03-3586-3361, FAX 81-3-3584-4710.

614 312.3 JPN ISSN 0911-8489
JAPAN. MINISTRY OF HEALTH AND WELFARE. STATISTICS AND INFORMATION DEPARTMENT. STATISTICAL REPORT ON COMMUNICABLE DISEASES. Key Title: Densenbyo Tokei. Text in English, Japanese. a. JPY 3,150 (effective 1998). **Document type:** *Government.*
Supersedes in part (in 1981): Japan. Ministry of Health and Welfare. Statistics and Information Department. Statistical Report on Communicable Diseases and Food Poisonings
Published by: Ministry of Health and Welfare, Statistics and Information Department/Koseisho Daijin Kanbo Tokei Johobu, 1-2-3 Kasumigaseki, Chiyoda-ku, Tokyo 100-0013, Japan. TEL 81-3-3260-3181, FAX 81-3-3595-1607. R&P Yoke Kanegae. **Subscr. to:** Health & Welfare Statistics Association, 5-13-14 Roppongi, Minato-ku, Tokyo 106-0032, Japan. TEL 81-3-3586-3361, FAX 81-3-3584-4710.

614 JPN ISSN 0911-8497
JAPAN. MINISTRY OF HEALTH AND WELFARE. STATISTICS AND INFORMATION DEPARTMENT. STATISTICAL REPORT ON FOOD POISONINGS. Key Title: Shokuchudoku Tokei. Text in English, Japanese. a. JPY 3,360 (effective 1998). **Document type:** *Government.*
Supersedes in part (in 1981): Japan. Ministry of Health and Welfare. Statistics and Information Department. Statistical Report on Communicable Diseases and Food Poisonings
Published by: Ministry of Health and Welfare, Statistics and Information Department/Koseisho Daijin Kanbo Tokei Johobu, 1-2-3 Kasumigaseki, Chiyoda-ku, Tokyo 100-0013, Japan. TEL 81-3-3503-1711, FAX 81-3-3595-1607. R&P Yoke Kanegae. **Subscr. to:** Health & Welfare Statistics Association, 5-13-14 Roppongi, Minato-ku, Tokyo 106-0032, Japan. TEL 81-3-3586-3361, FAX 81-3-3584-4710.

614 315 JPN ISSN 0448-3952
JAPAN. MINISTRY OF HEALTH AND WELFARE. STATISTICS AND INFORMATION DEPARTMENT. STATISTICAL REPORT ON PUBLIC HEALTH ADMINISTRATION AND SERVICES/EISEI GYOSEI GYOMU HOKOKU. Text in Japanese. 1960. a. JPY 6,720 (effective 1998). **Document type:** *Government.*
Formerly: Eisei Nenpo
Published by: Ministry of Health and Welfare, Statistics and Information Department/Koseisho Daijin Kanbo Tokei Johobu, 1-2-3 Kasumigaseki, Chiyoda-ku, Tokyo 100-0013, Japan. TEL 81-3-3503-1700, FAX 81-3-3595-1607. R&P Yoke Kanegae. **Subscr. to:** Health & Welfare Statistics Association, 5-13-14 Roppongi, Minato-ku, Tokyo 106-0032, Japan. TEL 81-3-3586-3361, FAX 81-3-3584-4710.

JOURNAL OF PREVENTION AND INTERVENTION IN THE COMMUNITY. see *PSYCHOLOGY—Abstracting, Bibliographies, Statistics*

614.1 USA
KENTUCKY ANNUAL VITAL STATISTICS REPORT. Text in English. 1911. a. USD 10 (effective 1999). back issues avail. **Document type:** *Government.* **Description:** Presents birth, death, marriage, and divorce statistics in the state of Kentucky for the year.
Former titles: Kentucky. Cabinet for Health Services. Vital Statistics Report; Kentucky. Cabinet for Human Resources. Vital Statistics Report; Kentucky. Department for Human Resources. Selected Vital Statistics and Planning Data (0145-5990); Kentucky Vital Statistics (0098-6739); Kentucky Vital Statistics Report
Indexed: SRI.
Published by: Department for Public Health, 275 E Main St, Frankfort, KY 40621. TEL 502-564-2757, FAX 502-564-6533. Ed. George Robertson. Circ: 600.

614 NLD ISSN 0075-6954
RA412.5.N4
KOSTEN EN FINANCIERING VAN DE GEZONDHEIDSZORG IN NEDERLAND/COST OF HEALTH CARE IN THE NETHERLANDS. Text in Dutch, English. 1953. irreg. NLG 25. **Document type:** *Government.*
—KNAW.
Published by: Centraal Bureau voor de Statistiek, Prinses Beatrixlaan 428, PO Box 4000, Voorburg 2270 JM, Netherlands. TEL 31-70-337-3800, FAX 31-70-387-7429, infoservice@cbs.nl, http://www.cbs.nl. **Orders to:** SDU-Publishers, Christoffel Plantijnstraat 2, The Hague 2500 EA, Netherlands.

614 016 USA ISSN 1077-5587
RA410.A1 CODEN: MCRRFH
MEDICAL CARE RESEARCH AND REVIEW. Text in English. 1944. q. USD 75 to individuals; USD 265 to institutions; USD 25 newsstand/cover to individuals; USD 75 newsstand/cover to institutions (effective 2002). adv. bk.rev. bibl, illus, abstr. back issues avail.; reprint service avail. from PQC. *Refereed.* **Document type:** *Academic/Scholarly.* **Description:** Analyzes, critiques, and synthesizes literature and research in the field of health care.
Former titles (until Mar. 1995): Medical Care Review (0025-7087); Public Health Economics and Medical Care Abstracts
Related titles: Microform ed.: (from PQC); Online - full text ed.: (from EBSCO Publishing, O C L C Online Computer Library Center, Inc., RoweCom Information Quest, ProQuest Information & Learning, ingenta, Swets Blackwell, Institute for Scientific Information).
Indexed: ASSIA, Abstr.Soc.Geront., AgeLine, CINAHL, Curr.Cont., Human Resour.Abstr., Ind.Med. (1995-), Int.Nurs.Ind., P.A.I.S., PsycInfo, SSCI, e-psyche.

—BLDSC (5526.908000), CISTI, GNLM, IDS, ingenta.
CCC.
Published by: (Foundation of the American College of Healthcare Executives), Sage Publications, Inc., 2455 Teller Rd, Thousand Oaks, CA 91320. TEL 805-499-0721, FAX 805-499-0871, order@sagepub.com, info@sagepub.com, http://www.sagepub.com. Eds. Jeffrey Alexander, Thomas Rice. R&P Tanya Udin. Adv. contact DeAnna Vega Hammersley. Circ: 1,300. **Overseas subscr. to:** Sage Publications Ltd., 6 Bonhill St, London EC2A 4PU, United Kingdom; Sage Publications India Pvt. Ltd., 4215, New Delhi 110 048, India.

614 362.1 BGR
MEDITSINSKI PREGLED. MEDITSINSKI MENIDZHMENT I ZDRAVNA POLITIKA. Text in Bulgarian. 1970. q., latest vol.32, 2001. BGL 14 domestic; USD 30 foreign (effective 2001 - 2002). adv. bk.rev. abstr. bibl. index. 48 p./no. *Refereed.* **Document type:** *Journal, Academic/Scholarly, Abstract/Index, Bibliography.* **Description:** Contains original articles and abstracts of foreign publications in the field of public health planning and administration.
Formerly: Informatsiia za Rakovodni Kadri v Zdraveopazvaneto i Meditsinskata Nauka (0204-9791)
Published by: Meditsinski Universitet - Sofia, Tsentur za Informatsiia po Meditsina/Medical University - Sofia, Medical Information Center, 1 Sv Georgi Sofiiski ul, Sofia 1431, Bulgaria. TEL 359-2-9522342, FAX 359-2-9522393, mutafov@sun.medun.acad.bg, http://www.medun.acad.bg. Ed. Dr. V Borissovv. R&P, Adv. contact Dr. Christo Mutafov. B&W page USD 50, color page USD 150; trim 160 x 110. Circ: 350. **Dist. by:** Sofia Books, Ul Silivria 16, Sofia 1404, Bulgaria. TEL 359-2-9586257, sofiabooks@hotmail.com, http://www.sofiabooks.hit.bg.

614 310 USA ISSN 0539-7413
RA407.4.M5
MICHIGAN HEALTH STATISTICS. Text in English. 1898. a. illus. **Document type:** *Government.* **Description:** Statistical tables, graphs, and text containing natality, mortality, life expectancy, infant mortality, marriage and divorce information for the residents of Michigan.
Formerly: Michigan Public Health Statistics
Related titles: Microfiche ed.
Published by: Department of Community Health, Division for Vital Records and Health Statistics, 3423 N Martin Luther King Jr Blvd, Box 30619, Lansing, MI 48909. TEL 517-335-8705, FAX 517-335-8711, sandbornJoy@state.mi.us, http://www.mdch.state.mi.us. Ed. Kathy Humphrys. Circ: 1,000.

362.1 USA ISSN 0094-5641
RA407.4.M6
MINNESOTA HEALTH STATISTICS. Text in English. 1972. a. USD 10.95. **Document type:** *Government.*
Indexed: SRI.
Published by: Department of Health, Center for Health Statistics, 717 Delaware St, S E, Box 9441, Minneapolis, MN 55440-9441. TEL 612-297-3000, FAX 612-623-5264. Ed. Linda Salkowicz. R&P Angie Sechler. Circ: 900. **Subscr. to:** Minnesota Bookstore, Print Communications Division, 117 University Ave., St. Paul, MN 55155.

MISSOURI MONTHLY VITAL STATISTICS. see *POPULATION STUDIES—Abstracting, Bibliographies, Statistics*

317.78 USA ISSN 0098-1974
HA471
MISSOURI VITAL STATISTICS. Text in English. a. free per issue. **Document type:** *Government.* **Description:** Contains tables and graphs.
Related titles: Microfiche ed.: (from CIS).
Indexed: SRI.
Published by: Department of Health, Center for Health Information Management & Epidemiology, PO Box 570, Jefferson City, MO 65102. TEL 314-751-6272. Ed. Garland Land. Circ: 900.

317.86 USA ISSN 0077-1198
HA481
MONTANA VITAL STATISTICS. Text in English. 1954. a. free per issue. **Document type:** *Government.*
Former titles: Montana. State Department of Health. Annual Statistical Supplement (0097-9120); Montana State Board of Health. Annual Statistical Supplement (0097-9112)
Indexed: SRI.
Published by: Department of Public Health and Human Services, Vital Statistics Bureau, 111 N Sanders, Helena, MT 59604. TEL 406-444-2614, FAX 406-444-2606. Circ: 850 (controlled).

NARCOTIC DRUGS: ESTIMATED WORLD REQUIREMENTS FOR (YEAR). see *PHARMACY AND PHARMACOLOGY—Abstracting, Bibliographies, Statistics*

362.1 NLD
NETHERLANDS. CENTRAAL BUREAU VOOR DE STATISTIEK. LEEFSITUATIE VAN DE NEDERLANDSE BEVOLKING, DEEL 1: GEZONDHEID EN KWALITEIT VAN DE ARBEID. Key Title: Leefsituatie van de Nederlandse Bevolking, Deel 1: Gezondheid en Kwaliteit van de Arbeid. Text in Dutch. 1975. a. NLG 24.50, EUR 11.12 per issue. charts. **Document type:** *Government.* **Description:** Surveys the current situation and trends regarding overall public health and working conditions, analyzed by age, gender, race, level of education and professional or vocational training completed, socioeconomic status, and household composition.
—KNAW.
Published by: Centraal Bureau voor de Statistiek, Prinses Beatrixlaan 428, PO Box 4000, Voorburg 2270 JM, Netherlands. TEL 31-70-337-3800, FAX 31-70-387-7429, infoservice@cbs.nl, http://www.cbs.nl.

362.1021 304.6 NZL
NEW ZEALAND. STATISTICS NEW ZEALAND. HOUSEHOLD HEALTH SURVEY. Text in English. irreg., latest 1996-97. stat. **Document type:** *Government.* **Description:** Contains information about the health status of New Zealanders, their use and perception of health related behaviors such as smoking, alcohol consumption and exercise.
Related titles: Online - full content ed.
Published by: Statistics New Zealand/Te Tari Tatau, PO Box 2922, Wellington, New Zealand. TEL 64-4-495-4600, FAX 64-4-473-2626, info@stats.govt.nz, http://www.stats.govt.nz.

362.1021 NOR ISSN 0332-7906
HA1501
NORWAY. STATISTISK SENTRALBYRAA. HELSESTATISTIKK/STATISTICS NORWAY. HEALTH STATISTICS. Text in Norwegian; Summaries in English. 1962. a. NOK 80. **Document type:** *Government.*
Published by: Statistisk Sentralbyraa, Postboks 8131, Dep, Oslo 0033, Norway. TEL 47-22-86-45-00, FAX 47-22-86-49-73. Circ: 1,200.

362.9489 DNK ISSN 0906-3013
NYHEDSINFORMATION FOR SOCIAL-, SYGEHUS- OG SUNDHEDSSEKTOR. Text in Danish. 1982. m. DKK 395 (effective 1998). adv. illus. **Document type:** *Newspaper.*
Former titles (until 1990): Informationstidsskrift for Social- og Sundhedssektor (0901-8565); (until 1984): Informationskatalog for Social- og Sundhedssektor (0109-3487)
Published by: Visholm Media AS, Sydvestvej 49, PO Box 221, Glostrup 2600, Denmark. TEL 45-43-63-02-22, FAX 45-43-63-01-13, nyhedsinfo@visholm.dk, http://www.nyhedsinformation.dk. Adv. contact Svend Windahl.

304.6 USA ISSN 0098-5651
RA407.4.O6
OKLAHOMA HEALTH STATISTICS. Text in English. a. free per issue. illus.
Formerly (1943-1971): Public Health Statistics, State of Oklahoma (0099-118X)
Published by: Department of Health, Public Health Statistics Division, N E Tenth and Stonewall, Box 53551, Oklahoma City, OK 73105. TEL 405-271-5600.

304.6 614 USA ISSN 1524-377X
OREGON PUBLIC HEALTH STATISTICS REPORT. Cover title: Oregon Health Division, Vital Statistics Annual Report. Variant title: Oregon Vital Statistics. Text in English. 1960. a. single copies free. stat. **Description:** Consists of Oregon health statistics collected from death, birth, marriage and divorce certificates, adolescent suicide attempt reports, and induced termination of pregnancy reports. Includes tables, graphs, and narrative.
Indexed: SRI.
Published by: Oregon Department of Human Services Center for Health Statistics, Center for Disease Prevention and Epidemiology, Health Division, 800 N E Oregon St, Portland, OR 97232-2109. TEL 503-731-4354, FAX 503-731-3076, http://www.ohd.hr.state.or.us/cdpe/chs/statinfo.htm. Circ: 2,000.

304.6021 614 USA ISSN 1524-3796
▼ **OREGON VITAL STATISTICS COUNTY DATA.** Text in English. 1999. a. stat. **Description:** Consists of Oregon Health Statistics collected from Death, Birth, Marriage and Divorce Certificates, Adolescent Suicide Attempt Reports, and Induced Termination of Pregnancy Reports. Includes tables of information for each Oregon County.
Published by: Oregon Department of Human Services Center for Health Statistics, Center for Disease Prevention and Epidemiology, Health Division, 800 N E Oregon St, Portland, OR 97232-2109. TEL 503-731-4354, FAX 503-731-3076, http://www.ohd.hr.state.or.us/cdpe/chs/statinfo.htm.

614 USA ISSN 0079-7588
PUBLIC HEALTH CONFERENCE ON RECORDS AND STATISTICS. PROCEEDINGS. Text in English. 1950 (no.2). irreg., latest 1995. **Document type:** *Proceedings, Government.*
Published by: U.S. National Center for Health Statistics, 6525 Belcrest Rd, Hyattsville, MD 20782. TEL 301-458-4636, http://www.cdc.gov/nchs/.

614 360 PRI
PUERTO RICO. DEPARTMENT OF HEALTH. BOLETIN ESTADISTICO. Text in Spanish. 1979. irreg. price varies. **Document type:** *Government.*
Incorporates (in 2000): Puerto Rico. Department of Health. Informe de Recursos Humanos de la Salud; Which was formerly (until 1979): Puerto Rico. Department of Health. Informe del Registro de Professionales de la Salud
Published by: Department of Health, Auxiliary Secretariat for Planning, Evaluation, Statistics and Information Systems, Division of Statistics, P O Box 70184, San Juan, PR 00936. TEL 787-274-7875, FAX 787-274-7877. Circ: 500.

RADIATION PROTECTION ABSTRACTS. see *PHYSICS—Abstracting, Bibliographies, Statistics*

016.614 RUS ISSN 0204-3823
REFERATIVNYI ZHURNAL. AVARIINO-SPASATELNYE SLUZHBY. Text in Russian. 1978. m. **Document type:** *Abstract/Index.*
Formerly (until 1990): Risk i Bezopasnost
Published by: Vserossiiskii Institut Nauchnoi i Tekhnicheskoi Informatsii (VINITI), Usievicha ul 20-a, Moscow 125315, Russian Federation. TEL 7-095-1526441, FAX 7-095-943-0060. **Dist. by:** Mezhdunarodnaya Kniga, B Yakimanka 39, Moscow 117049, Russian Federation. TEL 7-095-2384967, FAX 7-095-2384634.

REFERATIVNYI ZHURNAL. ORGANIZATSIYA I BEZOPASNOST' DOROZHNOGO DVIZHENIYA. see *TRANSPORTATION—Abstracting, Bibliographies, Statistics*

614.84 016 RUS ISSN 0202-9898
TH9111
REFERATIVNYI ZHURNAL. POZHARNAYA OKHRANA. Text in Russian. 1971. m. USD 375. **Document type:** *Abstract/Index.*
—East View.
Published by: Vserossiiskii Institut Nauchnoi i Tekhnicheskoi Informatsii (VINITI), Usievicha ul 20-a, Moscow 125315, Russian Federation. TEL 7-095-1526441, FAX 7-095-943-0060. Ed. V E Dedikov. **Dist. by:** Mezhdunarodnaya Kniga, B Yakimanka 39, Moscow 117049, Russian Federation. TEL 7-095-2384967, FAX 7-095-2384634; **US dist. addr.:** East View Publications, 3020 Harbor Ln N, Minneapolis, MN 55447. TEL 612-550-0961.

S.A.R. NEWS. see *PUBLIC HEALTH AND SAFETY*

363.1021 USA ISSN 1084-3744
SAFETY ABSTRACTS. Text in English. 1995. irreg. **Document type:** *Bulletin.*
Published by: Triodyne Inc., 5950 W Touhy Ave, Niles, IL 60714-4610. TEL 847-677-4730, FAX 847-647-2047, infoserv@triodyne.com, http://www.triodyne.com.

614 GBR
SCOTTISH HOME DEPARTMENT. STATISTICAL BULLETINS. Text in English. 1983. q. **Document type:** *Government.*
Formerly: Scottish Home and Health Department. Statistical Bulletin (0264-1178)
Published by: Scottish Home Department, St Andrews House, Rm 324B, Regent Rd, Edinburgh EH1 3DG, United Kingdom. TEL 44-131-244-2227.

P

614 USA
SISTER COMMUNITIES HEALTH PROFILES OF THE U S - MEXICO BORDER/PERFILES DE SALUD DE LAS COMUNIDADES HERMANAS DE LA FRONTERA MEXICO - ESTADOS UNIDOS. Text in English, Spanish. 1994. a. USD 75; USD 500 to corporations; includes all organization publications. **Document type:** *Monographic series.*
Published by: (United States Mexico Border Health Association), Pan American Health Organization, El Paso Field Office, 6006 N Mesa, Ste 600, El Paso, TX 79912. TEL 915-581-6645, FAX 915-833-4768, vilchish@paho.org. Ed. Dr. Hugo Vilchis Licon.

SOUTH AFRICA. STATISTICS SOUTH AFRICA. STATISTICAL RELEASE. ROAD TRAFFIC COLLISIONS. see *TRANSPORTATION—Abstracting, Bibliographies, Statistics*

614.42 NCL ISSN 1018-0893
SOUTH PACIFIC EPIDEMIOLOGICAL AND HEALTH INFORMATION SERVICE ANNUAL REPORT. Text in English, French. 1972. a. **Document type:** *Monographic series.*
Published by: Secretariat of the Pacific Community, PO Box D5, Noumea Cedex 98848, New Caledonia. TEL 687-262000, FAX 687-263818, spc@spc.int, http://www.spc.int.

614.8 610 SWE ISSN 0346-8992
RA407.5.S8
SWEDEN. STATISTISKA CENTRALBYRAAN. STATISTISKA MEDDELANDEN. SUBGROUP HS (PUBLIC HEALTH AND MEDICAL CARE). Text in Swedish; Summaries in English. 1976. irreg. SEK 500 (effective 1992). **Document type:** *Abstract/Index.*
Published by: Statistiska Centralbyraan, Publishing Unit, Orebro 70189, Sweden.

P

614 JPN
TOYAMA-KEN EISEI TOKEI NENPO/TOYAMA PREFECTURE. ANNUAL REPORT OF PUBLIC HEALTH. Text in Japanese. 1949. a. free per issue.
Published by: Toyama-ken Kosei-bu/Toyama Prefecture, Welfare Department, 1-7 Shin-Sogawa, Toyama 930, Japan. Circ: 400.

304.6 USA ISSN 0147-3956
RA407.3 CODEN: NADADR
U.S. NATIONAL CENTER FOR HEALTH STATISTICS. ADVANCE DATA FROM VITAL AND HEALTH STATISTICS. Text in English. 1979 (no.47). irreg. **Document type:** *Government.*
Indexed: AgeLine, Food Sci.& Tech.Abstr., Nutr.Abstr., Popul.Ind.
—GNLM.
Published by: U.S. National Center for Health Statistics, 6525 Belcrest Rd, Hyattsville, MD 20782. TEL 301-458-4636, http://www.cdc.gov/nchs/.

317 016 USA ISSN 0278-4912
Z7553.M43
U.S. NATIONAL CENTER FOR HEALTH STATISTICS. CATALOG OF PUBLICATIONS. Text in English. a. free per issue. **Document type:** *Catalog, Government.*
Formerly: U.S. National Center for Health Statistics. Current Listing and Topical Index to the Vital and Health Statistics Series (0092-7287)
Published by: U.S. National Center for Health Statistics, 6525 Belcrest Rd, Hyattsville, MD 20782. TEL 301-458-4636, http://www.cdc.gov/nchs/.

304.6 USA ISSN 0083-2014
RA409
U.S. NATIONAL CENTER FOR HEALTH STATISTICS. VITAL AND HEALTH STATISTICS. SERIES 1. PROGRAMS AND COLLECTION PROCEDURES. Text in English. 1963. irreg., latest vol.37. price varies. **Document type:** *Monographic series, Government.*
Indexed: Chic.Per.Ind., Excerp.Med., Ind.Med. (1963-).
Published by: U.S. National Center for Health Statistics, Data Dissemination Branch, 6525 Belcrest Rd, Hyattsville, MD 20782. TEL 301-458-4636, http://www.cdc.gov/nchs/. **Orders to:** U.S. Government Printing Office, Superintendent of Documents.

614 USA ISSN 0083-1972
U.S. NATIONAL CENTER FOR HEALTH STATISTICS. VITAL AND HEALTH STATISTICS. SERIES 10. DATA FROM THE HEALTH INTERVIEW SURVEY. Text in English. 1963. irreg., latest vol.199. price varies. **Document type:** *Government.*
Indexed: Excerp.Med., Ind.Med. (1963-).
Published by: U.S. National Center for Health Statistics, Data Dissemination Branch, 6525 Belcrest Rd, Hyattsville, MD 20782. TEL 301-458-4636, http://www.cdc.gov/nchs/. **Orders to:** U.S. Government Printing Office, Superintendent of Documents.

614 USA
U.S. NATIONAL CENTER FOR HEALTH STATISTICS. VITAL AND HEALTH STATISTICS. SERIES 11. DATA FROM THE HEALTH AND NUTRITION EXAMINATION SURVEY. Variant title: Data from the Health Examination Survey and the National Health and Nutrition Examination Survey. Text in English. 1964. irreg., latest vol.242. price varies. **Document type:** *Government.*
Formerly: U.S. National Center for Health Statistics. Vital and Health Statistics. Series 11. Data from the Health Examination Survey (0083-1980)
Indexed: Excerp.Med., Ind.Med. (1964-).
Published by: U.S. National Center for Health Statistics, Data Dissemination Branch, 6525 Belcrest Rd, Hyattsville, MD 20782. TEL 301-458-4636, http://www.cdc.gov/nchs/. **Orders to:** U.S. Government Printing Office, Superintendent of Documents.

614 USA
U.S. NATIONAL CENTER FOR HEALTH STATISTICS. VITAL AND HEALTH STATISTICS. SERIES 14. DATA ON HEALTH RESOURCES. Text in English. 1968. irreg., latest vol.34. price varies. **Document type:** *Government.*
Formerly: U.S. National Center for Health Statistics. Vital and Health Statistics. Series 14. Data on Health Resources: Manpower and Facilities (0083-1999)
Indexed: Excerp.Med., Ind.Med. (coverage dropped).
Published by: U.S. National Center for Health Statistics, Data Dissemination Branch, 6525 Belcrest Rd, Hyattsville, MD 20782. TEL 301-458-4636, http://www.cdc.gov/nchs/. **Orders to:** U.S. Government Printing Office, Superintendent of Documents. TEL 202-574-1800, FAX 202-574-2250.

304.6 USA ISSN 0083-2057
RA409 CODEN: VHSBA
U.S. NATIONAL CENTER FOR HEALTH STATISTICS. VITAL AND HEALTH STATISTICS. SERIES 2. DATA EVALUATION AND METHODS RESEARCH. Text in English. 1963. irreg., latest vol.125. price varies. **Document type:** *Government.*
Indexed: Excerp.Med., Ind.Med. (1963-), Popul.Ind.
Published by: U.S. National Center for Health Statistics, Data Dissemination Branch, 6525 Belcrest Rd, Hyattsville, MD 20782. TEL 301-458-4636, http://www.cdc.gov/nchs/. **Orders to:** U.S. Government Printing Office, Superintendent of Documents.

304.6 USA ISSN 0083-2022
U.S. NATIONAL CENTER FOR HEALTH STATISTICS. VITAL AND HEALTH STATISTICS. SERIES 20. DATA ON MORTALITY. Text in English. 1965. irreg., latest vol.31. price varies. **Document type:** *Government.*
Supersedes in part (in 1973): U.S. National Center for Health Statistics. Vital and Health Statistics. Series 22. Data on Natality and Mortality Surveys (0083-2049)
Indexed: Excerp.Med., Ind.Med. (1965-).
Published by: (Data Dissemination Branch), U.S. National Center for Health Statistics, Data Dissemination Branch, 6525 Belcrest Rd, Hyattsville, MD 20782. TEL 301-458-4636, http://www.cdc.gov/nchs/. **Orders to:** U.S. Government Printing Office, Superintendent of Documents.

304.6 USA ISSN 1057-7629
HB3505
U.S. NATIONAL CENTER FOR HEALTH STATISTICS. VITAL AND HEALTH STATISTICS. SERIES 21. DATA ON NATALITY, MARRIAGE, AND DIVORCE. Key Title: Vital and Health Statistics. Series 21. Data on Natality, Marriage, and Divorce. Variant title: Data on Natality, Marriage, and Divorce. Text in English. 1964. irreg., latest vol.55. price varies. **Document type:** *Government.*
Formerly (until 1989): U.S. National Center for Health Statistics. Vital and Health Statistics. Series 21. Data from the National Vital Statistics System (0083-2030); Which incorporated in part (in 1973): U.S. National Center for Health Statistics. Vital and Health Statistics. Series 22. Data on Natality and Mortality Surveys (0083-2049)
Indexed: Excerp.Med., Ind.Med. (1989-), Popul.Ind.
Published by: U.S. National Center for Health Statistics, Data Dissemination Branch, 6525 Belcrest Rd, Hyattsville, MD 20782. TEL 301-458-4636, http://www.cdc.gov/nchs/. **Orders to:** U.S. Government Printing Office, Superintendent of Documents.

304.6 USA ISSN 0278-5234
U.S. NATIONAL CENTER FOR HEALTH STATISTICS. VITAL AND HEALTH STATISTICS. SERIES 23. DATA FROM THE NATIONAL SURVEY OF FAMILY GROWTH. Text in English. 1976. irreg., latest vol.20. **Document type:** *Government.*
Indexed: Ind.Med. (1977-), Popul.Ind.
Published by: U.S. National Center for Health Statistics, Data Dissemination Branch, 6525 Belcrest Rd, Hyattsville, MD 20782. TEL 301-458-4636, http://www.cdc.gov/nchs/. **Subscr. to:** U.S. Government Printing Office, Superintendent of Documents.

304.6 USA
U.S. NATIONAL CENTER FOR HEALTH STATISTICS. VITAL AND HEALTH STATISTICS. SERIES 24. COMPILATIONS OF DATA ON NATALITY, MORTALITY, DIVORCE, AND INDUCED TERMINATIONS OF PREGNANCY. Text in English. 1989. irreg., latest vol.8. price varies. **Document type:** *Monographic series, Government.* **Description:** Reports on trends of births, deaths, marriages and divorces, along with abortions.
Indexed: Excerp.Med.
Published by: U.S. National Center for Health Statistics, Data Dissemination Branch, 6525 Belcrest Rd, Hyattsville, MD 20782. TEL 301-458-4636, http://www.cdc.gov/nchs/. **Orders to:** U.S. Government Printing Office, Superintendent of Documents.

304.6 USA ISSN 0083-2065
U.S. NATIONAL CENTER FOR HEALTH STATISTICS. VITAL AND HEALTH STATISTICS. SERIES 3. ANALYTICAL STUDIES. Text in English. 1964. irreg., latest vol.31. price varies. **Document type:** *Government.*
Indexed: Excerp.Med., Ind.Med. (coverage dropped).
Published by: U.S. National Center for Health Statistics, Data Dissemination Branch, 6525 Belcrest Rd, Hyattsville, MD 20782. TEL 301-458-4636, http://www.cdc.gov/nchs/. **Orders to:** U.S. Government Printing Office, Superintendent of Documents.

304.6 USA ISSN 0083-2073
HA37
U.S. NATIONAL CENTER FOR HEALTH STATISTICS. VITAL AND HEALTH STATISTICS. SERIES 4. DOCUMENTS AND COMMITTEE REPORT. Text in English. 1965. irreg., latest vol.30. price varies. **Document type:** *Government.*
Indexed: Excerp.Med., Ind.Med. (1965-).
Published by: U.S. National Center for Health Statistics, Data Dissemination Branch, 6525 Belcrest Rd, Hyattsville, MD 20782. TEL 301-458-4636, http://www.cdc.gov/nchs/. **Orders to:** U.S. Government Printing Office, Superintendent of Documents.

304.6 USA ISSN 0892-8959
U.S. NATIONAL CENTER FOR HEALTH STATISTICS. VITAL AND HEALTH STATISTICS. SERIES 5. COMPARATIVE INTERNATIONAL VITAL AND HEALTH STATISTICS REPORTS. Text in English. 1984. irreg., latest vol.9. price varies. **Document type:** *Monographic series, Government.* **Description:** Comprises analytical and descriptive reports comparing U.S. vital and health statistics with those of other countries.
Indexed: Excerp.Med., Ind.Med. (1984-).
Published by: U.S. National Center for Health Statistics, Data Dissemination Branch, 6525 Belcrest Rd, Hyattsville, MD 20782. TEL 301-458-4636, http://www.cdc.gov/nchs/. **Orders to:** U.S. Government Printing Office, Superintendent of Documents.

U.S. NATIONAL CENTER FOR HEALTH STATISTICS. VITAL AND HEALTH STATISTICS. SERIES 6. COGNITION AND SURVEY MEASUREMENT. see *PSYCHOLOGY—Abstracting, Bibliographies, Statistics*

THE UNIVERSAL HEALTHCARE ALMANAC. see *STATISTICS*

614.109 USA ISSN 0083-6710
HA203
VITAL STATISTICS OF THE UNITED STATES. Text in English. 1937. a. (in 2 vols.). price varies. **Document type:** *Government.*
Indexed: Russ.Acad.Sci.Bibl.
—GNLM.
Published by: U.S. National Center for Health Statistics, Data Dissemination Branch, 6525 Belcrest Rd, Hyattsville, MD 20782. TEL 301-458-4636, http://www.cdc.gov/nchs/. **Orders to:** U.S. Government Printing Office, Superintendent of Documents.

628 016 AUT ISSN 0083-761X
WASTE MANAGEMENT RESEARCH ABSTRACTS. Text in English. 1965. biennial. free per issue. **Document type:** *Abstract/Index.*
Related titles: Online - full text ed.
Indexed: GeoRef.
Published by: International Atomic Energy Agency/Agence Internationale de l'Energie Atomique, Division of Conference and Document Services, Wagramer Str 5, Postfach 100, Vienna, W 1400, Austria. TEL 43-1-2600-0, FAX 43-1-2600-7, ron.shani@iaea.org, http://www.iaea.org/cgi-bin/irais.showwmt.pl?wmwmra.wmt, http://www.iaea.org/programmes/irais/. Circ: 2,100.

614 CHE ISSN 0250-3794
RA651
WORLD HEALTH STATISTICS ANNUAL. Text in English, French. a. USD 99 (effective 1999). **Description:** Contains life tables, changing morbidity and mortality rates for virtually every country in the world.
Formerly (until 1965): Annual Epidemiological and Vital Statistics (0509-2531)
Related titles: Microfiche ed.: (from CIS); ♦ Russian ed.: Ezhegodnik Mirovoi Sanitarnoi Statistiki. ISSN 0250-8664.
Indexed: IIS.
—BLDSC (9356.050000), GNLM.
Published by: World Health Organization, Marketing and Dissemination, Geneva, 27 1211, Switzerland. TEL 41-22-791-2476, FAX 41-22-791-4857, publications@who.ch, http://www.who.int. Circ: 4,800.

614.7 310 JPN ISSN 0915-048X
CODEN: YKSNDQ
YAMAGUCHIKEN EISEI KOGAI KENKYU SENTA NENPO. Text in Japanese. 1987. a. per issue exchange basis. **Description:** Annual report of the center. Reports on pollution control for air, water, noise, vibration, and offensive odors, as well as food safety and public health-related issues.
Formed by the merger of (1958-1987): Yamaguchiken Eisei Kenkyujo Nenpo (0288-7436); (1974-1987): Yamaguchi (0914-031X)
Indexed: Abstr.Hyg., Anal.Abstr.
—CASDDS.
Published by: Yamaguchiken Eisei Kogai Kenkyu Senta/Yamaguchi Prefectural Research Institute of Health, 5-67 Aoi 2-chome, Yamaguchi-shi 753-0821, Japan. TEL 81-839-22-7630, FAX 81-839-22-7632. Circ: 500.

PUBLISHING AND BOOK TRADE

see also BIBLIOGRAPHIES; JOURNALISM; LIBRARY AND INFORMATION SCIENCES; PATENTS, TRADEMARKS AND COPYRIGHTS

A M P A NEWSLETTER. see *MEDICAL SCIENCES*

090 GBR
ANNUAL REGISTER OF BOOK VALUES - SCIENCES & MEDICINE. Text in English. 1987. a. GBP 22, USD 38 (effective 1998). back issues avail. **Document type:** *Bibliography.* **Description:** Provides information on the market values of old and used scientific and medical books.
Formerly (until 1996): International Rare Book Prices - Sciences and Medicine (0952-2999)
Published by: Clique, Ltd., 7 Pulleyn Dr., York YO2 2DY, United Kingdom. TEL 44-1904-631752, FAX 44-1904-651325. Ed. Michael Cole.

BRAILLE BOOK REVIEW (LARGE PRINT EDITION). see *HANDICAPPED—Visually Impaired*

570 USA
C B E VIEWS* . Text in English. 1978. bi-m. USD 38. adv. bk.rev. **Document type:** *Newsletter.* **Description:** Forum for the exchange of information among authors, editors, and publishers in the life sciences.
Formerly (until 1977): Council of Biology Editors. Newsletter (0164-5609)
Published by: Council of Biology Editors Inc., 11250 Roger Bacon Dr, Ste 8, Reston, VA 20190-5202. TEL 847-480-4349. Ed. Martha Tacker. Adv. contact Alison C Brown. Circ: 1,200.

ELSEVIER SCIENCE. CATALOGUE - BOOKS. see *SCIENCES: COMPREHENSIVE WORKS*

ELSEVIER SCIENCE. CATALOGUE - JOURNALS. see *SCIENCES: COMPREHENSIVE WORKS*

ELSEVIER SCIENCE. CATALOGUE ON CD-ROM. see *SCIENCES: COMPREHENSIVE WORKS*

ELSEVIER SCIENCE. DISPATCH LIST FOR JOURNALS, BOOK SERIES AND PROCEEDINGS. see *SCIENCES: COMPREHENSIVE WORKS*

ELSEVIER SCIENCE. NEW AND FORTHCOMING PUBLICATIONS. see *SCIENCES: COMPREHENSIVE WORKS*

READINGS; a journal of reviews and commentary in mental health. see *MEDICAL SCIENCES—Psychiatry And Neurology*

PUBLISHING AND BOOK TRADE—Computer Applications

070.5797 AUT ISSN 1609-2775
▼ **ONLINE PUBLISHING IN MEDICINE.** Text in English. 2000. q. USD 75 domestic; USD 115 foreign; USD 35 newsstand/cover (effective 2001). adv. back issues avail. *Refereed.* **Document type:** *Journal, Academic/Scholarly.* **Description:** Publishes articles, case reports, reviews, and letters with the aim of improving communications in understanding the multidisciplinary field of modern online publishing involving basic science and clinical research in medicine and biomedicine.
Related titles: Online - full text ed.
Published by: V I C E R Publishing, PO Box 14, Vienna A-1097, Austria. TEL 43-676-9568085, FAX 43-676-9568086, vicer@vicer.org, http://www.vicer.org. Ed., R&P Roland Hofbauer. adv.: B&W page USD 1,700, color page USD 2,200. Circ: 1,000 (paid and controlled).

RADIO

see COMMUNICATIONS—Radio

RADIOLOGY AND NUCLEAR MEDICINE

see MEDICAL SCIENCES—Radiology And Nuclear Medicine

RAILROADS

see TRANSPORTATION—Railroads

REAL ESTATE

see also ARCHITECTURE; BUILDING AND CONSTRUCTION; BUSINESS AND ECONOMICS; BUSINESS AND ECONOMICS—Investments; HOUSING AND URBAN PLANNING; LAW

TAX, ESTATE & FINANCIAL PLANNING FOR THE ELDERLY. see *GERONTOLOGY AND GERIATRICS*

REAL ESTATE—Abstracting, Bibliographies, Statistics

333.33 316.8 ZAF
SOUTH AFRICA. STATISTICS SOUTH AFRICA. CENSUS OF ESTATE AGENCIES, RENT COLLECTORS, APPRAISERS AND VALUERS. Text in English. irreg., latest 1990. ZAR 10 domestic; ZAR 11 foreign (effective 2000). **Document type:** *Government.*
Formerly (until Aug. 1998): South Africa. Central Statistical Service. Census of Estate Agencies, Rent Collectors, Appraisers and Valuers
Published by: Statistics South Africa/Statistieke Suid-Afrika, Private Bag X44, Pretoria 0001, South Africa. TEL 27-12-310-8911, FAX 27-12-310-8500, info@statssa.pwv.gov.za, http://www.statssa.gov.za.

333.33 ZAF
SOUTH AFRICA. STATISTICS SOUTH AFRICA. CENSUS OF LETTING OF OWN FIXED PROPERTY. Text in English. irreg., latest 1993. Free. **Document type:** *Government.*
Formerly (until Aug. 1998): South Africa. Central Statistical Service. Census of Letting of Own Fixed Property
Published by: Statistics South Africa/Statistieke Suid-Afrika, Private Bag X44, Pretoria 0001, South Africa. TEL 27-12-310-8911, FAX 27-12-310-8500, info@statssa.pwv.gov.za, http://www.statssa.gov.za.

RELIGIONS AND THEOLOGY

see also RELIGIONS AND THEOLOGY—Hindu; RELIGIONS AND THEOLOGY—Islamic; RELIGIONS AND THEOLOGY—Judaic; RELIGIONS AND THEOLOGY—Other Denominations And Sects; RELIGIONS AND THEOLOGY—Protestant; RELIGIONS AND THEOLOGY—Roman Catholic

AMERICAN JOURNAL OF PASTORAL COUNSELING. see *PSYCHOLOGY*

AMERICAN LEPROSY MISSIONS ANNUAL REPORT. see *MEDICAL SCIENCES—Communicable Diseases*

200 150 DEU ISSN 0084-6724
ARCHIV FUER RELIGIONSPSYCHOLOGIE. Text in German. 1929 (vol.4). irreg., latest vol.23, 2000. price varies. **Document type:** *Monographic series, Academic/Scholarly.*
Indexed: IBR, IBZ, Ind.Philos., Rel.Ind.One, Rel.Ind.Two, Russ.Acad.Sci.Bibl., e-psyche.
Published by: (Internationale Gesellschaft fuer Religionspsychologie und Religionswissenschaft), Vandenhoeck und Ruprecht, Robert-Bosch-Breite 6, Goettingen 37079, Germany. TEL 49-551-6959-0, FAX 49-551-695917.

291.5642 174.2 NLD ISSN 0926-261X
R725.55
BIOETHICS YEARBOOK. Text in English. 1991. a. NLG 200. *Refereed.* **Document type:** *Monographic series.* **Description:** Discusses and interprets recent theological issues, governmental policies, and general bioethics concerns.
—CCC.
Published by: (Center for Ethics, Medicine and Public Issues), Kluwer Academic Publishers Group (Subsidiary of: Wolters Kluwer N.V.), Spuiboulevard 50, PO Box 17, Dordrecht 3300 AA, Netherlands. FAX 31-78-639-2254, services@wkap.nl, http://www.wkap.nl. **Dist. by:** Journals Department, PO Box 322, Dordrecht 3300 AH, Netherlands. FAX 31-78-654-6474.

200 150 USA
C A P S REPORT NEWSLETTER; fellowship, personal news, membership, convention. Text in English. 1956. q. membership. bibl. **Document type:** *Newsletter.* **Description:** Covers information about and schedules of conventions, activities and decisions of the board; applying Christian beliefs to psychological professions; human interest stories about noteworthy members.
Formerly: EnCAPSulate Newsletter
Indexed: e-psyche.
Published by: Christian Association for Psychological Studies, Inc., PO Box 310400, New Braunfels, TX 78131-0400. TEL 830-629-2277, FAX 830-629-2342. Ed. Randolph K Sanders. Circ: 2,500.

C B M FREUNDESBRIEF. see *SOCIAL SERVICES AND WELFARE*

C H I L D NEWSLETTER. see *CHILDREN AND YOUTH—About*

CHRISTIAN BIOETHICS; non-ecumenical studies in medical morality. see *MEDICAL SCIENCES*

CHRISTIAN CHIROPRACTOR. see *MEDICAL SCIENCES—Chiropractic, Homeopathy, Osteopathy*

CHRISTIAN CHIROPRACTORS ASSOCIATION JOURNAL. see *MEDICAL SCIENCES—Chiropractic, Homeopathy, Osteopathy*

CHRISTIAN MEDICAL JOURNAL OF INDIA. see *MEDICAL SCIENCES*

268 USA ISSN 0009-5575
CHRISTIAN RECORD; for adult blind. Text in English. 1900. q. free to persons with visual impairments. **Document type:** *Magazine.* **Description:** Provides devotional and inspirational reading for adults with visual impairments.
Media: Braille.
Published by: Christian Record Services, PO Box 6097, Lincoln, NE 68506. TEL 402-488-0981, 905-436-6938, FAX 402-488-7582, 905-436-7102, 74617.236@compuserve.com, info@christianrecord.org, http://www.christianrecord.org. Ed. Gaylena Gibson. Circ: 2,900.

CHURCH OF SCOTLAND BRAILLE MAGAZINE. see *HANDICAPPED—Visually Impaired*

R

COMMON BOUNDARY; exploring spirituality, psychotherapy, and creativity. see *PSYCHOLOGY*

200 610 IND
CONTACT; the health & community development magazine of the W C C. Text in English, French, Portuguese, Spanish. q. USD 15, CHF 24. **Document type:** *Bulletin.*
Published by: World Council of Churches, c/o Christian Medical Assocation of India, Plot 2 A-3 Local Shopping Centre, Janak Puri, New Delhi 110 058, India. TEL 91-11-559-9991, FAX 91-11-559-8150, TELEX 415730-OIK-CH, cmaidel@giasdl01.vsnl.net.in, http://www.wcc-coe.org/health. Ed. Darlena David. Circ: 15,000.

DARSHANA INTERNATIONAL; an international quarterly of philosophy, psychology, sociology, psychical research, religion and mysticism. see *PHILOSOPHY*

DIRECTORY OF RESOURCES FOR THE BLIND AND VISUALLY IMPAIRED. see *HANDICAPPED—Visually Impaired*

EVANGELISCHE IMPULSE; Zeitschrift fuer die Arbeit mit alten Menschen. see *GERONTOLOGY AND GERIATRICS*

291.72 610 DEU
GESUNDHEIT IN DER EINEN WELT; Nachrichten aus der Aerzlichen Mission. Text in German. 1950. q. free per issue. bk.rev. illus. **Document type:** *Newsletter, Trade.*
Formerly: Nachrichen aus der Aerztlichen Mission (0027-7398)
Published by: Deutsches Institut fuer Aerztliche Mission/German Institute for Medical Mission, Paul-Lechler-Str 24, Tuebingen 72076, Germany. TEL 49-7071-206-512, FAX 49-7071-27125, difaem@cityinfonetz.de. Ed. Rainward Bastian. R&P Claudia Sander. Circ: 15,000.

GOSPEL MESSENGER. see *HANDICAPPED—Visually Impaired*

200 USA ISSN 1087-1586
HEALING MINISTRY. Text in English. 1995. bi-m. USD 71 domestic to individuals; USD 93 in Canada to individuals; USD 108 elsewhere to individuals; USD 110 domestic to institutions; USD 154 in Canada to institutions; USD 179 elsewhere to institutions (effective 2001). *Refereed.* **Document type:** *Academic/Scholarly.* **Description:** Publishes articles, poems, and commentary on the power of faith and prayer to spiritually heal and/or comfort the ill and dying.
Published by: Prime National Publishing Corp., 470 Boston Post Rd, Weston, MA 02493. TEL 781-899-2702, FAX 781-899-4900, healingministry@pnpco.com, http://www.pnpco.com. Ed., R&P Dennis N Ricci. Pub. Richard A DeVito Sr. TEL 781-899-2702 ext. 107.

R

200 150 USA ISSN 1050-8619
BL53.A1 CODEN: IPRLEB
THE INTERNATIONAL JOURNAL FOR THE PSYCHOLOGY OF RELIGION. Text in English. 1991. q. USD 40 in US & Canada to individuals; USD 70 elsewhere to individuals; USD 320 in US & Canada to institutions; USD 350 elsewhere to institutions (effective 2002). adv. bk.rev. illus. reprints avail. *Refereed.* **Document type:** *Journal, Academic/Scholarly.* **Description:** Forum for reporting specific results and encouraging discussion of the methods, theories, and applications of psychological research, in the broadest sense, to religions.
Related titles: Online - full text ed.: ISSN 1532-7582. USD 36 to individuals; USD 288 to institutions (effective 2002) (from CatchWord Ltd., EBSCO Publishing, O C L C Online Computer Library Center, Inc., RoweCom Information Quest, Swets Blackwell).
Indexed: ASSIA, Lang.& Lang.Behav.Abstr., PsycInfo, Psychol.Abstr. (1991-), Rel.& Theol.Abstr., Rel.Ind.One, Rel.Ind.Two, SOPODA, Soc.Serv.Abstr., Sociol.Abstr., e-psyche.
—BLDSC (4542.506200), CatchWord, ingenta. **CCC.**
Published by: Lawrence Erlbaum Associates, Inc., 10 Industrial Ave, Mahwah, NJ 07430-2262. TEL 201-760-3735, 800-926-6579, FAX 201-236-0072, journals@erlbaum.com, http://www.erlbaum.com/Journals/journals/IJPR/ijpr.htm. Ed. Raymond F Paloutzian TEL 805-565-6233. adv.: page USD 350; trim 5 x 8.

INTERNATIONAL JOURNAL OF CHILDREN'S SPIRITUALITY. see *PSYCHOLOGY*

INTERNATIONAL JOURNAL OF TRANSPERSONAL STUDIES. see *PSYCHOLOGY*

291 150 NLD ISSN 0925-4153
INTERNATIONAL SERIES IN THE PSYCHOLOGY OF RELIGIONS. Text in English, German. 1990. irreg., latest vol.8, 1998. price varies. back issues avail. **Document type:** *Monographic series, Academic/Scholarly.* **Description:** Examines religion from a psychological perspective.
Indexed: e-psyche.
—BLDSC (4549.270500).
Published by: Rodopi, Tijnmuiden 7, Amsterdam 1046 AK, Netherlands. TEL 31-20-611-4821, FAX 31-20-447-2979, F.van.der.Zee@Rodopi.nl, orders-queries@Rodopi.nl, http://www.rodopi.nl. Eds. J M van der Lans, Dr. Jaap A Belzen. **Dist in France by:** Nordeal; **Dist in N America by:** Rodopi (USA), One Rockefeller Plaza, Ste. 1420, New York, NY 10020. TEL 212-265-6360, 800-225-3998, FAX 212-265-6402.

230 362.4 USA
JOHN MILTON MAGAZINE. Text in English. 1933. q. free. **Document type:** *Newspaper.* **Description:** Contains stories, poetry, and informative, educational and devotional reading material from more than 50 religious periodicals.
Related titles: Online - full text ed.; Large type ed. 18 pt.; ♦ Supplement: World Day of Prayer Service.
Published by: John Milton Society for the Blind, 475 Riverside Dr, Rm 455, New York, NY 10115. TEL 212-870-3335, 212-870-3336, FAX 212-870-3229, order@jmsblind.org, http://www.jmsblind.org/jmsmag/index.htm. Ed. Darcy Quigley. Circ: 2,372.

230 150 USA ISSN 1063-2166
JOURNAL OF BIBLICAL COUNSELING. Text in English. 1978. 3/yr. (Academic calender: Fall - Spring). USD 21 domestic to individuals; USD 24 foreign to individuals (effective 2000). bk.rev. Religion Index One: Periodicals by American Theological Library Association. 60 p./no. 2 cols./p. back issues avail. **Document type:** *Journal, Academic/Scholarly.* **Description:** Publishes articles that both advance biblical counseling theoretically and provide concrete "how-to's" for pastors and laymen.
Formerly (until vol.11, no.1, 1992): Journal of Pastoral Practice (0196-9072)
Indexed: CCR, Chr.Per.Ind., Past.Care & Couns.Abstr., Rel.& Theol.Abstr., Rel.Ind.One, Rel.Ind.Two, e-psyche.
Published by: Christian Counseling & Educational Foundation, 1803 E Willow Grove Ave, Glenside, PA 19038. TEL 215-884-7676, FAX 215-884-9435, mailjbc@aol.com, ccefmail@aol.com, http://www.ccef.org. Ed. David Powlison. R&P Susan Gingrich. Circ: 3,000.

JOURNAL OF BIBLICAL ETHICS IN MEDICINE. see *MEDICAL SCIENCES*

JOURNAL OF CHRISTIAN NURSING. see *MEDICAL SCIENCES—Nurses And Nursing*

JOURNAL OF HEALTH CARE CHAPLAINCY. see *PHYSICAL FITNESS AND HYGIENE*

200 157.63 USA ISSN 1053-8755
BV4460.3 CODEN: JMARE2
JOURNAL OF MINISTRY IN ADDICTION & RECOVERY. Text in English. 1994. s-a. USD 50 to individuals; USD 68 in Canada to individuals; USD 73 elsewhere to individuals; USD 95 to institutions; USD 128 in Canada to institutions; USD 138 elsewhere to institutions; USD 185 to libraries; USD 250 in Canada to libraries; USD 268 elsewhere to libraries (effective Aug. 2001). adv. bk.rev. back issues avail.; reprint service avail. from HAW. *Refereed.* **Document type:** *Journal, Academic/Scholarly.* **Description:** Offers pastoral caregivers and others in the addiction field innovative approaches to treating a variety of addictive behaviors.
Related titles: Microform ed.: (from PQC).
Indexed: ASSIA, CINAHL, G.Soc.Sci.& Rel.Per.Lit., Human Resour.Abstr., IMFL, Lang.& Lang.Behav.Abstr., Past.Care & Couns.Abstr., Per.Islam. (1993-), Ref.Zh., Rel.& Theol.Abstr., Rel.Ind.One, Rel.Ind.Two, SOPODA, Sociol.Abstr.
—BLDSC (5020.320000), Haworth.
Published by: Haworth Press, Inc., 10 Alice St, Binghamton, NY 13904-1580. TEL 607-722-5857, 800-429-6784, FAX 607-722-6362, 800-895-0582, getinfo@haworthpressinc.com, http://www.haworthpress.com/journals/journallist.asp. Ed. Rev. Richard Wallace. Pub. William Cohen. R&P Ruthann Heath TEL 607-723-5857 ext 316. Adv. contact Jackie Blakeslee TEL 607-722-5857 ext 346. B&W page USD 315, color page USD 550; trim 6 x 8.5.

250 USA ISSN 0022-3409
BV4000 CODEN: JPACA8
THE JOURNAL OF PASTORAL CARE. Text in English. 1947. q. USD 25.95 domestic to individuals; USD 28.25 foreign to individuals; USD 27.95 domestic to institutions; USD 30.75 foreign to institutions (effective 2000). adv. bk.rev. index. reprint service avail. from PSC,SCH. **Document type:** *Academic/Scholarly.* **Description:** Includes articles that reflect the cutting edges of clinical pastoral education and the pastoral counseling movements.
Related titles: Microfilm ed.: (from PQC).
Indexed: ASSIA, CCR, CERDIC, Int.Nurs.Ind., Mid.East: Abstr.& Ind., Past.Care & Couns.Abstr., Psychol.Abstr., Rel.& Theol.Abstr. (1968-), Rel.Ind.One, Rel.Ind.Two, Soc.Work Res.& Abstr., e-psyche.
—BLDSC (5029.500000), ingenta.
Published by: Journal of Pastoral Care Publications, Inc., 1549 Clairmont Rd, Ste 103, Decatur, GA 30033-4635. TEL 404-320-0195, FAX 404-320-0849, jpcp@jpcp.org, http://www.jpcp.org. Ed. Orlo C Strunk Jr. Adv. contact Janet H Emerson. Circ: 10,000. **Subscr. to:** Journal of Pastoral Care, Subscription Dept, c o Kutztown Publishing Co, Box 346, Kutztown, PA 19530.

JOURNAL OF PSYCHOLOGY AND CHRISTIANITY. see *PSYCHOLOGY*

JOURNAL OF PSYCHOLOGY AND THEOLOGY; an evangelical forum for the integration of psychology and theology. see *PSYCHOLOGY*

200 150 USA ISSN 0022-4197
RC321 CODEN: JRHEAT
JOURNAL OF RELIGION AND HEALTH. Text in English. 1961. q. USD 480, EUR 479 to institutions for print or online ed.; USD 576, EUR 574.80 to institutions for print & online eds.combined (effective 2002). adv. bk.rev. charts, illus. index. reprint service avail. from PQC,ISI. *Refereed.* **Document type:** *Journal, Academic/Scholarly.* **Description:** Explores contemporary modes of religious thought with emphasis on its relevance to current medical and psychological research.
Related titles: Microform ed.: (from PQC); Online - full text ed.: (from EBSCO Publishing, O C L C Online Computer Library Center, Inc., Swets Blackwell, Kluwer Online, Institute for Scientific Information, RoweCom Information Quest).
Indexed: ASCA, AgeLine, Arts & Hum.Cit.Ind., Curr.Cont., Excerp.Med., G.Soc.Sci.& Rel.Per.Lit., Ind.Jew.Per., Mid.East: Abstr.& Ind., Past.Care & Couns.Abstr., Psychol.Abstr., Rel.& Theol.Abstr. (1969-), Rel.Ind.One, Rel.Ind.Two, SSCI.
—BLDSC (5049.350000), IDS, Infotrieve, ingenta. **CCC.**
Published by: (Institute of Religion), Kluwer Academic - Plenum Publishers (Subsidiary of: Wolters Kluwer N.V.), 233 Spring St, New York, NY 10013-1578. TEL 212-620-8000, 800-221-9369, FAX 212-463-0742, info@plenum.com, http://www.wkap.nl/journalhome.htm/0022-4197. Ed. Barry Ulanov. **Subscr. outside the Americas to:** Kluwer Academic Publishers Group, Journals Department, PO Box 322, Dordrecht 3300 AH, Netherlands. TEL 31-78-639-2392, FAX 31-78-654-6474. **Co-sponsor:** Institute of Health.

200 362.4 USA ISSN 1522-8967
BV4460 CODEN: JRDRFJ
JOURNAL OF RELIGION, DISABILITY & HEALTH; bridging clinical practice and spiritual supports. Text in English. 1993. q. USD 60 to individuals; USD 81 in Canada to individuals; USD 87 elsewhere to individuals; USD 140 to institutions; USD 189 in Canada to institutions; USD 203 elsewhere to institutions; USD 160 to libraries; USD 216 in Canada to libraries; USD 232 elsewhere to libraries (effective Aug. 2001). adv. bk.rev. back issues avail.; reprint service avail. from HAW. *Refereed.* **Document type:** *Journal, Academic/Scholarly.* **Description:** Provides an interfaith, interdisciplinary forum that will reflect and support the growing dialogue between religious/spiritual perspectives and clinical/scientific perspectives in supporting people with disabilities and their families.
Formerly (until 1998): Journal of Religion in Disability and Rehabilitation (1059-9258)
Related titles: Microfiche ed.; Microform ed.
Indexed: AMED, ASSIA, Abstr.Anthropol., CINAHL, Human Resour.Abstr., IMFL, Ind.Philos., Lang.& Lang.Behav.Abstr., Past.Care & Couns.Abstr., Per.Islam. (1993-), Rel.& Theol.Abstr., SOPODA, Sage Fam.Stud.Abstr., Soc.Work Res.& Abstr., Sociol.Abstr.
—Haworth.

Published by: Haworth Press, Inc., Haworth Pastoral Press, 10 Alice St, Binghamton, NY 13904-1580. TEL 607-722-5857, 800-429-6784, FAX 607-722-6362, 800-895-0582, getinfo@haworthpressinc.com, http://www.haworthpress.com/journals/journallist.asp. Eds. David Coulter, William C Gaventa. Pub. William Cohen. Adv. contact Jackie Blakeslee TEL 607-722-5857 ext 346. B&W page USD 315, color page USD 550; trim 6 x 8.5. Circ: 600 (paid).

JOURNAL OF RELIGIOUS GERONTOLOGY; the interdisiplinary journal of practice, theory & applied research. see *GERONTOLOGY AND GERIATRICS*

JOURNAL OF SPIRITUAL BODYWORK. see *ALTERNATIVE MEDICINE*

200 150 CAN ISSN 1192-3830
JOURNAL OF THE PSYCHOLOGY OF RELIGION. Text in English. 1992. a. CND 15. **Document type:** *Academic/Scholarly.* **Description:** Forum for drawing impartially on all branches of psychology to shed light on religious phenomena to overcome current compartmentalizations.
Indexed: Rel.& Theol.Abstr., e-psyche.
Published by: McGill University, Faculty of Religious Studies, 3520 University St, Montreal, PQ H3A 2A7, Canada. TEL 514-398-6138. Eds. Arvind Sharma, Kaisa Puhakka.

291 616.89 GBR
LINGDALE PAPERS. Text in English. irreg., latest vol.26. GBP 2 per issue (effective 2001). **Document type:** *Monographic series.* **Description:** Covers topics in psychological therapy from a theological perspective.
Indexed: e-psyche.
—BLDSC (5221.141000).
Published by: Bridge Pastoral Foundation, Queen's College, Somerset Road, Birmingham B15 2QH, United Kingdom.

LINK (MARKET HARBOROUGH). see *HANDICAPPED—Visually Impaired*

200.19 SWE ISSN 1103-5757
LUND STUDIES IN PSYCHOLOGY OF RELIGION. Text in English. 1993. irreg. price varies. **Document type:** *Academic/Scholarly.*
Indexed: e-psyche.
Published by: University of Lund, Department of Theology and Religious Studies, Allhelgma Kyrog 8, Lund 22362, Sweden.

MEDICINE, RELIGION TOGETHER. see *MEDICAL SCIENCES*

MENTAL HEALTH, RELIGION & CULTURE. see *PSYCHOLOGY*

NATIONAL CENTER FOR SCIENCE EDUCATION. REPORTS. see *SCIENCES: COMPREHENSIVE WORKS*

NEW CRUCIBLE; a magazine about man and his environment. see *PSYCHOLOGY*

266.025 GBR
NEW DAY. Text in English. 1896. 2/yr. free per issue. **Document type:** *Bulletin.*
Formerly: Without the Camp (0043-7018)
—CCC.
Published by: Leprosy Mission, Goldhay Way, Orton Goldhay, Peterborough PE2 5GZ, United Kingdom. TEL 44-1733-370505, FAX 44-1733-404880, post@tlmew.org.uk, http://www.leprosymission.org. Ed., R&P Fiona Todd. Circ: 165,000.

THE PARK RIDGE CENTER. BULLETIN. see *MEDICAL SCIENCES*

PASTORAL PSYCHOLOGY. see *PSYCHOLOGY*

RELIGIEUSES DANS LES PROFESSIONS DE SANTE. see *HEALTH FACILITIES AND ADMINISTRATION*

RES MEDICAE. see *MEDICAL SCIENCES*

▼ **RESEARCH NEWS & OPPORTUNITIES IN SCIENCE AND THEOLOGY.** see *SCIENCES: COMPREHENSIVE WORKS*

THE RESHAPING OF PSYCHOANALYSIS; from Sigmund Freud to Ernest Becker. see *PSYCHOLOGY*

SHAMAN; journal of the international society for shamanistic research. see *ALTERNATIVE MEDICINE*

DER SONNTAGSBRIEF. see *GERONTOLOGY AND GERIATRICS*

230 150 USA
SPECIAL INSIGHT. Text in English. 1958. bi-m. USD 18; includes Psychology for Living.
Indexed: e-psyche.
Published by: Narramore Christian Foundation, 250 W Colorado Blvd, Arcadia, CA 91066. TEL 626-821-8400, FAX 626-821-8409, ncf@pacbell.net. R&P Ruth Narramore. Circ: 12,000.

SPIRITUAL MASSAGE MINISTRY NEWSLETTER. see *ALTERNATIVE MEDICINE*

220 USA ISSN 0039-2677
THE STUDENT (LINCOLN). Text in English. 1927. m. free to persons with visual impairments. **Description:** Provides daily helps for the serious adult Bible student with a visual impairment.
Media: Audio cassette/tape. **Related titles:** Braille ed.
Indexed: Curr.Ind.Stat.
Published by: Christian Record Services, PO Box 6097, Lincoln, NE 68506. TEL 402-488-0981, FAX 402-488-7582, info@christianrecord.org, http://www.christianrecord.org. Ed. Doug Kittleson. Circ: 1,500.

290 150 USA
STUDIES IN THE PSYCHOLOGY OF RELIGION. Text in English. irreg., latest vol.7. USD 49.95 per issue (effective 2001). *Refereed.* **Document type:** *Monographic series, Academic/Scholarly.*
Indexed: e-psyche.
—BLDSC.
Published by: Edwin Mellen Press, 415 Ridge St, Box 450, Lewiston, NY 14092. TEL 716-754-2788, FAX 716-754-4056, mellen@wzrd.com, http://www.mellenpress.com/.

291.21 ITA
TESTIMONI; quindicinale di informazione e aggiornamento per istituti di vita consacrata. Text in Italian. 1978. fortn. ITL 50,000, ITL 88,000 foreign (effective 1999). adv. bk.rev. **Description:** Informs consecrated men and women on psychology and spiritual life.
Published by: Centro Editoriale Dehoniano, Via Nosadella, 6, Bologna, BO 40123, Italy. TEL 39-051-306811, FAX 39-051-341706, ced-amm@dehoniane.it. Circ: 11,000.

200 174.2 NLD ISSN 0928-8783
THEOLOGY AND MEDICINE. Text in English. 1992. irreg., latest vol.8, 1995. price varies. back issues avail. *Refereed.* **Document type:** *Monographic series.*
—BLDSC (8814.541220).
Published by: Kluwer Academic Publishers Group (Subsidiary of: Wolters Kluwer N.V.), Spuiboulevard 50, PO Box 17, Dordrecht 3300 AA, Netherlands. FAX 31-78-639-2254, services@wkap.nl, http://www.wkap.nl. **Dist. by:** Journals Department, PO Box 322, Dordrecht 3300 AH, Netherlands. FAX 31-78-654-6474.

TODAY'S CHRISTIAN DOCTOR. see *MEDICAL SCIENCES*

291.432 AUS ISSN 1324-9878
TRANSNATIONAL NETWORK FOR THE STUDY OF PHYSICAL, PSYCHOLOGICAL & SPIRITUAL WELL-BEING. NEWSLETTER. Variant title: Newsletter : Relaxation and Meditation. Text in English. 1989. s-a. AUD 20 domestic; USD 20 foreign (effective 2000). bk.rev. **Document type:** *Newsletter, Academic/Scholarly.* **Description:** Contains topical issues in the field of study; placing articles and book reviews in content of the current issues; emphasizing coming events.
Published by: Linking Publications, 16 Campbell Rd, Kenthurst, NSW 2156, Australia. TEL 61-2-9654-9262, FAX 61-2-9654-9409, mjblows@tig.com.au. Ed., R&P Mark Blows. Circ: 200 (controlled).

V.E. BULLETIN. (Voluntary Euthanasia) see *PHILOSOPHY*

230 615.852 GBR
WHOLENESS. Text in English. 1991. bi-m. GBP 14.40; GBP 16.50 in Europe; GBP 18 elsewhere (effective 2000). adv. bk.rev. **Document type:** *Consumer.* **Description:** Provides news and information on the Christian healing ministry and related topics.
Formerly: Healing and Wholeness (0962-0893)
Published by: Monarch C C P Ltd, PO Box 17911, London SW1E 5ZR, United Kingdom. TEL 44.20-7316-1450, FAX 44-20-7316-1453, monarchccp@premier.org.uk, http://www.premier.org.uk/. Ed. Jane Collins. Adv. contact Robin Jones. B&W page GBP 395, color page GBP 455; trim 210 x 297. Circ: 5,500.

WOMEN TODAY MAGAZINE. see *WOMEN'S INTERESTS*

WORD & DEED. see *MEDICAL SCIENCES—Communicable Diseases*

RELIGIONS AND THEOLOGY—Buddhist

see also ORIENTAL STUDIES

RELIGIONS AND THEOLOGY—Hindu

see also ORIENTAL STUDIES

294.5 IND
ARUT PERUM JOTHI. Text in English, Tamil. 1970 (vol.11). m. INR 6. adv.
Address: Arumbakkam, Chennai, Tamil Nadu 600 029, India.

RELIGIONS AND THEOLOGY—Islamic

297.5642 SAU ISSN 0950-4567
ISLAMIC WORLD MEDICAL JOURNAL. Text in English. 1984. bi-m.
Published by: Islamic Press Agency, P O Box 4288, Jeddah, Saudi Arabia.

RELIGIONS AND THEOLOGY—Judaic

see also ETHNIC INTERESTS

296.3642 ISR ISSN 0793-2952
ASSIA - JEWISH MEDICAL ETHICS. Text in English. 1988. irreg. (2 nos./vol.). USD 20 per vol.. adv. *Refereed.* **Document type:** *Academic/Scholarly.*
Published by: Shaare Zadek Medical Center, Falk Schlesinger Institute for Medical Halachic Research, P O Box 3235, Jerusalem 91031, Israel. TEL 972-2-6555266, FAX 972-2-6523295, medhal@szmc.org.il, http://www.szmc.org.il/machon. Ed. Rabbi Dr Mordechai Halperin. Circ: 500.

296 ISR
BISHVILEI HAREFUAH. Text in Hebrew. a. USD 3 (effective 1998).
Published by: Laniado Hospital, Netanya 42150, Israel. TEL 053-21666. Ed. Rabbi Schwartz.

JEWISH BRAILLE REVIEW. see *HANDICAPPED—Visually Impaired*

JEWISH GUILD FOR THE BLIND. NEWSLETTER. see *HANDICAPPED—Visually Impaired*

296.3 USA ISSN 0700-9801
BF51 CODEN: JPJUD8
JOURNAL OF PSYCHOLOGY AND JUDAISM. (Journal of Psycology and Judaism will cease after completion of vol.24.) Text in English. 1976. q. USD 410, EUR 409.50 to institutions for print or online ed.; USD 492, NLG 1,082.40, EUR 491.40 to institutions for print & online eds.combined (effective 2001). adv. bk.rev. reprint service avail. from PQC,ISI. *Refereed.* **Document type:** *Journal, Academic/Scholarly.* **Description:** Explores the relationship between modern psychology and Judaism on philosophical and clinical levels.
Incorporates (1986-1991): Journal of Aging and Judaism (0884-8688)
Related titles: Microform ed.: (from PQC); Online - full text ed.: (from O C L C Online Computer Library Center, Inc., Swets Blackwell, Kluwer Online).
Indexed: AgeLine, Curr.Cont. (coverage dropped), Excerp.Med., G.Soc.Sci.& Rel.Per.Lit., IBR, Ind.Jew.Per., Ind.Philos., Lang.& Lang.Behav.Abstr., M.L.A., Mid.East: Abstr.& Ind., Past.Care & Couns.Abstr., Psychol.Abstr., Rel.& Theol.Abstr. (1979-), Rel.Ind.One, Rel.Ind.Two, SOPODA, SSCI (coverage dropped), Soc.Serv.Abstr., Sociol.Abstr., Viol.& Abuse Abstr., e-psyche.
—BLDSC (5043.410000), ingenta. **CCC.**
Published by: Kluwer Academic - Plenum Publishers (Subsidiary of: Wolters Kluwer N.V.), 233 Spring St, New York, NY 10013-1578. TEL 212-620-8000, 800-221-9369, FAX 212-463-0742, info@plenum.com, http://www.wkap.nl/journalhome.htm/0700-9801. Ed. Dr. Reuven P Bulka. Circ: 1,000. **Subscr. outside the Americas to:** Kluwer Academic Publishers Group, Journals Department, PO Box 322, Dordrecht 3300 AH, Netherlands. TEL 31-78-639-2392, FAX 31-78-654-6474.

R

296 USA
OUR WAY*. Text in English. 1970. irreg. (3-4/yr.). USD 6. adv. **Description:** News and information about the Jewish deaf community, with emphasis on the youth.
Published by: National Conference of Synagogue Youth, 11 Broadway, New York, NY 10004. TEL 212-613-8233, FAX 212-613-0633, ncsy@ou.org. Ed. Rabbi E Lederfeind. Circ: 2,000.

RELIGIONS AND THEOLOGY—Protestant

280.4 DEU
B I M S. (Blaukreuz Information - Meinungen - Szene) Text in German. 1986. q. DEM 10. adv. bk.rev.
Published by: Blaues Kreuz in der Evangelischen Kirche, Dieterichsstr 17A, Hannover 30159, Germany. TEL 0511-651917. Ed. Guenter Blueder. Circ: 1,500.

283 362.41 GBR ISSN 0009-1529
CHANNELS OF BLESSING. Text in English. 1893. bi-m. GBP 9 (effective 2000). **Document type:** *Bulletin.* **Description:** Digests articles from the Evangelical Christian Press; material includes news, overseas developments, commentary on current issues, personal experiences, Bible study, and devotional thought.
Media: Braille.
Published by: Royal National Institute for the Blind, PO Box 173, Peterborough, Cambs PE2 6WX, United Kingdom. TEL 44-1733-370-777, FAX 44-1733-317555, webmaster@rnib.org.ukk, http://www.rnib.org. Circ: 150. **Co-sponsor:** Torch Trust for the Blind.

DAILY DEVOTIONS FOR THE DEAF. see *HANDICAPPED—Hearing Impaired*

266 GBR
HEALTHSERVE. Text in English. 1962. q. donations only. adv. bk.rev. illus. 20 p./no. back issues avail. *Refereed.* **Document type:** *Magazine, Consumer.* **Description:** Contains articles by Christian doctors, nurses, journalists and medical-health workers in the developing world working through church agencies.
Formerly (until March 2001): Saving Health (0036-5106)
Indexed: CERDIC.
Published by: Medical Missionary Association, 106-110 Watney St, London E1W 2QE, United Kingdom. TEL 44-20-7790-1336, FAX 44-20-7790-1384, magazines@mmahealthserve.org.uk, info@mmahealthserve.org.uk, http://mmahealthserve.org.uk. Eds. Dr. D Clegg, Steven Fouch. Adv. contact Steven Fouch. Circ: 1,000; 1,000 (controlled).

280.4 DEU ISSN 0343-4591
LEBENDIGE SEELSORGE; Zeitschrift fuer alle Fragen der Seelsorge. Text in German. 1949. s-m. DEM 51; DEM 38 to students (effective 1999). adv. bk.rev. **Document type:** *Bulletin.*
Related titles: ♦ Supplement: Lebendige Katechese. ISSN 0171-4171.
Indexed: IBZ, Ind.Philos., e-psyche.
Published by: Seelsorge Verlag Echter, Postfach 5560, Wuerzburg 97005, Germany. TEL 49-931-6671-0, FAX 49-931-6671151. Ed. Lothar Roos. Adv. contact Thomas Haeussner. page DEM 1,500; trim 105 x 139. Circ: 4,000.

LUTHERAN MESSENGER FOR THE BLIND. see *HANDICAPPED—Visually Impaired*

287.6 USA ISSN 0025-6021
BV4580.A1
MATURE YEARS. Text in English. 1954. q. USD 4.50 newsstand/cover; USD 16 (effective 2001). illus. **Document type:** *Consumer.* **Description:** Contains articles of interest to elderly persons, written from a religious perspective.
Related titles: Microform ed.: (from PQC); Large type ed. 14 pt.
Indexed: AgeLine, Meth.Per.Ind.
Published by: (United Methodist Church), United Methodist Publishing House, Cokesbury TEL 615-749-6292, 800-672-1789, FAX 615-749-6512, http://www.umph.org, http://www.umph.org; http://www.gbod.org/. Ed. Marvin Cropsey. Circ: 55,000.

TRACT MESSENGER. see *HANDICAPPED—Visually Impaired*

287.6 USA ISSN 0042-0735
BV4800
THE UPPER ROOM; daily devotional guide, interdenominational, international. Text in English. 1935. bi-m. USD 7.95 domestic; USD 11.95 foreign (effective 2002). **Description:** Contains meditation, prayer, suggested scripture reading, and a prayer focus for each day.
Related titles: Audio cassette/tape ed.: USD 35; Braille ed.: free; Large type ed. 18 pt.: USD 8.95 domestic; USD 12.45 foreign (effective 2002); ♦ Spanish ed.: El Aposento Alto. ISSN 0003-6552.
Published by: (United Methodist Church, General Board of Discipleship), The Upper Room, 1908 Grand Ave, P O Box 340004, Nashville, TN 37203-0004. TEL 615-340-7250, FAX 615-340-7267, theupperroomMagazine@upperroom.org, http://www.upperroom.org. Circ: 2,000,000 (paid).

RELIGIONS AND THEOLOGY—Roman Catholic

C H A C INFO/INFO A C C S. see *HEALTH FACILITIES AND ADMINISTRATION*

C H A C REVIEW. see *HEALTH FACILITIES AND ADMINISTRATION*

C P F I NEWSLETTER. see *PHARMACY AND PHARMACOLOGY*

282 USA ISSN 8756-4068
CATHOLIC HEALTH WORLD. Text in English. 1985. s-m. (22/yr.). USD 35 domestic; USD 40 foreign (effective 2001). adv. 8 p./no. back issues avail. **Document type:** *Newspaper.* **Description:** Contains national and regional news, features, human interest items, articles on people and health care legislation, and reports of events.
Related titles: Online - full text ed.
Published by: Catholic Health Association of the United States, 4455 Woodson Rd., St. Louis, MO 63134-3797. TEL 314-427-2500, FAX 314-427-0029. Ed. Terry Van Schaik. Pub. Rev. Michael D Place. Adv. contact Donna Troy TEL 314-253-3450. Circ: 11,500.

261.561 GBR ISSN 0008-8226
CATHOLIC MEDICAL QUARTERLY. Text in English. 1923. q. GBP 15 to non-members; USD 30 foreign to non-members (effective 2001); Plus 5 British Pounds ($10) postage to addresses outside Europe. adv. bk.rev. bibl. index. back issues avail. **Document type:** *Directory.* **Description:** Consists of information about bio-ethics, the Guild's activities and letters.
Indexed: P C I.
Published by: Guild of Catholic Doctors, 60 Grove End Rd, London NW8 9NH, United Kingdom. TEL 44-20-7266-4246, FAX 44-20-7266-4813. Circ: 2,000.

THE CATHOLIC PHARMACIST. see *PHARMACY AND PHARMACOLOGY*

253.5 USA ISSN 0160-7960
LC461 CODEN: COVADQ
COUNSELING AND VALUES. Text in English. 1956. 3/yr. USD 35 domestic to institutions; USD 47 foreign to institutions (effective 2001). adv. bk.rev. abstr, bibl, illus. 80 p./no. back issues avail.; reprint service avail. from PQC. *Refereed.* **Document type:** *Journal, Academic/Scholarly.* **Description:** Focused on the role of values and religion in counseling and psychology.
Formerly: National Catholic Guidance Conference Journal (0027-8912)
Related titles: Microform ed.: (from PQC); Online - full text ed.: (from ProQuest Information & Learning, H. W. Wilson).
Indexed: AgeLine, C.I.J.E., Cath.Ind., Educ.Ind. (Jan.2001-), High.Educ.Abstr., PsycInfo, Psychol.Abstr. (1971-), Rel.Ind.One, Rel.Ind.Two, Soc.Work Res.& Abstr., e-psyche.
—BLDSC (3481.320000), ingenta. **CCC.**
Published by: (Association for Religious and Value Issues in Counseling), American Counseling Association, 5999 Stevenson Ave, Alexandria, VA 22304-3300. TEL 703-823-9800, FAX 703-823-0252, http://www.counselling.org, http://www.counseling.org, http://www.ncda.org. Ed. Dennis Engels. R&P Cynthia Peay TEL 703-823-9800 x 249. Adv. contact Kathy Maguire TEL 703-823-9800 ext 207. Circ: 3,400.

261.561 USA ISSN 1071-3778
ETHICS AND MEDICS. Text in English. 1976. m. USD 18 domestic; USD 20 foreign (effective 1999). cum.index: 1976-1996. back issues avail. *Refereed.* **Document type:** *Newsletter, Academic/Scholarly.* **Description:** Catholic perspective on moral issues in the health and life sciences.
Related titles: Online - full text ed.: (from EBSCO Publishing).
Indexed: Cath.Ind.
Published by: National Catholic Bioethics Center, 159 Washington St, Brighton, MA 02135-4325. TEL 617-787-1900, FAX 617-787-4900, postmaster@ncbcenter.org, http://www.ncbcenter.org. Ed., R&P Edward J Furton. Pub. John M Haas. Circ: 25,500 (paid).

KATHOLISCHER BERUFSVERBAND FUER PFLEGEBERUFE. MITTEILUNGSBLATT. see *MEDICAL SCIENCES*

266.2 USA
MEDICAL MISSION NEWS. Text in English. 1931. q. free per issue. *Refereed.* **Description:** Distribution of medicines to 6,000 mission units in 60 countries, placement of healthcare professionals and para-professionals in clinical facilities the world over, and indigenous training.
Incorporates (1962-1992): Professional Placement Newsnotes
Published by: Catholic Medical Mission Board, Inc., 10 W 17th St, New York, NY 10011. TEL 212-242-7757, FAX 212-807-9161. Ed. Shirley Stephenson. Circ: 55,000.

NATIONAL FEDERATION OF CATHOLIC PHYSICIANS' GUILDS. NEWSLETTER. see *MEDICAL SCIENCES*

282.0872 DEU
RING DES WORTES; Seelsorgebrief fuer Hoergeschaedigte, Kranke und Senioren. Text in German. 1958. bi-m. free per issue. **Document type:** *Newsletter.* **Description:** Devotional material for hearing impaired and hospitalized people and seniors.
Published by: Erzbischoefliches Generalvikariat, Hauptabteilung Seelsorge, Marzellenstr 32, Cologne 50668, Germany. Ed. Karl Heinz Stockhausen. Circ: 10,500.

RELIGIONS AND THEOLOGY—Other Denominations And Sects

289.3 USA
AFFINITY. Text in English. 1977. m. USD 25 (effective 2001). **Description:** Publication in support of gay and lesbian Mormons; focuses on education of authorities and lay members regarding homosexuality.
Published by: Affirmation: Gay & Lesbian Mormons, PO Box 46022, Los Angeles, CA 90046. TEL 213-255-7251, http://www.affirmation.org. Circ: 750.

299.934 USA ISSN 0006-8918
BRAILLE STAR THEOSOPHIST. Text in English. 1926. s-a. free per issue. **Document type:** *Newsletter, Newspaper.*
Published by: Theosophical Book Association for the Blind, Inc., 54 Krotona Hill, Ojai, CA 93023. TEL 805-646-2121, TBAB@compuserve.com. Circ: 2,500.

289.5 USA ISSN 0145-7365
BX6901
CHRISTIAN SCIENCE QUARTERLY. BIBLE LESSONS (CITATION EDITION). Text in English. 1890. q. USD 18; USD 5 newsstand/cover (effective 2002). adv.
Incorporates (198?-2000): Christian Science Quarterly. Bible Lessons (Study Edition) (1061-6713)

Media: Large Type (13 pt.). **Related titles:** French ed.: Livret Trimestriel de la Christian Science. Lecons Bibliques. ISSN 1520-4170; German ed.: Christian Science Vierteljahrsheft. Bibellektionen. ISSN 1520-4189; Italian ed.: Libretto Trimestrale della Christian Science. Lezioni Bibliche. ISSN 1520-6955; Portuguese ed.: Livrete Trimestral da Christian Science. Licoes Biblicas. ISSN 1520-698X; Spanish ed.: Cuaderno Trimestral de la Christian Science. Lecciones Biblicas. ISSN 1520-7013; Czech ed.: Ctvrtletnik Christian Science. Biblicke Lecke. ISSN 1520-3433; Danish ed.: Christian Science Kvartalshaefte. Bibelstudium; Dutch ed.: Christian Science Kwartaalboekje. Bijbellessen. ISSN 1520-345X; Greek ed.: Trimeniaio Periodiko tes Christian Science. Biblika Mathemata. ISSN 1520-4197; Japanese ed.: Christian Science Kotari. Seisho Kyokar. ISSN 1520-7048; Norwegian ed.: Christian Science Kvartalshefte. ISSN 1520-6963; Russian ed.: Ezhekvartal'nik Christian Science. Bibleiskie Uroki. ISSN 1520-703X; Swedish ed.: Christian Science Kvartalshaefte. Bibelstudium; Polish ed.: Kwartalnik Christian Science. Lekcje Biblijne. ISSN 1520-6971; Indonesian ed.: Buku Triwulanan Christian Science; ♦ Special ed. of: Christian Science Quarterly. Bible Lessons (Full Text Edition). ISSN 1053-251X.
Published by: (First Church of Christ, Scientist), The Christian Science Publishing Society, One Norway St, Boston, MA 02115-3122. TEL 617-450-2213, 800-288-7090, FAX 617-450-2930, fischerm@csps.com, http://www.tfccs.com/GV/CSPS/Quarterly.jhtml. Ed. John Selover. Pub. Noel Fischer. R&P Alex Roth TEL 617-450-3746. Adv. contact Carol Humphry. **Subscr. to:** CDS Subscriver Services, PO Box 37304, Boone, IA 50037-2304. TEL 800-456-4851.

299.934 DEU ISSN 0935-798X
DER MERKURSTAB. Text in German. 1950. bi-m. bk.rev. **Document type:** *Academic/Scholarly.*
—GNLM.
Published by: Gesellschaft Anthroposophischer Aerzte in Deutschland e.V., Roggenstr 82, Filderstadt 70794, Germany. TEL 49-711-7799711, FAX 49-711-7799712, ges.anth.aerzte@t-online.de.

RESPIRATORY DISEASES

see *MEDICAL SCIENCES—Respiratory Diseases*

RHEUMATOLOGY

see *MEDICAL SCIENCES—Rheumatology*

ROADS AND TRAFFIC

see *TRANSPORTATION—Roads And Traffic*

ROBOTICS

see *COMPUTERS—Artificial Intelligence; COMPUTERS—Robotics*

ROMAN CATHOLICISM

see *RELIGIONS AND THEOLOGY—Roman Catholic*

RUBBER

see also *ENGINEERING—Chemical Engineering; PLASTICS*

SCHOOL ORGANIZATION AND ADMINISTRATION

see *EDUCATION—School Organization And Administration*

SCIENCES: COMPREHENSIVE WORKS

A F P SCIENCES; bulletin information scientifique, technique, medicale. see *MEDICAL SCIENCES*

500 570 YUG ISSN 0352-5740
CODEN: BASNA6
ACADEMIE SERBE DES SCIENCES ET DES ARTS. CLASSE DES SCIENCES MATHEMATIQUES ET NATURELLES. BULLETIN SCIENCES NATURELLES. Text in French. 1952. s-a. price varies.
Supersedes in part: Academie Serbe des Sciences et des Arts. Classe des Sciences Mathematiques et Naturelles. Bulletin. Nouvelle Serie (0001-4184)
Related titles: ♦ Serbo-Croatian ed.: Srpska Akademija Nauka i Umetnosti. Odeljenje Prirodno-Matematickih Nauka. Glas. ISSN 0374-7956.
Indexed: Biol.Abstr., Chem.Abstr., Chem.Indus.Notes, Chem.Titles, Deep Sea Res.& Oceanogr.Abstr., Zoo.Rec.
—CASDDS, KNAW, Linda Hall.
Published by: Srpska Akademija Nauka i Umetnosti/Serbian Academy of Arts and Sciences, Knez Mihailova 35, Belgrade 11000, Yugoslavia. TEL 381-11-187144, FAX 381-11-182825, TELEX 72593 SANU. Ed. Vladimir Pantic. Circ: 1,000.

500 BRA ISSN 0044-5967
QH111 CODEN: AAMZAZ
ACTA AMAZONICA. Text in English, Portuguese, Spanish. 1971. irreg. (1-3/yr.). USD 100 (effective 2000). bk.rev. *Refereed.* **Document type:** *Academic/Scholarly.* **Description:** Publication in pure and applied sciences including botany, agronomy, aquatic biology, tropical pathology, forest research, zoology and wood technology.
Related titles: Microfilm ed.: (from OMN).
Indexed: Abstr.Hyg., Agroforest.Abstr., Apic.Abstr., Appl.Ecol.Abstr., Aqua.Sci.& Fish.Abstr., Bio-Contr.News & Info., Biol.Abstr., Chem.Abstr., Chem.Indus.Notes, Chem.Titles, Crop Physiol.Abstr., Curr.Adv.Ecol.Sci., Deep Sea Res.& Oceanogr.Abstr., Entomol.Abstr., Environ.Sci.Poll.Mgmt., Field Crop Abstr., Forest Prod.Abstr., Forest.Abstr., GeoRef, Helminthol.Abstr., Hort.Abstr., INIS Atomind., Irr.& Drain.Abstr., Mass Spectr.Bull., Nutr.Abstr., Plant Breed.Abstr., Protozool.Abstr., Rev.Appl.Entomol., Rev.Med.& Vet.Mycol., Rev.Plant Path., Seed Abstr., Sel.Water Res.Abstr., Soils & Fert., Sport Fish.Abstr., Vet.Bull., Wild.Rev., Zoo.Rec.
—BLDSC (0593.100000), CASDDS, CISTI.
Published by: Instituto Nacional de Pesquisas da Amazonia, Av Andre Araujo, N 2936 Petropolis, PO Box 478, Manaus, AM 69083-000, Brazil. TEL 55-92-643-3220, FAX 55-92-6433030, TELEX 0922269, biblio@inpa.gov.br. Ed. Ozorio Jose de Menezes Fonseca. Circ: 1,500.

500.9 610 DEU ISSN 0001-5857
CODEN: ACHLAG
ACTA HISTORICA LEOPOLDINA. Text in German. 1963. irreg., latest vol.22, 1993. price varies. bibl, charts, illus. **Document type:** *Academic/Scholarly.*
Related titles: ♦ Supplement to: Acta Historica Leopoldina. Supplement. ISSN 0232-8615.
Indexed: BHA, Biol.Abstr., C.C.M.J., IBZ, Math.R., Zent.Math.
—CISTI, Linda Hall.
Published by: (Archiv fuer Geschichte der Naturforschung und Medizin, Deutsche Akademie der Naturforscher Leopoldina), Johann Ambrosius Barth Verlag in Medizinverlage Heidelberg GmbH & Co. KG, Ruedigerstr 14, Stuttgart 70469, Germany. TEL 49-711-8931-0, FAX 49-711-8931422, fuchsm@huethig.de, http://www.huethig.de, http://www.thieme.de. Circ: 1,200.

500.9 DEU ISSN 0232-8615
ACTA HISTORICA LEOPOLDINA. SUPPLEMENT. Text in English. 1977. irreg.
Related titles: ♦ Supplement: Acta Historica Leopoldina. ISSN 0001-5857.
Published by: Johann Ambrosius Barth Verlag in Medizinverlage Heidelberg GmbH & Co. KG, Ruedigerstr 14, Stuttgart 70469, Germany. TEL 49-6221-489251, FAX 49-711-8931422. Ed. S Hofmann von Kap-herr.

509 610.9 DNK ISSN 0065-1311
CODEN: AHSMA7
ACTA HISTORICA SCIENTIARUM NATURALIUM ET MEDICINALIUM. Text in English, German. ceased; resumed 1942. irreg. price varies. back issues avail. **Document type:** *Monographic series.*
Indexed: GeoRef, Ind.Med. (coverage dropped).
—CISTI, GNLM, Infotrieve, Linda Hall. **CCC.**
Published by: (Denmark. Danish National Library of Science and Medicine), Blackwell Munksgaard, Book Division, Noerre Soegade 35, PO Box 2148, Copenhagen K 1016, Denmark. FAX 45-77-33-33-77, subscription.service@mail.munksgaard.dk, http://www.munksgaard.dk. Ed. Poul Aagaard Christiansen.

500 610 MEX ISSN 0188-6266
CODEN: ACUNFO
ACTA UNIVERSITARIA. Text in Spanish; Summaries in English, Spanish. 1991. 3/yr. MXP 20 domestic; USD 10 foreign (effective 2000). adv. bk.rev. abstr, bibl, charts, illus. *Refereed.* **Document type:** *Academic/Scholarly.* **Description:** Publishes research and commentary on social, agricultural, and engineering sciences.
Published by: Universidad de Guanajuato, Direccion de Investigacion, Lascurain de Retana 5, Col Centro, Guanajuato, GTO 36000, Mexico. TEL 52-4-7320006, FAX 52-4-7329312, vargase@quijote.ugto.mx, http://www.ugto.mx/ugto/acta/actuani.html. Ed., R&P, Adv. contact Esperanza Vargas-Pacheco. Circ: 1,500.

500 610 SWE ISSN 0346-5462
ACTA UNIVERSITATIS UPSALIENSIS. Text in Multiple languages. 1861. irreg. price varies. bibl, charts, illus. index. **Document type:** *Monographic series.*
Formerly (until 1960): Uppsala Universitets Aarsskrift (0372-4654)
Indexed: AgBiotech, Bibl.Ling., GeoRef, M.L.A., MLA Intl.Bibl. (coverage dropped), Russ.Acad.Sci.Bibl., Soils & Fert.
—CISTI, KNAW, Linda Hall.
Published by: (Kungliga Vetenskaps-Societeten, Uppsala Universitet), Acta Universitatis Upsaliensis (Subsidiary of: Uppsala University), PO Box 256, Uppsala 75105, Sweden. Ed. Bengt Landgren. **Dist. by:** Almqvist & Wiksell International.

590 USA
ANIMAL NATURAL HISTORY SERIES. Text in English. 1996. irreg. price varies. **Document type:** *Monographic series, Academic/Scholarly.*
Indexed: Zoo.Rec.
Published by: University of Oklahoma Press, 4100 28th Ave N W, Norman, OK 73069. TEL 405-325-2000, FAX 405-364-5798.

577 USA ISSN 1523-0430
G575 CODEN: AAAПГO
ARCTIC, ANTARCTIC AND ALPINE RESEARCH. Text in English. 1969. q. USD 80 domestic to individuals; USD 90 foreign to individuals; USD 125 domestic to institutions; USD 135 foreign to institutions; USD 60 domestic to students; USD 70 foreign to students (effective 2002). adv. bk.rev. bibl, charts, illus, stat, maps. index. back issues avail.; reprint service avail. from PSC,SCH. *Refereed.* **Document type:** *Academic/Scholarly.* **Description:** Presents original research pertaining to cold environments, both past and present.
Formerly: Arctic and Alpine Research (0004-0851)
Related titles: Microform ed.: (from PQC); Online - full text ed.: (from Institute for Scientific Information).
Indexed: ASCA, Abstr.Anthropol., Agricola, Appl.Ecol.Abstr., Aqua.Sci.& Fish.Abstr., Biol.Abstr., Chem.Abstr., Curr.Adv.Ecol.Sci., Curr.Adv.Gen.& Molec.Biol., Curr.Cont., Deep Sea Res.& Oceanogr.Abstr., Ecol.Abstr., Environ.Abstr., Environ.Ind., Environ.Per.Bibl. (1989-), Environ.Sci.Poll.Mgmt., Field Crop Abstr., Forest Prod.Abstr., Forest.Abstr., Geo.Abstr.P.G., GeoRef, Geol.Abstr., Helminthol.Abstr., Herb.Abstr., IDA, INIS Atomind., Ind.Sci.Rev., Int.Abstr.Biol.Sci., Irr.& Drain.Abstr., Key Word Ind.Wildl.Res., Meteor.& Geoastrophys.Abstr., Microbiol.Abstr., Pollut.Abstr., Ref.Zh., Rev.Appl.Entomol., Rev.Med.& Vet.Mycol., Sci.Cit.Ind., Seed Abstr., Sel.Water Res.Abstr., Soils & Fert., Sport Fish.Abstr., Weed Abstr., Wild.Rev., World Ag.Econ.& Rur.Soc.Abstr., Zoo.Rec.
—BLDSC (1663.068000), CASDDS, CISTI, EMDOCS, IDS, Infotrieve, ingenta, Linda Hall. **CCC.**
Published by: University of Colorado, Institute of Arctic and Alpine Research, UCB 450, Boulder, CO 80309-0450. TEL 303-492-3765, FAX 303-492-6388, salzberg@spot.colorado.edu., http://www.colorado.edu/INSTAAR/arcticalpine/. Ed. James P Syvitski. R&P Kathleen Salzberg. Circ: 800.

▼ **BEHAVIORAL & COGNITIVE NEUROSCIENCE REVIEWS.** see *PSYCHOLOGY*

500 IND ISSN 0006-7903
CODEN: TBICAQ
BOSE INSTITUTE. TRANSACTIONS*. Text in English. 1918. q. INR 32, USD 7.50. back issues avail.
Indexed: Biol.Abstr., Chem.Abstr., Field Crop Abstr., Herb.Abstr., INIS Atomind., INSPEC (pre-1969-1991, dropped).
—AskIEEE, CASDDS, CISTI, Linda Hall.
Published by: Bose Institute, 93-1 Acharya Prafulla Chandra Rd., Kolkata, West Bengal 700 009, India. Ed. Dr. D M Bose.

S

CARIBBEAN JOURNAL OF SCIENCE. see *BIOLOGY*

508 USA ISSN 0097-4463
AS36 CODEN: CIMUAU
CARNEGIE MUSEUM OF NATURAL HISTORY. ANNALS. Key Title: Annals of Carnegie Museum. Text in English. 1901. q. USD 35 to individuals; USD 75 foreign to individuals; USD 75 to institutions (effective 1999). charts, illus. index. back issues avail. *Refereed.* **Document type:** *Academic/Scholarly.* **Description:** Contributions in organismal biology, earth sciences and anthropology.
Related titles: Online - full text ed.: (from Institute for Scientific Information).
Indexed: ASCA, Anthropol.Lit. (coverage dropped), Biol.Abstr., Curr.Cont., Deep Sea Res.& Oceanogr.Abstr., Ecol.Abstr., Geo.Abstr.H.G., GeoRef, Geol.Abstr., IBR, Ind.Sci.Rev., Poult.Abstr., Ref.Zh., Rev.Appl.Entomol., Rev.Med.& Vet.Mycol., Sci.Cit.Ind., Sport Fish.Abstr., Wild.Rev., Zoo.Rec.
—BLDSC (1022.000000), CISTI, IDS, ingenta, Linda Hall.
Published by: Carnegie Museum of Natural History, Office of Scientific Publications, 4400 Forbes Ave, Pittsburgh, PA 15213-4080. TEL 412-622-3287, FAX 412-622-8837, scipubs@clpgh.org, http://www.clpgh.org/cmnh/scipub. R&P Mary Ann Schmidt. Circ: 900.

508 USA ISSN 0145-9058
CODEN: BCMHD9
CARNEGIE MUSEUM OF NATURAL HISTORY. BULLETIN. Text in English. 1976. irreg., latest vol.34, 1998. price varies. bibl, charts, illus. index. back issues avail. **Document type:** *Academic/Scholarly.* **Description:** Contains monographs in organismal biology, earth sciences and anthropology.
Indexed: Biol.Abstr., GeoRef, Sport Fish.Abstr., Wild.Rev., Zoo.Rec.
—Linda Hall.
Published by: Carnegie Museum of Natural History, Office of Scientific Publications, 4400 Forbes Ave, Pittsburgh, PA 15213-4080. TEL 412-622-3287, FAX 412-622-8837, scipubs@clpgh.org, http://www.clpgh.org/cmnh/scipub. R&P Mary Ann Schmidt. Circ: (controlled).

CELLULAR AND MOLECULAR LIFE SCIENCES. see *BIOLOGY*

CUADERNOS VALENCIANOS DE HISTORIA DE LA MEDICINA Y DE LA CIENCIA. see *MEDICAL SCIENCES*

EARLY SCIENCE AND MEDICINE; a journal for the study of science, technology and medicine in the pre-modern period. see *MEDICAL SCIENCES*

500 600 610 USA
Q145
EAST ASIAN SCIENCE, TECHNOLOGY, AND MEDICINE. Text in English. 1975. a. FRF 330 to individuals; FRF 410 to institutions; FRF 220 to students (effective 1999). adv. bk.rev. *Refereed.* **Document type:** *Academic/Scholarly.* **Description:** Dedicated to the study of traditional and modern East Asian science, technology and medicine.
Formerly: Chinese Science (0361-9001)
Indexed: Amer.Hist.& Life, Bibl.Asian Stud. (1977-1996), Hist.Abstr. (1995-).
—BLDSC (3645.941000), CISTI, ingenta.
Published by: International Society for the History of East Asian Science, Technology and Medicine, Seminar Fur Sinologie und Koreanistik, Eberhard-Karls-Universitat Tubingen, Wilhelmstr. 133, Tubingen 72074, Germany. FAX 49-7071-295733, eastm@uni-tuebingen.de; hans-ulrich.vogel@uni-tuebingen. Ed. Hans Ulrich Vogel. Circ: 500.

017.8 NLD
ELSEVIER SCIENCE. CATALOGUE - BOOKS. Text in English. a. **Document type:** *Catalog.* **Description:** Complete listing of all Elsevier scientific books and book series published throughout the world, including the Excerpta Medica, North-Holland and Pergamon imprints.
Formerly (until 1994): Elsevier Science Publishers. Catalogue - Books
Related titles: CD-ROM ed.; Online - full text ed.; ♦ Supplement: Elsevier Science. New and Forthcoming Publications.
Published by: Elsevier Science BV, PO Box 211, Amsterdam 1000 AE, Netherlands. TEL 31-20-485-2911, FAX 31-20-485-2457, nlinfo-f@elsevier.nl; usinfo-f@elsevier.com; forinfo-kyf04035@niftyserve.or.jp, http://www.elsevier.nl/. **Subscr. in Australasia and the Far East to:** Elsevier Science (Singapore) Pte Ltd, No.1 Temasek Ave, 17-01 Millenia Tower, Singapore 039192, Singapore. TEL 65-434-3727, FAX 65-337-2230; **Subscr. in Japan to:** Elsevier Science Inc - Japan Regional Office, 9-15 Higashi-Azabu 1-chome, Minato-ku, Tokyo 106-0044, Japan. TEL 81-3-5561-5033, FAX 81-3-5561-5047; **Subscr. in the Americas to:** Elsevier Science, PO Box 945, New York, NY 10159-0945. TEL 212-633-3730, FAX 212-633-3680, usinfo-f@elsevier.com, http://www.elsevier.com.

017.8 NLD
ELSEVIER SCIENCE. CATALOGUE - JOURNALS. Text in English. a. **Document type:** *Catalog.* **Description:** Complete listing, ordered by subject areas, of all scientific, technical and academic journals, newsletters and abstracting journals published worldwide under the Elsevier name, including the North-Holland, Pergamon and Excerpta Medica imprints, and affiliated publishing companies in 7 countries.
Formerly (until 1994): Elsevier Science Publishers. Catalogue - Journals
Related titles: CD-ROM ed.; Online - full text ed.; ♦ Supplement: Elsevier Science. New and Forthcoming Publications.
Published by: Elsevier Science BV, PO Box 211, Amsterdam 1000 AE, Netherlands. TEL 31-20-485-2911, FAX 31-20-485-2457, nlinfo-f@elsevier.nl; usinfo-f@elsevier.coml forinfo-kyf04035@niftyserve.or.jp, http://www.elsevier.nl/. **Subscr. in Australasia and the Far East to:** Elsevier Science (Singapore) Pte Ltd, No.1 Temasek Ave, 17-01 Millenia Tower, Singapore 039192, Singapore. TEL 65-434-3727, FAX 65-337-2230; **Subscr. in Japan to:** Elsevier Science Inc - Japan Regional Office, 9-15 Higashi-Azabu 1-chome, Minato-ku, Tokyo 106-0044, Japan. TEL 81-3-5561-5033, FAX 81-3-5561-5047; **Subscr. in the Americas to:** Elsevier Science, PO Box 945, New York, NY 10159-0945. TEL 212-633-3730, FAX 212-633-3680, http://www.elsevier.com.

017.8 NLD
ELSEVIER SCIENCE. CATALOGUE ON CD-ROM. Text in English. 1993. a. **Document type:** *Catalog.* **Description:** Complete, fully searchable listing of all Elsevier scientific book and journal publications, including book series, software and other products. Provides complete descriptions and contents lists, independent reviews of published books, and forthcoming title information. Also lists journal editors and editorial boards, recently published papers, and coverage by abstracting services.
Formerly (until 1994): Elsevier Science Publishers. Catalogue on CD-ROM
Media: CD-ROM.
Published by: Elsevier Science BV, PO Box 211, Amsterdam 1000 AE, Netherlands. TEL 31-20-485-2911, FAX 31-20-485-2457, nlinfo-f@elsevier.nl; usinfo-f@elsevier.com; forinfo-kyf04035@niftyserve.or.jp, http://www.elsevier.nl/. **Subscr. in Australasia and the Far East to:** Elsevier Science (Singapore) Pte Ltd, No.1 Temasek Ave, 17-01 Millenia Tower, Singapore 039192, Singapore. TEL 65-434-3727, FAX 65-337-2230; **Subscr. in Japan to:** Elsevier Science Inc - Japan Regional Office, 9-15 Higashi-Azabu 1-chome, Minato-ku, Tokyo 106-0044, Japan. TEL 81-3-5561-5033, FAX 81-3-5561-5047; **Subscr. in the Americas to:** Elsevier Science, PO Box 945, New York, NY 10159-0945. TEL 212-633-3730, FAX 212-633-3680, usinfo-f@elsevier.com, http://www.elsevier.com.

017.8 NLD
ELSEVIER SCIENCE. DISPATCH LIST FOR JOURNALS, BOOK SERIES AND PROCEEDINGS. Text in English. m. **Document type:** *Catalog.* **Description:** Provides news of most recent publications, including volume, number and date, for all Elsevier book series, journals, and proceedings worldwide.
Formerly (until Nov. 1993): Elsevier Science Publishers. Dispatch List for Journals, Book Series and Proceedings.
Published by: Elsevier Science BV, PO Box 211, Amsterdam 1000 AE, Netherlands. TEL 31-20-485-2911, FAX 31-20-485-2457, nlinfo-f@elsevier.nl; usinfo-f@elsevier.com; forinfo-kyf04035@niftyserve.or.jp, http://www.elsevier.nl/. **Subscr. in Australasia and the Far East to:** Elsevier Science (Singapore) Pte Ltd, No.1 Temasek Ave, 17-01 Millenia Tower, Singapore 039192, Singapore. TEL 65-434-3727, FAX 65-337-2230; **Subscr. in Japan to:** Elsevier Science Inc - Japan Regional Office, 9-15 Higashi-Azabu 1-chome, Minato-ku, Tokyo 106-0044, Japan. TEL 81-3-5561-5033, FAX 81-3-5561-5047; **Subscr. in the Americas to:** Elsevier Science, PO Box 945, New York, NY 10159-0945. TEL 212-633-3730, FAX 212-633-3680, usinfo-f@elsevier.com, http://www.elsevier.com.

017.8 NLD
ELSEVIER SCIENCE. NEW AND FORTHCOMING PUBLICATIONS. Text in English. 1992 (no.283). m. **Document type:** *Catalog.* **Description:** Contains all new and forthcoming book and journal publications worldwide from Elsevier and its imprints and affiliated companies in 7 countries, including Pergamon, Excerpta Medica and North-Holland.
Former titles (until 1994): Elsevier Science Publishers. New and Forthcoming Publications; (until July 1993): Elsevier Science Publishers. New and Forthcoming Books and Journals; Supersedes: Pergamon New Publications Booklet
Related titles: ♦ Supplement to: Elsevier Science. Catalogue - Books; ♦ Supplement to: Elsevier Science. Catalogue - Journals.
Published by: Elsevier Science BV, PO Box 211, Amsterdam 1000 AE, Netherlands. TEL 31-20-485-2911, FAX 31-20-485-2457, nlinfo-f@elsevier.nl; usinfo-f@elsevier.com; forinfo-kyf04035@niftyserve.or.jp, http://www.elsevier.nl/. **Subscr. in Australasia and the Far East to:** Elsevier Science (Singapore) Pte Ltd, No.1 Temasek Ave, 17-01 Millenia Tower, Singapore 039192, Singapore. TEL 65-434-3727, FAX 65-337-2230; **Subscr. in Japan to:** Elsevier Science Inc - Japan Regional Office, 9-15 Higashi-Azabu 1-chome, Minato-ku, Tokyo 106-0044, Japan. TEL 81-3-5561-5033, FAX 81-3-5561-5047; **Subscr. in the Americas to:** Elsevier Science, PO Box 945, New York, NY 10159-0945. TEL 212-633-3730, FAX 212-633-3680, usinfo-f@elsevier.com, http://www.elsevier.com.

500 GBR ISSN 1062-7987
AS9 CODEN: EURREK
EUROPEAN REVIEW. Text in English. 1993. q. GBP 58 to individuals; USD 166 to institutions (effective 2002). back issues avail. *Refereed.* **Document type:** *Academic/Scholarly.* **Description:** Promotes intra-European studies relating to society, education, and research from an interdisciplinary approach, including the humanities, law, economics, social sciences, cognitive science, mathematics, medicine, natural sciences, and technological sciences.
Related titles: Microform ed.: (from PQC); Online - full text ed.: (from Swets Blackwell, RoweCom Information Quest).
Indexed: Ecol.Abstr., Geo.Abstr.H.G., Geo.Abstr.P.G., Geol.Abstr., IDA, Int.Polit.Sci.Abstr., Soc.Serv.Abstr., Sociol.Abstr.
—BLDSC (3829.935100). **CCC.**
Published by: (Academia Europaea), Cambridge University Press, Edinburgh Bldg, Shaftesbury Rd, Cambridge CB2 2RU, United Kingdom. FAX 44-1223-315052, information@cup.cam.ac.uk, information@cambridge.org, http://www.cup.cam.ac.uk, http://www.uk.cambridge.org/journals/pmu. Eds. Arnold Burgen, Henk Wesseling. adv.: B&W page GBP 595, color page GBP 1,495; trim 165 x 248. Circ: 2,000.

GESNERUS; Swiss journal of the history of medicine and sciences. see *MEDICAL SCIENCES*

GESNERUS. SUPPLEMENT. see *MEDICAL SCIENCES*

GEWINA; tijdschrift voor de geschiedenis der geneeskunde, natuurwetenschappen, wiskunde en techniek. see *MEDICAL SCIENCES*

GLASGOW NATURALIST. see *BIOLOGY*

550 570 560 ITA
CODEN: GMFNDF
GORTANIA; atti del Museo Friulano di Storia Naturale. Text in English, French, German, Italian; Summaries in English, French, German, Italian, Slovenian. 1979. a. per issue exchange basis. *Refereed.* **Document type:** *Bulletin.*

S

Indexed: Biol.Abstr., Ecol.Abstr., Geo.Abstr.P.G., GeoRef, Geol.Abstr., Herb.Abstr., Irr.& Drain.Abstr., Soils & Fert., Weed Abstr., Zoo.Rec.

Published by: Comune di Udine, Museo Friulano di Storia Naturale, Via Lionello, 1, Udine, UD 33100, Italy. TEL 39-0432-510221, FAX 39-0432-504109, mfsn@comune.udine.it, http://www.comune.udine.it. Ed. Carlo Morandini. Circ: 600.

HISTORIA, CIENCIAS, SAUDE - MANGUINHOS. see *HISTORY*

ILLINOIS. NATURAL HISTORY SURVEY. REPORTS. see *CONSERVATION*

500 USA ISSN 0019-2252
Q11 CODEN: TISAAH

ILLINOIS STATE ACADEMY OF SCIENCE. TRANSACTIONS. Text in English. 1908. q. USD 50 (effective 1999 & 2000). charts, illus. *Refereed.* **Document type:** *Academic/Scholarly.*

Related titles: Microform ed.: (from PQC).

Indexed: Aqua.Sci.& Fish.Abstr., Biol.Abstr., Chem.Abstr., Chem.Indus.Notes, Chem.Titles, Crop Physiol.Abstr., Environ.Sci.Poll.Mgmt., Excerp.Med., Field Crop Abstr., Forest.Abstr., GeoRef, Helminthol.Abstr., Herb.Abstr., Ind.Vet., Irr.& Drain.Abstr., Key Word Ind.Wildl.Res., Math.R., Nutr.Abstr., Plant Breed.Abstr., Pollut.Abstr., Poult.Abstr., Protozool.Abstr., Ref.Zh., Rev.Appl.Entomol., Rev.Med.& Vet.Mycol., Rev.Plant Path., Russ.Acad.Sci.Bibl., SASA (1947-), Seed Abstr., Sel.Water Res.Abstr., Soils & Fert., Soyabean Abstr., Sport Fish.Abstr., Weed Abstr., Wild.Rev., World Ag.Econ.& Rur.Soc.Abstr., Zent.Math., Zoo.Rec.

—CASDDS, CISTI, ingenta, Linda Hall.

Published by: Illinois State Academy of Sciences, 502 South Spring Street, Illinois State Museum, Springfield, IL 62706. TEL 217-782-6436, FAX 217-782-1254, il-st-acad-sci.org, http://www.museum.state.il.us/isas/. Ed. Teresa L North. Circ: 1,100 (paid).

557 970 570 USA ISSN 0445-3395

ILLINOIS. STATE MUSEUM. SCIENTIFIC PAPERS SERIES. Text in English. 1940. irreg., latest vol.26, 1996. price varies. illus. *Refereed.* **Document type:** *Monographic series.*

Indexed: GeoRef, Sport Fish.Abstr., Zoo.Rec.

Published by: Illinois State Museum, Springfield, IL 62706. TEL 217-782-7386, FAX 217-782-1254, editor@museum.state.il.us, http://www.museum.state.il.us.

500 600 610 DNK ISSN 0281-9341

ILLUSTRERAD VETENSKAP. Text in Swedish. 1984. 16/yr. DKK 48.75 newsstand/cover (effective 2002). adv. illus. 84 p./no. 4 cols./p. **Document type:** *Magazine, Consumer.*

Related titles: ♦ Danish ed.: Illustreret Videnskab. ISSN 0109-2456; ♦ German ed.: Illustrierte Wissenschaft. ISSN 0942-7090; Finnish ed.: Tieteen Kuvalehti. ISSN 0903-5583; Norwegian ed.: Illustrert Vitenskap. ISSN 0800-3955.

Published by: Bonnier Publications A-S, Strandboulevarden 130, Copenhagen 2100, Denmark. TEL 45-39-17-20-00, FAX 45-39-17-23-00, kundtjanst@bp.bonnier.dk, http://www.illustreradvetenskap.com. Eds. Jens Erik Mathiesen, Sture Axelsson. Pub. Lars Engstroem. adv.: color page SEK 34,600; trim 185 x 250. Circ: 378,000 (paid and controlled).

500 NLD ISSN 0531-5131
CODEN: EXMDA4

INTERNATIONAL CONGRESS SERIES. Variant title: Excerpta Medica International Congress Series. Text in Dutch. irreg., latest 1997 (approx. 30/yr.). price varies. back issues avail. *Refereed.* **Document type:** *Monographic series, Proceedings.*

Related titles: Online - full text ed.: (from Institute for Scientific Information).

Indexed: AgeLine, Agri.& Environ.Biotech.Abstr., Anim.Breed.Abstr., Biol.Abstr., Chem.Abstr., Chem.Indus.Notes, Chem.Titles, Immun.Abstr., Med.& Pharm.Biotech.Abstr., Oncog.G.F.Abstr., Zoo.Rec.

—BLDSC (4539.356050), CASDDS, CISTI, IDS, Infotrieve, KNAW. **CCC.**

Published by: Elsevier Science BV, PO Box 211, Amsterdam 1000 AE, Netherlands. nlinfo-f@elsevier.nl; usinfo-f@elsevier.com; forinfo-kyf04035@niftyserve.or.jp; asiainfo@elsevier.com.sg, http://www.elsevier.nl/. **Subscr. in Australasia and the Far East to:** Elsevier Science (Singapore) Pte Ltd, No.1 Temasek Ave, 17-01 Millenia Tower, Singapore 039192, Singapore. TEL 65-434-3727, FAX 65-337-2230; **Subscr. in Japan to:** Elsevier Science Inc - Japan Regional Office, 9-15 Higashi-Azabu 1-chome, Minato-ku, Tokyo 106-0044, Japan. TEL 81-3-5561-5033, FAX 81-3-5561-5047; **Subscr. in the Americas to:** Elsevier Science, PO Box 945, New York, NY 10159-0945. TEL 212-633-3730, FAX 212-633-3680, http://www.elsevier.com.

INTERNATIONAL JOURNAL OF RADIATION BIOLOGY. see *MEDICAL SCIENCES—Oncology*

500 610 TUR
Q80.T8

ISLAMIC ACADEMY OF SCIENCES. MEDICAL JOURNAL. Text in English. 1988. q. USD 40 (effective 1999). adv. bk.rev., Website rev. abstr, charts, illus, stat. back issues avail. *Refereed.* **Document type:** *Journal, Academic/Scholarly.* **Description:** Presents results of original research in different scientific disciplines.

Formerly (Until Aug. 2000): Islamic Academy of Sciences. Journal (1016-3360)

Related titles: CD-ROM ed.; Diskette ed.; E-mail ed.; Fax ed.; Microfilm ed.; Online - full text ed.

Indexed: Per.Islam. (1992-).

—CISTI.

Published by: (Islamic Academy of Sciences JOR), Anadolu Health and Research Foundation, Kizilay, Mithatpasa Caddesi 66-5, Ankara 06420, Turkey. TEL 90-312-4250319, FAX 90-312-4259487, nacibor@bir.net.tr, http://www.medicaljournal-jas.corg. Ed. Naci M Bor. Circ: 1,000 (paid). **Co-sponsor:** Organization of Islamic Conference, Standing Committee on Scientific Cooperation.

500 610 CHN ISSN 1000-9965
CODEN: JDXUET

JINAN DAXUE XUEBAO (ZIRAN KEXUE YU YIXUE BAN)/JOURNAL OF JINAN UNIVERSITY(NATURAL SCIENCE AND MEDICINE EDITION). (First and third issues cover natural science; second and fourth issues cover medical science.) Text in Chinese; Contents page in English. 1980. bi-m. CNY 4 newsstand/cover domestic (effective 2000). **Document type:** *Academic/Scholarly.*

Formerly (until 1989): Jinan Li-yi Xuebao - Jinan University. Journal of Science and Medicine (1000-5064)

Related titles: Online - full content ed.: (from WanFang Data Corp.).

Indexed: Chem.Abstr., Chem.Indus.Notes, Chem.Titles, Zoo.Rec.

—BLDSC (4809.599000), CASDDS.

Published by: Jinan Daxue, Xuebao Bianjibu/Jinan University, Journal Editorial Department, Rm. 217, 2nd Fl, Bldg. 75, Shipai, Guangzhou, Guangdong 510632, China. TEL 81-20-8522-0281, oxb@jnu.edu.cn. Ed., R&P Weiliang Wang. **Dist. outside China by:** China International Book Trading Corp, 35 Chegongzhuang Xilu, Haidian District, Beijing 100044, China.

JOURNAL OF CONSCIOUSNESS STUDIES; controversies in science & the humanities. see *PSYCHOLOGY*

JOURNAL OF SCIENTIFIC RESEARCH IN PLANTS & MEDICINES. see *PHARMACY AND PHARMACOLOGY*

LABORATORY PRACTICE; research techniques and equipment. see *MEDICAL SCIENCES—Experimental Medicine, Laboratory Technique*

500 LVA ISSN 1407-009X
AS262 CODEN: LZAVEP

LATVIJAS ZINATNU AKADEMIJAS VETIS. B DALA. DABASZINATNES/LATVIAN ACADEMY OF SCIENCES. SECTION B. NATURAL SCIENCES. PROCEEDINGS. Text in Latvian, English. 1947. m. USD 54 (effective 1998). bk.rev. abstr, bibl, charts, illus. index. **Document type:** *Proceedings.*

Supersedes in part (in 1992): Latvijas Zinatnu Akademijas Vestis (0868-6556); Formerly (until 1990): Latvijas P.S.R. Zinatnu Akademijas Vestis (0132-6422)

Indexed: Abstr.Bull.Inst.Pap.Chem., Anim.Breed.Abstr., Aqua.Sci.& Fish.Abstr., Aquacult.Abstr., Biol.Abstr., C.C.M.J., Chem.Abstr., Chem.Indus.Notes, Chem.Titles, Crop Physiol.Abstr., Dairy Sci.Abstr., Derwent Biotech.Abstr., Environ.Sci.Poll.Mgmt., Field Crop Abstr., Forest Prod.Abstr., Forest.Abstr., Hist.Abstr. (coverage dropped), Hort.Abstr., INIS Atomind., INSPEC (pre-1969-1994, 1997-), Ind.Vet., Irr.& Drain.Abstr., M.L.A., MLA Intl.Bibl. (coverage dropped), Mass Spectr.Bull., Math.R., Numis.Lit., Nutr.Abstr., Ornam.Hort., Plant Breed.Abstr., Plant Grow.Reg.Abstr., Poult.Abstr., Rev.Appl.Entomol., Rev.Plant Path., Russ.Acad.Sci.Bibl., Soils & Fert., Sugar Ind.Abstr., Weed Abstr., World Ag.Econ.& Rur.Soc.Abstr., Zent.Math., Zoo.Rec.

—BLDSC (6746.880000), AskIEEE, CASDDS, CISTI, Linda Hall.

Published by: Latvijas Zinatny Akademijas/Latvian Academy of Sciences, Akademijas Laukums 1, Riga 1524, Latvia. TEL 371-7229830, vestis@ac.iza.lv. Ed. Inta Rozenvalde. Circ: 1,400. **Dist. by:** Mezhdunarodnaya Kniga, B Yakimanka 39, Moscow 117049, Russian Federation. TEL 7-095-2384967, FAX 7-095-2384634; **US dist. addr.:** East View Publications, 3020 Harbor Ln N, Minneapolis, MN 55447. TEL 612-550-0961.

508 CAN ISSN 0823-2911

MANITOBA NATURALISTS SOCIETY BULLETIN. Text in English. 1975. m. (11/yr.). CND 40 to members. adv. bk.rev. back issues avail. **Document type:** *Bulletin.* **Description:** Covers natural history topics, outdoor recreation activities, natural history lectures and workshops and environmental protection issues.

Published by: Manitoba Naturalists Society, 401 63 Albert St, Winnipeg, MB R3B 1G4, Canada. TEL 204-943-9029, FAX 204-943-9029. Ed. Margaret Kapinga. Adv. contact Paul Vonwichert. page CND 200; trim 7.25 x 9.5. Circ: 1,500.

508 ARG ISSN 0539-3027

MUSEO MUNICIPAL DE HISTORIA NATURAL DE SAN RAFAEL. INSTITUTO DE CIENCIAS NATURALES. NOTAS. Text in Spanish. 1957. irreg. on exchange basis. **Document type:** *Bulletin.*

Formerly: Museo de Historia Natural de San Rafael. Instituto de Ciencias Naturales. Notas

Indexed: GeoRef.

Published by: Museo Municipal de Historia Natural de San Rafael, Parque Mariano Moreno, San Rafael, Mendoza 5600, Argentina. FAX 54-0627-21244. Ed. Humberto A Lagiglia. Circ: 1,200.

NATIONAL ACADEMY OF SCIENCES, INDIA. PROCEEDINGS. SECTION B. BIOLOGICAL SCIENCES. see *BIOLOGY*

505 USA ISSN 0027-8424
Q11

NATIONAL ACADEMY OF SCIENCES OF THE UNITED STATES OF AMERICA. PROCEEDINGS. Text in English. 1914. bi-w. USD 165 to individuals Print & Online eds.; USD 290 foreign to individuals Print & Online eds.; USD 800 to institutions Print & Online eds.; USD 995 foreign to institutions Print & Online eds. (effective 1999). adv. charts, illus, pat, stat. index, cum.index: vol.1-50. reprints avail. *Refereed.* **Document type:** *Proceedings, Academic/Scholarly.* **Description:** Publishes brief reports that describe the results of original research of exceptional importance.

Former titles (until 1985): National Academy of Sciences of the United States of America. Proceedings. Physical Sciences (0273-1142); National Academy of Sciences of the United States of America. Proceedings. Biological Sciences (0273-1134); Which superseded in part: National Academy of Sciences. Proceedings

Related titles: Microfilm ed.: (from PQC); Online - full text ed.: ISSN 1091-6490. USD 100 (effective 1999) (from HighWire Pr., JSTOR (Web-based Journal Archive), EBSCO Publishing, Gale Group, Factiva, Institute for Scientific Information, RoweCom Information Quest).

S

Indexed: AIDS Abstr., ASCA, Abstr.Hyg., AgBiotech, Agricola, Anim.Behav.Abstr., Anim.Breed.Abstr., Appl.Ecol.Abstr., Aqua.Sci.& Fish.Abstr., Aquacult.Abstr., Arts & Hum.Cit.Ind. (coverage dropped), BBCI, Bibl.Agri., Bio-Contr.News & Info., Biol.& Agr.Ind. (Aug.1989-), Biol.Abstr., CEABA, Cal.Tiss.Abstr. (coverage dropped), Chem.Abstr., Chem.Cit.Ind., Chem.Indus.Notes, Chem.Titles, Chemorec.Abstr., Compumath, Crop Physiol.Abstr., Curr.Adv.Biochem., Curr.Adv.Cancer Res., Curr.Adv.Cell & Devel.Biol., Curr.Adv.Ecol.Sci., Curr.Adv.Gen.& Molec.Biol., Curr.Biotech.Abstr., Curr.Cont., Curr.Ind.Stat., Curr.Ref.Fish Res., Dairy Sci.Abstr., Deep Sea Res.& Oceanogr.Abstr., Derwent Biotech.Abstr., Eng.Ind., Entomol.Abstr., Environ.Sci.Poll.Mgmt., Excerp.Med., Field Crop Abstr., Food Sci.& Tech.Abstr., Forest Prod.Abstr., Forest.Abstr., Gen.Sci.Ind. (Jun.1992-), Genet.Abstr., GeoRef, Helminthol.Abstr., Herb.Abstr., Hort.Abstr., Hum.Gen.Abstr., INIS Atomind., INSPEC (pre-1969-Dec.1985, dropped), Immun.Abstr. (coverage dropped), Ind.Med. (1915-), Ind.Sci.Rev., Ind.Vet., Inpharma, Int.Abstr.Biol.Sci., Irr.& Drain.Abstr., Jrnl.Watch Inf.Dis., Kidney, Maize Abstr., Mass Spectr.Bull., Mat.Sci.Cit.Ind. (coverage dropped), Math.R., Med.& Surg.Dermat., Microbiol.Abstr., NRN, Neurosci.Abstr., Neurosci.Cit.Ind., Nuc.Acids Abstr., Nutr.Abstr., Ocean.Abstr., Ornam.Hort., Pharm.&Out.News, Plant Breed.Abstr., Plant Gen.Res.Abstr., Plant Grow.Reg.Abstr., Postharvest, Potato Abstr., Poult.Abstr., Protozool.Abstr., Reac., Ref.Zh., Rev.Appl.Entomol., Rev.Arom.& Med.Plants, Rev.Med.& Vet.Mycol., Rev.Plant Path., Rice Abstr., Russ.Acad.Sci.Bibl., SSCI (coverage dropped), Sci.Cit.Ind., Seed Abstr., Soils & Fert., Sorghum & Millets Abstr., Soyabean Abstr., Sport Fish.Abstr., Sugar Ind.Abstr., THA, Telegen, Tox.Abstr. (coverage dropped), Triticale Abstr., Trop.Dis.Bull., VITIS, Vet.Bull., Virol.Abstr. (coverage dropped), Weed Abstr., Wild.Rev., World Ag.Econ.& Rur.Soc.Abstr., Zent.Math., Zoo.Rec.
—BLDSC (6762.000000), CASDDS, CINDOC, CISTI, Ei, GNLM, IDS, ingenta, KNAW, Linda Hall. **CCC.**

Published by: National Academy of Sciences, Proceedings Office, 2101 Constitution Ave, Washington, DC 20418. TEL 202-334-2672, FAX 202-334-2738, pnas@nas.edu, subspnas@nas.edu, http://www.pnas.org. Ed. Nicholas R Cozzarelli. Pub. Kenneth R Fulton. R&P Barbara Bacon. adv.: B&W page USD 1,840, color page USD 2,935; trim 10 x 7. Circ: 10,132. **Subscr. in Japan to:** Usaco Corp., Tsutsumi Bldg, 13-12 Shinbashi 1-chome, Minato-ku, Tokyo 105-0004, Japan.

500 USA
QH359

NATIONAL CENTER FOR SCIENCE EDUCATION. REPORTS. Text in English. 1997. bi-m. USD 30 domestic; USD 37 foreign; USD 7 newsstand/cover (effective 2001). adv. bk.rev. bibl. cum.index: nos.1-31 on diskette. back issues avail.; reprints avail. *Refereed.* **Document type:** *Academic/Scholarly.* **Description:** Discusses issues and current events in science education, focusing on evolutionary science and the evolution-creation controversy.

Formed by the merger of (1980-1997): Creation - Evolution (0738-6001); (1981-1997): N C S E Reports (1064-2358)

Indexed: C.I.J.E., GeoRef, Zoo.Rec.
—BLDSC (7560.199000), ingenta.

Published by: National Center for Science Education, Inc., P O Box 9477, Berkeley, CA 94709-0477. TEL 510-526-1674, 800-290-6006, FAX 510-526-1675, ncse@natcenscied.org, editor@ncseweb.org, http://www.natcenscied.org, http://www.ncseweb.org. Ed., Adv. contact Andrew J Petto. Pub., R&P Eugenie C Scott. Circ: 4,000 (paid and free).

S

500 BLR
Q60 CODEN: DBLRAC

NATIONALNAYA AKADEMIYA NAVUK BELARUSI. DOKLADY/NATIONAL ACADEMY OF SCIENCES OF BELARUS. PAPERS. Text in Russian; Abstracts and contents page in English. 1957. m. BYB 120,000 (effective 1999). bibl, charts, illus. index. **Document type:** *Academic/Scholarly.* **Description:** Publishes scientific results in mathematics, natural sciences and engineering.

Formerly (until 1992): Akademiya Navuk Belarusskai S.S.R. Doklady (0002-354X)

Indexed: Alloys Ind., Biol.Abstr., C.C.M.J., Chem.Abstr., Chem.Indus.Notes, Chem.Titles, Crop Physiol.Abstr., Curr.Cont. (coverage dropped), Curr.Ind.Stat., Deep Sea Res.& Oceanogr.Abstr., Eng.Mat.Abstr., Field Crop Abstr., GeoRef, Helminthol.Abstr., INIS Atomind., Mat.Sci.Cit.Ind. (coverage dropped), Met.Abstr., Met.Abstr.Ind., Nonfer.Met.Alert, PCC Alert, Russ.Acad.Sci.Bibl., Steels Alert, Triticale Abstr., World Alum.Abstr.
—CASDDS, CISTI, IDS, Linda Hall. **CCC.**

Published by: (Nationalnaya Akademiya Navuk Belarusi/National Academy of Sciences of Belarus), Vydavetstvo Belaruskaya Navuka, Kuprevicha 18, Minsk 220141, Belarus. TEL 375-172-2841801, FAX 375-172-284252494, TELEX 252277 NAUKA. Ed. A P Voitovich. Circ: 400.

500 GBR ISSN 0028-0836
Q1 CODEN: NATUAS

NATURE; international weekly journal of science. Text in English. 1869. w. USD 159 in United States to individuals; GBP 109 elsewhere to individuals; USD 775 in United States to institutions; GBP 360 elsewhere to institutions (effective 2001). adv. bk.rev. abstr, bibl, charts, illus, tr.lit. index. back issues avail.; reprints avail. *Refereed.* **Document type:** *Magazine, Academic/Scholarly.* **Description:** Publishes original scientific research reports, review articles surveying recent developments in specific disciplines, short contributions, letters, and commentary.

Related titles: Braille ed.; CD-ROM ed.: (from Ovid Technologies, Inc.); Microform ed.: (from PQC,PMC); Online - full text ed.: (from Ovid Technologies, Inc., EBSCO Publishing, ingenta, Gale Group, Factiva, Institute for Scientific Information); Talking Book ed.; ♦ Supplement: Nature Genetics. ISSN 1061-4036.

Indexed: ABC, AESIS, A.I.Abstr., A.I.C.P. (1938-), AIDS Abstr., AMED, Abstr.Bull.Inst.Pap.Chem., Abstr.Hyg., Acad.Ind., Acid Pre.Dig., AgBiotech, Agri.& Environ.Biotech.Abstr. (coverage dropped), Agricola, Agroforest.Abstr., Alloys Ind., Anal.Abstr., Anim.Behav.Abstr., Anim.Breed.Abstr., Anthropol.Lit., Appl.Ecol.Abstr., Appl.Mech.Rev., Aqua.Sci.& Fish.Abstr., Art & Archaeol.Tech.Abstr., Arts & Hum.Cit.Ind. (coverage dropped), Bibl.Agri., Bibl.Asian Stud. (1971), Bibl.Dev.Med.& Child Neur., Bio-Contr.News & Info., Bioeng.Abstr., Biol.& Agr.Ind. (Jan.1996-), Biol.Abstr., Biol.Dig., Biostat., Biwk.Pap.Rad.Chem.& Photochem., Bk.Rev.Ind. (1982-), Br.Archaeol.Abstr., Br.Ceram.Abstr., Br.Educ.Ind., Br.Geol.Lit., Br.Tech.Ind., CEABA, C.I.S. Abstr., CSNB, Cadscan, Cal.Tiss.Abstr., Chem.Abstr., Chem.Cit.Ind., Chem.Indus.Notes, Chem.Titles, Chemorec.Abstr., Child.Bk.Rev.Ind. (1982-), Comput.& Info.Sys., Crop Physiol.Abstr., Curr.Adv.Biochem., Curr.Adv.Ecol.Sci., Curr.Biotech.Abstr., Curr.Chem.React., Curr.Cont., Curr.Ind.Stat., Curr.Ref.Fish Res., Curr.Tit.Dent., Dairy Sci.Abstr., Deep Sea Res.& Oceanogr.Abstr., Dent.Ind., Derwent Biotech.Abstr., Diab.Cont., Diar.Dis.Res., Ecol.Abstr., Electron.& Communic.Abstr.J., Energy Info.Abstr., Eng.Ind., Eng.Mat.Abstr., Entomol.Abstr., Environ.Abstr., Environ.Ind., Environ.Sci.Poll.Mgmt., Excerp.Med., Field Crop Abstr., Fluidex, Focus on: Vet.Sci.& Med., Food Sci.& Tech.Abstr., Forest Prod.Abstr., Forest.Abstr., Fut.Surv., Gen.Sci.Ind. (Mar.1984-), Genet.Abstr. (coverage dropped), Geo.Abstr.H.G., Geo.Abstr.P.G., GeoRef, Geol.Abstr., Geomech.Abstr., Helminthol.Abstr., Herb.Abstr., High.Educ.Curr.Aware.Bull., Hort.Abstr., Hum.Gen.Abstr., IDA, I.M.M.Abstr., INIS Atomind., INSPEC (pre-1969-), I.P.A., ISMEC, Immun.Abstr. (coverage dropped), Ind.Chem., Ind.Med. (1869-), Ind.Sci.Rev., Ind.Vet., Inpharma, Int.Abstr.Biol.Sci., Int.Aerosp.Abstr., Int.Nurs.Ind., Irr.& Drain.Abstr., Jrnl.Watch Derm., Jrnl.Watch Inf.Dis., Jrnl.Watch Neuro., Jrnl.Watch Psych., Kidney, Lab.Haz.Bull., Lead Abstr., Ling.Abstr., Maize Abstr., Mass Spectr.Bull., Mat.Sci.Cit.Ind. (coverage dropped), Math.R., Met.Abstr., Met.Abstr.Ind., Meteor.& Geoastrophys.Abstr., Microbiol.Abstr., Mid.East: Abstr.& Ind., Mineral.Abstr., NRN, Neurosci.Abstr., Neurosci.Cit.Ind., Nonfer.Met.Alert, Nuc.Acids Abstr., Numis.Lit., Nutr.Abstr., Ocean.Abstr., Oncog.G.F.Abstr. (coverage dropped), PCC Alert, PMR, Peace Res.Abstr., Petrol.Abstr., Pharm.&Out.News, Pig News & Info., Plant Breed.Abstr., Plant Gen.Res.Abstr., Plant Grow.Reg.Abstr., Pollut.Abstr., Postharvest, Potato Abstr., Poult.Abstr., Protozool.Abstr., PsycInfo, Psychol.Abstr. (1928-), RAPRA, RCI, Reac., Ref.Zh., Res.High.Educ.Abstr., Rev.Appl.Entomol., Rev.Arom.& Med.Plants, Rev.Med.& Vet.Mycol., Rev.Plant Path., Rice Abstr., Risk Abstr., Rural Devel.Abstr., Russ.Acad.Sci.Bibl., SSCI (coverage dropped), Saf.Sci.Abstr., Sci.Cit.Ind., Seed Abstr., Sel.Water Res.Abstr., So.Pac.Per.Ind., Soils & Fert., Solid St.Abstr., Sport Fish.Abstr., Steels Alert, Telegen, Tox.Abstr. (coverage dropped), Triticale Abstr., Trop.Dis.Bull., VITIS, Vet.Bull., Virol.Abstr. (coverage dropped), WMB, W.R.C.Inf., Weed Abstr., Wild.Rev., World Ag.Econ.& Rur.Soc.Abstr., World Alum.Abstr., World Text.Abstr., Zincscan, Zoo.Rec., e-psyche.
—BLDSC (6045.000000), AskIEEE, CASDDS, CINDOC, CIS, CISTI, Ei, EMDOCS, GNLM, IDS, ingenta, KNAW, Linda Hall, PADDS. **CCC.**

Published by: Macmillan Magazines Ltd, 4-7 Porters South, Crinan St, London N1 9XW, United Kingdom. TEL 44-20-7833-4000, 800-524-0384, FAX 44-20-7843-4998, 615-377-0525, nature@nature.com, subscriptions@natureny.com, http://www.nature.com/nature. Ed. Philip Campbell. adv.: B&W page GBP 4,680, color page GBP 5,625; trim 215 x 278. Circ: 60,185. **Subscr. to:** Brunel Rd., Basingstoke, Hants RG21 2XS, United Kingdom. TEL 44-1256-29242, FAX 44-1256-842084.

NATURE STRUCTURAL BIOLOGY. see *BIOLOGY*

500 USA ISSN 0077-8923
Q11 CODEN: ANYAA9

NEW YORK ACADEMY OF SCIENCES. ANNALS. Text in English. 1823. irreg., latest vol.882, 1999. bibl, charts, illus. index, cum.index: 1960-1974. back issues avail.; reprint service avail. from PQC. *Refereed.* **Document type:** *Academic/Scholarly.*

Related titles: Microfilm ed.: (from PMC); Online - full text ed.: (from Ovid Technologies, Inc., Institute for Scientific Information).

Indexed: AESIS, ASCA, Abstr.Anthropol., Abstr.Health Care Manage.Stud., Abstr.Hyg., Agri.& Environ.Biotech.Abstr. (coverage dropped), Anim.Behav.Abstr. (coverage dropped), Anim.Breed.Abstr., Anthropol.Lit. (coverage dropped), Aqua.Sci.& Fish.Abstr., Bio-Contr.News & Info., Biodet.Abstr., Biol.Abstr., C.C.M.J., C.I.S. Abstr., Cadscan, Chem.Abstr., Chem.Cit.Ind., Chem.Indus.Notes, Chem.Titles, Chemorec.Abstr., Curr.Adv.Cell & Devel.Biol., Curr.Adv.Ecol.Sci., Dairy Sci.Abstr., Deep Sea Res.& Oceanogr.Abstr., Derwent Biotech.Abstr., Environ.Sci.Poll.Mgmt., Excerp.Med., Field Crop Abstr., GeoRef, Helminthol.Abstr., Herb.Abstr., Hort.Abstr., INIS Atomind., INSPEC (coverage dropped), Ind.Med. (1877-), Ind.Vet., Int.Aerosp.Abstr., Lead Abstr., M.L.A., MLA Intl.Bibl., Mass Spectr.Bull., Math.R., Neurosci.Abstr. (coverage dropped), Nutr.Abstr., Ocean.Abstr., Pollut.Abstr., Protozool.Abstr., Psychol.Abstr., RCI, Rev.Appl.Entomol., Rev.Med.& Vet.Mycol., Rev.Plant Path., Risk Abstr., SSCI (coverage dropped), Saf.Sci.Abstr., Sci.Cit.Ind., Soils & Fert., Soyabean Abstr., Sport Fish.Abstr., Sugar Ind.Abstr., THA, Telegen, Trop.Dis.Bull., Vet.Bull., Weed Abstr., Wild.Rev., World Ag.Econ.& Rur.Soc.Abstr., Zent.Math., Zincscan, Zoo.Rec.
—BLDSC (1031.000000), ADONIS, CASDDS, CINDOC, CISTI, EMDOCS, GNLM, IDS, ingenta, KNAW, Linda Hall. **CCC.**

Published by: New York Academy of Sciences, 2 E 63rd St, New York, NY 10021. TEL 212-838-0230, 800-443-6927, FAX 212-888-2894, publications@nyas.org, http://www.nyas.org. Circ: 1,000.

577 USA ISSN 0550-1067
CODEN: NOGAB2

NOTICIAS DE GALAPAGOS. Text in English. 1963. s-a. USD 25. adv. bk.rev. **Document type:** *Academic/Scholarly.* **Description:** Covers science and conservation in Galapagos, the Galapagos National Park Service, and the Charles Darwin Research Station.

Indexed: Biol.Abstr., Curr.Tit.Ocean, Deep Sea Res.& Oceanogr.Abstr., Sport Fish.Abstr., Wild.Rev., Zoo.Rec.

Published by: Charles Darwin Foundation Inc., 100 N Washington St, Ste 311, Falls Church, VA 22046. FAX 703-538-6835. Ed., R&P Howard L Snell. Adv. contact Johannah Barry. Circ: 6,000.

500 ROM ISSN 0253-1879
CODEN: OCRNAM

OCROTIREA NATURII SI A MEDIULUI INCONJURATOR. Text in Romanian; Summaries in English, French, German, Russian. 1955. s-a. bk.rev. charts, illus, bibl. index, cum.index.

Formerly (until 1975): Ocrotirea Naturii (0029-8263)

Indexed: Biol.Abstr., GeoRef, Russ.Acad.Sci.Bibl., Sport Fish.Abstr., Wild.Rev., Zoo.Rec.
—CISTI, KNAW, Linda Hall.

Published by: (Academia Romana), Editura Academiei Romane, Calea 13 Septembrie 13, Bucharest 76117, Romania. TEL 407680. Ed. Nicolae Botnariuc. **Dist. by:** Rodipet S.A.. TEL 401-618-5103, FAX 401-222-6407.

500 570 USA ISSN 1044-6753
CODEN: JPSCEY

PENNSYLVANIA ACADEMY OF SCIENCE. JOURNAL. Text in English. 1924. 3/yr. USD 45 (effective 2001). bk.rev. abstr. back issues avail. *Refereed.* **Document type:** *Journal, Academic/Scholarly.* **Description:** Presents papers from the natural, engineering and social sciences.

Formerly: Pennsylvania Academy of Science. Proceedings (0096-9222)

Related titles: Online - full text ed.

Indexed: Biol.Abstr., Chem.Abstr., Chem.Indus.Notes, Chem.Titles, GeoRef, Meteor.& Geoastrophys.Abstr., SASA (1946-), Sel.Water Res.Abstr., Sport Fish.Abstr., Wild.Rev., Zoo.Rec.
—BLDSC (4839.645000), CASDDS, CISTI, ingenta, KNAW, Linda Hall.
Published by: Pennsylvania Academy of Science, c/o Dr S K Majumdar, Ed, Dept of Biology, Lafayette College, Easton, PA 18042. TEL 610-330-5464, FAX 610-330-5705, majumdas@lafayette.edu. Ed. S K Majumdar. R&P S.K. Majumdar. Circ: 700.

PITTSBURGH SERIES IN PHILOSOPHY & HISTORY OF SCIENCE. see *PHILOSOPHY*

500 574 VAT
PONTIFICIA ACADEMIA SCIENTIARUM. DOCUMENTA. Text in English, French. irreg.
Indexed: Biol.Abstr.
Published by: Pontificia Academia Scientiarum, Casina Pio IV 00120, Vatican City. TEL 39-066-9883195, FAX 39-066-9885218, TELEX 2040 DIRIGENTEL VA, academy.sciences@acdscience.va.

500 574 VAT ISSN 0377-9971
CODEN: PASVAE
PONTIFICIA ACADEMIA SCIENTIARUM. SCRIPTA VARIA. Text in English, French. irreg.
Indexed: Biol.Abstr., C.C.M.J., Meteor.& Geoastrophys.Abstr.
—CASDDS, Linda Hall.
Published by: Pontificia Academia Scientiarum, Casina Pio IV 00120, Vatican City. TEL 39-066-9883195, FAX 39-066-9885218, TELEX 2024 DIRGENTEL VA, academy.sciences@acdscience.va.

500 070 USA ISSN 1062-4155
PROBE; David Zimmerman's newsletter on science, media, policy and health. Text in English. 1991. m. USD 65 to individuals; USD 75 foreign to individuals; USD 95 to institutions (effective 2000). bk.rev. back issues avail. **Document type:** *Newsletter.* **Description:** Explores the links between science, reason, and democracy.
Published by: Probe Newsletter, Inc., 139 W 13th St, 6, New York, NY 10011-7856. TEL 212-647-0200, FAX 212-463-8002, http://www.probenewsletter.com. Ed., R&P David R Zimmerman. Circ: 750. **Subscr. to:** PO Box 1321, Cathedral Sta, New York, NY 10025-1321.

616.8 610 200 500 USA
▼ **RESEARCH NEWS & OPPORTUNITIES IN SCIENCE AND THEOLOGY.** Text and summaries in English. 2000. m. (except Jul.-Aug. combined). USD 10 domestic; USD 15 foreign (effective 2001). adv. bk.rev., film rev., Website rev. abstr, illus, stat, tr.lit. 36 p./no. back issues avail. *Refereed.* **Document type:** *Newspaper, Consumer, Academic/Scholarly, Newspaper-distributed.*
Published by: Research News & Opportunities in Science and Theology, Inc., 415 Clarion Dr, Durham, NC 27705. jgodfrey@nc.rr.com, http://www.researchnewsonline.org. Ed. Karl Giberson. Pub. Harold Koenig. R&P Janet Calhoun TEL 617-745-3931. Adv. contact Jocelyn Godfrey TEL 919-309-7775. B&W page USD 1,200, color page USD 1,560; trim 9.75 x 12.125. Circ: 2,100 (paid); 25,900 (controlled).

RESOURCE DIRECTORY OF SCIENTISTS AND ENGINEERS WITH DISABILITIES. see *BIOGRAPHY*

500 RUS ISSN 0869-5652
AS262 CODEN: DAKNEQ
ROSSIISKAYA AKADEMIYA NAUK. DOKLADY; svodnyi vypusk. Text in Russian; Contents page in English. 1933. 36/yr. RUR 750 per month (effective 2001). charts, illus. index. reprint service avail. from PSC. *Refereed.* **Document type:** *Academic/Scholarly.* **Description:** Includes material from the areas of mathematics, physics, computer science, and control theory. Publishes important new research in mathematics and its applications.
Formerly (until no.4, 1992): Akademiya Nauk S.S.S.R. Doklady (0002-3264)
Related titles: Microform ed.: (from BHP); Online - full text ed.; ♦ Partial English Translation: Doklady Earth Sciences. ISSN 1028-334X; ♦ Partial English Translation: Doklady Biological Sciences. ISSN 0012-4966; ♦ Partial English Translation: Doklady Chemistry. ISSN 0012-5008; ♦ Partial English Translation: Doklady Physical Chemistry. ISSN 0012-5016; ♦ Partial English Translation: Doklady Mathematics. ISSN 1064-5624; ♦ Partial English Translation: Doklady Physics. ISSN 1028-3358; ♦ Partial English Translation: Environmental Geoscience; ♦ Partial English Translation: Doklady Biochemistry and Biophysics. ISSN 1607-6729.
Indexed: Alloys Ind., Anal.Abstr., Aqua.Sci.& Fish.Abstr., Aquacult.Abstr., Art & Archaeol.Tech.Abstr., Biol.Abstr., C.C.M.J., Chem.Abstr., Comput.Rev., Cott.& Trop.Fibr.Abstr., Crop Physiol.Abstr., Curr.Cont. (coverage dropped), Curr.Ind.Stat., Cyb.Abstr., Deep Sea Res.& Oceanogr.Abstr., Dent.Ind., Eng.Ind., Environ.Sci.Poll.Mgmt., Field Crop Abstr., GeoRef, Geotech.Abstr., Helminthol.Abstr., Hort.Abstr., INIS Atomind., INSPEC (pre-1969-1992), Ind.Med. (coverage dropped), Maize Abstr., Mass Spectr.Bull., Math.R., Met.Abstr., Met.Abstr.Ind., Meteor.& Geoastrophys.Abstr., Nonfer.Met.Alert, Nutr.Abstr., PCC Alert, Petrol.Abstr., Psychol.Abstr., RCI (coverage dropped), Ref.Zh., Sci.Cit.Ind. (coverage dropped), Solid St.Abstr., Soyabean Abstr., Steels Alert, Triticale Abstr., Vet.Bull., World Alum.Abstr., Zent.Math., Zoo.Rec.
—BLDSC (0053.900000), AskIEEE, CASDDS, CINDOC, CISTI, East View, GNLM, IDS, Infotrieve, KNAW, Linda Hall, PADDS. **CCC.**
Published by: (Rossiiskaya Akademiya Nauk/Russian Academy of Sciences), M A I K Nauka - Interperiodica, Mezhdunarodnyi Otdel, Profsoyuznaya ul 90, Moscow 117864, Russian Federation. TEL 7-095-3347380, FAX 7-095-336-0666, compmg@maik.ru, http://www.maik.rssi.ru/. Ed. Victor A. Kabanov. Circ: 5,250. **Dist. by:** Mezhdunarodnaya Kniga, B Yakimanka 39, Moscow 117049, Russian Federation; **US dist. addr.:** East View Publications, 3020 Harbor Ln N, Minneapolis, MN 55447. TEL 612-550-0961.

SCANDINAVIAN JOURNAL OF MEDICINE & SCIENCE IN SPORTS. see *MEDICAL SCIENCES—Sports Medicine*

SCANDINAVIAN JOURNAL OF MEDICINE & SCIENCE IN SPORTS ONLINE. see *MEDICAL SCIENCES—Sports Medicine*

507.1 GBR ISSN 0036-6811
Q1 CODEN: SSCRAD
SCHOOL SCIENCE REVIEW. Text in English. 1919. q. GBP 66 (effective 2001). adv. bk.rev. charts, illus. cum.index: vols.48-57 (1967-1977). reprint service avail. from PQC. *Refereed.* **Document type:** *Academic/Scholarly.*
Related titles: Microform ed.: (from PQC); Online - full text ed.: (from Gale Group).
Indexed: Br.Educ.Ind., C.I.J.E., CSNB, Chem.Abstr., Chem.Titles, Cont.Pg.Educ., Dairy Sci.Abstr., ERA, Educ.Tech.Abstr., Environ.Abstr., Excerp.Med., High.Educ.Curr.Aware.Bull., INSPEC (pre-1969-Jun.1974, dropped), Lab.Haz.Bull., Russ.Acad.Sci.Bibl., Stud.Wom.Abstr., Tech.Educ.Abstr.
—BLDSC (8093.000000), CASDDS, CIS, ingenta.
Published by: Association for Science Education, College Ln, Hatfield, Herts AL10 9AA, United Kingdom. TEL 44-1707-283000, FAX 44-1707-266532, sharonrolland@ase.org.uk, http://www.ase.org.uk/. Ed. Mick Nott. R&P Jane Hanrott. Adv. contact Tracy Hague. Circ: 19,000.

500 GBR ISSN 0950-5431
Q175.4
SCIENCE AS CULTURE. Text in English. 1974. q. GBP 47, USD 76 to individuals; GBP 155, USD 254 to institutions (effective 2002). adv. bk.rev. abstr, bibl. index. back issues avail.; reprint service avail. from PQC. *Refereed.* **Document type:** *Academic/Scholarly.* **Description:** Explores all the ways in which science, technology and medicine are involved in shaping society's values and priorities.
Former titles (until 1987): Radical Science Series; (until 1974): Radical Science Journal (0305-0963)
Related titles: Microform ed.: (from PQC); Online - full text ed.: ISSN 1470-1189 (from CatchWord Ltd., EBSCO Publishing, O C L C Online Computer Library Center, Inc., RoweCom Information Quest, Swets Blackwell).
Indexed: Alt.Press Ind., Curr.Cont. (coverage dropped), Intl.Bibl.Soc.Sci., Lang.& Lang.Behav.Abstr., Left Ind. (1987-), Russ.Acad.Sci.Bibl., SOPODA, Soc.Serv.Abstr., Sociol.Abstr.
—BLDSC (8142.250000), CatchWord, Infotrieve, ingenta. **CCC.**
Published by: Carfax Publishing Limited (Subsidiary of: Taylor & Francis Group), PO Box 25, Abingdon, Oxon OX14 3UE, United Kingdom. TEL 44-1235-401000, FAX 44-1235-401550, enquiries@carfax.co.uk, enquiry@tandf.co.uk, http://www.carfax.co.uk; http://www.shef.ac.uk. Ed. Robert M Young. Adv. contact Jody Falco. Circ: 750.

SHIMANE IKA DAIGAKU KIYO/SHIMANE MEDICAL UNIVERSITY. BULLETIN. see *MEDICAL SCIENCES*

500 DEU ISSN 0039-4564
Q3 CODEN: SZWBAC
SUDHOFFS ARCHIV; Zeitschrift fuer Wissenschaftsgeschichte. Text in English, French, German. 1908. s-a. EUR 135.40 domestic; EUR 139 in Europe; EUR 146 elsewhere; EUR 75 newsstand/cover (effective 2002). adv. bk.rev. bibl, illus. index. back issues avail. **Document type:** *Journal, Academic/Scholarly.*
Formerly: Sudhoffs Archiv fuer Geschichte der Medizin und der Naturwissenschaften
Indexed: Amer.Hist.& Life, BHA, Chem.Abstr., Excerp.Med., Hist.Abstr. (1963-73, 1979-80, 1993-), IBZ, Ind.Med. (1969-), Int.Nurs.Ind., Math.R., Russ.Acad.Sci.Bibl.
—CISTI, GNLM, Infotrieve, Linda Hall. **CCC.**
Published by: Franz Steiner Verlag Stuttgart GmbH, Birkenwaldstr 44, Stuttgart 70191, Germany. TEL 49-711-2582-0, FAX 49-711-2582390, service@steiner-verlag.de, http://www.steiner-verlag.de. Ed. Paul Unschuld. R&P Sabine Koerner. Adv. contact Susanne Szoradi. Circ: 500.

500 610 DEU ISSN 0341-0773
SUDHOFFS ARCHIV. BEIHEFTE. Text in German. irreg., latest vol.41, 1999. price varies. **Document type:** *Monographic series, Academic/Scholarly.*
Indexed: GeoRef, Ind.Med. (1970-).
Published by: Franz Steiner Verlag Stuttgart GmbH, Birkenwaldstr 44, Stuttgart 70191, Germany. TEL 49-711-2582-0, FAX 49-711-2582390, franz.steiner.verlag@t-online.de, http://www.steiner-verlag.de. R&P Sabine Koerner.

UNIVERSITY OF KANSAS. MUSEUM OF NATURAL HISTORY. PUBLIC EDUCATION SERIES. see *BIOLOGY*

UNIVERSITY OF KANSAS. MUSEUM OF NATURAL HISTORY. SPECIAL PUBLICATIONS. see *BIOLOGY*

500 GBR ISSN 0083-7989
CODEN: WGCSA
WENNER GREN CENTER INTERNATIONAL SYMPOSIUM SERIES. Variant title: Wenner-Gren International Series. Text in English. 1962. irreg., latest 1995. price varies. **Document type:** *Monographic series, Proceedings.*
Indexed: Biol.Abstr., Chem.Abstr., Chem.Indus.Notes.
—BLDSC, CASDDS, CISTI.
Published by: Pergamon (Subsidiary of: Elsevier Science), The Boulevard, Langford Ln, East Park, Kidlington, Oxford OXB 1GB, United Kingdom. FAX 44-1865-843010, nlinfo-f@elsevier.nl; usinfo-f@elsevier.com; forinfo-kyf04035@niftyserve.or.jp, nlinfo-f@elsevier/nl; usinfo-f@elsevier.com; forinfo-kyf04035@niftyserve.or.jp, http://www.elsevier.nl/. **Subscr. in Australasia and the Far East to:** Elsevier Science (Singapore) Pte Ltd, No.1 Temasek Ave, 17-01 Millenia Tower, Singapore 039192, Singapore. TEL 65-434-3727, FAX 65-337-2230; **Subscr. in the Americas to:** Elsevier Science, PO Box 945, New York, NY 10159-0945. TEL 212-633-3730, FAX 212-633-3680, usinfo-f@elsevier.com, http://www.elsevier.com; **Subscr. to:** Elsevier Science BV, PO Box 211, Amsterdam 1000 AE, Netherlands. TEL 31-20-485-3757, FAX 31-20-485-3432, nlinfo-f@elsevier.nl, http://www.elsevier.nl.

500 600 POL ISSN 0137-8929
WIEDZA I ZYCIE. Text in Polish. 1926. m. PLZ 3.30 per issue; PLZ 4.40 newsstand/cover (effective 1999). adv. **Document type:** *Academic/Scholarly.* **Description:** Offers a popular science magazine covering science, technology and medicine. Each issues contains a supplement, devoted to the humanities.
Indexed: AgroLibrex, Russ.Acad.Sci.Bibl.
Published by: Proszynski i S-ka S.A., Ul Garazowa 7, Warsaw 02651, Poland. TEL 48-22-6077700, FAX 48-22-6077704, wiedzizycie@proszynski.com.pl, http://www.proszynski.com.pl. Adv. contact Grzegorz Kosior. Circ: 107,183.

YOGA AND TOTAL HEALTH. see *PHILOSOPHY*

S

SCIENCES: COMPREHENSIVE WORKS—Abstracting, Bibliographies, Statistics

016.5 YUG ISSN 0352-5945
Z7409
BIBLIOGRAFIJA JUGOSLAVIJE. CLANCI I PRILOZI U SERIJSKIM PUBLIKACIJAMA. SERIJA B: PRIRODNE, PRIMENJENE, MEDICINSKE I TEHNICKE NAUKE. Text in Serbo-Croatian. 1950. bi-m., latest vol.52, 2001. DEM 426 (effective 2001 - 2002). 80 p./no. 2 cols./p. **Description:** Bibliography of articles in books and serials, covering various scientific branches.
Former titles (until 1985): Bibliografija Jugoslavije. Naucni i Strucni Radovi u Serijskim Publikacijama. Serija B: Prirodne, Primenjene, Medicinske i Tehnicke Nauke (0352-2393); Bibliografija Jugoslavije. Serija B: Prirodne i Primenjene Nauke. Clanci i Prilozi u Casopisima, Listovima i Zbornicima (0523-218X)
Related titles: Online - full text ed.
Published by: Jugoslovenski Bibliografsko-Informacijski Institut (YUBIN)/Yugoslav Institute for Bibliography and Information, Terazije 26, Belgrade, Yugoslavia. FAX 381-11-687760, yubin@jbi.bg.ac.yu, http://www.yugoslavia.com/culture/yubin. Ed. Radomir Glavicki. Adv. contact Tanja Ostojic.

500 600 016 USA ISSN 0012-3293
Z7409 CODEN: DPPSAV
DIRECTORY OF PUBLISHED PROCEEDINGS. SERIES S E M T - SCIENCE, ENGINEERING, MEDICINE AND TECHNOLOGY. Text in English. 1965. 10/yr. USD 585. bibl. index, cum.index. **Document type:** *Directory, Abstract/Index.* **Description:** Contains an index of conferences and the published proceedings in the fields of science, engineering, medicine and technology. Domestic and foreign conferences are cited.
Related titles: Online - full text ed.: (from Institute for Scientific Information).
—BLDSC (3594.930000), CASDDS, CISTI, GNLM, Linda Hall.
Published by: InterDok Corp., 173 Halstead Ave, Box 326, Harrison, NY 10528. TEL 914-835-3506, FAX 914-835-6757, http://www.interdok.com.

NITRIC OXIDE. see *BIOLOGY—Abstracting, Bibliographies, Statistics*

061 005 UKR ISSN 1561-1086
H8.U45
UKRAINSKII REFERATIVNYI ZURNAL. SERIA 1. PRIRODNICHI NAUKI, MEDICINA/UKRAINIAN JOURNAL OF ABSTRACTS. SER. 1. PRIRODNICI NAUKI, MEDICINE. Text and summaries in English, Russian, Ukrainian. 1995. q. UAK 250 domestic; USD 200 foreign (effective 2000). **Document type:** *Monographic series, Abstract/Index, Government.*
Published by: Natsional'na Akademiya Nauk Ukrainy, Institut Problem Reestratsii Informatsii/National Academy of Sciences of Ukraine, Institute for Information Recording, Vul Shpaka 2, Kiev 03113, Ukraine. TEL 380-44-4468389, FAX 380-44-2417233, djerelo@cki.ipri.kiev.ua, http://www.nbuv.gov.ua. Ed., Pub. V Petrov. Circ: 150 (paid); 100 (controlled).

SECURITY

see CRIMINOLOGY AND LAW ENFORCEMENT—Security

SHIPS AND SHIPPING

see TRANSPORTATION—Ships And Shipping

SINGLES' INTERESTS AND LIFESTYLES

SCARLET LETTER. see *WOMEN'S INTERESTS*

SMALL BUSINESS

see BUSINESS AND ECONOMICS—Small Business

SOCIAL SCIENCES: COMPREHENSIVE WORKS

001.3 IND ISSN 0970-2385
HD70.I4
ABHIGYAN; the journal of foundation for organization research and education. Text in English. 1983. q. INR 250, USD 50 (effective Jan. 2000). adv. bk.rev. back issues avail. *Refereed.* **Document type:** *Academic/Scholarly.* **Description:** Expression of the changing management scenario and organization.
Indexed: Indian Psychol.Abstr., PsycInfo, Psychol.Abstr. (1983-), Pub.Admin.Abstr.
—BLDSC (0549.392000).
Published by: Foundation for Organisational Research and Education, Adhitam Kendra, B-18, Qutab Institutional Area, New Delhi 110 016, India. TEL 91-11-6863396, FAX 91-11-6964229, TELEX 031-73215 FORE IN. Ed. Vinayshil Gautam. Pub. Deepa Verma. R&P, Adv. contact Mereena Mathew. B&W page INR 15,000. Circ: 700.

300 610 CHE ISSN 0275-5742
ADVANCES IN MEDICAL SOCIAL SCIENCE; health and illness as viewed by anthropology, geography, history, psychology and sociology. Text in English. 1983. irreg., latest vol.2, 1984. price varies. *Refereed.* **Document type:** *Monographic series.*
Indexed: Anthropol.Lit. (coverage dropped).
—CCC.
Published by: Gordon and Breach - Harwood Academic (Subsidiary of: Taylor & Francis Group), PO Box 531, Lausanne 1000, Switzerland. Ed. Julio L Ruffini. **Subscr. addr. in US:** International Publishers Direct, PO Box 32160, Newark, NJ 07102. FAX 215-750-6343.

AGEING AND SOCIETY. see *GERONTOLOGY AND GERIATRICS*

320 300 USA ISSN 0002-7642
H1
AMERICAN BEHAVIORAL SCIENTIST. Text in English. 1957. m. USD 125 to individuals; USD 775 to institutions; USD 20 newsstand/cover to individuals; USD 70 newsstand/cover to institutions (effective 2002). adv. index. back issues avail.; reprints avail. *Refereed.* **Document type:** *Academic/Scholarly.* **Description:** Focuses, in theme-organized issues prepared under guest editors, on emerging cross-disciplinary interests, research and problems in the social and behavioral sciences.
Related titles: Microform ed.: (from PQC); Online - full text ed.: (from Gale Group, EBSCO Publishing, O C L C Online Computer Library Center, Inc., RoweCom Information Quest, ProQuest Information & Learning, ingenta, Swets Blackwell, Institute for Scientific Information).
Indexed: A.B.C.Pol.Sci., ASCA, ASSIA, Abstr.Crim.& Pen., Acad.Ind., Adol.Ment.Hlth.Abstr., AgeLine, Art.Hosp.& Tour., Bibl.Asian Stud. (1973-1983), Bibl.Engl.Lang.& Lit., Bibl.Ind., Bk.Rev.Ind., C.I.J.E., Chic.Per.Ind., Commun.Abstr., Cont.Pg.Manage., Crim.Just.Abstr., Curr.Cont., Educ.Admin.Abstr., Ekist.Ind., Fam.Ind., Fut.Surv., Hist.Abstr. (1970-1988, dropped), Human Resour.Abstr., IBR, IBZ, IDA, IMFL, Int.Polit.Sci.Abstr., Intl.Bibl.Soc.Sci., Mid.East: Abstr.& Ind., P.A.I.S., Peace Res.Abstr., Pers.Lit., Polit.Sci.Abstr., PsycInfo, Psychol.Abstr. (1962-), Russ.Acad.Sci.Bibl., SSCI, Sage Pub.Admin.Abstr., Sage Race Rel.Abstr., Sage Urb.Stud.Abstr., Soc.Sci.Ind. (Sep.1982-), Soc.Serv.Abstr., Sociol.Abstr., THA, Urb.Aff.Abstr., e-psyche.
—BLDSC (0810.780000), IDS, Infotrieve, ingenta. **CCC.**
Published by: Sage Publications, Inc., 2455 Teller Rd, Thousand Oaks, CA 91320. TEL 805-499-0721, FAX 805-499-0871, info@sagepub.com, http://www.sagepub.com. Eds. Kay Deaux, Martin Bulmer. R&P Tanya Udin. Adv. contact DeAnna Vega Hammersley. Circ: 1,750. **Overseas subscr. to:** Sage Publications Ltd., 6 Bonhill St, London EC2A 4PU, United Kingdom; Sage Publications India Pvt. Ltd., 4215, New Delhi 110 048, India.

ASSOCIATION FOR THE STUDY OF PLAY NEWSLETTER. see *PSYCHOLOGY*

BASIC AND APPLIED SOCIAL PSYCHOLOGY. see *PSYCHOLOGY*

300 USA ISSN 1015-082X
CHEIRON NEWSLETTER. Text in English. 1973. s-a. USD 20 to individuals; USD 30 to institutions. adv. bk.rev. bibl. back issues avail. **Document type:** *Newsletter.* **Description:** Summarizes on-going research of historians in psychology and the behavioral and social sciences who are largely members of the Cheiron Society.
Indexed: e-psyche.
Published by: International Society for History of the Behavioral and Social Sciences, c/o Psychology Office, Bulfinch 501, Massachusetts General Hospital, Boston, MA 02114. TEL 617-492-1130. Ed. Eugene Taylor. Circ: 500. **Co-sponsor:** Cheiron Society.

301 616.89 USA
CLINICAL SOCIOLOGY: RESEARCH AND PRACTICE. Text in English. 1996. irreg., latest 2000. price varies. *Refereed.* **Document type:** *Monographic series.* **Description:** Publishes studies in the field of clinical sociology, including ethical and legal issues, methods of intervention and evaluation, and the role of clinical sociology in specific settings.
Indexed: e-psyche.
Published by: Kluwer Academic - Plenum Publishers (Subsidiary of: Wolters Kluwer N.V.), 233 Spring St, New York, NY 10013-1578. TEL 212-620-8000, 800-221-9369, FAX 212-463-0742, info@plenum.com, http://www.plenum.com. Ed. John G Bruhn.

300 USA ISSN 1069-3971
H1 CODEN: CRCRE4
CROSS-CULTURAL RESEARCH; the journal of comparative social science. Text in English. 1966. q. USD 65 to individuals; USD 270 to institutions; USD 25 newsstand/cover to individuals; USD 70 newsstand/cover to institutions (effective 2002). adv. bk.rev. bibl, charts, illus. index. back issues avail.; reprint service avail. from PQC. *Refereed.* **Document type:** *Academic/Scholarly.* **Description:** Studies cross-cultural or comparative issues in the social and behavioral sciences. Examines topics that span societies, nations and cultures, providing strategies for the systematic testing of theories about human society and behavior. Research reports, review articles, methodological studies, bibliographies and discussion pieces offer a wealth of information on cross-cultural issues providing a global perspective.
Former titles (until 1993): Behavior Science Research (0094-3673); Behavior Science Notes (0005-7886)
Related titles: Microform ed.: (from PQC); Online - full text ed.: (from EBSCO Publishing, O C L C Online Computer Library Center, Inc., RoweCom Information Quest, ProQuest Information & Learning, Gale Group, ingenta, Swets Blackwell, Institute for Scientific Information).
Indexed: A.I.C.P., ASSIA, Abstr.Anthropol., AgeLine, Amer.Bibl.Slavic & E.Eur.Stud., Anthropol.Lit., Bibl.Asian Stud. (1974, 1997-1998), Crim.Just.Abstr., Curr.Cont., E.I., ERA, Human Resour.Abstr., IBR, IBZ, IMFL, Indian Psychol.Abstr., Int.Polit.Sci.Abstr., Intl.Bibl.Soc.Sci., Lang.& Lang.Behav.Abstr., Peace Res.Abstr., PsycInfo, Psychol.Abstr. (1974-), SOPODA, SSCI, Soc.Sci.Ind. (Jul.1999-), Soc.Serv.Abstr., Sociol.Abstr., e-psyche.
—BLDSC (3488.825000), Infotrieve, ingenta. **CCC.**
Published by: (Society for Cross-Cultural Research), Sage Publications, Inc., 2455 Teller Rd, Thousand Oaks, CA 91320. TEL 805-499-0721, FAX 805-499-0871, libaries@sagepub.com, http://www.sagepub.com, http://www.sage.co.uk/. Ed. Melvin Ember. Adv. contact DeAnna Vega Hammersley. Circ: 500. **Overseas subscr. to:** Sage Publications Ltd., 6 Bonhill St, London EC2A 4PU, United Kingdom; Sage Publications India Pvt. Ltd., 4215, New Delhi 110 048, India. **Co-sponsor:** Human Relations Area Files, Inc.

EUROHEALTH. see *PUBLIC HEALTH AND SAFETY*

FREE ASSOCIATIONS; psychoanalysis, groups, politics, culture. see *PSYCHOLOGY*

HARYANA AGRICULTURAL UNIVERSITY. JOURNAL OF RESEARCH. see *AGRICULTURE*

HAWLIYAT KULLIYAT AL-A'DAAB/ANNALS OF THE FACULTY OF ARTS. see *HUMANITIES: COMPREHENSIVE WORKS*

▼ **HEALTH, RISK & SOCIETY.** see *PUBLIC HEALTH AND SAFETY*

▼ **HEALTH SERVICES AND OUTCOMES RESEARCH METHODOLOGY**; an international journal devoted to quantitative methods for the study of utilization, quality, cost and outcomes of health. see *MEDICAL SCIENCES*

304.2 USA
HUMAN ECOLOGY. ANNUAL REPORT. Text in English. a. **Document type:** *Corporate.*
Published by: New York State College of Human Ecology, 1150 Comstock Hall, Cornell University, Ithaca, NY 14850-0901. TEL 607-255-2216, FAX 607-255-3794, jcs6@cornell.edu.

156 DEU ISSN 1045-6767
GN365.9 CODEN: HNATER
HUMAN NATURE; an interdisciplinary biosocial perspective. Text in English. 1990. q. EUR 83.10 domestic to individuals; EUR 86.20 foreign to individuals; EUR 173.10 domestic to institutions; EUR 176.20 foreign to institutions; EUR 42 newsstand/cover (effective 2002). back issues avail.; reprint service avail. from PSC,SCH. *Refereed.* **Document type:** *Journal, Academic/Scholarly.* **Description:** Dedicated to advancing the interdisciplinary investigation of the biological, social, and environmental factors which underline human behavior.
Related titles: Online - full text ed.: (from Institute for Scientific Information).
Indexed: Crim.Just.Abstr., Curr.Cont., Indian Psychol.Abstr., Intl.Bibl.Soc.Sci., Lang.& Lang.Behav.Abstr., PsycInfo, Psychol.Abstr. (1990-), Russ.Acad.Sci.Bibl., SOPODA, SSCI, Soc.Serv.Abstr., Sociol.Abstr., e-psyche.
—BLDSC (4336.223500), GNLM, IDS, ingenta. **CCC.**
Published by: Walter de Gruyter und Co., Genthiner Str 13, Berlin 10785, Germany. TEL 49-30-26005-0, FAX 49-30-26005-251, wdg-info@degruyter.de, http://www.unm.edu/~humnat, http://www.degruyter.de. Ed. Jane B Lancaster. Circ: 250.

300 GBR ISSN 0018-7267
H1 CODEN: HUREAA
HUMAN RELATIONS; towards the integration of the social sciences. Text in English. 1947. m. GBP 65 to individuals; GBP 474 to institutions; GBP 6 newsstand/cover to individuals; GBP 41 newsstand/cover to institutions (effective 2002). adv. bk.rev. bibl, charts, illus. index. reprint service avail. from PSC,SCH. *Refereed.* **Document type:** *Academic/Scholarly.* **Description:** Provides an interdisciplinary forum for research into human relations among all the social sciences.
Related titles: Microfilm ed.: (from PQC); Online - full text ed.: (from ProQuest Information & Learning, CatchWord Ltd., Gale Group, Northern Light Technology, Inc., EBSCO Publishing, O C L C Online Computer Library Center, Inc., RoweCom Information Quest, ingenta, Swets Blackwell, Kluwer Online, Factiva, Institute for Scientific Information).
Indexed: ABI Inform. (Jul.1972-), A.I.C.P., ASCA, ASSIA, Abstr.Anthropol., Abstr.Crim.& Pen., AgeLine, Arts & Hum.Cit.Ind. (coverage dropped), B.P.I. (Jul.1995-May 1999), BPIA, Br.Hum.Ind., Bus.Ind., CINAHL, Chic.Per.Ind., Commun.Abstr., Cont.Pg.Manage., Crim.Just.Abstr., Curr.Cont., Curr.Ind.Stat., ERA, Educ.Admin.Abstr., Emerald, Ergon.Abstr., Fam.Ind., Human Resour.Abstr., IBR, IMFL, Indian Psychol.Abstr., Int.Lab.Doc., Intl.Bibl.Soc.Sci., Lang.& Lang.Behav.Abstr., Manage.Cont., Mark.Res.Abstr. (1964-), Mid.East: Abstr.& Ind., P C I, P.A.I.S., Peace Res.Abstr., Pers.Lit., PsycInfo, Psychol.Abstr. (1949-), Psycscan A.P., Russ.Acad.Sci.Bibl., SCIMP (1978-), SOMA, SOPODA, SSCI, Sage Race Rel.Abstr., Soc.Sci.Ind. (Nov.1982-Dec.1999), Soc.Serv.Abstr., Sociol.Abstr., Stud.Wom.Abstr., Viol.& Abuse Abstr., e-psyche.
—BLDSC (4336.400000), CatchWord, IDS, ingenta. **CCC.**
Published by: (Tavistock Institute of Human Relations), Sage Publications Ltd., 6 Bonhill St, London EC2A 4PU, United Kingdom. TEL 44-20-7374-0645, FAX 44-20-7374-8741, market@sagepub.co.uk, http://www.sage.co.uk/. Ed. Paul Willman. Circ: 2,000. **Subscr. to:** Sage Publications India Pvt. Ltd., P O Box 4215, New Delhi 110 048, India. TEL 91-11-641-9884, FAX 91-11-647-2426; Sage Publications, Inc., 2455 Teller Rd, Thousand Oaks, CA 91320.

301 058.7 SWE ISSN 1101-4431
INFORMATIONSBULLETINEN; tidskrift foer livskvalitet. Text in Swedish. 1986. bi-m. SEK 120 (effective 1997). adv. bk.rev. **Document type:** *Bulletin.*
Indexed: e-psyche.
Published by: Circulus, Fack 15057, Uppsala 75015, Sweden. TEL 46-295-43034, FAX 46-295-43018, Guy.Madison@psyk.uu.se. Ed. Guy Madison. Circ: 2,000.

INTERDISCIPLINARIA; revista de psicologia y ciencias afines/journal of psychology and related sciences. see *PSYCHOLOGY*

INTERFACES: LINGUISTICS, PSYCHOLOGY AND HEALTH THERAPEUTICS; an international journal of research, notes and commentary. see *LINGUISTICS*

JOURNAL FOR THE THEORY OF SOCIAL BEHAVIOUR. see *PSYCHOLOGY*

JOURNAL OF APPLIED HEALTH BEHAVIOUR. see *PSYCHOLOGY*

JOURNAL OF APPLIED SOCIAL PSYCHOLOGY. see *PSYCHOLOGY*

910.03 USA ISSN 0021-9347
E185.5
JOURNAL OF BLACK STUDIES. Text in English. 1970. bi-m. USD 80 to individuals; USD 400 to institutions; USD 20 newsstand/cover to individuals; USD 75 newsstand/cover to institutions (effective 2002). adv. bk.rev. illus. index. back issues avail.; reprint service avail. from PQC. *Refereed.* **Document type:** *Academic/Scholarly.* **Description:** Sustains full analytical discussion of economic, political, sociological, historical, literary, and philosophical issues related to African-Americans.
Related titles: Microform ed.: (from PQC); Online - full text ed.: (from JSTOR (Web-based Journal Archive), EBSCO Publishing, O C L C Online Computer Library Center, Inc., RoweCom Information Quest, ProQuest Information & Learning, Gale Group, ingenta, Swets Blackwell, Institute for Scientific Information).
Indexed: ASCA, ASSIA, AgeLine, Amer.Hist.& Life, Arts & Hum.Cit.Ind. (coverage dropped), BHA, Bk.Rev.Ind. (1984-), Br.Archaeol.Abstr., C.I.J.E., Chic.Per.Ind., Child.Bk.Rev.Ind. (1984-), Crim.Just.Abstr., Curr.Cont., Curr.Cont.Africa, Environ.Sci.Poll.Mgmt., Fam.Ind., High.Educ.Abstr., Hist.Abstr. (1970-), Human Resour.Abstr., IBR, IMFL, Ind.Per.Blacks, Int.Polit.Sci.Abstr., Intl.Bibl.Soc.Sci., Lang.& Lang.Behav.Abstr., Mult.Ed.Abstr., P C I, P.A.I.S., Peace Res.Abstr., Polit.Sci.Abstr., PsycInfo, Psychol.Abstr. (1991-), Risk Abstr., SOPODA, SSCI, Saf.Sci.Abstr., Sage Fam.Stud.Abstr., Sage Pub.Admin.Abstr., Sage Race Rel.Abstr., Soc.Sci.Ind. (Jan.1994-), Soc.Serv.Abstr., Soc.Work Res.& Abstr., Sociol.Abstr., Viol.& Abuse Abstr., e-psyche.
—BLDSC (4954.200000), IDS, Infotrieve, ingenta. **CCC.**
Published by: (Association of Black Psychologists), Sage Publications, Inc., 2455 Teller Rd, Thousand Oaks, CA 91320. TEL 805-499-0721, FAX 805-499-0871, info@sagepub.com, http://www.sagepub.co.uk/journals/usdetails/ioozo.html. Eds. Molefi Kete Asante, Terry Kershaw. R&P Tanya Udin. Adv. contact DeAnna Vega Hammersley. Circ: 1,750. **Overseas subscr. to:** Sage Publications Ltd., 6 Bonhill St, London EC2A 4PU, United Kingdom; Sage Publications India Pvt. Ltd., 4215, New Delhi 110 048, India.

JOURNAL OF SOCIAL BEHAVIOR AND PERSONALITY. see *PSYCHOLOGY*

L S E HEALTH DISCUSSION PAPER. see *PUBLIC HEALTH AND SAFETY*

LANTERNINO; trimestrale di storia della medicina e studi sociali. see *MEDICAL SCIENCES*

300 NLD ISSN 0924-4905
LONGITUDINAL RESEARCH IN THE BEHAVIORAL, SOCIAL AND MEDICAL SCIENCES. Text in English. 1981. irreg. price varies. *Refereed.* **Document type:** *Monographic series.*
Published by: Kluwer Academic Publishers Group (Subsidiary of: Wolters Kluwer N.V.), Spuiboulevard 50, PO Box 17, Dordrecht 3300 AA, Netherlands. FAX 31-78-639-2254, services@wkap.nl, http://www.wkap.nl. **Dist. by:** Journals Department, PO Box 322, Dordrecht 3300 AH, Netherlands. FAX 31-78-654-6474.

300 USA
LONGITUDINAL RESEARCH IN THE SOCIAL AND BEHAVIORAL SCIENCES; an interdisciplinary series. Text in English. 1995. irreg., latest 2000. price varies. **Document type:** *Monographic series.* **Description:** Focuses on key topics in the growing field of research methodology.
Indexed: e-psyche.
Published by: Kluwer Academic - Plenum Publishers (Subsidiary of: Wolters Kluwer N.V.), 233 Spring St, New York, NY 10013-1578. TEL 212-620-8035, 800-221-9369, FAX 212-463-0742, info@plenum.com, http://www.plenum.com.

MANAB MON; a journal depicting the modern trends in psychology, biology, and sociology. see *PSYCHOLOGY*

MEDDELELSER OM GROENLAND. MAN & SOCIETY. see *ANTHROPOLOGY*

300 610 DEU
MEDIZINSOZIOLOGIE. Text in German. irreg., latest vol.3, 1993. **Document type:** *Monographic series.*
Indexed: Russ.Acad.Sci.Bibl.
Published by: Lit Verlag, Grindelberg 15A, Hamburg 20144, Germany. TEL 49-40-446446, FAX 49-40-441422.

THE MILBANK QUARTERLY; a journal of public health and health care policy . see *POLITICAL SCIENCE*

300 150 BRA ISSN 0102-7484
MIMESIS (BAURU); revista da area de ciencias humanas. Text in Portuguese. 1979. s-a. BRL 20, USD 10 per issue (effective 2000). bk.rev. abstr, bibl, charts, illus, maps. back issues avail. **Document type:** *Journal, Academic/Scholarly.* **Description:** Contains original works of technical, didactic, and scientific character in the area of humanities. Promotes research directed to the academic community in general.
Indexed: MLA Intl.Bibl., Soc.Serv.Abstr., Sociol.Abstr.
Published by: (Universidade do Sagrado Coracao), Editora da Universidade do Sagrado Coracao, Rua Irma Arminda, 10-50, Bauru, SP 17044-160, Brazil. TEL 55-014-235-7111, FAX 55-14-235-7219, npu@usc.br, edusc@usc.br, http://www.usc.br. Ed. Marilene Cabello Di Flora. Pub. Lina Ana Santarosa. R&P Luis Eugenio Vescio TEL 55-14-2357378. Circ: 500.

MIND & HUMAN INTERACTION. see *PSYCHOLOGY*

N A T O ADVANCED SCIENCE INSTITUTES SERIES D: BEHAVIOURAL AND SOCIAL SCIENCES. see *PSYCHOLOGY*

300 363.3 USA
NATURAL HAZARDS CENTER. QUICK RESPONSE REPORTS. Text in English. 1986. irreg., latest vol.113, 1999. **Description:** Consists of reports presenting the results of research by social scientists conducted immediately following disasters. Covers immediate impact and response for a broad range of disasters - natural and caused by humans - in diverse settings, and affecting all types of human communities.
Media: Online - full text.
Published by: University of Colorado, Natural Hazards Center, Quick Response Program, Campus Box 482, Boulder, CO 80309. TEL 303-492-6819, FAX 903-492-2151, hazctr@colorado.edu, http://www.colorado.edu/hazards. R&P David L Butler TEL 303-492-4180. **Co-sponsor:** National Science Foundation.

508 AUT ISSN 1016-605X
NEUE DENKSCHRIFTEN DES NATURHISTORISCHEN MUSEUMS IN WIEN. Text in German. irreg. price varies. **Document type:** *Monographic series, Academic/Scholarly.*
Formerly (until 1977): Denkschriften des Naturhistorischen Museums in Wien
Indexed: Biol.Abstr., GeoRef, Zoo.Rec.
Published by: Verlag Ferdinand Berger und Soehne GmbH, Wienerstrasse 21-23, Horn, N 3580, Austria. TEL 43-2982-4161332, FAX 43-2982-4161382, druckerei.office@berger.at, http://www.berger.at. Eds. Friedrich Bachmayer, Ortwin Schultz. Circ: 500.

300 DEU ISSN 0077-801X
NEW BABYLON: STUDIES IN THE SOCIAL SCIENCES. Text in German. irreg., latest vol.50, 1993. price varies. back issues avail. **Document type:** *Monographic series, Academic/Scholarly.*
Indexed: e-psyche.
Published by: Walter de Gruyter und Co., Mouton de Gruyter, Genthiner Str 13, Berlin 10785, Germany. TEL 49-30-26005-0, FAX 49-30-26005222, 49-30-26005-251, wdg-info@degruyter.de, http://www.degruyter.de.

NEW GENETICS AND SOCIETY. see *BIOLOGY—Genetics*

NONLINEAR DYNAMICS, PSYCHOLOGY, AND LIFE SCIENCES. see *PSYCHOLOGY*

NURSING RESEARCH. see *MEDICAL SCIENCES—Nurses And Nursing*

PERSPECTIVES ON CULTURE AND MEDICINE. see *MEDICAL SCIENCES*

PSYCHOLOGY TODAY. see *PSYCHOLOGY*

SOCIAL SCIENCE & MEDICINE. see *MEDICAL SCIENCES*

SOCIOECONOMIC CHARACTERISTICS OF MEDICAL PRACTICE. see *MEDICAL SCIENCES*

SOTSIONIKA, MENTOLOGIYA I PSIKHOLOGIYA LICHNOSTI/SOCIONICS, MENTOLOGY AND PERSONALITY PSYCHOLOGY. see *SOCIOLOGY*

▼ **UNDERSTANDING STATISTICS**; statistical issues in psychology, education, and the social sciences. see *STATISTICS*

S

UNIVERSIDADE DO SAGRADO CORACAO. CADERNOS DE DIVULGACAO CULTURAL. see *MEDICAL SCIENCES*

300 001.3 PHL ISSN 0047-5742
AS539.5
UNIVERSITY OF SANTO TOMAS. GRADUATE SCHOOL. JOURNAL OF GRADUATE RESEARCH. Variant title: University of Santo Tomas Journal of Graduate Research. Text in English. 1971. s-a. PHP 280 domestic to individuals; USD 8.50 foreign to individuals; PHP 200 domestic to institutions; USD 6.50 foreign to institutions (effective 2000). bk.rev. bibl, illus, charts. **Document type:** *Academic/Scholarly.*
Indexed: Bibl.Asian Stud. (1985-1989), INIS Atomind., Ind.Phil.Per.
—ingenta.
Published by: (University Of Santo Tomas, Graduate School), Santo Tomas University Press, Espana St, Manila 1008, Philippines. TEL 632-731-3101, FAX 632-732-7486, 63-2-740-9732, odgs@ustcc.ust.edu.ph. Ed. Belen L Tangco. Pub. Rev. Jose Antonio E. Aureada. Circ: 1,500.

VERHALTENSTHERAPIE UND PSYCHOSOZIALE PRAXIS. see *PSYCHOLOGY*

VS; quaderni di studi semiotici. see *LINGUISTICS*

SOCIAL SCIENCES: COMPREHENSIVE WORKS—Abstracting, Bibliographies, Statistics

300.1 USA
METHODOLOGY IN THE SOCIAL SCIENCES. Text in English. irreg. **Document type:** *Monographic series.* **Description:** Introduces new methods to the practicing researcher.
Published by: Guilford Publications, Inc., 72 Spring St, New York, NY 10012. TEL 212-431-9800, 800-365-7006, FAX 212-966-6708, info@guilford.com, http://www.guilford.com. Ed. David Kenny.

SCITECH BOOK NEWS; an annotated bibliography of new books in science, technology, & medicine. see *BIBLIOGRAPHIES*

SOCIAL SERVICES AND WELFARE

see also DRUG ABUSE AND ALCOHOLISM; HANDICAPPED; PUBLIC HEALTH AND SAFETY

A B P CONTACT. see *HANDICAPPED*

A C A NEWS; the provincial newsletter for seniors. see *GERONTOLOGY AND GERIATRICS*

A F B NEWS. see *HANDICAPPED—Visually Impaired*

614 USA ISSN 0279-1692
A H C A NOTES. Text in English. 1972. m. USD 150 to non-members; USD 15 to members (effective 2000). illus. **Document type:** *Newsletter, Trade.*
Formerly: A H C A Weekly Notes (0146-6321)
—ingenta.
Published by: American Health Care Association, 1201 L St, N W, Washington, DC 20005. TEL 202-842-4444, FAX 202-842-3860. Ed., R&P Nathan Childs TEL 202-898-6327. Pub. Linda Keegan. Circ: 10,000.

A H R C CHRONICLE. see *MEDICAL SCIENCES—Psychiatry And Neurology*

A M S STUDIES IN MODERN SOCIETY. see *PUBLIC HEALTH AND SAFETY*

613 NLD ISSN 0168-2857
A S; maandblad voor de activiteitensector. (Activiteitensektor) Key Title: AS. Maandblad Aktiviteitensektor. Text in Dutch. 1980. m. (10/yr.). free to qualified personnel. adv. bk.rev. **Document type:** *Trade.* **Description:** Provides social service leaders at various mental-health, rehabilitative, and gerontological agencies (both in- and out-patient) with news and professional advice.
Incorporates (1956-1982): Ligament (0024-3264)
Published by: Elsevier Gezondheidszorg B.V., Tijdstroom (Subsidiary of: Reed Elsevier plc Group), Planetenbaan 1, Maarssen 3600 AK, Netherlands. TEL 31-346-577577, FAX 31-346-554287, http://www.tijdstroom.nl. Circ: 5,000 (controlled).

ABILITIES. see *HANDICAPPED—Hearing Impaired*

ACTIVITY DIRECTOR'S GUIDE; the complete guide of ideas, tips and techniques for the busy professional. see *GERONTOLOGY AND GERIATRICS*

360 AUS ISSN 1030-7451
ACTIVNEWS. Text in English. 1953. m. AUD 40 to membership (effective 2000). adv. bk.rev. back issues avail. *Refereed.* **Document type:** *Newsletter.* **Description:** Promotes the wide range of services for adults and children with developmental disabilities in Western Australia.
Formerly: Our Children (0048-2382)
Published by: Activ Foundation Inc., 116 Jersey St, Jolimont, W.A. 6014, Australia. TEL 61-9-3870555, FAX 61-9-3870599, active@wantree.com.au. Ed., R&P Heather Monteiro. Circ: 2,500.

ADVANCES IN CLINICAL REHABILITATION. see *MEDICAL SCIENCES—Physical Medicine And Rehabilitation*

ADVANCES IN LIFE COURSE RESEARCH. see *GERONTOLOGY AND GERIATRICS*

362.28 NLD ISSN 0922-3061
ADVANCES IN SUICIDOLOGY. Text in Dutch. 1989. irreg., latest vol.2, 1995. price varies. back issues avail. *Refereed.* **Document type:** *Monographic series.* **Description:** Scholarly treatment of issues pertaining to the prevention of suicide.
Indexed: e-psyche.
—BLDSC (0711.593800), CISTI.
Published by: Brill Academic Publishers, PO Box 9000, Leiden 2300 PA, Netherlands. TEL 31-71-535-3500, FAX 31-71-531-7532, cs@brill.nl. R&P Elizabeth Venekamp.

360 USA
ADVANCES (PRINCETON). Text in English. 1988. q. **Document type:** *Newsletter.* **Description:** Grants, programs sponsored by the Robert Wood Johnson Foundation.
Published by: Robert Wood Johnson Foundation, PO Box 2316, Princeton, NJ 08543-2316. TEL 609-452-8701, http://www.rwjf.org. Ed. Paul Tarini.

AFYA. see *MEDICAL SCIENCES*

362.1 616.9 GBR ISSN 0962-4171
AIDS ANALYSIS AFRICA. Text in English. 199?. bi-m. GBP 60, USD 100. **Document type:** *Newsletter.* **Description:** Reports economic, legislative, and political developments affecting persons with AIDS or social services on their behalf.
Supersedes in part: AIDS and Society (1055-0380)
Indexed: Ind.S.A.Per., Sugar Ind.Abstr.
Published by: AIDS Analysis Ltd., Ste 71, Ludgate House, 107-111 Fleet St, London EC4A 2AB, United Kingdom. TEL 44-171-955-0231, FAX 44-171-353-1516, mcr1: africa-analysis@geonet.com. Ed. Rex Winsbury.

362.1 616.9 GBR ISSN 1359-1452
AIDS ANALYSIS ASIA. Text in English. 1995. bi-m. GBP 60, USD 100. illus, maps. **Document type:** *Bulletin.*
Supersedes in part: AIDS and Society (1055-0380)
Published by: AIDS Analysis Ltd., Ste 71, Ludgate House, 107-111 Fleet St, London EC4A 2AB, United Kingdom. TEL 44-171-955-0231, FAX 44-171-353-1516, mcr1: africa-analysis@geonet.com. Ed. Rex Winsbury.

ALABAMA COUNSELING ASSOCIATION. JOURNAL. see *OCCUPATIONS AND CAREERS*

ALERT; maandblad voor rampenbestrijding en crisisbeheersing. see *CIVIL DEFENSE*

ALERT (ADELAIDE). see *MEDICAL SCIENCES—Endocrinology*

ALERT (EWING); news on alcoholism and drug addiction services for persons who are hard of hearing. see *DRUG ABUSE AND ALCOHOLISM*

ALL ABOUT MEDICARE. see *INSURANCE*

362.6 GBR
ALMSHOUSES GAZETTE. Text in English. 1950. q. **Document type:** *Bulletin.*
Published by: Almshouse Association, Billingbear Lodge, Carters Hill, Wokingham, Berks RG40 5RU, United Kingdom. TEL 44-1344-52922.

ALZHEIMER'S CARE GUIDE; published especially for those who care for people with Alzheimer's disease and related disorders. see *GERONTOLOGY AND GERIATRICS*

▼ **ALZHEIMER'S CARE QUARTERLY.** see *MEDICAL SCIENCES—Psychiatry And Neurology*

ALZHEIMER'S RESEARCH REVIEW. see *MEDICAL SCIENCES—Psychiatry And Neurology*

362.1 614 USA ISSN 0888-0352
RA973.5
AMERICAN HEALTH CARE ASSOCIATION. PROVIDER. Text in English. 1975. m. USD 48 (effective 2000). adv. illus. **Document type:** *Trade.*
Formerly: American Health Care Association. Journal (0360-4969)
Related titles: Online - full text ed.
Indexed: Abstr.Soc.Geront., AgeLine, I.P.A., Int.Nurs.Ind., Med.Care Rev.
—BLDSC (6937.687000), CISTI, GNLM, ingenta.
Published by: American Health Care Association, 1201 L St, N W, Washington, DC 20005. TEL 202-842-4444, FAX 202-842-3860. Ed., R&P Joanne Erickson TEL 202-898-2811. Pub. Linda Keegan. Adv. contact Mike Disanto. Circ: 36,000.

AMERICAN JOURNAL OF ORTHOPSYCHIATRY. see *PSYCHOLOGY*

362.6 USA
AMERICAN PARKINSON DISEASE ASSOCIATION. NEWSLETTER. Text in English. 1965. q. free per issue. **Document type:** *Newsletter.* **Description:** Informs recipients A.P.D.A. activities, how to cope with their disorder, and of developments in medical research.
Indexed: e-psyche.
Published by: American Parkinson Disease Association, Inc., 1250 Hylan Blvd, Ste 4B, Staten Island, NY 10305. TEL 800-223-2732. Ed. Paul Maestrone.

AMERICAN REHABILITATION. see *EDUCATION—Special Education And Rehabilitation*

AMERICANS WITH DISABILITIES ACT: PUBLIC ACCOMMODATIONS AND COMMERCIAL FACILITIES. see *HANDICAPPED*

306.461 AUS ISSN 1036-6733
ANNUAL REVIEW OF HEALTH SOCIAL SCIENCES. Text in English. 1991. a. *Refereed.* **Document type:** *Academic/Scholarly.*
Published by: University of New South Wales, School of Health Services Management, Sydney, NSW 2052, Australia. TEL 61-2-9385-2592, FAX 61-2-9385-1036.

ARAFMI NEWS; providing support for carers of people with mental disorders. see *MEDICAL SCIENCES—Psychiatry And Neurology*

362.3 USA
THE ARC INSIGHT. Text in English. 1952. q. USD 15 (effective 1998). adv. bk.rev. illus. reprint service avail. from PQC. **Document type:** *Newspaper.*
Former titles: The Arc Today; A R C (0199-9435); Mental Retardation News (0009-4072); Children Limited
Related titles: Microform ed.: (from PQC).
Indexed: e-psyche.
Published by: Arc, National Headquarters, 1010 Wayne Ave, Ste 650, Silver Spring, MD 20910. TEL 3015653842, info@thearc.org, http://www.thearc.org. Ed. Chris Privett. R&P Liz Moore. Adv. contact Jim Humphrey. Circ: 95,000.

ARIZONA MEDICINE. see *PUBLIC HEALTH AND SAFETY*

ARKANSAS. DIVISION OF REHABILITATION SERVICES. ANNUAL REPORT. see *EDUCATION—Special Education And Rehabilitation*

ASAHIGAWASO KENKYU NENPO/ASAHIGAWASO INSTITUTE OF MEDICAL WELFARE. ANNUAL REPORT. see *MEDICAL SCIENCES*

362.4 615.82 IND
ASIA PACIFIC DISABILITY REHABILITATION JOURNAL. Text in English. 1990. s-a. free. bk.rev. *Refereed.* **Document type:** *Academic/Scholarly.* **Description:** Covers policy development, concept clarification, development of methodology in areas of service delivery, training of manpower and programme evaluation, and development of technology related to rehabilitation.
Formerly: Actionaid Disability News (0971-9601)
—BLDSC.

S

Published by: (Shree Ramana Maharishi Academy for the Blind), Asia Pacific Disability Rehabilitation Journal, J-124 Ushas Apartments, 16 th Main, 4th Block, Jayanagar, Bangalore, Karnataka 560 011, India. http://www.dinf.ne.jp/doc/prdl/othr/apdrj/apdrj.html. Ed., Pub., R&P Dr. Maya Thomas. Circ: 2,000.

362.4 615.82 IND
▼ **ASIA PACIFIC DISABILITY REHABILITATION JOURNAL. SELECTED READINGS SERIES.** Text in English. 2000. irreg. **Document type:** *Monographic series, Academic/Scholarly.* **Description:** Covers basic concepts and outlines good practices and research activities for community based rehabilitation services.
Published by: Asia Pacific Disability Rehabilitation Journal, J-124 Ushas Apartments, 16 th Main, 4th Block, Jayanagar, Bangalore, Karnataka 560 011, India. FAX 91-80-6633762, thomasmaya@hotmail.com, http://www.dinf.ne.jp/doc/prdl/othr/apdrj/apdrj.html. Ed. Dr. Maya Thomas.

ASSOCIATION OF BEHAVIORAL HEALTH MANAGEMENT NEWSLETTER. see *PUBLIC HEALTH AND SAFETY*

ASSOCIATION OF GAY AND LESBIAN PSYCHIATRISTS. NEWSLETTER. see *HOMOSEXUALITY*

AUSTRALIAN AND NEW ZEALAND JOURNAL OF FAMILY THERAPY; innovative and contextual approaches to human problems. see *SOCIOLOGY*

AUTUMN SCHOOL OF STUDIES ON ALCOHOL & DRUGS. PROCEEDINGS OF SEMINARS. see *DRUG ABUSE AND ALCOHOLISM*

THE B V A BULLETIN. (Blinded Veterans Association) see *HANDICAPPED—Visually Impaired*

362 JPN ISSN 0912-8662
BANBU* /BAMBOO. Text in Japanese. m. JPY 900 per issue.
Published by: Nihon Iryo Kikaku, 4-14 Kanda-Iwamoto-cho, Chiyoda-ku, Tokyo 101-0033, Japan.

BEHAVIORAL HEALTHCARE TOMORROW. see *PSYCHOLOGY*

361.3 158 GBR ISSN 0268-2621
BEREAVEMENT CARE; an international journal for those who help bereaved people. Text in English. 1982. 3/yr. GBP 17 domestic to individuals; GBP 24 in Ireland to individuals; USD 33 in United States to individuals; USD 48 in Canada to individuals; AUD 49 in Australia to individuals; GBP 19 elsewhere to individuals; GBP 29 domestic to institutions; GBP 39 in Ireland to institutions; USD 54 in United States to institutions; USD 78 in Canada to institutions; AUD 80 in Australia to institutions; GBP 31 elsewhere to institutions (effective 2001). adv. bk.rev. abstr, charts, illus. index. 16 p./no. back issues avail. *Refereed.* **Document type:** *Journal, Academic/Scholarly.* **Description:** For all who wish to deepen their understanding of bereavement. Contains articles of importance to those who help bereaved persons, including counsellors, psychotherapists, psychologists, social workers, the clergy, funeral directors, doctors, and nurses.
Indexed: AMED, Brit.Nur.Ind., e-psyche.
—BLDSC (1893.880000).
Published by: Cruse Bereavement Care, 126 Sheen Rd, Richmond, Surrey TW9 1UR, United Kingdom. TEL 44-208- 940-4818, FAX 44-208-940-7638, info@crusebereavementcare.org.uk. Ed., R&P, Adv. contact Rosie Dalzell TEL 44-181-940-4818. Circ: 2,000 (paid).

BETHPHAGE MESSENGER. see *EDUCATION—Special Education And Rehabilitation*

304.6 KOR ISSN 1226-072X
BOGEON SAHOE YEONGU/HEALTH AND SOCIAL WELFARE REVIEW. Text in English, Korean. 1981. s-a. USD 10 newsstand/cover (effective 2001). 200 p./no. *Refereed.* **Document type:** *Journal, Academic/Scholarly.*
Former titles (until 1995): Bogeon Sahoe Nonjib / Journal of Population, Health and Social Welfare (1226-0282); (until 1989): In-gu Bo-geon Nonjib / Journal of Population and Health Studies (0259-9112)
Indexed: ExtraMED, Popul.Ind.
—BLDSC (42740882500).
Published by: Korea Institute for Health and Social Affairs, San 42-14 Bulgwang-Dong, Eunpyung-Ku, Seoul 122-705, Korea, S.. TEL 82-2-385-8149, 82-2-355-8003, FAX 82-2-355-9500, 82-2-352-2181, library@kihusa.re.kr, http://www.kihusa.re.kr. Ed. Hyun Ae Ahn. Circ: 500.

BRAILLE MONITOR (INKPRINT EDITION). see *HANDICAPPED—Visually Impaired*

BRAILLE SPORTING RECORD. see *HANDICAPPED—Visually Impaired*

BREAKTHROUGH; international mental health journal. see *PSYCHOLOGY*

BRIEFINGS ON J C A H O - A A A H C: AMBULATORY CARE. (Joint Commission on Accreditation of Healthcare Organizations - Accreditation Association for Ambula) see *HEALTH FACILITIES AND ADMINISTRATION*

BRITISH JOURNAL OF DEVELOPMENTAL DISABILITIES. see *EDUCATION—Special Education And Rehabilitation*

362.14 GBR ISSN 1462-1665
▼ **BRITISH JOURNAL OF HOMECARE.** Text in English. 1999. bi-m. GBP 40 domestic to individuals; GBP 60 in Europe to individuals; GBP 72 elsewhere to individuals; GBP 84 domestic to institutions; GBP 114 in Europe to institutions; GBP 132 elsewhere to institutions (effective 2000).
—BLDSC (2309.445000).
Published by: Greycoat Publishing, 1 Harley St, London W1N 1DA, United Kingdom. TEL 44-20-7637-1828, FAX 44-20-7637-3020, greycoat@compuserve.com. Ed. Michael Rennie. Pub. Ashley Wallis.

BRITISH JOURNAL OF VISUAL IMPAIRMENT. see *HANDICAPPED—Visually Impaired*

BRITISH POLIO FELLOWSHIP. BULLETIN. see *MEDICAL SCIENCES—Psychiatry And Neurology*

BROWN UNIVERSITY CHILD AND ADOLESCENT BEHAVIOR LETTER; monthly reports on the problems of children and adolescents growing up. see *CHILDREN AND YOUTH—About*

C A S CADE. see *MEDICAL SCIENCES—Pediatrics*

362.5 DEU
C B M FREUNDESBRIEF. Text in German. 1961. bi-m. free. **Document type:** *Bulletin, Consumer.*
Published by: Christoffel-Blindenmission e.V., Nibelungenstr 124, Bensheim 64625, Germany. TEL 49-6251-131-0, FAX 49-6251-131-122, communications@cbm-i.org, http://www.cbmi.de. Circ: 500,000. **U.S. subscr. to:** Christian Blind Mission International Inc., 450 E Park Ave, Greenville, SC 29601. TEL 864-239-0065, FAX 864-239-0069.

CANADIAN NATIONAL INSTITUTE FOR THE BLIND. NATIONAL ANNUAL REVIEW. see *HANDICAPPED—Visually Impaired*

THE CAPSTONE (TOWSON); news from the Council, and its accreditation and evaluation systems and ProLerna. see *HANDICAPPED*

CARE PLAN. see *PUBLIC HEALTH AND SAFETY*

360 AUS
CARERS IN VICTORIA. Text in English. 1995. q. members only. adv. charts, illus, stat, tr.lit. 16 p./no. back issues avail. **Document type:** *Newsletter.* **Description:** Provides information for care-givers, service providers, welfare workers, government and community seeking to improve the quality of life of care-givers.
Formerly (until Spring, 2001): Victorian Carer (1440-5040)
Published by: Carers Association Victoria, Level 5, 130 Lt Collins St, Melbourne, VIC 3000, Australia. TEL 61-3-9650-9966, FAX 61-3-9650-8066, cav@carersvic.org.au, http://www.carersvic.org.au/. Ed., Adv. contact Eileen Hayes. Circ: 7,000.

CARING (WASHINGTON). see *MEDICAL SCIENCES—Nurses And Nursing*

CHILD ABUSE & NEGLECT. see *CHILDREN AND YOUTH—About*

362.76 AUS ISSN 1320-2871
CHILD ABUSE PREVENTION; national child protection clearing house newsletter. Text in English. 1994. s-a. free per issue. bk.rev. abstr, bibl. back issues avail. **Document type:** *Newsletter.* **Description:** Provides information bulletin of research, practice, and policy for professionals working in areas related to child abuse prevention.
Related titles: CD-ROM ed.
Published by: Australian Institute of Family Studies, 300 Queen St, Melbourne, VIC 3000, Australia. TEL 61-3-9214-7888, FAX 61-3-9214-7839, fic@aifs.org.au, http://www.aifs.org.au. Ed. Judy Adams. Circ: 7,000.

362.7 155.4 GBR ISSN 0952-9136
CODEN: CABEEB
CHILD ABUSE REVIEW. Text in English. 1992. 6/yr. USD 285 in United Kingdom; USD 285 in Canada & Mexico; USD 285 elsewhere; USD 300 combined subscription in United States for print and online eds.; USD 300 combined subscription in Canada & Mexico for print and online eds.; USD 300 combined subscription elsewhere for print and online eds. (effective 2002). adv. **Document type:** *Academic/Scholarly.* **Description:** Reflects current child welfare issues and concerns.
Related titles: Online - full text ed.: ISSN 1099-0852. USD 285 in United States; USD 285 in Canada & Mexico; USD 285 elsewhere (effective 2002) (from EBSCO Publishing, ingenta, Wiley InterScience).
Indexed: ASSIA, Brit.Nur.Ind., Crim.Just.Abstr., Fam.Ind., Indian Psychol.Abstr., PsycInfo, Viol.& Abuse Abstr., e-psyche.
—BLDSC (3172.912700), GNLM, Infotrieve. **CCC.**
Published by: Wiley Europe Ltd., Baffins Ln, Chichester, W Sussex PO19 1UD, United Kingdom. TEL 44-1243-779777, FAX 44-1243-775878, cs-journals@wiley.co.uk, customer@wiley.co.uk, http://www.interscience.wiley.com/jpages/0952-9136/, http://www.wiley.co.uk. adv.: B&W page GBP 650, color page GBP 1,550; trim 200 x 260. Circ: 2,600. **Subscr. in the US to:** John Wiley & Sons, Inc., Journals, 605 Third Ave, New York, NY 10158. TEL 212-850-6645, FAX 212-850-6021, subinfo@wiley.com; **Subscr. to:** John Wiley & Sons Ltd., Baffins Ln, Chichester, Sussex PO19 IUD, United Kingdom. TEL 44-1243-779777, FAX 44-1243-843232, cs-journals@wiley.co.uk.

CHILD & ADOLESCENT HEALTH CARE. see *MEDICAL SCIENCES—Pediatrics*

CHILDREN AND YOUTH SERVICES REVIEW; an international multidisciplinary review of the welfare of young people. see *CHILDREN AND YOUTH—About*

CHRIS; Kinderzeitschrift der Christoffel-Blindenmission. see *CHILDREN AND YOUTH—For*

360 614.8 USA ISSN 0898-6339
HV99.C55
CLEVELAND FOUNDATION. ANNUAL REPORT. Text in English. a. **Document type:** *Corporate.* **Description:** The foundation exists to enhance the quality of life for all residents of Greater Cleveland. Using funds entrusted to its stewardship by thousands of people of various means, the foundation makes grants to non-profit organizations and governmental agencies to address the community's needs and opportunities.
Published by: Cleveland Foundation, 1422 Euclid Ave, Ste 1400, Cleveland, OH 44115. TEL 216-861-3810, FAX 216-861-1729. Ed. Lynne E Woodman.

CLINICAL CHILD PSYCHOLOGY & PSYCHIATRY. see *CHILDREN AND YOUTH—About*

CLINICAL GERONTOLOGIST; the journal of aging and mental health. see *GERONTOLOGY AND GERIATRICS*

361 158 GBR ISSN 1466-3651
THE COGNITIVE BEHAVIOURAL SOCIAL WORK REVIEW. Text in English. 1982. a. GBP 10 (effective 2000). bk.rev. **Document type:** *Academic/Scholarly.*
Formerly (until 1997): Behavioural Social Work Review (0269-9559)
Indexed: ERA.
—BLDSC (3292.873500).
Published by: Cognitive Behavioural Social Work Group, University of Hull, Hull HU6 7RX, United Kingdom. Ed. Jonathan Parker. R&P Rosemary Strange TEL 44-1455-845682.

COMMUNICATION (LONDON, 1967); the magazine of the National Autistic Society. see *EDUCATION—Special Education And Rehabilitation*

360 AUS
▼ **COMMUNITY CARE REVIEW NEWSLETTER.** Text in English. 2000 (Feb. 18th, no.1). **Document type:** *Newsletter, Government.*
Related titles: Online - full content ed.
Published by: Community Care Division (Subsidiary of: Department of Human Services), Level 13, 555 Collin St, Melbourne, VIC 3000, Australia. TEL 61-3-9616-7121, michael.aughton@dhs.vic.gov.au. Ed. Jan Carter.

301.1 362 USA ISSN 0010-3853
RA790.A1 CODEN: CMHJAY
COMMUNITY MENTAL HEALTH JOURNAL. Text in English. 1965. bi-m. USD 92 in the Americas to individuals for print or online ed.; EUR 92 elsewhere to individuals for print or online ed.; USD 583 in the Americas to institutions for print or online ed.; EUR 582 elsewhere to institutions for print or online ed.; USD 699.60 in the Americas to institutions for print & online eds. combined; EUR 698.40 elsewhere to institutions for print & online eds. combined (effective 2002). adv. bk.rev., film rev. abstr, bibl, charts, illus. index. back issues avail.; reprint service avail. from PQC,ISI. *Refereed.* **Document type:** *Journal, Academic/Scholarly.* **Description:** Coordinates emergent approaches to mental health and social well-being, covering crisis intervention, suicide prevention, family therapy, and social welfare.
Related titles: Microform ed.: (from PQC); Online - full text ed.: (from CatchWord Ltd., Northern Light Technology, Inc., EBSCO Publishing, O C L C Online Computer Library Center, Inc., RoweCom Information Quest, ProQuest Information & Learning, Gale Group, Swets Blackwell, Kluwer Online, Factiva, Institute for Scientific Information).
Indexed: AMED, ASCA, ASSIA, Abstr.Health Care Manage.Stud., Adol.Ment.Hlth.Abstr., AgeLine, Biol.Abstr., CERDIC, CINAHL, Curr.Adv.Ecol.Sci., Curr.Cont., ERA, Environ.Sci.Poll.Mgmt., Excerp.Med., Fam.Ind., High.Educ.Abstr., Hosp.Lit.Ind., Human Resour.Abstr., Ind.Med. (1965-), Int.Nurs.Ind., Lang.& Lang.Behav.Abstr., Media Rev.Dig. (Jan.1989-), Ment.Retard.Abstr., Mid.East: Abstr.& Ind., Mult.Ed.Abstr., P C I, Pollut.Abstr., Psyclnfo, Psychol.Abstr. (1973-), Risk Abstr., SOPODA, SSCI, Saf.Sci.Abstr., Sage Fam.Stud.Abstr., Sage Race Rel.Abstr., Sci.Cit.Ind. (coverage dropped), Soc.Sci.Ind. (Dec.1982-), Soc.Serv.Abstr., Soc.Work Res.& Abstr., Sociol.Abstr., Sp.Ed.Needs Abstr., e-psyche.
—BLDSC (3363.643000), CatchWord, CISTI, GNLM, IDS, Infotrieve, ingenta, KNAW. **CCC.**
Published by: (National Council of Community Mental Health Centers, Inc.), Kluwer Academic - Plenum Publishers (Subsidiary of: Wolters Kluwer N.V.), 233 Spring St, New York, NY 10013-1578. TEL 212-620-8000, 800-221-9369, FAX 212-463-0742, services@wkap.nl, info@plenum.com, http://www.wkap.nl/journalhome.htm/0010-3853. Ed. David L Cutler. **Subscr. outside the Americas to:** Kluwer Academic Publishers Group, Journals Department, PO Box 322, Dordrecht 3300 AH, Netherlands. TEL 31-78-639-2392, FAX 31-78-654-6474.

COMMUNITY PSYCHIATRIC NURSING. see *MEDICAL SCIENCES—Nurses And Nursing*

361 610 USA
CONCERN NEWS. Text in English. 1961. 4/yr. free or donation. illus. **Document type:** *Newsletter.* **Description:** News of projects and people working to ensure the survival of children whose lives are at risk and the access to health care for those in need, reporting on medical assistance & malnutrition issues, and efforts to build self-reliant health care systems in countries throughout the world.
Former titles: Project Concern News (0033-0906); Project Concern Newsletter
Related titles: Online - full text ed.
Published by: Project Concern International, 3550 Afton Rd, San Diego, CA 92123. TEL 619-279-9690, FAX 619-694-0294, postmaster@projcon.cts.com, http://www.serve.com/PCI. Ed. Charles Goldberg. Circ: 5,000.

CONTACT NEWS; voice of the Irish deaf. see *HANDICAPPED—Hearing Impaired*

CONTINUING CARE; supporting the transition into post hospital care. see *HEALTH FACILITIES AND ADMINISTRATION*

CONTINUUM (CHICAGO); an interdisciplinary journal on continuity of care. see *HEALTH FACILITIES AND ADMINISTRATION*

362 616.21 ITA
CORRIERE DEI LARINGECTOMIZZATI. Text in Italian. 1957. q. adv. illus. **Description:** Organizational news for laryngectomees and users of artificial speaking devices.
Published by: Associazione Italiana Laringectomizzati, Via Friuli, 28, Milan, MI 20135, Italy. TEL 02-5510819. Ed. Dr. Giuseppe Sapa.

361.3 COL
CUADERNOS DEL CIDS. (In 3 series) Text in Spanish. 1997. 6/yr. (2 per series). COP 157,000 domestic; USD 71 foreign; COP 142,500 domestic to libraries; USD 65 foreign to libraries (effective 2002). *Refereed.* **Description:** Presents the results of field work by the Center for Research on Social Dynamics, which embraces the methodological research perspective.
Published by: Universidad Externado de Colombia, Departamento de Publicaciones, Calle 12, 1-17 Este, Apartado Aereo 034141, Bogota, DC, Colombia. TEL 57-1-341-0288, FAX 57-1-3424948, pblccsns@impsat.net.co.

DEAF - BLIND PERSPECTIVES. see *HANDICAPPED—Visually Impaired*

DEAF SAN DIEGAN. see *HANDICAPPED—Hearing Impaired*

362.3 CAN ISSN 0383-8528
DIALECT. Text in English. 1977. bi-m. free per issue. adv. bk.rev., film rev. back issues avail. **Document type:** *Newsletter.* **Description:** Publishes writing that promotes the full inclusion, equality and dignity of people with intellectual disabilities.
Indexed: e-psyche.
Published by: Saskatchewan Association for Community Living, 3031 Louise St, Saskatoon, SK S7J 3L1, Canada. TEL 306-955-3344, FAX 306-373-3070, sacl.comm@home.com, http://www.members.home.net/sacl.com. Ed., R&P, Adv. contact Karin Melberg-Schwier. Circ: 5,900.

DIRECTORY OF AL-ANON AND ALATEEN MEETINGS IN AUSTRALIA. see *DRUG ABUSE AND ALCOHOLISM*

362.6 USA
DIRECTORY OF FEDERAL AID FOR THE AGING. Text in English. irreg. **Document type:** *Directory.*
Published by: Ready Reference Press, PO Box 5879, Santa Monica, CA 90405.

362.4 371 USA
DIRECTORY OF FEDERAL AID FOR THE HANDICAPPED. Text in English. irreg. **Document type:** *Directory.*
Published by: Ready Reference Press, PO Box 5879, Santa Monica, CA 90405.

360 USA ISSN 0888-7624
RA997.A2
DIRECTORY OF NURSING HOMES. Text in English. 1982. a. USD 249 (effective 1999). **Document type:** *Directory.* **Description:** Covers nearly 16,300 state licensed long-term care facilities, with complete profiles of each facility.
Formerly: Directory of Nursing Home Facilities
Published by: H C I A Inc., 300 E Lombard St, Baltimore, MD 21202. TEL 800-568-3282, FAX 410-547-8297.

DIRECTORY OF RESOURCES FOR THE BLIND AND VISUALLY IMPAIRED. see *HANDICAPPED—Visually Impaired*

DISABILITY, PREGNANCY & PARENTHOOD INTERNATIONAL; a forum for disabled parents and professionals to exchange information and experience. see *HANDICAPPED*

DISABILITY UPDATE. see *HANDICAPPED*

DYSTONIA DIALOGUE. see *MEDICAL SCIENCES*

ECHO DE L'UNION. see *GERONTOLOGY AND GERIATRICS*

EDUCATION FOR HEALTH; change in training and practice. see *MEDICAL SCIENCES*

EQUAL TIME: OUTREACH NEWSLETTER. see *HOMOSEXUALITY*

368 658.3 DEU ISSN 0014-0279
DIE ERSATZKASSE. Text in German. 1916. m. DEM 50.40 (effective 1998). adv. bk.rev. illus, stat. **Document type:** *Bulletin.*
Indexed: Excerp.Med., World Bibl.Soc.Sec.
—GNLM.
Published by: Verband der Angestellten-Krankenkassen e.V., Frankfurter Str 84, Siegburg 53721, Germany. Ed. Rainer Josten. Circ: 6,544.

▼ **ETHICAL HUMAN SCIENCES AND SERVICES**; an international journal of critical inquiry. see *MEDICAL SCIENCES—Psychiatry And Neurology*

F P A B HIGHLIGHTS. see *BIRTH CONTROL*

360 NLD ISSN 0920-6469
FACT SHEET ON THE NETHERLANDS. Text in Dutch, English, French, German. irreg. free per issue. **Document type:** *Government.* **Description:** Publishes information pertaining to social welfare and public health.
Published by: Ministerie van Volksgezondheid Welzijn en Sport, Publieksvoorlichting/Ministry of Health, Welfare and Sport, Public Information Office, Postbus 5406, Rijswijk (ZH) 2280 HK, Netherlands. TEL 31-70-3407890.

FAMILY PLANNING ASSOCIATION OF NEPAL. ANNUAL REPORT. see *BIRTH CONTROL*

FAMILY SUPPORT BULLETIN. see *HANDICAPPED—Physically Impaired*

FAMILY THERAPY; the journal of the California Graduate School of Family Psychology. see *MEDICAL SCIENCES—Psychiatry And Neurology*

FAMILY THERAPY NEWS. see *PSYCHOLOGY*

FEDERAL BENEFITS FOR VETERANS AND DEPENDENTS. see *MILITARY*

FIAPAS. see *HANDICAPPED—Hearing Impaired*

THE FITZHUGH DIRECTORY OF INDEPENDENT HEALTHCARE AND LONG TERM CARE. FINANCIAL INFORMATION. see *MEDICAL SCIENCES*

FOKUS PAA FAMILIEN; tidsskrift for familiebehandling. see *MEDICAL SCIENCES—Psychiatry And Neurology*

FONDAMENTAL. see *MEDICAL SCIENCES—Oncology*

FOR THOSE WHO GIVE AND GRIEVE; a quarterly newsletter for donor families. see *MEDICAL SCIENCES—Urology And Nephrology*

THE FUTURE OF CHILDREN. see *CHILDREN AND YOUTH—About*

GEISTIGE BEHINDERUNG; Fachzeitschrift der Lebenshilfe fuer geistig Behinderte. see *EDUCATION—Special Education And Rehabilitation*

GERIATRIC CARE. see *GERONTOLOGY AND GERIATRICS*

▼ **GERON**; tijdschrift ouder worden en maatsarry. see *GERONTOLOGY AND GERIATRICS*

360 DEU ISSN 0016-9153
GESICHERTES LEBEN. Text in German. 1954. bi-m. DEM 9.80 (effective 2000). adv. **Document type:** *Bulletin, Consumer.*
Published by: Wirtschaftsdienst Gesellschaft fuer Medien & Kommunikation mbH & Co. OHG, Siemensstr 6, Bad Homburg 61352, Germany. TEL 49-6172-670-0, FAX 49-6172-670144, vertrieb@wdv.de. Ed. Michael Kaschel. Adv. contact Walter Piezonka. B&W page DEM 25,400, color page DEM 40,640. Circ: 2,075,000.

360 610 JPN ISSN 0388-743X
GIFUKEN KOSEIREN IGAKU ZASSHI/GIFU WELFARE FEDERATION. JOURNAL. Text in Japanese. 1980. a.
Published by: Gifuken Koseiren Igaku Zasshi Henshushitsu, 13-1 Usa-Minami 4-chome, Gifu-shi 500-8367, Japan.

362.2 ITA ISSN 1120-9747
GIORNALE ITALIANO DI SUICIDOLOGIA/ITALIAN JOURNAL OF SUICIDOLOGY. Text in Italian. 1991. s-a. ITL 80,000; ITL 90,000 foreign (effective 1999). adv. bk.rev. abstr. back issues avail. *Refereed.* **Document type:** *Academic/Scholarly.* **Description:** Covers suicidal behavior, epidemiology, risk factor identification, psychology, sociology, biology of suicide, ethical issues and preventive strategies for health professionals.
Indexed: Environ.Sci.Poll.Mgmt., IBR, IBZ, Ind.Philos., Lang.& Lang.Behav.Abstr., Pollut.Abstr., Psyclnfo, Risk Abstr., SOPODA, Saf.Sci.Abstr., Soc.Serv.Abstr., Sociol.Abstr., e-psyche.
—BLDSC (4588.341550).
Published by: Associazione Italiana per lo Studio e la Prevenzione del Suicidio, c/o Servizio di Psicogeriatria, Universita di Padova, Via Elisabetta Suor Vendramini, 7, Padua, PD 35137, Italy. TEL 39-49-8216263, FAX 39-49-8216264, aispsuic@intercity.it. Ed. Diego De Leo. Circ: 900.

360 614 GBR
GOOD PRACTICE SERIES. Text in English. irreg., latest vol.9, 2001. **Document type:** *Monographic series, Academic/Scholarly.* **Description:** Explores topics of current concern to professionals working in social work, health care and the probation service.
—BLDSC (4201.351800).
Published by: Jessica Kingsley Publishers, 116 Pentonville Rd, London N1 9JB, United Kingdom. TEL 44-207-833-2307, FAX 44-20-7837-2917, post@jkp.com, http://www.jkp.com. Ed. Jacki Pritchard. **Dist. in US by:** Plymbridge Distributors Ltd, Plymbridge House, Estover Rd, Plymouth, Devon PL6 7PY, United Kingdom. TEL 44-1752-202300, FAX 44-1752-202330, enquiries@plymbridge.com, http://www.plymbridge.com.

GREAT BRITAIN. DEPARTMENT OF HEALTH AND SOCIAL SECURITY. HEALTH BUILDING NOTES. see *HEALTH FACILITIES AND ADMINISTRATION*

GREAT BRITAIN. DEPARTMENT OF HEALTH AND SOCIAL SECURITY. HEALTH EQUIPMENT NOTES. see *HEALTH FACILITIES AND ADMINISTRATION*

GREAT IDEAS FOR LONG-TERM CARE. see *GERONTOLOGY AND GERIATRICS*

360 GBR ISSN 0951-824X
GROUPWORK. Text in English. 1988. 3/yr. GBP 55 domestic; USD 90 in North America; GBP 60 elsewhere (effective 2000). index. back issues avail. **Document type:** *Academic/Scholarly.* **Description:** Covers social work with groups of all types.
Indexed: ASSIA, Abstr.Soc.Geront., Crim.Just.Abstr., ERA, IBR, IBZ, Ind.Philos., Intl.Bibl.Soc.Sci., Lang.& Lang.Behav.Abstr., Mult.Ed.Abstr., SOPODA, Sage Fam.Stud.Abstr., Soc.Serv.Abstr., Soc.Work Res.& Abstr., Sociol.Abstr., Stud.Wom.Abstr., e-psyche.
—BLDSC (4220.460000). **CCC.**
Published by: Whiting & Birch Ltd., PO Box 872, London SE23 3HL, United Kingdom. TEL 44-20-8244-2421, FAX 44-20-8244-2448, savpub@dircon.co.uk. Ed. Oded Manor. Circ: 750.

GUIDE TO HEALTH SERVICES OF THE WORLD. see *PUBLIC ADMINISTRATION*

GUIDE TO THE NURSING HOME INDUSTRY. see *HEALTH FACILITIES AND ADMINISTRATION*

HANDICAP & BELEID; tijdschrift voor beleidmakers en dienstverleners. see *HANDICAPPED*

HANDICAP NEWS. see *HANDICAPPED*

HANDISCOOP. see *HANDICAPPED*

HARICOT; newsletter for the renal patients of Australia. see *MEDICAL SCIENCES—Urology And Nephrology*

HARTMANNBUND IN BADEN - WUERTTEMBERG. see *PUBLIC HEALTH AND SAFETY*

362.7 USA ISSN 0362-6296
RJ501.H3
HAWAII. DEPARTMENT OF HEALTH. MENTAL HEALTH SERVICES FOR CHILDREN AND YOUTH; children's MH services branch. Key Title: Mental Health Services for Children and Youth. Text in English. 1970. a. stat. **Document type:** *Government.*
Published by: Department of Health, Child and Adolescent Mental Health Division, 3627 Kilauea Ave, Rm 101, Honolulu, HI 96816. TEL 808-548-6335. Circ: 300.

HAWAII'S NATIONAL GAY COMMUNITY NEWS; Hawaii and Western States. see *HOMOSEXUALITY*

HEALTH AND SOCIAL SERVICE WORKFORCE IN ALBERTA. see *PUBLIC HEALTH AND SAFETY*

360 USA ISSN 0360-7283
HV687.5.U5 CODEN: HSWODK
HEALTH & SOCIAL WORK. Text in English. 1976. q. USD 79.95 to non-members; USD 45 to members; USD 99.95 to institutions; USD 30 to student member (effective 2001). adv. bk.rev. illus. index. back issues avail.; reprint service avail. from PQC. *Refereed.* **Document type:** *Academic/Scholarly.* **Description:** Examines health-related social problems and issues dealing with the client and the community.
Related titles: Microfiche ed.: (from PQC); Online - full text ed.: (from ProQuest Information & Learning, Gale Group, Northern Light Technology, Inc., Factiva, Institute for Scientific Information).
Indexed: ASCA, ASSIA, Abstr.Anthropol., Abstr.Crim.& Pen., Abstr.Health Care Manage.Stud., Abstr.Soc.Geront., Adol.Ment.Hlth.Abstr., AgeLine, Behav.Med.Abstr., Biol.Abstr., C.I.J.E., CINAHL, Chic.Per.Ind., Crim.Just.Abstr., Curr.Cont., DSH Abstr., Dent.Ind., ERA, Environ.Sci.Poll.Mgmt., Except.Child Educ.Abstr., Excerp.Med., Fam.Ind., Human Resour.Abstr., IMFL, Ind.Med. (1976-), Int.Nurs.Ind., Intl.Bibl.Soc.Sci., Lang.& Lang.Behav.Abstr., Mult.Ed.Abstr., P C I, Pollut.Abstr., PsycInfo, Psychol.Abstr. (1976-), Rehabil.Lit., Risk Abstr., SOPODA, SSCI, Saf.Sci.Abstr., Soc.Sci.Ind. (Jan.1987-), Soc.Serv.Abstr., Soc.Work Res.& Abstr., Sociol.Abstr., Sp.Ed.Needs Abstr., World Bibl.Soc.Sec., e-psyche.
—BLDSC (4274.884000), GNLM, IDS, ingenta, KNAW. **CCC.**
Published by: (National Association of Social Workers), N A S W Press, 750 First St, N E, Ste 700, Washington, DC 20002-4241. TEL 202-408-8600, 800-227-3590, FAX 301-206-7989, press@naswdc.org, http://www.naswpress.org/publications/journals/health/hswintro.html. Ed. Sharon Keigher. R&P Lori Eatmon TEL 800-638-8799 ext.341. Circ: 6,500. **Subscr. to:** Allen Press Inc., PO Box 1897, Lawrence, KS 66044-8897. http://www.allenpress.com. **Dist. by:** NASW Press Distribution Center, Box 431, Annapolis JCT, MD 20701.

HEALTH CARE FINANCING REVIEW. see *MEDICAL SCIENCES*

HEALTH CARE FINANCING REVIEW. SUPPLEMENT. see *PUBLIC HEALTH AND SAFETY*

361 610 USA ISSN 0268-1153
CODEN: HRTPE2
HEALTH EDUCATION RESEARCH; theory and practice. Text in English. 1986. 6/yr. GBP 86, USD 152 to individuals; GBP 200, USD 310 to institutions; GBP 30, USD 38 to students (effective Feb. 2002). adv. bk.rev. index. back issues avail.; reprint service avail. from SWZ. *Refereed.* **Document type:** *Journal, Academic/Scholarly.* **Description:** Promotes understanding of the processes, rationale and philosophy underlying the work of practicing health educators in an international forum.
Related titles: Online - full text ed.: ISSN 1465-3648. GBP 180, USD 279 to institutions Online only (effective Feb. 2002) (from HighWire Pr., EBSCO Publishing, O C L C Online Computer Library Center, Inc., RoweCom Information Quest, ingenta, Swets Blackwell, Institute for Scientific Information).
Indexed: ASCA, ASSIA, Abstr.Anthropol., Addic.Abstr., AgeLine, Biol.Abstr., Br.Educ.Ind., Brit.Nur.Ind., CINAHL, Chic.Per.Ind., Cont.Pg.Educ., Curr.Cont., Curr.Tit.Dent., Environ.Sci.Poll.Mgmt., Excerp.Med., HRIS, Ind.Med. (coverage dropped), Mult.Ed.Abstr., Pollut.Abstr., PsycInfo, Psychol.Abstr. (1986-), Risk Abstr., SSCI, Saf.Sci.Abstr., Sci.Cit.Ind. (coverage dropped), Stud.Wom.Abstr., THA, Tech.Educ.Abstr., e-psyche.
—BLDSC (4275.011440), EMDOCS, GNLM, IDS, ingenta, KNAW. **CCC.**
Published by: Oxford University Press, Academic Division, Great Clarendon St, Oxford OX2 6DP, United Kingdom. TEL 44-1865-267907, FAX 44-1865-267835, jnl.info@oup.co.uk, http://her.oupjournals.org/, http://www.oup.co.uk/journals. Eds. J R Sorenson, K Tones. Pub. Janet Fox. R&P Fionna Willis. adv.: page GBP 240, page USD 430. Circ: 1,050. **Subscr. outside the Americas to:** Journals Marketing, Great Clarendon St, Oxford OX2 6DP, United Kingdom.

362.1 USA ISSN 0361-2929
RA981.C3
HEALTH FACILITIES DIRECTORY. Spine title: Directory of Health Facilities. Text in English. 1975. q. free per issue. **Document type:** *Government.*
Published by: Department of Health Services, Licensing and Certification Division, 714 744 P St, Box 942732, Sacramento, CA 94234-7320. TEL 916-322-2810.

HEALTH PROFESSIONS COUNCIL OF SOUTH AFRICA. REGISTER OF SUPPLEMENTARY HEALTH SERVICES PROFESSIONS. see *MEDICAL SCIENCES*

THE HEALTH SERVICE JOURNAL; for people involved in NHS management. see *HEALTH FACILITIES AND ADMINISTRATION*

362.5 USA ISSN 1036-4005
HEALTH TRANSITION REVIEW. Text in English. 1991. s-a. free per issue. **Description:** Covers health in poor countries (the social, cultural and behavioural determinants of health).
Related titles: Online - full text ed.
Indexed: A.I.C.P. (1991-), Intl.Bibl.Soc.Sci., Popul.Ind., Rural Devel.Abstr., Stat.Theor.Meth.Abstr. (1996-).
—GNLM.
Address: c/o Harvard School of Public Health, Dept of Population & International Health, 665 Huntington Ave, Boston, MA 02115. Ed. Alan G Hill. Circ: 2,000.

HEALTH WORKFORCE IN ALBERTA. ANNUAL REPORT. see *PUBLIC HEALTH AND SAFETY*

HEALTHCARE TRENDS REPORT; the monthly digest of business and public policy news. see *MEDICAL SCIENCES*

HEALTHY MINDS. see *CHILDREN AND YOUTH—About*

HERE'S HELP. see *GERONTOLOGY AND GERIATRICS*

HOME CARE EDUCATION MANAGEMENT. see *MEDICAL SCIENCES—Nurses And Nursing*

362.76 618.92 USA
HOME CARE FAMILY NEWSLETTER. Text in English. 1991. bi-m. free. **Document type:** *Newsletter.* **Description:** Informs parents of the Children's Hospital Home Care support group for parents of children with chronic illness. Alerts parents of special-needs children of services and other resources in the greater Philadelphia area.
Published by: Children's Hospital of Philadelphia, Home Care Department, Driscoll Bldg, 34th and Civic Center Blvd, Philadelphia, PA 19104-4399. TEL 215-590-3272. Ed., R&P Peggy MacGregor. Circ: 1,300.

HOME CARE QUALITY MANAGEMENT. see *MEDICAL SCIENCES—Nurses And Nursing*

HOME HEALTH FOCUS. see *MEDICAL SCIENCES—Nurses And Nursing*

HOSPICE MANAGEMENT ADVISOR. see *HEALTH FACILITIES AND ADMINISTRATION*

362 USA
HOSPICE TODAY. Text in English. 1981. q. free per issue. bk.rev. **Document type:** *Newsletter.* **Description:** Informs friends, volunteers, and financial supporters about the activities and programs of the agency, its services to the community, and its role as a resource and an advocate on issues related to death, grief and terminal illness.
Formerly (until 1987): Hospice Care Newsletter
Published by: Hospice of the Florida Suncoast, 300 E Bay Dr, Largo, FL 34640. TEL 813-586-4432, FAX 813-586-5213. Ed. Kimberly Walter. Circ: 65,000 (controlled).

HOUSING THE ELDERLY REPORT. see *HOUSING AND URBAN PLANNING*

363.8 USA ISSN 0740-1116
HUNGER NOTES. Text in English. 1976. q. USD 18 domestic to individuals; USD 45 foreign to individuals; USD 45 domestic to institutions; USD 51 foreign to institutions (effective 1999). adv. bk.rev. illus. **Document type:** *Academic/Scholarly.* **Description:** Presents facts and insights on hunger, poverty, grassroots self-help, and socioeconomic development for policy-makers, educators and activists. Acts as a guide to organizations and print resources on the specific focus of each issue.
Indexed: HR Rep., P.A.I.S.
Published by: World Hunger Education Service, PO Box 29056, Washington, DC 29056. TEL 202-269-6322, hungerno@aol.com, http://www.worldhunger.com. Ed. Lane Vanderslice. R&P, Adv. contact Paula Smith. Circ: 1,100 (paid).

HYGEIA; an online journal for pregnancy and neonatal loss. see *PSYCHOLOGY*

362.4 615.82 FIN ISSN 0356-7249
I T - INVALIDITYOE. Text in Finnish. 1941. m. FIM 275 (effective 2000). adv. bk.rev. illus. **Description:** Covers disability, social welfare, and rehabilitation.
Formerly: Suomen Invalidi (0049-2566)
Published by: Invalidiliitto r.y., Kumpulantie 1, Helsinki 00520, Finland. FAX 358-9-146-1443, it-lehti@invalidiliitto.fi, http://www.it-lehti.fi. Eds. Sirkkt Kivi, Voitto Korhonen. Circ: 60,162.

ILCO-PRAXIS. see *MEDICAL SCIENCES—Oncology*

INFORMATIONSDIENST ALTERSFRAGEN. see *GERONTOLOGY AND GERIATRICS*

S

INSIGHTS (BELLE MEAD). see *HEALTH FACILITIES AND ADMINISTRATION*

INTEGRA; boletin de noticias. see *HANDICAPPED*

INTERNATIONAL ASSOCIATION OF WORKERS FOR TROUBLED CHILDREN AND YOUTH. CONGRESS REPORTS. see *EDUCATION—Special Education And Rehabilitation*

360 GBR ISSN 0749-6753
CODEN: IJHMEO

INTERNATIONAL JOURNAL OF HEALTH PLANNING AND MANAGEMENT. Text in English. 1986. q. USD 1,180 in United States; USD 1,180 in Canada & Mexico; USD 1,180 elsewhere; USD 1,239 combined subscription in United States for print and online eds.; USD 1,239 combined subscription in Canada & Mexico for print and online eds.; USD 1,239 combined subscription elsewhere for print and online eds. (effective 2002). adv. back issues avail.; reprint service avail. from SWZ. *Refereed.* **Document type:** *Academic/Scholarly.* **Description:** Discusses major issues in health planning, management systems, and practices; maintains a balance between practice and theory from a variety of schools of thought.
Related titles: Online - full text ed.: ISSN 1099-1751. USD 1,180 in United States; USD 1,180 in Canada & Mexico; USD 1,180 elsewhere (effective 2002) (from EBSCO Publishing, Wiley InterScience, Institute for Scientific Information).
Indexed: ASCA, ASSIA, Abstr.Health Care Manage.Stud., Curr.Cont., Environ.Sci.Poll.Mgmt., Excerp.Med., Geo.Abstr.H.G., IDA, Lang.& Lang.Behav.Abstr., Pollut.Abstr., SOPODA, SSCI, Soc.Serv.Abstr., Sociol.Abstr.
—BLDSC (4542.277600), EMDOCS, GNLM, IDS, Infotrieve, ingenta. **CCC.**
Published by: Wiley Europe Ltd., Baffins Ln, Chichester, W Sussex PO19 1UD, United Kingdom. TEL 44-1243-779777, FAX 44-1243-775878, customer@wiley.co.uk, http://www.wiley.co.uk. adv.: B&W page GBP 650, color page GBP 1,550; trim 165 x 248. Circ: 550. **Subscr. in the Americas to:** John Wiley & Sons, Inc., Journals, 605 Third Ave, New York, NY 10158. TEL 212-850-6021, 212-850-6645, subinfo@jwiley.com.

363.34 USA ISSN 0280-7270
HV551.2

INTERNATIONAL JOURNAL OF MASS EMERGENCIES AND DISASTERS. Text in English. 1983. 3/yr., latest vol.19, 2001. USD 45 to individual members; USD 48 to institutional members; USD 20 to students (effective 2001); includes Unscheduled Events. adv. bk.rev., software rev., video rev. abstr. back issues avail. *Refereed.* **Document type:** *Journal, Academic/Scholarly.*
Indexed: EEA, Geo.Abstr.H.G., Geo.Abstr.P.G., Lang.& Lang.Behav.Abstr., SOPODA, Soc.Serv.Abstr., Sociol.Abstr. (1983-).
—BLDSC (4542.332000), CISTI.
Published by: International Research Committee on Disasters, P O Box 425557, Women s Studies Program, Texas Women s University, Denton, TX 76204. TEL 256-782-8053, brenda@jsucc.jsu.edu, http://www.udel.edu/drc/ircd/. Eds. Maureen Fordham, Ronald Perry. R&P, Adv. contact Brenda Phillips TEL 256-782-8053.

INTERNATIONAL JOURNAL OF MENTAL HEALTH. see *PSYCHOLOGY*

▼ **THE INTERNATIONAL JOURNAL OF MENTAL HEALTH PROMOTION**; promoting mental health, preventing mental disorders. see *PUBLIC HEALTH AND SAFETY*

INVENTORY OF HEALTH WORKFORCE IN ALBERTA. see *PUBLIC HEALTH AND SAFETY*

IRYO TO FUKUSHI/JAPANESE JOURNAL OF MEDICAL SOCIAL WORK. see *MEDICAL SCIENCES*

ISSUES IN CHILD ABUSE ACCUSATIONS. see *CHILDREN AND YOUTH—About*

302.76 AUS ISSN 1321-2540

ISSUES IN CHILD ABUSE PREVENTION. Text in English. 1994. s-a. free per issue. bk.rev. abstr. bibl. back issues avail. **Document type:** *Academic/Scholarly.* **Description:** Provides an information bulletin of research, practice, and policy for professionals working in areas related to child abuse prevention.
Related titles: CD-ROM ed.
Published by: Australian Institute of Family Studies, 300 Queen St, Melbourne, VIC 3000, Australia. TEL 61-3-9214-7888, FAX 61-3-9214-7839, fic@aifs.org.au, http://www.aifs.org.au. Ed. Judy Adams. Circ: 7,000.

J A O G NEWS. see *MEDICAL SCIENCES—Obstetrics And Gynecology*

J D C - BROOKDALE INSTITUTE OF GERONTOLOGY AND HUMAN DEVELOPMENT. ANNUAL REPORT. see *GERONTOLOGY AND GERIATRICS*

J D C - BROOKDALE INSTITUTE OF GERONTOLOGY AND HUMAN DEVELOPMENT. RESEARCH SERIES. see *GERONTOLOGY AND GERIATRICS*

JAHRBUCH KRITISCHE MEDIZIN. see *MEDICAL SCIENCES*

JOURNAL OF ADDICTIONS & OFFENDER COUNSELING. see *PSYCHOLOGY*

JOURNAL OF BEHAVIORAL HEALTH SERVICES AND RESEARCH. see *PUBLIC HEALTH AND SAFETY*

362.76 USA ISSN 1053-8712
HV6570 CODEN: JCABEK

JOURNAL OF CHILD SEXUAL ABUSE; research, treatment & program innovations for victims, survivors & offenders. Text in English. 1992. q. USD 60 to individuals; USD 81 in Canada to individuals; USD 87 elsewhere to individuals; USD 125 to institutions; USD 169 in Canada to institutions; USD 181 elsewhere to institutions; USD 225 to libraries; USD 304 in Canada to libraries; USD 326 elsewhere to libraries (effective Aug. 2001). adv. bk.rev. back issues avail.; reprint service avail. from HAW. *Refereed.* **Document type:** *Journal, Academic/Scholarly.* **Description:** Covers research issues, clinical issues, case studies and brief reports on young victims, adult survivors and the offenders.
Related titles: Microfiche ed.: (from PQC); Microform ed.; Online - full text ed.: (from ProQuest Information & Learning).
Indexed: ASSIA, Abstr.Anthropol., Behav.Med.Abstr., C.I.J.E., CINAHL, CJPI, Child Devel.Abstr., Crim.Just.Abstr., DNP, ERA, Educ.Admin.Abstr., Environ.Sci.Poll.Mgmt., Except.Child Educ.Abstr., Excerp.Med. (1993-), Fam.Ind., G.Soc.Sci.& Rel.Per.Lit., IBZ, IMFL, Ind.Per.Art.Relat.Law, Ind.Philos., Lang.& Lang.Behav.Abstr., Mult.Ed.Abstr., PsycInfo, Psychol.Abstr. (1992-), Ref.Zh., SOPODA, Sage Fam.Stud.Abstr., Sage Race Rel.Abstr., Sage Urb.Stud.Abstr., Soc.Serv.Abstr., Soc.Work Res.& Abstr., Sociol.Abstr., Sp.Ed.Needs Abstr., Stud.Wom.Abstr., Viol.& Abuse Abstr., e-psyche.
—BLDSC (4957.905000), EMDOCS, GNLM, Haworth, ingenta.
Published by: Haworth Press, Inc., 10 Alice St, Binghamton, NY 13904-1580. TEL 607-722-5857, 800-429-6784, FAX 607-722-6362, 800-895-0582, getinfo@haworthpressinc.com, http://www.haworthpress.com/journals/journallist.asp. Ed. Robert A Geffner. Pub. William Cohen. R&P Ruthann Heath TEL 607-723-5857 ext 316. Adv. contact Jackie Blakeslee TEL 607-722-5857 ext 346. B&W page USD 315, color page USD 550; trim 6 x 8.5.

JOURNAL OF GAY & LESBIAN PSYCHOTHERAPY. see *PSYCHOLOGY*

306.766 USA ISSN 1053-8720
HV1449 CODEN: JGLSEI

JOURNAL OF GAY & LESBIAN SOCIAL SERVICES; issues in practice, policy & research. Text in English. 1994. q. USD 50 domestic to individuals; USD 68 in Canada to individuals; USD 73 elsewhere to individuals; USD 90 domestic to institutions; USD 122 in Canada to institutions; USD 131 elsewhere to institutions; USD 150 domestic to libraries; USD 203 in Canada to libraries; USD 218 elsewhere to libraries (effective Aug. 2001). adv. illus. back issues avail.; reprint service avail. from HAW. *Refereed.* **Document type:** *Journal, Academic/Scholarly.* **Description:** Focuses on policy, program and practice issues aiming to promote the well-being of homosexuals and bisexuals in contemporary society.
Related titles: Microform ed.: (from PQC); Online - full text ed.: (from Northern Light Technology, Inc.).
Indexed: Abstr.Hyg., AgeLine, CWI, Crim.Just.Abstr., DNP, ERA, Environ.Sci.Poll.Mgmt., Fam.Ind., IBZ, IMFL, Ind.Per.Art.Relat.Law, Lang.& Lang.Behav.Abstr., P.A.I.S., Ref.Zh., Risk Abstr., SOPODA, Saf.Sci.Abstr., Sage Fam.Stud.Abstr., Soc.Serv.Abstr., Soc.Work Res.& Abstr., Sociol.Abstr., Sp.Ed.Needs Abstr., Stud.Wom.Abstr.
—BLDSC (4987.643000), Haworth, ingenta.
Published by: Haworth Press, Inc., 10 Alice St, Binghamton, NY 13904-1580. TEL 607-722-5857, 800-429-6784, FAX 607-722-6362, 800-895-0582, getinfo@haworthpressinc.com, http://www.haworthpress.com/journals/journallist.asp. Ed. James J Kelly. Pub. William Cohen. R&P Ruthann Heath TEL 607-723-5857 ext 316. Adv. contact Jackie Blakeslee TEL 607-722-5857 ext 346. B&W page USD 315, color page USD 550; trim 6 x 8.5.

360 614.8 USA ISSN 0897-7186
RA418 CODEN: JHSPEH

JOURNAL OF HEALTH & SOCIAL POLICY. Text in English. 1989. q. USD 75 to individuals; USD 101 in Canada to individuals; USD 109 elsewhere to individuals; USD 150 to institutions; USD 203 in Canada to institutions; USD 218 elsewhere to institutions; USD 360 to libraries; USD 486 in Canada to libraries; USD 522 elsewhere to libraries (effective Aug. 2001). adv. bk.rev. illus. back issues avail.; reprint service avail. from HAW. *Refereed.* **Document type:** *Journal, Academic/Scholarly.* **Description:** Addresses health and social policy issues, concerns, and questions.
Related titles: Microfiche ed.: (from PQC); Microform ed.; Online - full text ed.: free with subscr. to the print ed.
Indexed: Abstr.Anthropol., Abstr.Hyg., Abstr.Soc.Geront., Environ.Sci.Poll.Mgmt., Geo.Abstr.H.G., Helminthol.Abstr., IBZ, IDA, IMFL, Int.Nurs.Ind., Int.Polit.Sci.Abstr., Lang.& Lang.Behav.Abstr., Nutr.Abstr., P.A.I.S., Pollut.Abstr., Psychol.Abstr., Rev.Appl.Entomol., Rev.Plant Path., Risk Abstr., SOPODA, Saf.Sci.Abstr., Sage Urb.Stud.Abstr., Soc.Serv.Abstr., Soc.Work Res.& Abstr., Sociol.Abstr., THA, Viol.& Abuse Abstr., Weed Abstr., World Ag.Econ.& Rur.Soc.Abstr., e-psyche.
—BLDSC (4996.731000), GNLM, Haworth, KNAW.
Published by: Haworth Press, Inc., 10 Alice St, Binghamton, NY 13904-1580. TEL 607-722-5857, 800-429-6784, FAX 607-722-6362, 800-895-0582, getinfo@haworthpressinc.com, http://www.haworthpress.com/journals/journallist.asp. Eds. Marvin D Feit, Stanley Battle. Pub. William Cohen. R&P Ruthann Heath TEL 607-723-5857 ext 316. Adv. contact Jackie Blakeslee TEL 607-722-5857 ext 346. B&W page USD 315, color page USD 550; trim 6 x 8.5.

JOURNAL OF HEALTH CARE FOR THE POOR AND UNDERSERVED. see *MEDICAL SCIENCES*

360 USA ISSN 1091-1359
HM251 CODEN: JHBEF2

JOURNAL OF HUMAN BEHAVIOR IN THE SOCIAL ENVIRONMENT; a professional journal. Text in English. 1998. q. USD 50 to individuals; USD 68 in Canada to individuals; USD 73 elsewhere to individuals; USD 75 to institutions; USD 101 in Canada to institutions; USD 109 elsewhere to institutions; USD 105 to libraries; USD 142 in Canada to libraries; USD 152 elsewhere to libraries (effective Aug. 2001). adv. back issues avail.; reprint service avail. from HAW. **Document type:** *Journal, Academic/Scholarly.* **Description:** Helps social workers grasp developing issues in human behavior.
Related titles: Microform ed.
Indexed: CINAHL, Crim.Just.Abstr., IBZ, Lang.& Lang.Behav.Abstr., Pollut.Abstr., Ref.Zh., SOPODA, Sage Fam.Stud.Abstr., Soc.Serv.Abstr., Soc.Work Res.& Abstr., Sociol.Abstr.
—BLDSC (5003.413400), Haworth, ingenta.
Published by: Haworth Press, Inc., 10 Alice St, Binghamton, NY 13904-1580. TEL 607-722-5857, 800-429-6784, FAX 607-722-6362, 800-895-0582, getinfo@haworthpressinc.com, http://www.haworthpress.com/journals/journallist.asp. Eds. John S. Wodarski, Marvin D. Feit. Pub. William Cohen. R&P Ruthann Heath TEL 607-723-5857 ext 316. Adv. contact Jackie Blakeslee TEL 607-722-5857 ext 346. B&W page USD 315, color page USD 550; trim 6 x 8.5.

JOURNAL OF INTELLECTUAL DISABILITY RESEARCH. see *MEDICAL SCIENCES—Psychiatry And Neurology*

JOURNAL OF MARITAL AND FAMILY THERAPY. see *PSYCHOLOGY*

JOURNAL OF NEPHROLOGY SOCIAL WORK. see *MEDICAL SCIENCES—Urology And Nephrology*

JOURNAL OF OFFENDER REHABILITATION; a multidisciplinary journal of innovation in research, services, and programs in corrections and criminal justice. see *CRIMINOLOGY AND LAW ENFORCEMENT*

S

360 610.73 GBR ISSN 1460-6690
JOURNAL OF PRACTICE TEACHING IN HEALTH & SOCIAL WORK. Text in English. 1998. 3/yr. GBP 55 domestic; USD 90 in United States; GBP 60 elsewhere (effective 2000). adv. bk.rev. bibl. back issues avail. *Refereed.* **Document type:** *Academic/Scholarly.*
Description: Covers field education, workplace learning & training in social work, health education, etc.
Indexed: IBZ, Soc.Serv.Abstr., Sociol.Abstr.
Published by: Whiting & Birch Ltd., PO Box 872, London SE23 3HL, United Kingdom. TEL 44-20-8244-2421, FAX 44-20-8244-2448, savpub@dircon.co.uk. Ed. Lynda Deacon. Pub., R&P David Whiting. adv.: B&W page GBP 250.

JOURNAL OF PSYCHOSOCIAL NURSING AND MENTAL HEALTH SERVICES. see *MEDICAL SCIENCES—Nurses And Nursing*

360 614 GBR ISSN 0957-4832
CODEN: JPHME9
JOURNAL OF PUBLIC HEALTH MEDICINE. Text in English. 1979. q. GBP 103, USD 187 to individuals; GBP 166, USD 299 to institutions (effective Mar. 2002). adv. bk.rev. index. back issues avail. *Refereed.* **Document type:** *Journal, Academic/Scholarly.*
Description: Addresses the practice of community medicine.
Formerly: Community Medicine (0142-2456)
Related titles: Online - full text ed.: ISSN 1464-3782. GBP 150, USD 290 to institutions Online only (effective Mar. 2002) (from EBSCO Publishing, O C L C Online Computer Library Center, Inc., RoweCom Information Quest, ingenta, Swets Blackwell, Institute for Scientific Information).
Indexed: ASCA, ASSIA, Abstr.Hyg., Addic.Abstr., AgBiotech, AgeLine, Bibl.Dev.Med.& Child Neur., Curr.Adv.Ecol.Sci., Curr.Cont., Dairy Sci.Abstr., Excerp.Med., Fam.Ind., Hosp.Abstr., INIS Atomind., Ind.Med. (1990-), Inpharma, Med.Care Rev., Nutr.Abstr., Pharm.&Out.News, Protozool.Abstr., Reac., Rev.Med.& Vet.Mycol., Rev.Plant Path., Risk Abstr., SSCI, Sage Race Rel.Abstr., Sci.Cit.Ind., Trop.Dis.Bull.
—BLDSC (5043.560000), CISTI, EMDOCS, GNLM, IDS, ingenta, KNAW. **CCC.**
Published by: (Faculty of Public Health Medicine), Oxford University Press, Academic Division, Great Clarendon St, Oxford OX2 6DP, United Kingdom. TEL 44-1865-267907, FAX 44-1865-267835, jnl.info@oup.co.uk, http://www.pubmed.oupjournals.org, http://www.oup.co.uk/journals, http://www3.oup.co.uk/pubmed/. Eds. E G Jessop, Norman Vetter. Pub. Mandy Sketch. R&P Fionna Willis. adv.: B&W page GBP 380, B&W page USD 685; trim 178 x 255. Circ: 2,550.
Affiliate: Oxford University Press, Journals.

JOURNAL OF REHABILITATION. see *MEDICAL SCIENCES—Physical Medicine And Rehabilitation*

JOURNAL OF REHABILITATION ADMINISTRATION. see *MEDICAL SCIENCES—Physical Medicine And Rehabilitation*

362.1786 617.03 SWE ISSN 1650-1977
CODEN: SJRMAA
JOURNAL OF REHABILITATION MEDICINE. Text in English. 1969. 6/yr. GBP 79, USD 130 to individuals; GBP 155, USD 255 to institutions (effective 2002). adv. bk.rev. charts, illus. *Refereed.* **Document type:** *Journal, Academic/Scholarly.* **Description:** Publishes articles concerned with medical, psychological, social, economic and technological aspects of rehabilitation.
Formerly (until 2001): Scandinavian Journal of Rehabilitation Medicine (0036-5505)
Related titles: Online - full text ed.: (from EBSCO Publishing, O C L C Online Computer Library Center, Inc., RoweCom Information Quest, CatchWord Ltd., ingenta, Swets Blackwell, Institute for Scientific Information); ♦ Supplement: Journal of Rehabilitation Medicine. Supplement.
Indexed: AMED, ASSIA, Bibl.Dev.Med.& Child Neur., Biol.Abstr., CINAHL, Curr.Cont., Environ.Sci.Poll.Mgmt., Ergon.Abstr., Except.Child Educ.Abstr., Excerp.Med., Focus on: Sports Sci.& Med., Ind.Med. (1969-), Inpharma, Int.Nurs.Ind., Neurosci.Cit.Ind., Psychol.Abstr., Reac., SSCI (coverage dropped), Sportsearch.
—BLDSC (5048.954000), CISTI, GNLM, IDS, ingenta, KNAW. **CCC.**
Published by: (Information on Rehabilitation Foundation), Taylor & Francis AS (Subsidiary of: Taylor & Francis Group), Cort Adelersgt. 17, Solli, PO Box 2562, Oslo 0202, Norway. TEL 47-22-12-98-80, FAX 47-22-12-98-90, Journals@ tandf.no, http://www.tandf.co.uk/tfas. Ed. Gunnar Grimby. Circ: 1,200. **Subscr. to:** Taylor & Francis Inc.

362.1786 SWE
JOURNAL OF REHABILITATION MEDICINE. SUPPLEMENT. Text in English. 1970. irreg.
Formerly: Scandinavian Journal of Rehabilitation Medicine. Supplement (0346-8720)
Related titles: ♦ Supplement to: Journal of Rehabilitation Medicine. ISSN 1650-1977.
Indexed: CINAHL, Ind.Med. (1970-).
—BLDSC (8087.531000).
Published by: (Information on Rehabilitation Foundation), Taylor & Francis AB (Subsidiary of: Taylor & Francis Group), Hollaendargatan 20, PO Box 3255, Stockholm 11160, Sweden. TEL 46-8-4408040, FAX 46-8-4408050, journals@se.tandf.no, http://www.tandf.co.uk/journals/tfas.html. **Subscr. to:** Taylor & Francis Inc, 325 Chestnut St, Ste 800, Philadelphia, PA 19106.

302.17 USA ISSN 1053-0789
HN1 CODEN: JSDHET
JOURNAL OF SOCIAL DISTRESS AND THE HOMELESS. Text in English. 1992. q. USD 322, EUR 321 to institutions for print or online ed.; USD 386.40, EUR 385.20 to institutions for print & online eds.combined (effective 2002). adv. bk.rev. illus. Index. reprints avail. *Refereed.* **Document type:** *Journal, Academic/Scholarly.* **Description:** Explores the link between social distress and issues such as homelessness, violence, and racial tension and its institutionalization in modern society.
Related titles: Online - full text ed.: (from EBSCO Publishing, O C L C Online Computer Library Center, Inc., Swets Blackwell, Kluwer Online, Institute for Scientific Information, RoweCom Information Quest).
Indexed: ASSIA, AgeLine, Crim.Just.Abstr., Curr.Cont., Fam.Ind., IMFL, Intl.Bibl.Soc.Sci., Lang.& Lang.Behav.Abstr., Peace Res.Abstr., PsycInfo, Psychol.Abstr. (1992-), SOPODA, SSCI, Sage Urb.Stud.Abstr., Soc.Serv.Abstr., Soc.Work Res.& Abstr., Sociol.Abstr., Viol.& Abuse Abstr., e-psyche.
—BLDSC (5064.753000), IDS, Infotrieve, ingenta. **CCC.**
Published by: Kluwer Academic - Plenum Publishers (Subsidiary of: Wolters Kluwer N.V.), 233 Spring St, New York, NY 10013-1578. TEL 212-620-8000, 800-221-9369, FAX 212-463-0742, info@plenum.com, http://www.wkap.nl/journalhome.htm/1053-0789. Ed. Robert W Rieber. **Subscr. outside the Americas to:** Kluwer Academic Publishers Group, Journals Department, PO Box 322, Dordrecht 3300 AH, Netherlands. TEL 31-78-639-2392, FAX 31-78-654-6474.

360 369.4 GBR ISSN 0265-0533
CODEN: JSWPEC
JOURNAL OF SOCIAL WORK PRACTICE. Text in English. 1983. s-a. GBP 78, USD 130 to individuals; GBP 207, USD 340 to institutions (effective 2002). adv. bk.rev. index. back issues avail. *Refereed.* **Document type:** *Academic/Scholarly.*
Related titles: Microfiche ed.; Online - full text ed.: ISSN 1465-3885 (from CatchWord Ltd., Northern Light Technology, Inc., EBSCO Publishing, O C L C Online Computer Library Center, Inc., RoweCom Information Quest, ProQuest Information & Learning, Swets Blackwell, Institute for Scientific Information).
Indexed: ASCA, ASSIA, AgeLine, Brit.Nur.Ind., Curr.Cont., ERA, Fam.Ind., Intl.Bibl.Soc.Sci., Lang.& Lang.Behav.Abstr., Mult.Ed.Abstr., P C I, Psychol.Abstr., Res.High.Educ.Abstr., SOPODA, SSCI, Soc.Serv.Abstr., Soc.Work Res.& Abstr., Sociol.Abstr., Sp.Ed.Needs Abstr., Stud.Wom.Abstr.
—BLDSC (5064.919000), CatchWord, IDS. **CCC.**
Published by: Carfax Publishing Limited (Subsidiary of: Taylor & Francis Group), PO Box 25, Abingdon, Oxon OX14 3UE, United Kingdom. TEL 44-1235-401000, FAX 44-1235-401550, enquiries@carfax.co.uk, enquiry@tandf.co.uk, http://www.carfax.co.uk.

361.3 616.86 USA ISSN 1533-256X
▼ **JOURNAL OF SOCIAL WORK PRACTICE IN THE ADDICTIONS.** Text in English. 2001. q. (vol.1 triannual). USD 50 domestic to individuals; USD 68 in Canada to individuals; USD 73 elsewhere to individuals; USD 75 domestic to institutions; USD 101 in Canada to institutions; USD 109 elsewhere to institutions; USD 115 domestic to libraries; USD 155 in Canada to libraries; USD 167 foreign to libraries (effective Aug. 2001). adv. **Document type:** *Journal, Academic/Scholarly.*
Description: Features articles on innovative individual, family, group work, and community practice models for treating and preventing substance abuse and other addictions in diverse populations.
Related titles: Online - full text ed.: free with subscr. to the print ed.
Published by: Haworth Press, Inc., 10 Alice St, Binghamton, NY 13904-1580. TEL 607-722-5857, 800-342-9678, FAX 607-722-6362, 800-895-0582, getinfo@haworthpressinc.com, http://www.haworthpress.com/journals/journallist.asp. Ed. S Lala Ashenberg Straussner. Pub. William Cohen. R&P Ruthann Heath TEL 607-723-5857 ext 316. Adv. contact Jackie Blakeslee TEL 607-722-5857 ext 346. B&W page USD 315, color page USD 550; trim 6 x 8.5.

JUGENDROTKREUZ. see *CHILDREN AND YOUTH—For*

KATERN VROUWENZELFHULP. see *WOMEN'S HEALTH*

360 614.8 USA
KEEPING THE TRUST. Text in English. 1987. q. free per issue. illus. **Document type:** *Newsletter.*
Published by: Cleveland Foundation, 1422 Euclid Ave, Ste 1400, Cleveland, OH 44115. TEL 216-861-3810. Ed. Mary Frances Knuth. Circ: 5,000.

KETJU; professional periodical on mental retardation. see *MEDICAL SCIENCES—Pediatrics*

KINDEROPVANG. see *CHILDREN AND YOUTH—About*

KONTENRAHMEN FUER DIE TRAEGER DER GESETZLICHEN KRANKENVERSICHERUNG, KONTENRAHMEN FUER DIE TRAEGER DER SOZIALEN PFLEGEVERSICHERUNG UND DEN AUSGLEICHSFONDS. see *PUBLIC HEALTH AND SAFETY*

KRANKENDIENST; Zeitschrift fuer kath. Krankenhaeuser, Sozialstationen und Pflegeberufe. see *HEALTH FACILITIES AND ADMINISTRATION*

KUULOVIESTI/HEARING NEWS. see *HANDICAPPED—Hearing Impaired*

L A S NEWS. see *MEDICAL SCIENCES—Orthopedics And Traumatology*

LESBIAN AND GAY COUNSELLING NEWS. see *HOMOSEXUALITY*

362.4 DEU
LICHTBLICKE; Magazin der Christoffel-Blindenmission. Text in German. 1911. bi-m. free. illus. **Document type:** *Bulletin.* **Description:** Covers Christian missionary work and medical aid to the blind, the handicapped, and the hungry in Third World countries.
Former titles (until 1999): Weltweiten Christlichen Behindertendiakonte. Projekt-Berichte; (until 1997): Weltweiten Christlichen Behindertendiakonte. Berichte (0944-3118); Weltweiten Christlichen Armendiakonie. Bericht (0723-1539); (until 1979): Weltweiten Christlichen Behindertenhilfe. Bericht (0723-1512); Weltweiten Dienst Christlicher Blindennothilfe. Bericht (0723-1490); Evangelische Missionsarbeit an Blinden und Augenkranken in Asien und Afrika. Bericht (0723-1482); Evangelische Missionsarbeit an den Blinden in Asien und Afrika. Bericht (0723-1474); Evangelische Missionsarbeit an den Blinden Irans. Bericht (0723-1466); Christoffel-Blindenmission. Bericht (0009-580X)
Published by: Christoffel-Blindenmission e.V., Nibelungenstr 124, Bensheim 64625, Germany. TEL 49-6251-131-0, FAX 49-6251-131-122, 101666.2434@compuserve.com, communications@cbm-i.org, http://www.cbmi.de. Ed. Christian Osterhaus. Circ: 500,000. **U.S. subscr. to:** Christian Blind Mission International Inc., 450 E Park Ave, Greenville, SC 29601. TEL 864-239-0065, FAX 864-239-0069.

613.082 CAN
LIFE GUARDIAN. Text in English. 1971. bi-m. CND 10. adv. back issues avail. **Document type:** *Newsletter.*
Description: Articles on counselling, human interest, information on running a crisis pregnancy center.
Published by: Birthright, 777 Coxwell Ave, Toronto, ON M4C 3C6, Canada. TEL 416-469-4789, FAX 416-469-1772. Ed., R&P, Adv. contact Mary Berney. Circ: 1,600.

360 150 GBR ISSN 1366-6282
A LIFE IN THE DAY; work and daytime opportunities for people who use mental health services. Text in English. 1997. q. GBP 40 to individuals; GBP 55 to institutions. **Document type:** *Bulletin.* **Description:** Supports and promotes innovative work and daytime opportunities for people who use mental health services.
Indexed: Brit.Nur.Ind., e-psyche.

S

Published by: Pavilion Publishing Ltd., 8 St George's Pl, Brighton, East Sussex BN1 4GB, United Kingdom. TEL 44-1273-623222, FAX 44-1273-625526, pavpub@pavilion.co.uk, http://www.pavpub.com. Ed. Bob Grove.

LIGHT (WHEATON). see *HANDICAPPED—Visually Impaired*

LONDON DISABILITY NEWS. see *HANDICAPPED*

LONG TERM CARE. see *GERONTOLOGY AND GERIATRICS*

362.1 612 616.5 USA
LOOSE CONNECTIONS. Text in English. 1986. q. USD 25 domestic to membership; USD 30 in Canada & Mexico to membership; USD 35 elsewhere to membership. adv. bk.rev. **Document type:** *Newsletter, Consumer.* **Description:** Provides emotional support and information to persons who suffer from Ehlers Danlos syndrome and serves as communication link with the medical community.
Published by: Ehlers-Danlos National Foundation, 6399 Wilshire Blvd, Ste 510, Los Angeles, CA 90048. TEL 323-651-3038, FAX 323-651-3038, loosejoint@aol.com. Ed. Maggie Buckley. Pub. Keith Clarke. R&P, Adv. contact Linda Neuman-Potash. Circ: 2,000.

LOSINKA. see *PUBLIC ADMINISTRATION—Municipal Government*

360 610 CAN
M A P NEWS. Text in English. 1989. q. free per issue. bk.rev. illus. **Document type:** *Newsletter.* **Description:** Reports on the events and medical conditions in the Occupied Territories.
Related titles: French ed.: Info A M P.
Published by: Medical Aid for Palestine/Aide Medicale pour la Palestine, 356 Sherbrooke E, Montreal, PQ H2X 1E6, Canada. TEL 514-843-7875, FAX 514-843-3061. Circ: 2,000.

M G Z. (Maatschappelijke Gezondheidszorg) see *MEDICAL SCIENCES—Nurses And Nursing*

MAATGEVEND. see *HANDICAPPED*

MABAT SHELANU/OUR REVIEW. see *HANDICAPPED—Hearing Impaired*

MANAGEMENT ISSUES IN SOCIAL CARE. see *PUBLIC HEALTH AND SAFETY*

MANAGEMENT KINDEROPVANG. see *CHILDREN AND YOUTH—About*

361.73 361.8 ESP ISSN 0214-5979
MANOS UNIDAS. Text in Spanish. 1978 (Jul., no.44). q. ESP 1,000; USD 15 foreign. bk.rev. charts, illus, bibl. Supplement avail. **Document type:** *Bulletin.*
Published by: Campana Contra el Hambre en el Mundo, Barquillo, 38-2, Madrid 28004, Spain. TEL 91-308-2020, FAX 91-308-4208. Ed. Ana de Felipe. Pub. Javier Marmol. Circ: 60,000.

360 610 USA ISSN 0098-3616
HD7106.U5
MEDICAID RECIPIENT CHARACTERISTICS AND UNITS OF SELECTED MEDICAL SERVICES. Text in English. a.
Published by: U.S. National Center for Social Statistics, U S Department of Health, Education and Welfare, 330 Independence Ave, S W, Washington, DC 20201. TEL 301-436-7900.

362.4 GBR
MEDICAL AND DISABILITY APPEAL TRIBUNALS: THE LEGISLATION. Text in English. irreg., latest 1999. GBP 36 base vol(s). 3rd ed, 1998; GBP 17 updates 1999 supplement (effective 2000). **Document type:** *Trade.* **Description:** Discusses UK social welfare benefits legislation affecting persons with disabilities.
Published by: (Child Poverty Action Group), Sweet & Maxwell Ltd., 100 Avenue Rd, London NW3 3PF, United Kingdom. TEL 44-20-7393-7000, FAX 44-20-7449-1111, customer.services@sweetandmaxwell.co.uk, http://www.smlawpub.co.uk. Ed. Mark Rowland. **Subscr. outside the UK to:** Cheriton House, North Way, Andover, Hants SP10 5BE, United Kingdom. TEL 44-1264-342706, sminfo@itps.co.uk.

MENTAL HEALTH IN CHILDREN. see *PSYCHOLOGY*

362.2 USA ISSN 0191-6750
MENTAL HEALTH REPORT. Text in English. 1976. bi-w. USD 396; USD 412 out of North America (effective 2000). back issues avail. **Document type:** *Newsletter.* **Description:** Provides funding and operational tips for managers of mental health programs in public and private sectors.
Indexed: e-psyche.
—CCC.
Published by: Business Publishers, Inc., 8737 Colesville Rd, 11th Fl, Silver Spring, MD 20910-3928. TEL 301-587-6300, 800-274-6737, FAX 301-589-8493, bpinews@bpinews.com, http://www.bpinews.com. Ed. Brian Love. Pub. Leonard A Eiserer.

THE MENTAL HEALTH REVIEW. see *MEDICAL SCIENCES—Psychiatry And Neurology*

▼ **MENTAL HEALTH SERVICES RESEARCH.** see *PSYCHOLOGY*

MITEINANDER. see *MEDICAL SCIENCES*

MOTHER AND CHILD. see *WOMEN'S INTERESTS*

N H O NEWSLINE. see *ALTERNATIVE MEDICINE*

NATIONAL BOARD FOR NURSING, MIDWIFERY AND HEALTH VISITING FOR NORTHERN IRELAND. CONSOLIDATED ACCOUNTS (YEAR). see *MEDICAL SCIENCES—Nurses And Nursing*

NATIONAL COUNCIL NEWS. see *MEDICAL SCIENCES—Psychiatry And Neurology*

NATIONAL COUNCIL OF LA RAZA. AIDS NEWSLETTER. see *MEDICAL SCIENCES—Communicable Diseases*

360 USA ISSN 0164-7415
HQ767.15
NATIONAL RIGHT TO LIFE NEWS. Text in English. 1973. s-m. USD 16 domestic; USD 28 foreign (effective 2000). adv. bk.rev., film rev., play rev. charts, illus, pat, stat. index. back issues avail. **Document type:** *Newspaper.* **Description:** Covers issues of abortion, infanticide, and euthanasia from medical, ethical, social and public policy perspectives.
Related titles: Online - full text ed.: (from Gale Group).
Published by: National Right to Life Committee, Inc., 419 Seventh St, N W, Ste 500, Washington, DC 20004. TEL 202-626-8824, FAX 202-347-4754, dha1245@juno.com. Ed., R&P, Adv. contact Dave Andrusko. Pub. Wanda Franz. Circ: 390,000.

NATURAL HAZARDS CENTER. QUICK RESPONSE REPORTS. see *SOCIAL SCIENCES: COMPREHENSIVE WORKS*

NEW BEACON (INKPRINT EDITION); the journal of blind welfare. see *HANDICAPPED—Visually Impaired*

NEW CHOICES; the magazine for your health, money & travel. see *GERONTOLOGY AND GERIATRICS*

NEW YORK (STATE). COMMISSION ON QUALITY OF CARE FOR THE MENTALLY DISABLED. ANNUAL REPORT. see *HEALTH FACILITIES AND ADMINISTRATION*

NEWS ABOUT LIBRARY SERVICES FOR THE BLIND AND PHYSICALLY HANDICAPPED. see *HANDICAPPED*

NIEUWSBRIEF OF OUDERENZORG. see *GERONTOLOGY AND GERIATRICS*

NORCAL CENTER ON DEAFNESS NEWSLINE. see *HANDICAPPED—Hearing Impaired*

NURSE AIDE - V I P; published especially for those very important people who care for the elderly. see *GERONTOLOGY AND GERIATRICS*

OBEROENDE. see *DRUG ABUSE AND ALCOHOLISM*

OCCUPATIONAL THERAPY IN MENTAL HEALTH; a journal of psychosocial practice and research. see *MEDICAL SCIENCES—Psychiatry And Neurology*

614 AUT ISSN 0029-9901
OESTERREICHISCHES JUGENDROTKREUZ. ARBEITSBLAETTER. Text in German. 1947. q. free per issue. adv. bk.rev. illus. index. **Document type:** *Newsletter.* **Description:** News and information of the Austrian Youth Red Cross.
Published by: Oesterreichisches Jugendrotkreuz, Wiedner Hauptstrasse 32, Vienna, W 1041, Austria. FAX 43-1-58900179. Ed. Karl Zarhuber. Circ: 10,000 (controlled).

OKEE. see *MEDICAL SCIENCES—Psychiatry And Neurology*

OLD AGE: A REGISTER OF SOCIAL RESEARCH. see *GERONTOLOGY AND GERIATRICS*

306.38 USA ISSN 0146-3640
OLDER AMERICANS REPORT. Text in English. 1976. w. USD 417 in North America (effective 2001). back issues avail. **Document type:** *Newsletter.* **Description:** News for directors of senior citizens' programs; includes funding, nutrition and Social Security news.
Incorporates (1992-1997): Managing Senior Care (1063-035X); Formerly (until 198?): Aging Service News (0197-4025)
Related titles: Online - full text ed.: (from NewsNet).
—CCC.
Published by: Business Publishers, Inc., 8737 Colesville Rd, 11th Fl, Silver Spring, MD 20910-3928. TEL 301-587-6300, 800-274-6737, FAX 301-589-8493, bpinews@bpinews.com, http://www.bpinews.com. Ed. Nancy Aldrich. Pub. Leonard A Eiserer.

362 610.7 649 SWE ISSN 0280-4123
OMVAARDAREN. Text in Swedish. 1953. 5/yr. SEK 150. adv. 24 p./no. 3 cols./p.
Former titles (until 1974): Svensk Sjukskoeterskefoerening - Pedagogiska Sektionens Medlemsblad; (until 9182): Tidskrift foer Sjuksvaardspedagoger
Published by: Laerarfoerbundet, Fack 12239, Stockholm 10226, Sweden. TEL 46-8-737-65-00, FAX 46-8-657-97-48. Ed. Britta Morberger. Adv. contact Annelie Bjoernsdotter Lundqvist. B&W page SEK 5,300, color page SEK 8,000; trim 266 x 182. Circ: 3,600.

ONE IN SEVEN. see *HANDICAPPED—Hearing Impaired*

OP OOGHOOGTE. see *MEDICAL SCIENCES—Ophthalmology And Optometry*

OPENMIND; the mental health magazine. see *MEDICAL SCIENCES—Psychiatry And Neurology*

OUDERENZORG. see *GERONTOLOGY AND GERIATRICS*

360 614 USA
OVERVIEW (OLYMPIA). Text in English. 1973. m. free per issue. illus.
Published by: Department of Social and Health Services, MS OB 44Q, Olympia, WA 98504. TEL 206-753-7039. Ed. Mary Vaughn.

360 GBR ISSN 1350-4703
P S S R U BULLETIN. Text in English. 197?. irreg. free. **Document type:** *Bulletin.* **Description:** Covers policy research and analysis on equity and efficiency, and so of resources, needs and outcomes in community and long-term care and related areas. The researchers are from a wide range of disciplines and backrounds, including the caring profession.
Formerly (until 1985): P S S R U Newsletter (1351-9468)
Related titles: Online - full text ed.
—BLDSC (6945.964000).
Published by: Personal Social Services Research Unit, University of Canterbury at Kent, Cornwallis Bldg, University Rd, Canterbury, Kent CT2 7LJ, United Kingdom. TEL 44-1227-827773, FAX 44-1227-827038, pssru@ukc.ac.uk, http://www.ukc.ac.uk/pssru. Ed. Ken Judge. Circ: 5,000.

P W A C RESOURCE DIRECTORY. see *MEDICAL SCIENCES—Communicable Diseases*

P W A COALITION NEWSLINE. see *MEDICAL SCIENCES—Communicable Diseases*

PALLIATIVE CARE TODAY; the journal for today's palliative care team. see *MEDICAL SCIENCES—Oncology*

362.4 636.7 USA
PARTNERS (SYLMAR). Text in English. q. free per issue.
Former titles: I G E News; International Guiding Eyes. Newsletter
Published by: International Guiding Eyes, 13445 Glenoaks Blvd, Sylmar, CA 91342.

S

362 CAN ISSN 1194-8167
PEER COUNSELLOR JOURNAL. Text in English. 1983. s-a. CND 53.50 (effective 1999). bk.rev. back issues avail. **Document type:** *Academic/Scholarly.* **Description:** Studies peer helping in education, business and community agencies at all levels from children to senior citizens. Provides news, program ideas and resources.
Formerly: Peer Counsellor Newsletter (1180-470X)
Indexed: e-psyche.
Published by: Peer Resources, 1052 Davie St, Victoria, BC V8S 4E3, Canada. TEL 250-595-3503, FAX 250-595-3504, rcarr@islandnet.com, http://www.peer.ca/peer.html. Ed., R&P Rey A Carr. Circ: 7,000.

PEOPLE'S MEDICAL SOCIETY NEWSLETTER. see *CONSUMER EDUCATION AND PROTECTION*

PHOENIX SOCIETY NEWSLETTER. see *MEDICAL SCIENCES—Orthopedics And Traumatology*

360 GBR ISSN 0264-5033
PRIMARY HEALTH CARE. Text in English. 10/yr. GBP 80 in Europe to institutions; GBP 96 elsewhere to institutions (effective 2002). **Document type:** *Academic/Scholarly.* **Description:** Directed to members of staff in health centers, health clinics, and major group practices in the United Kingdom.
Indexed: Brit.Nur.Ind.
—BLDSC (6612.908900).
Published by: R C N Publishing Co. (Subsidiary of: B M J Publishing Group), R C N Direct, Copse Walk, Cardiff Gate Business Park, Cardiff CF23 8XG, United Kingdom. TEL 44-29-2054-6450, FAX 44-29-2054-6401, directjournalsteam@rcn.org.uk, http://www.rcn.org.uk/. Ed. J Sylvester. Circ: 13,000.

360 614 ITA ISSN 0393-9510
PROSPETTIVE SOCIALI E SANITARIE. Text in Italian. 1970. bi-w. (22/yr.). EUR 62 domestic; EUR 80 foreign (effective 2002). bk.rev. abstr, bibl, charts, stat. 22 p./no. 3 cols./p. back issues avail. *Refereed.* **Document type:** *Newsletter.*
Published by: Istituto per la Ricerca Sociale, Via Venti Settembre, 24, Milan, MI 20123, Italy. TEL 39-02-46764276, 39-02-467641, FAX 39-02-46764312, pss@hsn.it, http://www.irs-online.it. Eds. Emmanuele Ranci Ortigosa, Francesca Susani. R&P, Adv. contact Francesca Susani.

PSYCHIATRIC REHABILITATION JOURNAL. see *MEDICAL SCIENCES—Psychiatry And Neurology*

360 616.89 USA ISSN 1522-8878
HV40
PSYCHOANALYTIC SOCIAL WORK. Text in English. 1987. q. USD 60 to individuals; USD 81 in Canada to individuals; USD 87 elsewhere to individuals; USD 125 to institutions; USD 169 in Canada to institutions; USD 181 elsewhere to institutions; USD 225 to libraries; USD 304 in Canada to libraries; USD 326 elsewhere to libraries (effective Aug. 2001). adv. bk.rev. illus. back issues avail.; reprint service avail. from HAW. *Refereed.* **Document type:** *Journal, Academic/Scholarly.* **Description:** Provides social work clinicians and clinical educators with highly informative and stimulating articles relevant to the practice of psychoanalytic social work with the individual client.
Former titles (until 1999): Journal of Analytic Social Work (1052-9950); (until 1992): Journal of Independent Social Work (0883-7562)
Related titles: Microfiche ed.: (from PQC); Microform ed.
Indexed: ASSIA, Abstr.Anthropol., C.I.J.E. (coverage dropped), Crim.Just.Abstr., ERA, Human Resour.Abstr., IBZ, IMFL, Ind.Philos., Lang.& Lang.Behav.Abstr., Mult.Ed.Abstr., Per.Islam. (1990-), PsycInfo, Psychoanal.Abstr., Psychol.Abstr., Ref.Zh., SOPODA, Sage Fam.Stud.Abstr., Soc.Serv.Abstr., Soc.Work Res.& Abstr., Sociol.Abstr., Stud.Wom.Abstr., Viol.& Abuse Abstr., e-psyche.
—BLDSC (6946.274200), Haworth, ingenta.
Published by: Haworth Press, Inc., 10 Alice St, Binghamton, NY 13904-1580. TEL 607-722-5857, 800-429-6784, FAX 607-722-6362, 800-895-0582, getinfo@haworthpressinc.com, http://www.haworthpress.com/journals/journallist.asp. Ed. Jerrold R Brandell. Pub. William Cohen. R&P Ruthann Heath TEL 607-723-5857 ext 316. Adv. contact Jackie Blakeslee TEL 607-722-5857 ext 346. B&W page USD 315, color page USD 550; trim 6 x 8.5. Circ: 450.

PSYCHOSOZIALE UMSCHAU. see *MEDICAL SCIENCES—Psychiatry And Neurology*

PSYCHOTHERAPY NETWORKER. see *PSYCHOLOGY*

PUBLIC ASSISTANCE & WELFARE TRENDS - STATE CAPITALS. see *LAW*

PUERTO RICO. DEPARTMENT OF HEALTH. BOLETIN ESTADISTICO. see *PUBLIC HEALTH AND SAFETY—Abstracting, Bibliographies, Statistics*

PUERTO RICO. DEPARTMENT OF HEALTH. INFORME ESTADISTICO DE FACILIDADES DE SALUD. see *HEALTH FACILITIES AND ADMINISTRATION*

RAAKPUNT. see *MEDICAL SCIENCES—Psychiatry And Neurology*

REACH NEWSLETTER. see *EDUCATION—Special Education And Rehabilitation*

RECHTSPRAAK ZORGVERZEKERING. see *INSURANCE*

REFLECTIONS: NARRATIVES OF PROFESSIONAL HELPING. see *EDUCATION—Special Education And Rehabilitation*

REMEMBERING YESTERDAY; recalling those happy memories from the golden age of our past. see *GERONTOLOGY AND GERIATRICS*

RENALINK. see *MEDICAL SCIENCES—Urology And Nephrology*

362.4 USA ISSN 1043-1209
KF480.A15
REPORT ON DISABILITY PROGRAMS. Text in English. 1978. bi-w. USD 317 (effective 2001). back issues avail. **Document type:** *Newsletter.* **Description:** Focuses primarily on legislative changes on federal and state level. ALso provides networking information. Audience: policymaker, service providers, colleges, lawyers and state agencies.
Former titles (until 1989): Handicapped Americans Report (0276-2889); (until 1985): Handicapped Rights and Regulations (0191-6734)
Indexed: Rehabil.Lit.
—CCC.
Published by: Business Publishers, Inc., 8737 Colesville Rd, 11th Fl, Silver Spring, MD 20910-3928. TEL 301-587-6300, 800-274-6737, FAX 301-589-8493, bpinews@bpinews.com, http://www.bpinews.com. Ed. Robert Grupe. Pub. Leonard A Eiserer.

RESEARCH COMMUNICATIONS IN BEHAVIORAL PSYCHOLOGY AND PSYCHIATRY; including behavioral and neurosciences. see *PSYCHOLOGY*

RESEARCH ON SOCIAL WORK PRACTICE. see *SOCIOLOGY*

REVISTA VENEZOLANA DE SANIDAD Y ASISTENCIA SOCIAL. see *PUBLIC HEALTH AND SAFETY*

REVUE DE L'INFIRMIERE. see *MEDICAL SCIENCES—Nurses And Nursing*

362.41 GBR ISSN 0969-0468
ROYAL NATIONAL INSTITUTE FOR THE BLIND. UPDATE. Text in English. 10/yr. GBP 25. **Document type:** *Bulletin.* **Description:** Carries information on local society projects, RNIB services and developments, notices of forthcoming events, and general discussion articles. Aimed at RNIB staff and volunteers, along with central and local government agencies, libraries, and manufacturers of specialist equipment.
Related titles: Online - full text ed.
Published by: Royal National Institute for the Blind, Voluntary Agencies Link Unit, 224 Great Portland St, London W1N 6AA, United Kingdom. FAX 44-1733-371555, cgainsford@rnib.org.uk, http://www.rnib.org.uk. **Subscr. to:** RNIB Customer Services, PO Box 173, Peterborough, Cambs PE2 6WS, United Kingdom. FAX 44-1733-371555.

360 613 GBR ISSN 1466-4240
ROYAL SOCIETY FOR THE PROMOTION OF HEALTH. JOURNAL. Text in English. q. GBP 61; GBP 64 foreign (effective 1999). adv. bk.rev. bibl, charts, illus. index. *Refereed.* **Document type:** *Academic/Scholarly.* **Description:** Concerns all aspects of health and health-related issues; disciplines include medical, social services, environment, health and safety, sanitation, nutrition, construction, pharmeceuticals and health education.
Formerly (until 1998): Royal Society of Health Journal (0264-0325)
Related titles: Microform ed.: (from PQC); Online - full text ed.: (from Institute for Scientific Information).
Indexed: ASCA, ASSIA, Abstr.Hyg., Addic.Abstr., AgeLine, Archit.Per.Ind., Art.Hosp.& Tour., Biol.Abstr., Br.Tech.Ind., Brit.Nur.Ind., Chem.Abstr., Compumath, Curr.Adv.Ecol.Sci., Curr.Cont., Dairy Sci.Abstr., Dent.Ind., Excerp.Med., Food Sci.& Tech.Abstr., HRIS, Helminthol.Abstr., INIS Atomind., I.P.A., Ind.Med. (1983-), Ind.Vet., Int.Nurs.Ind., Lang.& Lang.Behav.Abstr., NRN, Nutr.Abstr., P C I, Ref.Zh., Rev.Arom.& Med.Plants, Rev.Med.& Vet.Mycol., Risk Abstr., SOPODA, SSCI, Sel.Water Res.Abstr., Soc.Work Res.& Abstr., Sociol.Abstr., THA, Trop.Dis.Bull., Vet.Bull., W.R.C.Inf., Weed Abstr.
—BLDSC (4864.700000), CISTI, EMDOCS, GNLM, IDS, ingenta, KNAW.
Published by: Royal Society for the Promotion of Health, R S H House, 38A St George's Dr, London SW1V 4BH, United Kingdom. TEL 44-20-7630-0121, FAX 44-20-7976-6847, rshealth@rshealth.org.uk. Ed. Prof G Jill Davies. Circ: 9,000.

S C I PSYCHOSOCIAL PROCESS. (Spinal Cord Injury) see *PSYCHOLOGY*

SANTE DE L'HOMME. see *MEDICAL SCIENCES*

SCANDINAVIAN JOURNAL OF PUBLIC HEALTH. see *MEDICAL SCIENCES*

SCANDINAVIAN JOURNAL OF PUBLIC HEALTH. SUPPLEMENT. see *MEDICAL SCIENCES*

SCARLET LETTER. see *WOMEN'S INTERESTS*

THE SEEING EYE ANNUAL REPORT. see *HANDICAPPED—Visually Impaired*

THE SEEING EYE GUIDE. see *HANDICAPPED—Visually Impaired*

360 614.8 MEX ISSN 0582-4001
SEGURIDAD SOCIAL. Text in Spanish. 1958. bi-m. MXP 330, USD 55. film rev. charts, illus, stat. Supplement avail. **Document type:** *Academic/Scholarly.*
Indexed: World Bibl.Soc.Sec.
Published by: Conferencia Interamericana de Seguridad Social, Apto. 99089, Calle San RAMON, Unidad Independencia Imss, Mexico City, DF 10100, Mexico. TEL 5950011, FAX 6838524. Ed. Maria Elvira Contreras Saucedo. R&P Juan Luis Soto Barzalobre. Circ: 700.
Co-sponsor: Instituto Mexicano del Seguro Social.

360 DEU
SELBSTHILFE SPEKTRUM RHEIN - MAIN. Text in German. 1984. a. back issues avail.
Published by: Koordination und Entwicklung von Selbsthilfe e.V. (KES), Theodor-Stern-Kai 7, Frankfurt Am Main 60596, Germany. TEL 069-63017603, FAX 069-63016301. Circ: 2,000.

361.8 614.58 USA
SELF-HELP AND PSYCHOLOGY MAGAZINE. Text in English. 1994. d. free per issue. adv. bk.rev. **Document type:** *Bulletin.*
Media: Online - full text.
Indexed: e-psyche.
Published by: Marlene Maheu, Ed. & Pub., 106 Thorn St, San Diego, CA 92103. TEL 619-277-2772, FAX 619-294-8181, drm@cybertowers.com, http://cybertowers.com/selfhelp. R&P, Adv. contact Marlene Maheu. Circ: 184,000.

361.8 614.58 USA ISSN 8756-1425
HV547
THE SELF-HELP SOURCEBOOK; your guide to community and online support group. Text in English. 1986. biennial. USD 12 (effective 1999). **Document type:** *Directory.* **Description:** Lists national, international and model groups, toll-free helplines and clearinghouses around the world for persons working in the health, mental health, and social service fields. Also contains a how-to section for starting up groups and accessing them via personal computer.
Former titles (until 1986): Self-Help Group Directory (0740-7548); Self-Help Group Sourcebook
Indexed: e-psyche.
Published by: American Self-Help Clearinghouse, Saint Clares Hospital Center, 25 Pocono Rd, Denville, NJ 07834. TEL 973-625-7101, http://www.mentalhelp.net/selfhelp. Ed. E Madara. R&P Ed Madara TEL 201-625-9565. Circ: 4,000.

362.6 USA ISSN 0199-7947
SENIOR CITIZEN SENTINEL* . Text in English. 1942. q. USD 5. adv. bk.rev. back issues avail.

S

Published by: California League of Senior Citizens, 1917 S Chestnut Ave, Apt 16E, Fresno, CA 93702-5552. TEL 213-386-7771. Ed. Kay Corbutt. Circ: 1,000.

SENIOR NEWS. see *GERONTOLOGY AND GERIATRICS*

SETTIMANA DEL SORDO; organo di informazione dei minorati dell'udito e della parola. see *HANDICAPPED—Hearing Impaired*

360 GBR
SHAFTESBURY PEOPLE. Text in English. 1848. s-a. membership. illus. **Document type:** *Newsletter.*
Former titles: Shaftesbury Review (0037-3168); Shaftesbury Newsletter
Published by: Shaftesbury Society, 16-20 Kingston Rd, London SW19 1JZ, United Kingdom. TEL 44-181-239-5555, FAX 44-181-239-5580. Ed. Jonathan Brewer. Circ: 10,000.

SIDA AHORA. see *MEDICAL SCIENCES—Communicable Diseases*

360 USA ISSN 0037-7317
HV1 CODEN: SMSWAW
SMITH COLLEGE STUDIES IN SOCIAL WORK. Text in English. 1930. 3/yr., latest vol.71, no.3. USD 20 domestic; USD 23 foreign (effective 2001). bk.rev. abstr. index. 150 p./no. back issues avail. *Refereed.* **Document type:** *Journal, Academic/Scholarly.* **Description:** Covers various clinical and research topics in social work.
Related titles: Online - full text ed.: (from Northern Light Technology, Inc., ProQuest Information & Learning, Institute for Scientific Information).
Indexed: ASCA, ASSIA, AgeLine, Curr.Cont., Fam.Ind., Hist.Abstr. (1969-1976, dropped), IMFL, Lang.& Lang.Behav.Abstr., Mid.East: Abstr.& Ind., P C I, P.A.I.S. (coverage dropped), PsycInfo, Psychol.Abstr. (1930-), SOPODA, SSCI, Sage Fam.Stud.Abstr., Soc.Serv.Abstr., Soc.Work Res.& Abstr., Sociol.Abstr., e-psyche.
—BLDSC (8311.200000), IDS, ingenta.
Published by: Smith College, School for Social Work, Lilly Hall, Northampton, MA 01063. TEL 413-585-7984, FAX 413-585-7994. Ed., R&P Gerald Schamess. Circ: 2,000 (paid).

SOCIAL SERVICE JOBS. see *OCCUPATIONS AND CAREERS*

360 362 USA ISSN 0098-1389
HV687.A2 CODEN: SWHCDO
SOCIAL WORK IN HEALTH CARE; the journal of health care work. Text in English. 1975. q. (2 vols./yr.). USD 75 to individuals; USD 101 in Canada to individuals; USD 109 elsewhere to individuals; USD 150 to institutions; USD 203 in Canada to institutions; USD 218 elsewhere to institutions; USD 250 to libraries; USD 338 in Canada to libraries; USD 363 elsewhere to libraries (effective Aug. 2001). adv. bk.rev. abstr, charts, illus. back issues avail.; reprint service avail. from HAW. *Refereed.* **Document type:** *Journal, Academic/Scholarly.* **Description:** Deals with social work, theory, practice, and administration in a wide variety of health care settings.
Related titles: Microfiche ed.: (from PQC); Microform ed.; Online - full text ed.: (from Institute for Scientific Information).
Indexed: ASCA, ASSIA, Abstr.Health Care Manage.Stud., Abstr.Soc.Geront., Adol.Ment.Hlth.Abstr., AgeLine, Behav.Abstr., Behav.Med.Abstr., Biol.Abstr., CINAHL, Chicago Psychoanal.Lit.Ind., Curr.Cont., ERA, Excerp.Med., Fam.Ind., Hosp.Abstr., Human Resour.Abstr., IBZ, IMFL, Ind.Med. (1975-), Int.Nurs.Ind., Lang.& Lang.Behav.Abstr., Med.Care Rev., PSI, Peace Res.Abstr., PsycInfo, Psychol.Abstr. (1975-), Ref.Zh., Rehabil.Lit., SOPODA, SSCI, Sage Fam.Stud.Abstr., Sage Pub.Admin.Abstr., Soc.Serv.Abstr., Soc.Work Res.& Abstr., Sociol.Abstr., Sp.Ed.Needs Abstr., Stud.Wom.Abstr., Viol.& Abuse Abstr., e-psyche.
—BLDSC (8318.225600), GNLM, Haworth, IDS, ingenta, KNAW.
Published by: Haworth Press, Inc., 10 Alice St, Binghamton, NY 13904-1580. TEL 607-722-5857, 800-429-6784, FAX 607-722-6362, 800-895-0582, TELEX 4932599 HAWORTH, getinfo@haworthpressinc.com, http://www.haworthpress.com/journals/journallist.asp. Ed. Gary Rosenburg. Pub. William Cohen. R&P Ruthann Heath TEL 607-723-5857 ext 316. Adv. contact Jackie Blakeslee TEL 607-722-5857 ext 346. B&W page USD 315, color page USD 550; trim 6 x 8.5. Circ: 2,025.

362.1 USA
SOCIAL WORK LEADER. Text in English. 10/yr. membership.
Formerly (until 1998): Social Work Administration
Published by: American Hospital Association, Society for Social Work Leadership in Health Care, 1 N Franklin, 31st Fl, Chicago, IL 60606. TEL 312-422-3770, FAX 312-422-3772, jbrody1@aha.org. Ed. Salvinija G Kernaghan.

362.8 USA ISSN 0160-9513
HV45 CODEN: SWGRDU
SOCIAL WORK WITH GROUPS; a journal of community and clinical practice. Text in English. 1978. q. USD 75 to individuals; USD 101 in Canada to individuals; USD 109 elsewhere to individuals; USD 175 to institutions; USD 236 in Canada to institutions; USD 254 elsewhere to institutions; USD 400 to libraries; USD 540 in Canada to libraries; USD 580 elsewhere to libraries (effective Aug. 2001). adv. bk.rev. bibl, illus. back issues avail.; reprint service avail. from PSC,SCH. *Refereed.* **Document type:** *Journal, Academic/Scholarly.* **Description:** Covers the areas of groupwork in psychiatric, rehabilitative, and multipurpose social work and social services agencies.
Related titles: Microfiche ed.: (from PQC); Microform ed.; Online - full text ed.: (from Gale Group, Factiva).
Indexed: ASCA, ASSIA, Abstr.Soc.Geront., Adol.Ment.Hlth.Abstr., AgeLine, Chic.Per.Ind., Crim.Just.Abstr., Curr.Cont. (coverage dropped), ERA, G.Soc.Sci.& Rel.Per.Lit., Human Resour.Abstr., IBZ, IMFL, Lang.& Lang.Behav.Abstr., Mult.Ed.Abstr., PsycInfo, Psychol.Abstr. (1979-), SOPODA, SSCI (coverage dropped), Soc.Sci.Ind. (Jan.1994-), Soc.Serv.Abstr., Soc.Work Res.& Abstr., Sociol.Abstr., Sp.Ed.Needs Abstr., Stud.Wom.Abstr., Viol.& Abuse Abstr., e-psyche.
—BLDSC (8318.225000), Haworth, IDS, ingenta.
Published by: Haworth Press, Inc., 10 Alice St, Binghamton, NY 13904-1580. TEL 607-722-5857, 800-429-6784, FAX 607-722-6362, 800-895-0582, getinfo@haworthpressinc.com, http://www.haworthpress.com/journals/journallist.asp. Eds. Andrew Malekoff, Roselle Kurland. Pub. William Cohen. R&P Ruthann Heath TEL 607-723-5857 ext 316. Adv. contact Jackie Blakeslee TEL 607-722-5857 ext 346. B&W page USD 315, color page USD 550; trim 6 x 8.5. Circ: 1,200.

SOCIALISM AND HEALTH. see *PUBLIC HEALTH AND SAFETY*

SOCIALMEDICINSK TIDSKRIFT. see *MEDICAL SCIENCES*

SOZIALPSYCHIATRISCHE INFORMATIONEN. see *PSYCHOLOGY*

SPRINGER SERIES ON REHABILITATION. see *MEDICAL SCIENCES—Physical Medicine And Rehabilitation*

361.6 153.1 USA ISSN 0743-5916
HV3006.P4
STATE PLAN FOR DEVELOPMENTAL DISABILITIES. Text in English. 1977. a. **Document type:** *Government.*
Formerly: Pennsylvania. Development Disabilities Planning Council. Pennsylvania State Plan (0193-1423)
Indexed: e-psyche.
Published by: Developmental Disabilities Planning Council, Health & Welfare Bldg, Harrisburg, PA 17120. Circ: 2,000.

DE STEM VAN DE OUDERS. see *HANDICAPPED*

361 ITA
LA STILLA; organo di stampa dell'A.V.I.S. provinciale di Mantova. Text in Italian. 1965. m.
Published by: Associazione Volontari Italiani Sangue (A.V.I.S.), c/o Ospedale "C. Poma", Via Albertoni, 1, Mantua, MN 46100, Italy.

STREETWIZE COMMUNICATIONS; youth rights comics. see *CHILDREN AND YOUTH—For*

STUDIENSTIFTUNG. JAHRESBERICHT. see *EDUCATION—Special Education And Rehabilitation*

SUIZIDPROPHYLAXE. see *MEDICAL SCIENCES—Psychiatry And Neurology*

SVENSK FAMILJETERAPI. see *MEDICAL SCIENCES—Psychiatry And Neurology*

362 SWE ISSN 0346-2129
SVENSK HANDIKAPPTIDSKRIFT. Text in Swedish. 1923. 10/yr. SEK 190. adv. 32 p./no. 3 cols./p.
Formerly (until 1966): Svensk Vanfoeretidskrift
Published by: Handikappades Riksfoerbund, Katrinebergsvaegen 6, Stockholm 11743, Sweden. TEL 46-8-18-91-00, FAX 46-8-645-65-41. Ed. Elisabet Geite. Pub. Folke Carlsson. Adv. contact Lars Goeran Andersson. B&W page SEK 11,700, color page SEK 16,700; trim 270 x 190. Circ: 28,100.

T C H I UPDATE. see *HANDICAPPED—Hearing Impaired*

TAPPING TECHNOLOGY. see *HANDICAPPED—Physically Impaired*

THERAPEUTIC COMMUNITIES. see *PHILOSOPHY*

THERAPY WEEKLY; the newspaper for the remedial professions. see *HEALTH FACILITIES AND ADMINISTRATION*

649.8 GBR ISSN 0268-4047
THIS CARING BUSINESS. Text in English. 1985. 10/yr. GBP 50 domestic; GBP 75 in Europe; GBP 80 elsewhere (effective 2001). adv. bk.rev. charts, stat, tr.lit. back issues avail. **Document type:** *Trade.* **Description:** Covers commercially oriented matters relating to long-stay health and residential care.
Published by: Careworld Publishing House Ltd., 1 St Thomas Rd, Hastings, E Sussex TN34 3LG, United Kingdom. TEL 44-1424-718406, FAX 44-1424-718460. Ed. Michael Monk. R&P, Adv. contact Jonathan Heyes TEL 44-1422-375317. Circ: 18,366.

▼ **TIDSSKRIFT FOR ARBEJDSLIV.** see *BUSINESS AND ECONOMICS—Labor And Industrial Relations*

TIJDSCHRIFT VOOR BEDRIJFS- EN VERZEKERINGSGENEESKUNDE. see *MEDICAL SCIENCES*

HET TIJDSCHRIFT VOOR VERZORGENDEN. see *MEDICAL SCIENCES—Nurses And Nursing*

TIMELINES. see *MEDICAL SCIENCES*

TINNITUS TODAY. see *MEDICAL SCIENCES—Otorhinolaryngology*

TREATING ABUSE TODAY; trauma, treatment and trends. see *PSYCHOLOGY*

TWIN SERVICES REPORTER. see *CHILDREN AND YOUTH—About*

U C S F MAGAZINE. see *MEDICAL SCIENCES*

360 GBR ISSN 1368-230X
UNIT COSTS OF HEALTH & SOCIAL CARE. Text in English. 1993. a. charts, stat. **Document type:** *Bulletin.*
Formerly (until 1996): Unit Costs of Community Care (0969-4226)
—BLDSC (9090.785418).
Published by: Personal Social Services Research Unit, University of Canterbury at Kent, Cornwallis Bldg, University Rd, Canterbury, Kent CT2 7LJ, United Kingdom. TEL 44-1227-827773, FAX 44-1227-827038, pssru@ukc.ac.uk, http://www.ukc.ac.uk/PSSRU, http://www.ukc.ac.uk/pssru. Ed. Ken Judge.

VIEWPOINT (LONDON, 1995). see *MEDICAL SCIENCES—Psychiatry And Neurology*

VIOLENCE AND VICTIMS. see *SOCIOLOGY*

VIVRE ENSEMBLE. see *EDUCATION—Special Education And Rehabilitation*

VOICE OF SILENCE NEWSLETTER. see *HANDICAPPED—Hearing Impaired*

LA VOIX DES PARENTS. see *HANDICAPPED*

VOLUNTEER AND VISTORS' GUIDE. see *GERONTOLOGY AND GERIATRICS*

VOLUNTEER LEADER. see *HEALTH FACILITIES AND ADMINISTRATION*

WASHINGTON COUNSELETTER. see *OCCUPATIONS AND CAREERS*

S

360 610 USA ISSN 0095-1609
HV86
WASHINGTON (STATE). DEPARTMENT OF SOCIAL AND HEALTH SERVICES. INCOME MAINTENANCE, COMMUNITY SOCIAL SERVICES AND MEDICAL ASSISTANCE. Text in English. 1974 (vol.27). m. free per issue. charts, stat. **Document type:** *Government.*
Published by: Department of Social and Health Services, Office of Program Analysis, MS OB 34F, Olympia, WA 98504. TEL 206-753-7039.

362.41 GBR
WELCOME TO THE WORLD OF... Text in English. m. free per issue. **Document type:** *Newsletter.* **Description:** Brings readers who are blind or visually impaired the latest in mainstream news and services, each issue focusing on a particular subject.
Media: Braille. **Related titles:** Diskette ed.; Online - full text ed.
Published by: Royal National Institute for the Blind, 224 Great Portland St, London W1N 6AA, United Kingdom. FAX 44-1733-371555, webmaster@rnib.org.uk, cservices@rnib.org.uk, http://www.rnib.org.uk. **Subscr. to:** RNIB Customer Services, PO Box 173, Peterborough, Cambs PE2 6WS, United Kingdom. TEL 44-1733-370777.

360 616.89 GBR ISSN 1365-9820
WELFARE WORLD. Text in English. 1980. q. GBP 20 (effective 1997). adv. bk.rev. illus. **Document type:** *Academic/Scholarly, Trade.* **Description:** Contains articles, courses, conference listings and diary dates, a letters page, news of the regional centres of the institute, and a student's page.
Former titles (until 1996): Welfare (0269-879X); (until 1990): Welfare Journal; Welfare and Social Services Journal (0261-4049); Welfare Officer
Indexed: e-psyche.
—BLDSC (9294.157300).
Published by: Institute of Welfare Officers, 3rd Fl, Newland House, 137-139 Hagley Rd, Edgbaston, Birmingham B16 8UA, United Kingdom. FAX 44-1235-469272. Ed., Adv. contact Brenda Baxter. R&P Peter Morgan. Circ: 2,000.

WORD FROM WASHINGTON (WASHINGTON, D.C.). see *HANDICAPPED*

WORLD DISASTERS REPORT. see *PUBLIC HEALTH AND SAFETY*

WORLD'S WOMAN'S CHRISTIAN TEMPERANCE UNION. TRIENNIAL REPORT. see *DRUG ABUSE AND ALCOHOLISM*

ZAGADNIENIA WYCHOWAWCZE A ZDROWIE PSYCHICZNE. see *MEDICAL SCIENCES—Psychiatry And Neurology*

360 NLD ISSN 1381-4664
ZORG & WELZIJN; opiniemagazine voor de sector zorg en welzijn. Text in Dutch. 1946. m. adv. bk.rev. index. **Document type:** *Journal, Academic/Scholarly.* **Description:** Examines issues of interest to caregivers and nurses.
Supersedes (in 1994): Welzijnsweekblad (0169-0639); Which incorporated in part (in 1980): T M W Welzijnsweekblad (0165-117X); (1976-1978): Welzijnsweekblad (0169-3697); And superseded in part (in 1981): Welzijnsmaandblad (0169-3190); Which was formerly (until 1981): T M W Welzijnsmaanblad (0165-1277); (until 1979): Tijdschrift voor Maatschappijvraagstukken en Welzijnwerk (0169-3247); (until 1972): Tijdschrift voor Mens en Welzijn
—KNAW.
Published by: Elsevier Gezondheidszorg B.V., Tijdstroom (Subsidiary of: Reed Elsevier plc Group), Planetenbaan 1, Maarssen 3600 AK, Netherlands. TEL 31-346-577577, FAX 31-346-554287, http://www.zorgwelzijn.nl, http://www.tijdstroom.nl. Circ: 9,000. **Subscr. to:** Elsevier Den Haag, Postbus 16500, The Hague 2500 BM, Netherlands. TEL 31-70-381-9900, FAX 31-70-333-8399.

SOCIAL SERVICES AND WELFARE—Abstracting, Bibliographies, Statistics

EXCERPTA MEDICA. SECTION 20: GERONTOLOGY AND GERIATRICS. see *GERONTOLOGY AND GERIATRICS—Abstracting, Bibliographies, Statistics*

EXCERPTA MEDICA. SECTION 40: DRUG DEPENDENCE, ALCOHOL ABUSE AND ALCOHOLISM. see *DRUG ABUSE AND ALCOHOLISM—Abstracting, Bibliographies, Statistics*

360 FIN ISSN 0784-8757
FINLAND. TILASTOKESKUS. ELINOLOT. Text in Finnish. irreg.
Published by: Tilastokeskus/Statistics Finland, Tyopajakatu 13, Statistics Finland, Helsinki 00022, Finland. TEL 358-9-17341.

360 GRC ISSN 0253-9454
RA407.5.G73
GREECE. NATIONAL STATISTICAL SERVICE. SOCIAL WELFARE AND HEALTH STATISTICS. Text in English, Greek. 1967. a., latest 1995. GRD 3,000. back issues avail. **Document type:** *Government.*
Formerly (until 1976): Greece. National Statistical Service. Bulletin of Social Welfare and Health Statistics
Published by: National Statistical Service of Greece, Statistical Information and Publications Division/Ethniki Statistiki Yperesia tes Ellados, 14-16 Lykourgou St, Athens 101 66, Greece. TEL 30-1-3289-397, FAX 30-1-3241-102.

HEALTH SERVICE ABSTRACTS. see *MEDICAL SCIENCES—Abstracting, Bibliographies, Statistics*

360 GBR ISSN 1361-3677
RA407.5.G7
HEALTH STATISTICS WALES. Text in English. a. GBP 12 (effective 2000). **Document type:** *Bulletin, Government.*
Formed by the merger of (1984-1995): Welsh Hospital Waiting List Bulletin (0266-0776); Health and Personal Social Services Statistics for Wales (0307-0840); (1982-1995): Key Statistical Indicators for Health in Wales (0969-3084); (1981-1995): Mental Health Statistics for Wales (0260-5252)
—BLDSC (4275.205500). **CCC.**
Published by: National Assembly of Wales, Statistical Directorate5, Publication Unit, Cathays Park, Cardiff CF1 3NP, United Kingdom. TEL 44-2920-825054, FAX 44-2920-825350, stats.pubs@wales.gsi.gov.uk.

361.65021 USA
IDAHO. DEPARTMENT OF HEALTH AND WELFARE. RESEARCH AND STATISTICS SECTION. QUARTERLY WELFARE STATISTICAL BULLETIN. Text in English. q. **Document type:** *Bulletin, Government.*
Former titles: Idaho. Department of Health and Welfare. Bureau of Research and Statistics. Quarterly Welfare Statistical Bulletin; Idaho. Department of Health and Welfare. Bureau of Research and Statistics. Research Report (0098-8561)
Indexed: SRI.
Published by: Department of Health and Welfare, Medicaid and Welfare Research Section, Statehouse, Boise, ID 83720. TEL 208-334-6900. Ed. Linda Caballero. Circ: 180.

362 USA
ILLINOIS. DEPARTMENT OF HUMAN SERVICES. DIVISION OF DISABILITY AND BEHAVIORAL HEALTH SERVICES. ILLINOIS STATISTICS. Text in English. 1930. a. free per issue. **Document type:** *Government.*
Former titles: Mental Health Statistics for Illinois (0076-6453); Illinois. Department of Mental Health. Administrator's Data Manual
Indexed: SRI.
Published by: Department of Human Services, Division of Disability and Behavioral Health Services, 100 Sount Grand Ave E, Lowest level, Springfield, IL 62762. TEL 217-785-9404. Ed. Jim Kane. Circ: 950.

362 310 ISR ISSN 0075-1014
HA1931
ISRAEL. CENTRAL BUREAU OF STATISTICS. DIAGNOSTIC STATISTICS OF HOSPITALIZATIONS. Text in English, Hebrew. 1950. irreg., latest 1987. ILS 18.50. **Document type:** *Government.*
Published by: Central Bureau of Statistics, PO Box 13015, Jerusalem 91130, Israel. TEL 972-2-6553364, FAX 972-2-6521340.

JAPAN. MINISTRY OF HEALTH AND WELFARE. STATISTICS AND INFORMATION DEPARTMENT. HANDBOOK OF HEALTH AND WELFARE STATISTICS. see *PUBLIC HEALTH AND SAFETY—Abstracting, Bibliographies, Statistics*

MALAWI. NATIONAL STATISTICAL OFFICE. SURVEY OF HANDICAPPED PERSONS. see *HANDICAPPED—Abstracting, Bibliographies, Statistics*

362.1 616.891 USA ISSN 0361-9311
RC443
MENTAL HEALTH STATISTICAL NOTES. Text in English. 1969. irreg. free per issue. back issues avail. **Document type:** *Government.* **Description:** Provides statistical information on mental health services in the U.S. for selected organizations, years, and patient populations.
Indexed: Ind.Med. (coverage dropped), e-psyche.
—BLDSC (5678.585750).
Published by: U.S. Center for Mental Health Services, Division of State and Community Systems Development, Survey and Analysis Branch, 5600 Fishers Ln, Rockville, MD 20857. TEL 301-443-3344, FAX 301-443-7926, msonnews@aoachms1.ssw.dhhs.gov. Ed. Mary Anne Sonnenschein. Circ: 6,000.

NEW LITERATURE ON VISUAL IMPAIRMENT. see *HANDICAPPED—Abstracting, Bibliographies, Statistics*

REFERATIVNYI ZHURNAL. GERONTOLOGIYA. GERIATRIYA. see *GERONTOLOGY AND GERIATRICS—Abstracting, Bibliographies, Statistics*

649.8021 GBR
RESIDENTIAL CARE HOMES SCOTLAND. STATISTICAL INFORMATION NOTE. Text in English. a.
Former titles: Residential Community Care Scotland. Statistical Information Note; (until 1997): Community Care, Scotland
—BLDSC.
Published by: Community Care Statistics, Room 52, James Craig Walk, Edinburgh EH1 3BA, United Kingdom. TEL 44-131-2443777. Ed. Steven Gillespie.

SOCIOLOGY

see also FOLKLORE; POPULATION STUDIES; SOCIAL SCIENCES: COMPREHENSIVE WORKS; SOCIAL SERVICES AND WELFARE

ACTA MEDICA ET SOCIOLOGICA. see *MEDICAL SCIENCES*

ADVANCES (CHICAGO); progress in Alzheimer research and care. see *MEDICAL SCIENCES—Psychiatry And Neurology*

302 USA ISSN 0065-2601
HM251 CODEN: AXSPAQ
ADVANCES IN EXPERIMENTAL SOCIAL PSYCHOLOGY. Text in English. 1964. irreg., latest vol.30, 1998. index. reprint service avail. from PSC,SCH,ISI. *Refereed.*
Related titles: Online - full text ed.: (from Institute for Scientific Information).
Indexed: ASCA, Biol.Abstr., P C I, Russ.Acad.Sci.Bibl., SSCI, e-psyche.
—BLDSC (0706.100000), ingenta. **CCC.**
Published by: Academic Press, Inc., Journal Division (Subsidiary of: Harcourt Brace & Company), 525 B St, Ste 1900, San Diego, CA 92101-4495. TEL 619-231-0926, FAX 619-699-6715. Ed. Leonard Berkowitz. **Subscr. to:** Order Dept., 6277 Sea Harbor Dr, 4th Fl, Orlando, FL 32887. TEL 800-321-5068.

301 USA ISSN 1057-6290
RA418 CODEN: AMSOEI
ADVANCES IN MEDICAL SOCIOLOGY. Text in English. 1990. irreg., latest vol.6, 1996. USD 78.50. **Document type:** *Monographic series.*
Indexed: Lang.& Lang.Behav.Abstr., SOPODA, Soc.Serv.Abstr., Sociol.Abstr.
—BLDSC (0709.376200), GNLM, Infotrieve. **CCC.**
Published by: J A I Press Inc., 100 Prospect St, Box 811, Stamford, CT 06904-0811. TEL 203-323-9606, FAX 203-357-8446, jai@jaipress.com. Ed. Gary Albrecht.

ADVANCES IN SUICIDOLOGY. see *SOCIAL SERVICES AND WELFARE*

AFTERLOSS; the monthly newsletter to comfort and care for those who mourn. see *MEDICAL SCIENCES—Psychiatry And Neurology*

AGROTROPICA. see *AGRICULTURE*

AMERICAN FAMILY THERAPY ACADEMY NEWSLETTER. see *PSYCHOLOGY*

S

302 USA ISSN 0091-0562
RA790.A1 CODEN: AJCPCK
AMERICAN JOURNAL OF COMMUNITY PSYCHOLOGY. Text in English. 1973. bi-m. USD 655, EUR 653 to institutions for print or online ed.; USD 134, EUR 134 to individuals for print or online ed.; USD 786, EUR 783.60 to institutions for print & online eds. combined (effective 2002). adv. illus. Index. back issues avail.; reprints avail. *Refereed.* **Document type:** *Journal, Academic/Scholarly.* **Description:** Publishes quantitative and qualitative research on community psychological interventions at the social, neighborhood, organizational, group, and individual levels.
Related titles: Microfilm ed.: (from PQC); Online - full text ed.: (from Gale Group, Northern Light Technology, Inc., EBSCO Publishing, O C L C Online Computer Library Center, Inc., RoweCom Information Quest, ProQuest Information & Learning, Swets Blackwell, Kluwer Online, Factiva, Institute for Scientific Information).
Indexed: ASCA, ASSIA, Abstr.Crim.& Pen., Adol.Ment.Hlth.Abstr., AgeLine, CINAHL, Chic.Per.Ind., Crim.Just.Abstr., Curr.Cont., ERA, Environ.Sci.Poll.Mgmt., Except.Child Educ.Abstr., Excerp.Med., Fam.Ind., IBZ, IMFL, INIS Atomind., Ind.Med. (1973-), Ind.Philos., Lang.& Lang.Behav.Abstr., Mid.East: Abstr.& Ind., Mult.Ed.Abstr., P C I, PSI, Peace Res.Abstr., Pollut.Abstr., Psyclnfo, Psychol.Abstr. (1974-), Ref.Zh., Risk Abstr., Russ.Acad.Sci.Bibl., SOPODA, SSCI, Saf.Sci.Abstr., Sage Fam.Stud.Abstr., Sage Pub.Admin.Abstr., Sage Race Rel.Abstr., Sage Urb.Stud.Abstr., Soc.Sci.Ind. (Feb.1987-), Soc.Serv.Abstr., Soc.Work Res.& Abstr., Sociol.Abstr., Sp.Ed.Needs Abstr., THA, e-psyche.
—BLDSC (0824.070000), GNLM, IDS, ingenta. **CCC.**
Published by: (American Psychological Association), Kluwer Academic - Plenum Publishers (Subsidiary of: Wolters Kluwer N.V.), 233 Spring St, New York, NY 10013-1578. TEL 212-620-8000, 800-221-9369, FAX 212-463-0742, http://www.wkap.nl/journalhome.htm/0091-0562. Ed. W S Davidson. R&P Rose Luongo TEL 781-871-6311.

AMERICAN JOURNAL OF FAMILY THERAPY. see *PSYCHOLOGY*

ANNUAL EDITIONS: DRUGS, SOCIETY & BEHAVIOR. see *DRUG ABUSE AND ALCOHOLISM*

ANNUAL EDITIONS: DYING, DEATH, AND BEREAVEMENT. see *PSYCHOLOGY*

ANNUAL EDITIONS: HUMAN SEXUALITY. see *BIOLOGY*

ANNUAL REVIEW OF SEX RESEARCH. see *PSYCHOLOGY*

APPLIED DEVELOPMENTAL SCIENCE. see *PSYCHOLOGY*

ARBEITEN ZUR SOZIALWISSENSCHAFTLICHEN PSYCHOLOGIE. see *PSYCHOLOGY*

ARCHIVOS HISPANOAMERICANOS DE SEXOLOGIA. see *PSYCHOLOGY*

ATMA JAYA RESEARCH CENTRE. SOCIO-MEDICAL RESEARCH REPORT/PUSAT PENELITIAN ATMA JAYA. PENELITIAN TENTANG KEBUTUHAN KESEHATAN MASYARAKAT DAN SISTEM PELEYANAN KESEHATAN DI KECAMATAN PENJARINGAN. see *MEDICAL SCIENCES*

306.85 AUS ISSN 0814-723X
HQ10 CODEN: ANZTE7
AUSTRALIAN AND NEW ZEALAND JOURNAL OF FAMILY THERAPY; innovative and contextual approaches to human problems. Text in English. 1979. q. AUD 88 in Australia to individuals; AUD 80 in New Zealand to individuals; AUD 140 in North America to individuals; AUD 120 elsewhere to individuals; AUD 126 in Australia to institutions; AUD 115 in New Zealand to institutions; AUD 205 in North America to institutions; AUD 180 elsewhere to institutions (effective 2001). adv. bk.rev. back issues avail. **Document type:** *Academic/Scholarly.* **Description:** Promotes theory and practice of family therapy.
Formerly: Australian Journal of Family Therapy
Related titles: Online - full text ed.: (from EBSCO Publishing, O C L C Online Computer Library Center, Inc., RoweCom Information Quest, ingenta, Swets Blackwell).
Indexed: ASSIA, Fam.Ind., IMFL, Lang.& Lang.Behav.Abstr., Psyclnfo, Psychol.Abstr. (1983-), SOPODA, Sage Fam.Stud.Abstr., Soc.Serv.Abstr., Soc.Work Res.& Abstr., Sociol.Abstr., Viol.& Abuse Abstr., e-psyche.
—BLDSC (1796.886500), Infotrieve, ingenta. **CCC.**
Address: PO Box 135, Moorebank, NSW 1875, Australia. FAX 61-2-9825-4885, journalsubs@start.com.au. Eds. Hugh Crago, Maureen Crago. Circ: 1,044 (paid).

BEHAVIOR AND SOCIAL ISSUES. see *PSYCHOLOGY*

BEITRAEGE ZUR PSYCHOLOGIE UND SOZIOLOGIE DES KRANKEN MENSCHEN. see *PSYCHOLOGY*

178 NLD ISSN 0921-3996
BLAUWE WEGWIJZER. Text in Dutch. 1963. bi-m. NLG 10 (effective 2001). adv. bk.rev. illus, stat. **Document type:** *Consumer.*
Formerly: Blauwe Kruis (0006-4653)
Published by: Christelijke Beweging voor Drankbestrijding, Groningensingel 677, Arnhem 6835 GA, Netherlands. TEL 31-26-3217889. Ed. H Ploeger. Circ: 3,400.

306.7 ISL ISSN 1021-7150
BLEIKT OG BLATT. Text in Icelandic. bi-m. ISK 3,294, USD 50; ISK 669 newsstand/cover (effective 1998). adv. **Description:** Focuses on issues and events related to sex and the relationship between the sexes. Contributors are chiefly physicians, psychologists, sex therapists, nurses and other members of the medical and health professions.
Indexed: e-psyche.
Published by: Frodi Ltd., Seljavegur 2, Reykjavik 101, Iceland. TEL 354-515-5648, FAX 354-515-5599, bogb@frodi.is. Ed. David Thor Jonsson. Adv. contact Sigrun Thorvardardottir. B&W page ISK 49,900, color page ISK 89,700; trim 20.5 x 28.4. Circ: 11,000.

CAHIERS CRITIQUES DE THERAPIE FAMILIALE ET DE PRATIQUES DE RESEAUX. see *PSYCHOLOGY*

CANADIAN JOURNAL OF BEHAVIOURAL SCIENCE/REVUE CANADIENNE DES SCIENCES DU COMPORTEMENT. see *PSYCHOLOGY*

302 USA ISSN 0738-0151
HV701 CODEN: CASWDD
CHILD AND ADOLESCENT SOCIAL WORK JOURNAL. Text in English. 1970. bi-m. USD 496 in the Americas to institutions for print or online ed.; EUR 495 elsewhere to institutions for print or online ed.; USD 595.20 in the Americas to institutions for print & online eds. combined; EUR 594 elsewhere to institutions for print & online eds. combined (effective 2002). adv. bk.rev. bibl, illus. reprints avail. *Refereed.* **Document type:** *Journal, Academic/Scholarly.* **Description:** Focuses on clinical social work practice with children, adolescents, and their families.
Supersedes (in 1982): Family and Child Mental Health Journal (0190-230X); Which was formerly (until 1980): Issues in Child Mental Health (0362-403X); (until vol.5, 1977): Psychosocial Process (0556-431X)
Related titles: Online - full text ed.: (from EBSCO Publishing, O C L C Online Computer Library Center, Inc., RoweCom Information Quest, Gale Group, Swets Blackwell, Kluwer Online, Factiva).
Indexed: ASSIA, Adol.Ment.Hlth.Abstr., Child Devel.Abstr., Environ.Sci.Poll.Mgmt., Fam.Ind., IMFL, Lang.& Lang.Behav.Abstr., Psyclnfo, Psychol.Abstr. (1984-), Risk Abstr., SOPODA, Saf.Sci.Abstr., Soc.Sci.Ind. (Jan.1994-), Soc.Serv.Abstr., Soc.Work Res.& Abstr., Sociol.Abstr., Stud.Wom.Abstr., e-psyche.
—BLDSC (3172.914000), GNLM, Infotrieve, ingenta. **CCC.**
Published by: Kluwer Academic - Plenum Publishers (Subsidiary of: Wolters Kluwer N.V.), 233 Spring St, New York, NY 10013-1578. TEL 212-620-8000, 800-221-9369, FAX 212-463-0742, services@wkap.nl, info@plenum.com, http://www.wkap.nl/journalhome.htm/0738-0151. Ed. Thomas K Kenemore. **Subscr. to:** Kluwer Academic Publishers Group, Journals Department, PO Box 322, Dordrecht 3300 AH, Netherlands. TEL 31-78-639-2392, FAX 31-78-654-6474.

305.8 GBR ISSN 1360-418X
COMPLEMENTARY CARE JOURNAL. Text in English. 1996. bi-m. **Document type:** *Consumer.* **Description:** Seeks to create a symposium for ideas and initiatives concerning social care, health and personal growth from an ethnic perspective.
Published by: Complementary Community Care Services Ltd., PO Box 7991, London SE15 3YB, United Kingdom. TEL 44-171-639-5226, FAX 44-171-732-5560. Ed. Phillip Makepeace.

CONNEXIONS. see *PSYCHOLOGY*

CONTEMPORARY FAMILY THERAPY; an international journal. see *PSYCHOLOGY*

CONTEMPORARY SEXUALITY; the international resource for educators, researchers and therapists. see *PSYCHOLOGY*

306 USA ISSN 1099-9809
RC455.4.E8 CODEN: CDEPFD
CULTURAL DIVERSITY & ETHNIC MINORITY PSYCHOLOGY. Text in English. 1995. q. USD 58 domestic to non-members; USD 73 foreign to non-members; USD 36 domestic to members; USD 46 foreign to members; USD 162 domestic to institutions; USD 194 foreign to institutions (2001). adv. back issues avail. *Refereed.* **Document type:** *Academic/Scholarly.* **Description:** For psychologists, social workers, psychiatrists, counselors and other mental health professionals. Explores the way age, ethnicity, gender, race, sexual orientation, socio-economic status, language, religion, and political and social ideology can have an impact on clinical assessment and the treatment process.
Formerly (until 1999): Cultural Diversity and Mental Health (1077-341X)
Related titles: Microform ed.: (from PQC).
Indexed: Agricola (coverage dropped), Curr.Cont. (coverage dropped), ERA, Educ.Ind., Ind.Med. (1999-), Mult.Ed.Abstr., Psyclnfo, SSCI (coverage dropped), Soc.Serv.Abstr., Sociol.Abstr., e-psyche.
—BLDSC (3491.662416), EMDOCS, GNLM, ingenta. **CCC.**
Published by: (American Psychological Association), John Wiley & Sons, Inc., Journals (Subsidiary of: Wiley InterScience), 750 First St, N E, Washington, DC 20002-4242. TEL 202-336-5600, FAX 202-336-5568, TELEX 12-7063, subinfo@jwiley.com, http://www.apa.org/journals/cdp.html. Eds. Gail E Wyatt, Lillian Comas Diaz. Adv. contact Jodi Ashcraft. B&W page GBP 175; trim 10 x 6.88. Circ: 1,200 (paid). **Subscr. outside the Americas to:** John Wiley & Sons Ltd., Baffins Ln, Chichester, Sussex PO19 IUD, United Kingdom. FAX 44-1243-776128.

CULTURE & PSYCHOLOGY. see *PSYCHOLOGY*

306.7 GBR ISSN 1369-1058
▼ **CULTURE, HEALTH AND SEXUALITY.** Text in English. 1999. q. GBP 71, USD 118 to individuals; GBP 164, USD 271 to institutions (effective 2002). *Refereed.* **Document type:** *Academic/Scholarly.* **Description:** Publishes scholarly papers in the fields of culture, health, human reproduction and sexuality.
Related titles: Online - full text ed.: ISSN 1464-5351 (from CatchWord Ltd., EBSCO Publishing, O C L C Online Computer Library Center, Inc., RoweCom Information Quest, Swets Blackwell).
Indexed: Addic.Abstr., Anthropol.Lit., Intl.Bibl.Soc.Sci.
—BLDSC (3491.669040), CatchWord.
Published by: (International Association for Study of Sexuality, Culture and Society), Taylor & Francis Group, Taylor & Francis Ltd., 11 New Fetter Ln, London EC4P 4EE, United Kingdom. TEL 44-20-7583-9855, FAX 44-20-7842-2298, info@tandf.co.uk, http://www.tandf.co.uk. Ed. Peter Aggleton. **Subscr. in N. America to:** Taylor & Francis Ltd., 325 Chestnut St, Suite 800, Philadelphia, PA 19016. TEL 800-354-1420, FAX 215-625-8914, info@taylorandfrancis.com, http://www.taylorandfrancis.com/.

CYBERPSYCHOLOGY & BEHAVIOR; the impact of the Internet, multi-media & virtual reality on behavior & society. see *COMPUTERS—Internet*

CZLOWIEK I SPOLECZENSTWO. see *EDUCATION*

D W D NEWSLETTER. see *GERONTOLOGY AND GERIATRICS*

305.42 BOL
DE TEXTOS. Text in Spanish. irreg., latest vol.10, 1985. price varies. **Document type:** *Monographic series, Academic/Scholarly.*
Published by: Centro de Investigaciones Sociales, Casilla 6931 - C.C., La Paz, Bolivia. TEL 591-2-352931. Ed. Antonio Cisneros.

▼ **DEATH & DYING SOURCEBOOK.** see *PHILOSOPHY*

DEATH STUDIES; education - counseling - care - law - ethics. see *PSYCHOLOGY*

301 CHE ISSN 0378-7931
HM291
DEVIANCE ET SOCIETE. Text in French; Abstracts in English, German. 1977. q. CHF 90, EUR 58.44 to individuals; CHF 160, EUR 103.89 to institutions (effective 2002). **Document type:** *Journal, Academic/Scholarly.*
Indexed: Abstr.Crim.& Pen., Crim.Just.Abstr., e-psyche.
—BLDSC (3579.099700). **CCC.**

S

Published by: Editions Medecine et Hygiene, Case Postale 456, Geneva, 4 1211, Switzerland. TEL 41-22-7029311, FAX 41-22-7029355, abonnements@medhyg.ch, http://www.medhyg.ch. Ed. Philippe Robert.

301 USA ISSN 0163-9625
HM1 CODEN: DEBEDF
DEVIANT BEHAVIOR. Text in English. 1979. bi-m. GBP 89, USD 147 to individuals; GBP 227, USD 375 to institutions (effective 2002). adv. bk.rev. bibl, charts, illus. index. back issues avail.; reprint service avail. from PQC,PSC,SCH. *Refereed.* **Document type:** *Academic/Scholarly.* **Description:** Presents scientific findings on cultural norm violations from a wide variety of perspectives.
Related titles: Microfiche ed.: (from PQC); Online - full text ed.: ISSN 1521-0456 (from CatchWord Ltd., EBSCO Publishing, O C L C Online Computer Library Center, Inc., RoweCom Information Quest, Swets Blackwell, Institute for Scientific Information).
Indexed: ASCA, Abstr.Anthropol., Abstr.Crim.& Pen., Arts & Hum.Cit.Ind. (coverage dropped), Biol.Abstr., Chic.Per.Ind., Crim.Just.Abstr., Curr.Cont., Educ.Admin.Abstr., Environ.Sci.Poll.Mgmt., Fam.Ind., Lang.& Lang.Behav.Abstr., Peace Res.Abstr., PsycInfo, Psychol.Abstr. (1981-), Risk Abstr., Russ.Acad.Sci.Bibl., SOPODA, SSCI, Saf.Sci.Abstr., Sage Fam.Stud.Abstr., Sage Urb.Stud.Abstr., Soc.Serv.Abstr., Sociol.Abstr., Viol.& Abuse Abstr., e-psyche.
—BLDSC (3579.099900), CatchWord, CISTI, IDS, ingenta. **CCC.**
Published by: Taylor & Francis Ltd. (Subsidiary of: Taylor & Francis Group), 325 Chestnut St, Suite 800, Philadelphia, PA 19016. TEL 215-625-8900, FAX 215-625-2940, info@taylorandfrancis.com, http://www.taylorandfrancis.com/. Ed. Craig J Forsyth. Circ: 300. **Subscr. addr. in Europe:** Taylor & Francis Group, Journals Customer Service, Rankine Rd, Basingstoke, Hants RG24 8PR, United Kingdom. TEL 44-1256-813000, FAX 44-1256-479438, enquiry@tanf.co.uk, http://www.tandf.co.uk/journals.

DISCOURSE & SOCIETY; an international journal for the study of discourse and communication in their social, political and cultural contexts. see *PSYCHOLOGY*

DOCTOR - PATIENT STUDIES. see *MEDICAL SCIENCES*

▼ **DOMESTIC VIOLENCE AND CHILD ABUSE SOURCEBOOK.** see *CRIMINOLOGY AND LAW ENFORCEMENT*

155.91 USA ISSN 0013-9165
HM206 CODEN: EVBHAF
ENVIRONMENT AND BEHAVIOR. Text in English. 1969. bi-m. USD 90 to individuals; USD 425 to institutions; USD 25 newsstand/cover to individuals; USD 75 newsstand/cover to institutions (effective 2002). adv. bk.rev. abstr, charts, illus. index. back issues avail.; reprint service avail. from PQC,PSC,SCH. *Refereed.* **Document type:** *Academic/Scholarly.* **Description:** Discusses the interaction of the physical environment and human behavioral systems and covers the study, design, and control of the physical environment. Analyses and records the influence of environment on individuals, groups and institutions.
Related titles: Microfilm ed.: (from PQC); Online - full text ed.: (from EBSCO Publishing, O C L C Online Computer Library Center, Inc., RoweCom Information Quest, ProQuest Information & Learning, Gale Group, ingenta, Swets Blackwell, Institute for Scientific Information).
Indexed: ASCA, ASSIA, AgeLine, Amer.Bibl.Slavic & E.Eur.Stud., Aqua.Sci.& Fish.Abstr., Art.Hosp.& Tour., Arts & Hum.Cit.Ind. (coverage dropped), Avery Ind.Archit.Per., C.I.J.E. (coverage dropped), Crim.Just.Abstr., Curr.Adv.Ecol.Sci., Curr.Cont., Curr.Cont.M.E., Curr.Ind.Stat., Diar.Dis.Res., E.I., Energy Rev., Environ.Abstr., Environ.Per.Bibl. (1972-), Environ.Sci.Poll.Mgmt., Excerp.Med., Geo.Abstr.H.G., GeoRef, HRIS, Human Resour.Abstr., IBR, IBZ, IDA, INIS Atomind., Intl.Bibl.Soc.Sci., Lang.& Lang.Behav.Abstr., Mag.Ind., Mar.Aff.Bibl., P C I, Peace Res.Abstr., Pollut.Abstr., PsycInfo, Psychol.Abstr. (1969-), Psycscan A.P., Res.High.Educ.Abstr., Risk Abstr., SOPODA, SSCI, Sage Fam.Stud.Abstr., Sage Urb.Stud.Abstr., Sel.Water Res.Abstr., Soc.Sci.Ind. (Jan.1983-), Soc.Serv.Abstr., Sociol.Abstr., Stud.Wom.Abstr., Wild.Rev., e-psyche.
—BLDSC (3791.097000), CISTI, IDS, ingenta. **CCC.**
Published by: (Environmental Design Research Association), Sage Publications, Inc., 2455 Teller Rd, Thousand Oaks, CA 91320. TEL 805-499-0721, FAX 805-499-0871, info@sagepub.com, http://www.sagepub.com. Ed. Robert B Bechtel. Pub. Sara Miller McCune. R&P Tanya Udin. Adv. contact DeAnna Vega Hammersley. Circ: 1,500. **Overseas subscr. to:** Sage Publications Ltd., 6 Bonhill St, London EC2A 4PU, United Kingdom; Sage Publications India Pvt. Ltd., 4215, New Delhi 110 048, India.

ETHNOPSYCHOANALYSE. see *PSYCHOLOGY*

EUROPEAN JOURNAL OF SOCIAL PSYCHOLOGY. see *PSYCHOLOGY*

FAMILIENDYNAMIK; interdisziplinaere Zeitschrift fuer systemorientierte Praxis und Forschung. see *PSYCHOLOGY*

FAMILY PROCESS. see *PSYCHOLOGY*

FAMILY THERAPY NEWS. see *PSYCHOLOGY*

▼ **GENES, BRAIN AND BEHAVIOR.** see *BIOLOGY—Genetics*

GRUPPENDYNAMIK UND ORGANISATIONSBERATUNG; Zeitschrift fuer angewandte Sozialpsychologie. see *PSYCHOLOGY*

GUILFORD FAMILY THERAPY SERIES. see *PSYCHOLOGY*

306 CHE ISSN 0891-7795
HEALTH, SOCIETY AND CULTURE. Text in English. 1987. irreg., latest vol.2. price varies. *Refereed.* **Document type:** *Monographic series.*
Indexed: Avery Ind.Archit.Per.
—CISTI.
Published by: Gordon and Breach - Harwood Academic (Subsidiary of: Taylor & Francis Group), PO Box 531, Lausanne 1000, Switzerland. Ed. H A Baer. **Subscr. addr. in US:** International Publishers Direct, PO Box 32160, Newark, NJ 07102. FAX 215-750-6343.

HUMAN NATURE; an interdisciplinary biosocial perspective. see *SOCIAL SCIENCES: COMPREHENSIVE WORKS*

HUMAN STRESS: CURRENT SELECTED RESEARCH. see *PSYCHOLOGY*

306.481 DEU ISSN 0933-1719
PN6149.P5 CODEN: HUMRES
HUMOR; international journal of humor research. Text in English. 1988. q. EUR 153.10 domestic; EUR 156.20 foreign; EUR 37 newsstand/cover (effective 2002). adv. bk.rev. illus. Index. back issues avail.; reprint service avail. from PSC,SCH. *Refereed.* **Document type:** *Journal, Academic/Scholarly.* **Description:** Scholarly journal for the publication of research papers on humor as an important and universal human faculty.
Former titles: World Humor and Irony Movement Serials Yearbook; World Humor and Irony Membership Serial Yearbook; Western Humor and Irony Membership Serial Yearbook (0737-0342)
Related titles: Online - full text ed.: (from Institute for Scientific Information).
Indexed: AgeLine, Arts & Hum.Cit.Ind., Bibl.Ling., Curr.Cont., IBZ, Ind.Philos., Intl.Bibl.Soc.Sci., Lang.& Lang.Behav.Abstr., MLA Intl.Bibl., PsycInfo, Psychol.Abstr. (1988-), SOPODA, SSCI, Sociol.Abstr., e-psyche.
—BLDSC (4336.730500), IDS, Infotrieve, ingenta. **CCC.**
Published by: Walter de Gruyter und Co., Mouton de Gruyter, Genthiner Str 13, Berlin 10785, Germany. TEL 49-30-26005-0, FAX 49-30-26005-251, wdg-info@degruyter.de, http://www.degruyter.de. Ed. Lawrence E Mintz. adv.: page DEM 500; trim 115 x 190. **U.S. subscr. to:** Walter de Gruyter Inc., 200 Saw Mill River Rd, Hawthorne, NY 10532. TEL 914-747-0110.

301 USA ISSN 1054-1373
R726.8
ILLNESS, CRISIS, AND LOSS. Text in English. 1991. q. USD 55 to individuals; USD 250 to institutions; USD 20 newsstand/cover to individuals; USD 65 newsstand/cover to institutions (effective 2002). **Description:** Based on the premise that research in the fields of life-threatening illness and thanatology will be advanced by bringing together the expertise of professionals in sociology, social work, nursing, and counseling.
Related titles: Online - full text ed.: (from EBSCO Publishing, O C L C Online Computer Library Center, Inc., RoweCom Information Quest, ingenta, Swets Blackwell).
Indexed: Abstr.Soc.Geront., IBZ, Soc.Serv.Abstr., Sociol.Abstr., Viol.& Abuse Abstr.
—BLDSC (4365.910000), Infotrieve. **CCC.**
Published by: Sage Publications, Inc., 2455 Teller Rd, Thousand Oaks, CA 91320. TEL 805-499-0721, FAX 805-499-0871, info@sagepub.com, http://www.sagepub.com. Ed. Robert Bendiksen. R&P Tanya Udin. Adv. contact DeAnna Vega Hammersley. **Foreign subscr. to:** Sage Publications Ltd., 6 Bonhill St, London EC2A 4PU, United Kingdom; **Subscr. to:** Sage Publications India Pvt. Ltd., 4215, New Delhi 110 048, India.

INSIDE M S. (Multiple Sclerosis) see *MEDICAL SCIENCES—Psychiatry And Neurology*

INTERNATIONAL ASSOCIATION FOR CROSS-CULTURAL PSYCHOLOGY. INTERNATIONAL CONFERENCE. SELECTED PAPERS. see *PSYCHOLOGY*

THE INTERNATIONAL JOURNAL OF ACTION METHODS; psychodrama, skill training and role playing. see *PSYCHOLOGY*

INTERNATIONAL JOURNAL OF BEHAVIORAL MEDICINE. see *PSYCHOLOGY*

INTERNATIONAL JOURNAL OF BEHAVIOURAL SCIENCES. see *PSYCHOLOGY*

INTERNATIONAL JOURNAL OF BIOSOCIAL AND MEDICAL RESEARCH; bridging the gap between the natural and social sciences to better understand human behavior. see *NUTRITION AND DIETETICS*

INTERNATIONAL JOURNAL OF GROUP TENSIONS; an interdisciplinary quarterly of behavioral sciences devoted to the study of conflict and violence in human relationships. see *PSYCHOLOGY*

JOURNAL OF AGING & SOCIAL POLICY; a journal devoted to aging & social policy. see *GERONTOLOGY AND GERIATRICS*

JOURNAL OF APPLIED BEHAVIORAL SCIENCE. see *PSYCHOLOGY*

JOURNAL OF APPLIED HEALTH BEHAVIOUR. see *PSYCHOLOGY*

▼ **JOURNAL OF APPLIED PSYCHOANALYTIC STUDIES.** see *PSYCHOLOGY*

156 GBR ISSN 0021-9320
HQ750.A1 CODEN: JBSLAR
JOURNAL OF BIOSOCIAL SCIENCE. Text in English. 1969. q. GBP 178 to institutions (effective 2002). adv. bk.rev. index, cum.index: 1969-1978. back issues avail. *Refereed.* **Document type:** *Academic/Scholarly.* **Description:** Contains material dealing with the common ground between biology and sociology, including reproduction and its control, gerontology, ecology, genetics, applied psychology, sociology, education, criminology, demography, health and epidemiology.
Related titles: Online - full text ed.: (from EBSCO Publishing, O C L C Online Computer Library Center, Inc., RoweCom Information Quest, Swets Blackwell, Institute for Scientific Information); Supplement: ISSN 0300-9645. 1969.
Indexed: A.I.C.P. (1969-), ASCA, Abstr.Anthropol., Abstr.Hyg., Adol.Ment.Hlth.Abstr., AgeLine, Anthropol.Lit. (coverage dropped), Arts & Hum.Cit.Ind. (coverage dropped), Bibl.Asian Stud. (1970, 1974-1991), Biol.Abstr., Brit.Nur.Ind., Curr.Cont., Curr.Lit.Fam.Plan., Dent.Ind., Diar.Dis.Res., Excerp.Med., Fam.Ind., IDA, Ind.Med. (1969-), Ind.Sci.Rev., Intl.Bibl.Soc.Sci., Lang.& Lang.Behav.Abstr., Mid.East: Abstr.& Ind., Mult.Ed.Abstr., Nutr.Abstr., P C I, Popul.Ind., PsycInfo, Psychol.Abstr. (1976-), Rural Recreat.Tour.Abstr., SOPODA, SSCI, Sci.Cit.Ind. (coverage dropped), Soc.Serv.Abstr., Sociol.Abstr., Stud.Wom.Abstr., THA, Trop.Dis.Bull., World Ag.Econ.& Rur.Soc.Abstr., e-psyche.
—BLDSC (4954.100000), GNLM, Infotrieve, ingenta, KNAW. **CCC.**

S

Published by: Cambridge University Press, Edinburgh Bldg, Shaftesbury Rd, Cambridge CB2 2RU, United Kingdom. FAX 44-1223-315052, information@cup.cam.ac.uk, information@cambridge.org, http://www.cup.cam.ac.uk, http://www.uk.cambridge.org/journals/pmu. Ed. C G N Mascie Taylor. R&P Linda Nicol. Adv. contact Rebecca Symons. Circ: 600.

302.23 USA ISSN 0196-8599
P87
JOURNAL OF COMMUNICATION INQUIRY. Text in English. 1974. q. USD 45 to individuals; USD 150 to institutions; USD 20 newsstand/cover to individuals; USD 50 newsstand/cover to institutions (effective 2002). adv. bk.rev. illus. back issues avail.; reprints avail. *Refereed.* **Document type:** *Academic/Scholarly.* **Description:** Emphasizes interdisciplinary inquiry into communication and mass communication phenomena within cultural and historical perspectives.
Related titles: Online - full text ed.: (from EBSCO Publishing, O C L C Online Computer Library Center, Inc., RoweCom Information Quest, Gale Group, ingenta, Swets Blackwell, Factiva).
Indexed: Amer.Hist.& Life, Commun.Abstr., ERA, Film Lit.Ind., Hist.Abstr. (1986-), Hum.Ind. (Jan.2000-), IBZ, Lang.& Lang.Behav.Abstr., MLA Intl.Bibl., Peace Res.Abstr., SOPODA, Sage Pub.Admin.Abstr., Soc.Serv.Abstr., Sociol.Abstr., Stud.Wom.Abstr.
—BLDSC (4961.620000), Infotrieve, ingenta. **CCC.**
Published by: Sage Publications, Inc., 2455 Teller Rd, Thousand Oaks, CA 91320. TEL 805-499-0721, FAX 805-499-0871, info@sagepub.com, http://www.uiowa.edu./~journal/misc/ices.html. Ed. Matthew Cecil. R&P Tanya Udin. Adv. contact DeAnna Vega Hammersley. Circ: 1,000 (paid).

JOURNAL OF COMMUNITY AND APPLIED SOCIAL PSYCHOLOGY. see *PSYCHOLOGY*

JOURNAL OF COMMUNITY PSYCHOLOGY. see *PSYCHOLOGY*

JOURNAL OF CROSS-CULTURAL PSYCHOLOGY. see *PSYCHOLOGY*

JOURNAL OF CULTURAL DIVERSITY; an interdisciplinary journal. see *MEDICAL SCIENCES—Nurses And Nursing*

JOURNAL OF EARLY ADOLESCENCE. see *CHILDREN AND YOUTH—About*

JOURNAL OF EXPERIMENTAL SOCIAL PSYCHOLOGY. see *PSYCHOLOGY*

JOURNAL OF FAMILY THERAPY. see *MEDICAL SCIENCES—Psychiatry And Neurology*

JOURNAL OF FAMILY VIOLENCE. see *CRIMINOLOGY AND LAW ENFORCEMENT*

JOURNAL OF FLUENCY DISORDERS. see *PSYCHOLOGY*

▼ **JOURNAL OF HAPPINESS STUDIES**; an interdisciplinary forum on subjective well-being. see *PSYCHOLOGY*

302 USA ISSN 0022-1465
R11 CODEN: JHSBA5
JOURNAL OF HEALTH AND SOCIAL BEHAVIOR. Text in English. 1960. q. USD 60 domestic to individuals non-members; USD 80 foreign to individuals non-members; USD 120 domestic to institutions non-members; USD 140 foreign to institutions non-members; USD 30 domestic to members; USD 50 foreign to members (effective 2001). adv. bk.rev. charts, illus. index. back issues avail.; reprint service avail. from PQC. *Refereed.* **Document type:** *Journal, Academic/Scholarly.* **Description:** Publishes reports of empirical studies, theoretical analyses, and synthesizing reviews that employ a sociological perspective to clarify aspects of social life bearing on human health and illness, both physical and mental.
Formerly (until 1967): Journal of Health and Human Behavior (0095-9006)
Related titles: Microform ed.: (from MIM,PQC); Online - full text ed.: (from ProQuest Information & Learning, JSTOR (Web-based Journal Archive), Gale Group, Factiva, Institute for Scientific Information).
Indexed: ASCA, ASSIA, Abstr.Anthropol., Addic.Abstr., AgeLine, Biol.Abstr., Brit.Nur.Ind., Crim.Just.Abstr., Curr.Cont., ERA, Environ.Sci.Poll.Mgmt., Excerp.Med., IBZ, Ind.Med. (1967-), Int.Nurs.Ind., Lang.& Lang.Behav.Abstr., Mult.Ed.Abstr., P C I, PsycInfo, Psychol.Abstr. (1960-), Risk Abstr., Russ.Acad.Sci.Bibl., SOPODA, SSCI, Saf.Sci.Abstr., Sage Race Rel.Abstr., Soc.Sci.Ind. (Mar.1982-), Soc.Serv.Abstr., Soc.Work Res.& Abstr., Sociol.Abstr. (1961-), Sp.Ed.Needs Abstr.
—BLDSC (4996.730000), CISTI, GNLM, IDS, ingenta.
Published by: American Sociological Association, 1307 New York Ave, N W, Ste 700, Washington, DC 20005-4701. publications@asanet.org, http://www.asanet.org, http://www.lemoyne.edu. Ed. Michael Hughes. Adv. contact India L Winstead. Circ: 4,300 (paid).

JOURNAL OF HOMOSEXUALITY. see *HOMOSEXUALITY*

JOURNAL OF INTERPERSONAL VIOLENCE; concerned with the study and treatment of victims and perpetrators of physical and sexual violence. see *CRIMINOLOGY AND LAW ENFORCEMENT*

JOURNAL OF LANGUAGE AND SOCIAL PSYCHOLOGY. see *PSYCHOLOGY*

JOURNAL OF MARITAL AND FAMILY THERAPY. see *PSYCHOLOGY*

302 USA ISSN 1529-3041
▼ **JOURNAL OF MUNDANE BEHAVIOR.** Text in English. 2000. irreg. (2-4/yr). free. bk.rev. illus. back issues avail. *Refereed.* **Document type:** *Journal, Academic/Scholarly.* **Description:** Explores and examines the "unmarked," those aspects, behaviors, and rituals of our everyday lives that typically go unnoticed. Poses the question what is mundane and what is unusual, and what makes them so.
Media: Online - full content.
Published by: California State University, Fullerton, Department of Sociology, PO Box 6846, Fullerton, CA 92834-6846. TEL 714-278-3531, FAX 714-278-2001, sschaffer@fullerton.edu, http://www.mundanebehavior.org, http://hss.fullerton.edu/sociology. Ed. Myron Orleans.

JOURNAL OF ORGANIZATIONAL BEHAVIOUR. see *PSYCHOLOGY*

THE JOURNAL OF RURAL HEALTH. see *MEDICAL SCIENCES*

JOURNAL OF SEX RESEARCH. see *PSYCHOLOGY*

JOURNAL OF SOCIAL DISTRESS AND THE HOMELESS. see *SOCIAL SERVICES AND WELFARE*

JOURNAL OF SOCIAL ISSUES. see *PSYCHOLOGY*

306.7 USA ISSN 1043-4070
HQ12 CODEN: JHSEEI
JOURNAL OF THE HISTORY OF SEXUALITY. Text in English. 1990. q. USD 41 domestic to individuals; USD 55 in Canada & Mexico to individuals; USD 63 rest of world to individuals; USD 125 domestic to institutions; USD 139 in Canada & Mexico to institutions; USD 147 rest of world to institutions (effective 2001 - 2002). adv. bk.rev. illus. reprints avail. *Refereed.* **Document type:** *Academic/Scholarly.* **Description:** Examines the history of sexuality in all its expressions, recognizing differences of class, culture, gender, race, and sexual orientation. Provides a forum for historical, critical and theoretical research in the field. Presents original articles and critical reviews from historians and social scientists worldwide.
Related titles: Online - full text ed.: (from Gale Group, Swets Blackwell, Institute for Scientific Information, RoweCom Information Quest).
Indexed: ASCA, AgeLine, Amer.Bibl.Slavic & E.Eur.Stud., Amer.Hist.& Life, Arts & Hum.Cit.Ind., BHA, Crim.Just.Abstr., Curr.Cont., Fam.Ind., Hist.Abstr. (1990-), Hum.Ind. (Jun.1995-), Int.Polit.Sci.Abstr., Intl.Bibl.Soc.Sci., Lang.& Lang.Behav.Abstr., MLA Intl.Bibl., Rel.Ind.One, Rel.Ind.Two, Russ.Acad.Sci.Bibl., SOPODA, SSCI, Sage Race Rel.Abstr., Soc.Serv.Abstr., Sociol.Abstr., Stud.Wom.Abstr., e-psyche.
—BLDSC (5002.050000), GNLM, IDS, Infotrieve, ingenta. **CCC.**
Published by: University of Texas Press, PO Box 7819, Austin, TX 78713-7819. TEL 512-471-4531, FAX 512-232-7178, utpress@uts.cc.utexas.edu, http://www.utexas.edu/utpress/. Eds. Barbara Loomis, Williams Bonds. R&P Juli Martin TEL 512-471-4531. Adv. contact Leah Dixon. page USD 320; trim 9 x 6.

JOURNAL OF YOUTH STUDIES. see *CHILDREN AND YOUTH—About*

302 DEU ISSN 0023-2653
HM5
KOELNER ZEITSCHRIFT FUER SOZIOLOGIE UND SOZIALPSYCHOLOGIE. Text in German. 1927. 4/yr. DEM 207 domestic; DEM 217 foreign; DEM 136 to students (effective 2001). adv. bk.rev. charts, illus. index, cum.index. reprint service avail. from SCH,PSC. *Refereed.* **Document type:** *Journal, Academic/Scholarly.*
Related titles: Online - full text ed.: (from Institute for Scientific Information).
Indexed: Abstr.Crim.& Pen., Curr.Cont., Curr.Ind.Stat., Ger.J.Psych., IBR, IBZ, INIS Atomind., Ind.Philos., Int.Polit.Sci.Abstr., Intl.Bibl.Soc.Sci., Lang.& Lang.Behav.Abstr., P.A.I.S., Phil.Ind., PsycInfo, Psychol.Abstr. (1948-), RILM, Russ.Acad.Sci.Bibl., SOPODA, SSCI, Soc.Serv.Abstr., Sociol.Abstr. (1952-53), e-psyche.
—BLDSC (5104.500000), IDS. **CCC.**
Published by: Westdeutscher Verlag GmbH (Wiesbaden) (Subsidiary of: BertelsmannSpringer), Postfach 1546, Wiesbaden 65173, Germany. TEL 49-611-7878151, FAX 49-611-7878423. Circ: 2,200.

THE LEADERSHIP QUARTERLY; an international journal of political, social and behavioral science. see *BUSINESS AND ECONOMICS—Management*

LESBIAN AND GAY COUNSELLING NEWS. see *HOMOSEXUALITY*

MATERIALIEN AUS DER BILDUNGSFORSCHUNG. see *EDUCATION*

▼ **MEDIA PSYCHOLOGY.** see *PSYCHOLOGY*

MEDIENPSYCHOLOGIE; Zeitschrift fuer Individual- und Massenkommunikation. see *PSYCHOLOGY*

302 150 ISR ISSN 0025-8679
HQ768
MEGAMOT; behavioural sciences journal. Text in Hebrew; Summaries in English. 1949. q. USD 45; ILS 160 to individuals; ILS 180 to institutions (effective 2001). adv. bk.rev. abstr, bibl, charts, illus, stat. cum.index. 150 p./no. 1 cols./p. back issues avail. *Refereed.* **Document type:** *Journal, Academic/Scholarly.*
Formerly: Child Welfare Research Quarterly
Indexed: Ind.Heb.Per. (1977-2000), Intl.Bibl.Soc.Sci., PsycInfo, Psychol.Abstr. (1985-), SSCI (coverage dropped), e-psyche.
Published by: Henrietta Szold Institute, Kiryat Menachem, 9 Columbia St, Jerusalem 96583, Israel. FAX 972-2-6437698, szold@szold.org.il, megamot@szold,org.il, http://www.szold.org.il. Ed. Y Yinon. adv.: page USD 80. Circ: 700 (paid).

MENTAL HEALTH, RELIGION & CULTURE. see *PSYCHOLOGY*

NEW DOCTOR. see *MEDICAL SCIENCES*

▼ **NORTH AMERICAN JOURNAL OF PSYCHOLOGY.** see *PSYCHOLOGY*

NOUVELLE REVUE D'ETHNOPSYCHIATRIE. see *MEDICAL SCIENCES—Psychiatry And Neurology*

OMEGA: JOURNAL OF DEATH AND DYING. see *PSYCHOLOGY*

306.77 NLD ISSN 0167-5907
PAIDIKA; the journal of paedophilia. Text in English. 1987. 2/yr. NLG 95, USD 57 to individuals; USD 110 to libraries. adv. bk.rev. illus. Index. back issues avail.; reprints avail. **Document type:** *Academic/Scholarly.* **Description:** Documents opposing viewpoints concerning paedophilia.
Indexed: e-psyche.
Published by: Stichting Paidika Foundation, Postbus 15463, Amsterdam 1001 ML, Netherlands. Ed. Joseph Geraci. Circ: 1,000.

PERSPECTIVES ON DEATH AND DYING SERIES. see *PSYCHOLOGY*

▼ **PLENUM SERIES ON HUMAN EXCEPTIONALITY.** see *PSYCHOLOGY*

PRO FAMILIA MAGAZIN; die Zeitschrift fuer Sexualpaedagogik, Sexualberatung und Familienplanung. see *PSYCHOLOGY*

S

306 POL ISSN 0552-2234
PROBLEMY RODZINY. Text in Polish; Summaries in English. 1961. bi-m. PLZ 60; PLZ 10 newsstand/cover (effective 2000). adv. bk.rev. abstr, bibl, stat. **Document type:** *Academic/Scholarly.* **Description:** Provides reports on scientific studies on marriages and family conducted in Poland or abroad. The marital and family problems are studied in the aspects of demography, health, economy, social policy, sociology, psychology, law, history, culture, religion, customs and medicine mainly sexology, contraception, obstetrics, pediatrics.
Indexed: Russ.Acad.Sci.Bibl.
Published by: Towarzystwo Rozwoju Rodziny, Zarzad Glowny, c/o Problemy Rodziny, Redakcja, Ul Schillera 4-35, Warsaw 00248, Poland. TEL 48-22-8319310. Ed. Zofia Dabrowska Caban. Circ: 1,200 (controlled).

PSYCHOLOGY AND SOCIOLOGY OF SPORT: CURRENT SELECTED RESEARCH. see *PSYCHOLOGY*

RELACIONES. see *PSYCHOLOGY*

REPRESENTATIVE RESEARCH IN SOCIAL PSYCHOLOGY. see *PSYCHOLOGY*

RESEARCH AND PRACTICE. see *MEDICAL SCIENCES—Psychiatry And Neurology*

RESEARCH IN THE SOCIOLOGY OF HEALTH CARE. see *MEDICAL SCIENCES*

361.3 USA ISSN 1049-7315
HV1 CODEN: RSWPEW
RESEARCH ON SOCIAL WORK PRACTICE. Text in English. 1990. bi-m. USD 80 to individuals; USD 325 to institutions; USD 20 newsstand/cover to individuals; USD 60 newsstand/cover to institutions (effective 2002). adv. bk.rev. abstr, illus. Index. back issues avail.; reprint service avail. from PSC,SCH. *Refereed.* **Document type:** *Journal, Academic/Scholarly.* **Description:** Devoted to the publication of empirical research concerning the methods and outcomes of social work practice. It carries regular features that include new methods of assessment, scholarly reviews, invited essays and book reviews.
Related titles: Online - full text ed.: (from EBSCO Publishing, O C L C Online Computer Library Center, Inc., RoweCom Information Quest, ProQuest Information & Learning, Gale Group, ingenta, Swets Blackwell, Institute for Scientific Information).
Indexed: ASCA, ASSIA, Abstr.Soc.Geront., AgeLine, Brit.Nur.Ind., C.I.J.E. (coverage dropped), Crim.Just.Abstr., Curr.Cont., Fam.Ind., Human Resour.Abstr., Lang.& Lang.Behav.Abstr., Peace Res.Abstr., PsycInfo, Psychol.Abstr. (1991-), SOPODA, SSCI, Sage Pub.Admin.Abstr., Sage Urb.Stud.Abstr., Soc.Sci.Ind. (Jul.1999-), Soc.Serv.Abstr., Soc.Work Res.& Abstr., Sociol.Abstr., Viol.& Abuse Abstr., e-psyche.
—BLDSC (7770.680000), IDS, ingenta. **CCC.**
Published by: Sage Publications, Inc., 2455 Teller Rd, Thousand Oaks, CA 91320. TEL 805-499-0721, FAX 805-499-0871, info@sagepub.com, http://www.sagepub.com. Ed. Bruce A Thyer. Pub. Sara Miller McCune. R&P Tanya Udin. Adv. contact DeAnna Vega Hammersley. page GBP 195; trim 193 x 119. Circ: 1,200. **Overseas subscr. to:** Sage Publications Ltd., 6 Bonhill St, London EC2A 4PU, United Kingdom. TEL 44-20-7374-0645, FAX 44-20-7374-8741; Sage Publications India Pvt. Ltd., 4215, New Delhi 110 048, India. TEL 91-11-641-9884, FAX 91-11-647-2426.

306.7 USA ISSN 0091-3995
HQ1
S I E C U S REPORT. Text in English. 1972. bi-m. USD 75. adv. bk.rev., film rev. bibl, illus. Index. back issues avail.; reprint service avail. from PQC,ISI. **Document type:** *Academic/Scholarly.* **Description:** Covers all aspects of human sexuality, including AIDS.
Formerly: S I E C U S Newsletter (0036-150X)
Related titles: Microfilm ed.; Online - full text ed.: (from ProQuest Information & Learning, Gale Group, Factiva).
Indexed: CWI, Curr.Lit.Fam.Plan., Educ.Ind. (Jan.1984-), IMFL, Media Rev.Dig. (Jan.1989-).
—BLDSC (8271.970000), ingenta.
Published by: Sexuality Information and Education Council of the U S, 130 W 42nd St, Ste 350, New York, NY 10036. TEL 212-819-9770, FAX 212-819-9776, siecus@siecus.org, http://www.siecus.org/pubs/srpt.html. Ed., R&P Mac Edwards. Circ: 3,500.

303.6 USA
SAGE SERIES ON VIOLENCE AGAINST WOMEN. Text in English. m. USD 417 (effective 2000). back issues avail. **Document type:** *Monographic series.* **Description:** Examines the legal, sociological, and psychological aspects of domestic violence against women.
Published by: Sage Publications, Inc., 2455 Teller Rd, Thousand Oaks, CA 91320. TEL 805-499-0721, FAX 805-499-0871, info@sagepub.com, http://www.sagepub.com. Ed. Claire M Renzetti. Pub. Sara Miller McCune. R&P Tanya Udin. Adv. contact DeAnna Vega Hammersley. **Overseas subscr. to:** Sage Publications Ltd., 6 Bonhill St, London EC2A 4PU, United Kingdom; Sage Publications India Pvt. Ltd., 4215, New Delhi 110 048, India.

SEX ROLES. see *PSYCHOLOGY*

SEXUAL ABUSE; a journal of research and treatment. see *PSYCHOLOGY*

SEXUAL SCIENCE. see *PSYCHOLOGY*

SEXUALITIES; studies in culture and society. see *PSYCHOLOGY*

SMALL GROUP RESEARCH; an international journal of theory, investigation and application. see *PSYCHOLOGY*

SOCIAL BEHAVIOR AND PERSONALITY; an international journal. see *PSYCHOLOGY*

SOCIAL PSYCHOLOGICAL APPLICATIONS TO SOCIAL ISSUES. see *PSYCHOLOGY*

302 USA ISSN 0190-2725
HM1
SOCIAL PSYCHOLOGY QUARTERLY. Text in English. 1937. q. USD 50 domestic to individuals; USD 65 foreign to individuals; USD 95 domestic to institutions; USD 110 foreign to institutions; USD 30 domestic to members; USD 50 foreign to members (effective 2001). adv. bibl, illus. index. back issues avail.; reprint service avail. from PQC,PSC,SCH. *Refereed.* **Document type:** *Academic/Scholarly.* **Description:** Publishes papers pertaining to the processes and products of social interaction. Includes the study of the primary relations of individuals to one another or to groups, collectives, or institutions, and the study of intra-individual processes insofar as they substantially influence, or are influenced by, social forces.
Former titles (until 1978): Social Psychology (0147-829X); (until 1977): Sociometry (0038-0431)
Related titles: Microform ed.: (from MIM,PQC); Online - full text ed.: (from JSTOR (Web-based Journal Archive), ProQuest Information & Learning, Gale Group, Factiva, Institute for Scientific Information).
Indexed: ASCA, ASSIA, Adol.Ment.Hlth.Abstr., AgeLine, Amer.Bibl.Slavic & E.Eur.Stud., Crim.Just.Abstr., Curr.Cont., ERA, Educ.Admin.Abstr., Environ.Sci.Poll.Mgmt., IMFL, Ind.Philos., Int.Polit.Sci.Abstr., Lang.& Lang.Behav.Abstr., M.L.A., MLA Intl.Bibl., Mid.East: Abstr.& Ind., P C I, PsycInfo, Psychol.Abstr. (1937-), Risk Abstr., Russ.Acad.Sci.Bibl., SOPODA, SSCI, Saf.Sci.Abstr., Sage Race Rel.Abstr., Soc.Sci.Ind. (Jun.1982-), Soc.Serv.Abstr., Sociol.Abstr. (1953-), Stud.Wom.Abstr., e-psyche.
—BLDSC (8318.146300), IDS, ingenta.
Published by: American Sociological Association, 1307 New York Ave, N W, Ste 700, Washington, DC 20005-4701. TEL 202-383-9005, FAX 202-638-0882, publications@asanet.org, http://www.asanet.org/Pubs/spqinfo.htm, http://www.lemoyne.edu. Ed. Cecelia Ridgeway. Circ: 5,000.

155.82 DEU ISSN 0038-0377
HM3
SOCIOLOGUS; Zeitschrift fuer empirische Ethnosoziologie und Ethnopsychologie. Text in English, German. 1951. s-a. EUR 72; EUR 57.60 to students; EUR 40 newsstand/cover (effective 2002). bk.rev. abstr, illus. index. reprint service avail. from PSC,SCH. **Document type:** *Journal, Academic/Scholarly.*
Indexed: A.I.C.P. (1925-1933, 1951-), Anthropol.Lit., Bibl.Asian Stud. (1970-1991), Bibl.Ling., Cott.& Trop.Fibr.Abstr., E.I., IBR, IBZ, Ind.Philos., Int.Polit.Sci.Abstr., Intl.Bibl.Soc.Sci., P C I, P.A.I.S., Rural Devel.Abstr., Russ.Acad.Sci.Bibl., World Ag.Econ.& Rur.Soc.Abstr.
—BLDSC (8319.660000), ingenta. **CCC.**
Published by: Duncker und Humblot GmbH, Postfach 410329, Berlin 12113, Germany. TEL 49-30-790006-0, FAX 49-30-79000631, info@duncker-humblot.de, http://www.duncker-humblot.de.

301 GBR ISSN 0141-9889
RA418
SOCIOLOGY OF HEALTH AND ILLNESS; a journal of medical sociology. Text in English. 1979. bi-m. (plus a. monograph). GBP 247 to institutions in UK & Europe; USD 477 to institutions in the Americas & Caribbean; GBP 331 elsewhere to institutions (effective 2002). adv. bk.rev. illus. index. reprints avail. *Refereed.* **Document type:** *Academic/Scholarly.* **Description:** An international journal which publishes sociological articles on all aspects of health, illness and medicine, focusing on empirical research of a qualitative kind. Provides a sociological perspective on the theory of medical knowledge, the practice of medical work, and the experience of receiving or giving medical care.
Incorporates (in 1999): Sociology of Health and Illness Monograph Series
Related titles: Microform ed.; Online - full text ed.: (from EBSCO Publishing, O C L C Online Computer Library Center, Inc., RoweCom Information Quest, ingenta, Gale Group, Swets Blackwell, Institute for Scientific Information).
Indexed: ASCA, ASSIA, Abstr.Health Care Manage.Stud., Abstr.Hyg., AgeLine, Arts & Hum.Cit.Ind. (coverage dropped), Brit.Nur.Ind., CINAHL, Curr.Cont., ERA, Excerp.Med., Fam.Ind., I.P.A., Intl.Bibl.Soc.Sci., Lang.& Lang.Behav.Abstr., Med.Care Rev., Mid.East: Abstr.& Ind., Mult.Ed.Abstr., P C I, Psychol.Abstr., Russ.Acad.Sci.Bibl., SOPODA, SSCI, Sage Race Rel.Abstr., Soc.Sci.Ind. (Jul.1999-), Soc.Serv.Abstr., Sociol.Abstr. (1979-), Sociol.Educ.Abstr., Stud.Wom.Abstr., Tech.Educ.Abstr., e-psyche.
—BLDSC (8319.692000), CISTI, GNLM, IDS, ingenta. **CCC.**
Published by: Blackwell Publishers Ltd., 108 Cowley Rd, Oxford OX4 1JF, United Kingdom. TEL 44-1865-791100, FAX 44-1865-791347, jnlinfo@blackwellpublishers.co.uk, http://www.blackwellpublishers.co.uk. Eds. Elizabeth Murphy, Robert Dingwall, Veronica James. Circ: 950.

790 USA ISSN 0741-1235
SOCIOLOGY OF SPORT JOURNAL. Short title: S S J. Text in English. 1984. q. USD 45 to individuals; USD 135 to institutions; USD 30 to students (effective 2001). adv. bk.rev. bibl, charts, stat, illus. index. back issues avail.; reprint service avail. from PSC,SCH. *Refereed.* **Document type:** *Academic/Scholarly.* **Description:** Focuses on the relationship between sport, society, and social institutions from the perspectives of social psychology, sociology and anthropology. Designed to communicate research, critical thought, and theory development.
Related titles: Online - full text ed.: (from Gale Group, Institute for Scientific Information).
Indexed: ASCA, AgeLine, Arts & Hum.Cit.Ind. (coverage dropped), CBCA Ref., C.I.J.E., Curr.Cont., Focus on: Sports Sci.& Med., IBZ, Lang.& Lang.Behav.Abstr., Phys.Ed.Ind., Rural Recreat.Tour.Abstr., SOPODA, SSCI, Sage Race Rel.Abstr., Soc.Sci.Ind. (Jul.1999-), Soc.Serv.Abstr., Sociol.Abstr. (1984-), Sportsearch (1984-).
—BLDSC (8319.696830), IDS, ingenta. **CCC.**
Published by: (North American Society for the Sociology of Sport), Human Kinetics Publishers, Inc., PO Box 5076, Champaign, IL 61825-5076. TEL 217-351-5076, 800-747-4457, FAX 217-351-2674, http://www.humankinetics.com. Ed. Christopher Stevenson. Pub. Rainer Martens. R&P Cheri Banks TEL 217-351-5076 ext 2275. Circ: 1,119 (paid).

302 300 UKR ISSN 1680-4325
SOTSIONIKA, MENTOLOGIYA I PSIKHOLOGIYA LICHNOSTI/SOCIONICS, MENTOLOGY AND PERSONALITY PSYCHOLOGY. Text in Russian; Summaries in English. 1995. bi-m. USD 48 domestic; USD 132 foreign; USD 22 newsstand/cover (effective 2002). index. back issues avail. **Document type:** *Journal, Academic/Scholarly.*
Related titles: Online - full text ed.
Published by: Institut Sotsioniki, a/s 23, Kiev 02206, Ukraine. Eds. A. V. Dr. Bukalov, E. A. Dr. Donchenko, Yu. I. Prof. Saenko. Circ: 600 (paid). **Dist. by:** East View Publications, 2030 Harbor Ln N, Minneapolis, MN 55447. TEL 612-550-0961, periodicals@eastview.com.

SOUTH PACIFIC JOURNAL OF PSYCHOLOGY. see *PSYCHOLOGY*

STRUCTURAL EQUATION MODELING; a multidisciplinary journal. see *PSYCHOLOGY*

STUDIEN UND BERICHTE. see *EDUCATION*

STUDIES IN FAMILY PLANNING. see *POPULATION STUDIES*

S

THEORETICAL POPULATION BIOLOGY; an international journal. see *BIOLOGY*

TOPIA REVISTA; psicoanalisis, sociedad y cultura. see *PSYCHOLOGY*

LE TRAVAIL HUMAIN. see *PSYCHOLOGY*

301 USA ISSN 0042-0468
UNSCHEDULED EVENTS; research committee on disasters newsletter. Text in English. 1967. q. USD 35 to individual members; USD 48 to institutional members; USD 20 to students (effective 1999); includes International Journal of Mass Emergencies and Disasters. adv. bk.rev. abstr. back issues avail. **Document type:** *Newsletter.*
Published by: International Research Committee on Disasters, c/o David Neal, Treas, Institute of Emergency Admin & Planning, Univ of North Texas, Box 13438, Denton, TX 76203. TEL 817-565-4267. Ed. George Rogers. Circ: 250.

VENEREOLOGY; the interdisciplinary international journal of sexual health. see *MEDICAL SCIENCES—Dermatology And Venereology*

303.6 USA ISSN 1077-8012
HV6250.4.W65 CODEN: VAWOFG
VIOLENCE AGAINST WOMEN; an international and interdisciplinary journal. Text in English. 1995. m. USD 165 to individuals; USD 475 to institutions; USD 20 newsstand/cover to individuals; USD 50 newsstand/cover to institutions (effective 2002). adv. bk.rev. bibl. illus. back issues avail.; reprints avail. *Refereed.* **Document type:** *Academic/Scholarly.* **Description:** Publishes empirical research, as well as cross-cultural and historical analyses, on all aspects of violence against women and girls.
Related titles: Online - full text ed.: (from EBSCO Publishing, O C L C Online Computer Library Center, Inc., RoweCom Information Quest, ProQuest Information & Learning, Gale Group, ingenta, Swets Blackwell, Institute for Scientific Information).
Indexed: ASSIA, Abstr.Soc.Geront., CJPI, Crim.Just.Abstr., Curr.Cont., ERA, Environ.Sci.Poll.Mgmt., Fam.Ind., Fem.Per. (1995-), Human Resour.Abstr., Indian Psychol.Abstr., Lang.& Lang.Behav.Abstr., Mult.Ed.Abstr., Pollut.Abstr., PsycInfo, Risk Abstr., SOPODA, SSCI, Saf.Sci.Abstr., Sage Fam.Stud.Abstr., Sage Urb.Stud.Abstr., Soc.Sci.Ind. (Jul.1999-), Soc.Serv.Abstr., Sociol.Abstr., Stud.Wom.Abstr., Viol.& Abuse Abstr., e-psyche.
—BLDSC (9237.750800), Infotrieve, ingenta. **CCC.**
Published by: Sage Publications, Inc., 2455 Teller Rd, Thousand Oaks, CA 91320. TEL 818-597-4867, FAX 818-597-4879, info@sagepub.com, http://www.sagepub.co.uk/journals/details/j0062.html, http://www.sagepub.com. Ed. Claire M Renzetti. Pub. Sara Miller McCune. R&P Tanya Udin. Adv. contact DeAnna Vega Hammersley. page USD 275. **Overseas subscr. to:** Sage Publications Ltd., 6 Bonhill St, London EC2A 4PU, United Kingdom; Sage Publications India Pvt. Ltd., 4215, New Delhi 110 048, India.

303.6 USA ISSN 0886-6708
HV6250
VIOLENCE AND VICTIMS. Text in English. 1986. 6/yr., latest vol.16, 2001, June. USD 72 in United States to individuals; USD 121 for 2 yrs. in United States to individuals; USD 84 foreign to individuals; USD 138 for 2 yrs. foreign to individuals; USD 148 in United States to institutions; USD 251 for 2 yrs. in United States to institutions; USD 169 foreign to institutions; USD 288 for 2 yrs. foreign to institutions (effective 2001). adv. bk.rev., software rev., video rev., Website rev. abstr, bibl. back issues avail.; reprints avail. *Refereed.* **Document type:** *Journal, Academic/Scholarly, Abstract/Index, Bibliography.* **Description:** Provides a forum for the latest developments in theory, research, policy, clinical practice and social services in the areas of interpersonal violence and victimization.
Related titles: Online - full text ed.: (from Gale Group).
Indexed: Abstr.Crim.& Pen., Crim.Just.Abstr., Educ.Admin.Abstr., Excerp.Med., Fam.Ind., IMFL, Ind.Med. (1986-), Lang.& Lang.Behav.Abstr., Peace Res.Abstr., PsycInfo, Psychol.Abstr. (1986-), Rel.Ind.One, Rel.Ind.Two, SOPODA, Sage Fam.Stud.Abstr., Sage Urb.Stud.Abstr., Soc.Sci.Ind. (Jul.1999-), Soc.Serv.Abstr., Soc.Work Res.& Abstr., Sociol.Abstr., Viol.& Abuse Abstr., e-psyche.
—BLDSC (9237.751000), EMDOCS, GNLM, ingenta, KNAW. **CCC.**
Published by: Springer Publishing Company, 536 Broadway, New York, NY 10012. TEL 212-431-4370, FAX 212-941-7842, springer@springerpub.com, http://www.springerpub.com. Ed. Roland Maiuro. Pub. Ursula Springer. R&P Dorothy Kouwenberg. adv.: B&W page USD 300; 5.5 x 8.5.

ZEITSCHRIFT FUER SOZIALPSYCHOLOGIE. see *PSYCHOLOGY*

SOCIOLOGY—Abstracting, Bibliographies, Statistics

016.30685 USA ISSN 1089-6147
HQ1
FAMILY INDEX. Text in English. 1996. m. USD 199 (effective 2001). **Document type:** *Abstract/Index, Academic/Scholarly, Bibliography.* **Description:** Guide to the world's family literature. Designed for students, researchers and practitioners. Includes 35000+ family-related articles published since 1995 from more than 1,100 journals representing many disciplines, such as family studies, psychology, sociology, social work, law, nursing, medicine, counseling, religion and gerontology.
Media: Online - full content.
Indexed: e-psyche.
Published by: Family Scholar Publications, 1001 University Ave, Ste 401, Columbia, MO 65201. TEL 573-449-8171, info@familyscholar.com, http://www.famindx.com, http://www.familyscholar.com. Ed. Jason D Hans. R&P Irina Gorokhova. Circ: 500.

HUMAN SEXUALITY. see *MEDICAL SCIENCES—Abstracting, Bibliographies, Statistics*

302.015195 JPN ISSN 0385-5481
KODO KEIRYOGAKU/JAPANESE JOURNAL OF BEHAVIORMETRICS. Text in Japanese; Summaries in English. 1974. s-a. JPY 2,100 (effective 2001). *Refereed.* **Document type:** *Academic/Scholarly.*
Indexed: Curr.Cont. (1990-, dropped), Curr.Ind.Stat., Lang.& Lang.Behav.Abstr., PsycInfo, Psychol.Abstr. (1983-), SOPODA, Sociol.Abstr., Stat.Theor.Meth.Abstr. (1990-), e-psyche.
—BLDSC (4651.013000).
Published by: Nihon Kodo Keiryo Gakkai/Behaviormetric Society of Japan, 6-7 Minami-Azabu 4-chome, Minato-ku, Tokyo 106-0047, Japan. TEL 81-3-5421-8766, fumih@toyoeiwa.ac.jp. Ed. Fumi Hayashi.

302.015195 JPN
NIHON KODO KEIRYO GAKKAI TAIKAI HAPPYO RONBUN SHOROKUSHU. Text in Japanese. 1973. a. abstr. **Document type:** *Proceedings.* **Description:** Contains abstracts from the annual meeting of the society.
Indexed: e-psyche.
Published by: Nihon Kodo Keiryo Gakkai/Behaviormetric Society of Japan, 6-7 Minami-Azabu 4-chome, Minato-ku, Tokyo 106-0047, Japan. TEL 81-3-5421-8766. Ed. Kazouo Shigemasu.

016.30685 USA ISSN 0164-0283
HQ536
SAGE FAMILY STUDIES ABSTRACTS. Text in English. 1979. q. USD 125 to individuals; USD 575 to institutions; USD 35 newsstand/cover to individuals; USD 150 newsstand/cover to institutions (effective 2002). adv. illus. back issues avail.; reprint service avail. from PSC,SCH. **Document type:** *Abstract/Index.* **Description:** Abstracts major articles, reports, books, and other materials on policy, theory, and research relating to the family, interpersonal relations, human development, therapy and counseling.
Related titles: Online - full text ed.: (from EBSCO Publishing, O C L C Online Computer Library Center, Inc., RoweCom Information Quest, ProQuest Information & Learning, ingenta, Swets Blackwell).
Indexed: e-psyche.
—CCC.
Published by: Sage Publications, Inc., 2455 Teller Rd, Thousand Oaks, CA 91320. TEL 805-499-0721, FAX 805-499-0871, info@sagepub.com, http://www.sagepub.com. Pub. Sara Miller McCune. R&P Tanya Udin. Adv. contact DeAnna Vega Hammersley. Circ: 500 (paid). **Overseas subscr. to:** Sage Publications Ltd., 6 Bonhill St, London EC2A 4PU, United Kingdom; Sage Publications India Pvt. Ltd., 4215, New Delhi 110 048, India.

016.3036 USA ISSN 1077-2197
HV6493
VIOLENCE & ABUSE ABSTRACTS; current literature in interpersonal violence. Text in English. 1995. q. USD 90 to individuals; USD 600 to institutions; USD 30 newsstand/cover to individuals; USD 160 newsstand/cover to institutions (effective 2002). adv. back issues avail.; reprints avail. **Document type:** *Abstract/Index.* **Description:** Abstract articles on the legal, medical, psychological, and social aspects of all types of interpersonal violence, including child abuse, domestic violence, rape and sexual harassment, gang violence, and elder abuse.
Related titles: Online - full text ed.: (from EBSCO Publishing, O C L C Online Computer Library Center, Inc., RoweCom Information Quest, ProQuest Information & Learning, ingenta, Swets Blackwell).
—CCC.
Published by: Sage Publications, Inc., 2455 Teller Rd, Thousand Oaks, CA 91320. TEL 805-499-0721, FAX 805-499-0871, info@sagepub.com, http://www.sagepub.com. Pub. Sara Miller McCune. R&P Tanya Udin. Adv. contact DeAnna Vega Hammersley. **Overseas subscr. to:** Sage Publications Ltd., 6 Bonhill St, London EC2A 4PU, United Kingdom; Sage Publications India Pvt. Ltd., 4215, New Delhi 110 048, India.

SOCIOLOGY—Computer Applications

BEHAVIOUR AND INFORMATION TECHNOLOGY; an international journal on the human aspects of computing. see *PSYCHOLOGY*

301 004 GBR ISSN 0747-5632
BF39.5 CODEN: CHBEEQ
COMPUTERS IN HUMAN BEHAVIOR. Text in English. 1985. 6/yr. EUR 195 in Europe to qualified personnel; JPY 25,900 in Japan to qualified personnel; USD 218 elsewhere to qualified personnel; EUR 859 in Europe to institutions; JPY 114,000 in Japan to institutions; USD 961 elsewhere to institutions (effective 2002). adv. bk.rev. back issues avail.; reprint service avail. from PSC,SCH. *Refereed.* **Document type:** *Academic/Scholarly.* **Description:** Scholarly journal dedicated to examining the use of computers from a psychological perspective.
Related titles: Microfilm ed.; Online - full text ed.: (from ingenta, Gale Group, Swets Blackwell, ScienceDirect, Institute for Scientific Information).
Indexed: ASCA, Abstr.Hum.Comp.Inter., AgeLine, C.I.J.E., Commun.Abstr., Compumath, Comput.Abstr., Curr.Cont., Eng.Ind., Environ.Sci.Poll.Mgmt., Ergon.Abstr., Excerp.Med., High.Educ.Abstr., INSPEC (1985-), Ind.Philos., Indian Psychol.Abstr., Inform.Sci.Abstr., Lang.& Lang.Behav.Abstr., Microcomp.Ind. (Apr.1998-), Pollut.Abstr., PsycInfo, Psychol.Abstr. (1985-), Risk Abstr., Russ.Acad.Sci.Bibl., SOPODA, SSCI, Saf.Sci.Abstr., Soc.Sci.Ind. (Jul.1999-), Soc.Serv.Abstr., Sociol.Abstr., e-psyche.
—BLDSC (3394.921600), AskIEEE, Ei, GNLM, IDS, ingenta, Linda Hall. **CCC.**
Published by: Pergamon (Subsidiary of: Elsevier Science), The Boulevard, Langford Ln, East Park, Kidlington, Oxford OXB 1GB, United Kingdom. FAX 44-1865-843010, nlinfo-f@elsevier.nl; usinfo-f@elsevier.com; forinfo-kyf04035@niftyserve.or.jp, nlinfo-f@elsevier/nl; usinfo-f@elsevier.com; forinfo-kyf04035@niftyserve.or.jp, http://www.elsevier.nl/inca/publications/store/7/5/9/. Ed. Robert D Tennyson. **Subscr. in Australasia and the Far East to:** Elsevier Science (Singapore) Pte Ltd, No.1 Temasek Ave, 17-01 Millenia Tower, Singapore 039192, Singapore. TEL 65-434-3727, FAX 65-337-2230; **Subscr. in the Americas to:** Elsevier Science, PO Box 945, New York, NY 10159-0945. TEL 212-633-3730, FAX 212-633-3680; **Subscr. to:** Elsevier Science BV, PO Box 211, Amsterdam 1000 AE, Netherlands. TEL 31-20-485-3757, FAX 31-20-485-3432, http://www.elsevier.nl.

SOFTWARE

see *COMPUTERS—Software*

SOUND

see *PHYSICS—Sound*

SOUND RECORDING AND REPRODUCTION

see also *MUSIC*

S

GOOD VIBRATIONS. see *HANDICAPPED—Visually Impaired*

SPECIAL EDUCATION AND REHABILITATION

see EDUCATION—Special Education And Rehabilitation

SPORTS AND GAMES

see also MEDICAL SCIENCES—Sports Medicine; SPORTS AND GAMES—Ball Games; SPORTS AND GAMES—Bicycles And Motorcycles; SPORTS AND GAMES—Horses And Horsemanship; SPORTS AND GAMES—Outdoor Life

A C H P E R HEALTHY LIFESTYLES JOURNAL. see *EDUCATION*

790.1 617.1 USA
A S M A NEWS. (American Sports Medicine Association) Text in English. a. USD 50 to members. adv. bk.rev. back issues avail. **Document type:** *Newsletter.* **Description:** Covers sports medicine, injury prevention, athletic training, sports medicine certification.
Published by: American Sports Medicine Association, Board of Certification, 660 W Duarte Rd, Arcadia, CA 91007. TEL 818-445-1978, FAX 818-574-1999. Ed. Steve Lewis. Circ: 3,500 (controlled).

ACTIVE MAGAZINE. see *WOMEN'S HEALTH*

ASSOCIATION FOR THE STUDY OF PLAY NEWSLETTER. see *PSYCHOLOGY*

797.21 AUS ISSN 1327-6085
AUSTRALIAN SWIMMING AND FITNESS. Text in English. 1996. 9/yr. AUD 40.05; AUD 60 in New Zealand; AUD 80 elsewhere. **Document type:** *Consumer.*
Published by: J P Publications, PO Box 2805, Taren Point, NSW 2229, Australia. TEL 62-2-9542-7335, FAX 62-2-9542-7323, jppublic@ozemail.com.au, http://www.magna.com.au/~iphala. Ed. Tracie Spicer.

BIOLOGY OF SPORT; a quarterly journal of sport and exercise sciences. see *MEDICAL SCIENCES—Sports Medicine*

794.1 362.41 GBR ISSN 0006-8756
BRAILLE CHESS MAGAZINE. Text in English. 1934. q. GBP 16 (effective 2000). index. **Document type:** *Consumer.* **Description:** Covers news of the current trends and chess competions.
Media: Braille. **Related titles:** Diskette ed.
Published by: Royal National Institute for the Blind, PO Box 173, Peterborough, Cambs PE2 6WX, United Kingdom. TEL 44-1733-370-777, FAX 44-1733-371555, webmaster@rnib.org.uk, http://www.rnib.org.uk. Ed. Hans Cohn. Circ: 113.

796 617.1 USA ISSN 1066-7814
GV557 CODEN: CJAPEY
CANADIAN JOURNAL OF APPLIED PHYSIOLOGY/ REVUE CANADIENNE DE PHYSIOLOGIE APPLIQUEE. Short title: C J A P - R C P A. Text in English, French. 1976. bi-m. USD 54 to individuals; USD 162 to institutions; USD 36 to students (effective 2001). adv. bk.rev. abstr, bibl, charts, stat, illus. index. back issues avail.; reprints avail. *Refereed.* **Document type:** *Journal, Academic/Scholarly.* **Description:** Offers forum for applied physiology topics contributing to understanding of physical activity, health, and fitness.
Former titles (until 1992): Canadian Journal of Sport Sciences (0833-1235); Canadian Journal of Applied Sport Science (0700-3978)
Related titles: Microfiche ed.: (from MML); Microform ed.: (from MML); Online - full text ed.: (from Institute for Scientific Information).
Indexed: AMED, ASCA, Biol.Abstr., CBCA Ref., CINAHL, Can.B.P.I., Chem.Abstr., Chem.Indus.Notes, Chem.Titles, Curr.Cont. (coverage dropped), Ergon.Abstr., Excerp.Med., Focus on: Sports Sci.& Med., IBZ, Ind.Med. (1993-), PsycInfo, Psychol.Abstr. (1976-), SSCI (coverage dropped), Sci.Cit.Ind. (coverage dropped), Sportsearch (1987-), e-psyche.
—BLDSC (3028.570000), CASDDS, GNLM, IDS, ingenta, KNAW. **CCC.**
Published by: (Canadian Society for Exercise Physiology CAN), Human Kinetics Publishers, Inc., PO Box 5076, Champaign, IL 61825-5076. TEL 217-351-5076, FAX 217-351-2674, http://www.humankinetics.com/products/journals/journal.cfm?id=CJAP. Ed. Terry Graham. Pub. Rainer Martens. R&P Cheri Banks TEL 217-351-5076 ext 2275. Adv. contact Patty Rodriguiz. Circ: 974 (paid and free).

COLLECTION PSYCHOLOGIE ET PEDAGOGIE DU SPORT. see *PSYCHOLOGY*

790.1 DEU ISSN 0946-3003
CONDITION; Ratgebermagazin fuer Lauf- und Ausdauersport. Text in German. 1969. 10/yr. EUR 40 domestic; EUR 4 newsstand/cover (effective 2002). 52 p./no. 3 cols./p. back issues avail. **Document type:** *Magazine, Consumer.* **Description:** Covers distance running and other endurance sports.
Former titles (until 1994): Sport Special - Condition (0940-192X); (until 1991): Condition (0340-2991)
Related titles: Supplement: Condition Aktuell.
Published by: (Interessengemeinschaft der Langstreckenlaeufer), Meyer und Meyer Fachverlag GmbH, Von-Coels-Str 390, Aachen 52080, Germany. TEL 49-241-95810-0, FAX 49-241-9581010, verlag@meyer-meyer-sports.com, marketing@meyer-meyer-sports.com, http://www.meyer-meyer-sports.com. Ed. Maike Masurat. Adv. contact Michael Friesing TEL 49-241-9581012. Circ: 15,000.

CORRICOLARI; el corredor y su mundo. see *PHYSICAL FITNESS AND HYGIENE*

CURATE REGENERATE. see *PHYSICAL FITNESS AND HYGIENE*

790.1 USA
DEAFSPORTZINE. Text in English. 1996. w.
Media: Online - full text.
Published by: Silent News, Inc., 133 Gaither Dr., Ste. E, Mt. Laurel, NJ 08054-1710. barry@clark.net, barry@deafdigest.com, http://www.yellowstar.com/DeafSportZine/sportzine.htm. Ed. Barry M Strassler.

EUROPEAN YEARBOOK OF SPORT PSYCHOLOGY. see *PSYCHOLOGY*

FIT FOR FUN. see *PHYSICAL FITNESS AND HYGIENE*

790.1 617.1 CHN
FUJIAN TIYU KEJI/FUJIAN SPORTS SCIENCE AND TECHNOLOGY. Text in Chinese. q. CNY 3. **Description:** Covers sports theory, training, psychology, medicine as well as sports biophysics and biochemistry.
Published by: Fujiansheng Tiyu Kexue Yanjiusuo/Fujian Sports Science Institute, No 17, Zhuangyuan Xiang, Wusi Lu, Fuzhou, Fujian 350005, China. TEL 554963. Ed. He Fangsheng. **Dist. overseas by:** Jiangsu Publications Import & Export Corp., 56 Gao Yun Ling, Nanjing, Jiangsu, China. **Co-sponsor:** Fujian Tiyu Kexue Xuehui.

▼ **GYM**; for the physical man. see *PHYSICAL FITNESS AND HYGIENE*

THE HONG KONG JOURNAL OF SPORTS MEDICINE AND SPORTS SCIENCE. see *MEDICAL SCIENCES—Sports Medicine*

371.7 ROM
INSTITUTUL DE SUBINGINERI ORADEA. LUCRARI STIINTIFICE: SERIA EDUCATIE FIZICA SI SPORT. Text in Romanian; Text occasionally in English, French; Summaries in Romanian, English, German. 1967. a. **Document type:** *Academic/Scholarly.*
Formerly: Institutul Pedagogic Oradea. Lucrari Stiintifice: Seria Educatie Fizica si Sport; Which superseded in part (in 1973): Institutul Pedagogic Oradea. Lucrari Stiintifice: Seria Educatie Fizica, Biologie, Stiinte Medicale; Which superseded in part (in 1971): Institutul Pedagogic Oradea. Lucrari Stiintifice: Seria A si Seria B; Which was formerly (until 1969): Institutul Pedagogic Oradea. Lucrari Stiintifice
Published by: Institutul de Subingineri Oradea, Calea Armatei Rosii 5, Oradea 3700, Romania.

613.7 ITA
JOGGING - LA GRANDE CORSA. Text in Italian. 1980. bi-m. ITL 30,000 domestic; ITL 60,000 in Europe; ITL 90,000 elsewhere. adv. back issues avail. *Refereed.* **Document type:** *Consumer.* **Description:** Reports news of long-distance races, marathons and adventure.
Formerly (until 1992): Jogging
Published by: Publimaster s.r.l., Via Giovanni Gioacchino Winckelmann, 2, Milan, MI 20146, Italy. TEL 39-2-424191, FAX 39-2-47710278. Ed. Amedeo Stevaraglia. Adv. contact Alessandro Zonca. color page ITL 7,000,000; trim 280 x 190. Circ: 25,000.

JOURNAL OF GAMBLING STUDIES. see *MEDICAL SCIENCES—Psychiatry And Neurology*

JOURNAL OF SPORT AND EXERCISE PSYCHOLOGY. see *PSYCHOLOGY*

790.1 150 USA ISSN 0162-7341
GV561
JOURNAL OF SPORT BEHAVIOR. Text in English. 1978. q. USD 30; USD 55 foreign (effective 2001). illus. Index. reprints avail. *Refereed.* **Document type:** *Academic/Scholarly.* **Description:** Deals with the sociological, psychological, anthropological and related applications to the science of sport.
Related titles: CD-ROM ed.: (from ProQuest Information & Learning); Microform ed.: (from PQC); Online - full text ed.: (from Gale Group, ProQuest Information & Learning, Northern Light Technology, Inc., Factiva).
Indexed: Environ.Sci.Poll.Mgmt., Nutr.Abstr., Phys.Ed.Ind., PsycInfo, Psychol.Abstr. (1980-), Risk Abstr., Rural Recreat.Tour.Abstr., Saf.Sci.Abstr., Sportsearch (1978-), e-psyche.
—BLDSC (5066.186000), ingenta. **CCC.**
Published by: University of South Alabama, Department of Psychology, Mobile, AL 36688-0008. TEL 334-460-7131, FAX 334-460-7252, WGilley@usamail.usouthal.edu, elabbe@usamail.usouthal.edu, cwelsh@usamail.usouthal.edu. Eds. Elise Labbe-Coldsmith, M Cay Welsh. Circ: 450.

790.1 GBR ISSN 0264-0414
GV561 CODEN: JSSCEL
JOURNAL OF SPORTS SCIENCES. Text in English. 1983. m. GBP 766, USD 1,230 to institutions (effective 2002). adv. bk.rev. illus. reprints avail. *Refereed.* **Document type:** *Academic/Scholarly.* **Description:** Provides a contact point among the separate disciplines in sports sciences. Includes contributions from the human sciences: anatomy, anthropology, behavioral sciences, physiology, and psychology. Papers cover technologies such as design of playing equipment and sports facilities, as well as applied research in training, team selection, performance prediction or modification, and stress reduction.
Related titles: Online - full text ed.: ISSN 1466-447X (from CatchWord Ltd., EBSCO Publishing, O C L C Online Computer Library Center, Inc., RoweCom Information Quest, Swets Blackwell, Institute for Scientific Information).
Indexed: AMED, ASCA, Appl.Mech.Rev., Environ.Sci.Poll.Mgmt., Ergon.Abstr., Excerp.Med. (1992-), Focus on: Sports Sci.& Med., IBZ, Ind.Med. (1983-), Inpharma, Nutr.Abstr., Pharm.&Out.News, Phys.Ed.Ind., Pollut.Abstr., Reac., Risk Abstr., Rural Recreat.Tour.Abstr., Saf.Sci.Abstr., Sportsearch (1983-).
—BLDSC (5066.350000), CatchWord, EMDOCS, GNLM, IDS, ingenta, KNAW. **CCC.**
Published by: (British Association of Sports Sciences), E. & F.N. Spon (Subsidiary of: Taylor & Francis Group), 11 New Fetter Ln, London EC4P 4EE, United Kingdom. TEL 44-20-7842-2344, FAX 44-20-7842-2391, journals@tandf.co.uk, http://www.tandf.co.uk/journals. Ed. D Kerwin. R&P Sally Sweet. **Subscr. in US & Canada to:** Routledge, Taylor & Francis Ltd, 29 W 35th St, New York, NY 10001-2299. TEL 212-216-7800; **Subscr. to:** Routledge, Subscriptions, PO Box 362, Abingdon, Oxon OX14 3WB, United Kingdom. TEL 44-1235-401060, FAX 44-1235-401075.

JOURNAL OF TEACHING IN PHYSICAL EDUCATION. see *EDUCATION—Teaching Methods And Curriculum*

JUOKSIJA. see *PHYSICAL FITNESS AND HYGIENE*

LEISURE SCIENCES; an interdisciplinary journal. see *LEISURE AND RECREATION*

THE MENTAL EDGE. see *PSYCHOLOGY*

MUSCULAR DEVELOPMENT. see *PHYSICAL FITNESS AND HYGIENE*

790.1 616.86 USA
N C A A DRUG TESTING PROGRAM* . Text in English. a. USD 1.50. **Description:** Establishes NCAA procedures and regulations for drug testing of student athletes, and includes a list of banned drugs.
Published by: National Collegiate Athletic Association, Circulation Department, PO Box 781046, Indianapolis, IN 46278. TEL 913-339-1900.

S

NATURAL DEVELOPMENT. see *PHYSICAL FITNESS AND HYGIENE*

613.713 ITA ISSN 1126-0874
OLYMPIAN'S NEWS. Text in Italian. bi-m. ITL 54,000; ITL 10,000, EUR 5.16 newsstand/cover (effective 1999). **Document type:** *Consumer.* **Description:** Contains articles on muscle and fitness strategies. For competitive body builders.
Address: Via Fiorentina, 72, Figline Valdarno, FI 50063, Italy. TEL 39-055-959530, FAX 39-055-9156982, olympian@ats.it, http://www.olympian.it. Ed. Sandro Ciccarelli. **Dist. by:** Italian Press Dist. Stampa, Via Ghisalba, 7, Ospiate di Bollate, MI 20021, Italy. TEL 39-02-38300940.

790.1 CAN ISSN 0226-1561
ONTARIO WRESTLER MAGAZINE✶. Text in English. 1981. bi-m. CND 20, USD 35 (effective 1991). adv. bk.rev. illus, stat. **Document type:** *Newsletter.* **Description:** Offers articles, tournament dates, coach and executive information, results.
Indexed: Ref.Zh., Sportsearch (1980-).
Published by: Ontario Amateur Wrestling Association, 1600 James Naismith Dr, Gloucester, ON K1B 5N4, Canada. TEL 416-495-4170, FAX 416-495-4165. Ed., Adv. contact Sean Norris. Circ: 2,500 (paid).

OXYGEN!; serious fitness for serious women. see *WOMEN'S HEALTH*

PALAESTRA; forum of sport, physical education and recreation for those with disabilities. see *EDUCATION—Special Education And Rehabilitation*

PHYSICAL EDUCATION NEW ZEALAND. JOURNAL. see *EDUCATION—Teaching Methods And Curriculum*

PSYCHOLOGIE UND SPORT. see *PSYCHOLOGY*

QIGONG. see *PHYSICAL FITNESS AND HYGIENE*

RECREATION - ACCESS IN THE '90'S. see *HANDICAPPED*

RESEARCH QUARTERLY FOR EXERCISE AND SPORT. see *PHYSICAL FITNESS AND HYGIENE*

797.21 613.7 USA ISSN 1083-6357
RODALE'S FITNESS SWIMMER; technique - nutrition - workouts. Text in English. 1991. bi-m. USD 19.94; CND 26 in Canada; USD 40 elsewhere; USD 2.95 newsstand/cover; GBP 2.50 newsstand/cover in United Kingdom. adv. bk.rev. reprints avail. **Document type:** *Consumer.* **Description:** Covers the aquatic lifestyle of year-round swimmers, cross trainers and water exercise enthusiasts.
Formerly (until 1995): Fitness Swimmer (1066-7105)
Published by: Rodale, 33 E Minor St, Emmaus, PA 18098. TEL 610-967-5171, FAX 610-967-8963, marybswim@aol.com, http://www.fitnessswimmer.com. Ed. Mary Bolster. Pub. Heidi Rodale. Adv. contact Derek Weatherford. B&W page USD 2,800, color page USD 3,587; trim 10.75 x 8. Circ: 60,000. **Subscr. to:** PO Box 7421, Red Oak, IA 51591-7421. **Dist. in UK by:** MarketForce UK Ltd, 247 Tottenham Court Rd, London, Middx W1T 7AU, United Kingdom. TEL 44-207-261-5199, FAX 44-207-261-7341.

796.07 DEU ISSN 0722-1088
ROLLSTUHLSPORT. Text in German. 1982. m. DEM 40. adv. illus. back issues avail. **Document type:** *Bulletin.*
Published by: Deutscher Rollstuhl Sportverband e.V., Friedrich-Alfred-Str 15, Duisburg 47226, Germany. Eds. Herbert Krah, Ralf Harperath. Circ: 5,000.

RUNNING & FITNEWS. see *PHYSICAL FITNESS AND HYGIENE*

SCANDINAVIAN JOURNAL OF MEDICINE & SCIENCE IN SPORTS. see *MEDICAL SCIENCES—Sports Medicine*

SCANDINAVIAN JOURNAL OF MEDICINE & SCIENCE IN SPORTS ONLINE. see *MEDICAL SCIENCES—Sports Medicine*

SOCIOLOGY OF SPORT JOURNAL. see *SOCIOLOGY*

790.1 613.7 USA
SPLASH! (COLORADO SPRINGS). Text in English. 1993. bi-m. free to members; USD 15 domestic to non-members; USD 25 foreign to non-members (effective 2000). **Document type:** *Consumer.* **Description:** Conceived in the hope of improving communication among clubs, coaches, local swimming committees, USA Swimming staff, and the Board of Directors. Provides information on programs and services of USA Swimming and the people and events of the sport of swimming.
Formed by the merger of (1976-1993): Lanelines; (1944-1993): U S Swimming News (0883-0347)
Published by: U S A Swimming, One Olympic Plaza, Colorado Springs, CO 80909. TEL 719-578-4578, FAX 719-575-4049, csnyder@usa-swimming.org, http://www.usa-swimming.org. Ed., R&P Charlie Snyder. Pub. Chuck Wielgus. Circ: 185,000.

SPORT & MEDICINA. see *MEDICAL SCIENCES—Sports Medicine*

THE SPORT PSYCHOLOGIST. see *PSYCHOLOGY*

790.1 617.1 DEU ISSN 0939-3706
SPORT SCIENCES INTERNATIONAL. Text in English. 1994. irreg. **Document type:** *Monographic series.*
Published by: Peter Lang GmbH Europaeischer Verlag der Wissenschaften, Eschborner Landstr 42-50, Frankfurt Am Main 60489, Germany. TEL 49-69-780705-0, FAX 49-69-78070543, 101622.27@compuserve.com, zentrale.frankfurt@peterlang.com, http://www.peterlang.de. Ed. Dieter Hackfort. R&P Ruediger Brunsch.

SPORTS DOCUMENTATION MONTHLY BULLETIN. see *EDUCATION—Abstracting, Bibliographies, Statistics*

SPORTS MEDICINE DIGEST. see *MEDICAL SCIENCES—Sports Medicine*

796.077 617.1 AUS ISSN 1032-5506
SPORTS TRAINERS DIGEST. Text in English. 1987. q. AUD 25 domestic (effective 1999); AUD 35 foreign. back issues avail. **Document type:** *Newsletter.* **Description:** Provides basic sports medicine including first aid, crisis management and injury prevention to sports participants.
Published by: Sports Medicine Australia, PO Box 897, Belconnen, ACT 2616, Australia. TEL 61-6-2516944, FAX 61-6-2531489. Ed. Matt Reid. Circ: 13,000.

SPORTVERLETZUNG - SPORTSCHADEN. see *MEDICAL SCIENCES*

790.1 578.77 770 910.09 DEU ISSN 0170-4001
TAUCHEN; internationales Unterwasser-Magazin. Text in German. 1978. m. DEM 103.20; DEM 8 newsstand/cover (effective 2001). adv. bk.rev. charts, illus. index. back issues avail. **Document type:** *Magazine, Consumer.*
Published by: Jahr Top Special Verlag, Jessenstr 1, Hamburg 22767, Germany. TEL 49-40-38906-0, FAX 49-40-38906302, plettner@jahr-tsv.de, http://www.jahr-tsv.de. Ed. Maike Gruetzedick. Adv. contact Waltraud Jante. B&W page DEM 5,220, color page DEM 9,396. Circ: 50,311 (paid).

790.1 CHN ISSN 1000-677X
TIYU KEXUE/SPORTS SCIENCE. Text in Chinese; Abstracts in English. 1981. bi-m. USD 27 (effective 2000). **Document type:** *Consumer.*
Indexed: Sportsearch (1985-).
—BLDSC (8419.839520).
Published by: (China Sports Science Society), Renmin Tiyu Chubanshe/People's Sports Publishing House, 8 Tiyuguan Lu, Chongwen-qu, Beijing 100061, China. TEL 86-1-6714-2466, FAX 86-1-6711-6129. Ed. Zhang Caizhen. Circ: 20,000. **Dist. in U.S. by:** China Books & Periodicals, Inc, 2929 24th St, San Francisco, CA 94110. TEL 415-282-2994.

613.7 USA ISSN 1058-3548
TRAINING AND CONDITIONING. Text in English. 1991. 9/yr., latest vol.11, no.4. USD 24 domestic; USD 30 in Canada (effective 2001). back issues avail. **Document type:** *Magazine, Trade.* **Description:** Provides pertinent information on the various training and conditioning techniques, trends, procedures and products to professionals involved in the training and conditioning of competitive athletes.
Published by: Momentum Media, 2488 N Triphammer Rd, Ithaca, NY 14850-1014. Ed., R&P Eleanor Frankel TEL 607-257-6970 ext 18. Pub., Adv. contact Mark Goldberg TEL 607-257-6970 ext 11. Circ: 28,126 (controlled).

790.1 052 USA
U S A B A AGENDA. Text in English. 1976. 12/yr. free per issue. bk.rev. 18 p./no. **Document type:** *Newspaper-distributed.*
Former titles: SportsScoop; U S A B A Newsletter
Related titles: Talking Book ed.
Published by: United States Association for Blind Athletes, 33 N Institute, Colorado Springs, CO 80903. TEL 719-630-0422, FAX 719-630-0616. Ed. Mark Lucas. Circ: 4,500.

U S TEAM SPOTLIGHT. see *HANDICAPPED—Hearing Impaired*

V A H P E R D JOURNAL. see *PHYSICAL FITNESS AND HYGIENE*

WEIGHTLIFTING U S A. see *PHYSICAL FITNESS AND HYGIENE*

Y M C A WEEKLY NEWS. (Young Men's Christian Association) see *PHYSICAL FITNESS AND HYGIENE*

SPORTS AND GAMES—Abstracting, Bibliographies, Statistics

790.1 616 CAN ISSN 1192-1420
DRUG FILE UPDATE; a current awareness index to publications on drugs and doping in sport. Text in English. a. USD 25. **Document type:** *Abstract/Index.* **Description:** Reflects the latest literature and concerns about drugs and doping in sport from around the world. References grouped by individual sport and country.
Published by: Sport Information Resource Centre (SIRC)/Centre de Documentation pour le Sport, 116 Albert St Ste 400, Ottawa, ON K1P 5G3, Canada. TEL 613-231-7472, FAX 613-231-3739, moreinfo@sirc.ca. **Co-sponsor:** Canadian Centre for Drug-Free Sport.

688.76 USA
FITNESS IN AMERICA. Text in English. 1987. biennial. USD 95 (effective 2000). **Document type:** *Trade.* **Description:** Analyzes adult participation in seven fitness activities, with geographical and demographic information.
Published by: National Sporting Goods Association, 1601 Feehanville Dr, Ste 300, Mt. Prospect, IL 60056-6305. TEL 847-296-6742, 800-815-5422, FAX 847-391-9827, http://www.nsga.org. Ed. Thomas B Doyle.

HEALTH, PHYSICAL EDUCATION AND RECREATION, EXERCISE AND SPORT SCIENCES MICROFORM PUBLICATIONS BULLETIN; a subject and author index of dissertations and theses including abstracts. see *PHYSICAL FITNESS AND HYGIENE—Abstracting, Bibliographies, Statistics*

SPORTS DOCUMENTATION MONTHLY BULLETIN. see *EDUCATION—Abstracting, Bibliographies, Statistics*

SPORTS AND GAMES—Ball Games

796.352 USA
AMPUTEE GOLFER. Text in English. a. **Document type:** *Consumer.* **Description:** Offers physical and mental therapy to amputees through involvement with golf.
Published by: National Amputee Golf Association, 11 Walnut Hill Rd, Amherst, NH 03031. TEL 800-633-6242, naga@execpc.com, b1naga@aol.com, http://www.nagagolf.org. Ed. Bob Wilson. R&P Jim Coombes. Adv. contact Patty Johnson.

610 IRL ISSN 0791-5357
GOLFER'S COMPANION. Text in English. 1973. 4/yr. IEP 5. adv. bk.rev.
Published by: Sports Enterprises Ltd., PO Box 14, Dun Laoghaire, Co. Dublin, Ireland. Ed. Pat Ruddy. Circ: 20,000.

796.352 USA
N A G A NEWSLETTER. Text in English. s-a. **Document type:** *Newsletter.*
Published by: National Amputee Golf Association, 11 Walnut Hill Rd, Amherst, NH 03031. TEL 800-633-6242, b1naga@aol.com, http://www.nagagolf.org. Ed. Bob Wilson. R&P Jim Coombes. Adv. contact Patty Johnson.

793.342 USA
TENNISPRO MAGAZINE. Text in English. 1988. bi-m. free per issue to members. adv. bk.rev. **Document type:** *Magazine, Trade.* **Description:** Geared for the tennis teaching professionals. Covers sports science, programming, sports medicine, new drills and product reviews.

Published by: U S Professional Tennis Registry, PO Box 4739, Hilton Head Island, SC 29938. TEL 843-785-7244, FAX 843-886-2033, ptr@ptrtennis.org, http://www.ptrtennis.org, http://www.usptr.org/. Ed., R&P Peggy Edwards. Adv. contact Julie Jilly. Circ: 11,200 (free).

SPORTS AND GAMES—Bicycles And Motorcycles

388.347 640.73 USA
MASS CYCLIST✶ . Text in English. 1979. q. USD 30; includes membership (effective 2000). bk.rev. charts, illus, tr.lit. back issues avail. **Document type:** *Newsletter.* **Description:** Newsletter of the Coalition, a bicycle advocacy group working to promote the safe and practical use of the bicycle for both transportation and recreation.
Former titles (until 1993): Boston Cyclist; Spoke 'n Word
Published by: Massachusetts Bicycle Coalition, 59 Temple Pl Ste 669, Boston, MA 02111-1307. TEL 617-491-RIDE, jack2bike@mediaone.net, http://www.massbike.org. Ed. Jack W Johnson. Adv. contact Larry Slotnick. Circ: 1,000.

SPORTS AND GAMES—Horses And Horsemanship

636.1 CAN ISSN 0840-6200
CANADIAN HORSEMAN. Text in English. 1982. 5/yr. CND 18.95 domestic; CND 20.37 Atlantic; USD 28.95 elsewhere Atlantic; CND 3.50 newsstand/cover Atlantic (effective 2000). adv. bk.rev. **Document type:** *Consumer.* **Description:** Offers general information about health care and training issues for all riders.
Formerly (until 1988): Horse Sense (0821-5073)
Related titles: ♦ Supplement: The Canadian Horse Annual.
Indexed: Sportsearch (1989-).
—CISTI.
Published by: Horse Publications, 225 Industrial Pkwy S, P O Box 670, Aurora, ON L4G 4J9, Canada. TEL 905-727-0107, FAX 905-841-1530, horsepower@horsenet.com. Ed., R&P Lee Benson. Pub. Susan Jane Anstey. Adv. contact Vicki Mosher Tessier. B&W page CND 1,150, color page CND 2,045. Circ: 6,000.

COUNTRY ROAD CHRONICLES. see *NATIVE AMERICAN STUDIES*

EQUINE ATHLETE; the equine sports medicine news journal. see *VETERINARY SCIENCE*

798 GBR
EQUINE BEHAVIOUR. Text in English. 1978. s-a. GBP 6. bk.rev. abstr, bibl, charts, illus. back issues avail. **Description:** Includes observations, reports and analyses on all aspects of equine behavior from worldwide sources.
Indexed: e-psyche.
Published by: Equine Behaviour Study Circle, Leyland Farm, Gawcott, Buckingham, Bucks, United Kingdom. Ed. Moyra Williams. Circ: 150.

798 636.089 CAN ISSN 0828-864X
EQUINEWS; serving the horse industry - all breeds, all disciplines. Text in English. 1980. m. CND 15 domestic; CND 22 foreign. adv. back issues avail.
Formerly (until 1984): Hoof Beats
Published by: John Whittle, Ed. & Pub. (Subsidiary of: Westview Publications), Site 15 C 5 R R 6, Vernon, BC V1T 6Y5, Canada. TEL 604-542-2002, FAX 604-549-7099.

EQUUS. see *BIOLOGY—Zoology*

HOOFCARE & LAMENESS; the journal of equine foot science. see *VETERINARY SCIENCE*

THE HORSE REPORT. see *VETERINARY SCIENCE*

798.2 362.4 USA ISSN 1067-5876
N A R H A NEWS. Text in English. 1970. 8/yr. USD 40 in North America to membership; USD 60 out of North America to membership (effective 2000). adv. bk.rev. **Document type:** *Newsletter.* **Description:** Provides news and technical information for people who assist the physically and mentally disabled to ride horses for therapy and recreation.
Indexed: InterActions Bibl., Sportsearch (1983-).
Published by: North American Riding for the Handicapped Association, Inc., PO Box 33150, Denver, CO 80233. TEL 303-452-1212, 800-369-7433, FAX 303-252-4610. Circ: 4,500.

798.2 362.4 USA
N A R H A STRIDES. Text in English. 1995. 4/yr. USD 40 in North America to membership; USD 60 elsewhere to membership (effective 2000). adv. bk.rev. illus. **Description:** Provides feature articles and news of interest for people who assist the mentally and physically disabled to ride horses for therapy and recreation.
Published by: North American Riding for the Handicapped Association, Inc., PO Box 33150, Denver, CO 80233. TEL 303-452-1212, 800-369-7433, FAX 303-252-4610, http://www.narha.org. Circ: 4,500.

798.2 615.8 DEU ISSN 0942-7546
THERAPEUTISCHES REITEN. Text in German. 1982. q. **Document type:** *Bulletin.*
Formerly (until 1992): Therapeutisches Reiten in Medizin, Paedagogik, Sport (0935-5804)
Indexed: InterActions Bibl. (1994-).
Published by: Deutsches Kuratorium fuer Therapeutisches Reiten e.V., Wasserfuhr 47D, Bielefeld 33619, Germany. TEL 44-521-160380, FAX 44-521-101487, thrdelius@aol.com, http://www.pferd-aktuell.de. Ed. Franziska Delius.

SPORTS AND GAMES—Outdoor Life

796.172 AUS ISSN 1321-2036
AUSTRALIAN SURF LIFESAVER. Text in English. 1994. bi-m. AUD 28. adv. back issues avail. **Document type:** *Consumer.* **Description:** Contains the latest info on Australia's top ironmen and ironwomen, surfboats and jurions, as well as health and exercise tips, the latest in beach apparel and equipment, travel ideas.
Published by: (Surf Life Saving Australia Ltd.), J P Publications, PO Box 2805, Taren Point, NSW 2229, Australia. TEL 61-2-9542-7335, FAX 61-2-9542-7323, jppublic@ozemail.com.au, http://www.magna.com.au/~iphala. Ed. Tracie Spicer. Adv. contact Sally Arnold. page AUD 1,500; trim 275 x 205. Circ: 50,000.

FITNESS. see *PHYSICAL FITNESS AND HYGIENE*

796.42 617.1 AUS ISSN 0047-7672
MODERN ATHLETE AND COACH. Text in English. 1962. q. AUD 25 domestic; AUD 32 foreign (effective 2000 - 2001). adv. bk.rev. **Document type:** *Trade.* **Description:** Covers coaching on all track and field events, as well as such related subjects as nutrition, physiology, psychology, and biomechanics.
Indexed: Phys.Ed.Ind., Sportsearch (1974-).
—BLDSC (5883.690000), ingenta.
Published by: Australian Track & Field Coaches Association, 1 Fox Ave, Athelstone, SA 5076, Australia. TEL 61-8-8337-4510, FAX 61-8-8337-4510. Ed., Adv. contact Jess Jarver. Circ: 3,200.

PSYCHOLOGY AND SOCIOLOGY OF SPORT: CURRENT SELECTED RESEARCH. see *PSYCHOLOGY*

797.21 613.7 USA
SWIMMING POOLS TODAY. Text in English. 1985. q. USD 5. bk.rev. **Document type:** *Newsletter.* **Description:** Featuring the swimming pool: safety, chemistry, cleaning, repair, and new products; swimming for fitness and health; entertainment at the poolside.
Published by: National Swimming Pool Owner's Association (NSPOA), 1213 Ridgecrest Circle, Denton, TX 76205-5421. Ed., Pub. Tom A Doron. Circ: 36,000.

WILDERNESS AND ENVIRONMENTAL MEDICINE; official publication of the wilderness medical society. see *MEDICAL SCIENCES*

SPORTS MEDICINE

see MEDICAL SCIENCES—Sports Medicine

STATISTICS

see also MATHEMATICS; POPULATION STUDIES; and also Abstracting, Bibliographies, Statistics subheadings under specific subjects

A A C O M ANNUAL STATISTICAL REPORT. see *MEDICAL SCIENCES—Abstracting, Bibliographies, Statistics*

A H A HOSPITAL STATISTICS (YEAR). see *HEALTH FACILITIES AND ADMINISTRATION—Abstracting, Bibliographies, Statistics*

A R L ACADEMIC LAW AND MEDICAL LIBRARY STATISTICS. see *LIBRARY AND INFORMATION SCIENCES—Abstracting, Bibliographies, Statistics*

ADVANCES IN RISK ANALYSIS. see *PUBLIC HEALTH AND SAFETY—Abstracting, Bibliographies, Statistics*

AUSTRALIA. BUREAU OF STATISTICS. AUSTRALIAN HEALTH TRENDS. see *PUBLIC HEALTH AND SAFETY—Abstracting, Bibliographies, Statistics*

AUSTRALIA. BUREAU OF STATISTICS. AUSTRALIAN HOSPITAL STATISTICS. see *HEALTH FACILITIES AND ADMINISTRATION—Abstracting, Bibliographies, Statistics*

AUSTRALIA. BUREAU OF STATISTICS. AUSTRALIA'S FOOD AND NUTRITION. see *NUTRITION AND DIETETICS—Abstracting, Bibliographies, Statistics*

AUSTRALIA. BUREAU OF STATISTICS. CANCER IN AUSTRALIA. see *MEDICAL SCIENCES—Oncology*

AUSTRALIA. BUREAU OF STATISTICS. CHILDREN'S HEALTH SCREENING. see *MEDICAL SCIENCES—Abstracting, Bibliographies, Statistics*

AUSTRALIA. BUREAU OF STATISTICS. CHILDREN'S IMMUNISATION, AUSTRALIA. see *MEDICAL SCIENCES—Abstracting, Bibliographies, Statistics*

AUSTRALIA. BUREAU OF STATISTICS. CHIROPRACTIC AND OSTEOPATHIC SERVICES, AUSTRALIA. see *MEDICAL SCIENCES—Abstracting, Bibliographies, Statistics*

AUSTRALIA. BUREAU OF STATISTICS. DEATHS DUE TO DISEASES AND CANCERS OF THE RESPIRATORY SYSTEM, AUSTRALIA. see *MEDICAL SCIENCES—Abstracting, Bibliographies, Statistics*

AUSTRALIA. BUREAU OF STATISTICS. DENTAL SERVICES, AUSTRALIA. see *MEDICAL SCIENCES—Abstracting, Bibliographies, Statistics*

AUSTRALIA. BUREAU OF STATISTICS. HEALTH IN AUSTRALIA - WHAT YOU SHOULD KNOW. see *PUBLIC HEALTH AND SAFETY—Abstracting, Bibliographies, Statistics*

AUSTRALIA. BUREAU OF STATISTICS. HOSPITALS, AUSTRALIA. see *HEALTH FACILITIES AND ADMINISTRATION—Abstracting, Bibliographies, Statistics*

AUSTRALIA. BUREAU OF STATISTICS. INFORMATION PAPER: NATIONAL NUTRITION SURVEY, CONFIDENTIALISED UNIT RECORD FILE. see *NUTRITION AND DIETETICS—Abstracting, Bibliographies, Statistics*

AUSTRALIA. BUREAU OF STATISTICS. INJURIES, AUSTRALIA. see *MEDICAL SCIENCES—Abstracting, Bibliographies, Statistics*

AUSTRALIA. BUREAU OF STATISTICS. MEDICAL LABOUR FORCE. see *MEDICAL SCIENCES—Abstracting, Bibliographies, Statistics*

AUSTRALIA. BUREAU OF STATISTICS. NATIONAL HEALTH INFORMATION MODEL. see *PUBLIC HEALTH AND SAFETY—Abstracting, Bibliographies, Statistics*

AUSTRALIA. BUREAU OF STATISTICS. NATIONAL HEALTH SURVEY: ABORIGINAL AND TORRES STRAIT ISLANDER RESULTS, AUSTRALIA. see *PUBLIC HEALTH AND SAFETY—Abstracting, Bibliographies, Statistics*

AUSTRALIA. BUREAU OF STATISTICS. NATIONAL HEALTH SURVEY: ASTHMA AND OTHER RESPIRATORY CONDITIONS, AUSTRALIA. see *MEDICAL SCIENCES—Abstracting, Bibliographies, Statistics*

AUSTRALIA. BUREAU OF STATISTICS. NATIONAL HEALTH SURVEY: CANCER SCREENING, AUSTRALIA. see *MEDICAL SCIENCES—Abstracting, Bibliographies, Statistics*

S

AUSTRALIA. BUREAU OF STATISTICS. NATIONAL HEALTH SURVEY: CARDIOVASCULAR AND RELATED CONDITIONS, AUSTRALIA. see *MEDICAL SCIENCES—Abstracting, Bibliographies, Statistics*

AUSTRALIA. BUREAU OF STATISTICS. NATIONAL HEALTH SURVEY: DIABETES, AUSTRALIA. see *MEDICAL SCIENCES—Abstracting, Bibliographies, Statistics*

AUSTRALIA. BUREAU OF STATISTICS. NATIONAL HEALTH SURVEY: HEALTH RISK FACTORS, AUSTRALIA. see *PUBLIC HEALTH AND SAFETY—Abstracting, Bibliographies, Statistics*

AUSTRALIA. BUREAU OF STATISTICS. NATIONAL HEALTH SURVEY: SUMMARY OF RESULTS. see *PUBLIC HEALTH AND SAFETY—Abstracting, Bibliographies, Statistics*

AUSTRALIA. BUREAU OF STATISTICS. NATIONAL HEALTH SURVEY: SUMMARY RESULTS, AUSTRALIAN STATES AND TERRITORIES. see *PUBLIC HEALTH AND SAFETY—Abstracting, Bibliographies, Statistics*

AUSTRALIA. BUREAU OF STATISTICS. NATIONAL HEALTH SURVEY: USE OF MEDICATIONS, AUSTRALIA. see *MEDICAL SCIENCES—Abstracting, Bibliographies, Statistics*

AUSTRALIA. BUREAU OF STATISTICS. NATIONAL HEALTH SURVEY: USERS' GUIDE. see *PUBLIC HEALTH AND SAFETY—Abstracting, Bibliographies, Statistics*

AUSTRALIA. BUREAU OF STATISTICS. NATIONAL NUTRITION SURVEY: FOODS EATEN, AUSTRALIA. see *NUTRITION AND DIETETICS—Abstracting, Bibliographies, Statistics*

AUSTRALIA. BUREAU OF STATISTICS. NATIONAL NUTRITION SURVEY: NUTRIENT INTAKES AND PHYSICAL MEASUREMENTS, AUSTRALIA. see *NUTRITION AND DIETETICS—Abstracting, Bibliographies, Statistics*

AUSTRALIA. BUREAU OF STATISTICS. NORTHERN TERRITORY OFFICE. NATIONAL HEALTH SURVEY: DARWIN-PALMERSTON AND ALICE SPRINGS. see *PUBLIC HEALTH AND SAFETY—Abstracting, Bibliographies, Statistics*

AUSTRALIA. BUREAU OF STATISTICS. OCCASIONAL PAPER: CIGARETTE SMOKING AMONG INDIGENOUS AUSTRALIANS. see *PHYSICAL FITNESS AND HYGIENE—Abstracting, Bibliographies, Statistics*

▼ **AUSTRALIA. BUREAU OF STATISTICS. OCCASIONAL PAPER: HOSPITAL STATISTICS, ABORIGINAL AND TORRES STRAIT ISLANDER AUSTRALIANS.** see *HEALTH FACILITIES AND ADMINISTRATION—Abstracting, Bibliographies, Statistics*

AUSTRALIA. BUREAU OF STATISTICS. OCCASIONAL PAPER: OVERWEIGHT AND OBESITY, INDIGENOUS AUSTRALIANS. see *PHYSICAL FITNESS AND HYGIENE—Abstracting, Bibliographies, Statistics*

AUSTRALIA. BUREAU OF STATISTICS. OCCASIONAL PAPER: SELF-ASSESSED HEALTH STATUS, INDIGENOUS AUSTRALIANS. see *PHYSICAL FITNESS AND HYGIENE—Abstracting, Bibliographies, Statistics*

AUSTRALIA. BUREAU OF STATISTICS. OPTOMETRY AND OPTICAL DISPENSING SERVICES, AUSTRALIA. see *MEDICAL SCIENCES—Abstracting, Bibliographies, Statistics*

AUSTRALIA. BUREAU OF STATISTICS. PHYSIOTHERAPY SERVICES, AUSTRALIA. see *MEDICAL SCIENCES—Abstracting, Bibliographies, Statistics*

AUSTRALIA. BUREAU OF STATISTICS. PRIVATE HOSPITALS, AUSTRALIA. see *HEALTH FACILITIES AND ADMINISTRATION—Abstracting, Bibliographies, Statistics*

AUSTRALIA. BUREAU OF STATISTICS. PRIVATE MEDICAL PRACTICE INDUSTRY, AUSTRALIA. see *MEDICAL SCIENCES—Abstracting, Bibliographies, Statistics*

AUSTRALIA. BUREAU OF STATISTICS. PRIVATE MEDICAL PRACTITIONERS, AUSTRALIA. see *MEDICAL SCIENCES—Abstracting, Bibliographies, Statistics*

319 AUS ISSN 0157-3713

AUSTRALIA. BUREAU OF STATISTICS. QUEENSLAND OFFICE. QUEENSLAND AT A GLANCE. Text in English. 1978. a. AUD 1.10 newsstand/cover per brochure (effective 2001). **Document type:** *Government.* **Description:** Provides statistics on all aspects of Queensland life: population, labor, wages, health, welfare services, law and crime, education, agriculture, mining, construction, transportation, communication, tourism, prices and finance.

Published by: Australian Bureau of Statistics, Queensland Office, 313 Adelaide St, Brisbane, QLD 4000, Australia. TEL 07-222-6022, FAX 07-229-6171.

AUSTRALIA. BUREAU OF STATISTICS. THE HEALTH AND WELFARE OF AUSTRALIA'S ABORIGINAL AND TORRES STRAIT ISLANDER PEOPLES. see *PHYSICAL FITNESS AND HYGIENE—Abstracting, Bibliographies, Statistics*

▼ **AUSTRALIA. BUREAU OF STATISTICS. VETERINARY SERVICES, AUSTRALIA.** see *VETERINARY SCIENCE—Abstracting, Bibliographies, Statistics*

AUSTRALIA. BUREAU OF STATISTICS. WESTERN AUSTRALIAN OFFICE. HOME SAFETY DEVICES, WESTERN AUSTRALIA. see *NUTRITION AND DIETETICS—Abstracting, Bibliographies, Statistics*

AUSTRALIA. BUREAU OF STATISTICS. WOMEN'S SAFETY SURVEY, UNIT RECORD FILE, AUSTRALIA. see *PUBLIC HEALTH AND SAFETY—Abstracting, Bibliographies, Statistics*

BELGIUM. INSTITUT NATIONAL DE STATISTIQUE. ACCIDENTS DE LA CIRCULATION SUR LA VOIE PUBLIQUE AVEC TUES ET BLESSES. see *PUBLIC HEALTH AND SAFETY—Abstracting, Bibliographies, Statistics*

BELGIUM. INSTITUT NATIONAL DE STATISTIQUE. STATISTIQUES DES CAUSES DE DECES. see *POPULATION STUDIES—Abstracting, Bibliographies, Statistics*

BELGIUM. MINISTERE DES AFFAIRES SOCIALES DE LA SANTE PUBLIQUE ET DE L'ENVIRONNEMENT. ADMINISTRATION DES SOINS DE SANTE. ANNUAIRE STATISTIQUE DES HOPITAUX/BELGIUM. MINISTERIE VAN VOLKSGEZONDHEID EN LEEFMILIEU. BESTUUR VOOR DE VERZORGINGSINSTELLINGEN. STATISTISCH JAARBOEK VAN DE ZIEKENHUIZEN. see *PUBLIC HEALTH AND SAFETY—Abstracting, Bibliographies, Statistics*

BELGIUM. NATIONAAL INSTITUUT VOOR DE STATISTIEK. STATISTIEK VAN DOODSOORZAKEN. see *POPULATION STUDIES—Abstracting, Bibliographies, Statistics*

BELGIUM. NATIONAAL INSTITUUT VOOR DE STATISTIEK. VERKEERSONGEVALLEN OP DE OPENBARE WEG MET DODEN OF GEWONDEN. see *PUBLIC HEALTH AND SAFETY—Abstracting, Bibliographies, Statistics*

BELIZE FAMILY HEALTH SURVEY. see *MEDICAL SCIENCES—Abstracting, Bibliographies, Statistics*

570.15195 USA ISSN 8750-0434

BIOMETRIC BULLETIN. Text in English. 1984. q. USD 20. abstr. back issues avail. **Document type:** *Newsletter.* —CCC.

Published by: International Biometric Society, 1444 I St, N W, Ste 700, Washington, DC 20005-2210. TEL 202-712-9049, FAX 202-216-9646, ibs@bostromdc.com, http://www.tibs.org. Ed. Geert Molenberghs. Circ: 6,400 (paid).

570.15195 USA ISSN 0006-341X CODEN: BIOMB6

BIOMETRICS. Text in English, French. 1945. q. USD 140 (effective 2001). adv. bk.rev. charts, illus, stat. index, cum.index: vols.1-20, 1945-1964. back issues avail.; reprints avail. *Refereed.* **Document type:** *Academic/Scholarly.* **Description:** Scientific journal emphasizing the role of statistics and mathematics in the biological sciences.

Formerly (until 1947): Biometrics Bulletin (0099-4987)

Related titles: Microfiche ed.: (from BHP); Microform ed.: (from PQC,PMC); Online - full text ed.: (from ProQuest Information & Learning, Institute for Scientific Information).

Indexed: A.S.& T.Ind. (Jan.2001-), ASCA, Abstr.Anthropol., AgBiotech, Agri.Eng.Abstr., Anim.Breed.Abstr., Appl.Mech.Rev., Biol.& Agr.Ind. (Mar.1983-), Biol.Abstr., Biostat., C.C.M.J., C.I.S. Abstr., Chem.Abstr., Compumath, Comput.Abstr., Comput.Cont., Curr.Adv.Ecol.Sci., Curr.Cont. (1961-), Curr.Ind.Stat., Deep Sea Res.& Oceanogr.Abstr., Dent.Ind., Ecol.Abstr., Eng.Ind., Excerp.Med., Food Sci.& Tech.Abstr., Forest Prod.Abstr., Forest.Abstr., Helminthol.Abstr., Herb.Abstr., Hort.Abstr., IDA, INIS Atomind., INSPEC (Jun.1982-Dec.1985, dropped), Ind.Med. (1945-), Ind.Sci.Rev., Ind.Vet., Inpharma, J.Cont.Quant.Meth., Maize Abstr., Math.R., Nutr.Abstr., Oper.Res.Manage.Sci., Plant Breed.Abstr., Qual.Contr.Appl.Stat., Reac., Rev.Appl.Entomol., Rev.Plant Path., Risk Abstr., SSCI (coverage dropped), Sci.Cit.Ind., Soils & Fert., Sorghum & Millets Abstr., Sport Fish.Abstr., Stat.Theor.Meth.Abstr. (1961-), Triticale Abstr., Vet.Bull., W.R.C.Inf., Wild.Rev., Zent.Math., Zoo.Rec.

—BLDSC (2088.000000), CISTI, Ei, EMDOCS, GNLM, IDS, ingenta, Linda Hall. **CCC.**

Published by: International Biometric Society, 1444 I St, N W, Ste 700, Washington, DC 20005-2210. TEL 202-712-9049, FAX 202-216-9646, ibs@bostromdc.com; orders@allenpress.com, http://stat.tamu.edu/Biometrics/, http://www.tibs.org. Ed. Raymond Carroll. Pub. David L Santini. R&P Moayad Zahralddin. Adv. contact Moayad Zahradralddin. Circ: 8,600. **Subscr. to:** Allen Press Inc., PO Box 1897, Lawrence, KS 66044-8897.

BIOMETRIKA. see *BIOLOGY—Abstracting, Bibliographies, Statistics*

BOTSWANA. CENTRAL STATISTICS OFFICE. DEMOGRAPHIC AND HEALTH SURVEY. see *BUSINESS AND ECONOMICS—Abstracting, Bibliographies, Statistics*

BOTSWANA. CENTRAL STATISTICS OFFICE. HEALTH STATISTICS REPORT. see *MEDICAL SCIENCES—Abstracting, Bibliographies, Statistics*

BRITISH COLUMBIA. DIVISION OF VITAL STATISTICS AGENCY. QUARTERLY DIGEST. see *PUBLIC HEALTH AND SAFETY—Abstracting, Bibliographies, Statistics*

BRITISH JOURNAL OF MATHEMATICAL AND STATISTICAL PSYCHOLOGY. see *PSYCHOLOGY*

C R C FACTSHEETS. (Cancer Research Campaign) see *MEDICAL SCIENCES—Abstracting, Bibliographies, Statistics*

CANCER INCIDENCE AND MORTALITY MICHIGAN. see *PUBLIC HEALTH AND SAFETY—Abstracting, Bibliographies, Statistics*

CHARTERED INSTITUTE OF PUBLIC FINANCE AND ACCOUNTANCY. CEMETERIES STATISTICS. ACTUALS. see *PUBLIC HEALTH AND SAFETY—Abstracting, Bibliographies, Statistics*

CHARTERED INSTITUTE OF PUBLIC FINANCE AND ACCOUNTANCY. CREMATORIA STATISTICS. ACTUALS. see *PUBLIC HEALTH AND SAFETY—Abstracting, Bibliographies, Statistics*

CHARTERED INSTITUTE OF PUBLIC FINANCE AND ACCOUNTANCY. ENVIRONMENTAL HEALTH STATISTICS. ACTUALS. see *PUBLIC HEALTH AND SAFETY—Abstracting, Bibliographies, Statistics*

CORNELL UNIVERSITY. NEW YORK STATE COLLEGE OF AGRICULTURE AND LIFE SCIENCES. BIOMETRICS UNIT. ANNUAL REPORT. see *BIOLOGY—Abstracting, Bibliographies, Statistics*

COST SURVEY. see *MEDICAL SCIENCES—Abstracting, Bibliographies, Statistics*

ENCUESTA NACIONAL DE NUTRICION. see *NUTRITION AND DIETETICS—Abstracting, Bibliographies, Statistics*

ETESIA STATISTIKE. EREVNA TOU KARKINOU/ANNUAL STATISTICAL SURVEY OF CANCER. see *MEDICAL SCIENCES—Abstracting, Bibliographies, Statistics*

EZHEGODNIK MIROVOI SANITARNOI STATISTIKI. see *PUBLIC HEALTH AND SAFETY—Abstracting, Bibliographies, Statistics*

S

S

SISTER COMMUNITIES HEALTH PROFILES OF THE U S - MEXICO BORDER/PERFILES DE SALUD DE LAS COMUNIDADES HERMANAS DE LA FRONTERA MEXICO - ESTADOS UNIDOS. see *PUBLIC HEALTH AND SAFETY—Abstracting, Bibliographies, Statistics*

316.8 ZAF
HA1991

SOUTH AFRICA. STATISTICS SOUTH AFRICA. BULLETIN OF STATISTICS. Text in Afrikaans, English. 1967. q. ZAR 80 per issue (effective 2000). **Document type:** *Bulletin, Government.*

Former titles (until Aug. 1998): South Africa. Central Statistical Service. Bulletin of Statistics (0034-5024); South Africa. Department of Statistics. Bulletin of Statistics; South Africa. Department of Statistics. Monthly Bulletin of Statistics

Indexed: Russ.Acad.Sci.Bibl.

Published by: Statistics South Africa/Statistieke Suid-Afrika, Private Bag X44, Pretoria 0001, South Africa. TEL 27-12-310-8911, FAX 27-12-310-8500, info@statssa.pwv.gov.za, http://www.statssa.gov.za. Circ: 1,200.

SOUTH AFRICA. STATISTICS SOUTH AFRICA. CENSUS OF ESTATE AGENCIES, RENT COLLECTORS, APPRAISERS AND VALUERS. see *REAL ESTATE—Abstracting, Bibliographies, Statistics*

SOUTH AFRICA. STATISTICS SOUTH AFRICA. CENSUS OF HOSPITALS, CLINICS AND OTHER HEALTH SERVICE ESTABLISHMENTS. see *HEALTH FACILITIES AND ADMINISTRATION—Abstracting, Bibliographies, Statistics*

SOUTH AFRICA. STATISTICS SOUTH AFRICA. CENSUS OF LETTING OF OWN FIXED PROPERTY. see *REAL ESTATE—Abstracting, Bibliographies, Statistics*

SOUTH AFRICA. STATISTICS SOUTH AFRICA. CENSUS OF MEDICAL, DENTAL AND OTHER HEALTH SERVICES - CHIROPRACTORS, HOMEOPATHS, NATUROPATHS, OSTEOPATHS AND HERBALISTS. see *MEDICAL SCIENCES—Abstracting, Bibliographies, Statistics*

SOUTH AFRICA. STATISTICS SOUTH AFRICA. CENSUS OF MEDICAL, DENTAL AND OTHER HEALTH SERVICES - DENTISTS. see *MEDICAL SCIENCES—Abstracting, Bibliographies, Statistics*

SOUTH AFRICA. STATISTICS SOUTH AFRICA. CENSUS OF MEDICAL, DENTAL AND OTHER HEALTH SERVICES - DOCTORS. see *MEDICAL SCIENCES—Abstracting, Bibliographies, Statistics*

SOUTH AFRICA. STATISTICS SOUTH AFRICA. CENSUS OF MEDICAL, DENTAL AND OTHER HEALTH SERVICES - SUPPLEMENTARY HEALTH SERVICES AND DENTAL TECHNICIANS. see *MEDICAL SCIENCES—Abstracting, Bibliographies, Statistics*

SOUTH AFRICA. STATISTICS SOUTH AFRICA. CENSUS OF PROFESSIONAL AND BUSINESS SERVICES - ACCOUNTING, AUDITING AND BOOK-KEEPING SERVICES. see *BUSINESS AND ECONOMICS—Abstracting, Bibliographies, Statistics*

SOUTH AFRICA. STATISTICS SOUTH AFRICA. CENSUS OF PROFESSIONAL AND BUSINESS SERVICES - ADVERTISING PRACTITIONERS AND ALLIED SERVICES AND MARKETING RESEARCH SERVICES. see *ADVERTISING AND PUBLIC RELATIONS—Abstracting, Bibliographies, Statistics*

SOUTH AFRICA. STATISTICS SOUTH AFRICA. CENSUS OF PROFESSIONAL AND BUSINESS SERVICES - DATA PROCESSING SERVICES. see *BUSINESS AND ECONOMICS—Abstracting, Bibliographies, Statistics*

SOUTH AFRICA. STATISTICS SOUTH AFRICA. ROAD TRAFFIC COLLISIONS. see *TRANSPORTATION—Abstracting, Bibliographies, Statistics*

SOUTH AFRICA. STATISTICS SOUTH AFRICA. STATISTICAL RELEASE. CENSUS OF AUXILIARY, HEALTH SERVICES AND DENTAL TECHNICIANS (YEAR). see *MEDICAL SCIENCES—Abstracting, Bibliographies, Statistics*

SOUTH AFRICA. STATISTICS SOUTH AFRICA. STATISTICAL RELEASE. CENSUS OF CHIROPRACTORS AND HOMEOPATHS. see *MEDICAL SCIENCES—Abstracting, Bibliographies, Statistics*

SOUTH AFRICA. STATISTICS SOUTH AFRICA. STATISTICAL RELEASE. CENSUS OF DENTISTS (YEAR). see *MEDICAL SCIENCES—Abstracting, Bibliographies, Statistics*

SOUTH AFRICA. STATISTICS SOUTH AFRICA. STATISTICAL RELEASE. CENSUS OF DOCTORS (YEAR). see *MEDICAL SCIENCES—Abstracting, Bibliographies, Statistics*

SOUTH AFRICA. STATISTICS SOUTH AFRICA. STATISTICAL RELEASE. CENSUS OF HOSPITALS, CLINICS AND OTHER HEALTH SERVICE ESTABLISHMENTS (YEAR). see *HEALTH FACILITIES AND ADMINISTRATION—Abstracting, Bibliographies, Statistics*

SOUTH AFRICA. STATISTICS SOUTH AFRICA. STATISTICAL RELEASE. ROAD TRAFFIC COLLISIONS. see *TRANSPORTATION—Abstracting, Bibliographies, Statistics*

310 618.202 GBR

SOUTH EAST THAMES PERINATAL MONITORING GROUP. PROVISIONAL STATISTICS. Text in English. a.

Published by: West Kent Health Authority, South East Thames Perinatal Monitoring Unit, Preston Hall, Aylesford, Kent ME20 7NJ, United Kingdom. Ed. Patricia Hanson.

SOUTH PACIFIC EPIDEMIOLOGICAL AND HEALTH INFORMATION SERVICE ANNUAL REPORT. see *PUBLIC HEALTH AND SAFETY—Abstracting, Bibliographies, Statistics*

519.502461 GBR ISSN 0962-2802
R853.S7 CODEN: SMMRFQ

STATISTICAL METHODS IN MEDICAL RESEARCH. Text in English. 1992. 6/yr. GBP 83 in Europe to individuals; USD 148 in North America to individuals; GBP 104 rest of world to individuals; GBP 229 in Europe to institutions; USD 428 in North America to institutions; GBP 263 rest of world to institutions; GBP 63 in Europe to members International Society for Clinical Biostatistics and International Biometric Society; USD 112 in North America to members International Society for Clinical Biostatistics and International Biometric Society; GBP 80 rest of world to members International Society for Clinical Biostatistics and International Biometric Society; GBP 131 in developing nations; GBP 64 newsstand/cover in Europe; USD 113 newsstand/cover in North America; GBP 72 newsstand/cover rest of world (effective 2002). adv. back issues avail.; reprints avail. *Refereed.* **Document type:** *Journal, Academic/Scholarly.* **Description:** Contains review articles covering all the main areas of medical statistics.

Related titles: Online - full text ed.: (from EBSCO Publishing, O C L C Online Computer Library Center, Inc., RoweCom Information Quest, ingenta, Swets Blackwell, Institute for Scientific Information).

Indexed: ASSIA, Curr.Cont. (1992-), Curr.Ind.Stat., Ind.Med. (1992-), Sci.Cit.Ind., Stat.Theor.Meth.Abstr. (1992-).

—BLDSC (8448.573050), GNLM, Infotrieve, KNAW. **CCC.**

Published by: Arnold Publishers (Subsidiary of: Hodder Headline plc.), 338 Euston Rd, London NW1 3BH, United Kingdom. TEL 44-20-7873-6337, FAX 44-20-7873-6325, arnoldjournals@hodder.co.uk, http://www.palliativemedjournal.com. Eds. Brian Everitt, Graham Dunn, Theodore Holford. Adv. contact Mary Attree. **Dist. by:** Turpin Distribution Services Ltd., Blackhorse Rd, Letchworth, Herts SG6 1HN, United Kingdom. TEL 44-1462-488900, FAX 44-1462-483011.

STATISTICAL RECORD OF HEALTH AND MEDICINE. see *MEDICAL SCIENCES—Abstracting, Bibliographies, Statistics*

STATISTICS IN MEDICINE. see *MEDICAL SCIENCES—Abstracting, Bibliographies, Statistics*

U.S. CENTERS FOR DISEASE CONTROL. REPORTED TUBERCULOSIS IN THE UNITED STATES. see *MEDICAL SCIENCES—Respiratory Diseases*

U.S. NATIONAL CENTER FOR HEALTH STATISTICS. VITAL AND HEALTH STATISTICS. SERIES 10. DATA FROM THE HEALTH INTERVIEW SURVEY. see *PUBLIC HEALTH AND SAFETY—Abstracting, Bibliographies, Statistics*

U.S. NATIONAL CENTER FOR HEALTH STATISTICS. VITAL AND HEALTH STATISTICS. SERIES 11. DATA FROM THE HEALTH AND NUTRITION EXAMINATION SURVEY. see *PUBLIC HEALTH AND SAFETY—Abstracting, Bibliographies, Statistics*

U.S. NATIONAL CENTER FOR HEALTH STATISTICS. VITAL AND HEALTH STATISTICS. SERIES 14. DATA ON HEALTH RESOURCES. see *PUBLIC HEALTH AND SAFETY—Abstracting, Bibliographies, Statistics*

U.S. NATIONAL CENTER FOR HEALTH STATISTICS. VITAL AND HEALTH STATISTICS. SERIES 2. DATA EVALUATION AND METHODS RESEARCH. see *PUBLIC HEALTH AND SAFETY—Abstracting, Bibliographies, Statistics*

U.S. NATIONAL CENTER FOR HEALTH STATISTICS. VITAL AND HEALTH STATISTICS. SERIES 20. DATA ON MORTALITY. see *PUBLIC HEALTH AND SAFETY—Abstracting, Bibliographies, Statistics*

U.S. NATIONAL CENTER FOR HEALTH STATISTICS. VITAL AND HEALTH STATISTICS. SERIES 21. DATA ON NATALITY, MARRIAGE, AND DIVORCE. see *PUBLIC HEALTH AND SAFETY—Abstracting, Bibliographies, Statistics*

U.S. NATIONAL CENTER FOR HEALTH STATISTICS. VITAL AND HEALTH STATISTICS. SERIES 23. DATA FROM THE NATIONAL SURVEY OF FAMILY GROWTH. see *PUBLIC HEALTH AND SAFETY—Abstracting, Bibliographies, Statistics*

U.S. NATIONAL CENTER FOR HEALTH STATISTICS. VITAL AND HEALTH STATISTICS. SERIES 24. COMPILATIONS OF DATA ON NATALITY, MORTALITY, DIVORCE, AND INDUCED TERMINATIONS OF PREGNANCY. see *PUBLIC HEALTH AND SAFETY—Abstracting, Bibliographies, Statistics*

U.S. NATIONAL CENTER FOR HEALTH STATISTICS. VITAL AND HEALTH STATISTICS. SERIES 3. ANALYTICAL STUDIES. see *PUBLIC HEALTH AND SAFETY—Abstracting, Bibliographies, Statistics*

U.S. NATIONAL CENTER FOR HEALTH STATISTICS. VITAL AND HEALTH STATISTICS. SERIES 5. COMPARATIVE INTERNATIONAL VITAL AND HEALTH STATISTICS REPORTS. see *PUBLIC HEALTH AND SAFETY—Abstracting, Bibliographies, Statistics*

U.S. NATIONAL CENTER FOR HEALTH STATISTICS. VITAL AND HEALTH STATISTICS. SERIES 6. COGNITION AND SURVEY MEASUREMENT. see *PSYCHOLOGY—Abstracting, Bibliographies, Statistics*

U.S. NATIONAL INSTITUTE ON DRUG ABUSE. STATISTICAL SERIES D. DATA FROM THE CLIENT ORIENTED DATA ACQUISITION PROCESS. QUARTERLY REPORT. PROVISIONAL DATA. see *PHYSICAL FITNESS AND HYGIENE—Abstracting, Bibliographies, Statistics*

001.433 USA ISSN 1534-844X

▼ **UNDERSTANDING STATISTICS;** statistical issues in psychology, education, and the social sciences. Text in English. forthcoming 2002. q. USD 40 in North America to individuals; USD 65 elsewhere to individuals; USD 150 in North America to institutions; USD 175 elsewhere to institutions (effective 2002). **Document type:** *Journal, Academic/Scholarly.* **Description:** Aims to make psychologists and other behavioral scientists aware of relevant recent developments in statistics, point out current poor practice in their use of statistics, illustrate innovative uses of software, highlight software inadequacies, and generally make non-statisticians in a variety of disciplines more aware of what modern statistics has to offer them.

Related titles: Online - full text ed.: ISSN 1532-8031. forthcoming 2002. USD 36 to individuals; USD 135 to institutions (effective 2002).

Published by: Lawrence Erlbaum Associates, Inc., 10 Industrial Ave, Mahwah, NJ 07430-2262. TEL 201-760-3735, 800-926-6579, FAX 201-236-0072, journals@erlbaum.com, http://www.erlbaum.com/Journals/journals/US/us.htm. Ed. Brian S Everitt.

S

362.1 USA ISSN 1069-6725
THE UNIVERSAL HEALTHCARE ALMANAC. Text in English. 1985. q. USD 195 (effective 2001). bk.rev. **Document type:** *Academic/Scholarly.* **Description:** Contains healthcare statistics covering national healthcare expenditures, hospitals, managed care, DRGs, health insurance, healthcare professionals, long-term care, and related topics.
Published by: Silver & Cherner Ltd., 10221 N 32nd St, Ste D, Phoenix, AZ 85028-3849. TEL 602-996-2220, FAX 602-996-2330, uhaeditor@aol.com. Ed., Pub. Linda L Cherner. Circ: 600 (paid).

VITAL STATISTICS OF THE UNITED STATES. see *PUBLIC HEALTH AND SAFETY—Abstracting, Bibliographies, Statistics*

WORLD HEALTH STATISTICS ANNUAL. see *PUBLIC HEALTH AND SAFETY—Abstracting, Bibliographies, Statistics*

YAMAGUCHIKEN EISEI KOGAI KENKYU SENTA NENPO. see *PUBLIC HEALTH AND SAFETY—Abstracting, Bibliographies, Statistics*

SURGERY

see MEDICAL SCIENCES—Surgery

TAXATION

see BUSINESS AND ECONOMICS—Public Finance, Taxation

TEACHING METHODS AND CURRICULUM

see EDUCATION—Teaching Methods And Curriculum

TECHNOLOGY: COMPREHENSIVE WORKS

A F P SCIENCES; bulletin information scientifique, technique, medicale. see *MEDICAL SCIENCES*

ADVANCES IN NATURAL AND TECHNOLOGICAL HAZARDS RESEARCH. see *PUBLIC HEALTH AND SAFETY*

APPLIED ERGONOMICS; human factors in technology and society. see *ENGINEERING*

▼ **BEHAVIORAL & COGNITIVE NEUROSCIENCE REVIEWS.** see *PSYCHOLOGY*

BIOPHARMACEUTICAL PROCESS VALIDATION. see *BIOLOGY*

CRYOLETTERS. see *BIOLOGY—Physiology*

CURRENT AWARENESS. S D I SERVICE. see *MEDICAL SCIENCES*

EAST ASIAN SCIENCE, TECHNOLOGY, AND MEDICINE. see *SCIENCES: COMPREHENSIVE WORKS*

EURO COURSES. HEALTH PHYSICS AND RADIATION PROTECTION. see *ENERGY—Nuclear Energy*

600 150 IND
FOCUS GROUP KIT. Text in English. (in 6 vols.). USD 99.95 (effective 2000); complete set. **Description:** Provides the reader with a systematic and readable approach to the design, implementation and analysis of focus group data.
Published by: Sage Publications India Pvt. Ltd., P O Box 4215, New Delhi 110 048, India. TEL 91-11-644-4958, FAX 91-11-6472426, http://www.sagepub.com. Eds. David L Morgan, Richard A Krueger.

FORMA. see *BIOLOGY*

HEALTH TECHNOLOGY MANAGEMENT. see *MEDICAL SCIENCES*

HOSPITAL TECHNOLOGY SERIES. see *HEALTH FACILITIES AND ADMINISTRATION*

I E E E ENGINEERING IN MEDICINE AND BIOLOGY MAGAZINE. see *BIOLOGY—Bioengineering*

ILLUSTRERAD VETENSKAP. see *SCIENCES: COMPREHENSIVE WORKS*

IN FOCUS (MOUNTAIN VIEW). see *HANDICAPPED—Visually Impaired*

INDEX AND ABSTRACTS OF A P I HEALTH-RELATED RESEARCH (YEARS). see *PUBLIC HEALTH AND SAFETY—Abstracting, Bibliographies, Statistics*

M T DIALOG. (Medizin-Technischer) see *MEDICAL SCIENCES*

MEDICAL DESIGN TECHNOLOGY; new products, materials & components for medical device designers. see *MEDICAL SCIENCES*

MEDIZIN, TECHNIK UND GESELLSCHAFT. see *MEDICAL SCIENCES*

NATURE BIOTECHNOLOGY. see *BIOLOGY—Biotechnology*

PHARMA TECHNOLOGIE JOURNAL. see *PHARMACY AND PHARMACOLOGY*

679.9 DEU
RECYCLING MAGAZIN; Fachblatt des gesamten Handels mit Alt- und Abfallstoffen. Text in German. 1938. s-m. DEM 219 (effective 1998). adv. illus, stat. index. **Document type:** *Trade.*
Formerly: Rohstoff Rundschau (0035-7863)
—**CCC.**
Published by: Reed Elsevier Deutschland GmbH (Subsidiary of: Reed Elsevier group), Gabrielenstr 9, Munich 80636, Germany. TEL 49-89-89817199, FAX 49-89-89817102, TELEX 522451. Ed. Erich Schweiger. Pub. Wolfram Haase. Adv. contact Hendrik Vandervliet.

600 FRA ISSN 1145-5217
TECHNOLOGIE & SANTE. Text in French. 1990. q. FRF 1,200 domestic; FRF 1,450 foreign (effective 2000). adv. back issues avail. *Refereed.* **Document type:** *Trade.* **Description:** Covers hospital organization, medical technology, and information systems.
Published by: C N E H, 9 rue Antoine Chantin, Paris 75014, France. TEL 33-1-40441515, FAX 33-1-40448724, http://www.cneh.fr. Ed., R&P, Adv. contact Veronique Douville. Circ: 1,000.

600 613.62 USA
TECHNOLOGY SPECIAL INTEREST SECTION QUARTERLY. Text in English. 1991. q. USD 20 (effective 1999). **Document type:** *Newsletter.*
Formerly: Technology Special Interest Section Newsletter (1059-0609)
Published by: American Occupational Therapy Association, Inc., 4720 Montgomery Lane, Bethesda, MD 20814-3425. TEL 301-652-2682, FAX 301-652-7711.

WIEDZA I ZYCIE. see *SCIENCES: COMPREHENSIVE WORKS*

XIBEI LINXUEYUAN XUEBAO/NORTHWESTERN FORESTRY UNIVERSITY. JOURNAL. see *FORESTS AND FORESTRY*

TECHNOLOGY: COMPREHENSIVE WORKS—Abstracting, Bibliographies, Statistics

SCITECH BOOK NEWS; an annotated bibliography of new books in science, technology, & medicine. see *BIBLIOGRAPHIES*

TELEPHONE AND TELEGRAPH

see COMMUNICATIONS—Telephone And Telegraph

TELEVISION AND CABLE

see COMMUNICATIONS—Television And Cable

TEXTILE INDUSTRIES AND FABRICS

see also CLOTHING TRADE

MEDICAL TEXTILES; an international newsletter. see *MEDICAL SCIENCES*

THEATER

see also DANCE

792 150 ITA ISSN 0392-2367
ATTI DELLO PSICODRAMMA. Text in Italian; Summaries in English. 1975. a. ITL 35,000 for 2 yrs.. adv. illus.
Indexed: Psychol.Abstr., e-psyche.
Published by: Casa Ediitrice Astrolabio-Ubaldini, Via Guido d'Arezzo 16, Rome, RM 00198, Italy. Ed. Ottavio Rosati. Circ: 5,000. **Co-sponsor:** Associazione Ricerche sullo Psicodramma Analitico di Roma.

TOBACCO

see also AGRICULTURE—Crop Production And Soil

ASHES TO DUST. see *PUBLIC HEALTH AND SAFETY*

157 616 GBR ISSN 1462-2203
CODEN: NTREF6
▼ **NICOTINE & TOBACCO RESEARCH.** Text in English. 1999. q. GBP 88, USD 145 to individuals; GBP 217, USD 360 to institutions (effective 2002). *Refereed.* **Document type:** *Academic/Scholarly.* **Description:** Aims to provide a forum for empirical findings on the many aspects of nicotine and tobacco, including research from a variety of arenas.
Related titles: Online - full content ed.: ISSN 1469-994X (from EBSCO Publishing, O C L C Online Computer Library Center, Inc., Swets Blackwell); Online - full text ed.: (from CatchWord Ltd., RoweCom Information Quest).
Indexed: Addic.Abstr., Environ.Sci.Poll.Mgmt., Ind.Med., Tox.Abstr.
—CatchWord.
Published by: (Society for Research on Nicotine and Tobacco), Carfax Publishing Limited (Subsidiary of: Taylor & Francis Group), PO Box 25, Abingdon, Oxon OX14 3UE, United Kingdom. TEL 44-1235-401000, FAX 44-1235-401550, enquiries@carfax.co.uk, enquiry@tandf.co.uk, http://www.carfax.co.uk. Ed. Gary E Swan.

NON-SMOKERS' UPDATE. see *PUBLIC HEALTH AND SAFETY*

679.7 USA ISSN 0897-9626
NONSMOKERS' VOICE. Text in English. 1977. biennial. USD 35 domestic; USD 50 foreign (effective 2000 - 2001). adv. **Document type:** *Newsletter.* **Description:** Contains new research on effects of secondhand smoke, smoke-free actions, local and state legislation, tactics of the tobacco industry.
Published by: Group to Alleviate Smoking Pollution (GASP), 2885 Aurora Ave, 37, Boulder, CO 80303-2252. TEL 303-444-9799, FAX 303-444-2399, gaspco@gaspforair.org, http://www.gaspforair.org. Ed. Peter Bialick. Pub., R&P, Adv. contact Pete Bialick. Circ: 1,000.

SMOKE; cigars, pipes and life's other burning desires. see *GENERAL INTEREST PERIODICALS—United States*

679.7 610 GBR ISSN 0964-4563
HV5725
TOBACCO CONTROL; an international journal. Text in English; Summaries in Chinese, French, Spanish. 1992. q. GBP 82, USD 215 combined subscription to individuals includes print & online eds.; GBP 162 to institutions for print only (effective 2002); USD 260 to institutions for print only (effective 2001). adv. bk.rev. charts, illus, stat. index. back issues avail. *Refereed.* **Document type:** *Academic/Scholarly.* **Description:** Studies the nature and extent of tobacco use worldwide, the effects of tobacco use on health, the economy, the environment and society, and the efforts of the health community to prevent its use.
Related titles: Online - full text ed.: Tobbacco Control Online. ISSN 1468-3318. GBP 50, USD 75 to individuals (effective 2001); Online free from January 2002. (from HighWire Pr., EBSCO Publishing, O C L C Online Computer Library Center, Inc., Swets Blackwell, SilverPlatter Information, Inc., Ovid Technologies, Inc., Institute for Scientific Information).
Indexed: Addic.Abstr., Curr.Cont., Hosp.Abstr., Ind.Med. (1992-), Int.Nurs.Ind., SSCI, Sci.Cit.Ind., World Ag.Econ.& Rur.Soc.Abstr.
—BLDSC (8859.576550), GNLM, IDS, Infotrieve. **CCC.**
Published by: B M J Publishing Group, B M A House, Tavistock Sq, London WC1H 9JR, United Kingdom. TEL 44-20-7387-4499, FAX 44-20-7383-6400, info.norththames@bma.org.uk, http://tc.bmjjournals.com/ , http://www.bma.org.uk, http:// www.tobbaccocontrol.com/. Ed. Simon Chapman. Pub. Alex Williamson. R&P Carol Torselli TEL 44-20-7383-6674. Adv. contact Euan Currer TEL 44-20-7383-6181.

T

TOBACCO—Abstracting, Bibliographies, Statistics

633.71 016 USA ISSN 0040-8298
SB273
TOBACCO ABSTRACTS; world literature on Nicotiana. Text in English. 1957. bi-m. USD 120 domestic; USD 200 foreign (effective 2001). index. back issues avail. **Document type:** *Abstract/Index.* **Description:** Covers tobacco culture, economics, genetics, chemistry, manufacture and distribution.
—BLDSC (8859.575000), CISTI, Linda Hall.
Published by: Tobacco Literature Service, 3210 Faucette Dr, Rm 204-206 Budler Bldg, Campus Box 7603, NC State University, Raleigh, NC 27695-760. TEL 919-513-3150, cbridges@cals1.cals.ncsu.edu (Internet) or Carolyn_Bridges@ncsu.edu. Ed. Pamela E Puryear. Circ: 500.

TOXICOLOGY AND ENVIRONMENTAL SAFETY

see ENVIRONMENTAL STUDIES—Toxicology And Environmental Safety

TRADE AND INDUSTRIAL DIRECTORIES

see BUSINESS AND ECONOMICS—Trade And Industrial Directories

TRANSPORTATION

see also TRANSPORTATION—Air Transport; TRANSPORTATION—Automobiles; TRANSPORTATION—Railroads; TRANSPORTATION—Roads And Traffic; TRANSPORTATION—Ships And Shipping; TRANSPORTATION—Trucks And Trucking

ARBEIT UND GESUNDHEIT. SONDERAUSGABE VERKEHR. see *PUBLIC HEALTH AND SAFETY*

343.09322 USA
CHEMICAL REGULATION REPORTER: HAZARDOUS MATERIALS TRANSPORTATION. Text in English. 1982 (Apr). m. USD 724 (effective 2000). **Document type:** *Trade.* **Description:** Contains rules and regulations governing shipment of hazardous material by rail, air, ship, highway and pipeline, including DOT's Harzardous Materials Tables and EPA's rules for it's hazardous waste tracking system.
Published by: The Bureau of National Affairs, Inc., 1231 25th St NW, Washington, DC 20037. TEL 202-452-4200, icrutre@bna.com, http://www.bna.com. Pub. Paul N Wojcik.

I C A D T S REPORTER. see *DRUG ABUSE AND ALCOHOLISM*

JOURNAL OF SAFETY RESEARCH. see *OCCUPATIONAL HEALTH AND SAFETY*

380.5 614.85 USA ISSN 1082-104X
KELLER'S TRANSPORTATION SAFETY TRAINING NEWSLETTER. Text in English. 1995. m. USD 125 (effective 2001). **Description:** Provides information on current training methods, DOT regulations, and other transportation related topics.
Published by: J.J. Keller & Associates, Inc., 3003 W Breezewood Lane, Box 368, Neenah, WI 54957-0368. TEL 920-722-2848, 800-327-6868, FAX 920-727-7526, http://www.jjkeller.com.

328 363.12 NZL
NEW ZEALAND. LAND TRANSPORT SAFETY AUTHORITY. RULES. Text in English. irreg. **Document type:** *Government.* **Description:** Includes the official rules and advisory updates of the Authority.
Published by: (New Zealand. Land Transport Safety Authority), GP Legislation Services, P.O. Box 12418, Thorndon, Wellington, New Zealand. TEL 64-4-496-5655, FAX 64-4-496-5698, http://www.gplegislation.co.nz.

NUCLEUS (CAMBRIDGE). see *ENERGY*

SOUTH AFRICA. STATISTICS SOUTH AFRICA. ROAD TRAFFIC COLLISIONS. see *TRANSPORTATION—Abstracting, Bibliographies, Statistics*

388 158.7 USA
QA76.87
▼ **TRANSPORTATION HUMAN FACTORS.** Text in English. 1999. q. adv. *Refereed.* **Document type:** *Journal, Academic/Scholarly.* **Description:** Examines the role of human factors in all areas of transportation.
Media: Online - full content.
Indexed: Environ.Sci.Poll.Mgmt., Ergon.Abstr., HRIS, Pollut.Abstr., Risk Abstr., Saf.Sci.Abstr., e-psyche.
—BLDSC (9026.237000), CatchWord.
Published by: Lawrence Erlbaum Associates, Inc., 10 Industrial Ave, Mahwah, NJ 07430-2262. TEL 201-760-3735, 800-926-6579, FAX 201-236-0072, journals@erlbaum.com, http://zerlina.catchword.com/vl=9142511/cl=26/nw=1/rpsv/cw/erlbaum/10939741/contp1.htm, http://www.erlbaum.com. Ed. Barry Kantowitz. adv.: page USD 275; trim 6 x 9.

TRANSPORTATION SAFETY RECOMMENDATIONS. see *PUBLIC HEALTH AND SAFETY*

TRANSPORTATION—Abstracting, Bibliographies, Statistics

BELGIUM. INSTITUT NATIONAL DE STATISTIQUE. ACCIDENTS DE LA CIRCULATION SUR LA VOIE PUBLIQUE AVEC TUES ET BLESSES. see *PUBLIC HEALTH AND SAFETY—Abstracting, Bibliographies, Statistics*

BELGIUM. NATIONAAL INSTITUUT VOOR DE STATISTIEK. VERKEERSONGEVALLEN OP DE OPENBARE WEG MET DODEN OF GEWONDEN. see *PUBLIC HEALTH AND SAFETY—Abstracting, Bibliographies, Statistics*

614 380.5 FRA
E C M T STATISTICAL REPORT ON ROAD ACCIDENTS. Text in French. a. price varies.
Indexed: IIS.
Published by: Organization for Economic Cooperation and Development, European Council of Ministers of Transport, 2 rue Andre Pascal, Paris Cedex 16 75775, France. TEL 33-1-45248200, FAX 33-1-49104276, sales@oecd.org, http://www.oecd.org. **U.S. orders to:** O.E.C.D. Publications and Information Center, 2001 L St, N W, Ste 650, Washington, DC 20036-4922. TEL 202-785-6323.

ITALY. ISTITUTO NAZIONALE DI STATISTICA. STATISTICA DEGLI INCIDENTI STRADALI. see *PUBLIC HEALTH AND SAFETY—Abstracting, Bibliographies, Statistics*

016.3883 016.614 RUS ISSN 0202-9952
REFERATIVNYI ZHURNAL. ORGANIZATSIYA I BEZOPASNOST' DOROZHNOGO DVIZHENIYA. Text in Russian. 1973. m. USD 120. **Document type:** *Abstract/Index.*
—East View. **CCC.**
Published by: Vserossiiskii Institut Nauchnoi i Tekhnicheskoi Informatsii (VINITI), Usievicha ul 20-a, Moscow 125315, Russian Federation. TEL 7-095-1526441, FAX 7-095-943-0060. Ed. Valentin Lukanin. **Dist. by:** Mezhdunarodnaya Kniga, B Yakimanka 39, Moscow 117049, Russian Federation. TEL 7-095-2384967, FAX 7-095-2384634; **US dist. addr.:** East View Publications, 3020 Harbor Ln N, Minneapolis, MN 55447. TEL 612-550-0961.

388.021 ZAF
SOUTH AFRICA. STATISTICS SOUTH AFRICA. ROAD TRAFFIC COLLISIONS. Text in English. a., latest 1999. ZAR 30 domestic; ZAR 33 foreign (effective 2000). **Document type:** *Government.*
Former titles (until Aug.1998): South Africa. Central Statistical Service. Road Traffic Collisions (0258-7793); South Africa. Department of Statistics. Road Traffic Accidents (0584-195X)
Published by: Statistics South Africa/Statistieke Suid-Afrika, Private Bag X44, Pretoria 0001, South Africa. TEL 27-12-310-8911, FAX 27-12-310-8500, info@statssa.pwv.gov.za, http://www.statssa.gov.za.

388 316.8 ZAF
SOUTH AFRICA. STATISTICS SOUTH AFRICA. STATISTICAL RELEASE. ROAD TRAFFIC COLLISIONS. Text in English. m. **Document type:** *Government.*
Formerly (until Aug. 1998): South Africa. Central Statistical Service. Statistical Release. Road Traffic Collisions
Published by: Statistics South Africa/Statistieke Suid-Afrika, Private Bag X44, Pretoria 0001, South Africa. TEL 27-12-310-8911, FAX 27-12-310-8500, info@statssa.pwv.gov.za, http://www.statssa.gov.za.

TRANSPORTATION—Air Transport

363.7 CAN
EMERGENCY RESPONSE GUIDANCE FOR AIRCRAFT INCIDENTS INVOLVING DANGEROUS GOODS. Text in English. biennial. USD 22 (effective 2002).
Related titles: French ed.; Russian ed.; Spanish ed.
Published by: International Civil Aviation Organization, Attn: Document Sales Unit, 999 University St, Montreal, PQ H3C 5H7, Canada. TEL 514-954-8022, FAX 514-954-6769, sales_unit@icao.org.

387.74 614.86 USA
FACTS AND ADVICE FOR AIRLINE PASSENGERS. Text in English. 1979. biennial. USD 5 (effective 2000). **Document type:** *Consumer.* **Description:** Shows how to avoid or minimize the inconvenience of airline service problems.
Published by: Aviation Consumer Action Project, PO Box 19029, Washington, DC 20036. TEL 202-638-4000. R&P Paul Hudson.

FLYING DOCTOR QUEENSLAND. see *HEALTH FACILITIES AND ADMINISTRATION*

370.19 USA ISSN 1050-8414
TL553.6
THE INTERNATIONAL JOURNAL OF AVIATION PSYCHOLOGY. Text in English. 1991. q. USD 50 in US & Canada to individuals; USD 80 elsewhere to individuals; USD 390 in US & Canada to individuals; USD 420 elsewhere to individuals (effective 2002). adv. bk.rev. *Refereed.* **Document type:** *Journal, Academic/Scholarly.* **Description:** Development and management of safe, effective aviation systems from the standpoint of the human operators.
Related titles: Online - full text ed.: ISSN 1532-7108. USD 45 to individuals; USD 351 to institutions (effective 2002) (from CatchWord Ltd., EBSCO Publishing, O C L C Online Computer Library Center, Inc., RoweCom Information Quest, Swets Blackwell, Institute for Scientific Information).
Indexed: ASCA, Curr.Cont., Environ.Sci.Poll.Mgmt., Ergon.Abstr., Int.Aerosp.Abstr., Pollut.Abstr., PsycInfo, Psychol.Abstr. (1991-), Risk Abstr., SSCI, Saf.Sci.Abstr., e-psyche.
—BLDSC (4542.125500), CatchWord, CISTI, Infotrieve, Linda Hall. **CCC.**
Published by: Lawrence Erlbaum Associates, Inc., 10 Industrial Ave, Mahwah, NJ 07430-2262. TEL 201-760-3735, 800-926-6579, FAX 201-236-0072, journals@erlbaum.com, http://www.erlbaum.com/Journals/journals/IJAP/ijap.htm. Ed. Richard S Jensen TEL 740-967-4030. adv.: page USD 325; trim 5 x 8.

387.7 DEU
MONATSBERICHT ANGEZEIGTER FLUGUNFAELLE. Text in German. 1983. m. DEM 80. **Document type:** *Government.*
Formerly: Monatsbericht der Angezeigten Flugunfallunteruntersuchungsstelle
Published by: Luftfahrt-Bundesamt, Flugunfalluntersuchungsstelle, Postfach 3054, Braunschweig 38020, Germany. TEL 0531-2355-0, FAX 0531-2355246. Circ: 100.

387.74 616.02 GBR ISSN 1365-6597
SHEPHARD'S AIR AMBULANCE HANDBOOK. Text in English. a. GBP 35 in United Kingdom; USD 60 foreign (effective 2000). adv. back issues avail.; reprints avail. **Document type:** *Magazine, Trade.* **Description:** Global guide to emergency and medical aviation.
Former titles (until 1995): Air Ambulance Handbook (1355-6061); (until 1994): E M S Helicopter Handbook (0968-6541)
Published by: Shephard Press Ltd., 111 High St, Burnham, Bucks SL1 7JZ, United Kingdom. TEL 44-1628-604311, 800-873-2147, FAX 44-1628-664334, 44-1628-664075, publishing@shephard.co.uk, http://www.shephard.co.uk. Ed. Sara Waddington. Adv. contact Merina Kanelias.

363.7 CAN
TECHNICAL INSTRUCTIONS FOR THE SAFE TRANSPORT OF DANGEROUS GOODS BY AIR. Text in English. biennial. USD 88 (effective 2001).
Related titles: French ed.; Spanish ed.; Russian ed.
Published by: International Civil Aviation Organization, Attn: Document Sales Unit, 999 University St, Montreal, PQ H3C 5H7, Canada. TEL 514-954-8022, FAX 514-954-6769, sales_unit@icao.org.

TRANSPORTATION—Automobiles

ARZT UND AUTO; der kraftfahrende Arzt. see *MEDICAL SCIENCES*

T

ASSOCIATION FOR THE ADVANCEMENT OF AUTOMOTIVE MEDICINE. PROCEEDINGS. see *MEDICAL SCIENCES*

EMERGENCY RESPONSE GUIDEBOOK. see *PUBLIC HEALTH AND SAFETY*

388 USA
FEDERAL MOTOR CARRIER SAFETY ADMINISTRATION REGISTER; a daily summary of motor carrier applications and of decisions and notices. Text in English. d. USD 995 (effective 2001). **Document type:** *Government.*
Published by: U.S. Department of Transportation, Federal Motor Carrier Safety Administration, 400 Seventh St SW, Washington, DC 20590. TEL 202-366-2519, http://www.fmcsa.dot.gov. **Subscr. to:** U.S. Government Printing Office, Superintendent of Documents, PO Box 371954, Pittsburgh, PA 15250-7954. TEL 202-512-1800, FAX 202-512-2250, orders@gpo.gov, http://www.access.gpo.gov.

629.283 614.8 USA ISSN 0164-1344
HE5614.3.C3
JOURNAL OF TRAFFIC SAFETY EDUCATION. Text in English. 1953. q. USD 8. adv. bk.rev.
Related titles: Online - full text ed.: (from H. W. Wilson).
Indexed: Educ.Ind. (Oct.1983-Apr.1991), HRIS.
Published by: California Association for Safety Education, 5151 State University Dr, Los Angeles, CA 90032. TEL 213-343-4622. Ed. William Cole. Circ: 2,800.

LOUISIANA. DEPARTMENT OF PUBLIC SAFETY. SUMMARY OF MOTOR VEHICLE TRAFFIC ACCIDENTS. KENNER. see *PUBLIC HEALTH AND SAFETY*

LOUISIANA. DEPARTMENT OF PUBLIC SAFETY. SUMMARY OF MOTOR VEHICLE TRAFFIC ACCIDENTS. RURAL. see *PUBLIC HEALTH AND SAFETY*

LOUISIANA. DEPARTMENT OF PUBLIC SAFETY. SUMMARY OF MOTOR VEHICLE TRAFFIC ACCIDENTS. SHREVEPORT. see *PUBLIC HEALTH AND SAFETY*

LOUISIANA. DEPARTMENT OF PUBLIC SAFETY. SUMMARY OF MOTOR VEHICLE TRAFFIC ACCIDENTS. STATEWIDE. see *PUBLIC HEALTH AND SAFETY*

MOTOR VEHICLE SAFETY; a report on activities under the National Traffic and Motor Vehicle Safety Act of 1966. see *PUBLIC HEALTH AND SAFETY*

REVUE AUTOMOBILE MEDICALE. see *MEDICAL SCIENCES*

388.3 FRA ISSN 0035-8568
ROUTE. Text in French. 1970 (no.33). q. FRF 40. adv. charts, illus, stat.
Published by: Comite National du Secours Routiers Francais, 50 quai Bleriot, Paris 75016, France. Ed. Pierre Merard. Circ: 7,000.

TRANSPORTATION—Railroads

385 614.85 GBR
SAFETYEXCHANGE; railway safety is everyone's business. Text in English. **Document type:** *Newsletter.*
Published by: Railway Safety, Evergreen House, 160 Euston Rd, London NW1 2DX, United Kingdom. enquiries@railwaysafety.org.uk, http://www.railwaysafety.org.uk/. Ed. Helen Goodman TEL 44-20-7904-7704.

614.8 AUT ISSN 0037-4539
SICHERHEIT ZUERST. Text in German. 1958. q. free per issue. **Document type:** *Trade.*
Indexed: C.I.S. Abstr.
Published by: Versicherungsanstalt der Oesterreichischen Eisenbahnen, Unfallverhuetungsdienst, Linke Wienzeile 48-52, Vienna, W 1060, Austria. TEL 43-1-58848237, FAX 43-1-58848332. Ed. Anton Schifter. Circ: 20,000.

TRANSPORTATION—Roads And Traffic

see also ENGINEERING—Civil Engineering

388.4131 GBR
CAMBRIDGESHIRE COUNTY COUNCIL. ROAD SAFETY PLAN (YEAR). Text in English. a. charts, stat. **Document type:** *Government.* **Description:** Reviews the previous year's road safety activity in Cambridgeshire and sets out action plans for the following year.
Published by: Cambridgeshire County Council, Shire Hall, Castle Hill, Cambridge CB3 0AP, United Kingdom. TEL 44-1223-717111, FAX 44-1223-717201, charterline@cambridgeshire.gov.uk, http://www.camcnty.gov.uk/sub/eandt/rdsafety/index.htm, http://www.cambridgeshire.gov.uk/.

CARE ON THE ROAD. see *PUBLIC HEALTH AND SAFETY*

CONCIENCIA VIAL. see *PUBLIC HEALTH AND SAFETY*

388 624 GBR ISSN 1464-1380
CURRENT TOPICS IN TRANSPORT. Text in English. 1992. irreg. price varies. **Document type:** *Monographic series, Government, Abstract/Index.*
—BLDSC (3504.931000).
Published by: T R L Limited, Old Wokingham Rd, Crowthorne, Berks RG45 6AU, United Kingdom. TEL 44-1344-770783, FAX 44-1344-770193, info@trl.co.uk, http://www.trl.co.uk. **Subscr. to:** .PO Box 303, Wokingham, Berks RG45 6YX, United Kingdom.

INSURANCE INSTITUTE FOR HIGHWAY SAFETY. STATUS REPORT. see *PUBLIC HEALTH AND SAFETY*

LOUISIANA. DEPARTMENT OF PUBLIC SAFETY. SUMMARY OF MOTOR VEHICLE TRAFFIC ACCIDENTS. RURAL. see *PUBLIC HEALTH AND SAFETY*

LOUISIANA. DEPARTMENT OF PUBLIC SAFETY. SUMMARY OF MOTOR VEHICLE TRAFFIC ACCIDENTS. SHREVEPORT. see *PUBLIC HEALTH AND SAFETY*

LOUISIANA. DEPARTMENT OF PUBLIC SAFETY. SUMMARY OF MOTOR VEHICLE TRAFFIC ACCIDENTS. STATEWIDE. see *PUBLIC HEALTH AND SAFETY*

388.4 NLD ISSN 0166-4654
MENSEN OP STRAAT. Text in Dutch. 1963. q. NLG 15, EUR 6.80 (effective 1999). bk.rev. illus. *Refereed.* **Document type:** *Academic/Scholarly.* **Description:** Discusses all aspects of pedestrian safety, including government road safety policies, society initiatives to improve road safety, with particular emphasis on urban areas.
Former titles (until 1977): Voetganger; Feiten, Cijfers, Meningen (0014-9721)
Published by: Voetgangersvereniging/Dutch Pedestrian Association, Emmapark 9, The Hague 2595 ES, Netherlands. TEL 31-70-347-1501, FAX 31-70-381-9654, Voetver@pz.nl. Ed. Sjoerd van Andel. Circ: 3,500.

388 USA
MISSOURI. DIVISION OF HIGHWAY SAFETY (YEAR). HIGHWAY SAFETY PLAN. Text in English. 1971. a. *Refereed.* **Document type:** *Government.*
Former titles: Missouri's Annual Highway Safety Program; Missouri Annual Highway Safety Work Program (0091-1097)
Published by: Division of Highway Safety, PO Box 104808, Jefferson City, MO 65110-4808. TEL 573-751-4161, FAX 573-634-5977, kshikles@mdhs.state.mo.us, http://www.dps.state.mo.us/dps/mdhs/hs.htm. Ed., R&P Vicky S Williams. Circ: 50 (controlled).

388.4131 AUS
MONASH UNIVERSITY ACCIDENT RESEARCH CENTRE. CONSULTANTS' REPORTS SERIES. Text in English. irreg.
Former titles: Australian Transport Safety Bureau. Road Safety Research Report (1445-4467); (until 199?): C R Canberra (0810-770X)
Related titles: Online - full content ed.
Published by: Monash University Accident Research Centre, Clayton Campus, Monash University, PO Box 70A, Monash, VIC 3800, Australia. TEL 61-3-9905-4371, FAX 61-3-9905-4363, muarc.enquire@general.monash.edu.au, http://www.atsb.gov.au/road/research/crreport.cfm, http://www.general.monash.edu.au/muarc.

388.4131 AUS
MONASH UNIVERSITY ACCIDENT RESEARCH CENTRE. MINOR REPORTS SERIES. Text in English. irreg.
Published by: Monash University Accident Research Centre, Clayton Campus, Monash University, PO Box 70A, Monash, VIC 3800, Australia. TEL 61-3-9905-4371, FAX 61-3-9905-4363, muarc.enquire@general.monash.edu.au, http://www.atsb.gov.au/road/research/mrreport.cfm, http://www.general.monash.edu.au/muarc.

388.4131 AUS
MONASH UNIVERSITY ACCIDENT RESEARCH CENTRE. OTHER REPORTS SERIES. Text in English. irreg.
Published by: Monash University Accident Research Centre, Clayton Campus, Monash University, PO Box 70A, Monash, VIC 3800, Australia. TEL 61-3-9905-4371, FAX 61-3-9905-4363, muarc.enquire@general.monash.edu.au, http://www.atsb.gov.au/road/research/orreport.cfm, http://www.general.monash.edu.au/muarc.

MOTOR VEHICLE SAFETY; a report on activities under the National Traffic and Motor Vehicle Safety Act of 1966. see *PUBLIC HEALTH AND SAFETY*

SIGNAL. see *OCCUPATIONAL HEALTH AND SAFETY*

388.31 GBR
T R L NEWS. (Transport Research Laboratory) Text in English. q. free per issue. **Document type:** *Newsletter.*
Related titles: Online - full text ed.
Indexed: Curr.Lit.Traf.& Trans., HRIS.
Published by: T R L Limited, Press and Public Relations Section, Old Wokingham Rd, Crowthorne, Berks RG45 6AU, United Kingdom. TEL 44-1344-773131, FAX 44-1344-770356, info@lib.trl.co.uk, http://www.trl.co.uk. Ed. Sarah Bailey. Circ: 7,000.

388.31 AUT ISSN 0042-4048
VERKEHRSPSYCHOLOGISCHER INFORMATIONSDIENST. Text in German. 1962. a. free per issue. **Document type:** *Corporate.*
Indexed: Dok.Str.
Published by: Kuratorium fuer Verkehrssicherheit, Verkehrspsychologisches Institut, Oelzeltgasse 3, Vienna, W 1031, Austria. TEL 43-1-71770145, FAX 43-1-717709, wernerklemenjak@kfv.or.at, http://www.kfv.or.at. Ed. Werner Klemenjak. Circ: 2,000.

TRANSPORTATION—Ships And Shipping

RECOMMENDATIONS ON THE SAFE USE OF PESTICIDES IN SHIPS. see *ENVIRONMENTAL STUDIES—Toxicology And Environmental Safety*

SHIP SAFETY AND POLLUTION PREVENTION - SHIP MANAGEMENT AND PORT STATE CONTROL. see *ENVIRONMENTAL STUDIES—Toxicology And Environmental Safety*

SOLAS - INTERNATIONAL CONVENTION FOR THE SAFETY OF LIFE AT SEA. AMENDMENTS. see *ENVIRONMENTAL STUDIES—Toxicology And Environmental Safety*

TRANSPORTATION—Trucks And Trucking

HAZARDOUS MATERIALS REGULATION GUIDE. see *ENVIRONMENTAL STUDIES—Toxicology And Environmental Safety*

388.324 614.85 USA ISSN 1092-3101
MOTOR CARRIER SAFETY REPORT. Text in English. 1974. m. USD 125 (effective 2002). **Description:** Covers federal and state motor carrier safety requirements and related subject.
Published by: J.J. Keller & Associates, Inc., 3003 W Breezewood Lane, Box 368, Neenah, WI 54957-0368. TEL 920-722-2848, 800-327-6868, FAX 920-727-7526, http://www.jjkeller.com.

TRAVEL AND TOURISM

see also GEOGRAPHY; HOTELS AND RESTAURANTS

AERZTLICHES JOURNAL REISE UND MEDIZIN. see *MEDICAL SCIENCES*

T

U

943 DEU ISSN 1434-6672
BAD TOELZ AKTUELL; Informationen und Veranstaltungen. Text in German. 1950. m. DEM 48 (effective 2001). adv. play rev. **Document type:** *Bulletin, Consumer.* **Description:** Information for visitors to Bad Toelz, including local events and health treatments.
Formerly: Kurjournal - Bad Toelz
Published by: Tourist-Information, Ludwigstr 11, Bad Toelz 83646, Germany. TEL 49-8041-7867-0, FAX 49-8041-786756, info@bad-toelz.de, http://www.bad-toelz.de. Ed. Corinna Ewerdwalbesloh. Adv. contact Stephanie Lackermeier TEL 49-8041-7551936. Circ: 6,000.

910.09 CAN ISSN 0821-5758
DOCTOR'S REVIEW; leisure-time journal for physicians. Text in English. 1983. m. CND 46, USD 90 domestic; CND 110 foreign.
Published by: Parkhurst Publishing, 400 McGill St, 3rd Fl, Montreal, PQ H2Y 2G1, Canada. FAX 514-397-0228, parkhurst@vir.com, http://www.bestmdsite.com. Ed. Madeleine Partous. Pub. David Elkins. Circ: 36,220 (controlled).

FACTS AND ADVICE FOR AIRLINE PASSENGERS. see *TRANSPORTATION—Air Transport*

FLUG- UND REISEMEDIZIN; Tropenmedizin - Tauchmedizin - Bergmedizin - Expeditionsmedizin - Polarmedizin. see *MEDICAL SCIENCES*

910.202 613.7 USA ISSN 1057-8048
RA802
FODOR'S HEALTHY ESCAPES. Text in English. 1989. irreg., latest vol.4, 1995. USD 15.
Formerly (until 1990): Fodor's Health and Fitness Vacations (1047-5052)
Published by: Fodor's Travel Publications, Inc. (Subsidiary of: Random House, Inc.), 201 E 50th St, New York, NY 10022. TEL 800-733-3000. Ed. Allison B Stern. **Dist. by:** Random House Inc., 400 Hahn Rd, Westminster, MD 21157.

910.91 614 USA
▼ **HEALTHY TRAVELER.** Text in English. 2002. q. free with subscr. to National Geographic Traveler. **Document type:** *Magazine, Consumer.* **Description:** Contains information on regional health alerts, list of English speaking Hospitals and health facilities, medical information on travelling with the elderly or children, and other related travel health topics.
Related titles: ♦ Supplement to: National Geographic Traveler. ISSN 0747-0932.
Published by: National Geographic Society, 1145 17th St, N W, Washington, DC 20036.

INTERNATIONAL TRAVEL HEALTH GUIDE. see *MEDICAL SCIENCES*

JOURNAL OF TRAVEL MEDICINE. see *MEDICAL SCIENCES*

LIFESTYLE AND TRAVEL FOR PHYSICIANS. see *LIFESTYLE*

MAENNER AKTUELL. see *HOMOSEXUALITY*

614.86 DEU
MEINE GESUNDHEIT. Text in German. 1981. 4/yr. adv. **Document type:** *Magazine, Consumer.*
Published by: Otto Hoffmanns Verlag GmbH, Arnulfstr 10, Munich 80335, Germany. TEL 49-89-545845-0, FAX 49-89-54584520. Ed. Kirsten Westphal. adv.: B&W page DEM 31,500, color page DEM 43,200. Circ: 7,400,000.

910.202 USA ISSN 0745-4554
PHYSICIANS' TRAVEL & MEETING GUIDE. Text in English. 1982. m. USD 70 in the Americas to individuals; USD 105 elsewhere to individuals; USD 111 in the Americas to institutions; USD 140 elsewhere to institutions (effective 2000). adv. tr.lit. **Document type:** *Trade.* **Description:** Helps physicians plan their attendance at medical meetings as well as their personal and business travel.
—CCC.
Published by: Quadrant HealthCom, 26 Main St, Ste A, Chatham, NJ 07928-2402. TEL 973-701-8900, FAX 973-701-8892. Ed. Bea Riemschneider. Pub. Terry Bean. Adv. contact Denise Labowicz. Circ: 113,000.

SPA FINDER. see *PHYSICAL FITNESS AND HYGIENE*

STUDIES IN PHYSICAL CULTURE AND TOURISM. see *PHYSICAL FITNESS AND HYGIENE*

TRAVEL MEDICINE ADVISOR. see *MEDICAL SCIENCES*

TRAVEL MEDICINE INTERNATIONAL. see *MEDICAL SCIENCES*

910 610 USA ISSN 0899-2169
TRAVELING HEALTHY. Text in English. 1988. bi-m. USD 45 domestic; USD 49 foreign (effective 2001). back issues avail. **Document type:** *Newsletter.* **Description:** Alerts travelers about health and medical issues.
Published by: Travel Medicine, Inc., 369 Pleasant St., Northampton, MA 01060-0795. TEL 413-584-0381, FAX 413-584-6656, travmed@travmed.com, http://www.travelinghealthy.com. Ed. Dr. Karl Neumann. Pub. Dr. Stuart R Rose. Circ: 1,250 (paid and free).

TRUCKS AND TRUCKING

see TRANSPORTATION—Trucks And Trucking

UROLOGY AND NEPHROLOGY

see MEDICAL SCIENCES—Urology And Nephrology

VETERINARY SCIENCE

A N Z C C A R T NEWS. see *ANIMAL WELFARE*

636.089 USA ISSN 1616-8771
▼ **A O RECOMMENDED LITERATURE. VETERINARY TRAUMA AND DISORDERS.** Text in English. 2001. 6/yr. EUR 165 to individuals; EUR 248 to institutions (effective 2002). **Document type:** *Journal, Academic/Scholarly.*
Related titles: Online - full text ed.
Published by: Thieme Medical Publishers, 333 Seventh Ave, New York, NY 10001. TEL 212-760-0888, 800-782-3488, FAX 212-947-1112, custserv@thieme.com, http://www.thieme.com.

636.089 USA
A V E A NEWSLETTER✱. Text in English. 1936. q. membership. **Document type:** *Newsletter.* **Description:** Concerns exhibiting at veterinary conventions.
Published by: American Veterinary Exhibitors Association, 106 W 11th St, Ste 1600, Kansas City, MO 64105-1806. TEL 805-683-0489. Ed. Fred Hamlin. Circ: 200.

636.089029 USA ISSN 0898-6657
SF611
A V M A DIRECTORY. Text in English. 1920. a. USD 100; USD 120 foreign (effective 2001). adv. charts, stat. **Document type:** *Directory.* **Description:** Provides historic and current guidance information about the profession, alphabetic and geographic listings of all AVMA members and many non-members, and listings for many governmental agencies, allied veterinary groups, and other organizations concerned with animal health and welfare.
Formerly (until 1984): American Veterinary Medical Association. Directory (0066-1147)
Indexed: Curr.Adv.Ecol.Sci., SRI.
—CISTI.
Published by: American Veterinary Medical Association, 1931 N Meacham Rd, Ste 100, Schaumburg, IL 60173-4360. TEL 847-925-8070, FAX 847-925-1329. Ed. Amy Voigt. R&P Anna Marie Garge. Circ: 62,400 (paid).

ABSTRACTS OF BULGARIAN SCIENTIFIC LITERATURE. AGRICULTURE AND FORESTRY. VETERINARY MEDICINE. see *VETERINARY SCIENCE—Abstracting, Bibliographies, Statistics*

636.089 FRA ISSN 0001-4192
CODEN: BAVFAV
ACADEMIE VETERINAIRE DE FRANCE. BULLETIN. Text in French. 1844. 4/yr. FRF 700 domestic; FRF 900 foreign (effective 2000). adv. bk.rev. abstr, bibl, charts, illus, stat. index. **Document type:** *Bulletin.*
Indexed: Agri.& Environ.Biotech.Abstr. (coverage dropped), Anim.Breed.Abstr., Biol.Abstr., Chem.Abstr., Curr.Adv.Ecol.Sci., Curr.Cont. (coverage dropped), Dairy Sci.Abstr., Derwent Biotech.Abstr., Food Sci.& Tech.Abstr., Helminthol.Abstr., Ind.Vet., Nutr.Abstr., Poult.Abstr., Rev.Plant Path., Vet.Bull.
—BLDSC (2378.000000), CASDDS, CISTI, GNLM, Linda Hall.
Published by: Academie Veterinaire de France, 60 bd. Latour-Maubourg, Paris 75007, France. FAX 33-3-20877132, TELEX 820 187 F. Ed. Marc V Catsaras. Circ: 800.

636.089 POL ISSN 0860-2840
CODEN: AAAVEZ
ACTA ACADEMIAE AGRICULTURAE AC TECHNICAE OLSTENENSIS. VETERINARIA/AGRICULTURAL AND TECHNICAL ACADEMY IN OLSZTYN. VETERINARY MEDICINE. Text in Polish; Summaries in English, Polish. 1972. irreg. price varies. adv. bibl, charts, illus. **Document type:** *Academic/Scholarly.*
Formerly (until 1985): Akademia Rolniczo-Techniczna. Zeszyty Naukowe. Weterynaria (0324-9220)
Indexed: AgroLibrex, Anim.Breed.Abstr., Chem.Abstr., Curr.Cont. (coverage dropped), Dairy Sci.Abstr., Ind.Vet., Pig News & Info., Vet.Bull.
—CASDDS, CISTI.
Published by: (Akademia Rolniczo-Techniczna im. M. Oczapowskiego), Wydawnictwo A R T Olsztyn, Blok 12, Olsztyn-Kortowo 10-957, Poland. TEL 48-89-5273310, artbib@moskit.art.olsztyn.pl. Ed. Barbara Grudniewska. R&P Jolanta Mieszkalska. Adv. contact Maciej Gajecki. Circ: 130 (controlled). **Dist. by:** Ars Polona, Krakowskie Przedmiescie 7, Warsaw, Poland. TEL 48-22-265334.

636.089 ITA ISSN 0001-6136
CODEN: AMVEAX
ACTA MEDICA VETERINARIA. Text in Italian; Summaries in English, French, German, Spanish. 1955. bi-m. USD 10. bk.rev. charts, illus, tr.lit. index.
Indexed: Anim.Breed.Abstr., Biol.Abstr., Chem.Abstr., Dairy Sci.Abstr., Excerp.Med., Food Sci.& Tech.Abstr., Helminthol.Abstr., Herb.Abstr., Ind.Med. (coverage dropped), Ind.Vet., Nutr.Abstr., Pig News & Info., Protozool.Abstr., Rev.Med.& Vet.Mycol., Small Anim.Abstr., Vet.Bull.
—CASDDS, CISTI, GNLM, Linda Hall.
Published by: Facolta di Medicina Veterinaria, Via Veterinaria, 1, Naples, NA 80137, Italy.

636.08 ESP ISSN 0214-039X
ACTA VETERINARIA. Text in Spanish. 1987. a. ESP 2,000.
Indexed: Curr.Cont. (coverage dropped), Helminthol.Abstr., Ind.SST.
—CINDOC.
Published by: Universidad de Extremadura, Servicio de Publicaciones, Ctra. de Trujillo, s-n, Caceres 10071, Spain.

636.08 YUG ISSN 0567-8315
CODEN: ACVTA8
ACTA VETERINARIA. Text in Serbo-Croatian. 1951. bi-m. USD 60 foreign (effective 2001). adv. abstr, bibl, charts, illus, stat. back issues avail. *Refereed.* **Document type:** *Academic/Scholarly.*
Related titles: Online - full text ed.: (from Institute for Scientific Information).
Indexed: Anim.Breed.Abstr., Bio-Contr.News & Info., Curr.Cont., Dairy Sci.Abstr., Field Crop Abstr., Focus on: Vet.Sci.& Med., Food Sci.& Tech.Abstr., Herb.Abstr., INIS Atomind., Ind.Vet., Maize Abstr., Nutr.Abstr., Pig News & Info., Poult.Abstr., Protozool.Abstr., Ref.Zh., Rev.Appl.Entomol., Rev.Med.& Vet.Mycol., Soyabean Abstr., Sugar Ind.Abstr., Triticale Abstr., Vet.Bull., Weed Abstr., Zoo.Rec.
—BLDSC (0670.880000), CASDDS, CISTI, IDS.
Published by: Veterinarski Fakultet, Bulevar J N A 18, Belgrade, Yugoslavia. vks@vet.bg.ac.yu. Ed., R&P Velibor Stojic. Adv. contact Jadranka Tijanic. Circ: 200.

636.089 CZE ISSN 0001-7213
CODEN: ACVTB9
ACTA VETERINARIA BRNO. Text in English; Summaries in Czech, English, Russian. 1922. q. USD 72 in Europe; USD 76 elsewhere (effective 2000). adv. bk.rev. bibl, charts, illus. index. cum.index. *Refereed.* **Document type:** *Academic/Scholarly.* **Description:** Publishes original research articles in basic and applied veterinary sciences and medicine, including food hygiene.
Formerly: Acta Universitatis Agriculturae. Facultas Veterinaria: Rada B
Related titles: Online - full text ed.: (from Institute for Scientific Information).

Indexed: ASCA, AgBiotech, Agri.Eng.Abstr., Anim.Breed.Abstr., Apic.Abstr., Aqua.Sci.& Fish.Abstr., Aquacult.Abstr., Biol.Abstr., Chem.Abstr., Chem.Indus.Notes, Chem.Titles, Crop Physiol.Abstr., Curr.Adv.Ecol.Sci., Curr.Cont., Dairy Sci.Abstr., Excerp.Med., Field Crop Abstr., Focus on: Vet.Sci.& Med., Food Sci.& Tech.Abstr., Helminthol.Abstr., Hort.Abstr., Ind.Vet., Nutr.Abstr., Pig News & Info., Poult.Abstr., Protozool.Abstr., Rev.Med.& Vet.Mycol., Sci.Cit.Ind. (coverage dropped), Sport Fish.Abstr., Triticale Abstr., Vet.Bull., Weed Abstr., Wild.Rev., Zoo.Rec.
—CASDDS, CISTI, IDS, ingenta, Linda Hall.
Published by: University of Veterinary and Pharmaceutical Sciences, Palackeho 1-3, Brno 61242, Czech Republic. TEL 420-5-4156-2505, FAX 420-5-412-1151, baranyi@dior.ics.muni.cz, actavet@vfu.cz, http://www.vfu.cz/acta-vet/actavet.html. Ed., R&P, Adv. contact Dr. Eva Baranyiova. Circ: 500.

636.089 HUN ISSN 0236-6290
CODEN: AVHUEA
ACTA VETERINARIA HUNGARICA. Text in English. 1951. q. USD 198 (effective 2002). adv. bk.rev. bibl, charts, illus, abstr. index. 120 p./no. back issues avail. *Refereed.* **Document type:** *Journal, Academic/Scholarly.* **Description:** Publishes studies concerned with research on morphology, physiology, biochemistry, microbiology, immunology, reproduction biology and clinical veterinary medicine, etiology, pathogenesis, diagnostics and control of infectious, parasitic and metabolic diseases.
Formerly (until 1982): Academiae Scientiarum Hungaricae. Acta Veterinaria (0001-7205)
Related titles: Online - full text ed.: (from Institute for Scientific Information).
Indexed: ASCA, AgBiotech, Agri.& Environ.Biotech.Abstr. (coverage dropped), Anim.Breed.Abstr., Biol.Abstr., Chem.Abstr., Chem.Indus.Notes, Chem.Titles, Curr.Adv.Ecol.Sci., Curr.Cont., Dairy Sci.Abstr., Derwent Biotech.Abstr., Excerp.Med., Focus on: Vet.Sci.& Med., Helminthol.Abstr., INIS Atomind., Ind.Med. (1983-), Ind.Vet., Nutr.Abstr., Pig News & Info., Postharvest, Poult.Abstr., Protozool.Abstr., Rev.Appl.Entomol., Rev.Med.& Vet.Mycol., Rev.Plant Path., Sci.Cit.Ind., Soils & Fert., Triticale Abstr., Vet.Bull., Weed Abstr., Zoo.Rec.
—BLDSC (0670.980000), CASDDS, CISTI, GNLM, IDS, Infotrieve, KNAW, Linda Hall. **CCC.**
Published by: (Magyar Tudomanyos Akademia, Magyar Tudomanyos Akademia, Acta Veterinaria/Hungarian Academy of Sciences), Akademiai Kiado Rt., PO Box 245, Budapest 1519, Hungary. TEL 36-1-4648233, FAX 36-1-4648297, journals@akkrt.hu, http://www.akkrt.hu. Ed. Janos Meszaros. adv.: B&W page HUF 40,000, color page HUF 100,000; trim 237 x 165.

636.089 DNK ISSN 0044-605X
CODEN: AVSCA7
ACTA VETERINARIA SCANDINAVICA. Text in English; Summaries in Danish, English. 1959. q. DKK 1,125 (effective 1999). bibl, charts, illus. *Refereed.* **Document type:** *Academic/Scholarly.*
Related titles: Online - full text ed.: (from Institute for Scientific Information); ♦ Supplement: Acta Veterinaria Scandinavica. Supplementum. ISSN 0065-1699.
Indexed: ASCA, AgBiotech, Agri.& Environ.Biotech.Abstr. (coverage dropped), Anim.Breed.Abstr., Bio-Contr.News & Info., Biol.Abstr., Chem.Abstr., Chem.Indus.Notes, Chem.Titles, Curr.Adv.Ecol.Sci., Curr.Cont., Dairy Sci.Abstr., Derwent Biotech.Abstr., Excerp.Med., Focus on: Vet.Sci.& Med., Food Sci.& Tech.Abstr., Helminthol.Abstr., INIS Atomind., Ind.Med. (1959-), Ind.Sci.Rev., Ind.Vet., Nutr.Abstr., Pig News & Info., Poult.Abstr., Protozool.Abstr., Ref.Zh., Rev.Appl.Entomol., Rev.Med.& Vet.Mycol., Rev.Plant Path., Sci.Cit.Ind., Small Anim.Abstr., Soils & Fert., Sport Fish.Abstr., Triticale Abstr., Vet.Bull., Wild.Rev., World Ag.Econ.& Rur.Soc.Abstr., Zoo.Rec.
—BLDSC (0671.300000), CASDDS, CISTI, GNLM, IDS, ingenta, Linda Hall.
Published by: (Societatum Veteranariarum Scandanivacarum), Danske Dyrlaegeforening, Rosenlunds Alle 8, Vanlose 2720, Denmark. TEL 45-38-71-08-88, FAX 45-38-71-03-22. Ed. Dr. J F Agger.

636.089 DNK ISSN 0065-1699
SF604 CODEN: AVSPAC
ACTA VETERINARIA SCANDINAVICA. SUPPLEMENTUM. Text in English, French, German; Summaries in English, German. 1961. irreg. DKK 1,125 (effective 1999). **Document type:** *Academic/Scholarly.*
Related titles: ♦ Supplement to: Acta Veterinaria Scandinavica. ISSN 0044-605X.
Indexed: Abstr.Hyg., Biol.Abstr., Dairy Sci.Abstr., Food Sci.& Tech.Abstr., INIS Atomind., Ind.Med. (1966-), Ind.Vet., Nutr.Abstr., Pig News & Info., Poult.Abstr., Ref.Zh., Vet.Bull., World Ag.Econ.& Rur.Soc.Abstr., Zoo.Rec.
—BLDSC (0671.301000), CASDDS, CISTI, ingenta, Linda Hall.
Published by: (Societatum Veteranariarum Scandanivacarum), Danske Dyrlaegeforening, Rosenlunds Alle 8, Vanlose 2720, Denmark. TEL 45-38-71-08-88, FAX 45-38-71-03-22. Ed. Dr. J F Agger.

636.089 MEX
ACTUALIDAD VETERINARIA. Text in Spanish. 1976. 6/yr.
Address: Via GUSTAVO BAZ 118, Bosque de Echegaray, Naucalpan, MEX 53310, Mexico. Ed. Alfonso Ortega Said. Circ: 5,000.

ADVANCES IN ANIMAL PHYSIOLOGY AND ANIMAL NUTRITION/FORTSCHRITTE IN DER TIERPHYSIOLOGIE UND TIERERNAEHRUNG. see *BIOLOGY—Physiology*

636.089 USA ISSN 1041-7826
ADVANCES IN SMALL ANIMAL MEDICINE AND SURGERY; a monthly review of current developments in veterinary medicine. Text in English. 1988. m. USD 92 domestic to individuals; USD 148 foreign to individuals; USD 140 domestic to institutions; USD 197 foreign to institutions; USD 57 domestic to students; USD 76 foreign to students; USD 17 per issue (effective 2001). *Refereed.* **Document type:** *Newsletter, Abstract/Index.* **Description:** Provides insight into specific topics and allows veterinarians and veterinary technicians to apply new tests and treatments in their practices. Abstracts material from recent publications and presentations.
—Infotrieve. **CCC.**
Published by: W.B. Saunders Co. (Subsidiary of: Harcourt Publishers Ltd.), 11830 Westline Industrial Dr, St Louis, MO 63146. TEL 800-325-4177, http://www.wbsaunders.com. Ed. C B Chastain. **Subscr. to:** Periodicals Fulfillment, W B Saunders Co, 6277 Sea Harbor Dr, 4th Fl, Orlando, FL 32891-4800.

636.089 GBR
ADVANCES IN VETERINARY DERMATOLOGY. Text in English. irreg., latest vol.2, 1993. price varies. *Refereed.* **Document type:** *Proceedings.*
—BLDSC (0711.755000).
Published by: Pergamon (Subsidiary of: Elsevier Science), The Boulevard, Langford Ln, East Park, Kidlington, Oxford OXB 1GB, United Kingdom. FAX 44-1865-843010, nlinfo-f@elsevier.nl; usinfo-f@elsevier.com; forinfo-kyf04035@niftyserve.or.jp, nlinfo-f@elsevier/nl; usinfo-f@elsevier.com; forinfo-kyf04035@niftyserve.or.jp, http://www.elsevier.nl/. **Subscr. in Australasia and the Far East to:** Elsevier Science (Singapore) Pte Ltd, No.1 Temasek Ave, 17-01 Millenia Tower, Singapore 039192, Singapore. TEL 65-434-3727, FAX 65-337-2230; **Subscr. in the Americas to:** Elsevier Science, PO Box 945, New York, NY 10159-0945. TEL 212-633-3730, FAX 212-633-3680, usinfo-f@elsevier.com, http://www.elsevier.com; **Subscr. to:** Elsevier Science BV, PO Box 211, Amsterdam 1000 AE, Netherlands. TEL 31-20-485-3757, FAX 31-20-485-3432, nlinfo-f@elsevier.nl, http://www.elsevier.nl.

636.089 USA
SF745 CODEN: AVSCB8
ADVANCES IN VETERINARY MEDICINE. Text in English. 1953. irreg., latest vol.40, 1997. index. reprint service avail. from ISI. *Refereed.* **Document type:** *Monographic series.*
Formerly: Advances in Veterinary Science and Comparative Medicine (0065-3519)
Related titles: Online - full text ed.: (from Institute for Scientific Information).
Indexed: ASCA, Agri.& Environ.Biotech.Abstr. (coverage dropped), Anim.Breed.Abstr., Biol.Abstr., Chem.Abstr., Chem.Indus.Notes, Chem.Titles, Dairy Sci.Abstr., Dent.Ind., Excerp.Med., Focus on: Vet.Sci.& Med., Helminthol.Abstr., INIS Atomind., Ind.Med. (1997-), Ind.Sci.Rev., Ind.Vet., Nutr.Abstr., Pig News & Info., Protozool.Abstr., Sci.Cit.Ind., Vet.Bull., Zoo.Rec.
—BLDSC (0711.780000), CASDDS, CISTI, GNLM, ingenta, Linda Hall. **CCC.**
Published by: Academic Press, Inc., Journal Division (Subsidiary of: Harcourt Brace & Company), 525 B St, Ste 1900, San Diego, CA 92101-4495. TEL 619-231-0926, FAX 619-699-6715. Eds. Charles E Cornelius, Charles F Simpson. **Subscr. to:** Order Dept., 6277 Sea Harbor Dr, 4th Fl, Orlando, FL 32887. TEL 800-321-5068.

AGBIOTECH REPORTER; agricultural research - business. see *AGRICULTURE*

THE AGRICULTURAL AND VETERINARY PHARMACIST. see *PHARMACY AND PHARMACOLOGY*

AGROTROPICA. see *AGRICULTURE*

636.089 POL ISSN 0137-1975
CODEN: ZNRWA9
AKADEMIA ROLNICZA WE WROCLAWIU. ZESZYTY NAUKOWE. WETERYNARIA. Text in Polish. 1955. irreg. price varies. **Document type:** *Academic/Scholarly.*
Formerly (until 1973): Wyzsza Szkola Rolnicza we Wroclawiu. Zeszyty Naukowe. Weterynaria (0520-9315)
Indexed: AgroLibrex.
—CASDDS, CISTI.
Published by: Akademia Rolnicza we Wroclawiu, Ul Norwida 25, Wroclaw 50375, Poland. FAX 48-71-229576, wyd@ozi.ar.wroc.pl. Circ: 350. **Subscr. to:** Wydawnictwo Akademii Rolniczej, ul Sopocka 23, Wroclaw 50344, Poland. TEL 48-71-3281277.

636.089 USA
(YEAR) ALLEN D. LEMAN SWINE CONFERENCE. PROCEEDINGS. Text in English. a. USD 45 (effective 2000). **Document type:** *Proceedings, Academic/Scholarly.*
Published by: University of Minnesota, College of Veterinary Medicine, 1365 Gortner Ave, 440 Veterinary Teaching Hospital, Saint Paul, MN 55108-1016. TEL 612-624-3434, FAX 612-625-5755, 800-380-8636, vop@tc.umn.edu, http://www.cvm.umn.edu/outreach.

590 636.089 ITA
ALLEVATORE* . Text in Italian. 1945. w. ITL 40,000.
Published by: Associazione Italiana Allevatori/Italian Breeders' Association, Via Tomasetti 9, Rome, RM 00161, Italy. TEL 39-6-8550207. Ed. Fortunato Tirelli. adv.: color page ITL 2,400,000. Circ: 76,000.

636.089 USA ISSN 0164-1999
SF605 CODEN: SPAHDN
AMERICAN ANIMAL HOSPITAL ASSOCIATION. ANNUAL MEETING SCIENTIFIC PROCEEDINGS. Text in English. a. USD 42 to non-members (effective 2000). adv. **Document type:** *Proceedings.*
—CASDDS.
Published by: American Animal Hospital Association, PO Box 150899, Denver, CO 80215-0899. TEL 303-986-2800, FAX 303-986-1700. R&P Linda Sears. Adv. contact Stephanie Pates.

636.089 USA ISSN 0587-2871
SF601 CODEN: JAAHBL
AMERICAN ANIMAL HOSPITAL ASSOCIATION. JOURNAL. Text in English. 1965. bi-m. USD 107 in US & Canada (effective 2001). adv. bk.rev. abstr, charts, illus, tr.lit. Index. back issues avail.; reprint service avail. from PQC. *Refereed.* **Document type:** *Journal, Academic/Scholarly.* **Description:** Contains accurate, timely, scientific, and technical information pertaining to the practice of small animal medicine and surgery.
Formerly: American Animal Hospital Association Bulletin (0002-7251)
Related titles: Microform ed.: (from PQC); Online - full text ed.: (from Institute for Scientific Information).
Indexed: ASCA, Agricola, Anim.Breed.Abstr., Biol.& Agr.Ind. (Mar.1983-), Biol.Abstr., Chem.Abstr., Curr.Cont., Derwent Biotech.Abstr., Excerp.Med., Focus on: Vet.Sci.& Med., Helminthol.Abstr., Ind.Med. (1965-), Ind.Sci.Rev., Ind.Vet., Nutr.Abstr., Protozool.Abstr., Ref.Zh., Rev.Appl.Entomol., Rev.Med.& Vet.Mycol., Rev.Plant Path., Sci.Cit.Ind., Small Anim.Abstr., Vet.Bull., Wild.Rev.
—BLDSC (4683.790000), CASDDS, CISTI, EMDOCS, GNLM, IDS, ingenta. **CCC.**
Published by: American Animal Hospital Association, 12575 W Bayaud Ave, Lakewood, CO 80228. TEL 303-986-2800, FAX 303-986-1700, jaaha@aahanet.com, http://www.aahanet.org/web/journal_overview.html. Ed. Dr. Walt Ingwersen. R&P Loraine Miller. Adv. contact Stephanie Pates. B&W page USD 1,200, color page USD 2,600. Circ: 14,100 (paid and controlled).

636.089 USA ISSN 1079-9737
AMERICAN ASSOCIATION OF BOVINE PRACTITIONERS CONFERENCE. Text in English. a. USD 35 (effective 2000). **Document type:** *Proceedings.*
Formerly (until 1991): American Association of Bovine Practitioners. Proceedings of the Annual Convention (0743-0450)
Indexed: Agricola.
—BLDSC (6840.583000).

Published by: American Association of Bovine Practitioners, c/o Dr Bob Smith, 3404 Live Oak Lane, Stillwater, OK 74075. TEL 405-372-3693, FAX 405-372-0939. R&P Bob Smith. Circ: 6,000.

636.089 USA ISSN 0065-7182
AMERICAN ASSOCIATION OF EQUINE PRACTITIONERS. PROCEEDINGS OF THE ANNUAL CONVENTION. Text in English. 1956 (2nd). a. USD 70 to non-members; USD 35 to members. back issues avail. *Refereed.* **Document type:** *Proceedings.* **Description:** Provides documentation of the scientific presentations in abstract and review paper form, available at the AAEP annual convention held the first weekend of December. Topics include EPM, equine orthopedic surgery and colic.
Related titles: Microfilm ed.: (from PQC).
Indexed: AgBiotech, Agricola, Anim.Breed.Abstr., Helminthol.Abstr., Ind.Vet., Protozool.Abstr., Rev.Med.& Vet.Mycol., Vet.Bull.
—BLDSC (6840.585000), CISTI.
Published by: American Association of Equine Practitioners, 4075 Iron Works Pike, Lexington, KY 40511-8434. TEL 606-233-0147, FAX 606-233-1968, rahelaaep@aol.com, http://www.aaep.org. Ed., R&P Rahel Klaphere. Circ: 6,000.

636.08 USA
AMERICAN ASSOCIATION OF ZOO VETERINARIANS. ANNUAL PROCEEDINGS. Text in English. 1968. a. USD 45 per issue (effective 2000). back issues avail. **Document type:** *Proceedings.* **Description:** Covers zoo and wildlife veterinary medicine.
Indexed: Derwent Biotech.Abstr., Sport Fish.Abstr., Wild.Rev., Zoo.Rec.
Published by: American Association of Zoo Veterinarians, 6 North Pennell Rd, Media, PA 19063. TEL 610-892-4812, FAX 610-892-4813, http:// www.worldzoo.org. Ed., R&P Wilbur B Amond. Circ: 1,250.

636.089 USA ISSN 0894-7708
CODEN: PAVME6
AMERICAN COLLEGE OF VETERINARY INTERNAL MEDICINE. PROCEEDINGS*. Text in English. 1983. a. USD 45; USD 50 foreign. adv. back issues avail. **Document type:** *Proceedings.* **Description:** Covers topics in internal medicine, cardiology, oncology, neurology, nutrition, clinical pathology, comparative endocrinology, comparative gastroenterology, urology and nephrology, and liver study.
Indexed: Zoo.Rec.
—BLDSC (6842.444000).
Published by: American College of Veterinary Internal Medicine, 1997 Wadsworth Blvd, No A, Lakewood, CO 80215-3327. TEL 303-980-7136, FAX 303-980-7137. Ed. Robert Denovo. R&P, Adv. contact June Johnson.

636.089 USA ISSN 1526-2499
AMERICAN FUND FOR ALTERNATIVES TO ANIMAL RESEARCH. NEWS ABSTRACTS. Text in English. 1978. 3/yr. USD 15 per academic year domestic to individuals; USD 20 per academic year foreign to individuals; USD 10 per academic year to students (effective 2001 - 2002). bk.rev. bibl. back issues avail. **Document type:** *Bulletin, Consumer.* **Description:** Provides financing for scientific programs to develop, evaluate or teach alternatives to animals in research, testing and education.
Related titles: Fax ed.; Online - full text ed.
Published by: American Fund for Alternatives to Animal Research, 175 W 12th St, No 16G, New York, NY 10011-8220. TEL 212-989-8073, FAX 212-989-8073, thurston@accesst.com. Ed., R&P, Adv. contact Ethel Thurston. Circ: 2,000 (paid); 5,000 (controlled).

We target and finance planned replacements for animals in research. The American Fund for Alternatives to Animal Research's science board consists only of active researchers currently publishing in the forefront of science. No animal is used on any AFAAR program. The 35 grants awarded since our founding in 1977 have saved hundreds of animals and opened up new fields of science. Thousands more must depend on your generous support. To plan a gift or bequest, contact: The American Fund for Alternatives to Animal Research (AFAAR), 175 W. 12th St., #16G, New York, NY 10011, 212-989-8073. *Publisher provided annotation.*

636.7 USA
AMERICAN HEARTWORM SOCIETY. BULLETIN. Text in English. 1974. q. USD 48. adv. **Document type:** *Bulletin, Proceedings.* **Description:** Keeping up on current research and commercial development on the prevention and treatment of heartworm disease in dogs.
Published by: American Heartworm Society, 161 S Lincolnway, Ste 302, N, Aurora, IL 60542. TEL 630-844-9676. Ed. Dr. R Lee Seward. R&P Eve C Larocca. Circ: 1,200.

636.089 USA ISSN 1053-5608
SF992.H4
AMERICAN HEARTWORM SOCIETY. SYMPOSIUM PROCEEDINGS. Text in English. 1977. triennial. USD 48 to non-members; USD 44 to members. **Document type:** *Proceedings.*
Published by: American Heartworm Society, 161 S Lincolnway, Ste 302, N, Aurora, IL 60542. TEL 630-844-9676.

636.087 USA
AMERICAN HOLISTIC VETERINARY MEDICAL ASSOCIATION. JOURNAL. Text in English. 1982. q. USD 65 domestic to membership; USD 90 foreign to membership (effective 2000). adv. bk.rev. **Document type:** *Trade.* **Description:** Promotes natural healing, preventive health care, nutrition and avoidance of drugs and medication in Veterinary medicine.
Formerly (until Sep. 1989): American Holistic Veterinary Medical Association. Newsletter
Indexed: Wild.Rev.
Published by: American Holistic Veterinary Medical Association, 2214 Old Emmorton Rd, Bel Air, MD 21015. TEL 410-569-0795, FAX 410-569-2346, ahvma@compuserve.com. Ed., R&P Jan A Bergeron TEL 732-671-7856. Pub. Carvel G Tiekert. Adv. contact Theresa Mall. page USD 375. Circ: 1,000.

AMERICAN JOURNAL OF PRIMATOLOGY. see *BIOLOGY—Zoology*

636.089 USA ISSN 0002-9645
SF601 CODEN: AJVRAH
AMERICAN JOURNAL OF VETERINARY RESEARCH. Text in English. 1940. m. USD 165 domestic; USD 175 foreign (effective 2001). bk.rev., software rev. charts, illus. stat. index. back issues avail.; reprints avail. *Refereed.* **Document type:** *Academic/Scholarly.* **Description:** Provides reports of basic research in veterinary medicine and associated biological sciences.
Related titles: Microform ed.: (from PQC,PMC); Online - full text ed.: (from Institute for Scientific Information).
Indexed: ASCA, Abstr.Anthropol., AgBiotech, Agricola, Anim.Breed.Abstr., Aqua.Sci.& Fish.Abstr., Bibl.Agri., Bio-Contr.News & Info., Biol.& Agr.Ind. (Mar.1983-), Biol.Abstr., Cal.Tiss.Abstr. (coverage dropped), Chem.Abstr., Chem.Indus.Notes, Chem.Titles, Curr.Adv.Cancer Res., Curr.Adv.Ecol.Sci., Curr.Cont., Dairy Sci.Abstr., Dent.Ind., Derwent Biotech.Abstr., Diar.Dis.Res., Environ.Sci.Poll.Mgmt., Excerp.Med., Focus on: Vet.Sci.& Med., Food Sci.& Tech.Abstr., Helminthol.Abstr., Herb.Abstr., INIS Atomind., Ind.Med. (1940-), Ind.Sci.Rev., Ind.Vet., Maize Abstr., Microbiol.Abstr., Neurosci.Cit.Ind., Nutr.Abstr., Pig News & Info., Poult.Abstr., Protozool.Abstr., Rev.Appl.Entomol., Rev.Arom.& Med.Plants, Rev.Med.& Vet.Mycol., SSCI (coverage dropped), Sci.Cit.Ind., Small Anim.Abstr., Soyabean Abstr., Sport Fish.Abstr., Tox.Abstr. (coverage dropped), Vet.Bull., Weed Abstr., Wild.Rev., Zoo.Rec.
—BLDSC (0840.000000), CASDDS, CISTI, EMDOCS, GNLM, IDS, ingenta, Linda Hall.
Published by: American Veterinary Medical Association, 1931 N Meacham Rd, Ste 100, Schaumburg, IL 60173-4360. TEL 847-925-8070, FAX 847-925-1329, http://www.avma.org. Ed., R&P Dr. Janis H Audin. Circ: 6,299 (paid).

AMERICAN LARYNGOLOGICAL ASSOCIATION. TRANSACTIONS. see *MEDICAL SCIENCES—Otorhinolaryngology*

636.089 USA ISSN 0003-1488
SF601 CODEN: JAVMA4
AMERICAN VETERINARY MEDICAL ASSOCIATION. JOURNAL. Text in English. 1877. s-m. USD 120; USD 140 foreign (effective 1999). adv. bk.rev., software rev., video rev. charts, illus. s-a. index. reprints avail. *Refereed.* **Document type:** *Journal, Academic/Scholarly.* **Description:** Provides news of the profession, reports of scientific research and opportunities for member dialogue through letters and special commentaries.
Related titles: Microfiche ed.: (from BHP); Microform ed.: (from PQC); Online - full text ed.: (from Institute for Scientific Information).
Indexed: ASCA, Abstr.Hyg., AgBiotech, Agri.& Environ.Biotech.Abstr. (coverage dropped), Agricola, Anim.Breed.Abstr., Aqua.Sci.& Fish.Abstr., Bibl.Agri., Biol.& Agr.Ind. (Jan.1983-), Biol.Abstr., Chem.Abstr., Chem.Indus.Notes, Chem.Titles, Chemorec.Abstr., Curr.Adv.Cancer Res., Curr.Cont., Dairy Sci.Abstr., Dent.Ind., Derwent Biotech.Abstr., Excerp.Med., Focus on: Vet.Sci.& Med., Food Sci.& Tech.Abstr., Helminthol.Abstr., INIS Atomind., Ind.Med. (1915-), Ind.Sci.Rev., Ind.Vet., Nutr.Abstr., Pig News & Info., Poult.Abstr., Protozool.Abstr., Rev.Appl.Entomol., Rev.Med.& Vet.Mycol., Rev.Plant Path., SRI, SSCI (coverage dropped), Sci.Cit.Ind., Small Anim.Abstr., Soils & Fert., Soyabean Abstr., Sport Fish.Abstr., Vet.Bull., Weed Abstr., Wild.Rev., World Ag.Econ.& Rur.Soc.Abstr., Zoo.Rec.
—BLDSC (4695.000000), CASDDS, CISTI, EMDOCS, GNLM, IDS, ingenta, Linda Hall.
Published by: American Veterinary Medical Association, 1931 N Meacham Rd, Ste 100, Schaumburg, IL 60173-4360. TEL 847-925-8070, FAX 847-925-1329, http://www.avma.org/publications. Ed. Dr. Janis H Audin. Circ: 61,083 (paid).

636.089 USA
AMERICAN VETERINARY MEDICAL ASSOCIATION. NEWS. Text in English. 1996. bi-w. charts, stat. **Document type:** *Newsletter, Trade.* **Description:** Covers all aspects of veterinary medicine, care and policy.
Media: Online - full text.
Published by: American Veterinary Medical Association, 1931 N Meacham Rd, Ste 100, Schaumburg, IL 60173-4360. TEL 847-925-8070, 800-248-2862, FAX 847-925-1329, 73711.555@compuserve.com, http://www.AVMA.org/onlnews/newsdefault.asp, http://www.AVMA.org/onlnews/newsindx.html.

636.089 ARG ISSN 1514-2590
ANALECTA VET. Text in Spanish. 1998. s-a.
Media: Online - full text. **Related titles:** ♦ Print ed.: Analecta Veterinaria. ISSN 0365-5148.
Published by: Universidad Nacional de la Plata, Facultad de Ciencias Veterinarias, Calle 60, Y 118, La Plata, Buenos Aires 1900, Argentina. analecta@fcv.medvet.unlp.edu.ar, http:// fcv.medvet.unlp.edu.ar/analecta.htm. Ed. Eduardo Marotta. Adv. contact Nestor Oscar Stnachi.

636.089 ARG ISSN 0365-5148
CODEN: ANVTAH
ANALECTA VETERINARIA. Text in Spanish; Summaries in English. 1969. 2/yr. USD 21 domestic; USD 32 foreign (effective 1999). adv. back issues avail. *Refereed.*
Related titles: ♦ Online - full text ed.: Analecta Vet. ISSN 1514-2590.
Indexed: Anim.Breed.Abstr., Biol.Abstr., Chem.Abstr., Food Sci.& Tech.Abstr., Ind.Vet., Nutr.Abstr., Vet.Bull., Zoo.Rec.
—BLDSC (0869.170000), CASDDS, Linda Hall.
Published by: Universidad Nacional de la Plata, Facultad de Ciencias Veterinarias, Calle 60, Y 118, La Plata, Buenos Aires 1900, Argentina. analecta@fcv.medvet.unlp.edu.ar, http:// fcv.medvet.unlp.edu.ar/analecta.htm. Ed. Eduardo Marotta. Adv. contact Nestor Oscar Stnachi. Circ: 800.

636.089 ESP ISSN 0213-5434
CODEN: AVMAE9
ANALES DE VETERINARIA DE MURCIA. Text in Spanish, English. 1985. a., latest vol.15, 1999. ESP 1,500 (effective 2001). bk.rev. abstr. back issues avail. **Document type:** *Academic/Scholarly.* **Description:** Contains original research and advances in all fields of veterinary science.
Indexed: Helminthol.Abstr., Ind.SST, Ind.Vet., Poult.Abstr. —CINDOC.
Published by: Universidad de Murcia, Servicio de Publicaciones, C Actor Isidoro Maiquez 9, Murcia 30007, Spain. TEL 34-68-363014, FAX 34-68-363414, vgm@um.es, http://www.um.es/spumweb. Ed. Francisco Laredo Alvarez. Circ: 160.

636.089 DEU ISSN 0340-2096
CODEN: AHEMA5
ANATOMIA, HISTOLOGIA, EMBRYOLOGIA. Text in English. 1972. bi-m. DEM 1,586.18 in Europe to institutions; DEM 676.72 in Europe to individuals; DEM 1,625.30 elsewhere to institutions; DEM 715.84 elsewhere to individuals; DEM 1,744.80 in Europe to institutions print & online eds. combined; DEM 744.39 in Europe to individuals print & online eds. combined; DEM 1,787.83, DEM 787.42 elsewhere to institutions print & online eds. combined (effective 2001). adv. bk.rev. illus, stat. back issues avail. *Refereed.* **Document type:** *Journal, Academic/Scholarly.* **Description:** Anatomical, histological and embryological investigations involving human, veterinary and zoological studies.
Formerly (until 1973): Zentralblatt fuer Veterinaermedizin. Reihe C: Anatomia, Histologia, Embryologica (0300-8649)
Related titles: ♦ Online - full text ed.: Anatomia, Histologia, Embryologia Online. ISSN 1439-0264; ♦ Supplement: Advances in Veterinary Medicine. ISSN 0301-2794.
Indexed: ASCA, Agri.& Environ.Biotech.Abstr. (coverage dropped), Anim.Breed.Abstr., Biol.Abstr., Curr.Adv.Ecol.Sci., Curr.Cont., Dairy Sci.Abstr., Dent.Ind., Derwent Biotech.Abstr., Excerp.Med., Focus on: Vet.Sci.& Med., Helminthol.Abstr., INIS Atomind., Ind.Med. (1973-), Ind.Vet., Nutr.Abstr., Pig News & Info., Poult.Abstr., Ref.Zh., Rev.Appl.Entomol., Sci.Cit.Ind. (coverage dropped), Sport Fish.Abstr., Vet.Bull., Wild.Rev., Zoo.Rec.
—BLDSC (0897.960000), ADONIS, CISTI, GNLM, IDS, Infotrieve, Linda Hall. **CCC.**
Published by: (World Association of Veterinary Anatomists IND), Blackwell Wissenschafts Verlag GmbH, Kurfuerstendamm 57, Berlin 10707, Germany. TEL 49-30-32790665, FAX 49-30-32790610, abo@blackwis.de, http://www.blackwell.de. Ed. Fred Sinowatz. adv.: B&W page DEM 560; trim 122 x 202.

636.089 DEU ISSN 1439-0264
ANATOMIA, HISTOLOGIA, EMBRYOLOGIA ONLINE. Text in English. 6/yr. DEM 610 to individuals; DEM 1,428 to institutions (effective 2001). *Refereed.* **Document type:** *Academic/Scholarly.*
Media: Online - full text (from EBSCO Publishing, O C L C Online Computer Library Center, Inc., ingenta, Munksgaard & Blackwell Science's Synergy, Swets Blackwell, Institute for Scientific Information). **Related titles:** ♦ Print ed.: Anatomia, Histologia, Embryologia. ISSN 0340-2096.
Published by: Blackwell Wissenschafts Verlag GmbH, Kurfuerstendamm 57, Berlin 10707, Germany. TEL 49-30-32790665, FAX 49-30-32790610, abo@blackwis.de, http://www.blackwell-science.com/~cgilib/jnlpage.bin?Journal=XAHE&File=XAHE&Page=aims, http://www.blackwell.de.

ANIMAL BEHAVIOUR. see *BIOLOGY—Zoology*

ANIMAL FEED SCIENCE AND TECHNOLOGY; an international scientific journal. see *AGRICULTURE—Feed, Flour And Grain*

636.089 USA
ANIMAL FEEDING AND NUTRITION. Text in English. 1977. irreg., latest 1995. back issues avail. *Refereed.* **Document type:** *Monographic series.*
Published by: Academic Press, Inc., Journal Division (Subsidiary of: Harcourt Brace & Company), 525 B St, Ste 1900, San Diego, CA 92101-4495. TEL 619-231-6616, FAX 619-699-6715. Ed. Tony J Cunha. **Subscr. to:** Order Dept., 6277 Sea Harbor Dr, 4th Fl, Orlando, FL 32887. TEL 800-321-5068.

636.089 NCL ISSN 1019-8458
ANIMAL HEALTH ADVISORY LEAFLET. Text in French. 1994. irreg., latest 1996. **Document type:** *Monographic series.*
Published by: Secretariat of the Pacific Community, PO Box D5, Noumea Cedex 98848, New Caledonia. TEL 687-262000, FAX 687-263818, spc@spc.int, http://www.spc.int.

636.089 AUS ISSN 1329-198X
ANIMAL HEALTH NEWSLETTER. Text in English. irreg. free per issue. **Document type:** *Newsletter.*
Formerly: A A H L Newsletter
—CISTI.
Published by: C S I R O Animal Health, Private Bag 24, Geelong, VIC 3220, Australia. TEL 61-3-5227-5000, FAX 61-3-5227-5555, aahl@dah.csiro.au, http://www.ah.csiro.au. Ed. Emma Homes. Circ: 10,000.

636.089 UGA
ANIMAL HEALTH RESEARCH CENTRE. ANNUAL REPORT. Text in English. a.
Indexed: Rev.Appl.Entomol.
Published by: Animal Health Research Centre, PO Box 24, Entebbe, Uganda.

636.089 GBR ISSN 1466-2523
▼ **ANIMAL HEALTH RESEARCH REVIEWS.** Text in English. 2000. s-a. GBP 130 to institutions; USD 225 in the Americas to institutions; GBP 145 to institutions includes online access; USD 245 in the Americas to institutions includes online access (effective 2002). adv. *Refereed.* **Document type:** *Journal, Academic/Scholarly.* **Description:** Contains review articles covering all aspects of animal health.
Related titles: Online - full text ed.: GBP 115 to institutions; USD 200 in the Americas to institutions (effective 2002) (from ingenta, Swets Blackwell, RoweCom Information Quest).
Indexed: Ind.Vet., Nutr.Abstr., Poult.Abstr., Protozool.Abstr., Vet.Bull.
—BLDSC (0904.006800).
Published by: CABI Publishing, CAB International, Wallingford, Oxon OC10 8DE, United Kingdom. TEL 44-1491-832111, FAX 44-1491-829292, cabi@cabi.org, http://www.cabi.org/Publishing/Products/Journals/Primary/AHRR/Index.asp. Ed. Robert Ellis. Pub., R&P Katie Deaton. Adv. contact Tania Fisher. B&W page GBP 550.

636.089 GBR
ANIMAL HEALTH TRUST. ANNUAL REVIEW. Text in English. 1963. a. free per issue. bk.rev. charts, illus. index. **Document type:** *Corporate.*
Formerly: Animal Health Trust. Annual Report (0142-6591); Formerly: Animal Health (0003-3502)
Indexed: Biol.Abstr.
—CISTI, Linda Hall.
Published by: Animal Health Trust, Lanwades Park, Kentford, PO Box 5, Newmarket, Suffolk CB8 7UU, United Kingdom. TEL 44-1638-751000, FAX 44-1638-555606, TELEX 818418 ANHLTH G, http://www.aht.org.uk, http://www.aht.org.uk. Ed., R&P Clare Phillips. Circ: 9,000.

ANIMAL HUSBANDRY AND BREEDING. see *AGRICULTURE—Poultry And Livestock*

636.089 GBR ISSN 0262-2238
ANIMAL PHARM; world animal health and nutrition news. Text in English. 1982. 2/m. GBP 445 in Europe and in Middle East; USD 870 in US & Canada; JPY 130,000 in Japan; GBP 460 rest of world (effective 2001). bk.rev. 2 cols./p. back issues avail.; reprints avail. **Document type:** *Newsletter.* **Description:** Includes regulations, companies, livestock and market trends, product news (introductions, R&D) and environmental issues for the international animal health and nutrition industry.
Related titles: Online - full text ed.: (from Data-Star, The Dialog Corporation, S T N International, Gale Group).
Indexed: ABC, P.N.I., PROMT.
—BLDSC (0905.030000), CISTI. **CCC.**
Published by: P J B Publications Ltd., 18-20 Hill Rise, Richmond, Surrey TW10 6UA, United Kingdom. TEL 44-20-8948-3262, FAX 44-20-8332-8990, info@pjbpubs.com, http://www.pjbpubs.com/animal/index.html. Ed. Mark Clements. Pub. Philip Brown. R&P Annette Watts TEL 44-20-8332-8961. Adv. contact Tom Jamison TEL 44-20-8332-8871. Circ: 1,100 (paid). **Subscr. addr. in N America:** Pharmabooks Ltd., 1775 Broadway, Ste 511, New York, NY 10019. TEL 212-262-8230, FAX 212-262-8234.

ANIMAL REPRODUCTION SCIENCE. see *AGRICULTURE—Poultry And Livestock*

636.089 GBR ISSN 0264-4754
ANIMAL TECHNOLOGY. Text in English. 1950. 3/yr. GBP 25. adv. bk.rev. charts, illus.
Formerly: Institute of Animal Technicians. Journal (0020-2711)
Indexed: AgBiotech, Agricola, Anim.Breed.Abstr., Bio-Contr.News & Info., Biol.Abstr., Dairy Sci.Abstr., Ind.Vet., Nutr.Abstr., Protozool.Abstr., Rev.Appl.Entomol., Rev.Med.& Vet.Mycol., Vet.Bull.
—BLDSC (0905.125000), CISTI.
Published by: Institute of Animal Technology of Great Britain, c/o Geoffrey E. Ward, Ed, Department of Biochemistry, University College, Box 78, Cathays Park, Cardiff, United Kingdom. Circ: 1,500. **Subscr. addr.:** c/o John A. Gregory, Zoology Department, Royal Postgraduate Medical School, Du Cane Rd, London W12 0HS, United Kingdom.

636.089 TUR ISSN 1300-0861
CODEN: VTFDAQ
ANKARA UNIVERSITESI VETERINER FAKULTESI DERGISI/UNIVERSITY OF ANKARA. FACULTY OF VETERINARY MEDICINE. JOURNAL. Text in Turkish; Summaries in English, French, German. 1954. q. TRL 1,500,000; USD 35 foreign (effective 1999). bk.rev. bibl, charts, illus. **Document type:** *Academic/Scholarly.*
Indexed: AgBiotech, Anim.Breed.Abstr., Bio-Contr.News & Info., Biol.Abstr., Chem.Abstr., Dairy Sci.Abstr., Helminthol.Abstr., INIS Atomind., Ind.Vet., Int.Polit.Sci.Abstr., Nutr.Abstr., Poult.Abstr., Protozool.Abstr., Rev.Appl.Entomol., Rev.Med.& Vet.Mycol., Small Anim.Abstr., Soyabean Abstr., Triticale Abstr., Vet.Bull.
Published by: University of Ankara, Faculty of Veterinary Medicine, 06110 Diskapi, Ankara, Turkey. TEL 90-312-3170315, FAX 90-312-3164422, TELEX 42045 IRB-TR, info@ankara.edu.tr. Ed. Attila Tanyolac. R&P Dr. Ergun Ozalp. Circ: 450.

636.089 BEL ISSN 0003-4118
CODEN: AMVRA4
ANNALES DE MEDECINE VETERINAIRE. Text in French. 1849. 6/yr. BEF 1,500. adv. bk.rev. charts, illus. index. *Refereed.* **Document type:** *Academic/Scholarly.*
Related titles: Online - full text ed.: (from Institute for Scientific Information).
Indexed: ASCA, AgBiotech, Agri.& Environ.Biotech.Abstr. (coverage dropped), Agri.Eng.Abstr., Anim.Breed.Abstr., Aqua.Sci.& Fish.Abstr., Biol.Abstr., Chem.Abstr., Curr.Adv.Ecol.Sci., Curr.Adv.Gen.& Molec.Biol., Curr.Cont., Dairy Sci.Abstr., Derwent Biotech.Abstr., Focus on: Vet.Sci.& Med., Helminthol.Abstr., INIS Atomind., Ind.Med. (coverage dropped), Ind.Sci.Rev., Ind.Vet., Key Word Ind.Wildl.Res., Nutr.Abstr., Pig News & Info., Poult.Abstr., Protozool.Abstr., Ref.Zh., Rev.Appl.Entomol., Rev.Med.& Vet.Mycol., Rev.Plant Path., Sci.Cit.Ind., Small Anim.Abstr., Vet.Bull.
—BLDSC (0982.000000), CASDDS, IDS.
Published by: Imprimerie Bietlot, Sart Tilman, 20 Bd de Colonster, B42, Liege 4000, Belgium. TEL 32-41-664020, FAX 32-41-662935. Ed. P P Pastoret. Pub. P Lekeux. R&P P. Lekeux. Circ: 1,500.

639.089 POL ISSN 0301-7737
SF604 CODEN: ACDDA6
ANNALES UNIVERSITATIS MARIAE CURIE-SKLODOWSKA. SECTIO DD. MEDICINA VETERINARIA. Text in Polish, English; Summaries in English. 1949. a. price varies. **Document type:** *Academic/Scholarly.*
Indexed: AgroLibrex, Anim.Breed.Abstr., Biol.Abstr., Chem.Abstr., INIS Atomind., Ind.Vet., Nutr.Abstr., Ornam.Hort., Poult.Abstr., Ref.Zh., Rev.Appl.Entomol., Rev.Med.& Vet.Mycol., Rev.Plant Path., Sport Fish.Abstr., Vet.Bull., Wild.Rev., Zoo.Rec.
—CASDDS, CISTI, KNAW, Linda Hall.
Published by: Uniwersytet Marii Curie-Sklodowskiej, Wydawnictwo, Pl M Curie Sklodowskiej 5, Lublin 20031, Poland. Ed. Zdzislaw Glinski. Circ: 500.

636.089 POL ISSN 0239-4243
SF84 CODEN: AUEZE3
ANNALES UNIVERSITATIS MARIAE CURIE-SKLODOWSKA. SECTIO EE. ZOOTECHNIKA. Text in English, Polish; Summaries in English. 1983. a. price varies. **Document type:** *Academic/Scholarly.*
Indexed: AgroLibrex, Anim.Breed.Abstr., Dairy Sci.Abstr., Herb.Abstr., Hort.Abstr., Ind.Vet., Maize Abstr., Nutr.Abstr., Pig News & Info., Poult.Abstr., Protozool.Abstr., Sport Fish.Abstr., Sugar Ind.Abstr., Triticale Abstr., Vet.Bull., Weed Abstr., Wild.Rev., World Ag.Econ.& Rur.Soc.Abstr., Zoo.Rec.
—CISTI, KNAW, Linda Hall.
Published by: Uniwersytet Marii Curie-Sklodowskiej, Wydawnictwo, Pl M Curie Sklodowskiej 5, Lublin 20031, Poland. TEL 48-81-375304, FAX 48-81-336699. Ed. Marian Budzynski. Circ: 650.

636.089 USA ISSN 0887-7386
CODEN: AHPDE3
APIS; the international journal bulletin for specialty livestock and pet-animal product development. Text in English. 1989. irreg. USD 165 (effective 1999). adv. bibl, charts, illus. index. back issues avail. **Document type:** *Trade.* **Description:** Covers research and development, manufacture, chemistry formulation and raw materials for veterinary products, animal health and allied industries.
—CCC.
Published by: C I T A International (USA), Industrial Journals Division, 3464 W Earll Dr, Ste E F, Phoenix, AZ 85017-5260. TEL 602-447-0480, FAX 602-447-0305. Ed. E M Morsy. R&P E Morsy. Circ: 2,000.

636.089 EGY ISSN 0003-746X
ARAB VETERINARY MEDICAL ASSOCIATION. JOURNAL. Text in Arabic, English. 1964 (vol.14). q. USD 10. bk.rev. charts, illus.
Published by: Arab Veterinary Medical Association, 8 Sh 26 July, Cairo, Egypt. Ed. K N Soliman.

636.089 CHE ISSN 0003-942X
CODEN: ARTIA2
ARCHIVES OF ANIMAL NUTRITION/ARCHIV FUER TIERERNAEHRUNG. Text and summaries in English, German. 1951. 12/yr. (in 2 vols.). USD 236, GBP 196 to individuals; USD 1,250, GBP 946 to institutions (effective 2002). bk.rev. charts, illus. index. *Refereed.* **Document type:** *Journal, Academic/Scholarly.*
Related titles: Online - full text ed.: (from Institute for Scientific Information).
Indexed: ASCA, Agri.& Environ.Biotech.Abstr. (coverage dropped), Anim.Breed.Abstr., Biodet.Abstr., Biol.Abstr., Chem.Abstr., Curr.Adv.Ecol.Sci., Curr.Cont., Dairy Sci.Abstr., Derwent Biotech.Abstr., Excerp.Med., Food Sci.& Tech.Abstr., Helminthol.Abstr., Herb.Abstr., INIS Atomind., Ind.Med. (1950-), Ind.Sci.Rev., Ind.Vet., Maize Abstr., Nutr.Abstr., Pig News & Info., Postharvest, Potato Abstr., Poult.Abstr., Protozool.Abstr., Rev.Med.& Vet.Mycol., Rice Abstr., Sci.Cit.Ind., Soils & Fert., Soyabean Abstr., Sugar Ind.Abstr., Triticale Abstr., Vet.Bull.
—BLDSC (1631.227000), CASDDS, CISTI, GNLM, Infotrieve, Linda Hall. **CCC.**
Published by: Gordon and Breach - Harwood Academic (Subsidiary of: Taylor & Francis Group), PO Box 531, Lausanne 1000, Switzerland. TEL 41-21-6411280, FAX 41-21-6411281, info@gbhap.com, http://www.gbhap.com. Ed. Ortwin Simon. **Subscr. addr. in US:** International Publishers Direct, PO Box 32160, Newark, NJ 07102. FAX 215-750-6343.

636.089 ITA ISSN 0004-0479
CODEN: AVEIAN
ARCHIVIO VETERINARIO ITALIANO. Text in English, Italian; Summaries in English, French, German. 1950. bi-m. ITL 50,000; ITL 70,000 foreign. adv. bk.rev. abstr, charts, illus. index. **Document type:** *Academic/Scholarly.*
Related titles: Microfilm ed.: (from PMC).
Indexed: Agri.& Environ.Biotech.Abstr. (coverage dropped), Agri.Eng.Abstr., Anim.Breed.Abstr., Biol.Abstr., Curr.Adv.Ecol.Sci., Curr.Cont. (coverage dropped), Dairy Sci.Abstr., Derwent Biotech.Abstr., Food Sci.& Tech.Abstr., Helminthol.Abstr., Ind.Sci.Rev., Ind.Vet., Nutr.Abstr., Sport Fish.Abstr., Vet.Bull., Wild.Rev., Zoo.Rec.
—CASDDS, CISTI, GNLM, Linda Hall.
Published by: (Universita degli Studi di Milano, Facolta di Veterinaria), U T E T SpA, Corso Raffaello 28, Turin 10125, Italy. TEL 39-2-29003555. Eds. Carlo Cantoni, G. Redaelli. Circ: 1,000. **Co-sponsor:** Istituto di Ispezione degli Alimenti di Origine Animale, Facolta Medica Veterinaria.

636.08 CHL ISSN 0301-732X
CODEN: AMVED2
ARCHIVOS DE MEDICINA VETERINARIA. Text in Spanish. 1969. s-a. USD 45 (effective 1997). *Refereed.* **Document type:** *Academic/Scholarly.* **Description:** Contains scientific review articles, original articles, and short communications.
Related titles: Online - full text ed.: (from SciELO, Institute for Scientific Information).
Indexed: ASCA, AgBiotech, Anim.Breed.Abstr., Chem.Indus.Notes, Chem.Titles, Curr.Cont., Dairy Sci.Abstr., Focus on: Vet.Sci.& Med., Helminthol.Abstr., Ind.Vet., Nutr.Abstr., Pig News & Info., Poult.Abstr., Protozool.Abstr., Rev.Appl.Entomol., Rev.Med.& Vet.Mycol., Sport Fish.Abstr., Sugar Ind.Abstr., Vet.Bull., Wild.Rev., Zoo.Rec.
—BLDSC (1655.410000), CASDDS, IDS.
Published by: Universidad Austral de Chile, Facultad de Ciencias Veterinarias, Casilla 567, Valdivia, Chile. TEL 56-63-221690, FAX 56-63-221459. Ed. Carmen Gallo S. R&P Manfred Max Neef. Circ: 400.

ARCHIVOS DE ZOOTECNIA. see *AGRICULTURE—Poultry And Livestock*

636.08 NLD ISSN 0923-3970
ARGOS. Text in Dutch, English, German; Summaries in English. 1989. 2/yr. NLG 27.50 (effective 1999). adv. bk.rev. bibl. cum.index: nos.1-10. back issues avail. **Document type:** *Bulletin, Academic/Scholarly.* **Description:** Covers topics in veterinary history, with emphasis on the Netherlands.
Indexed: Ind.Vet.
Published by: Veterinair Historisch Genootschap, c/o Bibliotheek Diergeneeskunde, Postbus 80159, Utrecht 3508 TD, Netherlands. Ed. A H H M Mathijsen. R&P A Mathijsen. Adv. contact P C Knijff. B&W page NLG 600; trim 200 x 280. Circ: 400.

636.089 BRA ISSN 0102-0935
CODEN: ABMZDB
ARQUIVO BRASILEIRO DE MEDICINA VETERINARIA E ZOOTECNIA/BRAZILIAN JOURNAL OF VETERINARY AND ANIMAL SCIENCES. Text and summaries in Portuguese, English. 1943. bi-m. BRL 60, USD 100 (effective 1998). adv. reprint service avail. from ISI. *Refereed.* **Document type:** *Academic/Scholarly.* **Description:** Contains articles on veterinary medicine, animal science, technology and inspection of products of animal origin.
Formerly (until vol.35, 1983): Universidade Federal de Minas Gerais. Escola de Veterinaria. Arquivos (0076-8863)
Related titles: Microform ed.; Online - full text ed.: (from SciELO, Institute for Scientific Information).
Indexed: ASCA, AgBiotech, Agrindex, Anim.Breed.Abstr., Bibl.Agri., Bio-Contr.News & Info., Biodet.Abstr., Biol.Abstr., Chem.Abstr., Dairy Sci.Abstr., Focus on: Vet.Sci.& Med., Food Sci.& Tech.Abstr., Helminthol.Abstr., Herb.Abstr., INIS Atomind., Ind.Med. (coverage dropped), Ind.Vet., Maize Abstr., Nutr.Abstr., Pig News & Info., Poult.Abstr., Protozool.Abstr., Ref.Zh., Rev.Appl.Entomol., Rev.Med.& Vet.Mycol., Soyabean Abstr., Sport Fish.Abstr., Sugar Ind.Abstr., Vet.Bull., Wild.Rev., Zoo.Rec.
—BLDSC (1695.100000), CISTI, IDS, ingenta.
Published by: Universidade Federal de Minas Gerais, Escola de Veterinaria, Ave. ANTONIO CARLOS, 6627, Centro, Caixa Postal 567, Belo Horizonte, MG 30161-970, Brazil. TEL 55-31-4992042, FAX 55-31-4992041, TELEX 0312308 UFMG, journal@vet.ufmg.br. Ed. Lygia Maria Friche Passos. Circ: 1,000.

636.089 BRA ISSN 0102-6380
CODEN: ARSVE6
ARS VETERINARIA. Text in Portuguese; Summaries in English. 1985-1988; resumed 1992. s-a. USD 30 or exchange basis. charts, illus, stat.
Indexed: AgBiotech, Anim.Breed.Abstr., Biodet.Abstr., Biol.Abstr., Dairy Sci.Abstr., Food Sci.& Tech.Abstr., Helminthol.Abstr., INIS Atomind., Ind.Vet., Maize Abstr., Nutr.Abstr., Pig News & Info., Poult.Abstr., Protozool.Abstr., Ref.Zh., Rev.Appl.Entomol., Rev.Med.& Vet.Mycol., Sport Fish.Abstr., Vet.Bull.
—CISTI.
Published by: (Departamento de Patologia Veterinaria, Universidade Estadual Paulista), Editora U N E S P, Rodovia Carlos Tonanni, km 5, Jaboticabal, SP 14870-000, Brazil. TEL 55-016-3232500, FAX 55-016-3224275, arsvet@fcav.unesp.br.

ASKO; dwumiesiecznik kynologiczny. see *PETS*

636.089 EGY ISSN 1012-5973
ASSIUT VETERINARY MEDICAL JOURNAL. Text and summaries in Arabic, English. 1974. 4/yr. EGP 20, USD 45. charts, illus, stat. *Refereed.* **Document type:** *Academic/Scholarly.*
Indexed: AgBiotech, Anim.Breed.Abstr., Bio-Contr.News & Info., Biodet.Abstr., Dairy Sci.Abstr., Helminthol.Abstr., Ind.Vet., Maize Abstr., Nutr.Abstr., Postharvest, Potato Abstr., Poult.Abstr., Protozool.Abstr., Rev.Appl.Entomol., Rev.Arom.& Med.Plants, Rev.Med.& Vet.Mycol., Rice Abstr., Small Anim.Abstr., Soyabean Abstr., Triticale Abstr., Vet.Bull., Zoo.Rec.
—BLDSC (1746.672100), KNAW.
Published by: Assiut University, Faculty of Veterinary Medicine, Assiut, Egypt. FAX 088-333938, TELEX 92863 ASUNV UN. Ed. A A Ismail. Circ: 30.

636.089 USA
ASSOCIATION FOR VETERINARY INFORMATICS NEWSLETTER. Abbreviated title: A V I Newsletter. Text in English. 1992. bi-m. bk.rev. back issues avail. **Document type:** *Newsletter.* **Description:** Includes association news, commentaries and short notes.
Related titles: Online - full text ed.
Published by: Association for Veterinary Informatics, 1590 Augusta St, Dixon, CA 95620. TEL 916-752-4408, FAX 916-852-5680, rd-smith@uiuc.edu, http://netvet.wustl.edu/avi.htm/. Ed. Ronald D Smith.

636.089 ITA ISSN 0004-5977
ASSOCIAZIONE ITALIANA VETERINARI PER PICCOLI ANIMALI. BOLLETTINO. Text in Italian. 1961. q. membership. adv. bk.rev. abstr, bibl, charts, illus, stat, tr.lit. index.
Indexed: Anim.Breed.Abstr., Ind.Vet., Rev.Med.& Vet.Mycol., Small Anim.Abstr., Vet.Bull.
Published by: Cartografica Artigiana, Via Bela Bartok 21-23, Ferrara, FE 44100, Italy. FAX 0532-92668. Ed. Cesare Pareschi. Circ: 300.

636.089 AUS ISSN 1032-6626
AUSTRALIAN EQUINE VETERINARIAN. Text in English. 1983. q. AUD 155 (effective 1998). adv. bk.rev.
Indexed: Anim.Breed.Abstr., Ind.Vet., Rev.Appl.Entomol., Vet.Bull.
—BLDSC (1798.868000).
Published by: Australian Equine Veterinary Association, PO Box 371, Artarmon, NSW 2064, Australia. TEL 02-94115342, FAX 02-94133765, aeva@ava.com.au. Ed. Neil Walton. R&P, Adv. contact Jan Eagleton.

AUSTRALIAN JOURNAL OF EXPERIMENTAL AGRICULTURE. see *AGRICULTURE—Crop Production And Soil*

636.089 AUS ISSN 1320-9582
AUSTRALIAN VETERINARY ASSOCIATION. ANNUAL REPORT. Text in English. 1981. a. AUD 33 (effective 2000). **Document type:** *Corporate.*
Formerly (until 1990): Australian Veterinary Association. Year Book (0812-9169)
Published by: Australian Veterinary Association, 134-136 Hampden Rd, Artarmon, NSW 2064, Australia. TEL 61-2-94112733, FAX 61-2-9411-5089, sandrew@ava.com.au. R&P Steve Andrews TEL 61-6-2853600. Adv. contact James Tonkin.

636.089 AUS
AUSTRALIAN VETERINARY ASSOCIATION CONFERENCE HANDBOOK. Text in English. 1981. a. AUD 33 to non-members (effective 2000). adv. **Document type:** *Proceedings.*
Formerly (until 1991): Australian Advances in Veterinary Science (0728-8425)
Published by: Australian Veterinary Association, 134-136 Hampden Rd, Artarmon, NSW 2064, Australia. TEL 61-2-94112733, FAX 61-2-9411-5089, avacos@ava.com.au. Ed. Kevin Doyle. R&P Steve Andrews TEL 61-6-2853600. Adv. contact James Tonkin. Circ: 6,000.

636.089 AUS ISSN 0005-0423
CODEN: AUVJA2
AUSTRALIAN VETERINARY JOURNAL. Text in English. 1925. m. AUD 341 (effective 2001). adv. bk.rev. illus. index. back issues avail.; reprints avail. *Refereed.* **Document type:** *Academic/Scholarly.*
Related titles: Online - full text ed.: (from Institute for Scientific Information).
Indexed: ASCA, Abstr.Hyg., AgBiotech, Agri.& Environ.Biotech.Abstr. (coverage dropped), Agricola, Agroforest.Abstr., Anim.Breed.Abstr., Bibl.Agri., Bio-Contr.News & Info., Biol.& Agr.Ind. (coverage dropped), Biol.Abstr., Biotech.& Bioeng.Abstr., Cadscan, Chem.Abstr., Chem.Indus.Notes, Chem.Titles, Curr.Adv.Ecol.Sci., Curr.Cont., Dairy Sci.Abstr., Dent.Ind., Derwent Biotech.Abstr., Entomol.Abstr. (coverage dropped), Environ.Sci.Poll.Mgmt., Excerp.Med., Field Crop Abstr., Focus on: Vet.Sci.& Med., Food Sci.& Tech.Abstr., Forest.Abstr., Helminthol.Abstr., Herb.Abstr., INIS Atomind., Ind.Med. (1927-), Ind.Sci.Rev., Ind.Vet., Key Word Ind.Wildl.Res., Lead Abstr., Nutr.Abstr., Ornam.Hort., Pig News & Info., Poult.Abstr., Protozool.Abstr., Rev.Appl.Entomol., Rev.Med.& Vet.Mycol., Rev.Plant Path., Risk Abstr., Saf.Sci.Abstr., Sci.Cit.Ind., Small Anim.Abstr., So.Pac.Per.Ind., Soils & Fert., Soyabean Abstr., Sport Fish.Abstr., Tox.Abstr., Triticale Abstr., Trop.Dis.Bull., Vet.Bull., Virol.Abstr., Weed Abstr., Wild.Rev., Zincscan, Zoo.Rec.
—BLDSC (1824.000000), CASDDS, CISTI, GNLM, IDS, Infotrieve, ingenta, Linda Hall. **CCC.**
Published by: Australian Veterinary Association, 134-136 Hampden Rd, Artarmon, NSW 2064, Australia. TEL 61-2-94112733, FAX 61-2-9411-5089, avahq@ava.com.au, editor@ava.com.au, http://www.farmwide.com.au/nff/vetasscn/aboutava/aboutavj.htm, http://www.ava.com.au. Ed. Dennis Ringrose. R&P Steve Andrews TEL 61-6-2853600. Adv. contact James Tonkin. Circ: 4,500.

636 AUS ISSN 0310-138X
AUSTRALIAN VETERINARY PRACTITIONER. Text in English. 1971. q. AUD 150 to non-members; AUD 155 to institutions (effective 2001). adv. bk.rev. *Refereed.* **Document type:** *Academic/Scholarly.*
Related titles: Online - full text ed.: (from Institute for Scientific Information).
Indexed: ASCA, Anim.Breed.Abstr., Biol.Abstr., Curr.Adv.Ecol.Sci., Curr.Cont., Focus on: Vet.Sci.& Med., Helminthol.Abstr., Ind.Sci.Rev., Ind.Vet., Nutr.Abstr., Poult.Abstr., Protozool.Abstr., Ref.Zh., Rev.Appl.Entomol., Rev.Med.& Vet.Mycol., Sci.Cit.Ind. (coverage dropped), Small Anim.Abstr., Vet.Bull., Wild.Rev.
—BLDSC (1824.100000), IDS, ingenta.
Published by: Australian Small Animal Veterinary Association, PO Box 674, Surry Hills, NSW 2010, Australia. TEL 61-2-93607189, FAX 61-2-9211-8851, asava@ava.com.au. Ed. R E Atwell. Adv. contact Jenny Wade. B&W page AUD 600, color page AUD 1,050; trim 21 x 27.5. Circ: 1,200.

614.343 USA ISSN 0005-2086
CODEN: AVDIAI
AVIAN DISEASES. Text in English. 1957. q. USD 120 domestic; USD 130 in Canada & Mexico; USD 130 elsewhere (effective 2002). adv. bibl, charts, illus. index. back issues avail.; reprints avail. *Refereed.* **Document type:** *Academic/Scholarly.* **Description:** Devoted to the dissemination of information on domestic, pet, and wild birds.
Related titles: Microfilm ed.: (from WSH,PMC); Microform ed.: (from PQC); Online - full text ed.: (from Institute for Scientific Information).
Indexed: ASCA, AgBiotech, Agri.& Environ.Biotech.Abstr. (coverage dropped), Agri.Eng.Abstr., Agricola, Anim.Breed.Abstr., Aqua.Sci.& Fish.Abstr., Bibl.Agri., Biol.Abstr., Chem.Abstr., Curr.Adv.Cancer Res., Curr.Adv.Ecol.Sci., Curr.Cont., Derwent Biotech.Abstr., Environ.Sci.Poll.Mgmt., Focus on: Vet.Sci.& Med., Helminthol.Abstr., INIS Atomind., Ind.Med. (1957-), Ind.Sci.Rev., Ind.Vet., Int.Abstr.Biol.Sci., Maize Abstr., Microbiol.Abstr., Nutr.Abstr., Poult.Abstr., Protozool.Abstr., Rev.Appl.Entomol., Rev.Med.& Vet.Mycol., Rev.Plant Path., Sci.Cit.Ind., Small Anim.Abstr., Sport Fish.Abstr., Vet.Bull., Virol.Abstr. (coverage dropped), Wild.Rev., Zoo.Rec.
—BLDSC (1837.890000), CASDDS, CISTI, EMDOCS, GNLM, IDS, ingenta, Linda Hall.
Published by: American Association of Avian Pathologists, Inc., University of Pennsylvania, 382 W. Street Rd., New Bolton Center, Kennett Sq., PA 19348-1692. TEL 610-444-4282, FAX 610-925-8106, aaap@vet.upenn.edu, http://cahpwww.nbc.upenn.edu/~aaap/index.html. Ed. Dr. L van der Heide. Circ: 1,900.

636.089 GBR ISSN 0307-9457
CODEN: AVPADN
AVIAN PATHOLOGY. Text in English; Summaries in French, German, Spanish. 1972. bi-m. GBP 94, USD 177 to individuals; GBP 266, USD 445 to institutions (effective 2002). adv. bk.rev. back issues avail. *Refereed.* **Document type:** *Academic/Scholarly.*
Related titles: Online - full text ed.: ISSN 1465-3338 (from CatchWord Ltd., Northern Light Technology, Inc., EBSCO Publishing, O C L C Online Computer Library Center, Inc., RoweCom Information Quest, ProQuest Information & Learning, Swets Blackwell, Institute for Scientific Information).
Indexed: ASCA, AgBiotech, Agri.& Environ.Biotech.Abstr. (coverage dropped), Agricola, Anim.Breed.Abstr., Bibl.Agri., Biol.Abstr., Chem.Abstr., Chem.Indus.Notes, Chem.Titles, Curr.Adv.Ecol.Sci., Curr.Cont., Derwent Biotech.Abstr., Focus on: Vet.Sci.& Med., Helminthol.Abstr., Ind.Sci.Rev., Ind.Vet., Int.Abstr.Biol.Sci., Nutr.Abstr., Poult.Abstr., Protozool.Abstr., Ref.Zh., Rev.Appl.Entomol., Rev.Med.& Vet.Mycol., Sci.Cit.Ind., Small Anim.Abstr., Sport Fish.Abstr., Vet.Bull., Wild.Rev., Zoo.Rec.
—BLDSC (1837.891000), CASDDS, CatchWord, CISTI, EMDOCS, IDS, Infotrieve, ingenta, Linda Hall. **CCC.**
Published by: (World Veterinary Poultry Association), Taylor & Francis Ltd. (Subsidiary of: Taylor & Francis Group), 11 New Fetter Ln, London EC4P 4EE, United Kingdom. TEL 44-20-7842-2344, FAX 44-20-7842-2391, journals@tandf.co.uk, http://www.tandf.co.uk/journals/tf/03079457.html. Ed. D Cavanagh. Circ: 700.

AZABU DAIGAKU JUIGAKUBU KENKYU HOKOKU/AZABU UNIVERSITY. VETERINARY MEDICINE. BULLETIN. see *BIOLOGY—Zoology*

BANGLADESH JOURNAL OF ANIMAL SCIENCE. see *AGRICULTURE—Poultry And Livestock*

636.089 BGD ISSN 0378-8113
CODEN: BVJODC
BANGLADESH VETERINARY JOURNAL. Text in Bengali. 1967. q. USD 10. adv. bk.rev. charts, illus.
Formerly (until 1969): Pakistan Journal of Veterinary Science (0030-9915)
Indexed: Anim.Breed.Abstr., Dairy Sci.Abstr., Helminthol.Abstr., Ind.Vet., Nutr.Abstr., Poult.Abstr., Protozool.Abstr., Rev.Appl.Entomol., Rice Abstr., Sugar Ind.Abstr., Vet.Bull.
—Linda Hall.
Published by: Bangladesh Veterinary Association, Agricultural University, Mymensingh, Bangladesh. Ed. M L Dewan. Circ: 1,000.

BEITRAEGE ZUR TROPISCHEN LANDWIRTSCHAFT UND VETERINAERMEDIZIN. see *AGRICULTURE*

636.089 DEU ISSN 0005-9366
CODEN: BEMTAM
BERLINER UND MUENCHENER TIERAERZTLICHE WOCHENSCHRIFT. Text in German, English. 1888. m. DEM 481.13 in Europe to individuals; DEM 514.38 elsewhere to individuals; DEM 852.74 in Europe to institutions; DEM 865.99 elsewhere to institutions; DEM 529.24 in Europe to individuals paper & online eds. combined; DEM 565.82 elsewhere to individuals paper & online eds. combined; DEM 938.01 in Europe to institutions paper & online eds. combined; DEM 952.59 elsewhere to institutions paper & online eds. combined (effective 2001). adv. bk.rev. abstr, illus, stat. index. back issues avail. *Refereed.* **Document type:** *Journal, Academic/Scholarly.*
Related titles: ♦ Online - full text ed.: Berliner und Muenchener Tieraerztliche Wochenschrift Online. ISSN 1439-0299.
Indexed: ASCA, AgBiotech, Agri.& Environ.Biotech.Abstr. (coverage dropped), Agri.Eng.Abstr., Anim.Breed.Abstr., Biodet.Abstr., Biol.Abstr., Chem.Abstr., Chem.Indus.Notes, Curr.Adv.Ecol.Sci., Curr.Cont., Dairy Sci.Abstr., Dent.Ind., Derwent Biotech.Abstr., Field Crop Abstr., Focus on: Vet.Sci.& Med., Food Sci.& Tech.Abstr., Helminthol.Abstr., Herb.Abstr., INIS Atomind., Ind.Med. (1938-), Ind.Sci.Rev., Ind.Vet., Key Word Ind.Wildl.Res., Nutr.Abstr., Pig News & Info., Poult.Abstr., Protozool.Abstr., Rev.Appl.Entomol., Rev.Med.& Vet.Mycol., Rev.Plant Path., Sci.Cit.Ind., Small Anim.Abstr., Soils & Fert., Vet.Bull., Wild.Rev., Zoo.Rec.
—BLDSC (1941.360000), CASDDS, GNLM, IDS, Infotrieve. **CCC.**
Published by: Blackwell Wissenschafts Verlag GmbH, Kurfuerstendamm 57, Berlin 10707, Germany. TEL 49-30-32790665, FAX 49-30-32790610, abo@blackwis.de, http://www.blackwell.de. Ed. H-J Sinell.

636.089 DEU ISSN 1439-0299
BERLINER UND MUENCHENER TIERAERZTLICHE WOCHENSCHRIFT ONLINE. Text in German, English. m. DEM 434 to individuals; DEM 768 to institutions (effective 2001). **Document type:** *Academic/Scholarly.*
Media: Online - full text (from Institute for Scientific Information). **Related titles:** ♦ Print ed.: Berliner und Muenchener Tieraerztliche Wochenschrift. ISSN 0005-9366.
Published by: Blackwell Wissenschafts Verlag GmbH, Kurfuerstendamm 57, Berlin 10707, Germany. TEL 49-30-32790665, FAX 49-30-32790610, abo@blackwis.de, http://www.blackwell.de/bmtw.htm.

636.089 DEU ISSN 0723-6212
BIOLOGISCHE TIERMEDIZIN. Text in German, Spanish. 1984. q. DEM 29; DEM 39 foreign (effective 1999). adv. **Document type:** *Academic/Scholarly.*
Indexed: Ind.Vet., Protozool.Abstr., Ref.Zh., Vet.Bull.
Published by: Aurelia Verlag GmbH, Dr.-Reckeweg-Str 2-4, Baden-Baden 76532, Germany. TEL 49-7221-50102, FAX 49-7221-501420, info@aurelia-verlag.de, http://www.aurelia-verlag.de. Ed. Dr. Erich Reinhart. adv.: B&W page DEM 3,000, B&W page XEU 1,533.88; trim 140 x 204. Circ: 12,000.

636 615.1 CZE
CODEN: BCZVDE
BIOPHARM. Text in Czech, Slovak, English. 1964. bi-m. CZK 54, USD 26.20. adv. bk.rev. bibl, charts, illus, stat. reprint service avail. from ISI.
Formerly (until 1991): Biologizace a Chemizace Zivocisne Vyroby - Veterinaria (0139-8571)
Indexed: Anim.Breed.Abstr., Cadscan, Chem.Abstr., Chem.Indus.Notes, Chem.Titles, Curr.Adv.Ecol.Sci., Curr.Cont. (coverage dropped), Dairy Sci.Abstr., Excerp.Med. (until 19??), Helminthol.Abstr., Ind.Sci.Rev., Ind.Vet., Lead Abstr., Nutr.Abstr., Pig News & Info., Poult.Abstr., Protozool.Abstr., Rev.Med.& Vet.Mycol., Sci.Cit.Ind. (coverage dropped), Vet.Bull., Zincscan.
—CASDDS, CISTI, IDS, Linda Hall.
Published by: (Spojene Podniky pro Zdravotnickou Vyrobu, Vyzkumny Ustav pro Biofaktory a Veterinarni Leciva, Odbor Vedeckych Informaci), Vetpres, Pohori-Chatoun, Jilove V Prague 254 49, Czech Republic. TEL 26 59 51. Ed. Bohumil Sevcik. **Subscr. to:** Artia, Ve Smeckach 30, Prague, 1 111 27, Czechoslovakia.

BLAA STJAERNAN; djurvaard inom totalfoersvaret. see *PETS*

636.089 SWE ISSN 0282-3926
BLADMAGEN. Text in Swedish. 1967. 5/yr. SEK 120 to members (effective 1990).
Published by: Veterinaermedicinska Foereningen, Fack 7074, Uppsala 75007, Sweden.

636.089 ARG ISSN 0379-0045
BOLETIN DE VIGILANCIA EPIDEMIOLOGICA DE LA RABIA PARA LAS AMERICAS. Text in Spanish. 1969. m. free per issue.
Supersedes in part (since vol.7, no.4, 1978): Vigilancia Epidemiologica
Related titles: ♦ English ed.: Bulletin of Epidemiological Surveillance of Rabies for the Americas.
Published by: Instituto Panamericano de Proteccion de Alimentos y Zoonosis/Panamerican Institute for Food Protection and Zoonoses, Casilla de correo 44, Martinez, BUENOS AIRES 1064, Argentina. TEL 54-11-8361000, FAX 54-11-8360927, TELEX 24577 AR PAZ, inppaz@inppaz.ops-oms.org, http://www.inppaz.org.ar. Ed. Eduardo Guarnera. Circ: 950.
Affiliate: World Health Organization.

636.089 USA ISSN 0524-1685
CODEN: BOVPBO
BOVINE PRACTITIONER. Text in English. 1969. s-a. USD 25 domestic; USD 31 foreign (effective 2000). adv. bk.rev. index. **Document type:** *Academic/Scholarly.* **Description:** Publishes manuscripts of interest to veterinarians engaged in cattle practice and research.
Indexed: Agri.Eng.Abstr., Anim.Breed.Abstr., Dairy Sci.Abstr., Ind.Vet., Nutr.Abstr., Protozool.Abstr., Rev.Appl.Entomol., Vet.Bull.
—BLDSC (2264.630000), CISTI.
Published by: American Association of Bovine Practitioners, c/o Dr Bob Smith, 3404 Live Oak Lane, Stillwater, OK 74075. TEL 405-372-8666, FAX 405-743-8422. R&P Bob Smith. Adv. contact James Jarrett. Circ: 6,000.

BOVINE VETERINARIAN. see *NUTRITION AND DIETETICS*

636.089 ESP ISSN 1130-4804
BOVIS. Text in Spanish. 1984. bi-m. ESP 7,175; ESP 9,700 foreign. **Document type:** *Trade.*
Indexed: Ind.SST.
—CINDOC.
Published by: Luzan 5 S.A. de Ediciones, Pasaje Virgen de la Alegria 14, Madrid 28027, Spain. TEL 34-1-4051595, FAX 34-1-4034907, luzan@luzan5.es, http://www.luzan5.es. Circ: 30,000.

636.089 590 BRA ISSN 1413-9596
BRAZILIAN JOURNAL OF VETERINARY RESEARCH AND ANIMAL SCIENCE. Text in English, Portuguese. 1938. bi-m., latest vol.38, 2001. USD 130 (effective 2001). abstr, bibl, illus, stat, maps. 100 p./no. back issues avail. *Refereed.* **Document type:** *Journal, Academic/Scholarly.* **Description:** Publishes full papers, short communications and review articles concerned with veterinary medicine, zootechny and related fields.
Former titles (until 1989): Universidade de Sao Paulo. Faculdade de Medicina Veterinaria e Zootecnia. Revista (0303-7525); (until 1971): Universidade de Sao Paulo. Faculdade de Medicina Veterinaria. Revista (0301-7273)
Related titles: Online - full text ed.: 1997. free (from SciELO).
Indexed: Anim.Breed.Abstr., Dairy Sci.Abstr., Helminthol.Abstr., Herb.Abstr., INIS Atomind., Ind.Vet., Pig News & Info., Sugar Ind.Abstr., Zoo.Rec.
—BLDSC (2277.419600).

V

Published by: Universidade do Sao Paulo, Faculdade de Medicina Veterinaria e Zootecnia, Av. Prof. Dr. O. Marques de Paiva, 87, Sao Paulo, SP 05508-000, Brazil. brazvet@fmvz.usp.br, brazvet@edu.usp.br, http://www.scielo.br/bjvras. Eds. Benjamin Eurico Malucelli, Joao Palermo-Neto.

BUFFALO JOURNAL; an international journal of buffalo science. see *AGRICULTURE—Poultry And Livestock*

BULGARIAN JOURNAL OF AGRICULTURAL SCIENCE. see *AGRICULTURE*

636.089 BGR ISSN 1311-1477
BULGARIAN JOURNAL OF VETERINARY MEDICINE. Text in English. q. USD 80 foreign (effective 2002). **Document type:** *Journal, Academic/Scholarly.* **Description:** Covers topics related to both fundamental and applied aspects of veterinary medicine; publishes original papers and reviews.
Published by: Thracian University, Faculty of Veterinary Medicine, Students' Campus, Stara Zagora 6000, Bulgaria. TEL 359-422801, FAX 359-4274112, info@uni-sz.bg, http://www.uni-sz.bg. **Dist. by:** Sofia Books, Ul Silivria 16, Sofia 1404, Bulgaria. TEL 359-2-9586257, sofiabooks@hotmail.com, http://www.sofiabooks.hit.bg.

V

BULLETIN OF ANIMAL HEALTH AND PRODUCTION IN AFRICA/BULLETIN DES SANTE ET PRODUCTION ANIMALES EN AFRIQUE. see *AGRICULTURE—Poultry And Livestock*

636.089 ARG
BULLETIN OF EPIDEMIOLOGICAL SURVEILLANCE OF RABIES FOR THE AMERICAS. Text in English. 1969. s-a. free per issue. **Document type:** *Monographic series.*
Related titles: ♦ Spanish ed.: Boletin de Vigilancia Epidemiologica de la Rabia para las Americas. ISSN 0379-0045.
Published by: Instituto Panamericano de Proteccion de Alimentos y Zoonosis/Panamerican Institute for Food Protection and Zoonoses, Casilla de Correos 44, Martinez, Buenos Aires 1640, Argentina. TEL 54-11-8361000, FAX 54-11-8360927, TELEX 24577 AR PAZ, inppaz@inppaz.ops-oms.org, http://www.inppaz.org.ar. Ed. Eduardo Guarnera. Circ: 450. **Affiliate:** World Health Organization.

636.08 CHE
BUNDESAMT FUER VETERINAERWESEN. MITTEILUNGEN. Text in German. 1900. 26/yr. CHF 26 (effective 2000). adv. **Document type:** *Newsletter, Government.* **Description:** Provides statistics and data concerning outbreaks of animal diseases. Also covers regulation of the exportation and importation of animals, meat and meat products to and from Switzerland.
Published by: Bundesamt fuer Veterinaerwesen, Schwarzenburgstr 161, Bern 3003, Switzerland. TEL 41-31-3238568, FAX 41-31-3248256, heinz.k.mueller@bvet.admin.ch, http://www.admin.ch/bvet/. Ed., R&P Heinz Mueller. Adv. contact Karin Reist. Circ: 13,000.

636.089 USA
C V M QUARTERLY. (College of Veterinary Medicine) Text in English. 1945. q. USD 5. adv. bk.rev. bibl, illus. **Document type:** *Newsletter.*
Formerly: Auburn Veterinarian
Indexed: Ind.Vet., Rev.Plant Path., Sport Fish.Abstr., Vet.Bull., Wild.Rev., Zoo.Rec. (until 19??).
Published by: Auburn University, College of Veterinary Medicine, 104 J E Greene Hall, Auburn, AL 36849. TEL 205-844-3698, FAX 334-844-3697. Ed. Gary Beard. Circ: 1,200.

636.089 USA ISSN 0008-1612
CALIFORNIA VETERINARIAN. Text in English. 1947. bi-m. USD 35; USD 45 in Canada; USD 55 elsewhere. adv. illus. index. back issues avail.; reprints avail. *Refereed.* **Document type:** *Academic/Scholarly.* **Description:** Includes business, legislative and regulatory information of interest to the veterinary profession; and association and allied organization news.
Related titles: Microform ed.: (from PQC).
Indexed: Agri.& Environ.Biotech.Abstr. (coverage dropped), Chem.Abstr., Derwent Biotech.Abstr., Ind.Vet., Rev.Med.& Vet.Mycol., Small Anim.Abstr., Sport Fish.Abstr., Vet.Bull., Wild.Rev., Zoo.Rec.
—BLDSC (3015.350000), CISTI, ingenta, Linda Hall.
Published by: California Veterinary Medical Association, 5231 Madison Ave, Sacramento, CA 95841. TEL 916-344-4985, FAX 916-344-6147. Ed., Pub., R&P, Adv. contact Laurie B Lynn. B&W page USD 800. Circ: 3,800.

CANADIAN HORSEMAN. see *SPORTS AND GAMES—Horses And Horsemanship*

636.089 610 CAN ISSN 0830-9000
CODEN: CJVRE9
CANADIAN JOURNAL OF VETERINARY RESEARCH/REVUE CANADIENNE DE RECHERCHE VETERINAIRE. Text in English, French. 1937. q. CND 107 domestic; USD 115 foreign (effective 2001). adv. bibl, charts, illus. index. reprints avail. *Refereed.* **Document type:** *Academic/Scholarly.*
Former titles: Canadian Journal of Comparative Medicine (0008-4050); Canadian Journal of Comparative Medicine and Veterinary Science
Related titles: Online - full text ed.: (from Institute for Scientific Information).
Indexed: ASCA, AgBiotech, Agri.& Environ.Biotech.Abstr. (coverage dropped), Agricola, Anim.Breed.Abstr., Bibl.Agri., Biol.Abstr., Chem.Abstr., Chem.Titles, Curr.Adv.Ecol.Sci., Curr.Cont., Dairy Sci.Abstr., Dent.Ind., Derwent Biotech.Abstr., Environ.Sci.Poll.Mgmt., Excerp.Med., Focus on: Vet.Sci.& Med., Food Sci.& Tech.Abstr., Helminthol.Abstr., INIS Atomind., Ind.Med. (1986-), Ind.Sci.Rev., Ind.Vet., Med.Care Rev., Microbiol.Abstr., Nutr.Abstr., Pig News & Info., Poult.Abstr., Protozool.Abstr., Rev.Med.& Vet.Mycol., Sci.Cit.Ind., Small Anim.Abstr., Sport Fish.Abstr., Triticale Abstr., Vet.Bull., Wild.Rev., World Ag.Econ.& Rur.Soc.Abstr., Zoo.Rec.
—BLDSC (3036.700000), CASDDS, CISTI, EMDOCS, GNLM, IDS, Infotrieve, ingenta, Linda Hall. **CCC.**
Published by: Canadian Veterinary Medical Association, 339 Booth St, Ottawa, ON K1R 7K1, Canada. TEL 613-236-1162, FAX 613-236-9681, kallen@cvma-acmv.org, http://www.cvma-acmv.org/vetjournals/. Ed. Dr. Eva Nagy. Adv. contact Laima Laffitte. Circ: 2,000 (paid).

636.089 CAN ISSN 0008-5286
CODEN: CNVJA9
CANADIAN VETERINARY JOURNAL/REVUE VETERINAIRE CANADIENNE. Text in English, French. 1960. m. CND 139.10 domestic; USD 140 foreign (effective 2001). adv. bk.rev. abstr, charts, illus. index. reprints avail. *Refereed.* **Document type:** *Academic/Scholarly.*
Related titles: Microform ed.: (from PQC,PMC); Online - full text ed.: (from Institute for Scientific Information).
Indexed: ASCA, AgBiotech, Agri.& Environ.Biotech.Abstr. (coverage dropped), Agri.Eng.Abstr., Agricola, Anim.Breed.Abstr., Aqua.Sci.& Fish.Abstr., Aquacult.Abstr., Bibl.Agri., Biol.Abstr., Chem.Abstr., Chem.Indus.Notes, Chem.Titles, Curr.Adv.Ecol.Sci., Curr.Cont., Dairy Sci.Abstr., Derwent Biotech.Abstr., Environ.Sci.Poll.Mgmt., Excerp.Med., Focus on: Vet.Sci.& Med., Helminthol.Abstr., Herb.Abstr., INIS Atomind., Ind.Med. (1960-), Ind.Sci.Rev., Ind.Vet., Nutr.Abstr., Pig News & Info., Poult.Abstr., Protozool.Abstr., Rev.Appl.Entomol., Rev.Med.& Vet.Mycol., SSCI (coverage dropped), Sci.Cit.Ind., Small Anim.Abstr., Sport Fish.Abstr., Vet.Bull., Wild.Rev., Zoo.Rec.
—BLDSC (3046.100000), CASDDS, CISTI, EMDOCS, GNLM, IDS, ingenta, Linda Hall. **CCC.**
Published by: Canadian Veterinary Medical Association, 339 Booth St, Ottawa, ON K1R 7K1, Canada. TEL 613-236-1162, FAX 613-236-9681, kallen@cvma-acmv.org, http://www.cvma-acmv.org/vetjournals/. Ed. Dr. Doug Hare. Adv. contact Laima Laffitte. Circ: 5,000 (paid).

636.089 ITA
CANI, GATTI E COMPAGNIA. Text in Italian. 1987. q. ITL 20,000 domestic; ITL 40,000 elsewhere; free to qualified personnel. adv.
Published by: Editore S.C.I.V.A.C., Via Pallavicino, 26, Cremona, CR 26100, Italy. TEL 0372-23501. Ed. Antonio Manfredi. adv.: page ITL 3,500,000. Circ: 90,000.

636.089 IND ISSN 0379-542X
CODEN: CHRNAR
CHEIRON; Tamil Nadu journal of veterinary science and animal husbandry. Text in English. 1972. bi-m. INR 40, USD 20. index. back issues avail.
Indexed: AgBiotech, Agri.Eng.Abstr., Anim.Breed.Abstr., Biodet.Abstr., Biol.Abstr., Chem.Abstr., Curr.Adv.Ecol.Sci., Dairy Sci.Abstr., Food Sci.& Tech.Abstr., Helminthol.Abstr., Herb.Abstr., Ind.Vet., Maize Abstr., Nutr.Abstr., Pig News & Info., Poult.Abstr., Protozool.Abstr., Rev.Appl.Entomol., Rev.Med.& Vet.Mycol., Rural Devel.Abstr., Sugar Ind.Abstr., Trop.Oil Seeds Abstr., Vet.Bull., World Ag.Econ.& Rur.Soc.Abstr.
—BLDSC (3133.430000), CASDDS.
Published by: Tamil Nadu Veterinary & Animal Science University, Chennai, Tamil Nadu 600 007, India. TEL 581-506, FAX 044-560114. Ed. M Mohamed Habibulla Khan. adv.: B&W page INR 1,000. Circ: 750.

CIENCIA RURAL. see *AGRICULTURE*

636.089 CUB ISSN 0253-5750
CODEN: CASVDA
CIENCIA Y TECNICA EN LA AGRICULTURA. SERIE: VETERINARIA. Abstracts and contents page in English. 1978. 2/yr. USD 14 in North America; USD 16 in Europe; USD 17 elsewhere.
Indexed: Agrindex, Ind.Vet., Vet.Bull.
—CASDDS.
Published by: Centro de Informacion y Documentacion Agropecuario, Gaveta Postal 4149, Havana 4, Cuba. **Dist. by:** Ediciones Cubanas, Obispo No. 527, Apdo. 605, Havana, Cuba.

636.089 CRI ISSN 0250-5649
CODEN: CIVEEV
CIENCIAS VETERINARIAS. Text in Spanish. 1979. s-a. USD 13. *Refereed.* **Document type:** *Academic/Scholarly.*
Indexed: Anim.Breed.Abstr., Dairy Sci.Abstr., Ind.Vet., Pig News & Info., Poult.Abstr., Protozool.Abstr., Rev.Appl.Entomol., Rev.Med.& Vet.Mycol., Sport Fish.Abstr., Vet.Bull., Wild.Rev., Zoo.Rec.
Published by: Escuela de Medicina Veterinaria, Biblioteca, Apdo. 86, Heredia, Costa Rica. TEL 506-2610025. Ed. Edwin Perez Chaverri.

CIGUATERA. see *FISH AND FISHERIES*

636.089 ITA ISSN 1120-7957
CINOLOGIA. Text in Italian. 1990. 4/yr. ITL 60,000; ITL 80,000 foreign.
Address: Via Trecchi, 20, Cremona, CR 26100, Italy. TEL 39-372-460440, FAX 39-372-457091. Ed. Mauriz Cornelli. adv.: color page ITL 2,000,000. Circ: 14,000.

636.089 USA ISSN 1096-2867
CODEN: SVMSEN
CLINICAL TECHNIQUES IN SMALL ANIMAL PRACTICE. Text in English. 1986. q. USD 116 domestic to individuals; USD 139 foreign to individuals; USD 168 domestic to institutions; USD 193 foreign to institutions; USD 69 domestic to students; USD 84 foreign to students; USD 49 per issue (effective 2001). adv. bibl, charts, illus. index. reprints avail. *Refereed.* **Document type:** *Journal, Academic/Scholarly.* **Description:** Each issue covers a specific theme of interest to small-animal veterinarians.
Formerly (until 1997): Seminars in Veterinary Medicine and Surgery: Small Animal (0882-0511)
Related titles: Online - full text ed.: (from Institute for Scientific Information).
Indexed: ASCA, Agricola, Curr.Cont., Derwent Biotech.Abstr., Focus on: Vet.Sci.& Med., INIS Atomind., Ind.Med. (1998-), Ind.Vet., Nutr.Abstr., Protozool.Abstr., Rev.Appl.Entomol., Small Anim.Abstr., Vet.Bull.
—BLDSC (3286.399350), GNLM, IDS, Infotrieve, ingenta. **CCC.**
Published by: W.B. Saunders Co. (Subsidiary of: Harcourt Publishers Ltd.), 11830 Westline Industrial Dr, St Louis, MO 63146. TEL 800-325-4177, http://www.wbsaunders.com. Ed. Dr. Robert J Murtaugh. Adv. contact Michael Goldberg. B&W page USD 640, color page USD 1,640; trim 10 x 7. Circ: 1,214. **Subscr. to:** Periodicals Fulfillment, W B Saunders Co, 6277 Sea Harbor Dr, 4th Fl, Orlando, FL 32891-4800.

636.089 CAN
COLLEGE OF VETERINARIANS OF ONTARIO. UPDATE. Text in English. 1983. 8/yr. USD 35. **Document type:** *Newsletter, Corporate.*
Formerly: Ontario Veterinary Association. Update (0821-6320)
—CISTI.
Published by: College of Veterinarians of Ontario, 2106 Gordon St, Guelph, ON N1L 1G6, Canada. FAX 519-824-6497. Ed., R&P Michele Fagan. Circ: 3,000.

636 JPN ISSN 0913-5316
COMPANION ANIMAL PRACTICE. Key Title: C A P. Companion Animal Practice. Text in Japanese. 1986. m. JPY 2,000 per issue. **Description:** Contains articles on small, companion animals.
Published by: Chikusan Publishing Co. Ltd. (Subsidiary of: Midori Group), Ikebukuro Nishiguchi Sky Bldg, 2-14-4 Ikebukuro, Toshima-ku, Tokyo 171-0014, Japan. TEL 03-3590-9454. Circ: 5,000.

636.089 USA ISSN 0193-1903
COMPENDIUM ON CONTINUING EDUCATION FOR THE PRACTICING VETERINARIAN. Text in English. 1979. m., latest vol.23. USD 58 domestic to individuals; USD 70 in Canada & Mexico to individuals; USD 99 elsewhere to individuals; USD 80 domestic to institutions; USD 105 in Canada & Mexico to institutions; USD 110 elsewhere to institutions (effective 2001). adv. bk.rev. illus, abstr, charts. index. 100 p./no. 3 cols./p. back issues avail.; reprints avail. *Refereed.* **Document type:** *Journal, Trade, Academic/Scholarly.*
Formerly: Compendium on Continuing Education for the Small Animal Practitioner (0164-5455)
Related titles: CD-ROM ed.; Microform ed.: (from PQC); Online - full text ed.: (from Institute for Scientific Information).
Indexed: ASCA, AgBiotech, Agri.Eng.Abstr., Agricola, Anim.Breed.Abstr., Bibl.Agri., Curr.Cont., Dairy Sci.Abstr., Focus on: Vet.Sci.& Med., Helminthol.Abstr., Herb.Abstr., Ind.Vet., Nutr.Abstr., Pig News & Info., Postharvest, Poult.Abstr., Protozool.Abstr., Rev.Appl.Entomol., Rev.Med.& Vet.Mycol., Small Anim.Abstr., Vet.Bull., Wild.Rev., World Ag.Econ.& Rur.Soc.Abstr.
—BLDSC (3363.967520), CISTI, IDS, ingenta.
Published by: Veterinary Learning Systems, 275 Phillips Blvd, Trenton, NJ 08618. TEL 609-882-5600, 800-426-9119, FAX 609-882-6357, info@vetlearn.com., http://www.vetlearn.com/compend.html. Ed. Antoinette Passaretti TEL 609-671-2022. Pub. Kenneth Senerth. R&P Anoinette Passaretti TEL 609-671-2022. Adv. contact Mark Reynolds. Circ: 35,000.

636.089 USA ISSN 1523-8652
▼ **COMPENDIUM'S STANDARDS OF CARE: EMERGENCY AND CRITICAL CARE MEDICINE.** Text in English. 1999. 11/yr. USD 69 domestic; USD 84 in Canada & Mexico to individuals (effective 2001); USD 116 foreign (effective 2000). bibl. yearly. 10 p./no. back issues avail.; reprints avail. *Refereed.* **Document type:** *Newsletter, Academic/Scholarly.* **Description:** Provides access to state-of-the-art information on how to treat specific emergency and critical conditions in dogs and cats.
Published by: Veterinary Learning Systems, 275 Phillips Blvd, Trenton, NJ 08618. TEL 609-882-5600, FAX 609-882-6357, http://www.vetlearn.com. Ed. Yvonne Stecher. Pub. Ken Senerth. R&P Antoinette Passarette TEL 609-672-2022. Circ: 1,400.

COMPLETING THE INTERNAL MARKET OF THE EUROPEAN COMMUNITY: 1992 LEGISLATION - VETERINARY & PHYTOSANITARY CONTROLS. see *LAW—International Law*

636.089 USA
THE CONFERENCE OF RESEARCH WORKERS IN ANIMAL DISEASES. PROCEEDINGS. Text in English. irreg. **Document type:** *Proceedings, Academic/Scholarly.*
Formerly: Conference of Research Workers in Animal Diseases. Abstracts
—BLDSC (6841.390000).
Published by: Conference of Research Workers in Animal Diseases, c/o Robert P Ellis, Colorado State University, Dept of Microbiology, Rm A102, Fort Collins, CO 80523-1677. TEL 970-491-5740, FAX 970-491-1815, rellis@cvmbs.colostate.edu, http://www.cvmbs.colostate.edu/microbiology/crwad/crwad.htm. **Dist. by:** Iowa State University Press, 2121 S State Ave, Ames, IA 50014-8300. TEL 515-294-5980.

636.089 CAN ISSN 0843-5634
CREST. Text in English. 1989. q. illus. **Document type:** *Newsletter.* **Description:** News of OVC's people, events and programs.
Published by: Ontario Veterinary College, Alumni Association, Dean s Office, University of Guelph, Guelph, ON N1G 2W1, Canada. TEL 519-823-8800, FAX 519-837-3230. Ed. Martha Leibbrandt. Circ: 5,100.

636.089 CUB ISSN 0138-8134
CUBA. CENTRO DE INFORMACION Y DOCUMENTACION AGROPECUARIO. BOLETIN DE RESENAS. SERIE: VETERINARIA. Abstracts in English. 1974. irreg. per issue exchange basis. stat.
Formerly: Cuba. Centro de Informacion y Divulgacion Agropecuario. Boletin de Resenas. Serie: Veterinaria
Indexed: Agrindex.
Published by: Centro de Informacion y Documentacion Agropecuario, Gaveta Postal 4149, Havana 4, Cuba. TEL 29-2227. **Dist. by:** Ediciones Cubanas, Obispo No. 461, Apdo. 605, Havana, Cuba.

636.089 NLD ISSN 0166-2333
CODEN: CTVSDD
CURRENT TOPICS IN VETERINARY MEDICINE AND ANIMAL SCIENCE. Text in English. 1978. irreg. price varies. *Refereed.* **Document type:** *Monographic series.*
Formerly (until 1979): Current Topics in Veterinary Medicine (0165-4586)
Indexed: Agricola, Chem.Abstr., Chem.Indus.Notes, Chem.Titles.
—CASDDS, CISTI, Infotrieve. **CCC.**
Published by: (Commission of the European Communities BEL), Kluwer Academic Publishers Group (Subsidiary of: Wolters Kluwer N.V.), Spuiboulevard 50, PO Box 17, Dordrecht 3300 AA, Netherlands. FAX 31-78-639-2254, services@wkap.nl, http://www.wkap.nl. **Dist. by:** Journals Department, PO Box 322, Dordrecht 3300 AH, Netherlands. FAX 31-78-654-6474.

636.089 DEU ISSN 0341-6593
CODEN: DDTWDG
D T W - DEUTSCHE TIERAERZTLICHE WOCHENSCHRIFT. Text in German; Summaries in English. 1893. 12/yr. DEM 365.50; DEM 389.40 foreign (effective 2000). adv. bk.rev. abstr, bibl, charts, illus. index. *Refereed.* **Document type:** *Trade.*
Former title: Deutsche Tieraerztliche Wochenschrift (0012-0847)
Related titles: Online - full text ed.: (from Institute for Scientific Information).
Indexed: Abstr.Hyg., AgBiotech, Agri.& Environ.Biotech.Abstr. (coverage dropped), Agri.Eng.Abstr., Anim.Breed.Abstr., Biol.Abstr., Chem.Abstr., Chem.Indus.Notes, Chem.Titles, Curr.Adv.Ecol.Sci., Curr.Cont., Dairy Sci.Abstr., Derwent Biotech.Abstr., Excerp.Med., Field Crop Abstr., Focus on: Vet.Sci.& Med., Food Sci.& Tech.Abstr., Helminthol.Abstr., Herb.Abstr., INIS Atomind., Ind.Med. (1971-), Ind.Sci.Rev., Ind.Vet., Key Word Ind.Wildl.Res., Maize Abstr., Nutr.Abstr., Pig News & Info., Potato Abstr., Poult.Abstr., Protozool.Abstr., Rev.Appl.Entomol., Rev.Med.& Vet.Mycol., Rev.Plant Path., SSCI (coverage dropped), Sci.Cit.Ind., Soils & Fert., Soyabean Abstr., Triticale Abstr., Vet.Bull., Weed Abstr., Wild.Rev., Zoo.Rec.
—BLDSC (3574.000000), CASDDS, CISTI, GNLM, IDS, Infotrieve, Linda Hall. **CCC.**
Published by: Verlag M. und H. Schaper GmbH, Borsigstr 5, Alfeld 31061, Germany. TEL 49-5181-8009-0, FAX 49-5181-8009-33, info@schaper-verlag.de, http://www.schaper-verlag.de. Ed. J Hartung. adv.: B&W page DEM 1,615, color page DEM 2,920; trim 274 x 184. Circ: 1,500.

636.089 USA ISSN 0012-7337
D V M; the newsmagazine of veterinary medicine. Text in English. 1970. m., latest vol.32. USD 39 in North America; USD 85 elsewhere; USD 4 newsstand/cover United States & Possessions (effective 2001). adv. bk.rev. abstr, illus, tr.lit. reprints avail. **Document type:** *Academic/Scholarly, Trade.* **Description:** Offers in-depth analysis of news affecting the ways in which veterinarians practice, along with practical and clinical management information.
Related titles: Microform ed.: (from PQC); Online - full text ed.: (from H. W. Wilson, ProQuest Information & Learning).
Indexed: Biol.& Agr.Ind. (Jan.1999-).
—Infotrieve. **CCC.**
Published by: Advanstar Communications Inc., Healthcare Group, 7500 Old Oak Blvd, Cleveland, OH 44130-3369. TEL 440-243-8100, FAX 440-891-2777, http://www.dvmnewsmagazine.com. Ed. Maureen Hrehocik. Circ: 45,320. **Subscr. to:** 131 W First St, Duluth, MN 55802. TEL 888-527-7008.

636.089 DNK ISSN 0106-6854
DANSK VETERINAERTIDSSKRIFT/DANISH VETERINARY JOURNAL. Text in Danish. 1918. 24/yr. DKK 975 (effective 1999). adv. bk.rev.
Formerly: Danske Dyrlaegeforening. Medlemsblad (0011-6564)
Indexed: AgBiotech, Agri.Eng.Abstr., Anim.Breed.Abstr., Biodet.Abstr., Biol.Abstr., Dairy Sci.Abstr., Food Sci.& Tech.Abstr., Helminthol.Abstr., Ind.Vet., Nutr.Abstr., Pig News & Info., Poult.Abstr., Protozool.Abstr., Ref.Zh., Rev.Appl.Entomol., Rev.Med.& Vet.Mycol., Small Anim.Abstr., Vet.Bull., Weed Abstr., World Ag.Econ.& Rur.Soc.Abstr.
—BLDSC (3533.035000).
Published by: Danske Dyrlaegeforening, Rosenlunds Alle 8, Vanlose 2720, Denmark. TEL 45-38-71-08-88, FAX 45-38-71-03-22. Ed. Borge Jorgensen. Circ: 4,000.

636.089 FRA ISSN 0180-3573
DEPECHE VETERINAIRE. Text in French. 1977. 44/yr. FRF 795 domestic to non-members; FRF 665 domestic to members; FRF 840 foreign to members (effective 2000). adv. bk.rev.
Published by: Syndicat National des Veterinaires Francais, 10 Place Leon Blum, Paris 75011, France. TEL 33-1-44933060, FAX 33-1-43797696. Ed. Claude Andrillon. Adv. contact F Chamari.

636.089 DEU ISSN 0340-1898
DEUTSCHES TIERAERZTEBLATT. Text in German. 1949. m. DEM 219; DEM 251 foreign (effective 2000). adv. bk.rev. stat. **Document type:** *Journal, Academic/Scholarly.*
Indexed: Ind.Vet., Vet.Bull.
—BLDSC (3578.160000), CISTI. **CCC.**
Published by: (Deutsche Tieraerzteschaft e.V.), Schluetersche GmbH und Co. KG, Hans-Boeckler-Allee 7, Hannover 30173, Germany. TEL 49-511-8550-0, FAX 49-511-85502405, anzeigen@schluetersche.de, http://www.schluetersche.de. Ed. Dr. Margund Mrozek. Circ: 29,465 (paid).

636.089 NLD ISSN 0167-5168
CODEN: DAVSDR
DEVELOPMENTS IN ANIMAL AND VETERINARY SCIENCES. Text in English. 1976. irreg., latest vol.25, 1991. price varies. back issues avail. *Refereed.* **Document type:** *Monographic series, Proceedings, Academic/Scholarly.* **Description:** Examines developments in various areas of the veterinary sciences.
Indexed: Zoo.Rec.
—BLDSC (3579.062000), CASDDS, CISTI, Infotrieve. **CCC.**
Published by: Elsevier Science BV, PO Box 211, Amsterdam 1000 AE, Netherlands. TEL 31-20-485-3757, 31-20-485-3911, FAX 31-20-485-3432, 31-20-485-3598, nlinfo-f@elsevier.nl; usinfo-f@elsevier.com; forinfo-kyf04035@niftyserve.or.jp, http://www.elsevier.nl/. **Subscr. in Australasia and the Far East to:** Elsevier Science (Singapore) Pte Ltd, No.1 Temasek Ave, 17-01 Millenia Tower, Singapore 039192, Singapore. TEL 65-434-3727, FAX 65-337-2230, asiainfo@elsevier.com.sg; **Subscr. in Japan to:** Elsevier Science Inc - Japan Regional Office, 9-15 Higashi-Azabu 1-chome, Minato-ku, Tokyo 106-0044, Japan. TEL 81-3-5561-5033, FAX 81-3-5561-5047, info@elsevier.co.jp; **Subscr. in the Americas to:** Elsevier Science, PO Box 945, New York, NY 10159-0945. TEL 212-633-3730, 212-633-3730, 888-437-4636, FAX 212-633-3680, usinfo-f@elsevier.com, http://www.elsevier.com

636.089 NLD
DEVELOPMENTS IN VETERINARY MEDICINE. Text in English. irreg. price varies. *Refereed.* **Document type:** *Monographic series.*
Published by: Kluwer Academic Publishers Group (Subsidiary of: Wolters Kluwer N.V.), Spuiboulevard 50, PO Box 17, Dordrecht 3300 AA, Netherlands. FAX 31-78-639-2254, services@wkap.nl, http://www.wkap.nl. **Dist. by:** Journals Department, PO Box 322, Dordrecht 3300 AH, Netherlands. FAX 31-78-654-6474.

636.089 NLD ISSN 0920-2412
DIER - EN - ARTS; wetenschappelijke praktijkgerichte informatie. Text in Dutch. 1986. 9/yr. NLG 90 domestic; NLG 125 foreign; NLG 47.50 to students; free. adv. bk.rev. abstr, bibl, charts, illus, stat. back issues avail. *Refereed.* **Document type:** *Journal, Academic/Scholarly.* **Description:** Provides information for practicing veterinary surgeons and includes examples of practical solutions to problems encountered in daily practice.
—KNAW.
Published by: Transmondial BV, Waalreseweg 17, Valkenswaard 5554 HA, Netherlands. TEL 31-40-203-0535, FAX 31-40-203-0535, transmondial@hetnet.nl. Ed., Pub., Adv. contact A M Beckers. B&W page NLG 1,950, color page NLG 3,650; trim 297 x 210. Circ: 3,200 (controlled).

636.089 FRA ISSN 1012-5329
DISEASE INFORMATION. Text in English. 1988. w. USD 120, EUR 120 (effective 2000). **Document type:** *Newsletter.* **Description:** Weekly reports on the status and outbreaks of e mergency animal diseases.
Related titles: Online - full text ed.; French ed.: Informations Sanitaires. ISSN 1012-5310; Spanish ed.: Informaciones Sanitarias. ISSN 1012-5337.
Indexed: Ind.Vet., Pig News & Info., Rev.Med.& Vet.Mycol., Vet.Bull.
—CISTI.
Published by: Office International des Epizooties, 12 rue de Prony, Paris 75017, France. FAX 33-1-42670987, oie@oie.int, http://www.oie.int. Ed. J Blancou. R&P Gill S Dilmitis TEL 33-1-44151888. **US subscr. to:** Scientific, Medical Publications of France, 100 E 42nd St, Ste 1002, New York, NY 10017. TEL 212-983-6278.

636.089 616.4 USA ISSN 0739-7240
CODEN: DANEEE
DOMESTIC ANIMAL ENDOCRINOLOGY. Text in English. 1984. 8/yr. EUR 117 in Europe to individuals; JPY 15,600 in Japan to individuals; USD 131 elsewhere to individuals; EUR 435 in Europe to institutions; JPY 57,600 in Japan to institutions; USD 486 elsewhere to institutions (effective 2002). adv. charts, illus, stat, abstr. index. back issues avail. *Refereed.* **Document type:** *Academic/Scholarly.* **Description:** Publishes papers on the endocrine physiology of domestic animal species, both in vivo and in vitro, from cellular to molecular.
Related titles: Online - full text ed.: (from ingenta, Swets Blackwell, ScienceDirect, Institute for Scientific Information).
Indexed: ASCA, AgBiotech, Agricola, Anim.Breed.Abstr., Aqua.Sci.& Fish.Abstr., Bibl.Agri., Biol.Abstr., Chem.Abstr., Chem.Indus.Notes, Chem.Titles, Curr.Cont., Dairy Sci.Abstr., Derwent Biotech.Abstr., Focus on: Vet.Sci.& Med., INSPEC (coverage dropped), Ind.Med. (1984-), Ind.Sci.Rev., Ind.Vet., Inpharma, Int.Abstr.Biol.Sci., Nutr.Abstr., Pig News & Info., Pollut.Abstr., Poult.Abstr., Protozool.Abstr., Reac., Sci.Cit.Ind., Small Anim.Abstr., Vet.Bull.
—BLDSC (3616.884000), CASDDS, CISTI, EMDOCS, GNLM, IDS, Infotrieve, ingenta, Linda Hall. **CCC.**
Published by: Elsevier Science, PO Box 945, New York, NY 10159-0945. TEL 212-989-5800, FAX 212-633-3990, usinfo-f@elsevier.com, http://www.elsevier.com/locate/domaniend. Ed. Dr. James L Sartin. **Subscr. in Australasia and the Far East to:** Elsevier Science (Singapore) Pte Ltd, No.1 Temasek Ave, 17-01 Millenia Tower, Singapore 039192, Singapore. TEL 65-434-3727, FAX 65-337-2230; **Subscr. in Japan to:** Elsevier Science Inc - Japan Regional Office, 9-15 Higashi-Azabu 1-chome, Minato-ku, Tokyo 106-0044, Japan. TEL 81-3-5561-5033; **Subscr. outside the Americas to:** Elsevier Science BV, PO Box 211, Amsterdam 1000 AE, Netherlands. TEL 31-20-485-3757.

DOSEI KYOKAI KAIHO/JAPANESE ASSOCIATION OF VETERINARY BIOLOGISTS. BULLETIN. see *BIOLOGY—Zoology*

636.089 ISL
DYRALAEKNARITID. Text in Icelandic. 1981. s-a. membership. **Description:** Features articles on veterinary medicine, hygiene, and the environment.
Published by: Dyralaeknafelag Islands, Lagmula 7, Reykjavik 108, Iceland. TEL 354-568-9545. Eds. Konrad Konardsson, Olafur Jonsson.

636.089 DNK ISSN 0906-1290
DYRENES RET - VOR PLIGT. Text in Danish. 1975. q. bk.rev. **Document type:** *Consumer.*
Formerly (until 1990): Komiteen mod Dyreforsoeg, Fonden til Sygdomsbekaempelse uden Dyreforsoeg (0109-3878)
Published by: Landsforeningen Komiteen Mod Dyreforsoeg, Valdemarsgade 67, 5 tv, PO Box 59, Charlottenlund 2920, Denmark. TEL 31-22-41-15. Ed. Henning Lobbe. adv.: B&W page DKK 2,300. Circ: 2,000.

636 EGY ISSN 1110-0222
CODEN: EJVSAU
EGYPTIAN JOURNAL OF VETERINARY SCIENCE. Text in English; Summaries in Arabic, English. 1964. a. USD 42 (effective 2000). reprint service avail. from IRC. **Document type:** *Academic/Scholarly.*
Former titles (until vol.9, 1972): United Arab Republic Journal of Veterinary Science (0041-7165); (until 1970): Journal of Veterinary Science of the United Arab Republic (0368-4709)
Related titles: CD-ROM ed.
Indexed: Anim.Breed.Abstr., Biol.Abstr., Chem.Abstr., Chem.Indus.Notes, Chem.Titles, Curr.Adv.Ecol.Sci., Dairy Sci.Abstr., Diar.Dis.Res., Excerp.Med. (until 19??), ExtraMED, Ind.Vet., Nutr.Abstr., Protozool.Abstr., Vet.Bull., Zoo.Rec.
—BLDSC (3664.425000), CASDDS, CISTI.
Published by: (Arabic Veterinary Medical Association), National Information and Documentation Centre (NIDOC), Tahrir St., Dokki, Awqaf P.O., Cairo, Egypt. TEL 20-2-3371696. Ed. M E Nawito. Circ: 1,500.

EMBRYO TRANSFER NEWSLETTER. see *BIOLOGY—Biotechnology*

636.089 FRA ISSN 1283-0828
ENCYCLOPEDIE VETERINAIRE. Text in French. 1998. base vol. updates 5/yr. bibl, charts, illus. back issues avail. **Document type:** *Academic/Scholarly.* **Description:** Provides an up-to-date reference on all topics in veterinary medicine.
Published by: Elsevier Paris, Editions Scientifiques et Medicales (Subsidiary of: Reed Elsevier plc. group), 23 rue Linois, Paris 75015, France. TEL 33-1-45589110, FAX 33-1-45589425, redaction-emc@elsevier.fr, http://www.elsevier.fr, http://www.elsevier.com. Ed. H Laforge.

636.089 GRC ISSN 0374-7417
CODEN: EEKSA
EPISTEMONIKE EPETERIS KTENIATRIKES SCHOLES. Text in Greek; Summaries in English. 1952. irreg. **Document type:** *Academic/Scholarly.*
Indexed: Biol.Abstr.
Published by: Aristotelian University of Thessaloniki, School of Veterinary Science, Thessaloniki 540 06, Greece. Ed. A G Spais. Circ: 500.

636 NLD ISSN 0923-3334
EQUATOR; newsletter on veterinary aspects of international development cooperation. Text in English. 1989. bi-m. free. bk.rev. bibl, illus, maps, abstr. back issues avail. **Document type:** *Newsletter.* **Description:** Covers developments, conference abstracts, calendar of events, and training courses. For professionals in animal health and production.
Published by: Utrecht University, Faculty of Veterinary Medicine, PO Box 80163, Utrecht 3508 TD, Netherlands. TEL 31-30-253-2116, FAX 31-30-253-1815, bic@bic.vet.uu.nl. Ed. Dr. R W Paling. R&P Jean H A Degooijer TEL 31-30-2537696.

636 USA ISSN 1047-8620
EQUINE ATHLETE; the equine sports medicine news journal. Text in English. 1988. bi-m. USD 19.95 domestic; USD 25.20 in Canada; USD 27.95 elsewhere; USD 3.95 newsstand/cover. adv. bk.rev. charts, illus. index. *Refereed.* **Document type:** *Consumer.* **Description:** Covers health and fitness for horses used for racing or dressage.
Indexed: ASCA, Agricola, Bibl.Agri., Focus on: Vet.Sci.& Med. (coverage dropped), Ind.Vet., Nutr.Abstr., Rev.Appl.Entomol., Vet.Bull.
—IDS.
Published by: Thoroughbred Times Company Inc., 496 Southland Dr, Box 8237, Lexington, KY 40503. TEL 606-260-9800, FAX 606-260-9812, equineathlete@fancypu. Ed. Denise Steffanus. Circ: 6,500. **Subscr. to:** PO Box 55946, Boulder, CO 80322-5946.

636.087 GBR ISSN 0957-7734
SF955
EQUINE VETERINARY EDUCATION. Text in English. 1989. 6/yr. GBP 92, USD 151.80 (effective 2000). adv. illus. *Refereed.* **Document type:** *Academic/Scholarly.* **Description:** Covers continuing education for equine veterinarians.
Related titles: Online - full text ed.: (from Institute for Scientific Information).
Indexed: ASCA, Anim.Breed.Abstr., Dairy Sci.Abstr., Focus on: Vet.Sci.& Med., Helminthol.Abstr., Ind.Vet., Nutr.Abstr., Protozool.Abstr., Rev.Appl.Entomol., Rev.Med.& Vet.Mycol., Vet.Bull.
—BLDSC (3794.519400), CISTI, IDS, ingenta.
Published by: Equine Veterinary Journal Ltd., Equine Veterinary Journal, 351 Exning Rd, Newmarket, Suffolk CB8 0AU, United Kingdom. TEL 44-1638-666160, FAX 44-1638-668665, evj.editorial@dial.pipex.com; evj.subs@dial.pipex.com. Ed. P D Rossdale. R&P Rachel Green. Adv. contact Tina Osbourne. Circ: 1,800.

636.089 GBR ISSN 0425-1644
CODEN: EQVJAI
EQUINE VETERINARY JOURNAL. Text in English. 1968. bi-m. GBP 72 domestic; GBP 87 foreign (effective 2001). adv. bk.rev. abstr, bibl, charts, illus, stat. index. back issues avail.; reprint service avail. from PQC. *Refereed.* **Document type:** *Trade, Academic/Scholarly.*
Related titles: Online - full text ed.: (from Institute for Scientific Information).
Indexed: ASCA, AgBiotech, Agri.Eng.Abstr., Agricola, Anim.Breed.Abstr., Bio-Contr.News & Info., Biol.Abstr., Curr.Adv.Ecol.Sci., Curr.Cont., Dairy Sci.Abstr., Dent.Ind., Derwent Biotech.Abstr., Focus on: Vet.Sci.& Med., Helminthol.Abstr., INIS Atomind., Ind.Med. (1968-), Ind.Sci.Rev., Ind.Vet., Nutr.Abstr., Protozool.Abstr., Rev.Med.& Vet.Mycol., Rev.Plant Path., Sci.Cit.Ind., Soyabean Abstr., Vet.Bull., Wild.Rev.
—BLDSC (3794.520000), CISTI, GNLM, IDS, ingenta.
Published by: (British Equine Veterinary Association), Equine Veterinary Journal Ltd., Equine Veterinary Journal, 351 Exning Rd, Newmarket, Suffolk CB8 0AU, United Kingdom. TEL 44-1638-666160, FAX 44-1638-668665, evj.editorial@dial.pipex.com; evj.subs@dial.pipex.com, http://www.evj.co.uk. Ed. P D Rossdale. R&P R Green. Adv. contact Tina Osbourne. color page GBP 1,400; trim 215 x 285. Circ: 2,000.

EQUINEWS; serving the horse industry - all breeds, all disciplines. see *SPORTS AND GAMES—Horses And Horsemanship*

EQUUS. see *BIOLOGY—Zoology*

636.08 ITA
EUROPEAN JOURNAL OF VETERINARY PATHOLOGY. Text in English. 1995. 3/yr. ITL 150,000.
Indexed: Agricola, Ind.Vet., Pig News & Info., Rev.Appl.Entomol., Rev.Med.& Vet.Mycol., Vet.Bull., Zoo.Rec.
—BLDSC (3829.747340).
Published by: S C I V A C, Palazzo Trecchi, Cremona, CR 26100, Italy. TEL 39-372-460440, FAX 39-372-457091. Ed. F Ehrensperger.

636.089 USA ISSN 1521-1363
▼ **EXOTIC D V M.** (Doctor Veterinary Medicine) Text in English. 1999. bi-m. USD 69 in North America; USD 89 elsewhere (effective 2001). adv. bk.rev. back issues avail. *Refereed.* **Document type:** *Magazine, Trade.* **Description:** Contains articles and features promoting the quality care of nontraditional companion animals.
Related titles: Online - full text ed.
Indexed: Pig News & Info., Protozool.Abstr., Rev.Med.& Vet.Mycol.
Published by: Zoological Education Network, PO Box 541749, Lake Worth, FL 33454-1749. TEL 561-641-6745, FAX 561-641-0234, subscribe@exoticdvm.com, http://www.exoticdvm.com. Ed., Pub., R&P, Adv. contact Linda Harrison.

F A S S VET; laekemedel foer veterinaermedicinsk bruk. see *PHARMACY AND PHARMACOLOGY*

636.089 USA ISSN 1057-6223
F D A VETERINARIAN. (Food & Drug Administration) Text in English. 1979. bi-m. USD 17 (effective 2001). charts. index. back issues avail. **Document type:** *Newsletter.*
Related titles: Microfiche ed.; Online - full text ed.
Indexed: Ind.Vet., Nutr.Abstr., Rev.Appl.Entomol.
Published by: U.S. Food & Drug Administration, Center for Veterinary Medicine, 7500 Standish Pl, Rockville, MD 20855. TEL 301-827-6513, FAX 301-594-1831, http://www.fda.gov/cvm/index/fdavet/fdavettoc.html. Ed. Karan A Kandra. Circ: 3,600. **Subscr. to:** U.S. Government Printing Office, Superintendent of Documents, PO Box 371954, Pittsburgh, PA 15250-7954. TEL 202-512-1800, FAX 202-512-2250, orders@gpo.gov, http://www.access.gpo.gov.

636.08 ESP ISSN 0373-1170
CODEN: AFVLA5
FACULTAD DE VETERINARIA DE LEON. ANALES. Text in Spanish. 1955. a. ESP 1,000. abstr. **Description:** Publishes original research on veterinary medicine, animal production, hygiene and food technology.
Indexed: Food Sci.& Tech.Abstr., Ind.SST, Ind.Vet.
—CASDDS, CISTI.
Published by: (Secretariado de Publicaciones), Universidad de Leon, Facultad de Veterinaria, Campus de Vegazana, Leon 24071, Spain. recpub@isidoro.unileon.es, http://www.unileon.es/vi/recpub/.

636.08 PAK
FARM SCIENTIST. Text in English, Urdu. 1990. m. USD 3 per issue.
Published by: Press Corporation of Pakistan, P O Box 3138, Karachi 75400, Pakistan. TEL 21-455-3703, FAX 21-7736198. Ed. Dr. M S Jaffery. Circ: 5,000.

636.039 614 USA ISSN 0164-6257
FEDERAL VETERINARIAN. Text in English. 1922. m. USD 40 in North America; USD 60 elsewhere (effective 2001). adv. bk.rev. back issues avail. **Document type:** *Newsletter, Trade.* **Description:** Federal regulatory news, meat inspection, animal disease control, human disease from animals and federal personnel issues.
Published by: National Association of Federal Veterinarians, 1101 Vermont Ave, NW, Ste 710, Washington, DC 20005-6308. TEL 202-289-6334, nafv@erols.com, http://users.erols.com/nafv/fedvet.htm. Ed., R&P, Adv. contact Dale D Boyle. B&W page USD 260; trim 9.5 x 7.5. Circ: 1,600 (paid and controlled).

636.089 USA
FELINE HEALTH TOPICS. Text in English. 1981. q. USD 30. back issues avail. **Document type:** *Newsletter.* **Description:** For veterinary professionals.
Indexed: Ref.Zh.

Published by: Cornell Feline Health Center, Cornell University, College of Veterinary Medicine, Ithaca, NY 14853-6401. TEL 607-253-3414, FAX 607-253-3419. Ed., R&P June Tuttle TEL 607-253-3093. Circ: 5,000 (paid and free).

636.089 SVK ISSN 0015-5748 CODEN: FVMCAW
FOLIA VETERINARIA. Text and summaries in English. 1956. q. SKK 200, USD 6 (effective 1999). adv. bk.rev. abstr, bibl. index.; cum.index. **Document type:** *Academic/Scholarly.*
Indexed: AgBiotech, Agri.Eng.Abstr., Anim.Breed.Abstr., Biol.Abstr., Chem.Abstr., Chem.Indus.Notes, Chem.Titles, Dairy Sci.Abstr., INIS Atomind., Ind.Vet., Nutr.Abstr., Pig News & Info., Poult.Abstr., Protozool.Abstr., Rev.Appl.Entomol., Small Anim.Abstr., Soyabean Abstr., Vet.Bull.
—CASDDS, CISTI.
Published by: Univerzita Veterinarskeho Lekarstva v Kosiciach/University of Veterinary Medicine, c/o Dir Sona Lemakova, Ustav Vedeckych Informacii a Kniznica, Komenskeho 73, Kosice 04181, Slovakia. TEL 421-95-6339689, FAX 421-95-6339689, TELEX 77322, lemakova@uvik.uvm.sk, http://www.uvm.sk. Ed. Dusan Magic. Circ: 550.

636.089 CHN ISSN 1003-4331
FUJIAN XUMU SHOUYI/FUJIAN JOURNAL OF ANIMAL HUSBANDRY AND VETERINARY SCIENCE. Text in Chinese; Abstracts and contents page in English. 1979. q. CNY 1.50 newsstand/cover. **Description:** Publishes investigative report, monographs, clinical information and productive experiences in the field of animal husbandry and veterinary sciences.
Published by: Fujina Xumu Shouyi Bianjibu, Pudang, Fuzhou Shijiao (Suburb), Fuzhou, Fujian 350013, China. TEL 0591-7593074, FAX 0591-7840650. Ed. Youquan Cheng. adv.: page CNY 1,000. **Dist. overseas by:** Jiangsu Publications Import & Export Corp., 56 Gao Yun Ling, Nanjing, Jiangsu, China.

636.089 FRA
G T V BULLETIN. (Groupements Techniques Veterinaires) Text in French. 1974. 5/yr. FRF 855; FRF 995 foreign (effective 1997). adv. bk.rev. **Document type:** *Bulletin.*
Indexed: Agri.Eng.Abstr., Anim.Breed.Abstr., Biodet.Abstr., Chem.Abstr., Dairy Sci.Abstr., Helminthol.Abstr., Ind.Vet., Nutr.Abstr., Poult.Abstr., Protozool.Abstr., Rev.Appl.Entomol., Rev.Med.& Vet.Mycol., Soyabean Abstr., Triticale Abstr., Vet.Bull., Weed Abstr., World Ag.Econ.& Rur.Soc.Abstr.
—BLDSC (2551.630000).
Published by: Groupements Techniques Veterinaires, Syndicat National des Groupements Techniques Veterinaires (SNGTV), 5 rue Moufle, Paris 75011, France. TEL 33-1-49295858, FAX 33-1-49297077. Ed. Dr. Faroult. Adv. contact Dr. Gauthey. Circ: 2,800.

GANAGRINCO; ganaderia - agricultura - industria - comercio. see *AGRICULTURE*

636.08 USA
GEORGIA EXTENSION NEWSLETTER. Text in English. m. **Document type:** *Newsletter.*
Published by: University of Georgia at Statesboro, Georgia Extension, Landrum Box 8112 G S U, Statesboro, GA 30460. TEL 912-681-5639, FAX 912-681-0376.

636.089 USA
GRAYSON GRAM. Text in English. 1984. q. free per issue.
Published by: Grayson Foundation, Inc., 821 Corporate Drive, Lexington, KY 40503. TEL 606-278-5243. Ed. Marc Allen Berry. Circ: 3,500.

636.089 DEU ISSN 1616-2315
▼ **GROSSTIERPRAXIS.** Text in German. 2000. m. EUR 93.90 domestic to institutions; EUR 98.90 in Europe to institutions; EUR 100.90 elsewhere to institutions; EUR 46 to students; EUR 8.90 newsstand/cover (effective 2002). **Document type:** *Journal, Academic/Scholarly.*
Published by: Georg Thieme Verlag, Ruedigerstr 14, Stuttgart 70469, Germany. TEL 49-711-8931-0, FAX 49-711-8931298, kunden.service@thieme.de, http://www.thieme.de.

GUOWAI XUMU KEJI/FOREIGN ANIMAL HUSBANDRY SCIENCE AND TECHNOLOGY. see *AGRICULTURE—Poultry And Livestock*

HARYANA AGRICULTURAL UNIVERSITY. JOURNAL OF RESEARCH. see *AGRICULTURE*

636.089 IND ISSN 0033-4359
HARYANA VETERINARIAN. Text in English. 1971 (vol.10). s-a. INR 20, USD 12. adv. bk.rev. abstr, charts, illus, stat. **Document type:** *Academic/Scholarly.*
Formerly: Punjab Veterinarian
Indexed: Dairy Sci.Abstr., Ind.Vet., Poult.Abstr., Rev.Med.& Vet.Mycol., Vet.Bull., Zoo.Rec.
—BLDSC (4271.150000).
Published by: Haryana Agricultural University, College of Veterinary Sciences, Hissar, Haryana 125 004, India. Ed. Dr. A R Rao. Circ: 500.

636.089 GRC ISSN 0257-2354
HELLENIC VETERINARY MEDICAL SOCIETY. BULLETIN/ELLINIKIS KTINIATRIKIS ETERIAS. DELTIO. Key Title: Deltion tes Ellenikes Ktiniatrikes Eterias. Text in Greek; Summaries in English. 1924. q. GRD 5,000, USD 120. adv. bk.rev. **Document type:** *Bulletin.*
Indexed: AgBiotech, Agri.Eng.Abstr., Anim.Breed.Abstr., Biodet.Abstr., Biol.Abstr., Dairy Sci.Abstr., Food Sci.& Tech.Abstr., Helminthol.Abstr., Ind.Vet., Nutr.Abstr., Pig News & Info., Poult.Abstr., Protozool.Abstr., Rev.Appl.Entomol., Rev.Med.& Vet.Mycol., Vet.Bull., Weed Abstr.
—BLDSC (2554.500000).
Published by: Hellenic Veterinary Medical Society, PO Box 18281, Athens 116 10, Greece. Ed. Dr. Agesilaus Tsagarakis. Circ: 1,000 (controlled). **Subscr. to:** Olga Sabatakou, PO Box 3546, Athens 102 10, Greece.

636.089 GBR ISSN 0268-4276
HENSTON VETERINARY VADE MECUM (LARGE ANIMAL). Text in English. 1984. a. GBP 39.50 (effective 2000). adv. index. back issues avail. **Document type:** *Trade.* **Description:** For veterinary surgeons or similarly qualified personnel. Covers diseases, conditions, and symptoms of large animals, as well as therapeutic products.
Published by: Veterinary Business Development Ltd., Olympus House, Werrington Centre, Peterborough Rd, Peterborough, Cambs PE7 3BY, United Kingdom. TEL 44-1733-325522, FAX 44-1733-325512, VBD@vetsonline.com. Ed. David Watson Bvetmed MRCVS. R&P Douglas Hutchison. Adv. contact Hutchison BVMS MRCVS. Circ: 4,200.

636.089 GBR ISSN 0268-4268
HENSTON VETERINARY VADE MECUM (SMALL ANIMAL). Text in English. 1984. a. GBP 39 (effective 2000). adv. index. back issues avail. **Document type:** *Trade.* **Description:** For veterinary surgeons or similarly qualified personnel. Covers diseases, conditions, and symptoms of small animals, as well as therapeutic products.
Published by: Veterinary Business Development Ltd., Olympus House, Werrington Centre, Peterborough Rd, Peterborough, Cambs PE7 3BY, United Kingdom. TEL 44-1733-325522, FAX 44-1733-325512, 100303.141@compuserve.com, VBD@vetsonline.com. Ed. David Watson Bvetmed MRCVS. Pub., R&P Douglas Hutchison. Circ: 5,000.

HIMACHAL JOURNAL OF AGRICULTURAL RESEARCH. see *AGRICULTURE*

636.089 DNK ISSN 0105-1423
SF615
HISTORIA MEDICINAE VETERINARIAE. Text and summaries in English, French, German. 1976. q. DKK 380 domestic; USD 89 foreign (effective 2001). adv. bk.rev. illus. index, cum.index every 5 years. 40 p./no. 2 cols./p. *Refereed.* **Document type:** *Proceedings, Academic/Scholarly.* **Description:** Covers veterinary science and history.
Indexed: IBZ, Ind.Vet., Vet.Bull.
—BLDSC (4316.056500), CISTI, Linda Hall.
Address: Soendergade 39, Viby, Sjaelland 4130, Denmark. Ed. Georg Theves. Circ: 250.

636.089 JPN ISSN 0018-3385
HOKKAIDO VETERINARY MEDICAL ASSOCIATION. JOURNAL/HOKKAIDO JUISHIKAI ZASSHI. Text in Japanese. 1967. m. JPY 350; JPY 350 foreign (effective 1999). adv. abstr, bibl, charts, illus, tr.lit. *Refereed.* **Document type:** *Academic/Scholarly.*
Indexed: Agrindex, Vet.Bull., Zoo.Rec.
Published by: Hokkaido Veterinary Medical Association, 24 Ken, 4-Jo, 5-chome, 9-3 Nishi-ku, Sapporo 063-0804, Japan. TEL 81-11-642-4826, FAX 81-11-642-4642, hokuju00@poplar.ocn.ne.jp. Ed., Pub., R&P, Adv. contact Hinoshi Kanagawa. B&W page JPY 30,000; trim 300 x 210. Circ: 2,600 (paid); 100 (controlled).

636.1 USA ISSN 1076-4704
HOOFCARE & LAMENESS; the journal of equine foot science. Text and summaries in English. 1985. q., latest vol.74, 2001. USD 59 domestic; USD 65 in Canada; USD 75 elsewhere; USD 15 newsstand/cover (effective 2001). adv. bk.rev., software rev., tel.rev., video rev., Website rev. charts, illus, tr.lit. index, cum.index: 1985-2000. 64 p./no. back issues avail.; reprints avail. *Refereed.* **Document type:** *Journal, Trade.* **Description:** Provides technical information related to the prevention and therapy of performance-related injuries, conformational challenges, and diseases of the foot that affect the world's horses.
Former titles (until 1992): Hoofcare and Lameness Quarterly Report (1062-3221); (until 1991): F Y I (1076-4690)
Published by: Hoofcare Publishing, 19 Harbor Loop, PO Box 660, Gloucester, MA 01930. TEL 978-281-3222, FAX 978-283-8775, franjurga@earthlink.net, editor@hoofcare.com, http://www.hoofcare.com. Ed., Pub., R&P, Adv. contact Fran Jurga. B&W page USD 700, color page USD 1,500; trim 8.5 x 11. Circ: 1,500 (paid).

636.1 USA
THE HORSE REPORT. Text in English. 1982. q. free per issue. back issues avail. **Document type:** *Newsletter.* **Description:** Covers recent research in equine health for horse owners, breeders, and veterinarians.
Indexed: Ind.Vet., Protozool.Abstr.
Published by: University of California at Davis, Center for Equine Health, School of Veterinary Medicine, One Shields Ave, Davis, CA 95616-8589. TEL 530-752-6433, FAX 530-752-9379, cehwebmaster@ucdavis.edu, http://www.vetmed.ucdavis.edu/ceh. Ed., R&P Laurie Fio. Circ: 17,000.

636.089 615 ZAF ISSN 0019-0918
I V S. (Index of Veterinary Specialists) Text in English. 1961. q. ZAR 90 domestic; ZAR 193 in United States; ZAR 175 in Europe; ZAR 212 in Australia & New Zealand (effective 2000). adv. back issues avail. **Description:** Indexes veterinary medicines available in South Africa in pharmacological order, alphabetically.
Published by: M I M S, Division of Times Media Limited, PO Box 2059, Pretoria 0001, South Africa. TEL 27-12-3485010, FAX 27-12-3617716. Ed. G Swan. Adv. contact Sandy Schoeman. Circ: 2,562.

636.089 ZAF
I V S DESK REFERENCE. (Index of Veterinary Specialists) Text in English. 1991. biennial. ZAR 100 domestic; ZAR 213 in United States; ZAR 220 in Europe; ZAR 232 in Australia & New Zealand. adv. **Description:** Provides full product information on veterinary medicines, including a generic-trade name index and a reference section.
Published by: M I M S, Division of Times Media Limited, PO Box 2059, Pretoria 0001, South Africa. TEL 27-12-3485010, FAX 27-12-3617716. Ed. G Swan. Adv. contact Sandy Schoeman. Circ: 2,800.

I W R C PROCEEDINGS. see *BIOLOGY—Zoology*

I W R C SKILLS SEMINARS. see *BIOLOGY—Zoology*

636.089 GBR ISSN 0263-841X CODEN: IPRCDH
IN PRACTICE (LONDON). Text in English. m. GBP 78.50 in United Kingdom; GBP 89 in Europe; GBP 78.50 in Africa; GBP 89 rest of world (effective 2001). adv. *Refereed.* **Document type:** *Trade.*
Related titles: Online - full text ed.: (from Institute for Scientific Information).
Indexed: Agri.Eng.Abstr., Agricola, Anim.Breed.Abstr., Biol.& Agr.Ind. (Jan.1983-Mar.1989), Biol.Abstr., Dairy Sci.Abstr., Dent.Ind., Derwent Biotech.Abstr., Excerp.Med., Focus on: Vet.Sci.& Med., Food Sci.& Tech.Abstr., Ind.Med. (coverage dropped), Ind.Vet., Pig News & Info., Protozool.Abstr., Small Anim.Abstr., Vet.Bull., Wild.Rev.
—BLDSC (4372.411000), CISTI, EMDOCS, GNLM, IDS, Infotrieve, ingenta, Linda Hall. **CCC.**
Published by: British Veterinary Association, 7 Mansfield St, London W1M 0AT, United Kingdom. TEL 0171-636-6541, FAX 0171-637-0620. Ed. Edward Boden. Circ: 10,000.

636.089 IND ISSN 0019-5057 CODEN: IJAHA4
INDIAN JOURNAL OF ANIMAL HEALTH. Text in English. 1960. s-a. USD 80; USD 40 elsewhere; USD 20 SAARC; INR 150 domestic (effective 2001). adv. bk.rev. abstr, bibl, charts, illus, stat. 90 p./no. 2 cols./p. back issues avail.; reprints avail. **Document type:** *Journal, Academic/Scholarly.* **Description:** Research and Original scientific publication on the subjects.

V

Indexed: AgBiotech, Agri.Eng.Abstr., Agroforest.Abstr., Anim.Breed.Abstr., Biol.Abstr., Chem.Abstr., Curr.Cont. (coverage dropped), Dairy Sci.Abstr., Food Sci.& Tech.Abstr., Helminthol.Abstr., Herb.Abstr., Hort.Abstr., Ind.Vet., Nutr.Abstr., Pig News & Info., Poult.Abstr., Protozool.Abstr., Rev.Appl.Entomol., Rev.Med.& Vet.Mycol., Rev.Plant Path., Soyabean Abstr., Vet.Bull., Zoo.Rec.
—CASDDS.
Address: 68, Kshudiram Bose Sarani, Kolkata 700 037, India. TEL 99-33-5571987, ijah.wb@hotmail.com. Ed. Dr. A. K. Bhattacharya. Pub. Dr. Swapan Kumar Roy. adv.: B&W page INR 600, color page INR 1,800; 20.5 x 15.2. Circ: 2,000. **Dist. by:** H P C Publishers Distributors Pvt. Ltd., 1st Fl., Flats 1 & 2, Darya Ganj, 4805-24 Bharat Ram Rd., New Delhi 110 002, India. TEL 91-11-325-4402, FAX 91-11-686-3511.

INDIAN JOURNAL OF ANIMAL NUTRITION. see *AGRICULTURE—Poultry And Livestock*

INDIAN JOURNAL OF ANIMAL RESEARCH; half-yearly research journal of animal, food, dairying and zoological sciences. see *AGRICULTURE—Poultry And Livestock*

V

636.089 IND ISSN 0367-8318
SF601 CODEN: IJLAA4
INDIAN JOURNAL OF ANIMAL SCIENCES. Text in English. 1931. m. USD 100 (effective 2001). adv. bk.rev. charts, illus. index. reprint service avail. from PQC. *Refereed.* **Document type:** *Journal, Academic/Scholarly, Government.* **Description:** Covers important original research work on animal breeding, diseases, physiology, nutrition, dairying, animal production technology and fisheries.
Formerly: Indian Journal of Veterinary Science and Animal Husbandry (0019-5715)
Related titles: Microform ed.: (from PQC); Online - full text ed.: (from Institute for Scientific Information).
Indexed: ASCA, AgBiotech, Agri.& Environ.Biotech.Abstr. (coverage dropped), Agri.Eng.Abstr., Agrindex, Agroforest.Abstr., Anim.Breed.Abstr., Aqua.Sci.& Fish.Abstr., Aquacult.Abstr., Biol.Abstr., Chem.Abstr., Chem.Indus.Notes, Chem.Titles, Chemorec.Abstr., Curr.Adv.Ecol.Sci., Curr.Adv.Gen.& Molec.Biol., Curr.Cont., Dairy Sci.Abstr., Derwent Biotech.Abstr., Diar.Dis.Res., Environ.Sci.Poll.Mgmt., Excerp.Med., Focus on: Vet.Sci.& Med., Food Sci.& Tech.Abstr., Forest.Abstr., Genet.Abstr., Helminthol.Abstr., Herb.Abstr., Hum.Gen.Abstr., INIS Atomind., Ind.Sci.Rev., Ind.Vet., Maize Abstr., Microbiol.Abstr., Nutr.Abstr., Pig News & Info., Plant Breed.Abstr., Postharvest, Poult.Abstr., Protozool.Abstr., Rev.Appl.Entomol., Rev.Med.& Vet.Mycol., Rev.Plant Path., Rice Abstr., Rural Recreat.Tour.Abstr., Sci.Cit.Ind. (coverage dropped), Small Anim.Abstr., Sorghum & Millets Abstr., Soyabean Abstr., Sport Fish.Abstr., Sugar Ind.Abstr., Triticale Abstr., Vet.Bull., Weed Abstr., Wild.Rev., World Ag.Econ.& Rur.Soc.Abstr., Zoo.Rec.
—BLDSC (4410.195000), CASDDS, CISTI, IDS, ingenta, Linda Hall.
Published by: (Indian Council of Agricultural Research), Scientific Publishers, 5-A New Pali Rd., P O Box 91, Jodhpur, Rajasthan 342 001, India. TEL 91-291-433323, FAX 91-291-512580, scienti@sancharnet.in, http://www.scientificpub.com. Ed. Aruna T Kumar. Adv. contact S K Joshi. Circ: 2,000.

636.089 611 IND ISSN 0971-1937
INDIAN JOURNAL OF VETERINARY ANATOMY. Text and summaries in English. 1989. s-a. INR 250, USD 50 (effective 1999). adv. bk.rev. back issues avail. *Refereed.* **Document type:** *Academic/Scholarly.* **Description:** Research articles on anatomy, histology, and embryology.
Indexed: Anim.Breed.Abstr., Dairy Sci.Abstr., Ind.Vet., Nutr.Abstr., Poult.Abstr., Vet.Bull.
—BLDSC (4421.850000).
Published by: Indian Association of Veterinary Anatomists (IAVA), c/o Dept. of Anatomy, College of Vet. Science and Animal Husbandry, C.S. Azad Univ. of Agriculture and Technology, Mathura, Uttar Pradesh 281 001, India. FAX 91-565-404819. Ed., R&P Dr. Chandra Pal TEL 91-565-408418. Adv. contact M M Farooqui. page USD 20. Circ: 200 (paid). **Affiliate:** World Association of Veterinary Anatomists.

639.089 IND ISSN 0970-051X
CODEN: IJVMDP
INDIAN JOURNAL OF VETERINARY MEDICINE. Text in English. 1981. s-a., latest vol.20, Dec. INR 400 domestic; USD 80 foreign (effective 2001). adv. bk.rev. author and subject indexes. 70 p./no. 2 cols./p. back issues avail. **Document type:** *Journal, Academic/Scholarly.*
Indexed: Dairy Sci.Abstr., Helminthol.Abstr., Ind.Vet., Nutr.Abstr., Poult.Abstr., Protozool.Abstr., Rev.Appl.Entomol., Rev.Med.& Vet.Mycol., Sport Fish.Abstr., Trop.Dis.Bull., Vet.Bull., Wild.Rev., Zoo.Rec.
—BLDSC (4421.880000), ingenta.
Published by: Indian Society for Veterinary Medicine, c/o Dr. D. Swarup, Ed., Div. of Medicine, Indian Veterinary Research Institute, Izatnagar, Uttar Pradesh 243 122, India. TEL 91-581-441587, 91-581-525541, FAX 91-581-447284, dswarup@iuri.up.nic.in. Ed. Dr. D Swarup. Adv. contact Dr. S Dey. B&W page INR 1,500. Circ: 50 (paid); 700 (controlled).

636.089 IND ISSN 0971-4251
THE INDIAN JOURNAL OF VETERINARY RESEARCH. Abbreviated title: I J V R. Text in English. 1992. biennial. INR 300, USD 30 (effective 2001). adv. bk.rev. *Refereed.* **Document type:** *Academic/Scholarly.*
Indexed: Anim.Breed.Abstr., Dairy Sci.Abstr., Ind.Vet., Nutr.Abstr., Poult.Abstr., Protozool.Abstr., Rev.Appl.Entomol., Vet.Bull.
—BLDSC (4421.950000).
Published by: (Indian Association for the Advancement of Veterinary Research), Indian Veterinary Research Institute, Division of Bacteriology and Mycology, Izatnagar, Uttar Pradesh 243 122, India. FAX 91-581-447284, TELEX VETEX. Ed. Rishendra Verma. Circ: 460.

636.089 IND ISSN 0254-4105
CODEN: IJVSD9
INDIAN JOURNAL OF VETERINARY SURGERY. Text in English. 1980. s-a. USD 60 to institutions (effective 2000). adv. bk.rev. **Document type:** *Academic/Scholarly.* **Description:** Publishes research results, clinical and review articles in Indian and foreign veterinary surgery and related subjects.
Indexed: Biol.Abstr., Ind.Vet., Indian Sci.Abstr., Rev.Arom.& Med.Plants, Sport Fish.Abstr., Vet.Bull., Wild.Rev.
Published by: Indian Society for Veterinary Surgery, Division of Surgery, Indian Veterinary Research Institute, Izatnagar, Uttar Pradesh 243 122, India. TEL 91-581-442870, TELEX 577 205 IN RI IN, ivri@x400nicgw.in. Ed. Dr. Gaj Raj Singh. R&P A P Singh. Adv. contact A.P. Singh. Circ: 1,000. **Dist. overseas by:** H P C Publishers Distributors Pvt. Ltd., 1st Fl., Flats 1 & 2, Darya Ganj, 4805-24 Bharat Ram Rd., New Delhi 110 002, India. TEL 91-11-686-3511, 91-11-3254401, FAX 91-11-686-3511.

INDIAN POULTRY INDUSTRY YEARBOOK. see *AGRICULTURE—Poultry And Livestock*

INDIAN POULTRY REVIEW. see *AGRICULTURE—Poultry And Livestock*

636.089 IND ISSN 0019-6479
SF604 CODEN: IVEJAC
INDIAN VETERINARY JOURNAL; a monthly record of veterinary science. (IVJ) Text in English. 1924. m. USD 110 (effective 2001). adv. bk.rev. abstr, illus, stat. index. 100 p./no. 2 cols./p. back issues avail.; reprint service avail. from ISI. *Refereed.* **Document type:** *Journal, Academic/Scholarly.* **Description:** Presents a monthly record of veterinary sciences, including animal husbandry, dairy, and poultry. Contains general research and clinical articles, short communications, editorial news, book reviews, flashback, and association news.
Related titles: Online - full content ed.; Online - full text ed.: (from Institute for Scientific Information).
Indexed: ASCA, AgBiotech, Agri.& Environ.Biotech.Abstr. (coverage dropped), Agri.Eng.Abstr., Agroforest.Abstr., Anim.Breed.Abstr., Biol.Abstr., Chem.Abstr., Chem.Indus.Notes, Chem.Titles, Curr.Adv.Cancer Res., Curr.Adv.Ecol.Sci., Curr.Adv.Gen.& Molec.Biol., Curr.Cont., Dairy Sci.Abstr., Derwent Biotech.Abstr., Field Crop Abstr., Focus on: Vet.Sci.& Med., Food Sci.& Tech.Abstr., Helminthol.Abstr., Herb.Abstr., Hort.Abstr., Ind.Med. (coverage dropped), Ind.Sci.Rev., Ind.Vet., Maize Abstr., Nutr.Abstr., Pig News & Info., Poult.Abstr., Protozool.Abstr., Rev.Appl.Entomol., Rev.Arom.& Med.Plants, Rev.Med.& Vet.Mycol., Rev.Plant Path., Rural Devel.Abstr., SSCI (coverage dropped), Sci.Cit.Ind. (coverage dropped), Small Anim.Abstr., Soyabean Abstr., Sport Fish.Abstr., Triticale Abstr., Trop.Dis.Bull., Trop.Oil Seeds Abstr., Vet.Bull., Weed Abstr., Wild.Rev., World Ag.Econ.& Rur.Soc.Abstr., Zoo.Rec.
—BLDSC (4431.000000), CASDDS, CISTI, GNLM, IDS, ingenta, Linda Hall.
Published by: Indian Veterinary Association, 11/7, Chamiers Rd., Chennai, Tamil Nadu 600 035, India. TEL 91-44-4351006, FAX 91-44-4338894, ivj@vsnl.com, http://www.indvetjournal.com. Ed., Pub., R&P, Adv. contact V D Padmanaban. B&W page USD 3,000; trim 18.2 x 24. Circ: 9,000 (paid).

590 IND ISSN 0250-5266
CODEN: IVMJDL
INDIAN VETERINARY MEDICAL JOURNAL. Text in English; Section in English, Hindi. 1977. q. USD 75 foreign (effective 2000). adv. bk.rev. bibl. **Document type:** *Academic/Scholarly.*
Supersedes (in 1977): U P Veterinary Journal
Related titles: Microfiche ed.
Indexed: Anim.Breed.Abstr., Biol.Abstr., Chem.Abstr., Chem.Indus.Notes, Chem.Titles, Dairy Sci.Abstr., Helminthol.Abstr., Hort.Abstr., Ind.Vet., Poult.Abstr., Protozool.Abstr., Rev.Med.& Vet.Mycol., Sport Fish.Abstr., Vet.Bull., Wild.Rev., Zoo.Rec.
—CASDDS, CISTI, ingenta.
Published by: Uttar Pradesh Veterinary Association, c/o Institute of Veterinary Biologicals, Badshahbagh, Lucknow, Uttar Pradesh 226 007, India. TEL 91-129-387352. Ed. J N S Yadava. R&P J.N.S. Yadava. Adv. contact S K Agarwal. page USD 120. Circ: 2,500. **Dist. by:** H P C Publishers Distributors Pvt. Ltd., 1st Fl., Flats 1 & 2, Darya Ganj, 4805-24 Bharat Ram Rd., New Delhi 110 002, India. TEL 91-11-325-4401, FAX 91-11-619-3511.

636.089 IND ISSN 0304-7067
SF779.M78
INDIAN VETERINARY RESEARCH INSTITUTE. ANNUAL REPORT. Text in English. 1947. a. per issue exchange basis.
Formerly: Muktesar, India. Imperial Veterinary Research Institute. Report
Indexed: Anim.Breed.Abstr.
—CISTI.
Published by: Indian Veterinary Research Institute, Mukteswar-Kumaon, Izatnagar, Uttar Pradesh 243 122, India. Circ: 1,500.

636.089 CUB ISSN 0138-7235
INFORMACION EXPRESS. SERIE: VETERINARIA. Text in Spanish. 1977. 4/yr. USD 9 in North America; USD 11 in South America; USD 13 in Europe; USD 18 elsewhere.
Indexed: Agrindex.
—CISTI.
Published by: Centro de Informacion y Documentacion Agropecuario, Gaveta Postal 4149, Havana 4, Cuba. **Dist. by:** Ediciones Cubanas, Obispo No. 527, Apdo. 605, Havana, Cuba.

636.089 ITA
INFORMATORE DI VETERINARIA E ZOOTECNIA. Text in Italian. 1986. a. ITL 145,000; ITL 156,000 in Europe; ITL 186,000 elsewhere. adv. *Refereed.* **Document type:** *Directory.* **Description:** Lists veterinary and zootechnical products and updates.
Related titles: CD-ROM ed.
Published by: Organizzazione Editoriale Medico Farmaceutica, Viale Zara, 69, Milan, MI 20124, Italy. TEL 39-2-332101, FAX 39-2-33210200, oemf@galactica.it. Ed. Carlo Marini. Adv. contact Guido Parazzoli. B&W page ITL 2,500,000. Circ: 45,000 (controlled).

636.089 ITA
L'INFORMATORE FARMACEUTICO DI VETERINARIA E ZOOTECNIA. Text in Italian. 1966. irreg., latest 2000. EUR 81.60 (effective 2001). **Document type:** *Directory, Consumer.*
Formerly: Guida di Veterinaria e Zootecnia (0391-1918)
Published by: O E M F SpA, Via Filippo Palizzi, 88, PO Box 10434, Milan, MI 20157, Italy. TEL 39-02-332101, FAX 39-02-3551731, info@oemf.it, http://www.oemf.it. Ed. Dr. G Panagia. Adv. contact Delia Weissy.

INSTITUT RAZI. ARCHIVES. see *MEDICAL SCIENCES—Communicable Diseases*

636.089 NPL ISSN 1018-6182
CODEN: JOISEP
INSTITUTE OF AGRICULTURE AND ANIMAL SCIENCE. JOURNAL. Text in English. 1980. a. **Document type:** *Academic/Scholarly.*
Indexed: Helminthol.Abstr., Rice Abstr., Sport Fish.Abstr., Wild.Rev., Zoo.Rec.
Published by: Institute of Agriculture and Animal Science, Rampur, Chitwan, Nepal.

INSTITUTE OF MEDICAL AND VETERINARY SCIENCE. ANNUAL REPORT OF THE COUNCIL. see *MEDICAL SCIENCES*

636.08 664 ARG
INSTITUTO PANAMERICANO DE PROTECCION DE ALIMENTOS Y ZOONOSIS EN LAS AMERICAS. Abbreviated title: Inpaz en las Americas. Text in Spanish. 1994. irreg. free per issue. **Document type:** *Newsletter.*
Related titles: English ed.: Inpaz in the Americas.
Published by: Instituto Panamericano de Proteccion de Alimentos y Zoonosis/Panamerican Institute for Food Protection and Zoonoses, Casilla de Correos 44, Martinez, Buenos Aires 1640, Argentina. TEL 54-11-8361000, FAX 54-11-8360927, TELEX 24577 AT PAZ, inppaz@inppaz.ops-oms.org, http://www.inppaz.org.ar. **Affiliate:** World Health Organization.

636.08 664 ARG
INSTITUTO PANAMERICANO DE PROTECCION DE ALIMENTOS Y ZOONOSIS. PUBLICACION TECNICA. Text in Spanish. 1993. irreg., latest vol.3, 1994. free per issue. **Document type:** *Monographic series.*
Published by: Instituto Panamericano de Proteccion de Alimentos y Zoonosis/Panamerican Institute for Food Protection and Zoonoses, Casilla de correo 44, Martinez, BUENOS AIRES 1064, Argentina. TEL 54-11-8361000, FAX 54-11-8360927, inppaz@inppaz.ops-oms.org, http://www.inppaz.org.ar.

636.089 AUS
INTERNATIONAL CONGRESS ON ANIMAL REPRODUCTION. PROCEEDINGS. Text in English. 1948. quadrennial, latest 1996, 13th, Sydney. USD 100 (effective 1998). **Document type:** *Proceedings.*
Formerly: International Congress on Animal Reproduction and Artificial Insemination. Proceedings (0074-4026)
Indexed: Biol.Abstr.
—CISTI.
Published by: International Standing Committee on International Congress on Animal Reproduction, c/o Careth Evans, Dept. of Animal Science, University Of Sydney, NSW 2006, Australia. TEL 61-2-9351-3363, garethe@vetsci.usyd.edu.auu.oz.au. Eds. C Evans, C M Stone. Circ: 2,000.

636.7 USA
INTERNATIONAL SYMPOSIUM ON CANINE HEARTWORM DISEASE. PROCEEDINGS. Text in English. 1969. irreg., latest vol.2, 1971. USD 12 (effective 1999). bibl, illus. **Document type:** *Proceedings.*
Published by: University of Florida, Institute of Food & Agricultural Sciences, Department of Veterinary Science, McCarty Hall, Gainesville, FL 32611-0620. TEL 904-392-1733. Ed. Richard E Bradley.

INTERNATIONAL WILDLIFE REHABILITATION COUNCIL. INDIVIDUAL PAPERS. see *BIOLOGY—Zoology*

636.089 USA ISSN 0099-5851
CODEN: ISUVA5
IOWA STATE UNIVERSITY VETERINARIAN. Text in English. 1938. s-a. USD 15 domestic to non-members; USD 20 foreign to non-members (effective 1999). adv. bk.rev. index. reprint service avail. from PQC. *Refereed.* **Document type:** *Academic/Scholarly.* **Description:** Each issue presents 3 research papers, one law case feature, and x-ray section and alumni news.
Related titles: Microfiche ed.: (from PQC).
Indexed: Agricola, Dairy Sci.Abstr., Ind.Vet., Pig News & Info., Ref.Zh., Rev.Appl.Entomol., Small Anim.Abstr., Sport Fish.Abstr., Vet.Bull., Wild.Rev., Zoo.Rec.
—CISTI, Linda Hall.
Published by: (American Veterinary Medical Association), Iowa State University, College of Veterinary Medicine, c/o Dept of Pathology, Ames, IA 50011. Ed. Eric Vymyslicky. Adv. contact Kerry Young. B&W page USD 130. Circ: 2,500.

636.089 IRL ISSN 0368-0762
CODEN: IVTJAJ
IRISH VETERINARY JOURNAL. Text in English. 1980 (vol.34). m. IEP 6. adv. bk.rev. abstr. *Refereed.* **Document type:** *Academic/Scholarly.*
Related titles: Online - full text ed.: (from Institute for Scientific Information).
Indexed: ASCA, Agri.Eng.Abstr., Anim.Breed.Abstr., Chem.Abstr., Curr.Cont., Dairy Sci.Abstr., Derwent Biotech.Abstr., Excerp.Med., Focus on: Vet.Sci.& Med., Helminthol.Abstr., INIS Atomind., Ind.Sci.Rev., Ind.Vet., Nutr.Abstr., Pig News & Info., Poult.Abstr., Protozool.Abstr., Rev.Appl.Entomol., Rev.Med.& Vet.Mycol., Rev.Plant Path., Sci.Cit.Ind., Small Anim.Abstr., Soyabean Abstr., Sport Fish.Abstr., Vet.Bull., Wild.Rev., Zoo.Rec.
—BLDSC (4575.000000), CASDDS, CISTI, IDS, ingenta.
Published by: Irish Veterinary Association, 53 Lansdowne Rd., Ballsbridge, Dublin 4, Ireland. TEL 01-6685263, FAX 01-6604345. Ed. Dr. P J Hartigan. Circ: 1,300.

636.089 ISR ISSN 0334-9152
CODEN: RVETA5
ISRAEL JOURNAL OF VETERINARY MEDICINE. Text in English, Hebrew. 1943. q. USD 75 (effective 2000). adv. bk.rev. charts, illus.
Formerly (until 1986): Refuah Veterinarith (0034-3153)
Indexed: Agri.& Environ.Biotech.Abstr. (coverage dropped), Anim.Breed.Abstr., Biol.Abstr., Chem.Abstr., Curr.Cont. (coverage dropped), Dairy Sci.Abstr., Derwent Biotech.Abstr., Excerp.Med., Food Sci.& Tech.Abstr., Helminthol.Abstr., Ind.Vet., Nutr.Abstr., Pig News & Info., Poult.Abstr., Protozool.Abstr., Rev.Appl.Entomol., Rev.Med.& Vet.Mycol., Small Anim.Abstr., Soyabean Abstr., Sport Fish.Abstr., Trop.Dis.Bull., Vet.Bull., Wild.Rev., Zoo.Rec.
—BLDSC (4583.816000), CASDDS, CISTI, ingenta.
Published by: Israel Veterinary Medical Association, P O Box 3076, Rishon Le Zion 75130, Israel. FAX 972-3-9681753. Eds. G Simon, I Glass. Circ: 1,200.

636.089 TUR ISSN 0378-2352
CODEN: IUVDD7
ISTANBUL UNIVERSITESI. VETERINER FAKULTESI DERGISI/UNIVERSITY OF ISTANBUL. FACULTY OF VETERINARY MEDICINE. JOURNAL. Key Title: Veteriner Fakultesi Dergisi. Text in Turkish; Summaries in English, French, German. 1975. 2/yr., latest vol.27. USD 6. software rev. abstr. back issues avail.; reprints avail. *Refereed.* **Document type:** *Journal, Academic/Scholarly.*
Indexed: AgBiotech, Anim.Breed.Abstr., Biol.Abstr., Dairy Sci.Abstr., Ind.Vet., Nutr.Abstr., Poult.Abstr., Rev.Appl.Entomol., Rev.Med.& Vet.Mycol., Sugar Ind.Abstr., Vet.Bull.
Published by: Istanbul Universitesi, Veteriner Fakultesi/University of Istanbul, Faculty of Veterinary Medicine, Avcilar Campus, Avcilar - Istanbul 34851, Turkey. TEL 90-212-5912193, 90-212-5916985, FAX 90-212-5916991, gunes@istanbul.edu.tr. Ed. Dr. Halil Gunes. Circ: 750.

ISTITUTO SUPERIORE DI SANITA. ANNALI. see *PUBLIC HEALTH AND SAFETY*

636.08 JPN
J A H A SHOREI HAPPYOKAI/JAPANESE ANIMAL HOSPITAL ASSOCIATION. PROCEEDINGS. Text in Japanese. a. **Document type:** *Proceedings.*
Published by: Nihon Dobutsu Byoin Fukushi Kyokai/Japanese Animal Hospital Association, Ikeda Bldg 201, 1-15 Shinogawa-Machi, Shinjuku-ku, Tokyo 162-0814, Japan. TEL 03-3235-3251, FAX 03-3235-3277.

J N K V V NEWS. see *AGRICULTURE*

636.089 AUT ISSN 0075-2606
JAHRBUCH FUER DEN OESTERREICHISCHEN TIERARZT. Text in German. 1950. a. ATS 378. adv.
Published by: Alois Goeschl und Co., Trummelhofgasse 12, Vienna, W 1190, Austria. Ed. Hiltraud Lechner.

636.089 JPN ISSN 0388-7421
SF917 CODEN: DIKNAA
JAPAN. MINISTRY OF AGRICULTURE, FORESTRY AND FISHERIES. NATIONAL VETERINARY ASSAY LABORATORY. ANNUAL REPORT. Text and summaries in English, Japanese. 1960. a. free per issue. back issues avail.
Indexed: Ind.Vet., Pig News & Info., Poult.Abstr., Vet.Bull.
—BLDSC (1369.500000), CASDDS.
Published by: Ministry of Agriculture Forestry and Fisheries, National Veterinary Assay Laboratory, 1-15-1 Tokura, Kokubunji-shi, Tokyo-to 185-0003, Japan. TEL 423-21-1841, FAX 423-21-1769. Circ: 800.

636.089 JPN ISSN 0047-1917
CODEN: JJVRAE
JAPANESE JOURNAL OF VETERINARY RESEARCH. Text in English, Multiple languages. 1954. q. per issue exchange basis. bk.rev. illus. *Refereed.* **Document type:** *Academic/Scholarly.*
Formerly: Juigaku Kenkyu
Related titles: Microfiche ed.; Microfilm ed.; Online - full text ed.: (from Institute for Scientific Information).
Indexed: ASCA, Anim.Breed.Abstr., Aqua.Sci.& Fish.Abstr., Aquacult.Abstr., Biol.Abstr., Chem.Abstr., Curr.Cont. (coverage dropped), Dairy Sci.Abstr., Environ.Sci.Poll.Mgmt., Excerp.Med., Focus on: Vet.Sci.& Med., Helminthol.Abstr., INIS Atomind., Ind.Med. (1954-), Ind.Sci.Rev., Ind.Vet., Microbiol.Abstr., Nutr.Abstr., Pig News & Info., Poult.Abstr., Protozool.Abstr., Ref.Zh., Rev.Appl.Entomol., Sci.Cit.Ind. (coverage dropped), Sport Fish.Abstr., Vet.Bull., Wild.Rev., World Ag.Econ.& Rur.Soc.Abstr., Zoo.Rec.
—BLDSC (4659.090000), CISTI, GNLM, IDS, ingenta, Linda Hall.
Published by: Hokkaido University, Faculty of Veterinary Medicine/Hokkaido Daigaku Juigakubu, Nishi-9-chome, Kita-18-jo, Sapporo 060, Japan. TEL 81-11-706-5215, FAX 81-11-709-7198. Ed. Misao Onuma. Circ: 650.

JOURNAL OF ANIMAL PHYSIOLOGY AND ANIMAL NUTRITION/ZEITSCHRIFT FUER TIERPHYSIOLOGIE UND TIERERNAEHRUNG. see *BIOLOGY—Physiology*

JOURNAL OF ANIMAL PHYSIOLOGY AND ANIMAL NUTRITION ONLINE. see *BIOLOGY—Physiology*

JOURNAL OF AQUATIC ANIMAL HEALTH. see *FISH AND FISHERIES*

636.087 USA ISSN 1082-6742
JOURNAL OF AVIAN MEDICINE AND SURGERY. Text in English; Summaries in Dutch, French, German, Italian, Spanish. 1980. q. USD 110 domestic; USD 115 in Canada & Mexico; USD 125 in Europe; USD 145 elsewhere (effective 2001). adv. bk.rev. abstr, illus. Index. back issues avail.; reprints avail. *Refereed.* **Document type:** *Academic/Scholarly.* **Description:** Addresses avian research, bird medicine and surger conservation, aviculture, pharmaceuticals and biologicals and veterinary medical education.
Former titles (until 1995): Association of Avian Veterinarians. Journal (1044-8314); (until 1989): A A V Today (0892-9904); (until 1987): A A V Newsletter
Related titles: Online - full text ed.: (from BioOne, Institute for Scientific Information).
Indexed: ASCA, Anim.Breed.Abstr., Bibl.Agri., Focus on: Vet.Sci.& Med., Helminthol.Abstr., Ind.Vet., Nutr.Abstr., Poult.Abstr., Protozool.Abstr., Rev.Med.& Vet.Mycol., Small Anim.Abstr., Sport Fish.Abstr., Vet.Bull., Wild.Rev., Zoo.Rec.
—BLDSC (4949.960000), IDS, ingenta.
Published by: Association of Avian Veterinarians, PO Box 210732, Bedford, TX 76095. TEL 817-428-7900, FAX 817-485-4800, aavpubs@aol.com. Ed. Dr. James Carpenter. R&P, Adv. contact Kathy Lyon. Circ: 3,500. **Subscr. to:** AAV Box 811720, Boca Raton, FL 33481. **Dist. by:** AAV Central Office, PO Box 811720, Boca Raton, FL 33481. TEL 561-393-8901, FAX 561-393-8902.

636.089 JPN
JOURNAL OF CLINICAL VETERINARY MEDICINE. Text in Japanese. m. JPY 1,200 per issue. **Document type:** *Trade.* **Description:** Designed for large animal veterinarians. Covers clinical medicine for large animals.
Published by: Chikusan Publishing Co. Ltd. (Subsidiary of: Midori Group), Ikebukuro Nishiguchi Sky Bldg, 2-14-4 Ikebukuro, Toshima-ku, Tokyo 171-0014, Japan. TEL 03-3590-9454. Circ: 36,000.

636.089 USA ISSN 0737-0806
JOURNAL OF EQUINE VETERINARY SCIENCE. Text in English. 1981. m. USD 155 domestic to individuals; USD 165 in Canada & Mexico to individuals; USD 185 elsewhere to individuals; USD 210 domestic to institutions; USD 220 in Canada & Mexico to institutions; USD 240 elsewhere to institutions. adv. bk.rev. *Refereed.* **Document type:** *Academic/Scholarly.*
Incorporates (1980-1997): Equine Veterinary Data (0739-9065); Incorporates: Equine Sportsmedicine News (0890-0140)
Related titles: Online - full text ed.: (from Institute for Scientific Information).
Indexed: ASCA, Agricola, Anim.Breed.Abstr., Curr.Cont., Dairy Sci.Abstr., Derwent Biotech.Abstr., Focus on: Vet.Sci.& Med., Helminthol.Abstr., Herb.Abstr., Ind.Vet., Nutr.Abstr., Protozool.Abstr., Rev.Appl.Entomol., Rev.Med.& Vet.Mycol., Triticale Abstr., Vet.Bull., Weed Abstr.
—BLDSC (4979.492000), CISTI, IDS, ingenta.
Published by: Veterinary Data, PO Box 1209, Wildomar, CA 92595. TEL 909-678-1889, FAX 909-678-1885, vetdata@inland.net. Ed., Pub. Dr. William E Jones. Circ: 5,100.

636.089 GBR ISSN 1098-612X
SF985
▼ **JOURNAL OF FELINE MEDICINE AND SURGERY.** Text in English. 1999. q. GBP 72 to individuals; GBP 146 to institutions (effective 2002). adv. bk.rev. charts, illus. *Refereed.* **Document type:** *Academic/Scholarly.* **Description:** Publishes original papers and reviews on all aspects of feline medicine and surgery, including relevant basic research.
Related titles: Online - full text ed.: (from Swets Blackwell).
Indexed: Derwent Biotech.Abstr., Ind.Vet., Nutr.Abstr., Rev.Med.& Vet.Mycol., Vet.Bull.
—BLDSC (4983.933000).

V

Published by: (European Society for Feline Medicine), W.B. Saunders Co. Ltd. (Subsidiary of: Harcourt Publishers Ltd.), 24-28 Oval Rd, London NW1 7DX, United Kingdom. TEL 44-1714-244200, FAX 44-20-7485-4752, cservice@harcourt.com, http://www.harcourt-international.com/journals/jfms. Ed. A H Sparkes. Pub. Wendy Jones. R&P Sarah Owen. Adv. contact Greg Holt. B&W page GBP 500, color page GBP 895; trim 210 x 280. Circ: 1,000. **Subscr. to:** Harcourt Publishers Ltd., Foots Cray High St, Sidcup, Kent DA14 5HP, United Kingdom. TEL 44-20-8308-5700, FAX 44-20-8309-0807.

JOURNAL OF HERPETOLOGICAL MEDICINE AND SURGERY. see *BIOLOGY—Zoology*

V

636.089 JPN ISSN 0916-8818 CODEN: JREDEF
JOURNAL OF REPRODUCTION AND DEVELOPMENT. Text in English. 1955. bi-m. JPY 8,000 to members; JPY 9,000 to non-members (effective 2001). adv. bk.rev. back issues avail. *Refereed.* **Document type:** *Academic/Scholarly.* **Description:** Publishes new findings and concepts in reproductive biology, reproductive endocrinology, reproductive immunology, and developmental biology.
Formerly (until Feb. 1992): Japanese Journal of Animal Reproduction (0385-9932)
Indexed: AgBiotech, Anim.Breed.Abstr., Chem.Abstr., Chem.Indus.Notes, Chem.Titles, Dairy Sci.Abstr., INIS Atomind., Ind.Vet., Nutr.Abstr., Pig News & Info., Poult.Abstr., Rev.Appl.Entomol., Sugar Ind.Abstr., Vet.Bull.
—BLDSC (5049.570000), CASDDS, CISTI, Infotrieve. **CCC.**
Published by: (Japanese Society of Animal Reproduction), I P E C Inc., 1-24-11 Sugamo, Toshima-ku, Tokyo 170-0002, Japan. TEL 81-3-5978-4067, FAX 81-3-5978-4068, http://www.soc.nacsis.ac.jp/jsar/, http://www.soc.nacsis.ac.jp/jsar/. Ed., R&P Dr. Yuji Mori.

636.089 GBR ISSN 0022-4510 CODEN: JAPRAN
JOURNAL OF SMALL ANIMAL PRACTICE. Text in English. 1960. m. GBP 145 in United Kingdom; GBP 160 rest of world (effective 2001). adv. bk.rev. bibl, charts, illus. index. back issues avail.; reprint service avail. from ISI. *Refereed.* **Document type:** *Academic/Scholarly.* **Description:** Publishes original research, review articles, and clinical case histories on all aspects of small animal medicine and surgery.
Related titles: Online - full text ed.: (from Institute for Scientific Information).
Indexed: ASCA, Abstr.Hyg., AgBiotech, Agri.& Environ.Biotech.Abstr. (coverage dropped), Agricola, Anim.Breed.Abstr., Bibl.Agri., Biol.Abstr., Chem.Abstr., Curr.Adv.Ecol.Sci., Curr.Cont., Dairy Sci.Abstr., Derwent Biotech.Abstr., Excerp.Med., Focus on: Vet.Sci.& Med., Helminthol.Abstr., Ind.Med. (1960-), Ind.Sci.Rev., Ind.Vet., Nutr.Abstr., Protozool.Abstr., Ref.Zh., Rev.Appl.Entomol., Rev.Med.& Vet.Mycol., Rev.Plant Path., Rice Abstr., Sci.Cit.Ind., Small Anim.Abstr., Sport Fish.Abstr., Vet.Bull., Wild.Rev., Zoo.Rec.
—BLDSC (5064.700000), CISTI, GNLM, IDS, Infotrieve, ingenta. **CCC.**
Published by: (British Small Animal Veterinary Association), British Veterinary Association, 7 Mansfield St, London W1M 0AT, United Kingdom. TEL 44-171-636-6541, FAX 44-171-637-0620, adminoff@bsava.com, http://www.bsava.com./members/jsap/aboutjsap.htm. Ed. Dr. F J Barr. Pub. Martin Alder. R&P Lewis Millington. Adv. contact Gillian Notton. Circ: 4,500. **Subscr. to:** TGS Subscriber Services, 6 Bourne Enterprise Centre, Wrotham Rd, Borough Green, Kent, United Kingdom. TEL 44-1732-884023, FAX 44-1732-884034.

636.089 USA ISSN 1537-209X
JOURNAL OF SWINE HEALTH AND PRODUCTION. Text in English. 1993. bi-m., latest vol.9, 2001. USD 90 (effective 2001); USD 95 in North America; USD 107.50 elsewhere (effective 2002). *Refereed.* **Document type:** *Journal, Academic/Scholarly.* **Description:** Research articles dealing with swine health and production.
Formerly: Swine Health and Production (1066-4963)
Related titles: CD-ROM ed.: USD 50 with membership or subscription to print ed. (effective 2001); Online - full content ed.; Online - full text ed.: (from Institute for Scientific Information).
Indexed: AgBiotech, Agricola, Anim.Breed.Abstr., Focus on: Vet.Sci.& Med., Ind.Vet., Nutr.Abstr., Pig News & Info., Vet.Bull., World Ag.Econ.& Rur.Soc.Abstr.
Published by: American Association of Swine Veterinarians, 902 1st Ave, Perry, IA 50220. TEL 515-465-5255, FAX 515-465-3832, aasv@netins.net, http://www.aasv.org. Ed. Cate Dewey. Adv. contact Kim Smith TEL 515-465-7920. Circ: 1,800.

636.089 IND ISSN 0971-0701 SF604 CODEN: JVASEY
JOURNAL OF VETERINARY AND ANIMAL SCIENCES. Text in English. 1970. s-a. USD 25 (effective 2000). *Refereed.* **Document type:** *Academic/Scholarly.*
Formerly (until vol.20, 1991): Kerala Journal of Veterinary Science (0374-8774)
Indexed: Anim.Breed.Abstr., Biol.Abstr., Chem.Abstr., Dairy Sci.Abstr., Helminthol.Abstr., Ind.Vet., Nutr.Abstr., Poult.Abstr., Rev.Appl.Entomol., Rural Ext.Educ.& Tr.Abstr., Rural Recreat.Tour.Abstr., Sport Fish.Abstr., Vet.Bull., Wild.Rev., World Ag.Econ.& Rur.Soc.Abstr., Zoo.Rec.
—CASDDS, CISTI.
Published by: Kerala Agricultural University, Faculty of Veterinary and Animal Sciences, Trichur, Kerala, India. TEL 91-487-370451, TELEX 887-268 KAU IN, kauhqr@ren.nic.in. Ed. C P N Iyer. Circ: 1,000. **Dist. overseas by:** HPC Publishers' Distributors Pvt. Ltd., 4805-24, 1st Bharat Ram Rd., Darya Ganj, New Delhi 110 002, India. TEL 91-11-325-4401, 91-11-686-3511.

636.087 USA ISSN 0898-7564
JOURNAL OF VETERINARY DENTISTRY. Text in English. 1984. q. USD 60 domestic; USD 70 in Canada & Mexico; USD 75 elsewhere (effective 2000). adv. *Refereed.* **Document type:** *Journal, Academic/Scholarly.* **Description:** Covers medical and surgical aspects of veterinary dentisty, including anatomy, crowns, restorations, endodontics, orthodontics, periodontics, and oral biology.
Formerly (until 1987): Veterinary Dentistry
Related titles: Online - full text ed.: (from Institute for Scientific Information); Includes: Animal Health Technician Dental Newsletter.
Indexed: Focus on: Vet.Sci.& Med., Wild.Rev.
—BLDSC (5072.355000), ingenta.
Published by: American Veterinary Dental Society, 530 Church St., Ste. 700, Nashville, TN 37219. TEL 615-254-3687, FAX 615-254-7047, vetdent@vet.upenn.edu, http://phl.vet.upenn.edu/jvd/index.html. Ed. Dr. Colin E. Harvey TEL 215-898-5903. Adv. contact Carolyn Schuster. B&W page USD 1,000, color page USD 1,650; trim 8.125 x 10.875. **Co-sponsors:** Academy of Veterinary Dentistry; American Veterinary Dental College.

636.089 USA ISSN 1040-6387
JOURNAL OF VETERINARY DIAGNOSTIC INVESTIGATION. Text in English. 1989. bi-m. USD 60 in US & Canada to individuals; USD 75 elsewhere to individuals; USD 50 to members; USD 100 to institutions (effective 2001). adv. back issues avail. *Refereed.* **Document type:** *Academic/Scholarly.* **Description:** Covers molecular biology, immunology, microbiology, clinical pathology, parasitology, anatomical pathology, toxicology, computer science and public health.
Related titles: Online - full text ed.: (from Institute for Scientific Information).
Indexed: ASCA, AgBiotech, Agricola, Bibl.Agri., Curr.Cont., Dairy Sci.Abstr., Focus on: Vet.Sci.& Med., Helminthol.Abstr., Herb.Abstr., Ind.Med. (1989-), Ind.Vet., Neurosci.Cit.Ind., Nutr.Abstr., Pig News & Info., Poult.Abstr., Protozool.Abstr., Rev.Appl.Entomol., Rev.Med.& Vet.Mycol., Sci.Cit.Ind., Sport Fish.Abstr., Triticale Abstr., Vet.Bull., Wild.Rev., Zoo.Rec.
—BLDSC (5072.360000), GNLM, IDS, ingenta.
Published by: American Association of Veterinary Laboratory Diagnosticians, PO Box 1522, Turlock, CA 95381. TEL 209-634-5837, FAX 209-667-4261, abickfor@cvdls.ucdavis.edu, http://www.aavld.org. Ed., R&P, Adv. contact John M Kreeger. B&W page USD 400, color page USD 750. Circ: 1,500.

636.089 617.1 USA ISSN 1056-6392
JOURNAL OF VETERINARY EMERGENCY AND CRITICAL CARE* . Text in English. 1991. q. USD 50 domestic to individuals; USD 55 in Canada & Mexico to individuals; USD 65 elsewhere to individuals; USD 35 domestic to institutions; USD 40 in Canada & Mexico to institutions; USD 50 elsewhere to institutions. adv. *Refereed.* **Document type:** *Academic/Scholarly.* **Description:** Covers clinical and nonclinical problems and solutions, case reports, and guest editorials.
Indexed: Ind.Vet., Vet.Bull.
—BLDSC (5072.362000).
Address: V E C C S Administration Office, 6335 Camp Bullis Rd, Ste 23, San Antonio, TX 78257-9722. TEL 210-826-1488. Ed. Dr. Marc Raffe. R&P, Adv. contact Mickey Debner. B&W page USD 450, color page USD 850. Circ: 2,500.

636.089 USA ISSN 0891-6640 CODEN: JVIMEM
JOURNAL OF VETERINARY INTERNAL MEDICINE. Text in English. 1987. bi-m. USD 60 domestic to individuals; USD 100 domestic to institutions; USD 30 domestic to students; USD 20 newsstand/cover (effective 2001). adv. illus. index. back issues avail.; reprints avail. *Refereed.* **Document type:** *Academic/Scholarly.* **Description:** Covers small- and large-animal internal medicine, cardiology, neurology, pathophysiology, and the disease process.
Related titles: Online - full text ed.: (from Institute for Scientific Information).
Indexed: ASCA, Agricola, Anim.Breed.Abstr., Curr.Cont., Dairy Sci.Abstr., Derwent Biotech.Abstr., Focus on: Vet.Sci.& Med., INIS Atomind., Ind.Med. (1987-), Ind.Vet., Nutr.Abstr., Protozool.Abstr., Rev.Appl.Entomol., Rev.Med.& Vet.Mycol., Rice Abstr., Sci.Cit.Ind., Small Anim.Abstr., Soyabean Abstr., Triticale Abstr., Vet.Bull.
—BLDSC (5072.365000), CASDDS, GNLM, ingenta.
Published by: American College of Veterinary Internal Medicine, 1997 Wadsworth Blvd, Ste A, Lakewood, CO 80215-3327 . TEL 303-231-9933, 800-245-9081, FAX 303-231-0880, acvim@acvim.org, http://www.acvim.org/wwwfp/jvim/jvim.htm. Eds. Kenneth W Hinchcliff, Stephen P DiBartola. adv.: B&W page USD 675, color page USD 1,540; trim 10 x 7. Circ: 1,000 (paid).

636.0890711 USA ISSN 0748-321X
JOURNAL OF VETERINARY MEDICAL EDUCATION. Text in English. 1974. 3/yr. USD 30 domestic to individuals; USD 40 domestic to institutions; USD 60 foreign to institutions (effective 2001). adv. bk.rev. illus. back issues avail.; reprint service avail. from PQC. *Refereed.* **Document type:** *Academic/Scholarly.* **Description:** Includes papers describing educational programs in veterinary educational institutions throughout the world.
Related titles: Microform ed.: (from PQC); Online - full text ed.: (from Institute for Scientific Information).
Indexed: ASCA, C.I.J.E. (coverage dropped), Cont.Pg.Educ., Focus on: Vet.Sci.& Med., Ind.Vet., Pig News & Info., SSCI (coverage dropped), Vet.Bull.
—BLDSC (5072.370000), CISTI, IDS, ingenta.
Published by: Association of American Veterinary Medical Colleges, 1101 Vermont Ave, NW, Ste 710, Washington, DC 20005. TEL 202-371-9195, FAX 202-842-0773, journals@utpress.utoronto.edu, http://www.utpjournals.com/jvme/jvme.html, http://aavmc.org/. Ed. Dr. Donald Walsh. Adv. contact Audrey Greenwood. Circ: 3,400 (paid).

636.089 JPN ISSN 0916-7250 CODEN: JVMSEQ
JOURNAL OF VETERINARY MEDICAL SCIENCE. Text in English. 1939. 6/yr. JPY 25,000 (effective 1994). adv. bk.rev. *Refereed.* **Document type:** *Academic/Scholarly.* **Description:** International journal on basic and applied veterinary medical sciences.
Formerly (until 1991): Japanese Journal of Veterinary Science (0021-5295)
Related titles: Online - full text ed.: (from Institute for Scientific Information).
Indexed: ASCA, AgBiotech, Agri.& Environ.Biotech.Abstr. (coverage dropped), Anim.Breed.Abstr., Biol.Abstr., Chem.Abstr., Chem.Titles, Curr.Cont., Dairy Sci.Abstr., Dent.Ind., Derwent Biotech.Abstr., Diar.Dis.Res., Focus on: Vet.Sci.& Med., Helminthol.Abstr., Herb.Abstr., INIS Atomind., Ind.Med. (1991-), Ind.Vet., Neurosci.Abstr. (coverage dropped), Nutr.Abstr., Pig News & Info., Plant Breed.Abstr., Poult.Abstr., Protozool.Abstr., Rev.Appl.Entomol., Rev.Arom.& Med.Plants, Rev.Med.& Vet.Mycol., Sci.Cit.Ind., Small Anim.Abstr., Soils & Fert., Sport Fish.Abstr., Triticale Abstr., Trop.Dis.Bull., Vet.Bull., Weed Abstr., Wild.Rev., Zoo.Rec.
—BLDSC (5072.375000), CASDDS, CISTI, GNLM, IDS, Infotrieve, ingenta. **CCC.**
Published by: (Japanese Society of Veterinary Science), Maruzen Co. Ltd./Maruzen Kabushikikaisha, 3-10 Nihonbashi 2-chome, Chuo-ku, Tokyo 103-0027, Japan. Ed. Hideaki Karaki. Circ: 5,000.

636.089 DEU ISSN 0931-184X CODEN: JVMAE6
JOURNAL OF VETERINARY MEDICINE. SERIES A; physiology, pathology, clinical medicine. Text in English, German. 1953. 10/yr. DEM 1,936.28 in Europe; DEM 1,979.30 elsewhere; DEM 2,129.91 in Europe print & online eds. combined; DEM 2,177.23 elsewhere print & online eds. combined (effective 2001). adv. bk.rev. illus. index, cum.index. back issues avail. *Refereed.* **Document type:** *Journal, Academic/Scholarly.* **Description:** Encompasses contributions on physiology, biochemistry, pharmacology, toxicology, etc.
Formerly: Zentralblatt fuer Veterinaermedizin. Reihe A (0300-8711); Supersedes in part (in 1969): Zentralblatt fuer Veterinaermedizin (0044-4294)

Related titles: ♦ Online - full text ed.: Journal of Veterinary Medicine. Series A Online. ISSN 1439-0442; ♦ Supplement: Advances in Veterinary Medicine. ISSN 0301-2794.
Indexed: ASCA, AgBiotech, Agri.& Environ.Biotech.Abstr. (coverage dropped), Anim.Breed.Abstr., Biol.Abstr., Chem.Abstr., Chem.Indus.Notes, Chem.Titles, Curr.Adv.Biochem., Curr.Adv.Ecol.Sci., Curr.Cont., Dairy Sci.Abstr., Derwent Biotech.Abstr., Excerp.Med. (until 1993), Focus on: Vet.Sci.& Med., Food Sci.& Tech.Abstr., Helminthol.Abstr., Herb.Abstr., Ind.Med. (2000-), Ind.Vet., Maize Abstr., Nutr.Abstr., Pig News & Info., Poult.Abstr., Protozool.Abstr., Ref.Zh., Rev.Appl.Entomol., Rev.Med.& Vet.Mycol., Sci.Cit.Ind., Small Anim.Abstr., Sport Fish.Abstr., Sugar Ind.Abstr., Triticale Abstr., Vet.Bull., Weed Abstr., Wild.Rev., Zoo.Rec.
—BLDSC (5072.385000), CASDDS, CISTI, GNLM, IDS, Infotrieve, ingenta, Linda Hall. **CCC.**
Published by: Blackwell Wissenschafts Verlag GmbH, Kurfuerstendamm 57, Berlin 10707, Germany. TEL 49-30-32790665, FAX 49-30-32790610, abo@blackwis.de, http://www.blackwell.de. Ed. Erwin Scharrer. adv.: B&W page DEM 560; trim 122 x 202. Circ: 400.

636.089 DEU ISSN 1439-0442
JOURNAL OF VETERINARY MEDICINE. SERIES A ONLINE. Text in English. 10/yr. DEM 1,743 (effective 2001). **Document type:** *Academic/Scholarly.*
Media: Online - full text (from EBSCO Publishing, O C L C Online Computer Library Center, Inc., RoweCom Information Quest, ingenta, Munksgaard & Blackwell Science's Synergy, Swets Blackwell, Institute for Scientific Information). **Related titles:** ♦ Print ed.: Journal of Veterinary Medicine. Series A. ISSN 0931-184X.
Published by: Blackwell Wissenschafts Verlag GmbH, Kurfuerstendamm 57, Berlin 10707, Germany. TEL 49-30-32790665, FAX 49-30-32790610, abo@blackwis.de, http://www.blackwell.de.

636.089 DEU ISSN 0931-1793
CODEN: ZVRBA2
JOURNAL OF VETERINARY MEDICINE. SERIES B; infectious diseases and veterinary public health. Text in English. 1953. 10/yr. DEM 1,946.28 in Europe; DEM 1,989.30 elsewhere; DEM 2,140.91 in Europe print & online eds. combined; DEM 2,188.23 elsewhere print & online eds. combined (effective 2001). adv. bk.rev. illus, stat. index; cum.index. back issues avail. *Refereed.* **Document type:** *Journal, Academic/Scholarly.* **Description:** Covers all aspects of veterinary microbiology and parasitology.
Formerly: Zentralblatt fuer Veterinaermedizin. Reihe B (0514-7166); Supersedes in part (in 1963): Zentralblatt fuer Veterinaermedizin (0044-4294)
Related titles: ♦ Online - full text ed.: Journal of Veterinary Medicine. Series B Online. ISSN 1439-0450; ♦ Supplement: Advances in Veterinary Medicine. ISSN 0301-2794.
Indexed: ASCA, AgBiotech, Agri.& Environ.Biotech.Abstr. (coverage dropped), Anim.Breed.Abstr., Biol.Abstr., Chem.Abstr., Chem.Titles, Curr.Adv.Ecol.Sci., Curr.Cont., Dairy Sci.Abstr., Derwent Biotech.Abstr., Environ.Sci.Poll.Mgmt., Focus on: Vet.Sci.& Med., Food Sci.& Tech.Abstr., Helminthol.Abstr., INIS Atomind., Ind.Med. (2000-), Ind.Vet., Nutr.Abstr., Pig News & Info., Poult.Abstr., Protozool.Abstr., Ref.Zh., Rev.Appl.Entomol., Rev.Arom.& Med.Plants, Rev.Med.& Vet.Mycol., Rev.Plant Path., Sci.Cit.Ind., Sport Fish.Abstr., Vet.Bull., Wild.Rev., Zoo.Rec.
—BLDSC (5072.386000), CASDDS, GNLM, IDS, Infotrieve, ingenta, Linda Hall. **CCC.**
Published by: Blackwell Wissenschafts Verlag GmbH, Kurfuerstendamm 57, Berlin 10707, Germany. TEL 49-30-32790665, FAX 49-30-32790610, abo@blackwis.de, http://www.blackwell.de. Ed. Oskar Kaaden. adv.: B&W page DEM 560; trim 122 x 190. Circ: 450.

636.089 DEU ISSN 1439-0450
JOURNAL OF VETERINARY MEDICINE. SERIES B ONLINE. Text in English. 10/yr. DEM 1,752 (effective 2001). **Document type:** *Academic/Scholarly.*
Media: Online - full text (from EBSCO Publishing, O C L C Online Computer Library Center, Inc., RoweCom Information Quest, ingenta, Munksgaard & Blackwell Science's Synergy, Swets Blackwell, Institute for Scientific Information). **Related titles:** ♦ Print ed.: Journal of Veterinary Medicine. Series B. ISSN 0931-1793.
Published by: Blackwell Wissenschafts Verlag GmbH, Kurfuerstendamm 57, Berlin 10707, Germany. TEL 49-30-32790665, FAX 49-30-32790610, abo@blackwis.de, http://www.blackwell.de.

636.08 IND ISSN 0971-1031
JOURNAL OF VETERINARY PARASITOLOGY. Text in English. 1987. s-a., latest vol.13, 1999. USD 100 (effective 2000). **Document type:** *Academic/Scholarly.*
Indexed: Bio-Contr.News & Info., Dairy Sci.Abstr., Helminthol.Abstr., Ind.Vet., Pig News & Info., Poult.Abstr., Protozool.Abstr., Rev.Appl.Entomol., Rev.Arom.& Med.Plants, Rev.Med.& Vet.Mycol., Sugar Ind.Abstr., Vet.Bull., Zoo.Rec.
Published by: (Indian Association for the Advancement of Veterinary Parasitology (IAAVP)), H P C Publishers Distributors Pvt. Ltd., 1st Fl., Flats 1 & 2, Darya Ganj, 4805-24 Bharat Ram Rd., New Delhi 110 002, India. TEL 91-11-3254401, FAX 91-11-619-3511, hpcpd@nda.vsnl.net.in, hpcpd@hpc.cc, http://www.hpc.cc, http://www.bizdelhi.com/publisher/hpc.

JOURNAL OF VETERINARY PHARMACOLOGY AND THERAPEUTICS. see *PHARMACY AND PHARMACOLOGY*

▼ **JOURNAL OF VETERINARY PHARMACOLOGY AND THERAPEUTICS ONLINE.** see *PHARMACY AND PHARMACOLOGY*

333.95416 USA ISSN 0090-3558
CODEN: JWIDAW
JOURNAL OF WILDLIFE DISEASES. Text in English. 1965. q. USD 62 to individuals; USD 105 to institutions; USD 31 to students (effective 2001). adv. bk.rev. abstr. charts, illus. index. back issues avail.; reprints avail. *Refereed.* **Document type:** *Journal, Academic/Scholarly.* **Description:** Publishes the results of original research and observations dealing with all aspects of infectious, parasitic, toxic, nutritional. physiologic, developmental and neoplastic diseases.
Former titles: Wildlife Disease Association. Journal (0043-5473); Wildlife Disease Association. Bulletin
Related titles: Online - full text ed.: (from Institute for Scientific Information).
Indexed: ASCA, Agricola, Aqua.Sci.& Fish.Abstr., Bio-Contr.News & Info., Biol.& Agr.Ind. (Jan.1990-), Biol.Abstr., Biol.Dig., Chem.Abstr., Chem.Titles, Curr.Adv.Ecol.Sci., Curr.Cont., Curr.Ref.Fish Res., Dairy Sci.Abstr., Dent.Ind., Derwent Biotech.Abstr., Entomol.Abstr., Environ.Per.Bibl., Environ.Sci.Poll.Mgmt., Focus on: Vet.Sci.& Med., Genet.Abstr., Helminthol.Abstr., Herb.Abstr., Hum.Gen.Abstr., INIS Atomind., Ind.Med. (1970-), Ind.Sci.Rev., Ind.Vet., Key Word Ind.Wildl.Res., Maize Abstr., Microbiol.Abstr., Nutr.Abstr., Ocean.Abstr. (coverage dropped), Pig News & Info., Pollut.Abstr., Postharvest, Poult.Abstr., Protozool.Abstr., Rev.Appl.Entomol., Rev.Med.& Vet.Mycol., Rev.Plant Path., Sci.Cit.Ind., Small Anim.Abstr., Soils & Fert., Sport Fish.Abstr., Vet.Bull., Wild Life Rev., Wild.Rev., Zoo.Rec.
—BLDSC (5072.620000), CASDDS, CISTI, GNLM, ingenta, Linda Hall.
Published by: Wildlife Disease Association, Inc., PO Box 1897, Lawrence, KS 66044-8897. TEL 785-843-1235, FAX 785-843-1274, wda@allenpress.com, orders@allenpress.com, http://www.wildlifedisease.org/, http://www.vet.uga.edu/wda; http://www.allenpress.com. Circ: 1,350 (paid).

JOURNAL OF WILDLIFE REHABILITATION. see *BIOLOGY—Zoology*

636 USA ISSN 1042-7260
CODEN: JZWMEI
JOURNAL OF ZOO AND WILDLIFE MEDICINE. Text in English. 1971. q. USD 195 in North America to institutions; USD 210 elsewhere to institutions (effective 2001). adv. bk.rev. charts, illus, stat, abstr. cum.index: 1970-1987. back issues avail.; reprints avail. *Refereed.* **Document type:** *Academic/Scholarly.* **Description:** Publishes original research findings and clinical observations as well as case reports in the field of veterinary medicine dealing with captive and free-ranging wild animals.
Formerly: Journal of Zoo Animal Medicine (0093-4526)
Media: Duplicated (not offset). **Related titles:** Online - full text ed.: (from BioOne, Institute for Scientific Information).
Indexed: ASCA, AgBiotech, Curr.Adv.Ecol.Sci., Curr.Cont., Dairy Sci.Abstr., Derwent Biotech.Abstr., Environ.Abstr., Focus on: Vet.Sci.& Med., Forest.Abstr., Helminthol.Abstr., Ind.Med. (1989-), Ind.Sci.Rev., Ind.Vet., Nutr.Abstr., Poult.Abstr., Protozool.Abstr., Rev.Appl.Entomol., Rev.Med.& Vet.Mycol., Sci.Cit.Ind., Small Anim.Abstr., Soyabean Abstr., Sport Fish.Abstr., Vet.Bull., Wild.Rev., Zoo.Rec.
—BLDSC (5072.765000), IDS, ingenta.
Published by: American Association of Zoo Veterinarians, 6 North Pennell Rd, Media, PA 19063. TEL 610-892-4812, FAX 610-892-4813, aazv@allnepress.com, http://www.worldzoo.org/aazv/journal.htm. Ed., R&P Wilbur B Amond. Circ: 1,200. **Subscr. to:** Allen Press Inc., PO Box 1897, Lawrence, KS 66044-8897.

636.089 KEN
KENYA AGRICULTURAL RESEARCH INSTITUTE. VETERINARY RESEARCH DEPARTMENT. ANNUAL REPORT. Text in English. 1977. a. **Document type:** *Corporate.*
Indexed: Field Crop Abstr., Herb.Abstr., Rev.Appl.Entomol., Weed Abstr.
Published by: Kenya Agricultural Research Institute, Veterinary Research Department, PO Box 30148, Nairobi, Kenya.

636.089 KEN ISSN 0256-5161
KENYA VETERINARIAN. Text in English. 1977. s-a. USD 10. adv. **Document type:** *Trade.*
Indexed: Ind.Vet., Soils & Fert., Vet.Bull.
Published by: Kenya Veterinary Association, PO Box 29089, Nairobi, Kenya. Ed. Dr. Thomas T Dolan. Circ: 500.

636.089 DEU ISSN 1434-9132
KLEINTIER KONKRET. Text in German. 1998. bi-m. EUR 102.90 domestic to institutions; EUR 108.90 in Europe to institutions; EUR 117.90 elsewhere to institutions (effective 2002). **Document type:** *Journal, Academic/Scholarly.*
Related titles: Online - full text ed.: ISSN 1439-3832.
Published by: Ferdinand Enke Verlag, Ruedigerstr 14, Stuttgart 70469, Germany. TEL 49-711-25520-0, FAX 49-711-2552030, enke@compuserve.com, http://www.thieme.de.

636.089 DEU ISSN 0023-2076
KLEINTIER-PRAXIS; Archiv fuer kleine Haus- und Nutztiere sowie Laboratoriums- und Zoo-Tiere. Text in German; Summaries in English. 1956. 12/yr. DEM 241.40; DEM 264.40 foreign (effective 2000). adv. bk.rev. bibl, charts, illus. index. *Refereed.* **Document type:** *Trade.*
Related titles: Online - full text ed.: (from Institute for Scientific Information).
Indexed: ASCA, Agri.& Environ.Biotech.Abstr. (coverage dropped), Anim.Breed.Abstr., Biol.Abstr., Chem.Abstr., Curr.Adv.Ecol.Sci., Curr.Cont., Dairy Sci.Abstr., Derwent Biotech.Abstr., Focus on: Vet.Sci.& Med., Helminthol.Abstr., INIS Atomind., Ind.Sci.Rev., Ind.Vet., Nutr.Abstr., Pig News & Info., Poult.Abstr., Protozool.Abstr., Rev.Appl.Entomol., Rev.Med.& Vet.Mycol., Rev.Plant Path., SSCI (coverage dropped), Small Anim.Abstr., Soils & Fert., Vet.Bull., Zoo.Rec.
—BLDSC (5099.121000), IDS, Infotrieve, Linda Hall. **CCC.**
Published by: (World Small Animal Veterinary Association, Deutsche Gruppe), Verlag M. und H. Schaper GmbH, Borsigstr 5, Alfeld 31061, Germany. TEL 49-5181-8009-0, FAX 49-5181-8009-33, info@schaper-verlag.de, http://www.schaper-verlag.de. Circ: 6,000.

636.089 DEU ISSN 1434-6400
KLEINTIERMEDIZIN. Text in German. 1998. 8/yr. EUR 50 domestic; EUR 66 foreign (effective 2002). adv. abstr, illus. **Document type:** *Magazine, Trade.*
Published by: Terra Verlag GmbH, Neuhauser Str 21, Postfach 1222, Konstanz 78464, West Germany. TEL 49-7531-812233, FAX 49-7531-812299, http://www.terra-verlag.de. Ed. Dieter Mueller. Adv. contact Martina Nock. B&W page XEU 1,620, color page XEU 3,400; trim 180 x 248. Circ: 1,800 (paid); 7,300 (controlled).

KONGELIGE VETERINAER- OG LANDBOHOEJSKOLE. HAANDBOG. see *AGRICULTURE*

LEBENDIGE TIERWELT; tieraerztlicher Ratgeber fuer Tierfreunde. see *ANIMAL WELFARE*

LLAMAS MAGAZINE; information for camelid lovers everywhere. see *BIOLOGY—Zoology*

636.589 POL ISSN 1425-6770
MAGAZYN - DROBIARSTWO. Text in Polish. 1995. m. USD 65 (effective 1998). adv. illus. reprints avail. **Description:** Publishes scientific and practical articles for poultry breeders and producers.
Indexed: AgroLibrex.

V

Published by: Wydawnictwo Medyczne Sanmedica Sp. z o.o., Ul Nowy Zjazd 1, Warsaw 00301, Poland. TEL 48-22-8262287, FAX 48-22-8263182. Ed. Piotr Szeleszczuk. Adv. contact Agnieszka Pawlowska. B&W page USD 650, color page USD 750. Circ: 2,500.

636.08 POL ISSN 1230-4425
MAGAZYN WETERYNARYJNY. Text in Polish. 1992. bi-m. USD 49 (effective 1998). adv. bibl, illus, tr.lit. index. **Document type:** *Academic/Scholarly.* **Description:** Clinical journal for veterinary surgeons and students.
Indexed: AgroLibrex, Anim.Breed.Abstr., Bio-Contr.News & Info., Dairy Sci.Abstr., Helminthol.Abstr., Ind.Vet., Nutr.Abstr., Pig News & Info., Poult.Abstr., Protozool.Abstr., Rev.Appl.Entomol., Rev.Med.& Vet.Mycol., Small Anim.Abstr., Vet.Bull.
—BLDSC (5334.255000).
Published by: Wydawnictwo Medyczne Sanmedica Sp. z o.o., Ul Nowy Zjazd 1, Warsaw 00301, Poland. TEL 48-22-8262287, FAX 48-22-8263182. Ed. Roman Lechowski. Adv. contact Agnieszka Pawlowska. B&W page USD 700, color page USD 950. Circ: 5,000.

V

636.089 HUN ISSN 0025-004X
CODEN: MGALA5
MAGYAR ALLATORVOSOK LAPJA/HUNGARIAN VETERINARY JOURNAL. Text in Hungarian; Summaries in English. 1878. m. HUF 3,960 (effective 1999). adv. bk.rev. abstr, bibl, charts, illus. index. back issues avail. *Refereed.* **Document type:** *Academic/Scholarly, Bibliography, Corporate, Abstract/Index.* **Description:** Provides information on the professional, social, educational and organizational lives of veterinarians in Hungary, for a readership primarily of veterinarians.
Related titles: Online - full text ed.: (from Institute for Scientific Information).
Indexed: Abstr.Hyg., AgBiotech, Agri.& Environ.Biotech.Abstr. (coverage dropped), Agri.Eng.Abstr., Anim.Breed.Abstr., Aqua.Sci.& Fish.Abstr., Aquacult.Abstr., Biol.Abstr., Cal.Tiss.Abstr., Chem.Abstr., Chem.Indus.Notes, Chem.Titles, Curr.Adv.Ecol.Sci., Curr.Cont., Dairy Sci.Abstr., Derwent Biotech.Abstr., Environ.Sci.Poll.Mgmt., Focus on: Vet.Sci.& Med., Food Sci.& Tech.Abstr., Helminthol.Abstr., INIS Atomind., Ind.Sci.Rev., Ind.Vet., Maize Abstr., Nutr.Abstr., Pig News & Info., Poult.Abstr., Protozool.Abstr., Rev.Appl.Entomol., Rev.Med.& Vet.Mycol., Rev.Plant Path., SSCI (coverage dropped), Small Anim.Abstr., Soyabean Abstr., Vet.Bull., World Ag.Econ.& Rur.Soc.Abstr.
—BLDSC (5340.300000), CASDDS, CISTI, IDS.
Published by: (India. Ministry of Agriculture IND), Magyar Mezogazdasag Ltd., Kossuth Lajos ter 11, Budapest 1055, Hungary. TEL 36-1-301-4324, FAX 36-1-301-4827. Ed. Laszlo Visnyei. Circ: 4,300.

636.089 IRN ISSN 1022-646X
CODEN: JVFTDR
MAJALLAH-I DANISHKADAH-I DAMPIZISHKI/JOURNAL OF THE FACULTY OF VETERINARY MEDICINE. Text in Persian, Modern; Contents page in English, Persian, Modern. 1937. q. IRR 2,500, USD 20; IRR 20,000 foreign (effective 1999). adv. bk.rev. abstr, bibl, illus, charts, stat. 100 p./no. **Document type:** *Academic/Scholarly.* **Description:** Publishes original research results in all branches of veterinary medicine.
Formerly (until 1993): Namah-i Danishkadah-i Dampizishki (0042-0123)
Related titles: CD-ROM ed.
Indexed: AgBiotech, Anim.Breed.Abstr., Aqua.Sci.& Fish.Abstr., Aquacult.Abstr., Dairy Sci.Abstr., ExtraMED, Food Sci.& Tech.Abstr., Ind.Vet., Nutr.Abstr., Postharvest, Poult.Abstr., Protozool.Abstr., Rev.Appl.Entomol., Rev.Med.& Vet.Mycol., Tox.Abstr., Vet.Bull., Virol.Abstr., World Ag.Econ.& Rur.Soc.Abstr., Zoo.Rec.
—BLDSC (4912.243000), CASDDS.
Published by: (Faculty of Veterinary Medicine/ Danishkadah-i Dampizishki, University of Teheran), Tehran University Printing and Publishing Institute, P O Box 14155-6453, Tehran, Iran. TEL 98-21-923510, FAX 98-21-933222, dsharibi@chamram.au.ut.ir. Ed. I Nowrouzian. Circ: 1,000 (paid).

636.089 MWI ISSN 0076-3365
MALAWI. DEPARTMENT OF VETERINARY SERVICES AND ANIMAL INDUSTRY. ANNUAL REPORT. Text in English. a. **Document type:** *Government.*
Indexed: Anim.Breed.Abstr., Field Crop Abstr., Herb.Abstr.
Published by: (Malawi. Department of Veterinary Services and Animal Industry), Government Printer, PO Box 37, Zomba, Malawi.

MARINE TURTLE NEWSLETTER. see *BIOLOGY—Zoology*

636.089 CAN ISSN 0225-9591
CODEN: MVEQDC
MEDECIN VETERINAIRE DU QUEBEC. Text in French. 1971. q. CND 30, USD 40. adv.
Indexed: Anim.Breed.Abstr., Biol.Abstr., Dairy Sci.Abstr., Helminthol.Abstr., Ind.Vet., Nutr.Abstr., Pig News & Info., Poult.Abstr., Pt.de Rep. (1983-), Rev.Med.& Vet.Mycol., Small Anim.Abstr., Sport Fish.Abstr., Vet.Bull., Wild.Rev.
—BLDSC (5487.670000), CISTI. **CCC.**
Published by: Ordre des Medecins Veterinaires du Quebec/Order of Veterinarians of Quebec, 800 ave Ste Anne, Ste 200, St Hyacinthe, PQ J2S 5G7, Canada. TEL 450-774-1427, FAX 450-774-7635. Ed. Jean Pierard. Circ: 2,600.

636.08 ESP ISSN 0212-8292
SF604 CODEN: MEVEEB
MEDICINA VETERINARIA. Text in Spanish; Summaries in English. 1984. m. ESP 9,600 domestic; ESP 14,000 foreign (effective 2000). adv. bk.rev. bibl, illus. back issues avail. *Refereed.* **Document type:** *Academic/Scholarly.*
Related titles: E-mail ed.; Fax ed.
Indexed: AgBiotech, Anim.Breed.Abstr., Apic.Abstr., Dairy Sci.Abstr., Derwent Biotech.Abstr., Excerp.Med. (1993-), Helminthol.Abstr., Ind.Vet., Nutr.Abstr., Pig News & Info., Poult.Abstr., Protozool.Abstr., Rev.Appl.Entomol., Rev.Med.& Vet.Mycol., Sport Fish.Abstr., Vet.Bull., Wild.Rev., Zoo.Rec.
—CINDOC, EMDOCS.
Published by: Pulso Ediciones S.A., Rambla del Celler 117-119, Sant Cugat Del Valles, Barcelona 08190, Spain. TEL 34-3-5896264, pulso@pulso.com, http://www.pulso.com/. Ed., R&P Beatriz Gallart. Pub. Josep Reixach. Adv. contact Albert Gallart. B&W page ESP 110,250, color page ESP 132,300; trim 297 x 210. Circ: 5,000 (paid).

636.08 PRT ISSN 0870-4295
MEDICO VETERINARIO. Text in Portuguese. 1986. q. PTE 7,800 in the European Union; PTE 9,000 elsewhere. adv. **Description:** Publishes veterinary articles. Includes information on new products and services, meetings and congresses.
Published by: Edicoes Vade-mecum Lda., Calcada do Tijolo, 45, Lisbon 1200, Portugal. TEL 351-1-3420518, FAX 351-1-3420682. Ed. Dr. Jose Paulo Sales Luis. Adv. contact Joaquim Azevedo. Circ: 3,000.

636.089 POL ISSN 0025-8628
CODEN: MDWTAG
MEDYCYNA WETERYNARYJNA. Text in Polish; Summaries in English. 1945. m. PLZ 144 domestic to individuals; PLZ 180 domestic to institutions; PLZ 84 domestic to students; USD 120 foreign to students (effective 2002). adv. bk.rev. abstr, bibl, charts, illus, mkt. index, cum.index. 80 p./no. 2 cols./p. *Refereed.* **Document type:** *Monographic series, Academic/Scholarly.* **Description:** Devoted to the problems of veterinary science and practice, and applied biology.
Related titles: Online - full text ed.: (from Institute for Scientific Information).
Indexed: ASCA, Abstr.Hyg., AgBiotech, Agri.Eng.Abstr., AgroLibrex, Anim.Breed.Abstr., Biol.Abstr., Chem.Abstr., Curr.Cont., Dairy Sci.Abstr., Derwent Biotech.Abstr., Excerp.Med., Focus on: Vet.Sci.& Med., Food Sci.& Tech.Abstr., Helminthol.Abstr., INIS Atomind., Ind.Vet., Maize Abstr., Nutr.Abstr., Pig News & Info., Poult.Abstr., Protozool.Abstr., Rev.Appl.Entomol., Rev.Med.& Vet.Mycol., Rev.Plant Path., Small Anim.Abstr., Soyabean Abstr., Vet.Bull., Weed Abstr.
—BLDSC (5536.050000), CASDDS, IDS, Linda Hall.
Published by: (Polskie Towarzystwo Nauk Weterynaryjnych), Medycyna Weterynaryjna, Ul Akademicka 12, Lubin 30-033, Poland. TEL 48-81-5332912, FAX 48-81-5332912, http://www.medwet.lublin.pl. Ed., R&P Dr. Edmund K Prost. Adv. contact Dr. Krzysztof Szkucik. Circ: 3,300 (controlled).

636.089 USA ISSN 0076-6542
SF748
MERCK VETERINARY MANUAL: A HANDBOOK OF DIAGNOSIS AND THERAPY FOR THE VETERINARIAN. Text in English. 1955. irreg., latest vol.8, 1998. USD 32 (effective 2000). adv. **Document type:** *Directory.*
—CISTI.
Published by: Merck Publishing Group, RY-7-220, P.O. Box 2000, Rahway, NJ 07065. TEL 732-594-4600, FAX 732-388-9778. Ed., R&P Susan Aiello. Adv. contact Pamela J Barnes.

MONOGRAFIE PARAZYTOLOGICZNE. see *BIOLOGY—Microbiology*

636.089 USA ISSN 0277-3015
NEW METHODS; the journal of animal health technology. Text in English. 1977-1984 (Jan.); resumed 1984. irreg. USD 32; USD 45 foreign (effective 1998). adv. bk.rev. bibl, charts, illus. index. back issues avail. **Document type:** *Newsletter.* **Description:** Information source that represents basic interests in the animal health profession.
Formerly: Methods: The Journal of Animal Health Technology
—Infotrieve. **CCC.**
Published by: New Methods Co., PO Box 22605, San Francisco, CA 94122-0605. TEL 415-379-9065. Ed., Pub., R&P, Adv. contact Ronald S Lippert. page USD 320; trim 11 x 8.5. Circ: 5,600 (controlled).

636.089 NZL ISSN 0048-0169
CODEN: NEZTAF
NEW ZEALAND VETERINARY JOURNAL. Text in English. 1952. 6/yr. NZD 125 to individuals; USD 110 in Australia to individuals; USD 85 in the Americas to individuals; USD 95 elsewhere to individuals; NZD 240 to institutions; USD 200 in Australia to institutions; USD 165 in the Americas to institutions; USD 185 elsewhere to institutions (effective 1999). adv. bk.rev. illus. *Refereed.* **Document type:** *Academic/Scholarly.* **Description:** Publishes original research and clinical observations in all aspects of veterinary science.
Related titles: Online - full text ed.: (from Institute for Scientific Information).
Indexed: ASCA, AgBiotech, Agri.& Environ.Biotech.Abstr. (coverage dropped), Anim.Behav.Abstr. (coverage dropped), Anim.Breed.Abstr., Bio-Contr.News & Info., Biol.Abstr., Cadscan, Chem.Abstr., Chem.Indus.Notes, Chem.Titles, Curr.Adv.Ecol.Sci., Curr.Cont., Dairy Sci.Abstr., Derwent Biotech.Abstr., Excerp.Med., Field Crop Abstr., Focus on: Vet.Sci.& Med., GeoRef, Helminthol.Abstr., Herb.Abstr., Ind.Med. (coverage dropped), Ind.Sci.Rev., Ind.Vet., Lead Abstr., Maize Abstr., Nutr.Abstr., Pig News & Info., Poult.Abstr., Protozool.Abstr., Rev.Appl.Entomol., Rev.Med.& Vet.Mycol., Rev.Plant Path., Sci.Cit.Ind., Small Anim.Abstr., Soils & Fert., Sport Fish.Abstr., Vet.Bull., Weed Abstr., Wild.Rev., Zincscan, Zoo.Rec.
—BLDSC (6099.900000), CASDDS, CISTI, GNLM, IDS, Infotrieve, ingenta, Linda Hall. **CCC.**
Published by: New Zealand Veterinary Association, Manners St, 11-212, Wellington, New Zealand. nzvj@massey.ac.nz, http://www.vetjournal.org.nz. Ed., R&P Peter Jolly. adv.: B&W page AUD 850, color page AUD 1,700; trim 210 x 297. Circ: 1,750.

NIGERIA. NATIONAL ANIMAL PRODUCTION RESEARCH INSTITUTE. JOURNAL; Journal of Animal Production Research. see *AGRICULTURE—Poultry And Livestock*

630 636.089 JPN ISSN 0373-8361
CODEN: NIPDAD
NIPPON JUI CHIKUSAN DAIGAKU KENKYU HOKOKU/NIPPON VETERINARY AND ANIMAL SCIENCE UNIVERSITY. BULLETIN. Text in English, Japanese; Summaries in English. 1953. a. USD 20 (effective 2000). reprints avail. *Refereed.* **Document type:** *Academic/Scholarly.*
Formerly: Nippon Jui Chikusan Daigaku Kiyo (0078-0839)
Related titles: Online - full text ed.
Indexed: AgBiotech, Anim.Breed.Abstr., Aqua.Sci.& Fish.Abstr., Aquacult.Abstr., Biol.Abstr., Chem.Abstr., Chem.Indus.Notes, Chem.Titles, Dairy Sci.Abstr., Environ.Sci.Poll.Mgmt., Food Sci.& Tech.Abstr., GeoRef, Helminthol.Abstr., INIS Atomind., Ind.Vet., Plant Breed.Abstr., Poult.Abstr., Protozool.Abstr., Rev.Appl.Entomol., Rev.Arom.& Med.Plants, Rev.Med.& Vet.Mycol., Soils & Fert., Vet.Bull., Zoo.Rec.
—BLDSC (2655.649000), CASDDS, CISTI.
Published by: Nippon Jui Chikusan Daigaku, 7-1 Kyonan-cho 1-chome, Musashino-shi, Tokyo-to 180-0023, Japan. TEL 81-422-31-4151, FAX 81-422-33-2094. Ed. Soichi Imai. Circ: 550 (controlled).

636.089 NOR ISSN 0029-2273
CODEN: NOVDAH
NORSK VETERINAERTIDSSKRIFT/NORWEGIAN VETERINARY MEDICAL JOURNAL. Text in Norwegian. 1888. m. NOK 700 in Scandinavia; NOK 900 in Europe; NOK 1,000 elsewhere (effective 1999). adv. bk.rev. charts, illus. index. reprints avail. *Refereed.* **Document type:** *Academic/Scholarly, Corporate.* **Description:** Prints information of interest to veterinarians and others with interest in public health, hygiene and meat control.
Indexed: Agri.& Environ.Biotech.Abstr. (coverage dropped), Anim.Breed.Abstr., Aqua.Sci.& Fish.Abstr., Biol.Abstr., Dairy Sci.Abstr., Food Sci.& Tech.Abstr., Helminthol.Abstr., Herb.Abstr., Ind.Vet., Nutr.Abstr., Pig News & Info., Protozool.Abstr., Rev.Appl.Entomol., Rev.Med.& Vet.Mycol., Small Anim.Abstr., Vet.Bull.
—BLDSC (6147.200000), CISTI, Linda Hall.

Published by: Norske Veterinaerforening/Norwegian Veterinary Association, General Birchs Gate 16, Oslo 0454, Norway. TEL 47-22-59-16-50, FAX 47-22-69-04-50. Eds. Ulf Erik Gustavsen, Vibeke Olsen. adv.: B&W page NOK 4,000, color page NOK 9,680; trim 185 x 260. Circ: 2,009.

NOVOSTI VETERINARNOI FARMATSII I MEDITSINY. see *PHARMACY AND PHARMACOLOGY*

636.089 RUS
NOVYE PROMYSHLENNYE KATALOGI. MEDITSINSKAYA TEKHNIKA. TEKHNIKA BEZOPASNOSTI. VETERINARNOE OBORUDOVANIE. Text in Russian. m. USD 345 in United States.
Published by: Rossiiskii N.I.I. Problem Transporta, Lubyanskii pr 5, Moscow 101820, Russian Federation. TEL 7-095-9254609, FAX 7-095-2002203. **US dist. addr.:** East View Publications, 3020 Harbor Ln N, Minneapolis, MN 55447. TEL 612-550-0961.

636.08969 FRA ISSN 0300-9823
SF781 CODEN: OTEBA6
O I E BULLETIN. Text in English, French, Spanish. bi-m. USD 90, EUR 90 (effective 2000). **Document type:** *Newsletter.* **Description:** Presents monthly evolution of the major epizootic diseases throughout the world.
Indexed: Ind.Vet., Rev.Appl.Entomol., Rev.Med.& Vet.Mycol., Vet.Bull.
—CISTI, GNLM.
Published by: Office International des Epizooties, 12 rue de Prony, Paris 75017, France. FAX 33-1-42670987, oie@oie.int, http://www.oie.int. Ed. J Blancou. R&P Gill S Dilmitis TEL 33-1-44151888. **US subscr. to:** Scientific, Medical Publications of France, 100 E 42nd St, Ste 1002, New York, NY 10017. TEL 212-983-6278.

636.08969 FRA ISSN 0253-1933
SF781 CODEN: RTOEDX
O I E REVUE SCIENTIFIQUE ET TECHNIQUE/O I E SCIENTIFIC AND TECHNICAL REVIEW. Text in English, French, Spanish; Summaries in English, French, Spanish. 1982. 3/yr. USD 80, EUR 80, FRF 540 (effective 2000). adv. *Refereed.* **Document type:** *Academic/Scholarly.* **Description:** Promotes experimental or other research work on diagnosis and control of contagious diseases of livestock. Also includes documents of importance to Chief Veterinary Officers of 155 member countries and to the world medical and veterinary scientific communities.
Related titles: Online - full text ed.: (from Institute for Scientific Information).
Indexed: Abstr.Hyg., Anim.Breed.Abstr., Bio-Contr.News & Info., Curr.Cont., Dairy Sci.Abstr., Derwent Biotech.Abstr., Focus on: Vet.Sci.& Med., Food Sci.& Tech.Abstr., Helminthol.Abstr., Ind.Med. (1982-), Ind.Vet., Pig News & Info., Poult.Abstr., Protozool.Abstr., Ref.Zh., Rev.Appl.Entomol., Rev.Med.& Vet.Mycol., Small Anim.Abstr., Trop.Dis.Bull., Vet.Bull., Wild.Rev., World Ag.Econ.& Rur.Soc.Abstr., Zoo.Rec.
—BLDSC (7950.029000), CISTI, GNLM, IDS, ingenta, KNAW.
Published by: Office International des Epizooties, 12 rue de Prony, Paris 75017, France. TEL 33-1-44151888, FAX 33-1-42670987, TELEX EPIZOTI 642 285 F, oie@oie.int, http://www.oie.int. Ed. J Blancou. R&P, Adv. contact Gill S Dilmitis TEL 33-1-44151888. **US subscr. to:** Scientific, Medical Publications of France, 100 E 42nd St, Ste 1002, New York, NY 10017. TEL 212-983-6278.

636.089 ITA ISSN 0392-1913
OBIETTIVI E DOCUMENTI VETERINARI. Short title: O D V. Text in Italian. 1980. m. (11/yr.). ITL 100,000 (effective 2000). adv. **Description:** Covers the veterinary sciences. Provides professional training information.
Indexed: Agroforest.Abstr., Anim.Breed.Abstr., Dairy Sci.Abstr., Helminthol.Abstr., Ind.Vet., Nutr.Abstr., Pig News & Info., Postharvest, Poult.Abstr., Protozool.Abstr., Rev.Appl.Entomol., Rev.Med.& Vet.Mycol., Rural Recreat.Tour.Abstr., Small Anim.Abstr., Trop.Dis.Bull., Vet.Bull., Weed Abstr., World Ag.Econ.& Rur.Soc.Abstr.
—BLDSC (6196.955000), CISTI.
Published by: Edagricole S.p.A., Via Emilia Levante 31, Bologna, BO 40139, Italy. TEL 39-51-62267, FAX 39-51-493660. Ed. Giovanni Ballarini. adv.: B&W page ITL 1,410,000, color page ITL 2,200,000; 210 x 280. Circ: 13,600.

636.08 AUT ISSN 1029-5313
OESTERREICHISCHE FREIBERUFS TIERARZT. Text in German. 1961. q. ATS 300; ATS 90 newsstand/cover (effective 2001). adv. **Document type:** *Magazine, Trade.*
Published by: (Berufverband Freiberuflich Taetiger Tieraerzte Oesterreichs), B W K Public Relations, Grossmannstr 30, Vienna 1220, Austria. TEL 43-1-7747094, FAX 43-1-7747095, office@bwk.at, http://www.bwk.at. Pub. Brigitte Weber-Kraus. adv.: B&W page ATS 8,640, color page ATS 17,580; trim 170 x 242. Circ: 3,400 (controlled).

636.089 AUT ISSN 0029-9766
OESTERREICHISCHER KLEINTIERZUECHTER. Text in German. 1946. m. ATS 500 (effective 1998). adv. bk.rev. illus. **Document type:** *Newsletter.*
Published by: (Rassezuchtverband Oesterreichischer Kleintierzuechter), Druck und Verlag Hammerer, Riedauerstrasse 48, Ried A-4910, Austria. TEL 43-7752-87011. Ed., R&P Fritz Marhann. Adv. contact Johann Ohlicher. page ATS 8,000; 255 x 192. Circ: 6,000.

636.089 USA
OHIO VETERINARY MEDICAL ASSOCIATION. NEWSLETTER. Text in English. 1952. m. USD 2 to members. adv. illus. **Document type:** *Newsletter.*
Formerly (until 1970): Ohio Veterinarian (0030-1213)
—CCC.
Published by: Ohio Veterinary Medical Association, 3168 Riverside Dr, Columbus, OH 43221. TEL 614-486-7253, FAX 614-486-1325. Ed. George Kukor. Circ: 1,930.

636.089 JPN ISSN 0911-5137
OKINAWA-KEN KACHIKU EISEI SHIKENJO NENPO/OKINAWA PREFECTURAL INSTITUTE OF ANIMAL HEALTH. ANNUAL REPORT. Text in Japanese; Summaries in English. 1958. a. free per issue. back issues avail. **Description:** Covers research on animal diseases.
Published by: Okinawa-ken Kachiku Eisei Shikenjo/Okinawa Prefectural Institute of Animal Health, 112 Kohagura, Naha-shi, Okinawa-ken 900-0000, Japan. TEL 0988-32-1515. Circ: 300.

636.089 ZAF ISSN 0030-2465
SF601 CODEN: OJVRAZ
ONDERSTEPOORT JOURNAL OF VETERINARY RESEARCH. Text in English. 1933. q., latest vol.68. ZAR 400 domestic; USD 100 foreign (effective 2002). adv. bk.rev. bibl, charts, illus. index, cum.index: 1933-1968, 1969-1973. reprint service avail. from PQC. *Refereed.* **Document type:** *Academic/Scholarly.* **Description:** Publishes papers reporting on original research covering all aspects of veterinary science, with particular emphasis on diseases and disease vectors of livestock and wildlife on the African continent of more than local interest.
Related titles: Microform ed.: (from PQC,PMC); Online - full text ed.: (from Northern Light Technology, Inc., ProQuest Information & Learning, Institute for Scientific Information).
Indexed: ASCA, AgBiotech, Agri.& Environ.Biotech.Abstr. (coverage dropped), Agri.Eng.Abstr., Anim.Breed.Abstr., Aqua.Sci.& Fish.Abstr., Aquacult.Abstr., Bio-Contr.News & Info., Biol.& Agr.Ind. (coverage dropped), Biol.Abstr., Chem.Abstr., Curr.Adv.Ecol.Sci., Curr.Cont., Dairy Sci.Abstr., Derwent Biotech.Abstr., Entomol.Abstr., Environ.Sci.Poll.Mgmt., Field Crop Abstr., Focus on: Vet.Sci.& Med., Food Sci.& Tech.Abstr., Helminthol.Abstr., Herb.Abstr., INIS Atomind., Ind.Med. (1951-), Ind.S.A.Per., Ind.Vet., Microbiol.Abstr., Nutr.Abstr., Pig News & Info., Poult.Abstr., Protozool.Abstr., Rev.Appl.Entomol., Rev.Arom.& Med.Plants, Rev.Med.& Vet.Mycol., Rev.Plant Path., Sci.Cit.Ind., Sport Fish.Abstr., Trop.Dis.Bull., Vet.Bull., Wild.Rev., Zoo.Rec.
—BLDSC (6258.000000), CASDDS, CISTI, GNLM, IDS, ingenta, Linda Hall.
Published by: Agricultural Research Council, Onderstepoort Veterinary Institute, Private Bag X5, Onderstepoort 0110, South Africa. TEL 27-12-5299111, FAX 27-12-5299318, 27-12-5299277, library@moon.ovi.ac.za, erna@moon.ovi.ac.za, http://www.ovi.ac.za. Ed., Pub. J Boomker. R&P D Swanepoel TEL 27-12-5299279. Circ: 400 (controlled).

636.089 AUS ISSN 1328-925X
ONLINE JOURNAL OF VETERINARY RESEARCH. Abbreviated title: O J V R. Text in English. 1996. 3/yr. USD 100 to individuals; USD 360 to institutions; USD 55 to students. adv. illus. reprints avail. *Refereed.* **Document type:** *Journal, Academic/Scholarly.* **Description:** Focuses primarily on comparative pathobiology, pharmacology-pharmacokinetics, toxicology and parasitology.
Media: Online - full text.
Indexed: Zoo.Rec.
Published by: Pestsearch International Pty. Ltd., 173 Chatswood Rd, Daisy Hill, QLD 4127, Australia. v.guerrini@mailbox.uq.edu.au, http://www.cpb.uokhsc.edu/ojvr/jvet196a.htm. Ed. V H Guerrini.

ONS VEE; maandblad voor de veehouderij. see *AGRICULTURE—Poultry And Livestock*

636.08 FRA
ORDRE DES VETERINAIRES. REVUE. Text in French. 4/yr. **Document type:** *Bulletin.*
Address: 34 rue Breguet, Paris 75011, France. TEL 47-00-12-27, FAX 47-00-09-25. Ed. V Bianchetti. Circ: 8,500.

PAKISTAN JOURNAL OF AGRICULTURE, AGRICULTURAL ENGINEERING AND VETERINARY SCIENCES. see *AGRICULTURE*

PAKISTAN JOURNAL OF ANIMAL SCIENCES. see *AGRICULTURE—Poultry And Livestock*

636.089 PAK
PAKISTAN VETERINARIAN; animal sciences. Text in English. 1988. m. USD 5 per issue.
Published by: Press Corporation of Pakistan, P O Box 3138, Karachi 75400, Pakistan. TEL 21-455-3703, FAX 21-7736198. Ed. Saeed Hafeez. Circ: 5,000.

636.089 PAK ISSN 0253-8318
CODEN: PVJODU
PAKISTAN VETERINARY JOURNAL. Text in English. 1981. q. PKR 200 domestic; USD 100 foreign (effective 2000). adv. bk.rev. *Refereed.* **Document type:** *Academic/Scholarly.*
Indexed: AgBiotech, Anim.Breed.Abstr., Bio-Contr.News & Info., Biol.Abstr., Chem.Abstr., Chem.Indus.Notes, Chem.Titles, Dairy Sci.Abstr., Helminthol.Abstr., Ind.Vet., Maize Abstr., Nutr.Abstr., Poult.Abstr., Protozool.Abstr., Rev.Appl.Entomol., Rev.Arom.& Med.Plants, Rev.Med.& Vet.Mycol., Small Anim.Abstr., Sport Fish.Abstr., Vet.Bull., Wild.Rev., World Ag.Econ.& Rur.Soc.Abstr., Zoo.Rec.
—BLDSC (6343.170000), CASDDS.
Published by: University of Agriculture, Faculty of Veterinary Science, Faisalabad 38040, Pakistan. TEL 92-41-624607, FAX 92-41-610200, nawazn@paknetl.ptc.pk; akhan@pjbs.org, ahrar@fsd.paknet.com.pk. Ed., R&P Muhammad Nawaz. Pub. Sikandar Hayat. Adv. contact Ahrar Khan. Circ: 1,000.

636.089 IRL
PEGASUS. Text in English. 1954. a. IEP 1 (effective 2001). adv. bk.rev. **Document type:** *Newsletter.* **Description:** Concerned with up-to-date developments and opportunities for recent graduates in Ireland and the world.
Formerly: A V S Journal (0066-9768)
Published by: Veterinary Student's Union of Ireland, c/o Student's Consultative Forum, Library Bldg., Belfield, Dublin 4, Ireland. TEL 353-1-7067109, FAX 353-1-7061151. Eds. Anne Parker, Barry O'Mahony. Adv. contact Barry O'Mahony. Circ: 1,500.

636.089 179 579 TUR ISSN 1300-1515
PENDIK VETERINER MIKROBIYOLOJI DERGISI. Text in Turkish; Summaries in English. 1967. 2/yr.
Indexed: Dairy Sci.Abstr., Ind.Vet., Nutr.Abstr., Poult.Abstr., Rev.Appl.Entomol., Vet.Bull., World Ag.Econ.& Rur.Soc.Abstr.
—BLDSC (6419.270500).
Published by: Pendik Veteriner Kontrol ve Arastirma Enstitusu, Ankara Caddesi 10, Pendik-Istanbul 81480, Turkey. TEL 90-216-3901280, FAX 90-216-3540249, administrator@istanbul.tagem.gov.tr, http://www.ahis.gov.tr. Ed. Dr. Kaya Demirozu. Circ: 1,000 (paid).

636.089 BRA ISSN 0100-736X
PESQUISA VETERINARIA BRASILEIRA/BRAZILIAN JOURNAL OF VETERINARY RESEARCH. Text and summaries in Portuguese, English. 1981. q. BRL 28 domestic to individuals; BRL 56 domestic to institutions; USD 50 foreign (effective 2002). Supplement avail.; back issues avail. *Refereed.* **Document type:** *Journal, Academic/Scholarly.* **Description:** Publishes original articles and review papers on all aspects of veterinary sciences. Includes contributions on animal pathology and related subjects, mainly diseases of economic importance and interest to public health.
Related titles: Online - full text ed.: (from SciELO, Institute for Scientific Information).

V

Indexed: Curr.Cont. (coverage dropped), Dairy Sci.Abstr., Focus on: Vet.Sci.& Med., Food Sci.& Tech.Abstr., Herb.Abstr., Ind.Vet., Nutr.Abstr., Pig News & Info., Poult.Abstr., Protozool.Abstr., Rev.Med.& Vet.Mycol., Vet.Bull., Weed Abstr., Wild.Rev.
—BLDSC (6428.246000), CISTI, IDS.
Published by: Colegio Brasileiro de Patologia Animal, Embrapa - CNPAB - PSA, Seropedica, RJ 23851970, Brazil. TEL 55-21-2682-1081, FAX 55-21-2682-1081, colegio@cbpa.org.br, http://www.scielo.br/pvb, http://www.cbpa.org.br/. Ed. Dr. Jurgen Dobereiner. Circ: 1,000.

636.089 DEU ISSN 0177-7726
PFERDEHEILKUNDE. Text in English, German; Summaries in English. 1985. bi-m. EUR 170 in Europe; EUR 60 to students (effective 2002). back issues avail. **Document type:** *Journal, Academic/Scholarly.*
Related titles: Online - full text ed.: (from Institute for Scientific Information).
Indexed: ASCA, AgBiotech, Anim.Breed.Abstr., Curr.Cont., Dairy Sci.Abstr., Helminthol.Abstr., Herb.Abstr., Ind.Vet., Nutr.Abstr., Rev.Appl.Entomol., Rev.Med.& Vet.Mycol., Vet.Bull.
—BLDSC (6437.519000), IDS. **CCC.**
Published by: Hippiatrika Verlag GmbH, Postfach 102251, Stuttgart 70018, Germany. TEL 49-711-2366332, FAX 49-711-2366337, berlin@pferdeheilkunde.de, http://www.pferdeheilkunde.de. Eds. B Huskamp, E Deegen, H D Lauk TEL 49-30-28040451.

636.089 PHL ISSN 0115-2173
CODEN: PJVSDI
PHILIPPINE JOURNAL OF VETERINARY AND ANIMAL SCIENCES. Text and summaries in English. 1975. q. PHP 350 domestic; USD 50 foreign (effective 2000). adv. bk.rev. charts, illus. back issues avail. **Document type:** *Academic/Scholarly.* **Description:** Covers veterinary and animal science subjects intended for academics, researchers, scientists.
Formerly: Philippine Journal of Animal Science
Indexed: Biol.Abstr., Chem.Abstr., Dairy Sci.Abstr., Food Sci.& Tech.Abstr., Nutr.Abstr.
—CASDDS, CISTI.
Published by: Philippine Society of Animal Sciences, c/o Institute of Animal Science, University of the, College of Agriculture, Los Banos, Laguna 4031, Philippines. ass@mudspring.uplb.edu.ph. Ed. Jazie A Acorda. R&P Annabelle S Sarabia TEL 63-49-536-2729. Circ: 1,000.

636.089 PHL ISSN 0031-7705
CODEN: PJVMAV
PHILIPPINE JOURNAL OF VETERINARY MEDICINE. Abbreviated title: P J V M. Text in English. 1962. s-a. PHP 200, USD 50 (effective 2000). adv. bk.rev. bibl, charts, illus. back issues avail. *Refereed.* **Document type:** *Journal, Academic/Scholarly.* **Description:** Publishes original research, review articles, abstracts of proceedings, short communications and research notes on all aspects of veterinary medicine.
Indexed: AgBiotech, Anim.Breed.Abstr., Biol.Abstr., Chem.Abstr., Curr.Cont. (coverage dropped), Dairy Sci.Abstr., Helminthol.Abstr., Ind.Vet., Nutr.Abstr., Pig News & Info., Poult.Abstr., Rev.Appl.Entomol., Vet.Bull., Zoo.Rec.
—BLDSC (6456.050000), CASDDS, CISTI.
Published by: University of the Philippines at Los Banos, College of Veterinary Medicine, Los Banos, Laguna 4031, Philippines. TEL 63-49-536-2730, FAX 63-49-536-2760, vetmed@laguna.net. Ed., R&P Conrado A Valdez. Circ: 300 (paid).

636.089 GBR ISSN 1352-9749
THE PIG JOURNAL. Text in English. 1976. s-a. GBP 35, USD 55; GBP 19.50, USD 30 newsstand/cover (effective 2001). bk.rev. abstr. back issues avail.; reprints avail. *Refereed.* **Document type:** *Proceedings.* **Description:** Discusses topics on pig diseases and treatment presented at national and international meetings or those submitted to the editor.
Former titles (until 1994): Pig Veterinary Journal (0956-0939); (until 1989): Pig Veterinary Society. Proceedings (0141-3074)
Related titles: CD-ROM ed.
Indexed: Agri.Eng.Abstr., Anim.Breed.Abstr., Dairy Sci.Abstr., Derwent Biotech.Abstr., Ind.Vet., Nutr.Abstr., Pig News & Info., Poult.Abstr., Rev.Med.& Vet.Mycol., Triticale Abstr., Vet.Bull., World Ag.Econ.& Rur.Soc.Abstr.
—BLDSC (6500.040000), CISTI.
Published by: Pig Veterinary Society, Southview, E. Tytherton, Chippenham, Wilts SN15 4LX, United Kingdom. TEL 44-1249-740380, FAX 44-1249-740380, pig-journal@talk21.com, http://www.pigjournal.co.uk. Eds. D Basinger, D.J. Taylor, S.H. Done. R&P D G S Burch TEL 44-1753-831886. Circ: 900.

636.089 FRA ISSN 0335-4997
CODEN: POVTEN
POINT VETERINAIRE. Text in French. 1973. 8/yr. FRF 810 (effective 1997). adv. bk.rev. *Refereed.* **Document type:** *Catalog.*
Related titles: Online - full text ed.: (from Institute for Scientific Information).
Indexed: ASCA, Agri.Eng.Abstr., Anim.Breed.Abstr., Bio-Contr.News & Info., Dairy Sci.Abstr., Focus on: Vet.Sci.& Med., Helminthol.Abstr., Ind.Vet., Nutr.Abstr., Pig News & Info., Poult.Abstr., Protozool.Abstr., Rev.Appl.Entomol., Rev.Med.& Vet.Mycol., Small Anim.Abstr., Vet.Bull., Weed Abstr., World Ag.Econ.& Rur.Soc.Abstr.
—BLDSC (6541.862000), IDS, Infotrieve. **CCC.**
Published by: Editions du Point Veterinaire S.A., 9 rue Alexandre, BP 233, Maisons Alfort Cedex 94702, France. TEL 33-1-45170225, FAX 33-1-45170274. Ed. Maryvonne Barbaray. Adv. contact Nadege Humbert. Circ: 6,000.

636.089 ESP ISSN 1130-8451
PORCI. Text in Spanish. 1991. 6/yr. ESP 7,175; ESP 9,700 foreign (effective 1999). adv.
Indexed: Ind.SST.
—CINDOC.
Published by: Luzon S.A. de Ediciones, Virgen de la Alegria, 9, Madrid 28027, Spain. TEL 1-4051505, FAX 1-403-49-07, veterinaria@luzan5.es, http://www.luzan5.es.

636.089 DEU ISSN 0032-681X
CODEN: PRTIAV
DER PRAKTISCHE TIERARZT. Text in German. 1921. 13/yr. DEM 202; DEM 238 foreign (effective 2000). adv. bk.rev. charts, illus. index. *Refereed.* **Document type:** *Journal, Trade.*
Related titles: Online - full text ed.: (from Institute for Scientific Information).
Indexed: ASCA, AgBiotech, Agri.& Environ.Biotech.Abstr. (coverage dropped), Agri.Eng.Abstr., Anim.Breed.Abstr., Aqua.Sci.& Fish.Abstr., Aquacult.Abstr., Chem.Abstr., Curr.Adv.Cancer Res., Curr.Adv.Ecol.Sci., Curr.Cont., Dairy Sci.Abstr., Derwent Biotech.Abstr., Focus on: Vet.Sci.& Med., Helminthol.Abstr., Herb.Abstr., INIS Atomind., Ind.Vet., Key Word Ind.Wildl.Res., Nutr.Abstr., Pig News & Info., Poult.Abstr., Protozool.Abstr., Rev.Appl.Entomol., Rev.Med.& Vet.Mycol., SSCI (coverage dropped), Small Anim.Abstr., Vet.Bull., World Ag.Econ.& Rur.Soc.Abstr.
—BLDSC (6601.200000), CASDDS, IDS, Infotrieve, Linda Hall. **CCC.**
Published by: (Bundesverbandes praktischer Tieraerzte e.V.), Schluetersche GmbH und Co. KG, Hans-Boeckler-Allee 7, Hannover 30173, Germany. TEL 49-511-8550-0, FAX 49-511-85502405, anzeigen@schluetersche.de, http://www.schluetersche.de. Ed. Dr. Leopold Temmler. Circ: 8,413 (paid); 8,985 (controlled).

636.089 FRA ISSN 0758-1882
PRATIQUE MEDICALE ET CHIRURGICALE DE L'ANIMAL DE COMPAGNIE. Text in French. 1966. 7/yr. FRF 1,200. adv. bk.rev. *Refereed.*
Formerly (until 1983): Animal de Compagnie (0245-9302)
Related titles: Online - full text ed.: (from Institute for Scientific Information).
Indexed: ASCA, Anim.Breed.Abstr., Derwent Biotech.Abstr., Focus on: Vet.Sci.& Med., Ind.Vet., Nutr.Abstr., Protozool.Abstr., Rev.Appl.Entomol., Rev.Med.& Vet.Mycol., Vet.Bull.
—BLDSC (6602.160000), IDS.
Published by: Conference Nationale des Veterinaires Specialises en Petits Animaux 82, avenue de Villiers, Paris 75017, France. TEL 42-67-72-96, FAX 42-67-51-76. Ed. Dr. J P Pages. Circ: 3,000.

636.089 NLD ISSN 0167-5877
PREVENTIVE VETERINARY MEDICINE; an international journal on research and development in veterinary epidemiology, animal disease prevention and control, and animal health economics. Text in English. 1983. 20/yr. EUR 1,295 in Europe to institutions; JPY 172,000 in Japan to institutions; USD 1,449 elsewhere to institutions (effective 2002). bk.rev. illus. index. reprints avail. *Refereed.* **Document type:** *Academic/Scholarly.* **Description:** Aims to disseminate, on a worldwide basis, information and reports of significance in the field of animal (mammalian, aquatic and avian) health programs and preventive veterinary medicine.
Related titles: Microform ed.: (from PQC); Online - full text ed.: (from ingenta, Swets Blackwell, Institute for Scientific Information, ScienceDirect).
Indexed: ASCA, AgBiotech, Agri.Eng.Abstr., Agricola, Anim.Breed.Abstr., Biol.Abstr., Curr.Adv.Ecol.Sci., Curr.Cont., Dairy Sci.Abstr., Derwent Biotech.Abstr., Focus on: Vet.Sci.& Med., Helminthol.Abstr., Ind.Med. (1982-), Ind.Vet., Maize Abstr., Nutr.Abstr., Pig News & Info., Poult.Abstr., Protozool.Abstr., Rev.Appl.Entomol., Rev.Arom.& Med.Plants, Rev.Med.& Vet.Mycol., SSCI (coverage dropped), Sci.Cit.Ind., Small Anim.Abstr., Sport Fish.Abstr., Vet.Bull., Wild.Rev., World Ag.Econ.& Rur.Soc.Abstr., Zoo.Rec.
—BLDSC (6612.795000), CISTI, IDS, Infotrieve, ingenta, Linda Hall. **CCC.**
Published by: Elsevier Science BV, PO Box 211, Amsterdam 1000 AE, Netherlands. TEL 31-20-485-2911, FAX 31-20-485-2457, http://www.elsevier.com/locate/prevetmed. Ed. H N Erb. Circ: 800. **Subscr. in Australasia and the Far East to:** Elsevier Science (Singapore) Pte Ltd, No.1 Temasek Ave, 17-01 Millenia Tower, Singapore 039192, Singapore. TEL 65-434-3727, FAX 65-337-2230; **Subscr. in Japan to:** Elsevier Science Inc - Japan Regional Office, 9-15 Higashi-Azabu 1-chome, Minato-ku, Tokyo 106-0044, Japan. TEL 81-3-5561-5033; **Subscr. in the Americas to:** Elsevier Science. TEL 212-633-3730, FAX 212-633-3680, usinfo-f@elsevier.com.

636.089 FRA ISSN 0990-0632
CODEN: PROAEK
PRODUCTIONS ANIMALES. Text in French. 1970. 5/yr. FRF 400; FRF 100 newsstand/cover (effective 1999). bk.rev. *Refereed.* **Document type:** *Academic/Scholarly.* **Description:** Deals with all species of zootechnical interest, covering feed and nutrition, physiology, pathology, genetics, production techniques, product quality and production economics.
Formerly (until 1988): Centre de Recherches Zootechniques et Veterinaires de Theix. Bulletin Technique (0395-7519)
Related titles: Online - full text ed.: (from Institute for Scientific Information).
Indexed: ASCA, AgBiotech, Anim.Breed.Abstr., Dairy Sci.Abstr., Focus on: Vet.Sci.& Med., Helminthol.Abstr., Herb.Abstr., Ind.Vet., Irr.& Drain.Abstr., Maize Abstr., Nutr.Abstr., Pig News & Info., Poult.Abstr., Protozool.Abstr., Ref.Zh., Rev.Appl.Entomol., SSCI (coverage dropped), Soils & Fert., Sugar Ind.Abstr., Vet.Bull., World Ag.Econ.& Rur.Soc.Abstr.
—BLDSC (6853.247000), IDS, Linda Hall.
Published by: I N R A Editions, RD 10, Versailles Cedex 78026, France. TEL 33-1-30833406, FAX 33-1-30833449, farce@ensam.inra.fr, http://www.inra.fr/PA/index.htm. Ed. Marie Helene Farce.

636.089 USA ISSN 1080-7446
PROFESSIONAL ANIMAL SCIENTIST. Text in English. 1985. q. USD 30. adv. bibl, charts, illus, stat, tr.lit. back issues avail. **Document type:** *Journal, Academic/Scholarly, Trade.* **Description:** Designed for researchers and professional practitioners of animal science.
Related titles: Online - full text ed.
Indexed: Agricola.
—BLDSC (6857.242500).
Published by: American Registry of Professional Animal Scientists, 1111 N Dunlap Ave, Savoy, IL 61874. FAX 217-398-4119, arpas@assochq.org, http://www.arpas.uiuc.edu. Ed. William Flatt. Pub. Bill Baumgardt. R&P Ann Mester TEL 217-356-3182.

636.089 MEX
PRONTUARIO DE ESPECIALIDADES VETERINARIAS. Text in Spanish. 1971. a.
Published by: Ediciones P L M S.A. de C.V., San Bernadino 17, Col del Valle, Mexico City, DF 03100, Mexico. TEL 687-1766, FAX 536-5027. Ed. Luis Hochenstein. Circ: 5,000.

636.08 USA
PULSE (PICO RIVERA). Text in English. 195?. m. membership. adv. illus. **Document type:** *Trade.* **Description:** Publishes case studies and other scientific and medical news of interest to doctors of veterinary medicine.
Published by: Southern California Veterinary Medical Association, 8338 Rosemead Blvd, Pico Rivera, CA 90660. TEL 310-948-4979. Ed. Richard L Holden. Adv. contact Marilyn Jensen. Circ: 1,100 (controlled).

R F L. (Rundschau Fleischhygiene und Lebensmittelueberwachung) see *FOOD AND FOOD INDUSTRIES*

636.089 FRA ISSN 1022-1050
RAPPORTS DE SYNTHESE SUR LES THEMES TECHNIQUES PRESENTES AU COMITE INTERNATIONAL OU AUX COMMISSIONS REGIONALES/COMPREHENSIVE REPORTS ON TECHNICAL ITEMS PRESENTED TO THE INTERNATIONAL COMMITTEE OR TO REGIONAL COMMISSIONS. Text in Multiple languages. 1993. a. EUR 25 newsstand/cover (effective 2000).
Published by: Office International des Epizooties, 12 rue de Prony, Paris 75017, France. TEL 33-1-44151888, FAX 33-1-42670987, oie@oie.int, http://www.oie.int.

RASSEGNA DI DIRITTO, LEGISLAZIONE E MEDICINA LEGALE VETERINARIA. see *LAW*

636.089 FRA ISSN 0034-1843
CODEN: RMVEAG
RECUEIL DE MEDECINE VETERINAIRE D'ALFORT. Text in French; Summaries in English, Spanish. 1824. 9/yr. FRF 1,050. adv. bk.rev. abstr, illus. index. reprint service avail. from PQC.
Indexed: ASCA, Anim.Breed.Abstr., Aqua.Sci.& Fish.Abstr., Aquacult.Abstr., Biol.Abstr., Chem.Abstr., Chem.Indus.Notes, Chem.Titles, Curr.Adv.Ecol.Sci., Curr.Cont. (coverage dropped), Derwent Biotech.Abstr., Excerp.Med., Focus on: Vet.Sci.& Med. (coverage dropped), Food Sci.& Tech.Abstr., Helminthol.Abstr., Ind.Vet., Key Word Ind.Wildl.Res., Maize Abstr., Nutr.Abstr., Poult.Abstr., Protozool.Abstr., Rev.Appl.Entomol., Rev.Med.& Vet.Mycol., SSCI (coverage dropped), Sport Fish.Abstr., Vet.Bull., Wild.Rev., Zoo.Rec.
—BLDSC (7329.000000), CASDDS, GNLM, IDS.
Published by: Association pour la Publication du Recueil de Medecine Veterinaire, Ecole Nationale Veterinaire, 7 av. du General de Gaulle, Maisons Alfort Cedex 94704, France. TEL 33-1-43967176, FAX 33-1-43751210. Ed. M Paragon. Circ: 25,000.

636.089 GBR
REGISTERS & DIRECTORY OF VETERINARY SURGEONS. Text in English. 1870. a. GBP 30 (effective 1999). adv. **Document type:** *Directory.*
Published by: Royal College of Veterinary Surgeons, Belgravia House, Royal College Of Veterinary Surgeons, 62 Horseferry Rd, London SW1P 2AF, United Kingdom. TEL 44-171-222-2001, FAX 44-171-222-2004, register@rcvs.org.uk, http://www.rcvs.org.uk/rcvs/. Eds. John Collins, Michael Sibley. Adv. contact T G Scott. Circ: 18,000.

636.089 DEU ISSN 0936-6768
S494 CODEN: RDANEF
REPRODUCTION IN DOMESTIC ANIMALS; physiology, pathology, biotechnology. Text in English. 1966. 6/yr. DEM 941.71 in Europe; DEM 978.87 elsewhere; DEM 1,035.88 in Europe print & online eds. combined; DEM 1,076.76 elsewhere print & online eds. combined (effective 2001). adv. bk.rev. illus, stat. index. *Refereed.* **Document type:** *Journal, Academic/Scholarly.* **Description:** Offers comprehensive information concerning physiology, pathology, and biotechnology of reproduction.
Formerly: Zuchthygiene (0044-5371)
Related titles: ♦ Online - full text ed.: Reproduction in Domestic Animals Online. ISSN 1439-0531.
Indexed: ASCA, AgBiotech, Agri.& Environ.Biotech.Abstr. (coverage dropped), Agricola, Anim.Breed.Abstr., Biol.Abstr., Chem.Abstr., Chem.Indus.Notes, Chem.Titles, Curr.Adv.Cell & Devel.Biol., Curr.Adv.Ecol.Sci., Curr.Adv.Gen.& Molec.Biol., Curr.Cont., Dairy Sci.Abstr., Derwent Biotech.Abstr., Focus on: Vet.Sci.& Med., Food Sci.& Tech.Abstr., Ind.Sci.Rev., Ind.Vet., Nutr.Abstr., Pig News & Info., Protozool.Abstr., Rev.Med.& Vet.Mycol., Sci.Cit.Ind., Soyabean Abstr., Vet.Bull., Wild.Rev.
—BLDSC (7713.599600), CASDDS, CISTI, IDS, Infotrieve, ingenta, Linda Hall. **CCC.**
Published by: Blackwell Wissenschafts Verlag GmbH, Kurfuerstendamm 57, Berlin 10707, Germany. TEL 49-30-32790665, FAX 49-30-32790610, abo@blackwis.de, http://www.blackwell.de. Ed. Heriberto Rodriguez-Martinez. adv.: B&W page DEM 540; trim 125 x 200. Circ: 500.

636.089 DEU ISSN 1439-0531
REPRODUCTION IN DOMESTIC ANIMALS ONLINE. Text in English. 6/yr. DEM 848 (effective 2001). **Document type:** *Academic/Scholarly.*
Media: Online - full text (from EBSCO Publishing, O C L C Online Computer Library Center, Inc., ingenta, Munksgaard & Blackwell Science's Synergy, Swets Blackwell, Institute for Scientific Information). **Related titles:** ♦ Print ed.: Reproduction in Domestic Animals. ISSN 0936-6768.
Published by: Blackwell Wissenschafts Verlag GmbH, Kurfuerstendamm 57, Berlin 10707, Germany. TEL 49-30-32790665, FAX 49-30-32790610, abo@blackwis.de, http://www.blackwell.de.

636.089 GBR ISSN 0034-5288
SF601 CODEN: RVTSA9
RESEARCH IN VETERINARY SCIENCE. Text in English. 1960. bi-m. GBP 131 to individuals; GBP 215 to institutions (effective 2002). adv. bibl, charts, illus, abstr. index. back issues avail.; reprint service avail. from PQC,SWZ. *Refereed.* **Document type:** *Academic/Scholarly.*
Related titles: Microform ed.: (from PQC,PMC); Online - full text ed.: (from EBSCO Publishing, RoweCom Information Quest, Swets Blackwell, IDEAL Online Library, Institute for Scientific Information).
Indexed: ASCA, AgBiotech, Agri.& Environ.Biotech.Abstr. (coverage dropped), Agricola, Anim.Breed.Abstr., Aqua.Sci.& Fish.Abstr., Aquacult.Abstr., Bibl.Agri., Biol.Abstr., Chem.Abstr., Chem.Indus.Notes, Chem.Titles, Curr.Adv.Ecol.Sci., Curr.Cont., Dairy Sci.Abstr., Dent.Ind., Derwent Biotech.Abstr., Excerp.Med., Focus on: Vet.Sci.& Med., Food Sci.& Tech.Abstr., Helminthol.Abstr., INIS Atomind., Ind.Med. (1960-), Ind.Sci.Rev., Ind.Vet., Nutr.Abstr., Pig News & Info., Poult.Abstr., Protozool.Abstr., Rev.Appl.Entomol., Rev.Med.& Vet.Mycol., Rev.Plant Path., Risk Abstr., SSCI (coverage dropped), Sci.Cit.Ind., Soils & Fert., Soyabean Abstr., Sport Fish.Abstr., Triticale Abstr., Vet.Bull., Wild.Rev., Zoo.Rec.
—BLDSC (7774.100000), CASDDS, CISTI, GNLM, IDS, ingenta, Linda Hall. **CCC.**
Published by: (British Veterinary Association), W.B. Saunders Co. Ltd. (Subsidiary of: Harcourt Publishers Ltd.), 24-28 Oval Rd, London NW1 7DX, United Kingdom. TEL 44-20-7424-4200, FAX 44-20-7424-4515, http://www.harcourt-international.com/journals/rvsc. Ed. E N Boden. Circ: 945. **Subscr. to:** Harcourt Publishers Ltd., Foots Cray High St, Sidcup, Kent DA14 5HP, United Kingdom. TEL 44-20-8308-5700, FAX 44-20-8309-0807.

636.08 591.2 BRA ISSN 0103-846X
CODEN: RBPVEW
REVISTA BRASILEIRA DE PARASITOLOGIA VETERINARIA/BRAZILIAN JOURNAL OF VETERINARY PARASITOLOGY. Text in Portuguese. 1991. s-a. USD 40. *Refereed.* **Document type:** *Academic/Scholarly.* **Description:** Presents original articles on basic or applied research in helminthology, protozoology and entomology, as related to animal health.
Indexed: Bio-Contr.News & Info., Dairy Sci.Abstr., Helminthol.Abstr., Ind.Vet., Poult.Abstr., Protozool.Abstr., Rev.Appl.Entomol., Vet.Bull., Zoo.Rec.
—BLDSC (7845.430000).
Published by: Colegio Brasileiro de Parasitologia Veterinaria, Av. Prof. Lineu Prestes, 1374, Edif. Biomedicas II, Cidade Univer., Sao Paulo, SP 05508-900, Brazil. TEL 55-11-8187336, FAX 55-11-8187417, rbpv@hotmail.com. Ed. Ney Kramer Amaral. Circ: 500.

636.089 BRA
CODEN: RSBZBM
REVISTA BRASILEIRA DE ZOOTECNIA/BRAZILIAN JOURNAL OF ANIMAL SCIENCE. Text in Portuguese; Summaries in English. 1972. bi-m. BRL 100, USD 100 (effective 1999). bk.rev. back issues avail. **Document type:** *Academic/Scholarly.*
Formerly: Sociedade Brasileira de Zootecnia. Revista (0100-4859)
Related titles: Online - full text ed.: (from Institute for Scientific Information).
Indexed: AgBiotech, Agri.Eng.Abstr., Agroforest.Abstr., Anim.Breed.Abstr., Biol.Abstr., Chem.Abstr., Chem.Titles, Crop Physiol.Abstr., Dairy Sci.Abstr., Field Crop Abstr., Focus on: Vet.Sci.& Med., Forest.Abstr., Herb.Abstr., Ind.Vet., Maize Abstr., Nutr.Abstr., Pig News & Info., Plant Breed.Abstr., Plant Gen.Res.Abstr., Postharvest, Poult.Abstr., Ref.Zh., Rev.Appl.Entomol., Rev.Med.& Vet.Mycol., Rev.Plant Path., Rice Abstr., Seed Abstr., Soils & Fert., Sorghum & Millets Abstr., Soyabean Abstr., Sport Fish.Abstr., Sugar Ind.Abstr., Triticale Abstr., Vet.Bull., Weed Abstr., Wild.Rev., World Ag.Econ.& Rur.Soc.Abstr., Zoo.Rec.
—BLDSC, CASDDS, CINDOC, CISTI, IDS.
Published by: Sociedade Brasileira de Zootecnia, Departamento de Zootecnia, Universidade Federal de Vicosa, Vicosa, MG 36570-000, Brazil. TEL 55-31-899-2271, FAX 55-31-8992270, TELEX 031-1587, rsbz@mail.ufv.br. Ed. Martinho de Almeida Esilva. Circ: 2,000.

REVISTA CERES; orgao de divulgacao tecnico-cientifica em ciencias agrarias. see *AGRICULTURE*

636.089 COL ISSN 0120-0690
REVISTA COLOMBIANA DE CIENCIAS PECUARIAS. Text in Spanish. 1978. s-a. USD 10 (effective 2000). **Document type:** *Journal, Academic/Scholarly.*
Published by: Universidad de Antioquia, Facultad de Medicina Veterinaria y de Zootecnia, Apartado Postal 1226, Medellin, Colombia.

636.089 CUB ISSN 0048-7678
REVISTA CUBANA DE CIENCIAS VETERINARIAS. Text in Spanish; Summaries in Spanish, English. 1970. 3/yr. USD 28 in South America; USD 30 in North America; USD 34 elsewhere. bk.rev. bibl, charts, illus.
Related titles: Microfilm ed.
Indexed: Anim.Breed.Abstr., Apic.Abstr., Biol.Abstr., Dairy Sci.Abstr., Helminthol.Abstr., Ind.Vet., Maize Abstr., Nutr.Abstr., Pig News & Info., Poult.Abstr., Protozool.Abstr., Rev.Med.& Vet.Mycol., Vet.Bull.
—Linda Hall.
Published by: (Consejo Cientifico Veterinario), Ediciones Cubanas, Obispo No. 527, Apdo. 605, Havana, Cuba. Circ: 3,000.

636.08 ESP ISSN 1130-2739
REVISTA DE EXPERIMENTACION ANIMAL. Text in Spanish. 1990. s-a. ESP 3,000.
Indexed: Ind.SST.
—CINDOC.
Published by: Universidad de Leon, Facultad de Veterinaria, Departamento de Medicina Animal, Campus de Vegazana, s-n, Leon 24007, Spain. Ed. Dr. Carlos Cesar Perez Garcia.

636.089 PER ISSN 0376-4370
SF604 CODEN: RIPEDT
REVISTA DE INVESTIGACIONES PECUARIAS. Text in English; Summaries in English. 1972. 3/yr. USD 40.
Indexed: Aqua.Sci.& Fish.Abstr., Vet.Bull.
—CISTI, Linda Hall.
Published by: Universidad Nacional Mayor de San Marcos, Instituto Veterinario de Investigaciones Tropicales y de Altura, Apdo. 41-0068, Lima 41, Peru. TEL 51-14-353059, FAX 51-14-353064. Ed. C Novoa. Circ: 1,500.

636.089 CUB ISSN 0253-570X
CODEN: RSANDH
REVISTA DE SALUD ANIMAL. Text in Spanish; Summaries in English. 1979. 4/yr. USD 21 in the Americas; USD 26 in Europe. charts, bibl.
Indexed: Agri.Eng.Abstr., Anim.Breed.Abstr., Biol.Abstr., Chem.Abstr., Chem.Indus.Notes, Chem.Titles, Dairy Sci.Abstr., Food Sci.& Tech.Abstr., Helminthol.Abstr., Herb.Abstr., Ind.Vet., Nutr.Abstr., Pig News & Info., Poult.Abstr., Protozool.Abstr., Rev.Appl.Entomol., Rev.Arom.& Med.Plants, Rev.Med.& Vet.Mycol., Soyabean Abstr., Sugar Ind.Abstr., Vet.Bull.
—BLDSC (7870.518000), CASDDS.
Published by: (Centro Nacional de Sanidad Agropecuaria), Ediciones Cubanas, Obispo No. 527, Apdo. 605, Havana, Cuba.

636.089 PRT ISSN 0035-0389
REVISTA PORTUGUESA DE CIENCIAS VETERINARIAS. Text in Portuguese. 1902. q. PTE 4,500, USD 80 (effective 1998). adv. bk.rev. abstr, bibl. index. **Document type:** *Academic/Scholarly.* **Description:** Papers from Portuguese researchers on all areas of veterinary science.
Indexed: Anim.Breed.Abstr., Aqua.Sci.& Fish.Abstr., Aquacult.Abstr., Biol.Abstr., Dairy Sci.Abstr., Environ.Sci.Poll.Mgmt., Food Sci.& Tech.Abstr., Helminthol.Abstr., Ind.Vet., Maize Abstr., Nutr.Abstr., Pig News & Info., Poult.Abstr., Protozool.Abstr., Rev.Appl.Entomol., Rev.Med.& Vet.Mycol., Vet.Bull.
—BLDSC (7869.880000), CISTI.
Published by: Sociedade Portuguesa de Ciencias Veterinarias, Rua D. Dinis 2-A, Lisbon 1250, Portugal. Ed. Luis Tavares. Circ: 1,100.

636.089 VEN ISSN 0484-8284
REVISTA VETERINARIA VENEZOLANA. Text in Spanish. m.
Formerly (until 1956): Revista Grancolombiana de Zootecnia Higiene y Medicina Veterinaria
Published by: Federacion de Colegios de Medicos Veterinarios de Venezuela, Qta. Marilina, Av. Paez, Calle Stolk, El Paraiso, Apdo. 2921, Caracas 102, Venezuela. Ed. Dr. C Ruiz Martinez.

V

636.089 COL ISSN 0120-4114
REVISTA VETERINARIA Y ZOOTECNICA DE CALDAS. Text in Spanish. 1982. 2/yr. COP 5,000, USD 5 (effective 1998). adv. back issues avail. *Refereed.* **Document type:** *Academic/Scholarly.* **Description:** Contains research articles on animal medicine and husbandry.
Published by: University of Caldas, School of Veterinary Medicine & Animal Husbandry, Apartado Aereo 275, Manizales, CAL, Colombia. TEL 57-968-852139, FAX 57-968-862520, ajjmillo@col2.telecom.com.co, http://www.ucaldas.edu.co/~ciagropc. Ed. Alberto Jaramillo J. Circ: 1,000.

V

636.089 FRA ISSN 0035-1555
CODEN: RVMVAH
REVUE DE MEDECINE VETERINAIRE. Text and summaries in French, English. 1838. m. FRF 780; FRF 945 foreign (effective 1999). adv. bk.rev. abstr, illus. index. reprint service avail. from PQC,ISI. *Refereed.* **Document type:** *Academic/Scholarly.* **Description:** Provides reviews, original reports, clinical reports.
Related titles: Online - full text ed.: (from Institute for Scientific Information).
Indexed: ASCA, Abstr.Hyg., AgBiotech, Agri.& Environ.Biotech.Abstr. (coverage dropped), Anim.Breed.Abstr., Aqua.Sci.& Fish.Abstr., Aquacult.Abstr., Biol.Abstr., Chem.Abstr., Chem.Indus.Notes, Chem.Titles, Curr.Adv.Ecol.Sci., Curr.Cont., Dairy Sci.Abstr., Derwent Biotech.Abstr., Entomol.Abstr., Excerp.Med., Focus on: Vet.Sci.& Med., Food Sci.& Tech.Abstr., Helminthol.Abstr., Ind.Sci.Rev., Ind.Vet., Nutr.Abstr., Pig News & Info., Poult.Abstr., Protozool.Abstr., Psychol.Abstr., Ref.Zh., Rev.Appl.Entomol., Rev.Med.& Vet.Mycol., Rev.Plant Path., Rural Recreat.Tour.Abstr., Sci.Cit.Ind., Small Anim.Abstr., Soils & Fert., Sport Fish.Abstr., Sugar Ind.Abstr., Triticale Abstr., Trop.Dis.Bull., Vet.Bull., Wild.Rev., World Ag.Econ.& Rur.Soc.Abstr., Zoo.Rec.
—BLDSC (7932.000000), CASDDS, CISTI, GNLM, IDS, Linda Hall.
Published by: Revue detionale Veterinaire, 23 Chemin des Capelles, Toulouse Cedex 3 31076, France. TEL 33-561-193835, FAX 33-561-193835, jy.jovglar@envt.fr. Ed. J P Euzeby. Circ: 3,300.

636.089 FRA ISSN 0035-1865
REVUE D'ELEVAGE ET DE MEDECINE VETERINAIRE DES PAYS TROPICAUX. Text in English, French; Summaries in English, French, Spanish. 1947. 4/yr. FRF 420 in France; FRF 560 in Europe; FRF 600 elsewhere (effective 1999). adv. bk.rev. abstr, bibl, charts. index, cum.index: 1947-1977. **Document type:** *Academic/Scholarly.*
Related titles: Microfiche ed.
Indexed: AgBiotech, Agri.& Environ.Biotech.Abstr. (coverage dropped), Anim.Breed.Abstr., Aqua.Sci.& Fish.Abstr., Aquacult.Abstr., Biol.Abstr., Curr.Adv.Ecol.Sci., Curr.Cont. (coverage dropped), Dairy Sci.Abstr., Derwent Biotech.Abstr., Entomol.Abstr. (coverage dropped), Environ.Sci.Poll.Mgmt., Excerp.Med., Field Crop Abstr., Food Sci.& Tech.Abstr., Helminthol.Abstr., Herb.Abstr., Ind.Med. (coverage dropped), Ind.Vet., Irr.& Drain.Abstr., Nutr.Abstr., Pig News & Info., Pollut.Abstr., Poult.Abstr., Protozool.Abstr., Ref.Zh., Rev.Appl.Entomol., Rev.Arom.& Med.Plants, Rev.Med.& Vet.Mycol., Rev.Plant Path., Rice Abstr., Risk Abstr., Saf.Sci.Abstr., So.Pac.Per.Ind., Trop.Oil Seeds Abstr., Vet.Bull., Zoo.Rec.
—BLDSC (7900.000000), CISTI, GNLM.
Published by: (Institut d'Elevage et de Medecine Veterinaire des Pays Tropicaux), Expansion Scientifique Francaise, 31 bd. de la Tour Maubourg, Paris Cedex 7 75343, France. TEL 33-1-40626400, FAX 33-1-45556920. Ed. A H Robinet. Circ: (controlled).

RIVISTA DI ZOOTECNIA E VETERINARIA; rassegna di informazione e aggiornamento. see *AGRICULTURE—Poultry And Livestock*

SANS LAISSE; magazine de l'education et des sports canins. see *PETS*

636.089 CHE ISSN 0036-7281
CODEN: SATHAA
SCHWEIZER ARCHIV FUER TIERHEILKUNDE. Text in German. 12/yr. CHF 240 domestic; CHF 268 foreign (effective 2001). adv. 64 p./no. *Refereed.* **Document type:** *Journal, Academic/Scholarly.*
Related titles: Online - full text ed.: (from Institute for Scientific Information).
Indexed: ASCA, AgBiotech, Agri.& Environ.Biotech.Abstr. (coverage dropped), Anim.Breed.Abstr., Biol.Abstr., Chem.Abstr., Curr.Adv.Ecol.Sci., Curr.Cont., Dairy Sci.Abstr., Derwent Biotech.Abstr., Excerp.Med., Focus on: Vet.Sci.& Med., Food Sci.& Tech.Abstr., Helminthol.Abstr., Ind.Med. (1859-), Ind.Sci.Rev., Ind.Vet., Key Word Ind.Wildl.Res., Nutr.Abstr., Pig News & Info., Poult.Abstr., Protozool.Abstr., Rev.Appl.Entomol., Rev.Med.& Vet.Mycol., Rev.Plant Path., SSCI (coverage dropped), Sci.Cit.Ind., Small Anim.Abstr., Soils & Fert., Vet.Bull., Wild.Rev.
—CASDDS, CISTI, GNLM, IDS, Infotrieve. **CCC.**
Published by: (Gesellschaft Schweizerischer Tieraerzte), Hans Huber AG, Laengassstr 76, Bern, 9 3000, Switzerland. TEL 41-31-3004500, FAX 41-31-3004591, zeitschriften@hanshuber.com, http://www.hanshuber.com. Ed. Dr. Rico Thun. Adv. contact Rene Waelchli. color page CHF 2,648; trim 216 x 303. Circ: 2,900.

636.089 FRA ISSN 0750-7682
CODEN: SVMCD8
SCIENCES VETERINAIRES - MEDECINE COMPAREE. Text in French. 1898. a. FRF 150 domestic; FRF 170 foreign (effective 2001). adv. bk.rev. **Document type:** *Bulletin, Monographic series.*
Formerly (until 1982): Societe des Sciences Veterinaires et de Medecine Comparee de Lyon. Bulletin (0301-1194)
Indexed: Agroforest.Abstr., Biol.Abstr., Chem.Abstr., Helminthol.Abstr., Ind.Vet., Nutr.Abstr., Poult.Abstr., Protozool.Abstr., Rice Abstr., Vet.Bull., Zoo.Rec.
—BLDSC (8167.600000), CASDDS.
Published by: Societe des Sciences Veterinaires et de Medecine Comparee de Lyon, Ecole Nationale Veterinaire de Lyon, BP 83, Marcy l'Etoile 69280, France. TEL 33-4-78872665, FAX 33-4-78872667. Ed. Michel Franck.

636.089 ITA ISSN 0037-1521
CODEN: SVETDJ
LA SELEZIONE VETERINARIA. Text in Italian. 1960. m. ITL 96,000, USD 80 (effective 2000). adv. bk.rev. reprints avail. **Description:** Articles on veterinary sciences with emphasis on infectious diseases, microbiology, parasitology, reproduction and breeding.
Indexed: AgBiotech, Anim.Breed.Abstr., Dairy Sci.Abstr., Ind.Vet., Key Word Ind.Wildl.Res., Nutr.Abstr., Pig News & Info., Poult.Abstr., Protozool.Abstr., Rev.Appl.Entomol., Rev.Arom.& Med.Plants, Rev.Med.& Vet.Mycol., Sugar Ind.Abstr., Vet.Bull.
—BLDSC (8235.340000), CASDDS.
Published by: Istituto Zooprofilattico Sperimentale della Lombardia e dell'Emilia Romagna "Bruno Ubertini", Via Antonio Bianchi, 9, Brescia, BS 25124, Italy. TEL 39-30-2290379, FAX 39-30-225613. Ed. Exio Lodetti. Adv. contact Frosi Grazia. Circ: 3,000.

636.089 FRA ISSN 0396-5015
SEMAINE VETERINAIRE. Text in French. 1976. 40/yr. FRF 1,200 (effective 1997). adv. **Document type:** *Newspaper.*
Incorporates: Eurovet
—CISTI. **CCC.**
Published by: Editions du Point Veterinaire S.A., 9 rue Alexandre, BP 233, Maisons Alfort Cedex 94702, France. TEL 33-1-45170225, FAX 33-1-45170274. Ed. Maryvonne Barbaray. Adv. contact Nadege Humbert. Circ: 5,000.

636.089 USA ISSN 1055-937X
SF994.2.A1
SEMINARS IN AVIAN AND EXOTIC PET MEDICINE. Text in English. 1992. q. USD 120 domestic to individuals; USD 157 foreign to individuals; USD 168 domestic to institutions; USD 207 foreign to institutions; USD 68 domestic to students; USD 94 foreign to students; USD 52 newsstand/cover (effective 2001). adv. illus. Index. reprints avail. *Refereed.* **Document type:** *Academic/Scholarly.* **Description:** Covers a single topic in avian and exotic-pet medicine in each issue.
Related titles: Online - full text ed.: (from Institute for Scientific Information).
Indexed: ASCA, Derwent Biotech.Abstr., Focus on: Vet.Sci.& Med., Wild.Rev., Zoo.Rec.
—BLDSC (8239.448200), IDS, Infotrieve, ingenta. **CCC.**
Published by: W.B. Saunders Co. (Subsidiary of: Harcourt Publishers Ltd.), 11830 Westline Industrial Dr, St Louis, MO 63146. TEL 800-325-4177, http://www.wbsaunders.com. Ed. Dr. Alan M Fudge. Adv. contact Michael Goldberg. B&W page USD 680, color page USD 1,655; trim 10 x 7. Circ: 1,530. **Subscr. to:** Periodicals Fulfillment, W B Saunders Co, 6277 Sea Harbor Dr, 4th Fl, Orlando, FL 32891-4800.

636.089 CHN ISSN 1000-7725
SHANGHAI XUMU SHOUYI TONGXUN/SHANGHAI BULLETIN OF VETERINARY SCIENCE. Text in Chinese. 1956. bi-m. CNY 4.80. adv. bk.rev.
Published by: Shanghai Nongye Kexueyuan, Xumu Shouyi Yanjiusuo/Shanghai Academy of Agricultural Science, Institute of Veterinary Science, 2451 Xietu Lu, Shanghai 200030, China. TEL 4383161. Ed. Liu Ruisan.

636.089 JPN ISSN 0912-2494
SHODOBUTSU HIFUKA RINSHO/JAPANESE JOURNAL OF SMALL ANIMAL DERMATOLOGY. Text in English, Japanese. 1973. irreg.
Published by: Shodobutsu Hifuka Kenkyukai/Japanese Society for Small Animal Dermatology, c/o Daigaku Nogakubu Kachiku, Naikagaku Kyoshitsu, 1-1 Yayoi 1-Chome, Bunkyo-ku, Tokyo 113-0032, Japan.

SINGAPORE JOURNAL OF PRIMARY INDUSTRIES. see *AGRICULTURE*

636.089 SVN ISSN 1580-4003
SLOVENIAN VETERINARY RESEARCH/SLOVENSKI VETERINARSKI ZBORNIK. Text in Slovenian, English. 1960. q., latest vol.38, 2001. SIT 6,000 domestic; USD 37 foreign (effective 2001). back issues avail. **Document type:** *Journal, Academic/Scholarly.* **Description:** Publishes scientific papers, review articles, professional papers, summaries of thesis, and other items such as critical reviews of articles published in research reports, letters to the editors and such others.
Former titles (until 2000): University of Ljubljana. Veterinary Faculty. Research Reports (1408-8495); Univerza v Ljubljani. Veterinarska Fakulteta. Zbornik (0353-8044); (until 1990): Univerza E. Kardelja v Ljubljani. Biotehniska Fakulteta. Zbornik. Veterinarstvo (0300-0362)
Indexed: Biol.Abstr., Hort.Abstr., Ind.Vet., Maize Abstr., Nutr.Abstr., Pig News & Info., Poult.Abstr., Rev.Med.& Vet.Mycol., Seed Abstr., Soyabean Abstr., Sport Fish.Abstr., Triticale Abstr., Vet.Bull., Weed Abstr., Wild.Rev., Zoo.Rec.
—BLDSC (8309.635000).
Published by: Univerza v Ljubljani, Veterinarska Fakulteta/University of Ljubljana, Veterinary Faculty, Gerbiceva 60, Ljubljana 1000, Slovenia. TEL 386-61-1779100, FAX 386-61-2832243, http://www.vf.uni-lj.si. Ed., R&P Srdan V Bavdek TEL 386-61-1779129. Adv. contact Matjaz Ursic. Circ: 500.

SMALL RUMINANT RESEARCH. see *AGRICULTURE—Poultry And Livestock*

636.089 FRA ISSN 1620-8706
SOCIETE VETERINAIRE PRACTIQUE DE FRANCE. BULLETIN BIMESTRIEL. Text in French. 1881. bi-m. FRF 190 domestic; FRF 210 foreign (effective 2000).
Former titles (unitl 1999): Societe Veterinaire Pratique de France. Bulletin Mensuel (0395-7500); (until 1924): Societe de Medecine Veterinaire Pratique. Bulletin Mensuel (1268-7022); (until 1903): Societe de Medecine Veterinaire Pratique. Bulletin (1268-7014)
Indexed: Abstr.Hyg., Anim.Breed.Abstr., Ind.Vet., Protozool.Abstr., Rev.Med.& Vet.Mycol., Vet.Bull.
—BLDSC (2924.948600).
Published by: Societe Veterinaire Pratique de France, 10 Placee Leon Blum, Paris 75011, France.

SODOBNO KMETIJSTVO. see *AGRICULTURE*

SOUTH AFRICAN JOURNAL OF ANIMAL SCIENCE. see *AGRICULTURE—Poultry And Livestock*

636.089 ZAF
CODEN: JAVTAP
SOUTH AFRICAN VETERINARY ASSOCIATION. SCIENTIFIC JOURNAL. Text in English. 1929. q. USD 357 (effective 1998). adv. bk.rev. abstr, charts, illus. index. back issues avail. *Refereed.* **Document type:** *Academic/Scholarly.*
Former titles: South African Veterinary Association. Journal (1019-9128); (until 1972): South African Veterinary Medical Association. Journal (0038-2809)
Related titles: Online - full text ed.: (from Institute for Scientific Information).

Indexed: ASCA, AgBiotech, Agri.& Environ.Biotech.Abstr. (coverage dropped), Agroforest.Abstr., Anim.Breed.Abstr., Bio-Contr.News & Info., Chem.Abstr., Chem.Indus.Notes, Chem.Titles, Curr.Adv.Ecol.Sci., Curr.Cont., Dairy Sci.Abstr., Dent.Ind., Derwent Biotech.Abstr., Excerp.Med., Field Crop Abstr., Focus on: Vet.Sci.& Med., Forest.Abstr., Helminthol.Abstr., Herb.Abstr., INIS Atomind., Ind.Med. (coverage dropped), Ind.S.A.Per., Ind.Vet., Nutr.Abstr., Pig News & Info., Poult.Abstr., Protozool.Abstr., Ref.Zh., Rev.Appl.Entomol., Rev.Arom.& Med.Plants, Rev.Med.& Vet.Mycol., Small Anim.Abstr., Sport Fish.Abstr., Vet.Bull., Weed Abstr., Wild.Rev., World Ag.Econ.& Rur.Soc.Abstr., Zoo.Rec.
—BLDSC (4901.950000), CASDDS, CISTI, GNLM, IDS, Infotrieve, ingenta. **CCC.**
Published by: South African Veterinary Association, Monument Park, PO Box 25033, Pretoria 0105, South Africa. TEL 27-12-3461150, FAX 27-12-3462929. Ed. Dr. M Penrith. Adv. contact K S Harpur. Circ: 1,600.

636.089 LKA
SRI LANKA VETERINARY JOURNAL. Text in English. 1953. s-a. USD 10. adv. bk.rev. abstr, charts, illus. index.
Formerly (until 1982): Ceylon Veterinary Journal (0009-0891)
Indexed: Anim.Breed.Abstr., Biol.Abstr., Chem.Abstr., Dairy Sci.Abstr., Field Crop Abstr., Helminthol.Abstr., Herb.Abstr., Ind.Vet., Nutr.Abstr., Pig News & Info., Poult.Abstr., Protozool.Abstr., Rev.Appl.Entomol., Small Anim.Abstr., Soils & Fert., Sri Lanka Sci.Ind., Vet.Bull.
—CISTI, Linda Hall.
Published by: Veterinary Research Institute, Peradeniya, Sri Lanka. Ed. S T Fernando. Circ: 1,000.

636.08 ROM ISSN 1224-7685
STUDIES AND RESEARCHES IN VETERINARY MEDICINE. Text in English. 1992. a. free per issue or exchange basis. *Refereed.* **Document type:** *Academic/Scholarly.* **Description:** Covers bacteriology, virology, immunology, morphopathology, toxicology, parasitology, metabolic and nutritional diseases, molecular biology, biotechnology, and pharmacology.
Indexed: Anim.Breed.Abstr., Ind.Vet., Pig News & Info., Poult.Abstr., Protozool.Abstr., Rev.Med.& Vet.Mycol., Vet.Bull.
—BLDSC.
Published by: Pasteur National Institute of Veterinary Medicine, Str. Giulesti 333, Bucharest 77826, Romania. TEL 40-1-2206920, FAX 40-1-2206915. Ed. Dr. Marius Pirvulescu. Circ: 150.

636.089 ITA
SUMMA (MILAN); mensile di formazione permanente per il medico veterinario. Text in Italian. 10/yr. ITL 115,000; ITL 95,000 to students.
Indexed: Helminthol.Abstr., Nutr.Abstr., Poult.Abstr., Protozool.Abstr.
—BLDSC.
Published by: Point Veterinaire Italie s.r.l, Via Francesco Melzi D'Eril, 26, Milan, MI 20154, Italy. TEL 39-2-336035, FAX 39-2-33606655. Ed. Dr. J P Dagneauz.

636.089 FIN ISSN 0039-5501
SUOMEN ELAINLAAKARILEHTI/FINSK VETERINAERTIDSKRIFT. Text in Finnish, Swedish; Summaries in English. 1893. m. FIM 450. adv. bk.rev. bibl, charts, illus. **Document type:** *Academic/Scholarly.*
Indexed: Abstr.Hyg., AgBiotech, Anim.Breed.Abstr., Apic.Abstr., Biol.Abstr., Dairy Sci.Abstr., Food Sci.& Tech.Abstr., Helminthol.Abstr., Ind.Vet., Nutr.Abstr., Pig News & Info., Poult.Abstr., Protozool.Abstr., Rev.Appl.Entomol., Rev.Med.& Vet.Mycol., Small Anim.Abstr., Vet.Bull.
—BLDSC (8541.800000).
Published by: Suomen Elainlaakariliitto/Finnish Veterinary Association, Maekelaenkatu 2 C, Helsinki 00500, Finland. pirkko.nousiainen@sell.fi. Ed. Marjut Hamalainen. Adv. contact Pirkko Nousiainen. Circ: 2,100.

636.089 SWE ISSN 0346-2250
SVENSK VETERINAERTIDNING. Text in Swedish. 1896. 15/yr. SEK 765 in Europe; SEK 1,090 elsewhere; SEK 50 newsstand/cover. adv. bk.rev. Supplement avail. *Refereed.* **Document type:** *Magazine, Trade.* **Description:** Articles of interest to veterinarians and news about the association.
Former titles (until 1964): Medlemsblad foer Sveriges Veterinaerfoerbund; (until 1950): Svenska Veterinaerlaekarefoereningens Medlemsblad
Indexed: Agri.Eng.Abstr., Anim.Breed.Abstr., Bio-Contr.News & Info., Dairy Sci.Abstr., Food Sci.& Tech.Abstr., Helminthol.Abstr., INIS Atomind., Ind.Vet., Nutr.Abstr., Pig News & Info., Poult.Abstr., Protozool.Abstr., Ref.Zh., Rev.Appl.Entomol., Rev.Med.& Vet.Mycol., Soyabean Abstr., Vet.Bull., World Ag.Econ.& Rur.Soc.Abstr.
—BLDSC (8562.598000).
Published by: Sveriges Veterinaerfoerbund/Swedish Veterinary Association, Box 12709, Stockholm 11294, Sweden. TEL 46-8-654-24-80, FAX 46-8-651-70-82, office@svf.se, http://www.svf.se/huvudram/frm3.html, http://www.svf.se/frame/frm3.html. Ed., Pub. Johan Beck-Friis. Adv. contact Birgitta Ahlkvist. B&W page SEK 7,850, color page SEK 13,850; trim 176 x 257. Circ: 2,700 (controlled).

636.089 USA
SWINE PRACTITIONER. Text in English. 1988. 8/yr. USD 25 domestic; USD 50 foreign (effective 2001). illus. **Document type:** *Trade.* **Description:** Serves veterinarians working with swine herds.
Indexed: Dairy Sci.Abstr., Ind.Vet., Nutr.Abstr., Pig News & Info., Rev.Appl.Entomol.
—BLDSC.
Published by: Vance Publishing Corporation (Lenexa), Livestock Division, 10901 W. 84th Terr., Ste. 200, Lenexa, KS 66210-1821. TEL 913-438-8700, FAX 913-438-0695. Ed. Jim Carlton. Pub. Bill Newham. Circ: 4,000 (controlled).

636.089 USA ISSN 1071-0566
TEXAS VETERINARIAN. Text in English. 1939. bi-m. USD 50 to individuals; USD 30 to institutions. adv. bk.rev. charts, illus, stat. **Document type:** *Trade.*
Formerly (until Apr. 1993): Texas Veterinary Medical Journal (0040-4756)
Published by: Texas Veterinary Medical Association, 6633 Hwy, 290 E, 201, Austin, TX 78723-1134. TEL 512-452-4224, FAX 512-452-6633. Ed. Donald M Ward. Adv. contact Ellen Smith. Circ: 3,000.

636.089 USA ISSN 0093-691X
CODEN: THGNBO
THERIOGENOLOGY; an international journal of animal reproduction. Text in English. 1974. 18/yr. EUR 235 in Europe to individuals; JPY 31,200 in Japan to individuals; USD 263 elsewhere to individuals; EUR 874 in Europe to institutions; JPY 116,000 in Japan to institutions; USD 978 elsewhere to institutions (effective 2002). abstr. back issues avail. *Refereed.* **Document type:** *Academic/Scholarly.* **Description:** Serves as an international forum for researchers, clinicians, and industry professionals involved in animal reproduction biology.
Related titles: Microfiche ed.: (from PQC); Online - full text ed.: (from ingenta, Swets Blackwell, Institute for Scientific Information, ScienceDirect).
Indexed: ASCA, AgBiotech, Agricola, Anim.Breed.Abstr., Bibl.Agri., Bibl.Repro., Biol.Abstr., Chem.Abstr., Chem.Indus.Notes, Chem.Titles, Curr.Adv.Cell & Devel.Biol., Curr.Adv.Ecol.Sci., Curr.Adv.Gen.& Molec.Biol., Curr.Cont., Dairy Sci.Abstr., Derwent Biotech.Abstr., Focus on: Vet.Sci.& Med., Helminthol.Abstr., Ind.Med. (1974-), Ind.Sci.Rev., Ind.Vet., Inpharma, Int.Abstr.Biol.Sci., Nutr.Abstr., Pig News & Info., Poult.Abstr., Protozool.Abstr., Reac., Rev.Appl.Entomol., Rev.Med.& Vet.Mycol., Sci.Cit.Ind., Small Anim.Abstr., Soyabean Abstr., Sport Fish.Abstr., Sugar Ind.Abstr., Vet.Bull., Weed Abstr., Wild.Rev., Zoo.Rec.
—BLDSC (8814.773000), CASDDS, CISTI, EMDOCS, IDS, ingenta, Linda Hall. **CCC.**
Published by: Elsevier Science, 655 Ave of the Americas, New York, NY 10010. TEL 212-989-5800, FAX 212-633-3990, http://www.elsevier.nl/inca/publications/store/5/2/5/0/2/4/. Eds. L F Archibald, Dr. Victor M Shille. **Subscr. in Australasia and the Far East to:** Elsevier Science (Singapore) Pte Ltd, No.1 Temasek Ave, 17-01 Millenia Tower, Singapore 039192, Singapore. TEL 65-434-3727, FAX 65-337-2230; **Subscr. in Japan to:** Elsevier Science Inc - Japan Regional Office, 9-15 Higashi-Azabu 1-chome, Minato-ku, Tokyo 106-0044, Japan. TEL 81-3-5561-5033; **Subscr. outside the Americas to:** Elsevier Science BV, PO Box 211, Amsterdam 1000 AE, Netherlands. TEL 31-20-485-3757, nlinfo-f@elsevier.nl.

636.089 DEU ISSN 1434-1220
TIERAERZTLICHE PRAXIS. AUSGABE G: GROSSTIERE - NUTZTIERE. Text in German. 1973. bi-m. DEM 174 to individuals; DEM 252 to institutions; DEM 116 to students (effective 2001). adv. **Document type:** *Journal, Academic/Scholarly.*
Supersedes in part (in 1997): Tieraerztliche Praxis (0303-6286)
Related titles: Online - full text ed.: (from Institute for Scientific Information).
Indexed: Anim.Breed.Abstr., Dairy Sci.Abstr., Derwent Biotech.Abstr., Focus on: Vet.Sci.& Med., GeoRef, Ind.Med. (until 1999, dropped), Ind.Vet., Maize Abstr., Nutr.Abstr., Pig News & Info., Poult.Abstr., Rev.Med.& Vet.Mycol., Triticale Abstr., Vet.Bull., Weed Abstr.
—BLDSC (8831.820000), GNLM, IDS, Infotrieve. **CCC.**
Published by: Schattauer GmbH, Hoelderlinstr 3, Stuttgart 70174, Germany. TEL 49-711-22987-0, FAX 49-711-2298775, info@schattauer.de, http://www.schattauer.com. Ed. Hartwig Bostedt. Pub. Dieter Bergemann. R&P Annika Schmidt TEL 49-711-2298713. Adv. contact Claudia Hartmann TEL 49-711-2298727. B&W page DEM 2,359, color page DEM 3,429; trim 176 x 240. Circ: 3,500 (controlled). **Subscr. to:** CSJ, Postfach 140220, Munich 80452, Germany. TEL 49-89-20959129, schattauer@csj.de.

636.089 DEU ISSN 1434-1239
CODEN: TAZPB8
TIERAERZTLICHE PRAXIS. AUSGABE K: KLEINTIERE - HEIMTIERE. Text in German. 1973. 6/yr. DEM 284 to individuals; DEM 460 to institutions; DEM 116 to students (effective 2001). adv. *Refereed.* **Document type:** *Journal, Academic/Scholarly.*
Supersedes in part (in 1997): Tieraerztliche Praxis (0303-6286)
Related titles: Online - full text ed.: (from Institute for Scientific Information).
Indexed: ASCA, Anim.Breed.Abstr., Derwent Biotech.Abstr., Focus on: Vet.Sci.& Med., Ind.Med. (until 1999, dropped), Ind.Vet., Key Word Ind.Wildl.Res., Nutr.Abstr., Poult.Abstr., Protozool.Abstr., Rev.Appl.Entomol., Rev.Med.& Vet.Mycol., Small Anim.Abstr., Vet.Bull., Zoo.Rec.
—BLDSC (8831.821000), GNLM, IDS, Infotrieve. **CCC.**
Published by: Schattauer GmbH, Hoelderlinstr 3, Stuttgart 70174, Germany. TEL 49-711-22987-0, FAX 49-711-2298750, info@schattauer.de, http://www.schattauer.com. Ed. Wilfried Kraft. Pub. Dieter Bergemann. R&Ps Annika Schmidt TEL 49-711-2298713, Hannelore Hensen. Adv. contact Claudia Hartmann TEL 49-711-2298727. B&W page DEM 2,354, color page DEM 3,429; 176 x 240. Circ: 4,500 (controlled). **Subscr. to:** CSJ, Postfach 140220, Munich 80452, Germany. TEL 49-89-20959129, schattauer@csj.de.

636.089 DEU ISSN 0049-3864
CODEN: MVMZA8
TIERAERZTLICHE UMSCHAU; Zeitschrift fuer alle Gebiete der Veterinaermedizin. Text in German. 1946. m. EUR 89 (effective 2002). adv. bk.rev. abstr. *Refereed.* **Document type:** *Magazine, Trade.*
Incorporates (1946-1994): Monatshefte fuer Veterinaermedizin (0026-9263)
Related titles: Online - full text ed.: (from Institute for Scientific Information).
Indexed: ASCA, Abstr.Hyg., AgBiotech, Agri.& Environ.Biotech.Abstr. (coverage dropped), Agri.Eng.Abstr., Anim.Breed.Abstr., Apic.Abstr., Aqua.Sci.& Fish.Abstr., Aquacult.Abstr., Biol.Abstr., Chem.Abstr., Curr.Adv.Ecol.Sci., Curr.Cont., Dairy Sci.Abstr., Derwent Biotech.Abstr., Environ.Sci.Poll.Mgmt., Focus on: Vet.Sci.& Med., Food Sci.& Tech.Abstr., Helminthol.Abstr., INIS Atomind., Ind.Vet., Key Word Ind.Wildl.Res., Nutr.Abstr., Pig News & Info., Poult.Abstr., Protozool.Abstr., Rev.Appl.Entomol., Rev.Med.& Vet.Mycol., Rev.Plant Path., Sci.Cit.Ind., Small Anim.Abstr., Soils & Fert., Vet.Bull., Wild.Rev., Zoo.Rec.
—BLDSC (8832.000000), CASDDS, GNLM, IDS, Infotrieve, Linda Hall. **CCC.**
Published by: Terra Verlag GmbH, Neuhauser Str 21, Postfach 1222, Konstanz 78464, West Germany. TEL 49-7531-812222, FAX 49-7531-812299, http://www.terra-verlag.de. Ed. O C Straub. Circ: 7,500.

636.08 DEU ISSN 0720-2237
TIERARZTLICHE-HOCHSCHULE-ANZEIGER. Key Title: TiHo-Anzeiger. Text in German. 1972. 8/yr. DEM 32 (effective 2001). adv. bk.rev., Website rev. 16 p./no. 3 cols./p. back issues avail. **Document type:** *Newspaper, Academic/Scholarly.*
Related titles: Online - full text ed.
Published by: Tieraerztliche Hochschule Hannover, Buenteweg 2, Hannover 30559, Germany. TEL 49-511-9538002, FAX 49-511-953828002, http://www.tiho-hannover.de/presse/anzeiger/index.htm. Ed., R&P Judith McAlister-Hermann. Adv. contact Birgit Bohn TEL 49-511-85502222.

636.08 DEU ISSN 0947-0956
TIERARZTLICHE HOCHSCHULE-FORSCHUNG FUERS LEBEN. Key Title: TiHo-Forschung fuers Leben. Text in German. 1994. a. DEM 8 (effective 2000). **Document type:** *Academic/Scholarly.*

V

Published by: Tieraerztliche Hochschule Hannover, Buenteweg 2, Hannover 30559, Germany. TEL 49-511-9538002, FAX 49-511-953828002, awegner@vw.tiho-hannover.de, http://www.tiho-hannover.de. Ed. Dr. Annette Wegner.

636.089 NLD ISSN 0040-7453
CODEN: TIDIAY

TIJDSCHRIFT VOOR DIERGENEESKUNDE/ NETHERLANDS JOURNAL OF VETERINARY SCIENCE. Text in Dutch; Summaries in Dutch, English. 1863. 24/yr. NLG 295 domestic; NLG 315 foreign (effective 2000). adv. bk.rev. abstr, bibl, charts, illus. index. *Refereed.* **Document type:** *Academic/Scholarly.*
Related titles: Online - full text ed.: (from Institute for Scientific Information).
Indexed: ASCA, Abstr.Hyg., Agri.Eng.Abstr., Anim.Breed.Abstr., Bibl.Agri., Biol.Abstr., Chem.Abstr., Curr.Adv.Cancer Res., Curr.Adv.Ecol.Sci., Curr.Cont., Dairy Sci.Abstr., Derwent Biotech.Abstr., Focus on: Vet.Sci.& Med., Food Sci.& Tech.Abstr., Helminthol.Abstr., INIS Atomind., Ind.Med. (1916-), Ind.Vet., Nutr.Abstr., Pig News & Info., Poult.Abstr., Protozool.Abstr., Rev.Appl.Entomol., Rev.Med.& Vet.Mycol., Rev.Plant Path., Rural Recreat.Tour.Abstr., SSCI (coverage dropped), Small Anim.Abstr., Sport Fish.Abstr., Trop.Dis.Bull., Vet.Bull., Wild.Rev., World Ag.Econ.& Rur.Soc.Abstr., Zoo.Rec.
—BLDSC (8838.000000), CASDDS, CISTI, GNLM, IDS, KNAW.
Published by: Koninklijke Nederlandse Maatschappij voor Diergeneeskunde/Royal Netherlands Veterinary Association, Julianalaan 10, Postbus 14031, Utrecht 3508 SB, Netherlands. TEL 31-30-2510111, FAX 31-30-2519847, tijdschrift@knmud.nl, tijdschrift@knmvd.nl. Ed. W Edel. R&P, Adv. contact S H Umans. B&W page NLG 1,825; 297 x 210. Circ: 5,200.

636.089 USA ISSN 1064-5101

TOPICS IN VETERINARY MEDICINE. Text in English. 1926. 3/yr. free per issue to qualified personnel. adv. **Document type:** *Consumer.* **Description:** Includes product development and application articles, company news, and educational articles on diseases and disease syndromes.
Formerly (until 1990): Norden News (0890-3727)
Indexed: Ind.Vet., Sport Fish.Abstr., Vet.Bull., Wild.Rev.
—Linda Hall.
Published by: Pfizer Animal Health, 812 Springdale Dr, Exton, PA 19341-2803. TEL 610-363-3100, FAX 610-968-5771, etchik00@pfizer.com, http://www.pfizer.com/ah. Ed. Kathleen M Etchison. R&P Kathleen Etchison TEL 610-363-3771. Circ: 55,000.

TRENDS IN PARASITOLOGY. see *BIOLOGY—Microbiology*

636.089 USA ISSN 1062-8266

TRENDS MAGAZINE. Text in English. 1985. bi-m. USD 60 domestic; USD 70 foreign (effective 2000). adv. **Document type:** *Trade.*
Published by: American Animal Hospital Association, PO Box 150899, Denver, CO 80215-0899. TEL 303-986-2800, FAX 303-986-1700. Ed. Kristin Stark. R&P Loraine Miller. Adv. contact Stephanie Pates. Circ: 14,200.

636.089 NLD ISSN 0049-4747
SF601 CODEN: TAHPAJ

TROPICAL ANIMAL HEALTH AND PRODUCTION. Text in Dutch. 1969. bi-m. EUR 440 to institutions for print or online ed.; EUR 528 to institutions print & online eds.combined (effective 2002). adv. bk.rev. charts, illus, stat. back issues avail. *Refereed.* **Description:** Publishes research, investigation, and observation in all fields of animal health and production that may lead to improved health and productivity of livestock, as well as better use of animal resources in developing nations.
Related titles: Online - full text ed.: (from EBSCO Publishing, O C L C Online Computer Library Center, Inc., RoweCom Information Quest, Swets Blackwell, Kluwer Online, Institute for Scientific Information).
Indexed: ASCA, Abstr.Hyg., AgBiotech, Agri.& Environ.Biotech.Abstr. (coverage dropped), Agricola, Agroforest.Abstr., Anim.Breed.Abstr., Bibl.Agri., Bio-Contr.News & Info., Biol.Abstr., Chem.Abstr., Curr.Adv.Ecol.Sci., Curr.Cont., Dairy Sci.Abstr., Derwent Biotech.Abstr., Excerp.Med., Field Crop Abstr., Focus on: Vet.Sci.& Med., Food Sci.& Tech.Abstr., Helminthol.Abstr., Herb.Abstr., Ind.Med. (1969-), Ind.Vet., Maize Abstr., Nutr.Abstr., Poult.Abstr., Protozool.Abstr., Rev.Appl.Entomol., Rev.Med.& Vet.Mycol., Rice Abstr., Sci.Cit.Ind., Small Anim.Abstr., So.Pac.Per.Ind., Sugar Ind.Abstr., Trop.Dis.Bull., Vet.Bull., Wild.Rev., World Ag.Econ.& Rur.Soc.Abstr.
—BLDSC (9054.300000), CASDDS, CISTI, GNLM, IDS, Infotrieve, ingenta. **CCC.**
Published by: Kluwer Academic Publishers Group (Subsidiary of: Wolters Kluwer N.V.), Spuiboulevard 50, PO Box 17, Dordrecht 3300 AA, Netherlands. FAX 31-78-939-2254, 31-78-639-2254, services@wkap.nl, http://www.wkap.nl/journalhome.htm/0049-4747. Ed. M M H Sewell. Pub. Vivian C Bone. Adv. contact Kathryn MacLean. Circ: 500. **Dist. by:** Journals Department, PO Box 322, Dordrecht 3300 AH, Netherlands. TEL 781-871-6600, FAX 31-78-654-6474.

636.089 NGA ISSN 0794-4845
CODEN: TRVTDJ

TROPICAL VETERINARIAN. Text in English. 1983. q., latest vol.19. NGN 1,000 domestic to individuals; USD 80 foreign to individuals; NGN 5,000, USD 120 domestic to institutions (effective 2001). adv. 75 p./no. back issues avail. *Refereed.* **Document type:** *Journal, Academic/Scholarly.* **Description:** Publishes research articles devoted to all aspects of health and disease of animals in the tropics.
Indexed: Curr.Cont. (coverage dropped), Ind.Vet., Pig News & Info., Poult.Abstr., Protozool.Abstr., Sport Fish.Abstr., Wild.Rev., Zoo.Rec.
Published by: University of Ibadan, Faculty of Veterinary Medicine, Editors, Ibadan, Oyo State, Nigeria. TEL 234-2-810-3043, tropivet@skannet.com, library@kdl.ui.edu.ng, dean.vetmedicine@vi.edu.org. Ed. Helen Nottidge. Adv. contact Dr. M O Abatan. page NGN 5,000.

636 TUR ISSN 1300-0128
SF604 CODEN: TVHAEN

TURK VETERINERLIK VE HAYVANCILIK DERGISI/TURKISH JOURNAL OF VETERINARY AND ANIMAL SCIENCES. Text in English, Turkish. 1976. bi-m. USD 150 (effective 1999). *Refereed.* **Document type:** *Journal, Academic/Scholarly.*
Former titles (until 1994): Doga Turkish Journal of Veterinary and Animal Sciences - Doga Turk Veterinerlik ve Hayvancilik Dergisi (1010-7592); Formerly: Doga Bilim Dergisi. Series D: Veterinary and Animal Sciences
Related titles: Online - full text ed.: (from Institute for Scientific Information).
Indexed: ASCA, AgBiotech, Agri.Eng.Abstr., Anim.Breed.Abstr., Biol.Abstr., Chem.Abstr., Dairy Sci.Abstr., Focus on: Vet.Sci.& Med., Food Sci.& Tech.Abstr., Helminthol.Abstr., INIS Atomind., Ind.Vet., Maize Abstr., Nutr.Abstr., Postharvest, Poult.Abstr., Protozool.Abstr., Rev.Appl.Entomol., Rev.Med.& Vet.Mycol., Soyabean Abstr., Triticale Abstr., Vet.Bull., Weed Abstr.
—BLDSC (9072.497000), CASDDS, IDS.
Published by: Scientific and Technical Research Council of Turkey - TUBITAK/Turkiye Bilimsel ve Teknik Arastirma Kurumu, Ataturk Bulvari No. 221, Kavaklidere, Ankara 06100, Turkey. TEL 90-312-468-5300, FAX 90-312-426-8073, bdym@tubitak.gov.tr, http://www.tubitak.gov.tr/journals/veterinary/. Ed. Sevinc Turker.

636.089 USA

U.S. DEPARTMENT OF AGRICULTURE. ANIMAL AND PLANT HEALTH INSPECTION SERVICE. REPORTED ARTHROPOD-BORNE ENCEPHALITIDES IN HORSES AND OTHER EQUIDAE✱ . Text in English. 1966. a. free per issue. illus, stat.
Indexed: Bibl.Agri.
Published by: U.S. Animal and Plant Health Inspection Service, U S Department of Agriculture Health Inspection Service, 4700 River Rd, Riverdale, MD 20737-1228. TEL 301-734-5240.

636.089 USA ISSN 0082-8750
SF601

UNITED STATES ANIMAL HEALTH ASSOCIATION. PROCEEDINGS OF THE ANNUAL MEETING. Text in English. 1969 (no.73). a. USD 30. back issues avail. **Document type:** *Proceedings.*
Supersedes: United States Livestock Sanitary Association. Proceedings
Indexed: Ind.Med. (coverage dropped), Ind.Vet., Pig News & Info., Poult.Abstr., Rev.Appl.Entomol., Vet.Bull., Zoo.Rec.
—BLDSC (6841.958000).
Published by: United States Animal Health Association, 8100 Three Chopt Rd, Ste 203, Box K227, Richmond, VA 23288-0001. TEL 804-285-3210, FAX 804-285-3367. Circ: 1,400.

636.089 VEN ISSN 0258-6576

UNIVERSIDAD CENTRAL DE VENEZUELA. FACULTAD DE CIENCIAS VETERINARIAS. REVISTA. Text in Spanish; Summaries in English, Spanish. 1939-1992; resumed 1998. 4/yr. free per issue to qualified personnel.
Formerly: Revista de Medicina Veterinaria y Parasitologia (0048-7724)
Indexed: Biol.Abstr., Chem.Abstr., Ind.Vet., Protozool.Abstr., Rev.Appl.Entomol., Vet.Bull.
—CISTI, Linda Hall.
Published by: Universidad Central de Venezuela, Facultad de Ciencias Veterinarias, Apdo. de Correos 4563, Maracay, Edo. Aragua, Venezuela. revisfcv@camelot.rect.ucv.ve, http://bibliovet.veter.ucv.ve/Revistafcv/index.htm. Eds. Donatella Tamburini, Harry Almela. Circ: 1,800.

636.089 GTM ISSN 0375-0884

UNIVERSIDAD DE SAN CARLOS DE GUATEMALA. FACULTAD DE MEDICINA VETERINARIA Y ZOOTECNIA REVISTA. Text in Spanish; Summaries in English, Spanish. 1962. irreg. per issue exchange basis.
Indexed: Biol.Abstr.
Published by: Universidad de San Carlos de Guatemala, Facultad de Medicina, Veterinaria y Zootecnia, Ciudad Universitaria, Zona 12, Edificio de Rectoria, Of 307, Guatemala City, Guatemala. TEL 502-760790.

636.089 VEN ISSN 0798-2259

UNIVERSIDAD DE ZULIA. FACULTAD DE CIENCIAS VETERINARIAS. REVISTA CIENTIFICA. (Includes off-prints) Text in Spanish; Abstracts in English, Spanish. 1990. q. VEB 8,000, USD 40 (effective 2000). bk.rev. bibl, charts, illus. *Refereed.* **Document type:** *Academic/Scholarly.* **Description:** Contains scientific papers and reviews in veterinary science.
Related titles: Online - full text ed.: (from Institute for Scientific Information).
Indexed: Abstr.Hyg., AgBiotech, Anim.Breed.Abstr., Dairy Sci.Abstr., Focus on: Vet.Sci.& Med., Herb.Abstr., Ind.Vet., Maize Abstr., Nutr.Abstr., Pig News & Info., Poult.Abstr., Protozool.Abstr., Rev.Appl.Entomol., Rev.Arom.& Med.Plants, Rev.Med.& Vet.Mycol., Sci.Cit.Ind. (coverage dropped), Seed Abstr., Soyabean Abstr., Triticale Abstr., Trop.Dis.Bull., Vet.Bull., Wild.Rev., World Ag.Econ.& Rur.Soc.Abstr.
—BLDSC (7851.137000), IDS.
Published by: Universidad del Zulia, Facultad de Ciencias Veterinarias, Apdo. 15252,, C.C. Galerias 1er Nivel, Local 45-E, Maracaibo, Zulia 4005-A, Venezuela. TEL 58-61-596158, FAX 58-61-425176, raromero@telcel.net.ve, revistacientific@cantv.net. Ed. Dr. Osiris Castejon Sandoval. Circ: 1,000 (paid).

636.089 ITA ISSN 0365-4729
SF604 CODEN: AMVPAW

UNIVERSITA DEGLI STUDI DI PISA. FACOLTA DI MEDICINA VETERINARIA DI PISA. ANNALI. Key Title: Annali della Facolta di Medicina Veterinaria di Pisa. Text in Italian. 1947. a. per issue exchange basis only. **Document type:** *Academic/Scholarly.* **Description:** Publishes original research articles in areas of veterinary medicine and animal production. Reports on faculty members.
Indexed: Dairy Sci.Abstr., Ind.Vet., Poult.Abstr., Rev.Appl.Entomol., Sport Fish.Abstr., Wild.Rev., Zoo.Rec.
—BLDSC (1006.300000), CASDDS, Linda Hall.
Published by: Universita degli Studi di Pisa, Biblioteca di Medicina Veterinaria di Pisa, Viale delle Piagge 2, Pisa, PI 56100, Italy. TEL 39-50-570270, FAX 39-50-581107, fazi@vet.unipi.it. Ed. Tito Livio Frateschi.

UNIVERSITATEA AGRONOMICA ION IONESCU DE LA BRAD. LUCRARI STIINTIFICE. SERIA ZOOTECHNIE - MEDICINA VETERINARIA. see *AGRICULTURE—Poultry And Livestock*

UNIVERSITATEA DE STIINTE AGRICOLE CLUJ-NAPOCA. BULETINUL. SERIA ZOOTEHNIE SI MEDICINA VETERINARA. see *AGRICULTURE—Poultry And Livestock*

636.08 ROM

UNIVERSITATEA DE STIINTE AGRONOMICE SI MEDICINA VETERINARA. LUCRARI STIINTIFICE. SERIA C, MEDICINA VETERINARA. Text in Romanian; Summaries in English. 1960. a. per issue exchange basis only. **Document type:** *Academic/Scholarly.*
Former titles: Universitatea de Stiinte Agronomice. Lucrari Stiintifice. Seria C, Medicina Veterinara; (until 1992): Institutul Agronomic Nicolae Balcescu. Lucrari Stiintifice. Seria C, Medicina Veterinara (0254-0509); Which superseded in part (in 1970): Institutul Agronomic Nicolae Balcescu. Lucrari Stiintifice. Seria C, Zootehnie si Medicina Veterinara (0524-8108); Which superseded in part: Institutul Agronomic Nicolae Balcescu. Anuarul Lucrarilor Stiintifice (1220-1987)
Indexed: Food Sci.& Tech.Abstr., Poult.Abstr., Protozool.Abstr., Rev.Appl.Entomol.
—CISTI.

Published by: Universitatea de Stiinte Agronomice si Medicina Veterinara, B-dul. Marasti 59, Sector 1, Bucharest 71331, Romania.

636 CAN ISSN 0383-8455
UNIVERSITE DE MONTREAL. FACULTE DE MEDECINE VETERINAIRE. ANNUAIRE. Text in English. 1968. a. free per issue. **Document type:** *Academic/Scholarly.*
Formerly: Ecole de Medecine Veterinaire, Saint-Hyacinthe, Quebec. Annuaire (0383-8447)
Published by: Universite de Montreal, Faculte de Medecine Veterinaire, C P 6128, succ A, Montreal, PQ H3C 3J7, Canada. TEL 514-343-6111, FAX 514-778-8114.

UNIVERSITY OF DAR ES SALAAM. FACULTY OF AGRICULTURE, FORESTRY AND VETERINARY SCIENCE. ANNUAL RECORD OF RESEARCH. see *AGRICULTURE*

636 USA ISSN 0076-9711
UNIVERSITY OF MISSOURI AT COLUMBIA. VETERINARY MEDICAL DIAGNOSTIC LABORATORY. ANNUAL REPORT. Text in English. 1967. a. USD 5. **Document type:** *Corporate.*
Published by: University of Missouri at Columbia, Veterinary Medical Diagnostic Laboratory, PO Box 6023, Columbia, MO 65205. TEL 314-882-6811, FAX 314-882-1411. Ed. H S Gosser. Circ: 800.

VACCINE. see *MEDICAL SCIENCES—Allergology And Immunology*

636.089 AUT ISSN 1029-5321
VET JOURNAL; Fachjournal der Oesterreichische Tieraerztinnen und Tieraerzte. Text in German. 1949. m. ATS 400 domestic; ATS 450 foreign (effective 2000). adv. bk.rev. **Document type:** *Magazine, Trade.*
Formerly (until 1995): Oesterreichische Tieraerztezeitung (0048-1475)
Indexed: Ind.Vet., Pig News & Info., Ref.Zh., Vet.Bull.
Published by: (Bundeskammer der Tieraerzte Oesterreichs), Vet Press, Franz-Jous-Str 19, Stockerau 2000, Austria. Eds. Johannes Weik, Dr. Richard Elhenicky. adv.: B&W page ATS 9,260, color page ATS 18,200; trim 170 x 242. Circ: 3,100.

636.08 GBR ISSN 1360-1962
VET ON-LINE. Variant title: The International Journal of Veterinary Medicne. Text in English. 1995. q. free per issue. bk.rev., software rev., video rev. *Refereed.* **Document type:** *Journal, Academic/Scholarly.*
Media: Online - full text.
Published by: Priory Lodge Education Ltd., 2 Cornflower Way, Moreton, Wirral CH46 1SV, United Kingdom. TEL 44-151-606-1796, FAX 44-151-606-1812, geoff@aldervet.demon.co.uk, solutions@priory.com, http://www.priory.com/journals/vet.htm. Ed. Dr. Stephen Baines. Circ: 35,000 (controlled).

636.08 DEU ISSN 0940-8711
VETERINAER SPIEGEL. Text in German. q. DEM 37.15, EUR 19 domestic; DEM 48.90, EUR 25 foreign (effective 2001). adv. **Document type:** *Journal, Trade.*
Published by: Beta Verlag und Marketinggesellschaft mbH, Postfach 140121, Bonn 53056, Germany. TEL 49-228-91937-0, FAX 49-228-252067, info@beta-publishing.com, http://www.veterinaerspiegel.de, http://www.beta-publishing.com. Ed. Thomas Steidl. R&P Heike Lange TEL 49-228-919370. Adv. contact Andreas Moll TEL 49-221-943691-0. Circ: 7,800.

636.089 BIH ISSN 0372-6827
CODEN: VTRNAE
VETERINARIA. Text in Serbo-Croatian; Summaries in English. 1951. q. USD 40. adv. bk.rev. index. back issues avail. **Document type:** *Academic/Scholarly.*
Description: Covers the field of animal production.
Indexed: Chem.Abstr., Chem.Indus.Notes, Food Sci.& Tech.Abstr., Ind.Vet., Maize Abstr., Pig News & Info., Rev.Med.& Vet.Mycol., Small Anim.Abstr., Sport Fish.Abstr., Vet.Bull., Wild.Rev., Zoo.Rec.
—CASDDS, CISTI, Linda Hall.
Published by: Savez Udruzenja Veterinara i Veterinarskih Tehnicara, V Putnika 134, Sarajevo 71000, Bosnia Herzegovina. TEL 071 655-922.

636.089 ARG ISSN 0326-4629
VETERINARIA ARGENTINA. Text in Spanish; Summaries in English. 1984. 10/yr. USD 66 in South America; USD 106 in Central America; USD 106 in North America; USD 116 in Europe; USD 130 elsewhere (effective 2001). adv. bk.rev. abstr, bibl, illus, pat. index, cum.index. back issues avail. *Refereed.* **Document type:** *Bulletin.*
Supersedes (1939-1984): Gaceta Veterinaria (0367-3812)
Indexed: Agri.Eng.Abstr., Anim.Breed.Abstr., Biol.Abstr., Chem.Abstr., Dairy Sci.Abstr., Helminthol.Abstr., Ind.Vet., Nutr.Abstr., Pig News & Info., Poult.Abstr., Protozool.Abstr., Rev.Appl.Entomol., Rev.Med.& Vet.Mycol., Rev.Plant Path., Small Anim.Abstr., Trop.Dis.Bull., Vet.Bull., Weed Abstr., Wild.Rev.
—BLDSC (9223.350000), CISTI, Linda Hall.
Published by: Veterinaria Argentina s.r.l., Viamonte, 494 2, Capital Federal, Buenos Aires 1053, Argentina. TEL 54-114-3119997, FAX 54-114-3119997, veterarg@elsitio.net, speroni@impsat1.com.ar. Eds. Norberto A Speroni, Dr. Emilio Morini. R&P, Adv. contact Norberto Speroni. B&W page USD 435; 210 x 150. Circ: 4,500.

636 BRA ISSN 0102-5716
CODEN: VEZOEO
VETERINARIA E ZOOTECNIA. Text in Portuguese; Summaries in English, Portuguese. 1985. a., latest vol.10, 1998. USD 30 (effective 2001); or exchange basis. abstr, bibl, charts. *Refereed.* **Document type:** *Journal, Academic/Scholarly.* **Description:** Original papers in veterinary medicine and zoological research.
Indexed: Anim.Breed.Abstr., Aqua.Sci.& Fish.Abstr., Aquacult.Abstr., Dairy Sci.Abstr., Environ.Sci.Poll.Mgmt., Helminthol.Abstr., INIS Atomind., Ind.Vet., Nutr.Abstr., Pollut.Abstr., Poult.Abstr., Rev.Appl.Entomol., Vet.Bull.
—CISTI.
Published by: Universidade Estadual Paulista, Ave. VICENTE FERREIRA, 1278, Centro, Caixa Postal 71, Marilia, SP 17515-901, Brazil. TEL 55-144-222504, FAX 55-144-222504, cgb@marilia.unesp.br. Ed. Sony Dimas Bicudo.

636.089 MEX
CODEN: VTERBU
VETERINARIA MEXICO. Text in Spanish; Summaries in English, Spanish. 1970. q. MXP 100, USD 50 (effective 2000). adv. bk.rev. charts, illus, stat. index. back issues avail. *Refereed.* **Document type:** *Academic/Scholarly.* **Description:** Publishes original research articles and clinical case reports in the general field of veterinary and animal science, with emphasis on local and national events.
Formerly (until 1975): Veterinaria (0301-5092)
Indexed: ASCA, AgBiotech, Anim.Breed.Abstr., Aqua.Sci.& Fish.Abstr., Aquacult.Abstr., Biol.Abstr., Chem.Abstr., Chem.Indus.Notes, Chem.Titles, Dairy Sci.Abstr., Derwent Biotech.Abstr., Environ.Sci.Poll.Mgmt., Focus on: Vet.Sci.& Med. (coverage dropped), Helminthol.Abstr., Herb.Abstr., Ind.Vet., Maize Abstr., Nutr.Abstr., Pig News & Info., Pollut.Abstr., Poult.Abstr., Protozool.Abstr., Rev.Appl.Entomol., Rev.Med.& Vet.Mycol., Rural Recreat.Tour.Abstr., SSCI (coverage dropped), Small Anim.Abstr., Sport Fish.Abstr., Sugar Ind.Abstr., Vet.Bull., Wild.Rev., World Ag.Econ.& Rur.Soc.Abstr., Zoo.Rec.
—BLDSC (9225.040000), CASDDS, CISTI, IDS.
Published by: Universidad Nacional Autonoma de Mexico, Facultad de Medicina Veterinaria y Zootecnia, Circuito Exterior, Ciudad Universitaria, Mexico 04510, Mexico. TEL 52-5-6225875, FAX 52-5-5508697, rmp@servidor.unam.mx, http://www.veterin.unam.mx. Ed. Raymundo Martinez Pena. Adv. contact Silvia M Gamboa Ponce. Circ: 1,500.

636.089 VEN ISSN 0379-8275
CODEN: VETRE3
VETERINARIA TROPICAL. Text in Spanish; Summaries in English, Spanish. 1976. a. VEB 40, USD 8; or exchange basis. bibl, charts, illus. *Refereed.* **Document type:** *Government.*
Formerly (until 1976): Instituto de Investigaciones Veterinarias. Boletin
Related titles: CD-ROM ed.
Indexed: Helminthol.Abstr., Ind.Vet., Pig News & Info., Poult.Abstr., Protozool.Abstr., Rev.Appl.Entomol., Vet.Bull., Wild.Rev.
Published by: Fondo Nacional de Investigaciones Agropecuarias, Apdo. 2103, Maracay 2105, Venezuela. FAX 58-43-836312. Ed. Aydee Cabrera de Green. Circ: 800.

636.08 AUS
THE VETERINARIAN. Text in English. m. (11/yr.). AUD 75 (effective 1999). adv. **Document type:** *Trade.*
Description: Covers politics, news, veterinary profiles, in-depth features, diagnostics, practice management, product information, continuing education, competitions and lifestyle information.
Indexed: Anim.Breed.Abstr.
Published by: Reed Business Information Pty. Ltd. (Subsidiary of: Reed Elsevier plc), Locked Bag 2999, Chatswood, NSW 2067, Australia. TEL 61-2-9422-2914, FAX 61-2-9422-2911, kathy.hutton@reedbusiness.com.au, http://www.reedbusiness.com.au/. Ed. Kathy Hutton. Pub. Fadia Matouk. Adv. contact Jasmin Cabaday. Circ: 3,927.

636.089 ITA
VETERINARIO D'ITALIA. Text in Italian. m.
Published by: Medici Veterinari Italiani di Medicina Pubblica, Via Del Tritone, 125, Rome, RM 00187, Italy. Ed. Roberto Cicala. Circ: 9,000.

636.089 CAN ISSN 0830-1743
VETERINARIUS. Text in French. 1984. 6/yr. USD 20. adv.
Indexed: Ind.Vet.
Published by: Ordre des Medecins Veterinaires du Quebec/Order of Veterinarians of Quebec, 800 ave Ste Anne, Ste 200, St Hyacinthe, PQ J2S 5G7, Canada. TEL 514-774-1427, FAX 514-774-7635. Ed. Dr. Louise Laliberte. Circ: 2,600.

636.089 RUS ISSN 0042-4846
CODEN: VETNAL
VETERINARIYA. Text in Russian. 1924. m. USD 127. bk.rev. bibl, illus. index. **Document type:** *Academic/Scholarly.*
Related titles: Microfiche ed.: (from EVP).
Indexed: Agri.& Environ.Biotech.Abstr. (coverage dropped), Agri.Eng.Abstr., Anim.Breed.Abstr., Apic.Abstr., Biol.Abstr., Chem.Abstr., Chem.Indus.Notes, Dairy Sci.Abstr., Derwent Biotech.Abstr., Food Sci.& Tech.Abstr., Helminthol.Abstr., Ind.Med. (coverage dropped), Ind.Vet., Maize Abstr., Nutr.Abstr., Pig News & Info., Poult.Abstr., Protozool.Abstr., Ref.Zh., Rev.Appl.Entomol., Rev.Med.& Vet.Mycol., Small Anim.Abstr., Soyabean Abstr., Triticale Abstr., Vet.Bull., Weed Abstr., Zoo.Rec.
—CASDDS, CISTI, East View, GNLM, Infotrieve. **CCC.**
Address: Sadovaya-Spasskaya 18, Moscow 107087, Russian Federation. TEL 7-095-2071060, FAX 7-095-2072870. Ed. Vladimir A Gar'kavtsev. Circ: 20,000. **Dist. by:** Mezhdunarodnaya Kniga, B Yakimanka 39, Moscow 117049, Russian Federation. TEL 7-095-2384967, FAX 7-095-2384634; **US dist. addr.:** East View Publications, 3020 Harbor Ln N, Minneapolis, MN 55447. TEL 612-550-0961.

636.089 BGR ISSN 1310-5825
VETERINARNA MEDITSINA/VETERINARY MEDICINE. Text in Bulgarian; Summaries in English. q. USD 92 foreign (effective 2002).
Published by: National Center for Agrarian Sciences, Tsarigradsko shosse Blvd. 125, bl. 1, entry 1, room 215, Sofia 1113, Bulgaria. **Dist. by:** Sofia Books, Ul Silivria 16, Sofia 1404, Bulgaria. TEL 359-2-9586257, sofiabooks@hotmail.com, http://www.sofiabooks.hit.bg.

636.089 RUS
VETERINARNAYA GAZETA. Text in Russian. s-m. **Document type:** *Academic/Scholarly.*
Published by: Izdatel'stvo Avto, Butyrskii val 24, Moscow 125047, Russian Federation. TEL 7-095-9783257, FAX 7-095-9782104. Ed. V A Simonyan. **US dist. addr.:** East View Publications, 3020 Harbor Ln N, Minneapolis, MN 55447. TEL 612-550-0961.

636 CZE ISSN 0375-8427
CODEN: VTMDAR
VETERINARNI MEDICINA. Variant title: Veterinary Medicine. Text and summaries in Czech, Slovak, English. 1956. m. USD 159 in Europe; USD 167 elsewhere (effective 2000). adv. bibl, charts, illus, stat. *Refereed.* **Document type:** *Academic/Scholarly.*
Related titles: Online - full text ed.: (from Institute for Scientific Information).
Indexed: ASCA, AgBiotech, Agri.Eng.Abstr., Anim.Breed.Abstr., Apic.Abstr., Biol.Abstr., Chem.Abstr., Chem.Indus.Notes, Chem.Titles, Curr.Adv.Ecol.Sci., Curr.Cont., Dairy Sci.Abstr., Derwent Biotech.Abstr., Excerp.Med., Field Crop Abstr., Focus on: Vet.Sci.& Med., Food Sci.& Tech.Abstr., Helminthol.Abstr., Herb.Abstr., INIS Atomind., Ind.Med. (coverage dropped), Ind.Sci.Rev., Ind.Vet., Maize Abstr., Nutr.Abstr., Pig News & Info., Poult.Abstr., Protozool.Abstr., Ref.Zh., Rev.Appl.Entomol., Rev.Med.& Vet.Mycol., Rev.Plant Path., Rice Abstr., Sci.Cit.Ind., Small Anim.Abstr., Triticale Abstr., Vet.Bull., Weed Abstr.
—BLDSC (9225.550000), CASDDS, CISTI, GNLM, IDS.

V

Published by: Ustav Zemedelskych a Potravinarskych Informaci/Institute of Agricultural and Food Information, Slezska 7, Prague, 2 120 56, Czech Republic. TEL 420-2-24257939, FAX 420-2-24253938, editor@uzpi.cz, http://www.vri.cz, http://www.uzpi.cz. Ed. Zdena Radosova. Circ: 450. **Co-sponsor:** Ceska Akademie Zemedelskych Ved.

636.089 HRV ISSN 0372-5480
CODEN: VEARA6

VETERINARSKI ARHIV. Text in Croatian, English. 1931. bi-m. DEM 40 domestic; USD 50 foreign. index, cum.index. back issues avail. *Refereed.* **Description:** Scientific journal of veterinary and related sciences: microbiology, immunology, parasitology, clinical sciences, animal science, physiology, anatomy.
Related titles: Online - full text ed.: (from Institute for Scientific Information).
Indexed: ASCA, Agri.& Environ.Biotech.Abstr. (coverage dropped), Anim.Breed.Abstr., Bio-Contr.News & Info., Biol.Abstr., Chem.Abstr., Chem.Indus.Notes, Dairy Sci.Abstr., Derwent Biotech.Abstr., Focus on: Vet.Sci.& Med. (coverage dropped), Helminthol.Abstr., Herb.Abstr., Ind.Vet., Nutr.Abstr., Pig News & Info., Poult.Abstr., Protozool.Abstr., Ref.Zh., Rev.Appl.Entomol., Rev.Med.& Vet.Mycol., Small Anim.Abstr., Soyabean Abstr., Sport Fish.Abstr., Sugar Ind.Abstr., Vet.Bull., Weed Abstr., Zoo.Rec.
—BLDSC (9226.100000), CASDDS, IDS, Linda Hall.
Published by: Sveuciliste u Zagrebu, Veterinarski Fakultet/University of Zagreb, Veterinary Faculty, Heinzelova 55, PO Box 190, Zagreb 41001, Croatia. TEL 385-41-290111. Ed. Dubravko Timet. Circ: 900.

636.089 GBR ISSN 1467-2987

VETERINARY ANAESTHESIA AND ANALGESIA. Text in English. 1970. 2/yr., latest vol.29, 2002. GBP 76 in Europe to individuals; USD 121 in North America to individuals; GBP 84 elsewhere to individuals; GBP 167 in Europe to institutions; USD 265 in North America to institutions; GBP 184 elsewhere to institutions (effective 2002). bk.rev. back issues avail. *Refereed.* **Document type:** *Journal, Trade.* **Description:** Contains original articles covering all branches of anaesthesia and the relief of pain in animals. Articles concerned with the following subjects related to anaesthesia and analgesia are also included: the basic sciences; pathophysiology of disease as it relates to anaesthetic management; equipment; intensive care; chemical restraint of animals including wildlife and exotic animals; welfare issues associated with pain and distress; education in veterinary anaesthesia and analgesia.
Former titles (until 2000): Journal of Veterinary Anaesthesia (1351-6574); (until 1991): Association of Veterinary Anaesthetists of Great Britain and Ireland. Journal (0950-7817); (until 1984): Association of Veterninary Anaesthetists. Proceedings (0269-5243)
Related titles: Online - full text ed.: Veterinary Anaesthesia and Analgesia Online. ISSN 1467-2995. 2000. GBP 69 in Europe to individuals; USD 109 in North America to individuals; GBP 69 elsewhere to individuals; GBP 151 in Europe to institutions; USD 239 in North America to institutions; GBP 151 elsewhere to institutions (effective 2002) (from EBSCO Publishing, O C L C Online Computer Library Center, Inc., ingenta, Munksgaard & Blackwell Science's Synergy, Swets Blackwell, RoweCom Information Quest).
Indexed: Chem.Abstr., Derwent Biotech.Abstr., Ind.Vet., Pig News & Info., Vet.Bull.
—BLDSC (9226.528500).
Published by: (Association of Veterinary Anaesthetists, American College of Veterinary Anesthesiologists USA, European College of Veterinary Anaesthesia), Blackwell Science Ltd., Osney Mead, Oxford OX2 0EL, United Kingdom. TEL 44-1865-206206, FAX 44-1865-721205, journals.cs@blacksci.co.uk, http://www.blackwell-science.com/vaa. Eds. E Clutton, P Pascoe. Pub. Elaine Stott. R&P Sophie Savage. Adv. contact Jenny Applin. Circ: 1,500.

636.089 DEU ISSN 0932-0814
SF910.5

VETERINARY AND COMPARATIVE ORTHOPAEDICS AND TRAUMATOLOGY. Short title: V.C.O.T. Text in English. 1988. q. USD 182 to individuals outside Europe; USD 268 to institutions outside Europe; USD 68 to students outside Europe (effective 2001). adv. bk.rev. abstr. *Refereed.* **Document type:** *Journal, Academic/Scholarly.*
Related titles: Online - full text ed.: (from Institute for Scientific Information).
Indexed: ASCA, Agricola, Bibl.Agri., Curr.Cont., Focus on: Vet.Sci.& Med., Ind.Vet., Small Anim.Abstr., Vet.Bull.
—BLDSC (9226.600000), GNLM, IDS, Infotrieve, ingenta. **CCC.**
Published by: Schattauer GmbH, Hoelderlinstr 3, Stuttgart 70174, Germany. TEL 49-711-22987-0, FAX 49-711-2298750, info@schattauer.de, http://www.schattauer.com. Ed. G Sumner Smith. Pub. Dieter Bergemann. R&P Annika Schmidt TEL 49-711-2298713. Adv. contact Claudia Hartmann TEL 49-711-2298727. B&W page DEM 1,820, color page DEM 3,670; 184 x 243. Circ: 1,500. **Subscr. to:** CSJ, Postfach 140220, Munich 80452, Germany. TEL 49-89-20959129, schattauer@csj.de. **Co-sponsor:** Veterinary Orthopedic Society (North America), European Society of Veterinary Orthopaedics and Traumatology, British Veterinary Orthopaedic Association.

VETERINARY AND HUMAN TOXICOLOGY. see *ENVIRONMENTAL STUDIES—Toxicology And Environmental Safety*

636.08 USA ISSN 1076-3872

VETERINARY CLINICAL NUTRITION; a professional, educational resource in nutrition for veterinarians. Text in English. 1994. q. USD 50 domestic; USD 55.25 in Canada; USD 64 elsewhere; USD 15 newsstand/cover (effective 2000). adv. *Refereed.* **Document type:** *Trade.* **Description:** Serves as a professional educational resource in nutrition for veterinarians.
Indexed: Agricola, Dairy Sci.Abstr., Ind.Vet., Nutr.Abstr., Poult.Abstr., Vet.Bull., Wild.Rev.
Published by: Veterinary Practice Publishing Co. (Subsidiary of: Fancy Publications, Inc.), PO Box 6050, Mission Viejo, CA 92690. TEL 949-855-8822, FAX 949-855-3045. Eds. Nancy Becker, David A Dzanis. R&P Nancy Becker. adv.: B&W page USD 648. Circ: 6,000 (paid).

636.089 USA ISSN 0275-6382
CODEN: VCPADJ

VETERINARY CLINICAL PATHOLOGY. Text in English. 1972. q. USD 60; USD 75 foreign (effective 1999). adv. bk.rev. abstr. index. back issues avail.; reprint service avail. from PQC. *Refereed.* **Document type:** *Academic/Scholarly.* **Description:** Covers the news, developments and trends affecting companion animal, exotic, equine and livestock veterinary practices. Topic areas include medical, business and industry, practice management and demographics.
Former titles: American Society for Veterinary Clinical Pathology. Journal; (until 1977): American Society of Veterinary Clinical Pathologists. Bulletin (0147-0701)
Related titles: Online - full text ed.: (from Institute for Scientific Information).
Indexed: ASCA, Agricola, Chem.Abstr., Focus on: Vet.Sci.& Med., Helminthol.Abstr., Ind.Vet., Nutr.Abstr., Poult.Abstr., Protozool.Abstr., Rev.Appl.Entomol., Rev.Med.& Vet.Mycol., Small Anim.Abstr., Vet.Bull., Wild.Rev.
—BLDSC (9227.015500), CASDDS, CISTI, IDS, ingenta, Linda Hall.
Published by: (American Society for Veterinary Clinical Pathology), Veterinary Practice Publishing Co. (Subsidiary of: Fancy Publications, Inc.), PO Box 6050, Mission Viejo, CA 92690. sgaunt@vt8200.vetmed.lsu.edu; orders@allenpress.com, http://www.asvcp.org/asvcppublications.html. Circ: 1,500. **Subscr. to:** Allen Press Inc., PO Box 1897, Lawrence, KS 66044-8897. TEL 785-843-1235, FAX 785-843-1274.

636.089 USA ISSN 0749-0739
SF951

VETERINARY CLINICS OF NORTH AMERICA: EQUINE PRACTICE. Text in English. 1985. 3/yr. USD 122 domestic to individuals; USD 144 in Canada to individuals; USD 161 elsewhere to individuals; USD 170 domestic to institutions; USD 210 foreign to institutions; USD 71 per issue (effective 2001). illus. Index. back issues avail.; reprints avail. *Refereed.* **Document type:** *Academic/Scholarly.* **Description:** Each issue covers a single topic relating to the treatment of conditions and diseases of horses.
Related titles: Microfilm ed.; Online - full text ed.: (from Institute for Scientific Information).
Indexed: ASCA, Curr.Adv.Ecol.Sci., Curr.Cont., Derwent Biotech.Abstr., Focus on: Vet.Sci.& Med., Ind.Med. (1985-), Ind.Sci.Rev., Ind.Vet., Protozool.Abstr., Rev.Med.& Vet.Mycol., Vet.Bull.
—BLDSC (9227.017800), CISTI, GNLM, IDS, Infotrieve, ingenta, Linda Hall. **CCC.**
Published by: W.B. Saunders Co. (Subsidiary of: Harcourt Publishers Ltd.), 11830 Westline Industrial Dr, St Louis, MO 63146. TEL 800-325-4177, http://www.harcourthealth.com/fcgi-bin/displaypage.pl?isbn=07490739, http://www.wbsaunders.com. Ed. John Vassallo. **Subscr. to:** Periodicals Fulfillment, W B Saunders Co, 6277 Sea Harbor Dr, 4th Fl, Orlando, FL 32891-4800. TEL 800-654-2542.

636.089 USA ISSN 1094-9194

VETERINARY CLINICS OF NORTH AMERICA: EXOTIC ANIMAL PRACTICE. Text in English. 1998. 3/yr. USD 110 domestic to individuals; USD 129 in Canada to individuals; USD 137 elsewhere to individuals; USD 158 domestic to institutions; USD 188 foreign to institutions; USD 63 per issue (effective 2001). illus. Index. reprints avail. *Refereed.* **Description:** Devotes each issue to a single topic in veterinary medicine. Provides detailed information invaluable to treating to treat exotic animal populations. Year 200 issues to include therapeutics, respiratory medicine, and soft tissue surgery.
Indexed: Ind.Med., Wild.Rev.
Published by: W.B. Saunders Co. (Subsidiary of: Harcourt Publishers Ltd.), 11830 Westline Industrial Dr, St Louis, MO 63146. TEL 800-325-4177, http://www.harcourthealth.com/fcgi-bin/displaypage.pl?isbn=10949194, http://www.wbsaunders.com. Ed. John Vassallo.

636.089 USA ISSN 0749-0720

VETERINARY CLINICS OF NORTH AMERICA: FOOD ANIMAL PRACTICE. Text in English. 1985. 3/yr. USD 99 domestic to individuals; USD 116 in Canada to individuals; USD 141 elsewhere to individuals; USD 134 domestic to institutions; USD 180 foreign to institutions; USD 61 per issue (effective 2001). illus. Index. back issues avail.; reprints avail. *Refereed.* **Document type:** *Academic/Scholarly.* **Description:** Each issue discusses an aspect of the treatment of conditions in cows, pigs, and sheep.
Related titles: Microfilm ed.; Online - full text ed.: (from Institute for Scientific Information).
Indexed: ASCA, Agri.Eng.Abstr., Anim.Breed.Abstr., Curr.Adv.Ecol.Sci., Curr.Cont., Dairy Sci.Abstr., Derwent Biotech.Abstr., Focus on: Vet.Sci.& Med., INIS Atomind., Ind.Med. (1985-), Ind.Vet., Nutr.Abstr., Pig News & Info., Poult.Abstr., Protozool.Abstr., Vet.Bull., Weed Abstr., World Ag.Econ.& Rur.Soc.Abstr.
—BLDSC (9227.017900), CISTI, GNLM, IDS, Infotrieve, ingenta, Linda Hall. **CCC.**
Published by: W.B. Saunders Co. (Subsidiary of: Harcourt Publishers Ltd.), 11830 Westline Industrial Dr, St Louis, MO 63146. TEL 800-325-4177, http://www.harcourthealth.com/fcgi-bin/displaypage.pl?isbn=07490720, http://www.wbsaunders.com. Ed. John Vassallo. **Subscr. to:** Periodicals Fulfillment, W B Saunders Co, 6277 Sea Harbor Dr, 4th Fl, Orlando, FL 32891-4800.

636.089 USA ISSN 0195-5616
CODEN: VNAPDW

VETERINARY CLINICS OF NORTH AMERICA: SMALL ANIMAL PRACTICE. Text in English. 1971. bi-m. USD 145 domestic to individuals; USD 177 in Canada to individuals; USD 199 elsewhere to individuals; USD 195 domestic to institutions; USD 249 foreign to institutions; USD 42 per issue (effective 2001). illus. index. reprint service avail. from PQC,ISI. *Refereed.* **Document type:** *Journal, Academic/Scholarly.*
Supersedes in part (in 1979): Veterinary Clinics of North America (0091-0279)
Related titles: Microform ed.: (from MIM,PQC); Online - full text ed.: (from Institute for Scientific Information).
Indexed: ASCA, Anim.Breed.Abstr., Aqua.Sci.& Fish.Abstr., Biol.Abstr., Curr.Adv.Ecol.Sci., Curr.Cont., Dairy Sci.Abstr., Dent.Ind., Derwent Biotech.Abstr., Excerp.Med., Focus on: Vet.Sci.& Med., Helminthol.Abstr., Ind.Med. (1979-), Ind.Vet., Nutr.Abstr., Poult.Abstr., Protozool.Abstr., Rev.Med.& Vet.Mycol., SSCI (coverage dropped), Sci.Cit.Ind., Small Anim.Abstr., Sport Fish.Abstr., Vet.Bull., Zoo.Rec.
—BLDSC (9227.020000), CISTI, IDS, Infotrieve, ingenta, Linda Hall. **CCC.**
Published by: W.B. Saunders Co. (Subsidiary of: Harcourt Publishers Ltd.), 11830 Westline Industrial Dr, St Louis, MO 63146. TEL 800-325-4177, http://www.harcourthealth.com/fcgi-bin/displaypage.pl?isbn=01955616, http://www.wbsaunders.com. Ed. John Vassallo. **Subscr. to:** Periodicals Fulfillment, W B Saunders Co, 6277 Sea Harbor Dr, 4th Fl, Orlando, FL 32891-4800.

636.089 GBR ISSN 0959-4493
SF901 CODEN: VEDEEK

VETERINARY DERMATOLOGY; an international journal. Text in English. 1990. q., latest vol.13, 2002. GBP 96 in Europe to individuals; USD 153 in North America to individuals; GBP 106 elsewhere to individuals; GBP 383 in Europe to institutions; USD 608 in North America to institutions; GBP 422 elsewhere to institutions (effective 2002). adv. **Document type:** *Journal, Academic/Scholarly.* **Description:** Covers the study of dermatology over a wide variety of species and serves as a unifying discipline for veterinarians and research scientists.

V

Related titles: Microfilm ed.: (from PQC); ♦ Online - full text ed.: Veterinary Dermatology Online. ISSN 1365-3164.
Indexed: ASCA, Agricola, Curr.Cont., Dairy Sci.Abstr., Derwent Biotech.Abstr., Focus on: Vet.Sci.& Med., Ind.Vet., Nutr.Abstr., Protozool.Abstr., Rev.Appl.Entomol., Rev.Med.& Vet.Mycol., Sci.Cit.Ind., Vet.Bull.
—BLDSC (9227.026000), IDS, Infotrieve, ingenta. **CCC.**
Published by: (European Society of Veterinary Dermatology), Blackwell Science Ltd., Osney Mead, Oxford OX2 0EL, United Kingdom. TEL 44-1865-206206, FAX 44-1865-721205, journals.cs@blacksci.co.uk, http://www.blackwell-science.com. Eds. D Lloyd, I Mason. Pub. Elaine Stott. R&P Sophie Savage. Adv. contact Jenny Applin. Circ: 1,000. **Co-sponsors:** American College of Veterinary Dermatology; European College of Veterinary Dermatology.

636.089 GBR ISSN 1365-3164
▼ **VETERINARY DERMATOLOGY ONLINE.** Text in English. 1999. bi-m. GBP 87 in Europe to individuals; USD 138 in North America to individuals; GBP 87 elsewhere to individuals; GBP 345 in Europe to institutions; USD 548 in North America to institutions; GBP 345 elsewhere to institutions (effective 2002). *Refereed.* **Document type:** *Academic/Scholarly.*
Media: Online - full text (from EBSCO Publishing, ingenta, Munksgaard & Blackwell Science's Synergy, Swets Blackwell, Institute for Scientific Information, RoweCom Information Quest). **Related titles:** Microfilm ed.: (from PQC); ♦ Print ed.: Veterinary Dermatology. ISSN 0959-4493.
Published by: Blackwell Science Ltd., Osney Mead, Oxford OX2 0EL, United Kingdom. TEL 44-1685-206206, FAX 44-1685-721205, website@blacksci.com, journals.cs@blacksci.co.uk, http://www.blackwell-science.com/~cgilib/jnlpage.bin?Journal=vderm&File=vderm&Page=aims.

VETERINARY ECONOMICS; business solutions for practicing veterinarians. see *BUSINESS AND ECONOMICS—Small Business*

636.089 USA ISSN 1047-6326
VETERINARY FORUM. Text in English. 1982. m. USD 35 (effective 2001). adv. bk.rev. tr.lit. *Refereed.* **Document type:** *Trade.* **Description:** Presents an interactive journal promoting exchange of information and ideas among veterinary practitioners.
Formerly: Veterinary Classified
—ingenta.
Published by: Veterinary Learning Systems, 275 Phillips Blvd, Trenton, NJ 08618. TEL 800-426-9119, FAX 609-882-6357, http://www.vetlearn.com. Ed. Lantz Miller. Pub. Michael Sollars. R&P Antoinette Passeretti TEL 609-671-2022. Circ: 50,000 (controlled).

636.089 GBR ISSN 0301-6943
VETERINARY HISTORY. Text in English. 1978. s-a. GBP 4 domestic to individuals; GBP 6 foreign to individuals; GBP 6 domestic to institutions; GBP 8 foreign to institutions (effective 2000). adv. bk.rev. **Document type:** *Academic/Scholarly.*
Indexed: Ind.Vet.
Published by: Veterinary History Society, c/o E Barbour-Hill, Ed., Tan Y Coed, High St, Bangor, Gwynedd LL57 1PX, United Kingdom. ebhvet@aol.com. Circ: 200.

636.089 NLD ISSN 0165-2427
CODEN: VIIMDS
VETERINARY IMMUNOLOGY AND IMMUNOPATHOLOGY; an international journal of comparative immunology. Text in English. 1980. 24/yr. EUR 1,572 in Europe to institutions; JPY 208,800 in Japan to institutions; USD 1,759 elsewhere to institutions (effective 2002). adv. bk.rev. illus. index. back issues avail. *Refereed.* **Document type:** *Academic/Scholarly.* **Description:** Deals with the study of veterinary immunology and immunopathology as applied to domestic animals, laboratory animals and other species that are useful to man.
Related titles: Microform ed.: (from PQC); Online - full text ed.: (from ingenta, Swets Blackwell, Institute for Scientific Information, ScienceDirect).
Indexed: AIDS & Cancer Res., ASCA, AgBiotech, Agricola, Anim.Breed.Abstr., Aqua.Sci.& Fish.Abstr., Biol.Abstr., Chem.Abstr., Chem.Indus.Notes, Curr.Adv.Ecol.Sci., Curr.Cont., Dairy Sci.Abstr., Derwent Biotech.Abstr., Excerp.Med., Focus on: Vet.Sci.& Med., Helminthol.Abstr., Immun.Abstr., Ind.Med. (1979-), Ind.Sci.Rev., Ind.Vet., Inpharma, Int.Abstr.Biol.Sci., Nutr.Abstr., Pig News & Info., Poult.Abstr., Protozool.Abstr., Reac., Rev.Appl.Entomol., Rev.Med.& Vet.Mycol., Sci.Cit.Ind., Small Anim.Abstr., Soyabean Abstr., Sport Fish.Abstr., Triticale Abstr., Vet.Bull., Wild.Rev., Zoo.Rec.
—BLDSC (9228.200000), CASDDS, CISTI, GNLM, IDS, ingenta, Linda Hall. **CCC.**
Published by: Elsevier Science BV, PO Box 211, Amsterdam 1000 AE, Netherlands. TEL 31-20-485-2911, FAX 31-20-485-2457, http://www.elsevier.nl/locate/vetimm. Eds. C J Howard, C L Baldwin, Dr. J Naessens. **Subscr. in Australasia and the Far East to:** Elsevier Science (Singapore) Pte Ltd, No.1 Temasek Ave, 17-01 Millenia Tower, Singapore 039192, Singapore. TEL 65-434-3727, FAX 65-337-2230; **Subscr. in Japan to:** Elsevier Science Inc - Japan Regional Office, 9-15 Higashi-Azabu 1-chome, Minato-ku, Tokyo 106-0044, Japan. TEL 81-3-5561-5033; **Subscr. in the Americas to:** Elsevier Science, PO Box 945, New York, NY 10159-0945. TEL 212-633-3730, FAX 212-633-3680, usinfo-f@elsevier.com.

636.08 658.8 USA ISSN 1074-7796
VETERINARY INDUSTRY NEWSLETTER; reporting on the business of veterinary products and animal health biotech. Variant title: Vet. Industry Newsletter. Text in English. 1993. m. USD 295 (effective 2001). pat, stat. back issues avail. **Document type:** *Newsletter.* **Description:** Covers marketing and business news for top executives in the animal health, animal health biotech, and veterinary products businesses, including new products, strategies, and promotions.
Related titles: E-mail ed.
Published by: Good Communications, Inc., PO Box 10069, Austin, TX 78766. TEL 512-454-6090, 800-968-1738, FAX 512-454-3420, help@gooddogmagazine.com, http://www.gooddogmagazine.com. Ed., Pub. Ross Becker.

636.089 POL ISSN 0042-4870
CODEN: BVIPA7
VETERINARY INSTITUTE, PULAWY. BULLETIN. Text and summaries in English. 1957. s-a. PLZ 30 domestic; USD 50 foreign (effective 2002); or exchange basis. abstr, bibl. 100 p./no. 1 cols./p. back issues avail. *Refereed.* **Document type:** *Bulletin.* **Description:** Publishes original scientific papers of research performed in the institute.
Formerly (until 1962): Instytut Weterynarii w Pulawach. Biuletyn (0079-791X)
Related titles: Duplicated (not offset) ed.; Fax ed.; Online - full text ed.: (from Institute for Scientific Information).
Indexed: ASCA, AgBiotech, AgroAgen, AgroLibrex, Anim.Breed.Abstr., Biol.Abstr., Chem.Abstr., Curr.Adv.Ecol.Sci., Dairy Sci.Abstr., Focus on: Vet.Sci.& Med., Food Sci.& Tech.Abstr., Helminthol.Abstr., INIS Atomind., Ind.Vet., Nutr.Abstr., Pig News & Info., Poult.Abstr., Ref.Zh., Rev.Med.& Vet.Mycol., Small Anim.Abstr., Vet.Bull.
—BLDSC (2805.301000), CASDDS, IDS, ingenta.
Published by: (State Committee for Scientific Research), National Veterinary Research Institute, c/o Krystyna Ciemiega-Wilczynska, Sec., Al Partyzantow 57, Pulawy 24100, Poland. TEL 48-81-8863051, FAX 48-81-8862595, krywilcz@piwet.pulawy.pl, http://www.piwet.pulawy.pl. Ed. Marian Grundboeck. Pub. Marian Truszczynski. Adv. contact Krystyna Wilczynska-Ciemiega. Circ: 550.

636.089 GBR ISSN 1090-0233
SF601 CODEN: VTJRFP
THE VETERINARY JOURNAL. Text in English. 1875. bi-m. GBP 136 to individuals; GBP 263 to institutions (effective 2002). adv. bk.rev. abstr, charts, illus, stat. index. reprint service avail. from SWZ,PQC. *Refereed.* **Document type:** *Academic/Scholarly.* **Description:** Publishes worldwide contributions on all aspects of veterinary science and its related subjects.
Former titles (until 1997): British Veterinary Journal (0007-1935); (until 1949): Veterinary Journal (0372-5545); (until 1900): Veterinary Journal and Annals of Comparative Pathology
Related titles: Microform ed.: (from PQC,PMC); Online - full text ed.: (from EBSCO Publishing, RoweCom Information Quest, Swets Blackwell, IDEAL Online Library, Institute for Scientific Information).
Indexed: ASCA, AgBiotech, Agri.& Environ.Biotech.Abstr. (coverage dropped), Agri.Eng.Abstr., Agricola, Anim.Breed.Abstr., Aqua.Sci.& Fish.Abstr., Aquacult.Abstr., Bibl.Agri., Biol.Abstr., C.I.S. Abstr., Chem.Abstr., Chem.Indus.Notes, Chem.Titles, Curr.Adv.Ecol.Sci., Curr.Cont., Dairy Sci.Abstr., Derwent Biotech.Abstr., Diar.Dis.Res., Environ.Sci.Poll.Mgmt., Excerp.Med., Focus on: Vet.Sci.& Med., Food Sci.& Tech.Abstr., Helminthol.Abstr., INIS Atomind., Ind.Med. (1997-), Ind.Sci.Rev., Ind.Vet., Microbiol.Abstr., Nutr.Abstr., Pig News & Info., Poult.Abstr., Protozool.Abstr., Rev.Appl.Entomol., Rev.Med.& Vet.Mycol., Rev.Plant Path., Risk Abstr., Sci.Cit.Ind., Small Anim.Abstr., Sport Fish.Abstr., Vet.Bull., Wild.Rev., Zoo.Rec.
—BLDSC (9228.600000), CASDDS, CISTI, EMDOCS, GNLM, IDS, ingenta, Linda Hall. **CCC.**
Published by: Bailliere Tindall (Subsidiary of: Harcourt Publishers Ltd.), 24-28 Oval Rd, London NW1 7DX, United Kingdom. TEL 44-20-7485-4752, FAX 44—20-7267-4466, TELEX 25775 ACPRES G, tvj@aht.org.uk, http://www.harcourt-international.com/journals/tvjl. Ed. A J Higgins. **Subscr. to:** Harcourt Publishers Ltd., Foots Cray High St, Sidcup, Kent DA14 5HP, United Kingdom. TEL 44-20-8308-5700, FAX 44-20-8309-0807.

636.08 EGY
CODEN: VMJGEA
VETERINARY MEDICAL JOURNAL GIZA. Text in English. 1953. q. *Refereed.* **Document type:** *Academic/Scholarly.*
Formerly (until 1988): Veterinary Medical Journal (0506-8266)
Indexed: AgBiotech, Agri.Eng.Abstr., Anim.Breed.Abstr., Chem.Abstr., Chem.Indus.Notes, Chem.Titles, Dairy Sci.Abstr., Helminthol.Abstr., Ind.Vet., Nutr.Abstr., Poult.Abstr., Protozool.Abstr., Rev.Appl.Entomol., Rev.Med.& Vet.Mycol., Sport Fish.Abstr., Sugar Ind.Abstr., Vet.Bull., Wild.Rev., Zoo.Rec.
—BLDSC, CASDDS.
Published by: Cairo University, Faculty of Veterinary Medicine, Giza, Cairo, Egypt. Ed. M Refai.

636.089 USA ISSN 1059-0994
VETERINARY MEDICAL REVIEW. Text in English. 1971; N.S. 1980. s-a. free per issue. charts, illus, stat. back issues avail. **Description:** For alumni, faculty and students, as well as other practicing veterinarians in Missouri.
Incorporates (1950-1979): Missouri Veterinarian (0540-4517); Which was formerly: Veterinary Scope
Indexed: Agri.& Environ.Biotech.Abstr. (coverage dropped), Anim.Breed.Abstr., Chem.Abstr., Dairy Sci.Abstr., Helminthol.Abstr., Ind.Vet., Protozool.Abstr., Vet.Bull.
Published by: University of Missouri at Columbia, College of Veterinary Medicine, Veterinary Medical Library, W218 Veterinary Medicine, Columbia, MO 65211. TEL 314-882-2461. Ed. Deborah Beroset Diamond. Circ: 3,000.

636.089 USA ISSN 8750-7943
CODEN: VEMEEV
VETERINARY MEDICINE. Text in English. 1905. m. USD 59 domestic; USD 70 in Canada & Mexico; USD 95 elsewhere; USD 10 newsstand/cover (effective 2001). adv. bk.rev. abstr, bibl, charts, illus, stat, tr.lit. index. reprints avail. *Refereed.* **Document type:** *Journal, Trade.* **Description:** Provides practicing veterinarians with peer reviewed practical solutions to common diagnostic and therapeutic problems.
Formerly (until 1985): Veterinary Medicine - Small Animal Clinician (0042-4889)
Related titles: Microform ed.: (from PQC); Online - full text ed.: (from Northern Light Technology, Inc., ProQuest Information & Learning, Institute for Scientific Information).
Indexed: ASCA, Agri.& Environ.Biotech.Abstr. (coverage dropped), Agricola, Anim.Breed.Abstr., Bibl.Agri., Biol.& Agr.Ind. (Jan.1983-Dec.1984), Biol.Abstr., Curr.Adv.Ecol.Sci., Curr.Cont., Dairy Sci.Abstr., Derwent Biotech.Abstr., Focus on: Vet.Sci.& Med., Helminthol.Abstr., Herb.Abstr., Ind.Med. (coverage dropped), Ind.Vet., Nutr.Abstr., Pig News & Info., Poult.Abstr., Protozool.Abstr., Rev.Appl.Entomol., Rev.Med.& Vet.Mycol., Rev.Plant Path., Risk Abstr., Small Anim.Abstr., Sport Fish.Abstr., Vet.Bull., Weed Abstr., Wild.Rev., World Ag.Econ.& Rur.Soc.Abstr., Zoo.Rec.
—BLDSC (9229.000000), CISTI, GNLM, IDS, ingenta, Linda Hall. **CCC.**
Published by: Veterinary Medicine Publishing Group (Subsidiary of: Medical Economics Co., Inc.), 15333 W. 95th, Lenexa, KS 66219. TEL 913-492-4300, 800-255-6864, FAX 913-492-4157, vm@vetmedpub.com., http://www.vetmedpub.com/vm/index.html. Ed. Margaret Rampey. Pub., R&P Rebecca Turner Chapman. Adv. contact Doug Catt. Circ: 26,020.

V

VETERINARY MEDICINE GUIDANCE MANUAL. see *PUBLIC HEALTH AND SAFETY*

VETERINARY MICROBIOLOGY; an international journal. see *BIOLOGY—Microbiology*

636.089 USA ISSN 1526-2073
VETERINARY NEUROLOGY AND NEUROSURGERY. Text in English. q. *Refereed.*
Address: 1507 Alice St, Davis, CA 95616. taholliday@ucdavis.edu, http://www.neurovet.org. Ed. T A Holliday.

636.089 617.7 GBR ISSN 1463-5216
▼ **VETERINARY OPHTHALMOLOGY.** Text in English. 1999. q., latest vol.5, 2002. GBP 65 in Europe to individuals; USD 104 in North America to individuals; GBP 72 elsewhere to individuals; GBP 247 in Europe to institutions; USD 392 in North America to institutions; GBP 272 elsewhere to institutions (effective 2002). adv. *Refereed.* **Document type:** *Journal, Academic/Scholarly.* **Description:** Contains material relating to all aspects of clinical and investigational veterinary and comparative ophthalmology.
Related titles: Online - full text ed.: Veterinary Ophthalmology Online. ISSN 1463-5224. 1998. GBP 59 in Europe to individuals; USD 94 in North America to individuals; GBP 59 elsewhere to individuals; GBP 223 in Europe to institutions; USD 353 in North America to institutions; GBP 223 elsewhere to institutions (effective 2002) (from EBSCO Publishing, O C L C Online Computer Library Center, Inc., RoweCom Information Quest, ingenta, Munksgaard & Blackwell Science's Synergy, Swets Blackwell, Institute for Scientific Information).
Indexed: Ind.Vet., Pig News & Info., Protozool.Abstr., Vet.Bull., Zoo.Rec.
Published by: (American College of Veterinary Ophthalmologists), Blackwell Science Ltd., Osney Mead, Oxford OX2 0EL, United Kingdom. TEL 44-1865-206206, FAX 44-1865-721205, journals.cs@blacksci.co.uk, http://www.blackwell-science.com. Ed. Kirk N Gelatt. Pub. Elaine Stott. R&P Sophie Savage. Adv. contact Jenny Applin. B&W page GBP 370, color page GBP 895; 210 x 275. Circ: 220.

636.089 NLD ISSN 0304-4017
CODEN: VPARDI
VETERINARY PARASITOLOGY; an international scientific journal. Text in English. 1975. 32/yr. EUR 1,883 in Europe to institutions; JPY 249,600 in Japan to institutions; USD 2,106 elsewhere to institutions (effective 2002). back issues avail. *Refereed.* **Document type:** *Academic/Scholarly.* **Description:** Publishes papers dealing with all aspects of disease prevention, pathology, treatment, epidemiology, and control of parasites in all animals which can be regarded as being useful to man.
Related titles: Microform ed.: (from PQC); Online - full text ed.: (from ingenta, Swets Blackwell, Institute for Scientific Information, ScienceDirect).
Indexed: ASCA, Abstr.Hyg., AgBiotech, Agricola, Anim.Breed.Abstr., Aqua.Sci.& Fish.Abstr., Aquacult.Abstr., Bio-Contr.News & Info., Biol.Abstr., Chem.Abstr., Chem.Indus.Notes, Chem.Titles, Curr.Adv.Ecol.Sci., Curr.Cont., Dairy Sci.Abstr., Dent.Ind., Derwent Biotech.Abstr., Entomol.Abstr., Environ.Sci.Poll.Mgmt., Excerp.Med., Focus on: Vet.Sci.& Med., Helminthol.Abstr., INIS Atomind., Ind.Med. (1975-), Ind.Sci.Rev., Ind.Vet., Int.Abstr.Biol.Sci., Microbiol.Abstr., Nutr.Abstr., Pig News & Info., Poult.Abstr., Protozool.Abstr., Rev.Appl.Entomol., Rev.Med.& Vet.Mycol., Sci.Cit.Ind., Small Anim.Abstr., Sport Fish.Abstr., Trop.Dis.Bull., Vet.Bull., Wild.Rev., Zoo.Rec.
—BLDSC (9229.163000), ADONIS, CASDDS, CISTI, EMDOCS, GNLM, IDS, Infotrieve, ingenta, Linda Hall. **CCC.**
Published by: Elsevier Science BV, PO Box 211, Amsterdam 1000 AE, Netherlands. TEL 31-20-485-2911, FAX 31-20-485-2457, nlinfo-f@elsevier.nl; usinfo-f@elsevier.com; forinfo-kyf04035@niftyserve.or.jp, http://www.elsevier.nl/locate/vetpar. Eds. D J O'Brien, J C Williams, S M Taylor. **Subscr. in Australasia and the Far East to:** Elsevier Science (Singapore) Pte Ltd, No.1 Temasek Ave, 17-01 Millenia Tower, Singapore 039192, Singapore. TEL 65-434-3727, FAX 65-337-2230; **Subscr. in Japan to:** Elsevier Science Inc - Japan Regional Office, 9-15 Higashi-Azabu 1-chome, Minato-ku, Tokyo 106-0044, Japan. TEL 81-3-5561-5033, FAX 81-3-5561-5047; **Subscr. in the Americas to:** Elsevier Science, PO Box 945, New York, NY 10159-0945. TEL 212-633-3730, FAX 212-633-3680, usinfo-f@elsevier.com.

636.089 USA ISSN 0300-9858
SF769 CODEN: VTPHAK
VETERINARY PATHOLOGY. Text in English, German. 1964. bi-m. USD 98 domestic to individuals; USD 104 in Canada & Mexico to individuals; USD 115 elsewhere to individuals; USD 121 domestic to institutions; USD 130 in Canada & Mexico to institutions; USD 143 elsewhere to institutions; USD 55 domestic to students (effective 2001). adv. bk.rev. bibl, charts, illus. index. back issues avail.; reprints avail. *Refereed.* **Document type:** *Academic/Scholarly.* **Description:** An official publication of the American College of Veterinary Pathologists, this international journal publishes original observations on the pathology of animals, both from natural and experimentally-induced diseases.
Formerly: Pathologia Veterinaria (0031-2975)
Related titles: Online - full text ed.: (from Institute for Scientific Information).
Indexed: ASCA, AgBiotech, Agri.& Environ.Biotech.Abstr. (coverage dropped), Agricola, Agroforest.Abstr., Anim.Breed.Abstr., Aqua.Sci.& Fish.Abstr., Aquacult.Abstr., Bibl.Agri., Biol.Abstr., Chem.Abstr., Chem.Indus.Notes, Curr.Adv.Cancer Res., Curr.Adv.Ecol.Sci., Curr.Cont., Dairy Sci.Abstr., Dent.Ind., Derwent Biotech.Abstr., Excerp.Med., Focus on: Vet.Sci.& Med., Helminthol.Abstr., Herb.Abstr., Ind.Med. (1971-), Ind.Sci.Rev., Ind.Vet., Inpharma, Nutr.Abstr., Pig News & Info., Poult.Abstr., Protozool.Abstr., Reac., Rev.Appl.Entomol., Rev.Med.& Vet.Mycol., Rev.Plant Path., Sci.Cit.Ind., Small Anim.Abstr., So.Pac.Per.Ind., Sport Fish.Abstr., Vet.Bull., Wild.Rev., Zoo.Rec.
—BLDSC (9229.165000), CASDDS, CISTI, EMDOCS, GNLM, ingenta, Linda Hall.
Published by: American College of Veterinary Pathologists, c/o Box 1897, Lawrence, KS 66044-8897. TEL 785-843-1235, FAX 785-843-1274, acvp@allenpress.com, http://www.afip.org/vetpath/. Ed. Donna F. Kusewitt. Circ: 1,200.

636.089 USA ISSN 0272-4669
SF917
VETERINARY PHARMACEUTICALS AND BIOLOGICALS. Text in English. biennial. USD 79.95 (effective 2000). **Document type:** *Directory.* **Description:** Covers veterinary products, including pharmaceuticals, biologicals, parasiticides, therapeutic diets, nutritional supplements, diagnostic aids, and supplies.
Related titles: Microform ed.: (from PQC).
—BLDSC (9229.167000), Infotrieve. **CCC.**
Published by: Veterinary Medicine Publishing Group (Subsidiary of: Medical Economics Co., Inc.), 15333 W. 95th, Lenexa, KS 66219. TEL 913-492-4300. Ed. Dr. Theresa Entriken. Pub. Rebecca Turner Chapman.

636.089 GBR ISSN 0042-4897
VETERINARY PRACTICE. Text in English. 1966. m. GBP 16 domestic; GBP 21 foreign (effective 2002). adv. bk.rev. abstr, charts, illus. 16 p./no. 6 cols./p. back issues avail.; reprints avail. **Document type:** *Journal, Trade.* **Description:** Presents news and articles on products and developments in the veterinary profession.
Formerly: Veterinary News
Related titles: Microform ed.: (from PQC).
Indexed: Dairy Sci.Abstr., Ind.Vet., Rev.Appl.Entomol., Small Anim.Abstr., Vet.Bull.
—BLDSC.
Published by: A.E. Morgan Publications Ltd., Stanley House, 9 West St, Epsom, Surrey KT18 7RL, United Kingdom. TEL 44-1372-741411, FAX 44-1372-744493. Ed. Chris Cattrall. Pub. Terence Morgan. Adv. contact Geoff Donovan. color page GBP 1,790; 215 x 300.

636.089 USA ISSN 1528-6398
VETERINARY PRACTICE NEWS; the information leader for veterinary practice and business. Text in English. m. USD 48 domestic; USD 61 in Canada (effective 2000).
Address: Box 15189, North Hollywood, CA 91615. TEL 818-760-8984, FAX 818-855-1850. Ed. Ellyce Rothrock.

636.089 USA ISSN 1047-8639
VETERINARY PRACTICE STAFF; current ideas and new information regarding health, industry and business practices. Text in English. 1989. bi-m. free per issue to qualified personnel. **Document type:** *Trade.* **Description:** For employees of the veterinary clinic, including technicians, assistants, office personnel, and receptionists.
Related titles: Online - full text ed.: (from Institute for Scientific Information).
Indexed: ASCA, Focus on: Vet.Sci.& Med., Ind.Vet., SSCI (coverage dropped).
—IDS.
Published by: Veterinary Practice Publishing Co. (Subsidiary of: Fancy Publications, Inc.), PO Box 6050, Mission Viejo, CA 92690. TEL 949-855-8822, FAX 949-855-3045. Ed. Brian Hutchins. Circ: 16,000.

636.089 USA ISSN 1092-8324
VETERINARY PRODUCT NEWS (YEAR). Short title: V P N. Text in English. 1987. m. USD 48 (effective 1999); includes VPN Sourcebook. adv. **Document type:** *Trade.* **Description:** Covers the news, developments and trends affecting companion animal, exotic, equine and livestock veterinary practices, including medical, business and industry, practice management and demographics.
Formerly (until 1996): Veterinarian Product News (1051-4260)
Published by: Fancy Publications, Inc., 3 Burroughs, Irvine, CA 92618-2804. TEL 949-855-8822, FAX 949-855-3045, http://www.petchannel.com. Ed. Brian Hutchins. Adv. contact Ray Magney. Circ: 48,000 (controlled). **Subscr. to:** PO Box 9090, Mission Viejo, CA 92690. TEL 949-855-8822.

636.089 NLD ISSN 0165-2176
CODEN: VEQUDU
VETERINARY QUARTERLY. Text in English. 1979. q. NLG 295 (effective 2000). back issues avail.; reprint service avail. from SWZ. *Refereed.* **Document type:** *Journal, Academic/Scholarly.* **Description:** Publishes the results of applied veterinary research in a variety of specialties.
Related titles: Microform ed.: (from PQC); Online - full text ed.: (from Institute for Scientific Information).
Indexed: ASCA, AgBiotech, Agri.& Environ.Biotech.Abstr. (coverage dropped), Agricola, Anim.Breed.Abstr., Bibl.Agri., Biol.Abstr., Chem.Abstr., Chem.Indus.Notes, Chem.Titles, Curr.Adv.Ecol.Sci., Curr.Cont., Dairy Sci.Abstr., Derwent Biotech.Abstr., Excerp.Med., Focus on: Vet.Sci.& Med., Food Sci.& Tech.Abstr., Helminthol.Abstr., Ind.Med. (1979-), Ind.Sci.Rev., Ind.Vet., Nutr.Abstr., Pig News & Info., Poult.Abstr., Protozool.Abstr., Rev.Appl.Entomol., Rev.Med.& Vet.Mycol., SSCI (coverage dropped), Sci.Cit.Ind., Small Anim.Abstr., Sport Fish.Abstr., Vet.Bull., Wild.Rev., Zoo.Rec.
—BLDSC (9229.270000), CASDDS, CISTI, GNLM, IDS, ingenta.
Published by: Koninklijke Nederlandse Maatschappij voor Diergeneeskunde/Royal Netherlands Veterinary Association, Julianalaan 10, Postbus 14031, Utrecht 3508 SB, Netherlands. TEL 31-50-2510111, FAX 31-30-2519847, vet.quarterly@knmvd.nl, tijdschrift@knmvd.nl. Ed. W Edel. R&P A M Tummers. Circ: 750.

636.089 USA ISSN 1058-8183
SF757.8 CODEN: VRULED
VETERINARY RADIOLOGY & ULTRASOUND. Text in English. 1960. bi-m. USD 87 domestic to individuals; USD 97 foreign to individuals; USD 107 domestic to institutions; USD 117 foreign to institutions (effective 2000). adv. illus. index. *Refereed.* **Document type:** *Academic/Scholarly.* **Description:** Presents articles of interest to the practicing veterinarian. Covers radiologic and ultrasound techniques, diagnostic interpretation, radiologic therapy and current advances in the field.
Former titles (until 1992): Veterinary Radiology (0196-3627); (until 1980): American Veterinary Radiology Society. Journal (0066-1155)
Related titles: Microform ed.: (from PQC); Online - full text ed.: (from Institute for Scientific Information).
Indexed: ASCA, Agricola, Anim.Breed.Abstr., Biol.Abstr., Curr.Cont., Focus on: Vet.Sci.& Med., Helminthol.Abstr., INIS Atomind., Ind.Med. (1992-), Ind.Sci.Rev., Ind.Vet., Nutr.Abstr., Pig News & Info., Poult.Abstr., Rev.Med.& Vet.Mycol., Sci.Cit.Ind., Small Anim.Abstr., Sport Fish.Abstr., Vet.Bull., Wild.Rev., Zoo.Rec.
—BLDSC (9229.281000), IDS, ingenta.
Published by: American College of Veterinary Radiology, c/o Lucinda Ayres, 2520 Beechridge Rd, Raleigh, NC 27608. TEL 919-513-6292, FAX 919-510-0560, vetradus@aol.com, http://www.acvr.ucdavis.edu. Ed., R&P Donald E Thrall TEL 919-829-4292. Adv. contact Lucinda Ayres. Circ: 1,000. **Co-sponsors:** International Veterinary Radiology Association; European Veterinary Radiology Association.

636.089 GBR ISSN 0042-4900
CODEN: VETRAX
VETERINARY RECORD; journal of the British Veterinary Association. Text in English. 1888. w. GBP 135 for 6 mos. domestic vol.148 (Jan.-Jun. 2001); GBP 180 for 6 mos. in Europe vol.148 (Jan.-Jun. 2001); GBP 150 for 6 mos. in Africa vol.148 (Jan.-Jun. 2001); GBP 180 for 6 mos. elsewhere vol.148 (Jan.-Jun. 2001) (effective 2001). adv. bk.rev. illus. Index. reprint service avail. from PQC. *Refereed.* **Document type:** *Academic/Scholarly.*
Related titles: Microform ed.: (from PQC); Online - full text ed.: (from Institute for Scientific Information).

Indexed: ASCA, Abstr.Hyg., AgBiotech, Agri.& Environ.Biotech.Abstr. (coverage dropped), Agri.Eng.Abstr., Agricola, Anim.Breed.Abstr., Aqua.Sci.& Fish.Abstr., Aquacult.Abstr., Bibl.Agri., Biol.& Agr.Ind. (Dec.1982-), Biol.Abstr., Chem.Abstr., Curr.Adv.Biochem., Curr.Adv.Cancer Res., Curr.Adv.Ecol.Sci., Curr.Cont., Dairy Sci.Abstr., Dent.Ind., Derwent Biotech.Abstr., Environ.Sci.Poll.Mgmt., Excerp.Med., Focus on: Vet.Sci.& Med., Food Sci.& Tech.Abstr., Helminthol.Abstr., Herb.Abstr., INIS Atomind., Ind.Med. (1888-), Ind.Sci.Rev., Ind.Vet., Int.Nurs.Ind., Maize Abstr., Neurosci.Cit.Ind., Nutr.Abstr., Pig News & Info., Poult.Abstr., Protozool.Abstr., Rev.Appl.Entomol., Rev.Arom.& Med.Plants, Rev.Med.& Vet.Mycol., Rev.Plant Path., Risk Abstr., Rural Recreat.Tour.Abstr., SSCI (coverage dropped), Sci.Cit.Ind., Small Anim.Abstr., Sport Fish.Abstr., Sugar Ind.Abstr., Vet.Bull., W.R.C.Inf., Weed Abstr., Wild.Rev., World Ag.Econ.& Rur.Soc.Abstr., Zoo.Rec.

—BLDSC (9230.000000), CASDDS, CISTI, GNLM, IDS, ingenta. **CCC.**

Published by: British Veterinary Association, 7 Mansfield St, London W1M 0AT, United Kingdom. TEL 0171-636-6541, FAX 0171-637-0620, http://www.vetrecord.co.uk, http://www.bva.co.uk/. Ed. Edward Boden. Circ: 10,000.

636.089 FRA ISSN 0928-4249 CODEN: VEREEM

VETERINARY RESEARCH. Text in English; Summaries in English, French. 1968. bi-m. FRF 1,974 domestic; EUR 339 in the European Union; EUR 368 elsewhere (effective 2001). adv. reprint service avail. from ISI. *Refereed.* **Document type:** *Academic/Scholarly.* **Description:** Covers all scientific aspects of veterinary and comparitive medicine and related subjects. The principal areas of interest are: immunology, virology, parasitology, physiology and biochemistry.

Former titles (until 1993): Annales de Recherches Veterinaires (0003-4193); (until 1969): Recherches Veterinaires (0486-1418)

Related titles: Microform ed.; Online - full text ed.: Veterinary Research (Online Edition). ISSN 1297-9716 (from EBSCO Publishing, ingenta, Swets Blackwell, Institute for Scientific Information, RoweCom Information Quest).

Indexed: ASCA, AgBiotech, Agri.& Environ.Biotech.Abstr., Anim.Breed.Abstr., Aqua.Sci.& Fish.Abstr., Aquacult.Abstr., Bibl.Agri., Biol.Abstr., Chem.Abstr., Chem.Indus.Notes, Curr.Adv.Ecol.Sci., Curr.Cont., Dairy Sci.Abstr., Dent.Ind., Derwent Biotech.Abstr., Diar.Dis.Res., Entomol.Abstr., Environ.Sci.Poll.Mgmt., Excerp.Med., Field Crop Abstr., Focus on: Vet.Sci.& Med., Genet.Abstr., Helminthol.Abstr., Herb.Abstr., Hum.Gen.Abstr., Ind.Med. (1993-), Ind.Sci.Rev., Ind.Vet., Microbiol.Abstr., Nutr.Abstr., Pig News & Info., Poult.Abstr., Protozool.Abstr., Rev.Appl.Entomol., Rev.Med.& Vet.Mycol., Rev.Plant Path., Sci.Cit.Ind., Sport Fish.Abstr., Vet.Bull., Wild.Rev., World Ag.Econ.& Rur.Soc.Abstr.

—BLDSC (9230.090000), CASDDS, CISTI, EMDOCS, GNLM, IDS, Infotrieve, ingenta, Linda Hall. **CCC.**

Published by: (France. Institut National de la Recherche Agronomique), E D P Sciences, 7 av. du Hoggar, B.P. 112, P.A. de Courtaboeuf, Les Ulis Cedex A 91944, France. TEL 33-1-69187575, FAX 33-1-69288491, subscribers@edpsciences.org, http://www.edpsciences.org. Eds. J Charley Poulain, J M Aynaud. Circ: 2,000.

636.089 NLD ISSN 0165-7380 CODEN: VRCODX

VETERINARY RESEARCH COMMUNICATIONS; an international journal publishing topical reviews and research articles on all aspects of the veterinary sciences. Text in Dutch. 1977. 8/yr. EUR 490 to institutions for print or online ed.; EUR 588 to institutions print & online eds.combined (effective 2002). adv. bk.rev. abstr, bibl, charts, illus. index, cum.index. back issues avail.; reprint service avail. from SWZ. *Refereed.* **Document type:** *Academic/Scholarly.* **Description:** Forum for current research in all disciplines of veterinary sciences.

Formerly: Veterinary Science Communications (0378-4312)

Related titles: Microform ed.: (from PQC); Online - full text ed.: (from EBSCO Publishing, O C L C Online Computer Library Center, Inc., RoweCom Information Quest, Swets Blackwell, Kluwer Online, Institute for Scientific Information).

Indexed: ASCA, AgBiotech, Agricola, Agroforest.Abstr., Anim.Breed.Abstr., Aqua.Sci.& Fish.Abstr., Aquacult.Abstr., Biol.Abstr., Chem.Abstr., Curr.Adv.Ecol.Sci., Curr.Cont., Dairy Sci.Abstr., Derwent Biotech.Abstr., Entomol.Abstr., Excerp.Med., Focus on: Vet.Sci.& Med., Helminthol.Abstr., Ind.Med. (1980-), Ind.Sci.Rev., Ind.Vet., Nutr.Abstr., Pig News & Info., Poult.Abstr., Protozool.Abstr., Rev.Appl.Entomol., Rev.Med.& Vet.Mycol., Sci.Cit.Ind., Small Anim.Abstr., Soyabean Abstr., Sport Fish.Abstr., Vet.Bull., Weed Abstr., Wild.Rev., Zoo.Rec.

—BLDSC (9230.200000), CASDDS, CISTI, GNLM, IDS, Infotrieve, ingenta. **CCC.**

Published by: Kluwer Academic Publishers Group (Subsidiary of: Wolters Kluwer N.V.), Spuiboulevard 50, PO Box 17, Dordrecht 3300 AA, Netherlands. FAX 31-78-639-2254, services@wkap.nl, http://www.wkap.nl/journalhome.htm///0165-7380. Ed. M M H Sewell. **Dist. by:** Journals Department, PO Box 322, Dordrecht 3300 AH, Netherlands. TEL 781-871-6600, FAX 31-78-654-6474.

636.08 NPL ISSN 1021-5042

VETERINARY REVIEW; a half-year Nepalese publication of animal production & health. Text in English. 1986. s-a. **Description:** Publishes reviews, results of original research, investigation and observations, progress reports, news and letters which may lead to improve health and productivity of livestock and better utilization of animal resources in Nepal.

Indexed: Anim.Breed.Abstr., Dairy Sci.Abstr., Forest.Abstr., Helminthol.Abstr., Herb.Abstr., Ind.Vet., Poult.Abstr., Protozool.Abstr., Rev.Appl.Entomol., Vet.Bull., Weed Abstr.

—BLDSC (9230.715000).

Published by: Pakhribas Agricultural Centre, Veterinary Investigation & Analytical Services Section, c/o Chief Information Officer, BAPSO, P O Box 106, Kathmandu, Nepal.

636.089 USA ISSN 0161-3499 SF911 CODEN: VESUD6

VETERINARY SURGERY. Text in English. 1978. bi-m. USD 136 domestic to individuals; USD 174 foreign to individuals; USD 200 domestic to institutions; USD 259 foreign to institutions; USD 90 domestic to students; USD 96 foreign to students; USD 44 per issue (effective 2001). adv. bk.rev. illus. index. reprint service avail. from PQC. *Refereed.* **Document type:** *Journal, Academic/Scholarly.* **Description:** Covers clinical and research topics of interest to veterinary surgeons.

Incorporates: Veterinary Anesthesia (0149-3949); Formerly: Journal of Veterinary Surgery

Related titles: Online - full text ed.: (from IDEAL Online Library, Institute for Scientific Information).

Indexed: ASCA, AgBiotech, Agricola, Biol.Abstr., Curr.Cont., Dairy Sci.Abstr., Derwent Biotech.Abstr., Focus on: Vet.Sci.& Med., INIS Atomind., Ind.Med. (1978-), Ind.Sci.Rev., Ind.Vet., Pig News & Info., Poult.Abstr., Rev.Med.& Vet.Mycol., Sci.Cit.Ind., Small Anim.Abstr., Sport Fish.Abstr., Vet.Bull., Wild.Rev.

—BLDSC (9231.037000), CASDDS, IDS, ingenta.

Published by: (American College of Veterinary Surgeons), W.B. Saunders Co. (Subsidiary of: Harcourt Publishers Ltd.), 11830 Westline Industrial Dr, St Louis, MO 63146. TEL 800-325-4177, http://www.wbsaunders.com. Ed. Dr. Philip B Vasseur. Adv. contact Michael Goldberg. B&W page USD 770, color page USD 1,820; trim 10 x 7. Circ: 2,434. **Subscr. to:** Periodicals Fulfillment, W B Saunders Co, 6277 Sea Harbor Dr, 4th Fl, Orlando, FL 32891-4800. **Co-sponsor:** European College of Veterinary Surgeons.

636.089 USA ISSN 8750-8990

VETERINARY TECHNICIAN; The complete journal for the veterinary hospital staff. Text in English. 1980. m. USD 38 domestic to individuals; USD 46 in Canada & Mexico to individuals; USD 55 elsewhere to individuals; USD 54 domestic to institutions; USD 59 in Canada & Mexico to institutions; USD 92 elsewhere to institutions (effective 2001). adv. bibl, charts, illus, stat. index. 80 p./no. 3 cols./p. back issues avail.; reprints avail. *Refereed.* **Document type:** *Journal, Academic/Scholarly, Bibliography.* **Description:** Focuses on aspects of veterinary medicine that veterinary technicians need to know.

Related titles: Online - full text ed.: (from Institute for Scientific Information).

Indexed: Dairy Sci.Abstr., Focus on: Vet.Sci.& Med., Ind.Vet., Protozool.Abstr., Small Anim.Abstr., Wild.Rev.

—BLDSC (9231.038000), IDS.

Published by: Veterinary Learning Systems, 275 Phillips Blvd, Trenton, NJ 08618. TEL 609-882-5600, 800-426-9119, FAX 609-882-6357, info@vetlearn.com. Ed., R&P Antoinette Passaretti TEL 609-671-2022. Pub. Ken Senerth. Adv. contact Mark Reynolds. Circ: 25,000.

636.089 GBR ISSN 1352-9374

VETERINARY TIMES. Text in English. 1970. m. GBP 89 domestic; GBP 98 foreign (effective 2000); (free to qualified personnel). adv. bk.rev. **Document type:** *Trade.* **Description:** Covers new products, new techniques and news.

Formerly (until 1984): Veterinary Drug

Indexed: Agri.Eng.Abstr., Anim.Breed.Abstr., Dairy Sci.Abstr., Ind.Vet., Nutr.Abstr., Pig News & Info., Poult.Abstr., Rev.Appl.Entomol., Rev.Arom.& Med.Plants, Rev.Med.& Vet.Mycol., Small Anim.Abstr.

Published by: Veterinary Business Development Ltd., Olympus House, Werrington Centre, Peterborough Rd, Peterborough, Cambs PE7 3BY, United Kingdom. TEL 44-1733-325522, FAX 44-1733-325512, ver.times@aversenline.com, VBD@vetsonline.com. Ed. David Watson Bvetmed MRCVS. Pub. Douglas Hutchison. Adv. contact Joy Bevan. Circ: 12,681.

636.089 TUR ISSN 0377-6395

VETERINER HEKIMLERI DERNEGI DERGISI. Text in Turkish. 1930. 4/yr. free per issue. adv. bk.rev. *Refereed.* **Document type:** *Bulletin, Academic/Scholarly.* **Description:** Covers scientific publications and news about veterinary surgery.

Formerly: Turk Veteriner Hekimleri Dernegi Dergisi (0376-8104)

Indexed: Anim.Breed.Abstr., Dairy Sci.Abstr., Ind.Vet., Poult.Abstr., Rev.Appl.Entomol., World Ag.Econ.& Rur.Soc.Abstr.

—BLDSC (9231.050000).

Published by: Turk Veteriner Hekimleri Dernegi/Turkish Veterinary Medical Association, Saglik Sok. 21-3, Yenisehir, Ankara, Turkey. TEL 90-312-431-6274, FAX 90-312-435-7914. Ed. Dr. Selim Aslan.

636.08 NLD

VIRUS INFECTIONS OF VERTEBRATES. Text in English. 1987. irreg., latest vol.6, 1996. price varies. back issues avail. *Refereed.* **Document type:** *Monographic series, Academic/Scholarly.* **Description:** Closely examines pathogenic viruses in vertebrate animals.

Published by: Elsevier Science BV, PO Box 211, Amsterdam 1000 AE, Netherlands. TEL 31-20-485-2911, nlinfo-f@elsevier.nl; usinfo-f@elsevier.com; forinfo-kyf04035@niftyserve.or.jp, http://www.elsevier.nl/. Ed. M C Horzinek. **Subscr. in Australasia and the Far East to:** Elsevier Science (Singapore) Pte Ltd, No.1 Temasek Ave, 17-01 Millenia Tower, Singapore 039192, Singapore. TEL 65-434-3727, FAX 65-337-2230; **Subscr. in Japan to:** Elsevier Science Inc - Japan Regional Office, 9-15 Higashi-Azabu 1-chome, Minato-ku, Tokyo 106-0044, Japan. TEL 81-3-5561-5033, FAX 81-3-5561-5047; **Subscr. in the Americas to:** Elsevier Science, PO Box 945, New York, NY 10159-0945. TEL 212-633-3730, FAX 212-633-3680, usinfo-f@elsevier.com, http://www.elsevier.com; **Subscr. to:** TEL 31-20-485-3757, FAX 31-20-485-3432.

636.089 BEL ISSN 0303-9021 CODEN: VDTIAX

VLAAMS DIERGENEESKUNDIG TIJDSCHRIFT/FLEMISH VETERINARY JOURNAL. Text in Dutch, English; Summaries in English. 1932. bi-m. BEF 1,800 (effective 2000). adv. bk.rev. abstr, charts, illus. index. *Refereed.* **Document type:** *Journal, Academic/Scholarly.*

Related titles: Online - full text ed.: (from Institute for Scientific Information).

Indexed: ASCA, Agri.& Environ.Biotech.Abstr. (coverage dropped), Anim.Breed.Abstr., Biol.Abstr., Chem.Abstr., Chem.Indus.Notes, Chem.Titles, Curr.Adv.Ecol.Sci., Curr.Cont., Dairy Sci.Abstr., Derwent Biotech.Abstr., Focus on: Vet.Sci.& Med., Helminthol.Abstr., Ind.Vet., Maize Abstr., Nutr.Abstr., Pig News & Info., Poult.Abstr., Protozool.Abstr., Rev.Med.& Vet.Mycol., Rev.Plant Path., Small Anim.Abstr., Vet.Bull.

—BLDSC (9246.000000), CASDDS, IDS, Linda Hall.

Published by: Universiteit Gent, Faculty of Veterinary Medicine, Salisburylaan 133, Merelbeke 9820, Belgium. Ed. L Devriese. Circ: 1,550.

636.089 AUT ISSN 0253-9411 CODEN: WTMOA3

WIENER TIERAERZTLICHE MONATSSCHRIFT. Text in German; Summaries in English. 1913. m. ATS 1,300, EUR 94.47; ATS 150, EUR 10.40 newsstand/cover (effective 2001). adv. bk.rev. abstr, bibl, charts, illus. index. **Document type:** *Magazine, Trade.*

Supersedes: Berliner und Muenchener Tieraerztliche Wochenschrift und Wiener Tieraerztliche Monatschrift (0723-6956); Which supersedes (in 1943): Wiener Tieraerztliche Monatschrift (0043-535X)

Related titles: Online - full text ed.: (from Institute for Scientific Information).

V

Indexed: AgBiotech, Agri.& Environ.Biotech.Abstr. (coverage dropped), Anim.Breed.Abstr., Biol.Abstr., Chem.Abstr., Chem.Indus.Notes, Chem.Titles, Curr.Adv.Ecol.Sci., Curr.Cont., Dairy Sci.Abstr., Derwent Biotech.Abstr., Excerp.Med., Focus on: Vet.Sci.& Med., Food Sci.& Tech.Abstr., Helminthol.Abstr., INIS Atomind., Ind.Sci.Rev., Ind.Vet., Key Word Ind.Wildl.Res., Nutr.Abstr., Pig News & Info., Poult.Abstr., Protozool.Abstr., Ref.Zh., Rev.Appl.Entomol., Rev.Med.& Vet.Mycol., Rev.Plant Path., Sci.Cit.Ind., Soils & Fert., Soyabean Abstr., Triticale Abstr., Vet.Bull.
—BLDSC (9316.000000), CASDDS, Linda Hall.
Published by: (Oesterreichische Tieraerzteschaft), B W K Public Relations, Grossmannstr 30, Vienna 1220, Austria. TEL 43-1-7747094, FAX 43-1-7747095, redaktion-wtm@oegt.at, office@bwk.at, http://www.wtm.at, http://www.bwk.at. Ed. Karin Moestl. Pub. Brigitte Weber-Kraus. adv.: B&W page ATS 8,230, color page ATS 17,170; trim 170 x 242. Circ: 1,800 (paid and controlled). **Co-sponsor:** Oesterreichische Gesellschaft der Tieraerzte.

V

WILDLIFE REHABILITATION. see *CONSERVATION*

333.95416 USA ISSN 1044-2618
WILDLIFE REHABILITATION TODAY. Text in English. 1989. q. USD 15 domestic; USD 18 in Canada; USD 27 elsewhere (effective 1999). adv. bk.rev. back issues avail. **Document type:** *Consumer, Trade.* **Description:** Contains technical and non-technical veterinary, wildlife rescue, reintroduction to the wild, care and rehab education articles.
Indexed: Environ.Abstr., Wild.Rev.
—CIS.
Published by: Coconut Creek Publishing Co., 2300 W. Sampleld Rd., Ste. 314, Pampano Beach, FL 33073-3046. TEL 954-977-5058, 888-978-1020, FAX 954-977-5158, wrt@theshelf.com; orders@allenpress.com, http://www.theshelf.com; http://www.allenpress.com. Ed., Pub., R&P Dan Mackey. Circ: 7,509 (paid). **Subscr. to:** Allen Press Inc., PO Box 1897, Lawrence, KS 66044-8897.

636.089 FRA ISSN 1017-3102
WORLD ANIMAL HEALTH IN (YEAR). Text in English. a. FRF 90, USD 90 (effective 2000). back issues avail. **Document type:** *Bulletin.* **Description:** Disease status of more than 170 countries for 108 diseases of animals and fish.
Related titles: French ed.: Sante Animale Mondiale en (Year). ISSN 1011-9299; Spanish ed.: Sanidad Animal Mundial en (Year). ISSN 1017-4362.
Indexed: Ind.Vet., Pig News & Info., Vet.Bull.
Published by: Office International des Epizooties, 12 rue de Prony, Paris 75017, France. FAX 33-1-42670987, oie@oie.int, http://www.oie.int. Ed. J Blancou. R&P Gill S Dilmitis TEL 33-1-44151888. **US subscr. to:** Scientific, Medical Publications of France, 100 E 42nd St, Ste 1002, New York, NY 10017. TEL 212-983-6278.

636.089 BEL
WORLD BUIATRICS CONGRESS. (Each report published in the host country) Text in English, French, German, Spanish. 1960. biennial. **Document type:** *Proceedings.*
Formerly: International Meeting on Cattle Diseases. Reports. (0074-6975)
Published by: World Association for Buiatrics, c/o P Lekeux, Sec, Faculte de Medecine Veterinaire, Batiment B42, Sart Tilman, Liege 4000, Belgium. TEL 32-41-564030, FAX 32-41-562935.

636.089 636 CHN ISSN 0366-6964
XUMU SHOUYI XUEBAO/ACTA VETERINARIA ET ZOOTECHNICA SINICA. Text in Chinese. q. USD 24 (effective 1997). **Document type:** *Academic/Scholarly.*
Indexed: ASCA, AgBiotech, Anim.Breed.Abstr., Biol.Abstr., Curr.Leather Lit., Dairy Sci.Abstr., Helminthol.Abstr., Ind.Vet., Maize Abstr., Nutr.Abstr., Pig News & Info., Poult.Abstr., Protozool.Abstr., Rev.Appl.Entomol., Rev.Med.& Vet.Mycol., Soyabean Abstr., Vet.Bull., Zoo.Rec.
—BLDSC (0670.900000), CISTI, IDS.
Published by: Zhongguo Nongye Kexueyuan, Xumu Yanjiusuo/Chinese Academy of Agricultural Sciences, Institute of Animal Husbandry, Yuanminyuan Lu, Haidian-qu, Beijing 100094, China. TEL 81-10-6258-1177, FAX 86-10-6258-2594. Ed. Chen You Chun.

YOU & YOUR VET. see *PETS*

636.089 ZMB
ZAMBIA. DEPARTMENT OF VETERINARY AND TSETSE CONTROL SERVICES. ANNUAL REPORT. Text in English. a. ZMK 200. **Document type:** *Government.* **Description:** Reports on the year's veterinary research and diagnostic work in the identification of disease in Zambia.
Published by: (Zambia. Department of Veterinary and Tsetse Control Services), Government Printing Department, PO Box 30136, Lusaka, Zambia.

636.089 NGA ISSN 0794-5086
ZARIYA VETERINARIAN. Variant title: Zariya Veterinarian(Z V). Text in English. 1986. s-a. NGN 2,000 domestic; USD 120 foreign. adv. 150 p./no. back issues avail. *Refereed.* **Document type:** *Journal, Academic/Scholarly.*
Published by: Ahmadu Bello University, Faculty of Veterinary Medicine, Samaru-Zaria, Kaduna, Nigeria. Ed., Adv. contact Dr. Jacob Kwaga. Circ: 1,000.

636.089 DEU ISSN 0939-7868
SF745.5.Z34
ZEITSCHRIFT FUER GANZHEITLICHE TIERMEDIZIN. Text in German. 1986. q. EUR 54.40 domestic to institutions; EUR 58.90 in Europe to institutions; EUR 59.90 elsewhere to institutions; EUR 39 to students; EUR 15.90 newsstand/cover (effective 2002). **Document type:** *Journal, Academic/Scholarly.*
Formerly (until 1991): Deutsche Zeitschrift fuer Biologische Veterinaermedizin (0179-714X)
Related titles: Online - full text ed.
Indexed: Vet.Bull.
Published by: (Deutsche Gesellschaft fuer Biologische Veterinaer-Medizin e.V.), Georg Thieme Verlag, Ruedigerstr 14, Stuttgart 70469, Germany. TEL 49-711-8931-0, FAX 49-711-8931298, leser.service@thieme.de, http://www.thieme.de. Ed. Dr. H Krueger.

636 RUS
ZHIVOTNOVOD DLYA VSEKH. Text in Russian. 1987. m. USD 240 in North America (effective 2001). adv. charts, illus, stat. *Refereed.* **Document type:** *Academic/Scholarly.* **Description:** Reflects the experience of successful farms and introduces the most modern technologies in all farming fields.
Formerly: Zhivotnovod (0235-246X)
Indexed: Ref.Zh.
—CISTI, East View.
Published by: Zhivotnovod, Sadovaya-Spasskaya 20, Moscow 107807, Russian Federation. TEL 7-095-1657360, FAX 7-095-1657360, givotnov@postman.ru, animal@east.ru. Ed., Pub., R&P Lyudmila A Pervova TEL 8-902-6752475. Adv. contact Yaroslav Nemirovsky. B&W page USD 800, color page USD 900; trim 210 x 290. Circ: 70,000 (controlled). **Subscr. to:** Marshala Zhukova, Pr-t Marshala Zhukova 4, Moscow 123837, Russian Federation. TEL 7-095-1950340, FAX 7-095-1951431. **Dist. by:** Mezhdunarodnaya Kniga, B Yakimanka 39, Moscow 117049, Russian Federation. TEL 7-095-2384967, FAX 7-095-2384634.; **US dist. addr.:** East View Publications, 3020 Harbor Ln N, Minneapolis, MN 55447. TEL 612-550-0961.

614.46 CHN ISSN 1005-944X
ZHONGGUO DONGWU JIANYI/CHINESE JOURNAL OF ANIMAL QUARANTINE. Text in Chinese. 1982. bi-m. CNY 3.50 newsstand/cover domestic. **Document type:** *Journal, Academic/Scholarly.*
Formerly (until 1993): Dongwu Jianyi (1004-681X)
Indexed: Protozool.Abstr.
Published by: Nongyebu Dongwu Jianyisuo, 369 Nanjing Lu, Qingdao 266032, China. TEL 86-532-5623545, aqima@public.qd.sd.cn.

ZHONGGUO RENSHOU GONGHUANBING ZAZHI/CHINESE JOURNAL OF ZOONOSES. see *BIOLOGY—Microbiology*

636.08 CHN ISSN 1005-4545
CODEN: ZSXUF5
ZHONGGUO SHOUYI XUEBAO/CHINESE JOURNAL OF VETERINARY SCIENCE. Text in Chinese. q. 104 p./no. **Document type:** *Academic/Scholarly.* **Description:** Covers the latest research and developments in veterinary science and related disciplines.
Indexed: AgBiotech, Anim.Breed.Abstr., Bio-Contr.News & Info., Dairy Sci.Abstr., Helminthol.Abstr., Ind.Vet., Nutr.Abstr., Pig News & Info., Poult.Abstr., Protozool.Abstr., Ref.Zh., Rev.Appl.Entomol., Rev.Arom.& Med.Plants, Rev.Med.& Vet.Mycol., Vet.Bull., Weed Abstr., Zoo.Rec.
—BLDSC (3180.693480), CASDDS.

Published by: Changchun Nongmu Daxue, 153 Xi an Dalu, Changchun, Jilin 130062, China. Ed. Yang Bensheng. **Dist. overseas by:** China International Book Trading Corp, 35 Chegongzhuang Xilu, Haidian District, Beijing 100044, China.

636.089 CHN
ZHONGGUO SHOUYI ZAZHI/CHINESE JOURNAL OF VETERINARY MEDICINE. Text in Chinese. 1953. m. USD 20.28 (effective 2000).
Indexed: AgBiotech, Anim.Breed.Abstr., Dairy Sci.Abstr., Helminthol.Abstr., Ind.Vet., Maize Abstr., Nutr.Abstr., Pig News & Info., Poult.Abstr., Protozool.Abstr., Rev.Appl.Entomol., Rev.Med.& Vet.Mycol., Vet.Bull., World Ag.Econ.& Rur.Soc.Abstr.
—BLDSC (3180.693000).
Published by: Zhongguo Xumu Shouyi Xuehui/Chinese Society of Animal Husbandry and Veterinary Science, Beijing Nongye Daxue, Dongwu Yixueyuan, Beijing 100094, China. TEL 86-1-62893040, FAX 86-1-62893961. Ed. Zhengxing Lu. Adv. contact Wang Ming. **Dist. overseas by:** China International Book Trading Corp, 35 Chegongzhuang Xilu, Haidian District, Beijing 100044, China.

636.089 TWN ISSN 0253-9179
CODEN: CKSCDN
ZHONGHUA MINGUO SHOUYI XUEHUI ZAZHI/CHINESE SOCIETY OF VETERINARY SCIENCE. JOURNAL. Text in Chinese, English. 1975. q.
Indexed: AgBiotech, Anim.Breed.Abstr., Chem.Abstr., Chem.Indus.Notes, Chem.Titles, Dairy Sci.Abstr., Helminthol.Abstr., Ind.Vet., Nutr.Abstr., Pig News & Info., Poult.Abstr., Protozool.Abstr., Rev.Appl.Entomol., Rev.Arom.& Med.Plants, Rev.Med.& Vet.Mycol., Soyabean Abstr., Sport Fish.Abstr., Vet.Bull., Weed Abstr., Wild.Rev., Zoo.Rec.
—BLDSC (4729.330500), CASDDS.
Published by: Zhonghua Minguo Shouyi Xuehui/Chinese Society of Veterinary Science, 142 Chou San Rd, Taipei 107, Taiwan.

636.089 ZWE ISSN 1016-1511
CODEN: ZVJOD4
ZIMBABWE VETERINARY JOURNAL. Text and summaries in English. 1970. q., latest vol.32, 2001. ZWD 300, USD 60 (effective 2001). adv. bk.rev. abstr. index. 30 p./no. back issues avail.; reprints avail. *Refereed.* **Document type:** *Journal, Academic/Scholarly.* **Description:** Contains original and review papers on all aspects of animal health in Zimbabwe and SADCC countries, including articles by non-veterinarians.
Formerly (until 1980): Rhodesian Veterinary Journal (0253-3278)
Indexed: Dairy Sci.Abstr., Field Crop Abstr., Helminthol.Abstr., Herb.Abstr., Ind.Vet., Pig News & Info., Poult.Abstr., Protozool.Abstr., Rev.Appl.Entomol., Rev.Med.& Vet.Mycol., Soyabean Abstr., Sport Fish.Abstr., Vet.Bull., Wild.Rev., Zoo.Rec.
Published by: Zimbabwe Veterinary Association, Causeway, PO Box CY 168, Harare, Zimbabwe. TEL 263-4-495859, FAX 263-4-495859, bvickers@esanet.zw. Ed. S Mukaratirwa. Pub. D B Vickers. R&P, Adv. contact Brian Vickers. Circ: 400.

VETERINARY SCIENCE—Abstracting, Bibliographies, Statistics

016.636089 BGR ISSN 0324-1068
CODEN: VMDNAV
ABSTRACTS OF BULGARIAN SCIENTIFIC LITERATURE. AGRICULTURE AND FORESTRY. VETERINARY MEDICINE. Key Title: Veterinarno-Medicinski Nauki. Text in Bulgarian. 1956. q. BGL 1.30 per issue. bibl. index. reprint service avail. from IRC. **Document type:** *Abstract/Index.*
Indexed: Agri.Eng.Abstr., Anim.Breed.Abstr., Chem.Abstr., Dairy Sci.Abstr., Field Crop Abstr., Forest Prod.Abstr., Forest.Abstr., Helminthol.Abstr., Herb.Abstr., INIS Atomind., Ind.Med. (coverage dropped), Ind.Vet., Pig News & Info., Plant Breed.Abstr., Protozool.Abstr., Rev.Med.& Vet.Mycol., Rev.Plant Path., VITIS, Vet.Bull., Weed Abstr.
—CASDDS. **CCC.**
Published by: (Akademiia na Selskostopanskite Nauki), Publishing House of the Bulgarian Academy of Sciences, Akad G Bonchev 6, Sofia 1113, Bulgaria. Circ: 1,280. **Dist. by:** Hemus, 6 Rouski blvd, Sofia 1000, Bulgaria.

636.097 016 JPN ISSN 0001-7221
ACTA VETERINARIA JAPONICA✱. Text in English, Multiple languages. 1956. q. per issue exchange basis. bk.rev. index.
—CISTI, GNLM.

Published by: Nihon University, Research Institute for Veterinary Science/Nihon Daigaku Juigaku Kenkyujo, c/o Japanese Society of Veterinary Science, Rokuno-Kaikan Bldg, 1-37-20 Yoyogi, Shibuya-ku, Tokyo 151-0053, Japan. Ed. Ushio Tanaka. Circ: 650.

635.021 AUS
▼ **AUSTRALIA. BUREAU OF STATISTICS. VETERINARY SERVICES, AUSTRALIA.** Text in English. 2001 (Jun). irreg. AUD 18.50 (effective 2001). **Document type:** *Government.*
Published by: Australian Bureau of Statistics, PO Box 10, Belconnen, ACT 2616, Australia. TEL 61-2-6252-5249, FAX 61-2-6252-6778, http://www.abs.gov.au.

016.636 USA ISSN 1067-8964
FOCUS ON: VETERINARY SCIENCE AND MEDICINE. Text in English. 1993. m. USD 350 (effective 2001). illus. reprints avail. **Document type:** *Abstract/Index, Bibliography.* **Description:** Provides bibliographic data and English-language author abstracts from international scholarly research journals and conference proceedings.
Media: Diskette. **Related titles:** Cumulative ed.: USD 495 (effective 2001).
Published by: Institute for Scientific Information, 3501 Market St., Philadelphia, PA 19104. TEL 215-386-0100, FAX 215-386-2911, webmaster@isinet.com, http://www.isinet.com. **Dist. in Europe by:** ISI Europe, Brunel Science Park, Kingston Ln, Uxbridge, Mddx UB8 3PQ, United Kingdom. TEL 44-1895-270016, FAX 44-1895-256710.

636.089 AUS ISSN 1033-2863
I V S ANNUAL. (Index of Veterinary Specialties) Text in English. 1980. a. AUD 82.75 in New Zealand; AUD 87.75 in PNG, Asia & Pacific Region; AUD 92.75 in US & Middle East; AUD 96.50 elsewhere (effective 2000). adv. **Document type:** *Directory.* **Description:** Classified listing of all veterinary drugs available in Australia.
Related titles: CD-ROM ed.
Published by: M I M S Australia (Subsidiary of: Medimedia Australia), PO Box 3000, St Leonards, NSW 2065, Australia. TEL 02-99027700, FAX 02-99027701. Ed. Wendy Alexander. Pub. Chris Wills. R&P Amanda Caswell. Adv. contact Sue McElroy. Circ: 3,500.

016.636 GBR ISSN 0019-4123
Z6674
INDEX VETERINARIUS; comprehensive monthly subject and author index to the world's veterinary literature available in print and on the internet. Text in English. 1933. m. GBP 1,095 to institutions print only; USD 1,785 in the Americas to institutions print only; GBP 1,110 to institutions online & print; USD 1,840 in the Americas to institutions online & print (effective 2002). adv. bibl, illus. back issues avail.; reprints avail. **Document type:** *Abstract/Index.*
Related titles: Online - full text ed.: GBP 960 to institutions online only; USD 1,680 in the Americas to institutions online only (effective 2002) (from DIMDI, The Dialog Corporation, S T N International); Cumulative ed.
—BLDSC (4390.000000), CISTI, Linda Hall. **CCC.**
Published by: CABI Publishing, Wallingford, Oxon OX10 8DE, United Kingdom. TEL 44-1491-832111, FAX 44-1491-829198, publishing@cabi.org, http://www.cabi.org/Publishing/Products/Journals/Abstract/IV/Index.asp. Adv. contact S Harris. B&W page GBP 100; 170 x 267. Circ: 750. **U.S. subscr. to:** 10 E 40th St, Ste 3203, New York, NY 10016. TEL 212-481-7018, 800-528-4841, FAX 212-686-7993, cabi-nao@cabi.org.

636.089 PAK
PAKISTAN VETERINARY INDEX. Text in English. 1985. a. USD 15.
Published by: Press Corporation of Pakistan, P O Box 3138, Karachi 75400, Pakistan. TEL 21-455-3703, FAX 21-7736198. Ed. Saeed Hafeez. Circ: 5,000.

016.636089 GBR ISSN 0042-4854
SF601
VETERINARY BULLETIN; a monthly abstract journal on veterinary science. Text in English. 1931. m. GBP 890 to institutions; USD 1,550 in the Americas to institutions; GBP 900 to institutions print & online eds.; USD 1,580 in the Americas to institutions print & online eds. (effective 2002). adv. bk.rev. illus. back issues avail.; reprints avail. **Document type:** *Abstract/Index.* **Description:** Presents abstracts of the core literature in the whole field of animal health.
Related titles: Online - full text ed.: GBP 760 to institutions; USD 1,350 in the Americas to institutions (effective 2002) (from DIMDI, The Dialog Corporation, S T N International).
Indexed: Dairy Sci.Abstr., Ind.Vet.
—BLDSC (9227.000000), CISTI, Linda Hall. **CCC.**
Published by: CABI Publishing, Wallingford, Oxon OX10 8DE, United Kingdom. TEL 44-1491-832111, FAX 44-1491-829198, publishing@cabi.org, http://www.cabi.org/Publishing/Products/Journals/Abstract/VB/Index.asp, http://www.ingenta.com. Adv. contact S Harris. B&W page GBP 225; 170 x 267. **Subscr. to:** 10 E 40th St, Ste 3203, New York, NY 10016. TEL 212-481-7018, 800-528-4841, FAX 212-686-7993, cabi-nao@cabi.org.

VIDEO

see COMMUNICATIONS—Video

VISUALLY IMPAIRED

see HANDICAPPED—Visually Impaired

WASTE MANAGEMENT

see ENVIRONMENTAL STUDIES—Waste Management

WATER RESOURCES

see also AGRICULTURE; CONSERVATION; ENVIRONMENTAL STUDIES; PUBLIC HEALTH AND SAFETY

333.91 USA
A S D W A UPDATE. Text in English. 1986. bi-m. USD 40 to non-members (effective 2000). bk.rev. **Document type:** *Newsletter.* **Description:** Examines issues related to the protection of public health through the assurance of high-quality drinking water.
Published by: Association of State Drinking Water Administrators, 1025 Connecticut Ave, N W, Ste 903, Washington, DC 20036. TEL 202-293-7655, FAX 202-293-7656. Ed., R&P Brendan Shane. Circ: 400.

628 DEU ISSN 0323-4320
TD430 CODEN: AHCBAU
ACTA HYDROCHIMICA ET HYDROBIOLOGICA; journal for water and wastewater research. Text in German, English. 1967. bi-m. EUR 608 in Europe; CHF 1,008 in Switzerland & Liechtenstein; USD 748 elsewhere; EUR 639 in Europe for print and online eds.; CHF 1,059 in Switzerland & Liechtenstein, for print and online eds.; USD 786 elsewhere for print and online eds. (effective 2002). adv. bk.rev. abstr, charts, illus, stat. index. reprint service avail. from ISI. *Refereed.* **Document type:** *Journal, Academic/Scholarly.* **Description:** Reports on the latest from all areas of water and environmental research.
Formerly (until 1992): Zeitschrift fuer Wasser- und Abwasserforschung (0044-3727)
Related titles: Online - full text ed.: ISSN 1521-401X. EUR 608 in Europe; CHF 1,008 in Switzerland & Liechtenstein; USD 748 elsewhere (effective 2002) (from EBSCO Publishing, Wiley InterScience, Institute for Scientific Information).
Indexed: AESIS, Anal.Abstr., Aqua.Sci.& Fish.Abstr., Aquacult.Abstr., CEABA, Chem.Abstr., Chem.Indus.Notes, Chem.Titles, Curr.Adv.Ecol.Sci., Curr.Cont., Curr.Ref.Fish Res., Ecol.Abstr., Environ.Sci.Poll.Mgmt., Fluidex, Geo.Abstr.P.G., GeoRef, IBR, INIS Atomind., Irr.& Drain.Abstr., Mass Spectr.Bull., Pollut.Abstr., Rev.Appl.Entomol., Risk Abstr., Sel.Water Res.Abstr., Soils & Fert., Sport Fish.Abstr., W.R.C.Inf., Weed Abstr., Zoo.Rec.
—BLDSC (0624.520000), CASDDS, CISTI, IDS, Infotrieve, ingenta, Linda Hall. **CCC.**
Published by: (Gesellschaft Deutscher Chemiker, Wasserchemische Gesellschaft), Wiley - V C H, Postfach 101161, Weinheim 69451, Germany. FAX 49-6201-606-117, subservice@wiley-vch.de, http://www.wiley-vch.de. Ed. F Frimmel. Adv. contact Marion Schulz. **Subscr. in the Americas to:** John Wiley & Sons, Inc., Journals. TEL 44-1243-779777, 212-850-6645, FAX 212-850-6021; **Subscr. outside Germany, Austria & Switzerland to:** John Wiley & Sons Ltd., Baffins Ln, Chichester, Sussex PO19 IUD, United Kingdom. TEL 44-1243-779777, FAX 44-1243-843232.

ASIAN ENVIRONMENT; journal of environmental science and technology for balanced development. see *ENVIRONMENTAL STUDIES*

614 AUS
AUSTRALIAN FLUORIDATION NEWS. AQUA-PURA. Text in English. 1963. bi-m. USD 20 to membership (effective 1999). bk.rev. **Document type:** *Newsletter.*
Formerly: Aqua Pura
Published by: Anti-Fluoridation Association of Victoria, GPO Box 369, Sydney, NSW 2000, Australia. TEL 61-3-5925088. Ed. G Walker. Circ: 2,000.

333.91 USA
CALIFORNIA WATER RESOURCES DIRECTORY; a guide to organizations and information resources. Text in English. ceased 1991; resumed 1984. irreg. (2nd ed. 1991). USD 25. **Document type:** *Directory.* **Description:** Comprehensive guide to the nearly 1,000 governmental and non-governmental organizations in the state that deal with water policy, development, supply, and conservation, as well as related health, environmental protection, energy, and economic aspects.
Published by: California Institute of Public Affairs, PO Box 189040, Sacramento, CA 95818. TEL 916-442-CIPA, FAX 916-442-2478, cipa@igc.org, http://www.igc.org/cipa. Ed. Roberta Childers. Circ: 750. **Affiliate:** The Claremont Graduate School.

333.91 614 GBR ISSN 1360-4015
TD201 CODEN: JIWMEZ
CHARTERED INSTITUTION OF WATER AND ENVIRONMENTAL MANAGEMENT. JOURNAL. Text in English. 1987. q. GBP 170 (effective 2000). adv. bk.rev. charts, illus. index; cum.index. back issues avail. *Refereed.* **Document type:** *Academic/Scholarly.* **Description:** Covers water, including water resources, river management, pollution control, fisheries, sewerage, navigation, and environmental management, including land and air.
Formerly (until 1995): Institution of Water and Environmental Management. Journal (0951-7359); Which was formed by the 1987 merger of: Public Health Engineer (0300-5925); Water Pollution Control (0043-129X); Institution of Water Engineers and Scientists. Journal (0309-1600); Public Health Engineer superseded (in 1973): Institution of Public Health Engineers. Journal (0020-3513); Which was formerly (until 1955): Institution of Sanitary Engineers. Journal (0368-2765); (until 1943): Institution of Sanitary Engineers. Bulletin (0366-4376); (1916-1939): Institution of Sanitary Engineers.; Water Pollution Control superseded (in 1967): Institution of Sewage Purification. Journal and Proceedings (0368-0215); Which was formerly (until 1933): Institution of Sewage Purification. Proceedings (0370-0100); (1932-1933): Association of Managers of Sewage Disposal Works. Proceedings. Journal of the Institution of Water Engineers and Scientists; Institution of Water Engineers and Scientists. Journal superseded (in 1975): Institution of Water Engineers. Journal (0020-3556); Which was formerly (1896-1947): Institution of Water Engineers. Transactions
Related titles: Online - full text ed.: (from Institute for Scientific Information).
Indexed: A.S.& T.Ind. (Jan.1997-), ASCA, Abstr.Bull.Inst.Pap.Chem., Agricola, Aqua.Sci.& Fish.Abstr., Bioeng.Abstr., Br.Tech.Ind., Chem.Abstr., Chem.Indus.Notes, Chem.Titles, Curr.Cont., Derwent Biotech.Abstr., Ecol.Abstr., Energy Info.Abstr., Eng.Ind., Environ.Abstr., Environ.Per.Bibl. (1972-), Environ.Sci.Poll.Mgmt., Fluidex, Geo.Abstr.H.G., Geo.Abstr.P.G., GeoRef, Geol.Abstr., Geomech.Abstr., IDA, INIS Atomind., Intl.Civil Eng.Abstr., Pollut.Abstr., Ref.Zh., Repindex, Rev.Appl.Entomol., SSCI (coverage dropped), Sci.Cit.Ind., Sel.Water Res.Abstr., Sport Fish.Abstr., W.R.C.Inf., Wild.Rev.
—BLDSC (9267.575000), CASDDS, CISTI, Ei, EMDOCS, IDS, Infotrieve, ingenta, Linda Hall. **CCC.**
Published by: Terence Dalton Ltd., Arbons House, Water St, Lavenham, Suffolk C010 9RN, United Kingdom. TEL 44-1787-249290, FAX 44-1787-248267, postmaster@lavenhambroup.co.uk. Ed. M D F Haigh. R&P Nick Reeves. Adv. contact Jonathon Hankin. B&W page GBP 825, color page GBP 1,290; trim 180 x 270. Circ: 11,694.

ENVIRONMENTAL TOXICOLOGY; an international journal. see *ENVIRONMENTAL STUDIES—Toxicology And Environmental Safety*

INGEGNERIA AMBIENTALE. see *PUBLIC HEALTH AND SAFETY*

INGEGNERIA AMBIENTALE QUADERNI. see *PUBLIC HEALTH AND SAFETY*

INSTITUTION OF ENGINEERS (INDIA). ENVIRONMENTAL ENGINEERING DIVISION. JOURNAL. see *ENVIRONMENTAL STUDIES*

W

JOURNAL OF AQUARICULTURE AND AQUATIC SCIENCES. see *BIOLOGY*

628 POL ISSN 0079-3477
POLSKA AKADEMIA NAUK. KOMITET GOSPODARKI WODNEJ. PRACE I STUDIA. Text in Polish. 1956. irreg., latest vol.11, 1972. price varies.
Published by: Polska Akademia Nauk, Komitet Gospodarki Wodnej, Palac Kultury i Nauki, Pietro XX, pok 20 21, Warsaw 00901, Poland. **Dist. by:** Ars Polona, Krakowskie Przedmiescie 7, Warsaw, Poland.

333.91 BEL
LA RADIOACTIVITE DES PRINCIPALES SOURCES D'EAU MINERALE EN BELGIQUE.* . Text in French. a.
Related titles: Flemish ed.
Published by: Ministere de la Sante Publique et de la Famille, Institut d'Hygiene et d'Epidemiologie/Ministerie van Volksgezondheid en van het Gezin, Rue Juliette Wytsman 14, Brussels 1050, Belgium.

614.8 627.5 USA ISSN 0270-4447
T55.A1
SAFETY NEWS. Text in English. 1937. q. membership. charts, illus, stat.
Former titles: Reclamation Safety News (0034-1436); Reclamation Safety Record
Indexed: Bibl.Agri., C.I.S. Abstr., Environ.Sci.Poll.Mgmt., Pollut.Abstr., Sel.Water Res.Abstr.
—BLDSC (8067.248000).
Published by: Bureau of Reclamation, Safety Office, PO Box 25007, Denver, CO 80225. TEL 303-236-6774. Circ: 550.

627 628 USA ISSN 1051-709X
TEXAS WATER UTILITIES JOURNAL. Text in English. 1990. m. USD 20; USD 25 foreign. adv. back issues avail. **Document type:** *Trade.* **Description:** Covers essential information for all individuals working within the water utilities industry in Texas, including rules and regulations, certification, education, and communication.
Published by: Texas Water Utilities Association, 1106 Clayton Ave, Ste 101 E, Austin, TX 78793-1033. TEL 512-459-3124, FAX 512-459-7124. Ed., Adv. contact Christine Loven. Circ: 9,800.

VODOSNABZHENIE I SANITARNAYA TEKHNIKA. see *PUBLIC HEALTH AND SAFETY*

333.91 AUS
WATER QUALITY NEWS. Text in English. 1998. q. **Document type:** *Newsletter.* **Description:** Features current affairs in the water industry and research highlights.
Media: Online - full text.
Published by: University of South Australia, School of Chemical Technology, C R C for Water Quality and Treatment, The Levels Campus, Mawson Lakes, SA, SA 5108, Australia. TEL 61-8-8302-3068, FAX 61-8-8302-3668, fred.lijauco@unisa.edu.au, http://www.med.monash.edu.au/epidemiology/crc/crcpubs.htm. Ed. Fred Lijauco.

363.7284 ZAF ISSN 0257-8700
WATER SEWAGE AND EFFLUENT. Text in English. 1980. q. ZAR 110 domestic; ZAR 155 in Africa; ZAR 90 elsewhere (effective 2000). adv. illus. **Document type:** *Trade.* **Description:** Concerns itself with all aspects of water, from the management at its source to the treatmaent of effluent.
Indexed: Fluidex, Ind.S.A.Per., W.R.C.Inf.
—BLDSC (9275.480000).
Published by: Brooke Pattrick Publications, PO Box 422, Bedfordview, Transvaal 2008, South Africa. TEL 27-11-622-4666, FAX 27-11-616-7196, bestbook@brookepattrick.co.za, Bpattric@global.co.za. Ed. Edith Webster. Pub. John Pattrick. Adv. contact Bev Garside. B&W page ZAR 3,300, color page ZAR 4,800. Circ: 1,952 (controlled).

YEARS AHEAD. see *PUBLIC HEALTH AND SAFETY*

WOMEN'S HEALTH

see also MEDICAL SCIENCES—Obstetrics And Gynecology

A L R A NEWSLETTER. see *BIRTH CONTROL*

A N R E D. see *MEDICAL SCIENCES—Psychiatry And Neurology*

618 USA ISSN 1091-5923
A W H O N N LIFELINES; promoting the health of women and newborns. Text in English. 1997. bi-m. Included with an institutional subscription to Journal of Obstetric, Gynecologic and Neonatal Nursing.. adv. illus. Index. 72 p./no. back issues avail.; reprints avail. *Refereed.* **Document type:** *Magazine, Academic/Scholarly.*
Related titles: CD-ROM ed.: (from Ovid Technologies, Inc.); Online - full text ed.: (from ingenta).
Indexed: CINAHL.
Published by: (Association of Women's Health, Obstetric, and Neonatal Nurses), Sage Publications, Inc., Sage Science Press, 2455 Teller Rd, Thousand Oaks, CA 91320. TEL 805-499-0721, FAX 805-499-0871, info@sagepub.com, http://www.sagesciencepress.com. Ed. Barbara Peterson Sinclair. Pub. Susan Hanscom. R&P Peter Marino. Adv. contact David Baker TEL 410-638-6831. B&W page USD 2,494, color page USD 4,399; bleed 8.375 x 11.125. Circ: 20,200 (paid).

A W H O N N NEWSLETTER. see *MEDICAL SCIENCES—Nurses And Nursing*

613.9 GBR ISSN 0262-7299
ABORTION REVIEW. Text in English. 1981. q. GBP 25 domestic; GBP 35 foreign. bk.rev. stat. **Document type:** *Newsletter.* **Description:** Round-up of the medical, legal and social aspects of abortion in the U.K., Europe, and the U.S.
Incorporates (in 1995): Abortion Research Notes (0361-1116)
Published by: Birth Control Trust, 16 Mortimer St, London W1N 7RJ, United Kingdom. TEL 44-171-580-9360, FAX 44-171-637-1378, bct@birthcontroltrust.org.uk, http://www.easynet.co.uk/bct/. Ed. Ann Furedi. R&P David Nolan. Circ: 500.

613.7 GBR
ACTIVE MAGAZINE. Text in English. 1993. q. GBP 9.95 domestic; GBP 45 foreign; GBP 2.25 newsstand/cover. adv. video rev. back issues avail. **Document type:** *Consumer.*
Former titles: Get Active Magazine (1360-4031); (until 1995): Active Lifestyle (1351-0991)
Published by: Active Publishing Ltd., Centre for Fitness, 41 Overstone Rd, London W6 0AD, United Kingdom. TEL 44-181-741-0215, FAX 44-181-748-7812. Ed. Lydia Campbell. Pub. Steve Evans. Adv. contact Kate Jacobsen. page GBP 1,795. Circ: 55,000.

618.082 NGA ISSN 1118-4841
AFRICAN JOURNAL OF REPRODUCTIVE HEALTH/REVUE AFRICAINE DE LA SANTE REPRODUCTIVE. Text in English, French. q. USD 25 in Africa to individuals; USD 35 elsewhere to individuals; USD 30 in Africa to institutions; USD 50 elsewhere to institutions (effective 2001). adv. bk.rev. abstr, charts, maps. 120 p./no. 2 cols./p. back issues avail.; reprints avail. **Document type:** *Journal, Academic/Scholarly.* **Description:** Publishes original research, comprehensive review articles, short and commentaries on reproductive health in Africa. Strives to provide a forum for African authors, as well as others working in Africa, to share findings on all aspects of reproductive health and to disseminate innovative, relevant and useful information on reproductive health throughout the continent.
Indexed: Fem.Per. (1997-), Ind.Med. (1997-), Popul.Ind.
—BLDSC (0732.555200).
Published by: Women's Health and Action Research Centre, 4 Alofoje Ave, Off Uwasota St, Benin City, Edo State, Nigeria. wharc@hyperia.com. Eds. F E Okonofua, R C Snow TEL 234-52-602334.

613.042 CHL ISSN 0717-2311
AGENDA SALUD. Text in Spanish. 1995. q. USD 10 (effective 1999). **Description:** Provides information on specific issues, such as nutrition, quality of services, and AIDS.
Published by: Isis Internacional, Casilla 2067 Correo Central, Santiago, Chile. TEL 56-2-6382219, FAX 56-2-6383142.

THE AKWA LETTER. see *PHYSICAL FITNESS AND HYGIENE*

613.042 610 USA ISSN 0098-8421
R15
AMERICAN MEDICAL WOMEN'S ASSOCIATION. JOURNAL. Text in English. 1946. q., latest vol.56. USD 70 domestic to individuals; USD 80 foreign to individuals; USD 135 domestic to institutions; USD 145 foreign to institutions (effective 2001). adv. bk.rev. bibl, illus. Index. 48 p./no. 3 cols./p. back issues avail.; reprint service avail. from PQC. *Refereed.* **Document type:** *Journal, Academic/Scholarly.* **Description:** Focuses on medical and policy issues in women's health. Issues are thematically organized and feature scholarly articles about a particular area of women's health.
Formerly: Woman Physician (0002-7103)
Related titles: Microform ed.: (from PQC); Online - full text ed.
Indexed: Biol.Abstr., Environ.Sci.Poll.Mgmt., Ind.Med. (1972-), Mult.Ed.Abstr., NRN, Pollut.Abstr., Risk Abstr., Saf.Sci.Abstr., Stud.Wom.Abstr.
—BLDSC (4689.100000), CISTI, GNLM, ingenta, KNAW. **CCC.**
Published by: American Medical Women's Association, Inc., 801 N Fairfax St, Ste 400, Alexandria, VA 22314. TEL 703-838-0500, FAX 703-549-3864, jamwa@amwa-doc.org, info@amwa-doc.org, http://www.jamwa.org/, http://www.amwa-doc.org. Ed. Wendy Chavkin. R&P, Adv. contact Meredith Becker Buxton TEL 212-304-5552. B&W page USD 1,050. Circ: 10,000 (paid).

613.04244 USA
ANNUAL EDITIONS: WOMEN'S HEALTH. Text in English. 1998. a. USD 12.25. illus. **Document type:** *Academic/Scholarly.*
Published by: Dushkin - McGraw-Hill, Sluice Dock, Guilford, CT 06437-9989. TEL 203-453-4351, FAX 203-453-6000. Eds. Maureen Edwards, Nora L Howley.

618 USA ISSN 1073-1695
RA564.85
ANNUAL REVIEW OF WOMEN'S HEALTH* . Text in English. 1993. a. back issues avail.
Published by: National League for Nursing, 61 Broadway, New York, NY 10006-2701. TEL 800-669-1656. Eds. Beverly J McElmurry, Randy Spreen Parker.

613.082 616.89 AUT ISSN 1434-1816
CODEN: AWMHF4
ARCHIVES OF WOMEN'S MENTAL HEALTH. Text in English. 1998. q. EUR 194.10 domestic; EUR 189.80 in Germany; EUR 54 newsstand/cover foreign (effective 2002). adv. abstr. back issues avail.; reprints avail. *Refereed.* **Document type:** *Journal, Academic/Scholarly.* **Description:** Assists clinicians, teachers and researchers in incorporating knowledge of all aspects of women's mental health into current and future clinical care and research.
Related titles: Online - full text ed.: ISSN 1435-1102 (from EBSCO Publishing, RoweCom Information Quest, Swets Blackwell, Springer LINK).
Indexed: e-psyche.
—BLDSC (1643.700000).
Published by: Springer-Verlag Wien (Subsidiary of: BertelsmannSpringer), Sachsenplatz 4-6, PO Box 89, Vienna, W 1201, Austria. TEL 43-1-3302415-0, FAX 43-1-330242665, journals@springer.at; helpdesk@link.springer.de, http://www.springer.at/wom_health. Eds. Mario Lanczik, Meir Steiner. R&P Angela Foessl TEL 43-1-3302415517. Adv. contact Michael Katzenberger TEL 43-1-3302415220. B&W page XEU 1,000; 170 x 230. **Subscr. in N. America to:** Springer-Verlag, Journals, 175 Fifth Ave, New York, NY 10010. TEL 212-460-1500, FAX 212-473-6272, orders@springer-ny.com, http://www.springer-ny.com.

610 IND
ASSOCIATION OF MEDICAL WOMEN IN INDIA. JOURNAL. Text in English. 1920. bi-m. INR 15. adv.
Published by: Association of Medical Women in India, IMA Bldg., Keshavrao Khudye Marg, 16 Haji Ali Park, Mumbai, Maharashtra 400 034, India. Ed. Dr. Tara Ramarao. Circ: 500.

613.082 USA
BE HEALTHY* . Text in English. a. free per issue. adv. **Document type:** *Catalog.* **Description:** Lists products for pregnant women and new parents.
Published by: Be Healthy, Inc., 70 Messenger St, Saint Albans, VT 05478-1547. TEL 802-496-4944, 800-433-5523, FAX 802-496-5222. Ed., Pub., R&P, Adv. contact Bob Olkin.

613.082 DEU
BILD DER FRAU SCHLANK & FIT. Variant title: Schlank & Fit. Text in German. 3/yr. EUR 1.80 newsstand/cover (effective 2002). adv. **Document type:** *Magazine, Consumer.*
Related titles: ♦ Supplement to: Bild der Frau.
Published by: Axel Springer Verlag AG, Axel-Springer-Platz 1, Hamburg 20355, Germany. TEL 49-40-34722884, FAX 49-40-34725540, bmertin@asv.de, http://www.asv.de. Adv. contact Brit Brand TEL 49-40-34723415. color page XEU 6,880. Circ: 340,000 (paid and controlled).

THE BIRTHKIT. see *MEDICAL SCIENCES—Obstetrics And Gynecology*

BOOTS HEALTH & BEAUTY. see *WOMEN'S INTERESTS*

BREAST CANCER: DISEASE STATE MANAGEMENT RESEARCH. see *MEDICAL SCIENCES—Oncology*

BREAST DISEASE; an international journal. see *MEDICAL SCIENCES—Obstetrics And Gynecology*

613.082 CAN ISSN 1480-0039
CANADIAN WOMEN'S HEALTH NETWORK. Text in English, French. 1996. bi-m. CND 20 to individuals; CND 35 to institutions (effective 2000). **Document type:** *Magazine.*
Indexed: Gend.Watch.
Address: 419 Graham Ave, Ste 203, Winnipeg, MB R3C 0M3, Canada. TEL 204-942-5500, cwhn@cwhn.ca, http://www.cwhn.ca.

CANCER SOURCEBOOK FOR WOMEN. see *MEDICAL SCIENCES—Oncology*

613.082 FRA
CAPITAL SANTE. Text in French. 1997. m. FRF 180; FRF 295 in the European Union; FRF 345 elsewhere.
Published by: Bayard Presse, 3 rue Bayard, Paris Cedex 8 75393, France. TEL 33-1-44356060, FAX 33-1-44356029. **Subscr. to:** Bayard Presse International, BP 12, Paris Entreprise 99505, France. TEL 33-1-44216000, FAX 33-3-20274192.

CARERS IN VICTORIA. see *SOCIAL SERVICES AND WELFARE*

613.082 613.081 CAN
CITY WOMAN. Text in English. s-a. free per issue. adv. bk.rev. back issues avail. **Document type:** *Consumer.* **Description:** Promotes healthy and active living for women of all ages.
Published by: Warrenty Communications Inc., 1755 Woodward Dr, Ottawa, ON K2C 0P9, Canada. TEL 613-225-9207, warrenty@compmore.net. Ed. Patricia den Boer. Pub., Adv. contact Brian Warren. Circ: 40,000.

613.082 618.1 GBR ISSN 1369-7137
CODEN: CLIMFC
CLIMACTERIC. Text in English. 1998. q. GBP 85, USD 145 to individuals; GBP 145, USD 235 to institutions (effective 2000). adv. bk.rev. illus. index. reprints avail. *Refereed.* **Document type:** *Academic/Scholarly.*
Related titles: Online - full text ed.: ISSN 1473-0804 (from CatchWord Ltd.).
Indexed: Inpharma, Pharm.&Out.News, Reac.
—BLDSC (3278.760000), ADONIS.
Published by: (International Menopause Society IRL), Parthenon Publishing Group (Subsidiary of: C R C Press (New York)), Casterton Hall, Casterton, Carnforth, Lancs LA6 2LA, United Kingdom. TEL 44-1524-272084, FAX 44-1524-271587, mail@parthpub.com, http://www.parthpub.com/. Eds. Alistair Maclennan, David Sturdee. R&P Jean Wright.

▼ **THE CLINICAL JOURNAL OF WOMEN'S HEALTH.** see *MEDICAL SCIENCES*

CLINICAL UPDATE. see *MEDICAL SCIENCES—Oncology*

610 DEU ISSN 0933-0747
CLIO; die Zeitschrift fuer Frauengesundheit. Text in German. 1976. s-a. DEM 38, USD 20 (effective 2001). adv. bk.rev. illus. back issues avail. *Refereed.* **Document type:** *Magazine, Consumer.* **Description:** Topics covered include women's health, gynecological diseases and feminist critiques of medical care, self-help and reproductive technology.
Related titles: Online - full text ed.: (from Northern Light Technology, Inc.).
Indexed: Abstr.Engl.Stud.
Published by: Feministisches Frauen GesundheitsZentrum e.V., Bamberger Str 51, Berlin 10777, Germany. TEL 49-30-2139597, FAX 49-30-2141927, ffgzberlin@snafu.de, http://www.ffgz.de. Eds. Cornelia Burgert, Petra Bentz. Adv. contact Heike Werner. Circ: 3,000. **Subscr. to:** Umbreit GmbH und Co., Mundelsheimerstr 3, Bietigheim-Bissingen 74321, Germany. TEL 49-7142-596385, FAX 49-7142-596387.

CONTEMPORARY SEXUALITY; the international resource for educators, researchers and therapists. see *PSYCHOLOGY*

CUADERNOS DE SALUD DE LA MUJER. see *MEDICAL SCIENCES—Obstetrics And Gynecology*

618.082 CHL
CUADERNOS MUJER SALUD. Text in Spanish. 1996. a. USD 20 (effective 2000). back issues avail. *Refereed.* **Document type:** *Academic/Scholarly.* **Description:** Offers in-depth analysis of priority issues in women's health through contributions by groups and individual LACWHN-member researchers.
Related titles: English ed.: Women's Health Collection.
Published by: Fundacion Red de Salud de las Mujeres Latinoamericanas y del Caribe, Casilla 50610, Santiago 1, Santiago, Chile. TEL 56-2-2237077, FAX 56-2-2231066, rsmlac@mail.bellsouth.cl, http://www.reddesalud.web.cl. Ed. Adriana Gomez.

CURRENT MEDICAL LITERATURE. BREAST CANCER. see *MEDICAL SCIENCES—Abstracting, Bibliographies, Statistics*

DONNA MODERNA. see *WOMEN'S INTERESTS*

613 649 POL ISSN 1233-2984
DZIECKO. Text in Polish. 1995. m. PLZ 2.50 per issue; PLZ 3.50 newsstand/cover (effective 1999). adv. **Document type:** *Consumer.* **Description:** Covers mother and child health care, spouse relations, advice on pregnancy, bringing up children.
Published by: Proszynski i S-ka S.A., Ul Garazowa 7, Warsaw 02651, Poland. TEL 48-22-6077700, FAX 48-22-6077704, http://www.proszynski.com.pl.

EESTI NAINE; a magazine for women. see *WOMEN'S INTERESTS*

613.04244 USA ISSN 0897-1870
ENDOMETRIOSIS ASSOCIATION NEWSLETTER. Text in English. 1980. bi-m. USD 35 domestic; USD 47 in Canada (effective 2000). bk.rev. reprints avail. **Document type:** *Newsletter.* **Description:** Offers information about endometriosis, a chronic disease affecting women and girls primarily in their reproductive years. Includes medical research and patient news and information.
Formerly (until 1988): Endometriosis Association (0899-2967)
Published by: Endometriosis Association, Inc., 8585 N 76th Pl, Milwaukee, WI 53223. TEL 414-355-2200, FAX 414-355-6065, endo@endometriosisassn.org, http://www.endometriosisassn.org. Ed. Mary Lou Ballweg. R&P Crystal Grotberg. Circ: 10,000.

613.082 USA
▼ **ENERGY FOR WOMEN**; how to energize your life. Text in English. 2001. q. USD 17.99; USD 4.99 newsstand/cover; USD 6.99 newsstand/cover in Canada (effective 2002). adv. **Document type:** *Magazine, Consumer.* **Description:** Provides in-depth information for women on health, fitness, nutrition, and exercise.
Published by: Muscle Media, Inc., 555 Corporate Circle, Golden, CO 80401. TEL 303-271-1002, 800-967-3462, FAX 303-604-3462, info@musclemedia.com, http://www.musclemedia.com. Ed. Gretchen Ferraro.

EUROPEAN EATING DISORDERS REVIEW. see *PSYCHOLOGY*

618.082 USA ISSN 0888-2398
CODEN: FPPCE9
FEMALE PATIENT: PRACTICAL ADVICE FOR PRIMARY CARE; total health care for women. Text in English. 1976. m. USD 93 in the Americas to institutions; USD 140 elsewhere to institutions (effective 2000). adv. **Document type:** *Trade.*
Supersedes in part (in 1981): Female Patient (0364-1198)
Indexed: Inpharma, Pharm.&Out.News, Reac.
—BLDSC (3905.168200), CISTI, EMDOCS, GNLM. **CCC.**
Published by: Quadrant HealthCom, 26 Main St, Ste A, Chatham, NJ 07928-2402. TEL 973-701-8900, FAX 973-701-8892. Ed. Caroline Tredway. Pub. Kathy McShea. Adv. contact Denise Andrade. Circ: 67,000.

FIELD ADVOCATE. see *GERONTOLOGY AND GERIATRICS*

FITNESS; mind - body - spirit for women. see *PHYSICAL FITNESS AND HYGIENE*

613.082 CHE ISSN 1021-5697
▼ **FRAUENHEILKUNDE AKTUELL.** Text in German. 2000. q. CHF 96, EUR 68.20 in Europe to institutions; CHF 107.60, USD 79.50 elsewhere to institutions (effective 2002). **Document type:** *Journal, Academic/Scholarly.*
Published by: S. Karger AG, Allschwilerstr 10, PO Box, Basel 4009, Switzerland. TEL 41-61-306-1111, FAX 41-61-306-1234, karger@karger.ch, http://www.online.karger.com/journals/FHK, http://www.karger.com.

613.082 DEU ISSN 1434-9086
FRAUENHEILKUNDE PLUS. Text in German. 1998. m. DEM 99 to institutions (effective 2000). **Document type:** *Academic/Scholarly.*
—GNLM.
Published by: Demeter Verlag GmbH und Co. KG, Ruedigerstr 14, Stuttgart 70469, Germany. TEL 49-711-8931-0, FAX 49-711-89311322, custserv@thieme.de, http://www.demeter-verlag.de.

GLOS KOBIETY; dwumiesiecznik dla pan. see *HANDICAPPED—Visually Impaired*

618.082 AUT
DAS GRUENE HAUS. Text in German. 1981. m. ATS 300 (effective 2000). adv. **Document type:** *Magazine, Consumer.*
Related titles: Online - full text ed.: ISSN 1605-1238.
Published by: Gruene Haus, Tuttenhofstrasse 63, Langenzersdorf, N 2103, Austria. TEL 43-2244-292370, FAX 43-2244-292373, redaktion@gruenehaus.at, http://www.gruenehaus.at/gruenehaus/index.html. Ed. Dieter Altermiller. Adv. contact Gertraud Altermiller. B&W page ATS 20,900, color page ATS 36,900; trim 191 x 256. Circ: 75,000 (paid).

W

GYNECOLOGIE OBSTETRIQUE ET FERTILITE. see *MEDICAL SCIENCES—Obstetrics And Gynecology*

H E R S NEWSLETTER. see *MEDICAL SCIENCES—Obstetrics And Gynecology*

HANDLING PREGNANCY AND BIRTH CASES. see *LAW—Family And Matrimonial Law*

618.082 USA ISSN 1070-910X
HARVARD WOMEN'S HEALTH WATCH; information for enlightened choices from Harvard Medical School. Variant title: Women's Health Watch. Text in English. 1993. m. USD 24 domestic; USD 40 in Canada; USD 47 elsewhere (effective 2000). *Refereed.* **Document type:** *Newsletter, Consumer, Academic/Scholarly.* **Description:** Addresses issues unique to women's health, such as mammography and hormone replacement therapy. Provides concise information to help readers make informed decisions.
Related titles: Online - full text ed.: (from Gale Group, Northern Light Technology, Inc., Factiva).
Indexed: Biol.Dig., CHNI, CINAHL.
—BLDSC (4270.809000).
Published by: (Harvard Medical School), Harvard Health Publications Group (Subsidiary of: Harvard Medical School), 164 Longwood Ave, Boston, MA 02115. TEL 617-432-1485, 800-829-5921, FAX 617-432-1506, hhp@hms.harvard.edu, http://www.health.harvard.edu. Eds. Carolyn Schatz, Dr. Celeste Robb-Nicholson. Circ: 400,000. **Subscr. to:** PO Box 420099, Palm Coasat, FL 32142-0099.

HEALTH & FITNESS MAGAZINE FOR HEALTHY, SOUND LIVING. see *PHYSICAL FITNESS AND HYGIENE*

HEALTH AND STRESS; the newsletter of the American Institute of Stress. see *MEDICAL SCIENCES*

618 USA ISSN 0739-9332
RA564.85 CODEN: HCWIDQ
HEALTH CARE FOR WOMEN INTERNATIONAL. Text in English. 1979. 8/yr. GBP 87, USD 143 to individuals; GBP 261, USD 431 to institutions (effective 2002). adv. bk.rev., film rev. bibl, charts, illus. index. back issues avail.; reprint service avail. from PQC. *Refereed.* **Document type:** *Academic/Scholarly.* **Description:** Takes an interdisciplinary approach to health care and related topics that concern women.
Formerly (until 1983): Issues in Health Care of Women (0161-5246)

Related titles: Online - full text ed.: ISSN 1096-4665 (from CatchWord Ltd., EBSCO Publishing, O C L C Online Computer Library Center, Inc., RoweCom Information Quest, Swets Blackwell).
Indexed: CINAHL, ERA, Fam.Ind., Fem.Per. (1986-), Int.Nurs.Ind., Intl.Bibl.Soc.Sci., J.of Abstr.Int.Educ., Lang.& Lang.Behav.Abstr., Mult.Ed.Abstr., NRN, Nurs.Abstr., PsycInfo, Psychol.Abstr. (1992-), Sage Fam.Stud.Abstr., Soc.Serv.Abstr., Sociol.Abstr., Sp.Ed.Needs Abstr., Stud.Wom.Abstr., Wom.Stud.Ind., e-psyche.
—BLDSC (4274.950600), CatchWord, GNLM, ingenta. **CCC.**
Published by: Taylor & Francis Ltd. (Subsidiary of: Taylor & Francis Group), 325 Chestnut St, Suite 800, Philadelphia, PA 19016. TEL 215-625-8900, FAX 215-625-2940, info@taylorandfrancis.com, http://www.taylorandfrancis.com/. Ed. Phyllis Noerager Stern. Circ: 400. **Subscr. addr. in Europe:** Taylor & Francis Group, Journals Customer Service, Rankine Rd, Basingstoke, Hants RG24 8PR, United Kingdom. TEL 44-1256-813000, FAX 44-1256-479438, enquiry@tanf.co.uk, http://www.tandf.co.uk/journals.

613.082 CAN ISSN 1496-1636
▼ **HEALTHY WOMAN.** Text in English. 2000. bi-m. adv. **Document type:** *Magazine, Consumer.*
Related titles: French ed.: Sante Femme. ISSN 1496-1644. 2000.
Published by: Rogers Media Publishing Ltd, 777 Bay St, 6th Fl, Toronto, ON M5W 1A7, Canada. TEL 416-596-5000, FAX 416-596-5881, http://www.rogers.com. Ed. Beth Thompson TEL 416-596-2561. Pub. Marc Thibodeau.

HEARTBEAT (ORLANDO). see *BIRTH CONTROL*

HOOFDZAKEN; nieuwsblad over migraine, hoofd- en aangezichtspijnen. see *MEDICAL SCIENCES—Psychiatry And Neurology*

618.082 DEU
IDEAL - GESUENDER LEBEN. Text in German. 8/yr. adv. **Document type:** *Consumer.*
Published by: Atlantikpresse Verlagsgesellschaft mbH, Im Neudeck 1, Speyer 67346, Germany. TEL 06232-310-0, FAX 06232-310292. Ed. Norbert Pirzer. Adv. contact Andreas Werner. Circ: 250,000.

INNOVATIONS IN BREAST CANCER CARE. see *MEDICAL SCIENCES—Oncology*

J A M A CONTRACEPTION NEWSLINE. (Journal of the American Medical Association) see *BIRTH CONTROL*

613.082 USA
J A M A WOMEN'S HEALTH NEWSLINE. (Journal of the American Medical Association) Text in English. 1998. w. back issues avail.
Media: Online - full text.
Indexed: NRN.
Published by: American Medical Association, J A M A Information Centers, 515 N State St, Chicago, IL 60610. TEL 312-464-5000, 800-262-2350, FAX 312-464-4181, womenshealth@ama-assn.org, http://www.ama-assn.org/special/womh/womh/womh.htm.

JOURNAL FUER MENOPAUSE; Zeitschrift fuer diagnostische, therapeutische und prophylaktische Aspekte im Klimakterium. see *MEDICAL SCIENCES—Obstetrics And Gynecology*

JOURNAL OF PERINATAL EDUCATION. see *MEDICAL SCIENCES—Obstetrics And Gynecology*

JOURNAL OF SPIRITUAL BODYWORK. see *ALTERNATIVE MEDICINE*

618.082 USA ISSN 1524-6094
CODEN: JWHMFP
JOURNAL OF WOMEN'S HEALTH AND GENDER-BASED MEDICINE. Text in English. 1992. 10/yr., latest vol.11, 2002. USD 99 domestic to individuals; USD 247 foreign to individuals; USD 119 domestic to individuals print and online eds. combined; USD 267 foreign to individuals print and online eds. combined; USD 304 domestic to institutions; USD 445 foreign to institutions; USD 365 domestic to institutions print and online eds. combined; USD 506 foreign to institutions print and online eds. combined (effective 2002). adv. back issues avail.; reprints avail. *Refereed.* **Document type:** *Journal, Academic/Scholarly.* **Description:** Publishes papers on diseases or conditions that hold greater risk for, or are more prevalent among women.
Formerly (until 2000): Journal of Women's Health (1059-7115)
Related titles: Online - full text ed.: USD 99 to individuals; USD 304 to institutions (effective 2002) (from CatchWord Ltd., EBSCO Publishing, O C L C Online Computer Library Center, Inc., RoweCom Information Quest, Swets Blackwell, Institute for Scientific Information).
Indexed: AgeLine, CINAHL, Cal.Tiss.Abstr., Crim.Just.Abstr., Curr.Cont., Environ.Sci.Poll.Mgmt., Excerp.Med. (1993-), Ind.Med. (1999-), Inpharma, Int.Nurs.Ind., NRN, Nutr.Abstr., Pharm.&Out.News, Pollut.Abstr., PsycInfo, Reac., Risk Abstr., SSCI, Saf.Sci.Abstr., Sci.Cit.Ind., e-psyche.
—BLDSC (5072.634450), CatchWord, CISTI, EMDOCS, GNLM, IDS, Infotrieve, ingenta, KNAW. **CCC.**
Published by: (Society for the Advancement of Women's Health Research), Mary Ann Liebert, Inc. Publishers, 2 Madison Ave, Larchmont, NY 10538. TEL 914—834-3100, FAX 914-834-1388, info@liebertpub.com, www.liebertpub.com/jwh, http://www.liebertpub.com. Eds. Dr. Bernadine P Healy, Denise Faustman, Dr. Florence P Haseltine.

JOURNAL OF WOMEN'S IMAGING. see *MEDICAL SCIENCES—Radiology And Nuclear Medicine*

362.1 NLD
KATERN VROUWENZELFHULP. Text in Dutch. 1992. bi-m. NLG 25 (effective 2000). back issues avail. **Document type:** *Newsletter.* **Description:** Reports news and concerns relating to women's health care issues and self-help organizations.
Supersedes (in 1996): Federatie Vrouwenzelfhulp. Nieuwsbrief (1383-7958); Which was formerly (until 1995): L P V Z Nieuwsbrief (0927-5991)
Published by: Federatie Vrouwenzelfhulp, Nieuwegracht 24a, Utrecht 3512 LR, Netherlands. TEL 31-30-236-8262, FAX 31-30-236-8242, info@vrouwenzelfhulp.nl.

LIFE GUARDIAN. see *SOCIAL SERVICES AND WELFARE*

LONGEVITY. see *GERONTOLOGY AND GERIATRICS*

LUPUS BEACON. see *MEDICAL SCIENCES—Rheumatology*

618 USA
M O M MAGAZINE✱. Text in English. 1984. q. USD 12. adv. bk.rev. **Description:** Promotes women's choices in health care. Offers alternative birth and parenting information.
Published by: Mothers and Others for Midwives, PO Box 2864, Big Bear City, CA 92314-2864. TEL 714-585-4175. Ed. Jeriann Fairman. Circ: 2,000.

613.082 616.99 618 USA
MAMM; women, cancer and community. Text in English. 1997. 10/yr. USD 14.95 domestic; USD 24.95 foreign (effective 2001). adv. back issues avail. **Document type:** *Magazine, Consumer.* **Description:** Aims to provide lay information on breast cancer treatments, research and related issues.
Indexed: CINAHL, Fem.Per. (1997-).
Published by: MAMM LLC, 41 E 11th St, 11th Fl, New York, NY 10003. TEL 212-699-6480, 888-901-6266, FAX 212-699-6496, letters@mamm.com, elsieh@mamm.com, http://www.mamm.com. Ed. Gwen Darien.

MARGRIET. see *WOMEN'S INTERESTS*

618.082 USA ISSN 1091-0220
MAYO CLINIC WOMEN'S HEALTHSOURCE. Text in English. 1997. m. USD 24.
Published by: Mayo Clinic, PO Box 56931, Boulder, CO 80322-6931. TEL 800-867-8633. Ed. Dr. Julie A Abbott.

618.082 USA
MEDICAL MISSION SISTERS NEWS. Text in English. 1927. q. free per issue. illus. index, cum.index. **Document type:** *Newsletter.*
Supersedes: Medical Missionary (0025-7389)
Published by: Society of Catholic Medical Missionaries, Inc., 8400 Pine Rd, Philadelphia, PA 19111. TEL 215-742-6100, FAX 215-342-3948. Ed., R&P Monica M McGinley. Circ: 52,000.

MEDITSINSKI PREGLED. AKUSHERSTVO I GINEKOLOGIIA. see *MEDICAL SCIENCES—Obstetrics And Gynecology*

613.082 USA ISSN 1521-2076
MEDSCAPE WOMEN'S HEALTH. Text in English. 1996. 6/yr. *Refereed.* **Description:** Features clinical news and full-text articles on the prevention, diagnosis, and treatment of a broad scope of health problems in women.
Media: Online - full text (from Institute for Scientific Information).
Indexed: Curr.Cont.
Published by: Medscape, Inc., 134 W 29th St, New York, NY 10001-5399. TEL 212-631-1600, http://www.medscape.com.

613.7 USA ISSN 1043-8734
RA564.85
MELPOMENE JOURNAL; a journal for women's health research. Text in English. 1981. 3/yr. USD 40 domestic to individuals; USD 50 foreign to individuals; USD 75 domestic to institutions (effective 2001). bk.rev. illus. reprints avail. **Document type:** *Newsletter, Academic/Scholarly.* **Description:** Research articles with scientific bibliographies, personal profiles, news and updates, providing information about health and physically active women.
Formerly: Melpomene Report
Related titles: Online - full text ed.: (from Northern Light Technology, Inc.).
Indexed: CWI, Sportsearch (1988-).
—ingenta.
Published by: Melpomene Institute for Women's Health Research, 1010 University Ave W, Saint Paul, MN 55104-4706. TEL 651-642-1951, FAX 651-642-1871, health@melpomene.org, http://www.melpomene.org. Ed., R&P Evelyn Cottle Raedler. Pub. Judy Mahle Lutter. Circ: 2,500 (paid).

MENOPAUSE. see *MEDICAL SCIENCES—Obstetrics And Gynecology*

618.082 USA ISSN 1062-7332
MENOPAUSE MANAGEMENT✱. Text in English. 1992. bi-m. USD 95 (effective 2000). **Description:** Serves as the society's education publication for health care professionals.
—BLDSC (5678.457035), Infotrieve. **CCC.**
Published by: North American Menopause Society, University Hospitals of Cleveland, Department of Obstetrics & Gynecology, 11100 Euclid, Cleveland, OH 44106. TEL 973-361-1280.

612.67 618.1 155.67 USA ISSN 1061-4397
MENOPAUSE NEWS. Text in English. 1991. bi-m. USD 25 to individuals; USD 30 foreign to individuals. bk.rev. illus. back issues avail.; reprints avail. **Document type:** *Newsletter, Consumer.* **Description:** Contains the latest medical and psychological information, as well as first-person accounts, letters.
Related titles: Online - full text ed.: (from Gale Group, Northern Light Technology, Inc., ProQuest Information & Learning).
Indexed: CHNI.
Address: 2074 Union St, Ste 10, San Francisco, CA 94123. TEL 415-567-2368, 800-241-6366, FAX 415-567-2368, mnews@well.com, http://www.menopausenews.com. Ed. Judith Stiles Askew. R&P Judith Styles Askew.

MIDLIFE WOMAN. see *WOMEN'S INTERESTS*

618.082 USA
MIDLIFE WOMEN'S HEALTH SOURCEBOOK. Text in English. 1997. a. USD 249; USD 269 foreign (effective 1999). **Document type:** *Trade.*
Published by: American Health Consultants (Subsidiary of: Medical Economics Co., Inc.), 3525 Piedmont Rd, N E, 6 Piedmont Center, Ste 400, Atlanta, GA 30305. TEL 404-262-5476, custserv@ahcpub.com, http://www.ahcpub.com.

MIDWIFERY TODAY WITH INTERNATIONAL MIDWIFE. see *MEDICAL SCIENCES—Obstetrics And Gynecology*

MOTHER AND CHILD. see *WOMEN'S INTERESTS*

618 362.7 USA ISSN 0733-3013
MOTHERING; the magazine of natural family living. Text in English. 1976. bi-m. USD 18.95 domestic; USD 23.95 in Canada; USD 35.45 elsewhere (effective 2001). adv. bk.rev. illus. Index. back issues avail.; reprints avail. **Document type:** *Consumer.* **Description:** Articles and departments pertaining to progressive childrearing in the areas of health, learning, and emotional and personal development.
Related titles: Microfiche ed.: (from PQC); Online - full text ed.: (from Gale Group, Northern Light Technology, Inc., Factiva).
Indexed: Alt.Press Ind., Child.Lit.Abstr., Hlth.Ind.

—BLDSC (5968.925200), ingenta.
Published by: Mothering Magazine, PO Box 1690, Santa Fe, NM 87504. TEL 800-984-8116, FAX 505-986-8335, info@mothering.com, http://www.mothering.com. Ed., Pub. Peggy O'Mara. R&P Tara Maestas TEL 505-984-6299. Adv. contact Beth Stephens. B&W page USD 2,750, color page USD 3,400. Circ: 78,000 (paid); 7,000 (controlled).

MOTHER'S DAY REPORT. see *GERONTOLOGY AND GERIATRICS*

▼ **MUSCLE & FITNESS HERS.** see *PHYSICAL FITNESS AND HYGIENE*

N A B C O BREAST CANCER RESOURCE LIST. see *MEDICAL SCIENCES—Oncology*

N A B C O NEWS. see *MEDICAL SCIENCES—Oncology*

618.082 GBR
N H S BREAST SCREENING PROGRAMME. (National Health Service) Text in English. 1993. a. GBP 10 to non-members (effective 1999). stat. **Document type:** *Government.* **Description:** Reports on activity and provides statistics of the UK Breast Screening Programme.
Published by: National Health Service, Breast Screening Programme, The Manor House, 260 Ecclesall Rd S, Sheffield, S Yorks S11 9PS, United Kingdom. TEL 44-114-271-1060, FAX 44-114-271-1089. Ed. Julietta Patnick. Circ: 5,500.

613.82 GBR
N H S CERVICAL SCREENING PROGRAMME (YEAR). (National Health Service) Text in English. 1998. a., latest 2000. GBP 10 to non-members (effective 2001). back issues avail. **Document type:** *Government.*
Related titles: Online - full content ed.
Published by: National Health Service, N H S Cervical Screen Programme, The Manor House, 260 Ecclesall Rd S, Sheffield, S Yorks S11 9PS, United Kingdom. TEL 44-114-271-1060, FAX 44-114-271-1089, http://www.cancerscreening.nhs.uk. Ed. Julietta Patrick. Circ: 7,000.

613.082 USA
N P W H NEWSLETTER: THE MONTHLY CYCLE. (Nurse Practitioners in Women's Health) Text in English. m.
Formerly: National Association of Nurse Practitioners in Reproductive Health. Newsletter
Related titles: Online - full content ed.
Published by: National Association of Nurse Practitioners in Women's Health, 503 Capitol Court, NE, Ste 300, Washington, DC 20002. TEL 202-543-9693, FAX 202-543-9858, info@npwh.org, http://www.npwh.org/newsletter1.htm.

613.7 USA
NATIONAL WOMEN'S HEALTH NETWORK. Text in English. bi-m. USD 25 (effective 2000).
Indexed: CHNI.
Address: 514 10th St, N W, Ste 400, Washington, DC 20004. TEL 202-347-1140, FAX 202-347-1168, http://www.womenshealthnetwork.org.

618.082 USA ISSN 0741-9147
NATIONAL WOMEN'S HEALTH REPORT. Text in English. 1984. bi-m. USD 25 to individuals; USD 75 to institutions. bk.rev. index. back issues avail. **Document type:** *Newsletter, Consumer.* **Description:** Covers medical and consumer issues relating to women's health.
Related titles: Online - full text ed.; (from LexisNexis, Northern Light Technology, Inc.).
Indexed: CINAHL, CWI, Gend.Watch.
—BLDSC (6033.412000).
Published by: National Women's Health Resource Center, 2425 L St, N W, 3rd Fl, Washington, DC 20037. TEL 202-293-6045, FAX 202-778-6306, nwhrc02@pop.erols.com. Ed. Heidi Rosvold Brenholtz. R&P Elizabeth A Battaglino. Circ: 30,000.

613.7 USA ISSN 8755-867X
NETWORK NEWS (WASHINGTON, 1975). Key Title: Network News - National Women's Health Network. Text in English. 1975. 6/yr. USD 25 to membership (effective 2000). bk.rev. **Document type:** *Consumer.* **Description:** For women's health activists. The network is a consciousness-raising political watchdog organization. Covers controversial issues and includes product alerts and interviews.
Former titles (until 1982): National Women's Health Network Newsletter (0277-0385); Network News
Related titles: Online - full text ed.: (from ProQuest Information & Learning, Gale Group).
Published by: National Women's Health Network, 514 10th St, N W, Ste 400, Washington, DC 20004. TEL 202-347-1140, FAX 202-347-1168, http://www.womenshealthnetwork.org. Ed. Lean Thayer. R&P Cynthia Pearson. Circ: 12,000 (paid).

NYUGAN NO RINSHO/JAPANESE JOURNAL OF BREAST CANCER. see *MEDICAL SCIENCES—Oncology*

O W L OBSERVER. see *GERONTOLOGY AND GERIATRICS*

ON THE ISSUES; the progressive woman's quarterly. see *WOMEN'S INTERESTS*

ONLINE BIRTH CENTER NEWS. see *MEDICAL SCIENCES—Obstetrics And Gynecology*

OUR SPECIAL; magazine devoted to matters of interest to blind women. see *HANDICAPPED—Visually Impaired*

OVULATION METHOD TEACHERS ASSOCIATION (PUBLICATION). see *BIRTH CONTROL*

613.082 790.1 CAN
OXYGEN!; serious fitness for serious women. Text in English. 1997. bi-m. USD 22.50 in US & Canada; USD 28.50 elsewhere. adv. **Document type:** *Consumer.* **Description:** Devoted to women's fitness.
Published by: Canusa Products, 6465 Airport Rd, Mississauga, ON L4V 1E4, Canada. TEL 905-678-7312, http://www.getbig.com/magazine/oxygen. Ed. Pamela Cottrell. Pub. Robert Kennedy. Adv. contact Rebecca Hall.

PRACTISING MIDWIFE; the voice of clinical midwifery. see *MEDICAL SCIENCES—Obstetrics And Gynecology*

PRIMARY CARE UPDATE FOR OB - GYNS. see *MEDICAL SCIENCES—Obstetrics And Gynecology*

613.082 CAN
PRO-CHOICE FORUM. Text in English. 1975. 3/yr. CND 10, USD 13. bk.rev. **Document type:** *Newsletter.* **Description:** Provides a national forum for news and opinion on abortion rights.
Formerly (until Dec. 1998): Pro-Choice News (0836-7221)
Published by: Canadian Abortion Rights Action League/Association Canadienne pour le Droit a l'Avortement, 1 Nicholas St, Ste 726, Ottawa, ON K1N 7B7, Canada. TEL 613-789-9956, FAX 613-789-9960, caral@caral.ca, http://www.caral.ca. Circ: 12,000.

057.86 CZE ISSN 1211-7404
PULS. Text in Czech. 1997. m. adv. **Document type:** *Magazine, Consumer.*
Formerly (until 1997): Fit Magazin (1211-6939)
Indexed: Russ.Acad.Sci.Bibl.
Published by: Mona Praha v.o.s., Mala Stepanska 17, Prague, 2 12079, Czech Republic. TEL 420-2-96162111, FAX 420-2-299423, mona@mona.cz, http://puls.mona.cz, http://www.mona.cz.

PULSE (ORLANDO). see *BIRTH CONTROL*

RADIANCE ONLINE; the magazine for large women. see *WOMEN'S INTERESTS*

613.082 GBR ISSN 1465-2803
REAL HEALTH & BEAUTY. Text in English. 1998. bi-m. GBP 2.30 newsstand/cover (effective 2001). adv. **Document type:** *Magazine, Consumer.* **Description:** Provides articles on a variety of topics including nutrition, fitness, complementary health and real-life stories, with the aim of empowering readers to take charge of their own health.
Published by: Attic Futura Ltd., 16-18 Berners St, London W1P 3DD, United Kingdom. TEL 44-20-7664-6400, FAX 44-20-7323-1854, viviencotterill@atticfutura.co.uk, http://www.atticfutura.co.uk. Ed. Rose Shillito. Pub. Bridget Marrison. Adv. contact Caroline Brookes. Circ: 41,050 (paid).

REDE NACIONAL FEMINISTA DE SAUDE E DIREITOS REPRODUTIVOS. JORNAL. see *WOMEN'S STUDIES*

618.082 USA
REGARDING WOMEN AND HEALTHCARE. Text in English. 3/yr. free per issue. **Document type:** *Newsletter.* **Description:** Discusses the emotional and physical health and well-being of women.
Published by: Robert Wood Johnson University Hospital, One Robert Wood Johnson Pl, New Brunswick, NJ 08901. TEL 732-828-3000. Ed. Maryann N Swierczek.

618.082 GBR ISSN 0968-8080
RG103 CODEN: RHMAFV
REPRODUCTIVE HEALTH MATTERS. Text in English; Summaries in French, Spanish. 1993. s-a. USD 60 in North America to institutions; USD 30 in North America to individuals; GBP 36 elsewhere to institutions; GBP 20 elsewhere to individuals (effective 2001). bk.rev. back issues avail. **Document type:** *Academic/Scholarly.* **Description:** Promotes laws, policies, research and services that meet women's reproductive health needs. Written by and for researchers and scientists, health service providers, health policy makers, women's health advocates, and people in related fields.
Related titles: Online - full text ed.: (from Institute for Scientific Information, RoweCom Information Quest).
Indexed: Abstr.Anthropol., CWI, Curr.Cont., Environ.Sci.Poll.Mgmt., Fem.Per. (1994-), Intl.Bibl.Soc.Sci., Lang.& Lang.Behav.Abstr., P.A.I.S., Popul.Ind., Rural Devel.Abstr., SOPODA, SSCI, Soc.Serv.Abstr., Sociol.Abstr., Stud.Wom.Abstr.
—BLDSC (7713.705700), GNLM, Infotrieve. **CCC.**
Published by: Blackwell Science Ltd., Osney Mead, Oxford OX2 0EL, United Kingdom. TEL 44-1865-206206, FAX 44-1865-721205, journals.cs@blacksci.co.uk, http://www.blackwell-science.com. Ed. Marge Berer. Pub. Elaine Stott. R&P Sophie Savage. Adv. contact Jenny Applin. Circ: 800.

RETT SYNDROME ASSOCIATION OF AUSTRALIA NEWSLETTER. see *MEDICAL SCIENCES—Psychiatry And Neurology*

618.082 CHL
REVISTA MUJER SALUD. Text in Spanish. 1984. q. CLP 8,000 domestic; USD 40 foreign (effective 2000). illus. *Refereed.* **Document type:** *Journal, Academic/Scholarly.* **Description:** Network news, opinions, analysis and up-to-date information on women's health issues.
Former titles: Red de Salud de las Mujeres Latinoamericanas y del Caribe. Revista (0716-8381); (until 1990): Red de Salud de las Mujeres Latinoamericanas y del Caribe. Boletin (0716-8489)
Related titles: English ed.: Women's Health Journal.
Published by: Fundacion Red de Salud de las Mujeres Latinoamericanas y del Caribe, Casilla 50610, Santiago 1, Santiago, Chile. TEL 56-2-2237077, FAX 56-2-2231066, rsmlac@mail.bellsouth.cl, http://www.reddesalud.web.cl. Ed. Deborah Meacham. Pub. Amparo Claro.

SAGE SERIES ON VIOLENCE AGAINST WOMEN. see *SOCIOLOGY*

613.082 ITA ISSN 1120-446X
SALVE; la salute della donne. Text in Italian. 1977. m. ITL 2,500 newsstand/cover. adv. illus. **Document type:** *Consumer.* **Description:** Reports on important topics in every area of women's health in a scientifically accurate, yet accessible manner.
Related titles: ♦ Supplement to: Anna (Italian Edition). ISSN 1120-4346.
Published by: R C S Periodici S.p.A. (Subsidiary of: R C S, Rizzoli - Corriere della Sera), Via Angelo Rizzoli, 2, Milan, MI 20132, Italy. TEL 39-02-2584-3647, FAX 39-02-2584-3903, info@periodici.rcs.it, http://www.rcs.it/inforcs/uk/strutt/periodic/testate/salve/scheda.htm, http://www.rsc.it/periodici. Ed. Ricardo Renzi. Adv. contact Flavio Biondi. Circ: 278,000 (paid).

SCARLET LETTER. see *WOMEN'S INTERESTS*

SELF. see *WOMEN'S INTERESTS*

SEMINARS IN BREAST DISEASE; diagnostic imaging, medical oncology, pathology, radiation oncology, surgery. see *MEDICAL SCIENCES—Obstetrics And Gynecology*

618.082 613.7 USA ISSN 0744-5121
SHAPE. Cover title: Joe Weider's Shape. Text in English. 1981. m. USD 19.97; USD 2.99 newsstand/cover domestic; GBP 2.25 newsstand/cover in United Kingdom (effective 2000). adv. bk.rev. illus. reprints avail. **Document type:** *Magazine, Consumer.* **Description:** Discusses health and nutrition for active women.
Related titles: Online - full text ed.: (from Northern Light Technology, Inc., ProQuest Information & Learning, America Online, Inc., Gale Group, Factiva).
Indexed: Hlth.Ind., Phys.Ed.Ind., Sportsearch (1983-).
—ingenta.

Published by: Weider Publications, 21100 Erwin St, Woodland Hills, CA 91367. TEL 818-884-6800, 800-340-8953, FAX 818-704-5734, http://www.shapemag.com. Ed. Barbara Harris. Pub. Joseph Weider. R&P Fiona Maynard. Adv. contact Jennifer Shelling. B&W page USD 57,770, color page USD 72,000; trim 10.5 x 7.88. Circ: 1,500,000 (paid). **Subscr. to:** PO Box 37207, Boone, IA 50037.

618.082 DEU ISSN 1422-9188
SHAPE. Text in German. 1998. m. DEM 60 domestic; CHF 60 in Switzerland; ATS 456 in Austria; DEM 68.40 elsewhere; DEM 5 newsstand/cover (effective 2000). adv. **Document type:** *Magazine, Consumer.* **Description:** Contains articles and features on how to get and stay in shape in healthy and fun ways.
Published by: M V G - Medien Verlagsgesellschaft mbH, Arabellastr. 33, Munich 81925, Germany. TEL 49-89-92340, FAX 49-89-9234202, http://www.shape.de. Ed. Benita Cantieni. Adv. contact Knut G Mueller.

618.082 USA
▼ **SHAPE PRESENTS FIT HOLLYWOOD.** Text in English. 2001 (Oct.). a. USD 3.99 newsstand/cover; USD 4.99 newsstand/cover in Canada (effective 2001). **Document type:** *Magazine, Consumer.* **Description:** Presents articles and features on the health and fitness secrets of celebrities.
Published by: Weider Publications, 21100 Erwin St, Woodland Hills, CA 91367. TEL 818-884-6800, 800-998-0731, FAX 818-716-5626.

618.082 ZAF
▼ **SHAPE SOUTH AFRICA.** Text in English. 2000. m. adv. **Document type:** *Magazine, Consumer.* **Description:** Aimed at women ages 20-34 years who are interested in and concerned with ways to improve their lives and realize the benefits of a healthier lifestyle.
Published by: Touchline Media, PO Box 16368, Vlaeberg, Cape Town 8018, South Africa. TEL 27-21-217810, FAX 27-21-215118, http://www.touchline.co.za. **Co-publisher:** Weider Publications.

613.082 GBR ISSN 1355-1868
SHE MAGAZINE GUIDE TO HAVING A BABY. Text in English. 1994. q. GBP 2.50 newsstand/cover. **Document type:** *Consumer.* **Description:** Comprehensive guide to all aspects of pregnancy and birth.
Published by: National Magazine Company Ltd., National Magazine House, 72 Broadwick St, London W1V 2BP, United Kingdom. TEL 44-20-7439-5000, FAX 44-207-437-6886. **Dist. by:** Comag, Tavistock Works, Tavistock Rd, W Drayton, Middx UB7 7QX, United Kingdom. TEL 44-1895-433600, FAX 44-1895-433602.

613.082 GBR
▼ **SHINE**; for a happier, healthier, sexier you. Text in English. 1999. m. GBP 2.60 newsstand/cover (effective 2001). **Document type:** *Magazine, Consumer.* **Description:** Contains articles and features with a strong health and beauty focus which incorporates fashion, real life and relationships.
Published by: Attic Futura Ltd., 16-18 Berners St, London W1P 3DD, United Kingdom. TEL 44-20-7664-6400, FAX 44-20-7323-1854, viviencotterill@atticfutura.co.uk, http://www.atticfutura.co.uk. Ed. Lucy Bulmer. Pub. Bridget Marrison. Adv. contact Emma Greenhalgh. Circ: 102,002 (paid).

SOBERING THOUGHTS. see *DRUG ABUSE AND ALCOHOLISM*

SPECIAL DELIVERY. see *MEDICAL SCIENCES—Obstetrics And Gynecology*

618.082 155.3 USA ISSN 0272-202X
SPRINGER SERIES: FOCUS ON WOMEN. Text in English. 1980. irreg., latest vol.18, 1998. price varies. **Document type:** *Monographic series.* **Description:** Explores women's issues from a psychological perspective.
Indexed: e-psyche.
Published by: Springer Publishing Company, 536 Broadway, New York, NY 10012. TEL 212-431-4370, FAX 212-941-7842, springer@springerpub.com, http://www.springerpub.com. Ed. Violet Franks. R&P Dorothy Kouwenberg.

613.082 USA
▼ **STRIVE.** Text in English. 2001. 10/yr. USD 10 (effective 2001). adv. **Document type:** *Magazine, Consumer.* **Description:** Presents cutting-edge lifestyle information for women on health, fitness, beauty, and other related topics.
Related titles: Online - full text ed.; Supplement: Strive: Action, Sports & Supplements Issue.
Published by: StriveMedia, 1209 Manhattan Ave, Ste 218, Manhattan Beach, CA 90266. TEL 310-563-6200, FAX 310-563-6220, info@striveonline.com, advertise@striveonline.com, http://www.striveonline.com. Ed. Mary Monroe. Pubs. Brett Benning, Samie Benning. Adv. contact Adam Ginsberg.

T R A C NEWSLETTER. (Transvaal Rural Action Committee) see *POLITICAL SCIENCE—Civil Rights*

▼ **TODAY'S HEALTH AND WELLNESS.** see *PHYSICAL FITNESS AND HYGIENE*

618.082 052 GBR ISSN 0967-6678
TOP SANTE; health & beauty. Text in English. 1993. m. GBP 23; GBP 1.95 newsstand/cover (effective 1999). adv. bk.rev. illus. back issues avail. **Document type:** *Magazine, Consumer.* **Description:** Looks at health, beauty, and well-being. Covers everything from overcoming common ailments to medical reports.
Related titles: French ed.: ISSN 1152-7137.
Published by: Emap Elan Ltd. (Subsidiary of: Emap Consumer Magazines Ltd.), Endeavour House, 189 Shaftesbury Ave, London WC2H 8JG, United Kingdom. TEL 44-207-437-9011, FAX 44-207-208-3709, http://www.emap.com. Ed. Jane Garton. Pub. Elizabeth Rees Jones. Adv. contact Jacqui Elliot. Circ: 148,064 (paid). **Subscr. to:** Tower Publishing Services Ltd., Tower House, Sovereign Park, Lathkill St, Market Harborough, Leics LE16 9EF, United Kingdom. TEL 44-1858-438833, FAX 44-1858-434958.

▼ **TRADITIONAL KITCHENS PRESENT**; Mary Dee's quick and tasty recipes. see *NUTRITION AND DIETETICS*

613.7 CAN
TURNER'S SYNDROME NEWS. Text in English. 1982. q. CND 50 to individuals; CND 75 to institutions; CND 25 to students (effective 2000). **Document type:** *Newsletter.*
Published by: Turner's Syndrome Society, 814 Glencairn Ave, Toronto, ON M6B 2A3, Canada. TEL 416-781-2086, 800-465-6744, FAX 416-781-7245, tssincan@web.net, http://www.turnersyndrome.ca. Ed. Sandi Hofbauer. Circ: 500.

VENEREOLOGY; the interdisciplinary international journal of sexual health. see *MEDICAL SCIENCES—Dermatology And Venereology*

618.082 USA ISSN 1069-742X
VIA (WARREN)✶ ; a guide through menopause and beyond. Text in English. 1993. q. USD 19.97. bk.rev. **Document type:** *Consumer.* **Description:** Covers healthcare issues, particularly peri- and postmenopause for mature women.
Published by: (National Coalition for Consumer Education, Inc.), Carrington Communications, Inc., PO Box 4227, Warren, NJ 07059-0227. TEL 201-584-3040, FAX 201-584-8867. Ed. Dr. Karen Hutchinson. Pub. Pamela Boggs. adv.: B&W page USD 3,500, color page USD 5,600. Circ: 50,000 (paid).

VIOLENCE AGAINST WOMEN; an international and interdisciplinary journal. see *SOCIOLOGY*

618.082 USA
W O R L D; a newsletter by, for and about women facing HIV disease. (Women Organized to Respond to Life-Threatening Diseases) Text in English. 1991. m. (Spanish ed. q.). USD 20 to individuals; USD 50 to institutions. adv. **Document type:** *Newsletter.* **Description:** Discusses social and medical issues women facing HIV disease encounter and lists important forthcoming conferences throughout the world.
Related titles: Spanish ed.
Indexed: CWI.
Address: PO Box 11535, Oakland, CA 94611. TEL 510-986-0340, FAX 510-986-0341. Ed., R&P Rebecca Denison. Adv. contact Sandi Luna.

613.082 DEU ISSN 1617-1950
▼ **WELLFIT.** Text in German. 2000. m. DEM 106.80 domestic; DEM 145.20 in Europe; DEM 258 elsewhere; DEM 4.50 newsstand/cover (effective 2001). adv. **Document type:** *Magazine, Consumer.* **Description:** Contains a variety of articles and features for women on fitness, beauty, health, fashion, sex and travel.
Published by: Burda Verlag GmbH, Arabellastr 23, Munich 81925, Germany. TEL 49-89-9250-0, FAX 49-89-92503519, http://www.burda.de. Ed. Ulrike Schlueter. Adv. contact Wolfgang Plate. B&W page XEU 10,440, color page XEU 13,044. **Subscr. to:** Postfach 290, Offenburg 77649, Germany.

613 USA
WHAT'S HAPPENING IN A M W A. Text in English. bi-m. membership. back issues avail. **Document type:** *Newsletter.* **Description:** Aims to improve the professional development and personal well-being of its members and to promote women's health.
Published by: American Medical Women's Association, Inc., 801 N Fairfax Dr, Ste 400, Alexandria, VA 22314. TEL 703-838-0500, FAX 703-549-3864, kmills@amwa-doc.org. Ed. Kelli Mills. Circ: 10,000.

610 USA ISSN 0363-0242
RG1 CODEN: WOHEDI
WOMEN & HEALTH; the multidisciplinary journal of women's health issues. Text in English. 1976. q. (2 vols./yr.). USD 60 to individuals; USD 81 in Canada to individuals; USD 87 elsewhere to individuals; USD 120 to institutions; USD 162 in Canada to institutions; USD 174 elsewhere to institutions; USD 335 to libraries; USD 452 in Canada to libraries; USD 486 elsewhere to libraries (effective Aug. 2001). adv. bk.rev. illus. back issues avail.; reprint service avail. from HAW,ISI. *Refereed.* **Document type:** *Journal, Academic/Scholarly.* **Description:** Contains information that is useful for all women, consumers, and providers of health care.
Related titles: Microfiche ed.: (from PQC); Microform ed.; Online - full text ed.: (from LexisNexis, Gale Group, Factiva, Institute for Scientific Information).
Indexed: ASCA, Abstr.Anthropol., Abstr.Crim.& Pen., Abstr.Health Care Manage.Stud., Abstr.Hyg., Adol.Ment.Hlth.Abstr., AgeLine, Alt.Press Ind., Bibl.Asian Stud. (1998), Biol.Abstr., Biol.Dig., CINAHL, CWI, Child Devel.Abstr., Crim.Just.Abstr., Curr.Cont., Curr.Lit.Fam.Plan., Dairy Sci.Abstr., ERA, Environ.Sci.Poll.Mgmt., Excerp.Med., Fem.Per. (1981-), Gen.Sci.Ind. (Jun.1992-), Gend.Watch, High.Educ.Abstr., Hlth.Ind., IBZ, IMFL, INIS Atomind., Ind.Med. (1976-), Lang.& Lang.Behav.Abstr., Med.Care Rev., Mult.Ed.Abstr., NRN, Nutr.Abstr., P.A.I.S., Pollut.Abstr., PsycInfo, Psychol.Abstr. (1979-), Ref.Zh., Risk Abstr., Rural Devel.Abstr., SOPODA, SSCI, Saf.Sci.Abstr., Sage Fam.Stud.Abstr., Sage Race Rel.Abstr., Soc.Sci.Ind. (Mar.1987-), Soc.Serv.Abstr., Soc.Work Res.& Abstr., Sociol.Abstr., Stud.Wom.Abstr., Trop.Dis.Bull., Viol.& Abuse Abstr., Wom.Stud.Abstr. (1976-), Wom.Stud.Ind., e-psyche.
—BLDSC (9343.260000), EMDOCS, GNLM, Haworth, IDS, ingenta, KNAW.
Published by: Haworth Press, Inc., 10 Alice St, Binghamton, NY 13904-1580. TEL 607-722-5857, 800-429-6784, FAX 607-722-6362, 800-895-0582, getinfo@haworthpressinc.com, http://www.haworthpress.com/journals/journallist.asp. Ed. Jeanne M Stellman. Pub. William Cohen. R&P Ruthann Heath TEL 607-723-5857 ext 316. Adv. contact Jackie Blakeslee TEL 607-722-5857 ext 346. B&W page USD 315, color page USD 550; trim 6 x 8.5. Circ: 1,225.

WOMEN & THERAPY; a feminist quarterly. see *PSYCHOLOGY*

610 USA
WOMEN IN CONTEXT. Text in English. 1978. irreg., latest vol.1. price varies. back issues avail. *Refereed.* **Document type:** *Monographic series.*
Formerly: Women in Context: Development and Stresses
Indexed: MLA Intl.Bibl. (coverage dropped).
Published by: Kluwer Academic - Plenum Publishers (Subsidiary of: Wolters Kluwer N.V.), 233 Spring St, New York, NY 10013-1578. TEL 212-620-8000, 800-221-9369, FAX 212-463-0742, info@plenum.com, http://www.plenum.com. Eds. C Robinowitz, J Spurlock.

WOMEN TODAY MAGAZINE. see *WOMEN'S INTERESTS*

613.9 NLD ISSN 1021-173X
WOMEN'S GLOBAL NETWORK FOR REPRODUCTIVE RIGHTS. NEWSLETTER. Text in English, French, Spanish. 1978. q. NLG 90 (effective 2001). bk.rev. *Refereed.* **Document type:** *Newsletter.* **Description:** Contains worldwide news on abortion, contraception and women's health issues.
Formerly (until 1988): Women's Global Network on Reproductive Rights (0921-304X)
Related titles: French ed.: Reseau Mondial des Femmes pour les Droits sur la Reproduction. ISSN 1021-1748; Spanish ed.

Published by: Women's Global Network for Reproductive Rights/Red Mundial de Mujeres para los Derechos Reproductivos, NZ Voorburgwal 32, Amsterdam 1012 RZ, Netherlands. TEL 31-20-620-9672, FAX 31-20-622-2450, office@wgnrr.nl. Ed. Sumati Nair.

613.082 GBR ISSN 1463-9106
WOMEN'S HEALTH. Text in English. m. GBP 26; GBP 2.20 newsstand/cover (effective 1999). **Document type:** *Consumer.*
Indexed: Int.Nurs.Ind.
Published by: W V Publications and Exhibitions Ltd., 57-59 Rochester Pl, London NW1 9JG, United Kingdom. TEL 44-20-7485-0011, FAX 44-20-7482-6269, wvmags@computer.com. **Dist. by:** Comag, Tavistock Works, Tavistock Rd, W Drayton, Middx UB7 7QX, United Kingdom. TEL 44-1895-433600, FAX 44-1895-433602.

618.082 USA
WOMEN'S HEALTH ADVISOR. Text in English. 1998. m. USD 32 domestic; USD 42 foreign (effective 2000). *Refereed.* **Document type:** *Newsletter.* **Description:** Brings together important health tips from all fields of Women's medicine.
Published by: Weill Cornell Medical College, Center for Women's Healthcare, 1300 York Ave, New York, NY 10021. TEL 800-847-7131. Ed. Gabrielle I Weiner. Pub. Dr. Orli R Etingin. **Subscr. to:** PO Box 420235, Palm Coast, FL 32142-0235.

613 USA
▼ **WOMEN'S HEALTH & FITNESS.** Text in English. 2002 (Jan.). bi-m. USD 4.99 newsstand/cover (effective 2001). **Document type:** *Magazine, Consumer.* **Description:** Contains information on health, fitness, nutrition, diet, recipes, wellness, relationships, children, careers and financial matters.
Published by: Highbury House Communications, Inc., 1925 Vaughn Rd Ste 235, Kennesaw, GA 30411. TEL 770-422-3225, http://www.womenshealthfitnessmagazine.com, http://www.hhc.co.uk/. Ed. David Pritchard TEL 770-422-3225 (ext 229). Circ: 150,000.

618.082 USA ISSN 1078-7674
WOMEN'S HEALTH DIGEST. Text in English. 1994. q. USD 28. adv. bk.rev. **Document type:** *Consumer.* **Description:** Inclues coverage of how medical afflictions affect women, along with reviews of methods of diagnosis and various available treatments. Features "Updating the Updates" which reviews information and develops a consensus opinion on "medical breakthroughs" covered in previous issues.
Published by: National Menopause Foundation, Inc., 222 S W 36th Terrace, Gainesville, FL 32607. TEL 352-372-9990. Ed. Eugenia Scharf. Pub. Morris Notelovitz. R&P, Adv. contact Elizabeth Reyes.

618 USA ISSN 1049-3867
RG1 CODEN: WHISEH
WOMEN'S HEALTH ISSUES. Text in English. 1991. 6/yr. EUR 105 in Europe to individuals; JPY 14,500 in Japan to individuals; USD 118 elsewhere to individuals; EUR 218 in Europe to institutions; JPY 28,900 in Japan to institutions; USD 243 elsewhere to institutions (effective 2002). adv. illus. back issues avail.; reprints avail. *Refereed.* **Document type:** *Academic/Scholarly.* **Description:** For health professionals, social scientists, policy makers, and others concerned with developments affecting health care for women.
Related titles: Microform ed.: (from PQC); Online - full text ed.: (from ingenta, Swets Blackwell, Institute for Scientific Information, ScienceDirect).
Indexed: ASCA, AgeLine, CINAHL, Curr.Cont., Environ.Sci.Poll.Mgmt., Excerp.Med. (1993-), Fam.Ind., Ind.Med. (1990-), Inpharma, Int.Nurs.Ind., Jrnl.Watch Wom.Hlth., Lang.& Lang.Behav.Abstr., Pollut.Abstr., Reac., SOPODA, SSCI, Soc.Serv.Abstr., Sociol.Abstr., Stud.Wom.Abstr.
—BLDSC (9343.379010), EMDOCS, GNLM, IDS, Infotrieve, ingenta, KNAW. **CCC.**
Published by: (Jacobs Institute of Women's Health), Elsevier Science, 655 Ave of the Americas, New York, NY 10010. FAX 212-633-3990, usinfo-f@elsevier.com, http://www.elsevier.nl/locate/issn/10493867. Eds. C S Weisman, Warren Pearse. Adv. contact Hank Blaney. B&W page USD 985, color page USD 2,160. Circ: 3,000 (paid). **Subscr. in Australasia and the Far East to:** Elsevier Science (Singapore) Pte Ltd, No.1 Temasek Ave, 17-01 Millenia Tower, Singapore 039192, Singapore. TEL 65-434-3727, FAX 65-337-2230; **Subscr. in Japan to:** Elsevier Science Inc - Japan Regional Office, 9-15 Higashi-Azabu 1-chome, Minato-ku, Tokyo 106-0044, Japan. TEL 81-3-5561-5033; **Subscr. outside the Americas to:** Elsevier Science BV, PO Box 211, Amsterdam 1000 AE, Netherlands. TEL 31-20-485-3757.

618.082 USA ISSN 1062-4163
WOMEN'S HEALTH LETTER; the monthly review of women's health issues. Text in English. 1992. m. USD 39; USD 52 foreign. bk.rev. charts, illus. back issues avail. **Document type:** *Newsletter.* **Description:** Covers information and issues concerning women's health, including research findings and viewpoints of leading experts from around the world.
Published by: Soundview, 7100 Peachtree Dunwoody Rd, Ste 100, Atlanta, GA 30328. TEL 770-399-5617, FAX 770-669-0692. Ed. Kerri Bodmer. Pub. Wallis Wood. R&P Garret Wood. Circ: 30,000. **Subscr. to:** PO Box 467939, Atlanta, GA 31146-7939.

613.082 USA ISSN 1067-9340
WOMEN'S HEALTH MONITOR. Text in English. 1993. bi-m. **Document type:** *Newsletter, Consumer.*
Published by: Data Centrum Communications, Inc., 21 W 38th St, 4th fl, New York, NY 10018.

618.082 GBR ISSN 0954-6677
WOMEN'S HEALTH NEWSLETTER. Text in English. 1984. q. GBP 12 in United Kingdom to individuals; GBP 15 in Europe to individuals; GBP 17 elsewhere to individuals; GBP 2.50 newsstand/cover (effective 2001). bk.rev. abstr. 26 p./no. 2 cols./p. back issues avail. *Refereed.* **Document type:** *Newsletter, Consumer.* **Description:** Contains health news abstracted from medical journals and health information features.
Published by: Women's Health, 52 Featherstone St, London EC1Y 8RT, United Kingdom. TEL 44-20-7251-6333, FAX 44-20-7250-4152, womenshealth@pop3.poptel.org.uk, http://www.womenshealthlondon.org.uk. Ed., R&P Tamara Beus. Circ: 600 (paid).

618.082 USA
WOMEN'S HEALTH SOURCE BOOK. Text in English. 1995. a., latest vol.4, 1999. USD 295 domestic; USD 325 foreign (effective 2001). **Document type:** *Trade.*
Published by: American Health Consultants (Subsidiary of: Medical Economics Co., Inc.), 3525 Piedmont Rd, N E, 6 Piedmont Center, Ste 400, Atlanta, GA 30305. TEL 404-262-5476, 404-262-7436, 800-688-2421, FAX 404-262-7837, 800-284-3291, custserv@ahcpub.com, http://www.ahcpub.com.

613.082 USA ISSN 1078-7240
WOMEN'S HEALTH WEEKLY. Text in English. w. (43/yr.). USD 342; USD 367 foreign. cum.index: bi-m. **Document type:** *Newsletter.* **Description:** Reports current news of women's health issues, including news reports and research from wire services and conferences. Aims to present clinical and non-clinical perspectives which can be understood by persons without a medical degree.
Related titles: Online - full text ed.: (from Factiva).
Published by: SerialsSEARCH Publications, PO Box 709, Hartwell, GA 30643. TEL 706-376-1915, FAX 706-376-4214, whw@serialsearch.com, http://www.newsfile.com/1w.htm. Ed., Pub. Alan D Henderson.

613.082 616.89 USA
WOMEN'S MENTAL HEALTH & DEVELOPMENT. Abbreviated title: W M H & D. Text in English. irreg., latest vol.2, 1997.
Indexed: e-psyche.
—BLDSC.
Published by: Sage Publications, Inc., 2455 Teller Rd, Thousand Oaks, CA 91320. TEL 805-499-0721, FAX 805-499-0871, info@sagepub.com, http://www.sagepub.com. R&P Tanya Udin. **Overseas subscr. to:** Sage Publications Ltd., 6 Bonhill St, London EC2A 4PU, United Kingdom; Sage Publications India Pvt. Ltd., 4215, New Delhi 110 048, India.

613.7 USA ISSN 1069-4927
WOMEN'S PHYSIQUE WORLD. Text in English. q. USD 3.95 per issue. **Document type:** *Magazine, Consumer.* **Description:** Covers contests and features biographical articles on competitive women bodybuilders.
Published by: Women's Physique Magazine, PO Box 429, Midland Park, NJ 07432. TEL 201-825-7448, orders@wpwmagazine.com, http://www.wpwmagazine.com. Ed. Steve Wennerstrom.

613 305.4 USA ISSN 0890-9695
WOMENWISE. Text in English. 1978. q. USD 15 to individuals; USD 20 to institutions. adv. bk.rev. back issues avail. *Refereed.* **Document type:** *Consumer.* **Description:** Covers women's health issues from a feminist perspective. Includes political analyses.
Related titles: CD-ROM ed.; Online - full text ed.: (from Northern Light Technology, Inc.).
Indexed: Gend.Watch.
Published by: Concord Feminist Health Center, 38 S Main St, Concord, NH 03301. TEL 603-225-2739, FAX 603-668-6255. Ed. Luita D Spangler. Adv. contact Susanne Hendrick. Circ: 5,000.

WORLD MEDICAL JOURNAL. see *MEDICAL SCIENCES*

THE YEAR BOOK OF OBSTETRICS, GYNECOLOGY, AND WOMEN'S HEALTH. see *MEDICAL SCIENCES—Obstetrics And Gynecology*

613.082 GBR ISSN 1351-0207
YOUR COMPLETE GUIDE TO PREGNANCY & BIRTH. Text in English. 1993. m. GBP 2.10 newsstand/cover. adv. illus. **Document type:** *Consumer.* **Description:** For pregnant women. Covers health, relationships, fitness, fashion, emotion, shopping, and reader's experiences. Includes assurance from women who have been there and advise from trustworthy experts.
Published by: Emap Elan Ltd. (Subsidiary of: Emap Consumer Magazines Ltd.), Endeavour House, 189 Shaftesbury Ave, London WC2H 8JG, United Kingdom. TEL 44-207-437-9011, FAX 44-207-208-3709, http://www.emap.com. Ed. Valery McConnell. Adv. contact Roya Croudace. **Subscr. to:** Tower Publishing Services Ltd., Tower House, Sovereign Park, Lathkill St, Market Harborough, Leics LE16 9EF, United Kingdom. TEL 44-1858-435339, FAX 44-1858-434958. **Dist. by:** Frontline Ltd., Unit 6, Stockwell Centre, Stephenson Way, Crawley, W Sussex RH10 1TN, United Kingdom. TEL 44-1733-555161, FAX 44-1293-415009.

613.05 GBR ISSN 1367-9708
YOUR HEALTH. Text in English. 1991. bi-m. GBP 7.80; GBP 1.95 newsstand/cover (effective 1999). **Document type:** *Consumer.*
Former titles (until 1997): Your Healthcare (1364-8799); (until 1996): Healthcare (0964-8925)
Published by: W V Publications and Exhibitions Ltd., 57-59 Rochester Pl, London NW1 9JG, United Kingdom. TEL 44-20-7331-1000, FAX 44-20-7331-1242.

613.082 RUS
ZHENSKOE ZDOROV'E. Text in Russian. bi-m. USD 109 in United States.
Published by: Novosti Nauki, A-ya 446, Moscow 104014, Russian Federation. TEL 7-095-5541552, FAX 7-095-1465965. Ed. I I Mosin. **US dist. addr.:** East View Publications, 3020 Harbor Ln N, Minneapolis, MN 55447. TEL 612-550-0961.

WOMEN'S HEALTH—Abstracting, Bibliographies, Statistics

016.618 USA ISSN 1521-4710
JOURNAL WATCH WOMEN'S HEALTH. Text in English. 1996 (Apr.). m. USD 89. 8 p./no. **Document type:** *Newsletter.* **Description:** Presents concise summaries of important research appearing in the women's health literature.
Published by: Massachusetts Medical Society, P O Box 9085, Waltham, MA 02254-9085.

016.613082 NZL ISSN 1173-9282
L M S ALERT. WOMEN'S HEALTH. (Literature Monitoring and Evaluation Service) Text in English. 1996. m. charts. *Refereed.* **Document type:** *Abstract/Index.*
Related titles: CD-ROM ed.; Online - full text ed.
Published by: Adis International Limited, Mairangi Bay, Private Bag 65901, Auckland 1010, New Zealand. TEL 64-9-477-0700, natalie.avenell@adis.com, http://www.adis.com. Ed. Natalie Avenell. Pub. Christopher J Mellor.

WOMEN'S INTERESTS

96 INC. see *LITERATURE*

A M A ALLIANCE TODAY. (American Medical Association) see *MEDICAL SCIENCES*

AMERICAN ASSOCIATION OF WOMEN DENTISTS. CHRONICLE. see *MEDICAL SCIENCES—Dentistry*

618 MYS
ASIAN AND PACIFIC WOMEN'S RESOURCE AND ACTION SERIES. Text in English. 1989. irreg. free per issue. *Refereed.* **Document type:** *Newsletter.* **Description:** Provides a forum for women's experiences and thoughts on issues critical to women's health, the environment, work and law from a Third World perspective.
Indexed: Abstr.Rural Dev.Trop.
Published by: Asian and Pacific Development Centre, PO Box 12224, Kuala Lumpur 50770, Malaysia. TEL 60-3-254-8088, FAX 60-3-255-0316, info@apdc.po.my, http://www.apdc.co.my/apdc. Ed. Noeleen Heyzerc.

ASSOCIATION OF MEDICAL WOMEN IN INDIA. JOURNAL. see *WOMEN'S HEALTH*

BEGINNINGS (FLAGSTAFF); the official newslettr of the American holistic nurses' association. see *MEDICAL SCIENCES—Nurses And Nursing*

BEST DIET. see *NUTRITION AND DIETETICS*

613.082 646.72 GBR
BOOTS HEALTH & BEAUTY. Variant title: Health & Beauty. Text in English. q. **Document type:** *Magazine, Consumer.*
Published by: Redwood Publishing, 7 St Martin's Pl, London WC2N 4HA, United Kingdom. TEL 44-20-7747-0700, FAX 44-20-7747-0701, infohub@redwoodgroup.net, http://www.redwood-publishing.com. Circ: 1,916,790.

CLIO; die Zeitschrift fuer Frauengesundheit. see *WOMEN'S HEALTH*

305.4 613.082 USA ISSN 0885-4319
COMMITTEE ON SOUTH ASIAN WOMEN BULLETIN. Text in English. 1983. irreg. USD 25 per issue (effective 1999). bk.rev. back issues avail. **Document type:** *Bulletin, Academic/Scholarly.*
Published by: Committee on South Asian Women, c/o Texas A & M, Psychology Department, College Station, TX 77843-4235. TEL 409-845-2576, FAX 409-845-4727. Ed. J Vaid.

CURRENT RESEARCH IN FAMILY & COMMUNITY SCIENCES. see *HOME ECONOMICS*

DE TEXTOS. see *SOCIOLOGY*

DIANE. see *HANDICAPPED—Visually Impaired*

305.42 ITA ISSN 1120-5024
DONNA MODERNA. Text in Italian. 1988. w. ITL 75,900; ITL 365,200 foreign. illus. **Document type:** *Consumer.*
Published by: Arnoldo Mondadori Editore S.p.A., Casella Postale 1833, Milan, MI 20101, Italy. TEL 39-2-3199345, FAX 39-2-75422302, http://www.mondadori.com. Ed. Patrizia Avoledo. adv.: page ITL 64,800,000. Circ: 630,000.

371.822 EST ISSN 0235-7488
HQ1104
EESTI NAINE; a magazine for women. Text in Estonian. 1924. m. USD 134 in United States. adv. illus.
Formerly: Noukogude Naine (0134-2312)
Indexed: Russ.Acad.Sci.Bibl.
Address: Tartu 31, Tallinn, Estonia. TEL 370-6419211, FAX 370-6419212, katrin@eak.ee. Ed. Katrin Streimann. Adv. contact Reet Maran. Circ: 15,000. **Dist. by:** Mezhdunarodnaya Kniga, B Yakimanka 39, Moscow 117049, Russian Federation. TEL 7-095-2384967, FAX 7-095-2384934; **US dist. addr.:** East View Publications, 3020 Harbor Ln N, Minneapolis, MN 55447. TEL 612-550-0961.

ENDOMETRIOSIS ASSOCIATION NEWSLETTER. see *WOMEN'S HEALTH*

EQUAL TIME: OUTREACH NEWSLETTER. see *HOMOSEXUALITY*

305.4 USA
EVOLVING WOMAN; A Woman's Guide to Wholeness. Text in English. 1994. m. USD 24 (effective 2000). adv. bk.rev. illus. 40 p./no. 4 cols./p. back issues avail. **Document type:** *Consumer.* **Description:** Covers self-help, spirituality and women's empowerment.
Indexed: e-psyche.
Published by: Jill Dutton, Ed. & Pub., 9320 Haskins St., Lenexa, KS 66215-3611. TEL 913-438-1156, FAX 913-438-1156, evolving@thirdwave.net. R&P, Adv. contact Jill Dutton. B&W page USD 657, color page USD 857; trim 13 x 10. Circ: 20,000 (controlled).

FIELD ADVOCATE. see *GERONTOLOGY AND GERIATRICS*

FIT PREGNANCY. see *MEDICAL SCIENCES—Obstetrics And Gynecology*

▼ **FIT PREGNANCY EN ESPANOL.** see *MEDICAL SCIENCES—Obstetrics And Gynecology*

FITNESS; mind - body - spirit for women. see *PHYSICAL FITNESS AND HYGIENE*

GLOS KOBIETY; dwumiesiecznik dla pan. see *HANDICAPPED—Visually Impaired*

GREAT EXPECTATIONS. see *MEDICAL SCIENCES—Obstetrics And Gynecology*

IN VERWACHTING. see *CHILDREN AND YOUTH—About*

J A M A CONTRACEPTION NEWSLINE. (Journal of the American Medical Association) see *BIRTH CONTROL*

▼ **JOURNAL OF COUPLE & RELATIONSHIP THERAPY.** see *PSYCHOLOGY*

KATERN VROUWENZELFHULP. see *WOMEN'S HEALTH*

L F L REPORTS. see *BIRTH CONTROL*

MADAM. see *HANDICAPPED—Visually Impaired*

305.42 NLD ISSN 0025-2956
MARGRIET. Text in Dutch. 1938. w. NLG 161.20 (effective 2000); NLG 3.35 newsstand/cover. adv. bk.rev. illus. **Document type:** *Magazine, Consumer.* **Description:** Offers women articles on issues and trends in health, fitness, and living.
Related titles: Online - full content ed.: MargrietOnline.
Published by: V N U Tijdschriften B.V., Postbus 1900, Hoofddorp 2130 JH, Netherlands. TEL 31-23-556-6770, FAX 31-23-556-6771, redactie@margriet.nl, ServiceTeam@tijdschriften.vnu.com, http://www.margriet.nl, http://www.vnu.nl. Eds. Anneliese Bergman, Rob van Vuure. adv.: B&W page NLG 31,256, color page NLG 44,650. Circ: 478,000.

305.4 USA ISSN 1061-348X
MIDLIFE WOMAN. Text in English. 1991. bi-m. USD 30 domestic to individuals; USD 35 in Canada & Mexico to individuals; USD 40 elsewhere to individuals; USD 60 domestic to institutions; USD 65 in Canada & Mexico to institutions; USD 70 elsewhere to institutions. bk.rev. 12 p./no. **Document type:** *Newsletter.* **Description:** Presents in-depth information on menopause and midlife issues including hormone therapy and alternatives, diet, exercise and relaxation, dealing with aging parents, heart disease, osteoporosis, hysterectomy and more.
Related titles: CD-ROM ed.; Online - full text ed.: (from Northern Light Technology, Inc.).
Indexed: CWI, Fem.Per. (1996-1997).
Published by: MidLife Women's Network, 5129 Logan Ave S, Minneapolis, MN 55419-1019. TEL 612-915-0020, 800-886-4354, FAX 612-925-0020, mdlfwoman@aol.com, http://users.aol.com/mdlfwoman/info.htm. Ed. Sharon Roe. Pub. Sharon Slettehaugh.

362 PAK ISSN 0379-2617
MOTHER AND CHILD. Text in English. 1965-1972; resumed 1974. q. PKR 100, USD 15 per issue (effective 2001). adv. bk.rev. back issues avail. **Document type:** *Journal.*
Related titles: CD-ROM ed.
Indexed: ExtraMED.
Published by: Maternity & Child Welfare Association of Pakistan, MCH House, 30-F, Gulberg-II, Lahore 54666, Pakistan. TEL 92-42-5756959, FAX 92-42-5710839, mcwap@pol.com.pk. Eds. Akram Sheikh, Dr. N Rehan. Circ: 1,000.

MOTHER'S DAY REPORT. see *GERONTOLOGY AND GERIATRICS*

NEW PARENT. see *MEDICAL SCIENCES—Obstetrics And Gynecology*

NIGHTINGALE. see *MEDICAL SCIENCES—Nurses And Nursing*

O W L OBSERVER. see *GERONTOLOGY AND GERIATRICS*

323.4 USA ISSN 0895-6014
RA564.85
ON THE ISSUES; the progressive woman's quarterly. Text in English. 1983. q. USD 14.95 to individuals; USD 21.95 foreign to individuals; USD 24.95 to institutions; USD 31.95 foreign to institutions (effective 2000). adv. bk.rev. illus. back issues avail.; reprints avail. **Document type:** *Academic/Scholarly.* **Description:** Feminist, humanist magazine of critical thinking dedicated to fostering collective responsibility for positive social change.
Related titles: Online - full text ed.: (from Northern Light Technology, Inc., LexisNexis).
Indexed: Access (1993-), Alt.Press Ind., Amer.Bibl.Slavic & E.Eur.Stud., CWI, Fem.Per. (1987-), Gend.Watch, Stud.Wom.Abstr.
—ingenta.
Published by: (Choices Women's Medical Center), Merle Hoffman Enterprises, Ltd., 29-28, 41st Ave., 12th Fl., Long Island City, NY 11101-3303. FAX 718-349-9458, ontheissues@compuserve.com, http://www.choiceswomensmedical.com, http://www.echonyc.com/. Eds. Jan Goodwin, Merle Hoffman. Pub. Merle Hoffman. Adv. contact Lori Sokol. Circ: 50,000.

OUR SPECIAL; magazine devoted to matters of interest to blind women. see *HANDICAPPED—Visually Impaired*

OUTLOOK (SEATTLE); reproductive health. see *PUBLIC HEALTH AND SAFETY*

PARENTS PREGNANCY. see *MEDICAL SCIENCES—Obstetrics And Gynecology*

PSYCHOLOGIE UND GESELLSCHAFTSKRITIK. see *PSYCHOLOGY*

305.42 USA
RADIANCE ONLINE; the magazine for large women. Text in English. q. **Document type:** *Magazine, Consumer.*
Media: Online - full text (from LexisNexis). **Related titles:** ♦ Print ed.: Radiance. ISSN 0889-9495.
Published by: Radiance, PO Box 30246, Oakland, CA 94604. TEL 510-482-0680, FAX 510-482-1576, nfo@radiancemagazine.com, info@radiancemagazine.com, http://www.radiancemagazine.com, http://www.radiancemagazine.com.

363 AUS ISSN 0311-7057
SCARLET LETTER✱. Text in English. 1969. bi-m. adv. bk.rev.
Formerly (until May 1977): C S M C News
Published by: National Council of Single Mothers and their Children, 220 Victoria Sq, Torrens Bldg, Adelaide, SA 5000, Australia. TEL 61-8-82262505, FAX 61-8-82262509, ncsmc@adelaide.on.net. Ed. Sharon Good. Circ: 2,000.

305.42 USA ISSN 0149-0699
RA778.A1
SELF. Text in English. 1979. m. USD 16 domestic; USD 27 in Canada; USD 30 foreign; USD 2.99 newsstand/cover; USD 3.95 newsstand/cover in Canada (effective 2001). adv. illus. reprint service avail. from PQC. **Document type:** *Magazine, Consumer.* **Description:** Concentrates on women's total well-being, including beauty, fitness, fashion, nutrition, health, psychology, and business issues.
Related titles: Microform ed.: (from PQC); Online - full text ed.: (from Gale Group, Factiva).
Indexed: PMR.
Published by: Conde Nast Publications Inc., 4 Times Square 5th Fl, New York, NY 10036. TEL 212-286-2860, FAX 212-286-8110, http://www.self.com. Ed. Lucy Danziger. Pub. Beth Fuchs Brenner. adv.: B&W page USD 44,290, color page USD 66,140; trim 10.88 x 8. Circ: 1,142,683 (paid). **Subscr. to:** PO Box 55480, Boulder, CO 80328-5480.

SHE MAGAZINE GUIDE TO HAVING A BABY. see *WOMEN'S HEALTH*

SOBERING THOUGHTS. see *DRUG ABUSE AND ALCOHOLISM*

TOP SANTE; health & beauty. see *WOMEN'S HEALTH*

UNION MATTERS. see *LABOR UNIONS*

UNTER UNS; Zeitschrift fuer Frauen und Maedchen. see *HANDICAPPED—Visually Impaired*

W F S QUARTERLY. see *FIRE PREVENTION*

305.4 CAN
WOMEN TODAY MAGAZINE. Text in English. m. free per issue. **Document type:** *Newsletter.*
Media: Online - full text.
Address: 20385 64th Ave, Langley, BC V2Y 1N5, Canada. TEL 604-514-2000, FAX 604-514-2124, editor@womentodaymagazine.com, http://www.womentodaymagazine.com. Ed. Claire Colvin. Pub. Katherine Kehler.

WOMEN'S HEALTH ADVISOR. see *WOMEN'S HEALTH*

▼ **WOMEN'S HEALTH & FITNESS.** see *WOMEN'S HEALTH*

WOMEN'S HEALTH LETTER; the monthly review of women's health issues. see *WOMEN'S HEALTH*

305.4 GBR ISSN 1355-4255
ZEST; the health and beauty magazine. Text in English. 1994. 10/yr. GBP 2.30 newsstand/cover. **Document type:** *Consumer.* **Description:** Contains advice, tips and secrets on maintaining and enhancing one's health and beauty.
Published by: National Magazine Company Ltd., National Magazine House, 72 Broadwick St, London W1V 2BP, United Kingdom. TEL 44-20-7439-5000, FAX 44-207-437-6886, zest.mail@natmags.co.uk. Ed. Eve Cameron. Pub. Vivien Cotterill. **Dist. by:** Comag, Tavistock Works, Tavistock Rd, W Drayton, Middx UB7 7QX, United Kingdom. TEL 44-1895-433600, FAX 44-1895-433602.

WOMEN'S INTERESTS—Abstracting, Bibliographies, Statistics

AUSTRALIA. BUREAU OF STATISTICS. WOMEN'S SAFETY SURVEY, UNIT RECORD FILE, AUSTRALIA. see *PUBLIC HEALTH AND SAFETY—Abstracting, Bibliographies, Statistics*

WOMEN'S STUDIES

COMMITTEE ON SOUTH ASIAN WOMEN BULLETIN. see *WOMEN'S INTERESTS*

FEMINISM & PSYCHOLOGY; an international journal. see *PSYCHOLOGY*

305.412 616.89 USA ISSN 0895-2833
RC488.5
JOURNAL OF FEMINIST FAMILY THERAPY; an international forum. Text in English. 1989. q. USD 60 to individuals; USD 81 in Canada to individuals; USD 87 elsewhere to individuals; USD 125 to institutions; USD 169 in Canada to institutions; USD 181 elsewhere to institutions; USD 340 to libraries; USD 459 in Canada to libraries (effective Aug. 2001); USD 493 elsewhere to libraries (effective Apr. 2001). adv. bk.rev. illus. back issues avail.; reprint service avail. from HAW,PSC,SCH. *Refereed.* **Document type:** *Journal, Academic/Scholarly.* **Description:** Explores feminist theory in relation to family therapy practice and theory.
Related titles: Microfiche ed.: (from PQC); Microform ed.
Indexed: ASSIA, Alt.Press Ind., CWI, ERA, Fem.Per. (1989-), Gend.Watch, IBZ, IMFL, Ind.Per.Art.Relat.Law, Ind.Philos., Lang.& Lang.Behav.Abstr., Mult.Ed.Abstr., SOPODA, Sage Fam.Stud.Abstr., Soc.Work Res.& Abstr., Sociol.Abstr., Stud.Wom.Abstr., Wom.Stud.Abstr. (1989-), e-psyche.
—BLDSC (4983.937000), GNLM, Haworth, ingenta.
Published by: Haworth Press, Inc., 10 Alice St, Binghamton, NY 13904-1580. TEL 607-722-5857, 800-429-6784, FAX 607-722-6362, 800-895-0582, getinfo@haworthpressinc.com, http://www.haworthpress.com/journals/journallist.asp. Ed. Toni Schindler Zimmerman. Pub. William Cohen. R&P Ruthann Heath TEL 607-723-5857 ext 316. Adv. contact Jackie Blakeslee TEL 607-722-5857 ext 346. B&W page USD 315, color page USD 550; trim 6 x 8.5.

305.26 USA ISSN 0895-2841
HV1457 CODEN: JWAGE5
JOURNAL OF WOMEN AND AGING; the multidiciplinary quarterly of psychosocial practice, theory & research. Text in English. 1989. q. USD 60 to individuals; USD 81 in Canada to individuals; USD 87 elsewhere to individuals; USD 175 to institutions; USD 236 in Canada to institutions; USD 254 elsewhere to institutions; USD 275 to libraries; USD 371 in Canada to libraries; USD 399 elsewhere to libraries (effective Aug. 2001). adv. bk.rev. illus. back issues avail.; reprint service avail. from HAW. *Refereed.* **Document type:** *Journal, Academic/Scholarly.* **Description:** Aims to enhance the knowledge of a variety of professionals concerned with meeting the social, psychological, and health care needs of women as they mature.
Related titles: Microform ed.: (from PQC); Online - full text ed.: (from ProQuest Information & Learning, Gale Group, LexisNexis, Factiva, Institute for Scientific Information).
Indexed: ASCA, Abstr.Anthropol., Abstr.Soc.Geront., AgeLine, CINAHL, CWI, Curr.Cont., Educ.Admin.Abstr., Environ.Sci.Poll.Mgmt., Fam.Ind., Fem.Per. (1989-), Gend.Watch, IBZ, IMFL, Ind.Med. (1988-), Ind.Philos., Int.Nurs.Ind., Lang.& Lang.Behav.Abstr., Mult.Ed.Abstr., Pollut.Abstr., Risk Abstr., SOPODA, SSCI, Soc.Serv.Abstr., Soc.Work Res.& Abstr., Sociol.Abstr., Sp.Ed.Needs Abstr., Stud.Wom.Abstr., Wom.Stud.Abstr. (1991-), Wom.Stud.Ind.
—BLDSC (5072.632800), GNLM, Haworth, IDS, ingenta.
Published by: Haworth Press, Inc., 10 Alice St, Binghamton, NY 13904-1580. TEL 607-722-5857, 800-429-6784, FAX 607-722-6362, 800-895-0582, getinfo@haworthpressinc.com, http://www.haworthpress.com/journals/journallist.asp. Ed. J Dianne Garner. Pub. William Cohen. R&P Ruthann Heath TEL 607-723-5857 ext 316. Adv. contact Jackie Blakeslee TEL 607-722-5857 ext 346. B&W page USD 315, color page USD 550; trim 6 x 8.5. Circ: 610.

PSYCHOLOGY OF WOMEN QUARTERLY. see *PSYCHOLOGY*

305.4 618.082 BRA
REDE NACIONAL FEMINISTA DE SAUDE E DIREITOS REPRODUTIVOS. JORNAL. Short title: Jornal da Rede. Text in Portuguese. 1992. q. **Document type:** *Bulletin.* **Description:** Publicizes studies and political action towards changing laws and public health procedures referring to women's health and reproduction.
Published by: Rede Nacional Feminista de Saude e Direitos Reprodutivos, c/o SOS Corpo, Genero e Cidadania, Rua Major Codeceira, 37, S Amaro, Recife, PE 50100-070, Brazil. TEL 55-81-4233044, FAX 55-81-4233180. Ed. Maria Betania Avila. Circ: 10,000.

SAGE SERIES ON VIOLENCE AGAINST WOMEN. see *SOCIOLOGY*

VIOLENCE AGAINST WOMEN; an international and interdisciplinary journal. see *SOCIOLOGY*

WOMEN & THERAPY; a feminist quarterly. see *PSYCHOLOGY*

WOMENWISE. see *WOMEN'S HEALTH*

ZOOLOGY

see BIOLOGY—Zoology

Z

SERIALS

Online Service Listing/ Serials Online

America Online, Incorporated 22000 A O L Way, Dulles, VA 20166 TEL 703-448-8700, FAX 703-265-2206; 8619 Westwood Ctr. Dr., Vienna, VA 22182-2285 TEL 800-827-6364, http://www.aol.com
Fit Pregnancy (USA) *Online - full text edition.* **3950**
Flex (GBR) *Online - full text edition.* **4353**
Men's Fitness (USA) *Online - full text edition.* **4222**
Muscle & Fitness Hers (USA) *Online - full text edition.* **4358**
Natural Health (USA) *Online - full text edition.* **3168**
Shape (USA) *Online - full text edition.* **4565**

BioOne c/o Association for Research Libraries, 21 Dupont Circle, Ste. 800, Washington, DC 20036 TEL 202-296-2296, http://www.bioone.org
American Museum Novitates (USA) *Online - full text edition.* **3350**
BioScience (USA) *Online - full text edition.* **3187**
Cell Stress & Chaperones (USA) *Online - full text edition.* **3582**
Entomological Society of America. Annals Online(USA) *Online - full content.* **3295**
Environmental Entomology (USA) *Online - full text edition.* **3295**
Evolution (USA) *Online - full text edition.* **3302**
In Vitro Cellular & Developmental Biology - Animal (USA) *Online - full text edition.* **3618**
In Vitro Cellular & Developmental Biology - Plant (USA) *Online - full text edition.* **3280**
Journal of Avian Medicine and Surgery (USA) *Online - full text edition.* **4545**
Journal of Economic Entomology (USA) *Online - full text edition.* **3296**
Journal of Mammalogy (USA) *Online - full text edition.* **3354**
Journal of Medical Entomology (USA) *Online - full text edition.* **3296**
Journal of Parasitology (USA) *Online - full text edition.* **3802**
Journal of Zoo and Wildlife Medicine (USA) *Online - full text edition.* **4547**
Photochemistry and Photobiology (USA) *Online - full text edition.* **3374**

Bureau of National Affairs, Incorporated, (BNA), The 1231 25th St., NW, Washington, DC 20037 TEL 202-452-4200, FAX 202-452-4226, TELEX 285656 BNAI WSH FAX 800-253-0332, customercare@bna.com, http://www.bna.com
B N A's Federal Environment & Safety Regulatory Monitoring Report (USA) *Online - full text edition.* **3436**
B N A's Health Care Daily Report (E-mail) (USA) *Online - full text edition.* **3502**
B N A's Health Care Fraud Report (USA) *Online - full text edition.* **3502**
B N A's Health Care Policy Report (USA) *Online - full text edition.* **4463**
B N A's Health Law Reporter (USA) *Online - full text edition.* **3537**
B N A's Medicare Report (USA) *Online - full text edition.* **3573**
B N A's SafetyNet (USA) *Online - full text edition.* **4251**
B N A's State Environment & Safety Regulatory Monitoring Report (USA) *Online - full text edition.* **3436**
Occupational Safety & Health Reporter (USA) *Online - full text edition.* **4262**
Product Safety & Liability Reporter (USA) *Online - full text edition.* **4486**
State Health Care Regulatory Developments (USA) *Online - full text edition.* **3523**

Cambridge Scientific Abstracts 7200 Wisconsin Ave., Bethesda, MD 20814 TEL 301-961-6700, 301-961-6798, 800-843-7751, FAX 301-961-6720, 301-961-6799, TELEX 89-8452, journals@csa.com, http://www.csa.com/journals
A S F A Marine Biotechnology Abstracts (USA) *Online - full text edition.* **3225**
AIDS & Cancer Research(USA) *Online - full text.* **3715**
Animal Behavior Abstracts (USA) *Online - full text edition.* **3225**
C S A Neurosciences Abstracts (USA) *Online - full content edition.* **3718**
Calcium and Calcified Tissue Abstracts (USA) *Online - full text edition.* **3228**
E-psyche(USA) *Online - full text.* **4457**
Entomology Abstracts (USA) *Online - full text edition.* **3230**
Health and Safety Science Abstracts (USA) *Online - full text edition.* **4496**
Microbiology Abstracts: Section B. Bacteriology (USA) *Online - full text edition.* **3233**
Microbiology Abstracts: Section C. Algology, Mycology and Protozoology (USA) *Online - full text edition.* **3233**
Nucleic Acids Abstracts (USA) *Online - full text edition.* **3234**
Risk Abstracts (USA) *Online - full text edition.* **3443**
Toxicology Abstracts (USA) *Online - full text edition.* **3443**

Canadian Centre for Occupational Health & Safety 250 Main St., E., Hamilton, ON L8N 1H6, Canada TEL 905-570-8094, 800-668-4284, FAX 905-572-2206, custserv@ccohs.ca, http://www.ccohs.ca
N I O S H T I C(USA) *Online - full text.* **4259**
R T E C S(USA) *Online - full text.* **3453**
Safety and Health at Work (CHE) *Online - full text edition.* **4269**

CatchWord Ltd. 23-28 Hythe Bridge St., Ground Fl., Oxford OX1 2ET, United Kingdom TEL 44-1865-799000, FAX 44-1865-799111, sales@catchword.com, http:// www.catchword.com
A D H D Report (USA) *Online - full text edition. (guilford)* **4067**
Acta Dermato-Venereologica (NOR) *Online - full text edition. (tandf)* **3843**
Acta Odontologica Scandinavica (NOR) *Online - full text edition. (tandf)* **3813**
Acta Oncologica (NOR) *Online - full text edition. (tandf)* **3966**
Acta Oto-Laryngologica (NOR) *Online - full text edition. (tandf)* **4029**
Acta Paediatrica (NOR) *Online - full text edition. (tandf)* **4039**
Addiction (GBR) *Online - full text edition. (carfax)* **3396**
Addiction Biology (GBR) *Online - full text edition. (carfax)* **3397**
Advances in Physiotherapy (NOR) *Online - full text edition. (tandf)* **4058**
Ageing International (USA) *Online - full text edition. (tranpub)* **3466**
Aging & Mental Health (GBR) *Online - full text edition. (carfax)* **3466**
The Aging Male (GBR) *Online - full text edition. (ppg)* **4221**
AIDS Care (GBR) *Online - full text edition. (carfax)* **3791**
AIDS Education and Prevention (USA) *Online - full text edition. (guilford)* **4460**
AIDS Patient Care and S T Ds (USA) *Online - full text edition. (mal)* **3791**
AIDS Research and Human Retroviruses (USA) *Online - full text edition. (mal)* **3792**
Alternative & Complementary Therapies (USA) *Online - full text edition. (mal)* **3163**
American Academy of Psychoanalysis. Journal (USA) *Online - full text edition. (guilford)* **4373**
American Journal of Family Therapy (USA) *Online - full text edition. (brunner)* **4374**
American Journal on Addictions (USA) *Online - full text edition. (brunner)* **3399**
Amyotrophic Lateral Sclerosis and Other Motor Neuron Disorders (GBR) *Online - full text edition. (dunitz)* **4072**
Animal Learning & Behavior (USA) *Online - full text edition. (psocpubs)* **4376**
Annals of Behavioral Medicine (USA) *Online - full text edition. (erlbaum)* **3715**
Annals of Clinical Biochemistry (GBR) *Online - full text edition. (rsm)* **3240**
Annals of Human Biology (GBR) *Online - full text edition. (tandf)* **3181**
Annals of Medicine (GBR) *Online - full text edition. (tandf)* **3871**
Annals of Tropical Medicine and Parasitology (GBR) *Online - full text edition. (carfax)* **3793**
Annals of Tropical Paediatrics (GBR) *Online - full text edition. (carfax)* **4040**
Anthropology & Medicine (GBR) *Online - full text edition. (carfax)* **3172**
Antioxidants & Redox Signaling (USA) *Online - full text edition. (mal)* **3567**
Antisense and Nucleic Acid Drug Development (USA) *Online - full text edition. (mal)* **3298**
Aphasiology (GBR) *Online - full text edition. (psych)* **4073**
Applied Developmental Science (USA) *Online - full text edition. (erlbaum)* **4377**
Applied Neuropsychology (USA) *Online - full text edition. (erlbaum)* **4073**
Applied Occupational & Environmental Hygiene (USA) *Online - full text edition. (tandf)* **4250**
Applied Psychology (GBR) *Online - full text edition. (psych)* **4377**
Archives of Andrology (USA) *Online - full text edition. (tandf)* **3568**
Archives of Sexual Behavior (USA) *Online - full text edition. (plenum)* **3568**
Artificial Life (USA) *Online - full text edition. (mitpress)* **3389**
Astrobiology (USA) *Online - full text edition. (mal)* **3183**
Attachment and Human Development (GBR) *Online - full text edition. (routledg)* **4379**
Avian Pathology (GBR) *Online - full text edition. (tandf)* **4539**
Basic and Applied Social Psychology (USA) *Online - full text edition. (erlbaum)* **4380**
Behavior Research Methods, Instruments, and Computers (USA) *Online - full text edition. (psocpubs)* **4380**
Behaviour (NLD) *Online - full text edition. (brill)* **3351**
Behaviour and Information Technology (GBR) *Online - full text edition. (tandf)* **4381**
Biochemical Genetics (USA) *Online - full text edition. (plenum)* **3299**

Biocontrol Science and Technology (GBR) *Online - full text edition. (tandf)* **3157**
Biomarkers (GBR) *Online - full text edition. (tandf)* **3575**
BioScience (USA) *Online - full text edition. (aibs)* **3187**
Biotech Software and Internet Report (USA) *Online - full text edition. (mal)* **3270**
Biotechnic and Histochemistry (GBR) *Online - full text edition. (bios)* **3334**
Biotechnology Law Report (USA) *Online - full text edition. (mal)* **3272**
Blood Pressure (NOR) *Online - full text edition. (tandf)* **3764**
Brain Injury (GBR) *Online - full text edition. (tandf)* **4077**
British Journal of Audiology (GBR) *Online - full text edition. (whurr)* **3489**
British Journal of Clinical Psychology (GBR) *Online - full text edition. (bpsoc)* **4383**
British Journal of Developmental Psychology (GBR) *Online - full text edition. (bpsoc)* **4383**
British Journal of Educational Psychology (GBR) *Online - full text edition. (bpsoc)* **4383**
British Journal of Guidance and Counselling (GBR) *Online - full text edition. (carfax)* **4269**
British Journal of Health Psychology (GBR) *Online - full text edition. (bpsoc)* **4384**
British Journal of Mathematical and Statistical Psychology (GBR) *Online - full text edition. (bpsoc)* **4384**
British Journal of Medical Psychology (GBR) *Online - full text edition. (bpsoc)* **4384**
British Journal of Neurosurgery (GBR) *Online - full text edition. (tandf)* **4182**
British Journal of Psychology (GBR) *Online - full text edition. (bpsoc)* **4384**
British Journal of Social Psychology (GBR) *Online - full text edition. (bpsoc)* **4384**
British Medical Bulletin (GBR) *Online - full text edition. (rsm)* **3579**
Cancer Biotherapy & Radiopharmaceuticals (USA) *Online - full text edition. (mal)* **3970**
Cardiology in the Young (GBR) *Online - full text edition. (gmed)* **3766**
The Cerebellum (GBR) *Online - full text edition. (dunitz)* **4081**
Child and Adolescent Psychopharmacology News (USA) *Online - full text edition. (guilford)* **4081**
Climacteric (GBR) *Online - full text edition. (ppg)* **4563**
Clinical Intensive Care (GBR) *Online - full text edition. (bios)* **3908**
Clinical Linguistics & Phonetics (GBR) *Online - full text edition. (tandf)* **4082**
Clinical Medicine (GBR) *Online - full text edition. (rcop)* **3586**
Clinical Risk (GBR) *Online - full text edition. (rsm)* **3587**
The Clinician in Management (GBR) *Online - full text edition. (rmp)* **3587**
Clio Medica (NLD) *Online - full text edition. (rodopi)* **3588**
Cognition and Emotion (GBR) *Online - full text edition. (psych)* **4388**
Cognition and Instruction (USA) *Online - full text edition. (erlbaum)* **4388**
Cognitiva (ESP) *Online - full text edition. (fias)* **4389**
Cognitive, Affective, & Behavioral Neuroscience (USA) *Online - full text edition. (psocpubs)* **4389**
Cognitive Neuropsychiatry (GBR) *Online - full text edition. (psych)* **4389**
Cognitive Neuropsychology (GBR) *Online - full text edition. (psych)* **4083**
Cognitive Therapy and Research (USA) *Online - full text edition. (plenum)* **4390**
Communication Disorders Quarterly (USA) *Online - full text edition. (proed)* **3420**
Community Mental Health Journal (USA) *Online - full text edition. (plenum)* **4512**
Counselling Psychology Quarterly (GBR) *Online - full text edition. (carfax)* **4392**
Creativity Research Journal (USA) *Online - full text edition. (erlbaum)* **4392**
Criminal Behaviour and Mental Health (GBR) *Online - full text edition. (whurr)* **4084**
Critical Public Health (GBR) *Online - full text edition. (carfax)* **4466**
Culture, Health and Sexuality (GBR) *Online - full text edition. (tandf)* **4520**
Current Medical Research and Opinion (GBR) *Online - full text edition. (libra)* **3591**
Current Psychology (New Brunswick) (USA) *Online - full text edition. (tranpub)* **4393**
CyberPsychology & Behavior (USA) *Online - full text edition. (mal)* **3390**
Cytokines, Cellular & Molecular Therapy (GBR) *Online - full text edition. (dunitz)* **3900**
Cytotherapy (GBR) *Online - full text edition. (dunitz)* **3900**
D N A and Cell Biology (USA) *Online - full text edition. (mal)* **3248**
Death Studies (USA) *Online - full text edition. (tandf)* **4394**
Developmental Neuropsychology (USA) *Online - full text edition. (erlbaum)* **4394**
Deviant Behavior (USA) *Online - full text edition. (tandf)* **4521**
Diabetes Technology & Therapeutics (USA) *Online - full text edition. (mal)* **3859**
Digestive Diseases and Sciences (USA) *Online - full text edition. (plenum)* **3888**
Disability and Rehabilitation (GBR) *Online - full text edition. (tandf)* **3484**
Disability & Society (GBR) *Online - full text edition. (carfax)* **3494**
Disease Management (USA) *Online - full text edition. (mal)* **3595**
Drug and Alcohol Review (GBR) *Online - full text edition. (carfax)* **3400**
Drug Delivery (USA) *Online - full text edition. (tandf)* **4288**
Drugs: Education, Prevention & Policy (GBR) *Online - full text edition. (carfax)* **3401**
e-biomed(USA) *Online - full text. (mal)* **3596**
Eating Disorders (USA) *Online - full text edition. (brunner)* **4395**
Echocardiography (USA) *Online - full text edition. (futura)* **3771**
Ecological Psychology (USA) *Online - full text edition. (erlbaum)* **4396**
Education for Health (GBR) *Online - full text edition. (tandf)* **3597**
Education for Primary Care (GBR) *Online - full text edition. (rmp)* **3597**
Educational Gerontology (USA) *Online - full text edition. (tandf)* **3470**
Educational Psychologist (USA) *Online - full text edition. (erlbaum)* **4396**
Educational Psychology (GBR) *Online - full text edition. (carfax)* **3410**
Educational Psychology in Practice (GBR) *Online - full text edition. (carfax)* **3410**
Ergonomics (GBR) *Online - full text edition. (tandf)* **3432**
Estudios de Psicologia (ESP) *Online - full text edition. (fias)* **4397**
Ethics & Behavior (USA) *Online - full text edition. (erlbaum)* **4397**
Ethnicity and Health (GBR) *Online - full text edition. (carfax)* **4468**
European Journal of Cognitive Psychology (GBR) *Online - full text edition. (psych)* **4397**
European Journal of Contraception and Reproductive Health Care (GBR) *Online - full text edition. (ppg)* **3358**
European Journal of Psychotherapy, Counselling and Health (GBR) *Online - full text edition. (routledg)* **4089**
European Journal of Surgery (NOR) *Online - full text edition. (tandf)* **4188**
European Journal of Work and Organizational Psychology (GBR) *Online - full text edition. (psych)* **4398**
Experimental Aging Research (USA) *Online - full text edition. (tandf)* **4398**
Experimental Lung Research (USA) *Online - full text edition. (tandf)* **4160**
Focus on Autism and Other Developmental Disabilities (USA) *Online - full text edition. (proed)* **4091**
Food Additives and Contaminants (GBR) *Online - full text edition. (tandf)* **4296**
Food and Agricultural Immunology (GBR) *Online - full text edition. (tandf)* **3197**
Frontiers of Medical and Biological Engineering (NLD) *Online - full text edition. (vsp)* **3237**
Gene Therapy and Regulation (NLD) *Online - full text edition. (vsp)* **3303**
Genetic Testing (USA) *Online - full text edition. (mal)* **3304**
Geomicrobiology Journal (USA) *Online - full text edition. (tandf)* **3322**
Gestalt Review (USA) *Online - full text edition. (tap)* **4400**
Gynecological Endocrinology (GBR) *Online - full text edition. (ppg)* **3863**
H P B (GBR) *Online - full text edition. (dunitz)* **3891**
Haematologia (NLD) *Online - full text edition. (vsp)* **3901**
Health Affairs (USA) *Online - full text edition. (phope)* **4471**
Health Care for Women International (USA) *Online - full text edition. (tandf)* **4563**
Health Communication (USA) *Online - full text edition. (erlbaum)* **4472**
Health Information on the Internet (GBR) *Online - full text edition. (rsm)* **3611**
Health, Risk & Society (GBR) *Online - full text edition. (carfax)* **4474**
Health Services Management Research (GBR) *Online - full text edition. (rsm)* **3613**
High Ability Studies (GBR) *Online - full text edition. (carfax)* **3422**
High Altitude Medicine and Biology (USA) *Online - full text edition. (mal)* **3614**
Human - Computer Interaction (Mahwah) (USA) *Online - full text edition. (erlbaum)* **3389**
Human Ecology (New York) (USA) *Online - full text edition. (plenum)* **3173**
Human Gene Therapy (USA) *Online - full text edition. (mal)* **3307**
Human Performance (USA) *Online - full text edition. (erlbaum)* **4402**
Human Relations (USA) *Online - full text edition. (plenum)* **4509**
I U B M B Life (AUS) *Online - full text edition. (tandf)* **3251**
Infancia y Aprendizaje (ESP) *Online - full text edition. (fias)* **3411**
Infancy (USA) *Online - full text edition. (erlbaum)* **3383**
Infectious Diseases in Obstetrics and Gynecology (USA) *Online - full text edition. (ppg)* **3953**
Inflammopharmacology (NLD) *Online - full text edition. (vsp)* **4302**
Inhalation Toxicology (USA) *Online - full text edition. (tandf)* **3451**
Institution of Mechanical Engineers. Proceedings. Part H: Journal of Engineering in Medicine (GBR) *Online - full text edition. (pep)* **3238**
Integrative Physiological and Behavioral Science (USA) *Online - full text edition. (tranpub)* **4095**
International Forum of Psychoanalysis (NOR) *Online - full text edition. (tandf)* **4405**
The International Journal for the Psychology of Religion (USA) *Online - full text edition. (erlbaum)* **4500**
The International Journal of Aviation Psychology (USA) *Online - full text edition. (erlbaum)* **4532**
International Journal of Behavioral Development (GBR) *Online - full text edition. (psych)* **4405**
International Journal of Behavioral Medicine (USA) *Online - full text edition. (erlbaum)* **4405**
International Journal of Cardiovascular Interventions (GBR) *Online - full text edition. (dunitz)* **3775**
International Journal of Children's Spirituality (GBR) *Online - full text edition. (carfax)* **4406**
International Journal of Cognitive Ergonomics (USA) *Online - full text edition. (erlbaum)* **4406**
International Journal of Cosmetic Surgery and Aesthetic Dermatology (USA) *Online - full text edition. (mal)* **3850**
International Journal of Disability, Development and Education (GBR) *Online - full text edition. (carfax)* **3423**
International Journal of Environmental Health Research (GBR) *Online - full text edition. (tandf)* **3439**
International Journal of Food Sciences and Nutrition (GBR) *Online - full text edition. (tandf)* **4236**
International Journal of Group Psychotherapy (USA) *Online - full text edition. (guilford)* **4406**
International Journal of Hyperthermia (GBR) *Online - full text edition. (tandf)* **3980**
International Journal of Language and Communication Disorders (GBR) *Online - full text edition. (tandf)* **4033**
International Journal of Pest Management (GBR) *Online - full text edition. (tandf)* **3158**
International Journal of Psychiatry in Clinical Practice (GBR) *Online - full text edition. (dunitz)* **4096**
The International Journal of Psycho-Analysis (GBR) *Online - full text edition. (psycan)* **4406**
International Journal of Psychology (GBR) *Online - full text edition. (psych)* **4407**
International Journal of Psychotherapy (GBR) *Online - full text edition. (carfax)* **4096**
International Journal of Radiation Biology (GBR) *Online - full text edition. (tandf)* **3980**
International Journal of S T D & AIDS (GBR) *Online - full text edition. (rsm)* **3800**
International Journal of Testing (USA) *Online - full text edition. (erlbaum)* **3411**
International Journal of Toxicology (GBR) *Online - full text edition. (tandf)* **3451**
International Review of Psychiatry (GBR) *Online - full text edition. (carfax)* **4097**
Intervention in School and Clinic (USA) *Online - full text edition. (proed)* **3423**
Issues in Comprehensive Pediatric Nursing (USA) *Online - full text edition. (tandf)* **3922**
Issues in Mental Health Nursing (USA) *Online - full text edition. (tandf)* **3922**
Journal of Aerosol Medicine (USA) *Online - full text edition. (mal)* **4161**
Journal of Alternative & Complementary Medicine (USA) *Online - full text edition. (mal)* **3167**
Journal of Anti-Aging Medicine (USA) *Online - full text edition. (mal)* **3475**
Journal of Applied Animal Welfare Science (USA) *Online - full text edition. (erlbaum)* **3172**
Journal of Applied Sport Psychology (USA) *Online - full text edition. (tandf)* **4174**
Journal of Audio Visual Media in Medicine (GBR) *Online - full text edition. (tandf)* **3629**
Journal of Behavioral Medicine (USA) *Online - full text edition. (plenum)* **4099**
Journal of Biomolecular Screening (USA) *Online - full text edition. (mal)* **3253**
Journal of Bone and Joint Surgery: British Volume (GBR) *Online - full text edition. (jbjs)* **4017**
Journal of Bone and Joint Surgery: British Volume on CD-ROM (GBR) *Online - full text edition. (jbjs)* **4018**
Journal of Cardiovascular Electrophysiology (USA) *Online - full text edition. (futura)* **3777**
Journal of Child and Adolescent Psychopharmacology (USA) *Online - full text edition. (mal)* **4099**
Journal of Child Psychotherapy (GBR) *Online - full text edition. (routledg)* **4411**
Journal of Clinical Child and Adolescent Psychology (USA) *Online - full text edition. (erlbaum)* **4411**
Journal of Clinical Excellence (GBR) *Online - full text edition. (rmp)* **3630**
Journal of Clinical Governance (GBR) *Online - full text edition. (rmp)* **3631**
Journal of Clinical Laser Medicine & Surgery (USA) *Online - full text edition. (mal)* **4147**
Journal of Cognition and Culture (NLD) *Online - full text edition. (brill)* **4412**
Journal of Cognition and Development (USA) *Online - full text edition. (erlbaum)* **4412**
Journal of Cognitive Neuroscience (USA) *Online - full text edition. (mitpress)* **4100**
Journal of Community Health (USA) *Online - full text edition. (plenum)* **3631**
Journal of Community Health Nursing (USA) *Online - full text edition. (erlbaum)* **3924**
Journal of Congestive Hearth Failure & Circulatory Support (GBR) *Online - full text edition. (dunitz)* **3777**
Journal of Constructivist Psychology (USA) *Online - full text edition. (tandf)* **4413**
Journal of Consumer Psychology (USA) *Online - full text edition. (erlbaum)* **3153**
Journal of Cutaneous Laser Therapy (GBR) *Online - full text edition. (dunitz)* **3850**
Journal of Dermatological Treatment (GBR) *Online - full text edition. (dunitz)* **3851**
Journal of Disability Policy Studies (USA) *Online - full text edition. (proed)* **3485**
Journal of Educational and Psychological Consultation (USA) *Online - full text edition. (erlbaum)* **3412**
Journal of Emotional and Behavioral Disorders (USA) *Online - full text edition. (proed)* **4101**
Journal of Endourology (USA) *Online - full text edition. (mal)* **4214**
Journal of Epidemiology and Biostatistics (GBR) *Online - full text edition. (dunitz)* **4479**
Journal of Family Planning and Reproductive Health Care (GBR) *Online - full text edition. (ffp)* **3359**
Journal of Forensic Psychiatry (GBR) *Online - full text edition. (routledg)* **4101**
Journal of Gynecologic Surgery (USA) *Online - full text edition. (mal)* **3955**
Journal of Health Communication (USA) *Online - full text edition. (tandf)* **3633**

Journal of Health Services Research & Policy (GBR) *Online - full text edition. (rsm)* **3634**
Journal of Hematotherapy & Stem Cell Research (USA) *Online - full text edition. (mal)* **3903**
Journal of Intellectual and Developmental Disability (GBR) *Online - full text edition. (tandf)* **4102**
Journal of Interferon & Cytokine Research (USA) *Online - full text edition. (mal)* **3749**
Journal of Interprofessional Care (GBR) *Online - full text edition. (carfax)* **3634**
Journal of Investigative Surgery (USA) *Online - full text edition. (tandf)* **4193**
Journal of Laparoendoscopic & Advanced Surgical Techniques (USA) *Online - full text edition. (mal)* **4194**
Journal of Laryngology and Otology (GBR) *Online - full text edition. (rsm)* **4034**
Journal of Learning Disabilities (USA) *Online - full text edition. (proed)* **3424**
The Journal of Legal Medicine (USA) *Online - full text edition. (tandf)* **3634**
Journal of Loss & Trauma (USA) *Online - full text edition. (tandf)* **4418**
Journal of Mammary Gland Biology and Neoplasia (USA) *Online - full text edition. (plenum)* **3345**
Journal of Medical Engineering & Technology (GBR) *Online - full text edition. (tandf)* **3635**
Journal of Medicinal Food (USA) *Online - full text edition. (mal)* **3636**
Journal of Men's Health (USA) *Online - full text edition. (mal)* **4221**
Journal of Mental Health (GBR) *Online - full text edition. (carfax)* **4102**
Journal of Microencapsulation (GBR) *Online - full text edition. (tandf)* **4308**
Journal of Micromechatronics (NLD) *Online - full text edition. (vsp)* **3434**
Journal of Nanoscience and Nanotechnology (USA) *Online - full text edition. (asp)* **3391**
Journal of Natural History (GBR) *Online - full text edition. (tandf)* **3204**
Journal of Neurotrauma (USA) *Online - full text edition. (mal)* **4019**
Journal of NeuroVirology (GBR) *Online - full text edition. (tandf)* **4105**
Journal of Nutritional & Environmental Medicine (GBR) *Online - full text edition. (carfax)* **4237**
Journal of Obstetrics and Gynaecology (GBR) *Online - full text edition. (tandf)* **3956**
Journal of Occupational and Organizational Psychology (GBR) *Online - full text edition. (bpsoc)* **4419**
Journal of Ocular Pharmacology and Therapeutics (USA) *Online - full text edition. (mal)* **4000**
Journal of Palliative Medicine (USA) *Online - full text edition. (mal)* **3637**
Journal of Personality Assessment (USA) *Online - full text edition. (erlbaum)* **4420**
Journal of Personality Disorders (USA) *Online - full text edition. (guilford)* **4420**
Journal of Phenomenological Psychology (USA) *Online - full text edition. (brill)* **4420**
Journal of Positive Behavior Interventions (USA) *Online - full text edition. (proed)* **4420**
Journal of Psychology and Financial Markets (USA) *Online - full text edition. (erlbaum)* **4421**
Journal of Rehabilitation Medicine (NOR) *Online - full text edition. (tandf)* **4515**
Journal of Reproductive and Infant Psychology (GBR) *Online - full text edition. (carfax)* **4421**
Journal of Research on Adolescence (USA) *Online - full text edition. (erlbaum)* **3384**
Journal of Sex & Marital Therapy (USA) *Online - full text edition. (brunner)* **4422**
Journal of Social and Clinical Psychology (USA) *Online - full text edition. (guilford)* **4422**
Journal of Social Work Practice (GBR) *Online - full text edition. (carfax)* **4515**
The Journal of Special Education (USA) *Online - full text edition. (proed)* **3424**
Journal of Sports Sciences (GBR) *Online - full text edition. (tandf)* **4525**
Journal of Substance Use (GBR) *Online - full text edition. (rmp)* **3404**
Journal of Systemic Therapies (USA) *Online - full text edition. (guilford)* **4423**
Journal of Telemedicine and Telecare (GBR) *Online - full text edition. (rsm)* **3638**
Journal of the Learning Sciences (USA) *Online - full text edition. (erlbaum)* **3413**
Journal of Toxicology and Environmental Health. Part A (USA) *Online - full text edition. (tandf)* **3452**
Journal of Toxicology and Environmental Health. Part B: Critical Reviews (USA) *Online - full text edition. (tandf)* **3452**
Journal of Vascular Technology (USA) *Online - full text edition. (svt)* **3779**
Journal of Women's Health and Gender-Based Medicine (USA) *Online - full text edition. (mal)* **4564**
Journal of Youth Studies (GBR) *Online - full text edition. (carfax)* **3384**
Laboratory Animals (GBR) *Online - full text edition. (rsm)* **3355**
Language and Cognitive Processes (GBR) *Online - full text edition. (psych)* **3551**
Language and Speech (GBR) *Online - full text edition. (king)* **3551**
Laterality (GBR) *Online - full text edition. (psych)* **4107**
Learning Disabilities Research and Practice (USA) *Online - full text edition. (erlbaum)* **3424**
Legal and Criminological Psychology (GBR) *Online - full text edition. (bpsoc)* **4425**
Leisure Sciences (USA) *Online - full text edition. (tandf)* **3547**
Logopedics Phoniatrics Vocology (NOR) *Online - full text edition. (tandf)* **4035**
Loss Prevention Bulletin (GBR) *Online - full text edition. (icheme)* **3433**
Mathematical Cognition (GBR) *Online - full text edition. (psych)* **4426**
Mathematical Thinking and Learning (USA) *Online - full text edition. (erlbaum)* **3554**
Measurement in Physical Education and Exercise Science (USA) *Online - full text edition. (erlbaum)* **4358**
Media Psychology (USA) *Online - full text edition. (erlbaum)* **4426**
Mediators of Inflammation (GBR) *Online - full text edition. (tandf)* **3648**
Medical Informatics and the Internet in Medicine (GBR) *Online - full text edition. (tandf)* **3812**
Medical Mycology (GBR) *Online - full text edition. (bios)* **3803**
Medical Teacher (GBR) *Online - full text edition. (tandf)* **3654**
Memory (GBR) *Online - full text edition. (psych)* **4426**
Memory and Cognition (USA) *Online - full text edition. (psocpubs)* **4426**
Menninger Clinic. Bulletin (USA) *Online - full text edition. (guilford)* **4109**
Mental Health, Religion & Culture (GBR) *Online - full text edition. (carfax)* **4427**
Metaphor and Symbol (USA) *Online - full text edition. (erlbaum)* **3551**
Microbial Drug Resistance (USA) *Online - full text edition. (mal)* **3660**
Microbial Ecology in Health & Disease (NOR) *Online - full text edition. (tandf)* **3803**
Military Psychology (USA) *Online - full text edition. (erlbaum)* **4428**
Minimally Invasive Therapy and Allied Technologies (GBR) *Online - full text edition. (dunitz)* **3661**
Molecular Membrane Biology (GBR) *Online - full text edition. (tandf)* **3258**
Mortality (GBR) *Online - full text edition. (carfax)* **4482**
Multivariate Behavioral Research (USA) *Online - full text edition. (erlbaum)* **4428**
N B E R - Frontiers in Health Policy (USA) *Online - full text edition. (mitpress)* **3663**
Neural Computation (USA) *Online - full text edition. (mitpress)* **3389**
Neurological Research (USA) *Online - full text edition. (ffront)* **4114**
Neurology and Clinical Neurophysiology (USA) *Online - full text edition. (mitpress)* **4115**
Neuropsychological Rehabilitation (GBR) *Online - full text edition. (psych)* **4117**
New Genetics and Society (GBR) *Online - full text edition. (carfax)* **3313**
Nicotine & Tobacco Research (GBR) *Online - full text edition. (carfax)* **4531**
Nordic Journal of Psychiatry (NOR) *Online - full text edition. (tandf)* **4120**
Nutrition and Cancer (USA) *Online - full text edition. (erlbaum)* **4241**
Pacing and Clinical Electrophysiology (PACE) (USA) *Online - full text edition. (futura)* **3780**
The Pain Clinic (NLD) *Online - full text edition. (vsp)* **3759**
Pan American Journal of Public Health (USA) *Online - full text edition. (paho)* **4484**
Pathology (GBR) *Online - full text edition. (carfax)* **3673**
Peace and Conflict (USA) *Online - full text edition. (erlbaum)* **4432**
Pediatric Asthma, Allergy & Immunology (USA) *Online - full text edition. (mal)* **4052**
Pediatric Endosurgery & Innovative Techniques (USA) *Online - full text edition. (mal)* **4052**
Pediatric Hematology & Oncology (USA) *Online - full text edition. (tandf)* **4053**
Pediatric Pathology & Molecular Medicine (USA) *Online - full text edition. (tandf)* **4053**
Pediatric Rehabilitation (GBR) *Online - full text edition. (tandf)* **4064**
Perception & Psychophysics (USA) *Online - full text edition. (psocpubs)* **4432**
Personality and Social Psychology Review (USA) *Online - full text edition. (erlbaum)* **4432**
Philosophical Psychology (GBR) *Online - full text edition. (routledg)* **4433**
Physiotherapy Theory and Practice (GBR) *Online - full text edition. (tandf)* **4065**
Platelets (Abingdon) (GBR) *Online - full text edition. (tandf)* **3213**
Politics and the Life Sciences (USA) *Online - full text edition. (beech)* **4368**
Prenatal and Neonatal Medicine (GBR) *Online - full text edition. (ppg)* **3961**
Primary Care Psychiatry (USA) *Online - full text edition. (libra)* **4123**
Psychiatry (USA) *Online - full text edition. (guilford)* **4126**
Psychiatry Psychology and Law (AUS) *Online - full text edition. (aap)* **4127**
Psychoanalytic Dialogues (USA) *Online - full text edition. (tap)* **4436**
Psychoanalytic Inquiry (USA) *Online - full text edition. (tap)* **4436**
Psychoanalytic Psychotherapy (GBR) *Online - full text edition. (routledg)* **4437**
The Psychoanalytic Review (USA) *Online - full text edition. (guilford)* **4437**
Psychoanalytic Studies (GBR) *Online - full text edition. (carfax)* **4437**
Psychodynamic Counselling (GBR) *Online - full text edition. (routledg)* **4127**
Psychological Inquiry (USA) *Online - full text edition. (erlbaum)* **4438**
Psychology, Evolution and Gender (GBR) *Online - full text edition. (routledg)* **4440**
Psychology, Health & Medicine (GBR) *Online - full text edition. (carfax)* **4440**
Psychonomic Bulletin & Review (USA) *Online - full text edition. (psocpubs)* **4442**
Quarterly Journal of Experimental Psychology. Section A: Human Experimental Psychology (GBR) *Online - full text edition. (psych)* **4443**
Quarterly Journal of Experimental Psychology. Section B: Comparative and Physiological Psychology (GBR) *Online - full text edition. (psych)* **4443**
Reading Psychology (USA) *Online - full text edition. (tandf)* **3414**
Rehabilitation Counseling Bulletin (USA) *Online - full text edition. (proed)* **3486**
Remedial and Special Education (USA) *Online - full text edition. (proed)* **3426**
Revista de Psicologia Social (ESP) *Online - full text edition. (fias)* **4445**
Royal Chemical Society. Journal. Perkin Transactions 1 (GBR) *Online - full text edition. (rsc)* **3379**
Royal Society of London. Philosophical Transactions. Biological Sciences (GBR) *Online - full text edition. (rsl)* **3217**
Royal Society of London. Proceedings. Biological Sciences (GBR) *Online - full text edition. (rsl)* **3217**
Sarcoma (GBR) *Online - full text edition. (carfax)* **3990**
Scandinavian Audiology (NOR) *Online - full text edition. (tandf)* **4038**
Scandinavian Cardiovascular Journal (NOR) *Online - full text edition. (tandf)* **4202**
Scandinavian Journal of Behaviour Therapy (NOR) *Online - full text edition. (tandf)* **4447**
Scandinavian Journal of Caring Sciences (NOR) *Online - full text edition. (tandf)* **3690**
Scandinavian Journal of Clinical & Laboratory Investigation (NOR) *Online - full text edition. (tandf)* **3880**
Scandinavian Journal of Gastroenterology (NOR) *Online - full text edition. (tandf)* **3895**
Scandinavian Journal of Infectious Diseases (NOR) *Online - full text edition. (tandf)* **3806**
Scandinavian Journal of Occupational Therapy (NOR) *Online - full text edition. (tandf)* **3690**
Scandinavian Journal of Plastic and Reconstructive Surgery and Hand Surgery (NOR) *Online - full text edition. (tandf)* **4202**
Scandinavian Journal of Primary Health Care (NOR) *Online - full text edition. (tandf)* **3690**
Scandinavian Journal of Public Health (NOR) *Online - full text edition. (tandf)* **3690**
Scandinavian Journal of Rheumatology (NOR) *Online - full text edition. (tandf)* **4171**
Scandinavian Journal of Urology and Nephrology (NOR) *Online - full text edition. (tandf)* **4218**
School Psychology Quarterly (USA) *Online - full text edition. (guilford)* **4447**
Science as Culture (GBR) *Online - full text edition. (carfax)* **4507**
Self and Identity (USA) *Online - full text edition. (tandf)* **4448**
Sensory Neuron (NLD) *Online - full text edition. (vsp)* **4133**
Sex Education (GBR) *Online - full text edition. (carfax)* **3415**
Sex Roles (USA) *Online - full text edition. (plenum)* **4448**
Sexual Addiction & Compulsivity (USA) *Online - full text edition. (brunner)* **4448**
Sexual and Relationship Therapy (GBR) *Online - full text edition. (carfax)* **4448**
Social Cognition (USA) *Online - full text edition. (guilford)* **4449**
Society & Animals (GBR) *Online - full text edition. (brill)* **3172**
Somatosensory and Motor Research (GBR) *Online - full text edition. (tandf)* **3349**
Spatial Vision (NLD) *Online - full text edition. (vsp)* **3554**
Structural Equation Modeling (USA) *Online - full text edition. (erlbaum)* **4451**
Suicide and Life-Threatening Behavior (USA) *Online - full text edition. (guilford)* **4451**
Surgical Infections (USA) *Online - full text edition. (mal)* **4204**
Teaching and Learning in Medicine (USA) *Online - full text edition. (erlbaum)* **3698**
Teaching of Psychology (USA) *Online - full text edition. (erlbaum)* **4452**
Telemedicine Journal and e-Health (USA) *Online - full text edition. (mal)* **3812**
Theoretical Issues in Ergonomics Science (GBR) *Online - full text edition. (tandf)* **3433**
Thinking & Reasoning (GBR) *Online - full text edition. (psych)* **4452**
Thyroid (USA) *Online - full text edition. (mal)* **3869**
Tissue Engineering (USA) *Online - full text edition. (mal)* **3294**
Toxicologic Pathology (USA) *Online - full text edition. (tandf)* **3454**
Toxicology Methods (USA) *Online - full text edition. (tandf)* **3456**
Trauma Quarterly (NLD) *Online - full text edition. (vsp)* **4207**
Twin Research (GBR) *Online - full text edition. (aap)* **3315**
Ultrastructural Pathology (USA) *Online - full text edition. (tandf)* **3991**
Vector Borne and Zoonotic Diseases (USA) *Online - full text edition. (mal)* **3706**
Viral Immunology (USA) *Online - full text edition. (mal)* **3752**
Visual Cognition (GBR) *Online - full text edition. (psych)* **4454**
Work and Stress (GBR) *Online - full text edition. (tandf)* **4455**
Xenobiotica (GBR) *Online - full text edition. (tandf)* **3264**

Central Institute for Scientific & Technical Information 52 A.G. Nasser, Sofia 1040, Bulgaria TEL 359-271-91-91, http://www.naeld.nag.bg
Physical Therapy (USA) *Online - full text edition.* **4064**

CISTI (Subsidiary of: National Research Council of Canada) 1200 Montreal Rd., Bldg, M-55, Ottawa, ON K1A 0S2, Canada TEL 613-993-9251, 800-668-1222, FAX 613-993-7619, cisti.producthelp@nrc.ca, http://www.nrc.ca/cisti
A S F A Marine Biotechnology Abstracts (USA) *Online - full text edition.* **3225**
Biochemistry and Cell Biology (CAN) *Online - full text edition.* **3243**
CAB International. Bureau of Nutrition. Annotated Bibliographies (GBR) *Online - full text edition.* **4248**
Canadian Journal of Microbiology (CAN) *Online - full text edition.* **3319**
Canadian Journal of Physiology and Pharmacology (CAN) *Online - full text edition.* **3340**
Genome (CAN) *Online - full text edition.* **3306**

Merck Index: An Encyclopedia of Chemicals and Drugs (USA) *Online - full text edition.* **4345**

CompuServe, Incorporated 5000 Arlington Centre Blvd., Columbus, OH 43220 TEL 614-457-0802, 800-848-8199, FAX 614-538-4023, http://www.compuserve.com
BioVenture View (USA) *Online - full text edition.* **3272**
Blood Weekly (USA) *Online - full text edition.* **3899**
Cancer Weekly Plus (USA) *Online - full text edition.* **3973**
Japanese Journal of Ophthalmology (NLD) *Online - full text edition.* **4000**
Journal of Aquariculture and Aquatic Sciences (USA) *Online - full text edition.* **3202**
Product Alert (USA) *Online - full text edition.* **3462**
Tuberculosis & Airborne Disease Weekly (USA) *Online - full text edition.* **3808**

Data Arkiv A.B. PO Box 12079, Stockholm 102 22, Sweden TEL 46-8-165220
Japanese Journal of Ophthalmology (NLD) *Online - full text edition.* **4000**

Data-Star 114 Jermyn St, Plaza Ste, London SW1Y 6HJ, United Kingdom; Radio Suisse AG, Laupenstr. 18A, Berne 38008, Switzerland TEL 41-31-5609500, FAX 43-31-509675
AIDS Weekly Plus (USA) *Online - full text edition. (PTS NEWSLETTER DATABASE)* **3792**
Alcoholism & Drug Abuse Weekly (USA) *Online - full text edition.* **3398**
Analgesics: The International Market (GBR) *Online - full text edition.* **4275**
Animal Pharm (GBR) *Online - full text edition. (PHIC, PHID, PHIN)* **4537**
Applied Genetics News (USA) *Online - full text edition.* **3299**
Biological Abstracts (USA) *Online - full text edition.* **3226**
Biological Abstracts - R R M (USA) *Online - full text edition.* **3226**
Biotech Business (USA) *Online - full text edition.* **3270**
BioVenture View (USA) *Online - full text edition.* **3272**
Blood Weekly (USA) *Online - full text edition.* **3899**
Cancer Weekly Plus (USA) *Online - full text edition.* **3973**
Chemical Hazards in Industry (GBR) *Online - full text edition. (CSNB)* **4268**
Chemical Safety NewsBase(GBR) *Online - full text. (CSNB)* **4268**
Clinica (GBR) *Online - full text edition. (PHIC, PHID, PHIN)* **3585**
Cough and Cold Remedies: The International Market (GBR) *Online - full text edition.* **4285**
Cumulative Index to Nursing & Allied Health Literature (USA) *Online - full text edition. (NAHL)* **3720**
Current Biotechnology (GBR) *Online - full text edition. (CUBI)* **3229**
Digestive Remedies: The International Market (GBR) *Online - full text edition.* **4287**
Drug G M P Report (USA) *E-mail edition.* **4289**
Drug Information (USA) *Online - full text edition of* A H F S Drug Information. (DIFT) **4273**
E R A News (GBR) *Online - full text edition.* **4291**
Environment Abstracts (USA) *Online - full text edition.* **3392**
Europe Drug & Device Report (USA) *E-mail edition.* **4292**
Excerpta Medica. Abstract Journals (NLD) *Online - full text edition.* **3230**
Excerpta Medica. Section 1: Anatomy, Anthropology, Embryology & Histology (NLD) *Online - full text edition.* **3230**
Excerpta Medica. Section 10: Obstetrics and Gynecology (NLD) *Online - full text edition.* **3723**
Excerpta Medica. Section 11: Otorhinolaryngology (NLD) *Online - full text edition.* **3724**
Excerpta Medica. Section 12: Ophthalmology (NLD) *Online - full text edition.* **3724**
Excerpta Medica. Section 13: Dermatology and Venereology (NLD) *Online - full text edition.* **3724**
Excerpta Medica. Section 14: Radiology (NLD) *Online - full text edition.* **3724**
Excerpta Medica. Section 15: Chest Diseases, Thoracic Surgery and Tuberculosis (NLD) *Online - full text edition.* **3724**
Excerpta Medica. Section 16: Cancer (NLD) *Online - full text edition.* **3724**
Excerpta Medica. Section 17: Public Health, Social Medicine and Epidemiology (NLD) *Online - full text edition.* **4495**
Excerpta Medica. Section 18: Cardiovascular Diseases and Cardiovascular Surgery (NLD) *Online - full text edition.* **3724**
Excerpta Medica. Section 19: Rehabilitation and Physical Medicine (NLD) *Online - full text edition.* **3725**
Excerpta Medica. Section 2: Physiology (NLD) *Online - full text edition.* **3725**
Excerpta Medica. Section 20: Gerontology and Geriatrics (NLD) *Online - full text edition.* **3482**
Excerpta Medica. Section 21: Developmental Biology and Teratology (NLD) *Online - full text edition.* **3230**
Excerpta Medica. Section 22: Human Genetics (NLD) *Online - full text edition.* **3230**
Excerpta Medica. Section 23: Nuclear Medicine (NLD) *Online - full text edition.* **3725**
Excerpta Medica. Section 24: Anesthesiology (NLD) *Online - full text edition.* **3725**
Excerpta Medica. Section 25: Hematology (NLD) *Online - full text edition.* **3725**
Excerpta Medica. Section 26: Immunology, Serology and Transplantation (NLD) *Online - full text edition.* **3725**
Excerpta Medica. Section 27: Biophysics, Bio-Engineering and Medical Instrumentation (NLD) *Online - full text edition.* **3231**
Excerpta Medica. Section 28: Urology and Nephrology (NLD) *Online - full text edition.* **3726**
Excerpta Medica. Section 29: Clinical and Experimental Biochemistry (NLD) *Online - full text edition.* **3231**
Excerpta Medica. Section 3: Endocrinology (NLD) *Online - full text edition.* **3726**
Excerpta Medica. Section 30: Clinical and Experimental Pharmacology (NLD) *Online - full text edition.* **4344**
Excerpta Medica. Section 31: Arthritis and Rheumatism (NLD) *Online - full text edition.* **3726**
Excerpta Medica. Section 32: Psychiatry (NLD) *Online - full text edition.* **3726**
Excerpta Medica. Section 33: Orthopedic Surgery (NLD) *Online - full text edition.* **3726**
Excerpta Medica. Section 35: Occupational Health and Industrial Medicine (NLD) *Online - full text edition.* **3726**
Excerpta Medica. Section 36: Health Policy, Economics and Management (NLD) *Online - full text edition.* **3524**
Excerpta Medica. Section 38: Adverse Reactions Titles (NLD) *Online - full text edition.* **4344**
Excerpta Medica. Section 4: Microbiology: Bacteriology, Mycology, Parasitology and Virology (NLD) *Online - full text edition.* **3231**
Excerpta Medica. Section 40: Drug Dependence, Alcohol Abuse and Alcoholism (NLD) *Online - full text edition.* **3407**
Excerpta Medica. Section 46: Environmental Health and Pollution Control (NLD) *Online - full text edition.* **3443**
Excerpta Medica. Section 48: Gastroenterology (NLD) *Online - full text edition.* **3726**
Excerpta Medica. Section 49: Forensic Science Abstracts (NLD) *Online - full text edition.* **3727**
Excerpta Medica. Section 5: General Pathology and Pathological Anatomy (NLD) *Online - full text edition.* **3231**
Excerpta Medica. Section 52: Toxicology (NLD) *Online - full text edition.* **3443**
Excerpta Medica. Section 6: Internal Medicine (NLD) *Online - full text edition.* **3727**
Excerpta Medica. Section 7: Pediatrics and Pediatric Surgery (NLD) *Online - full text edition.* **3727**
Excerpta Medica. Section 8: Neurology and Neurosurgery (NLD) *Online - full text edition.* **3727**
Excerpta Medica. Section 9: Surgery (NLD) *Online - full text edition.* **3727**
Eyewear: The International Market (GBR) *Online - full text edition.* **4015**
F D A Medical Bulletin (USA) *Online - full text edition.* **4294**
G P (GBR) *Online - full text edition. (GPGP)* **3604**
Generic Line (USA) *E-mail edition.* **4298**
Genomika (GBR) *Online - full text edition.* **3251**
Hazards in the Office (GBR) *Online - full text edition. (CSNB)* **4268**
Health News Daily (USA) *Online - full text edition. (HNDO)* **3612**
Health Policy & Biomedical Research: The Blue Sheet (USA) *Online - full text edition. (FDCR)* **3612**
Health Service Abstracts (GBR) *Online - full text edition.* **3728**
Industrial Health & Hazards Update (USA) *Online - full text edition.* **4256**
Inpharma Weekly (NZL) *Online - full text edition. (PHD, IPHC, IPHA, IPZZ)* **4345**
International Pharmaceutical Abstracts (USA) *Online - full text edition. (IPAB)* **4345**
Laboratory Hazards Bulletin (GBR) *Online - full text edition. (CSNB)* **4269**
Martindale: the Complete Drug Reference (GBR) *Online - full text edition.* **4314**
Medeconomics (GBR) *Online - full text edition.* **3648**
Medical Devices, Diagnostics & Instrumentation Reports: The Gray Sheet (USA) *Online - full text edition. (FDCR)* **3649**
Medicated Skincare: The International Market (GBR) *Online - full text edition.* **4315**
Meyler's Side Effects of Drugs (NLD) *Online - full text edition. (SEDB)* **4316**
N D A Pipeline (USA) *Online - full text edition. (NDAP)* **4317**
National Report on Computers and Health (USA) *Online - full text edition.* **3812**
New Product Launch Letter (GBR) *Online - full text edition.* **4319**
Nonprescription Pharmaceuticals and Nutritionals: The Tan Sheet (USA) *Online - full text edition. (FDCR)* **4319**
Pharma Marketletter (GBR) *Online - full text edition.* **4322**
Pharmaceutical Approvals Monthly (USA) *Online - full text edition. (FDCR)* **4323**
Pharmacies and Drugstores: A World Survey (GBR) *Online - full text edition.* **4325**
Pharmacoeconomics and Outcomes News (NZL) *Online - full text edition.* **4345**
Prescription Pharmaceuticals and Biotechnology: The Pink Sheet (USA) *Online - full text edition. (FDCR)* **4331**
Product Alert (USA) *Online - full text edition.* **3462**
PsycINFO(USA) *Online - full text. (PSYC)* **4458**
R & D Focus (GBR) *Online - full text edition.* **4333**
Reactions Weekly (NZL) *Online - full text edition. (READ, REAC, REAA, REZZ)* **4346**
Salud Publica de Mexico Online (MEX) *Online - full text edition of* Salud Publica de Mexico. **4489**
Scrip - World Pharmaceutical News (GBR) *Online - full text edition. (PHIC, PHID, PHIN)* **4335**
Side Effects of Drugs Annual (NLD) *Online - full text edition. (SEDB)* **4336**
Toiletries, Fragrances and Skin Care: The Rose Sheet (USA) *Online - full text edition. (FDCR)* **3176**
Tuberculosis & Airborne Disease Weekly (USA) *Online - full text edition.* **3808**
Vitamins & Dietary Supplements: The International Market (GBR) *Online - full text edition.* **4340**
Worldwide Biotech (USA) *Online - full text edition.* **3278**

The Dialog Corporation 11000 Regency Parkway, Ste. 10, Cary, NC 27511 TEL 919-462-8600, 800-210-9768, FAX 919-468-9890, http://www.dialog.com, http://www.dialog.com
A P I EnCompass: Environment (USA) *Online - full text edition of* Technical Literature Abstracts: Health & Environment. (File nos.354, 954) **3443**
Abstracts on Hygiene and Communicable Diseases (GBR) *Online - full text edition.* **3715**
AgBiotech News and Information (GBR) *Online - full text edition.* **3225**
AIDS Weekly Plus (USA) *Online - full text edition. (File no.636)* **3792**
Alcoholism & Drug Abuse Weekly (USA) *Online - full text edition.* **3398**
American Fitness (USA) *Online - full text edition. (File no.149)* **4350**
Analgesics: The International Market (GBR) *Online - full text edition.* **4275**
Animal Behavior Abstracts (USA) *Online - full text edition. (File no.76, LIFE SCIENCES COLLECTION)* **3225**
Animal Breeding Abstracts (GBR) *Online - full text edition.* **3156**
Animal Pharm (GBR) *Online - full text edition. (File No.129&130)* **4537**
Applied Genetics News (USA) *Online - full text edition.* **3299**
Archives of Dermatology (USA) *Online - full text edition.* **3845**
Archives of Family Medicine (USA) *Online - full text edition.* **3568**
Archives of General Psychiatry (USA) *Online - full text edition.* **4074**
Archives of Internal Medicine (USA) *Online - full text edition.* **3907**
Archives of Neurology (USA) *Online - full text edition.* **4074**
Archives of Ophthalmology (USA) *Online - full text edition.* **3994**
Archives of Otolaryngology - Head & Neck Surgery (USA) *Online - full text edition.* **4030**
Archives of Pediatrics & Adolescent Medicine (USA) *Online - full text edition.* **4041**
Archives of Surgery (USA) *Online - full text edition.* **4182**
The B B I Newsletter (USA) *Online - full text edition.* **3573**
Bibliography of Bioethics (USA) *Online - full text edition.* **3717**
Biocontrol News and Information (GBR) *Online - full text edition.* **3156**
Biological Abstracts (USA) *Online - full text edition. (File nos.5, 55)* **3226**
Biological Abstracts - R R M (USA) *Online - full text edition. (File nos.5, 55)* **3226**
Biotech Business (USA) *Online - full text edition.* **3270**
Biotechnology Abstracts (GBR) *Online - full text edition. (File no.357)* **3227**
BioVenture View (USA) *Online - full text edition. (File no.636)* **3272**
Blood Weekly (USA) *Online - full text edition.* **3899**
C S A Neurosciences Abstracts (USA) *Online - full content edition. (File no.76, LIFE SCIENCES COLLECTION)* **3718**
CAB International. Bureau of Nutrition. Annotated Bibliographies (GBR) *Online - full text edition.* **4248**
Calcium and Calcified Tissue Abstracts (USA) *Online - full text edition. (File no.76, LIFE SCIENCES COLLECTION)* **3228**
Cancer Weekly Plus (USA) *Online - full text edition.* **3973**
Chemical Hazards in Industry (GBR) *Online - full text edition. (File no.317)* **4268**
Chemical Safety NewsBase(GBR) *Online - full text. (File no.317)* **4268**
Clinica (GBR) *Online - full text edition. (File No. 129&130)* **3585**
Consumer Reports on Health (USA) *Online - full text edition. (File no.646)* **4351**
Cough and Cold Remedies: The International Market (GBR) *Online - full text edition.* **4285**
Current Biotechnology (GBR) *Online - full text edition. (File no.358)* **3229**
Current Contents: Clinical Medicine (USA) *Online - full text edition. (File no.440)* **3720**
Current Contents: Life Sciences (USA) *Online - full text edition. (File no.440)* **3229**
Current Contents: Social & Behavioral Sciences (USA) *Online - full text edition. (File no.440)* **4457**
Dermatology Times (USA) *Online - full text edition.* **3848**
Devices & Diagnostics Letter (USA) *E-mail edition.* **3529**
The Dictionary of Substances and Their Effects (GBR) *Online - full text edition. (File no.307)* **3448**
Digestive Remedies: The International Market (GBR) *Online - full text edition.* **4287**
Directory of Biomedical and Health Care Grants (USA) *Online - full text edition.* **3418**
Directory of Healthcare Group Purchasing Organizations (USA) *Online - full text edition.* **3370**
Directory of Hospital Personnel (USA) *Online - full text edition.* **3370**
Drug Data Report (ESP) *Online - full text edition.* **4288**
Drug G M P Report (USA) *E-mail edition.* **4289**
Drug Information (USA) *Online - full text edition of* A H F S Drug Information. (File no.229) **4273**
Drug News & Perspectives (ESP) *Online - full text edition.* **4289**

Online Service

E R A News (GBR) *Online - full text edition. (File 129&130)* **4291**
Entomology Abstracts (USA) *Online - full text edition. (File no.76, LIFE SCIENCES COLLECTION)* **3230**
Environment Abstracts (USA) *Online - full text edition.* **3392**
Europe Drug & Device Report (USA) *E-mail edition.* **4292**
Excerpta Medica. Abstract Journals (NLD) *Online - full text edition.* **3230**
Excerpta Medica. Section 1: Anatomy, Anthropology, Embryology & Histology (NLD) *Online - full text edition.* **3230**
Excerpta Medica. Section 10: Obstetrics and Gynecology (NLD) *Online - full text edition.* **3723**
Excerpta Medica. Section 11: Otorhinolaryngology (NLD) *Online - full text edition.* **3724**
Excerpta Medica. Section 12: Ophthalmology (NLD) *Online - full text edition.* **3724**
Excerpta Medica. Section 13: Dermatology and Venereology (NLD) *Online - full text edition.* **3724**
Excerpta Medica. Section 14: Radiology (NLD) *Online - full text edition.* **3724**
Excerpta Medica. Section 15: Chest Diseases, Thoracic Surgery and Tuberculosis (NLD) *Online - full text edition.* **3724**
Excerpta Medica. Section 16: Cancer (NLD) *Online - full text edition.* **3724**
Excerpta Medica. Section 17: Public Health, Social Medicine and Epidemiology (NLD) *Online - full text edition.* **4495**
Excerpta Medica. Section 18: Cardiovascular Diseases and Cardiovascular Surgery (NLD) *Online - full text edition.* **3724**
Excerpta Medica. Section 19: Rehabilitation and Physical Medicine (NLD) *Online - full text edition.* **3725**
Excerpta Medica. Section 2: Physiology (NLD) *Online - full text edition.* **3725**
Excerpta Medica. Section 20: Gerontology and Geriatrics (NLD) *Online - full text edition.* **3482**
Excerpta Medica. Section 21: Developmental Biology and Teratology (NLD) *Online - full text edition.* **3230**
Excerpta Medica. Section 22: Human Genetics (NLD) *Online - full text edition.* **3230**
Excerpta Medica. Section 23: Nuclear Medicine (NLD) *Online - full text edition.* **3725**
Excerpta Medica. Section 24: Anesthesiology (NLD) *Online - full text edition.* **3725**
Excerpta Medica. Section 25: Hematology (NLD) *Online - full text edition.* **3725**
Excerpta Medica. Section 26: Immunology, Serology and Transplantation (NLD) *Online - full text edition.* **3725**
Excerpta Medica. Section 27: Biophysics, Bio-Engineering and Medical Instrumentation (NLD) *Online - full text edition.* **3231**
Excerpta Medica. Section 28: Urology and Nephrology (NLD) *Online - full text edition.* **3726**
Excerpta Medica. Section 29: Clinical and Experimental Biochemistry (NLD) *Online - full text edition.* **3231**
Excerpta Medica. Section 3: Endocrinology (NLD) *Online - full text edition.* **3726**
Excerpta Medica. Section 30: Clinical and Experimental Pharmacology (NLD) *Online - full text edition.* **4344**
Excerpta Medica. Section 31: Arthritis and Rheumatism (NLD) *Online - full text edition.* **3726**
Excerpta Medica. Section 32: Psychiatry (NLD) *Online - full text edition.* **3726**
Excerpta Medica. Section 33: Orthopedic Surgery (NLD) *Online - full text edition.* **3726**
Excerpta Medica. Section 35: Occupational Health and Industrial Medicine (NLD) *Online - full text edition.* **3726**
Excerpta Medica. Section 36: Health Policy, Economics and Management (NLD) *Online - full text edition.* **3524**
Excerpta Medica. Section 38: Adverse Reactions Titles (NLD) *Online - full text edition.* **4344**
Excerpta Medica. Section 4: Microbiology: Bacteriology, Mycology, Parasitology and Virology (NLD) *Online - full text edition.* **3231**
Excerpta Medica. Section 40: Drug Dependence, Alcohol Abuse and Alcoholism (NLD) *Online - full text edition.* **3407**
Excerpta Medica. Section 46: Environmental Health and Pollution Control (NLD) *Online - full text edition.* **3443**
Excerpta Medica. Section 48: Gastroenterology (NLD) *Online - full text edition.* **3726**
Excerpta Medica. Section 49: Forensic Science Abstracts (NLD) *Online - full text edition.* **3727**
Excerpta Medica. Section 5: General Pathology and Pathological Anatomy (NLD) *Online - full text edition.* **3231**
Excerpta Medica. Section 52: Toxicology (NLD) *Online - full text edition.* **3443**
Excerpta Medica. Section 6: Internal Medicine (NLD) *Online - full text edition.* **3727**
Excerpta Medica. Section 7: Pediatrics and Pediatric Surgery (NLD) *Online - full text edition.* **3727**
Excerpta Medica. Section 8: Neurology and Neurosurgery (NLD) *Online - full text edition.* **3727**
Excerpta Medica. Section 9: Surgery (NLD) *Online - full text edition.* **3727**
Eyewear: The International Market (GBR) *Online - full text edition.* **4015**
F D A Consumer (USA) *Online - full text edition.* **3392**
F D A Medical Bulletin (USA) *Online - full text edition.* **4294**
Food and Drug Letter (USA) *E-mail edition.* **4296**
The G M P Letter (USA) *E-mail edition.* **3530**
Generic Line (USA) *E-mail edition.* **4298**
Genetics Abstracts (USA) *Online - full text edition. (File no.76, LIFE SCIENCES COLLECTION)* **3231**
Genomika (GBR) *Online - full text edition.* **3251**
Global Cosmetic Industry (USA) *Online - full text edition.* **3176**
Handbook on Injectable Drugs (USA) *Online - full text edition. (File no.229)* **4299**
Hazards in the Office (GBR) *Online - full text edition. (File no. 317)* **4268**
Health Devices Sourcebook (USA) *Online - full text edition. (File no.188)* **3611**
Health Devices System (USA) *Online - full text edition. (File no.198)* **3728**
Health Forum (USA) *Online - full text edition.* **3509**
Health Management Technology (USA) *Online - full text edition.* **3810**
Health News Daily (USA) *Online - full text edition. (File no.43)* **3612**
Health Policy & Biomedical Research: The Blue Sheet (USA) *Online - full text edition. (File no.187)* **3612**
Healthcare Financial Management (USA) *Online - full text edition.* **3510**
Helminthological Abstracts (GBR) *Online - full text edition.* **3232**
Hospitalis (CHE) *Online - full text edition.* **3514**
Immunology Abstracts (USA) *Online - full text edition. (File no.76, LIFE SCIENCES COLLECTION)* **3729**
Index Veterinarius (GBR) *Online - full text edition.* **4561**
Industrial Health (JPN) *Online - full text edition.* **4256**
Inpharma Weekly (NZL) *Online - full text edition. (File nos.428, 429)* **4345**
International Pharmaceutical Abstracts (USA) *Online - full text edition. (File no.74)* **4345**
J A M A: The Journal of the American Medical Association (USA) *Online - full text edition.* **3626**
Journal of Psychology and Theology (USA) *Online - full text edition.* **4421**
Laboratory Hazards Bulletin (GBR) *Online - full text edition. (File no.317)* **4269**
Martindale: the Complete Drug Reference (GBR) *Online - full text edition. (File no.141)* **4314**
McGraw-Hill's Biotechnology Newswatch (USA) *Online - full text edition. (File no.624, McGRAW-HILL PUBLICATIONS ONLINE)* **3276**
Medical and Health Care Books and Serials in Print (USA) *Online - full text edition.* **3732**
Medical & Pharmaceutical Biotechnology Abstracts (USA) *Online - full text edition. (File no.76, LIFE SCIENCES COLLECTION)* **3732**
Medical Devices, Diagnostics & Instrumentation Reports: The Gray Sheet (USA) *Online - full text edition. (File no.187)* **3649**
Medical Economics (USA) *Online - full text edition.* **3650**
Medicated Skincare: The International Market (GBR) *Online - full text edition.* **4315**
Medline (USA) *Online - full text edition of* Index Medicus. (File nos.154, 155, MEDLINE) **3729**
Merck Index: An Encyclopedia of Chemicals and Drugs (USA) *Online - full text edition.* **4345**
Meyler's Side Effects of Drugs (NLD) *Online - full text edition. (File no.70, SEDBASE)* **4316**
Microbiology Abstracts: Section A. Industrial & Applied Microbiology (USA) *Online - full text edition. (File no.76, LIFE SCIENCES COLLECTION)* **3233**
Microbiology Abstracts: Section B. Bacteriology (USA) *Online - full text edition. (File no.76, LIFE SCIENCES COLLECTION)* **3233**
Microbiology Abstracts: Section C. Algology, Mycology and Protozoology (USA) *Online - full text edition. (File no.76, LIFE SCIENCES COLLECTION)* **3233**
Mount Sinai Journal of Medicine (USA) *Online - full text edition.* **3663**
N I O S H T I C(USA) *Online - full text.* **4259**
National Report on Computers and Health (USA) *Online - full text edition.* **3812**
Nematological Abstracts (GBR) *Online - full text edition.* **3233**
Nonprescription Pharmaceuticals and Nutritionals: The Tan Sheet (USA) *Online - full text edition. (File no.187)* **4319**
Nucleic Acids Abstracts (USA) *Online - full text edition. (File no.76, LIFE SCIENCES COLLECTION)* **3234**
Nursing Homes (USA) *Online - full text edition.* **3933**
Nutrition Abstracts and Reviews. Series A: Human and Experimental (GBR) *Online - full text edition.* **4249**
Nutrition Abstracts and Reviews. Series B: Livestock Feeds and Feeding (GBR) *Online - full text edition.* **3157**
Occupational Safety & Health Reporter (USA) *Online - full text edition. (Laborlaw, File no.244)* **4262**
Peterson's Graduate and Professional Programs: The Biological Sciences (Year) (Book 3) (USA) *Online - full text edition. (File no.273)* **3416**
Pharmaceutical Approvals Monthly (USA) *Online - full text edition. (File no.187)* **4323**
Pharmacies and Drugstores: A World Survey (GBR) *Online - full text edition.* **4325**
Pharmacoeconomics and Outcomes News (NZL) *Online - full text edition.* **4345**
The Physician and Sportsmedicine (USA) *Online - full text edition.* **4176**
Plant Breeding Abstracts (GBR) *Online - full text edition.* **3157**
Postgraduate Medicine (USA) *Online - full text edition. (PGM)* **3678**
Prescription Pharmaceuticals and Biotechnology: The Pink Sheet (USA) *Online - full text edition. (File no.187)* **4331**
Product Alert (USA) *Online - full text edition. (File no. 636)* **3462**
Protozoological Abstracts (GBR) *Online - full text edition.* **3234**
Psychology Today (USA) *Online - full text edition.* **4441**
PsycINFO(USA) *Online - full text. (File no.11)* **4458**
R & D Focus (GBR) *Online - full text edition.* **4333**
Reactions Weekly (NZL) *Online - full text edition. (File nos.428, 429)* **4346**
Review of Medical and Veterinary Entomology (GBR) *Online - full text edition.* **3736**
Review of Medical and Veterinary Mycology (GBR) *Online - full text edition.* **3236**
Review of Plant Pathology (GBR) *Online - full text edition.* **3236**
Salud Publica de Mexico Online (MEX) *Online - full text edition of* Salud Publica de Mexico. **4489**
Saturday Evening Post (USA) *Online - full text edition.* **3465**
Scholastic Choices (USA) *Online - full text edition.* **3429**
Scrip - World Pharmaceutical News (GBR) *Online - full text edition. (File no.129&130)* **4335**
Side Effects of Drugs Annual (NLD) *Online - full text edition. (File no.70, SEDBASE)* **4336**
Toiletries, Fragrances and Skin Care: The Rose Sheet (USA) *Online - full text edition. (File no.187)* **3176**
Toxicology Abstracts (USA) *Online - full text edition. (File no.76, LIFE SCIENCES COLLECTION)* **3443**
Tree Physiology (CAN) *Online - full text edition.* **3283**
Tropical Diseases Bulletin (GBR) *Online - full text edition.* **3737**
Tuberculosis & Airborne Disease Weekly (USA) *Online - full text edition.* **3808**
Urology Times (USA) *Online - full text edition.* **4220**
Veterinary Bulletin (GBR) *Online - full text edition.* **4561**
Virology and AIDS Abstracts (USA) *Online - full text edition. (File no.76, LIFE SCIENCES COLLECTION)* **3236**
Vitamins & Dietary Supplements: The International Market (GBR) *Online - full text edition.* **4340**
Washington Drug Letter (Washington, 1979) (USA) *E-mail edition.* **4340**
Worldwide Biotech (USA) *Online - full text edition.* **3278**
Zhongguo Xinli Weisheng Zazhi (CHN) *Online - full text edition.* **4456**
Zoological Record (USA) *Online - full text edition. (File no.185)* **3236**

DIMDI Weisshausstrasse 36-38a, Cologne D-50676, Germany TEL 49-221-47240, FAX 49-221-411429, http://www.dimdi.de
Abstracts on Hygiene and Communicable Diseases (GBR) *Online - full text edition.* **3715**
AgBiotech News and Information (GBR) *Online - full text edition.* **3225**
Animal Breeding Abstracts (GBR) *Online - full text edition.* **3156**
Biocontrol News and Information (GBR) *Online - full text edition.* **3156**
Biological Abstracts (USA) *Online - full text edition.* **3226**
Biological Abstracts - R R M (USA) *Online - full text edition.* **3226**
CAB International. Bureau of Nutrition. Annotated Bibliographies (GBR) *Online - full text edition.* **4248**
Excerpta Medica. Abstract Journals (NLD) *Online - full text edition.* **3230**
Excerpta Medica. Section 1: Anatomy, Anthropology, Embryology & Histology (NLD) *Online - full text edition.* **3230**
Excerpta Medica. Section 10: Obstetrics and Gynecology (NLD) *Online - full text edition.* **3723**
Excerpta Medica. Section 11: Otorhinolaryngology (NLD) *Online - full text edition.* **3724**
Excerpta Medica. Section 12: Ophthalmology (NLD) *Online - full text edition.* **3724**
Excerpta Medica. Section 13: Dermatology and Venereology (NLD) *Online - full text edition.* **3724**
Excerpta Medica. Section 14: Radiology (NLD) *Online - full text edition.* **3724**
Excerpta Medica. Section 15: Chest Diseases, Thoracic Surgery and Tuberculosis (NLD) *Online - full text edition.* **3724**
Excerpta Medica. Section 16: Cancer (NLD) *Online - full text edition.* **3724**
Excerpta Medica. Section 17: Public Health, Social Medicine and Epidemiology (NLD) *Online - full text edition.* **4495**
Excerpta Medica. Section 18: Cardiovascular Diseases and Cardiovascular Surgery (NLD) *Online - full text edition.* **3724**
Excerpta Medica. Section 19: Rehabilitation and Physical Medicine (NLD) *Online - full text edition.* **3725**
Excerpta Medica. Section 2: Physiology (NLD) *Online - full text edition.* **3725**
Excerpta Medica. Section 20: Gerontology and Geriatrics (NLD) *Online - full text edition.* **3482**
Excerpta Medica. Section 21: Developmental Biology and Teratology (NLD) *Online - full text edition.* **3230**
Excerpta Medica. Section 22: Human Genetics (NLD) *Online - full text edition.* **3230**
Excerpta Medica. Section 23: Nuclear Medicine (NLD) *Online - full text edition.* **3725**
Excerpta Medica. Section 24: Anesthesiology (NLD) *Online - full text edition.* **3725**
Excerpta Medica. Section 25: Hematology (NLD) *Online - full text edition.* **3725**
Excerpta Medica. Section 26: Immunology, Serology and Transplantation (NLD) *Online - full text edition.* **3725**
Excerpta Medica. Section 27: Biophysics, Bio-Engineering and Medical Instrumentation (NLD) *Online - full text edition.* **3231**
Excerpta Medica. Section 28: Urology and Nephrology (NLD) *Online - full text edition.* **3726**

Online Service

Excerpta Medica. Section 29: Clinical and Experimental Biochemistry (NLD) *Online - full text edition.* **3231**
Excerpta Medica. Section 3: Endocrinology (NLD) *Online - full text edition.* **3726**
Excerpta Medica. Section 30: Clinical and Experimental Pharmacology (NLD) *Online - full text edition.* **4344**
Excerpta Medica. Section 31: Arthritis and Rheumatism (NLD) *Online - full text edition.* **3726**
Excerpta Medica. Section 32: Psychiatry (NLD) *Online - full text edition.* **3726**
Excerpta Medica. Section 33: Orthopedic Surgery (NLD) *Online - full text edition.* **3726**
Excerpta Medica. Section 35: Occupational Health and Industrial Medicine (NLD) *Online - full text edition.* **3726**
Excerpta Medica. Section 36: Health Policy, Economics and Management (NLD) *Online - full text edition.* **3524**
Excerpta Medica. Section 38: Adverse Reactions Titles (NLD) *Online - full text edition.* **4344**
Excerpta Medica. Section 4: Microbiology: Bacteriology, Mycology, Parasitology and Virology (NLD) *Online - full text edition.* **3231**
Excerpta Medica. Section 40: Drug Dependence, Alcohol Abuse and Alcoholism (NLD) *Online - full text edition.* **3407**
Excerpta Medica. Section 46: Environmental Health and Pollution Control (NLD) *Online - full text edition.* **3443**
Excerpta Medica. Section 48: Gastroenterology (NLD) *Online - full text edition.* **3726**
Excerpta Medica. Section 49: Forensic Science Abstracts (NLD) *Online - full text edition.* **3727**
Excerpta Medica. Section 5: General Pathology and Pathological Anatomy (NLD) *Online - full text edition.* **3231**
Excerpta Medica. Section 52: Toxicology (NLD) *Online - full text edition.* **3443**
Excerpta Medica. Section 6: Internal Medicine (NLD) *Online - full text edition.* **3727**
Excerpta Medica. Section 7: Pediatrics and Pediatric Surgery (NLD) *Online - full text edition.* **3727**
Excerpta Medica. Section 8: Neurology and Neurosurgery (NLD) *Online - full text edition.* **3727**
Excerpta Medica. Section 9: Surgery (NLD) *Online - full text edition.* **3727**
Helminthological Abstracts (GBR) *Online - full text edition.* **3232**
Index Veterinarius (GBR) *Online - full text edition.* **4561**
Informationsdienst Krankenhauswesen (DEU) *Online - full text edition.* **3515**
International Pharmaceutical Abstracts (USA) *Online - full text edition.* **4345**
Nematological Abstracts (GBR) *Online - full text edition.* **3233**
Nutrition Abstracts and Reviews. Series A: Human and Experimental (GBR) *Online - full text edition.* **4249**
Nutrition Abstracts and Reviews. Series B: Livestock Feeds and Feeding (GBR) *Online - full text edition.* **3157**
Plant Breeding Abstracts (GBR) *Online - full text edition.* **3157**
Protozoological Abstracts (GBR) *Online - full text edition.* **3234**
PsycINFO(USA) *Online - full text.* **4458**
Review of Medical and Veterinary Entomology (GBR) *Online - full text edition.* **3736**
Review of Medical and Veterinary Mycology (GBR) *Online - full text edition.* **3236**
Review of Plant Pathology (GBR) *Online - full text edition.* **3236**
Salud Publica de Mexico Online (MEX) *Online - full text edition of* Salud Publica de Mexico. **4489**
Tropical Diseases Bulletin (GBR) *Online - full text edition.* **3737**
Veterinary Bulletin (GBR) *Online - full text edition.* **4561**

Dow Jones Interactive PO Box 300, Princeton, NJ 08543-0300 TEL 609-452-1511, 800-369-7466, FAX 609-520-4775, http://www.djinteractive.com
Biomedical Market Newsletter (USA) *Online - full text edition.* **3366**
BioVenture View (USA) *Online - full text edition.* **3272**
Blood Weekly (USA) *Online - full text edition.* **3899**
Cancer Weekly Plus (USA) *Online - full text edition.* **3973**
McGraw-Hill's Biotechnology Newswatch (USA) *Online - full text edition. (BIO)* **3276**
The Physician and Sportsmedicine (USA) *Online - full text edition.* **4176**
Postgraduate Medicine (USA) *Online - full text edition. (PGM)* **3678**
Product Alert (USA) *Online - full text edition.* **3462**
Tuberculosis & Airborne Disease Weekly (USA) *Online - full text edition.* **3808**

EBSCO Publishing (Subsidiary of: EBSCO Industries, Inc.) 10 Estes St, Box 682, Ipswich, MA 01938 TEL 508-356-6565, 508-356-6500, 800-653-2726, FAX 508-356-5640, ep@epnet.com, , http://www.epnet.com
A I H A J (USA) *Online - full text edition.* **4249**
A J P: Cell Physiology Online (USA) *Online - full text edition of* American Journal of Physiology: Cell Physiology. **3337**
A J P: Endocrinology and Metabolism Online (USA) *Online - full text edition of* American Journal of Physiology: Endocrinology and Metabolism. **3338**
A J P: Gastrointestinal and Liver Physiology Online (USA) *Online - full text edition of* American Journal of Physiology: Gastrointestinal and Liver Physiology. **3338**
A J P: Heart and Circulatory Physiology Online (USA) *Online - full text edition of* American Journal of Physiology: Heart and Circulatory Physiology. **3338**
A J P: Lung Cellular and Molecular Physiology Online (USA) *Online - full text edition of* American Journal of Physiology: Lung Cellular and Molecular Physiology. **3338**
A J P: Regulatory, Integrative and Comparative Physiology Online (USA) *Online - full text edition of* American Journal of Physiology: Regulatory, Integrative and Comparative Physiology. **3338**
A J P: Renal Physiology Online (USA) *Online - full text edition of* American Journal of Physiology: Renal Physiology. **3339**
A J R (USA) *Online - full text edition.* **4139**
A N Z Journal of Surgery (AUS) *Online - full text edition.* **4178**
A R D Online (GBR) *Online - full text edition of* Annals of the Rheumatic Diseases. **4167**
Abdominal Imaging (USA) *Online - full text edition.* **3885**
Abstracts in Social Gerontology (USA) *Online - full text edition.* **3482**
Academic Emergency Medicine (USA) *Online - full text edition.* **4009**
Academic Psychiatry (USA) *Online - full text edition.* **4067**
Acta Anaesthesiologica Scandinavica (DNK) *Online - full text edition.* **3753**
Acta Biotheoretica (NLD) *Online - full text edition.* **3178**
Acta Dermato-Venereologica (NOR) *Online - full text edition.* **3843**
Acta Diabetologica (DEU) *Online - full text edition.* **3855**
Acta Ethologica Online(DEU) *Online - full text.* **3179**
Acta Haematologica (CHE) *Online - full text edition.* **3897**
Acta Hydrochimica et Hydrobiologica (DEU) *Online - full text edition.* **4561**
Acta Neurochirurgica (AUT) *Online - full text edition.* **4179**
Acta Neurologica Scandinavica (DNK) *Online - full text edition.* **4068**
Acta Neuropathologica (DEU) *Online - full text edition.* **4068**
Acta Odontologica Scandinavica (NOR) *Online - full text edition.* **3813**
Acta Oncologica (NOR) *Online - full text edition.* **3966**
Acta Ophthamologica Scandinavica Online(DNK) *Online - full text.* **3993**
Acta Oto-Laryngologica (NOR) *Online - full text edition.* **4029**
Acta Paediatrica (NOR) *Online - full text edition.* **4039**
Acta Physiologica Scandinavica (GBR) *Online - full text edition.* **3337**
Acta Psychiatrica Scandinavica (DNK) *Online - full text edition.* **4068**
Acta Radiologica (DNK) *Online - full text edition.* **4139**
Acta Zoologica Online(GBR) *Online - full text.* **3350**
Addiction (GBR) *Online - full text edition.* **3396**
Addiction Biology (GBR) *Online - full text edition.* **3397**
Advances in Health Sciences Education (NLD) *Online - full text edition.* **3560**
Advances in Physiology Education Online (USA) *Online - full text edition of* Advances in Physiology Education. **3337**
Advances in Physiotherapy (NOR) *Online - full text edition.* **4058**
Advances in Psychiatric Treatment Online (GBR) *Online - full text edition of* Advances in Psychiatric Treatment. **4070**
Advances in Renal Replacement Therapy (USA) *Online - full text edition.* **4209**
Adverse Drug Reaction Bulletin (USA) *Online - full text edition.* **4274**
Aesthetic Plastic Surgery (USA) *Online - full text edition.* **4179**
Aesthetic Surgery Journal (USA) *Online - full text edition.* **4179**
Age and Ageing (GBR) *Online - full text edition.* **3466**
Ageing and Society (GBR) *Online - full text edition.* **3466**
Aggressive Behavior (USA) *Online - full text edition.* **4373**
Aging & Mental Health (GBR) *Online - full text edition.* **3466**
AIDS (USA) *Online - full text edition.* **3790**
AIDS & Behavior (USA) *Online - full text edition.* **3739**
AIDS Care (GBR) *Online - full text edition.* **3791**
AIDS Patient Care and S T Ds (USA) *Online - full text edition.* **3791**
AIDS Research and Human Retroviruses (USA) *Online - full text edition.* **3792**
Alcohol & Alcoholism (GBR) *Online - full text edition.* **3397**
Alimentary Pharmacology and Therapeutics (GBR) *Online - full text edition.* **3886**
Allergology International (AUS) *Online - full text edition.* **3739**
Allergy (DNK) *Online - full text edition.* **3739**
Alternative & Complementary Therapies (USA) *Online - full content edition.* **3163**
Ambulatory Child Health Online(GBR) *Online - full text.* **4040**
American Academy of Dermatology. Journal (USA) *Online - full text edition.* **3844**
American Association for Pediatric Ophthalmology and Strabismus. Journal (USA) *Online - full content edition.* **3993**
American Behavioral Scientist (USA) *Online - full text edition.* **4508**
American College of Physicians Observer (USA) *Online - full text edition.* **3563**
American Family Physician (USA) *Online - full text edition.* **3563**
American Heart Journal (USA) *Online - full text edition.* **3762**
American Imago (USA) *Online - full text edition.* **4071**
American Journal of Clinical Nutrition (USA) *Online - full text edition.* **4228**
American Journal of Clinical Pathology (USA) *Online - full text edition.* **3563**
American Journal of Community Psychology (USA) *Online - full text edition.* **4520**
American Journal of Dance Therapy (USA) *Online - full text edition.* **3396**
American Journal of Drug and Alcohol Abuse (USA) *Online - full text edition.* **3399**
American Journal of Family Therapy (USA) *Online - full text edition.* **4374**
American Journal of Geriatric Psychiatry (USA) *Online - full text edition.* **3468**
American Journal of Health-System Pharmacy (USA) *Online - full text edition.* **4275**
American Journal of Hematology (USA) *Online - full text edition.* **3897**
American Journal of Human Biology (USA) *Online - full text edition.* **3180**
American Journal of Human Genetics (USA) *Online - full text edition.* **3297**
American Journal of Industrial Medicine (USA) *Online - full text edition.* **4249**
American Journal of Infection Control (USA) *Online - full text edition.* **3792**
American Journal of Kidney Diseases (USA) *Online - full text edition.* **4209**
American Journal of Medical Genetics (USA) *Online - full text edition.* **3298**
The American Journal of Medicine (USA) *Online - full text edition.* **3564**
American Journal of Nephrology (CHE) *Online - full text edition.* **4209**
American Journal of Obstetrics and Gynecology (USA) *Online - full text edition.* **3944**
American Journal of Orthodontics and Dentofacial Orthopedics (USA) *Online - full text edition.* **3814**
American Journal of Pathology (USA) *Online - full text edition.* **3564**
American Journal of Perinatology (USA) *Online - full text edition.* **3944**
American Journal of Primatology (USA) *Online - full text edition.* **3350**
American Journal of Psychiatry (USA) *Online - full text edition.* **4071**
American Journal of Psychoanalysis (USA) *Online - full text edition.* **4374**
American Journal of Reproductive Immunology Online(DNK) *Online - full text.* **3740**
American Journal of Respiratory and Critical Care Medicine (USA) *Online - full text edition.* **4158**
American Journal of Respiratory Cell and Molecular Biology (USA) *Online - full text edition.* **4158**
American Journal of Therapeutics (GBR) *Online - full text edition.* **3565**
American Journal on Addictions (USA) *Online - full text edition.* **3399**
American Medical Informatics Association. Journal (USA) *Online - full text edition.* **3809**
American Medical News (USA) *Online - full text edition.* **3565**
The American Naturalist (USA) *Online - full text edition.* **3180**
American Society of Echocardiography. Journal (USA) *Online - full text edition.* **3762**
American Society of Nephrology. Journal (USA) *Online - full text edition.* **4209**
Amino Acids (AUT) *Online - full text edition.* **3240**
Anaerobe (GBR) *Online - full text edition.* **3317**
Anaesthesia (Oxford) (GBR) *Online - full text edition.* **3754**
Der Anaesthesist (DEU) *Online - full text edition.* **3754**
Analytical Biochemistry (USA) *Online - full text edition.* **3240**
Analytical Cellular Pathology (NLD) *Online - full text edition.* **3285**
Analytische Psychologie (CHE) *Online - full text edition.* **4375**
Anatomia, Histologia, Embryologia Online(DEU) *Online - full text.* **4537**
The Anatomical Record (USA) *Online - full text edition.* **3181**
Anatomy and Embryology (DEU) *Online - full text edition.* **3339**
Andrologia (DEU) *Online - full text edition.* **3565**
Anesthesia and Analgesia (USA) *Online - full text edition.* **3755**
Anesthesiology (USA) *Online - full text edition.* **3755**
Angiogenesis (GBR) *Online - full text edition.* **3967**
Animal Behavior Abstracts (USA) *Online - full text edition.* **3225**
Animal Behaviour (GBR) *Online - full text edition.* **3350**
Animal Cognition (DEU) *Online - full text edition.* **4375**
Animal Genetics (GBR) *Online - full text edition.* **3298**
Annals of Biomedical Engineering (USA) *Online - full text edition.* **3566**
Annals of Clinical Psychiatry (USA) *Online - full text edition.* **4073**
Annals of Emergency Medicine (USA) *Online - full text edition.* **4010**
Annals of Hematology (DEU) *Online - full text edition.* **3898**
Annals of Human Biology (GBR) *Online - full text edition.* **3181**
Annals of Human Genetics (GBR) *Online - full text edition.* **3298**
Annals of Internal Medicine (USA) *Online - full text edition.* **3907**
Annals of Medicine (GBR) *Online - full text edition.* **3871**
Annals of Nutrition and Metabolism (CHE) *Online - full text edition.* **4229**
Annals of Oncology (NLD) *Online - full text edition.* **3967**
Annals of Surgery (USA) *Online - full text edition.* **4181**
Annals of Thoracic Surgery (USA) *Online - full text edition.* **4181**
Annals of Tropical Medicine and Parasitology (GBR) *Online - full text edition.* **3793**
Annals of Tropical Paediatrics (GBR) *Online - full text edition.* **4040**

Annals of Vascular Surgery (USA) *Online - full text edition.* **4181**
Annual Review of Biochemistry (USA) *Online - full text edition.* **3240**
Annual Review of Biophysics and Biomolecular Structure (USA) *Online - full text edition.* **3264**
Annual Review of Cell and Developmental Biology (USA) *Online - full text edition.* **3285**
Annual Review of Genetics (USA) *Online - full text edition.* **3298**
Annual Review of Immunology (USA) *Online - full text edition.* **3740**
Annual Review of Medicine Online (USA) *Online - full text edition of* Annual Review of Medicine: Selected Topics in the Clinical Sciences. **3567**
Annual Review of Microbiology (USA) *Online - full text edition.* **3317**
Annual Review of Neuroscience (USA) *Online - full text edition.* **4073**
Annual Review of Nutrition (USA) *Online - full text edition.* **4229**
Annual Review of Pharmacology and Toxicology (USA) *Online - full text edition.* **4276**
Annual Review of Physiology (USA) *Online - full text edition.* **3339**
Annual Review of Psychology (USA) *Online - full text edition.* **4376**
Annual Review of Public Health (USA) *Online - full text edition.* **4461**
Antarctic Science (GBR) *Online - full text edition.* **3182**
Anthropology & Medicine (GBR) *Online - full content edition.* **3172**
Anti-Cancer Drug Design (GBR) *Online - full text edition.* **3967**
Anti-Cancer Drugs (USA) *Online - full text edition.* **3967**
Antimicrobial Agents and Chemotherapy (USA) *Online - full text edition.* **3317**
Antonie van Leeuwenhoek (NLD) *Online - full text edition.* **3268**
Aphasiology (GBR) *Online - full text edition.* **4073**
Apoptosis (USA) *Online - full text edition.* **3285**
Appetite (GBR) *Online - full text edition.* **4229**
Applied and Environmental Microbiology (USA) *Online - full text edition.* **3318**
Applied Cardiopulmonary Pathophysiology (NLD) *Online - full text edition.* **3339**
Applied Cognitive Psychology (GBR) *Online - full text edition.* **4377**
Applied Developmental Science (USA) *Online - full text edition.* **4377**
Applied Microbiology and Biotechnology (DEU) *Online - full text edition.* **3268**
Applied Neuropsychology (USA) *Online - full text edition.* **4073**
Applied Occupational & Environmental Hygiene (USA) *Online - full text edition.* **4250**
Applied Psycholinguistics (GBR) *Online - full text edition.* **3550**
Applied Psychological Measurement (USA) *Online - full text edition.* **4377**
Applied Psychology (GBR) *Online - full text edition.* **4377**
Applied Psychophysiology and Biofeedback (USA) *Online - full text edition.* **4378**
Aquatic Ecology (NLD) *Online - full text edition.* **3182**
Archiv der Pharmazie (DEU) *Online - full text edition.* **4277**
Archives of Andrology (USA) *Online - full text edition.* **3568**
Archives of Biochemistry and Biophysics (USA) *Online - full text edition.* **3241**
Archives of Dermatological Research (DEU) *Online - full text edition.* **3845**
Archives of Dermatology (USA) *Online - full text edition.* **3845**
Archives of Disease in Childhood (GBR) *Online - full text edition.* **4040**
Archives of Environmental Contamination and Toxicology (USA) *Online - full text edition.* **3445**
Archives of Family Medicine (USA) *Online - full text edition.* **3568**
Archives of General Psychiatry (USA) *Online - full text edition.* **4074**
Archives of Gynecology and Obstetrics (DEU) *Online - full text edition.* **3945**
Archives of Internal Medicine (USA) *Online - full text edition.* **3907**
Archives of Microbiology (DEU) *Online - full text edition.* **3318**
Archives of Neurology (USA) *Online - full text edition.* **4074**
Archives of Ophthalmology (USA) *Online - full text edition.* **3994**
Archives of Orthopaedic and Trauma Surgery (DEU) *Online - full text edition.* **4010**
Archives of Otolaryngology - Head & Neck Surgery (USA) *Online - full text edition.* **4030**
Archives of Pediatrics & Adolescent Medicine (USA) *Online - full text edition.* **4041**
Archives of Physiology and Biochemistry (NLD) *Online - full text edition.* **3339**
Archives of Sexual Behavior (USA) *Online - full text edition.* **3568**
Archives of Surgery (USA) *Online - full text edition.* **4182**
Archives of Toxicology (DEU) *Online - full text edition.* **3445**
Archives of Virology (AUT) *Online - full text edition.* **3318**
Archives of Women's Mental Health (AUT) *Online - full text edition.* **4562**
Arteriosclerosis, Thrombosis, and Vascular Biology (USA) *Online - full text edition.* **3763**
Arthritis and Rheumatism (USA) *Online - full text edition.* **4167**
Arthroscopy (USA) *Online - full text edition.* **4010**
Arthroskopie (DEU) *Online - full text edition.* **3569**
Artificial Intelligence in Medicine (NLD) *Online - full text edition.* **3389**
Artificial Life (USA) *Online - full content edition.* **3389**
Artificial Organs (USA) *Online - full text edition.* **3871**
Asia Pacific Journal of Clinical Nutrition (AUS) *Online - full text edition.* **4229**
Asian Journal of Social Psychology (GBR) *Online - full text edition.* **4378**
Attachment and Human Development (GBR) *Online - full content edition.* **4379**
Audiology and Neuro-Otology (CHE) *Online - full text edition.* **4031**
Austral Ecology (AUS) *Online - full text edition.* **3183**
Australasian Journal of Dermatology (AUS) *Online - full text edition.* **3845**
Australasian Psychiatry (AUS) *Online - full text edition.* **4075**
Australasian Radiology (AUS) *Online - full text edition.* **4140**
Australian and New Zealand Journal of Family Therapy (GBR) *Online - full text edition.* **4520**
Australian and New Zealand Journal of Mental Health Nursing (AUS) *Online - full text edition.* **4075**
Australian & New Zealand Journal of Psychiatry (AUS) *Online - full text edition.* **4075**
Australian Journal of Experimental Agriculture (AUS) *Online - full text edition.* **3157**
Australian Journal of Rural Health (AUS) *Online - full text edition.* **4463**
Australian Occupational Therapy Journal (AUS) *Online - full text edition.* **4059**
Autism (GBR) *Online - full text edition.* **4075**
Autoimmunity (CHE) *Online - full text edition.* **3741**
Autonomic & Autacoid Pharmacology (GBR) *Online - full text edition.* **4279**
Avian Pathology (GBR) *Online - full text edition.* **4539**
B B A - Bioenergetics (NLD) *Online - full text edition.* **3278**
B B A - Biomembranes (NLD) *Online - full text edition.* **3285**
B B A - Gene Structure and Expression (NLD) *Online - full text edition.* **3299**
B B A - General Subjects (NLD) *Online - full text edition.* **3241**
B B A - Molecular and Cell Biology of Lipids (NLD) *Online - full text edition.* **3242**
B B A - Molecular Basis of Disease (NLD) *Online - full text edition.* **3299**
B B A - Molecular Cell Research (NLD) *Online - full text edition.* **3285**
B B A - Protein Structure and Molecular Enzymology (NLD) *Online - full text edition.* **3242**
B B A - Reviews on Cancer (NLD) *Online - full text edition.* **3968**
B J O Online (GBR) *Online - full text edition of* British Journal of Ophthalmology. **3994**
B J S M Online (GBR) *Online - full text edition of* British Journal of Sports Medicine. **4173**
B J U International (GBR) *Online - full text edition.* **4210**
Bailliere's Best Practice & Research in Clinical Anaesthesiology (GBR) *Online - full text edition.* **3756**
Bailliere's Best Practice & Research in Clinical Endocrinology and Metabolism (GBR) *Online - full text edition.* **3855**
Bailliere's Best Practice & Research in Clinical Gastroenterology (GBR) *Online - full text edition.* **3886**
Bailliere's Best Practice & Research in Clinical Haematology (GBR) *Online - full text edition.* **3898**
Bailliere's Best Practice & Research in Clinical Obstetrics and Gynaecology (GBR) *Online - full text edition.* **3945**
Bailliere's Best Practice & Research in Clinical Rheumatology (GBR) *Online - full text edition.* **4167**
Basic and Applied Social Psychology (USA) *Online - full text edition.* **4380**
Basic Research in Cardiology (DEU) *Online - full text edition.* **3764**
Behavior Genetics (USA) *Online - full text edition.* **3299**
Behavior Modification (USA) *Online - full text edition.* **4380**
Behavioral and Brain Sciences (GBR) *Online - full text edition.* **4380**
Behavioral Ecology (USA) *Online - full text edition.* **3184**
Behavioral Ecology and Sociobiology (DEU) *Online - full text edition.* **3436**
Behavioral Interventions (GBR) *Online - full text edition.* **4076**
Behavioral Sciences and the Law (GBR) *Online - full text edition.* **4381**
Behaviour (NLD) *Online - full content edition.* **3351**
Behaviour and Information Technology (GBR) *Online - full text edition.* **4381**
Behavioural and Cognitive Psychotherapy (GBR) *Online - full text edition.* **4382**
Bio-Medical Materials and Engineering (NLD) *Online - full text edition.* **3237**
Biocatalysis and Biotransformation (CHE) *Online - full text edition.* **3269**
Biochemical and Biophysical Research Communications (USA) *Online - full text edition.* **3242**
Biochemical Genetics (USA) *Online - full text edition.* **3299**
Biochemical Journal (GBR) *Online - full text edition.* **3242**
Biochemical Pharmacology (USA) *Online - full text edition.* **4279**
Biochemistry (USA) *Online - full text edition.* **3243**
Biochemistry and Cell Biology (CAN) *Online - full text edition.* **3243**
Biochimica et Biophysica Acta (NLD) *Online - full text edition.* **3244**
Bioconjugate Chemistry (USA) *Online - full text edition.* **3244**
Biocontrol News and Information (GBR) *Online - full text edition.* **3156**
Biocontrol Science and Technology (GBR) *Online - full text edition.* **3157**
Biodegradation (NLD) *Online - full text edition.* **3456**
BioDrugs (NZL) *Online - full text edition.* **4280**
Bioelectromagnetics (USA) *Online - full text edition.* **3264**
BioEssays (GBR) *Online - full text edition.* **3184**
Bioethics (GBR) *Online - full text edition.* **4346**
BioFactors (NLD) *Online - full text edition.* **3244**
Biofouling (CHE) *Online - full text edition.* **3446**
Biogeochemistry (NLD) *Online - full text edition.* **3245**
Biogerontology (NLD) *Online - full text edition.* **3468**
Biological Chemistry (DEU) *Online - full text edition.* **3245**
Biological Control (USA) *Online - full text edition.* **3185**
Biological Research for Nursing (USA) *Online - full text edition.* **3914**
Biological Reviews (GBR) *Online - full text edition.* **3185**
Biologicals (GBR) *Online - full text edition.* **3186**
Biologie in Unserer Zeit (DEU) *Online - full text edition.* **3186**
Biology and Fertility of Soils (DEU) *Online - full text edition.* **3157**
Biology of Reproduction (USA) *Online - full text edition.* **3186**
Biology of the Neonate (CHE) *Online - full text edition.* **3945**
Biomarkers (GBR) *Online - full text edition.* **3575**
Biomedical Chromatography (GBR) *Online - full text edition.* **3872**
Biomedical Microdevices (USA) *Online - full text edition.* **3576**
Biometrical Journal (DEU) *Online - full text edition.* **3187**
Biometrika (GBR) *Online - full text edition.* **3226**
Bioorganic & Medicinal Chemistry (GBR) *Online - full text edition.* **3377**
Bioorganic & Medicinal Chemistry Letters (GBR) *Online - full text edition.* **3378**
Biopharmaceutics & Drug Disposition (GBR) *Online - full text edition.* **4280**
Biophysical Journal (USA) *Online - full text edition.* **3265**
Biorheology (NLD) *Online - full text edition.* **3265**
BioScience (USA) *Online - full text edition.* **3187**
Bioscience Reports (USA) *Online - full text edition.* **3286**
Biospectroscopy (USA) *Online - full text edition.* **3376**
Biotech Software and Internet Report (USA) *Online - full text edition.* **3270**
Biotechnology and Applied Biochemistry (GBR) *Online - full text edition.* **3271**
Biotechnology and Bioengineering (USA) *Online - full text edition.* **3271**
Biotechnology Law Report (USA) *Online - full content edition.* **3272**
Biotechnology Letters (NLD) *Online - full text edition.* **3272**
Biotechnology Progress (USA) *Online - full text edition.* **3272**
Bipolar Disorders Online(DNK) *Online - full text.* **4077**
Birth (USA) *Online - full text edition.* **3946**
Blood (USA) *Online - full text edition.* **3898**
Blood Cells, Molecules, and Diseases (USA) *Online - full text edition.* **3898**
Blood Coagulation and Fibrinolysis (USA) *Online - full text edition.* **3898**
Blood Pressure (NOR) *Online - full text edition.* **3764**
Blood Pressure Monitoring (USA) *Online - full text edition.* **3764**
Blood Purification (CHE) *Online - full text edition.* **3899**
Blood Reviews (GBR) *Online - full text edition.* **3899**
Bone Marrow Transplantation (GBR) *Online - full text edition.* **3872**
Brain (GBR) *Online - full text edition.* **4077**
Brain and Cognition (USA) *Online - full text edition.* **4383**
Brain and Language (USA) *Online - full text edition.* **4383**
Brain and Mind (USA) *Online - full text edition.* **4077**
Brain, Behavior and Evolution (CHE) *Online - full text edition.* **4077**
Brain, Behavior, and Immunity (USA) *Online - full text edition.* **3741**
Brain Injury (GBR) *Online - full text edition.* **4077**
Brain Research (NLD) *Online - full text edition.* **4078**
Brain Research Protocols (NLD) *Online - full text edition.* **4078**
Brain Research Reviews (NLD) *Online - full text edition.* **4078**
The Breast (GBR) *Online - full text edition.* **3946**
Breast Cancer Research and Treatment (USA) *Online - full text edition.* **3969**
Breast Disease (NLD) *Online - full text edition.* **3946**
The Breast Journal Online(USA) *Online - full text.* **3946**
British Dental Journal (GBR) *Online - full text edition.* **3816**
British Food Journal (GBR) *Online - full text edition.* **3460**
British Homeopathic Journal (GBR) *Online - full text edition.* **3786**
British Journal of Anaesthesia (GBR) *Online - full text edition.* **3756**
British Journal of Cancer (GBR) *Online - full text edition.* **3969**
British Journal of Clinical Governance (GBR) *Online - full text edition.* **3578**
British Journal of Clinical Pharmacology (GBR) *Online - full text edition.* **4281**
British Journal of Clinical Psychology (GBR) *Online - full text edition.* **4383**
The British Journal of Criminology (GBR) *Online - full text edition.* **3393**
British Journal of Dermatology (GBR) *Online - full text edition.* **3845**

Online Service

British Journal of Developmental Psychology (GBR) *Online - full text edition.* **4383**
British Journal of Educational Psychology (GBR) *Online - full text edition.* **4383**
British Journal of Guidance and Counselling (GBR) *Online - full content edition.* **4269**
British Journal of Haematology (GBR) *Online - full text edition.* **3899**
British Journal of Health Psychology (GBR) *Online - full text edition.* **4384**
British Journal of Learning Disabilities (GBR) *Online - full text edition.* **4079**
British Journal of Mathematical and Statistical Psychology (GBR) *Online - full text edition.* **4384**
British Journal of Medical Psychology (GBR) *Online - full text edition.* **4384**
British Journal of Neurosurgery (GBR) *Online - full text edition.* **4182**
The British Journal of Nutrition (GBR) *Online - full text edition.* **4230**
British Journal of Obstetrics & Gynaecology (GBR) *Online - full text edition.* **3946**
British Journal of Oral and Maxillofacial Surgery (GBR) *Online - full text edition.* **4183**
British Journal of Pharmacology (GBR) *Online - full text edition.* **4281**
British Journal of Plastic Surgery (GBR) *Online - full text edition.* **4183**
British Journal of Psychiatry (GBR) *Online - full text edition.* **4079**
British Journal of Psychology (GBR) *Online - full text edition.* **4384**
British Journal of Radiology (GBR) *Online - full text edition.* **4141**
British Journal of Social Psychology (GBR) *Online - full text edition.* **4384**
British Journal of Special Education (GBR) *Online - full text edition.* **3419**
British Journal of Surgery (GBR) *Online - full text edition.* **4183**
British Medical Bulletin (GBR) *Online - full text edition.* **3579**
Bulletin of Environmental Contamination and Toxicology (USA) *Online - full text edition.* **3446**
Bulletin of Mathematical Biology (GBR) *Online - full text edition.* **3188**
Bulletin of the History of Medicine (USA) *Online - full text edition.* **3579**
Bundesgesundheitsblatt - Gesundheitsforschung - Gesundheitsschutz Online(DEU) *Online - full content.* **4464**
C A - A Cancer Journal for Clinicians (USA) *Online - full text edition.* **3969**
C N S Drugs (NZL) *Online - full text edition.* **4282**
Calcified Tissue International (USA) *Online - full text edition.* **3855**
Calcium and Calcified Tissue Abstracts (USA) *Online - full text edition.* **3228**
Cambridge Quarterly of Healthcare Ethics (GBR) *Online - full text edition.* **3581**
Canadian Journal of Microbiology (CAN) *Online - full text edition.* **3319**
Canadian Journal of Physiology and Pharmacology (CAN) *Online - full text edition.* **3340**
The Canadian Journal of Psychiatry (CAN) *Online - full text edition.* **4080**
Cancer (USA) *Online - full text edition.* **3969**
Cancer and Metastasis Reviews (USA) *Online - full text edition.* **3969**
Cancer Biotherapy & Radiopharmaceuticals (USA) *Online - full content edition.* **3970**
Cancer Causes & Control (NLD) *Online - full text edition.* **3970**
Cancer Chemotherapy and Pharmacology (DEU) *Online - full text edition.* **3970**
Cancer Detection and Prevention (USA) *Online - full text edition.* **3970**
Cancer Gene Therapy (USA) *Online - full text edition.* **3971**
Cancer Immunology, Immunotherapy (DEU) *Online - full text edition.* **3971**
The Cancer Journal from Scientific American (English Edition) (USA) *Online - full text edition.* **3972**
Cancer Practice Online(USA) *Online - full text.* **3972**
Cancer Treatment Reviews (GBR) *Online - full text edition.* **3973**
Carbohydrate Letters (CHE) *Online - full text edition.* **3246**
Carcinogenesis (GBR) *Online - full text edition.* **3974**
Cardiac Electrophysiology Review (USA) *Online - full text edition.* **3765**
Cardiology (CHE) *Online - full text edition.* **3765**
Cardiovascular and Interventional Radiology (USA) *Online - full text edition.* **4141**
Cardiovascular Drugs and Therapy (USA) *Online - full text edition.* **3766**
Caries Research (CHE) *Online - full text edition.* **3817**
Catheterization and Cardiovascular Interventions (USA) *Online - full text edition.* **3767**
Cell Adhesion and Communication (CHE) *Online - full text edition.* **3189**
Cell and Tissue Research (DEU) *Online - full text edition.* **3287**
Cell Biochemistry and Function (GBR) *Online - full text edition.* **3246**
Cell Biology and Toxicology (NLD) *Online - full text edition.* **3446**
Cell Calcium (Edinburgh) (GBR) *Online - full text edition.* **3287**
Cell Death and Differentiation (GBR) *Online - full text edition.* **3287**
Cell Motility and the Cytoskeleton (USA) *Online - full text edition.* **3287**
Cell Proliferation (GBR) *Online - full text edition.* **3287**
Cell Stress & Chaperones (USA) *Online - full text edition.* **3582**
Cells, Tissues, Organs (CHE) *Online - full text edition.* **3583**
Cellular and Molecular Life Sciences (CHE) *Online - full text edition.* **3190**
Cellular & Molecular Neurobiology (USA) *Online - full text edition.* **4080**
Cellular Immunology (USA) *Online - full text edition.* **3742**
Cellular Physiology and Biochemistry (DEU) *Online - full text edition.* **3288**
Cellulose (NLD) *Online - full text edition.* **3378**
Cephalalgia (GBR) *Online - full text edition.* **4080**
Cerebral Cortex (USA) *Online - full text edition.* **4081**
Cerebrovascular Diseases (CHE) *Online - full text edition.* **4081**
Chemical Health and Safety (USA) *Online - full text edition.* **3446**
Chemical Research in Toxicology (USA) *Online - full text edition.* **3447**
Chemical Senses (GBR) *Online - full text edition.* **3340**
Chemistry & Biology (GBR) *Online - full text edition.* **3372**
Chemistry and Ecology (CHE) *Online - full text edition.* **3372**
Chemoecology (CHE) *Online - full text edition.* **3378**
Chemotherapy (CHE) *Online - full text edition.* **4283**
Chest (USA) *Online - full text edition.* **4159**
Child Abuse Review (GBR) *Online - full text edition.* **4511**
Child and Adolescent Social Work Journal (USA) *Online - full text edition.* **4520**
Child and Youth Care Forum (USA) *Online - full text edition.* **3381**
Child: Care, Health and Development (GBR) *Online - full text edition.* **4042**
Child Language Teaching and Therapy (GBR) *Online - full text edition.* **3420**
Child Maltreatment (USA) *Online - full text edition.* **3381**
Child Psychiatry and Human Development (USA) *Online - full text edition.* **4081**
Child Psychology and Psychiatry Review (GBR) *Online - full text edition.* **4387**
Childhood (GBR) *Online - full text edition.* **3382**
Children & Society (GBR) *Online - full text edition.* **3382**
Child's Nervous System (DEU) *Online - full text edition.* **4081**
Chirality (USA) *Online - full text edition.* **3246**
Der Chirurg (DEU) *Online - full text edition.* **4184**
Chirurgische Gastroenterologie (CHE) *Online - full text edition.* **3887**
Christian Bioethics (NLD) *Online - full text edition.* **3584**
Chromosoma (DEU) *Online - full text edition.* **3300**
Chronobiology International (USA) *Online - full text edition.* **3191**
Circulation (Baltimore) (USA) *Online - full text edition.* **3768**
Circulation Research (USA) *Online - full text edition.* **3768**
Cladistics (GBR) *Online - full text edition.* **3191**
Clinica Chimica Acta (NLD) *Online - full text edition.* **3585**
Clinical Anatomy (USA) *Online - full text edition.* **3585**
Clinical and Diagnostic Laboratory Immunology (USA) *Online - full text edition.* **3742**
Clinical and Experimental Allergy (GBR) *Online - full text edition.* **3742**
Clinical and Experimental Dermatology (GBR) *Online - full text edition.* **3846**
Clinical and Experimental Hypertension (USA) *Online - full text edition.* **3768**
Clinical and Experimental Immunology (GBR) *Online - full text edition.* **3742**
Clinical and Experimental Medicine (DEU) *Online - full text edition.* **3585**
Clinical and Experimental Metastasis (NLD) *Online - full text edition.* **3974**
Clinical and Experimental Nephrology Online(JPN) *Online - full text.* **4211**
Clinical and Experimental Ophthalmology (AUS) *Online - full text edition.* **3995**
Clinical and Experimental Pharmacology & Physiology (AUS) *Online - full text edition.* **3341**
Clinical and Laboratory Haematology (GBR) *Online - full text edition.* **3899**
Clinical Autonomic Research (USA) *Online - full text edition.* **3586**
Clinical Chemistry (USA) *Online - full text edition.* **3873**
Clinical Chemistry and Laboratory Medicine (DEU) *Online - full text edition.* **3247**
Clinical Child and Family Psychology Review (USA) *Online - full text edition.* **4387**
Clinical Child Psychology & Psychiatry (GBR) *Online - full text edition.* **3382**
Clinical Diabetes (USA) *Online - full text edition.* **3856**
Clinical Drug Investigation (NZL) *Online - full text edition.* **4283**
Clinical Dysmorphology (USA) *Online - full text edition.* **3191**
Clinical Endocrinology (GBR) *Online - full text edition.* **3856**
Clinical Genetics (DNK) *Online - full text edition.* **3300**
Clinical Hemorheology and Microcirculation (NLD) *Online - full text edition.* **3899**
Clinical Immunology (USA) *Online - full text edition.* **3743**
Clinical Infectious Diseases (USA) *Online - full text edition.* **3794**
Clinical Intensive Care (GBR) *Online - full content edition.* **3908**
Clinical Linguistics & Phonetics (GBR) *Online - full text edition.* **4082**
Clinical Microbiology and Infection (GBR) *Online - full text edition.* **3586**
Clinical Microbiology Reviews (USA) *Online - full text edition.* **3319**
Clinical Nursing Research (USA) *Online - full text edition.* **3916**
Clinical Nutrition (GBR) *Online - full text edition.* **4231**
Clinical Oncology (GBR) *Online - full text edition.* **3975**
Clinical Oral Implants Research (DNK) *Online - full text edition.* **3818**
Clinical Oral Investigations (DEU) *Online - full text edition.* **3818**
Clinical Orthodontics and Research Online(DNK) *Online - full text.* **3818**
Clinical Otolaryngology and Allied Sciences (GBR) *Online - full text edition.* **4031**
Clinical Performance and Quality Health Care (GBR) *Online - full text edition.* **3587**
Clinical Pharmacokinetics (NZL) *Online - full text edition.* **4284**
Clinical Physiology and Functional Imaging (GBR) *Online - full text edition.* **3587**
Clinical Psychology (USA) *Online - full text edition.* **4388**
Clinical Psychology & Psychotherapy (GBR) *Online - full text edition.* **4388**
Clinical Radiology (GBR) *Online - full text edition.* **4142**
Clinical Rehabilitation (GBR) *Online - full text edition.* **4060**
Clinical Rheumatology (BEL) *Online - full text edition.* **4168**
Clinical Science (GBR) *Online - full text edition.* **3587**
Clinical Transplantation (DNK) *Online - full text edition.* **4185**
Clio Medica (NLD) *Online - full text edition.* **3588**
Cloning and Stem Cells (USA) *Online - full text edition.* **3300**
Cognition and Emotion (GBR) *Online - full text edition.* **4388**
Cognition and Instruction (USA) *Online - full text edition.* **4388**
Cognition, Technology and Work (GBR) *Online - full text edition.* **4388**
Cognitive Brain Research (NLD) *Online - full text edition.* **4083**
Cognitive Linguistics (DEU) *Online - full text edition.* **3550**
Cognitive Neuropsychiatry (GBR) *Online - full text edition.* **4389**
Cognitive Neuropsychology (GBR) *Online - full text edition.* **4083**
Cognitive Psychology (USA) *Online - full text edition.* **4389**
Cognitive Therapy and Research (USA) *Online - full text edition.* **4390**
College of Surgeons Hong Kong. Annals (AUS) *Online - full text edition.* **4185**
Colorectal Disease Online(GBR) *Online - full text.* **3887**
Combustion Science and Technology (CHE) *Online - full text edition.* **3379**
Community Genetics (CHE) *Online - full text edition.* **3300**
Community Mental Health Journal (USA) *Online - full text edition.* **4512**
Comparative Haematology International (GBR) *Online - full text edition.* **3900**
Comparative Political Studies (USA) *Online - full text edition.* **4367**
Computer Aided Surgery (USA) *Online - full text edition.* **4185**
Concepts in Magnetic Resonance (USA) *Online - full text edition.* **4142**
Connective Tissue Research (CHE) *Online - full text edition.* **3288**
Consciousness and Cognition (USA) *Online - full text edition.* **4391**
Conservation Biology (USA) *Online - full text edition.* **3392**
Contact Dermatitis (DNK) *Online - full text edition.* **3846**
Contact Lens & Anterior Eye (GBR) *Online - full text edition.* **3995**
Contemporary Educational Psychology (USA) *Online - full text edition.* **3410**
Contemporary Family Therapy (USA) *Online - full text edition.* **4391**
Coronary Artery Disease (USA) *Online - full text edition.* **3769**
Coronary Health Care (GBR) *Online - full text edition.* **3917**
Counselling Psychology Quarterly (GBR) *Online - full content edition.* **4392**
Criminal Justice & Behavior (USA) *Online - full text edition.* **3394**
Critical Public Health (GBR) *Online - full content edition.* **4466**
Critical Reviews in Toxicology (USA) *Online - full text edition.* **3447**
Cross-Cultural Research (USA) *Online - full text edition.* **4508**
Cryobiology (USA) *Online - full text edition.* **3266**
Culture & Psychology (GBR) *Online - full text edition.* **4393**
Culture, Health and Sexuality (GBR) *Online - full text edition.* **4520**
Culture, Medicine and Psychiatry (NLD) *Online - full text edition.* **3173**
Cumulative Index to Nursing & Allied Health Literature (USA) *Online - full text edition.* **3720**
Current Anaesthesia and Critical Care (GBR) *Online - full text edition.* **3756**
Current Biology (GBR) *Online - full text edition.* **3229**
Current Diagnostic Pathology (GBR) *Online - full text edition.* **3908**
Current Directions in Psychological Science (USA) *Online - full text edition.* **4393**
Current Eye Research (USA) *Online - full text edition.* **3996**
Current Genetics (DEU) *Online - full text edition.* **3300**
Current Microbiology (USA) *Online - full text edition.* **3320**
Current Obstetrics and Gynaecology (GBR) *Online - full text edition.* **3948**
Current Opinion in Anaesthesiology (USA) *Online - full text edition.* **3756**
Current Opinion in Biotechnology (GBR) *Online - full text edition.* **3273**
Current Opinion in Cardiology (USA) *Online - full text edition.* **3770**
Current Opinion in Cell Biology (GBR) *Online - full text edition.* **3288**
Current Opinion in Clinical Nutrition and Metabolic Care (USA) *Online - full text edition.* **4231**
Current Opinion in Critical Care (USA) *Online - full text edition.* **4012**

Online Service

Current Opinion in Endocrinology & Diabetes (USA) *Online - full text edition.* **3857**
Current Opinion in Gastroenterology (USA) *Online - full text edition.* **3888**
Current Opinion in Genetics & Development (GBR) *Online - full text edition.* **3301**
Current Opinion in Hematology (USA) *Online - full text edition.* **3900**
Current Opinion in Immunology (GBR) *Online - full text edition.* **3722**
Current Opinion in Infectious Diseases (USA) *Online - full text edition.* **3794**
Current Opinion in Lipidology (GBR) *Online - full text edition.* **3770**
Current Opinion in Nephrology & Hypertension (USA) *Online - full text edition.* **4211**
Current Opinion in Neurobiology (GBR) *Online - full text edition.* **4084**
Current Opinion in Neurology (USA) *Online - full text edition.* **4085**
Current Opinion in Obstetrics & Gynecology (USA) *Online - full text edition.* **3948**
Current Opinion in Oncology (USA) *Online - full text edition.* **3976**
Current Opinion in Ophthalmology (USA) *Online - full text edition.* **3996**
Current Opinion in Orthopedics (USA) *Online - full text edition.* **4013**
Current Opinion in Otolaryngology & Head and Neck Surgery (USA) *Online - full text edition.* **4031**
Current Opinion in Pediatrics (USA) *Online - full text edition.* **4043**
Current Opinion in Psychiatry (USA) *Online - full text edition.* **4085**
Current Opinion in Rheumatology (USA) *Online - full text edition.* **4168**
Current Opinion in Structural Biology (GBR) *Online - full text edition.* **3248**
Current Opinion in Urology (USA) *Online - full text edition.* **4211**
Current Orthopaedics (GBR) *Online - full text edition.* **4013**
Current Paediatrics (GBR) *Online - full text edition.* **4043**
Current Psychology (New Brunswick) (USA) *Online - full text edition.* **4393**
CyberPsychology & Behavior (USA) *Online - full text edition.* **3390**
Cytogenetic and Genome Research (CHE) *Online - full text edition.* **3301**
Cytokine (GBR) *Online - full text edition.* **3301**
Cytometry (USA) *Online - full text edition.* **3289**
Cytopathology (GBR) *Online - full text edition.* **3289**
Cytotechnology (NLD) *Online - full text edition.* **3289**
D N A and Cell Biology (USA) *Online - full text edition.* **3248**
D N A Sequence (CHE) *Online - full text edition.* **3248**
Death Studies (USA) *Online - full text edition.* **4394**
Dementia and Geriatric Cognitive Disorders (CHE) *Online - full text edition.* **4085**
Dental Traumatology Online(DNK) *Online - full text.* **3821**
Dentomaxillofacial Radiology (GBR) *Online - full text edition.* **4143**
Depression and Anxiety (USA) *Online - full text edition.* **4394**
Dermatologic Surgery Online(USA) *Online - full text.* **4187**
Dermatology (CHE) *Online - full text edition.* **3847**
Dermatology and Psychosomatics (CHE) *Online - full text edition.* **3848**
Development and Psychopathology (GBR) *Online - full text edition.* **4394**
Development (Cambridge) (GBR) *Online - full text edition.* **3192**
Development, Genes and Evolution (DEU) *Online - full text edition.* **3192**
Development, Growth and Differentiation (AUS) *Online - full text edition.* **3192**
Developmental Biology (USA) *Online - full text edition.* **3193**
Developmental Brain Research (NLD) *Online - full text edition.* **4086**
Developmental Dynamics (USA) *Online - full text edition.* **3193**
Developmental Immunology (CHE) *Online - full text edition.* **3744**
Developmental Medicine and Child Neurology (GBR) *Online - full text edition.* **4043**
Developmental Neuropsychology (USA) *Online - full text edition.* **4394**
Developmental Neuroscience (CHE) *Online - full text edition.* **4086**
Developmental Psychobiology (USA) *Online - full text edition.* **3193**
Developmental Review (USA) *Online - full text edition.* **4394**
Developmental Science (GBR) *Online - full text edition.* **4394**
Deviant Behavior (USA) *Online - full text edition.* **4521**
Diabetes (USA) *Online - full text edition.* **3857**
Diabetes Care (USA) *Online - full text edition.* **3857**
Diabetes - Metabolism Research and Reviews (GBR) *Online - full text edition.* **3858**
Diabetes, Obesity and Metabolism Online(GBR) *Online - full text.* **3858**
Diabetes Reviews (USA) *Online - full text edition.* **3859**
Diabetes Spectrum (USA) *Online - full text edition.* **3859**
Diabetes Technology & Therapeutics (USA) *Online - full text edition.* **3859**
Diabetic Medicine Online(GBR) *Online - full text.* **3860**
Diabetologia (DEU) *Online - full text edition.* **3860**
Diagnostic and Therapeutic Endoscopy (CHE) *Online - full text edition.* **3874**
Diagnostic Cytopathology (USA) *Online - full text edition.* **3289**
Differentiation (DEU) *Online - full text edition.* **3193**
Digestion (CHE) *Online - full text edition.* **3888**
Digestive Diseases (CHE) *Online - full text edition.* **3888**
Digestive Diseases and Sciences (USA) *Online - full text edition.* **3888**
Digestive Endoscopy Online(AUS) *Online - full text.* **3889**
Digestive Surgery (CHE) *Online - full text edition.* **4187**
Disability and Rehabilitation (GBR) *Online - full text edition.* **3484**
Disability & Society (GBR) *Online - full text edition.* **3494**
Disaster Prevention and Management (GBR) *Online - full text edition.* **4466**
Discourse & Society (GBR) *Online - full text edition.* **4395**
Discourse Studies (GBR) *Online - full text edition.* **3550**
Disease Management (USA) *Online - full text edition.* **3595**
Disease Management & Health Outcomes (NZL) *Online - full text edition.* **3595**
Disease Markers (NLD) *Online - full text edition.* **3976**
Diseases of the Esophagus Online(AUS) *Online - full text.* **4032**
Documenta Ophthalmologica (NLD) *Online - full text edition.* **3997**
Dreaming (USA) *Online - full text edition.* **3342**
Drug and Alcohol Review (GBR) *Online - full text edition.* **3400**
Drug and Chemical Toxicology (USA) *Online - full text edition.* **4287**
Drug Delivery (USA) *Online - full text edition.* **4288**
Drug Design and Discovery (CHE) *Online - full text edition.* **4288**
Drug Development and Industrial Pharmacy (USA) *Online - full text edition.* **4288**
Drug Development Research (USA) *Online - full text edition.* **4288**
Drug Metabolism and Disposition (USA) *Online - full text edition.* **4289**
Drug Metabolism Reviews (USA) *Online - full text edition.* **3596**
Drug Resistance Update (GBR) *Online - full text edition.* **3596**
Drug Safety (NZL) *Online - full text edition.* **4289**
Drugs (NZL) *Online - full text edition.* **4290**
Drugs & Aging (NZL) *Online - full text edition.* **4290**
Drugs: Education, Prevention & Policy (GBR) *Online - full text edition.* **3401**
Dyslexia (GBR) *Online - full text edition.* **3421**
Dysphagia (USA) *Online - full text edition.* **4032**
e A D C - F & N (GBR) *Online - full text edition of* Archives of Disease in Childhood. Fetal and Neonatal Edition. **3945**
The E M B O Journal (GBR) *Online - full text edition.* **3249**
E M J Online (GBR) *Online - full text edition of* Emergency Medicine Journal. **4014**
E-psyche(USA) *Online - full text.* **4457**
Early Childhood Education Journal (USA) *Online - full text edition.* **3410**
Ecography (DNK) *Online - full text edition.* **3437**
Ecological Psychology (USA) *Online - full text edition.* **4396**
Ecotoxicology (USA) *Online - full text edition.* **3448**
Ecotoxicology and Environmental Safety - Online (USA) *Online - full text edition of* Ecotoxicology and Environmental Safety. **3448**
Education for Health (GBR) *Online - full text edition.* **3597**
Educational and Psychological Measurement (USA) *Online - full text edition.* **4396**
Educational Gerontology (USA) *Online - full text edition.* **3470**
Educational Psychologist (USA) *Online - full text edition.* **4396**
Educational Psychology (GBR) *Online - full text edition.* **3410**
Educational Psychology in Practice (GBR) *Online - full text edition.* **3410**
Educational Psychology Review (USA) *Online - full text edition.* **3411**
Electro- and Magnetobiology (USA) *Online - full text edition.* **3266**
Elektronische Ausgabe (DEU) *Online - full text edition of* Der Hautarzt. **3849**
Emergency Medicine (Carleton South) (AUS) *Online - full text edition.* **4013**
Emergency Radiology (DEU) *Online - full text edition.* **4143**
Endocrine - Related Cancer (GBR) *Online - full text edition.* **3861**
Endocrine Reviews (USA) *Online - full text edition.* **3861**
Endocrinology (USA) *Online - full text edition.* **3861**
Endothelium (CHE) *Online - full text edition.* **3194**
Entomology Abstracts (USA) *Online - full text edition.* **3230**
Environment and Behavior (USA) *Online - full text edition.* **4521**
Environmental and Molecular Mutagenesis (USA) *Online - full text edition.* **3302**
Environmental Management & Health (GBR) *Online - full text edition.* **3438**
Environmental Microbiology (GBR) *Online - full text edition.* **3321**
Environmental Research (USA) *Online - full text edition.* **3439**
Environmental Toxicology (USA) *Online - full text edition.* **3449**
Epidemiology and Infection (GBR) *Online - full text edition.* **3321**
Epilepsia (USA) *Online - full text edition.* **4087**
Epilepsy and Behavior (USA) *Online - full text edition.* **3598**
Ergonomics (GBR) *Online - full text edition.* **3432**
Ethics & Behavior (USA) *Online - full text edition.* **4397**
Ethics and Medics (USA) *Online - full text edition.* **4502**
Ethik in der Medizin (DEU) *Online - full text edition.* **4347**
Ethnicity and Health (GBR) *Online - full text edition.* **4468**
Ethology Online(DEU) *Online - full text.* **3352**
Europace (GBR) *Online - full text edition.* **3771**
European Academy of Dermatology and Venereology. Journal (BEL) *Online - full text edition.* **3848**
European Addiction Research (CHE) *Online - full text edition.* **3401**
European Archives of Oto-Rhino-Laryngology (DEU) *Online - full text edition.* **4032**
European Archives of Psychiatry and Clinical Neurosciences (DEU) *Online - full text edition.* **4088**
European Biophysics Journal (DEU) *Online - full text edition.* **3266**
European Child & Adolescent Psychiatry (DEU) *Online - full text edition.* **4089**
European Eating Disorders Review (GBR) *Online - full text edition.* **4397**
European Heart Journal (GBR) *Online - full text edition.* **3771**
European Journal of Anaesthesiology (GBR) *Online - full text edition.* **3757**
European Journal of Applied Physiology (DEU) *Online - full text edition.* **3342**
European Journal of Biochemistry (GBR) *Online - full text edition.* **3249**
European Journal of Cancer Care Online(GBR) *Online - full text.* **3977**
European Journal of Cancer Prevention (USA) *Online - full text edition.* **3977**
European Journal of Cardio-Thoracic Surgery (NLD) *Online - full text edition.* **3771**
European Journal of Clinical Investigation (GBR) *Online - full text edition.* **3599**
European Journal of Clinical Microbiology & Infectious Diseases (DEU) *Online - full text edition.* **3321**
European Journal of Clinical Nutrition (GBR) *Online - full text edition.* **4232**
European Journal of Clinical Pharmacology (DEU) *Online - full text edition.* **4292**
European Journal of Cognitive Psychology (GBR) *Online - full text edition.* **4397**
European Journal of Dental Education Online(DNK) *Online - full text.* **3822**
European Journal of Echocardiography (GBR) *Online - full text edition.* **3771**
European Journal of Emergency Medicine (GBR) *Online - full text edition.* **4014**
European Journal of Endocrinology (GBR) *Online - full text edition.* **3862**
European Journal of Epidemiology (NLD) *Online - full text edition.* **3599**
European Journal of Gastroenterology and Hepatology (USA) *Online - full text edition.* **3889**
European Journal of Haematology (DNK) *Online - full text edition.* **3900**
The European Journal of Health Economics (DEU) *Online - full content edition.* **3600**
European Journal of Health Law (NLD) *Online - full text edition.* **3600**
European Journal of Human Genetics (GBR) *Online - full text edition.* **3302**
European Journal of Immunogenetics (GBR) *Online - full text edition.* **3302**
European Journal of Immunology (DEU) *Online - full text edition.* **3744**
European Journal of Morphology (NLD) *Online - full text edition.* **3195**
European Journal of Neurology (USA) *Online - full text edition.* **4089**
European Journal of Neuroscience (GBR) *Online - full text edition.* **4089**
European Journal of Nuclear Medicine and Molecular Imaging (DEU) *Online - full text edition.* **4144**
European Journal of Nutrition (DEU) *Online - full text edition.* **4233**
European Journal of Oncology Nursing (GBR) *Online - full text edition.* **3919**
European Journal of Orthodontics (GBR) *Online - full content edition.* **3823**
European Journal of Orthopaedic Surgery & Traumatology (FRA) *Online - full text edition.* **4014**
European Journal of Paediatric Neurology (GBR) *Online - full text edition.* **4044**
European Journal of Pain (GBR) *Online - full text edition.* **3600**
European Journal of Pediatrics (DEU) *Online - full text edition.* **4044**
European Journal of Personality (GBR) *Online - full text edition.* **4398**
European Journal of Pharmaceutical Sciences (NLD) *Online - full text edition.* **4292**
European Journal of Pharmacology (NLD) *Online - full text edition.* **4293**
European Journal of Plastic Surgery (DEU) *Online - full text edition.* **4188**
European Journal of Psychotherapy, Counselling and Health (GBR) *Online - full content edition.* **4089**
European Journal of Public Health (GBR) *Online - full text edition.* **4468**
European Journal of Social Psychology (GBR) *Online - full text edition.* **4398**
European Journal of Surgery (NOR) *Online - full text edition.* **4188**
European Journal of Surgical Oncology (GBR) *Online - full text edition.* **3977**
European Journal of Vascular and Endovascular Surgery (GBR) *Online - full text edition.* **3771**
European Journal of Work and Organizational Psychology (GBR) *Online - full text edition.* **4398**
European Neurology (CHE) *Online - full text edition.* **4089**
European Radiology (DEU) *Online - full text edition.* **4144**
The European Respiratory Journal (CHE) *Online - full text edition.* **4159**
European Spine Journal (DEU) *Online - full text edition.* **4189**
European Surgical Research (CHE) *Online - full text edition.* **4189**
European Urology (CHE) *Online - full text edition.* **4212**
Evaluation and the Health Professions (USA) *Online - full text edition.* **3600**

Evidence - Based Cardiovascular Medicine (GBR) Online - full text edition. 3772
Evidence - Based Obstetrics & Gynaecology (GBR) Online - full text edition. 3949
Evidence - Based Oncology (GBR) Online - full text edition. 3978
Evolution & Development Online(USA) Online - full text. 3195
Experimental Aging Research (USA) Online - full text edition. 4398
Experimental & Applied Acarology (NLD) Online - full text edition. 3352
Experimental and Molecular Pathology (USA) Online - full text edition. 3600
Experimental Biology and Medicine (Maywood) (USA) Online - full text edition. 3195
Experimental Biology Online(DEU) Online - full content. 3195
Experimental Brain Research (DEU) Online - full text edition. 4090
Experimental Dermatology Online(DNK) Online - full text. 3849
Experimental Eye Research (GBR) Online - full text edition. 3997
Experimental Lung Research (USA) Online - full text edition. 4160
Experimental Nephrology (CHE) Online - full text edition. 4212
Experimental Neurology (USA) Online - full text edition. 4090
Experimental Parasitology (USA) Online - full text edition. 3796
Experimental Physiology (GBR) Online - full text edition. 3342
The F A S E B Journal (USA) Online - full text edition. 3196
F E B S Letters (NLD) Online - full text edition. 3250
F E M S Microbiology Ecology (NLD) Online - full text edition. 3321
F E M S Microbiology Reviews (NLD) Online - full text edition. 3322
The Family Journal (USA) Online - full text edition. 4399
Family Practice (GBR) Online - full text edition. 3601
Feminism & Psychology (GBR) Online - full text edition. 4399
Fetal and Maternal Medicine Review (GBR) Online - full text edition. 3950
Fetal Diagnosis and Therapy (CHE) Online - full text edition. 3950
Fibrinolysis & Proteolysis (GBR) Online - full text edition. 3875
Fish and Shellfish Immunology (GBR) Online - full text edition. 3196
Folia Phoniatrica et Logopaedica (CHE) Online - full text edition. 4032
Food Additives and Contaminants (GBR) Online - full text edition. 4296
Food and Agricultural Immunology (GBR) Online - full text edition. 3197
Food Microbiology (GBR) Online - full text edition. 3322
The Foot (GBR) Online - full text edition. 4015
Foot and Ankle Surgery (GBR) Online - full text edition. 4189
Forschende Komplementaermedizin und Klassische Naturheilkunde (CHE) Online - full text edition. 3165
Forum der Psychoanalyse (DEU) Online - full text edition. 4399
Free Radical Biology & Medicine (USA) Online - full text edition. 3197
Freshwater Biology Online(GBR) Online - full text. 3197
Frontiers in Neuroendocrinology (USA) Online - full text edition. 3862
Frontiers of Medical and Biological Engineering (NLD) Online - full content edition. 3237
Fuctional Plant Biology (AUS) Online - full text edition. 3280
Games and Economic Behavior (USA) Online - full text edition. 4400
Gastric Cancer (JPN) Online - full content edition. 3978
Gastroenterology (USA) Online - full text edition. 3890
Gastrointestinal Endoscopy (USA) Online - full text edition. 3891
Gay and Lesbian Medical Association. Journal (USA) Online - full text edition. 3605
Gefaesschirurgie (DEU) Online - full text edition. 4189
Gene - C O M B I S (NLD) Online - full text edition of Gene. 3274
Gene Therapy and Regulation (NLD) Online - full content edition. 3303
Gene Therapy (Basingstoke) (GBR) Online - full text edition. 3606
General and Comparative Endocrinology (USA) Online - full text edition. 3863
Genes & Development (USA) Online - full text edition. 3303
Genes, Chromosomes & Cancer (USA) Online - full text edition. 3303
Genes to Cells (GBR) Online - full text edition. 3303
Genescreen (GBR) Online - full text edition. 3304
Genesis: The Journal of Genetics and Development (USA) Online - full text edition. 3304
Genetic Epidemiology (USA) Online - full text edition. 3304
Genetic Resources and Crop Evolution (NLD) Online - full text edition. 3304
Genetic Testing (USA) Online - full text edition. 3304
Genetica (NLD) Online - full text edition. 3305
Genetical Research (GBR) Online - full text edition. 3305
Genetics (USA) Online - full text edition. 3305
Genetics, Selection, Evolution Online (FRA) Online - full text edition of Genetics, Selection, Evolution. 3305
Genome (CAN) Online - full text edition. 3306
Genome Research (USA) Online - full text edition. 3306
Genomics (USA) Online - full text edition. 3306
Geomicrobiology Journal (USA) Online - full text edition. 3322
Geriatric Nursing (USA) Online - full text edition. 3472
Geriatrics Today (CAN) Online - full text edition. 3472
Gerontology (CHE) Online - full text edition. 3473
Glia (USA) Online - full text edition. 4092
Glycobiology (GBR) Online - full text edition. 3251
Glycoconjugate Journal (USA) Online - full text edition. 3251
Graefe's Archive for Clinical and Experimental Ophthalmology (DEU) Online - full text edition. 3998
Group Analysis (GBR) Online - full text edition. 4401
Group & Organization Management (USA) Online - full text edition. 3411
Group (New York) (USA) Online - full text edition. 4401
Growth Hormone and I G F Research (GBR) Online - full text edition. 3863
Gut Online (GBR) Online - full text edition of Gut. 3891
Gynaecological Endoscopy (GBR) Online - full text edition. 3951
Der Gynaekologe (DEU) Online - full text edition. 3951
Gynaekologisch - Geburtshilfliche Rundschau (CHE) Online - full text edition. 3951
Gynecologic and Obstetric Investigation (CHE) Online - full text edition. 3952
Gynecologic Oncology (USA) Online - full text edition. 3952
H E C Forum (NLD) Online - full text edition. 3508
H I V Medicine (GBR) Online - full text edition. 3796
H N O (Berlin) (DEU) Online - full text edition. 4033
H P B Surgery (CHE) Online - full text edition. 4190
Haematologia (NLD) Online - full content edition. 3901
Haemophilia Online(GBR) Online - full text. 3901
Harvard Review of Psychiatry (GBR) Online - full text edition. 4093
Head & Neck (USA) Online - full text edition. 4190
Headache Online(USA) Online - full text. 4093
Health (GBR) Online - full text edition. 4471
Health and Safety Science Abstracts (USA) Online - full text edition. 4496
Health and Social Care in the Community Online(GBR) Online - full text. 4472
Health Care Analysis (NLD) Online - full text edition. 3610
Health Care for Women International (USA) Online - full text edition. 4563
Health Care Management Science (NLD) Online - full text edition. 3509
Health Communication (USA) Online - full text edition. 4472
Health Economics (GBR) Online - full text edition. 3611
Health Education (GBR) Online - full text edition. 4354
Health Education Research (GBR) Online - full text edition. 4513
Health Expectations (GBR) Online - full text edition. 4473
Health Information and Libraries Journal Online(GBR) Online - full text. 3547
Health Policy and Planning (GBR) Online - full text edition. 4473
Health Promotion International (GBR) Online - full text edition. 4474
Health Promotion Practice (USA) Online - full text edition. 4474
Health, Risk & Society (GBR) Online - full text edition. 4474
Health Services and Outcomes Research Methodology (USA) Online - full text edition. 3612
Heart Drug (CHE) Online - full text edition. 4299
Heart Failure Reviews (USA) Online - full text edition. 3773
Heart, Lung & Circulation Online(AUS) Online - full text. 3773
Heart Online (GBR) Online - full text edition of Heart. 3772
Helicobacter (USA) Online - full text edition. 3323
Hematological Oncology (GBR) Online - full text edition. 3902
Hematology and Cell Therapy (FRA) Online - full text edition. 3902
Hepatology (USA) Online - full text edition. 3892
Heredity (GBR) Online - full text edition. 3307
Hernia (DEU) Online - full text edition. 4190
Herz (DEU) Online - full text edition. 3773
Herzschrittmachertherapie und Elektrophysiologie (DEU) Online - full text edition. 3774
High Ability Studies (GBR) Online - full text edition. 3422
High Altitude Medicine and Biology (USA) Online - full content edition. 3614
The Hippocampus (USA) Online - full text edition. 3614
Hispanic Journal of Behavioral Sciences (USA) Online - full text edition. 4402
The Histochemical Journal (NLD) Online - full text edition. 3290
Histochemistry and Cell Biology (DEU) Online - full text edition. 3290
Histopathology (GBR) Online - full text edition. 3979
Home Care Provider (USA) Online - full text edition. 3920
Homicide Studies (USA) Online - full text edition. 3394
Hormone Research (CHE) Online - full text edition. 3863
Hormones and Behavior (USA) Online - full text edition. 3863
Hospital Infection Control (USA) Online - full text edition. 3797
Human & Experimental Toxicology (GBR) Online - full text edition. 3450
Human Brain Mapping (USA) Online - full text edition. 4094
Human - Computer Interaction (Mahwah) (USA) Online - full text edition. 3389
Human Development (CHE) Online - full text edition. 3616
Human Ecology (New York) (USA) Online - full text edition. 3173
Human Factors and Ergonomics in Manufacturing (USA) Online - full text edition. 3435
Human Gene Therapy (USA) Online - full text edition. 3307
Human Genetics (DEU) Online - full text edition. 3307
Human Heredity (CHE) Online - full text edition. 3307
Human Immunology (USA) Online - full text edition. 3744
Human Molecular Genetics (GBR) Online - full text edition. 3308
Human Mutation (USA) Online - full text edition. 3308
Human Performance (USA) Online - full text edition. 4402
Human Psychopharmacology: Clinical and Experimental (GBR) Online - full text edition. 4094
Human Relations (USA) Online - full text edition. 4509
Human Reproduction (GBR) Online - full text edition. 3953
Human Reproduction Update (GBR) Online - full text edition. 3232
Hybridoma (USA) Online - full text edition. 3251
Hydrobiologia (NLD) Online - full text edition. 3199
Hypertension (USA) Online - full text edition. 3774
Hypertension in Pregnancy (USA) Online - full text edition. 3774
I E E E Engineering in Medicine and Biology Magazine (USA) Online - full text edition. 3237
I E E E Transactions on Biomedical Engineering (USA) Online - full text edition. 3237
I E E E Transactions on Evolutionary Computation (USA) Online - full text edition. 3284
I E E E Transactions on Information Technology in Biomedicine (USA) Online - full text edition. 3274
I E E E Transactions on Medical Imaging (USA) Online - full text edition. 4145
I E E E Transactions on Neural Systems and Rehabilitation Engineering (USA) Online - full text edition. 3238
Illness, Crisis, and Loss (USA) Online - full text edition. 4521
Immunogenetics (DEU) Online - full text edition. 3308
Immunologie und Impfen (DEU) Online - full text edition. 3745
Immunology (GBR) Online - full text edition. 3746
Immunology and Cell Biology (AUS) Online - full text edition. 3746
In Vitro Cellular & Developmental Biology - Plant (USA) Online - full text edition. 3280
Indoor Air Online(DNK) Online - full text. 4476
Indoor and Built Environment (CHE) Online - full text edition. 3747
Infant and Child Development (GBR) Online - full text edition. 4404
Infant Mental Health Journal (USA) Online - full text edition. 4045
Infection and Immunity (USA) Online - full text edition. 3798
Infectious Diseases in Obstetrics and Gynecology (USA) Online - full text edition. 3953
Inflammation (USA) Online - full text edition. 3620
Inflammation Research (CHE) Online - full text edition. 4301
Inflammopharmacology (NLD) Online - full content edition. 4302
Infusion Therapy and Transfusion Medicine (CHE) Online - full text edition. 3620
Inhalation Toxicology (USA) Online - full text edition. 3451
Injury Prevention (GBR) Online - full text edition. 4045
Injury Prevention and Safety Promotion (NLD) Online - full text edition. 3393
Inpharma Weekly (NZL) Online - full text edition. 4345
Institution of Mechanical Engineers. Proceedings. Part H: Journal of Engineering in Medicine (GBR) Online - full text edition. 3238
Instrumentation Science & Technology (USA) Online - full text edition. 3376
Intensive Care Medicine (DEU) Online - full text edition. 3621
Intensivmedizin und Notfallmedizin (DEU) Online - full text edition. 3621
International Archives of Allergy and Immunology (CHE) Online - full text edition. 3747
International Archives of Occupational and Environmental Health (DEU) Online - full text edition. 4257
International Clinical Psychopharmacology (USA) Online - full text edition. 4405
International Endodontic Journal Online(GBR) Online - full text. 3826
International Forum of Psychoanalysis (NOR) Online - full text edition. 4405
International Immunology (GBR) Online - full text edition. 3747
International Journal for Quality in Health Care (GBR) Online - full text edition. 3622
The International Journal for the Psychology of Religion (USA) Online - full text edition. 4500
International Journal of Andrology (GBR) Online - full text edition. 4213
International Journal of Angiology (USA) Online - full text edition. 3775
The International Journal of Aviation Psychology (USA) Online - full text edition. 4532
International Journal of Behavioral Development (GBR) Online - full text edition. 4405

Online Service

International Journal of Behavioral Medicine (USA) *Online - full text edition.* **4405**
International Journal of Biochemistry & Cell Biology (GBR) *Online - full text edition.* **3252**
International Journal of Biometeorology (DEU) *Online - full text edition.* **4223**
International Journal of Cancer (USA) *Online - full text edition.* **3980**
International Journal of Cardiovascular Imaging (NLD) *Online - full text edition.* **3775**
International Journal of Children's Spirituality (GBR) *Online - full text edition.* **4406**
International Journal of Clinical Oncology Online(JPN) *Online - full text.* **3980**
International Journal of Cognitive Ergonomics (USA) *Online - full text edition.* **4406**
International Journal of Colorectal Disease (DEU) *Online - full text edition.* **4191**
International Journal of Cosmetic Science (GBR) *Online - full text edition.* **3176**
International Journal of Dermatology (GBR) *Online - full text edition.* **3850**
International Journal of Developmental Biology (ESP) *Online - full text edition.* **3201**
International Journal of Disability, Development and Education (GBR) *Online - full text edition.* **3423**
International Journal of Eating Disorders (USA) *Online - full text edition.* **4236**
International Journal of Environmental Health Research (GBR) *Online - full text edition.* **3439**
International Journal of Epidemiology (GBR) *Online - full text edition.* **3623**
International Journal of Experimental Pathology (GBR) *Online - full text edition.* **3623**
International Journal of Food Sciences and Nutrition (GBR) *Online - full text edition.* **4236**
International Journal of Geriatric Psychiatry (GBR) *Online - full text edition.* **3474**
International Journal of Group Tensions (USA) *Online - full text edition.* **4406**
International Journal of Gynecological Cancer (USA) *Online - full text edition.* **3953**
International Journal of Health Care Quality Assurance (GBR) *Online - full text edition.* **3623**
International Journal of Health Planning and Management (GBR) *Online - full text edition.* **4514**
International Journal of Hyperthermia (GBR) *Online - full text edition.* **3980**
International Journal of Impotence Research (GBR) *Online - full text edition.* **4213**
International Journal of Language and Communication Disorders (GBR) *Online - full text edition.* **4033**
International Journal of Legal Medicine (DEU) *Online - full text edition.* **3882**
International Journal of Neural Systems (SGP) *Online - full text edition.* **3389**
International Journal of Neuro-Psychopharmacology (GBR) *Online - full text edition.* **4303**
International Journal of Neuroscience (CHE) *Online - full text edition.* **4096**
International Journal of Nursing Practice (AUS) *Online - full text edition.* **3921**
International Journal of Obesity (GBR) *Online - full text edition.* **4236**
International Journal of Offender Therapy and Comparative Criminology (USA) *Online - full text edition.* **3394**
International Journal of Oral & Maxillofacial Surgery (DNK) *Online - full text edition.* **3827**
International Journal of Paediatric Dentistry Online(GBR) *Online - full text.* **3827**
International Journal of Pediatric Hematology - Oncology (CHE) *Online - full text edition.* **3980**
International Journal of Pest Management (GBR) *Online - full text edition.* **3158**
International Journal of Pharmaceutical Medicine (USA) *Online - full text edition.* **4303**
International Journal of Pharmaceutics (NLD) *Online - full text edition.* **4303**
The International Journal of Psycho-Analysis (GBR) *Online - full text edition.* **4406**
International Journal of Psychology (GBR) *Online - full text edition.* **4407**
International Journal of Psychotherapy (GBR) *Online - full content edition.* **4096**
International Journal of Radiation Biology (GBR) *Online - full text edition.* **3980**
International Journal of Rehabilitation Research (USA) *Online - full text edition.* **4061**
The International Journal of Risk and Safety in Medicine (NLD) *Online - full text edition.* **3532**
International Journal of S T D & AIDS (GBR) *Online - full text edition.* **3800**
International Journal of Stress Management (USA) *Online - full text edition.* **3624**
International Journal of Surgical Investigation (CHE) *Online - full text edition.* **4191**
International Journal of Systematic and Evolutionary Microbiology (GBR) *Online - full text edition.* **3324**
International Journal of Toxicology (GBR) *Online - full text edition.* **3451**
International Journal of Trauma Nursing (USA) *Online - full text edition.* **3922**
International Journal of Urology (AUS) *Online - full text edition.* **4213**
International Neuropsychological Society. Journal (GBR) *Online - full text edition.* **4097**
International Nursing Review Online(GBR) *Online - full text.* **3922**
International Ophthalmology (NLD) *Online - full text edition.* **3999**
International Orthopaedics (DEU) *Online - full text edition.* **4016**
International Pharmaceutical Abstracts (USA) *Online - full text edition.* **4345**
International Review of Hydrobiology (DEU) *Online - full text edition.* **3201**
International Review of Psychiatry (GBR) *Online - full text edition.* **4097**
International Reviews of Immunology (CHE) *Online - full text edition.* **3747**
International Urogynecology Journal (GBR) *Online - full text edition.* **3954**
International Urology and Nephrology (HUN) *Online - full text edition.* **4214**
Der Internist (DEU) *Online - full text edition.* **3909**
Intervirology (CHE) *Online - full text edition.* **3324**
Invertebrate Neuroscience Online(DEU) *Online - full text.* **3353**
Invertebrate Systomatics (Online Edition)(AUS) *Online - full text.* **3353**
Investigational New Drugs (USA) *Online - full text edition.* **4304**
Investigative Ophthalmology & Visual Science (IOVS) (USA) *Online - full text edition.* **3999**
Issues in Comprehensive Pediatric Nursing (USA) *Online - full text edition.* **3922**
Issues in Interdisciplinary Care (USA) *Online - full text edition.* **3625**
Issues in Mental Health Nursing (USA) *Online - full text edition.* **3922**
J A M A: The Journal of the American Medical Association (USA) *Online - full text edition.* **3626**
J C P Online (GBR) *Online - full text edition of* Journal of Clinical Pathology. **3631**
J E C H Online (GBR) *Online - full text edition of* Journal of Epidemiology & Community Health. **3632**
J M B Online (GBR) *Online - full text edition of* Journal of Molecular Biology. **3254**
J M E Online (GBR) *Online - full text edition of* Journal of Medical Ethics. **3635**
J M G Online (GBR) *Online - full text edition of* Journal of Medical Genetics. **3310**
J M S Online (GBR) *Online - full text edition of* Journal of Medical Screening. **3802**
Japanese Journal of Clinical Oncology (GBR) *Online - full text edition.* **3981**
Japanese Psychological Research (JPN) *Online - full text edition.* **4408**
Journal for the Theory of Social Behaviour (GBR) *Online - full text edition.* **4408**
Journal of Abnormal Child Psychology (USA) *Online - full text edition.* **4409**
Journal of Adolescence (GBR) *Online - full text edition.* **3383**
Journal of Adolescent Research (USA) *Online - full text edition.* **4409**
Journal of Adult Development (USA) *Online - full text edition.* **4409**
Journal of Advanced Nursing (GBR) *Online - full text edition.* **3923**
Journal of Aging and Health (USA) *Online - full text edition.* **3474**
Journal of Aging & Identity (USA) *Online - full text edition.* **3475**
The Journal of Allergy and Clinical Immunology (USA) *Online - full text edition.* **3748**
Journal of Alzheimer's Disease (NLD) *Online - full text edition.* **4098**
Journal of Analytical Psychology (GBR) *Online - full text edition.* **4409**
Journal of Anatomy (GBR) *Online - full text edition.* **3202**
Journal of Anesthesia (JPN) *Online - full content edition.* **3757**
Journal of Animal Ecology (GBR) *Online - full text edition.* **3202**
Journal of Animal Physiology and Animal Nutrition Online(DEU) *Online - full text.* **3344**
Journal of Antimicrobial Chemotherapy (GBR) *Online - full text edition.* **3800**
Journal of Applied Animal Welfare Science (USA) *Online - full text edition.* **3172**
Journal of Applied Microbiology (GBR) *Online - full text edition.* **3324**
Journal of Applied Psychoanalytic Studies (USA) *Online - full text edition.* **4410**
Journal of Applied Research in Intellectual Disabilities (GBR) *Online - full text edition.* **4098**
Journal of Applied Therapeutic Research (CHE) *Online - full text edition.* **4305**
Journal of Applied Toxicology (GBR) *Online - full text edition.* **3451**
Journal of Aquatic Animal Health (USA) *Online - full text edition.* **3459**
Journal of Artificial Organs (JPN) *Online - full text edition.* **3876**
Journal of Assisted Reproduction and Genetics (USA) *Online - full text edition.* **3955**
Journal of Audio Visual Media in Medicine (GBR) *Online - full text edition.* **3629**
Journal of Autism and Developmental Disorders (USA) *Online - full text edition.* **3423**
Journal of Autoimmunity (GBR) *Online - full text edition.* **3748**
Journal of Bacteriology (USA) *Online - full text edition.* **3325**
Journal of Basic Microbiology (DEU) *Online - full text edition.* **3325**
Journal of Behavioral Medicine (USA) *Online - full text edition.* **4099**
Journal of Biochemistry and Molecular Biology Online(HKG) *Online - full content.* **3253**
Journal of Biochemistry, Molecular Biology and Biophysics (CHE) *Online - full text edition.* **3253**
Journal of Bioenergetics and Biomembranes (USA) *Online - full text edition.* **3253**
Journal of Biological Chemistry (USA) *Online - full text edition.* **3253**
Journal of Biological Rhythms (USA) *Online - full text edition.* **4099**
Journal of Biomechanical Engineering (USA) *Online - full text edition.* **3629**
Journal of Biomedical Informatics (USA) *Online - full text edition.* **3811**
Journal of Biomedical Materials Research (USA) *Online - full text edition.* **3275**
Journal of Biomedical Optics (USA) *Online - full text edition.* **4366**
Journal of Biomedical Science (CHE) *Online - full text edition.* **3630**
Journal of Biopharmaceutical Statistics (USA) *Online - full text edition.* **4345**
Journal of Biosocial Science (GBR) *Online - full text edition.* **4521**
Journal of Black Studies (USA) *Online - full text edition.* **4509**
Journal of Bone and Joint Surgery: American Volume (USA) *Online - full text edition.* **4017**
Journal of Bone and Mineral Metabolism (JPN) *Online - full text edition.* **3864**
Journal of Bone and Mineral Research (USA) *Online - full text edition.* **4018**
Journal of Business & Psychology (USA) *Online - full text edition.* **4411**
Journal of Cancer Research and Clinical Oncology (DEU) *Online - full text edition.* **3981**
Journal of Cardiovascular Risk (USA) *Online - full text edition.* **3777**
Journal of Cell Science (GBR) *Online - full text edition.* **3291**
Journal of Cellular Biochemistry (USA) *Online - full text edition.* **3254**
Journal of Child and Family Studies (USA) *Online - full text edition.* **4411**
Journal of Child Language (GBR) *Online - full text edition.* **3384**
Journal of Child Psychology & Psychiatry & Allied Disciplines (GBR) *Online - full text edition.* **4411**
Journal of Child Psychotherapy (GBR) *Online - full text edition.* **4411**
Journal of Classification (USA) *Online - full text edition.* **3553**
Journal of Clinical Apheresis (USA) *Online - full text edition.* **3903**
Journal of Clinical Child and Adolescent Psychology (USA) *Online - full text edition.* **4411**
Journal of Clinical Endocrinology and Metabolism (USA) *Online - full text edition.* **3864**
Journal of Clinical Geropsychology (USA) *Online - full text edition.* **3475**
Journal of Clinical Immunology (USA) *Online - full text edition.* **3748**
Journal of Clinical Investigation (USA) *Online - full text edition.* **3631**
Journal of Clinical Laboratory Analysis (USA) *Online - full text edition.* **3876**
Journal of Clinical Microbiology (USA) *Online - full text edition.* **3631**
Journal of Clinical Monitoring and Computing (NLD) *Online - full text edition.* **3631**
Journal of Clinical Neuroscience (GBR) *Online - full text edition.* **4100**
Journal of Clinical Nursing (GBR) *Online - full text edition.* **3923**
Journal of Clinical Oncology (USA) *Online - full text edition.* **3982**
Journal of Clinical Periodontology (DNK) *Online - full text edition.* **3828**
Journal of Clinical Pharmacology (USA) *Online - full text edition.* **4306**
Journal of Clinical Pharmacy and Therapeutics (GBR) *Online - full text edition.* **4306**
Journal of Clinical Psychology (USA) *Online - full text edition.* **4412**
Journal of Clinical Psychology in Medical Settings (USA) *Online - full text edition.* **4412**
Journal of Clinical Ultrasound (USA) *Online - full text edition.* **4147**
Journal of Cognition and Development (USA) *Online - full text edition.* **4412**
Journal of Cognitive Neuroscience (USA) *Online - full text edition.* **4100**
Journal of Communication Inquiry (USA) *Online - full text edition.* **4522**
Journal of Community and Applied Social Psychology (GBR) *Online - full text edition.* **4413**
Journal of Community Health (USA) *Online - full text edition.* **3631**
Journal of Community Health Nursing (USA) *Online - full text edition.* **3924**
Journal of Community Psychology (USA) *Online - full text edition.* **4413**
The Journal of Comparative Neurology (USA) *Online - full text edition.* **4100**
Journal of Comparative Pathology (GBR) *Online - full text edition.* **3203**
Journal of Comparative Physiology. A: Sensory, Neural, and Behavioral Physiology (DEU) *Online - full text edition.* **3344**
Journal of Comparative Physiology. B: Biochemical, Systemic, and Environmental Physiology (DEU) *Online - full text edition.* **3344**
Journal of Computational Neuroscience (NLD) *Online - full text edition.* **4100**
Journal of Constructivist Psychology (USA) *Online - full text edition.* **4413**
Journal of Consumer Psychology (USA) *Online - full text edition.* **3153**
Journal of Contemporary Psychotherapy (USA) *Online - full text edition.* **4413**
Journal of Cranio-Maxillo-Facial Surgery (GBR) *Online - full text edition.* **4192**
Journal of Craniofacial Genetics and Developmental Biology Online(DNK) *Online - full text.* **3309**
Journal of Cross-Cultural Gerontology (NLD) *Online - full text edition.* **3475**
Journal of Cross-Cultural Psychology (USA) *Online - full text edition.* **4414**
Journal of Cutaneous Pathology (DNK) *Online - full text edition.* **3850**
The Journal of Deaf Studies and Deaf Education (USA) *Online - full text edition.* **3491**
Journal of Developmental and Physical Disabilities (USA) *Online - full text edition.* **3485**
Journal of Drug Targeting (CHE) *Online - full text edition.* **4307**
Journal of Early Adolescence (USA) *Online - full text edition.* **3384**
Journal of Ecology (GBR) *Online - full text edition.* **3203**
Journal of Educational and Psychological Consultation (USA) *Online - full text edition.* **3412**
Journal of Emergency Nursing (USA) *Online - full text edition.* **3924**

Journal of Endocrinology (GBR) *Online - full text edition.* **3865**
Journal of English Linguistics (USA) *Online - full text edition.* **3550**
Journal of Environmental Psychology (GBR) *Online - full text edition.* **4415**
Journal of Enzyme Inhibition (CHE) *Online - full text edition.* **3254**
Journal of Evaluation in Clinical Practice Online(GBR) *Online - full text.* **3632**
Journal of Evolutionary Biology (GBR) *Online - full text edition.* **3309**
Journal of Experimental Biology (GBR) *Online - full text edition.* **3203**
Journal of Experimental Child Psychology (USA) *Online - full text edition.* **4415**
Journal of Experimental Marine Biology and Ecology (NLD) *Online - full text edition.* **3203**
The Journal of Experimental Medicine (USA) *Online - full text edition.* **3876**
Journal of Experimental Social Psychology (USA) *Online - full text edition.* **4415**
Journal of Experimental Zoology (USA) *Online - full text edition.* **3354**
Journal of Exposure Analysis and Environmental Epidemiology (GBR) *Online - full text edition.* **3440**
Journal of Family and Economic Issues (USA) *Online - full text edition.* **4416**
Journal of Family Nursing (USA) *Online - full content edition.* **3924**
Journal of Family Therapy (GBR) *Online - full text edition.* **4101**
Journal of Family Violence (USA) *Online - full text edition.* **3395**
Journal of Forensic Psychiatry (GBR) *Online - full text edition.* **4101**
Journal of Gambling Studies (USA) *Online - full text edition.* **4101**
Journal of Gastroenterology (JPN) *Online - full text edition.* **3893**
Journal of Gastroenterology and Hepatology (AUS) *Online - full text edition.* **3893**
Journal of Gene Medicine (USA) *Online - full text edition.* **3309**
Journal of General Internal Medicine (USA) *Online - full text edition.* **3910**
Journal of General Physiology (USA) *Online - full text edition.* **3344**
Journal of General Virology (GBR) *Online - full text edition.* **3325**
Journal of Genetic Counseling (USA) *Online - full text edition.* **4416**
Journal of Hand Surgery: American Volume (USA) *Online - full content edition.* **4193**
Journal of Hand Surgery: British and European Volume (GBR) *Online - full text edition.* **4193**
Journal of Happiness Studies (NLD) *Online - full text edition.* **4417**
Journal of Health Communication (USA) *Online - full text edition.* **3633**
Journal of Health Economics (NLD) *Online - full text edition.* **4479**
Journal of Health Politics, Policy and Law (USA) *Online - full text edition.* **3633**
Journal of Health Psychology (GBR) *Online - full text edition.* **4417**
The Journal of Heart and Lung Transplantation (GBR) *Online - full text edition.* **4193**
Journal of Helminthology (GBR) *Online - full text edition.* **3801**
Journal of Hematotherapy & Stem Cell Research (USA) *Online - full text edition.* **3903**
Journal of Hepato - Biliary - Pancreatic Surgery (JPN) *Online - full content edition.* **4193**
Journal of Hepatology (DNK) *Online - full text edition.* **3893**
Journal of Histochemistry and Cytochemistry (USA) *Online - full text edition.* **3291**
Journal of Hospital Infection (GBR) *Online - full text edition.* **3801**
Journal of Human Evolution (GBR) *Online - full text edition.* **3309**
Journal of Human Genetics (JPN) *Online - full text edition.* **3310**
Journal of Human Hypertension (GBR) *Online - full text edition.* **3778**
Journal of Human Lactation (USA) *Online - full text edition.* **3955**
Journal of Human Nutrition and Dietetics (GBR) *Online - full text edition.* **4237**
Journal of Humanistic Psychology (USA) *Online - full text edition.* **4417**
Journal of Hypertension (USA) *Online - full text edition.* **3778**
Journal of Immigrant Health (USA) *Online - full text edition.* **3634**
Journal of Immunology (USA) *Online - full text edition.* **3748**
Journal of Industrial Microbiology and Biotechnology (GBR) *Online - full text edition.* **3276**
Journal of Infection (GBR) *Online - full text edition.* **3801**
Journal of Infection and Chemotherapy (JPN) *Online - full text edition.* **4307**
Journal of Infectious Diseases (USA) *Online - full text edition.* **3802**
Journal of Inherited Metabolic Disease (NLD) *Online - full text edition.* **4046**
Journal of Intellectual Disability Research (GBR) *Online - full text edition.* **4102**
Journal of Intensive Care Medicine (USA) *Online - full text edition.* **3634**
Journal of Interferon & Cytokine Research (USA) *Online - full text edition.* **3749**
Journal of Internal Medicine (GBR) *Online - full text edition.* **3910**
Journal of Interpersonal Violence (USA) *Online - full text edition.* **3395**
Journal of Interprofessional Care (GBR) *Online - full text edition.* **3634**
Journal of Interventional Cardiac Electrophysiology (NLD) *Online - full text edition.* **3778**
The Journal of Investigative Dermatology (USA) *Online - full text edition.* **3851**
Journal of Investigative Surgery (USA) *Online - full text edition.* **4193**
Journal of Language and Social Psychology (USA) *Online - full text edition.* **4417**
Journal of Laryngology and Otology (GBR) *Online - full content edition.* **4034**
The Journal of Legal Medicine (USA) *Online - full text edition.* **3634**
Journal of Leukocyte Biology (USA) *Online - full text edition.* **3204**
Journal of Lipid Research (USA) *Online - full text edition.* **3254**
Journal of Lower Genital Tract Disease Online(USA) *Online - full text.* **3956**
Journal of Magnetic Resonance Imaging (USA) *Online - full text edition.* **4148**
Journal of Mammalian Evolution (USA) *Online - full text edition.* **3354**
Journal of Mammary Gland Biology and Neoplasia (USA) *Online - full text edition.* **3345**
Journal of Management in Medicine (GBR) *Online - full text edition.* **3634**
Journal of Managerial Psychology (GBR) *Online - full text edition.* **3365**
Journal of Manipulative and Physiological Therapeutics (USA) *Online - full text edition.* **3788**
Journal of Materials Science: Materials in Medicine (USA) *Online - full text edition.* **3434**
Journal of Mathematical Biology (DEU) *Online - full text edition.* **3204**
Journal of Mathematical Psychology (USA) *Online - full text edition.* **4418**
Journal of Medical Engineering & Technology (GBR) *Online - full text edition.* **3635**
Journal of Medical Humanities (USA) *Online - full text edition.* **3635**
Journal of Medical Microbiology (USA) *Online - full text edition.* **3635**
Journal of Medical Systems (USA) *Online - full text edition.* **3812**
Journal of Medical Virology (USA) *Online - full text edition.* **3635**
Journal of Medicinal Chemistry (USA) *Online - full text edition.* **4308**
Journal of Medicinal Food (USA) *Online - full content edition.* **3636**
The Journal of Medicine and Philosophy (NLD) *Online - full text edition.* **3636**
Journal of Membrane Biology (USA) *Online - full text edition.* **3291**
Journal of Memory and Language (USA) *Online - full text edition.* **3550**
Journal of Mental Health (GBR) *Online - full text edition.* **4102**
Journal of Microencapsulation (GBR) *Online - full text edition.* **4308**
Journal of Micromechatronics (NLD) *Online - full content edition.* **3434**
Journal of Microscopy (GBR) *Online - full text edition.* **3334**
Journal of Microscopy Research and Technique (USA) *Online - full text edition.* **3334**
Journal of Molecular and Cellular Cardiology (GBR) *Online - full text edition.* **3778**
Journal of Molecular Endocrinology (GBR) *Online - full text edition.* **3865**
Journal of Molecular Evolution (USA) *Online - full text edition.* **3310**
Journal of Molecular Medicine (DEU) *Online - full text edition.* **3636**
Journal of Molecular Recognition (GBR) *Online - full text edition.* **3378**
Journal of Morphology (USA) *Online - full text edition.* **3204**
Journal of Muscle Research and Cell Motility (NLD) *Online - full text edition.* **4018**
Journal of Natural History (GBR) *Online - full text edition.* **3204**
Journal of Natural Products (USA) *Online - full text edition.* **4308**
Journal of Near-Death Studies (USA) *Online - full text edition.* **4347**
Journal of Neural Transmission - Basic Neurosciences and Genetics - Parkinson's Disease and Allied Conditions - Alzheimer's Disease and Related Disorders - Biological Psychiatry (AUT) *Online - full text edition.* **4102**
Journal of Neuro-Oncology (USA) *Online - full text edition.* **3982**
Journal of Neurobiology (USA) *Online - full text edition.* **3345**
Journal of Neurochemistry (USA) *Online - full text edition.* **3255**
Journal of Neurocytology (USA) *Online - full text edition.* **3291**
Journal of Neuroendocrinology Online(GBR) *Online - full text.* **4103**
Journal of Neurogenetics (CHE) *Online - full text edition.* **4103**
Journal of Neurology (DEU) *Online - full text edition.* **4103**
Journal of Neurology, Neurosurgery and Psychiatry (GBR) *Online - full text edition.* **4104**
Journal of Neurophysiology Online (USA) *Online - full text edition of* Journal of Neurophysiology. **3345**
Journal of Neuropsychiatry and Clinical Neurosciences (USA) *Online - full text edition.* **4104**
Journal of Neuroscience (USA) *Online - full text edition.* **4104**
Journal of Neuroscience Research (USA) *Online - full text edition.* **4104**
Journal of Neurosurgery (USA) *Online - full text edition.* **4104**
Journal of NeuroVirology (GBR) *Online - full text edition.* **4105**
Journal of Nonverbal Behavior (USA) *Online - full text edition.* **4418**
Journal of Nursing Management (GBR) *Online - full text edition.* **3925**
Journal of Nutrition (USA) *Online - full text edition.* **4237**
Journal of Nutritional & Environmental Medicine (GBR) *Online - full text edition.* **4237**
Journal of Obstetrics and Gynaecology (GBR) *Online - full text edition.* **3956**
Journal of Occupational and Organizational Psychology (GBR) *Online - full text edition.* **4419**
Journal of Occupational Rehabilitation (USA) *Online - full text edition.* **4258**
Journal of Oncology Pharmacy Practice (USA) *Online - full text edition.* **4308**
Journal of Oral Pathology & Medicine (DNK) *Online - full text edition.* **3829**
Journal of Oral Rehabilitation Online(GBR) *Online - full text.* **3829**
Journal of Organizational Behaviour (GBR) *Online - full text edition.* **4419**
The Journal of Orthodontics (GBR) *Online - full text edition.* **3830**
Journal of Orthopaedic Science (JPN) *Online - full text edition.* **4019**
Journal of Paediatrics and Child Health (AUS) *Online - full text edition.* **4047**
Journal of Palliative Medicine (USA) *Online - full text edition.* **3637**
Journal of Pathogenesis (CHE) *Online - full text edition.* **3637**
Journal of Pathology (GBR) *Online - full text edition.* **3637**
Journal of Pediatric and Adolescent Gynecology (NLD) *Online - full text edition.* **4047**
Journal of Pediatric Health Care (USA) *Online - full text edition.* **4047**
Journal of Pediatric Psychology (GBR) *Online - full text edition.* **4419**
The Journal of Pediatrics (USA) *Online - full text edition.* **4047**
Journal of Peptide Research (DNK) *Online - full text edition.* **3255**
Journal of Peptide Science (GBR) *Online - full text edition.* **3378**
Journal of Perinatal Medicine (DEU) *Online - full text edition.* **3956**
Journal of Perinatology (GBR) *Online - full text edition.* **3956**
Journal of Periodontal Research (DNK) *Online - full text edition.* **3830**
Journal of Personality (USA) *Online - full text edition.* **4419**
Journal of Personality Assessment (USA) *Online - full text edition.* **4420**
Journal of Pharmaceutical Medicine (GBR) *Online - full text edition.* **4309**
Journal of Pharmaceutical Sciences (USA) *Online - full text edition.* **4309**
Journal of Pharmacology and Experimental Therapeutics (USA) *Online - full text edition.* **4310**
Journal of Physiology (GBR) *Online - full text edition.* **3345**
Journal of Pineal Research (DNK) *Online - full text edition.* **4105**
Journal of Plankton Research (GBR) *Online - full text edition.* **3204**
The Journal of Primary Prevention (USA) *Online - full text edition.* **4420**
The Journal of Prosthetic Dentistry (USA) *Online - full text edition.* **3830**
Journal of Protein Chemistry (USA) *Online - full text edition.* **3255**
Journal of Psychiatric & Mental Health Nursing Online(GBR) *Online - full text.* **4105**
Journal of Psycholinguistic Research (USA) *Online - full text edition.* **3551**
Journal of Psychology and Financial Markets (USA) *Online - full content edition.* **4421**
Journal of Psychopathology and Behavioral Assessment (USA) *Online - full text edition.* **4421**
Journal of Psychopharmacology (GBR) *Online - full text edition.* **4310**
Journal of Public Health Medicine (GBR) *Online - full text edition.* **4515**
Journal of Quality in Clinical Practice (AUS) *Online - full text edition.* **3637**
Journal of Radiological Protection (GBR) *Online - full text edition.* **3431**
Journal of Radiosurgery (USA) *Online - full text edition.* **4194**
Journal of Rational - Emotive and Cognitive - Behavior Therapy (USA) *Online - full text edition.* **4421**
Journal of Rehabilitation Medicine (NOR) *Online - full text edition.* **4515**
Journal of Religion and Health (USA) *Online - full text edition.* **4500**
Journal of Reproductive and Infant Psychology (GBR) *Online - full text edition.* **4421**
Journal of Research in Personality (USA) *Online - full text edition.* **4422**
Journal of Risk and Uncertainty (USA) *Online - full text edition.* **3363**
Journal of Sex & Marital Therapy (USA) *Online - full text edition.* **4422**
Journal of Sleep Research Online(GBR) *Online - full text.* **3638**
Journal of Social and Personal Relationships (GBR) *Online - full content edition.* **4423**
Journal of Social Distress and the Homeless (USA) *Online - full text edition.* **4515**
Journal of Social Issues (USA) *Online - full content edition.* **4423**
Journal of Social Work Practice (GBR) *Online - full text edition.* **4515**
Journal of Sports Sciences (GBR) *Online - full text edition.* **4525**
Journal of Structural Biology (USA) *Online - full text edition.* **3205**
Journal of Structural Learning and Intelligent Systems (CHE) *Online - full text edition.* **4423**
Journal of Surgical Oncology (USA) *Online - full text edition.* **4195**
Journal of Surgical Research (USA) *Online - full text edition.* **4195**
Journal of Telemedicine and Telecare (GBR) *Online - full text edition.* **3638**
Journal of the History of Biology (NLD) *Online - full text edition.* **3205**
Journal of the History of Medicine and Allied Sciences (GBR) *Online - full text edition.* **3638**
Journal of the History of the Behavioral Sciences (USA) *Online - full text edition.* **4424**
Journal of the History of the Neurosciences (NLD) *Online - full content edition.* **4106**
Journal of the Learning Sciences (USA) *Online - full text edition.* **3413**
Journal of the Peripheral Nervous System Online(USA) *Online - full text.* **4107**

Online Service

Journal of Theoretical Biology (GBR) *Online - full text edition.* **3205**
Journal of Theoretical Medicine (CHE) *Online - full text edition.* **3638**
The Journal of Thoracic and Cardiovascular Surgery (USA) *Online - full text edition.* **4195**
Journal of Thrombosis and Thrombolysis (USA) *Online - full text edition.* **3779**
Journal of Toxicology and Environmental Health. Part A (USA) *Online - full text edition.* **3452**
Journal of Toxicology and Environmental Health. Part B: Critical Reviews (USA) *Online - full text edition.* **3452**
Journal of Toxicology. Clinical Toxicology (USA) *Online - full text edition.* **4311**
Journal of Toxicology. Toxin Reviews (USA) *Online - full text edition.* **4311**
The Journal of Trace Elements in Experimental Medicine (USA) *Online - full text edition.* **3877**
Journal of Transcultural Nursing (USA) *Online - full content edition.* **3927**
Journal of Traumatic Stress (USA) *Online - full text edition.* **4424**
Journal of Tropical Pediatrics (GBR) *Online - full text edition.* **4047**
Journal of Urology (USA) *Online - full text edition.* **4215**
Journal of Vascular Research (CHE) *Online - full text edition.* **3779**
Journal of Vascular Surgery (USA) *Online - full text edition.* **4195**
Journal of Veterinary Medicine. Series A Online(DEU) *Online - full text.* **4547**
Journal of Veterinary Medicine. Series B Online(DEU) *Online - full text.* **4547**
Journal of Veterinary Pharmacology and Therapeutics Online(GBR) *Online - full text.* **4311**
Journal of Viral Hepatitis (GBR) *Online - full text edition.* **3893**
Journal of Virology (USA) *Online - full text edition.* **3326**
Journal of Vocational Behavior (USA) *Online - full text edition.* **4424**
Journal of W O C N (USA) *Online - full text edition.* **4195**
Journal of Women's Health and Gender-Based Medicine (USA) *Online - full text edition.* **4564**
Journal of Youth and Adolescence (USA) *Online - full text edition.* **3384**
Journal of Youth Studies (GBR) *Online - full text edition.* **3384**
Journal of Zoological Systematics and Evolutionary Research Online(DEU) *Online - full text.* **3355**
Journal Watch Online (USA) *Online - full text edition of* Journal Watch. **3730**
Kennedy Institute of Ethics. Journal (USA) *Online - full text edition.* **3640**
Kidney and Blood Pressure Research (CHE) *Online - full text edition.* **4215**
Kidney International Online (USA) *Online - full text edition of* Kidney International. **4215**
Klinische Neuroradiologie (DEU) *Online - full text edition.* **4149**
Knee Surgery, Sports Traumatology, Arthroscopy (DEU) *Online - full text edition.* **4175**
Kognitionswissenschaft (DEU) *Online - full text edition.* **4425**
Le Lait (FRA) *Online - full text edition.* **3326**
The Lancet (North American Edition) (USA) *Online - full text edition.* **3643**
Langenbecks Archives of Surgery (DEU) *Online - full text edition.* **4196**
Language and Cognitive Processes (GBR) *Online - full text edition.* **3551**
Language and Speech (GBR) *Online - full text edition.* **3551**
Lasers in Medical Science (GBR) *Online - full text edition.* **3643**
Lasers in Surgery and Medicine (USA) *Online - full text edition.* **4196**
Laterality (GBR) *Online - full text edition.* **4107**
Law and Human Behavior (USA) *Online - full text edition.* **3541**
Learning & Memory (USA) *Online - full text edition.* **4108**
Learning and Motivation (USA) *Online - full text edition.* **3413**
Legal and Criminological Psychology (GBR) *Online - full text edition.* **4425**
Leisure Sciences (USA) *Online - full text edition.* **3547**
Letters in Applied Microbiology (GBR) *Online - full text edition.* **3326**
Leukemia (GBR) *Online - full text edition.* **3903**
Leukemia and Lymphoma (CHE) *Online - full text edition.* **3903**
Life Chemistry Reports (CHE) *Online - full text edition.* **3373**
Linnean Society. Biological Journal (GBR) *Online - full text edition.* **3206**
Literature & Medicine (USA) *Online - full text edition.* **3552**
Liver (DNK) *Online - full text edition.* **3894**
Liver Transplantation (USA) *Online - full text edition.* **3894**
Logopedics Phoniatrics Vocology (NOR) *Online - full text edition.* **4035**
Loss Prevention Bulletin (GBR) *Online - full content edition.* **3433**
Luminescence (GBR) *Online - full text edition.* **3380**
Lung (USA) *Online - full text edition.* **4162**
Lupus (GBR) *Online - full text edition.* **4169**
M P Online (GBR) *Online - full text edition of* Molecular Pathology. **3879**
Magnetic Resonance in Medicine (GBR) *Online - full text edition.* **4150**
Mammalian Genome (USA) *Online - full text edition.* **3310**
Manual Therapy (GBR) *Online - full text edition.* **4063**
Manuelle Medizin und Osteopathische Medizin (DEU) *Online - full text edition.* **4063**
Marine Biological Association of the United Kingdom. Journal (GBR) *Online - full text edition.* **3207**
Marine Biology (DEU) *Online - full text edition.* **3207**
Marine Ecology Online(DEU) *Online - full text.* **3207**
Maternal and Child Health Journal (USA) *Online - full text edition.* **3957**
Mathematical Biosciences (USA) *Online - full text edition.* **3554**
Mathematical Cognition (GBR) *Online - full text edition.* **4426**
Mathematical Thinking and Learning (USA) *Online - full text edition.* **3554**
Measurement in Physical Education and Exercise Science (USA) *Online - full text edition.* **4358**
Mechanisms of Development (IRL) *Online - full text edition.* **3292**
Media Psychology (USA) *Online - full text edition.* **4426**
Mediators of Inflammation (GBR) *Online - full text edition.* **3648**
Medical and Pediatric Oncology (USA) *Online - full text edition.* **3984**
Medical & Veterinary Entomology Online(GBR) *Online - full text.* **3648**
Medical Biochemistry (CHE) *Online - full text edition.* **3256**
Medical Care Research and Review (USA) *Online - full text edition.* **4496**
Medical Education (GBR) *Online - full text edition.* **3650**
Medical Electron Microscopy (JPN) *Online - full text edition.* **3334**
Medical Hypotheses (GBR) *Online - full text edition.* **3651**
Medical Image Analysis (GBR) *Online - full text edition.* **4150**
Medical Informatics and the Internet in Medicine (GBR) *Online - full text edition.* **3812**
Medical Law Review (GBR) *Online - full text edition.* **3542**
Medical Microbiology and Immunology (DEU) *Online - full text edition.* **3749**
Medical Mycology (GBR) *Online - full text edition.* **3803**
Medical Oncology (GBR) *Online - full text edition.* **3984**
Medical Physics (USA) *Online - full text edition.* **3652**
Medical Principles and Practice (CHE) *Online - full text edition.* **3652**
Medical Teacher (GBR) *Online - full text edition.* **3654**
Medicinal Research Reviews (USA) *Online - full text edition.* **4315**
Medicine, Health Care and Philosophy (NLD) *Online - full text edition.* **3656**
Medizinische Klinik (DEU) *Online - full text edition.* **3658**
Medizinrecht (DEU) *Online - full text edition.* **3884**
Melanoma Research (GBR) *Online - full text edition.* **3984**
Memory (GBR) *Online - full text edition.* **4426**
Mental Health, Religion & Culture (GBR) *Online - full content edition.* **4427**
Mental Health Services Research (USA) *Online - full text edition.* **4427**
Mental Retardation and Developmental Disabilities (New York, 1995) (USA) *Online - full text edition.* **4109**
Metabolic Engineering (USA) *Online - full text edition.* **3238**
Metaphor and Symbol (USA) *Online - full text edition.* **3551**
Methods: A Companion to Methods in Enzymology (USA) *Online - full text edition.* **3256**
Methods in Cell Science (NLD) *Online - full text edition.* **3292**
Microbial Ecology (USA) *Online - full text edition.* **3327**
Microbial Ecology in Health & Disease (NOR) *Online - full text edition.* **3803**
Microbial Pathogenesis (GBR) *Online - full text edition.* **3804**
Microbiology (GBR) *Online - full text edition.* **3327**
Microbiology and Molecular Biology Reviews (USA) *Online - full text edition.* **3328**
Microbiology Today (GBR) *Online - full text edition.* **3328**
Microcirculation (GBR) *Online - full text edition.* **3661**
Microsurgery (USA) *Online - full text edition.* **4197**
Microvascular Research (USA) *Online - full text edition.* **3780**
Midwifery (GBR) *Online - full text edition.* **3958**
The Milbank Quarterly (USA) *Online - full text edition.* **4368**
Military Psychology (USA) *Online - full text edition.* **4428**
Minimally Invasive Therapy and Allied Technologies (GBR) *Online - full text edition.* **3661**
Mitigation and Adaptation Strategies for Global Change (NLD) *Online - full text edition.* **3441**
Molecular and Cellular Biochemistry (USA) *Online - full text edition.* **3257**
Molecular and Cellular Biology (USA) *Online - full text edition.* **3257**
Molecular and Cellular Neurosciences (USA) *Online - full text edition.* **4110**
Molecular and Cellular Probes (GBR) *Online - full text edition.* **3879**
Molecular Biology and Evolution (USA) *Online - full text edition.* **3208**
Molecular Biology Reports (NLD) *Online - full text edition.* **3257**
Molecular Brain Research (NLD) *Online - full text edition.* **4110**
Molecular Carcinogenesis (USA) *Online - full text edition.* **3984**
Molecular Cell Biology Research Communications (USA) *Online - full text edition.* **3292**
Molecular Endocrinology (USA) *Online - full text edition.* **3866**
Molecular Genetics and Genomics (DEU) *Online - full text edition.* **3311**
Molecular Genetics and Metabolism (USA) *Online - full text edition.* **3662**
Molecular Human Reproduction (GBR) *Online - full text edition.* **3958**
Molecular Medicine (USA) *Online - full text edition.* **4317**
Molecular Membrane Biology (GBR) *Online - full text edition.* **3258**
Molecular Pharmacology (USA) *Online - full text edition.* **4317**
Molecular Phylogenetics and Evolution (USA) *Online - full text edition.* **3311**
Molecular Plant Pathology (GBR) *Online - full text edition.* **3281**
Molecular Psychiatry (GBR) *Online - full text edition.* **4110**
Molecular Reproduction and Development (USA) *Online - full text edition.* **3258**
Molecular Therapy (USA) *Online - full text edition.* **3984**
Monatsschrift Kinderheilkunde (DEU) *Online - full text edition.* **4049**
Morbidity and Mortality Weekly Report (USA) *Online - full text edition.* **4482**
Mortality (GBR) *Online - full content edition.* **4482**
Motivation and Emotion (USA) *Online - full text edition.* **4428**
Multiple Sclerosis (GBR) *Online - full text edition.* **4111**
Multivariate Behavioral Research (USA) *Online - full text edition.* **4428**
Mund-, Kiefer- und Gesichtschirurgie (DEU) *Online - full text edition.* **4035**
Muscle & Nerve (USA) *Online - full text edition.* **3663**
Mutagenesis (GBR) *Online - full text edition.* **3311**
Mutation Research - D N A Repair (NLD) *Online - full text edition.* **3258**
Mutation Research - Genetic Toxicology and Environmental Mutagenesis (NLD) *Online - full text edition.* **3312**
Mutation Research - Reviews in Mutation Research (NLD) *Online - full text edition.* **3312**
Mycopathologia (NLD) *Online - full text edition.* **3281**
Mycoses (DEU) *Online - full text edition.* **3663**
N M R in Biomedicine (GBR) *Online - full text edition.* **4151**
Nahrung (DEU) *Online - full text edition.* **4239**
National Academy of Sciences of the United States of America. Proceedings (USA) *Online - full text edition.* **4505**
National Cancer Institute. Journal (USA) *Online - full text edition.* **3985**
Natural Hazards Review (USA) *Online - full text edition.* **3441**
Natural Toxins (USA) *Online - full text edition.* **3453**
Nature (GBR) *Online - full text edition.* **4506**
Nature Biotechnology (USA) *Online - full text edition.* **3276**
Nature Genetics (USA) *Online - full text edition.* **3312**
Nature Medicine (GBR) *Online - full text edition.* **3665**
Nature Neuroscience (USA) *Online - full text edition.* **4111**
Nature Structural Biology (USA) *Online - full text edition.* **3210**
Naunyn-Schmiedeberg's Archives of Pharmacology (DEU) *Online - full text edition.* **4318**
NeoPlasia (USA) *Online - full text edition.* **3985**
Nephrology, Dialysis and Transplantation (GBR) *Online - full text edition.* **4216**
Nephrology Online (AUS) *Online - full text edition of* Nephrology. **4216**
Nephron (CHE) *Online - full text edition.* **4216**
Der Nervenarzt (DEU) *Online - full text edition.* **4112**
Neural Networks (GBR) *Online - full text edition.* **3390**
Neural Processing Letters (USA) *Online - full text edition.* **3390**
Neuro-Ophthalmology (NLD) *Online - full text edition.* **4112**
Neurobiology of Disease (USA) *Online - full text edition.* **4112**
Neurobiology of Learning and Memory (USA) *Online - full text edition.* **4112**
Neurocase (GBR) *Online - full text edition.* **4112**
Neurochemical Research (USA) *Online - full text edition.* **4113**
Neuroendocrinology (CHE) *Online - full text edition.* **3867**
Neuroepidemiology (CHE) *Online - full text edition.* **4113**
Neurogastroenterology and Motility Online(GBR) *Online - full text.* **3894**
Neurogenetics (DEU) *Online - full text edition.* **3312**
NeuroImage (USA) *Online - full text edition.* **4113**
NeuroImmunoModulation (CHE) *Online - full text edition.* **3750**
Neurological Sciences (ITA) *Online - full text edition.* **4114**
Neurology (USA) *Online - full text edition.* **4114**
Neurology and Clinical Neurophysiology (USA) *Online - full content edition.* **4115**
Neuromodulation Online(USA) *Online - full text.* **4115**
Neuropathology (AUS) *Online - full text edition.* **4116**
Neuropathology & Applied Neurobiology Online (GBR) *Online - full text edition of* Neuropathology and Applied Neurobiology. **4116**
Neuropeptides (Edinburgh) (GBR) *Online - full text edition.* **3259**
Neuropsychobiology (CHE) *Online - full text edition.* **4116**
Neuropsychological Rehabilitation (GBR) *Online - full text edition.* **4117**
Neuropsychology, Development and Cognition. Section A: Journal of Clinical and Experimental Neuropsychology (NLD) *Online - full text edition.* **4429**
Neuropsychology, Development and Cognition. Section B: Aging, Neuropsychology and Cognition (NLD) *Online - full text edition.* **4429**

Neuropsychology, Development, and Cognition. Section C: Child Neuropsychology (NLD) *Online - full text edition.* **4429**
Neuropsychology, Development and Cognition. Section D: The Clinical Neuropsychologist (NLD) *Online - full text edition.* **4429**
Neuropsychology Review (USA) *Online - full text edition.* **4117**
Neuropsychopharmacology (USA) *Online - full text edition.* **4117**
Neuroradiology (DEU) *Online - full text edition.* **4151**
NeuroReport (USA) *Online - full text edition.* **4117**
Neuroscience Research Communications (GBR) *Online - full text edition.* **4118**
The Neuroscientist (USA) *Online - full text edition.* **4118**
NeuroSignals (CHE) *Online - full text edition.* **3259**
Neurosurgery (Baltimore) (USA) *Online - full text edition.* **4119**
Neurosurgical Review (DEU) *Online - full text edition.* **4197**
Neurourology and Urodynamics (USA) *Online - full text edition.* **4216**
New England Journal of Medicine (USA) *Online - full text edition.* **3666**
New Genetics and Society (GBR) *Online - full content edition.* **3313**
News in Physiological Sciences Online (USA) *Online - full text edition of* News in Physiological Sciences. **3346**
Nicotine & Tobacco Research (GBR) *Online - full content edition.* **4531**
Nonlinear Dynamics, Psychology, and Life Sciences (USA) *Online - full text edition.* **4430**
Nordic Journal of Psychiatry (NOR) *Online - full text edition.* **4120**
Notfall und Rettungsmedizin (DEU) *Online - full text edition.* **4022**
Nuclear Medicine Communications (USA) *Online - full text edition.* **4152**
Nucleic Acids Research (GBR) *Online - full text edition.* **3259**
Nurse Education Today (GBR) *Online - full text edition.* **3931**
Nursing and Health Sciences (AUS) *Online - full text edition.* **3932**
Nursing Ethics (GBR) *Online - full text edition.* **3933**
Nursing Inquiry (AUS) *Online - full text edition.* **3933**
Nursing Outlook (USA) *Online - full text edition.* **3934**
Nursing Philosophy Online (GBR) *Online - full text edition of* Nursing Philosophy. **3934**
Nursing Science Quarterly (USA) *Online - full text edition.* **3934**
Nutrition and Cancer (USA) *Online - full text edition.* **4241**
Nutrition and Food Science (GBR) *Online - full text edition.* **4241**
Nutrition Bulletin Online (GBR) *Online - full text edition of* Nutrition Bulletin. **4241**
Nutrition in Clinical Care Online(USA) *Online - full text.* **4242**
Nutrition Research Reviews (GBR) *Online - full text edition.* **4243**
Nutrition Society. Proceedings (GBR) *Online - full text edition.* **4243**
Nutritional Neuroscience (CHE) *Online - full text edition.* **4120**
O E M Online (GBR) *Online - full text edition of* Occupational and Environmental Medicine. **4261**
O R L (CHE) *Online - full text edition.* **4036**
Obesity Research (USA) *Online - full text edition.* **3668**
Obesity Reviews Online(GBR) *Online - full text.* **4244**
Obesity Surgery (USA) *Online - full text edition.* **4198**
Occupational Medicine (GBR) *Online - full text edition.* **4262**
Ocular Immunology and Inflammation (NLD) *Online - full text edition.* **4002**
Oecologia (DEU) *Online - full text edition.* **3211**
Oncogene (GBR) *Online - full text edition.* **3986**
The Oncologist (USA) *Online - full text edition.* **3986**
Oncology (CHE) *Online - full content edition.* **3986**
Der Onkologe (DEU) *Online - full text edition.* **3987**
Onkologie (CHE) *Online - full text edition.* **3987**
The Online Journal of Current Clinical Trials(USA) *Online - full content.* **3670**
Online Journal of Knowledge Synthesis for Nursing(USA) *Online - full text.* **3936**
Operative Orthopaedie und Traumatologie (DEU) *Online - full text edition.* **4022**
Ophthalmic Epidemiology (NLD) *Online - full text edition.* **4003**
Ophthalmic Genetics (NLD) *Online - full text edition.* **4003**
Ophthalmic Research (CHE) *Online - full text edition.* **4003**
Der Ophthalmologe (DEU) *Online - full text edition.* **4004**
Ophthalmologica (CHE) *Online - full text edition.* **4004**
Ophthalmology (USA) *Online - full text edition.* **4004**
Oral Diseases (GBR) *Online - full text edition.* **3834**
Oral Microbiology and Immunology (DNK) *Online - full text edition.* **3329**
Oral Surgery, Oral Medicine, Oral Pathology, Oral Radiology, and Endodontics (USA) *Online - full text edition.* **3835**
Orbit (NLD) *Online - full text edition.* **4005**
Organization & Environment (USA) *Online - full text edition.* **4263**
Organizational Behavior and Human Decision Processes (USA) *Online - full text edition.* **3366**
Origins of Life and Evolution of the Biosphere (NLD) *Online - full text edition.* **3212**
Der Orthopaede (DEU) *Online - full text edition.* **4022**
Osteoarthritis and Cartilage (GBR) *Online - full text edition.* **4169**
Osteoporosis International (GBR) *Online - full text edition.* **3671**
Oto-Rhino-Laryngologia Nova (CHE) *Online - full text edition.* **4036**
Otolaryngology - Head and Neck Surgery (USA) *Online - full text edition.* **4036**
Paediatric Anaesthesia Online(GBR) *Online - full text.* **3759**
Paediatric & Perinatal Epidemiology Online(GBR) *Online - full text.* **4050**
Paediatric Drugs (NZL) *Online - full text edition.* **4321**
Paediatric Respiratory Reviews (GBR) *Online - full text edition.* **4162**
The Pain Clinic (NLD) *Online - full content edition.* **3759**
Pain Medicine Online(USA) *Online - full text.* **4121**
Pain Reviews (GBR) *Online - full text edition.* **3671**
Palliative Medicine (GBR) *Online - full text edition.* **3672**
Parasite Immunology Online (GBR) *Online - full text edition of* Parasite Immunology. **3804**
Parasitology (Cambridge) (GBR) *Online - full text edition.* **3804**
Parasitology Research (DEU) *Online - full text edition.* **3330**
Patent Fast-Alert(GBR) *Online - full text.* **4321**
Pathobiology (CHE) *Online - full text edition.* **3750**
Der Pathologe (DEU) *Online - full text edition.* **3672**
Pathology (GBR) *Online - full text edition.* **3673**
Pathology and Oncology Research (GBR) *Online - full text edition.* **3988**
Pathology International (AUS) *Online - full text edition.* **3673**
Pathophysiology of Haemostasis and Thrombosis (CHE) *Online - full text edition.* **3904**
Peace and Conflict (USA) *Online - full text edition.* **4432**
Pediatric Allergy and Immunology (DNK) *Online - full text edition.* **4051**
Pediatric and Developmental Pathology (USA) *Online - full text edition.* **4051**
Pediatric Cardiology (USA) *Online - full text edition.* **3781**
Pediatric Dermatology (USA) *Online - full text edition.* **3852**
Pediatric Hematology & Oncology (USA) *Online - full text edition.* **4053**
Pediatric Nephrology (DEU) *Online - full text edition.* **4217**
Pediatric Neurosurgery (CHE) *Online - full text edition.* **4122**
Pediatric Pathology & Molecular Medicine (USA) *Online - full text edition.* **4053**
Pediatric Pulmonology (USA) *Online - full text edition.* **4053**
Pediatric Radiology (DEU) *Online - full text edition.* **4053**
Pediatric Rehabilitation (GBR) *Online - full text edition.* **4064**
Pediatric Research (USA) *Online - full text edition.* **4054**
Pediatric Surgery International (DEU) *Online - full text edition.* **4200**
Pediatric Transplantation (DNK) *Online - full text edition.* **4054**
Pediatrics (English Edition) (USA) *Online - full text edition.* **4054**
Pediatrics in Review (USA) *Online - full text edition.* **4054**
Pediatrics International (AUS) *Online - full text edition.* **4054**
Perfusion (GBR) *Online - full text edition.* **3781**
Periodontology 2000 Online(DNK) *Online - full text.* **3836**
Personality and Social Psychology Review (USA) *Online - full text edition.* **4432**
Perspectives in Biology and Medicine (USA) *Online - full content edition.* **3674**
Perspectives on Developmental Neurobiology (CHE) *Online - full text edition.* **4122**
Pesticide Biochemistry and Physiology (USA) *Online - full text edition.* **3159**
Pfluegers Archiv (DEU) *Online - full text edition.* **3674**
Pharmaceutical Biology (NLD) *Online - full text edition.* **4323**
Pharmaceutical Development and Technology (USA) *Online - full text edition.* **4323**
Pharmaceutical Research (USA) *Online - full content edition.* **4324**
PharmacoEconomics (NZL) *Online - full text edition.* **4326**
Pharmacoeconomics and Outcomes News (NZL) *Online - full text edition.* **4345**
Pharmacoepidemiology and Drug Safety (GBR) *Online - full text edition.* **4326**
Pharmacogenetics (USA) *Online - full text edition.* **3313**
Pharmacological Research (GBR) *Online - full text edition.* **4326**
Pharmacological Reviews (USA) *Online - full text edition.* **4326**
Pharmacology (CHE) *Online - full text edition.* **4326**
Pharmacology Reviews and Communications (CHE) *Online - full text edition.* **4327**
Pharmacy World and Science (NLD) *Online - full content edition.* **4329**
Philosophical Psychology (GBR) *Online - full text edition.* **4433**
Philosophy, Psychiatry, and Psychology Online (USA) *Online - full text edition of* Philosophy, Psychiatry & Psychology. **4348**
Phlebology (GBR) *Online - full text edition.* **3781**
Photodermatology, Photoimmunology & Photomedicine Online(DNK) *Online - full text.* **3852**
Photosynthesis Research (NLD) *Online - full text edition.* **3260**
Physical Therapy (USA) *Online - full text edition.* **4064**
Physics in Medicine and Biology (GBR) *Online - full text edition.* **3267**
Physiological Genomics (USA) *Online - full text edition.* **3260**
Physiological Measurement (GBR) *Online - full text edition.* **3676**
Physiological Reviews Online (USA) *Online - full text edition of* Physiological Reviews. **3347**
Physiotherapy Theory and Practice (GBR) *Online - full text edition.* **4065**
Phytochemical Analysis (GBR) *Online - full text edition.* **3282**
Phytotherapy Research (GBR) *Online - full text edition.* **3282**
Pigment Cell Research (DNK) *Online - full text edition.* **3293**
Pituitary (NLD) *Online - full text edition.* **3867**
Placenta (GBR) *Online - full text edition.* **3676**
Plant, Cell and Environment Online (GBR) *Online - full text edition of* Plant, Cell and Environment. **3213**
Plant Cell, Tissue and Organ Culture (NLD) *Online - full text edition.* **3293**
Plant Foods for Human Nutrition (NLD) *Online - full text edition.* **4244**
Plant Molecular Biology (NLD) *Online - full text edition.* **3213**
Platelets (Abingdon) (GBR) *Online - full text edition.* **3213**
Polar Biology (DEU) *Online - full text edition.* **3213**
Policy, Politics & Nursing Practice (USA) *Online - full text edition.* **3937**
Political Psychology (USA) *Online - full text edition.* **4368**
Postgraduate Medical Journal (GBR) *Online - full text edition.* **3678**
Prenatal Diagnosis (GBR) *Online - full text edition.* **3962**
Prevention Science (USA) *Online - full text edition.* **3805**
Preventive Medicine (USA) *Online - full text edition.* **3679**
Primary Care Psychiatry (USA) *Online - full text edition.* **4123**
Primary Health Care Research and Development (GBR) *Online - full text edition.* **3679**
Prostaglandins, Leukotrienes and Essential Fatty Acids (GBR) *Online - full text edition.* **3868**
The Prostate (USA) *Online - full text edition.* **3680**
Prostate Cancer and Prostatic Diseases (GBR) *Online - full text edition.* **3989**
The Prostate Journal Online(USA) *Online - full text.* **3680**
Protein Engineering (GBR) *Online - full text edition.* **3261**
Protein Expression and Purification (USA) *Online - full text edition.* **3261**
Protein Science (USA) *Online - full text edition.* **3261**
Proteins: Structure, Function, and Genetics (USA) *Online - full text edition.* **3261**
Protist (DEU) *Online - full text edition.* **3214**
Psychiatric Bulletin (GBR) *Online - full text edition.* **4125**
Psychiatric Genetics (USA) *Online - full text edition.* **3313**
Psychiatric News (USA) *Online - full text edition.* **4125**
Psychiatric Quarterly (USA) *Online - full text edition.* **4126**
Psychiatric Services (USA) *Online - full text edition.* **4126**
Psychiatry and Clinical Neurosciences (AUS) *Online - full text edition.* **4126**
Psycho-Oncology (GBR) *Online - full text edition.* **3989**
Psychoanalytic Studies (GBR) *Online - full text edition.* **4437**
Psychodynamic Counselling (GBR) *Online - full text edition.* **4127**
Psychological Inquiry (USA) *Online - full text edition.* **4438**
Psychological Medicine (GBR) *Online - full text edition.* **4127**
Psychological Research (DEU) *Online - full text edition.* **4438**
Psychological Science (USA) *Online - full content edition.* **4438**
Psychology & Marketing (USA) *Online - full text edition.* **4440**
Psychology, Evolution and Gender (GBR) *Online - full text edition.* **4440**
Psychology, Health & Medicine (GBR) *Online - full text edition.* **4440**
Psychology in the Schools (USA) *Online - full text edition.* **4441**
Psychopathology (CHE) *Online - full text edition.* **4128**
Psychopharmacology (DEU) *Online - full text edition.* **4332**
Psychophysiology (GBR) *Online - full text edition.* **4128**
Psychosomatics (USA) *Online - full text edition.* **4128**
Psychotherapeut (DEU) *Online - full text edition.* **4128**
Psychotherapy and Psychosomatics (CHE) *Online - full text edition.* **4129**
PsycINFO(USA) *Online - full text.* **4458**
Public Health (Basingstoke) (GBR) *Online - full text edition.* **3681**
Public Health Nursing (USA) *Online - full text edition.* **3938**
Public Health Nutrition (GBR) *Online - full text edition.* **4245**
Public Health Reports (USA) *Online - full text edition.* **4486**
Pulmonary Pharmacology & Therapeutics (GBR) *Online - full text edition.* **4163**
Q J M (GBR) *Online - full text edition.* **3681**
Qualitative Health Research (USA) *Online - full text edition.* **3681**
Quality Assurance Journal (GBR) *Online - full text edition.* **3682**
Quality in Health Care (GBR) *Online - full content edition.* **3682**
Quality of Life Research (NLD) *Online - full text edition.* **3682**
Quantitative Structure-Activity Relationships (DEU) *Online - full text edition.* **4332**
Quarterly Journal of Experimental Psychology. Section A: Human Experimental Psychology (GBR) *Online - full text edition.* **4443**

Quarterly Journal of Experimental Psychology. Section B: Comparative and Physiological Psychology (GBR) *Online - full text edition.* **4443**
Quarterly Reviews of Biophysics (GBR) *Online - full text edition.* **3267**
R N A (GBR) *Online - full text edition.* **3261**
Radiation and Environmental Biophysics (DEU) *Online - full text edition.* **3267**
Radiographics (USA) *Online - full text edition.* **4153**
Radiography (GBR) *Online - full text edition.* **4153**
Der Radiologe (DEU) *Online - full text edition.* **4153**
Radiology (USA) *Online - full text edition.* **4154**
Radiotherapy and Oncology (IRL) *Online - full text edition.* **4154**
Reactions Weekly (NZL) *Online - full text edition.* **4346**
Reading and Writing (NLD) *Online - full text edition.* **3551**
Reading Psychology (USA) *Online - full text edition.* **3414**
Rechtsmedizin (DEU) *Online - full text edition.* **3884**
Regulatory Toxicology and Pharmacology (USA) *Online - full text edition.* **3453**
Renal Failure (USA) *Online - full text edition.* **4217**
Reproduction, Fertility and Development (AUS) *Online - full content edition.* **3215**
Reproduction in Domestic Animals Online(DEU) *Online - full text.* **4551**
Reproduction, Nutrition, Development (FRA) *Online - full text edition.* **3215**
Reproductive Medicine Review (GBR) *Online - full text edition.* **3962**
Reproduktionsmedizin (DEU) *Online - full text edition.* **3962**
Research in Nursing & Health (USA) *Online - full text edition.* **3939**
Research in Veterinary Science (GBR) *Online - full text edition.* **4551**
Research on Aging (USA) *Online - full text edition.* **3480**
Research on Social Work Practice (USA) *Online - full text edition.* **4523**
Respiration (CHE) *Online - full text edition.* **4164**
Respiratory Medicine (GBR) *Online - full text edition.* **4164**
Respirology (AUS) *Online - full text edition.* **4164**
Review of Plant Pathology (GBR) *Online - full text edition.* **3236**
Reviews in Clinical and Experimental Hematology (GBR) *Online - full text edition.* **3904**
Reviews in Clinical Gerontology (GBR) *Online - full text edition.* **3480**
Reviews in Endocrine & Metabolic Disorders (USA) *Online - full text edition.* **3868**
Reviews in Medical Microbiology (USA) *Online - full text edition.* **3684**
Reviews in Medical Virology (GBR) *Online - full text edition.* **3331**
Rheumatology (GBR) *Online - full text edition.* **4171**
Rheumatology International (DEU) *Online - full text edition.* **4171**
Royal Chemical Society. Journal. Perkin Transactions 1 (GBR) *Online - full text edition.* **3379**
Royal College of Surgeons of Edinburgh. Journal (GBR) *Online - full text edition.* **4202**
Royal Society of London. Proceedings. Biological Sciences (GBR) *Online - full text edition.* **3217**
S T I Online (GBR) *Online - full text edition of* Sexually Transmitted Infections. **3853**
Sage Family Studies Abstracts (USA) *Online - full text edition.* **4524**
Sarcoma (GBR) *Online - full text edition.* **3990**
Scandinavian Audiology (NOR) *Online - full text edition.* **4038**
Scandinavian Cardiovascular Journal (NOR) *Online - full text edition.* **4202**
Scandinavian Journal of Behaviour Therapy (NOR) *Online - full text edition.* **4447**
Scandinavian Journal of Caring Sciences (NOR) *Online - full text edition.* **3690**
Scandinavian Journal of Clinical & Laboratory Investigation (NOR) *Online - full text edition.* **3880**
Scandinavian Journal of Gastroenterology (NOR) *Online - full text edition.* **3895**
Scandinavian Journal of Immunology Online (GBR) *Online - full text edition of* Scandinavian Journal of Immunology. **3751**
Scandinavian Journal of Infectious Diseases (NOR) *Online - full text edition.* **3806**
Scandinavian Journal of Medicine & Science in Sports Online(DNK) *Online - full text.* **4176**
Scandinavian Journal of Occupational Therapy (NOR) *Online - full text edition.* **3690**
Scandinavian Journal of Plastic and Reconstructive Surgery and Hand Surgery (NOR) *Online - full text edition.* **4202**
Scandinavian Journal of Primary Health Care (NOR) *Online - full text edition.* **3690**
Scandinavian Journal of Psychology (GBR) *Online - full text edition.* **4447**
Scandinavian Journal of Public Health (NOR) *Online - full text edition.* **3690**
Scandinavian Journal of Rheumatology (NOR) *Online - full text edition.* **4171**
Scandinavian Journal of Urology and Nephrology (NOR) *Online - full text edition.* **4218**
Scanning (USA) *Online - full text edition.* **3335**
Der Schmerz (DEU) *Online - full text edition.* **3690**
School Psychology International (GBR) *Online - full text edition.* **3429**
Science as Culture (GBR) *Online - full text edition.* **4507**
Seizure (GBR) *Online - full text edition.* **4133**
Seminars in Cancer Biology (GBR) *Online - full text edition.* **3349**
Seminars in Cell and Developmental Biology (GBR) *Online - full text edition.* **3294**
Seminars in Dialysis (USA) *Online - full text edition.* **4218**
Seminars in Hearing (USA) *Online - full text edition.* **4038**
Seminars in Immunology (GBR) *Online - full text edition.* **3751**
Seminars in Liver Diseases (USA) *Online - full text edition.* **3896**
Seminars in Neonatology (GBR) *Online - full text edition.* **3964**
Seminars in Neurology (USA) *Online - full text edition.* **4133**
Seminars in Radiation Oncology (USA) *Online - full text edition.* **3990**
Seminars in Respiratory and Critical Care Medicine (USA) *Online - full text edition.* **4165**
Seminars in Speech and Language (USA) *Online - full text edition.* **4038**
Seminars in Surgical Oncology (USA) *Online - full text edition.* **3990**
Seminars in the Neurosciences (USA) *Online - full text edition.* **4133**
Seminars in Thrombosis and Hemostasis (USA) *Online - full text edition.* **3905**
Sensory Neuron (NLD) *Online - full content edition.* **4133**
Sepsis (USA) *Online - full text edition.* **3807**
Sex Roles (USA) *Online - full text edition.* **4448**
Sexual Abuse (USA) *Online - full text edition.* **4448**
Sexual and Relationship Therapy (GBR) *Online - full content edition.* **4448**
Sexualities (GBR) *Online - full text edition.* **4448**
Sexuality and Disability (USA) *Online - full text edition.* **3692**
Skeletal Radiology (DEU) *Online - full text edition.* **4155**
Skin Pharmacology and Applied Skin Physiology (CHE) *Online - full text edition.* **4336**
Skin Research and Technology (DNK) *Online - full text edition.* **3853**
Skull Base Surgery (USA) *Online - full text edition.* **4203**
Sleep Medicine Reviews (GBR) *Online - full text edition.* **4134**
Small Group Research (USA) *Online - full text edition.* **4449**
Social Psychiatry and Psychiatric Epidemiology (DEU) *Online - full text edition.* **4134**
Social Psychology of Education (NLD) *Online - full text edition.* **3415**
Society & Animals (GBR) *Online - full text edition.* **3172**
Society for Research in Child Development. Monographs (USA) *Online - full text edition.* **3386**
Sociology of Health and Illness (GBR) *Online - full text edition.* **4523**
Somatosensory and Motor Research (GBR) *Online - full text edition.* **3349**
Southern Medical Journal (USA) *Online - full text edition.* **3695**
Spatial Cognition and Computation (NLD) *Online - full text edition.* **4450**
Spatial Vision (NLD) *Online - full content edition.* **3554**
Speech Communication (NLD) *Online - full text edition.* **3552**
Spinal Cord (GBR) *Online - full text edition.* **4134**
Spine (Philadelphia, 1976) (USA) *Online - full text edition.* **4026**
Sports Medicine (NZL) *Online - full text edition.* **4177**
Springer Seminars in Immunopathology (DEU) *Online - full text edition.* **3751**
Statistical Methods in Medical Research (GBR) *Online - full text edition.* **4530**
Statistics in Medicine (GBR) *Online - full text edition.* **3737**
Stem Cells (USA) *Online - full text edition.* **3219**
Stereotactic and Functional Neurosurgery (CHE) *Online - full text edition.* **4204**
Strabismus (NLD) *Online - full text edition.* **4007**
Strahlentherapie und Onkologie (DEU) *Online - full text edition.* **4156**
Stress (CHE) *Online - full text edition.* **3696**
Stress and Health (GBR) *Online - full text edition.* **4135**
Stroke (USA) *Online - full text edition.* **3783**
Structural Equation Modeling (USA) *Online - full text edition.* **4451**
Structure (GBR) *Online - full text edition.* **3220**
Substance Abuse (USA) *Online - full text edition.* **3406**
Support for Learning (GBR) *Online - full text edition.* **3427**
Supportive Care in Cancer (DEU) *Online - full text edition.* **3990**
Surgery (USA) *Online - full text edition.* **4204**
Surgery Today (JPN) *Online - full text edition.* **4204**
Surgical and Radiologic Anatomy (FRA) *Online - full text edition.* **3697**
Surgical Endoscopy (USA) *Online - full text edition.* **4204**
Surgical Infections (USA) *Online - full content edition.* **4204**
Surgical Oncology (GBR) *Online - full text edition.* **3991**
Synapse (New York) (USA) *Online - full text edition.* **4135**
System Familie (DEU) *Online - full text edition.* **4135**
Systematic Parasitology (NLD) *Online - full text edition.* **3220**
Teaching and Learning in Medicine (USA) *Online - full text edition.* **3698**
Teaching of Psychology (USA) *Online - full text edition.* **4452**
Techniques in Coloproctology Online(ITA) *Online - full text.* **3896**
Technology and Health Care (NLD) *Online - full text edition.* **3698**
Telemedicine Journal and e-Health (USA) *Online - full text edition.* **3812**
Teratogenesis, Carcinogenesis, and Mutagenesis (USA) *Online - full text edition.* **3699**
Teratology (USA) *Online - full text edition.* **3220**
Theoretical and Applied Genetics (DEU) *Online - full text edition.* **3314**
Theoretical Issues in Ergonomics Science (GBR) *Online - full text edition.* **3433**
Theoretical Medicine and Bioethics (NLD) *Online - full text edition.* **3699**
Theoretical Population Biology (USA) *Online - full text edition.* **3221**
Theory & Psychology (GBR) *Online - full text edition.* **4452**
Theory in Biosciences (DEU) *Online - full text edition.* **3221**
Therapeutic Apheresis Online(USA) *Online - full text.* **4218**
Thinking & Reasoning (GBR) *Online - full text edition.* **4452**
Thorax Online (GBR) *Online - full text edition of* Thorax. **3700**
Thrombosis and Haemostasis (DEU) *Online - full text edition.* **3783**
Tissue & Cell (GBR) *Online - full text edition.* **3294**
Tissue Antigens (DNK) *Online - full text edition.* **3701**
Tissue Engineering (USA) *Online - full content edition.* **3294**
Tobbacco Control Online (GBR) *Online - full text edition of* Tobacco Control. **4531**
Topoi (NLD) *Online - full text edition.* **4348**
Toxicological and Environmental Chemistry (CHE) *Online - full text edition.* **3454**
Toxicological Sciences (USA) *Online - full text edition.* **3455**
Toxicology and Applied Pharmacology (USA) *Online - full text edition.* **3455**
Toxicology and Industrial Health (GBR) *Online - full text edition.* **3455**
Toxicology Methods (USA) *Online - full text edition.* **3456**
Traffic (DNK) *Online - full text edition.* **3294**
Transcultural Psychiatry (GBR) *Online - full text edition.* **4136**
Transfusion (USA) *Online - full text edition.* **3702**
Transfusion Medicine (GBR) *Online - full text edition.* **3905**
Transgenic Research (NLD) *Online - full text edition.* **3314**
Transplant Immunology (GBR) *Online - full text edition.* **3751**
Transplant Infectious Disease Online(DNK) *Online - full text.* **4206**
Transplant International (DEU) *Online - full text edition.* **3702**
Transplantation (USA) *Online - full text edition.* **4206**
Transplantation Proceedings (USA) *Online - full text edition.* **4206**
Trauma(GBR) *Online - full text.* **4027**
Trauma Quarterly (NLD) *Online - full content edition.* **4207**
Trauma und Berufskrankheit (DEU) *Online - full text edition.* **4027**
Trauma, Violence & Abuse (USA) *Online - full text edition.* **4491**
Trends in Immunology Online (GBR) *Online - full text edition of* Trends in Immunology. **3752**
Tropical Animal Health and Production (NLD) *Online - full text edition.* **4554**
Tropical Medicine & International Health Online (GBR) *Online - full text edition of* Tropical Medicine & International Health. **4491**
Tuberculosis (GBR) *Online - full text edition.* **4166**
Tumor Biology (CHE) *Online - full text edition.* **3991**
Twin Research (GBR) *Online - full text edition.* **3315**
Ultramicroscopy (NLD) *Online - full text edition.* **3336**
Ultrasonic Imaging (USA) *Online - full text edition.* **4156**
Ultrasound in Obstetrics & Gynecology (GBR) *Online - full text edition.* **3965**
Ultrastructural Pathology (USA) *Online - full text edition.* **3991**
Der Unfallchirurg (DEU) *Online - full text edition.* **4027**
Der Urologe. Section A (DEU) *Online - full text edition.* **4219**
Der Urologe. Section B (DEU) *Online - full text edition.* **4219**
Urologia Internationalis (CHE) *Online - full text edition.* **4219**
Urological Research (DEU) *Online - full text edition.* **4219**
Vaccine Online (GBR) *Online - full text edition of* Vaccine. **3752**
Value in Health (USA) *Online - full text edition.* **4339**
Vascular Medicine (GBR) *Online - full text edition.* **3784**
Verhaltenstherapie (CHE) *Online - full content edition.* **4137**
Veterinary Anaesthesia and Analgesia Online (GBR) *Online - full text edition of* Veterinary Anaesthesia and Analgesia. **4556**
Veterinary Dermatology Online(GBR) *Online - full text.* **4557**
The Veterinary Journal (GBR) *Online - full text edition.* **4557**
Veterinary Ophthalmology Online (GBR) *Online - full text edition of* Veterinary Ophthalmology. **4558**
Veterinary Research Communications (NLD) *Online - full text edition.* **4559**
Veterinary Research (Online Edition) (FRA) *Online - full text edition of* Veterinary Research. **4559**
Violence Against Women (USA) *Online - full text edition.* **4524**
Violence & Abuse Abstracts (USA) *Online - full text edition.* **4524**
Virchows Archiv (DEU) *Online - full text edition.* **3223**
Virology (USA) *Online - full text edition.* **3332**
Virus Genes (USA) *Online - full text edition.* **3332**
Visual Cognition (GBR) *Online - full text edition.* **4454**

Visual Impairment Research (NLD) Online - full text edition. 3500
Visual Neuroscience (GBR) Online - full text edition. 4137
Vox Sanguinis (CHE) Online - full text edition. 3752
W J M (USA) Online - full text edition. 3707
Western Journal of Nursing Research (USA) Online - full text edition. 3943
Work and Stress (GBR) Online - full text edition. 4455
World Journal of Microbiology and Biotechnology (GBR) Online - full text edition. 3278
World Journal of Surgery (USA) Online - full text edition. 4207
World Journal of Urology (DEU) Online - full text edition. 4220
Wound Repair and Regeneration (USA) Online - full text edition. 4028
Xenobiotica (GBR) Online - full text edition. 3264
Xenotransplantation (DNK) Online - full text edition. 4207
Yeast (GBR) Online - full text edition. 3283
Zeitschrift fuer Gerontologie und Geriatrie (DEU) Online - full text edition. 3482
Zeitschrift fuer Herz, Thorax- und Gefaesschirurgie (DEU) Online - full text edition. 3785
Zeitschrift fuer Kardiologie (DEU) Online - full text edition. 3785
Zeitschrift fuer Laermbekaempfung (DEU) Online - full text edition. 4367
Zeitschrift fuer Rheumatologie (DEU) Online - full text edition. 4172
Zoomorphology (DEU) Online - full text edition. 3225
Zygote (GBR) Online - full text edition. 3315

European Space Agency Via Galileo Galilei, Casella Postale 64, Frascati, RM 00044, Italy TEL 39-6-440-4568, http://www.esa.int
BioVenture View (USA) Online - full text edition. 3272
CAB International. Bureau of Nutrition. Annotated Bibliographies (GBR) Online - full text edition. 4248
N A T O Advanced Science Institutes Series D: Behavioural and Social Sciences (NLD) Online - full text edition. (File no.128) 4429
N A T O Advanced Science Institutes Series H: Cell Biology (NLD) Online - full text edition. (File no.128) 3293
N I O S H T I C(USA) Online - full text. 4259

F I Z Technik Ostbahnhofstrasse 13-15, Frankfurt a.M. 60314, Germany TEL 49-69-4308-0, FAX 49-69-4308200, http://www.fiz-technik.de
Cardiovascular and Interventional Radiology (USA) Online - full text edition. 4141
Chemical Safety NewsBase(GBR) Online - full text. 4268
Environment Abstracts (USA) Online - full text edition. 3392
Der Radiologe (DEU) Online - full text edition. 4153

Factiva PO Box 300, Princeton, NJ 08543-0300; Route 1 at Ridge Rd., South Brunswick, NJ 08852, TEL 609-452-1511, 800-369-7466, FAX 609-520-4775, solutions@factiva.com, http://www.factiva.com
A J P: Cell Physiology Online (USA) Online - full text edition of American Journal of Physiology: Cell Physiology. (IPHC) 3337
A J P: Endocrinology and Metabolism Online (USA) Online - full text edition of American Journal of Physiology: Endocrinology and Metabolism. (IPHE) 3338
A J P: Gastrointestinal and Liver Physiology Online (USA) Online - full text edition of American Journal of Physiology: Gastrointestinal and Liver Physiology. (IPHG) 3338
A J P: Heart and Circulatory Physiology Online (USA) Online - full text edition of American Journal of Physiology: Heart and Circulatory Physiology. (IPHH) 3338
A J P: Lung Cellular and Molecular Physiology Online (USA) Online - full text edition of American Journal of Physiology: Lung Cellular and Molecular Physiology. (IPHM) 3338
A J P: Regulatory, Integrative and Comparative Physiology Online (USA) Online - full text edition of American Journal of Physiology: Regulatory, Integrative and Comparative Physiology. (IPHR) 3338
Addictive Behaviors (GBR) Online - full text edition. (FADD) 3397
Adolescence (San Diego) (USA) Online - full text edition. (ADOL) 3380
Advances in Physiology Education Online (USA) Online - full text edition of Advances in Physiology Education. (IPHV) 3337
Age and Ageing (GBR) Online - full text edition. (AGEN) 3466
Ageing and Society (GBR) Online - full text edition. (PANS) 3466
AIDS Alert (USA) Online - full text edition. (AIDA) 3791
AIDS Patient Care and S T Ds (USA) Online - full text edition. (IAPC) 3791
Alcohol Research & Health (USA) Online - full text edition. (AHRW) 3398
Alcoholism & Drug Abuse Weekly (USA) Online - full text edition. (ADAW) 3398
American Academy of Child and Adolescent Psychiatry. Journal (USA) Online - full text edition. (JACA) 4071
American Annals of the Deaf (USA) Online - full text edition. (IAAD) 3488
American Dental Association. Journal (USA) Online - full text edition. (IADA) 3814
American Dietetic Association. Journal (USA) Online - full text edition. (JADA) 4228
American Druggist (USA) Online - full text edition. (ADRG) 4275
American Family Physician (USA) Online - full text edition. (AFP) 3563
American Fitness (USA) Online - full text edition. (AFIT) 4350
American Geriatrics Society. Journal (USA) Online - full text edition. (FGER) 3467
The American Journal of Cardiology (USA) Online - full text edition. (IACR) 3762
American Journal of Clinical Nutrition (USA) Online - full text edition. (IAJC) 4228
American Journal of Community Psychology (USA) Online - full text edition. (AJCP) 4520
American Journal of Drug and Alcohol Abuse (USA) Online - full text edition. (AJDA) 3399
American Journal of Law & Medicine (USA) Online - full text edition. (AJLM) 3536
The American Journal of Medicine (USA) Online - full text edition. (IAMD) 3564
American Journal of Nursing (USA) Online - full text edition. (GJON) 3913
American Journal of Ophthalmology (USA) Online - full text edition. (AJOP) 3993
American Journal of Orthopsychiatry (USA) Online - full text edition. (GJOO) 4374
American Journal of Psychiatry (USA) Online - full text edition. (GPSI) 4071
American Journal of Psychoanalysis (USA) Online - full text edition. (PAJO) 4374
American Journal of Psychology (USA) Online - full text edition. (AJSY) 4374
American Journal of Psychotherapy (USA) Online - full text edition. (IPST) 4072
American Journal of Public Health (USA) Online - full text edition. (GAPH) 4461
American Journal of Sports Medicine (USA) Online - full text edition. (IASM) 4172
The American Naturalist (USA) Online - full text edition. (IANA) 3180
American Psychologist (USA) Online - full text edition. (GAMP) 4375
Animal Behaviour (GBR) Online - full text edition. (IANB) 3350
Animal Learning & Behavior (USA) Online - full text edition. (UPALB) 4376
Annual Review of Microbiology (USA) Online - full text edition. (IARM) 3317
Annual Review of Psychology (USA) Online - full text edition. (ANRS) 4376
Antiviral Agents Bulletin (USA) Online - full text edition. (AVAB) 4276
Antiviral Weekly (USA) Online - full text edition. (ANTV) 3740
Applied and Environmental Microbiology (USA) Online - full text edition. (IAEM) 3318
Applied Ergonomics (GBR) Online - full text edition. (FAPE) 3431
Applied Genetics News (USA) Online - full text edition. (AGNW) 3299
Archives of Environmental Health (USA) Online - full text edition. (AREH) 3435
Archives of Sexual Behavior (USA) Online - full text edition. (PASB) 3568
Arthritis Today (USA) Online - full text edition. (IATY) 4167
Asbestos & Lead Abatement Report (USA) Online - full text edition. (ASBC) 3443
Australian and New Zealand Journal of Public Health (AUS) Online - full text edition. (AUP) 4462
Behavior Therapy (USA) Online - full text edition. (IBTH) 4380
Behavioral and Brain Sciences (GBR) Online - full text edition. (IBBS) 4380
Behavioral Health Management (USA) Online - full text edition. (BHMG) 3399
Behavioral Neuroscience (USA) Online - full text edition. (IBNE) 4381
Behaviour Research and Therapy (GBR) Online - full text edition. (UPBRT) 4382
Better Nutrition (USA) Online - full text edition. (BNUT) 4230
Biological Bulletin (USA) Online - full text edition. (BIBU) 3185
Biological Reviews (GBR) Online - full text edition. (PBIR) 3185
Biomedical Materials (GBR) Online - full text edition. (BIOM) 3576
BioPharm (USA) Online - full text edition. (BIOP) 4280
BioScience (USA) Online - full text edition. (BIOS) 3187
Biotech Business (USA) Online - full text edition. (BTBU) 3270
BioVenture View (USA) Online - full text edition. (BIOV) 3272
Blood Weekly (USA) Online - full text edition. (BLDW) 3899
The British Journal of Criminology (GBR) Online - full text edition. (BJC) 3393
British Journal of Psychology (GBR) Online - full text edition. (BJSY) 4384
C A - A Cancer Journal for Clinicians (USA) Online - full text edition. (CACA) 3969
Canadian Journal of Experimental Psychology (CAN) Online - full text edition. (PCSY) 4386
Canadian Mining Journal (CAN) Online - full text edition. (CNMJ) 4225
The Career Development Quarterly (USA) Online - full text edition. (GCDQ) 4269
Chain Drug Review (USA) Online - full text edition. (CHDR) 3364
Chemische Rundschau (CHE) Online - full text edition. (CMRN) 3372
Chest (USA) Online - full text edition. (CHST) 4159
Child Abuse & Neglect (GBR) Online - full text edition. (ICAN) 3381
Child and Adolescent Social Work Journal (USA) Online - full text edition. (FCAS) 4520
Child Health Alert (USA) Online - full text edition. (CHLT) 4042
Chimica Oggi (ITA) Online - full text edition. (CHIMOG) 3372
Chimie Hebdo (FRA) Online - full text edition. (CHIABC) 3372
Clinical Diabetes (USA) Online - full text edition. (CLDB) 3856
Clinical Nursing Research (USA) Online - full text edition. (FCNR) 3916
Cognitive Psychology (USA) Online - full text edition. (ICOG) 4389
Community Mental Health Journal (USA) Online - full text edition. (PCMH) 4512
Consultant (Greenwich) (USA) Online - full text edition. (CNSL) 3589
Consumer Reports on Health (USA) Online - full text edition. (ICRH) 4351
Contemporary Drug Problems (USA) Online - full text edition. (CDP) 3400
Current Health 2 (USA) Online - full text edition. (CRHL) 3428
Dental Economics (USA) Online - full text edition. (ADEN) 3820
Developmental Psychology (USA) Online - full text edition. (GDPS) 4394
Diabetes (USA) Online - full text edition. (DBTS) 3857
Diabetes Forecast (USA) Online - full text edition. (DBTF) 3858
Diabetes Spectrum (USA) Online - full text edition. (DSPC) 3859
Diagnostic Imaging (USA) Online - full text edition. (DIMG) 4143
Drug Detection Report (USA) Online - full text edition. (DRDR) 3368
Drug News & Perspectives (ESP) Online - full text edition. (DNP) 4289
Drug Topics (USA) Online - full text edition. (DRG) 4290
The Eastern Pharmacist (IND) Online - full text edition. (EASPH) 4291
Ecology (USA) Online - full text edition. (GECO) 3437
The Elementary School Journal (USA) Online - full text edition. (IESJ) 3411
Environmental Nutrition (USA) Online - full text edition. (ENUT) 4232
Ergonomics (GBR) Online - full text edition. (FERG) 3432
Ernaehrungsdienst (DEU) Online - full text edition. (ERDNST) 3159
European Journal of Clinical Nutrition (GBR) Online - full text edition. (IECN) 4232
Exceptional Children (USA) Online - full text edition. (EXKD) 3422
Exceptional Parent (USA) Online - full text edition. (EXPT) 3422
Executive Health's Good Health Report (USA) Online - full text edition. (EXHR) 4352
F D A Consumer (USA) Online - full text edition. (FDAC) 3392
Family Planning Perspectives (USA) Online - full text edition. (GFPP) 3949
Family Practice News (USA) Online - full text edition. (FMLY) 3602
Flying Safety (USA) Online - full text edition. (FFLY) 3153
Food & Drug Packaging (USA) Online - full text edition. (FDPK) 4271
Frontiers of Health Services Management (USA) Online - full text edition. (FHS) 3507
Gene Therapy Weekly (USA) Online - full text edition. (GENT) 3606
Genetic Engineering News (USA) Online - full text edition. (GENS) 3304
Genetics (USA) Online - full text edition. (IGNT) 3305
Geriatrics (USA) Online - full text edition. (GRIA) 3472
The Gerontologist (USA) Online - full text edition. (GGGT) 3473
Gifted Child Quarterly (USA) Online - full text edition. (IGCQ) 3422
Global Cosmetic Industry (USA) Online - full text edition. (DRGCI) 3176
Harvard Health Letter (USA) Online - full text edition. (HRHL) 4354
Harvard Heart Letter (USA) Online - full text edition. (HHRL) 3772
Harvard Women's Health Watch (USA) Online - full text edition. (HWHW) 4563
Hastings Center Report (USA) Online - full text edition. (HCTR) 3610
Health Affairs (USA) Online - full text edition. (HAF) 4471
Health & Safety at Work (GBR) Online - full text edition. (HSAW) 4255
Health & Social Work (USA) Online - full text edition. (HSW) 4513
Health Care Financing Review (USA) Online - full text edition. (HCFR) 3610
Health Care Management Review (USA) Online - full text edition. (HCMR) 3508
The Health Care Manager (USA) Online - full text edition. (HCS) 3509
Health Care Strategic Management (USA) Online - full text edition. (HLCS) 3509
Health Forum (USA) Online - full text edition. (HOS) 3509
Health Industry Today (USA) Online - full text edition. (HLIN) 3611
Health Letter on the C D C (USA) Online - full text edition. (HCDC) 3611
Health Letter (Washington) (USA) Online - full text edition. (IHLT) 3612
Health Management Technology (USA) Online - full text edition. (HMT) 3810
Health (San Francisco) (USA) Online - full text edition. (HLTH) 4355
Health Services Research (USA) Online - full text edition. (HLSR) 3510
Healthcare Advertising Review (USA) Online - full text edition. (HADR) 3152
Healthcare Executive (USA) Online - full text edition. (HEE) 3510
Healthcare Financial Management (USA) Online - full text edition. (HFM) 3510
Healthcare Marketing Report (USA) Online - full text edition. (HMRP) 4355
HealthFacts (USA) Online - full text edition. (HLFT) 3613
Healthy Weight Journal (CAN) Online - full text edition. (IONH) 4235
Hepatitis Weekly (USA) Online - full text edition. (HEPT) 3797
Hospital Materials Management (USA) Online - full text edition. (HOMG) 3514
Hospital Materiel Management Quarterly (USA) Online - full text edition. (HMM) 3514
Human Biology (Detroit) (USA) Online - full text edition. (PHBI) 3199
Human Development (CHE) Online - full text edition. (IHUD) 3616

Human Ecology (New York) (USA) *Online - full text edition. (PHEC)* **3173**
Human Factors (USA) *Online - full text edition. (HUFA)* **3432**
Human Relations (USA) *Online - full text edition. (HREL)* **4509**
I N F O R M: International News on Fats, Oils & Related Materials (USA) *Online - full text edition. (INFM)* **3373**
Industrial Health & Hazards Update (USA) *Online - full text edition. (INHH)* **4256**
Inquiry (Rochester) (USA) *Online - full text edition. (INQ)* **3620**
Inside M S (USA) *Online - full text edition. (INMS)* **4095**
Intelligence (Kidlington) (GBR) *Online - full text edition. (UINTL)* **4404**
International Journal of Conflict Management (USA) *Online - full text edition. (IJCM)* **3365**
International Journal of Food Sciences and Nutrition (GBR) *Online - full text edition. (IFSN)* **4236**
International Journal of Social Psychiatry (GBR) *Online - full text edition. (ISPY)* **4096**
Issues in Law and Medicine (USA) *Online - full text edition. (ILMD)* **3626**
J M E Online (GBR) *Online - full text edition of* Journal of Medical Ethics. (PJME) **3635**
Journal of Abnormal Child Psychology (USA) *Online - full text edition. (JACP)* **4409**
Journal of Abnormal Psychology (USA) *Online - full text edition. (GABP)* **4409**
Journal of Adolescence (GBR) *Online - full text edition. (IADL)* **3383**
Journal of Aging & Social Policy (USA) *Online - full text edition. (FASP)* **3475**
Journal of Applied Behavior Analysis (USA) *Online - full text edition. (JAB)* **4410**
Journal of Athletic Training (USA) *Online - full text edition. (IATT)* **4174**
Journal of Bacteriology (USA) *Online - full text edition. (IJBC)* **3325**
Journal of Cell Biology (USA) *Online - full text edition. (IJCB)* **3290**
Journal of Child and Family Studies (USA) *Online - full text edition. (FCFS)* **4411**
Journal of Child Psychology & Psychiatry & Allied Disciplines (GBR) *Online - full text edition. (FPPA)* **4411**
Journal of Clinical Child and Adolescent Psychology (USA) *Online - full text edition. (ICCP)* **4411**
Journal of Clinical Psychology (USA) *Online - full text edition. (ICPS)* **4412**
Journal of Cognitive Neuroscience (USA) *Online - full text edition. (JCN)* **4100**
Journal of Communication Inquiry (USA) *Online - full text edition. (ISCI)* **4522**
Journal of Community Health (USA) *Online - full text edition. (JCH)* **3631**
Journal of Comparative Psychology (USA) *Online - full text edition. (PJCP)* **4413**
Journal of Consulting and Clinical Psychology (USA) *Online - full text edition. (GCCP)* **4413**
Journal of Counseling & Development (USA) *Online - full text edition. (GCND)* **4414**
Journal of Counseling Psychology (USA) *Online - full text edition. (GCPS)* **4414**
The Journal of Critical Illness (USA) *Online - full text edition. (JCRT)* **3632**
Journal of Drug Issues (USA) *Online - full text edition. (GJDI)* **3403**
Journal of Ecology (GBR) *Online - full text edition. (PJEC)* **3203**
The Journal of Economic Psychology (NLD) *Online - full text edition. (JEP)* **3366**
Journal of Educational Psychology (USA) *Online - full text edition. (GESY)* **3412**
Journal of Elder Abuse & Neglect (USA) *Online - full text edition. (FELD)* **3476**
Journal of Environmental Health (USA) *Online - full text edition. (JENV)* **3440**
Journal of Experimental Child Psychology (USA) *Online - full text edition. (IECP)* **4415**
Journal of Experimental Psychology: General (USA) *Online - full text edition. (PXPG)* **4415**
Journal of Experimental Psychology: Human Perception and Performance (USA) *Online - full text edition. (PXPH)* **4415**
Journal of Experimental Psychology: Learning, Memory, and Cognition (USA) *Online - full text edition. (PXPL)* **4415**
Journal of Experimental Social Psychology (USA) *Online - full text edition. (IESP)* **4415**
Journal of Family Practice (USA) *Online - full text edition. (JFMP)* **3633**
Journal of Family Psychology (USA) *Online - full text edition. (FJFP)* **4416**
Journal of Family Violence (USA) *Online - full text edition. (IJFV)* **3395**
Journal of General Physiology (USA) *Online - full text edition. (IJGP)* **3344**
The Journal of General Psychology (USA) *Online - full text edition. (JGPS)* **4416**
The Journal of Genetic Psychology (USA) *Online - full text edition. (JGEP)* **3309**
Journal of Gerontological Social Work (USA) *Online - full text edition. (PGSW)* **3476**
Journal of Health and Social Behavior (USA) *Online - full text edition. (PHSB)* **4522**
Journal of Health Care Finance (USA) *Online - full text edition. (JHCF)* **3516**
Journal of Health Economics (NLD) *Online - full text edition. (JHE)* **4479**
Journal of Health Politics, Policy and Law (USA) *Online - full text edition. (JHP)* **3633**
Journal of Healthcare Management (USA) *Online - full text edition. (HHSA)* **3517**
Journal of Homosexuality (USA) *Online - full text edition. (PJHX)* **3528**
Journal of Mammalogy (USA) *Online - full text edition. (PJMA)* **3354**
Journal of Marital and Family Therapy (USA) *Online - full text edition. (JUD)* **4418**
Journal of Memory and Language (USA) *Online - full text edition. (IJML)* **3550**
The Journal of Musculoskeletal Medicine (USA) *Online - full text edition. (JMSC)* **4018**
Journal of Nonverbal Behavior (USA) *Online - full text edition. (PJNB)* **4418**
Journal of Nutrition (USA) *Online - full text edition. (IJNU)* **4237**
Journal of Nutrition Education (CAN) *Online - full text edition. (PJNU)* **4237**
Journal of Occupational and Environmental Medicine (USA) *Online - full text edition. (IOCM)* **3636**
Journal of Occupational and Organizational Psychology (GBR) *Online - full text edition. (JOOP)* **4419**
Journal of Organizational Behavior Management (USA) *Online - full text edition. (JOR)* **4419**
Journal of Organizational Behaviour (GBR) *Online - full text edition. (JBH)* **4419**
Journal of Parapsychology (USA) *Online - full text edition. (PJPA)* **4271**
Journal of Personality (USA) *Online - full text edition. (PJPY)* **4419**
Journal of Personality and Social Psychology (USA) *Online - full text edition. (GPSP)* **4419**
Journal of Psychology: Interdisciplinary & Applied (USA) *Online - full text edition. (JOPS)* **4421**
Journal of Rehabilitation (USA) *Online - full text edition. (JRHB)* **4062**
Journal of Rehabilitation Research and Development (USA) *Online - full text edition. (PJHB)* **4020**
Journal of Safety Research (GBR) *Online - full text edition. (IJSR)* **4258**
Journal of School Health (USA) *Online - full text edition. (JSHL)* **4479**
Journal of Sex Research (USA) *Online - full text edition. (PJSX)* **4422**
The Journal of Social Psychology (USA) *Online - full text edition. (ISPS)* **4423**
Journal of Speech, Language, and Hearing Research (USA) *Online - full text edition. (IJHR)* **3491**
Journal of Sport and Exercise Psychology (USA) *Online - full text edition. (IJSP)* **4423**
Journal of Sport Behavior (USA) *Online - full text edition. (JSB)* **4525**
Journal of Studies on Alcohol (USA) *Online - full text edition. (GSAL)* **3403**
Journal of Substance Abuse Treatment (USA) *Online - full text edition. (IJSA)* **3404**
Journal of the Experimental Analysis of Behavior (USA) *Online - full text edition. (IXAB)* **4423**
Journal of Toxicology. Clinical Toxicology (USA) *Online - full text edition. (JTCT)* **4311**
Journal of Women and Aging (USA) *Online - full text edition. (IJWA)* **4569**
Journal of Youth and Adolescence (USA) *Online - full text edition. (JYAA)* **3384**
Journals of Gerontology. Series A: Biological Sciences & Medical Sciences (USA) *Online - full text edition. (UPGNO)* **3477**
Journals of Gerontology. Series B: Psychological Sciences & Social Sciences (USA) *Online - full text edition. (UPGNT)* **3477**
The Lancet (GBR) *Online - full text edition. (LANT)* **3642**
Learning and Motivation (USA) *Online - full text edition. (ILMM)* **3413**
Let's Live (USA) *Online - full text edition. (ILLV)* **4358**
Life Science Today (GBR) *Online - full text edition. (PMR)* **4313**
Literature and Psychology (USA) *Online - full text edition. (PLNP)* **3552**
Lookout - Nonfoods (USA) *Online - full text edition. (LKNF)* **3176**
M L O (USA) *Online - full text edition. (MLO)* **3879**
Managed Care Week (USA) *Online - full text edition. (MNCR)* **3532**
Marine Biology (DEU) *Online - full text edition. (IMRB)* **3207**
Marketing Health Services (USA) *Online - full text edition. (JHCM)* **3367**
Mayo Clinic Health Letter (USA) *Online - full text edition. (IMCH)* **3647**
Mayo Clinic Proceedings (USA) *Online - full text edition. (MAYO)* **3647**
Med Ad News (USA) *Online - full text edition. (MDAD)* **3367**
Medical Device Approval Letter with G M P - Design Controls Reviews (USA) *Online - full text edition. (MDAL)* **3879**
Medical Economics (USA) *Online - full text edition. (MDEC)* **3650**
Medical Letter on Drugs and Therapeutics (English Edition) (USA) *Online - full text edition. (IDNT)* **4315**
Medical Marketing & Media (USA) *Online - full text edition. (MMMD)* **4315**
Medical Materials Update (USA) *Online - full text edition. (MEMA)* **3652**
Medical Textiles (GBR) *Online - full text edition. (MEDT)* **3654**
Medicine (Baltimore) (USA) *Online - full text edition. (MDCN)* **3656**
Memory and Cognition (USA) *Online - full text edition. (PMCO)* **4426**
Metropolitan Life Insurance Company. Statistical Bulletin S B (USA) *Online - full text edition. (SB)* **3533**
Microbiology and Molecular Biology Reviews (USA) *Online - full text edition. (IMBR)* **3328**
Modern Maturity (USA) *Online - full text edition. (GMOM)* **3478**
Morbidity and Mortality Weekly Report (USA) *Online - full text edition. (MMWR)* **4482**
Mothering (USA) *Online - full text edition. (MOTH)* **4564**
National Academy of Sciences of the United States of America. Proceedings (USA) *Online - full text edition. (IPNA)* **4505**
The Nation's Health (USA) *Online - full text edition. (INAH)* **4483**
Natural Health (USA) *Online - full text edition. (NHLT)* **3168**
Nature (GBR) *Online - full text edition. (GNAA)* **4506**
Nature Biotechnology (USA) *Online - full text edition. (NABIO)* **3276**
New Choices (USA) *Online - full text edition. (GFIF)* **3478**
New England Journal of Medicine (USA) *Online - full text edition. (GNEM)* **3666**
New Zealand Pharmacy (NZL) *Online - full text edition. (ABXNZP)* **4319**
Nursing Homes (USA) *Online - full text edition. (NHOM)* **3933**
Nursing Management (USA) *Online - full text edition. (NSM)* **3933**
Nursing (Year) (USA) *Online - full text edition. (INUR)* **3935**
Nutraceuticals International (GBR) *Online - full text edition. (NUTR)* **4320**
Nutrition Action Healthletter (USA) *Online - full text edition. (NUAH)* **4241**
Nutrition Forum (USA) *Online - full text edition. (NUFM)* **4242**
Nutrition Research Newsletter (USA) *Online - full text edition. (NRNL)* **4243**
Nutrition Reviews (USA) *Online - full text edition. (INUT)* **4243**
Nutrition Today (USA) *Online - full text edition. (NTDY)* **4243**
O H Online (USA) *Online - full text edition of* Occupational Hazards. (OHZ) **4261**
O H S Canada (CAN) *Online - full text edition. (OHC)* **4260**
Occupational Health & Safety (USA) *Online - full text edition. (OHS)* **4261**
Omega: Journal of Death and Dying (USA) *Online - full text edition. (IOMG)* **4431**
Ophthalmology Times (USA) *Online - full text edition. (OPTH)* **4004**
Organizational Behavior and Human Decision Processes (USA) *Online - full text edition. (OBP)* **3366**
Ostomy Quarterly (USA) *Online - full text edition. (OSTQ)* **3671**
Palaestra (USA) *Online - full text edition. (PLST)* **3425**
Paraplegia News (USA) *Online - full text edition. (PLNS)* **3494**
Patient Care (USA) *Online - full text edition. (PATC)* **3673**
Pediatrics (English Edition) (USA) *Online - full text edition. (PDTR)* **4054**
Pediatrics for Parents (USA) *Online - full text edition. (PDFP)* **4054**
People's Medical Society Newsletter (USA) *Online - full text edition. (IMSN)* **3393**
Perceptual and Motor Skills (USA) *Online - full text edition. (IPMS)* **4432**
Personnel Psychology (USA) *Online - full text edition. (PPS)* **4433**
Perspectives in Biology and Medicine (USA) *Online - full text edition. (IPBM)* **3674**
Pharma Marketletter (GBR) *Online - full text edition. (MKLT)* **4322**
Pharmaceutical Executive (USA) *Online - full text edition. (PREX)* **4323**
Pharmacy Practice Management Quarterly (USA) *Online - full text edition. (PPMQ)* **4328**
Pharmacy Trade (AUS) *Online - full text edition. (ABXPHA)* **4329**
Physical Therapy (USA) *Online - full text edition. (PTRP)* **4064**
Physiological Reviews Online (USA) *Online - full text edition of* Physiological Reviews. (BODY) **3347**
Politics and the Life Sciences (USA) *Online - full text edition. (FPLS)* **4368**
Population and Environment (USA) *Online - full text edition. (IPNE)* **4433**
Product Alert (USA) *Online - full text edition. (PDAL)* **3462**
Professional Psychology: Research and Practice (USA) *Online - full text edition. (FPRP)* **4434**
Professional Safety (USA) *Online - full text edition. (PFS)* **4263**
Psychiatry (USA) *Online - full text edition. (PPSY)* **4126**
Psychological Assessment (USA) *Online - full text edition. (FPAS)* **4437**
Psychological Bulletin (USA) *Online - full text edition. (GPSB)* **4437**
The Psychological Record (USA) *Online - full text edition. (PYRE)* **4438**
Psychological Review (USA) *Online - full text edition. (UGPSR)* **4438**
Psychological Science (USA) *Online - full text edition. (IPYS)* **4438**
Psychology and Aging (USA) *Online - full text edition. (FPAG)* **3479**
Psychology & Marketing (USA) *Online - full text edition. (PSY)* **4440**
Psychology of Women Quarterly (GBR) *Online - full text edition. (PPWQ)* **4441**
Psychology Today (USA) *Online - full text edition. (PSYT)* **4441**
Psychopharmacology Update (USA) *Online - full text edition. (PPOU)* **4332**
Public Health Reports (USA) *Online - full text edition. (PHLR)* **4486**
Quarterly Review of Biology (USA) *Online - full text edition. (PQRB)* **3214**
R N Web (USA) *Online - full text edition of* R N. (RNJ) **3938**
Real Living with Multiple Sclerosis (USA) *Online - full text edition. (RLMS)* **4129**
Research Quarterly for Exercise and Sport (USA) *Online - full text edition. (RQES)* **4360**
Review of Optometry (USA) *Online - full text edition. (REVO)* **4006**
S I E C U S Report (USA) *Online - full text edition. (ISIE)* **4523**
Safety and Health (USA) *Online - full text edition. (ISNH)* **4264**
Saturday Evening Post (USA) *Online - full text edition. (SEVP)* **3465**
Self (USA) *Online - full text edition. (GSEL)* **4568**
Sex Roles (USA) *Online - full text edition. (ISXR)* **4448**
Sexually Transmitted Diseases (USA) *Online - full text edition. (ISXT)* **3853**
Shape (USA) *Online - full text edition. (ISHP)* **4565**
Social Biology (USA) *Online - full text edition. (PSOB)* **3314**
Social Cognition (USA) *Online - full text edition. (ISOC)* **4449**
Social Psychology Quarterly (USA) *Online - full text edition. (PSOP)* **4523**

Social Science & Medicine (GBR) *Online - full text edition. (ISMD)* **3694**
Social Work with Groups (USA) *Online - full text edition. (FSWG)* **4518**
Studies in Family Planning (USA) *Online - full text edition. (ISFP)* **4369**
Suicide and Life-Threatening Behavior (USA) *Online - full text edition. (PSUI)* **4451**
Total Health (USA) *Online - full text edition. (THLT)* **4246**
Trends in Neurosciences (GBR) *Online - full text edition. (ITNS)* **4137**
Trustee (USA) *Online - full text edition. (TST)* **3523**
Urology Times (USA) *Online - full text edition. (UROL)* **4220**
Vaccine Weekly (USA) *Online - full text edition. (VACW)* **4339**
Vegetarian Times (USA) *Online - full text edition. (VEGT)* **4247**
Vibrant Life (USA) *Online - full text edition. (VBRL)* **4362**
W H O Drug Information (CHE) *Online - full text edition. (WHDG)* **4492**
Warning Letter Bulletin (USA) *Online - full text edition. (WWAB)* **3707**
Women & Health (USA) *Online - full text edition. (PWNH)* **4566**
Women & Therapy (USA) *Online - full text edition. (IWNT)* **4455**
Women's Health Weekly (USA) *Online - full text edition. (WHWK)* **4567**
Worklife Report (CAN) *Online - full text edition. (WOL)* **3364**
World Health Organization. Bulletin (CHE) *Online - full text edition. (BWHO)* **3709**

G B I Freischutzstrasse 96e, Munich 81927, Germany TEL 89-9570064, FAX 89-954229, http://www.gbi.de
Seibt Medizinische Technik (DEU) *Online - full text edition.* **3691**

Gale Group Box 9187, Farmington Hills, MI 48333-9187 TEL 248-699-8072, 800-877-4253, FAX 248-699-8035 , galeord@galegroup.com, http://www.galegroup.com
A J P Online (USA) *Online - full text edition of* American Journal of Physiology (Consolidated). **3337**
A O R N Journal (USA) *Online - full text edition.* **3912**
A R D Online (GBR) *Online - full text edition of* Annals of the Rheumatic Diseases. **4167**
A S H A Leader (USA) *Online - full text edition.* **3488**
Addictive Behaviors (GBR) *Online - full text edition.* **3397**
Adolescence (San Diego) (USA) *Online - full text edition.* **3380**
Advances in Nursing Science (USA) *Online - full text edition.* **3912**
Advances in Skin and Wound Care (USA) *Online - full text edition.* **3844**
Age and Ageing (GBR) *Online - full text edition.* **3466**
Ageing and Society (GBR) *Online - full text edition.* **3466**
Aggressive Behavior (USA) *Online - full text edition.* **4373**
AIDS Alert (USA) *Online - full text edition.* **3791**
AIDS & Public Policy Journal (USA) *Online - full text edition.* **3791**
AIDS Patient Care and S T Ds (USA) *Online - full text edition.* **3791**
AIDS Weekly Plus (USA) *Online - full text edition.* **3792**
Alcohol Research & Health (USA) *Online - full text edition.* **3398**
Alcoholism & Drug Abuse Weekly (USA) *Online - full text edition.* **3398**
American Academy of Child and Adolescent Psychiatry. Journal (USA) *Online - full text edition.* **4071**
American Academy of Physician Assistants. Journal (USA) *Online - full text edition.* **3562**
American Annals of the Deaf (USA) *Online - full text edition.* **3488**
American Behavioral Scientist (USA) *Online - full text edition.* **4508**
American Dental Association. Journal (USA) *Online - full text edition.* **3814**
American Dietetic Association. Journal (USA) *Online - full text edition.* **4228**
American Druggist (USA) *Online - full text edition.* **4275**
American Family Physician (USA) *Online - full text edition.* **3563**
American Fitness (USA) *Online - full text edition.* **4350**
American Geriatrics Society. Journal (USA) *Online - full text edition.* **3467**
American Heart Journal (USA) *Online - full text edition.* **3762**
American Imago (USA) *Online - full text edition.* **4071**
American Journal of Clinical Nutrition (USA) *Online - full text edition.* **4228**
American Journal of Community Psychology (USA) *Online - full text edition.* **4520**
American Journal of Drug and Alcohol Abuse (USA) *Online - full text edition.* **3399**
American Journal of Epidemiology (USA) *Online - full text edition.* **3563**
American Journal of Family Therapy (USA) *Online - full text edition.* **4374**
American Journal of Human Biology (USA) *Online - full text edition.* **3180**
American Journal of Human Genetics (USA) *Online - full text edition.* **3297**
American Journal of Law & Medicine (USA) *Online - full text edition.* **3536**
The American Journal of Medicine (USA) *Online - full text edition.* **3564**
American Journal of Nursing (USA) *Online - full text edition.* **3913**
American Journal of Obstetrics and Gynecology (USA) *Online - full text edition.* **3944**
American Journal of Ophthalmology (USA) *Online - full text edition.* **3993**
American Journal of Orthopsychiatry (USA) *Online - full text edition.* **4374**
American Journal of Psychiatry (USA) *Online - full text edition.* **4071**
American Journal of Psychoanalysis (USA) *Online - full text edition.* **4374**
American Journal of Psychology (USA) *Online - full text edition.* **4374**
American Journal of Psychotherapy (USA) *Online - full text edition.* **4072**
American Journal of Public Health (USA) *Online - full text edition.* **4461**
American Journal of Sports Medicine (USA) *Online - full text edition.* **4172**
American Journal of Surgery (USA) *Online - full text edition.* **4180**
American Medical News (USA) *Online - full text edition.* **3565**
The American Naturalist (USA) *Online - full text edition.* **3180**
American Psychologist (USA) *Online - full text edition.* **4375**
American Rehabilitation (USA) *Online - full text edition.* **3419**
Animal Behaviour (GBR) *Online - full text edition.* **3350**
Animal Learning & Behavior (USA) *Online - full text edition.* **4376**
Animal Pharm (GBR) *Online - full text edition.* **4537**
Annals of Health Law (USA) *Online - full text edition.* **3536**
Annals of Internal Medicine (USA) *Online - full text edition.* **3907**
Annual Review of Biochemistry (USA) *Online - full text edition.* **3240**
Annual Review of Genetics (USA) *Online - full text edition.* **3298**
Annual Review of Microbiology (USA) *Online - full text edition.* **3317**
Annual Review of Physiology (USA) *Online - full text edition.* **3339**
Annual Review of Psychology (USA) *Online - full text edition.* **4376**
Annual Review of Sex Research (USA) *Online - full text edition.* **4376**
Antiviral Weekly (USA) *Online - full text edition.* **3740**
Applied and Environmental Microbiology (USA) *Online - full text edition.* **3318**
Applied Ergonomics (GBR) *Online - full text edition.* **3431**
Applied Genetics News (USA) *Online - full text edition.* **3299**
Arbor Age (USA) *Online - full text edition.* **3463**
Archives of Dermatology (USA) *Online - full text edition.* **3845**
Archives of Environmental Health (USA) *Online - full text edition.* **3435**
Archives of Family Medicine (USA) *Online - full text edition.* **3568**
Archives of General Psychiatry (USA) *Online - full text edition.* **4074**
Archives of Internal Medicine (USA) *Online - full text edition.* **3907**
Archives of Neurology (USA) *Online - full text edition.* **4074**
Archives of Ophthalmology (USA) *Online - full text edition.* **3994**
Archives of Otolaryngology - Head & Neck Surgery (USA) *Online - full text edition.* **4030**
Archives of Pediatrics & Adolescent Medicine (USA) *Online - full text edition.* **4041**
Archives of Sexual Behavior (USA) *Online - full text edition.* **3568**
Archives of Surgery (USA) *Online - full text edition.* **4182**
Arthritis Today (USA) *Online - full text edition.* **4167**
Asbestos & Lead Abatement Report (USA) *Online - full text edition.* **3443**
Association of Nurses in AIDS Care. Journal (USA) *Online - full text edition.* **3793**
Australian and New Zealand Journal of Public Health (AUS) *Online - full text edition.* **4462**
Australian Journal of Forensic Sciences (AUS) *Online - full text edition.* **3881**
The B B I Newsletter (USA) *Online - full text edition.* **3573**
The Back Letter (USA) *Online - full text edition.* **4011**
Behavior Therapy (USA) *Online - full text edition.* **4380**
Behavioral and Brain Sciences (GBR) *Online - full text edition.* **4380**
Behavioral Health Management (USA) *Online - full text edition.* **3399**
Behavioral Medicine (USA) *Online - full text edition.* **4381**
Behavioral Neuroscience (USA) *Online - full text edition.* **4381**
Behavioral Sciences and the Law (GBR) *Online - full text edition.* **4381**
Behaviour Research and Therapy (GBR) *Online - full text edition.* **4382**
Better Nutrition (USA) *Online - full text edition.* **4230**
Biochemistry (USA) *Online - full text edition.* **3243**
BioEssays (GBR) *Online - full text edition.* **3184**
Bioethics (GBR) *Online - full text edition.* **4346**
Biological Bulletin (USA) *Online - full text edition.* **3185**
Biological Reviews (GBR) *Online - full text edition.* **3185**
Biomedical Market Newsletter (USA) *Online - full text edition.* **3366**
Biomedical Materials (GBR) *Online - full text edition.* **3576**
BioPharm (USA) *Online - full text edition.* **4280**
BioScience (USA) *Online - full text edition.* **3187**
Biotech Business (USA) *Online - full text edition.* **3270**
BioVenture View (USA) *Online - full text edition.* **3272**
Birder's World (USA) *Online - full text edition.* **3336**
Blood Weekly (USA) *Online - full text edition.* **3899**
bmj.com(GBR) *Online - full text.* **3577**
Body Bulletin Newsletter (USA) *Online - full text edition.* **4252**
The British Journal of Criminology (GBR) *Online - full text edition.* **3393**
British Journal of Psychology (GBR) *Online - full text edition.* **4384**
Brown University Child and Adolescent Behavior Letter (USA) *Online - full text edition.* **3381**
Brown University Digest of Addiction Theory & Application (USA) *Online - full text edition.* **3399**
C A - A Cancer Journal for Clinicians (USA) *Online - full text edition.* **3969**
C T D News (USA) *Online - full text edition.* **4252**
Canadian Journal of Experimental Psychology (CAN) *Online - full text edition.* **4386**
Canadian Journal of Human Sexuality (CAN) *Online - full text edition.* **4386**
Canadian Mining Journal (CAN) *Online - full text edition.* **4225**
Cancer (USA) *Online - full text edition.* **3969**
Cancer Weekly Plus (USA) *Online - full text edition.* **3973**
Cell (USA) *Online - full text edition.* **3286**
Chain Drug Review (USA) *Online - full text edition.* **3364**
Chemische Rundschau (CHE) *Online - full text edition.* **3372**
Chemist & Druggist (GBR) *Online - full text edition.* **4283**
Chest (USA) *Online - full text edition.* **4159**
Child Abuse & Neglect (GBR) *Online - full text edition.* **3381**
Child and Adolescent Social Work Journal (USA) *Online - full text edition.* **4520**
Child Development (USA) *Online - full text edition.* **3381**
Child Health Alert (USA) *Online - full text edition.* **4042**
Child Study Journal (USA) *Online - full text edition.* **3409**
Children and Youth Services Review (GBR) *Online - full text edition.* **3382**
Clinica (GBR) *Online - full text edition.* **3585**
Clinical Cardiology Alert (USA) *Online - full text edition.* **3768**
Clinical Diabetes (USA) *Online - full text edition.* **3856**
Clinical Nursing Research (USA) *Online - full text edition.* **3916**
Clinical Oncology Alert (USA) *Online - full text edition.* **3975**
Clinical Pediatrics (USA) *Online - full text edition.* **4042**
Clinician Reviews (USA) *Online - full text edition.* **3587**
Club Industry (USA) *Online - full text edition.* **4351**
Cognitive Psychology (USA) *Online - full text edition.* **4389**
Cognitive Science (GBR) *Online - full text edition.* **4389**
Community and Worker Right-to-Know News (USA) *Online - full text edition.* **4253**
Community Mental Health Journal (USA) *Online - full text edition.* **4512**
Community Pharmacy (GBR) *Online - full text edition.* **4284**
Comparative Political Studies (USA) *Online - full text edition.* **4367**
Computers in Human Behavior (GBR) *Online - full text edition.* **4524**
Conservation Biology (USA) *Online - full text edition.* **3392**
Consultant (Greenwich) (USA) *Online - full text edition.* **3589**
Consumer Reports on Health (USA) *Online - full text edition.* **4351**
Contemporary Drug Problems (USA) *Online - full text edition.* **3400**
Contemporary Longterm Care (USA) *Online - full text edition.* **3505**
Contemporary Ob-Gyn (USA) *Online - full text edition.* **3948**
Contemporary Pediatrics (USA) *Online - full text edition.* **4043**
Contraceptive Technology Update (USA) *Online - full text edition.* **3358**
The Counseling Psychologist (USA) *Online - full text edition.* **4392**
Criminal Justice & Behavior (USA) *Online - full text edition.* **3394**
Critical Care Nursing Quarterly (USA) *Online - full text edition.* **3918**
Cross-Cultural Research (USA) *Online - full text edition.* **4508**
Current Health 2 (USA) *Online - full text edition.* **3428**
Current Psychology (New Brunswick) (USA) *Online - full text edition.* **4393**
Death Studies (USA) *Online - full text edition.* **4394**
Dermatology Nursing (USA) *Online - full text edition.* **3848**
Dermatology Times (USA) *Online - full text edition.* **3848**
Developmental Biology (USA) *Online - full text edition.* **3193**
Developmental Psychology (USA) *Online - full text edition.* **4394**
Diabetes (USA) *Online - full text edition.* **3857**
Diabetes Care (USA) *Online - full text edition.* **3857**
Diabetes Forecast (USA) *Online - full text edition.* **3858**
Diabetes Spectrum (USA) *Online - full text edition.* **3859**
Discourse & Society (GBR) *Online - full text edition.* **4395**
Disease Weekly Plus (USA) *Online - full text edition.* **3795**
Drug Detection Report (USA) *Online - full text edition.* **3368**
Drug News & Perspectives (ESP) *Online - full text edition.* **4289**
Drug Topics (USA) *Online - full text edition.* **4290**
Drug Utilization Review (USA) *Online - full text edition.* **4290**
Ear, Nose & Throat Journal (USA) *Online - full text edition.* **4032**

Ecological Applications (USA) *Online - full text edition.* **3437**
Ecological Monographs (USA) *Online - full text edition.* **3437**
Ecology (USA) *Online - full text edition.* **3437**
Educational and Psychological Measurement (USA) *Online - full text edition.* **4396**
The Elementary School Journal (USA) *Online - full text edition.* **3411**
Emerging Infectious Diseases (Online Edition)(USA) *Online - full text.* **4467**
Environment and Behavior (USA) *Online - full text edition.* **4521**
Environmental Nutrition (USA) *Online - full text edition.* **4232**
Ergonomics (GBR) *Online - full text edition.* **3432**
European Journal of Clinical Nutrition (GBR) *Online - full text edition.* **4232**
Evolution (USA) *Online - full text edition.* **3302**
Exceptional Children (USA) *Online - full text edition.* **3422**
Exceptional Parent (USA) *Online - full text edition.* **3422**
Executive Health's Good Health Report (USA) *Online - full text edition.* **4352**
F D A Consumer (USA) *Online - full text edition.* **3392**
F D A Enforcement Report (USA) *Online - full text edition.* **3394**
F D A Medical Bulletin (USA) *Online - full text edition.* **4294**
Families, Systems & Health (USA) *Online - full text edition.* **3601**
Family and Community Health (USA) *Online - full text edition.* **4469**
Family Planning Perspectives (USA) *Online - full text edition.* **3949**
Family Practice News (USA) *Online - full text edition.* **3602**
Family Process (USA) *Online - full text edition.* **4399**
Fire Chief (USA) *Online - full text edition.* **3458**
Food and Drug Law Journal (USA) *Online - full text edition.* **3539**
Food & Drug Packaging (USA) *Online - full text edition.* **4271**
Food, Drug, Cosmetic, and Medical Device Law Digest (USA) *Online - full text edition.* **3539**
Food Nutrition and Agriculture (ITA) *Online - full text edition.* **4233**
Forensic Science International (IRL) *Online - full text edition.* **3882**
Gene Therapy Weekly (USA) *Online - full text edition.* **3606**
Generations (San Francisco) (USA) *Online - full text edition.* **3471**
Genes & Development (USA) *Online - full text edition.* **3303**
Genesis Report - Dx (USA) *Online - full text edition.* **3606**
Genesis Report - Rx (USA) *Online - full text edition.* **4298**
Genetic Engineering News (USA) *Online - full text edition.* **3304**
Genetic, Social, and General Psychology Monographs (USA) *Online - full text edition.* **4400**
Genetics (USA) *Online - full text edition.* **3305**
Geriatrics (USA) *Online - full text edition.* **3472**
The Gerontologist (USA) *Online - full text edition.* **3473**
Gifted Child Quarterly (USA) *Online - full text edition.* **3422**
Global Cosmetic Industry (USA) *Online - full text edition.* **3176**
Group & Organization Management (USA) *Online - full text edition.* **3411**
Harvard Health Letter (USA) *Online - full text edition.* **4354**
Harvard Heart Letter (USA) *Online - full text edition.* **3772**
The Harvard Mental Health Letter (USA) *Online - full text edition.* **4093**
Harvard Women's Health Watch (USA) *Online - full text edition.* **4563**
Hastings Center Report (USA) *Online - full text edition.* **3610**
Health & Safety at Work (GBR) *Online - full text edition.* **4255**
Health & Social Work (USA) *Online - full text edition.* **4513**
Health Care Financing Review (USA) *Online - full text edition.* **3610**
Health Care Management Review (USA) *Online - full text edition.* **3508**
Health Care Strategic Management (USA) *Online - full text edition.* **3509**
Health Data Management (New York) (USA) *Online - full text edition.* **3509**
Health Education Journal (GBR) *Online - full text edition.* **4473**
Health Forum (USA) *Online - full text edition.* **3509**
Health Industry Today (USA) *Online - full text edition.* **3611**
Health Law in Canada (CAN) *Online - full text edition.* **3882**
Health Law Journal (CAN) *Online - full text edition.* **3539**
Health Law Review (CAN) *Online - full text edition.* **3539**
Health Letter on the C D C (USA) *Online - full text edition.* **3611**
Health Management Technology (USA) *Online - full text edition.* **3810**
Health Marketing Quarterly (USA) *Online - full text edition.* **4473**
Health Matrix: Journal of Law-Medicine (USA) *Online - full text edition.* **3540**
Health Products Business (USA) *Online - full text edition.* **3461**
Health Psychology (USA) *Online - full text edition.* **4402**
Health (San Francisco) (USA) *Online - full text edition.* **4355**
Health Services Research (USA) *Online - full text edition.* **3510**
Healthcare Advertising Review (USA) *Online - full text edition.* **3152**
Healthcare Financial Management (USA) *Online - full text edition.* **3510**
Healthcare Marketing Report (USA) *Online - full text edition.* **4355**
Healthcare Purchasing News (USA) *Online - full text edition.* **3511**
HealthFacts (USA) *Online - full text edition.* **3613**
HealthInform (USA) *Online - full text edition.* **3166**
Healthline (USA) *Online - full text edition.* **4475**
Hearing Journal (USA) *Online - full text edition.* **3491**
Hepatitis Weekly (USA) *Online - full text edition.* **3797**
Heredity (GBR) *Online - full text edition.* **3307**
Hispanic Journal of Behavioral Sciences (USA) *Online - full text edition.* **4402**
Holistic Nursing Practice (USA) *Online - full text edition.* **3920**
Hospital Law's Regan Report (USA) *Online - full text edition.* **3513**
Hospital Materials Management (USA) *Online - full text edition.* **3514**
Hospital Materiel Management Quarterly (USA) *Online - full text edition.* **3514**
Hospital Practice (USA) *Online - full text edition.* **3616**
Hospital Topics (USA) *Online - full text edition.* **3514**
Human Biology (Detroit) (USA) *Online - full text edition.* **3199**
Human Communication Research (USA) *Online - full text edition.* **4402**
Human Development (CHE) *Online - full text edition.* **3616**
Human Ecology (New York) (USA) *Online - full text edition.* **3173**
Human Factors (USA) *Online - full text edition.* **3432**
Human Relations (USA) *Online - full text edition.* **4509**
I D E A Health & Fitness Source (USA) *Online - full text edition.* **4356**
I E E E Transactions on Biomedical Engineering (USA) *Online - full text edition.* **3237**
I E E E Transactions on Medical Imaging (USA) *Online - full text edition.* **4145**
I N F O R M: International News on Fats, Oils & Related Materials (USA) *Online - full text edition.* **3373**
Industrial Health & Hazards Update (USA) *Online - full text edition.* **4256**
Infectious Disease Alert (USA) *Online - full text edition.* **3798**
Inquiry (Rochester) (USA) *Online - full text edition.* **3620**
Inside M S (USA) *Online - full text edition.* **4095**
Intelligence (Kidlington) (GBR) *Online - full text edition.* **4404**
Internal Medicine (USA) *Online - full text edition.* **3908**
Internal Medicine Alert (USA) *Online - full text edition.* **3909**
The International Journal of Action Methods (USA) *Online - full text edition.* **4405**
International Journal of Aging & Human Development (USA) *Online - full text edition.* **3474**
International Journal of Eating Disorders (USA) *Online - full text edition.* **4236**
International Journal of Food Sciences and Nutrition (GBR) *Online - full text edition.* **4236**
International Journal of Law and Psychiatry (GBR) *Online - full text edition.* **3540**
International Journal of Mental Health (USA) *Online - full text edition.* **4406**
International Journal of Offender Therapy and Comparative Criminology (USA) *Online - full text edition.* **3394**
International Journal of Social Psychiatry (GBR) *Online - full text edition.* **4096**
International Journal of Sport Nutrition & Exercise Metabolism (USA) *Online - full text edition.* **4236**
Issues in Law and Medicine (USA) *Online - full text edition.* **3626**
J A M A: The Journal of the American Medical Association (USA) *Online - full text edition.* **3626**
J M E Online (GBR) *Online - full text edition of Journal of Medical Ethics.* **3635**
Journal of Abnormal Child Psychology (USA) *Online - full text edition.* **4409**
Journal of Abnormal Psychology (USA) *Online - full text edition.* **4409**
Journal of Adolescence (GBR) *Online - full text edition.* **3383**
Journal of Aging & Social Policy (USA) *Online - full text edition.* **3475**
Journal of Aging Studies (GBR) *Online - full text edition.* **3475**
Journal of American College Health (USA) *Online - full text edition.* **4357**
Journal of Applied Behavior Analysis (USA) *Online - full text edition.* **4410**
Journal of Applied Behavioral Science (USA) *Online - full text edition.* **4410**
Journal of Applied Gerontology (USA) *Online - full text edition.* **3475**
Journal of Applied Psychology (USA) *Online - full text edition.* **4410**
Journal of Applied Social Psychology (USA) *Online - full text edition.* **4410**
Journal of Athletic Training (USA) *Online - full text edition.* **4174**
Journal of Bacteriology (USA) *Online - full text edition.* **3325**
Journal of Biomechanical Engineering (USA) *Online - full text edition.* **3629**
Journal of Black Psychology (USA) *Online - full text edition.* **4410**
Journal of Black Studies (USA) *Online - full text edition.* **4509**
Journal of Cardiovascular Nursing (USA) *Online - full text edition.* **3777**
Journal of Child and Adolescent Psychiatric Nursing (USA) *Online - full text edition.* **3923**
Journal of Child and Family Studies (USA) *Online - full text edition.* **4411**
Journal of Child Psychology & Psychiatry & Allied Disciplines (GBR) *Online - full text edition.* **4411**
Journal of Clinical Child and Adolescent Psychology (USA) *Online - full text edition.* **4411**
Journal of Clinical Psychology (USA) *Online - full text edition.* **4412**
Journal of Cognitive Neuroscience (USA) *Online - full text edition.* **4100**
Journal of Communication Inquiry (USA) *Online - full text edition.* **4522**
Journal of Community Health (USA) *Online - full text edition.* **3631**
Journal of Comparative Psychology (USA) *Online - full text edition.* **4413**
Journal of Consulting and Clinical Psychology (USA) *Online - full text edition.* **4413**
Journal of Contemporary Health Law and Policy (USA) *Online - full text edition.* **3632**
Journal of Counseling Psychology (USA) *Online - full text edition.* **4414**
The Journal of Critical Illness (USA) *Online - full text edition.* **3632**
Journal of Cross-Cultural Psychology (USA) *Online - full text edition.* **4414**
Journal of Dental Hygiene (USA) *Online - full text edition.* **3828**
Journal of Drug Issues (USA) *Online - full text edition.* **3403**
Journal of Ecology (GBR) *Online - full text edition.* **3203**
The Journal of Economic Psychology (NLD) *Online - full text edition.* **3366**
Journal of Educational Psychology (USA) *Online - full text edition.* **3412**
Journal of Elder Abuse & Neglect (USA) *Online - full text edition.* **3476**
Journal of Environmental Health (USA) *Online - full text edition.* **3440**
Journal of Ethnicity in Substance Abuse (USA) *Online - full text edition.* **3403**
Journal of Experimental Biology (GBR) *Online - full text edition.* **3203**
Journal of Experimental Child Psychology (USA) *Online - full text edition.* **4415**
Journal of Experimental Psychology: Animal Behavior Processes (USA) *Online - full text edition.* **4415**
Journal of Experimental Psychology: General (USA) *Online - full text edition.* **4415**
Journal of Experimental Psychology: Human Perception and Performance (USA) *Online - full text edition.* **4415**
Journal of Experimental Psychology: Learning, Memory, and Cognition (USA) *Online - full text edition.* **4415**
Journal of Experimental Social Psychology (USA) *Online - full text edition.* **4415**
Journal of Family Practice (USA) *Online - full text edition.* **3633**
Journal of Family Psychology (USA) *Online - full text edition.* **4416**
Journal of Family Violence (USA) *Online - full text edition.* **3395**
Journal of Gay & Lesbian Psychotherapy (USA) *Online - full text edition.* **4416**
Journal of General Physiology (USA) *Online - full text edition.* **3344**
The Journal of General Psychology (USA) *Online - full text edition.* **4416**
The Journal of Genetic Psychology (USA) *Online - full text edition.* **3309**
Journal of Gerontological Social Work (USA) *Online - full text edition.* **3476**
Journal of Health and Social Behavior (USA) *Online - full text edition.* **4522**
Journal of Health Care Finance (USA) *Online - full text edition.* **3516**
Journal of Health Economics (NLD) *Online - full text edition.* **4479**
Journal of Health Politics, Policy and Law (USA) *Online - full text edition.* **3633**
Journal of Healthcare Management (USA) *Online - full text edition.* **3517**
Journal of Homosexuality (USA) *Online - full text edition.* **3528**
Journal of Humanistic Psychology (USA) *Online - full text edition.* **4417**
Journal of Interpersonal Violence (USA) *Online - full text edition.* **3395**
Journal of Law and Health (USA) *Online - full text edition.* **3540**
The Journal of Law, Medicine & Ethics (USA) *Online - full text edition.* **3540**
Journal of Learning Disabilities (USA) *Online - full text edition.* **3424**
The Journal of Legal Medicine (USA) *Online - full text edition.* **3634**
Journal of Mammalogy (USA) *Online - full text edition.* **3354**
Journal of Managerial Psychology (GBR) *Online - full text edition.* **3365**
Journal of Marital and Family Therapy (USA) *Online - full text edition.* **4418**
The Journal of Medicine and Philosophy (NLD) *Online - full text edition.* **3636**
Journal of Motor Behavior (USA) *Online - full text edition.* **4418**
The Journal of Musculoskeletal Medicine (USA) *Online - full text edition.* **4018**
Journal of Neuroscience Nursing (USA) *Online - full text edition.* **3925**
Journal of Nonverbal Behavior (USA) *Online - full text edition.* **4418**
Journal of Nursing Care Quality (USA) *Online - full text edition.* **3925**
Journal of Nursing Scholarship (USA) *Online - full text edition.* **3926**
Journal of Nutrition (USA) *Online - full text edition.* **4237**
Journal of Nutrition Education (CAN) *Online - full text edition.* **4237**
Journal of Occupational and Environmental Medicine (USA) *Online - full text edition.* **3636**
Journal of Occupational and Organizational Psychology (GBR) *Online - full text edition.* **4419**
Journal of Offender Rehabilitation (USA) *Online - full text edition.* **3395**
Journal of Organizational Behavior Management (USA) *Online - full text edition.* **4419**
Journal of Organizational Behaviour (GBR) *Online - full text edition.* **4419**

Journal of Parapsychology (USA) *Online - full text edition.* **4271**
Journal of Perinatal and Neonatal Nursing (USA) *Online - full text edition.* **3926**
Journal of Personality (USA) *Online - full text edition.* **4419**
Journal of Personality and Social Psychology (USA) *Online - full text edition.* **4419**
Journal of Pharmaceutical Marketing and Management (USA) *Online - full text edition.* **4309**
Journal of Products and Toxics Liability (GBR) *Online - full text edition.* **3540**
Journal of Psychiatry and Law (USA) *Online - full text edition.* **3541**
Journal of Psychology: Interdisciplinary & Applied (USA) *Online - full text edition.* **4421**
Journal of Rehabilitation (USA) *Online - full text edition.* **4062**
The Journal of Respiratory Diseases (USA) *Online - full text edition.* **4161**
Journal of Safety Research (GBR) *Online - full text edition.* **4258**
Journal of School Health (USA) *Online - full text edition.* **4479**
Journal of Sex Research (USA) *Online - full text edition.* **4422**
Journal of Social Issues (USA) *Online - full content edition.* **4423**
The Journal of Social Psychology (USA) *Online - full text edition.* **4423**
The Journal of Special Education (USA) *Online - full text edition.* **3424**
Journal of Speech, Language, and Hearing Research (USA) *Online - full text edition.* **3491**
Journal of Sport and Exercise Psychology (USA) *Online - full text edition.* **4423**
Journal of Sport Behavior (USA) *Online - full text edition.* **4525**
Journal of Studies on Alcohol (USA) *Online - full text edition.* **3403**
Journal of Substance Abuse Treatment (USA) *Online - full text edition.* **3404**
Journal of Symbolic Logic (USA) *Online - full text edition.* **3553**
Journal of the Experimental Analysis of Behavior (USA) *Online - full text edition.* **4423**
Journal of the History of Sexuality (USA) *Online - full text edition.* **4522**
Journal of Toxicology. Clinical Toxicology (USA) *Online - full text edition.* **4311**
Journal of Trauma Nursing (USA) *Online - full text edition.* **3927**
Journal of Women and Aging (USA) *Online - full text edition.* **4569**
Journal of Youth and Adolescence (USA) *Online - full text edition.* **3384**
Journals of Gerontology. Series A: Biological Sciences & Medical Sciences (USA) *Online - full text edition.* **3477**
Laboratory Equipment (USA) *Online - full text edition.* **3878**
The Lancet (GBR) *Online - full text edition.* **3642**
The Lancet (North American Edition) (USA) *Online - full text edition.* **3643**
Law and Human Behavior (USA) *Online - full text edition.* **3541**
Law and Psychology Review (USA) *Online - full text edition.* **3541**
Learning and Motivation (USA) *Online - full text edition.* **3413**
Let's Live (USA) *Online - full text edition.* **4358**
Life Science Today (GBR) *Online - full text edition.* **4313**
Literature and Psychology (USA) *Online - full text edition.* **3552**
Lookout - Nonfoods (USA) *Online - full text edition.* **3176**
M L O (USA) *Online - full text edition.* **3879**
Managed Care Outlook (USA) *Online - full text edition.* **3532**
Managed Care Week (USA) *Online - full text edition.* **3532**
Marine Biology (DEU) *Online - full text edition.* **3207**
Marketing Health Services (USA) *Online - full text edition.* **3367**
Mayo Clinic Health Letter (USA) *Online - full text edition.* **3647**
McGraw-Hill's Biotechnology Newswatch (USA) *Online - full text edition.* **3276**
McKnight's Long-Term Care News (USA) *Online - full text edition.* **3477**
Med Ad News (USA) *Online - full text edition.* **3367**
Medical Anthropology Quarterly (USA) *Online - full text edition.* **3174**
Medical Design Technology (USA) *Online - full text edition.* **3649**
Medical Device Approval Letter with G M P - Design Controls Reviews (USA) *Online - full text edition.* **3879**
Medical Economics (USA) *Online - full text edition.* **3650**
Medical Journal of Australia (AUS) *Online - full text edition.* **3651**
Medical Law's Regan Report (USA) *Online - full text edition.* **3651**
Medical Letter on Drugs and Therapeutics (English Edition) (USA) *Online - full text edition.* **4315**
Medical Marketing & Media (USA) *Online - full text edition.* **4315**
Medical Materials Update (USA) *Online - full text edition.* **3652**
Medical Outcomes and Guidelines Alert (USA) *Online - full text edition.* **3652**
Medical Textiles (GBR) *Online - full text edition.* **3654**
Medical Trial Technique Quarterly (USA) *Online - full text edition.* **3545**
Medical Update (USA) *Online - full text edition.* **4358**
Medical Utilization Management (USA) *Online - full text edition.* **3655**
Medicine and Science in Sports and Exercise (USA) *Online - full text edition.* **4175**
Medicine (Baltimore) (USA) *Online - full text edition.* **3656**
MedSurg Nursing (USA) *Online - full text edition.* **4196**
Memory and Cognition (USA) *Online - full text edition.* **4426**
Menopause News (USA) *Online - full text edition.* **4564**
Men's Fitness (USA) *Online - full text edition.* **4222**
Men's Health (United States Edition) (USA) *Online - full text edition.* **4222**
Mental and Physical Disability Law Reporter (USA) *Online - full text edition.* **3546**
Mental Health Weekly (USA) *Online - full text edition.* **4427**
Merrill - Palmer Quarterly (USA) *Online - full text edition.* **4427**
Metropolitan Life Insurance Company. Statistical Bulletin S B (USA) *Online - full text edition.* **3533**
Microbiology (GBR) *Online - full text edition.* **3327**
Microbiology and Molecular Biology Reviews (USA) *Online - full text edition.* **3328**
The Milbank Quarterly (USA) *Online - full text edition.* **4368**
Modern Healthcare (Year) (USA) *Online - full text edition.* **3519**
Modern Maturity (USA) *Online - full text edition.* **3478**
Morbidity and Mortality Weekly Report (USA) *Online - full text edition.* **4482**
Mothering (USA) *Online - full text edition.* **4564**
N C A H F Newsletter (USA) *Online - full text edition.* **4482**
National Academy of Sciences of the United States of America. Proceedings (USA) *Online - full text edition.* **4505**
National Cancer Institute. Journal (USA) *Online - full text edition.* **3985**
National Report on Computers and Health (USA) *Online - full text edition.* **3812**
National Right to Life News (USA) *Online - full text edition.* **4516**
The Nation's Health (USA) *Online - full text edition.* **4483**
Natural Health (USA) *Online - full text edition.* **3168**
Nature (GBR) *Online - full text edition.* **4506**
Nature Biotechnology (USA) *Online - full text edition.* **3276**
Nature Medicine (GBR) *Online - full text edition.* **3665**
Nephrology Nursing Journal (USA) *Online - full text edition.* **3930**
Network News (Washington, 1975) (USA) *Online - full text edition.* **4565**
Neurology Alert (USA) *Online - full text edition.* **4115**
New Choices (USA) *Online - full text edition.* **3478**
New England Journal of Medicine (USA) *Online - full text edition.* **3666**
New Zealand Journal of Psychology (NZL) *Online - full text edition.* **4430**
Notre Dame Journal of Law, Ethics & Public Policy (USA) *Online - full text edition.* **4459**
The Nurse Practitioner (USA) *Online - full text edition.* **3931**
Nursing Administration Quarterly (USA) *Online - full text edition.* **3932**
Nursing and Health Care Perspectives (USA) *Online - full text edition.* **3932**
Nursing Diagnosis (USA) *Online - full text edition.* **3932**
Nursing Economics (USA) *Online - full text edition.* **3932**
Nursing Forum (USA) *Online - full text edition.* **3933**
Nursing Homes (USA) *Online - full text edition.* **3933**
Nursing Law's Regan Report (USA) *Online - full text edition.* **3933**
Nursing Management (USA) *Online - full text edition.* **3933**
Nursing Times (GBR) *Online - full text edition.* **3935**
Nursing (Year) (USA) *Online - full text edition.* **3935**
Nutraceuticals International (GBR) *Online - full text edition.* **4320**
Nutrition Action Healthletter (USA) *Online - full text edition.* **4241**
Nutrition and Food Science (GBR) *Online - full text edition.* **4241**
Nutrition Forum (USA) *Online - full text edition.* **4242**
Nutrition Health Review (USA) *Online - full text edition.* **4242**
Nutrition Research Newsletter (USA) *Online - full text edition.* **4243**
Nutrition Reviews (USA) *Online - full text edition.* **4243**
Nutrition Today (USA) *Online - full text edition.* **4243**
O H Online (USA) *Online - full text edition of* Occupational Hazards. **4261**
Ob-Gyn News (USA) *Online - full text edition.* **3960**
Occupational Safety and Health (GBR) *Online - full text edition.* **4262**
Office Nurse (USA) *Online - full text edition.* **3935**
Omega: Journal of Death and Dying (USA) *Online - full text edition.* **4431**
Ophthalmology Times (USA) *Online - full text edition.* **4004**
Organizational Behavior and Human Decision Processes (USA) *Online - full text edition.* **3366**
Orthopaedic Nursing Journal (USA) *Online - full text edition.* **3936**
Ostomy Quarterly (USA) *Online - full text edition.* **3671**
Palaestra (USA) *Online - full text edition.* **3425**
Paraplegia News (USA) *Online - full text edition.* **3494**
Patient Care (USA) *Online - full text edition.* **3673**
Pediatric Nursing (USA) *Online - full text edition.* **3937**
Pediatrics (English Edition) (USA) *Online - full text edition.* **4054**
Pediatrics for Parents (USA) *Online - full text edition.* **4054**
People's Medical Society Newsletter (USA) *Online - full text edition.* **3393**
Personality and Social Psychology Bulletin (USA) *Online - full text edition.* **4432**
Personnel Psychology (USA) *Online - full text edition.* **4433**
Perspectives in Biology and Medicine (USA) *Online - full content edition.* **3674**
Perspectives in Psychiatric Care (USA) *Online - full text edition.* **3937**
Pharma Marketletter (GBR) *Online - full text edition.* **4322**
Pharmaceutical Business News (GBR) *Online - full text edition.* **4323**
Pharmaceutical Executive (USA) *Online - full text edition.* **4323**
Pharmaceutical Processing (USA) *Online - full text edition.* **4324**
Pharmaceutical Technology (USA) *Online - full text edition.* **4325**
Physical Therapy (USA) *Online - full text edition.* **4064**
The Physician and Sportsmedicine (USA) *Online - full text edition.* **4176**
Physician Assistant (Springhouse) (USA) *Online - full text edition.* **3675**
Physician Executive (USA) *Online - full text edition.* **3521**
Physiological Reviews Online (USA) *Online - full text edition of* Physiological Reviews. **3347**
Plastic Surgical Nursing (USA) *Online - full text edition.* **3937**
Politics and the Life Sciences (USA) *Online - full content edition.* **4368**
Population and Environment (USA) *Online - full text edition.* **4433**
Postgraduate Medicine (USA) *Online - full text edition.* **3678**
Preventing School Failure (USA) *Online - full text edition.* **3425**
Prevention (USA) *Online - full text edition.* **4360**
Product Alert (USA) *Online - full text edition.* **3462**
Professional Psychology: Research and Practice (USA) *Online - full text edition.* **4434**
Psychiatry (USA) *Online - full text edition.* **4126**
Psychological Assessment (USA) *Online - full text edition.* **4437**
Psychological Bulletin (USA) *Online - full text edition.* **4437**
The Psychological Record (USA) *Online - full text edition.* **4438**
Psychological Review (USA) *Online - full text edition.* **4438**
Psychological Science (USA) *Online - full content edition.* **4438**
Psychology and Aging (USA) *Online - full text edition.* **3479**
Psychology of Women Quarterly (GBR) *Online - full text edition.* **4441**
Psychology Today (USA) *Online - full text edition.* **4441**
Psychopharmacology Update (USA) *Online - full text edition.* **4332**
Public Health Reports (USA) *Online - full text edition.* **4486**
Quadrant (USA) *Online - full text edition.* **4443**
Quarterly Journal of Experimental Psychology. Section A: Human Experimental Psychology (GBR) *Online - full text edition.* **4443**
Quarterly Review of Biology (USA) *Online - full text edition.* **3214**
Quest (Tucson) (USA) *Online - full text edition.* **4129**
R N Web (USA) *Online - full text edition of* R N. **3938**
Radiologic Technology (USA) *Online - full text edition.* **4153**
Real Living with Multiple Sclerosis (USA) *Online - full text edition.* **4129**
Research on Aging (USA) *Online - full text edition.* **3480**
Research on Social Work Practice (USA) *Online - full text edition.* **4523**
Research Quarterly for Exercise and Sport (USA) *Online - full text edition.* **4360**
Review of Optometry (USA) *Online - full text edition.* **4006**
Risk: Health, Safety & Environment (USA) *Online - full text edition.* **4488**
S I E C U S Report (USA) *Online - full text edition.* **4523**
Safety and Health (USA) *Online - full text edition.* **4264**
Saturday Evening Post (USA) *Online - full text edition.* **3465**
School Science Review (GBR) *Online - full text edition.* **4507**
Science and Justice (GBR) *Online - full text edition.* **3885**
Scrip - World Pharmaceutical News (GBR) *Online - full text edition.* **4335**
Self (USA) *Online - full text edition.* **4568**
Sex Roles (USA) *Online - full text edition.* **4448**
Sexually Transmitted Diseases (USA) *Online - full text edition.* **3853**
Shape (USA) *Online - full text edition.* **4565**
Social Action and the Law (USA) *Online - full text edition.* **4449**
Social Biology (USA) *Online - full text edition.* **3314**
Social Cognition (USA) *Online - full text edition.* **4449**
Social Psychology Quarterly (USA) *Online - full text edition.* **4523**
Social Science & Medicine (GBR) *Online - full text edition.* **3694**
Social Work with Groups (USA) *Online - full text edition.* **4518**
Society of Pediatric Nurses. Journal (USA) *Online - full text edition.* **3941**
Sociology of Health and Illness (GBR) *Online - full text edition.* **4523**
Sociology of Sport Journal (USA) *Online - full text edition.* **4523**
Special Delivery (USA) *Online - full text edition.* **3964**
State Health Monitor (USA) *Online - full text edition.* **3534**
Studies in Family Planning (USA) *Online - full text edition.* **4369**

Substance Abuse Report (USA) *Online - full text edition.* **3406**
Suicide and Life-Threatening Behavior (USA) *Online - full text edition.* **4451**
Total Health (USA) *Online - full text edition.* **4246**
Trends in Neurosciences (GBR) *Online - full text edition.* **4137**
Trends in Pharmacological Sciences (GBR) *Online - full text edition.* **4338**
Tuberculosis & Airborne Disease Weekly (USA) *Online - full text edition.* **3808**
Tufts University Health & Nutrition Letter (USA) *Online - full text edition.* **4246**
U S P - D I, Volume 2. Advice for the Patient (USA) *Online - full text edition.* **4338**
University of California, Berkeley. Wellness Letter (USA) *Online - full text edition.* **4362**
Urology Times (USA) *Online - full text edition.* **4220**
Vaccine Weekly (USA) *Online - full text edition.* **4339**
Vegetarian Times (USA) *Online - full text edition.* **4247**
Vibrant Life (USA) *Online - full text edition.* **4362**
Violence Against Women (USA) *Online - full text edition.* **4524**
Violence and Victims (USA) *Online - full text edition.* **4524**
W H O Drug Information (CHE) *Online - full text edition.* **4492**
W J M (USA) *Online - full text edition.* **3707**
Warning Letter Bulletin (USA) *Online - full text edition.* **3707**
Weight Watchers Magazine (USA) *Online - full text edition.* **4248**
Western Journal of Nursing Research (USA) *Online - full text edition.* **3943**
Whole Life Times (USA) *Online - full text edition.* **4227**
Windhover's IN VIVO (USA) *Online - full text edition.* **3709**
Women & Health (USA) *Online - full text edition.* **4566**
Women & Therapy (USA) *Online - full text edition.* **4455**
Worklife Report (CAN) *Online - full text edition.* **3364**
World Health Organization. Bulletin (CHE) *Online - full text edition.* **3709**
Worldwide Biotech (USA) *Online - full text edition.* **3278**

HighWire Press (Subsidiary of: Stanford University Libraries) 102 Green Library, Stanford University, Stanford, CA 94305-6004 TEL 650-723-2019, FAX 650-723-9325, contact@highwire.stanford.edu, http://www.highwire.stanford.edu, http://www.intl.highwire.org
A J N R (USA) *Online - full content edition.* **4139**
A J P: Cell Physiology Online (USA) *Online - full text edition of* American Journal of Physiology: Cell Physiology. **3337**
A J P: Endocrinology and Metabolism Online (USA) *Online - full text edition of* American Journal of Physiology: Endocrinology and Metabolism. **3338**
A J P: Gastrointestinal and Liver Physiology Online (USA) *Online - full text edition of* American Journal of Physiology: Gastrointestinal and Liver Physiology. **3338**
A J P: Heart and Circulatory Physiology Online (USA) *Online - full text edition of* American Journal of Physiology: Heart and Circulatory Physiology. **3338**
A J P: Lung Cellular and Molecular Physiology Online (USA) *Online - full text edition of* American Journal of Physiology: Lung Cellular and Molecular Physiology. **3338**
A J P: Regulatory, Integrative and Comparative Physiology Online (USA) *Online - full text edition of* American Journal of Physiology: Regulatory, Integrative and Comparative Physiology. **3338**
A J P: Renal Physiology Online (USA) *Online - full text edition of* American Journal of Physiology: Renal Physiology. **3339**
A J R (USA) *Online - full text edition.* **4139**
A R D Online (GBR) *Online - full text edition of* Annals of the Rheumatic Diseases. **4167**
AAPNews.org (USA) *Online - full text edition of* A A P News. **4039**
Academic Emergency Medicine (USA) *Online - full text edition.* **4009**
Academic Medicine (USA) *Online - full text edition.* **3556**
Academic Psychiatry (USA) *Online - full text edition.* **4067**
Advances in Physiology Education Online (USA) *Online - full text edition of* Advances in Physiology Education. **3337**
Advances in Psychiatric Treatment Online (GBR) *Online - full text edition of* Advances in Psychiatric Treatment. **4070**
Age and Ageing (GBR) *Online - full text edition.* **3466**
Alcohol & Alcoholism (GBR) *Online - full text edition.* **3397**
American Journal of Clinical Nutrition (USA) *Online - full text edition.* **4228**
American Journal of Epidemiology (USA) *Online - full text edition.* **3563**
American Journal of Geriatric Psychiatry (USA) *Online - full text edition.* **3468**
American Journal of Kidney Diseases (USA) *Online - full text edition.* **4209**
American Journal of Pathology (USA) *Online - full text edition.* **3564**
American Journal of Psychiatry (USA) *Online - full text edition.* **4071**
American Journal of Respiratory and Critical Care Medicine (USA) *Online - full text edition.* **4158**
American Journal of Respiratory Cell and Molecular Biology (USA) *Online - full text edition.* **4158**
American Medical Informatics Association. Journal (USA) *Online - full text edition.* **3809**
American Podiatric Medical Association. Journal (USA) *Online - full text edition.* **4010**
American Society of Nephrology. Journal (USA) *Online - full text edition.* **4209**
Anesthesia and Analgesia (USA) *Online - full text edition.* **3755**
Annals of Thoracic Surgery (USA) *Online - full text edition.* **4181**
Annual Review of Biochemistry (USA) *Online - full text edition.* **3240**
Annual Review of Biophysics and Biomolecular Structure (USA) *Online - full text edition.* **3264**
Annual Review of Cell and Developmental Biology (USA) *Online - full text edition.* **3285**
Annual Review of Genetics (USA) *Online - full text edition.* **3298**
Annual Review of Immunology (USA) *Online - full text edition.* **3740**
Annual Review of Medicine Online (USA) *Online - full text edition of* Annual Review of Medicine: Selected Topics in the Clinical Sciences. **3567**
Annual Review of Microbiology (USA) *Online - full text edition.* **3317**
Annual Review of Neuroscience (USA) *Online - full text edition.* **4073**
Annual Review of Nutrition (USA) *Online - full text edition.* **4229**
Annual Review of Pharmacology and Toxicology (USA) *Online - full text edition.* **4276**
Annual Review of Physiology (USA) *Online - full text edition.* **3339**
Annual Review of Psychology (USA) *Online - full text edition.* **4376**
Annual Review of Public Health (USA) *Online - full text edition.* **4461**
Anti-Cancer Drug Design (GBR) *Online - full text edition.* **3967**
Antimicrobial Agents and Chemotherapy (USA) *Online - full text edition.* **3317**
Applied and Environmental Microbiology (USA) *Online - full text edition.* **3318**
Archives of Disease in Childhood (GBR) *Online - full text edition.* **4040**
Arteriosclerosis, Thrombosis, and Vascular Biology (USA) *Online - full text edition.* **3763**
Asian Cardiovascular & Thoracic Annals (SGP) *Online - full text edition.* **3763**
B J O Online (GBR) *Online - full text edition of* British Journal of Ophthalmology. **3994**
B J S M Online (GBR) *Online - full text edition of* British Journal of Sports Medicine. **4173**
Behavioral Ecology (USA) *Online - full text edition.* **3184**
Biology of Reproduction (USA) *Online - full text edition.* **3186**
Biophysical Journal (USA) *Online - full text edition.* **3265**
Blood (USA) *Online - full text edition.* **3898**
bmj.com(GBR) *Online - full text.* **3577**
Brain (GBR) *Online - full text edition.* **4077**
British Journal of Anaesthesia (GBR) *Online - full text edition.* **3756**
British Journal of Pharmacology (GBR) *Online - full text edition.* **4281**
British Journal of Psychiatry (GBR) *Online - full text edition.* **4079**
British Medical Bulletin (GBR) *Online - full text edition.* **3579**
C V Surgery Online(USA) *Online - full text.* **3718**
Cancer Epidemiology, Biomarkers & Prevention (USA) *Online - full text edition.* **3971**
Cancer Research (USA) *Online - full text edition.* **3973**
Carcinogenesis (GBR) *Online - full text edition.* **3974**
Cell (USA) *Online - full text edition.* **3286**
Cell Growth & Differentiation (USA) *Online - full text edition.* **3974**
Cerebral Cortex (USA) *Online - full text edition.* **4081**
Chemical Senses (GBR) *Online - full text edition.* **3340**
Chest (USA) *Online - full text edition.* **4159**
Circulation (Baltimore) (USA) *Online - full text edition.* **3768**
Circulation Research (USA) *Online - full text edition.* **3768**
Clinical and Diagnostic Laboratory Immunology (USA) *Online - full text edition.* **3742**
Clinical Cancer Research (USA) *Online - full text edition.* **3975**
Clinical Chemistry (USA) *Online - full text edition.* **3873**
Clinical Microbiology Reviews (USA) *Online - full text edition.* **3319**
Clinical Psychology (USA) *Online - full text edition.* **4388**
Drug Metabolism and Disposition (USA) *Online - full text edition.* **4289**
The E M B O Journal (GBR) *Online - full text edition.* **3249**
E M B O Reports Online (GBR) *Online - full text edition of* E M B O Reports. **3301**
E M B Online (GBR) *Online - full text edition of* Evidence - Based Medicine. **3600**
E M J Online (GBR) *Online - full text edition of* Emergency Medicine Journal. **4014**
Endocrine Reviews (USA) *Online - full text edition.* **3861**
Endocrinology (USA) *Online - full text edition.* **3861**
European Journal of Biochemistry (GBR) *Online - full text edition.* **3249**
European Journal of Cardio-Thoracic Surgery (NLD) *Online - full text edition.* **3771**
Evidence - Based Mental Health (GBR) *Online - full text edition.* **4090**
Evidence - Based Nursing (GBR) *Online - full text edition.* **3919**
Experimental Biology and Medicine (Maywood) (USA) *Online - full text edition.* **3195**
The F A S E B Journal (USA) *Online - full text edition.* **3196**
Family Practice (GBR) *Online - full text edition.* **3601**
Gastroenterology (USA) *Online - full text edition.* **3890**
Genes & Development (USA) *Online - full text edition.* **3303**
Genetics (USA) *Online - full text edition.* **3305**
Genome Research (USA) *Online - full text edition.* **3306**
The Gerontologist (USA) *Online - full text edition.* **3473**
Glycobiology (GBR) *Online - full text edition.* **3251**
Gut Online (GBR) *Online - full text edition of* Gut. **3891**
Harvard Review of Psychiatry (GBR) *Online - full text edition.* **4093**
Health Education Research (GBR) *Online - full text edition.* **4513**
Health Policy and Planning (GBR) *Online - full text edition.* **4473**
Health Promotion International (GBR) *Online - full text edition.* **4474**
Heart Online (GBR) *Online - full text edition of* Heart. **3772**
Hepatology (USA) *Online - full text edition.* **3892**
Human Molecular Genetics (GBR) *Online - full text edition.* **3308**
Human Reproduction (GBR) *Online - full text edition.* **3953**
Hypertension (USA) *Online - full text edition.* **3774**
Immunity (USA) *Online - full text edition.* **3745**
Infection and Immunity (USA) *Online - full text edition.* **3798**
International Immunology (GBR) *Online - full text edition.* **3747**
International Journal of Epidemiology (GBR) *Online - full text edition.* **3623**
International Journal of Systematic and Evolutionary Microbiology (GBR) *Online - full text edition.* **3324**
Investigative Ophthalmology & Visual Science (IOVS) (USA) *Online - full text edition.* **3999**
J C P Online (GBR) *Online - full text edition of* Journal of Clinical Pathology. **3631**
J E C H Online (GBR) *Online - full text edition of* Journal of Epidemiology & Community Health. **3632**
J M E Online (GBR) *Online - full text edition of* Journal of Medical Ethics. **3635**
J M G Online (GBR) *Online - full text edition of* Journal of Medical Genetics. **3310**
J M S Online (GBR) *Online - full text edition of* Journal of Medical Screening. **3802**
J N M Online (USA) *Online - full text edition of* The Journal of Nuclear Medicine. **4148**
Journal of Antimicrobial Chemotherapy (GBR) *Online - full text edition.* **3800**
Journal of Applied Physiology Online (USA) *Online - full text edition of* Journal of Applied Physiology. **3344**
Journal of Bacteriology (USA) *Online - full text edition.* **3325**
Journal of Biological Chemistry (USA) *Online - full text edition.* **3253**
Journal of Cell Biology (USA) *Online - full text edition.* **3290**
Journal of Clinical Endocrinology and Metabolism (USA) *Online - full text edition.* **3864**
Journal of Clinical Investigation (USA) *Online - full text edition.* **3631**
Journal of Clinical Microbiology (USA) *Online - full text edition.* **3631**
The Journal of Deaf Studies and Deaf Education (USA) *Online - full text edition.* **3491**
The Journal of Experimental Medicine (USA) *Online - full text edition.* **3876**
Journal of General Physiology (USA) *Online - full text edition.* **3344**
Journal of General Virology (GBR) *Online - full text edition.* **3325**
Journal of Histochemistry and Cytochemistry (USA) *Online - full text edition.* **3291**
Journal of Immunology (USA) *Online - full text edition.* **3748**
The Journal of Investigative Dermatology (USA) *Online - full text edition.* **3851**
Journal of Lipid Research (USA) *Online - full text edition.* **3254**
Journal of Neurochemistry (USA) *Online - full text edition.* **3255**
Journal of Neurology, Neurosurgery and Psychiatry (GBR) *Online - full text edition.* **4104**
Journal of Neurophysiology Online (USA) *Online - full text edition of* Journal of Neurophysiology. **3345**
Journal of Neuropsychiatry and Clinical Neurosciences (USA) *Online - full text edition.* **4104**
Journal of Neuroscience (USA) *Online - full text edition.* **4104**
Journal of Nuclear Medicine Technology (USA) *Online - full text edition.* **4148**
Journal of Nutrition (USA) *Online - full text edition.* **4237**
The Journal of Orthodontics (GBR) *Online - full text edition.* **3830**
Journal of Pediatric Psychology (GBR) *Online - full text edition.* **4419**
Journal of Pharmacology and Experimental Therapeutics (USA) *Online - full text edition.* **4310**
Journal of Physiology (GBR) *Online - full text edition.* **3345**
Journal of Plankton Research (GBR) *Online - full text edition.* **3204**
The Journal of Thoracic and Cardiovascular Surgery (USA) *Online - full text edition.* **4195**
Journal of Vascular and Interventional Radiology (USA) *Online - full text edition.* **4149**
Journal of Virology (USA) *Online - full text edition.* **3326**
Journal Watch Cardiology (USA) *Online - full text edition.* **3730**
Journal Watch Online (USA) *Online - full text edition of* Journal Watch. **3730**
Journals of Gerontology. Series A: Biological Sciences & Medical Sciences (USA) *Online - full text edition.* **3477**
Laboratory Investigation (USA) *Online - full text edition.* **3878**

Learning & Memory (USA) *Online - full text edition.* **4108**
Liver Transplantation (USA) *Online - full text edition.* **3894**
M P Online (GBR) *Online - full text edition of* Molecular Pathology. **3879**
Medical Humanities (GBR) *Online - full text edition.* **3651**
Microbiology (GBR) *Online - full text edition.* **3327**
Microbiology and Molecular Biology Reviews (USA) *Online - full text edition.* **3328**
Modern Pathology (USA) *Online - full text edition.* **3662**
Molecular and Cellular Biology (USA) *Online - full text edition.* **3257**
Molecular Biology and Evolution (USA) *Online - full text edition.* **3208**
Molecular Cancer Therapeutics(USA) *Online - full text.* **3984**
Molecular Cell (USA) *Online - full text edition.* **3292**
Molecular Endocrinology (USA) *Online - full text edition.* **3866**
Molecular Human Reproduction (GBR) *Online - full text edition.* **3958**
Molecular Pharmacology (USA) *Online - full text edition.* **4317**
Mutagenesis (GBR) *Online - full text edition.* **3311**
National Academy of Sciences of the United States of America. Proceedings (USA) *Online - full text edition.* **4505**
National Cancer Institute. Journal (USA) *Online - full text edition.* **3985**
National Cancer Institute. Journal. Monographs (USA) *Online - full text edition.* **3985**
NeoReviews.org(USA) *Online - full content.* **4049**
Nephrology, Dialysis and Transplantation (GBR) *Online - full text edition.* **4216**
Neural Computation (USA) *Online - full text edition.* **3389**
Neurocase (GBR) *Online - full text edition.* **4112**
Neurology (USA) *Online - full text edition.* **4114**
Neuron (USA) *Online - full text edition.* **4115**
News in Physiological Sciences Online (USA) *Online - full text edition of* News in Physiological Sciences. **3346**
Nucleic Acids Research (GBR) *Online - full text edition.* **3259**
O E M Online (GBR) *Online - full text edition of* Occupational and Environmental Medicine. **4261**
Obesity Research (USA) *Online - full text edition.* **3668**
Occupational Medicine (GBR) *Online - full text edition.* **4262**
The Oncologist (USA) *Online - full text edition.* **3986**
Pediatric Research (USA) *Online - full text edition.* **4054**
Pediatrics (English Edition) (USA) *Online - full text edition.* **4054**
Pediatrics in Review (USA) *Online - full text edition.* **4054**
Pharmacological Reviews (USA) *Online - full text edition.* **4326**
Physiological Genomics (USA) *Online - full text edition.* **3260**
Physiological Reviews Online (USA) *Online - full text edition of* Physiological Reviews. **3347**
Plant and Cell Physiology (GBR) *Online - full text edition.* **3293**
Postgraduate Medical Journal (GBR) *Online - full text edition.* **3678**
Protein Engineering (GBR) *Online - full text edition.* **3261**
Protein Science (USA) *Online - full text edition.* **3261**
Psychiatric Bulletin (GBR) *Online - full text edition.* **4125**
Psychiatric News (USA) *Online - full text edition.* **4125**
Psychiatric Services (USA) *Online - full text edition.* **4126**
Psychosomatics (USA) *Online - full text edition.* **4128**
Psychotherapy Research (USA) *Online - full text edition.* **4443**
Public Health Reports (USA) *Online - full text edition.* **4486**
Q J M (GBR) *Online - full text edition.* **3681**
Quality in Health Care (GBR) *Online - full content edition.* **3682**
R S N A Index Online (USA) *Online - full text edition of* R S N A Index to Imaging Literature. **3735**
Radiographics (USA) *Online - full text edition.* **4153**
Radiology (USA) *Online - full text edition.* **4154**
Royal Society of Medicine. Journal (GBR) *Online - full text edition.* **3688**
S T I Online (GBR) *Online - full text edition of* Sexually Transmitted Infections. **3853**
Stem Cells (USA) *Online - full text edition.* **3219**
Stroke (USA) *Online - full text edition.* **3783**
Thorax Online (GBR) *Online - full text edition of* Thorax. **3700**
Tobbacco Control Online (GBR) *Online - full text edition of* Tobacco Control. **4531**
Toxicological Sciences (USA) *Online - full text edition.* **3455**
Transfusion (USA) *Online - full text edition.* **3702**
W J M (USA) *Online - full text edition.* **3707**

Human Resources Information Network (Subsidiary of: Executive Telecom System International) 9585 Valparaiso Ct., College Park N., Indianapolis, IN 46268 TEL 317-872-2045, FAX 317-872-2059
AIDS Policy and Law (USA) *Online - full text edition. (CDD, HDD)* **3536**
B N A's Medicare Report (USA) *Online - full text edition. (File DD)* **3573**
B N A's SafetyNet (USA) *Online - full text edition. (CDD, HDD)* **4251**
Industrial Health & Hazards Update (USA) *Online - full text edition.* **4256**
Occupational Safety & Health Reporter (USA) *Online - full text edition. (CDD, HDD)* **4262**
Workplace Substance Abuse Advisor (USA) *Online - full text edition. (CDD, HDD)* **3406**

IDEAL Online Library (Subsidiary of: Reed Elsevier plc) c/o Academic Press, 525 B St., Ste. 1900, San Diego, CA 92101-4459 TEL 619-231-6616, http://www.idealibrary.com
Accident and Emergency Nursing (GBR) *Online - full text edition.* **3912**
Aesthetic Surgery Journal (USA) *Online - full text edition.* **4179**
American Academy of Dermatology. Journal (USA) *Online - full text edition.* **3844**
American Association for Pediatric Ophthalmology and Strabismus. Journal (USA) *Online - full text edition.* **3993**
American Heart Journal (USA) *Online - full text edition.* **3762**
American Journal of Contact Dermatitis (USA) *Online - full text edition.* **3844**
American Journal of Emergency Medicine (USA) *Online - full text edition.* **4010**
American Journal of Infection Control (USA) *Online - full text edition.* **3792**
American Journal of Kidney Diseases (USA) *Online - full text edition.* **4209**
American Journal of Obstetrics and Gynecology (USA) *Online - full text edition.* **3944**
American Journal of Orthodontics and Dentofacial Orthopedics (USA) *Online - full text edition.* **3814**
American Journal of Otolaryngology (USA) *Online - full text edition.* **4030**
American Psychiatric Nurses Association. Journal (USA) *Online - full text edition.* **3913**
American Society of Echocardiography. Journal (USA) *Online - full text edition.* **3762**
Anaerobe (GBR) *Online - full text edition.* **3317**
Analytical Biochemistry (USA) *Online - full text edition.* **3240**
Animal Behaviour (GBR) *Online - full text edition.* **3350**
Annals of Diagnostic Pathology (USA) *Online - full text edition.* **3566**
Annals of Emergency Medicine (USA) *Online - full text edition.* **4010**
Appetite (GBR) *Online - full text edition.* **4229**
Applied Nursing Research (USA) *Online - full text edition.* **3913**
Archives of Biochemistry and Biophysics (USA) *Online - full text edition.* **3241**
Archives of Physical Medicine and Rehabilitation (USA) *Online - full text edition.* **4058**
Archives of Psychiatric Nursing (USA) *Online - full text edition.* **3914**
Arthroscopy (USA) *Online - full text edition.* **4010**
Bailliere's Best Practice & Research in Clinical Anaesthesiology (GBR) *Online - full text edition.* **3756**
Bailliere's Best Practice & Research in Clinical Endocrinology and Metabolism (GBR) *Online - full text edition.* **3855**
Bailliere's Best Practice & Research in Clinical Gastroenterology (GBR) *Online - full text edition.* **3886**
Bailliere's Best Practice & Research in Clinical Haematology (GBR) *Online - full text edition.* **3898**
Bailliere's Best Practice & Research in Clinical Obstetrics and Gynaecology (GBR) *Online - full text edition.* **3945**
Bailliere's Best Practice & Research in Clinical Rheumatology (GBR) *Online - full text edition.* **4167**
Biochemical and Biophysical Research Communications (USA) *Online - full text edition.* **3242**
Biological Control (USA) *Online - full text edition.* **3185**
Biologicals (GBR) *Online - full text edition.* **3186**
Blood Cells, Molecules, and Diseases (USA) *Online - full text edition.* **3898**
Blood Reviews (GBR) *Online - full text edition.* **3899**
Brain and Cognition (USA) *Online - full text edition.* **4383**
Brain and Language (USA) *Online - full text edition.* **4383**
Brain, Behavior, and Immunity (USA) *Online - full text edition.* **3741**
The Breast (GBR) *Online - full text edition.* **3946**
British Journal of Cancer (GBR) *Online - full text edition.* **3969**
British Journal of Oral and Maxillofacial Surgery (GBR) *Online - full text edition.* **4183**
British Journal of Plastic Surgery (GBR) *Online - full text edition.* **4183**
Bulletin of Mathematical Biology (GBR) *Online - full text edition.* **3188**
Cancer Treatment Reviews (GBR) *Online - full text edition.* **3973**
The Case Manager (USA) *Online - full text edition.* **3582**
Cell Calcium (Edinburgh) (GBR) *Online - full text edition.* **3287**
Cell Stress & Chaperones (USA) *Online - full text edition.* **3582**
Cellular Immunology (USA) *Online - full text edition.* **3742**
Cladistics (GBR) *Online - full text edition.* **3191**
Clinical Effectiveness in Nursing (GBR) *Online - full text edition.* **3916**
Clinical Immunology (USA) *Online - full text edition.* **3743**
Clinical Nutrition (GBR) *Online - full text edition.* **4231**
Clinical Pharmacology & Therapeutics (USA) *Online - full text edition.* **4284**
Clinical Radiology (GBR) *Online - full text edition.* **4142**
Cognitive Psychology (USA) *Online - full text edition.* **4389**
Complementary Therapies in Medicine (GBR) *Online - full text edition.* **3787**
Complementary Therapies in Nursing & Midwifery (GBR) *Online - full text edition.* **3917**
Comprehensive Psychiatry (USA) *Online - full text edition.* **4083**
Consciousness and Cognition (USA) *Online - full text edition.* **4391**
Contemporary Educational Psychology (USA) *Online - full text edition.* **3410**
Coronary Health Care (GBR) *Online - full text edition.* **3917**
Cryobiology (USA) *Online - full text edition.* **3266**
Current Anaesthesia and Critical Care (GBR) *Online - full text edition.* **3756**
Current Diagnostic Pathology (GBR) *Online - full text edition.* **3908**
Current Obstetrics and Gynaecology (GBR) *Online - full text edition.* **3948**
Current Orthopaedics (GBR) *Online - full text edition.* **4013**
Current Paediatrics (GBR) *Online - full text edition.* **4043**
Cytokine (GBR) *Online - full text edition.* **3301**
Developmental Biology (USA) *Online - full text edition.* **3193**
Developmental Review (USA) *Online - full text edition.* **4394**
Drug Resistance Update (GBR) *Online - full text edition.* **3596**
Ecotoxicology and Environmental Safety - Online (USA) *Online - full text edition of* Ecotoxicology and Environmental Safety. **3448**
EndoTrends (USA) *Online - full text edition.* **3862**
Environmental Research (USA) *Online - full text edition.* **3439**
Epilepsy and Behavior (USA) *Online - full text edition.* **3598**
Europace (GBR) *Online - full text edition.* **3771**
European Heart Journal (GBR) *Online - full text edition.* **3771**
European Journal of Echocardiography (GBR) *Online - full text edition.* **3771**
European Journal of Oncology Nursing (GBR) *Online - full text edition.* **3919**
European Journal of Paediatric Neurology (GBR) *Online - full text edition.* **4044**
European Journal of Pain (GBR) *Online - full text edition.* **3600**
European Journal of Surgical Oncology (GBR) *Online - full text edition.* **3977**
European Journal of Vascular and Endovascular Surgery (GBR) *Online - full text edition.* **3771**
Evidence - Based Cardiovascular Medicine (GBR) *Online - full text edition.* **3772**
Evidence - Based Healthcare (GBR) *Online - full text edition.* **4468**
Evidence - Based Obstetrics & Gynaecology (GBR) *Online - full text edition.* **3949**
Evidence - Based Oncology (GBR) *Online - full text edition.* **3978**
Experimental and Molecular Pathology (USA) *Online - full text edition.* **3600**
Experimental Eye Research (GBR) *Online - full text edition.* **3997**
Experimental Neurology (USA) *Online - full text edition.* **4090**
Experimental Parasitology (USA) *Online - full text edition.* **3796**
Fibrinolysis & Proteolysis (GBR) *Online - full text edition.* **3875**
Fish and Shellfish Immunology (GBR) *Online - full text edition.* **3196**
Food Microbiology (GBR) *Online - full text edition.* **3322**
The Foot (GBR) *Online - full text edition.* **4015**
Frontiers in Neuroendocrinology (USA) *Online - full text edition.* **3862**
Games and Economic Behavior (USA) *Online - full text edition.* **4400**
Gastroenterology (USA) *Online - full text edition.* **3890**
Gastrointestinal Endoscopy (USA) *Online - full text edition.* **3891**
General and Comparative Endocrinology (USA) *Online - full text edition.* **3863**
Genomics (USA) *Online - full text edition.* **3306**
Geriatric Nursing (USA) *Online - full text edition.* **3472**
Growth Hormone and I G F Research (GBR) *Online - full text edition.* **3863**
Gynecologic Oncology (USA) *Online - full text edition.* **3952**
Hepatology (USA) *Online - full text edition.* **3892**
Home Care Provider (USA) *Online - full text edition.* **3920**
Hormones and Behavior (USA) *Online - full text edition.* **3863**
Human Pathology (USA) *Online - full text edition.* **3616**
Insight (St. Louis) (USA) *Online - full text edition.* **3999**
Intensive and Critical Care Nursing (GBR) *Online - full text edition.* **3921**
International Journal of Obstetric Anesthesia (GBR) *Online - full text edition.* **3954**
International Journal of Oral & Maxillofacial Surgery (DNK) *Online - full text edition.* **3827**
International Journal of Trauma Nursing (USA) *Online - full text edition.* **3922**
J M B Online (GBR) *Online - full text edition of* Journal of Molecular Biology. **3254**
Journal of Adolescence (GBR) *Online - full text edition.* **3383**
The Journal of Allergy and Clinical Immunology (USA) *Online - full text edition.* **3748**
Journal of Arthroplasty (USA) *Online - full text edition.* **4017**
Journal of Autoimmunity (GBR) *Online - full text edition.* **3748**
Journal of Biomedical Informatics (USA) *Online - full text edition.* **3811**
Journal of Bodywork & Movement Therapies (GBR) *Online - full text edition.* **4061**
Journal of Cardiac Failure (USA) *Online - full text edition.* **3776**
Journal of Cardiothoracic and Vascular Anesthesia (USA) *Online - full text edition.* **3777**
Journal of Clinical Forensic Medicine (GBR) *Online - full text edition.* **3883**
Journal of Clinical Neuroscience (GBR) *Online - full text edition.* **4100**
Journal of Comparative Pathology (GBR) *Online - full text edition.* **3203**

Journal of Cranio-Maxillo-Facial Surgery (GBR) *Online - full text edition.* **4192**
Journal of Electrocardiology (USA) *Online - full text edition.* **3777**
Journal of Emergency Nursing (USA) *Online - full text edition.* **3924**
Journal of Environmental Psychology (GBR) *Online - full text edition.* **4415**
Journal of Experimental Child Psychology (USA) *Online - full text edition.* **4415**
Journal of Experimental Social Psychology (USA) *Online - full text edition.* **4415**
Journal of Hand Surgery: American Volume (USA) *Online - full text edition.* **4193**
Journal of Hand Surgery: British and European Volume (GBR) *Online - full text edition.* **4193**
Journal of Hospital Infection (GBR) *Online - full text edition.* **3801**
Journal of Human Evolution (GBR) *Online - full text edition.* **3309**
Journal of Infection (GBR) *Online - full text edition.* **3801**
The Journal of Laboratory and Clinical Medicine (USA) *Online - full text edition.* **3876**
Journal of Manipulative and Physiological Therapeutics (USA) *Online - full text edition.* **3788**
Journal of Mathematical Psychology (USA) *Online - full text edition.* **4418**
Journal of Memory and Language (USA) *Online - full text edition.* **3550**
Journal of Molecular and Cellular Cardiology (GBR) *Online - full text edition.* **3778**
Journal of Nuclear Cardiology (USA) *Online - full text edition.* **4148**
Journal of Oral and Maxillofacial Surgery (USA) *Online - full text edition.* **3829**
Journal of Orthopaedic Nursing (GBR) *Online - full text edition.* **3926**
The Journal of Pain (GBR) *Online - full text edition.* **3636**
Journal of Pediatric Health Care (USA) *Online - full text edition.* **4047**
Journal of Pediatric Nursing (USA) *Online - full text edition.* **3926**
Journal of Pediatric Oncology Nursing (USA) *Online - full text edition.* **3982**
Journal of Pediatric Surgery (USA) *Online - full text edition.* **4194**
The Journal of Pediatrics (USA) *Online - full text edition.* **4047**
Journal of Perianesthesia Nursing (USA) *Online - full text edition.* **3926**
Journal of Professional Nursing (USA) *Online - full text edition.* **3926**
The Journal of Prosthetic Dentistry (USA) *Online - full text edition.* **3830**
Journal of Prosthodontics (USA) *Online - full text edition.* **3830**
Journal of Renal Nutrition (USA) *Online - full text edition.* **4238**
Journal of Research in Personality (USA) *Online - full text edition.* **4422**
Journal of Shoulder and Elbow Surgery (USA) *Online - full text edition.* **4195**
Journal of Stroke and Cerebrovascular Diseases (USA) *Online - full text edition.* **3778**
Journal of Structural Biology (USA) *Online - full text edition.* **3205**
Journal of Surgical Research (USA) *Online - full text edition.* **4195**
Journal of Theoretical Biology (GBR) *Online - full text edition.* **3205**
The Journal of Thoracic and Cardiovascular Surgery (USA) *Online - full text edition.* **4195**
Journal of Vascular Nursing (USA) *Online - full text edition.* **3927**
Journal of Vascular Surgery (USA) *Online - full text edition.* **4195**
Journal of Vocational Behavior (USA) *Online - full text edition.* **4424**
Journal of W O C N (USA) *Online - full text edition.* **4195**
Learning and Motivation (USA) *Online - full text edition.* **3413**
Linnean Society. Biological Journal (GBR) *Online - full text edition.* **3206**
Liver Transplantation (USA) *Online - full text edition.* **3894**
Manual Therapy (GBR) *Online - full text edition.* **4063**
Medical Hypotheses (GBR) *Online - full text edition.* **3651**
Metabolic Engineering (USA) *Online - full text edition.* **3238**
Metabolism: Clinical and Experimental (USA) *Online - full text edition.* **3866**
Methods: A Companion to Methods in Enzymology (USA) *Online - full text edition.* **3256**
Microbial Pathogenesis (GBR) *Online - full text edition.* **3804**
Microvascular Research (USA) *Online - full text edition.* **3780**
Midwifery (GBR) *Online - full text edition.* **3958**
Molecular and Cellular Neurosciences (USA) *Online - full text edition.* **4110**
Molecular and Cellular Probes (GBR) *Online - full text edition.* **3879**
Molecular Cell Biology Research Communications (USA) *Online - full text edition.* **3292**
Molecular Diagnosis (USA) *Online - full text edition.* **3662**
Molecular Genetics and Metabolism (USA) *Online - full text edition.* **3662**
Molecular Phylogenetics and Evolution (USA) *Online - full text edition.* **3311**
Molecular Therapy (USA) *Online - full text edition.* **3984**
Neurobiology of Disease (USA) *Online - full text edition.* **4112**
Neurobiology of Learning and Memory (USA) *Online - full text edition.* **4112**
NeuroImage (USA) *Online - full text edition.* **4113**
Neuropeptides (Edinburgh) (GBR) *Online - full text edition.* **3259**
Nurse Education in Practice (GBR) *Online - full text edition.* **3931**
Nurse Education Today (GBR) *Online - full text edition.* **3931**
Nursing Outlook (USA) *Online - full text edition.* **3934**
Oral Surgery, Oral Medicine, Oral Pathology, Oral Radiology, and Endodontics (USA) *Online - full text edition.* **3835**
Organizational Behavior and Human Decision Processes (USA) *Online - full text edition.* **3366**
Osteoarthritis and Cartilage (GBR) *Online - full text edition.* **4169**
Otolaryngology - Head and Neck Surgery (USA) *Online - full text edition.* **4036**
Paediatric Respiratory Reviews (GBR) *Online - full text edition.* **4162**
Pain Management Nursing (USA) *Online - full text edition.* **3759**
Pathology and Oncology Research (GBR) *Online - full text edition.* **3988**
Pesticide Biochemistry and Physiology (USA) *Online - full text edition.* **3159**
Pharmacological Research (GBR) *Online - full text edition.* **4326**
Physical Therapy in Sport (GBR) *Online - full text edition.* **4176**
Placenta (GBR) *Online - full text edition.* **3676**
Preventive Medicine (USA) *Online - full text edition.* **3679**
Prostaglandins, Leukotrienes and Essential Fatty Acids (GBR) *Online - full text edition.* **3868**
Protein Expression and Purification (USA) *Online - full text edition.* **3261**
Pulmonary Pharmacology & Therapeutics (GBR) *Online - full text edition.* **4163**
Radiography (GBR) *Online - full text edition.* **4153**
Regional Anesthesia and Pain Medicine (USA) *Online - full text edition.* **3759**
Regulatory Toxicology and Pharmacology (USA) *Online - full text edition.* **3453**
Research in Veterinary Science (GBR) *Online - full text edition.* **4551**
Respiratory Medicine (GBR) *Online - full text edition.* **4164**
Seizure (GBR) *Online - full text edition.* **4133**
Seminars in Arthritis & Rheumatism (USA) *Online - full text edition.* **4172**
Seminars in Cancer Biology (GBR) *Online - full text edition.* **3349**
Seminars in Cell and Developmental Biology (GBR) *Online - full text edition.* **3294**
Seminars in Immunology (GBR) *Online - full text edition.* **3751**
Seminars in Neonatology (GBR) *Online - full text edition.* **3964**
Seminars in the Neurosciences (USA) *Online - full text edition.* **4133**
Sleep Medicine Reviews (GBR) *Online - full text edition.* **4134**
Solid State Nuclear Magnetic Resonance (GBR) *Online - full text edition.* **3377**
Surgery (USA) *Online - full text edition.* **4204**
Theoretical Population Biology (USA) *Online - full text edition.* **3221**
Tissue & Cell (GBR) *Online - full text edition.* **3294**
Toxicological Sciences (USA) *Online - full text edition.* **3455**
Toxicology and Applied Pharmacology (USA) *Online - full text edition.* **3455**
Tuberculosis (GBR) *Online - full text edition.* **4166**
Ultrasonic Imaging (USA) *Online - full text edition.* **4156**
The Veterinary Journal (GBR) *Online - full text edition.* **4557**
Veterinary Surgery (USA) *Online - full text edition.* **4559**
Virology (USA) *Online - full text edition.* **3332**

Infomart Dialog 1450 Don Mills Rd., Don Mills, ON M3B 2X7, Canada TEL 416-442-2198, FAX 416-445-3508
Canadian Mining Journal (CAN) *Online - full text edition.* **4225**

ingenta 23-28 Hythe Bridge St., Ground Fl., Oxford OX1 2ET, United Kingdom TEL 44-1865-799000, FAX 44-1865-799111, sales@ingenta.com, http://www.ingenta.com
A C C Current Journal Review (USA) *Online - full text edition.* **3714**
A C O G Clinical Review (USA) *Online - full text edition.* **3714**
A N Z Journal of Surgery (AUS) *Online - full text edition.* **4178**
A P M I S (DNK) *Online - full text edition.* **3178**
A R D Online (GBR) *Online - full text edition of* Annals of the Rheumatic Diseases. **4167**
A W H O N N Lifelines (USA) *Online - full text edition.* **4562**
Abstracts in Social Gerontology (USA) *Online - full text edition.* **3482**
Accident Analysis & Prevention (GBR) *Online - full text edition.* **4460**
Acta Anaesthesiologica Scandinavica (DNK) *Online - full text edition.* **3753**
Acta Dermato-Venereologica (NOR) *Online - full text edition.* **3843**
Acta Neurologica Scandinavica (DNK) *Online - full text edition.* **4068**
Acta Obstetrica et Gynecologica Scandinavica (DNK) *Online - full text edition.* **3944**
Acta Odontologica Scandinavica (NOR) *Online - full text edition.* **3813**
Acta Oncologica (NOR) *Online - full text edition.* **3966**
Acta Ophthamologica Scandinavica Online(DNK) *Online - full text.* **3993**
Acta Oto-Laryngologica (NOR) *Online - full text edition.* **4029**
Acta Paediatrica. Supplement (NOR) *Online - full text edition.* **4039**
Acta Physiologica Scandinavica (GBR) *Online - full text edition.* **3337**
Acta Psychiatrica Scandinavica. Supplementum (DNK) *Online - full text edition.* **4069**
Acta Psychologica (NLD) *Online - full text edition.* **4372**
Acta Radiologica (DNK) *Online - full text edition.* **4139**
Acta Tropica (NLD) *Online - full text edition.* **3790**
Acta Zoologica Online(GBR) *Online - full text.* **3350**
Addictive Behaviors (GBR) *Online - full text edition.* **3397**
Advanced Drug Delivery Reviews (NLD) *Online - full text edition.* **4274**
Advances in Colloid and Interface Science (NLD) *Online - full text edition.* **3379**
Advances in Enzyme Regulation (GBR) *Online - full text edition.* **3239**
Advances in Physiotherapy (NOR) *Online - full text edition.* **4058**
Age and Ageing (GBR) *Online - full text edition.* **3466**
Aggression and Violent Behavior (GBR) *Online - full text edition.* **4373**
Alcohol & Alcoholism (GBR) *Online - full text edition.* **3397**
Alcohol (New York) (USA) *Online - full text edition.* **3398**
Alimentary Pharmacology and Therapeutics (GBR) *Online - full text edition.* **3886**
Allergology International (AUS) *Online - full text edition.* **3739**
Allergy. Supplementum (DNK) *Online - full text edition.* **3740**
Ambulatory Child Health Online(GBR) *Online - full text.* **4040**
Ambulatory Surgery (NLD) *Online - full text edition.* **4179**
American Behavioral Scientist (USA) *Online - full text edition.* **4508**
American College of Cardiology. Journal (USA) *Online - full text edition.* **3761**
American College of Surgeons. Journal (USA) *Online - full text edition.* **4179**
The American Journal of Cardiology (USA) *Online - full text edition.* **3762**
American Journal of Clinical Dermatology (USA) *Online - full text edition.* **3844**
American Journal of Hypertension (USA) *Online - full text edition.* **3762**
The American Journal of Medicine (USA) *Online - full text edition.* **3564**
American Journal of Ophthalmology (USA) *Online - full text edition.* **3993**
American Journal of Preventive Medicine (USA) *Online - full text edition.* **3564**
American Journal of Reproductive Immunology Online(DNK) *Online - full text.* **3740**
American Journal of Surgery (USA) *Online - full text edition.* **4180**
Anaerobe (GBR) *Online - full text edition.* **3317**
Anaesthesia (Oxford) (GBR) *Online - full text edition.* **3754**
Analytical Biochemistry (USA) *Online - full text edition.* **3240**
Analytical Cellular Pathology (NLD) *Online - full text edition.* **3285**
Anatomia, Histologia, Embryologia Online(DEU) *Online - full text.* **4537**
Andrologia (DEU) *Online - full text edition.* **3565**
Animal Behaviour (GBR) *Online - full text edition.* **3350**
Animal Feed Science and Technology (NLD) *Online - full text edition.* **3159**
Animal Genetics (GBR) *Online - full text edition.* **3298**
Animal Health Research Reviews (GBR) *Online - full text edition.* **4537**
Animal Reproduction Science (NLD) *Online - full text edition.* **3160**
Annales de Biologie Clinique (FRA) *Online - full text edition.* **3181**
Annales de Genetique (FRA) *Online - full text edition.* **3298**
Annales de Readaptation et de Medecine Physique (FRA) *Online - full text edition.* **4058**
Annales Francaises d'Anesthesie et de Reanimation (FRA) *Online - full text edition.* **3755**
Annals of Applied Biology (GBR) *Online - full text edition.* **3181**
Annals of Epidemiology (USA) *Online - full text edition.* **4461**
Annals of Occupational Hygiene (GBR) *Online - full text edition.* **4250**
Annals of Thoracic Surgery (USA) *Online - full text edition.* **4181**
L' Annee Biologique (FRA) *Online - full text edition.* **3182**
Anti-Cancer Drug Design (GBR) *Online - full text edition.* **3967**
Antimicrobics and Infectious Diseases Newsletter (USA) *Online - full text edition.* **3793**
Antiviral Research (NLD) *Online - full text edition.* **3317**
Appetite (GBR) *Online - full text edition.* **4229**
Applied Animal Behaviour Science (NLD) *Online - full text edition.* **3350**
Applied Behavioral Science Review (GBR) *Online - full text edition.* **4377**
Applied Ergonomics (GBR) *Online - full text edition.* **3431**
Applied Occupational & Environmental Hygiene (USA) *Online - full text edition.* **4250**
Applied Psychological Measurement (USA) *Online - full text edition.* **4377**
Applied Psychology (GBR) *Online - full text edition.* **4377**
Applied Radiation and Isotopes (GBR) *Online - full text edition.* **4365**
Aquatic Toxicology (NLD) *Online - full text edition.* **3445**
Archives de Pediatrie (FRA) *Online - full text edition.* **4040**
Archives of Biochemistry and Biophysics (USA) *Online - full text edition.* **3241**
Archives of Clinical Neuropsychology (GBR) *Online - full text edition.* **4074**
Archives of Disease in Childhood (GBR) *Online - full text edition.* **4040**
Archives of Gerontology and Geriatrics (IRL) *Online - full text edition.* **3468**
Archives of Medical Research (MEX) *Online - full text edition.* **3568**
Archives of Oral Biology (GBR) *Online - full text edition.* **3351**

Artificial Intelligence in Medicine (NLD) *Online - full text edition.* **3389**
Artificial Organs (USA) *Online - full text edition.* **3871**
The Arts in Psychotherapy (GBR) *Online - full text edition.* **4378**
Asia Pacific Journal of Clinical Nutrition (AUS) *Online - full text edition.* **4229**
Asian Journal of Social Psychology (GBR) *Online - full text edition.* **4378**
Association of Nurses in AIDS Care. Journal (USA) *Online - full text edition.* **3793**
Atherosclerosis (IRL) *Online - full text edition.* **3763**
Atmospheric Environment (GBR) *Online - full text edition.* **3443**
Auris, Nasus, Larynx (NLD) *Online - full text edition.* **4031**
Austral Ecology (AUS) *Online - full text edition.* **3183**
Australasian Journal of Dermatology (AUS) *Online - full text edition.* **3845**
Australasian Psychiatry (AUS) *Online - full text edition.* **4075**
Australasian Radiology (AUS) *Online - full text edition.* **4140**
Australian and New Zealand Journal of Family Therapy (GBR) *Online - full text edition.* **4520**
Australian and New Zealand Journal of Mental Health Nursing (AUS) *Online - full text edition.* **4075**
Australian & New Zealand Journal of Psychiatry (AUS) *Online - full text edition.* **4075**
Australian Journal of Rural Health (AUS) *Online - full text edition.* **4463**
Australian Occupational Therapy Journal (AUS) *Online - full text edition.* **4059**
Autism (GBR) *Online - full text edition.* **4075**
Autonomic & Autacoid Pharmacology (GBR) *Online - full text edition.* **4279**
Autonomic Neuroscience: Basic & Clinical (NLD) *Online - full text edition.* **4075**
B B A - Bioenergetics (NLD) *Online - full text edition.* **3278**
B B A - Biomembranes (NLD) *Online - full text edition.* **3285**
B B A - Gene Structure and Expression (NLD) *Online - full text edition.* **3299**
B B A - General Subjects (NLD) *Online - full text edition.* **3241**
B B A - Molecular and Cell Biology of Lipids (NLD) *Online - full text edition.* **3242**
B B A - Molecular Basis of Disease (NLD) *Online - full text edition.* **3299**
B B A - Molecular Cell Research (NLD) *Online - full text edition.* **3285**
B B A - Protein Structure and Molecular Enzymology (NLD) *Online - full text edition.* **3242**
B B A - Reviews on Cancer (NLD) *Online - full text edition.* **3968**
B J O Online (GBR) *Online - full text edition of* British Journal of Ophthalmology. **3994**
B J S M Online (GBR) *Online - full text edition of* British Journal of Sports Medicine. **4173**
B J U International (GBR) *Online - full text edition.* **4210**
Behavior Modification (USA) *Online - full text edition.* **4380**
Behavioral Ecology (USA) *Online - full text edition.* **3184**
Behaviour Research and Therapy (GBR) *Online - full text edition.* **4382**
Behavioural Brain Research (NLD) *Online - full text edition.* **4076**
Behavioural Processes (NLD) *Online - full text edition.* **4076**
Biochemical and Biophysical Research Communications (USA) *Online - full text edition.* **3242**
Biochemical Journal (GBR) *Online - full text edition.* **3242**
Biochemical Pharmacology (USA) *Online - full text edition.* **4279**
Biochemical Systematics and Ecology (GBR) *Online - full text edition.* **3243**
Biochemistry and Molecular Biology Education (GBR) *Online - full text edition.* **3243**
Biochimie (FRA) *Online - full text edition.* **3244**
BioDrugs (NZL) *Online - full text edition.* **4280**
Bioelectrochemistry (CHE) *Online - full text edition.* **3244**
Bioethics (GBR) *Online - full text edition.* **4346**
Biofutur (FRA) *Online - full text edition.* **3269**
Biological Control (USA) *Online - full text edition.* **3185**
Biological Psychiatry (USA) *Online - full text edition.* **4076**
Biological Psychology (NLD) *Online - full text edition.* **4382**
Biological Research for Nursing (USA) *Online - full text edition.* **3914**
Biologicals (GBR) *Online - full text edition.* **3186**
Biology of the Cell (FRA) *Online - full text edition.* **3286**
Biomaterials (GBR) *Online - full text edition.* **3575**
Biomedical Materials (GBR) *Online - full text edition.* **3576**
Biomedicine and Pharmacotherapy (FRA) *Online - full text edition.* **3577**
Biometrika (GBR) *Online - full text edition.* **3226**
Biomolecular Engineering (NLD) *Online - full text edition.* **3269**
Bioorganic & Medicinal Chemistry (GBR) *Online - full text edition.* **3377**
Bioorganic & Medicinal Chemistry Letters (GBR) *Online - full text edition.* **3378**
Biophysical Chemistry (NLD) *Online - full text edition.* **3265**
Biophysics (RUS) *Online - full text edition.* **3265**
Biorheology (NLD) *Online - full text edition.* **3265**
Biosensors and Bioelectronics (GBR) *Online - full text edition.* **3270**
Biosystems (IRL) *Online - full text edition.* **3187**
Biotechnology Advances (USA) *Online - full text edition.* **3271**
Bipolar Disorders Online(DNK) *Online - full text.* **4077**
Birth (USA) *Online - full text edition.* **3946**
Blood Cells, Molecules, and Diseases (USA) *Online - full text edition.* **3898**
Blood Pressure (NOR) *Online - full text edition.* **3764**
Bone (USA) *Online - full text edition.* **4011**
Bone Marrow Transplantation (GBR) *Online - full text edition.* **3872**
Brain (GBR) *Online - full text edition.* **4077**
Brain and Cognition (USA) *Online - full text edition.* **4383**
Brain and Development (NLD) *Online - full text edition.* **4077**
Brain and Language (USA) *Online - full text edition.* **4383**
Brain, Behavior, and Immunity (USA) *Online - full text edition.* **3741**
Brain Research (NLD) *Online - full text edition.* **4078**
Brain Research Bulletin (USA) *Online - full text edition.* **4078**
Brain Research Protocols (NLD) *Online - full text edition.* **4078**
Brain Research Reviews (NLD) *Online - full text edition.* **4078**
Breast Disease (NLD) *Online - full text edition.* **3946**
The Breast Journal Online(USA) *Online - full text.* **3946**
British Food Journal (GBR) *Online - full text edition.* **3460**
British Homeopathic Journal (GBR) *Online - full text edition.* **3786**
British Journal of Clinical Governance (GBR) *Online - full text edition.* **3578**
British Journal of Clinical Pharmacology (GBR) *Online - full text edition.* **4281**
The British Journal of Criminology (GBR) *Online - full text edition.* **3393**
British Journal of Dermatology (GBR) *Online - full text edition.* **3845**
British Journal of Haematology (GBR) *Online - full text edition.* **3899**
British Journal of Learning Disabilities (GBR) *Online - full text edition.* **4079**
The British Journal of Nutrition (GBR) *Online - full text edition.* **4230**
British Journal of Special Education (GBR) *Online - full text edition.* **3419**
British Journal of Surgery (GBR) *Online - full text edition.* **4183**
Bulletin of Mathematical Biology (GBR) *Online - full text edition.* **3188**
Burns (GBR) *Online - full text edition.* **4011**
C N S Drugs (NZL) *Online - full text edition.* **4282**
Cancer Detection and Prevention (USA) *Online - full text edition.* **3970**
Cancer Gene Therapy (USA) *Online - full text edition.* **3971**
Cancer Genetics & Cytogenetics (USA) *Online - full text edition.* **3971**
Cancer Letters (IRL) *Online - full text edition.* **3972**
Cancer Practice Online(USA) *Online - full text.* **3972**
Cancer - Radiotherapie (FRA) *Online - full text edition.* **3972**
Carcinogenesis (GBR) *Online - full text edition.* **3974**
Cardiovascular Pathology (USA) *Online - full text edition.* **3767**
Cardiovascular Radiation Medicine (USA) *Online - full text edition.* **3767**
Cardiovascular Research (NLD) *Online - full text edition.* **3767**
Cardiovascular Surgery (GBR) *Online - full text edition.* **3767**
Cell (USA) *Online - full text edition.* **3286**
Cell Death and Differentiation (GBR) *Online - full text edition.* **3287**
Cell Proliferation (GBR) *Online - full text edition.* **3287**
Cell Transplantation (USA) *Online - full text edition.* **3288**
Cellular Immunology (USA) *Online - full text edition.* **3742**
Cellular Signalling (USA) *Online - full text edition.* **3288**
Cephalalgia (GBR) *Online - full text edition.* **4080**
Cerebral Cortex (USA) *Online - full text edition.* **4081**
Chemical Health and Safety (USA) *Online - full text edition.* **3446**
Chemical Senses (GBR) *Online - full text edition.* **3340**
Chemico-Biological Interactions (IRL) *Online - full text edition.* **3447**
Chemistry & Biology (GBR) *Online - full text edition.* **3372**
Chemistry and Physics of Lipids (IRL) *Online - full text edition.* **3246**
Chemosphere (GBR) *Online - full text edition.* **3447**
Child Abuse & Neglect (GBR) *Online - full text edition.* **3381**
Child Abuse Review (GBR) *Online - full text edition.* **4511**
Child: Care, Health and Development (GBR) *Online - full text edition.* **4042**
Child Language Teaching and Therapy (GBR) *Online - full text edition.* **3420**
Child Maltreatment (USA) *Online - full text edition.* **3381**
Childhood (GBR) *Online - full text edition.* **3382**
Children & Society (GBR) *Online - full text edition.* **3382**
Children and Youth Services Review (GBR) *Online - full text edition.* **3382**
Chinese Journal of Digestive Diseases Online(AUS) *Online - full text.* **3887**
Cladistics (GBR) *Online - full text edition.* **3191**
Clinica Chimica Acta (NLD) *Online - full text edition.* **3585**
Clinical and Applied Immunology Reviews (USA) *Online - full text edition.* **3742**
Clinical and Experimental Allergy (GBR) *Online - full text edition.* **3742**
Clinical and Experimental Dermatology (GBR) *Online - full text edition.* **3846**
Clinical and Experimental Immunology (GBR) *Online - full text edition.* **3742**
Clinical and Experimental Ophthalmology (AUS) *Online - full text edition.* **3995**
Clinical and Experimental Pharmacology & Physiology (AUS) *Online - full text edition.* **3341**
Clinical and Laboratory Haematology (GBR) *Online - full text edition.* **3899**
Clinical Biochemistry (USA) *Online - full text edition.* **3247**
Clinical Biomechanics (GBR) *Online - full text edition.* **3787**
Clinical Child Psychology & Psychiatry (GBR) *Online - full text edition.* **3382**
Clinical Drug Investigation (NZL) *Online - full text edition.* **4283**
Clinical Endocrinology (GBR) *Online - full text edition.* **3856**
Clinical Genetics (DNK) *Online - full text edition.* **3300**
Clinical Hemorheology and Microcirculation (NLD) *Online - full text edition.* **3899**
Clinical Imaging (USA) *Online - full text edition.* **4141**
Clinical Immunology (USA) *Online - full text edition.* **3743**
Clinical Microbiology and Infection (GBR) *Online - full text edition.* **3586**
Clinical Microbiology Newsletter (USA) *Online - full text edition.* **3319**
Clinical Neurology and Neurosurgery (NLD) *Online - full text edition.* **4082**
Clinical Neurophysiology (IRL) *Online - full text edition.* **4082**
Clinical Neuroscience Research (NLD) *Online - full text edition.* **4082**
Clinical Nursing Research (USA) *Online - full text edition.* **3916**
Clinical Oral Implants Research (DNK) *Online - full text edition.* **3818**
Clinical Orthodontics and Research Online(DNK) *Online - full text.* **3818**
Clinical Otolaryngology and Allied Sciences (GBR) *Online - full text edition.* **4031**
Clinical Performance and Quality Health Care (GBR) *Online - full text edition.* **3587**
Clinical Pharmacokinetics (NZL) *Online - full text edition.* **4284**
Clinical Physiology and Functional Imaging (GBR) *Online - full text edition.* **3587**
Clinical Psychology (USA) *Online - full text edition.* **4388**
Clinical Psychology Review (GBR) *Online - full text edition.* **4388**
Clinical Rehabilitation (GBR) *Online - full text edition.* **4060**
Clinical Therapeutics (USA) *Online - full text edition.* **3587**
Clinical Transplantation (DNK) *Online - full text edition.* **4185**
Clinics in Dermatology (USA) *Online - full text edition.* **3846**
Cognition (NLD) *Online - full text edition.* **4388**
Cognitive Brain Research (NLD) *Online - full text edition.* **4083**
Cognitive Development (GBR) *Online - full text edition.* **4389**
Cognitive Psychology (USA) *Online - full text edition.* **4389**
Cognitive Science (GBR) *Online - full text edition.* **4389**
College of Surgeons Hong Kong. Annals (AUS) *Online - full text edition.* **4185**
Colorectal Disease Online(GBR) *Online - full text.* **3887**
Combinatorial Chemistry & High Throughput Screening (USA) *Online - full text edition.* **3372**
Comparative Biochemistry and Physiology. Part A: Molecular & Integrative Physiology (USA) *Online - full text edition.* **3341**
Comparative Biochemistry and Physiology. Part B: Biochemistry & Molecular Biology (USA) *Online - full text edition.* **3247**
Comparative Biochemistry and Physiology. Toxicology & Pharmacology (USA) *Online - full text edition.* **3247**
Comparative Immunology, Microbiology and Infectious Diseases (GBR) *Online - full text edition.* **3320**
Comparative Political Studies (USA) *Online - full text edition.* **4367**
Computer Methods and Programs in Biomedicine (IRL) *Online - full text edition.* **3809**
Computerized Medical Imaging and Graphics (GBR) *Online - full text edition.* **3809**
Computers in Biology and Medicine (GBR) *Online - full text edition.* **3284**
Computers in Human Behavior (GBR) *Online - full text edition.* **4524**
Connective Tissue Research (CHE) *Online - full text edition.* **3288**
Consciousness and Cognition (USA) *Online - full text edition.* **4391**
Consciousness & Emotion (NLD) *Online - full content edition.* **4391**
Conservation Biology (USA) *Online - full text edition.* **3392**
Contact Dermatitis (DNK) *Online - full text edition.* **3846**
Contact Lens & Anterior Eye (GBR) *Online - full text edition.* **3995**
Contemporary Educational Psychology (USA) *Online - full text edition.* **3410**
Contraception (USA) *Online - full text edition.* **3357**
Controlled Clinical Trials (USA) *Online - full text edition.* **3873**
The Counseling Psychologist (USA) *Online - full text edition.* **4392**
Criminal Justice & Behavior (USA) *Online - full text edition.* **3394**
Critical Reviews in Oncology - Hematology (IRL) *Online - full text edition.* **3975**
Cross-Cultural Research (USA) *Online - full text edition.* **4508**
Cryobiology (USA) *Online - full text edition.* **3266**
Culture & Psychology (GBR) *Online - full text edition.* **4393**
Current Biology (GBR) *Online - full text edition.* **3229**
Current Directions in Psychological Science (USA) *Online - full text edition.* **4393**

Current Opinion in Biotechnology (GBR) *Online - full text edition.* **3273**
Current Opinion in Cell Biology (GBR) *Online - full text edition.* **3288**
Current Opinion in Genetics & Development (GBR) *Online - full text edition.* **3301**
Current Opinion in Immunology (GBR) *Online - full text edition.* **3722**
Current Opinion in Neurobiology (GBR) *Online - full text edition.* **4084**
Current Opinion in Structural Biology (GBR) *Online - full text edition.* **3248**
Current Pharmaceutical Design (USA) *Online - full text edition.* **4286**
Current Surgery (USA) *Online - full text edition.* **4186**
Current Therapeutic Research (USA) *Online - full text edition.* **3592**
Cytokine (GBR) *Online - full text edition.* **3301**
Cytokine and Growth Factor Reviews (GBR) *Online - full text edition.* **3248**
Cytopathology (GBR) *Online - full text edition.* **3289**
D N A Sequence (CHE) *Online - full text edition.* **3248**
Dental Materials (USA) *Online - full text edition.* **3820**
Dental Traumatology Online(DNK) *Online - full text.* **3821**
Dentomaxillofacial Radiology (GBR) *Online - full text edition.* **4143**
Dermatologic Surgery Online(USA) *Online - full text.* **4187**
Dermatologic Therapy (DNK) *Online - full text edition.* **3847**
Development, Growth and Differentiation (AUS) *Online - full text edition.* **3192**
Developmental and Comparative Immunology (GBR) *Online - full text edition.* **3743**
Developmental Biology (USA) *Online - full text edition.* **3193**
Developmental Brain Research (NLD) *Online - full text edition.* **4086**
Developmental Review (USA) *Online - full text edition.* **4394**
Developmental Science (GBR) *Online - full text edition.* **4394**
Diabetes, Obesity and Metabolism Online(GBR) *Online - full text.* **3858**
Diabetes Research and Clinical Practice (IRL) *Online - full text edition.* **3858**
Diabetic Medicine Online(GBR) *Online - full text.* **3860**
Diagnostic Microbiology and Infectious Disease (USA) *Online - full text edition.* **3320**
Digestive Endoscopy Online(AUS) *Online - full text.* **3889**
Disaster Prevention and Management (GBR) *Online - full text edition.* **4466**
Discourse & Society (GBR) *Online - full text edition.* **4395**
Discourse Studies (GBR) *Online - full text edition.* **3550**
Disease Management and Clinical Outcomes (USA) *Online - full text edition.* **3595**
Disease Management & Health Outcomes (NZL) *Online - full text edition.* **3595**
Diseases of the Esophagus Online(AUS) *Online - full text.* **4032**
Domestic Animal Endocrinology (USA) *Online - full text edition.* **4542**
Drug and Alcohol Dependence (IRL) *Online - full text edition.* **3400**
Drug Discovery Today (GBR) *Online - full text edition.* **4288**
Drug Resistance Update (GBR) *Online - full text edition.* **3596**
Drug Safety (NZL) *Online - full text edition.* **4289**
Drugs (NZL) *Online - full text edition.* **4290**
Drugs & Aging (NZL) *Online - full text edition.* **4290**
Dyslexia (GBR) *Online - full text edition.* **3421**
e A D C - F & N (GBR) *Online - full text edition of* Archives of Disease in Childhood. Fetal and Neonatal Edition. **3945**
The E M B O Journal (GBR) *Online - full text edition.* **3249**
E M J Online (GBR) *Online - full text edition of* Emergency Medicine Journal. **4014**
Early Human Development (IRL) *Online - full text edition.* **3948**
Eating Behaviors (NLD) *Online - full text edition.* **4395**
Ecography (DNK) *Online - full text edition.* **3437**
Ecotoxicology and Environmental Safety - Online (USA) *Online - full text edition of* Ecotoxicology and Environmental Safety. **3448**
Educational and Psychological Measurement (USA) *Online - full text edition.* **4396**
Emergency Medicine (Carleton South) (AUS) *Online - full text edition.* **4013**
Emotional and Behavioural Difficulties (GBR) *Online - full text edition.* **3421**
Environment and Behavior (USA) *Online - full text edition.* **4521**
Environment International (GBR) *Online - full text edition.* **3438**
Environmental Management & Health (GBR) *Online - full text edition.* **3438**
Environmental Microbiology (GBR) *Online - full text edition.* **3321**
Environmental Research (USA) *Online - full text edition.* **3439**
Environmental Toxicology and Pharmacology (NLD) *Online - full text edition.* **3449**
Enzyme and Microbial Technology (USA) *Online - full text edition.* **3273**
Epilepsy and Behavior (USA) *Online - full text edition.* **3598**
Epilepsy Research (NLD) *Online - full text edition.* **4088**
Ethology Online(DEU) *Online - full text.* **3352**
European Academy of Dermatology and Venereology. Journal (BEL) *Online - full text edition.* **3848**
European Biotechnology Newsletter (FRA) *Online - full text edition.* **3274**
European Eating Disorders Review (GBR) *Online - full text edition.* **4397**
European Heart Journal (GBR) *Online - full text edition.* **3771**
European Journal of Anaesthesiology (GBR) *Online - full text edition.* **3757**
European Journal of Biochemistry (GBR) *Online - full text edition.* **3249**
European Journal of Cancer (GBR) *Online - full text edition.* **3977**
European Journal of Cancer Care Online(GBR) *Online - full text.* **3977**
European Journal of Cardio-Thoracic Surgery (NLD) *Online - full text edition.* **3771**
European Journal of Clinical Investigation (GBR) *Online - full text edition.* **3599**
European Journal of Clinical Nutrition (GBR) *Online - full text edition.* **4232**
European Journal of Dental Education Online(DNK) *Online - full text.* **3822**
European Journal of Haematology (DNK) *Online - full text edition.* **3900**
The European Journal of Heart Failure (NLD) *Online - full text edition.* **3771**
European Journal of Human Genetics (GBR) *Online - full text edition.* **3302**
European Journal of Immunogenetics (GBR) *Online - full text edition.* **3302**
European Journal of Internal Medicine (USA) *Online - full text edition.* **3908**
European Journal of Medicinal Chemistry (FRA) *Online - full text edition.* **3250**
European Journal of Neurology (USA) *Online - full text edition.* **4089**
European Journal of Neuroscience (GBR) *Online - full text edition.* **4089**
European Journal of Obstetrics & Gynecology and Reproductive Biology (IRL) *Online - full text edition.* **3949**
European Journal of Orthodontics (GBR) *Online - full content edition.* **3823**
European Journal of Personality (GBR) *Online - full text edition.* **4398**
European Journal of Pharmaceutical Sciences (NLD) *Online - full text edition.* **4292**
European Journal of Pharmaceutics and Biopharmaceutics (NLD) *Online - full text edition.* **4293**
European Journal of Pharmacology (NLD) *Online - full text edition.* **4293**
European Journal of Public Health (GBR) *Online - full text edition.* **4468**
European Journal of Radiology (IRL) *Online - full text edition.* **4144**
European Journal of Soil Biology (FRA) *Online - full text edition.* **3195**
European Journal of Surgery (NOR) *Online - full text edition.* **4188**
European Journal of Ultrasound (IRL) *Online - full text edition.* **4144**
European Neuropsychopharmacology (NLD) *Online - full text edition.* **4089**
European Psychiatry (FRA) *Online - full text edition.* **4089**
Evaluation and the Health Professions (USA) *Online - full text edition.* **3600**
Evidence - Based Dentistry (GBR) *Online - full text edition.* **3823**
Evolution & Development Online(USA) *Online - full text.* **3195**
L' Evolution Psychiatrique (FRA) *Online - full text edition.* **4090**
Excerpta Medica. Section 35: Occupational Health and Industrial Medicine (NLD) *Online - full text edition.* **3726**
Experimental and Molecular Pathology (USA) *Online - full text edition.* **3600**
Experimental Biology and Medicine (Maywood) (USA) *Online - full text edition.* **3195**
Experimental Dermatology Online(DNK) *Online - full text.* **3849**
Experimental Eye Research (GBR) *Online - full text edition.* **3997**
Experimental Gerontology (USA) *Online - full text edition.* **3471**
Experimental Hematology (USA) *Online - full text edition.* **3901**
Experimental Neurology (USA) *Online - full text edition.* **4090**
Experimental Parasitology (USA) *Online - full text edition.* **3796**
F E B S Letters (NLD) *Online - full text edition.* **3250**
F E M S Immunology and Medical Microbiology (NLD) *Online - full text edition.* **3321**
F E M S Microbiology Ecology (NLD) *Online - full text edition.* **3321**
F E M S Microbiology Letters (NLD) *Online - full text edition.* **3322**
F E M S Microbiology Reviews (NLD) *Online - full text edition.* **3322**
The Family Journal (USA) *Online - full text edition.* **4399**
Family Practice (GBR) *Online - full text edition.* **3601**
Il Farmaco (FRA) *Online - full text edition.* **4295**
Feminism & Psychology (GBR) *Online - full text edition.* **4399**
Fertility and Sterility (USA) *Online - full text edition.* **3949**
Fish and Shellfish Immunology (GBR) *Online - full text edition.* **3196**
Fitoterapia (ITA) *Online - full text edition.* **3279**
Food and Chemical Toxicology (GBR) *Online - full text edition.* **3449**
Food Microbiology (GBR) *Online - full text edition.* **3322**
Foot and Ankle Surgery (GBR) *Online - full text edition.* **4189**
Forensic Science International (IRL) *Online - full text edition.* **3882**
Free Radical Biology & Medicine (USA) *Online - full text edition.* **3197**
Freshwater Biology Online(GBR) *Online - full text.* **3197**
Frontiers in Neuroendocrinology (USA) *Online - full text edition.* **3862**
Fundamental and Clinical Pharmacology (FRA) *Online - full text edition.* **4297**
Gait and Posture (NLD) *Online - full text edition.* **3605**
Games and Economic Behavior (USA) *Online - full text edition.* **4400**
Gene - C O M B I S (NLD) *Online - full text edition of* Gene. **3274**
Gene Therapy (Basingstoke) (GBR) *Online - full text edition.* **3606**
General and Comparative Endocrinology (USA) *Online - full text edition.* **3863**
General Hospital Psychiatry (USA) *Online - full text edition.* **4091**
General Pharmacology (USA) *Online - full text edition.* **4297**
Genes and Immunity (GBR) *Online - full text edition.* **3303**
Genes to Cells (GBR) *Online - full text edition.* **3303**
Genescreen (GBR) *Online - full text edition.* **3304**
Genetics, Selection, Evolution Online (FRA) *Online - full text edition of* Genetics, Selection, Evolution. **3305**
Genomics (USA) *Online - full text edition.* **3306**
Glycobiology (GBR) *Online - full text edition.* **3251**
Group Analysis (GBR) *Online - full text edition.* **4401**
Group & Organization Management (USA) *Online - full text edition.* **3411**
Gut Online (GBR) *Online - full text edition of* Gut. **3891**
Gynaecological Endoscopy (GBR) *Online - full text edition.* **3951**
Gynecologic Oncology (USA) *Online - full text edition.* **3952**
Gynecologie Obstetrique et Fertilite (FRA) *Online - full text edition.* **3952**
H I V Medicine (GBR) *Online - full text edition.* **3796**
H P B Surgery (CHE) *Online - full text edition.* **4190**
Haemophilia Online(GBR) *Online - full text.* **3901**
Harvard Review of Psychiatry (GBR) *Online - full text edition.* **4093**
Hazardous Waste Consultant (USA) *Online - full text edition.* **3457**
Headache Online(USA) *Online - full text.* **4093**
Health (GBR) *Online - full text edition.* **4471**
Health & Place (GBR) *Online - full text edition.* **3465**
Health and Social Care in the Community Online(GBR) *Online - full text.* **4472**
Health Education (GBR) *Online - full text edition.* **4354**
Health Education & Behavior (USA) *Online - full text edition.* **4472**
Health Education Research (GBR) *Online - full text edition.* **4513**
Health Expectations (GBR) *Online - full text edition.* **4473**
Health Information and Libraries Journal Online(GBR) *Online - full text.* **3547**
Health Policy (IRL) *Online - full text edition.* **4473**
Health Policy and Planning (GBR) *Online - full text edition.* **4473**
Health Promotion Practice (USA) *Online - full text edition.* **4474**
Hearing Research (NLD) *Online - full text edition.* **4033**
Heart, Lung & Circulation Online(AUS) *Online - full text.* **3773**
Heart Online (GBR) *Online - full text edition of* Heart. **3772**
Helicobacter (USA) *Online - full text edition.* **3323**
The Hematology Journal (GBR) *Online - full text edition.* **3773**
Hepatology Research (IRL) *Online - full text edition.* **3892**
Heredity (GBR) *Online - full text edition.* **3307**
Hispanic Journal of Behavioral Sciences (USA) *Online - full text edition.* **4402**
Histopathology (GBR) *Online - full text edition.* **3979**
Homicide Studies (USA) *Online - full text edition.* **3394**
Hormones and Behavior (USA) *Online - full text edition.* **3863**
Human & Experimental Toxicology (GBR) *Online - full text edition.* **3450**
Human Immunology (USA) *Online - full text edition.* **3744**
Human Molecular Genetics (GBR) *Online - full text edition.* **3308**
Human Movement Science (NLD) *Online - full text edition.* **3616**
Human Relations (USA) *Online - full text edition.* **4509**
Human Reproduction (GBR) *Online - full text edition.* **3953**
Human Reproduction Update (GBR) *Online - full text edition.* **3232**
I T B M - R B M (FRA) *Online - full text edition.* **3275**
I T B M - R B M News (FRA) *Online - full text edition.* **3275**
Illness, Crisis, and Loss (USA) *Online - full text edition.* **4521**
Immunity (USA) *Online - full text edition.* **3745**
Immunoanalyse et Biologie Specialisee (FRA) *Online - full text edition.* **3200**
Immunology (GBR) *Online - full text edition.* **3746**
Immunology and Cell Biology (AUS) *Online - full text edition.* **3746**
Immunology Letters (NLD) *Online - full text edition.* **3746**
Immunotechnology (NLD) *Online - full text edition.* **3746**
In Vitro Cellular & Developmental Biology - Plant (USA) *Online - full text edition.* **3280**
Indoor Air Online(DNK) *Online - full text.* **4476**
Industrial Crops and Products (NLD) *Online - full text edition.* **3158**
Infant Behavior and Development (GBR) *Online - full text edition.* **4404**
Injury (GBR) *Online - full text edition.* **4016**
Injury Prevention (GBR) *Online - full text edition.* **4045**
Inpharma Weekly (NZL) *Online - full text edition.* **4345**
Institut Pasteur. Annales. Actualites (FRA) *Online - full text edition.* **3323**
Institution of Mechanical Engineers. Proceedings. Part H: Journal of Engineering in Medicine (GBR) *Online - full text edition.* **3238**

Intelligence (Kidlington) (GBR) *Online - full text edition.* **4404**
International Commission on Radiological Protection. Annals (GBR) *Online - full text edition.* **4145**
International Contact Lens Clinic (USA) *Online - full text edition.* **3999**
International Endodontic Journal Online(GBR) *Online - full text.* **3826**
International Forum of Psychoanalysis (NOR) *Online - full text edition.* **4405**
International Immunology (GBR) *Online - full text edition.* **3747**
International Immunopharmacology (GBR) *Online - full text edition.* **4302**
International Journal for Parasitology (GBR) *Online - full text edition.* **3799**
International Journal for Quality in Health Care (GBR) *Online - full text edition.* **3622**
The International Journal of Action Methods (USA) *Online - full text edition.* **4405**
International Journal of Andrology (GBR) *Online - full text edition.* **4213**
International Journal of Antimicrobial Agents (NLD) *Online - full text edition.* **3323**
International Journal of Biochemistry & Cell Biology (GBR) *Online - full text edition.* **3252**
International Journal of Biological Macromolecules (NLD) *Online - full text edition.* **3252**
International Journal of Cardiology (IRL) *Online - full text edition.* **3775**
International Journal of Cosmetic Science (GBR) *Online - full text edition.* **3176**
International Journal of Dermatology (GBR) *Online - full text edition.* **3850**
International Journal of Developmental Neuroscience (GBR) *Online - full text edition.* **4095**
International Journal of Drug Policy (NLD) *Online - full text edition.* **3402**
International Journal of Epidemiology (GBR) *Online - full text edition.* **3623**
International Journal of Experimental Pathology (GBR) *Online - full text edition.* **3623**
International Journal of Food Microbiology (NLD) *Online - full text edition.* **3324**
International Journal of Gynecological Cancer (USA) *Online - full text edition.* **3953**
International Journal of Gynecology and Obstetrics (IRL) *Online - full text edition.* **3954**
International Journal of Health Care Quality Assurance (GBR) *Online - full text edition.* **3623**
International Journal of Hematology (JPN) *Online - full text edition.* **3903**
International Journal of Impotence Research (GBR) *Online - full text edition.* **4213**
International Journal of Law and Psychiatry (GBR) *Online - full text edition.* **3540**
International Journal of Medical Informatics (IRL) *Online - full text edition.* **3811**
International Journal of Nursing Practice (AUS) *Online - full text edition.* **3921**
International Journal of Nursing Studies (GBR) *Online - full text edition.* **3922**
International Journal of Obesity (GBR) *Online - full text edition.* **4236**
International Journal of Offender Therapy and Comparative Criminology (USA) *Online - full text edition.* **3394**
International Journal of Pediatric Otorhinolaryngology (IRL) *Online - full text edition.* **4033**
International Journal of Pharmaceutics (NLD) *Online - full text edition.* **4303**
International Journal of Psychophysiology (NLD) *Online - full text edition.* **4407**
International Journal of Radiation: Oncology - Biology - Physics (USA) *Online - full text edition.* **4146**
International Journal of Urology (AUS) *Online - full text edition.* **4213**
International Nursing Review Online(GBR) *Online - full text.* **3922**
Interventional Cardiology Newsletter (USA) *Online - full text edition.* **3775**
Isokinetics and Exercise Science (NLD) *Online - full text edition.* **4174**
Issues in Interdisciplinary Care (USA) *Online - full text edition.* **3625**
J A H Online (USA) *Online - full text edition of* Journal of Adolescent Health. **3629**
J C P Online (GBR) *Online - full text edition of* Journal of Clinical Pathology. **3631**
J E C H Online (GBR) *Online - full text edition of* Journal of Epidemiology & Community Health. **3632**
J M B Online (GBR) *Online - full text edition of* Journal of Molecular Biology. **3254**
J M E Online (GBR) *Online - full text edition of* Journal of Medical Ethics. **3635**
J M G Online (GBR) *Online - full text edition of* Journal of Medical Genetics. **3310**
J M S Online (GBR) *Online - full text edition of* Journal of Medical Screening. **3802**
J O G N N (USA) *Online - full text edition.* **3923**
Japanese Journal of Cancer Research (GBR) *Online - full text edition.* **3981**
Japanese Journal of Clinical Oncology (GBR) *Online - full text edition.* **3981**
Japanese Journal of Ophthalmology (NLD) *Online - full text edition.* **4000**
Japanese Psychological Research (JPN) *Online - full text edition.* **4408**
Journal de Pediatrie et de Puericulture (FRA) *Online - full text edition.* **3628**
Journal for Specialists in Group Work (USA) *Online - full text edition.* **4408**
Journal for the Theory of Social Behaviour (GBR) *Online - full text edition.* **4408**
Journal Midwifery and Women's Health (USA) *Online - full text edition.* **3955**
Journal of Adolescence (GBR) *Online - full text edition.* **3383**
Journal of Adolescent Research (USA) *Online - full text edition.* **4409**
Journal of Advanced Nursing (GBR) *Online - full text edition.* **3923**
Journal of Affective Disorders (NLD) *Online - full text edition.* **4098**
Journal of Aging and Health (USA) *Online - full text edition.* **3474**
Journal of Aging Studies (GBR) *Online - full text edition.* **3475**
Journal of Analytical Psychology (GBR) *Online - full text edition.* **4409**
Journal of Analytical Toxicology (USA) *Online - full text edition.* **3451**
Journal of Animal Ecology (GBR) *Online - full text edition.* **3202**
Journal of Animal Physiology and Animal Nutrition Online(DEU) *Online - full text.* **3344**
Journal of Antimicrobial Chemotherapy (GBR) *Online - full text edition.* **3800**
Journal of Anxiety Disorders (GBR) *Online - full text edition.* **4409**
Journal of Applied Behavioral Science (USA) *Online - full text edition.* **4410**
Journal of Applied Developmental Psychology (GBR) *Online - full text edition.* **4410**
Journal of Applied Gerontology (USA) *Online - full text edition.* **3475**
Journal of Applied Microbiology (GBR) *Online - full text edition.* **3324**
Journal of Applied Research in Intellectual Disabilities (GBR) *Online - full text edition.* **4098**
Journal of Autoimmunity (GBR) *Online - full text edition.* **3748**
Journal of Back and Musculoskeletal Rehabilitation (NLD) *Online - full text edition.* **4017**
The Journal of Behavior Therapy and Experimental Psychiatry (GBR) *Online - full text edition.* **4099**
Journal of Biochemical and Biophysical Methods (NLD) *Online - full text edition.* **3252**
Journal of Biological Rhythms (USA) *Online - full text edition.* **4099**
The Journal of Biomechanics (GBR) *Online - full text edition.* **3629**
Journal of Biomedical Informatics (USA) *Online - full text edition.* **3811**
Journal of Bioscience and Bioengineering (JPN) *Online - full text edition.* **3238**
Journal of Biotechnology (NLD) *Online - full text edition.* **3275**
Journal of Black Psychology (USA) *Online - full text edition.* **4410**
Journal of Black Studies (USA) *Online - full text edition.* **4509**
Journal of Cataract and Refractive Surgery (USA) *Online - full text edition.* **4000**
Journal of Chemical Neuroanatomy (NLD) *Online - full text edition.* **4099**
Journal of Child Psychology & Psychiatry & Allied Disciplines (GBR) *Online - full text edition.* **4411**
Journal of Chromatography. B, Biomedical Sciences and Applications (NLD) *Online - full text edition.* **3373**
The Journal of Clinical Anesthesia (USA) *Online - full text edition.* **3758**
The Journal of Clinical Epidemiology (USA) *Online - full text edition.* **3630**
Journal of Clinical Nursing (GBR) *Online - full text edition.* **3923**
Journal of Clinical Periodontology (DNK) *Online - full text edition.* **3828**
Journal of Clinical Pharmacology (USA) *Online - full text edition.* **4306**
Journal of Clinical Pharmacy and Therapeutics (GBR) *Online - full text edition.* **4306**
Journal of Clinical Virology (NLD) *Online - full text edition.* **3801**
Journal of Communication Disorders (USA) *Online - full text edition.* **4412**
Journal of Communication Inquiry (USA) *Online - full text edition.* **4522**
Journal of Congestive Hearth Failure & Circulatory Support (GBR) *Online - full text edition.* **3777**
Journal of Controlled Release (NLD) *Online - full text edition.* **4306**
Journal of Craniofacial Genetics and Developmental Biology Online(DNK) *Online - full text.* **3309**
Journal of Cross-Cultural Psychology (USA) *Online - full text edition.* **4414**
Journal of Cutaneous Pathology (DNK) *Online - full text edition.* **3850**
The Journal of Deaf Studies and Deaf Education (USA) *Online - full text edition.* **3491**
The Journal of Dentistry (GBR) *Online - full text edition.* **3828**
Journal of Dermatological Science (IRL) *Online - full text edition.* **3850**
Journal of Diabetes and Its Complications (USA) *Online - full text edition.* **3864**
Journal of Diagnostic Medical Sonography (USA) *Online - full text edition.* **4147**
Journal of Early Adolescence (USA) *Online - full text edition.* **3384**
Journal of Ecology (GBR) *Online - full text edition.* **3203**
The Journal of Economic Psychology (NLD) *Online - full text edition.* **3366**
Journal of Electromyography and Kinesiology (GBR) *Online - full text edition.* **3266**
The Journal of Emergency Medicine (USA) *Online - full text edition.* **4018**
Journal of English Linguistics (USA) *Online - full text edition.* **3550**
Journal of Environmental Psychology (GBR) *Online - full text edition.* **4415**
Journal of Environmental Radioactivity (GBR) *Online - full text edition.* **3440**
Journal of Epidemiology and Biostatistics (GBR) *Online - full text edition.* **4479**
Journal of Ethnopharmacology (IRL) *Online - full text edition.* **4307**
Journal of Evaluation in Clinical Practice Online(GBR) *Online - full text.* **3632**
Journal of Evolutionary Biology (GBR) *Online - full text edition.* **3309**
Journal of Experimental Child Psychology (USA) *Online - full text edition.* **4415**
Journal of Experimental Marine Biology and Ecology (NLD) *Online - full text edition.* **3203**
Journal of Experimental Social Psychology (USA) *Online - full text edition.* **4415**
Journal of Exposure Analysis and Environmental Epidemiology (GBR) *Online - full text edition.* **3440**
Journal of Family Nursing (USA) *Online - full content edition.* **3924**
Journal of Family Therapy (GBR) *Online - full text edition.* **4101**
Journal of Fluency Disorders (USA) *Online - full text edition.* **4416**
Journal of Gastroenterology and Hepatology (AUS) *Online - full text edition.* **3893**
Journal of General Internal Medicine (USA) *Online - full text edition.* **3910**
Journal of Health Care for the Poor and Underserved (USA) *Online - full text edition.* **3633**
Journal of Health Economics (NLD) *Online - full text edition.* **4479**
Journal of Health Psychology (GBR) *Online - full text edition.* **4417**
The Journal of Heart and Lung Transplantation (GBR) *Online - full text edition.* **4193**
Journal of Helminthology (GBR) *Online - full text edition.* **3801**
Journal of Hepatology (DNK) *Online - full text edition.* **3893**
Journal of Holistic Nursing (USA) *Online - full text edition.* **3924**
Journal of Human Evolution (GBR) *Online - full text edition.* **3309**
Journal of Human Hypertension (GBR) *Online - full text edition.* **3778**
Journal of Human Lactation (USA) *Online - full text edition.* **3955**
Journal of Human Nutrition and Dietetics (GBR) *Online - full text edition.* **4237**
Journal of Humanistic Psychology (USA) *Online - full text edition.* **4417**
Journal of Immunological Methods (NLD) *Online - full text edition.* **3748**
Journal of Industrial Microbiology and Biotechnology (GBR) *Online - full text edition.* **3276**
Journal of Inorganic Biochemistry (USA) *Online - full text edition.* **3254**
Journal of Intellectual Disability Research (GBR) *Online - full text edition.* **4102**
Journal of Intensive Care Medicine (USA) *Online - full text edition.* **3634**
Journal of Internal Medicine (GBR) *Online - full text edition.* **3910**
Journal of Interpersonal Violence (USA) *Online - full text edition.* **3395**
The Journal of Investigative Dermatology (USA) *Online - full text edition.* **3851**
Journal of Language and Social Psychology (USA) *Online - full text edition.* **4417**
Journal of Learning Disabilities (GBR) *Online - full text edition.* **3423**
Journal of Lower Genital Tract Disease Online(USA) *Online - full text.* **3956**
Journal of Luminescence (NLD) *Online - full text edition.* **4366**
Journal of Management in Medicine (GBR) *Online - full text edition.* **3634**
Journal of Managerial Psychology (GBR) *Online - full text edition.* **3365**
Journal of Mathematical Psychology (USA) *Online - full text edition.* **4418**
Journal of Memory and Language (USA) *Online - full text edition.* **3550**
Journal of Microbiological Methods (NLD) *Online - full text edition.* **3325**
Journal of Microscopy (GBR) *Online - full text edition.* **3334**
Journal of Molecular and Cellular Cardiology (GBR) *Online - full text edition.* **3778**
Journal of Molecular Graphics and Modelling (USA) *Online - full text edition.* **3377**
Journal of Neuroendocrinology Online(GBR) *Online - full text.* **4103**
Journal of Neuroimaging (USA) *Online - full text edition.* **4103**
Journal of Neuroimmunology (NLD) *Online - full text edition.* **4103**
Journal of Neurolinguistics (GBR) *Online - full text edition.* **4103**
Journal of Neurology, Neurosurgery and Psychiatry (GBR) *Online - full text edition.* **4104**
Journal of Neuroscience Methods (NLD) *Online - full text edition.* **4104**
Journal of NeuroVirology (GBR) *Online - full text edition.* **4105**
Journal of Nursing Management (GBR) *Online - full text edition.* **3925**
Journal of Nutritional Biochemistry (USA) *Online - full text edition.* **4238**
Journal of Oncology Pharmacy Practice (USA) *Online - full text edition.* **4308**
Journal of Oral Pathology & Medicine (DNK) *Online - full text edition.* **3829**
The Journal of Orthodontics (GBR) *Online - full text edition.* **3830**
Journal of Paediatrics and Child Health (AUS) *Online - full text edition.* **4047**
Journal of Pain and Symptom Management (USA) *Online - full text edition.* **4105**
Journal of Pediatric and Adolescent Gynecology (NLD) *Online - full text edition.* **4047**
Journal of Pediatric Psychology (GBR) *Online - full text edition.* **4419**
Journal of Peptide Research (DNK) *Online - full text edition.* **3255**
Journal of Perinatology (GBR) *Online - full text edition.* **3956**
Journal of Periodontal Research (DNK) *Online - full text edition.* **3830**
Journal of Personality (USA) *Online - full text edition.* **4419**
Journal of Pharmaceutical and Biomedical Analysis (NLD) *Online - full text edition.* **4309**
Journal of Pharmacological and Toxicological Methods (USA) *Online - full text edition.* **3452**
Journal of Pharmacy and Pharmacology (GBR) *Online - full text edition.* **4310**
Journal of Photochemistry and Photobiology, B: Biology (CHE) *Online - full text edition.* **3255**

Journal of Physiology (Paris) (FRA) *Online - full text edition.* **4105**
Journal of Pineal Research (DNK) *Online - full text edition.* **4105**
Journal of Plankton Research (GBR) *Online - full text edition.* **3204**
Journal of Psychiatric & Mental Health Nursing Online(GBR) *Online - full text.* **4105**
Journal of Psychiatric Research (GBR) *Online - full text edition.* **4106**
Journal of Psychopharmacology (GBR) *Online - full text edition.* **4310**
Journal of Psychosomatic Research (USA) *Online - full text edition.* **4106**
Journal of Public Health Medicine (GBR) *Online - full text edition.* **4515**
Journal of Quality in Clinical Practice (AUS) *Online - full text edition.* **3637**
Journal of Rehabilitation Medicine (NOR) *Online - full text edition.* **4515**
Journal of Reproductive Immunology (IRL) *Online - full text edition.* **3749**
Journal of Research in Personality (USA) *Online - full text edition.* **4422**
Journal of Safety Research (GBR) *Online - full text edition.* **4258**
Journal of School Psychology (GBR) *Online - full text edition.* **4422**
Journal of Sleep Research Online(GBR) *Online - full text.* **3638**
Journal of Social and Evolutionary Systems (GBR) *Online - full text edition.* **4422**
Journal of Social and Personal Relationships (GBR) *Online - full content edition.* **4423**
Journal of Social Issues (USA) *Online - full content edition.* **4423**
Journal of Steroid Biochemistry and Molecular Biology (GBR) *Online - full text edition.* **3255**
Journal of Structural Biology (USA) *Online - full text edition.* **3205**
Journal of Substance Abuse (GBR) *Online - full text edition.* **3403**
Journal of Substance Abuse Treatment (USA) *Online - full text edition.* **3404**
Journal of Surgical Research (USA) *Online - full text edition.* **4195**
Journal of the Neurological Sciences (NLD) *Online - full text edition.* **4106**
Journal of the Peripheral Nervous System Online(USA) *Online - full text.* **4107**
Journal of Theoretical Biology (GBR) *Online - full text edition.* **3205**
Journal of Thermal Biology (GBR) *Online - full text edition.* **3267**
Journal of Transcultural Nursing (USA) *Online - full content edition.* **3927**
Journal of Tropical Pediatrics (GBR) *Online - full text edition.* **4047**
Journal of Vestibular Research: Equilibrium and Orientation (NLD) *Online - full text edition.* **3345**
Journal of Veterinary Medicine. Series A Online(DEU) *Online - full text.* **4547**
Journal of Veterinary Medicine. Series B Online(DEU) *Online - full text.* **4547**
Journal of Veterinary Pharmacology and Therapeutics Online(GBR) *Online - full text.* **4311**
Journal of Viral Hepatitis (GBR) *Online - full text edition.* **3893**
Journal of Virological Methods (NLD) *Online - full text edition.* **3326**
Journal of Vocational Behavior (USA) *Online - full text edition.* **4424**
Journal of Vocational Rehabilitation (NLD) *Online - full text edition.* **4258**
Journal of Zoological Systematics and Evolutionary Research Online(DEU) *Online - full text.* **3355**
Kidney International Online (USA) *Online - full text edition of* Kidney International. **4215**
The Knee (NLD) *Online - full text edition.* **3345**
Le Lait (FRA) *Online - full text edition.* **3326**
The Leadership Quarterly (USA) *Online - full text edition.* **3365**
Learning and Individual Differences (GBR) *Online - full text edition.* **3413**
Learning and Instruction (GBR) *Online - full text edition.* **3413**
Learning and Motivation (USA) *Online - full text edition.* **3413**
Letters in Applied Microbiology (GBR) *Online - full text edition.* **3326**
Leukemia (GBR) *Online - full text edition.* **3903**
Leukemia Research (GBR) *Online - full text edition.* **3904**
Linnean Society. Biological Journal (GBR) *Online - full text edition.* **3206**
Liver (DNK) *Online - full text edition.* **3894**
Logopedics Phoniatrics Vocology (NOR) *Online - full text edition.* **4035**
Lung Cancer (IRL) *Online - full text edition.* **3983**
Lupus (GBR) *Online - full text edition.* **4169**
Lyon Pharmaceutique (FRA) *Online - full text edition.* **4313**
M P Online (GBR) *Online - full text edition of* Molecular Pathology. **3879**
Magnetic Resonance Imaging (USA) *Online - full text edition.* **4150**
Magnetic Resonance Materials in Physics, Biology and Medicine (GBR) *Online - full text edition.* **4366**
Marine Ecology Online(DEU) *Online - full text.* **3207**
Marine Environmental Research (GBR) *Online - full text edition.* **3444**
Mathematical Biosciences (USA) *Online - full text edition.* **3554**
Matrix Biology (NLD) *Online - full text edition.* **3646**
Maturitas (IRL) *Online - full text edition.* **3958**
Mechanisms of Ageing and Development (IRL) *Online - full text edition.* **3478**
Mechanisms of Development (IRL) *Online - full text edition.* **3292**
Medecine et Droit (FRA) *Online - full text edition.* **3884**
Medecine et Maladies Infectieuses (FRA) *Online - full text edition.* **3803**
Medecine Nucleaire (FRA) *Online - full text edition.* **4150**
Medical & Veterinary Entomology Online(GBR) *Online - full text.* **3648**
Medical Care Research and Review (USA) *Online - full text edition.* **4496**
Medical Decision Making (USA) *Online - full text edition.* **3649**
Medical Dosimetry (USA) *Online - full text edition.* **4150**
Medical Education (GBR) *Online - full text edition.* **3650**
Medical Engineering & Physics (GBR) *Online - full text edition.* **3650**
Medical Humanities (GBR) *Online - full text edition.* **3651**
Medical Hypotheses (GBR) *Online - full text edition.* **3651**
Medical Image Analysis (GBR) *Online - full text edition.* **4150**
Medical Law Review (GBR) *Online - full text edition.* **3542**
Medical Mycology (GBR) *Online - full text edition.* **3803**
Medical Oncology (GBR) *Online - full text edition.* **3984**
Medical Update for Psychiatrists (USA) *Online - full text edition.* **4108**
Metabolic Engineering (USA) *Online - full text edition.* **3238**
Methods: A Companion to Methods in Enzymology (USA) *Online - full text edition.* **3256**
Microbes and Infection (FRA) *Online - full text edition.* **3327**
Microbial Ecology in Health & Disease (NOR) *Online - full text edition.* **3803**
Microbial Pathogenesis (GBR) *Online - full text edition.* **3804**
Microcirculation (GBR) *Online - full text edition.* **3661**
Micron (GBR) *Online - full text edition.* **3335**
Microvascular Research (USA) *Online - full text edition.* **3780**
The Milbank Quarterly (USA) *Online - full text edition.* **4368**
Minimally Invasive Therapy and Allied Technologies (GBR) *Online - full text edition.* **3661**
Molecular and Biochemical Parasitology (NLD) *Online - full text edition.* **3256**
Molecular and Cellular Endocrinology (IRL) *Online - full text edition.* **3866**
Molecular and Cellular Neurosciences (USA) *Online - full text edition.* **4110**
Molecular and Cellular Probes (GBR) *Online - full text edition.* **3879**
Molecular Aspects of Medicine (GBR) *Online - full text edition.* **3662**
Molecular Brain Research (NLD) *Online - full text edition.* **4110**
Molecular Cell (USA) *Online - full text edition.* **3292**
Molecular Cell Biology Research Communications (USA) *Online - full text edition.* **3292**
Molecular Genetics and Metabolism (USA) *Online - full text edition.* **3662**
Molecular Human Reproduction (GBR) *Online - full text edition.* **3958**
Molecular Imaging and Biology (NLD) *Online - full text edition.* **4151**
Molecular Immunology (GBR) *Online - full text edition.* **3257**
Molecular Microbiology Online (GBR) *Online - full text edition of* Molecular Microbiology. **3329**
Molecular Phylogenetics and Evolution (USA) *Online - full text edition.* **3311**
Molecular Plant Pathology (GBR) *Online - full text edition.* **3281**
Molecular Psychiatry (GBR) *Online - full text edition.* **4110**
Molecular Therapy (USA) *Online - full text edition.* **3984**
Multiple Sclerosis (GBR) *Online - full text edition.* **4111**
Mutagenesis (GBR) *Online - full text edition.* **3311**
Mutation Research - D N A Repair (NLD) *Online - full text edition.* **3258**
Mutation Research - Fundamental and Molecular Mechanisms of Mutagenesis (NLD) *Online - full text edition.* **3311**
Mutation Research - Genetic Toxicology and Environmental Mutagenesis (NLD) *Online - full text edition.* **3312**
Mutation Research Letters (NLD) *Online - full text edition.* **3312**
Mutation Research - Reviews in Mutation Research (NLD) *Online - full text edition.* **3312**
Mycoses (DEU) *Online - full text edition.* **3663**
National Cancer Institute. Journal (USA) *Online - full text edition.* **3985**
Nature (GBR) *Online - full text edition.* **4506**
Nature Biotechnology (USA) *Online - full text edition.* **3276**
Nature Genetics (USA) *Online - full text edition.* **3312**
Nature Medicine (GBR) *Online - full text edition.* **3665**
Nature Neuroscience (USA) *Online - full text edition.* **4111**
Nature Structural Biology (USA) *Online - full text edition.* **3210**
NeoPlasia (USA) *Online - full text edition.* **3985**
Nephrology, Dialysis and Transplantation (GBR) *Online - full text edition.* **4216**
Nephrology Online (AUS) *Online - full text edition of* Nephrology. **4216**
Netherlands Journal of Medicine (NLD) *Online - full text edition.* **3911**
Neural Networks (GBR) *Online - full text edition.* **3390**
Neurobiology of Aging (USA) *Online - full text edition.* **3346**
Neurobiology of Disease (USA) *Online - full text edition.* **4112**
Neurobiology of Learning and Memory (USA) *Online - full text edition.* **4112**
Neurocase (GBR) *Online - full text edition.* **4112**
Neurochemistry International (GBR) *Online - full text edition.* **4113**
Neurogastroenterology and Motility Online(GBR) *Online - full text.* **3894**
NeuroImage (USA) *Online - full text edition.* **4113**
Neuromodulation Online(USA) *Online - full text.* **4115**
Neuromuscular Disorders (GBR) *Online - full text edition.* **4115**
Neuron (USA) *Online - full text edition.* **4115**
Neuropathology (AUS) *Online - full text edition.* **4116**
Neuropathology & Applied Neurobiology Online (GBR) *Online - full text edition of* Neuropathology and Applied Neurobiology. **4116**
Neuropharmacology (GBR) *Online - full text edition.* **4318**
Neurophysiologie Clinique (FRA) *Online - full text edition.* **4116**
Neuropsychologia (GBR) *Online - full text edition.* **4116**
Neuropsychopharmacology (USA) *Online - full text edition.* **4117**
NeuroRehabilitation (NLD) *Online - full text edition.* **4117**
Neuroscience (GBR) *Online - full text edition.* **4117**
Neuroscience and Biobehavioral Reviews (GBR) *Online - full text edition.* **4118**
Neuroscience Letters (IRL) *Online - full text edition.* **4118**
Neuroscience Research (IRL) *Online - full text edition.* **4118**
The Neuroscientist (USA) *Online - full text edition.* **4118**
Neurotoxicology and Teratology (USA) *Online - full text edition.* **4119**
New Ideas in Psychology (GBR) *Online - full text edition.* **4430**
Noise & Health (GBR) *Online - full text edition.* **4035**
Nordic Journal of Psychiatry (NOR) *Online - full text edition.* **4120**
Nuclear Medicine and Biology (USA) *Online - full text edition.* **4152**
Nucleic Acids Research (GBR) *Online - full text edition.* **3259**
Nurse Education Today (GBR) *Online - full text edition.* **3931**
Nursing and Health Sciences (AUS) *Online - full text edition.* **3932**
Nursing Ethics (GBR) *Online - full text edition.* **3933**
Nursing Inquiry (AUS) *Online - full text edition.* **3933**
Nursing Philosophy Online (GBR) *Online - full text edition of* Nursing Philosophy. **3934**
Nursing Science Quarterly (USA) *Online - full text edition.* **3934**
Nutrition (USA) *Online - full text edition.* **4241**
Nutrition and Food Science (GBR) *Online - full text edition.* **4241**
Nutrition Bulletin Online (GBR) *Online - full text edition of* Nutrition Bulletin. **4241**
Nutrition in Clinical Care Online(USA) *Online - full text.* **4242**
Nutrition Research (USA) *Online - full text edition.* **4243**
Nutrition Research Reviews (GBR) *Online - full text edition.* **4243**
Nutrition Society. Proceedings (GBR) *Online - full text edition.* **4243**
O E M Online (GBR) *Online - full text edition of* Occupational and Environmental Medicine. **4261**
Obesity Reviews Online(GBR) *Online - full text.* **4244**
Obstetrics and Gynecology (USA) *Online - full text edition.* **3960**
Oncogene (GBR) *Online - full text edition.* **3986**
Ophthalmic and Physiological Optics (GBR) *Online - full text edition.* **4003**
Ophthalmic Literature (GBR) *Online - full text edition.* **3734**
Ophthalmology (USA) *Online - full text edition.* **4004**
Opportunistic Pathogens (NLD) *Online - full text edition.* **3804**
Option - Bio (FRA) *Online - full text edition.* **3212**
Oral Diseases (GBR) *Online - full text edition.* **3834**
Oral Microbiology and Immunology (DNK) *Online - full text edition.* **3329**
Oral Oncology (GBR) *Online - full text edition.* **3988**
Organization & Environment (USA) *Online - full text edition.* **4263**
Organizational Behavior and Human Decision Processes (USA) *Online - full text edition.* **3366**
Paediatric Anaesthesia Online(GBR) *Online - full text.* **3759**
Paediatric & Perinatal Epidemiology Online(GBR) *Online - full text.* **4050**
Paediatric Drugs (NZL) *Online - full text edition.* **4321**
Pain (NLD) *Online - full text edition.* **4121**
Pain Medicine Online(USA) *Online - full text.* **4121**
Pain Reviews (GBR) *Online - full text edition.* **3671**
Palliative Medicine (GBR) *Online - full text edition.* **3672**
Parasite Immunology Online (GBR) *Online - full text edition of* Parasite Immunology. **3804**
Parasitology International (NLD) *Online - full text edition.* **3805**
Parkinsonism and Related Disorders (GBR) *Online - full text edition.* **4122**
Pathology International (AUS) *Online - full text edition.* **3673**
Pathophysiology (NLD) *Online - full text edition.* **3347**
Patient Education and Counseling (IRL) *Online - full text edition.* **4484**
Pediatric Allergy and Immunology (DNK) *Online - full text edition.* **4051**
Pediatric Dermatology (USA) *Online - full text edition.* **3852**
Pediatric Diabetes Online(DNK) *Online - full text.* **4052**

Online Service

A J P: Cell Physiology Online (USA) *Online - full text edition of* American Journal of Physiology: Cell Physiology. **3337**
A J P: Endocrinology and Metabolism Online (USA) *Online - full text edition of* American Journal of Physiology: Endocrinology and Metabolism. **3338**
A J P: Gastrointestinal and Liver Physiology Online (USA) *Online - full text edition of* American Journal of Physiology: Gastrointestinal and Liver Physiology. **3338**
A J P: Heart and Circulatory Physiology Online (USA) *Online - full text edition of* American Journal of Physiology: Heart and Circulatory Physiology. **3338**
A J P: Lung Cellular and Molecular Physiology Online (USA) *Online - full text edition of* American Journal of Physiology: Lung Cellular and Molecular Physiology. **3338**
A J P: Regulatory, Integrative and Comparative Physiology Online (USA) *Online - full text edition of* American Journal of Physiology: Regulatory, Integrative and Comparative Physiology. **3338**
A J P: Renal Physiology Online (USA) *Online - full text edition of* American Journal of Physiology: Renal Physiology. **3339**
A J R (USA) *Online - full text edition.* **4139**
A N A E (FRA) *Online - full text edition.* **4067**
A N Z Journal of Surgery (AUS) *Online - full text edition.* **4178**
A P M I S (DNK) *Online - full text edition.* **3178**
A R D Online (GBR) *Online - full text edition of* Annals of the Rheumatic Diseases. **4167**
A S A I O Journal (USA) *Online - full text edition.* **3556**
A S M News (Washington) (USA) *Online - full text edition.* **3315**
Abdominal Imaging (USA) *Online - full text edition.* **3885**
Academic Emergency Medicine (USA) *Online - full text edition.* **4009**
Academic Medicine (USA) *Online - full text edition.* **3556**
Academic Psychiatry (USA) *Online - full text edition.* **4067**
Academic Radiology (USA) *Online - full text edition.* **4139**
Academie Nationale de Medecine. Bulletin (FRA) *Online - full text edition.* **3556**
Accident Analysis & Prevention (GBR) *Online - full text edition.* **4460**
Acta Anaesthesiologica Scandinavica (DNK) *Online - full text edition.* **3753**
Acta Bioquimica Clinica Latinoamericana (ARG) *Online - full text edition.* **3239**
Acta Biotechnologica (DEU) *Online - full text edition.* **3268**
Acta Biotheoretica (NLD) *Online - full text edition.* **3178**
Acta Cardiologica (BEL) *Online - full text edition.* **3761**
Acta Chirurgica Belgica (BEL) *Online - full text edition.* **4178**
Acta Chirurgica Italica (ITA) *Online - full text edition.* **4178**
Acta Clinica Belgica (BEL) *Online - full text edition.* **3557**
Acta Cytologica (USA) *Online - full text edition.* **3284**
Acta Dermato-Venereologica (NOR) *Online - full text edition.* **3843**
Acta Diabetologica (DEU) *Online - full text edition.* **3855**
Acta Gastro-Enterologica Belgica (BEL) *Online - full text edition.* **3885**
Acta Haematologica (CHE) *Online - full text edition.* **3897**
Acta Histochemica (DEU) *Online - full text edition.* **3239**
Acta Histochemica et Cytochemica (JPN) *Online - full text edition.* **3284**
Acta Hydrochimica et Hydrobiologica (DEU) *Online - full text edition.* **4561**
Acta Medica Austriaca Online(AUT) *Online - full text.* **3557**
Acta Medica Okayama (JPN) *Online - full text edition.* **3558**
Acta Neurobiologiae Experimentalis (POL) *Online - full text edition.* **3179**
Acta Neurochirurgica (AUT) *Online - full text edition.* **4179**
Acta Neurologica Belgica (BEL) *Online - full text edition.* **4068**
Acta Neurologica Scandinavica (DNK) *Online - full text edition.* **4068**
Acta Neuropathologica (DEU) *Online - full text edition.* **4068**
Acta Neuropsychiatrica (NLD) *Online - full text edition.* **4068**
Acta Obstetrica et Gynecologica Scandinavica (DNK) *Online - full text edition.* **3944**
Acta Odontologica Scandinavica (NOR) *Online - full text edition.* **3813**
Acta Oncologica (NOR) *Online - full text edition.* **3966**
Acta Ophthamologica Scandinavica Online(DNK) *Online - full text.* **3993**
Acta Orthopaedica Scandinavica (NOR) *Online - full text edition.* **4009**
Acta Oto-Laryngologica (NOR) *Online - full text edition.* **4029**
Acta Paediatrica (NOR) *Online - full text edition.* **4039**
Acta Parasitologica (POL) *Online - full text edition.* **3316**
Acta Physiologica Scandinavica (GBR) *Online - full text edition.* **3337**
Acta Protozoologica (POL) *Online - full text edition.* **3316**
Acta Psychiatrica Scandinavica (DNK) *Online - full text edition.* **4068**
Acta Psychologica (NLD) *Online - full text edition.* **4372**
Acta Radiologica (DNK) *Online - full text edition.* **4139**
Acta Tropica (NLD) *Online - full text edition.* **3790**
Acta Veterinaria (YUG) *Online - full text edition.* **4534**
Acta Veterinaria Brno (CZE) *Online - full text edition.* **4534**
Acta Veterinaria Hungarica (HUN) *Online - full text edition.* **4535**
Acta Veterinaria Scandinavica (DNK) *Online - full text edition.* **4535**
Acta Virologica (SVK) *Online - full text edition.* **3316**
Acta Zoologica Online(GBR) *Online - full text.* **3350**
Actas Espanolas de Psiquiatria (ESP) *Online - full text edition.* **4069**
Acupuncture and Electro-Therapeutics Research (USA) *Online - full text edition.* **3162**
Adapted Physical Activity Quarterly (USA) *Online - full text edition.* **3418**
Adaptive Behavior (USA) *Online - full text edition.* **3389**
Addiction (GBR) *Online - full text edition.* **3396**
Addiction Biology (GBR) *Online - full text edition.* **3397**
Addictive Behaviors (GBR) *Online - full text edition.* **3397**
Administration and Policy in Mental Health (USA) *Online - full text edition.* **3559**
Adolescence (San Diego) (USA) *Online - full text edition.* **3380**
Adolescent Psychiatry (USA) *Online - full text edition.* **4069**
Advanced Drug Delivery Reviews (NLD) *Online - full text edition.* **4274**
Advances in Anatomic Pathology (USA) *Online - full text edition.* **3559**
Advances in Anatomy, Embryology and Cell Biology (USA) *Online - full text edition.* **3179**
Advances in Applied Microbiology (USA) *Online - full text edition.* **3316**
Advances in Audiology (CHE) *Online - full text edition.* **4029**
Advances in Biochemical Psychopharmacology (USA) *Online - full text edition.* **4274**
Advances in Cancer Research (USA) *Online - full text edition.* **3966**
Advances in Carbohydrate Chemistry and Biochemistry (USA) *Online - full text edition.* **3559**
Advances in Cardiology (CHE) *Online - full text edition.* **3761**
Advances in Child Development and Behavior (USA) *Online - full text edition.* **4372**
Advances in Clinical Chemistry (USA) *Online - full text edition.* **3239**
Advances in Colloid and Interface Science (NLD) *Online - full text edition.* **3379**
Advances in Enzyme Regulation (GBR) *Online - full text edition.* **3239**
Advances in Enzymology and Related Areas of Molecular Biology (GBR) *Online - full text edition.* **3239**
Advances in Experimental Medicine and Biology (USA) *Online - full text edition.* **3179**
Advances in Experimental Social Psychology (USA) *Online - full text edition.* **4519**
Advances in Genetics (USA) *Online - full text edition.* **3297**
Advances in Human Genetics (USA) *Online - full text edition.* **3297**
Advances in Immunology (USA) *Online - full text edition.* **3739**
Advances in Internal Medicine (USA) *Online - full text edition.* **3907**
Advances in Marine Biology (USA) *Online - full text edition.* **3179**
Advances in Microbial Ecology (USA) *Online - full text edition.* **3316**
Advances in Microbial Physiology (USA) *Online - full text edition.* **3317**
Advances in Neurology (USA) *Online - full text edition.* **4069**
Advances in Nursing Science (USA) *Online - full text edition.* **3912**
Advances in Nutritional Research (USA) *Online - full text edition.* **4228**
Advances in Pain Research and Therapy (USA) *Online - full text edition.* **4070**
Advances in Physiology Education Online (USA) *Online - full text edition of* Advances in Physiology Education. **3337**
Advances in Prostaglandin, Thromboxane, and Leukotriene Research (USA) *Online - full text edition.* **4274**
Advances in Protein Chemistry (USA) *Online - full text edition.* **3240**
Advances in Psychosomatic Medicine (CHE) *Online - full text edition.* **4070**
Advances in Renal Replacement Therapy (USA) *Online - full text edition.* **4209**
Advances in Second Messenger and Phosphoprotein Research (USA) *Online - full text edition.* **3240**
Advances in the Study of Behavior (USA) *Online - full text edition.* **4373**
Advances in Therapy (USA) *Online - full text edition.* **3560**
Advances in Veterinary Medicine (USA) *Online - full text edition.* **4535**
Advances in Virus Research (USA) *Online - full text edition.* **3317**
Adverse Drug Reactions and Toxicological Reviews (GBR) *Online - full text edition.* **4274**
Aesthetic Plastic Surgery (USA) *Online - full text edition.* **4179**
Age and Ageing (GBR) *Online - full text edition.* **3466**
Ageing and Society (GBR) *Online - full text edition.* **3466**
Aggression and Violent Behavior (GBR) *Online - full text edition.* **4373**
Aggressive Behavior (USA) *Online - full text edition.* **4373**
Aging & Mental Health (GBR) *Online - full text edition.* **3466**
Aging - Clinical and Experimental Research (ITA) *Online - full text edition.* **3467**
AIDS (USA) *Online - full text edition.* **3790**
AIDS & Public Policy Journal (USA) *Online - full text edition.* **3791**
AIDS Care (GBR) *Online - full text edition.* **3791**
AIDS Education and Prevention (USA) *Online - full text edition.* **4460**
AIDS Patient Care and S T Ds (USA) *Online - full text edition.* **3791**
AIDS Research and Human Retroviruses (USA) *Online - full text edition.* **3792**
Aktuelle Neurologie (DEU) *Online - full text edition.* **4070**
Aktuelle Rheumatologie (DEU) *Online - full text edition.* **4166**
Aktuelle Urologie (DEU) *Online - full text edition.* **4209**
Alcohol & Alcoholism (GBR) *Online - full text edition.* **3397**
Alcohol (New York) (USA) *Online - full text edition.* **3398**
Alcohol Research & Health (USA) *Online - full text edition.* **3398**
Alcoholism: Clinical and Experimental Research (USA) *Online - full text edition.* **3398**
Alimentary Pharmacology and Therapeutics (GBR) *Online - full text edition.* **3886**
Allergologie (DEU) *Online - full text edition.* **3739**
Allergy (DNK) *Online - full text edition.* **3739**
Allergy and Asthma Proceedings (USA) *Online - full text edition.* **3740**
Alternative Therapies in Health and Medicine (USA) *Online - full text edition.* **3163**
Alternatives to Laboratory Animals (GBR) *Online - full text edition.* **3870**
Altex (DEU) *Online - full text edition.* **3870**
Alzheimer Disease and Associated Disorders (USA) *Online - full text edition.* **4070**
Alzheimer's Reports (GBR) *Online - full text edition.* **4071**
Amazoniana (DEU) *Online - full text edition.* **3180**
Ambulatory Pediatrics (USA) *Online - full text edition.* **4040**
American Academy of Child and Adolescent Psychiatry. Journal (USA) *Online - full text edition.* **4071**
American Academy of Dermatology. Journal (USA) *Online - full text edition.* **3844**
American Aging Association. Journal (USA) *Online - full text edition.* **3467**
American Animal Hospital Association. Journal (USA) *Online - full text edition.* **4535**
American Annals of the Deaf (USA) *Online - full text edition.* **3488**
American Association for Cancer Research. Proceedings of the Annual Meeting (USA) *Online - full text edition.* **3967**
American Association for Pediatric Ophthalmology and Strabismus. Journal (USA) *Online - full text edition.* **3993**
American Association of Gynecologic Laparoscopists. Journal (USA) *Online - full text edition.* **3944**
American Behavioral Scientist (USA) *Online - full text edition.* **4508**
American College of Cardiology. Journal (USA) *Online - full text edition.* **3761**
American College of Nutrition. Journal (USA) *Online - full text edition.* **4228**
American College of Surgeons. Journal (USA) *Online - full text edition.* **4179**
American Dental Association. Journal (USA) *Online - full text edition.* **3814**
American Dietetic Association. Journal (USA) *Online - full text edition.* **4228**
American Family Physician (USA) *Online - full text edition.* **3563**
American Geriatrics Society. Journal (USA) *Online - full text edition.* **3467**
American Heart Journal (USA) *Online - full text edition.* **3762**
American Imago (USA) *Online - full text edition.* **4071**
American Indian and Alaska Native Mental Health Research (USA) *Online - full text edition.* **4226**
American Journal of Art Therapy (USA) *Online - full text edition.* **4058**
The American Journal of Cardiology (USA) *Online - full text edition.* **3762**
American Journal of Cardiovascular Pathology (USA) *Online - full text edition.* **3762**
The American Journal of Chinese Medicine (USA) *Online - full text edition.* **3715**
American Journal of Clinical Hypnosis (USA) *Online - full text edition.* **3906**
American Journal of Clinical Nutrition (USA) *Online - full text edition.* **4228**
American Journal of Clinical Oncology (USA) *Online - full text edition.* **3967**
American Journal of Clinical Pathology (USA) *Online - full text edition.* **3563**
American Journal of Community Psychology (USA) *Online - full text edition.* **4520**
American Journal of Dentistry (USA) *Online - full text edition.* **3814**
American Journal of Dermatopathology (USA) *Online - full text edition.* **3563**
American Journal of Drug and Alcohol Abuse (USA) *Online - full text edition.* **3399**
American Journal of Electroneurodiagnostic Technology (USA) *Online - full text edition.* **4071**
American Journal of Emergency Medicine (USA) *Online - full text edition.* **4010**
American Journal of Epidemiology (USA) *Online - full text edition.* **3563**
American Journal of Family Therapy (USA) *Online - full text edition.* **4374**
American Journal of Forensic Medicine and Pathology (USA) *Online - full text edition.* **3881**
American Journal of Gastroenterology (NLD) *Online - full text edition.* **3886**
American Journal of Geriatric Psychiatry (USA) *Online - full text edition.* **3468**
American Journal of Health Behavior (USA) *Online - full text edition.* **4350**
American Journal of Health Promotion (USA) *Online - full text edition.* **4461**
American Journal of Health-System Pharmacy (USA) *Online - full text edition.* **4275**
American Journal of Hematology (USA) *Online - full text edition.* **3897**
American Journal of Human Biology (USA) *Online - full text edition.* **3180**
American Journal of Human Genetics (USA) *Online - full text edition.* **3297**
American Journal of Hypertension (USA) *Online - full text edition.* **3762**

American Journal of Industrial Medicine (USA) Online - full text edition. 4249
American Journal of Infection Control (USA) Online - full text edition. 3792
American Journal of Kidney Diseases (USA) Online - full text edition. 4209
American Journal of Law & Medicine (USA) Online - full text edition. 3536
The American Journal of Managed Care (USA) Online - full text edition. 3564
American Journal of Medical Genetics (USA) Online - full text edition. 3298
The American Journal of Medicine (USA) Online - full text edition. 3564
American Journal of Nephrology (CHE) Online - full text edition. 4209
American Journal of Nursing (USA) Online - full text edition. 3913
American Journal of Obstetrics and Gynecology (USA) Online - full text edition. 3944
American Journal of Occupational Therapy (USA) Online - full text edition. 4250
American Journal of Ophthalmology (USA) Online - full text edition. 3993
American Journal of Orthodontics and Dentofacial Orthopedics (USA) Online - full text edition. 3814
American Journal of Orthopsychiatry (USA) Online - full text edition. 4374
American Journal of Otolaryngology (USA) Online - full text edition. 4030
American Journal of Pathology (USA) Online - full text edition. 3564
American Journal of Perinatology (USA) Online - full text edition. 3944
American Journal of Pharmaceutical Education (USA) Online - full text edition. 4275
American Journal of Physical Medicine and Rehabilitation (USA) Online - full text edition. 4058
American Journal of Preventive Medicine (USA) Online - full text edition. 3564
American Journal of Primatology (USA) Online - full text edition. 3350
American Journal of Psychiatry (USA) Online - full text edition. 4071
American Journal of Psychology (USA) Online - full text edition. 4374
American Journal of Psychotherapy (USA) Online - full text edition. 4072
American Journal of Public Health (USA) Online - full text edition. 4461
American Journal of Reproductive Immunology Online(DNK) Online - full text. 3740
American Journal of Respiratory and Critical Care Medicine (USA) Online - full text edition. 4158
American Journal of Respiratory Cell and Molecular Biology (USA) Online - full text edition. 4158
American Journal of Rhinology (USA) Online - full text edition. 4030
American Journal of Speech - Language Pathology (USA) Online - full text edition. 3489
American Journal of Sports Medicine (USA) Online - full text edition. 4172
American Journal of Surgery (USA) Online - full text edition. 4180
American Journal of Surgical Pathology (USA) Online - full text edition. 3564
American Journal of the Medical Sciences (USA) Online - full text edition. 3564
American Journal of Tropical Medicine and Hygiene (USA) Online - full text edition. 3792
American Journal of Veterinary Research (USA) Online - full text edition. 4536
American Journal on Addictions (USA) Online - full text edition. 3399
American Journal on Mental Retardation (USA) Online - full text edition. 4072
American Medical Informatics Association. Journal (USA) Online - full text edition. 3809
American Mosquito Control Association. Journal (USA) Online - full text edition. 3157
The American Naturalist (USA) Online - full text edition. 3180
American Podiatric Medical Association. Journal (USA) Online - full text edition. 4010
American Psychoanalytic Association. Journal (USA) Online - full text edition. 4375
American Psychologist (USA) Online - full text edition. 4375
American Society of Echocardiography. Journal (USA) Online - full text edition. 3762
American Society of Nephrology. Journal (USA) Online - full text edition. 4209
American Surgeon (USA) Online - full text edition. 4180
American Veterinary Medical Association. Journal (USA) Online - full text edition. 4536
Amino Acids (AUT) Online - full text edition. 3240
Amyloid (GBR) Online - full text edition. 4166
Amyotrophic Lateral Sclerosis and Other Motor Neuron Disorders (GBR) Online - full text edition. 4072
Anaerobe (GBR) Online - full text edition. 3317
Anaesthesia and Intensive Care (AUS) Online - full text edition. 3753
Anaesthesia (Oxford) (GBR) Online - full text edition. 3754
Anaesthesiologie und Intensivmedizin Online(DEU) Online - full text. 3754
Der Anaesthesist (DEU) Online - full text edition. 3754
Anales Espanoles de Pediatria (ESP) Online - full text edition. 4040
Analytical and Quantitative Cytology and Histology (USA) Online - full text edition. 3285
Analytical Biochemistry (USA) Online - full text edition. 3240
Analytical Cellular Pathology (NLD) Online - full text edition. 3285
Anatomia, Histologia, Embryologia Online(DEU) Online - full text. 4537
The Anatomical Record (USA) Online - full text edition. 3181
Anatomy and Embryology (DEU) Online - full text edition. 3339
Andrologia (DEU) Online - full text edition. 3565
Anesthesia and Analgesia (USA) Online - full text edition. 3755
Anesthesiology (USA) Online - full text edition. 3755
Anesthesiology Clinics of North America (USA) Online - full text edition. 3755
Angiology (USA) Online - full text edition. 3763
Angle Orthodontist (USA) Online - full text edition. 3815
Animal Behaviour (GBR) Online - full text edition. 3350
Animal Biotechnology (USA) Online - full text edition. 3268
Animal Feed Science and Technology (NLD) Online - full text edition. 3159
Animal Genetics (GBR) Online - full text edition. 3298
Animal Learning & Behavior (USA) Online - full text edition. 4376
Animal Reproduction Science (NLD) Online - full text edition. 3160
Annales Chirurgiae et Gynaecologiae (FIN) Online - full text edition. 4180
Annales de Biologie Clinique (FRA) Online - full text edition. 3181
Annales de Cardiologie et d'Angeiologie (FRA) Online - full text edition. 3763
Annales de Chirurgie (FRA) Online - full text edition. 4180
Annales de Dermatologie et de Venereologie (FRA) Online - full text edition. 3844
Annales de Genetique (FRA) Online - full text edition. 3298
Annales de Medecine Interne (FRA) Online - full text edition. 3907
Annales de Medecine Veterinaire (BEL) Online - full text edition. 4537
Annales de Pathologie (FRA) Online - full text edition. 3181
Annales d'Endocrinologie (FRA) Online - full text edition. 3855
Annales d'Urologie (FRA) Online - full text edition. 4210
Annales Francaises d'Anesthesie et de Reanimation (FRA) Online - full text edition. 3755
Annales Medico-Psychologiques (FRA) Online - full text edition. 4376
Annals of Allergy, Asthma, & Immunology (USA) Online - full text edition. 3740
Annals of Anatomy (DEU) Online - full text edition. 3566
Annals of Applied Biology (GBR) Online - full text edition. 3181
Annals of Behavioral Medicine (USA) Online - full text edition. 3715
Annals of Biomedical Engineering (USA) Online - full text edition. 3566
Annals of Clinical and Laboratory Science (USA) Online - full text edition. 3871
Annals of Clinical Biochemistry (GBR) Online - full text edition. 3240
Annals of Dyslexia (USA) Online - full text edition. 3419
Annals of Emergency Medicine (USA) Online - full text edition. 4010
Annals of Epidemiology (USA) Online - full text edition. 4461
Annals of Hematology (DEU) Online - full text edition. 3898
Annals of Human Biology (GBR) Online - full text edition. 3181
Annals of Human Genetics (GBR) Online - full text edition. 3298
Annals of Internal Medicine (USA) Online - full text edition. 3907
Annals of Medicine (GBR) Online - full text edition. 3871
Annals of Neurology (USA) Online - full text edition. 4073
Annals of Nuclear Medicine (JPN) Online - full text edition. 4140
Annals of Nutrition and Metabolism (CHE) Online - full text edition. 4229
Annals of Occupational Hygiene (GBR) Online - full text edition. 4250
Annals of Oncology (NLD) Online - full text edition. 3967
Annals of Ophthalmology (USA) Online - full text edition. 3993
Annals of Otology, Rhinology and Laryngology (USA) Online - full text edition. 4030
The Annals of Pharmacotherapy (USA) Online - full text edition. 4275
Annals of Plastic Surgery (USA) Online - full text edition. 4181
Annals of Saudi Medicine (SAU) Online - full text edition. 3566
Annals of Surgery (USA) Online - full text edition. 4181
Annals of Surgical Oncology (USA) Online - full text edition. 4181
Annals of Thoracic Surgery (USA) Online - full text edition. 4181
Annals of Tropical Medicine and Parasitology (GBR) Online - full text edition. 3793
Annals of Tropical Paediatrics (GBR) Online - full text edition. 4040
Annals of Vascular Surgery (USA) Online - full text edition. 4181
L' Annee Psychologique (FRA) Online - full text edition. 4376
Annual Reports in Medicinal Chemistry (USA) Online - full text edition. 4276
Annual Review of Biochemistry (USA) Online - full text edition. 3240
Annual Review of Biophysics and Biomolecular Structure (USA) Online - full text edition. 3264
Annual Review of Cell and Developmental Biology (USA) Online - full text edition. 3285
Annual Review of Genetics (USA) Online - full text edition. 3298
Annual Review of Immunology (USA) Online - full text edition. 3740
Annual Review of Medicine Online (USA) Online - full text edition of Annual Review of Medicine: Selected Topics in the Clinical Sciences. 3567
Annual Review of Microbiology (USA) Online - full text edition. 3317
Annual Review of Neuroscience (USA) Online - full text edition. 4073
Annual Review of Nutrition (USA) Online - full text edition. 4229
Annual Review of Pharmacology and Toxicology (USA) Online - full text edition. 4276
Annual Review of Physiology (USA) Online - full text edition. 3339
Annual Review of Psychology (USA) Online - full text edition. 4376
Annual Review of Public Health (USA) Online - full text edition. 4461
Antarctic Science (GBR) Online - full text edition. 3182
Anthrozoos (USA) Online - full text edition. 3350
Anti-Cancer Drug Design (GBR) Online - full text edition. 3967
Anti-Cancer Drugs (USA) Online - full text edition. 3967
Anticancer Research (GRC) Online - full text edition. 3967
Antimicrobial Agents and Chemotherapy (USA) Online - full text edition. 3317
Antisense and Nucleic Acid Drug Development (USA) Online - full text edition. 3298
Antiviral Chemistry and Chemotherapy (GBR) Online - full text edition. 3241
Antiviral Research (NLD) Online - full text edition. 3317
Antiviral Therapy (GBR) Online - full text edition. 3793
Antonie van Leeuwenhoek (NLD) Online - full text edition. 3268
Anxiety, Stress and Coping (CHE) Online - full text edition. 4377
Aphasiology (GBR) Online - full text edition. 4073
Apoptosis (USA) Online - full text edition. 3285
Appetite (GBR) Online - full text edition. 4229
Applied and Environmental Microbiology (USA) Online - full text edition. 3318
Applied and Preventive Psychology (GBR) Online - full text edition. 4377
Applied Animal Behaviour Science (NLD) Online - full text edition. 3350
Applied Biochemistry and Biotechnology (USA) Online - full text edition. 3241
Applied Biochemistry and Microbiology (RUS) Online - full text edition. 3241
Applied Cognitive Psychology (GBR) Online - full text edition. 4377
Applied Ergonomics (GBR) Online - full text edition. 3431
Applied Immunohistochemistry (USA) Online - full text edition. 3567
Applied Microbiology and Biotechnology (DEU) Online - full text edition. 3268
Applied Nursing Research (USA) Online - full text edition. 3913
Applied Psycholinguistics (GBR) Online - full text edition. 3550
Applied Psychological Measurement (USA) Online - full text edition. 4377
Applied Psychology (GBR) Online - full text edition. 4377
Applied Psychophysiology and Biofeedback (USA) Online - full text edition. 4378
Applied Radiation and Isotopes (GBR) Online - full text edition. 4365
Aquatic Microbial Ecology Online(DEU) Online - full text. 3318
Aquatic Toxicology (NLD) Online - full text edition. 3445
Archiv der Pharmazie (DEU) Online - full text edition. 4277
Archiv fuer Hydrobiologie (DEU) Online - full text edition. 3182
Archives de Pediatrie (FRA) Online - full text edition. 4040
Archives des Maladies du Coeur et des Vaisseaux (FRA) Online - full text edition. 3763
Archives Italiennes de Biologie (ITA) Online - full text edition. 4073
Archives of Andrology (USA) Online - full text edition. 3568
Archives of Animal Nutrition (CHE) Online - full text edition. 4538
Archives of Biochemistry and Biophysics (USA) Online - full text edition. 3241
Archives of Clinical Neuropsychology (GBR) Online - full text edition. 4074
Archives of Dermatological Research (DEU) Online - full text edition. 3845
Archives of Dermatology (USA) Online - full text edition. 3845
Archives of Disease in Childhood (GBR) Online - full text edition. 4040
Archives of Environmental Contamination and Toxicology (USA) Online - full text edition. 3445
Archives of Environmental Health (USA) Online - full text edition. 3435
Archives of General Psychiatry (USA) Online - full text edition. 4074
Archives of Gerontology and Geriatrics (IRL) Online - full text edition. 3468
Archives of Gynecology and Obstetrics (DEU) Online - full text edition. 3945
Archives of Histology and Cytology (JPN) Online - full text edition. 3285
Archives of Internal Medicine (USA) Online - full text edition. 3907
Archives of Medical Research (MEX) Online - full text edition. 3568
Archives of Microbiology (DEU) Online - full text edition. 3318
Archives of Neurology (USA) Online - full text edition. 4074
Archives of Ophthalmology (USA) Online - full text edition. 3994
Archives of Oral Biology (GBR) Online - full text edition. 3351
Archives of Orthopaedic and Trauma Surgery (DEU) Online - full text edition. 4010
Archives of Otolaryngology - Head & Neck Surgery (USA) Online - full text edition. 4030
Archives of Pathology & Laboratory Medicine (USA) Online - full text edition. 3568

Online Service

Archives of Pediatrics & Adolescent Medicine (USA) *Online - full text edition.* **4041**
Archives of Pharmacal Research (KOR) *Online - full text edition.* **4277**
Archives of Physical Medicine and Rehabilitation (USA) *Online - full text edition.* **4058**
Archives of Physiology and Biochemistry (NLD) *Online - full text edition.* **3339**
Archives of Psychiatric Nursing (USA) *Online - full text edition.* **3914**
Archives of Sexual Behavior (USA) *Online - full text edition.* **3568**
Archives of Surgery (USA) *Online - full text edition.* **4182**
Archives of Toxicology (DEU) *Online - full text edition.* **3445**
Archives of Virology (AUT) *Online - full text edition.* **3318**
Archivos de Bronconeumologia (ESP) *Online - full text edition.* **4158**
Archivos de Medicina Veterinaria (CHL) *Online - full text edition.* **4538**
Archivos Latinoamericanos de Nutricion (VEN) *Online - full text edition.* **4229**
Archivum Immunologiae et Therapiae Experimentalis (POL) *Online - full text edition.* **3569**
Arctic, Antarctic and Alpine Research (USA) *Online - full text edition.* **4503**
Arquivo Brasileiro de Medicina Veterinaria e Zootecnia (BRA) *Online - full text edition.* **4538**
Arquivos de Neuro-Psiquiatria (BRA) *Online - full text edition.* **4074**
Arteriosclerosis, Thrombosis, and Vascular Biology (USA) *Online - full text edition.* **3763**
Arthritis and Rheumatism (USA) *Online - full text edition.* **4167**
Arthritis Research (GBR) *Online - full text edition.* **3569**
Arthroscopy (USA) *Online - full text edition.* **4010**
Artificial Cells, Blood Substitutes, and Immobilization Biotechnology (USA) *Online - full text edition.* **3871**
Artificial Intelligence in Medicine (NLD) *Online - full text edition.* **3389**
Artificial Life (USA) *Online - full text edition.* **3389**
Artificial Organs (USA) *Online - full text edition.* **3871**
The Arts in Psychotherapy (GBR) *Online - full text edition.* **4378**
Arzneimittel-Forschung (DEU) *Online - full text edition.* **4278**
Asia Pacific Journal of Clinical Nutrition (AUS) *Online - full text edition.* **4229**
Asia Pacific Journal of Pharmacology (SGP) *Online - full text edition.* **4278**
Asian - Australasian Journal of Animal Sciences (KOR) *Online - full text edition.* **3160**
Asian Pacific Journal of Allergy & Immunology (THA) *Online - full text edition.* **3741**
Assessment (USA) *Online - full text edition.* **4378**
Assistive Technology (USA) *Online - full text edition.* **3419**
Association of Physicians of India. Journal (IND) *Online - full text edition.* **3571**
Atherosclerosis (IRL) *Online - full text edition.* **3763**
Athletic Therapy Today (USA) *Online - full text edition.* **4173**
Atmospheric Environment (GBR) *Online - full text edition.* **3443**
Attention and Performance (USA) *Online - full text edition.* **4379**
Audiology and Neuro-Otology (CHE) *Online - full text edition.* **4031**
Auris, Nasus, Larynx (NLD) *Online - full text edition.* **4031**
Austral Ecology (AUS) *Online - full text edition.* **3183**
Australasian Biotechnology (AUS) *Online - full text edition.* **3269**
Australian and New Zealand Journal of Obstetrics and Gynecology (AUS) *Online - full text edition.* **3945**
Australian & New Zealand Journal of Psychiatry (AUS) *Online - full text edition.* **4075**
Australian and New Zealand Journal of Public Health (AUS) *Online - full text edition.* **4462**
Australian Dental Journal (AUS) *Online - full text edition.* **3816**
Australian Journal of Experimental Agriculture (AUS) *Online - full text edition.* **3157**
Australian Journal of Physiotherapy (AUS) *Online - full text edition.* **4059**
Australian Journal of Psychology (AUS) *Online - full text edition.* **4379**
Australian Psychologist (AUS) *Online - full text edition.* **4379**
Australian Veterinary Journal (AUS) *Online - full text edition.* **4538**
Australian Veterinary Practitioner (AUS) *Online - full text edition.* **4539**
Autoimmunity (CHE) *Online - full text edition.* **3741**
Autonomic & Autacoid Pharmacology (GBR) *Online - full text edition.* **4279**
Autonomic Neuroscience: Basic & Clinical (NLD) *Online - full text edition.* **4075**
Avian Diseases (USA) *Online - full text edition.* **4539**
Avian Pathology (GBR) *Online - full text edition.* **4539**
Aviation, Space, and Environmental Medicine (USA) *Online - full text edition.* **3572**
B B A - Bioenergetics (NLD) *Online - full text edition.* **3278**
B B A - Biomembranes (NLD) *Online - full text edition.* **3285**
B B A - Gene Structure and Expression (NLD) *Online - full text edition.* **3299**
B B A - General Subjects (NLD) *Online - full text edition.* **3241**
B B A - Molecular and Cell Biology of Lipids (NLD) *Online - full text edition.* **3242**
B B A - Molecular Basis of Disease (NLD) *Online - full text edition.* **3299**
B B A - Molecular Cell Research (NLD) *Online - full text edition.* **3285**
B B A - Protein Structure and Molecular Enzymology (NLD) *Online - full text edition.* **3242**
B B A - Reviews on Cancer (NLD) *Online - full text edition.* **3968**
B J O Online (GBR) *Online - full text edition of* British Journal of Ophthalmology. **3994**
B J S M Online (GBR) *Online - full text edition of* British Journal of Sports Medicine. **4173**
B J U International (GBR) *Online - full text edition.* **4210**
Bailliere's Best Practice & Research in Clinical Endocrinology and Metabolism (GBR) *Online - full text edition.* **3855**
Bailliere's Best Practice & Research in Clinical Gastroenterology (GBR) *Online - full text edition.* **3886**
Bailliere's Best Practice & Research in Clinical Haematology (GBR) *Online - full text edition.* **3898**
Bailliere's Best Practice & Research in Clinical Obstetrics and Gynaecology (GBR) *Online - full text edition.* **3945**
Bailliere's Best Practice & Research in Clinical Rheumatology (GBR) *Online - full text edition.* **4167**
Bangladesh Journal of Botany (BGD) *Online - full text edition.* **3278**
Basic and Applied Social Psychology (USA) *Online - full text edition.* **4380**
Basic Research in Cardiology (DEU) *Online - full text edition.* **3764**
The Behavior Analyst (USA) *Online - full text edition.* **4380**
Behavior and Philosophy (USA) *Online - full text edition.* **4380**
Behavior Genetics (USA) *Online - full text edition.* **3299**
Behavior Modification (USA) *Online - full text edition.* **4380**
Behavior Research Methods, Instruments, and Computers (USA) *Online - full text edition.* **4380**
Behavior Therapy (USA) *Online - full text edition.* **4380**
Behavioral and Brain Sciences (GBR) *Online - full text edition.* **4380**
Behavioral Disorders (USA) *Online - full text edition.* **3419**
Behavioral Ecology (USA) *Online - full text edition.* **3184**
Behavioral Ecology and Sociobiology (DEU) *Online - full text edition.* **3436**
Behavioral Healthcare Tomorrow (USA) *Online - full text edition.* **4381**
Behavioral Interventions (GBR) *Online - full text edition.* **4076**
Behavioral Medicine (USA) *Online - full text edition.* **4381**
Behavioral Neuroscience (USA) *Online - full text edition.* **4381**
Behavioral Sciences and the Law (GBR) *Online - full text edition.* **4381**
Behaviour (NLD) *Online - full text edition.* **3351**
Behaviour and Information Technology (GBR) *Online - full text edition.* **4381**
Behaviour Change (AUS) *Online - full text edition.* **4381**
Behaviour Research and Therapy (GBR) *Online - full text edition.* **4382**
Behavioural Brain Research (NLD) *Online - full text edition.* **4076**
Behavioural Neurology (NLD) *Online - full text edition.* **4076**
Behavioural Pharmacology (USA) *Online - full text edition.* **4279**
Behavioural Processes (NLD) *Online - full text edition.* **4076**
Berliner und Muenchener Tieraerztliche Wochenschrift Online(DEU) *Online - full text.* **4539**
Bibliotheca Psychiatrica (CHE) *Online - full text edition.* **4076**
Bio-Medical Materials and Engineering (NLD) *Online - full text edition.* **3237**
Biocatalysis and Biotransformation (CHE) *Online - full text edition.* **3269**
Biocell (ARG) *Online - full text edition.* **3285**
Biochemical and Biophysical Research Communications (USA) *Online - full text edition.* **3242**
Biochemical Genetics (USA) *Online - full text edition.* **3299**
Biochemical Journal (GBR) *Online - full text edition.* **3242**
Biochemical Pharmacology (USA) *Online - full text edition.* **4279**
Biochemical Society Symposium (GBR) *Online - full text edition.* **3242**
Biochemical Society Transactions (GBR) *Online - full text edition.* **3243**
Biochemical Systematics and Ecology (GBR) *Online - full text edition.* **3243**
Biochemistry (USA) *Online - full text edition.* **3243**
Biochemistry and Cell Biology (CAN) *Online - full text edition.* **3243**
Biochemistry and Molecular Biology Education (GBR) *Online - full text edition.* **3243**
Biochemistry (Moscow) (RUS) *Online - full text edition.* **3244**
Biochimie (FRA) *Online - full text edition.* **3244**
Bioconjugate Chemistry (USA) *Online - full text edition.* **3244**
Biocontrol Science and Technology (GBR) *Online - full text edition.* **3157**
Biodegradation (NLD) *Online - full text edition.* **3456**
BioDrugs (NZL) *Online - full text edition.* **4280**
Bioelectrochemistry (CHE) *Online - full text edition.* **3244**
Bioelectromagnetics (USA) *Online - full text edition.* **3264**
BioEssays (GBR) *Online - full text edition.* **3184**
Bioethics (GBR) *Online - full text edition.* **4346**
BioFactors (NLD) *Online - full text edition.* **3244**
Biofizika (RUS) *Online - full text edition.* **3265**
Biofouling (CHE) *Online - full text edition.* **3446**
Biofutur (FRA) *Online - full text edition.* **3269**
Biogenic Amines (NLD) *Online - full text edition.* **3245**
Biogeochemistry (NLD) *Online - full text edition.* **3245**
Biogerontology (NLD) *Online - full text edition.* **3468**
Biological & Pharmaceutical Bulletin (JPN) *Online - full text edition.* **4280**
Biological Bulletin (USA) *Online - full text edition.* **3185**
Biological Chemistry (DEU) *Online - full text edition.* **3245**
Biological Control (USA) *Online - full text edition.* **3185**
Biological Psychiatry (USA) *Online - full text edition.* **4076**
Biological Psychology (NLD) *Online - full text edition.* **4382**
Biological Research (CHL) *Online - full text edition.* **3185**
Biological Reviews (GBR) *Online - full text edition.* **3185**
Biological Society of Washington. Proceedings (USA) *Online - full text edition.* **3185**
Biological Trace Element Research (USA) *Online - full text edition.* **3245**
Biologicals (GBR) *Online - full text edition.* **3186**
Biologicheskie Membrany (RUS) *Online - full text edition.* **3265**
Biology and Environment (IRL) *Online - full text edition.* **3186**
Biology and Fertility of Soils (DEU) *Online - full text edition.* **3157**
Biology of Blood and Marrow Transplantation (USA) *Online - full text edition.* **3898**
Biology of Reproduction (USA) *Online - full text edition.* **3186**
Biology of Sport (POL) *Online - full text edition.* **4173**
Biology of the Cell (FRA) *Online - full text edition.* **3286**
Biology of the Neonate (CHE) *Online - full text edition.* **3945**
Biomarkers (GBR) *Online - full text edition.* **3575**
Biomaterials (GBR) *Online - full text edition.* **3575**
Biomedical and Environmental Sciences (CHN) *Online - full text edition.* **3575**
Biomedical Chromatography (GBR) *Online - full text edition.* **3872**
Biomedical Letters (GBR) *Online - full text edition.* **3186**
Biomedical Research (JPN) *Online - full text edition.* **3576**
Biomedicine and Pharmacotherapy (FRA) *Online - full text edition.* **3577**
Biomedizinische Technik (DEU) *Online - full text edition.* **3577**
Biometrical Journal (DEU) *Online - full text edition.* **3187**
Biometrics (USA) *Online - full text edition.* **4528**
Biometrika (GBR) *Online - full text edition.* **3226**
Biomolecular Engineering (NLD) *Online - full text edition.* **3269**
Bioorganic & Medicinal Chemistry (GBR) *Online - full text edition.* **3377**
Bioorganic & Medicinal Chemistry Letters (GBR) *Online - full text edition.* **3378**
BioPharm (USA) *Online - full text edition.* **4280**
Biopharmaceutics & Drug Disposition (GBR) *Online - full text edition.* **4280**
Biophysical Chemistry (NLD) *Online - full text edition.* **3265**
Biophysical Journal (USA) *Online - full text edition.* **3265**
Biorheology (NLD) *Online - full text edition.* **3265**
BioScience (USA) *Online - full text edition.* **3187**
Bioscience, Biotechnology, and Biochemistry (JPN) *Online - full text edition.* **3270**
Bioscience Reports (USA) *Online - full text edition.* **3286**
Biosensors and Bioelectronics (GBR) *Online - full text edition.* **3270**
Biosystems (IRL) *Online - full text edition.* **3187**
Biotech Software and Internet Report (USA) *Online - full text edition.* **3270**
Biotechnic and Histochemistry (GBR) *Online - full text edition.* **3334**
BioTechniques (USA) *Online - full text edition.* **3270**
Biotechnology Advances (USA) *Online - full text edition.* **3271**
Biotechnology and Applied Biochemistry (GBR) *Online - full text edition.* **3271**
Biotechnology and Bioengineering (USA) *Online - full text edition.* **3271**
Biotechnology and Biotechnological Equipment (BGR) *Online - full text edition.* **3271**
Biotechnology and Development Monitor (NLD) *Online - full text edition.* **3271**
Biotechnology and Genetic Engineering Reviews (GBR) *Online - full text edition.* **3271**
Biotechnology Law Report (USA) *Online - full text edition.* **3272**
Biotechnology Letters (NLD) *Online - full text edition.* **3272**
Biotechnology Progress (USA) *Online - full text edition.* **3272**
Biotropica (USA) *Online - full text edition.* **3188**
Bipolar Disorders Online(DNK) *Online - full text.* **4077**
Birth (USA) *Online - full text edition.* **3946**
Blood (USA) *Online - full text edition.* **3898**
Blood Cells, Molecules, and Diseases (USA) *Online - full text edition.* **3898**
Blood Coagulation and Fibrinolysis (USA) *Online - full text edition.* **3898**
Blood Pressure (NOR) *Online - full text edition.* **3764**
Blood Pressure Monitoring (USA) *Online - full text edition.* **3764**
Blood Purification (CHE) *Online - full text edition.* **3899**
Blood Reviews (GBR) *Online - full text edition.* **3899**
bmj.com(GBR) *Online - full text.* **3577**
Bone (USA) *Online - full text edition.* **4011**
Bone Marrow Transplantation (GBR) *Online - full text edition.* **3872**
Brain (GBR) *Online - full text edition.* **4077**
Brain and Cognition (USA) *Online - full text edition.* **4383**

Online Service

Clinical Cardiology (Mahwah) (USA) *Online - full text edition.* **3768**
Clinical Chemistry (USA) *Online - full text edition.* **3873**
Clinical Chemistry and Laboratory Medicine (DEU) *Online - full text edition.* **3247**
Clinical Drug Investigation (NZL) *Online - full text edition.* **4283**
Clinical Dysmorphology (USA) *Online - full text edition.* **3191**
Clinical Electroencephalography (USA) *Online - full text edition.* **4082**
Clinical Endocrinology (GBR) *Online - full text edition.* **3856**
Clinical Genetics (DNK) *Online - full text edition.* **3300**
Clinical Hemorheology and Microcirculation (NLD) *Online - full text edition.* **3899**
Clinical Imaging (USA) *Online - full text edition.* **4141**
Clinical Immunology (USA) *Online - full text edition.* **3743**
Clinical Infectious Diseases (USA) *Online - full text edition.* **3794**
Clinical Journal of Pain (USA) *Online - full text edition.* **4082**
Clinical Journal of Sport Medicine (USA) *Online - full text edition.* **4173**
Clinical Leadership & Management Review (USA) *Online - full text edition.* **3873**
Clinical Linguistics & Phonetics (GBR) *Online - full text edition.* **4082**
Clinical Medicine (GBR) *Online - full text edition.* **3586**
Clinical Microbiology and Infection (GBR) *Online - full text edition.* **3586**
Clinical Microbiology Reviews (USA) *Online - full text edition.* **3319**
Clinical Nephrology (DEU) *Online - full text edition.* **4211**
Clinical Neurology and Neurosurgery (NLD) *Online - full text edition.* **4082**
Clinical Neuropathology (DEU) *Online - full text edition.* **4082**
Clinical Neuropharmacology (USA) *Online - full text edition.* **4284**
Clinical Neurophysiology (IRL) *Online - full text edition.* **4082**
Clinical Nuclear Medicine (USA) *Online - full text edition.* **4142**
Clinical Nutrition (GBR) *Online - full text edition.* **4231**
Clinical Obstetrics and Gynecology (USA) *Online - full text edition.* **3947**
Clinical Oncology (GBR) *Online - full text edition.* **3975**
Clinical Oral Implants Research (DNK) *Online - full text edition.* **3818**
Clinical Orthopaedics and Related Research (USA) *Online - full text edition.* **4012**
Clinical Otolaryngology and Allied Sciences (GBR) *Online - full text edition.* **4031**
Clinical Pediatrics (USA) *Online - full text edition.* **4042**
Clinical Pharmacokinetics (NZL) *Online - full text edition.* **4284**
Clinical Pharmacology & Therapeutics (USA) *Online - full text edition.* **4284**
Clinical Physiology and Functional Imaging (GBR) *Online - full text edition.* **3587**
Clinical Psychology (USA) *Online - full text edition.* **4388**
Clinical Psychology & Psychotherapy (GBR) *Online - full text edition.* **4388**
Clinical Psychology Review (GBR) *Online - full text edition.* **4388**
Clinical Radiology (GBR) *Online - full text edition.* **4142**
Clinical Rehabilitation (GBR) *Online - full text edition.* **4060**
Clinical Research and Regulatory Affairs (USA) *Online - full text edition.* **4284**
Clinical Reviews in Allergy & Immunology (USA) *Online - full text edition.* **3743**
Clinical Rheumatology (BEL) *Online - full text edition.* **4168**
Clinical Science (GBR) *Online - full text edition.* **3587**
Clinical Techniques in Small Animal Practice (USA) *Online - full text edition.* **4540**
Clinical Therapeutics (USA) *Online - full text edition.* **3587**
Clinical Transplantation (DNK) *Online - full text edition.* **4185**
Clinics in Chest Medicine (USA) *Online - full text edition.* **4159**
Clinics in Dermatology (USA) *Online - full text edition.* **3846**
Clinics in Geriatric Medicine (USA) *Online - full text edition.* **3469**
Clinics in Laboratory Medicine (USA) *Online - full text edition.* **3873**
Clinics in Perinatology (USA) *Online - full text edition.* **3947**
Clinics in Plastic Surgery (USA) *Online - full text edition.* **4185**
Clinics in Sports Medicine (USA) *Online - full text edition.* **4173**
Cognition (NLD) *Online - full text edition.* **4388**
Cognition and Emotion (GBR) *Online - full text edition.* **4388**
Cognition and Instruction (USA) *Online - full text edition.* **4388**
Cognitive, Affective, & Behavioral Neuroscience (USA) *Online - full text edition.* **4389**
Cognitive and Behavioral Practice (USA) *Online - full text edition.* **4389**
Cognitive Brain Research (NLD) *Online - full text edition.* **4083**
Cognitive Development (GBR) *Online - full text edition.* **4389**
Cognitive Linguistics (DEU) *Online - full text edition.* **3550**
Cognitive Neuropsychology (GBR) *Online - full text edition.* **4083**
Cognitive Psychology (USA) *Online - full text edition.* **4389**
Cognitive Science (GBR) *Online - full text edition.* **4389**
Cognitive Therapy and Research (USA) *Online - full text edition.* **4390**
Cold Spring Harbor Laboratory. Symposia on Quantitative Biology (USA) *Online - full text edition.* **3191**
Combinatorial Chemistry & High Throughput Screening (USA) *Online - full text edition.* **3372**
Combustion Science and Technology (CHE) *Online - full text edition.* **3379**
Community Dental Health (GBR) *Online - full text edition.* **3818**
Community Dentistry and Oral Epidemiology Online(DNK) *Online - full text.* **3818**
Community Mental Health Journal (USA) *Online - full text edition.* **4512**
Comparative Biochemistry and Physiology. Part A: Molecular & Integrative Physiology (USA) *Online - full text edition.* **3341**
Comparative Biochemistry and Physiology. Part B: Biochemistry & Molecular Biology (USA) *Online - full text edition.* **3247**
Comparative Biochemistry and Physiology. Toxicology & Pharmacology (USA) *Online - full text edition.* **3247**
Comparative Haematology International (GBR) *Online - full text edition.* **3900**
Comparative Immunology, Microbiology and Infectious Diseases (GBR) *Online - full text edition.* **3320**
Comparative Medicine (Memphis) (USA) *Online - full text edition.* **3351**
Comparative Political Studies (USA) *Online - full text edition.* **4367**
Compendium on Continuing Education for the Practicing Veterinarian (USA) *Online - full text edition.* **4541**
Complementary Therapies in Medicine (GBR) *Online - full text edition.* **3787**
Comprehensive Psychiatry (USA) *Online - full text edition.* **4083**
Comprehensive Therapy (USA) *Online - full text edition.* **3589**
Computer Methods and Programs in Biomedicine (IRL) *Online - full text edition.* **3809**
Computerized Medical Imaging and Graphics (GBR) *Online - full text edition.* **3809**
Computers in Biology and Medicine (GBR) *Online - full text edition.* **3284**
Computers in Human Behavior (GBR) *Online - full text edition.* **4524**
Computers in Nursing (USA) *Online - full text edition.* **3810**
Concepts in Magnetic Resonance (USA) *Online - full text edition.* **4142**
Confinia Cephalalgica (ITA) *Online - full text edition.* **4083**
Connective Tissue Research (CHE) *Online - full text edition.* **3288**
Consciousness and Cognition (USA) *Online - full text edition.* **4391**
Conservation Biology (USA) *Online - full text edition.* **3392**
Contact Dermatitis (DNK) *Online - full text edition.* **3846**
Contemporary Educational Psychology (USA) *Online - full text edition.* **3410**
Contemporary Family Therapy (USA) *Online - full text edition.* **4391**
Contemporary Ob-Gyn (USA) *Online - full text edition.* **3948**
Contemporary Psychoanalysis (USA) *Online - full text edition.* **4391**
Contemporary Psychology: A P A Review of Books (USA) *Online - full text edition.* **4391**
Contemporary Topics in Laboratory Animal Science (USA) *Online - full text edition.* **3873**
Contraception (USA) *Online - full text edition.* **3357**
Contributions to Gynecology and Obstetrics (CHE) *Online - full text edition.* **3948**
Contributions to Nephrology (CHE) *Online - full text edition.* **4211**
Controlled Clinical Trials (USA) *Online - full text edition.* **3873**
Cornea (USA) *Online - full text edition.* **3996**
Coronary Artery Disease (USA) *Online - full text edition.* **3769**
Cortex (ITA) *Online - full text edition.* **4084**
The Counseling Psychologist (USA) *Online - full text edition.* **4392**
Cranio: Journal of Craniomandibular Practice (USA) *Online - full text edition.* **3590**
Creativity Research Journal (USA) *Online - full text edition.* **4392**
Criminal Justice & Behavior (USA) *Online - full text edition.* **3394**
Crisis Intervention and Time-Limited Treatment (CHE) *Online - full text edition.* **4392**
Critical Care (GBR) *Online - full text edition.* **3590**
Critical Care Clinics (USA) *Online - full text edition.* **3590**
Critical Care Medicine (USA) *Online - full text edition.* **3590**
Critical Reviews in Biochemistry and Molecular Biology (USA) *Online - full text edition.* **3248**
Critical Reviews in Biomedical Engineering (USA) *Online - full text edition.* **3237**
Critical Reviews in Biotechnology (USA) *Online - full text edition.* **3273**
Critical Reviews in Clinical Laboratory Sciences (USA) *Online - full text edition.* **3591**
Critical Reviews in Diagnostic Imaging (USA) *Online - full text edition.* **4142**
Critical Reviews in Eukaryotic Gene Expression (USA) *Online - full text edition.* **3300**
Critical Reviews in Immunology (USA) *Online - full text edition.* **3743**
Critical Reviews in Microbiology (USA) *Online - full text edition.* **3320**
Critical Reviews in Neurobiology (USA) *Online - full text edition.* **4084**
Critical Reviews in Oncogenesis (USA) *Online - full text edition.* **3975**
Critical Reviews in Oncology - Hematology (IRL) *Online - full text edition.* **3975**
Critical Reviews in Oral Biology and Medicine (USA) *Online - full text edition.* **3819**
Critical Reviews in Therapeutic Drug Carrier Systems (USA) *Online - full text edition.* **4285**
Critical Reviews in Toxicology (USA) *Online - full text edition.* **3447**
Croatian Medical Journal (DEU) *Online - full text edition.* **3591**
Cross-Cultural Research (USA) *Online - full text edition.* **4508**
Cryobiology (USA) *Online - full text edition.* **3266**
CryoLetters (GBR) *Online - full text edition.* **3341**
Culture & Psychology (GBR) *Online - full text edition.* **4393**
Culture, Medicine and Psychiatry (NLD) *Online - full text edition.* **3173**
Current Biology (GBR) *Online - full text edition.* **3229**
Current Directions in Psychological Science (USA) *Online - full text edition.* **4393**
Current Drug Metabolism (USA) *Online - full text edition.* **4285**
Current Eye Research (USA) *Online - full text edition.* **3996**
Current Genetics (DEU) *Online - full text edition.* **3300**
Current Medical Research and Opinion (GBR) *Online - full text edition.* **3591**
Current Microbiology (USA) *Online - full text edition.* **3320**
Current Opinion in Biotechnology (GBR) *Online - full text edition.* **3273**
Current Opinion in Cardiology (USA) *Online - full text edition.* **3770**
Current Opinion in Cell Biology (GBR) *Online - full text edition.* **3288**
Current Opinion in Gastroenterology (USA) *Online - full text edition.* **3888**
Current Opinion in Genetics & Development (GBR) *Online - full text edition.* **3301**
Current Opinion in Hematology (USA) *Online - full text edition.* **3900**
Current Opinion in Immunology (GBR) *Online - full text edition.* **3722**
Current Opinion in Infectious Diseases (USA) *Online - full text edition.* **3794**
Current Opinion in Lipidology (GBR) *Online - full text edition.* **3770**
Current Opinion in Molecular Therapeutics (GBR) *Online - full text edition.* **4285**
Current Opinion in Nephrology & Hypertension (USA) *Online - full text edition.* **4211**
Current Opinion in Neurobiology (GBR) *Online - full text edition.* **4084**
Current Opinion in Neurology (USA) *Online - full text edition.* **4085**
Current Opinion in Obstetrics & Gynecology (USA) *Online - full text edition.* **3948**
Current Opinion in Oncology (USA) *Online - full text edition.* **3976**
Current Opinion in Pediatrics (USA) *Online - full text edition.* **4043**
Current Opinion in Psychiatry (USA) *Online - full text edition.* **4085**
Current Opinion in Rheumatology (USA) *Online - full text edition.* **4168**
Current Opinion in Structural Biology (GBR) *Online - full text edition.* **3248**
Current Orthopaedics (GBR) *Online - full text edition.* **4013**
Current Pharmaceutical Design (USA) *Online - full text edition.* **4286**
Current Problems in Cancer (USA) *Online - full text edition.* **3976**
Current Problems in Cardiology (USA) *Online - full text edition.* **3770**
Current Problems in Dermatology (USA) *Online - full text edition.* **3847**
Current Problems in Surgery (USA) *Online - full text edition.* **4186**
Current Psychology (New Brunswick) (USA) *Online - full text edition.* **4393**
Current Studies in Hematology and Blood Transfusion (CHE) *Online - full text edition.* **3900**
Current Therapeutic Research (USA) *Online - full text edition.* **3592**
Current Therapeutics (AUS) *Online - full text edition.* **3592**
Current Topics in Bioenergetics (USA) *Online - full text edition.* **3266**
Current Topics in Cellular Regulation (USA) *Online - full text edition.* **3192**
Current Topics in Developmental Biology (USA) *Online - full text edition.* **3192**
Current Topics in Membranes (USA) *Online - full text edition.* **3288**
Current Topics in Microbiology and Immunology (USA) *Online - full text edition.* **3320**
Cutis (USA) *Online - full text edition.* **3847**
CyberPsychology & Behavior (USA) *Online - full text edition.* **3390**
Cytogenetic and Genome Research (CHE) *Online - full text edition.* **3301**
Cytokine (GBR) *Online - full text edition.* **3301**
Cytokine and Growth Factor Reviews (GBR) *Online - full text edition.* **3248**
Cytokines, Cellular & Molecular Therapy (GBR) *Online - full text edition.* **3900**
Cytometry (USA) *Online - full text edition.* **3289**
Cytopathology (GBR) *Online - full text edition.* **3289**
Cytotechnology (NLD) *Online - full text edition.* **3289**
Cytotherapy (GBR) *Online - full text edition.* **3900**
D M W Disk-Archiv (DEU) *Online - full text edition.* **3723**
D N A and Cell Biology (USA) *Online - full text edition.* **3248**
D N A Sequence (CHE) *Online - full text edition.* **3248**
D T W - Deutsche Tieraerztliche Wochenschrift (DEU) *Online - full text edition.* **4541**
Danish Medical Bulletin (DNK) *Online - full text edition.* **3593**
Deafness and Education International (GBR) *Online - full text edition.* **3490**
Death Studies (USA) *Online - full text edition.* **4394**
Dementia and Geriatric Cognitive Disorders (CHE) *Online - full text edition.* **4085**
Dental Materials (USA) *Online - full text edition.* **3820**
Dental Traumatology Online(DNK) *Online - full text.* **3821**

Online Service

Dentomaxillofacial Radiology (GBR) Online - full text edition. 4143
Depression and Anxiety (USA) Online - full text edition. 4394
Dermatologic Clinics (USA) Online - full text edition. 3847
Dermatologic Surgery Online(USA) Online - full text. 4187
Dermatology (CHE) Online - full text edition. 3847
Deutsche Medizinische Wochenschrift (DEU) Online - full text edition. 3593
Development and Psychopathology (GBR) Online - full text edition. 4394
Development (Cambridge) (GBR) Online - full text edition. 3192
Development, Genes and Evolution (DEU) Online - full text edition. 3192
Development, Growth and Differentiation (AUS) Online - full text edition. 3192
Developmental and Comparative Immunology (GBR) Online - full text edition. 3743
Developmental Biology (USA) Online - full text edition. 3193
Developmental Brain Research (NLD) Online - full text edition. 4086
Developmental Dynamics (USA) Online - full text edition. 3193
Developmental Medicine and Child Neurology (GBR) Online - full text edition. 4043
Developmental Neuropsychology (USA) Online - full text edition. 4394
Developmental Neuroscience (CHE) Online - full text edition. 4086
Developmental Psychobiology (USA) Online - full text edition. 3193
Developmental Psychology (USA) Online - full text edition. 4394
Developmental Review (USA) Online - full text edition. 4394
Developmental Science (GBR) Online - full text edition. 4394
Developments in Ophthalmology (CHE) Online - full text edition. 3996
Deviant Behavior (USA) Online - full text edition. 4521
Diabetes (USA) Online - full text edition. 3857
Diabetes & Metabolism (FRA) Online - full text edition. 3857
Diabetes Care (USA) Online - full text edition. 3857
The Diabetes Educator (USA) Online - full text edition. 3858
Diabetes - Metabolism Research and Reviews (GBR) Online - full text edition. 3858
Diabetes, Nutrition & Metabolism, Clinical and Experimental (ITA) Online - full text edition. 3858
Diabetes, Obesity and Metabolism Online(GBR) Online - full text. 3858
Diabetes Research and Clinical Practice (IRL) Online - full text edition. 3858
Diabetic Medicine Online(GBR) Online - full text. 3860
Diabetologia (DEU) Online - full text edition. 3860
Diagnostic Cytopathology (USA) Online - full text edition. 3289
Diagnostic Microbiology and Infectious Disease (USA) Online - full text edition. 3320
Diagnostic Molecular Pathology (USA) Online - full text edition. 3594
Diagnostica (DEU) Online - full text edition. 4395
Dialysis & Transplantation (USA) Online - full text edition. 4212
Differentiation (DEU) Online - full text edition. 3193
Digestion (CHE) Online - full text edition. 3888
Digestive and Liver Disease (ITA) Online - full text edition. 3888
Digestive Diseases (CHE) Online - full text edition. 3888
Digestive Diseases and Sciences (USA) Online - full text edition. 3888
Digestive Surgery (CHE) Online - full text edition. 4187
Directory of Published Proceedings. Series S E M T - Science, Engineering, Medicine and Technology (USA) Online - full text edition. 4508
Disability and Rehabilitation (GBR) Online - full text edition. 3484
Disability & Society (GBR) Online - full text edition. 3494
Discourse & Society (GBR) Online - full text edition. 4395
Disease-a-Month (USA) Online - full text edition. 3594
Disease Management & Health Outcomes (NZL) Online - full text edition. 3595
Disease Markers (NLD) Online - full text edition. 3976
Diseases of the Colon and Rectum (USA) Online - full text edition. 4187
Diseases of the Esophagus Online(AUS) Online - full text. 4032
Documenta Ophthalmologica (NLD) Online - full text edition. 3997
Domestic Animal Endocrinology (USA) Online - full text edition. 4542
Dreaming (USA) Online - full text edition. 3342
Drug and Alcohol Dependence (IRL) Online - full text edition. 3400
Drug and Alcohol Review (GBR) Online - full text edition. 3400
Drug and Chemical Toxicology (USA) Online - full text edition. 4287
Drug and Therapeutics Bulletin (GBR) Online - full text edition. 4287
Drug Delivery (USA) Online - full text edition. 4288
Drug Development and Industrial Pharmacy (USA) Online - full text edition. 4288
Drug Development Research (USA) Online - full text edition. 4288
Drug Discovery Today (GBR) Online - full text edition. 4288
Drug Information Journal (USA) Online - full text edition. 4289
Drug Metabolism and Disposition (USA) Online - full text edition. 4289
Drug Metabolism Reviews (USA) Online - full text edition. 3596
Drug News & Perspectives (ESP) Online - full text edition. 4289
Drug Resistance Update (GBR) Online - full text edition. 3596
Drug Safety (NZL) Online - full text edition. 4289
Drugs (NZL) Online - full text edition. 4290
Drugs & Aging (NZL) Online - full text edition. 4290
Drugs & Therapy Perspectives (NZL) Online - full text edition. 4290
Drugs: Education, Prevention & Policy (GBR) Online - full text edition. 3401
Drugs of the Future (ESP) Online - full text edition. 4291
Drugs of Today (ESP) Online - full text edition. 4291
Drugs under Experimental and Clinical Research (CHE) Online - full text edition. 4291
Dynamische Psychiatrie (DEU) Online - full text edition. 4087
Dysphagia (USA) Online - full text edition. 4032
E H P Supplements (USA) Online - full text edition. 3436
The E M B O Journal (GBR) Online - full text edition. 3249
E M B O Reports Online (GBR) Online - full text edition of E M B O Reports. 3301
E M J Online (GBR) Online - full text edition of Emergency Medicine Journal. 4014
Ear and Hearing (USA) Online - full text edition. 4032
Early Human Development (IRL) Online - full text edition. 3948
The East African Medical Journal (KEN) Online - full text edition. 3597
Echocardiography (USA) Online - full text edition. 3771
Ecography (DNK) Online - full text edition. 3437
Ecological Applications (USA) Online - full text edition. 3437
Ecological Monographs (USA) Online - full text edition. 3437
Ecological Psychology (USA) Online - full text edition. 4396
Ecology (USA) Online - full text edition. 3437
Ecology of Food and Nutrition (CHE) Online - full text edition. 4232
Ecotoxicology (USA) Online - full text edition. 3448
Ecotoxicology and Environmental Safety - Online (USA) Online - full text edition of Ecotoxicology and Environmental Safety. 3448
Education and Training in Mental Retardation and Developmental Disabilities (USA) Online - full text edition. 3421
Educational and Psychological Measurement (USA) Online - full text edition. 4396
Educational Gerontology (USA) Online - full text edition. 3470
Educational Psychologist (USA) Online - full text edition. 4396
Educational Psychology Review (USA) Online - full text edition. 3411
Eksperimental'naya Onkologiya (UKR) Online - full text edition. 3977
Electro- and Magnetobiology (USA) Online - full text edition. 3266
Elektronische Ausgabe (DEU) Online - full text edition of Der Hautarzt. 3849
The Elementary School Journal (USA) Online - full text edition. 3411
Emergency Medicine (USA) Online - full text edition. 4013
Emergency Medicine Clinics of North America (USA) Online - full text edition. 4014
Emerging Infectious Diseases (Online Edition)(USA) Online - full text. 4467
L' Encephale (FRA) Online - full text edition. 4087
Endocrine (USA) Online - full text edition. 3860
Endocrine Journal (JPN) Online - full text edition. 3861
Endocrine Pathology (USA) Online - full text edition. 3861
Endocrine - Related Cancer (GBR) Online - full text edition. 3861
Endocrine Research (USA) Online - full text edition. 3861
Endocrine Reviews (USA) Online - full text edition. 3861
The Endocrinologist (USA) Online - full text edition. 3861
Endocrinology (USA) Online - full text edition. 3861
Endocrinology and Metabolism Clinics of North America (USA) Online - full text edition. 3862
Endocytobiosis and Cell Research (DEU) Online - full text edition. 3289
Endoscopy (DEU) Online - full text edition. 3889
Endothelium (CHE) Online - full text edition. 3194
Enfermedades Infecciosas y Microbiologia Clinica (ESP) Online - full text edition. 3795
Entomological Society of America. Annals (USA) Online - full text edition. 3295
Entomological Society of America. Annals Online (USA) Online - full text edition. 3295
Environment and Behavior (USA) Online - full text edition. 4521
Environment International (GBR) Online - full text edition. 3438
Environmental and Molecular Mutagenesis (USA) Online - full text edition. 3302
Environmental Entomology (USA) Online - full text edition. 3295
Environmental Health Perspectives (USA) Online - full text edition. 3438
Environmental Microbiology (GBR) Online - full text edition. 3321
Environmental Research (USA) Online - full text edition. 3439
Environmental Toxicology (USA) Online - full text edition. 3449
Environmental Toxicology and Chemistry (USA) Online - full text edition. 3449
Environmental Toxicology and Pharmacology (NLD) Online - full text edition. 3449
Enzyme and Microbial Technology (USA) Online - full text edition. 3273
Epidemiologic Reviews (USA) Online - full text edition. 3598
Epidemiology (USA) Online - full text edition. 4468
Epidemiology and Infection (GBR) Online - full text edition. 3321
Epilepsia (USA) Online - full text edition. 4087
Epilepsy Research (NLD) Online - full text edition. 4088
Epileptic Disorders (FRA) Online - full text edition. 4088
Equine Veterinary Education (GBR) Online - full text edition. 4542
Equine Veterinary Journal (GBR) Online - full text edition. 4542
Ergonomics (GBR) Online - full text edition. 3432
Ernaehrungs Umschau (DEU) Online - full text edition. 4232
Essays in Biochemistry (GBR) Online - full text edition. 3249
Estuaries (USA) Online - full text edition. 3194
Ethics & Behavior (USA) Online - full text edition. 4397
Ethiopian Medical Journal (ETH) Online - full text edition. 3599
Ethnicity and Health (GBR) Online - full text edition. 4468
Ethology Online(DEU) Online - full text. 3352
Europace (GBR) Online - full text edition. 3771
European Academy of Dermatology and Venereology. Journal (BEL) Online - full text edition. 3848
European Addiction Research (CHE) Online - full text edition. 3401
European Archives of Oto-Rhino-Laryngology (DEU) Online - full text edition. 4032
European Archives of Psychiatry and Clinical Neurosciences (DEU) Online - full text edition. 4088
European Biophysics Journal (DEU) Online - full text edition. 3266
European Child & Adolescent Psychiatry (DEU) Online - full text edition. 4089
European Cytokine Network (FRA) Online - full text edition. 3302
European Eating Disorders Review (GBR) Online - full text edition. 4397
European Heart Journal (GBR) Online - full text edition. 3771
European Journal of Anaesthesiology (GBR) Online - full text edition. 3757
European Journal of Applied Physiology (DEU) Online - full text edition. 3342
European Journal of Biochemistry (GBR) Online - full text edition. 3249
European Journal of Cancer (GBR) Online - full text edition. 3977
European Journal of Cancer Care Online(GBR) Online - full text. 3977
European Journal of Cancer Prevention (USA) Online - full text edition. 3977
European Journal of Cardio-Thoracic Surgery (NLD) Online - full text edition. 3771
European Journal of Cell Biology (DEU) Online - full text edition. 3289
European Journal of Clinical Investigation (GBR) Online - full text edition. 3599
European Journal of Clinical Microbiology & Infectious Diseases (DEU) Online - full text edition. 3321
European Journal of Clinical Nutrition (GBR) Online - full text edition. 4232
European Journal of Clinical Pharmacology (DEU) Online - full text edition. 4292
European Journal of Cognitive Psychology (GBR) Online - full text edition. 4397
European Journal of Dermatology (FRA) Online - full text edition. 3848
European Journal of Drug Metabolism and Pharmacokinetics (CHE) Online - full text edition. 4292
European Journal of Endocrinology (GBR) Online - full text edition. 3862
European Journal of Entomology (CZE) Online - full text edition. 3296
European Journal of Epidemiology (NLD) Online - full text edition. 3599
European Journal of Gastroenterology and Hepatology (USA) Online - full text edition. 3889
European Journal of Gynecological Oncology (CAN) Online - full text edition. 3977
European Journal of Haematology (DNK) Online - full text edition. 3900
The European Journal of Heart Failure (NLD) Online - full text edition. 3771
European Journal of Histochemistry (ITA) Online - full text edition. 3249
European Journal of Human Genetics (GBR) Online - full text edition. 3302
European Journal of Immunogenetics (GBR) Online - full text edition. 3302
European Journal of Immunology (DEU) Online - full text edition. 3744
European Journal of Medical Research (DEU) Online - full text edition. 3600
European Journal of Medicinal Chemistry (FRA) Online - full text edition. 3250
European Journal of Morphology (NLD) Online - full text edition. 3195
European Journal of Neurology (USA) Online - full text edition. 4089
European Journal of Neuroscience (GBR) Online - full text edition. 4089
European Journal of Nuclear Medicine and Molecular Imaging (DEU) Online - full text edition. 4144
European Journal of Nutrition (DEU) Online - full text edition. 4233
European Journal of Obstetrics & Gynecology and Reproductive Biology (IRL) Online - full text edition. 3949
European Journal of Ophthalmology (ITA) Online - full text edition. 3997
European Journal of Oral Sciences Online(DNK) Online - full text. 3823
European Journal of Orthodontics (GBR) Online - full text edition. 3823

Online Service

European Journal of Pain (GBR) *Online - full text edition.* **3600**
European Journal of Pediatric Surgery (DEU) *Online - full text edition.* **4188**
European Journal of Pediatrics (DEU) *Online - full text edition.* **4044**
European Journal of Personality (GBR) *Online - full text edition.* **4398**
European Journal of Pharmaceutical Sciences (NLD) *Online - full text edition.* **4292**
European Journal of Pharmaceutics and Biopharmaceutics (NLD) *Online - full text edition.* **4293**
European Journal of Pharmacology (NLD) *Online - full text edition.* **4293**
European Journal of Protistology (DEU) *Online - full text edition.* **4271**
European Journal of Psychiatry (ESP) *Online - full text edition.* **4089**
European Journal of Psychological Assessment (USA) *Online - full text edition.* **4398**
European Journal of Psychology of Education (DEU) *Online - full text edition.* **3411**
European Journal of Public Health (GBR) *Online - full text edition.* **4468**
European Journal of Radiology (IRL) *Online - full text edition.* **4144**
European Journal of Social Psychology (GBR) *Online - full text edition.* **4398**
European Journal of Soil Biology (FRA) *Online - full text edition.* **3195**
European Journal of Sports Traumatology and Related Research (ITA) *Online - full text edition.* **4173**
European Journal of Surgery (NOR) *Online - full text edition.* **4188**
European Journal of Surgical Oncology (GBR) *Online - full text edition.* **3977**
European Journal of Vascular and Endovascular Surgery (GBR) *Online - full text edition.* **3771**
European Neurology (CHE) *Online - full text edition.* **4089**
European Neuropsychopharmacology (NLD) *Online - full text edition.* **4089**
European Radiology (DEU) *Online - full text edition.* **4144**
The European Respiratory Journal (CHE) *Online - full text edition.* **4159**
European Spine Journal (DEU) *Online - full text edition.* **4189**
European Surgical Research (CHE) *Online - full text edition.* **4189**
European Urology (CHE) *Online - full text edition.* **4212**
Evaluation and the Health Professions (USA) *Online - full text edition.* **3600**
Evolution (USA) *Online - full text edition.* **3302**
Evolution & Development Online(USA) *Online - full text.* **3195**
L' Evolution Psychiatrique (FRA) *Online - full text edition.* **4090**
Evolutionary Biology (USA) *Online - full text edition.* **3302**
Exceptional Children (USA) *Online - full text edition.* **3422**
Exercise Immunology Review (USA) *Online - full text edition.* **4173**
Exercise Standards and Malpractice Reporter (USA) *Online - full text edition.* **3538**
Experimental Aging Research (USA) *Online - full text edition.* **4398**
Experimental & Applied Acarology (NLD) *Online - full text edition.* **3352**
Experimental and Clinical Endocrinology and Diabetes (DEU) *Online - full text edition.* **3862**
Experimental and Clinical Psychopharmacology (USA) *Online - full text edition.* **4398**
Experimental and Molecular Medicine (KOR) *Online - full text edition.* **3250**
Experimental and Molecular Pathology (USA) *Online - full text edition.* **3600**
Experimental and Toxicologic Pathology (DEU) *Online - full text edition.* **3600**
Experimental Animals (JPN) *Online - full text edition.* **3874**
Experimental Biology and Medicine (Maywood) (USA) *Online - full text edition.* **3195**
Experimental Brain Research (DEU) *Online - full text edition.* **4090**
Experimental Dermatology Online(DNK) *Online - full text.* **3849**
Experimental Eye Research (GBR) *Online - full text edition.* **3997**
Experimental Gerontology (USA) *Online - full text edition.* **3471**
Experimental Hematology (USA) *Online - full text edition.* **3901**
Experimental Lung Research (USA) *Online - full text edition.* **4160**
Experimental Nephrology (CHE) *Online - full text edition.* **4212**
Experimental Neurology (USA) *Online - full text edition.* **4090**
Experimental Parasitology (USA) *Online - full text edition.* **3796**
Experimental Physiology (GBR) *Online - full text edition.* **3342**
Expert Opinion On Investigational Drugs (GBR) *Online - full text edition.* **4293**
Expert Opinion on Therapeutic Patents (GBR) *Online - full text edition.* **4293**
Eye (GBR) *Online - full text edition.* **3997**
The F A S E B Journal (USA) *Online - full text edition.* **3196**
F D A Consumer (USA) *Online - full text edition.* **3392**
F E B S Letters (NLD) *Online - full text edition.* **3250**
F E M S Immunology and Medical Microbiology (NLD) *Online - full text edition.* **3321**
F E M S Microbiology Ecology (NLD) *Online - full text edition.* **3321**
F E M S Microbiology Letters (NLD) *Online - full text edition.* **3322**
F E M S Microbiology Reviews (NLD) *Online - full text edition.* **3322**
Family and Community Health (USA) *Online - full text edition.* **4469**
Family Medicine (USA) *Online - full text edition.* **3601**
Family Planning Perspectives (USA) *Online - full text edition.* **3949**
Family Practice (GBR) *Online - full text edition.* **3601**
Family Process (USA) *Online - full text edition.* **4399**
Il Farmaco (FRA) *Online - full text edition.* **4295**
Feminism & Psychology (GBR) *Online - full text edition.* **4399**
Fertility and Sterility (USA) *Online - full text edition.* **3949**
Fetal Diagnosis and Therapy (CHE) *Online - full text edition.* **3950**
Fibrinolysis & Proteolysis (GBR) *Online - full text edition.* **3875**
Fish and Shellfish Immunology (GBR) *Online - full text edition.* **3196**
Fitoterapia (ITA) *Online - full text edition.* **3279**
Fluoride (NZL) *Online - full text edition.* **3728**
Focus on Exceptional Children (USA) *Online - full text edition.* **3422**
Folia Biologica (CZE) *Online - full text edition.* **3196**
Folia Biologica (POL) *Online - full text edition.* **3196**
Folia Histochemica et Cytobiologica (POL) *Online - full text edition.* **3290**
Folia Microbiologica (GBR) *Online - full text edition.* **3250**
Folia Neuropathologica (POL) *Online - full text edition.* **4091**
Folia Parasitologica (CZE) *Online - full text edition.* **3796**
Folia Pharmacologica Japonica (JPN) *Online - full text edition.* **4296**
Folia Phoniatrica et Logopaedica (CHE) *Online - full text edition.* **4032**
Food Additives and Contaminants (GBR) *Online - full text edition.* **4296**
Food and Agricultural Immunology (GBR) *Online - full text edition.* **3197**
Food and Chemical Toxicology (GBR) *Online - full text edition.* **3449**
Food and Drug Law Journal (USA) *Online - full text edition.* **3539**
Food Hygienic Society of Japan. Journal (JPN) *Online - full text edition.* **4469**
Food Microbiology (GBR) *Online - full text edition.* **3322**
Foot & Ankle International (USA) *Online - full text edition.* **4015**
Forensic Science International (IRL) *Online - full text edition.* **3882**
Formosan Medical Association. Journal (HKG) *Online - full text edition.* **3603**
Formulary (USA) *Online - full text edition.* **4297**
Forschende Komplementaermedizin und Klassische Naturheilkunde (CHE) *Online - full text edition.* **3165**
Fortschritte der Neurologie, Psychiatrie (DEU) *Online - full text edition.* **4091**
Forum der Psychoanalyse (DEU) *Online - full text edition.* **4399**
Forum of Nutrition (CHE) *Online - full text edition.* **4234**
Free Radical Biology & Medicine (USA) *Online - full text edition.* **3197**
Freshwater Biology Online(GBR) *Online - full text.* **3197**
Frontiers in Bioscience (USA) *Online - full text edition.* **3603**
Frontiers in Neuroendocrinology (USA) *Online - full text edition.* **3862**
Frontiers of Gastrointestinal Research (CHE) *Online - full text edition.* **3889**
Frontiers of Hormone Research (CHE) *Online - full text edition.* **3863**
Frontiers of Oral Biology (CHE) *Online - full text edition.* **3824**
Frontiers of Radiation Therapy and Oncology (CHE) *Online - full text edition.* **4144**
Fuctional Plant Biology (AUS) *Online - full text edition.* **3280**
Functional Neurology (ITA) *Online - full text edition.* **4091**
Fundamental and Clinical Pharmacology (FRA) *Online - full text edition.* **4297**
The Future of Children (USA) *Online - full text edition.* **3383**
Gait and Posture (NLD) *Online - full text edition.* **3605**
Games and Economic Behavior (USA) *Online - full text edition.* **4400**
Gastro-Enterologie Clinique et Biologique (FRA) *Online - full text edition.* **3890**
Gastroenterology (USA) *Online - full text edition.* **3890**
Gastroenterology Clinics of North America (USA) *Online - full text edition.* **3890**
Gastrointestinal Endoscopy (USA) *Online - full text edition.* **3891**
Geburtshilfe und Frauenheilkunde (DEU) *Online - full text edition.* **3950**
Gematologiya i Transfusiologiya (RUS) *Online - full text edition.* **3901**
Gene - C O M B I S (NLD) *Online - full text edition of* Gene. **3274**
Gene Expression (USA) *Online - full text edition.* **3303**
Gene Therapy (Basingstoke) (GBR) *Online - full text edition.* **3606**
General and Comparative Endocrinology (USA) *Online - full text edition.* **3863**
General Hospital Psychiatry (USA) *Online - full text edition.* **4091**
General Pharmacology (USA) *Online - full text edition.* **4297**
General Physiology and Biophysics (SVK) *Online - full text edition.* **3343**
Generations (San Francisco) (USA) *Online - full text edition.* **3471**
Genes & Development (USA) *Online - full text edition.* **3303**
Genes & Genetic Systems (JPN) *Online - full text edition.* **3303**
Genes and Immunity (GBR) *Online - full text edition.* **3303**
Genes, Chromosomes & Cancer (USA) *Online - full text edition.* **3303**
Genes to Cells (GBR) *Online - full text edition.* **3303**
Genesis: The Journal of Genetics and Development (USA) *Online - full text edition.* **3304**
Genetic Counseling (CHE) *Online - full text edition.* **3304**
Genetic Engineering News (USA) *Online - full text edition.* **3304**
Genetic Epidemiology (USA) *Online - full text edition.* **3304**
Genetic Resources and Crop Evolution (NLD) *Online - full text edition.* **3304**
Genetic, Social, and General Psychology Monographs (USA) *Online - full text edition.* **4400**
Genetic Testing (USA) *Online - full text edition.* **3304**
Genetica (NLD) *Online - full text edition.* **3305**
Genetical Research (GBR) *Online - full text edition.* **3305**
Genetics (USA) *Online - full text edition.* **3305**
Genetics and Molecular Biology (BRA) *Online - full text edition.* **3305**
Genetics In Medicine (USA) *Online - full text edition.* **3305**
Genetics, Selection, Evolution Online (FRA) *Online - full text edition of* Genetics, Selection, Evolution. **3305**
Genome (CAN) *Online - full text edition.* **3306**
Genome Research (USA) *Online - full text edition.* **3306**
Genomics (USA) *Online - full text edition.* **3306**
Geomicrobiology Journal (USA) *Online - full text edition.* **3322**
Geriatric Nursing (USA) *Online - full text edition.* **3472**
Geriatrics (USA) *Online - full text edition.* **3472**
The Gerontologist (USA) *Online - full text edition.* **3473**
Gerontology (CHE) *Online - full text edition.* **3473**
Das Gesundheitswesen (DEU) *Online - full text edition.* **4470**
Gifted Child Quarterly (USA) *Online - full text edition.* **3422**
Giornale di Neuropsicofarmacologia (ITA) *Online - full text edition.* **4092**
Glia (USA) *Online - full text edition.* **4092**
Glycobiology (GBR) *Online - full text edition.* **3251**
Glycoconjugate Journal (USA) *Online - full text edition.* **3251**
Graefe's Archive for Clinical and Experimental Ophthalmology (DEU) *Online - full text edition.* **3998**
Group & Organization Management (USA) *Online - full text edition.* **3411**
Group (New York) (USA) *Online - full text edition.* **4401**
Growth, Development & Aging (USA) *Online - full text edition.* **3198**
Growth Factors (CHE) *Online - full text edition.* **3343**
Growth Hormone and I G F Research (GBR) *Online - full text edition.* **3863**
Gruppendynamik und Organisationsberatung (DEU) *Online - full text edition.* **4401**
Gruppenpsychotherapie und Gruppendynamik (DEU) *Online - full text edition.* **4092**
Gut Online (GBR) *Online - full text edition of* Gut. **3891**
Gynaecological Endoscopy (GBR) *Online - full text edition.* **3951**
Der Gynaekologe (DEU) *Online - full text edition.* **3951**
Gynecologic and Obstetric Investigation (CHE) *Online - full text edition.* **3952**
Gynecologic Oncology (USA) *Online - full text edition.* **3952**
Gynecological Endocrinology (GBR) *Online - full text edition.* **3863**
Gynecologie Obstetrique et Fertilite (FRA) *Online - full text edition.* **3952**
H N O (Berlin) (DEU) *Online - full text edition.* **4033**
Haematologia (NLD) *Online - full text edition.* **3901**
Haematologica (ITA) *Online - full text edition.* **3901**
Haemophilia Online(GBR) *Online - full text.* **3901**
Hand Clinics (USA) *Online - full text edition.* **4016**
Han'gug Yujeon Haghoeji (KOR) *Online - full text edition.* **3306**
Harvard Review of Psychiatry (GBR) *Online - full text edition.* **4093**
Hastings Center Report (USA) *Online - full text edition.* **3610**
Hazardous Waste Consultant (USA) *Online - full text edition.* **3457**
Head & Neck (USA) *Online - full text edition.* **4190**
Headache Online(USA) *Online - full text.* **4093**
Headache Quarterly (USA) *Online - full text edition.* **3728**
Health Affairs (USA) *Online - full text edition.* **4471**
Health & Place (GBR) *Online - full text edition.* **3465**
Health and Social Care in the Community Online(GBR) *Online - full text.* **4472**
Health & Social Work (USA) *Online - full text edition.* **4513**
Health Care Analysis (NLD) *Online - full text edition.* **3610**
Health Care Financing Review (USA) *Online - full text edition.* **3610**
Health Care Management Review (USA) *Online - full text edition.* **3508**
Health Communication (USA) *Online - full text edition.* **4472**
Health Economics (GBR) *Online - full text edition.* **3611**
Health Education & Behavior (USA) *Online - full text edition.* **4472**
Health Education Research (GBR) *Online - full text edition.* **4513**
Health Forum (USA) *Online - full text edition.* **3509**
Health Physics (USA) *Online - full text edition.* **3612**
Health Policy (IRL) *Online - full text edition.* **4473**
Health Policy and Planning (GBR) *Online - full text edition.* **4473**

International Journal of Neuro-Psychopharmacology (GBR) *Online - full text edition.* **4303**
International Journal of Neuroscience (CHE) *Online - full text edition.* **4096**
International Journal of Nursing Studies (GBR) *Online - full text edition.* **3922**
International Journal of Obesity (GBR) *Online - full text edition.* **4236**
International Journal of Obstetric Anesthesia (GBR) *Online - full text edition.* **3954**
International Journal of Offender Therapy and Comparative Criminology (USA) *Online - full text edition.* **3394**
International Journal of Oncology (GRC) *Online - full text edition.* **3980**
International Journal of Oral & Maxillofacial Implants (USA) *Online - full text edition.* **3826**
International Journal of Oral & Maxillofacial Surgery (DNK) *Online - full text edition.* **3827**
International Journal of Pancreatology (USA) *Online - full text edition.* **3864**
International Journal of Pediatric Otorhinolaryngology (IRL) *Online - full text edition.* **4033**
International Journal of Periodontics & Restorative Dentistry (USA) *Online - full text edition.* **3827**
International Journal of Pest Management (GBR) *Online - full text edition.* **3158**
International Journal of Pharmaceutics (NLD) *Online - full text edition.* **4303**
International Journal of Prosthodontics (USA) *Online - full text edition.* **3827**
International Journal of Psychiatry in Clinical Practice (GBR) *Online - full text edition.* **4096**
International Journal of Psychiatry in Medicine (USA) *Online - full text edition.* **4096**
The International Journal of Psycho-Analysis (GBR) *Online - full text edition.* **4406**
International Journal of Psychology (GBR) *Online - full text edition.* **4407**
International Journal of Psychophysiology (NLD) *Online - full text edition.* **4407**
International Journal of Radiation Biology (GBR) *Online - full text edition.* **3980**
International Journal of Radiation: Oncology - Biology - Physics (USA) *Online - full text edition.* **4146**
International Journal of Rehabilitation Research (USA) *Online - full text edition.* **4061**
International Journal of S T D & AIDS (GBR) *Online - full text edition.* **3800**
International Journal of Social Psychiatry (GBR) *Online - full text edition.* **4096**
International Journal of Sport Nutrition & Exercise Metabolism (USA) *Online - full text edition.* **4236**
International Journal of Sport Psychology (ITA) *Online - full text edition.* **4174**
International Journal of Sports Medicine (DEU) *Online - full text edition.* **4174**
International Journal of Stress Management (USA) *Online - full text edition.* **3624**
International Journal of Surgical Pathology (USA) *Online - full text edition.* **4191**
International Journal of Systematic and Evolutionary Microbiology (GBR) *Online - full text edition.* **3324**
International Journal of Technology Assessment in Health Care (GBR) *Online - full text edition.* **3875**
International Journal of Toxicology (GBR) *Online - full text edition.* **3451**
International Journal of Tuberculosis and Lung Disease (FRA) *Online - full text edition.* **4160**
International Journal of Urology (AUS) *Online - full text edition.* **4213**
International Neuropsychological Society. Journal (GBR) *Online - full text edition.* **4097**
International Ophthalmology Clinics (USA) *Online - full text edition.* **3999**
International Orthopaedics (DEU) *Online - full text edition.* **4016**
International Psychogeriatrics (USA) *Online - full text edition.* **4097**
International Review of Cytology (USA) *Online - full text edition.* **3290**
International Review of Experimental Pathology (USA) *Online - full text edition.* **3624**
International Review of Hydrobiology (DEU) *Online - full text edition.* **3201**
International Review of Neurobiology (USA) *Online - full text edition.* **4097**
International Review of Psychiatry (GBR) *Online - full text edition.* **4097**
International Review of Research in Mental Retardation (USA) *Online - full text edition.* **4097**
International Surgery (ITA) *Online - full text edition.* **4191**
International Urogynecology Journal (GBR) *Online - full text edition.* **3954**
International Yearbook of Nephrology (DEU) *Online - full text edition.* **4214**
Der Internist (DEU) *Online - full text edition.* **3909**
Interscience Conference on Antimicrobial Agents and Chemotherapy. Program and Abstracts (USA) *Online - full text edition.* **3324**
Intervention in School and Clinic (USA) *Online - full text edition.* **3423**
Interventional Neuroradiology (ITA) *Online - full text edition.* **4146**
Intervirology (CHE) *Online - full text edition.* **3324**
Invertebrate Biology (USA) *Online - full text edition.* **3353**
Invertebrate Systematics (Online Edition)(AUS) *Online - full text.* **3353**
Investigational New Drugs (USA) *Online - full text edition.* **4304**
Investigative Ophthalmology & Visual Science (IOVS) (USA) *Online - full text edition.* **3999**
Investigative Radiology (USA) *Online - full text edition.* **4146**
Irish Journal of Medical Sciences (IRL) *Online - full text edition.* **3625**
Irish Journal of Psychological Medicine (IRL) *Online - full text edition.* **4097**
Irish Veterinary Journal (IRL) *Online - full text edition.* **4545**
Isokinetics and Exercise Science (NLD) *Online - full text edition.* **4174**
Israel Journal of Psychiatry and Related Sciences (ISR) *Online - full text edition.* **4097**
Issues in Law and Medicine (USA) *Online - full text edition.* **3626**
Italian Journal of Biochemistry (ITA) *Online - full text edition.* **3252**
Italian Journal of Mineral & Electrolyte Metabolism (ITA) *Online - full text edition.* **3252**
J A H Online (USA) *Online - full text edition of* Journal of Adolescent Health. **3629**
J A I D S (USA) *Online - full text edition.* **3800**
J A M A: The Journal of the American Medical Association (USA) *Online - full text edition.* **3626**
J A R O (USA) *Online - full text edition.* **4034**
J C P Online (GBR) *Online - full text edition of* Journal of Clinical Pathology. **3631**
J C R: Journal of Clinical Rheumatology (USA) *Online - full text edition.* **4168**
J E C H Online (GBR) *Online - full text edition of* Journal of Epidemiology & Community Health. **3632**
J M B Online (GBR) *Online - full text edition of* Journal of Molecular Biology. **3254**
J M E Online (GBR) *Online - full text edition of* Journal of Medical Ethics. **3635**
J M G Online (GBR) *Online - full text edition of* Journal of Medical Genetics. **3310**
J M S Online (GBR) *Online - full text edition of* Journal of Medical Screening. **3802**
J N: Journal of Nephrology (ITA) *Online - full text edition.* **4214**
J N M Online (USA) *Online - full text edition of* The Journal of Nuclear Medicine. **4148**
Japanese Circulation Journal (JPN) *Online - full text edition.* **3776**
Japanese Heart Journal (JPN) *Online - full text edition.* **3776**
Japanese Journal of Cancer Research (GBR) *Online - full text edition.* **3981**
Japanese Journal of Chemotherapy (JPN) *Online - full text edition.* **4304**
Japanese Journal of Clinical Oncology (GBR) *Online - full text edition.* **3981**
Japanese Journal of Educational Psychology (JPN) *Online - full text edition.* **4408**
Japanese Journal of Infectious Diseases (JPN) *Online - full text edition.* **3627**
Japanese Journal of Ophthalmology (NLD) *Online - full text edition.* **4000**
The Japanese Journal of Pharmacology (JPN) *Online - full text edition.* **4304**
Japanese Journal of Physical Fitness and Sports Medicine (JPN) *Online - full text edition.* **4356**
Japanese Journal of Physiology (JPN) *Online - full text edition.* **3343**
Japanese Journal of Veterinary Research (JPN) *Online - full text edition.* **4545**
Japanese Psychological Research (JPN) *Online - full text edition.* **4408**
Japanese Society of Internal Medicine. Journal (JPN) *Online - full text edition.* **3909**
Joint Bone Spine (FRA) *Online - full text edition.* **4017**
Journal de Chirurgie (FRA) *Online - full text edition.* **4192**
Journal de Mycologie Medicale (FRA) *Online - full text edition.* **3747**
Journal de Radiologie (FRA) *Online - full text edition.* **4147**
Journal des Maladies Vasculaires (FRA) *Online - full text edition.* **3776**
Journal for the Theory of Social Behaviour (GBR) *Online - full text edition.* **4408**
Journal Francais d'Ophtalmologie (FRA) *Online - full text edition.* **4000**
Journal Midwifery and Women's Health (USA) *Online - full text edition.* **3955**
Journal of Abnormal Child Psychology (USA) *Online - full text edition.* **4409**
Journal of Abnormal Psychology (USA) *Online - full text edition.* **4409**
Journal of Addictive Diseases (USA) *Online - full text edition.* **3402**
Journal of Adolescence (GBR) *Online - full text edition.* **3383**
Journal of Adolescent Research (USA) *Online - full text edition.* **4409**
Journal of Adult Development (USA) *Online - full text edition.* **4409**
Journal of Advanced Nursing (GBR) *Online - full text edition.* **3923**
Journal of Aerosol Medicine (USA) *Online - full text edition.* **4161**
Journal of Affective Disorders (NLD) *Online - full text edition.* **4098**
Journal of Aging and Health (USA) *Online - full text edition.* **3474**
Journal of Aging and Physical Activity (USA) *Online - full text edition.* **3475**
Journal of Aging Studies (GBR) *Online - full text edition.* **3475**
Journal of Alcohol and Drug Education (USA) *Online - full text edition.* **3402**
The Journal of Allergy and Clinical Immunology (USA) *Online - full text edition.* **3748**
Journal of Alternative & Complementary Medicine (USA) *Online - full text edition.* **3167**
Journal of American College Health (USA) *Online - full text edition.* **4357**
Journal of Analytical Psychology (GBR) *Online - full text edition.* **4409**
Journal of Analytical Toxicology (USA) *Online - full text edition.* **3451**
Journal of Anatomy (GBR) *Online - full text edition.* **3202**
Journal of Andrology (USA) *Online - full text edition.* **3629**
Journal of Animal Ecology (GBR) *Online - full text edition.* **3202**
Journal of Animal Physiology and Animal Nutrition Online(DEU) *Online - full text.* **3344**
Journal of Anti-Aging Medicine (USA) *Online - full text edition.* **3475**
Journal of Antibiotics (JPN) *Online - full text edition.* **3629**
Journal of Antimicrobial Chemotherapy (GBR) *Online - full text edition.* **3800**
Journal of Anxiety Disorders (GBR) *Online - full text edition.* **4409**
Journal of Applied Behavior Analysis (USA) *Online - full text edition.* **4410**
Journal of Applied Biobehavioral Research (USA) *Online - full text edition.* **4410**
Journal of Applied Biomechanics (USA) *Online - full text edition.* **3344**
Journal of Applied Developmental Psychology (GBR) *Online - full text edition.* **4410**
Journal of Applied Gerontology (USA) *Online - full text edition.* **3475**
Journal of Applied Microbiology (GBR) *Online - full text edition.* **3324**
Journal of Applied Physiology Online (USA) *Online - full text edition of* Journal of Applied Physiology. **3344**
Journal of Applied Psychology (USA) *Online - full text edition.* **4410**
Journal of Applied Research in Intellectual Disabilities (GBR) *Online - full text edition.* **4098**
Journal of Applied Social Psychology (USA) *Online - full text edition.* **4410**
Journal of Applied Sport Psychology (USA) *Online - full text edition.* **4174**
Journal of Applied Toxicology (GBR) *Online - full text edition.* **3451**
Journal of Aquatic Animal Health (USA) *Online - full text edition.* **3459**
Journal of Arthroplasty (USA) *Online - full text edition.* **4017**
Journal of Asian Natural Products Research (CHE) *Online - full text edition.* **3167**
Journal of Assisted Reproduction and Genetics (USA) *Online - full text edition.* **3955**
Journal of Asthma (New York) (USA) *Online - full text edition.* **4161**
Journal of Athletic Training (USA) *Online - full text edition.* **4174**
Journal of Autism and Developmental Disorders (USA) *Online - full text edition.* **3423**
Journal of Autoimmunity (GBR) *Online - full text edition.* **3748**
Journal of Avian Medicine and Surgery (USA) *Online - full text edition.* **4545**
Journal of Back and Musculoskeletal Rehabilitation (NLD) *Online - full text edition.* **4017**
Journal of Bacteriology (USA) *Online - full text edition.* **3325**
Journal of Basic Microbiology (DEU) *Online - full text edition.* **3325**
The Journal of Behavior Therapy and Experimental Psychiatry (GBR) *Online - full text edition.* **4099**
Journal of Behavioral Health Services and Research (USA) *Online - full text edition.* **4479**
Journal of Behavioral Medicine (USA) *Online - full text edition.* **4099**
Journal of Bioactive and Compatible Polymers (USA) *Online - full text edition.* **3252**
Journal of Biochemical and Biophysical Methods (NLD) *Online - full text edition.* **3252**
Journal of Biochemistry (JPN) *Online - full text edition.* **3253**
Journal of Biochemistry and Molecular Biology (HKG) *Online - full text edition.* **3253**
Journal of Biochemistry and Molecular Biology Online (HKG) *Online - full text edition.* **3253**
Journal of Bioenergetics and Biomembranes (USA) *Online - full text edition.* **3253**
Journal of Biological Chemistry (USA) *Online - full text edition.* **3253**
Journal of Biological Education (GBR) *Online - full text edition.* **3202**
Journal of Biological Regulators and Homeostatic Agents (ITA) *Online - full text edition.* **3202**
Journal of Biological Rhythms (USA) *Online - full text edition.* **4099**
Journal of Biological Systems (SGP) *Online - full text edition.* **3202**
Journal of Biomaterials Applications (USA) *Online - full text edition.* **4192**
Journal of Biomechanical Engineering (USA) *Online - full text edition.* **3629**
The Journal of Biomechanics (GBR) *Online - full text edition.* **3629**
Journal of Biomedical Informatics (USA) *Online - full text edition.* **3811**
Journal of Biomedical Materials Research (USA) *Online - full text edition.* **3275**
Journal of Biomedical Optics (USA) *Online - full text edition.* **4366**
Journal of Biomedical Science (CHE) *Online - full text edition.* **3630**
Journal of Biomolecular Screening (USA) *Online - full text edition.* **3253**
Journal of Bioscience and Bioengineering (JPN) *Online - full text edition.* **3238**
Journal of Biosciences (IND) *Online - full text edition.* **3203**
Journal of Biosocial Science (GBR) *Online - full text edition.* **4521**
Journal of Biotechnology (NLD) *Online - full text edition.* **3275**
Journal of Black Studies (USA) *Online - full text edition.* **4509**
Journal of Bone and Joint Surgery: American Volume (USA) *Online - full text edition.* **4017**
Journal of Bone and Joint Surgery: British Volume (GBR) *Online - full text edition.* **4017**
Journal of Bone and Joint Surgery: British Volume on CD-ROM (GBR) *Online - full text edition.* **4018**
Journal of Bone and Mineral Metabolism (JPN) *Online - full text edition.* **3864**
Journal of Bone and Mineral Research (USA) *Online - full text edition.* **4018**
Journal of Burn Care & Rehabilitation (USA) *Online - full text edition.* **3630**

Journal of Business & Psychology (USA) *Online - full text edition.* **4411**
Journal of Cancer Education (USA) *Online - full text edition.* **3981**
Journal of Cancer Research and Clinical Oncology (DEU) *Online - full text edition.* **3981**
Journal of Cardiac Failure (USA) *Online - full text edition.* **3776**
Journal of Cardiac Surgery (USA) *Online - full text edition.* **3776**
Journal of Cardiothoracic and Vascular Anesthesia (USA) *Online - full text edition.* **3777**
Journal of Cardiovascular Electrophysiology (USA) *Online - full text edition.* **3777**
Journal of Cardiovascular Magnetic Resonance (USA) *Online - full text edition.* **3777**
Journal of Cardiovascular Pharmacology (USA) *Online - full text edition.* **4305**
Journal of Cardiovascular Risk (USA) *Online - full text edition.* **3777**
The Journal of Cardiovascular Surgery (ITA) *Online - full text edition.* **3777**
Journal of Career Assessment (USA) *Online - full text edition.* **4411**
Journal of Cataract and Refractive Surgery (USA) *Online - full text edition.* **4000**
Journal of Cell Biology (USA) *Online - full text edition.* **3290**
Journal of Cell Science (GBR) *Online - full text edition.* **3291**
Journal of Cellular Biochemistry (USA) *Online - full text edition.* **3254**
Journal of Cerebral Blood Flow and Metabolism (USA) *Online - full text edition.* **4099**
Journal of Chemical Neuroanatomy (NLD) *Online - full text edition.* **4099**
Journal of Chemotherapy (ITA) *Online - full text edition.* **3982**
Journal of Child and Adolescent Psychopharmacology (USA) *Online - full text edition.* **4099**
Journal of Child & Adolescent Substance Abuse (USA) *Online - full text edition.* **3402**
Journal of Child Language (GBR) *Online - full text edition.* **3384**
Journal of Child Neurology (CAN) *Online - full text edition.* **4099**
Journal of Child Psychology & Psychiatry & Allied Disciplines (GBR) *Online - full text edition.* **4411**
Journal of Chromatography. B, Biomedical Sciences and Applications (NLD) *Online - full text edition.* **3373**
Journal of Classification (USA) *Online - full text edition.* **3553**
The Journal of Clinical Anesthesia (USA) *Online - full text edition.* **3758**
Journal of Clinical Apheresis (USA) *Online - full text edition.* **3903**
Journal of Clinical Biochemical and Nutrition (JPN) *Online - full text edition.* **3254**
Journal of Clinical Child and Adolescent Psychology (USA) *Online - full text edition.* **4411**
Journal of Clinical Densitometry (USA) *Online - full text edition.* **3630**
Journal of Clinical Endocrinology and Metabolism (USA) *Online - full text edition.* **3864**
The Journal of Clinical Epidemiology (USA) *Online - full text edition.* **3630**
Journal of Clinical Ethics (USA) *Online - full text edition.* **3630**
Journal of Clinical Gastroenterology (USA) *Online - full text edition.* **3893**
Journal of Clinical Immunology (USA) *Online - full text edition.* **3748**
Journal of Clinical Investigation (USA) *Online - full text edition.* **3631**
Journal of Clinical Laboratory Analysis (USA) *Online - full text edition.* **3876**
Journal of Clinical Laser Medicine & Surgery (USA) *Online - full text edition.* **4147**
Journal of Clinical Ligand Assay (USA) *Online - full text edition.* **3748**
Journal of Clinical Microbiology (USA) *Online - full text edition.* **3631**
Journal of Clinical Neurophysiology (USA) *Online - full text edition.* **4100**
Journal of Clinical Neuroscience (GBR) *Online - full text edition.* **4100**
Journal of Clinical Nursing (GBR) *Online - full text edition.* **3923**
Journal of Clinical Oncology (USA) *Online - full text edition.* **3982**
Journal of Clinical Periodontology (DNK) *Online - full text edition.* **3828**
Journal of Clinical Pharmacology (USA) *Online - full text edition.* **4306**
Journal of Clinical Pharmacy and Therapeutics (GBR) *Online - full text edition.* **4306**
Journal of Clinical Psychiatry (USA) *Online - full text edition.* **4100**
Journal of Clinical Psychology (USA) *Online - full text edition.* **4412**
Journal of Clinical Psychology in Medical Settings (USA) *Online - full text edition.* **4412**
Journal of Clinical Psychopharmacology (USA) *Online - full text edition.* **4306**
Journal of Clinical Ultrasound (USA) *Online - full text edition.* **4147**
Journal of Clinical Virology (NLD) *Online - full text edition.* **3801**
Journal of Cognitive Neuroscience (USA) *Online - full text edition.* **4100**
Journal of College Student Development (USA) *Online - full text edition.* **4412**
Journal of Communication Disorders (USA) *Online - full text edition.* **4412**
Journal of Community and Applied Social Psychology (GBR) *Online - full text edition.* **4413**
Journal of Community Health (USA) *Online - full text edition.* **3631**
Journal of Community Psychology (USA) *Online - full text edition.* **4413**
The Journal of Comparative Neurology (USA) *Online - full text edition.* **4100**
Journal of Comparative Pathology (GBR) *Online - full text edition.* **3203**
Journal of Comparative Physiology. A: Sensory, Neural, and Behavioral Physiology (DEU) *Online - full text edition.* **3344**
Journal of Comparative Physiology. B: Biochemical, Systemic, and Environmental Physiology (DEU) *Online - full text edition.* **3344**
Journal of Comparative Psychology (USA) *Online - full text edition.* **4413**
Journal of Computational Neuroscience (NLD) *Online - full text edition.* **4100**
Journal of Computer-Assisted Tomography (USA) *Online - full text edition.* **4147**
Journal of Consciousness Studies (GBR) *Online - full text edition.* **4413**
Journal of Constructivist Psychology (USA) *Online - full text edition.* **4413**
Journal of Consulting and Clinical Psychology (USA) *Online - full text edition.* **4413**
Journal of Consumer Psychology (USA) *Online - full text edition.* **3153**
Journal of Controlled Release (NLD) *Online - full text edition.* **4306**
Journal of Counseling & Development (USA) *Online - full text edition.* **4414**
Journal of Counseling Psychology (USA) *Online - full text edition.* **4414**
Journal of Cranio-Maxillo-Facial Surgery (GBR) *Online - full text edition.* **4192**
Journal of Craniofacial Surgery (USA) *Online - full text edition.* **4193**
The Journal of Creative Behavior (USA) *Online - full text edition.* **3412**
Journal of Critical Care (USA) *Online - full text edition.* **4018**
Journal of Cross-Cultural Psychology (USA) *Online - full text edition.* **4414**
Journal of Crustacean Biology (USA) *Online - full text edition.* **3354**
Journal of Cutaneous Pathology (DNK) *Online - full text edition.* **3850**
Journal of Dental Research (USA) *Online - full text edition.* **3828**
The Journal of Dentistry (GBR) *Online - full text edition.* **3828**
Journal of Dentistry for Children (USA) *Online - full text edition.* **3828**
Journal of Dermatological Science (IRL) *Online - full text edition.* **3850**
Journal of Dermatological Treatment (GBR) *Online - full text edition.* **3851**
Journal of Developmental and Behavioral Pediatrics (USA) *Online - full text edition.* **4046**
Journal of Developmental and Physical Disabilities (USA) *Online - full text edition.* **3485**
Journal of Diabetes and Its Complications (USA) *Online - full text edition.* **3864**
Journal of Digital Imaging (DEU) *Online - full text edition.* **4147**
Journal of Drug Education (USA) *Online - full text edition.* **3403**
Journal of Drug Issues (USA) *Online - full text edition.* **3403**
Journal of Drug Targeting (CHE) *Online - full text edition.* **4307**
Journal of Early Adolescence (USA) *Online - full text edition.* **3384**
Journal of Early Intervention (USA) *Online - full text edition.* **3423**
Journal of Ecology (GBR) *Online - full text edition.* **3203**
Journal of Economic Entomology (USA) *Online - full text edition.* **3296**
The Journal of Economic Psychology (NLD) *Online - full text edition.* **3366**
Journal of Educational and Psychological Consultation (USA) *Online - full text edition.* **3412**
Journal of Educational Psychology (USA) *Online - full text edition.* **3412**
Journal of Elder Abuse & Neglect (USA) *Online - full text edition.* **3476**
Journal of Electrocardiology (USA) *Online - full text edition.* **3777**
The Journal of Electroconvulsive Therapy (USA) *Online - full text edition.* **4101**
Journal of Electromyography and Kinesiology (GBR) *Online - full text edition.* **3266**
Journal of Electron Microscopy (GBR) *Online - full text edition.* **3334**
The Journal of Emergency Medicine (USA) *Online - full text edition.* **4018**
Journal of Emotional and Behavioral Disorders (USA) *Online - full text edition.* **4101**
Journal of Employment Counseling (USA) *Online - full text edition.* **4414**
Journal of Endocrinological Investigation (ITA) *Online - full text edition.* **3865**
Journal of Endocrinology (GBR) *Online - full text edition.* **3865**
The Journal of Endodontics (USA) *Online - full text edition.* **3828**
Journal of Endotoxin Research (GBR) *Online - full text edition.* **3865**
Journal of Endourology (USA) *Online - full text edition.* **4214**
Journal of Endovascular Therapy (USA) *Online - full text edition.* **4193**
Journal of Environmental Biology (IND) *Online - full text edition.* **3440**
Journal of Environmental Health (USA) *Online - full text edition.* **3440**
Journal of Environmental Psychology (GBR) *Online - full text edition.* **4415**
Journal of Environmental Radioactivity (GBR) *Online - full text edition.* **3440**
Journal of Environmental Science and Health. Part A: Toxic Hazardous Substances and Environmental Engineering (USA) *Online - full text edition.* **3452**
Journal of Environmental Science and Health. Part B: Pesticides, Food Contaminants, and Agricultural Wastes (USA) *Online - full text edition.* **3440**
Journal of Environmental Science and Health. Part C: Environmental Carcinogenesis & Ecotoxicology Reviews (USA) *Online - full text edition.* **3452**
Journal of Enzyme Inhibition (CHE) *Online - full text edition.* **3254**
Journal of Equine Veterinary Science (USA) *Online - full text edition.* **4545**
Journal of Ethnopharmacology (IRL) *Online - full text edition.* **4307**
Journal of Evaluation in Clinical Practice Online(GBR) *Online - full text.* **3632**
Journal of Evolutionary Biochemistry and Physiology (RUS) *Online - full text edition.* **3254**
Journal of Evolutionary Biology (GBR) *Online - full text edition.* **3309**
Journal of Experimental and Clinical Cancer Research (ITA) *Online - full text edition.* **3982**
Journal of Experimental Animal Science (DEU) *Online - full text edition.* **3876**
Journal of Experimental Biology (GBR) *Online - full text edition.* **3203**
Journal of Experimental Child Psychology (USA) *Online - full text edition.* **4415**
Journal of Experimental Marine Biology and Ecology (NLD) *Online - full text edition.* **3203**
The Journal of Experimental Medicine (USA) *Online - full text edition.* **3876**
Journal of Experimental Psychology: Animal Behavior Processes (USA) *Online - full text edition.* **4415**
Journal of Experimental Psychology: Applied (USA) *Online - full text edition.* **4415**
Journal of Experimental Psychology: General (USA) *Online - full text edition.* **4415**
Journal of Experimental Psychology: Human Perception and Performance (USA) *Online - full text edition.* **4415**
Journal of Experimental Psychology: Learning, Memory, and Cognition (USA) *Online - full text edition.* **4415**
Journal of Experimental Social Psychology (USA) *Online - full text edition.* **4415**
Journal of Experimental Zoology (USA) *Online - full text edition.* **3354**
Journal of Exposure Analysis and Environmental Epidemiology (GBR) *Online - full text edition.* **3440**
Journal of Family Practice (USA) *Online - full text edition.* **3633**
Journal of Family Psychology (USA) *Online - full text edition.* **4416**
Journal of Family Therapy (GBR) *Online - full text edition.* **4101**
Journal of Family Violence (USA) *Online - full text edition.* **3395**
Journal of Fluency Disorders (USA) *Online - full text edition.* **4416**
Journal of Food Protection (USA) *Online - full text edition.* **3461**
Journal of Forensic Psychiatry (GBR) *Online - full text edition.* **4101**
Journal of Forensic Sciences (USA) *Online - full text edition.* **3883**
Journal of Gastroenterology (JPN) *Online - full text edition.* **3893**
Journal of Gastroenterology and Hepatology (AUS) *Online - full text edition.* **3893**
Journal of Gastrointestinal Surgery (USA) *Online - full text edition.* **4193**
Journal of Gene Medicine (USA) *Online - full text edition.* **3309**
The Journal of General and Applied Microbiology (JPN) *Online - full text edition.* **3325**
Journal of General Internal Medicine (USA) *Online - full text edition.* **3910**
Journal of General Physiology (USA) *Online - full text edition.* **3344**
The Journal of General Psychology (USA) *Online - full text edition.* **4416**
Journal of General Virology (GBR) *Online - full text edition.* **3325**
The Journal of Genetic Psychology (USA) *Online - full text edition.* **3309**
Journal of Geriatric Psychiatry and Neurology (CAN) *Online - full text edition.* **3476**
Journal of Glaucoma (USA) *Online - full text edition.* **4000**
Journal of Gynecologic Surgery (USA) *Online - full text edition.* **3955**
Journal of Hand Surgery: American Volume (USA) *Online - full text edition.* **4193**
Journal of Hand Surgery: British and European Volume (GBR) *Online - full text edition.* **4193**
Journal of Head Trauma Rehabilitation (USA) *Online - full text edition.* **4018**
Journal of Health and Social Behavior (USA) *Online - full text edition.* **4522**
Journal of Health Care for the Poor and Underserved (USA) *Online - full text edition.* **3633**
Journal of Health Communication (USA) *Online - full text edition.* **3633**
Journal of Health Economics (NLD) *Online - full text edition.* **4479**
Journal of Health Politics, Policy and Law (USA) *Online - full text edition.* **3633**
Journal of Health Population and Nutrition (BGD) *Online - full text edition.* **3730**
Journal of Health Psychology (GBR) *Online - full text edition.* **4417**
Journal of Health Science (JPN) *Online - full text edition.* **3452**
Journal of Healthcare Management (USA) *Online - full text edition.* **3517**
The Journal of Heart and Lung Transplantation (GBR) *Online - full text edition.* **4193**
The Journal of Heart Valve Disease (GBR) *Online - full text edition.* **3778**
Journal of Helminthology (GBR) *Online - full text edition.* **3801**
Journal of Hematotherapy & Stem Cell Research (USA) *Online - full text edition.* **3903**
Journal of Hepatology (DNK) *Online - full text edition.* **3893**
Journal of Histochemistry and Cytochemistry (USA) *Online - full text edition.* **3291**
Journal of Histotechnology (USA) *Online - full text edition.* **3291**
Journal of Homosexuality (USA) *Online - full text edition.* **3528**

Journal of Hospital Infection (GBR) *Online - full text edition.* **3801**
Journal of Human Evolution (GBR) *Online - full text edition.* **3309**
Journal of Human Genetics (JPN) *Online - full text edition.* **3310**
Journal of Human Hypertension (GBR) *Online - full text edition.* **3778**
Journal of Human Movement Studies (GBR) *Online - full text edition.* **4417**
Journal of Human Nutrition and Dietetics (GBR) *Online - full text edition.* **4237**
Journal of Human Virology (USA) *Online - full text edition.* **3801**
Journal of Humanistic Psychology (USA) *Online - full text edition.* **4417**
Journal of Hypertension (USA) *Online - full text edition.* **3778**
Journal of Immunoassay and Immunochemistry (USA) *Online - full text edition.* **3376**
Journal of Immunological Methods (NLD) *Online - full text edition.* **3748**
Journal of Immunology (USA) *Online - full text edition.* **3748**
Journal of Immunotherapy (USA) *Online - full text edition.* **3749**
Journal of Industrial Microbiology and Biotechnology (GBR) *Online - full text edition.* **3276**
Journal of Infection (GBR) *Online - full text edition.* **3801**
Journal of Infectious Diseases (USA) *Online - full text edition.* **3802**
Journal of Inherited Metabolic Disease (NLD) *Online - full text edition.* **4046**
Journal of Inorganic Biochemistry (USA) *Online - full text edition.* **3254**
Journal of Intellectual and Developmental Disability (GBR) *Online - full text edition.* **4102**
Journal of Intellectual Disability Research (GBR) *Online - full text edition.* **4102**
Journal of Intensive Care Medicine (USA) *Online - full text edition.* **3634**
Journal of Interferon & Cytokine Research (USA) *Online - full text edition.* **3749**
Journal of Internal Medicine (GBR) *Online - full text edition.* **3910**
Journal of International Medical Research (GBR) *Online - full text edition.* **3634**
Journal of Interpersonal Violence (USA) *Online - full text edition.* **3395**
Journal of Interventional Cardiac Electrophysiology (NLD) *Online - full text edition.* **3778**
Journal of Investigational Allergology and Clinical Immunology (DEU) *Online - full text edition.* **3749**
The Journal of Investigative Dermatology (USA) *Online - full text edition.* **3851**
The Journal of Investigative Dermatology Symposium Proceedings (USA) *Online - full text edition.* **3851**
Journal of Investigative Medicine (USA) *Online - full text edition.* **3883**
Journal of Investigative Surgery (USA) *Online - full text edition.* **4193**
The Journal of Laboratory and Clinical Medicine (USA) *Online - full text edition.* **3876**
Journal of Language and Social Psychology (USA) *Online - full text edition.* **4417**
Journal of Laparoendoscopic & Advanced Surgical Techniques (USA) *Online - full text edition.* **4194**
Journal of Laryngology and Otology (GBR) *Online - full text edition.* **4034**
The Journal of Law, Medicine & Ethics (USA) *Online - full text edition.* **3540**
Journal of Learning Disabilities (USA) *Online - full text edition.* **3424**
The Journal of Legal Medicine (USA) *Online - full text edition.* **3634**
Journal of Leukocyte Biology (USA) *Online - full text edition.* **3204**
Journal of Lipid Research (USA) *Online - full text edition.* **3254**
Journal of Liposome Research (USA) *Online - full text edition.* **4307**
Journal of Loss & Trauma (USA) *Online - full text edition.* **4418**
Journal of Luminescence (NLD) *Online - full text edition.* **4366**
Journal of Magnetic Resonance Imaging (USA) *Online - full text edition.* **4148**
Journal of Mammalogy (USA) *Online - full text edition.* **3354**
Journal of Mammary Gland Biology and Neoplasia (USA) *Online - full text edition.* **3345**
Journal of Manipulative and Physiological Therapeutics (USA) *Online - full text edition.* **3788**
Journal of Marital and Family Therapy (USA) *Online - full text edition.* **4418**
Journal of Materials Science: Materials in Medicine (USA) *Online - full text edition.* **3434**
Journal of Mathematical Biology (DEU) *Online - full text edition.* **3204**
Journal of Mathematical Psychology (USA) *Online - full text edition.* **4418**
Journal of Medical Engineering & Technology (GBR) *Online - full text edition.* **3635**
Journal of Medical Entomology (USA) *Online - full text edition.* **3296**
Journal of Medical Microbiology (USA) *Online - full text edition.* **3635**
Journal of Medical Speech - Language Pathology (USA) *Online - full text edition.* **4034**
Journal of Medical Systems (USA) *Online - full text edition.* **3812**
Journal of Medical Virology (USA) *Online - full text edition.* **3635**
Journal of Medicinal Chemistry (USA) *Online - full text edition.* **4308**
The Journal of Medicine and Philosophy (NLD) *Online - full text edition.* **3636**
Journal of Membrane Biology (USA) *Online - full text edition.* **3291**
Journal of Memory and Language (USA) *Online - full text edition.* **3550**
Journal of Microbiological Methods (NLD) *Online - full text edition.* **3325**
Journal of Microbiology and Biotechnology (HKG) *Online - full text edition.* **3276**
Journal of Microencapsulation (GBR) *Online - full text edition.* **4308**
Journal of Microscopy (GBR) *Online - full text edition.* **3334**
Journal of Microscopy Research and Technique (USA) *Online - full text edition.* **3334**
Journal of Mind and Behavior (USA) *Online - full text edition.* **4418**
Journal of Molecular and Cellular Cardiology (GBR) *Online - full text edition.* **3778**
The Journal of Molecular Diagnostics (USA) *Online - full text edition.* **3636**
Journal of Molecular Endocrinology (GBR) *Online - full text edition.* **3865**
Journal of Molecular Evolution (USA) *Online - full text edition.* **3310**
Journal of Molecular Graphics and Modelling (USA) *Online - full text edition.* **3377**
Journal of Molecular Medicine (DEU) *Online - full text edition.* **3636**
Journal of Molecular Microbiology and Biotechnology (GBR) *Online - full text edition.* **3326**
Journal of Molecular Neuroscience (USA) *Online - full text edition.* **4102**
Journal of Molecular Recognition (GBR) *Online - full text edition.* **3378**
Journal of Morphology (USA) *Online - full text edition.* **3204**
Journal of Motor Behavior (USA) *Online - full text edition.* **4418**
Journal of Multicultural Counseling and Development (USA) *Online - full text edition.* **4418**
Journal of Muscle Foods (USA) *Online - full text edition.* **3462**
Journal of Muscle Research and Cell Motility (NLD) *Online - full text edition.* **4018**
Journal of Musculoskeletal Pain (USA) *Online - full text edition.* **4019**
Journal of Music Therapy (USA) *Online - full text edition.* **4062**
Journal of Natural History (GBR) *Online - full text edition.* **3204**
Journal of Natural Products (USA) *Online - full text edition.* **4308**
Journal of Natural Toxins (USA) *Online - full text edition.* **4308**
Journal of Nervous and Mental Disease (USA) *Online - full text edition.* **4102**
Journal of Neural Transmission - Basic Neurosciences and Genetics - Parkinson's Disease and Allied Conditions - Alzheimer's Disease and Related Disorders - Biological Psychiatry (AUT) *Online - full text edition.* **4102**
Journal of Neural Transmission. Supplement (AUT) *Online - full text edition.* **4102**
Journal of Neuro-Oncology (USA) *Online - full text edition.* **3982**
Journal of Neuro-Ophthalmology (USA) *Online - full text edition.* **4000**
Journal of Neurobiology (USA) *Online - full text edition.* **3345**
Journal of Neurochemistry (USA) *Online - full text edition.* **3255**
Journal of Neurocytology (USA) *Online - full text edition.* **3291**
Journal of Neuroendocrinology Online(GBR) *Online - full text.* **4103**
Journal of Neurogenetics (CHE) *Online - full text edition.* **4103**
Journal of Neuroimaging (USA) *Online - full text edition.* **4103**
Journal of Neuroimmunology (NLD) *Online - full text edition.* **4103**
Journal of Neurolinguistics (GBR) *Online - full text edition.* **4103**
Journal of Neurology (DEU) *Online - full text edition.* **4103**
Journal of Neurology, Neurosurgery and Psychiatry (GBR) *Online - full text edition.* **4104**
Journal of Neuropathology and Experimental Neurology (USA) *Online - full text edition.* **4104**
Journal of Neurophysiology Online (USA) *Online - full text edition of* Journal of Neurophysiology. **3345**
Journal of Neuropsychiatry and Clinical Neurosciences (USA) *Online - full text edition.* **4104**
Journal of Neuroradiology (FRA) *Online - full text edition.* **4148**
Journal of Neuroscience (USA) *Online - full text edition.* **4104**
Journal of Neuroscience Methods (NLD) *Online - full text edition.* **4104**
Journal of Neuroscience Research (USA) *Online - full text edition.* **4104**
Journal of Neurosurgery (USA) *Online - full text edition.* **4104**
Journal of Neurosurgical Anesthesiology (USA) *Online - full text edition.* **3758**
Journal of Neurotrauma (USA) *Online - full text edition.* **4019**
Journal of NeuroVirology (GBR) *Online - full text edition.* **4105**
Journal of Nonverbal Behavior (USA) *Online - full text edition.* **4418**
Journal of Nuclear Cardiology (USA) *Online - full text edition.* **4148**
Journal of Nursing Administration (USA) *Online - full text edition.* **3925**
Journal of Nursing Care Quality (USA) *Online - full text edition.* **3925**
Journal of Nursing Education (USA) *Online - full text edition.* **3925**
Journal of Nursing Scholarship (USA) *Online - full text edition.* **3926**
Journal of Nutrition (USA) *Online - full text edition.* **4237**
Journal of Nutrition Education (CAN) *Online - full text edition.* **4237**
Journal of Nutritional Biochemistry (USA) *Online - full text edition.* **4238**
Journal of Nutritional Science and Vitaminology (JPN) *Online - full text edition.* **4238**
Journal of Occupational and Environmental Medicine (USA) *Online - full text edition.* **3636**
Journal of Occupational and Organizational Psychology (GBR) *Online - full text edition.* **4419**
Journal of Occupational Health (JPN) *Online - full text edition.* **4258**
Journal of Occupational Rehabilitation (USA) *Online - full text edition.* **4258**
Journal of Ocular Pharmacology and Therapeutics (USA) *Online - full text edition.* **4000**
Journal of Oral and Maxillofacial Surgery (USA) *Online - full text edition.* **3829**
Journal of Oral Pathology & Medicine (DNK) *Online - full text edition.* **3829**
Journal of Oral Rehabilitation Online(GBR) *Online - full text.* **3829**
Journal of Organizational Behavior Management (USA) *Online - full text edition.* **4419**
Journal of Organizational Behaviour (GBR) *Online - full text edition.* **4419**
Journal of Orofacial Pain (USA) *Online - full text edition.* **3830**
Journal of Orthopaedic and Sports Physical Therapy (USA) *Online - full text edition.* **4174**
Journal of Orthopaedic Research (USA) *Online - full text edition.* **4019**
Journal of Orthopaedic Trauma (USA) *Online - full text edition.* **4019**
Journal of Otolaryngology (CAN) *Online - full text edition.* **4034**
Journal of Paediatrics and Child Health (AUS) *Online - full text edition.* **4047**
The Journal of Pain (GBR) *Online - full text edition.* **3636**
Journal of Pain and Symptom Management (USA) *Online - full text edition.* **4105**
Journal of Palliative Care (CAN) *Online - full text edition.* **3636**
Journal of Parapsychology (USA) *Online - full text edition.* **4271**
Journal of Parasitology (USA) *Online - full text edition.* **3802**
Journal of Parenteral and Enteral Nutrition (USA) *Online - full text edition.* **4238**
Journal of Pathology (GBR) *Online - full text edition.* **3637**
Journal of Pediatric Endocrinology & Metabolism (ISR) *Online - full text edition.* **3865**
Journal of Pediatric Gastroenterology and Nutrition (USA) *Online - full text edition.* **4238**
Journal of Pediatric Hematology - Oncology (USA) *Online - full text edition.* **3982**
Journal of Pediatric Ophthalmology and Strabismus (USA) *Online - full text edition.* **4001**
Journal of Pediatric Orthopaedics (USA) *Online - full text edition.* **4019**
Journal of Pediatric Orthopaedics, Part B (USA) *Online - full text edition.* **4020**
Journal of Pediatric Psychology (GBR) *Online - full text edition.* **4419**
Journal of Pediatric Surgery (USA) *Online - full text edition.* **4194**
The Journal of Pediatrics (USA) *Online - full text edition.* **4047**
Journal of Peptide Research (DNK) *Online - full text edition.* **3255**
Journal of Peptide Science (GBR) *Online - full text edition.* **3378**
Journal of Perinatal and Neonatal Nursing (USA) *Online - full text edition.* **3926**
Journal of Perinatal Medicine (DEU) *Online - full text edition.* **3956**
Journal of Periodontal Research (DNK) *Online - full text edition.* **3830**
Journal of Periodontology (USA) *Online - full text edition.* **3830**
Journal of Personality (USA) *Online - full text edition.* **4419**
Journal of Personality and Social Psychology (USA) *Online - full text edition.* **4419**
Journal of Personality Assessment (USA) *Online - full text edition.* **4420**
Journal of Personality Disorders (USA) *Online - full text edition.* **4420**
Journal of Pharmaceutical and Biomedical Analysis (NLD) *Online - full text edition.* **4309**
Journal of Pharmaceutical Sciences (USA) *Online - full text edition.* **4309**
Journal of Pharmacokinetics and Pharmacodynamics (USA) *Online - full text edition.* **4310**
Journal of Pharmacological and Toxicological Methods (USA) *Online - full text edition.* **3452**
Journal of Pharmacology and Experimental Therapeutics (USA) *Online - full text edition.* **4310**
Journal of Pharmacy and Pharmaceutical Sciences(CAN) *Online - full text.* **4310**
Journal of Pharmacy and Pharmacology (GBR) *Online - full text edition.* **4310**
Journal of Photochemistry and Photobiology, B: Biology (CHE) *Online - full text edition.* **3255**
Journal of Physiology (GBR) *Online - full text edition.* **3345**
Journal of Physiology and Biochemistry (ESP) *Online - full text edition.* **3637**
Journal of Physiology and Pharmacology (POL) *Online - full text edition.* **3345**
Journal of Physiology (Paris) (FRA) *Online - full text edition.* **4105**
Journal of Pineal Research (DNK) *Online - full text edition.* **4105**
Journal of Planar Chromatography - Modern TLC (JPC) (HUN) *Online - full text edition.* **3376**
Journal of Plankton Research (GBR) *Online - full text edition.* **3204**
Journal of Plant Nutrition and Soil Science (DEU) *Online - full text edition.* **3232**
Journal of Professional Nursing (USA) *Online - full text edition.* **3926**
The Journal of Prosthetic Dentistry (USA) *Online - full text edition.* **3830**
Journal of Prosthetics and Orthotics (USA) *Online - full text edition.* **4020**

Online Service

Journal of Protein Chemistry (USA) *Online - full text edition.* **3255**
Journal of Psychiatric Research (GBR) *Online - full text edition.* **4106**
Journal of Psychiatry and Neuroscience (CAN) *Online - full text edition.* **4106**
Journal of Psychoactive Drugs (USA) *Online - full text edition.* **3403**
Journal of Psychoeducational Assessment (USA) *Online - full text edition.* **3412**
Journal of Psychohistory (USA) *Online - full text edition.* **4420**
Journal of Psycholinguistic Research (USA) *Online - full text edition.* **3551**
Journal of Psychology and Theology (USA) *Online - full text edition.* **4421**
Journal of Psychology: Interdisciplinary & Applied (USA) *Online - full text edition.* **4421**
Journal of Psychopathology and Behavioral Assessment (USA) *Online - full text edition.* **4421**
Journal of Psychopharmacology (GBR) *Online - full text edition.* **4310**
Journal of Psychophysiology (USA) *Online - full text edition.* **4421**
Journal of Psychosocial Nursing and Mental Health Services (USA) *Online - full text edition.* **3926**
Journal of Psychosocial Oncology (USA) *Online - full text edition.* **3983**
Journal of Psychosomatic Obstetrics and Gynecology (GBR) *Online - full text edition.* **3957**
Journal of Psychosomatic Research (USA) *Online - full text edition.* **4106**
Journal of Public Health Dentistry (USA) *Online - full text edition.* **3830**
Journal of Public Health Medicine (GBR) *Online - full text edition.* **4515**
Journal of Public Health Policy (USA) *Online - full text edition.* **4479**
Journal of Radiation Research (JPN) *Online - full text edition.* **4148**
Journal of Range Management (USA) *Online - full text edition.* **3205**
Journal of Receptor and Signal Transduction Research (USA) *Online - full text edition.* **3205**
Journal of Reconstructive Microsurgery (USA) *Online - full text edition.* **4194**
Journal of Refractive Surgery (USA) *Online - full text edition.* **4195**
Journal of Rehabilitation (USA) *Online - full text edition.* **4062**
Journal of Rehabilitation Medicine (NOR) *Online - full text edition.* **4515**
Journal of Rehabilitation Research and Development (USA) *Online - full text edition.* **4020**
Journal of Religion and Health (USA) *Online - full text edition.* **4500**
Journal of Reproductive and Infant Psychology (GBR) *Online - full text edition.* **4421**
Journal of Reproductive Immunology (IRL) *Online - full text edition.* **3749**
Journal of Reproductive Medicine (USA) *Online - full text edition.* **3957**
Journal of Research in Personality (USA) *Online - full text edition.* **4422**
Journal of Research on Adolescence (USA) *Online - full text edition.* **3384**
Journal of Rheumatology (CAN) *Online - full text edition.* **4169**
Journal of Risk and Uncertainty (USA) *Online - full text edition.* **3363**
The Journal of Rural Health (USA) *Online - full text edition.* **3637**
Journal of Safety Research (GBR) *Online - full text edition.* **4258**
Journal of School Health (USA) *Online - full text edition.* **4479**
Journal of School Psychology (GBR) *Online - full text edition.* **4422**
Journal of Sensory Studies (USA) *Online - full text edition.* **4106**
Journal of Sex & Marital Therapy (USA) *Online - full text edition.* **4422**
Journal of Sex Research (USA) *Online - full text edition.* **4422**
Journal of Shoulder and Elbow Surgery (USA) *Online - full text edition.* **4195**
Journal of Sleep Research Online(GBR) *Online - full text.* **3638**
Journal of Small Animal Practice (GBR) *Online - full text edition.* **4546**
Journal of Social and Clinical Psychology (USA) *Online - full text edition.* **4422**
Journal of Social and Personal Relationships (GBR) *Online - full text edition.* **4423**
Journal of Social Behavior and Personality (USA) *Online - full text edition.* **4423**
Journal of Social Distress and the Homeless (USA) *Online - full text edition.* **4515**
Journal of Social Issues (USA) *Online - full text edition.* **4423**
The Journal of Social Psychology (USA) *Online - full text edition.* **4423**
Journal of Social Work Practice (GBR) *Online - full text edition.* **4515**
The Journal of Special Education (USA) *Online - full text edition.* **3424**
Journal of Speech, Language, and Hearing Research (USA) *Online - full text edition.* **3491**
Journal of Spinal Disorders (USA) *Online - full text edition.* **4020**
Journal of Sport and Exercise Psychology (USA) *Online - full text edition.* **4423**
Journal of Sport Rehabilitation (USA) *Online - full text edition.* **4174**
Journal of Sports Chiropractic and Rehabilitation (USA) *Online - full text edition.* **3788**
The Journal of Sports Medicine and Physical Fitness (ITA) *Online - full text edition.* **4175**
Journal of Sports Sciences (GBR) *Online - full text edition.* **4525**
Journal of Steroid Biochemistry and Molecular Biology (GBR) *Online - full text edition.* **3255**
Journal of Strength and Conditioning Research (USA) *Online - full text edition.* **4175**
Journal of Structural Biology (USA) *Online - full text edition.* **3205**
Journal of Studies on Alcohol (USA) *Online - full text edition.* **3403**
Journal of Substance Abuse (GBR) *Online - full text edition.* **3403**
Journal of Substance Abuse Treatment (USA) *Online - full text edition.* **3404**
Journal of Surgical Oncology (USA) *Online - full text edition.* **4195**
Journal of Surgical Research (USA) *Online - full text edition.* **4195**
Journal of Swine Health and Production (USA) *Online - full text edition.* **4546**
Journal of Symbolic Logic (USA) *Online - full text edition.* **3553**
Journal of Teaching in Physical Education (USA) *Online - full text edition.* **3429**
Journal of Telemedicine and Telecare (GBR) *Online - full text edition.* **3638**
Journal of Texture Studies (USA) *Online - full text edition.* **3435**
Journal of the Experimental Analysis of Behavior (USA) *Online - full text edition.* **4423**
Journal of the History of Biology (NLD) *Online - full text edition.* **3205**
Journal of the History of Medicine and Allied Sciences (GBR) *Online - full text edition.* **3638**
Journal of the History of Sexuality (USA) *Online - full text edition.* **4522**
Journal of the History of the Behavioral Sciences (USA) *Online - full text edition.* **4424**
Journal of the Learning Sciences (USA) *Online - full text edition.* **3413**
Journal of the Medical Library Association (USA) *Online - full text edition.* **3638**
Journal of the Neurological Sciences (NLD) *Online - full text edition.* **4106**
Journal of the Neuromusculoskeletal System (USA) *Online - full text edition.* **3788**
Journal of the Peripheral Nervous System Online(USA) *Online - full text.* **4107**
Journal of Theoretical Biology (GBR) *Online - full text edition.* **3205**
Journal of Thermal Biology (GBR) *Online - full text edition.* **3267**
The Journal of Thoracic and Cardiovascular Surgery (USA) *Online - full text edition.* **4195**
Journal of Thoracic Imaging (USA) *Online - full text edition.* **4148**
Journal of Thrombosis and Thrombolysis (USA) *Online - full text edition.* **3779**
Journal of Toxicology and Environmental Health. Part A (USA) *Online - full text edition.* **3452**
Journal of Toxicology and Environmental Health. Part B: Critical Reviews (USA) *Online - full text edition.* **3452**
Journal of Toxicology. Clinical Toxicology (USA) *Online - full text edition.* **4311**
Journal of Toxicology. Cutaneous and Ocular Toxicology (USA) *Online - full text edition.* **4311**
Journal of Toxicology. Toxin Reviews (USA) *Online - full text edition.* **4311**
The Journal of Trace Elements in Experimental Medicine (USA) *Online - full text edition.* **3877**
Journal of Trace Elements in Medicine and Biology (DEU) *Online - full text edition.* **3205**
Journal of Trauma - Injury, Infection and Critical Care (USA) *Online - full text edition.* **4020**
Journal of Traumatic Stress (USA) *Online - full text edition.* **4424**
Journal of Travel Medicine (CAN) *Online - full text edition.* **3639**
Journal of Tropical Pediatrics (GBR) *Online - full text edition.* **4047**
Journal of Tumor Marker Oncology (USA) *Online - full text edition.* **3983**
Journal of Ultrasound in Medicine (USA) *Online - full text edition.* **4149**
Journal of Urban Health (USA) *Online - full text edition.* **3639**
Journal of Urology (USA) *Online - full text edition.* **4215**
Journal of Vascular and Interventional Radiology (USA) *Online - full text edition.* **4149**
Journal of Vascular Research (CHE) *Online - full text edition.* **3779**
Journal of Vascular Surgery (USA) *Online - full text edition.* **4195**
Journal of Vector Ecology (USA) *Online - full text edition.* **3206**
Journal of Vestibular Research: Equilibrium and Orientation (NLD) *Online - full text edition.* **3345**
Journal of Veterinary Dentistry (USA) *Online - full text edition.* **4546**
Journal of Veterinary Diagnostic Investigation (USA) *Online - full text edition.* **4546**
Journal of Veterinary Internal Medicine (USA) *Online - full text edition.* **4546**
Journal of Veterinary Medical Education (USA) *Online - full text edition.* **4546**
Journal of Veterinary Medical Science (JPN) *Online - full text edition.* **4546**
Journal of Veterinary Medicine. Series A Online(DEU) *Online - full text.* **4547**
Journal of Veterinary Medicine. Series B Online(DEU) *Online - full text.* **4547**
Journal of Veterinary Pharmacology and Therapeutics Online(GBR) *Online - full text.* **4311**
Journal of Viral Hepatitis (GBR) *Online - full text edition.* **3893**
Journal of Virological Methods (NLD) *Online - full text edition.* **3326**
Journal of Virology (USA) *Online - full text edition.* **3326**
Journal of Visual Impairment & Blindness (USA) *Online - full text edition.* **3498**
Journal of Vocational Behavior (USA) *Online - full text edition.* **4424**
Journal of Voice (USA) *Online - full text edition.* **4034**
Journal of Wildlife Diseases (USA) *Online - full text edition.* **4547**
Journal of Wildlife Rehabilitation (USA) *Online - full text edition.* **3355**
Journal of Women and Aging (USA) *Online - full text edition.* **4569**
Journal of Women's Health and Gender-Based Medicine (USA) *Online - full text edition.* **4564**
Journal of Youth and Adolescence (USA) *Online - full text edition.* **3384**
Journal of Zoo and Wildlife Medicine (USA) *Online - full text edition.* **4547**
Journal of Zoological Systematics and Evolutionary Research Online(DEU) *Online - full text.* **3355**
Journals of Gerontology. Series A: Biological Sciences & Medical Sciences (USA) *Online - full text edition.* **3477**
Journals of Gerontology. Series B: Psychological Sciences & Social Sciences (USA) *Online - full text edition.* **3477**
Jugoslovenska Medicinska Biohemija (YUG) *Online - full text edition.* **3255**
Kansas Entomological Society. Journal (USA) *Online - full text edition.* **3297**
Kardiologiya (RUS) *Online - full text edition.* **3779**
Kennedy Institute of Ethics. Journal (USA) *Online - full text edition.* **3640**
Key Issues in Human Genetics (CHE) *Online - full text edition.* **3310**
Kidney and Blood Pressure Research (CHE) *Online - full text edition.* **4215**
Kidney International Online (USA) *Online - full text edition of* Kidney International. **4215**
Kleintier-Praxis (DEU) *Online - full text edition.* **4547**
Klinische Monatsblaetter fuer Augenheilkunde und Augenarztliche Fortbildung (DEU) *Online - full text edition.* **4001**
Klinische Neurophysiologie (DEU) *Online - full text edition.* **4107**
Klinische Paediatrie (DEU) *Online - full text edition.* **4048**
The Knee (NLD) *Online - full text edition.* **3345**
Knee Surgery, Sports Traumatology, Arthroscopy (DEU) *Online - full text edition.* **4175**
Koelner Zeitschrift fuer Soziologie und Sozialpsychologie (DEU) *Online - full text edition.* **4522**
Krankenhauspharmazie (DEU) *Online - full text edition.* **4313**
Lab Animal (USA) *Online - full text edition.* **3877**
Laboratory Animals (GBR) *Online - full text edition.* **3355**
Laboratory Investigation (USA) *Online - full text edition.* **3878**
Laboratory Medicine (USA) *Online - full text edition.* **3878**
Laekartidningen (SWE) *Online - full text edition.* **3642**
Le Lait (FRA) *Online - full text edition.* **3326**
The Lancet (GBR) *Online - full text edition.* **3642**
Langenbecks Archives of Surgery (DEU) *Online - full text edition.* **4196**
Language and Cognitive Processes (GBR) *Online - full text edition.* **3551**
Language and Speech (GBR) *Online - full text edition.* **3551**
Language, Speech and Hearing Services in Schools (USA) *Online - full text edition.* **4035**
Laryngoscope (USA) *Online - full text edition.* **4035**
Lasers in Medical Science (GBR) *Online - full text edition.* **3643**
Lasers in Surgery and Medicine (USA) *Online - full text edition.* **4196**
Laterality (GBR) *Online - full text edition.* **4107**
Law and Human Behavior (USA) *Online - full text edition.* **3541**
The Leadership Quarterly (USA) *Online - full text edition.* **3365**
Learning and Individual Differences (GBR) *Online - full text edition.* **3413**
Learning and Instruction (GBR) *Online - full text edition.* **3413**
Learning & Memory (USA) *Online - full text edition.* **4108**
Learning and Motivation (USA) *Online - full text edition.* **3413**
Leber Magen Darm (DEU) *Online - full text edition.* **3894**
Leisure Sciences (USA) *Online - full text edition.* **3547**
Leprosy Review (GBR) *Online - full text edition.* **3803**
Letters in Applied Microbiology (GBR) *Online - full text edition.* **3326**
Leukemia (GBR) *Online - full text edition.* **3903**
Leukemia and Lymphoma (CHE) *Online - full text edition.* **3903**
Leukemia Research (GBR) *Online - full text edition.* **3904**
Linnean Society. Biological Journal (GBR) *Online - full text edition.* **3206**
Lipids (USA) *Online - full text edition.* **3256**
Literature & Medicine (USA) *Online - full text edition.* **3552**
Literature and Psychology (USA) *Online - full text edition.* **3552**
Liver (DNK) *Online - full text edition.* **3894**
Liver Transplantation (USA) *Online - full text edition.* **3894**
Luminescence (GBR) *Online - full text edition.* **3380**
Lung (USA) *Online - full text edition.* **4162**
Lung Cancer (IRL) *Online - full text edition.* **3983**
Lupus (GBR) *Online - full text edition.* **4169**
Lymphology (USA) *Online - full text edition.* **3866**
M L A News (Chicago) (USA) *Online - full text edition.* **3645**
M M W - Fortschritte der Medizin (DEU) *Online - full text edition.* **3645**
M P Online (GBR) *Online - full text edition of* Molecular Pathology. **3879**
Magnesium Research (GBR) *Online - full text edition.* **3646**
Magnetic Resonance Imaging (USA) *Online - full text edition.* **4150**
Magnetic Resonance in Medicine (GBR) *Online - full text edition.* **4150**

Online Service

Magyar Allatorvosok Lapja (HUN) *Online - full text edition.* **4548**
Mammalian Genome (USA) *Online - full text edition.* **3310**
Mankind Quarterly (USA) *Online - full text edition.* **3174**
Manual Therapy (GBR) *Online - full text edition.* **4063**
Marine Biological Association of the United Kingdom. Journal (GBR) *Online - full text edition.* **3207**
Marine Biology (DEU) *Online - full text edition.* **3207**
Marine Ecology Online(DEU) *Online - full text.* **3207**
Marine Ecology - Progress Series Online(DEU) *Online - full text.* **3208**
Marine Environmental Research (GBR) *Online - full text edition.* **3444**
Marketing Health Services (USA) *Online - full text edition.* **3367**
Mathematical Biosciences (USA) *Online - full text edition.* **3554**
Matrix Biology (NLD) *Online - full text edition.* **3646**
Maturitas (IRL) *Online - full text edition.* **3958**
Mayo Clinic Proceedings (USA) *Online - full text edition.* **3647**
Measurement and Evaluation in Counseling and Development (USA) *Online - full text edition.* **3413**
Mechanisms of Ageing and Development (IRL) *Online - full text edition.* **3478**
Mechanisms of Development (IRL) *Online - full text edition.* **3292**
Medecine et Hygiene (CHE) *Online - full text edition.* **3648**
Medecine et Maladies Infectieuses (FRA) *Online - full text edition.* **3803**
Medecine - Sciences (FRA) *Online - full text edition.* **3648**
Media Psychology (USA) *Online - full text edition.* **4426**
Mediators of Inflammation (GBR) *Online - full text edition.* **3648**
Medical & Biological Engineering & Computing (GBR) *Online - full text edition.* **3284**
Medical and Pediatric Oncology (USA) *Online - full text edition.* **3984**
Medical & Veterinary Entomology Online(GBR) *Online - full text.* **3648**
Medical Anthropology Quarterly (USA) *Online - full text edition.* **3174**
Medical Care (USA) *Online - full text edition.* **3649**
Medical Care Research and Review (USA) *Online - full text edition.* **4496**
Medical Clinics of North America (USA) *Online - full text edition.* **3649**
Medical Decision Making (USA) *Online - full text edition.* **3649**
Medical Education (GBR) *Online - full text edition.* **3650**
Medical Engineering & Physics (GBR) *Online - full text edition.* **3650**
Medical History (GBR) *Online - full text edition.* **3650**
Medical Hypotheses (GBR) *Online - full text edition.* **3651**
Medical Image Analysis (GBR) *Online - full text edition.* **4150**
Medical Informatics and the Internet in Medicine (GBR) *Online - full text edition.* **3812**
Medical Journal of Australia (AUS) *Online - full text edition.* **3651**
Medical Letter on Drugs and Therapeutics (English Edition) (USA) *Online - full text edition.* **4315**
Medical Microbiology and Immunology (DEU) *Online - full text edition.* **3749**
Medical Mycology (GBR) *Online - full text edition.* **3803**
Medical Oncology (GBR) *Online - full text edition.* **3984**
Medical Physics (USA) *Online - full text edition.* **3652**
Medical Principles and Practice (CHE) *Online - full text edition.* **3652**
Medical Problems of Performing Artists (USA) *Online - full text edition.* **3652**
Medical Teacher (GBR) *Online - full text edition.* **3654**
Medicina (ARG) *Online - full text edition.* **3655**
Medicina Clinica (ESP) *Online - full text edition.* **3655**
Medicina dello Sport (ITA) *Online - full text edition.* **4175**
Medicinal Chemistry Research (USA) *Online - full text edition.* **3655**
Medicinal Research Reviews (USA) *Online - full text edition.* **4315**
Medicine and Science in Sports and Exercise (USA) *Online - full text edition.* **4175**
Medicine (Baltimore) (USA) *Online - full text edition.* **3656**
Medicine, Science and the Law (GBR) *Online - full text edition.* **3884**
Medizinische Klinik (DEU) *Online - full text edition.* **3658**
Die Medizinische Welt (DEU) *Online - full text edition.* **3659**
Medscape Women's Health(USA) *Online - full text.* **4564**
Medycyna Weterynaryjna (POL) *Online - full text edition.* **4548**
Melanoma Research (GBR) *Online - full text edition.* **3984**
Memory (GBR) *Online - full text edition.* **4426**
Memory and Cognition (USA) *Online - full text edition.* **4426**
Menninger Clinic. Bulletin (USA) *Online - full text edition.* **4109**
Menopause (USA) *Online - full text edition.* **3958**
Mental Retardation (USA) *Online - full text edition.* **3424**
Mental Retardation and Developmental Disabilities (New York, 1995) (USA) *Online - full text edition.* **4109**
Merrill - Palmer Quarterly (USA) *Online - full text edition.* **4427**
Metabolic Brain Disease (USA) *Online - full text edition.* **3660**
Metabolism: Clinical and Experimental (USA) *Online - full text edition.* **3866**
Methods: A Companion to Methods in Enzymology (USA) *Online - full text edition.* **3256**
Methods and Findings in Experimental and Clinical Pharmacology (ESP) *Online - full text edition.* **4316**
Methods in Cell Biology (USA) *Online - full text edition.* **3292**
Methods in Enzymology (USA) *Online - full text edition.* **3256**
Methods in Microbiology (USA) *Online - full text edition.* **3327**
Methods of Biochemical Analysis (USA) *Online - full text edition.* **3256**
Methods of Information in Medicine (DEU) *Online - full text edition.* **3660**
Microbes and Infection (FRA) *Online - full text edition.* **3327**
Microbial Drug Resistance (USA) *Online - full text edition.* **3660**
Microbial Ecology (USA) *Online - full text edition.* **3327**
Microbial Pathogenesis (GBR) *Online - full text edition.* **3804**
Microbiological Research (DEU) *Online - full text edition.* **3327**
Microbiology (GBR) *Online - full text edition.* **3327**
Microbiology (RUS) *Online - full text edition.* **3327**
Microbiology and Immunology (JPN) *Online - full text edition.* **3328**
Microbiology and Molecular Biology Reviews (USA) *Online - full text edition.* **3328**
Microbios (GBR) *Online - full text edition.* **3328**
Microcirculation (GBR) *Online - full text edition.* **3661**
Micron (GBR) *Online - full text edition.* **3335**
Microsurgery (USA) *Online - full text edition.* **4197**
Microvascular Research (USA) *Online - full text edition.* **3780**
Midwifery (GBR) *Online - full text edition.* **3958**
Mikologiya i Fitopatologiya (RUS) *Online - full text edition.* **3281**
The Milbank Quarterly (USA) *Online - full text edition.* **4368**
Military Medicine (USA) *Online - full text edition.* **3661**
Military Psychology (USA) *Online - full text edition.* **4428**
Minerva Chirurgica (ITA) *Online - full text edition.* **4197**
Minimally Invasive Neurosurgery (DEU) *Online - full text edition.* **4110**
Minimally Invasive Therapy and Allied Technologies (GBR) *Online - full text edition.* **3661**
Modern Pathology (USA) *Online - full text edition.* **3662**
Modern Problems of Pharmacopsychiatry (CHE) *Online - full text edition.* **4110**
Molecular and Biochemical Parasitology (NLD) *Online - full text edition.* **3256**
Molecular and Cellular Biochemistry (USA) *Online - full text edition.* **3257**
Molecular and Cellular Biology (USA) *Online - full text edition.* **3257**
Molecular and Cellular Endocrinology (IRL) *Online - full text edition.* **3866**
Molecular and Cellular Neurosciences (USA) *Online - full text edition.* **4110**
Molecular and Cellular Probes (GBR) *Online - full text edition.* **3879**
Molecular Biology (RUS) *Online - full text edition.* **3257**
Molecular Biology and Evolution (USA) *Online - full text edition.* **3208**
Molecular Biology Reports (NLD) *Online - full text edition.* **3257**
Molecular Biotechnology (USA) *Online - full text edition.* **3276**
Molecular Brain Research (NLD) *Online - full text edition.* **4110**
Molecular Carcinogenesis (USA) *Online - full text edition.* **3984**
Molecular Cell (USA) *Online - full text edition.* **3292**
Molecular Diagnosis (USA) *Online - full text edition.* **3662**
Molecular Endocrinology (USA) *Online - full text edition.* **3866**
Molecular Genetics and Genomics (DEU) *Online - full text edition.* **3311**
Molecular Genetics and Metabolism (USA) *Online - full text edition.* **3662**
Molecular Human Reproduction (GBR) *Online - full text edition.* **3958**
Molecular Immunology (GBR) *Online - full text edition.* **3257**
Molecular Medicine (USA) *Online - full text edition.* **4317**
Molecular Membrane Biology (GBR) *Online - full text edition.* **3258**
Molecular Microbiology Online (GBR) *Online - full text edition of* Molecular Microbiology. **3329**
Molecular Neurobiology (USA) *Online - full text edition.* **3258**
Molecular Pharmacology (USA) *Online - full text edition.* **4317**
Molecular Phylogenetics and Evolution (USA) *Online - full text edition.* **3311**
Molecular Plant - Microbe Interactions (USA) *Online - full text edition.* **3258**
Molecular Psychiatry (GBR) *Online - full text edition.* **4110**
Molecular Reproduction and Development (USA) *Online - full text edition.* **3258**
Molecular Therapy (USA) *Online - full text edition.* **3984**
Molecular Vision(USA) *Online - full text.* **3258**
Monatsschrift Kinderheilkunde (DEU) *Online - full text edition.* **4049**
Monographs in Allergy (CHE) *Online - full text edition.* **3750**
Monographs in Oral Science (CHE) *Online - full text edition.* **3832**
Monographs in Virology (CHE) *Online - full text edition.* **3329**
Motivation and Emotion (USA) *Online - full text edition.* **4428**
Motor Control (USA) *Online - full text edition.* **4063**
Mount Sinai Journal of Medicine (USA) *Online - full text edition.* **3663**
Movement Disorders (USA) *Online - full text edition.* **4111**
Multiple Sclerosis (GBR) *Online - full text edition.* **4111**
Multivariate Behavioral Research (USA) *Online - full text edition.* **4428**
Muscle & Nerve (USA) *Online - full text edition.* **3663**
Mutagenesis (GBR) *Online - full text edition.* **3311**
Mutation Research - D N A Repair (NLD) *Online - full text edition.* **3258**
Mutation Research - Fundamental and Molecular Mechanisms of Mutagenesis (NLD) *Online - full text edition.* **3311**
Mutation Research - Genetic Toxicology and Environmental Mutagenesis (NLD) *Online - full text edition.* **3312**
Mutation Research - Reviews in Mutation Research (NLD) *Online - full text edition.* **3312**
Mycopathologia (NLD) *Online - full text edition.* **3281**
Mycoses (DEU) *Online - full text edition.* **3663**
N M C D (ITA) *Online - full text edition.* **4239**
N M R in Biomedicine (GBR) *Online - full text edition.* **4151**
Nahrung (DEU) *Online - full text edition.* **4239**
National Academy of Sciences of the United States of America. Proceedings (USA) *Online - full text edition.* **4505**
National Cancer Institute. Journal (USA) *Online - full text edition.* **3985**
National Medical Association. Journal (USA) *Online - full text edition.* **3665**
National Medical Journal of India (IND) *Online - full text edition.* **3665**
Natural Toxins (USA) *Online - full text edition.* **3453**
Nature (GBR) *Online - full text edition.* **4506**
Nature Biotechnology (USA) *Online - full text edition.* **3276**
Nature Genetics (USA) *Online - full text edition.* **3312**
Nature Medicine (GBR) *Online - full text edition.* **3665**
Nature Neuroscience (USA) *Online - full text edition.* **4111**
Nature Structural Biology (USA) *Online - full text edition.* **3210**
Naunyn-Schmiedeberg's Archives of Pharmacology (DEU) *Online - full text edition.* **4318**
Nebraska Symposium on Motivation (Publication) (USA) *Online - full text edition.* **4429**
Nederlands Tijdschrift voor Geneeskunde (NLD) *Online - full text edition.* **3665**
Nefrologia (ESP) *Online - full text edition.* **4216**
NeoPlasia (USA) *Online - full text edition.* **3985**
Neoplasma (SVK) *Online - full text edition.* **3985**
Nephrologie (CHE) *Online - full text edition.* **4216**
Nephrology, Dialysis and Transplantation (GBR) *Online - full text edition.* **4216**
Nephrology Online (AUS) *Online - full text edition of* Nephrology. **4216**
Nephron (CHE) *Online - full text edition.* **4216**
Der Nervenarzt (DEU) *Online - full text edition.* **4112**
Nervenheilkunde (DEU) *Online - full text edition.* **4112**
Netherlands Journal of Medicine (NLD) *Online - full text edition.* **3911**
Neural Computation (USA) *Online - full text edition.* **3389**
Neural Networks (GBR) *Online - full text edition.* **3390**
Neural Processing Letters (USA) *Online - full text edition.* **3390**
Neuro-Chirurgie (FRA) *Online - full text edition.* **4197**
Neuro-Oncology (USA) *Online - full text edition.* **3985**
Neuro-Ophthalmology (NLD) *Online - full text edition.* **4112**
Neurobiology of Aging (USA) *Online - full text edition.* **3346**
Neurobiology of Disease (USA) *Online - full text edition.* **4112**
Neurobiology of Learning and Memory (USA) *Online - full text edition.* **4112**
Neurocase (GBR) *Online - full text edition.* **4112**
Neurochemical Research (USA) *Online - full text edition.* **4113**
Neurochemistry International (GBR) *Online - full text edition.* **4113**
Neurocirugia (ESP) *Online - full text edition.* **4113**
Neuroendocrinology (CHE) *Online - full text edition.* **3867**
Neuroendocrinology Letters (SWE) *Online - full text edition.* **4113**
Neuroepidemiology (CHE) *Online - full text edition.* **4113**
Neurogastroenterology and Motility Online(GBR) *Online - full text.* **3894**
Neurogenetics (DEU) *Online - full text edition.* **3312**
NeuroImage (USA) *Online - full text edition.* **4113**
Neuroimaging Clinics of North America (USA) *Online - full text edition.* **4151**
NeuroImmunoModulation (CHE) *Online - full text edition.* **3750**
Neurologia Croatica (HRV) *Online - full text edition.* **4114**
Neurologia Medico-Chirurgica (JPN) *Online - full text edition.* **4114**
Neurologic Clinics (USA) *Online - full text edition.* **4114**
Neurologic Rehabilitation and Repair (USA) *Online - full text edition.* **4114**
Neurological Research (USA) *Online - full text edition.* **4114**
Neurological Sciences (ITA) *Online - full text edition.* **4114**

Neurological Surgery (JPN) *Online - full text edition.* **4197**
The Neurologist (USA) *Online - full text edition.* **4114**
Neurology (USA) *Online - full text edition.* **4114**
Neurology India (IND) *Online - full text edition.* **4115**
Neurology, Psychiatry and Brain Research (DEU) *Online - full text edition.* **4115**
Neuromodulation Online(USA) *Online - full text.* **4115**
Neuromuscular Disorders (GBR) *Online - full text edition.* **4115**
Neuron (USA) *Online - full text edition.* **4115**
Neuropathology (AUS) *Online - full text edition.* **4116**
Neuropathology & Applied Neurobiology Online (GBR) *Online - full text edition of* Neuropathology and Applied Neurobiology. **4116**
Neuropediatrics (DEU) *Online - full text edition.* **4049**
Neuropeptides (Edinburgh) (GBR) *Online - full text edition.* **3259**
Neuropharmacology (GBR) *Online - full text edition.* **4318**
Neurophysiologie Clinique (FRA) *Online - full text edition.* **4116**
Neurophysiology (USA) *Online - full text edition.* **4116**
Neuropsychiatrie (DEU) *Online - full text edition.* **4116**
Neuropsychiatry, Neuropsychology and Behavioral Neurology (USA) *Online - full text edition.* **4116**
Neuropsychobiology (CHE) *Online - full text edition.* **4116**
Neuropsychologia (GBR) *Online - full text edition.* **4116**
Neuropsychological Rehabilitation (GBR) *Online - full text edition.* **4117**
Neuropsychology (USA) *Online - full text edition.* **4117**
Neuropsychology, Development and Cognition. Section A: Journal of Clinical and Experimental Neuropsychology (NLD) *Online - full text edition.* **4429**
Neuropsychology, Development and Cognition. Section B: Aging, Neuropsychology and Cognition (NLD) *Online - full text edition.* **4429**
Neuropsychology, Development, and Cognition. Section C: Child Neuropsychology (NLD) *Online - full text edition.* **4429**
Neuropsychology, Development and Cognition. Section D: The Clinical Neuropsychologist (NLD) *Online - full text edition.* **4429**
Neuropsychology Review (USA) *Online - full text edition.* **4117**
Neuropsychopharmacology (USA) *Online - full text edition.* **4117**
Neuroradiology (DEU) *Online - full text edition.* **4151**
NeuroRehabilitation (NLD) *Online - full text edition.* **4117**
NeuroReport (USA) *Online - full text edition.* **4117**
Neuroscience (GBR) *Online - full text edition.* **4117**
Neuroscience and Biobehavioral Reviews (GBR) *Online - full text edition.* **4118**
Neuroscience Letters (IRL) *Online - full text edition.* **4118**
Neuroscience Research (IRL) *Online - full text edition.* **4118**
Neuroscience Research Communications (GBR) *Online - full text edition.* **4118**
The Neuroscientist (USA) *Online - full text edition.* **4118**
NeuroSignals (CHE) *Online - full text edition.* **3259**
Neurosurgery (Baltimore) (USA) *Online - full text edition.* **4119**
Neurosurgery Clinics of North America (USA) *Online - full text edition.* **4197**
Neurosurgery Quarterly (USA) *Online - full text edition.* **4197**
Neurosurgical Review (DEU) *Online - full text edition.* **4197**
Neurotoxicology and Teratology (USA) *Online - full text edition.* **4119**
NeuroToxicology (Little Rock) (USA) *Online - full text edition.* **4119**
Neurourology and Urodynamics (USA) *Online - full text edition.* **4216**
New England Journal of Medicine (USA) *Online - full text edition.* **3666**
New Genetics and Society (GBR) *Online - full text edition.* **3313**
New Ideas in Psychology (GBR) *Online - full text edition.* **4430**
The New Microbiologica (ITA) *Online - full text edition.* **3329**
New York Academy of Sciences. Annals (USA) *Online - full text edition.* **4506**
New Zealand Journal of Ecology (NZL) *Online - full text edition.* **3210**
New Zealand Journal of Psychology (NZL) *Online - full text edition.* **4430**
New Zealand Medical Journal (NZL) *Online - full text edition.* **3667**
New Zealand Veterinary Journal (NZL) *Online - full text edition.* **4548**
News in Physiological Sciences Online (USA) *Online - full text edition of* News in Physiological Sciences. **3346**
Nippon Nogeikagaku Kaishi (JPN) *Online - full text edition.* **3276**
Nippon Noyaku Gakkaishi (JPN) *Online - full text edition.* **3434**
Nordic Journal of Psychiatry (NOR) *Online - full text edition.* **4120**
Nordisk Psykologi (DNK) *Online - full text edition.* **4430**
Nuclear Medicine and Biology (USA) *Online - full text edition.* **4152**
Nuclear Medicine Communications (USA) *Online - full text edition.* **4152**
Nuclear Plant Journal (USA) *Online - full text edition.* **3431**
Nucleic Acids Research (GBR) *Online - full text edition.* **3259**
Nuklearmedizin (DEU) *Online - full text edition.* **4152**
Nurse Education Today (GBR) *Online - full text edition.* **3931**
Nurse Practitioner Forum (USA) *Online - full text edition.* **3931**
Nursing and Health Care Perspectives (USA) *Online - full text edition.* **3932**
Nursing Clinics of North America (USA) *Online - full text edition.* **3932**
Nursing Economics (USA) *Online - full text edition.* **3932**
Nursing Ethics (GBR) *Online - full text edition.* **3933**
Nursing History Review (USA) *Online - full text edition.* **3933**
Nursing Outlook (USA) *Online - full text edition.* **3934**
Nursing Research (USA) *Online - full text edition.* **3934**
Nursing Science Quarterly (USA) *Online - full text edition.* **3934**
Nutrition (USA) *Online - full text edition.* **4241**
Nutrition and Cancer (USA) *Online - full text edition.* **4241**
Nutrition Research (USA) *Online - full text edition.* **4243**
Nutrition Research Reviews (GBR) *Online - full text edition.* **4243**
Nutrition Reviews (USA) *Online - full text edition.* **4243**
Nutrition Society. Proceedings (GBR) *Online - full text edition.* **4243**
Nutritional Neuroscience (CHE) *Online - full text edition.* **4120**
O E M Online (GBR) *Online - full text edition of* Occupational and Environmental Medicine. **4261**
O I E Revue Scientifique et Technique (FRA) *Online - full text edition.* **4549**
O R L (CHE) *Online - full text edition.* **4036**
Obesity Research (USA) *Online - full text edition.* **3668**
Obesity Surgery (USA) *Online - full text edition.* **4198**
Obstetrical & Gynecological Survey (USA) *Online - full text edition.* **3960**
Obstetrics and Gynecology (USA) *Online - full text edition.* **3960**
Obstetrics and Gynecology Clinics of North America (USA) *Online - full text edition.* **3960**
Occupational Medicine (GBR) *Online - full text edition.* **4262**
Occupational Medicine (Philadelphia) (USA) *Online - full text edition.* **4262**
Occupational Therapy Journal of Research (USA) *Online - full text edition.* **3669**
Oceanography and Marine Biology: an Annual Review (GBR) *Online - full text edition.* **3408**
Ocular Immunology and Inflammation (NLD) *Online - full text edition.* **4002**
Odonatologica (NLD) *Online - full text edition.* **3211**
Oecologia (DEU) *Online - full text edition.* **3211**
Omega: Journal of Death and Dying (USA) *Online - full text edition.* **4431**
Oncogene (GBR) *Online - full text edition.* **3986**
Oncology (USA) *Online - full text edition.* **3986**
Oncology (CHE) *Online - full text edition.* **3986**
Oncology Reports (GRC) *Online - full text edition.* **3987**
Oncology Research (USA) *Online - full text edition.* **3987**
Onderstepoort Journal of Veterinary Research (ZAF) *Online - full text edition.* **4549**
Onkologie (CHE) *Online - full text edition.* **3987**
Online Journal of Knowledge Synthesis for Nursing(USA) *Online - full text.* **3936**
Operative Dentistry (USA) *Online - full text edition.* **3834**
Operative Techniques in Sports Medicine (USA) *Online - full text edition.* **4175**
Ophelia (DNK) *Online - full text edition.* **3212**
Ophthalmic and Physiological Optics (GBR) *Online - full text edition.* **4003**
Ophthalmic Plastic and Reconstructive Surgery (USA) *Online - full text edition.* **4003**
Ophthalmic Research (CHE) *Online - full text edition.* **4003**
Ophthalmic Surgery and Lasers (USA) *Online - full text edition.* **4199**
Der Ophthalmologe (DEU) *Online - full text edition.* **4004**
Ophthalmologica (CHE) *Online - full text edition.* **4004**
Ophthalmology (USA) *Online - full text edition.* **4004**
Optometry and Vision Science (USA) *Online - full text edition.* **4005**
Oral Diseases (GBR) *Online - full text edition.* **3834**
Oral Microbiology and Immunology (DNK) *Online - full text edition.* **3329**
Oral Oncology (GBR) *Online - full text edition.* **3988**
Oral Surgery, Oral Medicine, Oral Pathology, Oral Radiology, and Endodontics (USA) *Online - full text edition.* **3835**
Organization & Environment (USA) *Online - full text edition.* **4263**
Organizational Behavior and Human Decision Processes (USA) *Online - full text edition.* **3366**
Origins of Life and Evolution of the Biosphere (NLD) *Online - full text edition.* **3212**
Der Orthopaede (DEU) *Online - full text edition.* **4022**
Orthopedic Clinics of North America (USA) *Online - full text edition.* **4023**
Orthopedics (USA) *Online - full text edition.* **4023**
Osteoarthritis and Cartilage (GBR) *Online - full text edition.* **4169**
Osteoporosis International (GBR) *Online - full text edition.* **3671**
Otolaryngologic Clinics of North America (USA) *Online - full text edition.* **4036**
Otolaryngology - Head and Neck Surgery (USA) *Online - full text edition.* **4036**
Otology & Neurotology (USA) *Online - full text edition.* **4036**
Oxford Reviews of Reproductive Biology (GBR) *Online - full text edition.* **3346**
P D A Journal of Pharmaceutical Science and Technology (USA) *Online - full text edition.* **4320**
P P M P (DEU) *Online - full text edition.* **4121**
Pacing and Clinical Electrophysiology (PACE) (USA) *Online - full text edition.* **3780**
Paediatric Anaesthesia Online(GBR) *Online - full text.* **3759**
Paediatric & Perinatal Epidemiology Online(GBR) *Online - full text.* **4050**
Pain (NLD) *Online - full text edition.* **4121**
The Pain Clinic (NLD) *Online - full text edition.* **3759**
Pain Medicine Online(USA) *Online - full text.* **4121**
Pain Reviews (GBR) *Online - full text edition.* **3671**
Palliative Medicine (GBR) *Online - full text edition.* **3672**
Pancreas (USA) *Online - full text edition.* **3867**
Panminerva Medica (ITA) *Online - full text edition.* **3672**
Parasite (FRA) *Online - full text edition.* **3330**
Parasite Immunology Online (GBR) *Online - full text edition of* Parasite Immunology. **3804**
Parasitology (Cambridge) (GBR) *Online - full text edition.* **3804**
Parasitology International (NLD) *Online - full text edition.* **3805**
Parasitology Research (DEU) *Online - full text edition.* **3330**
Parkinsonism and Related Disorders (GBR) *Online - full text edition.* **4122**
Particulate Science and Technology (USA) *Online - full text edition.* **3434**
Pathobiology (CHE) *Online - full text edition.* **3750**
Der Pathologe (DEU) *Online - full text edition.* **3672**
Pathologie et Biologie (FRA) *Online - full text edition.* **3672**
Pathology (GBR) *Online - full text edition.* **3673**
Pathology International (AUS) *Online - full text edition.* **3673**
Pathology, Research and Practice (DEU) *Online - full text edition.* **3673**
Pathophysiology of Haemostasis and Thrombosis (CHE) *Online - full text edition.* **3904**
Patient Care (USA) *Online - full text edition.* **3673**
Patient Education and Counseling (IRL) *Online - full text edition.* **4484**
Pediatric Allergy and Immunology (DNK) *Online - full text edition.* **4051**
Pediatric and Developmental Pathology (USA) *Online - full text edition.* **4051**
Pediatric Annals (USA) *Online - full text edition.* **4051**
Pediatric Cardiology (USA) *Online - full text edition.* **3781**
Pediatric Clinics of North America (USA) *Online - full text edition.* **4052**
Pediatric Dermatology (USA) *Online - full text edition.* **3852**
Pediatric Emergency Care (USA) *Online - full text edition.* **4052**
Pediatric Exercise Science (USA) *Online - full text edition.* **4052**
Pediatric Hematology & Oncology (USA) *Online - full text edition.* **4053**
The Pediatric Infectious Disease Journal (USA) *Online - full text edition.* **4053**
Pediatric Nephrology (DEU) *Online - full text edition.* **4217**
Pediatric Neurology (USA) *Online - full text edition.* **4053**
Pediatric Neurosurgery (CHE) *Online - full text edition.* **4122**
Pediatric Pathology & Molecular Medicine (USA) *Online - full text edition.* **4053**
Pediatric Pulmonology (USA) *Online - full text edition.* **4053**
Pediatric Radiology (DEU) *Online - full text edition.* **4053**
Pediatric Research (USA) *Online - full text edition.* **4054**
Pediatric Surgery International (DEU) *Online - full text edition.* **4200**
Pediatric Transplantation (DNK) *Online - full text edition.* **4054**
Pediatrics (English Edition) (USA) *Online - full text edition.* **4054**
Pediatrics International (AUS) *Online - full text edition.* **4054**
Pedobiologia (DEU) *Online - full text edition.* **3159**
Peptides (USA) *Online - full text edition.* **3260**
Perception (GBR) *Online - full text edition.* **4432**
Perception & Psychophysics (USA) *Online - full text edition.* **4432**
Perceptual and Motor Skills (USA) *Online - full text edition.* **4432**
Perfusion (GBR) *Online - full text edition.* **3781**
Perfusion (DEU) *Online - full text edition.* **3781**
Periodicum Biologorum (HRV) *Online - full text edition.* **3212**
Periodontology 2000 Online(DNK) *Online - full text.* **3836**
Peritoneal Dialysis International (CAN) *Online - full text edition.* **3674**
Personal Relationships (GBR) *Online - full text edition.* **4457**
Personality and Individual Differences (GBR) *Online - full text edition.* **4432**
Personality and Social Psychology Bulletin (USA) *Online - full text edition.* **4432**
Personality and Social Psychology Review (USA) *Online - full text edition.* **4432**
Personnel Psychology (USA) *Online - full text edition.* **4433**
Perspectives in Biology and Medicine (USA) *Online - full text edition.* **3674**
Perspectives in Psychiatric Care (USA) *Online - full text edition.* **3937**
Pesquisa Agropecuaria Brasileira (BRA) *Online - full text edition.* **3155**
Pesquisa Veterinaria Brasileira (BRA) *Online - full text edition.* **4549**
Pesticide Biochemistry and Physiology (USA) *Online - full text edition.* **3159**

Pferdeheilkunde (DEU) *Online - full text edition.* **4550**
Pfluegers Archiv (DEU) *Online - full text edition.* **3674**
Pharma Selecta (NLD) *Online - full text edition.* **4322**
Pharmaceutical Biology (NLD) *Online - full text edition.* **4323**
Pharmaceutical Development and Technology (USA) *Online - full text edition.* **4323**
Pharmaceutical Journal (GBR) *Online - full text edition.* **4324**
PharmacoEconomics (NZL) *Online - full text edition.* **4326**
Pharmacoeconomics and Outcomes News (NZL) *Online - full text edition.* **4345**
Pharmacoepidemiology and Drug Safety (GBR) *Online - full text edition.* **4326**
Pharmacogenetics (USA) *Online - full text edition.* **3313**
Pharmacological Research (GBR) *Online - full text edition.* **4326**
Pharmacological Reviews (USA) *Online - full text edition.* **4326**
Pharmacology (CHE) *Online - full text edition.* **4326**
Pharmacology and Therapeutics (USA) *Online - full text edition.* **4326**
Pharmacology & Toxicology Online(DNK) *Online - full text.* **4327**
Pharmacology, Biochemistry and Behavior (USA) *Online - full text edition.* **4327**
Pharmacopsychiatry (DEU) *Online - full text edition.* **4123**
Pharmacotherapy (USA) *Online - full text edition.* **4327**
Die Pharmazeutische Industrie (DEU) *Online - full text edition.* **4329**
Die Pharmazie (DEU) *Online - full text edition.* **4330**
Philosophical Psychology (GBR) *Online - full text edition.* **4433**
Phlebologie (DEU) *Online - full text edition.* **3675**
Phlebology (GBR) *Online - full text edition.* **3781**
Photochemistry and Photobiology (USA) *Online - full text edition.* **3374**
Photodermatology, Photoimmunology & Photomedicine Online(DNK) *Online - full text.* **3852**
Photosynthesis Research (NLD) *Online - full text edition.* **3260**
Physica Medica (ITA) *Online - full text edition.* **3675**
Physical Therapy (USA) *Online - full text edition.* **4064**
The Physician and Sportsmedicine (USA) *Online - full text edition.* **4176**
Physics in Medicine and Biology (GBR) *Online - full text edition.* **3267**
Physikalische Medizin Rehabilitationsmedizin Kurortmedizin (DEU) *Online - full text edition.* **3676**
Physiological Genomics (USA) *Online - full text edition.* **3260**
Physiological Measurement (GBR) *Online - full text edition.* **3676**
Physiological Research (CZE) *Online - full text edition.* **3347**
Physiological Reviews Online (USA) *Online - full text edition of* Physiological Reviews. **3347**
Physiology and Behavior (USA) *Online - full text edition.* **3347**
Phytochemical Analysis (GBR) *Online - full text edition.* **3282**
Phytomedicine (DEU) *Online - full text edition.* **3676**
Phytotherapy Research (GBR) *Online - full text edition.* **3282**
Pigment Cell Research (DNK) *Online - full text edition.* **3293**
Placenta (GBR) *Online - full text edition.* **3676**
Plant and Cell Physiology (GBR) *Online - full text edition.* **3293**
Plant, Cell and Environment Online (GBR) *Online - full text edition of* Plant, Cell and Environment. **3213**
Plant Cell, Tissue and Organ Culture (NLD) *Online - full text edition.* **3293**
Plant Foods for Human Nutrition (NLD) *Online - full text edition.* **4244**
Plant Molecular Biology (NLD) *Online - full text edition.* **3213**
Planta Medica (DEU) *Online - full text edition.* **4330**
Plastic and Reconstructive Surgery (USA) *Online - full text edition.* **4200**
Platelets (Abingdon) (GBR) *Online - full text edition.* **3213**
Point Veterinaire (FRA) *Online - full text edition.* **4550**
Polar Biology (DEU) *Online - full text edition.* **3213**
Polish Journal of Pharmacology (POL) *Online - full text edition.* **4331**
Political Psychology (USA) *Online - full text edition.* **4368**
Politics and the Life Sciences (USA) *Online - full text edition.* **4368**
Population and Environment (USA) *Online - full text edition.* **4433**
Postgraduate Medical Journal (GBR) *Online - full text edition.* **3678**
Postgraduate Medicine (USA) *Online - full text edition.* **3678**
Postharvest Biology and Technology (NLD) *Online - full text edition.* **3277**
The Practitioner (GBR) *Online - full text edition.* **3678**
Der Praktische Tierarzt (DEU) *Online - full text edition.* **4550**
Pratique Medicale et Chirurgicale de l'Animal de Compagnie (FRA) *Online - full text edition.* **4550**
Praxis der Kinderpsychologie und Kinderpsychiatrie (DEU) *Online - full text edition.* **4123**
Prenatal and Neonatal Medicine (GBR) *Online - full text edition.* **3961**
Prenatal Diagnosis (GBR) *Online - full text edition.* **3962**
Preparative Biochemistry and Biotechnology (USA) *Online - full text edition.* **3260**
Prescrire International (FRA) *Online - full text edition.* **4331**
La Presse Medicale (FRA) *Online - full text edition.* **3679**
Preventive Medicine (USA) *Online - full text edition.* **3679**
Preventive Veterinary Medicine (NLD) *Online - full text edition.* **4550**
Primary Care (USA) *Online - full text edition.* **3679**
Primary Care Psychiatry (USA) *Online - full text edition.* **4123**
Primates (JPN) *Online - full text edition.* **3355**
Process Biochemistry (GBR) *Online - full text edition.* **3277**
Productions Animales (FRA) *Online - full text edition.* **4550**
Professional Psychology: Research and Practice (USA) *Online - full text edition.* **4434**
Progres en Urologie (FRA) *Online - full text edition.* **4217**
Progress in Applied Microcirculation (CHE) *Online - full text edition.* **3781**
Progress in Basic and Clinical Pharmacology (CHE) *Online - full text edition.* **4331**
Progress in Biochemical Pharmacology (CHE) *Online - full text edition.* **4331**
Progress in Biophysics & Molecular Biology (GBR) *Online - full text edition.* **3267**
Progress in Brain Research (NLD) *Online - full text edition.* **4123**
Progress in Cardiovascular Diseases (USA) *Online - full text edition.* **3781**
Progress in Clinical and Biological Research (USA) *Online - full text edition.* **3680**
Progress in Experimental Tumor Research (CHE) *Online - full text edition.* **3988**
Progress in Histochemistry and Cytochemistry (DEU) *Online - full text edition.* **3261**
Progress in Medical Virology (CHE) *Online - full text edition.* **3805**
Progress in Neuro-Psychopharmacology and Biological Psychiatry (USA) *Online - full text edition.* **4331**
Progress in Neurobiology (GBR) *Online - full text edition.* **3348**
Progress in Neurological Surgery (CHE) *Online - full text edition.* **4124**
Progress in Nuclear Magnetic Resonance Spectroscopy (NLD) *Online - full text edition.* **3377**
Progress in Nucleic Acid Research and Molecular Biology (USA) *Online - full text edition.* **3214**
Progress in Psychobiology and Physiological Psychology (USA) *Online - full text edition.* **4434**
Progress in Respiratory Research (CHE) *Online - full text edition.* **4163**
Progress in Retinal and Eye Research (GBR) *Online - full text edition.* **4006**
Progress in Surgery (CHE) *Online - full text edition.* **4201**
Prostaglandins and Other Lipid Mediators (USA) *Online - full text edition.* **3868**
Prostaglandins, Leukotrienes and Essential Fatty Acids (GBR) *Online - full text edition.* **3868**
The Prostate (USA) *Online - full text edition.* **3680**
Prostate Cancer and Prostatic Diseases (GBR) *Online - full text edition.* **3989**
Prosthetics and Orthotics International (DNK) *Online - full text edition.* **4024**
Protein Engineering (GBR) *Online - full text edition.* **3261**
Protein Expression and Purification (USA) *Online - full text edition.* **3261**
Protein Science (USA) *Online - full text edition.* **3261**
Proteins: Structure, Function, and Genetics (USA) *Online - full text edition.* **3261**
Proteomics (DEU) *Online - full text edition.* **3261**
Protist (DEU) *Online - full text edition.* **3214**
Psicothema: Revista de Psicologia (ESP) *Online - full text edition.* **4435**
Psikhologicheskii Zhurnal (RUS) *Online - full text edition.* **4435**
Psyche (DEU) *Online - full text edition.* **4436**
Psychiatric Annals (USA) *Online - full text edition.* **4125**
Psychiatric Clinics of North America (USA) *Online - full text edition.* **4125**
Psychiatric Genetics (USA) *Online - full text edition.* **3313**
Psychiatric Quarterly (USA) *Online - full text edition.* **4126**
Psychiatric Services (USA) *Online - full text edition.* **4126**
La Psychiatrie de l'Enfant (FRA) *Online - full text edition.* **4055**
Psychiatrische Praxis (DEU) *Online - full text edition.* **4126**
Psychiatry (USA) *Online - full text edition.* **4126**
Psychiatry and Clinical Neurosciences (AUS) *Online - full text edition.* **4126**
Psychiatry Research (IRL) *Online - full text edition.* **4127**
Psychiatry Research: Neuroimaging Section (IRL) *Online - full text edition.* **4127**
Psycho-Oncology (GBR) *Online - full text edition.* **3989**
Psychoanalytic Dialogues (USA) *Online - full text edition.* **4436**
Psychoanalytic Inquiry (USA) *Online - full text edition.* **4436**
Psychoanalytic Psychology (USA) *Online - full text edition.* **4436**
Psychoanalytic Quarterly (USA) *Online - full text edition.* **4437**
Psychoanalytic Study of the Child (USA) *Online - full text edition.* **4437**
Psychologia (JPN) *Online - full text edition.* **4437**
Psychologica Belgica (BEL) *Online - full text edition.* **4437**
Psychological Assessment (USA) *Online - full text edition.* **4437**
Psychological Bulletin (USA) *Online - full text edition.* **4437**
Psychological Inquiry (USA) *Online - full text edition.* **4438**
Psychological Medicine (GBR) *Online - full text edition.* **4127**
Psychological Methods (USA) *Online - full text edition.* **4438**
The Psychological Record (USA) *Online - full text edition.* **4438**
Psychological Reports (USA) *Online - full text edition.* **4438**
Psychological Research (DEU) *Online - full text edition.* **4438**
Psychological Review (USA) *Online - full text edition.* **4438**
Psychological Science (USA) *Online - full text edition.* **4438**
Psychologische Rundschau (DEU) *Online - full text edition.* **4439**
The Psychologist (GBR) *Online - full text edition.* **4440**
Psychology and Aging (USA) *Online - full text edition.* **3479**
Psychology & Education (USA) *Online - full text edition.* **4440**
Psychology & Health (CHE) *Online - full text edition.* **4440**
Psychology & Marketing (USA) *Online - full text edition.* **4440**
Psychology, Crime and Law (CHE) *Online - full text edition.* **4440**
Psychology in the Schools (USA) *Online - full text edition.* **4441**
Psychology of Addictive Behaviors (USA) *Online - full text edition.* **3405**
Psychology of Learning and Motivation: Advances in Research and Theory (USA) *Online - full text edition.* **4441**
Psychology of Women Quarterly (GBR) *Online - full text edition.* **4441**
Psychology, Public Policy, and Law (USA) *Online - full text edition.* **4441**
Psychometrika (CAN) *Online - full text edition.* **4442**
Psychoneuroendocrinology (GBR) *Online - full text edition.* **4128**
Psychonomic Bulletin & Review (USA) *Online - full text edition.* **4442**
Psychopathology (CHE) *Online - full text edition.* **4128**
Psychopharmacology (DEU) *Online - full text edition.* **4332**
Psychopharmakotherapie (DEU) *Online - full text edition.* **4332**
Psychophysiology (GBR) *Online - full text edition.* **4128**
Psychosomatic Medicine (USA) *Online - full text edition.* **4128**
Psychosomatics (USA) *Online - full text edition.* **4128**
Psychotherapeut (DEU) *Online - full text edition.* **4128**
Psychotherapy (USA) *Online - full text edition.* **4442**
Psychotherapy and Psychosomatics (CHE) *Online - full text edition.* **4129**
Psychotherapy Research (USA) *Online - full text edition.* **4443**
Pteridines (GBR) *Online - full text edition.* **3377**
Public Health (Basingstoke) (GBR) *Online - full text edition.* **3681**
Public Health Nursing (USA) *Online - full text edition.* **3938**
Public Health Reports (USA) *Online - full text edition.* **4486**
Pulmonary Pharmacology & Therapeutics (GBR) *Online - full text edition.* **4163**
Q J M (GBR) *Online - full text edition.* **3681**
Qualitative Health Research (USA) *Online - full text edition.* **3681**
Quality in Health Care (GBR) *Online - full text edition.* **3682**
Quality of Life Research (NLD) *Online - full text edition.* **3682**
Quantitative Structure-Activity Relationships (DEU) *Online - full text edition.* **4332**
Quarterly Journal of Experimental Psychology. Section A: Human Experimental Psychology (GBR) *Online - full text edition.* **4443**
Quarterly Journal of Experimental Psychology. Section B: Comparative and Physiological Psychology (GBR) *Online - full text edition.* **4443**
Quarterly Review of Biology (USA) *Online - full text edition.* **3214**
Quarterly Reviews of Biophysics (GBR) *Online - full text edition.* **3267**
Quest (Champaign) (USA) *Online - full text edition.* **3429**
Quintessence International (USA) *Online - full text edition.* **3837**
R N A (GBR) *Online - full text edition.* **3261**
Radiation and Environmental Biophysics (DEU) *Online - full text edition.* **3267**
Radiation Protection Dosimetry (GBR) *Online - full text edition.* **4366**
Radiographics (USA) *Online - full text edition.* **4153**
Der Radiologe (DEU) *Online - full text edition.* **4153**
Radiologic Clinics of North America (USA) *Online - full text edition.* **4153**
Radiology (USA) *Online - full text edition.* **4154**
Radiotherapy and Oncology (IRL) *Online - full text edition.* **4154**
Reactions Weekly (NZL) *Online - full text edition.* **4346**
Reading and Writing (NLD) *Online - full text edition.* **3551**
Recent Progress in Hormone Research. Proceedings of the Laurentian Hormone Conference (USA) *Online - full text edition.* **3868**
Recent Results in Cancer Research (USA) *Online - full text edition.* **3989**
Redox Report (GBR) *Online - full text edition.* **4333**
Regional Anesthesia and Pain Medicine (USA) *Online - full text edition.* **3759**
Regulatory Peptides (NLD) *Online - full text edition.* **3262**
Regulatory Toxicology and Pharmacology (USA) *Online - full text edition.* **3453**
Rehabilitation Counseling Bulletin (USA) *Online - full text edition.* **3486**

Rehabilitation Psychology (USA) *Online - full text edition.* **4444**
Remedial and Special Education (USA) *Online - full text edition.* **3426**
Renal Failure (USA) *Online - full text edition.* **4217**
Reproduction (GBR) *Online - full text edition.* **3215**
Reproduction, Fertility and Development (AUS) *Online - full text edition.* **3215**
Reproduction in Domestic Animals Online(DEU) *Online - full text.* **4551**
Reproduction, Nutrition, Development (FRA) *Online - full text edition.* **3215**
Reproductive Health Matters (GBR) *Online - full text edition.* **4565**
Reproductive Toxicology (USA) *Online - full text edition.* **3348**
Research Communications in Molecular Pathology and Pharmacology (USA) *Online - full text edition.* **3684**
Research in Developmental Disabilities (GBR) *Online - full text edition.* **4130**
Research in Microbiology (FRA) *Online - full text edition.* **3330**
Research in Nursing & Health (USA) *Online - full text edition.* **3939**
Research in Organizational Behavior (USA) *Online - full text edition.* **4444**
Research in Veterinary Science (GBR) *Online - full text edition.* **4551**
Research on Aging (USA) *Online - full text edition.* **3480**
Research on Social Work Practice (USA) *Online - full text edition.* **4523**
Research Quarterly for Exercise and Sport (USA) *Online - full text edition.* **4360**
Respiration (CHE) *Online - full text edition.* **4164**
Respiration Physiology (NLD) *Online - full text edition.* **3348**
Respiratory Medicine (GBR) *Online - full text edition.* **4164**
Restorative Neurology and Neuroscience (NLD) *Online - full text edition.* **4130**
Resuscitation (IRL) *Online - full text edition.* **4165**
Retina (USA) *Online - full text edition.* **4006**
Reviews in Contemporary Pharmacotherapy (GBR) *Online - full text edition.* **4334**
Reviews in Medical Microbiology (USA) *Online - full text edition.* **3684**
Reviews in Medical Virology (GBR) *Online - full text edition.* **3331**
Reviews in the Neurosciences (ISR) *Online - full text edition.* **4130**
Reviews of Environmental Contamination and Toxicology (USA) *Online - full text edition.* **3454**
Reviews of Physiology, Biochemistry and Pharmacology (USA) *Online - full text edition.* **3348**
Revista Brasileira de Zootecnia (BRA) *Online - full text edition.* **4551**
Revista Clinica Espanola (ESP) *Online - full text edition.* **3685**
Revista de Biologia Tropical (CRI) *Online - full text edition.* **3216**
Revista de Investigacion Clinica (MEX) *Online - full text edition.* **3685**
Revista de Neurologia (ESP) *Online - full text edition.* **4130**
Revista de Saude Publica (BRA) *Online - full text edition.* **4488**
Revista Ecuatoriana de Neurologia (ECU) *Online - full text edition.* **4131**
Revista Espanola de Cardiologia (ESP) *Online - full text edition.* **3782**
Revista Espanola de Enfermedades Digestivas (ESP) *Online - full text edition.* **3895**
Revista Latinoamericana de Psicologia (COL) *Online - full text edition.* **4445**
Revista Medica de Chile (CHL) *Online - full text edition.* **3686**
Revista Mexicana de Psicologia (MEX) *Online - full text edition.* **4445**
Revue de Chirurgie Orthopedique et Reparatrice de l'Appareil Moteur (FRA) *Online - full text edition.* **4025**
La Revue de Medecine Interne (FRA) *Online - full text edition.* **3911**
Revue de Medecine Veterinaire (FRA) *Online - full text edition.* **4552**
Revue de Neuropsychologie (FRA) *Online - full text edition.* **4131**
Revue d'Epidemiologie et de Sante Publique (FRA) *Online - full text edition.* **4488**
Revue des Maladies Respiratoires (FRA) *Online - full text edition.* **4165**
Revue du Praticien (FRA) *Online - full text edition.* **3687**
Revue Francaise d'Allergologie et d'Immunologie Clinique (FRA) *Online - full text edition.* **3751**
Revue Neurologique (FRA) *Online - full text edition.* **4131**
Rheumatic Diseases. Bulletin (USA) *Online - full text edition.* **4171**
Rheumatic Diseases Clinics of North America (USA) *Online - full text edition.* **4171**
Rheumatology (GBR) *Online - full text edition.* **4171**
Rheumatology International (DEU) *Online - full text edition.* **4171**
Rhinology (NLD) *Online - full text edition.* **4037**
Rivista di Biologia (ITA) *Online - full text edition.* **3216**
Rivista di Neuroradiologia (ITA) *Online - full text edition.* **4154**
RoeFo. Fortschritte auf dem Gebiet der Roentgenstrahlen und der bildgebenden Verfahren (DEU) *Online - full text edition.* **4155**
Rossiiskaya Akademiya Nauk. Izvestiya. Seriya Biologicheskaya (RUS) *Online - full text edition.* **3216**
Royal Chemical Society. Journal. Perkin Transactions 1 (GBR) *Online - full text edition.* **3379**
Royal College of Surgeons of Edinburgh. Journal (GBR) *Online - full text edition.* **4202**
Royal College of Surgeons of England. Annals (GBR) *Online - full text edition.* **4202**
Royal Society for the Promotion of Health. Journal (GBR) *Online - full text edition.* **4517**
Royal Society of London. Philosophical Transactions. Biological Sciences (GBR) *Online - full text edition.* **3217**
Royal Society of London. Proceedings. Biological Sciences (GBR) *Online - full text edition.* **3217**
Royal Society of Medicine. International Congress and Symposium Series (GBR) *Online - full text edition.* **3688**
Royal Society of Medicine. Journal (GBR) *Online - full text edition.* **3688**
Royal Society of Tropical Medicine and Hygiene. Transactions (GBR) *Online - full text edition.* **3806**
Russian Journal of Bioorganic Chemistry (RUS) *Online - full text edition.* **3379**
Russian Journal of Genetics (RUS) *Online - full text edition.* **3314**
S A M J South African Medical Journal (ZAF) *Online - full text edition.* **3688**
S S A Journal (USA) *Online - full text edition.* **4264**
S T I Online (GBR) *Online - full text edition of* Sexually Transmitted Infections. **3853**
S T P Pharma Sciences (FRA) *Online - full text edition.* **4335**
Safety Science (NLD) *Online - full text edition.* **4265**
Saggi (ITA) *Online - full text edition.* **4132**
Salud Mental (MEX) *Online - full text edition.* **4132**
Salud Publica de Mexico Online (MEX) *Online - full text edition of* Salud Publica de Mexico. **4489**
Sarcoidosis Vasculitis and Diffuse Lung Diseases (ITA) *Online - full text edition.* **3989**
Saudi Medical Journal (SAU) *Online - full text edition.* **3690**
Scandinavian Audiology (NOR) *Online - full text edition.* **4038**
Scandinavian Cardiovascular Journal (NOR) *Online - full text edition.* **4202**
Scandinavian Journal of Caring Sciences (NOR) *Online - full text edition.* **3690**
Scandinavian Journal of Clinical & Laboratory Investigation (NOR) *Online - full text edition.* **3880**
Scandinavian Journal of Gastroenterology (NOR) *Online - full text edition.* **3895**
Scandinavian Journal of Immunology Online (GBR) *Online - full text edition of* Scandinavian Journal of Immunology. **3751**
Scandinavian Journal of Infectious Diseases (NOR) *Online - full text edition.* **3806**
Scandinavian Journal of Laboratory Animal Science (DNK) *Online - full text edition.* **3880**
Scandinavian Journal of Medicine & Science in Sports Online(DNK) *Online - full text.* **4176**
Scandinavian Journal of Plastic and Reconstructive Surgery and Hand Surgery (NOR) *Online - full text edition.* **4202**
Scandinavian Journal of Primary Health Care (NOR) *Online - full text edition.* **3690**
Scandinavian Journal of Psychology (GBR) *Online - full text edition.* **4447**
Scandinavian Journal of Public Health (NOR) *Online - full text edition.* **3690**
Scandinavian Journal of Rheumatology (NOR) *Online - full text edition.* **4171**
Scandinavian Journal of Urology and Nephrology (NOR) *Online - full text edition.* **4218**
Scandinavian Journal of Work, Environment & Health (FIN) *Online - full text edition.* **4265**
Scanning (USA) *Online - full text edition.* **3335**
Schizophrenia Bulletin (USA) *Online - full text edition.* **4132**
Schizophrenia Research (NLD) *Online - full text edition.* **4132**
Der Schmerz (DEU) *Online - full text edition.* **3690**
School Psychology International (GBR) *Online - full text edition.* **3429**
School Psychology Quarterly (USA) *Online - full text edition.* **4447**
School Psychology Review (USA) *Online - full text edition.* **4447**
Schweizer Archiv fuer Tierheilkunde (CHE) *Online - full text edition.* **4552**
Schweizerische Rundschau fuer Medizin Praxis (CHE) *Online - full text edition.* **3691**
Schweizerische Zeitschrift fuer Psychologie (CHE) *Online - full text edition.* **4447**
Science and Justice (GBR) *Online - full text edition.* **3885**
Science & Sports (FRA) *Online - full text edition.* **4176**
The Science of the Total Environment (NLD) *Online - full text edition.* **3442**
Sciences Sociales et Sante (FRA) *Online - full text edition.* **4489**
SciTech Book News (USA) *Online - full text edition.* **3177**
Scottish Medical Journal (GBR) *Online - full text edition.* **3691**
Seibutsu Kogaku Kaishi (JPN) *Online - full text edition.* **3331**
Seikagaku (JPN) *Online - full text edition.* **3262**
Seizure (GBR) *Online - full text edition.* **4133**
La Semaine des Hopitaux (FRA) *Online - full text edition.* **3691**
Seminars in Anesthesia, Perioperative Medicine and Pain (USA) *Online - full text edition.* **3760**
Seminars in Arthritis & Rheumatism (USA) *Online - full text edition.* **4172**
Seminars in Avian and Exotic Pet Medicine (USA) *Online - full text edition.* **4552**
Seminars in Cancer Biology (GBR) *Online - full text edition.* **3349**
Seminars in Cell and Developmental Biology (GBR) *Online - full text edition.* **3294**
Seminars in Cutaneous Medicine & Surgery (USA) *Online - full text edition.* **3853**
Seminars in Diagnostic Pathology (USA) *Online - full text edition.* **3692**
Seminars in Dialysis (USA) *Online - full text edition.* **4218**
Seminars in Hematology (USA) *Online - full text edition.* **3905**
Seminars in Immunology (GBR) *Online - full text edition.* **3751**
Seminars in Liver Diseases (USA) *Online - full text edition.* **3896**
Seminars in Nephrology (USA) *Online - full text edition.* **4218**
Seminars in Neurology (USA) *Online - full text edition.* **4133**
Seminars in Nuclear Medicine (USA) *Online - full text edition.* **4155**
Seminars in Oncology (USA) *Online - full text edition.* **3990**
Seminars in Perinatology (USA) *Online - full text edition.* **4056**
Seminars in Radiation Oncology (USA) *Online - full text edition.* **3990**
Seminars in Reproductive Medicine (USA) *Online - full text edition.* **3869**
Seminars in Respiratory and Critical Care Medicine (USA) *Online - full text edition.* **4165**
Seminars in Roentgenology (USA) *Online - full text edition.* **4155**
Seminars in Surgical Oncology (USA) *Online - full text edition.* **3990**
Seminars in Thrombosis and Hemostasis (USA) *Online - full text edition.* **3905**
Seminars in Ultrasound, C T and M R (USA) *Online - full text edition.* **4155**
Sex Roles (USA) *Online - full text edition.* **4448**
Sexuality and Disability (USA) *Online - full text edition.* **3692**
Sexually Transmitted Diseases (USA) *Online - full text edition.* **3853**
Shengwu Huaxue yu Shengwu Wuli Jinzhan (CHN) *Online - full text edition.* **3262**
Shengwu Huaxue yu Shengwu Wuli Xuebao (CHN) *Online - full text edition.* **3262**
Shock (USA) *Online - full text edition.* **3693**
Silvae Genetica (DEU) *Online - full text edition.* **3282**
Skeletal Radiology (DEU) *Online - full text edition.* **4155**
Skin Pharmacology and Applied Skin Physiology (CHE) *Online - full text edition.* **4336**
Skin Research and Technology (DNK) *Online - full text edition.* **3853**
Sleep (USA) *Online - full text edition.* **4134**
Sleep Medicine Reviews (GBR) *Online - full text edition.* **4134**
Small Group Research (USA) *Online - full text edition.* **4449**
Small Ruminant Research (NLD) *Online - full text edition.* **3161**
Smith College Studies in Social Work (USA) *Online - full text edition.* **4518**
Social Behavior and Personality (NZL) *Online - full text edition.* **4449**
Social Biology (USA) *Online - full text edition.* **3314**
Social Cognition (USA) *Online - full text edition.* **4449**
Social History of Medicine (GBR) *Online - full text edition.* **3694**
Social Psychiatry and Psychiatric Epidemiology (DEU) *Online - full text edition.* **4134**
Social Psychology Quarterly (USA) *Online - full text edition.* **4523**
Social Science & Medicine (GBR) *Online - full text edition.* **3694**
Social Work in Health Care (USA) *Online - full text edition.* **4518**
Societe de Pathologie Exotique. Bulletin (FRA) *Online - full text edition.* **3694**
Society & Animals (GBR) *Online - full text edition.* **3172**
Society for Gynecologic Investigation. Journal (USA) *Online - full text edition.* **3964**
Society for Research in Child Development. Monographs (USA) *Online - full text edition.* **3386**
Sociobiology (USA) *Online - full text edition.* **3219**
Sociology of Health and Illness (GBR) *Online - full text edition.* **4523**
Sociology of Sport Journal (USA) *Online - full text edition.* **4523**
Soil Biology & Biochemistry (GBR) *Online - full text edition.* **3263**
Solid State Nuclear Magnetic Resonance (GBR) *Online - full text edition.* **3377**
Somatic Cell and Molecular Genetics (USA) *Online - full text edition.* **3314**
Somatosensory and Motor Research (GBR) *Online - full text edition.* **3349**
South African Journal of Animal Science (ZAF) *Online - full text edition.* **3162**
South African Journal of Psychology (ZAF) *Online - full text edition.* **4450**
South African Journal of Surgery (ZAF) *Online - full text edition.* **4204**
South African Veterinary Association. Scientific Journal (ZAF) *Online - full text edition.* **4552**
Southern Medical Journal (USA) *Online - full text edition.* **3695**
Sozial- und Praeventivmedizin (CHE) *Online - full text edition.* **3695**
Spatial Vision (NLD) *Online - full text edition.* **3554**
Speech Communication (NLD) *Online - full text edition.* **3552**
Spinal Cord (GBR) *Online - full text edition.* **4134**
Spine (Philadelphia, 1976) (USA) *Online - full text edition.* **4026**
The Sport Psychologist (USA) *Online - full text edition.* **4450**
Sports Medicine (NZL) *Online - full text edition.* **4177**
Sports Medicine and Arthroscopy Review (USA) *Online - full text edition.* **4026**
Sports Medicine Standards & Malpractice Reporter (USA) *Online - full text edition.* **3544**
Sportverletzung - Sportschaden (DEU) *Online - full text edition.* **3695**

Online Service

Sprache & Kognition (CHE) *Online - full text edition.* **4450**
Springer Seminars in Immunopathology (DEU) *Online - full text edition.* **3751**
Statistical Methods in Medical Research (GBR) *Online - full text edition.* **4530**
Statistics in Medicine (GBR) *Online - full text edition.* **3737**
Stem Cells (USA) *Online - full text edition.* **3219**
Stereotactic and Functional Neurosurgery (CHE) *Online - full text edition.* **4204**
Steroids (USA) *Online - full text edition.* **3263**
Strahlentherapie und Onkologie (DEU) *Online - full text edition.* **4156**
Strength and Conditioning Journal (USA) *Online - full text edition.* **4361**
Stress and Health (GBR) *Online - full text edition.* **4135**
Stroke (USA) *Online - full text edition.* **3783**
Structure (GBR) *Online - full text edition.* **3220**
Studia Psychologica (SVK) *Online - full text edition.* **4451**
Studies in Family Planning (USA) *Online - full text edition.* **4369**
Substance Use and Misuse (USA) *Online - full text edition.* **3406**
Suicide and Life-Threatening Behavior (USA) *Online - full text edition.* **4451**
Supportive Care in Cancer (DEU) *Online - full text edition.* **3990**
Surgery (USA) *Online - full text edition.* **4204**
Surgery Today (JPN) *Online - full text edition.* **4204**
Surgical and Radiologic Anatomy (FRA) *Online - full text edition.* **3697**
Surgical Clinics of North America (USA) *Online - full text edition.* **4204**
Surgical Endoscopy (USA) *Online - full text edition.* **4204**
Surgical Laparoscopy, Endoscopy and Percutaneous Techniques (USA) *Online - full text edition.* **4205**
Surgical Neurology (USA) *Online - full text edition.* **4205**
Surgical Oncology (GBR) *Online - full text edition.* **3991**
Surgical Pathology (USA) *Online - full text edition.* **3697**
Survey of Ophthalmology (USA) *Online - full text edition.* **3737**
Swedish Dental Journal (SWE) *Online - full text edition.* **3840**
Swiss Medical Weekly (CHE) *Online - full text edition.* **3697**
Symbiosis (ISR) *Online - full text edition.* **3220**
Synapse (New York) (USA) *Online - full text edition.* **4135**
System Familie (DEU) *Online - full text edition.* **4135**
Systematic and Applied Microbiology (DEU) *Online - full text edition.* **3331**
Systematic Parasitology (NLD) *Online - full text edition.* **3220**
T A S H Journal (USA) *Online - full text edition.* **3487**
Teaching and Learning in Medicine (USA) *Online - full text edition.* **3698**
Teaching of Psychology (USA) *Online - full text edition.* **4452**
Techniques in Neurosurgery (USA) *Online - full text edition.* **4206**
Telemedicine Journal and e-Health (USA) *Online - full text edition.* **3812**
Terapevticheskii Arkhiv (RUS) *Online - full text edition.* **3699**
Teratogenesis, Carcinogenesis, and Mutagenesis (USA) *Online - full text edition.* **3699**
Teratology (USA) *Online - full text edition.* **3220**
Texas Heart Institute Journal (USA) *Online - full text edition.* **3783**
Theoretical and Applied Genetics (DEU) *Online - full text edition.* **3314**
Theoretical Medicine and Bioethics (NLD) *Online - full text edition.* **3699**
Theoretical Population Biology (USA) *Online - full text edition.* **3221**
Theory & Psychology (GBR) *Online - full text edition.* **4452**
Theory in Biosciences (DEU) *Online - full text edition.* **3221**
Therapeutic Drug Monitoring (USA) *Online - full text edition.* **4337**
Therapeutische Umschau (CHE) *Online - full text edition.* **3700**
Therapie (GBR) *Online - full text edition.* **3700**
Therapie und Erfolg (DEU) *Online - full text edition.* **3700**
Theriogenology (USA) *Online - full text edition.* **4553**
The Thoracic and Cardiovascular Surgeon (DEU) *Online - full text edition.* **4206**
Thorax Online (GBR) *Online - full text edition of* Thorax. **3700**
Thrombosis and Haemostasis (DEU) *Online - full text edition.* **3783**
Thrombosis Research (GBR) *Online - full text edition.* **3784**
Thyroid (USA) *Online - full text edition.* **3869**
Tieraerztliche Praxis. Ausgabe G: Grosstiere - Nutztiere (DEU) *Online - full text edition.* **4553**
Tieraerztliche Praxis. Ausgabe K: Kleintiere - Heimtiere (DEU) *Online - full text edition.* **4553**
Tieraerztliche Umschau (DEU) *Online - full text edition.* **4553**
Tijdschrift voor Diergeneeskunde (NLD) *Online - full text edition.* **4554**
Tissue & Cell (GBR) *Online - full text edition.* **3294**
Tissue Antigens (DNK) *Online - full text edition.* **3701**
Tissue Engineering (USA) *Online - full text edition.* **3294**
Tissue Reactions (CHE) *Online - full text edition.* **3294**
Tobbacco Control Online (GBR) *Online - full text edition of* Tobacco Control. **4531**
Tohoku Journal of Experimental Medicine (JPN) *Online - full text edition.* **3880**
Topics in Geriatric Rehabilitation (USA) *Online - full text edition.* **3481**
Topics in Language Disorders (USA) *Online - full text edition.* **3427**
Topoi (NLD) *Online - full text edition.* **4348**
Toxicologic Pathology (USA) *Online - full text edition.* **3454**
Toxicological Sciences (USA) *Online - full text edition.* **3455**
Toxicology (IRL) *Online - full text edition.* **3455**
Toxicology and Applied Pharmacology (USA) *Online - full text edition.* **3455**
Toxicology and Industrial Health (GBR) *Online - full text edition.* **3455**
Toxicology in Vitro (GBR) *Online - full text edition.* **3455**
Toxicology Letters (IRL) *Online - full text edition.* **3456**
Toxicology Methods (USA) *Online - full text edition.* **3456**
Toxicon (GBR) *Online - full text edition.* **4338**
Trace Elements and Electrolytes (DEU) *Online - full text edition.* **3702**
Traffic (DNK) *Online - full text edition.* **3294**
Transfusion (USA) *Online - full text edition.* **3702**
Transfusion and Apheresis Science (GBR) *Online - full text edition.* **3905**
Transfusion Clinique et Biologique (FRA) *Online - full text edition.* **3905**
Transfusion Medicine (GBR) *Online - full text edition.* **3905**
Transfusion Medicine Reviews (USA) *Online - full text edition.* **3905**
Transgenic Research (NLD) *Online - full text edition.* **3314**
Transplant Immunology (GBR) *Online - full text edition.* **3751**
Transplant International (DEU) *Online - full text edition.* **3702**
Transplantation (USA) *Online - full text edition.* **4206**
Transplantation Proceedings (USA) *Online - full text edition.* **4206**
Le Travail Humain (FRA) *Online - full text edition.* **4453**
Tree Physiology (CAN) *Online - full text edition.* **3283**
Trends in Biochemical Sciences (GBR) *Online - full text edition.* **3263**
Trends in Biotechnology (GBR) *Online - full text edition.* **3277**
Trends in Cardiovascular Medicine (USA) *Online - full text edition.* **3784**
Trends in Cell Biology (GBR) *Online - full text edition.* **3295**
Trends in Cognitive Sciences (GBR) *Online - full text edition.* **4453**
Trends in Ecology and Evolution (GBR) *Online - full text edition.* **3221**
Trends in Endocrinology and Metabolism (GBR) *Online - full text edition.* **3869**
Trends in Genetics (GBR) *Online - full text edition.* **3314**
Trends in Immunology Online (GBR) *Online - full text edition of* Trends in Immunology. **3752**
Trends in Microbiology (GBR) *Online - full text edition.* **3332**
Trends in Molecular Medicine (GBR) *Online - full text edition.* **3702**
Trends in Neurosciences (GBR) *Online - full text edition.* **4137**
Trends in Parasitology (GBR) *Online - full text edition.* **3332**
Trends in Pharmacological Sciences (GBR) *Online - full text edition.* **4338**
Tropical Animal Health and Production (NLD) *Online - full text edition.* **4554**
Tropical Doctor (GBR) *Online - full text edition.* **3807**
Tropical Medicine & International Health Online (GBR) *Online - full text edition of* Tropical Medicine & International Health. **4491**
Tuberculosis (GBR) *Online - full text edition.* **4166**
Tumor Biology (CHE) *Online - full text edition.* **3991**
Tumori (ITA) *Online - full text edition.* **3991**
Turk Psikoloji Dergisi (TUR) *Online - full text edition.* **4453**
Turk Veterinerlik ve Hayvancilik Dergisi (TUR) *Online - full text edition.* **4554**
Turkish Journal of Pediatrics (TUR) *Online - full text edition.* **4057**
Ugeskrift for Laeger (DNK) *Online - full text edition.* **3703**
Ulster Medical Journal (GBR) *Online - full text edition.* **3704**
Ultramicroscopy (NLD) *Online - full text edition.* **3336**
Ultraschall in der Medizin (DEU) *Online - full text edition.* **3704**
Ultrasonic Imaging (USA) *Online - full text edition.* **4156**
Ultrasound in Medicine & Biology (USA) *Online - full text edition.* **3222**
Ultrasound in Obstetrics & Gynecology (GBR) *Online - full text edition.* **3965**
Ultrastructural Pathology (USA) *Online - full text edition.* **3991**
Undersea & Hyperbaric Medicine (USA) *Online - full text edition.* **3704**
Der Unfallchirurg (DEU) *Online - full text edition.* **4027**
Universidad de Zulia. Facultad de Ciencias Veterinarias. Revista Cientifica (VEN) *Online - full text edition.* **4554**
Upsala Journal of Medical Sciences (NOR) *Online - full text edition.* **3706**
Der Urologe. Section A (DEU) *Online - full text edition.* **4219**
Urologia Internationalis (CHE) *Online - full text edition.* **4219**
Urologic Clinics of North America (USA) *Online - full text edition.* **4219**
Urologic Oncology (USA) *Online - full text edition.* **3992**
Urological Research (DEU) *Online - full text edition.* **4219**
Urology (USA) *Online - full text edition.* **4220**
Vaccine Online (GBR) *Online - full text edition of* Vaccine. **3752**
Vasa (CHE) *Online - full text edition.* **3784**
Vascular Medicine (GBR) *Online - full text edition.* **3784**
Vascular Surgery (Glen Head) (USA) *Online - full text edition.* **4207**
Venereology (AUS) *Online - full text edition.* **3854**
Verhaltenstherapie (CHE) *Online - full text edition.* **4137**
Veterinarni Medicina (CZE) *Online - full text edition.* **4555**
Veterinarski Arhiv (HRV) *Online - full text edition.* **4556**
Veterinary and Comparative Orthopaedics and Traumatology (DEU) *Online - full text edition.* **4556**
Veterinary and Human Toxicology (USA) *Online - full text edition.* **3456**
Veterinary Clinical Pathology (USA) *Online - full text edition.* **4556**
Veterinary Clinics of North America: Equine Practice (USA) *Online - full text edition.* **4556**
Veterinary Clinics of North America: Food Animal Practice (USA) *Online - full text edition.* **4556**
Veterinary Clinics of North America: Small Animal Practice (USA) *Online - full text edition.* **4556**
Veterinary Dermatology Online(GBR) *Online - full text.* **4557**
Veterinary Economics (USA) *Online - full text edition.* **3369**
Veterinary Immunology and Immunopathology (NLD) *Online - full text edition.* **4557**
Veterinary Institute, Pulawy. Bulletin (POL) *Online - full text edition.* **4557**
The Veterinary Journal (GBR) *Online - full text edition.* **4557**
Veterinary Medicine (USA) *Online - full text edition.* **4557**
Veterinary Microbiology (NLD) *Online - full text edition.* **3332**
Veterinary Ophthalmology Online (GBR) *Online - full text edition of* Veterinary Ophthalmology. **4558**
Veterinary Parasitology (NLD) *Online - full text edition.* **4558**
Veterinary Pathology (USA) *Online - full text edition.* **4558**
Veterinary Practice Staff (USA) *Online - full text edition.* **4558**
Veterinary Quarterly (NLD) *Online - full text edition.* **4558**
Veterinary Radiology & Ultrasound (USA) *Online - full text edition.* **4558**
Veterinary Record (GBR) *Online - full text edition.* **4558**
Veterinary Research Communications (NLD) *Online - full text edition.* **4559**
Veterinary Research (Online Edition) (FRA) *Online - full text edition of* Veterinary Research. **4559**
Veterinary Surgery (USA) *Online - full text edition.* **4559**
Veterinary Technician (USA) *Online - full text edition.* **4559**
Vie et Milieu (FRA) *Online - full text edition.* **3223**
Violence Against Women (USA) *Online - full text edition.* **4524**
Viral Immunology (USA) *Online - full text edition.* **3752**
Virchows Archiv (DEU) *Online - full text edition.* **3223**
Virology (USA) *Online - full text edition.* **3332**
Virus Genes (USA) *Online - full text edition.* **3332**
Virus Research (NLD) *Online - full text edition.* **3333**
Vision Research (GBR) *Online - full text edition.* **4008**
Visual Cognition (GBR) *Online - full text edition.* **4454**
Visual Neuroscience (GBR) *Online - full text edition.* **4137**
Vitamins and Hormones: Advances in Research and Applications (USA) *Online - full text edition.* **4340**
Vlaams Diergeneeskundig Tijdschrift (BEL) *Online - full text edition.* **4559**
The Volta Review (USA) *Online - full text edition.* **3493**
Voprosy Meditsinskoi Khimii (RUS) *Online - full text edition.* **3264**
Voprosy Psikhologii (RUS) *Online - full text edition.* **4454**
Vox Sanguinis (CHE) *Online - full text edition.* **3752**
W H O Technical Report Series (CHE) *Online - full text edition.* **3707**
W J M (USA) *Online - full text edition.* **3707**
West Indian Medical Journal (JAM) *Online - full text edition.* **3708**
Western Journal of Nursing Research (USA) *Online - full text edition.* **3943**
Wiener Klinische Wochenschrift (AUT) *Online - full text edition.* **3708**
Wiener Tieraerztliche Monatsschrift (AUT) *Online - full text edition.* **4559**
Wilderness and Environmental Medicine (USA) *Online - full text edition.* **3708**
Women & Health (USA) *Online - full text edition.* **4566**
Women & Therapy (USA) *Online - full text edition.* **4455**
Women's Health Issues (USA) *Online - full text edition.* **4567**
Work and Stress (GBR) *Online - full text edition.* **4455**
World Health Organization. Bulletin (CHE) *Online - full text edition.* **3709**
World Journal of Gastroenterology (CHN) *Online - full text edition.* **3897**
World Journal of Microbiology and Biotechnology (GBR) *Online - full text edition.* **3278**
World Journal of Surgery (USA) *Online - full text edition.* **4207**
World Journal of Urology (DEU) *Online - full text edition.* **4220**
Wound Repair and Regeneration (USA) *Online - full text edition.* **4028**
Wounds (USA) *Online - full text edition.* **4028**

Xenobiotica (GBR) *Online - full text edition.* **3264**
Xenotransplantation (DNK) *Online - full text edition.* **4207**
Yakugaku Zasshi (JPN) *Online - full text edition.* **4341**
Yakuri to Chiryo (JPN) *Online - full text edition.* **4341**
Yale Journal of Biology and Medicine (USA) *Online - full text edition.* **3709**
Yaowu Shipin Fenxi (TWN) *Online - full text edition.* **3463**
Yeast (GBR) *Online - full text edition.* **3283**
Yonsei Medical Journal (KOR) *Online - full text edition.* **3710**
Zeitschrift fuer Arbeits- und Organisationspsychologie (DEU) *Online - full text edition.* **4455**
Zeitschrift fuer Entwicklungspsychologie und Paedagogische Psychologie (DEU) *Online - full text edition.* **4456**
Zeitschrift fuer Experimentelle Psychologie (DEU) *Online - full text edition.* **4456**
Zeitschrift fuer Gastroenterologie (DEU) *Online - full text edition.* **3897**
Zeitschrift fuer Geburtshilfe und Neonatologie (DEU) *Online - full text edition.* **3965**
Zeitschrift fuer Gerontologie und Geriatrie (DEU) *Online - full text edition.* **3482**
Zeitschrift fuer Kardiologie (DEU) *Online - full text edition.* **3785**
Zeitschrift fuer Kinder- und Jugendpsychiatrie und Psychotherapie (CHE) *Online - full text edition.* **4138**
Zeitschrift fuer Klinische Psychologie, Psychopathologie und Psychotherapie (DEU) *Online - full text edition.* **4138**
Zeitschrift fuer Klinische Psychologie und Psychotherapie - Forschung und Praxis (DEU) *Online - full text edition.* **4456**
Zeitschrift fuer Naturforschung. Section C: A Journal of Biosciences (DEU) *Online - full text edition.* **3224**
Zeitschrift fuer Orthopaedie und Ihre Grenzgebiete (DEU) *Online - full text edition.* **4028**
Zeitschrift fuer Paedagogische Psychologie (CHE) *Online - full text edition.* **4456**
Zeitschrift fuer Psychologie (DEU) *Online - full text edition.* **4456**
Zeitschrift fuer Rheumatologie (DEU) *Online - full text edition.* **4172**
Zeitschrift fuer Sozialpsychologie (CHE) *Online - full text edition.* **4456**
Zentralblatt fuer Chirurgie (DEU) *Online - full text edition.* **4208**
Zentralblatt fuer Gynaekologie (DEU) *Online - full text edition.* **3965**
Zentralblatt fuer Neurochirurgie (DEU) *Online - full text edition.* **4138**
Zhongguo Yaoli Xuebao (CHN) *Online - full text edition.* **4342**
Zhongyang Yanjiuyuan Zhiwuxue Huikan (TWN) *Online - full text edition.* **3283**
Zhurnal Nevropatologii i Psikhiatrii im. S.S. Korsakova (RUS) *Online - full text edition.* **4139**
Zhurnal Obshchei Biologii (RUS) *Online - full text edition.* **3224**
Zhurnal Vysshei Nervnoi Deyatel'nosti (RUS) *Online - full text edition.* **3349**
Zoological Studies (TWN) *Online - full text edition.* **3357**
Zoology (DEU) *Online - full text edition.* **3357**
Zoomorphology (DEU) *Online - full text edition.* **3225**
Zygote (GBR) *Online - full text edition.* **3315**

JICST 5-3, Yonbancho, Chiyoda-Ku, Tokyo 102-0081, Japan TEL 81-3-5214-8413, FAX 81-3-5214-8410, overseas@mr.jst.go.jp, http://www.jst.go.jp
Brain and Nerve (JPN) *Online - full text edition.* **4077**
Current Bibliography on Science and Technology: Life Sciences (JPN) *Online - full text edition.* **3229**
Excerpta Medica. Abstract Journals (NLD) *Online - full text edition.* **3230**
Excerpta Medica. Section 1: Anatomy, Anthropology, Embryology & Histology (NLD) *Online - full text edition.* **3230**
Excerpta Medica. Section 10: Obstetrics and Gynecology (NLD) *Online - full text edition.* **3723**
Excerpta Medica. Section 11: Otorhinolaryngology (NLD) *Online - full text edition.* **3724**
Excerpta Medica. Section 12: Ophthalmology (NLD) *Online - full text edition.* **3724**
Excerpta Medica. Section 13: Dermatology and Venereology (NLD) *Online - full text edition.* **3724**
Excerpta Medica. Section 14: Radiology (NLD) *Online - full text edition.* **3724**
Excerpta Medica. Section 15: Chest Diseases, Thoracic Surgery and Tuberculosis (NLD) *Online - full text edition.* **3724**
Excerpta Medica. Section 16: Cancer (NLD) *Online - full text edition.* **3724**
Excerpta Medica. Section 17: Public Health, Social Medicine and Epidemiology (NLD) *Online - full text edition.* **4495**
Excerpta Medica. Section 18: Cardiovascular Diseases and Cardiovascular Surgery (NLD) *Online - full text edition.* **3724**
Excerpta Medica. Section 19: Rehabilitation and Physical Medicine (NLD) *Online - full text edition.* **3725**
Excerpta Medica. Section 2: Physiology (NLD) *Online - full text edition.* **3725**
Excerpta Medica. Section 20: Gerontology and Geriatrics (NLD) *Online - full text edition.* **3482**
Excerpta Medica. Section 21: Developmental Biology and Teratology (NLD) *Online - full text edition.* **3230**
Excerpta Medica. Section 22: Human Genetics (NLD) *Online - full text edition.* **3230**
Excerpta Medica. Section 23: Nuclear Medicine (NLD) *Online - full text edition.* **3725**
Excerpta Medica. Section 24: Anesthesiology (NLD) *Online - full text edition.* **3725**
Excerpta Medica. Section 25: Hematology (NLD) *Online - full text edition.* **3725**
Excerpta Medica. Section 26: Immunology, Serology and Transplantation (NLD) *Online - full text edition.* **3725**
Excerpta Medica. Section 27: Biophysics, Bio-Engineering and Medical Instrumentation (NLD) *Online - full text edition.* **3231**
Excerpta Medica. Section 28: Urology and Nephrology (NLD) *Online - full text edition.* **3726**
Excerpta Medica. Section 29: Clinical and Experimental Biochemistry (NLD) *Online - full text edition.* **3231**
Excerpta Medica. Section 3: Endocrinology (NLD) *Online - full text edition.* **3726**
Excerpta Medica. Section 30: Clinical and Experimental Pharmacology (NLD) *Online - full text edition.* **4344**
Excerpta Medica. Section 31: Arthritis and Rheumatism (NLD) *Online - full text edition.* **3726**
Excerpta Medica. Section 32: Psychiatry (NLD) *Online - full text edition.* **3726**
Excerpta Medica. Section 33: Orthopedic Surgery (NLD) *Online - full text edition.* **3726**
Excerpta Medica. Section 35: Occupational Health and Industrial Medicine (NLD) *Online - full text edition.* **3726**
Excerpta Medica. Section 36: Health Policy, Economics and Management (NLD) *Online - full text edition.* **3524**
Excerpta Medica. Section 38: Adverse Reactions Titles (NLD) *Online - full text edition.* **4344**
Excerpta Medica. Section 4: Microbiology: Bacteriology, Mycology, Parasitology and Virology (NLD) *Online - full text edition.* **3231**
Excerpta Medica. Section 40: Drug Dependence, Alcohol Abuse and Alcoholism (NLD) *Online - full text edition.* **3407**
Excerpta Medica. Section 46: Environmental Health and Pollution Control (NLD) *Online - full text edition.* **3443**
Excerpta Medica. Section 48: Gastroenterology (NLD) *Online - full text edition.* **3726**
Excerpta Medica. Section 49: Forensic Science Abstracts (NLD) *Online - full text edition.* **3727**
Excerpta Medica. Section 5: General Pathology and Pathological Anatomy (NLD) *Online - full text edition.* **3231**
Excerpta Medica. Section 52: Toxicology (NLD) *Online - full text edition.* **3443**
Excerpta Medica. Section 6: Internal Medicine (NLD) *Online - full text edition.* **3727**
Excerpta Medica. Section 7: Pediatrics and Pediatric Surgery (NLD) *Online - full text edition.* **3727**
Excerpta Medica. Section 8: Neurology and Neurosurgery (NLD) *Online - full text edition.* **3727**
Excerpta Medica. Section 9: Surgery (NLD) *Online - full text edition.* **3727**
I to Cho (JPN) *Online - full text edition.* **3892**
Industrial Health (JPN) *Online - full text edition.* **4256**
Japanese Journal of Clinical Oncology (GBR) *Online - full text edition.* **3981**
Japanese Journal of Ophthalmology (NLD) *Online - full text edition.* **4000**
Jibi Inkoka, Tokeibu Geka (JPN) *Online - full text edition.* **4034**
Kokyu to Junkan (JPN) *Online - full text edition.* **4161**
Neurological Surgery (JPN) *Online - full text edition.* **4197**
Nippon Medical School. Journal (JPN) *Online - full text edition.* **3668**
Rigaku Ryoho Janaru (JPN) *Online - full text edition.* **4066**
Rihabiriteshon Igaku (JPN) *Online - full text edition.* **4066**
Seishin Igaku (JPN) *Online - full text edition.* **4132**

JSTOR (Web-based Journal Archive) 120 Fifth Ave., 5th Fl., New York, NY 10011 TEL 212-229-3700, FAX 212-229-6841, clm@jstor.org, http://www.jstor.org
The American Naturalist (USA) *Online - full text edition.* **3180**
Biometrika (GBR) *Online - full text edition.* **3226**
Biotropica (USA) *Online - full text edition.* **3188**
Conservation Biology (USA) *Online - full text edition.* **3392**
Ecological Applications (USA) *Online - full text edition.* **3437**
Ecological Monographs (USA) *Online - full text edition.* **3437**
Ecology (USA) *Online - full text edition.* **3437**
Ergonomics Abstracts (GBR) *Online - full content edition.* **3433**
Evolution (USA) *Online - full text edition.* **3302**
Family Planning Perspectives (USA) *Online - full text edition.* **3949**
International Family Planning Perspectives (USA) *Online - full text edition.* **3953**
Journal of Animal Ecology (GBR) *Online - full text edition.* **3202**
Journal of Black Studies (USA) *Online - full text edition.* **4509**
Journal of Ecology (GBR) *Online - full text edition.* **3203**
Journal of Health and Social Behavior (USA) *Online - full text edition.* **4522**
Journal of Symbolic Logic (USA) *Online - full text edition.* **3553**
National Academy of Sciences of the United States of America. Proceedings (USA) *Online - full text edition.* **4505**
Quarterly Review of Biology (USA) *Online - full text edition.* **3214**
Royal Society of London. Philosophical Transactions. Biological Sciences (GBR) *Online - full text edition.* **3217**
Royal Society of London. Proceedings. Biological Sciences (GBR) *Online - full text edition.* **3217**
Social Psychology Quarterly (USA) *Online - full text edition.* **4523**
Studies in Family Planning (USA) *Online - full text edition.* **4369**

Kluwer Online Spuiboulevard 50, Dordrecht 3300 AA, Netherlands TEL 31-78-6392179, FAX 31-78-6392300, 101 Philip Dr., Assinippi Park, Norwell, MA 02061 TEL 781-871-6600, FAX 781-871-6528, Kluwer@wkap.com, http://www.wkap.nl/kaphtml.htm/KLUWERONLINE
Acta Biotheoretica (NLD) *Online - full text edition.* **3178**
Administration and Policy in Mental Health (USA) *Online - full text edition.* **3559**
Advances in Health Sciences Education (NLD) *Online - full text edition.* **3560**
AIDS & Behavior (USA) *Online - full text edition.* **3739**
American Journal of Community Psychology (USA) *Online - full text edition.* **4520**
American Journal of Dance Therapy (USA) *Online - full text edition.* **3396**
American Journal of Psychoanalysis (USA) *Online - full text edition.* **4374**
Angiogenesis (GBR) *Online - full text edition.* **3967**
Annals of Clinical Psychiatry (USA) *Online - full text edition.* **4073**
Annals of Oncology (NLD) *Online - full text edition.* **3967**
Antonie van Leeuwenhoek (NLD) *Online - full text edition.* **3268**
Apoptosis (GBR) *Online - full text edition.* **3225**
Apoptosis (USA) *Online - full text edition.* **3285**
Applied Biochemistry and Microbiology (RUS) *Online - full text edition.* **3241**
Applied Psychophysiology and Biofeedback (USA) *Online - full text edition.* **4378**
Aquatic Ecology (NLD) *Online - full text edition.* **3182**
Archives of Sexual Behavior (USA) *Online - full text edition.* **3568**
Behavior Genetics (USA) *Online - full text edition.* **3299**
Biochemical Genetics (USA) *Online - full text edition.* **3299**
Biochemistry (Moscow) (RUS) *Online - full text edition.* **3244**
Biodegradation (NLD) *Online - full text edition.* **3456**
Biogeochemistry (NLD) *Online - full text edition.* **3245**
Biogerontology (NLD) *Online - full text edition.* **3468**
Biomedical Engineering (NLD) *Online - full text edition.* **3576**
Biomedical Microdevices (USA) *Online - full text edition.* **3576**
Bioscience Reports (USA) *Online - full text edition.* **3286**
Biotechnology Letters (NLD) *Online - full text edition.* **3272**
Brain and Mind (USA) *Online - full text edition.* **4077**
Brain Topography (USA) *Online - full text edition.* **4078**
Breast Cancer Research and Treatment (USA) *Online - full text edition.* **3969**
Bulletin of Experimental Biology and Medicine (NLD) *Online - full text edition.* **3188**
Cancer and Metastasis Reviews (USA) *Online - full text edition.* **3969**
Cancer Causes & Control (NLD) *Online - full text edition.* **3970**
Cardiac Electrophysiology Review (USA) *Online - full text edition.* **3765**
Cardiovascular Drugs and Therapy (USA) *Online - full text edition.* **3766**
Cardiovascular Engineering (USA) *Online - full text edition.* **3766**
Cell and Tissue Banking (NLD) *Online - full text edition.* **3286**
Cell Biology and Toxicology (NLD) *Online - full text edition.* **3446**
Cellular & Molecular Neurobiology (USA) *Online - full text edition.* **4080**
Cellulose (NLD) *Online - full text edition.* **3378**
Child and Adolescent Social Work Journal (USA) *Online - full text edition.* **4520**
Child and Youth Care Forum (USA) *Online - full text edition.* **3381**
Child Psychiatry and Human Development (USA) *Online - full text edition.* **4081**
Clinical and Experimental Metastasis (NLD) *Online - full text edition.* **3974**
Clinical Child and Family Psychology Review (USA) *Online - full text edition.* **4387**
Cognitive Therapy and Research (USA) *Online - full text edition.* **4390**
Community Mental Health Journal (USA) *Online - full text edition.* **4512**
Conservation Genetics (NLD) *Online - full text edition.* **3300**
Contemporary Family Therapy (USA) *Online - full text edition.* **4391**
Culture, Medicine and Psychiatry (NLD) *Online - full text edition.* **3173**
Cytotechnology (NLD) *Online - full text edition.* **3289**
Digestive Diseases and Sciences (USA) *Online - full text edition.* **3888**
Documenta Ophthalmologica (NLD) *Online - full text edition.* **3997**
Dreaming (USA) *Online - full text edition.* **3342**
Early Childhood Education Journal (USA) *Online - full text edition.* **3410**
Ecotoxicology (USA) *Online - full text edition.* **3448**
Educational Psychology Review (USA) *Online - full text edition.* **3411**
European Journal of Epidemiology (NLD) *Online - full text edition.* **3599**
European Journal of Health Law (NLD) *Online - full text edition.* **3600**
Experimental & Applied Acarology (NLD) *Online - full text edition.* **3352**
Familial Cancer (NLD) *Online - full text edition.* **3978**
Gay and Lesbian Medical Association. Journal (USA) *Online - full text edition.* **3605**

Genetic Resources and Crop Evolution (NLD) *Online - full text edition.* **3304**
Genetica (NLD) *Online - full text edition.* **3305**
Global Change & Human Health (NLD) *Online - full text edition.* **4470**
Glycoconjugate Journal (USA) *Online - full text edition.* **3251**
Group (New York) (USA) *Online - full text edition.* **4401**
H E C Forum (NLD) *Online - full text edition.* **3508**
Health Care Analysis (NLD) *Online - full text edition.* **3610**
Health Care Management Science (NLD) *Online - full text edition.* **3509**
Health Services and Outcomes Research Methodology (USA) *Online - full text edition.* **3612**
Heart Failure Reviews (USA) *Online - full text edition.* **3773**
The Histochemical Journal (NLD) *Online - full text edition.* **3290**
Human Physiology (RUS) *Online - full text edition.* **3616**
Human Relations (USA) *Online - full text edition.* **4509**
Hydrobiologia (NLD) *Online - full text edition.* **3199**
Inflammation (USA) *Online - full text edition.* **3620**
International Journal of Group Tensions (USA) *Online - full text edition.* **4406**
International Journal of Health Care Finance and Economics (USA) *Online - full text edition.* **4477**
International Journal of Rehabilitation and Health (USA) *Online - full text edition.* **3485**
International Journal of Sexuality and Gender Studies (USA) *Online - full text edition.* **3527**
International Journal of Stress Management (USA) *Online - full text edition.* **3624**
International Ophthalmology (NLD) *Online - full text edition.* **3999**
International Urology and Nephrology (HUN) *Online - full text edition.* **4214**
Investigational New Drugs (USA) *Online - full text edition.* **4304**
Journal of Abnormal Child Psychology (USA) *Online - full text edition.* **4409**
Journal of Adult Development (USA) *Online - full text edition.* **4409**
Journal of Aging & Identity (USA) *Online - full text edition.* **3475**
Journal of Applied Psychoanalytic Studies (USA) *Online - full text edition.* **4410**
Journal of Assisted Reproduction and Genetics (USA) *Online - full text edition.* **3955**
Journal of Autism and Developmental Disorders (USA) *Online - full text edition.* **3423**
Journal of Behavioral Education (USA) *Online - full text edition.* **3412**
Journal of Behavioral Medicine (USA) *Online - full text edition.* **4099**
Journal of Bioenergetics and Biomembranes (USA) *Online - full text edition.* **3253**
Journal of Business & Psychology (USA) *Online - full text edition.* **4411**
Journal of Child and Family Studies (USA) *Online - full text edition.* **4411**
Journal of Clinical Geropsychology (USA) *Online - full text edition.* **3475**
Journal of Clinical Immunology (USA) *Online - full text edition.* **3748**
Journal of Clinical Monitoring and Computing (NLD) *Online - full text edition.* **3631**
Journal of Clinical Psychology in Medical Settings (USA) *Online - full text edition.* **4412**
Journal of Community Health (USA) *Online - full text edition.* **3631**
Journal of Computational Neuroscience (NLD) *Online - full text edition.* **4100**
Journal of Contemporary Psychotherapy (USA) *Online - full text edition.* **4413**
Journal of Cross-Cultural Gerontology (NLD) *Online - full text edition.* **3475**
Journal of Developmental and Physical Disabilities (USA) *Online - full text edition.* **3485**
Journal of Evolutionary Biochemistry and Physiology (RUS) *Online - full text edition.* **3254**
Journal of Family and Economic Issues (USA) *Online - full text edition.* **4416**
Journal of Family Violence (USA) *Online - full text edition.* **3395**
Journal of Gambling Studies (USA) *Online - full text edition.* **4101**
Journal of Genetic Counseling (USA) *Online - full text edition.* **4416**
Journal of Happiness Studies (NLD) *Online - full text edition.* **4417**
Journal of Immigrant Health (USA) *Online - full text edition.* **3634**
Journal of Inherited Metabolic Disease (NLD) *Online - full text edition.* **4046**
Journal of Interventional Cardiac Electrophysiology (NLD) *Online - full text edition.* **3778**
Journal of Mammalian Evolution (USA) *Online - full text edition.* **3354**
Journal of Mammary Gland Biology and Neoplasia (USA) *Online - full text edition.* **3345**
Journal of Materials Science: Materials in Medicine (USA) *Online - full text edition.* **3434**
Journal of Medical Humanities (USA) *Online - full text edition.* **3635**
Journal of Medical Systems (USA) *Online - full text edition.* **3812**
Journal of Muscle Research and Cell Motility (NLD) *Online - full text edition.* **4018**
Journal of Near-Death Studies (USA) *Online - full text edition.* **4347**
Journal of Neuro-Oncology (USA) *Online - full text edition.* **3982**
Journal of Neurocytology (USA) *Online - full text edition.* **3291**
Journal of Nonverbal Behavior (USA) *Online - full text edition.* **4418**
Journal of Occupational Rehabilitation (USA) *Online - full text edition.* **4258**
Journal of Pharmacokinetics and Pharmacodynamics (USA) *Online - full text edition.* **4310**
Journal of Poetry Therapy (USA) *Online - full text edition.* **3553**
The Journal of Primary Prevention (USA) *Online - full text edition.* **4420**
Journal of Protein Chemistry (USA) *Online - full text edition.* **3255**
Journal of Psycholinguistic Research (USA) *Online - full text edition.* **3551**
Journal of Psychology and Judaism (USA) *Online - full text edition.* **4501**
Journal of Psychopathology and Behavioral Assessment (USA) *Online - full text edition.* **4421**
Journal of Radiosurgery (USA) *Online - full text edition.* **4194**
Journal of Rational - Emotive and Cognitive - Behavior Therapy (USA) *Online - full text edition.* **4421**
Journal of Religion and Health (USA) *Online - full text edition.* **4500**
Journal of Risk and Uncertainty (USA) *Online - full text edition.* **3363**
Journal of Social Distress and the Homeless (USA) *Online - full text edition.* **4515**
Journal of the History of Biology (NLD) *Online - full text edition.* **3205**
Journal of Thrombosis and Thrombolysis (USA) *Online - full text edition.* **3779**
Journal of Traumatic Stress (USA) *Online - full text edition.* **4424**
Journal of Youth and Adolescence (USA) *Online - full text edition.* **3384**
Law and Human Behavior (USA) *Online - full text edition.* **3541**
Maternal and Child Health Journal (USA) *Online - full text edition.* **3957**
Medicine, Health Care and Philosophy (NLD) *Online - full text edition.* **3656**
Mental Health Services Research (USA) *Online - full text edition.* **4427**
Metabolic Brain Disease (USA) *Online - full text edition.* **3660**
Methods in Cell Science (NLD) *Online - full text edition.* **3292**
Microbiology (GBR) *Online - full text edition.* **3327**
Microbiology (RUS) *Online - full text edition.* **3327**
Mitigation and Adaptation Strategies for Global Change (NLD) *Online - full text edition.* **3441**
Molecular and Cellular Biochemistry (USA) *Online - full text edition.* **3257**
Molecular Biology (RUS) *Online - full text edition.* **3257**
Molecular Biology Reports (NLD) *Online - full text edition.* **3257**
Motivation and Emotion (USA) *Online - full text edition.* **4428**
Mycopathologia (NLD) *Online - full text edition.* **3281**
Neural Processing Letters (USA) *Online - full text edition.* **3390**
Neurochemical Research (USA) *Online - full text edition.* **4113**
Neurophysiology (USA) *Online - full text edition.* **4116**
Neurophysiology (GBR) *Online - full text edition.* **3233**
Neuropsychology Review (USA) *Online - full text edition.* **4117**
Neuroscience and Behavioral Physiology (USA) *Online - full text edition.* **4118**
Nonlinear Dynamics, Psychology, and Life Sciences (USA) *Online - full text edition.* **4430**
Origins of Life and Evolution of the Biosphere (NLD) *Online - full text edition.* **3212**
Pastoral Psychology (USA) *Online - full text edition.* **4431**
Pharmaceutical Chemistry Journal (USA) *Online - full text edition.* **4323**
Photosynthesis Research (NLD) *Online - full text edition.* **3260**
Pituitary (NLD) *Online - full text edition.* **3867**
Plant Cell, Tissue and Organ Culture (NLD) *Online - full text edition.* **3293**
Plant Foods for Human Nutrition (NLD) *Online - full text edition.* **4244**
Plant Molecular Biology (NLD) *Online - full text edition.* **3213**
Population and Environment (USA) *Online - full text edition.* **4433**
Prevention Science (USA) *Online - full text edition.* **3805**
Psychiatric Quarterly (USA) *Online - full text edition.* **4126**
Quality of Life Research (NLD) *Online - full text edition.* **3682**
Reading and Writing (NLD) *Online - full text edition.* **3551**
Reviews in Endocrine & Metabolic Disorders (USA) *Online - full text edition.* **3868**
Russian Journal of Bioorganic Chemistry (RUS) *Online - full text edition.* **3379**
Russian Journal of Developmental Biology (RUS) *Online - full text edition.* **3217**
Russian Journal of Genetics (RUS) *Online - full text edition.* **3314**
Russian Journal of Marine Biology (RUS) *Online - full text edition.* **3217**
Sepsis (USA) *Online - full text edition.* **3807**
Sex Roles (USA) *Online - full text edition.* **4448**
Sexual Abuse (USA) *Online - full text edition.* **4448**
Sexuality and Disability (USA) *Online - full text edition.* **3692**
Social Psychology of Education (NLD) *Online - full text edition.* **3415**
Somatic Cell and Molecular Genetics (USA) *Online - full text edition.* **3314**
Spatial Cognition and Computation (NLD) *Online - full text edition.* **4450**
Substance Abuse (USA) *Online - full text edition.* **3406**
Systematic Parasitology (NLD) *Online - full text edition.* **3220**
Theoretical Medicine and Bioethics (NLD) *Online - full text edition.* **3699**
Topoi (NLD) *Online - full text edition.* **4348**
Transgenic Research (NLD) *Online - full text edition.* **3314**
Tropical Animal Health and Production (NLD) *Online - full text edition.* **4554**
Veterinary Research Communications (NLD) *Online - full text edition.* **4559**
Virus Genes (USA) *Online - full text edition.* **3332**
World Journal of Microbiology and Biotechnology (GBR) *Online - full text edition.* **3278**

LexisNexis (Subsidiary of: LEXIS Publishing) 9443 Springboro Pike, Miamisburg, OH 45342 TEL 937-865-6800, 800-227-4908, 800-544-7390, FAX 937-865-1666, 800-227-9597 http://www.lexisnexis.com
Accreditation Manual for Hospitals. Vol. 1: Standards (USA) *Online - full text edition.* **3501**
AIDS Litigation Reporter (USA) *Online - full text edition. (AIDS Litigation Reporter)* **3536**
American Family Physician (USA) *Online - full text edition. (American Family Physician)* **3563**
American Journal of Law & Medicine (USA) *Online - full text edition. (American Journal of Law and Medicine)* **3536**
American Journal of Psychiatry (USA) *Online - full text edition. (American Journal of Psychiatry)* **4071**
Annals of Health Law (USA) *Online - full text edition. (Annals of Health Law)* **3536**
Antiviral Weekly (USA) *Online - full text edition. (Antiviral Weekly)* **3740**
Applied Genetics News (USA) *Online - full text edition. (Applied Genetics News)* **3299**
B N A's Health Care Fraud Report (USA) *Online - full text edition.* **3502**
Behavioral Medicine (USA) *Online - full text edition. (Behavioral Medicine)* **4381**
Biotech Business (USA) *Online - full text edition. (Biotech Business)* **3270**
The Birthkit (USA) *Online - full text edition. (Birthkit)* **3946**
Breast Implant Litigation Reporter (USA) *Online - full text edition. (Breast Implant Litigation Reporter)* **3537**
Cal - O S H A Reporter (USA) *Online - full text edition. (Cal-OSHA Reporter)* **4252**
Canadian Association of Radiologists Journal (CAN) *Online - full text edition. (Canadian Association of Radiologists' Journal)* **4141**
Canadian Government Programs and Services (CAN) *Online - full text edition. (Canadian Government Programs & Services Newsletter)* **4458**
Canadian Journal of Behavioural Science (CAN) *Online - full text edition. (Canadian Journal of Behavioural Science)* **4385**
Canadian Journal of Experimental Psychology (CAN) *Online - full text edition. (Canadian Journal of Experimental Psychology)* **4386**
Canadian Journal of Human Sexuality (CAN) *Online - full text edition. (Canadian Journal of Human Sexuality)* **4386**
Canadian Journal of Microbiology (CAN) *Online - full text edition. (Canadian Journal of Microbiology)* **3319**
Canadian Journal of Respiratory Therapy (CAN) *Online - full text edition. (Canadian Journal of Respiratory Therapy)* **4158**
The Canadian Journal of Rural Medicine (CAN) *Online - full text edition. (Canadian Journal of Rural Medicine)* **3582**
Canadian Journal of Surgery (CAN) *Online - full text edition. (Canadian Journal of Surgery)* **4183**
Canadian Pharmaceutical Journal (CAN) *Online - full text edition. (Canadian Pharmaceutical Journal)* **4282**
Clinical and Investigative Medicine (CAN) *Online - full text edition. (Clinical & Investigative Medicine)* **3586**
Clinical Pediatrics (USA) *Online - full text edition. (Clinical Pediatrics)* **4042**
Community Pharmacy (GBR) *Online - full text edition. (Community Pharmacy)* **4284**
Consumer Reports on Health (USA) *Online - full text edition. (Consumer Reports On Health)* **4351**
Disability Compliance Bulletin (USA) *Online - full text edition.* **3484**
Diseases of the Colon and Rectum (USA) *Online - full text edition. (Diseases of the Colon & Rectum)* **4187**
Electromagnetic Field Litigation Reporter (USA) *Online - full text edition. (Electromagnetic Field Litigation Reporter)* **3430**
Environmental Compliance & Litigation Strategy (USA) *Online - full text edition. (Environmental Compliance and Litigation Strategy)* **3538**
Environmental Laboratory Washington Report (USA) *Online - full text edition. (Environmental Laboratory Washington Report)* **3874**
The Expert and the Law (USA) *Online - full text edition. (Expert and the Law, The)* **3538**
Family Health (CAN) *Online - full text edition. (Family Health)* **4469**
Family Planning Perspectives (USA) *Online - full text edition. (Family Planning Perspectives)* **3949**
Far East Focus (GBR) *Online - full text edition. (Far East Focus)* **4294**
Food and Drug Law Journal (USA) *Online - full text edition. (Food and Drug Law Journal)* **3539**
Formulary (USA) *Online - full text edition. (Formulary)* **4297**
Genome (CAN) *Online - full text edition. (Genome)* **3306**
The Guttmacher Report on Public Policy (USA) *Online - full text edition. (Guttmacher Report on Public Policy, The)* **3358**
Health Affairs (USA) *Online - full text edition. (Health Affairs)* **4471**

Health Data Management (New York) (USA) *Online - full text edition. (Health Data Management)* **3509**
Health Facilities Management (USA) *Online - full text edition. (Health Facilities Management)* **3509**
Health Law Journal (CAN) *Online - full text edition. (Health Law Journal)* **3539**
Health Law Litigation Reporter (USA) *Online - full text edition. (Health Law Litigation Reporter)* **3545**
Health Management Technology (USA) *Online - full text edition. (Health Management Technology)* **3810**
Health Matrix: Journal of Law-Medicine (USA) *Online - full text edition. (Health Matrix)* **3540**
Health Products Business (USA) *Online - full text edition. (Health Foods Business)* **3461**
Hospital Topics (USA) *Online - full text edition. (Hospital Topics)* **3514**
International Family Planning Perspectives (USA) *Online - full text edition. (International Family Planning Perspectives)* **3953**
Issues in Law and Medicine (USA) *Online - full text edition. (Issues in Law & Medicine)* **3626**
The Journal of Addiction and Mental Health (CAN) *Online - full text edition. (Journal of Addiction & Mental Health)* **3402**
Journal of American College Health (USA) *Online - full text edition. (Journal of American College Health)* **4357**
Journal of Contemporary Health Law and Policy (USA) *Online - full text edition. (Journal of Contemporary Health Law and Policy)* **3632**
Journal of Health Law (USA) *Online - full text edition. (Journal of Health Law)* **3633**
Journal of Law and Health (USA) *Online - full text edition. (Journal of Law and Health)* **3540**
The Journal of Legal Medicine (USA) *Online - full text edition. (Journal of Legal Medicine, The)* **3634**
Journal of Lesbian Studies (USA) *Online - full text edition. (Journal of Lesbian Studies)* **3528**
The Journal of Social Psychology (USA) *Online - full text edition. (Journal of Social Psychology)* **4423**
Journal of Women and Aging (USA) *Online - full text edition. (Journal of Women & Aging)* **4569**
Law and Psychology Review (USA) *Online - full text edition. (Law and Psychology Review)* **3541**
Marketing Health Services (USA) *Online - full text edition. (Marketing Health Services)* **3367**
Materials Management in Health Care (USA) *Online - full text edition. (Materials Management in Health Care)* **3518**
McGraw-Hill's Biotechnology Newswatch (USA) *Online - full text edition. (Biotechnology Newswatch)* **3276**
Mealey's Litigation Report: Breast Implants (USA) *Online - full text edition. (MEALEY)* **3545**
Mealey's Litigation Report: Drugs and Medical Devices (USA) *Online - full text edition. (Mealey's Litigation Report: Norplant)* **3546**
Mealey's Litigation Report: Fen-Phen - Redux (USA) *Online - full text edition. (Mealey's Litigation Report: Fen-Phen/Redux)* **4315**
Mealey's Managed Care Liability Report (USA) *Online - full text edition.* **3541**
Medical and Healthcare Marketplace Guide (USA) *Online - full text edition. (Medical & Healthcare Marketplace Guide)* **3371**
Medical Device Technology (GBR) *Online - full text edition. (Medical Device Technology)* **3649**
Medical Devices, Diagnostics & Instrumentation Reports: The Gray Sheet (USA) *Online - full text edition. (Gray Sheet - Medical Devices and Diagnostics, The)* **3649**
Medical Malpractice Law & Strategy (USA) *Online - full text edition. (Medical Malpractice Law & Strategy)* **3545**
Medical Materials Update (USA) *Online - full text edition. (Medical Materials Update)* **3652**
The Medical Post (CAN) *Online - full text edition. (Medical Post)* **3652**
Medicare & Medicaid Law Bulletin (USA) *Online - full text edition. (Medicare and Medicaid Law Bulletin)* **3533**
Midwifery Today with International Midwife (USA) *Online - full text edition. (Midwifery Today)* **3958**
Modern Healthcare (Year) (USA) *Online - full text edition. (Modern Healthcare)* **3519**
Morbidity and Mortality Weekly Report (USA) *Online - full text edition. (Morbidity and Mortality Weekly Report)* **4482**
National Cancer Institute. Journal (USA) *Online - full text edition. (Journal of the National Cancer Institute)* **3985**
National Women's Health Report (USA) *Online - full text edition. (National Women's Health Report)* **4565**
Network (Durham) (USA) *Online - full text edition. (Network - Durham)* **3359**
New York Health Law Update (USA) *Online - full text edition. (New York Health Law Update)* **4483**
Notre Dame Journal of Law, Ethics & Public Policy (USA) *Online - full text edition. (Notre Dame Journal of Law, Ethics & Public Policy)* **4459**
On the Issues (USA) *Online - full text edition. (On the Issues)* **4568**
Pediatrics (English Edition) (USA) *Online - full text edition. (Pediatrics)* **4054**
Pharma Japan (JPN) *Online - full text edition. (Pharma Japan)* **4322**
Pharmaceutical Approvals Monthly (USA) *Online - full text edition. (Pharmaceutical Approval Monthly)* **4323**
Pharmaceutical Business News (GBR) *Online - full text edition. (Pharmaceutical Business News)* **4323**
Pharmaceutical Litigation Reporter (USA) *Online - full text edition. (Pharmaceutical Litigation Reporter)* **3546**
Pharmacy Today (GBR) *Online - full text edition. (Pharmacy Today)* **4329**
The Physician and Sportsmedicine (USA) *Online - full text edition. (Physician and Sportsmedicine)* **4176**
Postgraduate Medicine (USA) *Online - full text edition. (Post Graduate Medicine)* **3678**
Psychology, Public Policy, and Law (USA) *Online - full text edition. (Psychology, Public Policy, and Law)* **4441**
Public Health Reports (USA) *Online - full text edition. (Public Health Reports)* **4486**
Pulse (GBR) *Online - full text edition. (Pulse)* **3681**
Quality Control Reports: The Gold Sheet (USA) *Online - full text edition. (Gold Sheet, The)* **4332**
Radiance Online(USA) *Online - full text. (Radiance-The Magazine for Large Women)* **4568**
Repetitive Stress Injury Litigation Reporter (USA) *Online - full text edition. (Repetitive Stress Injury Litigation Reporter)* **3543**
Shepard's O S H A Citations (USA) *Online - full text edition.* **3547**
Women & Health (USA) *Online - full text edition. (Women's Health Journal)* **4566**
Women & Therapy (USA) *Online - full text edition. (Women & Therapy)* **4455**
Workplace Substance Abuse Advisor (USA) *Online - full text edition. (National Report on Substance Abuse)* **3406**

Munksgaard & Blackwell Science's Synergy
35 Noerre Soegade, Box 2148, Copenhagen K, Denmark TEL 45-77-333333, FAX 45-77-333377, http://www.munksgaard-synergy.com

A N Z Journal of Surgery (AUS) *Online - full text edition.* **4178**
Acta Anaesthesiologica Scandinavica (DNK) *Online - full text edition.* **3753**
Acta Chirurgica Austriaca Online(AUT) *Online - full text.* **4178**
Acta Medica Austriaca Online(AUT) *Online - full text.* **3557**
Acta Neurologica Scandinavica (DNK) *Online - full text edition.* **4068**
Acta Obstetrica et Gynecologica Scandinavica (DNK) *Online - full text edition.* **3944**
Acta Ophthamologica Scandinavica Online(DNK) *Online - full text.* **3993**
Acta Physiologica Scandinavica (GBR) *Online - full text edition.* **3337**
Acta Psychiatrica Scandinavica (DNK) *Online - full text edition.* **4068**
Acta Radiologica (DNK) *Online - full text edition.* **4139**
Acta Zoologica Online(GBR) *Online - full text.* **3350**
Alimentary Pharmacology and Therapeutics (GBR) *Online - full text edition.* **3886**
Allergology International (AUS) *Online - full text edition.* **3739**
Allergy (DNK) *Online - full text edition.* **3739**
Ambulatory Child Health Online(GBR) *Online - full text.* **4040**
American Journal of Transplantation Online(DNK) *Online - full text.* **4180**
Anaesthesia (Oxford) (GBR) *Online - full text edition.* **3754**
Anatomia, Histologia, Embryologia Online(DEU) *Online - full text.* **4537**
Andrologia (DEU) *Online - full text edition.* **3565**
Animal Genetics (GBR) *Online - full text edition.* **3298**
Artificial Organs (USA) *Online - full text edition.* **3871**
Asia Pacific Journal of Clinical Nutrition (AUS) *Online - full text edition.* **4229**
Austral Ecology (AUS) *Online - full text edition.* **3183**
Australasian Journal of Dermatology (AUS) *Online - full text edition.* **3845**
Australasian Psychiatry (AUS) *Online - full text edition.* **4075**
Australasian Radiology (AUS) *Online - full text edition.* **4140**
Australian and New Zealand Journal of Mental Health Nursing (AUS) *Online - full text edition.* **4075**
Australian & New Zealand Journal of Psychiatry (AUS) *Online - full text edition.* **4075**
Australian Journal of Rural Health (AUS) *Online - full text edition.* **4463**
Australian Occupational Therapy Journal (AUS) *Online - full text edition.* **4059**
Autonomic & Autacoid Pharmacology (GBR) *Online - full text edition.* **4279**
B J U International (GBR) *Online - full text edition.* **4210**
Bipolar Disorders Online(DNK) *Online - full text.* **4077**
Birth (USA) *Online - full text edition.* **3946**
The Breast Journal Online(USA) *Online - full text.* **3946**
British Journal of Clinical Pharmacology (GBR) *Online - full text edition.* **4281**
British Journal of Dermatology (GBR) *Online - full text edition.* **3845**
British Journal of Haematology (GBR) *Online - full text edition.* **3899**
British Journal of Learning Disabilities (GBR) *Online - full text edition.* **4079**
British Journal of Surgery (GBR) *Online - full text edition.* **4183**
Cancer Practice Online(USA) *Online - full text.* **3972**
Cell Proliferation (GBR) *Online - full text edition.* **3287**
Cephalalgia (GBR) *Online - full text edition.* **4080**
Child: Care, Health and Development (GBR) *Online - full text edition.* **4042**
Chinese Journal of Digestive Diseases Online(AUS) *Online - full text.* **3887**
Clinical and Experimental Allergy (GBR) *Online - full text edition.* **3742**
Clinical and Experimental Dermatology (GBR) *Online - full text edition.* **3846**
Clinical and Experimental Immunology (GBR) *Online - full text edition.* **3742**
Clinical and Experimental Ophthalmology (AUS) *Online - full text edition.* **3995**
Clinical and Experimental Pharmacology & Physiology (AUS) *Online - full text edition.* **3341**
Clinical and Laboratory Haematology (GBR) *Online - full text edition.* **3899**
Clinical Endocrinology (GBR) *Online - full text edition.* **3856**
Clinical Genetics (DNK) *Online - full text edition.* **3300**
Clinical Microbiology and Infection (GBR) *Online - full text edition.* **3586**
Clinical Oral Implants Research (DNK) *Online - full text edition.* **3818**
Clinical Otolaryngology and Allied Sciences (GBR) *Online - full text edition.* **4031**
Clinical Physiology and Functional Imaging (GBR) *Online - full text edition.* **3587**
Clinical Transplantation (DNK) *Online - full text edition.* **4185**
College of Surgeons Hong Kong. Annals (AUS) *Online - full text edition.* **4185**
Colorectal Disease Online(GBR) *Online - full text.* **3887**
Conservation Biology (USA) *Online - full text edition.* **3392**
Contact Dermatitis (DNK) *Online - full text edition.* **3846**
Cytopathology (GBR) *Online - full text edition.* **3289**
Dental Traumatology Online(DNK) *Online - full text.* **3821**
Dermatologic Surgery Online(USA) *Online - full text.* **4187**
Dermatologic Therapy (DNK) *Online - full text edition.* **3847**
Development, Growth and Differentiation (AUS) *Online - full text edition.* **3192**
Diabetes, Obesity and Metabolism Online(GBR) *Online - full text.* **3858**
Diabetic Medicine Online(GBR) *Online - full text.* **3860**
Differentiation (DEU) *Online - full text edition.* **3193**
Digestive Endoscopy Online(AUS) *Online - full text.* **3889**
Diseases of the Esophagus Online(AUS) *Online - full text.* **4032**
Emergency Medicine (Carleton South) (AUS) *Online - full text edition.* **4013**
Environmental Microbiology (GBR) *Online - full text edition.* **3321**
Ethology Online(DEU) *Online - full text.* **3352**
European Academy of Dermatology and Venereology. Journal (BEL) *Online - full text edition.* **3848**
European Journal of Anaesthesiology (GBR) *Online - full text edition.* **3757**
European Journal of Biochemistry (GBR) *Online - full text edition.* **3249**
European Journal of Cancer Care Online(GBR) *Online - full text.* **3977**
European Journal of Clinical Investigation (GBR) *Online - full text edition.* **3599**
European Journal of Haematology (DNK) *Online - full text edition.* **3900**
European Journal of Immunogenetics (GBR) *Online - full text edition.* **3302**
European Journal of Neurology (USA) *Online - full text edition.* **4089**
European Journal of Neuroscience (GBR) *Online - full text edition.* **4089**
The European Respiratory Journal (CHE) *Online - full text edition.* **4159**
Evolution & Development Online(USA) *Online - full text.* **3195**
Experimental Dermatology Online(DNK) *Online - full text.* **3849**
Foot and Ankle Surgery (GBR) *Online - full text edition.* **4189**
Freshwater Biology Online(GBR) *Online - full text.* **3197**
Genes to Cells (GBR) *Online - full text edition.* **3303**
Genescreen (GBR) *Online - full text edition.* **3304**
Gynaecological Endoscopy (GBR) *Online - full text edition.* **3951**
H I V Medicine (GBR) *Online - full text edition.* **3796**
Haemophilia Online(GBR) *Online - full text.* **3901**
Headache Online(USA) *Online - full text.* **4093**
Health and Social Care in the Community Online(GBR) *Online - full text.* **4472**
Health Expectations (GBR) *Online - full text edition.* **4473**
Health Information and Libraries Journal Online(GBR) *Online - full text.* **3547**
Heart, Lung & Circulation Online(AUS) *Online - full text.* **3773**
Helicobacter (USA) *Online - full text edition.* **3323**
Heredity (GBR) *Online - full text edition.* **3307**
Histopathology (GBR) *Online - full text edition.* **3979**
Immunology (GBR) *Online - full text edition.* **3746**
Immunology and Cell Biology (AUS) *Online - full text edition.* **3746**
International Endodontic Journal Online(GBR) *Online - full text.* **3826**
International Journal of Andrology (GBR) *Online - full text edition.* **4213**
International Journal of Cosmetic Science (GBR) *Online - full text edition.* **3176**
International Journal of Dermatology (GBR) *Online - full text edition.* **3850**
International Journal of Experimental Pathology (GBR) *Online - full text edition.* **3623**
International Journal of Gynecological Cancer (USA) *Online - full text edition.* **3953**
International Journal of Nursing Practice (AUS) *Online - full text edition.* **3921**
International Journal of Oral & Maxillofacial Surgery (DNK) *Online - full text edition.* **3827**
International Journal of Paediatric Dentistry Online(GBR) *Online - full text.* **3827**

International Journal of Urology (AUS) *Online - full text edition.* **4213**
International Nursing Review Online(GBR) *Online - full text.* **3922**
Journal of Advanced Nursing (GBR) *Online - full text edition.* **3923**
Journal of Animal Ecology (GBR) *Online - full text edition.* **3202**
Journal of Animal Physiology and Animal Nutrition Online(DEU) *Online - full text.* **3344**
Journal of Applied Microbiology (GBR) *Online - full text edition.* **3324**
Journal of Applied Research in Intellectual Disabilities (GBR) *Online - full text edition.* **4098**
Journal of Clinical Nursing (GBR) *Online - full text edition.* **3923**
Journal of Clinical Periodontology (DNK) *Online - full text edition.* **3828**
Journal of Clinical Pharmacy and Therapeutics (GBR) *Online - full text edition.* **4306**
Journal of Cutaneous Pathology (DNK) *Online - full text edition.* **3850**
Journal of Ecology (GBR) *Online - full text edition.* **3203**
Journal of Evaluation in Clinical Practice Online(GBR) *Online - full text.* **3632**
Journal of Evolutionary Biology (GBR) *Online - full text edition.* **3309**
Journal of Gastroenterology and Hepatology (AUS) *Online - full text edition.* **3893**
Journal of General Internal Medicine (USA) *Online - full text edition.* **3910**
Journal of Human Nutrition and Dietetics (GBR) *Online - full text edition.* **4237**
Journal of Intellectual Disability Research (GBR) *Online - full text edition.* **4102**
Journal of Intensive Care Medicine (USA) *Online - full text edition.* **3634**
Journal of Internal Medicine (GBR) *Online - full text edition.* **3910**
The Journal of Investigative Dermatology (USA) *Online - full text edition.* **3851**
Journal of Lower Genital Tract Disease Online(USA) *Online - full text.* **3956**
Journal of Microscopy (GBR) *Online - full text edition.* **3334**
Journal of Neurochemistry (USA) *Online - full text edition.* **3255**
Journal of Neuroendocrinology Online(GBR) *Online - full text.* **4103**
Journal of Nursing Management (GBR) *Online - full text edition.* **3925**
Journal of Oral Rehabilitation Online(GBR) *Online - full text.* **3829**
Journal of Paediatrics and Child Health (AUS) *Online - full text edition.* **4047**
Journal of Peptide Research (DNK) *Online - full text edition.* **3255**
Journal of Psychiatric & Mental Health Nursing Online(GBR) *Online - full text.* **4105**
Journal of Quality in Clinical Practice (AUS) *Online - full text edition.* **3637**
Journal of Sleep Research Online(GBR) *Online - full text.* **3638**
Journal of the Peripheral Nervous System Online(USA) *Online - full text.* **4107**
Journal of Veterinary Medicine. Series A Online(DEU) *Online - full text.* **4547**
Journal of Veterinary Medicine. Series B Online(DEU) *Online - full text.* **4547**
Journal of Veterinary Pharmacology and Therapeutics Online(GBR) *Online - full text.* **4311**
Journal of Viral Hepatitis (GBR) *Online - full text edition.* **3893**
Journal of Zoological Systematics and Evolutionary Research Online(DEU) *Online - full text.* **3355**
Kidney International Online (USA) *Online - full text edition of* Kidney International. **4215**
Liver (DNK) *Online - full text edition.* **3894**
Marine Ecology Online(DEU) *Online - full text.* **3207**
Medical & Veterinary Entomology Online(GBR) *Online - full text.* **3648**
Medical Education (GBR) *Online - full text edition.* **3650**
Medical Mycology (GBR) *Online - full text edition.* **3803**
Molecular Microbiology Online (GBR) *Online - full text edition of* Molecular Microbiology. **3329**
Molecular Plant Pathology (GBR) *Online - full text edition.* **3281**
Mycoses (DEU) *Online - full text edition.* **3663**
Nephrology Online (AUS) *Online - full text edition of* Nephrology. **4216**
Neurogastroenterology and Motility Online(GBR) *Online - full text.* **3894**
Neuromodulation Online(USA) *Online - full text.* **4115**
Neuropathology (AUS) *Online - full text edition.* **4116**
Neuropathology & Applied Neurobiology Online (GBR) *Online - full text edition of* Neuropathology and Applied Neurobiology. **4116**
Nursing and Health Sciences (AUS) *Online - full text edition.* **3932**
Nursing Inquiry (AUS) *Online - full text edition.* **3933**
Nursing Philosophy Online (GBR) *Online - full text edition of* Nursing Philosophy. **3934**
Nutrition Bulletin Online (GBR) *Online - full text edition of* Nutrition Bulletin. **4241**
Nutrition in Clinical Care Online(USA) *Online - full text.* **4242**
Obesity Reviews Online(GBR) *Online - full text.* **4244**
Oral Microbiology and Immunology (DNK) *Online - full text edition.* **3329**
Paediatric Anaesthesia Online(GBR) *Online - full text.* **3759**
Paediatric & Perinatal Epidemiology Online(GBR) *Online - full text.* **4050**
Pain Medicine Online(USA) *Online - full text.* **4121**
Parasite Immunology Online (GBR) *Online - full text edition of* Parasite Immunology. **3804**
Pathology International (AUS) *Online - full text edition.* **3673**
Pediatric Allergy and Immunology (DNK) *Online - full text edition.* **4051**
Pediatric Dermatology (USA) *Online - full text edition.* **3852**
Pediatric Diabetes Online(DNK) *Online - full text.* **4052**
Pediatric Transplantation (DNK) *Online - full text edition.* **4054**
Pediatrics International (AUS) *Online - full text edition.* **4054**
Periodontology 2000 Online(DNK) *Online - full text.* **3836**
Pigment Cell Research (DNK) *Online - full text edition.* **3293**
Plant, Cell and Environment Online (GBR) *Online - full text edition of* Plant, Cell and Environment. **3213**
The Prostate Journal Online(USA) *Online - full text.* **3680**
Psychiatry and Clinical Neurosciences (AUS) *Online - full text edition.* **4126**
Public Health Nursing (USA) *Online - full text edition.* **3938**
Reproduction in Domestic Animals Online(DEU) *Online - full text.* **4551**
Respirology (AUS) *Online - full text edition.* **4164**
Reviews in Clinical and Experimental Hematology (GBR) *Online - full text edition.* **3904**
Scandinavian Journal of Immunology Online (GBR) *Online - full text edition of* Scandinavian Journal of Immunology. **3751**
Seminars in Dialysis (USA) *Online - full text edition.* **4218**
Somnologie (DEU) *Online - full text edition.* **3694**
Therapeutic Apheresis Online(USA) *Online - full text.* **4218**
Tissue Antigens (DNK) *Online - full text edition.* **3701**
Traffic (DNK) *Online - full text edition.* **3294**
Transfusion Medicine (GBR) *Online - full text edition.* **3905**
Transplant Infectious Disease Online(DNK) *Online - full text.* **4206**
Tropical Medicine & International Health Online (GBR) *Online - full text edition of* Tropical Medicine & International Health. **4491**
Ultrasound in Obstetrics & Gynecology (GBR) *Online - full text edition.* **3965**
Value in Health (USA) *Online - full text edition.* **4339**
Veterinary Anaesthesia and Analgesia Online (GBR) *Online - full text edition of* Veterinary Anaesthesia and Analgesia. **4556**
Veterinary Dermatology Online(GBR) *Online - full text.* **4557**
Veterinary Ophthalmology Online (GBR) *Online - full text edition of* Veterinary Ophthalmology. **4558**
Wound Repair and Regeneration (USA) *Online - full text edition.* **4028**
Xenotransplantation (DNK) *Online - full text edition.* **4207**

National Library of Medicine 8600 Rockville Pike, Bethesda, MD 20209 TEL 301-496-6193, 800-638-8480, FAX 301-496-4000 http://www.nlm.nih.gov
Bibliography of Bioethics (USA) *Online - full text edition.* **3717**
Bibliography of the History of Medicine (USA) *Online - full text edition.* **3717**
International Pharmaceutical Abstracts (USA) *Online - full text edition.* **4345**
Issues in Law and Medicine (USA) *Online - full text edition.* **3626**
Journal of Magnetic Resonance Imaging (USA) *Online - full text edition.* **4148**
List of Serials Indexed for Online Users (USA) *Online - full text edition.* **3731**
Medline (USA) *Online - full text edition of* Index Medicus. **3729**
N I O S H T I C(USA) *Online - full text.* **4259**
Psychopharmacology Bulletin (USA) *Online - full text edition.* **4332**

NewsNet (Subsidiary of: Independent Publications) 945 Haverford Rd., Bryn Mawr, PA 19010 TEL 610-527-8030, 800-345-1301, FAX 610-527-0338, info@newsnet.com, http://www.newsnet.com
AIDS Weekly Plus (USA) *Online - full text edition. (HH14)* **3792**
Applied Genetics News (USA) *Online - full text edition. (BT03)* **3299**
Biotech Business (USA) *Online - full text edition. (BT06)* **3270**
Blood Weekly (USA) *Online - full text edition.* **3899**
Cancer Weekly Plus (USA) *Online - full text edition. (HH15)* **3973**
Health Care Strategic Management (USA) *Online - full text edition.* **3509**
Health Grants & Contracts Weekly (USA) *Online - full text edition. (HH10)* **4459**
Health Industry Today (USA) *Online - full text edition.* **3611**
Health News Daily (USA) *Online - full text edition. (HH01)* **3612**
Healthcare Advertising Review (USA) *Online - full text edition.* **3152**
Hospital Materials Management (USA) *Online - full text edition.* **3514**
Hospital Payment and Information Management (USA) *Online - full text edition.* **3514**
Industrial Health & Hazards Update (USA) *Online - full text edition. (LA04)* **4256**
Managed Care Outlook (USA) *Online - full text edition. (HH12)* **3532**
McGraw-Hill's Biotechnology Newswatch (USA) *Online - full text edition. (BT08)* **3276**
Medical Outcomes and Guidelines Alert (USA) *Online - full text edition.* **3652**
Medical Utilization Management (USA) *Online - full text edition.* **3655**
Morbidity and Mortality Weekly Report (USA) *Online - full text edition.* **4482**
Older Americans Report (USA) *Online - full text edition.* **4516**
The Physician and Sportsmedicine (USA) *Online - full text edition. (ME05)* **4176**
Postgraduate Medicine (USA) *Online - full text edition. (ME06)* **3678**
Product Alert (USA) *Online - full text edition. (AD24)* **3462**
Profiles in Healthcare Marketing (USA) *Online - full text edition.* **3153**
Tuberculosis & Airborne Disease Weekly (USA) *Online - full text edition.* **3808**

NISC 601 Wyman Towers, Ste 806, 3100 St Paul St, Baltimore, MD 21218 TEL 410-243-0797, FAX 410-243-0892, sales@nisc.com, http://www.nisc.com, http://www.nisc.com
African Health Anthology (USA) *Online - full text edition.* **3715**
AIDSearch(USA) *Online - full text.* **3715**
Biotechnology Abstracts (GBR) *Online - full text edition.* **3227**
Entomology Abstracts (USA) *Online - full text edition.* **3230**
Health and Safety Science Abstracts (USA) *Online - full text edition.* **4496**
N I O S H T I C(USA) *Online - full text.* **4259**
PsycINFO(USA) *Online - full text.* **4458**
R T E C S(USA) *Online - full text.* **3453**

Northern Light Technology, Inc. One Athenaeum St., Cambridge, MA 02142 TEL 617-621-5100, FAX 617-621-3459, adsales@northernlight.com, http://www.northernlight.com
A S H A Leader (USA) *Online - full text edition.* **3488**
Academic Psychiatry (USA) *Online - full text edition.* **4067**
Addiction (GBR) *Online - full text edition.* **3396**
Addiction Biology (GBR) *Online - full text edition.* **3397**
Adolescence (CHE) *Online - full text edition.* **4069**
Adolescent Psychiatry (USA) *Online - full text edition.* **4069**
Aging (GBR) *Online - full text edition.* **3225**
AIDS Alert (USA) *Online - full text edition.* **3791**
AIDS Care (GBR) *Online - full text edition.* **3791**
Alcoholism & Drug Abuse Weekly (USA) *Online - full text edition.* **3398**
American Annals of the Deaf (USA) *Online - full text edition.* **3488**
American Druggist (USA) *Online - full text edition.* **4275**
American Family Physician (USA) *Online - full text edition.* **3563**
American Fitness (USA) *Online - full text edition.* **4350**
American Journal of Art Therapy (USA) *Online - full text edition.* **4058**
American Journal of Community Psychology (USA) *Online - full text edition.* **4520**
American Journal of Critical Care (USA) *Online - full text edition.* **3913**
American Journal of Family Therapy (USA) *Online - full text edition.* **4374**
American Journal of Geriatric Psychiatry (USA) *Online - full text edition.* **3468**
American Journal of Knee Surgery (USA) *Online - full text edition.* **4180**
American Journal of Law & Medicine (USA) *Online - full text edition.* **3536**
American Journal of Nephrology (CHE) *Online - full text edition.* **4209**
American Journal of Ophthalmology (USA) *Online - full text edition.* **3993**
American Journal of Pharmaceutical Education (USA) *Online - full text edition.* **4275**
American Journal of Psychiatry (USA) *Online - full text edition.* **4071**
American Journal of Psychoanalysis (USA) *Online - full text edition.* **4374**
American Journal of Psychology (USA) *Online - full text edition.* **4374**
American Journal of Psychotherapy (USA) *Online - full text edition.* **4072**
American Journal of Public Health (USA) *Online - full text edition.* **4461**
American Journal of Sports Medicine (USA) *Online - full text edition.* **4172**
The American Nurse (USA) *Online - full text edition.* **3913**
American Rehabilitation (USA) *Online - full text edition.* **3419**
American Surgeon (USA) *Online - full text edition.* **4180**
Angiology (USA) *Online - full text edition.* **3763**
Annals of Vascular Surgery (USA) *Online - full text edition.* **4181**
Annual Review of Genetics (USA) *Online - full text edition.* **3298**
Annual Review of Microbiology (USA) *Online - full text edition.* **3317**
Annual Review of Psychology (USA) *Online - full text edition.* **4376**
Annual Review of Sex Research (USA) *Online - full text edition.* **4376**
Antiviral Agents Bulletin (USA) *Online - full text edition.* **4276**
Antiviral Weekly (USA) *Online - full text edition.* **3740**
Applied Genetics News (USA) *Online - full text edition.* **3299**
Archives of Environmental Health (USA) *Online - full text edition.* **3435**
Archives of Pathology & Laboratory Medicine (USA) *Online - full text edition.* **3568**
Arizona Nurse (USA) *Online - full text edition.* **3914**
Asbestos & Lead Abatement Report (USA) *Online - full text edition.* **3443**
Australian Nursing Journal (AUS) *Online - full text edition.* **3914**
Avian Pathology (GBR) *Online - full text edition.* **4539**
B J O Online (GBR) *Online - full text edition of* British Journal of Ophthalmology. **3994**
Behavioral Health Management (USA) *Online - full text edition.* **3399**
Behavioral Medicine (USA) *Online - full text edition.* **4381**
Biological Bulletin (USA) *Online - full text edition.* **3185**

Online Service

Biomedical Market Newsletter (USA) *Online - full text edition.* **3366**
BioPharm (USA) *Online - full text edition.* **4280**
Biophysical Journal (USA) *Online - full text edition.* **3265**
BioScience (USA) *Online - full text edition.* **3187**
BioVenture View (USA) *Online - full text edition.* **3272**
Blood Weekly (USA) *Online - full text edition.* **3899**
Bone Marrow Transplantation (GBR) *Online - full text edition.* **3872**
Brain (GBR) *Online - full text edition.* **4077**
Breast Cancer (USA) *Online - full text edition.* **3968**
British Journal of Biomedical Science (GBR) *Online - full text edition.* **3872**
British Journal of Clinical Psychology (GBR) *Online - full text edition.* **4383**
The British Journal of Criminology (GBR) *Online - full text edition.* **3393**
British Journal of Developmental Psychology (GBR) *Online - full text edition.* **4383**
British Journal of Educational Psychology (GBR) *Online - full text edition.* **4383**
British Journal of Medical Psychology (GBR) *Online - full text edition.* **4384**
British Journal of Neurosurgery (GBR) *Online - full text edition.* **4182**
British Journal of Nursing (GBR) *Online - full text edition.* **3915**
British Journal of Perioperative Nursing (GBR) *Online - full text edition.* **3915**
British Journal of Psychology (GBR) *Online - full text edition.* **4384**
British Journal of Social Psychology (GBR) *Online - full text edition.* **4384**
Canadian Journal of Experimental Psychology (CAN) *Online - full text edition.* **4386**
Canadian Journal of Public Health (CAN) *Online - full text edition.* **4464**
Canadian Mining Journal (CAN) *Online - full text edition.* **4225**
Carcinogenesis (GBR) *Online - full text edition.* **3974**
Carcinogenesis (USA) *Online - full text edition.* **3974**
The Career Development Quarterly (USA) *Online - full text edition.* **4269**
Chain Drug Review (USA) *Online - full text edition.* **3364**
The Challenge (PAK) *Online - full text edition.* **4159**
Chest (USA) *Online - full text edition.* **4159**
Child Health Alert (USA) *Online - full text edition.* **4042**
Circulation Research (USA) *Online - full text edition.* **3768**
Cleft Palate - Craniofacial Journal (CAN) *Online - full text edition.* **4185**
Clinical Diabetes (USA) *Online - full text edition.* **3856**
Clinical Laboratory Science (USA) *Online - full text edition.* **3873**
Clinical Pediatrics (USA) *Online - full text edition.* **4042**
Clio (DEU) *Online - full text edition.* **4563**
Closing the Gap (USA) *Online - full text edition.* **3420**
Community Mental Health Journal (USA) *Online - full text edition.* **4512**
Congestive Heart Failure (USA) *Online - full text edition.* **3769**
Connexions (FRA) *Online - full text edition.* **4391**
Contemporary Longterm Care (USA) *Online - full text edition.* **3505**
Contraceptive Technology Update (USA) *Online - full text edition.* **3358**
Cooking Light (USA) *Online - full text edition.* **3526**
Critical Care Alert (USA) *Online - full text edition.* **4012**
Critical Care Nurse (USA) *Online - full text edition.* **3917**
Critical Reviews in Toxicology (USA) *Online - full text edition.* **3447**
Current Health 1 (USA) *Online - full text edition.* **3428**
Current Health 2 (USA) *Online - full text edition.* **3428**
Cutis (USA) *Online - full text edition.* **3847**
Dairy Council Digest(USA) *Online - full text.* **4231**
Dental Economics (ESP) *Online - full text edition.* **3820**
Dental Economics (USA) *Online - full text edition.* **3820**
Dermatology Nursing (USA) *Online - full text edition.* **3848**
Dermatology Times (USA) *Online - full text edition.* **3848**
Diabetes (DNK) *Online - full text edition.* **3857**
Diabetes (SWE) *Online - full text edition.* **3857**
Diabetes (USA) *Online - full text edition.* **3857**
Diabetes (FIN) *Online - full text edition.* **3857**
Diabetes Care (USA) *Online - full text edition.* **3857**
Diabetes Forecast (USA) *Online - full text edition.* **3858**
Diabetes Spectrum (USA) *Online - full text edition.* **3859**
Digestion (CHE) *Online - full text edition.* **3888**
Disability & Society (GBR) *Online - full text edition.* **3494**
Drug Detection Report (USA) *Online - full text edition.* **3368**
Drug Information Journal (USA) *Online - full text edition.* **4289**
Drug Topics (USA) *Online - full text edition.* **4290**
Drug Utilization Review (USA) *Online - full text edition.* **4290**
Education for Health (GBR) *Online - full text edition.* **3597**
Educational Psychology (GBR) *Online - full text edition.* **3410**
Emergency Medicine (USA) *Online - full text edition.* **4013**
Emergency Medicine Alert (USA) *Online - full text edition.* **4013**
Emergency Medicine Reports (USA) *Online - full text edition.* **4014**
Emergency Nurse (GBR) *Online - full text edition.* **3918**
Environmental Nutrition (USA) *Online - full text edition.* **4232**
Europa Medicophysica (ITA) *Online - full text edition.* **4060**
European Journal of Neuroscience (GBR) *Online - full text edition.* **4089**
European Neurology (CHE) *Online - full text edition.* **4089**
Evolution (USA) *Online - full text edition.* **3302**
Exceptional Children (USA) *Online - full text edition.* **3422**
Exceptional Parent (USA) *Online - full text edition.* **3422**
Family Planning Perspectives (USA) *Online - full text edition.* **3949**
Family Practice Alert (USA) *Online - full text edition.* **4352**
Family Practice Management (USA) *Online - full text edition.* **3602**
Female Patient: Practical Ob-Gyn Medicine (USA) *Online - full text edition.* **3949**
Florida Nurse (USA) *Online - full text edition.* **3919**
Flying Safety (USA) *Online - full text edition.* **3153**
Focus on Exceptional Children (USA) *Online - full text edition.* **3422**
Food & Drug Packaging (USA) *Online - full text edition.* **4271**
Formulary (USA) *Online - full text edition.* **4297**
Frontiers of Health Services Management (USA) *Online - full text edition.* **3507**
The Future of Children (USA) *Online - full text edition.* **3383**
Gene Therapy Weekly (USA) *Online - full text edition.* **3606**
Genesis Report - Dx (USA) *Online - full text edition.* **3606**
Genesis Report - Rx (USA) *Online - full text edition.* **4298**
Georgia Nursing (USA) *Online - full text edition.* **3919**
Geriatrics (USA) *Online - full text edition.* **3472**
The Gerontologist (USA) *Online - full text edition.* **3473**
Gerontology (CHE) *Online - full text edition.* **3473**
Gerontology (ISR) *Online - full text edition.* **3473**
Global Cosmetic Industry (USA) *Online - full text edition.* **3176**
Gut Online (GBR) *Online - full text edition of* Gut. **3891**
Harvard Health Letter (USA) *Online - full text edition.* **4354**
Harvard Heart Letter (USA) *Online - full text edition.* **3772**
The Harvard Mental Health Letter (USA) *Online - full text edition.* **4093**
Harvard Women's Health Watch (USA) *Online - full text edition.* **4563**
Hastings Center Report (USA) *Online - full text edition.* **3610**
Headache Online(USA) *Online - full text.* **4093**
Health Affairs (USA) *Online - full text edition.* **4471**
Health & Social Work (USA) *Online - full text edition.* **4513**
Health Care Financing Review (USA) *Online - full text edition.* **3610**
Health Care Strategic Management (USA) *Online - full text edition.* **3509**
Health Industry Today (USA) *Online - full text edition.* **3611**
Health Management Technology (USA) *Online - full text edition.* **3810**
Health Progress (USA) *Online - full text edition.* **3510**
Health Services Research (USA) *Online - full text edition.* **3510**
Healthcare Benchmarks (USA) *Online - full text edition.* **3510**
Healthcare Executive (USA) *Online - full text edition.* **3510**
Healthcare Financial Management (USA) *Online - full text edition.* **3510**
Healthcare Forum Journal (USA) *Online - full text edition.* **3510**
Healthcare Risk Management (USA) *Online - full text edition.* **3511**
HealthFacts (USA) *Online - full text edition.* **3613**
Heart & Soul (USA) *Online - full text edition.* **4355**
Heart Online (GBR) *Online - full text edition of* Heart. **3772**
Hepatitis Weekly (USA) *Online - full text edition.* **3797**
High Ability Studies (GBR) *Online - full text edition.* **3422**
Home Health Business Report (USA) *Online - full text edition.* **3511**
Hospice Management Advisor (USA) *Online - full text edition.* **3512**
Hospital Access Management (USA) *Online - full text edition.* **3512**
Hospital Case Management (USA) *Online - full text edition.* **3513**
Hospital Development (GBR) *Online - full text edition.* **3513**
Hospital Employee Health (USA) *Online - full text edition.* **3513**
Hospital Home Health (USA) *Online - full text edition.* **3513**
Hospital Infection Control (USA) *Online - full text edition.* **3797**
Hospital Materials Management (USA) *Online - full text edition.* **3514**
Hospital Peer Review (USA) *Online - full text edition.* **3514**
Hospital Topics (USA) *Online - full text edition.* **3514**
Human Factors (USA) *Online - full text edition.* **3432**
Human Relations (USA) *Online - full text edition.* **4509**
Hypertension (USA) *Online - full text edition.* **3774**
In Vitro Cellular & Developmental Biology - Animal (USA) *Online - full text edition.* **3618**
Industrial Health & Hazards Update (USA) *Online - full text edition.* **4256**
Infection Control & Hospital Epidemiology (USA) *Online - full text edition.* **3798**
Infectious Disease Alert (USA) *Online - full text edition.* **3798**
Internal Medicine Alert (USA) *Online - full text edition.* **3909**
International Angiology (ITA) *Online - full text edition.* **3774**
International Family Planning Perspectives (USA) *Online - full text edition.* **3953**
International Immunology (GBR) *Online - full text edition.* **3747**
International Journal of Childbirth Education (USA) *Online - full text edition.* **3953**
International Journal of Conflict Management (USA) *Online - full text edition.* **3365**
International Journal of Epidemiology (GBR) *Online - full text edition.* **3623**
International Journal of Group Psychotherapy (USA) *Online - full text edition.* **4406**
International Journal of Psychotherapy (GBR) *Online - full content edition.* **4096**
International Journal of Social Psychiatry (GBR) *Online - full text edition.* **4096**
International Journal of Surgical Pathology (USA) *Online - full text edition.* **4191**
International Review of Psychiatry (GBR) *Online - full text edition.* **4097**
Intervirology (CHE) *Online - full text edition.* **3324**
J C P Online (GBR) *Online - full text edition of* Journal of Clinical Pathology. **3631**
J E C H Online (GBR) *Online - full text edition of* Journal of Epidemiology & Community Health. **3632**
J M E Online (GBR) *Online - full text edition of* Journal of Medical Ethics. **3635**
J M G Online (GBR) *Online - full text edition of* Journal of Medical Genetics. **3310**
Journal of Abnormal Child Psychology (USA) *Online - full text edition.* **4409**
Journal of Addictions & Offender Counseling (USA) *Online - full text edition.* **4409**
Journal of American College Health (USA) *Online - full text edition.* **4357**
Journal of Athletic Training (USA) *Online - full text edition.* **4174**
The Journal of Cardiovascular Surgery (ITA) *Online - full text edition.* **3777**
Journal of Career Assessment (USA) *Online - full text edition.* **4411**
Journal of Child Neurology (CAN) *Online - full text edition.* **4099**
Journal of Clinical Psychiatry (USA) *Online - full text edition.* **4100**
Journal of Community Health (USA) *Online - full text edition.* **3631**
Journal of Continuing Education in Nursing (USA) *Online - full text edition.* **3924**
Journal of Cultural Diversity (USA) *Online - full text edition.* **3924**
Journal of Dental Hygiene (JPN) *Online - full text edition.* **3828**
Journal of Dental Hygiene (USA) *Online - full text edition.* **3828**
Journal of Dental Research (USA) *Online - full text edition.* **3828**
Journal of Drug Issues (USA) *Online - full text edition.* **3403**
Journal of Electrocardiology (USA) *Online - full text edition.* **3777**
Journal of Employment Counseling (USA) *Online - full text edition.* **4414**
Journal of Environmental Health (USA) *Online - full text edition.* **3440**
Journal of Esthetic and Restorative Dentistry (CAN) *Online - full text edition.* **3828**
Journal of Family Practice (USA) *Online - full text edition.* **3633**
Journal of Forensic Identification (USA) *Online - full text edition.* **3883**
Journal of Gay & Lesbian Social Services (USA) *Online - full text edition.* **4514**
The Journal of General Psychology (USA) *Online - full text edition.* **4416**
The Journal of Genetic Psychology (USA) *Online - full text edition.* **3309**
Journal of Gerontological Nursing (USA) *Online - full text edition.* **3476**
Journal of Interprofessional Care (GBR) *Online - full text edition.* **3634**
Journal of Investigative Medicine (USA) *Online - full text edition.* **3883**
Journal of Mammalogy (USA) *Online - full text edition.* **3354**
Journal of Mental Health (GBR) *Online - full text edition.* **4102**
Journal of Mental Health Counseling (USA) *Online - full text edition.* **4418**
Journal of Motor Behavior (USA) *Online - full text edition.* **4418**
Journal of Neuroscience Nursing (USA) *Online - full text edition.* **3925**
Journal of Neurosurgical Sciences (ITA) *Online - full text edition.* **4194**
Journal of Nuclear Medicine Technology (USA) *Online - full text edition.* **4148**
Journal of Nursing Education (USA) *Online - full text edition.* **3925**
Journal of Nutrition (USA) *Online - full text edition.* **4237**
Journal of Nutrition Education (CAN) *Online - full text edition.* **4237**
Journal of Nutritional & Environmental Medicine (GBR) *Online - full text edition.* **4237**
Journal of Orthopaedic Research (USA) *Online - full text edition.* **4019**
Journal of Otolaryngology (CAN) *Online - full text edition.* **4034**
Journal of Palliative Care (CAN) *Online - full text edition.* **3636**
Journal of Parapsychology (USA) *Online - full text edition.* **4271**
Journal of Personality Disorders (USA) *Online - full text edition.* **4420**
Journal of Phenomenological Psychology (USA) *Online - full text edition.* **4420**
Journal of Psychoactive Drugs (USA) *Online - full text edition.* **3403**

Journal of Rehabilitation (USA) *Online - full text edition.* **4062**
Journal of School Health (USA) *Online - full text edition.* **4479**
Journal of Sex Research (USA) *Online - full text edition.* **4422**
The Journal of Social Psychology (USA) *Online - full text edition.* **4423**
Journal of Social Work Practice (GBR) *Online - full text edition.* **4515**
Journal of Sport Behavior (USA) *Online - full text edition.* **4525**
Journal of Studies on Alcohol (USA) *Online - full text edition.* **3403**
Journal of Trauma Nursing (USA) *Online - full text edition.* **3927**
Journal of Travel Medicine (CAN) *Online - full text edition.* **3639**
Journal of Vascular Research (CHE) *Online - full text edition.* **3779**
Kansas Nurse (USA) *Online - full text edition.* **3927**
The Lancet (GBR) *Online - full text edition.* **3642**
Life Science Today (GBR) *Online - full text edition.* **4313**
Mankind Quarterly (USA) *Online - full text edition.* **3174**
Marketing Health Services (USA) *Online - full text edition.* **3367**
Mayo Clinic Proceedings (USA) *Online - full text edition.* **3647**
Med Ad News (USA) *Online - full text edition.* **3367**
Medical Decision Making (USA) *Online - full text edition.* **3649**
Medical Economics (USA) *Online - full text edition.* **3650**
Medical Ethics Advisor (USA) *Online - full text edition.* **3650**
Medical History (GBR) *Online - full text edition.* **3650**
Medical Marketing & Media (USA) *Online - full text edition.* **4315**
Medical Materials Update (USA) *Online - full text edition.* **3652**
Medical Teacher (GBR) *Online - full text edition.* **3654**
Medical Textiles (GBR) *Online - full text edition.* **3654**
MedSurg Nursing (USA) *Online - full text edition.* **4196**
Melpomene Journal (USA) *Online - full text edition.* **4564**
Menopause News (USA) *Online - full text edition.* **4564**
MidLife Woman (USA) *Online - full text edition.* **4568**
The Milbank Quarterly (USA) *Online - full text edition.* **4368**
Military Medicine (USA) *Online - full text edition.* **3661**
Minority Nurse Newsletter (USA) *Online - full text edition.* **3929**
Mothering (USA) *Online - full text edition.* **4564**
Multicultural Education Abstracts (GBR) *Online - full content edition.* **3415**
National Women's Health Report (USA) *Online - full text edition.* **4565**
The Nation's Health (USA) *Online - full text edition.* **4483**
Navy Medicine (USA) *Online - full text edition.* **3665**
Nephron (CHE) *Online - full text edition.* **4216**
Neuroendocrinology (CHE) *Online - full text edition.* **3867**
Neuroepidemiology (CHE) *Online - full text edition.* **4113**
Neurological Research (USA) *Online - full text edition.* **4114**
Neurology Alert (USA) *Online - full text edition.* **4115**
Neuropsychobiology (CHE) *Online - full text edition.* **4116**
The New York State Dental Journal (USA) *Online - full text edition.* **3833**
New Zealand Journal of Psychology (NZL) *Online - full text edition.* **4430**
The Nurse Practitioner (USA) *Online - full text edition.* **3931**
Nurse Researcher (GBR) *Online - full text edition.* **3931**
Nursing (PRT) *Online - full text edition.* **3931**
Nursing Diagnosis (USA) *Online - full text edition.* **3932**
Nursing Economics (USA) *Online - full text edition.* **3932**
Nursing Forum (USA) *Online - full text edition.* **3933**
Nursing Homes (USA) *Online - full text edition.* **3933**
Nursing Law's Regan Report (USA) *Online - full text edition.* **3933**
Nursing Management (USA) *Online - full text edition.* **3933**
Nursing Management (GBR) *Online - full text edition.* **3934**
Nursing Standard (GBR) *Online - full text edition.* **3934**
Nutrition Forum (USA) *Online - full text edition.* **4242**
Nutrition Forum (CAN) *Online - full text edition.* **4242**
Nutrition Health Review (USA) *Online - full text edition.* **4242**
Nutrition in Clinical Practice (USA) *Online - full text edition.* **4242**
Nutrition Research Newsletter (USA) *Online - full text edition.* **4243**
Nutrition Reviews (USA) *Online - full text edition.* **4243**
Nutrition Today (USA) *Online - full text edition.* **4243**
O H Online (USA) *Online - full text edition of* Occupational Hazards. **4261**
Occupational Health & Safety (USA) *Online - full text edition.* **4261**
Occupational Therapy International (GBR) *Online - full text edition.* **4262**
On the Issues (USA) *Online - full text edition.* **4568**
Onderstepoort Journal of Veterinary Research (ZAF) *Online - full text edition.* **4549**
Ophthalmology Times (USA) *Online - full text edition.* **4004**
Optometric Management (USA) *Online - full text edition.* **4005**
Orthopedics (USA) *Online - full text edition.* **4023**
Ostomy Quarterly (USA) *Online - full text edition.* **3671**
Palaestra (USA) *Online - full text edition.* **3425**
Paraplegia News (USA) *Online - full text edition.* **3494**
Pathobiology (CHE) *Online - full text edition.* **3750**
Patient Care (USA) *Online - full text edition.* **3673**
Patient Care (CAN) *Online - full text edition.* **3673**
Pediatric Annals (USA) *Online - full text edition.* **4051**
Pediatric Emergency Medicine Reports (USA) *Online - full text edition.* **4024**
Pediatric Nursing (USA) *Online - full text edition.* **3937**
Pediatrics (ITA) *Online - full text edition.* **4054**
Pediatrics for Parents (USA) *Online - full text edition.* **4054**
People's Medical Society Newsletter (USA) *Online - full text edition.* **3393**
Personnel Psychology (USA) *Online - full text edition.* **4433**
Perspectives in Psychiatric Care (USA) *Online - full text edition.* **3937**
Pharma Japan (JPN) *Online - full text edition.* **4322**
Pharmaceutical Business News (GBR) *Online - full text edition.* **4323**
Pharmaceutical Executive (USA) *Online - full text edition.* **4323**
Pharmaceutical Technology (USA) *Online - full text edition.* **4325**
Philosophical Psychology (GBR) *Online - full text edition.* **4433**
Physical Therapy (USA) *Online - full text edition.* **4064**
Physician Executive (USA) *Online - full text edition.* **3521**
Physician's Managed Care Report (USA) *Online - full text edition.* **3533**
Physician's Payment Update (USA) *Online - full text edition.* **3521**
Physiological Reviews Online (USA) *Online - full text edition of* Physiological Reviews. **3347**
Physiotherapy Research International (GBR) *Online - full text edition.* **4065**
Plastic Surgical Nursing (USA) *Online - full text edition.* **3937**
Postgraduate Medical Journal (GBR) *Online - full text edition.* **3678**
Postgraduate Medicine (USA) *Online - full text edition.* **3678**
Professional Safety (USA) *Online - full text edition.* **4263**
Professional School Counseling (USA) *Online - full text edition.* **3414**
Progress in Cardiovascular Nursing (USA) *Online - full text edition.* **3781**
Psychiatric Annals (USA) *Online - full text edition.* **4125**
Psychiatry (USA) *Online - full text edition.* **4126**
Psychiatry (CAN) *Online - full text edition.* **4126**
The Psychoanalytic Review (USA) *Online - full text edition.* **4437**
The Psychological Record (USA) *Online - full text edition.* **4438**
The Psychologist (GBR) *Online - full text edition.* **4440**
Psychology Today (USA) *Online - full text edition.* **4441**
Psychopathology (CHE) *Online - full text edition.* **4128**
Psychosomatics (USA) *Online - full text edition.* **4128**
Psychotherapy Research (USA) *Online - full text edition.* **4443**
Public Health Reports (USA) *Online - full text edition.* **4486**
Qualitative Health Research (USA) *Online - full text edition.* **3681**
Radiologic Technology (USA) *Online - full text edition.* **4153**
Rehabilitation Nursing (USA) *Online - full text edition.* **3939**
Rheumatic Diseases. Bulletin (USA) *Online - full text edition.* **4171**
Rheumatology (GBR) *Online - full text edition.* **4171**
Rheumatology (CHE) *Online - full text edition.* **4171**
Sanitary Maintenance (USA) *Online - full text edition.* **4489**
Saturday Evening Post (USA) *Online - full text edition.* **3465**
Schizophrenia Bulletin (USA) *Online - full text edition.* **4132**
School Psychology Quarterly (USA) *Online - full text edition.* **4447**
School Psychology Review (USA) *Online - full text edition.* **4447**
Seminars in Headache Management (CAN) *Online - full text edition.* **4448**
Shape (USA) *Online - full text edition.* **4565**
Signal (DEU) *Online - full text edition.* **3990**
Signal (CAN) *Online - full text edition.* **4266**
Smith College Studies in Social Work (USA) *Online - full text edition.* **4518**
Social Cognition (USA) *Online - full text edition.* **4449**
Special Delivery (USA) *Online - full text edition.* **3964**
Special Educational Needs Abstracts (GBR) *Online - full content edition.* **3416**
State Health Monitor (USA) *Online - full text edition.* **3534**
State Reproductive Health Monitor (USA) *Online - full text edition.* **3964**
Stress (CHE) *Online - full text edition.* **3696**
Stroke (USA) *Online - full text edition.* **3783**
Studies in Family Planning (USA) *Online - full text edition.* **4369**
Surgical Services Management (USA) *Online - full text edition.* **4205**
Thorax Online (GBR) *Online - full text edition of* Thorax. **3700**
Today's Surgical Nurse (USA) *Online - full text edition.* **3942**
Total Health (USA) *Online - full text edition.* **4246**
Trustee (USA) *Online - full text edition.* **3523**
Undersea & Hyperbaric Medicine (USA) *Online - full text edition.* **3704**
Urologic Nursing (USA) *Online - full text edition.* **4219**
Urology Times (USA) *Online - full text edition.* **4220**
Vaccine Weekly (USA) *Online - full text edition.* **4339**
Vegetarian Times (USA) *Online - full text edition.* **4247**
Veterinary Economics (USA) *Online - full text edition.* **3369**
Veterinary Medicine (USA) *Online - full text edition.* **4557**
Vibrant Life (USA) *Online - full text edition.* **4362**
Vitamins (JPN) *Online - full text edition.* **4340**
Vox Sanguinis (CHE) *Online - full text edition.* **3752**
Warning Letter Bulletin (USA) *Online - full text edition.* **3707**
Weekly Epidemiological Record (CHE) *Online - full text edition.* **4493**
Women & Therapy (USA) *Online - full text edition.* **4455**
WomenWise (USA) *Online - full text edition.* **4567**
Worklife Report (CAN) *Online - full text edition.* **3364**

O C L C Online Computer Library Center, Inc. 6565 Frantz Rd, Dublin, OH 43017 TEL 614-764-6000, 614-764-6144, 800-848-5878, FAX 614-764-6096, abstractscomments@oclc.org, http://www.oclc.org
A N Z Journal of Surgery (AUS) *Online - full text edition.* **4178**
Abstracts in Social Gerontology (USA) *Online - full text edition.* **3482**
Acta Anaesthesiologica Scandinavica (DNK) *Online - full text edition.* **3753**
Acta Biotheoretica (NLD) *Online - full text edition.* **3178**
Acta Dermato-Venereologica (NOR) *Online - full text edition.* **3843**
Acta Haematologica (CHE) *Online - full text edition.* **3897**
Acta Odontologica Scandinavica (NOR) *Online - full text edition.* **3813**
Acta Oncologica (NOR) *Online - full text edition.* **3966**
Acta Oto-Laryngologica (NOR) *Online - full text edition.* **4029**
Acta Paediatrica (NOR) *Online - full text edition.* **4039**
Acta Physiologica Scandinavica (GBR) *Online - full text edition.* **3337**
Acta Psychiatrica Scandinavica (DNK) *Online - full text edition.* **4068**
Acta Zoologica Online(GBR) *Online - full text.* **3350**
Addiction (GBR) *Online - full text edition.* **3396**
Addiction Biology (GBR) *Online - full text edition.* **3397**
Administration and Policy in Mental Health (USA) *Online - full text edition.* **3559**
Advances in Health Sciences Education (NLD) *Online - full text edition.* **3560**
Advances in Physiotherapy (NOR) *Online - full text edition.* **4058**
Ageing and Society (GBR) *Online - full text edition.* **3466**
Aging & Mental Health (GBR) *Online - full text edition.* **3466**
AIDS & Behavior (USA) *Online - full text edition.* **3739**
AIDS & Cancer Research(USA) *Online - full text.* **3715**
AIDS Care (GBR) *Online - full text edition.* **3791**
AIDS Patient Care and S T Ds (USA) *Online - full text edition.* **3791**
AIDS Research and Human Retroviruses (USA) *Online - full text edition.* **3792**
Alcohol & Alcoholism (GBR) *Online - full text edition.* **3397**
Alimentary Pharmacology and Therapeutics (GBR) *Online - full text edition.* **3886**
Allergology International (AUS) *Online - full text edition.* **3739**
Allergy (DNK) *Online - full text edition.* **3739**
American Behavioral Scientist (USA) *Online - full text edition.* **4508**
American Imago (USA) *Online - full text edition.* **4071**
American Journal of Community Psychology (USA) *Online - full text edition.* **4520**
American Journal of Dance Therapy (USA) *Online - full text edition.* **3396**
American Journal of Drug and Alcohol Abuse (USA) *Online - full text edition.* **3399**
American Journal of Family Therapy (USA) *Online - full text edition.* **4374**
American Journal of Nephrology (CHE) *Online - full text edition.* **4209**
American Journal of Perinatology (USA) *Online - full text edition.* **3944**
American Journal of Psychoanalysis (USA) *Online - full text edition.* **4374**
American Journal on Addictions (USA) *Online - full text edition.* **3399**
Anaerobe (GBR) *Online - full text edition.* **3317**
Anaesthesia (Oxford) (GBR) *Online - full text edition.* **3754**
Analytical Biochemistry (USA) *Online - full text edition.* **3240**
Analytical Cellular Pathology (NLD) *Online - full text edition.* **3285**
Analytische Psychologie (CHE) *Online - full text edition.* **4375**
Anatomia, Histologia, Embryologia Online(DEU) *Online - full text.* **4537**
Andrologia (DEU) *Online - full text edition.* **3565**
Angiogenesis (GBR) *Online - full text edition.* **3967**

Online Service

Animal Behaviour (GBR) *Online - full text edition.* **3350**
Animal Genetics (GBR) *Online - full text edition.* **3298**
Annals of Clinical Psychiatry (USA) *Online - full text edition.* **4073**
Annals of Human Biology (GBR) *Online - full text edition.* **3181**
Annals of Human Genetics (GBR) *Online - full text edition.* **3298**
Annals of Nutrition and Metabolism (CHE) *Online - full text edition.* **4229**
Annals of Oncology (NLD) *Online - full text edition.* **3967**
Annals of Tropical Medicine and Parasitology (GBR) *Online - full text edition.* **3793**
Annals of Tropical Paediatrics (GBR) *Online - full text edition.* **4040**
Anthropology & Medicine (GBR) *Online - full content edition.* **3172**
Anti-Cancer Drug Design (GBR) *Online - full text edition.* **3967**
Antonie van Leeuwenhoek (NLD) *Online - full text edition.* **3268**
Aphasiology (GBR) *Online - full text edition.* **4073**
Apoptosis (USA) *Online - full text edition.* **3285**
Appetite (GBR) *Online - full text edition.* **4229**
Applied Biochemistry and Biotechnology (USA) *Online - full text edition.* **3241**
Applied Developmental Science (USA) *Online - full text edition.* **4377**
Applied Neuropsychology (USA) *Online - full text edition.* **4073**
Applied Occupational & Environmental Hygiene (USA) *Online - full text edition.* **4250**
Applied Psycholinguistics (GBR) *Online - full text edition.* **3550**
Applied Psychological Measurement (USA) *Online - full text edition.* **4377**
Applied Psychology (GBR) *Online - full text edition.* **4377**
Applied Psychophysiology and Biofeedback (USA) *Online - full text edition.* **4378**
Aquatic Ecology (NLD) *Online - full text edition.* **3182**
Archives of Andrology (USA) *Online - full text edition.* **3568**
Archives of Biochemistry and Biophysics (USA) *Online - full text edition.* **3241**
Archives of Disease in Childhood (GBR) *Online - full text edition.* **4040**
Archives of Physiology and Biochemistry (NLD) *Online - full text edition.* **3339**
Archives of Sexual Behavior (USA) *Online - full text edition.* **3568**
Artificial Life (USA) *Online - full content edition.* **3389**
Artificial Organs (USA) *Online - full text edition.* **3871**
Asia Pacific Journal of Clinical Nutrition (AUS) *Online - full text edition.* **4229**
Asian Journal of Social Psychology (GBR) *Online - full text edition.* **4378**
Attachment and Human Development (GBR) *Online - full content edition.* **4379**
Audiology and Neuro-Otology (CHE) *Online - full text edition.* **4031**
Austral Ecology (AUS) *Online - full text edition.* **3183**
Australasian Journal of Dermatology (AUS) *Online - full text edition.* **3845**
Australasian Psychiatry (AUS) *Online - full text edition.* **4075**
Australasian Radiology (AUS) *Online - full text edition.* **4140**
Australian and New Zealand Journal of Family Therapy (GBR) *Online - full text edition.* **4520**
Australian and New Zealand Journal of Mental Health Nursing (AUS) *Online - full text edition.* **4075**
Australian & New Zealand Journal of Psychiatry (AUS) *Online - full text edition.* **4075**
Australian Journal of Rural Health (AUS) *Online - full text edition.* **4463**
Australian Occupational Therapy Journal (AUS) *Online - full text edition.* **4059**
Autism (GBR) *Online - full text edition.* **4075**
Autonomic & Autacoid Pharmacology (GBR) *Online - full text edition.* **4279**
Avian Pathology (GBR) *Online - full text edition.* **4539**
B J U International (GBR) *Online - full text edition.* **4210**
Bailliere's Best Practice & Research in Clinical Anaesthesiology (GBR) *Online - full text edition.* **3756**
Bailliere's Best Practice & Research in Clinical Endocrinology and Metabolism (GBR) *Online - full text edition.* **3855**
Bailliere's Best Practice & Research in Clinical Gastroenterology (GBR) *Online - full text edition.* **3886**
Bailliere's Best Practice & Research in Clinical Haematology (GBR) *Online - full text edition.* **3898**
Bailliere's Best Practice & Research in Clinical Obstetrics and Gynaecology (GBR) *Online - full text edition.* **3945**
Bailliere's Best Practice & Research in Clinical Rheumatology (GBR) *Online - full text edition.* **4167**
Basic and Applied Social Psychology (USA) *Online - full text edition.* **4380**
Behavior Genetics (USA) *Online - full text edition.* **3299**
Behavior Modification (USA) *Online - full text edition.* **4380**
Behavioral and Brain Sciences (GBR) *Online - full text edition.* **4380**
Behavioral Ecology (USA) *Online - full text edition.* **3184**
Behaviour (NLD) *Online - full content edition.* **3351**
Behaviour and Information Technology (GBR) *Online - full text edition.* **4381**
Behavioural and Cognitive Psychotherapy (GBR) *Online - full text edition.* **4382**
Bio-Medical Materials and Engineering (NLD) *Online - full text edition.* **3237**
Biochemical and Biophysical Research Communications (USA) *Online - full text edition.* **3242**
Biochemical Genetics (USA) *Online - full text edition.* **3299**
Biochemistry and Cell Biology (CAN) *Online - full text edition.* **3243**
Biocontrol Science and Technology (GBR) *Online - full text edition.* **3157**
Biodegradation (NLD) *Online - full text edition.* **3456**
BioDrugs (NZL) *Online - full text edition.* **4280**
Bioethics (GBR) *Online - full text edition.* **4346**
BioFactors (NLD) *Online - full text edition.* **3244**
Biogeochemistry (NLD) *Online - full text edition.* **3245**
Biogerontology (NLD) *Online - full text edition.* **3468**
Biological Chemistry (DEU) *Online - full text edition.* **3245**
Biological Control (USA) *Online - full text edition.* **3185**
Biological Research for Nursing (USA) *Online - full text edition.* **3914**
Biological Reviews (GBR) *Online - full text edition.* **3185**
Biologicals (GBR) *Online - full text edition.* **3186**
Biology of the Neonate (CHE) *Online - full text edition.* **3945**
Biomarkers (GBR) *Online - full text edition.* **3575**
Biomedical Microdevices (USA) *Online - full text edition.* **3576**
Biometrika (GBR) *Online - full text edition.* **3226**
Biorheology (NLD) *Online - full text edition.* **3265**
Bioscience Reports (USA) *Online - full text edition.* **3286**
Biotech Software and Internet Report (USA) *Online - full text edition.* **3270**
Biotechnology Law Report (USA) *Online - full content edition.* **3272**
Biotechnology Letters (NLD) *Online - full text edition.* **3272**
Bipolar Disorders Online(DNK) *Online - full text.* **4077**
Birth (USA) *Online - full text edition.* **3946**
Blood Cells, Molecules, and Diseases (USA) *Online - full text edition.* **3898**
Blood Pressure (NOR) *Online - full text edition.* **3764**
Blood Purification (CHE) *Online - full text edition.* **3899**
Blood Reviews (GBR) *Online - full text edition.* **3899**
Bone Marrow Transplantation (GBR) *Online - full text edition.* **3872**
Brain (GBR) *Online - full text edition.* **4077**
Brain and Cognition (USA) *Online - full text edition.* **4383**
Brain and Language (USA) *Online - full text edition.* **4383**
Brain and Mind (USA) *Online - full text edition.* **4077**
Brain, Behavior and Evolution (CHE) *Online - full text edition.* **4077**
Brain, Behavior, and Immunity (USA) *Online - full text edition.* **3741**
Brain Injury (GBR) *Online - full text edition.* **4077**
Brain Topography (USA) *Online - full text edition.* **4078**
The Breast (GBR) *Online - full text edition.* **3946**
Breast Cancer Research and Treatment (USA) *Online - full text edition.* **3969**
The Breast Journal Online(USA) *Online - full text.* **3946**
British Food Journal (GBR) *Online - full text edition.* **3460**
British Homeopathic Journal (GBR) *Online - full text edition.* **3786**
British Journal of Clinical Governance (GBR) *Online - full text edition.* **3578**
British Journal of Clinical Pharmacology (GBR) *Online - full text edition.* **4281**
The British Journal of Criminology (GBR) *Online - full text edition.* **3393**
British Journal of Dermatology (GBR) *Online - full text edition.* **3845**
British Journal of Guidance and Counselling (GBR) *Online - full content edition.* **4269**
British Journal of Haematology (GBR) *Online - full text edition.* **3899**
British Journal of Learning Disabilities (GBR) *Online - full text edition.* **4079**
British Journal of Neurosurgery (GBR) *Online - full text edition.* **4182**
British Journal of Oral and Maxillofacial Surgery (GBR) *Online - full text edition.* **4183**
British Journal of Pharmacology (GBR) *Online - full text edition.* **4281**
British Journal of Special Education (GBR) *Online - full text edition.* **3419**
British Journal of Surgery (GBR) *Online - full text edition.* **4183**
British Medical Bulletin (GBR) *Online - full text edition.* **3579**
Bulletin of Mathematical Biology (GBR) *Online - full text edition.* **3188**
Bulletin of the History of Medicine (USA) *Online - full text edition.* **3579**
C N S Drugs (NZL) *Online - full text edition.* **4282**
Cambridge Quarterly of Healthcare Ethics (GBR) *Online - full text edition.* **3581**
Canadian Journal of Microbiology (CAN) *Online - full text edition.* **3319**
Canadian Journal of Physiology and Pharmacology (CAN) *Online - full text edition.* **3340**
Cancer and Metastasis Reviews (USA) *Online - full text edition.* **3969**
Cancer Causes & Control (NLD) *Online - full text edition.* **3970**
Cancer Detection and Prevention (USA) *Online - full text edition.* **3970**
Cancer Gene Therapy (USA) *Online - full text edition.* **3971**
Carcinogenesis (GBR) *Online - full text edition.* **3974**
Cardiac Electrophysiology Review (USA) *Online - full text edition.* **3765**
Cardiology (CHE) *Online - full text edition.* **3765**
Cardiovascular Drugs and Therapy (USA) *Online - full text edition.* **3766**
Caries Research (CHE) *Online - full text edition.* **3817**
Cell Biology and Toxicology (NLD) *Online - full text edition.* **3446**
Cell Death and Differentiation (GBR) *Online - full text edition.* **3287**
Cell Proliferation (GBR) *Online - full text edition.* **3287**
Cells, Tissues, Organs (CHE) *Online - full text edition.* **3583**
Cellular & Molecular Neurobiology (USA) *Online - full text edition.* **4080**
Cellular Immunology (USA) *Online - full text edition.* **3742**
Cellulose (NLD) *Online - full text edition.* **3378**
Cephalalgia (GBR) *Online - full text edition.* **4080**
Cerebral Cortex (USA) *Online - full text edition.* **4081**
Cerebrovascular Diseases (CHE) *Online - full text edition.* **4081**
Chemical Senses (GBR) *Online - full text edition.* **3340**
Chemotherapy (CHE) *Online - full text edition.* **4283**
Child and Adolescent Social Work Journal (USA) *Online - full text edition.* **4520**
Child and Youth Care Forum (USA) *Online - full text edition.* **3381**
Child: Care, Health and Development (GBR) *Online - full text edition.* **4042**
Child Language Teaching and Therapy (GBR) *Online - full text edition.* **3420**
Child Maltreatment (USA) *Online - full text edition.* **3381**
Child Psychiatry and Human Development (USA) *Online - full text edition.* **4081**
Child Psychology and Psychiatry Review (GBR) *Online - full text edition.* **4387**
Childhood (GBR) *Online - full text edition.* **3382**
Chirurgische Gastroenterologie (CHE) *Online - full text edition.* **3887**
Christian Bioethics (NLD) *Online - full text edition.* **3584**
Chronobiology International (USA) *Online - full text edition.* **3191**
Cladistics (GBR) *Online - full text edition.* **3191**
Clinical and Experimental Allergy (GBR) *Online - full text edition.* **3742**
Clinical and Experimental Dermatology (GBR) *Online - full text edition.* **3846**
Clinical and Experimental Hypertension (USA) *Online - full text edition.* **3768**
Clinical and Experimental Immunology (GBR) *Online - full text edition.* **3742**
Clinical and Experimental Metastasis (NLD) *Online - full text edition.* **3974**
Clinical and Experimental Ophthalmology (AUS) *Online - full text edition.* **3995**
Clinical and Experimental Pharmacology & Physiology (AUS) *Online - full text edition.* **3341**
Clinical and Laboratory Haematology (GBR) *Online - full text edition.* **3899**
Clinical Chemistry and Laboratory Medicine (DEU) *Online - full text edition.* **3247**
Clinical Child and Family Psychology Review (USA) *Online - full text edition.* **4387**
Clinical Child Psychology & Psychiatry (GBR) *Online - full text edition.* **3382**
Clinical Drug Investigation (NZL) *Online - full text edition.* **4283**
Clinical Endocrinology (GBR) *Online - full text edition.* **3856**
Clinical Genetics (DNK) *Online - full text edition.* **3300**
Clinical Hemorheology and Microcirculation (NLD) *Online - full text edition.* **3899**
Clinical Immunology (USA) *Online - full text edition.* **3743**
Clinical Linguistics & Phonetics (GBR) *Online - full text edition.* **4082**
Clinical Microbiology and Infection (GBR) *Online - full text edition.* **3586**
Clinical Nursing Research (USA) *Online - full text edition.* **3916**
Clinical Nutrition (GBR) *Online - full text edition.* **4231**
Clinical Otolaryngology and Allied Sciences (GBR) *Online - full text edition.* **4031**
Clinical Pharmacokinetics (NZL) *Online - full text edition.* **4284**
Clinical Physiology and Functional Imaging (GBR) *Online - full text edition.* **3587**
Clinical Psychology (USA) *Online - full text edition.* **4388**
Clinical Radiology (GBR) *Online - full text edition.* **4142**
Clinical Rehabilitation (GBR) *Online - full text edition.* **4060**
Clinical Transplantation (DNK) *Online - full text edition.* **4185**
The Clinician in Management (GBR) *Online - full text edition.* **3587**
Cloning and Stem Cells (USA) *Online - full text edition.* **3300**
Cognition and Emotion (GBR) *Online - full text edition.* **4388**
Cognition and Instruction (USA) *Online - full text edition.* **4388**
Cognitive Linguistics (DEU) *Online - full text edition.* **3550**
Cognitive Neuropsychiatry (GBR) *Online - full text edition.* **4389**
Cognitive Neuropsychology (GBR) *Online - full text edition.* **4083**
Cognitive Psychology (USA) *Online - full text edition.* **4389**
Cognitive Therapy and Research (USA) *Online - full text edition.* **4390**
College of Surgeons Hong Kong. Annals (AUS) *Online - full text edition.* **4185**
Colorectal Disease Online(GBR) *Online - full text.* **3887**
Community Genetics (CHE) *Online - full text edition.* **3300**
Community Mental Health Journal (USA) *Online - full text edition.* **4512**

Online Service

Comparative Political Studies (USA) *Online - full text edition.* **4367**
Conflict Resolution Quarterly (USA) *Online - full text edition.* **4390**
Consciousness and Cognition (USA) *Online - full text edition.* **4391**
Conservation Biology (USA) *Online - full text edition.* **3392**
Conservation Genetics (NLD) *Online - full text edition.* **3300**
Contact Dermatitis (DNK) *Online - full text edition.* **3846**
Contact Lens & Anterior Eye (GBR) *Online - full text edition.* **3995**
Contemporary Educational Psychology (USA) *Online - full text edition.* **3410**
Contemporary Family Therapy (USA) *Online - full text edition.* **4391**
Coronary Health Care (GBR) *Online - full text edition.* **3917**
Counselling Psychology Quarterly (GBR) *Online - full content edition.* **4392**
Creativity Research Journal (USA) *Online - full text edition.* **4392**
Criminal Justice & Behavior (USA) *Online - full text edition.* **3394**
Critical Public Health (GBR) *Online - full content edition.* **4466**
Critical Reviews in Biochemistry and Molecular Biology (USA) *Online - full text edition.* **3248**
Critical Reviews in Biotechnology (USA) *Online - full text edition.* **3273**
Critical Reviews in Clinical Laboratory Sciences (USA) *Online - full text edition.* **3591**
Critical Reviews in Diagnostic Imaging (USA) *Online - full text edition.* **4142**
Critical Reviews in Microbiology (USA) *Online - full text edition.* **3320**
Critical Reviews in Toxicology (USA) *Online - full text edition.* **3447**
Cross-Cultural Research (USA) *Online - full text edition.* **4508**
Cryobiology (USA) *Online - full text edition.* **3266**
Culture & Psychology (GBR) *Online - full text edition.* **4393**
Culture, Health and Sexuality (GBR) *Online - full text edition.* **4520**
Culture, Medicine and Psychiatry (NLD) *Online - full text edition.* **3173**
Current Anaesthesia and Critical Care (GBR) *Online - full text edition.* **3756**
Current Diagnostic Pathology (GBR) *Online - full text edition.* **3908**
Current Directions in Psychological Science (USA) *Online - full text edition.* **4393**
Current Eye Research (USA) *Online - full text edition.* **3996**
Current Obstetrics and Gynaecology (GBR) *Online - full text edition.* **3948**
Current Orthopaedics (GBR) *Online - full text edition.* **4013**
Current Paediatrics (GBR) *Online - full text edition.* **4043**
CyberPsychology & Behavior (USA) *Online - full text edition.* **3390**
Cytogenetic and Genome Research (CHE) *Online - full text edition.* **3301**
Cytokine (GBR) *Online - full text edition.* **3301**
Cytopathology (GBR) *Online - full text edition.* **3289**
Cytotechnology (NLD) *Online - full text edition.* **3289**
D N A and Cell Biology (USA) *Online - full text edition.* **3248**
Death Studies (USA) *Online - full text edition.* **4394**
Dementia and Geriatric Cognitive Disorders (CHE) *Online - full text edition.* **4085**
Dentomaxillofacial Radiology (GBR) *Online - full text edition.* **4143**
Dermatologic Surgery Online(USA) *Online - full text.* **4187**
Dermatologic Therapy (DNK) *Online - full text edition.* **3847**
Dermatology (CHE) *Online - full text edition.* **3847**
Dermatology and Psychosomatics (CHE) *Online - full text edition.* **3848**
Development and Psychopathology (GBR) *Online - full text edition.* **4394**
Development, Growth and Differentiation (AUS) *Online - full text edition.* **3192**
Developmental Biology (USA) *Online - full text edition.* **3193**
Developmental Medicine and Child Neurology (GBR) *Online - full text edition.* **4043**
Developmental Neuropsychology (USA) *Online - full text edition.* **4394**
Developmental Neuroscience (CHE) *Online - full text edition.* **4086**
Developmental Review (USA) *Online - full text edition.* **4394**
Developmental Science (GBR) *Online - full text edition.* **4394**
Deviant Behavior (USA) *Online - full text edition.* **4521**
Diabetes, Obesity and Metabolism Online(GBR) *Online - full text.* **3858**
Diabetes Technology & Therapeutics (USA) *Online - full text edition.* **3859**
Diabetic Medicine Online(GBR) *Online - full text.* **3860**
Digestion (CHE) *Online - full text edition.* **3888**
Digestive Diseases (CHE) *Online - full text edition.* **3888**
Digestive Diseases and Sciences (USA) *Online - full text edition.* **3888**
Digestive Endoscopy Online(AUS) *Online - full text.* **3889**
Digestive Surgery (CHE) *Online - full text edition.* **4187**
Disability and Rehabilitation (GBR) *Online - full text edition.* **3484**
Disability & Society (GBR) *Online - full text edition.* **3494**
Disaster Prevention and Management (GBR) *Online - full text edition.* **4466**
Discourse & Society (GBR) *Online - full text edition.* **4395**
Discourse Studies (GBR) *Online - full text edition.* **3550**
Disease Management & Health Outcomes (NZL) *Online - full text edition.* **3595**
Disease Markers (NLD) *Online - full text edition.* **3976**
Diseases of the Esophagus Online(AUS) *Online - full text.* **4032**
Documenta Ophthalmologica (NLD) *Online - full text edition.* **3997**
Dreaming (USA) *Online - full text edition.* **3342**
Drug and Alcohol Review (GBR) *Online - full text edition.* **3400**
Drug and Chemical Toxicology (USA) *Online - full text edition.* **4287**
Drug Delivery (USA) *Online - full text edition.* **4288**
Drug Development and Industrial Pharmacy (USA) *Online - full text edition.* **4288**
Drug Metabolism Reviews (USA) *Online - full text edition.* **3596**
Drug Safety (NZL) *Online - full text edition.* **4289**
Drugs (NZL) *Online - full text edition.* **4290**
Drugs & Aging (NZL) *Online - full text edition.* **4290**
Drugs: Education, Prevention & Policy (GBR) *Online - full text edition.* **3401**
e A D C - F & N (GBR) *Online - full text edition of* Archives of Disease in Childhood. Fetal and Neonatal Edition. **3945**
e-biomed(USA) *Online - full text.* **3596**
The E M B O Journal (GBR) *Online - full text edition.* **3249**
E M J Online (GBR) *Online - full text edition of* Emergency Medicine Journal. **4014**
Early Childhood Education Journal (USA) *Online - full text edition.* **3410**
Ecological Psychology (USA) *Online - full text edition.* **4396**
Ecotoxicology (USA) *Online - full text edition.* **3448**
Ecotoxicology and Environmental Safety - Online (USA) *Online - full text edition of* Ecotoxicology and Environmental Safety. **3448**
Education for Health (GBR) *Online - full text edition.* **3597**
Educational and Psychological Measurement (USA) *Online - full text edition.* **4396**
Educational Gerontology (USA) *Online - full text edition.* **3470**
Educational Psychologist (USA) *Online - full text edition.* **4396**
Educational Psychology (GBR) *Online - full text edition.* **3410**
Educational Psychology in Practice (GBR) *Online - full text edition.* **3410**
Educational Psychology Review (USA) *Online - full text edition.* **3411**
Electro- and Magnetobiology (USA) *Online - full text edition.* **3266**
Emergency Medicine (Carleton South) (AUS) *Online - full text edition.* **4013**
Emotional and Behavioural Difficulties (GBR) *Online - full text edition.* **3421**
Environment and Behavior (USA) *Online - full text edition.* **4521**
Environmental Management & Health (GBR) *Online - full text edition.* **3438**
Environmental Microbiology (GBR) *Online - full text edition.* **3321**
Environmental Research (USA) *Online - full text edition.* **3439**
Epidemiology and Infection (GBR) *Online - full text edition.* **3321**
Ergonomics (GBR) *Online - full text edition.* **3432**
Ergonomics Abstracts (GBR) *Online - full content edition.* **3433**
Ethics & Behavior (USA) *Online - full text edition.* **4397**
Ethnicity and Health (GBR) *Online - full text edition.* **4468**
Ethology Online(DEU) *Online - full text.* **3352**
Europace (GBR) *Online - full text edition.* **3771**
European Academy of Dermatology and Venereology. Journal (BEL) *Online - full text edition.* **3848**
European Addiction Research (CHE) *Online - full text edition.* **3401**
European Heart Journal (GBR) *Online - full text edition.* **3771**
European Journal of Anaesthesiology (GBR) *Online - full text edition.* **3757**
European Journal of Biochemistry (GBR) *Online - full text edition.* **3249**
European Journal of Cancer Care Online(GBR) *Online - full text.* **3977**
European Journal of Clinical Investigation (GBR) *Online - full text edition.* **3599**
European Journal of Clinical Nutrition (GBR) *Online - full text edition.* **4232**
European Journal of Cognitive Psychology (GBR) *Online - full text edition.* **4397**
European Journal of Echocardiography (GBR) *Online - full text edition.* **3771**
European Journal of Epidemiology (NLD) *Online - full text edition.* **3599**
European Journal of Health Law (NLD) *Online - full text edition.* **3600**
European Journal of Human Genetics (GBR) *Online - full text edition.* **3302**
European Journal of Immunogenetics (GBR) *Online - full text edition.* **3302**
European Journal of Morphology (NLD) *Online - full text edition.* **3195**
European Journal of Neurology (USA) *Online - full text edition.* **4089**
European Journal of Neuroscience (GBR) *Online - full text edition.* **4089**
European Journal of Oncology Nursing (GBR) *Online - full text edition.* **3919**
European Journal of Orthodontics (GBR) *Online - full content edition.* **3823**
European Journal of Paediatric Neurology (GBR) *Online - full text edition.* **4044**
European Journal of Pain (GBR) *Online - full text edition.* **3600**
European Journal of Surgery (NOR) *Online - full text edition.* **4188**
European Journal of Work and Organizational Psychology (GBR) *Online - full text edition.* **4398**
European Neurology (CHE) *Online - full text edition.* **4089**
The European Respiratory Journal (CHE) *Online - full text edition.* **4159**
European Surgical Research (CHE) *Online - full text edition.* **4189**
European Urology (CHE) *Online - full text edition.* **4212**
Evaluation and the Health Professions (USA) *Online - full text edition.* **3600**
Evidence - Based Cardiovascular Medicine (GBR) *Online - full text edition.* **3772**
Evidence - Based Nursing (GBR) *Online - full text edition.* **3919**
Evidence - Based Obstetrics & Gynaecology (GBR) *Online - full text edition.* **3949**
Evidence - Based Oncology (GBR) *Online - full text edition.* **3978**
Evolution & Development Online(USA) *Online - full text.* **3195**
Experimental Aging Research (USA) *Online - full text edition.* **4398**
Experimental & Applied Acarology (NLD) *Online - full text edition.* **3352**
Experimental and Molecular Pathology (USA) *Online - full text edition.* **3600**
Experimental Biology and Medicine (Maywood) (USA) *Online - full text edition.* **3195**
Experimental Eye Research (GBR) *Online - full text edition.* **3997**
Experimental Lung Research (USA) *Online - full text edition.* **4160**
Experimental Nephrology (CHE) *Online - full text edition.* **4212**
Experimental Neurology (USA) *Online - full text edition.* **4090**
Experimental Parasitology (USA) *Online - full text edition.* **3796**
Experimental Physiology (GBR) *Online - full text edition.* **3342**
Familial Cancer (NLD) *Online - full text edition.* **3978**
The Family Journal (USA) *Online - full text edition.* **4399**
Family Practice (GBR) *Online - full text edition.* **3601**
Feminism & Psychology (GBR) *Online - full text edition.* **4399**
Fetal and Maternal Medicine Review (GBR) *Online - full text edition.* **3950**
Fetal Diagnosis and Therapy (CHE) *Online - full text edition.* **3950**
Fibrinolysis & Proteolysis (GBR) *Online - full text edition.* **3875**
Fish and Shellfish Immunology (GBR) *Online - full text edition.* **3196**
Folia Phoniatrica et Logopaedica (CHE) *Online - full text edition.* **4032**
Food Additives and Contaminants (GBR) *Online - full text edition.* **4296**
Food and Agricultural Immunology (GBR) *Online - full text edition.* **3197**
Food Microbiology (GBR) *Online - full text edition.* **3322**
The Foot (GBR) *Online - full text edition.* **4015**
Foot and Ankle Surgery (GBR) *Online - full text edition.* **4189**
Forschende Komplementaermedizin und Klassische Naturheilkunde (CHE) *Online - full text edition.* **3165**
Freshwater Biology Online(GBR) *Online - full text.* **3197**
Frontiers in Neuroendocrinology (USA) *Online - full text edition.* **3862**
Games and Economic Behavior (USA) *Online - full text edition.* **4400**
Gay and Lesbian Medical Association. Journal (USA) *Online - full text edition.* **3605**
Gene Therapy (Basingstoke) (GBR) *Online - full text edition.* **3606**
General and Comparative Endocrinology (USA) *Online - full text edition.* **3863**
Genes to Cells (GBR) *Online - full text edition.* **3303**
Genetic Resources and Crop Evolution (NLD) *Online - full text edition.* **3304**
Genetic Testing (USA) *Online - full text edition.* **3304**
Genetica (NLD) *Online - full text edition.* **3305**
Genetical Research (GBR) *Online - full text edition.* **3305**
Genome (CAN) *Online - full text edition.* **3306**
Genomics (USA) *Online - full text edition.* **3306**
Geomicrobiology Journal (USA) *Online - full text edition.* **3322**
Gerontology (CHE) *Online - full text edition.* **3473**
Glycobiology (GBR) *Online - full text edition.* **3251**
Glycoconjugate Journal (USA) *Online - full text edition.* **3251**
Group Analysis (GBR) *Online - full text edition.* **4401**
Group & Organization Management (USA) *Online - full text edition.* **3411**
Group (New York) (USA) *Online - full text edition.* **4401**
Gynaecological Endoscopy (GBR) *Online - full text edition.* **3951**
Gynaekologisch - Geburtshilfliche Rundschau (CHE) *Online - full text edition.* **3951**
Gynecologic and Obstetric Investigation (CHE) *Online - full text edition.* **3952**
Gynecologic Oncology (USA) *Online - full text edition.* **3952**
H E C Forum (NLD) *Online - full text edition.* **3508**
H I V Medicine (GBR) *Online - full text edition.* **3796**
Haemophilia Online(GBR) *Online - full text.* **3901**
Harvard Review of Psychiatry (GBR) *Online - full text edition.* **4093**
Headache Online(USA) *Online - full text.* **4093**
Health (GBR) *Online - full text edition.* **4471**
Health Affairs (USA) *Online - full text edition.* **4471**
Health and Social Care in the Community Online(GBR) *Online - full text.* **4472**
Health Care Analysis (NLD) *Online - full text edition.* **3610**
Health Care for Women International (USA) *Online - full text edition.* **4563**

Health Care Management Science (NLD) *Online - full text edition.* **3509**
Health Communication (USA) *Online - full text edition.* **4472**
Health Education (GBR) *Online - full text edition.* **4354**
Health Education Research (GBR) *Online - full text edition.* **4513**
Health Expectations (GBR) *Online - full text edition.* **4473**
Health Information and Libraries Journal Online(GBR) *Online - full text.* **3547**
Health Policy and Planning (GBR) *Online - full text edition.* **4473**
Health Promotion International (GBR) *Online - full text edition.* **4474**
Health Promotion Practice (USA) *Online - full text edition.* **4474**
Health, Risk & Society (GBR) *Online - full text edition.* **4474**
Health Services and Outcomes Research Methodology (USA) *Online - full text edition.* **3612**
Heart Failure Reviews (USA) *Online - full text edition.* **3773**
Heart, Lung & Circulation Online(AUS) *Online - full text.* **3773**
Heart Online (GBR) *Online - full text edition of* Heart. **3772**
Helicobacter (USA) *Online - full text edition.* **3323**
Heredity (GBR) *Online - full text edition.* **3307**
High Altitude Medicine and Biology (USA) *Online - full content edition.* **3614**
Hispanic Journal of Behavioral Sciences (USA) *Online - full text edition.* **4402**
The Histochemical Journal (NLD) *Online - full text edition.* **3290**
Histopathology (GBR) *Online - full text edition.* **3979**
Homicide Studies (USA) *Online - full text edition.* **3394**
Hormone Research (CHE) *Online - full text edition.* **3863**
Hormones and Behavior (USA) *Online - full text edition.* **3863**
Human & Experimental Toxicology (GBR) *Online - full text edition.* **3450**
Human - Computer Interaction (Mahwah) (USA) *Online - full text edition.* **3389**
Human Development (CHE) *Online - full text edition.* **3616**
Human Ecology (New York) (USA) *Online - full text edition.* **3173**
Human Gene Therapy (USA) *Online - full text edition.* **3307**
Human Heredity (CHE) *Online - full text edition.* **3307**
Human Molecular Genetics (GBR) *Online - full text edition.* **3308**
Human Performance (USA) *Online - full text edition.* **4402**
Human Relations (USA) *Online - full text edition.* **4509**
Human Reproduction (GBR) *Online - full text edition.* **3953**
Human Reproduction Update (GBR) *Online - full text edition.* **3232**
Hybridoma (USA) *Online - full text edition.* **3251**
Hydrobiologia (NLD) *Online - full text edition.* **3199**
Hypertension in Pregnancy (USA) *Online - full text edition.* **3774**
I U B M B Life (AUS) *Online - full text edition.* **3251**
Illness, Crisis, and Loss (USA) *Online - full text edition.* **4521**
Immunology (GBR) *Online - full text edition.* **3746**
Immunology and Cell Biology (AUS) *Online - full text edition.* **3746**
Indoor and Built Environment (CHE) *Online - full text edition.* **3747**
Inflammation (USA) *Online - full text edition.* **3620**
Infusion Therapy and Transfusion Medicine (CHE) *Online - full text edition.* **3620**
Inhalation Toxicology (USA) *Online - full text edition.* **3451**
Injury Prevention (GBR) *Online - full text edition.* **4045**
Injury Prevention and Safety Promotion (NLD) *Online - full text edition.* **3393**
Institution of Mechanical Engineers. Proceedings. Part H: Journal of Engineering in Medicine (GBR) *Online - full text edition.* **3238**
Instrumentation Science & Technology (USA) *Online - full text edition.* **3376**
International Archives of Allergy and Immunology (CHE) *Online - full text edition.* **3747**
International Endodontic Journal Online(GBR) *Online - full text.* **3826**
International Forum of Psychoanalysis (NOR) *Online - full text edition.* **4405**
International Immunology (GBR) *Online - full text edition.* **3747**
International Journal for Quality in Health Care (GBR) *Online - full text edition.* **3622**
The International Journal for the Psychology of Religion (USA) *Online - full text edition.* **4500**
International Journal of Andrology (GBR) *Online - full text edition.* **4213**
The International Journal of Aviation Psychology (USA) *Online - full text edition.* **4532**
International Journal of Behavioral Development (GBR) *Online - full text edition.* **4405**
International Journal of Behavioral Medicine (USA) *Online - full text edition.* **4405**
International Journal of Cardiovascular Imaging (NLD) *Online - full text edition.* **3775**
International Journal of Cognitive Ergonomics (USA) *Online - full text edition.* **4406**
International Journal of Cosmetic Science (GBR) *Online - full text edition.* **3176**
International Journal of Dermatology (GBR) *Online - full text edition.* **3850**
International Journal of Disability, Development and Education (GBR) *Online - full text edition.* **3423**
International Journal of Environmental Health Research (GBR) *Online - full text edition.* **3439**
International Journal of Epidemiology (GBR) *Online - full text edition.* **3623**
International Journal of Experimental Pathology (GBR) *Online - full text edition.* **3623**
International Journal of Food Sciences and Nutrition (GBR) *Online - full text edition.* **4236**
International Journal of Group Tensions (USA) *Online - full text edition.* **4406**
International Journal of Gynecological Cancer (USA) *Online - full text edition.* **3953**
International Journal of Health Care Quality Assurance (GBR) *Online - full text edition.* **3623**
International Journal of Hyperthermia (GBR) *Online - full text edition.* **3980**
International Journal of Impotence Research (GBR) *Online - full text edition.* **4213**
International Journal of Language and Communication Disorders (GBR) *Online - full text edition.* **4033**
International Journal of Neuro-Psychopharmacology (GBR) *Online - full text edition.* **4303**
International Journal of Nursing Practice (AUS) *Online - full text edition.* **3921**
International Journal of Obesity (GBR) *Online - full text edition.* **4236**
International Journal of Offender Therapy and Comparative Criminology (USA) *Online - full text edition.* **3394**
International Journal of Oral & Maxillofacial Surgery (DNK) *Online - full text edition.* **3827**
International Journal of Pest Management (GBR) *Online - full text edition.* **3158**
International Journal of Psychology (GBR) *Online - full text edition.* **4407**
International Journal of Psychotherapy (GBR) *Online - full content edition.* **4096**
International Journal of Radiation Biology (GBR) *Online - full text edition.* **3980**
International Journal of Rehabilitation and Health (USA) *Online - full text edition.* **3485**
The International Journal of Risk and Safety in Medicine (NLD) *Online - full text edition.* **3532**
International Journal of S T D & AIDS (GBR) *Online - full text edition.* **3800**
International Journal of Stress Management (USA) *Online - full text edition.* **3624**
International Journal of Toxicology (GBR) *Online - full text edition.* **3451**
International Journal of Urology (AUS) *Online - full text edition.* **4213**
International Neuropsychological Society. Journal (GBR) *Online - full text edition.* **4097**
International Nursing Review Online(GBR) *Online - full text.* **3922**
International Ophthalmology (NLD) *Online - full text edition.* **3999**
International Review of Psychiatry (GBR) *Online - full text edition.* **4097**
International Urology and Nephrology (HUN) *Online - full text edition.* **4214**
Intervirology (CHE) *Online - full text edition.* **3324**
Investigational New Drugs (USA) *Online - full text edition.* **4304**
Issues in Comprehensive Pediatric Nursing (USA) *Online - full text edition.* **3922**
Issues in Interdisciplinary Care (USA) *Online - full text edition.* **3625**
Issues in Mental Health Nursing (USA) *Online - full text edition.* **3922**
J C P Online (GBR) *Online - full text edition of* Journal of Clinical Pathology. **3631**
J E C H Online (GBR) *Online - full text edition of* Journal of Epidemiology & Community Health. **3632**
J M B Online (GBR) *Online - full text edition of* Journal of Molecular Biology. **3254**
J M E Online (GBR) *Online - full text edition of* Journal of Medical Ethics. **3635**
J M G Online (GBR) *Online - full text edition of* Journal of Medical Genetics. **3310**
J M S Online (GBR) *Online - full text edition of* Journal of Medical Screening. **3802**
Japanese Journal of Clinical Oncology (GBR) *Online - full text edition.* **3981**
Japanese Psychological Research (JPN) *Online - full text edition.* **4408**
Journal for the Theory of Social Behaviour (GBR) *Online - full text edition.* **4408**
Journal of Abnormal Child Psychology (USA) *Online - full text edition.* **4409**
Journal of Adolescence (GBR) *Online - full text edition.* **3383**
Journal of Adolescent Research (USA) *Online - full text edition.* **4409**
Journal of Adult Development (USA) *Online - full text edition.* **4409**
Journal of Advanced Nursing (GBR) *Online - full text edition.* **3923**
Journal of Aging and Health (USA) *Online - full text edition.* **3474**
Journal of Aging & Identity (USA) *Online - full text edition.* **3475**
Journal of Analytical Psychology (GBR) *Online - full text edition.* **4409**
Journal of Anatomy (GBR) *Online - full text edition.* **3202**
Journal of Animal Ecology (GBR) *Online - full text edition.* **3202**
Journal of Animal Physiology and Animal Nutrition Online(DEU) *Online - full text.* **3344**
Journal of Antimicrobial Chemotherapy (GBR) *Online - full text edition.* **3800**
Journal of Applied Animal Welfare Science (USA) *Online - full text edition.* **3172**
Journal of Applied Microbiology (GBR) *Online - full text edition.* **3324**
Journal of Applied Psychoanalytic Studies (USA) *Online - full text edition.* **4410**
Journal of Applied Research in Intellectual Disabilities (GBR) *Online - full text edition.* **4098**
Journal of Assisted Reproduction and Genetics (USA) *Online - full text edition.* **3955**
Journal of Audio Visual Media in Medicine (GBR) *Online - full text edition.* **3629**
Journal of Autism and Developmental Disorders (USA) *Online - full text edition.* **3423**
Journal of Autoimmunity (GBR) *Online - full text edition.* **3748**
Journal of Behavioral Education (USA) *Online - full text edition.* **3412**
Journal of Behavioral Medicine (USA) *Online - full text edition.* **4099**
Journal of Bioenergetics and Biomembranes (USA) *Online - full text edition.* **3253**
Journal of Biological Rhythms (USA) *Online - full text edition.* **4099**
Journal of Biomedical Informatics (USA) *Online - full text edition.* **3811**
Journal of Biomedical Science (CHE) *Online - full text edition.* **3630**
Journal of Biopharmaceutical Statistics (USA) *Online - full text edition.* **4345**
Journal of Biosocial Science (GBR) *Online - full text edition.* **4521**
Journal of Black Studies (USA) *Online - full text edition.* **4509**
Journal of Business & Psychology (USA) *Online - full text edition.* **4411**
Journal of Child and Family Studies (USA) *Online - full text edition.* **4411**
Journal of Child Language (GBR) *Online - full text edition.* **3384**
Journal of Child Psychology & Psychiatry & Allied Disciplines (GBR) *Online - full text edition.* **4411**
Journal of Child Psychotherapy (GBR) *Online - full text edition.* **4411**
Journal of Clinical Child and Adolescent Psychology (USA) *Online - full text edition.* **4411**
Journal of Clinical Geropsychology (USA) *Online - full text edition.* **3475**
Journal of Clinical Immunology (USA) *Online - full text edition.* **3748**
Journal of Clinical Monitoring and Computing (NLD) *Online - full text edition.* **3631**
Journal of Clinical Neuroscience (GBR) *Online - full text edition.* **4100**
Journal of Clinical Nursing (GBR) *Online - full text edition.* **3923**
Journal of Clinical Pharmacology (USA) *Online - full text edition.* **4306**
Journal of Clinical Pharmacy and Therapeutics (GBR) *Online - full text edition.* **4306**
Journal of Clinical Psychology in Medical Settings (USA) *Online - full text edition.* **4412**
Journal of Cognition and Development (USA) *Online - full text edition.* **4412**
Journal of Cognitive Neuroscience (USA) *Online - full text edition.* **4100**
Journal of Communication Inquiry (USA) *Online - full text edition.* **4522**
Journal of Community Health (USA) *Online - full text edition.* **3631**
Journal of Community Health Nursing (USA) *Online - full text edition.* **3924**
Journal of Computational Neuroscience (NLD) *Online - full text edition.* **4100**
Journal of Constructivist Psychology (USA) *Online - full text edition.* **4413**
Journal of Consumer Psychology (USA) *Online - full text edition.* **3153**
Journal of Contemporary Psychotherapy (USA) *Online - full text edition.* **4413**
Journal of Cranio-Maxillo-Facial Surgery (GBR) *Online - full text edition.* **4192**
Journal of Cross-Cultural Gerontology (NLD) *Online - full text edition.* **3475**
The Journal of Deaf Studies and Deaf Education (USA) *Online - full text edition.* **3491**
Journal of Developmental and Physical Disabilities (USA) *Online - full text edition.* **3485**
Journal of Early Adolescence (USA) *Online - full text edition.* **3384**
Journal of Ecology (GBR) *Online - full text edition.* **3203**
Journal of Educational and Psychological Consultation (USA) *Online - full text edition.* **3412**
Journal of English Linguistics (USA) *Online - full text edition.* **3550**
Journal of Environmental Psychology (GBR) *Online - full text edition.* **4415**
Journal of Evaluation in Clinical Practice Online(GBR) *Online - full text.* **3632**
Journal of Evolutionary Biology (GBR) *Online - full text edition.* **3309**
Journal of Experimental Child Psychology (USA) *Online - full text edition.* **4415**
Journal of Experimental Social Psychology (USA) *Online - full text edition.* **4415**
Journal of Exposure Analysis and Environmental Epidemiology (GBR) *Online - full text edition.* **3440**
Journal of Family and Economic Issues (USA) *Online - full text edition.* **4416**
Journal of Family Nursing (USA) *Online - full content edition.* **3924**
Journal of Family Therapy (GBR) *Online - full text edition.* **4101**
Journal of Family Violence (USA) *Online - full text edition.* **3395**
Journal of Forensic Psychiatry (GBR) *Online - full text edition.* **4101**
Journal of Gambling Studies (USA) *Online - full text edition.* **4101**
Journal of Gastroenterology and Hepatology (AUS) *Online - full text edition.* **3893**
Journal of General Internal Medicine (USA) *Online - full text edition.* **3910**
Journal of Genetic Counseling (USA) *Online - full text edition.* **4416**
Journal of Hand Surgery: American Volume (USA) *Online - full content edition.* **4193**
Journal of Hand Surgery: British and European Volume (GBR) *Online - full text edition.* **4193**
Journal of Health Communication (USA) *Online - full text edition.* **3633**
Journal of Health Politics, Policy and Law (USA) *Online - full text edition.* **3633**

Online Service

Journal of Health Psychology (GBR) *Online - full text edition.* **4417**
Journal of Hematotherapy & Stem Cell Research (USA) *Online - full text edition.* **3903**
Journal of Hospital Infection (GBR) *Online - full text edition.* **3801**
Journal of Human Evolution (GBR) *Online - full text edition.* **3309**
Journal of Human Hypertension (GBR) *Online - full text edition.* **3778**
Journal of Human Lactation (USA) *Online - full text edition.* **3955**
Journal of Human Nutrition and Dietetics (GBR) *Online - full text edition.* **4237**
Journal of Humanistic Psychology (USA) *Online - full text edition.* **4417**
Journal of Immigrant Health (USA) *Online - full text edition.* **3634**
Journal of Industrial Microbiology and Biotechnology (GBR) *Online - full text edition.* **3276**
Journal of Infection (GBR) *Online - full text edition.* **3801**
Journal of Inherited Metabolic Disease (NLD) *Online - full text edition.* **4046**
Journal of Intellectual Disability Research (GBR) *Online - full text edition.* **4102**
Journal of Intensive Care Medicine (USA) *Online - full text edition.* **3634**
Journal of Interferon & Cytokine Research (USA) *Online - full text edition.* **3749**
Journal of Internal Medicine (GBR) *Online - full text edition.* **3910**
Journal of Interpersonal Violence (USA) *Online - full text edition.* **3395**
Journal of Interprofessional Care (GBR) *Online - full text edition.* **3634**
Journal of Interventional Cardiac Electrophysiology (NLD) *Online - full text edition.* **3778**
The Journal of Investigative Dermatology (USA) *Online - full text edition.* **3851**
Journal of Investigative Surgery (USA) *Online - full text edition.* **4193**
Journal of Language and Social Psychology (USA) *Online - full text edition.* **4417**
Journal of Laryngology and Otology (GBR) *Online - full content edition.* **4034**
The Journal of Legal Medicine (USA) *Online - full text edition.* **3634**
Journal of Lower Genital Tract Disease Online(USA) *Online - full text.* **3956**
Journal of Mammalian Evolution (USA) *Online - full text edition.* **3354**
Journal of Mammary Gland Biology and Neoplasia (USA) *Online - full text edition.* **3345**
Journal of Management in Medicine (GBR) *Online - full text edition.* **3634**
Journal of Managerial Psychology (GBR) *Online - full text edition.* **3365**
Journal of Materials Science: Materials in Medicine (USA) *Online - full text edition.* **3434**
Journal of Mathematical Psychology (USA) *Online - full text edition.* **4418**
Journal of Medical Engineering & Technology (GBR) *Online - full text edition.* **3635**
Journal of Medical Humanities (USA) *Online - full text edition.* **3635**
Journal of Medical Systems (USA) *Online - full text edition.* **3812**
The Journal of Medicine and Philosophy (NLD) *Online - full text edition.* **3636**
Journal of Memory and Language (USA) *Online - full text edition.* **3550**
Journal of Mental Health (GBR) *Online - full text edition.* **4102**
Journal of Microencapsulation (GBR) *Online - full text edition.* **4308**
Journal of Microscopy (GBR) *Online - full text edition.* **3334**
Journal of Molecular and Cellular Cardiology (GBR) *Online - full text edition.* **3778**
Journal of Molecular Neuroscience (USA) *Online - full text edition.* **4102**
Journal of Muscle Research and Cell Motility (NLD) *Online - full text edition.* **4018**
Journal of Natural History (GBR) *Online - full text edition.* **3204**
Journal of Near-Death Studies (USA) *Online - full text edition.* **4347**
Journal of Neuro-Oncology (USA) *Online - full text edition.* **3982**
Journal of Neurocytology (USA) *Online - full text edition.* **3291**
Journal of Neuroendocrinology Online(GBR) *Online - full text.* **4103**
Journal of Neurology, Neurosurgery and Psychiatry (GBR) *Online - full text edition.* **4104**
Journal of NeuroVirology (GBR) *Online - full text edition.* **4105**
Journal of Nonverbal Behavior (USA) *Online - full text edition.* **4418**
Journal of Nursing Management (GBR) *Online - full text edition.* **3925**
Journal of Nutritional & Environmental Medicine (GBR) *Online - full text edition.* **4237**
Journal of Obstetrics and Gynaecology (GBR) *Online - full text edition.* **3956**
Journal of Occupational Rehabilitation (USA) *Online - full text edition.* **4258**
Journal of Oncology Pharmacy Practice (USA) *Online - full text edition.* **4308**
The Journal of Orthodontics (GBR) *Online - full text edition.* **3830**
Journal of Paediatrics and Child Health (AUS) *Online - full text edition.* **4047**
Journal of Pediatric Psychology (GBR) *Online - full text edition.* **4419**
Journal of Peptide Research (DNK) *Online - full text edition.* **3255**
Journal of Perinatal Medicine (DEU) *Online - full text edition.* **3956**
Journal of Perinatology (GBR) *Online - full text edition.* **3956**
Journal of Personality (USA) *Online - full text edition.* **4419**
Journal of Personality Assessment (USA) *Online - full text edition.* **4420**
Journal of Pharmacokinetics and Pharmacodynamics (USA) *Online - full text edition.* **4310**
Journal of Physiology (GBR) *Online - full text edition.* **3345**
Journal of Plankton Research (GBR) *Online - full text edition.* **3204**
Journal of Poetry Therapy (USA) *Online - full text edition.* **3553**
The Journal of Primary Prevention (USA) *Online - full text edition.* **4420**
Journal of Protein Chemistry (USA) *Online - full text edition.* **3255**
Journal of Psychiatric & Mental Health Nursing Online(GBR) *Online - full text.* **4105**
Journal of Psycholinguistic Research (USA) *Online - full text edition.* **3551**
Journal of Psychology and Financial Markets (USA) *Online - full content edition.* **4421**
Journal of Psychology and Judaism (USA) *Online - full text edition.* **4501**
Journal of Psychopathology and Behavioral Assessment (USA) *Online - full text edition.* **4421**
Journal of Psychopharmacology (GBR) *Online - full text edition.* **4310**
Journal of Public Health Medicine (GBR) *Online - full text edition.* **4515**
Journal of Quality in Clinical Practice (AUS) *Online - full text edition.* **3637**
Journal of Radiosurgery (USA) *Online - full text edition.* **4194**
Journal of Rational - Emotive and Cognitive - Behavior Therapy (USA) *Online - full text edition.* **4421**
Journal of Rehabilitation Medicine (NOR) *Online - full text edition.* **4515**
Journal of Religion and Health (USA) *Online - full text edition.* **4500**
Journal of Reproductive and Infant Psychology (GBR) *Online - full text edition.* **4421**
Journal of Research in Personality (USA) *Online - full text edition.* **4422**
Journal of Risk and Uncertainty (USA) *Online - full text edition.* **3363**
Journal of Sex & Marital Therapy (USA) *Online - full text edition.* **4422**
Journal of Social and Personal Relationships (GBR) *Online - full content edition.* **4423**
Journal of Social Distress and the Homeless (USA) *Online - full text edition.* **4515**
Journal of Social Issues (USA) *Online - full content edition.* **4423**
Journal of Social Work Practice (GBR) *Online - full text edition.* **4515**
Journal of Sports Sciences (GBR) *Online - full text edition.* **4525**
Journal of Structural Biology (USA) *Online - full text edition.* **3205**
Journal of Surgical Research (USA) *Online - full text edition.* **4195**
Journal of Telemedicine and Telecare (GBR) *Online - full text edition.* **3638**
Journal of the History of Biology (NLD) *Online - full text edition.* **3205**
Journal of the History of Medicine and Allied Sciences (GBR) *Online - full text edition.* **3638**
Journal of the History of the Neurosciences (NLD) *Online - full content edition.* **4106**
Journal of the Learning Sciences (USA) *Online - full text edition.* **3413**
Journal of the Peripheral Nervous System Online(USA) *Online - full text.* **4107**
Journal of Theoretical Biology (GBR) *Online - full text edition.* **3205**
Journal of Thrombosis and Thrombolysis (USA) *Online - full text edition.* **3779**
Journal of Toxicology and Environmental Health. Part B: Critical Reviews (USA) *Online - full text edition.* **3452**
Journal of Toxicology. Clinical Toxicology (USA) *Online - full text edition.* **4311**
Journal of Toxicology. Toxin Reviews (USA) *Online - full text edition.* **4311**
Journal of Transcultural Nursing (USA) *Online - full content edition.* **3927**
Journal of Traumatic Stress (USA) *Online - full text edition.* **4424**
Journal of Tropical Pediatrics (GBR) *Online - full text edition.* **4047**
Journal of Vascular Research (CHE) *Online - full text edition.* **3779**
Journal of Veterinary Medicine. Series A Online(DEU) *Online - full text.* **4547**
Journal of Veterinary Medicine. Series B Online(DEU) *Online - full text.* **4547**
Journal of Viral Hepatitis (GBR) *Online - full text edition.* **3893**
Journal of Vocational Behavior (USA) *Online - full text edition.* **4424**
Journal of Women's Health and Gender-Based Medicine (USA) *Online - full text edition.* **4564**
Journal of Youth and Adolescence (USA) *Online - full text edition.* **3384**
Journal of Youth Studies (GBR) *Online - full text edition.* **3384**
Journal of Zoological Systematics and Evolutionary Research Online(DEU) *Online - full text.* **3355**
Kennedy Institute of Ethics. Journal (USA) *Online - full text edition.* **3640**
Kidney and Blood Pressure Research (CHE) *Online - full text edition.* **4215**
Kidney International Online (USA) *Online - full text edition of* Kidney International. **4215**
Language and Cognitive Processes (GBR) *Online - full text edition.* **3551**
Laterality (GBR) *Online - full text edition.* **4107**
Law and Human Behavior (USA) *Online - full text edition.* **3541**
Learning and Motivation (USA) *Online - full text edition.* **3413**
Leisure Sciences (USA) *Online - full text edition.* **3547**
Letters in Applied Microbiology (GBR) *Online - full text edition.* **3326**
Leukemia (GBR) *Online - full text edition.* **3903**
Linnean Society. Biological Journal (GBR) *Online - full text edition.* **3206**
Literature & Medicine (USA) *Online - full text edition.* **3552**
Liver (DNK) *Online - full text edition.* **3894**
Logopedics Phoniatrics Vocology (NOR) *Online - full text edition.* **4035**
Loss Prevention Bulletin (GBR) *Online - full content edition.* **3433**
Lupus (GBR) *Online - full text edition.* **4169**
M P Online (GBR) *Online - full text edition of* Molecular Pathology. **3879**
Manual Therapy (GBR) *Online - full text edition.* **4063**
Marine Biological Association of the United Kingdom. Journal (GBR) *Online - full text edition.* **3207**
Maternal and Child Health Journal (USA) *Online - full text edition.* **3957**
Mathematical Cognition (GBR) *Online - full text edition.* **4426**
Mathematical Thinking and Learning (USA) *Online - full text edition.* **3554**
Measurement in Physical Education and Exercise Science (USA) *Online - full text edition.* **4358**
Media Psychology (USA) *Online - full text edition.* **4426**
Mediators of Inflammation (GBR) *Online - full text edition.* **3648**
Medical & Veterinary Entomology Online(GBR) *Online - full text.* **3648**
Medical Care Research and Review (USA) *Online - full text edition.* **4496**
Medical Education (GBR) *Online - full text edition.* **3650**
Medical Informatics and the Internet in Medicine (GBR) *Online - full text edition.* **3812**
Medical Law Review (GBR) *Online - full text edition.* **3542**
Medical Mycology (GBR) *Online - full text edition.* **3803**
Medical Oncology (GBR) *Online - full text edition.* **3984**
Medical Principles and Practice (CHE) *Online - full text edition.* **3652**
Medical Teacher (GBR) *Online - full text edition.* **3654**
Medicine, Health Care and Philosophy (NLD) *Online - full text edition.* **3656**
Memory (GBR) *Online - full text edition.* **4426**
Mental Health, Religion & Culture (GBR) *Online - full content edition.* **4427**
Mental Health Services Research (USA) *Online - full text edition.* **4427**
Metabolic Brain Disease (USA) *Online - full text edition.* **3660**
Metabolic Engineering (USA) *Online - full text edition.* **3238**
Metaphor and Symbol (USA) *Online - full text edition.* **3551**
Methods: A Companion to Methods in Enzymology (USA) *Online - full text edition.* **3256**
Methods in Cell Science (NLD) *Online - full text edition.* **3292**
Microbial Ecology in Health & Disease (NOR) *Online - full text edition.* **3803**
Microbial Pathogenesis (GBR) *Online - full text edition.* **3804**
Microcirculation (GBR) *Online - full text edition.* **3661**
Microvascular Research (USA) *Online - full text edition.* **3780**
Midwifery (GBR) *Online - full text edition.* **3958**
The Milbank Quarterly (USA) *Online - full text edition.* **4368**
Military Psychology (USA) *Online - full text edition.* **4428**
Mitigation and Adaptation Strategies for Global Change (NLD) *Online - full text edition.* **3441**
Molecular and Cellular Biochemistry (USA) *Online - full text edition.* **3257**
Molecular and Cellular Neurosciences (USA) *Online - full text edition.* **4110**
Molecular and Cellular Probes (GBR) *Online - full text edition.* **3879**
Molecular Biology Reports (NLD) *Online - full text edition.* **3257**
Molecular Biotechnology (USA) *Online - full text edition.* **3276**
Molecular Cell Biology Research Communications (USA) *Online - full text edition.* **3292**
Molecular Genetics and Metabolism (USA) *Online - full text edition.* **3662**
Molecular Human Reproduction (GBR) *Online - full text edition.* **3958**
Molecular Membrane Biology (GBR) *Online - full text edition.* **3258**
Molecular Phylogenetics and Evolution (USA) *Online - full text edition.* **3311**
Molecular Plant Pathology (GBR) *Online - full text edition.* **3281**
Molecular Psychiatry (GBR) *Online - full text edition.* **4110**
Molecular Therapy (USA) *Online - full text edition.* **3984**
Mortality (GBR) *Online - full content edition.* **4482**
Motivation and Emotion (USA) *Online - full text edition.* **4428**
Multiple Sclerosis (GBR) *Online - full text edition.* **4111**
Multivariate Behavioral Research (USA) *Online - full text edition.* **4428**
Mutagenesis (GBR) *Online - full text edition.* **3311**
Mycopathologia (NLD) *Online - full text edition.* **3281**
Mycoses (DEU) *Online - full text edition.* **3663**
National Cancer Institute. Journal (USA) *Online - full text edition.* **3985**
NeoPlasia (USA) *Online - full text edition.* **3985**
Nephrology, Dialysis and Transplantation (GBR) *Online - full text edition.* **4216**
Nephron (CHE) *Online - full text edition.* **4216**
Neural Processing Letters (USA) *Online - full text edition.* **3390**
Neuro-Ophthalmology (NLD) *Online - full text edition.* **4112**
Neurobiology of Disease (USA) *Online - full text edition.* **4112**
Neurobiology of Learning and Memory (USA) *Online - full text edition.* **4112**

Social Psychology of Education (NLD) *Online - full text edition.* **3415**
Sociology of Health and Illness (GBR) *Online - full text edition.* **4523**
Somatic Cell and Molecular Genetics (USA) *Online - full text edition.* **3314**
Somatosensory and Motor Research (GBR) *Online - full text edition.* **3349**
Spatial Cognition and Computation (NLD) *Online - full text edition.* **4450**
Spinal Cord (GBR) *Online - full text edition.* **4134**
Sports Medicine (NZL) *Online - full text edition.* **4177**
Statistical Methods in Medical Research (GBR) *Online - full text edition.* **4530**
Stereotactic and Functional Neurosurgery (CHE) *Online - full text edition.* **4204**
Strabismus (NLD) *Online - full text edition.* **4007**
Structural Equation Modeling (USA) *Online - full text edition.* **4451**
Substance Abuse (USA) *Online - full text edition.* **3406**
Support for Learning (GBR) *Online - full text edition.* **3427**
Surgical Infections (USA) *Online - full content edition.* **4204**
Systematic Parasitology (NLD) *Online - full text edition.* **3220**
Teaching and Learning in Medicine (USA) *Online - full text edition.* **3698**
Teaching of Psychology (USA) *Online - full text edition.* **4452**
Technology and Health Care (NLD) *Online - full text edition.* **3698**
Telemedicine Journal and e-Health (USA) *Online - full text edition.* **3812**
Theoretical Issues in Ergonomics Science (GBR) *Online - full text edition.* **3433**
Theoretical Medicine and Bioethics (NLD) *Online - full text edition.* **3699**
Theoretical Population Biology (USA) *Online - full text edition.* **3221**
Theory & Psychology (GBR) *Online - full text edition.* **4452**
Theory in Biosciences (DEU) *Online - full text edition.* **3221**
Therapeutic Apheresis Online(USA) *Online - full text.* **4218**
Thinking & Reasoning (GBR) *Online - full text edition.* **4452**
Thorax Online (GBR) *Online - full text edition of* Thorax. **3700**
Tissue Antigens (DNK) *Online - full text edition.* **3701**
Tissue Engineering (USA) *Online - full content edition.* **3294**
Tobbacco Control Online (GBR) *Online - full text edition of* Tobacco Control. **4531**
Topoi (NLD) *Online - full text edition.* **4348**
Toxicology and Applied Pharmacology (USA) *Online - full text edition.* **3455**
Toxicology and Industrial Health (GBR) *Online - full text edition.* **3455**
Toxicology Methods (USA) *Online - full text edition.* **3456**
Traffic (DNK) *Online - full text edition.* **3294**
Transcultural Psychiatry (GBR) *Online - full text edition.* **4136**
Transfusion Medicine (GBR) *Online - full text edition.* **3905**
Transgenic Research (NLD) *Online - full text edition.* **3314**
Transplant Infectious Disease Online(DNK) *Online - full text.* **4206**
Trauma(GBR) *Online - full text.* **4027**
Trauma, Violence & Abuse (USA) *Online - full text edition.* **4491**
Tropical Animal Health and Production (NLD) *Online - full text edition.* **4554**
Tropical Medicine & International Health Online (GBR) *Online - full text edition of* Tropical Medicine & International Health. **4491**
Tumor Biology (CHE) *Online - full text edition.* **3991**
Twin Research (GBR) *Online - full text edition.* **3315**
Ultrasound in Obstetrics & Gynecology (GBR) *Online - full text edition.* **3965**
Ultrastructural Pathology (USA) *Online - full text edition.* **3991**
Urologia Internationalis (CHE) *Online - full text edition.* **4219**
Value in Health (USA) *Online - full text edition.* **4339**
Vascular Medicine (GBR) *Online - full text edition.* **3784**
Verhaltenstherapie (CHE) *Online - full content edition.* **4137**
Veterinary Anaesthesia and Analgesia Online (GBR) *Online - full text edition of* Veterinary Anaesthesia and Analgesia. **4556**
Veterinary Ophthalmology Online (GBR) *Online - full text edition of* Veterinary Ophthalmology. **4558**
Veterinary Research Communications (NLD) *Online - full text edition.* **4559**
Violence Against Women (USA) *Online - full text edition.* **4524**
Violence & Abuse Abstracts (USA) *Online - full text edition.* **4524**
Virology (USA) *Online - full text edition.* **3332**
Virus Genes (USA) *Online - full text edition.* **3332**
Visual Cognition (GBR) *Online - full text edition.* **4454**
Visual Impairment Research (NLD) *Online - full text edition.* **3500**
Visual Neuroscience (GBR) *Online - full text edition.* **4137**
Vox Sanguinis (CHE) *Online - full text edition.* **3752**
Western Journal of Nursing Research (USA) *Online - full text edition.* **3943**
Work and Stress (GBR) *Online - full text edition.* **4455**
World Journal of Microbiology and Biotechnology (GBR) *Online - full text edition.* **3278**
Wound Repair and Regeneration (USA) *Online - full text edition.* **4028**
Xenobiotica (GBR) *Online - full text edition.* **3264**
Xenotransplantation (DNK) *Online - full text edition.* **4207**
Zygote (GBR) *Online - full text edition.* **3315**

Ovid Technologies, Incorporated 333 Seventh Ave., New York, NY 10001 TEL 212-563-3006, 800-950-2035, FAX 212-563-3784, http://www.ovid.com
A A C N Clinical Issues (USA) *Online - full text edition.* **3555**
A N Z Journal of Surgery (AUS) *Online - full text edition.* **4178**
A O R N Journal (USA) *Online - full text edition.* **3912**
A P M I S (DNK) *Online - full text edition.* **3178**
A P M I S Supplementum (DNK) *Online - full text edition.* **3178**
A R D Online (GBR) *Online - full text edition of* Annals of the Rheumatic Diseases. **4167**
A S A I O Journal (USA) *Online - full text edition.* **3556**
Acta Anaesthesiologica Scandinavica (DNK) *Online - full text edition.* **3753**
Acta Anaesthesiologica Scandinavica. Supplementum (DNK) *Online - full text edition.* **3753**
Acta Neurologica Scandinavica (DNK) *Online - full text edition.* **4068**
Acta Neurologica Scandinavica. Supplementum (DNK) *Online - full text edition.* **4068**
Acta Obstetrica et Gynecologica Scandinavica (DNK) *Online - full text edition.* **3944**
Acta Obstetrica et Gynecologica Scandinavica. Supplement (DNK) *Online - full text edition.* **3944**
Acta Physiologica Scandinavica (GBR) *Online - full text edition.* **3337**
Acta Physiologica Scandinavica. Supplementum (GBR) *Online - full text edition.* **3337**
Acta Psychiatrica Scandinavica (DNK) *Online - full text edition.* **4068**
Acta Psychiatrica Scandinavica. Supplementum (DNK) *Online - full text edition.* **4069**
Acta Radiologica (DNK) *Online - full text edition.* **4139**
Acta Radiologica. Supplementum (DNK) *Online - full text edition.* **4139**
Advances in Nursing Science (USA) *Online - full text edition.* **3912**
AIDS (USA) *Online - full text edition.* **3790**
AIDS Patient Care and S T Ds (USA) *Online - full text edition.* **3791**
Alcoholism: Clinical and Experimental Research (USA) *Online - full text edition.* **3398**
Alimentary Pharmacology and Therapeutics (GBR) *Online - full text edition.* **3886**
Alimentary Pharmacology and Therapeutics. Supplement (GBR) *Online - full text edition.* **3886**
Allergy (DNK) *Online - full text edition.* **3739**
Allergy. Supplementum (DNK) *Online - full text edition.* **3740**
Alzheimer Disease and Associated Disorders (USA) *Online - full text edition.* **4070**
American Academy of Child and Adolescent Psychiatry. Journal (USA) *Online - full text edition.* **4071**
American Academy of Dermatology. Journal (USA) *Online - full text edition.* **3844**
American Board of Family Practice. Journal (USA) *Online - full text edition.* **3562**
American Heart Journal (USA) *Online - full text edition.* **3762**
The American Journal of Cardiology (USA) *Online - full text edition.* **3762**
American Journal of Cardiovascular Drugs (NZL) *Online - full text edition.* **3762**
American Journal of Clinical Dermatology (USA) *Online - full text edition.* **3844**
American Journal of Clinical Oncology (USA) *Online - full text edition.* **3967**
American Journal of Dermatopathology (USA) *Online - full text edition.* **3563**
American Journal of Emergency Medicine (USA) *Online - full text edition.* **4010**
American Journal of Epidemiology (USA) *Online - full text edition.* **3563**
American Journal of Forensic Medicine and Pathology (USA) *Online - full text edition.* **3881**
American Journal of Health-System Pharmacy (USA) *Online - full text edition.* **4275**
American Journal of Infection Control (USA) *Online - full text edition.* **3792**
The American Journal of Medicine (USA) *Online - full text edition.* **3564**
American Journal of Nursing (USA) *Online - full text edition.* **3913**
American Journal of Obstetrics and Gynecology (USA) *Online - full text edition.* **3944**
American Journal of Perinatology (USA) *Online - full text edition.* **3944**
American Journal of PharmacoGenomics (NZL) *Online - full text edition.* **3298**
American Journal of Physical Medicine and Rehabilitation (USA) *Online - full text edition.* **4058**
American Journal of Psychiatry (USA) *Online - full text edition.* **4071**
American Journal of Public Health (USA) *Online - full text edition.* **4461**
American Journal of Surgery (USA) *Online - full text edition.* **4180**
American Journal of Surgical Pathology (USA) *Online - full text edition.* **3564**
American Journal of the Medical Sciences (USA) *Online - full text edition.* **3564**
American Society of Echocardiography. Journal (USA) *Online - full text edition.* **3762**
Anaesthesia (Oxford) (GBR) *Online - full text edition.* **3754**
Anesthesia and Analgesia (USA) *Online - full text edition.* **3755**
Anesthesiology (USA) *Online - full text edition.* **3755**
Angiology (USA) *Online - full text edition.* **3763**
Animal Genetics (GBR) *Online - full text edition.* **3298**
Annals of Allergy, Asthma, & Immunology (USA) *Online - full text edition.* **3740**
Annals of Emergency Medicine (USA) *Online - full text edition.* **4010**
Annals of Internal Medicine (USA) *Online - full text edition.* **3907**
Annals of Medicine (GBR) *Online - full text edition.* **3871**
Annals of Oncology (NLD) *Online - full text edition.* **3967**
Annals of Surgery (USA) *Online - full text edition.* **4181**
Annals of Surgical Oncology (USA) *Online - full text edition.* **4181**
Annual Review of Psychology (USA) *Online - full text edition.* **4376**
Anti-Cancer Drugs (USA) *Online - full text edition.* **3967**
Applied Immunohistochemistry (USA) *Online - full text edition.* **3567**
Archives of Dermatology (USA) *Online - full text edition.* **3845**
Archives of Disease in Childhood (GBR) *Online - full text edition.* **4040**
Archives of Environmental Health (USA) *Online - full text edition.* **3435**
Archives of Facial Plastic Surgery (USA) *Online - full text edition.* **4182**
Archives of Family Medicine (USA) *Online - full text edition.* **3568**
Archives of General Psychiatry (USA) *Online - full text edition.* **4074**
Archives of Internal Medicine (USA) *Online - full text edition.* **3907**
Archives of Neurology (USA) *Online - full text edition.* **4074**
Archives of Ophthalmology (USA) *Online - full text edition.* **3994**
Archives of Otolaryngology - Head & Neck Surgery (USA) *Online - full text edition.* **4030**
Archives of Pediatrics & Adolescent Medicine (USA) *Online - full text edition.* **4041**
Archives of Surgery (USA) *Online - full text edition.* **4182**
Arteriosclerosis, Thrombosis, and Vascular Biology (USA) *Online - full text edition.* **3763**
Arthritis and Rheumatism (USA) *Online - full text edition.* **4167**
Artificial Organs (USA) *Online - full text edition.* **3871**
B J O Online (GBR) *Online - full text edition of* British Journal of Ophthalmology. **3994**
B J S M Online (GBR) *Online - full text edition of* British Journal of Sports Medicine. **4173**
B J U International (GBR) *Online - full text edition.* **4210**
B J U International. Supplement (GBR) *Online - full text edition.* **4210**
Behavior Genetics (USA) *Online - full text edition.* **3299**
Behavioral Medicine (USA) *Online - full text edition.* **4381**
Behavioural Pharmacology (USA) *Online - full text edition.* **4279**
BioDrugs (NZL) *Online - full text edition.* **4280**
BioScience (USA) *Online - full text edition.* **3187**
Birth (USA) *Online - full text edition.* **3946**
Blood Coagulation and Fibrinolysis (USA) *Online - full text edition.* **3898**
Blood Pressure Monitoring (USA) *Online - full text edition.* **3764**
Breast Cancer Research and Treatment (USA) *Online - full text edition.* **3969**
British Journal of Clinical Pharmacology (GBR) *Online - full text edition.* **4281**
British Journal of Dermatology (GBR) *Online - full text edition.* **3845**
British Journal of Dermatology. Supplement (GBR) *Online - full text edition.* **3846**
British Journal of Haematology (GBR) *Online - full text edition.* **3899**
British Journal of Haematology. Supplement (GBR) *Online - full text edition.* **3899**
British Journal of Psychiatry (GBR) *Online - full text edition.* **4079**
British Journal of Surgery (GBR) *Online - full text edition.* **4183**
British Medical Bulletin (GBR) *Online - full text edition.* **3579**
C M A J (CAN) *Online - full text edition.* **3580**
C N S Drugs (NZL) *Online - full text edition.* **4282**
C N S: The Journal for Advanced Nursing Practice (USA) *Online - full text edition.* **3915**
Cancer Detection and Prevention (USA) *Online - full text edition.* **3970**
Cancer Nursing (USA) *Online - full text edition.* **3916**
Cardiovascular Drugs and Therapy (USA) *Online - full text edition.* **3766**
Chest (USA) *Online - full text edition.* **4159**
Child: Care, Health and Development (GBR) *Online - full text edition.* **4042**
Circulation (Baltimore) (USA) *Online - full text edition. (JWAT)* **3768**
Circulation Research (USA) *Online - full text edition.* **3768**
Clinical and Experimental Allergy (GBR) *Online - full text edition.* **3742**
Clinical and Experimental Allergy. Supplement (GBR) *Online - full text edition.* **3742**
Clinical and Experimental Dermatology (GBR) *Online - full text edition.* **3846**
Clinical and Experimental Immunology (GBR) *Online - full text edition.* **3742**
Clinical and Experimental Immunology. Supplement (GBR) *Online - full text edition.* **3742**
Clinical and Experimental Pharmacology & Physiology (AUS) *Online - full text edition.* **3341**
Clinical and Laboratory Haematology (GBR) *Online - full text edition.* **3899**
Clinical Diabetes (USA) *Online - full text edition.* **3856**
Clinical Drug Investigation (NZL) *Online - full text edition.* **4283**
Clinical Endocrinology (GBR) *Online - full text edition.* **3856**
Clinical Genetics (DNK) *Online - full text edition.* **3300**

Clinical Journal of Pain (USA) *Online - full text edition.* **4082**
Clinical Journal of Sport Medicine (USA) *Online - full text edition.* **4173**
Clinical Medicine (GBR) *Online - full text edition.* **3586**
Clinical Neuropharmacology (USA) *Online - full text edition.* **4284**
Clinical Nuclear Medicine (USA) *Online - full text edition.* **4142**
Clinical Obstetrics and Gynecology (USA) *Online - full text edition.* **3947**
Clinical Oral Implants Research (DNK) *Online - full text edition.* **3818**
Clinical Orthopaedics and Related Research (USA) *Online - full text edition.* **4012**
Clinical Otolaryngology and Allied Sciences (GBR) *Online - full text edition.* **4031**
Clinical Pediatrics (USA) *Online - full text edition.* **4042**
Clinical Pharmacokinetics (NZL) *Online - full text edition.* **4284**
Clinical Pharmacology & Therapeutics (USA) *Online - full text edition.* **4284**
Clinical Transplantation (DNK) *Online - full text edition.* **4185**
Computers in Nursing (USA) *Online - full text edition.* **3810**
Conservation Biology (USA) *Online - full text edition.* **3392**
Contact Dermatitis (DNK) *Online - full text edition.* **3846**
Cornea (USA) *Online - full text edition.* **3996**
Coronary Artery Disease (USA) *Online - full text edition.* **3769**
Critical Care Medicine (USA) *Online - full text edition.* **3590**
Critical Care Nursing Quarterly (USA) *Online - full text edition.* **3918**
Current Opinion in Anaesthesiology (USA) *Online - full text edition.* **3756**
Current Opinion in Cardiology (USA) *Online - full text edition.* **3770**
Current Opinion in Clinical Nutrition and Metabolic Care (USA) *Online - full text edition.* **4231**
Current Opinion in Critical Care (USA) *Online - full text edition.* **4012**
Current Opinion in Endocrinology & Diabetes (USA) *Online - full text edition.* **3857**
Current Opinion in Gastroenterology (USA) *Online - full text edition.* **3888**
Current Opinion in Hematology (USA) *Online - full text edition.* **3900**
Current Opinion in Infectious Diseases (USA) *Online - full text edition.* **3794**
Current Opinion in Lipidology (GBR) *Online - full text edition.* **3770**
Current Opinion in Nephrology & Hypertension (USA) *Online - full text edition.* **4211**
Current Opinion in Neurology (USA) *Online - full text edition.* **4085**
Current Opinion in Obstetrics & Gynecology (USA) *Online - full text edition.* **3948**
Current Opinion in Oncology (USA) *Online - full text edition.* **3976**
Current Opinion in Ophthalmology (USA) *Online - full text edition.* **3996**
Current Opinion in Organ Transplantation (USA) *Online - full text edition.* **3591**
Current Opinion in Orthopedics (USA) *Online - full text edition.* **4013**
Current Opinion in Otolaryngology & Head and Neck Surgery (USA) *Online - full text edition.* **4031**
Current Opinion in Pediatrics (USA) *Online - full text edition.* **4043**
Current Opinion in Psychiatry (USA) *Online - full text edition.* **4085**
Current Opinion in Pulmonary Medicine (USA) *Online - full text edition.* **4159**
Current Opinion in Rheumatology (USA) *Online - full text edition.* **4168**
Current Opinion in Urology (USA) *Online - full text edition.* **4211**
Dermatologic Therapy (DNK) *Online - full text edition.* **3847**
Dermatology Nursing (USA) *Online - full text edition.* **3848**
Diabetes (USA) *Online - full text edition.* **3857**
Diabetes Care (USA) *Online - full text edition.* **3857**
Diagnostic Molecular Pathology (USA) *Online - full text edition.* **3594**
Digestive Diseases and Sciences (USA) *Online - full text edition.* **3888**
Disease Management & Health Outcomes (NZL) *Online - full text edition.* **3595**
Diseases of the Colon and Rectum (USA) *Online - full text edition.* **4187**
Drug and Market Development Newsletter (USA) *Online - full text edition.* **3596**
Drug Safety (NZL) *Online - full text edition.* **4289**
Drugs (NZL) *Online - full text edition.* **4290**
Drugs & Aging (NZL) *Online - full text edition.* **4290**
e A D C - F & N (GBR) *Online - full text edition of* Archives of Disease in Childhood. Fetal and Neonatal Edition. **3945**
The E M B O Journal (GBR) *Online - full text edition.* **3249**
E M J Online (GBR) *Online - full text edition of* Emergency Medicine Journal. **4014**
Ear and Hearing (USA) *Online - full text edition.* **4032**
Endocrine Reviews (USA) *Online - full text edition.* **3861**
The Endocrinologist (USA) *Online - full text edition.* **3861**
Endocrinology (USA) *Online - full text edition.* **3861**
Epidemiologic Reviews (USA) *Online - full text edition.* **3598**
Epidemiology (USA) *Online - full text edition.* **4468**
Epilepsia (USA) *Online - full text edition.* **4087**
European Journal of Anaesthesiology (GBR) *Online - full text edition.* **3757**
European Journal of Anaesthesiology. Supplement (GBR) *Online - full text edition.* **3757**
European Journal of Cancer Prevention (USA) *Online - full text edition.* **3977**
European Journal of Clinical Investigation (GBR) *Online - full text edition.* **3599**
European Journal of Gastroenterology and Hepatology (USA) *Online - full text edition.* **3889**
European Journal of Haematology (DNK) *Online - full text edition.* **3900**
European Journal of Haematology. Supplementum (DNK) *Online - full text edition.* **3901**
European Journal of Immunogenetics (GBR) *Online - full text edition.* **3302**
Evidence - Based Healthcare (GBR) *Online - full text edition.* **4468**
Experimental Biology and Medicine (Maywood) (USA) *Online - full text edition.* **3195**
Family and Community Health (USA) *Online - full text edition.* **4469**
Fertility and Sterility (USA) *Online - full text edition.* **3949**
Gastroenterology Nursing (USA) *Online - full text edition.* **3891**
Genetics In Medicine (USA) *Online - full text edition.* **3305**
Genomika (GBR) *Online - full text edition.* **3251**
Geriatric Nursing (USA) *Online - full text edition.* **3472**
Gut Online (GBR) *Online - full text edition of* Gut. **3891**
Gynaecological Endoscopy (GBR) *Online - full text edition.* **3951**
Health Care Management Review (USA) *Online - full text edition.* **3508**
Health Forum (USA) *Online - full text edition.* **3509**
Health Physics (USA) *Online - full text edition.* **3612**
Heart Online (GBR) *Online - full text edition of* Heart. **3772**
Heredity (GBR) *Online - full text edition.* **3307**
Histopathology (GBR) *Online - full text edition.* **3979**
Holistic Nursing Practice (USA) *Online - full text edition.* **3920**
Hospital Pharmacy (USA) *Online - full text edition.* **4300**
Hospital Topics (USA) *Online - full text edition.* **3514**
Hypertension (USA) *Online - full text edition.* **3774**
Immunological Reviews (DNK) *Online - full text edition.* **3745**
Immunology (GBR) *Online - full text edition.* **3746**
Immunology and Cell Biology (AUS) *Online - full text edition.* **3746**
International Anesthesiology Clinics (USA) *Online - full text edition.* **3757**
International Journal of Andrology (GBR) *Online - full text edition.* **4213**
International Journal of Andrology. Supplement (GBR) *Online - full text edition.* **4213**
International Journal of Dermatology (GBR) *Online - full text edition.* **3850**
International Journal of Experimental Pathology (GBR) *Online - full text edition.* **3623**
International Journal of Gynecological Cancer (USA) *Online - full text edition.* **3953**
International Journal of Gynecological Pathology (USA) *Online - full text edition.* **3953**
International Journal of Nursing Practice (AUS) *Online - full text edition.* **3921**
International Journal of Oral & Maxillofacial Surgery (DNK) *Online - full text edition.* **3827**
International Journal of S T D & AIDS (GBR) *Online - full text edition.* **3800**
International Journal of Surgical Pathology (USA) *Online - full text edition.* **4191**
International Ophthalmology Clinics (USA) *Online - full text edition.* **3999**
Investigative Radiology (USA) *Online - full text edition.* **4146**
J A I D S (USA) *Online - full text edition.* **3800**
J A M A: The Journal of the American Medical Association (USA) *Online - full text edition. (JWAR)* **3626**
J C P Online (GBR) *Online - full text edition of* Journal of Clinical Pathology. **3631**
J E C H Online (GBR) *Online - full text edition of* Journal of Epidemiology & Community Health. **3632**
J M E Online (GBR) *Online - full text edition of* Journal of Medical Ethics. **3635**
J M G Online (GBR) *Online - full text edition of* Journal of Medical Genetics. **3310**
Journal for Nurses in Staff Development (USA) *Online - full text edition.* **3923**
Journal of Advanced Nursing (GBR) *Online - full text edition.* **3923**
The Journal of Allergy and Clinical Immunology (USA) *Online - full text edition.* **3748**
Journal of Ambulatory Care Management (USA) *Online - full text edition.* **3516**
Journal of Applied Microbiology (GBR) *Online - full text edition.* **3324**
Journal of Assisted Reproduction and Genetics (USA) *Online - full text edition.* **3955**
Journal of Autism and Developmental Disorders (USA) *Online - full text edition.* **3423**
Journal of Behavioral Medicine (USA) *Online - full text edition.* **4099**
Journal of Bioenergetics and Biomembranes (USA) *Online - full text edition.* **3253**
Journal of Bone and Joint Surgery: American Volume (USA) *Online - full text edition.* **4017**
Journal of Bone and Joint Surgery: British Volume (GBR) *Online - full text edition.* **4017**
Journal of Bone and Joint Surgery: British Volume on CD-ROM (GBR) *Online - full text edition.* **4018**
Journal of Cardiopulmonary Rehabilitation (USA) *Online - full text edition.* **3776**
Journal of Cardiovascular Nursing (USA) *Online - full text edition.* **3777**
Journal of Cardiovascular Pharmacology (USA) *Online - full text edition.* **4305**
Journal of Cerebral Blood Flow and Metabolism (USA) *Online - full text edition.* **4099**
Journal of Clinical Endocrinology and Metabolism (USA) *Online - full text edition.* **3864**
Journal of Clinical Gastroenterology (USA) *Online - full text edition.* **3893**
Journal of Clinical Immunology (USA) *Online - full text edition.* **3748**
Journal of Clinical Investigation (USA) *Online - full text edition.* **3631**
Journal of Clinical Neurophysiology (USA) *Online - full text edition.* **4100**
Journal of Clinical Nursing (GBR) *Online - full text edition.* **3923**
Journal of Clinical Periodontology (DNK) *Online - full text edition.* **3828**
Journal of Clinical Pharmacology (USA) *Online - full text edition.* **4306**
Journal of Clinical Pharmacy and Therapeutics (GBR) *Online - full text edition.* **4306**
Journal of Clinical Psychopharmacology (USA) *Online - full text edition.* **4306**
Journal of Computer-Assisted Tomography (USA) *Online - full text edition.* **4147**
Journal of Cutaneous Pathology (DNK) *Online - full text edition.* **3850**
The Journal of Electroconvulsive Therapy (USA) *Online - full text edition.* **4101**
Journal of Emergency Nursing (USA) *Online - full text edition.* **3924**
The Journal of Endodontics (USA) *Online - full text edition.* **3828**
Journal of Family Practice (USA) *Online - full text edition.* **3633**
Journal of Gastroenterology and Hepatology (AUS) *Online - full text edition.* **3893**
Journal of General Internal Medicine (USA) *Online - full text edition.* **3910**
Journal of Head Trauma Rehabilitation (USA) *Online - full text edition.* **4018**
Journal of Health Care Finance (USA) *Online - full text edition.* **3516**
Journal of Healthcare Management (USA) *Online - full text edition.* **3517**
Journal of Human Nutrition and Dietetics (GBR) *Online - full text edition.* **4237**
Journal of Hypertension (USA) *Online - full text edition.* **3778**
Journal of Immunotherapy (USA) *Online - full text edition.* **3749**
Journal of Infusion Nursing (USA) *Online - full text edition.* **3924**
Journal of Inherited Metabolic Disease (NLD) *Online - full text edition.* **4046**
Journal of Intellectual Disability Research (GBR) *Online - full text edition.* **4102**
Journal of Internal Medicine (GBR) *Online - full text edition.* **3910**
Journal of Internal Medicine. Supplement (GBR) *Online - full text edition.* **3910**
The Journal of Investigative Dermatology (USA) *Online - full text edition.* **3851**
The Journal of Laboratory and Clinical Medicine (USA) *Online - full text edition.* **3876**
Journal of Medical Microbiology (USA) *Online - full text edition.* **3635**
Journal of Microscopy (GBR) *Online - full text edition.* **3334**
Journal of Nervous and Mental Disease (USA) *Online - full text edition.* **4102**
Journal of Neuro-Oncology (USA) *Online - full text edition.* **3982**
Journal of Neurology, Neurosurgery and Psychiatry (GBR) *Online - full text edition.* **4104**
Journal of Neurosurgical Anesthesiology (USA) *Online - full text edition.* **3758**
Journal of Nursing Administration (USA) *Online - full text edition.* **3925**
Journal of Nursing Care Quality (USA) *Online - full text edition.* **3925**
Journal of Nursing Management (GBR) *Online - full text edition.* **3925**
Journal of Occupational and Environmental Medicine (USA) *Online - full text edition.* **3636**
Journal of Oral Pathology & Medicine (DNK) *Online - full text edition.* **3829**
Journal of Orthopaedic Trauma (USA) *Online - full text edition.* **4019**
Journal of Paediatrics and Child Health (AUS) *Online - full text edition.* **4047**
Journal of Pediatric Gastroenterology and Nutrition (USA) *Online - full text edition.* **4238**
Journal of Pediatric Hematology - Oncology (USA) *Online - full text edition.* **3982**
Journal of Pediatric Orthopaedics (USA) *Online - full text edition.* **4019**
The Journal of Pediatrics (USA) *Online - full text edition.* **4047**
Journal of Peptide Research (DNK) *Online - full text edition.* **3255**
Journal of Perinatal and Neonatal Nursing (USA) *Online - full text edition.* **3926**
Journal of Periodontal Research (DNK) *Online - full text edition.* **3830**
Journal of Spinal Disorders (USA) *Online - full text edition.* **4020**
The Journal of Thoracic and Cardiovascular Surgery (USA) *Online - full text edition.* **4195**
Journal of Thoracic Imaging (USA) *Online - full text edition.* **4148**
Journal of Trauma - Injury, Infection and Critical Care (USA) *Online - full text edition.* **4020**
Journal of Urology (USA) *Online - full text edition.* **4215**
Journal of Vascular and Interventional Radiology (USA) *Online - full text edition.* **4149**
Journal of Vascular Surgery (USA) *Online - full text edition.* **4195**
Journal of Viral Hepatitis (GBR) *Online - full text edition.* **3893**
Kidney International Online (USA) *Online - full text edition of* Kidney International. **4215**
Kidney International. Supplement (USA) *Online - full text edition.* **4215**
Laboratory Investigation (USA) *Online - full text edition.* **3878**
Laryngoscope (USA) *Online - full text edition.* **4035**
Letters in Applied Microbiology (GBR) *Online - full text edition.* **3326**
Lippincott's Case Management (USA) *Online - full text edition.* **3928**

Liver (DNK) *Online - full text edition.* **3894**
M C N: American Journal of Maternal Child Nursing (USA) *Online - full text edition.* **3928**
M P Online (GBR) *Online - full text edition of* Molecular Pathology. **3879**
Mayo Clinic Proceedings (USA) *Online - full text edition.* **3647**
Medical Care (USA) *Online - full text edition.* **3649**
Medical Education (GBR) *Online - full text edition.* **3650**
Medicine and Science in Sports and Exercise (USA) *Online - full text edition.* **4175**
Medicine (Baltimore) (USA) *Online - full text edition.* **3656**
Melanoma Research (GBR) *Online - full text edition.* **3984**
Menopause (USA) *Online - full text edition.* **3958**
The Milbank Quarterly (USA) *Online - full text edition.* **4368**
Modern Pathology (USA) *Online - full text edition.* **3662**
Molecular Endocrinology (USA) *Online - full text edition.* **3866**
Molecular Microbiology Online (GBR) *Online - full text edition of* Molecular Microbiology. **3329**
Nature (GBR) *Online - full text edition.* **4506**
Neurology (USA) *Online - full text edition.* **4114**
Neurosurgery (Baltimore) (USA) *Online - full text edition.* **4119**
New England Journal of Medicine (USA) *Online - full text edition. (NEJM)* **3666**
New York Academy of Sciences. Annals (USA) *Online - full text edition.* **4506**
Nuclear Medicine Communications (USA) *Online - full text edition.* **4152**
Nurse Educator (USA) *Online - full text edition.* **3931**
Nurse Researcher (GBR) *Online - full text edition.* **3931**
Nursing Administration Quarterly (USA) *Online - full text edition.* **3932**
Nursing and Health Care Perspectives (USA) *Online - full text edition.* **3932**
Nursing Management (GBR) *Online - full text edition.* **3934**
Nursing Research (USA) *Online - full text edition.* **3934**
Nursing Standard (GBR) *Online - full text edition.* **3934**
Nutrition Reviews (USA) *Online - full text edition.* **4243**
O E M Online (GBR) *Online - full text edition of* Occupational and Environmental Medicine. **4261**
Obstetrical & Gynecological Survey (USA) *Online - full text edition.* **3960**
Occupational Medicine (GBR) *Online - full text edition.* **4262**
Ophthalmic Plastic and Reconstructive Surgery (USA) *Online - full text edition.* **4003**
Optometry and Vision Science (USA) *Online - full text edition.* **4005**
Oral Microbiology and Immunology (DNK) *Online - full text edition.* **3329**
Oral Surgery, Oral Medicine, Oral Pathology, Oral Radiology, and Endodontics (USA) *Online - full text edition.* **3835**
Otolaryngology - Head and Neck Surgery (USA) *Online - full text edition.* **4036**
Otology & Neurotology (USA) *Online - full text edition.* **4036**
Outcomes Management (USA) *Online - full text edition.* **3936**
Paediatric Drugs (NZL) *Online - full text edition.* **4321**
Pan American Journal of Public Health (USA) *Online - full text edition.* **4484**
Pancreas (USA) *Online - full text edition.* **3867**
Pathology International (AUS) *Online - full text edition.* **3673**
Pediatric Allergy and Immunology (DNK) *Online - full text edition.* **4051**
Pediatric Allergy and Immunology. Supplementum (DNK) *Online - full text edition.* **4051**
Pediatric Dermatology (USA) *Online - full text edition.* **3852**
Pediatric Emergency Care (USA) *Online - full text edition.* **4052**
The Pediatric Infectious Disease Journal (USA) *Online - full text edition.* **4053**
Pediatric Research (USA) *Online - full text edition.* **4054**
PharmacoEconomics (NZL) *Online - full text edition.* **4326**
Pharmacogenetics (USA) *Online - full text edition.* **3313**
Pharmacology & Toxicology Online(DNK) *Online - full text.* **4327**
Pharmacology & Toxicology. Supplementum (DNK) *Online - full text edition.* **4327**
Pharmacy Practice Management Quarterly (USA) *Online - full text edition.* **4328**
Plastic and Reconstructive Surgery (USA) *Online - full text edition.* **4200**
Postgraduate Medical Journal (GBR) *Online - full text edition.* **3678**
Psychological Medicine (GBR) *Online - full text edition.* **4127**
Psychosomatic Medicine (USA) *Online - full text edition.* **4128**
Public Health Nursing (USA) *Online - full text edition.* **3938**
Q J M (GBR) *Online - full text edition.* **3681**
R N Web (USA) *Online - full text edition of* R N. **3938**
Royal Society of Medicine. Journal (GBR) *Online - full text edition.* **3688**
Royal Society of Medicine. Journal. Supplement (GBR) *Online - full text edition.* **3688**
S G I M Forum (USA) *Online - full text edition.* **3911**
S T I Online (GBR) *Online - full text edition of* Sexually Transmitted Infections. **3853**
Scandinavian Journal of Immunology Online (GBR) *Online - full text edition of* Scandinavian Journal of Immunology. **3751**
Seminars in Dialysis (USA) *Online - full text edition.* **4218**
Seminars in Liver Diseases (USA) *Online - full text edition.* **3896**
Seminars in Neurology (USA) *Online - full text edition.* **4133**
Seminars in Respiratory and Critical Care Medicine (USA) *Online - full text edition.* **4165**
Seminars in Thrombosis and Hemostasis (USA) *Online - full text edition.* **3905**
Sexually Transmitted Diseases (USA) *Online - full text edition.* **3853**
Skin Research and Technology (DNK) *Online - full text edition.* **3853**
Skull Base Surgery (USA) *Online - full text edition.* **4203**
Spine (Philadelphia, 1976) (USA) *Online - full text edition.* **4026**
Sports Medicine (NZL) *Online - full text edition.* **4177**
Stroke (USA) *Online - full text edition.* **3783**
Surgery (USA) *Online - full text edition.* **4204**
Surgical Laparoscopy, Endoscopy and Percutaneous Techniques (USA) *Online - full text edition.* **4205**
Texas Heart Institute Journal (USA) *Online - full text edition.* **3783**
Therapeutic Drug Monitoring (USA) *Online - full text edition.* **4337**
Thorax Online (GBR) *Online - full text edition of* Thorax. **3700**
Tissue Antigens (DNK) *Online - full text edition.* **3701**
Tobbacco Control Online (GBR) *Online - full text edition of* Tobacco Control. **4531**
Topics in Emergency Medicine (USA) *Online - full text edition.* **4027**
Topics in Geriatric Rehabilitation (USA) *Online - full text edition.* **3481**
Topics in Health Information Management (USA) *Online - full text edition.* **3523**
Topics in Magnetic Resonance Imaging (USA) *Online - full text edition.* **4156**
Transfusion Medicine (GBR) *Online - full text edition.* **3905**
Transplantation (USA) *Online - full text edition.* **4206**
Tropical Medicine & International Health Online (GBR) *Online - full text edition of* Tropical Medicine & International Health. **4491**
Vascular Surgery (Glen Head) (USA) *Online - full text edition.* **4207**
Xenotransplantation (DNK) *Online - full text edition.* **4207**

Oxford University Press Online Journals (Subsidiary of: Oxford University Press) Great Clarendon St, Oxford OX2 6DP, United Kingdom TEL 44-1865 267907, FAX 44-1865-267485, jnl.info@oup.co.uk, http://www3.oup.co.uk/jnls/online/
Journal of Urban Health (USA) *Online - full content edition.* **3639**

Project MUSE (Subsidiary of: Johns Hopkins University Press) 2715 N. Charles St., Baltimore, MD 21218-4319 TEL 410-516-6989, FAX 410-516-6968, http://muse.jhu.edu
American Imago (USA) *Online - full text edition.* **4071**
Bulletin of the History of Medicine (USA) *Online - full text edition.* **3579**
Journal of Health Politics, Policy and Law (USA) *Online - full text edition.* **3633**
Journal of the History of Medicine and Allied Sciences (GBR) *Online - full text edition.* **3638**
Kennedy Institute of Ethics. Journal (USA) *Online - full text edition.* **3640**
Literature & Medicine (USA) *Online - full text edition.* **3552**
Perspectives in Biology and Medicine (USA) *Online - full content edition.* **3674**
Philosophy, Psychiatry, and Psychology Online (USA) *Online - full text edition of* Philosophy, Psychiatry & Psychology. **4348**

ProQuest Information & Learning 300 N. Zeeb Rd., Ann Arbor, MI 48106-1346 TEL 734-761-4700, 800-521-0600, FAX 734-997-4040 info@proquest.com, http://www.umi.com
A B N F Journal (USA) *Online - full text edition. (38579)* **3912**
A O R N Journal (USA) *Online - full text edition. (35897)* **3912**
A R D Online (GBR) *Online - full text edition of* Annals of the Rheumatic Diseases. (28112) **4167**
A S H A (USA) *Online - full text edition. (17690)* **3488**
Abstracts in Social Gerontology (USA) *Online - full text edition. (35709)* **3482**
Addiction (GBR) *Online - full text edition. (17071)* **3396**
Addiction Abstracts (GBR) *Online - full text edition. (38683)* **3397**
Addiction Biology (GBR) *Online - full text edition. (38664)* **3397**
Adolescence (San Diego) (USA) *Online - full text edition. (26960)* **3380**
Adolescent Psychiatry (USA) *Online - full text edition. (36504)* **4069**
Advances in Nursing Science (USA) *Online - full text edition. (35665)* **3912**
AIDS Abstracts (GBR) *Online - full text edition. (38685)* **3715**
AIDS Care (GBR) *Online - full text edition. (9953)* **3791**
AIDS Education and Prevention (USA) *Online - full text edition. (37943)* **4460**
Alternative Therapies in Health and Medicine (USA) *Online - full text edition. (38441)* **3163**
American Academy of Audiology. Journal (CAN) *Online - full text edition. (36491)* **4029**
American Academy of Nurse Practitioners. Journal (USA) *Online - full text edition. (39096)* **3913**
American Academy of Psychoanalysis. Journal (USA) *Online - full text edition. (37944)* **4373**
American Annals of the Deaf (USA) *Online - full text edition. (27282)* **3488**
American Association of Occupational Health Nurses Journal (USA) *Online - full text edition. (39312)* **3913**
American Behavioral Scientist (USA) *Online - full text edition. (27862)* **4508**
American Chiropractic Association. Journal (USA) *Online - full text edition. (37328)* **3786**
American College of Surgeons. Journal (USA) *Online - full text edition. (27217)* **4179**
American Dietetic Association. Journal (USA) *Online - full text edition. (18999)* **4228**
American Druggist (USA) *Online - full text edition. (36525)* **4275**
American Family Physician (USA) *Online - full text edition. (24034)* **3563**
American Fitness (USA) *Online - full text edition. (11458)* **4350**
American Indian and Alaska Native Mental Health Research (USA) *Online - full text edition. (37877)* **4226**
American Journal of Art Therapy (USA) *Online - full text edition. (27666)* **4058**
American Journal of Audiology (USA) *Online - full text edition. (36486)* **3488**
American Journal of Clinical Nutrition (USA) *Online - full text edition. (27518)* **4228**
American Journal of Community Psychology (USA) *Online - full text edition. (18028)* **4520**
American Journal of Critical Care (USA) *Online - full text edition. (36637)* **3913**
American Journal of Family Therapy (USA) *Online - full text edition. (21029)* **4374**
American Journal of Geriatric Psychiatry (USA) *Online - full text edition. (37469)* **3468**
American Journal of Knee Surgery (USA) *Online - full text edition. (37945)* **4180**
American Journal of Law & Medicine (USA) *Online - full text edition. (18339)* **3536**
American Journal of Nephrology (CHE) *Online - full text edition. (10268)* **4209**
American Journal of Pathology (USA) *Online - full text edition. (21318)* **3564**
American Journal of Pharmaceutical Education (USA) *Online - full text edition. (36531)* **4275**
American Journal of Psychiatry (USA) *Online - full text edition. (28648)* **4071**
American Journal of Psychoanalysis (USA) *Online - full text edition. (27115)* **4374**
American Journal of Psychology (USA) *Online - full text edition. (29197)* **4374**
American Journal of Psychotherapy (USA) *Online - full text edition. (12495)* **4072**
American Journal of Public Health (USA) *Online - full text edition. (8)* **4461**
American Journal of Respiratory Cell and Molecular Biology (USA) *Online - full text edition. (12432)* **4158**
American Journal of Speech - Language Pathology (USA) *Online - full text edition. (36485)* **3489**
American Journal of Sports Medicine (USA) *Online - full text edition. (14418)* **4172**
American Journal on Addictions (USA) *Online - full text edition. (37448)* **3399**
The American Nurse (USA) *Online - full text edition. (38445)* **3913**
American Rehabilitation (USA) *Online - full text edition. (18305)* **3419**
American Surgeon (USA) *Online - full text edition. (35779)* **4180**
Anaesthesia and Intensive Care (AUS) *Online - full text edition. (37181)* **3753**
Angiology (USA) *Online - full text edition. (36630)* **3763**
Annals of Allergy, Asthma, & Immunology (USA) *Online - full text edition. (27067)* **3740**
Annals of Dyslexia (USA) *Online - full text edition. (17628)* **3419**
Annals of Otology, Rhinology and Laryngology (USA) *Online - full text edition. (26397)* **4030**
Annals of Tropical Paediatrics (GBR) *Online - full text edition. (38656)* **4040**
Annals of Vascular Surgery (USA) *Online - full text edition. (37001)* **4181**
Annual Review of Sex Research (USA) *Online - full text edition. (37741)* **4376**
Applied Psychological Measurement (USA) *Online - full text edition. (37364)* **4377**
Archives of Disease in Childhood (GBR) *Online - full text edition. (28110)* **4040**
Archives of Environmental Health (USA) *Online - full text edition. (24517)* **3435**
Archives of Pathology & Laboratory Medicine (USA) *Online - full text edition. (30163)* **3568**
Archives of Sexual Behavior (USA) *Online - full text edition. (19481)* **3568**
Arizona Nurse (USA) *Online - full text edition. (38433)* **3914**
Arteriosclerosis, Thrombosis, and Vascular Biology (USA) *Online - full text edition. (17151)* **3763**
Assessment (USA) *Online - full text edition. (38479)* **4378**
Association of Nurses in AIDS Care. Journal (USA) *Online - full text edition. (35937)* **3793**
Audiology and Neuro-Otology (CHE) *Online - full text edition. (33512)* **4031**
Augmentative and Alternative Communication (CAN) *Online - full text edition. (37661)* **3572**
Australian and New Zealand Journal of Public Health (AUS) *Online - full text edition. (16273)* **4462**
Australian Journal of Clinical Hypnotherapy and Hypnosis (AUS) *Online - full text edition. (37742)* **3906**
Australian Journal of Otolaryngology (AUS) *Online - full text edition. (38208)* **4031**
Australian Nursing Journal (AUS) *Online - full text edition. (36024)* **3914**

Avian Pathology (GBR) *Online - full text edition. (34447)* **4539**
B J O Online (GBR) *Online - full text edition of* British Journal of Ophthalmology. (28109) **3994**
Balance (Alexandria) (USA) *Online - full text edition. (40564)* **3468**
Behavior and Social Issues (USA) *Online - full text edition. (38079)* **4380**
Behavior Modification (USA) *Online - full text edition. (16524)* **4380**
Behavioral Disorders (USA) *Online - full text edition. (17560)* **3419**
Behavioral Health Management (USA) *Online - full text edition. (13860)* **3399**
Behavioral Medicine (USA) *Online - full text edition. (36031)* **4381**
Behavioral Research in Accounting (USA) *Online - full text edition. (11404)* **3362**
Biochemistry and Cell Biology (CAN) *Online - full text edition. (36120)* **3243**
Biocontrol Science and Technology (GBR) *Online - full text edition. (38651)* **3157**
Biological Bulletin (USA) *Online - full text edition. (21371)* **3185**
Biomedical Safety & Standards Newsletter (USA) *Online - full text edition. (13019)* **3576**
Biomedical Technology Information Service (USA) *Online - full text edition. (13020)* **3576**
Biometrics (USA) *Online - full text edition. (37041)* **4528**
BioPharm (USA) *Online - full text edition. (36036)* **4280**
Biophysical Journal (USA) *Online - full text edition. (36123)* **3265**
BioScience (USA) *Online - full text edition. (22908)* **3187**
Biotech Business (USA) *Online - full text edition. (33194)* **3270**
Blood Cells, Molecules, and Diseases (USA) *Online - full text edition. (17333)* **3898**
Body Bulletin Newsletter (USA) *Online - full text edition. (36040)* **4252**
Brain, Behavior and Evolution (CHE) *Online - full text edition. (37870)* **4077**
British Journal of Anaesthesia (GBR) *Online - full text edition. (28118)* **3756**
British Journal of Audiology (GBR) *Online - full content edition. (39404)* **3489**
British Journal of Biomedical Science (GBR) *Online - full text edition. (37186)* **3872**
British Journal of Clinical Psychology (GBR) *Online - full text edition. (37365)* **4383**
British Journal of Developmental Psychology (GBR) *Online - full text edition. (37366)* **4383**
British Journal of Educational Psychology (GBR) *Online - full text edition. (33217)* **4383**
British Journal of Guidance and Counselling (GBR) *Online - full content edition. (34449)* **4269**
British Journal of Mathematical and Statistical Psychology (GBR) *Online - full text edition. (36127)* **4384**
British Journal of Medical Psychology (GBR) *Online - full text edition. (37367)* **4384**
British Journal of Neurosurgery (GBR) *Online - full text edition. (34451)* **4182**
British Journal of Nursing (GBR) *Online - full text edition. (39049)* **3915**
British Journal of Perioperative Nursing (GBR) *Online - full text edition. (38804)* **3915**
British Journal of Psychology (GBR) *Online - full text edition. (15882)* **4384**
British Journal of Social Psychology (GBR) *Online - full text edition. (37369)* **4384**
C M A J (CAN) *Online - full text edition. (33824)* **3580**
Canadian Chiropractic Association. Journal (CAN) *Online - full text edition. (37253)* **3786**
Canadian Journal of Behavioural Science (CAN) *Online - full text edition. (41564)* **4385**
Canadian Journal of Dietetic Practice and Research (CAN) *Online - full text edition. (38819)* **4230**
Canadian Journal of Experimental Psychology (CAN) *Online - full text edition. (20379)* **4386**
Canadian Journal of Human Sexuality (CAN) *Online - full text edition. (38217)* **4386**
Canadian Journal of Microbiology (CAN) *Online - full text edition. (36143)* **3319**
Canadian Journal of Occupational Therapy (CAN) *Online - full text edition. (40569)* **4059**
Canadian Journal of Physiology and Pharmacology (CAN) *Online - full text edition. (37382)* **3340**
Canadian Journal of Public Health (CAN) *Online - full text edition. (37869)* **4464**
The Canadian Journal of Rural Medicine (CAN) *Online - full text edition. (39285)* **3582**
Canadian Journal of Surgery (CAN) *Online - full text edition. (33539)* **4183**
Canadian Mining Journal (CAN) *Online - full text edition. (12031)* **4225**
Canadian Psychology (CAN) *Online - full text edition. (41565)* **4386**
The Cancer Journal from Scientific American (English Edition) (USA) *Online - full text edition. (38531)* **3972**
The Career Development Quarterly (USA) *Online - full text edition. (26420)* **4269**
Caries Research (CHE) *Online - full text edition. (26453)* **3817**
Chart (USA) *Online - full text edition. (39178)* **3916**
Chemist & Druggist (GBR) *Online - full text edition. (34589)* **4283**
Chest (USA) *Online - full text edition. (28929)* **4159**
Child Health Alert (USA) *Online - full text edition. (11503)* **4042**
Child Maltreatment (USA) *Online - full text edition. (32457)* **3381**
Circulation (Baltimore) (USA) *Online - full text edition. (27249)* **3768**
Circulation Research (USA) *Online - full text edition. (27245)* **3768**
Clinical and Investigative Medicine (CAN) *Online - full text edition. (33540)* **3586**
Clinical Diabetes (USA) *Online - full text edition. (36050)* **3856**
Clinical Lab Letter (USA) *Online - full text edition. (13021)* **3873**
Clinical Laboratory Science (USA) *Online - full text edition. (36487)* **3873**
Clinical Microbiology and Infection (GBR) *Online - full text edition. (38223)* **3586**
Clinical Nursing Research (USA) *Online - full text edition. (32456)* **3916**
Clinical Pediatrics (USA) *Online - full text edition. (36052)* **4042**
Communication Disorders Quarterly (USA) *Online - full text edition. (40602)* **3420**
Community Mental Health Journal (USA) *Online - full text edition. (19197)* **4512**
Community Pharmacy (GBR) *Online - full text edition. (34596)* **4284**
Comparative Political Studies (USA) *Online - full text edition. (24724)* **4367**
Connecticut Nursing News (USA) *Online - full text edition. (38435)* **3917**
Contemporary Drug Problems (USA) *Online - full text edition. (23292)* **3400**
Contemporary Hypnosis (GBR) *Online - full text edition. (37743)* **3906**
Contemporary Longterm Care (USA) *Online - full text edition. (36071)* **3505**
Contemporary Surgery (USA) *Online - full text edition. (37021)* **4186**
Cooking Light (USA) *Online - full text edition. (36167)* **3526**
Counseling and Values (USA) *Online - full text edition. (37295)* **4502**
The Counseling Psychologist (USA) *Online - full text edition. (19416)* **4392**
Counselling Psychology Quarterly (GBR) *Online - full content edition. (34457)* **4392**
Counselor Education and Supervision (USA) *Online - full text edition. (27031)* **3410**
Criminal Behaviour and Mental Health (GBR) *Online - full content edition. (38039)* **4084**
Criminal Justice & Behavior (USA) *Online - full text edition. (17816)* **3394**
Critical Care Nurse (USA) *Online - full text edition. (36633)* **3917**
Critical Care Nursing Quarterly (USA) *Online - full text edition. (36080)* **3918**
Critical Reviews in Toxicology (USA) *Online - full text edition. (38195)* **3447**
Cross-Cultural Research (USA) *Online - full text edition. (27400)* **4508**
Current Health 1 (USA) *Online - full text edition. (32974)* **3428**
Current Health 2 (USA) *Online - full text edition. (18757)* **3428**
Current Medical Research and Opinion (GBR) *Online - full content edition. (37296)* **3591**
Cutis (USA) *Online - full text edition. (37972)* **3847**
Cytogenetic and Genome Research (CHE) *Online - full text edition. (27434)* **3301**
D V M (USA) *Online - full text edition. (36134)* **4541**
Dairy Council Digest(USA) *Online - full text. (36083)* **4231**
Death Studies (USA) *Online - full text edition. (19217)* **4394**
Dementia and Geriatric Cognitive Disorders (CHE) *Online - full text edition. (37871)* **4085**
Dental Economics (USA) *Online - full text edition. (27174)* **3820**
Dermatology Times (USA) *Online - full text edition. (35694)* **3848**
Diabetes (USA) *Online - full text edition. (23769)* **3857**
Diabetes Care (USA) *Online - full text edition. (17598)* **3857**
Diabetes Forecast (USA) *Online - full text edition. (11457)* **3858**
Diabetes Spectrum (USA) *Online - full text edition. (37201)* **3859**
Diagnostic Imaging (USA) *Online - full text edition. (37375)* **4143**
Digestion (CHE) *Online - full text edition. (26836)* **3888**
Dimensions of Critical Care Nursing (USA) *Online - full text edition. (37202)* **3918**
Disability & Society (GBR) *Online - full text edition. (37468)* **3494**
Drug and Alcohol Review (GBR) *Online - full text edition. (37603)* **3400**
Drug Information Journal (USA) *Online - full text edition. (38240)* **4289**
Drug Topics (USA) *Online - full text edition. (22506)* **4290**
Drugs: Education, Prevention & Policy (GBR) *Online - full text edition. (37601)* **3401**
Ear, Nose & Throat Journal (USA) *Online - full text edition. (37298)* **4032**
Ecological Monographs (USA) *Online - full text edition. (28833)* **3437**
Ecology (USA) *Online - full text edition. (23845)* **3437**
Education for Health (GBR) *Online - full text edition. (37559)* **3597**
Educational and Psychological Measurement (USA) *Online - full text edition. (27959)* **4396**
Educational Psychology (GBR) *Online - full text edition. (34460)* **3410**
The Elementary School Journal (USA) *Online - full text edition. (29196)* **3411**
Emergency Medicine (USA) *Online - full text edition. (37975)* **4013**
Environment and Behavior (USA) *Online - full text edition. (19375)* **4521**
Ethnicity and Health (GBR) *Online - full text edition. (37602)* **4468**
European Neurology (CHE) *Online - full text edition. (26835)* **4089**
Evaluation and the Health Professions (USA) *Online - full text edition. (16525)* **3600**
Exceptional Children (USA) *Online - full text edition. (17896)* **3422**
Exceptional Parent (USA) *Online - full text edition. (23148)* **3422**
F D A Consumer (USA) *Online - full text edition. (26588)* **3392**
Family and Community Health (USA) *Online - full text edition. (35986)* **4469**
The Family Journal (USA) *Online - full text edition. (36000)* **4399**
Family Planning Perspectives (USA) *Online - full text edition. (23177)* **3949**
Family Practice Management (USA) *Online - full text edition. (37668)* **3602**
Family Process (USA) *Online - full text edition. (39292)* **4399**
Female Patient: Practical Ob-Gyn Medicine (USA) *Online - full text edition. (37979)* **3949**
Fire Chief (USA) *Online - full text edition. (36567)* **3458**
Florida Nurse (USA) *Online - full text edition. (37205)* **3919**
Flying Safety (USA) *Online - full text edition. (23689)* **3153**
Focus on Exceptional Children (USA) *Online - full text edition. (19960)* **3422**
Focus on Geriatric Care and Rehabilitation (USA) *Online - full text edition. (37206)* **3471**
Folia Phoniatrica et Logopaedica (CHE) *Online - full text edition. (37872)* **4032**
Food and Agricultural Immunology (GBR) *Online - full text edition. (38654)* **3197**
Formulary (USA) *Online - full text edition. (36005)* **4297**
Frontiers of Health Services Management (USA) *Online - full text edition. (15980)* **3507**
The Future of Children (USA) *Online - full text edition. (38606)* **3383**
Generations (San Francisco) (USA) *Online - full text edition. (11455)* **3471**
Genetic, Social, and General Psychology Monographs (USA) *Online - full text edition. (37208)* **4400**
Genome (CAN) *Online - full text edition. (37377)* **3306**
Georgia Nursing (USA) *Online - full text edition. (38437)* **3919**
Geriatrics (USA) *Online - full text edition. (17521)* **3472**
The Gerontologist (USA) *Online - full text edition. (27214)* **3473**
Gerontology (CHE) *Online - full text edition. (10181)* **3473**
Global Cosmetic Industry (USA) *Online - full text edition. (26967)* **3176**
Group & Organization Management (USA) *Online - full text edition. (19427)* **3411**
Gut Online (GBR) *Online - full text edition of* Gut. (28089) **3891**
Hastings Center Report (USA) *Online - full text edition. (21451)* **3610**
Headache Online(USA) *Online - full text.* **4093**
Health Affairs (USA) *Online - full text edition. (15986)* **4471**
Health and Hygiene (GBR) *Online - full text edition. (37983)* **4471**
Health & Social Work (USA) *Online - full text edition. (18747)* **4513**
The Health Care Collector (USA) *Online - full text edition. (37551)* **3508**
Health Care Financing Review (USA) *Online - full text edition. (14925)* **3610**
Health Care Management Review (USA) *Online - full text edition. (17776)* **3508**
Health Care Strategic Management (USA) *Online - full text edition. (12636)* **3509**
Health Data Management (New York) (USA) *Online - full text edition. (34954)* **3509**
Health Education & Behavior (USA) *Online - full text edition. (22101)* **4472**
Health Forum (USA) *Online - full text edition. (28608)* **3509**
Health Industry Today (USA) *Online - full text edition. (20363)* **3611**
Health Letter (Washington) (USA) *Online - full text edition. (10838)* **3612**
Health Management Technology (USA) *Online - full text edition. (17789)* **3810**
Health Marketing Quarterly (USA) *Online - full text edition. (7976)* **4473**
Health Progress (USA) *Online - full text edition. (37123)* **3510**
Health (San Francisco) (USA) *Online - full text edition. (12318)* **4355**
Health Services Research (USA) *Online - full text edition. (26127)* **3510**
Health World (USA) *Online - full text edition. (10829)* **3166**
Healthcare Executive (USA) *Online - full text edition. (14232)* **3510**
Healthcare Financial Management (USA) *Online - full text edition. (17804)* **3510**
HealthFacts (USA) *Online - full text edition. (11602)* **3613**
Healthy Weight Journal (CAN) *Online - full text edition. (11429)* **4235**
Heart Online (GBR) *Online - full text edition of* Heart. (28113) **3772**
High Ability Studies (GBR) *Online - full text edition. (37556)* **3422**
Hispanic Journal of Behavioral Sciences (USA) *Online - full text edition. (17901)* **4402**
Holistic Nursing Practice (USA) *Online - full text edition. (36014)* **3920**
Hospital Development (GBR) *Online - full text edition. (36021)* **3513**
Hospital Law Newsletter (USA) *Online - full text edition. (37215)* **3513**
Hospital Materials Management (USA) *Online - full text edition. (12422)* **3514**
Hospital Materiel Management Quarterly (USA) *Online - full text edition. (17711)* **3514**
Hospital Practice (USA) *Online - full text edition. (26787)* **3616**
Hospital Topics (USA) *Online - full text edition. (29060)* **3514**
Human Biology (Detroit) (USA) *Online - full text edition. (27986)* **3199**
Human Communication Research (USA) *Online - full text edition. (19361)* **4402**
Human Ecology (New York) (USA) *Online - full text edition. (19489)* **3173**
Human Factors (USA) *Online - full text edition. (19745)* **3432**
Human Factors and Ergonomics Society Annual Meeting. Proceedings (USA) *Online - full text edition. (37218)* **3432**

Online Service

Human Relations (USA) *Online - full text edition. (28426)* **4509**
Hypertension (USA) *Online - full text edition. (18021)* **3774**
I T Health Care Strategist (USA) *Online - full text edition. (39258)* **3515**
In Vitro Cellular & Developmental Biology - Animal (USA) *Online - full text edition. (37220)* **3618**
Infants and Young Children (USA) *Online - full text edition. (36575)* **4045**
Infection Control & Hospital Epidemiology (USA) *Online - full text edition. (16982)* **3798**
Inquiry (Rochester) (USA) *Online - full text edition. (23871)* **3620**
Inside Ambulatory Care (USA) *Online - full text edition. (37438)* **3515**
Inside M S (USA) *Online - full text edition. (11469)* **4095**
Instituto de Medicina Tropical de Sao Paulo. Revista (BRA) *Online - full text edition. (38663)* **3799**
International Angiology (ITA) *Online - full text edition. (38262)* **3774**
International Family Planning Perspectives (USA) *Online - full text edition. (37240)* **3953**
The International Journal of Action Methods (USA) *Online - full text edition. (37326)* **4405**
International Journal of Childbirth Education (USA) *Online - full text edition. (38720)* **3953**
International Journal of Conflict Management (USA) *Online - full text edition. (32493)* **3365**
International Journal of Food Sciences and Nutrition (GBR) *Online - full text edition. (30322)* **4236**
International Journal of Group Psychotherapy (USA) *Online - full text edition. (37928)* **4406**
International Journal of Infectious Diseases (CAN) *Online - full text edition. (37435)* **3799**
International Journal of Leprosy and Other Mycobacterial Diseases (USA) *Online - full text edition. (18181)* **3799**
International Journal of Offender Therapy and Comparative Criminology (USA) *Online - full text edition. (20262)* **3394**
International Journal of Psychotherapy (GBR) *Online - full content edition. (34470)* **4096**
International Journal of S T D & AIDS (GBR) *Online - full text edition. (38467)* **3800**
International Journal of Social Psychiatry (GBR) *Online - full text edition. (12523)* **4096**
International Journal of Surgical Pathology (USA) *Online - full text edition. (38744)* **4191**
International Review of Psychiatry (GBR) *Online - full text edition. (34475)* **4097**
International Seminars in Paediatric Gastroenterology and Nutrition (CAN) *Online - full text edition. (37445)* **3892**
Intervention in School and Clinic (USA) *Online - full text edition. (23624)* **3423**
Intervirology (CHE) *Online - full text edition. (22467)* **3324**
Israel Journal of Psychiatry and Related Sciences (ISR) *Online - full text edition. (37243)* **4097**
Issues in Law and Medicine (USA) *Online - full text edition. (30263)* **3626**
J C P Online (GBR) *Online - full text edition of* Journal of Clinical Pathology. (28111) **3631**
J E C H Online (GBR) *Online - full text edition of* Journal of Epidemiology & Community Health. (28088) **3632**
J M E Online (GBR) *Online - full text edition of* Journal of Medical Ethics. (12511) **3635**
J M G Online (GBR) *Online - full text edition of* Journal of Medical Genetics. (38446) **3310**
J N M Online (USA) *Online - full text edition of* The Journal of Nuclear Medicine. (27354) **4148**
Journal for Specialists in Group Work (USA) *Online - full text edition. (36026)* **4408**
Journal of Abnormal Child Psychology (USA) *Online - full text edition. (19470)* **4409**
Journal of Addictions & Offender Counseling (USA) *Online - full text edition. (37246)* **4409**
Journal of Adolescent Research (USA) *Online - full text edition. (14330)* **4409**
Journal of Aging and Health (USA) *Online - full text edition. (13685)* **3474**
Journal of Alcohol and Drug Education (USA) *Online - full text edition. (19768)* **3402**
Journal of Ambulatory Care Management (USA) *Online - full text edition. (36990)* **3516**
Journal of American College Health (USA) *Online - full text edition. (27257)* **4357**
Journal of Applied Behavioral Science (USA) *Online - full text edition. (26803)* **4410**
Journal of Applied Gerontology (USA) *Online - full text edition. (13686)* **3475**
Journal of Athletic Training (USA) *Online - full text edition. (19516)* **4174**
Journal of Audio Visual Media in Medicine (GBR) *Online - full text edition. (38662)* **3629**
Journal of Behavioral Health Services and Research (USA) *Online - full text edition. (12423)* **4479**
Journal of Biological Rhythms (USA) *Online - full text edition. (13317)* **4099**
Journal of Black Psychology (USA) *Online - full text edition. (18065)* **4410**
Journal of Black Studies (USA) *Online - full text edition. (23378)* **4509**
Journal of Bone and Joint Surgery: American Volume (USA) *Online - full text edition. (28967)* **4017**
Journal of Cardiovascular Nursing (USA) *Online - full text edition. (35850)* **3777**
The Journal of Cardiovascular Surgery (ITA) *Online - full text edition. (36628)* **3777**
Journal of Career Assessment (USA) *Online - full text edition. (38480)* **4411**
Journal of Child and Adolescent Psychiatric Nursing (USA) *Online - full text edition. (35858)* **3923**
Journal of Child Neurology (CAN) *Online - full text edition. (14627)* **4099**
Journal of Child Sexual Abuse (USA) *Online - full text edition. (7856)* **4514**
Journal of Clinical Psychiatry (USA) *Online - full text edition. (27772)* **4100**
Journal of College Student Development (USA) *Online - full text edition. (22023)* **4412**
Journal of Community Health (USA) *Online - full text edition. (19174)* **3631**
Journal of Continuing Education in Nursing (USA) *Online - full text edition. (23906)* **3924**
Journal of Continuing Education in the Health Professions (CAN) *Online - full text edition. (37988)* **3632**
Journal of Cross-Cultural Psychology (USA) *Online - full text edition. (18453)* **4414**
Journal of Cultural Diversity (USA) *Online - full text edition. (38581)* **3924**
Journal of Cutaneous Medicine and Surgery (CAN) *Online - full text edition. (37436)* **3850**
Journal of Dental Research (USA) *Online - full text edition. (19555)* **3828**
Journal of Drug Issues (USA) *Online - full text edition. (22622)* **3403**
Journal of Early Adolescence (USA) *Online - full text edition. (16998)* **3384**
Journal of Elder Abuse & Neglect (USA) *Online - full text edition. (7961)* **3476**
Journal of Electrocardiology (USA) *Online - full text edition. (37009)* **3777**
Journal of Emotional and Behavioral Disorders (USA) *Online - full text edition. (37003)* **4101**
Journal of Employment Counseling (USA) *Online - full text edition. (35867)* **4414**
Journal of Environmental Health (USA) *Online - full text edition. (23855)* **3440**
Journal of Esthetic and Restorative Dentistry (CAN) *Online - full text edition. (38284)* **3828**
Journal of Family Nursing (USA) *Online - full content edition. (30423)* **3924**
Journal of Forensic Identification (USA) *Online - full text edition. (37247)* **3883**
Journal of Forensic Sciences (USA) *Online - full text edition. (19820)* **3883**
The Journal of General Psychology (USA) *Online - full text edition. (14345)* **4416**
The Journal of Genetic Psychology (USA) *Online - full text edition. (26603)* **3309**
Journal of Geriatric Psychiatry and Neurology (CAN) *Online - full text edition. (37439)* **3476**
Journal of Gerontological Nursing (USA) *Online - full text edition. (36484)* **3476**
Journal of Hand Surgery: American Volume (USA) *Online - full content edition. (36981)* **4193**
Journal of Head Trauma Rehabilitation (USA) *Online - full text edition. (36997)* **4018**
Journal of Health and Social Behavior (USA) *Online - full text edition. (27047)* **4522**
Journal of Health Care Finance (USA) *Online - full text edition. (17716)* **3516**
Journal of Health Care for the Poor and Underserved (USA) *Online - full text edition. (12307)* **3633**
Journal of Health Politics, Policy and Law (USA) *Online - full text edition. (19228)* **3633**
Journal of Healthcare Management (USA) *Online - full text edition. (23545)* **3517**
Journal of Holistic Nursing (USA) *Online - full text edition. (32453)* **3924**
Journal of Humanistic Psychology (USA) *Online - full text edition. (26495)* **4417**
Journal of Infectious Diseases (USA) *Online - full text edition. (29194)* **3802**
Journal of Interpersonal Violence (USA) *Online - full text edition. (13772)* **3395**
Journal of Interprofessional Care (GBR) *Online - full text edition. (37665)* **3634**
Journal of Investigative Medicine (USA) *Online - full text edition. (24033)* **3883**
Journal of Language and Social Psychology (USA) *Online - full text edition. (32452)* **4417**
Journal of Laryngology and Otology (GBR) *Online - full content edition. (33369)* **4034**
The Journal of Law, Medicine & Ethics (USA) *Online - full text edition. (18317)* **3540**
Journal of Learning Disabilities (USA) *Online - full text edition. (14092)* **3424**
Journal of Mammalogy (USA) *Online - full text edition. (28669)* **3354**
Journal of Marital and Family Therapy (USA) *Online - full text edition. (19058)* **4418**
Journal of Mental Health (GBR) *Online - full text edition. (34485)* **4102**
Journal of Mental Health Counseling (USA) *Online - full text edition. (35888)* **4418**
Journal of Motor Behavior (USA) *Online - full text edition. (37013)* **4418**
Journal of Multicultural Counseling and Development (USA) *Online - full text edition. (21928)* **4418**
Journal of Neurology, Neurosurgery and Psychiatry (GBR) *Online - full text edition. (28090)* **4104**
Journal of Neuropathology and Experimental Neurology (USA) *Online - full text edition. (29222)* **4104**
Journal of Neuropsychiatry and Clinical Neurosciences (USA) *Online - full text edition. (37249)* **4104**
Journal of Neuroscience Nursing (USA) *Online - full text edition. (38810)* **3925**
Journal of Neurosurgical Sciences (ITA) *Online - full text edition. (37990)* **4194**
Journal of Nonverbal Behavior (USA) *Online - full text edition. (19199)* **4418**
Journal of Nuclear Medicine Technology (USA) *Online - full text edition. (39290)* **4148**
Journal of Nursing Care Quality (USA) *Online - full text edition. (35900)* **3925**
Journal of Nursing Education (USA) *Online - full text edition. (23497)* **3925**
Journal of Nutrition (USA) *Online - full text edition. (23412)* **4237**
Journal of Nutrition Education (CAN) *Online - full text edition. (21825)* **4237**
Journal of Nutritional & Environmental Medicine (GBR) *Online - full text edition. (34487)* **4237**
Journal of Obstetrics and Gynaecology (GBR) *Online - full text edition. (34488)* **3956**
Journal of Occupational and Organizational Psychology (GBR) *Online - full text edition. (15880)* **4419**
Journal of Ophthalmic Nursing & Technology (USA) *Online - full text edition. (39314)* **3926**
Journal of Organizational Behavior Management (USA) *Online - full text edition. (7921)* **4419**
Journal of Orthopaedic Research (USA) *Online - full text edition. (12068)* **4019**
Journal of Orthopaedic Surgery (HKG) *Online - full text edition. (38286)* **4019**
Journal of Otolaryngology (CAN) *Online - full text edition. (37019)* **4034**
Journal of Palliative Care (CAN) *Online - full text edition. (36999)* **3636**
Journal of Parapsychology (USA) *Online - full text edition. (29287)* **4271**
Journal of Parenteral and Enteral Nutrition (USA) *Online - full text edition. (12704)* **4238**
Journal of Pediatric Ophthalmology and Strabismus (USA) *Online - full text edition. (37042)* **4001**
Journal of Perinatal and Neonatal Nursing (USA) *Online - full text edition. (35925)* **3926**
Journal of Personality Disorders (USA) *Online - full text edition. (37932)* **4420**
Journal of Phenomenological Psychology (USA) *Online - full text edition. (36987)* **4420**
Journal of Positive Behavior Interventions (USA) *Online - full text edition. (39291)* **4420**
Journal of Psychiatry and Neuroscience (CAN) *Online - full text edition. (39284)* **4106**
Journal of Psychoactive Drugs (USA) *Online - full text edition. (38472)* **3403**
Journal of Psychology and Theology (USA) *Online - full text edition. (39414)* **4421**
Journal of Psychology: Interdisciplinary & Applied (USA) *Online - full text edition. (14346)* **4421**
Journal of Psychosocial Nursing and Mental Health Services (USA) *Online - full text edition. (36635)* **3926**
Journal of Public Health Management and Practice (USA) *Online - full text edition. (37449)* **4479**
Journal of Rehabilitation (USA) *Online - full text edition. (13136)* **4062**
Journal of Rehabilitation Research and Development (USA) *Online - full text edition. (20977)* **4020**
Journal of Reproductive and Infant Psychology (GBR) *Online - full text edition. (34490)* **4421**
Journal of School Health (USA) *Online - full text edition. (26287)* **4479**
Journal of Sex Research (USA) *Online - full text edition. (22854)* **4422**
Journal of Social and Clinical Psychology (USA) *Online - full text edition. (36169)* **4422**
The Journal of Social Psychology (USA) *Online - full text edition. (14224)* **4423**
Journal of Social Work Practice (GBR) *Online - full text edition. (37604)* **4515**
The Journal of Special Education (USA) *Online - full text edition. (14093)* **3424**
Journal of Speech, Language, and Hearing Research (USA) *Online - full text edition. (17692)* **3491**
Journal of Sport Behavior (USA) *Online - full text edition. (11618)* **4525**
Journal of Theory Construction and Testing (USA) *Online - full text edition. (38580)* **3926**
Journal of Trauma Nursing (USA) *Online - full text edition. (37460)* **3927**
Journal of Travel Medicine (CAN) *Online - full text edition. (38289)* **3639**
Journal of Vascular Research (CHE) *Online - full text edition. (27452)* **3779**
Journal of Women and Aging (USA) *Online - full text edition. (7902)* **4569**
Journal of Youth and Adolescence (USA) *Online - full text edition. (19466)* **3384**
Journals of Gerontology. Series A: Biological Sciences & Medical Sciences (USA) *Online - full text edition. (9697)* **3477**
Kansas Nurse (USA) *Online - full text edition. (39095)* **3927**
Kidney and Blood Pressure Research (CHE) *Online - full text edition. (10188)* **4215**
The Lancet (GBR) *Online - full text edition. (28154)* **3642**
Language and Speech (GBR) *Online - full text edition. (38017)* **3551**
Language, Speech and Hearing Services in Schools (USA) *Online - full text edition. (17693)* **4035**
Literature and Psychology (USA) *Online - full text edition. (27927)* **3552**
M L O (USA) *Online - full text edition. (37122)* **3879**
The Managed Care Payment Advisor (USA) *Online - full text edition. (39054)* **3518**
Managed Care Quarterly (USA) *Online - full text edition. (37441)* **3518**
Mankind Quarterly (USA) *Online - full text edition. (35981)* **3174**
Marketing Health Services (USA) *Online - full text edition. (15686)* **3367**
Mayo Clinic Proceedings (USA) *Online - full text edition. (18188)* **3647**
Measurement and Evaluation in Counseling and Development (USA) *Online - full text edition. (22059)* **3413**
Medical Care Research and Review (USA) *Online - full text edition. (15957)* **4496**
Medical Decision Making (USA) *Online - full text edition. (32219)* **3649**
Medical Economics (USA) *Online - full text edition. (27473)* **3650**
Medical History (GBR) *Online - full text edition. (16707)* **3650**

Medical Letter on Drugs and Therapeutics (English Edition) (USA) *Online - full text edition. (27220)* **4315**

Medical Marketing & Media (USA) *Online - full text edition. (23956)* **4315**

Medical Oncology (GBR) *Online - full text edition. (38745)* **3984**

Medical Outcomes and Guidelines Alert (USA) *Online - full text edition. (33429)* **3652**

Medical Teacher (GBR) *Online - full text edition. (9875)* **3654**

Menninger Clinic. Bulletin (USA) *Online - full text edition. (37966)* **4109**

Menopause News (USA) *Online - full text edition. (38751)* **4564**

Men's Health (United States Edition) (USA) *Online - full text edition. (13006)* **4222**

Mental Health Nursing Journal (GBR) *Online - full text edition. (38729)* **4109**

Merrill - Palmer Quarterly (USA) *Online - full text edition. (20026)* **4427**

Military Medicine (USA) *Online - full text edition. (38133)* **3661**

Minority Nurse Newsletter (USA) *Online - full text edition. (38582)* **3929**

Modern Healthcare (Year) (USA) *Online - full text edition. (20762)* **3519**

Modern Maturity (USA) *Online - full text edition. (22606)* **3478**

Morbidity and Mortality Weekly Report (USA) *Online - full text edition. (15976)* **4482**

Mortality (GBR) *Online - full content edition. (38475)* **4482**

Multicultural Education Abstracts (GBR) *Online - full content edition. (37554)* **3415**

National Cancer Institute. Journal (USA) *Online - full text edition. (27377)* **3985**

National Medical Association. Journal (USA) *Online - full text edition. (36998)* **3665**

The Nation's Health (USA) *Online - full text edition. (23425)* **4483**

Navy Medicine (USA) *Online - full text edition. (37336)* **3665**

Nephron (CHE) *Online - full text edition. (27426)* **4216**

Network News (Washington, 1975) (USA) *Online - full text edition. (11369)* **4565**

Neuroendocrinology (CHE) *Online - full text edition. (27427)* **3867**

Neuroepidemiology (CHE) *Online - full text edition. (37873)* **4113**

Neurological Research (USA) *Online - full text edition. (38000)* **4114**

Neuropsychobiology (CHE) *Online - full text edition. (37874)* **4116**

New Genetics and Society (GBR) *Online - full content edition. (38661)* **3313**

The New York State Dental Journal (USA) *Online - full text edition. (37337)* **3833**

New Zealand Journal of Psychology (NZL) *Online - full text edition. (38530)* **4430**

Nurse Author and Editor (USA) *Online - full text edition. (40565)* **3535**

The Nurse Practitioner (USA) *Online - full text edition. (39399)* **3931**

Nurse Researcher (GBR) *Online - full text edition. (39056)* **3931**

Nursing Administration Quarterly (USA) *Online - full text edition. (36020)* **3932**

Nursing B C (CAN) *Online - full text edition. (38544)* **3932**

Nursing Diagnosis (USA) *Online - full text edition. (36028)* **3932**

Nursing Economics (USA) *Online - full text edition. (36025)* **3932**

Nursing Forum (USA) *Online - full text edition. (36030)* **3933**

Nursing Homes (USA) *Online - full text edition. (27339)* **3933**

Nursing Management (USA) *Online - full text edition. (23247)* **3933**

Nursing Management (GBR) *Online - full text edition. (37458)* **3934**

Nursing Science Quarterly (USA) *Online - full text edition. (38765)* **3934**

Nursing (Year) (USA) *Online - full text edition. (20469)* **3935**

Nutrition Action Healthletter (USA) *Online - full text edition. (11581)* **4241**

Nutrition Forum (USA) *Online - full text edition. (13287)* **4242**

Nutrition Health Review (USA) *Online - full text edition. (11481)* **4242**

Nutrition in Clinical Practice (USA) *Online - full text edition. (37000)* **4242**

Nutrition Reviews (USA) *Online - full text edition. (28287)* **4243**

O E M Online (GBR) *Online - full text edition of* Occupational and Environmental Medicine. (28086) **4261**

O H Online (USA) *Online - full text edition of* Occupational Hazards. (28592) **4261**

O H S Canada (CAN) *Online - full text edition. (12002)* **4260**

O R Manager (USA) *Online - full text edition. (40571)* **3520**

Occupational Health & Safety (USA) *Online - full text edition. (28654)* **4261**

Occupational Therapy International (GBR) *Online - full text edition. (38040)* **4262**

Occupational Therapy Journal of Research (USA) *Online - full text edition. (39316)* **3669**

Onderstepoort Journal of Veterinary Research (ZAF) *Online - full text edition. (38653)* **4549**

Ophthalmic Surgery and Lasers (USA) *Online - full text edition. (37008)* **4199**

Ophthalmology Times (USA) *Online - full text edition. (36035)* **4004**

Optometric Management (USA) *Online - full text edition. (27732)* **4005**

Orthopaedic Nursing Journal (USA) *Online - full text edition. (36037)* **3936**

Orthopedics (USA) *Online - full text edition. (36483)* **4023**

P T - Magazine of Physical Therapy (USA) *Online - full text edition. (38766)* **4064**

Palaestra (USA) *Online - full text edition. (11332)* **3425**

Pathobiology (CHE) *Online - full text edition. (10191)* **3750**

Patient Care (USA) *Online - full text edition. (26582)* **3673**

Patient Care Management (USA) *Online - full text edition. (37182)* **3936**

Pediatric Annals (USA) *Online - full text edition. (37016)* **4051**

Pediatric Nursing (USA) *Online - full text edition. (36049)* **3937**

Pediatrics (English Edition) (USA) *Online - full text edition. (23202)* **4054**

Pediatrics for Parents (USA) *Online - full text edition. (36054)* **4054**

People's Medical Society Newsletter (USA) *Online - full text edition. (11489)* **3393**

Personality and Social Psychology Bulletin (USA) *Online - full text edition. (19655)* **4432**

Personnel Psychology (USA) *Online - full text edition. (16486)* **4433**

Perspectives in Psychiatric Care (USA) *Online - full text edition. (36055)* **3937**

Pharmaceutical Executive (USA) *Online - full text edition. (13756)* **4323**

Pharmaceutical Representative (USA) *Online - full text edition. (38313)* **4324**

Pharmaceutical Technology (USA) *Online - full text edition. (37261)* **4325**

Pharmacy Practice Management Quarterly (USA) *Online - full text edition. (36670)* **4328**

Philosophical Psychology (GBR) *Online - full text edition. (34497)* **4433**

Photochemistry and Photobiology (USA) *Online - full text edition. (38649)* **3374**

Physical Education New Zealand. Journal (NZL) *Online - full text edition. (37327)* **3429**

Physical Therapy (USA) *Online - full text edition. (28675)* **4064**

The Physician and Sportsmedicine (USA) *Online - full text edition. (21539)* **4176**

Physician Assistant (Springhouse) (USA) *Online - full text edition. (39434)* **3675**

Physiotherapy Research International (GBR) *Online - full text edition. (38041)* **4065**

Plastic Surgical Nursing (USA) *Online - full text edition. (36061)* **3937**

Postgraduate Medical Journal (GBR) *Online - full text edition. (38447)* **3678**

The Practitioner (GBR) *Online - full text edition. (34622)* **3678**

Preventing School Failure (USA) *Online - full text edition. (23961)* **3425**

Prevention (USA) *Online - full text edition. (23645)* **4360**

Professional Medical Assistant (USA) *Online - full text edition. (40562)* **3938**

Professional Safety (USA) *Online - full text edition. (20380)* **4263**

Professional School Counseling (USA) *Online - full text edition. (34879)* **3414**

Progress in Cardiovascular Nursing (USA) *Online - full text edition. (36608)* **3781**

Promotion & Education (FRA) *Online - full text edition. (36193)* **4486**

Psychiatric Annals (USA) *Online - full text edition. (37014)* **4125**

Psychiatry (USA) *Online - full text edition. (28651)* **4126**

The Psychoanalytic Review (USA) *Online - full text edition. (37929)* **4437**

The Psychological Record (USA) *Online - full text edition. (26132)* **4438**

Psychologische Beitraege (DEU) *Online - full text edition. (40567)* **4439**

The Psychologist (GBR) *Online - full text edition. (38004)* **4440**

Psychology, Health & Medicine (GBR) *Online - full text edition. (37667)* **4440**

Psychology Today (USA) *Online - full text edition. (26257)* **4441**

Psychopathology (CHE) *Online - full text edition. (37875)* **4128**

Psychopharmacology Bulletin (USA) *Online - full text edition. (23652)* **4332**

Psychosomatics (USA) *Online - full text edition. (37033)* **4128**

Psychotherapy and Psychosomatics (CHE) *Online - full text edition. (37876)* **4129**

Psychotherapy Research (USA) *Online - full text edition. (38005)* **4443**

Public Health Reports (USA) *Online - full text edition. (28013)* **4486**

Pulse (GBR) *Online - full text edition. (34625)* **3681**

Q R C Advisor (USA) *Online - full text edition. (37270)* **3521**

Qualitative Health Research (USA) *Online - full text edition. (30413)* **3681**

Quality Management in Health Care (USA) *Online - full text edition. (37662)* **3521**

R N Web (USA) *Online - full text edition of* R N. (27477) **3938**

Radiology and Imaging Letter (USA) *Online - full text edition. (13024)* **4154**

Real Living with Multiple Sclerosis (USA) *Online - full text edition. (39400)* **4129**

Reclaiming Children and Youth (USA) *Online - full text edition. (37561)* **4444**

Regional Anesthesia and Pain Medicine (USA) *Online - full text edition. (36489)* **3759**

Rehabilitation Counseling Bulletin (USA) *Online - full text edition. (26229)* **3486**

Rehabilitation Nursing (USA) *Online - full text edition. (38576)* **3939**

Reimbursement Advisor (USA) *Online - full text edition. (37276)* **3522**

Remedial and Special Education (USA) *Online - full text edition. (17736)* **3426**

Research on Aging (USA) *Online - full text edition. (16532)* **3480**

Research on Social Work Practice (USA) *Online - full text edition. (32449)* **4523**

Research Quarterly for Exercise and Sport (USA) *Online - full text edition. (28631)* **4360**

Review (Washington) (USA) *Online - full text edition. (21507)* **3499**

Rheumatic Diseases. Bulletin (USA) *Online - full text edition. (37288)* **4171**

S I E C U S Report (USA) *Online - full text edition. (23228)* **4523**

S T I Online (GBR) *Online - full text edition of* Sexually Transmitted Infections. (28072) **3853**

The Safety & Health Practitioner (GBR) *Online - full text edition. (11728)* **4489**

Sage Family Studies Abstracts (USA) *Online - full text edition. (37039)* **4524**

Sanitary Maintenance (USA) *Online - full text edition. (38431)* **4489**

Saskatchewan Conce R N (CAN) *Online - full text edition. (38783)* **3940**

Saturday Evening Post (USA) *Online - full text edition. (22579)* **3465**

Schizophrenia Bulletin (USA) *Online - full text edition. (18315)* **4132**

Scholastic Choices (USA) *Online - full text edition. (34839)* **3429**

School Psychology Quarterly (USA) *Online - full text edition. (37933)* **4447**

School Psychology Review (USA) *Online - full text edition. (17559)* **4447**

Seminars in Headache Management (CAN) *Online - full text edition. (37446)* **4448**

Sex Roles (USA) *Online - full text edition. (19186)* **4448**

Sexual and Relationship Therapy (GBR) *Online - full content edition. (37625)* **4448**

Shape (USA) *Online - full text edition. (11553)* **4565**

Small Group Research (USA) *Online - full text edition. (13204)* **4449**

Smith College Studies in Social Work (USA) *Online - full text edition. (38078)* **4518**

Social Behavior and Personality (NZL) *Online - full text edition. (36980)* **4449**

Social Cognition (USA) *Online - full text edition. (16691)* **4449**

Social Psychology Quarterly (USA) *Online - full text edition. (28293)* **4523**

Society of Pediatric Nurses. Journal (USA) *Online - full text edition. (36687)* **3941**

Special Educational Needs Abstracts (GBR) *Online - full content edition. (38513)* **3416**

Stroke (USA) *Online - full text edition. (23419)* **3783**

Suicide and Life-Threatening Behavior (USA) *Online - full text edition. (19183)* **4451**

Surgical Services Management (USA) *Online - full text edition. (37459)* **4205**

Telemedicine & Telehealth Network (USA) *Online - full text edition. (38324)* **3699**

Thorax Online (GBR) *Online - full text edition of* Thorax. (28091) **3700**

Today's Surgical Nurse (USA) *Online - full text edition. (37280)* **3942**

Topics in Clinical Chiropractic (USA) *Online - full text edition. (37442)* **3789**

Topics in Clinical Nutrition (USA) *Online - full text edition. (37281)* **4246**

Topics in Emergency Medicine (USA) *Online - full text edition. (36481)* **4027**

Topics in Geriatric Rehabilitation (USA) *Online - full text edition. (36482)* **3481**

Topics in Health Information Management (USA) *Online - full text edition. (37282)* **3523**

Topics in Language Disorders (USA) *Online - full text edition. (17719)* **3427**

Topics in Stroke Rehabilitation (USA) *Online - full text edition. (37443)* **3784**

Total Health (USA) *Online - full text edition. (11446)* **4246**

Trustee (USA) *Online - full text edition. (22495)* **3523**

Undersea & Hyperbaric Medicine (USA) *Online - full text edition. (37285)* **3704**

Urologic Nursing (USA) *Online - full text edition. (37457)* **4219**

Urology Times (USA) *Online - full text edition. (36124)* **4220**

Vascular Surgery (Glen Head) (USA) *Online - full text edition. (38339)* **4207**

Vegetarian Times (USA) *Online - full text edition. (18695)* **4247**

Veterinary Economics (USA) *Online - full text edition. (19938)* **3369**

Veterinary Medicine (USA) *Online - full text edition. (36222)* **4557**

Vibrant Life (USA) *Online - full text edition. (36129)* **4362**

Violence Against Women (USA) *Online - full text edition. (30426)* **4524**

Violence & Abuse Abstracts (USA) *Online - full text edition. (37605)* **4524**

Vox Sanguinis (CHE) *Online - full text edition. (27420)* **3752**

W H O Drug Information (CHE) *Online - full text edition. (38546)* **4492**

W J M (USA) *Online - full text edition. (36053)* **3707**

Weekly Epidemiological Record (CHE) *Online - full text edition. (38549)* **4493**

Western Journal of Nursing Research (USA) *Online - full text edition. (13649)* **3943**

Women & Therapy (USA) *Online - full text edition. (7906)* **4455**

Worklife Report (CAN) *Online - full text edition. (14805)* **3364**

World Health Organization. Bulletin (CHE) *Online - full text edition. (15654)* **3709**

Questel Orbit Incorporated (Subsidiary of: France Telecom, Incorporated) 8000 Westpark Dr., McLean, VA 22102 TEL 703-442-0900, FAX 703-893-4632, http://www.questel.orbit.com

A P I EnCompass: Environment (USA) *Online - full text edition of* Technical Literature Abstracts: Health & Environment. (APILIT) **3443**

Biotechnology Abstracts (GBR) *Online - full text edition. (BIOT)* **3227**

Chemical Hazards in Industry (GBR) *Online - full text edition. (CSNB)* **4268**

Chemical Safety NewsBase(GBR) *Online - full text. (CSNB)* **4268**

Environment Abstracts (USA) *Online - full text edition.* **3392**

Health and Safety Science Abstracts (USA) *Online - full text edition. (ORBIT)* **4496**

Laboratory Hazards Bulletin (GBR) *Online - full text edition. (CSNB)* **4269**

PsycINFO(USA) *Online - full text.* **4458**

Safety and Health at Work (CHE) *Online - full text edition.* **4269**

Securite et Sante au Travail (CHE) *Online - full text edition.* **4269**

RoweCom Information Quest (Subsidiary of: RoweCom, Inc.) 5838 Edison Place, Carlsbad, CA 92008-6596 TEL 760-431-7474, 800-422-3223, FAX 760-431-8860, iqsales@eiq.com, iqcontent@eiq.com, http://www.informationquest.com

A D H D Report (USA) *Online - full text edition.* **4067**
A N Z Journal of Surgery (AUS) *Online - full text edition.* **4178**
A R D Online (GBR) *Online - full text edition of* Annals of the Rheumatic Diseases. **4167**
Abdominal Imaging (USA) *Online - full text edition.* **3885**
Abstracts in Social Gerontology (USA) *Online - full text edition.* **3482**
Academic Psychiatry (USA) *Online - full text edition.* **4067**
Acta Anaesthesiologica Scandinavica (DNK) *Online - full text edition.* **3753**
Acta Biotheoretica (NLD) *Online - full text edition.* **3178**
Acta Dermato-Venereologica (NOR) *Online - full text edition.* **3843**
Acta Diabetologica (DEU) *Online - full text edition.* **3855**
Acta Ethologica Online(DEU) *Online - full text.* **3179**
Acta Haematologica (CHE) *Online - full text edition.* **3897**
Acta Neurochirurgica (AUT) *Online - full text edition.* **4179**
Acta Neuropathologica (DEU) *Online - full text edition.* **4068**
Acta Odontologica Scandinavica (NOR) *Online - full text edition.* **3813**
Acta Oncologica (NOR) *Online - full text edition.* **3966**
Acta Oto-Laryngologica (NOR) *Online - full text edition.* **4029**
Acta Paediatrica (NOR) *Online - full text edition.* **4039**
Acta Physiologica Scandinavica (GBR) *Online - full text edition.* **3337**
Acta Zoologica Online(GBR) *Online - full text.* **3350**
Addiction (GBR) *Online - full text edition.* **3396**
Addiction Biology (GBR) *Online - full text edition.* **3397**
Administration and Policy in Mental Health (USA) *Online - full text edition.* **3559**
Advances in Health Sciences Education (NLD) *Online - full text edition.* **3560**
Advances in Physiotherapy (NOR) *Online - full text edition.* **4058**
Aesthetic Plastic Surgery (USA) *Online - full text edition.* **4179**
Aesthetic Surgery Journal (USA) *Online - full text edition.* **4179**
Age and Ageing (GBR) *Online - full text edition.* **3466**
Ageing and Society (GBR) *Online - full text edition.* **3466**
Aging & Mental Health (GBR) *Online - full text edition.* **3466**
AIDS & Behavior (USA) *Online - full text edition.* **3739**
AIDS Care (GBR) *Online - full text edition.* **3791**
AIDS Education and Prevention (USA) *Online - full text edition.* **4460**
AIDS Patient Care and S T Ds (USA) *Online - full text edition.* **3791**
AIDS Research and Human Retroviruses (USA) *Online - full text edition.* **3792**
Alcohol & Alcoholism (GBR) *Online - full text edition.* **3397**
Alimentary Pharmacology and Therapeutics (GBR) *Online - full text edition.* **3886**
Allergology International (AUS) *Online - full text edition.* **3739**
Allergy (DNK) *Online - full text edition.* **3739**
Alternative & Complementary Therapies (USA) *Online - full text edition.* **3163**
American Academy of Dermatology. Journal (USA) *Online - full text edition.* **3844**
American Academy of Psychoanalysis. Journal (USA) *Online - full text edition.* **4373**
American Association for Pediatric Ophthalmology and Strabismus. Journal (USA) *Online - full text edition.* **3993**
American Behavioral Scientist (USA) *Online - full text edition.* **4508**
American Geriatrics Society. Journal (USA) *Online - full text edition.* **3467**
American Heart Journal (USA) *Online - full text edition.* **3762**
American Imago (USA) *Online - full text edition.* **4071**
American Journal of Clinical Dermatology (USA) *Online - full text edition.* **3844**
American Journal of Community Psychology (USA) *Online - full text edition.* **4520**
American Journal of Dance Therapy (USA) *Online - full text edition.* **3396**
American Journal of Drug and Alcohol Abuse (USA) *Online - full text edition.* **3399**
American Journal of Family Therapy (USA) *Online - full text edition.* **4374**
American Journal of Geriatric Psychiatry (USA) *Online - full text edition.* **3468**
American Journal of Infection Control (USA) *Online - full text edition.* **3792**
American Journal of Nephrology (CHE) *Online - full text edition.* **4209**
American Journal of Obstetrics and Gynecology (USA) *Online - full text edition.* **3944**
American Journal of Orthodontics and Dentofacial Orthopedics (USA) *Online - full text edition.* **3814**
American Journal of Perinatology (USA) *Online - full text edition.* **3944**
American Journal of Psychoanalysis (USA) *Online - full text edition.* **4374**
American Journal on Addictions (USA) *Online - full text edition.* **3399**
American Psychiatric Nurses Association. Journal (USA) *Online - full text edition.* **3913**
American Society of Echocardiography. Journal (USA) *Online - full text edition.* **3762**
Amino Acids (AUT) *Online - full text edition.* **3240**
Anaerobe (GBR) *Online - full text edition.* **3317**
Anaesthesia (Oxford) (GBR) *Online - full text edition.* **3754**
Der Anaesthesist (DEU) *Online - full text edition.* **3754**
Analytical Biochemistry (USA) *Online - full text edition.* **3240**
Analytical Cellular Pathology (NLD) *Online - full text edition.* **3285**
Analytische Psychologie (CHE) *Online - full text edition.* **4375**
Anatomy and Embryology (DEU) *Online - full text edition.* **3339**
Andrologia (DEU) *Online - full text edition.* **3565**
Angiogenesis (GBR) *Online - full text edition.* **3967**
Animal Behaviour (GBR) *Online - full text edition.* **3350**
Animal Biotechnology (USA) *Online - full text edition.* **3268**
Animal Cognition (DEU) *Online - full text edition.* **4375**
Animal Genetics (GBR) *Online - full text edition.* **3298**
Animal Health Research Reviews (GBR) *Online - full text edition.* **4537**
Annales de Dermatologie et de Venereologie (FRA) *Online - full text edition.* **3844**
Annales de Kinesitherapie (FRA) *Online - full text edition.* **4172**
Annales de Medecine Interne (FRA) *Online - full text edition.* **3907**
Annales de Pathologie (FRA) *Online - full text edition.* **3181**
Annales d'Endocrinologie (FRA) *Online - full text edition.* **3855**
Annales d'Oto-Laryngologie (FRA) *Online - full text edition.* **4030**
Annals of Behavioral Medicine (USA) *Online - full text edition.* **3715**
Annals of Biomedical Engineering (USA) *Online - full text edition.* **3566**
Annals of Clinical Psychiatry (USA) *Online - full text edition.* **4073**
Annals of Emergency Medicine (USA) *Online - full text edition.* **4010**
Annals of Hematology (DEU) *Online - full text edition.* **3898**
Annals of Human Biology (GBR) *Online - full text edition.* **3181**
Annals of Human Genetics (GBR) *Online - full text edition.* **3298**
Annals of Nutrition and Metabolism (CHE) *Online - full text edition.* **4229**
Annals of Oncology (NLD) *Online - full text edition.* **3967**
Annals of Tropical Medicine and Parasitology (GBR) *Online - full text edition.* **3793**
Annals of Tropical Paediatrics (GBR) *Online - full text edition.* **4040**
Annals of Vascular Surgery (USA) *Online - full text edition.* **4181**
Anthropology & Medicine (GBR) *Online - full text edition.* **3172**
Anti-Cancer Drug Design (GBR) *Online - full text edition.* **3967**
Antioxidants & Redox Signaling (USA) *Online - full text edition.* **3567**
Antisense and Nucleic Acid Drug Development (USA) *Online - full text edition.* **3298**
Antonie van Leeuwenhoek (NLD) *Online - full text edition.* **3268**
Aphasiology (GBR) *Online - full text edition.* **4073**
Apoptosis (USA) *Online - full text edition.* **3285**
Appetite (GBR) *Online - full text edition.* **4229**
Applied Biochemistry and Microbiology (RUS) *Online - full text edition.* **3241**
Applied Developmental Science (USA) *Online - full text edition.* **4377**
Applied Microbiology and Biotechnology (DEU) *Online - full text edition.* **3268**
Applied Neuropsychology (USA) *Online - full text edition.* **4073**
Applied Occupational & Environmental Hygiene (USA) *Online - full text edition.* **4250**
Applied Psycholinguistics (GBR) *Online - full text edition.* **3550**
Applied Psychological Measurement (USA) *Online - full text edition.* **4377**
Applied Psychology (GBR) *Online - full text edition.* **4377**
Applied Psychophysiology and Biofeedback (USA) *Online - full text edition.* **4378**
Aquatic Ecology (NLD) *Online - full text edition.* **3182**
Archives des Maladies Professionnelles (FRA) *Online - full text edition.* **4251**
Archives of Andrology (USA) *Online - full text edition.* **3568**
Archives of Biochemistry and Biophysics (USA) *Online - full text edition.* **3241**
Archives of Dermatological Research (DEU) *Online - full text edition.* **3845**
Archives of Disease in Childhood (GBR) *Online - full text edition.* **4040**
Archives of Environmental Contamination and Toxicology (USA) *Online - full text edition.* **3445**
Archives of Gynecology and Obstetrics (DEU) *Online - full text edition.* **3945**
Archives of Microbiology (DEU) *Online - full text edition.* **3318**
Archives of Orthopaedic and Trauma Surgery (DEU) *Online - full text edition.* **4010**
Archives of Physiology and Biochemistry (NLD) *Online - full text edition.* **3339**
Archives of Sexual Behavior (USA) *Online - full text edition.* **3568**
Archives of Toxicology (DEU) *Online - full text edition.* **3445**
Archives of Virology (AUT) *Online - full text edition.* **3318**
Archives of Women's Mental Health (AUT) *Online - full text edition.* **4562**
Arthroskopie (DEU) *Online - full text edition.* **3569**
Artificial Cells, Blood Substitutes, and Immobilization Biotechnology (USA) *Online - full text edition.* **3871**
Artificial Life (USA) *Online - full text edition.* **3389**
Artificial Organs (USA) *Online - full text edition.* **3871**
Asia Pacific Journal of Clinical Nutrition (AUS) *Online - full text edition.* **4229**
Asian Journal of Social Psychology (GBR) *Online - full text edition.* **4378**
Asian Journal of Surgery (SGP) *Online - full text edition.* **4182**
Astrobiology (USA) *Online - full text edition.* **3183**
Attachment and Human Development (GBR) *Online - full text edition.* **4379**
Audiology and Neuro-Otology (CHE) *Online - full text edition.* **4031**
Austral Ecology (AUS) *Online - full text edition.* **3183**
Australasian Journal of Dermatology (AUS) *Online - full text edition.* **3845**
Australasian Psychiatry (AUS) *Online - full text edition.* **4075**
Australasian Radiology (AUS) *Online - full text edition.* **4140**
Australian and New Zealand Journal of Family Therapy (GBR) *Online - full text edition.* **4520**
Australian and New Zealand Journal of Mental Health Nursing (AUS) *Online - full text edition.* **4075**
Australian & New Zealand Journal of Psychiatry (AUS) *Online - full text edition.* **4075**
Australian Journal of Rural Health (AUS) *Online - full text edition.* **4463**
Australian Occupational Therapy Journal (AUS) *Online - full text edition.* **4059**
Autism (GBR) *Online - full text edition.* **4075**
Autoimmunity (CHE) *Online - full text edition.* **3741**
Autonomic & Autacoid Pharmacology (GBR) *Online - full text edition.* **4279**
Avian Pathology (GBR) *Online - full text edition.* **4539**
B J O Online (GBR) *Online - full text edition of* British Journal of Ophthalmology. **3994**
B J S M Online (GBR) *Online - full text edition of* British Journal of Sports Medicine. **4173**
B J U International (GBR) *Online - full text edition.* **4210**
Bailliere's Best Practice & Research in Clinical Anaesthesiology (GBR) *Online - full text edition.* **3756**
Bailliere's Best Practice & Research in Clinical Endocrinology and Metabolism (GBR) *Online - full text edition.* **3855**
Bailliere's Best Practice & Research in Clinical Gastroenterology (GBR) *Online - full text edition.* **3886**
Bailliere's Best Practice & Research in Clinical Haematology (GBR) *Online - full text edition.* **3898**
Bailliere's Best Practice & Research in Clinical Obstetrics and Gynaecology (GBR) *Online - full text edition.* **3945**
Bailliere's Best Practice & Research in Clinical Rheumatology (GBR) *Online - full text edition.* **4167**
Basic and Applied Social Psychology (USA) *Online - full text edition.* **4380**
Basic Research in Cardiology (DEU) *Online - full text edition.* **3764**
Behavior Genetics (USA) *Online - full text edition.* **3299**
Behavior Modification (USA) *Online - full text edition.* **4380**
Behavioral and Brain Sciences (GBR) *Online - full text edition.* **4380**
Behavioral Ecology (USA) *Online - full text edition.* **3184**
Behavioral Ecology and Sociobiology (DEU) *Online - full text edition.* **3436**
Behaviour and Information Technology (GBR) *Online - full text edition.* **4381**
Behavioural and Cognitive Psychotherapy (GBR) *Online - full text edition.* **4382**
Behavioural Neurology (NLD) *Online - full text edition.* **4076**
Bio-Medical Materials and Engineering (NLD) *Online - full text edition.* **3237**
Biocatalysis and Biotransformation (CHE) *Online - full text edition.* **3269**
Biochemical and Biophysical Research Communications (USA) *Online - full text edition.* **3242**
Biochemical Genetics (USA) *Online - full text edition.* **3299**
Biochemical Journal (GBR) *Online - full text edition.* **3242**
Biochemistry and Cell Biology (CAN) *Online - full text edition.* **3243**
Biochemistry (Moscow) (RUS) *Online - full text edition.* **3244**
BioComplexity (NLD) *Online - full text edition.* **3340**
Biocontrol Science and Technology (GBR) *Online - full text edition.* **3157**
Biodegradation (NLD) *Online - full text edition.* **3456**
BioDrugs (NZL) *Online - full text edition.* **4280**
Bioethics (GBR) *Online - full text edition.* **4346**
BioFactors (NLD) *Online - full text edition.* **3244**
Biofouling (CHE) *Online - full text edition.* **3446**
Biogeochemistry (NLD) *Online - full text edition.* **3245**
Biogerontology (NLD) *Online - full text edition.* **3468**
Biological Control (USA) *Online - full text edition.* **3185**
Biological Research for Nursing (USA) *Online - full text edition.* **3914**
Biological Reviews (GBR) *Online - full text edition.* **3185**
Biologicals (GBR) *Online - full text edition.* **3186**
Biology and Fertility of Soils (DEU) *Online - full text edition.* **3157**
Biology of the Neonate (CHE) *Online - full text edition.* **3945**
Biomarkers (GBR) *Online - full text edition.* **3575**
Biomedical Engineering (NLD) *Online - full text edition.* **3576**
Biomedical Microdevices (USA) *Online - full text edition.* **3576**
Biometrika (GBR) *Online - full text edition.* **3226**
Biophysical Journal (USA) *Online - full text edition.* **3265**

Developmental Immunology (CHE) *Online - full text edition.* **3744**
Developmental Medicine and Child Neurology (GBR) *Online - full text edition.* **4043**
Developmental Neuropsychology (USA) *Online - full text edition.* **4394**
Developmental Neuroscience (CHE) *Online - full text edition.* **4086**
Developmental Review (USA) *Online - full text edition.* **4394**
Developmental Science (GBR) *Online - full text edition.* **4394**
Deviant Behavior (USA) *Online - full text edition.* **4521**
Diabetes & Metabolism (FRA) *Online - full text edition.* **3857**
Diabetes, Obesity and Metabolism Online(GBR) *Online - full text.* **3858**
Diabetes Technology & Therapeutics (USA) *Online - full text edition.* **3859**
Diabetic Medicine Online(GBR) *Online - full text.* **3860**
Diabetologia (DEU) *Online - full text edition.* **3860**
Diagnostic and Therapeutic Endoscopy (CHE) *Online - full text edition.* **3874**
Differentiation (DEU) *Online - full text edition.* **3193**
Digestion (CHE) *Online - full text edition.* **3888**
Digestive Diseases (CHE) *Online - full text edition.* **3888**
Digestive Diseases and Sciences (USA) *Online - full text edition.* **3888**
Digestive Surgery (CHE) *Online - full text edition.* **4187**
Disability and Rehabilitation (GBR) *Online - full text edition.* **3484**
Disability & Society (GBR) *Online - full text edition.* **3494**
Disaster Prevention and Management (GBR) *Online - full text edition.* **4466**
Discourse & Society (GBR) *Online - full text edition.* **4395**
Discourse Studies (GBR) *Online - full text edition.* **3550**
Disease Management & Health Outcomes (NZL) *Online - full text edition.* **3595**
Disease Markers (NLD) *Online - full text edition.* **3976**
Diseases of the Esophagus Online(AUS) *Online - full text.* **4032**
Documenta Ophthalmologica (NLD) *Online - full text edition.* **3997**
Doklady Biological Sciences (RUS) *Online - full text edition.* **3193**
Dreaming (USA) *Online - full text edition.* **3342**
Drug and Alcohol Review (GBR) *Online - full text edition.* **3400**
Drug and Chemical Toxicology (USA) *Online - full text edition.* **4287**
Drug Delivery (USA) *Online - full text edition.* **4288**
Drug Design and Discovery (CHE) *Online - full text edition.* **4288**
Drug Development and Industrial Pharmacy (USA) *Online - full text edition.* **4288**
Drug Metabolism Reviews (USA) *Online - full text edition.* **3596**
Drug Safety (NZL) *Online - full text edition.* **4289**
Drugs (NZL) *Online - full text edition.* **4290**
Drugs & Aging (NZL) *Online - full text edition.* **4290**
Drugs: Education, Prevention & Policy (GBR) *Online - full text edition.* **3401**
Dysphagia (USA) *Online - full text edition.* **4032**
e A D C - F & N (GBR) *Online - full text edition of* Archives of Disease in Childhood. Fetal and Neonatal Edition. **3945**
e-biomed(USA) *Online - full text.* **3596**
The E M B O Journal (GBR) *Online - full text edition.* **3249**
E M B O Reports Online (GBR) *Online - full text edition of* E M B O Reports. **3301**
E M J Online (GBR) *Online - full text edition of* Emergency Medicine Journal. **4014**
Early Childhood Education Journal (USA) *Online - full text edition.* **3410**
Ecological Psychology (USA) *Online - full text edition.* **4396**
Ecotoxicology (USA) *Online - full text edition.* **3448**
Ecotoxicology and Environmental Safety - Online (USA) *Online - full text edition of* Ecotoxicology and Environmental Safety. **3448**
Education for Health (GBR) *Online - full text edition.* **3597**
Educational and Psychological Measurement (USA) *Online - full text edition.* **4396**
Educational Gerontology (USA) *Online - full text edition.* **3470**
Educational Psychologist (USA) *Online - full text edition.* **4396**
Educational Psychology (GBR) *Online - full text edition.* **3410**
Educational Psychology in Practice (GBR) *Online - full text edition.* **3410**
Educational Psychology Review (USA) *Online - full text edition.* **3411**
Electro- and Magnetobiology (USA) *Online - full text edition.* **3266**
Electronic Journal of Pathology and Histology (GBR) *Online - full text edition.* **3598**
Elektronische Ausgabe (DEU) *Online - full text edition of* Der Hautarzt. **3849**
Emergency Medicine (Carleton South) (AUS) *Online - full text edition.* **4013**
Emergency Radiology (DEU) *Online - full text edition.* **4143**
Emotional and Behavioural Difficulties (GBR) *Online - full text edition.* **3421**
L' Encephale (FRA) *Online - full text edition.* **4087**
Endothelium (CHE) *Online - full text edition.* **3194**
Environment and Behavior (USA) *Online - full text edition.* **4521**
Environmental Management & Health (GBR) *Online - full text edition.* **3438**
Environmental Microbiology (GBR) *Online - full text edition.* **3321**
Environmental Research (USA) *Online - full text edition.* **3439**
Epidemiology and Infection (GBR) *Online - full text edition.* **3321**
Epilepsy and Behavior (USA) *Online - full text edition.* **3598**
Ergonomics (GBR) *Online - full text edition.* **3432**
Ergonomics Abstracts (GBR) *Online - full text edition.* **3433**
Ethics & Behavior (USA) *Online - full text edition.* **4397**
Ethik in der Medizin (DEU) *Online - full text edition.* **4347**
Ethnicity and Health (GBR) *Online - full text edition.* **4468**
Ethology Online(DEU) *Online - full text.* **3352**
European Addiction Research (CHE) *Online - full text edition.* **3401**
European Archives of Oto-Rhino-Laryngology (DEU) *Online - full text edition.* **4032**
European Archives of Psychiatry and Clinical Neurosciences (DEU) *Online - full text edition.* **4088**
European Biophysics Journal (DEU) *Online - full text edition.* **3266**
European Child & Adolescent Psychiatry (DEU) *Online - full text edition.* **4089**
European Heart Journal (GBR) *Online - full text edition.* **3771**
European Journal of Anaesthesiology (GBR) *Online - full text edition.* **3757**
European Journal of Applied Physiology (DEU) *Online - full text edition.* **3342**
European Journal of Biochemistry (GBR) *Online - full text edition.* **3249**
European Journal of Cancer Care Online(GBR) *Online - full text.* **3977**
European Journal of Clinical Investigation (GBR) *Online - full text edition.* **3599**
European Journal of Clinical Microbiology & Infectious Diseases (DEU) *Online - full text edition.* **3321**
European Journal of Clinical Nutrition (GBR) *Online - full text edition.* **4232**
European Journal of Clinical Pharmacology (DEU) *Online - full text edition.* **4292**
European Journal of Cognitive Psychology (GBR) *Online - full text edition.* **4397**
European Journal of Epidemiology (NLD) *Online - full text edition.* **3599**
The European Journal of Health Economics (DEU) *Online - full text edition.* **3600**
European Journal of Health Law (NLD) *Online - full text edition.* **3600**
European Journal of Human Genetics (GBR) *Online - full text edition.* **3302**
European Journal of Immunogenetics (GBR) *Online - full text edition.* **3302**
European Journal of Morphology (NLD) *Online - full text edition.* **3195**
European Journal of Neurology (USA) *Online - full text edition.* **4089**
European Journal of Neuroscience (GBR) *Online - full text edition.* **4089**
European Journal of Nuclear Medicine and Molecular Imaging (DEU) *Online - full text edition.* **4144**
European Journal of Nutrition (DEU) *Online - full text edition.* **4233**
European Journal of Orthodontics (GBR) *Online - full text edition.* **3823**
European Journal of Orthopaedic Surgery & Traumatology (FRA) *Online - full text edition.* **4014**
European Journal of Pediatrics (DEU) *Online - full text edition.* **4044**
European Journal of Plastic Surgery (DEU) *Online - full text edition.* **4188**
European Journal of Psychotherapy, Counselling and Health (GBR) *Online - full text edition.* **4089**
European Journal of Public Health (GBR) *Online - full text edition.* **4468**
European Journal of Surgery (NOR) *Online - full text edition.* **4188**
European Journal of Surgical Oncology (GBR) *Online - full text edition.* **3977**
European Journal of Trauma (DEU) *Online - full text edition.* **4014**
European Journal of Vascular and Endovascular Surgery (GBR) *Online - full text edition.* **3771**
European Journal of Work and Organizational Psychology (GBR) *Online - full text edition.* **4398**
European Neurology (CHE) *Online - full text edition.* **4089**
European Radiology (DEU) *Online - full text edition.* **4144**
The European Respiratory Journal (CHE) *Online - full text edition.* **4159**
European Review (GBR) *Online - full text edition.* **4504**
European Spine Journal (DEU) *Online - full text edition.* **4189**
European Surgical Research (CHE) *Online - full text edition.* **4189**
European Urology (CHE) *Online - full text edition.* **4212**
Evaluation and the Health Professions (USA) *Online - full text edition.* **3600**
Evidence - Based Dentistry (GBR) *Online - full text edition.* **3823**
Evolution & Development Online(USA) *Online - full text.* **3195**
Experimental Aging Research (USA) *Online - full text edition.* **4398**
Experimental & Applied Acarology (NLD) *Online - full text edition.* **3352**
Experimental and Molecular Pathology (USA) *Online - full text edition.* **3600**
Experimental Biology and Medicine (Maywood) (USA) *Online - full text edition.* **3195**
Experimental Biology Online (DEU) *Online - full text edition.* **3195**
Experimental Brain Research (DEU) *Online - full text edition.* **4090**
Experimental Eye Research (GBR) *Online - full text edition.* **3997**
Experimental Lung Research (USA) *Online - full text edition.* **4160**
Experimental Nephrology (CHE) *Online - full text edition.* **4212**
Experimental Neurology (USA) *Online - full text edition.* **4090**
Experimental Parasitology (USA) *Online - full text edition.* **3796**
Experimental Physiology (GBR) *Online - full text edition.* **3342**
The F A S E B Journal (USA) *Online - full text edition.* **3196**
Facial Plastic Surgery (USA) *Online - full text edition.* **4189**
Familial Cancer (NLD) *Online - full text edition.* **3978**
The Family Journal (USA) *Online - full text edition.* **4399**
Family Practice (GBR) *Online - full text edition.* **3601**
Feminism & Psychology (GBR) *Online - full text edition.* **4399**
Fetal and Maternal Medicine Review (GBR) *Online - full text edition.* **3950**
Fetal Diagnosis and Therapy (CHE) *Online - full text edition.* **3950**
Feuillets de Radiologie (FRA) *Online - full text edition.* **4144**
Fish and Shellfish Immunology (GBR) *Online - full text edition.* **3196**
Focus on Alternative and Complementary Therapies (GBR) *Online - full text edition.* **4296**
Folia Phoniatrica et Logopaedica (CHE) *Online - full text edition.* **4032**
Food Additives and Contaminants (GBR) *Online - full text edition.* **4296**
Food and Agricultural Immunology (GBR) *Online - full text edition.* **3197**
Food Microbiology (GBR) *Online - full text edition.* **3322**
Foot and Ankle Surgery (GBR) *Online - full text edition.* **4189**
Forschende Komplementaermedizin und Klassische Naturheilkunde (CHE) *Online - full text edition.* **3165**
Forum der Psychoanalyse (DEU) *Online - full text edition.* **4399**
Freshwater Biology Online(GBR) *Online - full text.* **3197**
Frontiers in Neuroendocrinology (USA) *Online - full text edition.* **3862**
Fundamental and Clinical Pharmacology (FRA) *Online - full text edition.* **4297**
G I Cancer (CHE) *Online - full text edition.* **3978**
Games and Economic Behavior (USA) *Online - full text edition.* **4400**
Gastric Cancer (JPN) *Online - full text edition.* **3978**
Gastro-Enterologie Clinique et Biologique (FRA) *Online - full text edition.* **3890**
Gastrointestinal Endoscopy (USA) *Online - full text edition.* **3891**
Gay and Lesbian Medical Association. Journal (USA) *Online - full text edition.* **3605**
Gefaesschirurgie (DEU) *Online - full text edition.* **4189**
Gene Therapy (Basingstoke) (GBR) *Online - full text edition.* **3606**
General and Comparative Endocrinology (USA) *Online - full text edition.* **3863**
Genes and Immunity (GBR) *Online - full text edition.* **3303**
Genes to Cells (GBR) *Online - full text edition.* **3303**
Genetic Resources and Crop Evolution (NLD) *Online - full text edition.* **3304**
Genetic Testing (USA) *Online - full text edition.* **3304**
Genetica (NLD) *Online - full text edition.* **3305**
Genetical Research (GBR) *Online - full text edition.* **3305**
Genetics (USA) *Online - full text edition.* **3305**
Genetics, Selection, Evolution Online (FRA) *Online - full text edition of* Genetics, Selection, Evolution. **3305**
Genome (CAN) *Online - full text edition.* **3306**
Genomics (USA) *Online - full text edition.* **3306**
Geomicrobiology Journal (USA) *Online - full text edition.* **3322**
Geriatric Nursing (USA) *Online - full text edition.* **3472**
Gerontology (CHE) *Online - full text edition.* **3473**
Global Change & Human Health (NLD) *Online - full text edition.* **4470**
Glycobiology (GBR) *Online - full text edition.* **3251**
Glycoconjugate Journal (USA) *Online - full text edition.* **3251**
Graefe's Archive for Clinical and Experimental Ophthalmology (DEU) *Online - full text edition.* **3998**
Graft (USA) *Online - full text edition.* **4190**
Group Analysis (GBR) *Online - full text edition.* **4401**
Group & Organization Management (USA) *Online - full text edition.* **3411**
Group (New York) (USA) *Online - full text edition.* **4401**
Growth Factors (CHE) *Online - full text edition.* **3343**
Growth Hormone and I G F Research (GBR) *Online - full text edition.* **3863**
Gut Online (GBR) *Online - full text edition of* Gut. **3891**
Gynaecological Endoscopy (GBR) *Online - full text edition.* **3951**
Der Gynaekologe (DEU) *Online - full text edition.* **3951**
Gynaekologisch - Geburtshilfliche Rundschau (CHE) *Online - full text edition.* **3951**
Gynecologic and Obstetric Investigation (CHE) *Online - full text edition.* **3952**
Gynecologic Oncology (USA) *Online - full text edition.* **3952**
H E C Forum (NLD) *Online - full text edition.* **3508**
H I V Medicine (GBR) *Online - full text edition.* **3796**
H N O (Berlin) (DEU) *Online - full text edition.* **4033**
H P B Surgery (CHE) *Online - full text edition.* **4190**
Haemophilia Online(GBR) *Online - full text.* **3901**

Online Service

Online Service

Western Journal of Nursing Research (USA) *Online - full text edition.* **3943**
Work (NLD) *Online - full text edition.* **4267**
Work and Stress (GBR) *Online - full text edition.* **4455**
World Journal of Microbiology and Biotechnology (GBR) *Online - full text edition.* **3278**
World Journal of Surgery (USA) *Online - full text edition.* **4207**
World Journal of Urology (DEU) *Online - full text edition.* **4220**
Wound Repair and Regeneration (USA) *Online - full text edition.* **4028**
Xenobiotica (GBR) *Online - full text edition.* **3264**
Xenotransplantation (DNK) *Online - full text edition.* **4207**
Zeitschrift fuer Gerontologie und Geriatrie (DEU) *Online - full text edition.* **3482**
Zeitschrift fuer Herz, Thorax- und Gefaesschirurgie (DEU) *Online - full text edition.* **3785**
Zeitschrift fuer Kardiologie (DEU) *Online - full text edition.* **3785**
Zeitschrift fuer Laermbekaempfung (DEU) *Online - full text edition.* **4367**
Zeitschrift fuer Rheumatologie (DEU) *Online - full text edition.* **4172**
Zoomorphology (DEU) *Online - full text edition.* **3225**
Zygote (GBR) *Online - full text edition.* **3315**

S T N International c/o Chemical Abstracts Service, 2540 Olentengy River Rd., PO Box 3012, Columbus, OH 43210-0012 TEL 614-447-3600, 800-753-4227, FAX 614-447-3751, TELEX 6842086 CHMAB, help@cas.org, http://www.cas.org
A P I EnCompass: Environment (USA) *Online - full text edition of* Technical Literature Abstracts: Health & Environment. (APILIT) **3443**
Abstracts on Hygiene and Communicable Diseases (GBR) *Online - full text edition.* **3715**
AgBiotech News and Information (GBR) *Online - full text edition.* **3225**
Animal Behavior Abstracts (USA) *Online - full text edition. (LIFESCI)* **3225**
Animal Breeding Abstracts (GBR) *Online - full text edition.* **3156**
Animal Pharm (GBR) *Online - full text edition.* **4537**
Biocontrol News and Information (GBR) *Online - full text edition.* **3156**
Biological Abstracts (USA) *Online - full text edition. (BIOSIS)* **3226**
Biological Abstracts - R R M (USA) *Online - full text edition. (BIOSIS)* **3226**
C S A Neurosciences Abstracts (USA) *Online - full content edition. (LIFESCI)* **3718**
Calcium and Calcified Tissue Abstracts (USA) *Online - full text edition. (LIFESCI)* **3228**
Chemical Abstracts - Biochemistry Sections (USA) *Online - full text edition. (CA)* **3228**
Chemical Hazards in Industry (GBR) *Online - full text edition. (CSNB)* **4268**
Chemical Safety NewsBase(GBR) *Online - full text. (CSNB)* **4268**
Clinica (GBR) *Online - full text edition.* **3585**
E R A News (GBR) *Online - full text edition.* **4291**
Entomology Abstracts (USA) *Online - full text edition. (LIFESCI)* **3230**
Genetics Abstracts (USA) *Online - full text edition. (LIFESCI)* **3231**
Genomika (GBR) *Online - full text edition.* **3251**
Hazards in the Office (GBR) *Online - full text edition. (CSNB)* **4268**
Health and Safety Science Abstracts (USA) *Online - full text edition.* **4496**
Helminthological Abstracts (GBR) *Online - full text edition.* **3232**
Immunology Abstracts (USA) *Online - full text edition. (LIFESCI)* **3729**
Index Veterinarius (GBR) *Online - full text edition.* **4561**
Laboratory Hazards Bulletin (GBR) *Online - full text edition. (CSNB)* **4269**
Medical & Pharmaceutical Biotechnology Abstracts (USA) *Online - full text edition. (LIFESCI)* **3732**
Medline (USA) *Online - full text edition of* Index Medicus. (MEDLINE) **3729**
Merck Index: An Encyclopedia of Chemicals and Drugs (USA) *Online - full text edition.* **4345**
Microbiology Abstracts: Section A. Industrial & Applied Microbiology (USA) *Online - full text edition. (LIFESCI)* **3233**
Microbiology Abstracts: Section B. Bacteriology (USA) *Online - full text edition. (LIFESCI)* **3233**
Microbiology Abstracts: Section C. Algology, Mycology and Protozoology (USA) *Online - full text edition. (LIFESCI)* **3233**
Nematological Abstracts (GBR) *Online - full text edition.* **3233**
Nucleic Acids Abstracts (USA) *Online - full text edition. (LIFESCI)* **3234**
Nutrition Abstracts and Reviews. Series A: Human and Experimental (GBR) *Online - full text edition.* **4249**
Nutrition Abstracts and Reviews. Series B: Livestock Feeds and Feeding (GBR) *Online - full text edition.* **3157**
Plant Breeding Abstracts (GBR) *Online - full text edition.* **3157**
Protozoological Abstracts (GBR) *Online - full text edition.* **3234**
Review of Medical and Veterinary Entomology (GBR) *Online - full text edition.* **3736**
Review of Medical and Veterinary Mycology (GBR) *Online - full text edition.* **3236**
Review of Plant Pathology (GBR) *Online - full text edition.* **3236**
Scrip - World Pharmaceutical News (GBR) *Online - full text edition.* **4335**
Toxicology Abstracts (USA) *Online - full text edition. (LIFESCI)* **3443**
Tropical Diseases Bulletin (GBR) *Online - full text edition.* **3737**
Veterinary Bulletin (GBR) *Online - full text edition.* **4561**
Virology and AIDS Abstracts (USA) *Online - full text edition. (LIFESCI)* **3236**

SciELO (Scientific Electronic Library Online) FAPESP - BIREME, Rue Botucatu 862, Sao Paulo SP 04023-901, Brazil TEL 55-11-576-9863, scielo@bireme.br, http://www.scielo.br http://www.scielo.br
Acta Cirurgica Brasileira (BRA) *Online - full text edition.* **4178**
Archivos de Medicina Veterinaria (CHL) *Online - full text edition.* **4538**
Arquivo Brasileiro de Medicina Veterinaria e Zootecnia (BRA) *Online - full text edition.* **4538**
Arquivos de Neuro-Psiquiatria (BRA) *Online - full text edition.* **4074**
Associacao Medica Brasileira. Revista (BRA) *Online - full text edition.* **3571**
Biological Research (CHL) *Online - full text edition.* **3185**
Bragantia (BRA) *Online - full text edition.* **3154**
Brazilian Journal of Biology (BRA) *Online - full text edition.* **3188**
Brazilian Journal of Medical and Biological Research (BRA) *Online - full text edition.* **3578**
Brazilian Journal of Microbiology (BRA) *Online - full text edition.* **3319**
Brazilian Journal of Veterinary Research and Animal Science (BRA) *Online - full text edition.* **4539**
Electronic Journal of Biotechnology (CHL) *Online - full text edition.* **3273**
Electronic Journal of Biotechnology(CHL) *Online - full content.* **3273**
Genetics and Molecular Biology (BRA) *Online - full text edition.* **3305**
Historia, Ciencias, Saude - Manguinhos (BRA) *Online - full text edition.* **3526**
Instituto de Medicina Tropical de Sao Paulo. Revista (BRA) *Online - full text edition.* **3799**
Instituto Oswaldo Cruz, Rio de Janeiro. Memorias (BRA) *Online - full text edition.* **3200**
Journal of Venomous Animals and Toxins (BRA) *Online - full text edition.* **3354**
Parasitologia al Dia (CHL) *Online - full text edition.* **3330**
Pesquisa Odontologica Brasileira (BRA) *Online - full text edition.* **3836**
Pesquisa Veterinaria Brasileira (BRA) *Online - full text edition.* **4549**
Psicologia: Reflexao e Critica (BRA) *Online - full text edition.* **4435**
Psicologia U S P (BRA) *Online - full text edition.* **4435**
Revista Brasileira de Cirurgia Cardiovascular (BRA) *Online - full text edition.* **3782**
Revista Brasileira de Psiquiatria (BRA) *Online - full text edition.* **4130**
Revista Chilena de Anatomia (CHL) *Online - full text edition.* **3685**
Revista Chilena de Pediatria (CHL) *Online - full text edition.* **4056**
Revista de Saude Publica (BRA) *Online - full text edition.* **4488**
Revista Medica de Chile (CHL) *Online - full text edition.* **3686**
Salud Publica de Mexico Online (MEX) *Online - full text edition of* Salud Publica de Mexico. **4489**
Sao Paulo Medical Journal (BRA) *Online - full text edition.* **3689**
Universidade de Sao Paulo. Hospital das Clinicas. Revista (BRA) *Online - full text edition.* **3704**

ScienceDirect (Division of Elsevier Science), PO Box 945, New York, NY 10159-0945 TEL 212-462-1978, 888-615-4500, FAX 212-633-3680, usinfo@sciencedirect.com, http://www.sciencedirect.com http://www.sciencedirect.com/
A C C Current Journal Review (USA) *Online - full text edition.* **3714**
A C O G Clinical Review (USA) *Online - full text edition.* **3714**
Accident Analysis & Prevention (GBR) *Online - full text edition.* **4460**
Acta Psychologica (NLD) *Online - full text edition.* **4372**
Acta Tropica (NLD) *Online - full text edition.* **3790**
Addictive Behaviors (GBR) *Online - full text edition.* **3397**
Advanced Drug Delivery Reviews (NLD) *Online - full text edition.* **4274**
Advances in Colloid and Interface Science (NLD) *Online - full text edition.* **3379**
Advances in Enzyme Regulation (GBR) *Online - full text edition.* **3239**
Aggression and Violent Behavior (GBR) *Online - full text edition.* **4373**
Alcohol (New York) (USA) *Online - full text edition.* **3398**
Ambulatory Surgery (NLD) *Online - full text edition.* **4179**
American College of Cardiology. Journal (USA) *Online - full text edition.* **3761**
American College of Surgeons. Journal (USA) *Online - full text edition.* **4179**
The American Journal of Cardiology (USA) *Online - full text edition.* **3762**
American Journal of Hypertension (USA) *Online - full text edition.* **3762**
The American Journal of Medicine (USA) *Online - full text edition.* **3564**
American Journal of Ophthalmology (USA) *Online - full text edition.* **3993**
American Journal of Preventive Medicine (USA) *Online - full text edition.* **3564**
American Journal of Surgery (USA) *Online - full text edition.* **4180**
Animal Feed Science and Technology (NLD) *Online - full text edition.* **3159**
Animal Reproduction Science (NLD) *Online - full text edition.* **3160**
Annales de Genetique (FRA) *Online - full text edition.* **3298**
Annales de Readaptation et de Medecine Physique (FRA) *Online - full text edition.* **4058**
Annales Francaises d'Anesthesie et de Reanimation (FRA) *Online - full text edition.* **3755**
Annals of Epidemiology (USA) *Online - full text edition.* **4461**
Annals of Occupational Hygiene (GBR) *Online - full text edition.* **4250**
Annals of Thoracic Surgery (USA) *Online - full text edition.* **4181**
L' Annee Biologique (FRA) *Online - full text edition.* **3182**
Antimicrobics and Infectious Diseases Newsletter (USA) *Online - full text edition.* **3793**
Antiviral Research (NLD) *Online - full text edition.* **3317**
Applied Animal Behaviour Science (NLD) *Online - full text edition.* **3350**
Applied Behavioral Science Review (GBR) *Online - full text edition.* **4377**
Applied Ergonomics (GBR) *Online - full text edition.* **3431**
Applied Radiation and Isotopes (GBR) *Online - full text edition.* **4365**
Applied Radiology (USA) *Online - full text edition.* **4140**
Aquatic Toxicology (NLD) *Online - full text edition.* **3445**
Archives of Clinical Neuropsychology (GBR) *Online - full text edition.* **4074**
Archives of Gerontology and Geriatrics (IRL) *Online - full text edition.* **3468**
Archives of Medical Research (MEX) *Online - full text edition.* **3568**
Archives of Oral Biology (GBR) *Online - full text edition.* **3351**
Artificial Intelligence in Medicine (NLD) *Online - full text edition.* **3389**
The Arts in Psychotherapy (GBR) *Online - full text edition.* **4378**
Atherosclerosis (IRL) *Online - full text edition.* **3763**
Atmospheric Environment (GBR) *Online - full text edition.* **3443**
Auris, Nasus, Larynx (NLD) *Online - full text edition.* **4031**
Autonomic Neuroscience: Basic & Clinical (NLD) *Online - full text edition.* **4075**
B B A - Bioenergetics (NLD) *Online - full text edition.* **3278**
B B A - Biomembranes (NLD) *Online - full text edition.* **3285**
B B A - Gene Structure and Expression (NLD) *Online - full text edition.* **3299**
B B A - General Subjects (NLD) *Online - full text edition.* **3241**
B B A - Molecular and Cell Biology of Lipids (NLD) *Online - full text edition.* **3242**
B B A - Molecular Basis of Disease (NLD) *Online - full text edition.* **3299**
B B A - Molecular Cell Research (NLD) *Online - full text edition.* **3285**
B B A - Protein Structure and Molecular Enzymology (NLD) *Online - full text edition.* **3242**
B B A - Reviews on Cancer (NLD) *Online - full text edition.* **3968**
Behaviour Research and Therapy (GBR) *Online - full text edition.* **4382**
Behavioural Brain Research (NLD) *Online - full text edition.* **4076**
Behavioural Processes (NLD) *Online - full text edition.* **4076**
Biochemical Pharmacology (USA) *Online - full text edition.* **4279**
Biochemical Systematics and Ecology (GBR) *Online - full text edition.* **3243**
Biochemistry and Molecular Biology Education (GBR) *Online - full text edition.* **3243**
Biochimie (FRA) *Online - full text edition.* **3244**
Bioelectrochemistry (CHE) *Online - full text edition.* **3244**
Biofutur (FRA) *Online - full text edition.* **3269**
Biological Psychiatry (USA) *Online - full text edition.* **4076**
Biological Psychology (NLD) *Online - full text edition.* **4382**
Biology of the Cell (FRA) *Online - full text edition.* **3286**
Biomaterials (GBR) *Online - full text edition.* **3575**
Biomedicine and Pharmacotherapy (FRA) *Online - full text edition.* **3577**
Biomolecular Engineering (NLD) *Online - full text edition.* **3269**
Bioorganic & Medicinal Chemistry (GBR) *Online - full text edition.* **3377**
Bioorganic & Medicinal Chemistry Letters (GBR) *Online - full text edition.* **3378**
Biophysical Chemistry (NLD) *Online - full text edition.* **3265**
Biosensors and Bioelectronics (GBR) *Online - full text edition.* **3270**
Biosystems (IRL) *Online - full text edition.* **3187**
Biotechnology Advances (USA) *Online - full text edition.* **3271**
Bone (USA) *Online - full text edition.* **4011**
Brain and Development (NLD) *Online - full text edition.* **4077**
Brain Research (NLD) *Online - full text edition.* **4078**
Brain Research Bulletin (USA) *Online - full text edition.* **4078**
Brain Research Protocols (NLD) *Online - full text edition.* **4078**
Brain Research Reviews (NLD) *Online - full text edition.* **4078**
British Journal of Obstetrics & Gynaecology (GBR) *Online - full text edition.* **3946**
Burns (GBR) *Online - full text edition.* **4011**
Cancer Genetics & Cytogenetics (USA) *Online - full text edition.* **3971**
Cancer Letters (IRL) *Online - full text edition.* **3972**
Cancer - Radiotherapie (FRA) *Online - full text edition.* **3972**

Cardiovascular Pathology (USA) *Online - full text edition.* **3767**
Cardiovascular Radiation Medicine (USA) *Online - full text edition.* **3767**
Cardiovascular Research (NLD) *Online - full text edition.* **3767**
Cardiovascular Surgery (GBR) *Online - full text edition.* **3767**
Cell Transplantation (USA) *Online - full text edition.* **3288**
Cellular Signalling (USA) *Online - full text edition.* **3288**
Chemical Health and Safety (USA) *Online - full text edition.* **3446**
Chemico-Biological Interactions (IRL) *Online - full text edition.* **3447**
Chemistry & Biology (GBR) *Online - full text edition.* **3372**
Chemistry and Physics of Lipids (IRL) *Online - full text edition.* **3246**
Chemosphere (GBR) *Online - full text edition.* **3447**
Child Abuse & Neglect (GBR) *Online - full text edition.* **3381**
Children and Youth Services Review (GBR) *Online - full text edition.* **3382**
Clinica Chimica Acta (NLD) *Online - full text edition.* **3585**
Clinical and Applied Immunology Reviews (USA) *Online - full text edition.* **3742**
Clinical Biochemistry (USA) *Online - full text edition.* **3247**
Clinical Biomechanics (GBR) *Online - full text edition.* **3787**
Clinical Imaging (USA) *Online - full text edition.* **4141**
Clinical Microbiology Newsletter (USA) *Online - full text edition.* **3319**
Clinical Neurology and Neurosurgery (NLD) *Online - full text edition.* **4082**
Clinical Neurophysiology (IRL) *Online - full text edition.* **4082**
Clinical Neuroscience Research (NLD) *Online - full text edition.* **4082**
Clinical Psychology Review (GBR) *Online - full text edition.* **4388**
Clinical Therapeutics (USA) *Online - full text edition.* **3587**
Clinics in Dermatology (USA) *Online - full text edition.* **3846**
Cognition (NLD) *Online - full text edition.* **4388**
Cognitive Brain Research (NLD) *Online - full text edition.* **4083**
Cognitive Development (GBR) *Online - full text edition.* **4389**
Cognitive Science (GBR) *Online - full text edition.* **4389**
Comparative Biochemistry and Physiology. Part A: Molecular & Integrative Physiology (USA) *Online - full text edition.* **3341**
Comparative Biochemistry and Physiology. Part B: Biochemistry & Molecular Biology (USA) *Online - full text edition.* **3247**
Comparative Biochemistry and Physiology. Toxicology & Pharmacology (USA) *Online - full text edition.* **3247**
Comparative Immunology, Microbiology and Infectious Diseases (GBR) *Online - full text edition.* **3320**
Computer Methods and Programs in Biomedicine (IRL) *Online - full text edition.* **3809**
Computerized Medical Imaging and Graphics (GBR) *Online - full text edition.* **3809**
Computers in Biology and Medicine (GBR) *Online - full text edition.* **3284**
Computers in Human Behavior (GBR) *Online - full text edition.* **4524**
Contraception (USA) *Online - full text edition.* **3357**
Controlled Clinical Trials (USA) *Online - full text edition.* **3873**
Critical Reviews in Biochemistry and Molecular Biology (USA) *Online - full text edition.* **3248**
Critical Reviews in Biotechnology (USA) *Online - full text edition.* **3273**
Critical Reviews in Clinical Laboratory Sciences (USA) *Online - full text edition.* **3591**
Critical Reviews in Diagnostic Imaging (USA) *Online - full text edition.* **4142**
Critical Reviews in Microbiology (USA) *Online - full text edition.* **3320**
Critical Reviews in Oncology - Hematology (IRL) *Online - full text edition.* **3975**
Critical Reviews in Toxicology (USA) *Online - full text edition.* **3447**
Current Biology (GBR) *Online - full text edition.* **3229**
Current Opinion in Biotechnology (GBR) *Online - full text edition.* **3273**
Current Opinion in Cell Biology (GBR) *Online - full text edition.* **3288**
Current Opinion in Genetics & Development (GBR) *Online - full text edition.* **3301**
Current Opinion in Immunology (GBR) *Online - full text edition.* **3722**
Current Opinion in Neurobiology (GBR) *Online - full text edition.* **4084**
Current Opinion in Pharmacology (GBR) *Online - full text edition.* **4285**
Current Opinion in Structural Biology (GBR) *Online - full text edition.* **3248**
Current Surgery (USA) *Online - full text edition.* **4186**
Current Therapeutic Research (USA) *Online - full text edition.* **3592**
Cytokine and Growth Factor Reviews (GBR) *Online - full text edition.* **3248**
Dental Materials (USA) *Online - full text edition.* **3820**
Developmental and Comparative Immunology (GBR) *Online - full text edition.* **3743**
Developmental Brain Research (NLD) *Online - full text edition.* **4086**
Diabetes Research and Clinical Practice (IRL) *Online - full text edition.* **3858**
Diagnostic Microbiology and Infectious Disease (USA) *Online - full text edition.* **3320**
Domestic Animal Endocrinology (USA) *Online - full text edition.* **4542**
Drug and Alcohol Dependence (IRL) *Online - full text edition.* **3400**
Drug Discovery Today (GBR) *Online - full text edition.* **4288**
Early Human Development (IRL) *Online - full text edition.* **3948**
Eating Behaviors (NLD) *Online - full text edition.* **4395**
Environment International (GBR) *Online - full text edition.* **3438**
Environmental Toxicology and Pharmacology (NLD) *Online - full text edition.* **3449**
Enzyme and Microbial Technology (USA) *Online - full text edition.* **3273**
Epilepsy Research (NLD) *Online - full text edition.* **4088**
European Academy of Dermatology and Venereology. Journal (BEL) *Online - full text edition.* **3848**
European Journal of Cancer (GBR) *Online - full text edition.* **3977**
European Journal of Cardio-Thoracic Surgery (NLD) *Online - full text edition.* **3771**
The European Journal of Heart Failure (NLD) *Online - full text edition.* **3771**
European Journal of Internal Medicine (USA) *Online - full text edition.* **3908**
European Journal of Medicinal Chemistry (FRA) *Online - full text edition.* **3250**
European Journal of Obstetrics & Gynecology and Reproductive Biology (IRL) *Online - full text edition.* **3949**
European Journal of Pharmaceutical Sciences (NLD) *Online - full text edition.* **4292**
European Journal of Pharmaceutics and Biopharmaceutics (NLD) *Online - full text edition.* **4293**
European Journal of Pharmacology (NLD) *Online - full text edition.* **4293**
European Journal of Radiology (IRL) *Online - full text edition.* **4144**
European Journal of Soil Biology (FRA) *Online - full text edition.* **3195**
European Journal of Ultrasound (IRL) *Online - full text edition.* **4144**
European Neuropsychopharmacology (NLD) *Online - full text edition.* **4089**
European Psychiatry (FRA) *Online - full text edition.* **4089**
Experimental Gerontology (USA) *Online - full text edition.* **3471**
Experimental Hematology (USA) *Online - full text edition.* **3901**
F E B S Letters (NLD) *Online - full text edition.* **3250**
F E M S Immunology and Medical Microbiology (NLD) *Online - full text edition.* **3321**
F E M S Microbiology Ecology (NLD) *Online - full text edition.* **3321**
F E M S Microbiology Letters (NLD) *Online - full text edition.* **3322**
F E M S Microbiology Reviews (NLD) *Online - full text edition.* **3322**
Il Farmaco (FRA) *Online - full text edition.* **4295**
Fertility and Sterility (USA) *Online - full text edition.* **3949**
Fitoterapia (ITA) *Online - full text edition.* **3279**
Food and Chemical Toxicology (GBR) *Online - full text edition.* **3449**
Forensic Science International (IRL) *Online - full text edition.* **3882**
Free Radical Biology & Medicine (USA) *Online - full text edition.* **3197**
Gait and Posture (NLD) *Online - full text edition.* **3605**
Gene - C O M B I S (NLD) *Online - full text edition of* Gene. **3274**
General Hospital Psychiatry (USA) *Online - full text edition.* **4091**
General Pharmacology (USA) *Online - full text edition.* **4297**
Health & Place (GBR) *Online - full text edition.* **3465**
Health Policy (IRL) *Online - full text edition.* **4473**
Hearing Research (NLD) *Online - full text edition.* **4033**
Hepatology Research (IRL) *Online - full text edition.* **3892**
Human Immunology (USA) *Online - full text edition.* **3744**
Human Movement Science (NLD) *Online - full text edition.* **3616**
I T B M - R B M (FRA) *Online - full text edition.* **3275**
I T B M - R B M News (FRA) *Online - full text edition.* **3275**
Immunology Letters (NLD) *Online - full text edition.* **3746**
Immunotechnology (NLD) *Online - full text edition.* **3746**
Industrial Crops and Products (NLD) *Online - full text edition.* **3158**
Infant Behavior and Development (GBR) *Online - full text edition.* **4404**
Injury (GBR) *Online - full text edition.* **4016**
Institut Pasteur. Annales. Actualites (FRA) *Online - full text edition.* **3323**
Intelligence (Kidlington) (GBR) *Online - full text edition.* **4404**
International Commission on Radiological Protection. Annals (GBR) *Online - full text edition.* **4145**
International Contact Lens Clinic (USA) *Online - full text edition.* **3999**
International Immunopharmacology (GBR) *Online - full text edition.* **4302**
International Journal for Parasitology (GBR) *Online - full text edition.* **3799**
International Journal of Antimicrobial Agents (NLD) *Online - full text edition.* **3323**
International Journal of Biochemistry & Cell Biology (GBR) *Online - full text edition.* **3252**
International Journal of Biological Macromolecules (NLD) *Online - full text edition.* **3252**
International Journal of Cardiology (IRL) *Online - full text edition.* **3775**
International Journal of Developmental Neuroscience (GBR) *Online - full text edition.* **4095**
International Journal of Drug Policy (NLD) *Online - full text edition.* **3402**
International Journal of Food Microbiology (NLD) *Online - full text edition.* **3324**
International Journal of Gynecology and Obstetrics (IRL) *Online - full text edition.* **3954**
International Journal of Law and Psychiatry (GBR) *Online - full text edition.* **3540**
International Journal of Medical Informatics (IRL) *Online - full text edition.* **3811**
International Journal of Neural Systems (SGP) *Online - full text edition.* **3389**
International Journal of Nursing Studies (GBR) *Online - full text edition.* **3922**
International Journal of Pediatric Otorhinolaryngology (IRL) *Online - full text edition.* **4033**
International Journal of Pharmaceutics (NLD) *Online - full text edition.* **4303**
International Journal of Psychophysiology (NLD) *Online - full text edition.* **4407**
International Journal of Radiation: Oncology - Biology - Physics (USA) *Online - full text edition.* **4146**
Interventional Cardiology Newsletter (USA) *Online - full text edition.* **3775**
J A H Online (USA) *Online - full text edition of* Journal of Adolescent Health. **3629**
Japanese Journal of Ophthalmology (NLD) *Online - full text edition.* **4000**
Journal de Pediatrie et de Puericulture (FRA) *Online - full text edition.* **3628**
Journal Midwifery and Women's Health (USA) *Online - full text edition.* **3955**
Journal of Affective Disorders (NLD) *Online - full text edition.* **4098**
Journal of Aging Studies (GBR) *Online - full text edition.* **3475**
Journal of Anxiety Disorders (GBR) *Online - full text edition.* **4409**
Journal of Applied Developmental Psychology (GBR) *Online - full text edition.* **4410**
The Journal of Behavior Therapy and Experimental Psychiatry (GBR) *Online - full text edition.* **4099**
Journal of Biochemical and Biophysical Methods (NLD) *Online - full text edition.* **3252**
Journal of Biological Systems (SGP) *Online - full text edition.* **3202**
The Journal of Biomechanics (GBR) *Online - full text edition.* **3629**
Journal of Biotechnology (NLD) *Online - full text edition.* **3275**
Journal of Cataract and Refractive Surgery (USA) *Online - full text edition.* **4000**
Journal of Chemical Neuroanatomy (NLD) *Online - full text edition.* **4099**
Journal of Chromatography. B, Biomedical Sciences and Applications (NLD) *Online - full text edition.* **3373**
The Journal of Clinical Anesthesia (USA) *Online - full text edition.* **3758**
The Journal of Clinical Epidemiology (USA) *Online - full text edition.* **3630**
Journal of Clinical Virology (NLD) *Online - full text edition.* **3801**
Journal of Cognitive Systems Research (USA) *Online - full text edition.* **4412**
Journal of Communication Disorders (USA) *Online - full text edition.* **4412**
Journal of Controlled Release (NLD) *Online - full text edition.* **4306**
The Journal of Dentistry (GBR) *Online - full text edition.* **3828**
Journal of Dermatological Science (IRL) *Online - full text edition.* **3850**
Journal of Diabetes and Its Complications (USA) *Online - full text edition.* **3864**
The Journal of Economic Psychology (NLD) *Online - full text edition.* **3366**
Journal of Electromyography and Kinesiology (GBR) *Online - full text edition.* **3266**
The Journal of Emergency Medicine (USA) *Online - full text edition.* **4018**
Journal of Environmental Radioactivity (GBR) *Online - full text edition.* **3440**
Journal of Ethnopharmacology (IRL) *Online - full text edition.* **4307**
Journal of Experimental Marine Biology and Ecology (NLD) *Online - full text edition.* **3203**
Journal of Fluency Disorders (USA) *Online - full text edition.* **4416**
Journal of Health Economics (NLD) *Online - full text edition.* **4479**
The Journal of Heart and Lung Transplantation (GBR) *Online - full text edition.* **4193**
Journal of Hepatology (DNK) *Online - full text edition.* **3893**
Journal of Immunological Methods (NLD) *Online - full text edition.* **3748**
Journal of Inorganic Biochemistry (USA) *Online - full text edition.* **3254**
Journal of Luminescence (NLD) *Online - full text edition.* **4366**
Journal of Microbiological Methods (NLD) *Online - full text edition.* **3325**
Journal of Molecular Graphics and Modelling (USA) *Online - full text edition.* **3377**
Journal of Musculoskeletal Research (SGP) *Online - full text edition.* **4019**
Journal of Neuroimmunology (NLD) *Online - full text edition.* **4103**
Journal of Neurolinguistics (GBR) *Online - full text edition.* **4103**
Journal of Neuroscience Methods (NLD) *Online - full text edition.* **4104**
Journal of Nutritional Biochemistry (USA) *Online - full text edition.* **4238**
Journal of Orthopaedic Research (USA) *Online - full text edition.* **4019**
Journal of Pain and Symptom Management (USA) *Online - full text edition.* **4105**
Journal of Pediatric and Adolescent Gynecology (NLD) *Online - full text edition.* **4047**
Journal of Pharmaceutical and Biomedical Analysis (NLD) *Online - full text edition.* **4309**
Journal of Pharmacological and Toxicological Methods (USA) *Online - full text edition.* **3452**
Journal of Photochemistry and Photobiology, B: Biology (CHE) *Online - full text edition.* **3255**

Online Service

Journal of Physiology (Paris) (FRA) *Online - full text edition.* **4105**
Journal of Psychiatric Research (GBR) *Online - full text edition.* **4106**
Journal of Psychosomatic Research (USA) *Online - full text edition.* **4106**
Journal of Reproductive Immunology (IRL) *Online - full text edition.* **3749**
Journal of Safety Research (GBR) *Online - full text edition.* **4258**
Journal of School Psychology (GBR) *Online - full text edition.* **4422**
Journal of Steroid Biochemistry and Molecular Biology (GBR) *Online - full text edition.* **3255**
Journal of Substance Abuse (GBR) *Online - full text edition.* **3403**
Journal of Substance Abuse Treatment (USA) *Online - full text edition.* **3404**
Journal of the Neurological Sciences (NLD) *Online - full text edition.* **4106**
Journal of Thermal Biology (GBR) *Online - full text edition.* **3267**
Journal of Virological Methods (NLD) *Online - full text edition.* **3326**
The Knee (NLD) *Online - full text edition.* **3345**
The Lancet (GBR) *Online - full text edition.* **3642**
The Lancet Oncology (GBR) *Online - full text edition.* **3983**
The Leadership Quarterly (USA) *Online - full text edition.* **3365**
Learning and Individual Differences (GBR) *Online - full text edition.* **3413**
Learning and Instruction (GBR) *Online - full text edition.* **3413**
Legal Medicine (NLD) *Online - full text edition.* **3884**
Leukemia Research (GBR) *Online - full text edition.* **3904**
Lung Cancer (IRL) *Online - full text edition.* **3983**
Magnetic Resonance Imaging (USA) *Online - full text edition.* **4150**
Magnetic Resonance Materials in Physics, Biology and Medicine (GBR) *Online - full text edition.* **4366**
Marine Environmental Research (GBR) *Online - full text edition.* **3444**
Mathematical Biosciences (USA) *Online - full text edition.* **3554**
Matrix Biology (NLD) *Online - full text edition.* **3646**
Maturitas (IRL) *Online - full text edition.* **3958**
Mechanisms of Ageing and Development (IRL) *Online - full text edition.* **3478**
Mechanisms of Development (IRL) *Online - full text edition.* **3292**
Medecine et Droit (FRA) *Online - full text edition.* **3884**
Medical Dosimetry (USA) *Online - full text edition.* **4150**
Medical Engineering & Physics (GBR) *Online - full text edition.* **3650**
Medical Image Analysis (GBR) *Online - full text edition.* **4150**
Medical Update for Psychiatrists (USA) *Online - full text edition.* **4108**
Microbes and Infection (FRA) *Online - full text edition.* **3327**
Micron (GBR) *Online - full text edition.* **3335**
Molecular and Biochemical Parasitology (NLD) *Online - full text edition.* **3256**
Molecular and Cellular Endocrinology (IRL) *Online - full text edition.* **3866**
Molecular Aspects of Medicine (GBR) *Online - full text edition.* **3662**
Molecular Brain Research (NLD) *Online - full text edition.* **4110**
Molecular Imaging and Biology (NLD) *Online - full text edition.* **4151**
Molecular Immunology (GBR) *Online - full text edition.* **3257**
Mutation Research - D N A Repair (NLD) *Online - full text edition.* **3258**
Mutation Research - Fundamental and Molecular Mechanisms of Mutagenesis (NLD) *Online - full text edition.* **3311**
Mutation Research - Genetic Toxicology and Environmental Mutagenesis (NLD) *Online - full text edition.* **3312**
Mutation Research - Reviews in Mutation Research (NLD) *Online - full text edition.* **3312**
Netherlands Journal of Medicine (NLD) *Online - full text edition.* **3911**
Neural Networks (GBR) *Online - full text edition.* **3390**
Neurobiology of Aging (USA) *Online - full text edition.* **3346**
Neurochemistry International (GBR) *Online - full text edition.* **4113**
Neuromuscular Disorders (GBR) *Online - full text edition.* **4115**
Neuropharmacology (GBR) *Online - full text edition.* **4318**
Neurophysiologie Clinique (FRA) *Online - full text edition.* **4116**
Neuropsychologia (GBR) *Online - full text edition.* **4116**
Neuropsychopharmacology (USA) *Online - full text edition.* **4117**
Neuroscience (GBR) *Online - full text edition.* **4117**
Neuroscience and Biobehavioral Reviews (GBR) *Online - full text edition.* **4118**
Neuroscience Letters (IRL) *Online - full text edition.* **4118**
Neuroscience Research (IRL) *Online - full text edition.* **4118**
Neurotoxicology and Teratology (USA) *Online - full text edition.* **4119**
NeuroToxicology (Little Rock) (USA) *Online - full text edition.* **4119**
New Ideas in Psychology (GBR) *Online - full text edition.* **4430**
Nuclear Medicine and Biology (USA) *Online - full text edition.* **4152**
Nutrition (USA) *Online - full text edition.* **4241**
Nutrition Research (USA) *Online - full text edition.* **4243**
Obstetrics and Gynecology (USA) *Online - full text edition.* **3960**
Ophthalmic and Physiological Optics (GBR) *Online - full text edition.* **4003**
Ophthalmology (USA) *Online - full text edition.* **4004**
Opportunistic Pathogens (NLD) *Online - full text edition.* **3804**
Option - Bio (FRA) *Online - full text edition.* **3212**
Oral Oncology (GBR) *Online - full text edition.* **3988**
Pain (NLD) *Online - full text edition.* **4121**
Parasitology International (NLD) *Online - full text edition.* **3805**
Parkinsonism and Related Disorders (GBR) *Online - full text edition.* **4122**
Pathophysiology (NLD) *Online - full text edition.* **3347**
Patient Education and Counseling (IRL) *Online - full text edition.* **4484**
Pediatric Neurology (USA) *Online - full text edition.* **4053**
Peptides (USA) *Online - full text edition.* **3260**
Personality and Individual Differences (GBR) *Online - full text edition.* **4432**
Pharmacology and Therapeutics (USA) *Online - full text edition.* **4326**
Pharmacology, Biochemistry and Behavior (USA) *Online - full text edition.* **4327**
Physiology and Behavior (USA) *Online - full text edition.* **3347**
Postharvest Biology and Technology (NLD) *Online - full text edition.* **3277**
Preventive Veterinary Medicine (NLD) *Online - full text edition.* **4550**
Primary Care Update for Ob - Gyns (USA) *Online - full text edition.* **3962**
Process Biochemistry (GBR) *Online - full text edition.* **3277**
Progress in Biophysics & Molecular Biology (GBR) *Online - full text edition.* **3267**
Progress in Neuro-Psychopharmacology and Biological Psychiatry (USA) *Online - full text edition.* **4331**
Progress in Neurobiology (GBR) *Online - full text edition.* **3348**
Progress in Nuclear Magnetic Resonance Spectroscopy (NLD) *Online - full text edition.* **3377**
Progress in Pediatric Cardiology (IRL) *Online - full text edition.* **3782**
Progress in Retinal and Eye Research (GBR) *Online - full text edition.* **4006**
Prostaglandins and Other Lipid Mediators (USA) *Online - full text edition.* **3868**
Psychiatry Research (IRL) *Online - full text edition.* **4127**
Psychiatry Research: Neuroimaging Section (IRL) *Online - full text edition.* **4127**
Psychology of Sport & Exercise (NLD) *Online - full text edition.* **4441**
Psychoneuroendocrinology (GBR) *Online - full text edition.* **4128**
Radiotherapy and Oncology (IRL) *Online - full text edition.* **4154**
Regulatory Peptides (NLD) *Online - full text edition.* **3262**
Reproductive Toxicology (USA) *Online - full text edition.* **3348**
Research in Developmental Disabilities (GBR) *Online - full text edition.* **4130**
Research in Microbiology (FRA) *Online - full text edition.* **3330**
Respiration Physiology (NLD) *Online - full text edition.* **3348**
Resuscitation (IRL) *Online - full text edition.* **4165**
Revue du Rhumatisme (Edition Francaise) (FRA) *Online - full text edition.* **4170**
Revue Francaise des Laboratoires (FRA) *Online - full text edition.* **3216**
Safety Science (NLD) *Online - full text edition.* **4265**
Schizophrenia Research (NLD) *Online - full text edition.* **4132**
The Science of the Total Environment (NLD) *Online - full text edition.* **3442**
Sleep Medicine (NLD) *Online - full text edition.* **4134**
Small Ruminant Research (NLD) *Online - full text edition.* **3161**
Social Science & Medicine (GBR) *Online - full text edition.* **3694**
Society for Gynecologic Investigation. Journal (USA) *Online - full text edition.* **3964**
Soil Biology & Biochemistry (GBR) *Online - full text edition.* **3263**
Solid State Nuclear Magnetic Resonance (GBR) *Online - full text edition.* **3377**
Speech Communication (NLD) *Online - full text edition.* **3552**
Steroids (USA) *Online - full text edition.* **3263**
Structure (GBR) *Online - full text edition.* **3220**
Surgical Neurology (USA) *Online - full text edition.* **4205**
Surgical Oncology (GBR) *Online - full text edition.* **3991**
Survey of Ophthalmology (USA) *Online - full text edition.* **3737**
Theriogenology (USA) *Online - full text edition.* **4553**
Thrombosis Research (GBR) *Online - full text edition.* **3784**
Toxicology (IRL) *Online - full text edition.* **3455**
Toxicology in Vitro (GBR) *Online - full text edition.* **3455**
Toxicology Letters (IRL) *Online - full text edition.* **3456**
Toxicon (GBR) *Online - full text edition.* **4338**
Transfusion and Apheresis Science (GBR) *Online - full text edition.* **3905**
Transfusion Clinique et Biologique (FRA) *Online - full text edition.* **3905**
Transplant Immunology (GBR) *Online - full text edition.* **3751**
Transplantation Proceedings (USA) *Online - full text edition.* **4206**
Trends in Biochemical Sciences (GBR) *Online - full text edition.* **3263**
Trends in Biotechnology (GBR) *Online - full text edition.* **3277**
Trends in Cardiovascular Medicine (USA) *Online - full text edition.* **3784**
Trends in Cell Biology (GBR) *Online - full text edition.* **3295**
Trends in Cognitive Sciences (GBR) *Online - full text edition.* **4453**
Trends in Ecology and Evolution (GBR) *Online - full text edition.* **3221**
Trends in Endocrinology and Metabolism (GBR) *Online - full text edition.* **3869**
Trends in Genetics (GBR) *Online - full text edition.* **3314**
Trends in Immunology Online (GBR) *Online - full text edition of* Trends in Immunology. **3752**
Trends in Microbiology (GBR) *Online - full text edition.* **3332**
Trends in Molecular Medicine (GBR) *Online - full text edition.* **3702**
Trends in Neurosciences (GBR) *Online - full text edition.* **4137**
Trends in Parasitology (GBR) *Online - full text edition.* **3332**
Trends in Pharmacological Sciences (GBR) *Online - full text edition.* **4338**
Ultramicroscopy (NLD) *Online - full text edition.* **3336**
Ultrasound in Medicine & Biology (USA) *Online - full text edition.* **3222**
Urologic Oncology (USA) *Online - full text edition.* **3992**
Urology (USA) *Online - full text edition.* **4220**
Vaccine Online (GBR) *Online - full text edition of* Vaccine. **3752**
Veterinary Immunology and Immunopathology (NLD) *Online - full text edition.* **4557**
Veterinary Microbiology (NLD) *Online - full text edition.* **3332**
Veterinary Parasitology (NLD) *Online - full text edition.* **4558**
Virus Research (NLD) *Online - full text edition.* **3333**
Vision Research (GBR) *Online - full text edition.* **4008**
Women's Health Issues (USA) *Online - full text edition.* **4567**

SilverPlatter Information, Incorporated 100 River Ridge Dr., Norwood, MA 02062 TEL 781-769-2599, 800-343-0064, FAX 781-769-8763, info@silverplatter.com, http://www.silverplatter.com
A R D Online (GBR) *Online - full text edition of* Annals of the Rheumatic Diseases. **4167**
B J O Online (GBR) *Online - full text edition of* British Journal of Ophthalmology. **3994**
B J S M Online (GBR) *Online - full text edition of* British Journal of Sports Medicine. **4173**
EMBASE Alert (USA) *Online - full text edition.* **3723**
EMBASE List of Journals Indexed (Year) (NLD) *Online - full text edition.* **3723**
Gut Online (GBR) *Online - full text edition of* Gut. **3891**
J M S Online (GBR) *Online - full text edition of* Journal of Medical Screening. **3802**
O E M Online (GBR) *Online - full text edition of* Occupational and Environmental Medicine. **4261**
S T I Online (GBR) *Online - full text edition of* Sexually Transmitted Infections. **3853**
Thorax Online (GBR) *Online - full text edition of* Thorax. **3700**
Tobbacco Control Online (GBR) *Online - full text edition of* Tobacco Control. **4531**

Springer LINK Springer-Verlag, Tiergartenstr.17, Heidelberg 69121, Germany FAX 49-6221-487-120; Springer-Verlag, 175 Fifth Ave., New York, NY 10010 FAX 212-539-1719, http://link.springer.de
Abdominal Imaging (USA) *Online - full text edition. (261)* **3885**
Acta Diabetologica (DEU) *Online - full text edition. (592)* **3855**
Acta Ethologica Online(DEU) *Online - full text. (10211)* **3179**
Acta Neurochirurgica (AUT) *Online - full text edition. (701)* **4179**
Acta Neuropathologica (DEU) *Online - full text edition. (401)* **4068**
Aesthetic Plastic Surgery (USA) *Online - full text edition. (266)* **4179**
Amino Acids (AUT) *Online - full text edition. (726)* **3240**
Der Anaesthesist (DEU) *Online - full text edition. (101)* **3754**
Anatomy and Embryology (DEU) *Online - full text edition. (429)* **3339**
Annals of Hematology (DEU) *Online - full text edition. (277)* **3898**
Annals of Vascular Surgery (USA) *Online - full text edition. (10016)* **4181**
Applied Microbiology and Biotechnology (DEU) *Online - full text edition. (253)* **3268**
Archives of Dermatological Research (DEU) *Online - full text edition. (403)* **3845**
Archives of Environmental Contamination and Toxicology (USA) *Online - full text edition. (244)* **3445**
Archives of Gynecology and Obstetrics (DEU) *Online - full text edition. (404)* **3945**
Archives of Microbiology (DEU) *Online - full text edition. (203)* **3318**
Archives of Orthopaedic and Trauma Surgery (DEU) *Online - full text edition. (402)* **4010**
Archives of Toxicology (DEU) *Online - full text edition. (204)* **3445**
Archives of Virology (AUT) *Online - full text edition. (705)* **3318**
Archives of Women's Mental Health (AUT) *Online - full text edition. (737)* **4562**
Arthroskopie (DEU) *Online - full text edition. (142)* **3569**
Asian Journal of Surgery (SGP) *Online - full text edition. (10116)* **4182**
Basic Research in Cardiology (DEU) *Online - full text edition. (395)* **3764**
Behavioral Ecology and Sociobiology (DEU) *Online - full text edition. (265)* **3436**
Biology and Fertility of Soils (DEU) *Online - full text edition. (374)* **3157**
Brain Tumor Pathology (JPN) *Online - full text edition. (10014)* **3968**

Zeitschrift fuer Rheumatologie (DEU) *Online - full text edition. (393)* **4172**
Zoomorphology (DEU) *Online - full text edition. (435)* **3225**

Swets Blackwell PO Box 800, Lisse 2160 SZ, Netherlands TEL 31-252-435111, FAX 31-252-415888, swetsnetnavigator@nl.swetsblackwell.com, http://www.swetsblackwell.com
A C C Current Journal Review (USA) *Online - full text edition. (2271184)* **3714**
A C O G Clinical Review (USA) *Online - full text edition. (1679880)* **3714**
A N Z Journal of Surgery (AUS) *Online - full text edition. (684759)* **4178**
A P M I S (DNK) *Online - full text edition. (1661981)* **3178**
A R D Online (GBR) *Online - full text edition of* Annals of the Rheumatic Diseases. (458538) **4167**
Abdominal Imaging (USA) *Online - full text edition. (396141)* **3885**
Abstracts in Social Gerontology (USA) *Online - full text edition. (1992260)* **3482**
Accident Analysis & Prevention (GBR) *Online - full text edition. (376213)* **4460**
Accident and Emergency Nursing (GBR) *Online - full text edition. (2267381)* **3912**
Acta Anaesthesiologica Scandinavica (DNK) *Online - full text edition. (1127985)* **3753**
Acta Biotheoretica (NLD) *Online - full text edition. (256935)* **3178**
Acta Dermato-Venereologica (NOR) *Online - full text edition. (1107461)* **3843**
Acta Dermato-Venereologica. Supplementum (NOR) *Online - full text edition. (1107488)* **3843**
Acta Diabetologica (DEU) *Online - full text edition. (293652)* **3855**
Acta Ethologica Online(DEU) *Online - full text. (4065905)* **3179**
Acta Haematologica (CHE) *Online - full text edition. (695327)* **3897**
Acta Histochemica (DEU) *Online - full text edition. (364541)* **3239**
Acta Neurochirurgica (AUT) *Online - full text edition. (798789)* **4179**
Acta Neurologica Scandinavica (DNK) *Online - full text edition. (1099892)* **4068**
Acta Neuropathologica (DEU) *Online - full text edition. (677388)* **4068**
Acta Obstetrica et Gynecologica Scandinavica (DNK) *Online - full text edition. (1088637)* **3944**
Acta Odontologica Scandinavica (NOR) *Online - full text edition. (538833)* **3813**
Acta Oncologica (NOR) *Online - full text edition. (668141)* **3966**
Acta Ophthamologica Scandinavica Online(DNK) *Online - full text. (1119664)* **3993**
Acta Oto-Laryngologica (NOR) *Online - full text edition. (1086987)* **4029**
Acta Oto-Laryngologica. Supplement (NOR) *Online - full text edition. (1086995)* **4029**
Acta Paediatrica (NOR) *Online - full text edition. (1096192)* **4039**
Acta Paediatrica. Supplement (NOR) *Online - full text edition. (654868)* **4039**
Acta Physiologica Scandinavica (GBR) *Online - full text edition. (1088084)* **3337**
Acta Psychiatrica Scandinavica (DNK) *Online - full text edition. (1084933)* **4068**
Acta Psychiatrica Scandinavica. Supplementum (DNK) *Online - full text edition. (1084941)* **4069**
Acta Psychologica (NLD) *Online - full text edition. (449725)* **4372**
Acta Radiologica (DNK) *Online - full text edition. (2256215)* **4139**
Acta Radiologica. Supplementum (DNK) *Online - full text edition. (139807)* **4139**
Acta Tropica (NLD) *Online - full text edition. (456713)* **3790**
Acta Zoologica Online(GBR) *Online - full text. (112763)* **3350**
Addiction (GBR) *Online - full text edition. (363235)* **3396**
Addiction Abstracts (GBR) *Online - full content edition. (2384132)* **3397**
Addiction Biology (GBR) *Online - full text edition. (3507858)* **3397**
Addictive Behaviors (GBR) *Online - full text edition. (430315)* **3397**
Administration and Policy in Mental Health (USA) *Online - full text edition. (1537903)* **3559**
Advanced Drug Delivery Reviews (NLD) *Online - full text edition. (1501119)* **4274**
Advances in Colloid and Interface Science (NLD) *Online - full text edition. (207063)* **3379**
Advances in Enzyme Regulation (GBR) *Online - full text edition. (392618)* **3239**
Advances in Health Sciences Education (NLD) *Online - full text edition. (2997509)* **3560**
Advances in Physiotherapy (NOR) *Online - full text edition. (3993779)* **4058**
Aesthetic Plastic Surgery (USA) *Online - full text edition. (240222)* **4179**
Age and Ageing (GBR) *Online - full text edition. (71838)* **3466**
Ageing and Society (GBR) *Online - full text edition. (1061380)* **3466**
Aggression and Violent Behavior (GBR) *Online - full text edition. (3317706)* **4373**
Aging & Mental Health (GBR) *Online - full text edition. (3225429)* **3466**
AIDS (USA) *Online - full text edition. (1579576)* **3790**
AIDS & Behavior (USA) *Online - full text edition. (3232956)* **3739**
AIDS Care (GBR) *Online - full text edition. (1742523)* **3791**
AIDS Patient Care and S T Ds (USA) *Online - full text edition. (1652060)* **3791**
AIDS Research and Human Retroviruses (USA) *Online - full text edition. (1323997)* **3792**
Alcohol & Alcoholism (GBR) *Online - full text edition. (415650)* **3397**
Alcohol (New York) (USA) *Online - full text edition. (1363158)* **3398**
Alimentary Pharmacology and Therapeutics (GBR) *Online - full text edition. (1578731)* **3886**
Allergology International (AUS) *Online - full text edition. (3006727)* **3739**
Allergy (DNK) *Online - full text edition. (276898)* **3739**
Allergy. Supplementum (DNK) *Online - full text edition. (2888084)* **3740**
Alternative & Complementary Therapies (USA) *Online - full content edition. (2721155)* **3163**
Ambulatory Child Health Online(GBR) *Online - full text. (2658267)* **4040**
Ambulatory Surgery (NLD) *Online - full text edition. (2273357)* **4179**
American Behavioral Scientist (USA) *Online - full text edition. (718394)* **4508**
American College of Cardiology. Journal (USA) *Online - full text edition. (1206001)* **3761**
American College of Surgeons. Journal (USA) *Online - full text edition. (386723)* **4179**
American Geriatrics Society. Journal (USA) *Online - full text edition. (127272)* **3467**
American Imago (USA) *Online - full text edition. (102601)* **4071**
The American Journal of Cardiology (USA) *Online - full text edition. (99821)* **3762**
American Journal of Cardiovascular Drugs (NZL) *Online - full text edition. (4455940)* **3762**
American Journal of Clinical Dermatology (USA) *Online - full text edition. (4067290)* **3844**
American Journal of Community Psychology (USA) *Online - full text edition. (673951)* **4520**
American Journal of Dance Therapy (USA) *Online - full text edition. (960292)* **3396**
American Journal of Drug and Alcohol Abuse (USA) *Online - full text edition. (314145)* **3399**
American Journal of Epidemiology (USA) *Online - full text edition. (1123807)* **3563**
American Journal of Family Therapy (USA) *Online - full text edition. (998672)* **4374**
American Journal of Hypertension (USA) *Online - full text edition. (1389823)* **3762**
The American Journal of Medicine (USA) *Online - full text edition. (373230)* **3564**
American Journal of Nephrology (CHE) *Online - full text edition. (1107372)* **4209**
American Journal of Ophthalmology (USA) *Online - full text edition. (383678)* **3993**
American Journal of Preventive Medicine (USA) *Online - full text edition. (1400231)* **3564**
American Journal of Psychoanalysis (USA) *Online - full text edition. (646156)* **4374**
American Journal of Reproductive Immunology Online(DNK) *Online - full text. (1051709)* **3740**
American Journal of Surgery (USA) *Online - full text edition. (474827)* **4180**
American Journal of Surgical Pathology (USA) *Online - full text edition. (677264)* **3564**
American Journal of Transplantation Online(DNK) *Online - full text. (4512162)* **4180**
American Journal on Addictions (USA) *Online - full text edition. (2137100)* **3399**
Amino Acids (AUT) *Online - full text edition. (2140268)* **3240**
Anaerobe (GBR) *Online - full text edition. (2726416)* **3317**
Anaesthesia (Oxford) (GBR) *Online - full text edition. (455059)* **3754**
Der Anaesthesist (DEU) *Online - full text edition. (557005)* **3754**
Analytical Biochemistry (USA) *Online - full text edition. (285552)* **3240**
Analytical Cellular Pathology (NLD) *Online - full text edition. (1753363)* **3285**
Analytische Psychologie (CHE) *Online - full text edition. (112690)* **4375**
Anatomia, Histologia, Embryologia Online(DEU) *Online - full text. (616273)* **4537**
Anatomy and Embryology (DEU) *Online - full text edition. (64130)* **3339**
Andrologia (DEU) *Online - full text edition. (592560)* **3565**
Anesthesia and Analgesia (USA) *Online - full text edition. (35653)* **3755**
Anesthesiology (USA) *Online - full text edition. (162760)* **3755**
Angiogenesis (GBR) *Online - full text edition. (3541916)* **3967**
Animal Behaviour (GBR) *Online - full text edition. (248878)* **3350**
Animal Cognition (DEU) *Online - full text edition. (3603423)* **4375**
Animal Feed Science and Technology (NLD) *Online - full text edition. (490547)* **3159**
Animal Genetics (GBR) *Online - full text edition. (317829)* **3298**
Animal Health Research Reviews (GBR) *Online - full text edition. (4060970)* **4537**
Animal Reproduction Science (NLD) *Online - full text edition. (483966)* **3160**
Annales de Readaptation et de Medecine Physique (FRA) *Online - full text edition. (1057871)* **4058**
Annals of Biomedical Engineering (USA) *Online - full text edition. (708054)* **3566**
Annals of Clinical Psychiatry (USA) *Online - full text edition. (1799479)* **4073**
Annals of Epidemiology (USA) *Online - full text edition. (2005697)* **4461**
Annals of Hematology (DEU) *Online - full text edition. (104051)* **3898**
Annals of Human Biology (GBR) *Online - full text edition. (425826)* **3181**
Annals of Human Genetics (GBR) *Online - full text edition. (237221)* **3298**
Annals of Medicine (GBR) *Online - full text edition. (1123297)* **3871**
Annals of Nutrition and Metabolism (CHE) *Online - full text edition. (39608)* **4229**
Annals of Occupational Hygiene (GBR) *Online - full text edition. (693944)* **4250**
Annals of Oncology (NLD) *Online - full text edition. (1846701)* **3967**
Annals of Surgery (USA) *Online - full text edition. (365068)* **4181**
Annals of Thoracic Surgery (USA) *Online - full text edition. (9040)* **4181**
Annals of Tropical Medicine and Parasitology (GBR) *Online - full text edition. (779393)* **3793**
Annals of Tropical Paediatrics (GBR) *Online - full text edition. (1051733)* **4040**
Annals of Vascular Surgery (USA) *Online - full text edition. (3461564)* **4181**
L' Annee Biologique (FRA) *Online - full text edition. (325171)* **3182**
Anthropology & Medicine (GBR) *Online - full content edition. (3270122)* **3172**
Anti-Cancer Drug Design (GBR) *Online - full text edition. (1422111)* **3967**
Antioxidants & Redox Signaling (USA) *Online - full content edition. (3925307)* **3567**
Antiviral Research (NLD) *Online - full text edition. (1038850)* **3317**
Antonie van Leeuwenhoek (NLD) *Online - full text edition. (2018411)* **3268**
Aphasiology (GBR) *Online - full text edition. (1572547)* **4073**
Apoptosis (USA) *Online - full text edition. (3307891)* **3285**
Appetite (GBR) *Online - full text edition. (1039253)* **4229**
Applied Animal Behaviour Science (NLD) *Online - full text edition. (304646)* **3350**
Applied Biochemistry and Microbiology (RUS) *Online - full text edition. (145815)* **3241**
Applied Developmental Science (USA) *Online - full text edition. (3241939)* **4377**
Applied Ergonomics (GBR) *Online - full text edition. (90425)* **3431**
Applied Microbiology and Biotechnology (DEU) *Online - full text edition. (578649)* **3268**
Applied Neuropsychology (USA) *Online - full text edition. (2387948)* **4073**
Applied Occupational & Environmental Hygiene (USA) *Online - full text edition. (1527886)* **4250**
Applied Psycholinguistics (GBR) *Online - full text edition. (965103)* **3550**
Applied Psychological Measurement (USA) *Online - full text edition. (3258610)* **4377**
Applied Psychology (GBR) *Online - full text edition. (258725)* **4377**
Applied Psychophysiology and Biofeedback (USA) *Online - full text edition. (172294)* **4378**
Applied Radiation and Isotopes (GBR) *Online - full text edition. (186996)* **4365**
Aquatic Ecology (NLD) *Online - full text edition. (751111)* **3182**
Aquatic Toxicology (NLD) *Online - full text edition. (1046756)* **3445**
Archives of Andrology (USA) *Online - full text edition. (59315)* **3568**
Archives of Biochemistry and Biophysics (USA) *Online - full text edition. (760374)* **3241**
Archives of Clinical Neuropsychology (GBR) *Online - full text edition. (1570587)* **4074**
Archives of Dermatological Research (DEU) *Online - full text edition. (821756)* **3845**
Archives of Disease in Childhood (GBR) *Online - full text edition. (411884)* **4040**
Archives of Environmental Contamination and Toxicology (USA) *Online - full text edition. (723975)* **3445**
Archives of Gerontology and Geriatrics (IRL) *Online - full text edition. (1191039)* **3468**
Archives of Gynecology and Obstetrics (DEU) *Online - full text edition. (465631)* **3945**
Archives of Medical Research (MEX) *Online - full text edition. (707198)* **3568**
Archives of Microbiology (DEU) *Online - full text edition. (314374)* **3318**
Archives of Oral Biology (GBR) *Online - full text edition. (406295)* **3351**
Archives of Orthopaedic and Trauma Surgery (DEU) *Online - full text edition. (445177)* **4010**
Archives of Physiology and Biochemistry (NLD) *Online - full text edition. (777692)* **3339**
Archives of Sexual Behavior (USA) *Online - full text edition. (305103)* **3568**
Archives of Toxicology (DEU) *Online - full text edition. (1114743)* **3445**
Archives of Virology (AUT) *Online - full text edition. (752746)* **3318**
Archives of Women's Mental Health (AUT) *Online - full text edition. (3779963)* **4562**
Arthroskopie (DEU) *Online - full text edition. (1650165)* **3569**
Artificial Intelligence in Medicine (NLD) *Online - full text edition. (1714791)* **3389**
Artificial Life (USA) *Online - full content edition. (2261863)* **3389**
Artificial Organs (USA) *Online - full text edition. (944564)* **3871**
The Arts in Psychotherapy (GBR) *Online - full text edition. (1030418)* **4378**
Asia Pacific Family Medicine Online(AUS) *Online - full text. (4513010)* **3570**
Asia Pacific Journal of Clinical Nutrition (AUS) *Online - full text edition. (2797100)* **4229**
Asian Journal of Social Psychology (GBR) *Online - full text edition. (3012832)* **4378**
Asian Journal of Surgery (SGP) *Online - full text edition. (1046209)* **4182**
Atherosclerosis (IRL) *Online - full text edition. (155039)* **3763**
Atmospheric Environment (GBR) *Online - full text edition. (1921878)* **3443**
Attachment and Human Development (GBR) *Online - full content edition. (3879828)* **4379**
Audiology and Neuro-Otology (CHE) *Online - full text edition. (2978695)* **4031**
Auris, Nasus, Larynx (NLD) *Online - full text edition. (998354)* **4031**
Austral Ecology (AUS) *Online - full text edition. (110531)* **3183**
Australasian Journal of Dermatology (AUS) *Online - full text edition. (735671)* **3845**
Australasian Psychiatry (AUS) *Online - full text edition. (2791609)* **4075**
Australasian Radiology (AUS) *Online - full text edition. (475874)* **4140**

Australian and New Zealand Journal of Family Therapy (GBR) *Online - full text edition. (1609327)* **4520**
Australian and New Zealand Journal of Mental Health Nursing (AUS) *Online - full text edition. (2730235)* **4075**
Australian & New Zealand Journal of Psychiatry (AUS) *Online - full text edition. (647519)* **4075**
Australian Journal of Experimental Agriculture (AUS) *Online - full text edition. (768375)* **3157**
Australian Journal of Rural Health (AUS) *Online - full text edition. (2752751)* **4463**
Australian Occupational Therapy Journal (AUS) *Online - full text edition. (1235559)* **4059**
Autism (GBR) *Online - full text edition. (3246191)* **4075**
Autonomic & Autacoid Pharmacology (GBR) *Online - full text edition. (1076485)* **4279**
Autonomic Neuroscience: Basic & Clinical (NLD) *Online - full text edition. (938882)* **4075**
Avian Pathology (GBR) *Online - full text edition. (384747)* **4539**
B B A - Bioenergetics (NLD) *Online - full text edition. (539287)* **3278**
B B A - Biomembranes (NLD) *Online - full text edition. (624470)* **3285**
B B A - Gene Structure and Expression (NLD) *Online - full text edition. (45446)* **3299**
B B A - General Subjects (NLD) *Online - full text edition. (721425)* **3241**
B B A - Molecular and Cell Biology of Lipids (NLD) *Online - full text edition. (792896)* **3242**
B B A - Molecular Basis of Disease (NLD) *Online - full text edition. (2002531)* **3299**
B B A - Molecular Cell Research (NLD) *Online - full text edition. (1154583)* **3285**
B B A - Protein Structure and Molecular Enzymology (NLD) *Online - full text edition. (1154567)* **3242**
B B A - Reviews on Cancer (NLD) *Online - full text edition. (730882)* **3968**
B J O Online (GBR) *Online - full text edition of* British Journal of Ophthalmology. (770450) **3994**
B J S M Online (GBR) *Online - full text edition of* British Journal of Sports Medicine. (733873) **4173**
B J U International (GBR) *Online - full text edition. (129941)* **4210**
Bailliere's Best Practice & Research in Clinical Anaesthesiology (GBR) *Online - full text edition. (1603396)* **3756**
Bailliere's Best Practice & Research in Clinical Endocrinology and Metabolism (GBR) *Online - full text edition. (1603418)* **3855**
Bailliere's Best Practice & Research in Clinical Gastroenterology (GBR) *Online - full text edition. (1603426)* **3886**
Bailliere's Best Practice & Research in Clinical Haematology (GBR) *Online - full text edition. (1603434)* **3898**
Bailliere's Best Practice & Research in Clinical Obstetrics and Gynaecology (GBR) *Online - full text edition. (1603450)* **3945**
Bailliere's Best Practice & Research in Clinical Rheumatology (GBR) *Online - full text edition. (1603485)* **4167**
Basic and Applied Social Psychology (USA) *Online - full text edition. (1036599)* **4380**
Basic Research in Cardiology (DEU) *Online - full text edition. (827231)* **3764**
Behavior Genetics (USA) *Online - full text edition. (709905)* **3299**
Behavior Modification (USA) *Online - full text edition. (527181)* **4380**
Behavioral and Brain Sciences (GBR) *Online - full text edition. (181587)* **4380**
Behavioral Ecology (USA) *Online - full text edition. (1992147)* **3184**
Behavioral Ecology and Sociobiology (DEU) *Online - full text edition. (378089)* **3436**
Behaviour (NLD) *Online - full content edition. (270261)* **3351**
Behaviour and Information Technology (GBR) *Online - full text edition. (1103512)* **4381**
Behaviour Research and Therapy (GBR) *Online - full text edition. (450170)* **4382**
Behavioural and Cognitive Psychotherapy (GBR) *Online - full text edition. (1091794)* **4382**
Behavioural Brain Research (NLD) *Online - full text edition. (951412)* **4076**
Behavioural Neurology (NLD) *Online - full text edition. (1686186)* **4076**
Behavioural Processes (NLD) *Online - full text edition. (636266)* **4076**
Bio-Medical Materials and Engineering (NLD) *Online - full text edition. (1935933)* **3237**
Biochemical and Biophysical Research Communications (USA) *Online - full text edition. (559652)* **3242**
Biochemical Genetics (USA) *Online - full text edition. (189022)* **3299**
Biochemical Journal (GBR) *Online - full text edition. (204250)* **3242**
Biochemical Pharmacology (USA) *Online - full text edition. (688258)* **4279**
Biochemical Society Transactions (GBR) *Online - full text edition. (293539)* **3243**
Biochemical Systematics and Ecology (GBR) *Online - full text edition. (104825)* **3243**
Biochemistry and Cell Biology (CAN) *Online - full text edition. (796239)* **3243**
Biochemistry and Molecular Biology Education (GBR) *Online - full text edition. (115223)* **3243**
Biochemistry (Moscow) (RUS) *Online - full text edition. (114898)* **3244**
Biochimie (FRA) *Online - full text edition. (1316362)* **3244**
Biocontrol Science and Technology (GBR) *Online - full text edition. (2033968)* **3157**
Biodegradation (NLD) *Online - full text edition. (1860097)* **3456**
BioDrugs (NZL) *Online - full text edition. (2406330)* **4280**
Bioelectrochemistry (CHE) *Online - full text edition. (107921)* **3244**
Bioethics (GBR) *Online - full text edition. (1579266)* **4346**
BioFactors (NLD) *Online - full text edition. (1640712)* **3244**
Biofutur (FRA) *Online - full text edition. (1201220)* **3269**
Biogeochemistry (NLD) *Online - full text edition. (1371185)* **3245**
Biogerontology (NLD) *Online - full text edition. (4224574)* **3468**
Biological Chemistry (DEU) *Online - full text edition. (58211)* **3245**
Biological Control (USA) *Online - full text edition. (2025523)* **3185**
Biological Psychiatry (USA) *Online - full text edition. (98175)* **4076**
Biological Psychology (NLD) *Online - full text edition. (238813)* **4382**
Biological Research for Nursing (USA) *Online - full text edition. (3821552)* **3914**
Biological Reviews (GBR) *Online - full text edition. (670391)* **3185**
Biologicals (GBR) *Online - full text edition. (274836)* **3186**
Biology and Fertility of Soils (DEU) *Online - full text edition. (1395335)* **3157**
Biology of the Cell (FRA) *Online - full text edition. (183156)* **3286**
Biology of the Neonate (CHE) *Online - full text edition. (291889)* **3945**
Biomarkers (GBR) *Online - full text edition. (2984121)* **3575**
Biomaterials (GBR) *Online - full text edition. (1024221)* **3575**
Biomedical Engineering (NLD) *Online - full text edition. (141100)* **3576**
Biomedical Microdevices (USA) *Online - full text edition. (3598802)* **3576**
Biomedicine and Pharmacotherapy (FRA) *Online - full text edition. (1085212)* **3577**
Biometrika (GBR) *Online - full text edition. (256277)* **3226**
Biomolecular Engineering (NLD) *Online - full text edition. (1212893)* **3269**
Bioorganic & Medicinal Chemistry (GBR) *Online - full text edition. (2400995)* **3377**
Bioorganic & Medicinal Chemistry Letters (GBR) *Online - full text edition. (2091410)* **3378**
Biophysical Chemistry (NLD) *Online - full text edition. (8001)* **3265**
Biorheology (NLD) *Online - full text edition. (608890)* **3265**
Bioscience Reports (USA) *Online - full text edition. (1087940)* **3286**
Biosensors and Bioelectronics (GBR) *Online - full text edition. (1396285)* **3270**
Biosystems (IRL) *Online - full text edition. (31623)* **3187**
Biotech Software and Internet Report (USA) *Online - full text edition. (1420488)* **3270**
Biotechnology Advances (USA) *Online - full text edition. (1231162)* **3271**
Biotechnology and Applied Biochemistry (GBR) *Online - full text edition. (1005707)* **3271**
Biotechnology Law Report (USA) *Online - full content edition. (1595334)* **3272**
Biotechnology Letters (NLD) *Online - full text edition. (1633252)* **3272**
Bipolar Disorders Online(DNK) *Online - full text. (3828603)* **4077**
Birth (USA) *Online - full text edition. (60690)* **3946**
Blood Cells, Molecules, and Diseases (USA) *Online - full text edition. (272922)* **3898**
Blood Pressure (NOR) *Online - full text edition. (2215373)* **3764**
Blood Purification (CHE) *Online - full text edition. (1207369)* **3899**
Blood Reviews (GBR) *Online - full text edition. (1621173)* **3899**
Bone (USA) *Online - full text edition. (189863)* **4011**
Bone Marrow Transplantation (GBR) *Online - full text edition. (2262053)* **3872**
Brain (GBR) *Online - full text edition. (600865)* **4077**
Brain and Cognition (USA) *Online - full text edition. (1134434)* **4383**
Brain and Development (NLD) *Online - full text edition. (1029509)* **4077**
Brain and Language (USA) *Online - full text edition. (331732)* **4383**
Brain and Mind (USA) *Online - full text edition. (4006623)* **4077**
Brain, Behavior and Evolution (CHE) *Online - full text edition. (820563)* **4077**
Brain, Behavior, and Immunity (USA) *Online - full text edition. (1578855)* **3741**
Brain Injury (GBR) *Online - full text edition. (1604309)* **4077**
Brain Research (NLD) *Online - full text edition. (1083430)* **4078**
Brain Research Bulletin (USA) *Online - full text edition. (721476)* **4078**
Brain Research Protocols (NLD) *Online - full text edition. (3478386)* **4078**
Brain Research Reviews (NLD) *Online - full text edition. (920096)* **4078**
Brain Topography (USA) *Online - full text edition. (1693336)* **4078**
The Breast (GBR) *Online - full text edition. (2137003)* **3946**
Breast Cancer Research and Treatment (USA) *Online - full text edition. (1060228)* **3969**
Breast Disease (NLD) *Online - full text edition. (1603256)* **3946**
The Breast Journal Online(USA) *Online - full text. (2723212)* **3946**
British Food Journal (GBR) *Online - full text edition. (397660)* **3460**
British Homeopathic Journal (GBR) *Online - full text edition. (1045040)* **3786**
British Journal of Cancer (GBR) *Online - full text edition. (2022079)* **3969**
British Journal of Clinical Governance (GBR) *Online - full text edition. (3983617)* **3578**
British Journal of Clinical Pharmacology (GBR) *Online - full text edition. (392103)* **4281**
British Journal of Clinical Psychology (GBR) *Online - full text edition. (1107933)* **4383**
The British Journal of Criminology (GBR) *Online - full text edition. (575771)* **3393**
British Journal of Dermatology (GBR) *Online - full text edition. (1128965)* **3845**
British Journal of Dermatology. Supplement (GBR) *Online - full text edition. (1128973)* **3846**
British Journal of Developmental Psychology (GBR) *Online - full text edition. (1197177)* **4383**
British Journal of Educational Psychology (GBR) *Online - full text edition. (203440)* **4383**
British Journal of Guidance and Counselling (GBR) *Online - full content edition. (218316)* **4269**
British Journal of Haematology (GBR) *Online - full text edition. (65080)* **3899**
British Journal of Health Psychology (GBR) *Online - full text edition. (3260194)* **4384**
British Journal of Learning Disabilities (GBR) *Online - full text edition. (1154303)* **4079**
British Journal of Mathematical and Statistical Psychology (GBR) *Online - full text edition. (578665)* **4384**
British Journal of Medical Psychology (GBR) *Online - full text edition. (296627)* **4384**
British Journal of Neurosurgery (GBR) *Online - full text edition. (1565974)* **4182**
The British Journal of Nutrition (GBR) *Online - full text edition. (1673157)* **4230**
British Journal of Oral and Maxillofacial Surgery (GBR) *Online - full text edition. (656453)* **4183**
British Journal of Plastic Surgery (GBR) *Online - full text edition. (587214)* **4183**
British Journal of Psychology (GBR) *Online - full text edition. (743291)* **4384**
British Journal of Radiology (GBR) *Online - full text edition. (261882)* **4141**
British Journal of Social Psychology (GBR) *Online - full text edition. (1107941)* **4384**
British Journal of Special Education (GBR) *Online - full text edition. (181986)* **3419**
British Journal of Surgery (GBR) *Online - full text edition. (709050)* **4183**
British Medical Bulletin (GBR) *Online - full text edition. (456411)* **3579**
Bulletin of Environmental Contamination and Toxicology (USA) *Online - full text edition. (14478)* **3446**
Bulletin of Experimental Biology and Medicine (NLD) *Online - full text edition. (215104)* **3188**
Bulletin of Mathematical Biology (GBR) *Online - full text edition. (507857)* **3188**
Bulletin of the History of Medicine (USA) *Online - full text edition. (612057)* **3579**
Bundesgesundheitsblatt - Gesundheitsforschung - Gesundheitsschutz Online(DEU) *Online - full content. (57940)* **4464**
Burns (GBR) *Online - full text edition. (115819)* **4011**
C N S Drugs (NZL) *Online - full text edition. (2406357)* **4282**
Calcified Tissue International (USA) *Online - full text edition. (387584)* **3855**
Cambridge Quarterly of Healthcare Ethics (GBR) *Online - full text edition. (2143658)* **3581**
Canadian Journal of Microbiology (CAN) *Online - full text edition. (141046)* **3319**
Canadian Journal of Physiology and Pharmacology (CAN) *Online - full text edition. (425494)* **3340**
Cancer and Metastasis Reviews (USA) *Online - full text edition. (1126652)* **3969**
Cancer Biotherapy & Radiopharmaceuticals (USA) *Online - full content edition. (1399756)* **3970**
Cancer Causes & Control (NLD) *Online - full text edition. (2016109)* **3970**
Cancer Chemotherapy and Pharmacology (DEU) *Online - full text edition. (1301799)* **3970**
Cancer Detection and Prevention (USA) *Online - full text edition. (787132)* **3970**
Cancer Gene Therapy (USA) *Online - full text edition. (2372215)* **3971**
Cancer Genetics & Cytogenetics (USA) *Online - full text edition. (932450)* **3971**
Cancer Immunology, Immunotherapy (DEU) *Online - full text edition. (1301772)* **3971**
Cancer Letters (IRL) *Online - full text edition. (192740)* **3972**
Cancer Practice Online(USA) *Online - full text. (2275201)* **3972**
Cancer Treatment Reviews (GBR) *Online - full text edition. (567876)* **3973**
Carcinogenesis (GBR) *Online - full text edition. (1013068)* **3974**
Cardiac Electrophysiology Review (USA) *Online - full text edition. (3305880)* **3765**
Cardiology (CHE) *Online - full text edition. (654469)* **3765**
Cardiovascular and Interventional Radiology (USA) *Online - full text edition. (397458)* **4141**
Cardiovascular Drugs and Therapy (USA) *Online - full text edition. (1577565)* **3766**
Cardiovascular Pathology (USA) *Online - full text edition. (2122928)* **3767**
Cardiovascular Radiation Medicine (USA) *Online - full text edition. (3933989)* **3767**
Cardiovascular Research (NLD) *Online - full text edition. (170100)* **3767**
Cardiovascular Surgery (GBR) *Online - full text edition. (2273047)* **3767**
Caries Research (CHE) *Online - full text edition. (242675)* **3817**
Cell and Tissue Banking (NLD) *Online - full text edition. (4174917)* **3286**
Cell and Tissue Research (DEU) *Online - full text edition. (464538)* **3287**
Cell Biology and Toxicology (NLD) *Online - full text edition. (1536672)* **3446**
Cell Calcium (Edinburgh) (GBR) *Online - full text edition. (961191)* **3287**
Cell Death and Differentiation (GBR) *Online - full text edition. (2476312)* **3287**
Cell Proliferation (GBR) *Online - full text edition. (681954)* **3287**
Cells, Tissues, Organs (CHE) *Online - full text edition. (561770)* **3583**
Cellular and Molecular Life Sciences (CHE) *Online - full text edition. (813257)* **3190**
Cellular & Molecular Neurobiology (USA) *Online - full text edition. (1064959)* **4080**

Cellular Immunology (USA) *Online - full text edition. (566667)* **3742**
Cellular Physiology and Biochemistry (DEU) *Online - full text edition. (1957325)* **3288**
Cellular Signalling (USA) *Online - full text edition. (1689940)* **3288**
Cellulose (NLD) *Online - full text edition. (2337525)* **3378**
Cephalalgia (GBR) *Online - full text edition. (1068008)* **4080**
Cerebral Cortex (USA) *Online - full text edition. (2021293)* **4081**
Cerebrovascular Diseases (CHE) *Online - full text edition. (1957309)* **4081**
Chemical Health and Safety (USA) *Online - full text edition. (2758172)* **3446**
Chemical Senses (GBR) *Online - full text edition. (645362)* **3340**
Chemico-Biological Interactions (IRL) *Online - full text edition. (482935)* **3447**
Chemistry & Biology (GBR) *Online - full text edition. (2508834)* **3372**
Chemistry and Physics of Lipids (IRL) *Online - full text edition. (657921)* **3246**
Chemoecology (CHE) *Online - full text edition. (1961411)* **3378**
Chemosphere (GBR) *Online - full text edition. (124648)* **3447**
Chemotherapy (CHE) *Online - full text edition. (240826)* **4283**
Child Abuse & Neglect (GBR) *Online - full text edition. (702196)* **3381**
Child and Adolescent Social Work Journal (USA) *Online - full text edition. (2025922)* **4520**
Child and Youth Care Forum (USA) *Online - full text edition. (961841)* **3381**
Child: Care, Health and Development (GBR) *Online - full text edition. (127345)* **4042**
Child Language Teaching and Therapy (GBR) *Online - full text edition. (1367692)* **3420**
Child Maltreatment (USA) *Online - full text edition. (2956047)* **3381**
Child Psychiatry and Human Development (USA) *Online - full text edition. (1643509)* **4081**
Child Psychology and Psychiatry Review (GBR) *Online - full text edition. (3273075)* **4387**
Childhood (GBR) *Online - full text edition. (2273810)* **3382**
Children and Youth Services Review (GBR) *Online - full text edition. (935131)* **3382**
Child's Nervous System (DEU) *Online - full text edition. (370908)* **4081**
Chinese Journal of Digestive Diseases Online(AUS) *Online - full text. (4542509)* **3887**
Der Chirurg (DEU) *Online - full text edition. (380687)* **4184**
Chirurgische Gastroenterologie (CHE) *Online - full text edition. (1724282)* **3887**
Christian Bioethics (NLD) *Online - full text edition. (2746476)* **3584**
Chromosoma (DEU) *Online - full text edition. (556882)* **3300**
Chronobiology International (USA) *Online - full text edition. (1370340)* **3191**
Cladistics (GBR) *Online - full text edition. (1542044)* **3191**
Clinica Chimica Acta (NLD) *Online - full text edition. (386782)* **3585**
Clinical and Applied Immunology Reviews (USA) *Online - full text edition. (1035436)* **3742**
Clinical and Experimental Allergy (GBR) *Online - full text edition. (456489)* **3742**
Clinical and Experimental Dermatology (GBR) *Online - full text edition. (4219)* **3846**
Clinical and Experimental Hypertension (USA) *Online - full text edition. (1208438)* **3768**
Clinical and Experimental Immunology (GBR) *Online - full text edition. (299316)* **3742**
Clinical and Experimental Medicine (DEU) *Online - full text edition. (265489)* **3585**
Clinical and Experimental Metastasis (NLD) *Online - full text edition. (1248855)* **3974**
Clinical and Experimental Nephrology Online(JPN) *Online - full text. (3244164)* **4211**
Clinical and Experimental Ophthalmology (AUS) *Online - full text edition. (1409069)* **3995**
Clinical and Experimental Pharmacology & Physiology (AUS) *Online - full text edition. (1208802)* **3341**
Clinical and Laboratory Haematology (GBR) *Online - full text edition. (907847)* **3899**
Clinical Biochemistry (USA) *Online - full text edition. (293687)* **3247**
Clinical Biomechanics (GBR) *Online - full text edition. (1549324)* **3787**
Clinical Chemistry and Laboratory Medicine (DEU) *Online - full text edition. (416266)* **3247**
Clinical Child and Family Psychology Review (USA) *Online - full text edition. (3518930)* **4387**
Clinical Child Psychology & Psychiatry (GBR) *Online - full text edition. (3911632)* **3382**
Clinical Drug Investigation (NZL) *Online - full text edition. (1807234)* **4283**
Clinical Effectiveness in Nursing (GBR) *Online - full text edition. (3244172)* **3916**
Clinical Endocrinology (GBR) *Online - full text edition. (125598)* **3856**
Clinical Genetics (DNK) *Online - full text edition. (273422)* **3300**
Clinical Hemorheology and Microcirculation (NLD) *Online - full text edition. (1050362)* **3899**
Clinical Imaging (USA) *Online - full text edition. (964484)* **4141**
Clinical Immunology (USA) *Online - full text edition. (29483)* **3743**
Clinical Linguistics & Phonetics (GBR) *Online - full text edition. (1604317)* **4082**
Clinical Microbiology and Infection (GBR) *Online - full text edition. (2910489)* **3586**
Clinical Microbiology Newsletter (USA) *Online - full text edition. (1042300)* **3319**
Clinical Neurology and Neurosurgery (NLD) *Online - full text edition. (807672)* **4082**
Clinical Neurophysiology (IRL) *Online - full text edition. (1405810)* **4082**
Clinical Nursing Research (USA) *Online - full text edition. (2127881)* **3916**
Clinical Nutrition (GBR) *Online - full text edition. (1611836)* **4231**
Clinical Oncology (GBR) *Online - full text edition. (1866494)* **3975**
Clinical Oral Implants Research (DNK) *Online - full text edition. (1994522)* **3818**
Clinical Oral Investigations (DEU) *Online - full text edition. (3247392)* **3818**
Clinical Orthodontics and Research Online(DNK) *Online - full text. (3558185)* **3818**
Clinical Orthopaedics and Related Research (USA) *Online - full text edition. (105708)* **4012**
Clinical Otolaryngology and Allied Sciences (GBR) *Online - full text edition. (225975)* **4031**
Clinical Performance and Quality Health Care (GBR) *Online - full text edition. (2318512)* **3587**
Clinical Pharmacokinetics (NZL) *Online - full text edition. (1838407)* **4284**
Clinical Physiology and Functional Imaging (GBR) *Online - full text edition. (1098470)* **3587**
Clinical Psychology (USA) *Online - full text edition. (2384795)* **4388**
Clinical Psychology Review (GBR) *Online - full text edition. (1113100)* **4388**
Clinical Radiology (GBR) *Online - full text edition. (350591)* **4142**
Clinical Rehabilitation (GBR) *Online - full text edition. (1619616)* **4060**
Clinical Rheumatology (BEL) *Online - full text edition. (545112)* **4168**
Clinical Risk (GBR) *Online - full text edition. (2793377)* **3587**
Clinical Science (GBR) *Online - full text edition. (1221558)* **3587**
Clinical Therapeutics (USA) *Online - full text edition. (401692)* **3587**
Clinical Transplantation (DNK) *Online - full text edition. (1604465)* **4185**
Clinics in Dermatology (USA) *Online - full text edition. (1352598)* **3846**
Clio Medica (NLD) *Online - full text edition. (599131)* **3588**
Cloning and Stem Cells (USA) *Online - full text edition. (3803376)* **3300**
Cognition (NLD) *Online - full text edition. (509094)* **4388**
Cognition and Emotion (GBR) *Online - full text edition. (1621572)* **4388**
Cognition and Instruction (USA) *Online - full text edition. (1352989)* **4388**
Cognition, Technology and Work (GBR) *Online - full text edition. (3822419)* **4388**
Cognitive Brain Research (NLD) *Online - full text edition. (2154048)* **4083**
Cognitive Development (GBR) *Online - full text edition. (1558307)* **4389**
Cognitive Linguistics (DEU) *Online - full text edition. (1865730)* **3550**
Cognitive Neuropsychiatry (GBR) *Online - full text edition. (2961504)* **4389**
Cognitive Neuropsychology (GBR) *Online - full text edition. (1374206)* **4083**
Cognitive Psychology (USA) *Online - full text edition. (378143)* **4389**
Cognitive Science (GBR) *Online - full text edition. (306452)* **4389**
Cognitive Therapy and Research (USA) *Online - full text edition. (134910)* **4390**
College of Surgeons Hong Kong. Annals (AUS) *Online - full text edition. (4023234)* **4185**
ColoProctology (DEU) *Online - full text edition. (1804200)* **3887**
Colorectal Disease Online(GBR) *Online - full text. (3796167)* **3887**
Combinatorial Chemistry & High Throughput Screening (USA) *Online - full text edition. (3490009)* **3372**
Community Dentistry and Oral Epidemiology Online(DNK) *Online - full text. (461377)* **3818**
Community Genetics (CHE) *Online - full text edition. (3498387)* **3300**
Community Mental Health Journal (USA) *Online - full text edition. (1519611)* **4512**
Comparative Biochemistry and Physiology. Part A: Molecular & Integrative Physiology (USA) *Online - full text edition. (186988)* **3341**
Comparative Biochemistry and Physiology. Part B: Biochemistry & Molecular Biology (USA) *Online - full text edition. (525588)* **3247**
Comparative Biochemistry and Physiology. Toxicology & Pharmacology (USA) *Online - full text edition. (457507)* **3247**
Comparative Haematology International (GBR) *Online - full text edition. (2033305)* **3900**
Comparative Political Studies (USA) *Online - full text edition. (801356)* **4367**
Complementary Therapies in Medicine (GBR) *Online - full text edition. (2266903)* **3787**
Complementary Therapies in Nursing & Midwifery (GBR) *Online - full text edition. (2652285)* **3917**
Computer Methods and Programs in Biomedicine (IRL) *Online - full text edition. (392766)* **3809**
Computerized Medical Imaging and Graphics (GBR) *Online - full text edition. (199974)* **3809**
Computers in Biology and Medicine (GBR) *Online - full text edition. (34452)* **3284**
Computers in Human Behavior (GBR) *Online - full text edition. (1386689)* **4524**
Consciousness and Cognition (USA) *Online - full text edition. (2097109)* **4391**
Conservation Biology (USA) *Online - full text edition. (1578774)* **3392**
Conservation Genetics (NLD) *Online - full text edition. (4006674)* **3300**
Contact Dermatitis (DNK) *Online - full text edition. (245070)* **3846**
Contact Lens & Anterior Eye (GBR) *Online - full text edition. (1348329)* **3995**
Contemporary Educational Psychology (USA) *Online - full text edition. (1052853)* **3410**
Contemporary Family Therapy (USA) *Online - full text edition. (1748238)* **4391**
Contraception (USA) *Online - full text edition. (526029)* **3357**
Controlled Clinical Trials (USA) *Online - full text edition. (920193)* **3873**
Coronary Artery Disease (USA) *Online - full text edition. (2258374)* **3769**
Coronary Health Care (GBR) *Online - full text edition. (3244199)* **3917**
Counselling Psychology Quarterly (GBR) *Online - full content edition. (1670239)* **4392**
Creativity Research Journal (USA) *Online - full text edition. (2165112)* **4392**
Criminal Justice & Behavior (USA) *Online - full text edition. (634891)* **3394**
Critical Care Medicine (USA) *Online - full text edition. (724432)* **3590**
Critical Public Health (GBR) *Online - full content edition. (1143441)* **4466**
Critical Reviews in Biochemistry and Molecular Biology (USA) *Online - full text edition. (231215)* **3248**
Critical Reviews in Biotechnology (USA) *Online - full text edition. (1337726)* **3273**
Critical Reviews in Clinical Laboratory Sciences (USA) *Online - full text edition. (578843)* **3591**
Critical Reviews in Diagnostic Imaging (USA) *Online - full text edition. (545023)* **4142**
Critical Reviews in Microbiology (USA) *Online - full text edition. (705020)* **3320**
Critical Reviews in Oncology - Hematology (IRL) *Online - full text edition. (1338358)* **3975**
Critical Reviews in Toxicology (USA) *Online - full text edition. (229733)* **3447**
Cross-Cultural Research (USA) *Online - full text edition. (277975)* **4508**
Cryobiology (USA) *Online - full text edition. (154040)* **3266**
Culture & Psychology (GBR) *Online - full text edition. (2718537)* **4393**
Culture, Health and Sexuality (GBR) *Online - full text edition. (3869679)* **4520**
Culture, Medicine and Psychiatry (NLD) *Online - full text edition. (689203)* **3173**
Current Anaesthesia and Critical Care (GBR) *Online - full text edition. (1864998)* **3756**
Current Diagnostic Pathology (GBR) *Online - full text edition. (2403765)* **3908**
Current Directions in Psychological Science (USA) *Online - full text edition. (2143682)* **4393**
Current Drug Metabolism (USA) *Online - full text edition. (4017536)* **4285**
Current Drug Targets (USA) *Online - full text edition. (4017692)* **4285**
Current Eye Research (USA) *Online - full text edition. (1044354)* **3996**
Current Genetics (DEU) *Online - full text edition. (969338)* **3300**
Current Genomics (USA) *Online - full text edition. (4017617)* **3300**
Current Medicinal Chemistry - Anti-Inflammatory & Anti-Allergy Agents (NLD) *Online - full text edition. (4464788)* **4285**
Current Microbiology (USA) *Online - full text edition. (497207)* **3320**
Current Obstetrics and Gynaecology (GBR) *Online - full text edition. (2012812)* **3948**
Current Opinion in Allergy and Clinical Immunology (GBR) *Online - full content edition. (4515919)* **3743**
Current Opinion in Anaesthesiology (USA) *Online - full text edition. (1689169)* **3756**
Current Opinion in Biotechnology (GBR) *Online - full text edition. (1980343)* **3273**
Current Opinion in Cardiology (USA) *Online - full text edition. (1510401)* **3770**
Current Opinion in Cell Biology (GBR) *Online - full text edition. (1808729)* **3288**
Current Opinion in Clinical Nutrition and Metabolic Care (USA) *Online - full text edition. (3550427)* **4231**
Current Opinion in Critical Care (USA) *Online - full text edition. (2384809)* **4012**
Current Opinion in Endocrinology & Diabetes (USA) *Online - full text edition. (2384825)* **3857**
Current Opinion in Gastroenterology (USA) *Online - full text edition. (1426273)* **3888**
Current Opinion in Genetics & Development (GBR) *Online - full text edition. (2082845)* **3301**
Current Opinion in Hematology (USA) *Online - full text edition. (2334488)* **3900**
Current Opinion in Immunology (GBR) *Online - full text edition. (1689150)* **3722**
Current Opinion in Infectious Diseases (USA) *Online - full text edition. (1689037)* **3794**
Current Opinion in Lipidology (GBR) *Online - full text edition. (1879839)* **3770**
Current Opinion in Nephrology & Hypertension (USA) *Online - full text edition. (2264293)* **4211**
Current Opinion in Neurobiology (GBR) *Online - full text edition. (2082837)* **4084**
Current Opinion in Neurology (USA) *Online - full text edition. (1689177)* **4085**
Current Opinion in Obstetrics & Gynecology (USA) *Online - full text edition. (1879847)* **3948**
Current Opinion in Oncology (USA) *Online - full text edition. (1879820)* **3976**
Current Opinion in Ophthalmology (USA) *Online - full text edition. (1927477)* **3996**
Current Opinion in Organ Transplantation (USA) *Online - full text edition. (3307867)* **3591**
Current Opinion in Orthopedics (USA) *Online - full text edition. (1879863)* **4013**
Current Opinion in Otolaryngology & Head and Neck Surgery (USA) *Online - full text edition. (2384841)* **4031**
Current Opinion in Pediatrics (USA) *Online - full text edition. (1878492)* **4043**
Current Opinion in Psychiatry (USA) *Online - full text edition. (1681680)* **4085**
Current Opinion in Pulmonary Medicine (USA) *Online - full text edition. (2384868)* **4159**
Current Opinion in Rheumatology (USA) *Online - full text edition. (1841343)* **4168**
Current Opinion in Structural Biology (GBR) *Online - full text edition. (2023407)* **3248**
Current Opinion in Urology (USA) *Online - full text edition. (2160358)* **4211**

Current Orthopaedics (GBR) *Online - full text edition. (1559133)* **4013**
Current Paediatrics (GBR) *Online - full text edition. (2012820)* **4043**
Current Pharmaceutical Biotechnology (USA) *Online - full text edition. (4017684)* **3273**
Current Pharmaceutical Design (USA) *Online - full text edition. (2946254)* **4286**
Current Protein and Peptide Science (USA) *Online - full text edition. (4017641)* **3248**
Current Surgery (USA) *Online - full text edition. (655945)* **4186**
Current Therapeutic Research (USA) *Online - full text edition. (27871)* **3592**
CyberPsychology & Behavior (USA) *Online - full text edition. (3597172)* **3390**
Cytogenetic and Genome Research (CHE) *Online - full text edition. (616621)* **3301**
Cytokine (GBR) *Online - full text edition. (1929534)* **3301**
Cytokine and Growth Factor Reviews (GBR) *Online - full text edition. (1769197)* **3248**
Cytopathology (GBR) *Online - full text edition. (1910809)* **3289**
Cytotechnology (NLD) *Online - full text edition. (1645501)* **3289**
D N A and Cell Biology (USA) *Online - full text edition. (1079409)* **3248**
Death Studies (USA) *Online - full text edition. (42382)* **4394**
Dementia and Geriatric Cognitive Disorders (CHE) *Online - full text edition. (1850075)* **4085**
Dental Materials (USA) *Online - full text edition. (1380478)* **3820**
Dental Traumatology Online(DNK) *Online - full text. (1380443)* **3821**
Dentomaxillofacial Radiology (GBR) *Online - full text edition. (324361)* **4143**
Dermatologic Surgery Online(USA) *Online - full text. (157783)* **4187**
Dermatologic Therapy (DNK) *Online - full text edition. (2953390)* **3847**
Dermatology (CHE) *Online - full text edition. (418153)* **3847**
Dermatology and Psychosomatics (CHE) *Online - full text edition. (4013247)* **3848**
Development and Psychopathology (GBR) *Online - full text edition. (1772031)* **4394**
Development (Cambridge) (GBR) *Online - full text edition. (645508)* **3192**
Development, Genes and Evolution (DEU) *Online - full text edition. (109576)* **3192**
Development, Growth and Differentiation (AUS) *Online - full text edition. (717835)* **3192**
Developmental and Comparative Immunology (GBR) *Online - full text edition. (542059)* **3743**
Developmental Biology (USA) *Online - full text edition. (34150)* **3193**
Developmental Brain Research (NLD) *Online - full text edition. (1046764)* **4086**
Developmental Medicine and Child Neurology (GBR) *Online - full text edition. (755036)* **4043**
Developmental Neuropsychology (USA) *Online - full text edition. (1498452)* **4394**
Developmental Neuroscience (CHE) *Online - full text edition. (712442)* **4086**
Developmental Review (USA) *Online - full text edition. (1083058)* **4394**
Developmental Science (GBR) *Online - full text edition. (3525406)* **4394**
Deviant Behavior (USA) *Online - full text edition. (995355)* **4521**
Diabetes, Obesity and Metabolism Online(GBR) *Online - full text. (3807568)* **3858**
Diabetes Research and Clinical Practice (IRL) *Online - full text edition. (1387383)* **3858**
Diabetes Technology & Therapeutics (USA) *Online - full text edition. (3827763)* **3859**
Diabetic Medicine Online(GBR) *Online - full text. (1377248)* **3860**
Diabetologia (DEU) *Online - full text edition. (431869)* **3860**
Diagnostic Microbiology and Infectious Disease (USA) *Online - full text edition. (1212885)* **3320**
Differentiation (DEU) *Online - full text edition. (27987)* **3193**
Digestion (CHE) *Online - full text edition. (667390)* **3888**
Digestive Diseases (CHE) *Online - full text edition. (1207393)* **3888**
Digestive Diseases and Sciences (USA) *Online - full text edition. (167770)* **3888**
Digestive Endoscopy Online(AUS) *Online - full text. (2865734)* **3889**
Digestive Surgery (CHE) *Online - full text edition. (1347721)* **4187**
Disability and Rehabilitation (GBR) *Online - full text edition. (912425)* **3484**
Disability & Society (GBR) *Online - full text edition. (1430793)* **3494**
Disaster Prevention and Management (GBR) *Online - full text edition. (2213265)* **4466**
Discourse & Society (GBR) *Online - full text edition. (1927094)* **4395**
Discourse Studies (GBR) *Online - full text edition. (3789349)* **3550**
Disease Management (USA) *Online - full text edition. (3598020)* **3595**
Disease Management and Clinical Outcomes (USA) *Online - full text edition. (3256073)* **3595**
Disease Management & Health Outcomes (NZL) *Online - full text edition. (3235823)* **3595**
Disease Markers (NLD) *Online - full text edition. (1176986)* **3976**
Diseases of the Esophagus Online(AUS) *Online - full text. (2406225)* **4032**
Documenta Ophthalmologica (NLD) *Online - full text edition. (340979)* **3997**
Doklady Biological Sciences (RUS) *Online - full content edition. (707163)* **3193**
Domestic Animal Endocrinology (USA) *Online - full text edition. (1319620)* **4542**
Dreaming (USA) *Online - full text edition. (2025310)* **3342**
Drug and Alcohol Dependence (IRL) *Online - full text edition. (74314)* **3400**
Drug and Alcohol Review (GBR) *Online - full text edition. (1561502)* **3400**
Drug and Chemical Toxicology (USA) *Online - full text edition. (350540)* **4287**
Drug Delivery (USA) *Online - full text edition. (2147165)* **4288**
Drug Development and Industrial Pharmacy (USA) *Online - full text edition. (342394)* **4288**
Drug Discovery Today (GBR) *Online - full text edition. (3612287)* **4288**
Drug Metabolism Reviews (USA) *Online - full text edition. (670855)* **3596**
Drug Resistance Update (GBR) *Online - full text edition. (3572242)* **3596**
Drug Safety (NZL) *Online - full text edition. (1525956)* **4289**
Drugs (NZL) *Online - full text edition. (343994)* **4290**
Drugs & Aging (NZL) *Online - full text edition. (2031442)* **4290**
Drugs: Education, Prevention & Policy (GBR) *Online - full text edition. (2355035)* **3401**
Dysphagia (USA) *Online - full text edition. (1509284)* **4032**
e A D C - F & N (GBR) *Online - full text edition of* Archives of Disease in Childhood. Fetal and Neonatal Edition. (3246329) **3945**
The E M B O Journal (GBR) *Online - full text edition. (1116231)* **3249**
E M B O Reports Online (GBR) *Online - full text edition of* E M B O Reports. (4274709) **3301**
E M J Online (GBR) *Online - full text edition of* Emergency Medicine Journal. (1338048) **4014**
Early Childhood Education Journal (USA) *Online - full text edition. (1426885)* **3410**
Early Human Development (IRL) *Online - full text edition. (573493)* **3948**
Ecography (DNK) *Online - full text edition. (908797)* **3437**
Ecological Psychology (USA) *Online - full text edition. (1729799)* **4396**
Ecotoxicology (USA) *Online - full text edition. (2186691)* **3448**
Ecotoxicology and Environmental Safety - Online (USA) *Online - full text edition of* Ecotoxicology and Environmental Safety. (290017) **3448**
Education for Health (GBR) *Online - full text edition. (1795791)* **3597**
Educational and Psychological Measurement (USA) *Online - full text edition. (255890)* **4396**
Educational Gerontology (USA) *Online - full text edition. (342408)* **3470**
Educational Psychologist (USA) *Online - full text edition. (213233)* **4396**
Educational Psychology (GBR) *Online - full text edition. (1039067)* **3410**
Educational Psychology in Practice (GBR) *Online - full text edition. (1600915)* **3410**
Educational Psychology Review (USA) *Online - full text edition. (1735020)* **3411**
Electro- and Magnetobiology (USA) *Online - full text edition. (1154818)* **3266**
Elektronische Ausgabe (DEU) *Online - full text edition of* Der Hautarzt. (681784) **3849**
Emergency Medicine (Carleton South) (AUS) *Online - full text edition. (3835707)* **4013**
Emergency Radiology (DEU) *Online - full text edition. (2380641)* **4143**
Endocrine - Related Cancer (GBR) *Online - full text edition. (2366045)* **3861**
Environment and Behavior (USA) *Online - full text edition. (91448)* **4521**
Environment International (GBR) *Online - full text edition. (37850)* **3438**
Environmental Management & Health (GBR) *Online - full text edition. (1841998)* **3438**
Environmental Microbiology (GBR) *Online - full text edition. (3795977)* **3321**
Environmental Research (USA) *Online - full text edition. (170666)* **3439**
Environmental Toxicology and Pharmacology (NLD) *Online - full text edition. (2955156)* **3449**
Enzyme and Microbial Technology (USA) *Online - full text edition. (901938)* **3273**
Epidemiology and Infection (GBR) *Online - full text edition. (211761)* **3321**
Epilepsia (USA) *Online - full text edition. (654221)* **4087**
Epilepsy and Behavior (USA) *Online - full text edition. (4051858)* **3598**
Epilepsy Research (NLD) *Online - full text edition. (1776207)* **4088**
Ergonomics (GBR) *Online - full text edition. (269840)* **3432**
Ergonomics Abstracts (GBR) *Online - full content edition. (83151)* **3433**
Ethics & Behavior (USA) *Online - full text edition. (2019736)* **4397**
Ethik in der Medizin (DEU) *Online - full text edition. (1650211)* **4347**
Ethnicity and Health (GBR) *Online - full text edition. (2932148)* **4468**
Ethology Online(DEU) *Online - full text. (672149)* **3352**
Europace (GBR) *Online - full text edition. (3821455)* **3771**
European Academy of Dermatology and Venereology. Journal (BEL) *Online - full text edition. (2174820)* **3848**
European Addiction Research (CHE) *Online - full text edition. (2506726)* **3401**
European Archives of Oto-Rhino-Laryngology (DEU) *Online - full text edition. (387975)* **4032**
European Archives of Psychiatry and Clinical Neurosciences (DEU) *Online - full text edition. (677310)* **4088**
European Biophysics Journal (DEU) *Online - full text edition. (700398)* **3266**
European Child & Adolescent Psychiatry (DEU) *Online - full text edition. (2169029)* **4089**
European Heart Journal (GBR) *Online - full text edition. (1362844)* **3771**
European Journal of Anaesthesiology (GBR) *Online - full text edition. (1338056)* **3757**
European Journal of Applied Physiology (DEU) *Online - full text edition. (816884)* **3342**
European Journal of Biochemistry (GBR) *Online - full text edition. (634018)* **3249**
European Journal of Cancer (GBR) *Online - full text edition. (1710486)* **3977**
European Journal of Cancer Care Online(GBR) *Online - full text. (2121743)* **3977**
European Journal of Cardio-Thoracic Surgery (NLD) *Online - full text edition. (1635697)* **3771**
European Journal of Cell Biology (DEU) *Online - full text edition. (1304720)* **3289**
European Journal of Clinical Investigation (GBR) *Online - full text edition. (259993)* **3599**
European Journal of Clinical Microbiology & Infectious Diseases (DEU) *Online - full text edition. (1196367)* **3321**
European Journal of Clinical Nutrition (GBR) *Online - full text edition. (1703773)* **4232**
European Journal of Clinical Pharmacology (DEU) *Online - full text edition. (99929)* **4292**
European Journal of Cognitive Psychology (GBR) *Online - full text edition. (1740768)* **4397**
European Journal of Dental Education Online(DNK) *Online - full text. (3262294)* **3822**
European Journal of Echocardiography (GBR) *Online - full text edition. (4059964)* **3771**
European Journal of Endocrinology (GBR) *Online - full text edition. (1100947)* **3862**
European Journal of Epidemiology (NLD) *Online - full text edition. (1503782)* **3599**
European Journal of Haematology (DNK) *Online - full text edition. (1096265)* **3900**
The European Journal of Health Economics (DEU) *Online - full content edition. (4134028)* **3600**
European Journal of Health Law (NLD) *Online - full text edition. (2362279)* **3600**
The European Journal of Heart Failure (NLD) *Online - full text edition. (3885925)* **3771**
European Journal of Human Genetics (GBR) *Online - full text edition. (2260352)* **3302**
European Journal of Immunogenetics (GBR) *Online - full text edition. (156531)* **3302**
European Journal of Internal Medicine (USA) *Online - full text edition. (1781820)* **3908**
European Journal of Medicinal Chemistry (FRA) *Online - full text edition. (257788)* **3250**
European Journal of Morphology (NLD) *Online - full text edition. (3282112)* **3195**
European Journal of Neurology (USA) *Online - full text edition. (2491516)* **4089**
European Journal of Neuroscience (GBR) *Online - full text edition. (1766244)* **4089**
European Journal of Nuclear Medicine and Molecular Imaging (DEU) *Online - full text edition. (591637)* **4144**
European Journal of Nutrition (DEU) *Online - full text edition. (800546)* **4233**
European Journal of Obstetrics & Gynecology and Reproductive Biology (IRL) *Online - full text edition. (540641)* **3949**
European Journal of Oncology Nursing (GBR) *Online - full text edition. (3244261)* **3919**
European Journal of Oral Sciences Online(DNK) *Online - full text. (518948)* **3823**
European Journal of Orthodontics (GBR) *Online - full content edition. (949892)* **3823**
European Journal of Orthopaedic Surgery & Traumatology (FRA) *Online - full text edition. (2140322)* **4014**
European Journal of Paediatric Neurology (GBR) *Online - full text edition. (3330605)* **4044**
European Journal of Pain (GBR) *Online - full text edition. (3351963)* **3600**
European Journal of Pediatrics (DEU) *Online - full text edition. (755214)* **4044**
European Journal of Pharmaceutical Sciences (NLD) *Online - full text edition. (2278960)* **4292**
European Journal of Pharmaceutics and Biopharmaceutics (NLD) *Online - full text edition. (95141)* **4293**
European Journal of Pharmacology (NLD) *Online - full text edition. (2154234)* **4293**
European Journal of Plastic Surgery (DEU) *Online - full text edition. (302058)* **4188**
European Journal of Psychotherapy, Counselling and Health (GBR) *Online - full content edition. (3526151)* **4089**
European Journal of Public Health (GBR) *Online - full text edition. (2037912)* **4468**
European Journal of Radiology (IRL) *Online - full text edition. (1076124)* **4144**
European Journal of Soil Biology (FRA) *Online - full text edition. (206784)* **3195**
European Journal of Surgery (NOR) *Online - full text edition. (2017628)* **4188**
European Journal of Surgery. Supplement (NOR) *Online - full text edition. (1084062)* **4188**
European Journal of Surgical Oncology (GBR) *Online - full text edition. (511765)* **3977**
European Journal of Trauma (DEU) *Online - full text edition. (1147676)* **4014**
European Journal of Ultrasound (IRL) *Online - full text edition. (2382318)* **4144**
European Journal of Vascular and Endovascular Surgery (GBR) *Online - full text edition. (1619608)* **3771**
European Journal of Work and Organizational Psychology (GBR) *Online - full text edition. (2075784)* **4398**
European Neurology (CHE) *Online - full text edition. (821632)* **4089**
European Neuropsychopharmacology (NLD) *Online - full text edition. (2060787)* **4089**
European Radiology (DEU) *Online - full text edition. (2056895)* **4144**
The European Respiratory Journal (CHE) *Online - full text edition. (1661361)* **4159**
European Review (GBR) *Online - full text edition. (2273136)* **4504**
European Spine Journal (DEU) *Online - full text edition. (2140276)* **4189**
European Surgical Research (CHE) *Online - full text edition. (49468)* **4189**
European Urology (CHE) *Online - full text edition. (566330)* **4212**
Evaluation and the Health Professions (USA) *Online - full text edition. (373672)* **3600**

Evidence - Based Cardiovascular Medicine (GBR) *Online - full text edition. (3244202)* **3772**
Evidence - Based Dentistry (GBR) *Online - full text edition. (4496337)* **3823**
Evidence - Based Obstetrics & Gynaecology (GBR) *Online - full text edition. (3244237)* **3949**
Evidence - Based Oncology (GBR) *Online - full text edition. (4055187)* **3978**
Evolution & Development Online(USA) *Online - full text. (3827860)* **3195**
Experimental Aging Research (USA) *Online - full text edition. (255904)* **4398**
Experimental & Applied Acarology (NLD) *Online - full text edition. (1387510)* **3352**
Experimental and Molecular Pathology (USA) *Online - full text edition. (593885)* **3600**
Experimental Biology and Medicine (Maywood) (USA) *Online - full text edition. (367818)* **3195**
Experimental Biology Online(DEU) *Online - full content. (3850625)* **3195**
Experimental Brain Research (DEU) *Online - full text edition. (1109030)* **4090**
Experimental Dermatology Online(DNK) *Online - full text. (2147866)* **3849**
Experimental Eye Research (GBR) *Online - full text edition. (440140)* **3997**
Experimental Gerontology (USA) *Online - full text edition. (631558)* **3471**
Experimental Hematology (USA) *Online - full text edition. (1381628)* **3901**
Experimental Lung Research (USA) *Online - full text edition. (919616)* **4160**
Experimental Nephrology (CHE) *Online - full text edition. (2260360)* **4212**
Experimental Neurology (USA) *Online - full text edition. (4429923)* **4090**
Experimental Parasitology (USA) *Online - full text edition. (188425)* **3796**
Experimental Physiology (GBR) *Online - full text edition. (652288)* **3342**
F E B S Letters (NLD) *Online - full text edition. (459224)* **3250**
F E M S Immunology and Medical Microbiology (NLD) *Online - full text edition. (1653458)* **3321**
F E M S Microbiology Ecology (NLD) *Online - full text edition. (1391100)* **3321**
F E M S Microbiology Letters (NLD) *Online - full text edition. (1391097)* **3322**
F E M S Microbiology Reviews (NLD) *Online - full text edition. (1391119)* **3322**
Familial Cancer (NLD) *Online - full text edition. (4006690)* **3978**
The Family Journal (USA) *Online - full text edition. (3814963)* **4399**
Family Practice (GBR) *Online - full text edition. (1346423)* **3601**
Il Farmaco (FRA) *Online - full text edition. (1832034)* **4295**
Feminism & Psychology (GBR) *Online - full text edition. (1936387)* **4399**
Fertility and Sterility (USA) *Online - full text edition. (432814)* **3949**
Fetal and Maternal Medicine Review (GBR) *Online - full text edition. (1763733)* **3950**
Fetal Diagnosis and Therapy (CHE) *Online - full text edition. (1554115)* **3950**
Fibrinolysis & Proteolysis (GBR) *Online - full text edition. (1579940)* **3875**
Fish and Shellfish Immunology (GBR) *Online - full text edition. (2025507)* **3196**
Fitoterapia (ITA) *Online - full text edition. (2257351)* **3279**
Folia Phoniatrica et Logopaedica (CHE) *Online - full text edition. (647209)* **4032**
Food Additives and Contaminants (GBR) *Online - full text edition. (1330608)* **4296**
Food and Agricultural Immunology (GBR) *Online - full text edition. (1742582)* **3197**
Food and Chemical Toxicology (GBR) *Online - full text edition. (234605)* **3449**
Food Microbiology (GBR) *Online - full text edition. (1326430)* **3322**
The Foot (GBR) *Online - full text edition. (2012901)* **4015**
Foot and Ankle Surgery (GBR) *Online - full text edition. (2473542)* **4189**
Forensic Science International (IRL) *Online - full text edition. (692883)* **3882**
Forum der Psychoanalyse (DEU) *Online - full text edition. (1509306)* **4399**
Free Radical Biology & Medicine (USA) *Online - full text edition. (1640488)* **3197**
Freshwater Biology Online(GBR) *Online - full text. (569364)* **3197**
Frontiers in Neuroendocrinology (USA) *Online - full text edition. (520195)* **3862**
Frontiers of Medical and Biological Engineering (NLD) *Online - full content edition. (1672010)* **3237**
Fuctional Plant Biology (AUS) *Online - full text edition. (15660)* **3280**
Fundamental and Clinical Pharmacology (FRA) *Online - full text edition. (1570692)* **4297**
Gait and Posture (NLD) *Online - full text edition. (2273373)* **3605**
Games and Economic Behavior (USA) *Online - full text edition. (1790862)* **4400**
Gastric Cancer (JPN) *Online - full content edition. (3798119)* **3978**
Gay and Lesbian Medical Association. Journal (USA) *Online - full text edition. (4343921)* **3605**
Gefaesschirurgie (DEU) *Online - full text edition. (2939207)* **4189**
Gene - C O M B I S (NLD) *Online - full text edition of* Gene. (545031) **3274**
Gene Therapy and Regulation (NLD) *Online - full content edition. (4027604)* **3303**
Gene Therapy (Basingstoke) (GBR) *Online - full text edition. (2352869)* **3606**
General and Comparative Endocrinology (USA) *Online - full text edition. (217107)* **3863**
General Hospital Psychiatry (USA) *Online - full text edition. (932310)* **4091**
General Pharmacology (USA) *Online - full text edition. (238651)* **4297**
Genes and Immunity (GBR) *Online - full text edition. (4028201)* **3303**
Genes to Cells (GBR) *Online - full text edition. (2923092)* **3303**
Genescreen (GBR) *Online - full text edition. (4046447)* **3304**
Genetic Resources and Crop Evolution (NLD) *Online - full text edition. (2126443)* **3304**
Genetic Testing (USA) *Online - full text edition. (3316580)* **3304**
Genetica (NLD) *Online - full text edition. (398950)* **3305**
Genetical Research (GBR) *Online - full text edition. (283908)* **3305**
Genetics, Selection, Evolution Online (FRA) *Online - full text edition of* Genetics, Selection, Evolution. (237493) **3305**
Genome (CAN) *Online - full text edition. (246093)* **3306**
Genomics (USA) *Online - full text edition. (1590812)* **3306**
Geomicrobiology Journal (USA) *Online - full text edition. (166065)* **3322**
Geriatrics & Gerontology International Online(AUS) *Online - full text. (4513029)* **3472**
Gerontology (CHE) *Online - full text edition. (33820)* **3473**
Global Change & Human Health (NLD) *Online - full text edition. (4014200)* **4470**
Glycobiology (GBR) *Online - full text edition. (2026171)* **3251**
Glycoconjugate Journal (USA) *Online - full text edition. (1395475)* **3251**
Graefe's Archive for Clinical and Experimental Ophthalmology (DEU) *Online - full text edition. (328618)* **3998**
Graft (USA) *Online - full text edition. (4030524)* **4190**
Group Analysis (GBR) *Online - full text edition. (85197)* **4401**
Group & Organization Management (USA) *Online - full text edition. (310786)* **3411**
Group (New York) (USA) *Online - full text edition. (1582348)* **4401**
Growth Hormone and I G F Research (GBR) *Online - full text edition. (2405121)* **3863**
Gut Online (GBR) *Online - full text edition of* Gut. (649139) **3891**
Gynaecological Endoscopy (GBR) *Online - full text edition. (2152061)* **3951**
Der Gynaekologe (DEU) *Online - full text edition. (541761)* **3951**
Gynaekologisch - Geburtshilfliche Rundschau (CHE) *Online - full text edition. (582123)* **3951**
Gynecologic and Obstetric Investigation (CHE) *Online - full text edition. (175501)* **3952**
Gynecologic Oncology (USA) *Online - full text edition. (143057)* **3952**
H E C Forum (NLD) *Online - full text edition. (1850326)* **3508**
H I V Medicine (GBR) *Online - full text edition. (4046498)* **3796**
H N O (Berlin) (DEU) *Online - full text edition. (250120)* **4033**
Haematologia (NLD) *Online - full content edition. (159670)* **3901**
Haemophilia Online(GBR) *Online - full text. (2489848)* **3901**
Hand Surgery (SGP) *Online - full text edition. (2976730)* **4190**
Handbook of Practice Management (GBR) *Online - full content edition. (2601958)* **3609**
Harvard Review of Psychiatry (GBR) *Online - full text edition. (2318458)* **4093**
Hazardous Waste Consultant (USA) *Online - full text edition. (1604015)* **3457**
Headache Online(USA) *Online - full text. (715956)* **4093**
Health (GBR) *Online - full text edition. (3226735)* **4471**
Health & Place (GBR) *Online - full text edition. (2658399)* **3465**
Health and Social Care in the Community Online(GBR) *Online - full text. (2264188)* **4472**
Health Care Analysis (NLD) *Online - full text edition. (2273152)* **3610**
Health Care for Women International (USA) *Online - full text edition. (1403753)* **4563**
Health Care Management Science (NLD) *Online - full text edition. (3496295)* **3509**
Health Communication (USA) *Online - full text edition. (1729802)* **4472**
Health Education (GBR) *Online - full text edition. (2224690)* **4354**
Health Education Research (GBR) *Online - full text edition. (1502077)* **4513**
Health Expectations (GBR) *Online - full text edition. (3538397)* **4473**
Health Information and Libraries Journal Online(GBR) *Online - full text. (1366807)* **3547**
Health Policy (IRL) *Online - full text edition. (920002)* **4473**
Health Policy and Planning (GBR) *Online - full text edition. (1517422)* **4473**
Health Promotion International (GBR) *Online - full text edition. (1517430)* **4474**
Health Promotion Practice (USA) *Online - full text edition. (4005015)* **4474**
Health, Risk & Society (GBR) *Online - full text edition. (3815994)* **4474**
Health Services and Outcomes Research Methodology (USA) *Online - full text edition. (3815595)* **3612**
Hearing Research (NLD) *Online - full text edition. (57347)* **4033**
Heart and Vessels (JPN) *Online - full text edition. (1416073)* **3772**
Heart Drug (CHE) *Online - full text edition. (4019741)* **4299**
Heart Failure Reviews (USA) *Online - full text edition. (2929651)* **3773**
Heart, Lung & Circulation Online(AUS) *Online - full text. (3218368)* **3773**
Heart Online (GBR) *Online - full text edition of* Heart. (127094) **3772**
Helicobacter (USA) *Online - full text edition. (2973375)* **3323**
Hematology and Cell Therapy (FRA) *Online - full text edition. (782505)* **3902**
The Hematology Journal (GBR) *Online - full text edition. (4121309)* **3773**
Hepatology Research (IRL) *Online - full text edition. (2267217)* **3892**
Heredity (GBR) *Online - full text edition. (92940)* **3307**
Hernia (DEU) *Online - full text edition. (3443817)* **4190**
Herz (DEU) *Online - full text edition. (394866)* **3773**
Herzschrittmachertherapie und Elektrophysiologie (DEU) *Online - full text edition. (2117444)* **3774**
High Ability Studies (GBR) *Online - full text edition. (2268434)* **3422**
High Altitude Medicine and Biology (USA) *Online - full content edition. (4115821)* **3614**
Hispanic Journal of Behavioral Sciences (USA) *Online - full text edition. (1878573)* **4402**
The Histochemical Journal (NLD) *Online - full text edition. (117358)* **3290**
Histochemistry and Cell Biology (DEU) *Online - full text edition. (209481)* **3290**
Histopathology (GBR) *Online - full text edition. (488968)* **3979**
Homicide Studies (USA) *Online - full text edition. (3228746)* **3394**
Hormone Research (CHE) *Online - full text edition. (394971)* **3863**
Hormones and Behavior (USA) *Online - full text edition. (772569)* **3863**
Human & Experimental Toxicology (GBR) *Online - full text edition. (1128655)* **3450**
Human Antibodies (NLD) *Online - full text edition. (1864130)* **3744**
Human Biology (Detroit) (USA) *Online - full text edition. (625809)* **3199**
Human - Computer Interaction (Mahwah) (USA) *Online - full text edition. (1379488)* **3389**
Human Development (CHE) *Online - full text edition. (455571)* **3616**
Human Ecology (New York) (USA) *Online - full text edition. (331899)* **3173**
Human Gene Therapy (USA) *Online - full text edition. (1850938)* **3307**
Human Genetics (DEU) *Online - full text edition. (481459)* **3307**
Human Heredity (CHE) *Online - full text edition. (622745)* **3307**
Human Immunology (USA) *Online - full text edition. (960861)* **3744**
Human Molecular Genetics (GBR) *Online - full text edition. (2266504)* **3308**
Human Movement Science (NLD) *Online - full text edition. (1177222)* **3616**
Human Performance (USA) *Online - full text edition. (1669419)* **4402**
Human Physiology (RUS) *Online - full text edition. (204315)* **3616**
Human Relations (USA) *Online - full text edition. (288640)* **4509**
Human Reproduction (GBR) *Online - full text edition. (1506080)* **3953**
Human Reproduction Update (GBR) *Online - full text edition. (2669277)* **3232**
Hybridoma (USA) *Online - full text edition. (1079387)* **3251**
Hydrobiologia (NLD) *Online - full text edition. (1763903)* **3199**
Hypertension in Pregnancy (USA) *Online - full text edition. (1208446)* **3774**
I T B M - R B M News (FRA) *Online - full text edition. (3020541)* **3275**
I U B M B Life (AUS) *Online - full text edition. (1051997)* **3251**
Illness, Crisis, and Loss (USA) *Online - full text edition. (3814971)* **4521**
Illustrated Case Reports in Gastroenterology (GBR) *Online - full text edition. (2461900)* **3892**
Immunoanalyse et Biologie Specialisee (FRA) *Online - full text edition. (1794329)* **3200**
Immunogenetics (DEU) *Online - full text edition. (137065)* **3308**
Immunological Reviews (DNK) *Online - full text edition. (125784)* **3745**
Immunologie und Impfen (DEU) *Online - full text edition. (3801985)* **3745**
Immunology (GBR) *Online - full text edition. (254215)* **3746**
Immunology and Cell Biology (AUS) *Online - full text edition. (34002)* **3746**
Immunology Letters (NLD) *Online - full text edition. (927147)* **3746**
Immunotechnology (NLD) *Online - full text edition. (2658275)* **3746**
In Vitro Cellular & Developmental Biology - Plant (USA) *Online - full text edition. (2080486)* **3280**
Indoor Air Online(DNK) *Online - full text. (2029979)* **4476**
Indoor and Built Environment (CHE) *Online - full text edition. (2035766)* **3747**
Industrial Crops and Products (NLD) *Online - full text edition. (2080079)* **3158**
Infant Behavior and Development (GBR) *Online - full text edition. (618780)* **4404**
Infection (DEU) *Online - full text edition. (601268)* **3619**
Inflammation (USA) *Online - full text edition. (82716)* **3620**
Inflammation Research (CHE) *Online - full text edition. (175994)* **4301**
Inflammopharmacology (NLD) *Online - full content edition. (2014025)* **4302**
Infusion Therapy and Transfusion Medicine (CHE) *Online - full text edition. (8044)* **3620**
Inhalation Toxicology (USA) *Online - full text edition. (1646826)* **3451**
Injury (GBR) *Online - full text edition. (131628)* **4016**
Injury Prevention and Safety Promotion (NLD) *Online - full text edition. (2388081)* **3393**
Inpharma Weekly (NZL) *Online - full text edition. (1149571)* **4345**
Institut Pasteur. Annales. Actualites (FRA) *Online - full text edition. (2003880)* **3323**
Institution of Mechanical Engineers. Proceedings. Part H: Journal of Engineering in Medicine (GBR) *Online - full text edition. (1783521)* **3238**
Instrumentation Science & Technology (USA) *Online - full text edition. (107247)* **3376**
Intensive and Critical Care Nursing (GBR) *Online - full text edition. (1412981)* **3921**
Intensive Care Medicine (DEU) *Online - full text edition. (210617)* **3621**

Intensivmedizin und Notfallmedizin (DEU) *Online - full text edition. (178160)* **3621**
Internal Medicine Journal Online(AUS) *Online - full text. (4680685)* **3909**
International Archives of Allergy and Immunology (CHE) *Online - full text edition. (381470)* **3747**
International Archives of Occupational and Environmental Health (DEU) *Online - full text edition. (374075)* **4257**
International Commission on Radiological Protection. Annals (GBR) *Online - full text edition. (679828)* **4145**
International Contact Lens Clinic (USA) *Online - full text edition. (1508725)* **3999**
International Endodontic Journal Online(GBR) *Online - full text. (547573)* **3826**
International Forum of Psychoanalysis (NOR) *Online - full text edition. (2215403)* **4405**
International Immunology (GBR) *Online - full text edition. (1766473)* **3747**
International Immunopharmacology (GBR) *Online - full text edition. (919411)* **4302**
International Journal for Parasitology (GBR) *Online - full text edition. (536830)* **3799**
International Journal for Quality in Health Care (GBR) *Online - full text edition. (1730444)* **3622**
The International Journal for the Psychology of Religion (USA) *Online - full text edition. (2019760)* **4500**
International Journal of Andrology (GBR) *Online - full text edition. (1086715)* **4213**
International Journal of Angiology (USA) *Online - full text edition. (3876349)* **3775**
International Journal of Antimicrobial Agents (NLD) *Online - full text edition. (2021412)* **3323**
The International Journal of Aviation Psychology (USA) *Online - full text edition. (2019752)* **4532**
International Journal of Behavioral Development (GBR) *Online - full text edition. (50377)* **4405**
International Journal of Behavioral Medicine (USA) *Online - full text edition. (2367955)* **4405**
International Journal of Biochemistry & Cell Biology (GBR) *Online - full text edition. (400556)* **3252**
International Journal of Biological Macromolecules (NLD) *Online - full text edition. (956244)* **3252**
International Journal of Biometeorology (DEU) *Online - full text edition. (249092)* **4223**
International Journal of Cardiology (IRL) *Online - full text edition. (715115)* **3775**
International Journal of Cardiovascular Imaging (NLD) *Online - full text edition. (1330004)* **3775**
International Journal of Children's Spirituality (GBR) *Online - full text edition. (3326454)* **4406**
International Journal of Clinical Oncology Online(JPN) *Online - full text. (3285294)* **3980**
International Journal of Cognitive Ergonomics (USA) *Online - full text edition. (3241955)* **4406**
International Journal of Colorectal Disease (DEU) *Online - full text edition. (1509314)* **4191**
International Journal of Cosmetic Science (GBR) *Online - full text edition. (12025)* **3176**
International Journal of Cosmetic Surgery and Aesthetic Dermatology (USA) *Online - full content edition. (3868761)* **3850**
International Journal of Dermatology (GBR) *Online - full text edition. (315192)* **3850**
International Journal of Developmental Neuroscience (GBR) *Online - full text edition. (1276689)* **4095**
International Journal of Disability, Development and Education (GBR) *Online - full text edition. (132918)* **3423**
International Journal of Drug Policy (NLD) *Online - full text edition. (1859900)* **3402**
International Journal of Environmental Health Research (GBR) *Online - full text edition. (2016788)* **3439**
International Journal of Epidemiology (GBR) *Online - full text edition. (406635)* **3623**
International Journal of Experimental Pathology (GBR) *Online - full text edition. (402923)* **3623**
International Journal of Food Microbiology (NLD) *Online - full text edition. (1334379)* **3324**
International Journal of Food Sciences and Nutrition (GBR) *Online - full text edition. (198080)* **4236**
International Journal of Group Tensions (USA) *Online - full text edition. (1454757)* **4406**
International Journal of Gynecological Cancer (USA) *Online - full text edition. (2032716)* **3953**
International Journal of Gynecology and Obstetrics (IRL) *Online - full text edition. (162310)* **3954**
International Journal of Health Care Quality Assurance (GBR) *Online - full text edition. (2148471)* **3623**
International Journal of Hyperthermia (GBR) *Online - full text edition. (1390139)* **3980**
International Journal of Impotence Research (GBR) *Online - full text edition. (1876759)* **4213**
International Journal of Language and Communication Disorders (GBR) *Online - full text edition. (540994)* **4033**
International Journal of Law and Psychiatry (GBR) *Online - full text edition. (162000)* **3540**
International Journal of Legal Medicine (DEU) *Online - full text edition. (756199)* **3882**
International Journal of Medical Informatics (IRL) *Online - full text edition. (88951)* **3811**
International Journal of Neural Systems (SGP) *Online - full text edition. (1846140)* **3389**
International Journal of Neuro-Psychopharmacology (GBR) *Online - full text edition. (3614816)* **4303**
International Journal of Nursing Practice (AUS) *Online - full text edition. (3018245)* **3921**
International Journal of Nursing Studies (GBR) *Online - full text edition. (94102)* **3922**
International Journal of Obesity (GBR) *Online - full text edition. (438650)* **4236**
International Journal of Offender Therapy and Comparative Criminology (USA) *Online - full text edition. (3258602)* **3394**
International Journal of Oral & Maxillofacial Surgery (DNK) *Online - full text edition. (785814)* **3827**
International Journal of Paediatric Dentistry Online(GBR) *Online - full text. (1439979)* **3827**
International Journal of Pediatric Otorhinolaryngology (IRL) *Online - full text edition. (952060)* **4033**
International Journal of Pest Management (GBR) *Online - full text edition. (804851)* **3158**
International Journal of Pharmaceutics (NLD) *Online - full text edition. (521175)* **4303**
The International Journal of Psycho-Analysis (GBR) *Online - full text edition. (21814)* **4406**
International Journal of Psychology (GBR) *Online - full text edition. (485675)* **4407**
International Journal of Psychophysiology (NLD) *Online - full text edition. (1254235)* **4407**
International Journal of Psychotherapy (GBR) *Online - full content edition. (2951118)* **4096**
International Journal of Radiation Biology (GBR) *Online - full text edition. (584010)* **3980**
International Journal of Radiation: Oncology - Biology - Physics (USA) *Online - full text edition. (394769)* **4146**
International Journal of Rehabilitation and Health (USA) *Online - full text edition. (2380757)* **3485**
The International Journal of Risk and Safety in Medicine (NLD) *Online - full text edition. (1980106)* **3532**
International Journal of S T D & AIDS (GBR) *Online - full text edition. (1838164)* **3800**
International Journal of Sexuality and Gender Studies (USA) *Online - full text edition. (2940299)* **3527**
International Journal of Stress Management (USA) *Online - full text edition. (2354179)* **3624**
International Journal of Technology Assessment in Health Care (GBR) *Online - full text edition. (1398504)* **3875**
International Journal of Toxicology (GBR) *Online - full text edition. (1174711)* **3451**
International Journal of Urology (AUS) *Online - full text edition. (2651386)* **4213**
International Neuropsychological Society. Journal (GBR) *Online - full text edition. (2668556)* **4097**
International Nursing Review Online(GBR) *Online - full text. (6181)* **3922**
International Ophthalmology (NLD) *Online - full text edition. (916390)* **3999**
International Orthopaedics (DEU) *Online - full text edition. (46086)* **4016**
International Review of Psychiatry (GBR) *Online - full text edition. (1742612)* **4097**
International Urogynecology Journal (GBR) *Online - full text edition. (2019949)* **3954**
International Urology and Nephrology (HUN) *Online - full text edition. (548626)* **4214**
Der Internist (DEU) *Online - full text edition. (215023)* **3909**
Interventional Cardiology Newsletter (USA) *Online - full text edition. (2271214)* **3775**
Intervirology (CHE) *Online - full text edition. (513504)* **3324**
Invertebrate Neuroscience Online(DEU) *Online - full text. (2955164)* **3353**
Invertebrate Systomatics (Online Edition)(AUS) *Online - full text. (1642308)* **3353**
Investigational New Drugs (USA) *Online - full text edition. (1202456)* **4304**
Investigative Radiology (USA) *Online - full text edition. (564052)* **4146**
Isokinetics and Exercise Science (NLD) *Online - full text edition. (1985701)* **4174**
Issues in Comprehensive Pediatric Nursing (USA) *Online - full text edition. (106976)* **3922**
Issues in Interdisciplinary Care (USA) *Online - full text edition. (3765911)* **3625**
Issues in Mental Health Nursing (USA) *Online - full text edition. (1458086)* **3922**
J A H Online (USA) *Online - full text edition of* Journal of Adolescent Health. (1715100) **3629**
J A I D S (USA) *Online - full text edition. (1655655)* **3800**
J A R O (USA) *Online - full content edition. (4051661)* **4034**
J C P Online (GBR) *Online - full text edition of* Journal of Clinical Pathology. (802077) **3631**
J E C H Online (GBR) *Online - full text edition of* Journal of Epidemiology & Community Health. (297119) **3632**
J M B Online (GBR) *Online - full text edition of* Journal of Molecular Biology. (6661) **3254**
J M E Online (GBR) *Online - full text edition of* Journal of Medical Ethics. (504211) **3635**
J M G Online (GBR) *Online - full text edition of* Journal of Medical Genetics. (524867) **3310**
J O G N N (USA) *Online - full text edition. (169684)* **3923**
Japanese Journal of Clinical Oncology (GBR) *Online - full text edition. (793302)* **3981**
Japanese Journal of Ophthalmology (NLD) *Online - full text edition. (114189)* **4000**
Japanese Psychological Research (JPN) *Online - full text edition. (259861)* **4408**
Journal de Pediatrie et de Puericulture (FRA) *Online - full text edition. (264555)* **3628**
Journal for the Theory of Social Behaviour (GBR) *Online - full text edition. (468630)* **4408**
Journal Midwifery and Women's Health (USA) *Online - full text edition. (678287)* **3955**
Journal of Abnormal Child Psychology (USA) *Online - full text edition. (121541)* **4409**
Journal of Adolescence (GBR) *Online - full text edition. (405426)* **3383**
Journal of Adolescent Research (USA) *Online - full text edition. (1623125)* **4409**
Journal of Adult Development (USA) *Online - full text edition. (2316528)* **4409**
Journal of Advanced Nursing (GBR) *Online - full text edition. (552135)* **3923**
Journal of Aerosol Medicine (USA) *Online - full content edition. (1651595)* **4161**
Journal of Affective Disorders (NLD) *Online - full text edition. (916404)* **4098**
Journal of Aging and Health (USA) *Online - full text edition. (1731173)* **3474**
Journal of Aging & Identity (USA) *Online - full text edition. (2940272)* **3475**
Journal of Aging Studies (GBR) *Online - full text edition. (1582410)* **3475**
Journal of Alternative & Complementary Medicine (USA) *Online - full content edition. (2721201)* **3167**
Journal of Alzheimer's Disease (NLD) *Online - full text edition. (3637956)* **4098**
Journal of Analytical Psychology (GBR) *Online - full text edition. (632872)* **4409**
Journal of Anatomy (GBR) *Online - full text edition. (740322)* **3202**
Journal of Anesthesia (JPN) *Online - full content edition. (2383268)* **3757**
Journal of Animal Ecology (GBR) *Online - full text edition. (7641)* **3202**
Journal of Animal Physiology and Animal Nutrition Online(DEU) *Online - full text. (429643)* **3344**
Journal of Anti-Aging Medicine (USA) *Online - full content edition. (3597180)* **3475**
Journal of Antimicrobial Chemotherapy (GBR) *Online - full text edition. (1146394)* **3800**
Journal of Anxiety Disorders (GBR) *Online - full text edition. (1577158)* **4409**
Journal of Applied Animal Welfare Science (USA) *Online - full text edition. (2930145)* **3172**
Journal of Applied Behavioral Science (USA) *Online - full text edition. (142182)* **4410**
Journal of Applied Developmental Psychology (GBR) *Online - full text edition. (913278)* **4410**
Journal of Applied Microbiology (GBR) *Online - full text edition. (1497693)* **3324**
Journal of Applied Psychoanalytic Studies (USA) *Online - full text edition. (3849422)* **4410**
Journal of Applied Research in Intellectual Disabilities (GBR) *Online - full text edition. (1694294)* **4098**
Journal of Assisted Reproduction and Genetics (USA) *Online - full text edition. (1340468)* **3955**
Journal of Audio Visual Media in Medicine (GBR) *Online - full text edition. (251399)* **3629**
Journal of Autism and Developmental Disorders (USA) *Online - full text edition. (472158)* **3423**
Journal of Autoimmunity (GBR) *Online - full text edition. (1696866)* **3748**
Journal of Back and Musculoskeletal Rehabilitation (NLD) *Online - full text edition. (2120216)* **4017**
The Journal of Behavior Therapy and Experimental Psychiatry (GBR) *Online - full text edition. (501611)* **4099**
Journal of Behavioral Education (USA) *Online - full text edition. (2025272)* **3412**
Journal of Behavioral Medicine (USA) *Online - full text edition. (829722)* **4099**
Journal of Biochemical and Biophysical Methods (NLD) *Online - full text edition. (913685)* **3252**
Journal of Biochemistry and Molecular Biology Online(HKG) *Online - full content. (1192019)* **3253**
Journal of Bioenergetics and Biomembranes (USA) *Online - full text edition. (225851)* **3253**
Journal of Biological Rhythms (USA) *Online - full text edition. (1750887)* **4099**
Journal of Biological Systems (SGP) *Online - full text edition. (2804638)* **3202**
Journal of Biomechanical Engineering (USA) *Online - full text edition. (269034)* **3629**
The Journal of Biomechanics (GBR) *Online - full text edition. (605905)* **3629**
Journal of Biomedical Informatics (USA) *Online - full text edition. (460206)* **3811**
Journal of Biomedical Science (CHE) *Online - full text edition. (2381753)* **3630**
Journal of Biomolecular Screening (USA) *Online - full content edition. (3236684)* **3253**
Journal of Biopharmaceutical Statistics (USA) *Online - full text edition. (2026554)* **4345**
Journal of Biosocial Science (GBR) *Online - full text edition. (486280)* **4521**
Journal of Biotechnology (NLD) *Online - full text edition. (1339648)* **3275**
Journal of Black Studies (USA) *Online - full text edition. (411027)* **4509**
Journal of Bodywork & Movement Therapies (GBR) *Online - full text edition. (3244253)* **4061**
Journal of Bone and Mineral Metabolism (JPN) *Online - full text edition. (2955563)* **3864**
Journal of Business & Psychology (USA) *Online - full text edition. (2246074)* **4411**
Journal of Cancer Research and Clinical Oncology (DEU) *Online - full text edition. (761176)* **3981**
Journal of Cataract and Refractive Surgery (USA) *Online - full text edition. (1287214)* **4000**
Journal of Cell Science (GBR) *Online - full text edition. (1548948)* **3291**
Journal of Chemical Neuroanatomy (NLD) *Online - full text edition. (1668609)* **4099**
Journal of Child and Family Studies (USA) *Online - full text edition. (2137151)* **4411**
Journal of Child Language (GBR) *Online - full text edition. (757845)* **3384**
Journal of Child Psychology & Psychiatry & Allied Disciplines (GBR) *Online - full text edition. (112372)* **4411**

Online Service

Journal of Child Psychotherapy (GBR) *Online - full text edition. (491217)* **4411**
Journal of Chromatography. B, Biomedical Sciences and Applications (NLD) *Online - full text edition. (687219)* **3373**
Journal of Classification (USA) *Online - full text edition. (2171570)* **3553**
The Journal of Clinical Anesthesia (USA) *Online - full text edition. (1712357)* **3758**
Journal of Clinical Child and Adolescent Psychology (USA) *Online - full text edition. (211591)* **4411**
The Journal of Clinical Epidemiology (USA) *Online - full text edition. (236675)* **3630**
Journal of Clinical Forensic Medicine (GBR) *Online - full text edition. (2480603)* **3883**
Journal of Clinical Gastroenterology (USA) *Online - full text edition. (1063448)* **3893**
Journal of Clinical Geropsychology (USA) *Online - full text edition. (2653591)* **3475**
Journal of Clinical Immunology (USA) *Online - full text edition. (1064967)* **3748**
Journal of Clinical Monitoring and Computing (NLD) *Online - full text edition. (1386662)* **3631**
Journal of Clinical Neuroscience (GBR) *Online - full text edition. (3011356)* **4100**
Journal of Clinical Nursing (GBR) *Online - full text edition. (2121794)* **3923**
Journal of Clinical Periodontology (DNK) *Online - full text edition. (409634)* **3828**
Journal of Clinical Pharmacology (USA) *Online - full text edition. (613878)* **4306**
Journal of Clinical Pharmacy and Therapeutics (GBR) *Online - full text edition. (416355)* **4306**
Journal of Clinical Psychology in Medical Settings (USA) *Online - full text edition. (2380749)* **4412**
Journal of Clinical Virology (NLD) *Online - full text edition. (2267225)* **3801**
Journal of Cognition and Development (USA) *Online - full text edition.* **4412**
Journal of Cognitive Neuroscience (USA) *Online - full text edition. (1758071)* **4100**
Journal of Communication Disorders (USA) *Online - full text edition. (787965)* **4412**
Journal of Communication Inquiry (USA) *Online - full text edition. (1593447)* **4522**
Journal of Community Health (USA) *Online - full text edition. (1527576)* **3631**
Journal of Community Health Nursing (USA) *Online - full text edition. (1363085)* **3924**
Journal of Comparative Pathology (GBR) *Online - full text edition. (110388)* **3203**
Journal of Comparative Physiology. A: Sensory, Neural, and Behavioral Physiology (DEU) *Online - full text edition. (1363344)* **3344**
Journal of Comparative Physiology. B: Biochemical, Systemic, and Environmental Physiology (DEU) *Online - full text edition. (1363352)* **3344**
Journal of Computational Neuroscience (NLD) *Online - full text edition. (2442531)* **4100**
Journal of Computer-Assisted Tomography (USA) *Online - full text edition. (223794)* **4147**
Journal of Constructivist Psychology (USA) *Online - full text edition. (1646834)* **4413**
Journal of Consumer Psychology (USA) *Online - full text edition. (2212269)* **3153**
Journal of Contemporary Psychotherapy (USA) *Online - full text edition. (183830)* **4413**
Journal of Controlled Release (NLD) *Online - full text edition. (1357212)* **4306**
Journal of Cranio-Maxillo-Facial Surgery (GBR) *Online - full text edition. (159328)* **4192**
Journal of Craniofacial Genetics and Developmental Biology Online(DNK) *Online - full text. (1050400)* **3309**
Journal of Cross-Cultural Gerontology (NLD) *Online - full text edition. (1535366)* **3475**
Journal of Cross-Cultural Psychology (USA) *Online - full text edition. (621943)* **4414**
Journal of Cutaneous Medicine and Surgery (CAN) *Online - full text edition. (3017524)* **3850**
Journal of Cutaneous Pathology (DNK) *Online - full text edition. (707031)* **3850**
The Journal of Deaf Studies and Deaf Education (USA) *Online - full text edition. (2960575)* **3491**
The Journal of Dentistry (GBR) *Online - full text edition. (494267)* **3828**
Journal of Dermatological Science (IRL) *Online - full text edition. (1837427)* **3850**
Journal of Developmental and Physical Disabilities (USA) *Online - full text edition. (1651854)* **3485**
Journal of Diabetes and Its Complications (USA) *Online - full text edition. (1467085)* **3864**
Journal of Early Adolescence (USA) *Online - full text edition. (1459775)* **3384**
Journal of Ecology (GBR) *Online - full text edition. (372633)* **3203**
The Journal of Economic Psychology (NLD) *Online - full text edition. (1067184)* **3366**
Journal of Educational and Psychological Consultation (USA) *Online - full text edition. (1856189)* **3412**
Journal of Electromyography and Kinesiology (GBR) *Online - full text edition. (2013517)* **3266**
The Journal of Emergency Medicine (USA) *Online - full text edition. (1302051)* **4018**
Journal of Endocrinology (GBR) *Online - full text edition. (1763296)* **3865**
Journal of Endourology (USA) *Online - full content edition. (1677675)* **4214**
Journal of English Linguistics (USA) *Online - full text edition. (120227)* **3550**
Journal of Environmental Psychology (GBR) *Online - full text edition. (1051725)* **4415**
Journal of Environmental Radioactivity (GBR) *Online - full text edition. (1385674)* **3440**
Journal of Ethnopharmacology (IRL) *Online - full text edition. (906484)* **4307**
Journal of Evaluation in Clinical Practice Online(GBR) *Online - full text. (2944391)* **3632**
Journal of Evolutionary Biochemistry and Physiology (RUS) *Online - full text edition. (811971)* **3254**
Journal of Evolutionary Biology (GBR) *Online - full text edition. (1624032)* **3309**
Journal of Experimental Biology (GBR) *Online - full text edition. (812269)* **3203**
Journal of Experimental Child Psychology (USA) *Online - full text edition. (612944)* **4415**
Journal of Experimental Marine Biology and Ecology (NLD) *Online - full text edition. (538868)* **3203**
Journal of Experimental Social Psychology (USA) *Online - full text edition. (61638)* **4415**
Journal of Experimental Therapeutics and Oncology Online(USA) *Online - full text. (2994836)* **3982**
Journal of Exposure Analysis and Environmental Epidemiology (GBR) *Online - full text edition. (2115603)* **3440**
Journal of Family and Economic Issues (USA) *Online - full text edition. (1546724)* **4416**
Journal of Family Nursing (USA) *Online - full content edition. (2718340)* **3924**
Journal of Family Therapy (GBR) *Online - full text edition. (915637)* **4101**
Journal of Family Violence (USA) *Online - full text edition. (1506145)* **3395**
Journal of Feline Medicine and Surgery (GBR) *Online - full text edition. (3814564)* **4545**
Journal of Fluency Disorders (USA) *Online - full text edition. (300861)* **4416**
Journal of Forensic Psychiatry (GBR) *Online - full text edition. (1877313)* **4101**
Journal of Gambling Studies (USA) *Online - full text edition. (1611771)* **4101**
Journal of Gastroenterology (JPN) *Online - full text edition. (244856)* **3893**
Journal of Gastroenterology and Hepatology (AUS) *Online - full text edition. (1511505)* **3893**
Journal of General Internal Medicine (USA) *Online - full text edition. (1554018)* **3910**
Journal of Genetic Counseling (USA) *Online - full text edition. (2137186)* **4416**
Journal of Hand Surgery: American Volume (USA) *Online - full content edition. (76643)* **4193**
Journal of Hand Surgery: British and European Volume (GBR) *Online - full text edition. (1087827)* **4193**
Journal of Happiness Studies (NLD) *Online - full text edition. (4006828)* **4417**
The Journal of Headache and Pain Online(ITA) *Online - full content. (4414144)* **4102**
Journal of Health Communication (USA) *Online - full text edition. (3215520)* **3633**
Journal of Health Economics (NLD) *Online - full text edition. (1119079)* **4479**
Journal of Health Politics, Policy and Law (USA) *Online - full text edition. (621919)* **3633**
Journal of Health Psychology (GBR) *Online - full text edition. (2802880)* **4417**
The Journal of Heart and Lung Transplantation (GBR) *Online - full text edition. (1532200)* **4193**
Journal of Helminthology (GBR) *Online - full text edition. (509922)* **3801**
Journal of Hematotherapy & Stem Cell Research (USA) *Online - full text edition. (2256169)* **3903**
Journal of Hepato - Biliary - Pancreatic Surgery (JPN) *Online - full content edition. (3802809)* **4193**
Journal of Hepatology (DNK) *Online - full text edition. (1379739)* **3893**
Journal of Hospital Infection (GBR) *Online - full text edition. (998516)* **3801**
Journal of Human Evolution (GBR) *Online - full text edition. (396516)* **3309**
Journal of Human Genetics (JPN) *Online - full text edition. (150827)* **3310**
Journal of Human Hypertension (GBR) *Online - full text edition. (1620347)* **3778**
Journal of Human Lactation (USA) *Online - full text edition. (2025418)* **3955**
Journal of Human Nutrition and Dietetics (GBR) *Online - full text edition. (1659529)* **4237**
Journal of Humanistic Psychology (USA) *Online - full text edition. (467030)* **4417**
Journal of Immigrant Health (USA) *Online - full text edition. (3518949)* **3634**
Journal of Immunological Methods (NLD) *Online - full text edition. (717584)* **3748**
Journal of Industrial Microbiology and Biotechnology (GBR) *Online - full text edition. (1504495)* **3276**
Journal of Infection (GBR) *Online - full text edition. (934356)* **3801**
Journal of Infection and Chemotherapy (JPN) *Online - full text edition. (2906090)* **4307**
Journal of Inherited Metabolic Disease (NLD) *Online - full text edition. (917834)* **4046**
Journal of Inorganic Biochemistry (USA) *Online - full text edition. (346527)* **3254**
Journal of Intellectual and Developmental Disability (GBR) *Online - full text edition. (363952)* **4102**
Journal of Intellectual Disability Research (GBR) *Online - full text edition. (681350)* **4102**
Journal of Intensive Care Medicine (USA) *Online - full text edition. (1623656)* **3634**
Journal of Interferon & Cytokine Research (USA) *Online - full text edition. (2803984)* **3749**
Journal of Internal Medicine (GBR) *Online - full text edition. (1096230)* **3910**
Journal of Interpersonal Violence (USA) *Online - full text edition. (1535412)* **3395**
Journal of Interprofessional Care (GBR) *Online - full text edition. (1377256)* **3634**
Journal of Interventional Cardiac Electrophysiology (NLD) *Online - full text edition. (3035662)* **3778**
The Journal of Investigative Dermatology (USA) *Online - full text edition. (332097)* **3851**
Journal of Investigative Surgery (USA) *Online - full text edition. (1646753)* **4193**
Journal of Language and Social Psychology (USA) *Online - full text edition. (1153811)* **4417**
Journal of Laparoendoscopic & Advanced Surgical Techniques (USA) *Online - full content edition. (2077620)* **4194**
Journal of Laryngology and Otology (GBR) *Online - full content edition. (1137417)* **4034**
Journal of Learning Disabilities (GBR) *Online - full text edition. (3244660)* **3423**
The Journal of Legal Medicine (USA) *Online - full text edition. (1460196)* **3634**
Journal of Lower Genital Tract Disease Online(USA) *Online - full text. (3256537)* **3956**
Journal of Luminescence (NLD) *Online - full text edition. (217417)* **4366**
Journal of Mammalian Evolution (USA) *Online - full text edition. (2272172)* **3354**
Journal of Mammary Gland Biology and Neoplasia (USA) *Online - full text edition. (2940310)* **3345**
Journal of Management in Medicine (GBR) *Online - full text edition. (1191381)* **3634**
Journal of Managerial Psychology (GBR) *Online - full text edition. (1517538)* **3365**
Journal of Materials Science: Materials in Medicine (USA) *Online - full text edition. (1878212)* **3434**
Journal of Mathematical Biology (DEU) *Online - full text edition. (828432)* **3204**
Journal of Mathematical Psychology (USA) *Online - full text edition. (469297)* **4418**
Journal of Medical Engineering & Technology (GBR) *Online - full text edition. (188646)* **3635**
Journal of Medical Humanities (USA) *Online - full text edition. (1606530)* **3635**
Journal of Medical Systems (USA) *Online - full text edition. (144258)* **3812**
Journal of Medicinal Food (USA) *Online - full content edition. (3764656)* **3636**
The Journal of Medicine and Philosophy (NLD) *Online - full text edition. (110108)* **3636**
Journal of Membrane Biology (USA) *Online - full text edition. (300276)* **3291**
Journal of Memory and Language (USA) *Online - full text edition. (130109)* **3550**
Journal of Mental Health (GBR) *Online - full text edition. (2150271)* **4102**
Journal of Microbiological Methods (NLD) *Online - full text edition. (1205773)* **3325**
Journal of Microencapsulation (GBR) *Online - full text edition. (1330594)* **4308**
Journal of Micromechatronics (NLD) *Online - full content edition. (4027612)* **3434**
Journal of Microscopy (GBR) *Online - full text edition. (313769)* **3334**
Journal of Molecular and Cellular Cardiology (GBR) *Online - full text edition. (321737)* **3778**
Journal of Molecular Endocrinology (GBR) *Online - full text edition. (1913174)* **3865**
Journal of Molecular Evolution (USA) *Online - full text edition. (203122)* **3310**
Journal of Molecular Graphics and Modelling (USA) *Online - full text edition. (1230948)* **3377**
Journal of Molecular Medicine (DEU) *Online - full text edition. (1698052)* **3636**
Journal of Muscle Research and Cell Motility (NLD) *Online - full text edition. (1005146)* **4018**
Journal of Musculoskeletal Research (SGP) *Online - full text edition. (3243656)* **4019**
Journal of Natural History (GBR) *Online - full text edition. (58440)* **3204**
Journal of Near-Death Studies (USA) *Online - full text edition. (2246090)* **4347**
Journal of Neural Transmission - Basic Neurosciences and Genetics - Parkinson's Disease and Allied Conditions - Alzheimer's Disease and Related Disorders - Biological Psychiatry (AUT) *Online - full text edition. (1842781)* **4102**
Journal of Neuro-Oncology (USA) *Online - full text edition. (1129910)* **3982**
Journal of Neurochemistry (USA) *Online - full text edition. (687278)* **3255**
Journal of Neurocytology (USA) *Online - full text edition. (642924)* **3291**
Journal of Neuroendocrinology Online(GBR) *Online - full text. (1766589)* **4103**
Journal of Neuroimaging (USA) *Online - full text edition. (2030349)* **4103**
Journal of Neuroimmunology (NLD) *Online - full text edition. (1250302)* **4103**
Journal of Neurolinguistics (GBR) *Online - full text edition. (1553798)* **4103**
Journal of Neurology (DEU) *Online - full text edition. (756636)* **4103**
Journal of Neurology, Neurosurgery and Psychiatry (GBR) *Online - full text edition. (139602)* **4104**
Journal of Neuroscience Methods (NLD) *Online - full text edition. (483354)* **4104**
Journal of Neurotrauma (USA) *Online - full content edition. (1331434)* **4019**
Journal of NeuroVirology (GBR) *Online - full text edition. (2728672)* **4105**
Journal of Nonverbal Behavior (USA) *Online - full text edition. (1537881)* **4418**
Journal of Nursing Management (GBR) *Online - full text edition. (2264196)* **3925**
Journal of Nutritional & Environmental Medicine (GBR) *Online - full text edition. (1874292)* **4237**
Journal of Nutritional Biochemistry (USA) *Online - full text edition. (592315)* **4238**
Journal of Obstetrics and Gynaecology (GBR) *Online - full text edition. (1056336)* **3956**
Journal of Occupational and Organizational Psychology (GBR) *Online - full text edition. (579351)* **4419**
Journal of Occupational Rehabilitation (USA) *Online - full text edition. (2014041)* **4258**
Journal of Oncology Pharmacy Practice (USA) *Online - full text edition. (2968193)* **4308**
Journal of Oral Pathology & Medicine (DNK) *Online - full text edition. (449830)* **3829**
Journal of Oral Rehabilitation Online(GBR) *Online - full text. (235571)* **3829**
Journal of Orofacial Orthopedics (DEU) *Online - full text edition. (532916)* **4019**
The Journal of Orthodontics (GBR) *Online - full text edition. (457175)* **3830**
Journal of Orthopaedic Nursing (GBR) *Online - full text edition. (3195384)* **3926**

Journal of Orthopaedic Science (JPN) *Online - full text edition. (2961687)* **4019**
Journal of Paediatrics and Child Health (AUS) *Online - full text edition. (53201)* **4047**
Journal of Pain and Symptom Management (USA) *Online - full text edition. (1553410)* **4105**
Journal of Palliative Medicine (USA) *Online - full text edition. (3764621)* **3637**
Journal of Pediatric Orthopaedics (USA) *Online - full text edition. (1028405)* **4019**
Journal of Pediatric Psychology (GBR) *Online - full text edition. (551821)* **4419**
Journal of Peptide Research (DNK) *Online - full text edition. (461156)* **3255**
Journal of Perinatal Medicine (DEU) *Online - full text edition. (799165)* **3956**
Journal of Perinatology (GBR) *Online - full text edition. (1713566)* **3956**
Journal of Periodontal Research (DNK) *Online - full text edition. (759465)* **3830**
Journal of Personality (USA) *Online - full text edition. (686050)* **4419**
Journal of Personality Assessment (USA) *Online - full text edition. (448508)* **4420**
Journal of Pharmaceutical and Biomedical Analysis (NLD) *Online - full text edition. (1188623)* **4309**
Journal of Pharmacokinetics and Pharmacodynamics (USA) *Online - full text edition. (94706)* **4310**
Journal of Pharmacological and Toxicological Methods (USA) *Online - full text edition. (826340)* **3452**
Journal of Photochemistry and Photobiology, B: Biology (CHE) *Online - full text edition. (1639870)* **3255**
Journal of Physiology (Paris) (FRA) *Online - full text edition. (358509)* **4105**
Journal of Pineal Research (DNK) *Online - full text edition. (1387189)* **4105**
Journal of Plankton Research (GBR) *Online - full text edition. (477605)* **3204**
Journal of Poetry Therapy (USA) *Online - full text edition. (1639293)* **3553**
The Journal of Primary Prevention (USA) *Online - full text edition. (959154)* **4420**
Journal of Protein Chemistry (USA) *Online - full text edition. (1138332)* **3255**
Journal of Psychiatric & Mental Health Nursing Online(GBR) *Online - full text. (2388677)* **4105**
Journal of Psychiatric Research (GBR) *Online - full text edition. (453625)* **4106**
Journal of Psycholinguistic Research (USA) *Online - full text edition. (539457)* **3551**
Journal of Psychology and Financial Markets (USA) *Online - full content edition. (3806499)* **4421**
Journal of Psychology and Judaism (USA) *Online - full text edition. (560715)* **4501**
Journal of Psychopathology and Behavioral Assessment (USA) *Online - full text edition. (939358)* **4421**
Journal of Psychopharmacology (GBR) *Online - full text edition. (1609017)* **4310**
Journal of Psychosomatic Research (USA) *Online - full text edition. (516953)* **4106**
Journal of Public Health Medicine (GBR) *Online - full text edition. (921114)* **4515**
Journal of Quality in Clinical Practice (AUS) *Online - full text edition. (1434012)* **3637**
Journal of Radiosurgery (USA) *Online - full text edition. (3518957)* **4194**
Journal of Rational - Emotive and Cognitive - Behavior Therapy (USA) *Online - full text edition. (2246112)* **4421**
Journal of Rehabilitation Medicine (NOR) *Online - full text edition. (1406965)* **4515**
Journal of Religion and Health (USA) *Online - full text edition. (1748327)* **4500**
Journal of Reproductive and Infant Psychology (GBR) *Online - full text edition. (1644785)* **4421**
Journal of Reproductive Immunology (IRL) *Online - full text edition. (906034)* **3749**
Journal of Research in Personality (USA) *Online - full text edition. (766917)* **4422**
Journal of Risk and Uncertainty (USA) *Online - full text edition. (1651234)* **3363**
Journal of Safety Research (GBR) *Online - full text edition. (616958)* **4258**
Journal of School Psychology (GBR) *Online - full text edition. (253588)* **4422**
Journal of Sex & Marital Therapy (USA) *Online - full text edition. (1582305)* **4422**
Journal of Sleep Research Online(GBR) *Online - full text. (2152096)* **3638**
Journal of Social and Personal Relationships (GBR) *Online - full content edition. (1312774)* **4423**
Journal of Social Distress and the Homeless (USA) *Online - full text edition. (2025337)* **4515**
Journal of Social Issues (USA) *Online - full content edition. (168661)* **4423**
Journal of Social Work Practice (GBR) *Online - full text edition. (1477897)* **4515**
Journal of Sports Sciences (GBR) *Online - full text edition. (1231049)* **4525**
Journal of Steroid Biochemistry and Molecular Biology (GBR) *Online - full text edition. (35033)* **3255**
Journal of Structural Biology (USA) *Online - full text edition. (221740)* **3205**
Journal of Substance Abuse (GBR) *Online - full text edition. (1693271)* **3403**
Journal of Substance Abuse Treatment (USA) *Online - full text edition. (1353543)* **3404**
Journal of Surgical Pathology (GBR) *Online - full text edition. (3507580)* **3638**
Journal of Surgical Research (USA) *Online - full text edition. (752037)* **4195**
Journal of Telemedicine and Telecare (GBR) *Online - full text edition. (2674254)* **3638**
Journal of the History of Biology (NLD) *Online - full text edition. (745561)* **3205**
Journal of the History of Medicine and Allied Sciences (GBR) *Online - full text edition. (307742)* **3638**
Journal of the History of Sexuality (USA) *Online - full text edition. (1840770)* **4522**
Journal of the History of the Neurosciences (NLD) *Online - full content edition. (2884380)* **4106**
Journal of the Learning Sciences (USA) *Online - full text edition. (2019787)* **3413**
Journal of the Neurological Sciences (NLD) *Online - full text edition. (324124)* **4106**
Journal of the Peripheral Nervous System Online(USA) *Online - full text. (3442500)* **4107**
Journal of Theoretical Biology (GBR) *Online - full text edition. (742775)* **3205**
Journal of Thermal Biology (GBR) *Online - full text edition. (134767)* **3267**
Journal of Thrombosis and Thrombolysis (USA) *Online - full text edition. (2442523)* **3779**
Journal of Toxicology and Environmental Health. Part A (USA) *Online - full text edition. (673900)* **3452**
Journal of Toxicology and Environmental Health. Part B: Critical Reviews (USA) *Online - full text edition. (3547418)* **3452**
Journal of Toxicology. Clinical Toxicology (USA) *Online - full text edition. (679631)* **4311**
Journal of Toxicology. Toxin Reviews (USA) *Online - full text edition. (1162632)* **4311**
Journal of Transcultural Nursing (USA) *Online - full content edition. (1960199)* **3927**
Journal of Trauma - Injury, Infection and Critical Care (USA) *Online - full text edition. (49417)* **4020**
Journal of Traumatic Stress (USA) *Online - full text edition. (1651870)* **4424**
Journal of Tropical Pediatrics (GBR) *Online - full text edition. (257869)* **4047**
Journal of Urology (USA) *Online - full text edition. (487732)* **4215**
Journal of Vascular Research (CHE) *Online - full text edition. (516902)* **3779**
Journal of Vestibular Research: Equilibrium and Orientation (NLD) *Online - full text edition. (1869167)* **3345**
Journal of Veterinary Medicine. Series A Online(DEU) *Online - full text. (460362)* **4547**
Journal of Veterinary Medicine. Series B Online(DEU) *Online - full text. (566373)* **4547**
Journal of Veterinary Pharmacology and Therapeutics Online(GBR) *Online - full text. (330515)* **4311**
Journal of Viral Hepatitis (GBR) *Online - full text edition. (2428547)* **3893**
Journal of Virological Methods (NLD) *Online - full text edition. (956457)* **3326**
Journal of Vocational Behavior (USA) *Online - full text edition. (680745)* **4424**
Journal of Vocational Rehabilitation (NLD) *Online - full text edition. (2040719)* **4258**
Journal of Women's Health and Gender-Based Medicine (USA) *Online - full text edition. (2243318)* **4564**
Journal of Youth and Adolescence (USA) *Online - full text edition. (258628)* **3384**
Journal of Youth Studies (GBR) *Online - full text edition. (3538087)* **3384**
Journal of Zoological Systematics and Evolutionary Research Online(DEU) *Online - full text. (802557)* **3355**
Kennedy Institute of Ethics. Journal (USA) *Online - full text edition. (2112264)* **3640**
Kidney and Blood Pressure Research (CHE) *Online - full text edition. (679127)* **4215**
Kidney International Online (USA) *Online - full text edition of* Kidney International. (1200712) **4215**
Kidney International. Supplement (USA) *Online - full text edition. (1200720)* **4215**
Klinische Neuroradiologie (DEU) *Online - full text edition. (2119714)* **4149**
The Knee (NLD) *Online - full text edition. (2347970)* **3345**
Knee Surgery, Sports Traumatology, Arthroscopy (DEU) *Online - full text edition. (2263076)* **4175**
Kognitionswissenschaft (DEU) *Online - full text edition. (2020963)* **4425**
Laboratory Animals (GBR) *Online - full text edition. (300071)* **3355**
Le Lait (FRA) *Online - full text edition. (703931)* **3326**
The Lancet (GBR) *Online - full text edition. (522279)* **3642**
Langenbecks Archives of Surgery (DEU) *Online - full text edition. (1100998)* **4196**
Language and Cognitive Processes (GBR) *Online - full text edition. (1386654)* **3551**
Language and Speech (GBR) *Online - full text edition. (684562)* **3551**
Laryngoscope (USA) *Online - full text edition. (82643)* **4035**
Lasers in Medical Science (GBR) *Online - full text edition. (1525913)* **3643**
Laterality (GBR) *Online - full text edition. (2952920)* **4107**
Law and Human Behavior (USA) *Online - full text edition. (432644)* **3541**
Learning and Individual Differences (GBR) *Online - full text edition. (1784242)* **3413**
Learning and Instruction (GBR) *Online - full text edition. (1935976)* **3413**
Learning and Motivation (USA) *Online - full text edition. (181382)* **3413**
Legal and Criminological Psychology (GBR) *Online - full text edition. (2668882)* **4425**
Leisure Sciences (USA) *Online - full text edition. (132268)* **3547**
Letters in Applied Microbiology (GBR) *Online - full text edition. (1497707)* **3326**
Leukemia (GBR) *Online - full text edition. (1576283)* **3903**
Leukemia Research (GBR) *Online - full text edition. (332941)* **3904**
Linnean Society. Biological Journal (GBR) *Online - full text edition. (405914)* **3206**
Literature & Medicine (USA) *Online - full text edition. (1471066)* **3552**
Liver (DNK) *Online - full text edition. (1044826)* **3894**
Logopedics Phoniatrics Vocology (NOR) *Online - full text edition. (2231557)* **4035**
Loss Prevention Bulletin (GBR) *Online - full content edition. (902063)* **3433**
Lung (USA) *Online - full text edition. (73563)* **4162**
Lung Cancer (IRL) *Online - full text edition. (1506005)* **3983**
Lupus (GBR) *Online - full text edition. (2084015)* **4169**
M P Online (GBR) *Online - full text edition of* Molecular Pathology. (2803364) **3879**
Magnetic Resonance Imaging (USA) *Online - full text edition. (1188615)* **4150**
Magnetic Resonance Materials in Physics, Biology and Medicine (GBR) *Online - full text edition. (2191164)* **4366**
Mammalian Genome (USA) *Online - full text edition. (2020998)* **3310**
Manual Therapy (GBR) *Online - full text edition. (2923106)* **4063**
Manuelle Medizin und Osteopathische Medizin (DEU) *Online - full text edition. (1128825)* **4063**
Marine Biological Association of the United Kingdom. Journal (GBR) *Online - full text edition. (704954)* **3207**
Marine Biology (DEU) *Online - full text edition. (196894)* **3207**
Marine Ecology Online(DEU) *Online - full text. (1092367)* **3207**
Marine Environmental Research (GBR) *Online - full text edition. (912042)* **3444**
Maternal and Child Health Journal (USA) *Online - full text edition. (3232980)* **3957**
Mathematical Biosciences (USA) *Online - full text edition. (296899)* **3554**
Mathematical Cognition (GBR) *Online - full text edition. (2669129)* **4426**
Mathematical Thinking and Learning (USA) *Online - full text edition. (3806464)* **3554**
Matrix Biology (NLD) *Online - full text edition. (1040421)* **3646**
Maturitas (IRL) *Online - full text edition. (320056)* **3958**
Measurement in Physical Education and Exercise Science (USA) *Online - full text edition. (3216896)* **4358**
Mechanisms of Ageing and Development (IRL) *Online - full text edition. (460907)* **3478**
Mechanisms of Development (IRL) *Online - full text edition. (231967)* **3292**
Medecine et Droit (FRA) *Online - full text edition. (2403455)* **3884**
Media Psychology (USA) *Online - full text edition. (3806472)* **4426**
Mediators of Inflammation (GBR) *Online - full text edition. (2152347)* **3648**
Medical & Veterinary Entomology Online(GBR) *Online - full text. (1568566)* **3648**
Medical Care (USA) *Online - full text edition. (205028)* **3649**
Medical Care Research and Review (USA) *Online - full text edition. (233595)* **4496**
Medical Decision Making (USA) *Online - full text edition. (1079484)* **3649**
Medical Dosimetry (USA) *Online - full text edition. (1711555)* **4150**
Medical Education (GBR) *Online - full text edition. (45160)* **3650**
Medical Electron Microscopy (JPN) *Online - full text edition. (3247740)* **3334**
Medical Engineering & Physics (GBR) *Online - full text edition. (910600)* **3650**
Medical Hypotheses (GBR) *Online - full text edition. (585394)* **3651**
Medical Image Analysis (GBR) *Online - full text edition. (3929833)* **4150**
Medical Informatics and the Internet in Medicine (GBR) *Online - full text edition. (733776)* **3812**
Medical Law Review (GBR) *Online - full text edition. (2306131)* **3542**
Medical Microbiology and Immunology (DEU) *Online - full text edition. (308595)* **3749**
Medical Mycology (GBR) *Online - full text edition. (703559)* **3803**
Medical Oncology (GBR) *Online - full text edition. (1317717)* **3984**
Medical Physics (USA) *Online - full text edition. (634077)* **3652**
Medical Principles and Practice (CHE) *Online - full text edition. (1757318)* **3652**
Medical Teacher (GBR) *Online - full text edition. (991562)* **3654**
Medical Update for Psychiatrists (USA) *Online - full text edition. (2954281)* **4108**
Medicine and Science in Sports and Exercise (USA) *Online - full text edition. (186074)* **4175**
Medicine, Health Care and Philosophy (NLD) *Online - full text edition. (3489868)* **3656**
Medizinische Klinik (DEU) *Online - full text edition. (725595)* **3658**
Medizinrecht (DEU) *Online - full text edition. (1282174)* **3884**
Memory (GBR) *Online - full text edition. (2265443)* **4426**
Mental Health, Religion & Culture (GBR) *Online - full content edition. (3538095)* **4427**
Mental Health Services Research (USA) *Online - full text edition. (3814688)* **4427**
Merrill - Palmer Quarterly (USA) *Online - full text edition. (395323)* **4427**
Metabolic Brain Disease (USA) *Online - full text edition. (1506129)* **3660**
Metabolic Engineering (USA) *Online - full text edition. (3544656)* **3238**
Metaphor and Symbol (USA) *Online - full text edition. (1561375)* **3551**
Methods: A Companion to Methods in Enzymology (USA) *Online - full text edition. (2147157)* **3256**
Methods in Cell Science (NLD) *Online - full text edition. (964719)* **3292**
Microbes and Infection (FRA) *Online - full text edition. (1027530)* **3327**
Microbial Drug Resistance (USA) *Online - full content edition. (2721236)* **3660**
Microbial Ecology (USA) *Online - full text edition. (145033)* **3327**
Microbial Ecology in Health & Disease (NOR) *Online - full text edition. (1668641)* **3803**
Microbial Pathogenesis (GBR) *Online - full text edition. (1520768)* **3804**
Microbiology (RUS) *Online - full text edition. (24392)* **3327**

Online Service

Microcirculation (GBR) *Online - full text edition. (914797)* **3661**
Micron (GBR) *Online - full text edition. (340030)* **3335**
Microvascular Research (USA) *Online - full text edition. (727938)* **3780**
Midwifery (GBR) *Online - full text edition. (1415263)* **3958**
The Milbank Quarterly (USA) *Online - full text edition. (49336)* **4368**
Military Psychology (USA) *Online - full text edition. (1729829)* **4428**
Minimally Invasive Therapy and Allied Technologies (GBR) *Online - full text edition. (2121328)* **3661**
Mitigation and Adaptation Strategies for Global Change (NLD) *Online - full text edition. (2658623)* **3441**
Molecular and Biochemical Parasitology (NLD) *Online - full text edition. (956430)* **3256**
Molecular and Cellular Biochemistry (USA) *Online - full text edition. (371076)* **3257**
Molecular and Cellular Endocrinology (IRL) *Online - full text edition. (567612)* **3866**
Molecular and Cellular Neurosciences (USA) *Online - full text edition. (1863207)* **4110**
Molecular and Cellular Probes (GBR) *Online - full text edition. (1579479)* **3879**
Molecular Aspects of Medicine (GBR) *Online - full text edition. (725234)* **3662**
Molecular Biology (RUS) *Online - full text edition. (296864)* **3257**
Molecular Biology Reports (NLD) *Online - full text edition. (149683)* **3257**
Molecular Brain Research (NLD) *Online - full text edition. (1502743)* **4110**
Molecular Cell Biology Research Communications (USA) *Online - full text edition. (3914895)* **3292**
Molecular Genetics and Genomics (DEU) *Online - full text edition. (100013)* **3311**
Molecular Genetics and Metabolism (USA) *Online - full text edition. (827045)* **3662**
Molecular Human Reproduction (GBR) *Online - full text edition. (2994976)* **3958**
Molecular Imaging and Biology (NLD) *Online - full text edition. (3535940)* **4151**
Molecular Immunology (GBR) *Online - full text edition. (268917)* **3257**
Molecular Medicine (USA) *Online - full text edition. (2723263)* **4317**
Molecular Membrane Biology (GBR) *Online - full text edition. (656925)* **3258**
Molecular Microbiology Online (GBR) *Online - full text edition of* Molecular Microbiology. (1611755) **3329**
Molecular Phylogenetics and Evolution (USA) *Online - full text edition. (2147122)* **3311**
Molecular Plant Pathology (GBR) *Online - full text edition. (4027345)* **3281**
Molecular Psychiatry (GBR) *Online - full text edition. (2967367)* **4110**
Molecular Therapy (USA) *Online - full text edition. (4051890)* **3984**
Monatsschrift Kinderheilkunde (DEU) *Online - full text edition. (610216)* **4049**
Mortality (GBR) *Online - full content edition. (2951126)* **4482**
Motivation and Emotion (USA) *Online - full text edition. (168335)* **4428**
Multiple Sclerosis (GBR) *Online - full text edition. (2506041)* **4111**
Multivariate Behavioral Research (USA) *Online - full text edition. (674699)* **4428**
Mund-, Kiefer- und Gesichtschirurgie (DEU) *Online - full text edition. (3360261)* **4035**
Mutagenesis (GBR) *Online - full text edition. (1506099)* **3311**
Mutation Research - D N A Repair (NLD) *Online - full text edition. (1275895)* **3258**
Mutation Research - Fundamental and Molecular Mechanisms of Mutagenesis (NLD) *Online - full text edition. (1807579)* **3311**
Mutation Research - Genetic Toxicology and Environmental Mutagenesis (NLD) *Online - full text edition. (140074)* **3312**
Mutation Research - Reviews in Mutation Research (NLD) *Online - full text edition. (25240)* **3312**
Mycopathologia (NLD) *Online - full text edition. (774189)* **3281**
Mycoses (DEU) *Online - full text edition. (289876)* **3663**
National Cancer Institute. Journal (USA) *Online - full text edition. (2410400)* **3985**
Naunyn-Schmiedeberg's Archives of Pharmacology (DEU) *Online - full text edition. (165158)* **4318**
NeoPlasia (USA) *Online - full text edition. (3987116)* **3985**
Nephrology, Dialysis and Transplantation (GBR) *Online - full text edition. (1560751)* **4216**
Nephrology Online (AUS) *Online - full text edition of* Nephrology. (3900843) **4216**
Nephron (CHE) *Online - full text edition. (193046)* **4216**
Der Nervenarzt (DEU) *Online - full text edition. (598089)* **4112**
Netherlands Journal of Medicine (NLD) *Online - full text edition. (244120)* **3911**
Neural Computation (USA) *Online - full text edition. (1758098)* **3389**
Neural Networks (GBR) *Online - full text edition. (1650394)* **3390**
Neural Processing Letters (USA) *Online - full text edition. (2753251)* **3390**
Neuro-Ophthalmology (NLD) *Online - full text edition. (1031678)* **4112**
Neurobiology of Aging (USA) *Online - full text edition. (1392417)* **3346**
Neurobiology of Disease (USA) *Online - full text edition. (3780082)* **4112**
Neurobiology of Learning and Memory (USA) *Online - full text edition. (57851)* **4112**
Neurocase (GBR) *Online - full text edition. (2670739)* **4112**
Neurochemical Research (USA) *Online - full text edition. (764035)* **4113**
Neurochemistry International (GBR) *Online - full text edition. (1039156)* **4113**
Neuroendocrinology (CHE) *Online - full text edition. (242373)* **3867**
Neuroepidemiology (CHE) *Online - full text edition. (1129465)* **4113**
Neurogastroenterology and Motility Online(GBR) *Online - full text. (1894250)* **3894**
Neurogenetics (DEU) *Online - full text edition. (3250121)* **3312**
NeuroImage (USA) *Online - full text edition. (2147149)* **4113**
NeuroImmunoModulation (CHE) *Online - full text edition. (2381737)* **3750**
Neurological Sciences (ITA) *Online - full text edition. (1585967)* **4114**
Neurology and Clinical Neurophysiology (USA) *Online - full content edition. (4536495)* **4115**
Neuromodulation Online(USA) *Online - full text. (3542785)* **4115**
Neuromuscular Disorders (GBR) *Online - full text edition. (2051753)* **4115**
Neuropathology (AUS) *Online - full text edition. (2796708)* **4116**
Neuropathology & Applied Neurobiology Online (GBR) *Online - full text edition of* Neuropathology and Applied Neurobiology. (53791) **4116**
Neuropeptides (Edinburgh) (GBR) *Online - full text edition. (961167)* **3259**
Neuropharmacology (GBR) *Online - full text edition. (322989)* **4318**
Neurophysiologie Clinique (FRA) *Online - full text edition. (612987)* **4116**
Neurophysiology (USA) *Online - full text edition. (78034)* **4116**
Neuropsychobiology (CHE) *Online - full text edition. (813303)* **4116**
Neuropsychologia (GBR) *Online - full text edition. (48097)* **4116**
Neuropsychological Rehabilitation (GBR) *Online - full text edition. (2018608)* **4117**
Neuropsychology, Development and Cognition. Section A: Journal of Clinical and Experimental Neuropsychology (NLD) *Online - full text edition. (907839)* **4429**
Neuropsychology, Development and Cognition. Section B: Aging, Neuropsychology and Cognition (NLD) *Online - full text edition. (2372134)* **4429**
Neuropsychology, Development, and Cognition. Section C: Child Neuropsychology (NLD) *Online - full text edition. (2483211)* **4429**
Neuropsychology, Development and Cognition. Section D: The Clinical Neuropsychologist (NLD) *Online - full text edition. (1565745)* **4429**
Neuropsychology Review (USA) *Online - full text edition. (1763008)* **4117**
Neuroradiology (DEU) *Online - full text edition. (812242)* **4151**
NeuroRehabilitation (NLD) *Online - full text edition. (2076470)* **4117**
Neuroscience (GBR) *Online - full text edition. (778354)* **4117**
Neuroscience and Behavioral Physiology (USA) *Online - full text edition. (11517)* **4118**
Neuroscience and Biobehavioral Reviews (GBR) *Online - full text edition. (476455)* **4118**
Neuroscience Letters (IRL) *Online - full text edition. (1119621)* **4118**
Neuroscience Research (IRL) *Online - full text edition. (1735756)* **4118**
The Neuroscientist (USA) *Online - full text edition. (2651572)* **4118**
NeuroSignals (CHE) *Online - full text edition. (2035758)* **3259**
Neurosurgical Review (DEU) *Online - full text edition. (939978)* **4197**
Neurotoxicology and Teratology (USA) *Online - full text edition. (1019198)* **4119**
New Genetics and Society (GBR) *Online - full content edition. (1715348)* **3313**
New Ideas in Psychology (GBR) *Online - full text edition. (1188658)* **4430**
Nicotine & Tobacco Research (GBR) *Online - full content edition. (3816052)* **4531**
Nonlinear Dynamics, Psychology, and Life Sciences (USA) *Online - full text edition. (3233014)* **4430**
Nordic Journal of Psychiatry (NOR) *Online - full text edition. (448117)* **4120**
Notfall und Rettungsmedizin (DEU) *Online - full text edition. (3602729)* **4022**
Nuclear Medicine and Biology (USA) *Online - full text edition. (677493)* **4152**
Nucleic Acids Research (GBR) *Online - full text edition. (2222531)* **3259**
Nurse Education in Practice (GBR) *Online - full text edition. (4529065)* **3931**
Nurse Education Today (GBR) *Online - full text edition. (1114336)* **3931**
Nursing and Health Sciences (AUS) *Online - full text edition. (4002350)* **3932**
Nursing Ethics (GBR) *Online - full text edition. (2383438)* **3933**
Nursing Inquiry (AUS) *Online - full text edition. (2784106)* **3933**
Nursing Philosophy Online (GBR) *Online - full text edition of* Nursing Philosophy. (4046625) **3934**
Nursing Science Quarterly (USA) *Online - full text edition. (1661760)* **3934**
Nutrition (USA) *Online - full text edition. (1644556)* **4241**
Nutrition and Cancer (USA) *Online - full text edition. (927910)* **4241**
Nutrition and Food Science (GBR) *Online - full text edition. (343927)* **4241**
Nutrition Bulletin Online (GBR) *Online - full text edition of* Nutrition Bulletin. (552259) **4241**
Nutrition in Clinical Care Online(USA) *Online - full text. (4057767)* **4242**
Nutrition Research (USA) *Online - full text edition. (1050249)* **4243**
Nutrition Research Reviews (GBR) *Online - full text edition. (2790483)* **4243**
Nutrition Society. Proceedings (GBR) *Online - full text edition. (406392)* **4243**
O E C D Guidelines for the Testing of Chemicals(FRA) *Online - full content. (1658638)* **3453**
O E M Online (GBR) *Online - full text edition of* Occupational and Environmental Medicine. (255599) **4261**
O M I C S: A Journal of Integrative Biology (USA) *Online - full text edition. (2984741)* **3313**
O R L (CHE) *Online - full text edition. (772747)* **4036**
Obesity Reviews Online(GBR) *Online - full text. (4046641)* **4244**
Obstetrical & Gynecological Survey (USA) *Online - full text edition. (0)* **3960**
Obstetrics and Gynecology (USA) *Online - full text edition. (447692)* **3960**
Occupational Ergonomics (USA) *Online - full text edition. (2929767)* **4261**
Occupational Medicine (GBR) *Online - full text edition. (31720)* **4262**
Ocular Immunology and Inflammation (NLD) *Online - full text edition. (2237407)* **4002**
Oecologia (DEU) *Online - full text edition. (763217)* **3211**
Oncogene (GBR) *Online - full text edition. (1620339)* **3986**
Oncology (CHE) *Online - full content edition. (630004)* **3986**
Der Onkologe (DEU) *Online - full text edition. (2901978)* **3987**
Onkologie (CHE) *Online - full text edition. (908932)* **3987**
Operative Orthopaedie und Traumatologie (DEU) *Online - full text edition. (1798227)* **4022**
Ophthalmic and Physiological Optics (GBR) *Online - full text edition. (418994)* **4003**
Ophthalmic Epidemiology (NLD) *Online - full text edition. (2388103)* **4003**
Ophthalmic Genetics (NLD) *Online - full text edition. (1115367)* **4003**
Ophthalmic Research (CHE) *Online - full text edition. (477834)* **4003**
Der Ophthalmologe (DEU) *Online - full text edition. (485780)* **4004**
Ophthalmologica (CHE) *Online - full text edition. (186260)* **4004**
Opportunistic Pathogens (NLD) *Online - full text edition. (1579495)* **3804**
Option - Bio (FRA) *Online - full text edition. (0)* **3212**
Oral Diseases (GBR) *Online - full text edition. (2728761)* **3834**
Oral Microbiology and Immunology (DNK) *Online - full text edition. (1580299)* **3329**
Oral Oncology (GBR) *Online - full text edition. (2160064)* **3988**
Orbit (NLD) *Online - full text edition. (1108751)* **4005**
Organisms Diversity and Evolution (DEU) *Online - full text edition. (4674324)* **3212**
Organization & Environment (USA) *Online - full text edition. (1761900)* **4263**
Organizational Behavior and Human Decision Processes (USA) *Online - full text edition. (722391)* **3366**
Origins of Life and Evolution of the Biosphere (NLD) *Online - full text edition. (205532)* **3212**
Der Orthopaede (DEU) *Online - full text edition. (320927)* **4022**
Osteoarthritis and Cartilage (GBR) *Online - full text edition. (2272121)* **4169**
Osteoporosis International (GBR) *Online - full text edition. (2021056)* **3671**
Oto-Rhino-Laryngologia Nova (CHE) *Online - full text edition. (2081164)* **4036**
Paediatric Anaesthesia Online(GBR) *Online - full text. (2121867)* **3759**
Paediatric & Perinatal Epidemiology Online(GBR) *Online - full text. (1578790)* **4050**
Paediatric Drugs (NZL) *Online - full text edition. (3909115)* **4321**
Paediatric Respiratory Reviews (GBR) *Online - full text edition. (4429907)* **4162**
Pain (NLD) *Online - full text edition. (337692)* **4121**
The Pain Clinic (NLD) *Online - full content edition. (1418912)* **3759**
Pain Medicine Online(USA) *Online - full text. (4057783)* **4121**
Pain Practice Online(USA) *Online - full text. (4542762)* **4122**
Pain Reviews (GBR) *Online - full text edition. (2383446)* **3671**
Palliative Medicine (GBR) *Online - full text edition. (1590855)* **3672**
Pancreatology (CHE) *Online - full text edition. (4474392)* **3867**
Parasite Immunology Online (GBR) *Online - full text edition of* Parasite Immunology. (615307) **3804**
Parasitology (Cambridge) (GBR) *Online - full text edition. (186945)* **3804**
Parasitology International (NLD) *Online - full text edition. (3256456)* **3805**
Parasitology Research (DEU) *Online - full text edition. (654264)* **3330**
Parkinsonism and Related Disorders (GBR) *Online - full text edition. (2658402)* **4122**
Pastoral Psychology (USA) *Online - full text edition. (2246120)* **4431**
Pathobiology (CHE) *Online - full text edition. (268496)* **3750**
Der Pathologe (DEU) *Online - full text edition. (951226)* **3672**
Pathology (GBR) *Online - full text edition. (429139)* **3673**
Pathology and Oncology Research (GBR) *Online - full text edition. (3581853)* **3988**
Pathology International (AUS) *Online - full text edition. (724947)* **3673**
Pathology, Research and Practice (DEU) *Online - full text edition. (399949)* **3673**
Pathophysiology (NLD) *Online - full text edition. (2317230)* **3347**
Pathophysiology of Haemostasis and Thrombosis (CHE) *Online - full text edition. (157961)* **3904**
Patient Education and Counseling (IRL) *Online - full text edition. (902217)* **4484**
Peace and Conflict (USA) *Online - full text edition. (2816172)* **4432**
Pediatric Allergy and Immunology (DNK) *Online - full text edition. (1894188)* **4051**
Pediatric and Developmental Pathology (USA) *Online - full text edition. (3506479)* **4051**

Pediatric Asthma, Allergy & Immunology (USA) *Online - full content edition. (1535226)* **4052**
Pediatric Cardiology (USA) *Online - full text edition. (969427)* **3781**
Pediatric Dermatology (USA) *Online - full text edition. (1225499)* **3852**
Pediatric Diabetes Online(DNK) *Online - full text. (4055160)* **4052**
Pediatric Hematology & Oncology (USA) *Online - full text edition. (1337858)* **4053**
The Pediatric Infectious Disease Journal (USA) *Online - full text edition. (1175459)* **4053**
Pediatric Nephrology (DEU) *Online - full text edition. (1571990)* **4217**
Pediatric Neurology (USA) *Online - full text edition. (1575678)* **4053**
Pediatric Neurosurgery (CHE) *Online - full text edition. (1539574)* **4122**
Pediatric Pathology & Molecular Medicine (USA) *Online - full text edition. (1375431)* **4053**
Pediatric Radiology (DEU) *Online - full text edition. (451223)* **4053**
Pediatric Rehabilitation (GBR) *Online - full text edition. (3264831)* **4064**
Pediatric Surgery International (DEU) *Online - full text edition. (1509322)* **4200**
Pediatric Transplantation (DNK) *Online - full text edition. (3449602)* **4054**
Pediatrics International (AUS) *Online - full text edition. (1885707)* **4054**
Pedobiologia (DEU) *Online - full text edition. (547514)* **3159**
Peptides (USA) *Online - full text edition. (1248650)* **3260**
Perfusion (GBR) *Online - full text edition. (1510843)* **3781**
Periodontology 2000 Online(DNK) *Online - full text. (2147874)* **3836**
Personality and Individual Differences (GBR) *Online - full text edition. (959669)* **4432**
Personality and Social Psychology Review (USA) *Online - full text edition. (3241963)* **4432**
Perspectives in Biology and Medicine (USA) *Online - full content edition. (263990)* **3674**
Pesticide Biochemistry and Physiology (USA) *Online - full text edition. (814148)* **3159**
Pfluegers Archiv (DEU) *Online - full text edition. (142751)* **3674**
Pharmaceutical Biology (NLD) *Online - full text edition. (590797)* **4323**
Pharmaceutical Chemistry Journal (USA) *Online - full text edition. (556602)* **4323**
Pharmaceutical Development and Technology (USA) *Online - full text edition. (2946432)* **4323**
Pharmaceutical Research (USA) *Online - full content edition. (1326368)* **4324**
PharmacoEconomics (NZL) *Online - full text edition. (2124289)* **4326**
Pharmacoeconomics and Outcomes News (NZL) *Online - full text edition. (2489554)* **4345**
Pharmacological Research (GBR) *Online - full text edition. (398640)* **4326**
Pharmacology (CHE) *Online - full text edition. (546968)* **4326**
Pharmacology and Therapeutics (USA) *Online - full text edition. (781053)* **4326**
Pharmacology & Toxicology Online(DNK) *Online - full text. (1977717)* **4327**
Pharmacology, Biochemistry and Behavior (USA) *Online - full text edition. (1106236)* **4327**
Pharmacy World and Science (NLD) *Online - full content edition. (1848623)* **4329**
Die Pharmazie (DEU) *Online - full text edition. (376752)* **4330**
Philosophical Psychology (GBR) *Online - full text edition. (1670247)* **4433**
Philosophy, Psychiatry, and Psychology Online (USA) *Online - full text edition of* Philosophy, Psychiatry & Psychology. (2384787) **4348**
Phlebology (GBR) *Online - full text edition. (1676342)* **3781**
Photodermatology, Photoimmunology & Photomedicine Online(DNK) *Online - full text. (1324039)* **3852**
Photosynthesis Research (NLD) *Online - full text edition. (997412)* **3260**
Physical Therapy in Sport (GBR) *Online - full text edition. (1141937)* **4176**
Physics in Medicine and Biology (GBR) *Online - full text edition. (532509)* **3267**
Physiological Measurement (GBR) *Online - full text edition. (960926)* **3676**
Physiology and Behavior (USA) *Online - full text edition. (570389)* **3347**
Physiotherapy Theory and Practice (GBR) *Online - full text edition. (1516817)* **4065**
Phytomedicine (DEU) *Online - full text edition. (2401827)* **3676**
Pigment Cell Research (DNK) *Online - full text edition. (1608754)* **3293**
Pituitary (NLD) *Online - full text edition. (3463435)* **3867**
Placenta (GBR) *Online - full text edition. (958042)* **3676**
Plant and Cell Physiology (GBR) *Online - full text edition. (1206311)* **3293**
Plant, Cell and Environment Online (GBR) *Online - full text edition of* Plant, Cell and Environment. (1740) **3213**
Plant Cell, Tissue and Organ Culture (NLD) *Online - full text edition. (1060252)* **3293**
Plant Foods for Human Nutrition (NLD) *Online - full text edition. (784648)* **4244**
Plant Molecular Biology (NLD) *Online - full text edition. (1060198)* **3213**
Plastic and Reconstructive Surgery (USA) *Online - full text edition. (396826)* **4200**
Platelets (Abingdon) (GBR) *Online - full text edition. (1997904)* **3213**
Polar Biology (DEU) *Online - full text edition. (1128809)* **3213**
Policy, Politics & Nursing Practice (USA) *Online - full text edition. (4052714)* **3937**
Political Psychology (USA) *Online - full text edition. (1002619)* **4368**
Population and Environment (USA) *Online - full text edition. (1628380)* **4433**
Postgraduate Medical Journal (GBR) *Online - full text edition. (1095617)* **3678**
Postharvest Biology and Technology (NLD) *Online - full text edition. (2021439)* **3277**
Prevention Science (USA) *Online - full text edition. (4012496)* **3805**
Preventive Medicine (USA) *Online - full text edition. (825417)* **3679**
Preventive Veterinary Medicine (NLD) *Online - full text edition. (1119044)* **4550**
Primary Care Update for Ob - Gyns (USA) *Online - full text edition. (2382326)* **3962**
Primary Health Care Research and Development (GBR) *Online - full text edition. (4049586)* **3679**
Process Biochemistry (GBR) *Online - full text edition. (549118)* **3277**
Progress in Biophysics & Molecular Biology (GBR) *Online - full text edition. (584835)* **3267**
Progress in Neuro-Psychopharmacology and Biological Psychiatry (USA) *Online - full text edition. (548561)* **4331**
Progress in Neurobiology (GBR) *Online - full text edition. (67075)* **3348**
Progress in Nuclear Magnetic Resonance Spectroscopy (NLD) *Online - full text edition. (606588)* **3377**
Progress in Orthodontics Online(DNK) *Online - full text. (4125452)* **3837**
Progress in Pediatric Cardiology (IRL) *Online - full text edition. (2201321)* **3782**
Progress in Retinal and Eye Research (GBR) *Online - full text edition. (1400789)* **4006**
Prostaglandins and Other Lipid Mediators (USA) *Online - full text edition. (1742345)* **3868**
Prostaglandins, Leukotrienes and Essential Fatty Acids (GBR) *Online - full text edition. (1726374)* **3868**
Prostate Cancer and Prostatic Diseases (GBR) *Online - full text edition. (3275973)* **3989**
The Prostate Journal Online(USA) *Online - full text. (3542793)* **3680**
Protein Engineering (GBR) *Online - full text edition. (1568558)* **3261**
Protein Expression and Purification (USA) *Online - full text edition. (1926535)* **3261**
Protein Science (USA) *Online - full text edition. (2142341)* **3261**
Protist (DEU) *Online - full text edition. (630020)* **3214**
Psychiatric Quarterly (USA) *Online - full text edition. (665932)* **4126**
Psychiatry and Clinical Neurosciences (AUS) *Online - full text edition. (663948)* **4126**
Psychiatry Research (IRL) *Online - full text edition. (938750)* **4127**
Psychiatry Research: Neuroimaging Section (IRL) *Online - full text edition. (2023334)* **4127**
Psychoanalytic Studies (GBR) *Online - full text edition. (3816060)* **4437**
Psychodynamic Counselling (GBR) *Online - full text edition. (2679426)* **4127**
Psychological Inquiry (USA) *Online - full text edition. (1842609)* **4438**
Psychological Medicine (GBR) *Online - full text edition. (1196073)* **4127**
Psychological Research (DEU) *Online - full text edition. (819042)* **4438**
Psychological Science (USA) *Online - full content edition. (4448669)* **4438**
Psychology, Evolution and Gender (GBR) *Online - full text edition. (3864413)* **4440**
Psychology, Health & Medicine (GBR) *Online - full text edition. (3826058)* **4440**
Psychoneuroendocrinology (GBR) *Online - full text edition. (112364)* **4128**
Psychopathology (CHE) *Online - full text edition. (234893)* **4128**
Psychopharmacology (DEU) *Online - full text edition. (80837)* **4332**
Psychophysiology (GBR) *Online - full text edition. (208280)* **4128**
Psychotherapeut (DEU) *Online - full text edition. (406791)* **4128**
Psychotherapy and Psychosomatics (CHE) *Online - full text edition. (108006)* **4129**
Psychotherapy Research (USA) *Online - full text edition. (1877372)* **4443**
Public Health (Basingstoke) (GBR) *Online - full text edition. (780715)* **3681**
Public Health Nursing (USA) *Online - full text edition. (1371215)* **3938**
Public Health Nutrition (GBR) *Online - full text edition. (3551482)* **4245**
Public Health Reports (USA) *Online - full text edition. (255939)* **4486**
Pulmonary Pharmacology & Therapeutics (GBR) *Online - full text edition. (1668242)* **4163**
Q J M (GBR) *Online - full text edition. (673463)* **3681**
Qualitative Health Research (USA) *Online - full text edition. (2127423)* **3681**
Quality in Health Care (GBR) *Online - full content edition. (2152533)* **3682**
Quality of Life Research (NLD) *Online - full text edition. (2149508)* **3682**
Quarterly Journal of Experimental Psychology. Section A: Human Experimental Psychology (GBR) *Online - full text edition. (1074733)* **4443**
Quarterly Journal of Experimental Psychology. Section B: Comparative and Physiological Psychology (GBR) *Online - full text edition. (1074741)* **4443**
Quarterly Reviews of Biophysics (GBR) *Online - full text edition. (791830)* **3267**
R N A (GBR) *Online - full text edition. (2724405)* **3261**
Radiation and Environmental Biophysics (DEU) *Online - full text edition. (502006)* **3267**
Radiography (GBR) *Online - full text edition. (2778858)* **4153**
Der Radiologe (DEU) *Online - full text edition. (297097)* **4153**
Radiotherapy and Oncology (IRL) *Online - full text edition. (1325582)* **4154**
Reactions Weekly (NZL) *Online - full text edition. (1747592)* **4346**
Reading and Writing (NLD) *Online - full text edition. (1764101)* **3551**
Reading Psychology (USA) *Online - full text edition. (1080431)* **3414**
Rechtsmedizin (DEU) *Online - full text edition. (2021102)* **3884**
Regulatory Peptides (NLD) *Online - full text edition. (1007483)* **3262**
Regulatory Toxicology and Pharmacology (USA) *Online - full text edition. (1082981)* **3453**
Renal Failure (USA) *Online - full text edition. (494593)* **4217**
Reproduction, Fertility and Development (AUS) *Online - full content edition. (1767399)* **3215**
Reproduction in Domestic Animals Online(DEU) *Online - full text. (754749)* **4551**
Reproduction, Nutrition, Development (FRA) *Online - full text edition. (551139)* **3215**
Reproductive Medicine Review (GBR) *Online - full text edition. (2143704)* **3962**
Reproductive Toxicology (USA) *Online - full text edition. (1640801)* **3348**
Reproduktionsmedizin (DEU) *Online - full text edition. (1509292)* **3962**
Research in Developmental Disabilities (GBR) *Online - full text edition. (1038958)* **4130**
Research in Veterinary Science (GBR) *Online - full text edition. (794325)* **4551**
Research on Aging (USA) *Online - full text edition. (907758)* **3480**
Research on Social Work Practice (USA) *Online - full text edition. (2077167)* **4523**
Respiration (CHE) *Online - full text edition. (465445)* **4164**
Respiration Physiology (NLD) *Online - full text edition. (499668)* **3348**
Respiratory Medicine (GBR) *Online - full text edition. (708135)* **4164**
Respirology (AUS) *Online - full text edition. (3080293)* **4164**
Resuscitation (IRL) *Online - full text edition. (536466)* **4165**
Reviews in Clinical and Experimental Hematology (GBR) *Online - full text edition. (3336727)* **3904**
Reviews in Clinical Gerontology (GBR) *Online - full text edition. (2028891)* **3480**
Reviews in Endocrine & Metabolic Disorders (USA) *Online - full text edition. (4006860)* **3868**
La Revue de Medecine Interne (FRA) *Online - full text edition. (115266)* **3911**
Rheumatology (GBR) *Online - full text edition. (1785508)* **4171**
Rheumatology International (DEU) *Online - full text edition. (969443)* **4171**
Royal Chemical Society. Journal. Perkin Transactions 1 (GBR) *Online - full text edition. (470244)* **3379**
Royal Society of London. Philosophical Transactions. Biological Sciences (GBR) *Online - full text edition. (337587)* **3217**
Royal Society of London. Proceedings. Biological Sciences (GBR) *Online - full text edition. (438456)* **3217**
Russian Academy of Sciences. Biology Bulletin (RUS) *Online - full text edition. (421901)* **3217**
Russian Journal of Bioorganic Chemistry (RUS) *Online - full text edition. (127175)* **3379**
Russian Journal of Developmental Biology (RUS) *Online - full text edition. (612014)* **3217**
Russian Journal of Genetics (RUS) *Online - full text edition. (273139)* **3314**
Russian Journal of Marine Biology (RUS) *Online - full text edition. (467960)* **3217**
S T I Online (GBR) *Online - full text edition of* Sexually Transmitted Infections. (415758) **3853**
Safety Science (NLD) *Online - full text edition. (481203)* **4265**
Sage Family Studies Abstracts (USA) *Online - full text edition. (907766)* **4524**
Sarcoma (GBR) *Online - full text edition. (3507874)* **3990**
Scandinavian Audiology (NOR) *Online - full text edition. (1089056)* **4038**
Scandinavian Cardiovascular Journal (NOR) *Online - full text edition. (2017636)* **4202**
Scandinavian Journal of Behaviour Therapy (NOR) *Online - full text edition. (916234)* **4447**
Scandinavian Journal of Caring Sciences (NOR) *Online - full text edition. (1590731)* **3690**
Scandinavian Journal of Clinical & Laboratory Investigation (NOR) *Online - full text edition. (1088920)* **3880**
Scandinavian Journal of Clinical and Laboratory Investigation. Supplement (NOR) *Online - full text edition. (1088939)* **3880**
Scandinavian Journal of Gastroenterology (NOR) *Online - full text edition. (1123947)* **3895**
Scandinavian Journal of Gastroenterology. Supplement (SWE) *Online - full text edition. (1123955)* **3895**
Scandinavian Journal of Immunology Online (GBR) *Online - full text edition of* Scandinavian Journal of Immunology. (463523) **3751**
Scandinavian Journal of Infectious Diseases (NOR) *Online - full text edition. (1119613)* **3806**
Scandinavian Journal of Medicine & Science in Sports Online(DNK) *Online - full text. (2029995)* **4176**
Scandinavian Journal of Occupational Therapy (NOR) *Online - full text edition. (2406586)* **3690**
Scandinavian Journal of Plastic and Reconstructive Surgery and Hand Surgery (NOR) *Online - full text edition. (2017644)* **4202**
Scandinavian Journal of Primary Health Care (NOR) *Online - full text edition. (1326546)* **3690**
Scandinavian Journal of Psychology (GBR) *Online - full text edition. (546135)* **4447**
Scandinavian Journal of Public Health (NOR) *Online - full text edition. (1151436)* **3690**
Scandinavian Journal of Rheumatology (NOR) *Online - full text edition. (1088149)* **4171**
Scandinavian Journal of Rheumatology. Supplement (NOR) *Online - full text edition. (745480)* **4172**

Scandinavian Journal of Urology and Nephrology (NOR) *Online - full text edition. (2016435)* **4218**
Scandinavian Journal of Urology and Nephrology. Supplement (SWE) *Online - full text edition. (700738)* **4218**
Schizophrenia Research (NLD) *Online - full text edition. (1652354)* **4132**
Der Schmerz (DEU) *Online - full text edition. (1644912)* **3690**
School Psychology International (GBR) *Online - full text edition. (1037439)* **3429**
Science as Culture (GBR) *Online - full text edition. (1144588)* **4507**
The Science of the Total Environment (NLD) *Online - full text edition. (736643)* **3442**
Seizure (GBR) *Online - full text edition. (2155729)* **4133**
Seminars in Cancer Biology (GBR) *Online - full text edition. (1928880)* **3349**
Seminars in Cell and Developmental Biology (GBR) *Online - full text edition. (1878123)* **3294**
Seminars in Dialysis (USA) *Online - full text edition. (1693425)* **4218**
Seminars in Immunology (GBR) *Online - full text edition. (1920227)* **3751**
Seminars in Neonatology (GBR) *Online - full text edition. (2960400)* **3964**
Seminars in the Neurosciences (USA) *Online - full text edition. (1920235)* **4133**
Sensory Neuron (NLD) *Online - full content edition. (2801035)* **4133**
Sepsis (USA) *Online - full text edition. (3211401)* **3807**
Sex Roles (USA) *Online - full text edition. (487805)* **4448**
Sexual Abuse (USA) *Online - full text edition. (1879871)* **4448**
Sexual and Relationship Therapy (GBR) *Online - full content edition. (1430807)* **4448**
Sexualities (GBR) *Online - full text edition. (3401960)* **4448**
Sexuality and Disability (USA) *Online - full text edition. (1749153)* **3692**
Sign Language Studies (USA) *Online - full text edition. (585238)* **3551**
Skeletal Radiology (DEU) *Online - full text edition. (547034)* **4155**
Skin Pharmacology and Applied Skin Physiology (CHE) *Online - full text edition. (1650106)* **4336**
Skin Research and Technology (DNK) *Online - full text edition. (2718197)* **3853**
Sleep Medicine (NLD) *Online - full text edition. (4049799)* **4134**
Sleep Medicine Reviews (GBR) *Online - full text edition. (3330613)* **4134**
Small Group Research (USA) *Online - full text edition. (158380)* **4449**
Small Ruminant Research (NLD) *Online - full text edition. (1652362)* **3161**
Social Psychiatry and Psychiatric Epidemiology (DEU) *Online - full text edition. (620211)* **4134**
Social Psychology of Education (NLD) *Online - full text edition. (2907453)* **3415**
Social Science & Medicine (GBR) *Online - full text edition. (374024)* **3694**
Society & Animals (GBR) *Online - full text edition. (2232340)* **3172**
Society for Gynecologic Investigation. Journal (USA) *Online - full text edition. (2423413)* **3964**
Sociology of Health and Illness (GBR) *Online - full text edition. (910791)* **4523**
Soil Biology & Biochemistry (GBR) *Online - full text edition. (439932)* **3263**
Solid State Nuclear Magnetic Resonance (GBR) *Online - full text edition. (2154005)* **3377**
Somatic Cell and Molecular Genetics (USA) *Online - full text edition. (6459)* **3314**
Spatial Cognition and Computation (NLD) *Online - full text edition. (3769453)* **4450**
Spatial Vision (NLD) *Online - full content edition. (1398008)* **3554**
Speech Communication (NLD) *Online - full text edition. (1119206)* **3552**
Spinal Cord (GBR) *Online - full text edition. (478016)* **4134**
Spine (Philadelphia, 1976) (USA) *Online - full text edition. (608319)* **4026**
Sports Medicine (NZL) *Online - full text edition. (1341839)* **4177**
Springer Seminars in Immunopathology (DEU) *Online - full text edition. (773654)* **3751**
Statistical Methods in Medical Research (GBR) *Online - full text edition. (2143577)* **4530**
Stereotactic and Functional Neurosurgery (CHE) *Online - full text edition. (276057)* **4204**
Steroids (USA) *Online - full text edition. (450561)* **3263**
Strabismus (NLD) *Online - full text edition. (2237377)* **4007**
Strahlentherapie und Onkologie (DEU) *Online - full text edition. (420484)* **4156**
Structural Equation Modeling (USA) *Online - full text edition. (2381672)* **4451**
Structure (GBR) *Online - full text edition. (2368307)* **3220**
Substance Abuse (USA) *Online - full text edition. (1889184)* **3406**
Support for Learning (GBR) *Online - full text edition. (642908)* **3427**
Supportive Care in Cancer (DEU) *Online - full text edition. (2263106)* **3990**
Surgery Today (JPN) *Online - full text edition. (312088)* **4204**
Surgical and Radiologic Anatomy (FRA) *Online - full text edition. (227897)* **3697**
Surgical Endoscopy (USA) *Online - full text edition. (1563971)* **4204**
Surgical Infections (USA) *Online - full content edition. (3598276)* **4204**
Surgical Neurology (USA) *Online - full text edition. (755508)* **4205**
Surgical Oncology (GBR) *Online - full text edition. (2152126)* **3991**
Survey of Ophthalmology (USA) *Online - full text edition. (688738)* **3737**
System Familie (DEU) *Online - full text edition. (1650289)* **4135**
Systematic Parasitology (NLD) *Online - full text edition. (932264)* **3220**
Teaching and Learning in Medicine (USA) *Online - full text edition. (1729810)* **3698**
Teaching of Psychology (USA) *Online - full text edition. (389005)* **4452**
Techniques in Coloproctology Online(ITA) *Online - full text. (3185087)* **3896**
Technology and Disability (NLD) *Online - full text edition. (2120151)* **3487**
Technology and Health Care (NLD) *Online - full text edition. (2343304)* **3698**
Telemedicine Journal and e-Health (USA) *Online - full text edition. (2785919)* **3812**
Theoretical and Applied Genetics (DEU) *Online - full text edition. (808296)* **3314**
Theoretical Issues in Ergonomics Science (GBR) *Online - full text edition. (4060830)* **3433**
Theoretical Medicine and Bioethics (NLD) *Online - full text edition. (1002597)* **3699**
Theoretical Population Biology (USA) *Online - full text edition. (512974)* **3221**
Theory & Psychology (GBR) *Online - full text edition. (2012162)* **4452**
Theory in Biosciences (DEU) *Online - full text edition. (91464)* **3221**
Therapeutic Apheresis Online(USA) *Online - full text. (3256626)* **4218**
Theriogenology (USA) *Online - full text edition. (458643)* **4553**
Thinking & Reasoning (GBR) *Online - full text edition. (2599414)* **4452**
Thorax Online (GBR) *Online - full text edition of* Thorax. (235792) **3700**
Thrombosis Research (GBR) *Online - full text edition. (1329987)* **3784**
Tissue & Cell (GBR) *Online - full text edition. (756202)* **3294**
Tissue Antigens (DNK) *Online - full text edition. (19488)* **3701**
Tissue Engineering (USA) *Online - full content edition. (2721244)* **3294**
Tobbacco Control Online (GBR) *Online - full text edition of* Tobacco Control. (2152843) **4531**
Topoi (NLD) *Online - full text edition. (1203754)* **4348**
Toxicological Sciences (USA) *Online - full text edition. (1061399)* **3455**
Toxicology (IRL) *Online - full text edition. (688010)* **3455**
Toxicology and Applied Pharmacology (USA) *Online - full text edition. (232114)* **3455**
Toxicology and Industrial Health (GBR) *Online - full text edition. (1539728)* **3455**
Toxicology in Vitro (GBR) *Online - full text edition. (1570617)* **3455**
Toxicology Letters (IRL) *Online - full text edition. (792209)* **3456**
Toxicology Methods (USA) *Online - full text edition. (2031078)* **3456**
Toxicon (GBR) *Online - full text edition. (372870)* **4338**
Traffic (DNK) *Online - full text edition. (3939820)* **3294**
Transcultural Psychiatry (GBR) *Online - full text edition. (624179)* **4136**
Transfusion and Apheresis Science (GBR) *Online - full text edition. (992062)* **3905**
Transfusion Medicine (GBR) *Online - full text edition. (2030926)* **3905**
Transgenic Research (NLD) *Online - full text edition. (2149583)* **3314**
Transplant Immunology (GBR) *Online - full text edition. (2275112)* **3751**
Transplant Infectious Disease Online(DNK) *Online - full text. (3828638)* **4206**
Transplant International (DEU) *Online - full text edition. (1650297)* **3702**
Transplantation Proceedings (USA) *Online - full text edition. (1730150)* **4206**
Trauma(GBR) *Online - full text. (3823431)* **4027**
Trauma Quarterly (NLD) *Online - full content edition. (1883372)* **4207**
Trauma und Berufskrankheit (DEU) *Online - full text edition. (3506517)* **4027**
Trauma, Violence & Abuse (USA) *Online - full text edition. (4052757)* **4491**
Trends in Biochemical Sciences (GBR) *Online - full text edition. (1176625)* **3263**
Trends in Biotechnology (GBR) *Online - full text edition. (1315668)* **3277**
Trends in Cardiovascular Medicine (USA) *Online - full text edition. (2021455)* **3784**
Trends in Cell Biology (GBR) *Online - full text edition. (2129221)* **3295**
Trends in Cognitive Sciences (GBR) *Online - full text edition. (3256685)* **4453**
Trends in Ecology and Evolution (GBR) *Online - full text edition. (1542842)* **3221**
Trends in Endocrinology and Metabolism (GBR) *Online - full text edition. (1858750)* **3869**
Trends in Genetics (GBR) *Online - full text edition. (1507443)* **3314**
Trends in Immunology Online (GBR) *Online - full text edition of* Trends in Immunology. (1088874) **3752**
Trends in Microbiology (GBR) *Online - full text edition. (2273489)* **3332**
Trends in Molecular Medicine (GBR) *Online - full text edition. (2801507)* **3702**
Trends in Neurosciences (GBR) *Online - full text edition. (920045)* **4137**
Trends in Parasitology (GBR) *Online - full text edition. (1500724)* **3332**
Trends in Pharmacological Sciences (GBR) *Online - full text edition. (1088823)* **4338**
Tropical Animal Health and Production (NLD) *Online - full text edition. (453080)* **4554**
Tropical Medicine & International Health Online (GBR) *Online - full text edition of* Tropical Medicine & International Health. (406058) **4491**
Tuberculosis (GBR) *Online - full text edition. (2137054)* **4166**
Tumor Biology (CHE) *Online - full text edition. (959464)* **3991**
Twin Research (GBR) *Online - full text edition. (3619702)* **3315**
Ultramicroscopy (NLD) *Online - full text edition. (746193)* **3336**
Ultrasound in Medicine & Biology (USA) *Online - full text edition. (183903)* **3222**
Ultrasound in Obstetrics & Gynecology (GBR) *Online - full text edition. (2042436)* **3965**
Ultrastructural Pathology (USA) *Online - full text edition. (995398)* **3991**
Der Unfallchirurg (DEU) *Online - full text edition. (630144)* **4027**
Der Urologe. Section A (DEU) *Online - full text edition. (592765)* **4219**
Der Urologe. Section B (DEU) *Online - full text edition. (783404)* **4219**
Urologia Internationalis (CHE) *Online - full text edition. (105104)* **4219**
Urologic Oncology (USA) *Online - full text edition. (2934930)* **3992**
Urological Research (DEU) *Online - full text edition. (642959)* **4219**
Urology (USA) *Online - full text edition. (705519)* **4220**
Vaccine Online (GBR) *Online - full text edition of* Vaccine. (1289233) **3752**
Value in Health (USA) *Online - full text edition. (3827852)* **4339**
Vascular Medicine (GBR) *Online - full text edition. (1877615)* **3784**
Verhaltenstherapie (CHE) *Online - full content edition. (2011727)* **4137**
Veterinary Anaesthesia and Analgesia Online (GBR) *Online - full text edition of* Veterinary Anaesthesia and Analgesia. (4046684) **4556**
Veterinary Dermatology Online(GBR) *Online - full text. (1891820)* **4557**
Veterinary Immunology and Immunopathology (NLD) *Online - full text edition. (920088)* **4557**
The Veterinary Journal (GBR) *Online - full text edition. (722685)* **4557**
Veterinary Microbiology (NLD) *Online - full text edition. (316369)* **3332**
Veterinary Ophthalmology Online (GBR) *Online - full text edition of* Veterinary Ophthalmology. (2215918) **4558**
Veterinary Parasitology (NLD) *Online - full text edition. (407933)* **4558**
Veterinary Research Communications (NLD) *Online - full text edition. (294276)* **4559**
Veterinary Research (Online Edition) (FRA) *Online - full text edition of* Veterinary Research. (253928) **4559**
Violence Against Women (USA) *Online - full text edition. (2727641)* **4524**
Violence & Abuse Abstracts (USA) *Online - full text edition. (2718545)* **4524**
Virchows Archiv (DEU) *Online - full text edition. (2798)* **3223**
Virology (USA) *Online - full text edition. (239364)* **3332**
Virus Genes (USA) *Online - full text edition. (1624741)* **3332**
Virus Research (NLD) *Online - full text edition. (1339605)* **3333**
Vision Research (GBR) *Online - full text edition. (152196)* **4008**
Visual Cognition (GBR) *Online - full text edition. (2363704)* **4454**
Visual Impairment Research (NLD) *Online - full text edition. (3812995)* **3500**
Visual Neuroscience (GBR) *Online - full text edition. (1668722)* **4137**
Vox Sanguinis (CHE) *Online - full text edition. (516252)* **3752**
Western Journal of Nursing Research (USA) *Online - full text edition. (1489690)* **3943**
Wilderness and Environmental Medicine (USA) *Online - full text edition. (1892762)* **3708**
Women's Health Issues (USA) *Online - full text edition. (2018187)* **4567**
Work and Stress (GBR) *Online - full text edition. (1604376)* **4455**
World Journal of Microbiology and Biotechnology (GBR) *Online - full text edition. (1346431)* **3278**
World Journal of Surgery (USA) *Online - full text edition. (545813)* **4207**
World Journal of Urology (DEU) *Online - full text edition. (1200879)* **4220**
Wound Repair and Regeneration (USA) *Online - full text edition. (2318431)* **4028**
Xenobiotica (GBR) *Online - full text edition. (107689)* **3264**
Xenotransplantation (DNK) *Online - full text edition. (2415399)* **4207**
Zeitschrift fuer Gerontologie und Geriatrie (DEU) *Online - full text edition. (295744)* **3482**
Zeitschrift fuer Herz, Thorax- und Gefaesschirurgie (DEU) *Online - full text edition. (1590707)* **3785**
Zeitschrift fuer Kardiologie (DEU) *Online - full text edition. (167436)* **3785**
Zeitschrift fuer Rheumatologie (DEU) *Online - full text edition. (1123920)* **4172**
Zoomorphology (DEU) *Online - full text edition. (411493)* **3225**
Zygote (GBR) *Online - full text edition. (2274124)* **3315**

Telesystemes-Questel 83-85 blvd. Vincent-Auriol, Paris 75013, France TEL 33-144236464, FAX 33-144236465
Bibliography of Bioethics (USA) *Online - full text edition. (BIOETHICS)* **3717**
Merck Index: An Encyclopedia of Chemicals and Drugs (USA) *Online - full text edition.* **4345**
N I O S H T I C(USA) *Online - full text.* **4259**

WanFang Data Corp. Rm 432, 15 Fu Xing lu, Beijing 100038, China TEL 86-1-68515544 ext 2432, 86-1-68515544 ext 2430, 86-1-68511818, FAX 86-1-68514021, chinainfo@chinainfo.gov.cn, http://www.chinainfo.gov.cn/periodical
Acta Pharmacologica Sinica (CHN) *Online - full content edition.* **4273**
Aizheng (CHN) *Online - full content edition.* **3966**
Anhui Yike Daxue Xuebao (CHN) *Online - full content edition.* **3565**
Anquan (CHN) *Online - full content edition.* **4462**
Baiqiuen Yike Daxue Xuebao (CHN) *Online - full content edition.* **3574**

Baixuebing (CHN) *Online - full content edition.* **3898**
Bangbu Yixueyuan Xuebao (CHN) *Online - full content edition.* **3574**
Beijing Daxue Xuebao (Yixue Ban) (CHN) *Online - full text edition.* **3574**
Beijing Shengwu Yixue Gongcheng (CHN) *Online - full content edition.* **3574**
Beijing Yixue (CHN) *Online - full content edition.* **3574**
Bingdu Xuebao (CHN) *Online - full content edition.* **3575**
Biomedical and Environmental Sciences (CHN) *Online - full content edition.* **3575**
Chinese Academic Journal. Medicine & Hygiene (CHN) *Online - full text edition.* **3584**
Chinese Academic Journal. Medicine & Hygiene (CHN) *Online - full content edition.* **3584**
Chinese Journal of Cancer Research (CHN) *Online - full content edition.* **3974**
Chinese Journal of Integrated Traditional and Western Medicine (CHN) *Online - full content edition.* **3584**
Chinese Medical Journal (CHN) *Online - full content edition.* **3584**
Chinese Medical Sciences Journal (CHN) *Online - full content edition.* **3584**
Dizhen Kanan Anquan (CHN) *Online - full content edition.* **3408**
Dongwu Fenlei Xuebao (CHN) *Online - full content edition.* **3351**
Dongwu Xuebao (CHN) *Online - full content edition.* **3352**
Hangtian Yixue yu Yixue Gongcheng (CHN) *Online - full content edition.* **3153**
Hebei Zhongyiyao Xuebao (CHN) *Online - full content edition.* **3613**
Jiangsu Yiyao (CHN) *Online - full content edition.* **3628**
Jiankang Shijie (CHN) *Online - full content edition.* **4357**
Jiankang Zhinan (Zhong Lao Nan) (CHN) *Online - full content edition.* **4357**
Jiefangjun Yixue Zazhi (CHN) *Online - full content edition.* **3628**
Jinan Daxue Xuebao (Ziran Kexue yu Yixue Ban) (CHN) *Online - full content edition.* **4505**
Jizhen Yixue (CHN) *Online - full content edition.* **4017**
Junshi Yixue Kexueyuan Yuankan (CHN) *Online - full content edition.* **3639**
Linye Laodong Anquan (CHN) *Online - full content edition.* **3463**
Meiguo Yixuehui Zazhi (Zhongwen Ban) (CHN) *Online - full content edition.* **3660**
Shandong Yiyao (CHN) *Online - full content edition.* **3692**
World Journal of Gastroenterology (CHN) *Online - full content edition.* **3897**
Xian Medical University. Journal (CHN) *Online - full content edition.* **3709**
Xiaoer Jijiu Yixue (CHN) *Online - full content edition.* **4057**
Xibao yu Fenzi Mianyixue Zazhi (CHN) *Online - full content edition.* **3752**
Xibei Linxueyuan Xuebao (CHN) *Online - full content edition.* **3464**
Yaowu Fenxi Zazhi (CHN) *Online - full content edition.* **4341**
Yaoxue Xuebao (CHN) *Online - full content edition.* **4341**
Yingguo Yixue Zazhi (Zhongwen Ban) (CHN) *Online - full content edition.* **3710**
Yingyang Xuebao (CHN) *Online - full content edition.* **4248**
Yixue yu Zhexue (CHN) *Online - full content edition.* **4349**
Yiyong Shengwu Lixue (CHN) *Online - full content edition.* **3710**
Youjiang Minzu Yixueyuan Xuebao (CHN) *Online - full content edition.* **3710**
Yunnan Zhongyi Xueyuan Xuebao (CHN) *Online - full content edition.* **3711**
Yunyang Yixueyuan Xuebao (CHN) *Online - full content edition.* **3711**
Zhejiang Linchuang Yixue (CHN) *Online - full content edition.* **3711**
Zhejiang Yufang Yixue (CHN) *Online - full content edition.* **3712**
Zhejiang Zhongxiyi Jiehe Zazhi (CHN) *Online - full content edition.* **3712**
Zhiwu Baohu Xuebao (CHN) *Online - full content edition.* **3283**
Zhongcaoyao (CHN) *Online - full content edition.* **3712**
Zhongfeng yu Shenjing Jibing Zazhi (CHN) *Online - full content edition.* **4138**
Zhonggou Dongmai Yinghua Zazhi (CHN) *Online - full content edition.* **3712**
Zhongguo Bingduxue (CHN) *Online - full content edition.* **3333**
Zhongguo Bingli Shengli Zazhi (CHN) *Online - full content edition.* **3712**
Zhongguo Chuji Weisheng Baojian (CHN) *Online - full content edition.* **3712**
Zhongguo Dangdai Erke Zazhi (CHN) *Online - full content edition.* **4057**
Zhongguo Fanglao Tongxun (CHN) *Online - full content edition.* **4166**
Zhongguo Feiyan Zazhi (CHN) *Online - full content edition.* **4166**
Zhongguo Gongye Yixue Zazhi (CHN) *Online - full content edition.* **4268**
Zhongguo Gushang (CHN) *Online - full content edition.* **4028**
Zhongguo Guzhi Shusong Zazhi (CHN) *Online - full content edition.* **3482**
Zhongguo Jiguang Yixue Zazhi (CHN) *Online - full content edition.* **3712**
Zhongguo Jijiu Yixue (CHN) *Online - full content edition.* **3712**
Zhongguo Jishengchongbing Fangzhi Zazhi (CHN) *Online - full content edition.* **3808**
Zhongguo Jizhu Jisui Zazhi (CHN) *Online - full content edition.* **4028**
Zhongguo Kangfu Lilun Yu Shijian (CHN) *Online - full content edition.* **4067**
Zhongguo Kangfu Yixue Zazhi (CHN) *Online - full content edition.* **3712**
Zhongguo Linchuang Yaolixue Zazhi (CHN) *Online - full content edition.* **4341**
Zhongguo Mianyixue Zazhi (CHN) *Online - full content edition.* **3752**
Zhongguo Minjian Liaofa (CHN) *Online - full content edition.* **3171**
Zhongguo Renshou Gonghuanbing Zazhi (CHN) *Online - full content edition.* **3333**
Zhongguo Shenghua Yaowu Zazhi (CHN) *Online - full content edition.* **4342**
Zhongguo Shengwu Huaxue yu Fenzi Shengwu Xuebao (CHN) *Online - full content edition.* **3264**
Zhongguo Shenjing Mianyixue he Shenjingbingxue Zazhi (CHN) *Online - full content edition.* **4138**
Zhongguo Weisheng Tongji (CHN) *Online - full content edition.* **4364**
Zhongguo Xiandai Yingyong Yaoxue (CHN) *Online - full content edition.* **4342**
Zhongguo Xinli Weisheng Zazhi (CHN) *Online - full text edition.* **4456**
Zhongguo Xinyao Zazhi (CHN) *Online - full content edition.* **4342**
Zhongguo Yaoke Daxue Xuebao (CHN) *Online - full content edition.* **4342**
Zhongguo Yaolixue yu Dulixue Zazhi (CHN) *Online - full content edition.* **3456**
Zhongguo Yaoshi (Beijing) (CHN) *Online - full content edition.* **4342**
Zhongguo Yaoshi (Wuyi) (CHN) *Online - full content edition.* **4342**
Zhongguo Yaowu Yilaixing Zazhi (CHN) *Online - full content edition.* **3406**
Zhongguo Yaowuhuaxue Zazhi (CHN) *Online - full content edition.* **4342**
Zhongguo Yikan (CHN) *Online - full content edition.* **3713**
Zhongguo Yixue Kexueyuan Xuebao (CHN) *Online - full content edition.* **3713**
Zhongguo Yixue Yingxiang Jishu (CHN) *Online - full content edition.* **4157**
Zhongguo Yiyuan Yaoxue Zazhi (CHN) *Online - full content edition.* **4343**
Zhongguo Yundong Yixue Zazhi (CHN) *Online - full content edition.* **4178**
Zhongguo Zhongxiyi Jiehe Zazhi (CHN) *Online - full content edition.* **3713**
Zhongguo Zhongyao Zazhi (CHN) *Online - full content edition.* **4343**
Zhongguo Zhongyi Jichu Yixue Zazhi (CHN) *Online - full content edition.* **3713**
Zhonghua Binglixue Zazhi (CHN) *Online - full content edition.* **3713**
Zhonghua Chuangshang Zazhi (CHN) *Online - full content edition.* **4028**
Zhonghua Chuanranbing Zazhi (CHN) *Online - full content edition.* **3713**
Zhonghua Er-Bi-Yanhouke Zazhi (CHN) *Online - full content edition.* **4039**
Zhonghua Erke Zazhi (CHN) *Online - full content edition.* **4057**
Zhonghua Fangshe Yixue yu Fanghu Zazhi (CHN) *Online - full content edition.* **4157**
Zhonghua Fangshexua Zazhi (CHN) *Online - full content edition.* **4157**
Zhonghua Fengshibingxue Zazhi (CHN) *Online - full content edition.* **4172**
Zhonghua Fuchanke Zazhi (CHN) *Online - full content edition.* **3966**
Zhonghua Guke Zazhi (CHN) *Online - full content edition.* **4029**
Zhonghua Huli Zazhi (CHN) *Online - full content edition.* **3943**
Zhonghua Jiehe he Huxi Zazhi (CHN) *Online - full content edition.* **4166**
Zhonghua Jingshenke Zazhi (CHN) *Online - full content edition.* **4138**
Zhonghua Laonian Yixue Zazhi (CHN) *Online - full content edition.* **3482**
Zhonghua Liliao Zazhi (CHN) *Online - full content edition.* **4067**
Zhonghua Liuxingbingxue Zazhi (CHN) *Online - full content edition.* **3713**
Zhonghua Neifenmi Daixie Zazhi (CHN) *Online - full content edition.* **3870**
Zhonghua Qigong (CHN) *Online - full content edition.* **4364**
Zhonghua Qiguan Yizhi Zazhi (CHN) *Online - full content edition.* **4208**
Zhonghua Shenjingke Zazhi (CHN) *Online - full content edition.* **4139**
Zhonghua Shiyan he Linchuang Bingduxue Zazhi (CHN) *Online - full text edition.* **3808**
Zhonghua Waike Zazhi (CHN) *Online - full content edition.* **4208**
Zhonghua Weishengwuxue he Mianyixue Zazhi (CHN) *Online - full content edition.* **3753**
Zhonghua Xiaohua Zazhi (CHN) *Online - full content edition.* **3897**
Zhonghua Xin-Xueguanbing Zazhi (CHN) *Online - full content edition.* **3785**
Zhonghua Xueyexue Zazhi (CHN) *Online - full content edition.* **3906**
Zhonghua Yanke Zazhi (CHN) *Online - full content edition.* **4008**
Zhonghua Yixue Jianyan Zazhi (CHN) *Online - full content edition.* **3881**
Zhonghua Yixue Zazhi (CHN) *Online - full content edition.* **3714**
Zhonghua Yiyuan Guanli Zazhi (CHN) *Online - full content edition.* **3524**
Zhonghua Zhengxing Shaoshang Waike Zazhi (CHN) *Online - full content edition.* **4208**
Zhonghua Zhongliu Zazhi (CHN) *Online - full content edition.* **3992**
Zhongliu Fangzhi Yanjiu (CHN) *Online - full content edition.* **3992**
Zhongyao Xinyao yu Lingchuang Yaoli (CHN) *Online - full content edition.* **4343**

West Group (Subsidiary of: Thomson Corporation, The) 620 Opperman Dr., Eagan, MN 55123 TEL 651-687-7000, 800-328-4880, http://www.westgroup.com
American Journal of Law & Medicine (USA) *Online - full text edition.* **3536**
Forensic Services Directory (USA) *Online - full text edition.* **3539**
Issues in Law and Medicine (USA) *Online - full text edition.* **3626**
The Journal of Law, Medicine & Ethics (USA) *Online - full text edition.* **3540**
Mealey's Litigation Report: Breast Implants (USA) *Online - full text edition.* **3545**
Mealey's Litigation Report: Drugs and Medical Devices (USA) *Online - full text edition.* **3546**
Mealey's Litigation Report: Fen-Phen - Redux (USA) *Online - full text edition.* **4315**
Risk: Health, Safety & Environment (USA) *Online - full text edition.* **4488**

Wiley InterScience (Subsidiary of: John Wiley & Sons, Inc., Journals) 605 Third Ave., New York, NY 10158 TEL 212-850-6000, FAX 212-850-6088, http://www.interscience.wiley.com/
Acta Biotechnologica (DEU) *Online - full text edition.* **3268**
Acta Hydrochimica et Hydrobiologica (DEU) *Online - full text edition.* **4561**
Aggressive Behavior (USA) *Online - full text edition.* **4373**
American Journal of Hematology (USA) *Online - full text edition.* **3897**
American Journal of Human Biology (USA) *Online - full text edition.* **3180**
American Journal of Industrial Medicine (USA) *Online - full text edition.* **4249**
American Journal of Medical Genetics (USA) *Online - full text edition.* **3298**
American Journal of Primatology (USA) *Online - full text edition.* **3350**
The Anatomical Record (USA) *Online - full text edition.* **3181**
Annals of Neurology (USA) *Online - full text edition.* **4073**
Applied Cognitive Psychology (GBR) *Online - full text edition.* **4377**
Archiv der Pharmazie (DEU) *Online - full text edition.* **4277**
Arthritis and Rheumatism (USA) *Online - full text edition.* **4167**
Behavioral Interventions (GBR) *Online - full text edition.* **4076**
Behavioral Sciences and the Law (GBR) *Online - full text edition.* **4381**
Bioelectromagnetics (USA) *Online - full text edition.* **3264**
BioEssays (GBR) *Online - full text edition.* **3184**
Biologie in Unserer Zeit (DEU) *Online - full text edition.* **3186**
Biomedical Chromatography (GBR) *Online - full text edition.* **3872**
Biometrical Journal (DEU) *Online - full text edition.* **3187**
Biopharmaceutics & Drug Disposition (GBR) *Online - full text edition.* **4280**
Biospectroscopy (USA) *Online - full text edition.* **3376**
Biotechnology and Bioengineering (USA) *Online - full text edition.* **3271**
C I T Plus (DEU) *Online - full text edition.* **3433**
Cancer (USA) *Online - full text edition.* **3969**
Catheterization and Cardiovascular Interventions (USA) *Online - full text edition.* **3767**
Cell Biochemistry and Function (GBR) *Online - full text edition.* **3246**
Cell Motility and the Cytoskeleton (USA) *Online - full text edition.* **3287**
Chemie-Ingenieur-Technik (DEU) *Online - full text edition.* **3433**
Child Abuse Review (GBR) *Online - full text edition.* **4511**
Children & Society (GBR) *Online - full text edition.* **3382**
Chirality (USA) *Online - full text edition.* **3246**
Clinical Anatomy (USA) *Online - full text edition.* **3585**
Clinical Psychology & Psychotherapy (GBR) *Online - full text edition.* **4388**
Computer Aided Surgery (USA) *Online - full text edition.* **4185**
Concepts in Magnetic Resonance (USA) *Online - full text edition.* **4142**
Cytometry (USA) *Online - full text edition.* **3289**
Depression and Anxiety (USA) *Online - full text edition.* **4394**
Developmental Dynamics (USA) *Online - full text edition.* **3193**
Developmental Psychobiology (USA) *Online - full text edition.* **3193**
Diabetes - Metabolism Research and Reviews (GBR) *Online - full text edition.* **3858**
Diagnostic Cytopathology (USA) *Online - full text edition.* **3289**
Drug Development Research (USA) *Online - full text edition.* **4288**
Dyslexia (GBR) *Online - full text edition.* **3421**
Environmental and Molecular Mutagenesis (USA) *Online - full text edition.* **3302**
Environmental Toxicology (USA) *Online - full text edition.* **3449**
European Eating Disorders Review (GBR) *Online - full text edition.* **4397**
European Journal of Immunology (DEU) *Online - full text edition.* **3744**
European Journal of Personality (GBR) *Online - full text edition.* **4398**
European Journal of Social Psychology (GBR) *Online - full text edition.* **4398**
Gene Function and Disease (DEU) *Online - full text edition.* **3606**
Genes, Chromosomes & Cancer (USA) *Online - full text edition.* **3303**
Genesis: The Journal of Genetics and Development (USA) *Online - full text edition.* **3304**
Genetic Epidemiology (USA) *Online - full text edition.* **3304**
Glia (USA) *Online - full text edition.* **4092**
Head & Neck (USA) *Online - full text edition.* **4190**
Health Economics (GBR) *Online - full text edition.* **3611**
Hematological Oncology (GBR) *Online - full text edition.* **3902**
The Hippocampus (USA) *Online - full text edition.* **3614**
Human Brain Mapping (USA) *Online - full text edition.* **4094**
Human Factors and Ergonomics in Manufacturing (USA) *Online - full text edition.* **3435**
Human Mutation (USA) *Online - full text edition.* **3308**

Human Psychopharmacology: Clinical and Experimental (GBR) *Online - full text edition.* **4094**
Infant and Child Development (GBR) *Online - full text edition.* **4404**
Infant Mental Health Journal (USA) *Online - full text edition.* **4045**
Infectious Diseases in Obstetrics and Gynecology (USA) *Online - full text edition.* **3953**
International Journal of Cancer (USA) *Online - full text edition.* **3980**
International Journal of Eating Disorders (USA) *Online - full text edition.* **4236**
International Journal of Geriatric Psychiatry (GBR) *Online - full text edition.* **3474**
International Journal of Health Planning and Management (GBR) *Online - full text edition.* **4514**
International Review of Hydrobiology (DEU) *Online - full text edition.* **3201**
Journal of Applied Toxicology (GBR) *Online - full text edition.* **3451**
Journal of Basic Microbiology (DEU) *Online - full text edition.* **3325**
Journal of Biomedical Materials Research (USA) *Online - full text edition.* **3275**
Journal of Cellular Biochemistry (USA) *Online - full text edition.* **3254**
Journal of Clinical Apheresis (USA) *Online - full text edition.* **3903**
Journal of Clinical Laboratory Analysis (USA) *Online - full text edition.* **3876**
Journal of Clinical Psychology (USA) *Online - full text edition.* **4412**
Journal of Clinical Ultrasound (USA) *Online - full text edition.* **4147**
Journal of Community and Applied Social Psychology (GBR) *Online - full text edition.* **4413**
Journal of Community Psychology (USA) *Online - full text edition.* **4413**
The Journal of Comparative Neurology (USA) *Online - full text edition.* **4100**
Journal of Environmental Medicine (GBR) *Online - full text edition.* **3632**
Journal of Experimental Zoology (USA) *Online - full text edition.* **3354**
Journal of Gene Medicine (USA) *Online - full text edition.* **3309**
Journal of Magnetic Resonance Imaging (USA) *Online - full text edition.* **4148**
Journal of Medical Virology (USA) *Online - full text edition.* **3635**
Journal of Microscopy Research and Technique (USA) *Online - full text edition.* **3334**
Journal of Molecular Recognition (GBR) *Online - full text edition.* **3378**
Journal of Morphology (USA) *Online - full text edition.* **3204**
Journal of Neurobiology (USA) *Online - full text edition.* **3345**
Journal of Neuroscience Research (USA) *Online - full text edition.* **4104**
Journal of Organizational Behaviour (GBR) *Online - full text edition.* **4419**
Journal of Pathology (GBR) *Online - full text edition.* **3637**
Journal of Peptide Science (GBR) *Online - full text edition.* **3378**
Journal of Pharmaceutical Sciences (USA) *Online - full text edition.* **4309**
Journal of Plant Nutrition and Soil Science (DEU) *Online - full text edition.* **3232**
Journal of Surgical Oncology (USA) *Online - full text edition.* **4195**
Journal of the History of the Behavioral Sciences (USA) *Online - full text edition.* **4424**
The Journal of Trace Elements in Experimental Medicine (USA) *Online - full text edition.* **3877**
Lasers in Surgery and Medicine (USA) *Online - full text edition.* **4196**
Lebensmittelchemie (DEU) *Online - full text edition.* **3462**
Luminescence (GBR) *Online - full text edition.* **3380**
Magnetic Resonance in Medicine (GBR) *Online - full text edition.* **4150**
Medical and Pediatric Oncology (USA) *Online - full text edition.* **3984**
Medicinal Research Reviews (USA) *Online - full text edition.* **4315**
Mental Retardation and Developmental Disabilities (New York, 1995) (USA) *Online - full text edition.* **4109**
Microsurgery (USA) *Online - full text edition.* **4197**
Molecular Carcinogenesis (USA) *Online - full text edition.* **3984**
Molecular Reproduction and Development (USA) *Online - full text edition.* **3258**
Movement Disorders (USA) *Online - full text edition.* **4111**
Muscle & Nerve (USA) *Online - full text edition.* **3663**
N M R in Biomedicine (GBR) *Online - full text edition.* **4151**
Nahrung (DEU) *Online - full text edition.* **4239**
Natural Toxins (USA) *Online - full text edition.* **3453**
Neuroscience Research Communications (GBR) *Online - full text edition.* **4118**
Neurourology and Urodynamics (USA) *Online - full text edition.* **4216**
Pediatric Pulmonology (USA) *Online - full text edition.* **4053**
Pharmacoepidemiology and Drug Safety (GBR) *Online - full text edition.* **4326**
Pharmazie in Unserer Zeit (DEU) *Online - full text edition.* **4330**
Phytochemical Analysis (GBR) *Online - full text edition.* **3282**
Phytotherapy Research (GBR) *Online - full text edition.* **3282**
Practical Diabetes International (GBR) *Online - full text edition.* **3867**
Prenatal Diagnosis (GBR) *Online - full text edition.* **3962**
The Prostate (USA) *Online - full text edition.* **3680**
Proteins: Structure, Function, and Genetics (USA) *Online - full text edition.* **3261**
Proteomics (DEU) *Online - full text edition.* **3261**
Psycho-Oncology (GBR) *Online - full text edition.* **3989**
Psychology & Marketing (USA) *Online - full text edition.* **4440**
Psychology in the Schools (USA) *Online - full text edition.* **4441**
Quality Assurance Journal (GBR) *Online - full text edition.* **3682**
Quantitative Structure Activity Relationships (DEU) *Online - full text edition.* **4332**
Research in Nursing & Health (USA) *Online - full text edition.* **3939**
Reviews in Medical Virology (GBR) *Online - full text edition.* **3331**
Seminars in Surgical Oncology (USA) *Online - full text edition.* **3990**
Statistics in Medicine (GBR) *Online - full text edition.* **3737**
Stress and Health (GBR) *Online - full text edition.* **4135**
Synapse (New York) (USA) *Online - full text edition.* **4135**
Teratogenesis, Carcinogenesis, and Mutagenesis (USA) *Online - full text edition.* **3699**
Teratology (USA) *Online - full text edition.* **3220**
Yeast (GBR) *Online - full text edition.* **3283**

H. W. Wilson 950 University Ave., Bronx, NY 10452-4224 TEL 718-588-8400, 800-367-6770, FAX 718-681-1511, 800-590-1617, intlsales@hwwilson.com, http://www.hwwilson.com
A I H A J (USA) *Online - full text edition.* **4249**
Adolescence (San Diego) (USA) *Online - full text edition.* **3380**
Alcohol Research & Health (USA) *Online - full text edition.* **3398**
American Academy of Child and Adolescent Psychiatry. Journal (USA) *Online - full text edition.* **4071**
American Annals of the Deaf (USA) *Online - full text edition.* **3488**
American Family Physician (USA) *Online - full text edition.* **3563**
American Geriatrics Society. Journal (USA) *Online - full text edition.* **3467**
American Journal of Art Therapy (USA) *Online - full text edition.* **4058**
American Journal of Epidemiology (USA) *Online - full text edition.* **3563**
American Journal of Law & Medicine (USA) *Online - full text edition.* **3536**
American Journal of Psychotherapy (USA) *Online - full text edition.* **4072**
American Journal of Public Health (USA) *Online - full text edition.* **4461**
American Journal on Mental Retardation (USA) *Online - full text edition.* **4072**
Annals of Dyslexia (USA) *Online - full text edition.* **3419**
Annals of Health Law (USA) *Online - full text edition.* **3536**
Annual Review of Biochemistry (USA) *Online - full text edition.* **3240**
Annual Review of Cell and Developmental Biology (USA) *Online - full text edition.* **3285**
Annual Review of Genetics (USA) *Online - full text edition.* **3298**
Annual Review of Immunology (USA) *Online - full text edition.* **3740**
Annual Review of Microbiology (USA) *Online - full text edition.* **3317**
Annual Review of Nutrition (USA) *Online - full text edition.* **4229**
Annual Review of Physiology (USA) *Online - full text edition.* **3339**
Annual Review of Psychology (USA) *Online - full text edition.* **4376**
Annual Review of Sex Research (USA) *Online - full text edition.* **4376**
Archives of Environmental Health (USA) *Online - full text edition.* **3435**
BioScience (USA) *Online - full text edition.* **3187**
The British Journal of Nutrition (GBR) *Online - full text edition.* **4230**
British Journal of Psychology (GBR) *Online - full text edition.* **4384**
Business and Health (USA) *Online - full text edition.* **3531**
The Career Development Quarterly (USA) *Online - full text edition.* **4269**
Child Study Journal (USA) *Online - full text edition.* **3409**
Club Industry (USA) *Online - full text edition.* **4351**
Counseling and Values (USA) *Online - full text edition.* **4502**
Counselor Education and Supervision (USA) *Online - full text edition.* **3410**
Creative Child and Adult Quarterly (USA) *Online - full text edition.* **4270**
Current Health 1 (USA) *Online - full text edition.* **3428**
Current Health 2 (USA) *Online - full text edition.* **3428**
D V M (USA) *Online - full text edition.* **4541**
Drug Discovery & Development (USA) *Online - full text edition.* **4288**
E H P Supplements (USA) *Online - full text edition.* **3436**
Education and Training in Mental Retardation and Developmental Disabilities (USA) *Online - full text edition.* **3421**
Educational and Psychological Measurement (USA) *Online - full text edition.* **4396**
Emerging Infectious Diseases (Online Edition)(USA) *Online - full text.* **4467**
Environmental Health Perspectives (USA) *Online - full text edition.* **3438**
Evolution (USA) *Online - full text edition.* **3302**
Exceptional Children (USA) *Online - full text edition.* **3422**
Exceptional Parent (USA) *Online - full text edition.* **3422**
F D A Consumer (USA) *Online - full text edition.* **3392**
Focus on Exceptional Children (USA) *Online - full text edition.* **3422**
Generations (San Francisco) (USA) *Online - full text edition.* **3471**
Geriatrics (USA) *Online - full text edition.* **3472**
Global Cosmetic Industry (USA) *Online - full text edition.* **3176**
Growth, Development & Aging (USA) *Online - full text edition.* **3198**
Hastings Center Report (USA) *Online - full text edition.* **3610**
Health Care Financing Review (USA) *Online - full text edition.* **3610**
Health Forum (USA) *Online - full text edition.* **3509**
Health Management Technology (USA) *Online - full text edition.* **3810**
Health Matrix: Journal of Law-Medicine (USA) *Online - full text edition.* **3540**
Healthcare Financial Management (USA) *Online - full text edition.* **3510**
HealthInform (USA) *Online - full text edition.* **3166**
Human Biology (Detroit) (USA) *Online - full text edition.* **3199**
Human Factors (USA) *Online - full text edition.* **3432**
International Journal of Disability, Development and Education (GBR) *Online - full text edition.* **3423**
International Journal of Mental Health (USA) *Online - full text edition.* **4406**
International Journal of Social Psychiatry (GBR) *Online - full text edition.* **4096**
Intervention in School and Clinic (USA) *Online - full text edition.* **3423**
Issues in Law and Medicine (USA) *Online - full text edition.* **3626**
Job Safety and Health Quarterly (USA) *Online - full text edition.* **4257**
Journal of Addictions & Offender Counseling (USA) *Online - full text edition.* **4409**
Journal of Aging Studies (GBR) *Online - full text edition.* **3475**
Journal of Alcohol and Drug Education (USA) *Online - full text edition.* **3402**
Journal of American College Health (USA) *Online - full text edition.* **4357**
Journal of Applied Behavior Analysis (USA) *Online - full text edition.* **4410**
Journal of Biological Education (GBR) *Online - full text edition.* **3202**
Journal of Continuing Education in Nursing (USA) *Online - full text edition.* **3924**
Journal of Counseling & Development (USA) *Online - full text edition.* **4414**
Journal of Drug Issues (USA) *Online - full text edition.* **3403**
Journal of Employment Counseling (USA) *Online - full text edition.* **4414**
Journal of Environmental Health (USA) *Online - full text edition.* **3440**
The Journal of General Psychology (USA) *Online - full text edition.* **4416**
The Journal of Genetic Psychology (USA) *Online - full text edition.* **3309**
Journal of Humanistic Counseling, Education and Development (USA) *Online - full text edition.* **4417**
Journal of Instructional Psychology (USA) *Online - full text edition.* **3412**
The Journal of Law, Medicine & Ethics (USA) *Online - full text edition.* **3540**
Journal of Learning Disabilities (USA) *Online - full text edition.* **3424**
Journal of Marital and Family Therapy (USA) *Online - full text edition.* **4418**
Journal of Multicultural Counseling and Development (USA) *Online - full text edition.* **4418**
Journal of Music Therapy (USA) *Online - full text edition.* **4062**
Journal of Nursing Education (USA) *Online - full text edition.* **3925**
Journal of Parapsychology (USA) *Online - full text edition.* **4271**
Journal of Parasitology (USA) *Online - full text edition.* **3802**
Journal of Psychology: Interdisciplinary & Applied (USA) *Online - full text edition.* **4421**
Journal of Rehabilitation (USA) *Online - full text edition.* **4062**
Journal of School Health (USA) *Online - full text edition.* **4479**
Journal of Sex Research (USA) *Online - full text edition.* **4422**
The Journal of Social Psychology (USA) *Online - full text edition.* **4423**
The Journal of Special Education (USA) *Online - full text edition.* **3424**
Journal of Speech, Language, and Hearing Research (USA) *Online - full text edition.* **3491**
Journal of Studies on Alcohol (USA) *Online - full text edition.* **3403**
Journal of Traffic Safety Education (USA) *Online - full text edition.* **4533**
Journal of Visual Impairment & Blindness (USA) *Online - full text edition.* **3498**
Language, Speech and Hearing Services in Schools (USA) *Online - full text edition.* **4035**
Literature and Psychology (USA) *Online - full text edition.* **3552**
Managed Healthcare (USA) *Online - full text edition.* **3518**
Marketing Health Services (USA) *Online - full text edition.* **3367**
Measurement and Evaluation in Counseling and Development (USA) *Online - full text edition.* **3413**
Medical Anthropology Quarterly (USA) *Online - full text edition.* **3174**
Medicine and Science in Sports and Exercise (USA) *Online - full text edition.* **4175**
Mental Retardation (USA) *Online - full text edition.* **3424**
Merrill - Palmer Quarterly (USA) *Online - full text edition.* **4427**
Modern Healthcare (Year) (USA) *Online - full text edition.* **3519**

New Choices (USA) *Online - full text edition.* **3478**
Notre Dame Journal of Law, Ethics & Public Policy (USA) *Online - full text edition.* **4459**
Nutrition Research Reviews (GBR) *Online - full text edition.* **4243**
Nutrition Today (USA) *Online - full text edition.* **4243**
O H Online (USA) *Online - full text edition of* Occupational Hazards. **4261**
Personnel Psychology (USA) *Online - full text edition.* **4433**
Pharmaceutical Executive (USA) *Online - full text edition.* **4323**
Politics and the Life Sciences (USA) *Online - full text edition.* **4368**
Preventing School Failure (USA) *Online - full text edition.* **3425**
Professional Safety (USA) *Online - full text edition.* **4263**
Professional School Counseling (USA) *Online - full text edition.* **3414**
The Psychological Record (USA) *Online - full text edition.* **4438**
Psychology Today (USA) *Online - full text edition.* **4441**
Public Health Reports (USA) *Online - full text edition.* **4486**
R N Web (USA) *Online - full text edition of* R N. **3938**
Rehabilitation Counseling Bulletin (USA) *Online - full text edition.* **3486**
Remedial and Special Education (USA) *Online - full text edition.* **3426**
Review (Washington) (USA) *Online - full text edition.* **3499**
Risk: Health, Safety & Environment (USA) *Online - full text edition.* **4488**
Saturday Evening Post (USA) *Online - full text edition.* **3465**
Scholastic Choices (USA) *Online - full text edition.* **3429**
School Psychology Review (USA) *Online - full text edition.* **4447**
T A S H Journal (USA) *Online - full text edition.* **3487**
Teacher Education and Special Education (USA) *Online - full text edition.* **3427**

Online Service

SERIALS

Title Index

A C S Digest (American Cryonics Society) (USA) **3870**
• A C S M's Health & Fitness Journal (American College of Sports Medicine) (USA ISSN 1091-5397) **4349**, 4172
A C S P Selection Sante *see* C P H A Health Digest **4464**, 4351
A C T International Cytogenetics Laboratory Directory (Association of Cytogenetic Technologists) (USA ISSN 0732-8753) **3870**, 3284
A D A A Reporter (Anxiety Disorders Association of America) (USA) **4371**
A.D.A. Forecast *see* Diabetes Forecast **3858**
A D A Legal Advisor (American Dental Association) (USA) **3813**, 3535
A D A M H A News (Alcohol, Drug Abuse, and Mental Health Administration) (USA) **3396**, 4371
A D A News (American Dental Association) (USA ISSN 0895-2930) **3813**
A D A Newsletter *see* Alberta Dental Association. Updater **3814**
A D A R A Journal (American Deafness & Rehabilitation Association) (USA ISSN 0899-9228) **3488**
A D A R A Newsletter (American Deafness & Rehabilitation Association) (USA) **3488**
A D A R D S New Zealand News *see* Alzheimers News **4071**
➤ A D C News (DEU) **3966**, 3239
A D D - up (Attention Deficit Disorder) (USA ISSN 1084-5518) **4067**
A D H A Access *see* Access (Chicago) **3813**
• A D H D Report (Attention Deficit Hyperactivity Disorder) (USA ISSN 1065-8025) **4067**
A D I News *see* Effective School Practices **3428**
• ➤ A D M (Asociacion Dental Mexicana, A.C.) (MEX ISSN 0001-0944) **3813**
A D T A Newsletter (American Dance Therapy Association) (USA) **4058**, 3396
➤ A E C A Research in Practice (Australian Early Childhood Association) (AUS) **3380**, 4371
A E C A Resource Book Series *see* A E C A Research in Practice **3380**, 4371
A E C C (Asociacion Espanola Contra el Cancer) (ESP ISSN 1133-3871) **3966**
A E P Appointments Broadsheet (Association of Educational Psychologists) (GBR) **4269**, 4371
A E R Report (Association for Education and Rehabilitation of the Blind and Visually Impaired) (USA) **3495**
A E T F A T Index (Association pour l'Etude Taxonomique de la Flore d'Afrique Tropicale) (BEL ISSN 0066-9784) **3225**, 3145, 3278
A F A R Annual Report (American Foundation for AIDS Research) (USA) **3790**
A F B Action *see* A W H P Action **4349**, 3361
A F B Directory of Services for Blind and Visually Impaired Persons in the United States *see* A F B Directory of Services for Blind and Visually Impaired Persons in the United States and Canada **3495**
• A F B Directory of Services for Blind and Visually Impaired Persons in the United States and Canada (American Foundation for the Blind Press) (USA ISSN 1067-5833) **3495**
• A F B News (American Foundation for the Blind Press) (USA) **3495**, 4510
A F H H A Insider (American Federation of Home Health Agencies) (USA) **3912**, 3785
A F I P Atlas of Tumor Pathology (Armed Forces Institute of Pathology) (USA) **3966**
A F P Sciences (Agence France Presse) (FRA) **3555**, 4503, 4531
• A G A News (American Gastroenterological Association) (USA) **3885**
A G D Impact (Academy of General Dentistry) (USA ISSN 0194-729X) **3813**
A G H E Exchange (Association for Gerontology in Higher Education) (USA ISSN 0890-278X) **3465**, 3417
A G P A Newsletter *see* Group Circle **4401**
A H *see* American Health **4350**
➤ A H A F Journal (American Handwriting Analysis Foundation) (USA ISSN 1041-956X) **4371**
• A H A Guide to the Health Care Field (American Hospital Association) (USA ISSN 0094-8969) **3524**, 4460
A H A Hospital Statistics (Year) (American Hospital Association) (USA) **3524**, 4527
A H A News (American Hospital Association) (USA ISSN 0891-6608) **3500**
A H A News (American Hippotherapy Association) (USA) **3483**
A H C A Notes (American Health Care Association) (USA ISSN 0279-1692) **4510**, 4460
• A H F S Drug Information (American Hospital Formulary Service) (USA ISSN 1063-8792) **4273**
A H I L Quarterly *see* Interface (Chicago, 1978) **3548**, 4061
• ➤ A H P Perspective (Association for Humanistic Psychology) (USA) **4371**
A H R *see* Australian Health Review **3502**
A H R A Announcement *see* A H R A Link **4139**
A H R A Link (American Healthcare Radiology Administrators) (USA) **4139**
A H R A Record (Alberta Health Records Association) (CAN) **3555**, 3500
A H R C Chronicle (Association for the Help of Retarded Children, New York City Chapter) (USA ISSN 0001-1436) **4067**, 3418, 4510
• A H R Q Research Activities (Agency for Healthcare Research and Quality) (USA) **3500**
➤ A I Ch E Equipment Testing Procedures Series (Equipment Testing Procedures Committee) (USA ISSN 0569-5473) **3433**, 3870
A I D Verbraucherdienst *see* Ernaehrung im Fokus **4232**, 3460
• ➤ A I H A J (USA) **4249**
A I H P Notes (American Institute of the History of Pharmacy) (USA) **4273**, 3526
A I M S Newsletter *see* Australian Journal of Medical Science **3572**, 3871
A I M S Self Assessment Programmes Series (Australian Institute of Medical Scientists) (AUS) **3870**
• ➤ A I N S - Anaesthesiologie Intensivmedizin Notfallmedizin Schmerztherapie (DEU) **3753**
A I U M Reporter (American Institute for Ultrasound in Medicine) (USA) **4139**, 3236, 3943
A J A S *see* Asian - Australasian Journal of Animal Sciences **3160**, 3269
A J D C - American Journal of Diseases of Children *see* Archives of Pediatrics & Adolescent Medicine **4041**
A J H P *see* American Journal of Health Promotion **4461**, 4228, 4350
A J I C *see* American Journal of Infection Control **3792**
A J K S *see* American Journal of Knee Surgery **4180**, 4058, 4172
➤ A J N Guide (American Journal of Nursing Co.) (USA) **3912**
• ➤ A J N R (American Journal of Neuroradiology) (USA ISSN 0195-6108) **4139**
A J O D O *see* American Journal of Orthodontics and Dentofacial Orthopedics **3814**
A J P: Cell Physiology Online *see* American Journal of Physiology: Cell Physiology **3337**, 3284
A J P: Endocrinology and Metabolism Online *see* American Journal of Physiology: Endocrinology and Metabolism **3338**, 3855
A J P: Gastrointestinal and Liver Physiology Online *see* American Journal of Physiology: Gastrointestinal and Liver Physiology **3338**, 3886
A J P: Heart and Circulatory Physiology Online *see* American Journal of Physiology: Heart and Circulatory Physiology **3338**, 3762
A J P: Lung Cellular and Molecular Physiology Online *see* American Journal of Physiology: Lung Cellular and Molecular Physiology **3338**, 3240, 3285
A J P Online *see* American Journal of Physiology (Consolidated) **3337**, 3564
A J P: Regulatory, Integrative and Comparative Physiology Online *see* American Journal of Physiology: Regulatory, Integrative and Comparative Physiology **3338**
A J P: Renal Physiology Online *see* American Journal of Physiology: Renal Physiology **3339**, 4209
• ➤ A J R (American Journal of Roentgenology) (USA ISSN 0361-803X) **4139**
A J S Informationen *see* Aktion Jugendschutz. Informationen **3380**, 3397
A K F Newsletter for Health Professionals *see* Clinical Strategies: A K F Newsletter for Nephrology Professionals **4211**
A L L-O-Grams (Affiliated Leadership League of and for the Blind of America) (USA ISSN 0195-363X) **3495**
A L R A Newsletter (Abortion Law Reform Association) (GBR) **3357**, 3545, 3966, 4562
A L S Newsletter (USA) **4067**
A M A Alliance Today (American Medical Association) (USA) **3555**, 4568
A M A List of Medical Services and Fees (Australian Medical Association) (AUS ISSN 1329-1955) **3555**
A M A Victoria Branch News (Australian Medical Association) (AUS ISSN 0813-6394) **3555**
A M B *see* Acta Medica Bulgarica **3870**
A M C R A's Managed Care Monitor *see* Monitor (Washington, 1970) **3533**, 3519, 3662
▼ A M D A Advocacy in Action (American Medical Directors Association) (USA) **3555**
A M D A Reports (American Medical Directors Association) (USA) **3465**
• A M E D (GBR) **3171**, 3145, 3714
A M H C Scoring Guidelines *see* Accreditation Manual for Home Care. Vol. 2: Scoring Guidelines **3501**, 3557
A M H C Standards *see* Accreditation Manual for Home Care. Vol. 1: Standards **3501**, 3557
A M I A - Annual Fall Symposium. Proceedings *see* A M I A Symposium. Proceedings **3808**
➤ A M I A Symposium. Proceedings (American Medical Informatics Association) (USA) **3808**
A M I News (Association of Medical Illustrators) (USA) **3555**
A M P A Newsletter (American Medical Publishers' Association) (USA) **3555**, 4499
A M P R A Review (American Medical Peer Review Association) *see* Quality Advocate **3681**
A M R O: The Journal for Health Care Information and Medical Records *see* Institute of Health Record Information & Management. Journal **3621**, 3515
A M S A Focus *see* The New Physician **3666**
A M S E C T Today (American Society of Extra-Corporeal Technology, Inc.) (USA) **3555**
A M S Studies in Modern Society (USA ISSN 0275-8407) **4460**, 4371, 4510
A M T *see* Arzneimitteltherapie **4278**
A M T Chronicle (Association of Medical Technologists) (IND) **3870**
A M T Events *see* Journal of Continuing Education Topics & Issues **3632**
A M U News (American Malacological Union, Inc.) (USA ISSN 1041-5300) **3349**
• A M W A Freelance Directory (American Medical Writers Association) (USA ISSN 0194-004X) **3556**
A M W A Journal (American Medical Writers Association) (USA ISSN 1075-6361) **3556**
A N A D: Working Together (National Association of Anorexia Nervosa and Associated Disorders) (USA) **4371**, 3556
• ➤ A N A E (Approche Neuropsychologique des Apprentissages chez l'Enfant) (FRA ISSN 0999-792X) **4067**
A N D I News (Autism Network for Dietary Intervention) (USA) **4067**, 4227
A N E C (Asociacion Nacional de Enfermeras de Colombia) (COL ISSN 0120-1832) **3912**
A N N A Journal *see* Nephrology Nursing Journal **3930**, 4216
A N P H I Papers (Academy of Nursing of the Philippines) (PHL ISSN 0065-0676) **3912**
• ➤ A N R E D (Anorexia Nervosa & Related Eating Disorders, Inc.) (USA) **4067**, 4371, 4562
A N R E D Alert (Print) *see* A N R E D **4067**, 4371, 4562
A N Z C C A R T News (Australian and New Zealand Council for the Care of Animals in Research and Teaching Limited) (AUS ISSN 1039-9089) **3171**, 4534
• ➤ A N Z Journal of Surgery (AUS ISSN 1445-1433) **4178**
A O A Yearbook and Directory of Osteopathic Physicians (American Osteopathic Association) (USA) **3785**
A O H A Progress *see* Osteopathic Progress **3520**, 3789
• ➤ A O R N Journal (Association of periOperative Registered Nurses, Inc.) (USA) **3912**
▼ • A O Recommended Literature. Craniomaxillofacial Trauma and Disorders (USA ISSN 1616-8747) **4009**
▼ • A O Recommended Literature. General and Orthopedic Trauma (USA ISSN 1616-8755) **4009**
▼ • A O Recommended Literature. Spine Trauma and Disorders (USA ISSN 1616-8763) **4009**
▼ • A O Recommended Literature. Veterinary Trauma and Disorders (USA ISSN 1616-8771) **4534**
A O T A Self Study Series (American Occupational Therapy Association, Inc.) (USA ISSN 1059-1753) **4249**
A O T Journal *see* Australian Occupational Therapy Journal **4059**
A P A I T (Asian Pacific AIDS Intervention Team) (USA) **3457**, 3790
A P A Monitor *see* Monitor on Psychology **4428**
A P A Q *see* Adapted Physical Activity Quarterly **3418**, 4349
• A P A Research Psychology Funding Bulletin (American Psychological Association) (USA) **4371**
• ➤ A P C D Journal (Associacao Paulista de Cirurgioes Dentistas) (BRA) **3813**
A P C O Bulletin *see* Public Safety Communications **4487**, 3388
A P F News (American Physicians Fellowship for Medicine in Israel) (USA) **3556**
A P H Slate (American Printing House for the Blind, Inc.) (USA ISSN 1081-5198) **3495**
• A P H Technology Update (American Printing House for the Blind, Inc.) (USA) **3391**, 3495
A P I Abstracts - Health and Environment *see* Technical Literature Abstracts: Health & Environment **3443**, 3152, 3442
A P I EnCompass: Environment *see* Technical Literature Abstracts: Health & Environment **3443**, 3152, 3442
A P M A News (American Podiatric Medical Association) (USA ISSN 8750-2585) **4009**
• ➤ A P M I S (Acta Pathologica Microbiologica et Immunologica Scandinavica) (DNK ISSN 0903-4641) **3178**, 3556
• A P M I S Supplementum (DNK ISSN 0903-465X) **3178**, 3556
A P N J *see* Australia Paediatric Nurse Journal **3914**, 4041
A P R C Journal of Experimental Psychology (Agra Psychological Research Cell) (IND) **4371**
A P R T Newsletter *see* Association for Past-Life Research and Therapies. Newsletter **4379**
• A P S Bulletin (American Pain Society) (USA ISSN 1057-1590) **3753**, 4067, 4273
A P S Journal *see* Pain Forum **4121**
A P S Observer (American Psychological Society) (USA ISSN 1050-4672) **4371**
A P V News (Arbeitsgemeinschaft fuer Pharmazeutische Verfahrenstechnik) (DEU) **4273**
A Propos *see* Candid Facts **3582**
A Q I S Bulletin (Australian Quarantine and Inspection Service) (AUS ISSN 1033-9280) **3153**, 3459, 4460
A R B M *see* Annuaire de la Recherche Bio-Medicale **3182**, 3567
A R C *see* The Arc Insight **4510**, 3380, 4073
A R D Online *see* Annals of the Rheumatic Diseases **4167**
A R L Academic Law and Medical Library Statistics (Association of Research Libraries) (USA ISSN 1088-1093) **3549**, 3544, 3714, 4527
A R N N Access *see* A R N N L Access **3912**
A R N N L Access (Association of Registered Nurses of Newfoundland and Labrador) (CAN) **3912**
A R N Network (Association of Rehabilitation Nurses) (USA) **3912**
A R N News *see* A R N Network **3912**
A R T A *see* Assisted Reproductive Technology - Andrology **3571**
A S (Activiteitensektor) (NLD ISSN 0168-2857) **4510**, 3465, 3495
• ➤ A S A I O Journal (American Society for Artificial Internal Organs, Inc.) (USA ISSN 1058-2916) **3556**, 3870
• ➤ A S A M News (American Society of Addiction Medicine) (USA) **3396**
A S A Refresher Courses in Anesthesiology (American Society of Anesthesiologists) (USA ISSN 0363-471X) **3753**
A S B Bulletin (Association of Southeastern Biologists, Inc.) (USA ISSN 0001-2386) **3178**
A S C L S Today (American Society for Clinical Laboratory Science) (USA ISSN 1073-466X) **3870**
• A S C P Update (American Society of Consultant Pharmacists) (USA ISSN 1050-5725) **4273**

Title

Title

Accreditation Manual for Hospitals. Vol. 2: Scoring Guidelines (USA ISSN 1083-1770) **3501**, 3557
Accreditation Manual for Long Term Care (USA ISSN 1084-4376) **3501**, 3557
➤ Accredited Professional Programs of Colleges and Schools of Pharmacy (USA) **4273**
• Acheronta (ARG ISSN 0329-9147) **4371**
• Acimed (CUB ISSN 1024-9435) **3557**, 3501
Acoustic Neuroma Association Notes (USA) **4029**, 3966, 4178
Acquired Immune Deficiency Syndrome *see* AIDS **3790**
Acquired Immune Deficiency Syndrome Alert *see* AIDS Alert **3791**, 3739
Acquired Immune Deficiency Syndrome & Hepatitus Digest *see* AIDS & Hepatitus Digest **3791**
Acquired Immune Deficiency Syndrome & Public Policy Journal *see* AIDS & Public Policy Journal **3791**, 3536, 4460
Acquired Immune Deficiency Syndrome Education and Prevention *see* AIDS Education and Prevention **4460**, 4349
Acquired Immune Deficiency Syndrome Information Exchange *see* AIDS Information Exchange **3791**, 3844, 4460
Acquired Immune Deficiency Syndrome Legal Bibliography *see* AIDS Legal Bibliography **3544**, 3176, 3547, 3715, 3791
Acquired Immune Deficiency Syndrome Litigation Reporter *see* AIDS Litigation Reporter **3536**, 3791
Acquired Immune Deficiency Syndrome Policy and Law *see* AIDS Policy and Law **3536**, 3791, 4460
Acta Academiae Agriculturae ac Technicae Olstenensis. Veterinaria/Agricultural and Technical Academy in Olsztyn. Veterinary Medicine (POL ISSN 0860-2840) **4534**
Acta Academiae Medicinae Bengbu *see* Bangbu Yixueyuan Xuebao **3574**
Acta Academiae Medicinae Sinica *see* Zhongguo Yixue Kexueyuan Xuebao **3713**
Acta Agraria et Silvestria. Series Zootechnica (POL ISSN 0065-0935) **3160**
➤ Acta Amazonica (BRA ISSN 0044-5967) **4503**
Acta Anaesthesiologica Belgica (BEL ISSN 0001-5164) **3753**
Acta Anaesthesiologica Italica *see* Acta Anaesthesiologica Italica & Anaesthesia and Intensive Care in Italy **3753**
Acta Anaesthesiologica Italica & Anaesthesia and Intensive Care in Italy (ITA ISSN 1124-8882) **3753**
• ➤ Acta Anaesthesiologica Scandinavica (DNK ISSN 0001-5172) **3753**
• Acta Anaesthesiologica Scandinavica. Supplementum (DNK ISSN 0515-2720) **3753**
Acta Anatomica *see* Cells, Tissues, Organs **3583**, 3288
Acta Anatomica Nipponica/Kaibogaku Zasshi (JPN ISSN 0022-7722) **3178**, 3172, 3284, 3557
Acta Bio-medica de l'Ateneo Parmense *see* Ateneo Parmense. Acta Bio-Medica **3571**, 3183
Acta Biochimica et Biophysica Hungarica *see* Neurobiology **4151**
Acta Biochimica et Biophysica Sinica *see* Shengwu Huaxue yu Shengwu Wuli Xuebao **3262**, 3268
Acta Biologiae Experimentalis Sinica *see* Shiyan Shengwu Xuebao **3294**
Acta Biologica (DEU ISSN 0722-4192) **3178**, 3785
Acta Biologica (HRV ISSN 0448-0147) **3178**
➤ Acta Biologica Colombiana (COL ISSN 0120-548X) **3278**
Acta Biologica Cracoviensia. Zoologia (POL ISSN 0001-530X) **3350**
Acta Biologica Debrecina (HUN ISSN 0567-7327) **3178**
Acta Biologica et Medica (POL ISSN 0065-1087) **3178**, 3557
Acta Biologica Iugoslavica. Serija A: Zemljiste i Biljka (YUG ISSN 0514-6658) **3178**
Acta Biologica Iugoslavica. Serija B: Mikrobiologija (YUG ISSN 0581-1538) **3316**
Acta Biologica Iugoslavica. Serija C: Iugoslavica Physiologica et Pharmacologica Acta (YUG ISSN 0021-3225) **3178**, 4273
Acta Biologica Iugoslavica. Serija D: Ekologija (YUG ISSN 0531-9110) **3178**, 3435
Acta Biologica Iugoslavica. Serija F: Genetika (YUG ISSN 0534-0012) **3297**
Acta Biologica Leopoldensia (BRA ISSN 0101-5354) **3178**
Acta Biologica Silesiana *see* Uniwersytet Slaski w Katowicach. Prace Naukowe. Acta Biologica Silesiana **3223**
➤ Acta Biologica Venezuelica (VEN ISSN 0001-5326) **3178**
Acta Biomedica Lovaniensia (BEL) **3557**
• Acta Biophysica Sinica (CHN ISSN 1000-6737) **3264**, 3239, 3377
• ➤ Acta Bioquimica Clinica Latinoamericana (ARG ISSN 0325-2957) **3239**
• ➤ Acta Biotechnologica (DEU ISSN 0138-4988) **3268**
• ➤ Acta Biotheoretica (NLD ISSN 0001-5342) **3178**
➤ Acta Botanica Croatica (HRV ISSN 0365-0588) **3278**
Acta Botanica Yunnanica *see* Yunnan Zhiwu Yanjiu **3283**
Acta Cancerologica (PER ISSN 1013-5545) **3966**
• ➤ Acta Cardiologica (BEL ISSN 0001-5385) **3761**
Acta Cardiologica Mediterranea (ITA ISSN 0392-9698) **3761**
Acta Cardiologica. Supplementum (BEL ISSN 0373-7934) **3761**
Acta Cardiomyologica *see* Acta Myologica **3761**, 3870
Acta Chemica Scandinavica *see* Royal Chemical Society. Journal. Perkin Transactions 1 **3379**, 3262
➤ Acta Chirurgiae Plasticae (CZE ISSN 0001-5423) **4178**
Acta Chirurgica *see* European Journal of Surgery **4188**
• Acta Chirurgica Austriaca (AUT ISSN 0001-544X) **4178**
• Acta Chirurgica Austriaca Online (AUT ISSN 1563-2563) **4178**
• ➤ Acta Chirurgica Belgica (BEL ISSN 0001-5458) **4178**
Acta Chirurgica Belgica. Supplementum (BEL ISSN 0515-2763) **4178**
• Acta Chirurgica Italica (ITA ISSN 0001-5466) **4178**
Acta Chirurgica Mediterranea (ITA ISSN 0393-6376) **4178**, 3943
Acta Chirurgica. Supplement *see* European Journal of Surgery. Supplement **4188**
• Acta Cirurgica Brasileira (BRA ISSN 0102-8650) **4178**
Acta Cirurgica Brasileira. Suplemento (BRA ISSN 0102-9592) **4179**
• ➤ Acta Clinica Belgica (BEL ISSN 0001-5512) **3557**
• ➤ Acta Clinica Croatica (HRV ISSN 0353-9466) **3557**
• Acta Clinica Croatica. Supplement (HRV ISSN 0353-9474) **3557**
Acta Concilium Ophthalmologicum *see* International Congress of Ophthalmology. Abstracts **3999**
Acta Criminologiae et Medicinae Legalis Japonica/Hanzaigaku Zasshi (JPN ISSN 0302-0029) **3393**, 3881
• ➤ Acta Cytologica (USA ISSN 0001-5547) **3284**
Acta de Odontologia Pediatrica (DOM ISSN 0252-1032) **3813**, 4039
• ➤ Acta Dermato-Venereologica (NOR ISSN 0001-5555) **3843**
• Acta Dermato-Venereologica. Supplementum (NOR ISSN 0365-8341) **3843**
➤ Acta Dermatovenerologica Alpina, Pannonica et Adriatica (SVN ISSN 1318-4458) **3843**
➤ Acta Dermatovenerologica Croatica (HRV ISSN 1330-027X) **3843**
Acta Dermatovenerologica Iugoslavica *see* Acta Dermatovenerologica Alpina, Pannonica et Adriatica **3843**
• ➤ Acta Diabetologica (DEU ISSN 0940-5429) **3855**
Acta Embryologiae et Morphologiae Experimentalis *see* Animal Biology **3181**
Acta Endocrinologica Panamericana (ARG ISSN 0065-1192) **3855**
Acta Endoscopica (FRA ISSN 0240-642X) **3885**
➤ Acta Endoscopica Polona (POL ISSN 0867-4140) **3885**
Acta Entomologica Bohemoslovaca *see* European Journal of Entomology **3296**
Acta Entomologica Sinica *see* Kunchong Xuebao **3297**
• ➤ Acta Ethologica (DEU ISSN 0873-9749) **3350**, 4372
• ➤ Acta Ethologica Online (DEU ISSN 1437-9546) **3179**, 4372
Acta Facultatis Medicae Fluminensis (HRV ISSN 0065-1206) **3557**
Acta Facultatis Medicae Universitatis Brunensis (CZE ISSN 0521-2561) **3557**, 3179
Acta Facultatis Medicinae Skopiensis *see* Medicinska Misla **3657**
Acta Facultatis Pharmaceuticae Bohemoslovenicae *see* Universitas Comeniana. Acta Facultatis Pharmaceuticae **4339**
• ➤ Acta Fisiatrica (BRA ISSN 0104-7795) **4009**
• ➤ Acta Gastro-Enterologica Belgica (BEL ISSN 0001-5644) **3885**
• ➤ Acta Gastroenterologica Latinoamericana (ARG ISSN 0300-9033) **3885**
Acta Genetica et Teratologica (URY ISSN 0797-6852) **3297**
Acta Genetica Sinica *see* Yichuan Xuebao **3315**
Acta Geneticae Medicae et Gemellologiae: Twin Research (ITA ISSN 0001-5660) **3297**, 3557
Acta Gerontologica (ITA ISSN 0001-5741) **3465**
Acta Ginecologica (ESP ISSN 0001-5776) **3943**
• ➤ Acta Haematologica (CHE ISSN 0001-5792) **3897**
➤ Acta Haematologica Polonica (POL ISSN 0001-5814) **3897**
Acta Hepatologica Japonica *see* Kanzo **3893**
• ➤ Acta Histochemica (DEU ISSN 0065-1281) **3239**
• ➤ Acta Histochemica et Cytochemica/Nihon Soshiki Saibo Kagakkai Gakkaishi (JPN ISSN 0044-5991) **3284**, 3239
Acta Historica Leopoldina (DEU ISSN 0001-5857) **4503**, 3557
Acta Historica Leopoldina. Supplement (DEU ISSN 0232-8615) **4503**, 3557
Acta Historica Scientiarum Naturalium et Medicinalium (DNK ISSN 0065-1311) **4503**, 3557
Acta Hospitalia (BEL ISSN 0044-6009) **3501**
➤ Acta Hydrobiologica (POL ISSN 0065-132X) **3179**
Acta Hydrobiologica Sinica *see* Shuisheng Shengwu Xuebao **3218**, 3408, 3409
• ➤ Acta Hydrochimica et Hydrobiologica (DEU ISSN 0323-4320) **4561**, 4460
Acta Leprologica (CHE ISSN 0001-5938) **3790**
Acta Medica (CUB ISSN 0864-3210) **3557**
➤ Acta Medica (CZE ISSN 1211-4286) **3557**
Acta Medica *see* Igaku Kenkyu **3618**
Acta Medica (MEX ISSN 0001-5997) **3557**
• ➤ Acta Medica Austriaca (AUT ISSN 0303-8173) **3557**
• Acta Medica Austriaca Online (AUT ISSN 1563-2571) **3557**
➤ Acta Medica Auxologica (ITA ISSN 0001-6004) **3855**, 3380, 3912, 3943
➤ Acta Medica Baltica (DEU ISSN 0946-3445) **3558**
➤ Acta Medica Bulgarica (BGR ISSN 0324-1750) **3870**
Acta Medica Costarricense (CRI ISSN 0001-6012) **3558**
Acta Medica Croatica (HRV ISSN 1330-0164) **3558**
Acta Medica Dominicana (DOM ISSN 0379-4857) **3558**
Acta Medica Empirica *see* Erfahrungsheilkunde **3599**
Acta Medica et Biologica/Igaku Seibutsugaku Kenkyu Kiyo (JPN ISSN 0567-7734) **3558**, 3179
Acta Medica et Sociologica (BGR ISSN 0515-2925) **3558**, 4519
➤ Acta Medica Iranica (IRN ISSN 0044-6025) **3558**
Acta Medica Iugoslavica *see* Acta Medica Croatica **3558**
Acta Medica Iugoslavica (English Edition) *see* Acta Medica Croatica **3558**
➤ Acta Medica Kinki University (JPN ISSN 0386-6092) **3558**
Acta Medica Lituanica (LTU ISSN 1392-0138) **3558**
Acta Medica Medianae (YUG ISSN 0365-4478) **3558**
Acta Medica Mediterranea (ITA ISSN 0393-6384) **3558**
➤ Acta Medica Nagasakiensia (JPN ISSN 0001-6055) **3558**
• ➤ Acta Medica Okayama (JPN ISSN 0386-300X) **3558**
Acta Medica Peruana (PER ISSN 1018-8800) **3558**
Acta Medica Philippina (PHL ISSN 0001-6071) **3558**
Acta Medica Romana (ITA ISSN 0001-6098) **3558**, 3179, 4372
➤ Acta Medica. Supplementum (CZE ISSN 1211-247X) **3558**
Acta Medica Veterinaria (ITA ISSN 0001-6136) **4534**
Acta Medicinae Legalis (CHE) **3881**
Acta Medicinae Legalis et Socialis *see* Acta Medicinae Legalis **3881**
Acta Mediterranea di Patologia Infettiva e Tropicale (ITA ISSN 0392-9515) **3790**
• Acta Microbiologica et Immunologica Hungarica (HUN ISSN 1217-8950) **3316**, 3739
Acta Microbiologica Hungarica *see* Acta Microbiologica et Immunologica Hungarica **3316**, 3739
• Acta Microbiologica Polonica (POL ISSN 0137-1320) **3316**
Acta Microbiologica Sinica *see* Weishengwu Xuebao **3333**
Acta Micropalaeontologica Sinica *see* Weiti Gushengwu Xuebao **3333**
Acta Musei Moraviae. Supplementum: Folia Mendeliana (CZE ISSN 0085-0748) **3297**
➤ Acta Myologica (ITA ISSN 1128-2460) **3761**, 3870
Acta Neonatologica Japonica *see* Nihon Shinseiji Gakkai Zasshi **4049**
• ➤ Acta Neurobiologiae Experimentalis (POL ISSN 0065-1400) **3179**
• ➤ Acta Neurochirurgica (AUT ISSN 0001-6268) **4179**, 4068
➤ Acta Neurochirurgica. Supplementum (AUT ISSN 0065-1419) **4068**, 4179
• ➤ Acta Neurologica Belgica (BEL ISSN 0300-9009) **4068**
• ➤ Acta Neurologica Scandinavica (DNK ISSN 0001-6314) **4068**
• ➤ Acta Neurologica Scandinavica. Supplementum (DNK ISSN 0065-1427) **4068**
Acta Neurologica Sinica *see* Acta Neurologica Taiwanica **4068**
Acta Neurologica Taiwanica (TWN ISSN 1028-768X) **4068**
• ➤ Acta Neuropathologica (DEU ISSN 0001-6322) **4068**
Acta Neuropathologica. Supplement (DEU ISSN 0065-1435) **4068**
• ➤ Acta Neuropsychiatrica (NLD ISSN 0924-2708) **4068**
Acta Obstetrica et Gynaecologica Japonica *see* Nihon Sanka Fujinka Gakkai Zasshi **3959**
Acta Obstetrica et Gynecologica (ESP) **3943**
• ➤ Acta Obstetrica et Gynecologica Scandinavica (DNK ISSN 0001-6349) **3944**
Acta Obstetrica et Gynecologica Scandinavica (Edicion Espanola) *see* Acta Obstetrica et Gynecologica **3943**
• Acta Obstetrica et Gynecologica Scandinavica. Supplement (DNK ISSN 0300-8835) **3944**
• ➤ Acta Odontologica Scandinavica (NOR ISSN 0001-6357) **3813**
▼ ➤ Acta of Bioengineering and Biomechanics (POL ISSN 1509-409X) **3236**, 4058
• ➤ Acta Oncologica (NOR ISSN 0284-186X) **3966**
Acta Oncologica. Supplement (NOR ISSN 1100-1704) **3966**
Acta Ophthalmologica *see* Acta Ophthalmologica Scandinavica **3992**
Acta Ophthalmologica Iugoslavica (HRV ISSN 0001-6403) **3992**
• ➤ Acta Ophthalmologica Scandinavica (DNK ISSN 1395-3907) **3992**
Acta Ophthalmologica Scandinavica. Supplementum (DNK ISSN 1395-3931) **3993**
Acta Ophthalmologica. Supplementum *see* Acta Ophthalmologica Scandinavica. Supplementum **3993**
• Acta Ophthamologica Scandinavica Online (DNK ISSN 1600-5465) **3993**
Acta Orthopaedica Belgica (BEL ISSN 0001-6462) **4009**
Acta Orthopaedica Belgica. Supplementum (BEL ISSN 0772-7623) **4009**
➤ Acta Orthopaedica Iugoslavica (YUG ISSN 0350-2309) **4009**
• ➤ Acta Orthopaedica Scandinavica (NOR ISSN 0001-6470) **4009**
Acta Orthopaedica Scandinavica. Supplementum (NOR ISSN 0300-8827) **4009**
• ➤ Acta Oto-Laryngologica (NOR ISSN 0001-6489) **4029**
• Acta Oto-Laryngologica. Supplement (NOR ISSN 0365-5237) **4029**

Title

Title

• ➤ Adolescence (San Diego) (USA ISSN 0001-8449) **3380**, 3409, 4372
Adolescent and Pediatric Gynecology *see* Journal of Pediatric and Adolescent Gynecology **4047**, 3956
➤ Adolescent Medicine (Philadelphia) (USA ISSN 1041-3499) **4039**
• Adolescent Medicine (Washington) (USA ISSN 0044-6335) **3559**
• ➤ Adolescent Psychiatry (USA ISSN 0065-2008) **4069**, 3380, 4372
➤ Adorerian/Adlerian (JPN ISSN 0918-1490) **4372**
Adult Day Care Letter *see* Adult Day Services Letter **3466**, 3364, 3501
• Adult Day Services Letter (USA) **3466**, 3364, 3501
▼ ➤ Adultspan (USA ISSN 1524-6817) **4372**, 3380
Advance *see* Advance for Occupational Therapy Practitioners **4058**, 4249
Advance *see* Advance for Physical Therapists and P T Assistants **4058**
Advance Data from Vital and Health Statistics *see* U.S. National Center for Health Statistics. Advance Data from Vital and Health Statistics **4498**
➤ Advance for Administrators in Radiology and Radiation Oncology (USA ISSN 1096-6285) **4140**
➤ Advance for Administrators of the Laboratory (USA ISSN 1096-6269) **3870**
• Advance for Audiologists (USA) **3559**
Advance for Directors in Rehabilitation (USA) **3559**
• Advance for Health Information Executives (USA) **3390**, 3501
➤ Advance for Health Information Professionals (USA ISSN 1061-3269) **3559**, 3547
• ➤ Advance for Imaging and Radiation Therapy Professionals (USA) **4140**
➤ Advance for Managers of Respiratory Care (USA ISSN 1096-6307) **4157**
• ➤ Advance for Medical Laboratory Professionals (USA ISSN 1088-5676) **3870**
Advance for Medical Record Professionals *see* Advance for Health Information Professionals **3559**, 3547
Advance for Medical Technologists *see* Advance for Medical Laboratory Professionals **3870**
➤ Advance for Nurse Practitioners (USA ISSN 1096-6293) **3912**
• Advance for Nurses (USA) **3912**
➤ Advance for Occupational Therapy Practitioners (USA ISSN 1099-9507) **4058**, 4249
Advance for Physical Therapists *see* Advance for Physical Therapists and P T Assistants **4058**
• ➤ Advance for Physical Therapists and P T Assistants (Physical Therapy) (USA ISSN 1099-9493) **4058**
➤ Advance for Physician Assistants (USA ISSN 1096-6315) **3559**
• Advance for Providers of Post-Acute Care (USA) **3912**
Advance for Radiologic Science Professionals *see* Advance for Imaging and Radiation Therapy Professionals **4140**
➤ Advance for Respiratory Care Practitioners (USA ISSN 1074-2301) **4158**
➤ Advance for Speech - Language Pathologists and Audiologists (USA ISSN 1062-5747) **4029**
Advanced Cardiac Life Support Alert *see* Emergency Medicine Alert **4013**
• ➤ Advanced Drug Delivery Reviews (NLD ISSN 0169-409X) **4274**, 3179
Advanced Psychology Texts (USA) **4372**
➤ Advanced Rescue Technology (USA) **4009**, 4460
Advanced Series in Neuroscience (SGP) **4069**
Advanced Technology in Surgical Care *see* Same-Day Surgery **4202**
➤ Advanced Traditional Chinese Medicine Series (NLD ISSN 1382-6883) **3162**, 3559
➤ Advances and Technical Standards in Neurosurgery (AUT ISSN 0095-4829) **4069**, 4179
Advances (Chicago) (USA) **4069**, 3466, 4519
Advances in A L S - M N D (Amyotrophic Lateral Sclerosis - Motor Neuron Disease) (GBR ISSN 0965-1802) **4069**
Advances in Amino Acid Mimetics and Peptidomimetics (USA) **3239**
• ➤ Advances in Anatomic Pathology (USA ISSN 1072-4109) **3559**
• ➤ Advances in Anatomy, Embryology and Cell Biology (USA ISSN 0301-5556) **3179**, 3284
Advances in Anesthesia (USA ISSN 0737-6146) **3753**
Advances in Animal Physiology and Animal Nutrition/Fortschritte in der Tierphysiologie und Tierernaehrung (DEU ISSN 0301-2743) **3337**, 3350, 4535
Advances in Antiviral Drug Design (USA ISSN 1075-8593) **4274**, 3239
Advances in Applied Developmental Psychology (USA) **4372**
Advances in Applied Lipid Research (USA) **3239**
• ➤ Advances in Applied Microbiology (USA ISSN 0065-2164) **3316**
• ➤ Advances in Audiology (CHE ISSN 0254-8747) **4029**
➤ Advances in Behavioral Biology (USA ISSN 0099-6246) **4372**, 3179
Advances in Behavioral Economics (USA ISSN 0890-0159) **4372**, 3363
Advances in Behaviour Research and Therapy *see* Behaviour Research and Therapy **4382**
Advances in Biochemical Engineering - Biotechnology (USA ISSN 0724-6145) **3268**, 3236, 3239
• ➤ Advances in Biochemical Psychopharmacology (USA ISSN 0065-2229) **4274**, 4069
Advances in Bioengineering *see* Advances in Computational Bioengineering **3236**
➤ Advances in Bioengineering (USA ISSN 0360-9960) **3236**
▼ Advances in Bioengineering Series (GBR) **3236**
Advances in Bioethics (USA) **4346**, 3179
• ➤ Advances in Biological Psychiatry (CHE ISSN 0378-7354) **4069**
➤ Advances in Biomaterials (NLD ISSN 0272-3840) **3239**
Advances in Biophysical Chemistry (USA ISSN 1057-8943) **3379**, 3239
Advances in Blood Disorders (CHE ISSN 1074-3944) **3897**
• ➤ Advances in Cancer Research (USA ISSN 0065-230X) **3966**
• ➤ Advances in Carbohydrate Chemistry and Biochemistry (USA ISSN 0065-2318) **3559**, 3239
Advances in Cardiac Surgery (USA ISSN 0889-5074) **3761**, 4179
• ➤ Advances in Cardiology (CHE ISSN 0065-2326) **3761**
Advances in Cardiovascular Disease *see* Xinxueguanbingxue Jinzhan **3785**
Advances in Cell Biology *see* Postepy Biologii Komorki **3293**, 3677
• ➤ Advances in Child Development and Behavior (USA ISSN 0065-2407) **4372**, 4039
Advances in Child Neuropsychology (USA ISSN 0940-8606) **4372**, 4069
➤ Advances in Clinical and Experimental Medicine/Postepy Medycyny Klinicznej i Doswiadczalnej (POL ISSN 1230-025X) **3870**
• ➤ Advances in Clinical Chemistry (USA ISSN 0065-2423) **3239**
Advances in Clinical Neuropsychology (USA ISSN 0748-4410) **4069**, 4372
➤ Advances in Clinical Pathology (ITA ISSN 1125-5552) **3559**
➤ Advances in Clinical Pharmacology (USA) **4274**
Advances in Clinical Rehabilitation (USA ISSN 0892-8878) **4058**, 4510
Advances in Cognition and Educational Practice (USA) **3409**, 4372
• ➤ Advances in Colloid and Interface Science (NLD ISSN 0001-8686) **3379**, 3179, 4365
Advances in Combustion Toxicology (USA ISSN 0899-7195) **3445**, 4274
Advances in Comparative Psychology (USA) **4372**
➤ Advances in Computational Bioengineering (GBR ISSN 1465-3222) **3236**
➤ Advances in Consciousness Research (NLD ISSN 1381-589X) **4372**, 4069
➤ Advances in Contraceptive Delivery Systems (USA ISSN 1012-8689) **3357**
Advances in Dental Research (USA ISSN 0895-9374) **3814**
Advances in Dermatology (USA ISSN 0882-0880) **3844**
Advances in Developmental Biology (USA) **3179**
Advances in Disease Vector Research (USA ISSN 0934-6112) **3790**
➤ Advances in Drug Research (USA ISSN 0065-2490) **4274**
➤ Advances in Echo-Contrast (NLD ISSN 0925-5206) **3809**, 4140
➤ Advances in Electromagnetic Fields in Living Systems (USA) **3264**, 3337, 3560
• ➤ Advances in Enzyme Regulation (GBR ISSN 0065-2571) **3239**
• ➤ Advances in Enzymology and Related Areas of Molecular Biology (GBR ISSN 0065-258X) **3239**
➤ Advances in Epileptology (USA ISSN 0892-726X) **4069**
• ➤ Advances in Experimental Medicine and Biology (USA ISSN 0065-2598) **3179**, 3560
• ➤ Advances in Experimental Social Psychology (USA ISSN 0065-2601) **4519**, 4372
Advances in Food and Nutrition Research (USA ISSN 1043-4526) **4227**, 3459
Advances in Food Research *see* Advances in Food and Nutrition Research **4227**, 3459
Advances in Food Sciences (DEU ISSN 1431-7737) **3459**
• ➤ Advances in Genetics (USA ISSN 0065-2660) **3297**
Advances in Genetics. Supplement (USA ISSN 0065-2679) **3297**
Advances in Genome Biology (USA ISSN 1067-5701) **3297**, 3240
Advances in Gerontological Nursing (USA) **3466**, 3912
➤ Advances in Health Economics and Health Services Research (USA ISSN 0731-2199) **4349**
Advances in Health Economics and Health Services Research. Supplement (USA ISSN 1054-1888) **3560**
Advances in Health Education and Promotion (USA ISSN 0896-1255) **4349**, 4221
➤ Advances in Health Education: Current Research (USA ISSN 0890-4073) **3428**, 4349, 4372
• ➤ Advances in Health Sciences Education (NLD ISSN 1382-4996) **3560**, 3417
▼ • Advances in Hepatitis C (NZL ISSN 1530-5767) **3790**
Advances in Host Defense Mechanisms (USA ISSN 0732-0566) **3790**, 3739
➤ Advances in Human Factors - Ergonomics (NLD ISSN 0921-2647) **4372**, 4069
• ➤ Advances in Human Genetics (USA ISSN 0065-275X) **3297**
• ➤ Advances in Immunology (USA ISSN 0065-2776) **3739**
➤ Advances in Infancy Research (USA ISSN 0732-9598) **4039**, 4373
➤ Advances in Inflammation Research (USA ISSN 0197-8322) **3560**
• Advances in Internal Medicine (USA ISSN 0065-2822) **3907**
Advances in Laser Medicine (DEU) **4140**
➤ Advances in Learning and Behavioral Disabilities (USA ISSN 0735-004X) **3418**, 3380, 4373
Advances in Lectin Research (USA ISSN 0941-3472) **3240**
Advances in Life Course Research (USA) **3466**, 4510
Advances in Life Sciences (CHE) **3179**
Advances in Lipobiology (USA) **3240**
➤ Advances in M R I - Contrast (Magnetic Resonance Imaging) (NLD ISSN 0925-9848) **4140**, 3809
• ➤ Advances in Marine Biology (USA ISSN 0065-2881) **3179**, 3408
➤ Advances in Medical Social Science (CHE ISSN 0275-5742) **4508**, 3560
Advances in Medical Sociology (USA ISSN 1057-6290) **4519**, 3560
Advances in Medicinal Chemistry (USA ISSN 1067-5698) **3560**, 3371
Advances in Mental Retardation and Developmental Disabilities (USA ISSN 0742-6313) **3418**, 4069
Advances in Metabolic Disorders *see* Advances in Metabolism **3855**
➤ Advances in Metabolism (USA) **3855**
• ➤ Advances in Microbial Ecology (USA ISSN 0147-4863) **3316**
• ➤ Advances in Microbial Physiology (USA ISSN 0065-2911) **3317**
• Advances in Mind - Body Medicine (GBR ISSN 1470-3556) **3560**, 3162
➤ Advances in Modern Biotechnology/Avances en Biotecnologia Moderna (CUB ISSN 1027-2860) **3268**
Advances in Molecular Biology *see* Uspehi na Moleculiarnata Biologia **3223**
Advances in Motivation and Achievement (USA ISSN 0749-7423) **4373**
➤ Advances in Motor Development Research (USA ISSN 0888-9287) **4349**, 3380, 3466
➤ Advances in Natural and Technological Hazards Research (NLD) **4460**, 4223, 4531
Advances in Nephrology (USA) **4209**
Advances in Nephrology from the Necker Hospital *see* Advances in Nephrology **4209**
Advances in Neural Science (USA ISSN 1074-7575) **4069**
➤ Advances in Neurochemistry (USA ISSN 0098-6089) **3240**, 4069
Advances in Neurological Sciences *see* Shinkei Kenkyu no Shinpo **4133**
• ➤ Advances in Neurology (USA ISSN 0091-3952) **4069**
➤ Advances in Neuropsychiatry and Psychopharmacology (USA ISSN 1057-6592) **4070**, 4274
➤ Advances in Neuroscience (USA ISSN 1059-1540) **4070**
Advances in Neurotrauma Research (JPN ISSN 0916-698X) **4070**, 4179
Advances in Noise Research (GBR) **4029**, 3443, 3488, 4249
• ➤ Advances in Nursing Science (USA ISSN 0161-9268) **3912**
• ➤ Advances in Nutritional Research (USA ISSN 0149-9483) **4228**
Advances in Occupational Ergonomics and Safety (NLD ISSN 1384-2269) **4249**, 3431, 4058
Advances in Occupational Medicine & Rehabilitation/Aggiornamenti in Medicina Occupazionale e Riabilitazione (ITA ISSN 1123-8364) **4249**, 4058
Advances in Oncobiology (USA) **3966**
Advances in Oncology (USA) **3966**
Advances in Organ Biology (NLD) **3337**
• ➤ Advances in Oto-Rhino-Laryngology (CHE ISSN 0065-3071) **4029**
Advances in Otolaryngology - Head and Neck Surgery (USA ISSN 0887-6916) **4029**, 4179
• ➤ Advances in Pain Research and Therapy (USA ISSN 0146-0722) **4070**, 3560
Advances in Pediatrics (USA ISSN 0065-3101) **4039**
Advances in Perinatal Medicine (USA ISSN 0731-1400) **3944**
• ➤ Advances in Pharmaceutical Sciences (USA ISSN 0065-3136) **4274**
Advances in Pharmacological Sciences (CHE) **4274**
➤ Advances in Pharmacology (USA ISSN 1054-3589) **4274**
Advances in Pharmacology and Chemotherapy *see* Advances in Pharmacology **4274**
• ➤ Advances in Physiology Education (USA ISSN 1043-4046) **3337**, 3409
Advances in Physiology Education Online *see* Advances in Physiology Education **3337**, 3409
▼ • Advances in Physiotherapy (NOR ISSN 1403-8196) **4058**
Advances in Plastic and Reconstructive Surgery *see* Key Issues in Plastic and Cosmetic Surgery **4196**
• ➤ Advances in Prostaglandin, Thromboxane, and Leukotriene Research (USA ISSN 0732-8141) **4274**
• ➤ Advances in Protein Chemistry (USA ISSN 0065-3233) **3240**
• Advances in Psychiatric Treatment (GBR ISSN 1355-5146) **4070**
Advances in Psychiatric Treatment Online *see* Advances in Psychiatric Treatment **4070**
➤ Advances in Psychology (NLD ISSN 0166-4115) **4373**
• ➤ Advances in Psychosomatic Medicine (CHE ISSN 0065-3268) **4070**
➤ Advances in Regulation of Cell Growth Series (USA ISSN 1053-9506) **3179**
Advances in Rehabilitation *see* Postepy Rehabilitacji **4065**
• Advances in Renal Replacement Therapy (USA ISSN 1073-4449) **4209**, 4179
Advances in Reproductive Endocrinology (GBR ISSN 1362-9670) **3855**
➤ Advances in Reproductive Health Care (NLD) **3944**, 4209
➤ Advances in Risk Analysis (USA) **4494**, 4527
• ➤ Advances in Second Messenger and Phosphoprotein Research (USA ISSN 1040-7952) **3240**
• ➤ Advances in Skin and Wound Care (USA ISSN 1527-7941) **3844**
➤ Advances in Small Animal Medicine and Surgery (USA ISSN 1041-7826) **4535**
Advances in Stroke *see* Current Medical Literature. Advances in Stroke **3720**, 3770

Title

Title

AIDS Surveillance in Europe. Quarterly Report *see* HIV - AIDS Surveillance in Europe. **3797**
• AIDS Therapies (USA) **3792**, 4460
• AIDS Treatment Data Network Information Bulletin (USA) **3792**
AIDS Treatment Update (GBR ISSN 0969-4706) **3792**, 4275
AIDS Weekly *see* AIDS Weekly Plus **3792**, 3180, 3361, 4460
• AIDS Weekly Plus (USA) **3792**, 3180, 3361, 4460
AIDS (Year) (GBR ISSN 1350-2840) **3715**, 3792
• AIDSearch (USA) **3715**, 3145
AIDSida Info (USA) **3527**, 3457, 3792
Aiiku Tsushin/Letters of Human Growth (JPN) **3409**, 4373
Ain Shams Medical Journal (EGY ISSN 0002-2144) **3561**
Air Ambulance Handbook *see* Shephard's Air Ambulance Handbook **4532**, 4025
➤ Air Medical Journal (USA ISSN 1067-991X) **3561**, 3153
Aira County Medical Association. Journal *see* Airagun Ishikai Igakkaishi **3561**
Airagun Ishikai Igakkaishi/Aira County Medical Association. Journal (JPN ISSN 0917-9267) **3561**
Airone (ITA) **3180**
Airone Junio *see* Do Do **3193**, 3386
Airwave (CAN ISSN 1187-9106) **4158**
• Aizheng/Chinese Journal of Cancer (CHN ISSN 1000-467X) **3966**
Akademia Rolnicza we Wroclawiu. Zeszyty Naukowe. Weterynaria (POL ISSN 0137-1975) **4535**
Akademie fuer Oeffentliches Gesundheitswesen. Schriftenreihe (DEU ISSN 0172-2131) **4460**
Akademiya Meditsinskikh Nauk S.S.S.R. Vestnik *see* Rossiiskaya Akademiya Meditsinskikh Nauk. Vestnik **3687**
➤ Akademiya Medychnykh Nauk Ukrainy. Zhurnal (UKR) **3561**
Akademiya Nauk Gruzinskoi S.S.R. Izvestiya. Seriya Biologicheskaya (GEO) **3180**
Akademiya Nauk Kazakhskoi S.S.R. Izvestiya. Seriya Biologicheskaya *see* Akademiya Nauk Kazakhstana. Izvestiya. Seriya Biologicheskaya **3180**
Akademiya Nauk Kazakhstana. Izvestiya. Seriya Biologicheskaya (KAZ) **3180**
Akademiya Nauk S.S.S.R. Doklady *see* Rossiiskaya Akademiya Nauk. Doklady **4507**
Akademiya Nauk S.S.S.R. Izvestiya. Seriya Biologicheskaya *see* Rossiiskaya Akademiya Nauk. Izvestiya. Seriya Biologicheskaya **3216**
Akademiya Nauk Turkmenistana. Izvestiya. Seriya Biologicheskikh Nauk (TKM) **3180**
Akademiya Nauk Turkmenskoi S.S.R. Izvestiya. Seriya Biologicheskikh Nauk *see* Akademiya Nauk Turkmenistana. Izvestiya. Seriya Biologicheskikh Nauk **3180**
Akademiya Navuk Belarusskai S.S.R. Doklady *see* Nationalnaya Akademiya Navuk Belarusi. Doklady **4506**
Akademiya Zdorov'ya (UKR) **3562**
Akahige/Takko Town Hospital. Annual Report (JPN ISSN 0911-1549) **3501**
➤ Akita Igaku/Akita Journal of Medicine (JPN ISSN 0386-6106) **3562**
Akita Journal of Medicine *see* Akita Igaku **3562**
Akita Journal of Obstetricians and Gynecologists *see* Akita Sanfujinka Iho **3944**
Akita Journal of Rural Medicine/Akitaken Noson Igakkai Zasshi (JPN ISSN 0002-368X) **3562**
Akita Medical Journal *see* Akitaken Ishikai Zasshi **3562**
Akita Sanfujinka Iho/Akita Journal of Obstetricians and Gynecologists (JPN) **3944**
Akitaken Ishikai Zasshi/Akita Medical Journal (JPN ISSN 0286-7656) **3562**
Akitaken Noson Igakkai Zasshi *see* Akita Journal of Rural Medicine **3562**
• Akos - Encyclopedie Pratique de Medecine (FRA ISSN 1293-2973) **3562**
Akron Dental Society. Bulletin (USA ISSN 0002-3701) **3814**
Aktion Jugendschutz. Informationen (DEU ISSN 0720-3551) **3380**, 3397
Aktiv (AUT) **4349**, 4228
Aktuell Optik och Optometri (SWE ISSN 0348-5730) **3993**
Aktuell Sikkerhet (NOR ISSN 0808-6567) **4249**
Aktuelle Chirurgie *see* Viszeralchirurgie **4207**
• ➤ Aktuelle Dermatologie (DEU ISSN 0340-2541) **3844**
• Aktuelle Ernaehrungsmedizin (DEU ISSN 0341-0501) **4228**, 3562
Aktuelle Immunologie (DEU ISSN 0931-2579) **3739**
• ➤ Aktuelle Neurologie (DEU ISSN 0302-4350) **4070**
Aktuelle Onkologie (DEU ISSN 0174-2744) **3967**
Aktuelle Radiologie *see* RoeFo. Fortschritte auf dem Gebiet der Roentgenstrahlen und der bildgebenden Verfahren **4155**
• ➤ Aktuelle Rheumatologie (DEU ISSN 0341-051X) **4166**
• Aktuelle Traumatologie (DEU ISSN 0044-6173) **4009**
• ➤ Aktuelle Urologie (DEU ISSN 0001-7868) **4209**
Aktuellt (SWE) **3397**, 4275
Akupunktur: Theorie und Praxis (DEU ISSN 0340-3130) **3163**, 3562
Der Akupunkturarzt - Aurikulotherapeut (DEU ISSN 0172-9322) **3562**
Akusherstvo i Ginekologiya/Obstetrics and Gynecology (RUS ISSN 0300-9092) **3944**
The Akwa Letter (USA) **4349**, 4221, 4562
Al-Ahram Medical Guide *see* Dalil al-Ahram al-Tibbi **3592**
Al-Anon Speaks Out (USA ISSN 1054-1446) **3397**
Al-Magallat al-Iskandiriyyah li-Tibb al-Asnan *see* Alexandria Dental Journal **3814**
Al-Majallah Al-Misriyyah li-Jirahat al-'Itham *see* Egyptian Orthopaedic Journal **4013**
Al-Majallah al-Misriyyah li-Ulum al-Aghdhiya *see* Egyptian Journal of Food Science **3460**
Al-Majallah al-Tibbiyyah *see* United Arab Emirates. Al-Qiyadah al-Aamah lil-Quwwat al-Musallihah. Majallah al-Tibbiyyah **3704**, 4224
➤ Alabama Counseling Association. Journal (USA) **4269**, 4373, 4510
Alabama Epic (USA) **3562**
Alabama Medicine *see* M A S A Review **3644**
Alabama Nurse (USA ISSN 0002-4317) **3913**
Alabama's Health (USA ISSN 0145-6857) **4460**
Alam Tib al-Asnan *see* Arab Dental **3815**
Alameda-Contra Costa Medical Association. Bulletin (USA ISSN 0002-4414) **3562**
Alaska. Department of Health and Social Services. Division of Alcoholism and Drug Abuse. Report (USA) **3397**
Alaska. Department of Health and Social Services. Office of Alcoholism. Report *see* Alaska. Department of Health and Social Services. Division of Alcoholism and Drug Abuse. Report **3397**
➤ Alaska Medicine (USA ISSN 0002-4538) **3562**
Alaska Nurse (USA ISSN 0002-4546) **3913**
Alateen Talk (USA ISSN 1054-1411) **3386**, 3397, 3495
• Albert Hofmann's Strange Mistake (USA) **3870**
Alberta Council on Aging News *see* A C A News **3465**, 4510
Alberta Dental Association. Updater (CAN) **3814**
Alberta Health Records Association Record *see* A H R A Record **3555**, 3500
Alberta R N (Registered Nurses) (CAN ISSN 1481-9988) **3913**
➤ Alces (CAN ISSN 0835-5851) **3350**
• ➤ Alcohol & Alcoholism (GBR ISSN 0735-0414) **3397**
Alcohol and Other Drugs *see* Alkohol och Narkotika **3399**
Alcohol, Drug Abuse, and Mental Health Administration News *see* A D A M H A News **3396**, 4371
Alcohol Health & Research World *see* Alcohol Research & Health **3398**
Alcohol Issues Insights (USA ISSN 1067-3105) **3176**, 3397, 3536
• ➤ Alcohol (New York) (USA ISSN 0741-8329) **3398**
• ➤ Alcohol Research & Health (USA) **3398**
• ➤ Alcoholism (HRV ISSN 0002-502X) **3398**
• Alcoholism & Drug Abuse Weekly (USA ISSN 1042-1394) **3398**
• ➤ Alcoholism: Clinical and Experimental Research (USA ISSN 0145-6008) **3398**
➤ Alcoholism. Supplement (HRV ISSN 1330-6170) **3398**
➤ Alcoholism Treatment Quarterly (USA ISSN 0734-7324) **3398**
Alcologia (ITA ISSN 0394-9826) **3398**
Alcool ou Sante (FRA ISSN 0002-5054) **3398**
Alcoologie *see* Alcoologie et Addictologie **3398**
Alcoologie et Addictologie (FRA ISSN 1620-4522) **3398**
Aldring og Eldre (NOR ISSN 0801-9991) **3467**
➤ Alergia (MEX ISSN 0002-5151) **3739**
Alergologija i Klinicka Imunologija (YUG ISSN 0354-3978) **3739**
Alert (NLD ISSN 0920-3168) **3387**, 4460, 4510
➤ Alert (Adelaide) (AUS ISSN 0706-1870) **3855**, 4510
Alert (Ewing) (USA) **3398**, 3488, 4510
Alerte au S I D A Oceanie *see* Pacific AIDS Alert Bulletin **3804**
Alexandria Dental Journal/Al-Magallat al-Iskandiriyyah li-Tibb al-Asnan (EGY) **3814**
Alexandria Faculty of Medicine Bulletin *see* University of Alexandria. Faculty of Medicine. Bulletin **3705**
Alexandria Medical Journal (EGY ISSN 0516-5849) **3562**
Alfred Benzon Symposium. Proceedings (DNK ISSN 0105-3639) **3337**
Algologia (ITA ISSN 0392-9116) **4070**, 3761
Algological Studies (DEU ISSN 0342-1120) **3180**, 3278, 3408
Alimarket. No Alimentacion (ESP ISSN 1139-6903) **4228**
Alimentacion Nutricion y Agricultura *see* Food Nutrition and Agriculture **4233**
Alimentacion, Nutricion y Salud (ESP ISSN 1136-4815) **4228**, 3459
Alimentacion y Nutricion *see* Food Nutrition and Agriculture **4233**
• ➤ Alimentary Pharmacology and Therapeutics (GBR ISSN 0269-2813) **3886**
• Alimentary Pharmacology and Therapeutics. Supplement (GBR ISSN 0953-0673) **3886**
Alimentation et la Vie *see* Alimentation et la Vie - Nouvelle Presentation **4228**
Alimentation et la Vie - Nouvelle Presentation (FRA) **4228**
Alimentation Nutrition et Agriculture *see* Food Nutrition and Agriculture **4233**
Alimentazione Nutrizione Metabolismo (ITA ISSN 0392-7512) **4228**
➤ Alimentos e Nutricao (BRA ISSN 0103-4235) **4228**, 3459
Aliments du Pacifique Sud *see* South Pacific Foods Leaflet **3462**, 4246
➤ Alive (CAN ISSN 0228-586X) **4350**, 4228
➤ The Alkaloids (USA ISSN 0099-9598) **3377**, 4275
Alkohol och Narkotika/Alcohol and Other Drugs (SWE ISSN 0345-0732) **3399**
All About AIDS *see* AIDSearch **3715**, 3145
All About Issues *see* Celebrate Life (Stafford) **3357**, 4369
All about Medicare (USA ISSN 1044-9426) **3530**, 4510
All about Weight Loss, Health, and Fitness *see* Greg Landry's Fitness Newsletter **4354**
All India Institute of Speech and Hearing. Journal (IND ISSN 0377-0524) **3488**, 3419
All India Ophthalmological Society. Proceedings *see* Indian Ophthalmology - Year Book **3998**
All Natural Muscular Development *see* Muscular Development **4358**, 4525
Allegheny County Medical Society. Bulletin (USA ISSN 0098-3772) **3562**
Allegheny County Pharmacist (USA ISSN 0002-5690) **4275**
(Year) Allen D. Leman Swine Conference. Proceedings (USA) **4535**
Allergia (SWE ISSN 0002-5747) **3739**
Allergic Disease and Therapy (USA ISSN 1053-1092) **3739**
Allergie et Immunologie (FRA ISSN 0397-9148) **3739**
Allergie Konkret (DEU) **3739**
➤ Allergo Journal (DEU ISSN 0941-8849) **3739**
• ➤ Allergologia et Immunopathologia/International Journal for Clinical and Investigative Allergology and Clinical Immunology (ESP ISSN 0301-0546) **3739**
• ➤ Allergologie (DEU ISSN 0344-5062) **3739**
Allergology & Immunology *see* Arerugi, Men'eki **3740**
• ➤ Allergology International (AUS ISSN 1323-8930) **3739**
• ➤ Allergy (DNK ISSN 0105-4538) **3739**
Allergy & Asthma Advocate (USA) **3740**, 4158
▼ Allergy and Asthma Health (USA) **3740**
• ➤ Allergy and Asthma Proceedings (USA ISSN 1088-5412) **3740**
• ➤ Allergy & Clinical Immunology International (USA) **3740**
Allergy and Clinical Immunology News *see* Allergy & Clinical Immunology International **3740**
Allergy Hotline (USA) **3740**, 3459
Allergy Proceedings *see* Allergy and Asthma Proceedings **3740**
• Allergy. Supplementum (DNK ISSN 0108-1675) **3740**
Allevatore (ITA) **4535**
Der Allgemeinarzt (DEU ISSN 0172-7249) **3562**
Allgemeine Homoeopathische Zeitung (DEU ISSN 0002-5887) **3785**
Alliance (Charleston) (USA) **3387**, 3562
• Alliance (Wisconsin) (USA) **4070**
Allied and Complementary Medicine *see* A M E D **3171**, 3145, 3714
Allied Health and Rehabilitation Professions Education Directory *see* Health Professions Career and Education Directory **3612**, 3416
Allied Health Education Directory *see* Health Professions Career and Education Directory **3612**, 3416
Allied Health Trends *see* Trends (Washington, 1969) **4491**
Allt om Hjaelpmedel (SWE ISSN 1103-8063) **3483**
Almshouses Gazette (GBR) **4510**, 3467
Aloe, Cactus & Succulent Society of Zimbabwe. Ingens Bulletin (ZWE ISSN 1016-524X) **3278**, 3464
Alon Lemoreh Habiologia/Pamphlet for Biology Teachers (ISR ISSN 0333-9815) **3180**
➤ Alpe Adria Microbiology Journal (ITA ISSN 1121-9750) **3317**, 3792
Alpha Omegan (USA ISSN 0002-6417) **3814**
• Alt-Health Watch (USA) **3171**, 3145
Altenburger Naturwissenschaftliche Forschungen (DEU ISSN 0232-5381) **3180**, 3407, 4271
Altenheim (DEU ISSN 0002-6573) **3913**
Altenhilfe *see* Informationsdienst Altersfragen **3474**, 4513
Altenpflege (DEU ISSN 0341-0455) **3913**
Alternativ Medicin (SWE ISSN 1100-7079) **3163**, 3785
• Alternative & Complementary Therapies (USA ISSN 1076-2809) **3163**
Alternative Health Practitioner *see* Complementary Health Practice Review **3164**, 3787
Alternative Medicine Alert (USA) **3163**
Alternative Medicine Digest *see* Alternative Medicine Magazine **3163**
Alternative Medicine Magazine (USA) **3163**
➤ Alternative Medicine Review (USA ISSN 1089-5159) **3163**
▼ Alternative Medicine Sourcebook (USA) **3163**
• ➤ Alternative Therapies in Health and Medicine (USA ISSN 1078-6791) **3163**
Alternatives for the Health Conscious Individual *see* Alternatives (Ingram) **3562**
Alternatives (Ingram) (USA ISSN 0893-5025) **3562**
• ➤ Alternatives to Laboratory Animals (GBR ISSN 0261-1929) **3870**
• Altex (DEU ISSN 0946-7785) **3870**, 3171
Altlasten - Spektrum (DEU ISSN 0942-3818) **3456**, 3445
Altschul Symposia Series (USA) **3562**
Alumnae Magazine *see* The Academic Nurse **3912**
Alumnus (New York) (USA) **4009**, 3388
• ➤ Alzheimer Disease and Associated Disorders (USA ISSN 0893-0341) **4070**, 3467
Alzheimerfoereningen (SWE ISSN 1100-0899) **4070**
Alzheimer's Association Newsletter *see* Advances (Chicago) **4069**, 3466, 4519
Alzheimer's Care Guide (USA ISSN 1070-5112) **3467**, 4070, 4510
▼ Alzheimer's Care Quarterly (USA ISSN 1525-3279) **4070**, 4510
• ➤ Alzheimer's Disease Review (USA) **4071**
Alzheimer's Disease Sourcebook (USA) **4071**, 3467
Alzheimer's Home Companion (USA) **3467**
Alzheimers News (NZL ISSN 1173-4361) **4071**
• ➤ Alzheimer's Reports (GBR ISSN 1461-6130) **4071**
Alzheimer's Research Review (USA) **4071**, 4510
Alzheimer's, Stroke and 29 Other Neurological Disorders *see* Alzheimer's Disease Sourcebook **4071**, 3467
Am F A R Annual Report *see* A F A R Annual Report **3790**
Amakusa Marine Biological Laboratory. Publications (JPN ISSN 0065-6682) **3180**
• ➤ Amazoniana (DEU ISSN 0065-6755) **3180**
Ambiente e Sicurezza sul Lavoro (ITA ISSN 0393-7054) **4249**
Ambiente Energia Lavoro (ITA ISSN 1122-4991) **4461**

Title

Title

Blind and Visually Impaired Persons in the United States and Canada **3495**
American Foundation for the Blind Press News *see* A F B News **3495**, 4510
• American Fund for Alternatives to Animal Research. News Abstracts (USA ISSN 1526-2499) **4536**
American Gastroenterological Association News *see* A G A News **3885**
• ➤ American Geriatrics Society. Journal (USA ISSN 0002-8614) **3467**
American Geriatrics Society Newsletter (USA) **3467**
➤ American Group Psychotherapy Monograph Series (USA ISSN 0742-3187) **4374**
American Handwriting Analysis Foundation Journal *see* A H A F Journal **4371**
• American Health (USA ISSN 1523-3359) **4350**
American Health Care Association. Journal *see* American Health Care Association. Provider **4510**, 4461
American Health Care Association Notes *see* A H C A Notes **4510**, 4460
• American Health Care Association. Provider (USA ISSN 0888-0352) **4510**, 4461
American Health Consultants. Phase III Report (USA) **4275**
American Health for Women *see* American Health **4350**
American Health Information Management Association. Journal (USA ISSN 1060-5487) **3563**
• American Health Line (USA) **4461**
American Healthcare Radiology Administrators Link *see* A H R A Link **4139**
➤ American Heart Association. Scientific Sessions. Abstracts (USA ISSN 0065-8502) **3715**, 3761
• ➤ American Heart Journal (USA ISSN 0002-8703) **3762**
American Heartworm Society. Bulletin (USA) **4536**
American Heartworm Society. Symposium Proceedings (USA ISSN 1053-5608) **4536**
American Herb Association Newsletter (USA) **3464**, 4275
American Hippotherapy Association News *see* A H A News **3483**
American Holistic Veterinary Medical Association. Journal (USA) **4536**
American Holistic Veterinary Medical Association. Newsletter *see* American Holistic Veterinary Medical Association. Journal **4536**
American Hospital Association Guide to the Health Care Field *see* A H A Guide to the Health Care Field **3524**, 4460
American Hospital Association Hospital Statistics (Year) *see* A H A Hospital Statistics (Year) **3524**, 4527
American Hospital Association News *see* A H A News **3500**
American Hospital Formulary Service Drug Information *see* A H F S Drug Information **4273**
• ➤ American Imago (USA ISSN 0065-860X) **4071**, 3552, 3552, 4374
• ➤ American Indian and Alaska Native Mental Health Research (USA ISSN 0893-5394) **4226**, 3457, 4374
American Industrial Hygiene Association. Conference Abstracts (USA) **4268**
American Industrial Hygiene Association Journal *see* A I H A J **4249**
American Institute for Cancer Research Newsletter (USA ISSN 1044-4580) **3967**, 4228
American Institute for Ultrasound in Medicine Reporter *see* A I U M Reporter **4139**, 3236, 3943
American Institute of Gerontology and Human Development. Brookdale Institute of Gerontology and Human Development. Discussion Papers *see* American Institute of Gerontology and Human Development. Brookdale Institute of Gerontology and Human Development. Research Reports **3467**, 4374
American Institute of Gerontology and Human Development. Brookdale Institute of Gerontology and Human Development. Research Reports (ISR) **3467**, 4374
American Institute of Homeopathy. Journal (USA ISSN 0002-8967) **3786**
American Institute of Stress. Newsletter *see* Health and Stress **3610**, 4221, 4563
American Institute of the History of Pharmacy Notes *see* A I H P Notes **4273**, 3526
American Institute of the History of Pharmacy. Publications (USA ISSN 0270-0611) **4275**
American Institute of Ultrasound in Medicine. Annual Scientific Conference. Proceedings (USA) **4140**
American International Journal of Arts, Sciences, Engineering and Medicine (IRL ISSN 0743-0884) **3175**, 3431, 3563
➤ American Journal of Acupuncture (USA ISSN 0091-3960) **3163**, 3563
American Journal of Alzheimer's Care and Related Disorders and Research *see* American Journal of Alzheimer's Disease **3467**
➤ American Journal of Alzheimer's Disease (USA ISSN 1082-5207) **3467**
American Journal of Anatomy *see* Developmental Dynamics **3193**, 3594
The American Journal of Anesthesiology (USA ISSN 1078-4500) **3753**
• ➤ American Journal of Art Therapy (USA ISSN 0007-4764) **4058**, 3175, 3419
• American Journal of Audiology (USA ISSN 1059-0889) **3488**
American Journal of Bariatric Medicine *see* Bariatrician **3908**, 3855
• ➤ The American Journal of Cardiology (USA ISSN 0002-9149) **3762**
▼ • American Journal of Cardiovascular Drugs (NZL ISSN 1175-3277) **3762**, 4275
• ➤ American Journal of Cardiovascular Pathology (USA ISSN 0887-8005) **3762**
• ➤ The American Journal of Chinese Medicine (USA ISSN 0192-415X) **3715**, 3163
▼ • ➤ American Journal of Clinical Dermatology (USA ISSN 1175-0561) **3844**
• ➤ American Journal of Clinical Hypnosis (USA ISSN 0002-9157) **3906**
• ➤ American Journal of Clinical Nutrition (USA ISSN 0002-9165) **4228**, 3563
• ➤ American Journal of Clinical Oncology (USA ISSN 0277-3732) **3967**
• ➤ American Journal of Clinical Pathology (USA ISSN 0002-9173) **3563**, 3180
• ➤ American Journal of Community Psychology (USA ISSN 0091-0562) **4520**, 4374
• ➤ American Journal of Contact Dermatitis (USA ISSN 1046-199X) **3844**
➤ American Journal of Cosmetic Surgery (USA ISSN 0748-8068) **4180**
• ➤ American Journal of Critical Care (USA ISSN 1062-3264) **3913**, 4010
• ➤ American Journal of Dance Therapy (USA ISSN 0146-3721) **3396**, 4374
• ➤ American Journal of Dentistry (USA ISSN 0894-8275) **3814**
• ➤ American Journal of Dermatopathology (USA ISSN 0193-1091) **3563**, 3844
• ➤ American Journal of Drug and Alcohol Abuse (USA ISSN 0095-2990) **3399**
American Journal of E E G Technology *see* American Journal of Electroneurodiagnostic Technology **4071**
➤ American Journal of Electromedicine (USA ISSN 0894-8291) **3563**
• ➤ American Journal of Electroneurodiagnostic Technology (USA ISSN 1086-508X) **4071**
• ➤ American Journal of Emergency Medicine (USA ISSN 0735-6757) **4010**, 3871
• ➤ American Journal of Epidemiology (USA ISSN 0002-9262) **3563**
• ➤ American Journal of Family Therapy (USA ISSN 0192-6187) **4374**, 4520
• ➤ American Journal of Forensic Medicine and Pathology (USA ISSN 0195-7910) **3881**
➤ American Journal of Forensic Psychiatry (USA ISSN 0163-1942) **3881**, 3536, 4071
➤ American Journal of Forensic Psychology (USA ISSN 0733-1290) **4374**, 3536
• ➤ American Journal of Gastroenterology (NLD ISSN 0002-9270) **3886**
➤ American Journal of Geriatric Cardiology (USA ISSN 1076-7460) **3762**, 3468
• ➤ American Journal of Geriatric Psychiatry (USA ISSN 1064-7481) **3468**, 4071
• ➤ American Journal of Health Behavior (USA ISSN 1087-3244) **4350**
• ➤ American Journal of Health Promotion (USA ISSN 0890-1171) **4461**, 4228, 4350
• ➤ American Journal of Health-System Pharmacy (USA ISSN 1079-2082) **4275**, 3501
• ➤ American Journal of Hematology (USA ISSN 0361-8609) **3897**
➤ The American Journal of Hospice and Palliative Care (USA ISSN 1049-9091) **3564**, 3468
American Journal of Hospital Pharmacy *see* American Journal of Health-System Pharmacy **4275**, 3501
• ➤ American Journal of Human Biology (USA ISSN 1042-0533) **3180**
• ➤ American Journal of Human Genetics (USA ISSN 0002-9297) **3297**
• ➤ American Journal of Hypertension (USA ISSN 0895-7061) **3762**
American Journal of Hypertension. Edicion en Espanol (ESP) **3762**
• ➤ American Journal of Industrial Medicine (USA ISSN 0271-3586) **4249**
• ➤ American Journal of Infection Control (USA ISSN 0196-6553) **3792**
• ➤ American Journal of Kidney Diseases (USA ISSN 0272-6386) **4209**, 3284, 3855, 3898
• ➤ American Journal of Knee Surgery (USA ISSN 0899-7403) **4180**, 4058, 4172
• ➤ American Journal of Law & Medicine (USA ISSN 0098-8588) **3536**, 3564
• ➤ The American Journal of Managed Care (USA ISSN 1096-1860) **3564**
American Journal of Managed Healthcare *see* The American Journal of Managed Care **3564**
American Journal of Maternal Child Nursing *see* M C N: American Journal of Maternal Child Nursing **3928**
• ➤ American Journal of Medical Genetics (USA ISSN 0148-7299) **3298**, 3564
American Journal of Medical Genetics. Supplement (USA ISSN 1040-3787) **3298**, 3564
• ➤ The American Journal of Medicine (USA ISSN 0002-9343) **3564**
▼ ➤ American Journal of Medicine and Sports (USA ISSN 1524-2196) **4172**
American Journal of Natural Medicine *see* The International Journal of Integrative Medicine **3167**
• ➤ American Journal of Nephrology (CHE ISSN 0250-8095) **4209**
American Journal of Neuroradiology *see* A J N R **4139**
• ➤ American Journal of Nursing (USA ISSN 0002-936X) **3913**
American Journal of Nursing Co. Guide *see* A J N Guide **3912**
• ➤ American Journal of Obstetrics and Gynecology (USA ISSN 0002-9378) **3944**
• ➤ American Journal of Occupational Therapy (USA ISSN 0272-9490) **4250**, 3564
• ➤ American Journal of Ophthalmology (USA ISSN 0002-9394) **3993**
American Journal of Optometry and Physiological Optics *see* Optometry and Vision Science **4005**
• ➤ American Journal of Orthodontics and Dentofacial Orthopedics (USA ISSN 0889-5406) **3814**
➤ The American Journal of Orthopedics (USA ISSN 1078-4519) **4010**
• ➤ American Journal of Orthopsychiatry (USA ISSN 0002-9432) **4374**, 3380, 4510
• ➤ American Journal of Otolaryngology (USA ISSN 0196-0709) **4030**
American Journal of Otology *see* Otology & Neurotology **4036**
➤ American Journal of Pain Management (USA ISSN 1059-1494) **3564**
➤ American Journal of Pastoral Counseling (USA ISSN 1094-6098) **4374**, 4499
• ➤ American Journal of Pathology (USA ISSN 0002-9440) **3564**
The American Journal of Pathology, Part B *see* The Journal of Molecular Diagnostics **3636**
American Journal of Pediatric Hematology - Oncology *see* Journal of Pediatric Hematology - Oncology **3982**, 3903, 4047
• ➤ American Journal of Perinatology (USA ISSN 0735-1631) **3944**
• ➤ American Journal of Pharmaceutical Education (USA ISSN 0002-9459) **4275**, 3417
▼ • American Journal of PharmacoGenomics (NZL ISSN 1175-2203) **3298**, 3240, 3268
American Journal of Physical Medicine *see* American Journal of Physical Medicine and Rehabilitation **4058**
• ➤ American Journal of Physical Medicine and Rehabilitation (USA ISSN 0894-9115) **4058**
• ➤ American Journal of Physiology: Cell Physiology (USA ISSN 0363-6143) **3337**, 3284
• ➤ American Journal of Physiology (Consolidated) (USA ISSN 0002-9513) **3337**, 3564
• ➤ American Journal of Physiology: Endocrinology and Metabolism (USA ISSN 0193-1849) **3338**, 3855
• ➤ American Journal of Physiology: Gastrointestinal and Liver Physiology (USA ISSN 0193-1857) **3338**, 3886
• ➤ American Journal of Physiology: Heart and Circulatory Physiology (USA ISSN 0363-6135) **3338**, 3762
• ➤ American Journal of Physiology: Lung Cellular and Molecular Physiology (USA ISSN 1040-0605) **3338**, 3240, 3285
• ➤ American Journal of Physiology: Regulatory, Integrative and Comparative Physiology (USA ISSN 0363-6119) **3338**
American Journal of Physiology: Renal, Fluid and Electrolyte Physiology *see* American Journal of Physiology: Renal Physiology **3339**, 4209
• ➤ American Journal of Physiology: Renal Physiology (USA) **3339**, 4209
• ➤ American Journal of Preventive Medicine (USA ISSN 0749-3797) **3564**, 4461
• ➤ American Journal of Primatology (USA ISSN 0275-2565) **3350**, 3172, 4374, 4536
• ➤ American Journal of Psychiatry (USA ISSN 0002-953X) **4071**
• ➤ American Journal of Psychoanalysis (USA ISSN 0002-9548) **4374**, 4072
• ➤ American Journal of Psychology (USA ISSN 0002-9556) **4374**
• ➤ American Journal of Psychotherapy (USA ISSN 0002-9564) **4072**
• ➤ American Journal of Public Health (USA ISSN 0090-0036) **4461**
• ➤ American Journal of Reproductive Immunology (DNK ISSN 1046-7408) **3740**, 3945
• American Journal of Reproductive Immunology Online (DNK ISSN 1600-0897) **3740**, 3945
• ➤ American Journal of Respiratory and Critical Care Medicine (USA ISSN 1073-449X) **4158**
• ➤ American Journal of Respiratory Cell and Molecular Biology (USA ISSN 1044-1549) **4158**
• ➤ American Journal of Rhinology (USA ISSN 1050-6586) **4030**
American Journal of Roentgenology *see* A J R **4139**
• American Journal of Speech - Language Pathology (USA ISSN 1058-0360) **3489**, 3550, 3564
• ➤ American Journal of Sports Medicine (USA ISSN 0363-5465) **4172**
• ➤ American Journal of Surgery (USA ISSN 0002-9610) **4180**
• ➤ American Journal of Surgical Pathology (USA ISSN 0147-5185) **3564**, 4180
American Journal of Surgical Pathology. Part B: Diagnostic Molecular Pathology *see* Diagnostic Molecular Pathology **3594**
• ➤ American Journal of the Medical Sciences (USA ISSN 0002-9629) **3564**
• ➤ American Journal of Therapeutics (GBR ISSN 1075-2765) **3565**, 4275
➤ American Journal of Therapy (USA) **3565**
▼ • ➤ American Journal of Transplantation (DNK ISSN 1600-6135) **4180**, 3740
▼ • ➤ American Journal of Transplantation Online (DNK ISSN 1600-6143) **4180**, 3740
• ➤ American Journal of Tropical Medicine and Hygiene (USA ISSN 0002-9637) **3792**
• ➤ American Journal of Veterinary Research (USA ISSN 0002-9645) **4536**
• ➤ American Journal on Addictions (USA ISSN 1055-0496) **3399**, 4072
• ➤ American Journal on Mental Retardation (USA ISSN 0895-8017) **4072**
American Kennel Club Puppies (USA) **4272**
American Kidney Fund. Annual Report (USA) **4209**
American Laryngological Association. Transactions (USA) **4030**, 4536
American Leprosy Missions Annual Report (USA) **3792**, 4499
American Malacological Union, Inc. News *see* A M U News **3349**
American Medical Association Alliance Today *see* A M A Alliance Today **3555**, 4568
American Medical Association. Council on Ethical and Judicial Affairs. Code of Medical Ethics. Current Opinions with Annotations (USA) **3565**
American Medical Association. Council on Ethical and Judicial Affairs. Current Opinions *see* American Medical Association. Council on Ethical and Judicial Affairs. Code of

Title

Anaesthesia and Intensive Care in Italy *see* Acta Anaesthesiologica Italica & Anaesthesia and Intensive Care in Italy **3753**
Anaesthesia Essays and Researches (JOR ISSN 0259-1162) **3753**
• ➤ Anaesthesia On-Line (GBR ISSN 1361-8245) **3754**
• ➤ Anaesthesia (Oxford) (GBR ISSN 0003-2409) **3754**
Anaesthesie - Intensivtherapie - Notfallmedizin - Schmerztherapie *see* A I N S - Anaesthesiologie Intensivmedizin Notfallmedizin Schmerztherapie **3753**
Anaesthesie Journal (CHE) **3754**
• ➤ Anaesthesiologie und Intensivmedizin (DEU ISSN 0170-5334) **3754**
Anaesthesiologie und Intensivmedizin/ Anaesthesiology and Intensive Care Medicine (USA ISSN 0171-1814) **3754**
• Anaesthesiologie und Intensivmedizin Online (DEU ISSN 1439-0256) **3754**
Anaesthesiologie und Reanimation (DEU ISSN 0323-4983) **3754**
Anaesthesiology and Intensive Care Medicine *see* Anaesthesiologie und Intensivmedizin **3754**
• ➤ Der Anaesthesist (DEU ISSN 0003-2417) **3754**
Der Anaesthesist. Supplement (DEU ISSN 1437-4943) **3754**
➤ Anais Brasileiros de Dermatologia (BRA ISSN 0365-0596) **3844**
Anais de Enfermagen *see* Revista Brasileira de Enfermagem **3939**
Anais Paulistas de Medicina e Cirurgia (BRA ISSN 0003-245X) **4180**
• Analecta Vet (ARG ISSN 1514-2590) **4536**
• ➤ Analecta Veterinaria (ARG ISSN 0365-5148) **4536**
Anales Cuidados Intensivos (ESP) **3565**
Anales de Anatomia *see* European Journal of Anatomy **3599**, 3342
Anales de Anatomia Normal *see* Revista Chilena de Anatomia **3685**, 3215
Anales de Cirugia (ARG ISSN 0066-1465) **4180**
Anales de Cirugia Cardiaca y Cirugia Vascular (ESP ISSN 1135-2760) **3762**, 4180
Anales de la Escuela Nacional de Ciencias Biologicas (Mexico) *see* Instituto Politecnico Nacional. Escuela Nacional de Ciencias Biologicas. Anales **3200**
➤ Anales de Medicina Interna (ESP ISSN 0212-7199) **3907**
➤ Anales de Medicina Interna. Seminarios (ESP) **3907**
Anales de Ortopedia y Traumatologia (MEX ISSN 0044-8184) **4010**
➤ Anales de Psicologia (ESP ISSN 0212-9728) **4375**
➤ Anales de Psiquiatria (ESP ISSN 0213-0599) **4072**
Anales de Veterinaria de Murcia (ESP ISSN 0213-5434) **4537**
Anales del Desarrollo *see* International Journal of Developmental Biology **3201**
Anales del Instituto Corachan (ESP ISSN 0003-2530) **3565**
Anales del Sistema Sanitario de Navarra (ESP ISSN 1137-6627) **4461**
Anales del Sistema Sanitario de Navarra. Suplemento (ESP ISSN 1137-814X) **4461**
• Anales Espanoles de Pediatria (ESP ISSN 0302-4342) **4040**
Anales Espanoles de Pediatria. Suplemento (ESP ISSN 0213-9146) **4040**
➤ Anales Otorrinolaringologicos Ibero-Americanos (ESP ISSN 0303-8874) **4030**
➤ Analgesia (USA ISSN 1071-569X) **3754**, 4072
Analgesic Guidelines *see* Therapeutic Guidelines. Analgesic **3760**
• Analgesics: The International Market (GBR) **4275**, 3366
Anali Klinicke Bolnice. Suplement *see* Acta Clinica Croatica. Supplement **3557**
Analise Psicologica (PRT ISSN 0870-8231) **4375**
Analogues in Cancer and Human Reproduction (NLD) **3967**
• ➤ Analyse (NLD ISSN 0166-7688) **3871**
▼ Analyse Freudienne (FRA ISSN 1253-1472) **4072**
Analyses of Hazardous Substances in Biological Materials (DEU ISSN 0179-7247) **3445**, 3376
Analytic Psychotherapy and Psychopathology *see* Psichiatria e Psicoterapia Analitica **4124**, 4435
• ➤ Analytical and Quantitative Cytology and Histology (USA ISSN 0884-6812) **3285**
• ➤ Analytical Biochemistry (USA ISSN 0003-2697) **3240**
• ➤ Analytical Cellular Pathology (NLD ISSN 0921-8912) **3285**
Analytical Instrumentation *see* Instrumentation Science & Technology **3376**, 3875
➤ Analytical Profiles of Drug Substances (USA ISSN 0099-5428) **4275**
Analytical Psychology Club of New York. Bulletin (USA) **4375**, 3552
Analytical Trilogy *see* Revista de Psicanalise Integral **4445**
Analytische Kinder- und Jugendlichen-Psychotherapie (DEU ISSN 0945-6740) **4375**
• ➤ Analytische Psychologie (CHE ISSN 0301-3006) **4375**
• ➤ Anatomia, Histologia, Embryologia (DEU ISSN 0340-2096) **4537**
• ➤ Anatomia, Histologia, Embryologia Online (DEU ISSN 1439-0264) **4537**
• ➤ The Anatomical Record (USA ISSN 0003-276X) **3181**, 3565
Anatomical Society of India. Journal *see* Journal of the Anatomical Society of India. **3205**, 3638
Anatomical Society of Southern Africa. Proceedings of Annual Congress *see* Anatomiese Vereniging van Suider-Afrika. Kongresverrigtinge **3339**, 3565
Anatomiese Vereniging van Suider-Afrika. Kongresverrigtinge/Anatomical Society of Southern Africa. Proceedings of Annual Congress (ZAF) **3339**, 3565
Anatomische Gesellschaft. Verhandlungen (DEU ISSN 0066-1562) **3565**
Anatomischer Anzeiger *see* Annals of Anatomy **3566**, 3181
Anatomy (AUS) **3814**
• ➤ Anatomy and Embryology (DEU ISSN 0340-2061) **3339**, 3565
Anch'Io (ITA) **3565**
Anchor Point Magazine (USA ISSN 0895-366X) **4375**, 3550
Ancient Science of Life (IND ISSN 0257-7941) **3163**, 3565
Anda (IDN ISSN 0126-1215) **4375**
• Anderson's Ohio E P A on CD-ROM (Ohio Environmental Protection Agency) (USA) **3445**, 4458
• ➤ Andrologia (DEU ISSN 0303-4569) **3565**
Andrologie (FRA ISSN 1166-2654) **3565**
Andros Digest (USA) **4375**
L'Ane (FRA ISSN 0294-653X) **4375**
➤ Anestesia en Mexico (MEX ISSN 1405-0056) **3754**
Anestesia - Rianimazione *see* Encyclopedie Medico-Chirurgicale. Anestesia - Rianimazione **3756**, 4187
Anestesista (ITA ISSN 0392-5854) **3754**
➤ Anesteziologie a Neodkladna Pece (CZE ISSN 0862-4968) **3754**
Anesteziologiia i Intensivno Lechenie (BGR ISSN 1310-4284) **3754**, 3906
Anesteziologiya i Reanimatologiya/ Anesthesiology and Intensive Care (RUS ISSN 0201-7563) **3755**, 4180
• ➤ Anesthesia and Analgesia (USA ISSN 0003-2999) **3755**
• Anesthesia and Critical Care Resources on the Internet (USA ISSN 1090-3577) **3755**
Anesthesia and Resuscitation *see* Masui to Sosei **3758**
• Anesthesia Malpractice Prevention (USA ISSN 1085-6897) **3755**, 3536
Anesthesia Patient Safety Foundation. Newsletter (USA) **3755**
➤ Anesthesia Progress (USA ISSN 0003-3006) **3815**, 3755
Anesthesie - Reanimation *see* Encyclopedie Medico-Chirurgicale. Anesthesie - Reanimation **3757**, 4187
Anesthesie - Reanimation Pratique (FRA ISSN 0996-8296) **3755**
• ➤ Anesthesiology (USA ISSN 0003-3022) **3755**
Anesthesiology and Intensive Care *see* Anesteziologiya i Reanimatologiya **3755**, 4180
• Anesthesiology Clinics of North America (USA ISSN 0889-8537) **3755**
• Anesthesiology News (USA ISSN 0747-4679) **3755**
Anesthesiology Review *see* The American Journal of Anesthesiology **3753**
Angewandte Arbeitswissenschaft (DEU ISSN 0341-0900) **3364**, 4250
Angina: Disease State Management Resource (USA) **3762**
• ➤ Angiogenesis (GBR ISSN 0969-6970) **3967**, 3762
Angiogenesis Research *see* Angiogenesis **3967**, 3762
Angiologia *see* Anales de Cirugia Cardiaca y Cirugia Vascular **3762**, 4180
➤ Angiologie (FRA ISSN 0765-4871) **3762**
Angiologiya i Sosudistaya Khirurgiya (RUS) **4180**
• ➤ Angiology (USA ISSN 0003-3197) **3763**
• ➤ Angle Orthodontist (USA ISSN 0003-3219) **3815**
Anhoerig (SWE ISSN 0280-512X) **3399**
Anhui Institute of Traditional Chinese Medicine. Journal *see* Anhui Zhongyi Xueyuan Xuebao **3565**
Anhui Medical Sciences *see* Anhui Yixue **3565**
• Anhui Yike Daxue Xuebao/Acta Universitatis Medicinalis Anhui (CHN ISSN 1000-1492) **3565**
Anhui Yixue/Anhui Medical Sciences (CHN ISSN 1000-0399) **3565**
Anhui Yixueyuan Xuebao *see* Anhui Yike Daxue Xuebao **3565**
Anhui Zhongyi Xueyuan Xuebao/Anhui Institute of Traditional Chinese Medicine. Journal (CHN ISSN 1000-2219) **3565**
Anima (ITA) **4375**, 3529
• Animal Behavior Abstracts (USA ISSN 0301-8695) **3225**, 3145, 3350
• ➤ Animal Behaviour (GBR ISSN 0003-3472) **3350**, 4375, 4537
Animal Biology (ITA ISSN 1121-1431) **3181**
• ➤ Animal Biotechnology (USA ISSN 1049-5398) **3268**, 3160
• Animal Breeding Abstracts (GBR ISSN 0003-3499) **3156**, 3145, 3154
• ➤ Animal Cognition (DEU ISSN 1435-9448) **4375**
Animal Experimentation. Improvements and Alternatives *see* Alternatives to Laboratory Animals **3870**
• ➤ Animal Feed Science and Technology (NLD ISSN 0377-8401) **3159**, 4537
➤ Animal Feeding and Nutrition (USA) **4537**
• ➤ Animal Genetics (GBR ISSN 0268-9146) **3298**, 3350
Animal Health *see* Animal Health Trust. Annual Review **4537**
Animal Health Advisory Leaflet (NCL ISSN 1019-8458) **4537**
Animal Health Newsletter (AUS ISSN 1329-198X) **4537**
Animal Health Research Centre. Annual Report (UGA) **4537**
▼ • ➤ Animal Health Research Reviews (GBR ISSN 1466-2523) **4537**
Animal Health Technician Dental Newsletter *see* Journal of Veterinary Dentistry **4546**
Animal Health Trust. Annual Report *see* Animal Health Trust. Annual Review **4537**
Animal Health Trust. Annual Review (GBR) **4537**
Animal Husbandry and Breeding (GRC) **3160**, 4537
• ➤ Animal Learning & Behavior (USA ISSN 0090-4996) **4376**
Animal Natural History Series (USA) **4503**, 3350
Animal Nutrition Association of Canada. Eastern Nutrition Conference. Proceedings (CAN) **3160**, 4228
• Animal Pharm (GBR ISSN 0262-2238) **4537**
Animal Production and Health Newsletter (AUT ISSN 1011-2529) **4140**
• ➤ Animal Reproduction Science (NLD ISSN 0378-4320) **3160**, 4537
Animal Research Resources *see* Comparative Medicine Research Resources **3719**, 3147, 3873
Animal Technology (GBR ISSN 0264-4754) **4537**
• Animal Welfare Information Center Bulletin (USA) **3171**
Animal Welfare Information Center Newsletter *see* Animal Welfare Information Center Bulletin **3171**
Animalia (ESP ISSN 0214-3151) **4272**
Animal's Eye Research *see* Hikaku Ganka Kenkyu **3998**
Animals News *see* Animaruzu Nyusu **3871**
Animaruzu Nyusu/Animals News (JPN ISSN 0910-0911) **3871**
Anitekkusu/Laboratory Animal Technology and Science (JPN ISSN 0915-3667) **3871**
Ankara Medical School. Journal (TUR ISSN 1300-5464) **3565**
➤ Ankara Universitesi. Tip Fakultesi. Mecmuasi/University of Ankara. Faculty of Medicine. Journal (TUR ISSN 0365-8104) **3566**
Ankara Universitesi. Tip Fakultesi. Mecmuasi. Supplementum *see* Ankara Universitesi. Tip Fakultesi. Mecmuasi **3566**
Ankara Universitesi Veteriner Fakultesi Dergisi/University of Ankara. Faculty of Veterinary Medicine. Journal (TUR ISSN 1300-0861) **4537**
Anleitung fuer die Chemische Laboratoriumspraxis *see* Anleitung fuer die Chemische Laboratoriumspraxis - Chemical Laboratory Practice **3371**, 3871
Anleitung fuer die Chemische Laboratoriumspraxis - Chemical Laboratory Practice (USA ISSN 0172-4967) **3371**, 3871
Anmeldte Arbejdsbetingede Lidelser. Aarsopgoerelse *see* Anmeldte Arbejdsulykker og Arbejdsbetingede Lidelser **4250**
Anmeldte Arbejdsulykker og Arbejdsbetingede Lidelser (DNK ISSN 1396-6715) **4250**
Anmeldte Arbejdsulykker. Yearbook *see* Anmeldte Arbejdsulykker og Arbejdsbetingede Lidelser **4250**
Annales Academiae Medicae Cracoviensis *see* Annales Collegii Medici Universitatis Iagiellonicae Cracoviensis **3715**, 3145
Annales Academiae Medicae Gedanensis (POL ISSN 0303-4135) **3566**
Annales Academiae Medicae Stetinensis *see* Pomorska Akademia Medyczna w Szczecinie. Roczniki **3677**
➤ Annales Academiae Medicae Stetinensis. Suplement (POL ISSN 1427-4930) **3566**
• ➤ Annales Chirurgiae et Gynaecologiae (FIN ISSN 0355-9521) **4180**, 3945
Annales Collegii Medici Antverpiensis (BEL ISSN 0003-3863) **3566**
Annales Collegii Medici Universitatis Iagiellonicae Cracoviensis (POL ISSN 1232-9371) **3715**, 3145
➤ Annales de Biochimie Clinique du Quebec (CAN ISSN 0709-8502) **3871**, 3376
• ➤ Annales de Biologie Clinique (FRA ISSN 0003-3898) **3181**, 3566
• Annales de Cardiologie et d'Angeiologie (FRA ISSN 0003-3928) **3763**
• ➤ Annales de Chirurgie (FRA ISSN 0003-3944) **4180**
Annales de Chirurgie de la Main et du Membre Superieur *see* Chirurgie de la Main **4184**
Annales de Chirurgie Plastique *see* Annales de Chirurgie Plastique et Esthetique **4181**
Annales de Chirurgie Plastique et Esthetique (FRA ISSN 0294-1260) **4181**
Annales de Chirurgie Thoracique et Cardio-Vasculaire (FRA ISSN 0066-2054) **3763**, 4181
• ➤ Annales de Dermatologie et de Venereologie (FRA ISSN 0151-9638) **3844**
➤ Annales de Gastroenterologie et d'Hepatologie (FRA ISSN 0066-2070) **3886**
• ➤ Annales de Genetique (FRA ISSN 0003-3995) **3298**
• Annales de Kinesitherapie (FRA ISSN 0302-427X) **4172**, 3786
Annales de l'Institut Pasteur - Actualites *see* Institut Pasteur. Annales. Actualites **3323**, 3251, 3308
• ➤ Annales de Medecine Interne (FRA ISSN 0003-410X) **3907**
• ➤ Annales de Medecine Veterinaire (BEL ISSN 0003-4118) **4537**
Annales de Parasitologie Humaine et Comparee *see* Parasite **3330**, 3804
• ➤ Annales de Pathologie (FRA ISSN 0242-6498) **3181**, 3566
➤ Annales de Pediatrie (FRA ISSN 0066-2097) **4040**
▼ Annales de Psychiatrie (FRA ISSN 0768-7559) **4072**
Annales de Radiologie (FRA ISSN 0003-4185) **4140**
• ➤ Annales de Readaptation et de Medecine Physique (FRA ISSN 0168-6054) **4058**
• ➤ Annales d'Endocrinologie (FRA ISSN 0003-4266) **3855**
Annales des Cliniques Psychologiques *see* Clinique Psychanalitique et Psycho-Pathologie **4388**
Annales des Falsifications de l'Expertise Chimique et Toxicologique (FRA ISSN 0242-6110) **3445**
Annales des Falsifications et de l'Expertise Chimique *see* Annales des Falsifications de l'Expertise Chimique et Toxicologique **3445**

Title

Title

• ➤ Annual Review of Physiology (USA ISSN 0066-4278) **3339**
• ➤ Annual Review of Psychology (USA ISSN 0066-4308) **4376**
• ➤ Annual Review of Public Health (USA ISSN 0163-7525) **4461**
• Annual Review of Sex Research (USA ISSN 1053-2528) **4376**, 4520
Annual Review of Women's Health (USA ISSN 1073-1695) **4562**, 4462
Annual Review. Respiratory Organ *see* Annual Review Kokyuki **4158**
Annual Review Saibo Seibutsugaku/Annual Review of Cell Biology (JPN) **3285**
Annual Review Shinkei/Annual Review. Nerve (JPN) **4073**
Annual Statistical Survey of Cancer *see* Etesia Statistike. Erevna tou Karkinou **3723**, 3977, 4528
Annual Summary of Vital Statistics (Boise) *see* Idaho. Department of Health and Welfare. Vital Statistics (Year) **4496**, 4475, 4529
• Annuario dei Fornitori della Sanita in Italia (ITA) **3501**, 3369
• Annuario Ottico Italiano (ITA) **3369**, 3993
Anonyma Alkoholister. Bulletin (SWE ISSN 0281-577X) **3399**
Anorexia Nervosa & Related Eating Disorders, Inc. *see* A N R E D **4067**, 4371, 4562
• Anquan/Safety (CHN ISSN 1002-3631) **4462**
• ➤ Antarctic Science (GBR ISSN 0954-1020) **3182**, 3407, 3465
Anthologia Medica Santoriana (ITA ISSN 0365-4621) **3567**
• Anthropology & Medicine (GBR ISSN 1364-8470) **3172**, 3567
➤ Anthropology of Consciousness (USA ISSN 1053-4202) **3172**, 4376
Anthropology of Food and Nutrition (GBR) **3459**, 3172, 4229
• ➤ Anthrozoos (USA ISSN 0892-7936) **3350**, 3871
• ➤ Anti-Cancer Drug Design (GBR ISSN 0266-9536) **3967**, 3241
• ➤ Anti-Cancer Drugs (USA ISSN 0959-4973) **3967**
▼ Anti-Infectives Today (NZL ISSN 1174-5924) **4276**
Antibacterial Products and Markets (GBR) **4276**, 3369
Antibiotic Guidelines *see* Therapeutic Guidelines. Antibiotic **3700**
Antibiotic Resistance Sourcebook (USA) **4276**
➤ Antibiotics and Chemotherapy (CHE ISSN 0066-4758) **4276**
Antibiotics and Chemotherapy *see* Kagaku Ryoho no Ryoiki **3910**
Antibiotics and Chemotherapy *see* Antibiotiki i Khimioterapiya **4276**
Antibiotics Chemotherapy (GBR ISSN 1366-5146) **3567**, 3793
Antibiotiki i Khimioterapiya/Antibiotics and Chemotherapy (RUS ISSN 0235-2990) **4276**
Antibiotiki i Meditsinskaya Biotekhnologiya *see* Antibiotiki i Khimioterapiya **4276**
Antibody, Immunoconjugates, and Radiopharmaceuticals *see* Cancer Biotherapy & Radiopharmaceuticals **3970**, 4282
• ➤ Anticancer Research (GRC ISSN 0250-7005) **3967**
Antiinfective Drugs and Chemotherapy *see* A D C News **3966**, 3239
• ➤ Antimicrobial Agents and Chemotherapy (USA ISSN 0066-4804) **3317**, 3968
Antimicrobial Evaluation, Development & Clinical Application *see* Journal of Infectious Disease Pharmacotherapy **4307**, 3802
Antimicrobial Newsletter *see* Lablink **3802**
Antimicrobic Newsletter *see* Antimicrobics and Infectious Diseases Newsletter **3793**
• ➤ Antimicrobics and Infectious Diseases Newsletter (USA ISSN 1069-417X) **3793**
Antioquia Medica (COL ISSN 0044-8389) **3567**
▼ • ➤ Antioxidants & Redox Signaling (USA ISSN 1523-0864) **3567**, 3241
• ➤ Antisense and Nucleic Acid Drug Development (USA ISSN 1087-2906) **3298**, 3241
Antisense Research and Development *see* Antisense and Nucleic Acid Drug Development **3298**, 3241
The Antiseptic (IND ISSN 0003-5998) **4182**
• Antiviral Agents Bulletin (USA ISSN 0897-9871) **4276**, 3268, 3793
• ➤ Antiviral Chemistry and Chemotherapy (GBR ISSN 0956-3202) **3241**, 3793, 4276
• ➤ Antiviral Research (NLD ISSN 0166-3542) **3317**, 3793
• ➤ Antiviral Therapy (GBR ISSN 1359-6535) **3793**, 3241, 3317
• Antiviral Weekly (USA ISSN 1086-0207) **3740**, 3317
• ➤ Antonie van Leeuwenhoek (NLD ISSN 0003-6072) **3268**, 3317
➤ Antropo-ekologiia (BGR) **3435**, 4229, 4250, 4350
Anuario de Psicologia (ESP ISSN 0066-5126) **4377**
Anuario de Psicologia Juridica (ESP ISSN 1133-0740) **4377**, 3536
Anuario Enfermedades de Notificacion Obligatoria (CHL) **3567**
Anxiety *see* Depression and Anxiety **4394**, 4086
Anxiety Disorders Association of America Reporter *see* A D A A Reporter **4371**
• Anxiety Disorders Foundation of Australia. Newsletter (AUS ISSN 1328-7761) **4073**, 4377
Anxiety Research *see* Anxiety, Stress and Coping **4377**
• ➤ Anxiety, Stress and Coping (CHE ISSN 1061-5806) **4377**
Anzccart News *see* A N Z C C A R T News **3171**, 4534
Aomori City Hospital. Medical Journal *see* Aomori Shimin Byoin Ishi **3567**
Aomori Kenritsu Byoin Nenpo/Aomori Prefectural Hospitals. Annual Reports (JPN) **3502**
Aomori Kenritsu Chuo Byoin Ishi/Aomori Prefectural Central Hospital. Medical Journal (JPN ISSN 0387-0138) **3502**
Aomori Medical Association. Journal *see* Aomoriken Ishikaiho **3567**
Aomori Municipal Hospital Establishment Association. Journal *see* Aomoriken Jichitai Igakkaishi **3567**, 3502
Aomori Prefectural Central Hospital. Medical Journal *see* Aomori Kenritsu Chuo Byoin Ishi **3502**
Aomori Prefectural Hospitals. Annual Reports *see* Aomori Kenritsu Byoin Nenpo **3502**
Aomori Rosai Byoin Ishi/Aomori Rosai Medical Journal (JPN ISSN 0918-1369) **3567**
Aomori Rosai Medical Journal *see* Aomori Rosai Byoin Ishi **3567**
Aomori Shimin Byoin Ishi/Aomori City Hospital. Medical Journal (JPN ISSN 0914-7500) **3567**
Aomori Society of Obstetricians and Gynecologists. Journal *see* Aomoriken Rinsho Sanfujinka Ikaishi **3945**
Aomori Society of Rural Medicine. Journal *see* Aomoriken Noson Igakkai Zasshi **3567**
Aomori Society of Sports Medicine. Journal *see* Aomoriken Supotsu Igaku Kenkyukaishi **4172**
Aomoriken Ishikaiho/Aomori Medical Association. Journal (JPN ISSN 0914-6873) **3567**
Aomoriken Jichitai Igakkaishi/Aomori Municipal Hospital Establishment Association. Journal (JPN ISSN 0913-4581) **3567**, 3502
Aomoriken Noson Igakkai Zasshi/Aomori Society of Rural Medicine. Journal (JPN ISSN 0916-0450) **3567**
Aomoriken Rinsho Sanfujinka Ikaishi/Aomori Society of Obstetricians and Gynecologists. Journal (JPN ISSN 0913-8307) **3945**
Aomoriken Sagyo Ryoho Kenkyukaishi/Bulletin of Aomori Occupational Therapy (JPN ISSN 0918-1431) **4058**, 4250
Aomoriken Supotsu Igaku Kenkyukaishi/Aomori Society of Sports Medicine. Journal (JPN ISSN 0918-0257) **4172**
APA-Journal. Gesundheit (AUT) **4350**, 4462
Aparato Locomotor *see* Encyclopedie Medico-Chirurgicale. Aparato Locomotor **4168**, 4014
Apex (Leeds) (GBR ISSN 1460-1729) **3815**
• ➤ Aphasiology (GBR ISSN 0268-7038) **4073**
Apis (USA ISSN 0887-7386) **4538**, 3160, 3171
Apka Swasthya (IND ISSN 0003-6498) **4350**
Aplastic Anemia & M D S International Foundation. Newsletter (USA) **3898**
Aplastic Anemia Foundation of America. Newsletter *see* Aplastic Anemia & M D S International Foundation. Newsletter **3898**
• Apoptosis (GBR ISSN 1350-4541) **3225**, 3145, 3182
• ➤ Apoptosis (USA ISSN 1360-8185) **3285**, 3567
Apoteket (SWE ISSN 0349-2516) **4276**
Apotekstjaenstemannen *see* Farmacifacket **4295**
• ➤ Apothecary (USA ISSN 0003-6560) **4276**
➤ Apotheekmanagement (NLD ISSN 0921-0288) **4276**
Die Apotheke (AUT) **4276**
Apotheke (DEU) **4350**
Apotheke Aktuell (DEU) **4276**
Apotheke Heute (DEU ISSN 0173-1882) **3152**, 4277
Apotheke und Krankenhaus (DEU ISSN 0177-9591) **4277**, 3502
Apotheken Journal Reise und Pharmazie (DEU) **4277**
Apotheken Kurier (DEU) **4277**
Apotheken-Magazin (DEU ISSN 0724-9950) **4277**
Apotheken-Magazin fuer Senioren & Diabetiker (DEU) **4350**, 3855
Apotheken-Praxis (DEU ISSN 0721-8370) **4277**, 3364
Apotheken Umschau (DEU ISSN 0402-7108) **4350**, 3567
Der Apotheker-Berater (DEU ISSN 0720-549X) **4277**
Apotheker - Jahrbuch (DEU ISSN 0066-5347) **4277**
Apotheker Journal *see* Apotheken Journal Reise und Pharmazie **4277**
Apotheker-Zeitung (DEU ISSN 0178-4862) **4277**
Apothekersblad (BEL ISSN 0003-6579) **4277**
Appareil Locomoteur *see* Encyclopedie Medico-Chirurgicale. Appareil Locomoteur **4168**, 4014
• The Appeal Letter (USA) **3530**
• ➤ Appetite (GBR ISSN 0195-6663) **4229**
• ➤ Applied and Environmental Microbiology (USA ISSN 0099-2240) **3318**, 3268, 3459
• ➤ Applied and Preventive Psychology (GBR ISSN 0962-1849) **4377**
• ➤ Applied Animal Behaviour Science (NLD ISSN 0168-1591) **3350**, 4377
• Applied Behavioral Science Review (GBR ISSN 1068-8595) **4377**
• ➤ Applied Biochemistry and Biotechnology (USA ISSN 0273-2289) **3241**, 3268
Applied Biochemistry and Biotechnology Part B *see* Molecular Biotechnology **3276**, 3662
• ➤ Applied Biochemistry and Microbiology (RUS ISSN 0003-6838) **3241**, 3318
• ➤ Applied Cardiopulmonary Pathophysiology (NLD ISSN 0920-5268) **3339**, 3763, 4158
➤ Applied Clinical Trials (USA ISSN 1064-8542) **3567**
• ➤ Applied Cognitive Psychology (GBR ISSN 0888-4080) **4377**
Applied Cytogenetics (USA ISSN 1056-5191) **3299**, 3268, 3285
• Applied Developmental Science (USA ISSN 1088-8691) **4377**, 4520
• ➤ Applied Ergonomics (GBR ISSN 0003-6870) **3431**, 4377, 4531
• Applied Genetics News (USA ISSN 0271-7107) **3299**, 3268
➤ Applied H.R.M. Research (Human Resources Management) (USA ISSN 1055-9094) **4377**, 3368
Applied Health Physics Abstracts and Notes *see* Radiation Protection Abstracts **4365**, 3151, 4497
Applied Human Science (JPN ISSN 1341-3473) **3339**, 3172
• ➤ Applied Immunohistochemistry (USA ISSN 1062-3345) **3567**
Applied Industrial Psychology *see* Psychologie v Ekonomicke Praxi **4439**
• ➤ Applied Microbiology and Biotechnology (DEU ISSN 0175-7598) **3268**, 3299, 3318
• ➤ Applied Neuropsychology (USA ISSN 0908-4282) **4073**, 4377
• ➤ Applied Nursing Research (USA ISSN 0897-1897) **3913**, 3871
• ➤ Applied Occupational & Environmental Hygiene (USA ISSN 1047-322X) **4250**, 4462
• ➤ Applied Psycholinguistics (GBR ISSN 0142-7164) **3550**, 4073, 4377
➤ Applied Psycholinguistics and Communication Disorders (USA) **3550**, 4377
• ➤ Applied Psychological Measurement (USA ISSN 0146-6216) **4377**
• ➤ Applied Psychology (GBR ISSN 0269-994X) **4377**
Applied Psychology (USA) **4377**
• ➤ Applied Psychophysiology and Biofeedback (USA ISSN 1090-0586) **4378**, 4226
• ➤ Applied Radiation and Isotopes (GBR ISSN 0969-8043) **4365**, 3871, 4140
• ➤ Applied Radiology (USA ISSN 0160-9963) **4140**
➤ Applied Virology Research (USA ISSN 1041-245X) **3318**
Approche Neuropsychologique des Apprentissages chez l'Enfant *see* A N A E **4067**
Approved Bioequivalency Codes (USA) **4277**
Approved Drug Products with Therapeutic Equivalence Evaluations (USA ISSN 1048-5996) **4277**
Approved Providers of Continuing Pharmaceutical Education (USA) **4277**, 3416
• APStracts (USA ISSN 1080-4757) **3225**, 3145
Apteka (UKR) **4277**
Apuntes de Medicina Deportiva *see* Apunts **4173**, 4010
➤ Apuntes de Psicologia (ESP ISSN 0213-3334) **4378**
Apunts (ESP ISSN 0212-4009) **4173**, 4010
Aqua Pura *see* Australian Fluoridation News. Aqua-Pura **4561**, 4463
Aquaristik - Fachmagazin (DEU ISSN 1437-4854) **3459**, 3464
• Aquatic Biology, Aquaculture & Fisheries Resources (ZAF ISSN 1083-883X) **3225**, 3145
• ➤ Aquatic Ecology (NLD ISSN 1386-2588) **3182**
• ➤ Aquatic Microbial Ecology (DEU ISSN 0948-3055) **3318**
• ➤ Aquatic Microbial Ecology Online (DEU ISSN 1616-1564) **3318**
Aquatic Sciences & Fisheries Abstracts Marine Biotechnology Abstracts *see* A S F A Marine Biotechnology Abstracts **3225**, 3145, 3268, 3407, 3408
• ➤ Aquatic Toxicology (NLD ISSN 0166-445X) **3445**, 3241
➤ Aquilo. Serie Botanica (FIN ISSN 0570-5169) **3278**, 3435
Arab Dental/Alam Tib al-Asnan (DEU) **3815**
• ➤ Arab Journal of Biotechnology (EGY ISSN 1110-6875) **3269**
Arab Medical Bulletin (SDN ISSN 0254-9492) **3567**
Arab Medico (DEU ISSN 0723-5100) **3567**
Arab Veterinary Medical Association. Journal (EGY ISSN 0003-746X) **4538**
Arachnologia *see* Arachnologia - Bulletin d'Information et de Liaison du C I D A **3351**
Arachnologia - Bulletin d'Information et de Liaison du C I D A (FRA ISSN 0763-1901) **3351**
Arafmi News (AUS) **4073**, 4510
Arbeidervern (NOR ISSN 0332-7124) **4250**
Arbeidsmiljoe (NOR ISSN 0800-2088) **4250**
Arbeidsomstandigheden-actueel *see* Arbeidsomstandigheden Concreet **4250**
Arbeidsomstandigheden Concreet (NLD ISSN 0929-1105) **4250**
Arbeidsveiligheid (BEL ISSN 0770-7649) **4250**
Arbeit Betrieb Organisation Aktuell *see* Wirtschaftspsychologie **4455**
Arbeit und Gesundheit (DEU ISSN 0946-7599) **4250**
Arbeit und Gesundheit. Sonderausgabe Verkehr (DEU ISSN 0948-0935) **4462**, 4532
Arbeit und Sicherheit *see* A S Vorort **4225**, 4249
Arbeit und Sicherheit Vorort *see* A S Vorort **4225**, 4249
Arbeiten aus dem Paul-Ehrlich-Institut, dem Georg-Speyer-Haus und dem Ferdinand-Blum-Institut *see* Bundesamt fuer Sera und Impfstoffe. Paul-Ehrlich-Institut. Arbeiten **3579**, 3188
Arbeiten zur Geschichte der Medizin in Giessen (DEU ISSN 0174-268X) **3568**
Arbeiten zur Sozialwissenschaftlichen Psychologie (DEU) **4378**, 4520
Arbeitsgemeinschaft fuer Klinische Nephrologie. Mitteilungen *see* Deutsche Arbeitsgemeinschaft fuer Klinische Nephrologie. Mitteilungen **4211**
Arbeitsgemeinschaft fuer Pharmazeutische Verfahrenstechnik News *see* A P V News **4273**
Arbeitshefte Gruppenanalyse (DEU) **4378**
Arbeitshefte Kinderpsychoanalyse (DEU ISSN 0721-9628) **4378**
Arbeitsmedizin, Sozialmedizin, Praeventivmedizin *see* Arbeitsmedizin, Sozialmedizin, Umweltmedizin **4462**, 3568, 4250
Arbeitsmedizin, Sozialmedizin, Praeventivmedizin. Sonderheft *see* Arbeitsmedizin, Sozialmedizin, Umweltmedizin. Supplement **4462**, 3568, 4250
Arbeitsmedizin, Sozialmedizin, Umweltmedizin (DEU ISSN 0944-6052) **4462**, 3568, 4250

Title

Title

➤ Army Medical Services Magazine (GBR) **4223**, 3569
Arnoldia Zimbabwe (ZWE ISSN 0250-6386) **3183**
Arogya (IND ISSN 0253-682X) **4350**, 3569
• Aroma-Chology Review (USA ISSN 1098-044X) **3175**, 4378
▼ Aromatherapy (GBR ISSN 1470-4056) **3163**
Aromatherapy Today (AUS) **3163**
Aromatic Thymes (USA) **3163**
• ➤ Arquivo Brasileiro de Medicina Veterinaria e Zootecnia/Brazilian Journal of Veterinary and Animal Sciences (BRA ISSN 0102-0935) **4538**
Arquivo de Patologia (PRT ISSN 0004-2714) **3569**
• ➤ Arquivos Brasileiros de Cirurgia Digestiva (BRA ISSN 0102-6720) **3886**, 4182
Arquivos Brasileiros de Endocrinologia e Metabologia (BRA ISSN 0004-2730) **3855**
Arquivos Brasileiros de Medicina (BRA ISSN 0365-0723) **3907**
Arquivos Brasileiros de Oftalmologia (BRA ISSN 0004-2749) **3994**
Arquivos Brasileiros de Tuberculose e Doencas do Torax (BRA ISSN 0004-2765) **4158**
Arquivos Catarinenses de Medicina (BRA ISSN 0004-2773) **3569**
Arquivos de Cirurgia Clinica e Experimental (BRA ISSN 0066-7846) **4182**, 3871
➤ Arquivos de Gastroenterologia (BRA ISSN 0004-2803) **3886**
Arquivos de Geriatria e Gerontologia (BRA ISSN 1413-7615) **3468**
Arquivos de Medicina (PRT ISSN 0871-3413) **3569**
• ➤ Arquivos de Neuro-Psiquiatria (BRA ISSN 0004-282X) **4074**
➤ Arquivos de Saude Mental do Estado de Sao Paulo (BRA ISSN 0103-0809) **4074**, 4378
Arquivos de Saude Mental do Estado de Sao Paulo. Suplemento (BRA ISSN 0103-0817) **4074**, 4378
Arquivos do Centro de Estudos do Curso de Odontologia *see* Universidade Federal de Minas Gerais. Faculdade de Odontologia. Arquivos em Odontologia **3842**
Arquivos dos Hospitais e da Faculdade de Ciencias Medicas da Santa Casa de Sao Paulo (BRA ISSN 0018-5442) **3502**, 3569
Arquivos em Odontologia *see* Universidade Federal de Minas Gerais. Faculdade de Odontologia. Arquivos em Odontologia **3842**
Arquivos Portugueses de Cirurgia (PRT ISSN 0872-2226) **4182**
➤ Ars Curandi. Clinica Medica (BRA ISSN 0571-1320) **3907**
Ars Medici (CHE ISSN 0004-2897) **3569**
• Ars Pharmaceutica (ESP ISSN 0004-2927) **4278**
Ars Veterinaria (BRA ISSN 0102-6380) **4538**
Arshiv-i Mu'assasah-i Razi *see* Institut Razi. Archives **3799**, 4544
Art & Understanding *see* A & U **3552**, 3175, 3790
Art & Understanding *see* A & U **3552**, 3175, 3790
Art Dentaire Liberal (FRA ISSN 0571-1525) **3815**
Art et Technique Dentaires (FRA ISSN 1146-0717) **3815**
Art Hazards News (USA ISSN 0197-7903) **4251**, 3175
Art Therapy (USA ISSN 0742-1656) **4059**, 3175
• Artemisa (MEX ISSN 1405-0242) **3716**, 3145
Artere (CAN ISSN 0823-4124) **3502**, 4278
Arteres et Veines (FRA ISSN 0293-5090) **3763**
Arteriosclerosi News (ITA ISSN 1123-1378) **3907**
Arteriosclerosis and Thrombosis *see* Arteriosclerosis, Thrombosis, and Vascular Biology **3763**
• ➤ Arteriosclerosis, Thrombosis, and Vascular Biology (USA ISSN 1079-5642) **3763**
➤ Artery (USA ISSN 0098-6127) **3763**
Arthritis Action *see* On the Move (Ashford) **4169**
• ➤ Arthritis and Rheumatism (USA ISSN 0004-3591) **4167**
Arthritis Care and Research *see* Arthritis and Rheumatism **4167**
Arthritis: Disease State Management Resource (USA) **4167**
Arthritis Foundation Annual Report (USA ISSN 0191-2836) **4167**
Arthritis Health Monitor (USA ISSN 1067-9421) **4167**
Arthritis Hotline (USA) **4167**, 3786
Arthritis News (CAN ISSN 0820-9006) **4167**
Arthritis News (GBR ISSN 0144-6339) **3494**
Arthritis News (NZL ISSN 1171-8986) **4167**
▼ • Arthritis Research (GBR ISSN 1465-9905) **3569**
Arthritis Self-Management (USA) **4167**
Arthritis Today (GBR ISSN 0969-7039) **4167**
• Arthritis Today (USA ISSN 0890-1120) **4167**
Arthro Express *see* Arthritis News **4167**
• Arthropod Endocrinology News (USA ISSN 1522-4120) **3855**
• ➤ Arthropod Management Tests (USA) **3157**
Arthroscopy (JPN ISSN 0910-223X) **4011**, 4167, 4182
• ➤ Arthroscopy (USA ISSN 0749-8063) **4010**, 4182
• ➤ Arthroskopie (DEU ISSN 0933-7946) **3569**
Arthur Andersen Washington Healthcare Newsletter (USA) **3502**, 3536
➤ Articulata (DEU ISSN 0171-4090) **3183**
➤ Articulator (USA ISSN 0272-9067) **3815**
• ➤ Artificial Cells, Blood Substitutes, and Immobilization Biotechnology (USA ISSN 1073-1199) **3871**, 3269
• ➤ Artificial Intelligence in Medicine (NLD ISSN 0933-3657) **3389**, 3569
• Artificial Life (USA ISSN 1064-5462) **3389**, 3183
• ➤ Artificial Organs (USA ISSN 0160-564X) **3871**, 4182
Der Artikulator (DEU ISSN 0720-972X) **3815**
Arts Access News (AUS ISSN 1329-0517) **3483**, 3175
Arts Assistent (NLD ISSN 0928-611X) **3569**
• ➤ The Arts in Psychotherapy (GBR ISSN 0197-4556) **4378**, 3175
▼ ➤ Arts Therapies Research Library (GBR) **3569**, 3175, 4225
ArtsenZaken (NLD ISSN 1387-1870) **3569**
Arukoru Iryo Kenkyu/Japanese Studies on Alcoholism Treatment (JPN ISSN 0910-495X) **3399**
Arukoru Kenkyu to Yakubutsu Izon/Japanese Journal of Alcohol Studies and Drug Dependence (JPN ISSN 0389-4118) **3399**
Arumeida Iho/Oita City Medical Association. Journal (JPN ISSN 0913-7343) **3570**
Arut Perum Jothi (IND) **4501**, 3570
Arznei-Telegramm (DEU ISSN 0066-8192) **4278**
• ➤ Arzneimittel-Forschung/Drug Research (DEU ISSN 0004-4172) **4278**
Arzneimittel, Rezeptpruefung, Regress (DEU ISSN 0933-1859) **4278**
Arzneimittel Zeitung (DEU ISSN 0935-2767) **4278**, 3361
Der Arzneimittelbrief (DEU) **4278**
Arzneimitteltherapie (DEU ISSN 0723-6913) **4278**
Arzt in Niederoesterreich (AUT ISSN 0004-4180) **3570**, 4462
Arzt und Auto (DEU ISSN 0341-4434) **3570**, 4532
Arzt und Krankenhaus (DEU ISSN 0341-9754) **3570**
Arzt und Praxis (AUT ISSN 1026-8421) **3570**
Arzt und Praxis (CHE ISSN 1016-8400) **3570**
Der Arzt und Sein Recht (DEU ISSN 0935-5553) **3570**, 3536
Arzthaftpflicht - Rechtsprechung (DEU ISSN 0933-1352) **3570**, 3536
Arzthaftungsrecht (DEU) **3570**, 3536
Die Arzthelferin (DEU ISSN 0931-5853) **3914**
Arzthelferin Aktuell *see* Praxis Nah **4200**, 3938
Arztrecht (DEU ISSN 0343-5733) **3570**, 3536
As *see* ASko **4272**, 3171, 4538
AS. Maandblad Aktiviteitensektor *see* A S **4510**, 3465, 3495
Asahi Chuo Byoin Iho/Asahi General Hospital. Medical Journal (JPN ISSN 0285-9017) **3570**
Asahi General Hospital. Medical Journal *see* Asahi Chuo Byoin Iho **3570**
Asahigawaso Institute of Medical Welfare. Annual Report *see* Asahigawaso Kenkyu Nenpo **3570**, 4510
Asahigawaso Kenkyu Nenpo/Asahigawaso Institute of Medical Welfare. Annual Report (JPN ISSN 0913-4603) **3570**, 4510
Asahikawa City Hospital. Journal *see* Asahikawa Shiritsu Byoin Ishi **3570**, 3502
Asahikawa Ika Daigaku Nenpo/Asahikawa Medical College. Annual Report (JPN ISSN 0918-7022) **3570**
Asahikawa Medical College. Annual Report *see* Asahikawa Ika Daigaku Nenpo **3570**
Asahikawa Red Cross Hospital. Medical Journal *see* Asahikawa Sekijuji Byoin Igaku Zasshi **3570**
Asahikawa Sekijuji Byoin Igaku Zasshi/Asahikawa Red Cross Hospital. Medical Journal (JPN ISSN 0913-4417) **3570**
Asahikawa Shiritsu Byoin Ishi/Asahikawa City Hospital. Journal (JPN ISSN 0287-024X) **3570**, 3502
Asamblea Mundial de la Salud y del Consejo Ejecutivo. Manual de Resoluciones y Decisiones *see* World Health Organization. Handbook of Resolutions and Decisions of the World Health Assembly and the Executive Board. **4493**
• Asbestos & Lead Abatement Report (USA ISSN 1068-2643) **3443**
Asbestos Victims of America Advisor *see* A V A Advisor **3966**, 3536
Asclepio (ESP ISSN 0210-4466) **3570**, 3172
Asepsis (USA ISSN 1062-0281) **3570**
Ashes to Dust (AUS ISSN 0816-4347) **4462**, 3392, 3399, 4531
Asia - Oceania Journal of Obstetrics and Gynaecology *see* Journal of Obstetrics and Gynaecology **3956**
Asia - Pacific Dental News (HKG) **3815**
➤ Asia Pacific Disability Rehabilitation Journal (IND) **4510**, 4059
▼ Asia Pacific Disability Rehabilitation Journal. Selected Readings Series (IND) **4511**, 4059
▼ • Asia Pacific Family Medicine (AUS ISSN 1444-1683) **3570**
▼ • Asia Pacific Family Medicine Online (AUS) **3570**
The Asia Pacific Heart Journal *see* Heart, Lung & Circulation **3773**
Asia Pacific Hospital *see* Hospital and Healthcare **3512**
• ➤ Asia Pacific Journal of Clinical Nutrition (AUS ISSN 0964-7058) **4229**
➤ Asia - Pacific Journal of Ophthalmology (SGP ISSN 0129-1653) **3994**
• Asia Pacific Journal of Pharmacology (SGP ISSN 0217-9687) **4278**
Asia Pacific Journal of Speech, Language and Hearing (GBR ISSN 1361-3286) **4030**, 3489
Asian American and Pacific Islander Journal of Health (USA) **4462**, 3570
➤ Asian and Pacific Women's Resource and Action Series (MYS) **4568**, 3357, 3945
Asian Archives of Anaesthesiology and Resuscitation (IND ISSN 0301-0368) **3755**
• ➤ Asian - Australasian Journal of Animal Sciences (KOR ISSN 1011-2367) **3160**, 3269
• Asian Cardiovascular & Thoracic Annals (SGP ISSN 0218-4923) **3763**
Asian Dentist (SGP) **3815**
Asian Environment (PHL ISSN 0116-2993) **3436**, 4251, 4462, 4561
Asian Hospital (HKG ISSN 1011-596X) **3502**
Asian Hospital & Healthcare Management (GBR) **3502**
Asian Hospital NewsFax (HKG) **3502**
▼ Asian Journal of Andrology (CHN) **3570**
Asian Journal of Oral and Maxillofacial Surgery (JPN ISSN 0915-6992) **3815**, 4182
Asian Journal of Physical Education (TWN ISSN 1015-1990) **4350**
Asian Journal of Psychology and Education (IND ISSN 0971-2909) **3409**, 4378
• Asian Journal of Social Psychology (GBR ISSN 1367-2223) **4378**, 3526
• ➤ Asian Journal of Surgery (HKG ISSN 1015-9584) **4182**
Asian Medical News (HKG ISSN 0250-3328) **3570**
Asian Pacific AIDS Intervention Team *see* A P A I T **3457**, 3790
Asian Pacific Congress of Cardiology. Symposia (IDN ISSN 0587-5471) **3763**
• ➤ Asian Pacific Journal of Allergy & Immunology (THA ISSN 0125-877X) **3741**
• Asian - Pacific Newsletter on Occupational Health and Safety (FIN ISSN 1237-0843) **4251**
Asian - Pacific Newsletter on Occupational Health and Safety - Online *see* Asian - Pacific Newsletter on Occupational Health and Safety **4251**
Askew *see* Lacanian Studies **4425**
ASko (POL ISSN 1231-6857) **4272**, 3171, 4538
Asociacion Bioquimica Argentina. Revista (ARG ISSN 0004-4768) **3241**
Asociacion Dental Mexicana, A.C. *see* A D M **3813**
Asociacion Espanola Contra el Cancer *see* A E C C **3966**
Asociacion Espanola Contra el Cancer. Memoria (ESP) **3968**
Asociacion Espanola Contra el Cancer. Memoria Tecnico-Administrativa *see* Asociacion Espanola Contra el Cancer. Memoria **3968**
Asociacion Medica de Puerto Rico. Boletin (PRI ISSN 0004-4849) **3570**
Asociacion Mexicana de Facultades y Escuelas de Medicina. Boletin (MEX ISSN 0004-4857) **3570**
Asociacion Nacional de Enfermeras de Colombia *see* A N E C **3912**
➤ Asociacion Odontologica Argentina. Revista (ARG ISSN 0004-4881) **3815**
Asociacion para Evitar la Ceguera en Mexico. Archivos (MEX ISSN 0004-489X) **3570**
Asociacion Venezolana de Psicologia Social. Boletin *see* Asociacion Venezolana de Psicologia Social. Revista **4378**
Asociacion Venezolana de Psicologia Social Fasciculo *see* A V E P S O Fasciculo **4371**
Asociacion Venezolana de Psicologia Social. Revista (VEN) **4378**
Aspel's Gazette (GBR ISSN 0958-8167) **3502**
Aspen's Nurse Executive Network *see* Patient Care Management **3936**
• ➤ Assessment (USA ISSN 1073-1911) **4378**, 4074
➤ Assia (ISR ISSN 0334-3871) **3570**
➤ Assia - Jewish Medical Ethics (ISR ISSN 0793-2952) **4501**, 3570
Assistance et le Prothesiste Dentaires (FRA) **3815**
Assisted Living Business Report (USA) **3502**, 3468
Assisted Living Success (USA) **3502**, 3468
Assisted Reproduction *see* Reproductive Technologies **3962**
➤ Assisted Reproductive Technology - Andrology (USA) **3571**
Assistenti di Studio Medico (CHE) **3571**
Assistenza Infermieristica e Ricerca (ITA ISSN 1592-5986) **3914**
• ➤ Assistive Technology (USA ISSN 1040-0435) **3419**, 3571
➤ Assistive Technology Research Series (NLD ISSN 1383-813X) **3488**, 3388
➤ Assiut Veterinary Medical Journal (EGY ISSN 1012-5973) **4538**
Associacao Brasileira de Endodontia Seccao Sao Paulo Boletim *see* A B E S P Boletim **3813**
Associacao Brasileira de Psiquiatria e Asociacion Psiquiatrica de la America Latina. Revista *see* Revista Brasileira de Psiquiatria **4130**
Associacao Medica Brasileira. Jornal (BRA ISSN 0004-5233) **3571**
• Associacao Medica Brasileira. Revista (BRA ISSN 0004-5241) **3571**
Associacao Medica de Minas Gerais. Revista (BRA ISSN 0004-525X) **3571**
Associacao Paulista de Cirurgioes Dentistas Journal *see* A P C D Journal **3813**
• ➤ Associacao Paulista de Cirurgioes Dentistas. Revista (BRA ISSN 0004-5276) **3815**
Associated Bodywork and Massage Professionals News *see* Massage and Bodywork **4358**
Association Belge des Paralyses Contact *see* A B P Contact **3483**, 4067, 4510
Association Canadienne des Enseignants(es) des Sourds(es) et des Malentendants(es). Revue *see* C A E D H H Journal **3489**, 3420
Association Canadienne des Radiologistes. Journal *see* Canadian Association of Radiologists Journal **4141**
Association Canadienne pour la Sante Mentale. Rapport Annuel *see* Canadian Mental Health Association. Annual Report **4386**, 4465
Association Catholique Canadienne de la Sante. Revue *see* C H A C Review **3503**, 3580, 4502
Association Dentaire Canadienne. Journal *see* Canadian Dental Association. Journal **3817**
Association des Anatomistes. Bulletin *see* Morphologie **3662**, 3209
Association des Medecins de Langue Francaise du Canada. Bulletin (CAN ISSN 0004-539X) **3571**
Association des Medecins Israelites de France. Revue Medicale *see* J A M I F **3627**
Association des Morphologistes. Bulletin *see* Morphologie **3662**, 3209
Association des Pharmaciens de l'Industrie. Bulletin (FRA) **4278**
Association des Sages-Femmes de la Maternite de Nancy. Bulletin (FRA) **3945**
• Association for Applied Psychophysiology and Biofeedback. Proceedings of the Annual Meeting (USA) **4379**, 4074

Title

➤ Augenblick (DEU) **3495**
Augenlicht (DEU) **3994**
Der Augenoptiker (DEU ISSN 0004-7929) **3994**
Der Augenspiegel (DEU ISSN 0004-7937) **3994**
• ➤ Augmentative and Alternative Communication (CAN ISSN 0743-4618) **3572**
Aural News (GBR ISSN 0004-8054) **3489**
Auris (SWE ISSN 0045-0030) **3489**
• Auris, Nasus, Larynx (NLD ISSN 0385-8146) **4031**
Austin Dental News *see* Tenth Times **3841**
➤ Austra-Link (AUS ISSN 0726-4607) **3399**
• Austral Ecology (AUS ISSN 1442-9985) **3183**
• ➤ Australasian Biotechnology (AUS ISSN 1036-7128) **3269**
➤ Australasian College of Nutritional and Environmental Medicine. Journal (AUS ISSN 1328-8040) **3572**, 3446, 4229
Australasian Health and Healing *see* Health & Healing **3165**
• ➤ Australasian Journal of Dermatology (AUS ISSN 0004-8380) **3845**
• ➤ Australasian Journal of Disaster and Trauma Studies (NZL ISSN 1174-4707) **4011**
➤ Australasian Journal of Ecotoxicology (AUS ISSN 1323-3475) **3446**
➤ Australasian Journal of Emergency Care (AUS ISSN 1328-3626) **4011**, 3914, 4182
➤ Australasian Journal of Psychotherapy (AUS) **4379**, 4075
➤ Australasian Journal on Ageing (AUS) **3468**
• ➤ Australasian Physical & Engineering Sciences in Medicine (AUS ISSN 0158-9938) **3871**, 4365
• Australasian Psychiatry (AUS ISSN 1039-8562) **4075**
• ➤ Australasian Radiology (AUS ISSN 0004-8461) **4140**
▼ ➤ Australasian Rehabilitation Nurses Association. Official Journal (AUS ISSN 1440-3994) **4059**
Australia and New Zealand Journal of Developmental Disabilities *see* Journal of Intellectual and Developmental Disability **4102**
Australia. Bureau of Statistics. Australian Health Trends (AUS) **4494**, 4527
Australia. Bureau of Statistics. Australian Hospital Statistics (AUS ISSN 1036-613X) **3524**, 4527
Australia. Bureau of Statistics. Australia's Food and Nutrition (AUS) **4248**, 4527
Australia. Bureau of Statistics. Australia's Health (AUS ISSN 1032-6138) **4462**
Australia. Bureau of Statistics. Cancer in Australia (AUS) **3968**, 3716, 4527
Australia. Bureau of Statistics. Children's Health Screening (AUS) **3716**, 4041, 4527
Australia. Bureau of Statistics. Children's Immunisation *see* Australia. Bureau of Statistics. Children's Immunisation, Australia **3716**, 3741, 4041, 4527
Australia. Bureau of Statistics. Children's Immunisation, Australia (AUS) **3716**, 3741, 4041, 4527
Australia. Bureau of Statistics. Chiropractic and Osteopathic Services, Australia (AUS) **3716**, 4527
Australia. Bureau of Statistics. Deaths Due to Diseases and Cancers of the Respiratory System, Australia (AUS) **3716**, 4158, 4527
Australia. Bureau of Statistics. Dental Services, Australia (AUS) **3716**, 3816, 4527
Australia. Bureau of Statistics. Health in Australia - What You Should Know (AUS) **4494**, 4527
Australia. Bureau of Statistics. Hospitals, Australia (AUS) **3524**, 4527
Australia. Bureau of Statistics. Information Paper: National Nutrition Survey, Confidentialised Unit Record File (AUS) **4248**, 4229, 4527
Australia. Bureau of Statistics. Injuries, Australia (AUS) **3716**, 4527
Australia. Bureau of Statistics. Medical Labour Force (AUS) **3716**, 4527
Australia. Bureau of Statistics. National Health Information Model (AUS) **4494**, 4527
Australia. Bureau of Statistics. National Health Survey: Aboriginal and Torres Strait Islander Results, Australia (AUS) **4494**, 4527
Australia. Bureau of Statistics. National Health Survey: Asthma and Other Respiratory Conditions, Australia (AUS) **3716**, 4158, 4527
Australia. Bureau of Statistics. National Health Survey: Cancer Screening, Australia (AUS) **3716**, 3968, 4527
Australia. Bureau of Statistics. National Health Survey: Cardiovascular and Related Conditions, Australia (AUS) **3716**, 3764, 4528
Australia. Bureau of Statistics. National Health Survey: Diabetes, Australia (AUS) **3716**, 3855, 4528
Australia. Bureau of Statistics. National Health Survey: Health Risk Factors, Australia (AUS) **4494**, 4528
Australia. Bureau of Statistics. National Health Survey: Summary of Results (AUS) **4494**, 4528
Australia. Bureau of Statistics. National Health Survey: Summary Results, Australian States and Territories (AUS) **4495**, 4528
Australia. Bureau of Statistics. National Health Survey: Use of Medications, Australia (AUS) **3716**, 4528
Australia. Bureau of Statistics. National Health Survey: Users' Guide (AUS) **4495**, 4528
Australia. Bureau of Statistics. National Nutrition Survey: Foods Eaten, Australia (AUS) **4248**, 4528
Australia. Bureau of Statistics. National Nutrition Survey: Nutrient Intake, Australia *see* Australia. Bureau of Statistics. National Nutrition Survey: Nutrient Intakes and Physical Measurements, Australia **4248**, 4528
Australia. Bureau of Statistics. National Nutrition Survey: Nutrient Intakes and Physical Measurements, Australia (AUS) **4248**, 4528
Australia. Bureau of Statistics. Northern Territory Office. National Health Survey: Darwin-Palmerston and Alice Springs (AUS) **4495**, 4528
Australia. Bureau of Statistics. Occasional Paper: Cigarette Smoking among Indigenous Australians (AUS) **4364**, 4528
▼ Australia. Bureau of Statistics. Occasional Paper: Hospital Statistics, Aboriginal and Torres Strait Islander Australians (AUS) **3524**, 4528
Australia. Bureau of Statistics. Occasional Paper: Overweight and Obesity, Indigenous Australians (AUS) **4364**, 4528
Australia. Bureau of Statistics. Occasional Paper: Self-Assessed Health Status, Indigenous Australians (AUS) **4364**, 4528
Australia. Bureau of Statistics. Optometry and Optical Dispensing Services, Australia (AUS) **3716**, 3994, 4528
Australia. Bureau of Statistics. Physiotherapy Services, Australia (AUS) **3716**, 4059, 4528
Australia. Bureau of Statistics. Private Hospitals, Australia (AUS ISSN 1039-3005) **3524**, 4528
Australia. Bureau of Statistics. Private Medical Practice Industry, Australia (AUS) **3716**, 4528
Australia. Bureau of Statistics. Private Medical Practitioners, Australia (AUS) **3716**, 4528
Australia. Bureau of Statistics. Queensland Office. Queensland at a Glance (AUS ISSN 0157-3713) **4528**
Australia. Bureau of Statistics. The Health and Welfare of Australia's Aboriginal and Torres Strait Islander Peoples (AUS ISSN 1441-2004) **4364**, 4528
▼ Australia. Bureau of Statistics. Veterinary Services, Australia (AUS) **4561**, 4528
Australia. Bureau of Statistics. Western Australian Office. Home Safety Devices, Western Australia (AUS) **4248**, 4528
Australia. Bureau of Statistics. Women's Safety Survey, Unit Record File, Australia (AUS) **4495**, 4528, 4569
• Australia. Department of the Treasury. Advisory Panel on the Marketing of Infant Formula. Annual Report (AUS) **4462**
Australia Paediatric Nurse Journal (AUS ISSN 1036-5060) **3914**, 4041
Australian Advances in Veterinary Science *see* Australian Veterinary Association Conference Handbook **4538**
• Australian Adverse Drug Reactions Bulletin (AUS ISSN 1325-8540) **4278**
Australian and New Zealand Biotechnology Directory *see* Directory of Australian Biotechnology Companies **3369**, 3273
Australian and New Zealand Council for the Care of Animals in Research and Teaching Limited News *see* A N Z C C A R T News **3171**, 4534
➤ Australian and New Zealand Directory of Genetics Support Groups, Services and Information (AUS) **3226**, 3145, 3299
• Australian and New Zealand Journal of Family Therapy (AUS ISSN 0814-723X) **4520**, 4379, 4511
Australian and New Zealand Journal of Medicine *see* Internal Medicine Journal **3909**
• ➤ Australian and New Zealand Journal of Mental Health Nursing (AUS ISSN 1324-3780) **4075**, 3914
• ➤ Australian and New Zealand Journal of Obstetrics and Gynecology (AUS ISSN 0004-8666) **3945**
Australian and New Zealand Journal of Ophthalmology *see* Clinical and Experimental Ophthalmology **3995**
• ➤ Australian & New Zealand Journal of Psychiatry (AUS ISSN 0004-8674) **4075**
• ➤ Australian and New Zealand Journal of Public Health (AUS ISSN 1326-0200) **4462**, 3793
Australian and New Zeland Journal of Surgery *see* A N Z Journal of Surgery **4178**
Australian Association of Occupational Therapists. Journal *see* Australian Occupational Therapy Journal **4059**
Australian Biochemical Society. Proceedings (AUS ISSN 0067-1703) **3241**
Australian Chiropractors' Association. Journal *see* Chiropractic Journal of Australia **3786**
Australian Chiropractor's Association. Membership Directory *see* Chiropractors' Association of Australia. Membership Directory **3787**
Australian College of Midwives Incorporated Journal *see* A C M I Journal **3943**
Australian College of Nutritional and Environmental Medicine. Journal *see* Australasian College of Nutritional and Environmental Medicine. Journal **3572**, 3446, 4229
Australian Continence Journal (AUS ISSN 1324-2989) **4210**, 4059
Australian Council for Health Physical Education and Recreation Inc. Healthy Lifestyles Journal *see* A C H P E R Healthy Lifestyles Journal **3409**, 4349, 4525
• Australian Council on Smoking and Health Newsletter (AUS ISSN 1329-6884) **4350**, 3399
➤ Australian Critical Care (AUS ISSN 1036-7314) **3914**
Australian Dental Association. News Bulletin (AUS ISSN 0810-7440) **3816**
• ➤ Australian Dental Journal (AUS ISSN 0045-0421) **3816**
Australian Dental Practice Magazine (AUS ISSN 1320-2340) **3816**, 3364, 3366
• Australian Department of Health & Aged Care. Annual Report (AUS) **4462**
• Australian Department of Health & Aged Care. Budget Papers (AUS) **4462**
Australian Department of Health & Aged Care. Chief Medical Officer's Report (AUS) **4462**
• Australian Department of Health & Aged Care. Corporate Plan (AUS) **4462**
Australian Department of Health & Aged Care. Health and Aged Care Occasional Papers New Series (AUS) **4463**
Australian Department of Health & Aged Care. Health and Aged Care Occasional Papers Series *see* Australian Department of Health & Aged Care. Health and Aged Care Occasional Papers New Series **4463**
• Australian Department of Health & Aged Care. Health Financing Series Occasional papers (AUS) **4463**
Australian Doctor (AUS ISSN 1039-7116) **3572**, 4463
Australian Dr Weekly *see* Australian Doctor **3572**, 4463
Australian Early Childhood Association Research in Practice *see* A E C A Research in Practice **3380**, 4371
➤ Australian Endodontic Journal (AUS ISSN 1329-1947) **3816**
Australian Equine Veterinarian (AUS ISSN 1032-6626) **4538**
• Australian Family Physician (AUS ISSN 0300-8495) **3572**
Australian Fluoridation News. Aqua-Pura (AUS) **4561**, 4463
Australian Health and Aged Care Journal *see* International Hospital & Aged Care Journal **3515**, 3365, 3474, 4257
Australian Health and Medical Exports *see* Australian Health and Medical Industry Guide **3369**, 3572
Australian Health and Medical Industry Guide (AUS ISSN 1323-0824) **3369**, 3572
➤ Australian Health Review (AUS ISSN 0156-5788) **3502**
• Australian Indigenous Health Bulletin (AUS ISSN 1445-7253) **4463**
Australian Institute of Medical Scientists Self Assessment Programmes Series *see* A I M S Self Assessment Programmes Series **3870**
Australian Institute of Parapsychological Research Bulletin *see* Australian Parapsychological Review **4271**, 4379
Australian Institute of Pharmacy Management Newsletter (AUS ISSN 0706-3202) **4278**
Australian Institute of Psychic Research Bulletin *see* Australian Parapsychological Review **4271**, 4379
➤ Australian Journal of Advanced Nursing (AUS ISSN 0813-0531) **3914**
Australian Journal of Audiology (AUS ISSN 0157-1532) **3489**, 4031
Australian Journal of Biological Sciences *see* Reproduction, Fertility and Development **3215**
Australian Journal of Clinical and Experimental Hypnosis (AUS ISSN 0156-0417) **3906**
• Australian Journal of Clinical Hypnotherapy and Hypnosis (AUS ISSN 0810-0713) **3906**
Australian Journal of Ecology *see* Austral Ecology **3183**
Australian Journal of Emergency Care *see* Australasian Journal of Emergency Care **4011**, 3914, 4182
➤ The Australian Journal of Emergency Management (AUS ISSN 1324-1540) **3387**, 4463
• ➤ Australian Journal of Experimental Agriculture (AUS ISSN 0816-1089) **3157**, 4538
• ➤ Australian Journal of Forensic Sciences (AUS ISSN 0045-0618) **3881**
Australian Journal of Guidance & Counselling (AUS ISSN 1037-2911) **4379**
➤ Australian Journal of Hospital Pharmacy (AUS ISSN 0310-6810) **4278**, 3502
➤ Australian Journal of Learning Disabilities (AUS ISSN 1324-8928) **3419**
• ➤ Australian Journal of Management and Organisational Behaviour (AUS ISSN 1440-4567) **4379**, 3364
Australian Journal of Marriage and Family *see* Journal of Family Studies **3554**, 4416
➤ Australian Journal of Medical Herbalism (AUS ISSN 1033-8330) **3163**
➤ Australian Journal of Medical Science (AUS ISSN 1038-1643) **3572**, 3871
• Australian Journal of Otolaryngology (AUS ISSN 1037-2105) **4031**, 4182
Australian Journal of Pharmacy (AUS ISSN 0004-8399) **4278**
• ➤ Australian Journal of Physiotherapy (AUS ISSN 0004-9514) **4059**
Australian Journal of Plant Physiology *see* Fuctional Plant Biology **3280**
➤ Australian Journal of Primary Health - Interchange (AUS ISSN 1324-2296) **3572**
• ➤ Australian Journal of Psychology (AUS ISSN 0004-9530) **4379**
Australian Journal of Psychotherapy *see* Australasian Journal of Psychotherapy **4379**, 4075
Australian Journal of Public Health *see* Australian and New Zealand Journal of Public Health **4462**, 3793
Australian Journal of Remedial Education *see* Australian Journal of Learning Disabilities **3419**
• Australian Journal of Rural Health (AUS ISSN 1038-5282) **4463**, 3914
Australian Journal of Science and Medicine in Sport *see* Journal of Science and Medicine in Sport **4174**
Australian Journal of Transpersonal Psychology *see* International Journal of Transpersonal Studies **4407**, 4347, 4500
Australian Journal on Ageing *see* Australasian Journal on Ageing **3468**
Australian Marine Conservation Society. Bulletin *see* Turning the Tide **3392**
Australian Medical Association List of Medical Services and Fees *see* A M A List of Medical Services and Fees **3555**
Australian Medical Association. Victoria Branch. Monthly Paper *see* A M A Victoria Branch News **3555**
Australian Medical Association Victoria Branch News *see* A M A Victoria Branch News **3555**
Australian Medical Record Journal *see* Health Information Management **3611**, 3548
• Australian Medicine (AUS) **3572**, 4463

• B N A's Medicare Report (USA ISSN 1049-7986) **3573**, 3537
• B N A's Safety Library on C D (USA) **4251**
• B N A's SafetyNet (USA ISSN 1091-2894) **4251**
• B N A's State Environment & Safety Regulatory Monitoring Report (USA ISSN 1065-8076) **3436**, 3537
B N F Annual Conference Proceedings (British Nutrition Foundation) (GBR) **4229**
B N F Briefing Papers (British Nutrition Foundation) (GBR ISSN 1350-6854) **4229**
B N F Nutrition Bulletin *see* Nutrition Bulletin **4241**, 3462
B N F Task Force Reports (British Nutrition Foundation) (GBR) **4230**
B P I Jahresbericht (Bundesverband der Pharmazeutischen Industrie e.V.) (DEU) **4279**
B R H S Newsletter (British Regional Heart Study) (GBR) **3573**
B T I *see* Biotech Tech International **3270**
B T I A (Bulletin Technique de l'Insemination Artificielle) (FRA ISSN 0153-6281) **3299**
B T - L M & S (Building Technology - Land Management & Safety) (LCA ISSN 1010-5700) **3361**, 4463
B U M C Proceedings *see* Baylor University Medical Center Proceedings **3574**
• The B V A Bulletin (Blinded Veterans Association) (USA ISSN 0005-3430) **3495**, 4223, 4511
Babraham Institute. Corporate Plan (GBR ISSN 1359-1533) **3340**, 3177, 3299, 3357
• Babraham Institute. Report (GBR ISSN 1354-8425) **3340**, 3177, 3299
▼ Baby (Kennesaw) (USA) **3380**, 4041
Baby Magazine Infant Care Guide (USA) **4041**, 3380
Baby on the Way: Basics *see* Parenting's Healthy Pregnancy **3961**, 3385
Baby Post (DEU ISSN 0724-1119) **3380**, 4041
Baby - Unser Glueck (DEU) **3380**, 4041
Babycare Book (AUS ISSN 1326-1665) **4041**, 3380
BabyFirst (USA) **4041**, 3380
• The Back Letter (USA ISSN 0894-7376) **4011**
Back to Work (CAN) **4251**, 3419
Backletter *see* The Back Letter **4011**
The BackLetter (USA) **4011**
Bacon's Medical & Health Media Directory (USA ISSN 1520-2674) **3573**, 3388
➤ Bacteriologia, Virusologia, Parazitologia, Epidemiologia (ROM ISSN 1220-3696) **3318**, 3793
Bad Toelz Aktuell (DEU ISSN 1434-6672) **4534**, 4463
Badischer Landesverein fuer Naturkunde und Naturschutz, Freiburg. Mitteilungen. Neue Folge (DEU ISSN 0067-2858) **3183**, 3407
Bahamas Pharmaceutical Association. Newsletter (BHS) **4279**
• Bahrain Medical Bulletin (BHR ISSN 1012-7666) **3573**
• ➤ Bahrain Medical Society. Journal (BHR ISSN 1015-6321) **3573**
• ➤ Bailliere's Best Practice & Research in Clinical Anaesthesiology (GBR ISSN 1521-6896) **3756**
• ➤ Bailliere's Best Practice & Research in Clinical Endocrinology and Metabolism (GBR ISSN 1521-690X) **3855**
• ➤ Bailliere's Best Practice & Research in Clinical Gastroenterology (GBR ISSN 1521-6918) **3886**
• ➤ Bailliere's Best Practice & Research in Clinical Haematology (GBR ISSN 1521-6926) **3898**
• ➤ Bailliere's Best Practice & Research in Clinical Obstetrics and Gynaecology (GBR ISSN 1521-6934) **3945**
• ➤ Bailliere's Best Practice & Research in Clinical Rheumatology (GBR ISSN 1521-6942) **4167**
Bailliere's Clinical Anaesthesiology *see* Bailliere's Best Practice & Research in Clinical Anaesthesiology **3756**
Bailliere's Clinical Endocrinology and Metabolism *see* Bailliere's Best Practice & Research in Clinical Endocrinology and Metabolism **3855**
Bailliere's Clinical Gastroenterology *see* Bailliere's Best Practice & Research in Clinical Gastroenterology **3886**
Bailliere's Clinical Haematology *see* Bailliere's Best Practice & Research in Clinical Haematology **3898**
➤ Bailliere's Clinical Infectious Diseases (GBR ISSN 1071-6564) **3793**
Bailliere's Clinical Obstetrics and Gynaecology *see* Bailliere's Best Practice & Research in Clinical Obstetrics and Gynaecology **3945**
➤ Bailliere's Clinical Paediatrics (GBR ISSN 0963-6714) **4041**
➤ Bailliere's Clinical Psychiatry (GBR ISSN 1074-8806) **4075**
Bailliere's Clinical Rheumatology *see* Bailliere's Best Practice & Research in Clinical Rheumatology **4167**
➤ Bailliere's Handbook of First Aid (GBR) **3574**
Bailliere's Midwives' Dictionary (GBR) **3945**
Bailliere's Nurses' Dictionary (GBR) **3914**
Baioenjiniaringu Shinpojumu Ronbunju/Bioengineering Symposium (JPN) **3237**
Baiofidobakku Kenkyu/Japanese Journal of Biofeedback Research (JPN ISSN 0386-1856) **4380**
Baioindasutori Nenkan/Yearbook of Bioindustry (JPN) **3269**
Baiomedikaru/Japanese Biomedical Forum. Journal (JPN ISSN 0917-4915) **3574**
• Baiqiuen Yike Daxue Xuebao/Norman Bethune University of Medical Sciences. Journal (CHN ISSN 0253-3707) **3574**
Baisho Igaku/Journal of Compensation Medicine (JPN ISSN 0910-5816) **3574**
• Baixuebing/Journal of Leukemia (CHN ISSN 1006-6934) **3898**
Balance (GBR ISSN 0005-4216) **3855**
• Balance (Alexandria) (USA ISSN 1094-6195) **3468**, 3914
Balans (NLD ISSN 0005-4259) **3393**
➤ Balcan Medical Union. Archives (ROM) **3574**
▼ • Balint-Journal (DEU ISSN 1439-5142) **4075**
Balkan Journal of Medical Genetics (BGR ISSN 1311-0160) **3299**
Balkan Union of Oncology. Journal (GRC ISSN 1107-0625) **3968**
Balneoklimatologiia i Fizikalna Terapiia *see* Healed Tourist **4061**
Balneologia Polska (POL ISSN 0005-4402) **3574**
➤ Baltic Journal of Laboratory Animal Science (LVA ISSN 1407-0944) **3872**
Balto Alternative *see* Baltimore Alternative **0**
Bamah (Givatayim) (ISR) **3968**
Bamboo *see* Banbu **4511**, 3574
Banbu/Bamboo (JPN ISSN 0912-8662) **4511**, 3574
Banbury Reports (USA ISSN 0198-0068) **3183**
Banbury Reports Series *see* Banbury Reports **3183**
Band *see* Ja! - Wir Atmen **3747**
Das Band (DEU ISSN 0170-902X) **3419**, 3483
Bandelette *see* I A O Straight Talk **3825**
Bandolier (GBR ISSN 1353-9906) **3574**
Banff International Behavioral Sciences Series (USA) **4380**
• Bangbu Yixueyuan Xuebao/Acta Academiae Medicinae Bengbu (CHN ISSN 1000-2200) **3574**
Bangladesh Journal of Animal Science (BGD ISSN 0379-430X) **3160**, 4539
Bangladesh Journal of Biological Sciences (BGD ISSN 1016-4057) **3183**, 3154
• ➤ Bangladesh Journal of Botany (BGD ISSN 0253-5416) **3278**
Bangladesh Journal of Dermatology, Venereology and Leprology (BGD) **3845**
Bangladesh Journal of Psychology (BGD ISSN 1022-7466) **4380**
Bangladesh Medical Journal (BGD ISSN 0301-035X) **3574**
• Bangladesh Medical Research Council Bulletin (BGD ISSN 0377-9238) **3574**
• Bangladesh Pharmaceutical Journal (BGD ISSN 0301-4606) **4279**
Bangladesh Veterinary Journal (BGD ISSN 0378-8113) **4539**
Baptist Medical Centers News *see* B M C News **3502**
Bar Associations in Focus on Aging and the Law *see* B I F O C A L **3536**, 3468
Barbados. Ministry of Health. Chief Medical Officer. Annual Report (BRB) **4463**
Barbados Nursing Journal (BRB ISSN 0572-6042) **3914**
Barcelona Quirurgica (ESP) **4182**
Barclays Health Law Bulletin (California Edition) (USA) **3537**, 3574
• ➤ Barents Newsletter on Occupational Health and Safety (FIN ISSN 1455-8459) **4251**
➤ Bariatrician (USA ISSN 1099-4521) **3908**, 3855
Barnbladet (SWE ISSN 0349-1994) **4041**, 3914
▼ Barts and the London Chronicle (GBR ISSN 1470-2282) **3502**
Bart's Journal *see* Barts and the London Chronicle **3502**
Basel Institute for Immunology. Annual Report (CHE ISSN 0301-3782) **3741**
Baseline (GBR ISSN 0964-0185) **3468**
➤ Le Basi Razionali della Terapia (ITA) **4279**
➤ Basic and Applied Myology (ITA ISSN 1120-9992) **3183**
• ➤ Basic and Applied Social Psychology (USA ISSN 0197-3533) **4380**, 4508
➤ Basic and Clinical Cardiology Series (USA) **3764**
➤ Basic & Clinical Endocrinology (USA ISSN 0891-2068) **3855**
Basic and Clinical Immunology (USA ISSN 0891-2076) **3741**
Basic and Clinical Oncology (USA ISSN 1073-0028) **3968**
Basic and Clinical Pharmacology (USA ISSN 0891-2033) **4279**
Basic Histology (USA ISSN 0891-2106) **3285**
➤ Basic Life Sciences (USA ISSN 0090-5542) **3183**
Basic Medical Science and Clinics *see* Jichu Yixue yu Linchuang **3628**
• ➤ Basic Research in Cardiology (DEU ISSN 0300-8428) **3764**
Basic Research in Cardiology. Supplement (DEU ISSN 1433-0946) **3764**
Basis (NOR) **3914**
Basler Beitraege zur Chirurgie (CHE ISSN 1013-7459) **4182**
Basler Veroeffentlichungen zur Geschichte der Medizin und der Biologie. Neue Folge (CHE) **3574**, 3183
Basque Region. Departamento de Sanidad. Presupuesto *see* Basque Region. Osasun Saileko. Aurrekontua **3716**
Basque Region. Osasun Saileko. Aurrekontua/Basque Region. Departamento de Sanidad. Presupuesto (ESP) **3716**
Bat Kol (ISR) **3489**
Batiment - Entretien (FRA) **4251**, 3436
Batting the Breeze (USA ISSN 0005-6367) **4158**
Bau (DEU ISSN 0341-096X) **4251**
Bau-Berufsgenossenschaft Hannover. Mitteilungsblatt (DEU ISSN 0931-2862) **4251**
Baum-Zeitung (DEU ISSN 0341-3624) **3279**
Bayer Alkalizer (USA) **3183**, 3368
Bayer Berichte *see* Bayer Report **4279**, 3372
Bayer Report (DEU) **4279**, 3372
Bayerisches Aerzteblatt (DEU ISSN 0005-7126) **3574**
Baylor Dental Journal (USA ISSN 0005-7258) **3816**
Baylor Medicine (USA) **3574**
Baylor Progress (USA) **3502**, 3574
• ➤ Baylor University Medical Center Proceedings (USA ISSN 0899-8280) **3574**
Be Healthy (USA) **4562**
Be Slim (GBR ISSN 0956-5345) **4350**
• Be Your Own Therapist Newsletter (USA) **4380**
The Beacon (AUS) **3968**
Beacon (Davenport) (USA) **3786**
Beacon House Bulletin *see* Mental Health Matters **4427**, 4481
Beau (USA) **3527**, 4222
Beauty Handbook (USA) **4350**
➤ Bechterew-Brief (DEU) **4167**
• Before Birth and Beyond (USA ISSN 1520-7730) **3380**, 4041
Beginnings (Flagstaff) (USA ISSN 1071-2984) **3914**, 4568
• ➤ The Behavior Analyst (USA ISSN 0738-6729) **4380**
• ➤ Behavior and Philosophy (USA ISSN 1053-8348) **4380**
• ➤ Behavior and Social Issues (USA ISSN 1064-9506) **4380**, 4520
• ➤ Behavior Genetics (USA ISSN 0001-8244) **3299**, 3574
• ➤ Behavior Modification (USA ISSN 0145-4455) **4380**
• ➤ Behavior Research Methods, Instruments, and Computers (USA ISSN 0743-3808) **4380**
Behavior Science Research *see* Cross-Cultural Research **4508**, 4393
The Behavior Therapist (USA ISSN 0278-8403) **4380**
• ➤ Behavior Therapy (USA ISSN 0005-7894) **4380**
• ➤ Behavioral and Brain Sciences (GBR ISSN 0140-525X) **4380**, 3184, 4076
▼ • ➤ Behavioral & Cognitive Neuroscience Reviews (USA ISSN 1534-5823) **4381**, 4076, 4503, 4531
Behavioral and Neural Biology *see* Neurobiology of Learning and Memory **4112**, 3210, 4429
• ➤ Behavioral Disorders (USA ISSN 0198-7429) **3419**
• ➤ Behavioral Ecology (USA ISSN 1045-2249) **3184**
• ➤ Behavioral Ecology and Sociobiology (DEU ISSN 0340-5443) **3436**, 3184, 4381
Behavioral Educator (USA) **3428**, 4381
• Behavioral Health Accreditation & Accountability Alert (USA ISSN 1529-7055) **4076**, 4381
Behavioral Health Business News (USA) **3531**, 3399, 4076
• Behavioral Health Management (USA ISSN 1075-6701) **3399**
Behavioral Health Outcomes *see* Behavioral Health Accreditation & Accountability Alert **4076**, 4381
Behavioral Health Section Newsletter (USA) **4076**
• ➤ Behavioral Healthcare Tomorrow (USA ISSN 1063-8490) **4381**, 4511
• ➤ Behavioral Interventions (GBR ISSN 1072-0847) **4076**
• ➤ Behavioral Medicine (USA ISSN 0896-4289) **4381**, 4076
• ➤ Behavioral Neuroscience (USA ISSN 0735-7044) **4381**, 4076
Behavioral Psychology *see* Psicologia Conductual **4435**
• Behavioral Research in Accounting (USA ISSN 1050-4753) **3362**, 4381
Behavioral Residential Treatment *see* Behavioral Interventions **4076**
• ➤ Behavioral Sciences and the Law (GBR ISSN 0735-3936) **4381**, 3537
▼ Behavioral Sleep Medicine (USA) **4381**
➤ Behaviormetrika (JPN ISSN 0385-7417) **4457**
➤ Behaviorology (USA ISSN 1047-8663) **4381**, 3409
• ➤ Behaviour (NLD ISSN 0005-7959) **3351**, 4381
• ➤ Behaviour and Information Technology (GBR ISSN 0144-929X) **4381**, 4524
• ➤ Behaviour Change (AUS ISSN 0813-4839) **4381**
• ➤ Behaviour Research and Therapy (GBR ISSN 0005-7967) **4382**
• Behavioural and Cognitive Psychotherapy (GBR ISSN 1352-4658) **4382**
• ➤ Behavioural Brain Research (NLD ISSN 0166-4328) **4076**
• ➤ Behavioural Neurology (NLD ISSN 0953-4180) **4076**
• ➤ Behavioural Pharmacology (USA ISSN 0955-8810) **4279**, 4382
• ➤ Behavioural Processes (NLD ISSN 0376-6357) **4076**
Behavioural Psychotherapist (GBR ISSN 0953-7074) **4382**
Behavioural Psychotherapy *see* Behavioural and Cognitive Psychotherapy **4382**
Behavioural Social Work Review *see* The Cognitive Behavioural Social Work Review **4511**, 4389
Behindertenhilfe Durch Erziehung, Unterricht und Therapie (DEU ISSN 0171-9718) **3419**
Behindertensport *see* Plusport News **4176**
Behindertenzeitschrift *see* Deutsche Behindertenzeitschrift **3420**, 4086
Beijing Biomedical Engineering *see* Beijing Shengwu Yixue Gongcheng **3574**
• ➤ Beijing Daxue Xuebao (Yixue Ban)/Peking University. Journal (Health Sciences) (CHN ISSN 1671-167X) **3574**
Beijing Medical Journal *see* Beijing Yixue **3574**
• Beijing Shengwu Yixue Gongcheng/Beijing Biomedical Engineering (CHN ISSN 1002-3208) **3574**
Beijing Traditional Chinese Medicine *see* Beijing Zhongyi **3164**, 3574
Beijing University of Traditional Chinese Medicine. Journal *see* Beijing Zhongyi Daxue Xuebao **3574**
Beijing Yike Daxue Xuebao *see* Beijing Daxue Xuebao (Yixue Ban) **3574**
• Beijing Yixue/Beijing Medical Journal (CHN ISSN 0253-9713) **3574**
Beijing Zhongyi/Beijing Traditional Chinese Medicine (CHN ISSN 0476-0247) **3164**, 3574
Beijing Zhongyi Daxue Xuebao/Beijing University of Traditional Chinese Medicine. Journal (CHN ISSN 1006-2157) **3574**

Title

Title

Bioelectromagnetics Society Newsletter (USA ISSN 0889-4191) **3265**
Bioengineering *see* Northeast Bioengineering Conference. Proceedings **3238**, 3433
Bioengineering Symposium *see* Baioenjiniaringu Shinpojumu Ronbunju **3237**
• ➤ BioEssays (GBR ISSN 0265-9247) **3184**
• ➤ Bioethics (GBR ISSN 0269-9702) **4346**, 3184
➤ Bioethics Forum (USA ISSN 1065-7274) **3529**, 3172, 3575, 4346
Bioethics Literature Review (USA ISSN 0886-8913) **3717**, 3146, 3545
Bioethics Outlook (AUS ISSN 1037-6410) **4346**, 3575
➤ Bioethics Yearbook (NLD ISSN 0926-261X) **4499**, 3575, 4347
• ➤ BioFactors (NLD ISSN 0951-6433) **3244**
Biofeedback and Self Regulation *see* Applied Psychophysiology and Biofeedback **4378**, 4226
Biofeedback (Cincinnati) (USA ISSN 1060-2488) **3184**, 3547
Biofeedback Clinicians (USA) **3575**
Biofeedback Society of America. Proceedings of the Annual Meeting *see* Association for Applied Psychophysiology and Biofeedback. Proceedings of the Annual Meeting **4379**, 4074
• Biofeedback (Wheat Ridge) (USA ISSN 1081-5937) **4382**, 4076
• ➤ Biofizika (RUS ISSN 0006-3029) **3265**
➤ Biofizika Zhivoi Kletki/Biophysics of Living Cells (RUS ISSN 0301-2425) **3265**
Bioforum (DEU ISSN 0940-0079) **3184**, 3319
Bioforum International (DEU) **3184**, 3269
• ➤ Biofouling (CHE ISSN 0892-7014) **3446**
• ➤ Biofutur (FRA ISSN 0294-3506) **3269**
• ➤ Biogenic Amines (NLD ISSN 0168-8561) **3245**
• ➤ Biogeochemistry (NLD ISSN 0168-2563) **3245**
Biogeographica (FRA ISSN 1165-6638) **3184**
Biogeographical Society of Japan. Bulletin/Nihon Seibutsu Chiri Gakkai Kaiho (JPN ISSN 0067-8716) **3184**
▼ • ➤ Biogerontology (NLD ISSN 1389-5729) **3468**, 3184
Bioimaging *see* Cytometry **3289**
Bioindustry Directory *see* Biotechnology News **3272**
• The BioInformer (GBR ISSN 1462-1355) **3283**
Bioingenioeren (NOR ISSN 0801-6828) **3379**
• Biokhimiya (RUS ISSN 0320-9725) **3245**
Biokhimiya Zhivotnykh i Cheloveka (UKR ISSN 0136-9377) **3245**
BioLaw: A Legal and Ethical Reporter on Medicine, Health Care, and Bioengineering (USA) **3237**, 3537
➤ Biologi Italiani (ITA ISSN 0392-2510) **3184**
Biologia (MEX ISSN 0185-2000) **3185**
Biologia. D: Biochemia a Molekularna Biologia *see* Biologia. Section: Cellular and Molecular Biology **3245**
Biologia e Etologia (ITA) **3185**
Biologia. Section: Cellular and Molecular Biology (SVK ISSN 1335-6399) **3245**
Biologia w Szkole (POL ISSN 0137-8031) **3185**
• Biological Abstracts (USA ISSN 0006-3169) **3226**, 3146, 3185
Biological Abstracts Cumulative Indexes (USA) **3226**, 3146, 3185
• Biological Abstracts - R R M (Reports, Reviews, Meetings) (USA ISSN 0192-6985) **3226**, 3146, 3185
Biological Abstracts - R R M Cumulative Index (Reports, Reviews, and Meetings) (USA) **3226**, 3146, 3185
• Biological & Agricultural Index (USA ISSN 0006-3177) **3226**, 3146, 3156
• Biological and Cultural Tests for Control of Plant Diseases (USA ISSN 0887-2236) **3279**
• ➤ Biological & Pharmaceutical Bulletin (JPN ISSN 0918-6158) **4280**, 3245
• ➤ Biological Bulletin (USA ISSN 0006-3185) **3185**
Biological Bulletin of Poznan (POL ISSN 1426-5656) **3185**
• ➤ Biological Chemistry (DEU ISSN 1431-6730) **3245**
Biological Chemistry Hoppe-Seyler *see* Biological Chemistry **3245**
• ➤ Biological Control (USA ISSN 1049-9644) **3185**
Biological Effects of Low Level Exposures Newsletter *see* B E L L E Newsletter **3446**, 4463
Biological Journal of the Linnean Society *see* Linnean Society. Biological Journal **3206**
Biological Nursing Research *see* Biological Research for Nursing **3914**
• ➤ Biological Psychiatry (USA ISSN 0006-3223) **4076**, 3185, 3245
• ➤ Biological Psychology (NLD ISSN 0301-0511) **4382**, 3185
➤ Biological Regulation & Development (USA ISSN 0271-9355) **3245**
• ➤ Biological Research (CHL ISSN 0716-9760) **3185**, 3872
▼ • ➤ Biological Research for Nursing (USA ISSN 1099-8004) **3914**
Biological Research in Norwich *see* Norwich Research Park Newsletter **3313**
Biological Research Reports from the University of Jyvaskyla (FIN ISSN 0356-1062) **3185**
• ➤ Biological Reviews (GBR ISSN 1464-7931) **3185**
• Biological Rhythms (GBR ISSN 0142-8004) **3226**, 3146, 3717
Biological Science/Seibutsu Kagaku (JPN ISSN 0045-2033) **3185**
Biological Science News *see* Seibutsu Kagaku Nyusu **3218**
➤ Biological Sciences Review (GBR ISSN 0953-5365) **3185**
Biological Signals and Receptors *see* NeuroSignals **3259**
• ➤ Biological Society of Washington. Proceedings (USA ISSN 0006-324X) **3185**, 3279, 3351
Biological Therapies in Dentistry (CAN ISSN 0882-1852) **3816**, 3575
Biological Therapies in Psychiatry *see* Biological Therapies in Psychiatry Newsletter **4077**
• Biological Therapies in Psychiatry Newsletter (USA ISSN 1044-422X) **4077**
Biological Therapy *see* Biomedical Therapy **3577**
• ➤ Biological Trace Element Research (USA ISSN 0163-4984) **3245**
• ➤ Biologicals (GBR ISSN 1045-1056) **3186**
• ➤ Biologicheskie Membrany (RUS ISSN 0233-4755) **3265**, 3286
Biologicheskii Zhurnal Armenii *see* Hayastany Kensabanakan Andes **3198**
• Biologie in Unserer Zeit (DEU ISSN 0045-205X) **3186**
Biologische Arbeitsstoff Toleranz Werte und Expositionsaequivalente fuer Krebserzeugende Arbeitsstoffe (DEU ISSN 0930-195X) **4252**
➤ Biologische Medizin (DEU ISSN 0340-8671) **3786**
Biologische Tiermedizin (DEU ISSN 0723-6212) **4539**, 3186
Biologische Zeitschrift (DEU ISSN 0179-5295) **3295**
Biologisches Zentralblatt *see* Theory in Biosciences **3221**
Biologist (GBR ISSN 0006-3347) **3186**
Biologiya Morya/Marine Biology (RUS ISSN 0134-3475) **3186**, 3408
Biologizace a Chemizace Zivocisne Vyroby - Veterinaria *see* Biopharm **4539**, 4280
• ➤ Biology and Environment (IRL ISSN 0791-7945) **3186**, 3407
• ➤ Biology and Fertility of Soils (DEU ISSN 0178-2762) **3157**, 3186
Biology Bulletin of the Russian Academy of Sciences *see* Russian Academy of Sciences. Biology Bulletin **3217**
• Biology Digest (USA ISSN 0095-2958) **3226**, 3146, 3186
Biology Forum *see* Rivista di Biologia **3216**
Biology International: I U B S Newsmagazine (International Union of Biological Sciences) (FRA ISSN 0253-2069) **3186**
• Biology of Blood and Marrow Transplantation (USA ISSN 1083-8791) **3898**
Biology of Extracellular Matrix (USA ISSN 0887-3224) **3286**
• ➤ Biology of Reproduction (USA ISSN 0006-3363) **3186**
Biology of Reproduction. Supplement (USA ISSN 0523-6754) **3340**, 3575
• ➤ Biology of Sport (POL ISSN 0860-021X) **4173**, 3340, 4280, 4525
• ➤ Biology of the Cell (FRA ISSN 0248-4900) **3286**
• ➤ Biology of the Neonate (CHE ISSN 0006-3126) **3945**, 3186
• ➤ Biomarkers (GBR ISSN 1354-750X) **3575**, 3186
▼ ➤ BIOmaterialen (DEU ISSN 1616-0177) **3816**
• ➤ Biomaterials (GBR ISSN 0142-9612) **3575**, 3245, 3269, 3434
Biomaterials, Artificial Cells and Artificial Organs *see* Artificial Cells, Blood Substitutes, and Immobilization Biotechnology **3871**, 3269
Biomaterials, Artificial Cells and Immobilization Biotechnology *see* Artificial Cells, Blood Substitutes, and Immobilization Biotechnology **3871**, 3269
Biomathematics (USA ISSN 0067-8821) **3186**, 3553
Biomechanics *see* Biomekhanika **3265**, 4365
• ➤ Biomedical and Environmental Sciences (CHN ISSN 0895-3988) **3575**, 4280
Biomedical & Health Research (BEL ISSN 0778-4910) **3575**
Biomedical and Health Research Series (NLD ISSN 0929-6743) **3575**
Biomedical Business International Newsletter *see* The B B I Newsletter **3573**, 3363
Biomedical Business International Newsletter Medical Device Week *see* B B I N: Medical Device Week **3573**, 3363
• ➤ Biomedical Chromatography (GBR ISSN 0269-3879) **3872**, 3376
Biomedical Engineering *see* Biomedizinische Technik **3577**
• ➤ Biomedical Engineering (NLD ISSN 0006-3398) **3576**
• Biomedical Engineering Citation Index (USA) **3717**
Biomedical Engineering Society Bulletin *see* B M E S Bulletin **3573**, 3431
Biomedical Ethics Reviews (USA ISSN 0742-1796) **3576**, 4347
Biomedical Fuzzy Systems Bulletin (JPN ISSN 0915-9274) **3576**
Biomedical Gerontology *see* Kiso Roka Kenkyu **3255**
Biomedical Gerontology Circular *see* Kiso Roka Gakkai Sakyura **3477**, 3255
Biomedical Informatics. Journal (USA) **3576**, 3872
• ➤ Biomedical Letters (GBR ISSN 0961-088X) **3186**, 3576
• ➤ Biomedical Market Newsletter (USA ISSN 1064-4180) **3366**, 3576
• Biomedical Materials (GBR ISSN 0955-7717) **3576**, 4367
Biomedical Meetings Index (USA ISSN 1083-8104) **4220**, 3186, 3576, 4280
• Biomedical Microdevices (USA ISSN 1387-2176) **3576**
Biomedical Perspectives (JPN ISSN 0918-6514) **3576**, 3186
• Biomedical Products (USA ISSN 0192-1266) **3576**, 3872
➤ Biomedical Progress (DEU ISSN 0934-0734) **3898**
▼ • ➤ Biomedical Research (AUS ISSN 1442-830X) **3576**, 3187
• ➤ Biomedical Research (JPN ISSN 0388-6107) **3576**, 3187, 3436
Biomedical Research on Trace Elements (JPN ISSN 0916-717X) **3245**
Biomedical Research Technology Resources *see* Biomedical Technology Research Resources **3576**, 3187
• Biomedical Safety & Standards Newsletter (USA ISSN 1080-9775) **3576**
➤ Biomedical Sciences Instrumentation (USA ISSN 0067-8856) **3576**, 3529
Biomedical Scientist (GBR ISSN 1352-7673) **3872**
• Biomedical Technology Information Service (USA ISSN 0147-2682) **3576**
• Biomedical Technology Research Resources (USA) **3576**, 3187
• Biomedical Therapy (USA) **3577**
• Biomedicas (MEX ISSN 1607-6788) **3187**, 3577
Biomedicine (IND ISSN 0970-2067) **3577**
• ➤ Biomedicine and Pharmacotherapy (FRA ISSN 0753-3322) **3577**, 4280
Biomeditsina *see* Meditsinski Pregled. Klinika i Predklinika **3732**, 3150, 4345
Biomeditsinskaya Radioelektronika (RUS) **3577**
• ➤ Biomedizinische Technik/Biomedical Engineering (DEU ISSN 0013-5585) **3577**
Biomekhanika/Biomechanics (BGR ISSN 0204-7594) **3265**, 4365
➤ Biomembranes (USA ISSN 0067-8864) **3286**
Biometeorology (USA ISSN 0067-8902) **4223**, 3187
Biometeorology Bulletin (AUS ISSN 1022-9205) **4223**, 3154, 3187, 3577
Biometric Bulletin (USA ISSN 8750-0434) **4528**, 3187
• ➤ Biometrical Journal (DEU ISSN 0323-3847) **3187**
Biometrical Letters *see* Listy Biometryczne **3207**
• ➤ Biometrics (USA ISSN 0006-341X) **4528**, 3187, 3553
Biometrie Humaine et Anthropologie (FRA ISSN 1279-7863) **3172**
• ➤ Biometrika (GBR ISSN 0006-3444) **3226**, 3187, 4528
• ➤ Biomolecular Engineering (NLD ISSN 1389-0344) **3269**, 3299
Bionics (USA) **3872**, 3363
Bionieuws (NLD ISSN 0924-7734) **3187**
Bionika (UKR ISSN 0374-6569) **3265**
Bionomica (DEU ISSN 0006-3487) **4351**
BioNyt/Bio-News (DNK ISSN 0107-4415) **3187**, 3436, 3577
• ➤ Bioorganic & Medicinal Chemistry (GBR ISSN 0968-0896) **3377**, 3577
• ➤ Bioorganic & Medicinal Chemistry Letters (GBR ISSN 0960-894X) **3378**, 3577
• ➤ Bioorganicheskaya Khimiya (RUS ISSN 0132-3423) **3378**, 3245
Biopharm (CZE) **4539**, 4280
• ➤ BioPharm (USA ISSN 1040-8304) **4280**
➤ Biopharmaceutical Process Validation (USA) **3187**, 4531
• ➤ Biopharmaceutics & Drug Disposition (GBR ISSN 0142-2782) **4280**
• Biophoenix Database on CD-ROM (GBR) **3577**, 3187, 3270, 3361, 4280
Biophotonics International (USA ISSN 1081-8693) **3577**, 3270
• ➤ Biophysical Chemistry (NLD ISSN 0301-4622) **3265**, 3245
• ➤ Biophysical Journal (USA ISSN 0006-3495) **3265**
➤ Biophysical Society. Annual Meeting. Abstracts (USA ISSN 0523-6800) **3226**, 3146, 3265
• ➤ Biophysics (RUS ISSN 0006-3509) **3265**
Biophysics of Living Cells *see* Biofizika Zhivoi Kletki **3265**
Bioprocess Technology Series *see* Biopharmaceutical Process Validation **3187**, 4531
➤ Biopsy Interpretation Series (USA ISSN 0895-2140) **3577**, 3872
Biopsyche (ITA ISSN 0392-2529) **3173**
• Bioresearch Monitoring Alert (USA) **3529**, 3537, 3577
• ➤ Biorheology (NLD ISSN 0006-355X) **3265**
• ➤ BioScience (USA ISSN 0006-3568) **3187**
• ➤ Bioscience, Biotechnology, and Biochemistry (JPN ISSN 0916-8451) **3270**, 3245
• ➤ Bioscience Reports (USA ISSN 0144-8463) **3286**, 3245
Biosciences (FRA ISSN 1158-467X) **3187**
Biosciences Appliquees *see* Biosciences **3187**
• ➤ Biosensors and Bioelectronics (GBR ISSN 0956-5663) **3270**, 3265
• BIOSIS Evolutions (USA ISSN 1081-8669) **3226**, 3146, 3187
BIOSIS Previews Search Guide (Year) *see* BIOSIS Search Guide (Year) **3226**, 3146, 3187
BIOSIS Search Guide (Year) (USA) **3226**, 3146, 3187
• BIOSIS Serial Sources (USA ISSN 1086-2951) **3227**, 3146, 3187
• ➤ Biospectroscopy (USA ISSN 1075-4261) **3376**, 3266
Biostatistica (USA ISSN 1041-7648) **3227**
• ➤ Biostatistics (GBR ISSN 1465-4644) **3577**
• ➤ Biosystems (IRL ISSN 0303-2647) **3187**
BioTec (DEU ISSN 0937-2725) **3270**
Biotech & Histochem *see* Biotechnic and Histochemistry **3334**, 3270, 3286
• Biotech Business (USA ISSN 0899-5702) **3270**
Biotech Daily *see* Washington Drug Letter (Washington, 1979) **4340**, 3369
Biotech Equipment Update (USA) **3270**, 3529
Biotech-Info *see* Biotechnology Information **3227**, 3146, 3272
BioTech Market News & Legal Strategies (USA) **3270**, 3361, 3537
BioTech Market News and Strategies *see* BioTech Market News & Legal Strategies **3270**, 3361, 3537
• BioTech Navigator (USA ISSN 1092-8995) **3363**, 3270
Biotech Products International *see* Biotech Tech International **3270**
Biotech Reporter *see* AgBiotech Reporter **3153**, 3268, 4535
• ➤ Biotech Software and Internet Report (USA ISSN 1527-9162) **3270**, 3391, 3872
Biotech Tech International (BEL) **3270**
• Biotech Watch (USA) **3270**
• ➤ Biotechnic and Histochemistry (GBR ISSN 1052-0295) **3334**, 3270, 3286

Title

Title

• ➤ Brain and Language (USA ISSN 0093-934X) **4383**, 3550
▼ • Brain and Mind (NLD ISSN 1389-1987) **4077**
• Brain and Nerve/No to Shinkei (JPN ISSN 0006-8969) **4077**
• ➤ Brain, Behavior and Evolution (CHE ISSN 0006-8977) **4077**
• ➤ Brain, Behavior, and Immunity (USA ISSN 0889-1591) **3741**
Brain Damage, Behaviour and Cognition (USA ISSN 0967-9944) **4077**
▼ Brain Disorders Sourcebook (USA) **4077**
• ➤ Brain Injury (GBR ISSN 0269-9052) **4077**
Brain Injury Association. Catalogue of Educational Materials (USA) **4011**
Brain Injury Source (USA ISSN 1094-3439) **4011**
Brain Injury Update (USA ISSN 1084-5968) **3717**, 4078
• Brain - Mind (USA ISSN 1072-3927) **4078**, 4383
Brain - Mind and Common Sense *see* Brain - Mind **4078**, 4383
Brain News (IND ISSN 0006-8985) **4078**
• ➤ Brain Pathology (USA ISSN 1015-6305) **4078**, 3872
• ➤ Brain Research (NLD ISSN 0006-8993) **4078**
• ➤ Brain Research Bulletin (USA ISSN 0361-9230) **4078**
Brain Research Foundation Annual Report (USA) **4078**
• ➤ Brain Research Protocols (NLD ISSN 1385-299X) **4078**
• ➤ Brain Research Reviews (NLD ISSN 0165-0173) **4078**
Brain Science *see* Burein Saiensu **4079**, 3340
• ➤ Brain Topography (USA ISSN 0896-0267) **4078**
• Brain Tumor Pathology (JPN ISSN 1433-7398) **3968**, 4079
BrainScan (NLD ISSN 1380-3980) **4079**
Brainwaves Newsletter *see* Brain Research Foundation Annual Report **4078**
Brandeis University. Institute for Health Policy. Research News (USA) **3578**, 3537
Brandenburgisches Aerzteblatt (DEU ISSN 0939-3471) **3578**
Brandschutz (DEU ISSN 0006-9094) **3458**, 3526
Brasil-Medico (BRA ISSN 0006-9205) **3578**
• Brasilia Medica (BRA ISSN 0524-2053) **3578**
Bratislava Medical Journal *see* Bratislavske Lekarske Listy **3578**
• ➤ Bratislavske Lekarske Listy/Bratislava Medical Journal (SVK ISSN 0006-9248) **3578**
Braunschweiger Veroeffentlichungen zur Geschichte der Pharmazie und Naturwissenschaften (DEU ISSN 0722-7159) **4281**
Brazil. Conselho Federal de Farmacia. Relatorio *see* Infarma **4301**
• ➤ Brazilian Dental Journal (BRA ISSN 0103-6440) **3816**
Brazilian Journal of Agricultural Research *see* Pesquisa Agropecuaria Brasileira **3155**
Brazilian Journal of Animal Science *see* Revista Brasileira de Zootecnia **4551**, 3159
• Brazilian Journal of Biology/Revista Brasileira de Biologia (BRA ISSN 1519-6984) **3188**
➤ Brazilian Journal of Epilepsy and Clinical Neurophysiology/Jornal Brasileiro de Epilepsia e Neurofisiologia Clinica (BRA ISSN 0104-9275) **4079**
➤ Brazilian Journal of Food Technology (BRA) **3460**, 4230
Brazilian Journal of Genetics *see* Genetics and Molecular Biology **3305**
• ➤ Brazilian Journal of Medical and Biological Research (BRA ISSN 0100-879X) **3578**, 3188
• ➤ Brazilian Journal of Microbiology (BRA ISSN 1517-8382) **3319**
Brazilian Journal of Rheumatology *see* Revista Brasileira de Reumatologia **4170**
Brazilian Journal of School Health *see* Revista Brasileira de Saude Escolar **4487**, 3418
Brazilian Journal of Veterinary and Animal Sciences *see* Arquivo Brasileiro de Medicina Veterinaria e Zootecnia **4538**
Brazilian Journal of Veterinary Parasitology *see* Revista Brasileira de Parasitologia Veterinaria **4551**, 3215
Brazilian Journal of Veterinary Research *see* Pesquisa Veterinaria Brasileira **4549**
• ➤ Brazilian Journal of Veterinary Research and Animal Science (BRA ISSN 1413-9596) **4539**, 3351

Breaking Chains *see* A L R A Newsletter **3357**, 3545, 3966, 4562
Breakthrough (GBR ISSN 1363-898X) **4383**, 4079, 4463, 4511
• ➤ The Breast (GBR ISSN 0960-9776) **3946**
• ➤ Breast Cancer (USA ISSN 1074-6900) **3968**, 3946
Breast Cancer: Disease State Management Research (USA) **3968**, 4563
• Breast Cancer Newsletter (USA) **3968**
▼ • Breast Cancer Research (GBR ISSN 1465-5411) **3968**
• ➤ Breast Cancer Research and Treatment (USA ISSN 0167-6806) **3969**
• ➤ Breast Disease (NLD ISSN 0888-6008) **3946**, 3969, 4563
Breast Diseases (USA ISSN 1043-321X) **3946**, 3717
• Breast Implant Litigation Reporter (USA ISSN 1062-1814) **3537**, 3578
• ➤ The Breast Journal (USA ISSN 1075-122X) **3946**, 3340
• The Breast Journal Online (USA ISSN 1524-4741) **3946**, 3340
• Breast News (AUS ISSN 1324-7077) **3969**, 3946
➤ Breastfeeding Abstracts (USA ISSN 0896-4572) **3717**, 3146, 3386
➤ Breastfeeding Review (AUS ISSN 0729-2759) **4230**
Breath Series (USA) **4226**, 4347, 4383
Breathline (USA) **3756**, 3915
• ➤ Breeding Science (JPN) **3154**
Bref Info (FRA) **3816**
Brief Bibliography Series: Selective Annotated Bibliographies for Gerontology Instruction *see* Association for Gerontology in Higher Education. Brief Bibliography **3482**, 3176
Briefings on Ambulatory Care Accrediation *see* Briefings on J C A H O - A A A H C: Ambulatory Care **3503**, 4511
Briefings on Hospital Safety (USA ISSN 1076-5972) **3503**, 4464
Briefings on J C A H O (Joint Commission on Accreditation of Healthcare Organizations) (USA ISSN 1054-6995) **3503**
Briefings on J C A H O - A A A H C: Ambulatory Care (Joint Commission on Accreditation of Healthcare Organizations - Accreditation Association for Ambula) (USA ISSN 1098-0598) **3503**, 4511
Briefings on J C A H O Long - Term and Subacute Care (Joint Commission on Accreditation of Healthcare Organizations) (USA) **3578**
Briefings on Long-Term Care Regulations (USA ISSN 1076-6014) **3503**, 3578
Briefings on Subacute Care *see* Briefings on J C A H O Long - Term and Subacute Care **3578**
Briggs Update: Drugs in Pregnancy and Lactation (USA ISSN 0897-6112) **3946**, 4281
➤ Brill's Studies in Epistemology, Psychology and Psychiatry (NLD ISSN 0924-0314) **4347**, 4079
Bristol-Meyers Cancer Symposia. Proceedings *see* Bristol-Myers - Squibb Cancer Symposia **3969**
Bristol-Myers - Squibb Cancer Symposia (USA) **3969**
Bristol-Myers Squibb - Mead Johnson Nutrition Symposia (USA ISSN 1057-6606) **4230**
Bristol-Myers Squibb Symposium on Pain Research Series (USA) **3756**
Bristol-Myers - Zimmer Orthopaedic Symposium Series (USA) **4011**
British Acupuncture Association. Newsletter (GBR ISSN 0260-5996) **3164**, 3578
British Association for Behavioural Psychotherapy. Newsletter *see* Behavioural Psychotherapist **4382**
British Association for Psychopharmacology. Monograph (GBR ISSN 0264-2689) **4281**, 4079
British Association of Dermatologists. Newsletter *see* B A D News **3845**
British Association of Psychotherapists. Journal (GBR ISSN 0954-0350) **4383**
British Association of Teachers of the Deaf. Association Magazine (GBR) **3489**, 3419
British Association of Teachers of the Deaf. Journal *see* Deafness and Education International **3490**, 3420
British Columbia Cancer Research Centre. Annual Report (CAN ISSN 1185-1031) **3969**
British Columbia. Division of Vital Statistics Agency. Quarterly Digest (CAN ISSN 1188-1437) **4495**, 4528

➤ British Columbia Medical Journal (CAN ISSN 0007-0556) **3578**
British Columbia. Ministry of Health. Annual Report (CAN ISSN 0706-4810) **4464**
British Contact Lens Association. Journal *see* Contact Lens & Anterior Eye **3995**
• ➤ British Dental Journal (GBR ISSN 0007-0610) **3816**
British Dental Nurses' Journal (GBR ISSN 1356-3807) **4182**, 3816
British Dental Surgery Assistant *see* British Dental Nurses' Journal **4182**, 3816
British Fertility Society. Journal *see* Human Fertility **3952**, 3864
• British Food Journal (GBR ISSN 0007-070X) **3460**
British Heart Journal *see* Heart **3772**
• ➤ British Homeopathic Journal (GBR ISSN 0007-0785) **3786**
British Homeopathy Review *see* British Homeopathic Journal **3786**
British Institute of Learning Disabilities. Current Awareness Service (GBR) **3415**, 3177, 3419
British Institute of Radiology Reports (GBR) **4140**
British Journal of Addiction *see* Addiction **3396**
• ➤ British Journal of Anaesthesia (GBR ISSN 0007-0912) **3756**
British Journal of Anaesthesia International Journal of Anaesthesia (South African Edition) *see* B J A: International Journal of Anaesthesia (South African Edition) **3755**
• ➤ British Journal of Audiology (GBR ISSN 0300-5364) **3489**
• ➤ British Journal of Biomedical Science (GBR ISSN 0967-4845) **3872**
• ➤ British Journal of Cancer (GBR ISSN 0007-0920) **3969**
The British Journal of Cardiology (GBR ISSN 0969-6113) **3764**
The British Journal of Chiropractic (GBR ISSN 1466-2108) **3786**
• British Journal of Clinical Governance (GBR ISSN 1466-4100) **3578**, 3364
• ➤ British Journal of Clinical Pharmacology (GBR ISSN 0306-5251) **4281**
British Journal of Clinical Pharmacology. Supplement (GBR ISSN 0264-3774) **4281**
British Journal of Clinical Practice *see* International Journal of Clinical Practice **3622**
British Journal of Clinical Practice. Symposium Supplement *see* International Journal of Clinical Practice. Symposium Supplement **3623**
• ➤ British Journal of Clinical Psychology (GBR ISSN 0144-6657) **4383**
British Journal of Clinical Research *see* Journal of Clinical Research **4306**, 3631
British Journal of Community Health Nursing *see* British Journal of Community Nursing **3915**
British Journal of Community Nursing (GBR ISSN 1462-4753) **3915**
• ➤ The British Journal of Criminology (GBR ISSN 0007-0955) **3393**, 4383
• ➤ British Journal of Dermatology (GBR ISSN 0007-0963) **3845**
British Journal of Dermatology Nursing (GBR) **3845**
• British Journal of Dermatology. Supplement (GBR ISSN 0366-077X) **3846**
• ➤ British Journal of Developmental Disabilities (GBR ISSN 0969-7950) **3419**, 4079, 4383, 4511
• ➤ British Journal of Developmental Psychology (GBR ISSN 0261-510X) **4383**
▼ The British Journal of Diabetes and Vascular Disease (GBR ISSN 1474-6514) **3855**
• ➤ British Journal of Educational Psychology (GBR ISSN 0007-0998) **4383**, 3409
British Journal of Experimental and Clinical Hypnosis *see* Contemporary Hypnosis **3906**, 4391
British Journal of Family Planning *see* Journal of Family Planning and Reproductive Health Care **3359**
▼ ➤ The British Journal of Forensic Practice (GBR ISSN 1463-6646) **3881**
• ➤ British Journal of General Practice (GBR ISSN 0960-1643) **3578**
• ➤ British Journal of Guidance and Counselling (GBR ISSN 0306-9885) **4269**, 4383
• ➤ British Journal of Haematology (GBR ISSN 0007-1048) **3899**
• British Journal of Haematology. Supplement (GBR ISSN 0963-1860) **3899**

➤ The British Journal of Hand Therapy (GBR ISSN 1369-9571) **4059**, 4011
• ➤ British Journal of Health Psychology (GBR ISSN 1359-107X) **4384**, 3578
British Journal of Healthcare Computing *see* British Journal of Healthcare Computing & Information Management **3809**
British Journal of Healthcare Computing & Information Management (GBR) **3809**
▼ British Journal of Homecare (GBR ISSN 1462-1665) **4511**, 3915
British Journal of Hospital Medicine *see* Hospital Medicine (London, 1998) **3615**, 3514
British Journal of Hospital Medicine (Edicion Espanola) *see* Hospital Medicine (London, 1998) **3615**, 3514
British Journal of Industrial Medicine *see* Occupational and Environmental Medicine **4261**
▼ ➤ The British Journal of Infection Control (GBR) **3793**
British Journal of Intensive Care (GBR ISSN 0961-7930) **3578**
• British Journal of Learning Disabilities (GBR ISSN 1354-4187) **4079**
• ➤ British Journal of Mathematical and Statistical Psychology (GBR ISSN 0007-1102) **4384**, 3553, 4528
British Journal of Medical Economics *see* Journal of Medical Economics **3635**, 3517
• ➤ British Journal of Medical Psychology (GBR ISSN 0007-1129) **4384**, 4079
British Journal of Midwifery (GBR ISSN 0969-4900) **3946**
British Journal of Music Therapy (GBR) **4059**, 4225
• ➤ British Journal of Neurosurgery (GBR ISSN 0268-8697) **4182**
• British Journal of Nursing (GBR ISSN 0966-0461) **3915**
• ➤ The British Journal of Nutrition (GBR ISSN 0007-1145) **4230**
• ➤ British Journal of Obstetrics & Gynaecology (GBR ISSN 0306-5456) **3946**
British Journal of Obstetrics & Gynaecology. Supplement (GBR ISSN 0140-7686) **3947**
➤ British Journal of Occupational Therapy (GBR ISSN 0308-0226) **3579**
• ➤ British Journal of Ophthalmology (GBR ISSN 0007-1161) **3994**
British Journal of Optometry and Dispensing (GBR ISSN 1351-6736) **3995**
• ➤ British Journal of Oral and Maxillofacial Surgery (GBR ISSN 0266-4356) **4183**, 3816
British Journal of Orthodontics *see* The Journal of Orthodontics **3830**
• ➤ British Journal of Perioperative Nursing (GBR) **3915**, 4183
• ➤ British Journal of Pharmacology (GBR ISSN 0007-1188) **4281**
➤ British Journal of Physical Education. Research Supplement (GBR) **3428**, 4364
➤ British Journal of Phytotherapy (GBR ISSN 0959-6879) **3164**, 3279
• ➤ British Journal of Plastic Surgery (GBR ISSN 0007-1226) **4183**
British Journal of Podiatric Medicine and Surgery *see* British Journal of Podiatry **4011**
British Journal of Podiatric Medicine and Surgery *see* Podiatry Now **4024**
➤ British Journal of Podiatry (GBR ISSN 1460-7328) **4011**
British Journal of Projective Psychology (GBR ISSN 0309-7757) **4384**, 4079
British Journal of Projective Psychology and Personality Study *see* British Journal of Projective Psychology **4384**, 4079
• ➤ British Journal of Psychiatry (GBR ISSN 0007-1250) **4079**
• ➤ British Journal of Psychology (GBR ISSN 0007-1269) **4384**
➤ British Journal of Psychotherapy (GBR ISSN 0265-9883) **4079**
• ➤ British Journal of Radiology (GBR ISSN 0007-1285) **4141**
British Journal of Renal Medicine (GBR ISSN 1365-5604) **4210**
British Journal of Rheumatology *see* Rheumatology **4171**
British Journal of Sexual Medicine (GBR ISSN 0301-5572) **3579**
• ➤ British Journal of Social Psychology (GBR ISSN 0144-6665) **4384**
• British Journal of Special Education (GBR ISSN 0952-3383) **3419**, 4384
• ➤ British Journal of Sports Medicine (GBR ISSN 0306-3674) **4173**
• ➤ British Journal of Surgery (GBR ISSN 0007-1323) **4183**

Title

Title

Cambridge Medical Reviews. Neurology and Psychiatry (GBR ISSN 1350-1461) **4080**
Cambridge Medicine (GBR ISSN 0952-1119) **3581**
Cambridge Philosophical Society. Biological Reviews *see* Biological Reviews **3185**
• ➤ Cambridge Quarterly of Healthcare Ethics (GBR ISSN 0963-1801) **3581**
Cambridge Scientific Abstracts Neurosciences Abstracts *see* C S A Neurosciences Abstracts **3718**, 3147
Cambridge Scientific Biochemistry Abstracts: Part 2. Nucleic Acids *see* Nucleic Acids Abstracts **3234**, 3150, 3259
Cambridge Studies in Biotechnology (GBR ISSN 0957-0330) **3273**
Cambridge Studies in Mathematical Biology (GBR ISSN 0263-9424) **3189**, 3553
Cambridge Texts in the Physiological Sciences (GBR ISSN 0951-077X) **3340**
Cambridgeshire County Council. Road Safety Plan (Year) (GBR) **4533**, 4458, 4464
Cameo Newsletter *see* Aging News **3467**
Canada Communicable Disease Report/Releve des Maladies Transmissibles au Canada (CAN ISSN 1188-4169) **4464**
Canada Diseases Weekly Report *see* Canada Communicable Disease Report **4464**
Canadian Academy of Sport Medicine Review *see* Clinical Journal of Sport Medicine **4173**, 4012, 4351
Canadian Association for Health, Physical Education and Recreation. Journal *see* Canadian Association for Health, Physical Education, Recreation and Dance. Journal **4364**
Canadian Association for Health, Physical Education, Recreation and Dance. Journal (CAN ISSN 1201-2319) **4364**
Canadian Association for Laboratory Animal Science Newsletter (CAN ISSN 0045-4354) **3872**
Canadian Association of Critical Care Nurses. Official Journal *see* Dynamics **3596**
Canadian Association of Educators of the Deaf and Hard of Hearing Journal *see* C A E D H H Journal **3489**, 3420
Canadian Association of Nephrology Nurses and Technologists Journal *see* C A N N T Journal **3915**, 4210
Canadian Association of Pathologists. Newsletter (CAN ISSN 0703-8372) **3581**
• ➤ Canadian Association of Radiologists Journal/Association Canadienne des Radiologistes. Journal (CAN ISSN 0846-5371) **4141**
Canadian Association of the Deaf Chat *see* C A D Chat **4031**, 3489
Canadian (Belleville) (CAN ISSN 0008-2805) **3489**
Canadian Biochemical Society. Bulletin *see* Canadian Society of Biochemistry, Molecular and Cellular Biology. Bulletin **3246**
Canadian Biotech News (CAN ISSN 1188-455X) **3273**
Canadian Biotech Research (CAN) **3273**
Canadian Bulletin of Fisheries and Aquatic Sciences (CAN ISSN 0706-6503) **3459**, 3189
➤ Canadian Bulletin of Medical History/Bulletin Canadien d'Histoire de la Medecine (CAN ISSN 0823-2105) **3581**
Canadian Childbirth Educator *see* Pre & Post Natal News **3938**
• ➤ Canadian Chiropractic Association. Journal (CAN ISSN 0008-3194) **3786**
Canadian Dental Assistants Association. Journal (CAN ISSN 1199-1666) **3817**
➤ Canadian Dental Association. Journal/Association Dentaire Canadienne. Journal (CAN ISSN 0709-8936) **3817**
➤ Canadian Dental Hygienists Association. Probe (CAN ISSN 0834-1494) **3817**
Canadian Dietetic Association. Journal *see* Canadian Journal of Dietetic Practice and Research **4230**
• Canadian Directory of Health Care Conferences/Repertoire Canadien des Conferences de Soins de Sante (CAN ISSN 1193-6452) **4220**, 3581
➤ Canadian Emergency News (CAN ISSN 0847-947X) **4012**
Canadian Employment Safety and Health Guide (CAN) **4252**, 3537
• ➤ Canadian Family Physician/Medecin de Famille Canadien (CAN ISSN 0008-350X) **3581**
Canadian Federation of Biological Societies. Annual Meeting. Programme, Proceedings (CAN ISSN 0845-5066) **3189**
• Canadian Federation of Biological Societies. Newsletter (CAN ISSN 0068-8681) **3189**
Canadian Feed Industry Association. Eastern Nutrition Conference. Proceedings *see* Animal Nutrition Association of Canada. Eastern Nutrition Conference. Proceedings **3160**, 4228
• Canadian Government Programs and Services (CAN ISSN 0045-4893) **4458**
Canadian Health Care Management (CAN) **3581**, 3531
Canadian Health Facilities Law Guide (CAN) **3537**, 4464
Canadian Healthcare Business News (CAN) **4059**
• Canadian Healthcare Manager (CAN ISSN 1202-9718) **3504**
Canadian Healthcare Source Book (CAN ISSN 1201-530X) **3582**
Canadian Heart Foundation. Annual Report *see* Heart and Stroke Foundation of Canada. Annual Report **3772**
Canadian HIV - AIDS Policy & Law Newsletter *see* Canadian HIV - AIDS Policy & Law Review **3537**, 3794
• Canadian HIV - AIDS Policy & Law Review (CAN ISSN 1496-399X) **3537**, 3794
Canadian Horseman (CAN ISSN 0840-6200) **4527**, 4540
Canadian Intramural Recreation Association. Bulletin (CAN ISSN 1187-0818) **4351**, 3381, 3428
Canadian Intravenous Nurses Association *see* C I N A **3915**
• ➤ The Canadian Journal of Adlerian Psychology (CAN) **4385**
Canadian Journal of Allergy and Clinical Immunology (CAN ISSN 1203-844X) **3741**
• ➤ Canadian Journal of Anaesthesia/Journal Canadien d'Anesthesie (CAN ISSN 0832-610X) **3756**
• ➤ Canadian Journal of Applied Physiology/Revue Canadienne de Physiologie Appliquee (USA ISSN 1066-7814) **4525**, 4173
• ➤ Canadian Journal of Behavioural Science/Revue Canadienne des Sciences du Comportement (CAN ISSN 0008-400X) **4385**, 3409, 4520
• ➤ Canadian Journal of Cardiology (CAN ISSN 0828-282X) **3764**, 3872, 4183
➤ Canadian Journal of Cardiovascular Nursing (CAN ISSN 0843-6096) **3915**, 3765
Canadian Journal of Clinical Pharmacology/Journal Canadien de Pharmacologie Clinique (CAN ISSN 1198-581X) **4282**
Canadian Journal of Community Mental Health/Revue Canadienne de Sante Mentale Communautaire (CAN ISSN 0713-3936) **4385**, 4464
Canadian Journal of Continuing Medical Education (CAN ISSN 0843-994X) **3582**, 3416
➤ Canadian Journal of Counselling/Revue Canadienne de Counseling (CAN ISSN 0828-3893) **4386**, 3409
➤ Canadian Journal of Diabetes Care (CAN) **3856**, 4351
Canadian Journal of Diagnosis (CAN ISSN 0839-1866) **3582**
• ➤ Canadian Journal of Dietetic Practice and Research/Revue canadienne de la Practique et de la Recherche en Dietetique (CAN ISSN 1486-3847) **4230**
• ➤ Canadian Journal of Experimental Psychology/Revue Canadienne de Psychologie Experimentale (CAN ISSN 1196-1961) **4386**
• ➤ Canadian Journal of Gastroenterology (CAN ISSN 0835-7900) **3886**
Canadian Journal of Genetics and Cytology - Journal Canadien de Genetique et de Cytologie *see* Genome **3306**, 3290
Canadian Journal of Herbalism (CAN ISSN 0848-9629) **3164**, 3279, 4282
• ➤ Canadian Journal of Hospital Pharmacy (CAN ISSN 0008-4123) **4282**, 3504
• ➤ Canadian Journal of Human Sexuality (CAN ISSN 1188-4517) **4386**
Canadian Journal of Medical Laboratory Science (CAN ISSN 1207-5833) **3872**
Canadian Journal of Medical Radiation Technology/Journal Canadien des Techniques en Radiation Medicale (CAN ISSN 0820-5930) **4141**
Canadian Journal of Medical Technology *see* Canadian Journal of Medical Laboratory Science **3872**
• ➤ Canadian Journal of Microbiology/Journal Canadien de Microbiologie (CAN ISSN 0008-4166) **3319**
➤ Canadian Journal of Music Therapy/Revue Canadienne de Musicotherapie (CAN) **4225**, 4386
• ➤ Canadian Journal of Neurological Sciences (CAN ISSN 0317-1671) **4080**
Canadian Journal of Nursing Administration *see* Canadian Journal of Nursing Leadership **3915**
➤ Canadian Journal of Nursing Leadership (CAN) **3915**
➤ The Canadian Journal of Nursing Research/Revue Canadienne de Recherche en Sciences Infirmieres (CAN ISSN 0844-5621) **3915**
• ➤ Canadian Journal of Occupational Therapy/Revue Canadienne d'Ergotherapie (CAN ISSN 0008-4174) **4059**
• ➤ Canadian Journal of Ophthalmology/ Journal Canadien d'Ophtalmologie (CAN ISSN 0008-4182) **3995**
Canadian Journal of Optometry/Revue Canadienne d'Optometrie (CAN ISSN 0045-5075) **3995**
• ➤ Canadian Journal of Physiology and Pharmacology/Journal Canadien de Physiologie et Pharmacologie (CAN ISSN 0008-4212) **3340**, 4282
• ➤ Canadian Journal of Plant Pathology (CAN ISSN 0706-0661) **3279**, 3286
Canadian Journal of Plastic Surgery (CAN ISSN 1195-2199) **4183**
• ➤ The Canadian Journal of Psychiatry/Revue Canadienne de Psychiatrie (CAN ISSN 0706-7437) **4080**
➤ Canadian Journal of Psychoanalysis/Revue Canadienne de Psychanalyse (CAN ISSN 1195-3330) **4080**
Canadian Journal of Psychology *see* Canadian Journal of Experimental Psychology **4386**
• ➤ Canadian Journal of Public Health/Revue Canadienne de Sante Publique (CAN ISSN 0008-4263) **4464**
Canadian Journal of Radiography, Radiation Therapy, Nuclear Medicine *see* Canadian Journal of Medical Radiation Technology **4141**
• ➤ Canadian Journal of Respiratory Therapy/Revue Canadienne de la Therapie Respiratoire (CAN ISSN 1205-9838) **4158**
• ➤ The Canadian Journal of Rural Medicine/Journal Canadien de la Medecine Rurale (CAN ISSN 1203-7796) **3582**
Canadian Journal of School Psychology (CAN ISSN 0829-5735) **3409**, 4386
Canadian Journal of Special Education (BRN ISSN 0827-3391) **3420**
Canadian Journal of Sport Sciences *see* Canadian Journal of Applied Physiology **4525**, 4173
• ➤ Canadian Journal of Surgery/Journal Canadien de Chirurgie (CAN ISSN 0008-428X) **4183**
➤ Canadian Journal of Urology (CAN ISSN 1195-9479) **4210**
• ➤ Canadian Journal of Veterinary Research/Revue Canadienne de Recherche Veterinaire (CAN ISSN 0830-9000) **4540**, 3582
• ➤ Canadian Journal on Aging/Revue Canadienne du Vieillissement (CAN ISSN 0714-9808) **3469**
Canadian Medical Association Journal *see* C M A J **3580**
Canadian Medical Directory (CAN ISSN 0068-9203) **3582**
Canadian Mental Health Association. Annual Report/Association Canadienne pour la Sante Mentale. Rapport Annuel (CAN ISSN 0068-9211) **4386**, 4465
• ➤ Canadian Mining Journal (CAN ISSN 0008-4492) **4225**, 3408, 4252
Canadian National Institute for the Blind. National Annual Report *see* Canadian National Institute for the Blind. National Annual Review **3496**, 4511
Canadian National Institute for the Blind. National Annual Review (CAN) **3496**, 4511
Canadian Nurse *see* Canadian Nurse **3915**, 4465
Canadian Nurse/L'Infirmiere Canadienne (CAN) **3915**, 4465
Canadian Nurses Association. Helen K. Mussallem Library. Periodical Holdings *see* Helen K. Mussallem. Periodical Holdings List **3729**, 3919
Canadian Nursing Home (CAN ISSN 0847-5520) **3504**
Canadian Nursing Management (CAN) **3915**
Canadian Occupational Health & Safety News (CAN ISSN 0709-5252) **4252**
Canadian Occupational Safety & Health Law (CAN ISSN 0704-3724) **4252**, 3537
Canadian Occupational Safety and Health Law Monthly Report (CAN ISSN 0825-608X) **4252**, 3537
➤ Canadian Oncology Nursing Journal/Revue Canadienne de Nursing Oncologique (CAN ISSN 1181-912X) **3915**, 3969
Canadian Operating Room Nursing Journal (CAN ISSN 0712-6778) **3915**, 4183
Canadian Paediatric Society. Annual Report (CAN ISSN 1199-7044) **4042**
Canadian Paediatric Society News *see* C P S News **4041**
Canadian Paediatric Society. News Bulletin *see* C P S News **4041**
• ➤ Canadian Pharmaceutical Journal/Revue Pharmaceutique Canadienne (CAN ISSN 0828-6914) **4282**
• Canadian Psychiatric Association Bulletin (CAN) **4080**
• ➤ Canadian Psychology (CAN ISSN 0708-5591) **4386**
Canadian Public Health Association Health Digest *see* C P H A Health Digest **4464**, 4351
Canadian Red Cross Blood Transfusion Service. Annual Report *see* Canadian Red Cross Society. Blood Services. Annual Report **3899**
Canadian Red Cross Society. Blood Services. Annual Report (CAN ISSN 0840-5360) **3899**
Canadian Rehabilitation Council for the Disabled. Annual Report *see* Easter Seals - March of Dimes National Council. Annual Report **3421**, 3484
➤ Canadian Respiratory Journal (CAN ISSN 1198-2241) **4159**
Canadian Society for Immunology. Bulletin (CAN ISSN 0068-9653) **3741**
Canadian Society of Biochemistry and Molecular Biology. Bulletin *see* Canadian Society of Biochemistry, Molecular and Cellular Biology. Bulletin **3246**
Canadian Society of Biochemistry, Molecular and Cellular Biology. Bulletin (CAN) **3246**
• ➤ Canadian Veterinary Journal/Revue Veterinaire Canadienne (CAN ISSN 0008-5286) **4540**
Canadian Women's Health Network (CAN ISSN 1480-0039) **4563**
Cancer *see* Syopa **3991**
• ➤ Cancer (USA ISSN 0008-543X) **3969**
• ➤ Cancer and Metastasis Reviews (USA ISSN 0167-7659) **3969**
➤ Cancer Biochemistry Biophysics (CHE ISSN 0305-7232) **3970**, 3246, 3266
Cancer Biology and Medicine (NLD) **3970**
Cancer Biotherapy *see* Cancer Biotherapy & Radiopharmaceuticals **3970**, 4282
• ➤ Cancer Biotherapy & Radiopharmaceuticals (USA ISSN 1084-9785) **3970**, 4282
Cancer Case Presentations: The Tumor Board (USA ISSN 1090-7491) **3970**
• ➤ Cancer Causes & Control (NLD ISSN 0957-5243) **3970**
Cancer Challenge *see* Live Well with Cancer **3983**
➤ Cancer Chemotherapy and Biological Response Modifiers (NLD ISSN 0921-4410) **3970**
• ➤ Cancer Chemotherapy and Pharmacology (DEU ISSN 0344-5704) **3970**, 4282
Cancer Chemotherapy and Pharmacology. Supplement (DEU ISSN 0943-9404) **3970**, 4282
Cancer Communications *see* Oncology Research **3987**
• ➤ Cancer Control (USA ISSN 1073-2748) **3970**
Cancer Control Journal (USA ISSN 0191-3794) **3970**
Cancer Cytopathology *see* Cancer **3969**
• ➤ Cancer Detection and Prevention (USA ISSN 0361-090X) **3970**
➤ Cancer Drug Discovery and Development (USA) **3971**, 3899
• Cancer Drug News (C D N) (GBR ISSN 1369-7129) **3971**
Cancer Economics (USA ISSN 1053-9611) **3971**
• Cancer Epidemiology (GBR ISSN 1365-330X) **3718**, 3147, 3971
• ➤ Cancer Epidemiology, Biomarkers & Prevention (USA ISSN 1055-9965) **3971**

Title

Cancer Facts and Figures (USA ISSN 0069-0147) **3971**
• ➤ Cancer Forum (AUS ISSN 0311-306X) **3971**
▼ • Cancer Futures (DEU) **3971**
• ➤ Cancer Gene Therapy (USA ISSN 0929-1903) **3971**, 3300
• ➤ Cancer Genetics & Cytogenetics (USA ISSN 0165-4608) **3971**, 3300
Cancer Growth and Progression (NLD) **3971**
• ➤ Cancer Immunology, Immunotherapy (DEU ISSN 0340-7004) **3971**
➤ Cancer in Focus (CAN) **3971**
Cancer in Puerto Rico (PRI ISSN 0896-9035) **3971**
Cancer Incidence and Mortality Michigan (USA) **4495**, 3718, 3971, 4528
Cancer Incidence in Slovenia *see* Incidenca Raka v Sloveniji **3979**
Cancer Incidence in Sweden (SWE ISSN 0280-7165) **3718**, 3971
• ➤ Cancer Investigation (USA ISSN 0735-7907) **3972**
Cancer Journal *see* The Cancer Journal from Scientific American (English Edition) **3972**
• ➤ The Cancer Journal from Scientific American (English Edition) (USA ISSN 1081-4442) **3972**
The Cancer Journal from Scientific American (Spanish Edition) *see* The Cancer Journal from Scientific American (English Edition) **3972**
• The Cancer Journal (Online Edition)/Le Journal du Cancer (FRA ISSN 1292-8658) **3582**
The Cancer Journal (Print Edition) *see* The Cancer Journal (Online Edition) **3582**
Cancer Letter (USA ISSN 0096-3917) **3972**
• ➤ Cancer Letters (IRL ISSN 0304-3835) **3972**
➤ Cancer Molecular Biology (EGY) **3972**
• ➤ Cancer Nursing (USA ISSN 0162-220X) **3916**, 3972
Cancer Nursing Practice (GBR) **3916**, 3972
Cancer on Disk *see* Cancer **3969**
• Cancer Pain Release (USA ISSN 1013-3097) **3972**
Cancer Pharmacology Annual (NLD ISSN 0920-7848) **3972**
• ➤ Cancer Practice (USA ISSN 1065-4704) **3972**
• Cancer Practice Online (USA ISSN 1523-5394) **3972**
• ➤ Cancer - Radiotherapie (FRA ISSN 1278-3218) **3972**, 4141
• ➤ Cancer Research (USA ISSN 0008-5472) **3973**
Cancer Research Campaign. Annual Report *see* Cancer Research Campaign. Scientific Yearbook **3973**
Cancer Research Campaign Factsheets *see* C R C Factsheets **3718**, 3969, 4528
Cancer Research Campaign. Scientific Yearbook (GBR) **3973**
Cancer Research Monographs (USA ISSN 0892-0001) **3973**
Cancer Research News *see* Cancer in Focus **3971**
Cancer Research on Prevention and Treatment *see* Zhongliu Fangzhi Yanjiu **3992**
Cancer Research, Therapy and Control (CHE ISSN 1064-0525) **3973**
Cancer Researcher Weekly *see* Cancer Weekly Plus **3973**
Cancer Review (USA) **3973**
Cancer Sourcebook (USA) **3973**
Cancer Sourcebook for Women (USA) **3973**, 4563
Cancer Statistics Registrations. England and Wales. *see* Great Britain. Government Statistical Service. Cancer Statistics Registrations. England and Wales **3728**, 3978, 4529
➤ Cancer Surveys (USA ISSN 0261-2429) **3973**
Cancer Therapy and Control *see* Cancer Research, Therapy and Control **3973**
▼ Cancer Today (NZL ISSN 1174-5916) **3973**
➤ Cancer Topics (GBR ISSN 0265-1319) **3973**
Cancer Topics Abstracts *see* Cancer Topics **3973**
➤ Cancer Treatment and Research (NLD ISSN 0927-3042) **3973**
• ➤ Cancer Treatment Reviews (GBR ISSN 0305-7372) **3973**
Cancer Watch (USA ISSN 1059-3802) **3973**
• Cancer Weekly Plus (USA) **3973**
CancerCare Manitoba Report (CAN) **3973**
• Cancerologie Aujourd'hui (FRA ISSN 1140-9916) **3974**
Cancerweekly *see* Cancer Weekly Plus **3973**
Cancro (ITA ISSN 0008-5480) **3974**
Candid Facts/A Propos (CAN ISSN 0226-2347) **3582**
Candlelighters Childhood Cancer Foundation Quarterly Newsletter (USA) **3974**, 4042
Candlelighters Childhood Cancer Foundation Youth Newsletter (USA) **3974**, 3381
Cani, Gatti e Compagnia (ITA) **4540**
Cannabis Canada *see* Cannabis Culture **3549**, 3164
Cannabis Culture (CAN) **3549**, 3164
The Cape Doctor (ZAF) **3582**
Capital Nursing (USA) **3916**
Capital Sante (FRA) **4563**
Capital University of Medical Sciences. Journal *see* Shoudu Yike Daxue **3693**
Capitation Management Report (USA ISSN 1083-7183) **4465**, 3504
Capitation Rates and Data (USA ISSN 1090-1574) **4465**, 3504
The Capstone (Towson) (USA) **3483**, 3420, 4511
Capsule *see* Kapuseru **4312**
Capsule *see* The Medicare Advisory Capsule **3519**
Caption (USA) **3388**, 3489
• ➤ Carbohydrate Letters (CHE ISSN 1073-5070) **3246**, 3340
• ➤ Carcinogenesis (GBR ISSN 0143-3334) **3974**
• ➤ Carcinogenesis (USA ISSN 0147-4006) **3974**
Carcinogensis, Teratogensis and Mutagenesis *see* Yanbian - Jibian - Tubian **3992**, 3224, 3456
Carcinological Society of Japan. Cancer (JPN ISSN 0918-1989) **3974**
Cardarelli (ITA ISSN 0576-7202) **3582**
Cardiac Alert (USA ISSN 0194-2557) **4351**, 3765
▼ Cardiac and Vascular Regeneration (USA ISSN 1527-7917) **3765**
• Cardiac Electrophysiology Review (USA ISSN 1385-2264) **3765**
Cardiac Imaging Monitor *see* Current Medical Literature. Cardiac Imaging Monitor **3721**, 3147, 3770, 4142
Cardiac Practice (JPN ISSN 0915-874X) **3765**
Cardiac Surgery (USA ISSN 1072-9798) **4183**, 3765
Cardio Intervention (USA) **3765**
Cardio News (DEU ISSN 1437-1073) **3765**
Cardio-Vascular Clinical Trials (GBR ISSN 1368-731X) **3765**
Cardiologia *see* Italian Heart Journal **3775**
➤ La Cardiologia nella Pratica Clinica (ITA ISSN 0945-8298) **3765**
Cardiologie (FRA ISSN 0983-4532) **3765**
Cardiologie (NLD ISSN 0929-7456) **3765**
Cardiologie Pratique (FRA ISSN 0766-3633) **3765**
Cardiologie Pratique. Supplement (FRA ISSN 1240-3318) **3765**
Le Cardiologue (FRA ISSN 0769-0819) **3765**
• ➤ Cardiology (CHE ISSN 0008-6312) **3765**
Cardiology *see* Kardiologiya **3779**
Cardiology (Bethesda) (USA) **3765**
Cardiology Board Review *see* Cardiology Review **3766**
• Cardiology Clinics (USA ISSN 0733-8651) **3765**
Cardiology Clinics: Annual of Drug Therapy (USA ISSN 1089-408X) **3765**
Cardiology - Critical Care Technology *see* M E N Cardiology - Critical Care Technology **4149**, 3780
Cardiology Health Monitor (USA ISSN 1067-9332) **3765**
Cardiology in Practice (CAN ISSN 0844-5575) **3765**
• Cardiology in Review (USA ISSN 1061-5377) **3766**
Cardiology in the Elderly *see* Coronary Artery Disease **3769**
• ➤ Cardiology in the Young (GBR ISSN 1047-9511) **3766**
Cardiology News (GBR ISSN 1368-8979) **3766**
Cardiology Practice Advisor (USA) **3504**, 3766
➤ Cardiology Review (USA ISSN 1092-6607) **3766**
Cardiology Special Edition (USA) **3766**
Cardiology Today (USA) **3766**
➤ Cardiology Update (USA ISSN 0163-1675) **3766**
Cardioscience *see* Cardiovascular Research **3767**
▼ ➤ Cardiovasc (DEU ISSN 1617-4933) **3766**
Cardiovascular (ESP ISSN 1133-6846) **3766**
• ➤ Cardiovascular and Interventional Radiology (USA ISSN 0174-1551) **4141**, 3766
Cardiovascular Device Update (USA ISSN 1084-3930) **3766**
Cardiovascular Disease *see* Today in Medicine. Cardiovascular Disease **3784**
▼ Cardiovascular Disease in Practice (GBR ISSN 1466-4992) **3766**
• Cardiovascular Disease Management (USA ISSN 1086-041X) **3766**
Cardiovascular Drug Alerts *see* Primary Care Medicine Drug Alerts **4331**, 3679
• ➤ Cardiovascular Drug Reviews (USA ISSN 0897-5957) **4282**, 3766
• ➤ Cardiovascular Drugs and Therapy (USA ISSN 0920-3206) **3766**, 4282
▼ • Cardiovascular Engineering (USA ISSN 1567-8822) **3766**
Cardiovascular Guidelines *see* Therapeutic Guidelines. Cardiovascular **3783**
Cardiovascular Imaging *see* C I - Cardiovascular Imaging **3764**
Cardiovascular Journal of Southern Africa (ZAF ISSN 1015-9657) **3766**
➤ Cardiovascular Pathobiology (USA ISSN 1088-7180) **3767**
• ➤ Cardiovascular Pathology (USA ISSN 1054-8807) **3767**
• Cardiovascular Pharmacology (GBR ISSN 0263-7243) **4344**, 3147, 3767
Cardiovascular Pulmonary Digest *see* C P Digest **3764**
▼ • ➤ Cardiovascular Radiation Medicine (USA ISSN 1522-1865) **3767**, 4141
• ➤ Cardiovascular Research (NLD ISSN 0008-6363) **3767**
➤ Cardiovascular Reviews & Reports (USA ISSN 0197-3118) **3767**
Cardiovascular Reviews and Reports (Edicion Espanola) *see* Cardiovascular **3766**
• ➤ Cardiovascular Risk Factors (ESP ISSN 1133-9160) **3767**
• ➤ Cardiovascular Surgery (GBR ISSN 0967-2109) **3767**, 4183
➤ Cardiovascular Surgery (USA ISSN 0069-0406) **3767**, 4183
Cardiovascular Surgery Online *see* C V Surgery Online **3718**
Cardiovascularia *see* Cardio News **3765**
Care (GBR) **3469**
Care Connection (CAN ISSN 0843-9966) **3916**
Care in the Home *see* Staying Alive **4490**
Care Konkret (DEU ISSN 1435-9286) **3469**
Care Magazine (USA) **3582**, 3164
▼ ➤ Care Management Journals (USA ISSN 1521-0987) **3916**
Care of the Elderly *see* Geriatric Medicine **3471**
Care of the Surgical Patient *see* Scientific American Surgery **4202**
Care on the Road (GBR) **4465**, 4533
Care Plan (GBR ISSN 1355-0454) **4465**, 4511
Career Development for Exceptional Individuals (USA ISSN 0885-7288) **3420**, 4269
• ➤ The Career Development Quarterly (USA ISSN 0889-4019) **4269**, 4386
➤ Career Planning and Adult Development Journal (USA ISSN 0736-1920) **3416**, 4270
Career Planning and Adult Development Network Newsletter (USA ISSN 0898-1353) **3416**, 4270
Career Planning and Adult Development Newsletter *see* Career Planning and Adult Development Network Newsletter **3416**, 4270
Careers for Disabled Graduates *see* Disabled Graduates Casebook **3417**, 3484
Caregiver (USA) **3469**
Carers in Victoria (AUS) **4511**, 3483, 4221, 4563
Caribbean Chronicle (VIR) **3916**
Caribbean Diet Digest (VIR) **4231**
Caribbean Family Planning Affiliation. Annual Report (ATG) **3357**
Caribbean Health (GBR ISSN 1462-8120) **4465**
➤ Caribbean Journal of Criminology & Social Psychology (TTO ISSN 1025-5591) **3394**, 4386
• ➤ Caribbean Journal of Science (PRI ISSN 0008-6452) **3189**, 4504
Caribbean Nurses Organization. Newsletter (USA) **3916**
Caribbean Research Institute. Report (VIR) **3526**, 3189, 3392
• ➤ Caries Research (CHE ISSN 0008-6568) **3817**
Caring (CAN) **3916**
▼ Caring for the Ages (USA ISSN 1526-4114) **3504**
Caring Notes (USA) **4386**, 3947
Caring (Washington) (USA ISSN 0738-467X) **3916**, 4511
Caritas-Gemeinschaft. Publication *see* Caritas und Pflege **3916**
Caritas und Pflege (DEU ISSN 0948-003X) **3916**
Carnation Nutrition Education Series (USA ISSN 1049-4901) **4231**
Carnegie-Mellon Symposia on Cognition Series (USA) **4386**, 3381
• ➤ Carnegie Museum of Natural History. Annals (USA ISSN 0097-4463) **4504**, 3173, 3189, 4271
Carnegie Museum of Natural History. Bulletin (USA ISSN 0145-9058) **4504**, 3173, 3189, 4271
Carnegie Symposium on Cognition *see* Carnegie-Mellon Symposia on Cognition Series **4386**, 3381
Carolina Journal of Pharmacy (USA ISSN 0528-1725) **4282**
• Carolina Tips (USA ISSN 0045-5865) **3189**, 3428
Carotenoids Other Than Vitamin A (USA ISSN 0069-0732) **3246**
Carotid and Neurovascular Intervention (GBR ISSN 1465-1327) **3767**
• ➤ Caryologia (ITA ISSN 0008-7114) **3286**
Cascade *see* C A S Code **4041**, 4511
Case Management Advisor (USA ISSN 1053-5500) **3582**
• The Case Manager (USA ISSN 1061-9259) **3582**, 3531
Case Studies (AUS ISSN 1321-9324) **4386**
Case Western Reserve University. School of Dentistry. Alumni Magazine (USA) **3817**
Case Western Reserve University. School of Dentistry. Dental Alumni News *see* Case Western Reserve University. School of Dentistry. Alumni Magazine **3817**
➤ Casopis Lekaru Ceskych (CZE ISSN 0008-7335) **3582**
➤ Casualty Simulation (GBR ISSN 0008-7580) **4465**
Catalog of Captioned Films for the Deaf (USA ISSN 0093-7215) **4225**, 3177, 3489
Catalogo de Trabajos de Investigacion en Salud (ESP) **3582**
➤ Catalogue of Palaearctic Diptera (NLD) **3295**
Category Report - Health & Beauty Aids (USA ISSN 1086-119X) **3175**, 4282
Category Report - Household, Pet & Miscellaneous Products (USA ISSN 1086-1203) **3175**, 4282
Catering and Health *see* Hygiene and Nutrition in Food Service and Catering **3461**, 4235
Cath Lab Digest (USA) **3767**
Catheterization and Cardiovascular Diagnosis *see* Catheterization and Cardiovascular Interventions **3767**
• ➤ Catheterization and Cardiovascular Interventions (USA ISSN 1522-1946) **3767**
Catholic Health Association of Canada Info *see* C H A C Info **3503**, 3580, 4502
Catholic Health Association of Canada Review *see* C H A C Review **3503**, 3580, 4502
• Catholic Health World (USA ISSN 8756-4068) **4502**
Catholic Medical Quarterly (GBR ISSN 0008-8226) **4502**, 3582
The Catholic Pharmacist (USA) **4282**, 4502
Catholic University Medical College Journal (KOR) **3582**
➤ Catnap (GBR ISSN 1357-8944) **4080**
Cause di Morte (ITA ISSN 1121-0958) **4370**
Causes of Death in Denmark *see* Doedsaarsagerne **4370**
Cedars-Sinai Compass *see* Cedars - Sinai Medical Center Compass **3504**
Cedars - Sinai Medical Center Compass (USA ISSN 0008-8684) **3504**
Celebrate Life (Stafford) (USA) **3357**, 4369
Celebrate the Self (USA) **4222**
Celiac News (CAN ISSN 0833-1464) **3846**
• ➤ Cell (USA ISSN 0092-8674) **3286**
• ➤ Cell Adhesion and Communication (CHE ISSN 1061-5385) **3189**
Cell Analysis (USA ISSN 0737-1233) **3286**
➤ Cell and Chromosome Research Journal (IND ISSN 0254-2935) **3286**
▼ • ➤ Cell and Tissue Banking (NLD ISSN 1389-9333) **3286**
• ➤ Cell and Tissue Research (DEU ISSN 0302-766X) **3287**
• ➤ Cell Biochemistry and Biophysics (USA ISSN 1085-9195) **3287**, 3246, 3266
• ➤ Cell Biochemistry and Function (GBR ISSN 0263-6484) **3246**, 3287
• ➤ Cell Biology and Toxicology (NLD ISSN 0742-2091) **3446**, 3287

Title

Title

Chinese Journal of Ophthalmology *see* Zhonghua Yanke Zazhi **4008**
Chinese Journal of Organ Transplantation *see* Zhonghua Qiguan Yizhi Zazhi **4208**
Chinese Journal of Orthopedics *see* Zhonghua Guke Zazhi **4029**
Chinese Journal of Osteoporosis *see* Zhongguo Guzhi Shusong Zazhi **3482**, 4028
Chinese Journal of Otorhinolaryngology *see* Zhonghua Er-Bi-Yanhouke Zazhi **4039**
Chinese Journal of Parasitic Disease Control *see* Zhongguo Jishengchongbing Fangzhi Zazhi **3808**, 3224, 4494
Chinese Journal of Parasitology and Parasitic Diseases *see* Zhongguo Jishengchongxue yu Jishengchongbing Zazhi **3333**
Chinese Journal of Parasitology and Parasitic Diseases *see* Zhongguo Jishengchong yu Jishengchongbing Zazhi **3808**, 3224, 4494
Chinese Journal of Pathology *see* Zhonghua Binglixue Zazhi **3713**
Chinese Journal of Pathophysiology *see* Zhongguo Bingli Shengli Zazhi **3712**
Chinese Journal of Pediatrics *see* Zhonghua Erke Zazhi **4057**
Chinese Journal of Pharmaceuticals *see* Zhongguo Yiyao Gongye Zazhi **4342**
Chinese Journal of Pharmacology and Toxicology *see* Zhongguo Yaolixue yu Dulixue Zazhi **3456**, 4342
Chinese Journal of Physical Medicine and Rehabilitation *see* Zhonghua Wuli yu Kangfu Zazhi **4067**
Chinese Journal of Physical Therapy *see* Zhonghua Liliao Zazhi **4067**
➤ Chinese Journal of Physiological Sciences (CHN ISSN 0258-6428) **3340**
• Chinese Journal of Physiology/Chung-kuo Sheng Li Hsueh Tsa Chih (TWN ISSN 0304-4920) **3340**, 3584
Chinese Journal of Plastic Surgery and Burns *see* Zhonghua Zhengxing Shaoshang Waike Zazhi **4208**
Chinese Journal of Practical Gynecology and Obstetrics *see* Zhongguo Shiyong Fuke yu Chanke Zazhi **3966**
Chinese Journal of Practical Internal Medicine *see* Zhongguo Shiyong Neike Zazhi **3911**
Chinese Journal of Practical Ophthalmology *see* Zhongguo Shiyong Yanke Zazhi **4008**
Chinese Journal of Practical Pediatrics *see* Zhongguo Shiyong Erke Zazhi **4057**
Chinese Journal of Practical Surgery *see* Zhongguo Shiyong Waike Zazhi **4208**
Chinese Journal of Prevention and Control of STD & AIDS *see* Zhongguo Xingbing Aizibing Fangzhi **3808**
Chinese Journal of Preventive Medicine *see* Zhonghua Yufang Yixue Zazhi **3714**
Chinese Journal of Psychiatry *see* Zhonghua Jingshenke Zazhi **4138**
➤ Chinese Journal of Psychology (TWN ISSN 1013-9656) **4387**
Chinese Journal of Public Health *see* Zhongguo Gonggong Weisheng Xuebao **4494**
Chinese Journal of Radiological Medicine and Protection *see* Zhonghua Fangshe Yixue yu Fanghu Zazhi **4157**, 3431
Chinese Journal of Radiology *see* Zhonghua Fangshexua Zazhi **4157**
Chinese Journal of Rehabilitation *see* Zhongguo Kangfu **4364**
Chinese Journal of Rehabilitation Medicine *see* Zhongguo Kangfu Yixue Zazhi **3712**
Chinese Journal of Rehabilitation Theory & Practice *see* Zhongguo Kangfu Lilun Yu Shijian **4067**
Chinese Journal of Reparative and Reconstructive Surgery *see* Zhongguo Xiufu Chongjian Waike Zazhi **4208**, 3295, 4028
Chinese Journal of Rheumatology *see* Zhonghua Fengshibingxue Zazhi **4172**, 3224, 4343
Chinese Journal of Spine and Spinal Cord *see* Zhongguo Jizhu Jisui Zazhi **4028**
Chinese Journal of Sports Medical Science *see* Zhongguo Yundong Yixue Zazhi **4178**
Chinese Journal of Stomatology *see* Zhonghua Kouqiang Yixue Zazhi **3897**
Chinese Journal of Surgery *see* Zhonghua Waike Zazhi **4208**
Chinese Journal of Surgery of Integrated Traditional Chinese and Western Medicine *see* Zhongguo Zhongxiyi Jiehe Waike Zazhi **4208**
Chinese Journal of Thoracic and Cardiovascular Surgery *see* Zhonghua Xiong-xin Xueguan Waike Zazhi **3785**
Chinese Journal of Traditional Medical Science and Technology *see* Zhongguo Zhongyiyao Keji **3713**
Chinese Journal of Traumatology *see* Zhonghua Chuangshang Zazhi **4028**
Chinese Journal of Traumatology (CHN ISSN 1008-1275) **4012**
Chinese Journal of Tuberculosis and Respiratory Diseases *see* Zhonghua Jiehe he Huxi Zazhi **4166**
Chinese Journal of Ultrasonography *see* Zhonghua Chaosheng Yingxiangxue Zazhi **4157**
Chinese Journal of Ultrasound in Medicine *see* Zhongguo Chaosheng Yixue Zazhi **4157**
Chinese Journal of Urology *see* Zhonghua Miniao Waike Zazhi **4220**
Chinese Journal of Veterinary Medicine *see* Zhongguo Shouyi Zazhi **4560**
Chinese Journal of Veterinary Science *see* Zhongguo Shouyi Xuebao **4560**
Chinese Journal of Virology *see* Bingdu Xuebao **3575**
Chinese Journal of Zoonoses *see* Zhongguo Renshou Gonghuanbing Zazhi **3333**, 3808, 4560
Chinese Medical Digest (Hygienics) *see* Zhongguo Yixue Wenzhai (Weishengxue) **4364**, 3152
• ➤ Chinese Medical Journal/Zhonghua Yixue Zazhi Yingwen Ban (CHN ISSN 0366-6999) **3584**
Chinese Medical Journal (TWN ISSN 0578-1337) **3584**
• ➤ Chinese Medical Sciences Journal (CHN ISSN 1001-9294) **3584**, 3190, 4283
Chinese Medicine *see* Kanpo Igaku **3167**
Chinese Medicine Information News *see* Zhongguo Yiyue Bao **3713**
Chinese Mental Health Journal *see* Zhongguo Xinli Weisheng Zazhi **4456**
Chinese New Drugs Journal *see* Zhongguo Xinyao Zazhi **4342**
Chinese Pharmaceutical Abstracts *see* Zhongguo Yaoxue Wenzhai **3171**, 3152
Chinese Pharmaceutical Affairs *see* Zhongguo Yaoshi (Beijing) **4342**
Chinese Pharmaceutical Journal *see* Zhonghua Yixue Zazhi **3714**
Chinese Pharmaceutical Journal *see* Zhongguo Yaoxue Zazhi **4342**
Chinese Pharmacological Bulletin *see* Zhongguo Yaolixue Tongbao **4342**
Chinese Primary Health Care *see* Zhongguo Chuji Weisheng Baojian **3712**
Chinese Rural Doctors *see* Zhongguo Xiangcun Yisheng **3713**
Chinese Safety Science Journal *see* Zhongguo Anquan Kexue Xuebao **4268**
Chinese Science *see* East Asian Science, Technology, and Medicine **4504**, 3597, 4531
Chinese Society of Veterinary Science. Journal *see* Zhonghua Minguo Shouyi Xuehui Zazhi **4560**
Chinese Traditional and Herbal Drugs *see* Zhongcaoyao **3712**, 3171
Chinese Traditional Patent Medicine *see* Zhongchenyao **4341**
Chinese Women and Children's Health *see* Zhongguo Fuyou Baojian **3966**
• ➤ Chinesische Medizin (DEU ISSN 0930-2786) **3164**
• ➤ Chirality (USA ISSN 0899-0042) **3246**
➤ Chiropody Review (GBR ISSN 0009-4714) **4183**
Chiropractic Economics (USA ISSN 1087-1985) **3786**
Chiropractic Health Ways (USA) **3786**
➤ Chiropractic History (USA ISSN 0736-4377) **3786**, 3177, 3526
The Chiropractic Journal (USA) **3786**
• ➤ Chiropractic Journal of Australia (AUS ISSN 1036-0913) **3786**
• Chiropractic OnLine Today (USA) **3786**
Chiropractic Products (USA ISSN 1041-2360) **3787**
The Chiropractic Report (CAN ISSN 0836-1444) **3787**
➤ Chiropractic Research Journal (USA ISSN 0899-6938) **3787**
Chiropractic Sports Medicine *see* Journal of Sports Chiropractic and Rehabilitation **3788**, 4175
➤ Chiropractic Technique (USA ISSN 0899-3467) **3787**
Chiropractors' Association of Australia. Membership Directory (AUS ISSN 1037-8839) **3787**
• ➤ Der Chirurg (DEU ISSN 0009-4722) **4184**
Chirurgia (BGR ISSN 0450-2167) **4184**
➤ Chirurgia (ITA ISSN 0394-9508) **4184**
Chirurgia (ROM ISSN 1221-9118) **4184**
Chirurgia degli Organi di Movimento (ITA ISSN 0009-4749) **4184**
➤ Chirurgia del Piede (ITA ISSN 0392-0771) **4184**
Chirurgia e Patologia Sperimentale (ITA ISSN 0009-4757) **4184**
Chirurgia Gastroenterologica (ITA ISSN 0009-4765) **3887**, 4184
Chirurgia Italiana (ITA ISSN 0009-4773) **4184**
• Chirurgia Maxillofacialis et Plastica/Maxillofacial and Plastic Surgery (HRV ISSN 0009-4781) **4184**, 3817
Chirurgia Svizzera *see* Swiss Surgery **4205**, 4026
Chirurgie *see* Annales de Chirurgie **4180**
▼ Chirurgie de la Main (FRA ISSN 1297-3203) **4184**
Chirurgie Endoscopique (FRA ISSN 1240-3156) **3584**
Chirurgie Suisse *see* Swiss Surgery **4205**, 4026
Chirurgie Vasculaire *see* Encyclopedie Medico-Chirurgicale. Techniques Chirurgicales. Chirurgie Vasculaire **4187**, 3771
Chirurgien-Dentiste de France (FRA ISSN 0009-4838) **3817**
• ➤ Chirurgische Gastroenterologie (CHE ISSN 0177-9990) **3887**
Chirurgische Praxis (DEU ISSN 0009-4846) **4184**
Chiryo *see* Journal of Therapy **3638**
Chiryo Kyoiku Kenkyu Kiyo/Gifu University. Department of Remedial Education. Report (JPN ISSN 0916-2682) **3420**
Chisholm Health Ethics Bulletin (AUS ISSN 1443-3591) **3584**
• Chloroplasts (GBR ISSN 0264-9640) **3228**, 3147, 3288
Choice (Chula Vista) (USA) **3974**
Choice Health Reader (AUS ISSN 1324-8065) **4351**, 3392
• Choices (BEL) **4369**, 3357, 3584
Choices (Washington) *see* Voices (Washington) **3393**, 3706
Chojugaku Kenkyu/Research of Longevity Science (JPN ISSN 0910-3058) **3469**, 3164
Chokaku Gengo Shogai/Communication Disorder Research (JPN ISSN 0300-0338) **3341**, 4081
• Cholesterol & Lipoproteins (GBR ISSN 0964-7597) **3228**, 3147, 3247
Cholesterol News (ITA ISSN 1120-0030) **3584**
Chongqing Medicine *see* Chongqing Yiyao **3584**
Chongqing Yiyao/Chongqing Medicine (CHN ISSN 1000-7911) **3584**
Chono Gengogaku Kenkyu/Japanese Journal of Communication Disorders (JPN) **4031**
➤ Choonpa Igaku/Japanese Journal of Medical Ultrasonics (JPN ISSN 0287-0592) **4141**
Choonpa Kensa Gijutsu/Japan Society of Sonographers. Journal (JPN) **4141**
Chot Mai Het Thang Phaet *see* Medical Association of Thailand. Journal **3649**
Chovekat i Negovata Zhiznena Sreda *see* Antropo-ekologiia **3435**, 4229, 4250, 4350
➤ Chowanna (POL ISSN 0137-706X) **3410**, 4387
Chris (DEU) **3386**, 3584, 4511
Christian Association for Psychological Studies, Inc. Report Newsletter *see* C A P S Report Newsletter **4499**, 4385
• ➤ Christian Bioethics (NLD ISSN 1380-3603) **3584**, 4347, 4499
Christian Chiropractor (USA) **3787**, 4499
Christian Chiropractors Association Journal (USA) **3787**, 4499
Christian Medical and Dental Society Journal *see* Today's Christian Doctor **3701**, 4501
Christian Medical Association of India. Journal *see* Christian Medical Journal of India **3584**, 4499
• ➤ Christian Medical College Vellore Alumni Journal (IND ISSN 0009-5451) **3584**, 3388
Christian Medical Journal of India (IND ISSN 0970-5007) **3584**, 4499
Christian Pharmacists Fellowship International Newsletter *see* C P F I Newsletter **4282**, 4502
Christian Record (USA ISSN 0009-5575) **4499**, 3496
Christian Science Kotari. Seisho Kyokar *see* Christian Science Quarterly. Bible Lessons (Citation Edition) **4502**
Christian Science Kvartalshaefte. Bibelstudium *see* Christian Science Quarterly. Bible Lessons (Citation Edition) **4502**
Christian Science Kvartalshaefte. Bibelstudium *see* Christian Science Quarterly. Bible Lessons (Citation Edition) **4502**
Christian Science Kvartalshefte *see* Christian Science Quarterly. Bible Lessons (Citation Edition) **4502**
Christian Science Kwartaalboekje. Bijbellessen *see* Christian Science Quarterly. Bible Lessons (Citation Edition) **4502**
Christian Science Quarterly. Bible Lessons (Citation Edition) (USA ISSN 0145-7365) **4502**
Christian Science Quarterly. Bible Lessons (Study Edition) *see* Christian Science Quarterly. Bible Lessons (Citation Edition) **4502**
Christian Science Vierteljahrsheft. Bibellektionen *see* Christian Science Quarterly. Bible Lessons (Citation Edition) **4502**
Christoffel-Blindenmission e.V. Freundesbrief *see* C B M Freundesbrief **4511**, 4499
Chrome - Dome (USA) **4221**
• ➤ Chromosoma (DEU ISSN 0009-5915) **3300**
Chronic Disease Prevention File *see* C D P File **4464**
Chronic Diseases Notes & Reports (USA ISSN 1041-5513) **4465**, 4369
➤ Chronica Dermatologica (ITA ISSN 0011-1759) **3846**
Chronobiologia (ITA ISSN 0390-0037) **3190**, 3856
• ➤ Chronobiology International (USA ISSN 0742-0528) **3191**, 3585
Chuangshang Zazhi *see* Zhonghua Chuangshang Zazhi **4028**
Chubu Byoin Igaku Zasshi/Okinawa Chubu Hospital. Bulletin (JPN ISSN 0913-8684) **3585**, 3504
Chubu Geka Gakkai Sokaigo/Chubu Surgical Society. Proceedings of Annual Meeting (JPN) **4184**
Chubu Nippon Seikei Geka Saigai Geka Gakkai Shoroku/Central Japan Association of Orthopaedic and Traumatic Surgery. Abstracts (JPN) **3718**, 4012
Chubu Nippon Seikei Geka Saigai Geka Gakkai Zasshi/Central Japan Journal of Orthopaedic Surgery & Traumatology (JPN ISSN 0008-9443) **4012**
Chubu Surgical Society. Proceedings of Annual Meeting *see* Chubu Geka Gakkai Sokaigo **4184**
Chudoku Kenkyu *see* Japanese Journal of Toxicology **3451**, 4305
Chugoku-Shikoku Orthopaedic Association. Journal *see* Chugoku Shikoku Seikei Geka Gakkai Zasshi **4012**
Chugoku Shikoku Seikei Geka Gakkai Zasshi/Chugoku-Shikoku Orthopaedic Association. Journal (JPN ISSN 0915-2695) **4012**
Chui Rinsho/Clinical Journal of Traditional Chinese Medicine (JPN ISSN 0389-4843) **3164**, 3585
Chuju Kagaku Sogo Kenkyu Hokoku/Comprehensive Studies on Science of Aging (JPN) **3469**
Chung-Hua Erh Pi Yen Hou K'o Tsa Chih *see* Zhonghua Er-Bi-Yanhouke Zazhi **4039**
Chung-Hua K'ou Ch'iang K'o Tsa Chih *see* Zhonghua Kouqiang Yixue Zazhi **3897**
Chung-Hua Yen K'o Tsa Chih *see* Zhonghua Yanke Zazhi **4008**
Chung-kuo Sheng Li Hsueh Tsa Chih *see* Chinese Journal of Physiology **3340**, 3584
Chuoju Kagaku Koenkai Kirokushu/Lectures on Science of Aging (JPN ISSN 0918-533X) **3469**
Church of Scotland Braille Magazine (GBR) **3496**, 4499
Chusei General Hospital. Journal *see* Chusei Sogo Byoin Zasshi **3504**
Chusei Sogo Byoin Zasshi/Chusei General Hospital. Journal (JPN ISSN 0389-4894) **3504**
▼ Ciencia Forense (ESP ISSN 1575-6793) **3881**
➤ Ciencia Ginecologika (ESP ISSN 1137-2273) **3947**
Ciencia Pediatrika *see* Pediatrika **4055**
Ciencia Pharmaceutica *see* Ciencia y Tecnologia Pharmaceutica **4283**
Ciencia Psicologica (ESP ISSN 1135-5956) **4387**
➤ Ciencia Rural (BRA ISSN 0103-8478) **3154**, 4540
Ciencia y Enfermeria (CHL ISSN 0717-2079) **3916**

Title

● ➤ Clinical Nursing Research (USA ISSN 1054-7738) **3916**
● ➤ Clinical Nutrition (GBR ISSN 0261-5614) **4231**, 3887
● ➤ Clinical Obstetrics and Gynecology (USA ISSN 0009-9201) **3947**
● Clinical Oncology (GBR ISSN 0936-6555) **3975**
● ➤ Clinical Oncology Alert (USA ISSN 0886-7186) **3975**
● ➤ Clinical Oral Implants Research (DNK ISSN 0905-7161) **3818**
● ➤ Clinical Oral Investigations (DEU ISSN 1432-6981) **3818**, 3586
● Clinical Orthodontics and Research (DNK ISSN 1397-5927) **3818**
● Clinical Orthodontics and Research Online (DNK) **3818**
➤ Clinical Orthopaedic Society. Journal (USA ISSN 1069-6970) **4012**
Clinical Orthopaedic Surgery *see* Rinsho Seikei Geka **4025**
● ➤ Clinical Orthopaedics and Related Research (USA ISSN 0009-921X) **4012**
● ➤ Clinical Otolaryngology and Allied Sciences (GBR ISSN 0307-7772) **4031**
▼ Clinical Pediatric Emergency Medicine (GBR ISSN 1522-8401) **4042**, 4012
Clinical Pediatric Endocrinology (JPN ISSN 0918-5739) **4042**, 3856
Clinical Pediatrics *see* Shonika **4057**
● ➤ Clinical Pediatrics (USA ISSN 0009-9228) **4042**
➤ Clinical Pediatrics Series (USA) **4043**
● ➤ Clinical Performance and Quality Health Care (GBR ISSN 1063-0279) **3587**
▼ Clinical Perspectives in Gastroenterology (USA ISSN 1098-8351) **3887**
Clinical Perspectives in Obstetrics and Gynecology (USA ISSN 0178-0328) **3947**
Clinical Pharmacokinetic Newsletter (USA ISSN 0886-7879) **4284**
● ➤ Clinical Pharmacokinetics (NZL ISSN 0312-5963) **4284**
● ➤ Clinical Pharmacology & Therapeutics (USA ISSN 0009-9236) **4284**
Clinical Pharmacology Research *see* International Journal of Clinical Pharmacology Research **4302**
Clinical Pharmacology Series (USA) **4284**
Clinical Pharmacy *see* American Journal of Health-System Pharmacy **4275**, 3501
Clinical Physics and Physiological Measurement *see* Physiological Measurement **3676**, 4365
Clinical Physiology *see* Clinical Physiology and Functional Imaging **3587**, 3341
● ➤ Clinical Physiology and Functional Imaging (GBR ISSN 1475-0961) **3587**, 3341
Clinical Physiology Series (USA) **3341**
Clinical Positron Imaging *see* Molecular Imaging and Biology **4151**
Clinical Practice in Urology (USA ISSN 0177-8994) **4211**
➤ Clinical Practice of Alternative Medicine (USA ISSN 1527-4772) **3587**
➤ Clinical Practice of Gynecology (USA ISSN 1043-3198) **3947**
Clinical Practice Recommendations (USA) **3856**
▼ Clinical Prosthodontics and Implant Dentistry (SGP) **3818**
Clinical Psychiatry *see* Seishin Igaku **4132**
Clinical Psychiatry News (USA ISSN 0270-6644) **4083**
➤ The Clinical Psychologist (USA ISSN 0009-9244) **4387**
➤ Clinical Psychology (GBR ISSN 1473-8279) **4387**
● ➤ Clinical Psychology (USA ISSN 0969-5893) **4388**
● ➤ Clinical Psychology & Psychotherapy (GBR ISSN 1063-3995) **4388**
Clinical Psychology Forum *see* Clinical Psychology **4387**
● ➤ Clinical Psychology Review (GBR ISSN 0272-7358) **4388**
Clinical Pulmonary Medicine (USA ISSN 1068-0640) **4159**
● ➤ Clinical Radiology (GBR ISSN 0009-9260) **4142**, 3975
Clinical Radiology *see* Rinsho Hoshasen **4154**
● ➤ Clinical Rehabilitation (GBR ISSN 0269-2155) **4060**
Clinical Reproduction and Fertility *see* Reproduction, Fertility and Development **3215**
Clinical Research *see* Journal of Investigative Medicine **3883**
● ➤ Clinical Research and Regulatory Affairs (USA ISSN 1060-1333) **4284**
Clinical Research Practices and Drug Regulatory Affairs *see* Clinical Research and Regulatory Affairs **4284**
● Clinical Research Resources Directory (USA) **3719**, 3873
Clinical Respiratory Physiology *see* The European Respiratory Journal **4159**
Clinical Reviews (USA) **3587**
Clinical Reviews in Allergy *see* Clinical Reviews in Allergy & Immunology **3743**
● ➤ Clinical Reviews in Allergy & Immunology (USA ISSN 1080-0549) **3743**
● ➤ Clinical Rheumatology (BEL ISSN 0770-3198) **4168**
● Clinical Risk (GBR ISSN 1356-2622) **3587**, 3537
● ➤ Clinical Science (GBR ISSN 0143-5221) **3587**, 3191
Clinical Series *see* N S S L H A Clinical Series **4035**
➤ Clinical Sociology: Research and Practice (USA) **4508**, 4388
Clinical Strategies: A K F Newsletter for Nephrology Professionals (USA) **4211**
Clinical Study *see* Kurinikaru Sutadi **3928**
Clinical Surgery International (GBR ISSN 0263-4422) **4185**
➤ Clinical Surveys in Endocrinology (USA ISSN 1050-3374) **3856**
● ➤ Clinical Techniques in Small Animal Practice (USA ISSN 1096-2867) **4540**
● ➤ Clinical Therapeutics (USA ISSN 0149-2918) **3587**
● ➤ Clinical Transplantation (DNK ISSN 0902-0063) **4185**
Clinical Trials *see* Clinical Trials Monitor **3587**, 4284
● Clinical Trials Monitor (USA) **3587**, 4284
● Clinical Trials News (USA) **3975**
● Clinical Update (AUS ISSN 1328-9454) **3975**, 4185, 4563
Clinical Vision Science *see* Vision Research **4008**
Clinician (IND ISSN 0009-9341) **3587**
Clinician *see* Kurinishian **3641**
● The Clinician in Management (GBR ISSN 0965-5751) **3587**, 3364, 3504
● Clinician News (USA) **3587**
● ➤ Clinician Reviews (USA ISSN 1052-0627) **3587**
Clinician's Manual on Hyperlipidemia (Year) (GBR ISSN 0958-1650) **3719**, 3769
Clinician's Manual on Hypertension and Concomitant Hyperlipidaemia (GBR ISSN 0964-5969) **3719**, 3769
➤ Clinician's Research Digest (USA ISSN 8756-3207) **4388**
Clinician's Toolbox (USA) **4388**
Clinicien (CAN ISSN 0832-9184) **3587**
Clinics Atlas of Office Procedures (USA ISSN 1094-0626) **3588**, 3908
● ➤ Clinics in Chest Medicine (USA ISSN 0272-5231) **4159**
● ➤ Clinics in Colon & Rectal Surgery (USA ISSN 1531-0043) **4185**, 3887
● ➤ Clinics in Dermatology (USA ISSN 0738-081X) **3846**
Clinics in Developmental Medicine (GBR ISSN 0069-4835) **4043**, 4083
Clinics in Diagnostic Ultrasound (USA ISSN 0193-743X) **4142**, 4367
Clinics in Family Practice (USA ISSN 1522-5720) **3588**
● ➤ Clinics in Geriatric Medicine (USA ISSN 0749-0690) **3469**
● ➤ Clinics in Laboratory Medicine (USA ISSN 0272-2712) **3873**
Clinics in Liver Disease (USA ISSN 1089-3261) **3887**
▼ Clinics in Occupational and Environmental Medicine (USA ISSN 1526-0046) **3588**, 3436, 4253
● ➤ Clinics in Perinatology (USA ISSN 0095-5108) **3947**
● ➤ Clinics in Plastic Surgery (USA ISSN 0094-1298) **4185**
Clinics in Podiatric Medicine & Surgery (USA ISSN 0891-8422) **4012**
● ➤ Clinics in Sports Medicine (USA ISSN 0278-5919) **4173**
CliniCum (AUT) **3504**
Clinique (FRA ISSN 0009-935X) **3588**
La Clinique Lacanienne (FRA ISSN 1288-6629) **4083**
Clinique Psychanalitique et Psycho-Pathologie (FRA ISSN 1281-6124) **4388**
Cliniques Mediterraneennes (FRA ISSN 0762-7491) **4083**
ClinPsyc *see* PsycINFO **4458**, 3151
ClinPsyc *see* Psychological Abstracts **4458**, 3151
● ➤ Clio (DEU ISSN 0933-0747) **4563**, 3947, 4568
● Clio Medica (NLD ISSN 0045-7183) **3588**
Clipping Monthly Report *see* Gekkan Igaku Joho **3605**
Cloning *see* Cloning and Stem Cells **3300**, 3273
▼ ● ➤ Cloning and Stem Cells (USA ISSN 1536-2302) **3300**, 3273
Closed-Head Injury (USA) **3588**, 3537
● Closing the Gap (USA ISSN 0886-1935) **3420**, 3416, 3488
Clot and Hematologic Malignancies (ITA ISSN 0393-487X) **3900**
● Club Industry (USA ISSN 0747-8283) **4351**
Club News (GBR) **3547**, 4465
● cma.ca (Canadian Medical Association) (CAN) **3588**
Co M B Revista *see* Colegio Medico de Barcelona. Revista **3588**
Co-Op News (Hanover) (USA) **3463**, 4231
Coalition on Sexuality and Disability, Inc. Newsletter *see* C S D Newsletter **3483**
Coatings, Regulations and the Environment (GBR ISSN 0967-2508) **4271**, 4253
▼ Cochlear Implants International (GBR ISSN 1467-0100) **4185**
➤ Cocuk Sagligi ve Hastaliklari Dergisi (TUR ISSN 0010-0161) **4043**
Codex Committee on Pesticide Residues. Report on the Meeting *see* Pesticide Residues in Food **4485**, 3462
Coding Clinic for ICD-9-CM (USA ISSN 0742-9800) **3504**
Coeur et Sante (FRA ISSN 0335-5306) **4351**, 3769
cognitio (DEU) **3550**, 4388
● ➤ Cognition (NLD ISSN 0010-0277) **4388**
Cognition and Brain Sciences Unit. Annual Report (GBR ISSN 1467-5919) **4083**
● ➤ Cognition and Emotion (USA ISSN 0269-9931) **4388**
● ➤ Cognition and Instruction (USA ISSN 0737-0008) **4388**, 3410
➤ Cognition and Language (USA) **3550**, 3410, 4388
▼ ● Cognition, Technology and Work (GBR ISSN 1435-5558) **4388**, 4347
● ➤ Cognitiva (ESP ISSN 0214-3550) **4389**
● ➤ Cognitive, Affective, & Behavioral Neuroscience (USA ISSN 1530-7026) **4389**
● ➤ Cognitive and Behavioral Practice (USA ISSN 1077-7229) **4389**
The Cognitive Behavioural Social Work Review (GBR ISSN 1466-3651) **4511**, 4389
● ➤ Cognitive Brain Research (NLD ISSN 0926-6410) **4083**, 3809
● ➤ Cognitive Development (GBR ISSN 0885-2014) **4389**
● ➤ Cognitive Linguistics (DEU ISSN 0936-5907) **3550**, 4389
Cognitive Linguistics Research (DEU) **3550**, 4389
● Cognitive Neuropsychiatry (GBR ISSN 1354-6805) **4389**
● ➤ Cognitive Neuropsychology (USA ISSN 0264-3294) **4083**
● ➤ Cognitive Psychology (USA ISSN 0010-0285) **4389**
● ➤ Cognitive Science (GBR ISSN 0364-0213) **4389**, 3550
▼ Cognitive Science Quarterly (FRA ISSN 1466-6553) **4389**
➤ Cognitive Science Series (Cambridge) (USA ISSN 0732-1295) **4389**
➤ Cognitive Science Series: Technical Monographs and Edited Collections (USA) **4389**
Cognitive Science Society. Annual Conference. Proceedings (USA) **4389**
Cognitive Science Society. Annual Conference. Program *see* Cognitive Science Society. Annual Conference. Proceedings **4389**
Cognitive Systems (NLD ISSN 0256-663X) **4390**, 3550
● ➤ Cognitive Therapy and Research (USA ISSN 0147-5916) **4390**
Cold Spring Harbor Laboratory. Abstracts of Papers Presented at Meetings (USA ISSN 0084-8824) **3191**, 3147
Cold Spring Harbor Laboratory. Annual Report (USA ISSN 0069-5009) **3191**
● ➤ Cold Spring Harbor Laboratory. Symposia on Quantitative Biology (USA ISSN 0091-7451) **3191**
Cold Spring Harbor Monograph Series (USA ISSN 0270-1847) **3191**
Coleccion Ciencias Biologicas (ESP) **3191**
Coleccion Ciencias Medicas de Bolsillo (ESP) **3588**
Coleccion F A O, Alimentacion y Nutricion *see* F A O Food and Nutrition Series **4233**
Coleccion Libros de Enfermeria (ESP) **3917**
Coleccion Libros de Medicina (ESP) **3588**
➤ Colegio Brasileiro de Cirurgioes. Revista (BRA ISSN 0100-6991) **4185**
Colegio Medico de Barcelona. Revista (ESP) **3588**
Colegio Medico de El Salvador. Archivos (SLV ISSN 0010-0641) **3588**
Colegio Nacional de Enfermeras. Revista *see* Enfermeras **3918**
Colegio Oficial de Psicologos de Madrid. Documentacion Psicologica (ESP) **4457**, 3177
● Colegio Oficial de Psicologos de Madrid. Monografia (ESP) **4390**
Colegio Oficial de Psicologos de Madrid. Selecciones de Prensa (ESP) **4457**, 3147
➤ Colexio Oficial de Psicologos de Galicia. Cadernos de Psicolxia (ESP ISSN 0213-5973) **4390**
Colimpex Medical Execupad (ZAF) **3588**
Colimpex Paediatric Execupad (ZAF) **3917**
Collection F A O, Alimentation et Nutrition *see* F A O Food and Nutrition Series **4233**
Collection Orientations (FRA ISSN 0246-4950) **3410**, 4390
Collection Pathologie, Sciences, Formation (FRA ISSN 1271-9145) **3588**
Collection Psychologie (FRA ISSN 0993-7536) **4390**
Collection Psychologie et Pedagogie du Sport (FRA) **4390**, 4525
Collection Psychologie et Pedagogie du Travail (FRA ISSN 0981-7727) **4390**
Collection Tests Psychologiques (FRA ISSN 1242-5028) **4390**
● Collegamento (ITA ISSN 0390-8739) **4284**
College des Medecins du Quebec. Annuaire Medical (CAN) **3588**
College des Medecins du Quebec. Bulletin *see* College des Medecins du Quebec. Le College **3588**
College des Medecins du Quebec. Le College (CAN) **3588**
College Information Booklet (USA) **3787**, 3417
College of American Pathologists Today *see* C A P Today **3580**, 3189
▼ ● College of Maharishi Vedic Medicine News (USA) **3164**
College of Physicians and Surgeons of British Columbia. Annual Report (CAN) **3588**
College of Physicians and Surgeons of British Columbia. Medical Directory (CAN ISSN 0069-5726) **3588**
College of Physicians & Surgeons Pakistan. Index of Dissertations. (PAK) **3588**
● ➤ College of Physicians and Surgeons Pakistan. Journal (PAK ISSN 1022-386X) **3588**
College of Physicians of Philadelphia. Transactions & Studies (USA ISSN 0010-1087) **3588**
College of Psychologists of Ontario. Bulletin (CAN) **4390**
College of Speech and Language Therapists. Bulletin *see* Royal College of Speech and Language Therapists. Bulletin **3426**
● ➤ College of Surgeons Hong Kong. Annals (AUS ISSN 1028-4001) **4185**
College of Veterinarians of Ontario. Update (CAN) **4540**
College of Veterinary Medicine Quarterly *see* C V M Quarterly **4540**
College Royal des Medecins et Chirurgiens du Canada. Annales *see* Royal College of Physicians and Surgeons of Canada. Annals **3688**
Colleges of Medicine of South Africa. Transactions (ZAF ISSN 0375-3220) **3589**
➤ Collegian (AUS ISSN 1322-7696) **3917**
Collettivita - Convivenze (ITA ISSN 1120-639X) **3504**, 4465
Colloquium Mosbach (USA ISSN 0366-5887) **3247**
Colombia Medica (COL ISSN 0120-8322) **3589**
Colon and Rectal Surgery Outlook (USA ISSN 0894-8062) **3719**, 3887, 4185
● ➤ ColoProctology (DEU ISSN 0174-2442) **3887**
➤ Colorado Dental Association. Journal (USA ISSN 0010-1559) **3818**
Colorado Journal of Pharmacy (USA ISSN 0010-163X) **4284**
➤ Colorado Medicine (USA ISSN 0199-7343) **3589**
Colorado Nurse (USA ISSN 0010-1680) **3917**

Title

Title

Congenital Malformations Surveillance *see* U.S. Centers for Disease Control. Congenital Malformations Surveillance **3236**, 3152, 3222
• ➤ Congestive Heart Failure (USA ISSN 1079-7998) **3769**
Congestive Heart Failure: Disease State Management Resource (USA) **3769**
Congregation News (USA) **3489**, 3457
Congres de Psychanalyse des Langues Romanes. Rapports *see* Revue Francaise de Psychanalyse **4446**
Congres International de la Population. Proceedings *see* International Population Conference. Proceedings **4369**, 3359
Congresso Europeo di Storia Ospitaliera. Atti (ITA ISSN 0589-3267) **3504**
Connecticut. Commission on the Deaf and Hearing-Impaired. Annual Report (USA) **3489**
Connecticut. Commission to Study and Investigate the Problems of Deaf and Hearing-Impaired Persons. Annual Report *see* Connecticut. Commission on the Deaf and Hearing-Impaired. Annual Report **3489**
Connecticut Hospice Newsletter (USA) **4351**, 4391
• ➤ Connecticut Medicine (USA ISSN 0010-6178) **3589**
• Connecticut Nursing News (USA ISSN 0278-4092) **3917**
Connecticut Pharmacist (USA) **4284**
Connecticut State Dental Association. Journal (USA ISSN 0010-6232) **3818**
Connections (CAN ISSN 0828-301X) **4168**
Connections (Largo) (USA) **3504**, 3589
Connections Newsletter (New York) (USA) **3589**
Connective Issues (USA ISSN 8756-9086) **3769**, 3496
Connective Tissue (JPN ISSN 0916-572X) **3589**
Connective Tissue Diseases/Malattie del Tessuto Connettivo (ITA ISSN 0394-0748) **4168**
• ➤ Connective Tissue Research (CHE ISSN 0300-8207) **3288**
Connelly Report (USA) **4231**, 4351
Connexions *see* Connections **4168**
• Connexions (FRA ISSN 0337-3126) **4391**, 4520
Connexions Psychosociologie Sciences Humaines *see* Connexions **4391**, 4520
• Conrad Notes (USA) **3975**
• Conscious Choice (USA) **3436**, 4231
• ➤ Consciousness and Cognition (USA ISSN 1053-8100) **4391**
▼ • ➤ Consciousness & Emotion (NLD ISSN 1566-5836) **4391**
➤ Consciousness and Self-Regulation: Advances in Research and Theory (USA ISSN 0146-5457) **4391**
Conseil de Recherches Medicales. Communique *see* Medical Research Council Newsletter **3653**
Consejo General de Ondotologos y Estomatologos. Revista (ESP ISSN 1136-4319) **3818**
Conservation and Land Management Science *see* C A L M Science **3391**, 3189, 3436, 3463
• ➤ Conservation Biology (USA ISSN 0888-8892) **3392**, 3191
▼ • ➤ Conservation Genetics (NLD ISSN 1566-0621) **3300**, 3392
Conservative Medical Society Bulletin *see* C M S Bulletin **3580**
Consolidated Omnibus Budget Reconciliation Act Advisory *see* C O B R A Advisory **3503**, 3531
▼ Construction & Engineering Magazine (USA ISSN 1533-1490) **4253**, 3361, 3431
Construction Safety *see* Jianzhu Anquan **4257**, 3361
Constructive Criticism (USA ISSN 1052-8164) **4391**, 3175, 3552
Consultant (GBR) **4351**
• ➤ Consultant (Greenwich) (USA ISSN 0010-7069) **3589**
• ➤ The Consultant Pharmacist (USA ISSN 0888-5109) **4285**
Consulting Medical Laboratories. Bulletin (JOR ISSN 0254-7147) **3590**
➤ Consulting Psychology Journal: Practice and Research (USA ISSN 1061-4087) **4391**
Consumer Pharmacist (USA ISSN 0738-0615) **4285**
• Consumer Product Safety Review (USA) **3392**, 4465
• Consumer Reports on Health (USA ISSN 1058-0832) **4351**, 3392
Consumers' Guide to Hospitals (USA ISSN 1070-2644) **3392**, 3504
• Consumers Reference Disc (USA ISSN 1053-1424) **3393**, 3147
Contact (IND) **4500**, 3590
Contact *see* Contact News **3490**, 4512
• ➤ Contact Dermatitis (DNK ISSN 0105-1873) **3846**
Contact Dermatitis. Supplement (DNK ISSN 1396-6669) **3846**
Contact (Hank) *see* Global Contact **3998**
Contact Lens *see* Contact Lens Journal **3995**
• ➤ Contact Lens & Anterior Eye (GBR ISSN 1367-0484) **3995**
Contact Lens Association of Ophthalmologists Journal *see* C L A O Journal **3995**
Contact Lens Journal (GBR ISSN 0306-9575) **3995**
Contact Lens Spectrum (USA ISSN 0885-9175) **3995**
Contact Lens Update (USA ISSN 0885-9264) **3719**, 3996
Contact Magazine (GBR) **3787**
Contact News (IRL ISSN 1393-4805) **3490**, 4512
Contact Point (USA ISSN 0010-7301) **3819**
Contacto (USA) **3719**, 3996
Contacto: Mini-Abstracts *see* Contacto **3719**, 3996
Contemporary Administrator for Long-Term Care *see* Contemporary Longterm Care **3505**
➤ Contemporary Biomedicine (USA) **3248**
➤ Contemporary Cancer Research (USA) **3975**
➤ Contemporary Cardiology (USA) **3769**
▼ ➤ Contemporary Clinical Neuroscience (USA) **4083**
• Contemporary Diagnostic Radiology (USA ISSN 0149-9009) **4142**
Contemporary Dialysis & Nephrology (USA ISSN 0899-837X) **4211**
• Contemporary Drug Problems (USA ISSN 0091-4509) **3400**, 3537
• ➤ Contemporary Educational Psychology (USA ISSN 0361-476X) **3410**, 4391
➤ Contemporary Endocrinology (USA ISSN 0196-8653) **3856**
Contemporary Ergonomics (GBR ISSN 0267-4718) **3431**, 4391
Contemporary Esthetics and Restorative Practice (USA ISSN 1523-2581) **3819**
• ➤ Contemporary Family Therapy (USA ISSN 0892-2764) **4391**, 4520
➤ Contemporary Geriatric Medicine (USA ISSN 0748-2760) **3470**
➤ Contemporary Gerontology (USA ISSN 1069-0840) **3470**
Contemporary Health Digest (JPN) **4351**
➤ Contemporary Hematology (USA) **3900**
Contemporary Hematology - Oncology *see* Contemporary Hematology **3900**
• ➤ Contemporary Hypnosis (GBR ISSN 0960-5290) **3906**, 4391
➤ Contemporary Immunology (USA) **3743**
➤ Contemporary Internal Medicine (USA ISSN 1042-9646) **3908**
Contemporary Issues in Biomedicine, Ethics, and Society *see* Contemporary Biomedicine **3248**
Contemporary Issues in Communication Science & Disorders (USA) **4031**
Contemporary Issues in Computed Tomography (USA ISSN 0266-0601) **4142**, 3810
➤ Contemporary Issues in Genetics and Evolution (NLD ISSN 0929-712X) **3300**
Contemporary Issues in Infectious Diseases (USA ISSN 0888-7756) **3794**
Contemporary Issues in Nephrology (USA ISSN 0161-9934) **4211**
➤ Contemporary Issues in Risk Analysis (USA ISSN 1040-4376) **4465**
Contemporary Issues in Surgical Pathology (USA ISSN 0743-510X) **3590**, 4185
Contemporary Long-Term Care Payment and Regulatory Alert (USA ISSN 1521-3447) **3504**
Contemporary Long-Term Care Reimbursement Bulletin *see* Contemporary Long-Term Care Payment and Regulatory Alert **3504**
• Contemporary Longterm Care (USA ISSN 8750-9652) **3505**
➤ Contemporary Metabolism (USA ISSN 0193-340X) **3856**
➤ Contemporary Nephrology (USA ISSN 0278-1700) **4211**
Contemporary Neurology *see* Neurology and Clinical Neurophysiology **4115**
➤ Contemporary Neurology Series (GBR ISSN 0069-9446) **4083**
Contemporary Neuroscience (USA ISSN 1061-5954) **4084**, 3248
• Contemporary Neurosurgery (USA ISSN 0163-2108) **4186**, 4084
➤ Contemporary Nurse (AUS ISSN 1037-6178) **3917**
Contemporary Ob-Gyn (CAN ISSN 1194-7519) **3948**
• ➤ Contemporary Ob-Gyn (USA ISSN 0090-3159) **3948**
Contemporary Ophthalmic Forum (USA ISSN 0893-8733) **3996**
▼ Contemporary Oral Hygiene (USA) **3819**
Contemporary Pediatrics (CAN ISSN 1182-7076) **4043**
• Contemporary Pediatrics (USA ISSN 8750-0507) **4043**
Contemporary Perspectives in Rehabilitation (USA ISSN 1040-2217) **4060**
• ➤ Contemporary Psychoanalysis (USA ISSN 0010-7530) **4391**
Contemporary Psychology *see* Contemporary Psychology: A P A Review of Books **4391**
• ➤ Contemporary Psychology: A P A Review of Books (USA) **4391**
Contemporary Psychology Series (GBR) **4391**
➤ Contemporary Reviews in Obstetrics and Gynaecology (GBR ISSN 0953-9182) **3948**
Contemporary Sexuality (USA ISSN 1094-5725) **4391**, 4221, 4520, 4563
➤ Contemporary Social Psychology (USA ISSN 1041-3030) **4391**
▼ • Contemporary Spine Surgery (USA ISSN 1527-4268) **4186**, 4012
• ➤ Contemporary Surgery (USA ISSN 0045-8341) **4186**
➤ Contemporary Topics in Immunobiology (USA ISSN 0093-4054) **3743**, 3191
• ➤ Contemporary Topics in Laboratory Animal Science (USA ISSN 1060-0558) **3873**
Contemporary Topics in Vocational Psychology (USA) **4391**
Contemporary Urology (USA ISSN 1042-2250) **4211**
Contents (JPN ISSN 0385-6747) **4344**, 3147
Context (Canterbury) (GBR ISSN 0969-1936) **4391**
• ➤ Continua Neurologica (ESP ISSN 1139-515X) **4084**
• Continuing Care (USA ISSN 1057-428X) **3505**, 4512
Continuing Care News (USA) **3531**, 3505
Continuing Education Matters for O M P (Opthalmic Medical Personnel) (USA) **3996**, 4270
Continuing Medical Education *see* C M E **3580**, 3416
Continuing Medical Education Bulletin Dermatology *see* C M E Bulletin Dermatology **3846**
Continuing Medical Education Bulletin Oncology *see* C M E Bulletin Oncology **3969**
Continuing Medical Education Bulletin. Oncology *see* C M E Bulletin Oncology **3969**
Continuing Medical Education Directory (USA ISSN 1077-209X) **3590**, 3416
Continuing Medical Education Journal - Geriatric Medicine *see* C M E Journal - Geriatric Medicine **3580**, 3469
Continuing Medical Education Supplement to Clinics in Perinatology *see* Clinics in Perinatology **3947**
Continuing Medical Education Supplement to Emergency Medicine Clinics of North America *see* Emergency Medicine Clinics of North America **4014**
Continuing Medical Education Supplement to Magnetic Resonance Imaging Clinics of North America *see* Magnetic Resonance Imaging Clinics of North America **4150**
Continuing Medical Education Supplement to Medical Clinics of North America *see* Medical Clinics of North America **3649**
Continuing Medical Education Supplement to Neuroimaging Clinics of North America *see* Neuroimaging Clinics of North America **4151**
Continuing Medical Education Supplement to Pediatric Clinics of North America *see* Pediatric Clinics of North America **4052**
Continuing Medical Education Supplement to Radiologic Clinics of Norht America *see* Radiologic Clinics of North America **4153**
Continuing Medical Education Supplement to Urologic Clinics of North America *see* Urologic Clinics of North America **4219**
Continuing Professional Development Anaesthesia *see* C P D Anaesthesia **3756**
Continuing Professional Development Bulletin. Immunology and Allergy *see* C P D Bulletin. Immunology and Allergy **3741**
Continuing Professional Development Bulletin. Psychiatry *see* C P D Bulletin. Psychiatry **4080**
Continuous Home Evaluation of Clinical Knowledge *see* C H E C K **3580**
Continuum *see* Balance (Alexandria) **3468**, 3914
Continuum (Baltimore) (USA ISSN 1080-2371) **4084**
➤ Continuum (Chicago) (USA ISSN 1082-8419) **3505**, 4512
Continuum of Care *see* S A H O News **3522**, 4488
• ➤ Contraception (USA ISSN 0010-7824) **3357**, 3948
Contraception - Fertilite - Sexualite *see* Gynecologie Obstetrique et Fertilite **3952**, 3358, 4563
Contraceptive Education Bulletin (GBR) **3358**, 4465
Contraceptive Technology (USA ISSN 0091-9721) **3358**
• ➤ Contraceptive Technology Update (USA ISSN 0274-726X) **3358**
Contraceptives *see* Key Note Market Report: Contraceptives **3359**
Contract Pharma (USA) **4285**
Contrappunto (ITA ISSN 1590-0223) **4084**
Contribuicoes em Psicologia, Psiquiatria e Psicanalise (BRA) **4392**, 4084
➤ Contributions in Marine Science (USA ISSN 0082-3449) **3191**, 3407, 3436, 3459
Contributions in Medical History *see* Contributions in Medical Studies **3590**
Contributions in Medical Studies (USA ISSN 0886-8220) **3590**
Contributions in Psychology (USA ISSN 0736-2714) **4392**
• ➤ Contributions to Gynecology and Obstetrics (CHE ISSN 0304-4246) **3948**
➤ Contributions to Microbiology (CHE ISSN 1420-9519) **3320**
Contributions to Microbiology and Immunology *see* Contributions to Microbiology **3320**
• ➤ Contributions to Nephrology (CHE ISSN 0302-5144) **4211**
➤ Contributions to Oncology/Beitraege zur Onkologie (CHE ISSN 0250-3220) **3975**
Contributions to Residential Treatment (USA) **4392**, 3382
Contributions to the Study of Aging (USA ISSN 0732-085X) **3470**
Contributions to the Study of Music and Dance (USA ISSN 0193-9041) **4225**, 3396
Control of Communicable Diseases in Man (USA ISSN 8755-4046) **3794**
• ➤ Controlled Clinical Trials (USA ISSN 0197-2456) **3873**
• Controlled Release Society. International Symposium on Controlled Release of Bioactive Materials. Proceedings (USA ISSN 1022-0178) **3378**, 4285
Controlled Substances Handbook *see* Controlled Substances Regulation **3400**, 3394
Controlled Substances Regulation (USA) **3400**, 3394
Controversies in Cardiology (ITA) **3769**
➤ Controversies in Clinical Ophthalmology (USA) **3996**
Convulsive Therapy *see* The Journal of Electroconvulsive Therapy **4101**
• Cooking Light (USA ISSN 0886-4446) **3526**, 4231
• Cooking News (USA) **4231**
Cooperador Dental (ARG ISSN 0069-9799) **3819**
Coordination Council on Deafness of Nova Scotia. News *see* Atlantic Silent News **3489**
Coping *see* Coping with Cancer **3975**
➤ Coping with Allergies and Asthma (USA) **4159**
➤ Coping with Cancer (USA) **3975**
• ➤ Cor et Vasa (CZE ISSN 0010-8650) **3769**
• Core Journals in Cardiology (NLD ISSN 0165-9405) **3719**, 3147, 3769
• Core Journals in Clinical Neurology (NLD ISSN 0165-1056) **3719**, 3147
• Core Journals in Dermatology (NLD ISSN 0167-5796) **3719**, 3147, 3846
• Core Journals in Gastroenterology (NLD ISSN 0165-8719) **3719**, 3147, 3887
• Core Journals in Obstetrics - Gynecology (NLD ISSN 0376-5059) **3719**, 3147
• Core Journals in Ophthalmology (NLD ISSN 0165-1005) **3719**, 3147
• Core Journals in Pediatrics (NLD ISSN 0376-5040) **3720**, 3147
Core Medline (USA ISSN 1040-4066) **3720**, 3147

Title

▼ • Current Atherosclerosis Reports (USA ISSN 1523-3804) **3769**
• Current Awareness in Biological Sciences (NLD ISSN 0733-4443) **3229**, 3147, 3191
• Current Awareness in Health Education (USA) **4351**
Current Awareness. S D I Service (GBR) **3591**, 3192, 4531
Current Bibliographies in Medicine *see* National Library of Medicine. Current Bibliographies in Medicine **3733**
Current Bibliographies on Science and Technology: Biology, Pharmacy and Food Science (KOR) **3229**, 3147, 3192
• Current Bibliography on Science and Technology: Life Sciences/Kagaku Gijutsu Bunken Sokuho. Raifusaiensu Hen (JPN ISSN 0285-5100) **3229**, 3177, 3192
• ➤ Current Biology (USA ISSN 0960-9822) **3229**, 3147, 3192
• Current Biotechnology (DEU ISSN 0960-5037) **3229**, 3147, 3273
Current Canadian Ophthalmic Practice *see* Ophthalmic Practice **4003**
▼ Current Cancer Drug Targets (NLD ISSN 1568-0096) **3975**
Current Cancer Research (DEU ISSN 0940-0745) **3976**
Current Cancer Therapeutics (USA ISSN 1074-2816) **3976**
• Current Cardiology Reports (USA ISSN 1523-3782) **3769**
Current Cardiovascular Drugs (Year) (USA ISSN 1070-4345) **3769**, 4285
▼ ➤ Current Clinical Oncology (USA) **3976**, 3900
➤ Current Clinical Practice (USA ISSN 0168-6917) **3591**
• Current Clinical Trials: Oncology (USA ISSN 1070-9576) **3720**
▼ ➤ Current Clinical Urology (USA) **4211**
Current Comments (USA ISSN 0892-5798) **3874**, 3192
Current Communications in Cell and Molecular Biology Series (USA ISSN 1063-8806) **3248**, 3288
Current Concepts in Hospital Pharmacy/Byoin Yakkyoku (JPN ISSN 0911-2847) **4285**
Current Concepts in Magnesium Metabolism/Maguneshumu Taisha Konnichi no Kanaekata (JPN ISSN 0912-2249) **3856**
• Current Contents: Clinical Medicine (USA ISSN 0891-3358) **3720**, 3147
• Current Contents: Life Sciences (USA ISSN 0011-3409) **3229**, 3147, 3192
• Current Contents: Social & Behavioral Sciences (USA ISSN 0092-6361) **4457**, 3147, 4393
▼ Current Controlled Trials In Cardio Vascular Medicine (GBR ISSN 1468-6708) **3769**
Current Critical Care Diagnosis and Treatment (USA ISSN 1071-3964) **3591**
Current Critical Problems in Vascular Surgery (USA ISSN 1052-4436) **4186**, 3770
Current Diagnosis and Treatment in Cardiology (USA ISSN 1079-1051) **3770**
• Current Diagnostic Pathology (GBR ISSN 0968-6053) **3908**
Current Directions in Autoimmunity (CHE ISSN 1422-2132) **3743**, 3300
• ➤ Current Directions in Psychological Science (USA ISSN 0963-7214) **4393**
▼ Current Drug Discovery (GBR) **4285**
▼ • ➤ Current Drug Metabolism (USA ISSN 1389-2002) **4285**
▼ • ➤ Current Drug Targets (USA ISSN 1389-4501) **4285**
Current Emergency Diagnosis and Treatment (USA ISSN 0894-2293) **4012**, 3591
Current Emergency Therapy (USA ISSN 0739-8573) **4012**, 3591
• ➤ Current Eye Research (NLD ISSN 0271-3683) **3996**
Current Gastroenterology (USA ISSN 0198-8085) **3887**
• Current Gastroenterology Reports (USA ISSN 1522-8037) **3887**
• ➤ Current Genetics (DEU ISSN 0172-8083) **3300**
▼ • ➤ Current Genomics (USA ISSN 1389-2029) **3300**
• Current Health 1 (USA ISSN 0199-820X) **3428**, 4351
• Current Health 2 (USA ISSN 0163-156X) **3428**, 4351
Current Hepatology (USA ISSN 0198-8093) **3888**
➤ Current Histopathology (NLD ISSN 0272-1465) **3908**
• Current Hypertension Reports (USA ISSN 1522-6417) **3770**
Current Index to Journals in Science and Technology: Biology, Agriculture, Pharmacy *see* Current Bibliographies on Science and Technology: Biology, Pharmacy and Food Science **3229**, 3147, 3192
Current Infectious Disease Drugs (USA ISSN 1082-8877) **3794**, 4285
• Current Infectious Disease Reports (USA ISSN 1523-3847) **3743**
Current Insights in Ophthalmic Surgery *see* Ganka Shujutsu Konnichi no Kangaekata **3998**
• Current Interventional Cardiology Reports (USA ISSN 1523-3839) **3770**
Current Issues in Food Safety (USA) **3460**, 4253
▼ • ➤ Current Issues in Intestinal Microbiology (GBR ISSN 1466-531X) **3320**
Current Issues in Intestinal Microbiology Online *see* Current Issues in Intestinal Microbiology **3320**
• ➤ Current Issues in Molecular Biology (GBR ISSN 1467-3037) **3248**, 3273, 3300, 3320
Current Issues in Neurodegenerative Diseases (NLD ISSN 1380-7730) **4084**
Current Issues in Psychoanalytic Practice. Journal *see* Current Issues in Psychoanalytic Practice. Monographs **4393**
Current Issues in Psychoanalytic Practice. Monographs (USA) **4393**
• Current Issues in Public Health (GBR ISSN 1076-7762) **4466**
Current Issues in Toxicology (USA) **3447**, 4285
Current Literature on Aging *see* Abstracts in Social Gerontology **3482**, 3145
➤ Current Management of Pain (NLD ISSN 0923-2354) **4084**
• Current Medical Diagnosis and Treatment (USA ISSN 0092-8682) **3591**
Current Medical Literature. Advances in Stroke (GBR) **3720**, 3770
Current Medical Literature. Allergy (GBR ISSN 0968-5626) **3720**, 3743
Current Medical Literature. Anaesthesiology (GBR ISSN 0269-6959) **3720**, 3756
Current Medical Literature. Breast and Prostate Cancer *see* Current Medical Literature. Prostatic Disease **3722**, 4211
Current Medical Literature. Breast and Prostate Cancer *see* Current Medical Literature. Breast Cancer **3721**, 3976, 4563
Current Medical Literature. Breast Cancer (GBR ISSN 0956-6511) **3721**, 3976, 4563
Current Medical Literature. Cardiac Imaging Monitor (GBR ISSN 1364-4858) **3721**, 3147, 3770, 4142
Current Medical Literature. Cardiology (GBR ISSN 1354-0122) **3721**, 3770
Current Medical Literature. Cardiovascular Medicine *see* Current Medical Literature. Cardiology **3721**, 3770
Current Medical Literature. Clinical Nutrition (GBR ISSN 0965-7126) **4248**, 3147, 4231
Current Medical Literature. Colorectal Cancer (GBR ISSN 1364-4831) **3721**, 3147, 3888, 3976
Current Medical Literature. Critical Care Monitor (GBR) **3721**, 4012
Current Medical Literature. Dermatology (GBR ISSN 1361-4215) **3721**, 3846
• Current Medical Literature. Diabetes (GBR ISSN 0265-797X) **3721**, 3856
Current Medical Literature. Epilepsy Monitor (GBR ISSN 1359-8384) **3721**, 4084
Current Medical Literature. Focus on Depression *see* Current Medical Literature. Perspectives in Depression **3722**, 4084
Current Medical Literature. G H and Growth Factors (GBR ISSN 0269-185X) **3591**, 3341
Current Medical Literature. Gastroenterology (GBR ISSN 0263-2659) **3721**, 3888
Current Medical Literature. General Surgery (GBR ISSN 0966-0224) **3721**, 4186
Current Medical Literature. Geriatrics *see* Current Medical Literature. Health Care of Older People **3482**, 3148, 3721
Current Medical Literature. Gynaecology and Obstetrics (GBR ISSN 1356-742X) **3721**, 3948
Current Medical Literature. Health Care of Older People (GBR ISSN 1366-8544) **3482**, 3148, 3721
Current Medical Literature. Hospital Pharmacy *see* Current Medical Literature. International Hospital Pharmacy **4344**, 3721, 4285
Current Medical Literature. Infectious Diseases (GBR ISSN 0951-9602) **3721**, 3794
Current Medical Literature. Intensive Care Monitor *see* Current Medical Literature. Critical Care Monitor **3721**, 4012
Current Medical Literature. International Hospital Pharmacy (GBR ISSN 1354-5337) **4344**, 3721, 4285
Current Medical Literature. Interventional Cardiology Monitor (GBR ISSN 1352-738X) **3721**, 3770
Current Medical Literature. Leukaemia and Lymphoma (GBR ISSN 0969-7063) **3721**, 3976
Current Medical Literature. Medical Imaging (GBR) **3721**, 4142
Current Medical Literature. Nephrology and Hypertension (GBR ISSN 1357-1540) **3722**, 4211
Current Medical Literature. Nephrology and Urology *see* Current Medical Literature. Nephrology and Hypertension **3722**, 4211
Current Medical Literature. Nephrology and Urology *see* Current Medical Literature. Urology **3722**, 4211
Current Medical Literature. Neurology *see* Current Medical Literature. Neurology & Neurosurgery **3722**, 4084
Current Medical Literature. Neurology & Neurosurgery (GBR) **3722**, 4084
Current Medical Literature. Ophthalmology (GBR ISSN 0963-0112) **3722**, 3996
Current Medical Literature. Paediatrics (GBR ISSN 0951-9610) **3722**, 4043
Current Medical Literature. Perspectives in Depression (GBR ISSN 1361-634X) **3722**, 4084
Current Medical Literature. Prostatic Disease (GBR ISSN 1366-8552) **3722**, 4211
Current Medical Literature. Psychiatry (GBR ISSN 0957-770X) **3722**, 4084
Current Medical Literature. Psychiatry Reviews (GBR ISSN 1363-7339) **3722**, 3148, 4084
Current Medical Literature. Radiology *see* Current Medical Literature. Medical Imaging **3721**, 4142
Current Medical Literature. Respiratory Medicine (GBR ISSN 1361-6706) **3722**, 4159
Current Medical Literature. Reversible Obstructive Airways Disease *see* Current Medical Literature. Respiratory Medicine **3722**, 4159
Current Medical Literature. Rheumatology (GBR ISSN 0261-3360) **3722**, 4168
Current Medical Literature. Surgical Infection (GBR ISSN 0969-1537) **3722**, 4186
Current Medical Literature. Urology (GBR ISSN 1357-1532) **3722**, 4211
Current Medical Literature. Year in Stroke *see* Current Medical Literature. Advances in Stroke **3720**, 3770
Current Medical Practice (IND ISSN 0011-3700) **3591**
• ➤ Current Medical Research and Opinion (GBR ISSN 0300-7995) **3591**
▼ • Current Medicinal Chemistry - Anti-Inflammatory & Anti-Allergy Agents (NLD ISSN 1568-0142) **4285**
Current Medicine (GBR ISSN 0953-9352) **3591**
Current Medicine *see* Gendai Igaku **3605**
• ➤ Current Microbiology (USA ISSN 0343-8651) **3320**
➤ Current Neurology (NLD ISSN 0161-780X) **4084**
▼ • ➤ Current News in Medicine (AUT ISSN 1608-2222) **3591**
• Current Obstetrics and Gynaecology (GBR ISSN 0957-5847) **3948**
Current Obstetrics and Gynaecology - Edizione Italiana (ITA) **3948**
• Current Oncology Reports (USA ISSN 1523-3790) **3976**
➤ Current Oncology (Toronto) (CAN ISSN 1198-0052) **3976**
▼ • Current Opinion in Allergy and Clinical Immunology (GBR ISSN 1528-4050) **3743**
• Current Opinion in Anaesthesiology (USA ISSN 0952-7907) **3756**
Current Opinion in Anti-Inflammatory & Immunomodulatory Investigational Drugs *see* Current Opinion in Investigational Drugs **4285**
• ➤ Current Opinion in Biotechnology (GBR ISSN 0958-1669) **3273**
• ➤ Current Opinion in Cardiology (USA ISSN 0268-4705) **3770**
Current Opinion in Cardiology. Supplement (USA ISSN 1354-7232) **3770**
• ➤ Current Opinion in Cell Biology (GBR ISSN 0955-0674) **3288**
▼ • ➤ Current Opinion in Clinical Experimental Research (AUT ISSN 1563-311X) **3874**
• ➤ Current Opinion in Clinical Nutrition and Metabolic Care (USA ISSN 1363-1950) **4231**
• Current Opinion in Critical Care (USA ISSN 1070-5295) **4012**
Current Opinion in Dentistry *see* Current Opinion in Periodontology **3819**
• Current Opinion in Dermatology (GBR ISSN 1068-381X) **3847**
Current Opinion in Drug Discovery & Development (GBR ISSN 1367-6733) **4285**, 3376
• Current Opinion in Endocrinology & Diabetes (USA ISSN 1068-3097) **3857**
▼ ➤ Current Opinion in European Medicine (AUT ISSN 1607-6524) **3591**
• ➤ Current Opinion in Gastroenterology (USA ISSN 0267-1379) **3888**
• ➤ Current Opinion in Genetics & Development (GBR ISSN 0959-437X) **3301**
• Current Opinion in Hematology (USA ISSN 1065-6251) **3900**
• ➤ Current Opinion in Immunology (GBR ISSN 0952-7915) **3722**, 3148, 3743
• ➤ Current Opinion in Infectious Diseases (USA ISSN 0951-7375) **3794**
Current Opinion in Infectious Diseases. Supplement (USA) **3794**
Current Opinion in Investigational Drugs *see* Expert Opinion On Investigational Drugs **4293**
Current Opinion in Investigational Drugs (GBR ISSN 1472-4472) **4285**
• ➤ Current Opinion in Lipidology (GBR ISSN 0957-9672) **3770**
▼ • Current Opinion in Molecular Therapeutics (GBR ISSN 1464-8431) **4285**
• ➤ Current Opinion in Nephrology & Hypertension (USA ISSN 1062-4821) **4211**
• ➤ Current Opinion in Neurobiology (GBR ISSN 0959-4388) **4084**, 3341
• ➤ Current Opinion in Neurology (USA ISSN 1350-7540) **4085**
Current Opinion in Neurology and Neurosurgery *see* Current Opinion in Neurology **4085**
• ➤ Current Opinion in Obstetrics & Gynecology (USA ISSN 1040-872X) **3948**
• Current Opinion in Oncology (USA ISSN 1040-8746) **3976**
• Current Opinion in Ophthalmology (USA ISSN 1040-8738) **3996**
• Current Opinion in Organ Transplantation (USA ISSN 1087-2418) **3591**
Current Opinion in Orthodontics and Pedodontics *see* Current Opinion in Periodontology **3819**
• Current Opinion in Orthopedics (USA ISSN 1041-9918) **4013**
• Current Opinion in Otolaryngology & Head and Neck Surgery (USA ISSN 1068-9508) **4031**, 4186
• Current Opinion in Pediatrics (USA ISSN 1040-8703) **4043**
• ➤ Current Opinion in Periodontology (GBR ISSN 1065-626X) **3819**
▼ • Current Opinion in Pharmacology (GBR ISSN 1471-4892) **4285**
• ➤ Current Opinion in Psychiatry (USA ISSN 0951-7367) **4085**
• Current Opinion in Pulmonary Medicine (USA ISSN 1070-5287) **4159**
• Current Opinion in Rheumatology (USA ISSN 1040-8711) **4168**
• ➤ Current Opinion in Structural Biology (GBR ISSN 0959-440X) **3248**
• Current Opinion in Urology (USA ISSN 0963-0643) **4211**
Current Opinion on Therapeutic Patents *see* Expert Opinion on Therapeutic Patents **4293**, 4272
• ➤ Current Orthopaedics (GBR ISSN 0268-0890) **4013**
➤ Current Paediatric Research (IND ISSN 0971-9032) **4043**
• Current Paediatrics (GBR ISSN 0957-5839) **4043**
• Current Pain and Headache Reports (USA ISSN 1531-3433) **4085**
Current Pediatric Diagnosis and Treatment (USA ISSN 0093-8556) **4043**
Current Perspectives on Aging and Life Cycle *see* Advances in Life Course Research **3466**, 4510
▼ • ➤ Current Pharmaceutical Biotechnology (USA ISSN 1389-2010) **3273**, 4286
• ➤ Current Pharmaceutical Design (USA ISSN 1381-6128) **4286**

Title

Title

Title

Title

Dyslexia Handbook (GBR) **3421**, 4087
• ➤ Dysphagia (USA ISSN 0179-051X) **4032**
Dystonia Dialogue (USA) **3596**, 4512
Dziecko (POL ISSN 1233-2984) **4563**, 3358, 3382
e A D C - F & N *see* Archives of Disease in Childhood. Fetal and Neonatal Edition **3945**, 4041
E A P Digest (Employee Assistance Programs) (USA ISSN 0273-8910) **3401**, 4395
E A P P G *see* Australian Prescription Products Guide **4279**
• E & P Health, Safety and Environment (Exploration and Production) (USA ISSN 1067-1013) **4272**, 3148, 3443, 4268
▼ • e-biomed (USA ISSN 1524-8909) **3596**
E C C Newsletter (European Cancer Centre) (NLD ISSN 0927-328X) **3976**
➤ E C E T O C Document (European Centre for Ecotoxicology and Toxicology of Chemicals) (BEL ISSN 1013-9516) **3448**
➤ E C E T O C Monograph (European Centre for Ecotoxicology and Toxicology of Chemicals) (BEL ISSN 0773-6347) **3448**
➤ E C E T O C Special Report (New Series) (European Centre for Ecotoxicology and Toxicology of Chemicals) (BEL ISSN 1373-7244) **3448**
➤ E C E T O C Technical Report (European Centre for Ecotoxicology and Toxicology of Chemicals) (BEL ISSN 0773-8072) **3448**
E C M T Statistical Report on Road Accidents (European Council of Ministers of Transport) (FRA) **4532**, 3148, 4495
E C T *see* The Journal of Electroconvulsive Therapy **4101**
• ➤ E-chocardiography (USA) **3771**
E D I M E D (ITA) **4291**
E D Legal Letter (USA ISSN 1087-7347) **3538**, 3596
E D Management *see* Emergency Department Management **4013**, 3506
▼ E D News (ITA) **4212**, 3860
E D Nursing (Emergency Department) (USA) **3918**
➤ E D T N A - E R C A Journal (European Dialysis and Transplant Nurses Association, European Renal Care Association) (CHE ISSN 1019-083X) **4212**, 3918
E E G - E M G *see* Klinische Neurophysiologie **4107**
E E G Labor *see* Neurophysiologie - Labor **3780**, 4116
E H *see* Environmental Health **4467**, 3438
• E H & S Products (Environmental, Health & Safety) (USA) **4253**, 3444
E H N *see* Environmental Health News **4467**
➤ E H P (European Hospital Pharmacy) (DEU ISSN 1381-4060) **4291**
E H P *see* Environmental Health Perspectives **3438**, 4467
E H P *see* E H P Supplements **3436**, 4467
• ➤ E H P Supplements (Environmental Health Perspectives) (USA ISSN 1078-0475) **3436**, 4467
e-Health *see* Pharmaceutical Executive **4323**
• e-Health & Telemedicine News (USA) **3810**, 3538
▼ e-Healthcare Market Reporter (USA ISSN 1526-6052) **3361**, 3388, 3596
E I B *see* Environment Information Bulletin **4467**, 3448
E I R E C Kenkyu Hokokushu (Rehabilitation Engineering Center for Employment Injuries) (JPN ISSN 0919-5602) **4060**, 3364
E J B *see* Electronic Journal of Biotechnology **3273**, 3249
E J H *see* European Journal of Histochemistry **3249**, 3290
E J P R D *see* European Journal of Prosthodontics and Restorative Dentistry **3823**
E M A News (Environmental Management Association) (USA) **4467**
• ➤ The E M B O Journal (European Molecular Biology Organization) (GBR ISSN 0261-4189) **3249**, 3289
▼ • ➤ E M B O Reports (European Molecular Biology Organization) (GBR ISSN 1469-221X) **3301**, 3596
E M B O Reports Online *see* E M B O Reports **3301**, 3596
E M B Online *see* Evidence - Based Medicine **3600**
E M F Health & Safety Digest (Electric and Magnetic Field) (USA ISSN 1062-5526) **4253**, 3434, 3437, 4467
E M F Health Report (Electric and Magnetic Field) (USA ISSN 1070-4027) **4253**
E M J Online *see* Emergency Medicine Journal **4014**
E M S Communicator *see* E M S Insider **4013**, 3596
E M S Insider (USA ISSN 1081-4507) **4013**, 3596
• E M S Manager and Supervisor (Emergency Medical Service) (USA ISSN 1532-1576) **4013**
E M S Rescue Technology *see* Advanced Rescue Technology **4009**, 4460
E N B Link CD-ROM *see* E N B News **3918**, 3948
• E N B News (English National Board for Nursing, Midwifery, and Health Visiting) (GBR) **3918**, 3948
E N L B *see* Emergency Nurse Legal Bulletin **3918**, 3538
E N S B A N A Cahiers *see* Ecole Nationale Superieure de Biologie Appliquee a la Nutrition et a l'Alimentation. Cahiers **3460**, 4232
• ➤ E N T News (GBR ISSN 1368-8944) **4032**
E O R T C Monograph Series *see* European Organization for Research on Treatment of Cancer. Monograph Series **3977**
E P D A Magazine (European Parkinson's Disease Association) (NLD ISSN 1387-9340) **4087**
E P F P R (Egyptian Population and Family Planning Review) (EGY) **3358**
E P I B *see* European Pharmaceutical Intelligence Bulletin **4293**
E P I C Journal *see* Journal of Evidence Photography **4349**, 3883
E P L B *see* Emergency Physician Legal Bulletin **3598**, 3538
• E P P I C Information Sheet (Early Psychosis Prevention and Intervention Centre) (AUS ISSN 1326-2610) **4087**
• E-psyche (USA) **4457**, 3148
• E R A News (European Regulatory Affairs) (GBR ISSN 1462-3129) **4291**
E S A Newsletter (Entomological Society of America) (USA ISSN 0273-7353) **3295**
E S C Magazine (Every Second Counts) (USA) **4013**
E S E M News (European Society for Engineering and Medicine) (BEL) **3596**, 3237
E S - H W G - Entscheidungssammlung Heilmittelwerbegesetz (DEU) **4291**, 3538
E S J *see* The Elementary School Journal **3411**, 4396
E S N *see* European Safety Newsletter **4468**
• E-Streams (Contoocook) (USA ISSN 1098-4399) **3154**, 3596
E U Informationsbrief Gesundheit (European Union) (DEU ISSN 0949-8567) **4467**
▼ E&F - Eyewear & Fashion (ITA ISSN 1590-9638) **3997**
• ➤ Ear and Hearing (USA ISSN 0196-0202) **4032**
• ➤ Ear, Nose & Throat Journal (USA ISSN 0145-5613) **4032**
Ear, Nose and Throat News *see* E N T News **4032**
➤ Early Child Development and Care (CHE ISSN 0300-4430) **3382**, 4044
• ➤ Early Childhood Education Journal (USA ISSN 1082-3301) **3410**, 3382
▼ • ➤ Early Childhood Research & Practice (USA ISSN 1524-5039) **3410**, 3382, 4395
Early Childhood Update (USA) **4395**, 3410
Early Development and Parenting *see* Infant and Child Development **4404**, 3383
Early Education and Development (USA ISSN 1040-9289) **3410**, 4395
• ➤ Early Human Development (IRL ISSN 0378-3782) **3948**, 4044
Early Intervention (USA ISSN 1058-8396) **3421**, 3382
• Early Psychosis News (AUS ISSN 1326-0871) **4087**
Early Psychosis Prevention and Intervention Centre Information Sheet *see* E P P I C Information Sheet **4087**
• ➤ Early Science and Medicine (NLD ISSN 1383-7427) **3596**, 3526, 4504
East African Institute of Malaria and Vectorborne Diseases. Annual Report (TZA) **3795**
• ➤ The East African Medical Journal (KEN ISSN 0012-835X) **3597**
East African Newsletter on Occupational Health and Safety *see* African Newsletter on Occupational Health and Safety **4249**
➤ East and Central African Journal of Surgery (ZMB ISSN 1024-297X) **4187**
➤ East Asian Science, Technology, and Medicine (USA) **4504**, 3597, 4531
East Bay Vegan News *see* The Vegan News **4247**, 3172
➤ East European Medical Journal (ROM ISSN 1220-8795) **3597**
East European Medical Journal Supplement *see* East European Medical Journal **3597**
East Texas Medicine (USA ISSN 1050-6675) **3597**
Easter Seals - March of Dimes National Council. Annual Report (CAN ISSN 1482-8383) **3421**, 3484
Eastern Dental Society Bulletin (USA ISSN 0012-8759) **3822**
Eastern Japan Journal of Clinical Orthopaedics *see* Higashinihon Rinsho Seikei Geka Gakkai Zasshi **4016**
Eastern Mediterranean Health Journal/La Revue de Sante de la Mediterranee Orientale (EGY ISSN 1020-3397) **4467**
• ➤ The Eastern Pharmacist (IND ISSN 0012-8872) **4291**
EastWest Natural Health *see* Natural Health **3168**, 4227, 4359
• Eating and Weight Disorders (ITA ISSN 1124-4909) **4087**, 4232, 4395
▼ • Eating Behaviors (NLD ISSN 1471-0153) **4395**
• ➤ Eating Disorders (USA ISSN 1064-0266) **4395**
Eating Disorders Review (USA ISSN 1048-6984) **4087**, 4232
eB M J *see* bmj.com **3577**
Echo de l'Union (FRA ISSN 0243-0738) **3470**, 4512
• Echo Magazine (USA ISSN 1045-2346) **3527**
• ➤ Echocardiography (USA ISSN 0742-2822) **3771**
Echocardiography Journal *see* E-chocardiography **3771**
Echocardiography Journal of Cardiac Ultrasound *see* E-chocardiography **3771**
Eco News (ITA ISSN 1123-8399) **3948**
• ➤ Ecography (DNK ISSN 0906-7590) **3437**, 3194
Ecole Nationale Superieure de Biologie Appliquee a la Nutrition et a l'Alimentation. Cahiers (FRA ISSN 0221-0347) **3460**, 4232
➤ Ecologia (ESP ISSN 0214-0896) **3194**, 3392
Ecologia della Mente (ITA ISSN 0394-1310) **4396**
➤ Ecologia en Bolivia (BOL) **3194**, 3407
• ➤ Ecological Applications (USA ISSN 1051-0761) **3437**, 3194
• ➤ Ecological Monographs (USA ISSN 0012-9615) **3437**, 3194
• ➤ Ecological Psychology (USA ISSN 1040-7413) **4396**, 3392
Ecological Society of America. Bulletin (USA ISSN 0012-9623) **3437**, 3194
Ecological Studies: Analysis and Synthesis (USA ISSN 0070-8356) **3194**
The Ecologists (IND) **3194**, 3392
• ➤ Ecology (USA ISSN 0012-9658) **3437**, 3194
• ➤ Ecology of Food and Nutrition (CHE ISSN 0367-0244) **4232**
Ecology U S A (USA ISSN 0098-6615) **3437**, 3194
➤ Economic Microbiology (USA) **3320**
Economic Trends (Chicago) (USA ISSN 0882-5807) **3506**
Economics, Medicines, & Health (GBR ISSN 1356-9007) **3369**, 3597, 4291, 4467
• ➤ Ecotoxicology (USA ISSN 0963-9292) **3448**
• ➤ Ecotoxicology and Environmental Safety (USA ISSN 0147-6513) **3448**, 4467
Ecotoxicology and Environmental Safety - Online *see* Ecotoxicology and Environmental Safety **3448**, 4467
• Ecuador. Instituto Nacional de Estadistica y Censos. Anuario de Estadisticas Hospitalarias (ECU ISSN 0070-8895) **3506**
Ecuador. Instituto Nacional de Estadistica y Censos. Cuentas Nacionales de la Salud (ECU) **3369**, 3362, 3506
Editorials in Cardiology *see* L'information Cardiologique **3774**
Edogawa (JPN ISSN 0915-9061) **3597**
Edogawa City Medical Association. Journal *see* Edogawa **3597**
Edogawa City Medical Association. Proceedings *see* Edogawa Igakkaishi **3597**
Edogawa Igakkaishi/Edogawa City Medical Association. Proceedings (JPN ISSN 0915-8693) **3597**
Educacao Medica (PRT ISSN 0871-7958) **3597**
Educacion Continua en Salud (Year) Temas Escogidos (COL) **3597**
Educacion Medica (ESP) **3597**, 3410
Educacion Sanitaria (ESP) **4467**
• ➤ Education and Ageing (GBR ISSN 1352-8580) **3470**, 3410
➤ Education and Health (GBR ISSN 0265-1602) **3418**, 3597
Education and Psychology of the Gifted Series (USA) **3421**, 4396
Education and Psychology Review (IND ISSN 0046-1385) **3410**, 4396
Education and Training in Mental Retardation *see* Education and Training in Mental Retardation and Developmental Disabilities **3421**, 4087
• Education and Training in Mental Retardation and Developmental Disabilities (USA ISSN 1079-3917) **3421**, 4087
Education for General Practice *see* Education for Primary Care **3597**, 3417
• Education for Health (GBR ISSN 1357-6283) **3597**, 4512
• Education for Primary Care (GBR ISSN 1473-9879) **3597**, 3417
Education for the Handicapped *see* Practical Education for the Handicapped **3425**
Education of the Handicapped *see* Special Education Report **3427**, 3487
Education of Traditional Chinese Medicine *see* Zhongyi Jiaoyu **3171**, 3415
Education Sanitaire et Nutritionnelle d'Afrique Centrale (BEL ISSN 0004-5144) **4232**, 4467
Education Special Interest Section Newsletter *see* Education Special Interest Section Quarterly **3416**, 4254
Education Special Interest Section Quarterly (USA) **3416**, 4254
➤ Educational & Child Psychology (GBR) **4396**
Educational and Psychological Interactions (SWE ISSN 0070-9263) **3410**, 4396
• ➤ Educational and Psychological Measurement (USA ISSN 0013-1644) **4396**, 3410
Educational Commission for Foreign Medical Graduates. Annual Report (USA ISSN 0145-2037) **3597**
• ➤ Educational Gerontology (USA ISSN 0360-1277) **3470**, 3416
• ➤ Educational Psychologist (USA ISSN 0046-1520) **4396**, 3410
• ➤ Educational Psychology (GBR ISSN 0144-3410) **3410**, 4396
• ➤ Educational Psychology in Practice (USA ISSN 0266-7363) **3410**, 4396
• ➤ Educational Psychology Review (USA ISSN 1040-726X) **3411**, 4396
Educational Software Selector *see* T E S S **3416**, 3391
• Educational Synopses in Anesthesiology and Critical Care Medicine (USA ISSN 1080-3521) **3597**
➤ The Educational Therapist (USA) **3421**
Educational Therapy & Therapeutic Teaching (GBR ISSN 0964-8690) **3421**, 4060
Educator's Update (USA ISSN 1092-2687) **3358**
Educazione dei Sordi (ITA ISSN 1120-5393) **3490**, 3421
Eesti Naine (EST ISSN 0235-7488) **4568**, 3175, 3463, 4563
Eesti Teaduste Akadeemia. Toimetised. Bioloogia *see* Estonian Academy of Sciences. Proceedings. Biology - Ecology **3194**, 3439
Eesti Teaduste Akadeemia. Toimetised. Bioloogia. Okoloogia *see* Estonian Academy of Sciences. Proceedings. Biology - Ecology **3194**, 3439
Eesti Teaduste Akadeemia. Toimetised. Okoloogia *see* Estonian Academy of Sciences. Proceedings. Biology - Ecology **3194**, 3439
• ➤ Effective Clinical Practice (USA ISSN 1099-8128) **3597**
• ➤ Effective Health Care (GBR ISSN 0965-0288) **3597**
Effective School Practices (USA ISSN 1068-7378) **3428**
• Effeta (ITA ISSN 0013-2195) **3490**
Egeszsegneveles Szakkonyvtara (HUN ISSN 0073-4012) **4467**
➤ Egeszsegugyi Gazdasagi Szemle (HUN ISSN 0013-2276) **3506**
Egyptian Dental Journal (EGY ISSN 0070-9484) **3822**
Egyptian Journal of Bilharziasis (EGY ISSN 0301-8849) **3795**
Egyptian Journal of Biomedical Engineering (EGY ISSN 1012-5558) **3874**
• Egyptian Journal of Food Science/Al-Majallah al-Misriyyah li-Ulum al-Aghdhiya (EGY ISSN 1110-0192) **3460**

Title

➤ Encyclopedie Medico-Chirurgicale. Endocrinologie - Nutrition (FRA ISSN 1155-1941) **3860**, 4232
Encyclopedie Medico-Chirurgicale. Estomac - Intestin *see* Encyclopedie Medico-Chirurgicale. Gastro-Enterologie **3889**
Encyclopedie Medico-Chirurgicale. Foie - Pancreas *see* Encyclopedie Medico-Chirurgicale. Hepatologie **3889**
➤ Encyclopedie Medico-Chirurgicale. Gastro-Enterologie (FRA ISSN 1155-1968) **3889**
Encyclopedie Medico-Chirurgicale. Ginecologia - Obstetricia (FRA ISSN 1283-081X) **3948**
Encyclopedie Medico-Chirurgicale. Ginecologia - Ostetricia (FRA ISSN 1293-2639) **3949**
Encyclopedie Medico-Chirurgicale. Glandes Endocrines, Maladies de la Nutrition, Pathologie Generale *see* Encyclopedie Medico-Chirurgicale. Endocrinologie - Nutrition **3860**, 4232
➤ Encyclopedie Medico-Chirurgicale. Gynecologie (FRA ISSN 0246-1064) **3949**
Encyclopedie Medico-Chirurgicale. Gynecologie - Mamelle *see* Encyclopedie Medico-Chirurgicale. Gynecologie **3949**
Encyclopedie Medico-Chirurgicale. Hematologie *see* Traite d'Hematologie **3905**
➤ Encyclopedie Medico-Chirurgicale. Hepatologie (FRA ISSN 1155-1976) **3889**
Encyclopedie Medico-Chirurgicale, Instantanes Medicaux. Anesthesie - Reanimation *see* Encyclopedie Medico-Chirurgicale. Anesthesie - Reanimation **3757**, 4187
Encyclopedie Medico-Chirurgicale, Instantanes Medicaux. Appareil Locomoteur *see* Encyclopedie Medico-Chirurgicale. Appareil Locomoteur **4168**, 4014
Encyclopedie Medico-Chirurgicale, Instantanes Medicaux. Cardiologie *see* Encyclopedie Medico-Chirurgicale. Cardiologie **3771**
Encyclopedie Medico-Chirurgicale, Instantanes Medicaux. Coeur, Poumon, Larynx *see* Encyclopedie Medico-Chirurgicale. Traite de Radiodiagnostic: Coeur - Poumon **4143**, 4159
Encyclopedie Medico-Chirurgicale, Instantanes Medicaux. Dermatologie *see* Encyclopedie Medico-Chirurgicale. Dermatologie **3848**
Encyclopedie Medico-Chirurgicale, Instantanes Medicaux. Gastro-Enterologie *see* Encyclopedie Medico-Chirurgicale. Gastro-Enterologie **3889**
Encyclopedie Medico-Chirurgicale, Instantanes Medicaux. Gynecologie *see* Encyclopedie Medico-Chirurgicale. Gynecologie **3949**
Encyclopedie Medico-Chirurgicale, Instantanes Medicaux. Hematologie *see* Traite d'Hematologie **3905**
Encyclopedie Medico-Chirurgicale, Instantanes Medicaux. Nephrologie - Urologie *see* Encyclopedie Medico-Chirurgicale. Nephrologie - Urologie **4212**
Encyclopedie Medico-Chirurgicale, Instantanes Medicaux. Neurologie *see* Encyclopedie Medico-Chirurgicale. Neurologie **4087**
Encyclopedie Medico-Chirurgicale, Instantanes Medicaux. Ophtalmologie *see* Encyclopedie Medico-Chirurgicale. Ophtalmologie **3997**
Encyclopedie Medico-Chirurgicale, Instantanes Medicaux. Oto-Rhino-Laryngologie *see* Encyclopedie Medico-Chirurgicale. Oto-Rhino-Laryngologie **4032**
Encyclopedie Medico-Chirurgicale, Instantanes Medicaux. Pediatrie *see* Encyclopedie Medico-Chirurgicale. Pediatrie **4044**
Encyclopedie Medico-Chirurgicale, Instantanes Medicaux. Pneumologie *see* Encyclopedie Medico-Chirurgicale. Pneumologie **4159**
Encyclopedie Medico-Chirurgicale, Instantanes Medicaux. Psychiatrie *see* Traite de Psychiatrie **4136**
Encyclopedie Medico-Chirurgicale, Instantanes Medicaux, Radiodiagnostic: Tome 4 *see* Encyclopedie Medico-Chirurgicale. Traite de Radiodiagnostic: Appareil Digestif **4143**, 3889
Encyclopedie Medico-Chirurgicale, Instantanes Medicaux. Sang, Organes Hematopoietiques *see* Traite d'Hematologie **3905**
Encyclopedie Medico-Chirurgicale, Instantanes Medicaux. Techniques Chirurgicales - Appareil Digestif *see* Encyclopedie Medico-Chirurgicale. Techniques Chirurgicales. Appareil Digestif **4187**, 3889
Encyclopedie Medico-Chirurgicale, Instantanes Medicaux. Techniques Chirurgicales - Thorax *see* Encyclopedie Medico-Chirurgicale. Techniques Chirurgicales. Thorax **4187**, 4032
Encyclopedie Medico-Chirurgicale, Instantanes Medicaux. Techniques Chirurgicales - Chirurgie Vasculaire *see* Encyclopedie Medico-Chirurgicale. Techniques Chirurgicales. Chirurgie Vasculaire **4187**, 3771
Encyclopedie Medico-Chirurgicale, Instantanes Medicaux. Toxicologie - Pathologie Professionelle *see* Encyclopedie Medico-Chirurgicale. Traite de Toxicologie - Pathologie Professionelle **3448**, 4254
Encyclopedie Medico-Chirurgicale, Instantanes Medicaux. Urgences *see* Encyclopedie Medico-Chirurgicale. Urgences **4014**
Encyclopedie Medico-Chirurgicale. Intoxications, Pathologie du Travail, Maladies par Agents Physiques *see* Encyclopedie Medico-Chirurgicale. Traite de Toxicologie - Pathologie Professionelle **3448**, 4254
▼ ➤ Encyclopedie Medico-Chirurgicale. Kinesiterapia - Medicina Fisica (FRA ISSN 1293-2965) **4060**
Encyclopedie Medico-Chirurgicale. Kinesitherapie - Medecine Physique - Readaptation (FRA ISSN 1283-0887) **4060**
Encyclopedie Medico-Chirurgicale. Kinesitherapie, Reeducation Fonctionelle *see* Encyclopedie Medico-Chirurgicale. Kinesitherapie - Medecine Physique - Readaptation **4060**
Encyclopedie Medico-Chirurgicale. Maladies Infectieuses *see* Encyclopedie Medico-Chirurgicale. Traite des Maladies Infectieuses **3795**
Encyclopedie Medico-Chirurgicale. Maladies Infectieuses et Parasitaires *see* Encyclopedie Medico-Chirurgicale. Traite des Maladies Infectieuses **3795**
➤ Encyclopedie Medico-Chirurgicale. Medicina Riabilitativa (FRA ISSN 1283-078X) **4060**
➤ Encyclopedie Medico-Chirurgicale. Nephrologie - Urologie (FRA ISSN 1155-1917) **4212**
➤ Encyclopedie Medico-Chirurgicale. Neurologie (FRA ISSN 0246-0378) **4087**
➤ Encyclopedie Medico-Chirurgicale. Obstetrique (FRA ISSN 0246-0335) **3949**
Encyclopedie Medico-Chirurgicale. Odontologie (FRA ISSN 1283-0860) **3822**
Encyclopedie Medico-Chirurgicale. Odontologie et Stomatologie. Tome 1 *see* Encyclopedie Medico-Chirurgicale. Stomatologie **3822**
Encyclopedie Medico-Chirurgicale. Odontologie et Stomatologie. Tome 2 *see* Encyclopedie Medico-Chirurgicale. Odontologie **3822**
➤ Encyclopedie Medico-Chirurgicale. Ophtalmologie (FRA ISSN 0246-0343) **3997**
➤ Encyclopedie Medico-Chirurgicale. Oto-Rhino-Laryngologie (FRA ISSN 0246-0351) **4032**
Encyclopedie Medico-Chirurgicale. Pathologie du Travail, Intoxications, Maladies par Agents Physiques *see* Encyclopedie Medico-Chirurgicale. Traite de Toxicologie - Pathologie Professionelle **3448**, 4254
➤ Encyclopedie Medico-Chirurgicale. Pediatria/Encyclopedie Medico-Quirurgica. Pediatria (FRA ISSN 1245-1789) **4044**
➤ Encyclopedie Medico-Chirurgicale. Pediatrie (FRA ISSN 0246-0513) **4044**
➤ Encyclopedie Medico-Chirurgicale. Pneumologie (FRA ISSN 1155-195X) **4159**
➤ Encyclopedie Medico-Chirurgicale. Podologie (FRA) **4014**
Encyclopedie Medico-Chirurgicale. Poumon, Plevre, Mediastin *see* Encyclopedie Medico-Chirurgicale. Pneumologie **4159**
Encyclopedie Medico-Chirurgicale. Psychiatrie *see* Traite de Psychiatrie **4136**
Encyclopedie Medico-Chirurgicale. Psychiatrie Clinique et Therapeutique *see* Traite de Psychiatrie **4136**
Encyclopedie Medico-Chirurgicale. Radiodiagnostic, 1-2 *see* Encyclopedie Medico-Chirurgicale. Traite de Radiodiagnostic: Squelette Normal - Neuroradiologie - Appareil Locomoteur **4143**, 4014, 4087, 4168
Encyclopedie Medico-Chirurgicale. Radiodiagnostic, 5: Appareil Urinaire - Appareil Genital *see* Encyclopedie Medico-Chirurgicale. Traite de Radiodiagnostic: Urologie - Gynecologie **4144**, 3949, 4212
Encyclopedie Medico-Chirurgicale. Radiodiagnostic, 5: Urologie - Gynecologie *see* Encyclopedie Medico-Chirurgicale. Traite de Radiodiagnostic: Urologie - Gynecologie **4144**, 3949, 4212
Encyclopedie Medico-Chirurgicale. Radiodiagnostic, Tome 1: Squelette Normal *see* Encyclopedie Medico-Chirurgicale. Traite de Radiodiagnostic: Squelette Normal - Neuroradiologie - Appareil Locomoteur **4143**, 4014, 4087, 4168
Encyclopedie Medico-Chirurgicale. Radiodiagnostic: Tome 3, Appareil Cardio-vasculaire, Appareil Pulmonaire *see* Encyclopedie Medico-Chirurgicale. Traite de Radiodiagnostic: Coeur - Poumon **4143**, 4159
Encyclopedie Medico-Chirurgicale. Radiodiagnostic. Tome 3: Coeur, Poumon *see* Encyclopedie Medico-Chirurgicale. Traite de Radiodiagnostic: Coeur - Poumon **4143**, 4159
Encyclopedie Medico-Chirurgicale. Radiodiagnostic: Tome 4 *see* Encyclopedie Medico-Chirurgicale. Traite de Radiodiagnostic: Appareil Digestif **4143**, 3889
Encyclopedie Medico-Chirurgicale. Radiodiagnostic, Tomes 1 et 2, Squelette, Neuro-radiologie *see* Encyclopedie Medico-Chirurgicale. Traite de Radiodiagnostic: Squelette Normal - Neuroradiologie - Appareil Locomoteur **4143**, 4014, 4087, 4168
Encyclopedie Medico-Chirurgicale. Radiodiagnostic, Tomes 1 et 2: Squelette Normal, Neuroradiologie, Appareil Locomoteur *see* Encyclopedie Medico-Chirurgicale. Traite de Radiodiagnostic: Squelette Normal - Neuroradiologie - Appareil Locomoteur **4143**, 4014, 4087, 4168
Encyclopedie Medico-Chirurgicale. Rein, Organes Genito-urinaires *see* Encyclopedie Medico-Chirurgicale. Nephrologie - Urologie **4212**
➤ Encyclopedie Medico-Chirurgicale. Stomatologie (FRA ISSN 1283-0852) **3822**
➤ Encyclopedie Medico-Chirurgicale. Techniques Chirurgicales. Appareil Digestif (FRA ISSN 0246-0424) **4187**, 3889
➤ Encyclopedie Medico-Chirurgicale. Techniques Chirurgicales. Chirurgie Vasculaire (FRA ISSN 0246-0459) **4187**, 3771
Encyclopedie Medico-Chirurgicale. Techniques Chirurgicales. Cou et Tete *see* Encyclopedie Medico-Chirurgicale. Techniques Chirurgicales. Tete et Cou **4187**, 4032
Encyclopedie Medico-Chirurgicale. Techniques Chirurgicales. Cou - Thorax *see* Encyclopedie Medico-Chirurgicale. Techniques Chirurgicales. Thorax **4187**, 4032
Encyclopedie Medico-Chirurgicale. Techniques Chirurgicales. Tete et Cou (FRA) **4187**, 4032
➤ Encyclopedie Medico-Chirurgicale. Techniques Chirurgicales. Thorax (FRA ISSN 1241-8226) **4187**, 4032
Encyclopedie Medico-Chirurgicale. Techniques Chirurgicales - Urologie - Gynecologie *see* Encyclopedie Medico-Chirurgicale. Traite de Techniques Chirurgicales. Urologie **4188**, 4212
➤ Encyclopedie Medico-Chirurgicale. Tecniche Chirurgiche. Chirurgia Addominale (FRA ISSN 1283-0798) **4188**, 3889
Encyclopedie Medico-Chirurgicale. Tecniche Chirurgiche. Chirurgia O R L e Cervico-facciale (Oto-Rhino-Laryngologia) (FRA ISSN 1292-3036) **4188**, 4032
➤ Encyclopedie Medico-Chirurgicale. Tecniche Chirurgiche. Chirurgia Vascolare (FRA ISSN 1283-0801) **4188**, 3771
➤ Encyclopedie Medico-Chirurgicale. Tecniche Chirurgiche. Torace (FRA ISSN 1288-3336) **4188**, 4032
Encyclopedie Medico-Chirurgicale. Tomes 1 et 2: Neuroradiologie, Appareil Locomoteur *see* Encyclopedie Medico-Chirurgicale. Traite de Radiodiagnostic: Squelette Normal - Neuroradiologie - Appareil Locomoteur **4143**, 4014, 4087, 4168
➤ Encyclopedie Medico-Chirurgicale. Traite de Radiodiagnostic: Appareil Digestif (FRA ISSN 0246-0610) **4143**, 3889
➤ Encyclopedie Medico-Chirurgicale. Traite de Radiodiagnostic: Coeur - Poumon (FRA ISSN 1169-7768) **4143**, 4159
➤ Encyclopedie Medico-Chirurgicale. Traite de Radiodiagnostic: Principes et Techniques (FRA) **4143**
➤ Encyclopedie Medico-Chirurgicale. Traite de Radiodiagnostic: Squelette Normal - Neuroradiologie - Appareil Locomoteur (FRA ISSN 1257-5143) **4143**, 4014, 4087, 4168
➤ Encyclopedie Medico-Chirurgicale. Traite de Radiodiagnostic: Urologie - Gynecologie (FRA ISSN 1241-8218) **4144**, 3949, 4212
➤ Encyclopedie Medico-Chirurgicale. Traite de Techniques Chirurgicales. Gynecologie (FRA) **4188**, 3949
➤ Encyclopedie Medico-Chirurgicale. Traite de Techniques Chirurgicales. Orthopedie - Traumatologie (FRA ISSN 0246-0467) **4188**, 4014
➤ Encyclopedie Medico-Chirurgicale. Traite de Techniques Chirurgicales. Urologie (FRA ISSN 1283-0879) **4188**, 4212
Encyclopedie Medico-Chirurgicale. Traite de Techniques Chirurgicales - Urologie - Gynecologie *see* Encyclopedie Medico-Chirurgicale. Traite de Techniques Chirurgicales. Gynecologie **4188**, 3949
➤ Encyclopedie Medico-Chirurgicale. Traite de Toxicologie - Pathologie Professionelle (FRA ISSN 1155-1925) **3448**, 4254
➤ Encyclopedie Medico-Chirurgicale. Traite des Maladies Infectieuses (FRA ISSN 1166-8598) **3795**
➤ Encyclopedie Medico-Chirurgicale. Tratado de Praxis Medica (FRA ISSN 1283-0836) **3908**
➤ Encyclopedie Medico-Chirurgicale. Urgences (FRA ISSN 1241-8234) **4014**
Encyclopedie Medico-Chirurgicale. Urgences Medicales et Chirurgicales *see* Encyclopedie Medico-Chirurgicale. Urgences **4014**
➤ Encyclopedie Medico-Chirurgicale. Urgenze (FRA ISSN 1286-9341) **4014**
Encyclopedie Medico-Quirurgica. Pediatria *see* Encyclopedie Medico-Chirurgicale. Pediatria **4044**
Encyclopedie Veterinaire (FRA ISSN 1283-0828) **4542**
The Endeavor (Gettysburg) (USA ISSN 1526-8721) **3490**
Endemic Diseases Bulletin *see* Difangbing Tongbao **3795**
Endo (FRA ISSN 1168-5476) **3822**
Endo-Praxis *see* Endopraxis **3889**
• Endocrine (USA ISSN 1355-008X) **3860**, 3342
Endocrine Development (CHE ISSN 1421-7082) **3860**, 4044
• ➤ Endocrine Journal (JPN ISSN 0918-8959) **3861**
Endocrine Journal *see* Endocrine **3860**, 3342
• ➤ Endocrine Pathology (USA ISSN 1046-3976) **3861**
Endocrine Regulations (SVK ISSN 1210-0668) **3861**
• ➤ Endocrine - Related Cancer (GBR ISSN 1351-0088) **3861**
• ➤ Endocrine Research (USA ISSN 0743-5800) **3861**
• ➤ Endocrine Reviews (USA ISSN 0163-769X) **3861**
➤ Endocrine Society of Australia. Proceedings (AUS ISSN 0312-4738) **3861**
Endocrine Surgery *see* Naibunpi Geka **3867**, 4197
Endocrinologia (ESP ISSN 0211-2299) **3861**
Endocrinologia Experimentalis *see* Endocrine Regulations **3861**
Endocrinologia Iugoslavica (SVN ISSN 0351-1677) **3861**
Endocrinologie *see* Romanian Journal of Endocrinology **3869**
Endocrinologie - Nutrition *see* Encyclopedie Medico-Chirurgicale. Endocrinologie - Nutrition **3860**, 4232
• ➤ The Endocrinologist (USA ISSN 1051-2144) **3861**
• ➤ Endocrinology (USA ISSN 0013-7227) **3861**
Endocrinology and Metabolism *see* Growth Hormone and I G F Research **3863**
• ➤ Endocrinology and Metabolism Clinics of North America (USA ISSN 0889-8529) **3862**
Endocrinology Guidelines *see* Therapeutic Guidelines. Endocrinology **3869**
Endocurietherapy - Hyperthermia Oncology *see* Journal of Brachytherapy International **3981**
• ➤ Endocytobiosis and Cell Research (DEU ISSN 0256-1514) **3289**, 3301
Endodoncia (ESP ISSN 1130-9903) **3822**
Endodontic Practice (GBR ISSN 1465-9417) **3822**
Endodontics & Dental Traumatology *see* Dental Traumatology **3821**
Endodontics Newsletter (USA) **3822**

Title

Title

Title

Exercise & Health (USA ISSN 1086-1122) **4221**, 4352
➤ Exercise and Sport Sciences Reviews (USA ISSN 0091-6331) **4173**
Exercise for Men Only (USA ISSN 0882-4657) **4352**, 4221, 4222
• ➤ Exercise Immunology Review (USA ISSN 1077-5552) **4173**, 3744
Exercise Physiology: Current Selected Research (USA ISSN 0748-3155) **4352**, 4233
• ➤ Exercise Standards and Malpractice Reporter (USA ISSN 0891-0278) **3538**, 4173, 4352
Existenzanalyse (AUT ISSN 1024-7033) **4090**, 4398
Exkies (NLD ISSN 0928-4109) **3823**
▼ • Exogenous Dermatology (CHE ISSN 1424-4616) **3849**
▼ • ➤ Exotic D V M (Doctor Veterinary Medicine) (USA ISSN 1521-1363) **4542**
Exotic Veterinary Magazine *see* Exotic D V M **4542**
Expectations (USA) **3496**, 3386
Expecting Our Baby (GBR) **3949**
Experience (Chicago) (USA ISSN 1054-3473) **3538**, 3471
Experientia *see* Cellular and Molecular Life Sciences **3190**, 4504
Experiment & Therapy *see* Jikken Chiryo **3876**
• ➤ Experimental Aging Research (USA ISSN 0361-073X) **4398**, 3471
• ➤ Experimental & Applied Acarology (NLD ISSN 0168-8162) **3352**
Experimental and Clinical Endocrinology *see* Experimental and Clinical Endocrinology and Diabetes **3862**
• ➤ Experimental and Clinical Endocrinology and Diabetes (DEU ISSN 0947-7349) **3862**
Experimental and Clinical Endocrinology & Diabetes. Supplement (DEU ISSN 0948-146X) **3862**
Experimental & Clinical Endocrinology - Life Science Advances *see* Life Science Advances: Experimental & Clinical Endocrinology **3865**
• ➤ Experimental and Clinical Psychopharmacology (USA ISSN 1064-1297) **4398**, 4293
• ➤ Experimental and Molecular Medicine (KOR ISSN 1226-3613) **3250**, 3600
• ➤ Experimental and Molecular Pathology (USA ISSN 0014-4800) **3600**, 3376
• ➤ Experimental and Toxicologic Pathology (DEU ISSN 0940-2993) **3600**, 3449, 4293
• ➤ Experimental Animals (JPN ISSN 1341-1357) **3874**
• ➤ Experimental Biology and Medicine (Maywood) (USA) **3195**, 3874
➤ Experimental Biology and Medicine (Totowa) (USA) **3874**, 3250
• ➤ Experimental Biology Online (DEU ISSN 1430-3418) **3195**
Experimental Biology (Year) Abstracts *see* The F A S E B Journal **3196**
• ➤ Experimental Brain Research (DEU ISSN 0014-4819) **4090**
Experimental Brain Research Series (DEU ISSN 0932-4011) **4090**
Experimental Brain Research. Supplementa (USA ISSN 0172-9039) **4090**
• ➤ Experimental Dermatology (DNK ISSN 0906-6705) **3849**
• Experimental Dermatology Online (DNK ISSN 1600-0625) **3849**
• ➤ Experimental Eye Research (GBR ISSN 0014-4835) **3997**
• ➤ Experimental Gerontology (USA ISSN 0531-5565) **3471**
• ➤ Experimental Hematology (USA ISSN 0301-472X) **3901**
Experimental Hematology. Supplement (USA ISSN 0256-9280) **3901**
• ➤ Experimental Lung Research (USA ISSN 0190-2148) **4160**
• ➤ Experimental Nephrology (CHE ISSN 1018-7782) **4212**
• ➤ Experimental Neurology (USA ISSN 0014-4886) **4090**
Experimental Oncology *see* Eksperimental'naya Onkologiya **3977**, 3874
• ➤ Experimental Parasitology (USA ISSN 0014-4894) **3796**, 3196
Experimental Pathology *see* Experimental and Toxicologic Pathology **3600**, 3449, 4293
• ➤ Experimental Physiology (GBR ISSN 0958-0670) **3342**
➤ Experimental Virology (USA) **3321**
Experimentelle und Klinische Hypnose (DEU ISSN 0933-1093) **3906**, 4090

• The Expert and the Law (USA ISSN 0737-8726) **3538**, 3882
▼ • ➤ Expert Opinion on Biological Therapy (GBR ISSN 1471-2598) **3601**, 3250
▼ ➤ Expert Opinion On Drug Safety (GBR) **4293**
• ➤ Expert Opinion On Emerging Drugs (GBR ISSN 1472-8214) **4293**
• ➤ Expert Opinion On Emerging Therapeutic Targets (GBR ISSN 1472-8222) **4293**
• ➤ Expert Opinion On Investigational Drugs (GBR ISSN 1354-3784) **4293**
▼ • ➤ Expert Opinion on Pharmacotherapy (GBR ISSN 1465-6566) **4293**
• ➤ Expert Opinion on Therapeutic Patents (GBR ISSN 1354-3776) **4293**, 4272
▼ • ➤ Expert Review of Anticancer Therapy (GBR ISSN 1473-7140) **4294**, 3978
▼ • ➤ Expert Review of Molecular Diagnostics (GBR ISSN 1473-7159) **4294**
▼ • ➤ Expert Review of Neurotherapeutics (GBR ISSN 1473-7175) **4294**, 4090
▼ • ➤ Expert Review of Pharmacoeconomics & Outcomes Research (GBR ISSN 1473-7167) **4294**
• Expert Reviews in Molecular Medicine (GBR ISSN 1462-3994) **3908**
Exploration and Production Health, Safety and Environment *see* E & P Health, Safety and Environment **4272**, 3148, 3443, 4268
Explorer (Falls Church) (USA ISSN 0894-7929) **3823**
➤ Explorer (Lake Worth) (USA) **3823**
• Express Bulletins (GBR) **3231**, 3149, 3196
Express (Montreal) (CAN ISSN 0834-129X) **4090**
Expressions *see* Southwest Journal on Aging **3481**
Extended Care Product News (USA ISSN 0895-2906) **4352**, 4233
• Extracellular Matrix (GBR ISSN 0268-1617) **3231**, 3149, 3290
Extracta Dermatologica (DEU ISSN 0342-2828) **3727**, 3849, 4189
Extracta Orthopaedica (DEU ISSN 0344-5046) **3727**, 4015, 4189
Extracta Urologica (DEU ISSN 0344-5038) **4212**
Extracts from European Patent Specifications. Part 2. Electricity, Physics, Precision Engineering, Optics and Acoustics (DEU ISSN 0941-0031) **4272**, 4365
• ➤ ExtraMED (GBR) **3727**, 3149, 3601
• ➤ Eye (GBR ISSN 0950-222X) **3997**
Eye Care (IND ISSN 0255-4062) **3997**
Eye News (GBR ISSN 1368-8952) **3997**
➤ Eye on Improvement (USA) **3506**
Eye on Oregon (USA) **3997**
Eye on Psi Chi (USA ISSN 1092-0803) **4398**
➤ Eye Science/Yanke Xuebao (CHN ISSN 1000-4432) **3997**
Eye to Eye (USA) **3997**, 4468
Eyecare Business (USA ISSN 0885-9167) **3997**
EyeNet (USA ISSN 1097-2986) **3998**
Eyewear (USA ISSN 1098-0946) **3998**
• Eyewear: The International Market (GBR) **4015**, 3366
Ezhegodnik Mirovoi Sanitarnoi Statistiki (CHE ISSN 0250-8664) **4495**, 4528
Ezhekvartal'nik Christian Science. Bibleiskie Uroki *see* Christian Science Quarterly. Bible Lessons (Citation Edition) **4502**
F A B Bulletin *see* F A B Journal **3171**, 4272
F A B Journal (Feline Advisory Bureau) (GBR) **3171**, 4272
➤ F A C E (Facial Aesthetic Communication in Europe) (NLD ISSN 1240-3237) **3601**
F A C: Revista Practica de Medicina (ESP ISSN 0210-8852) **3601**
F A C: Revista Practica del Estudiante de Medicina *see* F A C: Revista Practica de Medicina **3601**
F A C T *see* Focus on Alternative and Complementary Therapies **4296**, 3165
F A O Food and Nutrition Series (Food and Agriculture Organization of the United Nations) (USA ISSN 1014-3181) **4233**
F A R M Report (Farm Animal Report Movement) (USA) **4233**
• ➤ The F A S E B Journal (Federation of American Societies for Experimental Biology) (USA ISSN 0892-6638) **3196**
F A S S *see* F A S S - Laekemedel i Sverige **4294**
F A S S - Farmacevtiska Specialiteter i Sverige *see* F A S S - Laekemedel i Sverige **4294**
F A S S - Laekemedel i Sverige (SWE ISSN 1400-6588) **4294**
F A S S Vet (SWE ISSN 0347-1136) **4294**, 4542

F & W - Fuehren und Wirtschaften im Krankenhaus (DEU ISSN 0175-4548) **3506**, 3365, 3368
F D A Compliance Policy Guidance. Manual (U.S. Food and Drug Administration) (USA) **3460**, 4294
F D A Compliance Policy Guide *see* F D A Compliance Policy Guidance. Manual **3460**, 4294
• F D A Consumer (Food and Drug Administration) (USA ISSN 0362-1332) **3392**, 3460, 4294
F D A Drug Bulletin *see* F D A Medical Bulletin **4294**
F D A Enforcement Manual (Food and Drug Administration) (USA) **3460**, 4294
• F D A Enforcement Report (Food and Drug Administration) (USA ISSN 1057-9397) **3394**, 4294
F D A Inspection. Basic Manual *see* F D A Inspection Operations Manual **3460**, 4294
F D A Inspection Operations Manual (Food and Drug Administration) (USA) **3460**, 4294
• F D A Medical Bulletin (Food and Drug Administration) (USA ISSN 1063-8067) **4294**
• F D A News (Food and Drug Administration) (USA ISSN 1069-5109) **4294**
F D A Papers *see* F D A Consumer **3392**, 3460, 4294
• F D A Veterinarian (Food & Drug Administration) (USA ISSN 1057-6223) **4542**
• F D A Week (Food and Drug Administration) (USA) **3393**, 3460, 4294
F D C Control Newsletter (Food, Drug, and Cosmetics) (USA) **3460**, 3369, 4223, 4294
F D I Dental World *see* F D I World **3823**
F D I News *see* F D I World **3823**
F D I World (Federation Dentaire Internationale) (GBR) **3823**
• ➤ F E B S Letters (Federation of European Biochemical Societies) (NLD ISSN 0014-5793) **3250**, 3266
• ➤ F E M S Immunology and Medical Microbiology (Federation of European Microbiological Societies) (NLD ISSN 0928-8244) **3321**, 3744
➤ F E M S Microbiology (Federation of European Microbiological Societies) (NLD ISSN 0921-8254) **3321**, 3274
• ➤ F E M S Microbiology Ecology (Federation of European Microbiological Societies) (NLD ISSN 0168-6496) **3321**, 3439
F E M S Microbiology Immunology *see* F E M S Immunology and Medical Microbiology **3321**, 3744
• ➤ F E M S Microbiology Letters (Federation of European Microbiological Societies) (NLD ISSN 0378-1097) **3322**
• ➤ F E M S Microbiology Reviews (Federation of European Microbiological Societies) (NLD ISSN 0168-6445) **3322**
▼ • F E M S Yeast Research (Federation of European Microbiological Societies) (NLD ISSN 1567-1356) **3322**, 3302, 3342
▼ • F H M Bionic (For Him Magazine) (GBR ISSN 1468-974X) **4221**, 4352
F I O D S Revue (Federation Internationale des Organisations de Donneurs de Sang Benevoles) (FRA ISSN 0253-1321) **3772**
F M A Today (Florida Medical Association, Inc.) (USA) **3601**, 3538
F M S Foundation Newsletter (False Memory Syndrome) (USA ISSN 1069-0484) **4399**, 3538
F.N.I.B. - Info (Federation Nationale Neutre des Infirmieres de Belgique) (BEL ISSN 0774-935X) **3919**
F P A B Highlights (Family Planning Association of Bangladesh) (BGD) **3358**, 3949, 4512
F P A C Monthly Report (Family Planning Association of China) (TWN) **3358**
F P A P Annual Report (Family Planning Association of Pakistan) (PAK) **3358**
F P A P Biennial Report *see* F P A P Annual Report **3358**
The F P O P Bulletin (Family Planning Organization of the Philippines) (PHL) **3358**
F P Report (Family Physician) (USA) **3601**
F R A M E News (Fund for the Replacement of Animals in Medical Experiments) (GBR ISSN 0268-4306) **3171**
F R C H Newsletter (Foundation for Research in Community Health) (IND) **4468**
F S M B Handbook (Federation of State Medical Boards) (USA ISSN 0888-5656) **3601**
F S M B Newsline (Federation of State Medical Boards) (USA ISSN 1062-5380) **3601**

• F T Biotechnology & Pharmaceutical Companies Database CD-ROM (Years) (Financial Times) (GBR) **3274**, 3369, 3370, 4294
F T M Newsletter (Female to Male) (USA) **3527**
Facets (Chicago) *see* A M A Alliance Today **3555**, 4568
Facets (San Diego) (USA) **3823**
Fachbuchverzeichnis Medizin (DEU) **3727**, 3177, 3601
Fachschwester - Fachpfleger (USA ISSN 0172-5238) **3919**
Facial Aesthetic Communication in Europe *see* F A C E **3601**
Facial Nerve Research (JPN ISSN 0914-790X) **4144**
• ➤ Facial Plastic Surgery (USA ISSN 0736-6825) **4189**
Facial Plastic Surgery Clinics of North America (USA ISSN 1064-7406) **4189**
Facility Care *see* FacilityCare **3507**
FacilityCare (USA) **3507**
Fact Sheet on the Netherlands (NLD ISSN 0920-6469) **4512**, 4468
Facts about Family Practice (USA ISSN 1074-8849) **3727**, 4529
Facts and Advice for Airline Passengers (USA) **4532**, 4468, 4534
Facts and Research in Gerontology (FRA ISSN 1163-0450) **3471**
➤ Facts and Research in Gerontology Newsletter (FRA ISSN 1167-4911) **3471**
Facts, Medicine and Health Care, Denmark *see* Tal og Data, Medicin og Sundhedsvaesen **4337**, 4362
Faculdade de Odontologia de Bauru. Revista (BRA) **3823**
Faculdade de Odontologia de Lins. Revista (BRA ISSN 0104-7582) **3823**
Faculdade de Odontologia de Pernambuco. Revista (BRA ISSN 0048-3419) **3823**
Faculdade de Odontologia de Porto Alegre. Revista (BRA ISSN 0566-1854) **3823**
Faculdade de Odontologia. Revista (BRA) **3823**
Facultad de Medicina de Barcelona. Revista de Psiquiatria (ESP ISSN 0213-7429) **4090**
Facultad de Veterinaria de Leon. Anales (ESP ISSN 0373-1170) **4542**
Facultad Nacional de Agronomia Medellin. Revista (COL ISSN 0304-2847) **3154**, 3196, 3463, 3553
Faire Face (FRA ISSN 0014-6951) **3494**
Faktor Arbeitsschutz (DEU ISSN 1433-7800) **3531**, 4254
➤ Falk Symposium (NLD ISSN 0161-5580) **3601**
Falling Leaf (GBR ISSN 0956-2400) **4223**, 4399
False Memory Syndrome Foundation Newsletter *see* F M S Foundation Newsletter **4399**, 3538
▼ • ➤ Familial Cancer (NLD ISSN 1389-9600) **3978**, 3302
• Familie & Co. (DEU ISSN 1431-9543) **4044**, 3383, 3483
Familien-Kalender (DEU) **3401**
Familiendynamik (DEU ISSN 0342-2747) **4399**, 4521
Familienmagazin (AUT) **3383**, 3411, 4399
• Families, Systems & Health (USA ISSN 1091-7527) **3601**
Family Almanac (USA) **3366**
• ➤ Family and Community Health (USA ISSN 0160-6379) **4469**
• Family and Neighbourhood Services Extra (AUS) **4469**
▼ Family Building (USA) **3949**
Family Care Health Monitor (USA) **3601**
➤ Family Economics and Nutrition Review (USA) **3527**, 3393, 4233
Family Economics Review *see* Family Economics and Nutrition Review **3527**, 3393, 4233
Family Focus (USA) **4212**
• Family Health (CAN ISSN 0830-0305) **4469**
• Family Index (USA ISSN 1089-6147) **4524**, 3149
• The Family Journal (USA ISSN 1066-4807) **4399**, 3554
• ➤ Family Medical Practice On-Line (GBR ISSN 1360-0176) **3601**
Family Medicine *see* Jiating Yixue **3628**
Family Medicine (GBR) **4044**, 3949
• Family Medicine (USA ISSN 0742-3225) **3601**, 3411
▼ • Family Medicine Net Guide (USA) **3601**, 3391
▼ • Family Medicine Net Guide eNewsletter (USA) **3601**, 3391
▼ • Family Medicine Net Guide Online (USA) **3601**, 3391

Title

Title

Title

Fukuoka Society for Clinical Surgery. Journal *see* Fukuokaken Rinsho Geka Igakkai Kaishi **4189**
Fukuoka Society of Hospital Pharmacy. Drug Information News (JPN) **4297**
Fukuoka University. Medical Bulletin *see* Fukuoka Daigaku Igaku Kiyo **3604**
Fukuoka University. Pharmaceutical Bulletin *see* Fukuoka Daigaku Yakugaku Kiyo **4297**
Fukuokaken Hoshasen Gishikaishi/Fukuoka Association of Radiological Technologists. Journal (JPN) **4144**
Fukuokaken Iho/Fukuoka Medical Association. Journal (JPN ISSN 0285-3418) **3604**
Fukuokaken Rinsho Geka Igakkai Kaishi/Fukuoka Society for Clinical Surgery. Journal (JPN) **4189**
Fukuroi Municipal Hospital. Journal *see* Fukuroi Shiritsu Fukuroi Shimin Byoin Kenkyushi **3604**
Fukuroi Shiritsu Fukuroi Shimin Byoin Kenkyushi/Fukuroi Municipal Hospital. Journal (JPN ISSN 0917-9011) **3604**
Fukushima Igaku Zasshi/Fukushima Medical Journal (JPN ISSN 0016-2582) **3604**
➤ Fukushima Journal of Medical Science (JPN ISSN 0016-2590) **3604**
Fukushima Journal of Psychology *see* Fukushima Shinrigaku Zasshi **4400**
Fukushima Kenritsu Byoin Igaku Kenkyushi/Fukushima Medical Bulletin (JPN ISSN 0913-2864) **3604**
Fukushima Medical Bulletin *see* Fukushima Kenritsu Byoin Igaku Kenkyushi **3604**
Fukushima Medical Journal *see* Fukushima Igaku Zasshi **3604**
Fukushima Shinrigaku Zasshi/Fukushima Journal of Psychology (JPN ISSN 0917-8163) **4400**
Fukuyama Akenohoshi Gakuin Eiyo Senmon Gakko Kenkyu Kiyo/Fukuyama Akenohoshi Gakuin School of Dietetics. Bulletin (JPN ISSN 0385-5880) **4234**
Fukuyama Akenohoshi Gakuin School of Dietetics. Bulletin *see* Fukuyama Akenohoshi Gakuin Eiyo Senmon Gakko Kenkyu Kiyo **4234**
Fukuyama Daigaku Yakugakubu Kenkyu Nenpo/Fukuyama University. Faculty of Pharmacy & Pharmaceutical Sciences. Annual Report (JPN ISSN 0288-724X) **4297**
Fukuyama Igaku/Fukuyama Medical Association. Journal (JPN ISSN 0917-1835) **3604**
Fukuyama Medical Association. Journal *see* Fukuyama Igaku **3604**
Fukuyama University. Faculty of Pharmacy & Pharmaceutical Sciences. Annual Report *see* Fukuyama Daigaku Yakugakubu Kenkyu Nenpo **4297**
Functional Foods *see* Functional Foods and Nutraceuticals **4234**, 3165
Functional Foods and Nutraceuticals (USA ISSN 1470-0336) **4234**, 3165
• ➤ Functional Neurology (ITA ISSN 0393-5264) **4091**
Functional Neurosurgery *see* Kinoteki No Shinkei Geka **4107**
Functional Orthodontist (USA ISSN 8756-3150) **3824**
Fund for the Replacement of Animals in Medical Experiments News *see* F R A M E News **3171**
Fundacentro *see* Revista Fundacentro **4263**
➤ Fundacion Espanola de Reumatologia. Seminarios (ESP) **4168**
Fundamenta Psychiatrica (DEU ISSN 0931-0428) **4091**
Fundamental and Applied Toxicology *see* Toxicological Sciences **3455**, 3702, 4338
Fundamental and Clinical Cardiology (USA ISSN 1067-5264) **3772**
• ➤ Fundamental and Clinical Pharmacology (GBR ISSN 0767-3981) **4297**
Fundamental Research Report of Pediatric Nutrition *see* Yoji Eiyo Kiso Chosa Kekka no Gaiyo **4057**
Funding Watch (USA) **4470**
• Fungal Genetics Newsletter (USA ISSN 0895-1942) **3197**
Funk und Elektronik (DEU) **3496**
Die Funktionskrankheiten des Bewegungsapparates *see* Die Funktionskrankheiten des Bewegungssystems **4015**, 3787, 4168
Die Funktionskrankheiten des Bewegungssystems (DEU ISSN 1433-1861) **4015**, 3787, 4168
Furi Rajikaru no Rinsho/Free Radicals in Clinical Medicine (JPN) **3604**
Fuss *see* Podologie **4200**
Futura (DEU ISSN 0179-6372) **3604**
Future Care *see* Long-Term Health Management **3518**
Future Health Scenarios (NLD) **4470**
• ➤ The Future of Children (USA ISSN 1054-8289) **3383**, 4470, 4512
Future Reflections (USA ISSN 0883-3419) **3497**, 3386, 3422
Fynske Laeger (DNK ISSN 0904-6895) **3604**
➤ Fysioterapeuten (NOR ISSN 0016-3384) **4060**
Fysioterapeuten (Copenhagen) (DNK) **4061**
➤ Fysioterapia (FIN ISSN 0789-5232) **4061**
➤ The G D P (GBR) **3824**
G e B *see* Le Basi Razionali della Terapia **4279**
G E D (Gastroenterologia e Endoscopia Digestiva) (BRA ISSN 0101-7772) **3890**
G E I Newsletter (Grief Education Institute) (USA) **4400**
G E N (VEN ISSN 0016-3503) **3890**
G H A A's National Directory of H M Os *see* National Directory of H M Os **3533**, 3664
• G H A Today Newsletter (Georgia Hospital Association) (USA) **3507**, 3604
• G I Cancer (Gastrointestinal) (CHE ISSN 1064-9700) **3978**, 3890
G I G Newsletter (Gluten Intolerance Group of North America) (USA ISSN 0890-507X) **4234**, 3890
G I - Gesundheits Ingenieur (DEU ISSN 0932-6200) **4470**, 3361, 3439
G I T (DEU ISSN 0016-3538) **3875**
G I T Laboratory Journal (DEU) **3604**, 3875
G I T Spezial Arbeitsschutz - Arbeitssicherheit *see* G I T Spezial Sicherheit und Management **4254**
G I T Spezial Sicherheit und Management (DEU) **4254**
G M D A Bulletin *see* G M D A Journal **3824**
G M D A Journal (Greater Milwaukee Dental Association) (USA) **3824**
G M H C Treatment Issues (Gay Men's Health Crisis) (USA ISSN 1077-1824) **3796**, 3539
• The G M P Letter (Good Manufacturing Practice) (USA ISSN 0196-626X) **3530**
G M P Regulations of Japan (JPN) **4297**, 3539
G N P *see* Guide National de Prescription des Medicaments **4298**
G O - Giovane Odontoiatra *see* Giovane Odontoiatra **3824**
• G P (General Practitioner) (GBR ISSN 0268-8417) **3604**
G P (General Practitioner) *see* Dental Implantology Update **3820**
G P I *see* Gesundheitspolitische Informationen **4470**
G P L C Update *see* E R A News **4291**
G P Weekly (General Practitioners) (NZL ISSN 1171-347X) **3604**
G R A C E *see* Genetic Resources and Crop Evolution **3304**, 3290
G R C Information Bulletin *see* G R C News **3471**
G R C News (Simon Fraser University, Gerontology Research Centre) (CAN ISSN 1188-181X) **3471**
G T V Bulletin (Groupements Techniques Veterinaires) (FRA) **4543**
G W G-Info *see* G W G - Zeitschrift **3422**
G W G - Zeitschrift (Gesellschaft fuer Wissenschaftliche Gespraechspsychotherapie e.V.) (DEU ISSN 0932-934X) **3422**
➤ G W U M C. Department of Biochemistry. Annual Spring Symposia Series (George Washington University Medical Center) (USA) **3250**
Gaceta Biomedicas *see* Biomedicas **3187**, 3577
Gaceta de la Facultad de Medicina *see* Universidad Nacional Autonona de Mexico. Facultad de Medicina. Gaceta **3704**
Gaceta de la Proteccion Laboral (ESP) **4254**
Gaceta Dental (ESP) **3824**
➤ Gaceta Medica (COL ISSN 0121-6309) **3604**
Gaceta Medica de Bilbao (ESP ISSN 0304-4858) **3604**
➤ Gaceta Medica de Caracas (VEN ISSN 0367-4762) **3604**
Gaceta Medica de Mexico (MEX ISSN 0016-3813) **3605**
• ➤ Gaceta Sanitaria (ESP ISSN 0213-9111) **4470**, 3605
Gaikoku Bunken Daijesuto. Kaku Igaku/Foreign Literature Digest. Nuclear Medicine (JPN ISSN 0911-2855) **4144**, 4297
• ➤ Gait and Posture (NLD ISSN 0966-6362) **3605**, 4015
Gakujutsu Zasshi/Kyoto College of Pharmacy. Scientific Journal (JPN ISSN 0288-349X) **4297**
Galathea Report (DNK ISSN 0416-704X) **3352**
Galicia Clinica (ESP ISSN 0304-4866) **3605**
Gallaudet Bulletin *see* Gallaudet Today **3490**
Gallaudet Today (USA ISSN 0016-4089) **3490**
The Gambia Family Planning Association Newsletter (GMB ISSN 0796-0174) **3358**
• ➤ Games and Economic Behavior (USA ISSN 0899-8256) **4400**, 3554
Gamete Research *see* Molecular Reproduction and Development **3258**, 3329
➤ Gamma (NLD ISSN 0016-4380) **4145**
Gamma Field Symposia (JPN ISSN 0435-1096) **3266**, 3155
Gan Kango/Japanese Journal of Cancer Care (JPN) **3978**
Gan Kanja to Taisho Ryoho/Symptom Control in Cancer Patients (JPN) **3978**
Gan Kenkyu, Jikken to Rinsho *see* Tumor Research: Experimental and Clinical **3991**
Gan No Rinsho *see* Japanese Journal of Cancer Clinics **3981**
➤ Gan To Kagaku Ryoho/Japanese Journal of Cancer and Chemotherapy (JPN ISSN 0385-0684) **3978**
Ganagrinco (VEN ISSN 0046-5399) **3155**, 4543
Ganka *see* Ophthalmology **4004**
Ganka Rinsho Iho/Japanese Review of Clinical Ophthalmology (JPN ISSN 0386-9601) **3998**
Ganka Shujutsu Konnichi no Kangaekata/Current Insights in Ophthalmic Surgery (JPN ISSN 0915-5066) **3998**
➤ Gann Monographs on Cancer Research (CHE ISSN 0072-0151) **3978**
Gaoxiong Yixue Kexue Zazhi *see* Kaohsiung Journal of Medical Sciences **3639**, 4312
Garcia de Orta: Serie de Antropobiologia (PRT ISSN 0870-0168) **3173**, 3197
Garden to Kitchen Newsletter (NCL ISSN 1022-9221) **4234**, 3155
Garlic Times (USA) **4234**, 3464
Gaslini (ITA ISSN 0390-5845) **4044**
▼ • Gastric Cancer (JPN ISSN 1436-3291) **3978**, 3890
Gastric Secretion *see* Gastrointestinal Hormones and Gastric Secretion **3728**, 3149, 3891, 4297
• ➤ Gastro-Enterologie Clinique et Biologique (FRA ISSN 0399-8320) **3890**
Gastro-Enterologie Pratique (FRA ISSN 0995-7278) **3890**
Gastro-Enterologie Quotidienne (FRA ISSN 0016-5077) **3890**
Gastroenterologia Clinica (ITA ISSN 1120-3757) **3890**
Gastroenterologia e Endoscopia Digestiva *see* G E D **3890**
Gastroenterologia Japonica *see* Journal of Gastroenterology **3893**
Gastroenterologia Oggi *see* Gli Specializzati. Gastroenterologia **3896**
Gastroenterologia y Hepatologia (ESP ISSN 0210-5705) **3890**
➤ Gastroenterological Endoscopy (JPN ISSN 0387-1207) **3890**
Gastroenterological Society of Taiwan. Journal *see* Zhonghua Minguo Xiaohua Xiyi Xuehui Zazhi **3897**
Gastroenterological Surgery *see* Shokaki Geka **3896**
➤ Gastroenterologie (FRA ISSN 0989-263X) **3890**
Gastroenterologiia *see* Meditsinski Pregled. Gastroenterologiia **3894**
The Gastroenterologist (USA ISSN 1065-2477) **3890**
Il Gastroenterologo (ITA ISSN 0391-8939) **3890**
• ➤ Gastroenterology (USA ISSN 0016-5085) **3890**
Gastroenterology *see* Today in Medicine. Gastroenterology **3896**
• ➤ Gastroenterology and Endoscopy News (USA ISSN 0883-8348) **3890**
• ➤ Gastroenterology Clinics of North America (USA ISSN 0889-8553) **3890**
Gastroenterology in Practice *see* International Journal of Gastroenterology **3892**, 4168
Gastroenterology International (International Edition) (ITA ISSN 0950-5911) **3891**
Gastroenterology International (Italian Edition) *see* Giornale di Gastroenterology **3891**
• Gastroenterology Nursing (USA ISSN 1042-895X) **3891**
Gastroenterology Nursing Buyer's Guide (USA) **3891**
Gastroenterology Today (GBR ISSN 0969-0131) **3891**
Gastroenteroloji *see* Turkish Journal of Gastroenterology **3896**
Gastrointestinal Cancer *see* G I Cancer **3978**, 3890
Gastrointestinal Drug Guidelines *see* Therapeutic Guidelines. Gastrointestinal **3896**
• ➤ Gastrointestinal Endoscopy (USA ISSN 0016-5107) **3891**
Gastrointestinal Endoscopy Clinics of North America (USA ISSN 1052-5157) **3891**
Gastrointestinal Hormones *see* Gastrointestinal Hormones and Gastric Secretion **3728**, 3149, 3891, 4297
• Gastrointestinal Hormones and Gastric Secretion (GBR ISSN 1461-5118) **3728**, 3149, 3891, 4297
Gastrointestinal Radiology *see* Abdominal Imaging **3885**, 4139
Gastronomie (DEU ISSN 0323-4762) **3527**
Gastrum Patologia del Aparato Digestivo (ESP ISSN 0211-058X) **3891**
Gateshead and South Tyneside Health Authority. Director of Public Health. Annual Report (GBR) **4470**
Gateway to Medicine *see* Iyaku no Mon **4304**
Gathered View (USA ISSN 1077-9965) **3605**, 3302 , 3422, 4234
Gaucher Disease Newsletter (USA) **3605**
• ➤ Gay and Lesbian Medical Association. Journal (USA ISSN 1090-7173) **3605**, 3527, 4368
Gay Archivist *see* Lesbian and Gay Archivist **3528**, 3526
Gay Community News (Honolulu) *see* Hawaii's National Gay Community News **3527**, 4513
Gay Counselling *see* Lesbian and Gay Counselling News **3528**, 4425, 4515, 4522
• Gay Men's Health Crisis (USA) **3875**, 3796
Gay Men's Health Crisis Treatment Issues *see* G M H C Treatment Issues **3796**, 3539
Gazet *see* Psy **4436**
• Gazeta dla Stomatologov, Zubnych Technikov... i ne Tolko (RUS) **3824**
• ➤ Gazeta Lekarska (POL ISSN 0867-2164) **3605**
Gazeta o Zdrowiu i Urodzie (POL ISSN 1232-1907) **4353**
Gazette Officielle du Thermalisme (FRA ISSN 0995-6301) **4353**
Gazette S C P *see* C P S News **4041**
Gazety Medikaly (MDG) **3605**
• ➤ Gazi Medical Journal/Gazi Tip Dergisi (TUR ISSN 1300-056X) **3605**
Gazi Tip Dergisi *see* Gazi Medical Journal **3605**
➤ Gazi Universitesi Eczacilik Fakultesi Dergisi (TUR ISSN 1015-9592) **4297**
Gazzetta Internazionale di Medicina e Chirurgia (ITA ISSN 0016-5662) **4189**
Gazzetta Medica Italiana - Aggiornamenti Clinicoterapeutici *see* Gazzetta Medica Italiana Archivio per le Scienze Mediche **3605**
Gazzetta Medica Italiana Archivio per le Scienze Mediche (ITA ISSN 0393-3660) **3605**
• ➤ Geburtshilfe und Frauenheilkunde (DEU ISSN 0016-5751) **3950**
Gedrag & Gezondheid (NLD ISSN 0921-5360) **4400**
Gedrag & Organisatie (NLD ISSN 0921-5077) **3507**, 3365
Gedragstherapie (NLD ISSN 0167-7454) **4400**, 3605
➤ Gedvernd (ISL ISSN 1022-4920) **4091**
• ➤ Gefaesschirurgie (DEU ISSN 0948-7034) **4189**, 3772
Gegengift (DEU) **4254**
Die Gegenwart (DEU ISSN 0016-5859) **3497**
➤ De Geheel-Onthouder (NLD ISSN 0166-2880) **3401**, 4470
Geistige Behinderung (DEU ISSN 0173-9573) **3422**, 4400, 4512
Geka *see* Surgery **4204**
Geka Chiryo/Surgical Therapy (JPN ISSN 0433-2644) **4189**
Geka Shudankai Shorokushu/Tokyo Surgical Society. Abstracts (JPN) **3728**, 4190
Geka to Taisha Eiyo/Japanese Journal of Surgical Metabolism and Nutrition (JPN ISSN 0389-5564) **4190**
➤ Gekkan Chiiki Igaku/Monthly Community Medicine (JPN ISSN 0914-4277) **3605**
Gekkan Hoken Shinryo/Monthly Review of Insurance Treatment (JPN ISSN 0385-8588) **3605**
Gekkan Igaku Joho/Clipping Monthly Report (JPN ISSN 0917-1061) **3605**
Gekkan Igaku to Iryo *see* Medical Science and Medical Care **3654**

Title

Title

Title

Title

H M O Practice *see* Effective Clinical Practice **3597**
• H M S Beagle (Her Majesty's Ship) (GBR) **3198**
H M T. Helsetjenesten - Medicinsk Teknikk (NOR ISSN 0803-2556) **3508**
H N O Aktuell (Hals - Nase - Ohren) (DEU ISSN 0943-0121) **4033**
• ➤ H N O (Berlin) (Hals-, Nasen-, Ohren-Heilkunde) (DEU ISSN 0017-6192) **4033**
H N O (Cologne) (Hals Nase Ohren) (DEU ISSN 0341-9746) **4033**
H N O Informationen (Hals - Nase - Ohren) (DEU ISSN 0344-9319) **4033**
H N O - Nachrichten (Hals Nase Ohren) (DEU ISSN 0177-1000) **4033**
H O P Nyusu/Hokkaido Hospital Pharmacists' Newsletter (JPN) **4298**
H P A Bulletin (Hospital Physicists Association) *see* Scope (York) **4365**, 3522
• H P B (GBR ISSN 1365-182X) **3891**
• ➤ H P B Surgery (CHE ISSN 0894-8569) **4190**
• H R Practitioners Guide (USA) **3368**, 3364
• H S R: Health Supplement Retailer (USA) **4234**, 3165, 3461, 4298
Ha-Gil He-Hadash (ISR) **3473**
Ha-Refuah (ISR ISSN 0017-7768) **3609**
Ha-Rokeach ha-Ivri *see* Israel Pharmaceutical Journal **4304**
Haandbog for Studerende ved Landbohoejskolen *see* Kongelige Veterinaer-og Landbohoejskole. Haandbog **3155**, 4547
Habilitative Mental Healthcare Newsletter *see* Mental Health Aspects of Developmental Disabilities **4109**, 4063
Habitechut (ISR) **4255**
➤ Hacettepe Dis Hekimligi Fakultesi Dergisi/Hacettepe Faculty of Dentistry Journal (TUR ISSN 0250-5207) **3824**
Hacettepe Faculty of Dentistry Journal *see* Hacettepe Dis Hekimligi Fakultesi Dergisi **3824**
Hacettepe Medical Journal (TUR ISSN 0259-2282) **3609**
Hacettepe Tip Dergisi *see* Hacettepe Medical Journal **3609**
Hachinohe City Hospital. Medical Journal *see* Hachinohe Shiritsu Shimin Byoin Ishi **3609**, 3508
Hachinohe Shiritsu Shimin Byoin Ishi/Hachinohe City Hospital. Medical Journal (JPN ISSN 0389-5122) **3609**, 3508
Hacia la Luz (ARG ISSN 0017-6478) **3497**, 3552
Hadshot Kuppot Holim (ISR) **3531**, 3364, 3609
➤ Haelsa (SWE ISSN 0345-4797) **4234**
Haelsokuriren (SWE ISSN 1102-3899) **4298**, 4354
• Haema (GRC ISSN 1108-2682) **3901**
• ➤ Haematologia (NLD ISSN 0017-6559) **3901**
Haematologica (ESP ISSN 1138-0381) **3901**
• ➤ Haematologica (ITA ISSN 0390-6078) **3901**
Haematologie und Bluttransfusion (USA ISSN 0440-0607) **3901**
• ➤ Haemophilia (GBR ISSN 1351-8216) **3901**
Haemophilia Foundation, Victoria. Newsletter (AUS) **3901**
• ➤ Haemophilia Online (GBR ISSN 1365-2516) **3901**
Haemophilia Society of Victoria. Newsletter *see* Haemophilia Foundation, Victoria. Newsletter **3901**
• Haemophilia. Supplement (GBR ISSN 1355-0691) **3902**
➤ Haemostaseologie (DEU ISSN 0720-9355) **3902**
Haemostasis *see* Pathophysiology of Haemostasis and Thrombosis **3904**, 3781
➤ Haessle Information (SWE ISSN 0346-9751) **4299**
Haeusliche Pflege (DEU ISSN 0935-8234) **4213**
Hagemi/Encouragement (JPN ISSN 0017-6605) **3494**
Haiti Sante (HTI) **4354**
Haixia Yufang Yixue Zazhi/Strait Journal of Preventive Medicine (CHN ISSN 1007-2705) **3609**
Hakko Kenkyujo Hokoku *see* Institute for Fermentation, Osaka. Research Communications **3323**, 3290
Hakkokogaku *see* Seibutsu Kogaku Kaishi **3331**
Hakodate Igakushi/Hokodate Medical Journal (JPN ISSN 0910-0725) **3609**
Hakoniwa Ryohogaku Kenkyu/Archives of Sandplay Therapy (JPN ISSN 0916-3662) **4092**

Hals - Nase - Ohren Aktuell *see* H N O Aktuell **4033**
Hals Nase Ohren (Cologne) *see* H N O (Cologne) **4033**
Hals - Nase - Ohren Informationen *see* H N O Informationen **4033**
Hals Nase Ohren Nachrichten *see* H N O - Nachrichten **4033**
Hals-, Nasen-, Ohren-Heilkunde (Berlin) *see* H N O (Berlin) **4033**
Hamamatsu Seikei Geka Kiyo/Hamamatsu University. Annual of Orthopaedic Surgery (JPN ISSN 0917-365X) **4015**, 4190
Hamamatsu University. Annual of Orthopaedic Surgery *see* Hamamatsu Seikei Geka Kiyo **4015**, 4190
Hamburger Aerzteblatt (DEU ISSN 0017-6915) **3609**
• Hamdard Medicus (PAK ISSN 0250-7188) **3609**
Hamdard Naunehal (PAK ISSN 0259-3734) **4234**
Hampden Hippocrat (USA) **3609**
Hanamaki City Medical Association. News *see* Iho Hanamaki **3618**
Hand *see* Journal of Hand Surgery: British and European Volume **4193**
The Hand and Upper Extremity (USA) **3609**
Hand and Upper Limb *see* The Hand and Upper Extremity **3609**
Hand and Wrist Pain (USA) **3609**, 3539
• ➤ Hand Clinics (USA ISSN 0749-0712) **4016**
Hand in Hand (CAN) **3919**
• Hand Surgery (SGP ISSN 0218-8104) **4190**
➤ Handbook of Behavioral Neurobiology (USA ISSN 0194-0880) **4092**, 3198
➤ Handbook of Chemical Neuroanatomy (NLD ISSN 0924-8196) **4092**, 3372
➤ Handbook of Clinical Neurology (NLD ISSN 0072-9752) **4092**
Handbook of Common Poisonings in Children (USA) **4044**
➤ Handbook of Electroencephalography and Clinical Neurophysiology (NLD ISSN 0304-4645) **4092**
Handbook of Experimental Pharmacology (USA ISSN 0171-2004) **4299**
Handbook of Feed Additives (GBR) **3160**, 3161
The Handbook of Health Assessment Tools (USA) **3609**
Handbook of Hyperlipidaemia (GBR) **3728**, 3772
➤ Handbook of Hypertension (NLD ISSN 0924-6541) **3772**
➤ Handbook of Lipid Research (USA ISSN 0163-9102) **3378**
Handbook of Medical Education (Year) (IND ISSN 0253-7621) **3609**, 3417
Handbook of Medical Treatment (USA ISSN 0072-9841) **3609**
Handbook of Medicinal Feed Additives *see* Handbook of Feed Additives **3160**, 3161
➤ Handbook of Natural Toxins (USA) **3609**, 4299
➤ Handbook of Neuropsychology (NLD) **4093**
Handbook of Non-Prescription Drugs (USA ISSN 0889-7816) **4299**
➤ Handbook of Physiology (USA ISSN 0072-9876) **3343**
• Handbook of Practice Management (GBR ISSN 0962-144X) **3609**
➤ Handbook of Psychology and Health Series (USA ISSN 0899-3122) **4401**, 4354
Handbook of Urology (USA ISSN 0932-2329) **4213**
• Handbook on Injectable Drugs (USA) **4299**
➤ Handbook on Synchrotron Radiation (NLD) **4365**
Handbuch der Medizinischen Radiologie *see* Medical Radiology **4150**
Handbuch fuer das Gesundheitswesen in Schleswig-Holstein (DEU) **3609**, 3370
• Handbuch fuer die Sanitaetsberufe Oesterreich (AUT ISSN 0073-0181) **3609**
Handchirurgie - Mikrochirurgie - Plastische Chirurgie (DEU ISSN 0722-1819) **4190**
Handgun Control. Semi-Annual Progress Report (USA) **3539**, 4471
Handhavingszakboekje (BEL) **3450**, 3539
Handicap & Beleid (NLD ISSN 1380-6661) **3484**, 4513
Handicap Idraet (DNK ISSN 0902-5618) **3484**
Handicap Idrett (NOR) **3422**, 3484
Handicap Information *see* Handicap Idraet **3484**
Handicap News (USA ISSN 0896-131X) **3484**, 4513
Handicapped Funding Directory *see* Directory of Grants for Organizations Serving People with Disabilities **3421**, 3418

Handikapp - Reflex (SWE ISSN 0348-8071) **4093**
Handiscoop (BEL ISSN 0779-3367) **3484**, 4513
Handling Pregnancy and Birth Cases (USA) **3546**, 3358, 4563
Handling Soft Tissue Injury Cases (USA) **3609**, 3539
Hanf! (DEU) **3549**, 3165
HanfBlatt (DEU) **3549**, 3165
• Hangtian Yixue yu Yixue Gongcheng/Space Medicine & Medical Engineering (CHN ISSN 1002-0837) **3153**, 3609
• ➤ Han'gug Sigpum Yeong'yang Gwahag Hoeji/Korean Society of Food Science and Nutrition. Journal (KOR ISSN 1226-3311) **4234**
Han'gug Yeong'yang Sigryang Haghoeji/Korean Society of Food and Nutrition. Journal *see* Han'gug Sigpum Yeong'yang Gwahag Hoeji **4234**
• ➤ Han'gug Yujeon Haghoeji/Korean Journal of Genetics (KOR ISSN 0254-5934) **3306**
Hannyan Nui-dai Hagsur Ji/Hanyang Medical College. Journal (KOR ISSN 0254-5942) **3609**
Hansten and Horn's Drug Interactions Analysis and Management (USA ISSN 1092-048X) **4299**
Hanyang Medical College. Journal *see* Hannyan Nui-dai Hagsur Ji **3609**
Hanzai Shinrigaku Kenkyu *see* Japanese Journal of Criminal Psychology **4408**
Hanzaigaku Zasshi *see* Acta Criminologiae et Medicinae Legalis Japonica **3393**, 3881
Happy, Healthy and Pregnant (ZAF ISSN 1023-4802) **3952**
Harbin Medicine *see* Harbin Yiyao **4299**
Harbin Yiyao/Harbin Medicine (CHN ISSN 1001-8131) **4299**
Haricot (AUS) **4213**, 4513
Harper-Grace Hospitals, Pharmacy and Therapeutics Newsletter *see* Harper Hospital, Pharmacy & Therapeutics Newsletter **4299**
Harper Hospital, Pharmacy & Therapeutics Newsletter (USA) **4299**
Harper's Biochemistry (USA ISSN 1043-9811) **3251**
Hartford Dental Society Newsletter (USA) **3825**
Hartmannbund in Baden - Wuerttemberg (DEU) **4471**, 4513
Hartmannbund Magazin (DEU ISSN 0944-7369) **3609**
➤ Harvard AIDS Institute Series on Gene Regulation of Human Retroviruses (USA ISSN 1063-0627) **3307**, 3796
➤ Harvard Books in Biophysics (USA ISSN 0073-0475) **3266**
• The Harvard Brain (USA) **4093**
Harvard Dental Bulletin (USA ISSN 1062-029X) **3825**
• ➤ Harvard Health Letter (USA ISSN 1052-1577) **4354**
• ➤ Harvard Heart Letter (USA ISSN 1051-5313) **3772**
Harvard Medical Alumni Bulletin (USA ISSN 0191-7757) **3388**, 3609
• Harvard Medical School. Center for Health and the Global Environment. Newsletter (USA) **4471**, 3439, 3609
Harvard Men's Health Watch (USA ISSN 1089-1102) **4221**
• The Harvard Mental Health Letter (USA ISSN 0884-3783) **4093**, 4401
• ➤ Harvard Review of Psychiatry (USA ISSN 1067-3229) **4093**
• ➤ Harvard Women's Health Watch (USA ISSN 1070-910X) **4563**
➤ Harvest (GBR ISSN 0266-4771) **4401**
Haryana Agricultural University. Journal of Research (IND ISSN 0379-4008) **3155**, 4508, 4543
Haryana Health Journal (IND ISSN 0017-8241) **4471**
Haryana Veterinarian (IND ISSN 0033-4359) **4543**
Hassei, Seicho, Bunka *see* Development, Growth and Differentiation **3192**
• ➤ Hastings Center Report (USA ISSN 0093-0334) **3610**, 3198, 4347
Hattatsu Shinrigaku Kenkyu/Japanese Journal of Developmental Psychology (JPN ISSN 0915-9029) **4401**
Hattatsu Yakuri Yakubutsu Chiryo Kenkyukai Zasshi/Japanese Journal of Developmental and Therapeutic Pharmacology (JPN ISSN 0914-9864) **4299**
Hausapotheke (DEU) **4299**
Der Hausarzt (DEU ISSN 1434-8950) **3610**

Hausarzt Bayern *see* Seminar Hausarztpraxis **3692**
Hausarzt Hessen *see* Seminar Hausarztpraxis **3692**
Hausarzt Nordrhein *see* Seminar Hausarztpraxis **3692**
Hausarzt Praxis Sachsen *see* Seminar Hausarztpraxis **3692**
Hausarzt Sachsen-Anhalt *see* Seminar Hausarztpraxis **3692**
Hausarzt Thueringen *see* Seminar Hausarztpraxis **3692**
• ➤ Der Hautarzt (DEU ISSN 0017-8470) **3849**
Der Hautarzt. Supplementum (DEU ISSN 0172-9713) **3849**
Hautfreund (DEU ISSN 0933-7385) **3849**
Hautnah Dermatologie (DEU ISSN 0938-0221) **3849**
Hautnah Gynaekologie und Geburtshilfe *see* Gynaekologie und Geburtshilfe **3951**
Hautnah Paediatrie *see* Paediatrie Hautnah **4050**, 3852
Having a Baby (GBR) **3383**, 3952
Hawaii Dental Association. Transactions (USA ISSN 0073-1021) **3825**
Hawaii Dental Journal (USA ISSN 0891-9933) **3825**
Hawaii. Department of Health. Mental Health Services for Children and Youth (USA ISSN 0362-6296) **4513**, 3383, 4471
Hawaii. Department of Health. Research and Statistics Office. R & S Report (USA ISSN 0093-3481) **4370**, 4364
Hawaii Health Messenger (USA ISSN 1053-9662) **4471**
➤ Hawaii Institute of Marine Biology. Technical Reports (USA ISSN 0073-1331) **3198**
➤ Hawaii Medical Journal (USA ISSN 0017-8594) **3610**
Hawaii's National Gay Community News (USA) **3527**, 4513
➤ Hawliyat Kulliyat al-A'daab/Annals of the Faculty of Arts (KWT ISSN 1560-5248) **3529**, 4347, 4402, 4508
Hayastani Bzhshkagitutyun/Armenian Medical Journal/Meditsinskaya Nauka Armenii (ARM) **3610**, 3875
Hayastany Kensabanakan Andes/Biologicheskii Zhurnal Armenii (ARM ISSN 0002-2918) **3198**
Hayes Directory of Dental Supply Houses (USA ISSN 0073-1404) **3825**
Hayes Directory of Medical Supply Houses (USA ISSN 0891-3242) **3508**
Hayes Druggist Directory (USA ISSN 0073-1420) **4299**
➤ Hazard (AUS ISSN 1320-0593) **4471**
Hazard Control Manager (USA) **4255**
Hazard Monthly *see* Hazard Technology **3387**, 3439, 4471
Hazard Prevention (USA ISSN 0743-8826) **4471**
• Hazard Technology (USA) **3387**, 3439, 4471
Hazardous Materials Newsletter (USA ISSN 0889-3454) **4471**, 3457
Hazardous Materials Regulation Guide (USA) **3450**, 4533
Hazardous Regulation Guide *see* Hazardous Materials Regulation Guide **3450**, 4533
Hazardous Substance Advisor *see* Keller's Industrial Safety Report **4258**
Hazardous Substances (GBR ISSN 0964-962X) **4255**
Hazardous Substances & Public Health (USA ISSN 1076-8920) **4471**, 3444, 3450
Hazardous Waste and Toxic Torts Law and Strategy *see* Environmental Compliance & Litigation Strategy **3538**, 3456, 3531, 4467
• ➤ Hazardous Waste Consultant (USA ISSN 0738-0232) **3457**, 3432, 4471
• Hazardous Waste Regulatory Analysis Service (USA ISSN 1087-0873) **3457**, 3432, 3450, 4471
• Hazards in the Office (GBR ISSN 0966-906X) **4268**, 3149
Hazards Magazine (GBR ISSN 0267-7296) **4255**, 4471
Hazelden News and Professional Update *see* Hazelden Voice **3401**
Hazelden Voice (USA) **3401**
HE-Xtra *see* H E - Xtra **4354**
• ➤ Head & Neck (USA ISSN 1043-3074) **4190**
Head Injury Update *see* Brain Injury Update **3717**, 4078
• ➤ Headache (USA ISSN 0017-8748) **4093**
Headache and Migraine Management Journal (USA) **3610**

Title

Title

Title

Title

Title

● ➤ The Immunologist (USA ISSN 1192-5612) **3745**
Immunologiya/Immunology (RUS ISSN 0206-4952) **3746**
● ➤ Immunology (GBR ISSN 0019-2805) **3746**
Immunology *see* Immunologiya **3746**
● Immunology Abstracts (USA ISSN 0307-112X) **3729**, 3149
● ➤ Immunology and Allergy Clinics of North America (USA ISSN 0889-8561) **3746**
● ➤ Immunology and Cell Biology (AUS ISSN 0818-9641) **3746**, 3200
➤ Immunology and Medicine (NLD) **3746**
Immunology Frontier *see* Men-Eki Immunoloji Furontia **3750**
● ➤ Immunology Letters (NLD ISSN 0165-2478) **3746**
➤ Immunology Series (USA) **3746**
Immunology. Supplement (GBR ISSN 0953-4954) **3746**
Immunology Today *see* Trends in Immunology **3752**
Immunomethods *see* Methods: A Companion to Methods in Enzymology **3256**
Immunonuclear Medicine *see* Men'eki Kaku Igaku **3750**, 4151
Immunopharmacology *see* International Immunopharmacology **4302**, 3747
● ➤ Immunopharmacology and Immunotoxicology (USA ISSN 0892-3973) **4300**
● ➤ Immunotechnology (NLD ISSN 1380-2933) **3746**, 3275
Immunotherapy *see* International Journal of Immunotherapy **3747**
● Immunotherapy Weekly (USA) **3746**
● Impact (Austin) (USA) **4094**, 4403
Impact Medecin (FRA) **3365**, 3618
Impact (Omaha) (USA) **3618**, 3417
● Imperial Cancer Research Fund. Scientific Report (GBR ISSN 0306-4905) **3979**
Implant (DEU ISSN 0948-5627) **3998**
Implant (FRA ISSN 1254-2431) **3825**
➤ Implant Dentistry (USA ISSN 1056-6163) **3825**
Implant Society (USA ISSN 1059-3489) **3825**
Implantologie (DEU ISSN 0943-9692) **3825**
Imprint (New York) (USA ISSN 0019-3062) **3921**
In Action *see* Frontline **3796**
● In Focus (Mountain View) (USA) **3497**, 4531
● ➤ In Practice (London) (GBR ISSN 0263-841X) **4543**
In Session: Psychotherapy in Practice *see* Journal of Clinical Psychology **4412**
In Sight (USA) **4476**
In the Family (USA ISSN 1083-4095) **3527**, 4403
In Touch (Calgary) *see* A Magazine of People and Possibilities **3168**
▼ In Touch (Melville) (USA ISSN 1522-7510) **3979**
In Verwachting (NLD) **3383**, 3953, 4568
● ➤ In Vitro Cellular & Developmental Biology - Animal (USA ISSN 1071-2690) **3618**, 3353
● ➤ In Vitro Cellular & Developmental Biology - Plant (USA ISSN 1054-5476) **3280**, 3275, 3308
In Vitro Diagnostic Technology *see* I V D Technology **3617**
In Vitro Diagnostics Industry Directory *see* Diagnostics Intelligence **4286**, 3594
➤ In Vitro Report (USA ISSN 1077-3975) **3343**, 3619
● ➤ In Vivo (GRC ISSN 0258-851X) **3875**
In Vivo *see* Windhover's IN VIVO **3709**, 3363
Incantesimo (ITA) **3175**, 3166
Incentive *see* Incitament **3619**, 3515
Incidenca Raka v Sloveniji/Cancer Incidence in Slovenia (SVN ISSN 0079-9580) **3979**
● ➤ Incitament/Incentive (SWE ISSN 1103-503X) **3619**, 3515
Inconscio e Cultura (ITA ISSN 0391-3198) **4403**
Indeks Biologi dan Pertanian de Indonesia *see* Indonesian Biological and Agricultural Index **3157**, 3149, 3155, 3200, 3232
The Independent Community Pharmacist (GBR ISSN 0963-0759) **4301**
Independent Health Facilities *see* Independent Healthcare Decisions **3515**
Independent Healthcare Association Focus *see* I H A Focus **3515**, 3474
Independent Healthcare Association. Initial Discussion Paper (GBR) **3515**, 3474
Independent Healthcare Decisions (GBR) **3515**
Independent Living (AUS ISSN 0815-2276) **3485**
Index and Abstracts of A P I Health-Related Research (Years) (USA) **4496**, 3149, 4272, 4531
Index Filicum (GBR) **3200**
Index Kewensis (GBR) **3200**, 3280
● Index Medicus (USA ISSN 0019-3879) **3729**, 3149
Index Medicus Indonesia (IDN ISSN 0853-9952) **3729**, 3149
Index Medicus Iugoslavicus *see* Bibliografija Medicinske Periodike Jugoslavije **3717**
Index Medicus Latinoamericano *see* L I L A C S - CD-ROM **3730**, 3177
Index of Current Medical Literature in the R F (RUS) **3729**
Index of Current Medical Literature in the U S S R *see* Index of Current Medical Literature in the R F **3729**
Index of Social Health (USA ISSN 1077-1212) **4496**
Index of Veterinary Specialists *see* I V S **4543**, 4300
Index of Veterinary Specialists Desk Reference *see* I V S Desk Reference **4543**, 4300
Index of Veterinary Specialties Annual *see* I V S Annual **4561**, 3149
Index Seminum (ISR) **3280**
● Index Veterinarius (GBR ISSN 0019-4123) **4561**, 3149
Indian Academy of Applied Psychology. Journal (IND ISSN 0019-4247) **4403**
➤ Indian Academy of Oral Medicine and Radiology. Journal (IND ISSN 0972-1363) **3825**, 4145
Indian & Eastern Pharmacy (IND ISSN 0019-4360) **4301**
Indian Anthropological Society. Journal (IND ISSN 0019-4387) **3173**
Indian Association of Occupational Medicine. Journal *see* Indian Journal of Industrial Medicine **3619**, 4256
Indian Biologist (IND ISSN 0302-7554) **3200**
Indian Chemicals and Pharmaceuticals Statistics (IND) **4344**
Indian Council of Medical Research Bulletin *see* I C M R Bulletin **3617**
Indian Dental Association. Journal (IND ISSN 0019-4611) **3825**
Indian Drug Manufacturers' Association Annual Publication *see* I D M A Annual Publication **4300**
Indian Drug Manufacturers' Association Bulletin *see* I D M A Bulletin **4300**
Indian Drugs (IND ISSN 0019-462X) **4301**
Indian Drugs and Pharmaceuticals Industry (IND ISSN 0019-4638) **4301**
Indian Health Trends and Services (USA ISSN 0885-9914) **4476**, 4369
● Indian Journal of Aerospace Medicine (IND ISSN 0970-6666) **3619**
Indian Journal of Anaesthesia (IND ISSN 0019-5049) **3757**
Indian Journal of Animal Health (IND ISSN 0019-5057) **4543**
➤ Indian Journal of Animal Nutrition (IND ISSN 0970-3209) **3161**, 4544
Indian Journal of Animal Research (IND ISSN 0367-6722) **3161**, 4544
● ➤ Indian Journal of Animal Sciences (IND ISSN 0367-8318) **4544**
Indian Journal of Applied Psychology (IND ISSN 0019-5073) **4403**
● ➤ Indian Journal of Biochemistry and Biophysics (IND ISSN 0301-1208) **3251**
● ➤ Indian Journal of Cancer (IND ISSN 0019-509X) **3979**
● ➤ The Indian Journal of Chest Diseases and Allied Sciences (IND ISSN 0377-9343) **3908**
Indian Journal of Clinical Psychology (IND ISSN 0303-2582) **4403**
➤ Indian Journal of Colo-Proctology (IND ISSN 0970-0935) **3892**, 4191
Indian Journal of Current Psychological Research (IND ISSN 0970-3748) **4403**
➤ Indian Journal of Dental Research (IND ISSN 0970-9290) **3825**
● ➤ Indian Journal of Dermatology (IND ISSN 0019-5154) **3850**
● Indian Journal of Dermatology, Venereology and Leprology (IND ISSN 0378-6323) **3850**, 3797
Indian Journal of Environmental Health (IND ISSN 0367-827X) **4476**, 3439
Indian Journal of Experimental Biology (IND ISSN 0019-5189) **3200**
● ➤ Indian Journal of Gastroenterology (IND ISSN 0254-8860) **3892**
Indian Journal of Genetics and Plant Breeding (IND ISSN 0019-5200) **3280**, 3308
Indian Journal of Gerontology (IND ISSN 0971-4189) **3474**
Indian Journal of Homoeopathic Medicine (IND ISSN 0019-5243) **3788**
● ➤ Indian Journal of Hospital Pharmacy (IND ISSN 0019-526X) **4301**
Indian Journal of Human Genetics (IND ISSN 0971-6866) **3308**
Indian Journal of Indigenous Medicines *see* PhytoMedica **3169**
Indian Journal of Industrial Medicine (IND ISSN 0019-5278) **3619**, 4256
● Indian Journal of Leprosy (IND ISSN 0254-9395) **3797**
➤ Indian Journal of Malariology (IND ISSN 0367-8326) **3797**
Indian Journal of Medical Microbiology (IND ISSN 0255-0857) **3746**
Indian Journal of Medical Photography (IND) **4349**, 3200, 3619
● ➤ The Indian Journal of Medical Research (IND ISSN 0971-5916) **3619**, 3200
Indian Journal of Medical Research. Section A, Infectious Diseases *see* The Indian Journal of Medical Research **3619**, 3200
Indian Journal of Medical Research. Section B, Biomedical Research other than Infectious Diseases *see* The Indian Journal of Medical Research **3619**, 3200
Indian Journal of Medical Research. Supplement (IND ISSN 0367-9012) **3619**
Indian Journal of Medical Sciences (IND ISSN 0019-5359) **3619**
Indian Journal of Mental Retardation (IND ISSN 0019-5375) **4094**
● Indian Journal of Microbiology (IND ISSN 0046-8991) **3323**
➤ Indian Journal of Mycology and Plant Pathology (IND) **3280**
● ➤ Indian Journal of Nutrition and Dietetics (IND ISSN 0022-3174) **4235**
Indian Journal of Occupational Therapy (IND ISSN 0445-7706) **4256**, 4061
● ➤ Indian Journal of Ophthalmology (IND ISSN 0301-4738) **3998**
Indian Journal of Orthopaedics (IND ISSN 0019-5413) **4016**
Indian Journal of Otolaryngology and Head and Neck *see* Indian Journal of Otolaryngology and Head and Neck Surgery **4033**
➤ Indian Journal of Otolaryngology and Head and Neck Surgery (IJO & HNS) (IND) **4033**
● ➤ Indian Journal of Pathology & Microbiology (IND ISSN 0377-4929) **3323**, 3619
Indian Journal of Pediatrics (IND ISSN 0019-5456) **4045**
● ➤ Indian Journal of Pharmaceutical Education (IND ISSN 0019-5464) **4301**
● ➤ Indian Journal of Pharmaceutical Sciences (IND ISSN 0250-474X) **4301**
● ➤ Indian Journal of Pharmacology (IND ISSN 0253-7613) **4301**
➤ Indian Journal of Physical Anthropology and Human Genetics (IND ISSN 0378-8156) **3308**, 3173
● ➤ Indian Journal of Physiology and Pharmacology (IND ISSN 0019-5499) **3343**, 4301
➤ Indian Journal of Plastic Surgery (IND ISSN 0970-0358) **4191**
● ➤ Indian Journal of Psychiatry (IND ISSN 0019-5545) **4094**
Indian Journal of Psychological Medicine (IND ISSN 0253-7176) **4094**
Indian Journal of Psychometry and Education (IND ISSN 0046-9009) **4404**, 3411
Indian Journal of Public Health (IND ISSN 0019-557X) **4476**
Indian Journal of Science and Industry *see* Indian Journal of Animal Research **3161**, 4544
Indian Journal of Surgery (IND ISSN 0019-5650) **4191**
➤ Indian Journal of Tuberculosis (IND ISSN 0019-5707) **4160**
Indian Journal of Unani Medicine (IND) **3166**
➤ Indian Journal of Veterinary Anatomy (IND ISSN 0971-1937) **4544**, 3619
Indian Journal of Veterinary Medicine (IND ISSN 0970-051X) **4544**
➤ The Indian Journal of Veterinary Research (IND ISSN 0971-4251) **4544**
Indian Journal of Veterinary Surgery (IND ISSN 0254-4105) **4544**
Indian Medical Association. Journal (IND ISSN 0019-5847) **3619**
Indian Medical Gazette (IND ISSN 0019-5863) **4191**, 3619
Indian Medicine/Indiyan Medisin (IND ISSN 0971-314X) **3166**
Indian Ophthalmology - Year Book (IND) **3998**
Indian Optometric Association. Journal *see* Optometry Today **4005**
Indian Pediatrics (IND ISSN 0019-6061) **4045**
Indian Pharmaceutical Directory (IND) **4301**
Indian Pharmaceutical Guide (IND ISSN 0073-6635) **4301**
➤ Indian Potato Association. Journal (IND ISSN 0970-8235) **3158**
Indian Poultry Industry Yearbook (IND ISSN 0970-9738) **3161**, 4544
Indian Poultry Review (IND ISSN 0019-6150) **3161**, 4544
The Indian Practitioner (IND ISSN 0019-6169) **3619**, 4476
Indian Psychological Abstracts *see* Indian Psychological Abstracts and Reviews **4457**, 3149
➤ Indian Psychological Abstracts and Reviews (IND ISSN 0971-524X) **4457**, 3149
Indian Psychological Review (IND ISSN 0019-6215) **4404**
Indian Society of Gastroenterology. Proceedings of the Annual Conference (IND) **3892**
Indian Society of Pedodontics and Preventive Dentistry. Journal (IND ISSN 0970-4388) **3825**
● ➤ Indian Veterinary Journal (IVJ) (IND ISSN 0019-6479) **4544**
Indian Veterinary Medical Journal (IND ISSN 0250-5266) **4544**
Indian Veterinary Research Institute. Annual Report (IND ISSN 0304-7067) **4544**
➤ Indiana Dental Association. Journal (USA ISSN 0019-6568) **3826**
Indiana Pharmacist (USA ISSN 1083-4974) **4301**
Indiana State Nursing Association Bulletin *see* I S N A Bulletin **3921**
Indianapolis District Dental Society. Newsletter (USA) **3826**
Indications in Antibiotic Therapy *see* Kosei Busshitsu Ryoho **4312**
● Indice de la Literatura Dental en Castellano (ARG ISSN 0325-0679) **3729**, 3149, 3826
● Indice Medico Espanol (ESP ISSN 0019-7068) **3729**, 3149
Individual Psychology *see* Journal of Individual Psychology **4417**
Individual Psychology News *see* Journal of Individual Psychology **4417**
Indiyan Medisin *see* Indian Medicine **3166**
Indonesian Association for Secure Contraception. Journal *see* Mantap: Majalah Ilmaih P K M I **3359**
Indonesian Biological and Agricultural Index/Indeks Biologi dan Pertanian de Indonesia (IDN) **3157**, 3149, 3155, 3200, 3232
Indonesian Journal of Bioanthropology/Berkala Bioanthropologi Indonesia (IDN ISSN 0216-7204) **3173**, 3200
Indonesian Journal of Industrial Hygiene, Occupational Health-Safety and Social Security/Majalah Higene Perusahaan, Kesehatan-Keselamatan Kerja, dan Jaminan Sosial (IDN ISSN 0126-0987) **4256**
Indonesian Journal of Public Health/Majalah Kesehatan Masyarakat Indonesia (IDN ISSN 0216-3527) **4476**
Indonesian Planned Parenthood Association Newsletter *see* I P P A Newsletter **3359**
Indonesian Public Health Association. Journal *see* Indonesian Journal of Public Health **4476**
● ➤ Indoor Air (DNK ISSN 0905-6947) **4476**
● Indoor Air Online (DNK ISSN 1600-0668) **4476**
Indoor Air Quality Update *see* I E Q Strategies **3444**, 3361, 4475
Indoor Air. Supplement (DNK ISSN 0908-5920) **4476**
● ➤ Indoor and Built Environment (CHE ISSN 1420-326X) **3747**
Indoor Environment *see* Indoor and Built Environment **3747**
▼ Indoor Environment Connections (indoor air quality) (USA ISSN 1526-8403) **3439**, 3525, 4476
Indoor Environmental Quality Strategies *see* I E Q Strategies **3444**, 3361, 4475
Indoor Pollution News *see* Asbestos & Lead Abatement Report **3443**
Industria Farmaceutica (ESP ISSN 0213-5574) **4301**
Industrial Accident Prevention Association. Annual Report *see* Industrial Accident Prevention Association. Annual Review **4256**

Title

Institut de Recherches Psychologiques. Bulletin (CAN ISSN 0832-7475) **4404**

Institut for Ferskvandsfiskeri og Fiskepleje. Aarsberetning *see* Danmarks Fiskeriundersoegelser. Aarsberetning **3459**, 3192

Institut National de la Sante et de la Recherche Medicale. Actualites (FRA ISSN 0755-4168) **4476**, 3620

Institut National de la Sante et de la Recherche Medicale. Bulletin d'Information *see* Institut National de la Sante et de la Recherche Medicale. Actualites **4476**, 3620

Institut National de la Sante et de la Recherche Medicale Symposia *see* I N S E R M Symposia **3617**

Institut National de Recherche et de Securite pour la Prevention des Accidents du Travail et des Mal Bulletin de Documentation *see* I N R S Bulletin de Documentation **4268**

Institut National de Statistique. Accidents de la Circulation sur la Voie Publique avec Tues et Blesses *see* Belgium. Institut National de Statistique. Accidents de la Circulation sur la Voie Publique avec Tues et Blesses **4495**, 4370, 4528, 4532

● ➤ Institut Pasteur. Annales. Actualites (FRA ISSN 0924-4204) **3323**, 3251, 3308

Institut Pasteur. Bulletin *see* Microbes and Infection **3327**, 3803

Institut Pasteur d'Algerie. Archives (DZA ISSN 0020-2460) **3323**

Institut Pasteur de Bangui. Rapport Annuel (CAF) **3621**

Institut Pasteur de Bangui. Rapport Bisannuel *see* Institut Pasteur de Bangui. Rapport Annuel **3621**

Institut Pasteur de Dakar. Rapport sur le Fonctionnement Technique (SEN ISSN 0377-3418) **3323**, 3747

● Institut Pasteur de Tunis. Archives (TUN ISSN 0020-2509) **3621**, 3200

Institut Pasteur Hellenique. Archives (GRC ISSN 0004-6620) **3323**, 3799

➤ Institut Razi. Archives (IRN ISSN 0365-3439) **3799**, 4544

Institut Royal des Sciences Naturelles de Belgique. Bulletin. Serie Entomologie (BEL ISSN 0374-6232) **3296**

Institute for Environment and Health Assessment *see* I E H Assessment **3439**, 3617

Institute for Environment and Health Assessment Indoor Air Quality in the Home: Carbon Monoxide *see* I E H Assessment Indoor Air Quality in the Home: Carbon Monoxide **3444**, 3450, 4475

Institute for Environment and Health Assessment on the Ecological Significance of Endocrine Disruption *see* I E H Assessment on the Ecological Significance of Endocrine Disruption **3444**, 3353

Institute for Environment and Health Report *see* I E H Report **3439**, 3617

Institute for Environment and Health Report on Approaches to Predicting Toxicity from Occupational Exposure to Dusts *see* I E H Report on Approaches to Predicting Toxicity from Occupational Exposure to Dusts **3450**, 4255, 4475

Institute for Environment and Health Report on Benzene In the Environment *see* I E H Report on Benzene In the Environment **3450**

Institute for Environment and Health Report on Factors Affecting the Absorption of Toxic Metals from the Diet *see* I E H Report on Factors Affecting the Absorption of Toxic Metals from the Diet **3450**, 3892, 4223, 4356

Institute for Environment and Health Report on Health Effects of Waste Combustion Products *see* I E H Report on Health Effects of Waste Combustion Products **3444**, 3457, 4356

Institute for Environment and Health Report on Perinatel Developmental Neurotoxcity *see* I E H Report on Perinatel Developmental Neurotoxcity **3450**, 4094, 4356

Institute for Environment and Health Report on U K Blood Lead Surveys *see* I E H Report on U K Blood Lead Surveys **3450**, 3902, 4475

Institute for Environment and Health Special Report *see* I E H Special Report **3439**, 3617

Institute for Environment and Health Special Report on Organophosphorus Esters *see* I E H Special Report on Organophosphorus Esters **3378**, 3450, 4475

Institute for Fermentation, Osaka. Research Communications/Hakko Kenkyujo Hokoku (JPN ISSN 0073-8751) **3323**, 3290

Institute for Laboratory Animal Research Journal *see* I L A R Journal **3353**, 3875

Institute for Studies in Psychological Testing Journal of Research in Educational & Psychological Testing & Measurement *see* I S P T Journal of Research in Educational & Psychological Testing & Measurement **3411**, 4403

Institute for Studies in Psychological Testing Quarterly Bulletin *see* I S P T Quarterly Bulletin **4403**

Institute of Agriculture and Animal Science. Journal (NPL ISSN 1018-6182) **4544**, 3155

Institute of Chemotherapy. Bulletin *see* Kagaku Ryoho Kenkyujo Kiyo **3957**

Institute of Economic Research. Publications on Family Planning (IND) **3359**

Institute of Electrical and Electronics Engineers, Inc. Transactions on Evolutionary Computation *see* I E E E Transactions on Evolutionary Computation **3284**, 3308

Institute of Electrical and Electronics Engineers, Inc. Transactions on Information Technology in Biomedicine *see* I E E E Transactions on Information Technology in Biomedicine **3274**, 3811

Institute of Environmental Sciences and Technology. Annual Technical Meeting. Proceedings (USA) **3439**, 3200, 3432

Institute of Environmental Sciences. Annual Technical Meeting. Proceedings *see* Institute of Environmental Sciences and Technology. Annual Technical Meeting. Proceedings **3439**, 3200, 3432

Institute of Environmental Sciences. Tutorial Series (USA ISSN 0073-9251) **3439**, 3200, 3432

Institute of Health Education. Journal *see* International Journal of Health Promotion and Education **4356**, 3411

Institute of Health Record Information & Management. Journal (GBR ISSN 1364-6974) **3621**, 3515

Institute of Health Sciences. Quarterly Medical News Bulletin (OMN) **3621**

Institute of Health Services Management Health & Social Services Yearbook *see* I H S M Health & Social Services Yearbook **4475**, 3515

Instytut Medycyny Morskiej i Tropikalnej w Gdyni. Bulletin Institute of Maritime and Tropical Medicine in Gdynia. Bulletin *see* International Maritime Health **3800**

Institute of Mathematics and Its Applications Journal of Mathematics Applied in Medicine & Biology *see* I M A Journal of Mathematics Applied in Medicine & Biology **3553**, 3199, 3617

Institute of Medical and Veterinary Science. Annual Report of the Council (AUS ISSN 0065-1907) **3621**, 4544

Institute of Medicine. Journal (NPL ISSN 0259-0972) **3621**

➤ Institute of Medicine of Chicago. Proceedings (USA ISSN 0091-746X) **3621**

Institute of Occupational Health. Proceedings (GBR) **4256**

Institute of Pharmacy Management International. Institute News *see* Institute of Pharmacy Management International. Institute News **4302**, 3365

Institute of Pharmacy Management International. Institute News (GBR ISSN 1369-8540) **4302**, 3365

Institute of Physical Sciences in Medicine. Report *see* Institute of Physics and Engineering in Medicine. Report **4145**, 4365

Institute of Physics and Engineering in Medicine. Report (GBR) **4145**, 4365

Institute of Postgraduate Medicine and Research. Journal (BGD ISSN 1017-9216) **3621**

Institute of Primate Research. Annual Report (KEN) **3353**, 3308

Institute of Psychophysical Research. Proceedings (GBR ISSN 0073-9561) **4404**

Institute of Public Health. Annual Report/Kokuritsu Koshu Eisei-in Nenpo (JPN) **4476**

➤ Institution of Chemists (India). Journal (IND ISSN 0020-3254) **3373**, 3875

Institution of Chemists (India). Proceedings (IND ISSN 0369-8599) **3373**, 3875

➤ Institution of Engineers (India). Environmental Engineering Division. Journal (IND ISSN 0251-110X) **3439**, 4476, 4561

● ➤ Institution of Mechanical Engineers. Proceedings. Part H: Journal of Engineering in Medicine (GBR ISSN 0954-4119) **3238**, 3435, 3621

Institution of Occupational Safety and Health. Journal (GBR ISSN 1366-1965) **4257**

Institution of Physics and Engineering in Medicine and Biology. Report *see* Institute of Physics and Engineering in Medicine. Report **4145**, 4365

Institution of Water and Environmental Management. Journal *see* Chartered Institution of Water and Environmental Management. Journal **4561**, 4465

Institutional Review Board A Review of Human Subjects Research *see* I R B: A Review of Human Subjects Research **3875**

➤ Instituto Adolfo Lutz. Revista (BRA ISSN 0073-9855) **3323**

Instituto Bacteriologico de Chile. Boletin *see* Instituto de Salud Publica de Chile. Boletin **4477**

➤ Instituto Barraquer. Anales (ESP ISSN 0020-3645) **3999**

Instituto Biologico da Bahia. Boletim (BRA ISSN 0020-3661) **3200**

Instituto de Biologia Marinha e Oceanografia. Trabalhos *see* Universidade Federal de Pernambuco. Departamento de Oceanografia. Centro de Tecnologia. Trabalhos Oceanograficos **3222**, 3409

Instituto de Higiene e Medicina Tropical. Anais (PRT ISSN 0303-7762) **4476**, 3799

Instituto de Investigacao Cientifica Tropical. Comunicacoes. Serie de Ciencias Biologicas (PRT ISSN 0871-1755) **3200**

Instituto de Investigaciones Biomedicas. Informe *see* Biomedicas **3187**, 3577

➤ Instituto de la Patagonia. Anales. Ciencias Sociales (CHL ISSN 0716-6478) **3526**, 3200

● Instituto de Medicina Tropical de Sao Paulo. Revista (BRA ISSN 0036-4665) **3799**

Instituto de Nutricion de Centro America y Panama (INCAP). Informe Anual (GTM ISSN 0533-4179) **4235**

Instituto de Salud Publica de Chile. Boletin (CHL ISSN 0716-1387) **4477**

Instituto de Tecnologia de Alimentos. Coletanea *see* Brazilian Journal of Food Technology **3460**, 4230

Instituto de Tecnologia de Alimentos. Instrucoes Praticas (BRA ISSN 0074-0144) **3461**, 4235

Instituto de Tecnologia de Alimentos. Instrucoes Tecnicas (BRA ISSN 0074-0152) **3461**, 4235

Instituto Estadual de Hematologia Arthur de Siqueira Cavalcanti. Revista (BRA ISSN 0103-3263) **3902**

Instituto Medico Beneficencia. Anales *see* Anales del Sistema Sanitario de Navarra **4461**

Instituto Medico "Sucre". Revista (BOL) **3621**

Instituto Mexicano del Seguro Social. Boletin Estadistico (MEX) **4477**

Instituto Mexicano del Seguro Social. Boletin sobre Morbilidad Hospitalaria (MEX) **4477**

Instituto Mexicano del Seguro Social. Boletin sobre Mortalidad (MEX) **4477**

Instituto Mexicano del Seguro Social. Boletin sobre Motivos de Consulta (MEX) **4477**

● ➤ Instituto Nacional de Cancerologia. Revista (MEX ISSN 0076-7131) **3980**

● ➤ Instituto Nacional de Enfermedades Respiratorias. Revista (MEX ISSN 0187-7585) **4160**

➤ Instituto Nacional de Medicina Legal de Colombia. Revista (COL ISSN 0120-0097) **3882**, 3394, 3546

Instituto Nacional de Neurologia y Neurocirugia. Archivos *see* Archivos de Neurociencias **4074**

● ➤ Instituto Oswaldo Cruz, Rio de Janeiro. Memorias (BRA ISSN 0074-0276) **3200**, 3621

Instituto Panamericano de Proteccion de Alimentos y Zoonosis en las Americas (ARG) **4545**, 3461

Instituto Panamericano de Proteccion de Alimentos y Zoonosis. Publicacion Tecnica (ARG) **4545**, 3461

➤ Instituto Politecnico Nacional. Escuela Nacional de Ciencias Biologicas. Anales (MEX ISSN 0365-1932) **3200**

Institutul Agronomic Cluj-Napoca. Buletinul. Seria Zootehnie si Medicina Veterinara *see* Universitatea de Stiinte Agricole Cluj-Napoca. Buletinul. Seria Zootehnie si Medicina Veterinara **3162**, 4554

Institutul Agronomic Ion Ionescu de la Brad. Lucrari Stiintifice. Seria Zootechnie - Medicina Veterinaria *see* Universitatea Agronomica Ion Ionescu de la Brad. Lucrari Stiintifice. Seria Zootechnie - Medicina Veterinaria **3162**, 4554

Institutul de Subingineri Oradea. Lucrari Stiintifice: Seria Biologic (ROM) **3200**

Institutul de Subingineri Oradea. Lucrari Stiintifice: Seria Educatie Fizica si Sport (ROM) **4525**, 4356

Institutul de Subingineri Oradea. Lucrari Stiintifice: Seria Pedagogie, Psihologie, Metodica (ROM) **3411**, 4404

Institutul Pedagogic Oradea. Lucrari Stiintifice Seria Biologic *see* Institutul de Subingineri Oradea. Lucrari Stiintifice: Seria Biologic **3200**

Institutul Pedagogic Oradea. Lucrari Stiintifice: Seria Educatie Fizica si Sport *see* Institutul de Subingineri Oradea. Lucrari Stiintifice: Seria Educatie Fizica si Sport **4525**, 4356

Institutul Pedagogic Oradea. Lucrari Stiintifice: Seria Pedagogie, Psihologie, Metodica *see* Institutul de Subingineri Oradea. Lucrari Stiintifice: Seria Pedagogie, Psihologie, Metodica **3411**, 4404

Instituut voor Perceptie Onderzoek Annual Progress Report *see* I P O Annual Progress Report **3550**, 4403

● ➤ Instrumentation Science & Technology (USA ISSN 1073-9149) **3376**, 3875

Insurance Directory (USA) **3532**

Insurance Handbook *see* Insurance Directory **3532**

Insurance Institute for Highway Safety. Status Report (USA ISSN 0018-988X) **4477**, 4533

Intand Newsletter (GBR ISSN 1461-5320) **4404**, 4365, 3368, 3416

● Integra (ESP) **3485**, 4514

Integral'noe Issledovanie Individual'nosti (RUS) **3411**, 4404

Integrated Pest Management Practitioner *see* I P M Practitioner **3158**

Integrated Traditional Chinese and Western Medicine in Practice of Critical Care Medicine *see* Zhongxiyi Jiehe Shiyong Linchuang Jijiu **3714**

● ➤ Integrative Physiological and Behavioral Science (USA ISSN 1053-881X) **4095**, 3343, 4404

Integrative Therapie (DEU ISSN 0342-6831) **4404**

● ➤ Intelligence (Kidlington) (GBR ISSN 0160-2896) **4404**

● ➤ Intensiv (DEU ISSN 0942-6035) **3621**

Intensiv- und Notfallbehandlung (DEU ISSN 0947-5362) **3621**

● ➤ Intensive and Critical Care Nursing (GBR ISSN 0964-3397) **3921**

Intensive Care Britain (Year) (GBR ISSN 0967-5728) **3621**

● ➤ Intensive Care Medicine (DEU ISSN 0342-4642) **3621**

Intensive Care Monitor (GBR ISSN 1360-306X) **3621**

➤ Intensive Care World (GBR ISSN 0266-7037) **3621**

Intensive Care World Monitor *see* Intensive Care Monitor **3621**

● ➤ Intensivmedizin und Notfallmedizin (DEU ISSN 0175-3851) **3621**

Inter-African Conference on Food and Nutrition. Programa e Informacoes (NER ISSN 0534-4700) **4235**

Inter-African Conference on Food and Nutrition. Report (NER ISSN 0538-2785) **4235**

Inter-African Conference on Medical Co-Operation. Meeting (NER ISSN 0534-4735) **3621**

● Interactive Healthcare Directory on CD-ROM (USA ISSN 1098-6049) **3811**

Interactive Healthcare Newsletter *see* Interactive Healthcare Report **3811**

Interactive Healthcare Report (USA) **3811**

Interactive Medicine (USA) **3621**

Interazioni (ITA) **4404**

The Interbehaviorist (USA ISSN 8755-612X) **4404**, 4347

Interbloc (FRA ISSN 0242-3960) **3921**

Intercellular and Intracellular Communications (GBR ISSN 0957-0799) **3290**

Intercon (ESP) **3622**

▼ ● Inter@ctiva (CHE) **3622**

Interdisciplinaria (ARG ISSN 0325-8203) **4405**, 4509

Interdisciplinaria Monographs (ARG ISSN 0326-1913) **4405**

➤ Interdisciplinary Topics in Gerontology (CHE ISSN 0074-1132) **3474**

Title

Title

see International Institute on the Prevention and Treatment of Dependencies. Selected Papers **3402**
International Journal for Clinical and Investigative Allergology and Clinical Immunology *see* Allergologia et Immunopathologia **3739**
International Journal for Consumer and Product Safety *see* Injury Prevention and Safety Promotion **3393**, 4476
➤ International Journal for Human Caring (USA ISSN 1091-5710) **3921**
• ➤ International Journal for Parasitology (GBR ISSN 0020-7519) **3799**, 3323
• ➤ International Journal for Quality in Health Care (GBR ISSN 1353-4505) **3622**
• ➤ The International Journal for the Psychology of Religion (USA ISSN 1050-8619) **4500**, 4405
• ➤ International Journal for Vitamin and Nutrition Research (USA ISSN 0300-9831) **4302**, 4235
• ➤ The International Journal of Action Methods (USA ISSN 1096-7680) **4405**, 4521
➤ International Journal of Adolescence and Youth (GBR ISSN 0267-3843) **3383**, 4405
International Journal of Adolescent Medicine and Health (ISR ISSN 0334-0139) **4046**
• ➤ International Journal of Adult Orthodontics and Orthognathic Surgery (USA ISSN 0742-1931) **3826**, 4191
International Journal of Aesthetic and Restorative Surgery *see* The International Journal of Cosmetic Surgery and Aesthetic Dermatology **4191**
• ➤ International Journal of Aging & Human Development (USA ISSN 0091-4150) **3474**
➤ International Journal of Alternative & Complementary Medicine (GBR ISSN 1357-9452) **3166**, 3747, 3788, 4235
International Journal of Anaesthesia *see* Anaesthesia On-Line **3754**
• ➤ International Journal of Andrology (GBR ISSN 0105-6263) **4213**
• International Journal of Andrology. Supplement (GBR ISSN 0106-1607) **4213**
• ➤ International Journal of Angiology (USA ISSN 1061-1711) **3775**, 4191
➤ International Journal of Animal Sciences (IND ISSN 0970-2857) **3161**, 3172, 3275
➤ International Journal of Anti-Aging Medicine (USA) **3474**, 3622
• ➤ International Journal of Antimicrobial Agents (NLD ISSN 0924-8579) **3323**
• ➤ International Journal of Aromatherapy (GBR ISSN 0962-4562) **3166**, 4227
• ➤ International Journal of Artificial Organs (ITA ISSN 0391-3988) **3622**, 3875
➤ International Journal of Arts Medicine (USA ISSN 1057-4263) **3622**, 3175
• ➤ The International Journal of Aviation Psychology (USA ISSN 1050-8414) **4532**, 3153, 4405
• ➤ International Journal of Behavioral Development (GBR ISSN 0165-0254) **4405**
• ➤ International Journal of Behavioral Medicine (USA ISSN 1070-5503) **4405**, 4521
International Journal of Behavioural Sciences (IND ISSN 0971-3190) **4406**, 4521
International Journal of Bio-Medical Computing *see* International Journal of Medical Informatics **3811**, 3284
International Journal of Biochemistry *see* International Journal of Biochemistry & Cell Biology **3252**, 3290
• ➤ International Journal of Biochemistry & Cell Biology (GBR ISSN 1357-2725) **3252**, 3290
• ➤ International Journal of Biological Macromolecules (NLD ISSN 0141-8130) **3252**
• ➤ International Journal of Biological Markers (ITA ISSN 0393-6155) **3201**
International Journal of Biology and Biochemistry *see* International Journal of Medical and Biological Frontiers **3623**, 3201
• ➤ International Journal of Biometeorology (DEU ISSN 0020-7128) **4223**, 3201, 3622
International Journal of Biosciences and the Law (GBR ISSN 1353-274X) **3201**, 3540
➤ International Journal of Biosocial and Medical Research (USA ISSN 1044-811X) **4235**, 4406, 4521
▼ • ➤ International Journal of Biotechnology (CHE ISSN 0963-6048) **3275**
• ➤ International Journal of Cancer/Journal International du Cancer (USA ISSN 0020-7136) **3980**
International Journal of Cancer. Supplement (USA ISSN 0898-6924) **3980**
International Journal of Cardiac Imaging *see* International Journal of Cardiovascular Imaging **3775**
• ➤ International Journal of Cardiology (IRL ISSN 0167-5273) **3775**
• ➤ International Journal of Cardiovascular Imaging (NLD) **3775**
• ➤ International Journal of Cardiovascular Interventions (GBR ISSN 1462-8848) **3775**
International Journal of Cell Cloning *see* Stem Cells **3219**
• ➤ International Journal of Childbirth Education (USA ISSN 0887-8625) **3953**, 4046
• International Journal of Children's Spirituality (GBR ISSN 1364-436X) **4406**, 3383, 3411, 4347, 4500
➤ International Journal of Circumpolar Health (FIN ISSN 1239-9736) **3622**, 4477
➤ International Journal of Clinical Acupuncture (USA ISSN 1047-1979) **3167**, 3622
• ➤ International Journal of Clinical and Experimental Hypnosis (USA ISSN 0020-7144) **3906**
International Journal of Clinical and Laboratory Research *see* Clinical and Experimental Medicine **3585**, 3872
International Journal of Clinical Monitoring and Computing *see* Journal of Clinical Monitoring and Computing **3631**, 3758
• International Journal of Clinical Oncology (JPN ISSN 1341-9625) **3980**
• International Journal of Clinical Oncology Online (JPN ISSN 1437-7772) **3980**
• ➤ International Journal of Clinical Pharmacology and Therapeutics (DEU ISSN 0946-1965) **4302**, 3451
• ➤ International Journal of Clinical Pharmacology Research (CHE ISSN 0251-1649) **4302**
International Journal of Clinical Pharmacology, Therapy and Toxicology *see* International Journal of Clinical Pharmacology and Therapeutics **4302**, 3451
• ➤ International Journal of Clinical Practice (GBR ISSN 1368-5031) **3622**
➤ International Journal of Clinical Practice. Symposium Supplement (GBR ISSN 1368-504X) **3623**
▼ • International Journal of Cognition & Technology (NLD ISSN 1569-2167) **4406**, 3389
International Journal of Cognitive Education and Mediated Learning *see* Journal of Cognitive Education **3412**, 4412
• International Journal of Cognitive Ergonomics (USA ISSN 1088-6362) **4406**
• ➤ International Journal of Colorectal Disease (DEU ISSN 0179-1958) **4191**
The International Journal of Communicative Psychoanalysis & Psychotherapy (USA ISSN 1062-3051) **4095**, 4406
▼ International Journal of Comparative Psychoanalysis (USA) **4406**
➤ International Journal of Comparative Psychology (USA ISSN 0889-3667) **4406**
International Journal of Computerized Dentistry (DEU ISSN 1463-4201) **3826**, 3811
• ➤ International Journal of Conflict Management (USA ISSN 1044-4068) **3365**
The International Journal of Cosmetic and Restorative Surgery *see* The International Journal of Cosmetic Surgery and Aesthetic Dermatology **4191**
• ➤ International Journal of Cosmetic Science (GBR ISSN 0142-5463) **3176**, 3875
▼ • ➤ International Journal of Cosmetic Surgery and Aesthetic Dermatology (USA ISSN 1530-8200) **3850**, 4191
➤ The International Journal of Cosmetic Surgery and Aesthetic Dermatology (USA) **4191**
International Journal of Dental Symposia (USA) **3826**
• ➤ International Journal of Dermatology (GBR ISSN 0011-9059) **3850**
• ➤ International Journal of Developmental Biology (ESP ISSN 0214-6282) **3201**
• ➤ International Journal of Developmental Neuroscience (GBR ISSN 0736-5748) **4095**
• ➤ International Journal of Disability, Development and Education (GBR ISSN 1034-912X) **3423**, 3485
• ➤ International Journal of Drug Policy (NLD ISSN 0955-3959) **3402**, 4302
• ➤ International Journal of Eating Disorders (USA ISSN 0276-3478) **4236**, 4406
▼ ➤ International Journal of Emergency Mental Health (USA ISSN 1522-4821) **4096**
• ➤ International Journal of Environmental Health Research (GBR ISSN 0960-3123) **3439**, 3623
• ➤ International Journal of Epidemiology (GBR ISSN 0300-5771) **3623**, 4477
• International Journal of Evolutionary Optimization (JPN) **3308**, 3284
International Journal of Experimental Diabetes Research (CHE ISSN 1560-4284) **3747**
• ➤ International Journal of Experimental Pathology (GBR ISSN 0959-9673) **3623**
International Journal of Fertility and Menopausal Studies *see* International Journal of Fertility and Women's Medicine **3623**, 3201
• ➤ International Journal of Fertility and Women's Medicine (USA) **3623**, 3201
• ➤ International Journal of Food Microbiology (NLD ISSN 0168-1605) **3324**, 3461
• International Journal of Food Properties (USA ISSN 1094-2912) **3201**
• ➤ International Journal of Food Sciences and Nutrition (GBR ISSN 0963-7486) **4236**
International Journal of Gastroenterology (GBR ISSN 1363-4534) **3892**, 4168
International Journal of General Practice and Primary Care *see* General Practice On-Line **3606**
International Journal of Genome Research (SGP ISSN 0218-1932) **3308**
• ➤ International Journal of Geriatric Psychiatry (GBR ISSN 0885-6230) **3474**, 4096
• ➤ International Journal of Group Psychotherapy (USA ISSN 0020-7284) **4406**, 4096
• ➤ International Journal of Group Tensions (USA ISSN 0047-0732) **4406**, 4368, 4521
• ➤ International Journal of Gynecological Cancer (USA ISSN 1048-891X) **3953**, 3980
• ➤ International Journal of Gynecological Pathology (USA ISSN 0277-1691) **3953**, 3623
• ➤ International Journal of Gynecology and Obstetrics (IRL ISSN 0020-7292) **3954**
▼ • International Journal of Health Care Finance and Economics (USA ISSN 1389-6563) **4477**, 3361, 3532
• International Journal of Health Care Quality Assurance (GBR ISSN 0952-6862) **3623**
• International Journal of Health Care Quality Assurance Incorporating Leadership in Health Services (GBR ISSN 1366-0756) **3516**
International Journal of Health Education *see* International Journal of Health Promotion and Education **4356**, 3411
• ➤ International Journal of Health Planning and Management (GBR ISSN 0749-6753) **4514**, 3623
➤ International Journal of Health Promotion and Education (GBR ISSN 1463-5240) **4356**, 3411
• ➤ International Journal of Health Services (USA ISSN 0020-7314) **4477**
▼ ➤ International Journal of Healthcare Technology and Management (CHE ISSN 1368-2156) **3811**, 3516
• ➤ International Journal of Hematology (JPN ISSN 0925-5710) **3903**
International Journal of Human Factors in Manufacturing *see* Human Factors and Ergonomics in Manufacturing **3435**, 4255, 4402
• ➤ International Journal of Hygiene and Environmental Health (DEU ISSN 1438-4639) **4477**
International Journal of Hypertension. Edicion Iberoamericana *see* Iberoamerican Journal of Hypertension **3774**
• ➤ International Journal of Hyperthermia (GBR ISSN 0265-6736) **3980**
• ➤ International Journal of Immunopathology and Pharmacology (ITA ISSN 0394-6320) **3747**, 4302
International Journal of Immunopharmacology *see* International Immunopharmacology **4302**, 3747
• ➤ International Journal of Immunotherapy (CHE ISSN 0255-9625) **3747**
• ➤ International Journal of Impotence Research (GBR ISSN 0955-9930) **4213**
International Journal of Infant Observation *see* Infant Observation **4045**
• ➤ International Journal of Infectious Diseases (CAN ISSN 1201-9712) **3799**, 4477
▼ ➤ The International Journal of Integrative Medicine (USA ISSN 1522-6255) **3167**
➤ International Journal of Intensive Care (GBR ISSN 1350-2794) **3623**
International Journal of Japanese Society of Pediatric Dentistry *see* Pediatric Dental Journal **3836**, 4052
• ➤ International Journal of Language and Communication Disorders (GBR ISSN 1368-2822) **4033**, 3423
• ➤ International Journal of Law and Psychiatry (GBR ISSN 0160-2527) **3540**, 4096
• ➤ International Journal of Legal Medicine (DEU ISSN 0937-9827) **3882**
• ➤ International Journal of Leprosy and Other Mycobacterial Diseases (USA ISSN 0148-916X) **3799**
➤ International Journal of Mass Emergencies and Disasters (USA ISSN 0280-7270) **4514**, 4477
International Journal of Medical and Biological Frontiers (USA) **3623**, 3201
• ➤ International Journal of Medical Informatics (IRL ISSN 1386-5056) **3811**, 3284
▼ • ➤ International Journal of Medical Marketing (GBR ISSN 1469-7025) **4303**, 3366
• ➤ International Journal of Medical Microbiology (DEU ISSN 1438-4221) **3800**, 3324
International Journal of Medical Practice and the Law *see* Medical Law International **3542**, 3651
International Journal of Medicine *see* Medicine On-Line **3656**
International Journal of Medicine and Biology *see* International Journal of Medical and Biological Frontiers **3623**, 3201
➤ International Journal of Medicine, Biology and the Environment (ITA ISSN 1128-935X) **3980**, 3440
▼ • ➤ International Journal of Men's Health (USA ISSN 1532-6306) **4221**
• ➤ International Journal of Mental Health (USA ISSN 0020-7411) **4406**, 4477, 4514
▼ ➤ The International Journal of Mental Health Promotion (GBR ISSN 1462-3730) **4477**, 4096, 4514
➤ International Journal of Methods in Psychiatric Research (GBR ISSN 1049-8931) **4096**
International Journal of Microcirculation: Clinical and Experimental *see* Journal of Vascular Research **3779**
International Journal of Microsurgery *see* Microsurgery **4197**, 3879
• ➤ International Journal of Molecular Medicine (GRC ISSN 1107-3756) **3623**
▼ ➤ International Journal of Nanoscience (SGP ISSN 0219-581X) **3391**, 3391, 3623
• International Journal of Neural Systems (SGP ISSN 0129-0657) **3389**
• ➤ International Journal of Neuro-Psychopharmacology (GBR ISSN 1461-1457) **4303**, 4406
International Journal of Neurology (URY ISSN 0020-7446) **4096**
International Journal of Neuropsychopharmacology (GBR) **4096**, 4303
• ➤ International Journal of Neuroscience (CHE ISSN 0020-7454) **4096**, 3252
• ➤ International Journal of Nursing Practice (AUS ISSN 1322-7114) **3921**
• ➤ International Journal of Nursing Studies (GBR ISSN 0020-7489) **3922**
• ➤ International Journal of Obesity (GBR ISSN 0307-0565) **4236**, 4356
• ➤ International Journal of Obstetric Anesthesia (GBR ISSN 0959-289X) **3954**, 3757
➤ International Journal of Occupational and Environmental Health (USA ISSN 1077-3525) **4257**
• ➤ International Journal of Occupational Medicine and Environmental Health (POL ISSN 1232-1087) **4257**, 4477
➤ International Journal of Occupational Safety and Ergonomics (POL ISSN 1080-3548) **4257**, 3373
• ➤ International Journal of Offender Therapy and Comparative Criminology (USA ISSN 0306-624X) **3394**, 4096
• ➤ International Journal of Oncology (GRC ISSN 1019-6439) **3980**
• ➤ International Journal of Oral & Maxillofacial Implants (USA ISSN 0882-2786) **3826**
• ➤ International Journal of Oral & Maxillofacial Surgery (GBR ISSN 0901-5027) **3827**, 4191

Title

International Symposium on Medical Virology. Proceedings *see* Medical Virology **3803**
International Symposium on Quality Control (JPN) **3624**
International System Safety Conference. Proceedings (USA) **4477**
International Tesla Society. Bulletin (USA) **4365**, 3624
➤ International Tinnitus Journal (USA ISSN 0946-5448) **4034**, 3491
International Travel and Health: Vaccination Requirements and Health Advice (CHE ISSN 1020-0169) **4478**
International Travel Health Guide (USA ISSN 1045-0572) **3624**, 4534
International Tremor Foundation Newsletter *see* I T F Newsletter **4094**
International Trends in Oncology (ITA ISSN 1125-632X) **3981**
International U S Surgeon (USA) **4191**
International Union Against Cancer. Proceedings of Congress (CHE ISSN 0074-9206) **3981**
International Union against Tuberculosis and Lung Disease. Conference Proceedings (FRA) **4161**, 4478
International Union against Tuberculosis and Lung Disease. Newsletter (FRA ISSN 1021-7754) **4161**
International Union against Tuberculosis and Lung Disease Newsletter (Edition Espanola) *see* I U A T L D Newsletter (Edition Espanola) **4160**
International Union against Tuberculosis and Lung Disease Newsletter (Edition Francaise) *see* I U A T L D Newsletter (Edition Francaise) **4160**
International Union against Tuberculosis. Conference Proceedings *see* International Union against Tuberculosis and Lung Disease. Conference Proceedings **4161**, 4478
International Union for the Scientific Study of Population Newsletter *see* I U S S P Newsletter **4369**, 3359
International Union for the Scientific Study of Population Papers *see* I U S S P Papers **4369**, 3359
International Union of Biochemistry and Molecular Biology Life *see* I U B M B Life **3251**
International Union of Biological Sciences. General Assemblies. Proceedings (FRA ISSN 0445-1333) **3201**
International Union of Biological Sciences. Reports of General Assemblies *see* International Union of Biological Sciences. General Assemblies. Proceedings **3201**
International Union of Pure and Applied Chemistry Series on Analytical and Physical Chemistry of Environmental Systems *see* I U P A C Series on Analytical and Physical Chemistry of Environmental Systems **3451**, 3373
International Universities Press, Inc. Stress and Health Series *see* I U P Stress and Health Series **4094**
International Update *see* AIDS Organisations Worldwide **3791**, 4275
• ➤ International Urogynecology Journal (GBR ISSN 0937-3462) **3954**, 4214
• ➤ International Urology and Nephrology (NLD ISSN 0301-1623) **4214**
International Ventilator Users Network News *see* I V U N News **3617**
International Wildlife Rehabilitation Council. Individual Papers (USA) **3353**, 4545
International Wildlife Rehabilitation Council Proceedings *see* I W R C Proceedings **3353**, 4543
International Wildlife Rehabilitation Council Skills Seminars *see* I W R C Skills Seminars **3353**, 4543
• International Yearbook of Nephrology (DEU ISSN 0921-9862) **4214**
Internationale Gesellschaft fuer Geschichte der Pharmazie. Veroeffentlichungen. Neue Folge (DEU) **4303**
Internationale Revue der Gesamten Hydrobiologie *see* International Review of Hydrobiology **3201**
Internationale Zeitschrift fuer Sozialpsychologie und Gruppendynamik (AUT ISSN 0254-928X) **4408**
Internationales Journal fuer Paradontologie und Restaurative Zahnheilkund (DEU ISSN 0721-0051) **3827**
Internationales Symposium gegen Drogen in der Schweiz (CHE) **3402**, 4408
• Internet Healthcare Strategies (USA ISSN 1528-7386) **3811**
• ➤ The Internet Journal of Advanced Nursing Practice (USA ISSN 1523-6064) **3922**
Internet Journal of Aeromedical Transportation *see* The Internet Journal of Rescue and Disaster Medicine **4016**
• ➤ The Internet Journal of Anesthesiology (USA ISSN 1092-406X) **3757**
▼ • ➤ The Internet Journal of Cardiology (USA) **3775**
Internet Journal of Disaster Medicine *see* The Internet Journal of Rescue and Disaster Medicine **4016**
• ➤ The Internet Journal of Emergency and Intensive Care Medicine (USA ISSN 1092-4051) **4016**
▼ • ➤ The Internet Journal of Family Practice (USA) **3909**
▼ • ➤ The Internet Journal of Gastroenterology (USA) **3893**
▼ • ➤ The Internet Journal of Gynecology and Obstetrics (USA) **3954**
▼ • ➤ The Internet Journal of Health (USA) **4478**
• ➤ Internet Journal of Health Promotion (AUS ISSN 1328-7443) **4478**
▼ • ➤ The Internet Journal of Infectious Diseases (USA) **3624**
▼ • ➤ The Internet Journal of Internal Medicine (USA) **3909**
▼ • ➤ The Internet Journal of Law, Healthcare and Ethics (USA ISSN 1528-8250) **3883**
The Internet Journal of Neonatology *see* The Internet Journal of Pediatrics and Neonatology **4046**
▼ • ➤ The Internet Journal of Neurology (USA) **4097**
▼ • The Internet Journal of Neurosurgery (USA) **4191**, 4097
▼ • ➤ The Internet Journal of Oncology (USA) **3981**
• ➤ The Internet Journal of Ophthalmology and Visual Science (USA) **3999**
▼ • ➤ The Internet Journal of Orthopedic Surgery (USA) **4016**, 4191
▼ • ➤ The Internet Journal of Otorhinolaryngology (USA) **4034**
▼ • The Internet Journal of Pain, Symptom Control and Palliative Care (USA) **3757**, 3981, 4061
▼ • ➤ The Internet Journal of Pathology (USA) **3624**
▼ • ➤ The Internet Journal of Pediatrics and Neonatology (USA ISSN 1528-8374) **4046**
▼ • ➤ The Internet Journal of Perfusionists (USA) **3775**, 4191
▼ • ➤ The Internet Journal of Plastic Surgery (USA) **4192**
▼ • ➤ The Internet Journal of Polish Anesthesiology and Surgery (USA) **4192**, 3757
▼ • Internet Journal of Public Health Education (DNK ISSN 1437-9619) **4478**
• ➤ The Internet Journal of Pulmonary Medicine (USA) **4161**, 3775
▼ • ➤ The Internet Journal of Radiology (USA) **4146**
• ➤ The Internet Journal of Rescue and Disaster Medicine (USA) **4016**
▼ • ➤ The Internet Journal of Rheumatology (USA) **4168**
• Internet Journal of Science - Biological Chemistry (GBR ISSN 1462-2149) **3252**
▼ • ➤ The Internet Journal of Surgery (USA) **4192**
• ➤ The Internet Journal of Thoracic and Cardiovascular Surgery (USA ISSN 1524-0274) **4192**, 3775
▼ ➤ The Internet Journal of Urology (USA) **4214**
➤ Internet - Medicina (ESP ISSN 1138-6215) **3811**, 3391
• Internet Medicine (USA ISSN 1086-5691) **3391**
• ➤ Der Internist (DEU ISSN 0020-9554) **3909**
Internist *see* The Original Internist **3789**, 3911
➤ L'Internista (ITA ISSN 1121-9017) **3909**
Internistische Praxis (DEU ISSN 0020-9570) **3909**
➤ Die Internistische Welt (DEU ISSN 0344-4201) **3909**
Internist's Intercom *see* I M Advantage **3908**
• ➤ InterNurse (GBR) **3922**
InterPsych Newsletter *see* PsychNews International **4436**, 4127
• ➤ Interscience Conference on Antimicrobial Agents and Chemotherapy. Program and Abstracts (USA ISSN 0733-6373) **3324**, 3981
Interstitial Cystitis Association Update (New York) *see* I C A Update (New York) **4213**
Intervencion Psicosocial (ESP ISSN 1132-0559) **4408**
Intervention (GBR) **4146**
• ➤ Intervention in School and Clinic (USA ISSN 1053-4512) **3423**, 4408
➤ Interventional Cardiology (NLD ISSN 0926-9649) **3775**
Interventional Cardiology Monitor *see* Current Medical Literature. Interventional Cardiology Monitor **3721**, 3770
• Interventional Cardiology Newsletter (USA ISSN 1063-4282) **3775**, 4192
• ➤ Interventional Neuroradiology (ITA ISSN 1123-9344) **4146**
Interventional Radiology Monitor *see* Intervention **4146**
▼ The Interventionalist (USA ISSN 1533-5364) **4146**
• ➤ Intervirology (CHE ISSN 0300-5526) **3324**
• Intestinal Function (GBR ISSN 0261-4995) **3729**, 3149, 3893
InTouch *see* In Touch (Melville) **3979**
Intoxications Alimentaires et Maladies d'Origine Hydrique au Canada *see* Foodborne and Waterborne Disease in Canada **3461**
Intravascular Imaging (GBR ISSN 1366-7122) **3775**
Intravenous Nurses Society Newsline *see* I N S Newsline **3921**
Intron - Canadian Molecular Biology *see* Canadian Biotech News **3273**
Intuition (USA ISSN 1085-3529) **4227**, 4097
Inventory of Health & Social Service Personnel *see* Inventory of Health Workforce in Alberta **4478**, 4514
Inventory of Health Workforce in Alberta (CAN) **4478**, 4514
• ➤ Invertebrate Biology (USA ISSN 1077-8306) **3353**
• Invertebrate Neurobiology (GBR ISSN 0261-4952) **3232**, 3149, 3343, 3729, 4097
• ➤ Invertebrate Neuroscience (DEU ISSN 1354-2516) **3353**
• Invertebrate Neuroscience Online (DEU ISSN 1439-1104) **3353**
• Invertebrate Systomatics (Online Edition) (AUS) **3353**
• ➤ Invertebrate Systomatics (Print Edition) (AUS ISSN 1445-5226) **3353**
• ➤ Investigacion Clinica (VEN ISSN 0535-5133) **3624**
Investigacion Clinica. Suplemento (VEN ISSN 0259-0395) **3625**
Investigacion y Educacion en Enfermeria (COL ISSN 0120-5307) **3922**
Investigational Drug Information. Medical and Dental *see* Chiken Ishiyaku Joho **4283**, 3817
Investigational Drug Patent Fast-Alert *see* Patent Fast-Alert **4321**, 4272
• ➤ Investigational New Drugs (USA ISSN 0167-6997) **4304**
• ➤ Investigative Ophthalmology & Visual Science (IOVS) (USA ISSN 0146-0404) **3999**
• ➤ Investigative Radiology (USA ISSN 0020-9996) **4146**
Iowa Board of Nursing. Newsletter (USA) **3922**
Iowa Comprehensive State Plan for Substance Abuse (Year) *see* Iowa Substance Abuse Report (Year) **3402**
Iowa Dental Journal (USA ISSN 0021-0498) **3827**
Iowa Medicine (USA ISSN 0746-8709) **3625**
Iowa Optometric Association News *see* I O A News **3998**
➤ The Iowa Orthopaedic Journal (USA) **4017**
Iowa Pharmacist (USA ISSN 0889-7735) **4304**
➤ Iowa State University Veterinarian (USA ISSN 0099-5851) **4545**
Iowa Substance Abuse Report (Year) (USA) **3402**
Iranian Dental Association. Bulletin *see* Jame'e Dandanpezeshki Iran. Namah-i **3827**
Iranian Dental Association. Journal - Jame'e-Ye Dandanpezeshkan-e Iran. Majalleh *see* Majda **3831**
➤ Iranian Journal of Medical Sciences (IRN ISSN 0253-0716) **3625**
• Iranian Journal of Public Health/Majalle-Ye Behdasht-e Iran (IRN ISSN 0304-4556) **4478**
Iraqi Medical Professions' Association. Journal (IRQ ISSN 0021-0927) **3625**
Ireland. Department of Agriculture and Food. Pesticide Residues in Food (IRL) **4478**, 3461
Ireland. National Disease Surveillance Centre. Report on the Epidemiology of Tuberculosis in Ireland (IRL) **3800**
Iri Sangyo Shinbun/Medical and Physical Instruments Newspaper (JPN) **3625**
• Irish Aid Annual Report (IRL) **3363**
➤ Irish Colleges of Physicians and Surgeons. Journal (IRL ISSN 0374-8405) **3625**
Irish Hospital (IRL) **3516**
• ➤ Irish Journal of Medical Sciences (IRL ISSN 0021-1265) **3625**
Irish Journal of Psychiatry (IRL ISSN 0790-1186) **4097**
• ➤ Irish Journal of Psychological Medicine (IRL ISSN 0790-9667) **4097**, 4408
➤ Irish Journal of Psychology (GBR ISSN 0303-3910) **4408**
• ➤ Irish Medical Journal (IRL ISSN 0332-3102) **3625**
Irish Medical News (IRL ISSN 0790-2905) **3625**
Irish Medical Times (GBR ISSN 0047-147X) **3625**
Irish Nursing Forum & Health Services (IRL ISSN 0790-7257) **3922**
Irish Pharmaceutical Union Review *see* I P U Review **4300**
➤ Irish Pharmacy Journal (IRL ISSN 0332-0707) **4304**
Irish Security News (IRL) **3396**, 4257
• ➤ Irish Veterinary Journal (IRL ISSN 0368-0762) **4545**
• Iron Metabolism (GBR ISSN 0142-8152) **3232**, 3149, 3252, 3729, 3864, 3903
Ironic Blood (USA ISSN 0895-7762) **3864**, 3903
Iryo Fukushi Gijutsu/Medical and Welfare Technology (JPN) **3625**
Iryo Hoshasen Bogo Newsletter/Newsletter on Radiological Protection in Medicine (JPN ISSN 0917-3056) **4146**
Iryo Jiko Joho Senta. Senta Nyusu/Medical Malpractice Information Center in Japan. Newsletter (JPN) **3545**, 3625
Iryo Joho Shisutemu Kenkyu Kaihatsu Hokokusho/Report of Research and Development of Medical Information System (JPN) **3625**, 3390
Iryo Johogaku/Japan Journal of Medical Informatics (JPN ISSN 0289-8055) **3625**
Iryo Kiki Gyosha Nenkan/Japanese Medical Industry Directory (JPN ISSN 1341-6162) **3370**, 3516
Iryo to Fukushi/Japanese Journal of Medical Social Work (JPN ISSN 0287-1521) **3625**, 4514
➤ Iryo to Shakai/Journal of Healthcare and Society (JPN ISSN 0916-9202) **3625**
Iryo to Shisetsu/Medical Service and Facility (JPN) **3625**
• isbi.com (Independent or Fee-paying Schools in the British Isles) (GBR ISSN 1472-0744) **3416**, 3423
Ishi Shikaishi Yakuzaishi Chosa/Survey on Physicians, Dentists and Pharmaceutists (JPN ISSN 0911-8470) **3625**, 3827, 4304
Ishikawa Kenritsu Chuo Byoin Igakushi/Ishikawa Prefectural Central Hospital. Medical Journal (JPN ISSN 0287-1777) **3625**, 3516
Ishikawa Prefectural Central Hospital. Medical Journal *see* Ishikawa Kenritsu Chuo Byoin Igakushi **3625**, 3516
Islamic Academy of Sciences. Journal *see* Islamic Academy of Sciences. Medical Journal **4505**, 3625
• ➤ Islamic Academy of Sciences. Medical Journal (TUR) **4505**, 3625
Islamic World Medical Journal (SAU ISSN 0950-4567) **4501**, 3625
• ➤ Isokinetics and Exercise Science (NLD ISSN 0959-3020) **4174**, 4017, 4356
Isotope and Radiation Research (EGY ISSN 0021-1907) **4146**
Isotope Technics, Diagnostics *see* Izotoptechnika, Diagnosztika **3373**, 4146
Isozyme *see* Gene Families and Isozymes Bulletin **3250**
Israel. Central Bureau of Statistics. Diagnostic Statistics of Hospitalizations (ISR ISSN 0075-1014) **4519**, 3525, 4529
Israel Institute for Biological Research. Publications (ISR) **3201**
Israel Institute for Biological Research. Scientific Activities *see* Israel Institute for Biological Research. Publications **3201**
Israel Journal of Medical Sciences *see* I M A J **3617**
Israel Journal of Physiotherapy (ISR ISSN 0021-2199) **4061**
• ➤ Israel Journal of Psychiatry and Related Sciences (ISR ISSN 0333-7308) **4097**
Israel Journal of Veterinary Medicine (ISR ISSN 0334-9152) **4545**

Title

Title

Title

Title

• Journal of Epidemiology and Biostatistics (GBR ISSN 1359-5229) **4479**, 3203
• ➤ Journal of Epidemiology & Community Health (GBR ISSN 0143-005X) **3632**, 4479
Journal of Epilepsy *see* Epilepsy Research **4088**, 4291
• ➤ Journal of Equine Veterinary Science (USA ISSN 0737-0806) **4545**
• ➤ Journal of Esthetic and Restorative Dentistry (CAN) **3828**, 4101
Journal of Esthetic Dentistry *see* Journal of Esthetic and Restorative Dentistry **3828**, 4101
Journal of Esthetic Dentistry (Edicion Espanola) (ESP) **3829**
Journal of Ethics, Law, and Aging *see* Ethics, Law, and Aging Review **3470**, 3538, 4347
• ➤ Journal of Ethnicity in Substance Abuse (USA ISSN 1533-2640) **3403**
➤ Journal of Ethnobiology (USA ISSN 0278-0771) **3203**, 3173, 3174
• ➤ Journal of Ethnopharmacology (IRL ISSN 0378-8741) **4307**
➤ Journal of Euromed Pharmacy (MLT ISSN 1023-3857) **4307**
• Journal of Evaluation in Clinical Practice (GBR ISSN 1356-1294) **3632**
▼ • Journal of Evaluation in Clinical Practice Online (GBR ISSN 1365-2753) **3632**
▼ • ➤ The Journal of Evidence-Based Dental Practice (USA ISSN 1532-3382) **3829**
Journal of Evidence Photography (USA) **4349**, 3883
• ➤ Journal of Evolutionary Biochemistry and Physiology (RUS ISSN 0022-0930) **3254**, 3344
• ➤ Journal of Evolutionary Biology (GBR ISSN 1010-061X) **3309**, 3281
• ➤ Journal of Evolutionary Psychology (USA ISSN 0737-4828) **4415**, 3552
• ➤ Journal of Excellence (CAN ISSN 1496-9955) **4415**
• ➤ Journal of Exercise Physiology (USA ISSN 1097-9751) **3344**
• ➤ Journal of Experimental and Clinical Cancer Research (ITA ISSN 0392-9078) **3982**
• ➤ Journal of Experimental Animal Science (DEU ISSN 0939-8600) **3876**
• ➤ Journal of Experimental Biology (GBR ISSN 0022-0949) **3203**
• ➤ Journal of Experimental Child Psychology (USA ISSN 0022-0965) **4415**, 3384
Journal of Experimental Hematology *see* Zhongguo Shiyan Xieyexue Zazhi **3905**
• ➤ Journal of Experimental Marine Biology and Ecology (NLD ISSN 0022-0981) **3203**
• ➤ The Journal of Experimental Medicine (USA ISSN 0022-1007) **3876**, 3982
Journal of Experimental Psychology *see* Journal of Experimental Psychology: General **4415**
• ➤ Journal of Experimental Psychology: Animal Behavior Processes (USA ISSN 0097-7403) **4415**
• ➤ Journal of Experimental Psychology: Applied (USA ISSN 1076-898X) **4415**
• ➤ Journal of Experimental Psychology: General (USA ISSN 0096-3445) **4415**
• ➤ Journal of Experimental Psychology: Human Perception and Performance (USA ISSN 0096-1523) **4415**
• ➤ Journal of Experimental Psychology: Learning, Memory, and Cognition (USA ISSN 0278-7393) **4415**
• ➤ Journal of Experimental Social Psychology (USA ISSN 0022-1031) **4415**, 4522
• ➤ Journal of Experimental Therapeutics and Oncology (USA ISSN 1359-4117) **3982**
▼ • Journal of Experimental Therapeutics and Oncology Online (USA) **3982**
• ➤ Journal of Experimental Zoology (USA ISSN 0022-104X) **3354**, 3876
➤ Journal of Experimental Zoology. Supplement (USA ISSN 1059-8324) **3354**, 3876
• ➤ Journal of Exposure Analysis and Environmental Epidemiology (GBR ISSN 1053-4245) **3440**, 3633
Journal of Extra-Corporeal Technology (USA ISSN 0022-1058) **3633**
➤ Journal of Eye Trauma (USA) **4000**, 4018
• ➤ Journal of Family and Economic Issues (USA ISSN 1058-0476) **4416**
Journal of Family Ecology and Consumer Science/Tydskrif vir Gesinekologie en Verbruikerswetenskappe (ZAF) **4237**, 3527
• ➤ Journal of Family Nursing (USA ISSN 1074-8407) **3924**
• ➤ Journal of Family Planning and Reproductive Health Care (GBR ISSN 1471-1893) **3359**
Journal of Family Planning Studies *see* Journal of Population and Health Studies **3359**
• ➤ Journal of Family Practice (USA ISSN 0094-3509) **3633**
• ➤ Journal of Family Psychology (USA ISSN 0893-3200) **4416**
• ➤ Journal of Family Psychotherapy (USA ISSN 0897-5353) **4416**, 4101
➤ Journal of Family Studies (AUS ISSN 1322-9400) **3554**, 4416
• ➤ Journal of Family Therapy (GBR ISSN 0163-4445) **4101**, 4416, 4522
• ➤ Journal of Family Violence (USA ISSN 0885-7482) **3395**, 4416, 4522
• Journal of Family Welfare (IND ISSN 0022-1074) **3359**
▼ • ➤ Journal of Feline Medicine and Surgery (GBR ISSN 1098-612X) **4545**, 4193
➤ Journal of Feminist Family Therapy (USA ISSN 0895-2833) **4569**, 4416
Journal of Fermentation and Bioengineering *see* Journal of Bioscience and Bioengineering **3238**, 3275
Journal of Fertilization and Implantation (JPN ISSN 0914-6776) **3955**
➤ Journal of Flow Visualization and Image Processing (USA ISSN 1065-3090) **3435**, 3153, 4365, 4365
• ➤ Journal of Fluency Disorders (USA ISSN 0094-730X) **4416**, 4522
Journal of Food and Drug Analysis *see* Yaowu Shipin Fenxi **3463**, 3881, 4248
• ➤ Journal of Food Mycology (USA ISSN 1369-1082) **3325**, 3276, 3461
• ➤ Journal of Food Protection (USA ISSN 0362-028X) **3461**, 3159, 4479
• ➤ Journal of Food Science and Nutrition (KOR ISSN 1226-332X) **4237**
• ➤ Journal of Foot and Ankle Surgery (USA ISSN 1067-2516) **4193**
Journal of Foot Surgery *see* Journal of Foot and Ankle Surgery **4193**
• ➤ Journal of Forensic Identification (USA ISSN 0895-173X) **3883**
➤ Journal of Forensic Medicine/Fayixue Zazhi (CHN ISSN 1004-5619) **3883**
➤ Journal of Forensic Neuropsychology (USA ISSN 1521-1029) **4101**
• ➤ Journal of Forensic Psychiatry (GBR ISSN 0958-5184) **4101**, 3883
▼ ➤ Journal of Forensic Psychology Practice (USA) **4416**, 3546
• ➤ Journal of Forensic Sciences (USA ISSN 0022-1198) **3883**
Journal of Gambling Behavior *see* Journal of Gambling Studies **4101**, 4525
• ➤ Journal of Gambling Studies (USA ISSN 1050-5350) **4101**, 4525
• ➤ Journal of Gastroenterology (JPN ISSN 0944-1174) **3893**
• ➤ Journal of Gastroenterology and Hepatology (AUS ISSN 0815-9319) **3893**
Journal of Gastrointestinal Motility *see* Neurogastroenterology and Motility **3894**
• ➤ Journal of Gastrointestinal Surgery (USA ISSN 1091-255X) **4193**
• ➤ Journal of Gay & Lesbian Psychotherapy (USA ISSN 0891-7140) **4416**, 3528, 4514
• ➤ Journal of Gay & Lesbian Social Services (USA ISSN 1053-8720) **4514**, 3528
Journal of Gay, Lesbian and Bisexual Identity *see* International Journal of Sexuality and Gender Studies **3527**, 4368, 4407
• The Journal of Gender-Specific Medicine (USA ISSN 1523-7036) **3633**, 3309
▼ • ➤ Journal of Gene Medicine (USA ISSN 1099-498X) **3309**, 3633
• ➤ The Journal of General and Applied Microbiology (JPN ISSN 0022-1260) **3325**
• ➤ Journal of General Internal Medicine (USA ISSN 0884-8734) **3910**
Journal of General Medicine (IND ISSN 0970-566X) **3633**
Journal of General Microbiology *see* Microbiology **3327**
Journal of General Orthodontics (USA ISSN 1048-1990) **3829**
• ➤ Journal of General Physiology (USA ISSN 0022-1295) **3344**, 3633
• ➤ The Journal of General Psychology (USA ISSN 0022-1309) **4416**
• ➤ Journal of General Virology (GBR ISSN 0022-1317) **3325**
• ➤ Journal of Genetic Counseling (USA ISSN 1059-7700) **4416**
• ➤ The Journal of Genetic Psychology (USA ISSN 0022-1325) **3309**, 4417
➤ Journal of Genetics & Breeding (ITA ISSN 0394-9257) **3309**
Journal of Geography of Health *see* Cahiers de Geographie de la Sante **3581**
Journal of Geriatric Dermatology *see* Skin & Aging **3481**, 3853
Journal of Geriatric Drug Therapy *see* Journal of Aging & Pharmacotherapy **4305**, 3475
➤ Journal of Geriatric Psychiatry (USA ISSN 0022-1414) **4101**, 3476
• ➤ Journal of Geriatric Psychiatry and Neurology (CAN ISSN 0891-9887) **3476**, 4101
Journal of Germfree Life and Gnotobiology *see* Mukin Seibutsu **3209**
• ➤ Journal of Gerontological Nursing (USA ISSN 0098-9134) **3476**, 3924
• ➤ Journal of Gerontological Social Work (USA ISSN 0163-4372) **3476**
Journal of Gerontology *see* Journals of Gerontology. Series A: Biological Sciences & Medical Sciences **3477**, 3639
Journal of Gerontology *see* Journals of Gerontology. Series B: Psychological Sciences & Social Sciences **3477**, 4424
Journal of Ginseng Research (KOR ISSN 1226-8453) **4307**, 3155
• ➤ Journal of Glaucoma (USA ISSN 1057-0829) **4000**
The Journal of Gnathology (DEU ISSN 0891-8171) **3829**
Journal of Graphoanalysis (USA ISSN 0022-1449) **4417**
Journal of Group Psychotherapy, Psychodrama and Sociometry *see* The International Journal of Action Methods **4405**, 4521
Journal of Gynaecology & Obstetrics *see* Acta Ginecologica **3943**
• ➤ Journal of Gynecologic Surgery (USA ISSN 1042-4067) **3955**, 4193
➤ Journal of Gynecologic Techniques (USA ISSN 1069-2673) **3955**
Journal of Gynecology and Obstetrics *see* Jinekoloji ve Obstetrik Dergisi **3954**
• ➤ Journal of Hand Surgery: American Volume (USA ISSN 0363-5023) **4193**
• ➤ Journal of Hand Surgery: British and European Volume (GBR ISSN 0266-7681) **4193**
➤ Journal of Hand Therapy (USA ISSN 0894-1130) **4062**
▼ • ➤ Journal of Happiness Studies (NLD ISSN 1389-4978) **4417**, 4522
• ➤ Journal of Head Trauma Rehabilitation (USA ISSN 0885-9701) **4018**
▼ • The Journal of Headache and Pain (ITA ISSN 1129-2369) **4101**
▼ • The Journal of Headache and Pain Online (ITA ISSN 1129-2377) **4102**
Journal of Health Administration Education (USA ISSN 0735-6722) **3516**, 3417
Journal of Health & Healing (USA ISSN 1044-2790) **4357**, 3633
Journal of Health and Hospital Law *see* Journal of Health Law **3633**, 3540
Journal of Health and Human Resources Administration *see* Journal of Health and Human Services Administration **3516**, 4479
➤ Journal of Health and Human Services Administration (USA ISSN 1079-3739) **3516**, 4479
Journal of Health and Place *see* Health & Place **3465**, 3610, 4472
Journal of Health & Population in Developing Countries (USA ISSN 1095-8940) **4479**, 4369
Journal of Health and Safety (GBR ISSN 0954-576X) **4257**
• ➤ Journal of Health and Social Behavior (USA ISSN 0022-1465) **4522**
• ➤ Journal of Health & Social Policy (USA ISSN 0897-7186) **4514**, 4479
Journal of Health Care Benefits (USA ISSN 1057-5073) **3368**
• ➤ Journal of Health Care Chaplaincy (USA ISSN 0885-4726) **4357**, 4500
Journal of Health Care Compliance (USA ISSN 1520-8303) **3633**, 3540
• ➤ Journal of Health Care Finance (USA ISSN 1078-6767) **3516**
• ➤ Journal of Health Care for the Poor and Underserved (USA ISSN 1049-2089) **3633**, 4514
Journal of Health Care Interior Design *see* Journal of Healthcare Design **3516**
Journal of Health Care Marketing *see* Marketing Health Services **3367**, 4358
• ➤ Journal of Health Communication (USA ISSN 1081-0730) **3633**, 3388
• ➤ Journal of Health Economics (NLD ISSN 0167-6296) **4479**, 3516
• Journal of Health Law (USA) **3633**, 3540
▼ • ➤ Journal of Health Management (IND ISSN 0972-0634) **3633**, 3516, 4459
• ➤ Journal of Health Politics, Policy and Law (USA ISSN 0361-6878) **3633**, 3516, 3540, 4367
• ➤ Journal of Health Population and Nutrition (BGD ISSN 1606-0997) **3730**, 3149, 3893
• ➤ Journal of Health Psychology (GBR ISSN 1359-1053) **4417**, 3633
• ➤ Journal of Health Science/Eisei Kagaku (JPN ISSN 1344-9702) **3452**, 3254, 4307, 4479
Journal of Health Science (USA) **4237**, 4357
Journal of Health Services Research *see* Journal of Health Services Research & Policy **3634**, 4479
• Journal of Health Services Research & Policy (GBR ISSN 1355-8196) **3634**, 4479
Journal of Healthcare and Society *see* Iryo to Shakai **3625**
Journal of Healthcare Design (USA ISSN 1068-1124) **3516**
• ➤ Journal of Healthcare Management (USA ISSN 1096-9012) **3517**
Journal of Healthcare Protection Management (USA ISSN 0891-7930) **3517**, 3396
➤ Journal of Healthcare Risk Management (USA ISSN 1074-4797) **3517**, 3532
➤ Journal of Healthcare Safety, Compliance & Infection Control (USA ISSN 1096-3707) **4258**, 3801
• ➤ The Journal of Heart and Lung Transplantation (GBR ISSN 1053-2498) **4193**
➤ Journal of Heart-Centered Therapies (USA ISSN 1520-5495) **3634**
Journal of Heart Failure (USA ISSN 1070-3837) **3778**
• ➤ The Journal of Heart Valve Disease (GBR ISSN 0966-8519) **3778**
Journal of Hebei Medicine *see* Hebei Yiyao **4299**
Journal of Hebei Traditional Chinese Medicine and Pharmacology *see* Hebei Zhongyiyao Xuebao **3613**
• ➤ Journal of Helminthology (GBR ISSN 0022-149X) **3801**
Journal of Hematotherapy *see* Journal of Hematotherapy & Stem Cell Research **3903**
• ➤ Journal of Hematotherapy & Stem Cell Research (USA ISSN 1525-8165) **3903**
• Journal of Hepato - Biliary - Pancreatic Surgery (JPN ISSN 0944-1166) **4193**
• ➤ Journal of Hepatology (NLD ISSN 0168-8278) **3893**
➤ Journal of Hepatology, Gastroenterology, Infectious Diseases (EGY) **3801**, 4479
Journal of Hepatology. Supplement (NLD ISSN 0169-5185) **3893**
▼ ➤ Journal of Herbal Pharmacotherapy (USA ISSN 1522-8940) **3910**, 3167
➤ Journal of Herbs, Spices & Medicinal Plants (USA ISSN 1049-6475) **3464**, 3281
➤ Journal of Herpetological Medicine and Surgery (USA) **3354**, 4546
• ➤ Journal of Histochemistry and Cytochemistry (USA ISSN 0022-1554) **3291**
• ➤ Journal of Histotechnology (USA ISSN 0147-8885) **3291**, 3254
➤ Journal of HIV - AIDS Prevention & Education for Adolescents & Children (USA ISSN 1069-837X) **3801**, 3384, 4479
Journal of HIV Combination Therapy *see* Journal of HIV Therapy **3801**
• ➤ Journal of HIV Therapy (GBR ISSN 1462-0308) **3801**
Journal of Hokkaido Radiological Technology *see* Hokkaido Hoshasen Gijutsu Zasshi **4145**
• Journal of Holistic Nursing (USA ISSN 0898-0101) **3924**
Journal of Home Health Care Practice *see* Home Health Care Management and Practice **3511**
• ➤ Journal of Homosexuality (USA ISSN 0091-8369) **3528**, 4522
▼ ➤ Journal of Hospice and Palliative Nursing (USA ISSN 1522-2179) **3924**
• ➤ Journal of Hospital Infection (GBR ISSN 0195-6701) **3801**
▼ • ➤ Journal of Hospital Librarianship (USA ISSN 1532-3269) **3548**, 3517
Journal of Hospital Marketing *see* Journal of Hospital Marketing & Public Relations **3367**, 3517
➤ Journal of Hospital Marketing & Public Relations (USA) **3367**, 3517

• ➤ Journal of Microscopy (GBR ISSN 0022-2720) **3334**

• ➤ Journal of Microscopy Research and Technique (USA ISSN 1059-910X) **3334**

Journal of Microsurgery *see* Microsurgery **4197**, 3879

Journal of Microwave Surgery (JPN ISSN 0917-7728) **4194**

Journal of Military Nursing & Research *see* J M N R **3923**, 4223

• ➤ Journal of Mind and Behavior (USA ISSN 0271-0137) **4418**, 4347

➤ Journal of Ministry in Addiction & Recovery (USA ISSN 1053-8755) **4500**, 3403

Journal of Modern Pharmacy (ZAF) **4308**

• ➤ Journal of Molecular and Cellular Cardiology (GBR ISSN 0022-2828) **3778**

• ➤ Journal of Molecular Biology (GBR ISSN 0022-2836) **3254**

▼ • ➤ The Journal of Molecular Diagnostics (USA ISSN 1525-1578) **3636**

• ➤ Journal of Molecular Endocrinology (GBR ISSN 0952-5041) **3865**

Journal of Molecular Epidemiology and Evolutionary Genetics and Infectious Diseases *see* Infection, Genetics and Evolution **3619**, 3308

• ➤ Journal of Molecular Evolution (USA ISSN 0022-2844) **3310**

Journal of Molecular Graphics *see* Journal of Molecular Graphics and Modelling **3377**, 3284

• ➤ Journal of Molecular Graphics and Modelling (USA ISSN 1093-3263) **3377**, 3284

• ➤ Journal of Molecular Medicine (DEU ISSN 0946-2716) **3636**

▼ • ➤ Journal of Molecular Microbiology and Biotechnology (GBR ISSN 1464-1801) **3326**, 3310

• ➤ Journal of Molecular Neuroscience (USA ISSN 0895-8696) **4102**

• ➤ Journal of Molecular Recognition (GBR ISSN 0952-3499) **3378**

• ➤ Journal of Morphology (USA ISSN 0362-2525) **3204**, 3636

• ➤ Journal of Motor Behavior (USA ISSN 0022-2895) **4418**, 3412

• ➤ Journal of Multicultural Counseling and Development (USA ISSN 0883-8534) **4418**, 3368, 3457

Journal of Multicultural Nursing *see* Journal of Multicultural Nursing and Health **3925**, 3457

➤ Journal of Multicultural Nursing and Health (USA ISSN 1526-8233) **3925**, 3457

▼ • ➤ Journal of Mundane Behavior (USA ISSN 1529-3041) **4522**, 3173, 4347, 4418

• ➤ Journal of Muscle Foods (USA ISSN 1046-0756) **3462**, 4237

• ➤ Journal of Muscle Research and Cell Motility (NLD ISSN 0142-4319) **4018**, 3291

• ➤ The Journal of Musculoskeletal and Neuronal Interactions (GRC) **4018**, 4102

Journal of Musculoskeletal Interactions *see* The Journal of Musculoskeletal and Neuronal Interactions **4018**, 4102

• ➤ The Journal of Musculoskeletal Medicine (USA ISSN 0899-2517) **4018**, 4168, 4174

• ➤ Journal of Musculoskeletal Pain (USA ISSN 1058-2452) **4019**, 3788, 4168

• ➤ Journal of Musculoskeletal Research (SGP ISSN 0218-9577) **4019**, 4168, 4174

Journal of Musculoskeletal System *see* Kotsu Kansetsu Jintai **4169**, 4021

• ➤ Journal of Music Therapy (USA ISSN 0022-2917) **4062**, 4225

Journal of Mycology and Plant Pathology *see* Indian Journal of Mycology and Plant Pathology **3280**

Journal of Myocardial Ischemia (USA ISSN 1045-7984) **3778**

▼ • ➤ Journal of Nanoscience and Nanotechnology (USA ISSN 1533-4880) **3391**, 3391, 3432, 3636

➤ Journal of Nara Medical Association (JPN ISSN 1345-0069) **3636**

• ➤ Journal of Natural History (GBR ISSN 0022-2933) **3204**

• ➤ Journal of Natural Products (USA ISSN 0163-3864) **4308**, 3254

• ➤ Journal of Natural Toxins (USA ISSN 1058-8108) **4308**, 3452

• ➤ Journal of Near-Death Studies (USA ISSN 0891-4494) **4347**, 4418

• ➤ The Journal of Neonatal Nursing (GBR ISSN 1355-1841) **3925**, 3956

Journal of Neonatal Nursing *see* Neonatal Network **3929**, 3959, 4049

Journal of Neonatology *see* Xinsheng Erke Zazhi **4057**

Journal of Nephrology *see* J N: Journal of Nephrology **4214**

Journal of Nephrology Social Work (USA) **4214**, 4514

• ➤ Journal of Nervous and Mental Disease (USA ISSN 0022-3018) **4102**

• ➤ Journal of Neural Transmission - Basic Neurosciences and Genetics - Parkinson's Disease and Allied Conditions - Alzheimer's Disease and Related Disorders - Biological Psychiatry (AUT) **4102**

Journal of Neural Transmission - Basic Neurosciences - Neurology Section - Psychiatry Section *see* Journal of Neural Transmission - Basic Neurosciences and Genetics - Parkinson's Disease and Allied Conditions - Alzheimer's Disease and Related Disorders - Biological Psychiatry **4102**

Journal of Neural Transmission. General Section *see* Journal of Neural Transmission - Basic Neurosciences and Genetics - Parkinson's Disease and Allied Conditions - Alzheimer's Disease and Related Disorders - Biological Psychiatry **4102**

Journal of Neural Transmission. Parkinson's Disease and Dementia Section *see* Journal of Neural Transmission - Basic Neurosciences and Genetics - Parkinson's Disease and Allied Conditions - Alzheimer's Disease and Related Disorders - Biological Psychiatry **4102**

• ➤ Journal of Neural Transmission. Supplement (AUT ISSN 0303-6995) **4102**

Journal of Neural Transplantation and Plasticity *see* Neural Plasticity **4112**

• ➤ Journal of Neuro-Oncology (USA ISSN 0167-594X) **3982**

• ➤ Journal of Neuro-Ophthalmology (USA ISSN 1070-8022) **4000**, 4103

• ➤ Journal of Neurobiology (USA ISSN 0022-3034) **3345**, 4103

• ➤ Journal of Neurochemistry (GBR ISSN 0022-3042) **3255**, 4103

• ➤ Journal of Neurocytology (USA ISSN 0300-4864) **3291**

• ➤ Journal of Neuroendocrinology (GBR ISSN 0953-8194) **4103**, 3865

• ➤ Journal of Neuroendocrinology Online (GBR ISSN 1365-2826) **4103**, 3865

• ➤ Journal of Neurogenetics (CHE ISSN 0167-7063) **4103**

• ➤ Journal of Neuroimaging (USA ISSN 1051-2284) **4103**, 4148

• ➤ Journal of Neuroimmunology (NLD ISSN 0165-5728) **4103**, 3749

• ➤ Journal of Neurolinguistics (GBR ISSN 0911-6044) **4103**, 3551

Journal of Neurologic Rehabilitation *see* Neurologic Rehabilitation and Repair **4114**

• ➤ Journal of Neurological Sciences/Norolojik Bilimler Dergisi (TUR ISSN 1300-1817) **4103**

• ➤ Journal of Neurology/Zeitschrift fuer Neurologie (DEU ISSN 0340-5354) **4103**

Journal of Neurology *see* Nevrologicheskii Zhurnal **4119**

Journal of Neurology and Psychiatry. S.S. Korsakov *see* Zhurnal Nevropatologii i Psikhiatrii im. S.S. Korsakova **4139**

• ➤ Journal of Neurology, Neurosurgery and Psychiatry (GBR ISSN 0022-3050) **4104**, 4194

Journal of Neurology. Supplement (DEU ISSN 0939-1517) **4104**

• ➤ Journal of Neuropathology and Experimental Neurology (USA ISSN 0022-3069) **4104**

• ➤ Journal of Neurophysiology (USA ISSN 0022-3077) **3345**, 4104

Journal of Neurophysiology Online *see* Journal of Neurophysiology **3345**, 4104

Journal of Neuroplasticity *see* Neural Plasticity **4112**

• ➤ Journal of Neuropsychiatry and Clinical Neurosciences (USA ISSN 0895-0172) **4104**

• ➤ Journal of Neuroradiology/Journal de Neuroradiologie (FRA ISSN 0150-9861) **4148**

• ➤ Journal of Neuroscience (USA ISSN 0270-6474) **4104**

Journal of Neuroscience *see* The Harvard Brain **4093**

• ➤ Journal of Neuroscience Methods (NLD ISSN 0165-0270) **4104**

• ➤ Journal of Neuroscience Nursing (USA ISSN 0888-0395) **3925**

• ➤ Journal of Neuroscience Research (USA ISSN 0360-4012) **4104**

• ➤ Journal of Neurosurgery (USA ISSN 0022-3085) **4104**, 4194

• ➤ Journal of Neurosurgical Anesthesiology (USA ISSN 0898-4921) **3758**, 4194

Journal of Neurosurgical Problems *see* Zhurnal Voprosy Neirokhirurgii im. N.N. Burdenko **4208**, 4139

• ➤ Journal of Neurosurgical Sciences (ITA ISSN 0390-5616) **4194**, 4104

• Journal of Neurotherapy (USA ISSN 1087-4208) **4105**

Journal of Neurotoxicology *see* NeuroToxicology (Little Rock) **4119**, 3453

• ➤ Journal of Neurotrauma (USA ISSN 0897-7151) **4019**, 4105

• ➤ Journal of NeuroVirology (USA ISSN 1355-0284) **4105**

• ➤ Journal of Nonverbal Behavior (USA ISSN 0191-5886) **4418**

Journal of Northern Occupational Health *see* Hoppo Sangyo Eisei **4255**

Journal of Nuclear Agriculture and Biology (IND ISSN 0379-5489) **3158**, 3204, 3431

Journal of Nuclear Biology and Medicine *see* The Quarterly Journal of Nuclear Medicine **4152**, 3214

• ➤ Journal of Nuclear Cardiology (USA ISSN 1071-3581) **4148**

• ➤ The Journal of Nuclear Medicine (USA ISSN 0161-5505) **4148**

• ➤ Journal of Nuclear Medicine Technology (USA ISSN 0091-4916) **4148**

Journal of Nurse - Midwifery *see* Journal Midwifery and Women's Health **3955**, 3923

➤ Journal of Nursing/Hu Li Tsa Chih (TWN ISSN 0047-262X) **3925**

• ➤ Journal of Nursing Administration (USA ISSN 0002-0443) **3925**

• ➤ Journal of Nursing Care Quality (USA ISSN 1057-3631) **3925**

• Journal of Nursing Education (USA ISSN 0022-3158) **3925**, 3417

➤ Journal of Nursing Law (USA ISSN 1073-7472) **3925**

• ➤ Journal of Nursing Management (GBR ISSN 0966-0429) **3925**, 3365

➤ Journal of Nursing Measurement (USA ISSN 1061-3749) **3925**

Journal of Nursing Quality Assurance *see* Journal of Nursing Care Quality **3925**

➤ Journal of Nursing Research (TWN) **3925**

• ➤ Journal of Nursing Scholarship (USA ISSN 1527-6546) **3926**, 3417

Journal of Nursing Staff Development *see* Journal for Nurses in Staff Development **3923**

➤ Journal of Nutraceuticals, Functional & Medical Foods (USA ISSN 1089-4179) **4308**, 4237

Journal of Nutrition *see* Yingyang Xuebao **4248**

• ➤ Journal of Nutrition (USA ISSN 0022-3166) **4237**

• ➤ Journal of Nutrition Education (CAN ISSN 0022-3182) **4237**, 3412

➤ Journal of Nutrition for the Elderly (USA ISSN 0163-9366) **3476**, 4237

Journal of Nutrition, Health and Aging (USA ISSN 1279-7707) **3910**, 4237

➤ Journal of Nutrition in Recipe & Menu Development (USA ISSN 1055-1379) **4237**

Journal of Nutritional and Environmental Medicine *see* Australasian College of Nutritional and Environmental Medicine. Journal **3572**, 3446, 4229

• ➤ Journal of Nutritional & Environmental Medicine (GBR ISSN 1359-0847) **4237**

• ➤ Journal of Nutritional Biochemistry (USA ISSN 0955-2863) **4238**, 3255

Journal of Nutritional Medicine *see* Journal of Nutritional & Environmental Medicine **4237**

• ➤ Journal of Nutritional Science and Vitaminology (JPN ISSN 0301-4800) **4238**

Journal of Obstetric, Gynecologic, and Neonatal Nursing *see* J O G N N **3923**, 3954

Journal of Obstetrics and Anesthesia *see* Bunben to Masui **3947**, 3756

• ➤ Journal of Obstetrics and Gynaecology (GBR ISSN 0144-3615) **3956**

• ➤ Journal of Obstetrics and Gynaecology (JPN ISSN 1341-8076) **3956**

• ➤ Journal of Obstetrics and Gynaecology of India (IND ISSN 0022-3190) **3956**

Journal of Obstetrics and Gynaecology of the British Commonwealth *see* British Journal of Obstetrics & Gynaecology **3946**

Journal of Obstetrics and Gynecology of the Republic of China *see* Taiwanese Journal of Obstetrics and Gynecology **3964**

• ➤ Journal of Occupational and Environmental Medicine (USA ISSN 1076-2752) **3636**, 3440, 4258

• ➤ Journal of Occupational and Organizational Psychology (GBR ISSN 0963-1798) **4419**

• ➤ Journal of Occupational Health (JPN ISSN 1341-9145) **4258**

➤ Journal of Occupational Health Psychology (USA ISSN 1076-8998) **4258**

• ➤ Journal of Occupational Rehabilitation (USA ISSN 1053-0487) **4258**, 4062

Journal of Ocular Pharmacology *see* Journal of Ocular Pharmacology and Therapeutics **4000**, 3476, 4308

• ➤ Journal of Ocular Pharmacology and Therapeutics (USA ISSN 1080-7683) **4000**, 3476, 4308

Journal of Ocular Trauma *see* Journal of Eye Trauma **4000**, 4018

• ➤ Journal of Offender Rehabilitation (USA ISSN 1050-9674) **3395**, 4419, 4514

Journal of Oncology Management (USA ISSN 1061-9364) **3982**

• ➤ Journal of Oncology Pharmacy Practice (USA ISSN 1078-1552) **4308**, 3982

➤ The Journal of One-Day Surgery (GBR) **4194**

Journal of Operative Dentistry *see* Operative Dentistry **3834**

• Journal of Ophthalmic Nursing & Technology (USA ISSN 0744-7132) **3926**, 4001

➤ Journal of Optometric Vision Development (USA ISSN 0149-886X) **4001**

Journal of Oral Anatomy *see* Koku Kaibo Kenkyu **3641**

• ➤ Journal of Oral and Maxillofacial Surgery (USA ISSN 0278-2391) **3829**, 4194

➤ Journal of Oral Implantology (USA ISSN 0160-6972) **3829**

▼ Journal of Oral Laser Applications (USA) **3829**

• ➤ Journal of Oral Pathology & Medicine (DNK ISSN 0904-2512) **3829**

• ➤ Journal of Oral Rehabilitation (GBR ISSN 0305-182X) **3829**

▼ • ➤ Journal of Oral Rehabilitation Online (GBR ISSN 1365-2842) **3829**

• ➤ Journal of Oral Science (JPN ISSN 1343-4934) **3829**

• ➤ Journal of Organizational Behavior Management (USA ISSN 0160-8061) **4419**, 3368

• ➤ Journal of Organizational Behaviour (GBR ISSN 0894-3796) **4419**, 4522

➤ Journal of Orgonomy (USA ISSN 0022-3298) **4105**, 4365

• ➤ Journal of Orofacial Orthopedics (DEU ISSN 1434-5293) **4019**

• ➤ Journal of Orofacial Pain (USA ISSN 1064-6655) **3830**

• ➤ The Journal of Orthodontics (GBR ISSN 1465-3125) **3830**

Journal of Orthomolecular Medicine (CAN ISSN 0834-4825) **4105**

• ➤ Journal of Orthopaedic and Sports Physical Therapy (USA ISSN 0190-6011) **4174**, 4019, 4062

• ➤ Journal of Orthopaedic Nursing (GBR ISSN 1361-3111) **3926**, 4019

• ➤ Journal of Orthopaedic Research (USA ISSN 0736-0266) **4019**

• Journal of Orthopaedic Science (JPN ISSN 0949-2658) **4019**

Journal of Orthopaedic Surgery *see* European Journal of Orthopaedic Surgery **4014**

• Journal of Orthopaedic Surgery (HKG ISSN 1022-5536) **4019**

• ➤ Journal of Orthopaedic Trauma (USA ISSN 0890-5339) **4019**

Journal of Orthopedic Surgical Techniques (GBR ISSN 0334-0236) **4194**, 4019

• ➤ Journal of Otolaryngology (CAN ISSN 0381-6605) **4034**

Journal of Otolaryngology, Head and Neck Surgery *see* J O H N S: Journal of Otolaryngology, Head and Neck Surgery **4034**, 4017

➤ Journal of Otolaryngology of Japan/Nihon Jibi Inkoka Gakkai Kaiho (JPN ISSN 0030-6622) **4034**

➤ Journal of Outcome Measurement (JOM) (USA ISSN 1090-655X) **3412**, 3424, 4223, 4419

➤ Journal of Outcomes Research (GBR ISSN 1369-698X) **4309**, 3517

• ➤ Journal of Paediatrics and Child Health (AUS ISSN 1034-4810) **4047**

Title

Title

Journal of Rehabilitation & Health *see* International Journal of Rehabilitation and Health **3485**, 4407
● ➤ Journal of Rehabilitation Medicine (SWE ISSN 1650-1977) **4515**, 3637
Journal of Rehabilitation Medicine. Supplement (SWE) **4515**, 3637
➤ Journal of Rehabilitation Outcomes Measurement (USA ISSN 1086-9654) **4062**
● ➤ Journal of Rehabilitation Research and Development (USA ISSN 0748-7711) **4020**, 3432
Journal of Religion and Aging *see* Journal of Religious Gerontology **3476**, 4501
● ➤ Journal of Religion and Health (USA ISSN 0022-4197) **4500**, 3637
➤ Journal of Religion, Disability & Health (USA ISSN 1522-8967) **4500**, 3485
Journal of Religion in Disability and Rehabilitation *see* Journal of Religion, Disability & Health **4500**, 3485
Journal of Religion in Psychotherapy *see* American Journal of Pastoral Counseling **4374**, 4499
➤ Journal of Religious Gerontology (USA ISSN 1050-2289) **3476**, 4501
● ➤ Journal of Renal Nutrition (USA ISSN 1051-2276) **4238**, 4214
➤ Journal of Reproduction and Development (JPN ISSN 0916-8818) **4546**
Journal of Reproduction and Fertility *see* Reproduction **3215**, 3684
Journal of Reproduction and Fertility (IND) **3205**, 3637
Journal of Reproduction and Fertility. Abstract Series *see* Reproduction. Abstract Series **3235**, 3152, 3348, 3736
Journal of Reproduction and Fertility. Supplement *see* Reproduction. Supplement **3348**, 3262, 3684
● ➤ Journal of Reproductive and Infant Psychology (GBR ISSN 0264-6838) **4421**
Journal of Reproductive Biology and Comparative Endocrinology *see* Journal of Endocrinology & Reproduction **3203**, 3865
● ➤ Journal of Reproductive Immunology (IRL ISSN 0165-0378) **3749**, 3957
● ➤ Journal of Reproductive Medicine (USA ISSN 0024-7758) **3957**
● ➤ Journal of Research in Personality (USA ISSN 0092-6566) **4422**
➤ Journal of Research in Pharmaceutical Economics (USA ISSN 0896-6621) **4310**, 3363
● ➤ Journal of Research on Adolescence (USA ISSN 1532-7795) **3384**, 4422
● ➤ The Journal of Respiratory Diseases (USA ISSN 0194-259X) **4161**
▼ ➤ Journal of Respiratory Diseases for Pediatricians (USA) **4047**, 4161
● ➤ Journal of Rheumatology (CAN ISSN 0315-162X) **4169**
Journal of Rheumatology and Medical Rehabilitation *see* Romatoloji ve Tibbi Rehabilitasyon Dergisi **4171**, 4066
● ➤ Journal of Risk and Uncertainty (USA ISSN 0895-5646) **3363**, 3365, 4422, 4529
● ➤ The Journal of Rural Health (USA ISSN 0890-765X) **3637**, 4479, 4522
➤ Journal of Russian and East European Psychology (USA ISSN 1061-0405) **4422**
● ➤ Journal of Safety Research (GBR ISSN 0022-4375) **4258**, 4532
● ➤ Journal of School Health (USA ISSN 0022-4391) **4479**, 3413
➤ Journal of School Nursing (USA ISSN 1059-8405) **3926**, 3413
Journal of School Psychology *see* Psykologisk Paedagogisk Raadgivning **4443**, 3414
● ➤ Journal of School Psychology (GBR ISSN 0022-4405) **4422**
➤ Journal of Science and Medicine in Sport (AUS ISSN 1440-2440) **4174**
Journal of Science of Labour *see* Rodo Kagaku (Kawasaki, 1924) **4264**
Journal of Scientific Research in Plants & Medicines (IND ISSN 0253-7249) **4311**, 3637, 4505
Journal of Senile Dementia *see* Ronenkichiho **4132**
● ➤ Journal of Sensory Studies (USA ISSN 0887-8250) **4106**, 3462, 4238
➤ Journal of Serotonin Research (GBR ISSN 1350-7702) **4106**, 3345
● ➤ Journal of Sex & Marital Therapy (GBR ISSN 0092-623X) **4422**
➤ Journal of Sex Education and Therapy (USA ISSN 0161-4576) **4357**, 4422
● ➤ Journal of Sex Research (USA ISSN 0022-4499) **4422**, 3637, 4522
Journal of Sexual Aggression (GBR ISSN 1355-2600) **4422**, 3395
● ➤ Journal of Shoulder and Elbow Surgery (USA ISSN 1058-2746) **4195**
● ➤ Journal of Sleep Research (GBR ISSN 0962-1105) **3637**, 4422
▼ ● ➤ Journal of Sleep Research Online (GBR ISSN 1365-2869) **3638**, 4422
Journal of Sleep Research. Supplement (GBR ISSN 0966-6826) **3638**, 4422
● ➤ Journal of Small Animal Practice (GBR ISSN 0022-4510) **4546**
Journal of Smooth Muscle Research/Nihon Heikatsukin Gakkai Kikanshi (JPN ISSN 0916-8737) **3638**, 4174
Journal of Snake *see* She Zhi **3692**, 3356
➤ Journal of Social and Administrative Pharmacy (SWE ISSN 0281-0662) **4311**
Journal of Social and Administrative Pharmacy. Supplement (SWE ISSN 0282-6607) **4311**
Journal of Social and Biological Structures *see* Journal of Social and Evolutionary Systems **4422**, 3205
● ➤ Journal of Social and Clinical Psychology (USA ISSN 0736-7236) **4422**
● ➤ Journal of Social and Evolutionary Systems (GBR ISSN 1061-7361) **4422**, 3205
● ➤ Journal of Social and Personal Relationships (GBR ISSN 0265-4075) **4423**
● ➤ Journal of Social Behavior and Personality (USA ISSN 0886-1641) **4423**, 4509
● ➤ Journal of Social Distress and the Homeless (USA ISSN 1053-0789) **4515**, 4423, 4522
● ➤ Journal of Social Issues (USA ISSN 0022-4537) **4423**, 4522
● ➤ The Journal of Social Psychology (USA ISSN 0022-4545) **4423**
● ➤ Journal of Social Work Practice (GBR ISSN 0265-0533) **4515**, 3384, 3403
▼ ● Journal of Social Work Practice in the Addictions (USA ISSN 1533-256X) **4515**, 3403
● ➤ The Journal of Special Education (USA ISSN 0022-4669) **3424**
Journal of Speech and Hearing Research *see* Journal of Speech, Language, and Hearing Research **3491**, 3551
● ➤ Journal of Speech, Language, and Hearing Research (USA ISSN 1092-4388) **3491**, 3551
➤ Journal of Spinal Cord Medicine (USA ISSN 1079-0268) **4062**, 4106
● ➤ Journal of Spinal Disorders (USA ISSN 0895-0385) **4020**, 4195
● ➤ Journal of Spiritual Bodywork (USA ISSN 1079-8390) **3167**, 4221, 4501, 4564
Journal of Spirochetal and Tickborne Diseases (USA) **3802**
● ➤ Journal of Sport and Exercise Psychology (USA ISSN 0895-2779) **4423**, 4174, 4525
● ➤ Journal of Sport Behavior (USA ISSN 0162-7341) **4525**, 4423
● ➤ Journal of Sport Rehabilitation (USA ISSN 1056-6716) **4174**, 4062
● ➤ Journal of Sports Chiropractic and Rehabilitation (USA ISSN 1084-1288) **3788**, 4175
● ➤ The Journal of Sports Medicine and Physical Fitness (ITA ISSN 0022-4707) **4175**, 4357
● ➤ Journal of Sports Sciences (GBR ISSN 0264-0414) **4525**, 4175
Journal of Sports Traumatology and Related Research *see* European Journal of Sports Traumatology and Related Research **4173**, 4014
Journal of Steroid Biochemistry *see* Journal of Steroid Biochemistry and Molecular Biology **3255**
● ➤ Journal of Steroid Biochemistry and Molecular Biology (GBR ISSN 0960-0760) **3255**
Journal of Strategic and Systematic Therapies *see* Journal of Systemic Therapies **4423**, 4106
● ➤ Journal of Strength and Conditioning Research (USA ISSN 1064-8011) **4175**, 4357
● ➤ Journal of Stroke and Cerebrovascular Diseases (USA ISSN 1052-3057) **3778**
● ➤ Journal of Structural Biology (USA ISSN 1047-8477) **3205**
Journal of Structural Learning *see* Journal of Structural Learning and Intelligent Systems **4423**, 3429, 3553
● ➤ Journal of Structural Learning and Intelligent Systems (CHE ISSN 1027-1015) **4423**, 3429, 3553
● ➤ Journal of Studies on Alcohol (USA ISSN 0096-882X) **3403**
➤ Journal of Submicroscopic Cytology and Pathology (ITA ISSN 1122-9497) **3291**, 3266
● ➤ Journal of Substance Abuse (GBR ISSN 0899-3289) **3403**
● ➤ Journal of Substance Abuse Treatment (USA ISSN 0740-5472) **3404**
Journal of Substance Misuse *see* Journal of Substance Use **3404**, 3926
● ➤ Journal of Substance Use (GBR ISSN 1465-9891) **3404**, 3926
● ➤ Journal of Surgical Oncology (USA ISSN 0022-4790) **4195**, 3983
➤ Journal of Surgical Outcomes (USA ISSN 1095-7340) **4195**
● ➤ Journal of Surgical Pathology (GBR ISSN 1078-9553) **3638**, 4195
Journal of Surgical Practice (USA ISSN 0161-9721) **4195**
● ➤ Journal of Surgical Research (USA ISSN 0022-4804) **4195**
● ➤ Journal of Swine Health and Production (USA ISSN 1537-209X) **4546**
● ➤ Journal of Symbolic Logic (USA ISSN 0022-4812) **3553**
● Journal of Systemic Therapies (USA ISSN 1195-4396) **4423**, 4106
● ➤ Journal of Teaching in Physical Education (USA ISSN 0273-5024) **3429**, 4525
▼ ● ➤ Journal of Technology in Counseling (USA) **4423**, 3391
● Journal of Telemedicine and Telecare (GBR ISSN 1357-633X) **3638**
● ➤ Journal of Texture Studies (USA ISSN 0022-4901) **3435**
Journal of Thanatology *see* Advances in Thanatology **4373**, 3501, 4460
Journal of the American Academy of Child and Adolescent Psychiatry *see* American Academy of Child and Adolescent Psychiatry. Journal **4071**, 3380
Journal of the American Academy of Nurse Practitioners *see* American Academy of Nurse Practitioners. Journal **3913**
Journal of the American Association of Forensic Dentists (USA ISSN 0743-491X) **3830**
Journal of the American Board of Family Practice *see* American Board of Family Practice. Journal **3562**
Journal of the American College of Cardiology *see* American College of Cardiology. Journal **3761**
Journal of the American College of Surgeons *see* American College of Surgeons. Journal **4179**
Journal of the American Dental Association *see* American Dental Association. Journal **3814**
Journal of the American Geriatrics Society *see* American Geriatrics Society. Journal **3467**
Journal of the American Medical Association *see* J A M A: The Journal of the American Medical Association **3626**
Journal of the American Medical Association Asthma Newsline *see* J A M A Asthma Newsline **4161**
Journal of the American Medical Association Brasil *see* J A M A Brasil **3626**
Journal of the American Medical Association Contraception Newsline *see* J A M A Contraception Newsline **3359**, 4564, 4568
Journal of the American Medical Association HIV - Aids Newsline *see* J A M A HIV - Aids Newsline **3800**
Journal of the American Medical Association Migraine Newsline *see* J A M A Migraine Newsline **4098**
Journal of the American Medical Association Sexually Transmitted Disease *see* J A M A Sexually Transmitted Disease **3800**
Journal of the American Medical Association Women's Health Newsline *see* J A M A Women's Health Newsline **4564**
▼ ● ➤ Journal of the American Medical Directors Association (USA ISSN 1525-8610) **3517**
Journal of the American Podiatric Medical Association *see* American Podiatric Medical Association. Journal **4010**
● ➤ Journal of the Anatomical Society of India. (IND) **3205**, 3638
Journal of the Association for Research in Otolaryngology *see* J A R O **4034**
Journal of the Association of Nurses in AIDS Care *see* Association of Nurses in AIDS Care. Journal **3793**, 3914
Journal of the Autonomic Nervous System *see* Autonomic Neuroscience: Basic & Clinical **4075**
Journal of the Bahrain Medical Society *see* Bahrain Medical Society. Journal **3573**
Journal of the British Homeopathic Society *see* British Homeopathic Journal **3786**
Journal of the Chemical Society. Perkin Transactions 1 *see* Royal Chemical Society. Journal. Perkin Transactions 1 **3379**, 3262
Journal of the College of Physicians and Surgeons Pakistan *see* College of Physicians and Surgeons Pakistan. Journal **3588**
Journal of the Diabetic Association of India. Education Section *see* Diabetic Association of India. Journal. Education Section **3859**
Journal of the Diabetic Association of India. Scientific Section *see* Diabetic Association of India. Journal. Scientific Section **3859**
Journal of the Egyptian Medical Association *see* Egyptian Medical Association. Journal **3597**
● ➤ Journal of the Experimental Analysis of Behavior (USA ISSN 0022-5002) **4423**
Journal of the Faculty of Veterinary Medicine *see* Majallah-i Danishkadah-i Dampizishki **4548**
Journal of the Formosan Medical Association *see* Formosan Medical Association. Journal **3603**
Journal of the Gay and Lesbian Medical Association *see* Gay and Lesbian Medical Association. Journal **3605**, 3527, 4368
● ➤ Journal of the History of Biology (NLD ISSN 0022-5010) **3205**, 3526
➤ Journal of the History of Dentistry (USA ISSN 1089-6287) **3830**
● ➤ Journal of the History of Medicine and Allied Sciences (USA ISSN 0022-5045) **3638**, 3526
● ➤ Journal of the History of Sexuality (USA ISSN 1043-4070) **4522**, 4424
● ➤ Journal of the History of the Behavioral Sciences (USA ISSN 0022-5061) **4424**, 3526
● ➤ Journal of the History of the Neurosciences (NLD ISSN 0964-704X) **4106**
● ➤ Journal of the Hong Kong College of Cardiology (AUS ISSN 1027-7811) **3779**
● ➤ Journal of the Hong Kong College of Cardiology Online (AUS) **3779**
Journal of the Hong Kong College of Radiologists (HKG) **4148**
▼ ➤ Journal of the I C R U (GBR ISSN 1473-6691) **4366**, 3440, 3638, 4480
Journal of the I S R P *see* International Society for Respiratory Protection. Journal **4160**, 4257
➤ Journal of the Indian Medical Association (GBR ISSN 1474-3655) **3638**
Journal of the Indian Medical Profession (IND) **3638**
Journal of the International Neuropsychological Society *see* International Neuropsychological Society. Journal **4097**
● ➤ Journal of the Learning Sciences (USA ISSN 1050-8406) **3413**, 4424
Journal of the Marine Biological Association of the United Kingdom *see* Marine Biological Association of the United Kingdom. Journal **3207**
Journal of the Medical and Dental Defence Unions (GBR) **3638**, 3830
Journal of the Medical Association of Thailand *see* Medical Association of Thailand. Journal **3649**
Journal of the Medical Defence Union *see* Journal of the Medical and Dental Defence Unions **3638**, 3830
● ➤ Journal of the Medical Library Association (USA) **3638**, 3548
Journal of the Medical Sciences/Berkala Ilmu Kedokteran (IDN ISSN 0126-1312) **3638**
Journal of the National Cancer Institute *see* National Cancer Institute. Journal **3985**
Journal of the National Cancer Institute. Monographs *see* National Cancer Institute. Journal. Monographs **3985**
● ➤ Journal of the Neurological Sciences (NLD ISSN 0022-510X) **4106**
● ➤ Journal of the Neuromusculoskeletal System (USA ISSN 1067-8239) **3788**, 4106
Journal of the Northamerican Association of Masters in Psyhcology *see* Journal of Psychological Practice **4420**
▼ ● ➤ Journal of the Pancreas (ITA ISSN 1590-8577) **3893**, 3865
Journal of the Pennsylvania Osteopathic Medical Association *see* Pennsylvania Osteopathic Medical Association. Journal **3674**, 3789

Title

Kagaku Ryoho no Ryoiki/Antibiotics and Chemotherapy (JPN ISSN 0913-2384) **3910**
Kagawa Colloquium on Neurosurgery. Journal *see* Kagawa No Shinkei Geka Danwakai Kaishi **4107**, 4195
Kagawa No Shinkei Geka Danwakai Kaishi/Kagawa Colloquium on Neurosurgery. Journal (JPN ISSN 0918-1172) **4107**, 4195
Kagawa Nutrition College. Journal *see* Joshi Eiyo Daigaku Kiyo **4237**
Kagoshima Association for Acute Medicine. Journal *see* Kagoshima Kyukyu Igakkaishi **3639**
Kagoshima Daigaku Igaku Zasshi/Medical Journal of Kagoshima University (JPN ISSN 0368-5063) **3639**
Kagoshima Kyukyu Igakkaishi/Kagoshima Association for Acute Medicine. Journal (JPN ISSN 0913-5073) **3639**
Kagoshima Society for Clinical Surgery. Journal *see* Kagoshimaken Rinsho Geka Ikaishi **4195**
Kagoshimaken Rinsho Geka Ikaishi/Kagoshima Society for Clinical Surgery. Journal (JPN ISSN 0913-459X) **4195**
➤ Kai Tiaki: Nursing New Zealand (NZL ISSN 1173-2032) **3927**
Kaibogaku Zasshi *see* Acta Anatomica Nipponica **3178**, 3172, 3284, 3557
Kaigai Ganka Bunken Joho/Ophthalmology Update (JPN) **4001**
Kaku Igaku/Japanese Journal of Nuclear Medicine (JPN ISSN 0022-7854) **4149**
Kaku Igaku Gazo Shindan/Imaging Diagnosis in Nuclear Medicine (JPN ISSN 0912-4195) **4149**
Kaku Igaku Gijutsu/Japanese Journal of Nuclear Medicine Technology (JPN ISSN 0289-100X) **4149**
Kaku Igaku Semina Shoreishu/Tokai Seminar in Nuclear Medicine (JPN ISSN 0912-6104) **4149**
Kaku Igaku Shorei Kentokai Shoreishu/Proceedings of Meeting on Case of Nuclear Medicine (JPN ISSN 0910-2213) **4149**
Kaleidoscope (Akron) (USA ISSN 0748-8742) **3485**, 3175, 3552
Kaleidoscope (Toronto) *see* The Hospital for Sick Children Journal **4045**, 3513
Kaleidoscope (Toronto) *see* Kids' Health **4048**
Kampo and Immuno-Allergy *see* Kanpo to Men'Eki Arerugi **3167**
Kanagawa Association of Psychiatry. Journal *see* Kanagawa-ken Seishin Igakkaishi **4107**
Kanagawa Dental College. Bulletin (JPN ISSN 0385-1443) **3830**
Kanagawa Hospital Pharmacists Association. Journal *see* Kanagawaken Byoin Yakuzaishikai Kaishi **4311**
Kanagawa Journal of Orthopedics and Traumatology *see* Kanagawa Seikei Saigai Geka Ikai Zasshi **4020**
Kanagawa Journal of Psychopharmacology *see* Kanagawa Seishin Yakuri **4424**, 4311
Kanagawa Kansetsu Geka Kenkyukaishi/Joint (JPN ISSN 0912-0904) **4196**
➤ Kanagawa-ken Seishin Igakkaishi/Kanagawa Association of Psychiatry. Journal (JPN ISSN 0288-9617) **4107**
Kanagawa Odontological Society. Journal *see* Kanagawa Shigaku **3830**
Kanagawa Physical Therapy Association. News *see* Kanagawaken Rigaku Ryohoshikai Nyusu **4062**
Kanagawa Rehabilitation Center. Journal *see* Kanagawaken Sogo Rihabiriteshon Senta Kiyo **4062**
Kanagawa Seikei Saigai Geka Ikai Zasshi/Kanagawa Journal of Orthopedics and Traumatology (JPN ISSN 0915-1451) **4020**
Kanagawa Seishin Yakuri/Kanagawa Journal of Psychopharmacology (JPN ISSN 0918-0354) **4424**, 4311
Kanagawa Shigaku/Kanagawa Odontological Society. Journal (JPN ISSN 0454-8302) **3830**
Kanagawaken Byoin Yakuzaishikai Kaishi/Kanagawa Hospital Pharmacists Association. Journal (JPN ISSN 0285-4775) **4311**
Kanagawaken Rigaku Ryohoshikai Nyusu/Kanagawa Physical Therapy Association. News (JPN) **4062**
Kanagawaken Sogo Rihabiriteshon Senta Kiyo/Kanagawa Rehabilitation Center. Journal (JPN ISSN 0285-3477) **4062**
Kanalen (SWE) **3927**
➤ Kanazawa Daigaku Igakubu Hokengakka Sagyo Ryohogakka Sotsugyo Kenkyu Ronbunshu/Kanazawa University. School of Health Sciences. Department of Occupational Therapy. Collection of Papers (JPN) **3639**
Kanazawa Daigaku Iryou Gijutsu Tanki Daigakubu Sagyo Ryohogakka Sotsugyo Kenkyu Ronbunshu *see* Kanazawa Daigaku Igakubu Hokengakka Sagyo Ryohogakka Sotsugyo Kenkyu Ronbunshu **3639**
Kanazawa University. School of Health Sciences. Department of Occupational Therapy. Collection of Papers *see* Kanazawa Daigaku Igakubu Hokengakka Sagyo Ryohogakka Sotsugyo Kenkyu Ronbunshu **3639**
Kandang Kerbau Hospital Bulletin *see* Singapore Journal of Obstetrics & Gynaecology **3964**, 3360, 3522
Kang Fu/Rehabilitation (CHN) **4062**
Kangli Shijie/Health and Happiness (CHN) **4357**
Kango/Nursing (JPN ISSN 0022-8362) **3927**
Kango Gakusei/Nurse Student (JPN ISSN 0385-5988) **3927**
Kango Gijutsu/Japanese Journal of Nursing Arts (JPN ISSN 0449-752X) **3927**
Kango Kenkyu/Japanese Journal of Nursing Research (JPN ISSN 0022-8370) **3927**
Kango Kyoiku/Japanese Journal of Nursing Education (JPN ISSN 0047-1895) **3927**
Kango Tenbo/Japanese Journal of Nursing Science (JPN ISSN 0385-549X) **3927**
Kangogaku Zasshi/Nursing Magazine (JPN ISSN 0387-351X) **3927**
Kanko Shikiso/Medical Researches for Photosensitizing Dyes (JPN ISSN 0461-5956) **4149**
Kanpo Igaku/Chinese Medicine (JPN ISSN 0288-2485) **3167**
Kanpo Kenkyu/Study on Chinese Medicine (JPN ISSN 0385-6526) **3167**
Kanpo no Rinsho/Journal of Kampo Medicine (JPN ISSN 0451-307X) **3167**
Kanpo to Men'Eki Arerugi/Kampo and Immuno-Allergy (JPN ISSN 0914-6407) **3167**
Kanpoyakuho/Chinese Drug News (JPN) **4312**
Kansai College of Acupuncture Medicine. Annual Report *see* Kansai Shinkyu Tanki Daigaku Nenpo **3167**
Kansai Ika Daigaku. Zasshi *see* Kansai Medical University. Journal **3639**
Kansai Kansetsukyo Hiza Kenkyukaishi/Journal of Kansai Arthroscopy and Knee (JPN ISSN 0915-7786) **4020**, 4196
Kansai Medical University. Journal/Kansai Ika Daigaku. Zasshi (JPN) **3639**
Kansai Shinkyu Tanki Daigaku Nenpo/Kansai College of Acupuncture Medicine. Annual Report (JPN ISSN 0912-9545) **3167**
Kansas Dental Association. Journal (USA ISSN 0888-7063) **3831**
• ➤ Kansas Entomological Society. Journal (USA ISSN 0022-8567) **3297**
• Kansas Nurse (USA ISSN 0022-8710) **3927**
Kansas Optometric Journal (USA ISSN 1063-1623) **4001**
Kansas Physician (USA) **3639**, 3541
Kansas State Board of Nursing. Newsletter (USA) **3927**
Kansenshogaku Zasshi *see* Japanese Association for Infectious Diseases. Journal **3800**
➤ Kansetsu Geka/Journal of Joint Surgery (JPN ISSN 0286-5394) **4020**
Kansetsu no Geka/Joint Surgery (JPN ISSN 0285-6255) **4020**
Kanto Journal of Orthopedics and Traumatology *see* Kanto Seikei Saigai Geka Gakkai Zasshi **4020**
Kanto Seikei Saigai Geka Gakkai Zasshi/Kanto Journal of Orthopedics and Traumatology (JPN ISSN 0389-7087) **4020**
Kanzo/Acta Hepatologica Japonica (JPN ISSN 0451-4203) **3893**
Kaohsiung Journal of Medical Sciences (TWN ISSN 0257-5655) **3639**, 4312
Kapuseru/Capsule (JPN ISSN 0287-2358) **4312**
• ➤ Kardiologia Polska/Polish Heart Journal (POL ISSN 0022-9032) **3779**
Kardiologie Assistenz (DEU ISSN 0938-7293) **3779**
• ➤ Kardiologiya/Cardiology (RUS ISSN 0022-9040) **3779**
Kardiovaskulaere Medizin/Medecine Cardiovasculaire (CHE ISSN 1423-5528) **3779**
Karnataka Medical Journal (IND ISSN 0377-9378) **3639**
➤ Karolinska Institute Nobel Conference Series (USA ISSN 1040-3353) **3639**
Kartei der Praktischen Medizin (DEU ISSN 0022-9113) **3730**, 3149
Karushumu Shinpojumu Koen Yoshi/Abstracts of Calcium Symposium (JPN) **3232**, 3149, 3206
Karyogram *see* Applied Cytogenetics **3299**, 3268, 3285
➤ Kasmera (VEN ISSN 0075-5222) **3639**
Kateiyaku Kenkyu/Research on Home Medicines (JPN ISSN 0289-4750) **4312**
Katern Vrouwenzelfhulp (NLD) **4564**, 4515, 4568
Katholischer Berufsverband fuer Pflegeberufe. Mitteilungsblatt (DEU) **3640**, 4502
Katsu/Japan Institute of Traditional Medicine. News (JPN ISSN 0912-0718) **3167**
Kawasaki Igakkai Shi (JPN ISSN 0386-5924) **3640**
Kawasaki Medical Journal (JPN ISSN 0385-0234) **3640**
Kawasaki Municipal Hospital. Annual Report *see* Kawasaki Shiritsu Kawasaki Byoin Nenpo **3517**
Kawasaki Municipal Ida Hospital. Annual Report *see* Kawasaki Shiritsu Ida Byoin Nenpo **3517**
Kawasaki Shiritsu Ida Byoin Nenpo/Kawasaki Municipal Ida Hospital. Annual Report (JPN) **3517**
Kawasaki Shiritsu Kawasaki Byoin Nenpo/Kawasaki Municipal Hospital. Annual Report (JPN) **3517**
Kazanskii Meditsinskii Zhurnal (RUS ISSN 0368-4814) **3640**
Keele Cognition Seminars (GBR ISSN 0952-1194) **4424**
Keele Papers in Geriatric Medicine and Gerontology (GBR ISSN 1365-9898) **3477**
Keeping the Trust (USA) **4515**, 4480
• ➤ Keio Journal of Medicine (JPN ISSN 0022-9717) **3640**
➤ Keiraku Chiryo/Japanese Society of Acupuncture. Journal (JPN) **3167**
Keisei Geka *see* Japanese Journal of Plastic & Reconstructive Surgery **4192**
Kekkaku/Tuberculosis (JPN ISSN 0022-9776) **4161**
Kekkaku No Kenkyu *see* Hokkaido University. Institute of Immunological Science. Bulletin **4160**, 3744
Kekkan/Japanese Journal of Circulation Research (JPN ISSN 0911-4637) **3779**
Kekkan to Naihi/Blood Vessel & Endothelium (JPN ISSN 0917-5318) **3779**
Keller's Compliance Focus (USA ISSN 1087-853X) **4258**
Keller's Industrial Safety Report (USA ISSN 1053-3826) **4258**
Keller's O S H A Safety Training Guide *see* Keller's O S H A Safety Training Newsletter **4258**
Keller's O S H A Safety Training Newsletter (USA ISSN 1077-7008) **4258**
Keller's Regulatory Update *see* Keller's Compliance Focus **4258**
Keller's Safety Management Today Newsletter (USA ISSN 1090-3445) **4258**
Keller's Transportation Safety Training Newsletter (USA ISSN 1082-104X) **4532**, 4258
Kenketsu Jigyo no Genkyo/Blood Donation in Nara Prefecture (JPN) **3903**
• ➤ Kennedy Institute of Ethics. Journal (USA ISSN 1054-6863) **3640**, 4347
Kennedy Institute of Ethics. Scope Note (USA) **3640**, 4347
Kennel and Cattery Management (GBR) **4272**
Kensa to Gijutsu/Modern Medical Laboratory (JPN ISSN 0301-2611) **3877**
Kensetsu Koji Saigai Boshi Teianshu/Proposals for Industrial Safety of Construction (JPN) **4258**, 3361
Kentucky Academy of Family Physicians Journal *see* K A F P Journal **3639**
Kentucky Annual Vital Statistics Report (USA) **4496**, 4529
Kentucky. Cabinet for Health Services. Vital Statistics Report *see* Kentucky Annual Vital Statistics Report **4496**, 4529
Kentucky Dental Association. Journal (USA ISSN 0744-396X) **3831**
➤ Kentucky Medical Association. Journal (USA ISSN 0023-0294) **3640**
Kentucky Medical News (USA) **3640**
Kentucky Nurse (USA ISSN 0742-8367) **3927**
The Kentucky Pharmacist (USA ISSN 0194-567X) **4312**
Kenya Agricultural Research Institute. Veterinary Research Department. Annual Report (KEN) **4547**
Kenya Medical Research Institute. Annual Report (KEN ISSN 0076-5988) **3640**
Kenya. Ministry of Health. Annual Report (KEN) **3640**
Kenya. Ministry of Health. Health Information Bulletin (KEN ISSN 0140-5071) **4480**, 3802
Kenya. Ministry of Health. Health Information System (KEN) **3640**
Kenya Nursing Journal (KEN ISSN 0301-0333) **3927**
Kenya Veterinarian (KEN ISSN 0256-5161) **4547**
Kerala Academy of Biology. Journal (IND ISSN 0374-860X) **3206**
Kerala Homoeo Journal (IND ISSN 0300-3957) **3789**
Kerala Medical Journal (IND ISSN 0301-4827) **3640**
Kern County Dental Society Newsletter *see* Kern County Dental Society Occlusal Register **3831**
Kern County Dental Society Occlusal Register (USA) **3831**
Kessei Hanno no Ayumi/Study Report of Serum Reaction (JPN ISSN 0913-9532) **3903**
➤ Ketju (FIN ISSN 0355-2918) **4048**, 4515
Ketsueki Frontier/Practical Hematology (JPN ISSN 1344-6940) **3903**
Ketsueki Jigyo/Blood Programme (JPN) **3903**
Ketsuekigaku Semina/Seminar in Hematology (JPN) **3903**
➤ Kevo Subarctic Research Institute. Reports (FIN ISSN 0453-7831) **3206**, 3407, 3441, 3465
• ➤ Key Issues in Human Genetics (CHE ISSN 1422-6251) **3310**
➤ Key Issues in Plastic and Cosmetic Surgery (CHE ISSN 1422-8408) **4196**
• Key Note Market Report: Contraceptives (GBR) **3359**
Key Note Market Report: Cosmetic Surgery (GBR) **4196**
Key Note Market Report: Equipment for the Disabled (GBR) **3485**
• Key Note Market Report: Medical Equipment (GBR) **3640**
Key Note Market Report: Nursing Care (GBR) **3927**
• Key Note Market Report: O T C Pharmaceuticals (Over The Counter) (GBR) **4312**
• Key Note Market Report: Ophthalmic Goods & Services (GBR) **4001**
• Key Note Market Report: Prescribed Pharmaceuticals (GBR) **4312**
• Key Note Market Report: Private Healthcare (GBR) **3640**
• Key Note Market Report: Retail Chemists & Drug Stores (GBR) **4312**
• Key Note Market Review: U K Healthcare (GBR ISSN 1356-6113) **3640**
• Key Note Market Review: U K Pharmaceutical Industry (GBR) **4312**, 3367
Key Note Report: Contraceptives *see* Key Note Market Report: Contraceptives **3359**
Key Note Report: Medical Equipment *see* Key Note Market Report: Medical Equipment **3640**
Key Note Report: O T C Pharmaceuticals *see* Key Note Market Report: O T C Pharmaceuticals **4312**
Key Note Report: Ophthalmic Goods and Services *see* Key Note Market Report: Ophthalmic Goods & Services **4001**
Key Note Report: Prescribed Pharmaceuticals *see* Key Note Market Report: Prescribed Pharmaceuticals **4312**
Key Note Report: Private Healthcare *see* Key Note Market Report: Private Healthcare **3640**
Key Note Report: Retail Chemists and Drug Stores *see* Key Note Market Report: Retail Chemists & Drug Stores **4312**
Key Statistical Indicators for Health in Wales *see* Health Statistics Wales **4519**, 4496
Key Topics in Brain Research (AUT ISSN 0934-1420) **4107**
Keystoner (USA ISSN 0886-7666) **4001**
• Khimiko-farmatsevticheskii Zhurnal (RUS ISSN 0023-1134) **4312**, 3373
Khirurgiya. Zhurnal im. N.I. Pirogova/Surgery (RUS ISSN 0023-1207) **4196**
• ➤ Kidney and Blood Pressure Research (CHE ISSN 1420-4096) **4215**
Kidney and Dialysis *see* Jin to Toseki **3628**, 4214

Title

Title

Title

Title

Title

Title

Medical Device Executive Portfolio *see* M X **3361**, 3645
Medical Device Problems Report from the D E N: Reports from Medical Device Users (Device Experience Network) (USA) **4481**, 3542, 3879
Medical Device Reporting from the D E N: Reports from Medical Device Manufacturers (Device Experience Network) (USA) **4481**, 3542, 3879
• Medical Device Technology (GBR ISSN 1048-6690) **3649**, 3542
• Medical Devices, Diagnostics & Instrumentation Reports: The Gray Sheet (USA ISSN 0163-2426) **3649**, 3530, 3542
Medical Devices Reporter *see* Medical Devices Reports **3650**
• Medical Devices Reports (USA) **3650**
Medical Digest (JPN ISSN 0543-2618) **3650**
• Medical Directory (GBR ISSN 0305-3342) **3518**, 3650
Medical Directory Database CD-ROM (Years) *see* Medical Directory **3518**, 3650
Medical Directory of New York State (USA ISSN 0273-0561) **3650**
Medical Doctor en Espanol *see* M D en Espanol **3645**
• ➤ Medical Dosimetry (USA ISSN 0958-3947) **4150**
• Medical Economics (USA ISSN 0025-7206) **3650**
Medical Economics for Surgeons *see* Medical Economics General Surgery - Orthopedic Surgery **4196**
Medical Economics General Surgery - Orthopedic Surgery (USA) **4196**
• Medical Economics Magazine (USA) **3361**, 3650
• ➤ Medical Education (GBR ISSN 0308-0110) **3650**, 3417
Medical Education *see* Igaku Kyoiku **3618**, 3411
• ➤ Medical Education Online (USA ISSN 1087-2981) **3650**, 3413
Medical Education. Supplement (GBR ISSN 1352-3929) **3650**, 3417
• Medical Electron Microscopy (JPN ISSN 0918-4287) **3334**
Medical Electronics and Equipment News *see* M E E N Cardiology - Critical Care Technology **4149**, 3780
Medical Electronics and Equipment News *see* M E E N Imaging Technology News **4149**
Medical Electronics Manufacturing (USA ISSN 1087-9447) **3430**, 3650
Medical Engineering *see* Meditsinskaya Tekhnika **3658**
• ➤ Medical Engineering & Physics (GBR ISSN 1350-4533) **3650**, 3256
Medical Equipment *see* Key Note Market Report: Medical Equipment **3640**
• Medical Equipment and Supply Guide (DEU ISSN 0946-5200) **3650**, 3879
• Medical Equipment Designer (USA ISSN 1055-4262) **3530**, 3650
• Medical Ethics Advisor (USA ISSN 0886-0653) **3650**, 4347
Medical Express Reports (GBR ISSN 0956-8298) **3650**, 4221
Medical Footwear *see* Kutsu no Igaku **3642**
Medical Forum Reporter (GBR ISSN 0958-3505) **3650**, 4221
Medical Gazette (PAK) **3650**
Medical Gazette *see* Santo Tomas Journal of Medicine **3689**
➤ Medical Grand Rounds (USA ISSN 0277-805X) **3650**
Medical Group Management Association Connexion *see* M G M A Connexion **3645**, 3518
Medical Group Management Journal *see* M G M A Connexion **3645**, 3518
Medical, Health and Welfare Libraries Group. Newsletter *see* Libraries Association. Health Libraries Group. Newsletter **3548**, 3644
The Medical Herald (USA ISSN 0891-799X) **3650**
• ➤ Medical History (GBR ISSN 0025-7273) **3650**
▼ • ➤ Medical Humanities (GBR ISSN 1468-215X) **3651**, 4347
➤ Medical Humanities Review (USA ISSN 0892-2772) **3529**, 3651
Medical Humanity *see* Medikaru Hyumaniti **3657**
Medical Hypnoanalysis Journal (USA ISSN 0894-5098) **3906**, 4108, 4426
• ➤ Medical Hypotheses (GBR ISSN 0306-9877) **3651**
• ➤ Medical Image Analysis (GBR ISSN 1361-8415) **4150**
Medical Imaging *see* Yingxiang Yixue **4157**
Medical Imaging (USA ISSN 1073-1202) **3651**
Medical Imaging International (USA) **3651**
Medical Imaging News (USA ISSN 1074-4819) **3651**
• ➤ Medical Imaging Technology (JPN ISSN 0288-450X) **4150**
Medical Industry Employment Opportunities (USA) **4270**, 3651
• Medical Industry Week (GBR) **3530**, 3651
Medical Informatics *see* Medical Informatics and the Internet in Medicine **3812**
• ➤ Medical Informatics and the Internet in Medicine (GBR ISSN 1463-9238) **3812**
• Medical Informatics Newsletter (CAN) **3812**
Medical Instrument News *see* Hoken Sangyo Jiho **3615**
Medical Intelligence (USA) **3812**
Medical Interface *see* Managed Care Interface **3518**, 3646
• ➤ Medical Journal Armed Forces India (IND ISSN 0377-1237) **3651**
• ➤ Medical Journal of Australia (AUS ISSN 0025-729X) **3651**
Medical Journal of Chinese People's Liberation Army *see* Jiefangjun Yixue Zazhi **3628**, 4224
Medical Journal of Kagoshima University *see* Kagoshima Daigaku Igaku Zasshi **3639**
Medical Journal of Kobe University *see* Kobe Daigaku Igakubu Kiyo **3641**
Medical Journal of Malaysia (MYS ISSN 0300-5283) **3651**
Medical Journal of the Chinese People's Armed Police Forces *see* Wujing Yixue **3709**, 3395
• ➤ Medical Journal of the Islamic Republic of Iran (IRN ISSN 1016-1430) **3651**
Medical Journal of Zambia (ZMB ISSN 0047-651X) **3651**
Medical Laboratory Observer *see* M L O **3879**
Medical Laboratory Sciences *see* British Journal of Biomedical Science **3872**
Medical Laboratory World (GBR ISSN 0140-3028) **3879**
Medical Laser Application (DEU ISSN 1615-1615) **3879**
Medical Laser Industrial Report *see* Medical Laser Report **4367**, 3651
Medical Laser Insight (USA) **4367**, 3651
Medical Laser Report (USA) **4367**, 3651
➤ Medical Law International (GBR ISSN 0968-5332) **3542**, 3651
• ➤ Medical Law Monitor (GBR ISSN 1351-6345) **3542**, 3651
Medical Law Reports (GBR ISSN 0957-9346) **3651**, 3542
• ➤ Medical Law Review (GBR ISSN 0967-0742) **3542**, 3651
• Medical Law's Regan Report (USA) **3651**, 3542
• ➤ Medical Letter on Drugs and Therapeutics (English Edition) (USA ISSN 0025-732X) **4315**
Medical Letter on Drugs and Therapeutics (French Edition) (CHE ISSN 0253-8512) **4315**
Medical Letter on Drugs and Therapeutics (Japanese Edition) (JPN ISSN 0910-6316) **4315**
Medical Liability Adisory Service *see* Emergency Department Law **3538**, 3598
➤ Medical Liability Monitor (USA ISSN 0732-9636) **3533**
Medical Liability Reporter (USA ISSN 0199-1833) **3545**, 3533
Medical Library Association. Bulletin *see* Journal of the Medical Library Association **3638**, 3548
Medical Library Association News (Chicago) *see* M L A News (Chicago) **3645**, 3548
Medical Literature Indexing Services in Pakistan (PAK) **3732**, 3150
Medical Malpractice (Charlottesville) (USA) **3545**, 3651
Medical Malpractice: Checklists and Discoveries (USA) **3651**, 3542
Medical Malpractice: Guide to Medical Issues (USA) **3542**, 3651
Medical Malpractice: Handling Dental Cases (USA) **3545**, 3831
Medical Malpractice: Handling Emergency Cases (USA) **3545**, 3651
Medical Malpractice: Handling Internal Medicine Cases (USA) **3545**, 3652
Medical Malpractice: Handling Obstetric and Neonatal Cases (USA) **3545**, 3958
Medical Malpractice Information Center in Japan. Newsletter *see* Iryo Jiko Joho Senta. Senta Nyusu **3545**, 3625
• Medical Malpractice Law & Strategy (USA ISSN 0747-8925) **3545**, 3652
• Medical Malpractice (New York) (USA) **3545**, 3652
Medical Malpractice - Ob-Gyn Litigation Reporter *see* Health Law Litigation Reporter **3545**, 3952
Medical Malpractice: Pharmacy Law (USA) **3545**, 4315
Medical Malpractice: Psychiatric Care (USA) **3545**, 4108
Medical Malpractice Reports (USA ISSN 1045-960X) **3545**, 3652
Medical Malpractice Verdicts, Settlements & Experts (USA ISSN 0888-658X) **3545**, 3652
Medical Management Network *see* C O R Clinical Excellence **3580**
Medical Manufacturing International *see* Medical Device Developments **4315**
• Medical Marketing & Media (USA ISSN 0025-7354) **4315**, 3367
• Medical Materials Update (USA ISSN 1077-3436) **3652**
Medical Microbiologist (GBR) **3652**, 3326
• ➤ Medical Microbiology and Immunology (DEU ISSN 0300-8584) **3749**
➤ Medical Mission News (USA) **4502**, 3652
Medical Mission Sisters News (USA) **4564**
Medical Monitor (GBR) **3652**
Medical Monitor Weekly *see* Medical Monitor **3652**
• ➤ Medical Mycology (GBR ISSN 1369-3786) **3803**, 3281
Medical News *see* Mejikaru Nyusu **3660**
Medical News, Medicine and Law (IND ISSN 0047-6536) **3884**
Medical News of the Month *see* Gekkan Iryo Joho **3605**
Medical News Report (USA ISSN 1054-3066) **3367**, 3153, 3652
The Medical Office Biller (USA ISSN 1078-1285) **3518**
Medical Office Manager (USA ISSN 1052-4894) **3365**, 3652
Medical Office Report (USA ISSN 0895-4313) **3652**, 3533
Medical Office Staff Management Strategies (USA) **3519**, 3365
• ➤ Medical Oncology (USA ISSN 1357-0560) **3984**
Medical Oncology and Tumor Pharmacotherapy *see* Medical Oncology **3984**
• Medical Outcomes and Guidelines Alert (USA ISSN 1067-4195) **3652**
Medical Parasitology and Parasitic Diseases *see* Meditsinskaya Parazitologiya i Parazitarnye Bolezni **3803**
Medical Pharmacy (JPN ISSN 0025-7427) **4315**
• ➤ Medical Physics (USA ISSN 0094-2405) **3652**, 4365
• The Medical Post (CAN ISSN 0025-7435) **3652**
Medical Practice (JPN ISSN 0910-1551) **3652**
• Medical Practice Communicator (USA ISSN 1074-1321) **3652**
Medical Practices Committee. Recruitment Survey (Year) (GBR) **3652**, 3364
Medical Practices Committee. Survey of G P Recruitment in England and Wales *see* Medical Practices Committee. Recruitment Survey (Year) **3652**, 3364
▼ Medical Prescription of Narcotics (CHE ISSN 1423-5765) **4315**, 3652
• ➤ Medical Principles and Practice (CHE ISSN 1011-7571) **3652**
• ➤ Medical Problems of Performing Artists (USA ISSN 0885-1158) **3652**, 3396, 4225
Medical Products of Japan (JPN ISSN 1341-6146) **3652**, 3371
Medical Products Sales (USA ISSN 0279-4802) **3652**, 3367, 3530
Medical Progress - Hong Kong Edition *see* Medical Progress (Southeast Asia Editions) **3653**
➤ Medical Progress (Indonesia Edition) (HKG ISSN 1015-4256) **3652**
➤ Medical Progress (Korea Edition) (HKG) **3652**
➤ Medical Progress (Malaysia Edition) (HKG ISSN 1015-4272) **3653**
➤ Medical Progress (Pakistan Edition) (HKG ISSN 1015-4280) **3653**
➤ Medical Progress (Philippines Edition) (HKG ISSN 1015-4299) **3653**
➤ Medical Progress (Singapore Edition) (HKG ISSN 1015-4302) **3653**
➤ Medical Progress (Southeast Asia Editions) (HKG ISSN 0377-9963) **3653**
➤ Medical Progress (Taiwan Edition) (HKG ISSN 1015-4310) **3653**
➤ Medical Progress (Thailand Edition) (HKG ISSN 1015-4329) **3653**
Medical Protection Society. Annual Report (GBR ISSN 0076-5961) **3653**
Medical Quarterly (MWI ISSN 1017-2920) **3653**
Medical Radiology (USA ISSN 0942-5373) **4150**
Medical Record Risks: Claims & Litigation (USA ISSN 1061-4192) **3533**, 3545, 3653
Medical Records Briefing (USA ISSN 1052-4924) **3519**, 3653
Medical Reform (CAN) **3653**
Medical Rehabilitation Review *see* N A R F Rehabilitation Report **4063**
Medical Research Centres (GBR) **3653**
Medical Research Centres in Ghana: Current Research Projects (GHA) **3653**
Medical Research Council News *see* M R C News **3645**
Medical Research Council News *see* M R C News **3645**
Medical Research Council Newsletter/Conseil de Recherches Medicales. Communique (CAN ISSN 0047-6560) **3653**
• Medical Research Council of Canada. Grants and Awards Guide/Guide de Subventions et Bourses (CAN ISSN 0839-8283) **3653**
Medical Research Council of Canada. Report of the President (CAN ISSN 0384-2029) **3653**
Medical Research Council Strategic Plan 1999 - 2003 *see* M R C Strategic Plan 1999 - 2003 **3645**
• Medical Research Funding Bulletin (USA) **3653**
Medical Researches for Photosensitizing Dyes *see* Kanko Shikiso **4149**
Medical review. Acupuncture *see* Meditsinski Pregled. Akupunktura **3168**
Medical Review. Allergology and Immunology *see* Meditsinski Pregled. Alergologiia i Klinichna Imunologiia **3750**
Medical Review. Children's Diseases *see* Meditsinski Pregled. Detski Bolesti **4048**, 4239
Medical School Admission Requirements, United States and Canada (USA ISSN 0066-9423) **3654**, 3417
Medical Science and Medical Care/Gekkan Igaku to Iryo (JPN ISSN 0019-1590) **3654**
Medical Science in Rural China *see* Zhongguo Nongcun Yixue **3712**
• ➤ Medical Science Monitor (POL ISSN 1234-1010) **3654**
Medical Science Series (USA) **3654**, 4365
➤ Medical Science Symposia Series (NLD ISSN 0928-9550) **3654**
Medical Scientific Update (USA) **4162**, 3749
Medical Service *see* Health Action **3508**, 3610
Medical Service and Facility *see* Iryo to Shisetsu **3625**
Medical Service Digest (USA ISSN 0041-7491) **3654**
Medical Society County of Kings, Inc. Bulletin *see* K C M S Bulletin **3639**
Medical Society of London. Transactions (GBR ISSN 0076-6011) **3654**
Medical Society of Milwaukee County. Membership Newsletter (USA) **3654**
Medical Society of Nova Scotia News *see* M S N S News **3645**
Medical Software Reviews (USA ISSN 1059-907X) **3812**, 3391
Medical Staff Briefing (USA ISSN 1076-6022) **3654**, 3519
Medical Staff Law Manual *see* Medical Staff Leader Handbook **3545**, 3654
Medical Staff Leader Handbook (USA) **3545**, 3654
Medical Student International (NLD) **3654**
• Medical Subject Headings - Annotated Alphabetic List (USA ISSN 0147-5711) **3732**
Medical Subject Headings (Black Book) (USA ISSN 0565-811X) **3654**
• Medical Subject Headings - Tree Structure (Year) (USA ISSN 0147-099X) **3732**
• ➤ Medical Teacher (GBR ISSN 0142-159X) **3654**, 3413
Medical Technology *see* Rinsho Kensagaku Zasshi **3687**
Medical Technology International (Year) (GBR) **3654**
Medical Technology Stock Letter (USA ISSN 1065-996X) **3363**, 3654
▼ Medical Tests Sourcebook (USA) **4150**
• Medical Textiles (GBR ISSN 0266-2078) **3654**, 4531

Title

Title

Medizinisch-Orthopaedische Technik (DEU ISSN 0340-5508) **4021**
Medizinisch-Pharmakologisches Kompendium (DEU ISSN 0934-9170) **4316**
Medizinisch-Technische Assistenten Fachzeitschrift der Technische Assistenten der Medizin *see* M T A - Fachzeitschrift der Technische Assistenten der Medizin **3645**, 3879
Medizinisch- Technische Assistenten Repetitorium *see* M T A - Repetitorium **3645**, 3879
➤ Medizinische Genetik (DEU ISSN 0936-5931) **3310**
Medizinische Hochschule Hannover Info *see* M H H - Info **3388**, 3645
Medizinische Informatik und Statistik (USA ISSN 0342-4103) **3658**
• ➤ Medizinische Klinik (DEU ISSN 0723-5003) **3658**
Medizinische Kongresse (DEU ISSN 0175-3053) **4221**, 3659
Medizinische Laenderkunde. Geomedical Monograph Series (USA ISSN 0076-6151) **3659**
Medizinische Monatsschrift fuer Pharmazeuten (DEU ISSN 0342-9601) **3659**
Der Medizinische Sachverstaendige (DEU ISSN 0025-8490) **3659**
• ➤ Die Medizinische Welt (DEU ISSN 0025-8512) **3659**
Medizinischer Literatur Anzeiger (DEU) **3732**
Medizinland (DEU ISSN 0944-1123) **3659**
Medizinprodukte Journal (DEU ISSN 0944-6885) **3659**
• ➤ Medizinrecht (DEU ISSN 0723-8886) **3884**
Medizinsoziologie (DEU) **4509**, 3659
Medizintechnik *see* M T - Medizintechnik **3645**
Medkalender (CHE) **3659**
Medlemsblad - A A F *see* A A F - Tidningen **4273**
Medline *see* Index Medicus **3729**, 3149
Medline CD *see* Index Medicus **3729**, 3149
• MedPro Month (USA) **3659**
MedR *see* Medizinrecht **3884**
• ➤ Medscape Mental Health (USA) **4109**
• Medscape Oncology (USA) **3984**
• ➤ Medscape Orthopedics & Sports Medicine (USA) **4021**, 4175
• ➤ Medscape Respiratory Care (USA) **4162**
• ➤ Medscape Women's Health (USA ISSN 1521-2076) **4564**
• ➤ MedSupport F S F Newsletter (Friends Supporting Friends) (USA) **3659**
• ➤ MedSurg Nursing (USA ISSN 1092-0811) **4196**, 3929
▼ • Meducator (CAN ISSN 0972-267X) **3659**, 3413
Medunsa Yearbook *see* Medical University of South Africa. Yearbook **3655**
Medycyna Doswiadczalna i Mikrobiologia (POL ISSN 0025-8601) **3327**, 3659
Medycyna Nowozytna/Modern Medicine - study on history of medicine (POL ISSN 1231-1960) **3659**
• Medycyna Pracy (POL ISSN 0465-5893) **3659**, 4259
Medycyna Praktyczna (POL ISSN 0867-499X) **3659**
Medycyna Praktyczna. Chirurgia (POL ISSN 1428-2712) **4197**
Medycyna Praktyczna. Ginekologia i Polozniclwo (POL) **3958**
Medycyna Praktyczna. Pediatria (POL) **4048**
Medycyna Praktyczna. Ultrasonografia (POL ISSN 1429-4966) **4151**
• ➤ Medycyna Weterynaryjna (POL ISSN 0025-8628) **4548**
Medycyna Wiejska/Rural Medicine (POL ISSN 0025-8636) **3659**
Medyk/Physician (POL ISSN 0867-3055) **3659**
MEEGID *see* Infection, Genetics and Evolution **3619**, 3308
• ➤ Megamot (ISR ISSN 0025-8679) **4522**, 3413, 4426
Meiguo Yixuehui Yanke Zazhi (CHN ISSN 1000-0348) **4001**
• Meiguo Yixuehui Zazhi (Zhongwen Ban)/J A M A: The Journal of the American Medical Association (Chinese Edition) (CHN ISSN 1000-842X) **3660**
Meiji Pharmaceutical University. Bulletin *see* Meiji Yakka Daigaku Kenkyu Kiyo **4316**
➤ Meiji Shinkyu Igaku/Meiji University of Oriental Medicine. Bulletin (JPN ISSN 0912-2419) **3168**
Meiji University of Oriental Medicine. Bulletin *see* Meiji Shinkyu Igaku **3168**
Meiji Yakka Daigaku Kenkyu Kiyo/Meiji Pharmaceutical University. Bulletin (JPN ISSN 0543-3975) **4316**
Meijo Daigaku Senkoka Yakugaku Senko Hokokushu (JPN ISSN 0911-9442) **4316**
➤ Meikai Daigaku Shigaku Zasshi/Meikai University Dental Journal/Meikai University School of Dentistry. Journal (JPN ISSN 0916-0701) **3832**, 3660
Meikai University Dental Journal *see* Meikai Daigaku Shigaku Zasshi **3832**, 3660
Meikai University School of Dentistry. Journal *see* Meikai Daigaku Shigaku Zasshi **3832**, 3660
Meine Gesundheit (DEU) **4534**, 4316
Mejikaru Nyusu/Medical News (JPN ISSN 0287-9085) **3660**
Melanoma Letter (USA) **3851**, 3984
• ➤ Melanoma Research (GBR ISSN 0960-8931) **3984**
• Melpomene Journal (USA ISSN 1043-8734) **4564**, 4358
Membrane *see* Maku **3292**
Membrane and Cell Biology *see* Biologicheskie Membrany **3265**, 3286
Membrane Oxygenator *see* Makugata Hai **4162**
➤ Membrane Science and Technology Series (NLD ISSN 0927-5193) **3292**
• ➤ Memisa Medisch (NLD ISSN 1381-3412) **3660**
Memisa Nieuws *see* Memisa Medisch **3660**
Memoirs of the Hourglass Cruises (USA ISSN 0085-0683) **3208**, 3408
Memorial Sloan-Kettering Cancer Center. Annual Report (USA) **3984**, 3519
Memorie dell Istituto Italiano di Idrobiologia "Dott. Marco de Marchi" *see* Journal of Limnology **3204**
Memorie di Biologia Marina e di Oceanografia (ITA ISSN 0390-492X) **3408**, 3208
• ➤ Memory (GBR ISSN 0965-8211) **4426**
• ➤ Memory and Cognition (USA ISSN 0090-502X) **4426**
Memphis Health Care News (USA ISSN 1043-8475) **4358**, 4239
Men-Eki Immunoloji Furontia/Immunology Frontier (JPN ISSN 0917-0774) **3750**
Mencap News *see* Viewpoint (London, 1995) **4137**, 4518
➤ Mendel (IND ISSN 0970-9649) **3311**
➤ Mendeliana (ARG ISSN 0325-223X) **3311**
Mendocino Medicine & Gazetteer (USA) **3660**
Men'eki Kaku Igaku/Immunonuclear Medicine (JPN ISSN 0914-8639) **3750**, 4151
• ➤ Menninger Clinic. Bulletin (USA ISSN 0025-9284) **4109**, 4427
Menninger Perspective (USA ISSN 0025-9292) **4109**, 4427
Menopausa News (ITA ISSN 1123-699X) **3958**
• ➤ Menopause (USA ISSN 1072-3714) **3958**, 3866, 4564
Menopause Management (USA ISSN 1062-7332) **4564**
• Menopause News (USA ISSN 1061-4397) **4564**, 3866
Men's Confidential Newsletter *see* Sex & Health **4222**, 4218, 4223, 4361
• Men's Fitness (USA ISSN 0893-4460) **4222**, 4358
▼ Men's Fitness en Espanol (USA ISSN 1531-457X) **4222**
▼ Men's Health (FRA ISSN 1294-971X) **4222**
Men's Health (RUS ISSN 1562-5117) **4222**
• Men's Health (Germany Edition) (DEU ISSN 1432-3818) **4222**
Men's Health Online *see* Men's Health (South Africa Edition) **4222**
▼ Men's Health (Portugal Edition) (PRT) **4222**
Men's Health (South Africa Edition) (ZAF) **4222**
▼ Men's Health (Spain Edition) (ESP) **4222**
Men's Health (United Kingdom Edition) (GBR) **4222**
• Men's Health (United States Edition) (USA ISSN 1054-4836) **4222**
Men's Health Watch *see* Harvard Men's Health Watch **4221**
Men's Workout (USA ISSN 1058-3041) **4222**, 4222
Mensa Research Journal (USA ISSN 0025-9551) **3424**
➤ Mensen op Straat (NLD ISSN 0166-4654) **4533**, 4481
Menstuff (Print) *see* Menstuff, The National Men's Resource **4223**, 4222, 4223
• Menstuff, The National Men's Resource (USA) **4223**, 4222, 4223
Mentaal *see* Psy **4436**
• Mental and Physical Disability Law Reporter (USA ISSN 0883-7902) **3546**, 4109
Mental Capacity: Medical and Legal Aspects of the Aging (USA) **3478**, 3546, 4427
Mental Disability Law: Civil and Criminal (USA) **3542**, 4109
The Mental Edge (USA) **4427**, 4525
Mental Handicap *see* British Journal of Learning Disabilities **4079**
Mental Handicap Bulletin *see* Learning Disability Bulletin **4108**
Mental Handicap Research *see* Journal of Applied Research in Intellectual Disabilities **4098**
Mental Health *see* Mielenterveys **4109**, 4481
Mental Health *see* Psykisk Haelsa **4443**, 4129
➤ Mental Health Aspects of Developmental Disabilities (USA) **4109**, 4063
➤ Mental Health Care (GBR ISSN 1368-1230) **4109**, 4427
Mental Health Data *see* New Zealand Health Information Service. Mental Health Data **3733**
Mental Health Directory (USA) **4481**
Mental Health Disorders Sourcebook (USA) **4427**
Mental Health in Children (USA) **4427**, 4109, 4516
Mental Health Law Bulletin (USA) **3546**, 4427
Mental Health Law News (USA ISSN 0889-017X) **3546**, 4427
• Mental Health Law Reporter (USA ISSN 0741-5141) **3546**, 4427
Mental Health Library Series (USA) **4427**
Mental Health Matters (AUS) **4109**, 4427
Mental Health Matters (CAN ISSN 1196-5304) **4427**
Mental Health Matters (GBR ISSN 0963-0201) **4427**, 4481
• ➤ Mental Health Nursing Journal (GBR ISSN 1353-0283) **4109**, 3929
Mental Health Practice (GBR ISSN 1465-8720) **4109**, 3929
• Mental Health, Religion & Culture (GBR ISSN 1367-4676) **4427**, 3174, 4501, 4522
Mental Health Report (USA ISSN 0191-6750) **4516**, 4109, 4427
Mental Health Research Review (GBR) **4427**
The Mental Health Review (GBR ISSN 1361-9322) **4109**, 4427, 4516
Mental Health Review Tribunal for England. Annual Report (Year) *see* Mental Health Review Tribunals for England and Wales. Annual Report **4481**, 4427
Mental Health Review Tribunal for Wales. Annual Report for (Year) *see* Mental Health Review Tribunals for England and Wales. Annual Report **4481**, 4427
Mental Health Review Tribunals for England and Wales. Annual Report (GBR) **4481**, 4427
Mental Health Section Newsletter *see* Behavioral Health Section Newsletter **4076**
Mental Health Services for Children and Youth *see* Hawaii. Department of Health. Mental Health Services for Children and Youth **4513**, 3383, 4471
▼ • ➤ Mental Health Services Research (USA ISSN 1522-3434) **4427**, 4516
Mental Health Special Interest Section Newsletter *see* Mental Health Special Interest Section Quarterly **4427**, 4259
Mental Health Special Interest Section Quarterly (USA) **4427**, 4259
Mental Health Statistical Notes (USA ISSN 0361-9311) **4519**, 3732, 4457, 4529
Mental Health Statistics for Illinois *see* Illinois. Department of Human Services. Division of Disability and Behavioral Health Services. Illinois Statistics **4519**, 4496, 4529
Mental Health Statistics for Wales *see* Health Statistics Wales **4519**, 4496
• Mental Health Weekly (USA ISSN 1058-1103) **4427**, 3542
➤ Mental Measurements Yearbook (USA ISSN 0076-6461) **4427**, 3429
• ➤ Mental Retardation (USA ISSN 0047-6765) **3424**, 4109
Mental Retardation and Developmental Disabilities Express *see* M R D D Express **3424**, 3385
• ➤ Mental Retardation and Developmental Disabilities (New York, 1995) (USA ISSN 1080-4013) **4109**, 3485
Mental Retardation and Learning Disability Bulletin *see* Developmental Disabilities Bulletin **4086**, 3420
Mentalites *see* Mentalities **3526**, 4427
➤ Mentalities/Mentalites (CAN ISSN 0111-8854) **3526**, 4427
Mente e Societa (ITA) **4427**
• Merck Index: An Encyclopedia of Chemicals and Drugs (USA ISSN 0076-6518) **4345**
• Merck Manual: A Handbook of Diagnosis and Therapy (USA ISSN 0076-6526) **3660**
The Merck Manual of Geriatrics (USA) **3478**
The Merck Manual of Medical Information - Home (USA) **3660**
Merck Veterinary Manual: A Handbook of Diagnosis and Therapy for the Veterinarian (USA ISSN 0076-6542) **4548**
Mere Nouvelle *see* New Mother **3385**, 3959
Meridian (DEU ISSN 0177-3852) **4227**, 4427
Meridians (Columbia) (USA) **3168**, 3660, 4270
Merkblaetter Gefaehrliche Arbeitsstoffe (DEU ISSN 0936-1197) **4259**
Merkur Magazin fuer Volksgesundheit (AUT ISSN 0026-010X) **4481**
Der Merkurstab (DEU ISSN 0935-798X) **4503**, 3660
• ➤ Merrill - Palmer Quarterly (USA ISSN 0272-930X) **4427**, 3385, 3413
Merrill - Palmer Quarterly of Behavior and Development *see* Merrill - Palmer Quarterly **4427**, 3385, 3413
Mertensiella (DEU ISSN 0934-6643) **3355**
• Message Line (USA ISSN 1060-233X) **3984**
Message (St. Paul) *see* The New Message **4119**
Messung von Gefahrstoffen (DEU ISSN 0936-4544) **3453**, 3542
• ➤ Metabolic Brain Disease (USA ISSN 0885-7490) **3660**
• Metabolic Engineering (USA ISSN 1096-7176) **3238**, 3292
➤ Metabolic, Pediatric and Systemic Ophthalmology (USA ISSN 0882-889X) **4001**
• ➤ Metabolism: Clinical and Experimental (USA ISSN 0026-0495) **3866**, 3208
➤ Metabolismes - Hormones - Nutrition (FRA) **3866**
Metal-Based Drugs (ISR ISSN 0793-0291) **3377**, 4316
• ➤ Metaphor and Symbol (USA ISSN 1092-6488) **3551**, 3552, 4428
Metaphor and Symbolic Activity *see* Metaphor and Symbol **3551**, 3552, 4428
Methodensammlung der Elektronenmikroskopie/ Methods of Electron Microscopy (DEU ISSN 0076-6771) **3335**
Methodologia (ITA ISSN 1120-3854) **3551**, 4428
Methodology in the Social Sciences (USA) **4510**
• ➤ Methods: A Companion to Methods in Enzymology (USA ISSN 1046-2023) **3256**
• ➤ Methods and Findings in Experimental and Clinical Pharmacology (ESP ISSN 0379-0355) **4316**
Methods and Principles in Medicinal Chemistry (DEU) **3660**
Methods - GenoMethods *see* Methods: A Companion to Methods in Enzymology **3256**
Methods - Immunomethods *see* Methods: A Companion to Methods in Enzymology **3256**
➤ Methods in Biotechnology (USA) **3276**, 3238
• ➤ Methods in Cell Biology (USA ISSN 0091-679X) **3292**
• ➤ Methods in Cell Science (NLD ISSN 1381-5741) **3292**
• ➤ Methods in Enzymology (USA ISSN 0076-6879) **3256**
• ➤ Methods in Microbiology (USA ISSN 0580-9517) **3327**
Methods in Molecular Biology (USA ISSN 1064-3745) **3208**
Methods in Molecular Genetics (USA ISSN 1067-2389) **3311**
• Methods in Molecular Medicine (USA) **3910**
Methods in Neurosciences (USA ISSN 1043-9471) **4109**
▼ ➤ Methods in Pharmacology and Toxicology (USA) **4316**
Methods in Toxicology (USA ISSN 1063-3677) **3453**, 4316
• ➤ Methods of Biochemical Analysis (USA ISSN 0076-6941) **3256**
Methods of Electron Microscopy *see* Methodensammlung der Elektronenmikroskopie **3335**
• ➤ Methods of Information in Medicine (DEU ISSN 0026-1270) **3660**
• Methods of Psychological Research (DEU) **4428**
Methods (San Diego) *see* Methods: A Companion to Methods in Enzymology **3256**
Metiers de la Petite Enfance (FRA ISSN 1258-780X) **3385**, 4048
▼ Metodologia de las Ciencias del Comportamiento (ESP) **4428**

Title

Title

Miyazaki Prefectural Institute for Public Health and Environment. Annual Report *see* Miyazakiken Eisei Kankyo Kenkyujo Nenpo **4481**
Miyazakiken Eisei Kankyo Kenkyujo Nenpo/Miyazaki Prefectural Institute for Public Health and Environment. Annual Report (JPN ISSN 0917-3331) **4481**
Miyazakiken Eisei Kenkyujoho *see* Miyazakiken Eisei Kankyo Kenkyujo Nenpo **4481**
Miyazakiken Kogai Senta Nenpo *see* Miyazakiken Eisei Kankyo Kenkyujo Nenpo **4481**
The Mobility Forum (USA) **4224**, 4481
Modan Media *see* Modern Media **3328**
Model for the Preparation of a Guidebook on Medical Discipline (USA ISSN 0888-6792) **3661**
Modell's Drugs in Current Use and New Drugs (USA ISSN 1044-0704) **4316**, 3662
• ➤ Modern Aging Research (USA ISSN 0275-360X) **3478**
Modern Athlete and Coach (AUS ISSN 0047-7672) **4527**, 4175
➤ Modern Biology Series (USA) **3208**
Modern Cell Biology (USA ISSN 0745-3000) **3292**
Modern Concepts in Immunology (USA ISSN 0891-3676) **3750**
Modern Diagnosis & Treatment *see* Xiandai Zhenduan yu Zhiliao **3709**
• Modern Drug Discovery (USA ISSN 1099-8209) **4317**, 3208
Modern Geriatrics (ESP ISSN 0214-378X) **3478**
• Modern Healthcare (Year) (USA ISSN 0160-7480) **3519**
Modern Hypertension Management (GBR ISSN 1465-5691) **3780**
• Modern Maturity (USA ISSN 0026-8046) **3478**
Modern Media/Modan Media (JPN ISSN 0026-8054) **3328**
Modern Medical Intelligence *see* Gendai Iryogaku **3605**
Modern Medical Laboratory *see* Kensa to Gijutsu **3877**
Modern Medical Practice *see* Pharmacy News **4328**
Modern Medicine *see* Modern Medicine of Australia **3662**
Modern Medicine *see* Suvremenna Medicina **3697**
➤ Modern Medicine of Australia (AUS ISSN 1030-3782) **3662**
Modern Medicine of South Africa (ZAF ISSN 0259-9333) **3662**
Modern Medicine - study on history of medicine *see* Medycyna Nowozytna **3659**
Modern Medicine Today *see* Medicina Moderna Oggi **3655**
➤ Modern Methods in Pharmacology (USA ISSN 0732-7218) **4317**
Modern Midwife *see* Practising Midwife **3961**, 3938, 4565
➤ Modern Neuroradiology Series (USA ISSN 1051-1369) **4151**
Modern Neurosurgery (USA ISSN 0723-0990) **4197**
• ➤ Modern Pathology (USA ISSN 0893-3952) **3662**, 3208
Modern Pharmacy *see* Journal of Modern Pharmacy **4308**
• Modern Physician (USA) **3662**
• ➤ Modern Problems of Pharmacopsychiatry (CHE ISSN 0077-0094) **4110**, 4317
➤ Modern Psychoanalysis (USA ISSN 0361-5227) **4428**
• ➤ Modern Rheumatology (JPN ISSN 1439-7595) **4169**
Modern Technics in Surgery. Head and Neck Surgery *see* Journal of Cardiac Surgery **3776**
Modern Technics in Surgery. Neurosurgery *see* Journal of Cardiac Surgery **3776**
Modern Technics in Surgery. Urologic Surgery *see* Journal of Cardiac Surgery **3776**
Moderna Laekare (SWE ISSN 1403-5502) **3535**, 3519, 3662
Moderne Unfallverhuetung (DEU ISSN 0544-7119) **4481**
Modus (ITA) **3866**
Modus (NLD ISSN 0927-2216) **3884**
• ➤ Molecular and Biochemical Parasitology (NLD ISSN 0166-6851) **3256**, 3328
Molecular and Cell Biology of Human Diseases (GBR) **3292**, 3804
• ➤ Molecular and Cellular Biochemistry (USA ISSN 0300-8177) **3257**, 3292
• ➤ Molecular and Cellular Biology (USA ISSN 0270-7306) **3257**, 3292
Molecular & Cellular Differentiation (USA ISSN 1065-3074) **3292**
• ➤ Molecular and Cellular Endocrinology (IRL ISSN 0303-7207) **3866**
• ➤ Molecular and Cellular Neurosciences (USA ISSN 1044-7431) **4110**
• ➤ Molecular and Cellular Probes (GBR ISSN 0890-8508) **3879**, 3373
Molecular and General Genetics *see* Molecular Genetics and Genomics **3311**
Molecular Andrology (USA) **3662**
• ➤ Molecular Aspects of Medicine (GBR ISSN 0098-2997) **3662**
• ➤ Molecular Biology (RUS ISSN 0026-8933) **3257**, 3292
• ➤ Molecular Biology and Evolution (USA ISSN 0737-4038) **3208**
Molecular Biology, Biochemistry and Biophysics (USA ISSN 0077-0221) **3257**, 3267
• ➤ Molecular Biology Reports (NLD ISSN 0301-4851) **3257**, 3292
• Molecular Biology Techniques (GBR ISSN 1356-1324) **3233**, 3150, 3257
▼ • ➤ Molecular Biology Today (GBR ISSN 1468-5698) **3281**, 3355
• ➤ Molecular Biotechnology (USA ISSN 1073-6085) **3276**, 3662
• ➤ Molecular Brain Research (NLD ISSN 0169-328X) **4110**, 3208
• Molecular Cancer Therapeutics (USA) **3984**
• ➤ Molecular Carcinogenesis (USA ISSN 0899-1987) **3984**, 3328
• ➤ Molecular Cell (USA ISSN 1097-2765) **3292**
• Molecular Cell Biology Research Communications (USA ISSN 1522-4724) **3292**
• ➤ Molecular Diagnosis (USA ISSN 1084-8592) **3662**, 3208
• ➤ Molecular Endocrinology (USA ISSN 0888-8809) **3866**
Molecular Genetic Medicine *see* Advances in Genetics **3297**
• ➤ Molecular Genetics and Genomics (DEU ISSN 1617-4615) **3311**
• ➤ Molecular Genetics and Metabolism (USA ISSN 1096-7192) **3662**, 3257
➤ Molecular Genetics, Microbiology and Virology (USA ISSN 0891-4168) **3329**, 3257, 3311
Molecular Genetics, Microbiology and Virusology *see* Molekulyarnaya Genetika, Mikrobiologiya i Virusologiya **3329**, 3311
• ➤ Molecular Human Reproduction (GBR ISSN 1360-9947) **3958**, 3208
• Molecular Imaging and Biology (NLD) **4151**
• ➤ Molecular Immunology (GBR ISSN 0161-5890) **3257**, 3750
▼ • Molecular Interventions (USA) **4317**
Molecular Medicine (JPN ISSN 0918-6557) **3866**
• ➤ Molecular Medicine (USA ISSN 1076-1551) **4317**
Molecular Medicine Today *see* Trends in Molecular Medicine **3702**
• ➤ Molecular Membrane Biology (GBR ISSN 0968-7688) **3258**, 3293
• ➤ Molecular Microbiology (GBR ISSN 0950-382X) **3329**
Molecular Microbiology Online *see* Molecular Microbiology **3329**
• ➤ Molecular Neurobiology (USA ISSN 0893-7648) **3258**, 3311, 4110
• ➤ Molecular Pathology (GBR ISSN 1366-8714) **3879**
• ➤ Molecular Pharmacology (USA ISSN 0026-895X) **4317**
• ➤ Molecular Phylogenetics and Evolution (USA ISSN 1055-7903) **3311**
• ➤ Molecular Plant - Microbe Interactions (USA ISSN 0894-0282) **3258**, 3281, 3329
▼ • Molecular Plant Pathology (GBR ISSN 1464-6722) **3281**, 3662
• ➤ Molecular Psychiatry (GBR ISSN 1359-4184) **4110**, 3208
• ➤ Molecular Reproduction and Development (USA ISSN 1040-452X) **3258**, 3329
• Molecular Therapy (USA ISSN 1525-0016) **3984**, 3258
• ➤ Molecular Vision (USA ISSN 1090-0535) **3258**, 3293
• Molekulyarnaya Biologiya (RUS ISSN 0026-8984) **3258**
Molekulyarnaya Fizika i Biofizika Vodnykh Sistem (RUS ISSN 0134-8485) **3267**
Molekulyarnaya Genetika, Mikrobiologiya i Virusologiya/Molecular Genetics, Microbiology and Virusology (RUS ISSN 0208-0613) **3329**, 3311
Momentum (Rochester) (USA) **3832**
Mon Enfant *see* Your Baby **3386**, 4057
➤ Monaldi Archives for Chest Disease (ITA ISSN 1122-0643) **4162**, 3293
Monash Bioethics Review (AUS ISSN 1321-2753) **4348**, 3542, 3662
• Monash University Accident Research Centre. Consultants' Reports Series (AUS) **4533**, 4482
Monash University Accident Research Centre. Minor Reports Series (AUS) **4533**, 4482
Monash University Accident Research Centre. Other Reports Series (AUS) **4533**, 4482
Monatsbericht Angezeigter Flugunfaelle (DEU) **4532**, 4482
Monatsbericht der Angezeigten Flugunfalluntersuchungsstelle *see* Monatsbericht Angezeigter Flugunfaelle **4532**, 4482
Monatshefte fuer Veterinaermedizin *see* Tieraerztliche Umschau **4553**
• ➤ Monatsschrift Kinderheilkunde (DEU ISSN 0026-9298) **4049**
Monday Morning Report (USA ISSN 0891-8651) **3404**
Monde Dentaire/Tandartsen Wereld (BEL) **3832**
Mondo Ortodontico (ITA ISSN 0391-2000) **3832**
Mongolian Medical Sciences *see* Mongolyn Anagaakh Ukhaan **3662**
Mongolyn Anagaakh Ukhaan/Mongolian Medical Sciences (MNG) **3662**
Moniteur des Pharmacies et des Laboratoires (FRA ISSN 0026-9689) **4317**
Moniteur Hospitalier (FRA ISSN 0993-9199) **4317**
Monitor *see* Ohio Monitor **4262**
• Monitor de la Farmacia y de la Terapeutica (ESP ISSN 0463-1536) **4317**
• ➤ Monitor on Psychology (USA ISSN 1529-4978) **4428**
Monitor (Washington, 1970) (USA) **3533**, 3519, 3662
• Monoclonal Antibodies (GBR ISSN 0261-4960) **3233**, 3150, 3750, 3879
Monografias de Dermatologia (ESP ISSN 0214-4735) **3851**
➤ Monografias de L.O.L.A. (Literature of Latin America) (ARG ISSN 0328-1620) **3208**
Monografias de Pediatria (ESP ISSN 0212-1603) **4049**
Monografias de Poblacion y Desarrollo (BOL) **3359**
Monografias de Psiquiatria (ESP ISSN 0214-4220) **4110**
Monografias de Salud Rural (ESP) **3662**
Monografie Biochemiczne (POL ISSN 0077-0485) **3258**
Monografie Parazytologiczne (POL ISSN 0540-6722) **3329**, 4548
➤ Monograph Series on Schizophrenia (USA ISSN 0077-0620) **4110**
➤ Monographiae Biologicae (NLD ISSN 0077-0639) **3208**
Monographien aus dem Gesamtgebiete der Psychiatrie - Psychiatry Series (USA ISSN 0077-0671) **4110**
• ➤ Monographs in Allergy (CHE ISSN 0077-0760) **3750**
➤ Monographs in Anaesthesiology (NLD ISSN 0303-254X) **3758**
➤ Monographs in Clinical Cytology (CHE ISSN 0077-0809) **3662**, 3293
➤ Monographs in Clinical Neuroscience (CHE ISSN 1420-2441) **4110**
Monographs in Clinical Pediatrics (CHE ISSN 1044-4882) **4049**
➤ Monographs in Epidemiology and Biostatistics (GBR ISSN 0740-0845) **4482**, 3208
Monographs in Human Genetics *see* Key Issues in Human Genetics **3310**
Monographs in Neural Sciences *see* Monographs in Clinical Neuroscience **4110**
➤ Monographs in Neuroscience (CHE ISSN 0737-3953) **4111**
➤ Monographs in Ophthalmology (NLD ISSN 0167-8612) **4001**
• ➤ Monographs in Oral Science (CHE ISSN 0077-0892) **3832**
➤ Monographs in Primatology (USA ISSN 0740-9729) **3355**
➤ Monographs in Psychobiology (CHE ISSN 0749-1190) **4428**, 3208
• ➤ Monographs in Virology (CHE ISSN 0077-0965) **3329**
Monographs on Endocrinology (USA ISSN 0077-1015) **3866**
Monographs on Pathology of Laboratory Animals (USA ISSN 0177-7475) **3879**
➤ Monographs on Physical Biochemistry (GBR ISSN 0309-0698) **3258**
Monographs on Theoretical and Applied Genetics (USA ISSN 0341-5376) **3311**
Monozine (USA) **3552**, 3662
➤ Monroe County Medical Society. Bulletin (USA) **3662**
Montana Comprehensive Chemical Dependency Plan (USA) **3404**
Montana State Plan for Alcohol Abuse and Alcoholism Prevention, Treatment and Rehabilitation *see* Montana Comprehensive Chemical Dependency Plan **3404**
Montana Vital Statistics (USA ISSN 0077-1198) **4497**
Monterrey Institute for the Sutdy of Alternative Healing Arts Newsletter *see* MISAHA Newsletter **3168**
Montgomery - Bucks Dental Society. Bulletin (USA ISSN 0027-0156) **3832**
Monthly Community Medicine *see* Gekkan Chiiki Igaku **3605**
▼ The Monthly D O S E (Development through Organization and Solidarity towards Excellence) (PHL) **3519**
Monthly Ethical Drug Index Complication *see* M E D I C **4345**, 3150
Monthly Index of Medical Specialities Africa *see* M I M S Africa **4314**
Monthly Index of Medical Specialities Caribbean *see* M I M S Caribbean **4314**
Monthly Index of Medical Specialities Middle East *see* M I M S Middle East **4314**
Monthly Index of Medical Specialties *see* M I M S **4314**, 3645
Monthly Index of Medical Specialties Medical Specialities *see* M I M S Medical Specialities **3732**, 3150, 4345
Monthly Medical & Fine *see* Gekkan Medikaru & Fain **3605**
Monthly Mini-Lessons in Care of the Aging (USA ISSN 0889-4744) **3478**
Monthly Prescribing Reference (USA ISSN 0883-0266) **4317**, 3542, 3662, 4482
Monthly Report on Adverse Reactions to Drugs *see* Iyakuhin Fukusayo Bunken Sokuho **4304**
Monthly Review of Insurance Treatment *see* Gekkan Hoken Shinryo **3605**
• Montrose Health E-Letter (USA) **4358**
Moon Magazine (GBR ISSN 0027-0911) **3498**, 3465
Moon Rainbow (GBR ISSN 0047-8083) **3498**, 3492
• ➤ Morbidity and Mortality Weekly Report (USA ISSN 0149-2195) **4482**, 4369
Morbidity & Mortality Weekly Report *see* Morbidity and Mortality Weekly Report **4482**, 4369
Morbidity and Mortality Weekly Report. Recommendations and Report *see* U.S. Centers for Disease Control. Morbidity and Mortality Weekly Report. Recommendations and Report **4491**, 4370
Morbilidad (URY) **4482**
• ➤ Morfologiya (RUS ISSN 1026-3543) **3209**, 3662
Morphologie (FRA ISSN 1286-0115) **3662**, 3209
Morphologie et Embryologie *see* Romanian Journal of Morphology and Embryology **3216**, 3687
• Mortality (GBR ISSN 1357-6275) **4482**, 3663
Moscow Society of Naturalists. Biological Series. Bulletin *see* Moskovskoe Obshchestvo Ispytatelei Priroda. Biologicheskii Otdel. Byulleten **3209**, 3408
➤ Moscow State University Biological Sciences Bulletin (USA ISSN 0096-3925) **3209**
Moskovskii Gosudarstvennyi Universitet. Vestnik. Seriya 14: Psikhologiya (RUS ISSN 0137-0936) **4428**
Moskovskii Gosudarstvennyi Universitet. Vestnik. Seriya 16: Biologiya (RUS ISSN 0137-0952) **3209**, 3159
Moskovskii Psikhoterapevticheskii Zhurnal (RUS ISSN 0135-2652) **4111**
Moskovskoe Obshchestvo Ispytatelei Priroda. Biologicheskii Otdel. Byulleten/Moscow Society of Naturalists. Biological Series. Bulletin (RUS ISSN 0027-1403) **3209**, 3408
Mosquito Systematics *see* American Mosquito Control Association. Journal **3157**
Motdrag (SWE ISSN 0280-3348) **3404**, 3385
Mother & Baby (AUS) **3959**, 3385, 4049
Mother and Child *see* Journal of Paediatrics, Obstetrics and Gynaecology (Hong Kong Edition) **3956**, 4047
• Mother and Child (PAK ISSN 0379-2617) **4568**, 3385, 4516, 4564
Mother of Asthmatics Report *see* The M A Report **3749**

Title

Title

N H E L P Health Advocate *see* Health Advocate **4354**, 3539
N H F Head Lines (National Headache Foundation) (USA ISSN 1521-2106) **4111**
N H I F Newsletter *see* T B I Challenge! **4026**
N H L A News *see* Health Lawyers News **3540**, 3611
N H O Newsline (National Hospice Organization) (USA ISSN 1081-5678) **3168**, 3519, 4516
N H S Breast Screening Programme (National Health Service) (GBR) **4565**
• N H S Cervical Screening Programme (Year) (National Health Service) (GBR) **4565**, 3959
N H S Confederation. Best Practice Papers (Publications Department) (GBR) **4482**
N H S Confederation. Research Papers (Publications Department) (GBR) **4482**
The N H S Handbook (Year) (National Health Service) (GBR ISSN 0953-8623) **4482**
N H S Health Advisory Service. Annual Report of the Director (National Health Service) (GBR) **4482**
N H S Information Authority. Occasional Paper (National Health Service) (GBR) **3519**
N H S Magazine (National Health Service) (GBR ISSN 1359-4443) **4482**
N H S Management Executive News *see* N H S News **4482**
N H S News (National Health Service) (GBR ISSN 1354-2362) **4482**
N.I.A.A.A. - R.U.C.A.S. Alcoholism Treatment Monographs *see* N I A A A - R U C A S Alcoholism Treatment Series **3404**
N I A A A - R U C A S Alcoholism Treatment Series (National Institute on Alcohol Abuse and Alcoholism - Rutgers University Center of Alcohol Studies) (USA ISSN 0147-0515) **3404**
N I C U: Japanese Journal of Neonatal Care *see* Neonatal Care **4049**
N I D A Research Monograph (U.S. National Institute on Drug Abuse) (USA ISSN 1046-9516) **3404**
N I F P General Series (National Institute of Health and Family Welfare) (IND ISSN 0077-4944) **3359**
N I F P Manual Series (National Institute of Health and Family Welfare) (IND ISSN 0077-4952) **3359**
N I F P Monograph Series (National Institute of Health and Family Welfare) (IND ISSN 0077-4960) **3359**
N I F P Report Series (National Institute of Health and Family Welfare) (IND ISSN 0077-4979) **3359**
N I F P Technical Paper Series (National Institute of Health and Family Welfare) (IND ISSN 0077-4987) **3359**
N I H Record (National Institutes of Health) (USA ISSN 1057-5871) **3664**
N.I.I. Sotsyal'noi Gigieny i Upravleniya Zdravookhraneniem. Byulleten' (RUS) **3664**
➤ N I M H A N S Journal (National Institute of Mental Health & Neuro Sciences) (IND ISSN 0254-0886) **4111**
N I O S H Manual of Analytical Methods (U.S. National Institute for Occupational Safety and Health) (USA) **4259**, 3453
• N I O S H Pocket Guide to Chemical Hazards (U.S. National Institute for Occupational Safety and Health) (USA) **4259**, 3453
• N I O S H T I C (U.S. National Institute for Occupational Safety and Health) (USA) **4259**
N I P R Symposium on Polar Biology. Proceedings *see* Polar Bioscience **3213**, 3465
N I P S *see* News in Physiological Sciences **3346**
N I R S Symposium. Proceedings *see* Hoiken Shinpojumu Shirizu **4145**
➤ N J A O P S Journal (New Jersey Association of Osteopathic Physicians and Surgeons) (USA ISSN 0892-0249) **3789**
N L M Newsline (Office of Public Information) (USA ISSN 1094-5970) **3548**, 3664
N L M Technical Bulletin (U.S. National Library of Medicine) (USA ISSN 0146-3055) **3548**, 3664
N M A M *see* N I O S H Manual of Analytical Methods **4259**, 3453
• ➤ N M C D (Nutrition, Metabolism and Cardiovascular Diseases) (ITA ISSN 0939-4753) **4239**, 3780
• ➤ N M R in Biomedicine (Nuclear Magnetic Resonance) (GBR ISSN 0952-3480) **4151**, 3377
N N F A Monitor *see* N N F A Today **3462**, 4239
N N F A Today (National Nutritional Foods Association) (USA) **3462**, 4239
N. Naturheilpraxis *see* Naturheilpraxis mit Naturmedizin **3169**, 3665
N O C I R C Annual Report (National Organization of Circumcision Information Resource Centers) (USA) **4049**
N O C I R C Newsletter *see* N O C I R C Annual Report **4049**
N O H A News (Nutrition for Optimal Health Association) (USA) **4239**, 3168, 3750
N P A Supplement (National Pharmaceutical Association) (GBR) **4317**
N P C H N *see* Neonatal, Paediatric and Child Health Nursing **3930**, 4049
N P G *see* N I O S H Pocket Guide to Chemical Hazards **4259**, 3453
N P R A National Safety Conference. Proceedings (National Petroleum Refiners Association) (USA) **4272**, 3435, 4259
N P R A Statistical Report. Annual Survey of Occupational Injuries & Injuries (National Petroleum Refiners Association) (USA) **4269**, 4272, 4529
• N P W H Newsletter: The Monthly Cycle (Nurse Practitioners in Women's Health) (USA) **4565**
N R C T L D Direct Radiation Monitoring Network (USA) **4366**, 4483
N R H A ENews (National Rural Health Association) (USA) **4483**, 3664
N R L News *see* National Right to Life News **4516**, 3542
N R P A Report *see* Straalevernrapport **4490**, 3442
N R T A Bulletin (National Retired Teachers Association) (USA ISSN 0027-6987) **3413**, 3478
N S C A Journal *see* Strength and Conditioning Journal **4361**
N S N A Newsletter *see* Imprint (New York) **3921**
N S S L H A Clinical Series (National Student Speech Language Hearing Association) (USA ISSN 0887-6584) **4035**
• ➤ N S W Public Health Bulletin (New South Wales) (AUS ISSN 1034-7674) **4483**
N T D *see* Nordisk Tidsskrift foer Doevundervisningen **3492**, 3425
N T I Bulletin (National Tuberculosis Institute) (IND) **4162**
N T I Newsletter *see* N T I Bulletin **4162**
N T I S Alerts: Biomedical Technology & Human Factors Engineering (U.S. National Technical Information Service) (USA) **3733**, 3150
N T I S Alerts: Health Care (U.S. National Technical Information Service) (USA) **4364**, 3150
N T Research (Nursing Times) (GBR ISSN 1361-4096) **3929**
N T S A Newsletter *see* Perspective (Silver Spring) **3674**
N T S R (Nederlands Tijdschrift voor Spoedeisende Medische Hulpverlening en Rampengeneeskunde) (NLD ISSN 1380-3522) **4021**
N U P E Journal *see* U N I S O N Magazine **3535**
N V F G Nuus *see* N A P W News **4317**, 3367
N V M Tijdschrift *see* Nederlands Tijdschrift voor Mondhygiene **3833**
N V V K Info (Nederlandse Vereniging voor Veiligheidskunde) (NLD ISSN 0928-4923) **4259**
N W D A Executive Newsletter (National Wholesale Druggists' Association) (USA) **4317**
N Y S S A Sphere (New York State Society of Anesthesiologists, Inc.) (USA ISSN 0095-2273) **3758**
N Y State Pharmacist (USA ISSN 0163-1586) **4317**
➤ N Z Family Physician (NZL ISSN 0110-022X) **3664**
N Z N U News *see* Kai Tiaki: Nursing New Zealand **3927**
Nachrichen aus der Aerztlichen Mission *see* Gesundheit in der Einen Welt **4500**, 3507, 4353
Naczelna Izba Aptekarska. Biuletyn (POL ISSN 1426-0514) **4318**
Naeringsforskning *see* Scandinavian Journal of Nutrition **4245**
Nagakura Kanpo Daijesuto/Nagakura Kanpo Digest (JPN ISSN 0911-9760) **3168**
Nagakura Kanpo Digest *see* Nagakura Kanpo Daijesuto **3168**
Nagano Association of Occupational Therapists. Journal *see* Naganoken Sagyo Ryohoshikai Gakujutsushi **4259**, 3664
Nagano Prefectural Society of Dialysis Therapy. Journal *see* Naganoken Jinko Toseki Kenkyukaishi **4216**
Naganoken Jinko Toseki Kenkyukaishi/Nagano Prefectural Society of Dialysis Therapy. Journal (JPN ISSN 0910-2329) **4216**
Naganoken Sagyo Ryohoshikai Gakujutsushi/Nagano Association of Occupational Therapists. Journal (JPN ISSN 0917-3617) **4259**, 3664
Naganoken Sanka Fujinka Ikaiho/Gynecological Society of Nagano. Bulletin (JPN) **3959**
Nagarjun (IND ISSN 0027-7576) **3664**
➤ Nagasaki Igakkai Zasshi/Nagasaki Medical Journal (JPN ISSN 0369-3228) **3664**
Nagasaki Medical Journal *see* Nagasaki Igakkai Zasshi **3664**
Nagoya City University. Faculty of Pharmaceutical Science. Annual Report *see* Nagoya Shiritsu Daigaku Yakugakubu Kenkyu Nenpo **4318**
Nagoya City University. Medical Association. Journal *see* Nagoya Shiritsu Daigaku Igakkai Zasshi **3664**
Nagoya Journal of Medical Science (JPN ISSN 0027-7622) **3664**
➤ Nagoya Medical Journal (JPN ISSN 0027-7649) **3664**
➤ Nagoya Shiritsu Daigaku Igakkai Zasshi/Nagoya City University. Medical Association. Journal (JPN ISSN 0027-7606) **3664**
Nagoya Shiritsu Daigaku Yakugakubu Kenkyu Nenpo/Nagoya City University. Faculty of Pharmaceutical Science. Annual Report (JPN ISSN 0369-5611) **4318**
• ➤ Nahrung/Food (DEU ISSN 0027-769X) **4239**
➤ Naibunpi Geka/Endocrine Surgery (JPN ISSN 0914-9953) **3867**, 4197
Naika/Internal Medicine (Tokyo, 1958) (JPN ISSN 0022-1961) **3910**
Naito Museum. Semi-Annual Report *see* Kusuri Hakubutsukan Dayori **4313**
Namah-i Danishkadah-i Dampizishki *see* Majallah-i Danishkadah-i Dampizishki **4548**
Nanjing Institute of Medical Sciences. Journal *see* Nanjing Yixueyuan Xuebao **3664**
Nanjing Institute of Traditional Chinese Medicine. Journal *see* Nanjing Zhongyi Xueyuan Xuebao **3664**
Nanjing Railway Medical College. Journal *see* Nanjing Tiedao Yixueyuan Xuebao **3664**
➤ Nanjing Tiedao Yixueyuan Xuebao/Nanjing Railway Medical College. Journal (CHN ISSN 1001-7275) **3664**
Nanjing Yixueyuan Xuebao/Nanjing Institute of Medical Sciences. Journal (CHN ISSN 1000-5331) **3664**
➤ Nanjing Zhongyi Xueyuan Xuebao/Nanjing Institute of Traditional Chinese Medicine. Journal (CHN ISSN 1000-5005) **3664**
Nantong Institute of Medical Sciences. Journal *see* Nantong Yixueyuan Xuebao **3664**
Nantong Yixueyuan Xuebao/Nantong Institute of Medical Sciences. Journal (CHN ISSN 1000-2057) **3664**
Napa-Solano Dental Society. District Six. Newsletter *see* Oracle (Fairfield) **3834**
• Napralert on CD-ROM (GBR ISSN 1360-3019) **4318**, 3209, 3373, 3664
Nara Igaku Zasshi *see* Journal of Nara Medical Association **3636**
Nara Joshi Daigaku Hoken Kanri Senta Nenpo/Nara Women's University. Health Administration Center. Archives of Health Care (JPN ISSN 0287-9549) **4483**, 3416
Nara Women's University. Health Administration Center. Archives of Health Care *see* Nara Joshi Daigaku Hoken Kanri Senta Nenpo **4483**, 3416
Narc Officer (USA ISSN 0889-7794) **3542**, 3395, 3404
Narconon-nytt (SWE ISSN 0281-3629) **3404**
Narcotic Drugs: Estimated World Requirements for (Year) (AUT ISSN 1013-3453) **4345**, 4497, 4529
Narcotics and Drug Abuse A to Z (USA ISSN 0094-3991) **3404**
Narcotics Anonymous Way Magazine *see* The N A Way Magazine **3404**, 4482
Naringsforskning. Supplement *see* Scandinavian Journal of Nutrition. Supplement **4245**
Naropa Institute Journal of Psychology *see* Journal of Contemplative Psychotherapy **4101**, 4413
Nas Glas *see* Savez Gluvih i Nagluvih Jugoslavije. Glas **3493**
Nase Liecive Rastliny (SVK ISSN 0323-2646) **3281**, 3664
Nash Malysh (RUS) **3664**
Nashe Zdorov'e (AZE) **3664**
Nashrat al-Mukhaddirat *see* Bulletin on Narcotics **3399**
Nasionale Veiligheid *see* National Safety **4483**
➤ Nassau County Dental Society. Newsletter (USA) **3833**
Nassau Dental News *see* Nassau County Dental Society. Newsletter **3833**
➤ Nat - Cent News (USA) **3492**, 3498
NAT. Norges Apotekerforenings Tidsskrift *see* Norges Apotekerforenings Tidsskrift **4319**
National Academies of Practice Forum *see* Issues in Interdisciplinary Care **3625**
National Academy of Indian Medicine. Annals (IND) **3664**
National Academy of Medical Sciences. Annals (IND ISSN 0379-038X) **3664**
National Academy of Sciences, India. Proceedings. Section B. Biological Sciences (IND ISSN 0369-8211) **3209**, 4505
National Academy of Sciences of Belarus. Papers *see* Nationalnaya Akademiya Navuk Belarusi. Doklady **4506**
National Academy of Sciences of Belarus. Proceedings. Biological Series *see* Nationalnaya Akademiya Navuk Belarusi. Vestsi. Seriya Biologichnykh Navuk **3210**
• ➤ National Academy of Sciences of the United States of America. Proceedings (USA ISSN 0027-8424) **4505**
National Accrediting Agency for Clinical Laboratory Sciences News *see* N A A C L S News **3663**
National Aids Treatment Advocacy Project Reports *see* N A T A P Reports **3804**
National Alliance for the Mentally Ill Advocate *see* N A M I Advocate **4111**
National Alliance of Breast Cancer Organizations News *see* N A B C O News **3985**, 3959, 4565
National Alopecia Areata Foundation Newsletter (USA ISSN 0894-1769) **3851**, 3175, 3867
National Amputee Golf Association Newsletter *see* N A G A Newsletter **4526**, 3494
National Animal Control Association News *see* N A C A News **4272**, 4482
National Association for Colitis and Crohn's Disease News *see* N A C C News **3894**
National Association for Home Care Report *see* N A H C Report **3663**
National Association for Special Educational Needs. Publications (GBR) **3425**
National Association for the Blind, India. Annual Report (IND) **3498**
National Association for the Care and Resettlement of Offenders Policy Paper *see* N A C R O Policy Paper **4111**
National Association for Visually Handicapped Update *see* N A V H Update **3498**
National Association of Anorexia Nervosa and Associated Disorders Working Together *see* A N A D: Working Together **4371**, 3556
National Association of Boards of Pharmacy Newsletter *see* N A B P Newsletter **4317**
• National Association of Boards of Pharmacy. Proceedings (USA ISSN 0077-3263) **4318**
National Association of Chain Drug Stores Annual Report *see* N A C D S Annual Report **3365**, 4317
National Association of Chain Drug Stores Chain Pharmacist Practice Memo *see* N A C D S Chain Pharmacist Practice Memo **4317**
National Association of Chain Drug Stores. Executive Newsletter (USA ISSN 1079-1116) **3366**, 4318
National Association of Chain Drug Stores Federal Report *see* N A C D S Federal Report **4317**
National Association of Chain Drug Stores. Legislative Newsletter *see* N A C D S Federal Report **4317**
National Association of Chain Drug Stores Sourcebook *see* N A C D S Sourcebook **3365**, 4317
National Association of Dental Laboratories. Membership Memo (USA) **3833**
National Association of Emergency Medical Technicians News *see* N A E M T News **3663**
National Association of Fire Officers Magazine *see* N A F O Magazine **4482**
National Association of Health Services Executives's Resume *see* N A H S E's Resume **4482**

Title

National Psychological Association for Psychoanalysis. Bulletin (USA ISSN 0077-5339) **4429**
National Psychological Association for Psychoanalysis. News and Reviews (USA) **4429**
National Register of Professional Hypnotherapists (USA) **3906**, 4429
National Register of Psychotherapists (GBR) **4111**
➤ National Rehabilitation Center for the Disabled. Research Bulletin (JPN ISSN 0285-1350) **3486**, 4063
● National Report on Computers and Health (USA ISSN 0273-4974) **3812**
National Report on Subacute Care (USA ISSN 1073-2551) **3665**, 3519
National Report on Substance Abuse *see* Workplace Substance Abuse Advisor **3406**
National Research Institute of Police Science. Report *see* Kagaku Keisatsu Kenkyujo Hokoku Hokagaku Hen **3883**
National Research Institute of Police Science. Report. Research of Forensic Science *see* Kagaku Keisatsu Kenkyujo Hokoku Hokagaku Hen **3883**
National Retired Teachers Association Bulletin *see* N R T A Bulletin **3413**, 3478
● National Right to Life News (USA ISSN 0164-7415) **4516**, 3542
National Rural Health Association ENews *see* N R H A ENews **4483**, 3664
National Safety/Nasionale Veiligheid (ZAF ISSN 0028-0097) **4483**
National Senior Citizens Law Center Washington Weekly (USA) **3542**, 3478
National Senior Citizens Law Center Weekly *see* National Senior Citizens Law Center Washington Weekly **3542**, 3478
National Society for Graphology Newsletter *see* Write-Up **4455**
National Society for the Prevention of Blindness. Report *see* Prevent Blindness America. Annual Report **4485**, 3499
National Society to Prevent Blindness. Annual Report *see* Prevent Blindness America. Annual Report **4485**, 3499
National Society to Prevent Blindness. Member News *see* Prevent Blindness News **4485**, 3499, 4006
National Spokesman *see* Epilepsy U S A **4088**
● National Strength & Conditioning Association Bulletin (USA) **4359**
National Student Speech Language Hearing Association Clinical Series *see* N S S L H A Clinical Series **4035**
National Student Speech Language Hearing Association. Journal *see* Contemporary Issues in Communication Science & Disorders **4031**
➤ National Taiwan University. College of Medicine. Memoirs (TWN ISSN 0028-0275) **3665**
National Tuberculosis Institute Bulletin *see* N T I Bulletin **4162**
➤ National Vital Statistics Reports (USA) **4370**, 4529
National Wholesale Druggists' Association Executive Newsletter *see* N W D A Executive Newsletter **4317**
National Women's Health Network (USA) **4565**
● National Women's Health Report (USA ISSN 0741-9147) **4565**
Nationalnaya Akademiya Navuk Belarusi. Doklady/National Academy of Sciences of Belarus. Papers (BLR) **4506**
Nationalnaya Akademiya Navuk Belarusi. Vestsi. Seriya Biologichnykh Navuk/National Academy of Sciences of Belarus. Proceedings. Biological Series (BLR) **3210**
● The Nation's Health (USA ISSN 0028-0496) **4483**
Natom. Farmacia Naturale *see* Farmacia Naturale **4295**
➤ Natuerlich Vegetarisch (DEU ISSN 1437-0735) **4240**
Natur *see* Natur und Kosmos **3441**, 3210, 3665
● ➤ Natur und Gesundheit (DEU ISSN 1433-9935) **3168**
Natur und Heilen (DEU ISSN 0932-3503) **4240**
● Natur und Kosmos (DEU) **3441**, 3210, 3665
Natur und Mensch: Jahresmitteilungen der Naturhistorischen Gesellschaft Nuernberg (DEU ISSN 0077-6025) **3210**, 3174, 3407, 3408
Natura (BRA) **3210**
Natura Jutlandica (DNK ISSN 0077-6033) **3210**
Natural Beauty & Health (USA) **4359**, 3168
Natural Bodybuilding and Fitness (USA ISSN 1071-555X) **4359**, 4223
Natural Business LOHAS Journal *see* L O H A S Journal **3361**, 3167, 4227
Natural Choice Magazine (GBR) **4359**
Natural Development (GBR ISSN 1369-9385) **4359**, 4526
Natural Environment Research Council. Report (GBR ISSN 0072-7008) **3441**
Natural Family Planning Council of Victoria. Bulletin *see* Ovulation Method Research and Reference Centre of Australia. Bulletin **3360**
Natural Food Trader (GBR) **4240**, 3462
● ➤ Natural Foods Merchandiser (USA ISSN 0164-338X) **3367**, 4240
● Natural Hazards Center. Quick Response Reports (USA) **4509**, 4516
● ➤ Natural Hazards Review (USA ISSN 1527-6988) **3441**, 3408, 4483
Natural Health (AUS ISSN 0816-2751) **4240**, 4359
Natural Health (GBR) **3168**, 4359
● Natural Health (USA ISSN 1067-9588) **3168**, 4227, 4359
▼ Natural Health Hollywood (USA) **3168**, 4359
Natural Health Review (AUS) **4359**, 3168
Natural Hygiene Society of New Jersey. Newsletter (USA) **4240**
● Natural Land News (USA) **4359**, 4240
Natural Living Today (USA ISSN 1087-5050) **3549**
Natural Medicines (JPN ISSN 1340-3443) **4318**
Natural Muscle Magazine (USA) **4359**, 4223
Natural Parent (GBR) **3385**, 3168
Natural Pharmacy (USA ISSN 1089-4853) **4318**, 3169
Natural Physique *see* Natural Bodybuilding and Fitness **4359**, 4223
Natural Product Sciences (KOR) **4318**
Natural Products Industry Insider (USA ISSN 1525-5301) **4240**, 3367
Natural Products News (GBR) **3379**, 4318
Natural Remedies (USA ISSN 1094-0189) **3169**, 4359
● ➤ Natural Toxins (USA ISSN 1056-9014) **3453**, 4318
● The Natural Way (USA ISSN 1082-0531) **3169**
➤ Naturalia (BRA ISSN 0101-1944) **3210**
➤ The Naturalist (GBR ISSN 0028-0771) **3210**, 3526
Naturalist *see* New Crucible **4430**, 4501
Naturamed (DEU ISSN 0931-1513) **3665**
Der Naturarzt (DEU ISSN 0028-081X) **3169**
● ➤ Nature (GBR ISSN 0028-0836) **4506**
Nature and Health (AUS ISSN 0815-7006) **3169**, 4227
● ➤ Nature Biotechnology (USA ISSN 1087-0156) **3276**, 3373, 3665, 4531
Nature et Progres (FRA ISSN 0182-7146) **3155**
● ➤ Nature Genetics (USA ISSN 1061-4036) **3312**
● ➤ Nature Medicine (GBR ISSN 1078-8956) **3665**, 3210
● ➤ Nature Neuroscience (USA ISSN 1097-6256) **4111**
▼ ● ➤ Nature Reviews Neuroscience (GBR) **4112**
● ➤ Nature Structural Biology (USA ISSN 1072-8368) **3210**, 4506
Naturheilpraxis mit Naturmedizin (DEU ISSN 0177-6754) **3169**, 3665
Naturismo (ITA ISSN 0392-4173) **4359**
Naturopath (USA ISSN 0028-100X) **3169**
Naturwissenschaften im Unterricht Biologie *see* Unterricht Biologie **3223**, 3430
➤ Naturwissenschaftlich - Medizinischen Vereins in Innsbruck. Berichte (AUT ISSN 0379-1416) **3210**, 3665
Naturwissenschaftliche Zeitschrift fuer Niederbayern (DEU ISSN 0932-9447) **3210**, 3407
Naturwissenschaftlicher Verein fuer Schwaben. Berichte (DEU ISSN 0720-3705) **3210**
Naturwissenschaftlicher Verein in Hamburg. Abhandlungen (DEU ISSN 0173-7481) **3355**, 4271
➤ Naturwissenschaftlicher Verein zu Bremen. Abhandlungen (DEU ISSN 0340-3718) **3210**, 3407, 4271
Natuurhistorisch Genootschap in Limburg. Publicaties (NLD ISSN 0374-955X) **3210**, 4271
Naucni Podmladak. Sveska za Medicinks Nauke (YUG ISSN 0352-5856) **3665**
Naukove Tovarystvo Imeni Shevchenka. Proceedings of the Section of Chemistry, Biology and Medicine (USA ISSN 0195-7198) **3373**, 3210, 3665
● ➤ Naunyn-Schmiedeberg's Archives of Pharmacology (DEU ISSN 0028-1298) **4318**, 3453
● Navy Medicine (USA ISSN 0895-8211) **3665**
Nebraska Journal (USA) **3413**, 4359
Nebraska Mortar and Pestle (USA ISSN 0028-1891) **4318**
Nebraska Nurse (USA ISSN 0028-1921) **3929**
Nebraska Statistical Report of Abortions (USA ISSN 0095-3105) **3360**
● Nebraska Symposium on Motivation (Publication) (USA ISSN 0146-7875) **4429**
Neck Pain (USA) **3665**, 3542
Nederlands Forensisch Tijdschrift *see* Modus **3884**
● ➤ Nederlands Militair Geneeskundig Tijdschrift (NLD ISSN 0028-2103) **3665**, 4224
Nederlands Tandartsenblad (NLD ISSN 0028-2111) **3833**
➤ Nederlands Tijdschrift voor Anesthesiologie (NLD ISSN 0921-8769) **3758**
Nederlands Tijdschrift voor Cardiologie *see* Cardiologie **3765**
Nederlands Tijdschrift voor de Psychologie en haar Grensgebieden (NLD ISSN 0028-2235) **4429**, 4112
➤ Nederlands Tijdschrift voor de Zorg aan Verstandelijk Gehandicapten (NLD) **3486**
Nederlands Tijdschrift voor Dermatologie en Venereologie (NLD ISSN 0925-8604) **3852**
Nederlands Tijdschrift voor Dietisten (NLD ISSN 0166-7203) **4240**
Nederlands Tijdschrift voor E H B O en Reddingwezen (NLD ISSN 0925-6040) **4483**
Nederlands Tijdschrift voor Ergotherapie (NLD ISSN 0166-4751) **4063**
● Nederlands Tijdschrift voor Geneeskunde (NLD ISSN 0028-2162) **3665**
Nederlands Tijdschrift voor Heelkunde (NLD ISSN 0926-7522) **3666**
Nederlands Tijdschrift voor Klinische Chemie (NLD ISSN 1380-3689) **3373**
➤ Nederlands Tijdschrift voor Medische Microbiologie (NLD ISSN 0929-0176) **3666**, 3329
Nederlands Tijdschrift voor Mondhygiene (NLD ISSN 1384-3966) **3833**
Nederlands Tijdschrift voor Obstetrie & Gynaecologie (NLD ISSN 0921-4011) **3959**
Nederlands Tijdschrift voor Osteoporose en Andere Botziekten (NLD ISSN 1386-1565) **3666**
Nederlands Tijdschrift voor Spoedeisende Medische Hulpverlening en Rampengeneeskunde *see* N T S R **4021**
● Nederlands Tijdschrift voor Tandheelkunde (NLD ISSN 0028-2200) **3833**
➤ Nederlands Tijdschrift voor Urologie (NLD ISSN 0929-0184) **4216**
Nederlands Tijdschrift voor Zwakzinnigenzorg *see* Nederlands Tijdschrift voor de Zorg aan Verstandelijk Gehandicapten **3486**
Nederlandse Cystic Fibrosis Stichting. Bericht *see* Nederlandse Cystic Fibrosis Stichting. C F Nieuws **4162**
Nederlandse Cystic Fibrosis Stichting. C F Nieuws (NLD ISSN 0925-1944) **4162**
Nederlandse Vereniging voor Klinische Chemie. Almanak (NLD) **3879**
Nederlandse Vereniging voor Klinische Chemie. Tijdschrift *see* Nederlands Tijdschrift voor Klinische Chemie **3373**
Nederlandse Vereniging voor Veiligheidskunde Info *see* N V V K Info **4259**
Needle Tips *see* Needle Tips and the Hepatitis B Coalition News **3750**, 4483
● Needle Tips and the Hepatitis B Coalition News (USA) **3750**, 4483
● ➤ Nefrologia (ESP ISSN 0211-6995) **4216**
➤ Nefrologiia, Hemodializa i Transplantatsiia (BGR ISSN 0204-6105) **4216**
● Negri News (ITA) **4318**, 3388
Nei Jing (CHN) **3666**
Neijing *see* Zhonghua Xiaohua Neijing Zazhi **3870**
Neike Xuezhi/Journal of Internal Medicine R O C (TWN ISSN 1016-7390) **3911**
Neirofiziologiya/Neurophysiology (UKR ISSN 0028-2561) **3346**, 4112
● Nematological Abstracts (GBR ISSN 0957-6797) **3233**, 3150, 3355
Nena dhe Femija (ALB) **4359**
Neodidagmata (POL ISSN 0077-653X) **3429**, 4429
Neonatal Care (JPN ISSN 1341-4577) **4049**
➤ Neonatal Intensive Care (USA ISSN 1062-2454) **3959**, 4049
➤ Neonatal Network (USA ISSN 0730-0832) **3929**, 3959, 4049
➤ Neonatal, Paediatric and Child Health Nursing (AUS ISSN 1441-6638) **3930**, 4049
Neoplasia (ESP ISSN 0212-9787) **3985**
▼ ● ➤ NeoPlasia (USA ISSN 1522-8002) **3985**
● ➤ Neoplasma (SVK ISSN 0028-2685) **3985**
▼ ● NeoReviews.org (USA ISSN 1526-9906) **4049**
Nepal. Department of Medicinal Plants. Annual Report (NPL) **3281**, 4318
➤ Nepal Medical Association. Journal (NPL ISSN 0028-2715) **3666**
● ➤ Nephrologie (CHE ISSN 0250-4960) **4216**
● ➤ Nephrology (AUS ISSN 1320-5358) **4216**
● ➤ Nephrology, Dialysis and Transplantation (GBR ISSN 0931-0509) **4216**
➤ Nephrology News & Issues (USA ISSN 0896-1263) **4216**
Nephrology News and Issues - Europe *see* Nephrology News & Issues **4216**
● ➤ Nephrology Nursing Journal (USA ISSN 1526-744X) **3930**, 4216
Nephrology Online *see* Nephrology **4216**
● ➤ Nephron (CHE ISSN 0028-2766) **4216**
● Nerve Cell Biology (GBR ISSN 0142-8225) **3233**, 3150, 3293, 3733, 4112
● ➤ Der Nervenarzt (DEU ISSN 0028-2804) **4112**
● ➤ Nervenheilkunde (DEU ISSN 0722-1541) **4112**
Nervni i Psikhichni Zaboliavaniia *see* Meditsinski Pregled. Nevrologiia i Psichiatriia **4109**, 3404
Nestle Foundation. Annual Report (CHE) **4240**
➤ Nestle Nutrition Series (USA ISSN 0742-2806) **4240**
Nestle Nutrition Workshop *see* Nestle Nutrition Series **4240**
▼ Nestle Nutrition Workshop Series Clinical and Performance Programme (CHE ISSN 1422-7584) **4240**
Netherlands. Centraal Bureau voor de Statistiek. Leefsituatie van de Nederlandse Bevolking, Deel 1: Gezondheid en Kwaliteit van de Arbeid (NLD) **4497**, 3362, 3363, 3364, 4269, 4529
Netherlands Journal of Aquatic Ecology *see* Aquatic Ecology **3182**
Netherlands Journal of Cardiology *see* Cardiologie **3765**
● ➤ Netherlands Journal of Medicine (NLD ISSN 0300-2977) **3911**, 3666
Netherlands Journal of Surgery *see* European Journal of Surgery **4188**
Netherlands Journal of Veterinary Science *see* Tijdschrift voor Diergeneeskunde **4554**
Netherlands Military Medical Review *see* Nederlands Militair Geneeskundig Tijdschrift **3665**, 4224
Netherlands. Ministerie van Binnenlandse Zaken. Inspectie voor het Brandweerwezen. Maandelijkse Mededelingen *see* Alert **3387**, 4460, 4510
● ➤ NetSci (USA) **4318**
Nettai Igaku *see* Tropical Medicine **3807**
● Network (Durham) (USA ISSN 0270-3637) **3359**, 3852, 3959
Network News - National Women's Health Network *see* Network News (Washington, 1975) **4565**
Network News (Sherman) (USA) **4368**, 3416
● Network News (Washington, 1975) (USA ISSN 8755-867X) **4565**
Neue Arzneimittel (DEU ISSN 0724-567X) **4318**
Neue B S (Betriebs Sicherheit) (AUT ISSN 1016-0515) **4260**, 3364
Neue Denkschriften des Naturhistorischen Museums in Wien (AUT ISSN 1016-605X) **4509**
Die Neue Sonderschule (DEU) **3413**, 3492, 3498
Neues Hoeren (DEU) **3492**
Neues von Synanon (DEU) **3404**
➤ Neumologia y Cirugia de Torax (MEX ISSN 1405-2938) **4197**
● ➤ Neural Computation (USA ISSN 0899-7667) **3389**, 4112
Neural Growth, Regeneration and Transplantation *see* Shinkei Soshiki no Seicho Saisei Ishoku **3294**
➤ Neural Network World (CZE ISSN 1210-0552) **3390**, 4112
● ➤ Neural Networks (GBR ISSN 0893-6080) **3390**, 4112
Neural Plasticity (ISR) **4112**
● ➤ Neural Processing Letters (USA ISSN 1370-4621) **3390**, 4112

Title

Title

Nishinihon Hifuka *see* Nishinihon Journal of Dermatology **3852**
Nishinihon Journal of Dermatology/Nishinihon Hifuka (JPN ISSN 0386-9784) **3852**
Nishinihon Journal of Urology/Nishi Nihon Hinyokika (JPN ISSN 0029-0726) **4217**
Nishinihon Sekitsui Kenkyukaishi/Western Japanese Research Society for Spine. Journal (JPN ISSN 0287-1092) **4022**
Nishinomiya Municipal Central Hospital. Bulletin *see* Nishinomiya Shiritsu Chuo Byoin Kiyo **3519**
Nishinomiya Shiritsu Chuo Byoin Kiyo/Nishinomiya Municipal Central Hospital. Bulletin (JPN ISSN 0914-8574) **3519**
Nissanfukai Tohoku Rengo Chiho Bukaiho/Tohoku Journal of Obstetrics and Gynecology (JPN) **3960**
Nisseiken Tayori/Nippon Institute for Biological Science. Journal (JPN ISSN 0029-0750) **3211**
• Nitric Oxide (GBR ISSN 1351-525X) **3234**, 3150 , 3259, 4508
No Cho Horumon Gakkai Nyusu/News of the Brain-Gut Hormone Research (JPN ISSN 0912-2532) **3867**
No no Igaku Seibutsugaku Konwakai Shoroku/Abstracts of Conference on Medicine and Biology of the Brain (JPN) **3234**, 3150, 3346
No Shinkei Geka *see* Neurological Surgery **4197**, 4114
No Shinkei Geka Janaru/Japanese Journal of Neurosurgery (JPN ISSN 0917-950X) **4430**, 4198
No Shinkei Geka Sokuho/Neurosurgery Letters (JPN ISSN 0917-1495) **4198**, 4120
No Sotchu no Geka/Surgery for Cerebral Stroke (JPN ISSN 0914-5508) **4198**, 4120
No to Hattatsu (JPN ISSN 0029-0831) **4120**
No to Shinkei *see* Brain and Nerve **4077**
Nobel Symposium Series (SWE ISSN 0078-0901) **3529**
Nocirc Newsletter *see* N O C I R C Annual Report **4049**
• ➤ The Noetic Journal (USA ISSN 1094-0359) **4365**, 3346, 4348, 4430
• Noetica (AUS ISSN 1324-6038) **4430**
Nogaku Kenkyu - Ohara Institute for Agricultural Biology. Report *see* Okayama Daigaku Shigen Seibutsu Kagaku Kenkyujo Hokoku **3211**
Nogyo Kankyo Gijutsu Kenkyusho Hokoku/National Institute of Agro-Environmental Sciences. Bulletin (JPN ISSN 0911-9450) **3155**, 3211
Nogyo Seibutsu Shigen Kenkyujo Kenkyu Hokoku/National Institute of Agrobiological Resources. Bulletin (JPN ISSN 0911-6575) **3211**
• ➤ Noise & Health (GBR ISSN 1463-1741) **4035**, 3444, 3492, 4260
Non-Prescription Drug Reference for Healthcare Professionals (CAN) **4319**
Non-Prescription Products Guide *see* Australian Prescription Products Guide **4279**
Non-Smokers' Update (AUS) **4484**, 4531
• ➤ Nonlinear Dynamics, Psychology, and Life Sciences (USA ISSN 1090-0578) **4430**, 3211, 3554, 4509
• Nonprescription Pharmaceuticals and Nutritionals: The Tan Sheet (USA ISSN 1068-5316) **4319**
Nonsmokers' Voice (USA ISSN 0897-9626) **4531**, 3444
Noodzaak *see* Alert **3387**, 4460, 4510
Noordernieuws (NLD) **3519**
NorCal Center on Deafness Newsline (USA) **3492**, 4516
NorCal Community Forum *see* NorCal Center on Deafness Newsline **3492**, 4516
Norden News *see* Topics in Veterinary Medicine **4554**
➤ Nordic Journal of Music Therapy/Nordisk Tidsskrift for Musikketerapi (NOR ISSN 0803-9828) **4064**, 4226
• ➤ Nordic Journal of Psychiatry (NOR ISSN 0803-9488) **4120**
Nordic Journal of Psychiatry. Supplement (NOR ISSN 0803-9496) **4120**
Nordic Studies on Alcohol and Drugs *see* Nordisk Alkohol- & Narkotikatidskrift **3404**
Nordisk Alkohol- & Narkotikatidskrift/Nordic Studies on Alcohol and Drugs (FIN ISSN 1455-0725) **3404**
Nordisk Alkoholtidskrift *see* Nordisk Alkohol- & Narkotikatidskrift **3404**
Nordisk Fysioterapi (NOR ISSN 1402-3024) **4064**
Nordisk Geriatrik (SWE ISSN 1403-2082) **3478**
Nordisk Hygienisk Tidskrift *see* Scandinavian Journal of Work, Environment & Health **4265**
Nordisk Psykiatrisk Tidsskrift *see* Nordic Journal of Psychiatry **4120**
Nordisk Psykiatrisk Tidsskrift. Supplement *see* Nordic Journal of Psychiatry. Supplement **4120**
• ➤ Nordisk Psykologi (DNK ISSN 0029-1463) **4430**
Nordisk Sexologi *see* Scandinavian Journal of Sexology **3690**
Nordisk Tidskrift foer Beteendeterapi *see* Scandinavian Journal of Behaviour Therapy **4447**
Nordisk Tidskrift foer Doevundervisningen (SWE ISSN 0029-1471) **3492**, 3425
Nordisk Tidsskrift for Musikketerapi *see* Nordic Journal of Music Therapy **4064**, 4226
Nordisk Tidsskrift for Spesialpedagogikk (NOR ISSN 0048-0509) **3425**, 4430
Nordwestdeutsche Gesellschaft fuer Innere Medizin. Kongressbericht (DEU ISSN 0029-1609) **3668**
Norges Apotekerforenings Tidsskrift (NOR ISSN 0802-8400) **4319**
Norman Bethune University of Medical Sciences. Journal *see* Baiqiuen Yike Daxue Xuebao **3574**
Normerede og Besatte Laegestillinger Samt Sengepladser paa Institutioner *see* Laegestillinger og Sengepladser paa Institutioner **3517**
Norolojik Bilimler Dergisi *see* Journal of Neurological Sciences **4103**
➤ Noropsikiyatri Arsivi/Archives of Neuropsychiatry (TUR ISSN 1300-0667) **4120**
Norsk Bedriftshelsetjeneste *see* Ramazzini **4263**
Norsk Tidsskrift for Arbeidsmedisin *see* Ramazzini **4263**
Norsk V V S (NOR ISSN 0029-2265) **3526**, 4484
➤ Norsk Veterinaertidsskrift/Norwegian Veterinary Medical Journal (NOR ISSN 0029-2273) **4548**
• ➤ Den Norske Tannlegeforenings Tidende/Norwegian Dental Journal (NOR ISSN 0029-2303) **3833**
▼ ➤ North American Journal of Psychology (USA ISSN 1527-7143) **4431**, 3413, 4522
North American Riding for the Handicapped Association, Inc. News *see* N A R H A News **4527**, 3486
North American Riding for the Handicapped Association, Inc. Strides *see* N A R H A Strides **4527**, 3486
North American Society of Adlerian Psychology. Newsletter (USA ISSN 0889-9428) **4431**
North Carolina Communicable Disease Morbidity Statistics (USA ISSN 0085-428X) **4369**
North Carolina Dental Review (USA) **3834**
➤ North Carolina Medical Journal (USA ISSN 0029-2559) **3668**
North Carolina Mental Health, Developmental Disabilities and Substance Abuse Laws (USA) **4120**, 3542
North Carolina Reported Pregnancies (USA) **4369**
North Carolina Vital Statistics (USA ISSN 0078-1371) **4370**, 4529
North Central Optometric Viewpoint (USA) **4002**
North Conway Institute, Inc. Catalyst *see* N C I Catalyst **3404**
North Dakota Society of Medical Technologists. Newsletter (USA ISSN 0048-069X) **3879**
North Dakota State Plan for Rehabilitation Facilities and Workshops (USA ISSN 0093-7843) **4064**, 3425
➤ North Eastern Doctors Calling (IND) **3668**
North Japanese Journal of Nuclear Medicine *see* Kita Nihon Kaku Igaku Danwakai **4149**
North Queensland Naturalist (AUS ISSN 0078-1630) **3211**
Northampton General Hospital Trust. Occasional Paper *see* N H S Information Authority. Occasional Paper **3519**
• Northeast Bioengineering Conference. Proceedings (USA ISSN 0277-1063) **3238**, 3433
Northern California Medicine *see* California Medicine **3581**
Northwest Dentistry (USA ISSN 0029-2915) **3834**
• Northwest Health (USA ISSN 1081-8928) **4359**
Northwestern Forestry University. Journal *see* Xibei Linxueyuan Xuebao **3464**, 3709, 4531
Northwestern University Cancer Center. Journal *see* Northwestern University. Robert H. Lurie Comprehensive Cancer Center. Journal **3985**
➤ Northwestern University. Robert H. Lurie Comprehensive Cancer Center. Journal (USA) **3985**
Norway. Direktoratet for Arbeidstilsynet. Forskrifter/Regulations (NOR) **4260**, 3417
Norway. Direktoratet for Brann og Eksplosjonsvern. Aarsberetning (NOR) **3458**, 4484
Norway. Statens Sprengstoffinspeksjon. Aarsberetning *see* Norway. Direktoratet for Brann og Eksplosjonsvern. Aarsberetning **3458**, 4484
Norway. Statistisk Sentralbyraa. Helsestatistikk/Statistics Norway. Health Statistics (NOR ISSN 0332-7906) **4497**, 4529
Norway. Statistisk Sentralbyraa. Pasientstatistikk (NOR ISSN 0806-0711) **3525**, 4529
Norwegian Dental Journal *see* Den Norske Tannlegeforenings Tidende **3833**
Norwegian Journal of Occupational Medicine *see* Ramazzini **4263**
Norwegian Radiation Protection Authority Report *see* Straalevernrapport **4490**, 3442
Norwegian Veterinary Medical Journal *see* Norsk Veterinaertidsskrift **4548**
Norwich Research Park Newsletter (GBR) **3313**
Notabene Medici (DEU ISSN 0340-5486) **3668**
• Der Notarzt (DEU ISSN 0177-2309) **3668**
Notes Pediatriques (FRA ISSN 0765-5010) **4049**
Notfall *see* Notfall und Rettungsmedizin **4022**
• ➤ Notfall und Rettungsmedizin (DEU ISSN 1434-6222) **4022**
Notfallmedizin (DEU ISSN 0341-2903) **4022**
Noticias de Galapagos (USA ISSN 0550-1067) **4506**, 3211, 3392
Noticias de Seguridad (USA ISSN 0888-1626) **4260**
Noticias Medicas (ESP ISSN 0029-4225) **3668**
Noticias Medicas (PRT ISSN 0870-2055) **3668**
Noticiero Cientifico. Serie: Biologia (CUB) **3211**
Noticiero de Tortugas Marinas *see* Marine Turtle Newsletter **3355**, 3392, 4548
Notivates *see* American Museum Novitates **3350**, 3465, 4271
Notizen zur Flora der Steiermark (AUT) **3281**
Notiziario Bibliografico di Audiologia *see* Notiziario Bibliografico di Audiologia O R L e Foniatria **3733**, 3150, 4035
Notiziario Bibliografico di Audiologia O R L e Foniatria (ITA ISSN 1121-4163) **3733**, 3150, 4035
Notiziario Chimico e Farmaceutico *see* N C F **4317**, 3373
Notiziario Chirurgico (ITA ISSN 0392-3584) **4198**
Notiziario Medico Farmaceutico *see* E D I M E D **4291**
Notiziaro della S I A A R T I *see* Societa Italiana di Anestesia, Analgesia, Rianimazione e Terapia Intensiva. Notizario **3760**
• Notre Dame Journal of Law, Ethics & Public Policy (USA ISSN 0883-3648) **4459**, 3542
Notre Temps (FRA ISSN 0029-456X) **3478**
Notulae Odonatologicae (NLD ISSN 0166-6584) **3211**
Nou to Jonkan/Brain and Circulation (JPN ISSN 1341-8440) **4120**, 3904
Noukogude Naine *see* Eesti Naine **4568**, 3175, 3463, 4563
Nouveau Biologiste (FRA ISSN 0181-3684) **3211**
Nouveau Centre de Sante (FRA ISSN 0292-384X) **3668**, 3535
Nouveau Genie Medical *see* N G M **3664**
Nouvel Hospitalier (FRA ISSN 1150-8116) **3519**
Nouvelle Revue d'Ethnopsychiatrie (FRA ISSN 0762-6819) **4120**, 4522
Nouvelles Dermatologiques (FRA ISSN 0752-5370) **3852**
Nova (CHE ISSN 1422-4178) **3930**
Nova Acta Paracelsica (CHE ISSN 0254-8712) **3668**
Nova Report on Lung Health and Wellness (USA) **4162**
Nova Scotia Dentist (CAN) **3834**
Nover (HUN ISSN 0864-7003) **3930**
Novinky Literatury: Zdravotnictvi *see* Novinky Literatury. Zdravotnictvi-Prirustky Fondu Narodni Lekarske Knihovny **3733**, 3177
Novinky Literatury. Zdravotnictvi-Prirustky Fondu Narodni Lekarske Knihovny (CZE ISSN 1212-3862) **3733**, 3177
Novoe v Oftal'mologii (RUS) **4002**
Novosti Farmatsii i Meditsiny/News in Pharmacology and Medicine (POL ISSN 0209-3928) **4319**, 3668
Novosti Veterinarnoi Farmatsii i Meditsiny (POL ISSN 0860-3847) **4319**, 4549
Novye Promyshlennye Katalogi. Meditsinskaya Tekhnika. Tekhnika Bezopasnosti. Veterinarnoe Oborudovanie (RUS) **4549**
➤ Nowotwory (POL ISSN 0029-540X) **3985**
Nuclear and Space Radiation Effects Conference. Proceedings (USA) **4162**
Nuclear Geophysics *see* Applied Radiation and Isotopes **4365**, 3871, 4140
Nuclear Lemons (USA) **3431**, 3430, 4484
Nuclear Magnetic Resonance in Biomedicine *see* N M R in Biomedicine **4151**, 3377
Nuclear Medicine *see* Nuklearmedizin **4152**
• ➤ Nuclear Medicine and Biology (USA ISSN 0969-8051) **4152**, 3211, 4366
➤ Nuclear Medicine Annual (USA ISSN 0272-0108) **4152**
• ➤ Nuclear Medicine Communications (USA ISSN 0143-3636) **4152**
• ➤ Nuclear Plant Journal (USA ISSN 0892-2055) **3431**, 3430, 4484
Nuclear Power Safety Report *see* Nuclear Lemons **3431**, 3430, 4484
Nuclear Regulatory Commission Thermoluminescence Dosimeters Direct Radiation Monitoring Network *see* N R C T L D Direct Radiation Monitoring Network **4366**, 4483
• Nucleic Acids Abstracts (USA ISSN 1070-2466) **3234**, 3150, 3259
Nucleic Acids and Molecular Biology (USA ISSN 0933-1891) **3259**
• ➤ Nucleic Acids Research (GBR ISSN 0305-1048) **3259**
➤ Nucleus (IND ISSN 0029-568X) **3293**, 3313
Nucleus (PHL ISSN 0115-2300) **3431**, 3155, 3374, 4152
• Nucleus (Cambridge) (USA ISSN 0888-5729) **3430**, 3441, 4484, 4532
Nucleus Science Journal *see* American Journal of Electromedicine **3563**
Nueva Cardiologia (MEX ISSN 1405-2229) **3780**
Nueva Enfermeria (ESP ISSN 0210-8275) **3930**
Nuffield Institute for Health. Working Papers (GBR) **4484**
Nukada Institute for Medical and Biological Research. Reports (JPN ISSN 0469-2071) **3668**, 3211
• ➤ Nuklearmedizin/Nuclear Medicine (DEU ISSN 0029-5566) **4152**
Der Nuklearmediziner (DEU ISSN 0723-7065) **4152**
Numark News (GBR ISSN 1358-6327) **4319**
Numark Newsline *see* Numark News **4319**
Nuova, Clinica Otorinolaringoiatrica (ITA) **4035**
Nuova Rivista di Neurologia (ITA ISSN 1122-035X) **4120**
Nuove Tecnologie in Medicina, Informatica, Telematica *see* Nuove Tecnologie in Medicina, Informatica, Telematica Applicazioni **3879**, 3389
▼ Nuove Tecnologie in Medicina, Informatica, Telematica Applicazioni (ITA) **3879**, 3389
Nuovi Annali di Igiene e Microbiologia *see* Annali di Igiene, Medicina Preventiva e di Comunita **4461**
Nuovi Argomenti di Medicina (ITA ISSN 0394-8889) **3668**
• ➤ Nuritinga (AUS ISSN 1440-1541) **3930**
Nurscene (CAN ISSN 0382-8476) **3930**
Nurse Aide - V I P (USA ISSN 1524-2900) **3479**, 3930, 4516
• Nurse Author and Editor (USA ISSN 1054-2353) **3535**, 3552, 3930
• Nurse - Beat (USA) **3930**
▼ • ➤ Nurse Education in Practice (GBR ISSN 1471-5953) **3931**, 3413
• ➤ Nurse Education Today (GBR ISSN 0260-6917) **3931**
• Nurse Educator (USA ISSN 0363-3624) **3931**, 3429
• ➤ The Nurse Practitioner (USA ISSN 0361-1817) **3931**
• ➤ Nurse Practitioner Forum (USA ISSN 1045-5485) **3931**
Nurse Practitioners in Women's Health Newsletter: The Monthly Cycle *see* N P W H Newsletter: The Monthly Cycle **4565**
➤ Nurse Practitioners' Prescribing Reference (USA ISSN 1074-3871) **4319**, 3668, 3931
• ➤ Nurse Researcher (GBR ISSN 1351-5578) **3931**, 3879
Nurse Student *see* Kango Gakusei **3927**
➤ The Nurse, the Patient and the Law (USA ISSN 0196-6790) **3931**, 3542

Title

Title

Title

Title

Title

Title

Pelagos (DZA ISSN 0031-4137) **3408**, 3212
Pelizza's Positive Principles for Better Living (USA ISSN 1070-6674) **4432**, 4359
Pendik Veteriner Mikrobiyoloji Dergisi (TUR ISSN 1300-1515) **4549**, 3172, 3330
Penn Dental Journal (USA ISSN 0031-4331) **3836**
• ➤ Pennsylvania Academy of Science. Journal (USA ISSN 1044-6753) **4506**, 3212
➤ Pennsylvania Dental Journal (USA ISSN 0031-4439) **3836**
Pennsylvania. Development Disabilities Planning Council. Pennsylvania State Plan *see* State Plan for Developmental Disabilities **4518**, 4450
• Pennsylvania Health & Fitness (USA) **3549**
Pennsylvania Medicine (USA ISSN 0031-4595) **3674**
Pennsylvania Message (USA ISSN 0031-4609) **3425**, 4122
➤ The Pennsylvania Nurse (USA ISSN 0031-4617) **3937**
➤ Pennsylvania Osteopathic Medical Association. Journal (USA ISSN 0479-9534) **3674**, 3789
Pennsylvania Pharmacist (USA ISSN 0031-4633) **4321**
Pennsylvania Society of Dentistry for Children Newsletter (USA) **3836**, 4055
People Plant Connection (USA ISSN 1067-4276) **4485**, 3464, 3674
People With AIDS Coalition of New York Coalition Newsline *see* P W A Coalition Newsline **3804**, 4516
People With AIDS Coalition of New York Resource Directory *see* P W A C Resource Directory **3804**, 4516
People with Disabilities (USA) **3486**
People with Special Needs - Down Syndrome Report (USA ISSN 0731-566X) **3425**
• People's Medical Society Newsletter (USA ISSN 0736-4873) **3393**, 3674, 4517
People's Public Security Review *see* Renmin Gongan Bao **4487**
Peptide Research *see* Journal of Peptide Research **3255**
• ➤ Peptides (USA ISSN 0196-9781) **3260**
• ➤ Perception (GBR ISSN 0301-0066) **4432**, 4005
Perception and Perceptual Development (USA ISSN 0191-2518) **4432**
• ➤ Perception & Psychophysics (USA ISSN 0031-5117) **4432**
• ➤ Perceptual and Motor Skills (USA ISSN 0031-5125) **4432**
Perfiles de Salud de las Comunidades Hermanas de la Frontera Mexico - Estados Unidos *see* Sister Communities Health Profiles of the U S - Mexico Border **4498**, 3736, 4530
• Performance and Practices of Successful Medical Groups (USA ISSN 1523-0465) **3674**
• ➤ Perfusion (DEU ISSN 0935-0020) **3781**, 3904
• ➤ Perfusion (GBR ISSN 0267-6591) **3781**
Perfusion Life *see* A M S E C T Today **3555**
Pergamon New Publications Booklet *see* Elsevier Science. New and Forthcoming Publications **4504**, 3547, 4499
Perianesthesia and Ambulatory Surgery Nursing Update (USA ISSN 1089-9480) **3937**, 4200
Perinatal Care (JPN ISSN 0910-8718) **3961**
Perinatal Medicine *see* Shusanki Igaku **3964**
Perinatal Practice (USA ISSN 0893-6293) **3961**
Perinatology Symposium (JPN ISSN 0910-3570) **3961**
• Periodicum Biologorum (HRV ISSN 0031-5362) **3212**, 3674
Periodoncia (ESP) **3836**
Periodontal Abstracts *see* Western Society of Periodontology. Journal. Periodontal Abstracts **3738**, 3152, 3842
➤ Periodontology (AUS ISSN 0726-5247) **3836**
• ➤ Periodontology 2000 (DNK ISSN 0906-6713) **3836**
• ➤ Periodontology 2000 Online (DNK) **3836**
Perioperative Services Management Resource (USA) **3937**, 4200
• ➤ Peritoneal Dialysis International (CAN ISSN 0896-8608) **3674**, 3880, 4217
Perkin 1 *see* Royal Chemical Society. Journal. Perkin Transactions 1 **3379**, 3262
Perkin Transactions 1 *see* Royal Chemical Society. Journal. Perkin Transactions 1 **3379**, 3262
Permanent Health Insurance *see* Kluwer Permanent Health Insurance **3532**, 3641
Permuted Medical Subject Headings (Year) (USA ISSN 1045-2338) **3734**

Persian Gulf Review *see* Gulf War Review **3450**, 4459
Persoenlichkeitsstoerungen - Theorie und Therapie (DEU ISSN 1433-6308) **4122**
Personal and Medical Injuries Law Letter (GBR ISSN 0267-3894) **3543**, 3674
• Personal Care News (USA) **4359**, 4244
Personal Fitness (USA ISSN 0738-7857) **4359**, 4175, 4244
Personal Health Reporter (USA ISSN 1061-4125) **3674**
Personal Injury State Verdict Survey (USA) **3543**, 3533
Personal Injury Verdict Survey *see* Personal Injury State Verdict Survey **3543**, 3533
• ➤ Personal Relationships (GBR ISSN 1350-4126) **4457**
Personal Social Services Research Unit Bulletin *see* P S S R U Bulletin **4516**, 4484
Personale- og Oekonomistatistik for Sygehusvaesenet (DNK ISSN 0107-1173) **3525**, 4529
Personale og Sengepladser ved de Sygedomsbehandlende Institutioner *see* Personale- og Oekonomistatistik for Sygehusvaesenet **3525**, 4529
Personalita - Dipendenze (ITA) **4122**
• ➤ Personality and Individual Differences (GBR ISSN 0191-8869) **4432**
Personality and Psychopathology (USA) **4432**
• ➤ Personality and Social Psychology Bulletin (USA ISSN 0146-1672) **4432**
• Personality and Social Psychology Review (USA ISSN 1088-8683) **4432**
Personality Psychology in Europe (NLD) **4432**
➤ Personality, Psychopathology and Psychotherapy (USA ISSN 0079-0931) **4433**
Personality Study and Group Behaviour (IND ISSN 0970-8111) **4433**
Personnel de la Sante au Canada *see* Health Personnel in Canada **3612**
• ➤ Personnel Psychology (USA ISSN 0031-5826) **4433**, 3368
Perspectivas en Psicologia (COL ISSN 0120-3878) **4433**
Perspectivas en Salud Publica (ESP ISSN 0188-0012) **4485**
Perspectivas Internacionales en Planificacion Familiar (USA ISSN 0190-3195) **3961**, 3360
Perspective on Aging *see* Innovations in Aging **3474**
Perspective (Silver Spring) (USA) **3674**
Perspectives (Baltimore) (USA) **4122**, 3425
• ➤ Perspectives in Biology and Medicine (USA ISSN 0031-5982) **3674**, 3212
➤ Perspectives in Biomechanics (CHE ISSN 0272-6327) **3212**
Perspectives in Cardiology (CAN ISSN 0828-6396) **3781**
Perspectives in Colon & Rectal Surgery *see* Clinics in Colon & Rectal Surgery **4185**, 3887
➤ Perspectives in Cytology & Genetics (IND) **3313**, 3293
Perspectives in Depression *see* Current Medical Literature. Perspectives in Depression **3722**, 4084
Perspectives in Education and Deafness *see* Odyssey: New Directions in Deaf Education **3425**
➤ Perspectives in Ethology (USA ISSN 0738-4394) **3355**
Perspectives in Healthcare Risk Management *see* Journal of Healthcare Risk Management **3517**, 3532
➤ Perspectives in Human Biology (AUS ISSN 1038-5762) **3212**, 3174
➤ Perspectives in Hypertension Series (USA ISSN 0898-6770) **3781**
➤ Perspectives in Immunology (USA) **3750**
➤ Perspectives in Law and Psychology (USA ISSN 0160-4422) **3543**, 4433
Perspectives in Neurological Surgery *see* Seminars in Neurosurgery **4203**, 4133
Perspectives in Nursing (USA ISSN 0894-1076) **3937**
Perspectives in Pediatric Cardiology (USA ISSN 1044-4157) **3781**, 4055
Perspectives in Plastic Surgery *see* Seminars in Plastic Surgery **4203**
• ➤ Perspectives in Psychiatric Care (USA ISSN 0031-5990) **3937**, 4122
Perspectives in Psychological Researches (IND ISSN 0971-1562) **3414**, 4433
➤ Perspectives in Psychotherapy (CHE ISSN 0735-4037) **4433**
Perspectives in Vascular Surgery *see* Perspectives in Vascular Surgery and Endovascular Therapy **4200**

• ➤ Perspectives in Vascular Surgery and Endovascular Therapy (USA ISSN 1531-0035) **4200**
Perspectives Internationales sur le Planning Familial (USA) **3961**, 3360
Perspectives on Culture and Medicine (NLD) **3674**, 4509
Perspectives on Death and Dying Series (USA ISSN 0733-6217) **4433**, 4522
• ➤ Perspectives on Developmental Neurobiology (CHE ISSN 1064-0517) **4122**, 3347
Perspectives on Dyslexia *see* Perspectives (Baltimore) **4122**, 3425
➤ Perspectives on Medical Research (USA ISSN 1053-8984) **3880**
Perspectives Psychiatriques (FRA ISSN 0031-6032) **4123**
Perspectives Sanitaire et Sociales (FRA ISSN 0757-0481) **3521**
➤ Perspectives (Toronto) (CAN ISSN 0831-7445) **3479**, 3937
Peru. Fuerzas Policiales. Revista de la Sanidad *see* Peru. Policia Nacional. Revista de la Sanidad **3674**, 4485
Peru. Policia Nacional. Revista de la Sanidad (PER ISSN 1018-6212) **3674**, 4485
Perugia Quadrennial International Conferences on Cancer. Proceedings (ITA ISSN 0069-8520) **3988**
• ➤ Pesquisa Agropecuaria Brasileira/Brazilian Journal of Agricultural Research (BRA ISSN 0100-204X) **3155**
Pesquisa Medica (BRA ISSN 0048-3567) **3674**
• Pesquisa Odontologica Brasileira (BRA ISSN 1517-7491) **3836**
• ➤ Pesquisa Veterinaria Brasileira/Brazilian Journal of Veterinary Research (BRA ISSN 0100-736X) **4549**
Pest Control Executive Reports *see* Executive Reports **4468**
Pesticide Analytical Manual (USA) **4485**, 3434
• ➤ Pesticide Biochemistry and Physiology (USA ISSN 0048-3575) **3159**, 3260
Pesticide Litigation Manual (USA) **3453**, 3159, 3543
Pesticide Residues in Food *see* Ireland. Department of Agriculture and Food. Pesticide Residues in Food **4478**, 3461
Pesticide Residues in Food (USA ISSN 0587-5943) **4485**, 3462
Pesticides Abstracts (USA ISSN 0093-3295) **3443**, 3150, 3444, 3453
Pesticides Monitor (GBR ISSN 1466-5670) **3453**, 3159, 4459
▼ Pesticides, People and Nature (USA ISSN 1520-9350) **3159**, 3453
Pesticides Register *see* Pesticides Monitor **3453**, 3159, 4459
• Peterson's Graduate and Professional Programs: The Biological Sciences (Year) (Book 3) (USA ISSN 1088-9434) **3416**, 3213
Peterson's Guide to Graduate Programs in the Biological and Agricultural Sciences (Year) (Book 3) *see* Peterson's Graduate and Professional Programs: The Biological Sciences (Year) (Book 3) **3416**, 3213
Peterson's Guide to Nursing Programs (USA ISSN 1073-7820) **3937**, 3416
Peterson's Job Opportunities in Health Care (USA ISSN 1071-0671) **4270**, 3674
Pfefferkorn Conference. Proceedings *see* Scanning Microscopy Supplement **3336**
• Pferdeheilkunde (DEU ISSN 0177-7726) **4550**
Pflege (CHE ISSN 1012-5302) **3937**
Pflege Aktuell (DEU ISSN 0944-8918) **3937**
Pflege- und Krankenhausrecht (DEU ISSN 1434-1212) **3546**, 3521, 4485
• Der Pflegebrief (Email Edition) (DEU ISSN 1433-1985) **3937**
Der Pflegebrief (Fax Edition) *see* Der Pflegebrief (Email Edition) **3937**
Der Pflegebrief (Fax Edition) *see* Der Pflegebrief (Online Edition) **3937**
• Der Pflegebrief (Online Edition) (DEU ISSN 1433-2795) **3937**
▼ ➤ Pflegemagazin (DEU ISSN 1439-7420) **4485**, 3521, 3937
Pflegen Ambulant (DEU ISSN 0937-0277) **4485**, 3674
Pflegezeitschrift (DEU ISSN 0945-1129) **3937**
• ➤ Pfluegers Archiv/European Journal of Physiology (DEU ISSN 0031-6768) **3674**, 3347
Pharma Brief (DEU) **4485**
• Pharma Business (GBR) **4322**, 3367
Pharma Daten (DEU) **4322**
Pharma-Flash (CHE ISSN 0378-7958) **4322**

Pharma Industry Directory *see* Biotechnology News **3272**
Pharma International (CHE ISSN 0301-1348) **4322**
• Pharma Japan (JPN ISSN 0285-4937) **4322**
Pharma Japan Yearbook (JPN) **4322**
Pharma Kodex (DEU ISSN 0948-7182) **4322**
➤ Pharma Kritik (CHE ISSN 1010-5409) **4322**
Pharma-Marketing Journal (DEU ISSN 0721-5665) **3367**, 3153, 4322
• Pharma Marketletter (GBR ISSN 1355-8501) **4322**
Pharma Medica (JPN ISSN 0289-5803) **4322**
➤ Pharma Patent Bulletin (GBR ISSN 1462-1428) **4322**
Pharma Recht (DEU ISSN 0172-6617) **4322**, 3543
• ➤ Pharma Selecta (NLD ISSN 0169-6882) **4322**
Pharma Technologie Journal (DEU ISSN 0931-9700) **4322**, 4531
Pharma Time (AUT) **4322**
• ➤ Pharma Times (IND ISSN 0031-6849) **4322**
Pharma und Food (DEU ISSN 1434-8942) **4322**, 4244
Pharma und Wir (DEU ISSN 0933-0909) **4322**
Pharmaca (HRV ISSN 0031-6857) **4322**
Pharmaceutica Acta Helvetiae *see* European Journal of Pharmaceutical Sciences **4292**
Pharmaceutical Activities Index - Directory (USA ISSN 1043-5905) **4345**
Pharmaceutical Administration in Japan (JPN) **4322**, 3543
Pharmaceutical and Biotech Daily *see* Washington Drug Letter (Washington, 1979) **4340**, 3369
Pharmaceutical and Cosmetic Equipment *see* Pharmaceutical Processing **4324**
Pharmaceutical & Cosmetic Quality *see* Pharmaceutical Formulation & Quality **4323**
Pharmaceutical & Cosmetic Review (ZAF ISSN 1015-4760) **3176**, 4322
• ➤ Pharmaceutical and Medical Device Litigation Bulletin (USA) **4323**, 3543
Pharmaceutical & Medical Packaging News (USA ISSN 1081-5481) **4271**, 4323
• Pharmaceutical Approvals Monthly (USA ISSN 1086-2218) **4323**
• ➤ Pharmaceutical Biology (NLD ISSN 1388-0209) **4323**
Pharmaceutical Biotechnology (USA) **3277**, 4323
• Pharmaceutical Business News (GBR ISSN 0956-0661) **4323**, 3361
• ➤ Pharmaceutical Chemistry Journal (USA ISSN 0091-150X) **4323**, 3374
• Pharmaceutical Companies Analysis (GBR ISSN 1359-625X) **4323**, 3363
• Pharmaceutical Company Profiles (GBR) **4323**, 3361
Pharmaceutical Daily *see* Washington Drug Letter (Washington, 1979) **4340**, 3369
• ➤ Pharmaceutical Development and Technology (USA ISSN 1083-7450) **4323**
Pharmaceutical Digest (USA) **4323**
➤ Pharmaceutical Engineering (USA ISSN 0273-8139) **3433**, 4323
• ➤ Pharmaceutical Executive (USA ISSN 0279-6570) **4323**
Pharmaceutical Formulation & Quality (USA ISSN 1531-2135) **4323**
• Pharmaceutical Formulation & Quality Buyers' Guide (USA) **4323**, 3176
Pharmaceutical Historian (GBR ISSN 0079-1393) **4323**
Pharmaceutical Industry Guide (USA ISSN 1085-4185) **4323**
• Pharmaceutical Journal (GBR ISSN 0031-6873) **4324**
Pharmaceutical Journal *see* Yakugaku Zasshi **4341**
Pharmaceutical Journal of Zimbabwe (ZWE) **4324**
Pharmaceutical Laboratory (USA) **4324**
Pharmaceutical: Latin American Industrial Report (USA) **4324**, 3363
Pharmaceutical Library Bulletin/Yakugaku Toshokan (JPN ISSN 0386-2062) **3548**, 4324
• Pharmaceutical Litigation Reporter (USA ISSN 0887-7815) **3546**, 4324
Pharmaceutical Manufacturers Association. Annual Survey Report (USA) **4345**, 4529
Pharmaceutical Manufacturers Association Statistical Factbook *see* P M A Statistical Factbook **4345**, 4529
Pharmaceutical Manufacturers of Japan (JPN) **3371**, 4324

Title

Title

Title

Pontificia Universidade Catolica do Rio Grande do Sul. Revista de Medicina (BRA ISSN 0103-2690) **3677**
Pontificia Universidade Catolica do Rio Grande do Sul. Revista Odontociencia (BRA ISSN 0102-9460) **3836**
Popular Medicine *see* Dazhong Yixue **3593**
Popular Psychology/Dazhong Xinlixue (CHN) **4433**
• ➤ Population and Environment (USA ISSN 0199-0039) **4433**, 4369
Porci (ESP ISSN 1130-8451) **4550**
Porphyre (FRA ISSN 0181-1169) **4331**
Portland Magazine (GBR ISSN 0048-4881) **3499**
➤ Portland Press Proceedings (GBR ISSN 0966-4068) **3880**
➤ Portland Press Research Monograph (GBR ISSN 0964-5845) **3260**
Positive Eating (GBR) **4245**, 3462
• Positive Health (GBR ISSN 1356-3963) **4360**, 3169, 4245
➤ Positive Outlook (ZAF ISSN 1022-5277) **3805**
➤ Post Acute Care Strategy Report (USA ISSN 1090-3909) **3938**, 3479, 4065
Post-Acute Data Report *see* Post-Acute Payment Report **4485**, 3521
Post-Acute Payment Report (USA) **4485**, 3521
• Post-Polio Directory (USA) **3677**
Post Traumatic Stress Disorder Research Quarterly *see* P T S D Research Quarterly **4121**, 4224
Postepy Biochemii (POL ISSN 0032-5422) **3260**
➤ Postepy Biologii Komorki/Advances in Cell Biology (POL ISSN 0324-833X) **3293**, 3677
Postepy Higieny i Medycyny Doswiadczalnej (POL ISSN 0032-5449) **3677**
Postepy Medycyny Klinicznej i Doswiadczalnej *see* Advances in Clinical and Experimental Medicine **3870**
Postepy Mikrobiologii (POL ISSN 0079-4252) **3330**
Postepy Nauk Medycznych (POL ISSN 0860-6196) **3677**, 3417
Postepy Pediatrii (POL ISSN 0079-4279) **4055**
Postepy Rehabilitacji/Advances in Rehabilitation (POL ISSN 0860-6161) **4065**
▼ Postgradualni Medicina (CZE ISSN 1212-4184) **3677**
Postgraduate Dentist: Middle East (GBR ISSN 0959-6666) **3836**
➤ Postgraduate Doctor: Caribbean (GBR ISSN 0267-0275) **3677**
Postgraduate Doctor: Middle East (GBR ISSN 0140-7724) **3677**
Postgraduate Institute of Medical Education and Research, Chandigarh. Bulletin (IND ISSN 0302-2404) **3677**, 3429
• ➤ Postgraduate Medical Journal (GBR ISSN 0032-5473) **3678**
Postgraduate Medical Journal. Supplement (GBR ISSN 0370-0593) **3678**
• ➤ Postgraduate Medicine (USA ISSN 0032-5481) **3678**
Postgraduate Medicine Hungary *see* Orvostovabbkepzo Szemle **3670**
Postgraduate Surgery: Middle East (GBR ISSN 0959-6674) **4200**, 3759
• ➤ Postharvest Biology and Technology (NLD ISSN 0925-5214) **3277**, 3156
Postscript *see* P S **4321**
Potomac View on Lung Health *see* Nova Report on Lung Health and Wellness **4162**
Potpourri from Herbal Acres (USA ISSN 0197-4084) **3464**, 3169, 3462
Potravinar (CZE ISSN 0032-566X) **3462**, 3535
Potravinarske Aktuality. Vyziva a Legislativa (CZE) **3462**, 4245
• Poz (USA ISSN 1075-5705) **3805**, 4485
Poz en Espanol (USA) **3805**
Pozar Eksplozija Preventiva (BIH ISSN 0351-4714) **3458**
Poznanskie Roczniki Medyczne (POL ISSN 0137-5350) **3678**
Poznanskie Towarzystwo Przyjaciol Nauk. Komisja Biologiczna. Prace (POL ISSN 0079-4619) **3214**
➤ Pracovni Lekarstvi (CZE ISSN 0032-6291) **3678**, 4263
Practica Odontologica (MEX ISSN 0185-5905) **3836**
Practica Otologica Kyoto/Jibi Inkoka Rinsho (JPN ISSN 0032-6313) **4037**
Practica Otologica Kyoto. Supplement/Jibi Inkoka Rinsho. Hosatsu (JPN ISSN 0912-1870) **4037**
Practica Pediatrica (MEX) **4055**
Practical Allergy and Immunology *see* Canadian Journal of Allergy and Clinical Immunology **3741**
Practical Diabetes *see* Practical Diabetes International **3867**
• Practical Diabetes International (GBR ISSN 1357-8170) **3867**
➤ Practical Diabetology (USA ISSN 0730-3491) **3868**
Practical Education for the Handicapped/Jissen Shogaiji Kyoiku (JPN) **3425**
• ➤ Practical Gastroenterology (USA ISSN 0277-4208) **3895**, 4169
A Practical Guide to Preventing Legal Malpractice (USA) **3543**, 3678
Practical Hematology *see* Ketsueki Frontier **3903**
➤ Practical Methods in Electron Microscopy (NLD ISSN 0165-201X) **3335**
➤ Practical Optometry (CAN ISSN 1181-6058) **4005**
➤ Practical Periodontics and Aesthetic Dentistry (USA ISSN 1042-2722) **3837**
Practical Pharmacy/Yakkyoku (JPN ISSN 0044-0035) **4331**
Practice Builder Association's What's Working *see* Practice Builders **3153**, 3367
Practice Builders (USA ISSN 1097-3389) **3153**, 3367
Practice in Prosthodontics/Hotetsu Rinsho (JPN ISSN 0018-6341) **3837**
Practice Nurse (GBR ISSN 0953-6612) **3938**
Practice Nursing (GBR ISSN 0964-9271) **3938**
Practice Nutrition *see* Nutrition in Practice **4242**
Practice Personnel Bulletin *see* Physicians Marketing & Management **3521**
Practice Standards of A S H P (Year) *see* Best Practices for Health-System Pharmacy **4279**, 3503
Practiciens et 3ieme Age *see* Practiciens et Troisieme Age **3479**
Practiciens et Troisieme Age (FRA ISSN 0242-9772) **3479**
Practicing Professional Series (USA) **4434**
➤ Practising Midwife (GBR ISSN 1461-3123) **3961**, 3938, 4565
• ➤ The Practitioner (GBR ISSN 0032-6518) **3678**
Practitioner *see* Tijdschrift voor Huisartsgeneeskunde **3700**
Der Praeparator (DEU ISSN 0032-6542) **3392**, 3214, 3678
Praevention und Rehabilitation (DEU ISSN 0937-552X) **3678**, 4065
Prairie Rose (USA ISSN 0032-6666) **3938**
Prakticke Zubni Lekarstvi *see* Ceska Stomatologie a Prakticke Zubni Lekarstvi **3817**
➤ Prakticky Lekar (CZE ISSN 0032-6739) **3678**
Praktijkmanagement (NLD ISSN 0169-1910) **3678**
Praktikan (SWE ISSN 1103-1727) **3837**, 4485
Praktische Arzt *see* Arzt und Praxis **3570**
Praktische Chirurgie (DEU ISSN 0079-4899) **4200**
Praktische Kieferorthopaedie *see* Kieferorthopaedie **3831**
Praktische Psychiatrie (DEU ISSN 0933-3851) **4123**
• ➤ Der Praktische Tierarzt (DEU ISSN 0032-681X) **4550**
Pratica Analitica (ITA ISSN 1120-9380) **4434**
Pratique (GBR ISSN 0269-1396) **3388**, 3526, 4485
• ➤ Pratique Medicale et Chirurgicale de l'Animal de Compagnie (FRA ISSN 0758-1882) **4550**, 4272
Praxis - Depesche (DEU ISSN 0948-8596) **3678**
• ➤ Praxis der Kinderpsychologie und Kinderpsychiatrie (DEU ISSN 0032-7034) **4123**, 4434
Praxis der Kinderpsychologie und Kinderpsychiatrie. Beihefte (DEU ISSN 0085-5073) **4434**, 4123
Praxis der Klinischen Verhaltensmedizin und Rehabilitation (DEU ISSN 0933-842X) **4065**
Praxis der Psychotherapie und Psychosomatik *see* Psychotherapeut **4128**, 4442
Praxis Ergotherapie (DEU ISSN 0932-9692) **4065**
Praxis Medica (Tomos I a VII) *see* Encyclopedie Medico-Chirurgicale. Tratado de Praxis Medica **3908**
Praxis Nah (DEU) **4200**, 3938
▼ • Praxis Post (USA) **3678**
Praxis Spiel und Gruppe (DEU ISSN 0934-5256) **3414**, 3385, 4434
➤ Praxisreport Psychologische Therapien und Psychotherapien (DEU ISSN 0941-7192) **4434**
Pre- and Perinatal Psychology Journal *see* Journal of Prenatal & Perinatal Psychology & Health **3956**, 3359, 4420
Pre & Post Natal News (CAN ISSN 1197-2297) **3938**
Predictive Oncology *see* International Journal of Cancer **3980**
Pregled Problema Mentalno Retardiranih Osoba (HRV ISSN 0032-7301) **4123**
Pregnancy (AUS ISSN 1035-5448) **3961**
Pregnancy (GBR ISSN 1368-6194) **3961**
▼ Pregnancy (USA) **3961**
Pregnancy & Birth (AUS) **3961**, 3385, 4055
Pregnancy, Birth and the Next 6 Months *see* Pregnancy **3961**
The Pregnancy Book (AUS ISSN 1328-5661) **3961**, 3385, 4055
➤ Prehospital Emergency Care (USA ISSN 1090-3127) **4024**
▼ Premier Hospital Services Report (USA ISSN 1523-4665) **3521**
• ➤ Prenatal and Neonatal Medicine (GBR ISSN 1359-8635) **3961**
• ➤ Prenatal Diagnosis (GBR ISSN 0197-3851) **3962**
Prensa Medica (BOL) **3678**
Prensa Medica (VEN) **3678**
➤ Prensa Medica Argentina (ARG ISSN 0032-745X) **3678**
Preparative Biochemistry *see* Preparative Biochemistry and Biotechnology **3260**, 3277
• ➤ Preparative Biochemistry and Biotechnology (USA ISSN 1082-6068) **3260**, 3277
Preparing and Winning Medical Negligence Cases (USA) **3543**, 3678
Prescribed Pharmaceuticals *see* Key Note Market Report: Prescribed Pharmaceuticals **4312**
➤ Prescriber (GBR ISSN 0959-6682) **4331**
➤ Prescriber's Letter (USA ISSN 1073-7219) **4331**
➤ Prescribing Reference for Obstetricians and Gynecologists (USA ISSN 1051-4171) **4331**, 3679, 3962
➤ Prescribing Reference for Pediatricians (USA ISSN 1051-3280) **4331**, 3679, 4055
Prescription and O T C Pharmaceuticals: The Pink Sheet *see* Nonprescription Pharmaceuticals and Nutritionals: The Tan Sheet **4319**
Prescription and O T C Pharmaceuticals: The Pink Sheet *see* Prescription Pharmaceuticals and Biotechnology: The Pink Sheet **4331**
• Prescription Pharmaceuticals and Biotechnology: The Pink Sheet (USA ISSN 1068-5324) **4331**
Prescription Products Guide *see* Australian Prescription Products Guide **4279**
• ➤ Prescrire International (FRA ISSN 1167-7422) **4331**, 3679
President's Letter *see* Arkansas Hospital Association. President's Letter **3502**
• ➤ La Presse Medicale (FRA ISSN 0755-4982) **3679**
La Presse Medicale (Edizione Italiana) (ITA ISSN 0393-0653) **3679**
Presse Thermale et Climatique (FRA ISSN 0032-7875) **3679**
Pressure (DEU) **3781**
Pressure (Bethesda) (USA ISSN 0889-0242) **3679**
Prevencion (San Sebastian) (ESP ISSN 0034-8732) **4485**
Prevenir les Risques du Metier (FRA ISSN 0982-443X) **4263**
Prevent (GBR ISSN 0300-2659) **4485**
Prevent Blindness America. Annual Report (USA) **4485**, 3499
Prevent Blindness News (USA) **4485**, 3499, 4006
Preventie (NLD ISSN 0169-0884) **4263**
• ➤ Preventing School Failure (USA ISSN 1045-988X) **3425**, 3486
• Prevention (USA ISSN 0032-8006) **4360**
• ➤ Prevention & Treatment (USA ISSN 1522-3736) **4123**, 4434
Prevention at Work *see* WorkSafe Magazine **4267**
Prevention au Canada *see* Safety Canada **4489**
Prevention in Human Services *see* Journal of Prevention and Intervention in the Community **4457**, 3149, 4496
Prevention in Practice Library (USA) **3679**, 4434
Prevention of Food Adulteration Cases (IND) **3543**, 3462, 4331
Prevention Pipeline (USA ISSN 1040-9882) **3405**
Prevention Routiere dans l'Entreprise (FRA ISSN 0032-8030) **4485**
▼ • ➤ Prevention Science (USA ISSN 1389-4986) **3805**
Prevention Weight Loss (USA) **4360**
Prevention's Quick & Healthy Cooking *see* Quick & Healthy Cooking **3527**
➤ Preventive Cardiology (USA ISSN 1520-037X) **3781**
• ➤ Preventive Medicine (USA ISSN 0091-7435) **3679**, 4485
▼ Preventive Medicine in Managed Care (USA) **3679**
Preventive Medicine Newsletter *see* A C P M News **3555**, 4460
• ➤ Preventive Veterinary Medicine (NLD ISSN 0167-5877) **4550**
Prevenzione & Assistenza Dentale (ITA ISSN 0393-9960) **3837**
Preview (Collinsville) (USA ISSN 1079-0187) **3837**
Previsions Glissantes Detaillees en Perspectives Sectorielles (Vol.19): Parachimie et Pharmacie *see* Previsions Glissantes Detaillees en Perspectives Sectorielles (Vol.22): Parachimie **3363**, 4331
Previsions Glissantes Detaillees en Perspectives Sectorielles (Vol.22): Parachimie (FRA) **3363**, 4331
Previsions Glissantes Detaillees en Perspectives Sectorielles (Vol.35): Sante *see* Previsions Glissantes Detaillees en Perspectives Sectorielles (Vol.38): Pharmacie - Sante **3363**, 3679
Previsions Glissantes Detaillees en Perspectives Sectorielles (Vol.38): Pharmacie - Sante (FRA) **3363**, 3679
Prevoyance (HTI) **4263**, 4485
• Prikladnaya Biokhimiya i Mikrobiologiya (RUS ISSN 0555-1099) **3260**, 3330
Prima Farma (NLD ISSN 1380-1775) **4331**
Primaer Sundhedstjenestestatistik *see* Sundhedsstatistikken (Year) **3525**, 3737
Primal Institute Newsletter (USA ISSN 0164-5056) **4434**
Primarily Nursing *see* Creative Nursing **3917**
Primary Cardiology (Edizione Italiana) (ITA ISSN 0393-6139) **3781**
Primary Care (JPN ISSN 0914-8426) **3679**
• ➤ Primary Care (USA ISSN 0095-4543) **3679**
• Primary Care & Cancer (USA ISSN 0743-8176) **3988**
Primary Care Case Reviews (USA ISSN 1096-8954) **3679**
Primary Care Medicine Drug Alerts (USA ISSN 1061-0359) **4331**, 3679
• Primary Care Medicine on CD-ROM (USA) **3679**
• Primary Care Optometry News (USA ISSN 1081-6437) **4006**
▼ • Primary Care Pharmacy (GBR ISSN 1469-1426) **4331**
• ➤ Primary Care Psychiatry (GBR ISSN 1355-2570) **4123**
Primary Care Reports (USA ISSN 1040-2497) **4055**
• Primary Care Respiratory Journal (GBR ISSN 1471-4418) **4163**
Primary Care Special Edition (USA) **3679**
• ➤ Primary Care Update for Ob - Gyns (USA ISSN 1068-607X) **3962**, 4565
• ➤ Primary Dental Care (GBR ISSN 1355-7610) **3837**
Primary Health Care (GBR ISSN 0264-5033) **4517**
Primary Health Care News (ZAF) **4485**, 3679
▼ • ➤ Primary Health Care Research and Development (GBR ISSN 1463-4236) **3679**
Primary Intention (AUS ISSN 1323-2495) **4024**
➤ Primary Psychiatry (USA ISSN 1082-6319) **4123**
Primary Sensory Neuron *see* Sensory Neuron **4133**, 3349
▼ • ➤ PrimaryCare (CHE ISSN 1424-3776) **3679**
Primate Eye (GBR ISSN 0305-8417) **3174**, 3172, 3355, 3392
• ➤ Primates (JPN ISSN 0032-8332) **3355**, 3174, 4434
Primatologie (FRA ISSN 1279-8304) **4123**
Prime Time (AUS ISSN 0729-5545) **3479**
Prime Times Magazine (Madison) (USA ISSN 0195-5934) **3393**, 3362, 4360

Title

• ➤ Prostaglandins, Leukotrienes and Essential Fatty Acids (GBR ISSN 0952-3278) **3868**
• ➤ The Prostate (USA ISSN 0270-4137) **3680**, 3989
Prostate Cancer (GBR) **3989**, 4217
• ➤ Prostate Cancer and Prostatic Diseases (GBR ISSN 1365-7852) **3989**, 4217
▼ • ➤ The Prostate Journal (USA ISSN 1095-5100) **3680**, 3989
• The Prostate Journal Online (USA ISSN 1525-1411) **3680**, 3989
• ➤ Prosthetics and Orthotics International (DNK ISSN 0309-3646) **4024**
Protease Inhibitor Reference (USA) **3261**, 3895, 4332
• ➤ Protein Engineering (GBR ISSN 0269-2139) **3261**
• ➤ Protein Expression and Purification (USA ISSN 1046-5928) **3261**
Protein, Nucleic Acid, Enzyme *see* Tanpakushitsu Kakusan Koso **3263**
▼ • Protein Profile Online (GBR ISSN 1369-4804) **3261**
• ➤ Protein Science (USA ISSN 0961-8368) **3261**
• Proteins: Post-Translational Processing (GBR ISSN 0952-0406) **3234**, 3150, 3261
• ➤ Proteins: Structure, Function, and Genetics (USA ISSN 0887-3585) **3261**
▼ • ➤ Proteomics (DEU ISSN 1615-9853) **3261**
• ➤ Protist (DEU ISSN 1434-4610) **3214**
• Protozoological Abstracts (GBR ISSN 0309-1287) **3234**, 3150, 3355
• Proven Trade Contacts (IND) **3680**, 3363
Provincial Drug Benefit Programs (CAN) **4332**
• Proving Medical Diagnosis and Prognosis (USA) **3543**, 3680
• Provizor (UKR) **4332**
Przeglad Dermatologiczny (POL ISSN 0033-2526) **3852**
Przeglad Epidemiologiczny (POL ISSN 0033-2100) **4486**
Przeglad Lekarski (POL ISSN 0033-2240) **3680**
Przeglad Psychologiczny/Psychological Review (POL ISSN 0048-5675) **4434**
Przeglad Zoologiczny (POL ISSN 0033-247X) **3356**
Przepisy Medycyny Ludowej (POL ISSN 1231-6652) **3169**
Psi Chi Newsletter *see* Eye on Psi Chi **4398**
➤ Psicanalise e Universidade/Psychoanalysis and University (BRA ISSN 1413-0556) **4434**
Psiche (ITA) **4434**
▼ Psiche Donna (ITA ISSN 1591-1209) **4124**
▼ Psichiatri Oggi (ITA ISSN 1129-0846) **4124**
Psichiatria dell'Infanzia e dell'Adolescenza (ITA ISSN 0393-361X) **4124**
Psichiatria di Consultazione (ITA ISSN 1127-395X) **4124**
Psichiatria e Psicoterapia (ITA) **4434**
➤ Psichiatria e Psicoterapia Analitica/Analytic Psychotherapy and Psychopathology (ITA ISSN 0393-9774) **4124**, 4435
Psichiatria e Territorio (ITA) **4124**
Psichiatria Generale e dell'Eta Evolutiva (ITA ISSN 0555-5299) **4124**
La Psichiatria nella Pratica Medica (ITA) **4124**
Psicoanalisi (ITA ISSN 1125-4963) **4435**
Psicoanalisi e Metodo (ITA) **4435**
• Psicodoc (ESP) **4458**, 3150
➤ Psicologia (VEN ISSN 0798-4308) **4435**
Psicologia Clinica dello Sviluppo (ITA) **4435**
Psicologia.Com *see* Revista Electronica de Psicologia **4445**
➤ Psicologia Conductual/Behavioral Psychology (ESP ISSN 1132-9483) **4435**
Psicologia Contemporanea (ITA ISSN 0390-346X) **4435**
➤ Psicologia desde el Caribe (COL ISSN 0123-417X) **4435**
Psicologia e Lavoro (ITA ISSN 0048-5691) **4435**, 3364
Psicologia e Scuola (ITA ISSN 0392-680X) **3414**, 4435
Psicologia em Revista (BRA) **4435**
Psicologia Iberoamericana (MEX ISSN 1405-0943) **4435**
Psicologia Italiana (ITA ISSN 0393-1064) **4435**
• Psicologia: Reflexao e Critica (BRA ISSN 0102-7972) **4435**
➤ Psicologia Revista (BRA) **4435**
• ➤ Psicologia: Teoria e Pesquisa/Psychology: Theory and Research (BRA ISSN 0102-3772) **4435**
• Psicologia U S P (BRA ISSN 0103-6564) **4435**
Psicologia - Universidade de Sao Paulo *see* Psicologia U S P **4435**
• ➤ Psicologica (ESP ISSN 0211-2159) **4435**
• ➤ Psicopatologia (ESP ISSN 0211-5549) **4124**
Psicoterapia (ITA ISSN 1123-766X) **4124**
Psicoterapia e Scienze Umane (ITA) **4124**, 3529
• ➤ Psicothema: Revista de Psicologia (ESP ISSN 0214-9915) **4435**
Psihologia (ROM ISSN 1220-689X) **4435**
Psikhologicheskie Issledovaniya (RUS) **4435**
• ➤ Psikhologicheskii Zhurnal (RUS ISSN 0205-9592) **4435**
Psikhologiia (BGR ISSN 0204-644X) **4436**
Psikhologiya v Biznese (RUS) **4436**
Psique (COL ISSN 0121-8913) **4124**
➤ Psiquiatria Biologica (BRA ISSN 0104-7787) **4124**
Psiquiatria Biologica (ESP ISSN 1134-5934) **4124**, 3214
Psiquiatria.Com *see* Revista Electronica de Psiquiatria **4131**
➤ Psiquiatria Publica (ESP ISSN 0213-8972) **4124**
➤ Psiquis (ESP ISSN 0210-8348) **4124**, 4436
➤ Pso Magazin (DEU ISSN 0931-1521) **3852**
Psori Newsletter (AUS) **3852**, 3750
Psoriasis Magazin *see* Pso Magazin **3852**
Psoriasis Newsletter (USA) **3852**
Psoriasis Resource (USA) **3852**, 4332
Psy (NLD ISSN 1385-7630) **4436**
PsycFirst *see* Psychological Abstracts **4458**, 3151
PsycFirst *see* PsycINFO **4458**, 3151
Psych Discourse (USA ISSN 1091-4781) **3414**, 4436
• ➤ Psych. Pflege Heute (DEU ISSN 0949-1619) **4125**
• ➤ Psyche (DEU ISSN 0033-2623) **4436**
Psyche (ITA) **4436**
• ➤ Psyche (Greenville, Online Edition) (USA) **4436**
Psychiatria Danubina (HRV ISSN 0353-5053) **4125**
Psychiatria et Neurologia Japonica/Seishin Shinkeigaku Zasshi (JPN ISSN 0033-2658) **4125**
Psychiatria Fennica (FIN ISSN 0079-7227) **4125**
Psychiatria Fennica. Julkaisusarja *see* Psychiatria Fennica. Reports **4125**
Psychiatria Fennica. Monografiasarja/Psychiatria Fennica. Monographs (FIN ISSN 0355-7707) **4125**
Psychiatria Fennica. Monographs *see* Psychiatria Fennica. Monografiasarja **4125**
Psychiatria Fennica. Reports (FIN ISSN 0359-3207) **4125**
• ➤ Psychiatria Polska (POL ISSN 0033-2674) **4125**
Psychiatric & Psychological Evidence (USA) **3543**, 4436
• ➤ Psychiatric Annals (USA ISSN 0048-5713) **4125**
• ➤ Psychiatric Bulletin (GBR ISSN 0955-6036) **4125**
• ➤ Psychiatric Care (GBR ISSN 1352-9579) **4125**
Psychiatric Clinics: Annual of Drug Therapy (USA ISSN 1068-3178) **4125**
• ➤ Psychiatric Clinics of North America (USA ISSN 0193-953X) **4125**
Psychiatric Forum (USA ISSN 0033-2690) **4125**
• ➤ Psychiatric Genetics (USA ISSN 0955-8829) **3313**, 4125
Psychiatric Journal of the University of Ottawa *see* Journal of Psychiatry and Neuroscience **4106**
Psychiatric Length of Stay Series (USA) **4125**
Psychiatric Length of Stay Series (Northcentral Edition) *see* Psychiatric Length of Stay Series **4125**
Psychiatric Length of Stay Series (Northeastern Edition) *see* Psychiatric Length of Stay Series **4125**
Psychiatric Length of Stay Series (Southern Edition) *see* Psychiatric Length of Stay Series **4125**
Psychiatric Length of Stay Series (Western Edition) *see* Psychiatric Length of Stay Series **4125**
Psychiatric Medicine (USA ISSN 0732-0868) **4125**
• Psychiatric News (USA ISSN 0033-2704) **4125**
• ➤ Psychiatric Quarterly (USA ISSN 0033-2720) **4126**
➤ Psychiatric Rehabilitation Journal (USA) **4126**, 4436, 4517
Psychiatric Rehabilitation Skills (USA ISSN 1097-3435) **4126**
• ➤ Psychiatric Services (USA ISSN 1075-2730) **4126**, 3521
• ➤ Psychiatric Times (USA ISSN 0893-2905) **4126**
➤ Psychiatrie (FRA) **4126**
Psychiatrie *see* Tijdschrift voor Psychiatrie **4136**
• ➤ La Psychiatrie de l'Enfant (FRA ISSN 0079-726X) **4055**, 4126
Psychiatrische Pflege Heute *see* Psych. Pflege Heute **4125**
• ➤ Psychiatrische Praxis (DEU ISSN 0303-4259) **4126**
• ➤ Psychiatrische Praxis. Supplement (DEU ISSN 0934-3008) **4126**
• Psychiatry (CAN ISSN 0838-7982) **4126**
• ➤ Psychiatry (USA ISSN 0033-2747) **4126**
• ➤ Psychiatry and Clinical Neurosciences (AUS ISSN 1323-1316) **4126**
Psychiatry Drug Alerts (USA ISSN 0894-4873) **4332**, 4127
Psychiatry in Practice (GBR ISSN 0262-5377) **4127**
Psychiatry in Progress (USA) **4127**
Psychiatry - Ireland (IRL) **4127**
• ➤ Psychiatry On-Line (GBR ISSN 1359-7620) **4127**
• ➤ Psychiatry Psychology and Law (AUS ISSN 1321-8719) **4127**, 3543, 4436
• ➤ Psychiatry Research (IRL ISSN 0165-1781) **4127**
• ➤ Psychiatry Research: Neuroimaging Section (IRL ISSN 0925-4927) **4127**
Psychiatry Reviews *see* Current Medical Literature. Psychiatry Reviews **3722**, 3148, 4084
• PsychNews International (USA ISSN 1366-9869) **4436**, 4127
Psycho (DEU ISSN 0340-7845) **4127**
➤ Psycho-analytic Psychotherapy in South Africa (ZAF ISSN 1023-0548) **4436**
➤ Psycho-Lingua (IND ISSN 0377-3132) **3551**, 4436
• ➤ Psycho-Oncology (GBR ISSN 1057-9249) **3989**, 4127, 4436
➤ Psychoanalyse en Cultuur/Psychoanalysis and Culture (NLD ISSN 0924-6290) **4436**, 3553, 4127
➤ Psychoanalysis and Contemporary Thought (USA ISSN 0161-5289) **4127**
Psychoanalysis and Culture *see* Psychoanalyse en Cultuur **4436**, 3553, 4127
➤ Psychoanalysis and History (GBR ISSN 1460-8235) **3526**, 4436
Psychoanalysis and Psychotherapy (USA ISSN 1057-5723) **4436**, 4127
Psychoanalysis and University *see* Psicanalise e Universidade **4434**
Psychoanalytic Abstracts (USA ISSN 1066-9884) **4458**, 3151
Psychoanalytic Books (USA ISSN 1044-2103) **4436**, 4127
Psychoanalytic Crosscurrents (USA) **4436**
• ➤ Psychoanalytic Dialogues (USA ISSN 1048-1885) **4436**
• ➤ Psychoanalytic Inquiry (USA ISSN 0735-1690) **4436**
• ➤ Psychoanalytic Psychology (USA ISSN 0736-9735) **4436**, 4127
• ➤ Psychoanalytic Psychotherapy (GBR ISSN 0266-8734) **4437**
• ➤ Psychoanalytic Quarterly (USA ISSN 0033-2828) **4437**
• ➤ The Psychoanalytic Review (USA ISSN 0033-2836) **4437**
➤ Psychoanalytic Social Work (USA ISSN 1522-8878) **4517**, 4437
▼ • ➤ Psychoanalytic Studies (GBR ISSN 1460-8952) **4437**
• Psychoanalytic Study of the Child (USA ISSN 0079-7308) **4437**
Psychoanalytische Blaetter zu Klinik, Forschung, Zeitgeschehen (DEU) **4127**, 4437
Psychobiology *see* Cognitive, Affective, & Behavioral Neuroscience **4389**
• Psychodynamic Counselling (GBR ISSN 1353-3339) **4127**
• ➤ Psychologia/Pushikorogia (JPN ISSN 0033-2852) **4437**
➤ Psychologia a Patopsychologia Dietata (SVK ISSN 0555-5574) **4437**, 3414, 3681
• ➤ Psychologica Belgica (BEL ISSN 0033-2879) **4437**
• Psychological Abstracts (USA ISSN 0033-2887) **4458**, 3151
• ➤ Psychological Assessment (USA ISSN 1040-3590) **4437**
Psychological Association of South Africa. Proceedings (ZAF) **4437**
• ➤ Psychological Bulletin (USA ISSN 0033-2909) **4437**
Psychological Cinema Register (USA ISSN 0272-0582) **4458**, 4225
• ➤ Psychological Inquiry (USA ISSN 1047-840X) **4438**
Psychological Institute of the Republic of South Africa. Proceedings *see* Psychological Association of South Africa. Proceedings **4437**
• ➤ Psychological Medicine (GBR ISSN 0033-2917) **4127**
Psychological Medicine. Monograph Supplement (GBR ISSN 0264-1801) **4438**
• ➤ Psychological Methods (USA ISSN 1082-989X) **4438**
Psychological Perspectives (USA ISSN 0033-2925) **4438**
• Psychological Perspectives on Lesbian and Gay Issues (USA ISSN 1072-7841) **3528**, 4438
• ➤ The Psychological Record (USA ISSN 0033-2933) **4438**
• ➤ Psychological Reports (USA ISSN 0033-2941) **4438**
• ➤ Psychological Research (DEU ISSN 0340-0727) **4438**
➤ Psychological Research Bulletin (SWE ISSN 0555-5620) **4438**
Psychological Research Journal (IND ISSN 0970-6097) **4438**
Psychological Research Reports *see* University of Turku. Psychological Research Reports **4454**
Psychological Review *see* Przeglad Psychologiczny **4434**
• ➤ Psychological Review (USA ISSN 0033-295X) **4438**
• ➤ Psychological Science (USA ISSN 0956-7976) **4438**
• Psychological Science Agenda (USA ISSN 1040-404X) **4439**
Psychological Studies *see* Pszichologiai Tanulmanyok **4443**
➤ Psychological Studies (IND ISSN 0033-2968) **4439**
Psychologie (NLD ISSN 0167-6598) **4439**
Psychologie Clinique et Projective (FRA ISSN 1265-5449) **4439**
➤ Psychologie en Maatschappij (NLD ISSN 0168-9223) **4439**
Psychologie & Education (FRA ISSN 1148-9502) **3414**, 4439
Psychologie et Psychometrie (FRA ISSN 0296-8770) **4439**
Psychologie Francaise (FRA ISSN 0033-2984) **4439**
Psychologie Heute (DEU ISSN 0340-1677) **4439**
Psychologie (Houten) *see* Nederlands Tijdschrift voor de Psychologie en haar Grensgebieden **4429**, 4112
Psychologie Preventive (CAN ISSN 0714-3494) **4439**
Psychologie Scolaire *see* Psychologie & Education **3414**, 4439
Psychologie und Gesellschaftskritik (DEU ISSN 0170-0537) **4439**, 4568
Psychologie und Person (DEU ISSN 0079-7405) **4439**
Psychologie und Sport (DEU ISSN 0945-6031) **4439**, 4526
Psychologie v Ekonomicke Praxi/Applied Industrial Psychology (CZE ISSN 0033-300X) **4439**
Psychologie Verstehen (DEU ISSN 0941-3049) **4439**
Psychologies (FRA) **4439**
• ➤ Psychologische Beitraege (DEU ISSN 0033-3018) **4439**
• ➤ Psychologische Rundschau (DEU ISSN 0033-3042) **4439**
• ➤ The Psychologist (GBR ISSN 0952-8229) **4440**
Psychologists for Social Responsibility. Newsletter (USA) **4440**, 4368
Psychology *see* Xinlixue **4455**
Psychology *see* Psychology & Education **4440**, 3414
• ➤ Psychology and Aging (USA ISSN 0882-7974) **3479**, 4440
➤ Psychology and Developing Societies (IND ISSN 0971-3336) **4440**
• ➤ Psychology & Education (USA) **4440**, 3414
• ➤ Psychology & Health (CHE ISSN 0887-0446) **4440**
Psychology and Health *see* Xinli yu Jiankang **4137**
Psychology and Health Series (GBR) **4440**
Psychology and Human Development *see* Social Behavior and Personality **4449**, 4523

Title

Title

The Quality Letter for Healthcare Leaders (USA ISSN 1047-5311) **3521**
• Quality Management in Health Care (USA ISSN 1063-8628) **3521**, 3543, 3682
Quality Matters (USA) **3682**
Quality of Care (USA) **4129**, 3426
Quality of Life (USA ISSN 1064-7988) **3682**, 3938
➤ Quality of Life Newsletter (FRA ISSN 1161-6407) **3682**, 4443, 4487
• ➤ Quality of Life Research (NLD ISSN 0962-9343) **3682**
➤ Quality Resource (USA) **3682**
Quality, Risk & Cost Advisor *see* Q R C Advisor **3521**, 3534
• ➤ Quantitative Structure-Activity Relationships (DEU ISSN 0931-8771) **4332**
Quarterly Injury & Illness Incidence Report *see* Western Wood Products Association. Quarterly Injury & Illness Incidence Report **4269**, 3464
Quarterly Journal of Dialysis *see* Toseki Furontia **4218**
Quarterly Journal of Experimental Physiology *see* Experimental Physiology **3342**
• ➤ Quarterly Journal of Experimental Psychology. Section A: Human Experimental Psychology (GBR ISSN 0272-4987) **4443**
• ➤ Quarterly Journal of Experimental Psychology. Section B: Comparative and Physiological Psychology (GBR ISSN 0272-4995) **4443**
Quarterly Journal of Medicine *see* Q J M **3681**
➤ The Quarterly Journal of Nuclear Medicine (ITA) **4152**, 3214
Quarterly Journal of Surgical Sciences (IND ISSN 0033-5657) **4201**
Quarterly Medical Review (IND ISSN 0481-2158) **3682**
• ➤ Quarterly Review of Biology (USA ISSN 0033-5770) **3214**
• ➤ Quarterly Reviews of Biophysics (GBR ISSN 0033-5835) **3267**, 3214
Quarterly Welfare Statistical Bulletin *see* Idaho. Department of Health and Welfare. Research and Statistics Section. Quarterly Welfare Statistical Bulletin **4519**, 4475
Quebec. Liquor Board. Annual Report *see* Societe des Alcools du Quebec. Rapport Annuel **3405**
Quebec (Province). Direction de la Recherche Scientifique et Technique. Activites (Year) *see* Quebec (Province). Direction de l'Innovation et des Technologies. Activites (Year) **3214**
Quebec (Province). Direction de l'Innovation et des Technologies. Activites (Year) (CAN) **3214**
Queen Alexandra Hospital for Children. Annual Report *see* Arbutus Society for Children. Annual Report **3502**
Queens County Dental Society. Bulletin (USA) **3837**
Queens Medical Magazine (GBR ISSN 0033-6033) **3682**
Queen's Medical Review (CAN ISSN 0079-8789) **3682**
Queensland Flying Doctor *see* Flying Doctor Queensland **3507**, 4532
➤ Queensland Naturalist (AUS ISSN 0079-8843) **3214**
Queensland Paediatric Nurses Association Journal *see* Australia Paediatric Nurse Journal **3914**, 4041
• ➤ Quekett Journal of Microscopy (GBR ISSN 0969-3823) **3335**
• ➤ Quest (Champaign) (USA ISSN 0033-6297) **3429**, 4176
Quest (Dallas) *see* Cancer Review **3973**
• Quest (Tucson) (USA ISSN 1087-1578) **4129**, 3494
Question and Answer Briefing (GBR) **4487**
Quick & Healthy Cooking (USA ISSN 0886-2338) **3527**
Quick Index of Medical Preparations Quarterly *see* Q I M P Quarterly **4332**
Quickening (USA ISSN 0196-3805) **3938**
Quintessence (Edicion Espanola) (ESP ISSN 0214-0985) **3837**
• ➤ Quintessence International (USA ISSN 0033-6572) **3837**
Quintessence of Dental Technology *see* Q D T **3837**
Quintessence Tecnica (Edicion Espanola) (ESP ISSN 1130-5339) **3837**
Die Quintessenz (Berlin) (DEU ISSN 0033-6580) **3837**
Quintessenz der Zahntechnik (DEU ISSN 0340-4641) **3837**
Quintessenz Journal *see* Quintessenz Team - Journal **3837**
Quintessenz Team - Journal (DEU) **3837**
➤ Quiron (ARG ISSN 0325-2345) **3682**
• Quit Smoking Report Ezine (USA) **4360**
Le Quotidien du Medecin (FRA) **3682**
Quotidien du Pharmacien (FRA ISSN 0764-5104) **4332**
R A C G P Training Program Victoria Newsletter (Royal Australian College of General Practitioners) (AUS) **3682**
R A C S Bulletin (Print Edition) *see* Surgical News (Online) **3418**, 3362
R A D A R Bulletin (Royal Association for Disability and Rehabilitation) (GBR ISSN 0954-237X) **3486**, 4065
R A J *see* Regulatory Affairs Journal **4333**
R A J Devices *see* Regulatory Affairs Journal. Devices **4333**
R A J Europe *see* Regulatory Affairs Journal Europe **4333**
▼ • R A J Europe (Regulatory Affairs Journals Ltd.) (USA) **4332**
• R & D Focus (GBR) **4333**
R and D Innovator *see* Innovative Leader (Online) **3365**, 3366, 3620
R & S Report (Honolulu) *see* Hawaii. Department of Health. Research and Statistics Office. R & S Report **4370**, 4364
R B M *see* Revista Brasileira de Medicina **3685**
R B M A Bulletin (Radiology Business Management Association) (USA) **4152**
R C *see* Respiratory Care **4164**
➤ R C M Midwives Journal (Royal College of Midwives) (GBR) **3962**
R C N Institute. Report (Royal College of Nursing) (GBR) **3938**, 3417
R C N National Health Manifesto. Annual Report (Royal College of Nursing) (GBR) **3938**
R C O E *see* Consejo General de Ondotologos y Estomatologos. Revista **3818**
R D A News (Riding for the Disabled Association of Australia) (AUS) **4065**
R D H (Registered Dental Hygienist) (USA ISSN 0279-7720) **3837**
R D I P *see* Respiratory Disease in Practice **4164**
R E R F Update (Radiation Effects Research Foundation) (JPN) **4152**
R E R Reports (USA) **3486**
R E S N A News (Rehabilitation Engineering and Assistive Technology Society of North America) (USA) **3426**, 3492, 3499
R F B & D Impact (Recording for the Blind & Dyslexic, Inc.) (USA) **3499**
R F B Issues *see* R F B & D Impact **3499**
R F L (Rundschau Fleischhygiene und Lebensmittelueberwachung) (DEU ISSN 0178-2010) **3462**, 4487, 4550
R F P D Actualites (Revue Francaise des Prothesistes Dentaires) (FRA ISSN 0997-3397) **3838**
R I T A *see* Research Initiative, Treatment Action! **3751**, 3806
R K W Kontakt (DEU) **3368**
R N *see* Registered Nurse **3939**
• ➤ R N (Registered Nurse) (USA ISSN 0033-7021) **3938**
• ➤ R N A (Ribonucleic Acid) (GBR ISSN 1355-8382) **3261**, 3313
R N A B C News *see* Nursing B C **3932**
R.N. Idaho (USA ISSN 0192-298X) **3939**
R N Web *see* R N **3938**
R O S P A Bulletin *see* O S & H Bulletin **4260**
R R S News (Radiation Research Society) (USA) **4152**
• R S N A Electronic Journal (Radiological Society of North America, Inc.) (USA ISSN 1090-7629) **4152**
R S N A Index Online *see* R S N A Index to Imaging Literature **3735**, 4152
• R S N A Index to Imaging Literature (Radiological Society of North America, Inc.) (USA) **3735**, 4152
➤ R S O Magazine (Radiation Safety Officer) (USA ISSN 1086-6353) **4263**, 4366, 4487
R S Rifiuti Solidi (ITA ISSN 0394-5391) **3457**
R T (USA ISSN 1040-6050) **4163**
R T D E *see* Research and Teaching in Developmental Education **3414**
• R T E C S (Registry of Toxic Effects of Chemical Substances) (USA) **3453**, 3374, 4487
R T Image (Radiologic Technology) (USA ISSN 1041-2182) **4152**
• R T International (Respiratory Therapy) (USA) **4163**
R T Magazine *see* R T **4163**
• R T Solutions E - Zine (USA) **4164**
R V S Fee Schedule (Relative Value Scale) (USA) **3534**, 3682
• Raakpunt (NLD ISSN 0166-4298) **4129**, 3426, 4444, 4517
• Rachel's Environment & Health Weekly (USA ISSN 1078-103X) **3441**, 3457, 3543
Rachel's Hazardous Waste News *see* Rachel's Environment & Health Weekly **3441**, 3457, 3543
Rachis (FRA ISSN 0997-7503) **4170**, 4025
Rad Magazine (GBR ISSN 0264-6412) **4152**
RadCureLetter (DEU ISSN 0945-8409) **4271**
• Radiance Online (USA) **4568**, 4360, 4565
Radiance Technique Journal (USA) **3169**, 4227
Radiance Technique Newsletter *see* Radiance Technique Journal **3169**, 4227
• ➤ Radiation and Environmental Biophysics (DEU ISSN 0301-634X) **3267**
Radiation Biology Research Communication *see* Hoshasen Seibutsu Kenkyu **3266**
Radiation Effects Research Foundation. Annual Report/Hoshasen Eikyo Kenkyusho Nenpo (JPN) **4152**
Radiation Effects Research Foundation. Commentary and Review Series/Hoshasen Eikyo Kenkyusho Kaisetsu Sosetsu Shu (JPN) **4152**
Radiation Effects Research Foundation Newsletter/Hoeiken Nyuzu Reta (JPN) **4153**
Radiation Effects Research Foundation Update *see* R E R F Update **4152**
Radiation Medicine (JPN ISSN 0288-2043) **4153**, 3989
Radiation Oncology Investigation *see* International Journal of Cancer **3980**
Radiation Oncology News (USA) **4153**
Radiation Protection Abstracts (GBR ISSN 1464-1437) **4365**, 3151, 4497
Radiation Protection and Environment (IND ISSN 0972-0464) **4487**
• ➤ Radiation Protection Dosimetry (GBR ISSN 0144-8420) **4366**, 3441, 3682, 4487
➤ Radiation Protection Management (USA ISSN 0740-0640) **4263**, 4366, 4487
Radiation Protection News and Notes (NZL ISSN 0113-4795) **4487**, 3457
Radiation Research Society News *see* R R S News **4152**
Radiation Safety Officer Magazine *see* R S O Magazine **4263**, 4366, 4487
➤ Radiation Therapist (USA ISSN 1084-1911) **4153**, 3989
Radiatsionnaya Biologiya, Radioekologiya (RUS ISSN 0869-8031) **4153**, 3267
Radical Community Medicine *see* Critical Public Health **4466**
La Radioactivite des Principales Sources d'Eau Minerale en Belgique. (BEL) **4562**, 4487
Radiobiologiya *see* Radiatsionnaya Biologiya, Radioekologiya **4153**, 3267
Radiographer (AUS ISSN 0033-8273) **4153**
• ➤ Radiographics (USA ISSN 0271-5333) **4153**
• Radiography (GBR ISSN 1078-8174) **4153**
Radiography Today *see* Synergy **4156**
Radioisotopes (JPN ISSN 0033-8303) **3374**
Radiokhimiya (RUS ISSN 0033-8311) **3380**, 4153
• ➤ Der Radiologe (DEU ISSN 0033-832X) **4153**
• ➤ Radiologia (ESP ISSN 0033-8338) **4153**
➤ Radiologia Brasileira (BRA ISSN 0100-3984) **4153**
➤ Radiologia Medica (ITA ISSN 0033-8362) **4153**
• ➤ Radiologic Clinics of North America (USA ISSN 0033-8389) **4153**
• ➤ Radiologic Technology (USA ISSN 0033-8397) **4153**, 3812
Radiologic Technology Image *see* R T Image **4152**
Radiological Sciences *see* Hoshasen Kagaku **4145**
Radiological Society of North America, Inc. Electronic Journal *see* R S N A Electronic Journal **4152**
Radiological Society of North America, Inc. Index to Imaging Literature *see* R S N A Index to Imaging Literature **3735**, 4152
Radiologie Assistent (DEU ISSN 0935-1779) **4153**
▼ • ➤ Radiologie up2date (DEU) **4154**
• The Radiologist (USA ISSN 1069-1286) **4154**
• ➤ Radiology (USA ISSN 0033-8419) **4154**
• Radiology and Imaging Letter (USA ISSN 0741-160X) **4154**
Radiology Business Management Association Bulletin *see* R B M A Bulletin **4152**
Radiology Management (USA ISSN 0198-7097) **3521**, 4154
➤ Radiology Now (GBR ISSN 1461-4650) **4154**
➤ Radionic Journal (GBR ISSN 1362-3958) **3682**
Radionic Quarterly *see* Radionic Journal **3682**
➤ Radionuclides in Nephrourology (USA) **4154**, 4217
➤ Radiopharmacy and Radiopharmacology Yearbook Series (CHE ISSN 0748-6111) **4333**
Radiosurgery (CHE ISSN 1024-2651) **4201**, 4129
• ➤ Radiotherapy and Oncology (IRL ISSN 0167-8140) **4154**, 3989
The Rag *see* Twelve Step Rag **3406**
• Ragged Edge (USA ISSN 1095-3949) **3499**, 3364, 4368
Ragiusan (ITA ISSN 1120-1762) **4487**
Railway Medical Journal *see* Tiedao Yixue **3700**
Rainbow Network *see* Rainbow News **3169**, 4227
Rainbow News (NZL ISSN 1174-3530) **3169**, 4227
Rainbow (Peterborough) (GBR) **3494**, 3492, 3499
Raioenjiniaringu Bumon Gakujutsu Koenkai Koen Ronbunshu/Japanese Society of Mechanical Engineers. Bioengineering Division Conference (JPN) **3238**
Ramazzini/Norwegian Journal of Occupational Medicine (NOR ISSN 0805-5238) **4263**
Ramsey Medical Society. Bulletin *see* MetroDoctors **3660**
Rapports de Synthese sur les Themes Techniques Presentes au Comite International ou aux Commissions Regionales/Comprehensive Reports on Technical Items Presented to the International Committee or to Regional Commissions (FRA ISSN 1022-1050) **4551**
Rassegna di Dermatologia e Sifilografia (ITA ISSN 0033-9490) **3852**
Rassegna di Diritto, Legislazione e Medicina Legale Veterinaria (ITA ISSN 0300-3485) **3543**, 4551
Rassegna di Patologia dell'Apparato Respiratorio (ITA ISSN 0033-9563) **4164**
Rassegna di Psicologia (ITA) **4444**
Rassegna di Urologia e Nefrologia (ITA ISSN 0033-992X) **3682**
Rassegna Geriatrica (ITA ISSN 0486-0306) **3480**
Rassegna Medica Sarda (ITA ISSN 0033-9776) **4201**
➤ Rassegna Medico-Chirurgica (ITA ISSN 1123-9166) **3682**
Rassegna Odontotecnica (ITA ISSN 0048-6787) **3838**
Rassegna Trimestrale di Odontoiatria (ITA ISSN 0033-9911) **3838**
Ratgeber aus der Apotheke *see* Ratgeber aus Ihrer Apotheke **4360**
Ratgeber aus Ihrer Apotheke (DEU ISSN 1438-2865) **4360**
Raum und Zeit (DEU ISSN 0722-7949) **3682**, 3441, 4365
Raumplanung und Umweltschutz im Kanton Zurich (CHE) **3529**, 4487
Raven Press Series in Physiology *see* Lippincott-Raven Press Series in Physiology **3346**
Ravintsara (MDG) **4487**
• Rawal Medical Journal (PAK ISSN 0303-5212) **3683**
Razza Bruna (ITA) **3161**
• Re Productions (NPL) **4360**, 3360, 4487
Reach Newsletter (GBR ISSN 1366-2031) **3426**, 4517
Reach Out (AUS) **3683**
Reaching Out (USA ISSN 1097-3052) **3486**, 3683
Reactions *see* Reactions Weekly **4346**, 3151
• Reactions Weekly (NZL ISSN 0114-9954) **4346**, 3151
• ➤ Reading and Writing (NLD ISSN 0922-4777) **3551**, 3414, 4129, 4444
• ➤ Reading Psychology (USA ISSN 0270-2711) **3414**, 4444
Readings (USA ISSN 0886-3784) **4129**, 4444, 4499
➤ Real Academia de Farmacia. Anales (ESP ISSN 0034-0618) **4333**
Real Academia Nacional de Medicina. Anales (ESP ISSN 0034-0634) **3683**
Real Health & Beauty (GBR ISSN 1465-2803) **4565**
▼ Real Healthcare (USA) **3522**, 3393, 3683, 4487
• Real Living with Multiple Sclerosis (USA ISSN 1079-4220) **4129**

Title

Title

Referatovy Vyber z Kardiologie/Abstracts of Cardiology (CZE ISSN 0139-6536) **3736**, 3151, 3782
Referatovy Vyber z Neurologie/Abstracts of Neurology (CZE ISSN 0034-2793) **3736**, 3151, 4130
Referatovy Vyber z Oftalmologie/Abstracts of Ophthalmology (CZE ISSN 0034-2807) **3736**, 3151, 4006
Referatovy Vyber z Ortopedie, Traumatologie a Pribuznych Oboru *see* Pohybove Ustroji **4024**, 3150, 3734
Referatovy Vyber z Pediatrie/Abstracts of Pediatrics (CZE ISSN 0034-2858) **3736**, 3152, 4056
Referatovy Vyber z Porodnictvi a Gynekologie/Abstracts of Obstetrics and Gynecology (CZE ISSN 0034-2866) **3736**, 3152
• Referatovy Vyber z Radiodiagnostiky/ Abstracts of Radiology (CZE ISSN 0862-2183) **3736**, 3152, 4154
• Referatovy Vyber z Revmatologie/Abstracts of Rheumatology (CZE ISSN 0034-2882) **3736**, 3152, 4170
Referatovy Vyber z Urologie *see* Referatovy Vyber a Aktuality z Urologie **3736**, 3151
Reference Circular Series *see* National Library Service. Reference Circular Series **3498**
➤ References en Gynecologie Obstetrique (FRA ISSN 1244-8168) **3962**
Referencias Medicas de Informacion Actualizada *see* Remedia **3177**, 3684
Reflections (Indianapolis) *see* Reflections on Nursing Leadership **3387**, 3939
Reflections (Long Beach) *see* Reflections: Narratives of Professional Helping **3426**, 4444, 4517
➤ Reflections: Narratives of Professional Helping (USA ISSN 1080-0220) **3426**, 4444, 4517
Reflections on Nursing Leadership (USA) **3387**, 3939
Refractive and Corneal Surgery *see* Journal of Refractive Surgery **4195**, 4001
Refuah *see* Ha-Refuah **3609**
Regan Report on Hospital Law *see* Hospital Law's Regan Report **3513**, 3540
Regan Report on Medical Law *see* Medical Law's Regan Report **3651**, 3542
Regan Report on Nursing Law *see* Nursing Law's Regan Report **3933**, 3542
Regarding Women and Healthcare (USA) **4565**
De Regenbooggids (NLD) **3528**
Regeneration: A Magazine of Left Green Social Thought *see* Synthesis - Regeneration: A Magazine of Green Social Thought **3442**, 3544, 4368
Regenerative Medicine *see* e-biomed **3596**
Regional Anesthesia *see* Regional Anesthesia and Pain Medicine **3759**
• ➤ Regional Anesthesia and Pain Medicine (USA ISSN 1098-7339) **3759**
Register of Authorized Laboratories *see* Register over Autoriserede Laboratorier **3880**
Register of Medical Practitioners, Interns and Dentists for the Republic of South Africa (ZAF) **3683**
Register over Autoriserede Laboratorier/Register of Authorized Laboratories (DNK ISSN 0105-9173) **3880**
Registered Dental Hygienist *see* R D H **3837**
Registered Nurse (CAN ISSN 1484-0863) **3939**
Registered Nurse *see* R N **3938**
Registered Nurse Journal *see* Registered Nurse **3939**
Registered Psychiatric Nurses' Association of Saskatchewan. R P News (CAN) **3939**
Registered Respiratory Therapist *see* Canadian Journal of Respiratory Therapy **4158**
Registers & Directory of Veterinary Surgeons (GBR) **4551**
Registro de Organismos de Salud (COL) **4487**
Registry of Interpreters for the Deaf. Professional interpreting journal. *see* Journal of Interpretation (Rockville) **3491**
Registry of Nurse-Midwifery Services and Practices *see* Directory of Nurse-Midwifery Practices (Year) **3918**
Registry of Toxic Effects of Chemical Substances *see* R T E C S **3453**, 3374, 4487
Regulations *see* Norway. Direktoratet for Arbeidstilsynet. Forskrifter **4260**, 3417
RegulationsMedizin (DEU ISSN 1430-7561) **3683**
• Regulatory Affairs Focus (USA ISSN 1097-2668) **3683**, 4459
• ➤ Regulatory Affairs Journal (GBR ISSN 0960-7889) **4333**
• ➤ Regulatory Affairs Journal. Devices (GBR ISSN 0969-4129) **4333**
• Regulatory Affairs Journal Europe (GBR) **4333**
Regulatory Affairs Journals Ltd. Europe *see* R A J Europe **4332**
• ➤ Regulatory Peptides (NLD ISSN 0167-0115) **3262**
• ➤ Regulatory Toxicology and Pharmacology (USA ISSN 0273-2300) **3453**, 3884, 4333
• Regulatory Update (USA ISSN 1065-1896) **4367**, 4487
Regulatory Watchdog Service (USA ISSN 0275-0902) **4459**, 4333, 4368
➤ Rehab & Community Care Management (CAN ISSN 1192-2508) **4065**, 3522
Rehab Continuum Report (USA) **3534**, 3683
• ➤ Rehab Management (USA ISSN 0899-6237) **3683**
Rehab Management International (USA ISSN 1056-6201) **3683**
Rehab Report (USA) **3486**, 4066
➤ Rehabilitace a Fyzikalni Lekarstvi (CZE ISSN 1211-2658) **4170**
➤ Rehabilitacia/Rehabilitation (SVK ISSN 0375-0922) **4066**
• ➤ Rehabilitacion (ESP ISSN 0048-7120) **4066**
Rehabilitacion: Prevencion y Integracion (USA) **4066**, 3486
Rehabilitation *see* Kang Fu **4062**
• ➤ Die Rehabilitation (DEU ISSN 0034-3536) **3683**
Rehabilitation *see* Rehabilitacia **4066**
• ➤ Rehabilitation Counseling Bulletin (USA ISSN 0034-3552) **3486**, 4130, 4270
➤ Rehabilitation Education (USA ISSN 0889-7018) **3426**
Rehabilitation Engineering and Assistive Technology Society of North America News *see* R E S N A News **3426**, 3492, 3499
Rehabilitation Engineering Center for Employment Injuries Kenkyu Hokokushu *see* E I R E C Kenkyu Hokokushu **4060**, 3364
Rehabilitation Gazette (USA ISSN 0361-4166) **3487**, 3426
• Rehabilitation Index (GBR ISSN 0955-0984) **3736**, 3152, 4066
Rehabilitation Industries Corporation. Annual Report (IND ISSN 0080-0724) **4066**, 3369, 3426
Rehabilitation International. World Congress. Proceedings (USA) **4066**
• Rehabilitation Nursing (USA ISSN 0278-4807) **3939**, 4066
• ➤ Rehabilitation Psychology (USA ISSN 0090-5550) **4444**
▼ Rehabilitation Sourcebook (USA) **4066**
Rehabilitation Technology Review *see* R E S N A News **3426**, 3492, 3499
Rehabilitation und Praevention (USA ISSN 0172-6412) **3683**
Reiki Magazin (DEU) **3169**
• Reimbursement Advisor (USA ISSN 0884-2795) **3522**, 3362, 3534
Reimbursement Update (USA ISSN 1075-7848) **3363**, 3522
Rejuvenation (BEL ISSN 0304-4408) **3480**
➤ Rejyonal Anestezi Bulten (TUR) **3759**
➤ Relaciones (URY ISSN 0797-9754) **4444**, 4523
Relative Value Scale Fee Schedule *see* R V S Fee Schedule **3534**, 3682
Relative Values for Physicians (USA ISSN 1065-7681) **3684**
Relazioni Clinico Scientifiche (ITA ISSN 0048-7198) **3684**, 3262
Relevant (NLD ISSN 1381-2866) **4348**, 3684
Releve des Maladies Transmissibles au Canada *see* Canada Communicable Disease Report **4464**
Religieuses d'Action Hospitaliere et Social *see* Religieuses dans les Professions de Sante **3522**, 4501
Religieuses dans les Professions de Sante (FRA ISSN 1146-3759) **3522**, 4501
Remedia (MEX ISSN 0304-1840) **3177**, 3684
• ➤ Remedial and Special Education (USA ISSN 0741-9325) **3426**
Remedy Magazine (USA) **4360**, 3684
Remembering Yesterday (USA ISSN 1524-2897) **3480**, 4517
The Remington Report (USA ISSN 1070-3411) **3684**
• ➤ Renal Failure (USA ISSN 0886-022X) **4217**
Renal Nursing and Technology Today *see* C N N T Newsletter **4210**, 3915
• Renal Physiology (GBR ISSN 0300-3434) **3235**, 3152, 3348, 3736, 3895
Renal Physiology and Biochemistry *see* Kidney and Blood Pressure Research **4215**
Renal Transplantation, Vascular Surgery *see* Jin Ishoku Kekkan Geka **4192**
Renalink (USA) **4217**, 4517
Renhold Vedligehold *see* Rent i Danmark **3366**, 4487
• Renin, Angiotensin & Kinins (GBR ISSN 0143-4284) **3235**, 3152, 3348, 3736, 3868, 4333
Renkouxue yu Jihua Shengyu/Demography and Family Planning (CHN ISSN 1005-4235) **4369**, 3360
Renmin Gongan Bao/People's Public Security Review (CHN) **4487**
Rent i Danmark (DNK ISSN 0906-270X) **3366**, 4487
Rentgenologia i Radiologia (BGR ISSN 0486-400X) **4154**
Repertoire Canadien des Conferences de Soins de Sante *see* Canadian Directory of Health Care Conferences **4220**, 3581
Repertoire International des Banques de Donnees Biomedicales (FRA ISSN 1169-6176) **3812**, 3177
Repertoire Mondial des Ecoles de Medecine *see* World Directory of Medical Schools **3709**, 3417
• Repetitive Stress Injury Litigation Reporter (USA ISSN 1067-0483) **3543**, 4263
• Repindex (PER ISSN 0252-7987) **3443**, 3152, 3441
Reponse a Tout Sante (FRA ISSN 1164-8961) **3684**
Report - Hastings Center *see* Hastings Center Report **3610**, 3198, 4347
Report (Latham) *see* New York State Nurses Association. Report **3930**
Report of National Nutritive Conditions *see* Kokumin Eiyo no Genjo **4238**
Report of Physiological Technology *see* Seirigaku Gijutsu Kenkyukai Hokoku **3348**
Report of Research and Development of Medical Information System *see* Iryo Joho Shisutemu Kenkyu Kaihatsu Hokokusho **3625**, 3390
Report on Alcohol, Drugs, and Disability (USA) **3405**, 3487
Report on Disability Programs (USA ISSN 1043-1209) **4517**, 3426, 3487, 4368
Report on Healthcare Information Management (USA) **3684**, 3548
Report on Medical Guidelines & Outcomes Research (USA ISSN 1050-5636) **3522**
Report on Medicare Compliance (USA ISSN 1089-6872) **3544**, 3684
Report on Nutritive Conditions in Tokyo *see* Tokyo Tomin no Eiyo Jokyo **4246**
Report on Patient Privacy (USA) **3522**
The Report on Pediatric Infectious Diseases (USA ISSN 1050-964X) **4056**
➤ Report Psychologie (DEU ISSN 0344-9602) **4444**
Report to Congress on Abnormal Occurrences *see* U.S. Nuclear Regulatory Commission. Report to Congress on Abnormal Occurrences **3431**, 3430
Reporter on Human Reproduction & the Law (USA ISSN 8756-2057) **3544**, 3360
Reportero Medico (ARG) **3684**
Reports in Public Health *see* Cadernos de Saude Publica **4464**
Reports of Investigations about Lake Biwa (JPN) **4487**, 3408
Reports of Psychiatria Fennica *see* Psychiatria Fennica. Reports **4125**
Reports on Rheumatic Diseases. Series 3. Practical Problems *see* Rheumatic Disease: In Practice (Series 4) **4170**
Reports on Rheumatic Diseases. Series 3. Topical Reviews *see* Rheumatic Disease Topical Reviews **4170**
Representations Books Series (USA) **4444**
➤ Representative Research in Social Psychology (USA ISSN 0034-4907) **4444**, 4523
▼ • Reproduction (GBR ISSN 1470-1626) **3215**, 3684
Reproduction. Abstract Series (GBR) **3235**, 3152, 3348, 3736
• Reproduction and Contraception (CHN ISSN 1001-7844) **3360**
• ➤ Reproduction, Fertility and Development (AUS ISSN 1031-3613) **3215**
• ➤ Reproduction in Domestic Animals (DEU ISSN 0936-6768) **4551**
• Reproduction in Domestic Animals Online (DEU ISSN 1439-0531) **4551**
• ➤ Reproduction, Nutrition, Development (FRA ISSN 0926-5287) **3215**, 3262, 3268
➤ Reproduction. Supplement (GBR) **3348**, 3262, 3684
Reproductions (PHL) **3215**, 4369
• Reproductive Health Matters (GBR ISSN 0968-8080) **4565**
• Reproductive Medicine Review (GBR ISSN 0962-2799) **3962**
• ➤ Reproductive Technologies (CAN ISSN 1528-4840) **3962**
• ➤ Reproductive Toxicology (USA ISSN 0890-6238) **3348**, 3262
• ➤ Reproduktionsmedizin (DEU ISSN 1434-6931) **3962**, 3360, 3880
• ➤ Republic of China. National Science Council. Proceedings. Part B: Life Sciences (TWN ISSN 0255-6596) **3684**, 3215
Res Medicae (ITA ISSN 0014-8784) **3684**, 4501
Research (DEU ISSN 0179-8618) **4333**, 3374
Research Alert (Philadelphia) (USA) **3152**
➤ Research and Clinical Center for Child Development. Annual Report (JPN ISSN 0386-8435) **3386**, 3684
Research and Clinical Forums (GBR ISSN 0143-3083) **3684**
Research and Practice (USA) **4130**, 3480, 4523
Research and Practice in Forensic Medicine *see* Hoigaku no Jissai to Kenkyu **3882**
➤ Research and Teaching in Developmental Education (USA ISSN 1046-3364) **3414**
Research Committee of Essential Amino Acids. Reports/Hissu Aminosan Kenkyu (JPN ISSN 0387-4141) **3262**
➤ Research Communications in Alcohol & Substances of Abuse (USA ISSN 1080-8388) **4333**, 3405
➤ Research Communications in Behavioral Psychology and Psychiatry (USA ISSN 1087-0695) **4444**, 4130, 4517
➤ Research Communications in Biochemistry and Cell & Molecular Biology (USA ISSN 1087-111X) **3262**, 3293, 3330
• ➤ Research Communications in Molecular Pathology and Pharmacology (USA ISSN 1078-0297) **3684**, 4333
Research Communications in Psychology, Psychiatry and Behavior *see* Research Communications in Behavioral Psychology and Psychiatry **4444**, 4130, 4517
Research Communications in Substances of Abuse *see* Research Communications in Alcohol & Substances of Abuse **4333**, 3405
Research. English Edition *see* Research **4333**, 3374
Research. English Edition *see* Research. Spanish Edition **4333**, 3374
Research in Community and Mental Health (USA ISSN 0192-0812) **4487**, 4444
Research in Complementary and Natural Classical Medicine *see* Forschende Komplementaermedizin und Klassische Naturheilkunde **3165**
• ➤ Research in Developmental Disabilities (GBR ISSN 0891-4222) **4130**, 3426
Research in Experimental Medicine *see* Clinical and Experimental Medicine **3585**, 3872
Research in Immunology *see* Microbes and Infection **3327**, 3803
• ➤ Research in Microbiology (FRA ISSN 0923-2508) **3330**
• ➤ Research in Nursing & Health (USA ISSN 0160-6891) **3939**
• ➤ Research in Organizational Behavior (USA ISSN 0191-3085) **4444**, 4368
Research in the Sociology of Health Care (USA ISSN 0275-4959) **3684**, 4487, 4523
• ➤ Research in Veterinary Science (GBR ISSN 0034-5288) **4551**
Research in Virology *see* Microbes and Infection **3327**, 3803
• ➤ Research Initiative, Treatment Action! (USA ISSN 1520-8745) **3751**, 3806
Research Institute of Industrial Safety. Annual Report *see* National Institute of Industrial Safety. Annual Report **4260**
➤ Research Methods in Neurochemistry (USA ISSN 0096-2902) **3262**, 4130
▼ ➤ Research News & Opportunities in Science and Theology (USA) **4507**, 3684, 4130, 4501
Research of Longevity Science *see* Chojugaku Kenkyu **3469**, 3164
• ➤ Research on Aging (USA ISSN 0164-0275) **3480**
Research on Drug Actions and Interactions *see* Iyakuhin Sogo Sayo Kenkyu **4304**, 3516
Research on Home Medicines *see* Kateiyaku Kenkyu **4312**

Title

Title

Title

Sante et Services Sociaux au Quebec (CAN ISSN 1203-3669) **4489**
Sante et Systemique *see* Health and System Science **3610**, 3508
Sante Femme *see* Healthy Woman **4564**
Sante Magazine (FRA ISSN 0397-0329) **4361**
Sante Mentale (FRA) **4132**
➤ Sante Mentale au Quebec (CAN ISSN 0383-6320) **4447**
Sante (Montrouge) *see* Cahiers d'Etudes et de Recherches Francophones. Sante **3581**, 4464
Sante Publique (FRA ISSN 0995-3914) **4489**
Sante Quebec (CAN ISSN 1180-3983) **3940**
• ➤ Santo Tomas Journal of Medicine (PHL ISSN 0115-1126) **3689**
Santo Tomas Nursing Journal (PHL ISSN 0048-9123) **3940**
Sanwa Kagaku Co. Medical Report *see* Byotai Seiri to Shindan Chiryo **3340**, 3580
Sao Paulo. Coordenadoria de Saude Mental. Arquivos *see* Arquivos de Saude Mental do Estado de Sao Paulo **4074**, 4378
• ➤ Sao Paulo Medical Journal (BRA ISSN 1516-3180) **3689**
Sapporo Igaku Zasshi/Sapporo Medical Journal (JPN ISSN 0036-472X) **3689**
Sapporo Medical Journal *see* Sapporo Igaku Zasshi **3689**
Sarcoidosis *see* Sarcoidosis Vasculitis and Diffuse Lung Diseases **3989**
• ➤ Sarcoidosis Vasculitis and Diffuse Lung Diseases (ITA ISSN 1124-0490) **3989**
• ➤ Sarcoma (GBR ISSN 1357-714X) **3990**
Saskatchewan Association of Health Organizations News *see* S A H O News **3522**, 4488
• Saskatchewan Conce R N (CAN ISSN 0836-7310) **3940**
Saskatchewan Drug Plan and Extended Benefits Branch. Annual Statistical Report (CAN ISSN 1487-198X) **4346**, 4335, 4529
Saskatchewan Health. Prescription Drug Services Branch. Annual Statistical Report *see* Saskatchewan Drug Plan and Extended Benefits Branch. Annual Statistical Report **4346**, 4335, 4529
Saskatchewan Health. Statistical Supplement to the Annual Report *see* Saskatchewan Drug Plan and Extended Benefits Branch. Annual Statistical Report **4346**, 4335, 4529
Saskatchewan. Laboratory and Disease Control Services Branch. Annual Statistical Report (CAN ISSN 1195-0307) **3534**, 3806
Saskatchewan Psychiatric Nurses' Association. Newsletter *see* Registered Psychiatric Nurses' Association of Saskatchewan. R P News **3939**
Saskatchewanan. Medical Services and Health Registration Branch. Annual Statistical Report (CAN ISSN 1486-1682) **3690**
• Saturday Evening Post (USA ISSN 0048-9239) **3465**, 3553, 4361
• Satya (USA) **4245**, 3172, 3442, 4368
Saude e Sociedade (BRA ISSN 0104-1290) **4489**
Saudi Heart Bulletin *see* Saudi Heart Journal **3782**
• ➤ Saudi Heart Journal (SAU ISSN 1018-077X) **3782**
➤ The Saudi Journal of Gastroenterology (SAU ISSN 1319-3767) **3895**
➤ Saudi Journal of Kidney Diseases and Transplantation (SAU ISSN 1319-2442) **4217**
• ➤ Saudi Medical Journal (SAU ISSN 0379-5284) **3690**
Savez Gluvih i Nagluvih Jugoslavije. Glas (YUG) **3493**
Saving Health *see* HealthServe **4502**, 3613
Sbornik Lekarsky (CZE ISSN 0036-5327) **3690**
Scalpel and Tongs (USA ISSN 0048-9255) **4346**, 3690
• ➤ Scandinavian Audiology (SWE ISSN 0105-0397) **4038**, 3493
Scandinavian Audiology. Supplement (SWE ISSN 0107-8593) **4038**, 3493
• ➤ Scandinavian Cardiovascular Journal (SWE ISSN 1401-7431) **4202**
Scandinavian Cardiovascular Journal. Supplementum (SWE ISSN 1401-7458) **4202**
Scandinavian Journal of Behavior Therapy. Supplementum (SWE ISSN 0346-8100) **4447**
• Scandinavian Journal of Behaviour Therapy/Nordisk Tidskrift foer Beteendeterapi (NOR ISSN 0284-5717) **4447**
• ➤ Scandinavian Journal of Caring Sciences (GBR ISSN 0283-9318) **3690**
• ➤ Scandinavian Journal of Clinical & Laboratory Investigation (NOR ISSN 0036-5513) **3880**, 3690
• Scandinavian Journal of Clinical and Laboratory Investigation. Supplement (NOR ISSN 0085-591X) **3880**, 3690
Scandinavian Journal of Dental Research *see* European Journal of Oral Sciences **3822**
• ➤ Scandinavian Journal of Gastroenterology (SWE ISSN 0036-5521) **3895**
• Scandinavian Journal of Gastroenterology. Supplement (SWE ISSN 0085-5928) **3895**
Scandinavian Journal of Haematology *see* European Journal of Haematology **3900**
Scandinavian Journal of Haematology. Supplementum *see* European Journal of Haematology. Supplementum **3901**
• ➤ Scandinavian Journal of Immunology (GBR ISSN 0300-9475) **3751**
Scandinavian Journal of Immunology Online *see* Scandinavian Journal of Immunology **3751**
Scandinavian Journal of Immunology. Supplement (GBR ISSN 0301-6323) **3751**
• ➤ Scandinavian Journal of Infectious Diseases (NOR ISSN 0036-5548) **3806**
Scandinavian Journal of Infectious Diseases. Supplementum (NOR ISSN 0300-8878) **3806**
• ➤ Scandinavian Journal of Laboratory Animal Science (DNK ISSN 0901-3393) **3880**
Scandinavian Journal of Logopedics and Phoniatrics *see* Logopedics Phoniatrics Vocology **4035**
• ➤ Scandinavian Journal of Medicine & Science in Sports (DNK ISSN 0905-7188) **4176**, 4507, 4526
• ➤ Scandinavian Journal of Medicine & Science in Sports Online (DNK ISSN 1600-0838) **4176**, 4507, 4526
• ➤ Scandinavian Journal of Nutrition/Naeringsforskning (SWE ISSN 1102-6480) **4245**
Scandinavian Journal of Nutrition. Supplement (SWE ISSN 1102-6510) **4245**
• ➤ Scandinavian Journal of Occupational Therapy (NOR ISSN 1103-8128) **3690**
Scandinavian Journal of Plastic and Reconstructive Surgery *see* Scandinavian Journal of Plastic and Reconstructive Surgery and Hand Surgery **4202**
• ➤ Scandinavian Journal of Plastic and Reconstructive Surgery and Hand Surgery (NOR ISSN 0284-4311) **4202**
Scandinavian Journal of Plastic and Reconstructive Surgery and Hand Surgery. Supplement (NOR ISSN 1235-662X) **4202**
• ➤ Scandinavian Journal of Primary Health Care (NOR ISSN 0281-3432) **3690**, 3522, 3940
Scandinavian Journal of Primary Health Care. Supplement (NOR ISSN 0284-6020) **3690**, 3522, 3940
• ➤ Scandinavian Journal of Psychology (GBR ISSN 0036-5564) **4447**
• ➤ Scandinavian Journal of Public Health (NOR ISSN 1403-4948) **3690**, 4517
Scandinavian Journal of Public Health. Supplement (NOR) **3690**, 4517
Scandinavian Journal of Rehabilitation Medicine *see* Journal of Rehabilitation Medicine **4515**, 3637
Scandinavian Journal of Rehabilitation Medicine. Supplement *see* Journal of Rehabilitation Medicine. Supplement **4515**, 3637
• ➤ Scandinavian Journal of Rheumatology (NOR ISSN 0300-9742) **4171**
• Scandinavian Journal of Rheumatology. Supplement (NOR ISSN 0301-3847) **4172**
➤ Scandinavian Journal of Sexology (DNK ISSN 1398-2966) **3690**
Scandinavian Journal of Social Medicine *see* Scandinavian Journal of Public Health **3690**, 4517
Scandinavian Journal of Thoracic and Cardiovascular Surgery *see* Scandinavian Cardiovascular Journal **4202**
Scandinavian Journal of Thoracic and Cardiovascular Surgery. Supplementum *see* Scandinavian Cardiovascular Journal. Supplementum **4202**
• ➤ Scandinavian Journal of Urology and Nephrology (SWE ISSN 0036-5599) **4218**
• Scandinavian Journal of Urology and Nephrology. Supplement (SWE ISSN 0300-8886) **4218**
• ➤ Scandinavian Journal of Work, Environment & Health (FIN ISSN 0355-3140) **4265**
Scandinavian Journal of Work, Environment and Health. Supplement (FIN ISSN 0356-6528) **4265**
➤ The Scandinavian Psychoanalytic Review (DNK ISSN 0106-2301) **4132**
• ➤ Scanning (USA ISSN 0161-0457) **3335**
Scanning Electron Microscopy *see* Scanning Microscopy **3335**, 3880, 4367
➤ Scanning Microscopy (USA ISSN 0891-7035) **3335**, 3880, 4367
Scanning Microscopy Supplement (USA ISSN 0892-953X) **3336**
Scarlet Letter (AUS ISSN 0311-7057) **4568**, 4508, 4517, 4565
Schering Annual Report (Year) (DEU) **4335**, 3238
Schiedsamtszeitung (DEU ISSN 0945-7097) **3544**, 4368
Schiffahrtmedizinisches Institut der Marine, Kiel. Veroeffentlichungen (DEU ISSN 0080-679X) **3690**
• ➤ Schizophrenia Bulletin (USA ISSN 0586-7614) **4132**
• ➤ Schizophrenia Research (NLD ISSN 0920-9964) **4132**
Schlank & Fit *see* Bild der Frau Schlank & Fit **4563**
Schlank und Fit (DEU) **4245**, 4361
Schleswig-Holsteinisches Aerzteblatt (DEU ISSN 0341-8707) **3690**
• ➤ Der Schmerz (DEU ISSN 0932-433X) **3690**
➤ Scholarly Inquiry for Nursing Practice (USA ISSN 0889-7182) **3940**
• Scholastic Choices (USA ISSN 0883-475X) **3429**, 3386, 3393, 3527
School Counselor *see* Professional School Counseling **3414**, 4434
School Food Service Journal *see* School Foodservice and Nutrition **3418**, 3462
School Food Service Research Review *see* Journal of Child Nutrition & Management **3418**, 3461
School Foodservice and Nutrition (USA ISSN 1075-3885) **3418**, 3462
School Health: A Guide for Health Professionals *see* School Health: Policy and Practice **4056**
➤ School Health Alert (USA ISSN 1048-3896) **3940**
School Health Bulletin *see* H E A P Journal **4471**
School Health: Policy and Practice (USA) **4056**
School Intervention Report (USA ISSN 0894-5152) **3386**, 3405
School Law Briefings (USA ISSN 1094-3749) **3426**, 3418
School Law Bulletin *see* School Law Briefings **3426**, 3418
School Nurse *see* Journal of School Nursing **3926**, 3413
School Nurse News (USA ISSN 1080-7543) **3940**, 3414
School of Education Annual Distinguished Lecture Series Monographs in Special Education and Rehabilitation *see* U S C Annual Distinguished Lecture Series Monographs in Special Education and Rehabilitation **3428**
School Practitioner Series *see* Guilford School Practitioner Series **4401**, 3383
• ➤ School Psychology International (GBR ISSN 0143-0343) **3429**, 4447
• ➤ School Psychology Quarterly (USA ISSN 1045-3830) **4447**, 3414
• ➤ School Psychology Review (USA ISSN 0279-6015) **4447**
• ➤ School Science Review (GBR ISSN 0036-6811) **4507**, 3429, 3690
Schools in the United States and Canada Offering Graduate Education in Pharmacology (USA) **4335**, 3417
Schrot und Korn (DEU ISSN 0931-1068) **4245**
Schulungsprofi Diabetes *see* Diabetesprofi **3859**
Schutz Aktuell (DEU ISSN 0937-2555) **3396**
Schweizer Apothekerzeitung/Giornale Svizzero di Farmacia/Journal Suisse de Pharmacie (CHE ISSN 1420-4932) **4335**
Schweizer Archiv fuer Neurologie und Psychiatrie (CHE ISSN 0258-7661) **4132**, 4202
• ➤ Schweizer Archiv fuer Tierheilkunde (CHE ISSN 0036-7281) **4552**
Schweizer Chirurgie *see* Swiss Surgery **4205**, 4026
Schweizer Hausapotheke (CHE ISSN 0258-6983) **4335**
➤ Schweizer Hebamme (CHE ISSN 1422-4526) **3940**
Schweizer Monatsschrift fuer Zahnmedizin *see* Schweizerische Monatsschrift fuer Zahnmedizin **3839**
Schweizer Optiker (CHE) **4007**
Schweizer Podologe (CHE) **4202**
➤ Schweizer Spital/Hopital Suisse/Ospedale Svizzero (CHE ISSN 0304-4432) **3522**
• ➤ Schweizerische Aerztezeitung/Bollettino dei Medici Svizzeri/Bulletin des Medecins Suisses (CHE ISSN 0036-7486) **3690**
Schweizerische Apotheker-Zeitung *see* Schweizer Apothekerzeitung **4335**
Schweizerische Laboratoriums Zeitschrift (CHE ISSN 0253-5211) **3880**
Schweizerische Medizinische Wochenschrift *see* Swiss Medical Weekly **3697**
Schweizerische Medizinische Wochenschrift (Supplementum) (CHE ISSN 0250-5525) **3691**
Schweizerische Monatsschrift fuer Zahnmedizin/Revue Mensuelle Suisse d'Odonto-Stomatologie/Rivista Mensile Svizzera di Odontologia e Stomatologia (CHE ISSN 0256-2855) **3839**
• Schweizerische Rundschau fuer Medizin Praxis/Revue Suisse de Medecine (CHE ISSN 1013-2058) **3691**
Schweizerische Zeitschrift fuer Pilzkunde/Bollettino Svizzero di Micologia/Bulletin Suisse de Mycologie (CHE ISSN 0373-2959) **3282**, 3331, 3336
• ➤ Schweizerische Zeitschrift fuer Psychologie/Revue Suisse de Psychologie/Swiss Journal of Psychology (CHE ISSN 1421-0185) **4447**
Schweizerische Zeitschrift fuer Sportmedizin *see* Schweizerische Zeitschrift fuer Sportmedizin und Sporttraumatologie **4176**
Schweizerische Zeitschrift fuer Sportmedizin und Sporttraumatologie/Revista Svizzera per Medicina e Traumatologia dello Sport/Revue Suisse pour Medecine et Traumatologie de Sports (CHE ISSN 1022-6699) **4176**
Schweizerischer Medizinalkalender *see* Medkalender **3659**
Schweizerisches Medizinisches Jahrbuch/Annuaire Medical Suisse (CHE ISSN 0080-7400) **3691**
Die Schwester - Der Pfleger (DEU ISSN 0340-5303) **3940**
Schwestern Revue *see* Krankenpflege Journal **3928**
• ➤ Science and Justice (GBR ISSN 1355-0306) **3885**
Science & Medicine (USA ISSN 1087-3309) **3880**
Science and Practice of Neuropsychology (USA) **4447**
• ➤ Science & Sports (FRA ISSN 0765-1597) **4176**
• ➤ Science as Culture (GBR ISSN 0950-5431) **4507**, 3691, 4368
➤ Science et Comportement (CAN ISSN 0841-7741) **4447**
Science of Fatigue and Rest *see* Hiro to Kyuyo no Kagaku **4093**
• ➤ The Science of the Total Environment (NLD ISSN 0048-9697) **3442**, 3444, 3454
Sciences et Techniques de l'Animal de Laboratoire *see* S T A L **3880**
Sciences et Techniques des Activites Physiques et Sportives *see* S T A P S **4176**, 4361
Sciences Medicales (FRA ISSN 0048-9727) **3691**
Sciences Orgonomiques (FRA ISSN 0767-6891) **3218**, 3691
• ➤ Sciences Sociales et Sante (FRA ISSN 0294-0337) **4489**
Sciences Techniques Pratiques Pharma Sciences *see* S T P Pharma Sciences **4335**
Sciences Veterinaires - Medecine Comparee (FRA ISSN 0750-7682) **4552**
• Scientia Pharmaceutica (AUT ISSN 0036-8709) **4335**
Scientific Affairs Division Advanced Science Institutes Series D: Behavioural and Social Sciences *see* N A T O Advanced Science Institutes Series D: Behavioural and Social Sciences **4429**, 4509
Scientific Affairs Division Advanced Science Institutes Series H: Cell Biology *see* N A T O Advanced Science Institutes Series H: Cell Biology **3293**
• ➤ Scientific American Medicine (USA ISSN 0194-9063) **3691**
▼ Scientific American Presents: The Quest to Beat Aging (USA) **3480**
Scientific American Science and Medicine *see* Science & Medicine **3880**
Scientific American Surgery (USA) **4202**

Title

Shodobutsu Hifuka Rinsho/Japanese Journal of Small Animal Dermatology (JPN ISSN 0912-2494) **4552**
Shojinkai Igakushi/Matsushita Medical Journal (JPN ISSN 0388-9734) **3693**
Shokaki Geka/Gastroenterological Surgery (JPN ISSN 0387-2645) **3896**
Shokaki Naishikyo/Endoscopia Digestiva (JPN ISSN 0915-3217) **3896**
Shokaki Naishikyo no Shinpo/Progress of Digestive Endoscopy (JPN ISSN 0389-9403) **3896**
Shokuchu Shokubutsu Kenkyukai Kaishi/Insectivorous Plant Society. Journal (JPN ISSN 0286-6102) **3282**, 3392
Shokuchudoku Tokei *see* Japan. Ministry of Health and Welfare. Statistics and Information Department. Statistical Report on Food Poisonings **4496**, 4529
Shokuhin Eiseigaku Zasshi *see* Food Hygienic Society of Japan. Journal **4469**, 4233
Shoni Geka/Japanese Journal of Pediatric Surgery (JPN ISSN 0385-6313) **4203**, 4056
Shoni Hoken Kenkyu/Journal of Child Health (JPN ISSN 0037-4113) **4361**, 4056
Shoni Naika/Japanese Journal of Pediatric Medicine (JPN ISSN 0385-6305) **4057**
Shonika/Clinical Pediatrics (JPN ISSN 0037-4121) **4057**
Shonika Rinsho *see* Japanese Journal of Pediatrics **4046**
➤ Shoudu Yike Daxue/Capital University of Medical Sciences. Journal (CHN) **3693**
Shoudu Yixueyuan Xuebao/Capital Institute of Medicine. Journal *see* Shoudu Yike Daxue **3693**
➤ Shoulei Xuebao/Acta Theriologica Sinica (CHN ISSN 1000-1050) **3356**
Shouwaike Zazhi/ Journal of Hand Surgery *see* Zhonghua Shouwaike Zazhi **4208**
Shoyakugaku Zasshi - Japanese Journal of Pharmacognosy *see* Natural Medicines **4318**
Shuangzu yu Baojian/China Reflexology Journal (CHN ISSN 1004-6569) **4026**
➤ Shuisheng Shengwu Xuebao/Acta Hydrobiologica Sinica (CHN ISSN 1000-3207) **3218**, 3408, 3409
Shujutsu/Operation (JPN ISSN 0037-4423) **4203**
Shukan Asahi Hyakka/Weekly Asahi Encyclopedia (JPN) **3356**
Shukan Igakkai Shinbun/New Medical World Weekly (JPN) **3693**
Shusanki Igaku/Perinatal Medicine (JPN ISSN 0386-9881) **3964**
Sibling Information Network Newsletter (USA) **3386**, 3499
Sichere Arbeit (AUT ISSN 0037-4512) **4266**
Sicherheit am Arbeitsplatz (DEU) **4266**
Sicherheit im Oeffentlichen Dienst *see* Faktor Arbeitsschutz **3531**, 4254
Sicherheit Zuerst (AUT ISSN 0037-4539) **4533**, 4490
Sicherheitsmagazin *see* Neue B S **4260**, 3364
Sicherheitsvorschriften fuer Medizinprodukte (DEU ISSN 0947-269X) **4336**, 3544
Sichuan Journal of Traditional Chinese Medicine *see* Sichuan Zhongyi **3170**, 3693
Sichuan Zhongyi/Sichuan Journal of Traditional Chinese Medicine (CHN ISSN 1000-3649) **3170**, 3693
SIDA (USA) **3807**, 3457
SIDA Ahora (USA) **3807**, 3457, 4518
➤ Sida: Botanical Miscellany (USA ISSN 0883-1475) **3282**
Sida Studies on Emergencies and Disaster Relief *see* Studies on Emergencies and Disaster Relief **3387**, 4490
SIDAahora (USA) **3807**
Sidafrique (FRA ISSN 1245-060X) **3807**, 3465
• ➤ Side Effects of Drugs Annual (NLD ISSN 0378-6080) **4336**, 3693
Sieboldia Acta Biologica/Shiborudia (JPN ISSN 0559-9822) **3218**
Siemens Electromedica *see* Electromedica (Deutsche Ausgabe) **3598**, 3430
Siete Dias Medicos (ESP ISSN 0214-3011) **3693**
Sight and Sound News (AUS) **3522**, 4007, 4038
Sight, Hearing and Dental Health (Persons Aged 2 to 14 Years) *see* Australia. Bureau of Statistics. Children's Health Screening **3716**, 4041, 4527
Sights and Sounds (USA) **3493**, 3426, 3499
• Sigletter (USA) **3693**
• Sign Language Studies (USA ISSN 0302-1475) **3551**, 3174
• Signal (CAN ISSN 0228-9091) **4266**, 4533
• Signal (DEU ISSN 0721-6831) **3990**
▼ • ➤ Signal Transduction (DEU ISSN 1615-4053) **3294**, 3262
• Signal Transduction & Cyclic Nucleotides (GBR ISSN 0964-7589) **3236**, 3152, 3262, 3736
Signal'naya Informatsiya. Fiziologiya i Morfologiya Cheloveka i Zhivotnykh: Krov' i Limfa (RUS ISSN 0233-6618) **3236**, 3152, 3349
Signal'naya Informatsiya. Ishimicheskaya Bolezn' Serdtsa (RUS ISSN 0234-9760) **3736**, 3783
Signal'naya Informatsiya. Neiropeptidy (RUS ISSN 0234-9752) **3736**, 3152, 4133
Signal'naya Informatsiya. Tekhnika Bezopasnosti. Sanitarnaya Tekhnika (RUS ISSN 0202-8905) **4269**, 3152
Signal'naya Informatsiya. Toksikologiya Lekarstvennaya (RUS ISSN 0233-6588) **4346**, 3152
Signature (Mahwah) (USA ISSN 1091-5222) **3839**
➤ Sigurnost/Safety (HRV ISSN 0350-6886) **4490**
Sihatak *see* Sehhatuk Alyoum **3691**
Sihhah *see* Health **4471**
Siksha (IND) **3415**, 4449
The Silent Advocate (USA ISSN 0037-5187) **3493**, 3427
Silent Messenger/Stille Boodskapper (ZAF ISSN 0037-5195) **3493**
Silent News (USA ISSN 0049-0490) **3493**
• ➤ Silvae Genetica (DEU ISSN 0037-5349) **3282**, 3314
Silver Sentinel (USA ISSN 1087-9366) **3481**
Silver Sheet (USA) **3693**
Simon Fraser University, Gerontology Research Centre News *see* G R C News **3471**
• Simply Better (AUS ISSN 1038-3514) **3549**, 4266, 4361
Simply Better, Your Choice, Your lifestyle *see* Simply Better **3549**, 4266, 4361
Simply Lite *see* SimplyLite **4361**, 4245
▼ SimplyLite (AUS) **4361**, 4245
Sindrome Down Notizie (ITA ISSN 1122-147X) **4133**
• Singapore Journal of Obstetrics & Gynaecology (SGP ISSN 0129-3273) **3964**, 3360, 3522
Singapore Journal of Primary Industries (SGP ISSN 0129-6485) **3156**, 3459, 4552
➤ Singapore Medical Journal (SGP ISSN 0037-5675) **3693**
Singapore Nursing Journal (SGP) **3940**
➤ Singapore Paediatric Journal (SGP ISSN 0218-9941) **4057**
Singapore Paediatric Society. Journal *see* Singapore Paediatric Journal **4057**
Singer Report on Healthcare Systems and Technology *see* Healthcare Perspective **3810**, 3532
Singer Report on Managed Care Systems and Technology *see* Healthcare Perspective **3810**, 3532
Sinistralian (USA) **3387**, 4449
Sinnets Helse (NOR ISSN 0049-0563) **4449**, 4490
Sino-Japanese Friendship Hospital. Journal *see* Zhongri Youhao Yiyuan Xuebao **3714**
Sister Communities Health Profiles of the U S - Mexico Border/Perfiles de Salud de las Comunidades Hermanas de la Frontera Mexico - Estados Unidos (USA) **4498**, 3736, 4530
Sistole (ESP) **3783**
➤ Sjogren's Syndrome Foundation Inc. (USA) **3751**
Sjukgymnasten (SWE ISSN 0037-6019) **3693**
Sjukhusfarmaci (SWE ISSN 0346-8453) **4336**, 3522
▼ Skandinavien Direkt (SWE) **3940**
• ➤ Skeletal Radiology (DEU ISSN 0364-2348) **4155**
➤ Skin & Aging (USA ISSN 1096-0120) **3481**, 3853
Skin & Allergy News (USA ISSN 0037-6337) **3853**
Skin Cancer Foundation Journal (USA ISSN 0898-6665) **3990**, 3853
Skin Inc. (USA ISSN 0898-6525) **3853**, 3176
Skin Pharmacology *see* Skin Pharmacology and Applied Skin Physiology **4336**, 3853
• ➤ Skin Pharmacology and Applied Skin Physiology (CHE ISSN 1422-2868) **4336**, 3853
Skin Research/Hifu (JPN ISSN 0018-1390) **3853**
• ➤ Skin Research and Technology (DNK ISSN 0909-752X) **3853**
• Skin Therapy Letter (CAN ISSN 1201-5989) **3853**
Skolhaelsan (SWE ISSN 0284-284X) **3941**
• ➤ Skull Base Surgery (USA ISSN 1052-1453) **4203**, 4007
Skyhopper (USA) **3356**, 3392
Slaa Tillbaka *see* Oberoende **3404**, 3542, 4516
• ➤ Sleep (USA ISSN 0161-8105) **4134**
• ➤ Sleep and Breathing (USA ISSN 1520-9512) **4134**
▼ • ➤ Sleep and Hypnosis (TUR ISSN 1302-1192) **4134**
▼ • ➤ Sleep Medicine (NLD ISSN 1389-9457) **4134**
• ➤ Sleep Medicine Reviews (GBR ISSN 1087-0792) **4134**
Sleep Research (USA ISSN 0093-0407) **4134**
▼ • Sleep Review (USA ISSN 1531-3034) **4449**
Slide Atlas of Current Dermatology *see* Current Opinion in Dermatology **3847**
Slide Atlas of Current Ophthalmology (Year) (GBR ISSN 1055-6575) **4007**
Slide Atlas of Current Orthopaedics (Year) (GBR ISSN 1055-6583) **4026**
Slide Atlas of Gastrointestinal Endoscopy (Year) (GBR) **3896**
Slim & Fit Diet & Exercise (USA ISSN 1058-2940) **4361**
Slimmer (GBR ISSN 0955-758X) **4245**, 4361
Slimming (AUS ISSN 1321-8824) **4246**
Slimming (GBR ISSN 0144-8129) **4246**, 4361
Slimming and Supplementary Nutrition: The International Market *see* Vitamins & Dietary Supplements: The International Market **4340**, 3367
Slimming Australia *see* Slimming **4246**
Slovak Academy of Sciences. Treatises on Biology *see* Slovenska Akademia Vied. Biologicke Prace **3218**
Slovenian Veterinary Research/Slovenski Veterinarski Zbornik (SVN ISSN 1580-4003) **4552**
Slovenska Akademia Vied. Biologicke Prace/Slovak Academy of Sciences. Treatises on Biology (SVK ISSN 0037-6930) **3218**
Slovenski Veterinarski Zbornik *see* Slovenian Veterinary Research **4552**
Slownik Biograficzny Polskich Nauk Medycznych XXX Wieku (POL) **3693**, 3177
Sluomen Virallinen Tilasto. 6 B, Kuolemansyyt *see* Finland. Tilastokeskus. Kuolemansyyt **4370**
Smaerta (SWE ISSN 1402-1048) **3941**
Small Group Behavior *see* Small Group Research **4449**, 4523
• ➤ Small Group Research (USA ISSN 1046-4964) **4449**, 4523
Small or Rural Hospitals Update (USA) **3522**
• ➤ Small Ruminant Research (NLD ISSN 0921-4488) **3161**, 4552
Smart Drug News (USA ISSN 1060-8427) **4336**, 4134
• ➤ Smith College Studies in Social Work (USA ISSN 0037-7317) **4518**, 4449
Smith - Kettlewell Technical File (USA) **3499**, 3427
Smith, Kline & French Laboratories Research Symposia Series *see* New Horizons in Therapeutics: Smith, Kline & French Laboratories Research Symposia Series **3666**
Smoking and Health Newsletter (USA) **4361**, 3405
Smoking or Health *see* Australian Council on Smoking and Health Newsletter **4350**, 3399
Snakeroot Extract (USA ISSN 0743-6033) **3526**, 3522, 3693
So Young! (USA ISSN 1088-7482) **4361**, 3176
Sober Times (USA ISSN 1059-6259) **3405**
Sobering Thoughts (USA ISSN 1071-4111) **3405**, 4566, 4568
• Social Action and the Law (USA ISSN 0272-765X) **4449**, 3544
• ➤ Social Behavior and Personality (NZL ISSN 0301-2212) **4449**, 4523
• ➤ Social Biology (USA ISSN 0037-766X) **3314**
• ➤ Social Cognition (USA ISSN 0278-016X) **4449**
• ➤ Social History of Medicine (GBR ISSN 0951-631X) **3694**
• ➤ Social Psychiatry and Psychiatric Epidemiology (DEU ISSN 0933-7954) **4134**
➤ Social Psychological Applications to Social Issues (USA) **4449**, 4523
• ➤ Social Psychology of Education (NLD ISSN 1381-2890) **3415**, 4449
• ➤ Social Psychology Quarterly (USA ISSN 0190-2725) **4523**, 4449
• ➤ Social Science & Medicine (GBR ISSN 0277-9536) **3694**, 4509
Social Service Jobs (USA) **4270**, 4449, 4518
Social Work Administration *see* Social Work Leader **4518**, 4490
• ➤ Social Work in Health Care (USA ISSN 0098-1389) **4518**, 4490
Social Work Leader (USA) **4518**, 4490
Social Work Practice with Children and Families (USA) **4449**
• ➤ Social Work with Groups (USA ISSN 0160-9513) **4518**
Socialism and Health (GBR ISSN 0037-8119) **4490**, 4518
Socialisticno Kmetijstvo *see* Sodobno Kmetijstvo **3156**, 3462, 4552
Socialmedicinsk Tidskrift (SWE ISSN 0037-833X) **3694**, 4518
Sociedad Americana de Oftalmologia y Optometria. Archivos/American Society for Ophthalmology and Optometry. Archives (COL ISSN 0037-8364) **4007**
• ➤ Sociedad Andaluza de Traumatologia y Ortopedia. Revista (ESP ISSN 0212-0771) **4026**
Sociedad Boliviana de Historia Natural. Revista (BOL) **3218**
Sociedad Colombiana de Endocrinologia. Revista (COL ISSN 0120-1182) **3869**
Sociedad de Biologia de Concepcion. Boletin (CHL ISSN 0037-850X) **3218**
Sociedad Espanola de Farmacia Hospitalaria. Boletin Informativo (ESP ISSN 1130-8230) **4336**, 3522
Sociedad Espanola de Historia de la Medicina. Boletin (ESP ISSN 0583-7480) **3694**
Sociedad Espanola de Medicina de Urgencias y Emergencias. Revista (ESP) **4026**
Sociedad Espanola de Medicina Rural y Generalista *see* S E M E R G E N **3689**
Sociedad Espanola de Oftalmologia. Archivos (ESP ISSN 0365-6691) **4007**
• ➤ Sociedad Espanola del Dolor. Revista (ESP ISSN 1134-8046) **3760**
Sociedad Espanola Interdisciplinaria de S I D A. Publicacion Oficial (Sindrome de Inmunodeficiencia Adquirida) (ESP ISSN 1130-1597) **3807**
Sociedad Espanola Interdisciplinaria del SIDA SIDA *see* S E I SIDA **3806**
• ➤ Sociedad Valenciana de Patologia Digestiva. Revista (ESP ISSN 0301-1143) **3896**
Sociedade Brasileira de Zootecnia. Revista *see* Revista Brasileira de Zootecnia **4551**, 3159
Sociedade das Ciencias Medicas de Lisboa. Jornal *see* Jornal das Ciencias Medicas **3628**
Sociedade de Medicina e Cirurgia de Sao Jose do Rio Preto. Revista (BRA) **4203**
Societa dei Naturalisti in Napoli. Bollettino (ITA ISSN 0366-2047) **3218**
Societa di Ortopedia e Traumatologia dell'Italia Meridionale ed Insulare. Atti e Memorie (ITA ISSN 0394-0713) **4026**
Societa Emiliana Romagnola Triveneta di Ortopedia e Traumatologia. Atti (ITA) **4026**
Societa Entomologica Italiana. Memorie (ITA ISSN 0037-8747) **3297**
Societa Italiana di Anestesia, Analgesia, Rianimazione e Terapia Intensiva. Notizario (ITA ISSN 1126-4683) **3760**
Societa Italiana di Biologia Sperimentale. Bollettino/Journal of Biological Research (ITA ISSN 0037-8771) **3219**
Societa Italiana di Chirurgia Oncologica. News (ITA ISSN 1123-7112) **3990**
Societa Italiana di Farmacia Ospedaliera. Bollettino (ITA ISSN 0037-8798) **4336**
Societa Italiana di Scienze Farmaceutiche Documenti *see* S.I.S.F. Documenti **4335**
Societa Lombarda di Medicina Legale e delle Assicurazioni. Archivio (ITA) **3885**, 3534
Societa Medico-Chirurgica della Provincia di Cremona. Bollettino (ITA ISSN 1121-1342) **4203**
Societa Medico-Chirurgica di Modena. Bollettino (ITA) **4203**
Societa Medico Chirurgica di Pavia. Bollettino (ITA ISSN 0390-8283) **3880**
Societas Internationalis Odontologica. Rapid Communications (NLD ISSN 0926-3551) **3219**
➤ Societas pro Fauna et Flora Fennica. Memoranda (FIN ISSN 0373-6873) **3219**
Societe Belge d'Ophtalmologie. Bulletin (BEL ISSN 0081-0746) **4007**

Title

Societe Canadienne de la Croix-Rouge. Services Transfusionnels. Rapport Annuel *see* Canadian Red Cross Society. Blood Services. Annual Report **3899**

Societe Canadienne de Pediatrie. Rapport Annuel *see* Canadian Paediatric Society. Annual Report **4042**

Societe Clinique des Hopitaux de Bruxelles. Bulletins et Comptes Rendus *see* Acta Clinica Belgica **3557**

Societe de Biogeographe. Compte Rendu des Seances *see* Biogeographica **3184**

Societe de Biologie et de Ses Filiales. Comptes Rendus des Seances *see* Societe de Biologie. Journal **3219**

Societe de Biologie. Journal (FRA ISSN 1295-0661) **3219**

• ➤ Societe de Pathologie Exotique. Bulletin (FRA) **3694**

Societe de Pathologie Exotique et de ses Filiales. Bulletin *see* Societe de Pathologie Exotique. Bulletin **3694**

Societe de Pharmacie de Bordeaux. Bulletin (FRA ISSN 0037-9093) **4336**

Societe de Pharmacie de Lille. Bulletin (FRA) **4336**

Societe de Pharmacie de Strasbourg. Bulletin (FRA ISSN 0037-9131) **4337**

Societe de Therapeutique. Bulletins et Memoires *see* Therapie **3700**

Societe des Alcools du Quebec. Rapport Annuel (CAN ISSN 0845-924X) **3405**

Societe des Amis des Sciences et des Lettres de Panan. Bulletin. Serie D: Sciences Biologiques *see* Biological Bulletin of Poznan **3185**

Societe des Naturalistes Luxembourgeois. Bulletin (LUX ISSN 0304-9620) **3219**, 3407

➤ Societe des Sciences Medicales du Grand-Duche de Luxembourg. Bulletin (LUX ISSN 0037-9247) **3694**

Societe d'Ophtalmologie de France. Bulletin (FRA ISSN 0081-1270) **4007**

Societe Francaise de Cancerologie Privee. Bulletin (FRA ISSN 0753-7417) **3990**

• Societe Francaise de Cardiologie. Bulletin d'Informations (FRA ISSN 0395-403X) **3783**

Societe Francaise de Chirurgie Orthopedique et Traumatologique. Conferences d'Enseignement (FRA ISSN 0081-1033) **4026**

Societe Francaise de Microbiologie. Annuaire (FRA ISSN 0081-1068) **3331**

Societe Francaise de Mycologie Medicale. Bulletin *see* Journal de Mycologie Medicale **3747**

Societe Francaise de Psycho-Prophylaxie Obstetricale. Bulletin Officiel (FRA) **3964**

Societe Francaise d'Ophtalmologie. Bulletins et Memoires *see* Ophtalmologie **4003**

Societe Francaise du Rorschach et des Methodes Projectives. Bulletin *see* Psychologie Clinique et Projective **4439**

Societe Linneenne de Bordeaux. Bulletin (FRA ISSN 0750-6848) **3356**, 3408

Societe Linneenne de Lyon. Bulletin Mensuel (FRA ISSN 0366-1326) **3219**

➤ Societe Linneenne de Provence. Bulletin (FRA ISSN 0373-0875) **3282**, 3356

Societe Royale Belge de Gynecologie et d'Obstetrique. Bulletin (BEL ISSN 0037-9522) **3964**

Societe Veterinaire Practique de France. Bulletin Bimestriel (FRA ISSN 1620-8706) **4552**

Societe Veterinaire Pratique de France. Bulletin Mensuel *see* Societe Veterinaire Practique de France. Bulletin Bimestriel **4552**

➤ Societe Zoologique de France. Memoires (FRA ISSN 0750-747X) **3356**

• ➤ Society & Animals (NLD ISSN 1063-1119) **3172**, 3442, 4449

Society for Antibacterial and Antifungal Agents, Japan. Abstracts of the Meeting *see* Nihon Bokin Bobai Gakkai. Nenji Taikai Yoshishu **3233**, 3150, 3329

Society for Applied Bacteriology. Symposium Series *see* Society for Applied Microbiology. Symposium Series **3331**

➤ Society for Applied Bacteriology. Technical Series (USA) **3331**

➤ Society for Applied Microbiology. Symposium Series (GBR ISSN 1467-4734) **3331**

Society for Companion Animal Studies. Journal (GBR ISSN 1363-464X) **3172**, 4449

Society for Cryobiology. News Notes (USA ISSN 1069-3610) **3219**

Society for Developmental Biology. Symposium (USA ISSN 0583-9009) **3219**

➤ Society for Existential Analysis. Journal (GBR ISSN 0958-0476) **4348**, 4449

Society for Experimental Biology and Medicine. Proceedings *see* Experimental Biology and Medicine (Maywood) **3195**, 3874

Society for Experimental Biology. Seminar Series (GBR ISSN 0309-6831) **3219**

Society for Experimental Biology. Symposia (GBR ISSN 0081-1386) **3219**

Society for General Microbiology. Quarterly *see* Microbiology Today **3328**

Society for General Microbiology. Symposium (GBR ISSN 0081-1394) **3331**

• ➤ Society for Gynecologic Investigation. Journal (USA ISSN 1071-5576) **3964**

Society for Health and Human Values. Bulletin *see* Of Value **4348**, 3238

Society for Health Systems. Journal (USA ISSN 1043-1721) **4266**

➤ Society for In Vitro Biology. Monograph Series (USA) **3277**, 3314

➤ Society for In Vitro Biology. Proceedings (USA) **3349**, 3694

Society for Mammary Glands and Lactation Research. Abstracts of the Meeting *see* Nyusen Hinyu Kenkyukai Koen Yoshishu **3733**, 3150, 3960

Society for Neuroscience. Abstracts (USA ISSN 0190-5295) **4134**, 3262

• ➤ Society for Research in Child Development. Monographs (USA ISSN 0037-976X) **3386**, 3415, 4449

Society for Research in Child Development Newsletter *see* S R C D Newsletter **3386**, 3414, 4056, 4446

Society for the Advancement of Anaesthesia in Dentistry Digest *see* S A A D Digest **3839**

Society for the Medical Application of Carbon Thirteen. Bulletin *see* 13C Igaku **3554**, 3336

Society for the Study of Human Biology. Symposia *see* Society for the Study of Human Biology. Symposium Series **3349**, 3174

➤ Society for the Study of Human Biology. Symposium Series (GBR ISSN 0954-7800) **3349**, 3174

Society for the Study of Inborn Errors of Metabolism. Symposia *see* Journal of Inherited Metabolic Disease **4046**

Society for Vector Ecology. Bulletin *see* Journal of Vector Ecology **3206**

Society Newsletter *see* Sexual Science **4448**, 4523

Society of Biological Chemists Newsletter *see* S B C Newsletter **3262**

Society of Biological Chemists. Proceedings (IND ISSN 0300-0486) **3262**

Society of General Internal Medicine Forum *see* S G I M Forum **3911**

Society of Health of Nigeria. Journal (NGA ISSN 0037-9905) **4490**

Society of Japanese Virologists. Bulletin *see* Nihon Uirusu Gakkai Kaiho **3329**

Society of Japanese Virologists. Hokkaido Branch. News *see* Nihon Uirusu Gakkai Hokkaido Shibu Kaiho **3329**

Society of Japanese Virologists. Proceedings of the Annual Meeting *see* Nihon Uirusu Gakkai Sokai Enzetsu Shoroku **3329**

Society of Laparoendoscopic Surgeons. Journal (USA ISSN 1086-8089) **4203**

Society of Magnetic Resonance in Medicine. Proceedings of Annual Conference *see* Jiki Kyomei Igakkai Puroguramu **4147**, 4365

Society of Nippon Dental College. Annual Publications *see* Nippon Dental University. Annual Publications **3833**

• ➤ Society of Pediatric Nurses. Journal (USA ISSN 1088-145X) **3941**, 4057

Society of Pediatric Psychology. Newsletter *see* Progress Notes **4434**

Society of Teachers of Family Medicine Messenger *see* S T F M Messenger **3689**

• ➤ Sociobiology (USA ISSN 0361-6525) **3219**

Socioeconomic Characteristics of Medical Practice (USA ISSN 0742-2709) **3694**, 4509

Sociologus (DEU ISSN 0038-0377) **4523**, 4449

• ➤ Sociology of Health and Illness (GBR ISSN 0141-9889) **4523**, 4134

Sociology of Health and Illness Monograph Series *see* Sociology of Health and Illness **4523**, 4134

• ➤ Sociology of Sport Journal (USA ISSN 0741-1235) **4523**, 4176, 4526

Socionics, Mentology and Personality Psychology *see* Sotsionika, Mentologiya i Psikhologiya Lichnosti **4523**, 4450, 4509

Sodobno Kmetijstvo (SVN ISSN 0350-1655) **3156**, 3462, 4552

Sofiiski Universitet. Biologicheski Fakultet. Godishnik (BGR ISSN 0081-1823) **3219**

Sogo Kango (JPN ISSN 0038-0660) **3941**

Sogo Rehabilitation (JPN ISSN 0386-9822) **4066**

Sogo Seikotsu/Synthesis Osteopathy (JPN ISSN 0910-1225) **3789**

• ➤ Soil Biology & Biochemistry (GBR ISSN 0038-0717) **3263**

Soins (FRA ISSN 0038-0814) **3941**

Soins - Chirurgie (FRA ISSN 0249-6429) **3941**, 4203

Soins - Encadrement, Formation (FRA ISSN 1163-4723) **3941**

Soins - Formation, Pedagogie, Encadrement *see* Soins - Encadrement, Formation **3941**

Soins Gerontologie (FRA ISSN 1268-6034) **3941**

Soins - Gynecologie, Obstetrique, Puericulture, Pediatrie *see* Soins - Pediatrie, Puericulture **3941**

Soins - Pediatrie, Puericulture (FRA ISSN 1259-4792) **3941**

Soins - Psychiatrie (FRA ISSN 0241-6972) **3941**, 4134

Solas - International Convention for the Safety of Life at Sea. Amendments (GBR) **3454**, 4533

• ➤ Solid State Nuclear Magnetic Resonance (GBR ISSN 0926-2040) **3377**, 3530, 4156

Solving Problems in the Teaching of Literacy (USA) **4449**

• ➤ Somatic Cell and Molecular Genetics (USA ISSN 0740-7750) **3314**, 3294

Somatics (USA ISSN 0147-5231) **4361**, 4176, 4227, 4449

• ➤ Somatosensory and Motor Research (GBR ISSN 0899-0220) **3349**, 4134

• Somnologie/Somnology (DEU ISSN 1432-9123) **3694**, 4450

Somnology *see* Somnologie **3694**, 4450

Sonderpaedagogik (DEU ISSN 0342-7366) **3427**

Sonderschule *see* Die Neue Sonderschule **3413**, 3492, 3498

Der Sonntagsbrief (DEU ISSN 0174-0350) **3481**, 3465, 4501

➤ Sonoma County Physician (USA ISSN 1087-8807) **3694**

➤ Soshiki Baiyo Kenkyu/Tissue Culture Research Communications (JPN ISSN 0912-3636) **3294**, 3263, 3277

Soshiki Saibo Kagaku Koshukai/Course Text of Histochemistry and Cytochemistry (JPN) **3294**

Soshiki Saibogaku Kiroku *see* Archives of Histology and Cytology **3285**, 3568

• Sotsionika, Mentologiya i Psikhologiya Lichnosti/Socionics, Mentology and Personality Psychology (UKR ISSN 1680-4325) **4523**, 4450, 4509

➤ Sotsyal'naya i Klinicheskaya Psikhyatriya (RUS ISSN 0869-4893) **4134**

• Sound Computing (USA) **3494**, 3499

Soundings *see* Good Vibrations **3497**, 4225, 4525

Sounds of Lexington (USA) **3493**

Sourcebook on Asbestos Diseases (USA) **3544**, 3694

South Africa Blind Workers Organisation News *see* S A B W O News **3499**

South Africa. Central Statistical Service. Bulletin of Statistics *see* South Africa. Statistics South Africa. Bulletin of Statistics **4530**

South Africa. Central Statistical Service. Census of Business Services - Accounting, Auditing and Book-keeping Services *see* South Africa. Statistics South Africa. Census of Professional and Business Services - Accounting, Auditing and Book-keeping Services **3362**, 4530

South Africa. Central Statistical Service. Census of Business Services - Advertising Practitioners and Allied Services and Marketing Research Services *see* South Africa. Statistics South Africa. Census of Professional and Business Services - Advertising Practitioners and Allied Services and Marketing Research Services **3153**, 4530

South Africa. Central Statistical Service. Census of Business Services - Data Processing Services *see* South Africa. Statistics South Africa. Census of Professional and Business Services - Data Processing Services **3362**, 3390, 4530

South Africa. Central Statistical Service. Census of Estate Agencies, Rent Collectors, Appraisers and Valuers *see* South Africa. Statistics South Africa. Census of Estate Agencies, Rent Collectors, Appraisers and Valuers **4499**, 4530

South Africa. Central Statistical Service. Census of Hospitals, Clinics and Other Health Service Establishments *see* South Africa. Statistics South Africa. Census of Hospitals, Clinics and Other Health Service Establishments **3525**, 4530

South Africa. Central Statistical Service. Census of Letting of Own Fixed Property *see* South Africa. Statistics South Africa. Census of Letting of Own Fixed Property **4499**, 4530

South Africa. Central Statistical Service. Census of Medical, Dental and Other Health Services - Chiropractors, Homeopaths, Naturopaths, Osteopaths and Herbalists *see* South Africa. Statistics South Africa. Census of Medical, Dental and Other Health Services - Chiropractors, Homeopaths, Naturopaths, Osteopaths and Herbalists **3736**, 3789, 4530

South Africa. Central Statistical Service. Census of Medical, Dental and Other Health Services - Dentists *see* South Africa. Statistics South Africa. Census of Medical, Dental and Other Health Services - Dentists **3736**, 3839, 4530

South Africa. Central Statistical Service. Census of Medical, Dental and Other Health Services - Doctors *see* South Africa. Statistics South Africa. Census of Medical, Dental and Other Health Services - Doctors **3737**, 4530

South Africa. Central Statistical Service. Census of Medical, Dental and Other Health Services - Supplementary Health Services and Dental Technicians *see* South Africa. Statistics South Africa. Census of Medical, Dental and Other Health Services - Supplementary Health Services and Dental Technicians **3737**, 4530

South Africa. Central Statistical Service. Road Traffic Collisions *see* South Africa. Statistics South Africa. Road Traffic Collisions **4532**, 4530, 4532

South Africa. Central Statistical Service. Statistical Release. Census of Auxiliary, Health Services and Dental Technicians (Year) *see* South Africa. Statistics South Africa. Statistical Release. Census of Auxiliary, Health Services and Dental Technicians (Year) **3737**, 3525, 4530

South Africa. Central Statistical Service. Statistical Release. Census of Chiropractors and Homeopaths *see* South Africa. Statistics South Africa. Statistical Release. Census of Chiropractors and Homeopaths **3737**, 4530

South Africa. Central Statistical Service. Statistical Release. Census of Dentists (Year) *see* South Africa. Statistics South Africa. Statistical Release. Census of Dentists (Year) **3737**, 4530

South Africa. Central Statistical Service. Statistical Release. Census of Doctors (Year) *see* South Africa. Statistics South Africa. Statistical Release. Census of Doctors (Year) **3737**, 3525, 4530

South Africa. Central Statistical Service. Statistical Release. Census of Hospitals, Clinics and Other Health Service. Establishments (Year) *see* South Africa. Statistics South Africa. Statistical Release. Census of Hospitals, Clinics and Other Health Service Establishments (Year) **3525**, 4530

South Africa. Central Statistical Service. Statistical Release. Road Traffic Collisions *see* South Africa. Statistics South Africa. Statistical Release. Road Traffic Collisions **4532**, 4498, 4530

South Africa. Statistics South Africa. Bulletin of Statistics (ZAF) **4530**

South Africa. Statistics South Africa. Census of Business Services - Accounting, Auditing and Book-keeping Services *see* South Africa. Statistics South Africa. Census of Professional and Business Services - Accounting, Auditing and Book-keeping Services **3362**, 4530

South Africa. Statistics South Africa. Census of Business Services - Advertising Practitioners and Allied Services and Marketing Research Services *see* South Africa. Statistics South Africa. Census of Professional and Business Services - Advertising Practitioners and Allied Services and Marketing Research Services **3153**, 4530

South Africa. Statistics South Africa. Census of Business Services - Data Processing Services *see* South Africa. Statistics South

Title

Title

• ➤ Sports Medicine Standards & Malpractice Reporter (USA ISSN 1041-696X) **3544**, 4177
• ➤ Sports Medicine, Training and Rehabilitation (CHE ISSN 1057-8315) **4177**
Sports Science *see* Tiyu Kexue **4526**
Sports Science Research *see* Tiyu Keyan **4177**, 4362
Sports Trainers Digest (AUS ISSN 1032-5506) **4526**, 4177
Sports Training, Medicine and Rehabilitation *see* Sports Medicine, Training and Rehabilitation **4177**
Sportsmedicine Digest *see* Sports Medicine Digest **4177**, 4526
SportsScoop *see* U S A B A Agenda **4526**, 3500
• Sportverletzung - Sportschaden (DEU ISSN 0932-0555) **3695**, 4526
Spotlight on AIDS (USA ISSN 0895-755X) **3807**
• Spotlight on Food (USA) **4246**
• ➤ Sprache & Kognition (CHE ISSN 0253-4533) **4450**
• ➤ Sprache - Stimme - Gehoer (DEU ISSN 0342-0477) **3427**, 4038
Die Sprachheilarbeit (DEU ISSN 0584-9470) **3427**, 3552
Sprechstunde (CHE) **3695**
➤ Spring Journal (USA ISSN 0362-0522) **4450**
Springer Handbook of Auditory Research (USA) **4038**
• ➤ Springer Seminars in Immunopathology (DEU ISSN 0344-4325) **3751**
Springer Series: Focus on Men (USA ISSN 0277-3422) **4222**, 4450
Springer Series: Focus on Women (USA ISSN 0272-202X) **4566**, 4450
Springer Series in Biophysics (USA ISSN 0932-2353) **3268**
Springer Series on Adulthood & Aging (USA ISSN 0272-5835) **3481**
Springer Series on Advanced Practice Nursing (USA) **3941**
Springer Series on Behavior Therapy and Behavioral Medicine (USA ISSN 0278-6729) **4450**, 4135
Springer Series on Comparative Treatments for Psychological Disorders (USA) **4450**
Springer Series on Death and Suicide (USA ISSN 0271-1192) **4450**
Springer Series on Ethics, Law, and Aging (USA) **3481**, 3544, 4348
Springer Series on Geriatric Nursing (USA) **3481**, 3941
Springer Series on Life Styles & Issues on Aging (USA) **3481**
Springer Series on Medical Education (USA ISSN 0277-4186) **3695**, 3417
Springer Series on Psychiatry (USA ISSN 0740-4212) **4135**
Springer Series on Rehabilitation (USA ISSN 0734-6522) **4066**, 4518
Springer Series on the Teaching of Nursing (USA ISSN 0272-1473) **3941**, 3417
Sprinkler Age (USA ISSN 0896-2685) **3458**
Sproutletter (USA ISSN 0744-9860) **4246**, 3463
➤ Sri Lanka Dental Journal (LKA ISSN 1391-0728) **3840**
Sri Lanka Pharmaceutical Association. Quarterly Newsletter (LKA) **4337**
Sri Lanka Veterinary Journal (LKA) **4553**
Srpska Akademija Nauka i Umetnosti. Odeljenje Medicinskih Nauka. Glas (YUG ISSN 0371-4039) **3695**
Srpska Akademija Nauka i Umetnosti. Odeljenje Medicinskih Nauka. Posebna Izdanja (YUG ISSN 0081-4016) **3695**
Srpski Arhiv za Celokupno Lekarstvo/Serbian Archives of Medicine (YUG ISSN 0370-8179) **3695**
St. Agnes News (USA) **3522**
St. Anthony's Coding for General Surgery Reimbursement (USA) **4204**, 3534
St. Anthony's Coding for Ophthalmology Reimbursement (USA) **4007**, 3534
St. Dunstan's Annual Brochure (GBR) **3500**
St. Dunstan's Annual Review *see* St. Dunstan's Annual Brochure **3500**
St. Dunstan's Review (GBR ISSN 0036-2808) **3500**
St. George's Hospital Medical School. Report (GBR) **3695**
St. John Hospital and Medical Center. Medical Bulletin (USA) **3695**
➤ St. John's Journal of Medicine (IND ISSN 0970-4221) **3695**
➤ St. Louis Metropolitan Medicine (USA ISSN 0892-1334) **3696**
St. Marianna University School of Medicine. Bulletin *see* Sei Marianna Ika Daigaku Kiyo **3691**, 3417
St. Patrick Hospital. Annual Report (USA) **3523**
St. Patrick Hospital Messenger (USA) **4361**
St Peter's News (GBR) **4218**
St. Thomas's Hospital Gazette (GBR) **3523**
➤ Stadler Genetics Symposium. Proceedings (USA ISSN 0081-4148) **3314**
Stain Technology *see* Biotechnic and Histochemistry **3334**, 3270, 3286
Stampa Medica (ITA ISSN 0038-9323) **3696**
➤ Standby (NLD ISSN 0922-310X) **3840**
➤ Stanford Nurse (USA) **3941**
The Star (Carville) (USA ISSN 0049-2116) **3807**
• Start-Up (USA ISSN 1090-4417) **3696**, 3363
Stat (Madison) (USA ISSN 0038-9986) **3941**
State-Approved Schools of Nursing - L.P.N. - L.V.N. (USA ISSN 0081-4423) **3941**, 3417
State-Approved Schools of Nursing - R.N. (USA ISSN 0081-4431) **3941**, 3417
State Bar of Wisconsin. Health Law Section. Newsletter *see* Health Law News **3539**, 3509 , 3611
State Capitals Newsletters. Public Assistance & Welfare Trends *see* Public Assistance & Welfare Trends - State Capitals **3543**, 4459, 4486 , 4517
State Capitals Newsletters. Public Health *see* Public Health - State Capitals **3543**, 3521, 4459, 4487
State Employment Relations Board Official Reporter *see* S E R B Official Reporter **3544**, 3880
• State Health Care Regulatory Developments (USA ISSN 1073-8886) **3523**, 3544
• State Health Monitor (USA ISSN 1522-5348) **3534**, 3696
State Health Notes (USA) **4490**, 3544, 3696
State of New York City's Municipal Hospital System (USA ISSN 0895-688X) **3523**
State Plan for Developmental Disabilities (USA ISSN 0743-5916) **4518**, 4450
• State Reproductive Health Monitor (USA ISSN 1046-6703) **3964**, 3546
Statens Seruminstitut, Centrale Afdeling for Sygehushygiejne Nyt *see* C A S Nyt **3503**, 3580
Station Biologique de Besse en Chandesse. Annales (FRA) **3297**
• ➤ Statistical Methods in Medical Research (GBR ISSN 0962-2802) **4530**, 3554, 3696
Statistical Record of Health and Medicine (USA ISSN 1078-6961) **3737**, 4530
• ➤ Statistics in Medicine (GBR ISSN 0277-6715) **3737**, 4530
Statistics Norway. Health Statistics *see* Norway. Statistisk Sentralbyraa. Helsestatistikk **4497**, 4529
Statistik om Legale Aborter *see* Statistik om Praevention og Aborter **3360**
Statistik om Praevention og Aborter (DNK ISSN 0106-7729) **3360**
Statistik om Sundhedsplejerskernes Virksomhed (DNK ISSN 0108-9714) **3737**
Statistische Nachrichten Bildungs- und Sozialeinrichtungen fuer Hoergeschaedigte in der Bundesrepublik Deutschland *see* Wer? Wo? Was? in der Hoergeschaedigtenpaedagogik **3488**
Status (SWE ISSN 0085-6738) **4490**
Status og Visioner - Sundhedsstyrelsen (DNK ISSN 0905-0035) **4490**
Status Report (Washington) *see* Insurance Institute for Highway Safety. Status Report **4477**, 4533
Staying Alive (GBR ISSN 1354-2249) **4490**
Staying Safe on the Job (USA ISSN 1080-0395) **4266**
Staying Well *see* Chiropractic Health Ways **3786**
• ➤ Stem Cells (USA ISSN 1066-5099) **3219**
De Stem van de Ouders (BEL ISSN 0776-5827) **3487**, 4135, 4518
Stent (GBR ISSN 1369-5339) **3783**
• ➤ Stereotactic and Functional Neurosurgery (CHE ISSN 1011-6125) **4204**, 4135
Sterilization in Australia (AUS ISSN 0725-7066) **4490**, 3523, 3544, 3696
• ➤ Steroids (USA ISSN 0039-128X) **3263**
Steuer-Brief fuer Aerzte und Zahnaerzte (DEU ISSN 0943-1896) **3696**, 3369
• Sticking Out Our Necks - The Thyroid Disease News Report (USA) **3869**
Stierenboek (NLD) **3162**
La Stilla (ITA) **4518**, 3905
Stille Boodskapper *see* Silent Messenger **3493**
Stitches (CAN ISSN 1199-1747) **3696**
Stockholms Universitet. Psykologiska Institutionen. Report Series (SWE ISSN 0345-0139) **4450**
Stoffmisbruk *see* Rus & Avhengighet **3405**
Stoma (PRT ISSN 0870-4287) **3840**
Stomach and Intestine *see* I to Cho **3892**
Stomatologia Mediterranea (ITA ISSN 1120-9402) **3840**
Stomatologichen Pregled (BGR ISSN 0204-6415) **3840**
• ➤ Stomatologie (AUT ISSN 0946-3151) **3840**
Stomatologija (BGR ISSN 0491-0982) **3840**
Stomatologiya/Stomatology (RUS ISSN 0039-1735) **3840**
Stomatologiya Rossii/Russian Stomatology (RUS) **3840**
Stomatology *see* Stomatologiya **3840**
Stomatoloski Glasnik Srbije (YUG ISSN 0039-1743) **3840**
• Straalevernrapport/N R P A Report (NOR ISSN 0804-4910) **4490**, 3442
• ➤ Strabismus (NLD ISSN 0927-3972) **4007**, 4135
Strahlenschutz (DEU ISSN 0935-4905) **4266**
StrahlenschutzPraxis (DEU ISSN 0947-434X) **4266**
Strahlentelex *see* Strahlentelex mit Elektrosmog-Report **3454**, 4490
Strahlentelex mit Elektrosmog-Report (DEU) **3454**, 4490
• ➤ Strahlentherapie und Onkologie (DEU ISSN 0179-7158) **4156**
Straight Talk (Pleasantville) (USA ISSN 1062-0095) **3387**, 3405
Strait Journal of Preventive Medicine *see* Haixia Yufang Yixue Zazhi **3609**
Strategic Commentary *see* Start-Up **3696**, 3363
• Strategic Commentary (USA) **3696**, 3363
Strategic Commentary Online *see* Start-Up **3696**, 3363
Strategic Health Care Marketing (USA ISSN 0749-5153) **3367**, 3523
• ➤ Strategic Orthopaedics (USA ISSN 1091-5915) **4026**
Strategic Outsourcing Report (USA ISSN 1521-2467) **4337**
Strategic Partners Report *see* Genetic Technology News **3304**
Strategies for Healthcare Excellence *see* C O R Clinical Excellence **3580**
➤ Strategies (Reston) (USA ISSN 0892-4562) **3430**, 4177
Strategy for Successful J C A H O Homecare Accreditation (Joint Commission on Accreditation of Healthcare Organizations) (USA) **3523**
Straub Foundation. Proceedings (USA ISSN 1080-5222) **3696**
Straub Pacific Health Foundation Proceedings *see* Straub Foundation. Proceedings **3696**
Street Pharmacologist (USA ISSN 0735-6544) **3405**, 4337
Streetwize Comics *see* Streetwize Communications **3387**, 3405, 3544, 4518
Streetwize Communications (AUS) **3387**, 3405, 3544, 4518
Strength and Conditioning *see* Strength and Conditioning Journal **4361**
• ➤ Strength and Conditioning Journal (USA ISSN 1524-1602) **4361**
• Stress (CHE ISSN 1025-3890) **3696**
Stress and Anxiety *see* Stress and Emotion **4450**
➤ Stress and Emotion (USA ISSN 1053-2161) **4450**
• ➤ Stress and Health (GBR ISSN 1532-3005) **4135**
▼ Stress & Trauma (FRA) **4451**
Stress et Trauma *see* Stress & Trauma **4451**
Stress Management for Law Enforcement (USA) **3395**, 4451
Stress Master *see* Health Master **4402**, 4355
Stress Medicine *see* Stress and Health **4135**
• ➤ Stressforskningsrapporter (SWE ISSN 0280-2783) **4451**, 4135
Stritch M.D. *see* Loyola Medicine **3388**, 3644
▼ • Strive (USA) **4566**, 3549
Strive: Action, Sports & Supplements Issue *see* Strive **4566**, 3549
• ➤ Stroke (USA ISSN 0039-2499) **3783**
Stroke Club International Bulletin (USA) **3783**
Stroke Connection Magazine (USA ISSN 1047-014X) **3783**
Stroke: Disease State Management Resource (USA) **3783**
Stroke News (GBR) **4066**
• Structural Equation Modeling (USA ISSN 1070-5511) **4451**, 4523
• ➤ Structure (USA ISSN 0969-2126) **3220**
Structure with Folding & Design *see* Structure **3220**
Strumenti di Riferimento *see* Istituto Superiore di Sanita. Notiziario **4478**
Stud Med (DNK ISSN 0039-2634) **3696**
Student Assistance Journal (USA ISSN 1042-6388) **3405**, 3386
• Student B M J (British Medical Journal) (GBR ISSN 0966-6494) **3696**
Student B M J (South African Edition) (British Medical Journal) (ZAF) **3696**
Student British Medical Journal *see* Student B M J **3696**
The Student (Lincoln) (USA ISSN 0039-2677) **4501**, 3500
Student National Medical Association. Journal *see* Journal for Minority Medical Students **3628**
Student und Praktikant (DEU ISSN 0721-8672) **4337**, 3430
Studi di Psicologia dell'Educazione (ITA ISSN 0393-6163) **3415**, 4451
Studi per l'Ecologia del Quaternario (ITA ISSN 0392-6788) **3174**, 4271
Studi Sassaresi (ITA ISSN 0371-3172) **3696**
Studia Psychologica (BEL) **4451**
• ➤ Studia Psychologica (SVK ISSN 0039-3320) **4451**
Studia Psychologica Clinica Upsaliensia (SWE ISSN 1100-3278) **4135**
Studia Psychologica et Paedagogica (SWE ISSN 0346-5926) **3415**, 4451
Studia Psychologica Upsaliensia (SWE ISSN 0586-8858) **4451**
➤ Studia Psychologiczne (POL ISSN 0081-685X) **4451**
Studia Societatis Scientiarum Torunensis. Sectio H. Medicina (POL ISSN 0860-9594) **3696**
Studia Universitatis "Babes-Bolyai". Biologia (ROM ISSN 1221-8103) **3220**
Studia Universitatis "Babes-Bolyai". Psychologia - Paedagogia (ROM ISSN 1221-8111) **3415**, 4451
Studien und Berichte (DEU ISSN 0076-5627) **3415**, 4451, 4523
➤ Studien zur Kinderpsychoanalyse. Jahrbuch (DEU ISSN 0255-6715) **4451**
Studienstiftung. Jahresbericht (DEU) **3427**, 4518
➤ Studies and Researches in Veterinary Medicine (ROM ISSN 1224-7685) **4553**
➤ Studies in Analytical Chemistry (NLD ISSN 0168-6461) **3377**
➤ Studies in Ancient Medicine (NLD ISSN 0925-1421) **3696**, 3526
Studies in Cognitive Systems (NLD ISSN 0924-0780) **4451**, 4348
Studies in Eating Disorders: An International Series (GBR) **4135**, 4246, 4451
Studies in Education and Psychology (SWE ISSN 0348-291X) **3415**, 4451
Studies in Educational Gerontology (GBR) **3481**
• ➤ Studies in Family Planning (USA ISSN 0039-3665) **4369**, 4523
➤ Studies in Fertility and Sterility (NLD) **3696**, 3220, 3349
Studies in Health and Human Values (USA) **3363**
➤ Studies in Health Technology and Informatics (NLD ISSN 0926-9630) **3696**, 3812
Studies in History of Medicine *see* Studies in History of Medicine and Science **3696**
➤ Studies in History of Medicine and Science (IND ISSN 0970-5562) **3696**
Studies in Human Biology (NLD ISSN 0926-9738) **3349**
➤ Studies in Infectious Diseases Research (USA) **3807**
➤ Studies in Linguistics and Philosophy (NLD ISSN 0924-4662) **4451**, 3552, 4348
Studies in Neuroscience (GBR ISSN 1351-8194) **4135**
Studies in Physical Culture and Tourism (POL ISSN 0867-1079) **4362**, 4534
➤ Studies in Physiology (GBR ISSN 0969-8116) **3349**
➤ Studies in Speech Pathology and Clinical Linguistics (NLD ISSN 0927-1813) **4135**, 3427, 3552
➤ Studies in the Psychology of Religion (USA) **4501**, 4451
➤ Studies in Visual Information Processing (NLD ISSN 0926-907X) **4135**, 3390, 4007
Studies of Nonlinear Phenomena in Life Science (SGP) **3220**
Studies on Current Health Problems (GBR ISSN 0473-8837) **3696**, 4490
Studies on Emergencies and Disaster Relief (SWE ISSN 1400-3120) **3387**, 4490

Title

T B V *see* Tijdschrift voor Bedrijfs- en Verzekeringsgeneeskunde **3700**, 3534, 4518
T B Weekly *see* Tuberculosis & Airborne Disease Weekly **3808**, 4491
T C (Terapia del Comportamento) (ITA) **3698**
T C A Report *see* In Vitro Report **3343**, 3619
T C H I Update (Tennessee Council for the Hearing Impaired) (USA) **3493**, 3427, 4518
T C J F S A *see* The Cancer Journal from Scientific American (English Edition) **3972**
T.C.P. *see* The Catholic Pharmacist **4282**, 4502
T D I National Directory of T T Y Numbers (Year) (Telecommunications for the Deaf, Inc.) (USA) **3493**, 3388
➤ The T E A C H Educator (Treatment Education Activists Combating HIV) (USA) **3807**
● T E S S (The Educational Software Selector) (USA) **3416**, 3391
● T G A News (Online Edition) (AUS ISSN 1325-8559) **4337**
● T G A News (Print Edition) (Therapeutic Goods Administration) (AUS) **4337**
T I *see* Aquaristik - Fachmagazin **3459**, 3464
T i B S *see* Trends in Biochemical Sciences **3263**
T I E S *see* Theoretical Issues in Ergonomics Science **3433**, 3369, 3434
T I N S Neurotoxins Supplement *see* Neurotoxins **4119**, 4271
T L C: The Waiting Room Magazine (ZAF) **3523**
T M I *see* Informatie & Zorg **3811**, 3620
T M J Update: A Current Review of Temporomandibular Joint Developments (USA ISSN 0885-9191) **3698**
T N T *see* Tandlaegernes Nye Tidsskrift **3841**, 3386
T N T *see* Telephone Nursing Telezine **3942**
T O I *see* Tecnica Ortopedica Internacional **4027**
T P A Speedletter (Texas Pharmacy Association) (USA ISSN 1096-9268) **4337**
T R A C Newsletter (Transvaal Rural Action Committee) (ZAF ISSN 1023-5310) **4368**, 3363, 3442, 4566
● T R L News (Transport Research Laboratory) (GBR) **4533**, 3434, 3454
T R T and R P A I Journal *see* Radiance Technique Journal **3169**, 4227
T S C A - T S C A T S *see* Toxic Substances Control Act - Test Submission Database **3454**
T S G *see* Tijdschrift voor Sociale Gezondheidszorg **3700**, 4491
T S P *see* The Sport Psychologist **4450**, 4526
T S Today *see* Reach Out **3683**
T T I Q *see* Tsetse and Trypanosomiasis Information Quarterly **3738**, 3152, 3703
T Ue - Technische Ueberwachung. Sicherheit Zuverlaessigheit und Umweltschutz in Wirtschaft und Verkehr *see* Technische Ueberwachung **4266**
T und E Dermatologie *see* Aerztliche Praxis. Dermatologie **3844**, 3175
T und E Gynaekologie *see* Aerztliche Praxis. Gynaekologie **3944**
T und E Neurologie Psychiatrie *see* Aerztliche Praxis. Neurologie Psychiatrie **4070**
T und E Paediatrie *see* Aerztliche Praxis. Paediatrie **4039**
T V B (Tijdschrift voor Verzorging en Beheer) (NLD ISSN 0167-0018) **3481**, 3698
T V - T S Tapestry *see* Transgender Tapestry **4453**, 3528
T v Z: Tijdschrift voor Verpleegkundigen (NLD ISSN 1380-3425) **3942**
T W Gynaekologie *see* Aerztliche Praxis. Gynaekologie **3944**
T W Neurologie - Psychiatrie *see* Aerztliche Praxis. Neurologie Psychiatrie **4070**
T W Paediatrie *see* Aerztliche Praxis. Paediatrie **4039**
▼ T Z Gesundheitsm@gazin (TagesZeitung) (DEU) **4362**
Ta'asiyot (ISR ISSN 0792-1322) **3553**
Tabac et Sante (FRA) **4362**, 3406
Tabachnaya Zavisimost i Kurenie Tabaka (RUS) **3737**, 3152
Tabibak Al-Khass (EGY) **3698**
Tabibok/Your Doctor (LBN) **3698**
Taegliche Praxis (DEU ISSN 0494-464X) **3698**
Taehan Kanho *see* Korean Nurse **3927**
Taehan Misaengmul Hakhoe Chi/Korean Society for Microbiology. Journal (KOR ISSN 0253-3162) **3331**
Taehan Sin'gyong Chongsin Uihak Hoeji *see* Korean Neuropsychiatric Association. Journal **4107**
TagesZeitung Gesundheitsm@gazin *see* T Z Gesundheitsm@gazin **4362**
Tai Chi & Alternative Health (GBR ISSN 1355-8307) **4270**, 3170, 4362
Taisha - Metabolism and Diseases *see* Molecular Medicine **3866**
Taiwan Medical & Health Equipment Buyers' Guide *see* Medical & Health Equipment Buyers' Guide **3371**, 3648
Taiwanese Journal of Obstetrics and Gynecology (TWN ISSN 1028-4559) **3964**
Takeda Research Laboratories. Journal (JPN ISSN 0371-5167) **3220**, 3374, 4337
Taking Sides: Clashing Views on Controversial Bioethical Issues (USA) **3698**, 4348
Taking Sides: Clashing Views on Controversial Issues in Drugs and Society (USA) **3406**
Taking Sides: Clashing Views on Controversial Issues in Health and Society (USA) **4490**
Taking Sides: Clashing Views on Controversial Issues in Human Sexuality (USA) **4452**
Taking Sides: Clashing Views on Controversial Moral Issues (USA) **4452**
Taking Sides: Clashing Views on Controversial Psychological Issues (USA) **4452**
Takko Town Hospital. Annual Report *see* Akahige **3501**
Tal og Data, Medicin og Sundhedsvaesen/Facts, Medicine and Health Care, Denmark (DNK ISSN 0107-1181) **4337**, 4362
Tal og Data om Medicin *see* Tal og Data, Medicin og Sundhedsvaesen **4337**, 4362
➤ TalentEd (AUS ISSN 0815-8150) **3427**
● Talking Book Topics (Large Print Edition) (USA ISSN 0039-9183) **3500**, 3548
Talking Books in the Public Library Systems of Metropolitan Toronto (CAN ISSN 0380-2973) **3549**, 3500
Talking Straight With Your Teenager *see* Straight Talk (Pleasantville) **3387**, 3405
Tallyboard *see* Ressource en Sante et en Securite **4263**, 4225
Tallyboard *see* Health & Safety Resource **3463**, 4255
Tan Sheet - Nonprescription Pharmaceuticals and Nutritionals *see* Nonprescription Pharmaceuticals and Nutritionals: The Tan Sheet **4319**
Tandartsen Wereld *see* Monde Dentaire **3832**
Tandartsen Wereld *see* Monde Dentaire **3832**
Tandartsenkrant (BEL) **3841**
Tandartspraktijk (NLD ISSN 0167-1685) **3841**
Tandhygienist Tidningen (SWE ISSN 1102-6146) **3841**
Tandlaegebladet/Danish Dental Journal (DNK ISSN 0039-9353) **3841**
Tandlaegernes Nye Tidsskrift (DNK ISSN 0901-9898) **3841**, 3386
Tandlaekartidningen (SWE ISSN 0039-6982) **3841**
Tandplejeren (DNK ISSN 0900-257X) **3841**, 3535
Tandskoetersketidningen (SWE ISSN 0346-2617) **3841**
Tandtechnisch Magazine (NLD ISSN 0929-2934) **3841**
Tandteknikern (SWE ISSN 0039-9361) **3841**
Tanpakushitsu Kakusan Koso/Protein, Nucleic Acid, Enzyme (JPN ISSN 0039-9450) **3263**
Tanzania Journal of Paediatrics (TZA ISSN 0856-311X) **4057**
Tape Medical Bulletin (GBR) **3698**, 3500
Tapping Technology (USA) **3495**, 3500, 4518
Tar Heel Nurse (USA ISSN 0039-9620) **3942**
The Tardieu Series (NLD ISSN 0924-610X) **3698**
Target M D (Muscular Dystrophy) (GBR) **3495**
Tarot Network News (USA) **4227**, 3459, 4348, 4452
Task Force Quarterly (USA) **3698**
➤ Tasmanian Naturalist (AUS ISSN 0819-6826) **3220**, 3442
Tauchen (DEU ISSN 0170-4001) **4526**, 3220, 4349
Tavricheskii Zhurnal Psikhyatrii/Acta Psychiatrica, Psychoterapeutica et Etologica Tavrica (UKR) **4136**
● Tax, Estate & Financial Planning for the Elderly (USA) **3481**, 3362, 4499
● Teacher Education and Special Education (USA ISSN 0888-4064) **3427**, 3430
● ➤ Teaching and Learning in Medicine (USA ISSN 1040-1334) **3698**, 3418
Teaching & Training (GBR ISSN 0040-0572) **3427**
● ➤ Teaching of Psychology (USA ISSN 0098-6283) **4452**, 3430
Team of Advocates for Special Kids Newsletter (USA) **3487**, 3387, 3427
Team Rehab Report *see* Rehab Report **3486**, 4066
Teamwork (DEU) **3841**
Teamwork (New York) (USA) **3869**
Teashi no Fujiyuuna Kodomotachi/Crippled Children (JPN ISSN 0040-0734) **3698**
Tech Sample (USA) **3698**
Techletter (USA ISSN 0883-8828) **4490**
Technical Instructions for the Safe Transport of Dangerous Goods by Air (CAN) **4532**, 3454
● Technical Literature Abstracts: Health & Environment (USA ISSN 1087-1411) **3443**, 3152, 3442
Technical Report of Medical Ultrasound Engineering *see* Kiso Gijutsu Kenkyu Bukai Shiryo **4149**
Techniek en Veiligheid *see* Voorkomen **4267**
Techniek in de Gezondheidszorg *see* Technologie in de Gezondheidszorg **3698**
Technique et Biologie (FRA ISSN 0766-5725) **3880**, 3220
Techniques Chirgicales. Tete et Cou *see* Encyclopedie Medico-Chirurgicale. Techniques Chirurgicales. Tete et Cou **4187**, 4032
Techniques Chirurgicales - Appareil Digestif *see* Encyclopedie Medico-Chirurgicale. Techniques Chirurgicales. Appareil Digestif **4187**, 3889
Techniques Chirurgicales - Chirurgie Vasculaire *see* Encyclopedie Medico-Chirurgicale. Techniques Chirurgicales. Chirurgie Vasculaire **4187**, 3771
Techniques Chirurgicales. Thorax *see* Encyclopedie Medico-Chirurgicale. Techniques Chirurgicales. Thorax **4187**, 4032
● ➤ Techniques in Coloproctology Online (ITA ISSN 1128-045X) **3896**
● Techniques in Colorproctology (ITA ISSN 1123-6337) **3896**
Techniques in Diagnostic Pathology (GBR ISSN 1066-5072) **3698**, 3220
▼ ● Techniques in Foot & Ankle Surgery (USA ISSN 1536-0644) **4205**, 4027
▼ ➤ Techniques in Gastrointestinal Endoscopy (USA ISSN 1096-2883) **3896**
● Techniques in Hand & Upper Extremity Surgery (USA ISSN 1089-3393) **4206**
▼ ● Techniques in Knee Surgery (USA ISSN 1536-0636) **4206**, 4027
● Techniques in Neurosurgery (USA ISSN 1077-2855) **4206**, 4136
● ➤ Techniques in Orthopaedics (USA ISSN 0885-9698) **4027**
➤ Techniques in Regional Anesthesia & Pain Management (USA ISSN 1084-208X) **3760**
▼ ● Techniques in Shoulder and Elbow Surgery (USA ISSN 1523-9896) **4206**
➤ Techniques in the Behavioral and Neural Sciences (NLD ISSN 0921-0709) **4136**
➤ Techniques in Urology (USA ISSN 1079-3259) **4218**
Techniques in Vascular and Interventional Radiology (USA ISSN 1089-2516) **4156**
➤ Techniques of Chemistry (USA ISSN 0082-2531) **3374**, 3880
Techniques Orthopediques (FRA ISSN 0397-3999) **4027**
Technische Ueberwachung (DEU) **4266**
➤ Technologie & Sante (FRA ISSN 1145-5217) **4531**, 3523
Technologie in de Gezondheidszorg (NLD ISSN 1567-861X) **3698**
● ➤ Technology and Disability (NLD ISSN 1055-4181) **3487**, 4066
● ➤ Technology and Health Care (NLD ISSN 0928-7329) **3698**, 3238
➤ Technology for Anesthesia (USA ISSN 8756-8578) **3760**
➤ Technology for Cardiology (USA ISSN 8756-8586) **3783**
➤ Technology for Respiratory Therapy (USA ISSN 8756-8616) **4165**
Technology Special Interest Section Newsletter *see* Technology Special Interest Section Quarterly **4531**, 4266
Technology Special Interest Section Quarterly (USA) **4531**, 4266
● Technomark Register. Contract Packagers & Manufacturers - Europe (GBR) **3371**, 4337
Technomark Register. Contract Research Organisations - North America (GBR) **3371**, 4337
● Technomark Register. European Contract Research Organisations. Clinical Research (GBR) **3371**, 4337
● Technomark Register. European Contract Research Organisations. Toxicology & Analysis (GBR) **3371**, 4337
Technoscope *see* Biofutur **3269**
● ➤ Tecnica Ortopedica Internacional/International Orthopaedic Technique (ESP ISSN 0214-4352) **4027**
Tecnica Ospedaliera (ITA ISSN 0392-4831) **3523**
Tecnica Sanitaria e Medicina di Comunita (ITA ISSN 0392-8144) **4490**
Tecnicas de Laboratorio (ESP ISSN 0371-5728) **3880**
Tecnicas Quirurgicas en Ortopedia y Traumatologia (ESP ISSN 1132-1954) **4027**
Tecniche Chirurgicale. Torace *see* Encyclopedie Medico-Chirurgicale. Tecniche Chirurgiche. Torace **4188**, 4032
Tecniche Chirurgiche Addominale *see* Encyclopedie Medico-Chirurgicale. Tecniche Chirurgiche. Chirurgia Addominale **4188**, 3889
Tecniche Chirurgiche. Chirurgia O R L e Cervico-Facciale *see* Encyclopedie Medico-Chirurgicale. Tecniche Chirurgiche. Chirurgia O R L e Cervico-facciale **4188**, 4032
Tecniche Chirurgiche. Chirurgia Vascolare *see* Encyclopedie Medico-Chirurgicale. Tecniche Chirurgiche. Chirurgia Vascolare **4188**, 3771
Teen Fag (USA) **3528**
Tegen de Tuberculose (NLD ISSN 0040-2125) **4165**
Tegenbericht *see* Proefdiervrij **3172**, 3880, 4348
Tehy (FIN ISSN 0358-4038) **3942**
Teion Igaku/Low Temperature Medicine (JPN ISSN 0285-4473) **3698**
Tele-Forum Kinderarzt (DEU) **4057**
Telecommunications for the Deaf, Inc. National Directory of T T Y Numbers (Year) *see* T D I National Directory of T T Y Numbers (Year) **3493**, 3388
Telemedicine (USA) **3523**
● Telemedicine & Telehealth Network (USA ISSN 1091-7853) **3699**, 3388
Telemedicine Business Newsletter (USA) **3699**, 3388
Telemedicine Journal *see* Telemedicine Journal and e-Health **3812**
● ➤ Telemedicine Journal and e-Health (USA ISSN 1530-5627) **3812**
● Telemedicine Today (USA ISSN 1078-0351) **3699**, 3388
● Telephone Nursing Telezine (USA) **3942**
Tell-a-Type (CAN) **4452**
Tema Farmacia (ITA) **4337**
Temas de Poblacion (PRY) **4370**, 4490
Temas Medicos *see* Temas de Poblacion **4370**, 4490
Tempo Medicina (PRT) **3699**
Tempo Medico (ITA ISSN 0492-6749) **3699**
Tennessee Council for the Hearing Impaired Update *see* T C H I Update **3493**, 3427, 4518
Tennessee Dental Association. Journal (USA ISSN 0040-3385) **3841**
Tennessee Journal of Health, Physical Education, Recreation and Dance (USA ISSN 0890-1597) **4362**
Tennessee Medical Association. Journal *see* Tennessee Medicine **3699**
Tennessee Medicine (USA ISSN 1088-6222) **3699**
Tennessee Medico-Legal Reporter (USA) **3544**, 3699
➤ Tennessee Nurse (USA ISSN 1055-3134) **3942**
Tennessee Pharmacist (USA ISSN 1047-0166) **4337**
Tennessee State Dental Association. Journal *see* Tennessee Dental Association. Journal **3841**
TennisPro Magazine (USA) **4526**, 4177
Tenth Times (USA) **3841**
● ➤ Terapevticheskii Arkhiv/Therapeutic Archives (RUS ISSN 0040-3660) **3699**
Terapia (POL ISSN 1230-3917) **3699**
Terapia del Comportamento *see* T C **3698**
Terapia Familiare (ITA ISSN 0391-2868) **3546**, 4452
Terapie Naturali e Erbe (ITA) **3170**
● ➤ Teratogenesis, Carcinogenesis, and Mutagenesis (USA ISSN 0270-3211) **3699**
● ➤ Teratology (USA ISSN 0040-3709) **3220**, 3454, 3699
Terme Europa (ITA) **4362**
Terminal Care Index *see* Palliative Care Index **3734**, 4431
TerraTech (DEU ISSN 0942-5675) **3442**
Terveys *see* Kotilaakari **4358**
Terviseleht (EST) **3699**
Test Gezondheid *see* Test Sante **4490**, 3393
Test Sante (BEL ISSN 1370-0650) **4490**, 3393

Title

Title

Title

Title

➤ Universita Karlova. Lekarska Fakulta. Lekarske Zpravy (CZE ISSN 0457-4206) **3705**
Universita Karlova. Lekarska Fakulta. Sbornik Vedeckych Praci *see* Acta Medica **3557**
Universita Karlova. Lekarska Fakulta. Sbornik Vedeckych Praci. Supplementum *see* Acta Medica. Supplementum **3558**
Universitaet Innsbruck. Alpin-Biologische Studien (AUT ISSN 0587-484X) **3222**
Universitaet Innsbruck. Medizinische Fakultaet. Arbeiten (AUT ISSN 0579-7772) **3705**
Universitaire Ziekenhuis Magazine *see* U Z Magazine **3523**, 4492
Universitas Comeniana. Acta Facultatis Pharmaceuticae (SVK ISSN 0041-9087) **4339**
Universitas Medica (COL ISSN 0041-9095) **3705**
Universitatea Agronomica Ion Ionescu de la Brad. Lucrari Stiintifice. Seria Zootechnie - Medicina Veterinaria (ROM) **3162**, 4554
Universitatea "Al. I. Cuza" din Iasi. Analele Stiintifice. Sectiunea 2a: Biologie (ROM ISSN 0041-9133) **3222**
Universitatea de Stiinte Agricole Cluj-Napoca. Buletinul. Seria Zootehnie si Medicina Veterinara (ROM ISSN 1221-3594) **3162**, 4554
Universitatea de Stiinte Agronomice. Lucrari Stiintifice. Seria C, Medicina Veterinara *see* Universitatea de Stiinte Agronomice si Medicina Veterinara. Lucrari Stiintifice. Seria C, Medicina Veterinara **4554**
Universitatea de Stiinte Agronomice. Lucrari Stiintifice. Seria F, Biotehnologii Vegetale, Biotehnologii Industriale, Biotehnologii Animale *see* Universitatea de Stiinte Agronomice si Medicina Veterinara. Lucrari Stiintifice. Seria F, Biotehnologii **3277**
Universitatea de Stiinte Agronomice si Medicina Veterinara. Lucrari Stiintifice. Seria C, Medicina Veterinara (ROM) **4554**
Universitatea de Stiinte Agronomice si Medicina Veterinara. Lucrari Stiintifice. Seria F, Biotehnologii (ROM ISSN 1224-7774) **3277**
Universitatea din Brasov. Buletinul. Seria C. Matematica, Fizica, Chimie *see* Transylvania University of Brasov. Bulletin. Series B **3554**, 3221, 4365
Universitatea din Craiova. Anale. Seria: Biologie, Agronomie, Horticultura (ROM ISSN 0254-7236) **3222**, 3156
Universitatea Transilvania din Brasov. Buletinul. Seria C. Matematica, Fizica, Chimie *see* Transylvania University of Brasov. Bulletin. Series B **3554**, 3221, 4365
Universite d'Abidjan. Annales. Serie B. Medecine (CIV ISSN 0253-441X) **3705**
Universite de Montreal. Faculte de Medecine Veterinaire. Annuaire (CAN ISSN 0383-8455) **4555**
Universite du Benin. Annales. Serie Science (TGO ISSN 1016-9210) **3222**
Universities Federation for Animal Welfare Handbook on the Care and Management of Laboratory Animals *see* U F A W Handbook on the Care and Management of Laboratory Animals **3172**
Universities Safety Association. Digest (GBR ISSN 1361-4266) **4492**, 3418
Universities Safety Association. Safety Digest *see* Universities Safety Association. Digest **4492**, 3418
• University College London. Eastman Academy. Newsletter (GBR) **3842**, 3388
University Health Sciences Librarians Newsletter *see* U H S L Newsletter **3549**, 3703
University - Industry Grants and Awards Guide *see* Medical Research Council of Canada. Grants and Awards Guide **3653**
➤ University of Alaska. Biological Papers (USA ISSN 0568-8604) **3222**
University of Alaska. Biological Papers. Special Reports (USA ISSN 0161-3243) **3222**
• University of Alexandria. Faculty of Medicine. Bulletin (EGY ISSN 1110-0834) **3705**
University of Ankara. Faculty of Medicine. Journal *see* Ankara Universitesi. Tip Fakultesi. Mecmuasi **3566**
University of Ankara. Faculty of Veterinary Medicine. Journal *see* Ankara Universitesi Veteriner Fakultesi Dergisi **4537**
University of Baghdad. Faculty of Medicine. Journal (IRQ ISSN 0041-9419) **3705**
University of Cairo. Faculty of Medicine. Gazette *see* University of Cairo. Faculty of Medicine. Medical Journal **3705**
➤ University of Cairo. Faculty of Medicine. Medical Journal (EGY ISSN 0045-3803) **3705**
University of Calcutta. University College of Medicine. Bulletin (IND ISSN 0008-0705) **3705**
University of California at San Francisco, Public Affairs Magazine *see* U C S F Magazine **3703**, 4491, 4518
• University of California, Berkeley. Wellness Letter (USA ISSN 0748-9234) **4362**, 4246
University of California. Lawrence Berkeley Laboratory. Biology and Medicine Division. Annual Report (USA ISSN 0272-9075) **3223**, 3705
University of Cape Town. Department of Obstetrics and Gynaecology. Annual Report (ZAF ISSN 0254-184X) **3965**
University of Chicago. Pritzker School of Medicine. Alumni Association. Bulletin *see* Medicine on the Midway **3388**, 3656
University of Chicago. Pritzker School of Medicine. Alumni Association. Magazine *see* Medicine on the Midway **3388**, 3656
University of Dar es Salaam. Faculty of Agriculture, Forestry and Veterinary Science. Annual Record of Research (TZA) **3156**, 3464, 4555
University of Delaware. Disaster Research Center. Miscellaneous Reports (USA) **3387**
➤ University of Delaware. Disaster Research Center. Report Series (USA) **3387**
University of Dundee. Tayside Centre for General Practice. Asthma Research Unit. Progress Report (GBR) **3752**
University of Ferdowsi. Faculty of Medicine. Letters/Daneshgah-e Ferdowsi. Daneshkade-Ye Pazeshki. Nameh (IRN) **3705**
University of Illinois at Chicago. College of Dentistry. Alumni Report (USA ISSN 1088-9108) **3388**, 3842
University of Istanbul. Faculty of Veterinary Medicine. Journal *see* Istanbul Universitesi. Veteriner Fakultesi Dergisi **4545**
University of Kansas. Museum of Natural History. Public Education Series (USA ISSN 0272-2658) **3223**, 4507
➤ University of Kansas. Museum of Natural History. Special Publications (USA ISSN 0193-7766) **3223**, 4507
University of Khartoum. Hydrobiological Research Unit. Annual Report (SDN ISSN 0379-9611) **3223**
University of Liberia. A.M. Dogliotti College of Medicine. Annual Report of the Dean (LBR) **3705**
University of Ljubljana. Veterinary Faculty. Research Reports *see* Slovenian Veterinary Research **4552**
University of Michigan. School of Dentistry. Alumni Bulletin (USA ISSN 0076-843X) **3842**
University of Missouri at Columbia. Veterinary Medical Diagnostic Laboratory. Annual Report (USA ISSN 0076-9711) **4555**
University of Nebraska Medical Center Discover *see* U N M C Discover **3703**, 4338
University of New South Wales. Faculty Handbooks: Medicine *see* University of New South Wales. Handbook: Medicine **3705**
University of New South Wales. Handbook: Medicine (AUS ISSN 1323-7926) **3705**
University of Occupational and Environmental Health. Journal (JPN ISSN 0387-821X) **4267**, 3705, 4492
University of Ondokuz Mayis Journal of Medicine *see* Ondokuz Mayis Universitesi Tip Dergisi **3669**
University of Osaka Prefecture. Bulletin. Series B: Agriculture and Life Sciences *see* University of Osaka Prefecture. College of Agriculture. Scientific Report **3156**, 3223
University of Osaka Prefecture. College of Agriculture. Scientific Report (JPN ISSN 1344-848X) **3156**, 3223
University of Osaka Prefecture. Series B Agriculture and Life Sciences Bulletin *see* University of Osaka Prefecture. College of Agriculture. Scientific Report **3156**, 3223
➤ University of Otago Medical School. Proceedings (NZL ISSN 0301-6331) **3705**
University of Santo Tomas. Graduate School. Journal of Graduate Research (PHL ISSN 0047-5742) **4510**, 3223, 3529
University of Santo Tomas Journal of Graduate Research *see* University of Santo Tomas. Graduate School. Journal of Graduate Research **4510**, 3223, 3529
University of Sheffield. School of Nursing and Midwifery. Research Report (GBR) **3942**
➤ University of South Florida. International Biomedical Symposia Series (USA) **3223**, 3705
University of Technology, Sydney. Faculty of Nursing Handbook *see* University of Technology, Sydney. Faculty of Nursing, Midwifery and Health Handbook **3942**, 3418
University of Technology, Sydney. Faculty of Nursing, Midwifery and Health Handbook (AUS ISSN 1442-617X) **3942**, 3418
University of Teheran. Faculty of Health. Institute of Research. List of Publications Received in the Library/Daneshgah-e Tehran. Daneshkade-Ye Bedasht va Anstitu Tahqiqat-e Behdashti. Akhbar-e Ketabkhaneh va Surat-e Nashriyat-e Resideh (IRN) **3738**
University of Teheran. Faculty of Medicine. Library Bulletin/Daneshgah-e Tehran. Daneshkade-Ye Pezeshki. Nashriye-Ye Ketabkhaneh (IRN) **3549**, 3705
University of Teheran. School of Pharmacy. Journal *see* Daru **4286**
University of Tehran. Faculty of Veterinary Medicine. Journal *see* Majallah-i Danishkadah-i Dampizishki **4548**
➤ The University of Texas Lifetime Health Letter (USA ISSN 0739-4217) **4362**, 4246
• University of Texas. M.D. Anderson Cancer Center. Research Report (USA) **3992**, 4157
University of the Sciences in Philadelphia Bulletin (USA) **4339**
University of Tokyo. Institute of Applied Microbiology. Reports (JPN ISSN 0082-481X) **3236**, 3152, 3332
➤ University of Toronto Medical Journal (CAN ISSN 0833-2207) **3705**
University of Turku. Psychological Research Reports (FIN ISSN 0359-0216) **4454**
University of Waikato. Antarctic Research Unit. Report (NZL ISSN 0110-2192) **3408**, 3223, 3283, 3332
University of Waterloo Biology Series (CAN ISSN 0317-3348) **3223**
➤ University of Western Ontario Medical Journal (CAN ISSN 0042-0336) **3705**
University of Wisconsin-Milwaukee. Field Station Bulletin (USA) **3223**, 3407
Univerza v Ljubljani. Veterinarska Fakulteta. Zbornik *see* Slovenian Veterinary Research **4552**
Univerzita Komenskeho. Filozoficka Fakulta. Zbornik: Psychologica (SVK ISSN 0083-419X) **4454**
Univerzita Komenskeho. Pedagogicka Fakulta v Trnave. Prirodne Vedy: Biologia-Genetika (SVK) **3315**
Uniwersytet im. Adama Mickiewicza. Biologia (POL ISSN 0554-811X) **3223**
Uniwersytet im. Adama Mickiewicza. Psychologia-Pedagogika (POL ISSN 0083-4254) **3415**, 4454
Uniwersytet Lodzki. Zeszyty Naukowe. Seria 2: Nauki Matematyczno-Przyrodnicze *see* Acta Universitatis Lodziensis: Folia Biochimica et Biophysica **3239**, 3264
Uniwersytet Mikolaja Kopernika, Torun. Nauki Matematyczno-Przyrodnicze. Biologia *see* Acta Universitatis Nicolai Copernici. Biologia **3179**
Uniwersytet Slaski w Katowicach. Prace Naukowe. Acta Biologica Silesiana (POL ISSN 0860-2441) **3223**
➤ Uniwersytet Slaski w Katowicach. Prace Naukowe. Psychologia. Badania i Aplikacje (POL ISSN 1428-8664) **4454**
Uniwersytet Slaski w Katowicach. Prace Naukowe. Psychologiczne Problemy Funkncjonowania Czlowieka w Sytuacji Pracy *see* Uniwersytet Slaski w Katowicach. Prace Naukowe. Psychologia. Badania i Aplikacje **4454**
Unlinked Anonymous HIV Seroprevalence Monitoring Programme in England and Wales *see* Unlinked Anonymous Prevalence Monitoring Programme in the United Kingdom **3808**
Unlinked Anonymous Prevalence Monitoring Programme in the United Kingdom (GBR) **3808**
Unlisted Drugs Index - Guide (USA ISSN 8755-7142) **4339**
Unscheduled Events (USA ISSN 0042-0468) **4524**, 4492
Unser Schaffen (AUT ISSN 0042-0492) **3500**
Unter Uns (DEU) **3500**, 4569
Unternehmer (AUT ISSN 0042-0581) **4492**
Unterricht Biologie (DEU ISSN 0341-5260) **3223**, 3430
Uomini e Idee (ITA ISSN 0042-0646) **3553**, 3175, 4454
Update (PRT ISSN 0871-620X) **3705**
Update (Birmingham) (USA) **4166**
• Update (Owings Mills) (USA) **4008**, 3500
Update Postgraduate Centre Series (GBR) **3705**
➤ Update (South African Edition) (ZAF ISSN 0258-929X) **3705**
Update (Sutton) (GBR ISSN 0301-5718) **3706**
The Upper Room (USA ISSN 0042-0735) **4502**, 3500
Uppsala Dissertations from the Faculty of Medicine (SWE ISSN 0282-8928) **3706**, 3738
• ➤ Upsala Journal of Medical Sciences (NOR ISSN 0300-9734) **3706**
Upsala Journal of Medical Sciences. Supplement (NOR ISSN 0300-9726) **3706**
Urban Health and Development Bulletin (ZAF) **4492**, 3706
Urbanisation and Health Newsletter *see* Urban Health and Development Bulletin **4492**, 3706
Uremia Investigation *see* Renal Failure **4217**
Urgenze *see* Encyclopedie Medico-Chirurgicale. Urgenze **4014**
➤ Uro-Gram (USA ISSN 1074-8687) **4218**
Uro News (DEU ISSN 1432-9026) **4219**
• Urodinamica (ITA ISSN 1120-5989) **4219**
➤ Urogynaecologia International Journal (ITA ISSN 1121-3086) **3965**, 4219
Urologe. Ausgabe A *see* Der Urologe. Section A **4219**
Urologe. Ausgabe B *see* Der Urologe. Section B **4219**
• ➤ Der Urologe. Section A (DEU ISSN 0340-2592) **4219**
• ➤ Der Urologe. Section B (DEU ISSN 0042-1111) **4219**
Urologia/Urology (ITA ISSN 0391-5603) **4219**
• ➤ Urologia Contemporanea (BRA ISSN 1413-0351) **4219**
• ➤ Urologia Integrada y de Investigacion (ESP ISSN 1136-7172) **4219**
• ➤ Urologia Internationalis (CHE ISSN 0042-1138) **4219**
Urologiai es Nephrologiai Szemle *see* Magyar Urologia **4215**
• ➤ Urologic Clinics of North America (USA ISSN 0094-0143) **4219**
• ➤ Urologic Nursing (USA ISSN 1053-816X) **4219**, 3942
• ➤ Urologic Oncology (USA ISSN 1078-1439) **3992**, 4219
Urologic Radiology *see* Abdominal Imaging **3885**, 4139
• ➤ Urological Research (DEU ISSN 0300-5623) **4219**
Urologiya/Urology (RUS) **4219**
Urologiya i Nefrologiya *see* Urologiya **4219**
Urology *see* Urologia **4219**
Urology *see* Urologiya **4219**
• ➤ Urology (USA ISSN 0090-4295) **4220**
Urology Digest (USA ISSN 0197-7709) **4220**
• ➤ Urology News (GBR ISSN 1368-8960) **4220**
• Urology Times (USA ISSN 0093-9722) **4220**
Uroloski Arhiv *see* Archivum Urologicum **4210**
UroOncology (CHE ISSN 1561-0950) **3992**, 4220
Usher Around the World (USA) **3500**, 3493
Uspehi na Moleculiarnata Biologia/Advances in Molecular Biology (BGR ISSN 0205-0625) **3223**
Uspekhi Sovremennoi Biologii (RUS ISSN 0042-1324) **3223**
Utah Nurse (USA) **3942**
Utano - Zimbabwe (ZWE ISSN 1021-5549) **3738**, 3177
➤ Uttar Pradesh Journal of Zoology (IND ISSN 0256-971X) **3356**
Uusi Optikko *see* Optometria **4005**
Uzbekskii Biologicheskii Zhurnal (UZB ISSN 0042-1685) **3223**
V A H P E R D Journal (Virginia Association for Health, Physical Education and Dance) (USA ISSN 0739-4586) **4362**, 4526
V A Medical Center Directory *see* Directory of Federal Health Care Facilities **3505**, 3594
V A Practitioner *see* Federal Practitioner **3602**
➤ V A T I S Update. Biotechnology (Value Added Technology Information Service) (IND ISSN 0971-5622) **3238**
V.C.O.T. *see* Veterinary and Comparative Orthopaedics and Traumatology **4556**, 4028
V C S Resource List (Vision Community Services) (USA) **3500**

Title

Title

Virginia Institute of Marine Science, Gloucester Point. Special Scientific Report (USA ISSN 0083-6443) **3224**
Virginia Mental Health, Mental Retardation, Substance Abuse and Related Law Annotated (USA) **4137**, 3544
Virginia Nurse *see* Virginia Nurses Today **3943**
Virginia Nurses Today (USA ISSN 1084-4740) **3943**
Virginia Pharmacist (USA ISSN 0042-6717) **4339**
Virginia's Health (USA ISSN 0199-1345) **4492**
Virksomheden ved Sygehuse (DNK ISSN 0903-8086) **3525**
Virologica Sinica *see* Zhongguo Bingduxue **3333**
• Virologie (FRA ISSN 1267-8694) **3332**
• ➤ Virology (USA ISSN 0042-6822) **3332**, 3808
• Virology and AIDS Abstracts (USA ISSN 0896-5919) **3236**, 3152, 3332
Virology Monographs/Virusforschung in Einzeldarstellungen (USA ISSN 0083-6591) **3332**, 3808
Virtual Journal of Clinical Orthodontics (Print) *see* Virtual Journal of Orthodontics (Online) **3842**
• ➤ Virtual Journal of Orthodontics (Online) (ITA ISSN 1128-6547) **3842**
Virus/Uirusu (JPN ISSN 0042-6857) **3332**, 3808
• ➤ Virus Genes (USA ISSN 0920-8569) **3332**, 3315
➤ Virus Infections of Vertebrates (NLD) **4559**
• ➤ Virus Research (NLD ISSN 0168-1702) **3333**
Virusforschung in Einzeldarstellungen *see* Virology Monographs **3332**, 3808
Vision Community Services Resource List *see* V C S Resource List **3500**
Vision Enhancement (USA ISSN 1094-8635) **3500**, 4008
Vision Monday (USA ISSN 0891-1770) **4008**, 3367
• ➤ Vision Research (GBR ISSN 0042-6989) **4008**
Vision Resource List *see* V C S Resource List **3500**
• Vision (Sheffield) (GBR ISSN 0142-8543) **3738**, 3152, 4008
Visionary (USA) **4008**, 3500, 4363
Visions Internationales (FRA ISSN 1149-5758) **4008**
Visions (San Francisco) (USA) **4454**
Visions (St. Louis) (USA) **4008**
Visiting Fireman (USA) **3458**
Visiting Nurse Association of Brooklyn Newsletter *see* V N A B Newsletter **3942**
Visitor Studies (USA ISSN 1064-5578) **4454**
• ➤ Visual Cognition (GBR ISSN 1350-6285) **4454**
▼ • ➤ Visual Impairment Research (NLD ISSN 1388-235X) **3500**
• ➤ Visual Neuroscience (GBR ISSN 0952-5238) **4137**, 4008
• Viszeralchirurgie (DEU ISSN 1435-3067) **4207**
Vita (GRC ISSN 1108-6033) **4363**
Vita dell'Infanzia (ITA ISSN 0042-7241) **3415**, 3387, 4454
Vita e Salute (ITA ISSN 0042-7268) **4363**
Vita Ospedaliera (ITA ISSN 0391-1470) **3523**, 3706
Vita Sana Magazin *see* Fuer Uns Vita Sana **4353**
Vita. Traditsii, Meditsina, Zdorov'e (RUS) **3706**
Vitae (COL ISSN 0121-4004) **4340**
Vital (DEU ISSN 0507-1747) **4363**
Vital and Health Statistics. Series 1. Programs and Collection Procedures *see* U.S. National Center for Health Statistics. Vital and Health Statistics. Series 1. Programs and Collection Procedures **4498**, 4370
Vital and Health Statistics. Series 10. Data from the Health Interview Survey *see* U.S. National Center for Health Statistics. Vital and Health Statistics. Series 10. Data from the Health Interview Survey **4498**, 4370, 4530
Vital and Health Statistics. Series 11. Data from the Health and Nutrition Examination Survey *see* U.S. National Center for Health Statistics. Vital and Health Statistics. Series 11. Data from the Health and Nutrition Examination Survey **4498**, 4370, 4530
Vital and Health Statistics. Series 13. Data on Health Resources Utilization *see* U.S. National Center for Health Statistics. Vital and Health Statistics. Series 13. Data on Health Resources Utilization **4492**, 3523
Vital and Health Statistics. Series 14. Data on Health Resources *see* U.S. National Center for Health Statistics. Vital and Health Statistics. Series 14. Data on Health Resources **4498**, 4370, 4530
Vital and Health Statistics. Series 2. Data Evaluation and Methods Research *see* U.S. National Center for Health Statistics. Vital and Health Statistics. Series 2. Data Evaluation and Methods Research **4498**, 4371, 4530
Vital and Health Statistics. Series 20. Data on Mortality *see* U.S. National Center for Health Statistics. Vital and Health Statistics. Series 20. Data on Mortality **4498**, 4371, 4530
Vital and Health Statistics. Series 21. Data on Natality, Marriage, and Divorce *see* U.S. National Center for Health Statistics. Vital and Health Statistics. Series 21. Data on Natality, Marriage, and Divorce **4498**, 4371, 4530
Vital and Health Statistics. Series 23. Data from the National Survey of Family Growth *see* U.S. National Center for Health Statistics. Vital and Health Statistics. Series 23. Data from the National Survey of Family Growth **4498**, 4371, 4530
Vital and Health Statistics. Series 24. Compilations of Data on Natality, Mortality, Divorce, and Induced Terminations of Pregnancy *see* U.S. National Center for Health Statistics. Vital and Health Statistics. Series 24. Compilations of Data on Natality, Mortality, Divorce, and Induced Terminations of Pregnancy **4498**, 4371, 4530
Vital and Health Statistics. Series 3. Analytical Studies *see* U.S. National Center for Health Statistics. Vital and Health Statistics. Series 3. Analytical Studies **4498**, 4371, 4530
Vital and Health Statistics. Series 4. Documents and Committee Report *see* U.S. National Center for Health Statistics. Vital and Health Statistics. Series 4. Documents and Committee Report **4498**, 4371
Vital and Health Statistics. Series 5. Comparative International Vital and Health Statistics Reports *see* U.S. National Center for Health Statistics. Vital and Health Statistics. Series 5. Comparative International Vital and Health Statistics Reports **4498**, 4371, 4530
Vital and Health Statistics. Series 6. Cognition and Survey Measurement *see* U.S. National Center for Health Statistics. Vital and Health Statistics. Series 6. Cognition and Survey Measurement **4458**, 4371, 4498, 4530
• ➤ Vital Signs (Cambridge) (USA) **4492**, 3431, 3706, 4224
➤ Vital Signs (Fresno) (USA) **3706**
Vital Signs Pharmacy Services Newsletter (USA ISSN 0739-9588) **4340**, 3943
Vital Statistics, Idaho *see* Idaho. Department of Health and Welfare. Vital Statistics (Year) **4496**, 4475, 4529
Vital Statistics of the United States (USA ISSN 0083-6710) **4498**, 4371, 4531
Vitalida Ahora (USA) **4363**
Vitality (ITA ISSN 1120-4591) **4247**, 4363
Vitality (USA ISSN 1074-5831) **4363**
Vitality Digest (USA) **3706**
Vitality Magazine (CAN ISSN 1180-0291) **3170**, 4227
Vitalstatistik *see* Sundhedsstatistikken (Year) **3525**, 3737
Vitamin B Research Committee. Report *see* Bitamin B Kenkyu Iikai Kiji **4280**
Vitamin B Research Committee. Short Note *see* Bitamin B Kenkyu Iinkai Hokokusho **4280**
Vitamin Information Centre Medical Update *see* V I C Medical Update **4246**
Vitamine, Mineralstoffe, Spurenelemente in Medizin, Ernaehrung und Umwelt *see* Vitaminspur **4340**
• Vitamins/Bitamin (JPN ISSN 0006-386X) **4340**
• Vitamins & Dietary Supplements: The International Market (GBR) **4340**, 3367
• ➤ Vitamins and Hormones: Advances in Research and Applications (USA ISSN 0083-6729) **4340**, 3706
➤ Vitaminspur (DEU ISSN 0943-3163) **4340**
Vitas (RUS) **3706**
Viva (ITA) **4363**
Viversani e Belli (ITA) **4363**, 3175
Vivir *see* Vivir con Salud **4363**
Vivir con Salud (ESP) **4363**
Vivre (FRA ISSN 0249-0358) **3992**
Vivre en Harmonie (FRA ISSN 0042-7608) **4247**
Vivre Ensemble (FRA ISSN 1152-6653) **3428**, 4518
• ➤ Vlaams Diergeneeskundig Tijdschrift/Flemish Veterinary Journal (BEL ISSN 0303-9021) **4559**
Vlees in Voeding (NLD ISSN 0168-8901) **4247**, 3463
➤ Vnitrni Lekarstvi (CZE ISSN 0042-773X) **3706**
Vocational Rehabilitation Review (USA) **3428**, 4067
Vodosnabzhenie i Sanitarnaya Tekhnika (RUS ISSN 0321-4044) **4492**, 4562
Voeding *see* Voeding Nu **4247**
Voeding en Voorlichting *see* Voeding Nu **4247**
Voeding Nu (NLD) **4247**
Voedingsmagazine (NLD ISSN 0922-8012) **4247**
Voedingsmiddelen Praktijk *see* Voedingsmiddelenpraktijk **3463**, 4492
▼ Voedingsmiddelenpraktijk (NLD ISSN 1566-3310) **3463**, 4492
Vogel und Umwelt (DEU ISSN 0173-0266) **3336**, 3392
Voi Hyvin (FIN ISSN 0780-1122) **4363**
Voice *see* Hearing Health **3491**
Voice Foundation. Newsletter (USA) **4166**
Voice (Ft. Lauderdale) (USA ISSN 1046-5642) **4067**
Voice of Naprapathy (USA) **3170**
Voice of Silence Newsletter (ITA) **3493**, 4518
Voice of the Diabetic (USA ISSN 1041-8490) **3500**, 3869
Voice of the Pharmacist (USA ISSN 0507-2379) **4340**
Voice of United Senior Citizens of Ontario (CAN ISSN 0382-0068) **3481**
➤ Voices (New Bern) (USA ISSN 0042-8272) **4454**
• Voices (Washington) (USA) **3393**, 3706
La Voix des Parents (BEL ISSN 0776-5835) **3487**, 4137, 4518
Voix du Diabete *see* Diabetes Voice **3859**
Voix du Retraite (FRA ISSN 0049-6707) **3481**
Voix du Silence *see* Voice of Silence Newsletter **3493**, 4518
➤ Vojenske Zdravotnicke Listy (CZE ISSN 0372-7025) **3707**, 4340
• Vojnosanitetski Pregled/Military Medical and Pharmaceutical (YUG ISSN 0042-8450) **3707**, 4224, 4340
Volksgesundheit (DEU ISSN 0042-8493) **4363**
• The Volta Review (USA ISSN 0042-8639) **3493**, 3428
Volta Voices (USA ISSN 1074-8016) **3493**, 3428
Voluntary Euthanasia Bulletin *see* V.E. Bulletin **4348**, 3706, 4501
Voluntary Euthanasia Society News *see* V E News **4349**, 3706
Volunteer and Vistors' Guide (USA ISSN 1524-2919) **3481**, 4518
Volunteer Leader (USA ISSN 0005-1861) **3523**, 4518
Von Hippel-Lindau Disease Family Forum *see* V H L Family Forum **4137**, 4008, 4220
Voorkomen (NLD ISSN 0926-4205) **4267**
Voprosy Biologicheskoi, Meditsinskoi, i Farmatsevticheskoi Khimii/Problems of Biological, Medical and Pharmacological (RUS) **3224**, 3707, 4340
Voprosy Kurortologii, Fizioterapii i Lechebnoi Fizicheskoi Kul'tury/Problems of Health Resorts, Physiotherapy and Exercise Therapy (RUS ISSN 0042-8787) **4067**
• ➤ Voprosy Meditsinskoi Khimii/Problems of Medical Chemistry (RUS ISSN 0042-8809) **3264**
Voprosy Okhrany Materinstva i Detstva *see* Rossiiskii Vestnik Perinatologii i Pediatrii **3963**, 4056
• ➤ Voprosy Onkologii/Problems in Oncology (RUS ISSN 0507-3758) **3992**
Voprosy Pitaniya/Problems of Nutrition (RUS ISSN 0042-8833) **4247**
• ➤ Voprosy Psikhologii (RUS ISSN 0042-8841) **4454**
Voprosy Radiobiologii i Biologicheskogo Deistviya Tsitostaticheskikh Preparatov (RUS ISSN 0302-556X) **4157**, 3224
Voprosy Virusologii/Problems of Virology (RUS ISSN 0507-4088) **3333**
Vordrucke fuer die Kassenaerztliche und Vertragsaerztliche Versorgung (DEU ISSN 0934-8794) **4492**
Vous *see* Vous et Votre Sante **3707**
Vous et Votre Sante (FRA ISSN 1241-9648) **3707**
Vox Hospitii *see* Tijdschrift voor Verpleeghuisgeneeskunde **3701**, 3523
• Vox Me D A L (CAN ISSN 0830-5315) **3388**, 3707
• ➤ Vox Sanguinis (GBR ISSN 0042-9007) **3752**, 3785
Voyages Internationaux et Sante. Vaccinations Exigees et Conseils d'Hygiene *see* International Travel and Health: Vaccination Requirements and Health Advice **4478**
Voz de Diabetes *see* Diabetes Voice **3859**
Vrach (RUS ISSN 0236-3054) **3707**
Vrachebnoe Delo *see* Likarska Sprava **3644**
Vrachebnye Tainy (RUS) **3707**
Vriend (NLD ISSN 0042-9139) **3493**, 3387
Vs (BEL ISSN 0393-8255) **3552**, 4349, 4454, 4510
Vsemirnaya Assambleya Zdravookhraneniya i Ispolnitel'nogo Komiteta. Sbornik Rezolyutsii i Reshenii *see* World Health Organization. Handbook of Resolutions and Decisions of the World Health Assembly and the Executive Board. **4493**
Vsemirnaya Organizatsiya Zdravookhraneniya. Byulleten' *see* World Health Organization. Bulletin **3709**
Vsemirnaya Organizatsiya Zdravookhraneniya. Seriya Tekhnicheskikh Dokladov (CHE ISSN 0250-8737) **3707**, 4492
➤ Vutreshni Bolesti (BGR ISSN 0506-2772) **3911**
Vychovavatel (SVK ISSN 0139-6919) **3415**, 4454
Vyziva *see* Vyziva a Potraviny **4247**
➤ Vyziva a Potraviny (CZE ISSN 1211-846X) **4247**
➤ Vyziva a Spotreba Potravin v Cislech (CZE ISSN 1212-0022) **4247**
Vyziva a Zdravie/Nutrition and Health (SVK ISSN 0042-9406) **4248**
Vyziva Lidu *see* Vyziva a Potraviny **4247**
W A News *see* Diabetes Path Finder **3858**
W A W Newsletter *see* William Alanson White Psychoanalytic Institute. Record **4455**
W C B News *see* WorkSafe Magazine **4267**
W D A Journal (Wisconsin Dental Association) (USA ISSN 1046-9338) **3842**
W F S Quarterly (Women in the Fire Service) (USA ISSN 1071-1767) **3458**, 4569
W H I N en Espanol *see* Workers' Health International Newsletter **4267**
W H M I S Compliance Manual (Workplace Hazardous Materials Information Systems) (CAN) **4267**
• W H O Drug Information (World Health Organization) (CHE ISSN 1010-9609) **4492**, 4340
• ➤ W H O Technical Report Series (World Health Organization) (CHE ISSN 0512-3054) **3707**, 4492
W I D H H News (Western Institute for the Deaf & Hard of Hearing) (CAN) **3493**
W I D News *see* W I D H H News **3493**
• ➤ W J M (USA) **3707**
W K W Magazin *see* Wiener Klinische Wochenschrift Magazin **3708**
W M H & D *see* Women's Mental Health & Development **4567**, 4455
W N Y F (With New York Firefighters) (USA ISSN 0042-9775) **3458**, 4492
W O R L D (Women Organized to Respond to Life-Threatening Diseases) (USA) **4566**, 3808
➤ W P S Professional Handbook Series (Western Psychological Services) (USA ISSN 0083-8977) **4454**
W S D A Membership Directory & Resource Guide (Washington State Dental Association) (USA) **3842**
W S D A News (Washington State Dental Association) (USA ISSN 1064-0835) **3842**
Wakayama Medical Reports (JPN ISSN 0511-084X) **3707**
Waksman Foundation of Japan. Report (JPN ISSN 0509-5832) **4340**
Walka z Alkoholizmem *see* Problemy Alkoholizmu **3405**
Walking Magazine (USA ISSN 1042-2102) **4363**
➤ Walter and Andree de Nottbeck Foundation Scientific Reports (FIN ISSN 0358-6758) **3333**, 3264
➤ Warm Earth (AUS ISSN 1320-3940) **3465**, 4248
• Warning Letter Bulletin (USA ISSN 1069-4218) **3707**, 4340
Warsaw Agricultural University. S G G W. Annals. Food Technology and Nutrition (POL) **3463**, 4248
Warta Dinas Kesehatan (IDN) **4492**
Wary Canary (USA ISSN 0899-1405) **3442**, 3707, 4492

Title

Title

Work Programs Special Interest Section Newsletter *see* Work Programs Special Interest Section Quarterly **4270**, 4267
Work Programs Special Interest Section Quarterly (USA) **4270**, 4267
Workers' Comp Advisor (USA ISSN 1054-7819) **3364**, 3544
Workers' Comp Managed Care (USA ISSN 1066-2669) **3534**, 3364
Workers' Compensation - Business Management Guide (USA) **3534**, 4267
Worker's Compensation Guide (USA) **3368**, 3544, 4267
Workers' Compensation Law Reporter *see* Workers' Compensation - Business Management Guide **3534**, 4267
Workers' Health International Newsletter (GBR ISSN 1351-4792) **4267**
Workers Life (Pretoria) (ZAF) **4267**, 3442
• Worklife Report (CAN ISSN 0834-292X) **3364**, 3368, 4267
▼ Workplace Ergonomics News (USA ISSN 1528-8013) **4267**
Workplace Hazardous Materials Information Systems Compliance Manual *see* W H M I S Compliance Manual **4267**
• Workplace Substance Abuse Advisor (USA) **3406**
• WorkSafe Magazine (CAN ISSN 1494-7412) **4267**
Worksite News (CAN ISSN 1203-3774) **4267**
Worksite Wellness Works (USA ISSN 1053-492X) **4493**, 3368
World Animal Health in (Year) (FRA ISSN 1017-3102) **4560**
➤ World Animal Science (NLD) **3356**
World Around You (USA ISSN 0199-8293) **3428**, 3494
World Around You. Teacher's Edition (USA ISSN 1059-9894) **3494**
World Book Health and Medical Annual (USA ISSN 0890-4480) **3430**, 3709, 4363
World Buiatrics Congress (BEL) **4560**, 3162
➤ World Catalogue of Insects (DNK ISSN 1398-8700) **3297**
World Chinese Journal of Digestology *see* Shijie Huaren Xiaohua Zazhi **3896**
World Congress of Music Therapy. Proceedings (ITA) **4226**, 4137
World Congress of Pain. Proceedings *see* Pain Research and Clinical Management **3671**
World Congress of Psychiatry. Proceedings (BEL ISSN 0084-1609) **4137**
World Congress on Fertility and Sterility. Proceedings (FRA ISSN 0084-1641) **3224**
World Congress on the Prevention of Occupational Accidents and Diseases. Proceedings (CHE ISSN 0084-165X) **4267**
World Council for Gifted and Talented Children. Yearbook (USA) **3428**
World Council of Enterostomal Therapists Journal (AUS ISSN 0819-4610) **3897**
▼ • World Dentistry (USA ISSN 1534-2530) **3842**
• World Diabetes/Diabete Mondial (CHE) **3785**
World Directory of Medical Schools (CHE ISSN 0512-2759) **3709**, 3417
World Disasters Report (NLD ISSN 0929-0850) **4493**, 4519
• World Drug Market Manual (GBR ISSN 0140-4806) **4340**
World Federation for Mental Health. Annual Report (USA) **4455**, 4493
World Federation for Mental Health. Newsletter (USA) **4455**, 4493
World Federation of Health Agencies for the Advancement of Voluntary Surgical Contraception. Communique (USA) **3360**
• ➤ World Health Organization. Bulletin (CHE ISSN 0042-9686) **3709**
World Health Organization Drug Information *see* W H O Drug Information **4492**, 4340
World Health Organization. Handbook of Resolutions and Decisions of the World Health Assembly and the Executive Board. (CHE ISSN 0301-0740) **4493**
World Health Organization. Regional Office for the Eastern Mediterranean. Annual Report of the Regional Director (EGY) **4493**
World Health Organization. Regional Office for the Eastern Mediterranean. Biennial Report of Regional Director *see* World Health Organization. Regional Office for the Eastern Mediterranean. Annual Report of the Regional Director **4493**
World Health Organization Technical Report Series *see* W H O Technical Report Series **3707**, 4492
World Health Organization. Technical Reports (CHE) **3808**
World Health Organization. Work of W H O *see* The World Health Report **4493**
• The World Health Report (CHE ISSN 1020-3311) **4493**
World Health Statistics Annual (CHE ISSN 0250-3794) **4499**, 4531
World Healthcare Marketing Directory (GBR) **3709**, 3367, 3371
• ➤ World Hospitals and Health Services (GBR ISSN 0512-3135) **3524**
World Industrial Safety and Hygiene Development *see* Shijie Laodong Anquan Weisheng Dongtai **4265**
• World Journal of Gastroenterology (CHN ISSN 1007-9327) **3897**
• ➤ World Journal of Microbiology and Biotechnology (GBR ISSN 0959-3993) **3278**, 3333
▼ • World Journal of Orthodontics (USA) **3842**
• ➤ World Journal of Surgery (USA ISSN 0364-2313) **4207**
• ➤ World Journal of Urology (DEU ISSN 0724-4983) **4220**
The World Market for Eyewear (GBR) **4028**, 3368
▼ The World Market for O T C Healthcare (Over the Counter) (GBR) **4341**, 3368, 3369
The World Market for Oral Hygiene (GBR) **3175**, 3368, 3842
The World Market for Skin Care and Sun Care (GBR) **3175**, 3368, 3854
World Medical Journal (DEU ISSN 0049-8122) **3709**, 3418, 3524, 4567
World Meetings: Medicine (USA ISSN 0161-2875) **4221**, 3709
World Notes on Antibiotics *see* Guowai Yiyao (Kangshengsu Fence) **4298**
World Notes on Herbal Medicine *see* Guowai Yiyao (Zhiwuyao Fence) **4298**
• World of Drug Information (USA) **4341**
World of Obstetrics and Gynecology *see* Sanfujinka no Sekai **3963**
World Pharmaceutical Developments (GBR) **4341**
World Pharmaceutical Directory (USA ISSN 0276-2277) **4341**, 3371
➤ World Psychology (USA ISSN 1078-8468) **4455**
World Rabbit Science (FRA ISSN 1257-5011) **3356**, 3162
• ➤ World Review of Nutrition and Dietetics (CHE ISSN 0084-2230) **4248**
• The World Wide Web Journal of Biology (USA) **3224**
• ➤ World Wide Wounds (GBR ISSN 1369-2607) **4028**
➤ Worldplast (USA ISSN 1075-3931) **4207**
World's Woman's Christian Temperance Union. Triennial Report (USA) **3406**, 4519
Worldwatch Reader (USA) **3442**, 3363, 4493
• Worldwide Biotech (USA) **3278**, 4341
➤ Wound Ballistics Review (USA ISSN 1055-0305) **3885**, 3395, 4225
Wound Care (USA) **3808**, 3854, 4028
Wound Care Products Resource *see* Resources in Wound Care **4025**
Wound Care Sourcebook (USA) **3854**, 4028
• ➤ Wound Repair and Regeneration (USA ISSN 1067-1927) **4028**
• ➤ Wounds (USA ISSN 1044-7946) **4028**
Write-Up (USA) **4455**
Wuerttembergische Bau-Berufsgenossenschaft. Mitteilungen (DEU ISSN 0172-2514) **3361**, 4267
➤ Wujing Yixue/Medical Journal of the Chinese People's Armed Police Forces (CHN ISSN 1004-3594) **3709**, 3395
Wyoming. Department of Health. Annual Report (USA) **4493**
Wyoming Fire News (USA) **3459**
Wyoming Nurse (USA) **3943**
Wyoming Physicians Newsletter *see* Physician Newsletter **3675**
Wyzsza Szkola Pedagogiczna im. Komisji Edukacji Narodowej w Krakowie. Rocznik Naukowo-Dydaktyczny. Prace Psychologiczne (POL) **4455**, 3430
Wyzsza Szkola Pedagogiczna im. Komisji Edukacji Narodowej w Krakowie. Rocznik Naukowo-Dydaktyczny. Prace z Dydaktyki Biologii (POL) **3224**, 3430
Xenobiotic Metabolism and Disposition *see* Yakubutsu Dotai **3709**
• ➤ Xenobiotica (GBR ISSN 0049-8254) **3264**
• ➤ Xenotransplantation (DNK ISSN 0908-665X) **4207**
Xi Psi Phi Quarterly (USA ISSN 0049-8262) **3842**
• Xian Medical University. Journal (CHN ISSN 1000-923X) **3709**
➤ Xiandai Zhenduan yu Zhiliao/Modern Diagnosis & Treatment (CHN ISSN 1001-8174) **3709**
Xianggang Huli Zazhi *see* Hong Kong Nursing Journal **3920**
• Xiaoer Jijiu Yixue/Pediatric Emergency Medicine (CHN ISSN 1007-9459) **4057**, 4028
Xibao Yanjiu *see* Cell Research **3189**
• Xibao yu Fenzi Mianyixue Zazhi/Journal of Cellular and Molecular Immunology (CHN ISSN 1007-8738) **3752**
• Xibei Linxueyuan Xuebao/Northwestern Forestry University. Journal (CHN ISSN 1001-7461) **3464**, 3709, 4531
Xin Xiaohuabingxueazhi - China National Journal of New Gastroenterology *see* Shijie Huaren Xiaohua Zazhi **3896**
Xin Yixue/New Medical Science (CHN ISSN 0253-9802) **3709**
Xin Yiyaoxue Zazhi *see* Zhongyi Zazhi **3171**, 3714, 4343
Xinli Kexue Tongxun/Information on Psychological Sciences (CHN ISSN 1000-6648) **4455**
➤ Xinli Xuebao/Acta Psychologica Sinica (CHN ISSN 0439-755X) **4455**
Xinli yu Jiankang/Psychology and Health (CHN ISSN 1005-7064) **4137**
Xinlixue/Psychology (CHN ISSN 1001-2532) **4455**
Xinsheng Erke Zazhi/Journal of Neonatology (CHN ISSN 1002-1213) **4057**
• ➤ Xinxueguanbingxue Jinzhan/Advances in Cardiovascular Disease (CHN) **3785**
Xinyao yu Linchuang - New Drugs and Clinical Remedies *see* Zhongguo Xinyao Yu Linchuang Zazhi **4342**, 3713
Xinzhongyi/New Journal of Traditional Chinese Medicine (CHN ISSN 0256-7415) **3170**, 3709, 4341
Xiong Xinxueguan Waike Zazhi *see* Zhonghua Xiong-xin Xueguan Waike Zazhi **3785**
Xumu Shouyi Xuebao/Acta Veterinaria et Zootechnica Sinica (CHN ISSN 0366-6964) **4560**, 3162
Xuzhou Institute of Medical Sciences. Journal *see* Xuzhou Yixueyuan Xuebao **3709**
Xuzhou Yixueyuan Xuebao/Xuzhou Institute of Medical Sciences. Journal (CHN ISSN 1000-2065) **3709**
Y M C A Weekly News (Young Men's Christian Association) (CAN) **4363**, 4248, 4526
Yakhak Hoeji *see* Pharmaceutical Society of Korea. Journal **4324**
Yakkyoku *see* Practical Pharmacy **4331**
Yakkyoku no Tomo (Tokyo, 1975)/Pharmacy Companion (JPN ISSN 0913-0683) **4341**
➤ Yakubutsu Dotai/Xenobiotic Metabolism and Disposition (JPN ISSN 0916-1139) **3709**
Yakugaku Toshokan *see* Pharmaceutical Library Bulletin **3548**, 4324
• ➤ Yakugaku Zasshi/Pharmaceutical Journal (JPN ISSN 0031-6903) **4341**
Yakugyo Shinbun *see* Japanese Weekly on Pharmacy and Chemistry **4305**, 3373
Yakup Shinmoon/Pharmaceutical News (KOR) **4341**
• Yakuri to Chiryo/Japanese Pharmacology and Therapeutics (JPN ISSN 0386-3603) **4341**
Yakuzaigaku *see* Journal of Pharmaceutical Science and Technology **4309**
Yale Children's Health Letter (USA ISSN 1078-5027) **4057**
• ➤ Yale Journal of Biology and Medicine (USA ISSN 0044-0086) **3709**, 3224
Yale Medicine (USA) **3710**
Yamaguchi Daigaku Igakubu Kiyo *see* Yamaguchi University. School of Medicine. Bulletin **3710**
Yamaguchi University. Drug Information News (JPN ISSN 0910-5247) **4341**
Yamaguchi University. School of Medicine. Bulletin/Yamaguchi Daigaku Igakubu Kiyo (JPN ISSN 0513-1812) **3710**
Yamaguchiken Eisei Kogai Kenkyu Senta Gyoseki Hokoku (JPN ISSN 0915-0498) **4493**, 3442, 3710
Yamaguchiken Eisei Kogai Kenkyu Senta Nenpo (JPN ISSN 0915-048X) **4499**, 4531
Yanbian - Jibian - Tubian/Carcinogensis, Teratogensis and Mutagenesis (CHN) **3992**, 3224, 3456
Yandi Bing/Ocular Fundus *see* Zhonghua Yandibing Zazhi **4008**
Yanke Xin Jinzhan *see* Recent Advances in Ophthalmology **4006**, 3939, 3989, 4201
Yanke Xuebao *see* Eye Science **3997**
• ➤ Yaowu Fenxi Zazhi/Journal of Pharmaceutical Analysis (CHN ISSN 0254-1793) **4341**
• ➤ Yaowu Shipin Fenxi/Journal of Food and Drug Analysis (TWN ISSN 1021-9498) **3463**, 3881, 4248
Yaoxue Tongbao - Chinese Pharmaceutical Bulletin *see* Zhongguo Yaoxue Zazhi **4342**
• Yaoxue Xuebao/Acta Pharmaceutica Sinica (CHN ISSN 0513-4870) **4341**
➤ Yati Yasui Yazhoubingxue Zazhi/Chinese Journal of Conservative Dentistry (CHN ISSN 1005-2593) **3843**
Year Book: Health Care in China *see* Zhongguo Weisheng Nianjian **3713**
Year Book of Allergy and Clinical Immunology *see* Year Book of Allergy, Asthma and Clinical Immunology **3752**
Year Book of Allergy, Asthma and Clinical Immunology (USA ISSN 1082-9776) **3752**
Year Book of Anesthesia and Pain Management *see* The Year Book of Anesthesiology and Pain Management **3760**
• The Year Book of Anesthesiology and Pain Management (USA ISSN 1073-5437) **3760**
• The Year Book of Cardiology (USA ISSN 0145-4145) **3785**
• Year Book of Chiropractic (USA ISSN 1066-484X) **3738**, 3790
Year Book of Clinical Microbiology (USA ISSN 1054-772X) **3333**
• Year Book of Critical Care Medicine (USA ISSN 0734-3299) **3710**
• The Year Book of Dentistry (USA ISSN 0084-3717) **3843**
Year Book of Dermatologic Surgery *see* The Year Book of Dermatology and Dermatologic Surgery **3738**, 3152, 3854
Year Book of Dermatology *see* The Year Book of Dermatology and Dermatologic Surgery **3738**, 3152, 3854
▼ • The Year Book of Dermatology and Dermatologic Surgery (USA) **3738**, 3152, 3854
• The Year Book of Diagnostic Radiology (USA ISSN 0098-1672) **4157**
Year Book of Digestive Diseases *see* The Year Book of Gastroenterology **3897**
• The Year Book of Emergency Medicine (USA ISSN 0271-7964) **4028**
• The Year Book of Endocrinology (USA ISSN 0084-3741) **3869**
• The Year Book of Family Practice (USA ISSN 0147-1996) **3710**
• The Year Book of Gastroenterology (USA ISSN 0739-5930) **3897**
• The Year Book of Hand Surgery (USA ISSN 0739-5949) **4207**, 4028
• The Year Book of Medicine (USA ISSN 0084-3873) **3710**
• The Year Book of Neonatal and Perinatal Medicine (USA ISSN 8756-5005) **3965**
Year Book of Nephrology *see* Year Book of Nephrology, Hypertension, and Mineral Metabolism **4220**
• Year Book of Nephrology, Hypertension, and Mineral Metabolism (USA ISSN 1086-7139) **4220**
• The Year Book of Neurology & Neurosurgery (USA ISSN 0513-5117) **4138**, 4208
• The Year Book of Nuclear Medicine (USA ISSN 0084-3903) **4157**
Year Book of Obstetrics and Gynecology *see* The Year Book of Obstetrics, Gynecology, and Women's Health **3965**, 4567
• The Year Book of Obstetrics, Gynecology, and Women's Health (USA ISSN 1090-798X) **3965**, 4567
• The Year Book of Oncology (USA ISSN 1040-1741) **3992**
The Year Book of Ophthalmology (USA ISSN 0084-392X) **4008**
• The Year Book of Orthopedics (USA ISSN 0276-1092) **3738**, 4028
• The Year Book of Otolaryngology - Head and Neck Surgery (USA ISSN 1041-892X) **4038**
Year Book of Pathology and Clinical Pathology *see* The Year Book of Pathology and Laboratory Medicine **3710**
• The Year Book of Pathology and Laboratory Medicine (USA ISSN 1077-9108) **3710**
• The Year Book of Pediatrics (USA ISSN 0084-3954) **4057**
• The Year Book of Plastic, Reconstructive, and Aesthetic Surgery (USA ISSN 1040-175X) **4208**
• The Year Book of Psychiatry and Applied Mental Health (USA ISSN 0084-3970) **4138**
• The Year Book of Pulmonary Disease (USA ISSN 8756-3452) **4166**

Title

• Zeitschrift fuer Klinische Psychologie und Psychotherapie - Forschung und Praxis (DEU ISSN 1616-3443) **4456**
• Zeitschrift fuer Laermbekaempfung (DEU ISSN 0174-1098) **4367**, 4494
Zeitschrift fuer Medizinische Ethik (DEU ISSN 0944-7652) **3711**, 4349
Zeitschrift fuer Medizinische Physik (DEU ISSN 0939-3889) **4067**
➤ Zeitschrift fuer Medizinische Psychologie (DEU ISSN 0940-5569) **4456**
Zeitschrift fuer Menschenkunde. Zentralblatt fuer Schriftpsychologie und Schriftvergleichung *see* Zeitschrift fuer Schriftpsychologie und Schriftvergleichung **4456**
Zeitschrift fuer Morphologie und Anthropologie (DEU ISSN 0044-314X) **3174**, 3224
• ➤ Zeitschrift fuer Naturforschung. Section C: A Journal of Biosciences (DEU ISSN 0939-5075) **3224**
Zeitschrift fuer Naturheilkunde (DEU ISSN 0044-3182) **3170**, 3711
Zeitschrift fuer Neurologie *see* Journal of Neurology **4103**
Zeitschrift fuer Neuropsychologie (CHE ISSN 1016-264X) **4456**
Zeitschrift fuer Onkologie *see* Deutsche Zeitschrift fuer Onkologie **3976**
• ➤ Zeitschrift fuer Orthopaedie und Ihre Grenzgebiete (DEU ISSN 0044-3220) **4028**
• ➤ Zeitschrift fuer Paedagogische Psychologie (CHE ISSN 1010-0652) **4456**
▼ Zeitschrift fuer Palliativmedizin (DEU ISSN 1615-2921) **3711**
Zeitschrift fuer Pflanzenernaehrung und Bodenkunde *see* Journal of Plant Nutrition and Soil Science **3232**, 3149, 3281
Zeitschrift fuer Physiotherapie *see* Physikalische Medizin Rehabilitationsmedizin Kurortmedizin **3676**
Zeitschrift fuer Phytotherapie (DEU ISSN 0722-348X) **3711**, 3283
Zeitschrift fuer Praktische Augenheilkunde *see* Z P A **4008**
• ➤ Zeitschrift fuer Psychologie (DEU ISSN 0044-3409) **4456**
Zeitschrift fuer Psychosomatische Medizin und Psychoanalyse *see* Zeitschrift fuer Psychosomatische Medizin und Psychotherapie **4138**
Zeitschrift fuer Psychosomatische Medizin und Psychoanalyse. Beihefte *see* Zeitschrift fuer Psychosomatische Medizin und Psychoanalyse. Monographien **4138**, 4456
Zeitschrift fuer Psychosomatische Medizin und Psychoanalyse. Monographien (DEU) **4138**, 4456
Zeitschrift fuer Psychosomatische Medizin und Psychotherapie (DEU) **4138**
• ➤ Zeitschrift fuer Rheumatologie (DEU ISSN 0340-1855) **4172**
Zeitschrift fuer Schriftpsychologie und Schriftvergleichung (AUT ISSN 1607-5579) **4456**
• Zeitschrift fuer Sexualforschung (DEU ISSN 0932-8114) **3711**, 4456
• ➤ Zeitschrift fuer Sozialpsychologie (CHE ISSN 0044-3514) **4456**, 4524
Zeitschrift fuer Stomatologie *see* Stomatologie **3840**
Zeitschrift fuer Stomatologie. Supplementem *see* Stomatologie **3840**
Zeitschrift fuer Systemische Therapie (DEU ISSN 0723-9505) **4456**
Zeitschrift fuer Tierphysiologie und Tierernaehrung *see* Journal of Animal Physiology and Animal Nutrition **3343**, 3354, 4545
Zeitschrift fuer Transaktionsanalyse in Theorie und Praxis (DEU ISSN 0176-9855) **4456**
Zeitschrift fuer Unfallchirurgie und Versicherungsmedizin *see* Swiss Surgery **4205**, 4026
Zeitschrift fuer Zahnaerztliche Implantologie (DEU) **3843**
Zeitschriftenbibliographie Gerontologie (DEU ISSN 0721-1872) **3483**, 3177
Zemljiste i Biljka *see* Acta Biologica Iugoslavica. Serija A: Zemljiste i Biljka **3178**
Zen Eishikyo Geppo/Japanese Association of Dietitian Training Institute. Monthly Bulletin (JPN) **4248**
Zensoku/Asthma (JPN ISSN 0914-7683) **4166**
Zentralblatt fuer Arbeitsmedizin, Arbeitsschutz und Ergonomie (DEU ISSN 0944-2502) **4268**
Zentralblatt fuer Bakteriologie *see* International Journal of Medical Microbiology **3800**, 3324
Zentralblatt fuer Bakteriologie, Mikrobiologie und Hygiene *see* Systematic and Applied Microbiology **3331**
• ➤ Zentralblatt fuer Chirurgie (DEU ISSN 0044-409X) **4208**
• ➤ Zentralblatt fuer Gynaekologie (DEU ISSN 0044-4197) **3965**
Zentralblatt fuer Hygiene und Umweltmedizin *see* International Journal of Hygiene and Environmental Health **4477**
• Zentralblatt fuer Kinderchirurgie (DEU ISSN 0940-9599) **4208**
Zentralblatt fuer Mikrobiologie *see* Microbiological Research **3327**
• ➤ Zentralblatt fuer Neurochirurgie (DEU ISSN 0044-4251) **4138**, 4208
Zentrales Nervensystem *see* Z N S - Zentrales Nervensystem **4138**
➤ Zentralsterilisation - Central Service (DEU ISSN 0942-6086) **3711**
Zero Population Growth, Inc. Reporter *see* The Z P G Reporter **4370**
Zest (GBR ISSN 1355-4255) **4569**, 3175, 4364
Zeszyty Naukowe Akademii Rolniczej we Wroclawiu. Weterynaria *see* Akademia Rolnicza we Wroclawiu. Zeszyty Naukowe. Weterynaria **4535**
Zhejiang Clinical Medical Journal *see* Zhejiang Linchuang Yixue **3711**
Zhejiang College of Traditional Chinese Medicine. Journal *see* Zhejiang Zhongyi Xueyuan Xuebao **3712**, 4341
Zhejiang Daxue Xuebao (Yixue Ban)/Zhejiang University. Journal (Medical Sciences Edition) (CHN ISSN 1008-9292) **3711**
Zhejiang Journal of Integrated Traditional Chinese and Western Medicine *see* Zhejiang Zhongxiyi Jiehe Zazhi **3712**
Zhejiang Journal of Traditional Chinese Medicine *see* Zhejiang Zhongyi Zazhi **3171**, 3712, 4341
▼ • Zhejiang Linchuang Yixue/Zhejiang Clinical Medical Journal (CHN ISSN 1008-7664) **3711**
Zhejiang Medical University. Journal *see* Zhejiang Yike Daxue Xuebao **3711**
Zhejiang University. Journal (Medical Sciences Edition) *see* Zhejiang Daxue Xuebao (Yixue Ban) **3711**
Zhejiang Yike Daxue Xuebao/Zhejiang Medical University. Journal (CHN ISSN 1000-1743) **3711**
• Zhejiang Yufang Yixue (CHN ISSN 1007-0931) **3712**
• Zhejiang Zhongxiyi Jiehe Zazhi/Zhejiang Journal of Integrated Traditional Chinese and Western Medicine (CHN ISSN 1005-4561) **3712**
Zhejiang Zhongyi Xueyuan Xuebao/Zhejiang College of Traditional Chinese Medicine. Journal (CHN ISSN 1005-5509) **3712**, 4341
• Zhejiang Zhongyi Zazhi/Zhejiang Journal of Traditional Chinese Medicine (CHN ISSN 0411-8421) **3171**, 3712, 4341
Zhenskoe Zdorov'e (RUS) **4567**
Zhivotnovod *see* Zhivotnovod dlya Vsekh **4560**, 3162
➤ Zhivotnovod dlya Vsekh (RUS) **4560**, 3162
• Zhiwu Baohu Xuebao/Acta Phytophylactica Sinica (CHN ISSN 0577-7518) **3283**
➤ Zhiwu Bingli Xuebao/Acta Phytopathologica Sinica (CHN ISSN 0412-0914) **3283**
Zhiwu Shenglixue Tongxun/Plant Physiology Communications (CHN ISSN 0412-0922) **3283**
➤ Zhiwu Shengtai Xuebao/Acta Phytoecologica Sinica (CHN ISSN 1005-264X) **3283**, 3442
Zhiwu Shengtaixue yu Diziwuxue Xuebao - Acta Phytoecologica et Geobotanica Sinica *see* Zhiwu Shengtai Xuebao **3283**, 3442
Zhiye Yixue/Occupational Medicine (CHN ISSN 1000-6486) **3712**
➤ Zhiye yu Jiankang/Occupation and Health (CHN ISSN 1004-1257) **4494**
Zhong Cao Yao/Chinese Herbal Medicine (CHN) **4341**, 3712
Zhong Lao Nian Baojian (CHN) **4364**
➤ Zhong Wai Yi Xue Zhe Zue/Chinese and International Philosophy of Medicine (NLD ISSN 1386-6354) **3712**, 4349
Zhong-Xiyi Jiehe Zazhi/Chinese Journal of Modern Developments in Traditional Medicine *see* Zhongguo Zhongxiyi Jiehe Zazhi **3713**
• Zhongcaoyao/Chinese Traditional and Herbal Drugs (CHN ISSN 0253-2670) **3712**, 3171
➤ Zhongchenyao/Chinese Traditional Patent Medicine (CHN ISSN 1001-1528) **4341**
• Zhongfeng yu Shenjing Jibing Zazhi/Journal of Apoplexy and Nervous Diseases (CHN ISSN 1003-2754) **4138**
• Zhonggou Dongmai Yinghua Zazhi/Chinese Journal of Arteriosclerosis (CHN ISSN 1007-3949) **3712**
Zhongguo Aizheng Yanjiu *see* Chinese Journal of Cancer Research **3974**
Zhongguo Anquan Kexue Xuebao/Chinese Safety Science Journal (CHN ISSN 1003-3033) **4268**
Zhongguo Baojian/Chinese Health Care (CHN ISSN 1005-2720) **4494**
Zhongguo Baojian Yingyang/China Health Nutrition (CHN ISSN 1004-7484) **4248**
• ➤ Zhongguo Bingduxue/Virologica Sinica (CHN ISSN 1003-5125) **3333**
• ➤ Zhongguo Bingli Shengli Zazhi/Chinese Journal of Pathophysiology (CHN ISSN 1000-4718) **3712**
Zhongguo Canjiren/Disability in China (CHN ISSN 1003-1081) **3487**
• ➤ Zhongguo Chaosheng Yixue Zazhi/Chinese Journal of Ultrasound in Medicine (CHN ISSN 1002-0101) **4157**
• Zhongguo Chuji Weisheng Baojian/Chinese Primary Health Care (CHN ISSN 1001-568X) **3712**
• Zhongguo Dangdai Erke Zazhi/Chinese Journal of Contemporary Pediatrics (CHN ISSN 1008-8830) **4057**
Zhongguo Difangbing Fangzhi Zazhi/Chinese Journal of Control of Endemic Diseases (CHN ISSN 1001-1889) **3712**
Zhongguo Difangbingxue Zazhi/Chinese Journal of Endemiology (CHN ISSN 1000-4955) **3712**
Zhongguo Dongwu Jianyi/Chinese Journal of Animal Quarantine (CHN ISSN 1005-944X) **4560**, 3712
• Zhongguo Fanglao Tongxun/Chinese Antituberculosis Association. Bulletin (CHN ISSN 1000-6621) **4166**
Zhongguo Fayixue Zazhi/Chinese Journal of Forensic Sciences (CHN ISSN 1001-5728) **3885**
• Zhongguo Feiyan Zazhi/Chinese Journal of Lung Cancer (CHN ISSN 1009-3419) **4166**
Zhongguo Fuyou Baojian/Chinese Women and Children's Health (CHN) **3966**
Zhongguo Gandan Waike Zazhi/Chinese Journal of Hepatobiliary Surgery (CHN) **3911**
➤ Zhongguo Gangchangbing Zazhi/Chinese Journal of Colo-Proctology (CHN ISSN 1000-1174) **3897**
Zhongguo Gonggong Weisheng/China's Public Health (CHN ISSN 1001-0580) **4494**
Zhongguo Gonggong Weisheng Xuebao/Chinese Journal of Public Health (CHN ISSN 1001-0572) **4494**
• Zhongguo Gongye Yixue Zazhi/Chinese Journal of Industrial Medicine (CHN ISSN 1002-221X) **4268**, 3712
• Zhongguo Gushang/China Journal of Orthopaedics and Traumatology (CHN ISSN 1003-0034) **4028**
• Zhongguo Guzhi Shusong Zazhi/Chinese Journal of Osteoporosis (CHN ISSN 1006-7108) **3482**, 4028
Zhongguo Haiyang Yaowu Zazhi/Chinese Journal of Marine Drugs (CHN ISSN 1002-3461) **4341**, 3224
• Zhongguo Jiguang Yixue Zazhi/Chinese Journal of Laser Medicine & Surgery (CHN ISSN 1003-9430) **3712**, 4367
Zhongguo Jihua Zhengyuxue Zazhi/Chinese Journal of Family Planning (CHN ISSN 1004-8189) **3360**
• ➤ Zhongguo Jijiu Yixue/Chinese Journal of Critical Care Medicine (CHN ISSN 1002-1949) **3712**
Zhongguo Jishengchong yu Jishengchongbing Zazhi/Chinese Journal of Parasitology and Parasitic Diseases (CHN) **3808**, 3224, 4494
• Zhongguo Jishengchongbing Fangzhi Zazhi/Chinese Journal of Parasitic Disease Control (CHN ISSN 1001-6627) **3808**, 3224, 4494
Zhongguo Jishengchongxue yu Jishengchongbing Zazhi/Chinese Journal of Parasitology and Parasitic Diseases (CHN ISSN 1000-7423) **3333**
• Zhongguo Jizhu Jisui Zazhi/Chinese Journal of Spine and Spinal Cord (CHN ISSN 1004-406X) **4028**
Zhongguo Kangfu/Chinese Journal of Rehabilitation (CHN ISSN 1001-2001) **4364**
• Zhongguo Kangfu Lilun Yu Shijian/Chinese Journal of Rehabilitation Theory & Practice (CHN ISSN 1006-9771) **4067**
• ➤ Zhongguo Kangfu Yixue Zazhi/Chinese Journal of Rehabilitation Medicine (CHN ISSN 1001-1242) **3712**
Zhongguo Laonian Bao/China Elderly Journal (CHN) **3482**
Zhongguo Linchuang Xinlixue Zazhi/Chinese Journal of Clinical Psychology (CHN ISSN 1005-3611) **4138**
• Zhongguo Linchuang Yaolixue Zazhi/The Chinese Journal of Clinical Pharmacology (CHN ISSN 1001-6821) **4341**
Zhongguo Mafeng Zazhi/Chinese Journal of Leprosy (CHN ISSN 1000-629X) **3712**
Zhongguo Meijie Shengwuxue ji Kongzhi Zazhi (CHN) **3752**
• ➤ Zhongguo Mianyixue Zazhi/Chinese Journal of Immunology (CHN ISSN 1000-484X) **3752**
• Zhongguo Minjian Liaofa/China's Naturopathy (CHN ISSN 1007-5798) **3171**
Zhongguo Minzu Minjian Yixue Zazhi/Chinese Journal of Ethnomedicine and Ethnopharmacy (CHN) **3712**
Zhongguo Nongcun Yixue/Medical Science in Rural China (CHN) **3712**
Zhongguo Qigong Kexue/China Qigong Science (CHN ISSN 1005-2569) **3171**, 4364
• ➤ Zhongguo Renshou Gonghuanbing Zazhi/Chinese Journal of Zoonoses (CHN ISSN 1002-2694) **3333**, 3808, 4560
• ➤ Zhongguo Shaoshang Chuangshang Zazhi/Chinese Journal of Burns, Wounds & Surface Ulcers (CHN ISSN 1001-0726) **4028**, 3854
• Zhongguo Shenghua Yaowu Zazhi (CHN ISSN 1005-1678) **4342**
Zhongguo Shenglixue Zazhi *see* Chinese Journal of Physiology **3340**, 3584
• ➤ Zhongguo Shengwu Huaxue yu Fenzi Shengwu Xuebao/Chinese Journal of Biochemistry and Molecular Biology (CHN ISSN 1007-7626) **3264**
Zhongguo Shengwu Yixue Gongcheng Xuebao/Chinese Journal of Biomedical Engineering (CHN ISSN 0258-8021) **3712**, 3239
Zhongguo Shenjin Kexue Zazhi/Chinese Journal of Neuroscience (CHN ISSN 1008-0872) **4138**
• Zhongguo Shenjing Mianyixue he Shenjingbingxue Zazhi/Chinese Journal of Neuroimmunology and Neurology (CHN ISSN 1006-2963) **4138**
Zhongguo Shiyan Fangjixue Zazhi/Chinese Journal of Experimental Traditional Medical Formulae (CHN ISSN 1005-9903) **4342**
Zhongguo Shiyan Xieyexue Zazhi/Journal of Experimental Hematology (CHN) **3905**
➤ Zhongguo Shiyong Erke Zazhi/Chinese Journal of Practical Pediatrics (CHN ISSN 1005-2224) **4057**
➤ Zhongguo Shiyong Fuke yu Chanke Zazhi/Chinese Journal of Practical Gynecology and Obstetrics (CHN ISSN 1005-2216) **3966**
➤ Zhongguo Shiyong Neike Zazhi/Chinese Journal of Practical Internal Medicine (CHN ISSN 1005-2194) **3911**
➤ Zhongguo Shiyong Waike Zazhi/Chinese Journal of Practical Surgery (CHN ISSN 1005-2208) **4208**
Zhongguo Shiyong Yanke Zazhi/Chinese Journal of Practical Ophthalmology (CHN ISSN 1006-4443) **4008**
Zhongguo Shouyi Xuebao/Chinese Journal of Veterinary Science (CHN ISSN 1005-4545) **4560**
Zhongguo Shouyi Zazhi/Chinese Journal of Veterinary Medicine (CHN) **4560**
Zhongguo Tangniaobing Zazhi/Chinese Diabetes Magazine (CHN) **3870**
Zhongguo Waike Nianjian *see* Zhongguo Weisheng Nianjian **3713**
Zhongguo Weisheng Nianjian/Year Book: Health Care in China (CHN) **3713**
• Zhongguo Weisheng Tongji/Chinese Journal of Health Statistics (CHN ISSN 1002-3674) **4364**
Zhongguo Weizhongbing Jijiu Yixue/Chinese Critical Care Medicine (CHN ISSN 1003-0603) **3713**
• Zhongguo Xiandai Yingyong Yaoxue/Chinese Journal of Modern Applied Pharmacy (CHN ISSN 1007-7693) **4342**
Zhongguo Xiangcun Yisheng/Chinese Rural Doctors (CHN) **3713**
➤ Zhongguo Xiaoduxue Zazhi/Chinese Journal of Disinfection Science (CHN ISSN 1001-7658) **3713**

Title

DATE DUE
